MEDICINES COMPENDIUM 2010

Published by

Datapharm Communications Ltd
Stocks House
9 North Street
Leatherhead
Surrey
KT22 7AX

Tel: +44 (0)1372 388381
Fax: +44 (0)1372 388384
Email: servicedesk@medicines.org.uk

DISCLAIMER

The Summaries of Product Characteristics (SPCs) and Data Sheets contained within this Compendium are prepare independently by each participating pharmaceutical company. The information is only applicable to the United Kingdon Neither Datapharm Communications Ltd (DCL) nor the Association of the British Pharmaceutical Industry (ABPI) giv any guarantee whatsoever as to the recency or accuracy of the information contained within this publication, includir that found in the SPCs or Data Sheets. A doctor or other appropriately qualified healthcare professional should always b consulted before taking or administering any of the products referred to within this book. To the maximum exte permitted by law neither DCL nor the ABPI accept any liability whatsoever in respect of any loss, damage or expense whatever kind arising from any information contained in this publication or for any error or omission in the Data Sheets SPCs.

Typeset by AJS DataSolutions Ltd, Huddersfield, West Yorkshire.
Printed in the UK by CPI William Clowes Beccles NR34 7TL.

ISSN 1475-326X
ISBN 978-0-907102-28-1

CKNOWLEDGEMENTS

'ith special thanks to:

- Those members of the pharmaceutical industry who regularly contribute information to the eMC (*electronic* Medicines Compendium, http://emc.medicines.org.uk)
- The Association of the British Pharmaceutical Industry (ABPI) for their continued support and enthusiasm.
- The Compendium team:

Julie Hayden	–	Operations Manager
Minoo Saggu	–	Operations Support
Millie Martin	–	Quality Control Executive
Doreen Camilleri- Novak	–	Quality Control
David Stevens	–	Quality Control
Julia Richardson	–	Typesetting Quality Control
Joan Terry	–	Customer Support
Fahad Bashir	–	Production Support
David Zak	–	Senior Software Developer

ARE YOU UP TO DATE?

There are over 20,000 changes to medicines information in the UK each year. The *electronic* Medicines Compendium (eMC) at http://emc.medicines.org.uk provides daily real time updates directly from the manufacturers. No registration is required and the information is provided free of charge. Patient Information Leaflets (PILs) are also available on the eMC, including PILs accessible for the blind and partially sighted.

Medicines information for patients

Medicines Guides www.medguides.medicines.org.uk are a leading source of online information about prescribed medicines for people who take medicines, their carers and the general public in the UK.

The resource is published under the governance of a multidisciplinary stakeholder group. This group of stakeholders is represented on the Medicines Information Project (MIP) Board and includes the Department of Health, NHS organisations including NHS Direct (www.nhsdirect.nhs.uk) and NHS Choices (www.nhs.uk), the pharmaceutical industry and its regulator (the MHRA) and patient and professional groups.

The MIP Board is a unique collaboration of groups with a shared vision to provide up to date, reliable information about medicines which is understandable to people.

Medicine Guides are also the source of medicines information available from the NHS Choices website, the NHS' online portal for patients and the general public in the UK (www.nhs.uk).

CONTENTS

NTRODUCTION

his is the twelfth edition of the Compendium in which ımmaries of Product Characteristics (SPCs) appear. New quirements came into effect in 1995 replacing Data Sheets ith SPCs for new products and those products coming up r licence renewal. Over the last fourteen years, the ajority of Data Sheets have been replaced with SPCs.

This edition is the ninth to be produced directly from the *ectronic* Medicines Compendium (*e*MC) which may be und at http://emc.medicines.org.uk.

'here the information comes from

'Cs and Data Sheets are prepared by the individual mpanies concerned and follow either the requirements ıd down by the European Commission's guideline on ımmary of Product Characteristics (for SPCs) or the "The edicines (Data Sheet) Regulations 1972", as amended ›r Data Sheets).

The SPCs and Data Sheets included in this Compendium ere the most up-to-date approved versions available as of th September 2009 and were sourced from the *e*MC which updated daily. Due to the constantly evolving nature of the formation contained within this book (there are an imated 20,000 changes a year to UK regulatory medicines formation) readers are advised to refer to the eMC for the ›st up-to-date approved versions. Patient Information aflets (PILs), where available, can also be found on the 1C. Access to the *e*MC is provided free of charge.

SPCs and Data Sheets are intended for members of the edical and pharmacy professions and are written with em in mind. Any member of the public who reads them ould bear in mind the need to take professional advice fore making any decision affecting his or her own edication based upon their contents.

evised SPCs/Data Sheets

dividual participating companies may issue loose-leaf Cs or Data Sheets which supersede those included in the edicines Compendium. It is advisable to retain any such vised SPCs/Data Sheets which are received and to indicate ıt fact on the corresponding documents within the ›mpendium.

egal category

ıe following abbreviations may be found under the ading 'Legal Category' in certain documents contained thin the Compendium.

L A preparation which is included in the General Sale List and can be sold from any retail outlet.

A Pharmacy sale medicine which can be sold only from a retail pharmacy. A Pharmacist must oversee the dispensing of this medicine although it can be purchased without a prescription.

)M A Prescription-Only Medicine.

) Controlled Drug: a preparation controlled by the Misuse of Drugs Act 1971 and Regulations. The CD is followed by (Sch 1), (Sch 2), (Sch 3), (Sch 4) or (Sch 5) depending on the schedule to the Misuse of Drugs Regulations 2001, as amended, in which the preparation is included.

Doctors are reminded that certain particulars must be in their own handwriting on prescriptions for certain preparations.

Adverse reactions to drugs

Any drug may produce unwanted or unexpected adverse reactions. Rapid detection and recording of adverse reactions is of vital importance so that unrecognised hazards are identified promptly and appropriate regulatory action is taken to ensure that medicines are used safely. Doctors, dentists, coroners, pharmacists, and nurses (see also self-reporting below) are urged to report suspected adverse reactions directly to the Medicines and Healthcare products Regulatory Agency (MHRA) through the Yellow Card Scheme using the electronic form at www.yellowcard.gov.uk. Alternatively, prepaid Yellow Cards for reporting are available bound in the inside back cover of this book or can be obtained from:

Medicines and Healthcare products Regulatory Agency
CHM FREEPOST
London
SW8 5BR
Tel: 0800 731 6789

Suspected adverse reactions to *any* therapeutic agent should be reported, including drugs (*self-medication* as well as those *prescribed*), blood products, vaccines, radiographic contrast media, complementary and herbal products.

A 24-hour Freephone service is available to all parts of the UK for advice and information on suspected adverse drug reactions; contact the National Yellow Card Information Service at the MHRA on 0800 731 6789. Outside office hours a telephone-answering machine will take messages.

Drug Safety Update is a monthly newsletter from the MHRA and the Commission on Human Medicines (CHM); it is available at www.mhra.gov.uk/mhra/drugsafetyupdate.

Self-reporting

Patients, parents, and carers can also report suspected adverse reactions to the MHRA. Reports can be submitted directly to the MHRA through the Yellow Card Scheme using the electronic form at www.yellowcard.gov.uk or by telephone on 0808 100 3352. Alternatively patient Yellow Cards are available from pharmacies and GP surgeries.

Newer drugs and vaccines

Only limited information is available from clinical trials on the safety of new medicines. Further understanding about the safety of medicines depends on the availability of information from routine clinical practice.

The black triangle symbol (▼) identifies newly licensed medicines that are monitored intensively by the MHRA. Such medicines include new active substances, biosimilar medicines, medicines that have been licensed for administration by a new route or drug delivery system, or for significant new indications which may alter the established risks and benefits of that drug, or that contain a new combination of active substances. There is no standard time for which products retain a black triangle; safety data are usually reviewed after 2 years.

Spontaneous reporting is particularly valuable for recognising possible new hazards rapidly. For medicines showing the black triangle symbol, the MHRA asks that **all** suspected reactions (including those considered non-serious) are reported through the Yellow Card Scheme. An adverse reaction should be reported even if it is not certain that the drug has caused it, or if the reaction is well recognised, or if other drugs have been given at the same time.

Established drugs and vaccines

Doctors, dentists, coroners, pharmacists and nurses are asked to report *all* serious suspected reactions, including those that are fatal, life-threatening, disabling, incapacitating, or which result in or prolong hospitalisation; they should be reported even if the effect is well recognised. Examples include anaphylaxis, blood disorders, endocri disturbances, effects on fertility, haemorrhage from an site, renal impairment, jaundice, ophthalmic disorder severe CNS effects, severe skin reactions, reactions i pregnant women, and any drug interactions. Reports o serious adverse reactions are required to enable compariso with other drugs of a similar class. Reports of overdos (deliberate or accidental) can complicate the assessment o adverse drug reactions, but provide important informatio on the potential toxicity of drugs.

For established drugs there is no need to report well-know relatively minor side-effects, such as dry mouth wi tricyclic antidepressants or constipation with opioids.

More detailed information on reporting can be found o the website at: www.yellowcard.gov.uk.

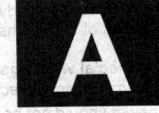

AA Sore Throat Spray

(Manx Healthcare)

NAME OF THE MEDICINAL PRODUCT
AA Sore Throat Spray

QUALITATIVE AND QUANTITATIVE COMPOSITION
enzocaine 1.5mg

PHARMACEUTICAL FORM
erosol spray with metered dose

CLINICAL PARTICULARS

1 Therapeutic indications
ymptomatic temporary relief of pain associated with sore roat pain and minor infections

2 Posology and method of administration
dults (including elderly):

pray two metered doses every two to three hours if equired (not more than sixteen doses in every 24 hours) r as directed by the physician.

hildren:

Children 6 – 12 years: One metered dose every two to three ours if required (not more than eight doses in every 24 ours) or as directed by the physician.

Not suitable for children under 6 years.

Route of administration
opical application to the mucosa of the mouth and throat y means of a metered dose aerosol.

Product should not be administered for more than 7 consecutive days.

Can be shaken before use.

4.3 Contraindications
Known hypersensitivity to benzocaine

4.4 Special warnings and precautions for use
This preparation should not be administered to children under 6 years or used for more than seven consecutive days unless directed by a physician.

If the sore throat is severe, persistent or accompanied by fever or headache, a physician should be consulted before the use of this product. Avoid spraying into the eyes.

Avoid inhalation of the product.

4.5 Interaction with other medicinal products and other forms of interaction
Benzocaine is an ester which on hydrolysis produces p-aminobenzoic acid, so it should not be used in patients being treated with sulphonamides.

4.6 Pregnancy and lactation
There is no evidence, at present, of hazard from benzocaine in pregnancy. However, only very limited data is available. Therefore it should not be used in pregnancy unless considered essential by a physician.

4.7 Effects on ability to drive and use machines
None

4.8 Undesirable effects
Hypersensitivity reactions to benzocaine have been reported.

4.9 Overdose
There have been no reports of overdosage with AAA Spray. Systemic effects are unlikely.

5. PHARMACOLOGICAL PROPERTIES

5.1 Pharmacodynamic properties
Benzocaine is a surface anaesthetic of the ester type. It has found frequent use as lozenges or solution to treat pain arising from various throat and mouth conditions.

5.2 Pharmacokinetic properties
Benzocaine is sparingly soluble in water with toxicity about a tenth that of cocaine. It is not readily absorbed from mucus membranes. It is an ester which on hydrolysis produced p-aminobenzoic acid.

5.3 Preclinical safety data
None stated

6. PHARMACEUTICAL PARTICULARS

6.1 List of excipients
Cetylpyridinium chloride

Glycerin

Ethanol

Clove bud oil

Menthol crystals

Sodium saccharin 450

Peppermint cremophor

Water

6.2 Incompatibilities
None

Figure 1

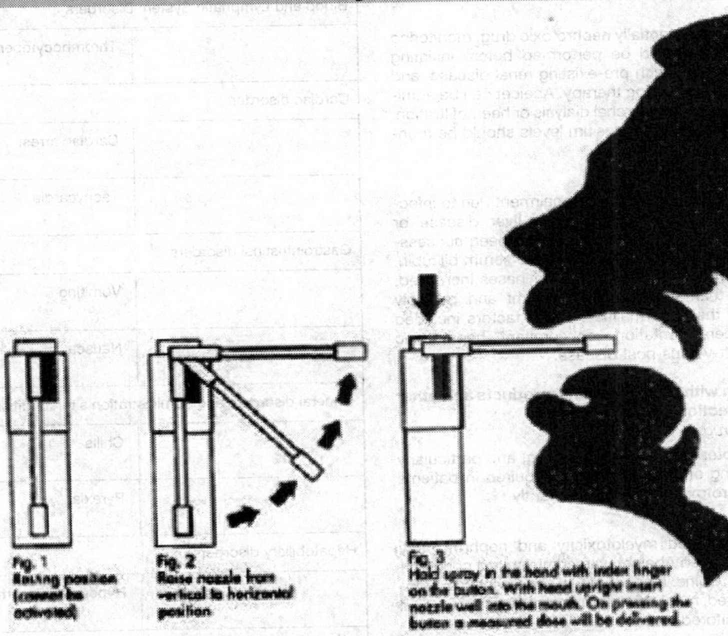
Fig. 1
Resting position (cannot be activated)
Fig. 2
Raise nozzle from vertical to horizontal position
Fig. 3
Hold spray in the hand with index finger on the button. With head upright insert nozzle well into the mouth. On pressing the button a measured dose will be delivered.

Pressing the plunger once delivers a single metered dose. (Before use it may be necessary to press the plunger 2-3 times to activate spray).

6.3 Shelf life
24 months

6.4 Special precautions for storage
Keep away from a naked flame. Store in a cool place

6.5 Nature and contents of container
White aluminium can with 100ml pumps, white high density polypropylene folding arm activator and white high density polyethylene cap.

6.6 Special precautions for disposal and other handling
(see Figure 1 above)

7. MARKETING AUTHORISATION HOLDER
Manx Pharma Ltd

Taylor Group House

Wedgnock Lane

Warwick

CV34 5YA

United Kingdom

8. MARKETING AUTHORISATION NUMBER(S)
PL 15833/0001

9. DATE OF FIRST AUTHORISATION/RENEWAL OF THE AUTHORISATION
1 September 1997

10. DATE OF REVISION OF THE TEXT
March 2008

Abelcet

(Cephalon Limited)

1. NAME OF THE MEDICINAL PRODUCT
Abelcet® 5mg/ml Concentrate for Solution for Infusion

2. QUALITATIVE AND QUANTITATIVE COMPOSITION
Amphotericin B Lipid Complex. Each vial contains 5mg Amphotericin B per ml.

For excipients, see 6.1.

3. PHARMACEUTICAL FORM
Concentrate for solution for infusion

4. CLINICAL PARTICULARS

4.1 Therapeutic indications
Abelcet is indicated for the treatment of severe invasive candidiasis.

Abelcet is also indicated as second line therapy for the treatment of severe systemic fungal infections in patients who have not responded to conventional amphotericin B or other systemic antifungal agents, in those who have renal impairment or other contra-indications to conventional amphotericin B, or in patients who have developed amphotericin B nephrotoxicity. Abelcet treatment is indicated as second line treatment for invasive aspergillosis, cryptococcal meningitis and disseminated cryptococcosis in HIV patients, fusariosis, coccidiomycosis, zygomycosis and blastomycosis.

4.2 Posology and method of administration
Abelcet is a sterile, pyrogen-free suspension which must be diluted for intravenous infusion only.

For severe systemic infections treatment is generally recommended at 5.0 mg/kg for at least 14 days. Abelcet should be administered by intravenous infusion at a rate of 2.5 mg/kg/hr. When commencing treatment with Abelcet for the first time it is recommended to administer a test dose immediately prior to the first infusion. The first infusion should be prepared according to the instructions then, over a period of approximately 15 minutes, 1mg of the infusion should be administered to the patient. After this amount has been administered the infusion should be stopped and the patient observed carefully for 30 minutes. If the patient shows no signs of hypersensitivity the infusion may be continued. As for use with all amphotericin B products, facilities for cardiopulmonary resuscitation should be readily at hand when administering Abelcet for the first time, due to the possible occurrence of anaphylactoid reactions. Abelcet has been administered for as long as 28 months, and cumulative doses have been as high as 73.6g without significant toxicity.

An in-line filter may be used for intravenous infusion of Abelcet. The mean pore diameter of the filter should be no less than 15 microns.

Abelcet may be administered to diabetic patients.

Paediatric use

Systemic fungal infections in children have been treated successfully with Abelcet at doses comparable to the recommended adult dose on a bodyweight basis. Adverse events seen in paediatric patients are similar to those seen in adults.

Use in elderly patients

Systemic fungal infections in elderly patients have been treated successfully with Abelcet at doses comparable to the recommended dose on a bodyweight basis.

Use in neutropenic patients

Abelcet has been used successfully to treat systemic fungal infections in patients who are severely neutropenic as a consequence of haematological malignancy or the use of cytotoxic or immunosuppressive drugs.

Use in patients with renal or liver disease

Systemic fungal infections in patients with renal or liver disease have been treated successfully with Abelcet at doses comparable to the recommended dose on a body weight basis (see special warnings and precautions for further information).

4.3 Contraindications
Abelcet is contraindicated in patients with known hypersensitivity to any of its constituents, unless in the opinion of

the physician the advantages of using Abelcet outweigh the risks of hypersensitivity.

4.4 Special warnings and precautions for use

Systemic Fungal Infections

Abelcet should not be used for treating common or superficial, clinically inapparent fungal infections that are detectable only by positive skin or serologic tests.

Renal Disease

Since Abelcet is a potentially nephrotoxic drug, monitoring of renal function should be performed before initiating treatment in patients with pre-existing renal disease, and at least once weekly during therapy. Abelcet can be administered to patients during renal dialysis or haemofiltration. Serum potassium and magnesium levels should be monitored regularly.

Liver Disease

Patients with concurrent hepatic impairment due to infection, graft-versus-host disease, other liver disease or administration of hepatotoxic drugs have been successfully treated with Abelcet. In cases where serum bilirubin, alkaline phosphatase or serum transaminases increased, factors other than Abelcet were present and possibly accounted for the abnormalities. These factors included infection, hyperalimentation, concomitant hepatotoxic drugs and graft-versus-host disease.

4.5 Interaction with other medicinal products and other forms of interaction

Nephrotoxic Drugs

Abelcet is a potentially nephrotoxic drug, and particularly close monitoring of renal function is required in patients receiving nephrotoxic drugs concomitantly.

Zidovudine

In dogs, exacerbated myelotoxicity and nephrotoxicity were observed when Abelcet was administered concomitantly with zidovudine. If concomitant treatment with zidovudine is required, renal and haematologic function should be closely monitored.

Cyclosporin

Preliminary data suggest that patients receiving Abelcet concomitantly with high dose cyclosporin experience an increase in serum creatinine. The data also suggest that the increase in serum creatinine is caused by cyclosporin and not Abelcet.

The interaction of Abelcet with other drugs has not been studied to date. Conventional amphotericin B has been reported to interact with antineoplastic agents, corticosteroids and corticotrophin (ACTH), digitalis glycosides and skeletal muscle relaxants.

Leukocyte transfusions

Acute pulmonary toxicity has been reported in patients receiving intravenous amphotericin B and leukocyte transfusions.

4.6 Pregnancy and lactation

Conventional amphotericin B has been used successfully to treat systemic fungal infections in pregnant women with no obvious effects on the foetus, but only a small number of cases have been reported. Reproductive toxicity studies of Abelcet in rats and rabbits showed no evidence of embryotoxicity, foetotoxicity or teratogenicity. However, safety for use in pregnant or lactating women has not been established for Abelcet. Therefore, Abelcet should be administered to pregnant or lactating women only for life-threatening disease when the likely benefit exceeds the risk to the mother and foetus.

4.7 Effects on ability to drive and use machines

Abelcet is unlikely to affect the ability of an individual to drive or use machines, since adverse reactions are usually infusion-related. However, the clinical condition of patients who require Abelcet generally precludes driving or operating machinery.

4.8 Undesirable effects

Related adverse events assessed by causality, severity and frequency have been tabulated in Table 1.

Table 1: Reports adverse events obtained from post-marketing surveillance (10.5 years data), the events are ranked by frequency within each system organ class

(see Table 1 opposite)

Adverse reactions that have been reported to occur with conventional amphotericin B may occur with Abelcet. In general, the physician should monitor the patient for any type of adverse event associated with conventional amphotericin B.

Patients in whom significant renal toxicity was observed following conventional amphotericin B frequently did not experience similar effects when Abelcet was substituted. Adverse reactions related to the administration of Abelcet have generally been mild or moderate, and have been most prevalent during the first 2 days of dosing.

Premedication (e.g. paracetamol) may be administered for the prevention of infusion related adverse events. The most common clinical adverse events have been chills, pyrexia, nausea and vomiting, which may occur during the first 2 days of treatment.

Table 1 Reports adverse events obtained from post-marketing surveillance (10.5 years data), the events are ranked by frequency within each system organ class

System Organ Class	**Adverse Event**	**Frequency**	
		%	**Category**
Blood and Lymphatic System Disorders			
	Thrombocytopenia	0.007	Very rare (< 0.01%)
Cardiac disorders			
	Cardiac arrest	0.008	Very rare (< 0.01%)
	Tachycardia	0.014	Rare (>0.01% and <0.1%)
Gastrointestinal disorders			
	Vomiting	0.005	Very rare (< 0.01%)
	Nausea	0.004	Very rare (< 0.01%)
General disorders and administration site conditions			
	Chills	0.058	Rare (>0.01% and <0.1%)
	Pyrexia	0.050	Rare (>0.01% and <0.1%)
Hepatobiliary disorders			
	Hyperbilirubinaemia	0.010	Rare (>0.01% and <0.1%)
Immune system disorders			
	Anaphylactic responses	0.011	Rare (>0.01% and <0.1%)
Investigations			
	Blood creatinine increased	0.019	Rare (>0.01% and <0.1%)
	Blood alkaline phosphatase increased	0.005	Very rare (< 0.01%)
	Liver test function abnormal	0.002	Very rare (< 0.01%)
Metabolism and Nutrition Disorders			
	Hypokalaemia	0.014	Rare (>0.01% and <0.1%)
Nervous system disorders			
	Convulsion	0.005	Very rare (< 0.01%)
	Encephalopathy	0.003	Very rare (< 0.01%)
	Neuropathy	0.002	Very rare (< 0.01%)
Renal and urinary disorders			
	Renal failure	0.006	Very rare (< 0.01%)
	Renal failure acute	0.005	Very rare (< 0.01%)
	Renal impairment	0.004	Very rare (< 0.01%)
Respiratory, thoracic and mediastinal disorders			
	Dyspnoea	0.016	Rare (>0.01% and <0.1%)
	Bronchospasm	0.010	Rare (>0.01% and <0.1%)
Skin and subcutaneous tissue disorders			
	Rash	0.006	Very rare (< 0.01%)
Vascular disorders			
	Hypertension	0.013	Rare (>0.01% and <0.1%)
	Hypotension	0.011	Rare (>0.01% and <0.1%)

›clines in renal function, shown by increased serum ›atinine and hypokalaemia, have not typically required ›scontinuation of treatment.

›normal liver function tests have been reported with ›elcet and other amphotericin B products. Although ›er factors such as infection, hyperalimentation, conco- ›tant hepatotoxic drugs and graft-versus-host disease ›y be contributory, a causal relationship with Abelcet ›nnot be excluded. Patients with abnormal liver function ›sts should be carefully monitored and cessation of treat- ›nt considered if liver function deteriorates.

Overdose

instance of toxicity due to overdose with Abelcet has ›en reported. One paediatric patient received a single ›se of 13.1mg/kg on one occasion, without adverse ›ects. Should an overdose occur, the patient should be ›ated as deemed appropriate by the physician.

PHARMACOLOGICAL PROPERTIES

elcet consists of the antifungal agent, amphotericin B, ›mplexed to two phospholipids. Amphotericin B is a ›crocyclic, polyene, broad-spectrum antifungal antibio- produced by *Streptomyces nodosus*. The lipophilic ›iety of amphotericin B allows molecules of the drug to complexed in a ribbon-like structure with the phospho- ›ds.

Pharmacodynamic properties

C Code

2A A01

›chanism of action

›photericin B, the active antifungal agent in Abelcet, may fungistatic or fungicidal, depending on its concentration d on fungal susceptibility. The drug probably acts by ›ding to ergosterol in the fungal cell membrane causing ›sequent membrane damage. As a result, cell contents k from the fungal cell, and, ultimately, cell death occurs. ›ding of the drug to sterols in human cell membranes ›y result in toxicity, although amphotericin B has greater ›nity for fungal ergosterol than for the cholesterol of ›man cells.

›crobiological activity

›photericin B is active against many fungal pathogens *in* *›o*, including *Candida* spp., *Cryptococcus neoformans*, *›ergillus* spp., *Mucor* spp., *Sporothrix schenckii*, *›stomyces dermatitidis*, *Coccidioides immitis* and *›toplasma capsulatum*. Most strains are inhibited by ›photericin B concentrations of 0.03-1.0 μg/ml. Ampho- ›cin B has little or no activity against bacteria or viruses. › activity of Abelcet against fungal pathogens *in vitro* is ›mparable to that of amphotericin B. However, activity of ›elcet *in vitro* may not predict activity in the infected host.

Pharmacokinetic properties

›photericin B is complexed to phospholipids in Abelcet. › pharmacokinetic properties of Abelcet and conven- ›al amphotericin B are different. Pharmacokinetic stu- s in animals showed that, after administration of ›elcet, amphotericin B levels were highest in the liver, ›een and lung. Amphotericin B in Abelcet was rapidly ›tributed to tissues. The ratio of drug concentrations in ›ues to those in blood increased disproportionately with ›reasing dose, suggesting that elimination of the drug ›m the tissues was delayed. Peak blood levels of ampho- ›icin B were lower after administration of Abelcet than ›er administration of equivalent amounts of conventional ›g. Administration of conventional amphotericin B ›ulted in much lower tissue levels than did dosing with ›elcet. However, in dogs, conventional amphotericin B ›duced 20-fold higher kidney concentrations than did ›elcet given at comparable doses.

› pharmacokinetics of Abelcet in whole blood were ›ermined in patients with mucocutaneous leishmaniasis. ›sults for mean pharmacokinetic parameters at 5.0 mg/ ›day were as follows:

	Abelcet
›ose: (mg/kg/day)	5.0
›eak blood level C_{max}: (μg/ml)	1.7
›rea under time-concentration curve ›UC_{0-24}: (μg.hr/ml)	9.5
›learance: (ml/hr.kg)	211.0
›olume of distribution Vd: (l/kg)	2286.0
›alf-life $T_{½}$: (hr)	173.4

› rapid clearance and large volume of distribution of ›elcet result in a relatively low AUC and are consistent › preclinical data showing high tissue concentrations. › kinetics of Abelcet are linear, the AUC increases ›portionately with dose.

›tails of the tissue distribution and metabolism of Abelcet ›umans, and the mechanisms responsible for reduced ›icity, are not well understood. The following data are ›ailable from necropsy in a heart transplant patient who received Abelcet at a dose of 5.3 mg/kg for 3 consecutive days immediately before death:

Organ	Abelcet tissue concentration expressed as amphotericin B content (mg/kg)
Spleen	290.0
Lung	222.0
Liver	196.0
Kidney	6.9
Lymph node	7.6
Heart	5.0
Brain	1.6

5.3 Preclinical safety data

Acute toxicity studies in rodents showed that Abelcet was 10-fold to 20-fold less toxic than conventional amphotericin B. Multiple-dose toxicity studies in dogs lasting 2-4 weeks showed that on a mg/kg basis, Abelcet was 8-fold to 10-fold less nephrotoxic than conventional amphotericin B. This decreased nephrotoxicity was presumably a result of lower drug concentrations in the kidney.

5.4 Carcinogenesis, mutagenesis and impairment of fertility

Since conventional amphotericin B first became available, there have been no reports of drug-related carcinogenicity, mutagenicity, teratogenicity or adverse effect on fertility. Abelcet has been shown not to be mutagenic by the *in vivo* mouse micronucleus assay, *in vitro* bacterial and lymphoma mutation assays, and an *in vivo* cytogenetic assay. It has been shown not to be teratogenic in mice and rabbits.

Phospholipids are essential constituents of human cell membranes. The average diet provides several grams of phospholipids each day. There is no evidence that phospholipids, including DMPC and DMPG, are carcinogenic, mutagenic or teratogenic.

6. PHARMACEUTICAL PARTICULARS

6.1 List of excipients

L-α-dimyristoylphosphatidylcholine (DMPC)

L-α-dimyristoylphosphatidylglycerol (sodium and ammonium salts) (DMPG)

Sodium Chloride

Water for Injection

6.2 Incompatibilities

Abelcet should not be mixed with other drugs or electrolytes.

6.3 Shelf life

24 months.

6.4 Special precautions for storage

Store at 2 - 8°C. Do not freeze. Keep vial in the outer carton.

6.5 Nature and contents of container

Abelcet is a sterile, pyrogen-free yellow suspension in a type I glass single use vial containing 10 or 20 ml (50 mg or 100 mg amphotericin B). The vial is sealed with a rubber stopper and aluminum seal. Vials are packaged in cartons of 10 vials. Not all pack sizes may be marketed.

6.6 Special precautions for disposal and other handling

Abelcet is a sterile, pyrogen-free suspension to be diluted for intravenous infusion only.

Preparation of the suspension for infusion

ASEPTIC TECHNIQUE MUST BE STRICTLY OBSERVED THROUGHOUT HANDLING OF ABELCET, SINCE NO BACTERIOSTATIC AGENT OR PRESERVATIVE IS PRESENT.

Allow the suspension to come to room temperature. Shake gently until there is no evidence of any yellow settlement at the bottom of the vial. Withdraw the appropriate dose of Abelcet from the required number of vials into one or more sterile 20 ml syringes using a 17 to 19 gauge needle. Remove the needle from each syringe filled with Abelcet and replace with the 5 micron high flow filter needle (supplied by B. Braun Medical, Inc.) provided with each vial. Insert the filter needle of the syringe into an IV bag containing 5.0% Dextrose for Injection and empty the contents of the syringe into the bag using either manual pressure or an infusion pump. The final infusion concentration should be 1 mg/ml. For paediatric patients and patients with cardiovascular disease the drug may be diluted with 5.0% Dextrose for Injection to a final infusion concentration of 2 mg/ ml. Do not use the agent after dilution with 5.0% Dextrose for Injection if there is any evidence of foreign matter. Vials are single use. Unused material should be discarded. The infusion is best administered by means of an infusion pump.

DO NOT DILUTE WITH SALINE SOLUTIONS OR MIX WITH OTHER DRUGS OR ELECTROLYTES. The compatibility of Abelcet with these materials has not been established. An existing intravenous line should be flushed with 5.0% Dextrose for Injection before infusion of Abelcet or a separate infusion line should be used.

The diluted ready for use suspension may be stored at 2°C - 8°C for up to 24 hours prior to use. Shake vigorously before use. Do not store for later use.

7. MARKETING AUTHORISATION HOLDER

Cephalon Limited
1 Albany Place
Hyde Way
Welwyn Garden City
Hertfordshire
AL7 3BT
UK

8. MARKETING AUTHORISATION NUMBER(S)

PL: 21799/0001

9. DATE OF FIRST AUTHORISATION/RENEWAL OF THE AUTHORISATION

16/02/2006

10. DATE OF REVISION OF THE TEXT

06/11/2007

Abraxane 5 mg/ml powder for suspension for infusion

(Abraxis BioScience Limited)

1. NAME OF THE MEDICINAL PRODUCT

Abraxane 5 mg/ml powder for suspension for infusion.

2. QUALITATIVE AND QUANTITATIVE COMPOSITION

Each vial contains 100 mg of paclitaxel (as paclitaxel albumin).

After reconstitution, each ml of suspension contains 5 mg of paclitaxel (as paclitaxel albumin).

Excipients

The reconstituted medicinal product contains approximately 425 mg sodium per dose.

For a full list of excipients, see section 6.1.

3. PHARMACEUTICAL FORM

Powder for suspension for infusion.

The reconstituted suspension has a pH of 6-7.5 and an osmolality of 300-360 mOsm/kg.

The powder is white to yellow.

4. CLINICAL PARTICULARS

4.1 Therapeutic indications

Abraxane monotherapy is indicated for the treatment of metastatic breast cancer in patients who have failed first-line treatment for metastatic disease and for whom standard, anthracycline containing therapy is not indicated (see section 4.4).

4.2 Posology and method of administration

Abraxane should only be administered under the supervision of a qualified oncologist in units specialised in the administration of cytotoxic agents.

The procedure for reconstitution is described in section 6.6.

The recommended dose of Abraxane is 260 mg/m^2 administered intravenously over 30 minutes every 3 weeks.

Dose adjustments during treatment:

Patients who experience severe neutropenia (neutrophil count < 0.50 × 10^9/l for a week or longer) or severe sensory neuropathy during Abraxane therapy should have the dose reduced to 220 mg/m^2 for subsequent courses. Following recurrence of severe neutropenia or severe sensory neuropathy, additional dose reduction should be made to 180 mg/m^2. Abraxane should not be administered until neutrophil counts recover to >1.5 × 10^9/l. For grade 3 sensory neuropathy withhold treatment until resolution to grade 1 or 2, followed by a dose reduction for all subsequent courses.

Patients with hepatic impairment:

Insufficient data are currently available to recommend dose modifications in patients with mild to moderate hepatic impairment that ensure acceptable toxicity while maintaining efficacy. Patients with severe hepatic impairment should not be treated with paclitaxel (see sections 4.4.and 5.2).

Patients with impaired renal function:

Studies in patients with impaired renal function have not been performed and insufficient data are currently available to recommend dose modifications in patients with renal impairment (see section 5.2).

Paediatric patients:

Abraxane is not recommended for use in children and adolescents below age 18 years due to insufficient data on safety and efficacy.

Elderly patients:

In the clinical studies, no toxicities occurred notably more frequently among elderly patients who received Abraxane.

Table 1: Adverse reactions reported with Abraxane at any dose in clinical studies.

Infections and infestations	*Common*: Infection, urinary tract infection, folliculitis, upper respiratory tract infection, candidiasis, sinusitis *Uncommon*: Oral candidiasis, nasopharyngitis, cellulitis, herpes simplex, viral infection, pneumonia, catheter-related infection, funga infection, herpes zoster, injection site infection
Neoplasms benign, malignant and unspecified (including cysts and polyps)	*Uncommon:* Metastatic pain, tumour necrosis
Blood and lymphatic system disorders	*Very Common*: Neutropenia, anaemia, leukopenia, thrombocytopenia, lymphopenia, bone marrow suppression *Common*: Febrile neutropenia
Immune system disorders	*Uncommon*[1]: Hypersensitivity *Rare:* Severe hypersensitivity
Metabolism and nutrition disorders	*Very common:* Anorexia *Common:* Dehydration, decreased appetite, hypokalaemia *Uncommon:* Hypophosphataemia, fluid retention, hypoalbuminaemia, polydipsia, hyperglycaemia, hypocalcaemia, hypoglycaemi hyponatraemia
Psychiatric disorders	*Common*: Insomnia, depression, anxiety *Uncommon*: Restlessness
Nervous system disorders	*Very Common*: Peripheral neuropathy, neuropathy, hypoaesthesia, paraesthesia. *Common*: Peripheral sensory neuropathy, headache, dysgeusia, dizziness, peripheral motor neuropathy, ataxia, sensory disturbanc somnolence. *Uncommon*: Polyneuropathy, areflexia, dyskinesia, hyporeflexia, neuralgia, sensory loss, syncope, postural dizziness, neuropathic pain, tremor
Eye disorders	*Common*: Increased lacrimation, blurred vision, dry eye, keratoconjunctivitis sicca, madarosis *Uncommon*: Eye irritation, eye pain, abnormal vision, reduced visual acuity, conjunctivitis, visual disturbance, eye pruritus, keratiti
Ear and labyrinth disorders	*Common*: Vertigo *Uncommon*: Ear pain, tinnitus
Cardiac disorders	*Common*: Tachycardia, arrhythmia, supraventricular tachycardia *Rare:* bradycardia, cardiac arrest
Vascular disorders	*Common*: Flushing, hot flushes, hypertension, lymphoedema *Uncommon*: Hypotension, peripheral coldness, orthostatic hypotension *Rare:* Thrombosis
Respiratory, thoracic and mediastinal disorders	*Common*: Dyspnoea, epistaxis, pharyngolaryngeal pain, cough, rhinitis, rhinorrhoea *Uncommon*: Productive cough, exertional dyspnoea, sinus congestion, decreased breath sounds, pleural effusion, allergic rhinitis hoarseness, nasal congestion, nasal dryness, wheezing, pulmonary emboli, pulmonary thromboembolism *Rare:* Interstitial pneumonitis
Gastrointestinal disorders	*Very Common*: Nausea, diarrhoea, vomiting, constipation, stomatitis *Common*: Abdominal pain, abdominal distension, upper abdominal pain, dyspepsia, gastrooesophageal reflux disease, oral hypoaesthesia *Uncommon*: Dysphagia, flatulence, glossodynia, dry mouth, gingival pain, loose stools, oesophagitis, lower abdominal pain, mout ulceration, oral pain, rectal haemorrhage
Hepatobiliary disorders	*Uncommon*: Hepatomegaly
Skin and subcutaneous tissue disorders	*Very Common*: Alopecia, rash *Common*: Nail disorder, pruritus, dry skin, erythema, nail pigmentation/discolouration, skin hyperpigmentation, onycholysis, nail changes *Uncommon*: Nail bed tenderness, urticaria, skin pain, photosensitivity reaction, pigmentation disorder, pruritic rash, skin disorder, hyperhidrosis, onychomadesis, erythematous rash, generalised rash, dermatitis, night sweats, maculo-papular rash, vitiligo, hypotrichosis, nail discomfort, generalized pruritus, macular rash, papular rash, skin lesion, swollen face
Musculoskeletal and connective tissue disorders	*Very Common*: Arthralgia, myalgia. *Common*: Pain in extremity, bone pain, back pain, muscle cramps, limb pain *Uncommon*: Chest wall pain, muscular weakness, neck pain, groin pain, muscle spasms, musculoskeletal pain, flank pain, limb discomfort, muscle weakness
Renal and urinary disorders	*Uncommon*: Dysuria, pollakiuria, haematuria, nocturia, polyuria, urinary incontinence
Reproductive system and breast disorders	*Uncommon*: Breast pain
General disorders and administration site conditions	*Very Common*: Fatigue, asthenia, pyrexia. *Common*: Peripheral oedema, mucosal inflammation, pain, rigors, oedema, weakness, decreased performance status, chest pai influenza-like illness, malaise, lethargy, hyperpyrexia *Uncommon*: Chest discomfort, abnormal gait, swelling, injection site reaction
Investigations	*Common*: Decreased weight, increased alanine aminotransferase, increased aspartate aminotransferase, decreased haematocrit, decreased red blood cell count, increased body temperature, increased gamma-glutamyltransferase, increased blood alkaline phosphatase *Uncommon*: Increased blood pressure, increased weight, increased blood lactate dehydrogenase, increased blood creatinine, increased blood glucose, increased blood phosphorus, decreased blood potassium, increased bilirubin
Injury, poisoning and procedural complications	*Uncommon*: Contusion *Rare*: Radiation recall phenomenon, radiation pneumonitis

[1] The frequency of hypersensitivity reactions is calculated based on one definitely related case in a population of 789 patients

Contraindications

persensitivity to the active substance or to any of the cipients.

ctation.

tients who have baseline neutrophil counts 1.5 × 10^9/l.

Special warnings and precautions for use

braxane is an albumin-bound nanoparticle formulation of aclitaxel, which may have substantially different pharma-logical properties compared to other formulations of aclitaxel (see sections 5.1 and 5.2). It should not be bstituted for or with other paclitaxel formulations.

ypersensitivity:

hypersensitivity occurs, the medicinal product should be scontinued immediately, symptomatic treatment should e initiated, and that patient should not be rechallenged th paclitaxel.

aematology:

one marrow suppression (primarily neutropenia) occurs equently with Abraxane. Neutropenia is dose-dependent nd a dose-limiting toxicity. Frequent monitoring of blood ell counts should be performed during Abraxane therapy. atients should not be retreated with subsequent cycles of braxane until neutrophils recover to > 1.5 × 10^9/l and latelets recover to > 100 × 10^9/l.

leuropathy:

ensory neuropathy occurs frequently with Abraxane, lthough development of severe symptoms is less com-mon. The occurrence of grade 1 or 2 sensory neuropathy loes not generally require dose reduction. If grade 3 sen-ory neuropathy develops, treatment should be withheld intil resolution to grade 1 or 2 followed by a dose reduction or all subsequent courses of Abraxane is recommended see section 4.2).

lepatic impairment:

Because the toxicity of paclitaxel can be increased with hepatic impairment, administration of Abraxane in patients with hepatic impairment should be performed with caution. Patients with hepatic impairment may be at increased risk of toxicity, particularly from myelosuppression, and such patients should be closely monitored for development of profound myelosuppression.

Patients with severe hepatic impairment (bilirubin > 5 × ULN or AST/ALT > 10 × ULN) have not been studied and should not be treated with Abraxane. The appropriate dose regimen in patients with less severe hepatic impairment is unknown. A dose reduction in patients with bilirubin > 2 ULN must be considered since paclitaxel clearance is decreased in patients with high bilirubin levels (see section 5.2).

Cardiotoxicity:

While cardiotoxicity unequivocally related to Abraxane has not been demonstrated, cardiac events are not uncommon in the indicated population, especially in patients who have previously received anthracyclines or have underlying car-diac or pulmonary disease. Thus patients receiving Abrax-ane should be vigilantly monitored by physicians for the occurrence of cardiac events.

CNS metastases:

The effectiveness and safety of Abraxane in patients with central nervous system (CNS) metastases has not been established. CNS metastases are generally not well con-trolled by systemic chemotherapy.

Gastrointestinal symptoms:

If patients experience nausea, vomiting and diarrhoea following the administration of Abraxane, they may be treated with commonly used anti-emetics and constipating agents.

Excipients:

When reconstituted, Abraxane contains approximately 425 mg sodium per dose. To be taken into consideration by patients on a controlled sodium diet.

4.5 Interaction with other medicinal products and other forms of interaction

No interaction studies have been performed.

The metabolism of paclitaxel is catalysed, in part, by cytochrome P450 isoenzymes CYP2C8 and CYP3A4 (see section 5.2). Therefore, caution should be exercised when administering paclitaxel concomitantly with medi-cines known to inhibit (e.g. ketoconazole and other imida-zole antifungals, erythromycin, fluoxetine, gemfibrozil, cimetidine, ritonavir, saquinavir, indinavir, and nelfinavir)) or induce (e.g. rifampicin, carbamazepine, phenytoin, efa-virenz, nevirapine) either CYP2C8 or CYP3A4.

Abraxane is indicated for mono-therapy. Abraxane should not be used in combination with other anticancer agents.

4.6 Pregnancy and lactation

Pregnancy:

There are very limited data on the use of paclitaxel in human pregnancy. Paclitaxel is suspected to cause ser-ious birth defects when administered during pregnancy. Studies in animals have shown reproductive toxicity (see section 5.3). Abraxane should not be used in pregnancy, and in women of childbearing potential not using effective contraception, unless the clinical condition of the mother requires treatment with paclitaxel.

Women of childbearing potential should use effective con-traception during and up to 1 month after receiving treat-ment with Abraxane. Male patients treated with Abraxane are advised not to father a child during and up to six months after treatment.

Lactation:

It is not known if paclitaxel is excreted in human milk. Because of potential serious adverse reactions in breast-feeding infants, Abraxane is contraindicated during lacta-tion. Breastfeeding must be discontinued for the duration of therapy.

Fertility:

Abraxane induced infertility in male rats (see section 5.3). Male patients should seek advice on conservation of sperm prior to treatment because of the possibility of irreversible infertility due to therapy with Abraxane.

Sexually active men and women should use effective methods of contraception during treatment and up to six months after treatment for men, and one month after treat-ment for women.

4.7 Effects on ability to drive and use machines

Abraxane has minor or moderate influence on the ability to drive and use machines. Abraxane may cause adverse reactions such as tiredness (very common) and dizziness (common) that may affect the ability to drive and use machinery. Patients should be advised not to drive and use machines if they feel tired or dizzy.

4.8 Undesirable effects

The following are the most common and important inci-dences of adverse reactions related to 229 patients with metastatic breast cancer who were treated with 260 mg/m^2 Abraxane once every three weeks in the pivotal phase III clinical study.

Blood and lymphatic system disorders: Neutropenia was the most notable important haematological toxicity (reported in 79% of patients), and was rapidly reversible and dose dependent; leukopenia was reported in 71% of patients. Grade 4 neutropenia (< 0.5 × 10^9/l) occurred in 9% of patients treated with Abraxane. Febrile neutropenia occurred in four patients on Abraxane. Anaemia (Hb < 10 g/dl) was observed in 46% of patients on Abraxane, and was severe (Hb < 8 g/dl) in three cases. Lymphopenia was observed in 45% of the patients.

Nervous system disorders: In general, the frequency and severity of neurotoxicity was dose-dependent in patients receiving Abraxane. Peripheral neuropathy (mostly Grade 1 or 2 sensory neuropathy) was observed in 68% of patients on Abraxane with 10% being Grade 3, and no cases of Grade 4.

Gastrointestinal disorders: Nausea occurred in 29% of the patients and diarrhoea in 25% of the patients.

Skin and subcutaneous tissue disorders: Alopecia was observed in 90% of the patients treated with Abraxane.

Musculoskeletal and connective tissue disorders: Arthral-gia occurred in 32% of patients on Abraxane and was severe in 6% of cases. Myalgia occurred in 24% of patients on Abraxane and was severe in 7% of cases. The symp-toms were usually transient, typically occurred three days after Abraxane administration and resolved within a week.

General disorders and administration site conditions: Asth-enia/Fatigue was reported in 40% of the patients.

Table 1 lists adverse reactions associated with the admin-istration of Abraxane to patients from studies in which Abraxane has been administered as a single agent at any dose in any indication (N = 789).

The frequency of undesirable effects listed in table 1 is defined using the following convention:

Very common (≥ 1/10); common (≥ 1/100 to < 1/10); uncommon (≥ 1/1,000 to < 1/100); rare (≥ 1/10,000 to < 1/1,000); very rare (< 1/10,000), not known (cannot be estimated from the available data).

Within each frequency grouping, undesirable effects are presented in order of decreasing seriousness.

(see Table 1 on previous page)

Post-marketing experience:

Cranial nerve palsies, vocal cord paresis, and rare reports of severe hypersensitivity reactions have been reported during post-marketing surveillance of Abraxane.

In some patients previously exposed to capecitabine, reports of palmar-plantar erythrodysaesthesiae have been reported as part of the continuing surveillance of Abraxane. Because these events have been reported voluntarily dur-ing clinical practice, true estimates of frequency cannot be made and a causal relationship to the events has not been established.

4.9 Overdose

There is no known antidote for paclitaxel overdose. In the event of an overdose, the patient should be closely mon-itored. Treatment should be directed at the major antici-pated toxicities, which are bone marrow suppression, mucositis and peripheral neuropathy.

5. PHARMACOLOGICAL PROPERTIES

5.1 Pharmacodynamic properties

Pharmacotherapeutic group: Taxanes, ATC Code: L01CD01

Paclitaxel is an antimicrotubule agent that promotes the assembly of microtubules from tubulin dimers and stabi-lises microtubules by preventing depolymerisation. This stability results in the inhibition of the normal dynamic reorganisation of the microtubule network that is essential for vital interphase and mitotic cellular functions. In addi-tion, paclitaxel induces abnormal arrays or "bundles" of microtubules throughout the cell cycle and multiple asters of microtubules during mitosis.

Abraxane contains human serum albumin-paclitaxel nano-particles, where the paclitaxel is present in a non-crystal-line, amorphous state. Albumin is known to mediate endothelial transcytosis of plasma constituents and *in vitro* studies demonstrated that the presence of albumin enhances transport of paclitaxel across endothelial cells. It is hypothesised that this enhanced transendothelial transport is mediated by the gp-60 albumin receptor, and that there is accumulation of paclitaxel in the area of tumour due to the albumin-binding protein SPARC (secreted protein acidic rich in cysteine).

Breast carcinoma:

Data from 106 patients accrued in two single-arm open-label studies and from 454 patients treated in a randomised Phase III comparative study are available to support the use of Abraxane in metastatic breast cancer. This informa-tion is presented below.

Single-arm open-label studies:

In one study, Abraxane was administered as a 30-minute infusion at a dose of 175 mg/m^2 to 43 patients with meta-static breast cancer. The second trial utilised a dose of 300 mg/m^2 as a 30 minute infusion in 63 patients with metastatic breast cancer. Patients were treated without steroid pre-treatment or planned G-CSF support. Cycles were administered at 3 week intervals. The response rates in all patients were 39.5% (95% CI: 24.9%-54.2%) and 47.6% (95% CI: 35.3%-60.0%), respectively. The median time to disease progression was 5.3 months (175 mg/m^2; 95% CI: 4.6-6.2 months) and 6.1 months (300 mg/m^2; 95% CI: 4.2-9.8 months).

Randomised comparative study:

This multi-centre trial was conducted in patients with meta-static breast cancer, who were treated every 3 weeks with single-agent paclitaxel, either as solvent-based paclitaxel 175 mg/m^2 given as a 3-hour infusion with premedication to prevent hypersensitivity (N = 225), or as Abraxane 260 mg/m^2 given as a 30 minute infusion without preme-dication (N = 229).

Sixty-four percent of patients had impaired performance status (ECOG 1 or 2) at study entry; 79% had visceral metastases; and 76% had > 3 sites of metastases. Four-teen percent of the patients had not received prior che-motherapy; 27% had received chemotherapy in the adjuvant setting only, 40% in the metastatic setting only, and 19% in both metastatic and adjuvant settings. Fifty-nine percent received study medicinal product as second or greater than second-line therapy. Seventy-seven per-cent of the patients had been previously exposed to anthracyclines.

Results for overall response rate and time to disease pro-gression, and progression-free survival and survival for patients receiving > 1st-line therapy, are shown below.

(see Table 2 on next page)

229 patients treated with Abraxane in the randomized, controlled clinical trial were evaluated for safety. Neuro-toxictiy to paclitaxel was evaluated through improvement by one grade for patients experiencing grade 3 peripheral neuropathy at any time during therapy. The natural course of peripheral neuropathy to resolution to baseline due to cumulative toxicity of Abraxane after > 6 courses of treat-ment was not evaluated and remains unknown.

5.2 Pharmacokinetic properties

The pharmacokinetics of total paclitaxel following 30- and 180-minute infusions of Abraxane at dose levels of 80 to 375 mg/m^2 were determined in clinical studies. The pacli-taxel exposure (AUC) increased linearly from 2653 to 16736 ng.hr/ml following dosing from 80 to 300 mg/m^2.

Following intravenous administration of Abraxane to patients with metastatic breast cancer at the recom-mended clinical dose of 260 mg/m^2, paclitaxel plasma concentrations declined in a multiphasic manner. The mean C_{max} of paclitaxel, which occurred at the end of the infusion, was 18.7 μg/ml. The mean total clearance was 15 l/hr/m^2. The terminal half-life was about 27 hours. The mean volume of distribution was 632 l/m^2; the large volume of distribution indicates extensive extravascular distribution and/or tissue binding of paclitaxel.

In a study in patients with advanced solid tumours, the pharmacokinetic characteristics of paclitaxel following Abraxane administered intravenously at 260 mg/m^2 over 30 minutes were compared with those following 175 mg/m^2 of the solvent-based paclitaxel injection administered over 3 hours. The clearance of paclitaxel with Abraxane was larger (43%) than that following a solvent-based pacli-taxel injection and its volume of distribution was also higher (53%). Differences in C_{max} and C_{max} corrected for dose reflected differences in total dose and rate of infusion. There were no differences in terminal half-lives.

In a repeat dose study with 12 patients receiving Abraxane administered intravenously at the approved

Table 2: Results for overall response rate, median time to disease progression, and progression-free survival as assessed by the investigator

Efficacy variable	Abraxane (260 mg/m²)	Solvent-based paclitaxel (175 mg/m²)	p-value
Response rate [95% CI] (%)			
> 1st-line therapy	26.5 [18.98, 34.05] (n = 132)	13.2 [7.54, 18.93] (n = 136)	0.006[a]
**Median time to disease progression [95% CI] (weeks)*			
> 1st-line therapy	20.9 [15.7, 25.9] (n = 131)	16.1 [15.0, 19.3] (n = 135)	0.011[b]
**Median Progression Free Survival [95% CI] (weeks)*			
> 1st-line therapy	20.6 [15.6, 25.9] (n = 131)	16.1 [15.0, 18.3] (n = 135)	0.010[b]
**Survival [95% CI] (weeks)*			
> 1st-line therapy	56.4 [45.1, 76.9] (n = 131)	46.7 [39.0, 55.3] (n = 136)	0.020[b]

* This data is based on Clinical Study Report: CA012-0 Addendum dated Final (23 March-2005)

[a] Chi-squared test

[b] Log-rank test

dose, intrapatient variability in systemic paclitaxel exposure (AUC_{int}) was 19% (range = 3.21%-27.70%). There was no evidence for accumulation of paclitaxel with multiple treatment courses.

The protein binding of paclitaxel following Abraxane was evaluated by ultrafiltration. The fraction of free paclitaxel was significantly higher with Abraxane (6.2%) than with solvent-based paclitaxel (2.3%). This resulted in significantly higher exposure to unbound paclitaxel with Abraxane compared with solvent-based paclitaxel, even though the total exposure is comparable. This is possibly due to paclitaxel not being trapped in Cremophor EL micelles as with solvent-based paclitaxel. Based on the published literature, *in vitro* studies of binding to human serum proteins, (using paclitaxel at 6μM) the presence of ranitidine, dexamethasone, or diphenhydramine did not affect protein binding of paclitaxel.

Based on the published literature, *in vitro* studies with human liver microsomes and tissue slices show that paclitaxel is metabolised primarily to 6α-hydroxypaclitaxel; and to two minor metabolites, 3'-p-hydroxypaclitaxel and 6α-3'-p-dihydroxypaclitaxel. The formation of these hydroxylated metabolites is catalysed by CYP2C8, -3A4, and both -2C8 and -3A4 respectively.

The pharmacokinetic profile of Abraxane administered as a 30 minute infusion was evaluated in 15 out of 30 patients with three levels of hepatic impairment based on serum bilirubin and liver enzyme levels. Figure 1 shows the correlation between paclitaxel clearance and total blood bilirubin as measured just prior to dosing.

Figure 1 Correlation between paclitaxel clearance and total blood bilirubin

(see Figure 1 below)

The effect of renal dysfunction on the disposition of paclitaxel has not been formally investigated.

In patients with metastatic breast cancer, after a 30 minute infusion of Abraxane at 260 mg/m², the mean value for cumulative urinary excretion of unchanged active substance accounted for 4% of the total administered dose with less than 1% as the metabolites 6α -hydroxypaclitaxel and 3'- *p* -hydroxypaclitaxel, indicating extensive non-renal clearance. Paclitaxel is principally eliminated by hepatic metabolism and biliary excretion.

Pharmacokinetics of paclitaxel in patients aged over 65 years seems comparable to that in patients less than 65 years. However, little information in patients over 75 years is available as only 3 patients over 75 years of age where included in the pharmacokinetic analysis.

5.3 Preclinical safety data

The carcinogenic potential of paclitaxel has not been studied. However, based on the published literature, paclitaxel is a potentially carcinogenic and genotoxic agent at clinical doses, based upon its pharmacodynamic mechanism of action. Paclitaxel has been shown to be clastogenic *in vitro* (chromosome aberrations in human lymphocytes) and *in vivo* (micronucleus test in mice). Paclitaxel has been shown to be genotoxic *in vivo* (micronucleus test in mice), but it did not induce mutagenicity in the Ames test or the Chinese hamster ovary/hypoxanthine-guanine phosphoribosyl transferase (CHO/HGPRT) gene mutation assay.

Paclitaxel at doses below the human therapeutic dose was associated with low fertility and foetal toxicity in rats. Animal studies with Abraxane showed non-reversible, toxic effects on the male reproductive organs at clinically relevant exposure levels.

6. PHARMACEUTICAL PARTICULARS

6.1 List of excipients

Human albumin solution (containing sodium, sodium caprylate and N-acetyl DL tryptophanate).

6.2 Incompatibilities

This medicinal product must not be mixed with other medicinal products except those mentioned in section 6.6.

6.3 Shelf life

Unopened vials: 3 years

Stability of reconstituted suspension in the vial:

After first reconstitution, the suspension should be filled into an infusion bag immediately. However, chemical and physical in use stability has been demonstrated for 8 hours at 2°C-8°C in the original carton, and protected from bright light. Alternative light-protection may be used in the clean room.

Stability of the reconstituted suspension in the infusion bag:

After reconstitution, the reconstituted suspension in the infusion bag should be used immediately. However chemical and physical in use stability has been demo strated for 8 hours not above 25°C.

6.4 Special precautions for storage

Unopened vials:

This medicinal product does not require any special te perature storage conditions.

Keep the vial in the outer carton in order to protect fro light.

Reconstituted suspension:

For storage conditions of the reconstituted medicinal pr duct, see section 6.3.

6.5 Nature and contents of container

50 ml vial (type 1 glass) with a stopper (butyl rubber), wi an overseal (aluminium), containing 100 mg paclitaxel.

Pack size of one vial.

6.6 Special precautions for disposal and other handlin

Preparation and administration precautions:

Paclitaxel is a cytotoxic anticancer medicinal product an as with other potentially toxic compounds, caution shoul be exercised in handling Abraxane. The use of glove goggles and protective clothing is recommended. If th suspension contacts the skin, the skin should be washe immediately and thoroughly with soap and water. If contacts mucous membranes, the membranes should b flushed thoroughly with water. Abraxane should only b prepared and administered by personnel appropriatel trained in the handling of cytotoxic agents. Pregnant sta should not handle Abraxane.

Reconstitution and administration of the product:

Abraxane is supplied as a sterile lyophilised powder fo reconstitution before use. After reconstitution, each ml o suspension contains 5 mg of paclitaxel.

Using a sterile syringe, 20 ml of sodium chloride 9 mg/m (0.9%) solution for infusion should slowly be injected into a vial of Abraxane over a minimum of 1 minute. The solutior should be directed onto the inside wall of the vial. The solution should not be injected directly onto the powder as this will result in foaming.

Once the addition is complete, the vial should be allowed to stand for a minimum of 5 minutes to ensure proper wetting of the solid. Then, the vial should gently and slowly be swirled and/or inverted for at least 2 minutes until complete resuspension of any powder occurs. The generation of foam must be avoided. If foaming or clumping occurs, the solution must stand for at least 15 minutes until foam subsides.

The reconstituted suspension should be milky and homogenous without visible precipitates. If precipitates or settling are visible, the vial should be gently inverted again to ensure complete resuspension prior to use. Some settling of the reconstituted suspension may occur. Complete resuspension should be ensured by mild agitation before use.

Discard the reconstituted suspension if precipitates are observed.

Calculate the exact total dosing volume of 5 mg/ml suspension required for the patient and inject the appropriate amount of reconstituted Abraxane into an empty, sterile, PVC or non-PVC type intravenous bag. The use of specialized DEHP-free solution containers or administration sets is not necessary to prepare or administer Abraxane infusions. In-line filters should not be used.

Any unused product or waste material should be disposed of in accordance with local requirements.

7. MARKETING AUTHORISATION HOLDER

Abraxis BioScience Limited

Rosanne House,

Parkway,

Welwyn Garden City,

Herts, AL8 6HG

United Kingdom

8. MARKETING AUTHORISATION NUMBER(S)

EU/1/07/428/001

9. DATE OF FIRST AUTHORISATION/RENEWAL OF THE AUTHORISATION

11 January 2008

10. DATE OF REVISION OF THE TEXT

08/2009

Detailed information on this product is available on the website of the European Medicines Agency (EMEA) http://www.emea.europa.eu

Figure 1 Correlation between paclitaxel clearance and total blood bilirubin

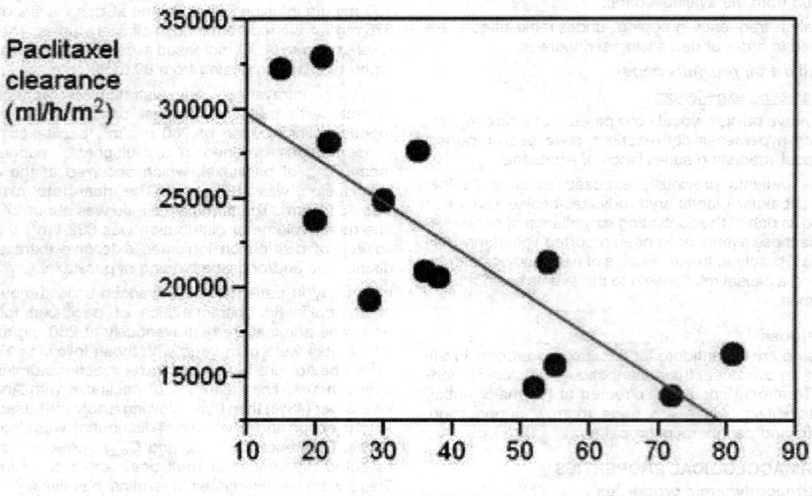

Abstral Sublingual Tablets

(ProStrakan)

1. NAME OF THE MEDICINAL PRODUCT

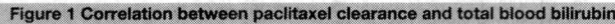

Abstral ▼ 100 microgram, 200 microgram, 300 microgram, 400 microgram, 600 microgram, 800 microgram sublingual tablets

QUALITATIVE AND QUANTITATIVE COMPOSITION

ach sublingual tablet contains:

00 micrograms fentanyl (as citrate)

00 micrograms fentanyl (as citrate)

00 micrograms fentanyl (as citrate)

00 micrograms fentanyl (as citrate)

00 micrograms fentanyl (as citrate)

00 micrograms fentanyl (as citrate)

or a full list of excipients, see section 6.1.

. PHARMACEUTICAL FORM

ublingual tablet

00 microgram sublingual tablet is a white round tablet

00 microgram sublingual tablet is a white oval-shaped ablet

00 microgram sublingual tablet is a white triangle-shaped ablet

00 microgram sublingual tablet is a white diamond-shaped tablet

00 microgram sublingual tablet is a white "D"-shaped ablet

00 microgram sublingual tablet is a white capsule-shaped ablet

. CLINICAL PARTICULARS

.1 Therapeutic indications

Management of breakthrough pain in adult patients using opioid therapy for chronic cancer pain. Breakthrough pain s a transient exacerbation of otherwise controlled chronic background pain.

4.2 Posology and method of administration

Abstral should only be administered to patients who are considered tolerant to their opioid therapy for persistent cancer pain. Patients can be considered opioid tolerant if they take at least 60 mg oral morphine per day, 25 micrograms transdermal fentanyl per hour, or an equianalgesic dose of another opioid for a week or longer.

Abstral sublingual tablets should be administered directly under the tongue at the deepest part. Abstral sublingual tablets should not be swallowed, but allowed to completely dissolve in the sublingual cavity without chewing or sucking. Patients should be advised not to eat or drink anything until the sublingual tablet is completely dissolved.

In patients who have a dry mouth water may be used to moisten the buccal mucosa before taking Abstral.

Dose titration:

The object of dose titration is to identify an optimal maintenance dose for ongoing treatment of breakthrough pain episodes. This optimal dose should provide adequate analgesia with an acceptable level of adverse reactions.

The optimal dose of Abstral will be determined by upward titration, on an individual patient basis. Several doses are available for use during the dose titration phase. The initial dose of Abstral used should be 100 micrograms, titrating upwards as necessary through the range of available dosage strengths.

Patients should be carefully monitored until an optimal dose is reached.

Switching from other fentanyl containing products to Abstral must not occur at a 1:1 ratio because of different absorption profiles. If patients are switched from another fentanyl containing product, a new dose titration with Abstral is required.

The following dose regimen is recommended for titration, although in all cases the physician should take into account the clinical need of the patient, age and concomitant illness.

All patients must start therapy with a single 100 microgram sublingual tablet. If adequate analgesia is not obtained within 15-30 minutes of administration of a single sublingual tablet, a supplemental (second) 100 microgram sublingual tablet may be administered. If adequate analgesia is not obtained within 15-30 minutes of the first dose, an increase in dose to the next highest tablet strength should be considered for the next episode of breakthrough pain. (Refer to figure below). Dose escalation should continue in a stepwise manner until adequate analgesia is achieved. The dose strength for the supplemental (second) sublingual tablet should be increased from 100 to 200 micrograms at doses of 400 micrograms and higher. This is illustrated in the schedule below. No more than two (2) sublingual tablets should be administered for a single episode of breakthrough pain during this titration phase.

(see Figure 1 below)

Strength (micrograms) of first sublingual tablet per episode of breakthrough pain	Strength (micrograms) of supplemental (second) sublingual tablet to be taken 15-30 minutes after first tablet, if required
100	100
200	100
300	100
400	200
600	200
800	-

If adequate analgesia is achieved at the higher dose, but undesirable effects are considered unacceptable, an intermediate dose (using the 100 microgram sublingual tablet where appropriate) may be administered.

Doses higher than 800 micrograms have not been evaluated in clinical studies.

In order to minimise the risk of opioid–related adverse reactions and to identify the appropriate dose, it is imperative that patients be monitored closely by health professionals during the titration process.

Maintenance therapy:

Once an appropriate dose has been established, which may be more than one tablet, patients should be maintained on this dose and should limit consumption to a maximum of four Abstral doses per day.

Dose re-adjustment:

If the response (analgesia or adverse reactions) to the titrated Abstral dose markedly changes, an adjustment of dose may be necessary to ensure that an optimal dose is maintained.

If more than four episodes of breakthrough pain are experienced per day over a period of more than four consecutive days, then the dose of the long acting opioid used for persistent pain should be re-evaluated. If the long acting opioid or dose of long acting opioid is changed the Abstral dose should be re-evaluated and re-titrated as necessary to ensure the patient is on an optimal dose.

It is imperative that any dose re-titration of any analgesic is monitored by a health professional.

Discontinuation of therapy:

For patients no longer requiring any opioid therapy, the Abstral dose should be taken into consideration before a gradual downward titration of opioids to minimise possible withdrawal effects.

In patients who continue to take their chronic opioid therapy for persistent pain but no longer require treatment for breakthrough pain, Abstral therapy may usually be discontinued immediately.

Use in children and adolescents:

Abstral must not be used in patients less than 18 years of age due to a lack of data on safety and efficacy.

Use in elderly patients

Dose titration needs to be approached with particular care and patients observed carefully for signs of fentanyl toxicity (see section 4.4).

Use in patients with renal and hepatic impairment

Patients with kidney or liver dysfunction should be carefully observed for signs of fentanyl toxicity during the Abstral titration phase (see section 4.4).

4.3 Contraindications

Hypersensitivity to the active substance or to any of the excipients.

Opioid-naïve patients because of the risk of life-threatening respiratory depression.

Severe respiratory depression or severe obstructive lung conditions.

4.4 Special warnings and precautions for use

Patients and their carers must be instructed that Abstral contains an active substance in an amount that can be fatal to a child, and therefore to keep all tablets out of the reach and sight of children.

Due to the potentially serious undesirable effects that can occur when taking an opioid therapy such as Abstral, patients and their carers should be made fully aware of the importance of taking Abstral correctly and what action to take should symptoms of overdose occur.

Before Abstral therapy is initiated, it is important that the patient's long-acting opioid treatment used to control their persistent pain has been stabilised.

Upon repeated administration of opioids such as fentanyl, tolerance and physical and/or psychological dependence may develop. Iatrogenic addiction following therapeutic use of opioids is rare.

In common with all opioids, there is a risk of clinically significant respiratory depression associated with the use of Abstral. Particular caution should be exercised during dose titration with Abstral in patients with chronic obstructive pulmonary disease or other medical conditions predisposing them to respiratory depression (e.g. myasthenia gravis) because of the risk of further respiratory depression, which could lead to respiratory failure.

Abstral should only be administered with extreme caution in patients who may be particularly susceptible to the intracranial effects of hyperkapnia, such as those showing evidence of raised intracranial pressure, reduced consciousness, coma or brain tumours. In patients with head injuries, the clinical course may be masked by the use of opioids. In such a case, opioids should be used only if absolutely necessary.

Intravenous fentanyl has been shown to cause bradycardia. Abstral should be used with caution in patients with bradyarrhythmias.

Data from intravenous studies with fentanyl suggest that elderly patients may have reduced clearance, a prolonged half-life and they may be more sensitive to the active substance than younger patients. Elderly, cachectic, or debilitated patients should be observed carefully for signs of fentanyl toxicity and the dose reduced if necessary.

Abstral should be administered with caution to patients with liver or kidney dysfunction, especially during the titration phase. The use of Abstral in patients with hepatic or renal impairment may increase the bioavailability of fentanyl and decrease its systemic clearance, which could lead to accumulation and increased and prolonged opioid effects.

Care should be taken in treating patients with hypovolaemia and hypotension.

Abstral has not been studied in patients with mouth wounds or mucositis. There may be a risk of increased systemic drug exposure in such patients and therefore extra caution is recommended during dose titration.

There should be no noticeable effects on cessation of treatment with Abstral, but possible symptoms of withdrawal are anxiety, tremor, sweating, paleness, nausea and vomiting.

Figure 1

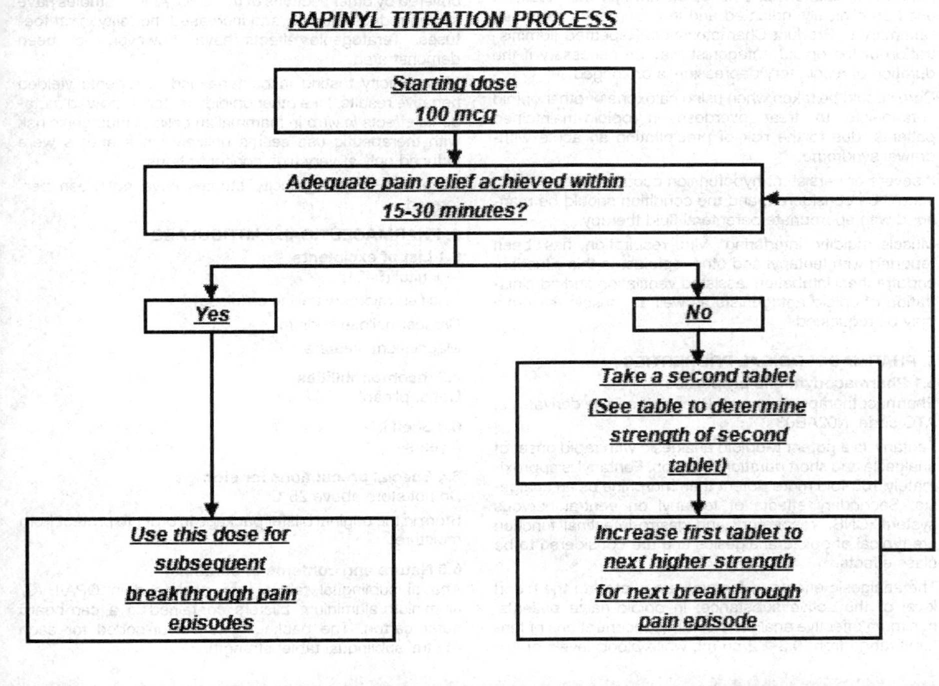
RAPINYL TITRATION PROCESS
Starting dose
100 mcg
Adequate pain relief achieved within
15-30 minutes?
Yes
No
Take a second tablet
(See table to determine
strength of second
tablet)
Use this dose for
subsequent
breakthrough pain
episodes
Increase first tablet to
next higher strength
for next breakthrough
pain episode

4.5 Interaction with other medicinal products and other forms of interaction

Fentanyl is metabolised by CYP3A4. Active substances that inhibit CYP3A4 activity such as macrolide antibiotics (e.g. erythromycin), azole antifungal agents (e.g. ketoconazole, itraconazole) or certain protease inhibitors (e.g. ritonavir) may increase the bioavailability of fentanyl by decreasing its systemic clearance, potentially enhancing or prolonging opioid effects. Grapefruit juice is also known to inhibit CYP3A4. Fentanyl should therefore be given to patients with caution if administered concomitantly with CYP3A4 inhibitors.

Concomitant use of other CNS depressants, such as other morphine derivatives (analgesics and antitussives), general anaesthetics, skeletal muscle relaxants, sedative antidepressants, sedative H1 antihistamines, barbiturates, anxiolytics (ie benzodiazepines), hypnotics, antipsychotics, clonidine and related substances may produce increased CNS depressant effects. Respiratory depression, hypotension and profound sedation may occur.

Alcohol potentiates the sedative effects of morphine-based analgesics, therefore concomitant administration of alcoholic beverages or medicinal products containing alcohol with Abstral is not recommended.

Abstral is not recommended for use in patients who have received monoamine oxidase (MAO) inhibitors within 14 days because severe and unpredictable potentiation by MAO inhibitors has been reported with opioid analgesics.

The concomitant use of partial opioid agonists/antagonists (e.g. buprenorphine, nalbuphine, pentazocine) is not recommended. They have high affinity to opioid receptors with relatively low intrinsic activity and therefore partially antagonise the analgesic effect of fentanyl and may induce withdrawal symptoms in opioid dependent patients.

4.6 Pregnancy and lactation

The safety of fentanyl in pregnancy has not been established. Studies in animals have shown reproductive toxicity (see section 5.3). The potential risk for humans is unknown. Fentanyl should only be used during pregnancy when clearly necessary.

Long-term treatment during pregnancy may cause withdrawal symptoms in the newborn infant.

Fentanyl should not be used during labour and delivery (including caesarean section) since fentanyl crosses the placenta and may cause respiratory depression in the foetus or in the newborn infant.

Fentanyl is excreted into breast milk and may cause sedation and respiratory depression in the breast-fed child. Fentanyl should only be used by breast-feeding women if the benefits clearly outweigh the potential risks for both mother and child.

4.7 Effects on ability to drive and use machines

No studies on the effects on the ability to drive and use machines have been performed.

However, fentanyl may impair the mental or physical ability to perform potentially hazardous tasks such as driving or operating machinery. Patients should be advised not to drive or operate machinery if they become dizzy or drowsy or experience blurred or double vision while taking Abstral.

4.8 Undesirable effects

Undesirable effects typical of opioids are to be expected with Abstral; they tend to decrease in intensity with continued use. The most serious potential adverse reactions associated with opioid use are respiratory depression (which could lead to respiratory arrest), hypotension and shock. Other very commonly reported adverse reactions include: nausea, vomiting, constipation, headache, somnolence/fatigue and dizziness.

Adverse reactions from clinical studies with Abstral in patients and volunteers, with a suspected relationship to treatment, are listed below by system organ class and frequency (very common ⩾ 1/10; common ⩾ 1/100 to < 1/10). Within each frequency grouping, undesirable effects are presented in order of decreasing seriousness.

Nervous system disorders

Very common: Dizziness, somnolence, headache

Common: Vasovagal reaction, hypoaesthesia, paraesthesia, hyperacusis

Eye disorders

Common: Vision abnormal

Respiratory, thoracic and mediastinal disorders

Common: Respiratory depression, rhinitis, pharyngitis

Gastrointestinal disorders

Very common: Nausea

Common: Vomiting, abdominal pain, diarrhoea, constipation, stomach discomfort, dyspepsia, dry mouth

Skin and subcutaneous tissue disorders

Common: Rash, pruritus

Vascular disorders

Common: Orthostatic hypotension, flushing, hot flush

General disorders and administration site conditions

Very common: Fatigue

Common: Asthenia, application site irritation

Psychiatric disorders

Common: Depression, anorexia, concentration impaired, euphoria

All the above adverse reactions were reported in opioid naïve volunteers administered with Abstral. Patients (n=23) treated with Abstral only experienced dizziness, nausea and vomiting.

The following adverse reactions associated with other medicinal products containing fentanyl have also been reported (very common ⩾ 1/10; common ⩾ 1/100 to < 1/10; uncommon ⩾ 1/1000 to < 1/100; rare ⩾ 1/10,000 to < 1/1000; very rare < 1/10,000; not known (cannot be estimated from available data)):

Cardiac disorders

Uncommon: Bradycardia, tachycardia, hypertension

Very rare: Arrhythmias

Nervous system disorders

Common: Myoclonus, insomnia, taste disorders

Uncommon: Abnormal gait/coordination, vertigo, amnesia, speech disorders, tremor

Respiratory thoracic and mediastinal disorders

Uncommon: Hypoventilation, asthma, dyspnoea,

Very rare: Apnoea, haemoptysis

Gastrointestinal disorders

Common: Gastro-intestinal occlusion, dysphagia, mouth ulcers/stomatitis, tongue disorder

Uncommon: Enlarged abdomen, flatulence, thirst

Rare: Hiccups

Renal and urinary disorders

Uncommon: Urinary retention, change in urinary frequency

Very rare: bladder spasm, oliguria

Skin and subcutaneous tissue disorders

Very common: Sweating

Injury, poisoning and procedural complications

Common: Accidental injuries

Vascular disorders

Common: Vasodilation

General disorders and administration site conditions

Uncommon: Malaise

Psychiatric disorders

Common: Hallucinations, confusion, anxiety, nervousness, abnormal thinking, abnormal dreams

Uncommon: Agitation, depersonalisation, emotional lability

4.9 Overdose

The symptoms of fentanyl overdose are an extension of its pharmacological actions, the most serious effect being respiratory depression, which may lead to respiratory arrest.

Management of opioid overdose in the immediate term includes removal of any remaining Abstral sublingual tablets from the mouth, physical and verbal stimulation of the patient and an assessment of the level of consciousness. A patent airway should be established and maintained. If necessary an oropharyngeal airway or endotracheal tube should be inserted, oxygen administered and mechanical ventilation initiated, as appropriate. Adequate body temperature and parenteral fluid intake should be maintained.

For the treatment of accidental overdose in opioid-naïve individuals, naloxone or other opioid antagonists should be used as clinically indicated and in accordance with their Summary of Product Characteristics. Repeated administration of the opioid antagonist may be necessary if the duration of respiratory depression is prolonged.

Care should be taken when using naloxone or other opioid antagonists to treat overdose in opioid-maintained patients, due to the risk of precipitating an acute withdrawal syndrome.

If severe or persistent hypotension occurs, hypovolaemia should be considered, and the condition should be managed with appropriate parenteral fluid therapy.

Muscle rigidity interfering with respiration has been reported with fentanyl and other opioids. In this situation, endotracheal intubation, assisted ventilation and administration of opioid antagonists as well as muscle relaxants may be requested.

5. PHARMACOLOGICAL PROPERTIES

5.1 Pharmacodynamic properties

Pharmacotherapeutic group: Phenylpiperidine derivatives, ATC code: N02AB03

Fentanyl is a potent µ-opioid analgesic with rapid onset of analgesia and short duration of action. Fentanyl is approximately 100-fold more potent than morphine as an analgesic. Secondary effects of fentanyl on central nervous system (CNS), respiratory and gastro-intestinal function are typical of opioid analgesics and are considered to be class effects.

The analgesic effects of fentanyl are related to the blood level of the active substance; in opioid-naïve patients, minimum effective analgesic serum concentrations of fentanyl range from 0.3-1.2 ng/ml, while blood levels of 10-20 ng/ml produce surgical anaesthesia and profour respiratory depression.

In patients with chronic cancer pain on stable maintenanc doses of opioids, Abstral has been shown to induce sig nificantly superior relief of breakthrough pain compared placebo from 15 minutes after administration onward with a significantly lower need for rescue analgesic the apy. The safety and efficacy of Abstral have been evalu ated in patients taking the drug at the onset of th breakthrough pain episode. Pre-emptive use of Abstra for predictable pain episodes was not investigated in th clinical trials.

Fentanyl, in common with all µ-opioid receptor agonists produces dose dependent respiratory depression. Thi risk is higher in opioid-naïve subjects than in patient experiencing severe pain or receiving chronic opioid ther apy. Long-term treatment with opioids typically leads t development of tolerance to their secondary effects.

While opioids generally increase the tone of urinary trac smooth muscle, the net effect tends to be variable, in som cases producing urinary urgency, in others, difficulty ir urination.

Opioids increase the tone and decrease the propulsive contractions of the smooth muscle of the gastrointestina tract leading to a prolongation in gastrointestinal transi time, which may be responsible for the constipating effec of fentanyl.

5.2 Pharmacokinetic properties

Fentanyl is a highly lipophilic drug absorbed very rapidly through the oral mucosa and more slowly through the gastrointestinal tract. Orally administered fentanyl undergoes pronounced hepatic and intestinal first pass effects.

Abstral is a quick dissolving sublingual tablet formulation. Rapid absorption of fentanyl occurs over about 30 minutes following administration of Abstral. The bioavailability of Abstral has not been studied but is estimated to be about 70%. Mean maximal plasma concentrations of fentanyl range from 0.2 to 1.3 ng/ml (after administration of 100 to 800 µg Abstral) and are reached within 22.5 to 240 minutes.

About 80-85% of fentanyl is bound by plasma proteins, mainly α1-glycoprotein and to a lesser extent albumin and lipoprotein. The volume of distribution of fentanyl at steady state is about 3-6 l/kg.

Fentanyl is metabolised primarily via CYP3A4 to a number of pharmacologically inactive metabolites, including norfentanyl. Within 72 hours of intravenous fentanyl administration around 75% of the dose is excreted into the urine, mostly as metabolites, with less than 10% as unchanged drug. About 9% of the dose is recovered in the faeces, primarily as metabolites. Total plasma clearance of fentanyl is about 0.5 l/h/kg. After Abstral administration, the main elimination half-life of fentanyl is about 7 hours (range 3-12.5 hours) and the terminal half-life is about 20 hours (range 11.5-25 hours).

The pharmacokinetics of Abstral have been shown to be dose proportional over the dose range of 100 to 800 µg.

Renal/hepatic impairment

Impaired hepatic or renal function could cause increased serum concentrations. Elderly, cachectic or generally impaired patients may have a lower fentanyl clearance, which could cause a longer terminal half-life for the compound (see sections 4.2 and 4.4).

5.3 Preclinical safety data

Safety pharmacology and repeated dose toxicity data reveal no special hazard for humans that is not already covered by other sections of this SPC. Animal studies have shown reduced fertility and increased mortality in rat foetuses. Teratogenic effects have, however, not been demonstrated.

Mutagenicity testing in bacteria and in rodents yielded negative results. Like other opioids fentanyl showed mutagenic effects *in vitro* in mammalian cells. A mutagenic risk with therapeutic use seems unlikely since effects were induced only at very high concentrations.

Long-term carcinogenicity studies have not been performed.

6. PHARMACEUTICAL PARTICULARS

6.1 List of excipients

Mannitol (E421)

Silicified microcrystalline cellulose

Croscarmellose sodium

Magnesium stearate

6.2 Incompatibilities

Not applicable.

6.3 Shelf life

2 years

6.4 Special precautions for storage

Do not store above 25°C.

Store in the original blister package in order to protect from moisture.

6.5 Nature and contents of container

Abstral sublingual tablets are packaged in OPA/PVC/aluminium/aluminium blisters contained in a cardboard outer carton. The packaging is colour-coded for each Abstral sublingual tablet strength.

ack size: Packs of 10 or 30 sublingual tablets. Not all pack zes may be marketed

6 Special precautions for disposal and other handling
aste material should be disposed of safely. Patients/ arers should be encouraged to return any unused product the Pharmacy, where it should be disposed of in accordance with national and local requirements.

MARKETING AUTHORISATION HOLDER
roStrakan Ltd
alabank Business Park
alashiels
D1 1QH
nited Kingdom

MARKETING AUTHORISATION NUMBER(S)
bstral 100 microgram sublingual tablets: PL 16508/0030
bstral 200 microgram sublingual tablets: PL 16508/0031
bstral 300 microgram sublingual tablets: PL 16508/0032
bstral 400 microgram sublingual tablets: PL 16508/0033
bstral 600 microgram sublingual tablets: PL 16508/0034
bstral 800 microgram sublingual tablets: PL 16508/0035

. DATE OF FIRST AUTHORISATION/RENEWAL OF HE AUTHORISATION
9/09/2008

0. DATE OF REVISION OF THE TEXT
ep 09

EGAL CATEGORY
CD (Sch2), POM

Accolate

(AstraZeneca UK Limited)

1. NAME OF THE MEDICINAL PRODUCT
ACCOLATE®

2. QUALITATIVE AND QUANTITATIVE COMPOSITION
'Accolate' contains 20 mg zafirlukast in each tablet.
For excipients, see 6.1.

3. PHARMACEUTICAL FORM
Film-coated tablet.
White to off white, round, biconvex film coated tablet.

4. CLINICAL PARTICULARS

4.1 Therapeutic indications
'Accolate' is indicated for the treatment of asthma.

4.2 Posology and method of administration
'Accolate' should be taken continuously.

Adults and children aged 12 years and over:

The dosage is one 20 mg tablet twice daily. This dosage should not be exceeded. Higher doses may be associated with elevations of one or more liver enzymes consistent with hepatotoxicity.

As food may reduce the bioavailability of zafirlukast, 'Accolate' should not be taken with meals.

Elderly:

The clearance of zafirlukast is significantly reduced in elderly patients (over 65 years old), and C_{max} and AUC are approximately double those of younger adults. However, accumulation of zafirlukast is no greater than that seen in multiple-dose trials conducted in adult subjects with asthma, and the consequences of the altered kinetics in the elderly are unknown.

Clinical experience with 'Accolate' in the elderly (over 65 years) is limited and caution is recommended until further information is available.

Children:

There is no clinical experience of the use of 'Accolate' in children under 12 years of age.

Until safety information is available, the use of 'Accolate' in children is contraindicated.

Renal impairment:

No dosage adjustment is necessary in patients with mild renal impairment. However, experience is limited in patients with moderate to severe renal impairment (see section 5.2) so clear dose recommendations cannot be given; 'Accolate' should be used with caution in this patient group.

4.3 Contraindications
'Accolate' should not be given to patients who have previously experienced hypersensitivity to the product or any of its ingredients.

'Accolate' is contraindicated in patients with hepatic impairment or cirrhosis; it has not been studied in patients with hepatitis or in long term studies of patients with cirrhosis.

'Accolate' is contraindicated in children under 12 years of age until safety information is available.

4.4 Special warnings and precautions for use
'Accolate' should be taken regularly to achieve benefit, even during symptom free periods. 'Accolate' therapy should normally be continued during acute exacerbations of asthma.

'Accolate' does not allow a reduction in existing steroid treatment.

As with inhaled steroids and cromones (disodium cromoglycate, nedocromil sodium), 'Accolate' is not indicated for use in the reversal of bronchospasm in acute asthma attacks.

'Accolate' has not been evaluated in the treatment of labile (brittle) or unstable asthma.

Cases of eosinophilic conditions, including Churg-Strauss Syndrome and eosinophilic pneumonia have been reported in association with Accolate usage. Presentations may involve various body systems including vasculitic rash, worsening pulmonary symptoms, cardiac complications or neuropathy. A causal relationship has neither been confirmed nor refuted. If a patient develops an eosinophilic condition, or a Churg-Strauss Syndrome type illness, Accolate should be stopped. A rechallenge test should not be performed and treatment should not be restarted.

Elevations in serum transaminases can occur during treatment with 'Accolate'. These are usually asymptomatic and transient but could represent early evidence of hepatotoxicity, and have very rarely been associated with more severe hepatocellular injury, fulminant hepatitis and liver failure, some of which resulted in a fatal outcome. Extremely rarely, cases of fulminant hepatitis and liver failure have been reported in patients in whom no previous clinical signs or symptoms suggestive of liver dysfunction were reported.

If clinical symptoms or signs suggestive of liver dysfunction occur (e.g. anorexia, nausea, vomiting, right upper quadrant pain, fatigue, lethargy, flu-like symptoms, enlarged liver, pruritus and jaundice), Accolate should be discontinued. The serum transaminases, in particular serum ALT, should be measured immediately and the patient managed accordingly.

Physicians may consider the value of routine liver function testing. Periodic serum transaminase testing has not proven to prevent serious injury but is generally believed that early detection of drug-induced hepatic injury along with immediate withdrawal of the suspect drug may enhance the likelihood of recovery. If liver function testing shows evidence of hepatotoxicity 'Accolate' should be discontinued immediately and the patient managed accordingly.

Patients in whom 'Accolate' was withdrawn because of hepatotoxicity should not be re-exposed to 'Accolate'.

4.5 Interaction with other medicinal products and other forms of interaction
'Accolate' may be administered with other therapies routinely used in the management of asthma and allergy. Inhaled steroids, inhaled and oral bronchodilator therapy, antibiotics and antihistamines are examples of agents which have been co-administered with 'Accolate' without adverse interaction.

'Accolate' may be administered with oral contraceptives without adverse interaction.

Co-administration with warfarin results in an increase in maximum prothrombin time by approximately 35%. It is therefore recommended that if 'Accolate' is co-administered with warfarin, prothrombin time should be closely monitored. The interaction is probably due to an inhibition by zafirlukast of the cytochrome P450 2C9 isoenzyme system.

In clinical trials co-administration with theophylline resulted in decreased plasma levels of zafirlukast, by approximately 30%, but with no effect on plasma theophylline levels. However, during post-marketing surveillance, there have been rare cases of patients experiencing increased theophylline levels when co-administered 'Accolate'.

Co-administration with terfenadine resulted in a 54% decrease in AUC for zafirlukast, but with no effect on plasma terfenadine levels.

Co-administration with acetylsalicylic acid ("aspirin", 650 mg four times a day) may result in increased plasma levels of zafirlukast, by approximately 45%.

Co-administration with erythromycin will result in decreased plasma levels of zafirlukast, by approximately 40%.

The clearance of zafirlukast in smokers may be increased by approximately 20%.

At concentrations of 10 microgram/ml and above, zafirlukast causes increases in the assay value for bilirubin in animal plasma. However, zafirlukast has not been shown to interfere with the 2,5-dichlorophenyl diazonium salt method of bilirubin analysis of human plasma.

4.6 Pregnancy and lactation
The safety of 'Accolate' in human pregnancy has not been established. In animal studies, zafirlukast did not have any apparent effect on fertility and did not appear to have any teratogenic or selective toxic effect on the foetus. The potential risks should be weighed against the benefits of continuing therapy during pregnancy and 'Accolate' should be used during pregnancy only if clearly needed.

Zafirlukast is excreted in human breast milk. 'Accolate' should not be administered to mothers who are breast-feeding.

4.7 Effects on ability to drive and use machines
There is no evidence that 'Accolate' affects the ability to drive and use machinery.

4.8 Undesirable effects
The following have been reported in association with the administration of 'Accolate':

Gastrointestinal:	nausea, vomiting, abdominal pain (common)
Hepatobiliary:	Symptomatic hepatitis with and without hyperbilirubinaemia (rare), hyperbilirubinaemia, without elevated liver function tests (rare), hepatic failure and fulminant hepatitis, sometimes with a fatal outcome (see section 4.4) (very rare)
General:	malaise (common)
Musculoskeletal:	arthralgia (rare), myalgia (rare)
Skin:	rash (including blistering), pruritus, hypersensitivity reactions including urticaria and angioedema (rare) and oedema (uncommon)
Neurological:	insomnia, headache (common)
Haematologic:	bruising (rare), bleeding disorders, including menorrhagia (rare), thrombocytopenia (rare), and agranulocytosis (very rare)

The above events have usually resolved following cessation of therapy. Headache and gastrointestinal disturbance are usually mild and do not necessitate withdrawal from therapy.

In placebo-controlled clinical trials, an increased incidence of infection has been observed in elderly patients given 'Accolate' (7.8% vs 1.4%). Infections were usually mild, predominantly affecting the respiratory tract.

4.9 Overdose
Limited information exists with regard to the effects of overdosage of 'Accolate' in humans.

Management should be supportive. Removal of excess medication by gastric lavage may be helpful.

5. PHARMACOLOGICAL PROPERTIES

5.1 Pharmacodynamic properties
ATC Code: R03D C01.

Pharmacotherapeutic Group: Leukotriene receptor antagonists.

The cysteinyl leukotrienes (LTC_4, LTD_4 and LTE_4) are potent inflammatory eicosanoids released from various cells including mast cells and eosinophils. These important pro-asthmatic mediators bind to cysteinyl leukotriene receptors found in the human airway. Leukotriene production and receptor occupation has been implicated in the pathophysiology of asthma. Effects include smooth muscle contraction, airway oedema and altered cell activity associated with the inflammatory process, including eosinophil influx to the lung.

'Accolate' is a competitive highly selective and potent oral peptide leukotriene antagonist of LTC_4, LTD_4 and LTE_4 components of slow reacting substance of anaphylaxis. In vitro studies have shown that 'Accolate' antagonises the contractile activity of all three peptide leukotrienes (leukotriene C_4, D_4, and E_4) in human conducting airway smooth muscle to the same extent. Animal studies have shown 'Accolate' to be effective in preventing peptide leukotriene-induced increases in vascular permeability, which give rise to oedema in the airways, and to inhibit peptide leukotriene-induced influx of eosinophils into airways.

The specificity of 'Accolate' has been shown by its action on leukotriene receptors and not prostaglandin, thromboxane, cholinergic and histamine receptors.

In a placebo-controlled study where segmental bronchoprovocation with allergen was followed by bronchoalveolar lavage 48 hours later, zafirlukast decreased the rise in basophils, lymphocytes and histamine, and reduced the stimulated production of superoxide by alveolar macrophages.

'Accolate' attenuated the increase in bronchial hyperresponsiveness that follows inhaled allergen challenge. Further, methacholine sensitivity was diminished by long-term dosing with 'Accolate' 20 mg twice daily.

Further, in clinical trials evaluating chronic therapy with 'Accolate', the lung function measured when plasma levels were at trough showed sustained improvements over baseline.

'Accolate' shows a dose dependent inhibition of bronchoconstriction induced by inhaled LTD_4. Asthmatic patients are approximately 10-fold more sensitive to the bronchoconstricting activity of inhaled LTD_4. A single oral dose of 'Accolate' can enable an asthmatic patient to inhale 100 times more LTD_4 and shows significant protection at 12 and 24 hours.

'Accolate' inhibits the bronchoconstriction caused by several kinds of challenge, such as the response to sulphur dioxide, exercise and cold air. 'Accolate' attenuates the early and late phase inflammatory reaction caused by various antigens such as grass, cat dander, ragweed and mixed antigens.

In asthmatic patients not adequately controlled by beta-agonist therapy (given as required) 'Accolate' improves symptoms (reducing daytime and nocturnal asthmatic symptoms), improves lung function, reduces the need for concomitant beta-agonist medication and reduces incidence of exacerbations. Similar benefits have been seen in patients with more severe asthma receiving high dose inhaled steroids.

In clinical studies, there was a significant first-dose effect on baseline bronchomotor tone observed within 2 hours of dosing, when peak plasma concentrations had not yet been achieved. Initial improvements in asthma symptoms occurred within the first week, and often the first few days, of treatment with 'Accolate'.

5.2 Pharmacokinetic properties

Peak plasma concentrations of zafirlukast are achieved approximately 3 hours after oral administration of 'Accolate'.

Administration of 'Accolate' with food increased the variability in the bioavailability of zafirlukast and reduced bioavailability in most (75%) subjects. The net reduction was approximately 40%.

Following twice-daily administration of 'Accolate' (30 to 80 mg bd), accumulation of zafirlukast in plasma was low (not detectable - 2.9 times first dose values; mean 1.45; median 1.27). The terminal half-life of zafirlukast is approximately 10 hours. Steady-state plasma concentrations of zafirlukast were proportional to the dose and predictable from single-dose pharmacokinetic data.

Zafirlukast is extensively metabolised. Following a radiolabelled dose the urinary excretion accounts for approximately 10% dose and faecal excretion for 89%. Zafirlukast is not detected in urine. The metabolites identified in human plasma were found to be at least 90-fold less potent than zafirlukast in a standard in-vitro test of activity.

Zafirlukast is approximately 99% protein bound to human plasma proteins, predominantly albumin, over the concentration range 0.25 to 4.0 microgram/ml.

Pharmacokinetic studies in special populations have been performed in a relatively small number of subjects, and the clinical significance of the following kinetic data is not established.

Pharmacokinetics of zafirlukast in adolescents and adults with asthma were similar to those of healthy adult males. When adjusted for body weight, the pharmacokinetics of zafirlukast are not significantly different between men and women.

Elderly subjects and subjects with stable alcoholic cirrhosis demonstrated an approximately two-fold increase in C_{max} and AUC compared to normal subjects given the same doses of 'Accolate'.

There are no significant differences in the pharmacokinetics of zafirlukast in patients with mild renal impairment and in normal subjects. However, there are no conclusive data available in patients with moderate or severe renal impairment, hence the recommendation for caution is used in this patient population.

5.3 Preclinical safety data

After multiple doses of greater than 40 mg/kg/day for up to 12 months, liver enlargement associated with degenerative/fatty change or glycogen deposition was seen in rats, mice and dogs. Histiocytic aggregates were seen in a number of tissues of dogs.

Male mice given 300 mg/kg zafirlukast daily had an increased incidence of hepatocellular adenomas compared to control animals. Rats given 2000 mg/kg zafirlukast daily had an increased incidence of urinary bladder papilloma compared to control animals. Zafirlukast was not mutagenic in a range of tests. The clinical significance of these findings during the long term use of 'Accolate' in man is uncertain.

There were no other notable findings from the pre-clinical testing.

6. PHARMACEUTICAL PARTICULARS

6.1 List of excipients

Croscarmellose sodium

Hypromellose E464

Lactose Monohydrate

Magnesium Stearate E572

Microcrystalline Cellulose E460

Povidone

Titanium Dioxide E171

6.2 Incompatibilities

None known

6.3 Shelf life

3 years

6.4 Special precautions for storage

Do not store above 30°C.

6.5 Nature and contents of container

Aluminium laminate/foil blister packs containing 56 or 100 tablets.

6.6 Special precautions for disposal and other handling

No special precautions.

7. MARKETING AUTHORISATION HOLDER

AstraZeneca UK Limited,

600 Capability Green,

Luton, LU1 3LU, UK.

8. MARKETING AUTHORISATION NUMBER(S)

PL 17901/0001

9. DATE OF FIRST AUTHORISATION/RENEWAL OF THE AUTHORISATION

1 June 2000

10. DATE OF REVISION OF THE TEXT

2nd May 2008

Accupro Tablets 5mg, 10mg, 20mg & 40mg

(Pfizer Limited)

1. NAME OF THE MEDICINAL PRODUCT

Accupro™ Tablets 5 mg

Accupro™ Tablets 10 mg

Accupro™ Tablets 20 mg

Accupro™ Tablets 40 mg

2. QUALITATIVE AND QUANTITATIVE COMPOSITION

Each 5mg tablet contains quinapril hydrochloride 5.416 mg (equivalent to 5 mg quinapril base)

Each 10mg tablet contains quinapril hydrochloride 10.832 mg (equivalent to 10 mg quinapril base)

Each 20mg tablet contains quinapril hydrochloride 21.664 mg (equivalent to 20 mg quinapril base)

Each 40mg tablet contains quinapril hydrochloride 43.328 mg (equivalent to 40 mg quinapril base)

3. PHARMACEUTICAL FORM

Reddish brown oval tablets scored on both sides and "5" embossed on both sides.

Reddish brown triangular tablets scored on both sides and "10" embossed on one side.

Reddish brown round tablets scored on both sides and "20" embossed on one side.

40mg tablet: Reddish-brown, oval, biconvex film-coated tablet with debossing '40' on one side and 'PD 535' on the other side.

4. CLINICAL PARTICULARS

4.1 Therapeutic indications

Hypertension

For the treatment of all grades of essential hypertension. Accupro is effective as monotherapy or concomitantly with diuretics in patients with hypertension.

Congestive Heart Failure

For the treatment of congestive heart failure when given concomitantly with a diuretic and/or cardiac glycoside. Treatment of congestive heart failure with Accupro should always be initiated under close medical supervision.

4.2 Posology and method of administration

For oral use

Adults

Hypertension

Monotherapy: The recommended initial dosage is 10 mg once daily in uncomplicated hypertension. Depending upon clinical response, patient's dosage may be titrated (by doubling the dose allowing adequate time for dosage adjustment) to a maintenance dosage of 20 to 40 mg/day given as a single dose or divided into 2 doses. Long-term control is maintained in most patients with a single daily dosage regimen. Patients have been treated with dosages up to 80 mg/day. Take either with or without food. The dose should always be taken at about the same time of day to help increase compliance.

Concomitant Diuretics: In order to determine if excess hypotension will occur, an initial dosage of 2.5 mg of Accupro is recommended in patients who are being treated with a diuretic. After this the dosage of Accupro should be titrated (as described above) to the optimal response. (See section 4.5 Interaction with other medicaments and other forms of interaction).

Congestive Heart Failure

In order to closely monitor patients for symptomatic hypotension, a single 2.5 mg initial dosage is recommended. After this, patients should be titrated to an effective dose: (up to 40 mg/day) given in 1 or 2 doses with concomitant diuretic and/or cardiac glycoside therapy. Patients are usually maintained effectively on doses of 10-20 mg/day given with concomitant therapy. Take either with or without food. The dose should always be taken at about the same time of day to help increase compliance.

Severe Heart Failure

In the treatment of severe or unstable congestive heart failure, Accupro should always be initiated in hospital under close medical supervision.

Other patients who may also be considered to be at higher risk and should have treatment initiated in hospital include: patients who are on high dose loop diuretics (e.g. > 80 mg furosemide) or on multiple diuretic therapy, have hypovolaemia, hyponatraemia (serum sodium < 130 mgEq/l) or systolic blood pressure < 90 mm Hg, are on high do vasodilator therapy, have a serum creatinine > 150 µmc or are aged 70 years or over.

Elderly/Renal Impairment

In elderly patients and in patients with a creatinine clea ance of less than 40 ml/min, an initial dosage in essenti hypertension of 2.5 mg is recommended followed by titra tion to the optimal response (see section 4.4 Special War ings and Precautions for Use).

Children and adolescents

There is limited clinical trial experience of the use of qu napril in hypertensive children aged 5 years and above (See section 5.1). There are no data regarding childre below 5 years of age. Therefore its use in children an adolescents is not recommended.

4.3 Contraindications

Accupro is contraindicated in patients with hypersensitivit to any of the ingredients.

Accupro is contraindicated during the second and thir trimesters of pregnancy (see sections 4.4 and 4.6).

Accupro is contraindicated in patients with a history o angioedema related to previous treatment with ACE inhi bitors.

Accupro is contraindicated in patients with hereditary/idiopathic angioneurotic oedema.

4.4 Special warnings and precautions for use

Accupro should not be used in patients with aortic stenosis or outflow obstruction.

Patients haemodialysed using high-flux polyacrylonitrile ('AN69') membranes are highly likely to experience anaphylactoid reactions if they are treated with ACE inhibitors. This combination should therefore be avoided, either by use of alternative antihypertensive drugs or alternative membranes for haemodialysis. Similar reactions have been observed during low density lipoprotein apheresis with dextran-sulphate. This method should therefore not be used in patients treated with ACE inhibitors.

Anaphylactoid reactions: Patients receiving ACE inhibitors during desensitising treatment with hymenoptera venom have experienced life threatening anaphylactoid reactions. These reactions were avoided by temporarily withholding ACE inhibitor therapy prior to each desensitisation.

In patients with renal insufficiency, monitoring of renal function during therapy should be performed as deemed appropriate; although in the majority renal function will not alter or may improve.

As a consequence of inhibiting the renin-angiotensin-aldosterone system, changes in renal function may be anticipated in susceptible individuals. In patients with severe heart failure whose renal function may depend on the activity of the renin-angiotensin-aldosterone system, treatment with ACE inhibitors, including quinapril, may be associated with oliguria and/or progressive azotemia and rarely acute renal failure and/or death.

The half-life of quinaprilat is prolonged as creatinine clearance falls. Patients with a creatinine clearance of <40 ml/min require a lower initial dosage of quinapril (see section 4.2 Posology and Method of Administration). These patients' dosage should be titrated upwards based upon therapeutic response, and renal function should be closely monitored although initial studies do not indicate that quinapril produces further deterioration in renal function.

In clinical studies in hypertensive patients with unilateral or bilateral renal artery stenosis, increases in blood urea nitrogen and serum creatinine have been observed in some patients following ACE inhibitor therapy. These increases were almost always reversible upon discontinuation of the ACE inhibitor and/or diuretic therapy. In such patients, renal function should be monitored during the first few weeks of therapy.

Some patients with hypertension or heart failure with no apparent pre-existing renal vascular disease have developed increases (>1.25 times the upper limit of normal) in blood urea and serum creatinine, usually minor and transient, especially when quinapril has been given concomitantly with a diuretic and has been observed in 4% and 3% respectively of patients on monotherapy. This is more likely to occur in patients with pre-existing renal impairment. Dosage reduction and/or discontinuation of a diuretic and/or quinapril may be required.

Angioedema: Angioedema has been reported in patients treated with angiotensin-converting enzyme inhibitors. If laryngeal stridor or angioedema of the face, tongue, or glottis occur, treatment should be discontinued immediately, the patient treated appropriately in accordance with accepted medical care, and carefully observed until the swelling disappears. In instances where swelling is confined to the face and lips, the condition generally resolves without treatment; antihistamines may be useful in relieving symptoms. Angioedema associated with laryngeal involvement may be fatal. Where there is involvement of the tongue, glottis, or larynx likely to cause airway obstruction, appropriate therapy e.g., subcutaneous adrenaline solution 1:1000 (0.3 to 0.5 ml) should be promptly administered.

Black patients receiving ACE inhibitor therapy generally have a higher incidence of angioedema than non-black patients.

testinal angioedema: Intestinal angioedema has been eported in patients treated with ACE inhibitors. These atients presented with abdominal pain (with or without ausea or vomiting); in some cases there was no prior istory of facial angioedema and C-1 esterase levels were ormal. The angioedema was diagnosed by procedures ncluding abdominal CT scan or ultrasound, or at surgery, nd symptoms resolved after stopping the ACE inhibitor. ntestinal angioedema should be included in the differential iagnosis of patients on ACE inhibitors presenting with bdominal pain.

Hypotension: Symptomatic hypotension was rarely seen in ypertensive patients treated with Accupro but it is a ossible consequence of ACE inhibition therapy particuarly in salt/volume depleted patients such as those preiously treated with diuretics, who have a dietary salt eduction, or who are on dialysis. If symptomatic hypotenion occurs, the patient should be placed in the supine osition and, if necessary, receive an intravenous infusion of normal saline. A transient hypotensive response is not a contraindication to further doses; however, lower doses of quinapril or any concomitant diuretic therapy should be considered if this event occurs.

Neutropenia/agranulocytosis: ACE inhibitors have been rarely associated with agranulocytosis and bone marrow depression in patients with uncomplicated hypertension but more frequently in patients with renal impairment, especially if they also have collagen vascular disease. As with other ACE inhibitors, monitoring of white blood cell counts in patients with collagen vascular disease and/or renal diseases should be considered.

Pregnancy: ACE inhibitors should not be initiated during pregnancy. Unless continued ACE inhibitor therapy is considered essential, patients planning pregnancy should be changed to alternative antihypertensive treatments which have an established safety profile for use in pregnancy. When pregnancy is diagnosed, treatment with ACE inhibitors should be stopped immediately, and, if appropriate, alternative therapy should be started (see sections 4.3 and 4.6).

4.5 Interaction with other medicinal products and other forms of interaction

Tetracycline and other drugs that interact with magnesium: Because of the presence of magnesium carbonate in the formulation, Accupro has been shown in healthy volunteers to reduce the absorption of tetracycline in concomitant administration by 28-37%. It is recommended that concomitant administration with tetracycline be avoided.

Concomitant diuretic therapy: Patients treated with diuretics may occasionally experience an excessive reduction of blood pressure after initiation of therapy with Accupro. This hypotensive effect may be effectively minimised by either discontinuing the diuretic or increasing the salt intake prior to the initial dose of Accupro. If discontinuation of the diuretic is not possible, medical supervision should be provided for up to two hours following administration of the initial dose (see section 4.4 Special Warnings and Precautions for Use and section 4.2 Posology and Method of Administration).

Agents increasing serum potassium: Quinapril is an angiotensin-converting enzyme inhibitor capable of lowering aldosterone levels, which in turn can result in elevation in serum potassium. Concomitant treatments with potassium sparing diuretics, potassium supplements or potassium salts should be used with caution and with appropriate monitoring of serum potassium. As with other ACE inhibitors, patients on quinapril alone may have increased serum potassium levels. When administered concomitantly, quinapril may reduce the hypokalaemia induced by thiazide diuretics.

Surgery/anaesthesia: Although no data are available to indicate there is an interaction between Accupro and anaesthetic agents that produces hypotension, caution should be exercised when patients undergo major surgery or anaesthesia since angiotensin converting enzyme inhibitors have been shown to block angiotensin II formation secondary to compensatory renin release. This may lead to hypotension which can be corrected by volume expansion.

Lithium: Increased serum lithium levels and symptoms of lithium toxicity have been reported in patients receiving concomitant lithium and ACE inhibitor therapy due to the sodium-losing effect of these agents. These drugs should be co-administered with caution and frequent monitoring of serum lithium levels is recommended. If a diuretic is also used, it may increase the risk of lithium toxicity.

Non-steroidal anti-inflammatory drugs: In some patients, the administration of a non-steroidal anti-inflammatory agent may reduce the antihypertensive effect of ACE inhibitors. Furthermore, it has been described that NSAIDs and ACE inhibitors exert an additive effect on the increase in serum potassium, whereas renal function may decrease. These effects are in principle reversible and occur especially in patients with compromised renal function.

Allopurinol, cytostatic and immunosuppressive agents, systemic corticosteroids or procainamide: Concomitant administration with ACE inhibitors may lead to an increased risk for leucopoenia.

Alcohol, barbiturates or narcotics: Potentiation of orthostatic hypotension may occur.

Other hypertensive drugs: There may be an additive effect or potentiation.

Antacids: May decrease the bioavailability of Accupro.

Antidiabetic drugs (oral hypoglycaemic agents and insulin): Dosage adjustments of the antidiabetic drug may be required.

4.6 Pregnancy and lactation

Pregnancy:

The use of ACE inhibitors is not recommended during the first trimester of pregnancy (see section 4.4). The use of ACE inhibitors is contraindicated during the 2nd and 3rd trimester of pregnancy (see sections 4.3 and 4.4).

Epidemiological evidence regarding the risk of teratogenicity following exposure to ACE inhibitors during the first trimester of pregnancy has not been conclusive; however a small increase in risk cannot be excluded. Unless continued ACE inhibitor therapy is considered essential, patients planning pregnancy should be changed to alternative antihypertensive treatments which have an established safety profile for use in pregnancy. When pregnancy is diagnosed, treatment with ACE inhibitors should be stopped immediately, and, if appropriate, alternative therapy should be started.

Exposure to ACE inhibitor therapy during the second and third trimesters is known to induce human foetotoxicity (decreased renal function, oligohydramnios, skull ossification retardation and/or death in the newborn) and neonatal toxicity (renal failure, hypotension, hyperkalaemia). (See section 5.3.). Should exposure to ACE inhibitor have occurred from the second trimester of pregnancy, ultrasound check of renal function and skull is recommended. Limb contractures, craniofacial deformities, hypoplastic lung development and intrauterine growth retardation have been reported in association with oligohydramnios.

Infants whose mothers have taken ACE inhibitors should be closely observed for hypotension, oliguria and hyperkalaemia. (see sections 4.3 and 4.4). If oliguria occurs, attention should be directed towards support of blood pressure and renal perfusion.

Lactation:

Limited pharmacokinetic data demonstrate very low concentrations in breast milk (see section 5.2). Although these concentrations seem to be clinically irrelevant, the use of Accupro in breastfeeding is not recommended for preterm infants and for the first few weeks after delivery, because of the hypothetical risk of cardiovascular and renal effects and because there is not enough clinical experience.

In the case of an older infant, the use of Accupro in a breast-feeding mother may be considered if this treatment is necessary for the mother and the child is observed for any adverse effect.

4.7 Effects on ability to drive and use machines

There are no studies on the effect of this medicine on the ability to drive. When driving vehicles or operating machines it should be taken into account that occasionally dizziness or weariness may occur.

4.8 Undesirable effects

The most frequent clinical adverse reactions in hypertension and congestive heart failure are headache, dizziness, rhinitis, coughing, upper respiratory tract infection, fatigue, nausea and vomiting. Other less frequent side effects are dyspepsia, myalgia, chest pain, abdominal pain, diarrhoea, back pain, sinusitis, insomnia, paraesthesia, nervousness, asthenia, pharyngitis, hypotension, palpitations, flatulence, depression, pruritus, rash, impotence, oedema, arthralgia, amblyopia.

Renal dysfunction, angioedema, hypotension, hyperkalaemia, neutropenia, agranulocytosis - see warnings and precautions.

The following side effects have been observed associated with ACE inhibitor therapy:

<u>Cardiac Disorders:</u> Tachycardia, myocardial infarction

<u>Nervous System Disorders:</u> Cerebral haemorrhage, disorders of balance, syncope, taste disturbances, transient ischaemic attacks

<u>Respiratory, Thoracic and Mediastinal Disorders</u>: Bronchitis, bronchospasm, dyspnoea

In individual cases angioneurotic oedema involving the upper airways has caused fatal airway obstruction.

<u>Gastrointestinal Disorders:</u> Constipation, dry mouth, glossitis, ileus, intestinal angioedema. Pancreatitis has been reported rarely in patients treated with ACE inhibitors; in some cases this has proved fatal.

<u>Hepatobiliary Disorders:</u> Cholestatic icterus, hepatitis

<u>Skin and Subcutaneous Tissue Disorders:</u> Alopecia, erythema multiforme, epidermic necrolysis, psoriasis-like efflorescences, Steven Johnson syndrome, urticaria. May be accompanied by fever, eosinophilia and/or increased ANA-titers.

<u>Psychiatric Disorders</u>: Confusion

<u>Eye Disorders:</u> Blurred vision

<u>Ear and Labyrinth Disorders:</u> Tinnitus

Investigations: Increases in blood urea and plasma creatinine may occur. Decreases in haematocrit, platelets and white cell count as well as elevation of liver enzymes and serum bilirubin. In patients with a congential deficiency concerning G-6-PDH individual cases of haemolytic anaemia have been reported.

4.9 Overdose

No data are available with respect to overdosage in humans. The most likely clinical manifestation would be symptoms attributable to severe hypotension, which should normally be treated by intravenous volume expansion.

Haemodialysis and peritoneal dialysis have little effect on the elimination of quinapril and quinaprilat.

Treatment is symptomatic and supportive consistent with established medical care.

5. PHARMACOLOGICAL PROPERTIES

5.1 Pharmacodynamic properties

Quinapril is rapidly de-esterified to quinaprilat (quinapril diacid, the principal metabolite) which is a potent angiotensin-converting enzyme (ACE) inhibitor.

ACE is a peptidyl dipeptidase that catalyses the conversion of angiotensin I to the vasoconstrictor angiotensin II which is involved in vascular control and function through many different mechanisms, including stimulation of aldosterone secretion by the adrenal cortex. The mode of action of quinapril in humans and animals is to inhibit circulating and tissue ACE activity, thereby decreasing vasopressor activity and aldosterone secretion.

In animal studies, the antihypertensive effect of quinapril outlasts its inhibitory effect on circulating ACE, whereas, tissue ACE inhibition more closely correlates with the duration of antihypertensive effects. Administration of 10-40 mg of quinapril to patients with mild to severe hypertension results in a reduction of both sitting and standing blood pressure with minimal effect on heart rate. Antihypertensive activity commences within one hour with peak effects usually achieved by two to four hours after dosing. Achievement of maximum blood pressure lowering effects may require two weeks of therapy in some patients. At the recommended doses, antihypertensive effects are maintained in most patients throughout the 24 hour dosing interval and continue during long term therapy. In a randomised clinical trial using target doses of 2.5, 5, 10 and 20 mg of quinapril, in 112 children and adolescents with hypertension or high normal blood pressure over 8 weeks (2 weeks double blind and 6 weeks extension), a reduction in systolic blood pressure alone was noted across all treatment groups at the end of 2 weeks only. A dose response effect between groups was not seen. The reduction in diastolic pressure overall, and for each group was similar to placebo in these subjects suggesting that a dose response effect was not established.

Long term effects of quinapril on growth, puberty and general development have not been studied.

5.2 Pharmacokinetic properties

Peak plasma Accupro concentrations are observed within 1 hour of oral administration. The extent of absorption is approximately 60%, and is not influenced by food. Following absorption, Accupro is de-esterified to its major active metabolite, quinaprilat, and to minor inactive metabolites. Accupro has an apparent half-life of approximately one hour. Peak plasma quinaprilat concentrations are observed approximately 2 hours following an oral dose of quinapril. Quinaprilat is eliminated primarily by renal excretion and has an effective accumulation half-life of 3 hours. In patients with renal insufficiency and creatinine clearance of $\leq$40ml/min, peak and trough quinaprilat concentrations increase, time to peak concentration increases, apparent half-life increases, and time to steady state may be delayed. The elimination of quinaprilat is also reduced in elderly patients (>65 years) and correlates well with the impaired renal function which frequently occurs in the elderly. Quinaprilat concentrations are reduced in patients with alcoholic cirrhosis due to impaired de-esterification of Accupro. Studies in rats indicate that Accupro and its metabolites do not cross the blood-brain barrier.

Lactation:

After a single oral dose of 20 mg of quinapril in six breast-feeding women, the M/P (milk to plasma ratio) for quinapril was 0.12. Quinapril was not detected in milk after 4 hours after the dose. Quinalapril milk levels were undetectable (<5 µg/L) at all time points. It is estimated that a breastfed infant would receive about 1.6% of the maternal weight-adjusted dosage of quinapril.

5.3 Preclinical safety data

The results of the preclinical tests do not add anything of further significance to the prescriber.

6. PHARMACEUTICAL PARTICULARS

6.1 List of excipients

Magnesium carbonate

Hydrous lactose

Gelatin

Crospovidone

Magnesium stearate

Candelilla wax

Colourings (Opadry Y-5-9020):

Hydroxypropylmethylcellulose

Hydroxypropylcellulose

Macrogol 400

Red iron oxide (E172)

Titanium Dioxide (E171)

6.2 Incompatibilities
None known

6.3 Shelf life
3 years

6.4 Special precautions for storage
Do not store above 25°C

6.5 Nature and contents of container
Tampertainer with dessicant containing 56 or 100 tablets

Polyamide/aluminium/PVC blister strip. Supplied in packs of 7, 28, 56 or 100 tablets

6.6 Special precautions for disposal and other handling
No special instructions needed

7. MARKETING AUTHORISATION HOLDER
Pfizer Limited
Ramsgate Road
Sandwich
Kent
CT13 9NJ
United Kingdom

8. MARKETING AUTHORISATION NUMBER(S)
PL 00057/0514
PL 00057/0515
PL 00057/0516
PL 00057/0517

9. DATE OF FIRST AUTHORISATION/RENEWAL OF THE AUTHORISATION
1 August 2003

10. DATE OF REVISION OF THE TEXT
June 2009

11 LEGAL STATUS
POM

Ref: AC9_5UK

Accuretic 10/12.5mg Tablets

(Pfizer Limited)

1. NAME OF THE MEDICINAL PRODUCT
Accuretic 10/12.5 mg

2. QUALITATIVE AND QUANTITATIVE COMPOSITION
Each tablet contains:

Quinapril hydrochloride 10.85 mg

(Equivalent to 10 mg quinapril base)

and

hydrochlorothiazide PhEur 12.5 mg

3. PHARMACEUTICAL FORM
Film-coated tablet

4. CLINICAL PARTICULARS

4.1 Therapeutic indications
For the treatment of all grades of essential hypertension in patients who have been stabilised on the individual components given in the same proportions.

4.2 Posology and method of administration
For oral use

Adults:

For patients currently not receiving a diuretic, whether or not they have been receiving quinapril monotherapy, the recommended initial dosage of quinapril/HCTZ is 10/12.5mg. Following initial therapy, the dose may be increased to 20/25mg. Effective blood pressure control is usually achieved with a dosage of 10/12.5mg. Effective blood pressure control is usually achieved with a dosage of 10/12.5mg.

Take either with or without food. The dose should always be taken at about the same time of day to help increase compliance.

In patients with congestive heart failure, with or without associated renal insufficiency, ACE inhibitor therapy for hypertension may cause an excessive drop in blood pressure. Accuretic therapy should be started under close medical supervision. Patients should be followed closely for the first two weeks of treatment and whenever the dosage is increased.

Renal Impairment:

Accuretic is not recommended for use in patients with creatinine clearance of less than 40 ml/min.

Elderly:

The dose should be kept as low as possible commensurate with achievement of adequate blood pressure control.

Children:

Not recommended. Safety and efficacy in children has not been established.

4.3 Contraindications
Accuretic is contra-indicated throughout pregnancy (see section 4.6).

Accuretic is contra-indicated in nursing mothers.

Accuretic is contra-indicated in patients with hypersensitivity to any of the ingredients.

Accuretic is contra-indicated in patients with anuria or hypersensitivity to quinapril, thiazides or any sulphonamide derived drug.

Accuretic is contra-indicated in patients with aortic stenosis or outflow obstruction.

Accuretic is contra-indicated in patients with a history of angioedema related to previous treatment with ACE inhibitors.

Accuretic is contra-indicated in patients with hereditary/idiopathic angioneurotic oedema.

4.4 Special warnings and precautions for use

Hypotension:

Accuretic can cause symptomatic hypotension, usually not more frequently than either drug as monotherapy. Symptomatic hypotension was rarely seen in uncomplicated hypertensive patients treated with quinapril but is a possible consequence of ACE inhibition therapy in salt/volume depleted patients such as those previously treated with diuretics, who have a dietary salt restriction, or who are on dialysis. The thiazide component of Accuretic may potentiate the action of other antihypertensive drugs. If symptomatic hypotension occurs, the patient should be placed in the supine position and, if necessary, receive an intravenous infusion of normal saline. A transient hypotensive response is not a contraindication to further doses; however, lower doses of the drug should be considered if this event occurs.

Sensitivity reactions:

Sensitivity reactions may occur in patients with or without a history of allergy or bronchial asthma, e.g. purpura, photosensitivity, urticaria, necrotising angitis, respiratory distress including pneumonitis and pulmonary oedema, anaphylactic reactions.

Renal Disease:

Accuretic should be used with caution in patients with renal disease. In severe renal disease thiazides may precipitate azotemia and in moderate renal impairment (creatinine clearance 10-20ml/min) thiazides are generally ineffective in such patients, and the effects of repeated dosing may be cumulative.

As a consequence of inhibiting the renin-angiotensin-aldosterone system, changes in renal function may be anticipated in susceptible individuals. In patients with severe heart failure, whose renal function may depend on the activity of the renin- angiotensin-aldosterone system, treatment with ACE inhibitors including quinapril, may be associated with oliguria and/or progressive azotemia and rarely acute renal failure and/or death.

The half-life of quinaprilat (the main active metabolite of quiniprii) is prolonged as creatinine clearance falls. Patients with a creatinine clearance of <40 ml/min require a lower initial dosage of quinapril. (see section 4.2 Posology and method of administration). These patients' dosage should be titrated upwards based upon therapeutic response, and renal function should be closely monitored although initial studies do not indicate that quinapril produces further deterioration in renal function.

In clinical studies in hypertensive patients with unilateral or bilateral renal artery stenosis, increases in blood urea nitrogen and serum creatinine have been observed in some patients following ACE inhibitor therapy. These increases were almost always reversible upon discontinuation of the ACE inhibitor and/or diuretic therapy. In such patients, renal function should be monitored during the first few weeks of therapy.

Some hypertensive patients with no apparent pre-existing renal vascular disease have developed increases in blood urea and serum creatinine, usually minor and transient, especially when quinapril has been given concomitantly with a diuretic. This is more likely to occur in patients with pre-existing renal impairment. Dosage reduction and/or discontinuation of any diuretic and/or quinapril may be required.

Anaphylactoid reactions:

Desensitisation: Patients receiving ACE inhibitors during desensitising treatment with hymenoptera venom have sustained life-threatening anaphylactoid reactions. In the same patients, these reactions have been avoided when ACE inhibitors were temporarily withheld, but they have reappeared upon inadvertant rechallenge.

LDL apheresis: Patients undergoing low-density lipoprotein apheresis with dextran-sulfate absorption when treated concomitantly with an ACE inhibitor, have reported anaphylactoid reactions.

Haemodialysis:

Patients haemodialysed using high-flux polyacrylonitrile ('AN69') membranes are highly likely to experience anaphylactoid reactions if they are treated with ACE inhibitors. This combination should therefore be avoided, either by use of alternative antihypertensive drugs or alternative membranes for haemodialysis.

Angioedema:

Angioedema has been reported in patients treated with angiotensin-converting enzyme inhibitors. If laryngeal stridor or angioedema of the face, tongue or glottis occurs, treatment with Accuretic should be discontinued immediately; the patient should be treated in accordance wit accepted medical care and carefully observed until th swelling disappears. In instances where the swelling i confined to the face and lips, the condition generall resolves without treatment; antihistamines may be usef in relieving symptoms. Angioedema associated with lar yngeal involvement may be fatal. Where there is involve ment of the tongue, glottis or larynx likely to cause airwa obstruction, emergency therapy including, but not limite to, subcutaneous adrenaline solution 1:1000 (0.3 to 0.5 m should be promptly administered.

Intestinal angioedema: Intestinal angioedema has bee reported in patients treated with ACE inhibitors. These patients presented with abdominal pain (with or withou nausea or vomiting); in some cases there was no prior history of facial angioedema and C-1 esterase levels were normal. The angioedema was diagnosed by procedures including abdominal CT scan or ultrasound, or at surgery and symptoms resolved after stopping the ACE inhibitor. Intestinal angioedema should be included in the differentia diagnosis of patients on ACE inhibitors presenting with abdominal pain.

Black patients receiving ACE inhibitor therapy have been reported to have a higher incidence of angioedema compared to non-black patients.

Liver Disease:

Accuretic should be used cautiously in patients with impaired hepatic function or progressive liver disease because of the known risks associated with alterations in fluid and electrolyte imbalance resulting from thiazide treatment. Quinaprilat concentrations are reduced in patients with alcoholic cirrhosis due to impaired de-esterification of quinapril.

Patients receiving Accuretic should be observed for clinical signs of thiazide induced fluid or electrolyte imbalance. In such patients periodic determination of serum electrolytes should be performed. Because quinapril reduces the production of aldosterone, its combination with hydrochlorothiazide may minimise diuretic induced hypokalaemia. However, some patients may still require potassium supplements.

Stevens-Johnson syndrome and exacerbations or activation of systemic lupus erythematosus have been reported with thiazides.

Hypoglycaemia and Diabetes:

ACE inhibitors have been associated with hypoglycaemia in diabetic patients on insulin or oral hypoglycaemic agents. Closer monitoring of diabetic patients may be required.

Cough:

Cough has been reported with the use of ACE inhibitors including quinapril. Characteristically, the cough is non-productive, persistent, and resolves after discontinuation of therapy. ACE inhibitor-induced cough should be considered as part of the differential diagnosis of cough.

Neutropenia/Agranulocytosis:

ACE inhibitors have been rarely associated with agranulocytosis and bone marrow depression in patients with uncomplicated hypertension but more frequently in patients with renal impairment, especially if they also have a collagen vascular disease. Agranulocytosis has been rarely reported during treatment with quinapril. As with other ACE inhibitors, periodic monitoring of the white blood cell counts in quinapril-treated patients with collagen vascular disease and/or renal disease should be considered.

4.5 Interaction with other medicinal products and other forms of interaction

Tetracycline and other drugs that interact with magnesium:

Because of the presence of magnesium carbonate in the formulation it is recommended that concomitant administration of Accuretic with tetracycline be avoided.

Agents increasing serum potassium:

Accuretic contains a thiazide diuretic, which tends to increase the urinary excretion of potassium but it also contains an ACE inhibitor, which tends to conserve potassium by lowering aldosterone levels. It is not advisable to routinely add potassium sparing diuretics or potassium supplements as this may result in elevated serum potassium

Other diuretics:

Accuretic contains a diuretic. Concomitant use of another diuretic may have an additive effect. Also, patients on diuretics, especially those who are volume and/or salt depleted, may experience an excessive reduction of blood pressure on initiation of therapy, or with increased dosage of an ACE inhibitor.

Surgery/anaesthesia:

Although no data are available to indicate that there is an interaction between Accuretic and anaesthetic agents that produce hypotension, caution should be exercised when patients undergo major surgery or anaesthesia since ACE inhibitors have been shown to block angiotensin II formation secondary to compensatory resin release. This may lead to hypotension which can be corrected by volume expansion.

Thiazides may decrease the arterial response to noradrenaline. In emergency surgery pre-anaesthetic and aesthetic agents should be administered in reduced ›ses. Thiazides may increase the response to tubocur- ne.

thium:

ɔreased serum lithium levels and symptoms of lithium ‹icity have been reported in patients receiving concomi- nt lithium and ACE inhibitor therapy or lithium and thia- de therapy. Lithium should not generally be given with ɔcuretic since the risk of lithium toxicity may be ɔreased.

orticosteroids, ACTH:

tensified electrolyte depletion, particularly hypokalaemia ıs been observed.

on-steroidal anti-inflammatory drugs:

some patients, the administration of a non-steroidal anti- flammatory agent can reduce the diuretic, natriuretic, and ntihypertensive effects of loop, potassium sparing, and ıiazide diuretics and may reduce the antihypertensive ffect of ACE inhibitors. Therefore, when Accuretic and on-steroidal anti-inflammatory agents are used concomi- ıntly the patients should be observed closely to determine the desired effect of Accuretic is obtained. Furthermore, it ıas been described that NSAIDs and ACE inhibitors exert n additive effect on the increase in serum potassium, vhereas renal function may decrease. These effects are ı principle reversible and occur especially in patients with ompromised renal function.

llopurinol, cytostatic and immunosuppressive agents, ystemic corticosteroids or procainamide:

Concomitant administration with ACE inhibitors may lead ɔ an increased risk for leucopenia.

lcohol, barbiturates or narcotics:

ᵓotentiation of orthostatic hypotension may occur.

Other antihypertensive drugs:

There may be an additive effect or potentiation.

Antacids:

May decrease the bioavailability of Accuretic.

Antidiabetic drugs (oral hypoglycaemic agents and nsulin):

Dosage adjustments of the antidiabetic drug may be required.

4.6 Pregnancy and lactation

Pregnancy:

Accuretic is contraindicated throughout pregnancy. Qui- napril has been shown to be foetoxic in rabbits. When ACE inhibitors have been used during the second and third trimesters of pregnancy, there have been reports of hypo- tension, renal failure, skull hypoplasia, and/or death in the newborn. Oligohydramnios has also been reported, presumably resulting from decreased renal function in the foetus; limb contractures, craniofacial deformities, hypoplastic lung development and intrauterine growth retardation have been reported in association with oligo- hydramnios. Should a woman become pregnant while receiving Accuretic, the drug should be discontinued as soon as possible. Infants exposed *in utero* to ACE inhibi- tors should be closely observed for hypotension, oliguria and hyperkalemia. If oliguria occurs, attention should be directed toward support of blood pressure and renal per- fusion.

Lactation:

ACE inhibitors, including quinapril, are secreted in human milk to a limited extent. Thiazides appear in human milk. Accuretic should therefore not be used in nursing mothers.

4.7 Effects on ability to drive and use machines

The ability to engage in activities such as operating machinery or operating a motor vehicle may be impaired due to dizziness and fatigue, especially when initiating quinapril therapy

4.8 Undesirable effects

The following adverse reactions have been reported in patients taking Accuretic. The adversereactions are clas- sified according to frequencies determined from clinical trials data.

Very common ≥ 1/10 (≥10%)

Common ≥ 1/100 and < 1/10 (≥1% and < 10%)

Uncommon ≥ 1/1000 and < 1/100 (≥0.1% and < 1%)

Rare ≥ 1/10,000 and < 1/1000 (≥0.01% and 0.1%)

Very rare < 1/10,000 (< 0.1%)

*If a listed adverse reaction term was not reported in clinical trials it was assumed to be rare, based on reporting rates versus estimated product use worldwide.

ADVERSE REACTIONS REPORTED IN PATIENTS TAK- ING QUINAPRIL

Infections and infestations

Uncommon Urinary tract infection

Blood and Lymphatic System disorders

Rare Agranulocytosis*, haemolytic anaemia*, neutrope- nia*, thrombocytopenia*

Immune System Disorders

Rare Anaphylactoid reaction*

Endocrine disorders

Uncommon Insulin requirements in diabetic patients may be altered by thiazides and latent diabetes mellitus may occur.

Metabolism and Nutrition Disorders

Common Hyperkalemia

Psychiatric Disorders

Common Insomnia

Uncommon Confusion, depression, nervousness

Nervous System Disorders Common Dizziness, headache, paresthesia

UncommonSomnolence, taste disturbances, transient ischaemic attacks

Rare Syncope*

Very rare Cerebral haemorrhage*

Eye Disorders

Uncommon Amblyopia

Very rare Blurred vision

Ear and Labyrinth Disorders

Uncommon Tinnitus, vertigo

Cardiac Disorders

Uncommon Angina pectoris, myocardial infarction, palpi- tations, tachycardia

Vascular Disorders

Common Hypotension, Postural hypotension*

Uncommon Vasodilatation

Respiratory, Thoracic and Mediastinal Disorders

Common Coughing, dyspnea, pharyngitis, rhinitis

Rare Bronchospasm*, eosinophilic pneumonitis

In individual cases angioneurotic oedema involving the upper airways has caused fatal airway instruction.

Gastrointestinal Disorders

Common Abdominal pains, diarrhoea, dyspepsia, nausea, vomiting

Uncommon Dry mouth or throat, flatulence, pancreatitis

Very rare Ileus

Hepato-biliary Disorders

Rare Hepatitis*, cholestatic icterus*

Skin and Subcutaneous Tissue Disorders

Uncommon Angioedema, increased perspiration, pruritus, rash

Rare Alopecia*, epidermic necrolysis*, eosinophilia* and/or increased ANA-titers*, exfoliative dermatitis*, pemphigus*, photosensitivity reaction*, urticaria

Very rare Psoriasis-like efflorescences

Musculoskeletal and Connective Tissue Disorders

Common Back pain, myalgia

Uncommon Arthralgia, hyperuricaemia may occur or frank gout be precipitated by thiazides in certain patients.

Renal and Urinary Disorders

Uncommon Renal dysfunction

Reproductive System and Breast Disorders

Uncommon Impotence

General Disorders and Administration Site Conditions

Common Chest pain, fatigue

Uncommon Fever, generalized oedema, peripheral oedema

Investigations

Common Increased serum creatinine, increased blood urea nitrogen.

Increases in cholesterol and triglyceride levels may be associated with thiazide diuretic therapy.

Decreases in hematocrit and white cell count as well as elevation of liver enzymes and serum bilirubin. In patients with a congenital deficiency concerning G-6-PDH, indivi- dual cases of hemolytic anaemia have been reported.

ADVERSE REACTIONS REPORTED IN PATIENTS TAKING QUINAPRIL/HYDROCHLOROTHIAZIDE

Infections and Infestations

Uncommon Urinary tract infection

Common Upper respiratory infection, viral infection

Blood and Lymphatic System Disorders

Rare Haemolytic anaemia*, thrombocytopenia*

Immune System Disorders

Rare Anaphylactoid reaction*

Endocrine disorders

Uncommon Insulin requirements in diabetic patients may be altered by thiazides and latent diabetes mellitus may occur.

Psychiatric Disorders

Common Insomnia

Uncommon Confusion, depression, nervousness

Nervous System Disorders

Common Dizziness, headache, somnolence

Uncommon Paresthesia, syncope, taste disturbances, transient ischaemic attacks

Rare Cerebral haemorrhage*

Eye Disorders Uncommon Amblyopia Very rare blurred vision

Ear and Labyrinth Disorders

Uncommon Tinnitus, vertigo

Cardiac Disorders

Common Myocardial infarction

Uncommon Palpitations, tachycardia

Vascular Disorders

Common Vasodilatation, Postural hypotension*

Uncommon Hypotension

Respiratory, Thoracic and Mediastinal Disorders

Common Bronchitis, coughing, pharyngitis, rhinitis,

Uncommon Dyspnea, sinusitis

Rare Bronchospasm*

In individual cases angioneurotic oedema involving the upper airways has caused fatal airway obstruction.

Gastrointestinal Disorders

Common Abdominal pains, diarrhoea, dyspepsia, nausea, vomiting

Uncommon Flatulence, dry mouth or throat

Rare Pancreatitis*

Very rare Ileus

Hepato-biliary Disorders

Rare Hepatitis*, Cholestatic icterus*

Skin and Subcutaneous Tissue Disorders

Uncommon Alopecia, photosensitivity reaction, pruritus, rash

Rare Epidermic necrolysis*, erythema multiforme*, exfolia- tive dermatitis*, pemphigus*, Stevens Johnson syndrome*, eosinophilia* and/or increased ANA-titers*, psoriasis-like efflorescences

Very rare Urticaria

Musculoskeletal and Connective Tissue Disorders

Common Back pain, myalgia, hyperuricaemia may occur or frank gout be precipitated by thiazides in certain patients

Uncommon Arthralgia

Renal and Urinary Disorders

Uncommon Renal dysfunction

Reproductive System and Breast Disorders

Uncommon Impotence

General Disorders and Administration Site Conditions

Common Asthenia, chest pain, fatigue

Uncommon Fever, peripheral oedema

Investigations

Uncommon Increased serum creatinine, increased blood urea nitrogen.

Increases in cholesterol and triglyceride levels may be associated with thiazide diuretic therapy.

Decreases in hematocrit and white cell count as well as elevation of liver enzymes and serum bilirubin. In patients with a congenital deficiency concerning G-6-PDH, indivi- dual cases of haemolytic anaemia have been reported.

4.9 Overdose

No data are available for Accuretic with respect to over- dosage in humans. The most likely clinical manifestation would be symptoms attributable to quinapril monotherapy overdosage such as severe hypotension, which would usually be treated by infusion of intravenous normal saline.

The most common signs and symptoms observed for HCTZ monotherapy overdosage are those caused by elec- trolyte depletion (hypokalemia, hypochloremia, hyponatre- mia) and dehydration resulting from excessive diuresis. If digitalis has also been administered, hypokalemia may accentuate cardiac arrythmias.

No specific information is available on the treatment of overdosage with quinapril/HCTZ. Haemodialysis and peri- toneal dialysis have little effect on the elimination of qui- napril and quinaprilat. Treatment is symptomatic and supportive consistent with established medical care.

5. PHARMACOLOGICAL PROPERTIES

5.1 Pharmacodynamic properties

Quinapril is rapidly de-esterified to quinaprilat (quinapril diacid, the principal metabolite), which is a potent angio- tensin-converting enzyme (ACE) inhibitor.

Quinapril and hydrochlorothiazide lower blood pressure by different, though complementary mechanisms. With diure- tic treatment, blood pressure and blood volume fall, result- ing in a rise in angiotensin II levels which tend to blunt the hypotensive effect. Quinapril blocks this rise in angiotensin II. The antihypertensive effects of quinapril and hydrochlor- othiazide are additive.

It should be noted that in controlled clinical trials, ACE inhibitors have an effect on blood pressure that is less in black patients than in non-blacks, although this difference is reported to disappear when a diuretic is added.

5.2 Pharmacokinetic properties

Quinapril:

Peak plasma quinapril concentrations are observed within 1 hour of oral administration. The extent of absorption is approximately 60%, and is not influenced by food.

Following absorption, quinapril is deesterified to its major active metabolite, quinaprilat, and to minor inactive metabolites. Quinapril has an apparent half-life of approximately one hour. Peak plasma quinaprilat concentrations are observed approximately 2 hours following an oral dose of quinapril. Quinaprilat is eliminated primarily by renal excretion and has an effective accumulation half-life of 7 hours. In patients with renal insufficiency and creatinine clearance of $\leq$40ml/min, peak and trough quinaprilat concentrations increase, time to peak concentration increases, apparent half-life increases, and time to steady state may be delayed. The elimination of quinaprilat is also reduced in elderly patients >65 years) and correlates well with the impaired renal function which frequently occurs in the elderly (see section 4.2 Posology and method of administration). Studies in rats indicate that Accuretic and its metabolites do not cross the blood-brain barrier.

Hydrochlorothiazide:

After oral administration of hydrochlorothiazide, diuresis begins within 2 hours, peaks in about 4 hours, and lasts about 6 to 12 hours. Hydrochlorothiazide is excreted unchanged by the kidney. When plasma levels have been followed for at least 24 hours, the plasma half-life has been observed to vary between 4 to 15 hours. At least 61% of the oral dose is eliminated unchanged within 24 hours. Hydrochlorothiazide crosses the placenta but not the blood-brain barrier.

5.3 Preclinical safety data
The results of the preclinical tests do not add anything of further significance to the prescriber.

6. PHARMACEUTICAL PARTICULARS
6.1 List of excipients
Accuretic tablets contain the following excipients:

Magnesium carbonate, lactose, povidone, crospovidone, magnesium stearate, candelilla wax, colourings: opadry pink OY-S-6937 (contains iron dioxide E172 and titanium dioxide E171 hydroxypropylmethyl cellulose, hydroxypropyl cellulose and polyethylene glycol).

6.2 Incompatibilities
None known.

6.3 Shelf life
3 years.

6.4 Special precautions for storage
Do not store above 25°C.

Store in the original package.

6.5 Nature and contents of container
Double sided aluminium foil blister enclosed in printed carton. Available in pack sizes of 7, 28, 30, 100 and 156.

6.6 Special precautions for disposal and other handling
No special instructions needed.

7. MARKETING AUTHORISATION HOLDER
Pfizer Limited
Ramsgate Road
Sandwich
Kent
CT13 9NJ
United Kingdom

8. MARKETING AUTHORISATION NUMBER(S)
PL 00057/0518

9. DATE OF FIRST AUTHORISATION/RENEWAL OF THE AUTHORISATION
1st May 2003.

10. DATE OF REVISION OF THE TEXT
November 2005.

Company Reference: AH 5_0.

Acnecide 5% w/w Gel

(Galderma (U.K) Ltd)

1. NAME OF THE MEDICINAL PRODUCT
Acnecide 5% w/w Gel

2. QUALITATIVE AND QUANTITATIVE COMPOSITION
Hydrous benzoyl peroxide equivalent to Benzoyl Peroxide 5% w/w

For excipients see 6.1

3. PHARMACEUTICAL FORM
Topical Gel

White, smooth gel

4. CLINICAL PARTICULARS
4.1 Therapeutic indications
Topical therapy for the treatment of acne vulgaris

4.2 Posology and method of administration
For external use only.

Adults and children:

After washing with a mild cleanser, apply once or twice daily or as directed to the affected areas. Initially Acnecide 5 should be used; treatment may be continued with Acnecide 10 provided Acnecide 5 has been well tolerated. The extent of any drying or peeling may be adjusted by modifying the dosage schedule.

4.3 Contraindications
Persons having known sensitivity to benzoyl peroxide.

4.4 Special warnings and precautions for use
A mild burning sensation will probably be felt on first application and some reddening and peeling of the skin will occur within a few days. During the first weeks of treatment a sudden increase in peeling will occur in most patients. This is not harmful and will normally subside within a day or two if treatment is temporarily discontinued. If severe irritation occurs, patients should be directed to use the medication less frequently, to temporarily discontinue use or to discontinue use altogether.

Benzoyl peroxide gel should not come into contact with the eyes, mouth, angles of the nose or mucous membranes. If the preparation enters the eye, wash thoroughly with water. Caution should be exercised when applying the drug to the neck and other sensitive areas.

Repeated exposure to sunlight or UV radiation should be avoided.

Contact with any coloured material including hair and dyed fabrics may result in bleaching or discoloration.

Due to the risk of sensitisation, benzoyl peroxide gel should not be applied on damaged skin.

4.5 Interaction with other medicinal products and other forms of interaction
There are no known interaction with other medications which might be used cutaneously and concurrently with benzoyl peroxide; however, drugs with desquamative, irritant and drying effects should not be used concurrently with benzoyl peroxide gel.

4.6 Pregnancy and lactation
There are no published reports relating to the effects of benzoyl peroxide on reproductive function, fertility, teratogenicity, embryotoxicity, or peri- and post- natal development in animals. In widespread clinical use for the cutaneous treatment of acne vulgaris, at concentrations up to 10% w/w for several decades, benzoyl peroxide has never been associated with effects on these parameters in humans. Caution should be exercised when prescribing to pregnant women.

It is not known whether benzoyl peroxide is excreted in animal or human milk. Because many drugs are excreted in human milk, caution should be exercised when benzoyl peroxide gel is administered to a nursing woman and the preparation should not be applied on the chest to avoid accidental transfer to the infant.

4.7 Effects on ability to drive and use machines
Based on the pharmacodynamic profile and extensive clinical experience, performance related to driving and using machines should not be affected during treatment with Benzoyl peroxide.

4.8 Undesirable effects
The major adverse reaction reported to date with benzoyl peroxide cutaneous therapy is irritation of the skin including erythema, burning, peeling, dryness, itching, stinging, feeling of skin tension locally at the site of application. This is reversible when treatment is reduced in frequency or discontinued. Allergic contact dermatitis, including face oedema, may occur.

4.9 Overdose
Benzoyl peroxide gel is a preparation indicated for topical treatment only. If the medication is applied excessively, no more rapid or better results will be obtained and severe irritation might develop. In this event, treatment must be discontinued and appropriate symptomatic therapy should be instituted.

5. PHARMACOLOGICAL PROPERTIES
5.1 Pharmacodynamic properties
Benzoyl peroxide is an established and effective keratolytic agent with antibacterial properties. It has been shown to be effective in reducing the local population of Propionibacterium acnes leading to a reduction in the production of irritant fatty acids in the sebaceous glands.

5.2 Pharmacokinetic properties
Not applicable. Acnecide is a topical preparation.

5.3 Preclinical safety data
In animal studies by the cutaneous route, benzoyl peroxide is associated with a minimal to moderate skin irritation potential including erythema and oedema. Phototoxic and photoallergic reactions have been reported for benzoyl peroxide therapy.

6. PHARMACEUTICAL PARTICULARS
6.1 List of excipients
Docusate sodium
Disodium edetate
Poloxamer 182
Carbomer 940
Propylene glycol
Acrylates copolymer or glycerol microsponge
Glycerol
Colloidal Anhydrous Silica
Purified water
Sodium hydroxide to adjust the pH.

6.2 Incompatibilities
Not applicable

6.3 Shelf life
3 Years

6.4 Special precautions for storage
Do not store above 25°C.

Do not freeze.

6.5 Nature and contents of container
White low density polyethylene tubes containing 60g ge

6.6 Special precautions for disposal and other handlin
No special requirements.

7. MARKETING AUTHORISATION HOLDER
Galderma (UK) Limited,
Meridien House
69-71 Clarendon Road
Watford
Herts.
WD17 1DS
UK

8. MARKETING AUTHORISATION NUMBER(S)
PL 10590/0006

9. DATE OF FIRST AUTHORISATION/RENEWAL O THE AUTHORISATION
13th July 1992

10. DATE OF REVISION OF THE TEXT
February 2006

Acnisal

(Alliance Pharmaceuticals

1. NAME OF THE MEDICINAL PRODUCT
Acnisal 2%w/w Cutaneous Solution

2. QUALITATIVE AND QUANTITATIVE COMPOSITION
Salicylic acid 2.0% w/w.

For excipients, see 6.1.

3. PHARMACEUTICAL FORM
Cutaneous solution

An opaque off-white cutaneous emollient solution.

4. CLINICAL PARTICULARS
4.1 Therapeutic indications
Acnisal is for the management of acne. It helps prevent ne comedones (blackheads and whiteheads) papules ar pustules (acne pimples).

4.2 Posology and method of administration
For topical administration.

Adults:

Acnisal is used to wash the affected area 2 to 3 times dail Lather with warm water, massage into skin, rinse and dr

Children:

As for adults.

Elderly:

As for adults.

4.3 Contraindications
Acnisal is contra-indicated in persons with a sensitivity salicylic acid.

4.4 Special warnings and precautions for use
For external use only. Avoid contact with the mouth, eye and other mucous membranes to avoid irritation.

As with other topical preparations containing salicylic aci excessive prolonged use may result in symptoms of sal cylism.

4.5 Interaction with other medicinal products and othe forms of interaction
None known.

4.6 Pregnancy and lactation
No limitations to the use of Acnisal during pregnancy lactation are known.

4.7 Effects on ability to drive and use machines
None known.

4.8 Undesirable effects
Salicylic acid is a mild irritant and may cause skin irritatio If undue skin irritation develops or increases adjust th usage schedule or consult your physician.

4.9 Overdose
Not applicable.

5. PHARMACOLOGICAL PROPERTIES
5.1 Pharmacodynamic properties
Human comedones, naturally or coal tar induced, are firml anchored and are dislodged with great difficulty. Mos classic "peeling" agents are ineffective: they are merel irritants which cause scaling, creating the illusion of come dolysis. While salicylic acid is an irritant its efficacy dependent on specific pharmacological effects. It seem to detach horny cells from each other by weakening th intercellular cement. As a result, the comedones tend

ındergo disorganisation. The effect is probably a good ɛal more complex. Salicylic acid penetrates skin readily ɪd increases turnover which also favours exfoliation of the ɔmedo. In concentrations of 0.5 to 2% it significantly ɛduces the formation of microcomedones, which are ɪe precursors of all other acne lesions.

2 Pharmacokinetic properties
here is no evidence of any systemic absorption from the se of Acnisal.

.3 Preclinical safety data
lone presented.

. PHARMACEUTICAL PARTICULARS

.1 List of excipients
urified water
enzyl alcohol
odium chloride
odium C14-C16 olefin sulphonate
auramide DEA (monoamide 716)
EG-7 Glyceryl cocoate
cusol OP301 (styrene/acrylate copolymer)

.2 Incompatibilities
lot applicable.

.3 Shelf life
years.

.4 Special precautions for storage
Store below 25°C.

.5 Nature and contents of container
Acnisal is supplied in a white HDPE bottle with a white olypropylene screw cap. Each bottle contains either 30ml or 177ml of Acnisal.

.6 Special precautions for disposal and other handling
No special requirements.

7. MARKETING AUTHORISATION HOLDER
Alliance Pharmaceuticals Ltd
Avonbridge House
Bath Road
Chippenham
Wiltshire
SN15 2BB

8. MARKETING AUTHORISATION NUMBER(S)
PL 16853/0070

9. DATE OF FIRST AUTHORISATION/RENEWAL OF THE AUTHORISATION
11th September 1998.

10. DATE OF REVISION OF THE TEXT
July 2008

Actidose-Aqua Advance

(Cambridge Laboratories)

1. NAME OF THE MEDICINAL PRODUCT
Actidose-Aqua Advance

2. QUALITATIVE AND QUANTITATIVE COMPOSITION
Actidose-Aqua Advance contains 1.04 g of Activated Charcoal/5 ml.

3. PHARMACEUTICAL FORM
Suspension for oral administration.

4. CLINICAL PARTICULARS

4.1 Therapeutic indications
For the emergency treatment of acute poisoning and drug overdosage where substances such as those listed in section 5.1 have been ingested. The list is not exhaustive and Actidose-Aqua Advance may be of benefit following ingestion of many other toxins.

Also indicated for a limited number of systemic poisonings resulting from parenteral overdosage or when the ingested toxin has been totally absorbed. This usually involves repeated doses of Actidose-Aqua Advance to remove compounds which undergo enterohepatic recycling or which can diffuse into the gastrointestinal tract along a concentration gradient. Under these circumstances multiple doses of Actidose-Aqua Advance adsorb the toxin thereby preventing its reabsorption and increasing the concentration gradient in favour of further diffusion of the toxin into the gastrointestinal tract. Compounds most effectively transferred by this mechanism are lipophilic, uncharged and not excessively protein-bound. Examples of compounds which can be eliminated more rapidly by "gastrointestinal dialysis" in this way are phenobarbitone and theophylline.

4.2 Posology and method of administration
The container should be shaken thoroughly prior to administration. If the dose of poison that has been ingested is known, a ratio of 10:1 (activated charcoal:toxin) may be used to determine the optimal dose of activated charcoal, subject to the limits of practicality. In the absence of any information regarding the amount of poison ingested, the following doses are recommended:

Adults (including the elderly) and children over 12 years of age:

For single dose therapy, 50-100 grams of activated charcoal (240-480 ml) taken as soon as possible after ingestion of the poison.

For multiple dose therapy, 25-50 grams of activated charcoal (120-240 ml) every 4-6 hours.

Children aged 1-12 years

For single dose therapy, 25-50 grams of activated charcoal (120-240 ml) taken as soon as possible after ingestion of the poison. For multiple dose therapy, the dose may be repeated every 4-6 hours.

Children under one year of age:

For single dose therapy, 1 g or 5 ml per kg bodyweight taken as soon as possible after ingestion of the poison. For multiple dose therapy, the dose may be repeated every 4-6 hours.

When syrup of ipecac is used to produce emesis, administration of Actidose-Aqua Advance should be delayed until 30-60 minutes after vomiting has ceased. If gastric lavage is being used to facilitate stomach evacuation a single dose of Actidose-Aqua Advance may be administered early in the procedure. This has the advantage of prompt administration of activated charcoal, but the gastric lavage returns will be black which may make it difficult to evaluate what the patient ingested by visual examination.

Actidose-Aqua Advance may be effective even when several hours have elapsed after ingestion of the poison if gastrointestinal motility is reduced by the toxin or if the drug is subject to enterohepatic or enteroenteric recycling.

4.3 Contraindications
Use of Actidose-Aqua Advance is contra-indicated in persons who are not fully conscious.

4.4 Special warnings and precautions for use
Actidose-Aqua Advance is not recommended for patients who have ingested corrosive agents such as strong acids or alkalis since the activated charcoal may obscure endoscopic visualisation of oesophageal and gastric lesions produced by the toxin. Actidose-Aqua Advance is of little or no value in the treatment of poisoning with cyanides, alcohols, iron salts, malathion and DDT.

Actidose-Aqua Advance is an adjunct in the management of poisoning emergencies. Prior to its use, proper basic life support measures must be implemented where required as well as the appropriate gastric emptying technique if indicated.

Actidose-Aqua Advance should be used with caution in patients who have been exposed to toxins which interfere with gastrointestinal motility (e.g. anticholinergics, opioids). Bowel sounds should be monitored frequently to assess peristaltic action, especially in patients undergoing multiple dose activated charcoal therapy.

4.5 Interaction with other medicinal products and other forms of interaction
Actidose-Aqua Advance will adsorb most medicaments and many other chemical substances. If a specific antidote is to be administered the likelihood of its adsorption by activated charcoal should be borne in mind, and a parenteral route of administration used if possible. Thus in the case of paracetamol, Actidose-Aqua Advance should not be given as well as oral methionine but may be used alone or in conjunction with intravenous N-acetylcysteine.

Other concurrent medications to counteract shock or associated infection should also be given parenterally since orally administered drugs may be bound to the activated charcoal in the gut.

4.6 Pregnancy and lactation
The safety of this medicinal product for use in human pregnancy has not been established. Experimental animal studies are insufficient to assess the safety with respect to the development of the embryo or foetus, the course of gestation and peri- and postnatal development.

Activated charcoal is however essentially inert pharmacologically and is not absorbed from the gastrointestinal tract. No hazard is therefore anticipated from its use during pregnancy or lactation.

4.7 Effects on ability to drive and use machines
None known

4.8 Undesirable effects
Both the patient and health care professionals should be aware that Actidose-Aqua Advance will produce black stools. A laxative may be given concurrently to accelerate the removal of the activated charcoal-toxin complex, but should be used with caution and only intermittently during multiple dose activated charcoal therapy since profuse and protracted diarrhoea may lead to fluid and electrolyte imbalance.

Aspiration of activated charcoal has been reported to produce airways obstruction and appropriate precautions should be taken. Gastrointestinal obstruction associated with the use of multiple dose activated charcoal therapy has been reported rarely.

4.9 Overdose
Actidose-Aqua Advance is well tolerated and due to its lack of toxicity overdosage requiring treatment is unlikely. A laxative may be administered to enhance elimination of the product.

5. PHARMACOLOGICAL PROPERTIES

5.1 Pharmacodynamic properties
Activated charcoal has a high adsorptive capacity for a wide range of compounds including many of those which are most commonly encountered in deliberate and accidental poisoning. Substances adsorbed include the following:

Aspirin and other salicylates
Barbiturates
Benzodiazepines
Chlormethiazole
Chloroquine
Chlorpromazine and related phenothiazines
Clonidine
Cocaine and other stimulants
Digoxin and digitoxin
Ibuprofen
Mefenamic acid
Mianserin
Nicotine
Paracetamol
Paraquat
Phenelzine and other monoamine oxidase inhibitors
Phenytoin
Propranolol and other beta-blockers
Quinine
Theophylline
Zidovudine

5.2 Pharmacokinetic properties
Activated charcoal is not absorbed from the gastrointestinal tract or subject to any metabolic processes. It is eliminated in the faeces.

5.3 Preclinical safety data
Activated charcoal is essentially inert pharmacologically and it would therefore be expected to be virtually devoid of toxicity, other than any ill effects arising from mechanical obstruction of the gut, or, if inhaled, the lungs.

The excipients in the product are all well known and widely used in medicinal products and should not give rise to any toxicological problems.

6. PHARMACEUTICAL PARTICULARS

6.1 List of excipients
Sucrose
Propylene glycol
Glycerine
Citric Acid
Purified water

6.2 Incompatibilities
None known.

6.3 Shelf life
Two years

6.4 Special precautions for storage
Store at 15 - 30°C. Do not refrigerate.

6.5 Nature and contents of container
(1) Low density polyethylene bottles containing 120 ml.
(2) Low density polyethylene bottles containing 240 ml.
(3) Low density polyethylene tubes containing 120 ml.

6.6 Special precautions for disposal and other handling
Shake well before use.

7. MARKETING AUTHORISATION HOLDER
Cambridge Laboratories Limited
Deltic House
Kingfisher Way
Silverlink Business Park
Wallsend
Tyne & Wear NE28 9NX

8. MARKETING AUTHORISATION NUMBER(S)
PL 12070/0011

9. DATE OF FIRST AUTHORISATION/RENEWAL OF THE AUTHORISATION
26 March 1996.

10. DATE OF REVISION OF THE TEXT
February 2000

Actilyse

(Boehringer Ingelheim Limited)

1. NAME OF THE MEDICINAL PRODUCT
Actilyse 10 mg
Powder and solvent for solution for injection and infusion

Actilyse 20 mg
Powder and solvent for solution for injection and infusion
Actilyse 50 mg
Powder and solvent for solution for injection and infusion

2. QUALITATIVE AND QUANTITATIVE COMPOSITION
1 vial with powder contains:

10 mg alteplase (corresponding to 5,800,000 IU) or
20 mg alteplase (corresponding to 11,600,000 IU) or
50 mg alteplase (corresponding to 29,000,000 IU), respectively.

Alteplase is produced by recombinant DNA technique using a Chinese hamster ovary cell-line. The specific activity of alteplase in-house reference material is 580,000 IU/mg. This has been confirmed by comparison with the second international WHO standard for t-PA. The specification for the specific activity of alteplase is 522,000 to 696,000 IU/mg.

For a full list of excipients, see section 6.1.

3. PHARMACEUTICAL FORM
Powder and solvent for solution for injection and infusion.

The powder is presented as a colourless to pale yellow lyophilizate cake.

4. CLINICAL PARTICULARS
4.1 Therapeutic indications
Thrombolytic treatment in acute myocardial infarction
- 90 minutes (accelerated) dose regimen (see section 4.2): for patients in whom treatment can be started within 6 h after symptom onset

- 3 h dose regimen (see section 4.2): for patients in whom treatment can be started between 6 - 12 h after symptom onset provided that the diagnosis has been clearly confirmed.

Actilyse has proven to reduce 30-day-mortality in patients with acute myocardial infarction.

Thrombolytic treatment in acute massive pulmonary embolism with haemodynamic instability

The diagnosis should be confirmed whenever possible by objective means such as pulmonary angiography or non-invasive procedures such as lung scanning. There is no evidence for positive effects on mortality and late morbidity related to pulmonary embolism.

Fibrinolytic treatment of acute ischaemic stroke

Treatment must be started within 3 hours of onset of the stroke symptoms and after prior exclusion of intracranial haemorrhage by means of appropriate imaging techniques.

4.2 Posology and method of administration
Actilyse should be given as soon as possible after symptom onset. The following dose guidelines apply.

Under aseptic conditions the content of an injection vial of Actilyse (10 mg or 20 mg or 50 mg) is dissolved with water for injections according to the following table to obtain either a final concentration of 1 mg alteplase/ml or 2 mg alteplase/ml:

(see Table 1 above)

The reconstituted solution should then be administered intravenously. It may be diluted further with sterile sodium chloride 9 mg/ml (0.9 %) solution for injection up to a minimal concentration of 0.2 mg/ml. A dilution of the reconstituted solution with sterilised water for injections or in general, the use of carbohydrate infusion solutions, e.g. dextrose is not recommended. Actilyse should not be mixed with other medicinal products neither in the same infusion-vial nor the same catheter (not even with heparin). For further practical instructions for preparation and handling see sections 6.2 and 6.6.

The experience in children and adolescents is limited. Actilyse is contraindicated for the treatment of acute stroke in children and adolescents (see section 4.3).

Myocardial infarction

a) 90 minutes (accelerated) dose regimen for patients with myocardial infarction, in whom treatment can be started within 6 hours after symptom onset:

	Concentration of alteplase	
	1 mg/ml	2 mg/ml
	ml	ml
15 mg as an intravenous bolus	15	7.5
50 mg as an infusion over 30 minutes	50	25
followed by an infusion of 35 mg over 60 minutes until the maximal dose of 100 mg	35	17.5

Table 1

Actilyse vial	10 mg	20 mg	50 mg
	Volume of water for injections to be added to dry powder:		
Final concentration (a) 1 mg alteplase/ml (ml)	10	20	50
(b) 2 mg alteplase/ml (ml)	5	10	25

In patients with a body weight below 65 kg the dose should be weight adjusted according to the following table:

	Concentration of alteplase	
	1 mg/ml	2 mg/ml
	ml	ml
15 mg as an intravenous bolus	15	7.5
	ml/kg bw	ml/kg bw
and 0.75 mg/kg body weight (bw) over 30 minutes (maximum 50 mg)	0.75	0.375
followed by an infusion of 0.5 mg/kg body weight (bw) over 60 minutes (maximum 35 mg)	0.5	0.25

b) 3 h dose regimen for patients, in whom treatment can be started between 6 and 12 hours after symptom onset:

	Concentration of alteplase	
	1 mg/ml	2 mg/ml
	ml	ml
10 mg as an intravenous bolus	10	5
50 mg as an infusion over the first hour	50	25
	ml/30 min	ml/ 30 min
followed by infusions of 10 mg over 30 minutes until the maximal dose of 100 mg over 3 hours	10	5

In patients with a body weight below 65 kg the total dose should not exceed 1.5 mg/kg.

The maximum dose of alteplase is 100 mg.

Adjunctive therapy:

Antithrombotic adjunctive therapy is recommended according to the current international guidelines for the management of patients with ST-elevation myocardial infarction; acetylsalicylic acid should be initiated as soon as possible after symptom onset and continued with life-long treatment unless it is contraindicated.

Pulmonary embolism

A total dose of 100 mg of alteplase should be administered in 2 hours. Most experience is available with the following dose regimen:

	Concentration of alteplase	
	1 mg/ml	2 mg/ml
	ml	ml
10 mg as an intravenous bolus over 1 - 2 minutes	10	5
followed by an intravenous infusion of 90 mg over 2 hours	90	45

The total dose should not exceed 1.5 mg/kg in patients with a body weight below 65 kg.

Adjunctive therapy:

After treatment with Actilyse heparin therapy should be initiated (or resumed) when aPTT values are less than twice the upper limit of normal. The infusion should be adjusted to maintain aPTT between 50-70 seconds (1.5 to 2.5 fold of the reference value).

Acute ischaemic stroke

Treatment must be performed by a physician specialised in neurological care. (See sections 4.3 and 4.4.)

The recommended dose is 0.9 mg alteplase/kg body weight (maximum of 90 mg) infused intravenously over 60 minutes with 10 % of the total dose administered as an initial intravenous bolus.

Treatment with Actilyse must be started within 3 hours c the onset of symptoms.

Adjunctive therapy:

The safety and efficacy of this regimen with concomitar administration of heparin and acetylsalicylic acid within th first 24 hours of onset of the symptoms have not bee sufficiently investigated.

Administration of acetylsalicylic acid or intravenou heparin should be avoided in the first 24 hours after treatment with Actilyse. If heparin is required for other indications (e.g. prevention of deep vein thrombosis) the dose should not exceed 10,000 IU per day, administered sub cutaneously.

4.3 Contraindications
Hypersensitivity to the active substance or to any of the excipients.

Actilyse is contraindicated in cases where there is a high risk of haemorrhage such as:

- significant bleeding disorder at present or within the past 6 months
- known haemorrhagic diathesis
- patients receiving oral anticoagulants, e.g. warfarin sodium
- manifest or recent severe or dangerous bleeding
- known history of or suspected intracranial haemorrhage
- suspected subarachnoid haemorrhage or condition after subarachnoid haemorrhage from aneurysm
- any history of central nervous system damage (i.e. neoplasm, aneurysm, intracranial or spinal surgery)
- recent (less than 10 days) traumatic external heart massage, obstetrical delivery, recent puncture of a non-compressible blood-vessel (e.g. subclavian or jugular vein puncture)
- severe uncontrolled arterial hypertension
- bacterial endocarditis, pericarditis
- acute pancreatitis
- documented ulcerative gastrointestinal disease during the last 3 months, oesophageal varices, arterial-aneurysm, arterial/venous malformations
- neoplasm with increased bleeding risk
- severe liver disease, including hepatic failure, cirrhosis, portal hypertension (oesophageal varices) and active hepatitis
- major surgery or significant trauma in past 3 months.

Additional contraindications in acute myocardial infarction:

- any known history of haemorrhagic stroke or stroke of unknown origin.
- known history of ischaemic stroke or transient ischaemic attack (TIA) in the preceding 6 months, except current acute ischaemic stroke within 3 hours.

Additional contraindications in acute pulmonary embolism:

- any known history of haemorrhagic stroke or stroke of unknown origin.
- known history of ischaemic stroke or transient ischaemic attack (TIA) in the preceding 6 months, except current acute ischaemic stroke within 3 hours.

Additional contraindications in acute ischaemic stroke:

- symptoms of ischaemic attack beginning more than 3 hours prior to infusion start or when time of symptom onset is unknown,
- minor neurological deficit or symptoms rapidly improving before start of infusion,
- severe stroke as assessed clinically (e.g. NIHSS >25) and/or by appropriate imaging techniques,
- seizure at onset of stroke,
- evidence of intracranial haemorrhage (ICH) on the CT-scan,
- symptoms suggestive of subarachnoid haemorrhage, even if CT-scan is normal,
- administration of heparin within the previous 48 hours and a thromboplastin time exceeding the upper limit of normal for laboratory,
- patients with any history of prior stroke and concomitant diabetes
- prior stroke within the last 3 months
- platelet count of below 100,000/mm^3
- systolic blood pressure > 185 or diastolic BP > 110 mm Hg, or aggressive management (intravenous pharmacotherapy) necessary to reduce BP to these limits
- blood glucose < 50 or > 400 mg/dl.

se in children, adolescents and elderly patients

ctilyse is not indicated for the treatment of acute stroke in aediatric patients under 18 years or adults over 80 years ' age.

4 Special warnings and precautions for use

hrombolytic/ fibrinolytic treatment requires adequate onitoring. Actilyse should only be used by physicians ained and experienced in the use of thrombolytic treatments and with the facilities to monitor that use. It is ecommended that when Actilyse is administered standard esuscitation equipment and pharmacotherapy be available in all circumstances.

he risk of intracranial haemorrhage is increased in elderly atients, therefore in these patients the risk/benefit evaluaon should be carried out carefully.

s yet, there is only limited experience with the use of ctilyse in children and adolescents.

s with all thrombolytic agents, the expected therapeutic enefit should be weighed up particularly carefully against he possible risk, especially in patients with

small recent traumas, such as biopsies, puncture of najor vessels, intramuscular injections, cardiac massage or resuscitation

conditions with an increased risk of haemorrhage which re not mentioned in section 4.3.

he use of rigid catheters should be avoided.

Additional special warnings and precautions in acute myocardial infarction:

A dose exceeding 100 mg of alteplase must not be given because it has been associated with an additional increase in intracranial bleeding.

Therefore special care must be taken to ensure that the dose of alteplase infused is as described in section 4.2.

There is limited experience with readministration of Actilyse. Actilyse is not suspected to cause anaphylactic reactions. If an anaphylactoid reaction occurs, the infusion should be discontinued and appropriate treatment initiated.

The expected therapeutic benefit should be weighed up particularly carefully against the possible risk, especially in patients with systolic blood pressure > 160 mm Hg.

GPIIb/IIIa antagonists:

Concomitant use of GPIIb/IIIa antagonists increases the risk of bleeding.

Additional special warnings and precautions in acute pulmonary embolism:

same as for acute myocardial infarction (see above)

Additional special warnings and precautions in acute ischaemic stroke:

Special precautions for use:

Treatment must be performed only by a physician trained and experienced in neurological care.

Special warnings / conditions with a decreased benefit/risk ratio:

Compared to other indications patients with acute ischaemic stroke treated with Actilyse have a markedly increased risk of intracranial haemorrhage as the bleeding occurs predominantly into the infarcted area. This applies in particular in the following cases:

- all situations listed in section 4.3. and in general all situations involving a high risk of haemorrhage
- small asymptomatic aneurysms of the cerebral vessels
- patients pre-treated with acetyl salicylic acid (ASA) may have a greater risk of intracerebral haemorrhage, particularly if Actilyse treatment is delayed. Not more than 0.9 mg alteplase/kg bodyweight (max. of 90 mg) should be administered in view of the increased risk of cerebral haemorrhage.

Treatment should not be initiated later than 3 hours after the onset of symptoms (see section 4.3) because of an unfavourable benefit/risk ratio mainly based on the following:

- positive treatment effects decrease over time
- mortality rate increases particularly in patients with prior ASA treatment
- risk increases with regard to symptomatic haemorrhages

Blood pressure (BP) monitoring during treatment administration and up to 24 hours seems justified; an intravenous antihypertensive therapy is also recommended if systolic BP > 180 mm Hg or diastolic BP > 105 mm Hg.

The therapeutic benefit is reduced in patients that had a prior stroke or in those with known uncontrolled diabetes, thus the benefit/risk ratio is considered less favourable, but still positive in these patients.

In patients with very mild stroke, the risks outweigh the expected benefit (see section 4.3).

Patients with very severe stroke are at higher risk for intracerebral haemorrhage and death and should not be treated (see section 4.3).

Patients with extensive infarctions are at greater risk of poor outcome including severe haemorrhage and death. In such patients, the benefit/risk ratio should be thoroughly considered.

In stroke patients the likelihood of good outcomes decreases with increasing age, increasing stroke severity and increased levels of blood glucose on admission while the likelihood of severe disability and death or relevant intracranial bleedings increases, independently from treatment. Patients over 80, patients with severe stroke (as assessed clinically and/or by appropriate imaging techniques) and patients with blood glucose levels < 50 mg/dl or > 400 mg/dl at baseline should not be treated with Actilyse (see section 4.3).

Other special warnings:

Reperfusion of the ischaemic area may induce cerebral oedama in the infarcted zone.

Due to an increased haemorrhagic risk, treatment with platelet aggregation inhibitors should not be initiated within the first 24 hours following thrombolysis with alteplase.

4.5 Interaction with other medicinal products and other forms of interaction

No formal interaction studies with Actilyse and medicinal products commonly administered in patients with acute myocardial infarction have been performed.

The risk of haemorrhage is increased if coumarine derivatives, oral anticoagulants, platelet aggregation inhibitors, unfractionated heparin or LMWH or other agents inhibiting coagulation are administered (before, during or within the first 24 hours after treatment with Actilyse) (see section 4.3).

Concomitant treatment with ACE inhibitors may enhance the risk of suffering an anaphylactoid reaction, as in the cases describing such reactions a relatively larger proportion of patients were receiving ACE inhibitors concomitantly.

Concomitant use of GPIIb/IIIa antagonists increases the risk of bleeding.

4.6 Pregnancy and lactation

There is very limited experience with the use of alteplase during pregnancy and lactation. Studies in animals have shown reproductive toxicity (see section 5.3). In cases of an acute life-threatening disease the benefit has to be evaluated against the potential risk.

It is not known if alteplase is excreted into breast milk.

4.7 Effects on ability to drive and use machines

Not relevant.

4.8 Undesirable effects

The frequency of the undesirable effects is described using the MedDRA frequency convention*.

*MedDRA frequency convention:

very common	>1/10
common	>1/100 and ⩽ 1/10
uncommon	>1/1,000 and ⩽ 1/100
rare	>1/10,000 and ⩽ 1/1,000
very rare	⩽ 1/10,000 including isolated reports

Except for intracranial haemorrhage as adverse reaction in the indication stroke and reperfusion arrhythmias in the indication myocardial infarction, there is no medical reason to assume that the qualitative and quantitative adverse reaction profile of Actilyse in the indications pulmonary embolism and acute ischaemic stroke is different from the profile in the indication myocardial infarction.

Haemorrhage

The most frequent adverse reaction associated with Actilyse is bleeding resulting in a fall in haematocrit and/or haemoglobin values:

very common: bleeding from damaged blood vessels (such as haematoma) injection site haemorrhage (puncture site haemorrhage, catheter site haematoma, catheter site haemorrhage)

common: intracranial haemorrhage (such as cerebral haemorrhage, cerebral haematoma, haemorrhagic stroke, haemorrhagic transformation of stroke, intracranial haematoma, subarachnoid haemorrhage) in the treatment of acute ischaemic stroke. Symptomatic intracerebral haemorrhage represents the major adverse reaction in the treatment of acute ischaemic stroke (up to 10 % of patients without any increase of overall mortality or morbidity). respiratory tract haemorrhage (such as pharyngeal haemorrhage, epistaxis, haemoptysis) gastrointestinal haemorrhage (such as gastric haemorrhage, gastric ulcer haemorrhage, haemorrhage rectum, haematemesis, melaena, mouth haemorrhage, gingival bleeding) ecchymosis urogenital haemorrhage (such as haematuria, haemorrhage urinary tract) blood transfusion (necessary)

uncommon: intracranial haemorrhage (such as cerebral haemorrhage, cerebral haematoma, haemorrhagic stroke, haemorrhagic transformation of stroke, intracranial haematoma, subarachnoid haemorrhage) in the treatment of acute myocardial infarction and acute pulmonary embolism haemopericardium retroperitoneal haemorrhage (such as retroperitoneal haematoma)

rare: bleeding in parenchymatous organs (such as hepatic haemorrhage, pulmonary haemorrhage)

very rare: eye haemorrhage

Death and permanent disability are reported in patients who have experienced stroke (including intracranial bleeding) and other serious bleeding episodes.

If a potentially dangerous haemorrhage occurs in particular cerebral haemorrhage, the fibrinolytic therapy must be discontinued. In general, however, it is not necessary to replace the coagulation factors because of the short half-life and the minimal effect on the systemic coagulation factors. Most patients who have bleeding can be managed by interruption of thrombolytic and anticoagulant therapy, volume replacement, and manual pressure applied to an incompetent vessel. Protamine should be considered if heparin has been administered within 4 hours of the onset of bleeding. In the few patients who fail to respond to these conservative measures, judicious use of transfusion products may be indicated. Transfusion of cryoprecipitate, fresh frozen plasma, and platelets should be considered with clinical and laboratory reassessment after each administration. A target fibrinogen level of 1 g/l is desirable with cryoprecipitate infusion. Antifibrinolytic agents are available as a last alternative.

Immune system disorders

uncommon: hypersensitivity reactions / anaphylactoid reactions (e.g. allergic reactions including rash, urticaria, bronchospasm, angio-oedema, hypotension, shock or any other symptom associated with allergic reactions)

very rare: serious anaphylaxis

Transient antibody formation to Actilyse has been observed in rare cases and with low titres, but a clinical relevance of this finding could not be established.

Nervous system disorders

very rare: events related to the nervous system (e.g. epileptic seizure, convulsion, aphasia, speech disorder, delirium, acute brain syndrome, agitation, confusion, depression, psychosis) often in association with concurrent ischaemic or haemorrhagic cerebrovascular events.

Cardiac disorders

As with other thrombolytic agents, the following events have been reported as sequelae of myocardial infarction and / or thrombolytic administration.

very common: recurrent ischaemia / angina, hypotension and heart failure / pulmonary oedema, reperfusion arrhythmias (such as arrhythmia, extrasystoles, AV block I° to complete, atrial fibrillation / flutter, bradycardia, tachycardia, ventricular arrhythmia, ventricular tachycardia/ fibrillation, electromechanical dissociation [EMD])

common: cardiac arrest, cardiogenic shock and reinfarction

uncommon: mitral regurgitation, pulmonary embolism, other systemic embolism / cerebral embolism, ventricular septal defect

These cardiac events can be life-threatening and may lead to death.

Vascular disorders

uncommon: embolism (thrombotic embolisation), which may lead to corresponding consequences in the organs concerned

Gastrointestinal disorders

common: nausea, vomiting

Investigations

very common: blood pressure decreased

common: body temperature increased

Injury and poisoning and procedural complications

rare: fat embolism (cholesterol crystal embolisation), which may lead to corresponding consequences in the organs concerned

4.9 Overdose

The relative fibrin specificity notwithstanding, a clinical significant reduction in fibrinogen and other blood coagulation components may occur after overdosage. In most cases, it is sufficient to await the physiological regeneration of these factors after the Actilyse therapy has been terminated. If, however, severe bleeding results, the infusion of fresh frozen plasma or fresh blood is recommended and if necessary, synthetic antifibrinolytics may be administered.

5. PHARMACOLOGICAL PROPERTIES

5.1 Pharmacodynamic properties

Pharmaco-therapeutic group: antithrombotic agent, ATC-code: B 01 A D 02

The active ingredient of Actilyse is alteplase, a recombinant human tissue-type plasminogen activator, a glycoprotein, which activates plasminogen directly to plasmin. When administered intravenously, alteplase remains relatively inactive in the circulatory system. Once bound to fibrin, it is activated, inducing the conversion of plasminogen to plasmin leading to the dissolution of the fibrin clot.

In a study including more than 40,000 patients with an acute myocardial infarction (GUSTO) the administration of 100 mg alteplase over 90 minutes, with concomitant iv. heparin infusion, led to a lower mortality after 30 days (6.3 %) as compared to the administration of streptokinase, 1.5 million U over 60 minutes, with s.c. or iv. heparin (7.3 %). Actilyse-treated patients showed higher infarct related vessel patency rates at 60 and 90 minutes after thrombolysis than the streptokinase-treated patients. No differences in patency rates were noted at 180 minutes or longer.

30-day-mortality is reduced as compared to patients not undergoing thrombolytic therapy.

The release of alpha-hydroxybutyrate-dehydrogenase (HBDH) is reduced. Global ventricular function as well as regional wall motion is less impaired as compared to patients receiving no thrombolytic therapy.

Myocardial infarction

A placebo controlled trial with 100 mg alteplase over 3 hours (LATE) showed a reduction of 30-day-mortality compared to placebo for patients treated within 6-12 hours after symptom onset. In cases, in which clear signs of myocardial infarction are present, treatment initiated up to 24 hours after symptom onset may still be beneficial.

Pulmonary embolism

In patients with acute massive pulmonary embolism with haemodynamic instability thrombolytic treatment with Actilyse leads to a fast reduction of the thrombus size and a reduction of pulmonary artery pressure. Mortality data are not available.

Acute stroke

In two USA studies (NINDS A/B) a significant higher proportion of patients, when compared to placebo, had a favourable outcome (no or minimal disability). These findings were not confirmed in two European studies and an additional USA study. In the latter studies however, the majority of patients were not treated within 3 hours of stroke onset. In a meta-analysis of all patients treated within 3 hours after stroke onset the beneficial effect of alteplase was confirmed. The risk difference versus placebo for a good recovery was 14.9 % (CI 95% 8.1 % to 21.7 %) despite an increased risk of severe and fatal intracranial haemorrhage. The data do not allow a definite conclusion to be drawn on the treatment effect on death. Nevertheless overall, the benefit/risk of alteplase, given within 3 hours of stroke onset and taking into account the precautions stated elsewhere in the SPC, is considered favourable.

Meta-analysis of all clinical data show that the agent is less effective in patients treated after 3 hours of onset (3 to 6 hours) compared with those treated within 3 hours of onset of symptoms, while the risks are higher, which makes the benefit/risk ratio of alteplase unfavourable outside the 0-3 h time frame.

Due to its relative fibrin-specificity alteplase at a dose of 100 mg leads to a modest decrease of the circulating fibrinogen levels to about 60 % at 4 hours, which is generally reverted to more than 80 % after 24 hours. Plasminogen and alpha-2-antiplasmin decrease to about 20 % and 35 % respectively after 4 hours and increase again to more than 80 % at 24 hours. A marked and prolonged decrease of the circulating fibrinogen level is only seen in few patients.

5.2 Pharmacokinetic properties

Alteplase is cleared rapidly from the circulating blood and metabolised mainly by the liver (plasma clearance 550 - 680 ml/min.). The relevant plasma half-life $t_{1/2}$ alpha is 4-5 minutes. This means that after 20 minutes less than 10% of the initial value is present in the plasma. For the residual amount remaining in a deep compartment, a beta-half-life of about 40 minutes was measured.

5.3 Preclinical safety data

In subchronic toxicity studies in rats and marmosets no unexpected undesirable effects were found.

No indications of a mutagenic potential were found in mutagenic tests.

In pregnant animals no teratogenic effects were observed after intravenous infusion of pharmacologically effective doses. In rabbits embryotoxicity (embryolethality, growth retardation) was induced by more than 3 mg/kg/day. No effects on peri-postnatal development or on fertility parameters were observed in rats with doses up to 10 mg/kg/day.

6. PHARMACEUTICAL PARTICULARS

6.1 List of excipients

Powder for solution:

Arginine

Phosphoric acid, dilute

Polysorbate 80

Solvent:

Water for injections

The pH of the reconstituted solution is 7.3 ± 0.5.

6.2 Incompatibilities

The reconstituted solution may be diluted with sterile sodium chloride 9 mg/ml (0.9 %) solution for injection up to a minimal concentration of 0.2 mg alteplase per ml.

Further dilution, the use of water for injections for dilution or in general the use of carbohydrate infusion solutions, e.g. dextrose, is not recommended due to increasing formation of turbidity of the reconstituted solution.

Actilyse should not be mixed with other medicinal products neither in the same infusion vial nor the same catheter (not even with heparin).

6.3 Shelf life

3 years

After reconstitution, an immediate use is recommended. However, the in-use stability has been demonstrated for 24 hours at 2 °C - 8 °C and for 8 hours at 25 °C.

6.4 Special precautions for storage

Do not store above 25°C. Store in the original package in order to protect from light.

For storage conditions of the reconstituted medicinal product, see section 6.3.

6.5 Nature and contents of container

Powder for solution:

10 ml, 20 ml or 50 ml sterilised glass vials, sealed with sterile siliconised grey butyl-type stoppers with aluminium/plastic flip-off caps.

Solvent:

The water for injections is filled into either 10 ml, 20 ml or 50 ml vials, depending on the size of the powder vials. The water for injections vials are sealed with rubber stoppers and aluminium/plastic flip-off caps.

Transfer cannulas (included with pack sizes of 20 mg and 50 mg only)

Pack sizes:

10 mg:

1 vial with 467 mg powder for solution for injection and infusion

1 vial with 10 ml of water for injections

20 mg:

1 vial with 933 mg powder for solution for injection and infusion

1 vial with 20 ml of water for injections

1 transfer cannula

50 mg:

1 vial with 2333 mg powder for solution for injection and infusion

1 vial with 50 ml of water for injections

1 transfer cannula

Not all pack sizes may be marketed.

6.6 Special precautions for disposal and other handling

For reconstitution to a final concentration of 1 mg alteplase per ml the full volume of solvent provided should be transferred to the vial containing the Actilyse powder. To this purpose a transfer cannula is included with the 20 mg and 50 mg pack sizes, which is to be used. For the 10 mg pack size a syringe should be used.

For reconstitution to a final concentration of 2 mg alteplase per ml only half of the solvent provided should be used. In these cases always a syringe should be used to transfer the required amount of solvent to the vial containing the Actilyse powder.

A table giving the volumes of solvent required for reconstitution to the final concentrations for each pack size is provided in section 4.2.

When reconstituting the product from the respective amount of powder and solvent, the mixture should only be agitated gently until complete dissolution. Any vigorous agitation should be avoided to prevent foam formation.

The reconstituted preparation is a clear and colourless to pale yellow solution. Prior to administration it should be inspected visually for particles and colour.

The reconstituted solution is for single use only. Any unused solution should be discarded.

7. MARKETING AUTHORISATION HOLDER

Boehringer Ingelheim Limited

Ellesfield Avenue

Bracknell

Berkshire RG12 8YS

8. MARKETING AUTHORISATION NUMBER(S)

PL 00015/0120

9. DATE OF FIRST AUTHORISATION/RENEWAL OF THE AUTHORISATION

Date of first authorisation: 12th October 1988

Date of last renewal: 26th April 2004

10. DATE OF REVISION OF THE TEXT

April 2009

LEGAL CATEGORY

POM

Actiq

(Cephalon (UK) Limited

1. NAME OF THE MEDICINAL PRODUCT

Actiq 200 micrograms compressed lozenge with integr oromucosal applicator.

Actiq 400 micrograms compressed lozenge with integr oromucosal applicator.

Actiq 600 micrograms compressed lozenge with integr oromucosal applicator.

Actiq 800 micrograms compressed lozenge with integr oromucosal applicator.

Actiq 1200 micrograms compressed lozenge with integr oromucosal applicator.

Actiq 1600 micrograms compressed lozenge with integr oromucosal applicator.

2. QUALITATIVE AND QUANTITATIVE COMPOSITION

One lozenge contains 200-400-600-800-1200-1600 micrograms fentanyl (as citrate).

Excipient(s):

Each lozenge contains dextrates (equivalent to approximately 2 grams of glucose), sucrose (approximately 30 milligrams confectioner's sugar) and propylene glycol (par of the artificial berry flavour and imprinting ink) as excipients.

For a full list of excipients, see section 6.1.

3. PHARMACEUTICAL FORM

Compressed lozenge with integral oromucosal applicator

Actiq is formulated as a white to off-white compressed powder drug matrix attached using edible glue to a fracture resistant radio opaque plastic applicator, marked with the dosage strength.

4. CLINICAL PARTICULARS

4.1 Therapeutic indications

Actiq is indicated for the management of breakthrough pain in patients already receiving maintenance opioid therapy for chronic cancer pain. Breakthrough pain is a transitory exacerbation of pain that occurs on a background of otherwise controlled persistent pain.

4.2 Posology and method of administration

In order to minimise the risks of opioid-related side-effects and to identify the "successful" dose, it is imperative that patients be monitored closely by health professionals during the titration process. Any unused Actiq units that the patient no longer requires must be disposed of properly. Patients must be reminded of the requirements to keep Actiq stored in a location away from children.

Method of administration

Actiq is intended for oromucosal administration, and therefore should be placed in the mouth against the cheek and should be moved around the mouth using the applicator, with the aim of maximising the amount of mucosal exposure to the product. The Actiq unit should be sucked, not chewed, as absorption of fentanyl via the buccal mucosa is rapid in comparison with systemic absorption via the gastrointestinal tract. Water may be used to moisten the buccal mucosa in patients with a dry mouth.

The Actiq unit should be consumed over a 15 minute period. If signs of excessive opioid effects appear before the Actiq unit is fully consumed it should be immediately removed, and consideration given to decreasing future dosages.

Dose titration and maintenance therapy

Actiq should be individually titrated to a "successful" dose that provides adequate analgesia and minimises side effects. In clinical trials the successful dose of Actiq for breakthrough pain was not predicted from the daily maintenance dose of opioid.

a) Titration

Before patients are titrated with Actiq, it is expected that their background persistent pain will be controlled by use of opioid therapy and that they are typically experiencing no more than 4 episodes of breakthrough pain per day.

The initial dose of Actiq used should be 200 micrograms, titrating upwards as necessary through the range of available dosage strengths (200, 400, 600, 800, 1200 and 1600 micrograms). Patients should be carefully monitored until a dose is reached that provides adequate analgesia with acceptable side effects using a single dosage unit per episode of breakthrough pain. This is defined as the successful dose.

During titration, if adequate analgesia is not obtained within 15 minutes after the patient completes consumption of a single Actiq unit, a second Actiq unit of the same strength may be consumed. No more than two Actiq units should be used to treat any individual pain episode. At 1600 micrograms, a second dose is only likely to be required by a minority of patients.

If treatment of consecutive breakthrough pain episodes requires more than one dosage unit per episode, an increase in dose to the next higher available strength should be considered.

Actiq® Titration Process

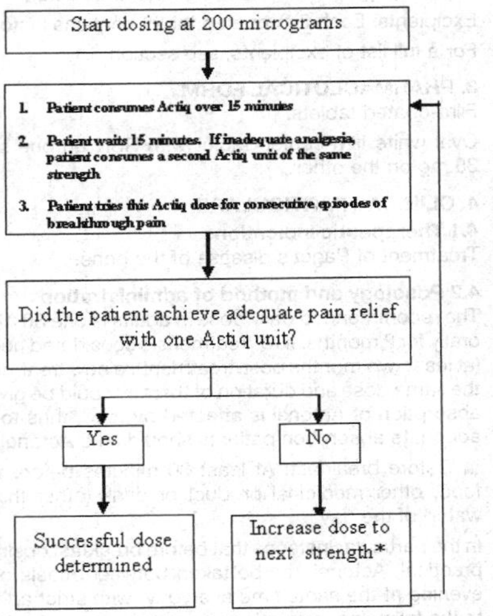
Start dosing at 200 micrograms
1. Patient consumes Actiq over 15 minutes
2. Patient waits 15 minutes. If inadequate analgesia, patient consumes a second Actiq unit of the same strength
3. Patient tries this Actiq dose for consecutive episodes of breakthrough pain
Did the patient achieve adequate pain relief with one Actiq unit?
Yes
No
Successful dose determined
Increase dose to next strength*

*Available dosage strengths include: 200, 400, 600, 800, 1200 and 1600 micrograms

laintenance

nce a successful dose has been established (i.e., on verage, an episode is effectively treated with a single nit), patients should be maintained on this dose and hould limit consumption to a maximum of four Actiq units er day.

atients should be monitored by a health professional to nsure that the maximum consumption of four units of ctiq per day is not exceeded.

Dose re-adjustment

more than four episodes of breakthrough pain are experienced per day, over a period of more than four consecutive days the dose of the long acting opioid used for persistent pain should be re-evaluated. If the dose of the long acting opioid is increased, the dose of Actiq to treat breakthrough pain may need to be reviewed.

t is imperative that any dose re-titration of any analgesic is monitored by a health professional.

Discontinuation of therapy

Actiq therapy may usually be immediately discontinued if no longer required for breakthrough pain only, in patients who continue to take their chronic opioid therapy for persistent pain.

For patients requiring discontinuation of all opioid therapy, account should be taken of the Actiq dose in consideration of a gradual downward opioid titration to avoid the possibility of abrupt withdrawal effects.

Use in children

The appropriate posology and safety of Actiq have not been established in children and adolescents.

Use in the elderly

Elderly patients have been shown to be more sensitive to the effects of fentanyl when administered intravenously. Therefore dose titration needs to be approached with particular care. In the elderly, elimination of fentanyl is slower and the terminal elimination half-life is longer, which may result in accumulation of the active substance and to a greater risk of undesirable effects.

Formal clinical trials with Actiq have not been conducted in the elderly. It has been observed, however, in clinical trials that patients over 65 years of age required lower doses of Actiq for successful relief of breakthrough pain.

Use in special patient populations

Special care should be taken during the titration process in patients with kidney or liver dysfunction.

4.3 Contraindications

Hypersensitivity to fentanyl or to any of the excipients.

Simultaneous use of monoamine-oxidase (MAO) inhibitors, or within 2 weeks after the cessation of the use of MAO inhibitors.

Severe respiratory depression or severe obstructive lung conditions.

4.4 Special warnings and precautions for use

It is important that the long acting opioid treatment used to treat the patient's persistent pain has been stabilised before Actiq therapy begins.

Tolerance and physical and/or psychological dependence may develop upon repeated administration of opioids such as fentanyl. However, iatrogenic addiction following therapeutic use of opioids is rare.

As with all opioids, there is a risk of clinically significant respiratory depression associated with the use of Actiq. Particular caution should be used when titrating Actiq in patients with non-severe chronic obstructive pulmonary disease or other medical conditions predisposing them to respiratory depression, as even normally therapeutic doses of Actiq may further decrease respiratory drive to the point of respiratory failure.

The product should not be given to opioid-naïve patients as there is an increased risk of respiratory depression and the appropriate dose in this patient population has not yet been determined.

Actiq should only be administered with extreme caution in patients who may be particularly susceptible to the intracranial effects of CO2 retention, such as those with evidence of increased intracranial pressure, or impaired consciousness. Opioids may obscure the clinical course of a patient with a head injury and should be used only if clinically warranted.

Intravenous fentanyl may produce bradycardia. Therefore, Actiq should be used with caution in patients with bradyarrhythmias.

In addition, Actiq should be administered with caution to patients with liver or kidney dysfunction. The influence of liver and renal impairment on the pharmacokinetics of the medicinal product has not been evaluated, however, when administered intravenously the clearance of fentanyl has been shown to be altered in hepatic and renal disease due to alterations in metabolic clearance and plasma proteins. After administration of Actiq, impaired liver and renal function may both increase the bioavailability of swallowed fentanyl and decrease its systemic clearance, which could lead to increased and prolonged opioid effects. Therefore, special care should be taken during the titration process in patients with moderate or severe hepatic or renal disease.

Careful consideration should be given to patients with hypovolaemia and hypotension.

Diabetic patients should be advised that the medicine product contains dextrates (dextrates are composed of 93% dextrose monohydrate and 7% maltodextrin. The total glucose load per dosage unit is approximately 1.89 grams per dose).

Patients with rare hereditary problems of fructose intolerance, glucose-galactose malabsorption or sucrase-isomaltase insufficiency should not take this medicine.

Normal oral hygiene is recommended to avoid any potential harm to the teeth

An evaluation of each out-patient concerning possible accidental child exposures should be undertaken.

Lozenges must be kept out of reach and sight of children and non-patients at all times before and after use. For instructions on handling and disposal, see Section 6.6.

4.5 Interaction with other medicinal products and other forms of interaction

Fentanyl is etabolized by the CYP3A4 isoenzyme in the liver and intestinal mucosa. Potent inhibitors of CYP3A4 such as macrolide antibiotics (e.g. erythromycin), azole antifungals (e.g. ketoconazole, itraconazole, and fluconazole) and certain protease inhibitors (e.g. ritonavir), may increase the bioavailability of swallowed fentanyl and may also decrease its systemic clearance which may result in increased or prolonged opioid effects. Similar effects could be seen after concurrent ingestion of grapefruit juice, which is known to inhibit CYP3A4. Hence caution is advised if fentanyl is given concomitantly with CYP3A4 inhibitors.

The concomitant use of other CNS depressants, including other opioids, sedatives or hypnotics, general anaesthetics, phenothiazines, tranquillisers, skeletal muscle relaxants, sedating antihistamines and alcohol may produce additive depressant effects.

Withdrawal symptoms may be precipitated through the administration of drugs with opioid antagonist activity, e.g., naloxone, or mixed agonist/antagonist analgesics (e.g., pentazocine, butorphanol, buprenorphine, nalbuphine).

4.6 Pregnancy and lactation

There are no adequate data from the use of fentanyl in pregnant women. Studies in animals have shown reproductive toxicity (see Section 5.3). Opioid analgesic agents can cause neonatal respiratory depression. With long-term use during pregnancy, there is a risk of neonatal withdrawal symptoms. Actiq should not be used in pregnancy unless clearly necessary.

It is advised not to use fentanyl during delivery because fentanyl passes through the placenta and may cause respiratory depression in the fœtus. The placental transfer ratio is 0.44 (fœtal:maternal ratio 1.00:2.27).

Fentanyl passes into breast milk, therefore women should not breast-feed while taking Actiq because of the possibility of sedation and/or respiratory depression in their infants. Breast feeding should not be restarted until at least 24 hours after the last administration of fentanyl.

4.7 Effects on ability to drive and use machines

No studies of the effects on the ability to drive and use machines have been performed. However, opioid analgesics may impair the mental and/or physical ability required for the performance of potentially dangerous tasks (e.g., driving a car or operating machinery). Patients should be advised not to drive or operate machinery if they experience somnolence, dizziness, blurred or double vision while taking Actiq.

4.8 Undesirable effects

Typical opioid side effects are to be expected with Actiq. Frequently, these will cease or decrease in intensity with continued use of the product, as the patient is titrated to the most appropriate dose. However, the most serious adverse events are respiratory depression (potentially leading to apnoea or respiratory arrest), circulatory depression, hypotension and shock and all patients should be closely monitored for these.

Application site reactions, including gum bleeding and irritation, have been reported in post-marketing use.

Because the clinical trials of Actiq were designed to evaluate safety and efficacy in treating breakthrough pain, all patients were also taking concomitant opioids, such as sustained-release morphine or transdermal fentanyl, for their persistent pain. Thus it is not possible to definitively separate the effects of Actiq alone.

The adverse events considered to be at least possibly-related to treatment, from clinical trials were as follows (very common>10%, common>1 - 10%, uncommon>0.1 - 1%):

Metabolism and nutrition disorders

Uncommon: anorexia

Psychiatric disorders

Common: confusion, anxiety, hallucinations, abnormal thinking

Uncommon: abnormal dreams, depersonalisation, depression, emotional lability, euphoria

Nervous system disorders

Very common: somnolence, dizziness

Common: headache, myoclonus, taste perversion

Uncommon: paraesthesia (including hyperaesthesia/circumoral paraesthesia), abnormal gait/incoordination

Eye disorders

Uncommon: abnormal vision (blurred, double vision)

Vascular disorders

Common: vasodilatation

Respiratory, thoracic and mediastinal disorders

Uncommon: dyspnoea

Gastrointestinal disorders

Very common: nausea, constipation

Common: vomiting, dry mouth, abdominal pain, dyspepsia, mouth ulcers/stomatitis, tongue disorder (for example, burning sensation, ulcers)

Uncommon: flatulence, abdomen enlarged

Skin and subcutaneous tissue disorders

Common: pruritus, sweating

Uncommon: rash

Renal and urinary disorders

Uncommon: urinary retention

General disorders and administration site conditions

Common: asthenia

Uncommon: malaise

Injury, poisoning and procedural complications

Common: accidental injury (for example, falls)

4.9 Overdose

The symptoms of fentanyl overdosage are expected to be similar in nature to those of intravenous fentanyl and other opioids, and are an extension of its pharmacological actions, with the most serious significant effect being respiratory depression.

Immediate management of opioid overdose includes removal of the Actiq unit via the applicator, if still in the mouth, ensuring a patent airway, physical and verbal stimulation of the patient, assessment of the level of consciousness, ventilatory and circulatory status, and assisted ventilation (ventilatory support) if necessary.

For treatment of overdosage (accidental ingestion) in the opioid naïve person, intravenous access should be obtained, and naloxone or other opioid antagonists should be employed as clinically indicated. The duration of respiratory depression following overdose may be longer than the effects of the opioid antagonist's action (e.g., the half-life of naloxone ranges from 30 to 81 minutes) and repeated administration may be necessary. Consult the Summary of Product Characteristics of the individual opioid antagonist for details about such use.

For treatment of overdose in opioid-maintained patients, intravenous access should be obtained. The judicious use of naloxone or another opioid antagonist may be warranted in some instances, but it is associated with the risk of precipitating an acute withdrawal syndrome.

Although muscle rigidity interfering with respiration has not been seen following the use of Actiq, this is possible with fentanyl and other opioids. If it occurs, it should be managed by the use of assisted ventilation, by an opioid antagonist, and as a final alternative, by a neuromuscular blocking agent.

5. PHARMACOLOGICAL PROPERTIES

5.1 Pharmacodynamic properties

Pharmacotherapeutic group: Opioid analgesic, phenylpiperidone derivative. ATC code N02A BO3.

Fentanyl, a pure opioid agonist, acts primarily through interaction with mu-opioid receptors located in the brain, spinal cord and smooth muscle. The primary site of therapeutic action is the central nervous system (CNS). The most clinically useful pharmacological effect of the interaction of fentanyl with mu-opioid receptors is analgesia. The analgesic effects of fentanyl are related to the blood level of the active substance, if proper allowance is made for the delay into and out of the CNS (a process with a 3-5 minute half-life). In opioid-naïve individuals, analgesia occurs at blood levels of 1 to 2 ng/ml, while blood levels of 10-20 ng/ml would produce surgical anaesthesia and profound respiratory depression.

In patients with chronic cancer pain on stable doses of regularly scheduled opioids to control their persistent pain, Actiq produced significantly more breakthrough pain relief compared with placebo at 15, 30, 45, and 60 minutes following administration.

Secondary actions include increase in the tone and decrease in the contractions of the gastrointestinal smooth muscle, which results in prolongation of gastrointestinal transit time and may be responsible for the constipatory effect of opioids.

While opioids generally increase the tone of urinary tract smooth muscle, the overall effect tends to vary, in some cases producing urinary urgency, in others difficulty in urination.

All opioid mu-receptor agonists, including fentanyl, produce dose dependent respiratory depression. The risk of respiratory depression is less in patients with pain and those receiving chronic opioid therapy who develop tolerance to respiratory depression and other opioid effects. In non-tolerant subjects, typically peak respiratory effects are seen 15 to 30 minutes following the administration of Actiq, and may persist for several hours.

5.2 Pharmacokinetic properties

General introduction

Fentanyl is highly lipophilic and can be absorbed very rapidly through the oral mucosa and more slowly by the conventional gastrointestinal route. It is subject to first-pass hepatic and intestinal metabolism and the metabolites do not contribute to fentanyl's therapeutic effects.

Absorption

The absorption pharmacokinetics of fentanyl from Actiq are a combination of rapid oromucosal absorption and slower gastrointestinal absorption of swallowed fentanyl. Approximately 25% of the total dose of Actiq is rapidly absorbed from the buccal mucosa. The remaining 75% of the dose is swallowed and slowly absorbed from the gastrointestinal tract. About 1/3 of this amount (25% of the total dose) escapes hepatic and intestinal first-pass elimination and becomes systemically available. Absolute bioavailability is about 50% compared to intravenous fentanyl, divided equally between rapid oromucosal and slower gastrointestinal absorption. C_{max} ranges from 0.39 to 2.51 ng/ml after consumption of Actiq (200 micrograms to 1600 micrograms). T_{max} is around 20 to 40 minutes after consumption of an Actiq unit (range 20 – 480 minutes).

Distribution

Animal data show that fentanyl is rapidly distributed to the brain, heart, lungs, kidneys and spleen followed by a slower redistribution to muscles and fat. The plasma protein binding of fentanyl is 80-85%. The main binding protein is alpha-1- acid glycoprotein, but both albumin and lipoproteins contribute to some extent. The free fraction of fentanyl increases with acidosis. The mean volume of distribution at steady state (V_{ss}) is 4 l/kg.

Biotransformation

Fentanyl is metabolised in the liver and in the intestinal mucosa to norfentanyl by CYP3A4 isoform. Norfentanyl is not pharmacologically active in animal studies. More than 90% of the administered dose of fentanyl is eliminated by biotransformation to N-dealkylated and hydroxylated inactive metabolites.

Elimination

Less than 7% of the dose is excreted unchanged in the urine, and only about 1% is excreted unchanged in the faeces. The metabolites are mainly excreted in the urine, while faecal excretion is less important. The total plasma clearance of fentanyl is 0.5 l/hr/kg (range 0.3-0.7 l/hr/kg). The terminal elimination half-life after Actiq administration is about 7 hours.

Linearity/non-linearity

Dose proportionality across the available range of dosages (200 micrograms to 1600 micrograms) of Actiq has been demonstrated.

5.3 Preclinical safety data

Non-clinical data reveal no special hazard for humans based on conventional studies of safety pharmacology, repeated dose toxicity and genotoxicity.

Studies with female rats revealed reduced fertility and enhanced embryonal mortality. More recent studies showed that effects on the embryo were due to maternal toxicity and not to direct effects of the substance on the developing embryo. In a study on pre- and postnatal development the survival rate of offspring was significantly reduced at doses which slightly reduced maternal weight. This effect could either be due to altered maternal care or a direct effect of fentanyl on the pups. Effects on somatic development and behaviour of the offspring were not observed. Teratogenic effects have not been demonstrated.

Long term carcinogenicity studies have not been performed.

6. PHARMACEUTICAL PARTICULARS

6.1 List of excipients

Lozenge:

Dextrates hydrated (containing glucose)

Citric acid, anhydrous

Disodium phosphate, anhydrous

Artificial berry flavour (maltodextrin, propylene glycol, artificial flavours and triethylcitrate)

Magnesium stearate

Edible glue used to attach the lozenge to the handle:

Modified maize based food starch (E1450)

Confectioner's sugar (sucrose and maize starch)

Water, purified

Imprinting ink:

Ethanol

De-ionised water

De-waxed white shellac

Propylene glycol

Blue synthetic coal tar dye (E133)

6.2 Incompatibilities

Not applicable.

6.3 Shelf life

3 years

6.4 Special precautions for storage

Do not store above 30°C.

6.5 Nature and contents of container

Each Actiq dosage unit is contained in a heat sealed blister package consisting of a paper/foil laminated lid, and a PVC/Aclar thermoformed blister, supplied in cartons of 3, 6, 15 or 30 individual units.

Not all pack sizes may be marketed.

6.6 Special precautions for disposal and other handling

Patients and their carers must be instructed that Actiq contains an active substance in an amount that can be fatal to a child. Patients and their carers must be instructed to keep all units out of the reach and sight of children and to discard open units appropriately.

Lozenges with residual active substance should at no time be discarded or misplaced. Any used or unused but no longer required product or waste material should be disposed of in accordance with local requirements.

7. MARKETING AUTHORISATION HOLDER

Cephalon UK Limited
1 Albany Place
Hyde Way
Welwyn Garden City
Hertdforshire
AL7 3BT
UK

8. MARKETING AUTHORISATION NUMBER(S)

Actiq 200 microgram compressed logenze with integral oromucosal applicator

PL 16260/003

Actiq 400 microgram compressed logenze with integral oromucosal applicator

PL 16260/004

Actiq 600 microgram compressed logenze with integral oromucosal applicator

PL 16260/005

Actiq 800 microgram compressed logenze with integral oromucosal applicator

PL 16260/006

Actiq 1200 microgram compressed logenze with integral oromucosal applicator

PL 16260/007

Actiq 1600 microgram compressed logenze with integral oromucosal applicator

PL 16260/008

9. DATE OF FIRST AUTHORISATION/RENEWAL OF THE AUTHORISATION

Date of first authorization: 10 August 2002

Date of renewal: 08 October 2005

10. DATE OF REVISION OF THE TEXT

July 2009

Actonel 30mg Film Coated Tablets

(Procter & Gamble Pharmaceuticals UK Limited)

1. NAME OF THE MEDICINAL PRODUCT

Actonel 30 mg film-coated tablets.

2. QUALITATIVE AND QUANTITATIVE COMPOSITIO

Each film-coated tablet contains 30 mg risedrona sodium (equivalent to 27.8 mg risedronic acid).

Excipients: Each film-coated tablet contains lactose.

For a full list of excipients, see section 6.1.

3. PHARMACEUTICAL FORM

Film-coated tablets.

Oval white film-coated tablet with RSN on one side a 30 mg on the other.

4. CLINICAL PARTICULARS

4.1 Therapeutic indications

Treatment of Paget's disease of the bone.

4.2 Posology and method of administration

The recommended daily dose in adults is one 30 mg tab orally for 2 months. If re-treatment is considered necessa (at least two months post-treatment), a new treatment wi the same dose and duration of therapy could be given. T absorption of Actonel is affected by food, thus to ensu adequate absorption patients should take Actonel:

■ Before breakfast: At least 30 minutes before the fi food, other medicinal product or drink (other than pla water) of the day.

In the particular instance that before breakfast dosing is n practical, Actonel can be taken between meals or in t evening at the same time everyday, with strict adheren to the following instructions, to ensure Actonel is taken an empty stomach:

■ Between meals: Actonel should be taken at least 2 hou before and at least 2 hours after any food, medici product or drink (other than plain water).

■ In the evening: Actonel should be taken at least 2 hou after the last food, medicinal product or drink (other th plain water) of the day. Actonel should be taken at least minutes before going to bed.

If an occasional dose is missed, Actonel can be tak before breakfast, between meals, or in the evening accor ing to the instructions above.

The tablet must be swallowed whole and not sucked chewed. To aid delivery of the tablet to the stoma Actonel is to be taken while in an upright position with glass of plain water (≥120 ml). Patients should not lie do for 30 minutes after taking the tablet (see section 4.4).

Physicians should consider the administration of supp mental calcium and vitamin D if dietary intake is inac quate, especially as bone turnover is significantly elevat in Paget's disease.

Elderly: No dosage adjustment is necessary since bioava ability, distribution and elimination were similar in elde (>60 years of age) compared to younger subjects.

Renal Impairment: No dosage adjustment is required those patients with mild to moderate renal impairment. T use of risedronate sodium is contraindicated in patie with severe renal impairment (creatinine clearance lov than 30 ml/min) (see sections 4.3 and 5.2).

Children: Safety and efficacy of Actonel have not be established in children and adolescents.

4.3 Contraindications

Hypersensitivity to risedronate sodium or to any of excipients.

Hypocalcaemia (see section 4.4).

Pregnancy and lactation.

Severe renal impairment (creatinine clearance <30 min).

4.4 Special warnings and precautions for use

Foods, drinks (other than plain water) and medicinal p ducts containing polyvalent cations (such as calcium, ma nesium, iron and aluminium) interfere with the absorpti of bisphosphonates and should not be taken at the sa time as Actonel (see section 4.5). In order to achieve intended efficacy, strict adherence to dosing recomme dations is necessary (see section 4.2).

Bisphosphonates have been associated with oesophagi gastritis, oesophageal ulcerations and gastroduode ulcerations. Thus, caution should be used:

• In patients who have a history of oesophageal disord which delay oesophageal transit or emptying e.g. strict or achalasia.

• In patients who are unable to stay in the upright posit for at least 30 minutes after taking the tablet.

• If risedronate is given to patients with active or rec oesophageal or upper gastrointestinal problems.

Prescribers should emphasise to patients the importar of paying attention to the dosing instructions and be aler any signs or symptoms of possible oesophageal reactic The patients should be instructed to seek timely medi attention if they develop symptoms of oesophageal irri tion such as dysphagia, pain on swallowing, retrosterı pain or new/worsened heartburn.

Hypocalcaemia should be treated before starting Acto therapy. Other disturbances of bone and mineral metab lism (e.g. parathyroid dysfunction, hypovitaminosis should be treated at the time of starting Actonel therap

Osteonecrosis of the jaw, generally associated with too extraction and/or local infection (including osteomyeli has been reported in patients with cancer receiv eatment regimens including primarily intravenously administered bisphosphonates. Many of these patients were so receiving chemotherapy and corticosteroids. Osteonecrosis of the jaw has also been reported in patients with steoporosis receiving oral bisphosphonates.

dental examination with appropriate preventive dentistry hould be considered prior to treatment with bisphosphoates in patients with concomitant risk factors (e.g. cancer, hemotherapy, radiotherapy, corticosteroids, poor oral ygiene).

Vhile on treatment, these patients should avoid invasive ental procedures if possible. For patients who develop steonecrosis of the jaw while on bisphosphonate therapy, ental surgery may exacerbate the condition. For patients equiring dental procedures, there are no data available to uggest whether discontinuation of bisphosphonate treatment reduces the risk of osteonecrosis of the jaw.

Clinical judgment of the treating physician should guide the nanagement plan of each patient based on individual enefit/risk assessment.

This medicine contains lactose. Patients with rare hereditary problems of galactose intolerance, the Lapp lactase deficiency or glucose-galactose malabsorption should not ake this medicine.

4.5 Interaction with other medicinal products and other forms of interaction

No formal interaction studies have been performed, however no clinically relevant interactions with other medicinal products were found during clinical trials.

Concomitant ingestion of medications containing polyvalent cations (e.g. calcium, magnesium, iron and aluminium) will interfere with the absorption of risedronate sodium (see section 4.4).

Risedronate sodium is not systemically metabolised, does not induce cytochrome P450 enzymes, and has low protein binding.

4.6 Pregnancy and lactation

There are no adequate data from the use of risedronate sodium in pregnant women. Studies in animals have shown reproductive toxicity (see section 5.3). The potential risk for humans is unknown. Studies in animal indicate that a small amount of risedronate sodium pass into breast milk.

Risedronate sodium must not be used during pregnancy or by breast-feeding women.

4.7 Effects on ability to drive and use machines

No effects on ability to drive and use machines have been observed.

4.8 Undesirable effects

Risedronate sodium has been studied in phase III clinical trials involving more than 15,000 patients. The majority of undesirable effects observed in clinical trials were mild to moderate in severity and usually did not require cessation of therapy.

Adverse experiences reported in phase III clinical trials in postmenopausal women with osteoporosis treated for up to 36 months with risedronate 5mg/day (n=5020) or placebo (n=5048) and considered possibly or probably related to risedronate are listed below using the following convention (incidences versus placebo are shown in brackets): very common ($\geq$1/10); common ($\geq$1/100; $<$1/10); uncommon ($\geq$1/1,000; $<$1/100); rare ($\geq$1/10,000; $<$1/1,000); very rare ($<$1/10,000).

Nervous system disorders:

Common: headache (1.8% vs. 1.4%)

Eye disorders:

Uncommon: iritis*

Gastrointestinal disorders:

Common: constipation (5.0% vs. 4.8%), dyspepsia (4.5% vs. 4.1%), nausea (4.3% vs. 4.0%), abdominal pain (3.5% vs. 3.3%), diarrhoea (3.0% vs. 2.7%)

Uncommon: gastritis (0.9% vs. 0.7%), oesophagitis (0.9% vs. 0.9%), dysphagia (0.4% vs. 0.2%), duodenitis (0.2% vs. 0.1%), oesophageal ulcer (0.2% vs. 0.2%)

Rare: glossitis ($<$0.1% vs. 0.1%), oesophageal stricture ($<$0.1% vs. 0.0%),

Musculoskeletal and connective tissues disorders:

Common: musculoskeletal pain (2.1% vs. 1.9%)

Investigations:

Rare: abnormal liver function tests*

* No relevant incidences from Phase III osteoporosis studies; frequency based on adverse event/laboratory/rechallenge findings in earlier clinical trials.

In a phase III Paget's Disease clinical trial comparing risedronate vs. etidronate (61 patients in each group), the following additional adverse experiences considered possibly or probably drug related by investigators have been reported (incidence greater in risedronate than in etidronate): arthralgia (9.8% vs. 8.2%); amblyopia, apnoea, bronchitis, colitis, corneal lesion, cramps leg, dizziness, dry eye, flu syndrome, hypocalcaemia, myasthenia, neoplasm, nocturia, oedema peripheral, pain bone, pain chest, rash, sinusitis, tinnitus, and weight decrease (all at 1.6% vs. 0.0%).

Laboratory findings: Early, transient, asymptomatic and mild decreases in serum calcium and phosphate levels have been observed in some patients.

The following additional adverse reactions have been reported during post-marketing use (frequency unknown):

Eye disorders:

iritis, uveitis

Muskuloskeletal and connective tissues disorders:

osteonecrosis of the jaw

Skin and subcutaneous tissue disorders:

hypersensitivity and skin reactions, including angioedema, generalised rash, urticaria and bullous skin reactions, some severe including isolated reports of Stevens-Johnson syndrome and toxic epidermal necrolysis.

hair loss.

Immune system disorders:

anaphylactic reaction

Hepatobiliary disorders:

serious hepatic disorders. In most of the reported cases the patients were also treated with other products known to cause hepatic disorders.

4.9 Overdose

No specific information is available on the treatment of overdose with risedronate sodium.

Decreases in serum calcium following substantial overdose may be expected. Signs and symptoms of hypocalcaemia may also occur in some of these patients.

Milk or antacids containing magnesium, calcium or aluminium should be given to bind risedronate and reduce absorption of risedronate sodium. In cases of substantial overdose, gastric lavage may be considered to remove unabsorbed risedronate sodium.

5. PHARMACOLOGICAL PROPERTIES

5.1 Pharmacodynamic properties

Pharmaco-therapeutic group: Bisphosphonates

ATC Code: M05 BA07

Risedronate sodium is a pyridinyl bisphosphonate that binds to bone hydroxyapatite and inhibits osteoclast-mediated bone resorption. The bone turnover is reduced while the osteoblast activity and bone mineralisation is preserved.

Paget's disease of the bone: In the clinical programme Actonel was studied in patients with Paget's disease. After treatment with Actonel 30 mg/day for 2 months the following was seen:

- serum alkaline phosphatase normalised in 77% of patients compared to 11% in the control group (etidronate 400 mg/day for 6 months). Significant reductions were observed in urinary hydroxyproline/creatinine and urinary deoxypyridinoline/creatinine
- radiographs taken at baseline and after 6 months demonstrated a decrease in the extent of osteolytic lesions in both the appendicular and axial skeleton. No new fractures were observed.

The observed response was similar in pagetic patients regardless of whether they had previously received other treatments for Paget's disease, or the severity of the disease.

53% of patients followed for 18 months after initiation of a single 2 month course of Actonel remained in biochemical remission.

In a trial comparing before-breakfast dosing and dosing at other times of the day in women with postmenopausal osteoporosis, lumbar spine BMD gains were statistically higher with before-breakfast dosing.

5.2 Pharmacokinetic properties

Absorption: Absorption after an oral dose is relatively rapid (t_{max} ~1 hour) and is independent of dose over the range studied (2.5 to 30 mg). Mean oral bioavailability of the tablet is 0.63% and is decreased when risedronate sodium is administered with food. Bioavailability was similar in men and women.

Distribution: The mean steady state volume of distribution is 6.3 l/kg in humans. Plasma protein binding is about 24%.

Metabolism: There is no evidence of systemic metabolism of risedronate sodium.

Elimination: Approximately half of the absorbed dose is excreted in urine within 24 hours, and 85% of an intravenous dose is recovered in the urine after 28 days. Mean renal clearance is 105 ml/min and mean total clearance is 122 ml/min, with the difference probably attributed to clearance due to adsorption to bone. The renal clearance is not concentration dependent, and there is a linear relationship between renal clearance and creatinine clearance. Unabsorbed risedronate sodium is eliminated unchanged in faeces. After oral administration the concentration-time profile shows three elimination phases with a terminal half-life of 480 hours.

Special Populations:

Elderly: no dosage adjustment is necessary.

5.3 Preclinical safety data

In toxicological studies in rat and dog dose dependent liver toxic effects of risedronate sodium were seen, primarily as enzyme increases with histological changes in rat. The clinical relevance of these observations is unknown. Testicular toxicity occurred in rat and dog at exposures considered in excess of the human therapeutic exposure. Dose related incidences of upper airway irritation were frequently noted in rodents. Similar effects have been seen with other bisphosphonates. Lower respiratory tract effects were also seen in longer term studies in rodents, although the clinical significance of these findings is unclear. In reproduction toxicity studies at exposures close to clinical exposure ossification changes were seen in sternum and/or skull of foetuses from treated rats and hypocalcemia and mortality in pregnant females allowed to deliver. There was no evidence of teratogenesis at 3.2mg/kg/day in rat and 10mg/kg/day in rabbit, although data are only available on a small number of rabbits. Maternal toxicity prevented testing of higher doses. Studies on genotoxicity and carcinogenesis did not show any particular risks for humans.

6. PHARMACEUTICAL PARTICULARS

6.1 List of excipients

Tablet core: Lactose monohydrate
Cellulose microcrystalline
Crospovidone
Magnesium stearate.

Film coating: Hypromellose
Macrogol
Hyprolose
Silicon dioxide
Titanium dioxide E171.

6.2 Incompatibilities

Not applicable.

6.3 Shelf life

5 years.

6.4 Special precautions for storage

This medicinal product does not require any special storage conditions.

6.5 Nature and contents of container

Opaque PVC/aluminium foil blister cards of 14 tablets in cardboard carton, tablet count 28 (2 × 14) and tablet count 14 (1 × 14).

Sample pack - Opaque PVC/aluminium foil blister cards of 3 tablets in cardboard carton, tablet count 3 (1 × 3).

Not all pack sizes may be marketed.

6.6 Special precautions for disposal and other handling

No special requirements.

7. MARKETING AUTHORISATION HOLDER

Procter & Gamble Pharmaceuticals UK Ltd.,
Rusham Park,
Whitehall Lane,
Egham,
Surrey,
TW20 9NW, UK

8. MARKETING AUTHORISATION NUMBER(S)

PL 00364/0071

9. DATE OF FIRST AUTHORISATION/RENEWAL OF THE AUTHORISATION

1999-10-07/2004-10-07

10. DATE OF REVISION OF THE TEXT

2008-09-19

Actonel 5mg Film Coated Tablets

(Procter & Gamble Pharmaceuticals UK Limited)

1. NAME OF THE MEDICINAL PRODUCT

Actonel 5 mg film-coated tablets.

2. QUALITATIVE AND QUANTITATIVE COMPOSITION

Each film-coated tablet contains 5 mg risedronate sodium (equivalent to 4.64 mg risedronic acid).

Excipients: Each film-coated tablet contains lactose.

For a full list of excipients, see section 6.1.

3. PHARMACEUTICAL FORM

Film-coated tablet.

Oval yellow film-coated tablet with RSN on one side and 5 mg on the other.

4. CLINICAL PARTICULARS

4.1 Therapeutic indications

Treatment of postmenopausal osteoporosis, to reduce the risk of vertebral fractures. Treatment of established postmenopausal osteoporosis, to reduce the risk of hip fractures. Prevention of osteoporosis in postmenopausal women with increased risk of osteoporosis (see section 5.1).

To maintain or increase bone mass in postmenopausal women undergoing long-term (more than 3 months), systemic corticosteroid treatment at doses $\geq$ 7.5mg/day prednisone or equivalent.

4.2 Posology and method of administration

The recommended daily dose in adults is one 5 mg tablet orally. The absorption of Actonel is affected by food, thus to ensure adequate absorption patients should take Actonel:

• Before breakfast: At least 30 minutes before the first food, other medicinal product or drink (other than plain water) of the day.

In the particular instance that before breakfast dosing is not practical, Actonel can be taken between meals or in the evening at the same time everyday, with strict adherence to the following instructions, to ensure Actonel is taken on an empty stomach:

• Between meals: Actonel should be taken at least 2 hours before and at least 2 hours after any food, medicinal product or drink (other than plain water).

• In the evening: Actonel should be taken at least 2 hours after the last food, medicinal product or drink (other than plain water) of the day. Actonel should be taken at least 30 minutes before going to bed.

If an occasional dose is missed, Actonel can be taken before breakfast, between meals, or in the evening according to the instructions above.

The tablets must be swallowed whole and not sucked or chewed. To aid delivery of the tablet to the stomach Actonel is to be taken while in an upright position with a glass of plain water (≥120 ml). Patients should not lie down for 30 minutes after taking the tablet (see section 4.4).

Supplemental calcium and vitamin D should be considered if the dietary intake is inadequate.

Elderly: No dosage adjustment is necessary since bioavailability, distribution and elimination were similar in elderly (>60 years of age) compared to younger subjects.

Renal Impairment: No dosage adjustment is required for those patients with mild to moderate renal impairment. The use of risedronate sodium is contraindicated in patients with severe renal impairment (creatinine clearance lower than 30 ml/min) (see sections 4.3 and 5.2).

Children: Safety and efficacy of Actonel have not been established in children and adolescents.

4.3 Contraindications

Hypersensitivity to risedronate sodium or to any of the excipients.

Hypocalcaemia (see section 4.4).

Pregnancy and lactation.

Severe renal impairment (creatinine clearance <30ml/min).

4.4 Special warnings and precautions for use

Foods, drinks (other than plain water) and medicinal products containing polyvalent cations (such as calcium, magnesium, iron and aluminium) interfere with the absorption of bisphosphonates and should not be taken at the same time as Actonel (see section 4.5) In order to achieve the intended efficacy, strict adherence to dosing recommendations is necessary (see section 4.2)

Efficacy of bisphosphonates in the treatment of postmenopausal osteoporosis is related to the presence of low bone mineral density (BMD T-score at hip or lumbar spine ≤-2.5 SD) and/or prevalent fracture.

High age or clinical risk factors for fracture alone are not reasons to initiate treatment of osteoporosis with a bisphosphonate.

The evidence to support efficacy of bisphosphonates including Actonel in very elderly women (>80 years) is limited (see section 5.1).

Bisphosphonates have been associated with oesophagitis, gastritis, oesophageal ulcerations and gastroduodenal ulcerations. Thus caution should be used:

• In patients who have a history of oesophageal disorders which delay oesophageal transit or emptying e.g. stricture or achalasia.

• In patients who are unable to stay in the upright position for at least 30 minutes after taking the tablet.

• If risedronate is given to patients with active or recent oesophageal or upper gastrointestinal problems.

Prescribers should emphasise to patients the importance of paying attention to the dosing instructions and be alert to any signs or symptoms of possible oesophageal reaction. The patients should be instructed to seek timely medical attention if they develop symptoms of oesophageal irritation such as dysphagia, pain on swallowing, retrosternal pain or new/worsened heartburn.

Hypocalcaemia should be treated before starting Actonel therapy. Other disturbances of bone and mineral metabolism (e.g. parathyroid dysfunction, hypovitaminosis D) should be treated at the time of starting Actonel therapy.

Osteonecrosis of the jaw, generally associated with tooth extraction and/or local infection (including osteomyelitis) has been reported in patients with cancer receiving treatment regimens including primarily intravenously administered bisphophonates. Many of these patients were also receiving chemotherapy and corticosteroids. Osteonecrosis of the jaw has also been reported in patients with osteoporosis receiving oral bisphosphonates.

A dental examination with appropriate preventive dentistry should be considered prior to treatment with bisphosphonates in patients with concomitant risk factors (e.g. cancer, chemotherapy, radiotherapy, corticosteroids, poor oral hygiene).

While on treatment, these patients should avoid invasive dental procedures if possible. For patients who develop osteonecrosis of the jaw while on bisphosphonate therapy, dental surgery may exacerbate the condition. For patients requiring dental procedures, there are no data available to suggest whether discontinuation of bisphosphonate treatment reduces the risk of osteonecrosis of the jaw.

Clinical judgment of the treating physician should guide the management plan of each patient based on individual benefit /risk assessment.

This medicine contains lactose. Patients with rare hereditary problems of galactose intolerance, the Lapp lactase deficiency or glucose-galactose malabsorption should not take this medicine.

4.5 Interaction with other medicinal products and other forms of interaction

No formal interaction studies have been performed, however no clinically relevant interactions with other medicinal products were found during clinical trials.

In the risedronate sodium Phase III osteoporosis studies, acetyl salicylic acid or NSAID use was reported by 33% and 45% of patients respectively.

If considered appropriate risedronate sodium may be used concomitantly with oestrogen supplementation.

Concomitant ingestion of medications containing polyvalent cations (e.g. calcium, magnesium, iron and aluminium) will interfere with the absorption of risedronate sodium (see section 4.4).

Risedronate sodium is not systemically metabolised, does not induce cytochrome P450 enzymes, and has low protein binding.

4.6 Pregnancy and lactation

There are no adequate data from the use of risedronate sodium in pregnant women. Studies in animals have shown reproductive toxicity (see section 5.3). The potential risk for humans is unknown. Studies in animal indicate that a small amount of risedronate sodium pass into breast milk.

Risedronate sodium must not be used during pregnancy or by breast-feeding women.

4.7 Effects on ability to drive and use machines

No effects on ability to drive and use machines have been observed.

4.8 Undesirable effects

Risedronate sodium has been studied in phase III clinical trials involving more than 15,000 patients. The majority of undesirable effects observed in clinical trials were mild to moderate in severity and usually did not require cessation of therapy.

Adverse experiences reported in phase III clinical trials in postmenopausal women with osteoporosis treated for up to 36 months with risedronate 5mg/day (n=5020) or placebo (n=5048) and considered possibly or probably related to risedronate are listed below using the following convention (incidences versus placebo are shown in brackets): very common (≥1/10); common (≥1/100; <1/10); uncommon (≥1/1,000; <1/100); rare (≥1/10,000; <1/1,000); very rare (<1/10,000).

Nervous system disorders:

Common: headache (1.8% vs. 1.4%)

Eye disorders:

Uncommon: iritis*

Gastrointestinal disorders:

Common: constipation (5.0% vs. 4.8%), dyspepsia (4.5% vs. 4.1%), nausea (4.3% vs. 4.0%), abdominal pain (3.5% vs. 3.3%), diarrhoea (3.0% vs. 2.7%)

Uncommon: gastritis (0.9% vs. 0.7%), oesophagitis (0.9% vs. 0.9%), dysphagia (0.4% vs. 0.2%), duodenitis (0.2% vs. 0.1%), oesophageal ulcer (0.2% vs. 0.2%)

Rare: glossitis (<0.1% vs. 0.1%), oesophageal stricture (<0.1% vs. 0.0%),

Musculoskeletal and connective tissues disorders:

Common: musculoskeletal pain (2.1% vs. 1.9%)

Investigations:

Rare: abnormal liver function tests*

* No relevant incidences from Phase III osteoporosis studies; frequency based on adverse event/laboratory/rechallenge findings in earlier clinical trials.

Laboratory findings: Early, transient, asymptomatic and mild decreases in serum calcium and phosphate levels have been observed in some patients.

The following additional adverse reactions have been reported during post-marketing use (frequency unknown):

Eye disorders:

iritis, uveitis

Muskuloskeletal and connective tissues disorders:

osteonecrosis of the jaw

Skin and subcutaneous tissue disorders:

hypersensitivity and skin reactions, including angioedema, generalised rash, urticaria and bullous skin reactions, some severe including isolated reports of Stevens-Johnson syndrome and toxic epidermal necrolysis.

hair loss.

Immune system disorders:

anaphylactic reaction

Hepatobiliary disorders:

serious hepatic disorders. In most of the reported case the patients were also treated with other products know to cause hepatic disorders.

4.9 Overdose

No specific information is available on the treatment overdose with risedronate sodium.

Decreases in serum calcium following substantial ove dose may be expected. Signs and symptoms of hypoca caemia may also occur in some of these patients.

Milk or antacids containing magnesium, calcium or alum nium should be given to bind risedronate and reduc absorption of risedronate sodium. In cases of substant overdose, gastric lavage may be considered to remo unabsorbed risedronate sodium.

5. PHARMACOLOGICAL PROPERTIES

5.1 Pharmacodynamic properties

Pharmaco-therapeutic group: Bisphosphonates

ATC Code: M05 BA07

Risedronate sodium is a pyridinyl bisphosphonate th binds to bone hydroxyapatite and inhibits osteoclas mediated bone resorption. The bone turnover is reduc while the osteoblast activity and bone mineralisation preserved. In preclinical studies risedronate sodiu demonstrated potent anti-osteoclast and antiresorpti activity, and dose dependently increased bone mass a biomechanical skeletal strength. The activity of risedrona sodium was confirmed by measuring biochemical marke for bone turnover during pharmacodynamic and clinic studies. Decreases in biochemical markers of bone tur over were observed within 1 month and reached a ma imum in 3-6 months.

Treatment and Prevention of Postmenopausal Oste porosis:

A number of risk factors are associated with postmen pausal osteoporosis including low bone mass, low bo mineral density, early menopause, a history of smoking a a family history of osteoporosis. The clinical consequen of osteoporosis is fractures. The risk of fractures increased with the number of risk factors.

The clinical programme studied the effect of risedrona sodium on the risk of hip and vertebral fractures a contained early and late postmenopausal women w and without fracture. Daily doses of 2.5 mg and 5 mg we studied and all groups, including the control grou received calcium and vitamin D (if baseline levels we low). The absolute and relative risk of new vertebral a hip fractures were estimated by use of a time-to-first eve analysis.

■ Two placebo-controlled trials (n=3,661) enrolled po menopausal women under 85 years with vertebral fra tures at baseline. Risedronate sodium 5 mg daily given 3 years reduced the risk of new vertebral fractures relat to the control group. In women with respectively at leas or at least 1 vertebral fractures, the relative risk reducti was 49% and 41% respectively (incidence of new verteb fractures with risedronate sodium 18.1% and 11.3%, w placebo 29.0% and 16.3%, respectively). The effect treatment was seen as early as the end of the first ye of treatment. Benefits were also demonstrated in wom with multiple fractures at baseline. Risedronate sodi 5 mg daily also reduced the yearly height loss compar to the control group.

■ Two further placebo controlled trials enrolled postm nopausal women above 70 years with or without verteb fractures at baseline. Women 70-79 years were enroll with femoral neck BMD T-score <-3 SD (manufacture range, i.e. -2.5 SD using NHANES III) and at least o additional risk factor. Women ≥80 years could be enroll on the basis of at least one non-skeletal risk factor for fracture or low bone mineral density at the femoral ne Statistical significance of the efficacy of risedrona sodium versus placebo is only reached when the t treatment groups 2.5 mg and 5 mg are pooled. The follo ing results are only based on *a-posteriori* analysis of su groups defined by clinical practice and current definiti of osteoporosis:

- In the subgroup of patients with femoral neck BMD score ≤-2.5SD (NHANES III) and at least one verteb fracture at baseline, risedronate sodium given for 3 yea reduced the risk of hip fractures by 46% relative to t control group (incidence of hip fractures in combined ris dronate sodium 2.5 and 5 mg groups 3.8%, placebo 7.4

- Data suggest that a more limited protection than this m be observed in the very elderly (≥80 years). This may due to the increasing importance of non-skeletal factors hip fracture with increasing age.

In these trials, data analysed as a secondary endpo indicated a decrease in the risk of new vertebral fractur in patients with low femoral neck BMD without verteb fracture and in patients with low femoral neck BMD with without vertebral fracture.

Risedronate sodium 5 mg daily given for 3 years increas bone mineral density (BMD) relative to control at the lum spine, femoral neck, trochanter and wrist and prevent bone loss at the mid-shaft radius.

In a one-year follow-up off therapy after three years eatment with risedronate sodium 5 mg daily there was oid reversibility of the suppressing effect of risedronate dium on bone turnover rate.

n postmenopausal women taking oestrogen, risedronate odium 5 mg daily increased bone mineral density (BMD) at e femoral neck and mid-shaft radius only, compared to estrogen alone.

Bone biopsy samples from postmenopausal women eated with risedronate sodium 5 mg daily for 2 to 3 years, nowed an expected moderate decrease in bone turnover. one formed during risedronate sodium treatment was of ormal lamellar structure and bone mineralisation. These ata together with the decreased incidence of osteoporo-s related fractures at vertebral sites in women with osteo-orosis appear to indicate no detrimental effect on bone uality.

Endoscopic findings from a number of patients with a umber of moderate to severe gastrointestinal complaints both risedronate sodium and control patients indicated o evidence of treatment related gastric, duodenal or esophageal ulcers in either group, although duodenitis as uncommonly observed in the risedronate sodium roup.

In a trial comparing before-breakfast dosing and dosing t other times of the day in women with postmenopausal steoporosis, lumbar spine BMD gains were statistically igher with before-breakfast dosing.

osteoepenic postmenopausal women, risedronate odium has shown superiority to placebo in increasing umbar spine BMD at 12 and 24 months.

orticosteroid Induced Osteoporosis: The clinical pro-ramme included patients initiating corticosteroid therapy ≥ 7.5 mg/day prednisone or equivalent) within the pre-ious 3 months or patients who had been taking corticos-eroids for more than 6 months. Results of these studies emonstrate that:

Risedronate sodium 5 mg daily given for one year main-ains or increases bone mineral density (BMD) relative to ontrol at the lumbar spine, femoral neck, and trochanter.

Risedronate sodium 5 mg daily reduced the incidence of ertebral fractures, monitored for safety, relative to control t 1 year in pooled studies.

histological examination of bone biopsies from patients aking corticosteroids and risedronate sodium 5 mg daily lid not show signs of disturbed mineralisation process.

5.2 Pharmacokinetic properties

Absorption: Absorption after an oral dose is relatively rapid (t_{max} ~1 hour) and is independent of dose over the range studied (2.5 to 30 mg). Mean oral bioavailability of the tablet s 0.63% and is decreased when risedronate sodium is administered with food. Bioavailability was similar in men and women.

Distribution: The mean steady state volume of distribution s 6.3 l/kg in humans. Plasma protein binding is about 24%.

Metabolism: There is no evidence of systemic metabolism of risedronate sodium.

Elimination: Approximately half of the absorbed dose is excreted in urine within 24 hours, and 85% of an intrave-nous dose is recovered in the urine after 28 days. Mean renal clearance is 105 ml/min and mean total clearance is 122 ml/min, with the difference probably attributed to clearance due to adsorption to bone. The renal clearance is not concentration dependent, and there is a linear rela-tionship between renal clearance and creatinine clearance. Unabsorbed risedronate sodium is eliminated unchanged in faeces. After oral administration the concentration-time profile shows three elimination phases with a terminal half-life of 480 hours.

Special Populations:

Elderly: no dosage adjustment is necessary.

Acetyl salicylic acid/NSAID users: Among regular acetyl salicylic acid or NSAID users (3 or more days per week) the incidence of upper gastrointestinal adverse events in rise-dronate sodium treated patients was similar to that in control patients.

5.3 Preclinical safety data

In toxicological studies in rat and dog dose dependent liver toxic effects of risedronate sodium were seen, primarily as enzyme increases with histological changes in rat. The clinical relevance of these observations is unknown. Tes-ticular toxicity occurred in rat and dog at exposures con-sidered in excess of the human therapeutic exposure. Dose related incidences of upper airway irritation were frequently noted in rodents. Similar effects have been seen with other bisphosphonates. Lower respiratory tract effects were also seen in longer term studies in rodents, although the clinical significance of these findings is unclear. In reproduction toxicity studies at exposures close to clinical exposure ossification changes were seen in sternum and/or skull of foetuses from treated rats and hypocalcemia and mortality in pregnant females allowed to deliver. There was no evidence of teratogenesis at 3.2mg/kg/day in rat and 10mg/kg/day in rabbit, although data are only available on a small number of rabbits. Maternal toxicity prevented testing of higher doses. Stu-dies on genotoxicity and carcinogenesis did not show any particular risks for humans.

6. PHARMACEUTICAL PARTICULARS

6.1 List of excipients

Tablet core: Lactose monohydrate
Cellulose microcrystalline
Crospovidone
Magnesium stearate.

Film coating: Iron oxide yellow E172
Hypromellose
Macrogol
Hyprolose
Silicon dioxide
Titanium dioxide E171.

6.2 Incompatibilities

Not applicable.

6.3 Shelf life

5 years.

6.4 Special precautions for storage

This medicinal product does not require any special sto-rage conditions.

6.5 Nature and contents of container

Opaque PVC/aluminium foil blister cards of 14 tablets in a cardboard carton, tablet count 14, 28 (2 × 14), 84 (6 × 14), 98 (7 × 14) or 10 × 14 (hospital bundle).

2 × 10 count perforated blister strip (hospital unit dose)

Not all pack sizes may be marketed.

6.6 Special precautions for disposal and other handling

No special requirements.

7. MARKETING AUTHORISATION HOLDER

Procter & Gamble Pharmaceuticals UK Ltd.,
Rusham Park,
Whitehall Lane,
Egham,
Surrey,
TW20 9NW, UK

8. MARKETING AUTHORISATION NUMBER(S)

PL 00364/0070

9. DATE OF FIRST AUTHORISATION/RENEWAL OF THE AUTHORISATION

1999-10-07/2004-10-07

10. DATE OF REVISION OF THE TEXT

2008-09-19

Actonel Combi film-coated tablets + effervescent granules

(Procter & Gamble Pharmaceuticals UK Limited)

1. NAME OF THE MEDICINAL PRODUCT

Actonel Combi 35 mg + 1000 mg / 880 IU film-coated tablets + effervescent granules

2. QUALITATIVE AND QUANTITATIVE COMPOSITION

Each film-coated tablet contains 35 mg risedronate sodium, (equivalent to 32.5 mg risedronic acid).

Each sachet of effervescent granules contains 2500 mg calcium carbonate equivalent to 1000 mg calcium and 22 micrograms (880 IU) colecalciferol (vitamin D_3).

Excipients: Each film-coated tablet contains lactose. Each sachet of effervescent granules contains potassium (163 mg), sucrose, soya-bean oil and sorbitol.

For a full list of excipients, see section 6.1.

3. PHARMACEUTICAL FORM

Film-coated tablet.

Risedronate tablets: Oval, light-orange, film-coated tablet with RSN on one side and 35 mg on the other.

Effervescent granules

Calcium carbonate/colecalciferol, white effervescent gran-ules.

4. CLINICAL PARTICULARS

4.1 Therapeutic indications

Treatment of postmenopausal osteoporosis, to reduce the risk of vertebral fractures.

Treatment of established postmenopausal osteoporosis, to reduce the risk of hip fractures (see section 5.1).

Actonel Combi is only intended for use in assessed patients for whom the amount of calcium and vitamin D_3 included is considered to provide adequate supplementa-tion.

4.2 Posology and method of administration

A weekly unit of Actonel Combi consists of 1 Actonel 35 mg film-coated tablet and 6 calcium/vitamin D_3 sachets in a box.

The recommended dose in adults is 1 Actonel 35 mg tablet on the first day followed on the next day by 1 calcium/vitamin D_3 sachet daily for 6 days. This 7-day sequence is then repeated each week starting with Actonel 35 mg tablet.

Actonel 35 mg (light-orange tablet):

The Actonel 35 mg tablet should be taken orally on the same day each week.

The absorption of risedronate sodium is affected by food, thus to ensure adequate absorption, patients should take the Actonel 35 mg tablet

- Before breakfast: at least 30 minutes before the first food, other medicinal product or drink (other than plain water) of the day.

The tablet must be swallowed whole and not sucked or chewed. To aid delivery of the tablet to the stomach the Actonel 35 mg tablet is to be taken while in an upright position with a glass of plain water (≥120 ml). Patients should not lie down for 30 minutes after taking the tablet (see section 4.4).

Calcium/vitamin D_3 (sachet):

Calcium/vitamin D_3 sachet should be taken each day for 6 days per week starting on the day after the Actonel 35 mg tablet is taken. The contents of the sachet should be poured into a glass of plain water, stirred and drunk imme-diately once the fizzing has subsided.

In case the Actonel 35 mg tablet dose is missed, patients should be instructed that the Actonel 35 mg tablet should be taken on the next day in the morning according to the dosing instructions. In this particular instance, patients should then take their calcium/vitamin D_3 sachet on the following day. Patients should be instructed that they should never take the tablet and the sachet the same day.

If the calcium/vitamin D_3 sachet dose is missed, the patient should be instructed to continue taking one sachet each day beginning on the day the missed dose is remembered. Patient should be instructed that they should not take two sachets on the same day. Any remaining calcium/vitamin D_3 sachet at the end of the weekly cycle should be dis-carded.

Elderly: No dosage adjustment is necessary since bioavail-ability, distribution and elimination were similar in elderly (>60 years of age) compared to younger subjects. This has also been shown in the very elderly, 75 years old and above in postmenopausal population.

Renal Impairment: No dosage adjustment is required for those patients with mild to moderate renal impairment. The use of risedronate sodium and calcium/vitamin D_3 is con-traindicated in patients with severe renal impairment (crea-tinine clearance lower than 30ml/min) (see sections 4.3 and 5.2).

Children: Safety and efficacy of Actonel Combi has not been established in children and adolescents.

4.3 Contraindications

Hypersensitivity to risedronate sodium, calcium carbonate, colecalciferol or to any of the excipients (in particular soya-bean oil).

Hypocalcaemia (see section 4.4)

Hypercalcaemia.

Hypercalciuria

Diseases and/or conditions (such as prolonged immobili-zation) associated with hypercalcaemia and/or hypercal-ciuria

Nephrolithiasis

Pregnancy and lactation.

Severe renal impairment (creatinine clearance <30ml/min).

Hypervitaminosis D

4.4 Special warnings and precautions for use

Risedronate sodium:

Foods, drinks (other than plain water) and medicinal pro-ducts containing polyvalent cations (such as calcium, mag-nesium, iron and aluminium) may interfere with the absorption of risedronate sodium and should not be taken at the same time (see section 4.5). Therefore the risedro-nate sodium tablet (light-orange tablet) should be taken at least 30 minutes before the first food, other medicinal product or drink of the day (see section 4.2).

Efficacy of bisphosphonates in the treatment of postme-nopausal osteoporosis is related to the presence of low bone mineral density (BMD) [T-score at hip or lumbar spine ≤-2.5 standard deviations (SD)] and/or prevalent fracture.

High age or clinical risk factors for fracture alone are not sufficient reasons to initiate treatment of osteoporosis with a bisphosphonate. The evidence to support efficacy of bisphosphonates including risedronate sodium in very elderly women (>80 years) is limited (see section 5.1).

Bisphosphonates have been associated with oesophagitis, gastritis, oesophageal ulcerations and gastroduodenal ulcerations. Thus, caution should be used:

- In patients who have a history of oesophageal disorders which delay oesophageal transit or emptying e.g. stricture or achalasia.
- In patients who are unable to stay in the upright position for at least 30 minutes after taking the tablet.
- If risedronate is given to patients with active or recent oesophageal or upper gastrointestinal problems.

Prescribers should emphasise to patients the importance of paying attention to the dosing instructions and be alert to any signs and symptoms of possible oesophageal reaction. The patients should be instructed to seek timely medical attention if they develop symptoms of oesophageal irritation such as dysphagia, pain on swallowing, retrosternal pain or new/worsened heartburn.

Hypocalcaemia should be treated before starting Actonel Combi therapy. Other disturbances of bone and mineral metabolism (i.e. parathyroid dysfunction, hypovitaminosis D) should be treated at the time of starting Actonel Combi therapy.

Osteonecrosis of the jaw, generally associated with tooth extraction and/or local infection (including osteomyelitis) has been reported in patients with cancer receiving treatment regimens including primarily intravenously administered bisphosphonates. Many of these patients were also receiving chemotherapy and corticosteroids. Osteonecrosis of the jaw has also been reported in patients with osteoporosis receiving oral bisphosphonates.

A dental examination with appropriate preventive dentistry should be considered prior to treatment with bisphosphonates in patients with concomitant risk factors (e.g. cancer, chemotherapy, radiotherapy, corticosteroids, poor oral hygiene).

While on treatment, these patients should avoid invasive dental procedures if possible. For patients who develop osteonecrosis of the jaw while on bisphosphonate therapy, dental surgery may exacerbate the condition. For patients requiring dental procedures, there are no data available to suggest whether discontinuation of bisphosphonate treatment reduces the risk of osteonecrosis of the jaw. Clinical judgment of the treating physician should guide the management plan of each patient based on individual benefit/risk assessment.

In patients with mild to moderate renal impairment or a history of absorptive or renal hypercalciuria, nephrocalcinosis, kidney stone formation, or hypophosphataemia, renal function, serum and urinary calcium and phosphate should be monitored regularly.

This medicinal product contains lactose. Patients with rare hereditary problems of galactose intolerance, the Lapp lactase deficiency or glucose-galactose malabsorption should not take this medicinal product.

Calcium carbonate/vitamin D_3:

Vitamin D_3 should be used with caution in patients with impairment of renal function and the effect on calcium and phosphate levels should be monitored. The risk of soft tissue calcification should be taken into account. In patients with severe renal insufficiency, vitamin D in the form of colecalciferol is not metabolised normally and another form of vitamin D should be used (see section 4.3)

During long-term treatment, serum and urinary calcium levels should be followed and renal function should be monitored through measurement of serum creatinine. Monitoring is especially important in elderly patients on concomitant treatment with cardiac glycosides or diuretics (see section 4.5) and in patients with a high tendency to calculus formation. Treatment must be reduced or suspended if urinary calcium exceeds 7.5 mmol/24 hour (300 mg/24 hour). In case of hypercalcaemia or signs of impaired renal function, treatment with calcium/vitamin D_3 sachets should be discontinued.

The dose of vitamin D_3 in the sachets should be considered when prescribing other drugs containing vitamin D. Additional doses of calcium or vitamin D should be taken under close medical supervision. In such cases it is necessary to monitor serum calcium levels and urinary calcium excretion frequently.

Calcium/vitamin D_3 sachets should be used with caution in patients suffering from sarcoidosis because of the risk of increased metabolism of vitamin D to its active metabolite. In these patients, serum calcium levels and urinary calcium excretion must be monitored.

Calcium/vitamin D_3 sachets should be used with caution in immobilised patients with osteoporosis due to the increased risk of hypercalcaemia. The calcium/vitamin D_3 treatment might be discontinued in prolonged immobilization and should only be resumed once the patient becomes mobile again.

This medicinal product contains sorbitol and sucrose. Patients with rare hereditary problems of fructose intolerance, glucose-galactose malabsorption or sucrase-isomaltase insufficiency should not take this medicinal product.

4.5 Interaction with other medicinal products and other forms of interaction

Risedronate sodium:

No formal interaction studies have been performed with risedronate sodium, however no clinically relevant interactions with other medicinal products were found during clinical trials. In the risedronate sodium Phase III osteoporosis studies with daily dosing, acetyl salicylic acid or non-steroidal anti-inflammatory drug (NSAID) use was reported by 33% and 45% of patients respectively. In the Phase III once a week study, acetyl salicylic acid or NSAID use was reported by 57% and 40% of patients respectively. Among regular acetyl salicylic acid or NSAID users (3 or more days per week) the incidence of upper gastrointestinal adverse events in risedronate sodium treated patients was similar to that in control patients.

If considered appropriate risedronate sodium may be used concomitantly with oestrogen supplementation.

Concomitant ingestion of medications containing polyvalent cations (e.g. calcium, magnesium, iron and aluminium) will interfere with the absorption of risedronate sodium (see section 4.4).

Risedronate sodium is not systemically metabolised, does not induce cytochrome P450 enzymes, and has low protein binding.

Calcium carbonate/vitamin D_3:

Thiazide diuretics reduce the urinary excretion of calcium. Due to increased risk of hypercalcaemia serum calcium should be regularly monitored during concomitant use of thiazide diuretics.

Systemic corticosteroids reduce calcium absorption. During concomitant use, it may be necessary to increase the dose of calcium.

Calcium carbonate may interfere with the absorption of concomitant administered tetracycline preparations. For this reason, tetracycline preparations should be administered at least two hours before or four to six hours after oral intake of calcium carbonate/vitamin D_3.

Hypercalcaemia may increase the toxicity of digitalis and other cardiac glycosides (risk of dysrhythmia) during treatment with calcium combined with vitamin D_3. Such patients should be monitored with regard to electrocardiogram (ECG) and serum calcium levels.

If sodium fluoride is used concomitantly, this preparation should be administered at least three hours before intake of calcium carbonate/vitamin D_3 since gastrointestinal absorption may be reduced.

Oxalic acid (found in spinach and rhubarb) and phytic acid (found in whole cereals) may inhibit calcium absorption through formation of insoluble compounds with calcium ions. The patient should not take calcium products within two hours of eating foods with high concentration of oxalic acid and phytic acid.

Simultaneous treatment with ion exchange resins such as cholestyramine or laxatives such as paraffin oil may reduce the gastrointestinal absorption of vitamin D.

4.6 Pregnancy and lactation

This medicinal product is contraindicated during pregnancy and lactation (see section 4.3).

Risedronate sodium:

There are no adequate data from use of risedronate sodium in pregnant women. Studies in animals have shown reproductive toxicity (see section 5.3). The potential risk to humans is unknown. Studies in animals indicate that a small amount of risedronate sodium pass into breast milk. Risedronate sodium must not be used during pregnancy or by breast-feeding women.

Calcium carbonate/vitamin D_3:

During pregnancy the daily intake should not exceed 1500 mg calcium and 600 IU colecalciferol (15μg vitamin D_3). There are no indications that vitamin D at therapeutic doses is teratogenic in humans. Studies in animals have shown reproductive toxicity with high doses of vitamin D. In pregnant women, overdoses of calcium and vitamin D should be avoided as permanent hypercalcaemia has been related to adverse effects on the developing foetus. Calcium and vitamin D 3 pass into breast milk. Calcium carbonate 2500 mg/vitamin D_3 880 IU dose granules must not be used during pregnancy and lactation.

4.7 Effects on ability to drive and use machines

No effects on ability to drive and use machines have been observed.

4.8 Undesirable effects

Risedronate sodium:

Risedronate sodium has been studied in phase III clinical trials involving more than 15,000 patients. The majority of undesirable effects observed in clinical trials were mild to moderate in severity and usually did not require cessation of therapy.

Adverse experiences reported in phase III clinical trials in postmenopausal women with osteoporosis treated for up to 36 months with risedronate sodium 5mg/day (n=5020) or placebo (n=5048) and considered possibly or probably related to risedronate sodium are listed below using the following convention (incidences versus placebo are shown in brackets): very common (≥1/10); common (≥1/100; <1/10); uncommon (≥1/1,000; <1/100); rare (≥1/10,000; <1/1,000); very rare (<1/10,000).

Nervous system disorders:

Common: headache (1.8% vs. 1.4%)

Eye disorders:

Uncommon: iritis*

Gastrointestinal disorders:

Common: constipation (5.0% vs. 4.8%), dyspepsia (4.5% vs. 4.1%), nausea (4.3% vs. 4.0%), abdominal pain (3.5% vs. 3.3%), diarrhoea (3.0% vs. 2.7%)

Uncommon: gastritis (0.9% vs. 0.7%), oesophagitis (0.9% vs. 0.9%), dysphagia (0.4% vs. 0.2%), duodenitis (0.2% vs. 0.1%), oesophageal ulcer (0.2% vs. 0.2%)

Rare: glossitis (<0.1% vs. 0.1%), oesophageal stricture (<0.1% vs. 0.0%),

Musculoskeletal and connective tissues disorders:

Common: musculoskeletal pain (2.1% vs. 1.9%)

Investigations:

Rare: abnormal liver function tests*

* No relevant incidences from Phase III osteoporosis st dies; frequency based on adverse event/laboratory/rech lenge findings in earlier clinical trials.

In a one-year, double-blind, multicentre study compari risedronate 5 mg daily (n= 480) and risedronate sodiu 35 mg weekly (n=485) in postmenopausal women w osteoporosis, the overall safety and tolerability profil were similar. The following additional adverse experienc considered possibly or probably drug related by inves gators have been reported (incidence greater in rised nate 35 mg than in risedronate sodium 5 mg grou gastrointestinal disorder (1.6% vs. 1.0%) and pain (1.2 vs. 0.8%).

Laboratory findings: Early, transient, asymptomatic a mild decreases in serum calcium and phosphate lev have been observed in some patients.

The following additional adverse reactions have be reported during post-marketing use (frequency unknow

Eye disorders:

iritis, uveitis

Muskuloskeletal and connective tissues disorders:

osteonecrosis of the jaw

Skin and subcutaneous tissue disorders:

hypersensitivity and skin reactions, including angioeder generalised rash, urticaria and bullous skin reactio some severe including isolated reports of Stevens-Jol son syndrome and toxic epidermal necrolysis.

hair loss.

Immune system disorders:

anaphylactic reaction

Hepatobiliary disorders:

serious hepatic disorders. In most of the reported cas the patients were also treated with other products kno to cause hepatic disorders.

Calcium carbonate/vitamin D_3

Adverse reactions are listed below, by system organ cl and frequency following convention: very common (≥ 10); common (≥1/100; <1/10); uncommon (≥1/1,0 <1/100); rare (≥1/10,000; <1/1,000); very rare (< 10,000).

Metabolism and nutrition disorders

Uncommon: Hypercalcaemia and hypercalciuria.

Gastrointestinal disorders

Rare: Constipation, flatulence, nausea, abdominal p and diarrhoea.

Skin and subcutaneous disorders

Rare: Pruritus, rash and urticaria.

4.9 Overdose

Risedronate sodium:

No specific information is available on the treatment acute overdose with risedronate sodium.

Decreases in serum calcium following substantial ov dose may be expected. Signs and symptoms of hypoc caemia may also occur in some of these patients.

Milk or antacids containing magnesium, calcium or alu nium should be given to bind risedronate sodium reduce absorption of risedronate sodium. In cases of s stantial overdose, gastric lavage may be considered remove unabsorbed risedronate sodium.

Calcium carbonate/vitamin D_3:

Overdose can lead to hypervitaminosis, hypercalciura hypercalcaemia. Symptoms of hypercalcaemia n include anorexia, thirst, nausea, vomiting, constipat abdominal pain, muscle weakness, fatigue, mental dis bances, polydipsia, polyuria, bone pain, nephrocalcino renal calculi and in severe cases, cardiac arrhythm Extreme hypercalcaemia may result in coma and de Persistently high calcium levels may lead to irrevers renal damage and soft tissue calcification.

Treatment of hypercalcaemia: The treatment with calc must be discontinued. Treatment with thiazide diuret lithium, vitamin A, vitamin D_3 and cardiac glycosides m also be discontinued. Emptying of the stomach in patie with impaired consciousness. Rehydration, and, accord to severity, isolated or combined treatment with loop di tics, bisphosphonates, calcitonin and corticostero Serum electrolytes, renal function and diuresis must monitored. In severe cases, ECG and central venous p sure should be followed.

5. PHARMACOLOGICAL PROPERTIES

5.1 Pharmacodynamic properties

Pharmaco-therapeutic group: Bisphosphonates, con nations,

ATC Code: M05BB04.

Risedronate sodium:

Risedronate sodium is a pyridinyl bisphosphonate binds to bone hydroxyapatite and inhibits osteocl mediated bone resorption. The bone turnover is redu while the osteoblast activity and bone mineralisatio eserved. In preclinical studies risedronate sodium emonstrated potent anti-osteoclast and antiresorptive ctivity, and dose dependently increased bone mass and omechanical skeletal strength. The activity of risedronate odium was confirmed by measuring biochemical markers r bone turnover during pharmacodynamic and clinical udies. Decreases in biochemical markers of bone turn-ver were observed within 1 month and reached a max-num in 3-6 months. Decreases in biochemical markers of one turnover were similar with risedronate sodium 35 mg eekly and risedronate sodium 5 mg daily at 12 months.

reatment of Postmenopausal Osteoporosis:

number of risk factors are associated with postmeno-ausal osteoporosis including low bone mass, low bone ineral density, early menopause, a history of smoking and family history of osteoporosis. The clinical consequence f osteoporosis is fractures. The risk of fractures is creased with the number of risk factors.

ased on effects on mean change in lumbar spine bone ineral density (BMD), risedronate sodium 35 mg weekly =485) was shown to be equivalent to risedronate sodium mg daily (n=480) in a one-year, double-blind, multicentre tudy of postmenopausal women with osteoporosis.

he clinical programme for risedronate sodium adminis-ered once daily studied the effect of risedronate sodium n the risk of hip and vertebral fractures and contained arly and late postmenopausal women with and without acture. Daily doses of 2.5 mg and 5 mg were studied and ll groups, including the control groups, received calcium nd vitamin D (if baseline levels were low). The absolute nd relative risk of new vertebral and hip fractures were stimated by use of a time-to-first event analysis.

Two placebo-controlled trials (n=3661) enrolled postme-opausal women under 85 years with vertebral fractures at aseline. Risedronate sodium 5 mg daily given for 3 years educed the risk of new vertebral fractures relative to the control group. In women with respectively at least 2 or at east 1 vertebral fractures, the relative risk reduction was 9% and 41% respectively (incidence of new vertebral ractures with risedronate sodium 18.1% and 11.3%, with lacebo 29.0% and 16.3%, respectively). The effect of eatment was seen as early as the end of the first year of treatment. Benefits were also demonstrated in women with multiple fractures at baseline. Risedronate sodium 5 mg daily also reduced the yearly height loss compared o the control group.

- Two further placebo controlled trials enrolled postmeno-pausal women above 70 years with or without vertebral ractures at baseline. Women 70-79 years were enrolled with femoral neck BMD T-score <-3 SD (manufacturer's ange, i.e. -2.5 SD using NHANES III) and at least one additional risk factor. Women ≥80 years could be enrolled on the basis of at least one non-skeletal risk factor for hip racture or low bone mineral density at the femoral neck. Statistical significance of the efficacy of risedronate sodium versus placebo is only reached when the two treatment groups 2.5 mg and 5 mg are pooled. The follow-ing results are only based on a-posteriori analysis of sub-groups defined by clinical practise and current definitions of osteoporosis:

- In the subgroup of patients with femoral neck BMD T-score ≤-2.5SD (NHANES III) and at least one vertebral fracture at baseline, risedronate sodium given for 3 years reduced the risk of hip fractures by 46% relative to the control group (incidence of hip fractures in combined rise-dronate sodium 2.5 and 5 mg groups 3.8%, placebo 7.4%);

- Data suggest that a more limited protection than this may be observed in the very elderly (≥80 years). This may be due to the increasing importance of non-skeletal factors for hip fracture with increasing age.

In these trials, data analysed as a secondary endpoint indicated a decrease in the risk of new vertebral fractures in patients with low femoral neck BMD without vertebral fracture and in patients with low femoral neck BMD with or without vertebral fracture.

- Risedronate sodium 5 mg daily given for 3 years increased BMD relative to control at the lumbar spine, femoral neck, trochanter and wrist and maintained bone density at the mid-shaft radius.

- In a one-year follow-up off therapy after three years treatment with risedronate sodium 5 mg daily there was rapid reversibility of the suppressing effect of risedronate sodium on bone turnover rate.

- Bone biopsy samples from postmenopausal women treated with risedronate sodium 5 mg daily for 2 to 3 years, showed an expected moderate decrease in bone turnover. Bone formed during risedronate sodium treatment was of normal lamellar structure and bone mineralisation. These data together with the decreased incidence of osteoporo-sis related fractures at vertebral sites in women with osteo-porosis appear to indicate no detrimental effect on bone quality.

- Endoscopic findings from a number of patients with a number of moderate to severe gastrointestinal complaints in both risedronate sodium and control patients indicated no evidence of treatment related gastric, duodenal or oesophageal ulcers in either group, although duodenitis was uncommonly observed in the risedronate sodium group.

Calcium carbonate/vitamin D_3:

In case of calcium deficiency, oral intake of calcium supplementation supports the remineralisation of the ske-leton. Vitamin D_3 increases the intestinal absorption of calcium.

Administration of calcium and vitamin D_3 counteracts the increase in parathyroid hormone (PTH) which is caused by calcium deficiency which causes increased bone resorp-tion.

A clinical study of institutionalised patients suffering from vitamin D deficiency indicated that a daily intake of effer-vescent granules of 1000 mg calcium/880 IU colecalciferol for six months normalised the value of the 25-hydoxylated metabolite of vitamin D_3 and reduced secondary hyperpar-athyroidism.

5.2 Pharmacokinetic properties

Risedronate sodium:

Absorption: risedronate sodium absorption after an oral dose is relatively rapid (t_{max} ~1 hour) and is independent of dose over the range studied (single dose study, 2.5 to 30 mg; multiple dose studies, 2.5 to 5 mg daily and up to 50 mg dosed weekly). Mean oral bioavailability of the tablet is 0.63% and is decreased when risedronate sodium is administered with food. Bioavailability was similar in men and women.

Distribution: The mean steady state volume of distribution of risedronate sodium is 6.3 l/kg in humans. Plasma protein binding is about 24%.

Metabolism: There is no evidence of systemic metabolism of risedronate sodium.

Elimination: Approximately half of the absorbed risedro-nate sodium dose is excreted in urine within 24 hours, and 85% of an intravenous dose is recovered in the urine after 28 days. Mean renal clearance is 105 ml/min and mean total clearance is 122 ml/min, with the difference probably attributed to clearance due to adsorption to bone. The renal clearance is not concentration dependent, and there is a linear relationship between renal clearance and crea-tinine clearance. Unabsorbed risedronate sodium is elimi-nated unchanged in faeces. After oral administration the concentration-time profile shows three elimination phases with a terminal half-life of 480 hours.

Special Populations

Elderly: no dosage adjustment is necessary.

Acetyl salicylic acid/ NSAID users: Among regular acetyl salicylic acid or NSAID users (3 or more days per week) the incidence of upper gastrointestinal adverse events in rise-dronate sodium treated patients was similar to that in control patients.

Calcium carbonate:

Absorption: During dissolution the calcium salt contained in the effervescent granules is transformed into calcium citrate. Calcium citrate is well absorbed, approximately 30% to 40% of the ingested dose.

Distribution and metabolism: 99% of calcium in the body is concentrated in the hard structure of bones and teeth. The remaining 1% is present in the intra- and extracellular fluids. About 50% of the total blood calcium content is physiologically active ionised form with approximately 10% being complexed to citrate, phosphate or other anions, the remaining 40% being bound to proteins, prin-cipally albumin.

Elimination: Calcium is eliminated through faeces, urine and sweat. Renal excretion depends on glomerular filtra-tion and calcium tubular reabsorption.

Vitamin D_3:

Absorption: Vitamin D is readily absorbed in the small intestine.

Distribution and metabolism: Colecalciferol and its meta-bolites circulate in the blood bound to a specific globulin. Colecalciferol is converted in the liver by hydroxylation to the active form 25-hydroxycolecalciferol. It is then further converted in the kidneys to 1,25 hydroxycolecalciferol. 1,25 hydroxycolecalciferol is the metabolite responsible for increasing calcium absorption. Vitamin D that is not metabolised is stored in adipose and muscle tissues.

Elimination: Vitamin D is excreted in faeces and urine.

5.3 Preclinical safety data

Risedronate sodium:

In toxicological studies in rat and dog dose dependent liver toxic effects of risedronate sodium were seen, primarily as enzyme increases with histological changes in rat. The clinical relevance of these observations is unknown. Tes-ticular toxicity occurred in rat and dog at exposures con-sidered in excess of the human therapeutic exposure. Dose related incidences of upper airway irritation were frequently noted in rodents. Similar effects have been seen with other bisphosphonates. Lower respiratory tract effects were also seen in longer term studies in rodents, but the clinical significance of these findings is unclear. In reproduction toxicity studies at exposures close to clinical exposure ossification changes were seen in sternum and/ or skull of foetuses from treated rats and hypocalcemia and mortality in pregnant females allowed to deliver. There was no evidence of teratogenesis at 3.2mg/kg/day in rat and 10mg/kg/day in rabbit, although data are only available on a small number of rabbits. Maternal toxicity prevented testing of higher doses. Studies on genotoxicity and carci-nogenesis did not show any particular risk for humans.

Calcium carbonate/vitamin D_3:

At doses far higher than the human therapeutic range, teratogenicity has been observed in animal studies (see section 4.6). There is no further information of relevance to the safety assessment in addition to what is stated in other parts of the SPC.

6. PHARMACEUTICAL PARTICULARS

6.1 List of excipients

Film-coated tablet:

Tablet core:	Lactose monohydrate, Cellulose microcrystalline, Crospovidone A, Magnesium stearate.
Film coating:	Hypromellose, Macrogol Hyprolose Silicon dioxide Titanium dioxide (E171), Iron oxide yellow (E172), Iron oxide red (E172).
Effervescent granules:	Citric acid anhydrous Malic acid, Gluconolactone, Maltodextrin, Sodium cyclamate, Saccharin sodium, Sorbitol E420, Mannitol E421, Gluconolactone, Dextrin, acacia, Lemon oils Lime flavour Rice starch, Potassium carbonate, All-rac-α-Tocopherol, Soya-bean oil, hydrogenated Gelatin, Sucrose, Maize starch.

6.2 Incompatibilities

Not applicable.

6.3 Shelf life

3 years.

6.4 Special precautions for storage

This medicinal product does not require any special sto-rage conditions.

6.5 Nature and contents of container

Combination pack constituted of an outer carton pack containing weekly unit(s) (carton boxes).

Each weekly unit contains:

Clear PVC/aluminium foil blister containing one tablet

Six sachets (laminated aluminium paper foil) containing effervescent granules

Pack sizes:

1 weekly unit: 1x(1 film-coated tablet + effervescent gran-ules in 6 sachets)

2 weekly units: 2x(1 film-coated tablet + effervescent gran-ules in 6 sachets)

4 weekly units: 4x(1 film-coated tablet + effervescent gran-ules in 6 sachets)

3x4 weekly units: 12x(1 film-coated tablet + effervescent granules in 6 sachets)

4x4 weekly units: 16x(1 film-coated tablet + effervescent granules in 6 sachets)

Not all pack sizes may be marketed.

6.6 Special precautions for disposal and other handling

No special requirements

7. MARKETING AUTHORISATION HOLDER

Procter & Gamble Pharmaceuticals UK Ltd.,
RushamPark,
Whitehall Lane,
Egham,
Surrey,
TW20 9NW, UK

8. MARKETING AUTHORISATION NUMBER(S)

PL 00364/0085

9. DATE OF FIRST AUTHORISATION/RENEWAL OF THE AUTHORISATION

2006-10-13

10. DATE OF REVISION OF THE TEXT

2008-09-19

Actonel Once a Week 35mg film coated tablets.

(Procter & Gamble Pharmaceuticals UK Limited)

1. NAME OF THE MEDICINAL PRODUCT

Actonel Once a Week 35 mg film-coated tablets.

2. QUALITATIVE AND QUANTITATIVE COMPOSITION

Each film-coated tablet contains 35 mg risedronate sodium (equivalent to 32.5 mg risedronic acid).

Excipients: Each film-coated tablet contains lactose.

For a full list of excipients, see section 6.1.

3. PHARMACEUTICAL FORM

Film-coated tablet.

Oval light-orange film-coated tablet with RSN on one side and 35 mg on the other.

4. CLINICAL PARTICULARS

4.1 Therapeutic indications

Treatment of postmenopausal osteoporosis, to reduce the risk of vertebral fractures. Treatment of established post-menopausal osteoporosis, to reduce the risk of hip fractures (see section 5.1).

Treatment of osteoporosis in men at high risk of fractures (see section 5.1).

4.2 Posology and method of administration

The recommended dose in adults is one 35 mg tablet orally once a week. The tablet should be taken on the same day each week.

The absorption of risedronate sodium is affected by food, thus to ensure adequate absorption patients should take Actonel Once a Week 35 mg:

- Before breakfast: At least 30 minutes before the first food, other medicinal product or drink (other than plain water) of the day.

Patients should be instructed that if a dose is missed, one Actonel Once a Week 35 mg tablet should be taken on the day that the tablet is remembered. Patients should then return to taking one tablet once a week on the day the tablet is normally taken. Two tablets should not be taken on the same day.

The tablet must be swallowed whole and not sucked or chewed. To aid delivery of the tablet to the stomach Actonel Once a Week 35 mg is to be taken while in an upright position with a glass of plain water ($\geq$120 ml). Patients should not lie down for 30 minutes after taking the tablet (see section 4.4).

Supplemental calcium and vitamin D should be considered if the dietary intake is inadequate.

Elderly: No dosage adjustment is necessary since bioavailability, distribution and elimination were similar in elderly (>60 years of age) compared to younger subjects.

This has also been shown in the very elderly, 75 years old and above postmenopausal population.

Renal Impairment: No dosage adjustment is required for those patients with mild to moderate renal impairment. The use of risedronate sodium is contraindicated in patients with severe renal impairment (creatinine clearance lower than 30ml/min) (see sections 4.3 and 5.2).

Children: Safety and efficacy of Actonel Once a Week 35 mg have not been established in children and adolescents.

4.3 Contraindications

Hypersensitivity to risedronate sodium or to any of the excipients.

Hypocalcaemia (see section 4.4).

Pregnancy and lactation.

Severe renal impairment (creatinine clearance <30ml/min).

4.4 Special warnings and precautions for use

Foods, drinks (other than plain water) and medicinal products containing polyvalent cations (such as calcium, magnesium, iron and aluminium) interfere with the absorption of bisphosphonates and should not be taken at the same time as Actonel Once a Week 35 mg (see section 4.5). In order to achieve the intended efficacy, strict adherence to dosing recommendations is necessary (see section 4.2).

Efficacy of bisphosphonates in the treatment of osteoporosis is related to the presence of low bone mineral density and/or prevalent fracture.

High age or clinical risk factors for fracture alone are not sufficient reasons to initiate treatment of osteoporosis with a bisphosphonate.

The evidence to support efficacy of bisphosphonates including risedronate in the very elderly (>80 years) is limited (see section 5.1).

Bisphosphonates have been associated with oesophagitis, gastritis, oesophageal ulcerations and gastroduodenal ulcerations. Thus, caution should be used:

- In patients who have a history of oesophageal disorders which delay oesophageal transit or emptying e.g. stricture or achalasia
- In patients who are unable to stay in the upright position for at least 30 minutes after taking the tablet.
- If risedronate is given to patients with active or recent oesophageal or upper gastrointestinal problems.

Prescribers should emphasise to patients the importance of paying attention to the dosing instructions and be alert to any signs and symptoms of possible oesophageal reaction. The patients should be instructed to seek timely medical attention if they develop symptoms of oesophageal irritation such as dysphagia, pain on swallowing, retrosternal pain or new/worsened heartburn.

Hypocalcaemia should be treated before starting Actonel Once a Week 35 mg therapy. Other disturbances of bone and mineral metabolism (i.e. parathyroid dysfunction, hypovitaminosis D) should be treated at the time of starting Actonel Once a Week 35 mg therapy.

Osteonecrosis of the jaw, generally associated with tooth extraction and/or local infection (including osteomyelitis) has been reported in patients with cancer receiving treatment regimens including primarily intravenously administered bisphosphonates. Many of these patients were also receiving chemotherapy and corticosteroids. Osteonecrosis of the jaw has also been reported in patients with osteoporosis receiving oral bisphosphonates.

A dental examination with appropriate preventive dentistry should be considered prior to treatment with bisphosphonates in patients with concomitant risk factors (e.g. cancer, chemotherapy, radiotherapy, corticosteroids, poor oral hygiene).

While on treatment, these patients should avoid invasive dental procedures if possible. For patients who develop osteonecrosis of the jaw while on bisphosphonate therapy, dental surgery may exacerbate the condition. For patients requiring dental procedures, there are no data available to suggest whether discontinuation of bisphosphonate treatment reduces the risk of osteonecrosis of the jaw.

Clinical judgment of the treating physician should guide the management plan of each patient based on individual benefit /risk assessment.

This medicine contains lactose. Patients with rare hereditary problems of galactose intolerance, the Lapp lactase deficiency or glucose-galactose malabsorption should not take this medicine.

4.5 Interaction with other medicinal products and other forms of interaction

No formal interaction studies have been performed, however no clinically relevant interactions with other medicinal products were found during clinical trials.

In the risedronate sodium Phase III osteoporosis studies with daily dosing, acetyl salicylic acid or NSAID use was reported by 33% and 45% of patients respectively. In the Phase III once a week study in postmenopausal women, acetyl salicylic acid or NSAID use was reported by 57% and 40% of patients respectively. Among regular acetyl salicylic acid or NSAID users (3 or more days per week) the incidence of upper gastrointestinal adverse events in risedronate sodium treated patients was similar to that in control patients.

If considered appropriate risedronate sodium may be used concomitantly with oestrogen supplementation (for women only).

Concomitant ingestion of medications containing polyvalent cations (e.g. calcium, magnesium, iron and aluminium) will interfere with the absorption of risedronate sodium (see section 4.4).

Risedronate sodium is not systemically metabolised, does not induce cytochrome P450 enzymes, and has low protein binding.

4.6 Pregnancy and lactation

There are no adequate data from the use of risedronate sodium in pregnant women. Studies in animals have shown reproductive toxicity (see section 5.3). The potential risk for humans is unknown. Studies in animal indicate that a small amount of risedronate sodium pass into breast milk.

Risedronate sodium must not be used during pregnancy or by breast-feeding women.

4.7 Effects on ability to drive and use machines

No effects on ability to drive and use machines have been observed.

4.8 Undesirable effects

Risedronate sodium has been studied in phase III clinical trials involving more than 15,000 patients. The majority of undesirable effects observed in clinical trials were mild to moderate in severity and usually did not require cessation of therapy.

Adverse experiences reported in phase III clinical trials in postmenopausal women with osteoporosis treated for up to 36 months with risedronate sodium 5mg/day (n=5020) or placebo (n=5048) and considered possibly or probably related to risedronate sodium are listed below using the following convention (incidences versus placebo are shown in brackets): very common ($\geqslant$1/10); common ($\geqslant$1/100; <1/10); uncommon ($\geqslant$1/1,000; <1/100); rare ($\geqslant$1/10,000; <1/1,000); very rare (<1/10,000).

Nervous system disorders:

Common: headache (1.8% vs. 1.4%)

Eye disorders:

Uncommon: iritis*

Gastrointestinal disorders:

Common: constipation (5.0% vs. 4.8%), dyspepsia (4.5% vs. 4.1%), nausea (4.3% vs. 4.0%), abdominal pain (3.5% vs. 3.3%), diarrhoea (3.0% vs. 2.7%)

Uncommon: gastritis (0.9% vs. 0.7%), oesophagitis (0.9% vs. 0.9%), dysphagia (0.4% vs. 0.2%), duodenitis (0.2% vs. 0.1%), oesophageal ulcer (0.2% vs. 0.2%)

Rare: glossitis (<0.1% vs. 0.1%), oesophageal strictu (<0.1% vs. 0.0%),

Musculoskeletal and connective tissues disorders:

Common: musculoskeletal pain (2.1% vs. 1.9%)

Investigations:

Rare: abnormal liver function tests*

* No relevant incidences from Phase III osteoporosis stu dies; frequency based on adverse event/laboratory/recha lenge findings in earlier clinical trials.

In a one-year, double-blind, multicentre study comparir risedronate sodium 5 mg daily (n= 480) and risedrona sodium 35 mg weekly (n=485) in postmenopausal wome with osteoporosis, the overall safety and tolerability profile were similar. The following additional adverse experience considered possibly or probably drug related by invest gators have been reported (incidence greater in risedr nate 35 mg than in risedronate sodium 5 mg grou gastrointestinal disorder (1.6% vs. 1.0%) and pain (1.2 vs. 0.8%).

In a 2-year study in men with osteoporosis, the overa safety and tolerability were similar between the treatme and the placebo groups. Adverse experiences were co sistent with those previously observed in women.

Laboratory findings: Early, transient, asymptomatic ar mild decreases in serum calcium and phosphate leve have been observed in some patients.

The following additional adverse reactions have be reported during post-marketing use (frequency unknow

Eye disorders:

iritis, uveitis

Muskuloskeletal and connective tissues disorders:

osteonecrosis of the jaw

Skin and subcutaneous tissue disorders:

hypersensitivity and skin reactions, including angioedem generalised rash, urticaria and bullous skin reactior some severe including isolated reports of Stevens Johns syndrome and toxic epidermal necrolysis.

hair loss

Immune system disorders:

anaphylactic reaction

Hepatobiliary disorders:

serious hepatic disorders. In most of the reported cas the patients were also treated with other products kno to cause hepatic disorders.

4.9 Overdose

No specific information is available on the treatment overdose with risedronate sodium.

Decreases in serum calcium following substantial ove dose may be expected. Signs and symptoms of hypoc caemia may also occur in some of these patients.

Milk or antacids containing magnesium, calcium or alu nium should be given to bind risedronate and redu absorption of risedronate sodium. In cases of substan overdose, gastric lavage may be considered to remo unabsorbed risedronate sodium.

5. PHARMACOLOGICAL PROPERTIES

5.1 Pharmacodynamic properties

Pharmaco-therapeutic group: Bisphosphonates

ATC Code: M05BA07.

Risedronate sodium is a pyridinyl bisphosphonate th binds to bone hydroxyapatite and inhibits osteocla mediated bone resorption. The bone turnover is reduc while the osteoblast activity and bone mineralisation preserved. In preclinical studies risedronate sodiu demonstrated potent anti-osteoclast and antiresorpti activity, and dose dependently increased bone mass a biomechanical skeletal strength. The activity of risedrona sodium was confirmed by measuring biochemical marke for bone turnover during pharmacodynamic and clini studies. In studies of post-menopausal women, decreas in biochemical markers of bone turnover were observ within 1 month and reached a maximum in 3-6 mont Decreases in biochemical markers of bone turnover we similar with Actonel Once a Week 35 mg and Actonel 5 r daily at 12 months.

In a study in men with osteoporosis, decreases in bioche ical markers of bone turnover were observed at the earlie time point of 3 months and continued to be observed at months.

Treatment of Postmenopausal Osteoporosis:

A number of risk factors are associated with postme pausal osteoporosis including low bone mass, low bo mineral density, early menopause, a history of smoking a a family history of osteoporosis. The clinical conseque of osteoporosis is fractures. The risk of fractures increased with the number of risk factors.

Based on effects on mean change in lumbar spine BM Actonel Once a Week 35 mg (n=485) was shown to quivalent to Actonel 5 mg daily (n=480) in a one-year, ouble-blind, multicentre study of postmenopausal omen with osteoporosis

he clinical programme for risedronate sodium adminis- ered once daily studied the effect of risedronate sodium n the risk of hip and vertebral fractures and contained arly and late postmenopausal women with and without acture. Daily doses of 2.5 mg and 5 mg were studied and ll groups, including the control groups, received calcium nd vitamin D (if baseline levels were low). The absolute nd relative risk of new vertebral and hip fractures were stimated by use of a time-to-first event analysis.

Two placebo-controlled trials (n=3661) enrolled postme- opausal women under 85 years with vertebral fractures at aseline. Risedronate sodium 5 mg daily given for 3 years educed the risk of new vertebral fractures relative to the ontrol group. In women with respectively at least 2 or at east 1 vertebral fractures, the relative risk reduction was 9% and 41% respectively (incidence of new vertebral ractures with risedronate sodium 18.1% and 11.3%, with lacebo 29.0% and 16.3%, respectively). The effect of reatment was seen as early as the end of the first year f treatment. Benefits were also demonstrated in women with multiple fractures at baseline. Risedronate sodium mg daily also reduced the yearly height loss compared o the control group.

Two further placebo controlled trials enrolled postmeno- ausal women above 70 years with or without vertebral ractures at baseline. Women 70-79 years were enrolled with femoral neck BMD T-score <-3 SD (manufacturer's ange, i.e. -2.5 SD using NHANES III) and at least one additional risk factor. Women ≥80 years could be enrolled on the basis of at least one non-skeletal risk factor for hip racture or low bone mineral density at the femoral neck. Statistical significance of the efficacy of risedronate versus lacebo is only reached when the two treatment groups 2.5 mg and 5 mg are pooled. The following results are only based on *a-posteriori* analysis of subgroups defined by clinical practise and current definitions of osteoporosis:

- In the subgroup of patients with femoral neck BMD T-score ≤-2.5SD (NHANES III) and at least one vertebral racture at baseline, risedronate sodium given for 3 years educed the risk of hip fractures by 46% relative to the control group (incidence of hip fractures in combined rise- dronate sodium 2.5 and 5 mg groups 3.8%, placebo 7.4%);
- Data suggest that a more limited protection than this may be observed in the very elderly (≥80 years). This may be due to the increasing importance of non-skeletal factors for hip fracture with increasing age.

In these trials, data analysed as a secondary endpoint indicated a decrease in the risk of new vertebral fractures in patients with low femoral neck BMD without vertebral fracture and in patients with low femoral neck BMD with or without vertebral fracture.

- Risedronate sodium 5 mg daily given for 3 years increased bone mineral density (BMD) relative to control at the lumbar spine, femoral neck, trochanter and wrist and maintained bone density at the mid-shaft radius.
- In a one-year follow-up off therapy after three years treatment with risedronate sodium 5 mg daily there was rapid reversibility of the suppressing effect of risedronate sodium on bone turnover rate.
- Bone biopsy samples from postmenopausal women treated with risedronate sodium 5 mg daily for 2 to 3 years, showed an expected moderate decrease in bone turnover. Bone formed during risedronate sodium treatment was of normal lamellar structure and bone mineralisation. These data together with the decreased incidence of osteoporo- sis related fractures at vertebral sites in women with osteo- porosis appear to indicate no detrimental effect on bone quality.

Endoscopic findings from a number of patients with a number of moderate to severe gastrointestinal complaints in both risedronate sodium and control patients indicated no evidence of treatment related gastric, duodenal or oesophageal ulcers in either group, although duodenitis was uncommonly observed in the risedronate sodium group.

Treatment of Osteoporosis in Men

Risedronate sodium 35mg once a week demonstrated efficacy in men with osteoporosis (age range 36 to 84 years) in a 2-year, double-blind, placebo-controlled study in 284 patients (risedronate sodium 35mg n = 191). All patients received supplemental calcium and vitamin D.

Increases in BMD were observed as early as 6 months following initiation of risedronate sodium treatment. Rise- dronate sodium 35mg once a week produced mean increases in BMD at the lumbar spine, femoral neck, tro- chanter and total hip compared to placebo after 2 years of treatment. Antifracture efficacy was not demonstrated in this study.

The bone effect (BMD increase and BTM decrease) of risedronate sodium is similar in males and females.

5.2 Pharmacokinetic properties

Absorption: Absorption after an oral dose is relatively rapid (t_{max} ~1 hour) and is independent of dose over the range studied (single dose study, 2.5 to 30 mg; multiple dose studies, 2.5 to 5 mg daily and up to 50 mg dosed weekly). Mean oral bioavailability of the tablet is 0.63% and is decreased when risedronate sodium is administered with food. Bioavailability was similar in men and women.

Distribution: The mean steady state volume of distribution is 6.3 l/kg in humans. Plasma protein binding is about 24%.

Metabolism: There is no evidence of systemic metabolism of risedronate sodium.

Elimination: Approximately half of the absorbed dose is excreted in urine within 24 hours, and 85% of an intrave- nous dose is recovered in the urine after 28 days. Mean renal clearance is 105 ml/min and mean total clearance is 122 ml/min, with the difference probably attributed to clearance due to adsorption to bone. The renal clearance is not concentration dependent, and there is a linear rela- tionship between renal clearance and creatinine clearance. Unabsorbed risedronate sodium is eliminated unchanged in faeces. After oral administration the concentration-time profile shows three elimination phases with a terminal half- life of 480 hours.

Special Populations

Elderly: no dosage adjustment is necessary.

Acetyl salicylic acid/NSAID users: Among regular acetyl salicylic acid or NSAID users (3 or more days per week) the incidence of upper gastrointestinal adverse events in rise- dronate sodium treated patients was similar to that in control patients.

5.3 Preclinical safety data

In toxicological studies in rat and dog dose dependent liver toxic effects of risedronate sodium were seen, primarily as enzyme increases with histological changes in rat. The clinical relevance of these observations is unknown. Tes- ticular toxicity occurred in rat and dog at exposures con- sidered in excess of the human therapeutic exposure. Dose related incidences of upper airway irritation were frequently noted in rodents. Similar effects have been seen with other bisphosphonates. Lower respiratory tract effects were also seen in longer term studies in rodents, although the clinical significance of these findings is unclear. In reproduction toxicity studies at exposures close to clinical exposure ossification changes were seen in sternum and/or skull of foetuses from treated rats and hypocalcemia and mortality in pregnant females allowed to deliver. There was no evidence of teratogenesis at 3.2mg/kg/day in rat and 10mg/kg/day in rabbit, although data are only available on a small number of rabbits. Maternal toxicity prevented testing of higher doses. Stu- dies on genotoxicity and carcinogenesis did not show any particular risks for humans.

6. PHARMACEUTICAL PARTICULARS

6.1 List of excipients

Tablet core: Lactose monohydrate,
Cellulose microcrystalline,
Crospovidone A,
Magnesium stearate.

Film coating: Iron oxide yellow E172
Iron oxide red E172
Hypromellose
Macrogol
Hyprolose
Silicon dioxide
Titanium dioxide E171

6.2 Incompatibilities

Not applicable.

6.3 Shelf life

3 years.

6.4 Special precautions for storage

This medicinal product does not require any special sto- rage conditions.

6.5 Nature and contents of container

Clear PVC/aluminium foil blisters in a cardboard carton.

Blisters in packs containing 1, 2, 4, 10, 12, or 16 tablets.

Not all pack sizes may be marketed.

6.6 Special precautions for disposal and other handling

No special requirements.

7. MARKETING AUTHORISATION HOLDER

Procter & Gamble Pharmaceuticals UK Ltd.,
Rusham Park,
Whitehall Lane,
Egham,
Surrey,
TW20 9NW, UK

8. MARKETING AUTHORISATION NUMBER(S)

PL 00364/0080

9. DATE OF FIRST AUTHORISATION/RENEWAL OF THE AUTHORISATION

3 December 2002/19 July 2007

10. DATE OF REVISION OF THE TEXT

19 September 2008

Actrapid 100 IU/ml, Solution for Injection in a vial

(Novo Nordisk Limited)

1. NAME OF THE MEDICINAL PRODUCT

Actrapid 100 IU/ml solution for injection in a vial

2. QUALITATIVE AND QUANTITATIVE COMPOSITION

Insulin human, rDNA (produced by recombinant DNA tech- nology in *Saccharomyces cerevisiae*).

1 ml contains 100 IU of insulin human

1 vial contains 10 ml equivalent to 1000 IU

One IU (International Unit) corresponds to 0.035 mg of anhydrous human insulin.

For a full list of excipients, see section 6.1.

3. PHARMACEUTICAL FORM

Solution for injection in a vial.

Clear, colourless, aqueous solution.

4. CLINICAL PARTICULARS

4.1 Therapeutic indications

Treatment of diabetes mellitus.

4.2 Posology and method of administration

Actrapid is a fast-acting insulin and may be used in com- bination with long-acting insulin products.

Dosage

Dosage is individual and determined in accordance with the needs of the patient. The individual insulin requirement is usually between 0.3 and 1.0 IU/kg/day. The daily insulin requirement may be higher in patients with insulin resis- tance (e.g. during puberty or due to obesity) and lower in patients with residual, endogenous insulin production.

In patients with diabetes mellitus optimised glycaemic control delays the onset of late diabetic complications. Close blood glucose monitoring is therefore recom- mended.

An injection should be followed within 30 minutes by a meal or snack containing carbohydrates.

Dosage adjustment

Concomitant illness, especially infections and feverish conditions, usually increases the patient's insulin require- ment.

Renal or hepatic impairment may reduce insulin require- ment.

Adjustment of dosage may also be necessary if patients change physical activity or their usual diet.

Dosage adjustment may be necessary when transferring patients from one insulin preparation to another (see sec- tion 4.4).

Administration

For subcutaneous or intravenous use. Actrapid may also be administered intravenously, which should only be car- ried out by health care professionals.

Actrapid is administered subcutaneously in the abdominal wall. The thigh, the gluteal region or the deltoid region may also be used.

Subcutaneous injection into the abdominal wall ensures a faster absorption than from other injection sites.

Injection into a lifted skin fold minimises the risk of unin- tended intramuscular injection.

The needle should be kept under the skin for at least 6 seconds to make sure the entire dose is injected.

Injection sites should be rotated within an anatomic region in order to avoid lipodystrophy.

The vials are for use with insulin syringes with a corre- sponding unit scale. When two types of insulin are mixed, draw the amount of fast-acting insulin first, followed by the amount of long-acting insulin.

Actrapid is accompanied by a package leaflet with detailed instruction for use to be followed.

4.3 Contraindications

Hypersensitivity to the active substance or to any of the excipients (see section 6.1).

Hypoglycaemia

4.4 Special warnings and precautions for use

Inadequate dosage or discontinuation of treatment, espe- cially in type 1 diabetes, may lead to **hyperglycaemia**.

Usually the first symptoms of hyperglycaemia set in gra- dually, over a period of hours or days. They include thirst, increased frequency of urination, nausea, vomiting, drow- siness, flushed dry skin, dry mouth, loss of appetite as well as acetone odour of breath.

In type 1 diabetes, untreated hyperglycaemic events even- tually lead to diabetic ketoacidosis, which is potentially lethal.

Hypoglycaemia may occur if the insulin dose is too high in relation to the insulin requirement (see sections 4.8 and 4.9).

Omission of a meal or unplanned, strenuous physical exer- cise may lead to hypoglycaemia.

Patients whose blood glucose control is greatly improved e.g. by intensified insulin therapy, may experience a change in their usual warning symptoms of hypoglycaemia and should be advised accordingly. Usual warning symptoms may disappear in patients with long-standing diabetes.

Transferring a patient to another type or brand of insulin should be done under strict medical supervision. Changes in strength, brand (manufacturer), type (fast-, dual-, long-acting insulin etc.), origin (animal, human or analogue insulin) and/or method of manufacture (recombinant DNA versus animal source insulin) may result in a need for a change in dosage. If an adjustment is needed when switching the patients to Actrapid, it may occur with the first dose or during the first several weeks or months.

As with any insulin therapy, injection site reactions may occur and include pain, itching, hives, swelling and inflammation. Continuous rotation of the injection site within a given area may help to reduce or prevent these reactions. Reactions usually resolve in a few days to a few weeks. On rare occasions, injection site reactions may require discontinuation of Actrapid.

A few patients who have experienced hypoglycaemic reactions after transfer from animal source insulin have reported that early warning symptoms of hypoglycaemia were less pronounced or different from those experienced with their previous insulin.

Before travelling between different time zones, the patient should be advised to consult the physician, since this may mean that the patient has to take insulin and meals at different times.

Due to the risk of precipitation in pump catheters, Actrapid should not be used in insulin pumps for continuous subcutaneous insulin infusion.

Actrapid contains metacresol, which may cause allergic reactions.

4.5 Interaction with other medicinal products and other forms of interaction

A number of medicinal products are known to interact with glucose metabolism. The physician must therefore take possible interactions into account and should always ask his patients about any medicinal products they take.

The following substances may reduce insulin requirement:

Oral hypoglycaemic agents (OHA), monoamine oxidase inhibitors (MAOI), non-selective beta-blocking agents, angiotensin converting enzyme (ACE) inhibitors, salicylates, alcohol, anabolic steroids and sulphonamides.

The following substances may increase insulin requirement:

Oral contraceptives, thiazides, glucocorticoids, thyroid hormones and beta-sympathomimetics, growth hormone and danazol.

Beta-blocking agents may mask the symptoms of hypoglycaemia and delay recovery from hypoglycaemia.

Octreotide/lanreotide may both decrease and increase insulin requirement.

Alcohol may intensify and prolong the hypoglycaemic effect of insulin.

4.6 Pregnancy and lactation

There are no restrictions on treatment of diabetes with insulin during pregnancy, as insulin does not pass the placental barrier.

Both hypoglycaemia and hyperglycaemia, which can occur in inadequately controlled diabetes therapy, increase the risk of malformations and death *in utero*. Intensified control in the treatment of pregnant women with diabetes is therefore recommended throughout pregnancy and when contemplating pregnancy.

Insulin requirements usually fall in the first trimester and subsequently increase during the second and third trimesters.

After delivery, insulin requirements return rapidly to pre-pregnancy values.

Insulin treatment of the nursing mother presents no risk to the baby. However, the Actrapid dosage may need to be adjusted.

4.7 Effects on ability to drive and use machines

The patient's ability to concentrate and react may be impaired as a result of hypoglycaemia. This may constitute a risk in situations where these abilities are of special importance (e.g. driving a car or operating machinery).

Patients should be advised to take precautions to avoid hypoglycaemia whilst driving. This is particularly important in those who have reduced or absent awareness of the warning signs of hypoglycaemia or have frequent episodes of hypoglycaemia. The advisability of driving should be considered in these circumstances.

4.8 Undesirable effects

As for other insulin products, in general, hypoglycaemia is the most frequently occurring undesirable effect. It may occur if the insulin dose is too high in relation to the insulin requirement. In clinical trials and during marketed use the frequency varies with patient population and dose regimens. Therefore, no specific frequency can be presented. Severe hypoglycaemia may lead to unconsciousness and/or convulsions and may result in temporary or permanent impairment of brain function or even death.

Frequencies of adverse drug reactions from clinical trials that are considered related to Actrapid, are listed below. The frequencies are defined as: uncommon (≥1/1000, < 1/100). Isolated spontaneous cases are presented as very rare defined as < 1/10,000, including isolated reports. Within each frequency grouping, undesirable effects are presented in order of decreasing seriousness.

Nervous system disorders

Uncommon – Peripheral neuropathy

Fast improvement in blood glucose control may be associated with a condition termed "acute painful neuropathy", which is usually reversible.

Eye disorders

Uncommon – Refraction disorders

Refraction anomalies may occur upon initiation of insulin therapy. These symptoms are usually of transitory nature.

Very rare – Diabetic retinopathy

Long-term improved glycaemic control decreases the risk of progression of diabetic retinopathy. However, intensification of insulin therapy with abrupt improvement in glycaemic control may be associated with temporary worsening of diabetic retinopathy.

Skin and subcutaneous tissue disorders

Uncommon – Lipodystrophy

Lipodystrophy may occur at the injection site as a consequence of failure to rotate injection sites within an area.

General disorders and administration site conditions

Uncommon – Injection site reactions

Injection site reactions (redness, swelling, itching, pain and haematoma at the injection site) may occur during treatment with insulin. Most reactions are transitory and disappear during continued treatment.

Uncommon – Oedema

Oedema may occur upon initiation of insulin therapy. These symptoms are usually of transitory nature.

Immune system disorders

Uncommon – Urticaria, rash

Very rare – Anaphylactic reactions

Symptoms of generalised hypersensitivity may include generalised skin rash, itching, sweating, gastrointestinal upset, angioneurotic oedema, difficulties in breathing, palpitation, reduction in blood pressure and fainting/loss of consciousness. Generalised hypersensitivity reactions are potentially life threatening.

4.9 Overdose

A specific overdose of insulin cannot be defined. However, hypoglycaemia may develop over sequential stages:

- Mild hypoglycaemic episodes can be treated by oral administration of glucose or sugary products. It is therefore recommended that the diabetic patients carry some sugar lumps, sweets, biscuits or sugary fruit juice.
- Severe hypoglycaemic episodes, where the patient has become unconscious, can be treated by glucagon (0.5 to 1 mg) given intramuscularly or subcutaneously by a person who has received appropriate instruction, or by glucose given intravenously by a medical professional. Glucose must also be given intravenously, if the patient does not respond to glucagon within 10 to 15 minutes.

Upon regaining consciousness, administration of oral carbohydrate is recommended for the patient in order to prevent relapse.

5. PHARMACOLOGICAL PROPERTIES

5.1 Pharmacodynamic properties

Pharmacotherapeutic group: insulins and analogues for injection, fast-acting, insulin (human). ATC code: A10A B01.

The blood glucose lowering effect of insulin is due to the facilitated uptake of glucose following binding of insulin to receptors on muscle and fat cells and to the simultaneous inhibition of glucose output from the liver.

A clinical trial in a single intensive care unit treating hyperglycaemia (blood glucose above 10 mmol/L) in 204 diabetic and 1344 non-diabetic patients undergoing major surgery showed that normoglycaemia (blood glucose 4.4 – 6.1 mmol/L) induced by intravenous Actrapid reduced mortality by 42% (8% versus 4.6%).

Actrapid is a fast-acting insulin.

Onset of action is within ½ hour, reaches a maximum effect within 1.5-3.5 hours and the entire time of duration is approximately 7-8 hours.

5.2 Pharmacokinetic properties

Insulin in the blood stream has a half-life of a few minutes. Consequently, the time-action profile of an insulin preparation is determined solely by its absorption characteristics.

This process is influenced by several factors (e.g. insulin dosage, injection route and site, thickness of subcutaneous fat, type of diabetes). The pharmacokinetics of insulin products are therefore affected by significant intra- and inter-individual variation.

Absorption

The maximum plasma concentration is reached within 1.5-2.5 hours after subcutaneous administration.

Distribution

No profound binding to plasma proteins, except circulatin insulin antibodies (if present) has been observed.

Metabolism

Human insulin is reported to be degraded by insulin pro tease or insulin-degrading enzymes and possibly protei disulfide isomerase. A number of cleavage (hydrolysis sites on the human insulin molecule have been proposed none of the metabolites formed following the cleavage ar active.

Elimination

The terminal half-life is determined by the rate of absorp tion from the subcutaneous tissue. The terminal half-lif ($t_{½}$) is therefore a measure of the absorption rather than c the elimination *per se* of insulin from plasma (insulin in th blood stream has a $t_{½}$ of a few minutes). Trials hav indicated a $t_{½}$ of about 2-5 hours.

Children and adolescents

The pharmacokinetic profile of Actrapid has been studie in a small number (n=18) of diabetic children (aged 6-1 years) and adolescents (aged 13-17 years). The data ar limited but suggest that the pharmacokinetic profile i children and adolescents may be similar to that in adults However, there were differences between age groups i C_{max}, stressing the importance of individual titration o human insulin.

5.3 Preclinical safety data

Non-clinical data reveal no special hazard for humans based on conventional studies of safety pharmacology repeated dose toxicity, genotoxicity, carcinogenic potential, toxicity to reproduction.

6. PHARMACEUTICAL PARTICULARS

6.1 List of excipients

Zinc chloride

Glycerol

Metacresol

Sodium hydroxide (for pH adjustment)

Hydrochloric acid (for pH adjustment)

Water for injections

6.2 Incompatibilities

Insulin products should only be added to compounds with which it is known to be compatible. Medicinal products added to the insulin solution may cause degradation of the insulin, e.g. if the medicinal products contain thiols or sulphites.

6.3 Shelf life

30 months when stored between 2°C-8°C.

6 weeks when used or stored at room temperature (below 25°C).

6.4 Special precautions for storage

Before use: Store in a refrigerator (2°C - 8°C).

Do not store them in or too near the freezer section or cooling element.

Do not freeze.

During use: do not refrigerate. Do not store above 25°C.

Keep the vial in the outer carton in order to protect from light.

Protect from excessive heat and sunlight.

6.5 Nature and contents of container

10 ml glass vial (type 1) closed with a bromobutyl/polyisoprene rubber stopper and a protective tamper-proof plastic cap.

Pack size: 1 × 10 ml.

6.6 Special precautions for disposal and other handling

For intravenous use, infusion systems with Actrapid at concentrations 0.05 IU/ml – 1.0 IU/ml insulin human in the following infusion fluids: 0.9% sodium chloride, 5% dextrose and 10% dextrose inclusive 40 mmol/l potassium chloride, using polypropylene infusion bags, are stable at room temperature for 24 hours. Although stable over time, a certain amount of insulin will initially be absorbed to the material of the infusion bag. Monitoring of blood glucose is necessary during the infusion.

Insulin preparations, which have been frozen must not be used.

Insulin solutions should not be used if they do not appear water clear and colourless.

Actrapid should not be used in insulin pumps for continuous subcutaneous insulin infusion.

Any unused product or waste material should be disposed of in accordance with local requirements.

7. MARKETING AUTHORISATION HOLDER

Novo Nordisk A/S

Novo Allé

DK-2880 Bagsværd

Denmark

8. MARKETING AUTHORISATION NUMBER(S)

Actrapid 100 IU/ml EU/1/02/230/003

9. DATE OF FIRST AUTHORISATION/RENEWAL OF THE AUTHORISATION

Date of first authorisation: 07 October 2002

Date of last renewal: 18 October 2007

. DATE OF REVISION OF THE TEXT

/2007

egal Status

OM

Acular

(Allergan Ltd)

NAME OF THE MEDICINAL PRODUCT

cular®.

QUALITATIVE AND QUANTITATIVE COMPOSITION

etorolac trometamol 0.5% w/v.

or excipients, see 6.1.

PHARMACEUTICAL FORM

ye drops, solution.

CLINICAL PARTICULARS

.1 Therapeutic indications

cular® is indicated for the prophylaxis and reduction of flammation and associated symptoms following ocular urgery.

.2 Posology and method of administration

oute of administration: Ocular.

ne drop instilled into the eye three times daily starting 24 ours pre-operatively and continuing for up to three weeks ost-operatively.

o special dosage for the elderly.

.3 Contraindications

cular® is contra-indicated in individuals hypersensitive to ny component of the medication.

he potential exists for cross-sensitivity to acetylsalicylic cid and other non-steroidal anti-inflammatory drugs. Acuar® is contra-indicated in individuals who have previously xhibited sensitivities to these drugs.

cular® is contra-indicated in children, and during pregancy or lactation.

.4 Special warnings and precautions for use

t is recommended that Acular® be used with caution in atients with known bleeding tendencies or who are eceiving other medications which may prolong bleeding ime, or patients with a known history of peptic ulceration.

n common with other anti-inflammatory drugs, Acular® may mask the usual signs of infection.

Concomitant use of Acular® and topical corticosteroids should be exercised with caution in patients susceptible to corneal epithelial breakdown.

Acular® contains benzalkonium chloride as a preservative and should not be used in patients continuing to wear soft (hydrophilic) contact lenses (since benzalkonium chloride is known to discolour this lens-type). Contact lenses should not be worn during instillation of the drug. After instillation there should be an interval of at least 15 minutes before reinsertion.

4.5 Interaction with other medicinal products and other forms of interaction

Acular® has been safely administered with systemic and ophthalmic medications such as antibiotics, sedatives, beta blockers, carbonic anhydrase inhibitors, miotics, mydriatics and cycloplegics.

Acular® may slow or delay healing. Topical corticosteroids are also known to slow or delay healing. Concomitant use of topical NSAIDs and topical corticosteroids may increase the potential for healing problems.

If Acular® is used concomitantly with other topical eye medications there must be an interval of at least 5 minutes between the two medications.

4.6 Pregnancy and lactation

There was no evidence of teratogenicity in rats or rabbits studied at maternally-toxic doses of ketorolac. Prolongation of the gestation period and/or delayed parturition were seen in the rat. Ketorolac and its metabolites have been shown to pass into the foetus and milk of animals. Ketorolac has been detected in human milk at low levels. Safety in human pregnancy has not been established. Ketorolac is therefore contra-indicated during pregnancy, labour or delivery, or in mothers who are breast feeding.

4.7 Effects on ability to drive and use machines

Transient blurring of vision may occur on instillation of eye drops. Do not drive or use hazardous machinery unless vision is clear.

4.8 Undesirable effects

a) The most frequent adverse events reported with the use of Acular® are transient stinging and burning on instillation.

The events below are classified according to their incidence in clinical trials.

b) Very Common (>1/10):

Ocular irritation or burning

Common (>1/100, <1/10):

Superficial punctate keratitis (SPK)

Eye pain or stinging

Hypersensitivity

Eye and/or eyelid oedema

Eye pruritus

Conjunctival / ocular hyperaemia

Rare (>1/10,000, <1/1,000):

Corneal ulcer (Ulcerative keratitis)

Corneal infiltrates

Blurred and/or diminished vision

Headache

Eye dryness

Lacrimation increased

c) Occasional post marketing reports of corneal damage including corneal thinning, corneal erosion, epithelial breakdown and corneal perforation have been received. These occurred mainly in patients using concomitant topical corticosteroids and/or with predisposing co-morbidity. See warnings and precautions section 4.4.

d) None of the typical adverse reactions reported with the use of systemic non-steroidal anti-inflammatory agents (including ketorolac trometamol) have been observed at the doses used in topical ophthalmic therapy.

4.9 Overdose

There is no experience of overdose by the ophthalmic route. Overdose is unlikely to occur via the recommended method of administration.

5. PHARMACOLOGICAL PROPERTIES

5.1 Pharmacodynamic properties

Pharmacotherapeutic classification (ATC) code: *S01BC* 05.

Acular® (ketorolac trometamol) is a non-steroidal anti-inflammatory agent demonstrating analgesic and anti-inflammatory activity. Ketorolac trometamol inhibits the cyclo-oxygenase enzyme essential for biosynthesis of prostaglandins. Acular® has been shown to reduce prostaglandin levels in the aqueous humour after topical ophthalmic administration.

Ketorolac trometamol given systemically does not cause pupil constriction. Results from clinical studies indicate that Acular® has no significant effect on intra-ocular pressure.

5.2 Pharmacokinetic properties

a) General characteristics

Absorption

Rabbit aqueous humor bioavailability:

Mean concentration of total radioactivity	0.856 μg-equiv./ml @ 0.5 hr 1.607 μg-equiv./ml @ 2 hr
T_{max}	3.38 hr
C_{max}	1.905 μg-equiv./ml
AUC (0-8 hr)	9.39 μg-equiv. hr/ml
Total AUC	13.53 μg-equiv. hr/ml
Half-life	3.77 hr
Absolute ocular bioavailability	3.7%

After topical ocular doses in the rabbit the half life of total radioactivity in aqueous humor was longer than after intracameral injection. This suggests that topical dosing may lead to a "reservoir" effect in the corneal epithelium and continued flux of drug from the reservoir into the aqueous humor.

Distribution

After ophthalmic doses were administered to rabbits, peak concentrations of radioactivity were achieved within 1 hour in the ocular tissues and were highest in the cornea (6.06 mcg-eq/ml). At 1 hour, the majority of the radioactivity (0.9% of administered dose) was recovered from the sclera (0.58%) and cornea (0.24%), and smaller amounts were recovered from the aqueous humor (0.026%), vitreous humor (0.023%), retina-choroid (0.018%), iris-ciliary body (0.007%) and lens (0.002%).

Relative to plasma AUC values, the AUC's in rabbits were higher for cornea (104 fold), sclera (27 fold), iris-ciliary body (5.8 fold), retina-choroid (5.6 fold) aqueous humor (3.3 fold) and approximately one-half in the vitreous humor and lens. After ophthalmic administration, concentrations of drug-related radioactivity were higher in the ocular tissues and lower in plasma compared with those after IV dosing.

Systemic Absorption

After ophthalmic doses in the rabbit, ketorolac was absorbed rapidly into the systemic circulation (T_{max}, 15 min). Plasma half-lives after ophthalmic doses (6.6 - 6.9 hr) were longer than those after IV administration (1.1 hr), suggesting that removal of drug from eye into the venous circulation may be rate-limiting. By comparison of drug levels in aqueous humor after intracameral injection vs. plasma levels after IV administration, ketorolac was shown to clear more rapidly from plasma (6 ml/min) than from the anterior chamber (11 mcl/min).

In the cynomolgus monkey, peak plasma levels of ketorolac occurred at 1.1 hr after the ophthalmic dose. The plasma half-life of ketorolac was similar after ophthalmic (1.8 hr) and IV doses (1.6 hr).

The majority of the ophthalmic dose was excreted in urine (66% in rabbit and 75% in monkey) and a small amount in faeces (11% in rabbit and 2% in monkey). The extent of systemic absorption after ophthalmic dosing averaged 73% in the rabbit and 76% in the cynomolgus monkey.

Metabolism

After ophthalmic administration in rabbits, ketorolac represented the major component (more than 90%) of radioactivity in aqueous humor and plasma and the p-hydroxy metabolite accounted for 5% of radioactivity in plasma. Ketorolac was also the major component (96%) of plasma radioactivity after ophthalmic dosing in monkeys.

After ophthalmic dosing in the rabbit, 72%, 17% and 6% of the total radioactivity in urine was comprised of intact ketorolac, p-hydroxy ketorolac and other polar metabolites, respectively. After IV dosing, the relative proportions of total radioactivity in urine averaged 6% as intact ketorolac, 68% as p-hydroxy ketorolac and 22% as polar metabolites.

In the monkey, intact ketorolac and its polar metabolite accounted for 32% and 65% of the total radioactivity in urine, respectively, after ophthalmic dosing, and 50% and 49% of the radioactivity in urine, respectively, after IV dosing. Thus, the metabolism of ketorolac was qualitatively similar after ophthalmic and IV administration in the monkey and rabbit.

b) Characteristics in patients

Ketorolac tromethamine solutions (0.1% or 0.5%) or vehicle were instilled into the eyes of patients approximately 12 hours and 1 hour prior to surgery. Concentrations of ketorolac in aqueous humor sampled at the time of surgery were at the lower limit of detection (40 ng/ml) in 1 patient and below the quantitation limit in 7 patients dosed with 0.1% ketorolac tromethamine. The average aqueous humor level of ketorolac in patients treated with 0.5% ketorolac tromethamine was 95 ng/ml. Concentrations of PGE_2 in aqueous humor were 80 pg/ml, 40 pg/ml and 28 pg/ml in patients treated with vehicle, 0.1% ketorolac tromethamine and 0.5% ketorolac tromethamine, respectively.

In the 21-day multiple dose (TID) tolerance study in healthy subjects, only 1 of 13 subjects had a detectable plasma level pre-dose (0.021 μg/ml). In another group of 13 subjects, only 4 subjects showed very low plasma levels of ketorolac (0.011 to 0.023 μg/ml) 15 minutes after the ocular dose.

Thus, higher levels of ketorolac in the aqueous humor and very low or no detectable plasma levels after ophthalmic doses, suggest that the use of ketorolac tromethamine by the ophthalmic route in treatment of ocular disorders results in quite low systemic absorption in patients.

5.3 Preclinical safety data

Acute, sub-acute and chronic studies of Acular® in experimental animals have established the safety of the drug. In addition, octoxynol 40 was separately evaluated for its ocular safety. Acular® was found to be non-irritating, it did not demonstrate a local anaesthetic effect, it did not influence the healing of experimental corneal wounds in rabbits, it did not enhance the spread of experimental ocular infections of Candida albicans, Herpes simplex virus type one, or Pseudomonas aeruginosa in rabbits, and it did not increase the ocular pressure of normal rabbit eyes.

6. PHARMACEUTICAL PARTICULARS

6.1 List of excipients

Sodium chloride Ph Eur

Benzalkonium chloride Ph Eur

Edetate disodium Ph Eur

Octoxynol 40

1N Sodium hydroxide Ph Eur or 1N Hydrochloric acid Ph Eur, to adjust pH

Purified water Ph Eur

6.2 Incompatibilities

None known.

6.3 Shelf life

24 months, unopened.

Discard any unused contents 28 days after opening the bottle.

6.4 Special precautions for storage

None.

6.5 Nature and contents of container

Bottle with dropper applicator, containing clear, colourless to slightly yellow, sterile ophthalmic solution. Pack sizes: 3, 5 and 10 ml.

6.6 Special precautions for disposal and other handling

None.

7. MARKETING AUTHORISATION HOLDER

Allergan Ltd.

Marlow International

The Parkway

Marlow

Bucks SL7 1YL

United Kingdom

8. MARKETING AUTHORISATION NUMBER(S)

PL 00426/0082

9. DATE OF FIRST AUTHORISATION/RENEWAL OF THE AUTHORISATION

27th July 2006

10. DATE OF REVISION OF THE TEXT

24th November 2006

ACWY Vax Vaccine

(GlaxoSmithKline UK)

1. NAME OF THE MEDICINAL PRODUCT

ACWY Vax ▼- powder and solvent for solution for injection in a pre-filled syringe

Meningococcal polysaccharide groups A, C, Y and W_{135} vaccine

2. QUALITATIVE AND QUANTITATIVE COMPOSITION

After reconstitution, 1 dose (0.5 ml) contains:

Neisseria meningitidis group A 50 µg

Neisseria meningitidis group C 50 µg

Neisseria meningitidis group Y 50 µg

Neisseria meningitidis group W_{135} 50 µg

For a full list of excipients, see section 6.1.

3. PHARMACEUTICAL FORM

Powder and solvent for solution for injection in a pre-filled syringe.

The powder is white. The solvent is clear and colourless.

4. CLINICAL PARTICULARS

4.1 Therapeutic indications

Active immunisation of children older than 2 years, adolescents and adults against invasive meningococcal disease caused by meningococci of groups A, C, W_{135} and Y.

ACWY Vax should be used in accordance with available official recommendations.

4.2 Posology and method of administration

Posology

One dose of 0.5 ml.

Subjects who remain at increased risk of invasive meningococcal disease may be revaccinated at intervals (see persistence of immune response in Section 5.1). Intervals should be in accordance with available official recommendations.

Method of administration

ACWY Vax is for deep subcutaneous injection only.

4.3 Contraindications

Hypersensitivity to the active substances or to any of the excipients.

Hypersensitivity after previous administration of ACWY Vax.

As with other vaccines, the administration of ACWY Vax should be postponed in subjects suffering from acute severe febrile illness. The presence of a minor infection, such as a cold, is not a contra-indication for immunisation.

4.4 Special warnings and precautions for use

As with all injectable vaccines, appropriate medical treatment should always be readily available in case of anaphylactic reactions following the administration of the vaccine.

Vaccination should be preceded by a review of the medical history (especially with regard to previous vaccination and possible occurrence of undesirable events) and a clinical examination.

ACWY Vax should under no circumstances be administered intravascularly or intradermally.

ACWY Vax will only confer protection against *Neisseria meningitidis* groups A, C, W_{135} and Y. Protection cannot be guaranteed in every individual vaccinated.

The vaccine may not elicit a protective immune response in subjects with impaired immune systems.

Group C, W_{135} and Y polysaccharides are poorly immunogenic in children less than 24 months of age. Group A polysaccharide induces an antibody response in children from the age of 6 months. However, the response is lower than that observed in older subjects and may be transient.

Group C polysaccharide may induce immunological hyporesponsiveness to further doses of polysaccharide C or to meningococcal group C conjugate vaccine. The clinical relevance of this phenomenon remains unknown.

4.5 Interaction with other medicinal products and other forms of interaction

There are no data on concomitant administration of ACWY Vax and other vaccines.

Different injection sites should be used when concomitant administration with other injectable vaccines can not be avoided.

4.6 Pregnancy and lactation

Pregnancy

Adequate human data on use during pregnancy and adequate animal reproduction studies are not available.

Nevertheless, vaccination during pregnancy may be considered when there is an increased risk for meningococcal disease.

Lactation

Adequate data on the administration of ACWY Vax to women who are breast-feeding are not available.

However, ACWY Vax may be administered to breast-feeding women when there is an increased risk of meningococcal disease.

4.7 Effects on ability to drive and use machines

The vaccine is unlikely to produce an effect on the ability to drive and use machines.

4.8 Undesirable effects

In recent clinical studies, ACWY Vax was administered to 502 subjects.

The most commonly reported adverse reactions were pain at the injection site and redness at the injection site.

Adverse reactions occurring during these studies were mostly reported within 48 hours following vaccination.

Adverse reactions considered as being at least possibly related to vaccination have been categorised by frequency as follows.

Frequencies are reported as:

Very common: (≥1/10)

Common: (≥1/100 to <1/10)

Uncommon: (≥ 1/1,000 to <1/100)

Within each frequency grouping, undesirable effects are presented in order of decreasing seriousness.

Nervous system disorders:

Very Common: headache

Common: drowsiness

Uncommon: dizziness

Gastrointestinal disorders:

Common: gastrointestinal symptoms e.g. nausea, vomiting and diarrhoea

Skin and subcutaneous tissue disorders:

Uncommon: urticaria, rash

Metabolism and nutrition disorders:

Common: loss of appetite

General disorders and administration site conditions:

Very common: pain, redness at the injection site, fatigue

Common: fever, swelling at the injection site

Psychiatric disorders:

Common: irritability

In a WHO study conducted in Ghana, ACWY Vax was administered to 177 adults. The following adverse reactions were observed in this trial:

Very common: tenderness at injection site

Common: induration at injection site.

In addition, the following adverse reactions have been reported during post-marketing surveillance:

Skin and subcutaneous tissue disorders:

Angioneurotic oedema

Musculoskeletal and connective tissue disorders:

Arthralgia, musculoskeletal stiffness

General disorders and administration site conditions:

Influenza-like symptoms, chills

Immune system disorders:

Allergic reactions, including anaphylactic and anaphylactoid reactions

4.9 Overdose

Cases of overdose (up to 10 times the recommended dose) have been reported during post-marketing surveillance. Adverse events reported following overdosage were similar to those reported with normal vaccine administration.

5. PHARMACOLOGICAL PROPERTIES

5.1 Pharmacodynamic properties

Pharmacotherapeutic group: Bacterial vaccines, ATC code: J07AH04

Immunogenicity data

ACWY Vax induces bactericidal antibodies against meningococci of groups A, C, W_{135} and Y.

The current formulation of ACWY Vax was shown immunologically non-inferior to the previous formulation of the vaccine in a trial conducted in Lebanon in 161 subjects aged 2-30 years.

The immunogenicity of the previous formulation of ACWY Vax was evaluated in four clinical studies conducted in Belgium, Lebanon, Poland and Taiwan (N =341) in subjects aged 2-30 years.

Antibody titres were measured with the serum bactericidal assay (SBA).

Vaccine response was defined as seroconversion for initially seronegative subjects (with SBA titre below 1:8) or as four-fold increase in SBA titre from pre to post vaccination for initially seropositive subjects.

The percentage of vaccine responders observed in the four clinical studies conducted with the previous formulation were as follows:

In children aged 2-5 years: Group A - 69.1%, Group C - 93.1%, Group W_{135} - 89.3%, Group Y - 79.2%.

In subjects aged 6-30 years: Group A - 72.2%, Group C 95.4%, Group W_{135} - 92.3%, Group Y -81.2%.

In initially seronegative subjects seroconversion rates we 100% for Group A and Y, and at least 92.9% for Group and W_{135}.

The risk of meningococcal disease is much higher in inc viduals with late complement component deficienc (LCCD) because of their inability to kill meningococci v the classical and alternative pathways. However, ACW Vax induces anti-capsular polysaccharide antibodie against each of the four groups in LCCD subjects. In spi of the complement deficiency, killing of meningococci A, (W_{135} and Y is observed when sera from LCCD subjec vaccinated with ACWY Vax are incubated with huma neutrophils.

Efficacy data

In response to a meningococcal disease epidemic in Bu kina Faso, a mass vaccination campaign with Menceva ACW was performed in more than 1.68 million children an adults aged from 2 to 29 years. The vaccine effectivenes against group A and W_{135} disease was 95.8% (95% C 81.8%-99.0%) for persons with reported vaccination.

Persistence of immune response

Literature data supports the persistence of vaccir induced antibody response for at least 3 years.

An ongoing clinical study has demonstrated that 100% subjects aged 18-25 years had bactericidal antibody titre ≥ 1:8 against meningococci of the groups A, W_{135} and and 96% for group C two years after vaccination.

In a study conducted in Ghana in 177 subjects aged 15-3 years, 100%, 88.4% and 93.5% of subjects had SBA titre ≥ 1:8 for group A, C and W_{135}, respectively at approx mately one year after vaccination with ACWY Vax.

In studies conducted among complement-deficient sul jects, the antibodies persisted for 3 years post vaccinatic with ACWY Vax and the revaccination restored antiboc concentrations.

5.2 Pharmacokinetic properties

Evaluation of pharmacokinetic properties is not require for vaccines.

5.3 Preclinical safety data

Preclinical data reveal no special hazard for humans base on general safety tests performed in animals.

6. PHARMACEUTICAL PARTICULARS

6.1 List of excipients

Powder:

Sucrose

Trometamol

Solvent:

Sodium chloride

Water for injections

6.2 Incompatibilities

In the absence of compatibility studies, this medicin product must not be mixed with other medicinal product

6.3 Shelf life

3 years.

After reconstitution, the vaccine should be used immec ately. However, chemical and physical in-use stability ha been demonstrated for 8 hours at 2-8°C.

6.4 Special precautions for storage

Store in a refrigerator (2°C – 8°C).

Do not freeze.

Store in the original package in order to protect from ligh

6.5 Nature and contents of container

Powder in a vial (type I glass) with a stopper and solve (0.5 ml) in a pre-filled syringe (type I glass) with a stopp with or without needles– pack size of 1.

Not all pack sizes may be marketed.

6.6 Special precautions for disposal and other handlir

The vaccine should be inspected visually for any foreig particulate matter and/or other coloration prior to admi istration. In the event of either being observed, discard th vaccine.

ACWY Vax must be reconstituted by adding the enti content of the supplied container of solvent to the vi containing the powder. The powder should be complete dissolved in the solvent.

The reconstituted vaccine is a clear colourless solution.

7. MARKETING AUTHORISATION HOLDER

SmithKline Beecham plc

Trading as:

GlaxoSmithKline UK

Stockley Park West

Uxbridge

Middlesex UB11 1BT

8. MARKETING AUTHORISATION NUMBER(S)

PL 10592/0301

9. DATE OF FIRST AUTHORISATION/RENEWAL C THE AUTHORISATION

23/06/2008

. DATE OF REVISION OF THE TEXT
/06/2008
)M

dartrel 0.25, 0.5, and 2.0 mg film-coated ablets

(GlaxoSmithKline UK)

NAME OF THE MEDICINAL PRODUCT
)ARTREL® 0.25, 0.5 or 2.0 mg film-coated tablets.

QUALITATIVE AND QUANTITATIVE COMPOSITION
ch film-coated tablet contains 0.25 / 0.5 / 2.0 mg of pinirole (as hydrochloride).

:cipient: 45.3 / 45.0 / 44.9 / 44.6 mg lactose

:cipient(s):

ctose

r a full list of excipients, see section 6.1.

PHARMACEUTICAL FORM
m-coated tablet.

25 mg: White oval-shaped, marked "GS" on one side and LE" on the other.

5 mg: Yellow oval-shaped, marked "GS" on one side and ES" on the other.

) mg: Pink oval-shaped, marked "GS" on one side and YG" on the other.

CLINICAL PARTICULARS

Therapeutic indications
)ARTREL is indicated for the symptomatic treatment of oderate to severe idiopathic Restless Legs Syndrome e section 5.1).

2 Posology and method of administration
al use.

ults

lividual dose titration against efficacy and tolerability is commended. Ropinirole should be taken just before dtime, however the dose can be taken up to 3 hours fore retiring. Ropinirole may be taken with food, to prove gastrointestinal tolerance.

eatment initiation (week 1)

e recommended initial dose is 0.25 mg once daily (admi-tered as above) for 2 days. If this dose is well tolerated e dose should be increased to 0.5 mg once daily for the nainder of week 1.

erapeutic regimen (week 2 onwards)

lowing treatment initiation, the daily dose should be reased until optimal therapeutic response is achieved. e average dose in clinical trials, in patients with moder- to severe Restless Legs Syndrome, was 2 mg once a y.

e dose may be increased to 1 mg once a day at week 2. e dose may then be increased by 0.5 mg per week over next two weeks to a dose of 2 mg once a day. In some tients, to achieve optimal improvement, the dose may be reased gradually up to a maximum of 4 mg once a day. clinical trials the dose was increased by 0.5 mg each ek to 3 mg once a day and then by 1 mg up to the ximum recommended dose of 4 mg once a day as own in table 1.

ses above 4 mg once daily have not been investigated in stless Legs Syndrome patients.

ble 1 Dose titration

/eek	2	3	4	5*	6*	7*
ose (mg)/ nce daily	1	1.5	2	2.5	3	4

o achieve optimal improvement in some patients.

e patient's response to ropinirole should be evaluated er 3 months treatment (see section 5.1). At this time the se prescribed and the need for continued treatment ould be considered. If treatment is interrupted for more n a few days it should be re-initiated by dose titration ried out as above.

ildren and adolescents

ARTREL is not recommended for use in children below years of age due to a lack of data on safety and efficacy.

lerly

e clearance of ropinirole is decreased in patients over 65 ars of age. Any increase in dosage should be gradual d titrated against the symptomatic response.

nal impairment

dosage adjustment is necessary in patients with mild to derate renal impairment (creatinine clearance between and 50 ml/min).

Contraindications

persensitivity to the active substance or to any of the cipients.

vere renal impairment (creatinine clearance <30 ml/ n)

vere hepatic impairment.

4.4 Special warnings and precautions for use

Ropinirole should not be used to treat neuroleptic akathisia, tasikinesia (neuroleptic-induced compulsive tendency to walk), or secondary Restless Legs Syndrome (e.g. caused by renal failure, iron deficiency anaemia or pregnancy).

During treatment with ropinirole, paradoxical worsening of Restless Legs Syndrome symptoms occurring with earlier onset (augmentation), and reoccurrence of symptoms in the early morning hours (early morning rebound), may be observed. If this occurs, treatment should be reviewed and dosage adjustment or discontinuation of treatment may be considered.

In Parkinson's disease, ropinirole has been associated uncommonly with somnolence and episodes of sudden sleep onset (see section 4.8) however, in Restless Legs Syndrome, this phenomenon is very rare. Nevertheless, patients must be informed of this phenomenon and advised to exercise caution while driving or operating machines during treatment with ropinirole. Patients who have experienced somnolence and/or an episode of sudden sleep onset must refrain from driving or operating machines. A reduction of dosage or termination of therapy may be considered.

Patients with major psychotic disorders should not be treated with dopamine agonists unless the potential benefits outweigh the risks.

Impulse control disorders including pathological gambling and hypersexuality, and increased libido, have been reported in patients treated with dopamine agonists, including ropinirole, principally for Parkinson's disease. Those disorders were reported especially at high doses and were generally reversible upon reduction of the dose or treatment discontinuation. Risk factors such as a history of compulsive behaviours were present in some cases (see section 4.8).

Ropinirole should be administered with caution to patients with moderate hepatic impairment. Undesirable effects should be closely monitored.

Patients with rare hereditary problems of galactose intolerance, the Lapp lactase deficiency or glucose-galactose malabsorption should not take this medicine.

Due to the risk of hypotension, patients with severe cardiovascular disease (in particular coronary insufficiency) should be treated with caution.

4.5 Interaction with other medicinal products and other forms of interaction

Ropinirole is principally metabolised by the cytochrome P450 isoenzyme CYP1A2. A pharmacokinetic study (with a ropinirole dose of 2 mg, three times a day) revealed that ciprofloxacin increased the C_{max} and AUC of ropinirole by 60% and 84% respectively, with a potential risk of adverse events. Hence, in patients already receiving ropinirole, the dose of ropinirole may need to be adjusted when medicinal products known to inhibit CYP1A2, e.g. ciprofloxacin, enoxacin or fluvoxamine, are introduced or withdrawn.

A pharmacokinetic interaction study between ropinirole (at a dose of 2 mg, three times a day) and theophylline, a substrate of CYP1A2, revealed no change in the pharmacokinetics of either ropinirole or theophylline. Therefore, it is not expected that ropinirole will compete with the metabolism of other medicinal products which are metabolised by CYP1A2.

Based on *in-vitro* data, ropinirole has little potential to inhibit cytochrome P450 at therapeutic doses. Hence, ropinirole is unlikely to affect the pharmacokinetics of other medicinal products, via a cytochrome P450 mechanism.

Smoking is known to induce CYP1A2 metabolism, therefore if patients stop or start smoking during treatment with ropinirole, dose adjustment maybe required.

Increased plasma concentrations of ropinirole have been observed in patients treated with hormone replacement therapy. In patients already receiving hormone replacement therapy, ropinirole treatment may be initiated in the usual manner. However, it may be necessary to adjust the ropinirole dose, in accordance with clinical response, if hormone replacement therapy is stopped or introduced during treatment with ropinirole.

No pharmacokinetic interaction has been seen between ropinirole and domperidone (a medicinal product used to treat nausea and vomiting) that would necessitate dosage adjustment of either medicinal product. Domperidone antagonises the dopaminergic actions of ropinirole peripherally and does not cross the blood-brain barrier. Hence its value as an anti-emetic in patients treated with centrally acting dopamine agonists.

Neuroleptics and other centrally active dopamine antagonists, such as sulpiride or metoclopramide, may diminish the effectiveness of ropinirole and, therefore, concomitant use of these medicinal products with ropinirole should be avoided.

4.6 Pregnancy and lactation

There are no adequate data from the use of ropinirole in pregnant women.

Studies in animals have shown reproductive toxicity (see section 5.3). As the potential risk for humans is unknown, it is recommended that ropinirole is not used during pregnancy unless the potential benefit to the patient outweighs the potential risk to the foetus.

Ropinirole should not be used in nursing mothers as it may inhibit lactation.

4.7 Effects on ability to drive and use machines

Patients being treated with ropinirole and presenting with somnolence and/or sudden sleep episodes must be informed to refrain from driving or engaging in activities where impaired alertness may put themselves or others at risk of serious injury or death (e.g. operating machines) until such effects have resolved (see also section 4.4).

4.8 Undesirable effects

Adverse drug reactions are listed below by system organ class and frequency. Frequencies from clinical trials are determined as excess incidence over placebo and are classed as very common (>1/10) or common (>1/100, <1/10) or uncommon (>1/1,000, <1/100).

Within each frequency grouping, undesirable effects are presented in order of decreasing seriousness.

Use of ropinirole in Restless Legs Syndrome

In Restless Legs Syndrome clinical trials the most common adverse drug reaction was nausea (approximately 30% of patients). Undesirable effects were normally mild to moderate and experienced at the start of therapy or on increase of dose and few patients withdrew from the clinical studies due to undesirable effects.

Table 2 lists the adverse drug reactions reported for ropinirole in the 12-week clinical trials at ⩾1.0% above the placebo rate or those reported uncommonly but known to be associated with ropinirole.

Table 2 Adverse drug reactions reported in 12-week Restless Legs Syndrome clinical trials (ropinirole n=309, placebo n=307)

Psychiatric disorders	
Common	Nervousness
Uncommon	Confusion
Nervous system disorders	
Common	Syncope, somnolence, dizziness (including vertigo)
Vascular disorders	
Uncommon	Postural hypotension, hypotension
Gastrointestinal disorders	
Very common	Vomiting, nausea
Common	Abdominal pain
General disorders and administration site conditions	
Common	Fatigue

Hallucinations were reported uncommonly in the open label long-term studies.

Paradoxical worsening of Restless Legs Syndrome symptoms occurring with earlier onset (augmentation), and reoccurrence of symptoms in the early morning hours (early morning rebound), may be observed during treatment with ropinirole.

Management of undesirable effects

Dose reduction should be considered if patients experience significant undesirable effects. If the undesirable effect abates, gradual up-titration can be re-instituted. Anti-nausea medicinal products that are not centrally active dopamine antagonists, such as domperidone, may be used, if required.

Other experience with ropinirole

Ropinirole is also indicated for the treatment of Parkinson's disease. The adverse drug reactions reported in patients with Parkinson's disease on ropinirole monotherapy and adjunct therapy at doses up to 24 mg/day at an excess incidence over placebo are described below.

Table 3 Adverse drug reactions reported in Parkinson's disease clinical trials at doses up to 24 mg/day

Psychiatric disorders	
Common	Hallucinations, confusion
Uncommon	Increased libido
Nervous system disorders	
Very common	Syncope, dyskinesia, somnolence
Gastrointestinal disorders	
Very common	Nausea
Common	Vomiting, abdominal pain, heartburn
General disorders and administration site conditions	
Common	Leg oedema

Post marketing reports

Hypersensitivity reactions (including urticaria, angioedema, rash, pruritus)

Psychotic reactions (other than hallucinations) including delirium, delusion, paranoia have been reported.

Impulse control disorders including pathological gambling and hypersexuality, and increased libido, have been reported (see section 4.4).

In Parkinson's disease, ropinirole is associated with somnolence and has been associated uncommonly (>1/1,000, <1/100) with excessive daytime somnolence and sudden sleep onset episodes, however, in Restless Legs Syndrome, this phenomenon is very rare (<1/10,000).

Following ropinirole therapy, postural hypotension or hypotension has been reported uncommonly (>1/1,000, <1/100), rarely severe.

Very rare cases of hepatic reactions (<1/10,000), mainly increase of liver enzymes, have been reported.

4.9 Overdose

It is anticipated that the symptoms of ropinirole overdose will be related to its dopaminergic activity. These symptoms may be alleviated by appropriate treatment with dopamine antagonists such as neuroleptics or metoclopramide.

5. PHARMACOLOGICAL PROPERTIES

5.1 Pharmacodynamic properties

Pharmacotherapeutic group: Dopamine agonist, ATC code: N04BC04.

Mechanism of action

Ropinirole is a non ergoline D2/D3 dopamine agonist which stimulates striatal dopamine receptors.

Clinical efficacy

ADARTREL should only be prescribed to patients with moderate to severe idiopathic Restless Legs Syndrome. Moderate to severe idiopathic Restless Legs Syndrome is typically represented by patients who suffer with insomnia or severe discomfort in the limbs.

In the four 12-week efficacy studies, patients with Restless Legs Syndrome were randomised to ropinirole or placebo, and the effects on the IRLS scale scores at week 12 were compared to baseline. The mean dose of ropinirole for the moderate to severe patients was 2.0 mg/day. In a combined analysis of moderate to severe Restless Legs Syndrome patients from the four 12-week studies, the adjusted treatment difference for the change from baseline in IRLS scale total score at week 12 Last Observation Carried Forward (LOCF) Intention To Treat population was -4.0 points (95% CI -5.6, -2.4, p<0.0001; baseline and week 12 LOCF mean IRLS points: ropinirole 28.4 and 13.5; placebo 28.2 and 17.4).

A 12-week placebo-controlled polysomnography study in Restless Legs Syndrome patients examined the effect of treatment with ropinirole on periodic leg movements of sleep. A statistically significant difference in the periodic leg movements of sleep was seen between ropinirole and placebo from baseline to week 12.

Although sufficient data are not available to adequately demonstrate the long term efficacy of ropinirole in Restless Legs Syndrome (see section 4.2), in a 36-week study, patients who continued on ropinirole demonstrated a significantly lower relapse rate compared with patients randomised to placebo (33% versus 58%, p=0.0156).

A combined analysis of data from moderate to severe Restless Legs Syndrome patients, in the four 12-week placebo-controlled studies, indicated that ropinirole-treated patients reported significant improvements over placebo on the parameters of the Medical Outcome Study Sleep Scale (scores on 0-100 range except sleep quantity). The adjusted treatment differences between ropinirole and placebo were: sleep disturbance (-15.2, 95% CI -19.37, -10.94; p<0.0001), sleep quantity (0.7 hours, 95% CI 0.49, 0.94); p<0.0001), sleep adequacy (18.6, 95% CI 13.77, 23.45; p<0.0001) and daytime somnolence (-7.5, 95% CI -10.86, -4.23; p<0.0001).

A rebound phenomenon following discontinuation of ropinirole treatment (end of treatment rebound) cannot be excluded. In clinical trials, although the average IRLS total scores 7-10 days after withdrawal of therapy were higher in ropinirole-treated patients than in placebo-treated patients, the severity of symptoms following withdrawal of therapy generally did not exceed the baseline assessment in ropinirole-treated patients.

In clinical studies most patients were of Caucasian origin.

Study of the effect of ropinirole on cardiac repolarisation

A thorough QT study conducted in male and female healthy volunteers who received doses of 0.5, 1, 2 and 4 mg of ropinirole film-coated (immediate release) tablets once daily showed a maximum increase of the QT interval duration at the 1mg dose of 3.46 milliseconds (point estimate) as compared to placebo. The upper bound of the one sided 95% confidence interval for the largest mean effect was less than 7.5 milliseconds. The effect of ropinirole at higher doses has not been systematically evaluated.

The available clinical data from a thorough QT study do no indicate a risk of QT prolongation at doses of ropinirole up to 4 mg/day.

5.2 Pharmacokinetic properties

Absorption

The bioavailability of ropinirole is about 50% (36% to 57%), with C_{max} reached on average 1.5 hours after the dose. A high fat meal decreases the rate of absorption of ropinirole, as shown by a delay in median Tmax by 2.6 hours and an average 25% decrease in Cmax.

Distribution

Plasma protein binding of ropinirole is low (10 – 40%). Consistent with its high lipophilicity, ropinirole exhibits a large volume of distribution (approx. 7 l/kg)

Metabolism

Ropinirole is primarily cleared by the cytochrome P450 enzyme, CYP1A2, and its metabolites are mainly excreted in the urine. The major metabolite is at least 100 times less potent than ropinirole in animal models of dopaminergic function.

Elimination

Ropinirole is cleared from the systemic circulation with an average elimination half-life of approximately 6 hours. No change in the oral clearance of ropinirole is observed following single and repeated oral administration. Wide inter-individual variability in the pharmacokinetic parameters has been observed.

Linearity

The pharmacokinetics of ropinirole are linear overall (C_{max} and AUC) in the therapeutic range between 0.25 mg and 4 mg, after a single dose and after repeated dosing.

Population-related characteristics

In patients over 65 years of age, a reduction in the systemic clearance of ropinirole by about 30% is possible.

In patients with mild to moderate renal impairment (creatinine clearance between 30 and 50 ml/min), no change in the pharmacokinetics of ropinirole is observed. No data are available in patients with severe renal impairment.

5.3 Preclinical safety data

Toxicology: The toxicology profile is principally determined by the pharmacological activity of ropinirole: behavioural changes, hypoprolactinaemia, decrease in blood pressure and heart rate, ptosis and salivation. In the albino rat only, retinal degeneration was observed in a long term study at the highest dose (50 mg/kg/day), and was probably associated with an increased exposure to light.

Genotoxicity: Genotoxicity was not observed in the usual battery of *in vitro* and *in vivo* tests.

Carcinogenicity: From two-year studies conducted in the mouse and rat at dosages up to 50 mg/kg/day there was no evidence of any carcinogenic effect in the mouse. In the rat, the only ropinirole-related lesions were Leydig cell hyperplasia and testicular adenoma resulting from the hypoprolactinaemic effect of ropinirole. These lesions are considered to be a species specific phenomenon and do not constitute a hazard with regard to the clinical use of ropinirole.

Reproductive Toxicity: Administration of ropinirole to pregnant rats at maternally toxic doses resulted in decreased foetal body weight at 60 mg/kg/day (approximately 15 times the AUC at the maximum dose in humans), increased foetal death at 90 mg/kg/day (approximately 25 times the AUC at the maximum dose in humans) and digit malformations at 150 mg/kg/day (approximately 40 times the AUC at the maximum dose in humans). There were no teratogenic effects in the rat at 120 mg/kg/day (approximately 30 times the AUC at the maximum dose in humans) and no indication of an effect on development in the rabbit.

Safety Pharmacology: *In vitro* studies have shown that ropinirole inhibits hERG-mediated currents. The IC_{50} is 5-fold higher than the expected maximum plasma concentration in patients treated at the highest recommended dose (4 mg/day), see section 5.1.

6. PHARMACEUTICAL PARTICULARS

6.1 List of excipients

Tablet cores:

Lactose monohydrate

Microcrystalline cellulose

Croscarmellose sodium

Magnesium stearate.

Film coating:

0.25mg: Hypromellose, Macrogol 400, Titanium dioxide (E171), Polysorbate 80 (E433).

0.5mg: Hypromellose, Macrogol 400, Titanium dioxide (E171), iron oxide yellow (E172), iron oxide red (E172), indigo carmine aluminium lake (E132)

2.0 mg: Hypromellose, Macrogol 400, Titanium dioxide (E171), iron oxide yellow (E172), iron oxide red (E172). Iron oxide red (E172).

6.2 Incompatibilities

Not applicable.

6.3 Shelf life

2 years.

6.4 Special precautions for storage

Do not store above 25 °C.

Store in the original package.

6.5 Nature and contents of container

0.25mg: PVC/PCTFE/Aluminium or PVC/PCTFE/PVC/Aluminium blister in cartons of 12 tablets

0.5mg: PVC/PCTFE/Aluminium or PVC/PCTFE/PVC/Aluminium blister in cartons of 28 or 84 tablets

2.0 mg: PVC/PCTFE/Aluminium or PVC/PCTFE/PVC/Aluminium blister in cartons of 28 or 84 tablets

6.6 Special precautions for disposal and other handling

No special requirements.

7. MARKETING AUTHORISATION HOLDER

GlaxoSmithKline UK Limited
980 Great West Road
Brentford
Middlesex
TW8 9GS
Trading as:
GlaxoSmithKline UK
Stockley Park West
Uxbridge
Middlesex
UB11 1BT

8. MARKETING AUTHORISATION NUMBER(S)

Adartrel 0.25 mg film coated tablets PL 19494/0033

Adartrel 0.5 mg film coated tablets PL 19494/0034

Adartrel 2.0 mg film coated tablets PL 19494/0036

9. DATE OF FIRST AUTHORISATION/RENEWAL OF THE AUTHORISATION

10 /05/2006

10. DATE OF REVISION OF THE TEXT

26 January 2009

Adcal 1500mg chewable tablets

(ProStrakan)

1. NAME OF THE MEDICINAL PRODUCT

Adcal 1500mg Chewable Tablets

2. QUALITATIVE AND QUANTITATIVE COMPOSITION

Per tablet:

Calcium carbonate: 1500mg

equivalent to 600mg of elemental calcium

3. PHARMACEUTICAL FORM

Chewable Tablet

4. CLINICAL PARTICULARS

4.1 Therapeutic indications

Adcal is a chewable tablet recommended as a supplementary source of calcium when normal requirements are high and in the correction of calcium deficiency in the diet. They can be used in osteoporosis therapy as an adjunct to more specific conventional treatments. Adcal chewable tablets can be used as a phosphate binding agent in the management of renal failure.

4.2 Posology and method of administration

Oral.

Adults, elderly and children

Dietary deficiency and as an adjunct in osteoporosis therapy; 2 chewable tablets per day, preferably one tablet each morning and evening.

For use in binding phosphate in the management of renal failure in patients on renal dialysis, the dose should be adjusted for the individual patient and is dependent on the serum phosphate level.

The tablets should be chewed, not swallowed whole and taken just prior to, during or immediately following a meal.

4.3 Contraindications

Absolute contra-indications are hypercalcaemia resulting for example from myeloma, bone metastases or other malignant bone disease, sarcoidosis; primary hyperparathyroidism and vitamin D overdosage. Severe renal failure untreated by renal dialysis. Hypersensitivity to any of the tablet ingredients.

Relative contra-indications are osteoporosis due to prolonged immobilisation, renal stones, severe hypercalciuria.

4.4 Special warnings and precautions for use

Patients with mild to moderate renal failure or mild hypercalciuria should be supervised carefully. Periodic checks of plasma calcium levels and urinary calcium excretion should be made in patients with mild to moderate renal failure or mild hypercalciuria.

Urinary calcium excretion should also be measured. In patients with a history of renal stones urinary calcium excretion should be measured to exclude hypercalciuria.

With long-term treatment it is advisable to monitor serum and urinary calcium levels and kidney function, and reduce or stop treatment temporarily if urinary calcium exceeds 7.5mmol/24 hours.

Allowances should be made for calcium and vitamin D supplements from other sources.

Patients with rare hereditary problems of fructose intolerance, glucose-galactose malabsorption or sucrase-isomaltase insufficiency should not take this medicine.

5 Interaction with other medicinal products and other rms of interaction

ne risk of hypercalcaemia should be considered in atients taking thiazide diuretics since these drugs can duce urinary calcium excretion. Hypercalcaemia must e avoided in digitalised patients.

he effects of digitalis and other cardiac glycosides may be ccentuated with the oral administration of calcium comined with Vitamin D. Strict medical supervision is needed nd, if necessary monitoring of ECG and calcium.

ertain foods (e.g. those containing oxalic acid, phosphate r phytinic acid) may reduce the absorption of calcium

alcium salts may reduce the absorption of thyroxine, isphosphonates, sodium fluoride, quinolone and tetracyline antibiotics or iron. It is advisable to allow a minimum eriod of four hours before taking the calcium.

alcium absorption is reduced in patients receiving sysemic corticosteroid therapy. This should be taken in to ccount when patients are receiving concomitant therapy.

.6 Pregnancy and lactation

During pregnancy and lactation treatment with Adcal hould be under the direction of a physician. During regnancy and lactation, requirements for calcium are ncreased but in deciding on the required supplementation allowances should be made for availability of these agents rom other sources. If Adcal and iron supplements are both equired to be administered to the patient, they should be aken at different times (see Section 4.5).

.7 Effects on ability to drive and use machines

None known

4.8 Undesirable effects

The use of calcium supplements has, rarely, given rise to mild gastro-intestinal disturbances, such as constipation, flatulence, nausea, gastric pain, diarrhoea.

4.9 Overdose

Overdosage may cause gastro-intestinal disturbances but would not be expected to cause hypercalcaemia except in patients treated with excessive doses of vitamin D. Treatment should be aimed at lowering serum calcium levels through a high fluid intake and low calcium diet. In severe cases treatments with corticosteroid and other specialist treatment may be necessary. Alkalosis is a potential but rare risk.

5. PHARMACOLOGICAL PROPERTIES

5.1 Pharmacodynamic properties

Calcium carbonate is a well established medicinal material and is used extensively for supplementation in deficiency states. Calcium carbonate is also widely used as an antacid.

5.2 Pharmacokinetic properties

The pharmacokinetic profiles of calcium and its salts are well known. Calcium carbonate is converted to calcium chloride by gastric acid. Calcium is absorbed to the extent of about 15-25% from the gastro-intestinal tract while the remainder reverts to insoluble calcium carbonate and calcium stearate, and is excreted in the faeces.

5.3 Preclinical safety data

Calcium carbonate is a well known and widely used material and has been used in clinical practice for many years. As such toxicity is only likely to occur in chronic overdosage where hypercalcaemia could result.

6. PHARMACEUTICAL PARTICULARS

6.1 List of excipients

Xylitol, polydextrose, pre-gelatinised starch, sodium saccharin, magnesium stearate, fruit flavour (contains propylene glycol and maltodextrin).

6.2 Incompatibilities

Not applicable, oral preparation.

6.3 Shelf life

24 months

6.4 Special precautions for storage

Do not store above 25°C.

Store in the original package. Keep container in the outer carton.

6.5 Nature and contents of container

PVC/PVdC aluminium foil blister packs of 10 (Physicians sample), or 100 tablets in a cardboard carton.

6.6 Special precautions for disposal and other handling

No special conditions

7. MARKETING AUTHORISATION HOLDER

ProStrakan Ltd.

Galabank Business Park

Galashiels

Scotland

TD1 1QH

8. MARKETING AUTHORISATION NUMBER(S)

PL16508/0005

9. DATE OF FIRST AUTHORISATION/RENEWAL OF THE AUTHORISATION

04/10/2005

10. DATE OF REVISION OF THE TEXT

November 2008

11 LEGAL CATEGORY

P

Adcal D3 chewable tablets

(ProStrakan)

1. NAME OF THE MEDICINAL PRODUCT

Adcal-D_3 Chewable tablets

2. QUALITATIVE AND QUANTITATIVE COMPOSITION

Per tablet:

Calcium carbonate: 1500mg equivalent to 600mg of elemental calcium

Colecalciferol: 400iu equivalent to 10μg vitamin D_3

This product also contains sucrose (part of the vitamin D3 concentrate: approximately 1.7 milligrams per tablet) and soya oil (also part of the vitamin D3 concentrate: approximately 0.3 milligrams per tablet).

For full list of excipients see 6.1

3. PHARMACEUTICAL FORM

Chewable Tablet

4. CLINICAL PARTICULARS

4.1 Therapeutic indications

As an adjunct to specific therapy for osteoporosis and in situations requiring therapeutic supplementation of malnutrition e.g. in pregnancy and established vitamin D dependent osteomalacia.

The prevention and treatment of calcium deficiency/vitamin D deficiency especially in the housebound and institutionalised elderly subjects. Deficiency of the active moieties is indicated by raised levels of PTH, lowered 25-hydroxy vitamin D and raised alkaline phosphatase levels which are associated with increased bone loss.

4.2 Posology and method of administration

Oral.

Adults and Elderly and children above 12 years of age:

2 chewable tablets per day, preferably one tablet each morning and evening.

Children:

Not recommended for children under 12 years.

4.3 Contraindications

Absolute contra-indications are hypercalcaemia resulting for example from myeloma, bone metastases or other malignant bone disease, sarcoidosis; primary hyperparathyroidism and vitamin D overdosage. Severe renal failure. Hypersensitivity to any of the tablet ingredients.

Relative contra-indications are osteoporosis due to prolonged immobilisation, renal stones, severe hypercalciuria.

Adcal-D_3 contains a small quantity of soya oil and is therefore contraindicated in patients who are allergic to peanuts or soya.

4.4 Special warnings and precautions for use

Patients with mild to moderate renal failure or mild hypercalciuria should be supervised carefully including periodic checks of plasma calcium levels and urinary calcium excretion.

In patients with a history of renal stones urinary calcium excretion should be measured to exclude hypercalciuria.

With long-term treatment it is advisable to monitor serum and urinary calcium levels and kidney function, and reduce or stop treatment temporarily if urinary calcium exceeds 7.5mmol/24 hours (300mg/24 hours).

Caution is required in patients receiving treatment for cardiovascular disease (see Section 4.5 – thiazide diuretics and cardiac glycosides including digitalis).

Adcal-D_3 should also be used with caution in other patients with increased risk of hypercalcaemia e.g. patients with sarcoidosis or those suffering from malignancies.

Patients with rare hereditary problems of fructose intolerance, glucose-galactose malabsorption or sucrase-isomaltase insufficiency should not take this medicine.

Each tablet contains a small amount of sugar (about 1.7 mg per tablet) and may be harmful to teeth if used for a prolonged period.

Allowances should be made for calcium and vitamin D supplements from other sources.

4.5 Interaction with other medicinal products and other forms of interaction

The risk of hypercalcaemia should be considered in patients taking thiazide diuretics since these drugs can reduce urinary calcium excretion. Hypercalcaemia must be avoided in digitalised patients.

Certain foods (e.g. those containing oxalic acid, phosphate or phytinic acid) may reduce the absorption of calcium.

Concomitant treatment with phenytoin or barbiturates can decrease the effect of vitamin D because of metabolic activation. Concomitant use of glucocorticoids can decrease the effect of vitamin D.

The effects of digitalis and other cardiac glycosides may be accentuated with the oral administration of calcium combined with Vitamin D. Strict medical supervision is needed and, if necessary monitoring of ECG and calcium.

Calcium salts may reduce the absorption of thyroxine, bisphosphonates, sodium fluoride, quinolone or tetracycline antibiotics or iron. It is advisable to allow a minimum period of four hours before taking the calcium.

4.6 Pregnancy and lactation

During pregnancy and lactation treatment with Adcal-D_3 should always be under the direction of a physician. During pregnancy and lactation, requirements for calcium and vitamin D are increased but in deciding on the required supplementation allowances should be made for availability of these agents from other sources. If Adcal-D_3 and iron supplements are both required to be administered to the patient, they should be taken at different times (see Section 4.5).

Overdoses of vitamin D have shown teratogenic effects in pregnant animals. However, there have been no studies on the use of this medicinal product in human pregnancy and lactation. In humans, long term hypercalcaemia can lead to physical and mental retardation, aortic stenosis and retinopathy in a new born child. Vitamin D and its metabolites pass into the breast milk.

4.7 Effects on ability to drive and use machines

None known.

4.8 Undesirable effects

The use of calcium supplements has, rarely, given rise to mild gastro-intestinal disturbances, such as constipation, flatulence, nausea, gastric pain, diarrhoea. Following administration of vitamin D supplements occasional skin rash has been reported. Hypercalciuria, and in rare cases hypercalcaemia have been seen with long term treatment at high dosages.

4.9 Overdose

The most serious consequence of acute or chronic overdose is hypercalcaemia due to vitamin D toxicity. Symptoms may include nausea, vomiting, polyuria, anorexia, weakness, apathy, thirst and constipation. Chronic overdoses can lead to vascular and organ calcification as a result of hypercalcaemia. Treatment should consist of stopping all intake of calcium and vitamin D and rehydration.

5. PHARMACOLOGICAL PROPERTIES

5.1 Pharmacodynamic properties

Strong evidence that supplemental calcium and vitamin D_3 can reduce the incidence of hip and other non-vertebral fractures derives from an 18 month randomised placebo controlled study in 3270 healthy elderly women living in nursing homes or apartments for elderly people. A positive effect on bone mineral density was also observed.

In patients treated with 1200mg elemental calcium and 800IU vitamin D_3 daily, i.e. the same dose delivered by two tablets of Adcal-D_3, the number of hip fractures was 43% lower ($p=0.043$) and the total number of non vertebral fractures was 32% lower than among those who received placebo. Proximal femur bone mineral density after 18 months of treatment increased 2.7% in the calcium/vitamin D_3 group and decreased 4.6% in the placebo group ($p < 0.001$). In the calcium/vitamin D_3 group, the mean serum PTH concentration decreased by 44% from baseline at 18 months and serum 25-hydroxy-vitamin D concentration had increased by 162% over baseline.

Analysis of the intention-to-treat results showed a decreased probability of both hip fractures ($p = 0.004$) and other fractures ($p < 0.001$) in the calcium/vitamin D_3 treatment group. Analysis of the other two populations (active treatment and those treated and followed for 18 months) revealed comparable results to the intention-to-treat analysis. The odds ratio for hip fractures among women in the placebo group compared with those in the calcium/vitamin D_3 group was 1.7 (95% CI 1.0 to 2.8) and that for other nonvertebral fractures was 1.4 (95% CI 1.4 to 2.1). In the placebo group, there was a marked increase in the incidence of hip fractures over time whereas the incidence in the calcium/vitamin D_3 group was stable. Thus treatment reduced the age-related risk of fracture at 18 months ($p = 0.007$ for hip fractures and $p = 0.009$ for all non-vertebral fractures). At 3 years follow-up, the decrease in fracture risk was maintained in the calcium/vitamin D_3 group.

5.2 Pharmacokinetic properties

The pharmacokinetic profiles of calcium and its salts are well known. Calcium carbonate is converted to calcium chloride by gastric acid. Calcium is absorbed to the extent of about 15-25% from the gastro-intestinal tract while the remainder reverts to insoluble calcium carbonate and calcium stearate, and is excreted in the faeces.

The pharmacokinetics of vitamin D is also well known. Vitamin D is well absorbed from the gastro-intestinal tract in the presence of bile. It is hydroxylated in the liver to form 25-hydroxycholecalciferol and then undergoes further hydroxylation in the kidney to form the active metabolite 1, 25 dihydroxycholecalciferol (calcitriol). The metabolites circulate in the blood bound to a specific α - globin, Vitamin D and its metabolites are excreted mainly in the bile and faeces.

5.3 Preclinical safety data

Calcium carbonate and vitamin D are well known and widely used materials and have been used in clinical practice for many years. As such toxicity is only likely to occur in chronic overdosage where hypercalcaemia could result.

6. PHARMACEUTICAL PARTICULARS

6.1 List of excipients

Xylitol, modified maize starch, sodium saccharin, magnesium stearate, DL-α-tocopherol, edible fats, gelatin, soya oil, sucrose and corn starch. 'Tutti-Frutti' flavour (contains propylene glycol).

6.2 Incompatibilities

Not applicable, oral preparation.

6.3 Shelf life

18 months

6.4 Special precautions for storage

Do not store above 25°C.

6.5 Nature and contents of container

Blister packs of 10 (physicians sample), 30, 56, 60, 90, 100 and 112 tablets in a cardboard carton.

6.6 Special precautions for disposal and other handling

No special conditions.

7. MARKETING AUTHORISATION HOLDER

ProStrakan Limited

Galabank Business Park

Galashiels

TD1 1QH

UK

8. MARKETING AUTHORISATION NUMBER(S)

PL 16508/0001

9. DATE OF FIRST AUTHORISATION/RENEWAL OF THE AUTHORISATION

1 December 1998

10. DATE OF REVISION OF THE TEXT

20 May 2009

Adcal D3 Lemon Chewable Tablets

(ProStrakan)

1. NAME OF THE MEDICINAL PRODUCT

Adcal-D_3 Lemon Chewable tablets

2. QUALITATIVE AND QUANTITATIVE COMPOSITION

Per tablet:

Calcium carbonate: 1500mg, equivalent to 600mg of elemental calcium

Colecalciferol: 400iu, equivalent to 10μg vitamin D_3

This product also contains sucrose (part of the vitamin D_3 concentrate: approximately 1.7 milligrams per tablet) and soya oil (also part of the vitamin D_3 concentrate: approximately 0.3 milligrams per tablet).

For full list of excipients see 6.1

3. PHARMACEUTICAL FORM

Chewable tablet

4. CLINICAL PARTICULARS

4.1 Therapeutic indications

As an adjunct to specific therapy for osteoporosis and in situations requiring therapeutic supplementation of malnutrition e.g. in pregnancy and established vitamin D dependent osteomalacia.

The prevention and treatment of calcium deficiency/vitamin D deficiency especially in the housebound and institutionalised elderly subjects. Deficiency of the active moieties is indicated by raised levels of PTH, lowered 25-hydroxy vitamin D and raised alkaline phosphatase levels which are associated with increased bone loss.

4.2 Posology and method of administration

Oral.

Adults and Elderly and Children above 12 years of age:

2 chewable tablets per day, preferably one tablet each morning and evening

Children:

Not recommended for children under 12 years.

4.3 Contraindications

Absolute contra-indications are hypercalcaemia resulting for example from myeloma, bone metastases or other malignant bone disease, sarcoidosis; primary hyperparathyroidism and vitamin D overdosage. Severe renal failure. Hypersensitivity to any of the tablet ingredients.

Relative contra-indications are osteoporosis due to prolonged immobilisation, renal stones, severe hypercalciuria.

Adcal-D_3 Lemon contains a small quantity of soya oil and is therefore contraindicated in patients who are allergic to peanuts or soya.

4.4 Special warnings and precautions for use

Patients with mild to moderate renal failure or mild hypercalciuria should be supervised carefully including periodic checks of plasma calcium levels and urinary calcium excretion.

In patients with a history of renal stones urinary calcium excretion should be measured to exclude hypercalciuria.

With long-term treatment it is advisable to monitor serum and urinary calcium levels and kidney function, and reduce or stop treatment temporarily if urinary calcium exceeds 7.5mmol/24 hours (300mg/24 hours).

Caution is required in patients receiving treatment for cardiovascular disease (see Section 4.5 – thiazide diuretics and cardiac glycosides including digitalis).

Adcal-D_3 Lemon should also be used with caution in other patients with increased risk of hypercalcaemia e.g. patients with sarcoidosis or those suffering from malignancies.

Patients with rare hereditary problems of fructose intolerance, glucose-galactose malabsorption or sucrose-isomaltase insufficiency should not take this medicine.

Each tablet contains a small amount of sugar (about 1.7 mg per tablet) and may be harmful to teeth if used for a prolonged period.

Allowances should be made for calcium and vitamin D supplements from other sources.

4.5 Interaction with other medicinal products and other forms of interaction

The risk of hypercalcaemia should be considered in patients taking thiazide diuretics since these drugs can reduce urinary calcium excretion. Hypercalcaemia must be avoided in digitalised patients.

Certain foods (e.g. those containing oxalic acid, phosphate or phytinic acid) may reduce the absorption of calcium.

Concomitant treatment with phenytoin or barbiturates can decrease the effect of vitamin D because of metabolic activation. Concomitant use of glucocorticoids can decrease the effect of vitamin D.

The effects of digitalis and other cardiac glycosides may be accentuated with the oral administration of calcium combined with Vitamin D. Strict medical supervision is needed and, if necessary monitoring of ECG and calcium.

Calcium salts may reduce the absorption of thyroxine, bisphosphonates, sodium fluoride, quinolone or tetracycline antibiotics or iron. It is advisable to allow a minimum period of four hours before taking the calcium.

4.6 Pregnancy and lactation

During pregnancy and lactation treatment with Adcal-D_3 Lemon should always be under the direction of a physician. During pregnancy and lactation, requirements for calcium and vitamin D are increased but in deciding on the required supplementation allowances should be made for availability of these agents from other sources. If Adcal-D_3 Lemon and iron supplements are both required to be administered to the patient, they should be taken at different times (see Section 4.5).

Overdoses of vitamin D have shown teratogenic effects in pregnant animals. However, there have been no studies on the use of this medicinal product in human pregnancy and lactation. In humans, long term hypercalcaemia can lead to physical and mental retardation, aortic stenosis and retinopathy in a new born child. Vitamin D and its metabolites pass into the breast milk.

4.7 Effects on ability to drive and use machines

None known.

4.8 Undesirable effects

The use of calcium supplements has, rarely, given rise to mild gastro-intestinal disturbances, such as constipation, flatulence, nausea, gastric pain, diarrhoea. Following administration of vitamin D supplements occasional skin rash has been reported. Hypercalciuria, and in rare cases hypercalcaemia have been seen with long term treatment at high dosages.

4.9 Overdose

The most serious consequence of acute or chronic overdose is hypercalcaemia due to vitamin D toxicity. Symptoms may include nausea, vomiting, polyuria, anorexia, weakness, apathy, thirst and constipation. Chronic overdoses can lead to vascular and organ calcification as a result of hypercalcaemia. Treatment should consist of stopping all intake of calcium and vitamin D and rehydration.

5. PHARMACOLOGICAL PROPERTIES

5.1 Pharmacodynamic properties

Strong evidence that supplemental calcium and vitamin D_3 can reduce the incidence of hip and other non-vertebral fractures derives from an 18 month randomised placebo controlled study in 3270 healthy elderly women living in nursing homes or apartments for elderly people. A positive effect on bone mineral density was also observed.

In patients treated with 1200mg elemental calcium and 800IU vitamin D daily, i.e. the same dose delivered by two tablets of Adcal-D_3 Lemon, the number of hip fractures was 43% lower ($p=0.043$) and the total number of non vertebral fractures was 32% lower than among those who received placebo. Proximal femur bone mineral density after 18 months of treatment increased 2.7% in the calcium/vitamin D_3 group and decreased 4.6% in the placebo group ($p < 0.001$). In the calcium/vitamin D_3 group, the mean serum PTH concentration decreased by 44% from baseline at 18 months and serum 25-hydroxyvitamin D concentration had increased by 162% over baseline.

Analysis of the intention-to-treat results showed a decreased probability of both hip fractures ($p = 0.004$) and other fractures ($p < 0.001$) in the calcium/vitamin D_3 treatment group. Analysis of the other two populatio (active treatment and those treated and followed for months) revealed comparable results to the intention-t treat analysis. The odds ratio for hip fractures amo women in the placebo group compared with those in th calcium/vitamin D_3 group was 1.7 (95% CI 1.0 to 2.8) ar that for other nonvertebral fractures was 1.4 (95% CI 1.4 2.1). In the placebo group, there was a marked increase the incidence of hip fractures over time whereas the inc dence in the calcium/vitamin D_3 group was stable. Th treatment reduced the age-related risk of fracture at months ($p = 0.007$ for hip fractures and $p = 0.009$ for a non-vertebral fractures). At 3 years follow-up, the decreas in fracture risk was maintained in the calcium/vitamin D group.

5.2 Pharmacokinetic properties

The pharmacokinetic profiles of calcium and its salts ar well known. Calcium carbonate is converted to calciur chloride by gastric acid. Calcium is absorbed to the exter of about 15-25% from the gastro-intestinal tract while th remainder reverts to insoluble calcium carbonate and cal cium stearate, and is excreted in the faeces.

The pharmacokinetics of vitamin D is also well known Vitamin D is well absorbed from the gastro-intestinal trac in the presence of bile. It is hydroxylated in the liver to forr 25-hydroxycholecalciferol and then undergoes furthe hydroxylation in the kidney to form the active metabolit 1, 25 dihydroxycholecalciferol (calcitriol). The metabolite circulate in the blood bound to a specific α– globin, Vitami D and its metabolites are excreted mainly in the bile anc faeces.

5.3 Preclinical safety data

Calcium carbonate and vitamin D are well known and widely used materials and have been used in clinical practice for many years. As such toxicity is only likely to occur in chronic overdosage where hypercalcaemia could result.

6. PHARMACEUTICAL PARTICULARS

6.1 List of excipients

Xylitol, modified maize starch, sodium saccharin, magnesium stearate, DL-α-tocopherol, edible fats, gelatin, soya oil, sucrose, corn starch and lemon flavour.

6.2 Incompatibilities

Not applicable, oral preparation.

6.3 Shelf life

18 months

6.4 Special precautions for storage

Do not store above 25°C.

6.5 Nature and contents of container

Blister packs of 10 (physicians sample), 30, 56, 60, 90, 100 and 112 tablets in a cardboard carton.

6.6 Special precautions for disposal and other handling

No special conditions.

Administrative Data

7. MARKETING AUTHORISATION HOLDER

ProStrakan Limited

Galabank Business Park

Galashiels

TD1 1QH

UK

8. MARKETING AUTHORISATION NUMBER(S)

PL 16508/0028

9. DATE OF FIRST AUTHORISATION/RENEWAL OF THE AUTHORISATION

19/07/2007

10. DATE OF REVISION OF THE TEXT

20/05/2009

Adcal-D3 Dissolve 1500mg/400IU Effervescent Tablets

(ProStrakan)

1. NAME OF THE MEDICINAL PRODUCT

Adcal-D_3 Dissolve 1500mg/400IU Effervescent Tablets

2. QUALITATIVE AND QUANTITATIVE COMPOSITION

One effervescent tablet contains:

1500 mg calcium carbonate (equivalent to 600 mg or 15 mmol elemental calcium)

400 I.U. or 10 micrograms colecalciferol (vitamin D_3) as colecalciferol concentrate 'powder form'

This product also contains sucrose (part of the vitamin D_3 concentrate: approximately 1.7 milligrams per tablet) and soya oil (also part of the vitamin D_3 concentrate: approximately 0.3 milligrams per tablet).

For a full list of excipients see Section 6.1

3. PHARMACEUTICAL FORM

White, round, lemon flavoured effervescent tablets.

CLINICAL PARTICULARS

1 Therapeutic indications

s an adjunct to specific therapy for osteoporosis and in tuations requiring therapeutic supplementation of malutrition e.g. in pregnancy and established vitamin D ependent osteomalacia.

ne prevention and treatment of calcium deficiency/vitain D deficiency especially in the housebound and institionalised elderly subjects. Deficiency of the active ioieties is indicated by raised levels of PTH, lowered 5-hydroxy vitamin D and raised alkaline phosphatase evels which are associated with increased bone loss.

.2 Posology and method of administration

ral.

Adults and elderly and children over 12 years of age:	Take 2 effervescent tablets daily, preferably one tablet each morning and evening. The effervescent tablets should be dissolved in a glass of water (approx. 200ml) and drunk immediately
Children:	Not recommended for children under 12 years.

.3 Contraindications

Absolute contra-indications are hypercalcaemia resulting or example from myeloma, bone metastases or other malignant bone disease, sarcoidosis; primary hyperparathyroidism and vitamin D overdosage. Severe renal failure. Hypersensitivity to any of the tablet excipients.

Relative contra-indications are osteoporosis due to prolonged immobilisation, renal stones, severe hypercalciuria.

Adcal-D_3 Dissolve contains a small quantity of soya oil and s therefore contraindicated in patients who are allergic to peanuts or soya.

.4 Special warnings and precautions for use

Patients with mild to moderate renal failure or mild hypercalciuria should be supervised carefully including periodic checks of plasma calcium levels and urinary calcium excretion.

In patients with a history of renal stones urinary calcium excretion should be measured to exclude hypercalciuria.

With long-term treatment it is advisable to monitor serum and urinary calcium levels and kidney function, and reduce or stop treatment temporarily if urinary calcium exceeds 7.5mmol/24 hours (300mg/24 hours).

Caution is required in patients receiving treatment for cardiovascular disease (see Section 4.5 – thiazide diuretics and cardiac glycosides including digitalis).

Adcal-D_3 Dissolve should also be used with caution in other patients with increased risk of hypercalcaemia e.g. patients with sarcoidosis or those suffering from malignancies.

Patients with rare hereditary problems of fructose intolerance, glucose-galactose malabsorption or sucrase-isomaltase insuffiency should not take this medicine.

Each tablet contains a small amount of sugar (about 1.7 mg per tablet) and may be harmful to teeth if used for a prolonged period.

Allowances should be made for calcium and vitamin D supplements from other sources.

__Information for diabetics__:

Patients who have diabetes mellitus or require a low-sugar diet should take account of the sucrose content of this medicinal product.

One effervescent tablet contains 1.672mg of sucrose.

4.5 Interaction with other medicinal products and other forms of interaction

The risk of hypercalcaemia should be considered in patients taking thiazide diuretics since these drugs can reduce urinary calcium excretion. Hypercalcaemia must be avoided in digitalised patients.

Certain foods (e.g. those containing oxalic acid, phosphate or phytinic acid) may reduce the absorption of calcium.

Concomitant treatment with phenytoin or barbiturates can decrease the effect of vitamin D because of metabolic activation. Concomitant use of glucocorticoids can decrease the effect of vitamin D.

The effects of digitalis and other cardiac glycosides may be accentuated with the oral administration of calcium combined with vitamin D. Strict medical supervision is needed and, if necessary monitoring of ECG and calcium.

Calcium salts may reduce the absorption of thyroxine, bisphosphonates, sodium fluoride, quinolone or tetracycline antibiotics or iron. It is advisable to allow a minimum period of four hours before taking the calcium.

4.6 Pregnancy and lactation

During pregnancy and lactation treatment with Adcal-D_3 Dissolve should always be under the direction of a physician. During pregnancy and lactation, requirements for calcium and vitamin D are increased but in deciding on the required supplementation allowances should be made for availability of these agents from other sources. If Adcal-D_3 Dissolve and iron supplements are both required to be administered to the patient, they should be taken at different times (see Section 4.5).

Overdoses of vitamin D have shown teratogenic effects in pregnant animals. However, there have been no studies on the use of this medicinal product in human pregnancy and lactation. In humans, long term hypercalcaemia can lead to physical and mental retardation, aortic stenosis and retinopathy in a new born child. Vitamin D and its metabolites pass into the breast milk.

4.7 Effects on ability to drive and use machines

No studies on the effects on the ability to drive and use machines have been performed.

4.8 Undesirable effects

The use of calcium supplements has, rarely, given rise to mild gastro-intestinal disturbances, such as constipation, flatulence, nausea, gastric pain, diarrhoea. Following administration of vitamin D supplements occasional skin rash has been reported. Hypercalciuria, and in rare cases, hypercalcaemia have been seen with long term treatment at high dosages.

4.9 Overdose

The most serious consequence of acute or chronic overdose is hypercalcaemia due to vitamin D toxicity. Symptoms may include nausea, vomiting, polyuria, anorexia, weakness, apathy, thirst and constipation. Chronic overdoses can lead to vascular and organ calcification as a result of hypercalcaemia. Treatment should consist of stopping all intake of calcium and vitamin D and rehydration.

5. PHARMACOLOGICAL PROPERTIES

5.1 Pharmacodynamic properties

Pharmacotherapeutic group: A12AX01 Calcium carbonate and colecalciferol

Strong evidence that supplemental calcium and vitamin D_3 can reduce the incidence of hip and other non-vertebral fractures derives from an 18 month randomised placebo controlled study in 3270 healthy elderly women living in nursing homes or apartments for elderly people. A positive effect on bone mineral density was also observed.

In patients treated with 1200mg elemental calcium and 800IU vitamin D_3 daily, i.e. the same dose delivered by two tablets of Adcal-D_3 Dissolve, the number of hip fractures was 43% lower ($p=0.043$) and the total number of non vertebral fractures was 32% lower than among those who received placebo. Proximal femur bone mineral density after 18 months of treatment increased 2.7% in the calcium/vitamin D_3 group and decreased 4.6% in the placebo group ($p < 0.001$). In the calcium/vitamin D_3 group, the mean serum PTH concentration decreased by 44% from baseline at 18 months and serum 25-hydroxy-vitamin D concentration had increased by 162% over baseline.

Analysis of the intention-to-treat results showed a decreased probability of both hip fractures ($p = 0.004$) and other fractures ($p < 0.001$) in the calcium/vitamin D_3 treatment group. Analysis of the other two populations (active treatment and those treated and followed for 18 months) revealed comparable results to the intention-to-treat analysis. The odds ratio for hip fractures among women in the placebo group compared with those in the calcium/vitamin D_3 group was 1.7 (95% CI 1.0 to 2.8) and that for other nonvertebral fractures was 1.4 (95% CI 1.4 to 2.1). In the placebo group, there was a marked increase in the incidence of hip fractures over time whereas the incidence in the calcium/vitamin D_3 group was stable. Thus treatment reduced the age-related risk of fracture at 18 months ($p = 0.007$ for hip fractures and $p = 0.009$ for all non-vertebral fractures). At 3 years follow-up, the decrease in fracture risk was maintained in the calcium/vitamin D_3 group.

5.2 Pharmacokinetic properties

The pharmacokinetic profiles of calcium and its salts are well known. Calcium carbonate is converted to calcium chloride by gastric acid. Calcium is absorbed to the extent of about 15-25% from the gastro-intestinal tract while the remainder reverts to insoluble calcium carbonate and calcium stearate, and is excreted in the faeces.

The pharmacokinetics of vitamin D is also well known. Vitamin D is well absorbed from the gastro-intestinal tract in the presence of bile. It is hydroxylated in the liver to form 25-hydroxycolecalciferol and then undergoes further hydroxylation in the kidney to form the active metabolite 1, 25 dihydroxycolecalciferol (calcitriol). The metabolites circulate in the blood bound to a specific α-globin. Vitamin D and its metabolites are excreted mainly in the bile and faeces.

5.3 Preclinical safety data

Calcium carbonate and vitamin D are well known and widely used materials and have been used in clinical practice for many years. As such, toxicity is only likely to occur in chronic overdosage where hypercalcaemia could result.

6. PHARMACEUTICAL PARTICULARS

6.1 List of excipients

citric acid anhydrous

malic acid

sodium hydrogen carbonate (E500)

sodium cyclamate (E953)

sodium carbonate anhydrous (E500)

maltodextrin

saccharin sodium (E954)

sucrose

gelatine

maize starch

hydrogenated soyabean oil

α-tocopherol

lemon flavour BSL Code 119 *containing* lemon oil, lime flavouring, sorbitol (E420), mannitol (E421), gluconolactone, maltodextrin and acacia

6.2 Incompatibilities

None

6.3 Shelf life

3 Years

6.4 Special precautions for storage

Do not store above 25°C.

Keep the container tightly closed.

6.5 Nature and contents of container

Packs of 4 × 14 effervescent tablets in a carton.

Each unit of 14 effervescent tablets is in an aluminium or polypropylene tube with a polyethylene stopper.

Contains a dessicant.

6.6 Special precautions for disposal and other handling

No special requirements

7. MARKETING AUTHORISATION HOLDER

ProStrakan Limited

Galabank Business Park

Galashiels

Scotland

TD1 1QH

8. MARKETING AUTHORISATION NUMBER(S)

PL 16508/0026

9. DATE OF FIRST AUTHORISATION/RENEWAL OF THE AUTHORISATION

22/11/2007

10. DATE OF REVISION OF THE TEXT

20/05/2009

Adenocor

(sanofi-aventis)

1. NAME OF THE MEDICINAL PRODUCT

Adenocor

2. QUALITATIVE AND QUANTITATIVE COMPOSITION

Each vial contains 6mg of adenosine per 2ml (3mg/ml).

For excipients, see 6.1

3. PHARMACEUTICAL FORM

Solution for injection

Clear, colourless solution

4. CLINICAL PARTICULARS

4.1 Therapeutic indications

Rapid conversion to a normal sinus rhythm of paroxysmal supraventricular tachycardias, including those associated with accessory by-pass tracts (Wolff-Parkinson-White Syndrome).

__Diagnostic Indications__

Aid to diagnosis of broad or narrow complex supraventricular tachycardias. Although Adenocor will not convert atrial flutter, atrial fibrillation or ventricular tachycardia to sinus rhythm, the slowing of AV conduction helps diagnosis of atrial activity.

Sensitisation of intra-cavitary electrophysiological investigations.

4.2 Posology and method of administration

Adenocor is intended for hospital use only with monitoring and cardiorespiratory resuscitation equipment available for immediate use. It should be administered by rapid IV bolus injection according to the ascending dosage schedule below. To be certain the solution reaches the systemic circulation administer either directly into a vein or into an IV line. If given into an IV line it should be injected as proximally as possible, and followed by a rapid saline flush.

Adenocor should only be used when facilities exist for cardiac monitoring. Patients who develop high-level AV block at a particular dose should not be given further dosage increments.

Therapeutic dose

Adult:

Initial dose: 3mg given as a rapid intravenous bolus (over 2 seconds).

Second dose: If the first dose does not result in elimination of the supraventricular tachycardia within 1 to 2 minutes, 6mg should be given also as a rapid intravenous bolus.

Third dose: If the second dose does not result in elimination of the supraventricular tachycardia within 1 to 2 minutes. 12mg should be given also as a rapid intravenous bolus.

Additional or higher doses are not recommended.

Children

No controlled paediatric study has been undertaken. Published uncontrolled studies show similar effects of adenosine in adults and children: effective doses for children were between 0.0375 and 0.25mg/kg.

Elderly

See dosage recommendations for adults.

Diagnostic dose

The above ascending dosage schedule should be employed until sufficient diagnostic information has been obtained.

Method of administration: Rapid intravenous injection only.

4.3 Contraindications

Adenocor is contraindicated for patients presenting:

– Known hypersensitivity to adenosine.

– Sick sinus syndrome, second or third degree Atrio-Ventricular block (except in patients with a functioning artificial pacemaker).

– Chronic obstructive lung disease (such as asthma)

– Long QT syndrome

– Severe hypotension; decompensated states of heart failure

4.4 Special warnings and precautions for use

Special warnings: Due to the possibility of transient cardiac arrhythmias arising during conversion of the supraventricular tachycardia to normal sinus rhythm, administration should be carried out in hospital with electrocardiographic monitoring.

Because it has the potential to cause significant hypotension, adenosine should be used with caution in patients with left main coronary stenosis, uncorrected hypovolemia, stenotic valvular heart disease, left to right shunt, pericarditis or pericardial effusion, autonomic dysfunction or stenotic carotid artery disease with cerebrovascular insufficiency.

Adenosine should be used with caution in patients with recent myocardial infarction, heart failure, or in patients with minor conduction defects (first degree A-V block, bundle branch block) that could be transiently aggravated during infusion. Adenosine should be used with caution in patients with atrial fibrillation or flutter and especially in those with an accessory by-pass tract since particularly the latter may develop increased conduction down the anomalous pathway.

Some cases of severe bradycardia have been reported. Some occurred in early post heart transplant patients; in the other cases, occult sino-atrial disease was present. The occurrence of severe bradycardia should be taken as a warning of underlying disease and could potentially favour the occurrence of torsades de pointes.

In patients with recent heart transplantation (less than 1 year) an increased sensitivity of the heart to adenosine has been observed.

Since neither the kidney nor the liver are involved in the degradation of exogenous adenosine, Adenocor's efficacy should be unaffected by hepatic or renal insufficiency.

As dipyridamole is a known inhibitor of adenosine uptake, it may potentiate the action of Adenocor. It is therefore suggested that Adenocor should not be administered to patients receiving dipyridamole; if use of Adenocor is essential, its dosage should be reduced (*see Section 4.5 Interactions with other Medicaments and other forms of Interaction*).

Precautions:

The occurrence of angina, severe bradycardia, severe hypotension, respiratory failure (potentially fatal), or asystole/cardiac arrest (potentially fatal), should lead to immediate discontinuation of administration.

In patients with history of convulsions/seizures, the administration of adenosine should be carefully monitored.

Because of the possible risk of torsades de pointes, Adenocor should be used with caution in patients with a prolonged QT interval, whether this is drug induced or of metabolic origin. Adenocor is contraindicated in patients with Long QT syndrome (see section 4.3).

Adenosine may precipitate or aggravate bronchospasm.

4.5 Interaction with other medicinal products and other forms of interaction

As dipyridamole is a known inhibitor of adenosine uptake, it may potentiate the action of Adenocor; in one study dipyridamole was shown to produce a 4 fold increase in adenosine actions. Asystole has been reported following concomitant administration. It is therefore suggested that Adenocor should not be administered to patients receiving dipyridamole; if use of Adenocor is essential, its dosage should be reduced. *See Section 4.4 Special Warnings and Precautions for Use.*

Theophylline and other xanthines such as caffeine are known strong inhibitors of adenosine.

Adenocor may interact with drugs tending to impair cardiac conduction.

4.6 Pregnancy and lactation

Pregnancy: In the absence of evidence that adenosine does not cause foetal harm, Adenocor should only be used during pregnancy where absolutely necessary.

Lactation: In the absence of clinical experience use of Adenocor during lactation should be considered only if essential.

4.7 Effects on ability to drive and use machines

Not applicable.

4.8 Undesirable effects

Adverse events are ranked under the heading of the frequency:

Very common ($>1/10$), Common ($\geq 1/100$, $<1/10$), Uncommon ($\geq 1/1000$, $<1/100$), Rare ($\geq 1/10000$, $<1/1000$), Very rare ($<1/10000$), Not known (cannot be estimated from available data).

These side effects are generally mild, of short duration (usually less than 1 minute) and well tolerated by the patient. However severe reactions can occur.

• **Nervous System disorders**

Common:

- Headache
- Dizziness / lightheadedness

Uncommon:

- Head pressure

Very rare:

- Transient, and spontaneously and rapidly reversible worsening of intracranial hypertension

Not known:

- Loss of consciousness / syncope
- Convulsions, especially in predisposed patients (see section 4.4)

• **Psychiatric disorders**

Common:

- Apprehension

• **Eye disorders**

Uncommon:

- Blurred vision

•**Gastrointestinal disorders**

Common:

- Nausea

Uncommon:

- Metallic taste

Not known:

- Vomiting

• **Cardiac Disorders:**

Very common:

- Asystole
- Bradycardia
- Sinus pause
- Atrioventricular block
- Atrial extrasystoles
- Skipped beats
- Ventricular excitability disorders such as ventricular extrasystoles, non-sustained ventricular tachycardia

Uncommon:

- Sinus tachycardia
- Palpitations

Very rare:

- Severe bradycardia which is not corrected by atropine and may require temporary pacing
- Atrial fibrillation
- Ventricular excitability disorders, including ventricular fibrillation and torsade de pointes (see section 4.4)

Not known:

- Hypotension sometimes severe
- Cardiac arrest, sometimes fatal especially in patients with underlying ischemic heart disease /cardiac disorder (see section 4.4)

• **Respiratory, thoracic and mediastinal disorders**

Very common:

- Dyspnoea (or the urge to take a deep breath)

Uncommon:

- Hyperventilation

Very rare:

- Bronchospasm (see section 4.4)

Not known:

- Respiratory failure (see section 4.4)
- Apnoea/Respiratory arrest

Cases with fatal outcome of respiratory failure, of bronc ospasm, and of apnea / respiratory arrest have bee reported.

• **Vascular disorders:**

Very common:

- Flushing

• **General disorders and Administration Site condition**

Very Common:

- Chest pressure/pain, feeling of thoracic constriction oppression

Common:

- Burning sensation

Uncommon:

- Sweating
- Feeling of general discomfort / weakness / pain

Very rare:

- Injection site reactions

4.9 Overdose

No cases of overdosage have been reported. As the ha life of adenosine in blood is very short, the duration of any effects is expected to be limited. Pharmacokinetic evalua tion indicates that methyl xanthines are competitive antagonists to adenosine, and that therapeutic concentra tions of theophylline block its exogenous effects.

5. PHARMACOLOGICAL PROPERTIES

5.1 Pharmacodynamic properties

ATC Code: Other Cardiac Preparations C01EB 10

Endogenous nucleoside with peripheral vasodilator/antiarrhythmic effect

Antiarrhythmic drug.

Adenosine is a purine nucleoside which is present in all cells of the body. Animal pharmacology studies have in several species shown that Adenosine has a negative dromotropic effect on the atrioventricular (AV) node.

In man Adenocor (Adenosine) administered by rapid intravenous injection slows conduction through the AV node. This action can interrupt re-entry circuits involving the AV node and restore normal sinus rhythm in patients with paroxysmal supraventricular tachycardias. Once the circuit has been interrupted, the tachycardia stops and normal sinus rhythm is re-established.

One acute interruption of the circuit is usually sufficient to arrest the tachycardia.

Since atrial fibrillation and atrial flutter do not involve the AV node as part of a re-entry circuit, Adenosine will not terminate these arrhythmias.

By transiently slowing AV conduction, atrial activity is easier to evaluate from ECG recordings and therefore the use of Adenosine can aid the diagnosis of broad or narrow complex tachycardias.

Adenosine may be useful during electrophysiological studies to determine the site of AV block or to determine in some cases of pre-excitation, whether conduction is occurring by an accessory pathway or via the AV node.

5.2 Pharmacokinetic properties

Adenosine is impossible to study via classical ADME protocols. It is present in various forms in all cells of the body where it plays an important role in energy production and utilisation systems. An efficient salvage and recycling system exists in the body, primarily in the erythrocytes and blood vessel endothelial cells. The half life in vitro is estimated to be <10 seconds. The in vivo half life may be even shorter.

5.3 Preclinical safety data

There are no pre-clinical data of relevance to the prescriber which are additional to that already included in other sections of the SPC.

6. PHARMACEUTICAL PARTICULARS

6.1 List of excipients

Sodium Chloride

Water for Injections

6.2 Incompatibilities

Compatibility with other medicines is not known.

6.3 Shelf life

36 months.

Any portion of the vial not used at once should be discarded.

6.4 Special precautions for storage

Do not refrigerate.

6.5 Nature and contents of container

Clear, type I glass vials with chlorobutyl rubber closures secured with aluminium caps. Packs of 6 vials in plastic trays in cardboard cartons.

6.6 Special precautions for disposal and other handling

None.

7. MARKETING AUTHORISATION HOLDER

Sanofi-aventis

One Onslow Street

Guildford

Surrey

GU1 4YS

UK

. MARKETING AUTHORISATION NUMBER(S)

'L 11723/0005

. DATE OF FIRST AUTHORISATION/RENEWAL OF HE AUTHORISATION

2th March 2002

0. DATE OF REVISION OF THE TEXT

0 March 2009

.egal Category

'OM

Adenoscan

(sanofi-aventis)

1. NAME OF THE MEDICINAL PRODUCT

ADENOSCAN® 30 mg/10 ml, solution for infusion

2. QUALITATIVE AND QUANTITATIVE COMPOSITION

Each 10 ml vial of Adenoscan® contains 30 mg of adenosine (3 mg/ml)

For excipients, see section 6.1.

3. PHARMACEUTICAL FORM

Solution for infusion.

Adenoscan® is a sterile clear, colourless solution.

4. CLINICAL PARTICULARS

4.1 Therapeutic indications

Intravenous Adenoscan® is a coronary vasodilator for use in conjunction with radionuclide myocardial perfusion imaging in patients who cannot exercise adequately or for whom exercise is inappropriate.

4.2 Posology and method of administration

Adenoscan® is intended for use in hospitals. It should be administered following the same procedure as for exercise testing where facilities for cardiac monitoring and cardiorespiratory resuscitation are available. During administration of Adenoscan® continuous ECG control is necessary as life-threatening arrhythmia might occur. Heart rate and blood pressure should be monitored every minute.

Adults:

1. Adenoscan® should be administered undiluted as a continuous peripheral intravenous infusion at a dose of 140 μg/kg/min for six minutes using an infusion pump. Separate venous sites for Adenoscan® and radionuclide administration are recommended to avoid an adenosine bolus effect.

2. After three minutes of Adenoscan® infusion, the radionuclide is injected to ensure sufficient time for peak coronary blood flow to occur. The optimal vasodilator protocol is achieved with six minutes of Adenoscan® infusion.

3. To avoid an adenosine bolus effect, blood pressure should be measured in the arm opposite to the Adenoscan® infusion.

The table below is given as a guide for adjustment of the infusion rate of undiluted Adenoscan®, in line with bodyweight (total dose 0.84 mg/kg).

Patient Weight (kg)	Infusion Rate (ml/min)
45 - 49	2.1
50 - 54	2.3
55 - 59	2.6
60 - 64	2.8
65 - 69	3.0
70 - 74	3.3
75 - 79	3.5
80 - 84	3.8
85 - 89	4.0
90 - 94	4.2
95 - 99	4.4
100 - 104	4.7

Children:

In the absence of data, the use of Adenoscan® in children cannot be recommended.

Elderly:

See dosage recommendations for adults.

4.3 Contraindications

Adenoscan® is contra-indicated in patients suffering from:

- Known hypersensitivity to adenosine
- Second or third degree AV block, sick sinus syndrome except in patients with a functioning artificial pacemaker
- Long QT syndrome
- Severe hypotension
- Unstable angina not successfully stabilised with medical therapy
- Decompensated states of heart failure
- Chronic obstructive lung disease with evidence of bronchospasm (e.g. asthma bronchiale)
- Concomitant use of dipyridamole.

4.4 Special warnings and precautions for use

Because it has the potential to cause significant hypotension, Adenoscan® should be used with caution in patients with left main coronary stenosis, uncorrected hypovolemia, stenotic valvular heart disease, left to right shunt, pericarditis or pericardial effusion, autonomic dysfunction or stenotic carotid artery disease with cerebrovascular insufficiency. Adenoscan® infusion should be discontinued in any patient who develops persistent or symptomatic hypotension.

Adenoscan® should be used with caution in patients with recent myocardial infarction or severe heart failure. Adenoscan® should be used with caution in patients with minor conduction defects (first degree AV block, bundle branch block) that could be transiently aggravated during infusion.

Adenosine may trigger convulsions in patients who are susceptible to convulsions.

Adenoscan® should be used with caution in patients with atrial fibrillation or flutter and especially in those with an accessory by-pass tract since particularly the latter may develop increased conduction down the anomalous pathway.

Rare cases of severe bradycardia have been reported. Some occurred in early post-transplant patients; in the other cases occult sino-atrial disease was present. The occurrence of severe bradycardia should be taken as a warning of underlying disease and should lead to treatment discontinuation. Severe bradycardia would favour the occurrence of torsades de pointes, especially in patients with prolonged QT intervals. But to date, no case of torsades de pointes has been reported when adenosine is continuously infused.

The occurrence of respiratory failure (potentially fatal), asystole/cardiac arrest (potentially fatal), angina, severe bradycardia or severe hypotension should also lead to treatment discontinuation.

In patients with recent heart transplantation (less than 1 year) an increased sensitivity of the heart to adenosine has been observed.

Adenosine may precipitate or aggravate bronchospasm (see sections 4.3 and 4.8).

Safety and effectiveness in paediatric patients have not been established. Therefore Adenoscan® is not recommended for use in children until further data become available.

Adenoscan® contains 9 mg Sodium per ml.

To be taken into consideration by patients on a controlled sodium diet.

4.5 Interaction with other medicinal products and other forms of interaction

Dipyridamole inhibits adenosine cellular uptake and metabolism, and potentiates the action of Adenoscan®. In one study dipyridamole was shown to produce a 4 fold increase in adenosine actions. It is therefore suggested that Adenoscan® should not be administered to patients receiving dipyridamole; if use of Adenoscan® is essential, dipyridamole should be stopped 24 hours before hand, or the dose of Adenoscan® should be greatly reduced.

Aminophylline, theophylline and other xanthines are competitive adenosine antagonists and should be avoided for 24 hours prior to use of Adenoscan®.

Food and drinks containing xanthines (tea, coffee, chocolate and cola) should be avoided for at least 12 hours prior to use of Adenoscan®.

Adenosine can safely be co-administered with other cardioactive or vasoactive drugs (*see Section 5.1*).

4.6 Pregnancy and lactation

It is not known whether Adenoscan® can cause harm when administered to pregnant or lactating women. Therefore the use during pregnancy is contraindicated unless the physician considers the benefits outweigh the risk. Adenoscan® should not be used during lactation period.

4.7 Effects on ability to drive and use machines

None known.

4.8 Undesirable effects

Effects related to the known pharmacology of adenosine are frequent, but usually self-limiting and of short duration. Discontinuation of infusion may be necessary if the effect is intolerable.

Methylxanthines, such as IV aminophylline or theophylline have been used to terminate persistent side effects (50-125 mg by slow intravenous injection).

Adverse events are ranked under the heading of the frequency:

Very common (>1/10), Common (≥1/100, <1/10), Uncommon (≥1/1000, <1/100), Rare (≥1/10000, <1/1000), Very rare (<1/10000).

Cardiac Disorders:

- common: Hypotension (see section 4.4), AV block, ST segment depression, sustained or non-sustained ventricular tachycardia.

If sustained second or third degree AV block develops the infusion should be discontinued. If first degree AV block occurs, the patient should be observed carefully as a quarter of patients will progress to a higher degree of block.

- rare: bradycardia sometimes severe (see section 4.4)
- not known: asystole /Cardiac arrest (some cases with fatal outcome, *see section 4.4*): sinus tachycardia, atrial fibrillation, ventricular fibrillation

Respiratory, thoracic and mediastinal disorders:

- very common: dyspnea (or the urge to breathe deeply)
- rare: bronchospasm (see section 4.4), nasal congestion
- very rare: respiratory failure (see section 4.4)
- not known: apnea/respiratory arrest

Cases with fatal outcome of respiratory failure, of bronchospasm, and of apnea / respiratory arrest have been reported

Nervous system disorders:

- very common: headache
- common: dizziness, light-headedness
- uncommon: paraesthesia,
- rare: tremor, drowsiness
- not known: loss of consciousness / syncope, convulsions, especially in predisposed patients (see section 4.4)

Eye disorders:

- rare: blurred vision

Ear and labyrinth disorders:

- rare: tinnitus

Psychiatric disorders:

- uncommon: nervousness

Gastro-intestinal disorders:

- common: nausea, vomiting, abdominal discomfort
- uncommon: metallic taste, dry mouth

Renal and Urinary disorders:

- rare: urinary urgency

Reproductive system and breast disorders:

- rare: nipple discomfort

Vascular disorders:

- very common: flushing

General disorders and administration site conditions:

- very common: chest pain or pressure
- common: throat, neck and jaw discomfort
- uncommon: sweating, discomfort in the leg, arm or back, weakness
- very rare: injection site reactions

4.9 Overdose

No cases of overdosage have been reported. Overdosage would cause severe hypotension, bradycardia or asystole. The half life of adenosine in blood is very short, and side effects of Adenoscan® (when they occur) would quickly resolve when the infusion is discontinued. Administration of IV aminophylline or theophylline may be needed.

5. PHARMACOLOGICAL PROPERTIES

5.1 Pharmacodynamic properties

ATC Code: Other Cardiac Preparations C01EB 10

Endogenous nucleoside with peripheral vasodilator / antiarrhythmic effect

Adenosine is a potent vasodilator in most vascular beds, except in renal afferent arterioles and hepatic veins where it produces vasoconstriction. Adenosine exerts its pharmacological effects through activation of purine receptors (cell-surface A_1 and A_2 adenosine receptors). Although the exact mechanism by which adenosine receptor activation relaxes vascular smooth muscle is not known, there is evidence to support both inhibition of the slow inward calcium current reducing calcium uptake, and activation of adenylate cyclase through A_2 receptors in smooth muscle cells. Adenosine may reduce vascular tone by modulating sympathetic neurotransmission. The intracellular uptake of adenosine is mediated by a specific transmembrane nucleoside transport system. Once inside the cell, adenosine is rapidly phosphorylated by adenosine kinase to adenosine monophosphate, or deaminated by adenosine deaminase to inosine. These intracellular metabolites of adenosine are not vasoactive.

Intracoronary Doppler flow catheter studies have demonstrated that intravenous Adenoscan® at 140 μg/kg/min produces maximum coronary hyperaemia (relative to intracoronary papaverine) in approximately 90% of cases within 2-3 minutes of the onset of the infusion. Coronary blood flow velocity returns to basal levels within 1-2 minutes of discontinuing the Adenoscan® infusion.

The increase in blood flow caused by Adenoscan® in normal coronary arteries is significantly more than that in stenotic arteries. Adenoscan® redirects coronary blood flow from the endocardium to the epicardium and may reduce collateral coronary blood flow thereby inducing regional ischaemia.

Continuous infusion of adenosine in man has been shown to produce a mild dose-dependent fall in mean arterial pressure and a dose-related positive chronotropic effect, most likely caused by sympathetic stimulation. The onset of this reflex increase in heart rate occurs later than the negative chronotropic/dromotropic effect. This differential effect is mostly observed after bolus injection thus explaining the potential use of adenosine as a treatment for supraventricular arrhythmias when administered as a bolus or as a coronary vasodilator when administered as an infusion.

Although Adenoscan® affects cardiac conduction, it has been safely and effectively administered in the presence of other cardioactive or vasoactive drugs such as beta adrenergic blocking agents, calcium channel antagonists, nitrates, ACE inhibitors, diuretics, digitalis or anti-arrhythmics.

5.2 Pharmacokinetic properties

It is impossible to study adenosine in classical pharmacokinetic studies. It is present in various forms in all the cells of the body where it plays an important role in energy production and utilisation systems. An efficient salvage and recycling system exists in the body, primarily in erythrocytes and blood vessel endothelial cells. The half-life *in vitro* is estimated to be less than 10 seconds. The *in vivo* half-life may be even shorter.

Since neither the kidney nor the liver are involved in the degradation of exogenous adenosine, the efficacy of Adenoscan® should be unaffected by hepatic or renal insufficiency.

5.3 Preclinical safety data

Because adenosine is naturally present in all living cells, studies in animals to evaluate the carcinogenic potential of Adenoscan® (adenosine) have not been performed.

6. PHARMACEUTICAL PARTICULARS

6.1 List of excipients

Sodium Chloride

Water for Injection

6.2 Incompatibilities

In the absence of compatibility studies, this medicinal product must not be mixed with other medicinal products.

6.3 Shelf life

The shelf life of the unopened product is 3 years.

The product should be used immediately after opening.

6.4 Special precautions for storage

Do not refrigerate.

See Section 6.3

6.5 Nature and contents of container

Type I glass vials with chlorobutyl rubber stoppers, packs with 6 vials

6.6 Special precautions for disposal and other handling

See section 4.2.

The product is for single use only.

Any portion of the vial not used at once should be discarded.

The product should be inspected visually for particulate matter and colouration prior to administration. Where the visual appearance of the product may have changed, the vial should be discarded.

7. MARKETING AUTHORISATION HOLDER

Sanofi-aventis

One Onslow Street

Guildford

Surrey

GU1 4YS

8. MARKETING AUTHORISATION NUMBER(S)

11723/0086

9. DATE OF FIRST AUTHORISATION/RENEWAL OF THE AUTHORISATION

26th September 2005

10. DATE OF REVISION OF THE TEXT

May 2008

Legal category

POM

Adizem-SR capsules

(Napp Pharmaceuticals Limited)

1. NAME OF THE MEDICINAL PRODUCT

ADIZEM®-SR capsules 90 mg, 120 mg, 180 mg

2. QUALITATIVE AND QUANTITATIVE COMPOSITION

Diltiazem hydrochloride 90 mg, 120 mg, 180 mg

For excipients, see section 6.1

3. PHARMACEUTICAL FORM

Prolonged release capsules

ADIZEM-SR capsules 90 mg are white capsules marked "90 mg"

ADIZEM-SR capsules 120 mg are white/brown capsules marked "120 mg"

ADIZEM-SR capsules 180 mg are white/pale brown capsules marked "180 mg"

The capsules contain prolonged release microgranules.

4. CLINICAL PARTICULARS

4.1 Therapeutic indications

For the management of angina pectoris.

For the treatment of mild to moderate hypertension.

4.2 Posology and method of administration

<u>Route of administration</u>

Oral.

Dosage may be taken with or without food, and should be swallowed whole and not chewed.

<u>Angina</u>

Adults: The usual initial dose is 90 mg twice daily. Dosage may be increased gradually to 120 mg twice daily, or 180 mg twice daily if required. Patients' responses may vary and dosage requirements can differ significantly between individual patients.

<u>Elderly and patients with impaired renal or hepatic function:</u>

In the elderly, dosage should commence at 60 mg diltiazem hydrochloride twice daily and the dose carefully titrated as required.

<u>Hypertension:</u>

Adults: the usual dose is one ADIZEM-SR 120 mg tablet or capsule twice daily. Patients may benefit by titrating from a lower total daily dose.

<u>Elderly and patients with impaired renal or hepatic function:</u>

The starting dose should be 60 mg diltiazem hydrochloride twice daily, increasing to one ADIZEM-SR 90 mg capsule twice daily and then to one ADIZEM-SR 120 mg tablet or capsule twice daily if clinically indicated.

<u>Children:</u>

The ADIZEM preparations are not recommended for children. Safety and efficacy in children has not been established.

In order to avoid confusion, it is suggested that patients once titrated to an effective dose using either ADIZEM-SR tablets or capsules should remain on this treatment and should not be changed between different presentations.

ADIZEM-SR capsules should not be taken at the same time as an alcoholic beverage (refer to section 4.5, Interactions with other Medicinal Products and Other Forms of Interaction).

4.3 Contraindications

Pregnancy and in women of child bearing capacity. Patients with bradycardia (less than 50 bpm), second or third degree heart block, sick sinus syndrome, decompensated cardiac failure, patients with left ventricular dysfunction following myocardial infarction. Concurrent use with dantrolene infusion because of the risk of ventricular fibrillation.

4.4 Special warnings and precautions for use

The product should be used with caution in patients with reduced left ventricular function. Patients with mild bradycardia, first degree AV block or prolonged PR interval should be observed closely. Diltiazem is considered unsafe in patients with acute porphyria.

4.5 Interaction with other medicinal products and other forms of interaction

Diltiazem is extensively metabolised by CYP3A4, and as a result serum levels of diltiazem may be:

- Increased by concomitant usage of CYP3A4 inhibitors such as H2 antagonists (e.g. cimetidine, ranitidine) and protease inhibitors (e.g. atazanavir, ritonavir)
- Decreased by concomitant usage of CYP3A4 inducers such as barbiturates (phenobarbital, primidone), phenytoin and rifampicin.

Diltiazem is also an inhibitor of CYP3A4, and may therefore increase serum levels of CYP3A4 substrates such as benzodiazepines (especially midazolam and triazolam), carbamazepine, ciclosporin, cilostazol, ivabradine, statins (simvastatin, atorvastatin, lovastatin), sirolimus, tacrolimus and theophylline. Care should be exercised in patients taking these drugs. Concomitant use of diltiazem with cilostazol and ivabradine should be avoided.

There may be an additive effect (increased depression of cardiac conduction with risk of bradycardia and AV block) when diltiazem is prescribed with drugs which may induce bradycardia or other anti-arrhythmic drugs (e.g. amiodarone and beta blockers). Patients with pre-existing conduction defects should not receive the combination of diltiazem and beta-blockers.

Enhanced antihypertensive effect may occur with concomitant use of other antihypertensive drugs (e.g. beta-blockers, diuretics, ACE-inhibitors) or drugs that cause hypotension such as aldesleukin and antipsychotics. Concomitant use with alpha-blockers (e.g. prazosin) should be strictly monitored because of the possible synergistic hypotensive effect of this combination.

Diltiazem hydrochloride may cause small increases in plasma levels of digoxin, requiring careful monitoring of AV conduction.

Diltiazem may increase serum levels of phenytoin.

Diltiazem may increase bioavailability of tricyclic antidepressants.

Treatment with diltiazem has been continued without problem during anaesthesia, but the anaesthetist should be made aware of the treatment regimen.

ADIZEM-SR capsules should not be taken at the same time as alcohol, as it may increase the rate of release of diltiazem from the prolonged release preparation. In addition the combination of alcohol and diltiazem may have an additive vasodilatory effect.

4.6 Pregnancy and lactation

Diltiazem hydrochloride is contraindicated in pregnar women or women of child bearing potential, and is nc recommended in nursing mothers.

4.7 Effects on ability to drive and use machines

Diltiazem may cause adverse reactions such as dizziness which may impair patients' ability to drive or operat machinery to a varying extent depending on the dosag and individual susceptibility. Therefore, patients should no drive or operate machinery if affected.

4.8 Undesirable effects

The adverse events listed below are classified by body system according to their incidence (common or uncommon). Common adverse events have an incidence of >1% and uncommon adverse events have an incidence o <1%.

Blood and the lymphatic system disorders	
Uncommon	thrombocytopenia
Nervous system disorders	
Common	dizziness
	headache
Uncommon	extrapyramidal disorder
Cardiac disorders	
Uncommon	atrioventricular block
	bradycardia
	palpitations
	sinoatrial block
Vascular disorders	
Common	facial flushing
	hypotension
Uncommon	vasculitis
Gastrointestinal disorders	
Common	gastrointestinal disorder
	nausea
Uncommon	gingival hyperplasia
Hepatobiliary disorders	
Uncommon	increased hepatic enzyme
	clinical hepatitis
Skin and subcutaneous tissue disorders	
Uncommon	allergic dermatitis
	erythema multiforme
	exfoliative dermatitis
	photosensitivity reaction
Reproductive system and breast disorders	
Uncommon	gynaecomastia
General disorders and administration site conditions	
Common	fatigue
	oedema legs

4.9 Overdose

The clinical symptoms of acute intoxication may include pronounced hypotension or even collapse and sinus bradycardia with or without atrioventricular conduction defects.

The patient should be closely monitored in hospital to exclude arrhythmias or atrioventricular conduction defects. Gastric lavage and osmotic diuresis should be undertaken when considered appropriate. Symptomatic bradycardia and high grade atrioventricular block may respond to atropine, isoprenaline or occasionally temporary cardiac pacing.

Hypotension may require correction with plasma volume expanders, intravenous calcium gluconate and positive inotropic agents. The formulation employs a prolonged release system which will continue to release diltiazem for some hours.

5. PHARMACOLOGICAL PROPERTIES

5.1 Pharmacodynamic properties

Pharmacotherapeutic group: Selective calcium channel blocker with direct cardiac effects

ATC Code: C08D B01

Diltiazem is an antianginal agent and calcium antagonist. Diltiazem inhibits transmembrane calcium entry in myocardial muscle fibres and in vascular smooth muscle fibres, thereby decreasing the quantity of intracellular calcium available to the contractile proteins.

5.2 Pharmacokinetic properties

ADIZEM-SR capsules is a form characterised by prolonged release of diltiazem hydrochloride in the digestive tract. Diltiazem is 80% bound to human plasma proteins (albumin, acid glucoproteins).

The biotransformation routes are:

- Deacetylation
- Oxidative o- and n-demethylation
- Conjugation of the phenolic metabolites.

The primary metabolites, n-demethyldiltiazem and desacetyldiltiazem exert less pharmacological activity than iltiazem. The other metabolites are pharmacologically active.

After administration of 180 to 300 mg of ADIZEM-SR capsules, a peak plasma concentration of 80 to 220 ng/ml, respectively, is obtained after about 5.5 hours.

The elimination half-life varies from 6 to 8 hours, depending on the strength.

5.3 Preclinical safety data
There are no pre-clinical data of relevance to the prescriber which are additional to that already included in other sections of the SPC.

6. PHARMACEUTICAL PARTICULARS

6.1 List of excipients

Capsule contents

Sucrose and maize starch SP microgranules

Povidone

Sucrose

Ethylcellulose

Talc

Aquacoat ECD 30

Dibutyl sebacate

Capsule shells

Titanium dioxide (E171)

Gelatin

Iron oxide (E172) – 120 mg and 180 mg capsules only.

Indigotine (E132) - 120 mg capsules only.

6.2 Incompatibilities
None known.

6.3 Shelf life
Three years.

6.4 Special precautions for storage
Do not store above 25°C.

6.5 Nature and contents of container
Blister packs (aluminium/PVC) boxed in cardboard cartons.

Pack sizes: 56 capsules

6.6 Special precautions for disposal and other handling
Not applicable

7. MARKETING AUTHORISATION HOLDER
Napp Pharmaceuticals Ltd
Cambridge Science Park
Milton Road
Cambridge CB4 0GW

8. MARKETING AUTHORISATION NUMBER(S)
PL 16950/0006-0008

9. DATE OF FIRST AUTHORISATION/RENEWAL OF THE AUTHORISATION
2 October 1992/23 September 2003

10. DATE OF REVISION OF THE TEXT
December 2008

11. LEGAL CATEGORY
POM

® The Napp device and ADIZEM are Registered Trade Marks

© Napp Pharmaceuticals Ltd 2008.

Adizem-SR tablets

(Napp Pharmaceuticals Limited)

1. NAME OF THE MEDICINAL PRODUCT
ADIZEM®-SR tablets 120 mg

2. QUALITATIVE AND QUANTITATIVE COMPOSITION
Diltiazem Hydrochloride 120 mg

For excipients see section 6.1

3. PHARMACEUTICAL FORM
White film-coated capsule-shaped, prolonged release tablets. The tablets are marked 120/DL on one side and with a scoreline on the other.

4. CLINICAL PARTICULARS

4.1 Therapeutic indications
For the management of angina pectoris. For the treatment of mild to moderate hypertension.

4.2 Posology and method of administration

Route of administration

Oral.

Dosage may be taken with or without food, and should be swallowed whole and not chewed.

Angina

Adults:

The usual initial dose is 90 mg twice-daily. Dosage may be increased gradually to 120 mg twice-daily, or 180 mg twice-daily if required. Patients' responses may vary and dosage requirements can differ significantly between individual patients.

Elderly and patients with impaired renal or hepatic function:
In the elderly, dosage should commence at 60 mg diltiazem hydrochloride twice-daily and the dose carefully titrated as required.

Hypertension

Adults:

The usual dose is one ADIZEM-SR 120 mg tablet or capsule twice-daily. Patients may benefit by titrating from a lower total daily dose.

Elderly and patients with impaired renal or hepatic function:
The starting dose should be 60 mg diltiazem hydrochloride twice-daily, increasing to one ADIZEM-SR 90 mg capsule twice-daily and then to one ADIZEM-SR 120 mg tablet or capsule twice-daily if clinically indicated.

Children:

The ADIZEM preparations are not recommended for children. Safety and efficacy in children has not been established.

In order to avoid confusion, it is suggested that patients, once titrated to an effective dose using either ADIZEM tablets or capsules, should remain on this treatment and should not be changed between different presentations.

4.3 Contraindications
Pregnancy and in women of child-bearing capacity. Patients with bradycardia (less than 50 bpm), second or third degree heart block, sick sinus syndrome, decompensated cardiac failure, patients with left ventricular dysfunction following myocardial infarction. Concurrent use with dantrolene infusion because of the risk of ventricular fibrillation.

4.4 Special warnings and precautions for use
The product should be used with caution in patients with reduced left ventricular function. Patients with mild bradycardia, first degree AV block or prolonged PR interval should be observed closely. Diltiazem is considered unsafe in patients with acute porphyria.

4.5 Interaction with other medicinal products and other forms of interaction
Diltiazem is extensively metabolised by CYP3A4, and as a result serum levels of diltiazem may be:

- Increased by concomitant usage of CYP3A4 inhibitors such as H2 antagonists (e.g. cimetidine, ranitidine) and protease inhibitors (e.g. atazanavir, ritonavir)

Decreased by concomitant usage of CYP3A4 inducers such as barbiturates (phenobarbital, primidone), phenytoin and rifampicin.

Diltiazem is also an inhibitor of CYP3A4, and may therefore increase serum levels of CYP3A4 substrates such as benzodiazepines (especially midazolam and triazolam), carbamazepine, ciclosporin, cilostazol, ivabradine, statins (simvastatin, atorvastatin, lovastatin), sirolimus, tacrolimus and theophylline. Care should be exercised in patients taking these drugs. Concomitant use of diltiazem with cilostazol and ivabradine should be avoided.

There may be an additive effect (increased depression of cardiac conduction with risk of bradycardia and AV block) when diltiazem is prescribed with drugs which may induce bradycardia or other anti-arrhythmic drugs (e.g. amiodarone and beta blockers). Patients with pre-existing conduction defects should not receive the combination of diltiazem and beta-blockers.

Enhanced antihypertensive effect may occur with concomitant use of other antihypertensive drugs (e.g. beta-blockers, diuretics, ACE-inhibitors) or drugs that cause hypotension such as aldesleukin and antipsychotics. Concomitant use with alpha-blockers (e.g. prazosin) should be strictly monitored because of the possible synergistic hypotensive effect of this combination.

Diltiazem hydrochloride may cause small increases in plasma levels of digoxin, requiring careful monitoring of AV conduction.

Diltiazem may increase serum levels of phenytoin.

Diltiazem may increase bioavailability of tricyclic antidepressants.

Treatment with diltiazem has been continued without problem during anaesthesia, but the anaesthetist should be made aware of the treatment regimen.

The combination of alcohol and diltiazem may have an additive vasodilatory effect

4.6 Pregnancy and lactation
Diltiazem hydrochloride is contra-indicated in pregnant women or women of child-bearing potential, and is not recommended in nursing mothers.

4.7 Effects on ability to drive and use machines
Diltiazem may cause adverse reactions such as dizziness, which may impair patients' ability to drive or operate machinery to a varying extent depending on the dosage and individual susceptibility. Therefore, patients should not drive or operate machinery if affected.

4.8 Undesirable effects
The adverse events listed below are classified by body system according to their incidence (common or uncommon). Common adverse events have an incidence of >1% and uncommon adverse events have an incidence of <1%.

Blood and the lymphatic system disorders

Uncommon	thrombocytopenia

Nervous system disorders

Common	dizziness
	headache
Uncommon	extrapyramidal disorder

Cardiac disorders

Uncommon	atrioventricular block
	bradycardia
	palpitations
	sinoatrial block

Vascular disorders

Common	facial flushing
	hypotension
Uncommon	vasculitis

Gastrointestinal disorders

Common	gastrointestinal disorder
	nausea
Uncommon	gingival hyperplasia

Hepatobiliary disorders

Uncommon	increased hepatic enzyme
	clinical hepatitis

Skin and subcutaneous tissue disorders

Uncommon	allergic dermatitis
	erythema multiforme
	exfoliative dermatitis
	photosensitivity reaction

Reproductive system and breast disorders

Uncommon	gynaecomastia

General disorders and administration site conditions

Common	fatigue
	oedema legs

4.9 Overdose
The clinical symptoms of acute intoxication may include pronounced hypotension or even collapse and sinus bradycardia with or without atrioventricular conduction defects.

The patient should be closely monitored in hospital to exclude arrhythmias or atrioventricular conduction defects. Gastric lavage and osmotic diuresis should be undertaken when considered appropriate. Symptomatic bradycardia and high grade atrioventricular block may respond to atropine, isoprenaline or occasionally temporary cardiac pacing.

Hypotension may require correction with plasma volume expanders, intravenous calcium gluconate and positive inotropic agents. The formulation employs a prolonged release system which will continue to release diltiazem for some hours.

5. PHARMACOLOGICAL PROPERTIES
Pharmacotherapeutic group: Selective calcium channel blocker with direct cardiac effects

ATC Code: C08D B01

5.1 Pharmacodynamic properties
Diltiazem is a calcium antagonist which restricts the slow channel entry of calcium ions into the cell and so reduces the liberation of calcium from stores in the endoplasmic reticulum. This results in a reduction in the amount of available intra-cellular calcium and consequently:

1) Reduction of myocardial oxygen consumption.

2) Dilation of small and large coronary arteries.

3) Mild peripheral vasodilation.

4) A negative dromotropic effect.

5) The reflex positive chronotropic and inotropic effects due to reflex sympathetic activity are partially inhibited. This results in a slight reduction or no change in heart rate.

The antianginal effect is due to a reduction in cardiac oxygen demand with maintenance of coronary blood flow. Cardiac contractility and ventricular ejection fraction are unchanged. Treatment with diltiazem increases exercise capacity, improves the indices of myocardial ischaemia in the angina patient and relieves the spasm of vasospastic (Prinzmetal's) angina.

5.2 Pharmacokinetic properties
An oral dose of diltiazem is almost completely absorbed. Despite this, diltiazem has a low bioavailability owing to hepatic first pass metabolism. Diltiazem is metabolised extensively and only 1.0 to 3.0% of the dose is excreted in the urine as unchanged diltiazem. The release of the drug has been prolonged in the 120 mg tablet by special pharmaceutical technology. The high peak concentrations of the absorption phase have been eliminated. This allows the tablet to be administered twice-daily.

5.3 Preclinical safety data
There are no pre-clinical data of relevance to the prescriber which are additional to that already included in other sections of the SPC.

6. PHARMACEUTICAL PARTICULARS

6.1 List of excipients

Lactose

Hydrogenated castor oil

Colloidal aluminium hydroxide

Acrylic resin

Talc

Magnesium stearate

Hypromellose

Sucrose

Glycerol 85%

Titanium dioxide (E171)

Polysorbate 80

6.2 Incompatibilities

None known.

6.3 Shelf life

36 months.

6.4 Special precautions for storage

Do not store above 30°C.

Store in the original package.

6.5 Nature and contents of container

Aluminium foil backed PVdC/PVC blister packs containing 56 tablets.

6.6 Special precautions for disposal and other handling

None.

7. MARKETING AUTHORISATION HOLDER

Napp Pharmaceuticals Ltd
Cambridge Science Park
Milton Road
Cambridge
CB4 0GW

8. MARKETING AUTHORISATION NUMBER(S)

PL 16950/0009

9. DATE OF FIRST AUTHORISATION/RENEWAL OF THE AUTHORISATION

21 December 1989/23 September 2003

10. DATE OF REVISION OF THE TEXT

December 2008

11. LEGAL CATEGORY

POM

® ADIZEM and the Napp device are Registered Trade Marks.

Adizem-XL capsules

(Napp Pharmaceuticals Limited)

1. NAME OF THE MEDICINAL PRODUCT

ADIZEM®-XL capsules 120, 180, 200, 240, 300 mg

2. QUALITATIVE AND QUANTITATIVE COMPOSITION

Diltiazem Hydrochloride 120, 180, 200, 240, 300 mg

For excipients, see section 6.1.

3. PHARMACEUTICAL FORM

Prolonged release capsules.

ADIZEM-XL capsules 120 mg have a pale pink body and a navy blue cap, marked DCR 120.

ADIZEM-XL capsules 180 mg have a dark pink body and a royal blue cap marked DCR 180.

ADIZEM-XL capsules 200 mg have a brown body and a brown cap marked DCR 200.

ADIZEM-XL capsules 240 mg have a dark red body and a blue cap marked DCR 240.

ADIZEM-XL capsules 300 mg have a dark maroon body and a pale blue cap marked DCR 300.

4. CLINICAL PARTICULARS

4.1 Therapeutic indications

Management of angina pectoris.

Treatment of mild to moderate hypertension.

4.2 Posology and method of administration

Route of administration

Oral

Posology

Dosage requirements may differ between patients with angina and patients with hypertension. In addition, individual patients' responses may vary necessitating careful titration. This range of capsule strengths facilitates titration to the optimal dose.

The capsules should be swallowed whole and not chewed.

Adults:

For patients new to diltiazem therapy the usual starting dose is one 240 mg capsule daily.

Patients currently receiving a total daily dose of 180 mg diltiazem (as 90 mg b.d. or 60 mg t.i.d.) and transferring to ADIZEM-XL capsules should be given the 240 mg capsule (o.d.). A patient receiving 240 mg/day of diltiazem (as 120 mg b.d.) should commence treatment on the 240 mg capsule (o.d.), titrating to the 300 mg capsule (o.d.) if required.

Elderly and patients with impaired hepatic and renal function:

For patients new to diltiazem therapy, the usual starting dose is one 120 mg capsule daily. If necessary the dose may be gradually increased but careful monitoring of this group of patients is advised.

Elderly patients transferring to ADIZEM-XL capsules should receive the same total daily dose of diltiazem, titrating upwards as required.

Children:

ADIZEM-XL capsules are not recommended for children. Safety and efficacy in children have not been established.

In order to avoid confusion, it is suggested that patients, once titrated to an effective dose using ADIZEM-XL capsules, should remain on this treatment and should not be changed between different presentations.

ADIZEM-XL capsules should not be taken at the same time as an alcoholic beverage (refer to Section 4.5, Interactions with other Medicinal Products and Other Forms of Interaction).

4.3 Contraindications

Pregnancy and in women of child bearing capacity. Patients with bradycardia (less than 50 bpm), second or third degree heart block, sick sinus syndrome, decompensated cardiac failure, patients with left ventricular dysfunction following myocardial infarction. Concurrent use with dantrolene infusion because of the risk of ventricular fibrillation. Peanut or soya allergies. Hypersensitivity to diltiazem or to any of the excipients.

4.4 Special warnings and precautions for use

The product should be used with caution in patients with reduced left ventricular function. Patients with mild bradycardia, first degree AV block or prolonged PR interval should be observed closely. Diltiazem is considered unsafe in patients with acute porphyria.

4.5 Interaction with other medicinal products and other forms of interaction

Diltiazem is extensively metabolised by CYP3A4, and as a result serum levels of diltiazem may be:

- Increased by concomitant usage of CYP3A4 inhibitors such as H2 antagonists (e.g. cimetidine, ranitidine) and protease inhibitors (e.g. atazanavir, ritonavir)
- Decreased by concomitant usage of CYP3A4 inducers such as barbiturates (phenobarbital, primidone), phenytoin and rifampicin.

Diltiazem is also an inhibitor of CYP3A4, and may therefore increase serum levels of CYP3A4 substrates such as benzodiazepines (especially midazolam and triazolam), carbamazepine, ciclosporin, cilostazol, ivabradine, statins (simvastatin, atorvastatin, lovastatin), sirolimus, tacrolimus and theophylline. Care should be exercised in patients taking these drugs. Concomitant use of diltiazem with cilostazol and ivabradine should be avoided.

There may be an additive effect (increased depression of cardiac conduction with risk of bradycardia and AV block) when diltiazem is prescribed with drugs which may induce bradycardia or other anti-arrhythmic drugs (e.g. amiodarone and beta blockers). Patients with pre-existing conduction defects should not receive the combination of diltiazem and beta-blockers.

Enhanced antihypertensive effect may occur with concomitant use of other antihypertensive drugs (e.g. beta-blockers, diuretics, ACE-inhibitors) or drugs that cause hypotension such as aldesleukin and antipsychotics. Concomitant use with alpha-blockers (e.g. prazosin) should be strictly monitored because of the possible synergistic hypotensive effect of this combination.

Diltiazem hydrochloride may cause small increases in plasma levels of digoxin, requiring careful monitoring of AV conduction.

Diltiazem may increase serum levels of phenytoin.

Diltiazem may increase bioavailability of tricyclic antidepressants.

Treatment with diltiazem has been continued without problem during anaesthesia, but the anaesthetist should be made aware of the treatment regimen.

ADIZEM-XL capsules should not be taken at the same time as alcohol, as it may increase the rate of release of diltiazem from the prolonged release preparation. In addition the combination of alcohol and diltiazem may have an additive vasodilatory effect.

4.6 Pregnancy and lactation

Diltiazem hydrochloride is contraindicated in pregnant women or women of child bearing potential, and is not recommended in nursing mothers.

4.7 Effects on ability to drive and use machines

Diltiazem may cause adverse reactions such as dizziness, which may impair patients' ability to drive or operate machinery to a varying extent depending on the dosage and individual susceptibility. Therefore, patients should not drive or operate machinery if affected.

4.8 Undesirable effects

The adverse events listed below are classified by boc system according to their incidence (common or uncom mon). Common adverse events have an incidence of >1 and uncommon adverse events have an incidence <1%.

Blood and the lymphatic system disorders	
Uncommon	thrombocytopenia
Nervous system disorders	
Common	dizziness
	headache
Uncommon	extrapyramidal disorder
Cardiac disorders	
Uncommon	atrioventricular block
	bradycardia
	palpitations
	sinoatrial block
Vascular disorders	
Common	facial flushing
	hypotension
Uncommon	vasculitis
Gastrointestinal disorders	
Common	gastrointestinal disorder
	nausea
Uncommon	gingival hyperplasia
Hepatobiliary disorders	
Uncommon	increased hepatic enzyme
	clinical hepatitis
Skin and subcutaneous tissue disorders	
Uncommon	allergic dermatitis
	erythema multiforme
	exfoliative dermatitis
	photosensitivity reaction
Reproductive system and breast disorders	
Uncommon	gynaecomastia
General disorders and administration site conditions	
Common	fatigue
	oedema legs

4.9 Overdose

The clinical symptoms of acute intoxication may include pronounced hypotension or even collapse and sinus bradycardia with or without atrioventricular conduction defects.

The patient should be closely monitored in hospital to exclude arrhythmias or atrioventricular conduction defects. Gastric lavage and osmotic diuresis should be undertaken when considered appropriate. Symptomatic bradycardia and high grade atrioventricular block may respond to atropine, isoprenaline or occasionally temporary cardiac pacing.

Hypotension may require correction with plasma volume expanders, intravenous calcium gluconate and positive inotropic agents. The formulation employs a prolonged release system which will continue to release diltiazem for some hours.

5. PHARMACOLOGICAL PROPERTIES

5.1 Pharmacodynamic properties

Pharmacotherapeutic group: Selective calcium channel blocker with direct cardiac effects

ATC Code: C08D B01

5.1 Pharmacodynamic Properties

Diltiazem is a calcium antagonist. It restricts the slow channel entry of calcium ions into the cell and so reduces the liberation of calcium from stores in the sarcoplasmic reticulum. This results in a reduction in the amount of vailable intra-cellular calcium and consequently a (1) eduction of myocardial oxygen consumption, (2) dilation f small and large coronary arteries, (3) mild peripheral asodilation, (4) negative dromotropic effects, (5) reflex ositive chronotropic and inotropic effects due to reflex ympathetic activity are partially inhibited and result in a light reduction or no change in heart rate.

'he antihypertensive effect is due to the reduction in perpheral vascular resistance.

'he antianginal effect is due to a reduction in the peripheral esistance, thereby decreasing the after-load, whilst a eduction in the vasomotor tone of the coronary circulation naintains the coronary blood flow. Cardiac contractility and ventricular ejection fraction are unchanged. Diltiazem ncreases exercise capacity and improves indices of myocardial ischaemia in the angina patient. Diltiazem relieves he spasm of vasospastic (Prinzmetal) angina.

5.2 Pharmacokinetic properties

An oral dose of diltiazem is almost completely absorbed. Despite this, diltiazem has a low bioavailability owing to extensive first pass metabolism. This process is saturable at higher doses of the drug resulting in a non-linear accumulation and higher blood concentrations at steady state than would be anticipated from those following a single dose.

ADIZEM-XL capsules reduce the degree of saturation by presenting diltiazem in a retarded fashion therefore eliminating the high peak concentrations of the absorption phase. This allows the capsule to be administered once daily.

In pharmacokinetic studies in healthy volunteers, diltiazem was well absorbed. The controlled release capsules provided prolonged absorption of the drug, producing peak steady state plasma concentrations between 4 and 14 hours post-dose. The availability of diltiazem from ADIZEM-XL capsules 120 mg (o.d.) relative to a prolonged release 60 mg diltiazem preparation (b.d.) was approximately 79% at steady state. Similarly, the availability of diltiazem from the 240 mg capsule (o.d.) relative to ADIZEM-SR tablets 120 mg (b.d.) was approximately 78%. The extent of absorption of diltiazem was not affected when ADIZEM-XL capsules were co-administered with a high-fat meal.

5.3 Preclinical safety data

There are no pre-clinical data of relevance to the prescriber which are additional to that already included in other sections of the SPC.

6. PHARMACEUTICAL PARTICULARS

6.1 List of excipients

Capsule Contents

Microcrystalline Cellulose

Ethylcellulose N10

Colloidal Anhydrous Silica

Polysorbate 80

Dibutyl Sebacate

Magnesium Stearate

Capsule shells

Iron oxide (E172)

Titanium dioxide (E171)

Sodium dodecylsulphate

Gelatin

Erythrosine (E127) (not present in the 200 mg capsule)

Indigo carmine (E132) (not present in the 200 mg capsule)

Patent blue V (E131) (300 mg capsule only)

Printing ink

Shellac

Soya lecithin

2-ethoxyethanol

Dimeticone

Titanium dioxide (E171)

6.2 Incompatibilities

None known

6.3 Shelf life

2 years

6.4 Special precautions for storage

Do not store above 25°C

6.5 Nature and contents of container

PVC/PVdC blister packs with aluminium foil (containing 28 capsules).

6.6 Special precautions for disposal and other handling

None.

Administrative Data

7. MARKETING AUTHORISATION HOLDER

Napp Pharmaceuticals Ltd

Cambridge Science Park

Milton Road

Cambridge CB4 0GW

8. MARKETING AUTHORISATION NUMBER(S)

PL 16950/0010-0013, 0121

9. DATE OF FIRST AUTHORISATION/RENEWAL OF THE AUTHORISATION

ADIZEM-XL capsules 120 mg, 180 mg, 240 mg, 300 mg:

11 August 1993 / 23 September 2003

ADIZEM-XL capsules 200 mg:

10 September 2001/23 September 2003

10. DATE OF REVISION OF THE TEXT

July 2009

11. Legal Category

POM

ADIZEM-XL capsules are the subject of UK Patent GB 2 258 613.

® The Napp device and ADIZEM are Registered Trade Marks.

Advagraf 0.5mg, 1mg, 3mg and 5mg Prolonged-release hard capsules

(Astellas Pharma Ltd)

1. NAME OF THE MEDICINAL PRODUCT

Advagraf 0.5 mg prolonged-release hard capsules

Advagraf 1 mg prolonged-release hard capsules

Advagraf 3 mg prolonged-release hard capsules

Advagraf 5 mg prolonged-release hard capsules

2. QUALITATIVE AND QUANTITATIVE COMPOSITION

Advagraf 0.5 mg prolonged-release hard capsules

Each prolonged-release hard capsule contains 0.5 mg tacrolimus (as monohydrate).

Excipients: Each capsule contains 53.64 mg lactose monohydrate.

The printing ink used to mark the capsule contains trace amounts of soya lecithin (0.48% of total printing ink composition).

Advagraf 1 mg prolonged-release hard capsules

Each prolonged-release hard capsule contains 1 mg tacrolimus (as monohydrate).

Excipients: Each capsule contains 107.28 mg lactose monohydrate.

The printing ink used to mark the capsule contains trace amounts of soya lecithin (0.48% of total printing ink composition).

Advagraf 3 mg prolonged-release hard capsules

Each prolonged-release hard capsule contains 3 mg tacrolimus (as monohydrate).

Excipients: Each capsule contains 321.84 mg lactose monohydrate.

The printing ink used to mark the capsule contains trace amounts of soya lecithin (0.48% of total printing ink composition).

Advagraf 5 mg prolonged-release hard capsules

Each prolonged-release hard capsule contains 5 mg tacrolimus (as monohydrate).

Excipients: Each capsule contains 536.4 mg lactose monohydrate.

The printing ink used to mark the capsule contains trace amounts of soya lecithin (0.48% of total printing ink composition).

For a full list of excipients, see section 6.1.

3. PHARMACEUTICAL FORM

Advagraf 0.5 mg prolonged-release hard capsules

Prolonged-release hard capsule.

Gelatin capsules imprinted in red with "0.5 mg" on the light yellow capsule cap and "* 647" on the orange capsule body, containing white powder.

Advagraf 1 mg prolonged-release hard capsules

Prolonged-release hard capsule.

Gelatin capsules imprinted in red with "1 mg" on the white capsule cap and "* 677" on the orange capsule body, containing white powder.

Advagraf 3 mg prolonged-release hard capsules

Prolonged-release hard capsule.

Gelatin capsules imprinted in red with "3 mg" on the orange capsule cap and "* 637" on the orange capsule body, containing white powder.

Advagraf 5 mg prolonged-release hard capsules

Prolonged-release hard capsule.

Gelatin capsules imprinted in red with "5 mg" on the greyish red capsule cap and "* 687" on the orange capsule body, containing white powder.

4. CLINICAL PARTICULARS

4.1 Therapeutic indications

Prophylaxis of transplant rejection in adult kidney or liver allograft recipients.

Treatment of allograft rejection resistant to treatment with other immunosuppressive medicinal products in adult patients.

4.2 Posology and method of administration

Advagraf is a once-a-day oral formulation of tacrolimus. Advagraf therapy requires careful monitoring by adequately qualified and equipped personnel. This medicinal product should only be prescribed, and changes in immunosuppressive therapy initiated, by physicians experienced in immunosuppressive therapy and the management of transplant patients.

Inadvertent, unintentional or unsupervised switching of immediate- or prolonged-release formulations of tacrolimus is unsafe. This can lead to graft rejection or increased incidence of side effects, including under- or overimmunosuppression, due to clinically relevant differences in systemic exposure to tacrolimus. Patients should be maintained on a single formulation of tacrolimus with the corresponding daily dosing regimen; alterations in formulation or regimen should only take place under the close supervision of a transplant specialist (see sections 4.4 and 4.8). Following conversion to any alternative formulation, therapeutic drug monitoring must be performed and dose adjustments made to ensure that systemic exposure to tacrolimus is maintained.

Posology

The recommended initial doses presented below are intended to act solely as a guideline. Advagraf is routinely administered in conjunction with other immunosuppressive agents in the initial post-operative period. The dose may vary depending upon the immunosuppressive regimen chosen. Advagraf dosing should primarily be based on clinical assessments of rejection and tolerability in each patient individually aided by blood level monitoring (see below under "Therapeutic drug monitoring"). If clinical signs of rejection are apparent, alteration of the immunosuppressive regimen should be considered.

In *de novo* kidney and liver transplant patients AUC_{0-24} of tacrolimus for Advagraf on Day 1 was 30% and 50% lower respectively, when compared with that for Prograf at equivalent doses. By Day 4, systemic exposure as measured by trough levels is similar for both kidney and liver transplant patients with both formulations. Careful and frequent monitoring of tacrolimus trough levels is recommended in the first two weeks post-transplant with Advagraf to ensure adequate drug exposure in the immediate post-transplant period. As tacrolimus is a substance with low clearance, adjustments to the Advagraf dose regimen may take several days before steady state is achieved.

To suppress graft rejection, immunosuppression must be maintained; consequently, no limit to the duration of oral therapy can be given.

Prophylaxis of kidney transplant rejection

Advagraf therapy should commence at a dose of 0.20 - 0.30 mg/kg/day administered once daily in the morning. Administration should commence within 24 hours after the completion of surgery.

Advagraf doses are usually reduced in the post-transplant period. It is possible in some cases to withdraw concomitant immunosuppressive therapy, leading to Advagraf monotherapy. Post-transplant changes in the condition of the patient may alter the pharmacokinetics of tacrolimus and may necessitate further dose adjustments.

Prophylaxis of liver transplant rejection

Advagraf therapy should commence at a dose of 0.10 - 0.20 mg/kg/day administered once daily in the morning. Administration should commence approximately 12-18 hours after the completion of surgery.

Advagraf doses are usually reduced in the post-transplant period. It is possible in some cases to withdraw concomitant immunosuppressive therapy, leading to Advagraf monotherapy. Post-transplant improvement in the condition of the patient may alter the pharmacokinetics of tacrolimus and may necessitate further dose adjustments.

Conversion of Prograf-treated patients to Advagraf

Allograft transplant patients maintained on twice daily Prograf capsules dosing requiring conversion to once daily Advagraf should be converted on a 1:1 (mg:mg) total daily dose basis. Advagraf should be administered in the morning.

In stable patients converted from Prograf capsules (twice daily) to Advagraf (once daily) on a 1:1 (mg:mg) total daily dose basis, the systemic exposure to tacrolimus (AUC_{0-24}) for Advagraf was approximately 10% lower than that for Prograf. The relationship between tacrolimus trough levels (C_{24}) and systemic exposure (AUC_{0-24}) for Advagraf is similar to that of Prograf. When converting from Prograf capsules to Advagraf, trough levels should be measured prior to conversion and within two weeks after conversion. Following conversion, tacrolimus trough levels should be monitored and if necessary dose adjustments made to maintain similar systemic exposure. Dose adjustments should be made to ensure that similar systemic exposure is maintained.

Conversion from ciclosporin to tacrolimus

Care should be taken when converting patients from ciclosporin-based to tacrolimus-based therapy (see sections 4.4 and 4.5). The combined administration of ciclosporin and tacrolimus is not recommended. Advagraf therapy should be initiated after considering ciclosporin blood concentrations and the clinical condition of the patient. Dosing should be delayed in the presence of elevated ciclosporin blood levels. In practice, tacrolimus-based therapy has been initiated 12 - 24 hours after discontinuation of ciclosporin. Monitoring of ciclosporin blood levels should be continued following conversion as the clearance of ciclosporin might be affected.

Treatment of allograft rejection

Increased doses of tacrolimus, supplemental corticosteroid therapy, and introduction of short courses of mono-/polyclonal antibodies have all been used to manage rejection episodes. If signs of toxicity such as severe adverse reactions are noted (see section 4.8), the dose of Advagraf may need to be reduced.

Treatment of allograft rejection after kidney or liver transplantation

For conversion from other immunosuppressants to once daily Advagraf, treatment should begin with the initial oral dose recommended in kidney and liver transplantation respectively for prophylaxis of transplant rejection.

Treatment of allograft rejection after heart transplantation

In adult patients converted to Advagraf, an initial oral dose of 0.15 mg/kg/day should be administered once daily in the morning.

Treatment of allograft rejection after transplantation of other allografts

Although there is no clinical experience with Advagraf in lung-, pancreas- or intestine-transplanted patients, Prograf has been used in lung-transplanted patients at an initial oral dose of 0.10 - 0.15 mg/kg/day, in pancreas-transplanted patients at an initial oral dose of 0.2 mg/kg/day and in intestinal transplantation at an initial oral dose of 0.3 mg/kg/day.

Dose adjustments in special populations

Hepatic impairment: Dose reduction may be necessary in patients with severe liver impairment in order to maintain the tacrolimus blood trough levels within the recommended target range.

Renal impairment: As the pharmacokinetics of tacrolimus are unaffected by renal function (see section 5.2), no dose adjustment is required. However, owing to the nephrotoxic potential of tacrolimus careful monitoring of renal function is recommended (including serial serum creatinine concentrations, calculation of creatinine clearance and monitoring of urine output).

Race: In comparison to Caucasians, black patients may require higher tacrolimus doses to achieve similar trough levels.

Gender: There is no evidence that male and female patients require different doses to achieve similar trough levels.

Elderly patients: There is no evidence currently available to indicate that dosing should be adjusted in elderly patients.

Therapeutic drug monitoring

Dosing should primarily be based on clinical assessments of rejection and tolerability in each individual patient aided by whole blood tacrolimus trough level monitoring.

As an aid to optimise dosing, several immunoassays are available for determining tacrolimus concentrations in whole blood. Comparisons of concentrations from the published literature to individual values in clinical practice should be assessed with care and knowledge of the assay methods employed. In current clinical practice, whole blood levels are monitored using immunoassay methods. The relationship between tacrolimus trough levels (C_{24}) and systemic exposure (AUC_{0-24}) is similar between the two formulations Advagraf and Prograf.

Blood trough levels of tacrolimus should be monitored during the post-transplantation period. Tacrolimus blood trough levels should be determined approximately 24 hours post-dosing of Advagraf, just prior to the next dose. Frequent trough level monitoring in the initial two weeks post transplantation is recommended, followed by periodic monitoring during maintenance therapy. Blood trough levels of tacrolimus should also be closely monitored following conversion from Prograf to Advagraf, dose adjustments, changes in the immunosuppressive regimen, or co-administration of substances which may alter tacrolimus whole blood concentrations (see section 4.5). The frequency of blood level monitoring should be based on clinical needs. As tacrolimus is a substance with low clearance, following adjustments to the Advagraf dose regimen it may take several days before the targeted steady state is achieved.

Data from clinical studies suggest that the majority of patients can be successfully managed if tacrolimus blood trough levels are maintained below 20 ng/ml. It is necessary to consider the clinical condition of the patient when interpreting whole blood levels. In clinical practice, whole blood trough levels have generally been in the range 5 - 20 ng/ml in liver transplant recipients and 10 - 20 ng/ml in kidney and heart transplant patients in the early post-transplant period. During subsequent maintenance therapy, blood concentrations have generally been in the range of 5 - 15 ng/ml in liver, kidney and heart transplant recipients.

Method of administration

Advagraf is a once-a-day oral formulation of tacrolimus. It is recommended that the oral daily dose of Advagraf be administered once daily in the morning. Advagraf prolonged-release hard capsules should be taken immediately following removal from the blister. Patients should be advised not to swallow the desiccant. The capsules should be swallowed ***whole*** with fluid (preferably water). Advagraf should generally be administered on an empty stomach or at least 1 hour before or 2 to 3 hours after a meal, to achieve maximal absorption (see section 5.2). A forgotten morning dose should be taken as soon as possible on the same day. A double dose should not be taken on the next morning.

In patients unable to take oral medicinal products during the immediate post-transplant period, tacrolimus therapy can be initiated intravenously (see Summary of Product Characteristics for Prograf 5 mg/ml concentrate for solution for infusion) at a dose approximately 1/5th of the recommended oral dose for the corresponding indication.

4.3 Contraindications

Hypersensitivity to tacrolimus, or to any of the excipients (see section 6.1)

Hypersensitivity to other macrolides

4.4 Special warnings and precautions for use

Medication errors, including inadvertent, unintentional or unsupervised substitution of immediate- or prolonged-release tacrolimus formulations, have been observed. This has led to serious adverse events, including graft rejection, or other side effects which could be a consequence of either under- or over-exposure to tacrolimus. Patients should be maintained on a single formulation of tacrolimus with the corresponding daily dosing regimen; alterations in formulation or regimen should only take place under the close supervision of a transplant specialist (see sections 4.2 and 4.8).

Advagraf is not recommended for use in children below 18 years due to limited data on safety and/or efficacy.

For treatment of allograft rejection resistant to treatment with other immunosuppressive medicinal products in adult patients clinical data are not yet available for the prolonged-release formulation Advagraf.

For prophylaxis of transplant rejection in adult heart allograft recipients clinical data are not yet available for Advagraf.

During the initial post-transplant period, monitoring of the following parameters should be undertaken on a routine basis: blood pressure, ECG, neurological and visual status, fasting blood glucose levels, electrolytes (particularly potassium), liver and renal function tests, haematology parameters, coagulation values, and plasma protein determinations. If clinically relevant changes are seen, adjustments of the immunosuppressive regimen should be considered.

When substances with a potential for interaction (see section 4.5) - particularly strong inhibitors of CYP3A4 (such as ketoconazole, voriconazole, itraconazole, telithromycin or clarithromycin) or inducers of CYP3A4 (such as rifampin, rifabutin) – are being combined with tacrolimus, tacrolimus blood levels should be monitored to adjust the tacrolimus dose as appropriate in order to maintain similar tacrolimus exposure.

Herbal preparations containing St. John's Wort (*Hypericum perforatum*) should be avoided when taking Advagraf due to the risk of interactions that lead to a decrease in both blood concentrations and the therapeutic effect of tacrolimus (see section 4.5).

The combined administration of ciclosporin and tacrolimus should be avoided and care should be taken when administering tacrolimus to patients who have previously received ciclosporin (see sections 4.2 and 4.5).

High potassium intake or potassium-sparing diuretics should be avoided (see section 4.5).

Certain combinations of tacrolimus with drugs known to have nephrotoxic or neurotoxic effects may increase the risk of these effects (see section 4.5).

Immunosuppressants may affect the response to vaccination and vaccination during treatment with tacrolimus may be less effective. The use of live attenuated vaccines should be avoided.

Since levels of tacrolimus in blood may significantly change during diarrhoea episodes, extra monitoring of tacrolimus concentrations is recommended during episodes of diarrhoea.

Cardiac disorders

Ventricular hypertrophy or hypertrophy of the septum, reported as cardiomyopathies, have been observed in Prograf treated patients on rare occasions and may also occur with Advagraf. Most cases have been reversible, occurring with tacrolimus blood trough concentrations much higher than the recommended maximum levels. Other factors observed to increase the risk of these clinical conditions included pre-existing heart disease, corticosteroid usage, hypertension, renal or hepatic dysfunction, infections, fluid overload, and oedema. Accordingly, high-risk patients receiving substantial immunosuppression should be monitored, using such procedures as echocardiography or ECG pre- and post-transplant (e.g. initially at 3 months and then at 9 -12 months). If abnormalities develop, dose reduction of Advagraf, or change of treatment to another immunosuppressive agent should be considered. Tacrolimus may prolong the QT interval but at this time lacks substantial evidence for causing *Torsades de Pointes*. Caution should be exercised in patients with diagnosed or suspected Congenital Long QT Syndrome.

Lymphoproliferative disorders and malignancies

Patients treated with tacrolimus have been reported to develop EBV-associated lymphoproliferative disorders (see section 4.8). A combination of immunosuppressives such as antilymphocytic antibodies (e.g. basiliximab, daclizumab) given concomitantly increases the risk of EBV-associated lymphoproliferative disorders. EBV-Viral Capsid Antigen (VCA)-negative patients have been reported to have an increased risk of developing lymphoproliferative disorders. Therefore, in this patient group, EBV-VCA serology should be ascertained before starting treatment with Advagraf. During treatment, careful monitoring with EBV-PCR is recommended. Positive EBV-PCR may persist for months and is *per se* not indicative of lymphoproliferative disease or lymphoma.

As with other potent immunosuppressive compounds, the risk of secondary cancer is unknown (see section 4.8).

As with other immunosuppressive agents, owing to the potential risk of malignant skin changes, exposure to sunlight and UV light should be limited by wearing protective clothing and using a sunscreen with a high protection factor.

Patients treated with immunosuppressants, including Advagraf are at increased risk for opportunistic infections (bacterial, fungal, viral and protozoal). Among these conditions are BK virus associated nephropathy and JC virus associated progressive multifocal leukoencephalopathy (PML). These infections are often related to a high total immunosuppressive burden and may lead to serious or fatal conditions that physicians should consider in the differential diagnosis in immunosuppressed patients with deteriorating renal function or neurological symptoms.

Patients treated with tacrolimus have been reported to develop posterior reversible encephalopathy syndrome (PRES). If patients taking tacrolimus present with symptoms indicating PRES such as headache, altered mental status, seizures, and visual disturbances, a radiological procedure (e.g. MRI) should be performed. If PRES is diagnosed, adequate blood pressure and seizure control and immediate discontinuation of systemic tacrolimus is advised. Most patients completely recover after appropriate measures are taken.

Special populations

There is limited experience in non-Caucasian patients and patients at elevated immunological risk (e.g. retransplantation, evidence of panel reactive antibodies, PRA).

Dose reduction may be necessary in patients with sever liver impairment (see section 4.2)

Advagraf capsules contain lactose. Patients with rare hereditary problems of galactose intolerance, the Lapp lactase deficiency or glucose-galactose malabsorption should not take this medicinal product.

The printing ink used to mark Advagraf capsules contains soya lecithin. In patients who are hypersensitive to peanut or soya, the risk and severity of hypersensitivity should be weighed against the benefit of using Advagraf.

4.5 Interaction with other medicinal products and other forms of interaction

Systemically available tacrolimus is metabolised by hepatic CYP3A4. There is also evidence of gastrointestinal metabolism by CYP3A4 in the intestinal wall. Concomitant use of substances known to inhibit or induce CYP3A4 may affect the metabolism of tacrolimus and thereby increase or decrease tacrolimus blood levels.

It is recommended to monitor tacrolimus blood levels whenever substances which have the potential to alter CYP3A metabolism or otherwise influence tacrolimus blood levels are used concomitantly, and to adjust the tacrolimus dose as appropriate in order to maintain similar tacrolimus exposure (see sections 4.2 and 4.4).

CYP3A4 inhibitors potentially leading to increased tacrolimus blood levels

Clinically the following substances have been shown to increase tacrolimus blood levels:

Strong interactions have been observed with antifungal agents such as ketoconazole, fluconazole, itraconazole and voriconazole, the macrolide antibiotic erythromycin or HIV protease inhibitors (e.g. ritonavir). Concomitant use of these substances may require decreased tacrolimus doses in nearly all patients. Pharmacokinetics studies have indicated that the increase in blood levels is mainly a result of increase in oral bioavailability of tacrolimus owing to the inhibition of gastrointestinal metabolism. Effect on hepatic clearance is less pronounced.

Weaker interactions have been observed with clotrimazole, clarithromycin, josamycin, nifedipine, nicardipine, diltiazem, verapamil, danazol, ethinylestradiol, omeprazole and nefazodone.

In vitro the following substances have been shown to be potential inhibitors of tacrolimus metabolism: bromocriptine, cortisone, dapsone, ergotamine, gestodene, lidocaine, mephenytoin, miconazole, midazolam, nilvadipine, norethindrone, quinidine, tamoxifen, (triacetyl)oleandomycin.

Grapefruit juice has been reported to increase the blood level of tacrolimus and should therefore be avoided.

ansoprazol and ciclosporin may potentially inhibit YP3A4-mediated metabolism of tacrolimus and thereby crease tacrolimus whole blood concentrations.

ther interactions potentially leading to increased tacroli-us blood levels

acrolimus is extensively bound to plasma proteins. Pos-ble interactions with other active substances known to ave high affinity for plasma proteins should be considered .g., NSAIDs, oral anticoagulants, or oral antidiabetics).

ther potential interactions that may increase systemic xposure of tacrolimus include prokinetic agents (such s metoclopramide and cisapride), cimetidine and magne-ium-aluminium-hydroxide.

CYP3A4 inducers potentially leading to decreased tacroli-nus blood levels

Clinically the following substances have been shown to decrease tacrolimus blood levels:

Strong interactions have been observed with rifampicin, phenytoin, St. John's Wort (*Hypericum perforatum*) which may require increased tacrolimus doses in almost all patients. Clinically significant interactions have also been observed with phenobarbital. Maintenance doses of corti-costeroids have been shown to reduce tacrolimus blood levels.

High dose prednisolone or methylprednisolone adminis-tered for the treatment of acute rejection have the potential to increase or decrease tacrolimus blood levels.

Carbamazepine, metamizole and isoniazid have the poten-tial to decrease tacrolimus concentrations.

Effect of tacrolimus on the metabolism of other medicinal products

Tacrolimus is a known CYP3A4 inhibitor; thus concomitant use of tacrolimus with medicinal products known to be metabolised by CYP3A4 may affect the metabolism of such medicinal products.

The half-life of ciclosporin is prolonged when tacrolimus is given concomitantly. In addition, synergistic/additive nephrotoxic effects can occur. For these reasons, the combined administration of ciclosporin and tacrolimus is not recommended and care should be taken when admin-istering tacrolimus to patients who have previously received ciclosporin (see sections 4.2 and 4.4).

Tacrolimus has been shown to increase the blood level of phenytoin.

As tacrolimus may reduce the clearance of steroid-based contraceptives leading to increased hormone exposure, particular care should be exercised when deciding upon contraceptive measures.

Limited knowledge of interactions between tacrolimus and statins is available. Clinical data suggest that the pharma-cokinetics of statins are largely unaltered by the co-admin-istration of tacrolimus.

Animal data have shown that tacrolimus could potentially decrease the clearance and increase the half-life of pen-tobarbital and antipyrine.

Other interactions leading to clinically detrimental effects

Concurrent use of tacrolimus with medicinal products known to have nephrotoxic or neurotoxic effects may increase these effects (e.g., aminoglycosides, gyrase inhi-bitors, vancomycin, cotrimoxazole, NSAIDs, ganciclovir or aciclovir).

Enhanced nephrotoxicity has been observed following the administration of amphotericin B and ibuprofen in conjunc-tion with tacrolimus.

As tacrolimus treatment may be associated with hyperka-laemia, or may increase pre-existing hyperkalaemia, high potassium intake, or potassium-sparing diuretics (e.g. amiloride, triamterene, or spironolactone) should be avoided (see section 4.4).

Immunosuppressants may affect the response to vaccina-tion and vaccination during treatment with tacrolimus may be less effective. The use of live attenuated vaccines should be avoided (see section 4.4).

4.6 Pregnancy and lactation

Pregnancy

Human data show that tacrolimus crosses the placenta. Limited data from organ transplant recipients show no evidence of an increased risk of adverse events on the course and outcome of pregnancy under tacrolimus treat-ment compared with other immunosuppressive medicinal products. To date, no other relevant epidemiological data are available. Tacrolimus treatment can be considered in pregnant women, when there is no safer alternative and when the perceived benefit justifies the potential risk to the foetus. In case of *in utero* exposure, monitoring of the newborn for the potential adverse events of tacrolimus is recommended (in particular effects on the kidneys). There is a risk for premature delivery (<37 week) (incidence of 66 of 123 births, i.e. 53.7%; however, data showed that the majority of the newborns had normal birth weight for their gestational age) as well as for hyperkalaemia in the new-born (incidence 8 of 111 neonates, i.e. 7.2 %) which, however normalises spontaneously.

In rats and rabbits, tacrolimus caused embryofoetal toxi-city at doses which demonstrated maternal toxicity (see section 5.3).

Lactation

Human data demonstrate that tacrolimus is excreted in breast milk. As detrimental effects on the newborn cannot be excluded, women should not breast-feed whilst receiv-ing Advagraf.

Fertility

A negative effect of tacrolimus on male fertility in the form of reduced sperm counts and motility was observed in rats (see section 5.3).

4.7 Effects on ability to drive and use machines

Tacrolimus may cause visual and neurological distur-bances. This effect may be enhanced if Advagraf is admi-nistered in association with alcohol.

No studies on the effects of tacrolimus (Advagraf) on the ability to drive and use machines have been performed.

4.8 Undesirable effects

The adverse reaction profile associated with immunosup-pressive agents is often difficult to establish owing to the underlying disease and the concurrent use of multiple medicinal products.

The most commonly reported adverse drug reactions (occurring in > 10% of patients) are tremor, renal impair-ment, hyperglycaemic conditions, diabetes mellitus, hyperkalaemia, infections, hypertension and insomnia.

Many of the adverse reactions stated below are reversible and/or respond to dose reduction. The frequency of adverse reactions is defined as follows: very common (⩾ 1/10); common (⩾ 1/100 to < 1/10); uncommon (⩾ 1/1,000 to < 1/100); rare (⩾ 1/10,000 to < 1/1,000); very rare (< 1/10,000), not known (cannot be estimated from the available data). Within each frequency grouping, undesirable effects are presented in order of decreasing seriousness.

Cardiac disorders

common: ischaemic coronary artery disorders, tachycar-dia

uncommon: heart failures, ventricular arrhythmias and cardiac arrest, supraventricular arrhythmias, cardiomyo-pathies, ECG investigations abnormal, ventricular hyper-trophy, palpitations, heart rate and pulse investigations abnormal

rare: pericardial effusion

very rare: echocardiogram abnormal

Blood and lymphatic system disorders

common: anaemia, thrombocytopenia, leukopenia, red blood cell analyses abnormal, leukocytosis

uncommon: coagulopathies, pancytopenia, neutropenia, coagulation and bleeding analyses, abnormal

rare: thrombotic thrombocytopenic purpura, hypopro-thrombinaemia

Nervous system disorders

very common: headache, tremor

common: nervous system disorders seizures, distur-bances in consciousness, peripheral neuropathies, dizzi-ness, paraesthesias and dysaesthesias, writing impaired

uncommon: encephalopathy, central nervous system hae-morrhages and cerebrovascular accidents, coma, speech and language abnormalities, paralysis and paresis, amne-sia

rare: hypertonia

very rare: myasthenia

Eye disorders

common: eye disorders, vision blurred, photophobia

uncommon: cataract

rare: blindness

Ear and labyrinth disorders

common: tinnitus

uncommon: hypoacusis

rare: deafness neurosensory

very rare: hearing impaired

Respiratory, thoracic and mediastinal disorders

common: parenchymal lung disorders, dyspnoea, pleural effusion, cough, pharyngitis, nasal congestion and inflam-mations

uncommon: respiratory failures, respiratory tract disor-ders, asthma

rare: acute respiratory distress syndrome

Gastrointestinal disorders

very common: diarrhoea, nausea

common: gastrointestinal signs and symptoms, vomiting, gastrointestinal and abdominal pains, gastrointestinal inflammatory conditions, gastrointestinal haemorrhages, gastrointestinal ulceration and perforation, ascites, stoma-titis and ulceration, constipation, dyspeptic signs and symptoms, flatulence, bloating and distension, loose stools

uncommon: acute and chronic pancreatitis, peritonitis, blood amylase increased, ileus paralytic, gastrooesopha-geal reflux disease, impaired gastric emptying

rare: pancreatic pseudocyst, subileus

Renal and urinary disorders

very common: renal impairment

common: renal failure, renal failure acute, nephropathy toxic, renal tubular necrosis, urinary abnormalities, oliguria, bladder and urethral symptoms

uncommon: haemolytic uraemic syndrome, anuria

very rare: nephropathy, cystitis haemorrhagic

Skin and subcutaneous tissue disorders

common: rash, pruritus, alopecias, acne, sweating increased

uncommon: dermatitis, photosensitivity

rare: toxic epidermal necrolysis (Lyell's syndrome)

very rare: Stevens Johnson syndrome

Musculoskeletal and connective tissue disorders

common: arthralgia, back pain, muscle cramps, pain in limb

uncommon: joint disorders

Endocrine disorders

rare: hirsutism

Metabolism and nutrition disorders

very common: diabetes mellitus, hyperglycaemic condi-tions, hyperkalaemia

common: anorexia, metabolic acidoses, other electrolyte abnormalities, hyponatraemia, fluid overload, hyperuricae-mia, hypomagnesaemia, hypokalaemia, hypocalcaemia, appetite decreased, hypercholesterolaemia, hyperlipidae-mia, hypertriglyceridaemia, hypophosphataemia

uncommon: dehydration, hypoglycaemia, hypoproteinae-mia, hyperphosphataemia

Infections and infestations

As is well known for other potent immunosuppressive agents, patients receiving tacrolimus are frequently at increased risk for infections (viral, bacterial, fungal, proto-zoal). The course of pre-existing infections may be aggra-vated. Both generalised and localised infections can occur.

Cases of BK virus associated nephropathy, as well as cases of JC virus associated progressive multifocal leu-koencephalopathy (PML), have been reported in patients treated with immunosuppressants, including Advagraf.

Injury, poisoning and procedural complications

common: primary graft dysfunction

Medication errors, including inadvertent, unintentional or unsupervised substitution of immediate- or prolonged-release tacrolimus formulations, have been observed. A number of associated cases of transplant rejection have been reported (frequency cannot be estimated from avail-able data).

Neoplasms benign, malignant and unspecified

Patients receiving immunosuppressive therapy are at increased risk of developing malignancies. Benign as well as malignant neoplasms including EBV-associated lym-phoproliferative disorders and skin malignancies have been reported in association with tacrolimus treatment.

Vascular disorders

very common: hypertension

common: thromboembolic and ischaemic events, vascular hypotensive disorders, haemorrhage, peripheral vascular disorders

uncommon: venous thrombosis deep limb, shock, infarc-tion

General disorders and administration site conditions

common: febrile disorders, pain and discomfort, asthenic conditions, oedema, body temperature perception dis-turbed, blood alkaline phosphatase increased, weight increased

uncommon: weight decreased, influenza like illness, blood lactate dehydrogenase increased, feeling jittery, feeling abnormal, multi-organ failure, chest pressure sensation, temperature intolerance

rare: fall, ulcer, chest tightness, mobility decreased, thirst

very rare: fat tissue increased

Immune system disorders

Allergic and anaphylactoid reactions have been observed in patients receiving tacrolimus (see section 4.4).

Hepatobiliary disorders

very common: liver function tests abnormal

common: bile duct disorders, hepatocellular damage and hepatitis, cholestasis and jaundice

rare: venoocclusive liver disease, hepatitic artery throm-bosis

very rare: hepatic failure

Reproductive system and breast disorders

uncommon: dysmenorrhoea and uterine bleeding

Psychiatric disorders

very common: insomnia

common: confusion and disorientation, depression, anxi-ety symptoms, hallucination, mental disorders, depressed mood, mood disorders and disturbances, nightmare

uncommon: psychotic disorder

4.9 Overdose

Experience with overdose is limited. Several cases of accidental overdose have been reported with tacrolimus; symptoms have included tremor, headache, nausea and vomiting, infections, urticaria, lethargy and increases in blood urea nitrogen, serum creatinine and alanine aminotransferase levels.

No specific antidote to tacrolimus therapy is available. If overdose occurs, general supportive measures and symptomatic treatment should be conducted.

Based on its high molecular weight, poor aqueous solubility, and extensive erythrocyte and plasma protein binding, it is anticipated that tacrolimus will not be dialysable. In isolated patients with very high plasma levels, haemofiltration or -diafiltration have been effective in reducing toxic concentrations. In cases of oral intoxication, gastric lavage and/or the use of adsorbents (such as activated charcoal) may be helpful, if used shortly after intake.

5. PHARMACOLOGICAL PROPERTIES

5.1 Pharmacodynamic properties

Pharmacotherapeutic group: Calcineurin inhibitors, ATC code: L04AD02

Mechanism of action

At the molecular level, the effects of tacrolimus appear to be mediated by binding to a cytosolic protein (FKBP12) which is responsible for the intracellular accumulation of the compound. The FKBP12-tacrolimus complex specifically and competitively binds to and inhibits calcineurin, leading to a calcium-dependent inhibition of T-cell signal transduction pathways, thereby preventing transcription of a discrete set of cytokine genes.

Tacrolimus is a highly potent immunosuppressive agent and has proven activity in both *in vitro* and *in vivo* experiments.

In particular, tacrolimus inhibits the formation of cytotoxic lymphocytes, which are mainly responsible for graft rejection. Tacrolimus suppresses T-cell activation and T-helper-cell dependent B-cell proliferation, as well as the formation of lymphokines (such as interleukins-2, -3, and γ-interferon) and the expression of the interleukin-2 receptor.

Results from clinical trials performed with once-daily tacrolimus Advagraf

Liver transplantation

The efficacy and safety of Advagraf and Prograf, both in combination with corticosteroids, was compared in 471 *de novo* liver transplant recipients. The event rate of biopsy confirmed acute rejection within the first 24 weeks after transplantation was 32.6% in the Advagraf group (N=237) and 29.3% in the Prograf group (N=234). The treatment difference (Advagraf – Prograf) was 3.3% (95% confidence interval [-5.7%, 12.3%]). The 12-month patient survival rates were 89.2% for Advagraf and 90.8% for Prograf; in the Advagraf arm 25 patients died (14 female, 11 male) and in the Prograf arm 24 patients died (5 female, 19 male). 12-month graft survival was 85.3% for Advagraf and 85.6% for Prograf.

Kidney transplantation

The efficacy and safety of Advagraf and Prograf, both in combination with mycophenolate mofetil (MMF) and corticosteroids, was compared in 667 *de novo* kidney transplant recipients. The event rate for biopsy-confirmed acute rejection within the first 24 weeks after transplantation was 18.6% in the Advagraf group (N=331) and 14.9% in the Prograf group (N=336). The treatment difference (Advagraf-Prograf) was 3.8% (95% confidence interval [-2.1%, 9.6%]). The 12-month patient survival rates were 96.9% for Advagraf and 97.5% for Prograf; in the Advagraf arm 10 patients died (3 female, 7 male) and in the Prograf arm 8 patients died (3 female, 5 male). 12-month graft survival was 91.5% for Advagraf and 92.8% for Prograf.

The efficacy and safety of Prograf, ciclosporin and Advagraf, all in combination with basiliximab antibody induction, MMF and corticosteroids, was compared in 638 *de novo* kidney transplant recipients. The incidence of efficacy failure at 12 months (defined as death, graft loss, biopsy-confirmed acute rejection, or lost to follow-up) was 14.0% in the Advagraf group (N=214), 15.1% in the Prograf group (N=212) and 17.0% in the ciclosporin group (N=212). The treatment difference was -3.0% (Advagraf-ciclosporin) (95.2% confidence interval [-9.9%, 4.0%]) for Advagraf vs. ciclosporin and -1.9% (Prograf-ciclosporin) (95.2% confidence interval [-8.9%, 5.2%]) for Prograf vs. ciclosporin. The 12-month patient survival rates were 98.6% for Advagraf, 95.7% for Prograf and 97.6% for ciclosporin; in the Advagraf arm 3 patients died (all male), in the Prograf arm 10 patients died (3 female, 7 male) and in the ciclosporin arm 6 patients died (3 female, 3 male). 12-month graft survival was 96.7% for Advagraf, 92.9% for Prograf and 95.7% for ciclosporin.

Clinical efficacy and safety of Prograf capsules bid in primary organ transplantation

In prospective studies oral Prograf was investigated as primary immunosuppressant in approximately 175 patients following lung, 475 patients following pancreas and 630 patients following intestinal transplantation. Overall, the safety profile of oral Prograf in these published studies appeared to be similar to what was reported in the large studies, where Prograf was used as primary treatment in liver, kidney and heart transplantation. Efficacy results of the largest studies in each indication are summarised below.

Lung transplantation

The interim analysis of a recent multicentre study using oral Prograf discussed 110 patients who underwent 1:1 randomisation to either tacrolimus or ciclosporin. Tacrolimus was started as continuous intravenous infusion at a dose of 0.01 to 0.03 mg/kg/day and oral tacrolimus was administered at a dose of 0.05 to 0.3 mg/kg/day. A lower incidence of acute rejection episodes for tacrolimus- versus ciclosporin-treated patients (11.5% versus 22.6%) and a lower incidence of chronic rejection, the bronchiolitis obliterans syndrome (2.86% versus 8.57%), was reported within the first year after transplantation. The 1-year patient survival rate was 80.8% in the tacrolimus and 83% in the ciclosporin group.

Another randomised study included 66 patients on tacrolimus versus 67 patients on ciclosporin. Tacrolimus was started as continuous intravenous infusion at a dose of 0.025 mg/kg/day and oral tacrolimus was administered at a dose of 0.15 mg/kg/day with subsequent dose adjustments to target trough levels of 10 to 20 ng/ml. The 1-year patient survival was 83% in the tacrolimus and 71% in the ciclosporin group, the 2-year survival rates were 76% and 66%, respectively. Acute rejection episodes per 100 patient-days were numerically fewer in the tacrolimus (0.85 episodes) than in the ciclosporin group (1.09 episodes). Obliterative bronchiolitis developed in 21.7% of patients in the tacrolimus group compared with 38.0% of patients in the ciclosporin group (p = 0.025). Significantly more ciclosporin-treated patients (n = 13) required a switch to tacrolimus than tacrolimus-treated patients to ciclosporin (n = 2) (p = 0.02) (Keenan et al., Ann Thoracic Surg 1995;60:580).

In an additional two-centre study, 26 patients were randomised to the tacrolimus versus 24 patients to the ciclosporin group. Tacrolimus was started as continuous intravenous infusion at a dose of 0.05 mg/kg/day and oral tacrolimus was administered at a dose of 0.1 to 0.3 mg/kg/day with subsequent dose adjustments to target trough levels of 12 to 15 ng/ml. The 1-year survival rates were 73.1% in the tacrolimus versus 79.2% in the ciclosporin group. Freedom from acute rejection was higher in the tacrolimus group at 6 months (57.7% versus 45.8%) and at 1 year after lung transplantation (50% versus 33.3%).

The three studies demonstrated similar survival rates. The incidences of acute rejection were numerically lower with tacrolimus in all three studies and one of the studies reported a significantly lower incidence of bronchiolitis obliterans syndrome with tacrolimus.

Pancreas transplantation

A multicentre study using oral Prograf included 205 patients undergoing simultaneous pancreas-kidney transplantation who were randomised to tacrolimus (n = 103) or to ciclosporin (n = 102). The initial oral per protocol dose of tacrolimus was 0.2 mg/kg/day with subsequent dose adjustments to target trough levels of 8 to 15 ng/ml by Day 5 and 5 to 10 ng/ml after Month 6. Pancreas survival at 1 year was significantly superior with tacrolimus: 91.3% versus 74.5% with ciclosporin ($p < 0.0005$), whereas renal graft survival was similar in both groups. In total 34 patients switched treatment from ciclosporin to tacrolimus, whereas only 6 tacrolimus patients required alternative therapy.

Intestinal transplantation

Published clinical experience from a single centre on the use of oral Prograf for primary treatment following intestinal transplantation showed that the actuarial survival rate of 155 patients (65 intestine alone, 75 liver and intestine, and 25 multivisceral) receiving tacrolimus and prednisone was 75% at 1 year, 54% at 5 years, and 42% at 10 years. In the early years the initial oral dose of tacrolimus was 0.3 mg/kg/day. Results continuously improved with increasing experience over the course of 11 years. A variety of innovations, such as techniques for early detection of Epstein-Barr (EBV) and CMV infections, bone marrow augmentation, the adjunct use of the interleukin-2 antagonist daclizumab, lower initial tacrolimus doses with target trough levels of 10 to 15 ng/ml, and most recently allograft irradiation were considered to have contributed to improved results in this indication over time.

5.2 Pharmacokinetic properties

Absorption

In man tacrolimus has been shown to be able to be absorbed throughout the gastrointestinal tract. Available tacrolimus is generally rapidly absorbed. Advagraf is a prolonged-release formulation of tacrolimus resulting in an extended oral absorption profile with an average time to maximum blood concentration (C_{max}) of approximately 2 hours (t_{max}).

Absorption is variable and the mean oral bioavailability of tacrolimus (investigated with the Prograf formulation) is in the range of 20% - 25% (individual range in adult patients 6% - 43%). The oral bioavailability of Advagraf was reduced when it was administered after a meal. Both the rate and extent of absorption of Advagraf were reduced when administered with food.

Bile flow does not influence the absorption of tacrolimus and therefore treatment with Advagraf may commence orally.

A strong correlation exists between AUC and whole blood trough levels at steady-state for Advagraf. Monitoring of whole blood trough levels therefore provides a good estimate of systemic exposure.

Distribution

In man, the disposition of tacrolimus after intravenous infusion may be described as biphasic.

In the systemic circulation, tacrolimus binds strongly to erythrocytes resulting in an approximate 20:1 distribution ratio of whole blood/plasma concentrations. In plasma, tacrolimus is highly bound (> 98.8%) to plasma proteins, mainly to serum albumin and α-1-acid glycoprotein.

Tacrolimus is extensively distributed in the body. The steady-state volume of distribution based on plasma concentrations is approximately 1300 l (healthy subjects). Corresponding data based on whole blood averaged 47.6 l.

Metabolism

Tacrolimus is widely metabolised in the liver, primarily by the cytochrome P450-3A4. Tacrolimus is also considerably metabolised in the intestinal wall. There are several metabolites identified. Only one of these has been shown *in vitro* to have immunosuppressive activity similar to that of tacrolimus. The other metabolites have only weak or no immunosuppressive activity. In systemic circulation only one of the inactive metabolites is present at low concentrations. Therefore, metabolites do not contribute to the pharmacological activity of tacrolimus.

Excretion

Tacrolimus is a low-clearance substance. In healthy subjects, the average total body clearance estimated from whole blood concentrations was 2.25 l/h. In adult liver, kidney and heart transplant patients, values of 4.1 l/h, 6.7 l/h and 3.9 l/h, respectively, have been observed. Factors such as low haematocrit and protein levels, which result in an increase in the unbound fraction of tacrolimus, or corticosteroid-induced increased metabolism, are considered to be responsible for the higher clearance rates observed following transplantation.

The half-life of tacrolimus is long and variable. In healthy subjects, the mean half-life in whole blood is approximately 43 hours.

Following intravenous and oral administration of ^{14}C-labelled tacrolimus, most of the radioactivity was eliminated in the faeces. Approximately 2% of the radioactivity was eliminated in the urine. Less than 1% of unchanged tacrolimus was detected in the urine and faeces, indicating that tacrolimus is almost completely metabolised prior to elimination: bile being the principal route of elimination.

5.3 Preclinical safety data

The kidneys and the pancreas were the primary organs affected in toxicity studies performed in rats and baboons. In rats, tacrolimus caused toxic effects to the nervous system and the eyes. Reversible cardiotoxic effects were observed in rabbits following intravenous administration of tacrolimus.

Embryofoetal toxicity was observed in rats and rabbits and was limited to doses that caused significant toxicity in maternal animals. In rats, female reproductive function including birth was impaired at toxic doses and the offspring showed reduced birth weights, viability and growth.

A negative effect of tacrolimus on male fertility in the form of reduced sperm counts and motility was observed in rats.

6. PHARMACEUTICAL PARTICULARS

6.1 List of excipients

Capsule content:

Hypromellose

Ethylcellulose

Lactose monohydrate

Magnesium stearate.

Capsule shell:

Titanium dioxide (E 171)

Yellow iron oxide (E 172)

Red iron oxide (E 172)

Sodium laurilsulfate

Gelatin.

Printing ink (Opacode S-1-15083):

Shellac

Lecithin (soya)

Simeticone

Red iron oxide (E 172)

Hydroxypropylcellulose.

6.2 Incompatibilities

Tacrolimus is not compatible with PVC (polyvinylchloride). Tubing, syringes and other equipment used to prepare a suspension of Advagraf capsule contents must not contain PVC.

6.3 Shelf life

3 years

After opening the aluminium wrapper: 1 year

6.4 Special precautions for storage

Store in the original package in order to protect from moisture.

6.5 Nature and contents of container

Transparent PVC/PVDC aluminium blister wrapped in an aluminium pouch with a desiccant containing 10 capsules per blister.

Advagraf 0.5 mg prolonged-release hard capsules
Pack sizes: 30, 50 and 100 prolonged-release hard capsules.

Advagraf 1 mg prolonged-release hard capsules
Pack sizes: 30, 50, 60 and 100 prolonged-release hard capsules.

Advagraf 3 mg prolonged-release hard capsules
Pack sizes: 30, 50 and 100 prolonged-release hard capsules.

Advagraf 5 mg prolonged-release hard capsules
Pack sizes: 30, 50 and 100 prolonged-release hard capsules.

Not all pack sizes may be marketed.

6.6 Special precautions for disposal and other handling
No special requirements.

7. MARKETING AUTHORISATION HOLDER
Astellas Pharma Europe B.V.
Elisabethhof 19
2353 EW Leiderdorp
Netherlands

8. MARKETING AUTHORISATION NUMBER(S)

Advagraf 0.5 mg prolonged-release hard capsules
EU/1/07/387/001
EU/1/07/387/002
EU/1/07/387/009

Advagraf 1 mg prolonged-release hard capsules
EU/1/07/387/003
EU/1/07/387/004
EU/1/07/387/005
EU/1/07/387/006

Advagraf 3 mg prolonged-release hard capsules
EU/1/07/387/011
EU/1/07/387/012
EU/1/07/387/013

Advagraf 5 mg prolonged-release hard capsules
EU/1/07/387/007
EU/1/07/387/008
EU/1/07/387/010

9. DATE OF FIRST AUTHORISATION/RENEWAL OF THE AUTHORISATION
23/04/07 (Advagraf 0.5 mg, 1 mg and 5 mg)
27/04/09 (Advagraf 3 mg)

10. DATE OF REVISION OF THE TEXT
27/04/2009

11. LEGAL CATEGORY
POM

AGGRASTAT solution for infusion and concentrate for solution for infusion

(Merck Sharp & Dohme Limited)

1. NAME OF THE MEDICINAL PRODUCT
AGGRASTAT ®* (50 micrograms/mL) Solution for infusion
AGGRASTAT ®* (250 micrograms/mL) Concentrate for solution for infusion

* in the following document the abbreviated terms detailed below are used.

- 'Aggrastat' means 'Aggrastat' Solution for Infusion or 'Aggrastat' Concentrate for Solution for Infusion.
- 'Aggrastat' Solution will be used when referring to 'Aggrastat' Solution for Infusion i.e. the 250 ml bag.
- 'Aggrastat' Concentrate will be used when referring to 'Aggrastat' Concentrate for Solution for Infusion i.e. the 50 ml vial.

2. QUALITATIVE AND QUANTITATIVE COMPOSITION
'Aggrastat' Solution:
1 ml of solution for infusion contains 56 micrograms of tirofiban hydrochloride monohydrate which is equivalent to 50 micrograms tirofiban.

'Aggrastat' Concentrate:
1 ml of concentrate for solution for infusion contains 281 micrograms of tirofiban hydrochloride monohydrate which is equivalent to 250 micrograms tirofiban.

For excipients, see section 6.1.

3. PHARMACEUTICAL FORM
'Aggrastat' Solution: Solution for Infusion
(250 ml bag)
A clear, colourless solution.
'Aggrastat' Concentrate: Concentrate for solution for infusion.
A clear, colourless concentrated solution.

4. CLINICAL PARTICULARS
4.1 Therapeutic indications
'Aggrastat' is indicated for the prevention of early myocardial infarction in patients presenting with unstable angina or non-Q-wave myocardial infarction with the last episode of chest pain occurring within 12 hours and with ECG changes and/or elevated cardiac enzymes.

Patients most likely to benefit from 'Aggrastat' treatment are those at high risk of developing myocardial infarction within the first 3-4 days after onset of acute angina symptoms including for instance those that are likely to undergo an early PTCA (see also 4.2 'Posology and method of administration' and 5.1 'Pharmacodynamic properties').

'Aggrastat' is intended for use with acetylsalicylic acid and unfractionated heparin.

4.2 Posology and method of administration
This product is for hospital use only, by specialist physicians experienced in the management of acute coronary syndromes.

'Aggrastat' concentrate for solution for infusion must be diluted before use.

'Aggrastat' is given intravenously at an initial infusion rate of 0.4 microgram/kg/min for 30 minutes. At the end of the initial infusion, 'Aggrastat' should be continued at a maintenance infusion rate of 0.1 microgram/kg/min. 'Aggrastat' should be given with unfractionated heparin (usually an intravenous bolus of 5,000 units [U] simultaneously with the start of 'Aggrastat' therapy, then approximately 1,000 U per hour, titrated on the basis of the activated thromboplastin time [APTT], which should be about twice the normal value) and ASA (see 5.1 'Pharmacodynamic properties', *PRISM-PLUS study*), unless contra-indicated.

No dosage adjustment is necessary for the elderly (see also 4.4 'Special warnings and precautions for use').

Patients with severe kidney failure
In severe kidney failure (creatinine clearance <30 ml/min) the dosage of 'Aggrastat' should be reduced by 50% (see also 4.4 'Special warnings and precautions for use' and 5.2 'Pharmacokinetic properties').

The following table is provided as a guide to dosage adjustment by weight.

'Aggrastat' Concentrate for Solution for Infusion must be diluted to the same strength as 'Aggrastat' Injection Premixed, as noted under *Instructions for Use.*

(see Table 1 below)

Start and duration of therapy with 'Aggrastat'
'Aggrastat' optimally should be initiated within 12 hours after the last anginal episode. The recommended duration should be at least 48 hours. Infusion of 'Aggrastat' and unfractionated heparin may be continued during coronary angiography and should be maintained for at least 12 hours and not more than 24 hours after angioplasty/atherectomy. Once a patient is clinically stable and no coronary intervention procedure is planned by the treating physician, the infusion should be discontinued. The entire duration of treatment should not exceed 108 hours.

Concurrent therapy (unfractionated heparin, ASA)
Treatment with unfractionated heparin is initiated with an i.v. bolus of 5,000 U and then continued with a maintenance infusion of 1,000 U per hour. The heparin dosage is titrated to maintain an APTT of approximately twice the normal value.

Unless contra-indicated, all patients should receive ASA orally before the start of 'Aggrastat' (see 5.1 'Pharmacodynamic properties', *PRISM-PLUS study*). This medication should be continued at least for the duration of the infusion of 'Aggrastat'.

If angioplasty (PTCA) is required, heparin should be stopped after PTCA, and the sheaths should be withdrawn once coagulation has returned to normal, e.g. when the activated clotting time (ACT) is less than 180 seconds (usually 2-6 hours after discontinuation of heparin).

AGGRASTAT SOLUTION

Instructions for use
Do not withdraw solution directly from the container with a syringe.

Directions for use of IntraVia®† containers
To open: Tear foil overpouch or plastic dust cover down side at slit and remove IntraVia® container. Some opacity of the plastic due to moisture absorption during the sterilisation process may be observed. This is normal and does not affect the solution quality or safety. The opacity will diminish gradually. Check for minute leaks by squeezing inner bag firmly. If leaks are found, discard solution as sterility may be impaired.

Do not use unless solution is clear and seal is intact.

Do not add supplementary medication or withdraw solution directly from the bag with a syringe.

CAUTION: Do not use plastic containers in series connections. Such use could result in air embolism due to residual air being drawn from the primary container before administration of the fluid from the secondary container is completed.

Preparation for administration
1. Suspend container from eyelet support.
2. Remove plastic protector from outlet port at bottom of container.
3. Attach administration set. Refer to complete directions accompanying set.

Use according to the dosage table above.

Where the solution and container permit, parenteral drugs should be inspected for visible particles or discoloration before use.

'Aggrastat' should only be given intravenously and may be administered with unfractionated heparin through the same infusion tube.

It is recommended that 'Aggrastat' be administered with a calibrated infusion set using sterile equipment.

Care should be taken to ensure that no prolongation of the infusion of the initial dose occurs and that miscalculation of the infusion rates for the maintenance dose on the basis of the patient's weight is avoided.

AGGRASTAT CONCENTRATE

Instructions for use
'Aggrastat' Concentrate must be diluted before use:
1. Draw 50 ml from a 250 ml container of sterile 0.9% saline or 5% glucose in water and replace with 50 ml 'Aggrastat' (from one 50 ml puncture vial) to make up a concentration of 50 microgram/ml. Mix well before use.
2. Use according to the dosage table above.

FOR BOTH FORMULATIONS
Where the solution and container permit, parenteral drugs should be inspected for visible particles or discoloration before use.

'Aggrastat' should only be given intravenously and may be administered with unfractionated heparin through the same infusion tube.

Table 1

	Most Patients		Severe Kidney Failure	
Patient Weight (kg)	30 min Loading Infusion Rate (ml/hr)	Maintenance Infusion Rate (ml/hr)	30 min Loading Infusion Rate (ml/hr)	Maintenance Infusion Rate (ml/hr)
30-37	16	4	8	2
38-45	20	5	10	3
46-54	24	6	12	3
55-62	28	7	14	4
63-70	32	8	16	4
71-79	36	9	18	5
80-87	40	10	20	5
88-95	44	11	22	6
96-104	48	12	24	6
105-112	52	13	26	7
113-120	56	14	28	7
121-128	60	15	30	8
129-137	64	16	32	8
138-145	68	17	34	9
146-153	72	18	36	9

It is recommended that 'Aggrastat' be administered with a calibrated infusion set using sterile equipment.

Care should be taken to ensure that no prolongation of the infusion of the initial dose occurs and that miscalculation of the infusion rates for the maintenance dose on the basis of the patient's weight is avoided.

4.3 Contraindications

'Aggrastat' is contra-indicated in patients who are hypersensitive to the active substance or to any of the excipients of the preparation or who developed thrombocytopenia during earlier use of a GP IIb/IIIa receptor antagonist.

Since inhibition of platelet aggregation increases the bleeding risk, 'Aggrastat' is contra-indicated in patients with:

• History of stroke within 30 days or any history of haemorrhagic stroke.

• Known history of intracranial disease (e.g. neoplasm, arteriovenous malformation, aneurysm).

• Active or recent (within the previous 30 days of treatment) clinically relevant bleeding (e.g. gastro-intestinal bleeding).

• Malignant hypertension.

• Relevant trauma or major surgical intervention within the past six weeks.

• Thrombocytopenia (platelet count $<100{,}000/mm^3$), disorders of platelet function.

• Clotting disturbances (e.g. prothrombin time >1.3 times normal or INR [International Normalised Ratio] >1.5).

• Severe liver failure.

4.4 Special warnings and precautions for use

The administration of 'Aggrastat' alone without unfractionated heparin is not recommended.

There is limited experience with concomitant administration of 'Aggrastat' with enoxaparin (see also 5.1 'Pharmacodynamic properties' and 5.2 'Pharmacokinetic properties'). The concomitant administration of 'Aggrastat' with enoxaparin is associated with a higher frequency of cutaneous and oral bleeding events, but not in TIMI bleeds**, when compared with the concomitant administration of 'Aggrastat' and unfractionated heparin. An increased risk of serious bleeding events associated with the concomitant administration of 'Aggrastat' and enoxaparin cannot be excluded, particularly in patients given additional unfractionated heparin in conjunction with angiography and/or PCI. The efficacy of 'Aggrastat' in combination with enoxaparin has not been established. The safety and efficacy of 'Aggrastat' with other low molecular weight heparins has not been investigated.

There is insufficient experience with the use of tirofiban hydrochloride in the following diseases and conditions, however, an increased risk of bleeding is suspected. Therefore, tirofiban hydrochloride is not recommended in:

• Traumatic or protracted cardiopulmonary resuscitation, organ biopsy or lithotripsy within the past two weeks

• Severe trauma or major surgery >6 weeks but <3 months previously

• Active peptic ulcer within the past three months

• Uncontrolled hypertension $>180/110$ mm Hg)

• Acute pericarditis

• Active or a known history of vasculitis

• Suspected aortic dissection

• Haemorrhagic retinopathy

• Occult blood in the stool or haematuria

• Thrombolytic therapy (see 4.5 'Interaction with other medicinal products and other forms of interaction').

• Concurrent use of drugs that increase the risk of bleeding to a relevant degree (see 4.5 'Interaction with other medicinal products and other forms of interaction').

There is no therapeutic experience with tirofiban hydrochloride in patients for whom thrombolytic therapy is indicated (e.g. acute transmural myocardial infarction with new pathological Q-waves or elevated ST-segments or left bundle-branch block in the ECG). Consequently, the use of tirofiban hydrochloride is not recommended in these circumstances.

'Aggrastat' infusion should be stopped immediately if circumstances arise that necessitate thrombolytic therapy (including acute occlusion during PTCA) or if the patient must undergo an emergency coronary artery bypass graft (CABG) operation or requires an intra-aortic balloon pump.

There are limited efficacy data in patients immediately undergoing PTCA.

There is no therapeutic experience with 'Aggrastat' in children, thus, the use of 'Aggrastat' is not recommended in these patients.

Other precautionary notes and measures

There are insufficient data regarding the re-administration of 'Aggrastat'.

Patients should be carefully monitored for bleeding during treatment with 'Aggrastat'. If treatment of haemorrhage is necessary, discontinuation of 'Aggrastat' should be considered (see also 4.9 'Overdose'). In cases of major or uncontrollable bleeding, tirofiban hydrochloride should be discontinued immediately.

'Aggrastat' should be used with special caution in the following conditions and patient groups:

• Recent clinically relevant bleeding (less than one year)

• Puncture of a non-compressible vessel within 24 hours before administration of 'Aggrastat'

• Recent epidural procedure (including lumbar puncture and spinal anaesthesia)

• Severe acute or chronic heart failure

• Cardiogenic shock

• Mild to moderate liver insufficiency

• Platelet count $<150{,}000/mm^3$, known history of coagulopathy or platelet function disturbance or thrombocytopenia

• Haemoglobin concentration less than 11 g/dl or haematocrit $<34\%$.

Special caution should be used during concurrent administration of, ticlopidine, clopidogrel, adenosine, dipyridamole, sulfinpyrazone, and prostacyclin.

Elderly patients, female patients, and patients with low body weight

Elderly and/or female patients had a higher incidence of bleeding complications than younger or male patients, respectively. Patients with a low body weight had a higher incidence of bleeding than patients with a higher body weight. For these reasons 'Aggrastat' should be used with caution in these patients and the heparin effect should be carefully monitored.

Impaired renal function

There is evidence from clinical studies that the risk of bleeding increases with decreasing creatinine clearance and hence also reduced plasma clearance of tirofiban. Patients with decreased renal function (creatinine clearance <60ml/min) should therefore be carefully monitored for bleeding during treatment with 'Aggrastat' and the heparin effect should be carefully monitored. In severe kidney failure the 'Aggrastat' dosage should be reduced (see also 4.2 'Posology and method of administration').

Femoral artery line

During treatment with 'Aggrastat' there is a significant increase in bleeding rates, especially in the femoral artery area, where the catheter sheath is introduced. Care should be taken to ensure that only the anterior wall of the femoral artery is punctured. Arterial sheaths may be removed when coagulation has returned to normal, e.g. when activated clotting time (ACT) is less than 180 seconds, (usually 2–6 hours after discontinuation of heparin).

After removal of the introducer sheath, careful haemostasis should be ensured under close observation.

General nursing care

The number of vascular punctures, and intramuscular injections should be minimised during the treatment with 'Aggrastat'. I.V. access should only be obtained at compressible sites of the body. All vascular puncture sites should be documented and closely monitored. The use of urinary catheters, nasotracheal intubation and nasogastric tubes should be critically considered.

Monitoring of laboratory values

Platelet count, haemoglobin and haematocrit levels should be determined before treatment with 'Aggrastat' as well as within 2-6 hours after start of therapy with 'Aggrastat' and at least once daily thereafter while on therapy (or more often if there is evidence of a marked decrease). In patients who have previously received GPIIb/IIIa receptor antagonists (cross reactivity can occur), the platelet count should be monitored immediately e.g. within the first hour of administration after re-exposure (see also 4.8 Undesirable effects). If the platelet count falls below $90{,}000/mm^3$, further platelet counts should be carried out in order to rule out pseudothrombocytopenia. If thrombocytopenia is confirmed, 'Aggrastat' and heparin should be discontinued. Patients should be monitored for bleeding and treated if necessary (see also 4.9 'Overdose').

In addition, activated thromboplastin time (APTT) should be determined before treatment and the anticoagulant effects of heparin should be carefully monitored by repeated determinations of APTT and the dose should be adjusted accordingly (see also 4.2 ('Posology and method of administration'). Potentially life-threatening bleeding may occur especially when heparin is administered with other products affecting haemostasis, such as GPIIb/IIIa receptor antagonists.

4.5 Interaction with other medicinal products and other forms of interaction

The use of several platelet aggregation inhibitors increases the risk of bleeding, likewise their combination with heparin, warfarin and thrombolytics. Clinical and biological parameters of haemostasis should be regularly monitored.

The concomitant administration of 'Aggrastat' and ASA (acetylsalicyclic acid or aspirin) increases the inhibition of platelet aggregation to a greater extent than aspirin alone, as measured by *ex vivo* APD-induced platelet aggregation test. The concomitant administration of 'Aggrastat' and unfractionated heparin increases the prolongation of the bleeding time to a greater extent as compared to unfractionated heparin alone.

With the concurrent use of 'Aggrastat' and unfractionated heparin and ASA there was a higher incidence of bleeding than when only unfractionated heparin and ASA were use together (see also 4.4 'Special warnings and special pre cautions for use' and 4.8 'Undesirable effects').

'Aggrastat' prolonged bleeding time; however, the com bined administration of 'Aggrastat' and ticlopidine did no additionally affect bleeding time.

Concomitant use of warfarin with 'Aggrastat' plus hepari was associated with an increased risk of bleeding.

'Aggrastat' is not recommended in thrombolytic therapy concurrent or less than 48 hours before administration o tirofiban hydrochloride or concurrent use of drugs tha increase the risk of bleeding to a relevant degree (e.g. ora anticoagulants, other parenteral GP IIb/IIIa inhibitors, dex tran solutions). There is insufficient experience with the use of tirofiban hydrochloride in these conditions; however, ar increased risk of bleeding is suspected.

4.6 Pregnancy and lactation

Pregnancy

For tirofiban hydrochloride, no clinical data on exposed pregnancies are available. Animal studies provide limited information with respect to effects on pregnancy, embryonal/foetal development, parturition, and postnatal development. 'Aggrastat' should not be used during pregnancy unless clearly necessary.

Lactation

It is not known whether 'Aggrastat' is excreted in human milk but it is known to be excreted in rat milk. Because of the potential for adverse effects on the nursing infant, a decision should be made whether to discontinue nursing or discontinue the drug, taking into account the importance of the drug to the mother.

4.7 Effects on ability to drive and use machines

No data are available on whether 'Aggrastat' impairs the ability to drive or operate machinery.

4.8 Undesirable effects

Bleeding

The adverse event causally related to 'Aggrastat' therapy (used concurrently with unfractionated heparin and ASA) most commonly reported was bleeding, which was usually of a milder nature.

In the PRISM-PLUS study, the overall incidence of major bleeding using the TIMI criteria (defined as a haemoglobin drop of >50 g/l with or without an identified site, intracranial haemorrhage, or cardiac tamponade) in patients treated with 'Aggrastat' in combination with heparin was not significantly higher than in the control group. The incidence of major bleeding using the TIMI criteria was 1.4% for 'Aggrastat' in combination with heparin and 0.8% for the control group (which received heparin). The incidence of minor bleeding using the TIMI criteria (defined as a haemoglobin drop of >30 g/l with bleeding from a known site, spontaneous gross haematuria, haematemesis or haemoptysis) was 10.5% for 'Aggrastat' in combination with heparin and 8.0% for the control group. There were no reports of intracranial bleeding for 'Aggrastat' in combination with heparin or in the control group. The incidence of retroperitoneal bleeding reported for 'Aggrastat' in combination with heparin was 0.0% and 0.1% for the control group. The percentage of patients who received a transfusion (including packed red blood cells, fresh frozen plasma, whole blood cryoprecipitates and platelets) was 4.0% for 'Aggrastat' and 2.8% for the control group.

'Aggrastat' given with unfractionated heparin and ASA was associated with gastro-intestinal, haemorrhoidal and postoperative bleeding, epistaxis, gum bleeds and surface dermatorrhagia as well as oozing haemorrhage (haematoma) in the area of intravascular puncture sites (e.g. in cardiac catheter examinations) significantly more often than was unfractionated heparin and ASA alone.

Non-bleeding-associated adverse reactions

The most common adverse drug reactions (incidence over 1%) associated with 'Aggrastat' given concurrently with heparin, apart from bleeding, were nausea (1.7%), fever (1.5%) and headache (1.1%); nausea, fever and headache occurred with incidences of 1.4%, 1.1% and 1.2%, respectively, in the control group.

The incidence of adverse non-bleeding-related events was higher in women (compared to men) and older patients (compared to younger patients). However, the incidences of non-bleeding-related adverse events in these patients were comparable for the 'Aggrastat' with heparin' group and the 'heparin alone' group.

[*Common*: ($>1/100$, $<1/10$)]

Nervous system and psychiatric disorders:

Common: headache

Gastro-intestinal disorders:

Common: nausea

General disorders and administration site conditions:

Common: fever

Investigations

The most common changes of laboratory parameters associated with 'Aggrastat' related to bleeding: reduction of haemoglobin and haematocrit levels and an increased occurrence of occult blood in urine and faeces.

Occasionally during 'Aggrastat' therapy an acute fall in the platelet count or thrombocytopenia occurred. The ercentage of patients in whom the platelet count fell to elow 90,000/mm^3 was 1.5%. The percentage of patients whom the platelet count fell to less than 50,000/mm^3 was .3%. These decreases were reversible upon discontinuation of 'Aggrastat'. Acute and severe platelet decreases ave been observed in patients with no prior history of hrombocytopenia upon re-administration of GPIIb/IIIa eceptor antagonists.

The following additional adverse reactions have been eported infrequently in post-marketing experience; they are derived from spontaneous reports for which precise ncidences cannot be determined:

Blood and lymphatic system disorders:

ntracranial bleeding, retroperitoneal bleding, haemopericardium, pulmonary (alveolar) haemorrhage, and epidural haematoma in the spinal region. Fatal bleedings have been eported rarely.

Acute and/or severe (<20,000/mm^3) decreases in platelet counts which may be associated with chills, low-grade fever or bleeding complications (see 'Investigations' above)

Immune system disorders:

Severe allergic reactions (e.g., bronchospasm, urticaria) including anaphylactic reactions. The reported cases have occurred during initial treatment (also on the first day) and during readministration of tirofiban. Some cases have been associated with severe thrombocytopenia (platelet counts <10,000/mm^3).

4.9 Overdose

Inadvertent overdosage with tirofiban hydrochloride occurred in the clinical studies, up to 50 microgram/kg as a three minute bolus or 1.2 microgram/kg/min as an initial infusion. Overdosage with up to 1.47 microgram/kg/min as a maintenance infusion rate has also occurred.

a) Symptoms of overdosage

The symptom of overdosage most commonly reported was bleeding, usually mucosal bleeding and localised bleeding at the arterial puncture site for cardiac catheterisation but also single cases of intracranial haemorrhages and retroperitoneal bleedings (see also 4.4 'Special warnings and precautions for use' and 5.1 'Pharmacodynamic properties', *PRISM-PLUS study*).

b) Measures

Overdosage with tirofiban hydrochloride should be treated in accordance with the patient's condition and the attending physician's assessment. If treatment of haemorrhage is necessary, the 'Aggrastat' infusion should be discontinued. Transfusions of blood and/or thrombocytes should also be considered. 'Aggrastat' can be removed by haemodialysis.

5. PHARMACOLOGICAL PROPERTIES

5.1 Pharmacodynamic properties

ATC-Code: B01A C17

Tirofiban hydrochloride is a non-peptidal antagonist of the GP IIb/IIIa receptor, an important platelet surface receptor involved in platelet aggregation. Tirofiban hydrochloride prevents fibrinogen from binding to the GP IIb/IIIa receptor, thus blocking platelet aggregation.

Tirofiban hydrochloride leads to inhibition of platelet function, evidenced by its ability to inhibit *ex vivo* ADP-induced platelet aggregation and to prolong bleeding time (BT). Platelet function returns to baseline within eight hours after discontinuation.

The extent of this inhibition runs parallel to the tirofiban hydrochloride plasma concentration.

In the target population the recommended dosage of 'Aggrastat', in the presence of unfractionated heparin and ASA, produced a more than 70% (median 89%) inhibition of *ex vivo* ADP-induced platelet aggregation in 93% of the patients, and a prolongation of the bleeding time by a factor of 2.9 during infusion. Inhibition was achieved rapidly with the 30-minute loading infusion and was maintained over the duration of the infusion.

PRISM-PLUS study

The double-blind, multicentre, controlled PRISM-PLUS study compared the efficacy of tirofiban and unfractionated heparin (n=773) versus unfractionated heparin (n=797) in patients with unstable angina or acute non-Q-wave myocardial infarction (NQWMI).

Patients had to have prolonged, repetitive anginal pain, or post-infarction angina within 12 hours prior to randomisation, accompanied by new transient or persistent ST-T wave changes (ST depression or elevation ⩾0.1 mV; T-wave inversions ⩾0.3 mV) or elevated cardiac enzymes (total CPK ⩾ 2 times upper limit of normal, or CK-MB fraction elevated at the time of enrollment (>5 % or greater than upper limit of normal]).

In this study, patients were randomised to either

– 'Aggrastat' (30 minute loading infusion of 0.4 microgram/kg/min followed by a maintenance infusion of 0.10 microgram/kg/min) and heparin (bolus of 5,000 units (U) followed by an infusion of 1,000 U/hr titrated to maintain an activated partial thromboplastin time (APTT) of approximately two times control),

– or heparin alone (bolus of 5,000 U followed by an infusion of 1,000 U/hr titrated to maintain an APTT of approximately two times control).

All patients received ASA unless contra-indicated; 300-325 mg orally per day were recommended for the first 48 hours and thereafter 80-325 mg orally per day (as determined by the physician). Study drug was initiated within 12 hours after the last anginal episode. Patients were treated for 48 hours, after which they underwent angiography and possibly angioplasty/atherectomy, if indicated, while tirofiban hydrochloride was continued. Tirofiban hydrochloride was infused for a mean period of 71.3 hours.

The combined primary study end-point was the occurrence of refractory ischaemia, myocardial infarction or death at seven days after the start of tirofiban hydrochloride.

The mean age of the population was 63 years; 32% of patients were female. At baseline approximately 58% of patients had ST segment depression; 53% had T-wave inversions; 46% of patients presented with elevated cardiac enzymes. During the study approximately 90% of patients underwent coronary angiography; 30% underwent early angioplasty and 23% underwent early coronary artery bypass surgery.

At the primary end-point, there was a 32% risk reduction (RR) (12.9% vs. 17.9%) in the tirofiban hydrochloride group for the combined end-point (p=0.004): this represents approximately 50 events avoided for 1,000 patients treated. Results of the primary end-point were principally attributed to the occurrence of myocardial infarction and refractory ischaemic conditions.

After 30 days the RR for the combined end-point (death/myocardial infarction/refractory ischaemic conditions/readmissions for unstable angina) was 22% (18.5% vs. 22.3%; p=0.029).

After six months the risk of the combined end-point (death/myocardial infarction/refractory ischaemic conditions/readmissions for unstable angina) was reduced by 19% (27.7% vs. 32.1%; p=0.024).

Regarding the most commonly used double combined end-point, death or myocardial infarction, the results at seven days, 30 days and six months were as follows: at seven days for the tirofiban group there was a 43% RR (4.9% vs. 8.3%; p=0.006); at 30 days the RR was 30% (8.7% vs. 11.9%; p=0.027) and at 6 months the RR was 23% (12.3% vs. 15.3%; p=0.063).

The reduction in the incidence of myocardial infarctions in patients receiving 'Aggrastat' appeared early during treatment (within the first 48 hours) and this reduction was maintained through six months, without significant effect on mortality.

In the 30% of patients who underwent angioplasty/atherectomy during initial hospitalisation, there was a 46% RR (8.8% vs. 15.2%) for the primary combined end-point at 30 days as well as a 43% RR (5.9% vs. 10.2%) for 'myocardial infarction or death'.

Based on a safety study, the concomitant administration of 'Aggrastat' with enoxaparin (n=315) was compared to the concomitant administration of 'Aggrastat' with unfractionated heparin (n=210) in patients presenting with unstable angina and non-Q-wave myocardial infarction. A 30 minute loading dose of tirofiban (0.4 microgram/kg/min) was followed by a maintenance infusion of 0.1 microgram/kg/min for up to 108 hours. Patients randomised to the enoxaparin group received a 1.0 mg/kg subcutaneous injection of enoxaparin every 12 hours for a period of at least 24 hours and a maximum duration of 96 hours. Patients randomised to the unfractionated heparin group received a 5000-unit intravenous bolus of unfractionated heparin followed by a maintenance infusion of 1000 units per hour for at least 24 hours and a maximum duration of 108 hours. The total TIMI bleed rate was 3.5% for the tirofiban/enoxaparin group and 4.8% for the tirofiban/unfractionated heparin group. Cutaneous bleeds and oral bleeds occurred more frequently in patients randomised to the enoxaparin group versus the unfractionated heparin group. Catheter site bleeds were more common in the enoxaparin group as compared to the unfractionated heparin group. Patients randomised to the enoxaparin group who subsequently required PCI were switched to unfractionated heparin peri-procedurally with the dose titrated to maintain an ACT of 250 seconds or higher. Although there was a signifcant difference in the rates of cutaneous bleeds between the two groups (29.2% in the enoxaparin converted to unfractionated heparin group and 15.2% in the unfractionated heparin group), there were no TIMI major bleeds (see also 4.4 'Special warnings and precautions for use') in either group. The efficacy of 'Aggrastat' in combination with enoxaparin has not been established.

Patients most likely to benefit from 'Aggrastat' treatment are those at high risk of developing myocardial infarction within the 3-4 days after onset of acute angina symptoms. According to epidemiological findings, a higher incidence of cardiovascular events has been associated with certain indicators, for instance: age, elevated heart rate or blood pressure, persistent or recurrent ischaemic cardiac pain, marked ECG changes (in particular ST-segment abnormalities), raised cardiac enzymes or markers (e.g. CK-MB, troponins) and heart failure.

5.2 Pharmacokinetic properties

Distribution

Tirofiban is not strongly bound to plasma protein, and protein binding is concentration-independent in the range of 0.01–25 microgram/ml. The unbound fraction in human plasma is 35%.

The distribution volume of tirofiban in the steady state is about 30 litres.

Biotransformation

Experiments with ^{14}C-labelled tirofiban showed the radioactivity in urine and faeces to be emitted chiefly by unchanged tirofiban. The radioactivity in circulating plasma originates mainly from unchanged tirofiban (up to 10 hours after administration). These data suggested limited metabolisation of tirofiban.

Elimination

After intravenous administration of ^{14}C-labelled tirofiban to healthy subjects, 66% of the radioactivity was recovered in the urine, 23% in the faeces. The total recovery of radioactivity was 91%. Renal and biliary excretion contribute significantly to the elimination of tirofiban.

In healthy subjects the plasma clearance of tirofiban is about 250 ml/min. Renal clearance is 39–69% of plasma clearance. The half-life is about 1.5 hours.

Gender

The plasma clearance of tirofiban in patients with coronary heart disease is similar in men and women.

Elderly patients

The plasma clearance of tirofiban is about 25% less in elderly >65 years) patients with coronary heart disease in comparison to younger (⩽65 years) patients.

Ethnic groups

No difference was found in the plasma clearance between patients of different ethnic groups.

Coronary Artery Disease

In patients with unstable angina pectoris or NQWMI the plasma clearance was about 200 ml/min, the renal clearance 39% of the plasma clearance. The half-life is about two hours.

Impaired renal function

In clinical studies, patients with decreased renal function showed a reduced plasma clearance of tirofiban depending on the degree of impairment of creatinine clearance. In patients with a creatinine clearance of less than 30 ml/min, including haemodialysis patients, the plasma clearance of tirofiban is reduced to a clinically relevant extent (over 50%) (see also 4.2 'Posology and method of administration'). Tirofiban is removed by haemodialysis.

Liver failure

There is no evidence of a clinically significant reduction of the plasma clearance of tirofiban in patients with mild to moderate liver failure. No data are available on patients with severe liver failure.

Effects of other drugs

The plasma clearance of tirofiban in patients receiving one of the following drugs was compared to that in patients not receiving that drug in a sub-set of patients (n=762) in the PRISM study. There were no substantial (>15%) effects of these drugs on the plasma clearance of tirofiban: acebutolol, alprazolam, amlodipine, aspirin preparations, atenolol, bromazepam, captopril, diazepam, digoxin, diltiazem, docusate sodium, enalapril, furosemide, glibenclamide, unfractionated heparin, insulin, isosorbide, lorazepam, lovastatin, metoclopramide, metoprolol, morphine, nifedipine, nitrate preparations, oxazepam, paracetamol, potassium chloride, propranolol, ranitidine, simvastatin, sucralfate and temazepam.

The pharmacokinetics and pharmacodynamics of 'Aggrastat' were investigated when concomitantly administered with enoxaparin (1mg/kg subcutaneously every 12 hours) and compared with the combination of 'Aggrastat' and unfractionated heparin. There was no difference in the clearance of 'Aggrastat' between the two groups.

5.3 Preclinical safety data

Preclinical data reveal no special hazard for humans based on conventional studies of safety pharmacology, repeated dose toxicity and genotoxicity.

Tirofiban crosses the placenta in rats and rabbits.

6. PHARMACEUTICAL PARTICULARS

6.1 List of excipients

Sodium chloride, sodium citrate dihydrate, citric acid anhydrous, water for injections, hydrochloric acid and/or sodium hydroxide (for pH adjustment).

6.2 Incompatibilities

Incompatibility has been found with diazepam. Therefore, 'Aggrastat' and diazepam should not be administered in the same intravenous line.

6.3 Shelf life

'Aggrastat' Solution: 2 years

'Aggrastat' Concentrate: 3 years.

From a microbiological point of view the diluted solution for infusion should be used immediately. If not used immediately, in use storage conditions are the responsibility of the user and would normally not be longer than 24 hours at 2-8°C, unless reconstitution has taken place in controlled and validated aseptic conditions.

6.4 Special precautions for storage

'Aggrastat' Solution:

Do not freeze. Keep container in foil overpouch to protect from light.

'Aggrastat' Concentrate:

Do not freeze. Keep container in outer carton to protect from light.

6.5 Nature and contents of container

'Aggrastat' Solution:

250 ml IntraVia™ container (PL 2408 plastic), colourless, 3-layer polyolefine film with outlet port and PVC tube with blue top. It is packed in a preprinted foil overpouch.

Pack sizes: 1 or 3 containers with 250 ml solution for infusion. Not all pack sizes may be marketed.

'Aggrastat' Concentrate:

50 ml Type I glass vial.

6.6 Special precautions for disposal and other handling

No incompatibilities have been found with 'Aggrastat' and the following intravenous formulations: atropine sulfate, dobutamine, dopamine, epinephrine HCl, furosemide, heparin, lidocaine, midazolam HCl, morphine sulfate, nitroglycerin, potassium chloride, propanolol HCl and famotidine injection.

'Aggrastat' Solution:

Some opacity of the plastic due to moisture absorption during the sterilisation process may be observed. This is normal and does not affect the solution quality or safety. The opacity will diminish gradually. Check for minute leaks by squeezing inner bag firmly. If leaks are found, discard solution as sterility may be impaired.

'Aggrastat' Concentrate:

'Aggrastat' concentrate for solution for infusion must be diluted before use.

See 4.2 'Posology and method of administration'.

Any unused solution should be discarded.

7. MARKETING AUTHORISATION HOLDER

Merck Sharp & Dohme Limited

Hertford Road, Hoddesdon, Hertfordshire EN11 9BU, UK

8. MARKETING AUTHORISATION NUMBER(S)

'Aggrastat' Solution: PL0025/0375

'Aggrastat' Concentrate: PL0025/0376

9. DATE OF FIRST AUTHORISATION/RENEWAL OF THE AUTHORISATION

First authorisation: 15 July 1999.

First renewal: 14 May 2003

10. DATE OF REVISION OF THE TEXT

September 2009

® denotes registered trademark of Merck & Co., Inc., Whitehouse Station, NJ, USA.

SPC.ARS-C.09.UK.3114 (IB-17)

† IntraVia is the tradename for the infusion bag used for 'Aggrastat' Solution. Trademark of Baxter International Inc.

**TIMI major bleeds are defined as a haemoglobin drop of > 50 g/l with or without an identified site, intracranial haemorrhage, or cardiac tamponade. TIMI minor bleeds are defined as a haemoglobin drop of > 30 g/l but ⩽ 50 g/l with bleeding from a known site or spontaneous gross haematuria, haematemesis, or haemoptysis. TIMI "loss no site" is defined as a haemoglobin drop > 40 g/l but < 50 g/l without an identified bleeding site.

Agrippal

(Novartis Vaccines)

1. NAME OF THE MEDICINAL PRODUCT

AGRIPPAL®

Suspension for injection in pre-filled syringe

Influenza vaccine (surface antigen, inactivated)

(2009/2010 season)

2. QUALITATIVE AND QUANTITATIVE COMPOSITION

Influenza virus surface antigens (haemagglutinin and neuraminidase), of the following strains*:

A/Brisbane/59/2007 (H1N1) – like strain (A/Brisbane/59/2007, IVR-148)

15 micrograms HA**

A/Brisbane/10/2007 (H3N2) – like strain (A/Uruguay/716/2007, NYMC X-175C)

15 micrograms HA**

B/Brisbane/60/2008 – like strain (B/Brisbane/60/2008)

15 micrograms HA**

Per 0.5 ml. dose

* propagated in fertilized hen's eggs from healthy chicken flocks

** haemagglutinin

This vaccine complies with the WHO recommendations (northern hemisphere) and EU decision for the 2009/2010 season.

For a full list of excipients see 6.1

3. PHARMACEUTICAL FORM

Suspension for injection in pre-filled syringe. The vaccine appears as a clear liquid.

4. CLINICAL PARTICULARS

4.1 Therapeutic indications

Prophylaxis of influenza, especially in those who run an increased risk of associated complications.

The use of Agrippal should be based on official recommendations.

4.2 Posology and method of administration

- Adults and children from 36 months: 0.5 ml

- Children from 6 months to 35 months: Clinical data are limited. Dosages of 0.25 ml or 0.5 ml have been used.

For children who have not previously been vaccinated, a second dose should be given after an interval of at least 4 weeks.

Immunisation should be carried out by intramuscular or deep subcutaneous injection.

For instructions for preparation, see section 6.6.

4.3 Contraindications

Hypersensitivity to the active substances, to any of the excipients and to residues (see below).

AGRIPPAL does not contain more than 0.2 µg of ovalbumin per 0.5 ml dose and 0.1 µg of ovalbumin per 0.25 ml dose.

The vaccine may contain residues of the following substances, e.g. eggs, chicken proteins, kanamycin and neomycin sulphate, formaldehyde, cetyltrimethylammonium bromide (CTAB) and polysorbate 80.

Immunisation shall be postponed in patients with febrile illness or acute infection.

4.4 Special warnings and precautions for use

As with all injectable vaccines, appropriate medical treatment and supervision should always be readily available in case of an anaphylactic event following the administration of the vaccine.

AGRIPPAL should under no circumstances be administered intravascularly.

Antibody response in patients with endogenous or iatrogenic immunosuppression may be insufficient.

4.5 Interaction with other medicinal products and other forms of interaction

AGRIPPAL may be given at the same time as other vaccines. Immunisation should be carried out on separate limbs. It should be noted that the adverse reactions may be intensified.

The immunological response may be diminished if the patient is undergoing immunosuppressant treatment.

Following influenza vaccination, false positive results in serology tests using the ELISA method to detect antibodies against HIV1, Hepatitis C and especially HTLV1 have been observed. The Western Blot technique disproves the false-positive ELISA results. The transient false positive reactions could be due to the IgM response to the vaccine.

4.6 Pregnancy and lactation

Limited data from vaccinations in pregnant women do not indicate that adverse foetal and maternal outcomes were attributable to the vaccine. The use of this vaccine may be considered from the second trimester of pregnancy. For pregnant women with medical conditions that increase their risk of complications from influenza, administration of the vaccine is recommended, irrespective of their stage of pregnancy.

AGRIPPAL may be used during lactation.

4.7 Effects on ability to drive and use machines

The vaccine is unlikely to produce an effect on the ability to drive and use machines.

4.8 Undesirable effects

ADVERSE REACTIONS OBSERVED FROM CLINICAL TRIALS

The safety of trivalent inactivated influenza vaccines is assessed in open label, uncontrolled clinical trials performed as annual update requirement, including at least 50 adults aged 18 – 60 years of age and at least 50 elderly aged 61 years or older. Safety evaluation is performed during the first 3 days following vaccination.

The following undesirable effects have been observed during clinical trials with the following frequencies:

Very common (⩾1/10); common (⩾1/100, <1/10); uncommon (⩾1/1,000, <1/100); rare (⩾1/10,000, <1/1,000); very rare (<1/10,000), including isolated reports.

Nervous system disorders

Common (⩾1/100, <1/10):

Headache*

Skin and subcutaneous tissue disorders

Common (⩾1/100, <1/10):

Sweating*

Musculoskeletal and connective tissue disorders

Common (⩾1/100, <1/10):

Myalgia, arthralgia*

General disorders and administration site conditions

Common (⩾1/100, <1/10):

Fever, malaise, shivering, fatigue. Local reactions: redness, swelling, pain, ecchymosis, induration.*

*These reactions usually disappear within 1-2 days without treatment.

ADVERSE REACTIONS REPORTED FROM POST MARKETING SURVEILLANCE

Adverse reactions reported from post marketing surveillance are, next to the reactions which have also been observed during the clinical trials, the following:

Blood and lymphatic system disorders:

Transient thrombocytopenia, transient lymphadenopathy

Immune system disorders:

Allergic reactions, in rare cases leading to shock, angioedema

Nervous system disorders:

Neuralgia, paraesthesiae, febrile convulsions, neurological disorders, such as encephalomyelitis, neuritis and Guillain-Barré syndrome.

Vascular disorders:

Vasculitis associated in very rare cases with transient renal involvement.

Skin and subcutaneous tissue disorders:

Generalised skin reactions including pruritus, urticaria or non-specific rash.

4.9 Overdose

Overdosage is unlikely to have any untoward effect.

5. PHARMACOLOGICAL PROPERTIES

5.1 Pharmacodynamic properties

Pharmacotherapeutic group: Influenza vaccine, ATC code: J07BB02 Seroprotection is generally obtained within 2 to 3 weeks. The duration of postvaccinal immunity to homologous strains or to strains closely related to the vaccine strains varies but is usually 6-12 months.

5.2 Pharmacokinetic properties

Not applicable.

5.3 Preclinical safety data

Not applicable.

6. PHARMACEUTICAL PARTICULARS

6.1 List of excipients

Sodium chloride, Potassium chloride, Potassium dihydrogen phosphate, Disodium phosphate dihydrate, Magnesium chloride, Calcium chloride, and Water for Injections.

6.2 Incompatibilities

In the absence of compatibility studies, this medicinal product must not be mixed with other medicinal products.

6.3 Shelf life

1 year.

6.4 Special precautions for storage

Store in a refrigerator (2°C – 8°C). Do not freeze. Keep the syringe in the outer carton in order to protect from light.

6.5 Nature and contents of container

0.5 ml of suspension in a pre-filled syringe (type I glass) with needle (23 G, 1" or 25 G, 1" or 25 G, 5/8") equipped with a rubber plunger stopper - pack size of 1 or 10.

0.5 ml of suspension in pre-filled syringe (type I glass) without needle, equipped with a rubber plunger stopper – pack size of 1 or 10.

Not all pack sizes may be marketed.

6.6 Special precautions for disposal and other handling

Unused vaccine and other waste material should be disposed of in compliance with local rules for the disposal of products of this nature. The vaccine should be allowed to reach room temperature before use.

Shake before use.

If half a dose (0.25 ml) is to be administered, discard half the contained volume (up to the mark indicated on the syringe barrel), before injection.

7. MARKETING AUTHORISATION HOLDER

Novartis Vaccines and Diagnostics S.r.l., Via Fiorentina 1, SIENA, Italy

8. MARKETING AUTHORISATION NUMBER(S)

PL 13767/0004

9. DATE OF FIRST AUTHORISATION/RENEWAL OF THE AUTHORISATION

8 March 1999/22 January 2009

10. DATE OF REVISION OF THE TEXT

June 2009

Aldactide 25mg and 50mg Tablets

(Pharmacia Limited)

1. NAME OF THE MEDICINAL PRODUCT

Aldactide 25.

Aldactide 50.

. QUALITATIVE AND QUANTITATIVE COMPOSITION

ach tablet contains 25mg spironolactone BP and 25mg ydroflumethiazide BP

ach tablet contains 50mg spironolactone BP and 50mg ydroflumethiazide BP

. PHARMACEUTICAL FORM

uff, film coated tablets engraved "SEARLE 101" on one ide.

uff, film coated tablets engraved "SEARLE 180" on one ide.

. CLINICAL PARTICULARS

.1 Therapeutic indications

Congestive cardiac failure.

.2 Posology and method of administration

Administration of Aldactide once daily with a meal is ecommended.

Adults

Most patients will require an initial dosage of 100mg spironolactone daily. The dosage should be adjusted as necessary and may range from 25mg to 200mg spironolactone daily.

Elderly

It is recommended that treatment is started with the lowest dose and titrated upwards as required to achieve maximum benefit. Care should be taken with severe hepatic and renal impairment which may alter drug metabolism and excretion.

Children

Although clinical trials using Aldactide have not been carried out in children, as a guide, a daily dosage providing 1.5 to 3mg of spironolactone per kilogram body weight given in divided doses, may be employed.

4.3 Contraindications

Aldactide is contraindicated in patients with anuria, acute renal insufficiency, rapidly deteriorating or severe impairment of renal function, hyperkalaemia, significant hypercalcaemia, Addison's disease and in patients who are hypersensitive to spironolactone, thiazide diuretics or to other sulphonamide derived drugs.

Aldactide should not be administered with other potassium conserving diuretics and potassium supplements should not be given routinely with Aldactide as hyperkalemia may be induced.

4.4 Special warnings and precautions for use

Warnings

Sulphonamide derivatives including thiazides have been reported to exacerbate or activate systemic lupus erythematosus.

Precautions

Fluid and electrolyte balance: Fluid and electrolyte status should be regularly monitored particularly in the elderly, in those with significant renal and hepatic impairment, and in patients receiving digoxin and drugs with pro-arrhythmic effects.

Hyperkalaemia may occur in patients with impaired renal function or excessive potassium intake and can cause cardiac irregularities which may be fatal. Should hyperkalaemia develop Aldactide should be discontinued, and if necessary, active measures taken to reduce the serum potassium to normal. *(See 4.3 Contraindications)*

Hypokalaemia may develop as a result of profound diuresis, particularly when Aldactide is used concomitantly with loop diuretics, glucocorticoids or ACTH.

Hyponatraemia may be induced especially when Aldactide is administered in combination with other diuretics.

Hepatic impairment: Caution should be observed in patients with acute or severe liver impairment as vigorous diuretic therapy may precipitate encephalopathy in susceptible patients. Regular estimation of serum electrolytes is essential in such patients.

Reversible hyperchloraemic metabolic acidosis usually in association with hyperkalaemia has been reported to occur in some patients with decompensated hepatic cirrhosis, even in the presence of normal renal function.

Urea and uric acid: Reversible increases in blood urea have been reported, particularly accompanying vigorous diuresis or in the presence of impaired renal function.

Thiazides may cause hyperuricaemia and precipitate attacks of gout in some patients.

Diabetes mellitus: Thiazides may aggravate existing diabetes and the insulin requirements may alter. Diabetes mellitus which has been latent may become manifest during thiazide administration.

Hyperlipidaemia: Caution should be observed as thiazides may raise serum lipids.

4.5 Interaction with other medicinal products and other forms of interaction

Spironolactone has been reported to increase serum digoxin concentration and to interfere with certain serum digoxin assays. In patients receiving digoxin and spironolactone the digoxin response should be monitored by means other than serum digoxin concentrations, unless the digoxin assay used has been proven not to be affected by spironolactone therapy. If it proves necessary to adjust the dose of digoxin, patients should be carefully monitored for evidence of enhanced or reduced digoxin effect. Potentiation of the effect of antihypertensive drugs occurs and their dosage may need to be reduced when Aldactide is added to the treatment regime and then adjusted as necessary. Since ACE inhibitors decrease aldosterone production they should not routinely be used with Aldactide, particularly in patients with marked renal impairment.

As carbenoxolone may cause sodium retention and thus decrease the effectiveness of Aldactide, concurrent use should be avoided.

Non-steroidal anti-inflammatory drugs may attentuate the natriuretic efficacy of diuretics due to inhibition of intrarenal synthesis of prostaglandins.

Concurrent use of lithium and thiazides may reduce lithium clearance leading to intoxication.

Spironolactone and thiazides may reduce vascular responsiveness to noradrenaline. Caution should be exercised in the management of patients subjected to regional or general anaesthesia while they are being treated with Aldactide.

Concomitant use of aldactide with other potassium-sparing diuretics, ACE inhibitors, angiotensin II antagonists, aldosterone blockers, potassium supplements, a diet rich in potassium, or salt substitutes containing potassium, may lead to severe hyperkalaemia.

In fluorimetric assays, spironolactone may interfere with the estimation of compounds with similar flourescence characteristics.

Spironolactone has been shown to increase the half-life of digoxin.

Aspirin, indometacin, and mefanamic acid have been shown to attenuate the diuretic effect of spironolactone.

Spironolactone enhances the metabolism of antipyrine.

Spironolactone can interfere with assays for plasma digoxin concentrations

The absorption of a number of drugs including thiazides is decreased when co-administered with colestyramine and colestipol.

Thiazide co-administered with calcium and/or vitamin D may increase the risk of hypercalcaemia. Thiazides may delay the elimination of quinidine.

4.6 Pregnancy and lactation

Pregnancy

Spironolactone or its metabolites may, and hydroflumethiazide does, cross the placental barrier. With spironolactone, feminisation has been observed in male rat foetuses, thiazides may decrease placental perfusion, increase uterine inertia and inhibit labour. In the foetus or neonate thiazides may cause jaundice, thrombocytopenia, hypoglycaemia, electrolyte imbalance and death from maternal complications. The use of Aldactide in pregnant women requires that the anticipated benefit be weighed against the possible hazards to the mother and foetus.

Lactation

Metabolites of spironolactone and hydroflumethiazide, have been detected in breast milk. If use of Aldactide is considered essential, an alternative method of infant feeding should be instituted.

4.7 Effects on ability to drive and use machines

Somnolence and dizziness have been reported to occur in some patients. Caution is advised when driving or operating machinery until the response to initial treatment has been determined.

4.8 Undesirable effects

Gynaecomastia may develop in association with the use of spironolactone. Development appears to be related to both dosage level and duration of therapy and is normally reversible when the drug is discontinued. In rare instances some breast enlargement may persist.

The following adverse events have been reported in association with spironolactone therapy:

Body as a Whole: malaise

Endocrine Disorders: benign breast neoplasm, breast pain

Gastrointestinal Disorders: gastrointestinal disturbances, nausea

Hematologic Disorders: leukopenia (including agranulocytosis), thrombocytopenia

Liver Disorders: hepatic function abnormal

Metabolic and Nutritional Disorders: electrolyte disturbances, hyperkalemia

Musculoskeletal Disorders: leg cramps

Nervous System Disorders: dizziness

Psychiatric Disorders: changes in libido, confusion

Reproductive Disorders: menstrual disorders

Skin and Appendages: alopecia, hypertrichosis, pruritus, rash, urticaria,

Urinary System Disorders: acute renal failure

The following isolated adverse event has been reported in association with spironolactone therapy:

Skin and Appendages: Stevens Johnson Syndrome

Adverse reactions reported in association with thiazides include: gastrointestinal upsets, skin rashes, photosensitivity, blood dyscrasias, raised serum lipids, aplastic anaemia, purpura muscle cramps, weakness, restlessness, headache, dizziness, vertigo, jaundice, orthostatic hypotension, impotence, paraesthesia, and rarely pancreatitis, necrotising vasculitis and xanthopsia. Rarely hypercalcaemia has been reported in association with thiazides, usually in patients with pre-existing metabolic bone disease or parathyroid dysfunction.

4.9 Overdose

Acute overdosage may be manifested by drowsiness, mental confusion, nausea, vomiting, dizziness or diarrhoea. Hyponatraemia, Hypokalaemia or hyperkalaemia may be induced or hepatic coma may be precipitated in patients with severe liver disease, but these effects are unlikely to be associated with acute overdosage. Symptoms of hyperkalaemia may manifest as paraesthesia, weakness, flaccid paralysis or muscle spasm and may be difficult to distinguish clinically from hypokalaemia. Electro-cardiographic changes are the earliest specific signs of potassium disturbances. No specific antidote has been identified. Improvement may be expected after withdrawal of the drug. General supportive measures including replacement of fluids and electrolytes may be indicated. For hyperkalaemia, reduce potassium intake, administer potassium-excreting diuretics, intravenous glucose with regular insulin or oral ion-exchange resins.

5. PHARMACOLOGICAL PROPERTIES

5.1 Pharmacodynamic properties

Spironolactone, as a competitive aldosterone antagonist, increases sodium excretion whilst reducing potassium loss at the distal renal tubule. It has a gradual and prolonged action.

Hydroflumethiazide is a thiazide diuretic. Diuresis is initiated usually within 2 hours and lasts for about 12-18 hours.

5.2 Pharmacokinetic properties

Spironolactone is well absorbed orally and is principally metabolised to active metabolites: sulphur containing metabolites (80%) and partly canrenone (20%). Although the plasma half life of spironolactone itself is short (1.3 hours) the half lives of the active metabolites are longer (ranging from 2.8 to 11.2 hours). Elimination of metabolites occurs primarily in the urine and secondarily through biliary excretion in the faeces.

Following the administration of 100 mg of spironolactone daily for 15 days in non-fasted healthy volunteers, time to peak plasma concentration (t_{max}), peak plasma concentration (C_{max}), and elimination half-life ($t_{1/2}$) for spironolactone is 2.6 hr., 80 ng/ml, and approximately 1.4 hr., respectively. For the 7-alpha-(thiomethyl) spironolactone and canrenone metabolites, t_{max} was 3.2 hr. and 4.3 hr., C_{max} was 391 ng/ml and 181 ng/ml, and $t_{1/2}$ was 13.8 hr. and 16.5 hr., respectively.

The renal action of a single dose of spironolactone reaches its peak after 7 hours, and activity persists for at least 24 hours

Hydroflumethiazide is incompletely but fairly rapidly absorbed from the gastro-intestinal tract. It appears to have a biphasic biological half-life with an estimated alpha-phase of about 2 hours and an estimated beta-phase of about 17 hours; it has a metabolite with a longer half-life, which is extensively bound to the red blood cells. Hydroflumethiazide is excreted in the urine; its metabolite has also been detected in the urine.

5.3 Preclinical safety data

Carcinogenicity: Spironolactone has been shown to produce tumours in rats when administered at high doses over a long period of time. The significance of these findings with respect to clinical use is not certain. However, the long term use of spironolactone in young patients requires careful consideration of the benefits and the potential hazard involved. Spironolactone or its metabolites may cross the placental barrier. With spironolactone, feminisation has been observed in male rat foetuses. The use of Aldactone in pregnant women requires that the anticipated benefit be weighed against the possible hazards to the mother and foetus.

6. PHARMACEUTICAL PARTICULARS

6.1 List of excipients

Aldactide 25 and 50 contains: Calcium sulphate dihydrate, corn starch, polyvinyl pyrrolidone, magnesium stearate, felocofix peppermint, hypromellose, polyethylene glycol and opaspray yellow (contains E172 and E171).

6.2 Incompatibilities

None stated.

6.3 Shelf life

The shelf life of Aldactide tablets is 5 years.

6.4 Special precautions for storage

Store in a dry place below 30°C.

6.5 Nature and contents of container

Aldactide 25mg and 50mg tablets may be packaged in the following containers: Amber glass bottles, HDPE containers or PVC/foil blister packs containing 100 and 500 tablets.

6.6 Special precautions for disposal and other handling

There are no special instructions for handling.

7. MARKETING AUTHORISATION HOLDER
Pharmacia Limited
Ramsgate Road
Sandwich CT13 9NJ
United Kingdom

8. MARKETING AUTHORISATION NUMBER(S)
Aldactide 25 - PL 00032/0391
Aldactide 50 - PL 00032/0392

9. DATE OF FIRST AUTHORISATION/RENEWAL OF THE AUTHORISATION
Aldactide 25 - 6 July 2002
Aldactide 50 – 23 May 2002

10. DATE OF REVISION OF THE TEXT
April 2007

11. LEGAL CATEGORY
POM.

Company Ref: AD 3_0

Aldactone 25mg, 50mg and 100mg Tablets

(Pharmacia Limited)

1. NAME OF THE MEDICINAL PRODUCT
Aldactone 25mg
Aldactone 50mg
Aldactone 100 mg

2. QUALITATIVE AND QUANTITATIVE COMPOSITION
Each tablet contains 25mg, 50mg or 100mg spironolactone BP

3. PHARMACEUTICAL FORM
Aldactone 25mg tablets are buff, film coated tablets engraved "SEARLE 39" on one side.

Aldactone 50mg tablets are white, film coated tablets engraved "SEARLE 916" on one side.

Aldactone 100 mg tablets are buff, film coated tablets engraved "SEARLE 134" on one side.

4. CLINICAL PARTICULARS
4.1 Therapeutic indications
Congestive cardiac failure.
Hepatic cirrhosis with ascites and oedema.
Malignant ascites
Nephrotic syndrome.
Diagnosis and treatment of primary aldosteronism.

4.2 Posology and method of administration
Administration of Aldactone once daily with a meal is recommended.

Adults

Congestive cardiac failure
Usual dose- 100mg/day. In difficult or severe cases the dosage may be gradually increased up to 400mg/day. When oedema is controlled, the usual maintenance level is 25mg-200mg/day.

Hepatic cirrhosis with ascites and oedema.
If urinary Na+/K+ ratio is greater than 1.0, 100mg/day. If the ratio is less than 1.0, 200-400mg/day. Maintenance dosage should be individually determined.

Malignant ascites
Initial dose usually 100-200mg/day. In severe cases the dosage may be gradually increased up to 400mg/day. When oedema is controlled, maintenance dosage should be individually determined.

Nephrotic syndrome
Usual dose 100-200mg/day. Spironolactone has not been shown to be anti-inflammatory, nor to affect the basic pathological process. Its use is only advised if glucocorticoids by themselves are insufficiently effective.

Diagnosis and treatment of primary aldosteronism.
Aldactone may be employed as an initial diagnostic measure to provide presumptive evidence of primary hyperaldosteronism while patients are on normal diets.

Long test: Aldactone is administered at a daily dosage of 400mg for three to four weeks. Correction of hypokalaemia and of hypertension provides presumptive evidence for the diagnosis of primary hyperaldosteronism.

Short test: Aldactone is administered at a daily dosage of 400mg for four days. If serum potassium increases during Aldactone administration but drops when Aldactone is discontinued, a presumptive diagnosis of primary hyperaldosteronism should be considered.

After the diagnosis of hyperaldosteronism has been established by more definitive testing procedures, Aldactone may be administered at doses of 100mg-400mg daily in preparation for surgery. For patients who are considered unsuitable for surgery, Aldactone may be employed for long-term maintenance therapy at the lowest effective dosage determined for the individual patient.

Elderly
It is recommended that treatment is started with the lowest dose and titrated upwards as required to achieve maximum benefit. Care should be taken with severe hepatic and renal impairment which may alter drug metabolism and excretion.

Children
Initial daily dosage should provide 3mg of spironolactone per kilogram body weight given in divided doses. Dosage should be adjusted on the basis of response and tolerance. If necessary a suspension may be prepared by crushing Aldactone tablets.

4.3 Contraindications
Aldactone is contraindicated in patients with anuria, acute renal insufficiency, rapidly deteriorating or severe impairment of renal function, hyperkalaemia, Addison's disease and in patients who are hypersensitive to spironolactone.

Aldactone should not be administered concurrently with other potassium conserving diuretics and potassium supplements should not be given routinely with Aldactone as hyperkalemia may be induced.

4.4 Special warnings and precautions for use
Warnings
None Stated.

Precautions
Fluid and electrolyte balance: Fluid and electrolyte status should be regularly monitored particularly in the elderly, in those with significant renal and hepatic impairment

Hyperkalaemia may occur in patients with impaired renal function or excessive potassium intake and can cause cardiac irregularities which may be fatal. Should hyperkalaemia develop Aldactone should be discontinued, and if necessary, active measures taken to reduce the serum potassium to normal. *(See 4.3 Contraindications)*

Hyponatremia may be induced, especially when Aldactone is administered in combination with other diuretics.

Reversible hyperchloraemic metabolic acidosis, usually in association with hyperkalaemia has been reported to occur in some patients with decompensated hepatic cirrhosis, even in the presence of normal renal function.

Urea: Reversible increases in blood urea have been reported in association with Aldactone therapy, particularly in the presence of impaired renal function.

4.5 Interaction with other medicinal products and other forms of interaction
Spironolactone has been reported to increase serum digoxin concentration and to interfere with certain serum digoxin assays. In patients receiving digoxin and spironolactone the digoxin response should be monitored by means other than serum digoxin concentrations, unless the digoxin assay used has been proven not to be affected by spironolactone therapy. If it proves necessary to adjust the dose of digoxin patients should be carefully monitored for evidence of enhanced or reduced digoxin effect.

Potentiation of the effect of antihypertensive drugs occurs and their dosage may need to be reduced when Aldactone is added to the treatment regime and then adjusted as necessary. Since ACE inhibitors decrease aldosterone production they should not routinely be used with Aldactone, particularly in patients with marked renal impairment.

As carbenoxolone may cause sodium retention and thus decrease the effectiveness of Aldactone concurrent use should be avoided.

Non-steroidal anti-inflammatory drugs may attenuate the natriuretic efficacy of diuretics due to inhibition of intrarenal synthesis of prostaglandins.

Spironolactone reduces vascular responsiveness to noradrenaline. Caution should be exercised in the management of patients subjected to regional or general anaesthesia while they are being treated with Aldactone.

Concomitant use of aldactone with other potassium-sparing diuretics, ACE inhibitors, angiotensin II antagonists, aldosterone blockers, potassium supplements, a diet rich in potassium, or salt substitutes containing potassium, may lead to severe hyperkalaemia.

In fluorimetric assays, spironolactone may interfere with the estimation of compounds with similar fluorescence characteristics.

Spironolactone has been shown to increase the half-life of digoxin.

Aspirin, indometacin, and mefanamic acid have been shown to attenuate the diuretic effect of spironolactone.

Spironolactone enhances the metabolism of antipyrine.

Spironolactone can interfere with assays for plasma digoxin concentrations

4.6 Pregnancy and lactation
Pregnancy
Spironolactone or its metabolites may cross the placental barrier. With spironolactone, feminisation has been observed in male rat foetuses. The use of Aldactone in pregnant women requires that the anticipated benefit be weighed against the possible hazards to the mother and foetus.

Lactation
Metabolites of spironolactone have been detected in breast milk. If use of Aldactone is considered essential, an alternative method of infant feeding should be instituted.

4.7 Effects on ability to drive and use machines
Somnolence and dizziness have been reported to occur i some patients. Caution is advised when driving or operat ing machinery until the response to initial treatment ha been determined.

4.8 Undesirable effects
Gynaecomastia may develop in association with the use c spironolactone. Development appears to be related tc both dosage level and duration of therapy and is normally reversible when the drug is discontinued. In rare instances some breast enlargement may persist.

The following adverse events have been reported in association with spironolactone therapy:

Body as a Whole: malaise
Endocrine Disorders: benign breast neoplasm, breast pair
Gastrointestinal Disorders: gastrointestinal disturbances, nausea
Hematologic Disorders: leukopenia (including agranulocytosis), thrombocytopenia
Liver Disorders: hepatic function abnormal
Metabolic and Nutritional Disorders: electrolyte disturbances, hyperkalemia
Musculoskeletal Disorders: leg cramps
Nervous System Disorders: dizziness
Psychiatric Disorders: changes in libido, confusion
Reproductive Disorders: menstrual disorders
Skin and Appendages: alopecia, hypertrichosis, pruritus, rash, urticaria,
Urinary System Disorders: acute renal failure

The following isolated adverse event has been reported in association with spironolactone therapy:

Skin & Appendages: Stevens Johnson Syndrome

4.9 Overdose
Acute overdosage may be manifested by drowsiness, mental confusion, nausea, vomiting, dizziness or diarrhoea. Hyponatraemia, or hyperkalaemia may be induced, but these effects are unlikely to be associated with acute overdosage. Symptoms of hyperkalaemia may manifest as paraesthesia, weakness, flaccid paralysis or muscle spasm and may be difficult to distinguish clinically from hypokalaemia. Electrocardiographic changes are the earliest specific signs of potassium disturbances. No specific antidote has been identified. Improvement may be expected after withdrawal of the drug. General supportive measures including replacement of fluids and electrolytes may be indicated. For hyperkalaemia, reduce potassium intake, administer potassium-excreting diuretics, intravenous glucose with regular insulin or oral ion-exchange resins.

5. PHARMACOLOGICAL PROPERTIES
5.1 Pharmacodynamic properties
Spironolactone, as a competitive aldosterone antagonist, increases sodium excretion whilst reducing potassium loss at the distal renal tubule. It has a gradual and prolonged action.

5.2 Pharmacokinetic properties
Spironolactone is well absorbed orally and is principally metabolised to active metabolites: sulphur containing metabolites (80%) and partly canrenone (20%). Although the plasma half life of spironolactone itself is short (1.3 hours) the half lives of the active metabolites are longer (ranging from 2.8 to 11.2 hours). Elimination of metabolites occurs primarily in the urine and secondarily through biliary excretion in the faeces.

Following the administration of 100 mg of spironolactone daily for 15 days in non-fasted healthy volunteers, time to peak plasma concentration (t_{max}), peak plasma concentration (C_{max}), and elimination half-life ($t_{1/2}$) for spironolactone is 2.6 hr., 80 ng/ml, and approximately 1.4 hr., respectively. For the 7-alpha-(thiomethyl) spironolactone and canrenone metabolites, t_{max} was 3.2 hr. and 4.3 hr., C_{max} was 391 ng/ml and 181 ng/ml, and $t_{1/2}$ was 13.8 hr. and 16.5 hr., respectively.

The renal action of a single dose of spironolactone reaches its peak after 7 hours, and activity persists for at least 24 hours

5.3 Preclinical safety data
Carcinogenicity: Spironolactone has been shown to produce tumours in rats when administered at high doses over a long period of time. The significance of these findings with respect to clinical use is not certain. However the long term use of spironolactone in young patients requires careful consideration of the benefits and the potential hazard involved. Spironolactone or its metabolites may cross the placental barrier. With spironolactone, feminisation has been observed in male rat foetuses. The use of Aldactone in pregnant women requires that the anticipated benefit be weighed against the possible hazards to the mother and foetus.

6. PHARMACEUTICAL PARTICULARS
6.1 List of excipients
Aldactone 25mg, 50mg & 100mg contain:

Calcium sulphate dihydrate, corn starch, polyvinyl pyrrolidone, magnesium stearate, felocofix peppermint, ypromellose, polyethylene glycol and opaspray yellow :ontains E171 and E172).

2 Incompatibilities

one stated.

.3 Shelf life

he shelf life of Aldactone tablets is 5 years.

.4 Special precautions for storage

tore in a dry place below 30°C.

5 Nature and contents of container

dactone 25mg, 50mg & 100mg tablets may be packaged the following containers:

mber glass or plastic bottles containing 100 or 500 ıblets.

DPE containers of 50 or 1,000 tablets.

VC/foil blister packs containing 100 or 500 tablets and VC/foil blister calender pack of 28 tablets.

6 Special precautions for disposal and other handling

one

MARKETING AUTHORISATION HOLDER

harmacia Limited

amsgate Road

andwich

ent, CT13 9NJ

nited Kingdom

MARKETING AUTHORISATION NUMBER(S)

dactone 25mg tablets: PL 00032/0394

dactone 50mg tablets: PL 00032/0395

dactone 100mg tablets: PL 00032/0393

DATE OF FIRST AUTHORISATION/RENEWAL OF IE AUTHORISATION

dactone 25mg tablets: 10 February 2002

dactone 50mg tablets: 14 February 2002

dactone 100mg tablets: 7 February 2002

. DATE OF REVISION OF THE TEXT

ay 2007

. LEGAL STATUS

)M

ef: AN3_0

limta 100mg/500mg powder for oncentrate for solution for infusion

(Eli Lilly and Company Limited)

NAME OF THE MEDICINAL PRODUCT

IMTA* 100mg and 500mg powder for concentrate for lution for infusion.

QUALITATIVE AND QUANTITATIVE COMPOSITION

ch 100mg vial contains 100mg of pemetrexed (as peme- xed disodium).

cipients: Each vial contains approximately 11 mg dium.

ch 500mg vial contains 500mg of pemetrexed (as peme- xed disodium).

cipients: Each vial contains approximately 54 mg dium.

ter reconstitution (see section 6.6), each vial contains mg/ml of pemetrexed.

r a full list of excipients see section 6.1.

PHARMACEUTICAL FORM

wder for concentrate for solution for infusion.

nite to either light yellow or green-yellow lyophilised wder.

CLINICAL PARTICULARS

Therapeutic indications

alignant pleural mesothelioma:

IMTA in combination with cisplatin is indicated for the atment of chemotherapy naive patients with unresect- le malignant pleural mesothelioma.

n-small cell lung cancer:

IMTA in combination with cisplatin is indicated for the t-line treatment of patients with locally advanced or etastatic non-small cell lung cancer other than predomi- ntly squamous cell histology (see section 5.1).

IMTA is indicated as monotherapy for the maintenance atment of locally advanced or metastatic non-small cell g cancer other than predominantly squamous cell his- ogy in patients whose disease has not progressed mediately following platinum-based chemotherapy. st-line treatment should be a platinum doublet with mcitabine, paclitaxel or docetaxel (see section 5.1).

IMTA is indicated as monotherapy for the second-line atment of patients with locally advanced or metastatic n-small cell lung cancer other than predominantly squa- us cell histology (see section 5.1).

4.2 Posology and method of administration

ALIMTA must only be administered under the supervision of a physician qualified in the use of anti-cancer chemotherapy.

ALIMTA in combination with cisplatin: The recommended dose of ALIMTA is 500mg/m² of body surface area (BSA) administered as an intravenous infusion over 10 minutes on the first day of each 21-day cycle. The recommended dose of cisplatin is 75mg/m² BSA infused over two hours approximately 30 minutes after completion of the pemetrexed infusion on the first day of each 21-day cycle. Patients must receive adequate anti-emetic treatment and appropriate hydration prior to and/or after receiving cisplatin (see also cisplatin Summary of Product Characteristics for specific dosing advice).

ALIMTA as single agent: In patients treated for non-small cell lung cancer after prior chemotherapy, the recommended dose of ALIMTA is 500mg/m² BSA administered as an intravenous infusion over 10 minutes on the first day of each 21-day cycle.

Pre-Medication Regimen

To reduce the incidence and severity of skin reactions, a corticosteroid should be given the day prior to, on the day of, and the day after pemetrexed administration. The corticosteroid should be equivalent to 4mg of dexamethasone administered orally twice a day (see section 4.4).

To reduce toxicity, patients treated with pemetrexed must also receive vitamin supplementation (see section 4.4). Patients must take oral folic acid or a multivitamin containing folic acid (350 to 1,000 micrograms) on a daily basis. At least five doses of folic acid must be taken during the seven days preceding the first dose of pemetrexed, and dosing must continue during the full course of therapy and for 21 days after the last dose of pemetrexed. Patients must also receive an intramuscular injection of vitamin B_{12} (1,000 micrograms) in the week preceding the first dose of pemetrexed and once every three cycles thereafter. Subsequent vitamin B_{12} injections may be given on the same day as pemetrexed.

Monitoring

Patients receiving pemetrexed should be monitored before each dose with a complete blood count, including a differential white cell count (WCC) and platelet count. Prior to each chemotherapy administration, blood chemistry tests should be collected to evaluate renal and hepatic function. Before the start of any cycle of chemotherapy, patients are required to have the following: absolute neutrophil count (ANC) should be ≥1,500 cells/mm³ and platelets should be ≥100,000 cells/mm³.

Creatinine clearance should be ≥45ml/min.

The total bilirubin should be ≤1.5-times upper limit of normal. Alkaline phosphatase (AP), aspartate transaminase (AST or SGOT), and alanine transaminase (ALT or SGPT) should be ≤3-times upper limit of normal. Alkaline phosphatase, AST, and ALT ≤5-times upper limit of normal is acceptable if liver has tumour involvement.

Dose Adjustments

Dose adjustments at the start of a subsequent cycle should be based on nadir haematologic counts or maximum non-haematologic toxicity from the preceding cycle of therapy. Treatment may be delayed to allow sufficient time for recovery. Upon recovery, patients should be re-treated using the guidelines in *Tables 1, 2, and 3*, which are applicable for ALIMTA used as a single agent or in combination with cisplatin.

Table 1. **Dose Modification Table for ALIMTA (as Single Agent or in Combination) and Cisplatin - Haematologic Toxicities**

Nadir ANC <500/mm³ and nadir platelets ≥50,000/mm³	75% of previous dose (both ALIMTA and cisplatin)
Nadir platelets <50,000/mm³ regardless of nadir ANC	75% of previous dose (both ALIMTA and cisplatin)
Nadir platelets <50,000/mm³ with bleeding[a], regardless of nadir ANC	50% of previous dose (both ALIMTA and cisplatin)

[a] These criteria meet the National Cancer Institute Common Toxicity Criteria (CTC v2.0; NCI 1998) definition of ≥CTC Grade 2 bleeding.

If patients develop non-haematologic toxicities ≥ Grade 3 (excluding neurotoxicity), ALIMTA should be withheld until resolution to less than or equal to the patient's pre-therapy value. Treatment should be resumed according to the guidelines in *Table 2*.

Table 2. **Dose Modification Table for ALIMTA (as Single Agent or in Combination) and Cisplatin - Non-Haematologic Toxicities[a, b]**

	Dose of ALIMTA (mg/m²)	Dose for Cisplatin (mg/m²)
Any Grade 3 or 4 toxicities except mucositis	75% of previous dose	75% of previous dose
Any diarrhoea requiring hospitalisation (irrespective of grade) or Grade 3 or 4 diarrhoea	75% of previous dose	75% of previous dose
Grade 3 or 4 mucositis	50% of previous dose	100% of previous dose

[a] National Cancer Institute Common Toxicity Criteria (CTC v2.0; NCI 1998)

[b] Excluding neurotoxicity

In the event of neurotoxicity, the recommended dose adjustment for ALIMTA and cisplatin is documented in *Table 3*. Patients should discontinue therapy if Grade 3 or 4 neurotoxicity is observed.

Table 3. **Dose Modification Table for ALIMTA (as Single Agent or in Combination) and Cisplatin - Neurotoxicity**

CTC[a] Grade	Dose of ALIMTA (mg/m²)	Dose for Cisplatin (mg/m²)
0-1	100% of previous dose	100% of previous dose
2	100% of previous dose	50% of previous dose

[a] National Cancer Institute Common Toxicity Criteria (CTC v2.0; NCI 1998)

Treatment with ALIMTA should be discontinued if a patient experiences any haematologic or non-haematologic Grade 3 or 4 toxicity after 2 dose reductions or immediately if Grade 3 or 4 neurotoxicity is observed.

Elderly: In clinical studies, there has been no indication that patients 65 years of age or older are at increased risk of adverse events compared to patients younger than 65 years old. No dose reductions other than those recommended for all patients are necessary.

Children and adolescents: ALIMTA is not recommended for use in children below 18 years of age due to insufficient data on safety and efficacy.

Patients with renal impairment (standard Cockcroft and Gault formula or glomerular filtration rate measured Tc99m-DPTA serum clearance method): Pemetrexed is primarily eliminated unchanged by renal excretion. In clinical studies, patients with creatinine clearance of ≥45ml/min required no dose adjustments other than those recommended for all patients. There are insufficient data on the use of pemetrexed in patients with creatinine clearance below 45ml/min; therefore, the use of pemetrexed is not recommended (see section 4.4).

Patients with hepatic impairment: No relationships between AST (SGOT), ALT (SGPT), or total bilirubin and pemetrexed pharmacokinetics were identified. However, patients with hepatic impairment, such as bilirubin >1.5-times the upper limit of normal and/or transaminase >3.0-times the upper limit of normal (hepatic metastases absent) or >5.0-times the upper limit of normal (hepatic metastases present), have not been specifically studied.

The ALIMTA solution must be prepared according to the instructions provided in section 6.6.

4.3 Contraindications

Hypersensitivity to the active substance or to any of the excipients.

Breast-feeding (see section 4.6).

Concomitant yellow fever vaccine (see section 4.5).

4.4 Special warnings and precautions for use

Pemetrexed can suppress bone marrow function as manifested by neutropenia, thrombocytopenia, and anaemia (or pancytopenia) (see section 4.8). Myelosuppression is usually the dose-limiting toxicity. Patients should be monitored for myelosuppression during therapy and pemetrexed should not be given to patients until absolute neutrophil count (ANC) returns to ≥1500 cells/mm³ and platelet count returns to ≥100,000 cells/mm³. Dose reductions for subsequent cycles are based on nadir ANC, platelet count, and maximum non-haematologic toxicity seen from the previous cycle (see section 4.2).

Less toxicity and reduction in Grade 3/4 haematologic and non-haematologic toxicities, such as neutropenia, febrile neutropenia, and infection with Grade 3/4 neutropenia, were reported when pre-treatment with folic acid and vitamin B_{12} was administered. Therefore, all patients treated with pemetrexed must be instructed to take folic acid and vitamin B_{12} as a prophylactic measure to reduce treatment-related toxicity (see section 4.2).

Skin reactions have been reported in patients not pre-treated with a corticosteroid. Pre-treatment with dexamethasone (or equivalent) can reduce the incidence and severity of skin reactions (see section 4.2).

An insufficient number of patients has been studied with creatinine clearance of below 45ml/min. Therefore, the use of pemetrexed in patients with creatinine clearance of < 45ml/min is not recommended (see section 4.2).

Patients with mild to moderate renal insufficiency (creatinine clearance from 45 to 79ml/min) should avoid taking non-steroidal anti-inflammatory drugs (NSAIDs), such as ibuprofen, and aspirin (>1.3g daily) for 2 days before, on the day of, and 2 days following pemetrexed administration (see section 4.5). All patients eligible for pemetrexed therapy should avoid taking NSAIDs with long elimination half-lives for at least 5 days prior to, on the day of, and at least 2 days following pemetrexed administration (see section 4.5).

Serious renal events, including acute renal failure, have been reported with pemetrexed alone or in association with other chemotherapeutic agents. Many of the patients in whom these occurred had underlying risk factors for the development of renal events, including dehydration or pre-existing hypertension or diabetes.

The effect of third-space fluid, such as pleural effusion or ascites, on pemetrexed is unknown. In patients with clinically significant third-space fluid, consideration should be given to draining the effusion prior to pemetrexed administration.

Due to the gastrointestinal toxicity of pemetrexed given in combination with cisplatin, severe dehydration has been observed. Therefore, patients should receive adequate anti-emetic treatment and appropriate hydration prior to and/or after receiving treatment.

Serious cardiovascular events, including myocardial infarction and cerebrovascular events, have been uncommonly reported during clinical studies with pemetrexed, usually when given in combination with another cytotoxic agent. Most of the patients in whom these events have been observed had pre-existing cardiovascular risk factors (see section 4.8).

Immunodepressed status is common in cancer patients. As a result, concomitant use of live attenuated vaccines is not recommended (see section 4.3 and section 4.5).

Pemetrexed can have genetically damaging effects. Sexually mature males are advised not to father a child during the treatment and up to 6 months thereafter. Contraceptive measures or abstinence are recommended. Owing to the possibility of pemetrexed treatment causing irreversible infertility, men are advised to seek counselling on sperm storage before starting treatment.

Women of childbearing potential must use effective contraception during treatment with pemetrexed (see section 4.6).

Cases of radiation pneumonitis have been reported in patients treated with radiation either prior, during, or subsequent to their pemetrexed therapy. Particular attention should be paid to these patients, and caution exercised with use of other radiosensitising agents.

Cases of radiation recall have been reported in patients who received radiotherapy weeks or years previously.

500 mg vial: This medicinal product contains approximately 54 mg of sodium per vial. To be taken into consideration by patients on a controlled sodium diet.

4.5 Interaction with other medicinal products and other forms of interaction

Pemetrexed is mainly eliminated unchanged renally by tubular secretion and to a lesser extent by glomerular filtration. Concomitant administration of nephrotoxic drugs (e.g., aminoglycoside, loop diuretics, platinum compounds, cyclosporin) could potentially result in delayed clearance of pemetrexed. This combination should be used with caution. If necessary, creatinine clearance should be closely monitored.

Concomitant administration of substances that are also tubularly secreted (e.g., probenecid, penicillin) could potentially result in delayed clearance of pemetrexed. Caution should be made when these drugs are combined with pemetrexed. If necessary, creatinine clearance should be closely monitored.

In patients with normal renal function (creatinine clearance ≥80ml/min), high doses of non-steroidal anti-inflammatory drugs (NSAIDs, such as ibuprofen >1600mg/day) and aspirin at higher doses (≥1.3g daily) may decrease pemetrexed elimination and, consequently, increase the occurrence of pemetrexed adverse events. Therefore, caution should be made when administering higher doses of NSAIDs or aspirin at higher doses concurrently with pemetrexed to patients with normal function (creatinine clearance ≥80ml/min).

In patients with mild to moderate renal insufficiency (creatinine clearance from 45 to 79ml/min), the concomitant administration of pemetrexed with NSAIDs (e.g., ibuprofen) or aspirin at higher doses should be avoided for 2 days before, on the day of, and 2 days following pemetrexed administration (see section 4.4).

In the absence of data regarding potential interaction with NSAIDs having longer half-lives, such as piroxicam or rofecoxib, the concomitant administration with pemetrexed should be avoided for at least 5 days prior to, on the day of, and at least 2 days following pemetrexed administration (see section 4.4).

Pemetrexed undergoes limited hepatic metabolism. Results from *in vitro* studies with human liver microsomes indicated that pemetrexed would not be predicted to cause clinically significant inhibition of the metabolic clearance of drugs metabolised by CYP3A, CYP2D6, CYP2C9, and CYP1A2.

Table 4

System organ class	Frequency	Event*	Pemetrexed/Cisplatin (N = 168)		Cisplatin (N = 163)	
			All grades toxicity (%)	Grade 3-4 toxicity (%)	All grades toxicity (%)	Grade 3-4 toxicity (%)
Blood and lymphatic system disorders	Very common	Neutrophils/ Granulocytes decreased	56.0	23.2	13.5	3.1
		Leucocytes decreased	53.0	14.9	16.6	0.6
		Haemoglobin decreased	26.2	4.2	10.4	0.0
		Platelets decreased	23.2	5.4	8.6	0.0
Metabolism and nutrition disorders	Common	Dehydration	6.5	4.2	0.6	0.6
Nervous system disorders	Very common	Neuropathy-sensory	10.1	0.0	9.8	0.6
	Common	Taste disturbance	7.7	0.0***	6.1	0.0***
Eye disorders	Common	Conjunctivitis	5.4	0.0	0.6	0.0
Gastrointestinal disorders	Very common	Diarrhoea	16.7	3.6	8.0	0.0
		Vomiting	56.5	10.7	49.7	4.3
		Stomatitis/ Pharyngitis	23.2	3.0	6.1	0.0
		Nausea	82.1	11.9	76.7	5.5
		Anorexia	20.2	1.2	14.1	0.6
		Constipation	11.9	0.6	7.4	0.6
	Common	Dyspepsia	5.4	0.6	0.6	0.0
Skin and subcutaneous tissue disorders	Very common	Rash	16.1	0.6	4.9	0.0
		Alopecia	11.3	0.0***	5.5	0.0***
Renal and urinary disorders	Very common	Creatinine elevation	10.7	0.6	9.8	1.2
		Creatinine clearance decreased**	16.1	0.6	17.8	1.8
General disorders and administration site conditions	Very common	Fatigue	47.6	10.1	42.3	9.2

* Refer to National Cancer Institute CTC version 2 for each grade of toxicity except the term "creatinine clearan decreased"** which is derived from the term "renal/genitourinary other".

*** According to National Cancer Institute CTC (v2.0; NCI 1998), taste disturbance and alopecia should only be reported Grade 1 or 2.

For the purpose of this table a cut off of 5% was used for inclusion of all events where the reporter considered a possil relationship to pemetrexed and cisplatin.

Interactions Common to all Cytotoxics

Due to the increased thrombotic risk in patients with cancer, the use of anticoagulation treatment is frequent. The high intra-individual variability of the coagulation status during diseases and the possibility of interaction between oral anticoagulants and anti-cancer chemotherapy require increased frequency of INR (International Normalised Ratio) monitoring, if it is decided to treat the patient with oral anticoagulants.

Concomitant Use Contraindicated

Yellow fever vaccine: Risk of fatal generalised vaccinale disease (see section 4.3).

Concomitant Use Not Recommended

Live attenuated vaccines (except yellow fever, for which concomitant use is contraindicated): Risk of systemic, possibly fatal, disease. The risk is increased in subjects who are already immunosuppressed by their underlying disease. Use an inactivated vaccine where it exists (poliomyelitis) (see section 4.4).

4.6 Pregnancy and lactation

There are no data from the use of pemetrexed in pregnant women; but pemetrexed, like other anti-metabolites, is suspected to cause serious birth defects when administered during pregnancy. Animal studies have shown reproductive toxicity (see section 5.3). Pemetrexed should not be used during pregnancy unless clearly necessary, after a careful consideration of the needs of the mother and the risk for the foetus (see section 4.4).

Women of childbearing potential must use effective contraception during treatment with pemetrexed. Pemetrexed can have genetically damaging effects. Sexually mature males are advised not to father a child during the treatment, and up to 6 months thereafter. Contraceptive measures or abstinence are recommended. Owing to the possibility of pemetrexed treatment causing irreversible infertility, m are advised to seek counselling on sperm storage bef starting treatment.

It is not known whether pemetrexed is excreted in hum milk, and adverse reactions on the suckling child cannot excluded. Breast-feeding must be discontinued duri pemetrexed therapy (see section 4.3).

4.7 Effects on ability to drive and use machines

No studies on the effects on the ability to drive and u machines have been performed. However, it has be reported that pemetrexed may cause fatigue. Therefo patients should be cautioned against driving or operati machines if this event occurs.

4.8 Undesirable effects

The table below provides the frequency and severity undesirable effects that have been reported in >5% of t patients with mesothelioma who were randomised receive cisplatin and pemetrexed, and 163 patients w mesothelioma randomised to receive single-agent cisp tin. In both treatment arms, these chemonaive patie were fully supplemented with folic acid and vitamin B_{12}

Adverse Reactions

Frequency estimate: Very common (≥1/10), common (≥ 100 and <1/10), uncommon (≥1/1,000 and <1/100), ra (≥1/10,000 and <1/1,000), very rare (<1/10,000) and r known (cannot be estimated from available data – spon neous reports).

Within each frequency grouping, undesirable effects a presented in order of decreasing seriousness.

(see Table 4 above)

Clinically relevant CTC toxicities that were repor in ≥1% and ≤5% of the patients that w randomly assigned to receive cisplatin and pemetre clude: renal failure, infection, pyrexia, febrile neutropenia, creased AST, ALT, and GGT, urticaria and chest pain.

linically relevant CTC toxicities that were reported in 1% of the patients that were randomly assigned to ceive cisplatin and pemetrexed include arrhythmia and otor neuropathy.

ne table below provides the frequency and severity of ndesirable effects that have been reported in >5% of 265 atients randomly assigned to receive single-agent pemetexed with folic acid and vitamin B_{12} supplementation, and 76 patients randomly assigned to receive single-agent ocetaxel. All patients were diagnosed with locally dvanced or metastatic non-small cell lung cancer and eceived prior chemotherapy.

see Table 5 opposite)

linically relevant CTC toxicities that were reported in ≥1% and ≤5% of the patients that were randomly ssigned to pemetrexed include: infection without neutroenia, febrile neutropenia, allergic reaction/hypersensitivy, increased creatinine, motor neuropathy, sensory europathy, erythema multiforme, and abdominal pain.

linically relevant CTC toxicities that were reported in <1% of the patients that were randomly assigned to emetrexed include supraventricular arrhythmias.

linically relevant Grade 3 and Grade 4 laboratory toxicities vere similar between integrated Phase 2 results from three ingle-agent pemetrexed studies (N = 164) and the Phase 3 ingle-agent pemetrexed study described above, with the xception of neutropenia (12.8% versus 5.3%, respecively) and alanine transaminase elevation (15.2% versus .9%, respectively). These differences were likely due to ifferences in the patient population, since the Phase 2 tudies included both chemonaive and heavily pre-treated reast cancer patients with pre-existing liver metastases nd/or abnormal baseline liver function tests.

he table below provides the frequency and severity of ndesirable effects considered possibly related to study rug that have been reported in >5% of 839 patients with SCLC who were randomised to receive cisplatin and emetrexed and 830 patients with NSCLC who were randomised to receive cisplatin and gemcitabine. All patients eceived study therapy as initial treatment for locally dvanced or metastatic NSCLC and patients in both treatment groups were fully supplemented with folic acid and itamin B_{12}.

see Table 6 opposite)

Clinically relevant toxicity that was reported in ≥1% and ≤5% of the patients that were randomly assigned to eceive cisplatin and pemetrexed include: AST increase, ALT increase, infection, febrile neutropenia, renal failure, pyrexia, dehydration, conjunctivitis, and creatinine clearance decrease.

Clinically relevant toxicity that was reported in <1% (uncommon) of the patients that were randomly assigned to receive cisplatin and pemetrexed include: GGT increase, chest pain, arrhythmia, and motor neuropathy.

Clinically relevant toxicities with respect to gender were similar to the overall population in patients receiving pemetrexed plus cisplatin.

The table below provides the frequency and severity of undesirable effects considered possibly related to study drug that have been reported in >5% of 441 patients randomly assigned to receive single-agent pemetrexed and 222 patients randomly assigned to receive placebo in the single-agent maintenance pemetrexed study (Study JMEN). All patients were diagnosed with Stage IIIB or IV NSCLC and had received prior platinum-based chemotherapy. Patients in both study arms were fully supplemented with folic acid and vitamin B_{12}.

(see Table 7 on next page)

Clinically relevant CTC toxicity of any grade that was reported in ≥1% and ≤5% of the patients that were randomly assigned to pemetrexed include: decreased platelets, decreased creatinine clearance, constipation, oedema, alopecia, increased creatinine, pruritus/itching, fever (in the absence of neutropenia), ocular surface disease (including conjunctivitis), increased lacrimation, and decreased glomerular filtration rate.

Clinically relevant CTC toxicity that was reported in <1% of the patients that were randomly assigned to pemetrexed include: febrile neutropenia, allergic reaction/hypersensitivity, motor neuropathy, erythema multiforme, renal failure, and supraventricular arrhythmia.

The incidence of adverse reactions was evaluated for patients who received ≤ 6 cycles of pemetrexed, and compared to patients who received > 6 cycles of pemetrexed. Increases in adverse reactions (all grades) were observed with longer exposure; however, no statistically significant differences in Grade 3/4 adverse reactions were seen.

Serious cardiovascular and cerebrovascular events, including myocardial infarction, angina pectoris, cerebrovascular accident, and transient ischaemic attack, have been uncommonly reported during clinical studies with pemetrexed, usually when given in combination with another cytotoxic agent. Most of the patients in whom these events have been observed had pre-existing cardiovascular risk factors.

Table 5

System organ class	Frequency	Event*	Pemetrexed (N = 265)		Docetaxel (N = 276)	
			All grades toxicity (%)	Grade 3-4 toxicity (%)	All grades toxicity (%)	Grade 3-4 toxicity (%)
Blood and lymphatic system disorders	Very common	Neutrophils/ Granulocytes decreased	10.9	5.3	45.3	40.2
		Leucocytes decreased	12.1	4.2	34.1	27.2
		Haemoglobin decreased	19.2	4.2	22.1	4.3
	Common	Platelets decreased	8.3	1.9	1.1	0.4
Gastrointestinal disorders	Very common	Diarrhoea	12.8	0.4	24.3	2.5
		Vomiting	16.2	1.5	12.0	1.1
		Stomatitis/ Pharyngitis	14.7	1.1	17.4	1.1
		Nausea	30.9	2.6	16.7	1.8
		Anorexia	21.9	1.9	23.9	2.5
	Common	Constipation	5.7	0.0	4.0	0.0
Hepatobiliary disorders	Common	SGPT (ALT) elevation	7.9	1.9	1.4	0.0
		SGOT (AST) elevation	6.8	1.1	0.7	0.0
Skin and subcutaneous tissue disorders	Very common	Rash/ desquamation	14.0	0.0	6.2	0.0
	Common	Pruritus	6.8	0.4	1.8	0.0
		Alopecia	6.4	0.4**	37.7	2.2**
General disorders and administration site conditions	Very common	Fatigue	34.0	5.3	35.9	5.4
	Common	Fever	8.3	0.0	7.6	0.0

* Refer to National Cancer Institute CTC version 2 for each grade of toxicity.

** According to National Cancer Institute CTC (v2.0; NCI 1998), alopecia should only be reported as Grade 1 or 2.

For the purpose of this table a cut off of 5% was used for inclusion of all events where the reporter considered a possible relationship to pemetrexed.

Table 6

System organ class	Frequency	Event**	Pemetrexed/Cisplatin (N = 839)		Gemcitabine/Cisplatin (N = 830)	
			All grades toxicity (%)	Grade 3 - 4 toxicity (%)	All grades toxicity (%)	Grade 3 - 4 toxicity (%)
Blood and lymphatic system disorders	Very common	Haemoglobin decreased	33.0*	5.6*	45.7*	9.9*
		Neutrophils/ Granulocytes decreased	29.0*	15.1*	38.4*	26.7*
		Leucocytes decreased	17.8	4.8*	20.6	7.6*
		Platelets decreased	10.1*	4.1*	26.6*	12.7*
Gastrointestinal disorders	Very common	Nausea	56.1	7.2*	53.4	3.9*
		Vomiting	39.7	6.1	35.5	6.1
		Anorexia	26.6	2.4*	24.2	0.7*
		Constipation	21.0	0.8	19.5	0.4
		Stomatitis/ Pharyngitis	13.5	0.8	12.4	0.1
		Diarrhoea without colostomy	12.4	1.3	12.8	1.6
	Common	Dyspepsia/ heartburn	5.2	0.1	5.9	0.0
General disorders and administration site conditions	Very common	Fatigue	42.7	6.7	44.9	4.9
Nervous system disorders	Common	Neuropathy-sensory	8.5*	0.0*	12.4*	0.6*
		Taste disturbance	8.1	0.0***	8.9	0.0***
Renal and urinary disorders	Very common	Creatinine elevation	10.1*	0.8	6.9*	0.5
Skin and subcutaneous tissue disorders	Very common	Alopecia	11.9*	0***	21.4*	0.5***
	Common	Rash/ desquamation	6.6	0.1	8.0	0.5

*p -values < 0.05 comparing pemetrexed/cisplatin to gemcitabine/cisplatin, using Fisher Exact test.

**Refer to National Cancer Institute CTC (v2.0; NCI 1998) for each Grade of Toxicity.

***According to National Cancer Institute CTC (v2.0; NCI 1998), taste disturbance and alopecia should only be reported as Grade 1 or 2.

For the purpose of this table, a cut off of 5% was used for inclusion of all events where the reporter considered a possible relationship to pemetrexed and cisplatin.

Table 7

System organ class	Frequency*	Event**	Pemetrexed (N = 441) All grades toxicity (%)	Pemetrexed (N = 441) Grade 3 - 4 toxicity (%)	Placebo (N = 222) All grades toxicity (%)	Placebo (N = 222) Grade 3 - 4 toxicity (%)
Infections and infestations	Common	Infection	5.2	1.6	1.8	0.0
Blood and lymphatic system disorders	Very common	Haemoglobin	15.2	2.7	5.4	0.5
	Common	Leucocytes	6.1	1.6	1.4	0.5
		Neutrophils	5.9	2.9	0.0	0.0
Nervous system disorders	Common	Neuropathy-sensory	8.8	0.7	4.1	0.0
Gastrointestinal disorders	Very common	Nausea	18.8	0.9	5.4	0.5
		Anorexia	18.6	1.8	5.0	0.0
	Common	Vomiting	8.6	0.2	1.4	0.0
		Mucositis/ Stomatitis	7.0	0.7	1.8	0.0
		Diarrhoea	5.2	0.5	2.7	0.0
Hepatobiliary disorders	Common	ALT (SGPT)	9.5	0.2	3.6	0.0
		AST (SGOT)	8.2	0.0	3.6	0.0
Skin and subcutaneous tissue disorders	Very common	Rash/ desquamation	10.0	0.0	3.2	0.0
General disorders and administration site conditions	Very common	Fatigue	24.5	5.0	10.4	0.5

Abbreviations: ALT = alanine transaminase; AST = aspartate transaminase; CTCAE = Common Terminology Criteria for Adverse Event; NCI = National Cancer Institute; SGOT = serum glutamic oxaloacectic transaminase; SGPT = serum glutamic pyruvic transaminase.

*Definition of frequency terms: Very common - ⩾ 10%; Common - > 5% and < 10%. For the purpose of this table, a cut off of 5% was used for inclusion of all events where the reporter considered a possible relationship to pemetrexed.

**Refer to NCI CTCAE Criteria (Version 3.0; NCI 2003) for each grade of toxicity.

Table 8 Efficacy of ALIMTA Plus cisplatin vs cisplatin in malignant pleural mesothelioma

Efficacy parameter	Randomised and treated patients: ALIMTA/Cisplatin (N = 226)	Randomised and treated patients: Cisplatin (N = 222)	Fully supplemented patients: ALIMTA/Cisplatin (N = 168)	Fully supplemented patients: Cisplatin (N = 163)
Median overall survival (months)	12.1	9.3	13.3	10.0
(95% CI)	(10.0-14.4)	(7.8-10.7)	(11.4-14.9)	(8.4-11.9)
Log rank *p*-value*	0.020		0.051	
Median time to tumour progression (months)	5.7	3.9	6.1	3.9
(95% CI)	(4.9-6.5)	(2.8-4.4)	(5.3-7.0)	(2.8-4.5)
Log rank *p*-value*	0.001		0.008	
Time to treatment failure (months)	4.5	2.7	4.7	2.7
(95% CI)	(3.9-4.9)	(2.1-2.9)	(4.3-5.6)	(2.2-3.1)
Log rank *p*-value*	0.001		0.001	
Overall response rate**	41.3%	16.7%	45.5%	19.6%
(95% CI)	(34.8-48.1)	(12.0-22.2)	(37.8-53.4)	(13.8-26.6)
Fisher's exact *p*-value*	<0.001		<0.001	

Abbreviation: CI = confidence interval.
**p*-value refers to comparison between arms.
**In the ALIMTA/cisplatin arm, randomised and treated (N = 225) and fully supplemented (N =167).

Rare cases of hepatitis, potentially serious, have been reported during clinical studies with pemetrexed.

Pancytopenia has been uncommonly reported during clinical trials with pemetrexed.

In clinical trials, cases of colitis (including intestinal and rectal bleeding, sometimes fatal, intestinal perforation, intestinal necrosis and typhlitis) have been reported uncommonly in patients treated with pemetrexed.

In clinical trials, cases of interstitial pneumonitis with respiratory insufficiency, sometimes fatal, have been reported uncommonly in patients treated with pemetrexed.

Uncommon cases of oedema have been reported in patients treated with pemetrexed.

Oesophagitis/ radiation oesophagitis has been uncommonly reported during clinical trials with pemetrexed.

During post-marketing surveillance, the following adverse reactions have been reported in patients treated with pemetrexed:

Cases of acute renal failure have been reported with pemetrexed alone or in association with other chemotherapeutic agents (see section 4.4).

Cases of radiation pneumonitis have been reported in patients treated with radiation either prior, during or subsequent to their pemetrexed therapy (see section 4.4).

Cases of radiation recall have been reported in patients who have received radiotherapy previously (see section 4.4).

Cases of peripheral ischaemia leading sometimes to extremity necrosis have been reported.

4.9 Overdose

Reported symptoms of overdose include neutropenia, anaemia, thrombocytopenia, mucositis, sensory polyneuropathy, and rash. Anticipated complications of overdose include bone marrow suppression as manifested by neutropenia, thrombocytopenia, and anaemia. In addition, infection with or without fever, diarrhoea, and/or mucositis may be seen. In the event of suspected overdose, patients should be monitored with blood counts and should receive supportive therapy as necessary. The use of calcium folinate/folinic acid in the management of pemetrexed overdose should be considered.

5. PHARMACOLOGICAL PROPERTIES

5.1 Pharmacodynamic properties

Pharmacotherapeutic group: Folic acid analogues. *ATC code:* L01BA04.

ALIMTA (pemetrexed) is a multi-targeted anti-cancer antifolate agent that exerts its action by disrupting crucial folate-dependent metabolic processes essential for cell replication.

In vitro studies have shown that pemetrexed behaves as multi-targeted antifolate by inhibiting thymidylate synthas (TS), dihydrofolate reductase (DHFR), and glycinamic ribonucleotide formyltransferase (GARFT), which are ke folate-dependent enzymes for the *de novo* biosynthesis thymidine and purine nucleotides. Pemetrexed is tran ported into cells by both the reduced folate carrier ar membrane folate binding protein transport systems. On in the cell, pemetrexed is rapidly and efficiently converte to polyglutamate forms by the enzyme folylpolyglutama synthetase. The polyglutamate forms are retained in ce and are even more potent inhibitors of TS and GARF Polyglutamation is a time- and concentration-depende process that occurs in tumour cells and, to a lesser exter in normal tissues. Polyglutamated metabolites have increased intracellular half-life resulting in prolonged dr action in malignant cells.

Clinical efficacy

Mesothelioma:

EMPHACIS, a multi-centre, randomised, single-bli Phase 3 study of ALIMTA plus cisplatin versus cispla in chemonaive patients with malignant pleural mesoth lioma, has shown that patients treated with ALIMTA a cisplatin had a clinically meaningful 2.8-month medi survival advantage over patients receiving cisplatin alor

During the study, low-dose folic acid and vitamin B supplementation was introduced to patients' therapy reduce toxicity. The primary analysis of this study w performed on the population of all patients random assigned to a treatment arm who received study dr (randomised and treated). A subgroup analysis was pe formed on patients who received folic acid and vitamin B supplementation during the entire course of study thera (fully supplemented). The results of these analyses of e cacy are summarised in the table below.

Efficacy of ALIMTA Plus cisplatin vs cisplatin in mali nant pleural mesothelioma

(see Table 8)

A statistically significant improvement of the clinically re vant symptoms (pain and dyspnoea) associated w malignant pleural mesothelioma in the ALIMTA/cispla arm (212 patients) versus the cisplatin arm alone (2 patients) was demonstrated using the Lung Cancer Sym tom Scale. Statistically significant differences in pulmona function tests were also observed. The separation betwe the treatment arms was achieved by improvement in lu function in the ALIMTA/cisplatin arm and deterioration lung function over time in the control arm.

There are limited data in patients with malignant pleu mesothelioma treated with ALIMTA alone. ALIMTA at dose of 500mg/m^2 was studied as a single agent in chemonaive patients with malignant pleural mesothelion The overall response rate was 14.1%.

NSCLC, second-line treatment:

A multi-centre, randomised, open-label Phase 3 study ALIMTA versus docetaxel in patients with locally advanc or metastatic NSCLC after prior chemotherapy has sho median survival times of 8.3 months for patients treat with ALIMTA (Intent-To-Treat [ITT] population N = 283) a 7.9 months for patients treated with docetaxel (ITT N = 28 Prior chemotherapy did not include ALIMTA. An analysis the impact of NSCLC histology on the treatment effect overall survival was in favour of ALIMTA versus doceta for other than predominantly squamous histolog (N=399, 9.3 versus 8.0 months, adjusted hazard ra (HR) = 0.78; 95% CI =0.61-1.00, p =0.047) and was favour of docetaxel for squamous cell carcinoma histolo (N =172, 6.2 versus 7.4 months, adjusted HR = 1.56; 95 CI =1.08-2.26, p =0.018). There were no clinically releva differences observed for the safety profile of ALIMTA wit the histology subgroups.

Limited clinical data from a separate randomised, Phase controlled trial, suggest that efficacy data (overall surviv progression free survival) for pemetrexed are simi between patients previously pre-treated with doceta (N = 41) and patients who did not receive previous do etaxel treatment (N = 540).

Efficacy of ALIMTA vs Docetaxel in NSCLC - I population

	ALIMTA	Docetaxel
Survival time (months)	(N = 283)	(N = 288)
• Median (m)	8.3	7.9
• 95% CI for median	(7.0-9.4)	(6.3-9.2)
• HR	0.99	
• 95% CI for HR	(0.82-1.20)	
• Non-inferiority *p*-value (HR)	0.226	
Progression-free survival (months)	(N = 283)	(N = 288)
• Median	2.9	2.9
• HR (95% CI)	0.97 (0.82-1.16)	

'ime to treatment 'ailure TTF - months)	(N = 283)	(N = 288)
• Median	2.3	2.1
• HR (95% CI)	0.84 (0.71-0.997)	
Response n: qualified for esponse)	(N = 264)	(N = 274)
• Response rate (%) 95% CI)	9.1 (5.9-13.2)	8.8 (5.7-12.8)
• Stable disease (%)	45.8	46.4

breviations: CI = confidence interval; HR = hazard ratio; ITT = intent treat; N = total population size.

SCLC, first-line treatment:

multi-centre, randomised, open-label, Phase 3 study of LIMTA plus cisplatin versus gemcitabine plus cisplatin in emonaive patients with locally advanced or metastatic tage IIIb or IV) non-small cell lung cancer (NSCLC) owed that ALIMTA plus cisplatin (Intent-To-Treat [ITT] opulation N = 862) met its primary endpoint and showed nilar clinical efficacy as gemcitabine plus cisplatin (ITT = 863) in overall survival (adjusted hazard ratio (HR) 0.94; % CI 0.84-1.05). All patients included in this study had ECOG performance status 0 or 1.

e primary efficacy analysis was based on the ITT population. Sensitivity analyses of main efficacy endpoints were so assessed on the Protocol Qualified (PQ) population. e efficacy analyses using PQ population are consistent th the analyses for the ITT population and support the n-inferiority of AC versus GC.

ogression-free survival (PFS) and overall response rate ere similar between treatment arms: median PFS was 4.8 onths for ALIMTA plus cisplatin versus 5.1 months for mcitabine plus cisplatin (adjusted hazard ratio (HR) 1.04; % CI= 0.94-1.15), and overall response rate was 30.6% % CI= 27.3- 33.9) for ALIMTA plus cisplatin versus .2% (95% CI 25.0-31.4) for gemcitabine plus cisplatin. S data were partially confirmed by an independent view (400/1725 patients were randomly selected for view).

e analysis of the impact of NSCLC histology on overall rvival demonstrated clinically relevant differences in survival according to histology, see table below.

icacy of ALIMTA + cisplatin vs gemcitabine + splatin in first-line non-small cell lung cancer – ITT pulation and histology subgroups

e Table 9 below)

plan Meier plots of overall survival by histology

e Figure 1 above)

ere were no clinically relevant differences observed for safety profile of ALIMTA plus cisplatin within the histology subgroups.

tients treated with ALIMTA and cisplatin required fewer nsfusions (16.4% versus 28.9%, p<0.001), red blood l transfusions (16.1% versus 27.3%, p<0.001) and telet transfusions (1.8% versus 4.5%, p=0.002). tients also required lower administration of erythropoie-'darbopoietin (10.4% versus 18.1%, p<0.001), G-CSF/ 1-CSF (3.1% versus 6.1%, p=0.004), and iron preparans (4.3% versus 7.0%, p=0.021).

CLC, maintenance treatment:

multi-centre, randomised, double-blind, placebo-conlled Phase 3 study (JMEN), compared the efficacy and ety of maintenance treatment with ALIMTA plus best oportive care (BSC) (N = 441) with that of placebo plus C (N = 222) in patients with locally advanced (Stage IIIB) metastatic (Stage IV) Non-Small Cell Lung Cancer SCLC) who did not progress after 4 cycles of first-line

Figure 1 Kaplan Meier plots of overall survival by histology

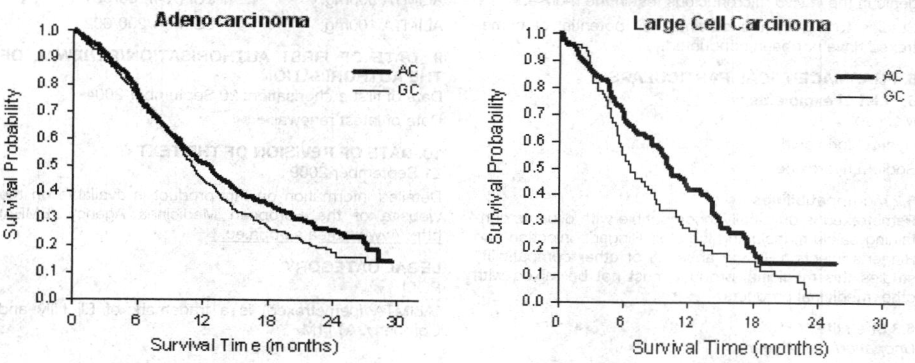

Figure 2 Kaplan Meier plots of progression-free survival (PFS) and overall survival ALIMTA versus placebo in patients with NSCLC other than predominantly squamous cell histology

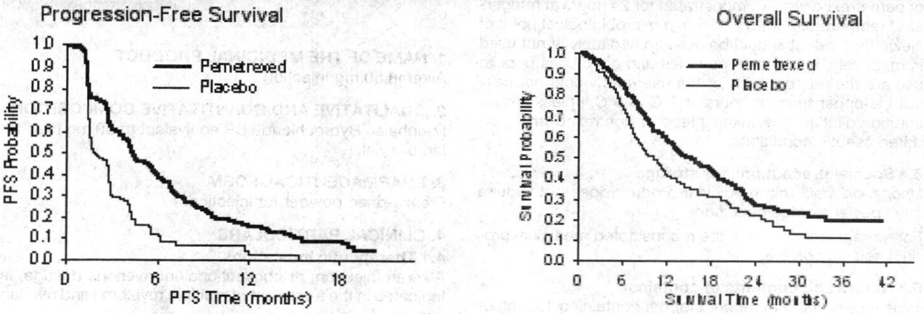

doublet therapy containing Cisplatin or Carboplatin in combination with Gemcitabine, Paclitaxel, or Docetaxel. First-line doublet therapy containing ALIMTA was not included. All patients included in this study had an ECOG performance status 0 or 1. Patients received maintenance treatment until disease progression. Efficacy and safety were measured from the time of randomisation after completion of first-line (induction) therapy. Patients received a median of 5 cycles of maintenance treatment with ALIMTA and 3.5 cycles of placebo. A total of 213 patients (48.3%) completed ⩾ 6 cycles and a total of 103 patients (23.4%) completed ⩾ 10 cycles of treatment with ALIMTA.

The study met its primary endpoint and showed a statistically significant improvement in PFS in the ALIMTA arm over the placebo arm (N = 581, independently reviewed population; median of 4.0 months and 2.0 months, respectively) hazard ratio = 0.60, (95% CI: 0.49-0.73, p < 0.00001). The independent review of patient scans confirmed the findings of the investigator assessment of PFS. The median OS for the overall population (N = 663) was 13.4 months for the ALIMTA arm and 10.6 months for the placebo arm, hazard ratio = 0.79 (95% CI: 0.65 to 0.95; p = 0.01192).

Consistent with other ALIMTA studies, a difference in efficacy according to NSCLC histology was observed in JMEN. For patients with NSCLC other than predominantly squamous cell histology (N = 430, independently reviewed population) median PFS was 4.4 months for the ALIMTA arm and 1.8 months for the placebo arm, hazard ratio = 0.47, (95% CI: 0.37-0.60, p= 0.00001). The median OS for patients with NSCLC other than predominantly squamous cell histology (N = 481) was 15.5 months for the ALIMTA arm and 10.3 months for the placebo arm hazard ratio = 0.70, (95% CI: 0.56-0.88, p=0.002). Including the induction phase the median OS for patients with NSCLC other than predominantly squamous cell histology was 18.6 months for the ALIMTA arm and 13.6 months for the placebo arm hazard ratio =0.71, (95% CI: 0.56-0.88, p=0.002).

The PFS and OS results in patients with squamous cell histology suggested no advantage for ALIMTA over placebo.

There were no clinically relevant differences observed for the safety profile of ALIMTA within the histology subgroups.

Kaplan Meier plots of progression-free survival (PFS) and overall survival ALIMTA versus placebo in patients with NSCLC other than predominantly squamous cell histology:

(see Figure 2 above)

5.2 Pharmacokinetic properties

The pharmacokinetic properties of pemetrexed following single-agent administration have been evaluated in 426 cancer patients with a variety of solid tumours at doses ranging from 0.2 to 838mg/m^2 infused over a 10-minute period. Pemetrexed has a steady-state volume of distribution of 9 l/m^2. *In vitro* studies indicate that pemetrexed is approximately 81% bound to plasma proteins. Binding was not notably affected by varying degrees of renal impairment. Pemetrexed undergoes limited hepatic metabolism. Pemetrexed is primarily eliminated in the urine, with 70% to 90% of the administered dose being recovered unchanged in urine within the first 24 hours following administration. Pemetrexed total systemic clearance is 91.8ml/min and the elimination half-life from plasma is 3.5 hours in patients with normal renal function (creatinine clearance of 90ml/min). Between patient variability in clearance is moderate at 19.3%. Pemetrexed total systemic exposure (AUC) and maximum plasma concentration increase proportionally with dose. The pharmacokinetics of pemetrexed are consistent over multiple treatment cycles.

The pharmacokinetic properties of pemetrexed are not influenced by concurrently administered cisplatin. Oral folic acid and intramuscular vitamin B_{12} supplementation do not affect the pharmacokinetics of pemetrexed.

5.3 Preclinical safety data

Administration of pemetrexed to pregnant mice resulted in decreased foetal viability, decreased foetal weight, incomplete ossification of some skeletal structures, and cleft palate.

Administration of pemetrexed to male mice resulted in reproductive toxicity characterised by reduced fertility rates and testicular atrophy. In a study conducted in beagle dog by intravenous bolus injection for 9 months, testicular findings (degeneration/necrosis of the seminiferous epithelium) have been observed. This suggests that pemetrexed may impair male fertility. Female fertility was not investigated.

Pemetrexed was not mutagenic in either the *in vitro* chromosome aberration test in Chinese hamster ovary cells, or

Table 9 Efficacy of ALIMTA + cisplatin vs gemcitabine + cisplatin in first-line non-small cell lung cancer – ITT population and histology subgroups

T population nd histology ıbgroups	Median overall survival in months (95% CI)				Adjusted hazard ratio (HR) (95% CI)	Superiority *p*-value
	ALIMTA + Cisplatin		Gemcitabine + Cisplatin			
T population = 1725)	10.3 (9.8 – 11.2)	N = 862	10.3 (9.6 – 10.9)	N = 863	0.94[a] (0.84 – 1.05)	0.259
denocarcinoma = 847)	12.6 (10.7 – 13.6)	N = 436	10.9 (10.2 –11.9)	N = 411	0.84 (0.71–0.99)	0.033
ırge cell = 153)	10.4 (8.6 – 14.1)	N = 76	6.7 (5.5 – 9.0)	N = 77	0.67 (0.48–0.96)	0.027
ther = 252)	8.6 (6.8 – 10.2)	N = 106	9.2 (8.1 – 10.6)	N = 146	1.08 (0.81–1.45)	0.586
quamous cell = 473)	9.4 (8.4 – 10.2)	N = 244	10.8 (9.5 – 12.1)	N = 229	1.23 (1.00–1.51)	0.050

previations: CI = confidence interval; ITT = Intent-To-Treat; N = total population size.

tatistically significant for non-inferiority, with the entire confidence interval for HR well below the 1.17645 non-inferiority rgin ($p < 0.001$).

the Ames test. Pemetrexed has been shown to be clastogenic in the *in vivo* micronucleus test in the mouse.

Studies to assess the carcinogenic potential of pemetrexed have not been conducted.

6. PHARMACEUTICAL PARTICULARS

6.1 List of excipients

Mannitol

Hydrochloric acid

Sodium hydroxide

6.2 Incompatibilities

Pemetrexed is physically incompatible with diluents containing calcium, including lactated Ringer's injection and Ringer's injection. In the absence of other compatibility studies this medicinal product must not be mixed with other medicinal products.

6.3 Shelf life

Unopened vial: 2 years

Reconstituted and infusion solutions: When prepared as directed, reconstituted and infusion solutions of ALIMTA contain no antimicrobial preservatives. Chemical and physical in-use stability of reconstituted and infusion solutions of pemetrexed were demonstrated for 24 hours at refrigerated temperature or 25°C. From a microbiological point of view, the product should be used immediately. If not used immediately, in-use storage times and conditions prior to use are the responsibility of the user and would normally not be longer than 24 hours at 2°C to 8°C, unless reconstitution/dilution has taken place in controlled and validated aseptic conditions.

6.4 Special precautions for storage

Unopened vial: This medicinal product does not require any special storage conditions.

For storage conditions of the reconstituted medicinal product see section 6.3.

6.5 Nature and contents of container

Type I glass vial with rubber stopper containing 100 mg or 500 mg of pemetrexed.

Pack of 1 vial.

Not all pack sizes may be marketed.

6.6 Special precautions for disposal and other handling

1. Use aseptic technique during the reconstitution and further dilution of pemetrexed for intravenous infusion administration.

2. Calculate the dose and the number of ALIMTA vials needed. Each vial contains an excess of pemetrexed to facilitate delivery of label amount.

3. Reconstitute 100mg vials with 4.2 ml of sodium chloride 9 mg/ml (0.9%) solution for injection, without preservative, resulting in a solution containing 25 mg/ml pemetrexed. Gently swirl each vial until the powder is completely dissolved. The resulting solution is clear and ranges in colour from colourless to yellow or green-yellow without adversely affecting product quality. The pH of the reconstituted solution is between 6.6 and 7.8. **Further dilution is required**.

Reconstitute 500mg vials with 20ml of sodium chloride 9mg/ml (0.9%) solution for injection, without preservative, resulting in a solution containing 25 mg/ml pemetrexed. Gently swirl each vial until the powder is completely dissolved. The resulting solution is clear and ranges in colour from colourless to yellow or green-yellow without adversely affecting product quality. The pH of the reconstituted solution is between 6.6 and 7.8. **Further dilution is required**.

4. The appropriate volume of reconstituted pemetrexed solution must be further diluted to 100ml with sodium chloride 9mg/ml (0.9%) solution for injection, without preservative, and administered as an intravenous infusion over 10 minutes.

5. Pemetrexed infusion solutions prepared as directed above are compatible with polyvinyl chloride- and polyolefin- lined administration sets and infusion bags.

6. Parenteral medicinal products must be inspected visually for particulate matter and discolouration prior to administration. If particulate matter is observed, do not administer.

7. Pemetrexed solutions are for single use only. Any unused product or waste material must be disposed of in accordance with local requirements.

Preparation and administration precautions: As with other potentially toxic anti-cancer agents, care should be exercised in the handling and preparation of pemetrexed infusion solutions. The use of gloves is recommended. If a pemetrexed solution contacts the skin, wash the skin immediately and thoroughly with soap and water. If pemetrexed solutions contact the mucous membranes, flush thoroughly with water. Pemetrexed is not a vesicant. There is not a specific antidote for extravasation of pemetrexed. There have been few reported cases of pemetrexed extravasation, which were not assessed as serious by the investigator. Extravasation should be managed by local standard practice as with other non-vesicants.

7. MARKETING AUTHORISATION HOLDER

Eli Lilly Nederland BV, Grootslag 1-5, NL-3991 RA Houten, The Netherlands.

8. MARKETING AUTHORISATION NUMBER(S)

ALIMTA 500mg: EU/1/04/290/001

ALIMTA 100mg: EU/1/04/290/002

9. DATE OF FIRST AUTHORISATION/RENEWAL OF THE AUTHORISATION

Date of first authorisation: 20 September 2004

Date of latest renewal:

10. DATE OF REVISION OF THE TEXT

21 September 2009

Detailed information on this product is available on the website of the European Medicines Agency (EMEA) http://www.emea.europa.eu.

LEGAL CATEGORY

POM

*ALIMTA (pemetrexed) is a trademark of Eli Lilly and Company. AT11M

Alkeran Injection 50 mg

(GlaxoSmithKline UK)

1. NAME OF THE MEDICINAL PRODUCT

Alkeran 50 mg Injection

2. QUALITATIVE AND QUANTITATIVE COMPOSITION

Melphalan Hydrochloride BP equivalent to 50 mg mephalan per vial.

3. PHARMACEUTICAL FORM

Freeze-dried powder for injection.

4. CLINICAL PARTICULARS

4.1 Therapeutic indications

Alkeran Injection, at conventional intravenous dosage, is indicated in the treatment of multiple myeloma and ovarian cancer.

Alkeran Injection, at high intravenous dosage, is indicated, with or without haematopoietic stem cell transplantation, for the treatment of multiple myeloma and childhood neuroblastoma.

Alkeran Injection, administered by regional arterial perfusion, is indicated in the treatment of localised malignant melanoma of the extremities and localised soft tissue sarcoma of the extremities.

In the above indications, Alkeran may be used alone or in combination with other cytotoxic drugs.

4.2 Posology and method of administration

Parenteral administration:

Alkeran Injection is for intravenous use and regional arterial perfusion only. Alkeran Injection should not be given without haematopoietic stem cell rescue at doses of above 140 mg/m^2.

For intravenous administration, it is recommended that Alkeran Injection solution is injected slowly into a fast-running infusion solution via a swabbed injection port.

If direct injection into a fast-running infusion is not appropriate, Alkeran Injection solution may be administered diluted in an infusion bag.

Alkeran is not compatible with infusion solutions containing dextrose and it is recommended that only sodium chloride intravenous infusion 0.9% w/v is used.

When further diluted in an infusion solution, Alkeran has reduced stability and the rate of degradation increases rapidly with rise in temperature. If Alkeran is infused at a room temperature of approximately 25°C, the total time from preparation of the injection solution to the completion of infusion should not exceed 1.5 hours.

Should any visible turbidity or crystallisation appear in the reconstituted or diluted solutions, the preparation must be discarded.

Care should be taken to avoid possible extravasation of Alkeran and in cases of poor peripheral venous access, consideration should be given to use of a central venous line.

If high dose Alkeran Injection is administered with or without autologous bone marrow transplantation, administration via a central venous line is recommended.

For regional arterial perfusion, the literature should be consulted for detailed methodology.

Multiple myeloma: Alkeran Injection is administered on an intermittent basis alone, or in combination with other cytotoxic drugs. Administration of prednisone has also been included in a number of regimens.

When used as a single agent, a typical intravenous Alkeran dosage schedule is 0.4 mg/kg body weight (16 mg/m^2 body surface area) repeated at appropriate intervals (e.g. once every 4 weeks), provided there has been recovery of the peripheral blood count during this period.

High-dose regimens generally employ single intravenous doses of between 100 and 200 mg/m^2 body surface area (approximately 2.5 to 5.0 mg/kg body weight), but haematopoietic stem cell rescue becomes essential following doses in excess of 140 mg/m^2 body surface area. Hydration and forced diuresis are also recommended.

Ovarian adenocarcinoma: When used intravenously as single agent, a dose of 1 mg/kg body weight (approx mately 40 mg/m^2 body surface area) given at intervals of weeks has often been used.

When combined with other cytotoxic drugs, intravenou doses of between 0.3 and 0.4 mg/kg body weight (12 t 16 mg/m^2 body surface area) have been used at intervals c 4 to 6 weeks.

Advanced neuroblastoma: Doses of between 100 an 240 mg/m^2 body surface area (sometimes divided equall over 3 consecutive days) together with haematopoieti stem cell rescue, have been used either alone or in com bination with radiotherapy and/or other cytotoxic drugs.

Malignant melanoma: Hyperthermic regional perfusio with Alkeran has been used as an adjuvant to surgery fo early malignant melanoma and as palliative treatment fo advanced but localised disease. The scientific literatur should be consulted for details of perfusion technique an dosage used. A typical dose range for upper extremit perfusions is 0.6-1.0 mg/kg bodyweight and for lowe extremity perfusions is 0.8-1.5 mg/kg body weight.

Soft tissue sarcoma: Hyperthermic regional perfusion wit Alkeran has been used in the management of all stages o localised soft tissue sarcoma, usually in combination wit surgery. A typical dose range for upper extremity perfu sions is 0.6-1.0 mg/kg body weight and for lower extremit perfusions is 1-1.4 mg/kg body weight.

Use in Children

Alkeran, at conventional dosage, is only rarely indicated ir children and dosage guidelines cannot be stated.

High dose Alkeran Injection, in association with haematopoietic stem cell rescue, has been used in childhoo neuroblastoma and dosage guidelines based on body surface area, as for adults, may be used.

Use in the elderly

Although Alkeran is frequently used at conventional dosage in the elderly, there is no specific information available relating to its administration to this patient subgroup.

Experience in the use of high dose Alkeran in elderly patients is limited. Consideration should therefore be given to ensure adequate performance status and organ function, before using high dose Alkeran Injection in elderly patients.

Dosage in renal impairment

Alkeran clearance, though variable, may be decreased in renal impairment.

Currently available pharmacokinetic data do not justify an absolute recommendation on dosage reduction when administering Alkeran Tablets to patients with renal impairment, but it may be prudent to use a reduced dosage initially until tolerance is established.

When Alkeran Injection is used at conventional intravenous dosage (16-40 mg/m^2 body surface area), it is recommended that the initial dose should be reduced by 50% and subsequent dosage determined according to the degree of haematological suppression.

For high intravenous doses of Alkeran (100 to 240 mg/m^2 body surface area), the need for dose reduction depends upon the degree of renal impairment, whether haematopoietic stem cells are re-infused, and therapeutic need. Alkeran Injection should not be given without haematopoietic stem cell rescue at doses of above 140 mg/m^2.

As a guide, for high dose Alkeran treatment without haematopoietic stem cell rescue in patients with moderate renal impairment (creatinine clearance 30 to 50 ml/min) a dose reduction of 50% is usual. High dose Alkeran (above 140 mg/m^2) without haematopoietic stem cell rescue should not be used in patients with more severe renal impairment.

High dose Alkeran with haematopoietic stem cell rescue has been used successfully even in dialysis dependent patients with end-stage renal failure. The relevant literature should be consulted for details.

4.3 Contraindications

Alkeran should not be given to patients who have suffered a previous hypersensitivity reaction to melphalan.

4.4 Special warnings and precautions for use

Alkeran is a cytotoxic drug, which falls into the general class of alkylating agents. It should be prescribed only by physicians experienced in the management of malignant disease with such agents. As with all high dose chemotherapy, precautions should be taken to prevent tumour lysis syndrome.

Immunisation using a live organism vaccine has the potential to cause infection in immunocompromised hosts. Therefore, immunisations with live organism vaccines are not recommended.

Since Alkeran is myelosuppressive, frequent blood counts are essential during therapy and the dosage should be delayed or adjusted if necessary.

Alkeran Injection solution can cause local tissue damage, should extravasation occur and consequently, it should not be administered by direct injection into a peripheral vein. It is recommended that Alkeran Injection solution is administered by injecting slowly into a fast-running intravenous infusion via a swabbed injection port, or via a central venous line.

view of the hazards involved and the level of supportive are required, the administration of high dose Alkeran jection should be confined to specialist centres, with e appropriate facilities and only be conducted by experinced clinicians.

patients receiving high dose Alkeran Injection, considration should be given to the prophylactic administration f anti-infective agents and the administration of blood roducts as required.

onsideration should be given to ensure adequate perforance status and organ function before using high dose lkeran Injection. Alkeran Injection should not be given ithout haematopoietic stem cell rescue at doses of above 40 mg/m^2.

s with all cytotoxic chemotherapy, adequate contracepve precautions should be practised when either partner is eceiving Alkeran.

afe handling of Alkeran

he handling of Alkeran formulations should follow guidenes for the handling of cytotoxic drugs according to the oyal Pharmaceutical Society of Great Britain Working arty on the handling of cytotoxic drugs.

Monitoring

ince Alkeran is a potent myelosuppressive agent, it is ssential that careful attention should be paid to the monoring of blood counts, to avoid the possibility of excessive nyelosuppression and the risk of irreversible bone marrow plasia. Blood counts may continue to fall after treatment is topped, so at the first sign of an abnormally large fall in eukocyte or platelet counts, treatment should be temporaily interrupted. Alkeran should be used with caution in atients who have undergone recent radiotherapy or chenotherapy in view of increased bone marrow toxicity.

Renal Impairment

lkeran clearance may be reduced in patients with renal npairment who may also have uraemic marrow suppresion. Dose reduction may therefore be necessary (see Posology and Method of Administration). See Undesirable Effects for elevation of blood urea.

Mutagenicity

Melphalan is mutagenic in animals and chromosome aberations have been observed in patients being treated with he drug.

Carcinogenicity

Melphalan, in common with other alkylating agents, has been reported to be leukaemogenic. There have been reports of acute leukaemia occurring after melphalan treatment for diseases such as amyloid, malignant melanoma, multiple myeloma, macroglobulinaemia, cold agglutinin syndrome and ovarian cancer.

A comparison of patients with ovarian cancer who received alkylating agents with those who did not, showed that the use of alkylating agents, including melphalan, significantly increased the incidence of acute leukaemia.

The leukaemogenic risk must be balanced against the potential therapeutic benefit when considering the use of melphalan.

Effects on Fertility

Alkeran causes suppression of ovarian function in premenopausal women resulting in amenorrhoea in a significant number of patients.

There is evidence from some animal studies that Alkeran can have an adverse effect on spermatogenesis. Therefore, it is possible that Alkeran may cause temporary or permanent sterility in male patients.

The label for the product will contain the following statements:

Keep out of the reach of children.

Store below 30° C

Do not refrigerate.

Protect from light

4.5 Interaction with other medicinal products and other forms of interaction

Vaccinations with live organism vaccines are not recommended in immunocompromised individuals (see Warnings and Precautions).

Nalidixic acid together with high-dose intravenous melphalan has caused deaths in children due to haemorrhagic entercolitis.

Impaired renal function has been described in bone marrow transplant patients who received high dose intravenous melphalan and who subsequently received ciclosporin to prevent graft-versus-host disease.

4.6 Pregnancy and lactation

The teratogenic potential of Alkeran has not been studied. In view of its mutagenic properties and structural similarity to known teratogenic compounds, it is possible that melphalan could cause congenital defects in the offspring of patients treated with the drug.

The use of melphalan should be avoided whenever possible during pregnancy, particularly during the first trimester. In any individual case, the potential hazard to the foetus must be balanced against the expected benefit to the mother.

Mothers receiving Alkeran should not breastfeed.

4.7 Effects on ability to drive and use machines

None known.

4.8 Undesirable effects

For this product there is no modern clinical documentation which can be used as support for determining the frequency of undesirable effects. Undesirable effects may vary in their incidence depending on the indication and dose received and also when given in combination with other therapeutic agents.

The following convention has been utilised for the classification of frequency:- Very common $\geq$1/10, common $\geq$1/100, $<$1/10, uncommon $\geq$1/1000 and $<$1/100, rare $\geq$1/10,000 and $<$1/1000, very rare $<$1/10,000.

Blood and Lymphatic System Disorders

Very common: bone marrow depression leading to leucopenia, thrombocytopenia and anaemia

Rare: haemolytic anaemia

Immune System Disorders

Rare: allergic reactions (see Skin and Subcutaneous Tissue Disorders)

Allergic reactions to melphalan such as urticaria, oedema, skin rashes and anaphylactic shock have been reported uncommonly following initial or subsequent dosing, particularly after intravenous administration. Cardiac arrest has also been reported rarely in association with such events.

Respiratory, Thoracic and Mediastinal Disorders

Rare: interstitial pneumonitis and pulmonary fibrosis (including fatal reports)

Gastrointestinal Disorders

Very common: nausea, vomiting and diarrhoea; stomatitis at high dose

Rare: stomatitis at conventional dose

The incidence of diarrhoea, vomiting and stomatitis becomes the dose-limiting toxicity in patients given high intravenous doses of melphalan in association with autologous bone marrow transplantation. Cyclophosphamide pretreatment appears to reduce the severity of gastrointestinal damage induced by high-dose melphalan and the literature should be consulted for details.

Hepatobiliary Disorders

Rare: hepatic disorders ranging from abnormal liver function tests to clinical manifestations such as hepatitis and jaundice; veno-occlusive disease following high dose treatment

Skin and Subcutaneous Tissue Disorders

Very common: alopecia at high dose

Common: alopecia at conventional dose

Rare: maculopapular rashes and pruritus (see Immune System Disorders)

Musculoskeletal and Connective Tissue Disorders

Injection, following isolated limb perfusion:

Very common: muscle atrophy, muscle fibrosis, myalgia, blood creatine phosphokinase increased.

Common: compartment syndrome

Not known: muscle necrosis, rhabdomyolysis

Renal and Urinary Disorders

Common: temporary significant elevation of the blood urea has been seen in the early stages of melphalan therapy in myeloma patients with renal damage

General Disorders and Administration Site Conditions

Very common: subjective and transient sensation of warmth and/or tingling

4.9 Overdose

Gastro-intestinal effects, including nausea, vomiting and diarrhoea are the most likely signs of acute oral overdosage. The immediate effects of acute intravenous overdosage are nausea and vomiting. Damage to the gastrointestinal mucosa may also ensue and diarrhoea, sometimes haemorrhagic, has been reported after overdosage. The principal toxic effect is bone marrow suppression, leading to leucopenia, thrombocytopenia and anaemia.

General supportive measures, together with appropriate blood and platelet transfusions, should be instituted if necessary and consideration given to hospitalisation, antibiotic cover, the use of haematological growth factors.

There is no specific antidote. The blood picture should be closely monitored for at least four weeks following overdosage until there is evidence of recovery.

5. PHARMACOLOGICAL PROPERTIES

5.1 Pharmacodynamic properties

Melphalan is a bifunctional alkylating agent. Formation of carbonium intermediates from each of the two bis-2-chloroethyl groups enables alkylation through covalent binding with the 7-nitrogen of guanine on DNA, cross-linking the two DNA strands and thereby preventing cell replication.

5.2 Pharmacokinetic properties

Absorption

The absorption of oral melphalan is highly variable with respect to both the time to first appearance of the drug in plasma and peak plasma concentration.

In studies of the absolute bioavailability of melphalan the mean absolute bioavailability ranged from 56 to 85%.

Intravenous administration can be used to avoid variability in absorption associated with myeloablative treatment.

Distribution

Melphalan is moderately bound to plasma proteins with reported percent binding ranging from 69% to 78%. There is evidence that the protein binding is linear in the range of plasma concentrations usually achieved in standard dose therapy, but that the binding may become concentration-dependent at the concentrations observed in high-dose therapy. Serum albumin is the major binding protein, accounting for about 55 to 60% the binding, and 20% is bound to α_1-acid glycoprotein. In addition, melphalan binding studies have revealed the existence of an irreversible component attributable to the alkylation reaction with plasma proteins.

Following administration of a two-minute infusion of doses ranging from 5 to 23 mg/m^2 body surface area (approximately 0.1 to 0.6 mg/kg bodyweight) to 10 patients with ovarian cancer or multiple myeloma, the mean volumes of distribution at steady state and central compartment were 29.1 ± 13.6 litres and 12.2 ± 6.5 litres, respectively.

In 28 patients with various malignancies who were given doses of between 70 and 200 mg/m^2 body surface area as a 2- to 20-min infusion, the mean volumes of distribution at steady state and central compartment were, respectively, 40.2 ± 18.3 litres and 18.2 ± 11.7 litres.

Melphalan displays limited penetration of the blood-brain barrier. Several investigators have sampled cerebrospinal fluid and found no measurable drug. Low concentrations (~10% of that in plasma) were observed in a single high-dose study in children.

Metabolism

In vivo and *in vitro* data suggest that spontaneous degradation rather than enzymatic metabolism is the major determinant of the drug's half-life in man.

Elimination

In 13 patients given oral melphalan at 0.6 mg/kg bodyweight, the plasma mean terminal elimination half-life was 90 ± 57 min with 11% of the drug being recovered in the urine over 24 h.

In 8 patients given a single bolus dose of 0.5 to 0.6 mg/kg bodyweight, the composite initial and terminal half-lives were reported to be 7.7 ± 3.3 min and 108 ± 20.8 min, respectively. Following injection of melphalan, monohydroxymelphalan and dihydroxymelphalan were detected in the patients' plasma, reaching peak levels at approximately 60 min and 105 min, respectively. A similar half-life of 126 ± 6 min was seen when melphalan was added to the patients' serum *in vitro* (37°C), suggesting that spontaneous degradation rather than enzymic metabolism may be the major determinant of the drug's half-life in man.

Following administration of a two-minute infusion of doses ranging from 5 to 23 mg/m^2 body surface area (approximately 0.1 to 0.6 mg/kg bodyweight) to 10 patients with ovarian cancer or multiple myeloma, the pooled initial and terminal half-lives were, respectively, 8.1 ± 6.6 min and 76.9 ± 40.7 min. A mean clearance of 342.7 ± 96.8 ml/min was recorded.

In 15 children and 11 adults given high-dose i.v. melphalan (140 mg/m^2 body surface area) with forced diuresis, the mean initial and terminal half-lives were found to be 6.5 ± 3.6 min and 41.4 ± 16.5 min, respectively. Mean initial and terminal half-lives of 8.8 ± 6.6 min and 73.1 ± 45.9 min, respectively, were recorded in 28 patients with various malignancies who were given doses of between 70 and 200 mg/m^2 body surface area as a 2- to 20-min infusion. The mean clearance was 564.6 159.1 ml/min.

Following hyperthermic (39°C) perfusion of the lower limb with 1.75 mg/kg bodyweight, mean initial and terminal half-lives of 3.6 ± 1.5 min and 46.5 ± 17.2 min, respectively, were recorded in 11 patients with advanced malignant melanoma. A mean clearance of 55.0 ± 9.4 ml/min was recorded.

Special Patient Populations

- **Renal impairment**

Melphalan clearance may be decreased in renal impairment *(see Dosage and Administration - Renal impairment and Warnings and Precautions - Renal impairment)*.

- **Elderly**

No correlation has been shown between age and melphalan clearance or with melphalan terminal elimination half-life *(see Dosage and Administration)*.

5.3 Preclinical safety data

There are no pre-clinical data of relevance to the prescriber which are additional to that already included in other sections of the SmPC.

6. PHARMACEUTICAL PARTICULARS

6.1 List of excipients

Hydrochloric Acid Ph.Eur.

Povidone K12 Ph.Eur.

Water for Injections BP

6.2 Incompatibilities

None known.

6.3 Shelf life

36 months.

6.4 Special precautions for storage
Store below 30° C

Protect from light

Do not refrigerate.

6.5 Nature and contents of container
Clear, neutral glass vial and bromobutyl rubber stopper with an aluminium collar.

Pack size: 50 mg

6.6 Special precautions for disposal and other handling
Preparation of Alkeran Injection Solution:

Alkeran Injection should be prepared at room temperature, by reconstituting the freeze-dried powder with the solvent-diluent provided. 10 ml of this vehicle should be added, as a single quantity, and the vial immediately shaken vigorously until solution is complete. The resulting solution contains the equivalent of 5 mg per ml anhydrous melphalan and has a pH of approximately 6.5.

Alkeran Injection solution has limited stability and should be prepared immediately before use. Any unused solution should be discarded according to standard guidelines for handling and disposal of cytotoxic drugs.

The reconstituted solution should not be refrigerated as this will cause precipitation.

7. MARKETING AUTHORISATION HOLDER
The Wellcome Foundation Limited

Greenford

Middlesex

UB6 0NN

trading as:

GlaxoSmithKline UK

Stockley Park West

Uxbridge

Middlesex

UB11 1BT

8. MARKETING AUTHORISATION NUMBER(S)
PL 00003/0323

9. DATE OF FIRST AUTHORISATION/RENEWAL OF THE AUTHORISATION
19 January 1999

10. DATE OF REVISION OF THE TEXT
30 October 2007

11 LEGAL STATUS
POM

Alkeran Injection Diluent

(GlaxoSmithKline UK)

1. NAME OF THE MEDICINAL PRODUCT
SOLVENT-DILUENT (for Alkeran Injection)

2. QUALITATIVE AND QUANTITATIVE COMPOSITION
No active ingredient present

3. PHARMACEUTICAL FORM
Liquid for reconstitution of Alkeran

4. CLINICAL PARTICULARS
4.1 Therapeutic indications
The Solvent-Diluent is used to reconstitute Alkeran Injection.

4.2 Posology and method of administration
The reconstituted injection is administered by infusion.

4.3 Contraindications
Not Applicable.

4.4 Special warnings and precautions for use
Not Applicable.

The label for this product will contain the following statements:

Keep out of the reach of children.

Store below 30° C

Do not refrigerate.

Protect from light

4.5 Interaction with other medicinal products and other forms of interaction
Not Applicable.

4.6 Pregnancy and lactation
Not Applicable.

4.7 Effects on ability to drive and use machines
Not Applicable.

4.8 Undesirable effects
Not Applicable.

4.9 Overdose
Not Applicable.

5. PHARMACOLOGICAL PROPERTIES
5.1 Pharmacodynamic properties
Not Applicable.

5.2 Pharmacokinetic properties
Not Applicable.

5.3 Preclinical safety data
Not Applicable.

6. PHARMACEUTICAL PARTICULARS
6.1 List of excipients

Excipient	Specification
Sodium citrate	Ph.Eur
Propylene glycol	Ph.Eur
Ethanol (96%)	BP
Water for injections	Ph.Eur

6.2 Incompatibilities
Not Applicable.

6.3 Shelf life
36 months

6.4 Special precautions for storage
Store below 30° C, protect from light, do not refrigerate.

6.5 Nature and contents of container
Clear neutral glass vial and chlorobutyl rubber stopper or fluoro-resin butyl rubber stopper with aluminium collar.

Pack size: 10 ml

6.6 Special precautions for disposal and other handling
Not Applicable.

Administrative Data
7. MARKETING AUTHORISATION HOLDER
The Wellcome Foundation Ltd

Greenford

Middlesex UB6 0NN

trading as:

GlaxoSmithKline UK

Stockley Park West

Uxbridge

Middlesex UB11 1BT

8. MARKETING AUTHORISATION NUMBER(S)
PL 00003/0324

9. DATE OF FIRST AUTHORISATION/RENEWAL OF THE AUTHORISATION
19 January 2005

10. DATE OF REVISION OF THE TEXT
08 July 2003

11. Legal Status
POM

Alkeran Tablets 2mg

(GlaxoSmithKline UK)

1. NAME OF THE MEDICINAL PRODUCT
Alkeran 2 mg Tablets

2. QUALITATIVE AND QUANTITATIVE COMPOSITION
Each tablet contains 2 mg melphalan.

3. PHARMACEUTICAL FORM
Film-coated tablets

ALKERAN are white to off-white film-coated, round, biconvex tablets engraved "GX EH3" on one side and "A" on the other.

4. CLINICAL PARTICULARS
4.1 Therapeutic indications
Alkeran Tablets are indicated in the treatment of multiple myeloma and advanced ovarian adenocarcinoma.

Alkeran either alone or in combination with other drugs has a significant therapeutic effect in a proportion of patients suffering from advanced breast carcinoma.

Alkeran is effective in the treatment of a proportion of patients suffering from polycythaemia vera.

4.2 Posology and method of administration
Since Alkeran is myelosuppressive, frequent blood counts are essential during therapy and the dosage should be delayed or adjusted if necessary (see *Special Warnings and Precautions for Use*).

Oral administration in Adults: The absorption of Alkeran after oral administration is variable. Dosage may need to be cautiously increased until myelosuppresion is seen, in order to ensure that potentially therapeutic levels have been reached.

Multiple Myleloma:

Numerous regimes have been used and the scientific literature should be consulted for details. The administration of Alkeran and prednisone is more effective than Alkeran alone. The combination is usually given on an intermittent basis, although the superiority of this technique over continuous therapy is not established. A typical oral dosage schedule is 0.15 mg/kg bodyweight/day in divided doses for 4 days repeated at intervals of six weeks. Prolonging treatment beyond one year in responders does not appear to improve results.

Ovarian adenocarcinoma:

A typical regimen is 0.2 mg/kg bodyweight/day orally for days. This is repeated every 4-8 weeks, or as soon as th bone marrow has recovered. Alkeran has also been us intravenously in the treatment of ovarian carcinoma.

Advanced carcinoma of the breast:

Alkeran has been given orally at a dose of 0.15 mg/k bodyweight or 6 mg/m^2 body surface area/day for 5 day and repeated every 6 weeks. The dose was decreased bone marrow toxicity was observed.

Polycythaemia vera:

For remission induction the usual dose is 6-10 mg daily f 5-7 days, after which 2-4 mg daily is given until satisfacto disease control is achieved. Therapy is maintained with dose of 2-6 mg per week. During maintenance therapy careful haematological control is essential with dosag adjustment according to the results of frequent bloo counts.

Children:

Alkeran is very rarely indicated in children and dosag guidelines cannot be stated.

Use in the elderly:

There is no specific information available on the use c Alkeran in elderly patients.

Dosage in renal impairment:

In patients with moderate to severe renal impairment cu rently available pharmacokinetic data do not justify a absolute recommendation on dosage reduction whe administering the oral preparation to these patients, b it may be prudent to use a reduced dose initially.

4.3 Contraindications
Alkeran should not be given to patients who have suffere a previous hypersensitivity reaction to melphalan.

4.4 Special warnings and precautions for use
Alkeran is an active cytotoxic agent for use only under th direction of physicians experienced in the administration such agents.

Immunisation using a live organism vaccine has the pote tial to cause infection in immunocompromised host Therefore, immunisations with live organism vaccines a not recommended.

Safe Handling of ALKERAN tablets:

See 6.6 Instructions for use/handling

Monitoring:

Since Alkeran is a potent myelosuppresive agent, it essential that careful attention should be paid to the mo itoring of blood counts to avoid the possibility of excessiv myelosuppression and the risk of irreversible bone marro aplasia. Blood counts may continue to fall after treatment stopped, so at the first sign of an abnormally large fall leucocyte or platelet counts, treatment should be tempora rily interrupted. Alkeran should be used with caution patients who have undergone recent radiotherapy or ch motherapy in view of increased bone marrow toxicity.

Renal impairment:

Patients with renal impairment should be closely observe as they may have uraemic marrow suppression. (S undesirable effects for elevation of blood urea Section 4.

Mutagenicity:

Alkeran is mutagenic in animals and chromosome aberr tions have been observed in patients being treated with th drug.

Carcinogenicity:

The evidence is growing that melphalan in common wi other alkylating agents has been reported to be leukaem genic. There have been reports of acute leukaemia occu ring after melphalan treatment for diseases such amyloid, malignant melanoma, macroglobulinaemia, co agglutinin syndrome and ovarian cancer.

A comparison of patients with ovarian cancer who receive alkylating agents with those who did not, showed that th use of alkylating agents, including melphalan, significan increased the incidence of acute leukaemia. The leuka mogenic risk must be balanced against the potential the apeutic benefit when considering the use of melphalan.

Alkeran causes suppression of ovarian function in prem nopausal women resulting in amenorrhoea in a significa number of patients.

4.5 Interaction with other medicinal products and oth forms of interaction
Vaccinations with live organism vaccines are not recor mended in immunocompromised individuals (see War ings and Precautions).

Nalidixic acid together with high-dose intravenous melph lan has caused deaths in children due to haemorrhag enterocolitis.

Impaired renal function has been described in bone ma row transplant patients who were pre-conditioned w high dose intravenous melphalan and who subsequen received ciclosporin to prevent graft-versus-host diseas

4.6 Pregnancy and lactation
As with all cytotoxic chemotherapy, adequate contrace tive precautions should be advised when either partner receiving Alkeran.

eratogenicity:

he teratogenic potential of Alkeran has not been studied. n view of its mutagenic properties and structural similarity o known teratogenic compounds, it is possible that melhalan could cause congenital defects in the offspring of atients treated with the drug.

regnancy:

he use of melphalan should be avoided whenever possile during pregnancy, particularly during the first trimester. n any individual case the potential hazard to the foetus nust be balanced against the expected benefit to the nother.

actation:

lother receiving Alkeran should not breast-feed.

.7 Effects on ability to drive and use machines

lot known.

.8 Undesirable effects

or this product there is no modern clinical documentation which can be used as support for determining the frequency of undesirable effects. Undesirable effects may vary in their incidence depending on the indication and lose received and also when given in combination with other therapeutic agents.

The following convention has been utilised for the classiication of frequency:- Very common ⩾1/10, common ⩾1/ 00, <1/10, uncommon ⩾1/1000 and <1/100, rare ⩾1/ 0,000 and <1/1000, very rare <1/10,000.

Blood and Lymphatic System Disorders

Very common: bone marrow depression leading to leucoenia, thrombocytopenia and anaemia

Rare: haemolytic anaemia

mmune System Disorders

Rare: allergic reactions (see Skin and Subcutaneous Tissue Disorders)

Allergic reactions to melphalan such as urticaria, oedema, skin rashes and anaphylactic shock have been reported uncommonly following initial or subsequent dosing, particularly after intravenous administration. Cardiac arrest has also been reported rarely in association with such events.

Respiratory, Thoracic and Mediastinal Disorders

Rare: interstitial pneumonitis and pulmonary fibrosis (including fatal reports)

Gastrointestinal Disorders

Very common: nausea, vomiting and diarrhoea; stomatitis at high dose

Rare: stomatitis at conventional dose

Gastrointestinal effects such as nausea and vomiting have been reported in up to 30% of patients receiving conventional oral doses of melphalan.

Hepatobiliary Disorders

Rare: hepatic disorders ranging from abnormal liver function tests to clinical manifestations such as hepatitis and jaundice

Skin and Subcutaneous Tissue Disorders

Very common: alopecia at high dose

Common: alopecia at conventional dose

Rare: maculopapular rashes and pruritus (see Immune System Disorders)

Renal and Urinary Disorders

Common: temporary significant elevation of the blood urea has been seen in the early stages of melphalan therapy in myeloma patients with renal damage

4.9 Overdose

Symptoms and signs:

Gastro-intestinal effects, including nausea, vomiting and diarrhoea are the most likely signs of acute oral overdosage. Diarrhoea, sometimes haemorrhagic, has been reported after intravenous overdosage. The principal toxic effect is bone marrow aplasia, leading to leucopoenia, thrombocytopenia and anaemia.

Treatment:

There is no specific antidote. The blood picture should be closely monitored for at least four weeks following overdosage until there is evidence of recovery.

General supportive measures, together with appropriate blood transfusion, should be instituted if necessary.

5. PHARMACOLOGICAL PROPERTIES

5.1 Pharmacodynamic properties

Melphalan is a bifunctional alkylating agent. Formation of carbonium intermediates from each of the two bis-2-chlorethyl groups enables alkylation through covalent binding with the 7-nitrogen of guanine on DNA, cross-linking two DNA strands and thereby preventing cell replication.

5.2 Pharmacokinetic properties

Absorption

The absorption of oral melphalan is highly variable with respect to both the time to first appearance of the drug in plasma and peak plasma concentration.

In studies of the absolute bioavailability of melphalan the mean absolute bioavailability ranged from 56 to 85%.

Intravenous administration can be used to avoid variability in absorption associated with myeloablative treatment.

In a study of 18 patients administered melphalan 0.2 to 0.25 mg/kg bodyweight orally, a maximum plasma concentration (range 87 to 350 nanograms/ml) was reached within 0.5 to 2.0 h.

The administration of melphalan tablets immediately after food delayed the time to achieving peak plasma concentrations and reduced the area under the plasma concentration-time curves by between 39 and 45%.

Distribution

Melphalan displays limited penetration of the blood-brain barrier. Several investigators have sampled cerebrospinal fluid and found no measurable drug. Low concentrations (~10% of that in plasma) were observed in a single high-dose study in children.

Elimination

In 13 patients given oral melphalan at 0.6 mg/kg bodyweight, the plasma mean terminal elimination half-life was 90 57 min with 11% of the drug being recovered in the urine over 24 h.

In 18 patients administered melphalan 0.2 to 0.25 mg/kg bodyweight orally, the mean elimination half-life was 1.12 0.15 h.

Special Patient Populations

Renal impairment

Melphalan clearance may be decreased in renal impairment *(see Dosage and Administration - Renal impairment and Warnings and Precautions - Renal impairment).*

Elderly

No correlation has been shown between age and melphalan clearance or with melphalan terminal elimination half-life *(see Dosage and Administration).*

5.3 Preclinical safety data

There are no preclinical data of relevance to the prescriber, which are additional to that in other sections of the SmPC.

6. PHARMACEUTICAL PARTICULARS

6.1 List of excipients

Tablet Core:

Microcrystalline cellulose

Crospovidone

Colloidal anhydrous silica

Magnesium stearate

Tablet Film Coating:

Hypromellose

Titanium dioxide

Macrogol

6.2 Incompatibilities

None known

6.3 Shelf life

24 months

6.4 Special precautions for storage

Store at 2°C to 8°C.

6.5 Nature and contents of container

Supplied in amber glass bottles with a child resistant closure containing 25 or 50 tablets.

6.6 Special precautions for disposal and other handling

Safe handling of ALKERAN tablets:

The handling of Alkeran tablets should follow guidelines for the handling of cytotoxic drugs according to prevailing local recommendations and/or regulations (for example Royal Pharmaceutical Society of Great Britain Working Party on the Handling of Cytotoxic Drugs).

Provided the outer coating of the tablet is intact, there is no risk in handling Alkeran tablets.

Alkeran tablets should not be divided.

Disposal:

Alkeran tablets should be destroyed in accordance with relevant local regulatory requirements concerning the disposal of cytotoxic drugs.

7. MARKETING AUTHORISATION HOLDER

The Wellcome Foundation Limited

Glaxo Wellcome House

Berkeley Avenue

Greenford

Middlesex, UB6 ONN

Trading as

GlaxoSmithKline UK

Stockley Park West

Uxbridge

Middlesex, UB11 1BT

8. MARKETING AUTHORISATION NUMBER(S)

PL 00003/5008R

9. DATE OF FIRST AUTHORISATION/RENEWAL OF THE AUTHORISATION

11 November 2002

10. DATE OF REVISION OF THE TEXT

9 July 2007

11 LEGAL STATUS

POM

ALLEGRON

(King Pharmaceuticals Ltd)

1. NAME OF THE MEDICINAL PRODUCT

ALLEGRON TABLETS

2. QUALITATIVE AND QUANTITATIVE COMPOSITION

Tablets containing Nortriptyline Hydrochloride EP equivalent to 10mg nortriptyline base tablets are white, unscored and have a diameter of 5.5mm. Marked 'KING'.

Tablets containing Nortriptyline Hydrochloride EP equivalent to 25mg nortriptyline base tablets are orange, scored and have a diameter of 8mm. Marked 'KING'.

3. PHARMACEUTICAL FORM

Tablet

4. CLINICAL PARTICULARS

4.1 Therapeutic indications

Allegron is indicated for the relief of symptoms of depression. It may also be used for the treatment of some cases of nocturnal enuresis.

4.2 Posology and method of administration

For oral administration.

Adults: The usual adult dose is 25mg three or four times daily. Dosage should begin at a low level and be increased as required. Alternatively, the total daily dose may be given once a day. When doses above 100mg daily are administered, plasma levels of nortriptyline should be monitored and maintained in the optimum range of 50 to 150ng/ml. Doses above 150mg per day are not recommended.

Lower than usual dosages are recommended for elderly patients and adolescents. Lower dosages are also recommended for outpatients than for hospitalised patients who will be under close supervision. The physician should initiate dosage at a low level and increase it gradually, noting carefully the clinical response and any evidence of intolerance. Following remission, maintenance medication may be required for a longer period of time at the lowest dose that will maintain remission.

If a patient develops minor side-effects, the dosage should be reduced. The drug should be discontinued promptly if adverse effects of a serious nature or allergic manifestations occur.

The elderly: 30 to 50mg/day in divided doses.

Adolescent patients: 30 to 50mg/day in divided doses.

Plasma levels: Optimal responses to nortriptyline have been associated with plasma concentrations of 50 to 150ng/ml. Higher concentrations may be associated with more adverse experiences. Plasma concentrations are difficult to measure, and physicians should consult the laboratory professional staff.

Many antidepressants (tricyclic antidepressants, including nortriptyline, selective serotonin re-uptake inhibitors and others) are metabolised by the hepatic cytochrome P450 isoenzyme P450IID6. Three to ten per cent of the population have reduced isoenzyme activity ('poor metabolisers') and may have higher than expected plasma concentrations at usual doses. The percentage of 'poor metabolisers' in a population is also affected by its ethnic origin.

Older patients have been reported to have higher plasma concentrations of the active nortriptyline metabolite 10-hydroxynortriptyline. In one case, this was associated with apparent cardiotoxicity, despite the fact that nortriptyline concentrations were within the 'therapeutic range'. Clinical findings should predominate over plasma concentrations as primary determinants of dosage changes.

Children: (for nocturnal enuresis only).

Age (years)	Weight		Dose (mg)
	kg	lb	
6-7	20-25	44-55	10
8-11	25-35	55-77	10-20
>11	35-54	77-119	25-35

The dose should be administered thirty minutes before bedtime.

The maximum period of treatment should not exceed three months. A further course of treatment should not be started until a full physical examination, including an ECG, has been made.

4.3 Contraindications

Hypersensitivity to nortriptyline.

Recent myocardial infarction, any degree of heart block or other cardiac arrhythmias.

Severe liver disease.

Mania.

Nortriptyline is contra-indicated for the nursing mother and for children under the age of six years.

Please also refer to 'Drug interactions' section.

4.4 Special warnings and precautions for use

Warnings: As improvement may not occur during the initial weeks of therapy, patients, especially those posing a high suicidal risk, should be closely monitored during this period.

Suicide/suicidal thoughts or clinical worsening. Depression is associated with an increased risk of suicidal thoughts, self harm and suicide (suicide-related events). This risk persists until significant remission occurs. As improvement may not occur during the first few weeks or more of treatment, patients should be closely monitored until such improvement occurs. It is general clinical experience that the risk of suicide may increase in the early stages of recovery

Patients with a history of suicide-related events, or this exhibiting a significant degree of suicidal ideation prior to commencement of treatment are known to be at greater risk of suicidal thoughts or suicide attempts, and should receive careful monitoring during treatment. A meta-analysis of placebo-controlled clinical trials of antidepressant drugs in adult patients with psychiatric disorders showed an increased risk of suicidal behaviour with antidepressants compared to placebo in patients less tan 25 years old.

Close supervision of patients and in particular those at high risk should accompany drug therapy in early treatment and following dose changes. Patients (an caregivers of patients) should be alerted about the need to monitor for any clinical worsening, suicidal behaviour or thoughts and unusual changes in behaviour and to seek medical advice immediately if these symptoms present.

Withdrawal symptoms, including insomnia, irritability and excessive perspiration, may occur on abrupt cessation of therapy.

The use of nortriptyline in schizophrenic patients may result in an exacerbation of the psychosis or may activate latent schizophrenic symptoms. If administered to overactive or agitated patients, increased anxiety and agitation may occur. In manic-depressive patients, nortriptyline may cause symptoms of the manic phase to emerge.

Cross sensitivity between nortriptyline and other tricyclic antidepressants is a possibility.

Patients with cardiovascular disease should be given nortriptyline only under close supervision because of the tendency of the drug to produce sinus tachycardia and to prolong the conduction time. Myocardial infarction, arrhythmia and strokes have occurred. Great care is necessary if nortriptyline is administered to hyperthyroid patients or to those receiving thyroid medication, since cardiac arrhythmias may develop.

The use of nortriptyline should be avoided, if possible, in patients with a history of epilepsy. If it is used, however, the patients should be observed carefully at the beginning of treatment, for nortriptyline is known to lower the convulsive threshold.

The elderly are particularly liable to experience adverse reactions, especially agitation, confusion and postural hypotension.

Troublesome hostility in a patient may be aroused by the use of nortriptyline.

Behavioural changes may occur in children receiving therapy for nocturnal enuresis.

If possible, the use of nortriptyline should be avoided in patients with narrow angle glaucoma or symptoms suggestive of prostatic hypertrophy.

The possibility of a suicide attempt by a depressed patient remains after the initiation of treatment. This possibility should be considered in relation to the quantity of drug dispensed at any one time.

When it is essential, nortriptyline may be administered with electroconvulsive therapy, although the hazards may be increased.

Both elevation and lowering of blood sugar levels have been reported. Significant hypoglycaemia was reported in a Type II diabetic patient maintained on chlorpropamide (250mg/day), after the addition of nortriptyline (125mg/day).

4.5 Interaction with other medicinal products and other forms of interaction

Drug interactions: Under no circumstances should nortriptyline be given concurrently with, or within two weeks of cessation of, therapy with monoamine oxidase inhibitors. Hyperpyretic crises, severe convulsions and fatalities have occurred when similar tricyclic antidepressants were used in such combinations.

Nortriptyline should not be given with sympathomimetic agents such as adrenaline, ephedrine, isoprenaline, noradrenaline, phenylephrine and phenylpropanolamine.

Nortriptyline may decrease the antihypertensive effect of guanethidine, debrisoquine, bethanidine and possibly clonidine. Concurrent administration of reserpine has been shown to produce a 'stimulating' effect in some depressed patients. It would be advisable to review all antihypertensive therapy during treatment with tricyclic antidepressants.

Barbiturates may increase the rate of metabolism of nortriptyline.

Anaesthetics given during tricyclic antidepressant therapy may increase the risk of arrhythmias and hypotension. If surgery is necessary, the drug should be discontinued, if possible, for several days prior to the procedure, or the anaesthetist should be informed if the patient is still receiving therapy.

Tricyclic antidepressants may potentiate the CNS depressant effect of alcohol.

The potentiating effect of excessive consumption of alcohol may lead to increased suicidal attempts or overdosage, especially in patients with histories of emotional disturbances or suicidal ideation.

Steady-state serum concentrations of the tricyclic antidepressants are reported to fluctuate significantly as cimetidine is either added to or deleted from the drug regimen. Higher than expected steady-state serum concentrations of the tricyclic antidepressant have been observed when therapy is initiated in patients already taking cimetidine. A decrease may occur when cimetidine therapy is discontinued.

Because nortriptyline's metabolism (like other tricyclic and SSRI antidepressants) involves the hepatic cytochrome P450IID6 isoenzyme system, concomitant therapy with drugs also metabolised by this system may lead to drug interactions. Lower doses than are usually prescribed for either the tricyclic antidepressant or the other drug may therefore be required.

Greater than two-fold increases in previously stable plasma levels of nortriptyline have occurred when fluoxetine was administered concomitantly. Fluoxetine and its active metabolite, norfluoxetine, have long half-lives (4-16 days for norfluoxetine).

Concomitant therapy with other drugs that are metabolised by this isoenzyme, including other antidepressants, phenothiazines, carbamazepine, propafenone, flecainide and encainide, or that inhibit this enzyme (eg, quinidine), should be approached with caution.

Supervision and adjustment of dosage may be required when nortriptyline is used with other anticholinergic drugs.

4.6 Pregnancy and lactation

Usage in pregnancy: The safety of nortriptyline for use during pregnancy has not been established, nor is there evidence from animal studies that it is free from hazard; therefore the drug should not be administered to pregnant patients or women of childbearing age unless the potential benefits clearly outweigh any potential risk.

Usage in nursing mothers: See 'Contra-indications'.

4.7 Effects on ability to drive and use machines

Nortriptyline may impair the mental and/or physical abilities required for the performance of hazardous tasks, such as operating machinery or driving a car; therefore the patient should be warned accordingly.

4.8 Undesirable effects

Included in the following list are a few adverse reactions that have not been reported with this specific drug. However, the pharmacological similarities among the tricyclic antidepressant drugs require that each of the reactions be considered when nortriptyline is administered.

Cardiovascular: Hypotension, hypertension, tachycardia, palpitation, myocardial infarction, arrhythmias, heart block, stroke.

Psychiatric: Confusional states (especially in the elderly) with hallucinations, disorientation, delusions; anxiety, restlessness, agitation; insomnia, panic, nightmares; hypomania; exacerbation of psychosis. Cases of suicidal ideation and suicidal behaviours have been reported during nortriptyline therapy or early treatment discontinuation (see Section 4.4).

Neurological: Numbness, tingling, paraesthesia of extremities; inco-ordination, ataxia, tremors; peripheral neuropathy; extrapyramidal symptoms; seizures, alteration of EEG patterns; tinnitus.

Anticholinergic: Dry mouth and, rarely, associated sublingual adenitis or gingivitis; blurred vision, disturbance of accommodation, mydriasis; constipation, paralytic ileus; urinary retention, delayed micturition, dilation of the urinary tract.

Allergic: Rash, petechiae, urticaria, itching, photosensitisation (avoid excessive exposure to sunlight); oedema (general or of face and tongue), drug fever, cross-sensitivity with other tricyclic drugs.

Haematological: Bone-marrow depression, including agranulocytosis; aplastic anaemia; eosinophilia; purpura; thrombocytopenia.

Gastro-intestinal: Nausea and vomiting, anorexia, epigastric distress, diarrhoea; peculiar taste, stomatitis, abdominal cramps, black tongue, constipation, paralytic ileus.

Endocrine: Gynaecomastia in the male; breast enlargement and galactorrhoea in the female; increased or decreased libido, impotence; testicular swelling; elevation or depression of blood sugar levels; syndrome of inappropriate secretion of antidiuretic hormone.

Other: Jaundice (simulating obstructive); altered liver function, hepatitis and liver necrosis; weight gain or loss; sweating; flushing; urinary frequency, nocturia; drowsiness, dizziness, weakness, fatigue; headache; parotid swelling; alopecia.

Withdrawal symptoms: Though these are not indicative of addiction, abrupt cessation of treatment after prolonged therapy may produce nausea, headache and malaise.

4.9 Overdose

Signs and symptoms: 50mg of a tricyclic antidepressant can be an overdose in a child. Of patients who are alive at presentation, mortality of 0-15% has been reported. Symptoms may begin within several hours and may include blurred vision, confusion, restlessness, dizziness, hypothermia, hyperthermia, agitation, vomiting, hyperactive reflexes, dilated pupils, fever, rapid heart rate, decreased bowel sounds, dry mouth, inability to void, myoclonic jerks, seizures, respiratory depression, myoglobinuric renal failure, nystagmus, ataxia, dysarthria, choreoathetosis, coma, hypotension and cardiac arrhythmias. Cardiac conduction may be slowed, with prolongation of QRS complex and QT intervals, right bundle branch and AV block, ventricular tachyarrhythmias (including Torsade de pointes and fibrillation) and death. Prolongation of QRS duration to more than 100msec is predictive of more severe toxicity. The absence of sinus tachycardia does not ensure a benign course. Hypotension may be caused by vasodilatation, central and peripheral alpha-adrenergic blockade and cardiac depression. In a healthy young person, prolonged resuscitation may be effective; one patient survived 5 hours of cardiac massage.

Treatment: Symptomatic and supportive therapy is recommended. Activated charcoal may be more effective than emesis or lavage to reduce absorption.

Ventricular arrhythmias, especially when accompanied by lengthened QRS intervals, may respond to alkalinisation by hyperventilation or administration of sodium bicarbonate. Serum electrolytes should be monitored and managed. Refractory arrhythmias may respond to propranolol, bretylium or lignocaine. Quinidine and procainamide usually should not be used because they may exacerbate arrhythmias and conduction already slowed by the overdose.

Seizures may respond to diazepam. Phenytoin may treat seizures and cardiac rhythm disturbances. Physostigmine may antagonise atrial tachycardia, gut immotility, myoclonic jerks and somnolence. The effects of physostigmine may be short-lived.

Diuresis and dialysis have little effect. Haemoperfusion is unproven. Monitoring should continue, at least until the QRS duration is normal.

5. PHARMACOLOGICAL PROPERTIES

5.1 Pharmacodynamic properties

Nortriptyline is a tricyclic antidepressant with actions and uses similar to these of Amitriptyline. It is the principal active metabolite of Amitriptyline.

In the treatment of depression Nortriptyline is given by mouth as the hydrochloride in doses equivalent to Nortriptyline 10mg 3 or 4 times daily initially, gradually increased to 25mg 4 times daily as necessary. A suggested initial dose for adolescents and the elderly is 10mg thrice daily. Inappropriately high plasma concentrations of Nortriptyline have been associated with deterioration in antidepressant response. Since Nortriptyline has prolonged half-life, once daily dosage regimens are also suitable, usually given at night.

5.2 Pharmacokinetic properties

Parts of metabolism of Nortriptyline include hydroxylation (possibly to active metabolites). N-oxidation and conjugation with glucuronic acid. Nortriptyline is widely distributed throughout the body and is extensively bound to plasma and tissue protein. Plasma concentrations of Nortriptyline vary very widely between individuals and no simple correlation with therapeutic response has been established.

5.3 Preclinical safety data

There are no preclinical data of relevance to the prescriber

6. PHARMACEUTICAL PARTICULARS

6.1 List of excipients

10mg Tablets: Maize Starch, Magnesium Stearate, Lactose Monohydrate, Calcium Phosphate, Purified Water. **Coat**: Glycerol, Methylhydroxypropyl Cellulose

25mg Tablets: Maize Starch, Magnesium Stearate, Lactose Monohydrate, Calcium Phosphate, Sunset Yellow, Purified Water. **Coat**: Glycerol, Methylhydroxypropyl Cellulose, Ethylcellulose, Methyl Alcohol, Isopropyl Alcohol, Methylene Chloride.

6.2 Incompatibilities

None Stated

6.3 Shelf life

36 months

6.4 Special precautions for storage

No special requirements

6.5 Nature and contents of container

High density polyethylene bottles containing 100 and 500 tablets

UPVC blister strips with aluminium foil backing containing 25 tablets

6.6 Special precautions for disposal and other handling

Not applicable

7. MARKETING AUTHORISATION HOLDER

King Pharmaceuticals Ltd

Donegal Street

Ballybofey

County Donegal

. MARKETING AUTHORISATION NUMBER(S)
0mg 14385/0001 25mg 14385/0002

. DATE OF FIRST AUTHORISATION/RENEWAL OF THE AUTHORISATION
30th March 1998

10. DATE OF REVISION OF THE TEXT
MARCH 2008

11. Legal Classification
POM

ALLERcalm Allergy Relief Tablets

(Actavis UK Ltd)

1. NAME OF THE MEDICINAL PRODUCT
1. CHLORPHENAMINE TABLETS BP 4mg
2. Alpharma Chlorphenamine Hayfever & Allergy Relief Tablets
3. Vantage Chlorphenamine Hayfever & Allergy Relief Tablets
4. ALLERcalm Allergy Relief Tablets

2. QUALITATIVE AND QUANTITATIVE COMPOSITION
Each tablet contains 4mg Chlorphenamine Maleate.

3. PHARMACEUTICAL FORM
Yellow uncoated tablets.

4. CLINICAL PARTICULARS
4.1 Therapeutic indications
1) For the symptomatic control of all allergic conditions which are responsive to antihistamines, including hay fever, urticaria, vasomotor rhinitis, angioneurotic oedema, food allergy, drug and serum reactions, insect bites.

4.2 Posology and method of administration
Posology
Adults: 1 tablet every four or six hours to a maximum daily dose of 24mg.

Not recommended for children under 12 years of age unless otherwise directed by a practitioner.

Elderly: As in adults, but the elderly are prone to confusional psychosis and other neurological anticholinergic effects.

Method of Administration
For oral administration.

4.3 Contraindications
Hypersensitivity to antihistamines; patients who have received therapy with MAOI's within the previous fourteen days.

4.4 Special warnings and precautions for use
In common with other drugs having anticholinergic effects, Chlorphenamine should be used with caution in epilepsy, prostatic hypertrophy, glaucoma, hepatic disease, bronchitis, bronchiectasis, thyrotoxicosis, raised intra-ocular pressure, severe hypertension or cardiovascular disease and bronchial asthma.

4.5 Interaction with other medicinal products and other forms of interaction
Chlorphenamine may have an additive effect when used concurrently with hypnotics and anxiolytics causing potentiation of drowsiness. A similar additive effect will result from concurrent usage of alcohol with Chlorphenamine. MAOI therapy intensifies the anticholinergic effects of Chlorphenamine. Chlorphenamine inhibits phenytoin metabolism and can lead to phenytoin toxicity.

4.6 Pregnancy and lactation
The safety of Chlorphenamine in pregnancy has not been established. Chlorphenamine should therefore only be used when clearly required and when potential benefits outweigh the potential unknown risks to the foetus. Use during the third trimester may result in reactions in the newborn or premature neonates.

Small amounts of antihistamines are excreted in breast milk. Use by nursing mothers is not recommended because of the risks of adverse effects in the infant.

Antihistamines may inhibit lactation.

4.7 Effects on ability to drive and use machines
The anticholinergic properties of Chlorphenamine may cause drowsiness, dizziness, blurred vision and psychomotor impairment, which can seriously hamper the patient's ability to drive and use machinery.

4.8 Undesirable effects
Sedation varying from slight drowsiness to deep sleep. Inability to concentrate, lassitude, blurred vision, GI disturbances such as nausea, vomiting and diarrhoea may occasionally occur. Urinary retention, headaches, dryness of the mouth. Dizziness, palpitation, tachycardia, arrhythmias, hypotension, tightness of the chest, abdominal pain, dyspepsia, anorexia, hepatic including jaundice, thickening of the bronchial secretions, haemolytic anaemia and other blood dyscrasias infrequently occur.

Allergic reactions including exfoliative dermatitis, photosensitivity and skin reactions. Urticaria, twitching, muscular weakness and in co-ordination. Tinnitus, depression, irritability and nightmares infrequently occur.

Paradoxical excitation in children and confusional psychosis in the elderly can occur.

The effects of alcohol may be increased. Children and the elderly are more likely to experience the neurological anticholinergic effects.

4.9 Overdose
The estimated lethal dose of Chlorphenamine is 25-50mg/kg body weight.

Symptoms and signs include sedation, paradoxical stimulation of the CNS, toxic psychosis, seizures, apnoea, convulsions, anticholinergic effects, dystonic reactions and cardiovascular collapse including arrhythmias.

Treatment includes gastric lavage or emesis using ipecacuanha syrup. Following these measures activated charcoal and cathartics may be administered to minimise absorption. Other symptomatic and supportive measures should be provided with special attention to cardiac, respiratory, renal and hepatic functions and fluid and electrolyte balance.

Treat hypotension and arrhythmias vigorously. CNS convulsions may be treated with IV diazepam or phenytoin. Haemoperfusion may be used in severe cases.

5. PHARMACOLOGICAL PROPERTIES
5.1 Pharmacodynamic properties
Chlorphenamine Maleate is an antihistamine.

5.2 Pharmacokinetic properties
Chlorphenamine Maleate is an alkylamine derivative with a plasma half-life of up to 42 hours which is extensively metabolised in the liver and excreted almost exclusively in the urine.

5.3 Preclinical safety data
There are no pre-clinical data of relevance to the prescriber which are additional to that already included in other sections of the SPC.

6. PHARMACEUTICAL PARTICULARS
6.1 List of excipients
Also contains: calcium sulphate, magnesium stearate, maize starch, E172, E460.

6.2 Incompatibilities
None known.

6.3 Shelf life
Shelf-life
Three years from the date of manufacture.

Shelf-life after dilution/reconstitution
Not applicable.

Shelf-life after first opening
Not applicable.

6.4 Special precautions for storage
Store below 25°C in a dry place.

6.5 Nature and contents of container
The product containers are rigid injection moulded polypropylene or injection blow-moulded polyethylene tablet containers with polyfoam wad or polyethylene ullage filler and snap-on polyethylene lids; in case any supply difficulties should arise the alternative is amber glass bottles with screw caps and polyfoam wad or cotton wool.

The product may also be supplied in blister packs in cartons:

a) Carton: Printed carton manufactured from white folding box board.

b) Blister pack: (i) 250μm white rigid PVC. (ii) Surface printed 20μm hard temper aluminium foil with 5-7g/M^2 PVC and PVdC compatible heat seal lacquer on the reverse side.

Pack sizes: 7, 28, 30, 50, 56, 60, 84, 90, 100, 112, 120, 168, 180, 250, 500, 1000.

Product may also be supplied in bulk packs, for reassembly purposes only, in polybags contained in tins, skillets or polybuckets filled with suitable cushioning material. Bulk packs are included for *temporary* storage of the finished product before final packaging into the proposed marketing containers.

Maximum size of bulk packs: 50,000.

6.6 Special precautions for disposal and other handling
Not applicable.

Administrative Data
7. MARKETING AUTHORISATION HOLDER
Name or style and permanent address of registered place of business of the holder of the Marketing Authorisation:

Actavis UK Limited
(Trading style: Actavis)
Whiddon Valley
BARNSTAPLE
N Devon EX32 8NS

8. MARKETING AUTHORISATION NUMBER(S)
PL 0142/0209

9. DATE OF FIRST AUTHORISATION/RENEWAL OF THE AUTHORISATION
9.5.86
Renewed: 20.10.02

10. DATE OF REVISION OF THE TEXT
June 2007

Alphaderm 1% & 10% w/w Cream

(Alliance Pharmaceuticals)

1. NAME OF THE MEDICINAL PRODUCT
Alphaderm 1% & 10%w/w Cream

2. QUALITATIVE AND QUANTITATIVE COMPOSITION
Alphaderm cream contains the active ingredients Hydrocortisone, PhEur 1% w/w and Urea, BP 10% w/w.

3. PHARMACEUTICAL FORM
Translucent white cream.

4. CLINICAL PARTICULARS
4.1 Therapeutic indications
For the treatment of all dry ichthyotic, eczematous conditions of the skin, including atopic, infantile, chronic allergic and irritant eczema, asteatotic, hyperkeratotic and lichenified eczema, neurodermatitis and prurigo.

4.2 Posology and method of administration
Adults, children and the elderly. A small amount should be applied topically to the preferably dry affected areas twice daily. In resistant lesions occlusive dressings may be used but this is usually unnecessary because of the self occlusive nature of the special base.

4.3 Contraindications
Primary bacterial, viral and fungal diseases of the skin and secondarily infected eczemas or intertrigo acne, perioral dermatitis, rosacea and, in general, should not be used on weeping surfaces.

Known hypersensitivity to the active ingredients or any of its excipients.

4.4 Special warnings and precautions for use
Caution should be exercised when using in children. In infants and children, long term continuous therapy should be avoided, as adrenal suppression can occur even without occlusion. Excessive absorption may occur when applied under napkins. Where possible treatment in infants should be limited to 5-7 days.

Application to moist or fissured skin may cause temporary irritation.

As with corticosteroids in general, prolonged application to the face and eyelids is undesirable and the cream should be kept away from the eyes.

4.5 Interaction with other medicinal products and other forms of interaction
None known.

4.6 Pregnancy and lactation
There is inadequate evidence for safety in human pregnancy. Topical administration of corticosteroids to pregnant animals can cause abnormalities of foetal development including cleft palate and intra-uterine growth retardation. There may, therefore, be a very small risk of such effects in the human foetus.

4.7 Effects on ability to drive and use machines
Alphaderm does not interfere with the ability to drive or use machines.

4.8 Undesirable effects
If used correctly Alphaderm is unlikely to cause side effects. However, the following events have been observed with topical steroids, and although are rare with hydrocortisone, may occur, especially with long-term use; spread and worsening of untreated infection; thinning of the skin; irreversible striae atrophicae and telangiectasia; contact dermatitis, perioral dermatitis; acne; mild depigmentation which may be reversible. Atrophic changes may occur in intertriginous areas or nappy areas in young children.

4.9 Overdose
Chronically, grossly excessive over-use on large areas of skin in, for example, children could result in adrenal suppression of the hypothalamic-pituitary axis (HPA) as well as topical and systemic signs and symptoms of high corticosteroid dosage. In such cases, treatment should not stop abruptly. Adrenal insufficiency may require treatment with systemic hydrocortisone. Ingestion of a large amount of Alphaderm would be expected to result in gastrointestinal irritation, nausea, and possibly vomiting. Symptomatic and supportive care should be given. Liberal oral administration of milk or water may be helpful.

5. PHARMACOLOGICAL PROPERTIES
5.1 Pharmacodynamic properties
Hydrocortisone is a naturally occurring glucocorticoid with proven anti-inflammatory and vasoconstrictive properties. Urea has been demonstrated to have hydrating, keratolytic and anti-pruritic properties. As such, urea has additional therapeutic effect in dry hyperkeratotic skin conditions. Alphaderm cream contains hydrocortisone and urea in a specially formulated base which assists the percutaneous

transportation of the active ingredients to the site of action. Due to this formulation, Alphaderm acts as a moderately potent topical corticosteroid. The base is self-occlusive and fulfils the functions of both an ointment and a cream.

5.2 Pharmacokinetic properties

Therapeutic activity of hydrocortisone depends upon the adequate penetration through the horny layer of the skin. The urea in the formulation solubilises part of the hydrocortisone and has a keratolytic effect. Both these factors increase penetration of the hydrocortisone

5.3 Preclinical safety data

None stated

6. PHARMACEUTICAL PARTICULARS

6.1 List of excipients

White soft paraffin, maize starch, isopropyl myristate, sycrowax HR-C, palmitic acid, sorbitan laurate and Arlatone G.

6.2 Incompatibilities

None known.

6.3 Shelf life

Two years

6.4 Special precautions for storage

Do not store above 25°C.

6.5 Nature and contents of container

Supplied in tubes of 30g and 100g.

6.6 Special precautions for disposal and other handling

A patient leaflet is provided with details of use and handling of the product.

7. MARKETING AUTHORISATION HOLDER

Alliance Pharmaceuticals Ltd

Avonbridge House

Bath Road

Chippenham

Wiltshire

SN15 2BB

8. MARKETING AUTHORISATION NUMBER(S)

PL 16853/0060.

9. DATE OF FIRST AUTHORISATION/RENEWAL OF THE AUTHORISATION

13 February 1990

10. DATE OF REVISION OF THE TEXT

August 2008

11. LEGAL STATUS

POM

Alphagan

(Allergan Ltd)

1. NAME OF THE MEDICINAL PRODUCT

Alphagan 0.2% w/v (2 mg/ml) eye drops, solution

2. QUALITATIVE AND QUANTITATIVE COMPOSITION

One ml solution contains 2.0 mg brimonidine tartrate, equivalent to 1.3 mg of brimonidine.

Excipient(s): Contains benzalkonium chloride 0.05 mg/ml.
For a full list of excipients, see section 6.1.

3. PHARMACEUTICAL FORM

Eye drops, solution.

Clear, greenish-yellow to light greenish-yellow solution.

4. CLINICAL PARTICULARS

4.1 Therapeutic indications

Reduction of elevated intraocular pressure (IOP) in patients with open angle glaucoma or ocular hypertension.

– As monotherapy in patients in whom topical beta-blocker therapy is contraindicated.

– As adjunctive therapy to other intraocular pressure lowering medications when the target IOP is not achieved with a single agent (see Section 5.1).

4.2 Posology and method of administration

Recommended dosage in adults (including the elderly)

The recommended dose is one drop of Alphagan in the affected eye(s) twice daily, approximately 12 hours apart. No dosage adjustment is required for the use in elderly patients.

As with any eye drops, to reduce possible systemic absorption, it is recommended that the lachrymal sac be compressed at the medial canthus (punctal occlusion) for one minute. This should be performed immediately following the instillation of each drop.

If more than one topical ophthalmic drug is to be used, the different drugs should be instilled 5-15 minutes apart.

Use in renal and hepatic impairment

Alphagan has not been studied in patients with hepatic or renal impairment (see section 4.4).

Use in paediatric subjects

No clinical studies have been performed in adolescents (12 to 17 years).

Alphagan is not recommended for use in children below 12 years and is contraindicated in neonates and infants (less than 2 years of age) (see sections 4.3, 4.4 and 4.9). It is known that severe adverse reactions can occur in neonates. The safety and efficacy of Alphagan have not been established in children.

4.3 Contraindications

– Hypersensitivity to the active substance or to any of the excipients.

– Neonates and infants (see section 4.8).

– Patients receiving monoamine oxidase (MAO) inhibitor therapy and patients on antidepressants which affect noradrenergic transmission (e.g. tricyclic antidepressants and mianserin).

4.4 Special warnings and precautions for use

Children of 2 years of age and above, especially those in the 2-7 age range and/or weighing < 20 Kg, should be treated with caution and closely monitored due to the high incidence of somnolence (see section 4.8).

Caution should be exercised in treating patients with severe or unstable and uncontrolled cardiovascular disease.

Some (12.7%)patients in clinical trials experienced an ocular allergic type reaction with Alphagan (see section 4.8 for details). If allergic reactions are observed, treatment with Alphagan should be discontinued.

Alphagan should be used with caution in patients with depression, cerebral or coronary insufficiency, Raynaud's phenomenon, orthostatic hypotension or thromboangiitis obliterans.

Alphagan has not been studied in patients with hepatic or renal impairment; caution should be used in treating such patients.

The preservative in Alphagan, benzalkonium chloride, may cause eye irritation. Avoid contact with soft contact lenses. Remove contact lenses prior to application and wait at least 15 minutes before reinsertion. Known to discolour soft contact lenses.

4.5 Interaction with other medicinal products and other forms of interaction

Although specific drug interactions studies have not been conducted with Alphagan, the possibility of an additive or potentiating effect with CNS depressants (alcohol, barbiturates, opiates, sedatives, or anaesthetics) should be considered.

No data on the level of circulating catecholamines after Alphagan administration are available. Caution, however, is advised in patients taking medications which can affect the metabolism and uptake of circulating amines e.g. chlorpromazine, methylphenidate, reserpine.

After the application of Alphagan, clinically insignificant decreases in blood pressure were noted in some patients. Caution is advised when using drugs such as antihypertensives and/or cardiac glycosides concomitantly with Alphagan.

Caution is advised when initiating (or changing the dose of) a concomitant systemic agent (irrespective of pharmaceutical form) which may interact with α-adrenergic agonists or interfere with their activity i.e. agonists or antagonists of the adrenergic receptor e.g. (isoprenaline, prazosin).

4.6 Pregnancy and lactation

The safety of use during human pregnancy has not been established. In animal studies, brimonidine tartrate did not cause any teratogenic effects. In rabbits, brimonidine tartrate, at plasma levels higher than are achieved during therapy in humans, has been shown to cause increased preimplantation loss and postnatal growth reduction. Alphagan should be used during pregnancy only if the potential benefit to the mother outweighs the potential risk to the foetus.

It is not known if brimonidine is excreted in human milk. The compound is excreted in the milk of the lactating rat. Alphagan should not be used by women nursing infants.

4.7 Effects on ability to drive and use machines

Alphagan may cause fatigue and/or drowsiness, which may impair the ability to drive or operate machinery. Alphagan may cause blurred and/or abnormal vision, which may impair the ability to drive or to use machinery, especially at night or in reduced lighting. The patient should wait until these symptoms have cleared before driving or using machinery.

4.8 Undesirable effects

The most commonly reported ADRs are oral dryness, ocular hyperaemia and burning/stinging, all occurring in 22 to 25% of patients. They are usually transient and not commonly of a severity requiring discontinuation of treatment.

Symptoms of ocular allergic reactions occurred in 12.7% of subjects (causing withdrawal in 11.5% of subjects) in clinical trials with the onset between 3 and 9 months in the majority of patients.

Within each frequency grouping, undesirable effects are presented in order of decreasing seriousness. The following terminologies have been used in order to classify the occurrence of undesirable effects: Very Common (≥1/10); Common (≥1/100 to <1/10); Uncommon (≥1/1,000 to <1/100); Rare (≥1/10,000 to <1/1,000); Very rare (<1/10,000), not known (cannot be estimated from the availabl data).

Cardiac disorders

Uncommon: palpitations/arrhythmias (including bradycar dia and tachycardia)

Nervous system disorders

Very common: headache, drowsiness

Common: dizziness, abnormal taste

Very rare: syncope

Eye disorders

Very common:

– ocular irritation including allergic reactions (hyperaemia burning and stinging, pruritus, foreign body sensatior conjunctival follicles)

– blurred vision

Common:

– local irritation (eyelid hyperaemia and oedema, blepha itis, conjunctival oedema and discharge, ocular pain an tearing)

– photophobia

– corneal erosion and staining

– ocular dryness

– conjunctival blanching

– abnormal vision

– conjunctivitis

Very rare:

– iritis (anterior uveitis)

– miosis

Respiratory, thoracic and mediastinal disorders

Common: upper respiratory symptoms

Uncommon: nasal dryness

Rare: dyspnoea

Gastrointestinal disorders

Very common: oral dryness

Common: gastrointestinal symptoms

Vascular disorders

Very rare: hypertension, hypotension

General disorders and administration site conditions

Very common: fatigue

Common: asthenia

Immune system disorders

Uncommon: systemic allergic reactions

Psychiatric disorders

Uncommon: depression

Very rare: insomnia

In cases where brimonidine has been used as part of th medical treatment of congenital glaucoma, symptoms brimonidine overdose such as loss of consciousnes hypotension, hypotonia, bradycardia, hypothermia, cyan sis and apnoea have been reported in neonates and infan receiving brimonidine (see section 4.3).

In a 3-month, phase 3 study in children aged 2-7 years wi glaucoma, inadequately controlled by beta-blockers, high prevalence of somnolence (55%) was reported wi Alphagan as adjunctive treatment. In 8% of children, th was severe and led to discontinuation of treatment in 13 The incidence of somnolence decreased with increasir age, being least in the 7-year-old age group (25%), but wa more affected by weight, occurring more frequently those children weighing ≤20 kg (63%) compared to thos weighing >20 kg (25%) (see section 4.4).

4.9 Overdose

<u>Ophthalmic overdose:</u>

There is no experience in adults with the unlikely case of a overdosage via the ophthalmic route. However, symptor of brimonidine overdose (including loss of consciousnes hypotension, hypotonia, bradycardia, hypothermia, cyan sis and apnoea) have been reported in neonates an infants receiving Alphagan as part of medical treatme of congenital glaucoma.

<u>Systemic overdose resulting from accidental ingestion:</u>

Two cases of adverse effects following inadvertent inge tion of 9-10 drops of Alphagan by adult subjects have bee received. The subjects experienced a hypotensive ep sode, followed in one instance by rebound hypertensic approximately 8 hours after ingestion. Both subjects we reported to have made a full recovery within 24 hours. N adverse effects were noted in a third subject who als ingested an unknown amount of Alphagan orally.

Reports of serious adverse effects following inadverte ingestion of Alphagan by paediatric subjects have bee published or reported to Allergan. The subjects exper enced symptoms of CNS depression, typically tempora coma or low level of consciousness, hypotonia, bradyca dia, hypothermia and apnoea, and required admission intensive care with intubation if indicated. All subjects we reported to have made a full recovery, usually within 6-2 hours.

Oral overdoses of other alpha-2-agonists have bee reported to cause symptoms such as hypotension, asth nia, vomiting, lethargy, sedation, bradycardia, arrhythmia miosis, apnoea, hypotonia, hypothermia, respiratory depression and seizure.

5. PHARMACOLOGICAL PROPERTIES

5.1 Pharmacodynamic properties

Pharmacotherapeutic group: Sympathomimetics in glaucoma therapy, ATC code = S01EA 05.

Brimonidine is an alpha-2 adrenergic receptor agonist that is 1000-fold more selective for the alpha-2 adrenoceptor than the alpha-1 adrenoreceptor.

This selectivity results in no mydriasis and the absence of vasoconstriction in microvessels associated with human retinal xenografts.

Topical administration of brimonidine tartrate decreases intraocular pressure (IOP) in humans with minimal effect on cardiovascular or pulmonary parameters.

Limited data are available for patients with bronchial asthma showing no adverse effects.

Alphagan has a rapid onset of action, with peak ocular hypotensive effect seen at two hours post-dosing. In two 1 year studies, Alphagan lowered IOP by mean values of approximately 4-6 mmHg.

Fluorophotometric studies in animals and humans suggest that brimonidine tartrate has a dual mechanism of action. It is thought that Alphagan may lower IOP by reducing aqueous humour formation and enhancing uveoscleral outflow.

Clinical trials show that Alphagan is effective in combination with topical beta-blockers. Shorter term studies also suggest that Alphagan has a clinically relevant additive effect in combination with travoprost (6 weeks) and latanoprost (3 months).

5.2 Pharmacokinetic properties

a) General characteristics

After ocular administration of a 0.2% solution twice daily for 10 days, plasma concentrations were low (mean Cmax was 0.06 ng/ml). There was a slight accumulation in the blood after multiple (2 times daily for 10 days) instillations. The area under the plasma concentration-time curve over 12 hours at steady state (AUC_{0-12h}) was 0.31 ng·hr/ml, as compared to 0.23 ng·hr/ml after the first dose. The mean apparent half-life in the systemic circulation was approximately 3 hours in humans after topical dosing.

The plasma protein binding of brimonidine after topical dosing in humans is approximately 29%.

Brimonidine binds reversibly to melanin in ocular tissues, in vitro and in vivo. Following 2 weeks of ocular instillation, the concentrations of brimonidine in iris, ciliary body and choroid-retina were 3- to 17-fold higher than those after a single dose. Accumulation does not occur in the absence of melanin.

The significance of melanin binding in humans is unclear. However, no significant ocular adverse reaction was found during biomicroscopic examination of eyes in patients treated with Alphagan for up to one year, nor was significant ocular toxicity found during a one year ocular safety study in monkeys given approximately four times the recommended dose of brimonidine tartrate.

Following oral administration to man, brimonidine is well absorbed and rapidly eliminated. The major part of the dose (around 75% of the dose) was excreted as metabolites in urine within five days; no unchanged drug was detected in urine. In vitro studies, using animal and human liver, indicate that the metabolism is mediated largely by aldehyde oxidase and cytochrome P450. Hence, the systemic elimination seems to be primarily hepatic metabolism.

Kinetics profile:

No great deviation from dose proportionality for plasma Cmax and AUC was observed following a single topical dose of 0.08%, 0.2% and 0.5%.

b) Characteristics in patients

Characteristics in elderly patients:

The C_{max}, AUC, and apparent half-life of brimonidine are similar in the elderly (subjects 65 years or older) after a single dose compared with young adults, indicating that its systemic absorption and elimination are not affected by age.

Based on data from a 3 month clinical study, which included elderly patients, systemic exposure to brimonidine was very low.

5.3 Preclinical safety data

Non-clinical data reveal no special hazard for humans based on conventional studies of safety pharmacology, repeated dose toxicity, genotoxicity, carcinogenic potential, toxicity to reproduction.

6. PHARMACEUTICAL PARTICULARS

6.1 List of excipients

Benzalkonium Chloride

Poly(vinyl alcohol)

Sodium chloride

Sodium citrate

Citric acid monohydrate

Purified water

Hydrochloric acid (for pH-adjustment) or

Sodium hydroxide (for pH-adjustment)

6.2 Incompatibilities

Not applicable.

6.3 Shelf life

Before first opening: 2 years for the 2.5 ml container.

3 years for the 5 ml and 10 ml containers.

After first opening: 28 days.

6.4 Special precautions for storage

Do not store above 25°C.

6.5 Nature and contents of container

White low density polyethylene dropper bottles with a 35 microlitre tip. The cap is either a conventional polystyrene screw cap or a Compliance Cap (C-Cap).

2.5 ml, 5 ml and 10 ml bottles in packs of 1, 3 or 6.

Not all pack sizes may be marketed.

6.6 Special precautions for disposal and other handling

No special requirements.

7. MARKETING AUTHORISATION HOLDER

Allergan Ltd

1st Floor Marlow International

The Parkway

Marlow

Buckinghamshire SL7 1YL

UK

8. MARKETING AUTHORISATION NUMBER(S)

PL 00426/0088

9. DATE OF FIRST AUTHORISATION/RENEWAL OF THE AUTHORISATION

Date of first authorisation: 18 March 1997

Date of last renewal: 17 September 2006

10. DATE OF REVISION OF THE TEXT

8th February 2008

Altargo 1% Ointment

(GlaxoSmithKline UK)

1. NAME OF THE MEDICINAL PRODUCT

Altargo▼ 1% ointment

2. QUALITATIVE AND QUANTITATIVE COMPOSITION

1 g contains 10 mg retapamulin (1% w/w).

For a full list of excipients, see section 6.1.

3. PHARMACEUTICAL FORM

Ointment

Smooth, off-white ointment.

4. CLINICAL PARTICULARS

4.1 Therapeutic indications

Short term treatment of the following superficial skin infections:

Impetigo.

Infected small lacerations, abrasions, or sutured wounds.

See sections 4.4 and 5.1 for important information regarding the clinical activity of retapamulin against different types of *Staphylococcus aureus*.

Consideration should be given to official guidance on the appropriate use of antibacterial agents.

4.2 Posology and method of administration

Retapamulin is for cutaneous use only.

Adults (aged 18-65 years), adolescents (aged 12-17 years), infants and children (aged from nine months to 11 years)

A thin layer of ointment should be applied to the affected area twice daily for five days.

The area treated may be covered with sterile bandage or gauze dressing.

Safety and efficacy have not been established in the following:

- Impetiginous lesions >10 in number and exceeding 100 cm^2 in total surface area.
- Infected lesions that exceed 10 cm in length or a total surface area >100 cm^2.

In patients aged less than 18 years the total surface area treated should be no more than 2% of the body surface area.

Patients not showing a clinical response within two to three days should be re-evaluated and alternative therapy should be considered (see section 4.4).

Infants under nine months of age

The safety and efficacy of retapamulin ointment has not been established in paediatric patients less than nine months of age.

Elderly (aged 65 and older)

No dosage adjustment is necessary.

Renal impairment

No dosage adjustment is necessary. See section 5.3.

Hepatic impairment

No dosage adjustment is necessary. See section 5.3.

4.3 Contraindications

Known or suspected hypersensitivity to retapamulin or to the excipient.

4.4 Special warnings and precautions for use

In the event of a sensitisation or severe local irritation from the use of retapamulin ointment, treatment should be discontinued, the ointment carefully wiped off, and appropriate alternative therapy for the infection instituted.

Retapamulin ointment must be kept away from the eyes and mucous membranes. Care must be taken to avoid ingestion.

Retapamulin should not be used to treat infections known or thought likely to be due to MRSA (see section 5.1).

In clinical studies of secondarily infected open wounds, the efficacy of retapamulin was inadequate in patients with infections caused by methicillin-resistant *Staphylococcus aureus* (MRSA). The reason for the reduced clinical efficacy observed in these patients is unknown.

Alternative therapy should be considered if there is no improvement or a worsening in the infected area after 2-3 days of treatment.

Retapamulin should not be used to treat abscesses.

Retapamulin ointment contains butylated hydroxytoluene, which may cause local skin reaction (e.g. contact dermatitis), or irritation to the eyes and mucous membranes.

As with other antibacterial agents, prolonged use of retapamulin may result in overgrowth of non-susceptible micro-organisms, including fungi.

4.5 Interaction with other medicinal products and other forms of interaction

The effect of concurrent application of retapamulin and other topical products to the same area of skin has not been studied, and is not recommended.

In human liver microsomes, retapamulin was a strong inhibitor of CYP3A4. Based on the low plasma concentration achieved in humans after topical application to abraded skin or infected superficial wounds, a clinically relevant inhibition is not expected *in vivo* (see section 5.2)

Co-administration of oral ketoconazole 200mg twice daily increased mean retapamulin $AUC_{(0-24)}$ and C_{max} by 81% after topical application of retapamulin 1% ointment on the abraded skin of healthy adult males.

Due to low systemic exposure following topical application in patients, dosage adjustments are considered to be unnecessary when topical retapamulin is applied during systemic treatment with CYP3A4 inhibitors.

4.6 Pregnancy and lactation

Pregnancy

No clinical data on exposed pregnancies are available. Animal studies have shown reproductive toxicity after oral administration and are insufficient with respect to effects on parturition and fetal/postnatal development (see Section 5.3).

Retapamulin ointment should only be used in pregnancy when topical antibacterial therapy is clearly indicated and the use of retapamulin is considered to be preferable to administration of a systemic antibacterial agent.

Lactation

It is unknown whether retapamulin is excreted in human breast milk. Minimal systemic exposure is observed in adults, therefore exposure of the breast-feeding infant is likely to be negligible. The excretion of retapamulin in milk has not been studied in animals. A decision on whether to continue/discontinue breast-feeding or to continue/discontinue therapy with Altargo should be made taking into account the benefit of breast-feeding to the child and the benefit of Altargo therapy to the woman.

4.7 Effects on ability to drive and use machines

No studies on the effects on the ability to drive and use machines have been performed. Altargo is administered topically and is unlikely to have an effect on the ability to drive or use machines.

4.8 Undesirable effects

In clinical studies in which 2150 patients with superficial skin infections applied Altargo, the most commonly reported adverse reaction was application site irritation, which affected approximately 1% of patients.

The following convention has been used for the classification of frequency:

Common ≥1/100 to <1/10

Uncommon ≥1/1000 to <1/100

Within each frequency grouping, undesirable effects are presented in order of decreasing seriousness.

Organ systems	Common	Uncommon
General disorders and administration site conditions	Application site reactions Irritation	Application site reactions Pain Pruritus Erythema
Skin and subcutaneous tissue disorders		Contact dermatitis

4.9 Overdose

Any signs or symptoms of overdose, either topically or by accidental ingestion, should be treated symptomatically.

No specific antidote is known.

5. PHARMACOLOGICAL PROPERTIES

5.1 Pharmacodynamic properties

Pharmacotherapeutic group: Dermatologicals ATC code: D06AX13

Mode of action

Retapamulin is a semi-synthetic derivative of the compound pleuromutilin, which is isolated through fermentation from *Clitopilus passeckerianus* (formerly *Pleurotus passeckerianus*).

Retapamulin selectively inhibits bacterial protein synthesis by interacting at a unique site on the 50S subunit of the bacterial ribosome that is distinct from the binding sites of other non-pleuromutilin antibacterial agents that interact with the ribosome.

Data indicate that the binding site involves ribosomal protein L3 and is in the region of the ribosomal P site and peptidyl transferase centre. By virtue of binding to this site, pleuromutilins inhibit peptidyl transfer, partially block P-site interactions, and prevent normal formation of active 50S ribosomal subunits. Therefore the pleuromutilins appear to inhibit bacterial protein synthesis by multiple mechanisms.

Retapamulin is predominantly bacteriostatic against *S. aureus* and *S. pyogenes*.

Mechanism of Resistance

Due to its distinct mechanism of action, retapamulin does not demonstrate target specific cross-resistance with other classes of antibacterial agents.

In vitro, two mechanisms have been identified which reduce susceptibility to retapamulin. One involves mutations in ribosomal protein L3, the other is a non-specific efflux mechanism (ABC transporter *vgaAv*). This non-target specific efflux mechanism has also been demonstrated to reduce the *in vitro* activity of streptogramin A.

No development of resistance was observed during treatment with retapamulin in the clinical study programme and all clinical isolates were inhibited by retapamulin concentrations of ≤2μg/ml.

Antibacterial spectrum

The prevalence of acquired resistance may vary geographically and with time for selected species, and local information on resistance is desirable, particularly when treating severe infections. As necessary, expert advice should be sought when the local prevalence of resistance is such that the utility of the agent in at least some types of infection is questionable.

Commonly susceptible species
Staphylococcus aureus$^{\$*}$
*Streptococcus pyogenes**
Streptococcus agalactiae
Inherently resistant organisms
Enterobacteriaceae
Pseudomonas aeruginosa
Enterococcus faecalis

$ *In vitro*, retapamulin was equally active against methicillin-susceptible and methicillin-resistant strains of *S. aureus*. However, see section 4.4 and below regarding clinical efficacy against MRSA. Retapamulin should not be used to treat infections known or thought likely to be due to MRSA.

* Activity has been satisfactorily demonstrated in clinical studies

Information from clinical trials

Very few MRSA were isolated in studies in impetigo and all were clinical successes(100%: 8/8).

In studies in impetigo and in two studies of secondarily infected open wounds (SIOW), clinical success rates were high for retapamulin in patients with mupirocin-resistant *S. aureus* (100%: 11/11) or fusidic acid-resistant *S. aureus* (96.7%: 29/30). However, in the two studies that enrolled patients with SIOW the efficacy of retapamulin in infections due to MRSA was inadequate (75.7%). No differences were observed in the *in vitro* activity of retapamulin versus *S. aureus* whether the isolates were susceptible or resistant to methicillin.

The explanation for lower clinical efficacy against MRSA in SIOW is unclear and it may have been influenced by the presence of a particular MRSA clone. In the case of treatment failure associated with *S. aureus*, the presence of strains possessing additional virulence factors (such as Panton-Valentine Leukocidin) should be considered.

(see Table 1 below)

5.2 Pharmacokinetic properties

Absorption

In a study of healthy adult subjects, 1% retapamulin ointment was applied daily to intact and to abraded skin under occlusion for up to 7 days. Systemic exposure following topical application of retapamulin through intact skin was very low. The geometric mean C_{max} value in plasma after application to 200 cm^2 of abraded skin was 9.75 ng/ml on day 1 and 8.79 ng/ml on day 7 and the maximum individual systemic exposure (C_{max}) recorded was 22.1 ng/ml.

Single plasma samples were obtained from 516 adult and paediatric patients who received topical treatment with retapamulin 1% ointment twice daily for 5 days for the treatment of secondarily infected traumatic lesions. Sampling occurred pre-dose for adult subjects on days 3 or 4, and between 0-12 hours after the last application for paediatric subjects on days 3 or 4. The majority of samples (89%) were below the lower limit of quantitation (0.5 ng/ml). Of the samples that had measurable concentrations 90% had retapamulin concentrations less than 2.5 ng/ml. The maximum measured plasma concentration of retapamulin was 10.7 ng/ml in adults and 18.5 ng/ml in paediatric patients.

Distribution

Due to the very low systemic exposures, tissue distribution of retapamulin has not been investigated in humans.

In vitro, retapamulin was shown to be a P-glycoprotein (Pgp) substrate and inhibitor.

However, the maximum individual systemic exposure in humans following topical application of 1% ointment on 200 cm^2 of abraded skin (C_{max}= 22 ng/ml; $AUC_{(0-24)}$ = 238 ng.h/ml) was 660-fold lower than the retapamulin IC_{50} for Pgp inhibition.

Retapamulin is approximately 94% bound to human plasma proteins.

Metabolism

The *in vitro* oxidative metabolism of retapamulin in human liver microsomes was primarily mediated by CYP3A4 with minor contributions from CYP2C8 and CYP2D6 (see section 4.5).

Elimination

Retapamulin elimination in humans has not been investigated.

Special Patient Populations

No pharmacokinetic data are available in children aged less than 2 years, or in patients with renal or hepatic impairment. However, due to the low systemic plasma levels that have been observed, no safety problems are foreseen.

5.3 Preclinical safety data

Repeated-dose toxicity

In 14-day (50, 150 or 450 mg/kg) oral toxicity studies in rats there was evidence of adaptive hepatic and thyroid changes. Neither of these findings is of clinical relevance.

In monkeys dosed orally (50, 150 or 450 mg/kg) for 14 days there was dose-related emesis.

Carcinogenesis, mutagenesis, reproductive toxicity

Long-term studies in animals to evaluate carcinogenic potential have not been conducted with retapamulin.

There was no evidence of genotoxicity when evaluated in *vitro* for gene mutation and/or chromosomal effects in the mouse lymphoma cell assay, in cultured human peripheral blood lymphocytes, or when evaluated *in vivo* for chromosomal effects in a rat micronucleus test.

There was no evidence of impaired fertility in male or female rats at oral doses of 50, 150, or 450 mg/kg/day, resulting in exposure margins of up to 5-times the highest human estimated exposure (topical application to 200 cm^2 abraded skin: AUC 238 ng.h/ml).

In an embryotoxicity study in rats, developmental toxicit (decreased fetal body weight and delayed skeletal ossifi cation) and maternal toxicity were observed at oral dose of ≥ 150 mg/kg/day (corresponding to ≥ 3 times th human estimated exposure (see above). There were n treatment-related malformations in rats.

Retapamulin was given as a continuous intravenous infu sion to pregnant rabbits from day 7 to day 19 of gestation Maternal toxicity was demonstrated at dosages o ≥ 7.2 mg/kg/day corresponding to ≥ 8 times the esti mated human exposure (see above). There was no treat ment-related effect on embryo-fetal development.

No studies to evaluate effects of retapamulin on pre-/post-natal development were performed. However, there were no systemic effects on juvenile rats with topical applicatior of retapamulin ointment.

6. PHARMACEUTICAL PARTICULARS

6.1 List of excipients

White soft paraffin.

Butylated hydroxytoluene

6.2 Incompatibilities

Not applicable.

6.3 Shelf life

Unopened: 2 years.

In-use: 7 days.

6.4 Special precautions for storage

Do not store above 25°C.

6.5 Nature and contents of container

0.5 g aluminium foil sachet. Carton of 12 sachets.

5 g, 10 g and 15 g aluminium tubes with a plastic screw cap. Carton of 1 tube.

Not all pack sizes may be marketed.

6.6 Special precautions for disposal and other handling

Any remaining ointment at the end of treatment should be discarded.

Any unused product or waste material should be disposed of in accordance with local requirements.

7. MARKETING AUTHORISATION HOLDER

Glaxo Group Ltd

Greenford Road

Greenford

Middlesex UB6 0NN

United Kingdom

8. MARKETING AUTHORISATION NUMBER(S)

EU/1/07/390/001

EU/1/07/390/002

EU/1/07/390/003

EU/1/07/390/004

9. DATE OF FIRST AUTHORISATION/RENEWAL OF THE AUTHORISATION

24 May 2007

10. DATE OF REVISION OF THE TEXT

24 May 2007

Detailed information on this medicine is available on the European Medicines Agency (EMEA) web site: http://www.emea.europa.eu/.

Alvedon Suppositories 60, 125, 250 mg

(AstraZeneca UK Limited)

1. NAME OF THE MEDICINAL PRODUCT

Alvedon Suppositories 60, 125, 250 mg.

2. QUALITATIVE AND QUANTITATIVE COMPOSITION

Each suppository contains Paracetamol 60, 125 or 250 mg.

For excipients see 6.1.

3. PHARMACEUTICAL FORM

Suppositories.

4. CLINICAL PARTICULARS

4.1 Therapeutic indications

For the treatment of mild to moderate pain and pyrexia in children:

up to the age of 1 year - 60 mg suppositories

aged 1-5 years - 125 mg suppositories

aged 6-12 years - 250 mg suppositories

Alvedon suppositories may be especially useful in patients unable to take oral forms of paracetamol, e.g. post-operatively or with nausea and vomiting.

4.2 Posology and method of administration

60 mg suppositories

Children 3 months to 1 year, 1-2 suppositories:

The dosage should be based on age and weight i.e.

Table 1 Clinical Success Rates at Follow up for SIOW patients with *S. aureus*

Phenotype/PFGE type	RETAPAMULIN			Cephalexin	
	n/N	Success Rate (%)	95% Exact CI	n/N	Success Rate (%)
S. aureus (all)	337/379	88.9	(85.3,91.9)	155/186	83.3
MRSA $	28/37	75.7	(58.8,88.2)	21/26	80.8
MSSA	309/342	90.4	(86.7,93.3)	133/159	83.6

CI: confidence interval. Exact CI is calculated using the F-distribution method.

$: the response rate for MRSA due to PVL+ MRSA was 8/13 (62%)

months (5 kg) - 60mg (1 suppository)

year (10 kg) - 120mg (2 suppositories)

nfants under 3 months:

One suppository (60 mg) is suitable for babies who develop fever following immunisation at 2 months. Otherwise only use in babies aged less than 3 months on a doctor's advice.

125 mg suppositories

Children 1-5 years, 1-2 suppositories:

The dosage should be based on age and weight i.e.

1 year (10 Kg) - 125mg (1 suppository)

5 years (20 Kg) -250mg (2 suppositories)

250 mg suppositories

Children 6 to 12 years 1-2 suppositories:

The dosage should be based on age and weight i.e.

6 years (20 Kg) - 250mg (1 suppository)

12 years (40 Kg) - 500mg (2 suppositories)

These doses may be repeated up to a maximum of 4 times in 24 hours. The dose should not be repeated more frequently than every 4 hours. The recommended dose should not be exceeded. Higher doses do not produce any increase in analgesic effect. Only whole suppositories should be administered – do not break suppository before administration.

4.3 Contraindications

Hypersensitivity to paracetamol or hard fat

4.4 Special warnings and precautions for use

Alvedon Suppositories should not be combined with other analgesic medications that contain paracetamol. Paracetamol should be given with care to patients with impaired kidney or liver function.

Label and Leaflet will state the following warnings:

Label:

"Immediate medical advice should be sought in the event of an overdose, even if the child seems well".

"Do not give with any other Paracetamol-containing products."

Leaflet:

"Immediate medical advice should be sought in the event of an overdose, even if the child seems well, because of the risk of delayed, serious liver damage."

4.5 Interaction with other medicinal products and other forms of interaction

Drugs which induce hepatic microsomal enzymes such as alcohol, barbiturates and other anticonvulsants, may increase the hepatotoxicity of paracetamol, particularly after overdosage.

The anti-coagulant effect of warfarin and other coumarins may be enhanced by prolonged regular use of paracetamol with increased risk of bleeding. The effect appears to increase as the dose of paracetamol is increased, but can occur with doses as low as 1.5 – 2 g paracetamol per day for at least 5 – 7 days. Occasional doses have no significant effect.

Enzyme-inducing medicines, such as some antiepileptic drugs (phenytoin, phenobarbital, carbamazepine) have been shown in pharmacokinetic studies to reduce the plasma AUC of paracetamol to approx. 60 %. Other substances with enzyme-inducing properties, e.g. rifampicin and St. John's wort (hypericum) are also suspected of causing lowered concentrations of paracetamol. In addition, the risk of liver damage during treatment with maximum recommended doses of paracetamol will be higher in patients being treated with enzyme-inducing agents.

4.6 Pregnancy and lactation

Not applicable.

4.7 Effects on ability to drive and use machines

None known.

4.8 Undesirable effects

Side-effects at therapeutic doses are rare.

Common >1/100	*Miscellaneous:*	Redness of the rectal mucous membranes
Rare <1/1000	*General:*	Allergic reactions
	Skin:	Exanthema, urticaria
	Liver:	Liver damage
	Genitourinary:	Increase in creatinine (mostly secondary to hepatorenal syndrome)

There have been reports of blood dyscrasias including thrombocytopenia and agranulocytosis, but these were not necessarily causally related to paracetamol.

Hepatic necrosis may occur after overdosage (see below).

4.9 Overdose

Immediate treatment is essential in the management of paracetamol overdose. Despite a lack of significant early symptoms, patients should be referred to a hospital urgently for immediate medical attention. Administration of oral methionine or intravenous N-acetylcysteine which may have a beneficial effect up to at least 48 hours after the overdose, may be required. General supportive measures must be available.

Symptoms of paracetamol overdose in the first 24 hours are pallor, nausea, vomiting, anorexia and abdominal pain. Liver damage may become apparent 12 to 48 hours after ingestion ingestion and clinical symptoms generally culminate after 4-6 days.

Abnormalities of glucose metabolism and metabolic acidosis may occur. In severe poisoning, hepatic failure may progress to encephalopathy, coma and death. Acute renal failure with acute tubular necrosis may develop even in the absence of severe liver damage. Cardiac arrhythmias and pancreatitis have been reported.

Toxicity: 5 g during 24 hours in a child aged 3 ½ years, 15-20 g in adults, caused fatal intoxication. The toxic dose for children and adults is generally >140 mg/kg. Malnutrition, dehydration, medication with enzyme-inducing drugs such as some antiepileptic drugs (phenytoin, phenobarbital, carbamazepine), rifampicin and St. John's wort (hypericum are risk factors, and even slight overdosage can then cause marked liver damage. Even subacute "therapeutic" overdose has resulted in severe intoxication with doses varying from 6 g/24 hours for a week, 20 g for 2-3 days, etc.

5. PHARMACOLOGICAL PROPERTIES

5.1 Pharmacodynamic properties

ATC code: N02BE01

Paracetamol is an aniline derivative with analgesic and antipyretic actions similar to those of aspirin but with no demonstrable anti-inflammatory activity. Paracetamol is less irritant to the stomach than aspirin. It does not affect thrombocyte aggregation or bleeding time. Paracetamol is generally well tolerated by patients hypersensitive to acetylsalicylic acid.

5.2 Pharmacokinetic properties

Paracetamol is well absorbed by both oral and rectal routes. Peak plasma concentrations occur about 2 to 3 hours after rectal administration. The plasma half life is about 2 hours.

Paracetamol is primarily metabolised in the liver by conjugation to glucuronide and sulphate. A small amount (about 3-10% of a therapeutic dose) is metabolised by oxidation and the reactive intermediate metabolite thus formed is bound preferentially to the liver glutathione and excreted as cystein and mercapturic acid conjugates. Excretion occurs via the kidneys. 2-3% of a therapeutic dose is excreted unchanged; 80-90% as glucuronide and sulphate and a smaller amount as cystein and mercapturic acid derivatives.

5.3 Preclinical safety data

Not applicable

6. PHARMACEUTICAL PARTICULARS

6.1 List of excipients

Hard fat (Witepsol H12)

6.2 Incompatibilities

None known.

6.3 Shelf life

3 years.

6.4 Special precautions for storage

Do not store above 25°C.

6.5 Nature and contents of container

PVC/polyethylene blister strips each containing 5 suppositories. Packs of 5 or 10 suppositories.

PVC/polyethylene blister strips each containing 1 suppository. Packs of 10 suppositories.

PVC/polyethylene blister strips each containing 1 suppository packed in high density polyethylene (HDPE) bottles with tamper-proof, child resistant, polypropylene (PP) lids. Packs of 10 suppositories.

Not all pack sizes may be marketed.

6.6 Special precautions for disposal and other handling

Peel the wrapper apart to remove the suppository, gently push into the rectum pointed end first.

7. MARKETING AUTHORISATION HOLDER

AstraZeneca UK Ltd.,

600 Capability Green,

Luton,

LU1 3LU,

UK

8. MARKETING AUTHORISATION NUMBER(S)

PL 17901/0096, 0097, 0098

9. DATE OF FIRST AUTHORISATION/RENEWAL OF THE AUTHORISATION

16th June 2002

10. DATE OF REVISION OF THE TEXT

14th September 2005

Alvesco 160 Inhaler

(Nycomed UK Ltd)

1. NAME OF THE MEDICINAL PRODUCT

Alvesco®▼ 160 Inhaler

2. QUALITATIVE AND QUANTITATIVE COMPOSITION

1 actuation (delivered dose from the mouthpiece) contains 160 micrograms of ciclesonide.

For excipients, see section 6.1.

3. PHARMACEUTICAL FORM

Pressurised inhalation, solution

Clear and colourless

4. CLINICAL PARTICULARS

4.1 Therapeutic indications

Treatment to control persistent asthma in adults and adolescents (12 years and older).

4.2 Posology and method of administration

The medicinal product is for inhalation use only.

Dosing recommendation for adults and adolescents:

The recommended dose of Alvesco is 160 micrograms once daily, which leads to asthma control in the majority of patients. However in severe asthmatics, a 12 week study has shown that a dose of 640 micrograms/day (given 320 micrograms twice daily) has demonstrated a reduction in the frequency of exacerbations but without an improvement in lung function (see section 5.1). Dose reduction to 80 micrograms once daily may be an effective maintenance dose for some patients.

Alvesco should preferably be administered in the evening although morning dosing of Alvesco has also been shown to be effective. The final decision on evening or morning dosing should be left to the discretion of the physician.

Symptoms start to improve with Alvesco within 24 hours of treatment. Once control is achieved, the dose of Alvesco should be individualised and titrated to the minimum dose needed to maintain good asthma control.

Patients with severe asthma are at risk of acute attacks and should have regular assessments of their asthma control including pulmonary function tests. Increasing use of short-acting bronchodilators to relieve asthma symptoms indicates deterioration of asthma control. If patients find that short-acting relief bronchodilator treatment becomes less effective, or they need more inhalations than usual, medical attention must be sought. In this situation, patients should be reassessed and consideration given to the need for increased anti-inflammatory treatment therapy (e.g. a higher dose of Alvesco for a short period [see section 5.1] or a course of oral corticosteroids). Severe asthma exacerbations should be managed the usual way.

To address specific patient needs, such as finding it difficult to press the inhaler and breathe in at the same time, Alvesco can be used with the AeroChamber Plus spacer device.

Specific patient groups:

There is no need to adjust the dose in elderly patients or those with hepatic or renal impairment.

To date, there are insufficient data available in the treatment of children under 12 years of age with ciclesonide.

Instructions for use / handling:

The patient needs to be instructed how to use the inhaler correctly.

If the inhaler is new or has not been used for one week or more, three puffs should be released into the air. No shaking is necessary as this is a solution aerosol.

During inhalation, the patient should preferably sit or stand, and the inhaler should be held upright with the thumb on the base, below the mouthpiece.

Instruct the patient to remove the mouthpiece cover, place the inhaler into their mouth, close their lips around the mouthpiece, and breathe in slowly and deeply. While breathing in through the mouth, the top of the inhaler should be pressed down. Then, patients should remove the inhaler from their mouth, and hold their breath for about 10 seconds, or as long as is comfortable. The patient is not to breathe out into the inhaler. Finally, patients should breathe out slowly and replace the mouthpiece cover.

The mouthpiece should be cleaned with a dry tissue or cloth weekly. The inhaler should not be washed or put in water.

For detailed instructions see Patient Information Leaflet.

4.3 Contraindications

Hypersensitivity to ciclesonide or any of the excipients.

4.4 Special warnings and precautions for use

As with all inhaled corticosteroids, Alvesco should be administered with caution in patients with active or quiescent pulmonary tuberculosis, fungal, viral or bacterial infections, and only if these patients are adequately treated.

As with all inhaled corticosteroids, Alvesco is not indicated in the treatment of status asthmaticus or other acute episodes of asthma where intensive measures are required.

As with all inhaled corticosteroids, Alvesco is not designed to relieve acute asthma symptoms for which an inhaled short-acting bronchodilator is required. Patients should be advised to have such rescue medication available.

Systemic effects of inhaled corticosteroids may occur, particularly at high doses prescribed for prolonged periods. These effects are much less likely to occur than with oral corticosteroids. Possible systemic effects include adrenal suppression, growth retardation in children and adolescents, decrease in bone mineral density, cataract and glaucoma. It is therefore important that the dose of inhaled corticosteroid is titrated to the lowest dose at which effective control of asthma is maintained.

It is recommended that the height of children and adolescents receiving prolonged treatment with inhaled corticosteroids is regularly monitored. If growth is slowed, therapy should be reviewed with the aim of reducing the dose of inhaled corticosteroid, if possible to the lowest dose at which effective control of asthma is maintained. In addition, consideration should be given to referring the patient to a paediatric respiratory specialist.

There is no data available in patients with severe hepatic impairment. An increased exposure in patients with severe hepatic impairment is expected and these patients should therefore be monitored for potential systemic effects.

The benefits of inhaled ciclesonide should minimise the need for oral steroids. However, patients transferred from oral steroids remain at risk of impaired adrenal reserve for a considerable time after transferring to inhaled ciclesonide. The possibility of respective symptoms may persist for some time.

These patients may require specialised advice to determine the extent of adrenal impairment before elective procedures. The possibility of residual impaired adrenal response should always be considered in an emergency (medical or surgical) and elective situations likely to produce stress, and appropriate corticosteroid treatment considered.

For the transfer of patients being treated with oral corticosteroids:

The transfer of oral steroid-dependent patients to inhaled ciclesonide, and their subsequent management, needs special care as recovery from impaired adrenocortical function, caused by prolonged systemic steroid therapy, may take a considerable time.

Patients who have been treated with systemic steroids for long periods of time, or at a high dose, may have adrenocortical suppression. With these patients adrenocortical function should be monitored regularly and their dose of systemic steroid reduced cautiously.

After approximately a week, gradual withdrawal of the systemic steroid is started by reducing the dose by 1 mg prednisolone per week, or its equivalent. For maintenance doses of prednisolone in excess of 10 mg daily, it may be appropriate to cautiously use larger reductions in dose at weekly intervals.

Some patients feel unwell in a non-specific way during the withdrawal phase despite maintenance or even improvement of respiratory function. They should be encouraged to persevere with inhaled ciclesonide and to continue withdrawal of systemic steroid, unless there are objective signs of adrenal insufficiency.

Patients transferred from oral steroids whose adrenocortical function is still impaired should carry a steroid warning card indicating that they need supplementary systemic steroid during periods of stress, e.g. worsening asthma attacks, chest infections, major intercurrent illness, surgery, trauma, etc.

Replacement of systemic steroid treatment with inhaled therapy sometimes unmasks allergies such as allergic rhinitis or eczema previously controlled by systemic drug.

Paradoxical bronchospasm with an immediate increase of wheezing or other symptoms of bronchoconstriction after dosing should be treated with an inhaled short-acting bronchodilator, which usually results in quick relief. The patient should be assessed and therapy with Alvesco should only be continued, if after careful consideration the expected benefit is greater than the possible risk. Correlation between severity of asthma and general susceptibility for acute bronchial reactions should be kept in mind (see section 4.8).

Patients inhaler technique should be checked regularly to make sure that inhaler actuation is synchronised with inhaling to ensure optimum delivery to the lungs.

Concomitant treatment with ketoconazole or other potent CYP3A4 inhibitors should be avoided unless the benefit outweighs the increased risk of systemic side effects of corticosteroids (see section 4.5).

4.5 Interaction with other medicinal products and other forms of interaction

In vitro data indicate that CYP3A4 is the major enzyme involved in the metabolism of the active metabolite of ciclesonide M1 in man.

In a drug-drug interaction study at steady state with ciclesonide and ketoconazole as a potent CYP3A4 inhibitor, the exposure to the active metabolite M1 increased approximately 3.5-fold, whereas the exposure to ciclesonide was not affected. Therefore the concomitant administration of potent inhibitors of CYP 3A4 (e.g. ketoconazole, itraconazole and ritonavir or nelfinavir) should be avoided unless the benefit outweighs the increased risk of systemic side effects of corticosteroids.

4.6 Pregnancy and lactation

There are no adequate and well-controlled studies in pregnant women.

In animal studies glucocorticoids have been shown to induce malformations (see section 5.3). This is not likely to be relevant for humans given recommended inhalation doses.

As with other glucocorticoids, ciclesonide should only be used during pregnancy if the potential benefit to the mother justifies the potential risk to the fetus. The lowest effective dose of ciclesonide needed to maintain adequate asthma control should be used.

Infants born of mothers who received corticosteroids during pregnancy are to be observed carefully for hypoadrenalism.

It is unknown whether inhaled ciclesonide is excreted in human breast milk. Administration of ciclesonide to women who are breast-feeding should only be considered if the expected benefit to the mother is greater than any possible risk to the child.

4.7 Effects on ability to drive and use machines

Inhaled ciclesonide has no or negligible influence on the ability to drive and use machines.

4.8 Undesirable effects

Approximately 5% of patients experienced adverse reactions in clinical trials with Alvesco given in the dose range 40 to 1280 micrograms per day. In the majority of cases, these were mild and did not require discontinuation of treatment with Alvesco.

(see Table 1 above)

Table 1

Frequency / System Organ Class	Uncommon (>1/1,000, <1/100)	Rare (1/10,000 – 1/,1000)
Cardiac Disorders		Palpitations**
Gastrointestinal Disorders	Nausea, vomiting* Bad taste	Abdominal pain* Dyspepsia*
General disorders and administration site conditions	Application site reactions Application site dryness	
Immune System Disorders		Angioedema Hypersensitivity
Infections and infestations	Oral fungal infections*	
Nervous System Disorders	Headache*	
Respiratory, thoracic and mediastinal disorders	Dysphonia Cough after inhalation* Paradoxical bronchospasm*	
Skin and subcutaneous tissue disorders	Eczema and rash	
Vascular disorders		Hypertension

* Similar or lower incidence when compared with placebo

** Palpitations were observed in clinical trials in cases mostly confounded with concomitant medication with known cardiac effects (e.g. theophylline or salbutamol).

Paradoxical bronchospasm may occur immediately after dosing and is an unspecific acute reaction to all inhaled medicinal products, which may be related to the active substance, the excipient, or evaporation cooling in the case of metered dose inhalers. In severe cases, withdrawal of Alvesco should be considered.

Systemic effects of inhaled corticosteroids may occur, particularly at high doses prescribed for prolonged periods. Possible systemic effects include Cushing's syndrome, Cushingoid features, adrenal suppression, growth retardation in children and adolescents, decrease in bone mineral density, cataract, glaucoma (see also section 4.4).

4.9 Overdose

Acute:

Inhalation by healthy volunteers of a single dose of 2880 micrograms of ciclesonide was well tolerated.

The potential for acute toxic effects following overdose of inhaled ciclesonide is low. After acute overdosage no specific treatment is necessary.

Chronic:

After prolonged administration of 1280 micrograms of ciclesonide, no clinical signs of adrenal suppression were observed. However, if higher than recommended dosage is continued over prolonged periods, some degree of adrenal suppression cannot be excluded. Monitoring of adrenal reserve may be necessary.

5. PHARMACOLOGICAL PROPERTIES

5.1 Pharmacodynamic properties

Pharmacotherapeutic group: Other drugs for obstructive airway diseases, Inhalants, Glucocorticoids, ATC Code: R03B A08

Ciclesonide exhibits low binding affinity to the glucocorticoid-receptor. Once orally inhaled, ciclesonide is enzymatically converted in the lungs to the principal metabolite (C21-des-methylpropionyl-ciclesonide) which has a pronounced anti-inflammatory activity and is thus considered as the active metabolite.

In four clinical trials, ciclesonide has been shown to reduce airway hyperresponsiveness to adenosine monophosphate in hyperreactive patients with maximal effect observed at the dose of 640 micrograms. In another trial, pretreatment with ciclesonide for seven days significantly attenuated the early and late phase reactions following inhaled allergen challenge. Inhaled ciclesonide treatment was also shown to attenuate the increase in inflammatory cells (total eosinophils) and inflammatory mediators in induced sputum.

A controlled study compared 24-hour plasma cortisol AUC in 26 adult asthmatic patients following 7 days of treatment. Compared to placebo, treatment with ciclesonide 320, 640, and 1,280 micrograms/day did not statistically significantly lower the 24-hour time averages of plasma cortisol ($AUC_{(0-24)}$/24 hours) nor was a dose-dependent effect seen.

In a clinical trial involving 164 adult male and female asthmatic patients, ciclesonide was given at doses of 320 micrograms or 640 micrograms/day over 12 weeks. After stimulation with 1 and 250 micrograms cosyntropin, no significant changes in plasma cortisol levels were observed versus placebo.

Double-blind placebo-controlled trials of 12-weeks duration in adults and adolescents have shown that treatment with ciclesonide resulted in improved lung function as measured by FEV_1 and peak expiratory flow, improved asthma symptom control, and decreased need for inhaled beta-2 agonist.

In a 12-week study of 680 severe asthmatics, previously treated with 500-1,000 micrograms fluticasone propionate per day or equivalent, 87.3% and 93.3% of patients remained exacerbation-free during treatment with 160 or 640 micrograms of ciclesonide, respectively. At the end of the 12 week study period, the results showed a statistically significant difference between the doses of 160 micrograms and 640 micrograms/day ciclesonide with regard to the occurrence of an exacerbation after the first day of the study: 43 patients/339 (= 12.7%) in the 160 micrograms/day group and 23 patients/341 (6.7%) in the 640 micrograms/day group (Hazard ratio=0.526; p= 0.0134). Both ciclesonide doses resulted in comparable FEV1 values at 12 weeks. Treatment-related adverse events were seen in 3.8% and 5% of patients treated with 160 or 640 micrograms per day of ciclesonide respectively. No study was performed to compare 160 micrograms, 320 micrograms and 640 micrograms daily dose in patients with severe asthma.

5.2 Pharmacokinetic properties

Ciclesonide is presented in HFA-134a propellant and ethanol as a solution aerosol, which demonstrates a linear relationship between different doses, puff strengths and systemic exposure.

Absorption:

Studies with oral and intravenous dosing of radiolabeled ciclesonide have shown an incomplete extent of oral absorption (24.5%). The oral bioavailability of both ciclesonide and the active metabolite is negligible (<0.5% for ciclesonide, <1% for the metabolite). Based on a γ-scintigraphy experiment, lung deposition in healthy subjects is 52%. In line with this figure, the systemic bioavailability for the active metabolite is >50% by using the ciclesonide metered dose inhaler. As the oral bioavailability for the active metabolite is <1%, the swallowed portion of the inhaled ciclesonide does not contribute to systemic absorption.

Distribution:

Following intravenous administration to healthy subjects, the initial distribution phase for ciclesonide was rapid and consistent with its high lipophilicity. The volume of distribution averaged 2.9 l/kg. The total serum clearance of ciclesonide is high (average 2.0 l/h/kg) indicating a high hepatic extraction. The percentage of ciclesonide bound to human plasma proteins averaged 99%, and that of the active metabolite 98-99%, indicating an almost complete binding of circulating ciclesonide/active metabolite to plasma proteins.

Metabolism:

Ciclesonide is primarily hydrolysed to its biologically active metabolite by esterase enzymes in the lung. Investigation of the enzymology of further metabolism by human liver microsomes showed that this compound is mainly metabolized to hydroxylated inactive metabolites by CYP3A4 catalysis. Furthermore, reversible lipophilic fatty acid ester conjugates of the active metabolite were detected in the lung.

Excretion:

Ciclesonide is predominantly excreted via the faeces (67%), after oral and intravenous administration, indicating that excretion via the bile is the major route of elimination.

Pharmacokinetic characteristics in patients:

Asthmatic patients

Ciclesonide shows no pharmacokinetic changes in mild asthmatic patients compared to healthy subjects.

Renal or hepatic insufficiency, elderly

According to population pharmacokinetics, age has no impact on the systemic exposure of the active metabolite.

Reduced liver function may affect the elimination of corticosteroids. In a study including patients with hepatic impairment suffering from liver cirrhosis, a higher systemic exposure to the active metabolite was observed.

Due to the lack of renal excretion of the active metabolite, studies on renal impaired patients have not been performed.

5.3 Preclinical safety data

Preclinical data with ciclesonide reveal no special hazard for humans based on conventional studies of safety pharmacology, repeated dose toxicity, genotoxicity, or carcinogenic potential.

In animal studies on reproductive toxicity, glucocorticosteroids have been shown to induce malformations (cleft palate, skeletal malformations). However, these animal results do not seem to be relevant for humans given recommended doses.

A treatment-related effect on the ovaries (namely atrophy) was observed at the top dose in two 12-month studies in dogs. This effect occurred at systemic exposures 5.27-8.34 times those noted at the 160 µg daily dose. The relevance of this finding to humans is unknown.

Animal studies with other glucocorticoids indicate that administration of pharmacological doses of glucocorticoids during pregnancy may increase the risk for intrauterine growth retardation, adult cardiovascular and/or metabolic disease and/or permanent changes in glucocorticoid receptor density, neurotransmitter turnover and behaviour. The relevance of these data to humans administered ciclesonide by inhalation is unknown.

6. PHARMACEUTICAL PARTICULARS

6.1 List of excipients

Norflurane (HFA-134a)

Ethanol, anhydrous

6.2 Incompatibilities

Not applicable.

6.3 Shelf life

30 metered actuations – 1 year

60 and 120 metered actuations – 3 years

6.4 Special precautions for storage

This medicinal product does not require any special storage conditions.

The container contains a pressurised liquid. Do not expose to temperatures higher than 50°C.

The container should not be punctured, broken or burnt even when apparently empty.

6.5 Nature and contents of container

The inhaler comprises a pressurised container made from aluminium and is sealed with a metering valve, mouthpiece, and cap.

30 metered actuations

60 metered actuations

120 metered actuations

Hospital packs:

10 × 30 metered actuations

10 × 60 metered actuations

10 × 120 metered actuations

Not all pack sizes may be marketed.

6.6 Special precautions for disposal and other handling

Patients should be carefully instructed in the proper use of their inhaler (see Patient Information Leaflet).

As with most inhaled medicinal products in pressurised containers, the therapeutic effect of this medicinal product may decrease when the container is cold. However, Alvesco delivers a consistent dose from –10°C to 40°C.

7. MARKETING AUTHORISATION HOLDER

Nycomed GmbH

Byk-Gulden-Str. 2

D-78467 Konstanz

Germany

8. MARKETING AUTHORISATION NUMBER(S)

PL 31752/0006

9. DATE OF FIRST AUTHORISATION/RENEWAL OF THE AUTHORISATION

16 April 2004

10. DATE OF REVISION OF THE TEXT

19 February 2009

Alvesco 80 Inhaler

(Nycomed UK Ltd)

1. NAME OF THE MEDICINAL PRODUCT

Alvesco®▼ 80 Inhaler

2. QUALITATIVE AND QUANTITATIVE COMPOSITION

1 actuation (delivered dose from the mouthpiece) contains 80 micrograms of ciclesonide.

For excipients, see section 6.1.

3. PHARMACEUTICAL FORM

Pressurised inhalation, solution

Clear and colourless

4. CLINICAL PARTICULARS

4.1 Therapeutic indications

Treatment to control persistent asthma in adults and adolescents (12 years and older).

4.2 Posology and method of administration

The medicinal product is for inhalation use only.

Dosing recommendation for adults and adolescents:

The recommended dose of Alvesco is 160 micrograms once daily, which leads to asthma control in the majority of patients. However in severe asthmatics, a 12 week study has shown that a dose of 640 micrograms/day (given 320 micrograms twice daily) has demonstrated a reduction in the frequency of exacerbations but without an improvement in lung function (see section 5.1). Dose reduction to 80 micrograms once daily may be an effective maintenance dose for some patients.

Alvesco should preferably be administered in the evening although morning dosing of Alvesco has also been shown to be effective. The final decision on evening or morning dosing should be left to the discretion of the physician.

Symptoms start to improve with Alvesco within 24 hours of treatment. Once control is achieved, the dose of Alvesco should be individualised and titrated to the minimum dose needed to maintain good asthma control.

Patients with severe asthma are at risk of acute attacks and should have regular assessments of their asthma control including pulmonary function tests. Increasing use of short-acting bronchodilators to relieve asthma symptoms indicates deterioration of asthma control. If patients find that short-acting relief bronchodilator treatment becomes less effective, or they need more inhalations than usual, medical attention must be sought. In this situation, patients should be reassessed and consideration given to the need for increased anti-inflammatory treatment therapy (e.g. a higher dose of Alvesco for a short period [see section 5.1] or a course of oral corticosteroids). Severe asthma exacerbations should be managed the usual way.

To address specific patient needs, such as finding it difficult to press the inhaler and breathe in at the same time, Alvesco can be used with the AeroChamber Plus spacer device.

Specific patient groups:

There is no need to adjust the dose in elderly patients or those with hepatic or renal impairment.

To date, there are insufficient data available in the treatment of children under 12 years of age with ciclesonide.

Instructions for use / handling:

The patient needs to be instructed how to use the inhaler correctly.

If the inhaler is new or has not been used for one week or more, three puffs should be released into the air. No shaking is necessary as this is a solution aerosol.

During inhalation, the patient should preferably sit or stand, and the inhaler should be held upright with the thumb on the base, below the mouthpiece.

Instruct the patient to remove the mouthpiece cover, place the inhaler into their mouth, close their lips around the mouthpiece, and breathe in slowly and deeply. While breathing in through the mouth, the top of the inhaler should be pressed down. Then, patients should remove the inhaler from their mouth, and hold their breath for about 10 seconds, or as long as is comfortable. The patient is not to breathe out into the inhaler. Finally, patients should breathe out slowly and replace the mouthpiece cover.

The mouthpiece should be cleaned with a dry tissue or cloth weekly. The inhaler should not be washed or put in water.

For detailed instructions see Patient Information Leaflet.

4.3 Contraindications

Hypersensitivity to ciclesonide or any of the excipients.

4.4 Special warnings and precautions for use

As with all inhaled corticosteroids, Alvesco should be administered with caution in patients with active or quiescent pulmonary tuberculosis, fungal, viral or bacterial infections, and only if these patients are adequately treated.

As with all inhaled corticosteroids, Alvesco is not indicated in the treatment of status asthmaticus or other acute episodes of asthma where intensive measures are required.

As with all inhaled corticosteroids, Alvesco is not designed to relieve acute asthma symptoms for which an inhaled short-acting bronchodilator is required. Patients should be advised to have such rescue medication available.

Systemic effects of inhaled corticosteroids may occur, particularly at high doses prescribed for prolonged periods. These effects are much less likely to occur than with oral corticosteroids. Possible systemic effects include adrenal suppression, growth retardation in children and adolescents, decrease in bone mineral density, cataract and glaucoma. It is therefore important that the dose of inhaled corticosteroid is titrated to the lowest dose at which effective control of asthma is maintained.

It is recommended that the height of children and adolescents receiving prolonged treatment with inhaled corticosteroids is regularly monitored. If growth is slowed, therapy should be reviewed with the aim of reducing the dose of inhaled corticosteroid, if possible to the lowest dose at which effective control of asthma is maintained. In addition, consideration should be given to referring the patient to a paediatric respiratory specialist.

There is no data available in patients with severe hepatic impairment. An increased exposure in patients with severe hepatic impairment is expected and these patients should therefore be monitored for potential systemic effects.

The benefits of inhaled ciclesonide should minimise the need for oral steroids. However, patients transferred from oral steroids remain at risk of impaired adrenal reserve for a considerable time after transferring to inhaled ciclesonide. The possibility of respective symptoms may persist for some time.

These patients may require specialised advice to determine the extent of adrenal impairment before elective procedures. The possibility of residual impaired adrenal response should always be considered in an emergency (medical or surgical) and elective situations likely to produce stress, and appropriate corticosteroid treatment considered.

For the transfer of patients being treated with oral corticosteroids:

The transfer of oral steroid-dependent patients to inhaled ciclesonide, and their subsequent management, needs special care as recovery from impaired adrenocortical function, caused by prolonged systemic steroid therapy, may take a considerable time.

Patients who have been treated with systemic steroids for long periods of time, or at a high dose, may have adrenocortical suppression. With these patients adrenocortical function should be monitored regularly and their dose of systemic steroid reduced cautiously.

After approximately a week, gradual withdrawal of the systemic steroid is started by reducing the dose by 1 mg prednisolone per week, or its equivalent. For maintenance doses of prednisolone in excess of 10 mg daily, it may be appropriate to cautiously use larger reductions in dose at weekly intervals.

Some patients feel unwell in a non-specific way during the withdrawal phase despite maintenance or even improvement of respiratory function. They should be encouraged to persevere with inhaled ciclesonide and to continue withdrawal of systemic steroid, unless there are objective signs of adrenal insufficiency.

Patients transferred from oral steroids whose adrenocortical function is still impaired should carry a steroid warning card indicating that they need supplementary systemic steroid during periods of stress, e.g. worsening asthma attacks, chest infections, major intercurrent illness, surgery, trauma, etc.

Replacement of systemic steroid treatment with inhaled therapy sometimes unmasks allergies such as allergic rhinitis or eczema previously controlled by systemic drug.

Paradoxical bronchospasm with an immediate increase of wheezing or other symptoms of bronchoconstriction after dosing should be treated with an inhaled short-acting bronchodilator, which usually results in quick relief. The patient should be assessed and therapy with Alvesco should only be continued, if after careful consideration the expected benefit is greater than the possible risk. Correlation between severity of asthma and general

Table 1

Frequency / System Organ Class	Uncommon (>1/1,000, <1/100)	Rare (1/10,000 – 1/,1000)
Cardiac Disorders		Palpitations**
Gastrointestinal Disorders	Nausea, vomiting* Bad taste	Abdominal pain* Dyspepsia*
General disorders and administration site conditions	Application site reactions Application site dryness	
Immune System Disorders		Angioedema Hypersensitivity
Infections and infestations	Oral fungal infections*	
Nervous System Disorders	Headache*	
Respiratory, thoracic and mediastinal disorders	Dysphonia Cough after inhalation* Paradoxical bronchospasm*	
Skin and subcutaneous tissue disorders	Eczema and rash	
Vascular disorders		Hypertension

* Similar or lower incidence when compared with placebo

** Palpitations were observed in clinical trials in cases mostly confounded with concomitant medication with known cardiac effects (e.g. theophylline or salbutamol).

susceptibility for acute bronchial reactions should be kept in mind (see section 4.8).

Patients inhaler technique should be checked regularly to make sure that inhaler actuation is synchronised with inhaling to ensure optimum delivery to the lungs.

Concomitant treatment with ketoconazole or other potent CYP3A4 inhibitors should be avoided unless the benefit outweighs the increased risk of systemic side effects of corticosteroids (see section 4.5).

4.5 Interaction with other medicinal products and other forms of interaction

In vitro data indicate that CYP3A4 is the major enzyme involved in the metabolism of the active metabolite of ciclesonide M1 in man.

In a drug-drug interaction study at steady state with ciclesonide and ketoconazole as a potent CYP3A4 inhibitor, the exposure to the active metabolite M1 increased approximately 3.5-fold, whereas the exposure to ciclesonide was not affected. Therefore the concomitant administration of potent inhibitors of CYP 3A4 (e.g. ketoconazole, itraconazole and ritonavir or nelfinavir) should be avoided unless the benefit outweighs the increased risk of systemic side effects of corticosteroids.

4.6 Pregnancy and lactation

There are no adequate and well-controlled studies in pregnant women.

In animal studies glucocorticoids have been shown to induce malformations (see section 5.3). This is not likely to be relevant for humans given recommended inhalation doses.

As with other glucocorticoids, ciclesonide should only be used during pregnancy if the potential benefit to the mother justifies the potential risk to the fetus. The lowest effective dose of ciclesonide needed to maintain adequate asthma control should be used.

Infants born of mothers who received corticosteroids during pregnancy are to be observed carefully for hypoadrenalism.

It is unknown whether inhaled ciclesonide is excreted in human breast milk. Administration of ciclesonide to women who are breast-feeding should only be considered if the expected benefit to the mother is greater than any possible risk to the child.

4.7 Effects on ability to drive and use machines

Inhaled ciclesonide has no or negligible influence on the ability to drive and use machines.

4.8 Undesirable effects

Approximately 5% of patients experienced adverse reactions in clinical trials with Alvesco given in the dose range 40 to 1280 micrograms per day. In the majority of cases, these were mild and did not require discontinuation of treatment with Alvesco.

(see Table 1 above)

Paradoxical bronchospasm may occur immediately after dosing and is an unspecific acute reaction to all inhaled medicinal products, which may be related to the active substance, the excipient, or evaporation cooling in the case of metered dose inhalers. In severe cases, withdrawal of Alvesco should be considered.

Systemic effects of inhaled corticosteroids may occur, particularly at high doses prescribed for prolonged periods. Possible systemic effects include Cushing's syndrome, Cushingoid features, adrenal suppression, growth retardation in children and adolescents, decrease in bone mineral density, cataract, glaucoma (see also section 4.4).

4.9 Overdose

Acute:

Inhalation by healthy volunteers of a single dose of 2880 micrograms of ciclesonide was well tolerated.

The potential for acute toxic effects following overdose of inhaled ciclesonide is low. After acute overdosage no specific treatment is necessary.

Chronic:

After prolonged administration of 1280 micrograms of ciclesonide, no clinical signs of adrenal suppression were observed. However, if higher than recommended dosage is continued over prolonged periods, some degree of adrenal suppression cannot be excluded. Monitoring of adrenal reserve may be necessary.

5. PHARMACOLOGICAL PROPERTIES

5.1 Pharmacodynamic properties

Pharmacotherapeutic group: Other drugs for obstructive airway diseases, Inhalants, Glucocorticoids, ATC Code: R03B A08

Ciclesonide exhibits low binding affinity to the glucocorticoid-receptor. Once orally inhaled, ciclesonide is enzymatically converted in the lungs to the principal metabolite (C21-des-methylpropionyl-ciclesonide) which has a pronounced anti-inflammatory activity and is thus considered as the active metabolite.

In four clinical trials, ciclesonide has been shown to reduce airway hyperresponsiveness to adenosine monophosphate in hyperreactive patients with maximal effect observed at the dose of 640 micrograms. In another trial, pretreatment with ciclesonide for seven days significantly attenuated the early and late phase reactions following inhaled allergen challenge. Inhaled ciclesonide treatment was also shown to attenuate the increase in inflammatory cells (total eosinophils) and inflammatory mediators in induced sputum.

A controlled study compared 24-hour plasma cortisol AUC in 26 adult asthmatic patients following 7 days of treatment. Compared to placebo, treatment with ciclesonide 320, 640, and 1,280 micrograms/day did not statistically significantly lower the 24-hour time averages of plasma cortisol ($AUC_{(0-24)}$/24 hours) nor was a dose-dependent effect seen.

In a clinical trial involving 164 adult male and female asthmatic patients, ciclesonide was given at doses of 320 micrograms or 640 micrograms/day over 12 weeks. After stimulation with 1 and 250 micrograms cosyntropin, no significant changes in plasma cortisol levels were observed versus placebo.

Double-blind placebo-controlled trials of 12-weeks duration in adults and adolescents have shown that treatment with ciclesonide resulted in improved lung function as measured by FEV_1 and peak expiratory flow, improved asthma symptom control, and decreased need for inhaled beta-2 agonist.

In a 12-week study of 680 severe asthmatics, previously treated with 500-1,000 micrograms fluticasone propionate per day or equivalent, 87.3% and 93.3% of patients remained exacerbation-free during treatment with 160 or 640 micrograms of ciclesonide, respectively. At the end of the 12 week study period, the results showed a statistically significant difference between the doses of 160 micrograms and 640 micrograms/day ciclesonide with regard to the occurrence of an exacerbation after the first day of the study: 43 patients/339 (= 12.7%) in the 160 micrograms/day group and 23 patients/341 (6.7%) in the 640 micrograms/day group (Hazard ratio=0.526; p= 0.0134). Both ciclesonide doses resulted in comparable FEV1 values at 12 weeks. Treatment-related adverse events were seen in 3.8% and 5% of patients treated with 160 or 640 micrograms per day of ciclesonide respectively. No study was performed to compare 160 micrograms, 320 micrograms and 640 micrograms daily dose in patients with severe asthma.

5.2 Pharmacokinetic properties

Ciclesonide is presented in HFA-134a propellant and ethanol as a solution aerosol, which demonstrates a linear relationship between different doses, puff strengths and systemic exposure.

Absorption:

Studies with oral and intravenous dosing of radiolabeled ciclesonide have shown an incomplete extent of oral absorption (24.5%). The oral bioavailability of both ciclesonide and the active metabolite is negligible (<0.5% for ciclesonide, <1% for the metabolite). Based on a γ-scintigraphy experiment, lung deposition in healthy subjects is 52%. In line with this figure, the systemic bioavailability for the active metabolite is >50% by using the ciclesonide metered dose inhaler. As the oral bioavailability for the active metabolite is <1%, the swallowed portion of the inhaled ciclesonide does not contribute to systemic absorption.

Distribution:

Following intravenous administration to healthy subjects, the initial distribution phase for ciclesonide was rapid and consistent with its high lipophilicity. The volume of distribution averaged 2.9 l/kg. The total serum clearance of ciclesonide is high (average 2.0 l/h/kg) indicating a high hepatic extraction. The percentage of ciclesonide bound to human plasma proteins averaged 99%, and that of the active metabolite 98-99%, indicating an almost complete binding of circulating ciclesonide/active metabolite to plasma proteins.

Metabolism:

Ciclesonide is primarily hydrolysed to its biologically active metabolite by esterase enzymes in the lung. Investigation of the enzymology of further metabolism by human liver microsomes showed that this compound is mainly metabolized to hydroxylated inactive metabolites by CYP3A4 catalysis. Furthermore, reversible lipophilic fatty acid ester conjugates of the active metabolite were detected in the lung.

Excretion:

Ciclesonide is predominantly excreted via the faeces (67%), after oral and intravenous administration, indicating that excretion via the bile is the major route of elimination.

Pharmacokinetic characteristics in patients:

Asthmatic patients

Ciclesonide shows no pharmacokinetic changes in mild asthmatic patients compared to healthy subjects.

Renal or hepatic insufficiency, elderly

According to population pharmacokinetics, age has no impact on the systemic exposure of the active metabolite.

Reduced liver function may affect the elimination of corticosteroids. In a study including patients with hepatic impairment suffering from liver cirrhosis, a higher systemic exposure to the active metabolite was observed.

Due to the lack of renal excretion of the active metabolite, studies on renal impaired patients have not been performed.

5.3 Preclinical safety data

Preclinical data with ciclesonide reveal no special hazard for humans based on conventional studies of safety pharmacology, repeated dose toxicity, genotoxicity, or carcinogenic potential.

In animal studies on reproductive toxicity, glucocorticosteroids have been shown to induce malformations (cleft palate, skeletal malformations). However, these animal results do not seem to be relevant for humans given recommended doses.

A treatment-related effect on the ovaries (namely atrophy) was observed at the top dose in two 12-month studies in dogs. This effect occurred at systemic exposures 5.27-8.34 times those noted at the 160 μg daily dose. The relevance of this finding to humans is unknown.

Animal studies with other glucocorticoids indicate that administration of pharmacological doses of glucocorticoids during pregnancy may increase the risk for intrauterine growth retardation, adult cardiovascular and/or metabolic disease and/or permanent changes in glucocorticoid receptor density, neurotransmitter turnover and behaviour. The relevance of these data to humans administered ciclesonide by inhalation is unknown.

6. PHARMACEUTICAL PARTICULARS

6.1 List of excipients

Norflurane (HFA-134a)

6.2 Incompatibilities
Not applicable.

6.3 Shelf life
30 metered actuations – 1 year
60 and 120 metered actuations – 3 years

6.4 Special precautions for storage
This medicinal product does not require any special storage conditions.

The container contains a pressurised liquid. Do not expose to temperatures higher than 50°C.

The container should not be punctured, broken or burnt even when apparently empty.

6.5 Nature and contents of container
The inhaler comprises a pressurised container made from aluminium and is sealed with a metering valve, mouthpiece, and cap.

30 metered actuations

60 metered actuations

120 metered actuations

Not all pack sizes may be marketed.

6.6 Special precautions for disposal and other handling
Patients should be carefully instructed in the proper use of their inhaler (see Patient Information Leaflet).

As with most inhaled medicinal products in pressurised containers, the therapeutic effect of this medicinal product may decrease when the container is cold. However, Alvesco delivers a consistent dose from –10°C to 40°C.

7. MARKETING AUTHORISATION HOLDER
Nycomed GmbH
Byk-Gulden-Str. 2
D-78467 Konstanz
Germany

8. MARKETING AUTHORISATION NUMBER(S)
PL 31752/0005

9. DATE OF FIRST AUTHORISATION/RENEWAL OF THE AUTHORISATION
16 April 2004

10. DATE OF REVISION OF THE TEXT
19 February 2009

Amaryl
(sanofi-aventis)

1. NAME OF THE MEDICINAL PRODUCT
Amaryl 1 mg, tablet
Amaryl 2 mg, tablet
Amaryl 3 mg, tablet
Amaryl 4 mg, tablet

2. QUALITATIVE AND QUANTITATIVE COMPOSITION
Each tablet contains 1mg, 2mg, 3mg or 4mg of glimepiride.

For a full list of excipients, see section6.1.

3. PHARMACEUTICAL FORM
Tablet

4. CLINICAL PARTICULARS

4.1 Therapeutic indications
Amaryl is indicated for the treatment of type 2 diabetes mellitus, when diet, physical exercise and weight reduction alone are not adequate.

4.2 Posology and method of administration
For oral administration

The basis for successful treatment of diabetes is a good diet, regular physical activity, as well as routine checks of blood and urine. Tablets or insulin cannot compensate if the patient does not keep to the recommended diet.

Dosage is determined by the results of blood and urinary glucose determinations.

The starting dose is 1 mg glimepiride per day. If good control is achieved this dosage should be used for maintenance therapy.

For the different dosage regimens appropriate strengths are available.

If control is unsatisfactory the dosage should be increased, based on the glycaemic control, in a stepwise manner with an interval of about 1 to 2 weeks between each step, to 2, 3 or 4 mg glimepiride per day.

A dosage of more than 4 mg glimepiride per day gives better results only in exceptional cases. The maximum recommended dose is 6 mg glimepiride per day.

In patients not adequately controlled with the maximum daily dose of metformin, concomitant glimepiride therapy can be initiated.

While maintaining the metformin dose, the glimepiride therapy is started with a low dose, and is then titrated up depending on the desired level of metabolic control up to the maximum daily dose. The combination therapy should

In patients not adequately controlled with the maximum daily dose of Amaryl, concomitant insulin therapy can be initiated if necessary. While maintaining the glimepiride dose, insulin treatment is started at low dose and titrated up depending on the desired level of metabolic control. The combination therapy should be initiated under close medical supervision.

Normally a single daily dose of glimepiride is sufficient. It is recommended that this dose be taken shortly before or during a substantial breakfast or - if none is taken - shortly before or during the first main meal.

If a dose is forgotten, this should not be corrected by increasing the next dose.

Tablets should be swallowed whole with some liquid.

If a patient has a hypoglycaemic reaction on 1 mg glimepiride daily, this indicates that they can be controlled by diet alone.

In the course of treatment, as an improvement in control of diabetes is associated with higher insulin sensitivity, glimepiride requirements may fall. To avoid hypoglycaemia timely dose reduction or cessation of therapy must therefore be considered. Change in dosage may also be necessary, if there are changes in weight or life style of the patient, or other factors that increase the risk of hypo-or hyperglycaemia.

Switch over from other oral hypoglycaemic agents to Amaryl

A switch over from other oral hypoglycaemic agents to Amaryl can generally be done. For the switch over to Amaryl the strength and the half-life of the previous medicinal product has to be taken into account. In some cases, especially in antidiabetics with a long half-life (e.g. chlorpropamide), a wash out period of a few days is advisable in order to minimise the risk of hypoglycaemic reactions due to the additive effect.

The recommended starting dose is 1 mg glimepiride per day. Based on the response the glimepiride dosage may be increased stepwise, as indicated earlier.

Switch over from Insulin to Amaryl

In exceptional cases, where type 2 diabetic patients are regulated on insulin, a changeover to Amaryl may be indicated. The changeover should be undertaken under close medical supervision.

Special Populations

Patients with renal or hepatic impairment:

See section 4.3.

Children and adolescents:

There are no data available on the use of glimepiride in patients under 8 years of age. For children aged 8 to 17 years, there are limited data on glimepiride as monotherapy (see sections 5.1 and 5.2).

The available data on safety and efficacy are insufficient in the paediatric population and therefore such use is not recommended.

4.3 Contraindications
Glimepiride is contraindicated in patients with the following conditions:

- hypersensitivity to glimepiride, other sulfonylureas or sulfonamides or to any of the excipients
- insulin dependent diabetes,
- diabetic coma,
- ketoacidosis,
- severe renal or hepatic function disorders. In case of severe renal or hepatic function disorders, a change over to insulin is required.

4.4 Special warnings and precautions for use
Amaryl must be taken shortly before or during a meal.

When meals are taken at irregular hours or skipped altogether, treatment with Amaryl may lead to hypoglycaemia. Possible symptoms of hypoglycaemia include: headache, ravenous hunger, nausea, vomiting, lassitude, sleepiness, disordered sleep, restlessness, aggressiveness, impaired concentration, alertness and reaction time, depression, confusion, speech and visual disorders, aphasia, tremor, paresis, sensory disturbances, dizziness, helplessness, loss of self-control, delirium, cerebral convulsions, somnolence and loss of consciousness up to and including coma, shallow respiration and bradycardia. In addition, signs of adrenergic counter-regulation may be present such as sweating, clammy skin, anxiety, tachycardia, hypertension, palpitations, angina pectoris and cardiac arrhythmias.

The clinical picture of a severe hypoglycaemic attack may resemble that of a stroke.

Symptoms can almost always be promptly controlled by immediate intake carbohydrates (sugar). Artificial sweeteners have no effect.

It is known from other sulfonylureas that, despite initially successful countermeasures, hypoglycaemia may recur.

Severe hypoglycaemia or prolonged hypoglycaemia, only temporarily controlled by the usual amounts of sugar, require immediate medical treatment and occasionally hospitalisation.

Factors favouring hypoglycaemia include:

- unwillingness or (more commonly in older patients) incapacity of the patient to cooperate,
- undernutrition, irregular mealtimes or missed meals or periods of fasting,
- alterations in diet,
- imbalance between physical exertion and carbohydrate intake,
- consumption of alcohol, especially in combination with skipped meals,
- impaired renal function,
- serious liver dysfunction,
- overdosage with Amaryl,
- certain uncompensated disorders of the endocrine system affecting carbohydrate metabolism or counterregulation of hypoglycaemia (as for example in certain disorders of thyroid function and in anterior pituitary or adrenocortical insufficiency),
- concurrent administration of certain other medicinal products (see section 4.5).

Treatment with Amaryl requires regular monitoring of glucose levels in blood and urine. In addition determination of the proportion of glycosylated haemoglobin is recommended.

Regular hepatic and haematological monitoring (especially leucocytes and thrombocytes) are required during treatment with Amaryl.

In stress-situations (e.g. accidents, acute operations, infections with fever, etc.) a temporary switch to insulin may be indicated.

No experience has been gained concerning the use of Amaryl in patients with severe impairment of liver function or dialysis patients. In patients with severe impairment of renal or liver function change over to insulin is indicated.

Treatment of patients with G6PD-deficiency with sulfonylurea agents can lead to hemolytic anaemia. Since glimepiride belongs to the class of sulfonylurea agents, caution should be used in patients with G6PD-deficiency and a non-sulfonylurea alternative should be considered.

Amaryl contains lactose monohydrate. Patients with rare hereditary problems of galactose intolerance, the Lapp lactase deficiency or glucose-galactose malabsorption should not take this medicine.

4.5 Interaction with other medicinal products and other forms of interaction
If glimepiride is taken simultaneously with certain other medicinal products, both undesired increases and decreases in the hypoglycaemic action of glimepiride can occur. For this reason, other medicinal products should only be taken with the knowledge (or at the prescription) of the doctor.

Glimepiride is metabolized by cytochrome P450 2C9 (CYP2C9). Its metabolism is known to be influenced by concomitant administration of CYP2C9 inducers (e.g. rifampicin) or inhibitors (e.g. fluconazole)

Results from an vivo interaction study reported in literature show that glimepiride AUC is increased approximately 2-fold by fluconazole, one of the most potent CYP2C9 inhibitors.

Based on the experience with glimepiride and with other sulfonylureas the following interactions have to be mentioned.

Potentiation of the blood-glucose-lowering effect and, thus, in some instances hypoglycaemia may occur when one of the following medicinal products is taken, for example:

- phenylbutazone, azapropazone and oxyfenbutazone,
- insulin and oral antidiabetic products, such as metformin,
- salicylates and p-amino-salicylic acid,
- anabolic steroids and male sex hormones,
- chloramphenicol, certain long acting sulfonamides, tetracyclines, quinolone antibiotics and clarithromycin
- coumarin anticoagulants,
- fenfluramine,
- fibrates,
- ACE inhibitors,
- fluoxetine, MAO-inhibitors
- allopurinol, probenicid, sulfinpyrazone,
- sympatholytics,
- cyclophosphamide, trophosphamide and iphosphamides,
- miconazol, fluconazole
- pentoxifylline (high dose parenteral),
- tritoqualine

Weakening of the blood-glucose-lowering effect and, thus raised blood glucose levels may occur when one of the following medicinal products is taken, for example:

- oestrogens and progestogens,
- saluretics, thiazide diuretics,
- thyroid stimulating agents, glucocorticoids,
- phenothiazine derivatives, chlorpromazine,
- adrenaline and sympathicomimetics,
- nicotinic acid (high dosages) and nicotinic acid derivatives,
- laxatives (long term use),
- phenytoin, diazoxide,

- glucagon, barbiturates and rifampicin,
- acetazolamide.

H_2 antagonists, betablockers, clonidine and reserpine may lead to either potentiation or weakening of the blood glucose lowering effect.

Under the influence of sympatholytic medicinal products such as betablockers, clonidine, guanethidine and reserpine, the signs of adrenergic counterregulation to hypoglycaemia may be reduced or absent.

Alcohol intake may potentiate or weaken the hypoglycaemic action of glimepiride in an unpredictable fashion.

Glimepiride may either potentiate or weaken the effects of coumarin derivatives.

4.6 Pregnancy and lactation

Pregnancy

Risk related to the diabetes

Abnormal blood glucose levels during pregnancy are associated with a higher incidence of congenital abnormalities and perinatal mortality. So the blood glucose level must be closely monitored during pregnancy in order to avoid the teratogenic risk. The use of insulin is required under such circumstances. Patients who consider pregnancy should inform their physician.

Risk related to glimepiride

There are no adequate data from the use of glimepiride in pregnant women. Animal studies have shown reproductive toxicity which likely was related to the pharmacologic action (hypoglycaemia) of glimepiride (see section 5.3).

Consequently, glimepiride should not be used during the whole pregnancy.

In case of treatment by glimepiride, if the patient plans to become pregnant or if a pregnancy is discovered, the treatment should be switched as soon as possible to insulin therapy.

Lactation

The excretion in human milk is unknown. Glimepiride is excreted in rat milk. As other sulfonylureas are excreted in human milk and because there is a risk of hypoglycaemia in nursing infants, breast-feeding is advised against during treatment with glimepiride.

4.7 Effects on ability to drive and use machines

No studies on the effects on the ability to drive and use machines have been performed.

The patient's ability to concentrate and react may be impaired as a result of hypoglycaemia or hyperglycaemia or, for example, as a result of visual impairment. This may constitute a risk in situations where these abilities are of special importance (e.g. driving a car or operating machinery).

Patients should be advised to take precautions to avoid hypoglycaemia whilst driving. This is particularly important in those who have reduced or absent awareness of the warning symptoms of hypoglycaemia or have frequent episodes of hypoglycaemia. It should be considered whether it is advisable to drive or operate machinery in these circumstances.

4.8 Undesirable effects

The following undesirable effects are based on experience with Amaryl and other sulfonylureas.

Blood and lymphatic system disorders

Rare: thrombocytopenia, leukopenia, granulocytopenia, agranulocytosis, erythropenia, haemolytic anaemia and pancytopenia, which are in general reversible upon discontinuation of medication.

Immune system disorders

Very rare: leukocytoclastic vasculitis, mild hypersensitivity reactions that may develop into serious reactions with dyspnoea, fall in blood pressure and sometimes shock.

Cross-allergenicity with sulfonylureas, sulfonamides or related substances is possible.

Metabolism and nutrition disorders

Rare: hypoglycaemia.

These hypoglycaemic reactions mostly occur immediately, may be severe and are not always easy to correct. The occurrence of such reactions depends, as with other hypoglycaemic therapies, on individual factors such as dietary habits and dosage (see further under section 4.4).

Eye disorders

Visual disturbances, transient, may occur especially on initiation of treatment, due to changes in blood glucose levels.

Gastrointestinal disorders

Very rare: nausea, vomiting, diarrhoea, abdominal distension, abdominal discomfort and abdominal pain, which seldom lead to discontinuation of therapy.

Hepato-biliary disorders

Hepatic enzymes increased.

Very rare: hepatic function abnormal (e.g. with cholestasis and jaundice), hepatitis and hepatic failure.

Skin and subcutaneous tissue disorders

Hypersensitivity reactions of the skin may occur as pruritus, rash, urticaria and photosensitivity.

Investigations

Very rare: blood sodium decrease.

4.9 Overdose

After ingestion of an overdosage hypoglycaemia may occur, lasting from 12 to 72 hours, and may recur after an initial recovery. Symptoms may not be present for up to 24 hours after ingestion. In general observation in hospital is recommended. Nausea, vomiting and epigastric pain may occur. The hypoglycaemia may in general be accompanied by neurological symptoms like restlessness, tremor, visual disturbances, co-ordination problems, sleepiness, coma and convulsions.

Treatment primarily consists of preventing absorption by inducing vomiting and then drinking water or lemonade with activated charcoal (adsorbent) and sodium-sulphate (laxative). If large quantities have been ingested, gastric lavage is indicated, followed by activated charcoal and sodium-sulphate. In case of (severe) overdosage hospitalisation in an intensive care department is indicated. Start the administration of glucose as soon as possible, if necessary by a bolus intravenous injection of 50 ml of a 50% solution, followed by an infusion of a 10% solution with strict monitoring of blood glucose. Further treatment should be symptomatic.

In particular when treating hypoglycaemia due to accidental intake of Amaryl in infants and young children, the dose of glucose given must be carefully controlled to avoid the possibility of producing dangerous hyperglycaemia. Blood glucose should be closely monitored.

5. PHARMACOLOGICAL PROPERTIES

5.1 Pharmacodynamic properties

Pharmacotherapeutic group: Oral blood glucose lowering drugs: Sulfonamides, urea derivatives. ATC Code: A10B B12.

Glimepiride is an orally active hypoglycaemic substance belonging to the sulfonylurea group. It may be used in non-insulin dependent diabetes mellitus.

Glimepiride acts mainly by stimulating insulin release from pancreatic beta cells.

As with other sulfonylureas this effect is based on an increase of responsiveness of the pancreatic beta cells to the physiological glucose stimulus. In addition, glimepiride seems to have pronounced extrapancreatic effects also postulated for other sulfonylureas.

Insulin release

Sulfonylureas regulate insulin secretion by closing the ATP-sensitive potassium channel in the beta cell membrane. Closing the potassium channel induces depolarisation of the beta cell and results - by opening of calcium channels - in an increased influx of calcium into the cell.

This leads to insulin release through exocytosis.

Glimepiride binds with a high exchange rate to a beta cell membrane protein which is associated with the ATP-sensitive potassium channel but which is different from the usual sulfonylurea binding site.

Extrapancreatic activity

The extrapancreatic effects are for example an improvement of the sensitivity of the peripheral tissue for insulin and a decrease of the insulin uptake by the liver.

The uptake of glucose from blood into peripheral muscle and fat tissues occurs via special transport proteins, located in the cells membrane. The transport of glucose in these tissues is the rate limiting step in the use of glucose. Glimepiride increases very rapidly the number of active glucose transport molecules in the plasma membranes of muscle and fat cells, resulting in stimulated glucose uptake.

Glimepiride increases the activity of the glycosyl-phosphatidylinositol-specific phospholipase C which may be correlated with the drug-induced lipogenesis and glycogenesis in isolated fat and muscle cells.

Glimepiride inhibits the glucose production in the liver by increasing the intracellular concentration of fructose-2,6-bisphosphate, which in its turn inhibits the gluconeogenesis.

General

In healthy persons, the minimum effective oral dose is approximately 0.6 mg. The effect of glimepiride is dose-dependent and reproducible. The physiological response to acute physical exercise, reduction of insulin secretion, is still present under glimepiride.

There was no significant difference in effect regardless of whether the medicinal product was given 30 minutes or immediately before a meal. In diabetic patients, good metabolic control over 24 hours can be achieved with a single daily dose.

Although the hydroxy metabolite of glimepiride caused a small but significant decrease in serum glucose in healthy persons, it accounts for only a minor part of the total drug effect.

Combination therapy with metformin

Improved metabolic control for concomitant glimepiride therapy compared to metformin alone in patients not adequately controlled with the maximum dosage of metformin has been shown in one study.

Combination therapy with insulin

Data for combination therapy with insulin are limited. In patients not adequately controlled with the maximum dosage of glimepiride, concomitant insulin therapy can be initiated. In two studies, the combination achieved the same improvement in metabolic control as insulin alone; however, a lower average dose of insulin was required in combination therapy.

Special populations

Children and adolescents

An active controlled clinical trial (glimepiride up to 8 mg daily or metformin up to 2,000 mg daily) of 24 weeks duration was performed in 285 children (8-17 years of age) with type 2 diabetes.

Both glimepiride and metformin exhibited a significant decrease from baseline in HbA_{1c} (glimepiride -0.95 (se 0.41); metformin -1.39 (se 0.40)). However, glimepiride did not achieve the criteria of non-inferiority to metformin in mean change from baseline of HbA_{1c}. The difference between treatments was 0.44% in favour of metformin. The upper limit (1.05) of the 95% confidence interval for the difference was not below the 0.3% non-inferiority margin.

Following glimepiride treatment, there were no new safety concerns noted in children compared to adult patients with type 2 diabetes mellitus. No long-term efficacy and safety data are available in paediatric patients.

5.2 Pharmacokinetic properties

Absorption: The bioavailability of glimepiride after oral administration is complete. Food intake has no relevant influence on absorption, only absorption rate is slightly diminished. Maximum serum concentrations (C_{max}) are reached approx. 2.5 hours after oral intake (mean 0.3 µg/ml during multiple dosing of 4 mg daily) and there is a linear relationship between dose and both C_{max} and AUC (area under the time/concentration curve).

Distribution: Glimepiride has a very low distribution volume (approx. 8.8 litres) which is roughly equal to the albumin distribution space, high protein binding (>99%), and a low clearance (approx. 48 ml/min).

In animals, glimepiride is excreted in milk. Glimepiride is transferred to the placenta. Passage of the blood brain barrier is low.

Biotransformation and elimination: Mean dominant serum half-life, which is of relevance for the serum concentrations under multiple-dose conditions, is about 5 to 8 hours. After high doses, slightly longer half-lives were noted.

After a single dose of radiolabelled glimepiride, 58% of the radioactivity was recovered in the urine, and 35% in the faeces. No unchanged substance was detected in the urine. Two metabolites - most probably resulting from hepatic metabolism (major enzyme is CYP2C9) - were identified both in urine and faeces: the hydroxy derivative and the carboxy derivative. After oral administration of glimepiride, the terminal half-lives of these metabolites were 3 to 6 and 5 to 6 hours respectively.

Comparison of single and multiple once-daily dosing revealed no significant differences in pharmacokinetics and the intraindividual variability was very low. There was no relevant accumulation.

Special populations

Pharmacokinetics were similar in males and females, as well as in young and elderly (above 65 years) patients. In patients with low creatinine clearance, there was a tendency for glimepiride clearance to increase and for average serum concentrations to decrease, most probably resulting from a more rapid elimination because of lower protein binding. Renal elimination of the two metabolites was impaired. Overall no additional risk of accumulation is to be assumed in such patients.

Pharmacokinetics in five non-diabetic patients after bile duct surgery were similar to those in healthy persons.

Children and adolescents

A fed study investigating the pharmacokinetics, safety, and tolerability of a 1 mg single dose of glimepiride in 30 paediatric patients (4 children aged 10-12 years and 26 children aged 12-17 years) with type 2 diabetes showed mean $AUC_{(0\text{-}last)}$, Cmax and $t_{1/2}$ similar to that previously observed in adults.

5.3 Preclinical safety data

Preclinical effects observed occurred at exposures sufficiently in excess of the maximum human exposure as to indicate little relevance to clinical use, or were due to the pharmacodynamic action (hypoglycaemia) of the compound. This finding is based on conventional safety pharmacology, repeated dose toxicity, genotoxicity, carcinogenicity, and reproduction toxicity studies. In the latter (covering embryotoxicity, teratogenicity and developmental toxicity), adverse effects observed were considered to be secondary to the hypoglycaemic effects induced by the compound in dams and in offspring.

6. PHARMACEUTICAL PARTICULARS

6.1 List of excipients

Lactose monohydrate

sodium starch glycollate (type A)

magnesium stearate,

microcrystalline cellulose

povidone 25000

Further as colouring agents:

Amaryl 1 mg: red iron oxide (E172)

Amaryl 2 mg: yellow iron oxide (E172), indigo-carmine aluminium lake (E132)

Amaryl 3 mg: yellow iron oxide (E172)

Amaryl 4 mg: indigo-carmine aluminium lake (E132)

.2 Incompatibilities
ot applicable

.3 Shelf life
years

.4 Special precautions for storage
o not store above 30°C.
tore in the original package.

.5 Nature and contents of container
VC/Aluminium blisters.
0 tablets

.6 Special precautions for disposal and other handling
o special requirements

. MARKETING AUTHORISATION HOLDER
Sanofi-aventis
PO Box 597
Guildford
Surrey

8. MARKETING AUTHORISATION NUMBER(S)
Amaryl Tablets, 1mg: PL 13402/0006
Amaryl Tablets, 2mg: PL 13402/0007
Amaryl Tablets, 3mg: PL 13402/0008
Amaryl Tablets, 4mg: PL 13402/0009

9. DATE OF FIRST AUTHORISATION/RENEWAL OF THE AUTHORISATION
8 November 1996

10. DATE OF REVISION OF THE TEXT
16 July 2008

Legal category: POM

Ambirix suspension for injection

(GlaxoSmithKline UK)

1. NAME OF THE MEDICINAL PRODUCT
Ambirix, suspension for injection▼

Hepatitis A (inactivated) and hepatitis B(rDNA) (HAB) vaccine (adsorbed).

2. QUALITATIVE AND QUANTITATIVE COMPOSITION
1 dose (1 ml) contains:

Hepatitis A virus (inactivated)[1,2]	720 ELISA Units
Hepatitis B surface antigen[3,4]	20 micrograms

[1]Produced on human diploid (MRC-5) cells

[2]Adsorbed on aluminium hydroxide, hydrated — 0.05 milligrams Al^{3+}

[3]Produced in yeast cells (*Saccharomyces cerevisiae*) by recombinant DNA technology

[4]Adsorbed on aluminium phosphate — 0.4 milligrams Al^{3+}

For a full list of excipients, see section 6.1.

3. PHARMACEUTICAL FORM
Suspension for injection.

Ambirix is a turbid white suspension.

4. CLINICAL PARTICULARS
4.1 Therapeutic indications
Ambirix is for use in non-immune persons from 1 year up to and including 15 years for protection against hepatitis A and hepatitis B infection.

Protection against hepatitis B infections may not be obtained until after the second dose (see section 5.1).

Therefore:

- Ambirix should be used only when there is a relatively low risk of hepatitis B infection during the vaccination course.

- It is recommended that Ambirix should be administered in settings where completion of the two-dose vaccination course can be assured.

4.2 Posology and method of administration
Posology

- Dosage

A dose of 1.0 ml is recommended for subjects from 1 year up to and including 15 years of age.

- Primary vaccination schedule

The standard primary course of vaccination with Ambirix consists of two doses, the first administered at the elected date and the second between six and twelve months after the first dose.

The recommended schedule should be adhered to. Once initiated, the primary course of vaccination should be completed with the same vaccine.

- Booster dose

In situations where a booster dose of hepatitis A and/or hepatitis B is desired, a monovalent or combined vaccine can be given. The safety and immunogenicity of Ambirix administered as a booster dose following a two dose primary course have not been evaluated.

The anti-hepatitis B surface antigen (anti-HBs) and anti-hepatitis A virus (anti-HAV) antibody titres observed following a primary vaccination course with Ambirix are in the range of what is seen following vaccination with the monovalent hepatitis A and B vaccines. General guidelines for booster vaccination can therefore be drawn from experience with the monovalent vaccines, as follows.

Hepatitis B

The need for a booster dose of hepatitis B vaccine in healthy individuals who have received a full primary vaccination course has not been established. However some official vaccination programmes currently include a recommendation for a booster dose of hepatitis B vaccine and these should be respected.

For some categories of subjects at risk of exposure to HBV (e.g. haemodialysis or immunocompromised patients) a precautionary attitude should be considered to ensure that a protective antibody level ⩾ 10 mIU/ml is maintained.

Hepatitis A

It is not yet fully established whether immunocompetent individuals who have responded to hepatitis A vaccination will require booster doses as protection in the absence of detectable antibodies may be ensured by immunological memory. Guidelines for boosting are based on the assumption that antibodies are required for protection. Anti-HAV antibodies have been predicted to persist for at least 10 years.

Method of administration

Ambirix is for intramuscular injection, usually into the deltoid muscle. However the anterolateral thigh may be used in very young subjects if preferred.

Exceptionally, the vaccine may be administered subcutaneously in patients with thrombocytopenia or bleeding disorders. However, this route of administration may result in suboptimal immune response to the vaccine. (see section 4.4)

4.3 Contraindications
Hypersensitivity to the active substances or to any of the excipients or neomycin.

Hypersensitivity after previous administration of hepatitis A and/or hepatitis B vaccines.

As with other vaccines, the administration of Ambirix should be postponed in subjects suffering from acute severe febrile illness.

4.4 Special warnings and precautions for use
As with all injectable vaccines, appropriate medical treatment and supervision should always be readily available in case of a rare anaphylactic event following the administration of the vaccine.

It is possible that subjects may be in the incubation period of a hepatitis A or hepatitis B infection at the time of vaccination. It is not known whether Ambirix will prevent hepatitis A and hepatitis B in such cases.

The vaccine will not prevent infection caused by other agents such as hepatitis C and hepatitis E and other pathogens known to infect the liver.

Ambirix is not recommended for postexposure prophylaxis (e.g. needle stick injury).

If rapid protection against hepatitis B is required, the standard three dose regimen of the combined vaccine containing 360 ELISA Units of formalin inactivated hepatitis A virus and 10 micrograms of recombinant hepatitis B surface antigen is recommended. This is because, a higher proportion of subjects are protected in the interval between the second and third dose of the three dose combined vaccine, than after a single dose of Ambirix. This difference is no longer present after the second dose of Ambirix (see section 5.1 for seroprotection rates).

It is recommended that the two-dose regimen of Ambirix be completed prior to start of sexual activity.

The vaccine has not been tested in patients with an impaired immune system. In haemodialysis patients and persons with an impaired immune system, adequate anti-HAV and anti-HBs antibody titers may not be obtained after the primary immunisation course.

Since intradermal injection or intramuscular administration into the gluteal muscle could lead to a suboptimal response to the vaccine, these routes should be avoided. However, exceptionally Ambirix can be administered subcutaneously to subjects with thrombocytopenia or bleeding disorders since bleeding may occur following an intramuscular administration to these subjects.

AMBIRIX SHOULD UNDER NO CIRCUMSTANCES BE ADMINISTERED INTRAVASCULARLY.

4.5 Interaction with other medicinal products and other forms of interaction
No data on concomitant administration of Ambirix with specific hepatitis A immunoglobulin or hepatitis B immunoglobulin have been generated. However, when the monovalent hepatitis A and hepatitis B vaccines were administered concomitantly with specific immunoglobulins there was no effect on seroconversion rates. Concomitant immunoglobulin administration may result in lower antibody titres.

When Ambirix was administered concomitantly with, but as a separate injection to a combined diphtheria, tetanus, acellular pertussis, inactivated poliomyelitis and *Haemophilus influenzae* type b vaccine (DTPa-IPV/Hib) or with a combined Measles-Mumps-Rubella vaccine in the second year of life, immune responses to all antigens were satisfactory (see section 5.1)

Concomitant administration of Ambirix and other vaccines than those listed above has not been studied. It is advised that Ambirix should not be administered at the same time as other vaccines unless absolutely necessary.

Concomitant vaccines should always be administered at separate injection sites and preferably into different limbs.

It may be expected that in patients receiving immunosuppressive treatment or patients with immunodeficiency, an adequate response may not be achieved.

4.6 Pregnancy and lactation
Pregnancy

The effect of Ambirix on foetal development has not been assessed. Ambirix should not be used during pregnancy unless it is clearly necessary.

Lactation

The effect on breastfed infants of Ambirix administered to the mothers has not been evaluated in clinical studies. Ambirix should not be used during lactation unless it is clearly necessary.

4.7 Effects on ability to drive and use machines
Drowsiness and dizziness can sometimes occur and may affect the ability to drive and use machines.

4.8 Undesirable effects
The current formulation of Ambirix does not contain thiomersal (an organomercuric compound) or any preservative. In a clinical study conducted with 3 doses of the current formulation in adults, the incidence of pain, redness, swelling, fatigue, gastro-enteritis, headache and fever was comparable to the incidence observed with the former thiomersal and preservative containing vaccine formulation. The following adverse reactions have been reported following the widespread use of the former formulation

Clinical trials involved the administration of 2029 doses of Ambirix to 1027 subjects from 1 year up to and including 15 years of age.

Local and general adverse reactions reported following primary vaccination with Ambirix were categorised by frequency.

Frequencies are reported below as:

Very common: ⩾ 1/10
Common: ⩾ 1/100 to < 1/10
Uncommon: ⩾ 1/1,000 to < 1/100
Rare: ⩾ 1/10,000 to < 1/1,000
Very rare: < 1/10,000

Nervous system disorders:
very common: headache
common: drowsiness

Gastrointestinal disorders:
common: gastrointestinal symptoms

Metabolism and nutrition disorders
very common: loss of appetite

General disorders and administration site conditions
very common: pain, redness, fatigue
common: swelling, fever

Psychiatric disorders:
very common: irritability/fussiness

In a study, in 300 subjects aged from 12 years up to and including 15 years, the reactogenicity profile of Ambirix was compared to that of the three-dose combined vaccine. The three-dose vaccine contained 360 ELISA Units of formalin inactivated hepatitis A virus and 10 micrograms of recombinant hepatitis B surface antigen in 0.5 ml. The incidence of local and general solicited symptoms after a two dose regimen of Ambirix was overall similar to that seen with the three dose combined vaccine, the only exceptions being a higher incidence of pain and fatigue on a per dose basis after Ambirix, but not on a per subject basis.

Pain was reported following 50.7% of doses in the Ambirix group, as compared to 39.1% of doses with the three dose combined vaccine. However, over the complete vaccination course, 66.4% of subjects who received Ambirix reported pain, as compared to 63.8% of subjects who received the three dose combined vaccine.

Fatigue was reported following 29.2% doses of Ambirix, as compared to 19.3% doses of the three dose combined vaccine. However, the incidence of fatigue was similar based on a per subject analysis (i.e. over the total vaccination course, 39.6% versus 36.2% of subjects for Ambirix and the three dose vaccine respectively).

The incidence of pain and fatigue graded as severe was low and similar to that observed with the three dose combined vaccine.

In a comparative trial in subjects aged 1-11 years, the incidences of local and general solicited symptoms in the Ambirix group were similar to those seen with the three-dose combined vaccine containing 360 ELISA Units of formalin inactivated hepatitis A virus and 10 micrograms of recombinant hepatitis B surface antigen. The exception was a higher incidence of pain after Ambirix in 6-11 year olds on a per dose basis, but not on a per subject basis.

The percentages of vaccinees reporting any solicited symptom graded as severe during a two-dose regimen of Ambirix or a three dose regimen with the combined vaccine containing 360 ELISA Units of formalin inactivated hepatitis A virus and 10 micrograms of recombinant hepatitis B surface antigen, were not statistically different.

During post-marketing surveillance with the three dose combined vaccine containing either 360 ELISA Units of formalin inactivated hepatitis A virus and 10 micrograms of recombinant hepatitis B surface antigen in a dose volume of 0.5 ml (recommended for subjects 1 year up to and including 15 years of age) or 720 ELISA Units of formalin inactivated hepatitis A virus and 20 micrograms of recombinant hepatitis B surface antigen in a dose volume of 1 ml (recommended from the age of 16 years onwards), the following adverse reactions have been reported.

Investigations

abnormal liver function tests

Blood and lymphatic system disorders

thrombocytopenia, thrombocytopenic purpura, lymphadenopathy

Nervous system disorders

syncope, dizziness, paresthesia, convulsions

Gastrointestinal disorders:

nausea, vomiting, diarrhoea, abdominal pain

Skin and subcutaneous tissue disorders

rash, pruritis, urticaria

Metabolism and nutrition disorders

decreased appetite

Vascular disorders

Hypotension

General disorders and administration site conditions

flu-like symptoms, fatigue

Immune system disorders

allergic reactions including anaphylactic and anaphylactoid reactions and serum sickness like disease

Following widespread use of the monovalent hepatitis A and/or hepatitis B vaccines, the following adverse reactions have additionally been reported.

Nervous system disorders

multiple sclerosis, myelitis, facial palsy, polyneuritis such as Guillain-Barré syndrome (with ascending paralysis), encephalitis, encephalopathy

Eye disorders

optic neuritis

Skin and subcutaneous tissue disorders

erythema exsudativum multiforme

Infections and infestations

meningitis

Vascular disorders

vasculitis

4.9 Overdose

No case of overdose has been reported.

5. PHARMACOLOGICAL PROPERTIES

5.1 Pharmacodynamic properties

Pharmaco-therapeutic group: Hepatitis vaccines, ATC code J07BC20.

Ambirix confers immunity against HAV and HBV infection by inducing specific anti-HAV and anti-HBs antibodies.

In clinical studies involving subjects from 1 year up to and including 15 years of age, seropositivity rates for anti-HAV antibodies were 99.1% one month after the first dose and 100% after the second dose given at month 6 (i.e month 7). Seropositivity rates for anti-HBs antibodies were 74.2% one month after the first dose and 100% after the second dose given at month 6 (i.e. month 7). The anti-HBs seroprotection rates (titers ≥ 10 mIU/ml) at these time points were 37.4% and 98.2% respectively.

In a comparative clinical trial conducted among subjects aged from 12 years up to and including 15 years of age, 142 received two doses of Ambirix and 147 received the standard three-dose combined vaccine. The latter contained 360 ELISA Units of formalin inactivated hepatitis A virus and 10 micrograms of recombinant hepatitis B surface antigen. For the 289 subjects evaluable for immunogenicity, seroprotection rates (SP in the table below) against hepatitis B were significantly higher at months 2 and 6 with the three-dose vaccine than with Ambirix.

(see Table 1 below)

Immune responses obtained one month after the full vaccination course (i.e at month 7) in a comparative clinical trial in children aged 1-11 years are presented in the following table. Also shown are the results reported in the comparative study performed in 12-15 year-olds. In both studies, subjects received either a two dose schedule of Ambirix or a three dose regimen of the combined vaccine containing 360 ELISA Units of formalin inactivated hepatitis A virus and 10 micrograms of recombinant hepatitis B surface antigen.

(see Table 2 below)

In a clinical study, 102 subjects aged from 12 years up to and including 15 years received the second dose of Ambirix at month 12, seropositivity rates for anti-HAV were 99.0% and seropositivity rates for anti-HBs were 99.0% at month 13 with seroprotection rates of 97.0%.

In subjects aged 12-15 years at the time of primary vaccination, anti-HAV and anti-HBs antibodies have been shown to persist for at least 24 months following the initiation of a 0, 6 month schedule of Ambirix. Seropositivity rates were 100% and 94.2% respectively for anti-HAV and anti-HBs antibodies at month 24. The seroprotection rate for anti-HBs at this time point was 93.3%. In this study, the immune response to both antigen components was comparable to that seen after a 3-dose regimen of the combined vaccine containing 360 ELISA Units of formalin inactivated hepatitis A virus and 10µg of recombinant hepatitis B surface antigen in a dose volume of 0.5 ml.

In a clinical study involving subjects from 12 years up to and including 15 years of age, the persistence of anti-HAV and anti-HBs antibodies at month 24 was shown to be similar following a 0, 6 month or a 0, 12 month schedule.

When the first dose of Ambirix was administered concomitantly with a booster dose of a combined diphtheria, tetanus, acellular pertussis, inactivated poliomyelitis and *Haemophilus influenzae* type b vaccine (DTPa-IPV/Hib) or with the first dose of a combined Measles-Mumps-Rubella vaccine in the second year of life, immune responses to all antigens were satisfactory.

These data were generated with the former Ambirix formulation containing thiomersal and a preservative. A clinical study conducted with 3 doses of the current formulation in adults showed that the current formulation elicited similar seroprotection and seroconversion rates as compared to the former formulation.

5.2 Pharmacokinetic properties

Evaluation of pharmacokinetic properties is not required for vaccines.

5.3 Preclinical safety data

Non-clinical data reveal no special hazard for humans based on general safety studies.

Table 1

Vaccine group	Anti-HBs Month 2 SP (%)	Anti-HBs Month 6 SP (%)	Anti-HBs Month 7 SP (%)
Ambirix	38	68.3	97.9
Combined HAB vaccine (360/10)	85.6	98.0	100

Table 2

Age group	Vaccine group	Anti-HAV		Anti-HBs	
		N	S+ (%)	N	SP (%)
1-5 yrs old	Ambirix	98	100	98	98
	Combined HAB vaccine (360/10)	92	100	92	100
6-11 yrs old	Ambirix	103	100	103	99
	Combined HAB vaccine (360/10)	96	100	96	100
12-15 yrs old	Ambirix	142	100	142	97.9
	Combined HAB vaccine (360/10)	147	100	147	100

6. PHARMACEUTICAL PARTICULARS

6.1 List of excipients

Sodium chloride

Water for injections

For adjuvants, see section 2.

6.2 Incompatibilities

Not applicable.

6.3 Shelf life

3 years.

6.4 Special precautions for storage

Store in a refrigerator (2°C - 8°C).

Do not freeze.

Store in the original package, in order to protect from light.

6.5 Nature and contents of container

1 ml of suspension in a prefilled syringe (type I glass) with a plunger stopper (rubber butyl).

Pack sizes of 1 and 10 with or without needles and pack size of 50 without needles.

Not all pack sizes may be marketed.

6.6 Special precautions for disposal and other handling

Upon storage, a fine white deposit with a clear colourless supernatant can be observed.

Before administration, the vaccine should be well shaken to obtain a slightly opaque, white suspension.

The vaccine should be visually inspected both before and after resuspension for any foreign particulate matter and/or change in physical appearance. The vaccine must not be used if any change in the appearance of the vaccine has taken place.

Any unused vaccine or waste material should be disposed of in accordance with local requirements.

7. MARKETING AUTHORISATION HOLDER

GlaxoSmithKline Biologicals s.a.

rue de l'Institut 89

B-1330 Rixensart, Belgium

8. MARKETING AUTHORISATION NUMBER(S)

EU/1/02/224/001

EU/1/02/224/002

EU/1/02/224/003

EU/1/02/224/004

EU/1/02/224/005

9. DATE OF FIRST AUTHORISATION/RENEWAL OF THE AUTHORISATION

Date of first authorisation: 30 August 2002

Date of latest renewal: 5 September 2007

10. DATE OF REVISION OF THE TEXT

30 August 2007

AmBisome

(Gilead Sciences Ltd)

1. NAME OF THE MEDICINAL PRODUCT

AmBisome 50 mg Powder for solution for infusion.

2. QUALITATIVE AND QUANTITATIVE COMPOSITION

Each vial contains 50 mg of amphotericin (50,000 units) encapsulated in liposomes. After reconstitution, the concentrate contains 4 mg/mL amphotericin B.

For a full list of excipients, see section 6.1.

3. PHARMACEUTICAL FORM

AmBisome is a sterile, Powder for solution for infusion. AmBisome is a yellow lyophilised cake or powder. After reconstitution, the product is an injectable intended to be administered by intravenous infusion.

4. CLINICAL PARTICULARS

4.1 Therapeutic indications

AmBisome is indicated in:

- the treatment of severe systemic and/or deep mycoses where toxicity (particularly nephrotoxicity) precludes the use of conventional systemic amphotericin B in effective dosages.
- the treatment of visceral leishmaniasis in immunocompetent patients including both adults and children.
- the empirical treatment of presumed fungal infections in febrile neutropenic patients, where the fever has failed to respond to broad spectrum antibiotics and appropriate investigations have failed to define a bacterial or viral cause.

Infections successfully treated with AmBisome include: disseminated candidiasis, aspergillosis, mucormycosis, chronic mycetoma, cryptococcal meningitis and visceral leishmaniasis.

This drug should not be used to treat the common clinically inapparent forms of fungal disease which show only positive skin or serologic tests.

4.2 Posology and method of administration

AmBisome should be administered by intravenous infusion over a 30 - 60 minute period. For doses greater than 5mg/

g/day, intravenous infusion over a 2 hour period is recommended (see section 4.4). The recommended concentration for intravenous infusion is 0.20 mg/ml to 2.00 mg/ml amphotericin B as AmBisome. AmBisome therapy has been administered for as long as three months, with a cumulative dose of 16.8 g of amphotericin B as AmBisome without significant toxicity.

Adult Patients

Treatment of mycoses:

Therapy is usually instituted at a daily dose of 1.0 mg/kg of body weight, and increased stepwise to 3.0 mg/kg, as required. Data are presently insufficient to define total dosage requirements and duration of treatment necessary for resolution of mycoses. However, a cumulative dose of 1.0 - 3.0 g of amphotericin B as AmBisome over 3 - 4 weeks has been typical. Dosage of amphotericin B as AmBisome must be adjusted to the specific requirements of each patient.

Treatment of visceral leishmaniasis:

A total dose of 21.0 - 30.0 mg/kg of body weight given over 10-21 days may be used in the treatment of visceral leishmaniasis. Particulars as to the optimal dosage and the eventual development of resistance are as yet incomplete. The product should be administered under strict medical supervision.

Empirical treatment of febrile neutropenia:

The recommended daily dose is 3 mg/kg body weight per day. Treatment should be continued until the recorded temperature is normalised for 3 consecutive days. In any event, treatment should be discontinued after a maximum of 42 days.

Paediatric Patients: Both systemic fungal infections in children and presumed fungal infections in children with febrile neutropenia have been successfully treated with AmBisome, without reports of unusual adverse events. Paediatric patients have received AmBisome at doses comparable to those used in adults on a per kilogram body weight basis.

AmBisome is not recommended for use in children below 1 month old due to a lack of data on safety and efficacy.

Elderly Patients: No alteration in dose or frequency of dosing is required.

Renal Impairment: AmBisome has been successfully administered to a large number of patients with pre-existing renal impairment at starting doses ranging from 1-3 mg/kg/day in clinical trials and no adjustment in dose or frequency of administration was required.

4.3 Contraindications

AmBisome is contraindicated in those patients who have shown hypersensitivity to the active substance or to any of the excipients unless, in the opinion of the physician, the condition requiring treatment is life-threatening and amenable only to AmBisome therapy.

4.4 Special warnings and precautions for use

Anaphylaxis and anaphylactoid reactions have been reported in association with AmBisome infusion. Allergic type reactions, including severe infusion-related reactions can occur during administration of amphotericin-containing products, including AmBisome (see section 4.8). Therefore, administration of a test dose is still advisable before a new course of treatment. For this purpose a small amount of an AmBisome infusion (e.g. 1 mg) can be administered for about 10 minutes, the infusion stopped and the patient observed carefully for the next 30 minutes. If there have been no severe allergic or anaphylactic/anaphylactoid reactions the infusion of AmBisome dose can be continued. If a severe allergic or anaphylactic/anaphylactoid reaction occurs, the infusion should be immediately discontinued and the patient should not receive further infusion of AmBisome.

Other severe infusion-related reactions can occur during administration of amphotericin B-containing products, including AmBisome (see section 4.8). Although infusion-related reactions are not usually serious, consideration of precautionary measures for the prevention or treatment of these reactions should be given to patients who receive AmBisome therapy. Slower infusion rates (over 2 hours) or routine doses of diphenhydramine, paracetamol, pethidine and/or hydrocortisone have been reported as successful in their prevention or treatment.

AmBisome has been shown to be substantially less toxic than conventional amphotericin B, particularly with respect to nephrotoxicity; however, adverse reactions including renal adverse reactions, may still occur.

In studies comparing AmBisome 3 mg/kg daily with higher doses (5, 6 or 10 mg/kg daily, it was found that the incidence rates of increased serum creatinine, hypokalaemia and hypomagnesaemia were notably higher in the high dose groups.

In particular, caution should be exercised when prolonged therapy is required. Regular laboratory evaluation of serum electrolytes, particularly potassium and magnesium as well as renal, hepatic and haematopoietic function should be performed, at least once weekly. This is particularly important in patients receiving concomitant nephrotoxic medications (see section 4.5). Renal function should be closely monitored in these patients. Due to the risk of hypokalaemia, appropriate potassium supplementation may be required during the course of AmBisome administration. If clinically significant reduction in renal function or worsening of other parameters occurs, consideration should be given to dose reduction, treatment interruption or discontinuation.

Acute pulmonary toxicity has been reported in patients given amphotericin B (as sodium deoxycholate complex) during or shortly after leukocyte transfusions. It is recommended that these infusions are separated by as long a period as possible and pulmonary function should be monitored.

In the Treatment of Diabetic Patients: It should be noted that AmBisome contains approximately 900 mg of sucrose in each vial.

4.5 Interaction with other medicinal products and other forms of interaction

No specific interaction studies have been performed with AmBisome. However, the following drugs are known to interact with amphotericin B and may interact with AmBisome:

Nephrotoxic medications: Concurrent administration of AmBisome with other nephrotoxic agents (for example ciclosporin, aminoglycosides, polymixins, tacrolimus and pentamidine) may enhance the potential for drug-induced renal toxicity in some patients. However, in patients receiving concomitant ciclosporin and/or aminoglycosides, AmBisome was associated with significantly less nephrotoxicity compared to amphotericin B. Regular monitoring of renal function is recommended in patients receiving AmBisome with any nephrotoxic medications.

Corticosteroids, corticotropin (ACTH) and diuretics: Concurrent use of corticosteroids, ACTH and diuretics (loop and thiazide) may potentiate hypokalemia.

Digitalis glycosides: AmBisome-induced hypokalemia may potentiate digitalis toxicity.

Skeletal muscle relaxants: AmBisome-induced hypokalemia may enhance the curariform effect of skeletal muscle relaxants (e.g. tubocurarine).

Antifungals: No evidence of benefit from the use of flucytosine with AmBisome has been observed. Whilst synergy between amphotericin and flucytosine has been reported, concurrent use may increase the toxicity of flucytosine by possibly increasing its cellular uptake and/or impairing its renal excretion.

Antineoplastic agents: Concurrent use of antineoplastic agents may enhance the potential for renal toxicity, bronchospasm and hypotension. Antineoplastic agents should be given concomitantly with caution.

Leukocyte transfusions: Acute pulmonary toxicity has been reported in patients given amphotericin B (as sodium deoxycholate complex) during or shortly after leukocyte transfusions. It is recommended these infusions are separated by as long a period as possible and pulmonary function should be monitored.

4.6 Pregnancy and lactation

Pregnancy

Teratogenicity studies in both rats and rabbits have concluded that AmBisome had no teratogenic potential in these species (See also section 5.3).

The safety of AmBisome in pregnant women has not been established. AmBisome should only be used during pregnancy if the possible benefits to be derived outweigh the potential risks to the mother and foetus.

Systemic fungal infections have been successfully treated in pregnant women with conventional amphotericin B without obvious effect on the foetus, but the number of cases reported is insufficient to draw any conclusions on the safety of AmBisome in pregnancy.

Lactation

It is unknown whether AmBisome is excreted in human breast milk. A decision on whether to breastfeed while receiving AmBisome should take into account the potential risk to the child as well as the benefit of breast feeding for the child and the benefit of AmBisome therapy for the mother.

4.7 Effects on ability to drive and use machines

No studies on the effects on the ability to drive and use machines have been performed. Some of the undesirable effects of AmBisome presented below may impact the ability to drive and use machines.

4.8 Undesirable effects

Fever and chills/rigors are the most frequent infusion-related reactions expected to occur during AmBisome administration. Less frequent infusion-related reactions may consist of one or more of the following symptoms: back pain, chest tightness or pain, dyspnoea, bronchospasm, flushing, tachycardia, and hypotension. These resolve rapidly on stopping the infusion and may not occur with every subsequent dose or when slower infusion rates (over 2 hours) are used. In addition, infusion-related reactions may also be prevented by the use of premedication. However, severe infusion-related reactions may necessitate the permanent discontinuation of AmBisome (see section 4.4).

In two double-blind, comparative studies, AmBisome treated patients experienced a significantly lower incidence of infusion-related reactions, as compared to patients treated with conventional amphotericin B or amphotericin B lipid complex.

In pooled study data from randomised, controlled clinical trials comparing AmBisome with conventional amphotericin B therapy in greater than 1,000 patients, reported adverse reactions were considerably less severe and less frequent in AmBisome treated patients as compared with conventional amphotericin B treated patients.

Nephrotoxicity occurs to some degree with conventional amphotericin B in most patients receiving the drug intravenously. In a double-blind study involving 687 patients, the incidence of nephrotoxicity with AmBisome (as measured by serum creatinine increase greater than 2.0 times baseline measurement), was approximately half that for conventional amphotericin B. In another double-blind study involving 244 patients, the incidence of nephrotoxicity with AmBisome (as measured by serum creatinine increase greater than 2.0 times baseline measurement) is approximately half that for Amphotericin B lipid complex.

The following adverse reactions have been attributed to AmBisome based on clinical trial data and post-marketing experience. The frequency is based on analysis from pooled clinical trials of 688 AmBisome treated patients; the frequency of adverse reactions identified from post-marketing experience is not known. Adverse reactions are listed below by body system organ class using MedDRA and are sorted by frequency. Within each frequency grouping, undesirable effects are presented in order of decreasing seriousness.

Frequencies are defined as:

Very common ($\geq$ 1/10)

Common ($\geq$ 1/100 to $<$ 1/10)

Uncommon ($\geq$ 1/1,000 to $<$ 1/100)

Very rare ($<$1/10,000), not known (cannot be estimated from the available data)

CARDIAC DISORDERS

Common: tachycardia

Not known: cardiac arrest, arrhythmia

BLOOD AND LYMPHATIC SYSTEM DISORDERS

Uncommon: thrombocytopenia

Not known: anemia

NERVOUS SYSTEM DISORDERS

Common: headache

Uncommon: convulsion

RESPIRATORY, THORACIC AND MEDIASTINAL DISORDERS

Common: dyspnoea

Uncommon: bronchospasm

GASTROINTESTINAL DISORDERS

Very common: nausea, vomiting

Common: diarrhoea, abdominal pain

RENAL AND URINARY DISORDERS

Common: increased creatinine, blood urea increased

Not known: renal failure, renal insufficiency

SKIN AND SUBCUTANEOUS DISORDERS

Common: rash

Not known: angioneurotic oedema

MUSCULOSKELETAL AND CONNECTIVE TISSUE DISORDERS

Common: back pain

METABOLISM AND NUTRITION DISORDERS

Very common: hypokalemia

Common: hypomagnesaemia, hypocalcemia, hyperglycemia, hyponatremia

VASCULAR DISORDERS

Common: vasodilatation, flushing, hypotension

GENERAL DISORDERS AND ADMINISTRATION SITE CONDITIONS

Very Common: pyrexia, rigors

Common: chest pain

IMMUNE SYSTEM DISORDERS

Uncommon: anaphylactoid reaction

Not known: anaphylactic reactions, hypersensitivity

HEPATOBILIARY DISORDERS

Common: liver function tests abnormal, hyperbilirubinaemia, alkaline phosphatase increased

4.9 Overdose

The toxicity of AmBisome due to acute overdose has not been defined. If overdose should occur, cease administration immediately. Carefully monitor clinical status including renal and hepatic function, serum electrolytes and haematological status. Haemodialysis or peritoneal dialysis does not appear to affect the elimination of AmBisome.

5. PHARMACOLOGICAL PROPERTIES

5.1 Pharmacodynamic properties

Pharmacotherapeutic group: Antimycotics for systemic use, antibiotics; ATC code: J02AA01.

Amphotericin B is a macrocyclic, polyene antifungal antibiotic produced by Streptomyces nodosus. Liposomes are closed, spherical vesicles formed from a variety of

Table 1

Diluent	Dilution	Concentration of Amphotericin B mg/mL	Maximum duration of storage at 2-8°C	Maximum duration of storage at 25±2°C
5% Dextrose	1:2	2.0	7 days	48 hours
	1:8	0.5	7 days	48 hours
	1:20	0.2	4 days	24 hours
10% Dextrose	1:2	2.0	48 hours	72 hours
20% Dextrose	1:2	2.0	48 hours	72 hours

amphiphilic substances such as phospholipids. Phospholipids arrange themselves into membrane bilayers when exposed to aqueous solutions. The lipophilic moiety of amphotericin allows the drug to be integrated into the lipid bilayer of the liposomes.

Amphotericin B is fungistatic or fungicidal depending on the concentration attained in body fluids and the susceptibility of the fungus. The drug is thought to act by binding to sterols in the fungal cell membrane, with a resulting change in membrane permeability, allowing leakage of a variety of small molecules. Mammalian cell membranes also contain sterols, and it has been suggested that the damage to human cells and fungal cells caused by amphotericin B may share common mechanisms.

Microbiology

Amphotericin B, the antifungal component of AmBisome, shows a high order of in vitro activity against many species of fungi. Most strains of *Histoplasma capsulatum, Coccidioides immitis, Candida spp., Blastomyces dermatitidis, Rhodotorula, Cryptococcus neoformans, Sporothrix schenkii, Mucor mucedo* and *Aspergillus fumigatus*, are inhibited by concentrations of amphotericin B ranging from 0.03 to 1.0 mcg/ml in vitro. Amphotericin has minimal or no effect on bacteria and viruses.

5.2 Pharmacokinetic properties

The pharmacokinetic profile of AmBisome, based upon total plasma concentrations of amphotericin B, was determined in cancer patients with febrile neutropenia and bone marrow transplant patients who received 1 hour infusions of 1.0 to 7.5mg/kg/day AmBisome for 3 to 20 days. AmBisome has a significantly different pharmacokinetic profile from that reported in the literature for conventional presentations of amphotericin B, with higher amphotericin B plasma concentrations (Cmax) and increased exposure (AUC_{0-24}) following administration of AmBisome as compared to conventional amphotericin B. After the first dose and last dose, the pharmacokinetic parameters of AmBisome (mean ± standard deviation) ranged from:

C max	7.3 μg/ml (± 3.8) to 83.7 μg/ml (± 43.0)
$T_{1/2}$	6.3 hr (± 2.0) to 10.7 hr (± 6.4)
AUC_{0-24}	27 μg.hr/ml (±14) to 555 μg.hr/ml (± 311)
Clearance (Cl)	11 ml/hr/kg (± 6) to 51 ml/hr/kg (± 44)
Volume of distribution (Vss)	0.10 L/kg (± 0.07) to 0.44 L/kg (±0.27)

Minimum and maximum pharmacokinetic values do not necessarily come from the lowest and highest doses, respectively. Following administration of AmBisome steady state was reached quickly (generally within 4 days of dosing). AmBisome pharmacokinetics following the first dose appear non-linear such that serum AmBisome concentrations are greater than proportional with increasing dose. This non-proportional dose response is believed to be due to saturation of reticuloendothelial AmBisome clearance. There was no significant drug accumulation in the plasma following repeated administration of 1 to 7.5mg/kg/day. Volume of distribution on day 1 and at steady state suggests that there is extensive tissue distribution of AmBisome. After repeated administration of AmBisome, the terminal elimination half-life ($t_{½β}$) for AmBisome was approximately 7 hours. The excretion of AmBisome has not been studied. The metabolic pathways of amphotericin B and AmBisome are not known. Due to the size of the liposomes, there is no glomerular filtration and renal elimination of AmBisome, thus avoiding interaction of amphotericin B with the cells of the distal tubuli and reducing the potential for nephrotoxicity seen with conventional amphotericin B presentations.

Renal Impairment

The effect of renal impairment on the pharmacokinetics of AmBisome has not been formally studied. Data suggest that no dose adjustment is required in patients undergoing haemodialysis or filtration procedures, however, AmBisome administration should be avoided during the procedure.

5.3 Preclinical safety data

In subchronic toxicity studies in dogs (1 month), rabbits (1 month) and rats (3 months) at doses equal to or, in some species, less than the clinical therapeutic doses of 1 to 3 mg/kg/day, the target organs for AmBisome toxicity were the liver and kidneys with thrombocytopenia also observed. All are known targets for amphotericin B toxicity.

AmBisome was found to be non-mutagenic in bacterial and mammalian systems.

Carcinogenicity studies have not been conducted with AmBisome.

No adverse effects on male or female reproductive function were noted in rats.

6. PHARMACEUTICAL PARTICULARS

6.1 List of excipients

Hydrogenated soy phosphatidylcholine

Cholesterol

Distearoylphosphatidylglycerol

Alpha tocopherol

Sucrose

Disodium succinate hexahydrate

Sodium hydroxide (for pH adjustment)

Hydrochloric acid (for pH adjustment)

6.2 Incompatibilities

AmBisome is incompatible with saline solutions and may not be mixed with other drugs or electrolytes.

This medicinal product must not be mixed with other medicinal products except those mentioned in section 6.6.

6.3 Shelf life

3 years

Shelf –life of AmBisome after first opening

As AmBisome does not contain any bacteriostatic agent, from a microbiological point of view, the reconstituted or diluted product should be used immediately.

In-use storage times and conditions prior to administration are the responsibility of the user and would normally not be longer than 24 hours at 2-8°C, unless reconstitution has taken place in controlled and validated aseptic conditions.

However, the following chemical and physical in-use stability data for AmBisome has been demonstrated:

Shelf-life after reconstitution:

Glass vials for 24 hours at 25±2°C exposed to ambient light

Glass vials and polypropylene syringes up to 7 days at 2-8°C

Do not freeze

DO NOT STORE partially used vials for future patient use.

Shelf-life after dilution with Dextrose:

PVC or Polyolefin infusion bags: 25±2°C exposed to ambient light or at 2-8°C. Do not freeze. See table below for recommendations.

(see Table 1 above)

6.4 Special precautions for storage

AmBisome: Unopened vials; Do not store above 25°C. Do not freeze. Keep container in the outer carton.

For storage conditions of the reconstituted and diluted medicinal product, see section 6.3.

6.5 Nature and contents of container

AmBisome is presented in 15 ml or 30ml sterile, Type I glass vials. The closure consists of a grey butyl rubber stopper and aluminium ring seal fitted with a removable plastic cap. Single-dose vials are packed ten per carton with 10 filters. Not all pack sizes may be marketed.

6.6 Special precautions for disposal and other handling

READ THIS ENTIRE SECTION CAREFULLY BEFORE BEGINNING RECONSTITUTION

AmBisome Must Be Reconstituted By Suitably Trained Staff.

AmBisome must be reconstituted using Sterile Water for Injection (without a bacteriostatic agent). After reconstitution with water for injections the concentrate is a translucent, yellow dispersion.

Vials of AmBisome Containing 50 mg of Amphotericin are Prepared as Follows:

1. Add 12 ml of Sterile Water for Injection to each AmBisome vial, to yield a preparation containing 4 mg/ml amphotericin.
2. IMMEDIATELY after the addition of water, SHAKE THE VIAL VIGOROUSLY for 30 seconds to completely disperse the AmBisome. Visually inspect the vial for particulate matter and continue shaking until complete dispersion is obtained.
3. Calculate the amount of reconstituted (4 mg/ml) AmBisome to be further diluted.
4. The infusion solution is obtained by dilution of the reconstituted AmBisome with between one (1) and nineteen (19) parts Dextrose Injection by volume, to give a final concentration in the recommended range c 2.00 mg/ml to 0.20 mg/ml amphotericin as AmBisome
5. Withdraw the calculated volume of reconstituted AmBisome into a sterile syringe. Using the 5 micron filter provided, instill the AmBisome preparation into a sterile container with the correct amount of Dextrose Injection.

Do not reconstitute the lyophilized powder/cake with salin or add saline to the reconstituted concentrate, or mix wit other drugs.

Use only Water for Injection to reconstitute the powde cake. Use only Dextrose Injection to dilute the reconst tuted product to the appropriate concentration for infusior

Aseptic technique must be strictly observed in all handlin since no preservative or bacteriostatic agent is present i AmBisome, or in the materials specified for reconstitutio and dilution. The use of any solution other than thos recommended, or the presence of a bacteriostatic ager (e.g. benzyl alcohol) in the solution, may cause precipita tion of AmBisome. Do not use material if there is an evidence of precipitation of foreign matter.

An in-line membrane filter may be used for intravenou infusion of AmBisome. However, the mean pore diamete of the filter should not be less than 1.0 micron.

NOTE: AMBISOME IS NOT PHYSICALLY COMPATIBL WITH SALINE SOLUTIONS AND SHOULD NOT BE MIXE WITH OTHER DRUGS OR ELECTROLYTES. AN EXISTIN INTRAVENOUS LINE MUST BE FLUSHED WITH DEX TROSE INJECTION PRIOR TO INFUSION OF AMBISOME IF THIS IS NOT FEASIBLE, AMBISOME SHOULD B ADMINISTERED THROUGH A SEPARATE LINE.

Any unused product or waste material should be dispose of in accordance with local requirements.

7. MARKETING AUTHORISATION HOLDER

Gilead Sciences International Limited,

Granta Park,

Abington,

Cambridge,

CB21 6GT.

8. MARKETING AUTHORISATION NUMBER(S)

PL: 16807/0001

9. DATE OF FIRST AUTHORISATION/RENEWAL O THE AUTHORISATION

11 September 1998/24 September 2004.

10. DATE OF REVISION OF THE TEXT

21/01/2009

Amilamont 5mg/5ml Oral Solution

(Rosemont Pharmaceuticals Limited)

1. NAME OF THE MEDICINAL PRODUCT

Amilamont 5mg/5ml Oral Solution

2. QUALITATIVE AND QUANTITATIVE COMPOSITION

Amiloride Hydrochloride BP 5.675mg equivalent to anhy drous Amiloride Hydrochloride 5mg

3. PHARMACEUTICAL FORM

Solution for oral administration

4. CLINICAL PARTICULARS

4.1 Therapeutic indications

Potassium - conserving agent; diuretic.

Although Amiloride Hydrochloride may be used alone, it principal indication is as concurrent therapy with thiazide or more potent diuretics to conserve potassium durin periods of vigorous diuresis and during long term main tenance therapy.

In hypertension, it is used as an adjunct to prolonge therapy with thiazides and similar agents to prevent potas sium depletion.

In congestive heart failure, Amiloride Hydrochloride may b effective alone, but its principal indication is for concomi tant use in patients receiving thiazides or more poter diuretic agents.

In hepatic cirrhosis with ascites, Amiloride Hydrochlorid usually provides adequate diuresis, with diminished potas sium loss and less risk of metabolic alkalosis, when use alone. It may be used with more potent diuretics when a greater diuresis is required while maintaining a mor balanced serum electrolyte pattern.

4.2 Posology and method of administration

Adults:

Amiloride Hydrochloride alone. The usual initial dosage is 10mg (as a single dose or 5mg twice a day). The total dail dose should not exceed 20mg (20ml) a day.

After diuresis has been achieved, the dosage may b reduced by 5mg (5ml) increments to the least amoun required.

miloride Hydrochloride with other diuretic therapy

Vhen Amiloride is used with a diuretic which is given on an ntermittent basis, it should be given at the same time as he diuretic.

Iypertension

Jsually 2.5mg (2.5ml) given once a day together with the sual antihypertensive dosage of the thiazide concurrently mployed. If necessary, increase to 5mg (5ml) given once a lay or in divided doses.

Congestive heart failure

nitially 2.5mg (2.5ml) a day together with the usual dosage of the diuretic concurrently employed, subsequently adjusted if required, but not exceeding 10mg (10ml) a day. Optimal dosage is determined by diuretic response and the plasma potassium level. Once an initial diuresis has been achieved, reduction in dosage may be attempted for maintenance therapy. Maintenance therapy may be on an intermittent basis.

Hepatic Cirrhosis with ascites

nitiate therapy with a low dose. A single daily dose of 5mg (5ml) plus a low dosage of the other diuretic agent may be increased gradually until there is an effective diuresis. The dosage of Amiloride Hydrochloride should not exceed 10mg (10ml) a day. Maintenance dosages may be lower than those required to initiate diuresis; dosage reduction should therefore be attempted when the patient's weight is stabilised. A gradual weight reduction is especially desirable in cirrhotic patients to reduce the likelihood of untoward reactions associated with diuretic therapy.

Children

The use of Amiloride Hydrochloride in children under 18 years of age is not recommended as safety and efficacy have not been established.

Elderly

The elderly are more susceptible to electrolyte imbalance, and are more likely to experience hyperkalaemia since renal reserve may be reduced. The dosage should be carefully adjusted according to renal function, blood electrolytes and diuretic response.

4.3 Contraindications

Hyperkalaemia (plasma potassium over 5.5mmol/l) other potassium-conserving agents or potassium supplements (see Precautions); Addison's disease; anuria; acute renal failure, severe progressive renal disease, diabetic nephropathy (see Precautions); prior sensitivity to this product. Safety for use in children is not established. See also 'Use in Pregnancy' and 'Use in the Breast Feeding mother'.

4.4 Special warnings and precautions for use

Diabetes Mellitus

To minimise the risk of hyperkalaemia in known or suspected diabetic patients, the status of renal function should be determined before initiating therapy. Amiloride Hydrochloride should be discontinued for at least three days before a glucose-tolerance test.

Metabolic or Respiratory Acidosis

Potassium-conserving therapy should be initiated only with caution in severely ill patients in whom metabolic or respiratory acidosis may occur e.g. patients with cardiopulmonary disease or decompensated diabetes. Shifts in acid-base balance alter the balance of extracellular-intracellular potassium, and the development of acidosis may be associated with rapid increases in plasma potassium.

Hyperkalaemia

This has been observed in patients receiving Amiloride Hydrochloride, alone or with other diuretics. These patients should be observed carefully for clinical, laboratory or ECG evidence of hyperkalaemia.

Some deaths have been reported in this group of patients. Hyperkalaemia has been noted particularly in the elderly and in hospital patients with hepatic cirrhosis or cardiac oedema who have known renal involvement, who were seriously ill, or were undergoing vigorous diuretic therapy.

Neither potassium-conserving agents nor a diet rich in potassium should be used with Amiloride Hydrochloride except in severe and/or refractory cases of hypokalaemia. If the combination is used, plasma potassium levels must be continuously monitored.

Impaired Renal Function

Patients with increases in blood urea over 10mmol/l, serum creatinine over 130μmol/l, or with diabetes mellitus, should not receive Amiloride Hydrochloride without careful, frequent monitoring of serum electrolytes and blood urea levels. In renal impairment, use of a potassium conserving agent may result in rapid development of hyperkalaemia.

Treatment of Hyperkalaemia

If hyperkalaemia occurs, Amiloride Hydrochloride should be discontinued immediately and, if necessary, active measures taken to reduce the plasma potassium level.

Electrolyte Imbalance and Reversible Blood Urea Increases.

Hyponatraemia and hypochloraemia may occur when Amiloride Hydrochloride is used with other diuretics. Reversible increases in blood urea levels have been reported accompanying vigorous diuresis, especially when diuretics were used in seriously ill patients, such as those with hepatic cirrhosis and metabolic alkalosis or those with resistant oedema. Careful monitoring of serum electrolytes and blood urea levels should therefore be carried out when Amiloride Hydrochloride is given with other diuretics to such patients.

Cirrhotic patients

Oral diuretic therapy is more frequently accompanied by side effects in patients with hepatic cirrhosis with or without ascites, because these patients are intolerant of acute shifts in electrolyte balance, and because they often already have hypokalaemia as a result of associated aldosteronism.

In patients with pre-existing severe liver disease, hepatic encephalopathy manifested by tremors, confusion and coma, and increased jaundice has been reported in association with diuretics, including Amiloride Hydrochloride.

Excipient Warnings

This product also contains liquid maltitol. Patients with rare hereditary problems of fructose should not take this medicine.

Methyl and propyl hydroxybenzoates are contained in this product which may cause allergic reactions (possibly delayed).

This product contains a flavouring agent which contains small amounts of ethanol, less than 100mg per 5ml.

4.5 Interaction with other medicinal products and other forms of interaction

Lithium should not be given with diuretics because they reduce its renal clearance and add a high risk of lithium toxicity.

When combined with thiazide diuretics, Amiloride can act synergistically with chlorpropamide to increase the risk of hyponatraemia.

Hyponatraemia and hypochloraemia may occur when Amiloride is used with other diuretics (See Section 4.4 Special warnings and precautions for use).

When Amiloride Hydrochloride is administered concomitantly with an angiotensin-converting enzyme inhibitor, angiotensin II receptor antagonist, trilostrane, ciclosporin or tacrolimus, the risk of hyperkalaemia may be increased. Therefore, if concomitant use of these agents is indicated because of demonstrated hypokalaemia, they should be used with caution and with frequent monitoring of serum potassium.

The concomitant administration of Amiloride and NSAIDs may lead to an increased risk of nephrotoxicity, an antagonism of the diuretic effect and possibly an increased risk of hyperkalaemia, particularly in elderly patients. Therefore, when amiloride hydrochloride is used concomitantly with NSAIDs, renal function and serum potassium levels should be carefully monitored.

4.6 Pregnancy and lactation

Because clinical experience is limited, Amiloride Hydrochloride is not recommended for use during pregnancy. The routine use of diuretics in otherwise healthy pregnant women with or without mild oedema is not indicated because they may be associated with hypovolaemia, increased blood viscosity and decreased placental perfusion.

Foetal and neonatal jaundice, foetal bone marrow depression and thrombocytopenia have also been described. The potential benefits of the drug must be weighed against the possible hazards to the foetus if it is administered to a woman of child bearing age.

It is not known whether Amiloride Hydrochloride is excreted in human milk. Because many drugs are excreted by this route, and because there is a risk that it might take this route of excretion and that it might then cause serious side effects in the breast feeding infant, the mother should either stop breast feeding or stop taking the drug. The decision depends on the importance of the drug to the mother.

4.7 Effects on ability to drive and use machines

None known

4.8 Undesirable effects

Amiloride Hydrochloride is normally well tolerated, although minor side effects are reported relatively frequently. Except for hyperkalaemia, significant side effects are infrequent. Nausea, anorexia, abdominal pain, flatulence and mild skin rash are probably due to Amiloride; but other side effects are generally associated with diuresis or with the underlying condition being treated.

Body as a whole

Headache, weakness, fatigue, back pain, chest pain, neck/shoulder ache, pain in the extremities.

Cardiovascular

Angina pectoris, orthostatic hypertension, arrhythmias, palpitation, one patient with partial heart block developed complete heartblock.

Digestive

Anorexia, nausea, vomiting, diarrhoea, constipation, abdominal pain, GI bleeding, jaundice, thirst, dyspepsia, flatulence.

Metabolism and nutrition disorders

Elevated plasma potassium levels above 5.5mmol/l, hyponatraemia. Serum uric acid levels may rise during treatment with Amiloride and acute attacks of gout may be precipitated.

Integumentary

Pruritus, rash, dryness of mouth, alopecia.

Musculoskeletal

Muscle cramps, joint pain. Serum uric acid levels may rise during treatment with Amiloride and acute attacks of gout may be precipitated.

Nervous

Dizziness, vertigo, paraesthesiae, tremors, encephalopathy.

Psychiatric

Nervousness, mental confusion, insomnia, decreased libido, depression, somnolence.

Respiratory

Cough, dyspnoea.

Special Senses

Nasal congestion, visual disturbances, increased intraocular pressure, tinnitus.

Urogenital

Impotence, polyuria, dysuria, bladder spasm, frequency of micturition.

Reactions in which no causal relationship could be established were activation of probable pre-existing peptic ulcer, aplastic anaemia, neutropenia and abnormal liver function tests. In a few cirrhotic patients, jaundice associated with the underlying disease had deepened but the drug relationship is uncertain.

4.9 Overdose

No data are available; and it is not known whether the drug is dialysable.

The most likely signs and symptoms are dehydration and electrolyte imbalance which should be treated by established methods. Therapy should be discontinued and the patient observed closely. No specific antidote is available. If ingestion is recent, emesis should be induced or gastric lavage performed. Treatment is symptomatic and supportive. If hyperkalaemia occurs, active measures should be taken to reduce plasma potassium levels.

The plasma half life of amiloride is about six hours.

5. PHARMACOLOGICAL PROPERTIES

5.1 Pharmacodynamic properties

Amiloride has mild diuretic and anti-hypertensive activity. It acts primarily in the distal tubule and does not require aldosterone for its action. Amiloride is a mild natriuretic which does not initiate a concomitant decrease in potassium levels. The mechanism of action includes inhibition of the electrogenic entry of sodium thus causing a fall in the electrical potential across the tubular epithelium. Since this potential is one of the main causes of the secretion of potassium, this mechanism is likely to be the basis of the potassium sparing effect. By blocking the sodium channels, Amiloride may also reduce exchange of $Na+$ ions and $H+$ ions. A combination of the Amiloride with a benzothiadazine diuretic will cause less magnesium excretion than the diuretic alone.

5.2 Pharmacokinetic properties

Amiloride is incompletely absorbed from the gastro-intestinal tract; only about 50% is recovered unchanged in the urine following an oral dose. The drug is not metabolised and can, therefore, be useful in patients with liver disease. Peak plasma concentrations are reached about 3 - 4 hours after oral administration and the plasma half-life is in the range of 6 - 9 hours.

In a 70Kg man, the distribution volume is about 5L/Kg, suggesting that the drug is widely distributed in the tissues. Amiloride appears to be weakly bound to plasma proteins as determined by electrophoretic and gel filtration studies. It is not known whether the drug is excreted in breast milk, although studies have shown the presence of Amiloride in the breast milk of rats.

Amiloride is excreted unchanged in the urine. In two studies in which single doses of 14C-Amiloride were used, approximately 50% was recovered in urine and 40% in the faeces within 72 hours. In radioactive studies, peak plasma levels of 38 - 40μg/L were seen three to four hours after a single 20mg oral dose. These low plasma levels are thought to be due to extravascular distribution as evidenced by the large volume of distribution.

In man, the calculate renal clearance of Amiloride exceed in the glomerular filtration, suggesting that there is a tubular secretory pathway. Renal clearance of the drug does not appear to be affected by probenecid, pH of the urine or urinary flow rate.

5.3 Preclinical safety data

None stated

6. PHARMACEUTICAL PARTICULARS

6.1 List of excipients

Citric Acid Monohydrate BP

Methyl Hydroxybenzoate BP

Propyl Hydroxybenzoate BP

Propylene Glycol BP

Vanillin BP

Compound Orange Spirit BP

Liquid Maltitol Ph Eur

Purified Water BP

6.2 Incompatibilities
None known

6.3 Shelf life
Shelf life in marketed pack 24 months

6.4 Special precautions for storage
Store at or below 25°C, out of reach of children

6.5 Nature and contents of container
Glass (Type III) amber bottle, with capacities of 125ml, 150ml, 200ml, 300ml

Closures: a) aluminium, EPE wadded ROPP caps

b) HDPE, EPE wadded, tamper evident

c) HDPE EPE wadded, tamper evident, child resistant

6.6 Special precautions for disposal and other handling
None stated

7. MARKETING AUTHORISATION HOLDER
Rosemont Pharmaceuticals Ltd

Rosemont House

Yorkdale Industrial park

Braithwaite Street

Leeds

LS11 9XE

8. MARKETING AUTHORISATION NUMBER(S)
PL 00427/0091

9. DATE OF FIRST AUTHORISATION/RENEWAL OF THE AUTHORISATION
21 November 1995

10. DATE OF REVISION OF THE TEXT
07 August 2009

Amiodarone Injection Minijet 30mg/ml (International Medication Systems)

(International Medication Systems (UK) Ltd)

1. NAME OF THE MEDICINAL PRODUCT
Amiodarone Injection Minijet 30mg/ml. Solution for injection.

2. QUALITATIVE AND QUANTITATIVE COMPOSITION
Amiodarone Hydrochloride 30mg/ml

(Each 10ml vial contains 300mg)

For excipients, see section 6.1.

3. PHARMACEUTICAL FORM
Solution for injection.

4. CLINICAL PARTICULARS

4.1 Therapeutic indications
Treatment should be initiated and normally monitored only under hospital or specialist supervision. Amiodarone injection is indicated only for the treatment of severe rhythm disorders not responding to other therapies or when other treatments cannot be used.

Tachyarrhythmias associated with Wolff-Parkinson-White Syndrome.

All types of tachyarrhythmias including: supraventricular, nodal and ventricular tachycardias; atrial flutter and fibrillation; ventricular fibrillation; when other drugs cannot be used. The injection is to be used where a rapid response is required.

4.2 Posology and method of administration
Amiodarone injection should only be used when facilities exist for cardiac monitoring, defibrillation and cardiac pacing.

In children, amiodarone injection normally should be given under the supervision of a paediatric cardiologist.

IV infusion is preferred to bolus due to the haemodynamic effects sometimes associated with rapid injection.

Amiodarone injection may be used prior to DC conversion.

Repeated or continuous infusion via peripheral veins may lead to local discomfort and inflammation. When repeated or continuous infusion is anticipated, administration by a central venous catheter is recommended.

The standard recommended dose is 5mg/kg bodyweight given by intravenous infusion over a period of 20 minutes to 2 hours. This should be administered as a dilute solution in 250ml 5% dextrose. This may be followed by repeat infusion up to 1,200mg (approximately 15mg/kg bodyweight) in up to 500ml 5% dextrose per 24 hours, the rate of infusion being adjusted on the basis of clinical response.

In extreme clinical emergency the drug may, at the discretion of the clinician, be given as a slow injection of 150-300mg in 10-20ml 5% dextrose over a minimum of 3 minutes. This should not be repeated for at least 15 minutes.

Patients treated with amiodarone injection must be continuously monitored e.g. in an intensive care unit.

When given by infusion amiodarone injection may reduce the drop size and, if appropriate, adjustments should be made to the rate of infusion.

Changeover from intravenous to oral therapy: as soon as an adequate response has been obtained, oral therapy should be initiated concomitantly at the usual loading dose (200mg three times a day). Amiodarone injection should then be phased out gradually.

Elderly: as with all patients it is important that the minimum effective dose is used. Whilst there is no evidence that dosage requirements are different for this group of patients they may be more susceptible to bradycardia and conduction effects if too high a dose is employed. Particular attentions should be paid to monitoring thyroid function. See Contraindications, Section 4.3 and Precautions, Section 4.4.

4.3 Contraindications
Sinus bradycardia and sino-atrial heart block. In patients with severe conduction disturbances (high grade AV block, bifascicular or trifascicular block) or sinus node disease, amiodarone injection should only be used in conjunction with a pacemaker.

Evidence or history of thyroid dysfunction. Thyroid function tests should be performed prior to therapy in all patients.

Severe respiratory failure, cardiovascular collapse, or severe arterial hypotension; congestive heart failure and cardiomyopathy are also contraindications when using amiodarone injection as a bolus injection.

Known hypersensitivity to iodine or to amiodarone (one ampoule contains approximately 112mg iodine).

The combination of amiodarone injection with drugs which may induce torsades de pointes is contraindicated (see Interactions, Section 4.5).

Lactation (see section 4.6 Lactation)

Amiodarone Injection Minijet contains benzyl alcohol. There have been reports of fatal "gasping syndrome" in neonates (hypotension, bradycardia and cardiovascular collapse) following the administration of intravenous solution containing this preservative. Amiodarone Injection Minijet is therefore contraindicated in infants or young children up to 3 years old.

4.4 Special warnings and precautions for use
Amiodarone Injection Minijet should only be used in a special care unit under continuous monitoring (ECG and blood pressure).

Too high a dose may lead to severe bradycardia and to conduction disturbances with the appearance of an idioventricular rhythm, particularly in elderly patients or during digitalis therapy. In these circumstances, amiodarone treatment should be withdrawn. If necessary beta-adrenostimulants or glucagon may be given.

Caution should be exercised in patients with hypotension and decompensated cardiomyopathy.

Amiodarone induces ECG changes; QT interval lengthening corresponding to prolonged repolarisation with the possible development of U and deformed T waves; these changes are evidence of its pharmacological action and do not reflect toxicity.

Although there have been no literature reports on the potentiation of hepatic adverse effects of alcohol, patients should be advised to moderate their alcohol intake while being treated with amiodarone.

Anaesthesia:

Before surgery, the anaesthetist should be informed that the patient is being treated with amiodarone (see section 4.5 Interactions with other Medicinal Products and other Forms of Interaction).

Increased plasma levels of flecainide have been reported with co-administration of amiodarone. The flecainide dose should be reduced accordingly and the patient closely monitored (see section 4.5 Interactions with other Medicinal Products and other Forms of Interaction).

4.5 Interaction with other medicinal products and other forms of interaction
Some of the more important drugs that interact with amiodarone include warfarin, digoxin, phenytoin and any drug which prolongs QT interval.

Amiodarone raises the plasma concentrations of highly protein bound drugs, for example oral anticoagulants and phenytoin. The dose of warfarin should be reduced accordingly. More frequent monitoring of prothrombin time both during and after amiodarone treatment is recommended. Phenytoin dosage should be reduced if signs of overdosage appear and plasma levels may be measured.

Administration of amiodarone injection to a patient already receiving digoxin will bring about an increase in the plasma digoxin concentration and thus precipitate symptoms and signs associated with high digoxin levels. Monitoring is recommended and digoxin dosage usually has to be reduced. A synergistic effect on heart rate and atrioventricular conduction is also possible.

Combined therapy with the following drugs which prolong the QT interval is contraindicated (see Contraindications, Section 4.3) due to the increased risk of torsades de pointes: for example:

- Class Ia anti-arrhythmic drugs e.g. quinidine, procainamide, disopyramide
- Class III anti-arrhythmic drugs e.g. sotalol, bretylium
- Intravenous erythromycin, co-trimoxazole or pentamidine injection
- Anti-psychotics e.g. chlorpromazine, thioridazine, pimc zide, haloperidol
- Lithium and tricyclic anti-depressants e.g. doxepi maprotiline, amitriptyline
- Certain antihistamines e.g. terfenadine, astemizole
- Anti-malarials e.g. quinine, mefloquine, chloroquin halofantrine

Combined therapy with the following drugs is not recom mended; beta blockers and certain calcium chann blockers (diltiazem, verapamil); potentiation of negativ chronotropic properties and conduction slowing effec may occur.

Stimulant laxatives may cause hypokalaemia thus increas ing the risk of torsades de pointes; other types of laxative should be used.

Caution should be exercised over combined therapy wi the following drugs which may cause hypokalaemia and/ hypomagnesaemia: diuretics, systemic corticosteroid tetracosactrin, intravenous amphotericin.

In case of hypokalaemia, corrective action should be tak and QT interval monitored. In case of torsades de point antiarrhythmic agents should not be given; pacing may b instituted and IV magnesium may be used.

Caution is advised in patients undergoing general anae thesia, or receiving high dose oxygen therapy.

Potentially severe complications have been reported patients taking amiodarone undergoing general anaesth sia: bradycardia unresponsive to atropine, hypotensic disturbances of conduction, decreased cardiac output.

A few cases of adult respiratory distress syndrome, mc often in the period immediately after surgery, have be observed. A possible interaction with high oxygen conce tration may be implicated. The anaesthetist should informed that the patient is taking amiodarone.

Amiodarone is an inhibitor of the hepatic microsomal cyt chrome 3A4 isoenzyme (CYP3A4). This inhibition can res in unexpectedly high plasma levels of other drugs whi are metabolized by CYP3A4 enzymes. Reported exampl of this interaction include immunosuppresives (ciclospor tacrolimus) and HMG-CoA Reductase Inhibitors (simva tatin, atorvastatin). Examples of other drugs known to metabolized by CYP3A4 are: fentanyl, lidocaine, macroli antibiotics (clarithromycin), midazolam, sildenafil, ergot mine.

Since amiodarone is a substrate for CYP3A4, drugs substances that inhibit these isoenzymes may decrea the metabolism and increase the serum concentration amiodarone.

Known inhibitors of CYP3A4 like protease inhibitors (in navir), histamine H2 antagonists (cimetidine), macroli antibiotics (clarithromycin), azol antifungals (ketoconazo itraconazole) can increase plasma levels of amiodaro When changing from intravenous amiodarone to oral am darone the consumption of grapefruit juice should avoided since it can increase the plasma levels of am darone.

Drugs and substances that stimulate the synthesis CYP3A4 (enzyme inducers) may lead to low amiodaro serum levels and potential decrease in efficacy. Report examples of this interaction include antibiotics (rifampic The use of St. John's Wort (Hypericum perforatum) patients receiving amiodarone could result in reduc amiodarone levels.

Amiodarone may supress other CYP450 enzymes, inclu ing CYP1A2, CYP2C9, CYP2D6. This inhibition can res in unexpectedly high plasma levels of other drugs wh are metabolized by those CYP450 enzymes like for exa ple flecainide, dextromethorphan, metoprolol.

4.6 Pregnancy and lactation
Pregnancy: Although no teratogenic effects have be observed in animals, there are insufficient data on t use of amiodarone during pregnancy in humans to jud any possible toxicity. However, in view of the pharmac logical properties of the drug on the foetus and its effe on the foetal thyroid gland, amiodarone is contraindicat during pregnancy, except in exceptional circumstances

Lactation: Amiodarone is excreted into the breast milk significant quantities and breast-feeding is contrain cated.

4.7 Effects on ability to drive and use machines
No studies on the effects on the ability to drive and u machines have been performed.

4.8 Undesirable effects
Following intravenous infusion, inflammation of veins possible. This may be avoided by the use of a cent venous catheter.

Rapid administration of amiodarone injection has be associated with hot flushes, sweating and nausea. A mc erate and transient reduction in blood pressure may occ Circulatory collapse may be precipitated by too ra administration or overdosage (atropine has been us successfully in such patients presenting with bradycard In case of respiratory failure, notably in asthmati bronchospasm and/or apnoea may also occur. Isolat cases of anaphylactic shock have been reported.

Amiodarone can cause serious adverse reactions affect the eyes, heart, lung, liver, thyroid gland, skin a eripheral nervous system (see below). Because these eactions can be delayed, patients on long term treatment hould be carefully supervised.

phthalmological: Patients on continuous therapy almost ways develop microdeposits in the cornea. The deposits re usually only discernable by slit-lamp examinations and ay rarely cause subjective symptoms such as visual aloes and blurring of vision. The deposits are considered ssentially benign, do not require discontinuation of amio-arone and regress following termination of treatment. are cases of impaired visual acuity due to optic neuritis ave been reported, although at present, the relationship ith amiodarone has not been established. Unless blurred r decreased vision occurs, opthalmological examination s recommended annually.

ardiac: Bradycardia, which is generally moderate and ose dependent, has been reported. In some cases (sinus ode disease, elderly patients) marked bradycardia or nore exceptionally sinus arrest has occurred. There have een rare instances of conduction disturbances (sino-atrial lock, various degrees of AV-block). Because of the long alf life of amiodarone, if bradycardia is severe and symp-omatic the insertion of a pacemaker should be consid-ered. Amiodarone has a low proarrhythmic effect. However rrhythmia (new occurrence or aggravation) followed in ome cases by cardiac arrest has been reported; with urrent knowledge it is not possible to differentiate a drug ffect from the underlying cardiac condition or lack of herapeutic efficacy. This has usually occurred in combi-ation with other precipitating factors particularly other antiarrhythmic agents, hypokalaemia and digoxin.

Pulmonary: Amiodarone can cause pulmonary toxicity hypersensitivity pneumonitis, alveolar/interstitial pneumo-nia or fibrosis, pleuritis, bronchiolitis obliterans organising pneumonia, pulmonary haemorrhage). Sometimes this toxicity can be fatal.

Presenting features can include dyspnoea (which may be severe and unexplained by the current cardiac status), non-productive cough and deterioration in general health (fatigue, weight loss and fever). The onset is usually slow but may be rapidly progressive. Whilst the majority of cases have been reported with long-term therapy, a few have occurred soon after starting treatment.

Patients should be carefully evaluated clinically and con-sideration given to chest X-ray before starting therapy. During treatment, if pulmonary toxicity is suspected, this should be repeated and associated with lung function testing including where possible measurement of transfer factor. Initial radiological changes may be difficult to dis-tinguish from pulmonary venous congestion. Pulmonary toxicity has usually been reversible following early with-drawal of amiodarone therapy, with or without corticoster-oid therapy. Clinical symptoms often resolve within a few weeks followed by slower radiological and lung function improvement. Some patients can deteriorate despite dis-continuing amiodarone. A few cases of adult respiratory distress syndrome, most often in the period after surgery, have been observed, resulting sometimes in fatalities (see Interactions, Section 4.5).

A few cases of bronchospasm have been reported in patients with severe respiratory failure and especially in asthmatic patients.

Hepatic: Amiodarone may be associated with a variety of hepatic effects, including cirrhosis, hepatitis and jaundice. Some fatalities have been reported, mainly following long-term therapy, although rarely they have occurred soon after starting treatment. It is advisable to monitor hepatic functions particularly transaminases before treatment and six monthly thereafter.

At the beginning of therapy, elevation of serum transami-nases which can be in isolation (1.5 to 3 times normal) may occur. These may return to normal with dose reduction, or sometimes spontaneously.

Isolated cases of acute liver disorders with elevated serum transaminases and/or jaundice may occur; in such cases treatment should be discontinued.

There have been reports of chronic liver disease. Alteration of of laboratory tests which may be minimal (transaminases elevated 1.5 to 5 times normal) or clinical signs (possible hepatomegaly) during treatment for longer than 6 months should suggest this diagnosis. Routine monitoring of liver function tests is therefore advised. Abnormal clinical and laboratory test results usually regress upon cessation of treatment. Histological findings may resemble pseudo-alcoholic hepatitis, but they can be variable and include chirrosis.

Thyroid: Both thyrotoxicosis and hypothyroidism have occurred during or soon after amiodarone treatment. Sim-ple monitoring of the usual biochemical tests is confusing because some tests such as free T4 and free T3 may be altered where the patient is euthyroid. Clinical monitoring is therefore recommended before start of treatment, then six monthly and should be continued for some months after discontinuation of treatment. This is particularly important in the elderly. In patients whose history indicates an increased risk of thyroid dysfunction, regular assessment is recommended.

Hyperthyroidism: Clinical features such as weight loss, asthenia, restlessness, increase in heart rate, recurrence of cardiac failure, should alert the clinician. The diagnosis may be sup-ported by an elevated serum T3, a low level of thyroid stimulating hormone (TSH) as measured by high sensitivity methods and a reduced TSH response to TRH. Elevation of reverse T3 (r T3) may also be found. In the case of hyperthyroidism, therapy should be withdrawn. Clinical recovery usually occurs within a few weeks, although severe cases, sometimes resulting in fatalities, have been reported.

Courses of anti-thyroid drugs have been used for the treatment of severe thyroid hyperactivity; large doses may be required initially. These may not always be effective and concomitant high dose corticosteroid therapy (eg 1mg/kg prednisolone) may be required for several weeks.

Hypothyroidism: Clinical features such as weight gain, reduced activity or excessive bradycardia should suggest the diagnosis. This may be supported by an elevated serum TSH level and an exaggerated TSH response to TRH. T_4 and T_3 levels may be low. Thyroid hypofunction usually resolves within 3 months of cessation of therapy; it may be treated cautiously with L-thyroxine. Concomitant use of amiodarone should be continued only in life threa-tening situations, when TSH levels may provide a guide to L-thyroxin dosage.

Dermatological: Patients taking amiodarone can become unduly sensitive to sunlight and should be warned of this possibility. In most cases, symptoms are limited to tingling, burning and erythema of sun exposed skin but severe phototoxic reactions with blistering may be seen. Photo-sensitivity may persist for several months after disconti-nuation of amiodarone. Photosensitivity may be minimised by limiting exposure to UV light, wearing suitable protective hats and clothing and by using a broad spectrum sun screening preparation. Rarely, a slate grey or bluish dis-colouration of light exposed skin, particularly on the face may occur. Resolution of this pigmentation may be very slow once the drug is discontinued. Other types of skin rashes including rash maculo-papular and isolated cases of exfoliative dermatitis have been reported. Cases of erythema have been reported during radiotherapy.

Neurological: Peripheral neuropathy can be caused by amiodarone. Myopathy has occasionally been reported. Both these conditions may be severe although they are usually reversible on drug withdrawal. Nightmares, vertigo, headaches, sleeplessness and paraesthesia may also occur. Tremor and ataxia have also infrequently been reported usually with complete regression after reduction of dose or withdrawal of the drug. Benign intracranial hypertension (pseudo-tumour cerebri) has been reported.

Other: Other unwanted effects occasionally reported include nausea, vomiting, metallic taste (which usually occur with loading dosage which regress on dose reduc-tion), fatigue, impotence, epididymo-orchitis, and alope-cia. Isolated cases suggesting a hypersensitivity reaction involving vasculitis, renal involvement with moderate ele-vation of creatinine levels or thrombocytopenia have been observed. Haemolytic or aplastic anaemia have rarely been reported. Isolated cases of anapylatic shock have been reported.

4.9 Overdose

Little information is available regarding acute overdosage with amiodarone. Few cases of sinus bradycardia, heart block, attacks of ventricular tachycardia, torsades de pointes, circulatory failure and hepatic injury have been reported.

In the event of overdose, treatment should be symptomatic in addition to general supportive measures. The patient should be monitored and if bradycardia occurs beta-adre-nostimulants or glucagon may be given. Spontaneously resolving attacks of ventricular tachycardia may also occur. Due to the pharmacokinetics of amiodarone, ade-quate and prolonged surveillance of the patient, particu-larly cardiac status, is recommended. Neither amiodarone nor its metabolites are dialysable.

5. PHARMACOLOGICAL PROPERTIES

5.1 Pharmacodynamic properties

Pharmacotherapeutic group: antiarrhythmic, Class III; ATC code: C01BD 01.

Amiodarone is a product for the treatment of tachyarryth-mias and has complex pharmacological actions. Its effects are anti-adrenergic (partial alpha and beta blockers). It has haemodynamic effects (increased blood flow and sys-tematic/coronary vasodilatation). The drug reduces myo-cardial oxygen consumption and has been shown to have a sparing effect of rat myocardial ATP utilisation, with decreased oxidative processes. Amiodarone inhibits the metallic and biochemical effects of catecholamines on the heart and inhibits Na+ and K+ activated ATP-ase.

5.2 Pharmacokinetic properties

Pharmacokinetics of amiodarone are unusual and com-plex, and have not been completely elucidated. Absorption following oral administration is variable and may be pro-longed, with enterohepatic cycling. The major metabolite is desethylamiodarone. Amiodarone is highly protein bound (> 95%). Renal excretion is minimal and faecal excretion is the major route. A study in both healthy volunteers and patients after intravenous administration of amiodarone reported that the calculated volumes of distribution and total blood clearance using a two-compartment open model were similar for both groups. Elimination of amio-darone after intravenous injection appeared to be biexpo-nential with a distribution phase lasting about 4 hours. The very high volume of distribution combined with a relatively low apparent volume for the central compartment sug-gests extensive tissue distribution. A bolus IV injection of 400mg gave a terminal T½ of approximately 11 hours.

5.3 Preclinical safety data

There are no pre-clinical data of relevance to the prescriber which are additional to that already included in other sec-tions of the SmPC.

6. PHARMACEUTICAL PARTICULARS

6.1 List of excipients

Benzyl alcohol

Polysorbate 80

Water for injections

6.2 Incompatibilities

Amiodarone Injection is incompatible with saline and when diluted should be administered solely in 5% dextrose solu-tion. Solutions containing less than 300mg amiodarone hydrochloride in 500ml dextrose 5% are unstable and should not be used.

The use of administration equipment or devices containing plasticizers such as DEHP (di-2-ethylhexyphthalate) in the presence of amiodarone may result in leaching out of DEHP. In order to minimise patient exposure to DEHP, the final amiodarone dilution for infusion should preferably be administered through non DEHP-containing sets.

6.3 Shelf life

36 months.

6.4 Special precautions for storage

Do not store above 25°C. Keep vial in the outer carton.

6.5 Nature and contents of container

The solution is contained in a type I glass vial with an elastomeric closure and a plastic vial cap.

An IMS Minijet® injector is supplied in the carton.

The product is available as 10ml.

6.6 Special precautions for disposal and other handling

The container is specially designed for use with the IMS Minijet® injector. The instructions for the use of the injector can be found on the side of the outer carton and are as follows;

- Remove the protective caps
- Carefully thread glass vial into injector 3 half turns or until the needle penetrates the stopper
- Remove the needle cap, point needle upwards and expel air.

All infusions longer than 2 hours should be made in glass containers.

7. MARKETING AUTHORISATION HOLDER

International Medication Systems (UK) Ltd

208 Bath Road

Slough

Berkshire

SL1 3WE

UK

8. MARKETING AUTHORISATION NUMBER(S)

PL 03265/0076

9. DATE OF FIRST AUTHORISATION/RENEWAL OF THE AUTHORISATION

28 January 2004

10. DATE OF REVISION OF THE TEXT

Approved: November 2007

Amoxil Capsules 250mg

(GlaxoSmithKline UK)

1. NAME OF THE MEDICINAL PRODUCT

Amoxil® Capsules 250 mg

2. QUALITATIVE AND QUANTITATIVE COMPOSITION

Amoxil Capsules 250 mg contain 250 mg amoxicillin per capsule

The amoxicillin is present as the trihydrate.

3. PHARMACEUTICAL FORM

Amoxil Capsules: maroon and gold capsules overprinted 'Amoxil 250'.

4. CLINICAL PARTICULARS

4.1 Therapeutic indications

Treatment of Infection: Amoxil is a broad spectrum anti-biotic indicated for the treatment of commonly occurring bacterial infections such as:

Upper respiratory tract infections

Otitis media

Acute and chronic bronchitis

Chronic bronchial sepsis

Lobar and bronchopneumonia

Cystitis, urethritis, pyelonephritis

Table 1 Prophylaxis of endocarditis

CONDITION		ADULTS' DOSAGE (INCLUDING ELDERLY)	CHILDREN'S DOSAGE	NOTES
Dental procedures: prophylaxis for patients undergoing extraction, scaling or surgery involving gingival tissues and who have not received a penicillin in the previous month. (N.B. Patients with prosthetic heart valves should be referred to hospital - see below).	Patient not having general anaesthetic.	3 g 'Amoxil' orally, 1 hour before procedure. A second dose may be given 6 hours later, if considered necessary.	Under 10: half adult dose. Under 5: quarter adult dose.	Note 1. If prophylaxis with 'Amoxil' is given twice within one month, emergence of resistant streptococc is unlikely to be a problem. Alternative antibiotics are recommended if more frequent prophylaxis is required, or if the patient has received a course of treatment with a penicillin during the previous month. Note 2. To minimise pain on injection, 'Amoxil' may be given as two injections of 500 mg dissolved in sterile 1% lidocaime solution (see *Administration*).
	Patient having general anaesthetic: if oral antibiotics considered to be appropriate.	Initially 3 g 'Amoxil' orally 4 hours prior to anaesthesia, followed by 3 g orally (or 1 g IV or IM if oral dose not tolerated) as soon as possible after the operation.		
	Patient having general anaesthetic: if oral antibiotics not appropriate.	1 g 'Amoxil' IV or IM immediately before induction; with 500 mg orally, 6 hours later.		
Dental procedures: patients for whom referral to hospital is recommended: a) Patients to be given a general anaesthetic who have been given a penicillin in the previous month. b) Patients to be given a general anaesthetic who have a prosthetic heart valve. c) Patients who have had one or more attacks of endocarditis.		Initially: 1 g 'Amoxil' IV or IM with 120 mg gentamicin IV or IM immediately prior to anaesthesia (if given) or 15 minutes prior to dental procedure. Followed by (6 hours later): 500 mg 'Amoxil' orally.	Under 10: the doses of 'Amoxil' should be half the adult dose; the dose of gentamicin should be 2 mg/kg. Under 5: the doses of 'Amoxil' should be quarter the adult dose; the dose of gentamicin should be 2 mg/kg.	See Note 2. Note 3. 'Amoxil' and gentamicin should not be mixed in the same syringe. Note 4. Please consult the appropriate data sheet for full prescribing information on gentamicin.
Genitourinary Surgery or Instrumentation: prophylaxis for patients who have no urinary tract infection and who are to have genito-urinary surgery or instrumentation under general anaesthesia. In the case of *Obstetric and Gynaecological Procedures* and *Gastrointestinal Procedures*– routine prophylaxis is recommended only for patients with prosthetic heart valves.		Initially: 1 g 'Amoxil' IV or IM with 120 mg gentamicin IV or IM, immediately before induction. Followed by (6 hours later): 500 mg 'Amoxil' orally or IV or IM according to clinical condition.		See Notes 2, 3 and 4 above.
Surgery or Instrumentation of the Upper Respiratory Tract	Patients other than those with prosthetic heart valves.	1 g 'Amoxil' IV or IM immediately before induction; 500 mg 'Amoxil' IV or IM 6 hours later.	Under 10: half adult dose. Under 5: quarter adult dose.	See Note 2 above. Note 5. The second dose of 'Amoxil' may be administered orally as 'Amoxil' Syrup SF/DF.
	Patients with prosthetic heart valves.	Initially: 1 g 'Amoxil' IV or IM with 120 mg gentamicin IV or IM, immediately before induction; followed by (6 hours later) 500 mg 'Amoxil' IV or IM.	Under 10: the dose of 'Amoxil' should be half the adult dose; the gentamicin dose should be 2 mg/kg. Under 5: the dose of 'Amoxil' should be quarter the adult dose; the dose of gentamicin should be 2 mg/kg.	See Notes 2, 3, 4 and 5 above.

Bacteriuria in pregnancy

Gynaecological infections including puerperal sepsis and septic abortion

Gonorrhoea

Peritonitis

Intra-abdominal sepsis

Septicaemia

Bacterial endocarditis

Typhoid and paratyphoid fever

Skin and soft tissue infections

Dental abscess (as an adjunct to surgical management)

Helicobacter pylori eradication in peptic (duodenal and gastric) ulcer disease.

In children with urinary tract infection the need for investigation should be considered.

Prophylaxis of endocarditis: Amoxil may be used for the prevention of bacteraemia, associated with procedures such as dental extraction, in patients at risk of developing bacterial endocarditis.

Consideration should be given to official local guidance (e.g. national requirements) on the appropriate use of antibacterial agents. "Susceptibility of the causative organisms to the treatment should be tested (if possible), although the therapy may be initiated before the results are available.

4.2 Posology and method of administration

Treatment of Infection:

Adult dosage (including elderly patients):

Standard adult dosage: 250 mg three times daily, increasing to 500 mg three times daily for more severe infections.

High dosage therapy (maximum recommended oral dosage 6 g daily in divided doses): A dosage of 3 g twice daily is recommended in appropriate cases for the treatment of severe or recurrent purulent infection of the respiratory tract.

Short course therapy: Simple acute urinary tract infection: two 3 g doses with 10-12 hours between the doses. Dental abscess: two 3 g doses with 8 hours between the doses. Gonorrhoea: single 3 g dose.

Renal impairement:

Glomerular filtration rate >30ml/min No adjustment necessary.

Glomerular filtration rate 10-30ml/min: Amoxicillin. max.500mg b.d

Glomerular filtration rate <10ml/min: Amoxicillin. Max. 500mg/day

Helicobacter eradication in peptic (duodenal and gastric) ulcer disease:

Amoxil is recommended at a dose of twice daily in association with a proton pump inhibitor and antimicrobial agents as detailed below:

Omeprazole 40 mg daily, Amoxicillin 1G BID, Clarithromycin 500mg BID × 7days

or

Omeprazole 40mg daily, Amoxicillin750mg-1G BID, Metronidazole 400mg TID × 7 days

Children's dosage (up to 10 years of age):

Standard children's dosage: 125 mg three times daily, increasing to 250 mg three times daily for more severe infections.

Renal impairement in children under 40 kg:

Creatnine clearance >30mL/min: No adjustment necessary.

Creatinine clearance 10-30mL/min: 15 mg/kg given b.i.d (maximum 500mg/twice daily).

Creatinine clearance <10mL/min: 15 mg/kg given as a single daily dose (maximum 500mg).

Amoxil Paediatric Suspension is recommended for children under six months of age.

In severe or recurrent acute otitis media, especially where compliance may be a problem, 750 mg twice a day for two days may be used as an alternative course of treatment in children aged 3 to 10 years.

In renal impairment the excretion of the antibiotic will be delayed and, depending on the degree of impairment, it may be necessary to reduce the total daily dosage.

Prophylaxis of endocarditis: see table on next page.

Administration: Oral:

Treatment should be continued for 2 to 3 days following the disappearance of symptoms. It is recommended that at least 10 days treatment be given for any infection caused by beta-haemolytic streptococci in order to achieve eradication of the organism.

Prophylaxis of endocarditis:

(see Table 1 above)

4.3 Contraindications

Amoxil is a penicillin and should not be given to penicillin-hypersensitive patients. Attention should be paid to possible cross-sensitivity with other beta-lactam antibiotics eg. cephalosporins.

4.4 Special warnings and precautions for use

Before initiating therapy with amoxicillin, careful enquiry should be made concerning previous hypersensitivity reactions to penicillins, cephalosporins.

Serious and occasionally fatal hypersensitivity (anaphylactoid) reactions have been reported in patients on penicillin therapy. These reactions are more likely to occur in individuals with a history of hypersensitivity to beta-lactam antibiotics (see 4.3).

Erythematous (morbilliform) rashes have been associated with glandular fever in patients receiving amoxicillin.

Prolonged use may also occasionally result in overgrowth of non-susceptible organisms.

In patients with reduced urine output, crystalluria has been observed very rarely, predominantly with parenteral therapy. During the administration of high doses of amoxicillin, it is advisable to maintain adequate fluid intake and urinary output in order to reduce the possibility of amoxicillin crystalluria (see Section 4.9 Overdose).

In patients with renal impairment, the rate of excretion of amoxicillin will be reduced depending on the degree of impairment and it may be necessary to reduce the total daily unit amoxicillin dosage accordingly (see section 4.2).

4.5 Interaction with other medicinal products and other forms of interaction

Probenecid decreases the renal tubular secretion of amoxicillin. Concurrent use with amoxicillin may result in increased and prolonged blood levels of amoxicillin.

In common with other antibiotics, amoxicillin may affect the gut flora, leading to lower oestrogen reabsorption and reduced efficacy of combined oral contraceptives.

Concurrent administration of allopurinol during treatment with amoxicillincan increase the likelihood of allergic skin reactions.

Prolongation of prothrombin time has been reported rarely in patients receiving amoxicillin. Appropriate monitoring should be undertaken when anticoagulants are prescribed concurrently.

It is recommended that when testing for the presence of glucose in urine during amoxicillin treatment, enzymatic glucose oxidase methods should be used. Due to the high urinary concentrations of amoxicillin, false positive readings are common with

6 Pregnancy and lactation

se in pregnancy:

nimal studies with Amoxil have shown no teratogenic ffects. The product has been in extensive clinical use nce 1972 and its suitability in human pregnancy has been vell documented in clinical studies. When antibiotic therpy is required during pregnancy, Amoxil may be considred appropriate when the potential benefits outweigh the otential risks associated with treatment.

Jse in lactation:

moxicillin may be given during lactation. With the excepon of the risk of sensitisation associated with the excreon of trace quantities of amoxicillinin breast milk, there are o known detrimental effects for the breast-fed infant.

.7 Effects on ability to drive and use machines

dverse effects on the ability to drive or operate machinery ave not been observed.

.8 Undesirable effects

he following convention has been utilised for the classiication of undesirable effects:-

/ery common (>1/10), common (>1/100, <1/10), ıncommon (>1/1000,<1/100), rare (>1/10,000, <1/1000), very rare (<1/10,000)

The majority of side effects listed below are not unique to amoxicillin and may occur when using other pencillins.

Jnless otherwise stated, the frequency of adverse events nas been derived from more than 30 years of post-marketng reports.

<u>nfections and infestations</u>

Very Rare: Mucocutaneous candidiasis

<u>Blood and lymphatic system disorders</u>

Very rare: Reversible leucopenia (including severe neutropenia or agranulocytosis), reversible thrombocytopenia and haemolytic anaemia.
Prolongation of bleeding time and prothrombin (see Section 4.5 - Interaction with other Medicinal Products and other Forms of Interaction)

<u>Immune system disorders</u>

Very rare: As with other antibiotics, severe allergic reactions, including angioneurotic oedema, anaphylaxis (see Section 4.4 Special Warnings and Precautions for Use), serum sickness and hypersensitivity vasculitis.
If a hypersensitivity reaction is reported, the treatment must be discontinued. (See also Skin and subcutaneous tissue disorders)

<u>Nervous system disorders</u>

Very rare: Hyperkinesia, dizziness and convulsions.
Convulsions may occur in patients with impaired renal function or in those receiving high doses.

<u>Gastrointestinal disorders</u>

<u>Clinical Trial Data</u>

***Common:** Diarrhoea and nausea.

***Uncommon:** Vomiting.

<u>Post-marketing Data</u>

Very rare: Antibiotic associated colitis (including pseudomembraneous colitis and haemorrhagic colitis).
Black hairy tongue
Superficial tooth discolouration has been reported in children. Good oral hygiene may help to prevent tooth discolouration as it can usually be removed by brushing.

<u>Hepato-biliary disorders</u>

Very rare: Hepatitis and cholestatic jaundice. A moderate rise in AST and/or ALT.
The significance of a rise in AST and/or ALT is unclear.

<u>Skin and subcutaneous tissue disorders</u>

<u>Clinical Trial Data</u>

***Common:** Skin rash

***Uncommon:** Urticaria and pruritus

<u>Post-marketing Data</u>

Very rare: Skin reactions such as erythema multiforme, Stevens Johnson syndrome, toxic epidermal necrolysis, bullous and exfoliative dermatitis and acute generalised exanthematous pustulosis (AGEP)
(See also Immune system disorders).

<u>Renal and urinary tract disorders</u>

Very rare: Interstitial nephritis.

Very rare: Crystalluria (see Section 4.9 Overdose).

*The incidence of these AEs was derived from clinical studies involving a total of approximately 6,000 adult and paediatric patients taking amoxicillin.

4.9 Overdose

Gastrointestinal effects such as nausea, vomiting and diarrhoea may be evident and should be treated symptomatically with attention to the water/electrolyte balance. Amoxicillin crystalluria, in some cases leading to renal failure, has been observed (see Section 4.4 Special warnings and special precautions for use).

Amoxicillin may be removed from the circulation by haemodialysis.

5. PHARMACOLOGICAL PROPERTIES

5.1 Pharmacodynamic properties

Amoxil is a broad spectrum antibiotic.

It is rapidly bactericidal and possesses the safety profile of a penicillin.

The wide range of organisms sensitive to the bactericidal action of Amoxil include:

Aerobes:

Gram positive	Gram negative
Streptococcus faecalis	*Haemophilus influenzae*
Streptococcus pneumoniae	*Escherichia coli*
Streptococcus pyogenes	*Proteus mirabilis*
Streptococcus viridans	*Salmonella* species
Staphylococcus aureus	*Shigella* species
(penicillin sensitive strains only)	*Bordetella pertussis*
	Brucella species
Corynebacterium species	*Neisseria gonorrhoeae*
Bacillus anthracis	*Neisseria meningitidis*
Listeria monocytogenes	*Vibrio cholerae*
	Pasteurella septica

Anaerobes:

Clostridium species

5.2 Pharmacokinetic properties

Amoxil is well absorbed by the oral and parenteral routes. Oral administration, usually at convenient t.d.s. dosage, produces high serum levels independent of the time at which food is taken. Amoxil gives good penetration into bronchial secretions and high urinary concentrations of unchanged antibiotic.

5.3 Preclinical safety data

Not applicable.

6. PHARMACEUTICAL PARTICULARS

6.1 List of excipients

Amoxil Capsules 250 Mg

Each capsule contains magnesium stearate (E572) and erythrosine (E127), indigo carmine (E132), titanium dioxide (E171), yellow iron oxide (E172) and gelatin.

6.2 Incompatibilities

None known.

6.3 Shelf life

Capsules 60M

6.4 Special precautions for storage

Amoxil Capsules should be stored in a dry place.

6.5 Nature and contents of container

Amoxil Capsules: 250 mg Original Pack of 21 with Patient Information Leaflet; also container of 500. Also packs of 3, 6, 12, 50, 100 and 50,000.

6.6 Special precautions for disposal and other handling

Not applicable.

Administrative Data

7. MARKETING AUTHORISATION HOLDER

Beecham Group plc

Great West Road, Brentford, Middlesex TW8 9GS

Trading as GlaxoSmithKline UK, Stockley Park West, Uxbridge, Middlesex UB11 1BT

And/or

Bencard or SmithKline Beecham Pharmaceuticals, Mundells, Welwyn Garden City, Hertfordshire, AL7 1EY.

8. MARKETING AUTHORISATION NUMBER(S)

Amoxil Capsules 250 mg 0038/0103

9. DATE OF FIRST AUTHORISATION/RENEWAL OF THE AUTHORISATION

19 April 1972 / 13 January 1998

10. DATE OF REVISION OF THE TEXT

30th September 2008

11. Legal Category

POM

Amoxil Capsules 500mg

(GlaxoSmithKline UK)

1. NAME OF THE MEDICINAL PRODUCT

Amoxil® Capsules 500 mg

2. QUALITATIVE AND QUANTITATIVE COMPOSITION

Amoxil Capsules 500 mg contain 500 mg amoxicillin per capsule

The amoxicillin is present as the trihydrate.

3. PHARMACEUTICAL FORM

Amoxil Capsules: maroon and gold capsules overprinted 'Amoxil 500'.

4. CLINICAL PARTICULARS

4.1 Therapeutic indications

Treatment of Infection: Amoxil is a broad spectrum antibiotic indicated for the treatment of commonly occurring bacterial infections such as:

Upper respiratory tract infections

Otitis media

Acute and chronic bronchitis

Chronic bronchial sepsis

Lobar and bronchopneumonia

Cystitis, urethritis, pyelonephritis

Bacteriuria in pregnancy

Gynaecological infections including puerperal sepsis and septic abortion

Gonorrhoea

Peritonitis

Intra-abdominal sepsis

Septicaemia

Bacterial endocarditis

Typhoid and paratyphoid fever

Skin and soft tissue infections

Dental abscess (as an adjunct to surgical management)

Helicobacter pylori eradication in peptic (duodenal and gastric) ulcer disease.

In children with urinary tract infection the need for investigation should be considered.

Prophylaxis of endocarditis: Amoxil may be used for the prevention of bacteraemia, associated with procedures such as dental extraction, in patients at risk of developing bacterial endocarditis.

Consideration should be given to official local guidance (e.g. national requirements) on the appropriate use of antibacterial agents."Susceptibility of the causative organism to the treatment should be tested (if possible), although the therapy may be initiated before the results are available.

4.2 Posology and method of administration

Treatment of Infection:

Adult dosage (including elderly patients):

Standard adult dosage: 250 mg three times daily, increasing to 500 mg three times daily for more severe infections.

High dosage therapy (maximum recommended oral dosage 6 g daily in divided doses): A dosage of 3 g twice daily is recommended in appropriate cases for the treatment of severe or recurrent purulent infection of the respiratory tract.

Short course therapy: Simple acute urinary tract infection: two 3 g doses with 10-12 hours between the doses. Dental abscess: two 3 g doses with 8 hours between the doses. Gonorrhoea: single 3 g dose.

Helicobacter eradication in peptic (duodenal and gastric) ulcer disease:

Amoxil is recommended at a dose of twice daily in association with a proton pump inhibitor and antimicrobial agents as detailed below:

Omeprazole 40 mg daily, Amoxicillin 1G BID, Clarithromycin 500mg BID × 7days

or

Omeprazole 40mg daily, Amoxicillin 750mg-1G BID, Metronidazole 400mg TID × 7 days

Renal impairment:

Glomerular filtration rate >30ml/min No adjustment necessary.

Glomerular filtration rate 10-30ml/min: Amoxicillin. max. 500mg b.d

Glomerular filtration rate <10ml/min: Amoxicillin. max. 500mg/day

Children's dosage (up to 10 years of age):

Standard children's dosage: 125 mg three times daily, increasing to 250 mg three times daily for more severe infections.

Renal impairment in children under 40 kg:

Creatinine clearance >30mL/min: No adjustment necessary.

Creatinine clearance 10-30mL/min: 15 mg/kg given b.i.d (maximum 500mg/twice daily).

Creatinine clearance <10mL/min: 15 mg/kg given as a single daily dose (maximum 500mg).

Amoxil Paediatric Suspension is recommended for children under six months of age.

In severe or recurrent acute otitis media, especially where compliance may be a problem, 750 mg twice a day for two days may be used as an alternative course of treatment in children aged 3 to 10 years.

Table 1 Prophylaxis of endocarditis

CONDITION		ADULTS' DOSAGE (INCLUDING ELDERLY)	CHILDREN'S DOSAGE	NOTES
Dental procedures: prophylaxis for patients undergoing extraction, scaling or surgery involving gingival tissues and who have not received a penicillin in the previous month. (N.B. Patients with prosthetic heart valves should be referred to hospital - see below).	Patient not having general anaesthetic.	3 g 'Amoxil' orally, 1 hour before procedure. A second dose may be given 6 hours later, if considered necessary.	Under 10: half adult dose. Under 5: quarter adult dose.	Note 1. If prophylaxis with 'Amoxil' is given twice within one month, emergence of resistant streptococci is unlikely to be a problem. Alternative antibiotics are recommended if more frequent prophylaxis is required, or if the patient has received a course of treatment with a penicillin during the previous month. Note 2. To minimise pain on injection, 'Amoxil' may be given as two injections of 500 mg dissolved in sterile 1% lidocaine solution (see *Administration*).
	Patient having general anaesthetic: if oral antibiotics considered to be appropriate.	Initially 3 g 'Amoxil' orally 4 hours prior to anaesthesia, followed by 3 g orally (or 1 g IV or IM if oral dose not tolerated) as soon as possible after the operation.		
	Patient having general anaesthetic: if oral antibiotics not appropriate.	1 g 'Amoxil' IV or IM immediately before induction; with 500 mg orally, 6 hours later.		
Dental procedures: patients for whom referral to hospital is recommended: a) Patients to be given a general anaesthetic who have been given a penicillin in the previous month. b) Patients to be given a general anaesthetic who have a prosthetic heart valve. c) Patients who have had one or more attacks of endocarditis.		Initially: 1 g 'Amoxil' IV or IM with 120 mg gentamicin IV or IM immediately prior to anaesthesia (if given) or 15 minutes prior to dental procedure. Followed by (6 hours later): 500 mg 'Amoxil' orally.	Under 10: the doses of 'Amoxil' should be half the adult dose; the dose of gentamicin should be 2 mg/kg. Under 5: the doses of 'Amoxil' should be quarter the adult dose; the dose of gentamicin should be 2 mg/kg.	See Note 2. Note 3. 'Amoxil' and gentamicin should not be mixed in the same syringe. Note 4. Please consult the appropriate data sheet for full prescribing information on gentamicin.
Genitourinary Surgery or Instrumentation: prophylaxis for patients who have no urinary tract infection and who are to have genito-urinary surgery or instrumentation under general anaesthesia. In the case of *Obstetric and Gynaecological Procedures* and *Gastrointestinal Procedures*– routine prophylaxis is recommended only for patients with prosthetic heart valves.		Initially: 1 g 'Amoxil' IV or IM with 120 mg gentamicin IV or IM, immediately before induction. Followed by (6 hours later): 500 mg 'Amoxil' orally or IV or IM according to clinical condition.		See Notes 2, 3 and 4 above.
Surgery or Instrumentation of the Upper Respiratory Tract	Patients other than those with prosthetic heart valves.	1 g 'Amoxil' IV or IM immediately before induction; 500 mg 'Amoxil' IV or IM 6 hours later.	Under 10: half adult dose. Under 5: quarter adult dose.	See Note 2 above. Note 5. The second dose of 'Amoxil' may be administered orally as 'Amoxil' Syrup SF/DF.
	Patients with prosthetic heart valves.	Initially: 1 g 'Amoxil' IV or IM with 120 mg gentamicin IV or IM, immediately before induction; followed by (6 hours later) 500 mg 'Amoxil' IV or IM.	Under 10: the dose of 'Amoxil' should be half the adult dose; the gentamicin dose should be 2 mg/kg. Under 5: the dose of 'Amoxil' should be quarter the adult dose; the dose of gentamicin should be 2 mg/kg.	See Notes 2, 3, 4 and 5 above.

In renal impairment the excretion of the antibiotic will be delayed and, depending on the degree of impairment, it may be necessary to reduce the total daily dosage.

Prophylaxis of endocarditis: see table on next page.

Administration: Oral:

Treatment should be continued for 2 to 3 days following the disappearance of symptoms. It is recommended that at least 10 days treatment be given for any infection caused by beta-haemolytic streptococci in order to achieve eradictaion of the organism.

Prophylaxis of endocarditis:

(see Table 1 above)

4.3 Contraindications

Amoxil is a penicillin and should not be given to penicillin-hypersensitive patients. Attention should be paid to possible cross-sensitivity with other beta-lactam antibiotics eg. cephalosporins.

4.4 Special warnings and precautions for use

Before initiating therapy with amoxicillin, careful enquiry should be made concerning previous hypersensitivity reactions to penicillins, cephalosporins.

Serious and occasionally fatal hypersensitivity (anaphylactoid) reactions have been reported in patients on penicillin therapy. These reactions are more likely to occur in individuals with a history of hypersensitivity to beta-lactam antibiotics (see 4.3).

Erythematous (morbilliform) rashes have been associated with glandular fever in patients receiving amoxicillin.

Prolonged use may also occasionally result in overgrowth of non-susceptible organisms.

In patients with reduced urine output, crystalluria has been observed very rarely, predominantly with parenteral therapy. During the administration of high doses of amoxicillin, it is advisable to maintain adequate fluid intake and urinary output in order to reduce the possibility of amoxicillin crystalluria (see Section 4.9 Overdose).

In patients with renal impairment, the rate of excretion of amoxicillin will be reduced depending on the degree of impairment and it may be necessary to reduce the total daily unit amoxicillin dosage accordingly (see section 4.2).

4.5 Interaction with other medicinal products and other forms of interaction

Probenecid decreases the renal tubular secretion of amoxicillin. Concurrent use with amoxicillin may result in increased and prolonged blood levels of amoxicillin.

In common with other antibiotics, amoxicillin may affect the gut flora, leading to lower oestrogen reabsorption and reduced efficacy of combined oral contraceptives.

Concurrent administration of allopurinol during treatment with amoxicillin can increase the likelihood of allergic skin reactions.

Prolongation of prothrombin time has been reported rarely in patients receiving amoxicillin. Appropriate monitoring should be undertaken when anticoagulants are prescribed concurrently.

It is recommended that when testing for the presence of glucose in urine during amoxicillin treatment, enzymatic glucose oxidase methods should be used. Due to the high urinary concentrations of amoxicillin, false positive readings are common with chemical methods.

4.6 Pregnancy and lactation

Use in pregnancy:

Animal studies with Amoxil have shown no teratogenic effects. The product has been in extensive clinical use since 1972 and its suitability in human pregnancy has been well documented in clinical studies. When antibiotic therapy is required during pregnancy, Amoxil may be considered appropriate when the potential benefits outweigh the potential risks associated with treatment.

Use in lactation:

Amoxicillin may be given during lactation. With the exception of the risk of sensitisation associated with the excretion of trace quantities of amoxicillin in breast milk, there are no known detrimental effects for the breast-fed infant.

4.7 Effects on ability to drive and use machines

Adverse effects on the ability to drive or operate machinery have not been observed.

4.8 Undesirable effects

The following convention has been utilised for the classification of undesirable effects:-

Very common (>1/10), common (>1/100, <1/10), uncommon (>1/1000,<1/100), rare (>1/10,000, <1/1000), very rare (<1/10,000)

The majority of side effects listed below are not unique to amoxicillin and may occur when using other penicillins.

Unless otherwise stated, the frequency of adverse events has been derived from more than 30 years of post-marketing reports.

Infections and infestations

Very Rare: Mucocutaneous candidiasis

Blood and lymphatic system disorders

Very rare: Reversible leucopenia (including severe neutropenia or agranulocytosis), reversible thrombocytopenia and haemolytic anaemia.
Prolongation of bleeding time and prothrombin (see Section 4.5 - Interaction with other Medicinal Products and other Forms of Interaction)

Immune system disorders

Very rare: As with other antibiotics, severe allergic reactions, including angioneurotic oedema, anaphylaxis (see Section 4.4 Special Warnings and Precautions for Use), serum sickness and hypersensitivity vasculitis.
If a hypersensitivity reaction is reported, the treatment must be discontinued. (See also Skin and subcutaneous tissue disorders)

Nervous system disorders

Very rare: Hyperkinesia, dizziness and convulsions. Convulsions may occur in patients with impaired renal function or in those receiving high doses.

Gastrointestinal disorders

Clinical Trial Data

***Common:** Diarrhoea and nausea.

***Uncommon:** Vomiting.

Post-marketing Data

Very rare: Antibiotic associated colitis (including pseudomembraneous colitis and haemorrhagic colitis).
Black hairy tongue
Superficial tooth discolouration has been reported in children. Good oral hygiene may help to prevent tooth discolouration as it can usually be removed by brushing.

Hepato-biliary disorders

Very rare: Hepatitis and cholestatic jaundice. A moderate rise in AST and/or ALT.
The significance of a rise in AST and/or ALT is unclear.

Skin and subcutaneous tissue disorders

Clinical Trial Data

***Common:** Skin rash

***Uncommon:** Urticaria and pruritus

Post-marketing Data

Very rare: Skin reactions such as erythema multiforme, Stevens Johnson syndrome, toxic epidermal necrolysis, bullous and exfoliative dermatitis and acute generalised exanthematous pustulosis (AGEP)
(See also Immune system disorders).

Renal and urinary tract disorders

Very rare: Interstitial nephritis.

Very rare: Crystalluria (see Section 4.9 Overdose).

'he incidence of these AEs was derived from clinical :udies involving a total of approximately 6,000 adult and aediatric patients taking amoxicillin.

.9 Overdose

astrointestinal effects such as nausea, vomiting and diar-oea may be evident and should be treated symptomati-ally with attention to the water/electrolyte balance. moxicillin crystalluria, in some cases leading to renal ilure, has been observed (see Section 4.4 Special warn-gs and special precautions for use).

moxicillin may be removed from the circulation by hae-odialysis.

PHARMACOLOGICAL PROPERTIES

1 Pharmacodynamic properties

moxil is a broad spectrum antibiotic.

is rapidly bactericidal and possesses the safety profile of penicillin.

ne wide range of organisms sensitive to the bactericidal :tion of Amoxil include:

erobes:

ram positive	Gram negative
reptococcus faecalis	*Haemophilus influenzae*
reptococcus pneumoniae	*Escherichia coli*
reptococcus pyogenes	*Proteus mirabilis*
reptococcus viridans	*Salmonella* species
aphylococcus aureus	*Shigella* species
enicillin sensitive strains only)	*Bordetella pertussis*
	Brucella species
orynebacterium species	*Neisseria gonorrhoeae*
acillus anthracis	*Neisseria meningitidis*
steria monocytogenes	*Vibrio cholerae*
	Pasteurella septica

naerobes:

ostridium species

2 Pharmacokinetic properties

moxil is well absorbed by the oral and parenteral routes. al administration, usually at convenient t.d.s. dosage, oduces high serum levels independent of the time at nich food is taken. Amoxil gives good penetration into onchial secretions and high urinary concentrations of changed antibiotic.

3 Preclinical safety data

ot applicable.

PHARMACEUTICAL PARTICULARS

1 List of excipients

noxil Capsules 500 Mg

ch capsule contains magnesium stearate (E572) and ythrosine (E127), indigo carmine (E132), titanium dioxide 171), yellow iron oxide (E172) and gelatin.

2 Incompatibilities

one known.

3 Shelf life

apsules 60M

4 Special precautions for storage

noxil Capsules should be stored in a dry place.

5 Nature and contents of container

noxil Capsules: 500 mg Original Pack of 21 with Patient ormation Leaflet; also container of 100. Also packs of 3, 12, 50 and 500.

6 Special precautions for disposal and other handling

ot applicable.

lministrative Data

MARKETING AUTHORISATION HOLDER

echam Group plc

eat West Road, Brentford, Middlesex TW8 9GS

ading as GlaxoSmithKline UK, Stockley Park West, bridge, Middlesex UB11 1BT

d/or

ncard or SmithKline Beecham Pharmaceuticals, ındells, Welwyn Garden City, Hertfordshire AL7 1EY.

MARKETING AUTHORISATION NUMBER(S)

noxil Capsules 500 mg 0038/0105

DATE OF FIRST AUTHORISATION/RENEWAL OF IE AUTHORISATION

April 1972 / 13 January 1998

DATE OF REVISION OF THE TEXT

th September 2008

. Legal Status

OM

moxil Paediatric Suspension

(GlaxoSmithKline UK)

NAME OF THE MEDICINAL PRODUCT

noxil® Paediatric Suspension

2. QUALITATIVE AND QUANTITATIVE COMPOSITION

Amoxil Paediatric Suspension contains 125 mg amoxicillin per 1.25 ml dose

The amoxicillin is present as the trihydrate.

3. PHARMACEUTICAL FORM

Amoxil Paediatric Suspension: citrus flavoured suspension. Presented as powder in bottles for preparing 20 ml.

4. CLINICAL PARTICULARS

4.1 Therapeutic indications

Treatment of Infection: Amoxil is a broad spectrum antibiotic indicated for the treatment of commonly occurring bacterial infections such as:

Upper respiratory tract infections

Otitis media

Acute and chronic bronchitis

Chronic bronchial sepsis

Lobar and bronchopneumonia

Cystitis, urethritis, pyelonephritis

Bacteriuria in pregnancy

Gynaecological infections including puerperal sepsis and septic abortion

Gonorrhoea

Peritonitis

Intra-abdominal sepsis

Septicaemia

Bacterial endocarditis

Typhoid and paratyphoid fever

Skin and soft tissue infections

Osteomyelitis

Dental abscess (as an adjunct to surgical management)

In children with urinary tract infection the need for investigation should be considered.

Prophylaxis of endocarditis: Amoxil may be used for the prevention of bacteraemia, associated with procedures such as dental extraction, in patients at risk of developing bacterial endocarditis.

Consideration should be given to official local guidance (e.g. national requirements) on the appropriate use of antibacterial agents."Susceptibility of the causative organism to the treatment should be tested (if possible), although the therapy may be initiated before the results are available.

4.2 Posology and method of administration

Treatment of Infection:

Adult dosage (including elderly patients):

Oral:

Standard adult dosage: 250 mg three times daily, increasing to 500 mg three times daily for more severe infections.

High dosage therapy (maximum recommended oral dosage 6 g daily in divided doses): A dosage of 3 g twice daily is recommended in appropriate cases for the treatment of severe or recurrent purulent infection of the respiratory tract.

Short course therapy: Simple acute urinary tract infection: two 3 g doses with 10-12 hours between the doses. Dental abscess: two 3 g doses with 8 hours between the doses. Gonorrhoea: single 3 g dose.

Renal impairment:

Glomerular filtration rate >30ml/min No adjustment necessary.

Glomerular filtration rate 10-30ml/min: Amoxicillin. max. 500mg b.d

Glomerular filtration rate <10ml/min: Amoxicillin. max. 500mg/day

Children's dosage (up to 10 years of age):

Oral:

Standard children's dosage: 125 mg three times daily, increasing to 250 mg three times daily for more severe infections.

Renal impairment in children under 40 kg:

Creatinine clearance >30mL/min: No adjustment necessary.

Creatinine clearance 10-30mL/min: 15 mg/kg given b.i.d (maximum 500mg/twice daily).

Creatinine clearance <10mL/min: 15 mg/kg given as a single daily dose (maximum 500mg).

Amoxil Paediatric Suspension is recommended for children under six months of age.

In severe or recurrent acute otitis media, especially where compliance may be a problem, 750 mg twice a day for two days may be used as an alternative course of treatment in children aged 3 to 10 years.

Prophylaxis of endocarditis:

(see Table 1 on next page)

In renal impairment the excretion of the antibiotic will be delayed and, depending on the degree of impairment, it may be necessary to reduce the total daily dosage.

Prophylaxis of endocarditis: see table on previous page.

Administration:

Oral.

Treatment should be continued for 2 to 3 days following the disappearance of symptoms. It is recommended that at least 10 days treatment be given for any infection caused by beta-haemolytic streptococci in order to achieve eradictaion of the organism.

4.3 Contraindications

Amoxil is a penicillin and should not be given to penicillin-hypersensitive patients. Attention should be paid to possible cross-sensitivity with other beta-lactam antibiotics eg. cephalosporins.

4.4 Special warnings and precautions for use

Before initiating therapy with amoxicillin, careful enquiry should be made concerning previous hypersensitivity reactions to penicillins, cephalosporins.

Serious and occasionally fatal hypersensitivity (anaphylactoid) reactions have been reported in patients on penicillin therapy. These reactions are more likely to occur in individuals with a history of hypersensitivity to beta-lactam antibiotics (see 4.3).

Erythematous (morbilliform) rashes have been associated with glandular fever in patients receiving amoxicillin.

Prolonged use may also occasionally result in overgrowth of non-susceptible organisms.

In patients with reduced urine output, crystalluria has been observed very rarely, predominantly with parenteral therapy. During the administration of high doses of amoxicillin, it is advisable to maintain adequate fluid intake and urinary output in order to reduce the possibility of amoxicillin crystalluria (see Section 4.9 Overdose).

In patients with renal impairment, the rate of excretion of amoxicillin will be reduced depending on the degree of impairment and it may be necessary to reduce the total daily unit amoxicillin dosage accordingly (see section 4.2).

4.5 Interaction with other medicinal products and other forms of interaction

Probenecid decreases the renal tubular secretion of amoxicillin. Concurrent use with Amoxil may result in increased and prolonged blood levels of amoxicillin.

In common with other antibiotics, amoxicillin may affect the gut flora, leading to lower oestrogen reabsorption and reduced efficacy of combined oral contraceptives.

Concurrent administration of allopurinol during treatment with amoxicillin can increase the likelihood of allergic skin reactions.

Prolongation of prothrombin time has been reported rarely in patients receiving amoxicillin. Appropriate monitoring should be undertaken when anticoagulants are prescribed concurrently.

It is recommended that when testing for the presence of glucose in urine during amoxicillin treatment, enzymatic glucose oxidase methods should be used. Due to the high urinary concentrations of amoxicillin, false positive readings are common with chemical methods.

4.6 Pregnancy and lactation

Use in pregnancy:

Animal studies with Amoxil have shown no teratogenic effects. The product has been in extensive clinical use since 1972 and its suitability in human pregnancy has been well documented in clinical studies. When antibiotic therapy is required during pregnancy, Amoxil may be considered appropriate when the potential benefits outweigh the potential risks associated with treatment.

Use in lactation:

Amoxicillin may be given during lactation. With the exception of the risk of sensitisation associated with the excretion of trace quantities of amoxicillin in breast milk, there are no known detrimental effects for the breast-fed infant.

4.7 Effects on ability to drive and use machines

Adverse effects on the ability to drive or operate machinery have not been observed.

4.8 Undesirable effects

The following convention has been utilised for the classification of undesirable effects:-

Very common (>1/10), common (>1/100, <1/10), uncommon (>1/1000,<1/100), rare (>1/10,000, <1/1000), very rare (<1/10,000)

The majority of side effects listed below are not unique to amoxicillin and may occur when using other penicillins.

Unless otherwise stated, the frequency of adverse events has been derived from more than 30 years of post-marketing reports.

Infections and infestations

Very Rare: Mucocutaneous candidiasis

Blood and lymphatic system disorders

Very rare: Reversible leucopenia (including severe neutropenia or agranulocytosis), reversible thrombocytopenia and haemolytic anaemia.
Prolongation of bleeding time and prothrombin (see Section 4.5 - Interaction with other Medicinal Products and other Forms of Interaction)

Table 1 Prophylaxis of endocarditis

CONDITION		ADULTS' DOSAGE (INCLUDING ELDERLY)	CHILDREN'S DOSAGE	NOTES
Dental procedures: prophylaxis for patients undergoing extraction, scaling or surgery involving gingival tissues and who have not received a penicillin in the previous month. (N.B. Patients with prosthetic heart valves should be referred to hospital - see below).	Patient not having general anaesthetic.	3 g 'Amoxil' orally, 1 hour before procedure. A second dose may be given 6 hours later, if considered necessary.	Under 10: half adult dose. Under 5: quarter adult dose.	Note 1. If prophylaxis with 'Amoxil' is given twice within one month, emergence of resistant streptococc is unlikely to be a problem. Alternative antibiotics are recommended if more frequent prophylaxis is required, or if the patient has received a course of treatment with a penicillin during the previous month. Note 2. To minimise pain on injection, 'Amoxil' may be given as two injections of 500 mg dissolved in sterile 1% lidocaine solution (see *Administration*).
	Patient having general anaesthetic: if oral antibiotics considered to be appropriate.	Initially 3 g 'Amoxil' orally 4 hours prior to anaesthesia, followed by 3 g orally (or 1 g IV or IM if oral dose not tolerated) as soon as possible after the operation.		
	Patient having general anaesthetic: if oral antibiotics not appropriate.	1 g 'Amoxil' IV or IM immediately before induction; with 500 mg orally, 6 hours later.		
Dental procedures: patients for whom referral to hospital is recommended: a) Patients to be given a general anaesthetic who have been given a penicillin in the previous month. b) Patients to be given a general anaesthetic who have a prosthetic heart valve. c) Patients who have had one or more attacks of endocarditis.		Initially: 1 g 'Amoxil' IV or IM with 120 mg gentamicin IV or IM immediately prior to anaesthesia (if given) or 15 minutes prior to dental procedure. Followed by (6 hours later): 500 mg 'Amoxil' orally.	Under 10: the doses of 'Amoxil' should be half the adult dose; the dose of gentamicin should be 2 mg/kg. Under 5: the doses of 'Amoxil' should be quarter the adult dose; the dose of gentamicin should be 2 mg/kg.	See Note 2. Note 3. 'Amoxil' and gentamicin should not be mixed in the same syringe. Note 4. Please consult the appropriate data sheet for full prescribing information on gentamicin.
Genitourinary Surgery or Instrumentation: prophylaxis for patients who have no urinary tract infection and who are to have genito-urinary surgery or instrumentation under general anaesthesia. In the case of *Obstetric and Gynaecological Procedures* and *Gastrointestinal Procedures*– routine prophylaxis is recommended only for patients with prosthetic heart valves.		Initially: 1 g 'Amoxil' IV or IM with 120 mg gentamicin IV or IM, immediately before induction. Followed by (6 hours later): 500 mg 'Amoxil' orally or IV or IM according to clinical condition.		See Notes 2, 3 and 4 above.
Surgery or Instrumentation of the Upper Respiratory Tract	Patients other than those with prosthetic heart valves.	1 g 'Amoxil' IV or IM immediately before induction; 500 mg 'Amoxil' IV or IM 6 hours later.	Under 10: half adult dose. Under 5: quarter adult dose.	See Note 2 above. Note 5. The second dose of 'Amoxil may be administered orally as 'Amoxil' Syrup SF/DF.
	Patients with prosthetic heart valves.	Initially: 1 g 'Amoxil' IV or IM with 120 mg gentamicin IV or IM, immediately before induction; followed by (6 hours later) 500 mg 'Amoxil' IV or IM.	Under 10: the dose of 'Amoxil' should be half the adult dose; the gentamicin dose should be 2 mg/kg. Under 5: the dose of 'Amoxil' should be quarter the adult dose; the dose of gentamicin should be 2 mg/kg.	See Notes 2, 3, 4 and 5 above.

<u>**Immune system disorders**</u>

Very rare: As with other antibiotics, severe allergic reactions, including angioneurotic oedema, anaphylaxis (see Section 4.4 Special Warnings and Precautions for Use), serum sickness and hypersensitivity vasculitis.
If a hypersensitivity reaction is reported, the treatment must be discontinued. (See also Skin and subcutaneous tissue disorders)

<u>**Nervous system disorders**</u>

Very rare: Hyperkinesia, dizziness and convulsions. Convulsions may occur in patients with impaired renal function or in those receiving high doses.

<u>**Gastrointestinal disorders**</u>

<u>Clinical Trial Data</u>

***Common:** Diarrhoea and nausea.

***Uncommon:** Vomiting.

<u>Post-marketing Data</u>

Very rare: Antibiotic associated colitis (including pseudomembraneous colitis and haemorrhagic colitis).
Black hairy tongue
Superficial tooth discolouration has been reported in children. Good oral hygiene may help to prevent tooth discolouration as it can usually be removed by brushing.

<u>**Hepato-biliary disorders**</u>

Very rare: Hepatitis and cholestatic jaundice. A moderate rise in AST and/or ALT.
The significance of a rise in AST and/or ALT is unclear.

<u>**Skin and subcutaneous tissue disorders**</u>

<u>Clinical Trial Data</u>

***Common:** Skin rash

***Uncommon:** Urticaria and pruritus

<u>Post-marketing Data</u>

Very rare: Skin reactions such as erythema multiforme, Stevens Johnson syndrome, toxic epidermal necrolysis, bullous and exfoliative dermatitis and acute generalised exanthematous pustulosis (AGEP)
(See also Immune system disorders).

<u>**Renal and urinary tract disorders**</u>

Very rare: Interstitial nephritis.

Very rare: Crystalluria (see Section 4.9 Overdose).

*The incidence of these AEs was derived from clinical studies involving a total of approximately 6,000 adult and paediatric patients taking amoxicillin.

4.9 Overdose

Gastrointestinal effects such as nausea, vomiting and diarrhoea may be evident and should be treated symptomatically with attention to the water/electrolyte balance. Amoxicillin crystalluria, in some cases leading to renal failure, has been observed (see Section 4.4 Special warnings and special precautions for use).

Amoxicillin may be removed from the circulation by haemodialysis.

5. PHARMACOLOGICAL PROPERTIES

5.1 Pharmacodynamic properties

Amoxil is a broad spectrum antibiotic.

It is rapidly bactericidal and possesses the safety profile of a penicillin.

The wide range of organisms sensitive to the bactericidal action of Amoxil include:

Aerobes:

Gram positive	Gram negative
Streptococcus faecalis	*Haemophilus influenzae*
Streptococcus pneumoniae	*Escherichia coli*
Streptococcus pyogenes	*Proteus mirabilis*
Streptococcus viridans	*Salmonella* species
Staphylococcus aureus	*Shigella* species
(penicillin sensitive strains only)	*Bordetella pertussis*
	Brucella species
Corynebacterium species	*Neisseria gonorrhoeae*
Bacillus anthracis	*Neisseria meningitidis*
Listeria monocytogenes	*Vibrio cholerae*
	Pasteurella septica

Anaerobes:

Clostridium species

5.2 Pharmacokinetic properties

Amoxil is well absorbed by the oral and parenteral routes. Oral administration, usually at convenient t.d.s. dosage, produces high serum levels independent of the time at which food is taken. Amoxil gives good penetration into bronchial secretions and high urinary concentrations o unchanged antibiotic.

5.3 Preclinical safety data

Not applicable.

6. PHARMACEUTICAL PARTICULARS

6.1 List of excipients

Amoxil Paediatric Suspension

The powder contains sodium benzoate (E211), sodiu carboxymethylcellulose (E466), quinoline yellow (E104 peach, strawberry and lemon dry flavours and sucros (0.6 g per 1.25 ml dose).

6.2 Incompatibilities

None known.

6.3 Shelf life

Paediatric Suspension 36M (once reconstituted: 14 days)

6.4 Special precautions for storage

Prior to use, Amoxil Paediatric Suspension should b stored in a dry place.

Once dispensed, Amoxil Paediatric Suspension should b stored at 25°C or below and used within 14 days. Amox Paediatric Suspension may be diluted with water or Syru BP.

6.5 Nature and contents of container

Amoxil Paediatric Suspension: 125 mg per 1.25 ml: Origin Pack of 20 ml with pipette and Patient Information Leafle

6.6 Special precautions for disposal and other handlin

None.

Administrative Data

7. MARKETING AUTHORISATION HOLDER

Beecham Group plc

Great West Road, Brentford, Middlesex TW8 9GS

Trading as GlaxoSmithKline UK Stockley Park Wes Uxbridge, Middlesex UB11 1BT

And/or

Bencard or SmithKline Beecham Pharmaceutical Mundells, Welwyn Garden City, Hertfordshire AL7 1EY

8. MARKETING AUTHORISATION NUMBER(S)

Amoxil Paediatric Suspension
125 mg per 1.25 ml 0038/0107

9. DATE OF FIRST AUTHORISATION/RENEWAL O THE AUTHORISATION

07 March 1972 / 13 January 1998

). DATE OF REVISION OF THE TEXT

)th September 2008

1. Legal Status

OM

Amoxil Sachets 3g Sucrose-Free

(GlaxoSmithKline UK)

. NAME OF THE MEDICINAL PRODUCT

moxil® Sachets 3 G Sucrose-Free

. QUALITATIVE AND QUANTITATIVE COMPOSITION

moxil Sachets 3 G Sucrose-Free contain 3 G amoxicillin er sachet

he amoxicillin is present as the trihydrate.

. PHARMACEUTICAL FORM

moxil Sachets SF: sucrose-free sachets in a sorbitol ase, for reconstitution in water.

ach sachet carries instructions for preparation.

. CLINICAL PARTICULARS

.1 Therapeutic indications

reatment of Infection: Amoxil is a broad spectrum antibiotic indicated for the treatment of commonly occurring acterial infections such as:

Jpper respiratory tract infections

Otitis media

Acute and chronic bronchitis

Chronic bronchial sepsis

Lobar and bronchopneumonia

Cystitis, urethritis, pyelonephritis

Bacteriuria in pregnancy

Gynaecological infections including puerperal sepsis and septic abortion

Gonorrhoea

Peritonitis

Intra-abdominal sepsis

Septicaemia

Bacterial endocarditis

Typhoid and paratyphoid fever

Skin and soft tissue infections

Osteomyelitis

Dental abscess (as an adjunct to surgical management)

In children with urinary tract infection the need for investigation should be considered.

Prophylaxis of endocarditis: Amoxil may be used for the prevention of bacteraemia, associated with procedures such as dental extraction, in patients at risk of developing bacterial endocarditis.

The wide range of organisms sensitive to the bactericidal action of Amoxil include:

Gram-positive	Gram-negative
Streptococcus faecalis	*Haemophilus influenzae*
Streptococcus pneumoniae	*Escherichia coli*
Streptococcus pyogenes	*Proteus mirabilis*
Streptococcus viridans	*Salmonella* species
Staphylococcus aureus	*Shigella* species
(penicillin-sensitive)	*Bordetella pertussis*
Clostridium species	*Brucella* species
Corynebacterium species	*Neisseria gonorrhoeae*
Bacillus anthracis	*Neisseria meningitidis*
Listeria monocytogenes	*Vibrio cholerae*
	Pasteurella septica

4.2 Posology and method of administration

Administration:

Oral:

Treatment of Infection:

Adult dosage (including elderly patients):

Standard adult dosage: 250 mg three times daily, increasing to 500 mg three times daily for more severe infections.

High dosage therapy (maximum recommended oral dosage 6 g daily in divided doses): A dosage of 3 g twice daily is recommended in appropriate cases for the treatment of severe or recurrent purulent infection of the respiratory tract.

Short course therapy: Simple acute urinary tract infection: two 3 g doses with 10-12 hours between the doses. Dental abscess: two 3 g doses with 8 hours between the doses. Gonorrhoea: single 3 g dose.

Children's dosage (up to 10 years of age):

Standard children's dosage: 125 mg three times daily, increasing to 250 mg three times daily for more severe infections.

Amoxil Paediatric Suspension is recommended for children under six months of age.

In severe or recurrent acute otitis media, especially where compliance may be a problem, 750 mg twice a day for two days may be used as an alternative course of treatment in children aged 3 to 10 years.

Prophylaxis of endocarditis:

(see Table 1 below)

In renal impairment the excretion of the antibiotic will be delayed and, depending on the degree of impairment, it may be necessary to reduce the total daily dosage.

Prophylaxis of endocarditis: see table on previous page.

4.3 Contraindications

Amoxil is a penicillin and should not be given to penicillin-hypersensitive patients. Attention should be paid to possible cross-sensitivity with other beta-lactam antibiotics eg. cephalosporins.

4.4 Special warnings and precautions for use

Serious and occasionally fatal hypersensitivity (anaphylactoid) reactions have been reported in patients on penicillin therapy. These reactions are more likely to occur in individuals with a history of hypersensitivity to beta-lactam antibiotics (see 4.3).

Erythematous (morbilliform) rashes have been associated with glandular fever in patients receiving amoxicillin.

Prolonged use may also occasionally result in overgrowth of non-susceptible organisms.

In patients with reduced urine output, crystalluria has been observed very rarely, predominantly with parenteral therapy. During the administration of high doses of amoxicillin, it is advisable to maintain adequate fluid intake and urinary output in order to reduce the possibility of amoxicillin crystalluria (see Section 4.9 Overdose).

Dosage should be adjusted in patients with renal impairment (see 4.2).

4.5 Interaction with other medicinal products and other forms of interaction

Probenecid decreases the renal tubular secretion of amoxicillin. Concurrent use with Amoxil may result in increased and prolonged blood levels of amoxicillin.

In common with other antibiotics, amoxicillin may affect the gut flora, leading to lower oestrogen reabsorption and reduced efficacy of combined oral contraceptives.

Concurrent administration of allopurinol during treatment with amoxicillin can increase the likelihood of allergic skin reactions.

Prolongation of prothrombin time has been reported rarely in patients receiving amoxicillin. Appropriate monitoring

Table 1 Prophylaxis of endocarditis

CONDITION		ADULTS' DOSAGE (INCLUDING ELDERLY)	CHILDREN'S DOSAGE	NOTES
Dental procedures: prophylaxis for patients undergoing extraction, scaling or surgery involving gingival tissues and who have not received a penicillin in the previous month. (N.B. Patients with prosthetic heart valves should be referred to hospital - see below).	Patient not having general anaesthetic.	3 g 'Amoxil' orally, 1 hour before procedure. A second dose may be given 6 hours later, if considered necessary.	Under 10: half adult dose. Under 5: quarter adult dose.	Note 1. If prophylaxis with 'Amoxil' is given twice within one month, emergence of resistant streptococci is unlikely to be a problem. Alternative antibiotics are recommended if more frequent prophylaxis is required, or if the patient has received a course of treatment with a penicillin during the previous month. Note 2. To minimise pain on injection, 'Amoxil' may be given as two injections of 500 mg dissolved in sterile 1% lidocaine solution (see *Administration*).
	Patient having general anaesthetic: if oral antibiotics considered to be appropriate.	Initially 3 g 'Amoxil' orally 4 hours prior to anaesthesia, followed by 3 g orally (or 1 g IV or IM if oral dose not tolerated) as soon as possible after the operation.		
	Patient having general anaesthetic: if oral antibiotics not appropriate.	1 g 'Amoxil' IV or IM immediately before induction; with 500 mg orally, 6 hours later.		
Dental procedures: patients for whom referral to hospital is recommended: a) Patients to be given a general anaesthetic who have been given a penicillin in the previous month. b) Patients to be given a general anaesthetic who have a prosthetic heart valve. c) Patients who have had one or more attacks of endocarditis.		Initially: 1 g 'Amoxil' IV or IM with 120 mg gentamicin IV or IM immediately prior to anaesthesia (if given) or 15 minutes prior to dental procedure. Followed by (6 hours later): 500 mg 'Amoxil' orally.	Under 10: the doses of 'Amoxil' should be half the adult dose; the dose of gentamicin should be 2 mg/kg. Under 5: the doses of 'Amoxil' should be quarter the adult dose; the dose of gentamicin should be 2 mg/kg.	See Note 2. Note 3. 'Amoxil' and gentamicin should not be mixed in the same syringe. Note 4. Please consult the appropriate data sheet for full prescribing information on gentamicin.
Genitourinary Surgery or Instrumentation: prophylaxis for patients who have no urinary tract infection and who are to have genito-urinary surgery or instrumentation under general anaesthesia. In the case of *Obstetric and Gynaecological Procedures* and *Gastrointestinal Procedures*– routine prophylaxis is recommended only for patients with prosthetic heart valves.		Initially: 1 g 'Amoxil' IV or IM with 120 mg gentamicin IV or IM, immediately before induction. Followed by (6 hours later): 500 mg 'Amoxil' orally or IV or IM according to clinical condition.		See Notes 2, 3 and 4 above.
Surgery or Instrumentation of the Upper Respiratory Tract	Patients other than those with prosthetic heart valves.	1 g 'Amoxil' IV or IM immediately before induction; 500 mg 'Amoxil' IV or IM 6 hours later.	Under 10: half adult dose. Under 5: quarter adult dose.	See Note 2 above. Note 5. The second dose of 'Amoxil' may be administered orally as 'Amoxil' Syrup SF/DF.
	Patients with prosthetic heart valves.	Initially: 1 g 'Amoxil' IV or IM with 120 mg gentamicin IV or IM, immediately before induction; followed by (6 hours later) 500 mg 'Amoxil' IV or IM.	Under 10: the dose of 'Amoxil' should be half the adult dose; the gentamicin dose should be 2 mg/kg. Under 5: the dose of 'Amoxil' should be quarter the adult dose; the dose of gentamicin should be 2 mg/kg.	See Notes 2, 3, 4 and 5 above.

should be undertaken when anticoagulants are prescribed concurrently.

It is recommended that when testing for the presence of glucose in urine during amoxicillin treatment, enzymatic glucose oxidase methods should be used. Due to the high urinary concentrations of amoxicillin, false positive readings are common with chemical methods.

4.6 Pregnancy and lactation
Use in pregnancy:

Animal studies with Amoxil have shown no teratogenic effects. The product has been in extensive clinical use since 1972 and its suitability in human pregnancy has been well documented in clinical studies. When antibiotic therapy is required during pregnancy, Amoxil may be considered appropriate when the potential benefits outweigh the potential risks associated with treatment.

Use in lactation:

Amoxicillin may be given during lactation. With the exception of the risk of sensitisation associated with the excretion of trace quantities of amoxicillin in breast milk, there are no known detrimental effects for the breast-fed infant.

4.7 Effects on ability to drive and use machines
Adverse effects on the ability to drive or operate machinery have not been observed.

4.8 Undesirable effects
The following convention has been utilised for the classification of undesirable effects:-

Very common (>1/10), common (>1/100, <1/10), uncommon (>1/1000,<1/100), rare (>1/10,000, <1/1000), very rare (<1/10,000)

The majority of side effects listed below are not unique to amoxicillin and may occur when using other penicillins.

Unless otherwise stated, the frequency of adverse events has been derived from more than 30 years of post-marketing reports.

Infections and infestations

Very Rare: Mucocutaneous candidiasis

Blood and lymphatic system disorders

Very rare: Reversible leucopenia (including severe neutropenia or agranulocytosis), reversible thrombocytopenia and haemolytic anaemia.

Prolongation of bleeding time and prothrombin (see Section 4.5 - Interaction with other Medicinal Products and other Forms of Interaction)

Immune system disorders

Very rare: As with other antibiotics, severe allergic reactions, including angioneurotic oedema, anaphylaxis (see Section 4.4 - Special Warnings and Precautions for Use), serum sickness and hypersensitivity vasculitis.

If a hypersensitivity reaction is reported, the treatment must be discontinued. (See also Skin and subcutaneous tissue disorders).

Nervous system disorders

Very rare: Hyperkinesia, dizziness and convulsions. Convulsions may occur in patients with impaired renal function or in those receiving high doses.

Gastrointestinal disorders

Clinical Trial Data

***Common:** Diarrhoea and nausea.

***Uncommon:** Vomiting.

Post-marketing Data

Very rare: Antibiotic associated colitis (including pseudomembranous colitis and haemorrhagic colitis).

Black hairy tongue

Superficial tooth discolouration has been reported in children. Good oral hygiene may help to prevent tooth discolouration as it can usually be removed by brushing.

Hepato-biliary disorders

Very rare: Hepatitis and cholestatic jaundice. A moderate rise in AST and/or ALT.

The significance of a rise in AST and/or ALT is unclear.

Skin and subcutaneous tissue disorders

Clinical Trial Data

***Common:** Skin rash

***Uncommon:** Urticaria and pruritus

Post-marketing Data

Very rare: Skin reactions such as erythema multiforme, Stevens-Johnson syndrome, toxic epidermal necrolysis, bullous and exfoliative dermatitis and acute generalised exanthematous pustulosis (AGEP)

(See also Immune system disorders).

Renal and urinary tract disorders

Very rare: Interstitial nephritis.

Very rare: Crystalluria (see Section 4.9 Overdose)

*The incidence of these AEs was derived from clinical studies involving a total of approximately 6,000 adult and paediatric patients taking amoxicillin.

4.9 Overdose
Gastrointestinal effects such as nausea, vomiting and diarrhoea may be evident and should be treated symptomatically with attention to the water/electrolyte balance.

Amoxicillin crystalluria, in some cases leading to renal failure, has been observed (see Section 4.4 Special warnings and special precautions for use).

Amoxicillin may be removed from the circulation by haemodialysis.

5. PHARMACOLOGICAL PROPERTIES
5.1 Pharmacodynamic properties
Amoxil is a broad spectrum antibiotic.

It is rapidly bactericidal and possesses the safety profile of a penicillin.

5.2 Pharmacokinetic properties
Amoxil is well absorbed by the oral and parenteral routes. Oral administration, usually at convenient t.d.s. dosage, produces high serum levels independent of the time at which food is taken. Amoxil gives good penetration into bronchial secretions and high urinary concentrations of unchanged antibiotic.

5.3 Preclinical safety data
Not applicable.

6. PHARMACEUTICAL PARTICULARS
6.1 List of excipients
Saccharin sodium

Xanthan gum (E415)

Peach dry flavour

Strawberry dry flavour

Lemon dry flavour

Sorbitol (E420)

6.2 Incompatibilities
None stated.

6.3 Shelf life
Sachet SF: 36 Months

6.4 Special precautions for storage
Amoxil Sachets SF should be stored in a dry place below 25°C.

6.5 Nature and contents of container
Amoxil Sachet 3 G Sucrose Free: Original packs of 2 and 14. Each sachet carries instructions for preparation and each pack contains a Patient Information Leaflet.

6.6 Special precautions for disposal and other handling
To be taken immediately following reconstitution.

Administrative Data
7. MARKETING AUTHORISATION HOLDER
Beecham Group plc

980 Great West Road

Brentford

Middlesex TW8 9GS

Trading as:

GlaxoSmithKline UK

Stockley Park West

Uxbridge

Middlesex UB11 1BT

8. MARKETING AUTHORISATION NUMBER(S)
Amoxil 3 G Sachet Sucrose-Free PL 00038/0334

9. DATE OF FIRST AUTHORISATION/RENEWAL OF THE AUTHORISATION
Amoxil 3 G Sachet Sucrose-Free 03 December 2002

10. DATE OF REVISION OF THE TEXT
24th September 2008

11. Legal Status
POM

Amoxil Syrup Sucrose-Free/Dye-Free 125mg/5ml

(GlaxoSmithKline UK)

1. NAME OF THE MEDICINAL PRODUCT
Amoxil® Syrup Sucrose-Free/Dye-Free 125 mg/5 ml

2. QUALITATIVE AND QUANTITATIVE COMPOSITION
Amoxil Syrup SF/DF 125 mg contains 125 mg amoxicillin per 5 ml dose.

The amoxicillin is present as the trihydrate.

3. PHARMACEUTICAL FORM
Amoxil Syrup SF/DF 125 mg/5 ml: citrus-flavoured sucrose-free/dye-free suspension in a sorbitol base. Presented as powder in bottles for preparing 100 ml.

4. CLINICAL PARTICULARS
4.1 Therapeutic indications
Treatment of Infection: Amoxil is a broad spectrum antibiotic indicated for the treatment of commonly occurring bacterial infections such as:

Upper respiratory tract infections

Otitis media

Acute and chronic bronchitis

Chronic bronchial sepsis

Lobar and bronchopneumonia

Cystitis, urethritis, pyelonephritis

Bacteriuria in pregnancy

Gynaecological infections including puerperal sepsis ar septic abortion

Gonorrhoea

Peritonitis

Intra-abdominal sepsis

Septicaemia

Bacterial endocarditis

Typhoid and paratyphoid fever

Skin and soft tissue infections

Osteomyelitis

Dental abscess (as an adjunct to surgical management)

In children with urinary tract infection the need for invest gation should be considered.

Prophylaxis of endocarditis: Amoxil may be used for th prevention of bacteraemia, associated with procedure such as dental extraction, in patients at risk of developin bacterial endocarditis.

The wide range of organisms sensitive to the bactericida action of Amoxil include:

Gram-positive	Gram-negative
Streptococcus faecalis	*Haemophilus influenzae*
Streptococcus pneumoniae	*Escherichia coli*
Streptococcus pyogenes	*Proteus mirabilis*
Streptococcus viridans	*Salmonella* species
Staphylococcus aureus	*Shigella* species
(penicillin-sensitive)	*Bordetella pertussis*
Clostridium species	*Brucella* species
Corynebacterium species	*Neisseria gonorrhoeae*
Bacillus anthracis	*Neisseria meningitidis*
Listeria monocytogenes	*Vibrio cholerae*
Pasteurella septica	

4.2 Posology and method of administration
Treatment of Infection:

Adult dosage (including elderly patients):

Oral:

Standard adult dosage: 250 mg three times daily, increasing to 500 mg three times daily for more severe infections.

High dosage therapy (maximum recommended oral dosage 6 g daily in divided doses): A dosage of 3 g twice daily is recommended in appropriate cases for the treatment of severe or recurrent purulent infection of the respiratory tract.

Short course therapy: Simple acute urinary tract infection: two 3 g doses with 10-12 hours between the doses. Dental abscess: two 3 g doses with 8 hours between the doses. Gonorrhoea: single 3 g dose.

Injectable:

500 mg IM eight hourly (or more frequently if necessary) in moderate infections. (This dose may be given by slow IV injection if more convenient.)

1 g IV six hourly in severe infections.

Children's dosage (up to 10 years of age):

Oral:

Standard children's dosage: 125 mg three times daily, increasing to 250 mg three times daily for more severe infections.

Amoxil Paediatric Suspension is recommended for children under six months of age.

Prophylaxis of endocarditis:

(see Table 1 on next page)

In severe or recurrent acute otitis media, especially where compliance may be a problem, 750 mg twice a day for two days may be used as an alternative course of treatment in children aged 3 to 10 years.

Injectable:

50-100 mg/kg body weight a day, in divided doses.

Parenteral therapy is indicated if the oral route is considered impracticable or unsuitable, and particularly for the urgent treatment of severe infection.

In renal impairment the excretion of the antibiotic will be delayed and, depending on the degree of impairment, it may be necessary to reduce the total daily dosage.

Prophylaxis of endocarditis: see table on previous page.

Administration:

Oral

4.3 Contraindications
Amoxil is a penicillin and should not be given to penicillin-hypersensitive patients. Attention should be paid to possible cross-sensitivity with other beta-lactam antibiotics eg. cephalosporins.

4.4 Special warnings and precautions for use
Serious and occasionally fatal hypersensitivity (anaphylactoid) reactions have been reported in patients on penicillin therapy. These reactions are more likely to occur in

Table 1 Prophylaxis of endocarditis

CONDITION		ADULTS' DOSAGE (INCLUDING ELDERLY)	CHILDREN'S DOSAGE	NOTES
Dental procedures : prophylaxis for patients undergoing extraction, scaling or surgery involving gingival tissues and who have not received a penicillin in the previous month. (N.B. Patients with prosthetic heart valves should be referred to hospital - see below).	Patient not having general anaesthetic.	3 g 'Amoxil' orally, 1 hour before procedure. A second dose may be given 6 hours later, if considered necessary.	Under 10: half adult dose. Under 5: quarter adult dose.	Note 1. If prophylaxis with 'Amoxil' is given twice within one month, emergence of resistant streptococci is unlikely to be a problem. Alternative antibiotics are recommended if more frequent prophylaxis is required, or if the patient has received a course of treatment with a penicillin during the previous month. Note 2. To minimise pain on injection, 'Amoxil' may be given as two injections of 500 mg dissolved in sterile 1% lignocaine solution (see *Administration*).
	Patient having general anaesthetic: if oral antibiotics considered to be appropriate.	Initially 3 g 'Amoxil' orally 4 hours prior to anaesthesia, followed by 3 g orally (or 1 g IV or IM if oral dose not tolerated) as soon as possible after the operation.		
	Patient having general anaesthetic: if oral antibiotics not appropriate.	1 g 'Amoxil' IV or IM immediately before induction; with 500 mg orally, 6 hours later.		
Dental procedures : patients for whom referral to hospital is recommended: a) Patients to be given a general anaesthetic who have been given a penicillin in the previous month. b) Patients to be given a general anaesthetic who have a prosthetic heart valve. c) Patients who have had one or more attacks of endocarditis.		Initially: 1 g 'Amoxil' IV or IM with 120 mg gentamicin IV or IM immediately prior to anaesthesia (if given) or 15 minutes prior to dental procedure. Followed by (6 hours later): 500 mg 'Amoxil' orally.	Under 10: the doses of 'Amoxil' should be half the adult dose; the dose of gentamicin should be 2 mg/kg. Under 5: the doses of 'Amoxil' should be quarter the adult dose; the dose of gentamicin should be 2 mg/kg.	See Note 2. Note 3. 'Amoxil' and gentamicin should not be mixed in the same syringe. Note 4. Please consult the appropriate data sheet for full prescribing information on gentamicin.
Genitourinary Surgery or Instrumentation : prophylaxis for patients who have no urinary tract infection and who are to have genito-urinary surgery or instrumentation under general anaesthesia. In the case of *Obstetric and Gynaecological Procedures* and *Gastrointestinal Procedures*– routine prophylaxis is recommended only for patients with prosthetic heart valves.		Initially: 1 g 'Amoxil' IV or IM with 120 mg gentamicin IV or IM, immediately before induction. Followed by (6 hours later): 500 mg 'Amoxil' orally or IV or IM according to clinical condition.		See Notes 2, 3 and 4 above.
Surgery or Instrumentation of the Upper Respiratory Tract	Patients other than those with prosthetic heart valves.	1 g 'Amoxil' IV or IM immediately before induction; 500 mg 'Amoxil' IV or IM 6 hours later.	Under 10: half adult dose. Under 5: quarter adult dose.	See Note 2 above. Note 5. The second dose of 'Amoxil' may be administered orally as 'Amoxil' Syrup SF/DF.
	Patients with prosthetic heart valves.	Initially: 1 g 'Amoxil' IV or IM with 120 mg gentamicin IV or IM, immediately before induction; followed by (6 hours later) 500 mg 'Amoxil' IV or IM.	Under 10: the dose of 'Amoxil' should be half the adult dose; the gentamicin dose should be 2 mg/kg. Under 5: the dose of 'Amoxil' should be quarter the adult dose; the dose of gentamicin should be 2 mg/kg.	See Notes 2, 3, 4 and 5 above.

individuals with a history of hypersensitivity to beta-lactam antibiotics (see 4.3).

Erythematous (morbilliform) rashes have been associated with glandular fever in patients receiving amoxicillin.

Prolonged use may also occasionally result in overgrowth of non-susceptible organisms.

In patients with reduced urine output, crystalluria has been observed very rarely, predominantly with parenteral therapy. During the administration of high doses of amoxicillin, it is advisable to maintain adequate fluid intake and urinary output in order to reduce the possibility of amoxicillin crystalluria (see Section 4.9 Overdose).

Dosage should be adjusted in patients with renal impairment (see 4.2).

4.5 Interaction with other medicinal products and other forms of interaction

In common with other broad spectrum antibiotics, amoxicillin may reduce the efficacy of oral contraceptives and patients should be warned accordingly.

Concurrent administration of allopurinol during treatment with amoxicillin can increase the likelihood of allergic skin reactions.

Prolongation of prothrombin time has been reported rarely in patients receiving amoxicillin. Appropriate monitoring should be undertaken when anticoagulants are prescribed concurrently.

It is recommended that when testing for the presence of glucose in urine during amoxicillin treatment, enzymatic glucose oxidase methods should be used. Due to the high urinary concentrations of amoxicillin, false positive readings are common with chemical methods.

4.6 Pregnancy and lactation

Use in pregnancy:

Animal studies with Amoxil have shown no teratogenic effects. The product has been in extensive clinical use since 1972 and its suitability in human pregnancy has been well documented in clinical studies. When antibiotic therapy is required during pregnancy, Amoxil may be considered appropriate when the potential benefits outweigh the potential risks associated with treatment.

Use in lactation:

Amoxicillin may be given during lactation. With the exception of the risk of sensitisation associated with the excretion of trace quantities of amoxicillin in breast milk, there are no known detrimental effects for the breast-fed infant.

4.7 Effects on ability to drive and use machines

Adverse effects on the ability to drive or operate machinery have not been observed.

4.8 Undesirable effects

The following convention has been utilised for the classification of undesirable effects:-

Very common (>1/10), common (>1/100, <1/10), uncommon (>1/1000,<1/100), rare (>1/10,000, <1/1000), very rare (<1/10,000)

The majority of side effects listed below are not unique to amoxicillin and may occur when using other pencillins.

Unless otherwise stated, the frequency of adverse events has been derived from more than 30 years of post-marketing reports.

__Blood and lymphatic system disorders__

Very rare: Reversible leucopenia (including severe neutropenia or agranulocytosis), reversible thrombocytopenia and haemolytic anaemia.

Prolongation of bleeding time and prothrombin (see Section 4.5 - Interaction with other Medicaments and other Forms of Interaction)

__Immune system disorders__

Very rare: As with other antibiotics, severe allergic reactions, including angioneurotic oedema, anaphylaxis (see Section 4.4 - Special Warnings and Precautions for Use), serum sickness and hypersensitivity vasculitis.

If a hypersensitivity reaction is reported, the treatment must be discontinued. (See also Skin and subcutaneous tissue disorders).

__Nervous system disorders__

Very rare: Hyperkinesia, dizziness and convulsions. Convulsions may occur in patients with impaired renal function or in those receiving high doses.

__Gastrointestinal disorders__

__Clinical Trial Data__

***Common:** Diarrhoea and nausea.

***Uncommon:** Vomiting.

__Post-marketing Data__

Very rare: Mucocutaneous candidiasis and antibiotic associated colitis (including pseudomembraneous colitis and haemorrhagic colitis).

Superficial tooth discolouration has been reported in children. Good oral hygiene may help to prevent tooth discolouration as it can usually be removed by brushing.

__Hepato-biliary disorders__

Very rare: Hepatitis and cholestatic jaundice. A moderate rise in AST and/or ALT.

The significance of a rise in AST and/or ALT is unclear.

__Skin and subcutaneous tissue disorders__

__Clinical Trial Data__

***Common:** Skin rash

***Uncommon:** Urticaria and pruritus

__Post-marketing Data__

Very rare: Skin reactions such as erythema multiforme, Stevens-Johnson syndrome, toxic epidermal necrolysis, bullous and exfoliative dermatitis and acute generalised exanthematous pustulosis (AGEP)

(See also Immune system disorders).

__Renal and urinary tract disorders__

Very rare: Interstitial nephritis.

Very rare: Crystalluria (see Section 4.9 Overdose).

*The incidence of these AE's was derived from clinical studies involving a total of approximately 6,000 adult and paediatric patients taking amoxicillin.

4.9 Overdose

Gastrointestinal effects such as nausea, vomiting and diarrhoea may be evident and should be treated symptomatically with attention to the water/electrolyte balance. Amoxicillin crystalluria, in some cases leading to renal failure, has been observed (see Section 4.4 Special warnings and special precautions for use).

Amoxicillin may be removed from the circulation by haemodialysis.

5. PHARMACOLOGICAL PROPERTIES

5.1 Pharmacodynamic properties

Amoxil is a broad spectrum antibiotic.

It is rapidly bactericidal and possesses the safety profile of a penicillin.

5.2 Pharmacokinetic properties

Amoxil is well absorbed by the oral and parenteral routes. Oral administration, usually at convenient t.d.s. dosage, produces high serum levels independent of the time at which food is taken. Amoxil gives good penetration into bronchial secretions and high urinary concentrations of unchanged antibiotic.

5.3 Preclinical safety data

Not applicable.

6. PHARMACEUTICAL PARTICULARS

6.1 List of excipients

Amoxil Syrup SF/DF 125 mg/5ml

The powder contains disodium edetate, sodium benzoate (E211), saccharin sodium, silica (E551), xanthan gum (E415), peach, strawberry and lemon dry flavours and sorbitol (E420).

6.2 Incompatibilities

None.

6.3 Shelf life

Amoxil Syrup SF/DF 125 mg /5 ml	60M (once reconstituted: 14 days)

6.4 Special precautions for storage
Store powder in a dry place. Once dispensed, Amoxil Syrup SF/DF should be used within 14 days. If dilution of the reconstituted SF/DF product is required, water should be used.

6.5 Nature and contents of container
Amoxil Syrup SF/DF 125 mg/5 ml: Original Pack of 100 ml with Patient InformationLeaflet.

6.6 Special precautions for disposal and other handling
None

Administrative Data
7. MARKETING AUTHORISATION HOLDER
Beecham Group plc
Great West Road
Brentford
Middlesex TW8 9GS
Trading as:
GlaxoSmithKline UK, Stockley Park West, Uxbridge, Middlesex UB11 1BT
And/or
Bencard or SmithKline Beecham Pharmaceuticals all at Mundells Welwyn Garden City, Hertfordshire AL7 1EY

8. MARKETING AUTHORISATION NUMBER(S)
Amoxil Syrup SF/DF 125 mg/5 ml 0038/0326

9. DATE OF FIRST AUTHORISATION/RENEWAL OF THE AUTHORISATION
14 May 1985 / 16 January 1998

10. DATE OF REVISION OF THE TEXT
5th July 2005

11. Legal Status
POM

Amoxil Syrup Sucrose-Free/Dye-Free 250mg/5ml

(GlaxoSmithKline UK)

1. NAME OF THE MEDICINAL PRODUCT
Amoxil® Syrup Sucrose-Free/Dye-Free 250 mg/5 ml

2. QUALITATIVE AND QUANTITATIVE COMPOSITION
Amoxil Syrup SF/DF 250 mg contains 250 mg amoxicillin per 5 ml dose.

The amoxicillin is present as the trihydrate.

3. PHARMACEUTICAL FORM
Amoxil Syrup SF/DF 250 mg/5 ml: citrus-flavoured sucrose-free/Dye Freesuspension in a sorbitol base. Presented as powder in bottles for preparing 100 ml.

4. CLINICAL PARTICULARS
4.1 Therapeutic indications
Treatment of Infection: Amoxil is a broad spectrum antibiotic indicated for the treatment of commonly occurring bacterial infections such as:

Upper respiratory tract infections
Otitis media
Acute and chronic bronchitis
Chronic bronchial sepsis
Lobar and bronchopneumonia
Cystitis, urethritis, pyelonephritis
Bacteriuria in pregnancy
Gynaecological infections including puerperal sepsis and septic abortion
Gonorrhoea
Peritonitis
Intra-abdominal sepsis
Septicaemia
Bacterial endocarditis
Typhoid and paratyphoid fever
Skin and soft tissue infections
Osteomyelitis
Dental abscess (as an adjunct to surgical management)

In children with urinary tract infection the need for investigation should be considered.

Prophylaxis of endocarditis: Amoxil may be used for the prevention of bacteraemia, associated with procedures such as dental extraction, in patients at risk of developing bacterial endocarditis.

The wide range of organisms sensitive to the bactericidal action of Amoxil include:

Gram-positive	Gram-negative
Streptococcus faecalis	*Haemophilus influenzae*
Streptococcus pneumoniae	*Escherichia coli*
Streptococcus pyogenes	*Proteus mirabilis*
Streptococcus viridans	*Salmonella* species
Staphylococcus aureus (penicillin-sensitive)	*Shigella* species
	Bordetella pertussis
Clostridium species	*Brucella* species
Corynebacterium species	*Neisseria gonorrhoeae*
Bacillus anthracis	*Neisseria meningitidis*
Listeria monocytogenes	*Vibrio cholerae*
Pasteurella septica	

4.2 Posology and method of administration
Treatment of Infection:

Adult dosage (including elderly patients):

Oral:

Standard adult dosage: 250 mg three times daily, increasing to 500 mg three times daily for more severe infections.

High dosage therapy (maximum recommended oral dosage 6 g daily in divided doses): A dosage of 3 g twice daily is recommended in appropriate cases for the treatment of severe or recurrent purulent infection of the respiratory tract.

Short course therapy: Simple acute urinary tract infection: two 3 g doses with 10-12 hours between the doses. Dental abscess: two 3 g doses with 8 hours between the doses. Gonorrhoea: single 3 g dose.

Injectable:

500 mg IM eight hourly (or more frequently if necessary) in moderate infections. (This dose may be given by slow IV injection if more convenient.)

1 g IV six hourly in severe infections.

Children's dosage (up to 10 years of age):

Oral:

Standard children's dosage: 125 mg three times daily, increasing to 250 mg three times daily for more severe infections.

Amoxil Paediatric Suspension is recommended for children under six months of age.

Prophylaxis of endocarditis:

(see Table 1)

In severe or recurrent acute otitis media, especially where compliance may be a problem, 750 mg twice a day for two days may be used as an alternative course of treatment in children aged 3 to 10 years.

Injectable:

50-100 mg/kg body weight a day, in divided doses.

Parenteral therapy is indicated if the oral route is considered impracticable or unsuitable, and particularly for the urgent treatment of severe infection.

In renal impairment the excretion of the antibiotic will be delayed and, depending on the degree of impairment, it may be necessary to reduce the total daily dosage.

Prophylaxis of endocarditis: see table on previous page.

Administration:

Oral

4.3 Contraindications
Amoxil is a penicillin and should not be given to penicillin-hypersensitive patients. Attention should be paid to possible cross-sensitivity with other beta-lactam antibiotics eg. cephalosporins.

4.4 Special warnings and precautions for use
Serious and occasionally fatal hypersensitivity (anaphylactoid) reactions have been reported in patients on penicillin therapy. These reactions are more likely to occur in individuals with a history of hypersensitivity to beta-lactam antibiotics (see 4.3).

Erythematous (morbilliform) rashes have been associated with glandular fever in patients receiving amoxicillin.

Prolonged use may also occasionally result in overgrowth of non-susceptible organisms.

In patients with reduced urine output, crystalluria has been observed very rarely, predominantly with parenteral therapy. During the administration of high doses of amoxicillin, it is advisable to maintain adequate fluid intake and urinary output in order to reduce the possibility of amoxicillin crystalluria (see Section 4.9 Overdose).

Dosage should be adjusted in patients with renal impairment (see 4.2).

4.5 Interaction with other medicinal products and other forms of interaction
In common with other broad spectrum antibiotics, amoxicillin may reduce the efficacy of oral contraceptives and patients should be warned accordingly.

Concurrent administration of allopurinol during treatment with amoxicillin can increase the likelihood of allergic skin reactions.

Prolongation of prothrombin time has been reported rarely in patients receiving amoxicillin. Appropriate monitoring should be undertaken when anticoagulants are prescribed concurrently.

It is recommended that when testing for the presence of glucose in urine during amoxicillin treatment, enzymatic glucose oxidase methods should be used. Due to the high urinary concentrations of amoxicillin, false positive readings are common with chemical methods.

4.6 Pregnancy and lactation
Use in pregnancy:

Animal studies with Amoxil have shown no teratogenic effects. The product has been in extensive clinical use since 1972 and its suitability in human pregnancy has bee[n] well documented in clinical studies. When antibiotic the[r]apy is required during pregnancy, Amoxil may be consid[er]ed appropriate when the potential benefits outweigh th[e] potential risks associated with treatment.

Use in lactation:

Amoxicillin may be given during lactation. With the excep[tion] of the risk of sensitisation associated with the excre[tion] of trace quantities of amoxicillin in breast milk, ther[e] are no known detrimental effects for the breast-fed infan[t].

4.7 Effects on ability to drive and use machines
Adverse effects on the ability to drive or operate machiner[y] have not been observed.

4.8 Undesirable effects
The following convention has been utilised for the classi[fi]fication of undesirable effects:-

Very common (>1/10), common (>1/100, <1/10) uncommon (>1/1000, <1/100), rare (>1/10,000, <1/1000), very rare (<1/10,000)

The majority of side effects listed below are not unique to amoxycillin and may occur when using other pencillins.

Unless otherwise stated, the frequency of adverse events has been derived from more than 30 years of post-marketing reports.

Blood and lymphatic system disorders
Very rare: Reversible leucopenia (including severe neutropenia or agranulocytosis), reversible thrombocytopenia and haemolytic anaemia.

Prolongation of bleeding time and prothrombin (see Section 4.5 - Interaction with other Medicaments and other Forms of Interaction)

Immune system disorders
Very rare: As with other antibiotics, severe allergic reactions, including angioneurotic oedema, anaphylaxis (see Section 4.4 - Special Warnings and Precautions for Use), serum sickness and hypersensitivity vasculitis.

If a hypersensitivity reaction is reported, the treatment must be discontinued. (See also Skin and subcutaneous tissue disorders).

Nervous system disorders
Very rare: Hyperkinesia, dizziness and convulsions. Convulsions may occur in patients with impaired renal function or in those receiving high doses.

Gastrointestinal disorders
Clinical Trial Data
***Common:** Diarrhoea and nausea.
***Uncommon:** Vomiting.
Post-marketing Data
Very rare: Mucocutaneous candidiasis and antibiotic associated colitis (including pseudomembraneous colitis and haemorrhagic colitis).

Superficial tooth discolouration has been reported in children. Good oral hygiene may help to prevent tooth discolouration as it can usually be removed by brushing.

Hepato-biliary disorders
Very rare: Hepatitis and cholestatic jaundice. A moderate rise in AST and/or ALT.

The significance of a rise in AST and/or ALT is unclear.

Skin and subcutaneous tissue disorders
Clinical Trial Data
***Common:** Skin rash
***Uncommon:** Urticaria and pruritus
Post-marketing Data
Very rare: Skin reactions such as erythema multiforme, Stevens-Johnson syndrome, toxic epidermal necrolysis, bullous and exfoliative dermatitis and acute generalised exanthematous pustulosis (AGEP)
(See also Immune system disorders).

Renal and urinary tract disorders
Very rare: Interstitial nephritis.
Very rare: Crystalluria (see Section 4.9 Overdose).
*The incidence of these AEs was derived from clinical studies involving a total of approximately 6,000 adult and paediatric patients taking amoxicillin.

4.9 Overdose
Gastrointestinal effects such as nausea, vomiting and diarrhoea may be evident and should be treated symptomatically with attention to the water/electrolyte balance. Amoxicillin crystalluria, in some cases leading to renal failure, has been observed (see Section 4.4 Special warnings and special precautions for use).

Amoxicillin may be removed from the circulation by haemodialysis.

5. PHARMACOLOGICAL PROPERTIES
5.1 Pharmacodynamic properties
Amoxil is a broad spectrum antibiotic.

It is rapidly bactericidal and possesses the safety profile of a penicillin.

5.2 Pharmacokinetic properties
Amoxil is well absorbed by the oral and parenteral routes. Oral administration, usually at convenient t.d.s. dosage, produces high serum levels independent of the time at

Table 1 Prophylaxis of endocarditis

CONDITION		ADULTS' DOSAGE (INCLUDING ELDERLY)	CHILDREN'S DOSAGE	NOTES
Dental procedures : prophylaxis for patients undergoing extraction, scaling or surgery involving gingival tissues and who have not received a penicillin in the previous month. (N.B. Patients with prosthetic heart valves should be referred to hospital - see below).	Patient not having general anaesthetic.	3 g 'Amoxil' orally, 1 hour before procedure. A second dose may be given 6 hours later, if considered necessary.	Under 10: half adult dose. Under 5: quarter adult dose.	Note 1. If prophylaxis with 'Amoxil' is given twice within one month, emergence of resistant streptococci is unlikely to be a problem. Alternative antibiotics are recommended if more frequent prophylaxis is required, or if the patient has received a course of treatment with a penicillin during the previous month. Note 2. To minimise pain on injection, 'Amoxil' may be given as two injections of 500 mg dissolved in sterile 1% lignocaine solution (see *Administration*).
	Patient having general anaesthetic: if oral antibiotics considered to be appropriate.	Initially 3 g 'Amoxil' orally 4 hours prior to anaesthesia, followed by 3 g orally (or 1 g IV or IM if oral dose not tolerated) as soon as possible after the operation.		
	Patient having general anaesthetic: if oral antibiotics not appropriate.	1 g 'Amoxil' IV or IM immediately before induction; with 500 mg orally, 6 hours later.		
Dental procedures : patients for whom referral to hospital is recommended: a) Patients to be given a general anaesthetic who have been given a penicillin in the previous month. b) Patients to be given a general anaesthetic who have a prosthetic heart valve. c) Patients who have had one or more attacks of endocarditis.		Initially: 1 g 'Amoxil' IV or IM with 120 mg gentamicin IV or IM immediately prior to anaesthesia (if given) or 15 minutes prior to dental procedure. Followed by (6 hours later): 500 mg 'Amoxil' orally.	Under 10: the doses of 'Amoxil' should be half the adult dose; the dose of gentamicin should be 2 mg/kg. Under 5: the doses of 'Amoxil' should be quarter the adult dose; the dose of gentamicin should be 2 mg/kg.	See Note 2. Note 3. 'Amoxil' and gentamicin should not be mixed in the same syringe. Note 4. Please consult the appropriate data sheet for full prescribing information on gentamicin.
Genitourinary Surgery or Instrumentation : prophylaxis for patients who have no urinary tract infection and who are to have genito-urinary surgery or instrumentation under general anaesthesia. In the case of *Obstetric and Gynaecological Procedures* and *Gastrointestinal Procedures*– routine prophylaxis is recommended only for patients with prosthetic heart valves.		Initially: 1 g 'Amoxil' IV or IM with 120 mg gentamicin IV or IM, immediately before induction. Followed by (6 hours later): 500 mg 'Amoxil' orally or IV or IM according to clinical condition.		See Notes 2, 3 and 4 above.
Surgery or Instrumentation of the Upper Respiratory Tract	Patients other than those with prosthetic heart valves.	1 g 'Amoxil' IV or IM immediately before induction; 500 mg 'Amoxil' IV or IM 6 hours later.	Under 10: half adult dose. Under 5: quarter adult dose.	See Note 2 above. Note 5. The second dose of 'Amoxil' may be administered orally as 'Amoxil' Syrup SF/DF.
	Patients with prosthetic heart valves.	Initially: 1 g 'Amoxil' IV or IM with 120 mg gentamicin IV or IM, immediately before induction; followed by (6 hours later) 500 mg 'Amoxil' IV or IM.	Under 10: the dose of 'Amoxil' should be half the adult dose; the gentamicin dose should be 2 mg/kg. Under 5: the dose of 'Amoxil' should be quarter the adult dose; the dose of gentamicin should be 2 mg/kg.	See Notes 2, 3, 4 and 5 above.

which food is taken. Amoxil gives good penetration into bronchial secretions and high urinary concentrations of unchanged antibiotic.

5.3 Preclinical safety data
Not applicable.

6. PHARMACEUTICAL PARTICULARS
6.1 List of excipients
Amoxil Syrup SF/DF 250 mg / 5ml

The powder contains disodium edetate, sodium benzoate (E211), saccharin sodium, silica (E551), xanthan gum (E415), peach, strawberry and lemon dry flavours and sorbitol (E420).

6.2 Incompatibilities
None.

6.3 Shelf life
Amoxil Syrup SF/DF 250 mg / 5 ml 60M (once reconstituted: 14 days)

6.4 Special precautions for storage
Store powder in a dry place. Once dispensed, Amoxil Syrup SF/DF should be used within 14 days. If dilution of the reconstituted SF/DF product is required, water should be used.

6.5 Nature and contents of container
Amoxil Syrup SF/DF 250 mg/5 ml: Original Pack of 100 ml with Patient InformationLeaflet.

6.6 Special precautions for disposal and other handling
None

Administrative Data
7. MARKETING AUTHORISATION HOLDER
Beecham Group plc
Great West Road, Brentford
Middlesex TW8 9GS

Trading as:

GlaxoSmithKline UK, Stockley Park West, Uxbridge, Middlesex UB11 1BT

And/or

Bencard or SmithKline Beecham Pharmaceuticals all at Mundells Welwyn Garden City, Hertfordshire AL7 1EY

8. MARKETING AUTHORISATION NUMBER(S)
Amoxil Syrup SF/DF 250 mg/5 ml 0038/0327

9. DATE OF FIRST AUTHORISATION/RENEWAL OF THE AUTHORISATION
14 May 1985 / 16 January 1998

10. DATE OF REVISION OF THE TEXT
5th July 2005

11. Legal Status
POM

Amoxil Vials for Injection 1g

(GlaxoSmithKline UK)

1. NAME OF THE MEDICINAL PRODUCT
Amoxil® Vials For Injection 1 G

2. QUALITATIVE AND QUANTITATIVE COMPOSITION
Amoxil Vials for Injection 1 g contain 1 g amoxicillin

The amoxicillin is present as the sodium salt in Amoxil injections (each 1 g vial contains approximately 3.3 mmol of sodium).

3. PHARMACEUTICAL FORM
Amoxil Vials: vials containing sterile powder for reconstitution.

4. CLINICAL PARTICULARS
4.1 Therapeutic indications
Treatment of Infection: Amoxil is a broad spectrum antibiotic indicated for the treatment of commonly occurring bacterial infections such as:

Upper respiratory tract infections
Otitis media
Acute and chronic bronchitis
Chronic bronchial sepsis
Lobar and bronchopneumonia
Cystitis, urethritis, pyelonephritis
Bacteriuria in pregnancy
Gynaecological infections including puerperal sepsis and septic abortion
Gonorrhoea
Peritonitis
Intra-abdominal sepsis
Septicaemia
Bacterial endocarditis
Typhoid and paratyphoid fever
Skin and soft tissue infections

In children with urinary tract infection the need for investigation should be considered.

Prophylaxis of endocarditis: Amoxil may be used for the prevention of bacteraemia, associated with procedures such as dental extraction, in patients at risk of developing bacterial endocarditis.

The wide range of organisms sensitive to the bactericidal action of Amoxil include:

Gram-positive	Gram-negative
Streptococcus faecalis	*Haemophilus influenzae*
Streptococcus pneumoniae	*Escherichia coli*
Streptococcus pyogenes	*Proteus mirabilis*
Streptococcus viridans	*Salmonella* species
Staphylococcus aureus (penicillin-sensitive)	*Shigella* species
	Bordetella pertussis
Clostridium species	*Brucella* species
Corynebacterium species	*Neisseria gonorrhoeae*
Bacillus anthracis	*Neisseria meningitidis*
Listeria monocytogenes	*Vibrio cholerae*
	Pasteurella septica

4.2 Posology and method of administration
Treatment of infection:
Adult dosage (including elderly patients):
Injectable:
500 mg IM eight hourly (or more frequently if necessary) in moderate infections. (This dose may be given by slow IV injection if more convenient.)
1 g IV six hourly in severe infections.
Children's dosage (up to 10 years of age):
Injectable:
50-100 mg/kg body weight a day, in divided doses.

Parenteral therapy is indicated if the oral route is considered impracticable or unsuitable, and particularly for the urgent treatment of severe infection.

In renal impairment the excretion of the antibiotic will be delayed and, depending on the degree of impairment, it may be necessary to reduce the total daily dosage.

Prophylaxis of endocarditis: see table on next page.
Prophylaxis of endocarditis:
(see Table 1 on next page)
Administration:
Intravenous Injection, Intravenous Infusion, Intramuscular:
Using vials for injection (See Section 6.6)

4.3 Contraindications
Amoxil is a penicillin and should not be given to penicillin-hypersensitive patients. Attention should be paid to possible cross-sensitivity with other beta-lactam antibiotics, e.g. cephalosporins.

4.4 Special warnings and precautions for use
Serious and occasionally fatal hypersensitivity (anaphylactoid) reactions have been reported in patients on penicillin

Table 1 Prophylaxis of endocarditis

CONDITION		ADULTS' DOSAGE (INCLUDING ELDERLY)	CHILDREN'S DOSAGE	NOTES
Dental procedures : prophylaxis for patients undergoing extraction, scaling or surgery involving gingival tissues and who have not received a penicillin in the previous month. (N.B. Patients with prosthetic heart valves should be referred to hospital - see below).	Patient not having general anaesthetic.	3 g 'Amoxil' orally, 1 hour before procedure. A second dose may be given 6 hours later, if considered necessary.	Under 10: half adult dose. Under 5: quarter adult dose.	Note 1. If prophylaxis with 'Amoxil' is given twice within one month, emergence of resistant streptococci is unlikely to be a problem. Alternative antibiotics are recommended if more frequent prophylaxis is required, or if the patient has received a course of treatment with a penicillin during the previous month. Note 2. To minimise pain on injection, 'Amoxil' may be given as two injections of 500 mg dissolved in sterile 1% lidocaine solution (see *Administration*).
	Patient having general anaesthetic: if oral antibiotics considered to be appropriate.	Initially 3 g 'Amoxil' orally 4 hours prior to anaesthesia, followed by 3 g orally (or 1 g IV or IM if oral dose not tolerated) as soon as possible after the operation.		
	Patient having general anaesthetic: if oral antibiotics not appropriate.	1 g 'Amoxil' IV or IM immediately before induction; with 500 mg orally, 6 hours later.		
Dental procedures : patients for whom referral to hospital is recommended: a) Patients to be given a general anaesthetic who have been given a penicillin in the previous month. b) Patients to be given a general anaesthetic who have a prosthetic heart valve. c) Patients who have had one or more attacks of endocarditis.		Initially: 1 g 'Amoxil' IV or IM with 120 mg gentamicin IV or IM immediately prior to anaesthesia (if given) or 15 minutes prior to dental procedure. Followed by (6 hours later): 500 mg 'Amoxil' orally.	Under 10: the doses of 'Amoxil' should be half the adult dose; the dose of gentamicin should be 2 mg/kg. Under 5: the doses of 'Amoxil' should be quarter the adult dose; the dose of gentamicin should be 2 mg/kg.	See Note 2. Note 3. 'Amoxil' and gentamicin should not be mixed in the same syringe. Note 4. Please consult the appropriate data sheet for full prescribing information on gentamicin.
Genitourinary Surgery or Instrumentation : prophylaxis for patients who have no urinary tract infection and who are to have genito-urinary surgery or instrumentation under general anaesthesia. In the case of *Obstetric and Gynaecological Procedures* and *Gastrointestinal Procedures*– routine prophylaxis is recommended only for patients with prosthetic heart valves.		Initially: 1 g 'Amoxil' IV or IM with 120 mg gentamicin IV or IM, immediately before induction. Followed by (6 hours later): 500 mg 'Amoxil' orally or IV or IM according to clinical condition.		See Notes 2, 3 and 4 above.
Surgery or Instrumentation of the Upper Respiratory Tract	Patients other than those with prosthetic heart valves.	1 g 'Amoxil' IV or IM immediately before induction; 500 mg 'Amoxil' IV or IM 6 hours later.	Under 10: half adult dose. Under 5: quarter adult dose.	See Note 2 above. Note 5. The second dose of 'Amoxil may be administered orally as 'Amoxil' Syrup SF/DF.
	Patients with prosthetic heart valves.	Initially: 1 g 'Amoxil' IV or IM with 120 mg gentamicin IV or IM, immediately before induction; followed by (6 hours later) 500 mg 'Amoxil' IV or IM.	Under 10: the dose of 'Amoxil' should be half the adult dose; the gentamicin dose should be 2 mg/kg. Under 5: the dose of 'Amoxil' should be quarter the adult dose; the dose of gentamicin should be 2 mg/kg.	See Notes 2, 3, 4 and 5 above.

therapy. These reactions are more likely to occur in individuals with a history of hypersensitivity to beta-lactam antibiotics (see Section 4.3).

Erythematous (morbilliform) rashes have been associated with glandular fever in patients receiving amoxicillin.

Prolonged use may also occasionally result in overgrowth of non-susceptible organisms.

In patients with reduced urine output, crystalluria has been observed very rarely, predominantly with parenteral therapy. During the administration of high doses of amoxicillin, it is advisable to maintain adequate fluid intake and urinary output in order to reduce the possibility of amoxicillin crystalluria (See Section 4.9 Overdose). Amoxicillin has been reported to precipitate in bladder catheters after intravenous administration of large doses. A regular check of patency should be maintained.

Dosage should be adjusted in patients with renal impairment (see Section 4.2).

When prepared for intramuscular or direct intravenous injection, Amoxil should be administered immediately after reconstitution. The stability of Amoxil in various infusion fluids is given in the Package Enclosure Leaflet.

4.5 Interaction with other medicinal products and other forms of interaction

In common with other broad spectrum antibiotics, amoxicillin may reduce the efficacy of oral contraceptives and patients should be warned accordingly.

Concurrent administration of allopurinol during treatment with amoxicillin can increase the likelihood of allergic skin reactions.

Prolongation of prothrombin time has been reported rarely in patients receiving amoxicillin. Appropriate monitoring should be undertaken when anticoagulants are prescribed concurrently.

It is recommended that when testing for the presence of glucose in urine during amoxicillin treatment, enzymatic glucose oxidase methods should be used. Due to the high urinary concentrations of amoxicillin, false positive readings are common with chemical methods.

4.6 Pregnancy and lactation

Use in pregnancy:

Animal studies with Amoxil have shown no teratogenic effects. The product has been in extensive clinical use since 1972 and its suitability in human pregnancy has been well documented in clinical studies. When antibiotic therapy is required during pregnancy, Amoxil may be considered appropriate when the potential benefits outweigh the potential risks associated with treatment.

Use in lactation:

Amoxicillin may be given during lactation. With the exception of the risk of sensitisation associated with the excretion of trace quantities of amoxicillin in breast milk, there are no known detrimental effects for the breast-fed infant.

4.7 Effects on ability to drive and use machines

Adverse effects on the ability to drive or operate machinery have not been observed.

4.8 Undesirable effects

The following convention has been utilised for the classification of undesirable effects:-

Very common (>1/10), common (>1/100, <1/10), uncommon (>1/1000,<1/100), rare (>1/10,000, <1/1000), very rare (<1/10,000)

The majority of side effects listed below are not unique to amoxicillin and may occur when using other penicillins.

Unless otherwise stated, the frequency of adverse events has been derived from more than 30 years of post-marketing reports.

Blood and lymphatic system disorders

Very rare: Reversible leucopenia (including severe neutropenia or agranulocytosis), reversible thrombocytopenia and haemolytic anaemia.

Prolongation of bleeding time and prothrombin (see Section 4.5 - Interaction with other Medicaments and other Forms of Interaction)

Immune system disorders

Very rare: As with other antibiotics, severe allergic reactions, including angioneurotic oedema, anaphylaxis (see Section 4.4 - Special Warnings and Precautions for Use), serum sickness and hypersensitivity vasculitis.

If a hypersensitivity reaction is reported, the treatment must be discontinued. (See also Skin and subcutaneous tissue disorders).

Nervous system disorders

Very rare: Hyperkinesia, dizziness and convulsions. Convulsions may occur in patients with impaired renal function or in those receiving high doses.

Gastrointestinal disorders

Clinical Trial Data

Common: Diarrhoea and nausea.

Uncommon: Vomiting.

Post-marketing Data

Very rare: Mucocutaneous candidiasis and antibiotic associated colitis (including pseudomembraneous colitis and haemorrhagic colitis).

Hepato-biliary disorders

Very rare: Hepatitis and cholestatic jaundice. A moderate rise in AST and/or ALT.

The significance of a rise in AST and/or ALT is unclear.

Skin and subcutaneous tissue disorders

Clinical Trial Data

Common: Skin rash

Uncommon: Urticaria and pruritus

Post-marketing Data

Very rare: Skin reactions such as erythema multiform Stevens-Johnson syndrome, toxic epidermal necrolysi bullous and exfoliative dermatitis and acute generalise exanthematous pustulosis (AGEP)

(See also Immune system disorders).

Renal and urinary tract disorders

Very rare: Interstitial nephritis, crystalluria (See Section 4 Overdose).

The incidence of these AEs was derived from clinic studies involving a total of approximately 6,000 adult ar paediatric patients taking amoxicillin.

4.9 Overdose

Gastrointestinal effects such as nausea, vomiting and dia rhoea may be evident and should be treated symptoma cally with attention to the water/electrolyte balanc Amoxicillin crystalluria, in some cases leading to ren failure, has been observed (see Section 4.4 Special war ings and special precautions for use).

Amoxicillin may be removed from the circulation by ha modialysis.

5. PHARMACOLOGICAL PROPERTIES

5.1 Pharmacodynamic properties

Amoxil is a broad spectrum antibiotic.

It is rapidly bactericidal and possesses the safety profile a penicillin.

5.2 Pharmacokinetic properties

Amoxil is well absorbed by the oral and parenteral route Amoxil gives good penetration into bronchial secretio and high urinary concentrations of unchanged antibiotic

5.3 Preclinical safety data

Not applicable.

6. PHARMACEUTICAL PARTICULARS

6.1 List of excipients

Amoxil Injection

None

6.2 Incompatibilities

Amoxil should not be mixed with blood products, oth proteinaceous fluids such as protein hydrolysates, or wi intravenous lipid emulsions.

If Amoxil is prescribed concurrently with an aminoglyco side, the antibiotics should not be mixed in the syring intravenous fluid container or giving set because loss

:tivity of the aminoglycoside can occur under these con-tions.

3 Shelf life

jection Vials 24 months

4 Special precautions for storage

noxil Vials for Injection should be stored at or below 25°c.

hen prepared for intramuscular or direct intravenous ection, Amoxil should be administered immediately after constitution. The stability of Amoxil in various infusion iids is dependent upon the concentration and tempera-re: stability times are given in the Package Enclosure aflet.

5 Nature and contents of container

noxil Vials for Injection: Clear Type I glass vials fitted with chlorobutyl rubber bung and an aluminium overseal. 1 g: cks of 5 or 10. Each pack carries instructions for use.

6 Special precautions for disposal and other handling

ravenous Injection:

ssolve 1 g in 20 ml Water for Injections BP (Final lume=20.8 ml).

noxil injection, suitably diluted, may be injected directly o a vein or the infusion line over a period of three to four nutes.

ravenous Infusion:

lutions may be prepared as described for intravenous ections and then added to an intravenous solution in a nibag or in-line burette and administered over a period of f to one hour. Alternatively, using a suitable reconstitu-n device, the appropriate volume of intravenous fluid y be transferred from the infusion bag into the vial and n drawn back into the bag after dissolution.

ramuscular:

g: Add 2.5 ml Water for Injections BP ‡ and shake orously (Final volume=3.3 ml).

he 1 g vial will not dissolve in sterile 1% solution of ocaine hydrochloride at the required concentration. To nimise pain on injection, 1 g of Amoxil may be given as separate injections of 500 mg dissolved in a sterile ution of 1% lidocaine hydrochloride.

ransient pink colouration or slight opalescence may pear during reconstitution. Reconstituted solutions are mally a pale straw colour.

ninistrative Data

MARKETING AUTHORISATION HOLDER

echam Group plc

at West Road, Brentford, Middlesex TW8 9GS

ding as GlaxoSmithKline UK, Stockley Park West, bridge, Middlesex UB11 1BT

l/or

card or SmithKline Beecham Pharmaceuticals at ndells Welwyn Garden City, Hertfordshire AL7 1 EY

MARKETING AUTHORISATION NUMBER(S)

oxil Vials for Injection 1 g 0038/0225

DATE OF FIRST AUTHORISATION/RENEWAL OF AUTHORISATION

oxil Vials for Injection 1 g 13.10.98

DATE OF REVISION OF THE TEXT

01/07

Legal Status

M

noxil Vials for Injection 500mg

(GlaxoSmithKline UK)

AME OF THE MEDICINAL PRODUCT

xil® Vials for Injection 500 Mg

UALITATIVE AND QUANTITATIVE COMPOSITION

xil Vials for Injection 500 mg contain 500 mg amox-

amoxicillin is present as the sodium salt in Amoxil tions (each 1 g vial contains approximately 3.3 mmol odium).

HARMACEUTICAL FORM

xil Vials: vials containing sterile powder for reconstitu-

LINICAL PARTICULARS

Therapeutic indications

tment of Infection: Amoxil is a broad spectrum anti-c indicated for the treatment of commonly occurring erial infections such as:

er respiratory tract infections

s media

e and chronic bronchitis

nic bronchial sepsis

r and bronchopneumonia

tis, urethritis, pyelonephritis

eriuria in pregnancy

Gynaecological infections including puerperal sepsis and septic abortion

Gonorrhoea

Peritonitis

Intra-abdominal sepsis

Septicaemia

Bacterial endocarditis

Typhoid and paratyphoid fever

Skin and soft tissue infections

In children with urinary tract infection the need for investigation should be considered.

Prophylaxis of endocarditis: Amoxil may be used for the prevention of bacteraemia, associated with procedures such as dental extraction, in patients at risk of developing bacterial endocarditis.

The wide range of organisms sensitive to the bactericidal action of Amoxil include:

Gram-positive	Gram-negative
Streptococcus faecalis	*Haemophilus influenzae*
Streptococcus pneumoniae	*Escherichia coli*
Streptococcus pyogenes	*Proteus mirabilis*
Streptococcus viridans	*Salmonella* species
Staphylococcus aureus	*Shigella* species
(penicillin-sensitive)	*Bordetella pertussis*
Clostridium species	*Brucella* species
Corynebacterium species	*Neisseria gonorrhoeae*
Bacillus anthracis	*Neisseria meningitidis*
Listeria monocytogenes	*Vibrio cholerae*
	Pasteurella septica

4.2 Posology and method of administration

Treatment of infection:

Adult dosage (including elderly patients):

Injectable:

500 mg IM eight hourly (or more frequently if necessary) in moderate infections. (This dose may be given by slow IV injection if more convenient.)

1 g IV six hourly in severe infections.

Children's dosage (up to 10 years of age):

Injectable:

50-100 mg/kg body weight a day, in divided doses.

Parenteral therapy is indicated if the oral route is considered impracticable or unsuitable, and particularly for the urgent treatment of severe infection.

In renal impairment the excretion of the antibiotic will be delayed and, depending on the degree of impairment, it may be necessary to reduce the total daily dosage.

Prophylaxis of endocarditis: see table on next page.

Prophylaxis of endocarditis:

(see Table 1 on next page)

Administration:

Intravenous Injection, Intravenous Infusion, Intramuscular: Using vials for injection (See Section 6.6)

4.3 Contraindications

Amoxil is a penicillin and should not be given to penicillin-hypersensitive patients. Attention should be paid to possible cross-sensitivity with other beta-lactam antibiotics, e.g. cephalosporins.

4.4 Special warnings and precautions for use

Serious and occasionally fatal hypersensitivity (anaphylactoid) reactions have been reported in patients on penicillin therapy. These reactions are more likely to occur in individuals with a history of hypersensitivity to beta-lactam antibiotics (see Section 4.3).

Erythematous (morbilliform) rashes have been associated with glandular fever in patients receiving amoxicillin.

Prolonged use may also occasionally result in overgrowth of non-susceptible organisms.

In patients with reduced urine output, crystalluria has been observed very rarely, predominantly with parenteral therapy. During the administration of high doses of amoxicillin, it is advisable to maintain adequate fluid intake and urinary output in order to reduce the possibility of amoxicillin crystalluria (see Section 4.9 Overdose). Amoxicillin has been reported to precipitate in bladder catheters after intravenous administration of large doses. A regular check of patency should be maintained.

Dosage should be adjusted in patients with renal impairment (see Section 4.2).

When prepared for intramuscular or direct intravenous injection, Amoxil should be administered immediately after reconstitution. The stability of Amoxil in various infusion fluids is given in the Package Enclosure Leaflet.

4.5 Interaction with other medicinal products and other forms of interaction

Probenecid decreases the renal tubular secretion of amoxicillin. Concurrent use with Amoxil may result in increased and prolonged blood levels of amoxicillin.

In common with other antibiotics, amoxicillin may affect the gut flora, leading to lower oestrogen reabsorption and reduced efficacy of combined oral contraceptives.

Concurrent administration of allopurinol during treatment with amoxicillin can increase the likelihood of allergic skin reactions.

Prolongation of prothrombin time has been reported rarely in patients receiving amoxicillin. Appropriate monitoring should be undertaken when anticoagulants are prescribed concurrently.

It is recommended that when testing for the presence of glucose in urine during amoxicillin treatment, enzymatic glucose oxidase methods should be used. Due to the high urinary concentrations of amoxicillin, false positive readings are common with chemical methods.

4.6 Pregnancy and lactation

Use in pregnancy

Animal studies with Amoxil have shown no teratogenic effects. The product has been in extensive clinical use since 1972 and its suitability in human pregnancy has been well documented in clinical studies. When antibiotic therapy is required during pregnancy, Amoxil may be considered appropriate when the potential benefits outweigh the potential risks associated with treatment.

Use in lactation:

Amoxicillin may be given during lactation. With the exception of the risk of sensitisation associated with the excretion of trace quantities of amoxicillin in breast milk, there are no known detrimental effects for the breast-fed infant.

4.7 Effects on ability to drive and use machines

Adverse effects on the ability to drive or operate machinery have not been observed.

4.8 Undesirable effects

The following convention has been utilised for the classification of undesirable effects:-

Very common (>1/10), common (>1/100, <1/10), uncommon (>1/1000,<1/100), rare (>1/10,000, <1/1000), very rare (<1/10,000)

The majority of side effects listed below are not unique to amoxicillin and may occur when using other penicillins.

Unless otherwise stated, the frequency of adverse events has been derived from more than 30 years of post-marketing reports.

Infections and infestations

Very Rare: Mucocutaneous candidiasis

Blood and lymphatic system disorders

Very rare: Reversible leucopenia (including severe neutropenia or agranulocytosis), reversible thrombocytopenia and haemolytic anaemia.

Prolongation of bleeding time and prothrombin (see Section 4.5 - Interaction with other Medicinal Products and other Forms of Interaction)

Immune system disorders

Very rare: As with other antibiotics, severe allergic reactions, including angioneurotic oedema, anaphylaxis (see Section 4.4 - Special Warnings and Precautions for Use), serum sickness and hypersensitivity vasculitis.

If a hypersensitivity reaction is reported, the treatment must be discontinued. (See also Skin and subcutaneous tissue disorders).

Nervous system disorders

Very rare: Hyperkinesia, dizziness and convulsions. Convulsions may occur in patients with impaired renal function or in those receiving high doses.

Gastrointestinal disorders

Clinical Trial Data

Common: Diarrhoea and nausea.

Uncommon: Vomiting.

Post-marketing Data

Very rare: Antibiotic associated colitis (including pseudomembraneous colitis and haemorrhagic colitis).

Hepato-biliary disorders

Very rare: Hepatitis and cholestatic jaundice. A moderate rise in AST and/or ALT.

The significance of a rise in AST and/or ALT is unclear.

Skin and subcutaneous tissue disorders

Clinical Trial Data

Common: Skin rash

Uncommon: Urticaria and pruritus

Post-marketing Data

Very rare: Skin reactions such as erythema multiforme, Stevens-Johnson syndrome, toxic epidermal necrolysis, bullous and exfoliative dermatitis and acute generalised exanthematous pustulosis (AGEP)

(See also Immune system disorders).

Renal and urinary tract disorders

Very rare: Interstitial nephritis, crystalluria (See Section 4.9 Overdose).

The incidence of these AEs was derived from clinical studies involving a total of approximately 6,000 adult and paediatric patients taking amoxicillin.

Table 1 Prophylaxis of endocarditis

CONDITION		ADULTS' DOSAGE (INCLUDING ELDERLY)	CHILDREN'S DOSAGE	NOTES
Dental procedures: prophylaxis for patients undergoing extraction, scaling or surgery involving gingival tissues and who have not received a penicillin in the previous month. (N.B. Patients with prosthetic heart valves should be referred to hospital - see below).	Patient not having general anaesthetic.	3 g 'Amoxil' orally, 1 hour before procedure. A second dose may be given 6 hours later, if considered necessary.	Under 10: half adult dose. Under 5: quarter adult dose.	Note 1. If prophylaxis with 'Amoxil' is given twice within one month, emergence of resistant streptococci is unlikely to be a problem. Alternative antibiotics are recommended if more frequent prophylaxis is required, or if the patient has received a course of treatment with a penicillin during the previous month. Note 2. To minimise pain on injection, 'Amoxil' may be given as two injections of 500 mg dissolved in sterile 1% lidocaine solution (see *Administration*).
	Patient having general anaesthetic: if oral antibiotics considered to be appropriate.	Initially 3 g 'Amoxil' orally 4 hours prior to anaesthesia, followed by 3 g orally (or 1 g IV or IM if oral dose not tolerated) as soon as possible after the operation.		
	Patient having general anaesthetic: if oral antibiotics not appropriate.	1 g 'Amoxil' IV or IM immediately before induction; with 500 mg orally, 6 hours later.		
Dental procedures: patients for whom referral to hospital is recommended: a) Patients to be given a general anaesthetic who have been given a penicillin in the previous month. b) Patients to be given a general anaesthetic who have a prosthetic heart valve. c) Patients who have had one or more attacks of endocarditis.		Initially: 1 g 'Amoxil' IV or IM with 120 mg gentamicin IV or IM immediately prior to anaesthesia (if given) or 15 minutes prior to dental procedure. Followed by (6 hours later): 500 mg 'Amoxil' orally.	Under 10: the doses of 'Amoxil' should be half the adult dose; the dose of gentamicin should be 2 mg/kg. Under 5: the doses of 'Amoxil' should be quarter the adult dose; the dose of gentamicin should be 2 mg/kg.	See Note 2. Note 3. 'Amoxil' and gentamicin should not be mixed in the same syringe. Note 4. Please consult the appropriate data sheet for full prescribing information on gentamicin.
Genitourinary Surgery or Instrumentation: prophylaxis for patients who have no urinary tract infection and who are to have genito-urinary surgery or instrumentation under general anaesthesia. In the case of *Obstetric and Gynaecological Procedures* and *Gastrointestinal Procedures*– routine prophylaxis is recommended only for patients with prosthetic heart valves.		Initially: 1 g 'Amoxil' IV or IM with 120 mg gentamicin IV or IM, immediately before induction. Followed by (6 hours later): 500 mg 'Amoxil' orally or IV or IM according to clinical condition.		See Notes 2, 3 and 4 above.
Surgery or Instrumentation of the Upper Respiratory Tract	Patients other than those with prosthetic heart valves.	1 g 'Amoxil' IV or IM immediately before induction; 500 mg 'Amoxil' IV or IM 6 hours later.	Under 10: half adult dose. Under 5: quarter adult dose.	See Note 2 above. Note 5. The second dose of 'Amox may be administered orally as 'Amoxil' Syrup SF/DF.
	Patients with prosthetic heart valves.	Initially: 1 g 'Amoxil' IV or IM with 120 mg gentamicin IV or IM, immediately before induction; followed by (6 hours later) 500 mg 'Amoxil' IV or IM.	Under 10: the dose of 'Amoxil' should be half the adult dose; the gentamicin dose should be 2 mg/kg. Under 5: the dose of 'Amoxil' should be quarter the adult dose; the dose of gentamicin should be 2 mg/kg.	See Notes 2, 3, 4 and 5 above.

4.9 Overdose
Gastrointestinal effects such as nausea, vomiting and diarrhoea may be evident and should be treated symptomatically with attention to the water/electrolyte balance. Amoxicillin crystalluria, in some cases leading to renal failure, has been observed (see Section 4.4 Special warnings and special precautions for use).

Amoxicillin may be removed from the circulation by haemodialysis.

5. PHARMACOLOGICAL PROPERTIES

5.1 Pharmacodynamic properties
Amoxil is a broad spectrum antibiotic.

It is rapidly bactericidal and possesses the safety profile of a penicillin.

5.2 Pharmacokinetic properties
Amoxil is well absorbed by the oral and parenteral routes. Amoxil gives good penetration into bronchial secretions and high urinary concentrations of unchanged antibiotic.

5.3 Preclinical safety data
Not applicable.

6. PHARMACEUTICAL PARTICULARS

6.1 List of excipients
Amoxil Injection: None

6.2 Incompatibilities
Amoxil should not be mixed with blood products, other proteinaceous fluids such as protein hydrolysates, or with intravenous lipid emulsions.

If Amoxil is prescribed concurrently with an aminoglycoside, the antibiotics should not be mixed in the syringe, intravenous fluid container or giving set because loss of activity of the aminoglycoside can occur under these conditions.

6.3 Shelf life
Injection Vials 24 months

6.4 Special precautions for storage
Amoxil Vials for Injection should be stored in a cool, dry place.

When prepared for intramuscular or direct intravenous injection, Amoxil should be administered immediately after reconstitution. The stability of Amoxil in various infusion fluids is dependent upon the concentration and temperature: stability times are given in the Package Enclosure Leaflet.

6.5 Nature and contents of container
Amoxil Vials for Injection: Clear Type I glass vials fitted with a chlorobutyl rubber bung and an aluminium overseal. 500 mg: packs of 5 or 10. Each pack carries instructions for use.

6.6 Special precautions for disposal and other handling
Intravenous Injection:
Dissolve 500 mg in 10 ml Water for Injections BP (Final volume=10.4 ml).

Amoxil injection, suitably diluted, may be injected directly into a vein or the infusion line over a period of three to four minutes.

Intravenous Infusion:
Solutions may be prepared as described for intravenous injections and then added to an intravenous solution in a minibag or in-line burette and administered over a period of half to one hour. Alternatively, using a suitable reconstitution device, the appropriate volume of intravenous fluid may be transferred from the infusion bag into the vial and then drawn back into the bag after dissolution.

Intramuscular:
500 mg: Add 2.5 ml Water for Injections BP † and shake vigorously (Final volume=2.9 ml).

If pain is experienced on intramuscular injection, a sterile 1% solution of lidocaine hydrochloride or 0.5% solution of procaine hydrochloride may be used in place of Water for Injections.

A transient pink colouration or slight opalescence may appear during reconstitution. Reconstituted solutions are normally a pale straw colour.

Administrative Data

7. MARKETING AUTHORISATION HOLDER
Beecham Group plc

Great West Road, Brentford, Middlesex TW8 9GS

Trading as GlaxoSmithKline UK Stockley Park West, Uxbridge, Middlesex UB11 1BT

And/or

Bencard or SmithKline Beecham Pharmaceuticals at Mundells Welwyn Garden City, Hertfordshire AL7 1 EY

8. MARKETING AUTHORISATION NUMBER(S)
Amoxil Vials for Injection 500 mg 0038/0222

9. DATE OF FIRST AUTHORISATION/RENEWAL OF THE AUTHORISATION
Amoxil Vials for Injection 500 mg 13.10.98

10. DATE OF REVISION OF THE TEXT
24th September 2008

11. Legal Status
POM

Anbesol Liquid

(SSL International pl

1. NAME OF THE MEDICINAL PRODUCT
Anbesol Liquid.

2. QUALITATIVE AND QUANTITATIVE COMPOSITIO
Lidocaine Hydrochloride Ph Eur 0.9% w/w; Chlorocre Ph Eur 0.1% w/w; and Cetylpyridinium Chloride Ph 0.02% w/w.

3. PHARMACEUTICAL FORM
Liquid for oral administration.

4. CLINICAL PARTICULARS

4.1 Therapeutic indications
For the temporary relief of pain caused by recurrent mo ulcers, denture irritation and teething.

4.2 Posology and method of administration
Adults, children and the elderly: apply undiluted to affected area with the fingertip. Two applications imme ately will normally be sufficient to obtain pain relief. Use to eight times a day. Babies teething: One application o Do not repeat for at least half an hour. Use up to eight tin a day.

4.3 Contraindications
Patients with a known history of hypersensitivity or alle type reactions to any of the constituents of the produc

4.4 Special warnings and precautions for use
If symptoms persist for more than 7 days, consult y doctor or dentist. For babies teething, do not repeat fc least half an hour. Keep all medicines out of the reach children. Do not exceed the stated dose.

4.5 Interaction with other medicinal products and ot forms of interaction
None known.

4.6 Pregnancy and lactation
No special precautions required.

4.7 Effects on ability to drive and use machines
None known.

4.8 Undesirable effects
There have been reports of non-specific ulceration foll ing oral cetylpyridinium chloride therapy.

4.9 Overdose
Ingestion of the complete contents of the marketed p would not be expected to cause any adverse effects.

. PHARMACOLOGICAL PROPERTIES

.1 Pharmacodynamic properties

idocaine hydrochloride: White crystalline powder soluble water and alcohol. Mechanism of action/effect: Lidoaine is a local anaesthetic of the amide type, which acts y reversible inhibition of nerve impulse generation and ansmission. Chlorocresol: Colourless crystals or a white ystalline powder slightly soluble in water and alcohol. hlorocresol has a disinfectant action. Cetylpyridinium hloride: A white unctuous powder soluble in water and cohol. Mechanism of action/effect: cetylpyridinium chlore has a disinfectant action.

2 Pharmacokinetic properties

docaine hydrochloride: Absorption and fate: Lidocaine is adily absorbed from mucous membranes and through amaged skin. Lidocaine undergoes first-pass metabolism the liver and about 90% is dealkylated to form monohylglycinexylidide and glycinexylidide. Further metabosm occurs and the metabolites are excreted in the urine ith less than 10% as unchanged lidocaine. Chlorocresol: bsorption: there is no significant absorption of chlorocreol through the skin or mucous. Cetylpyridinium chloride: bsorption: there is no significant absorption of cetylpyrinium chloride through the skin or mucous membranes.

3 Preclinical safety data

one stated.

PHARMACEUTICAL PARTICULARS

1 List of excipients

cohol 96% BP, Menthol BP, Glycerin Ph Eur, Caramel olour (containing colourants E110, E104, E123, E142), urified Water Ph Eur.

2 Incompatibilities

one known.

3 Shelf life

months.

4 Special precautions for storage

ore at a temperature not exceeding 25°C.

5 Nature and contents of container

5ml, 15 ml: glass bottles

6 Special precautions for disposal and other handling

ot applicable.

MARKETING AUTHORISATION HOLDER

SL International PLC. Venus, 1 Old Park Lane, Trafford rk, Manchester, M41 7HA.

MARKETING AUTHORISATION NUMBER(S)

. 17905/0074

DATE OF FIRST AUTHORISATION/RENEWAL OF IE AUTHORISATION

/08/2006

. DATE OF REVISION OF THE TEXT

/08/2006

nbesol Teething Gel

(SSL International plc)

NAME OF THE MEDICINAL PRODUCT

besol Teething Gel

QUALITATIVE AND QUANTITATIVE COMPOSITION

locaine Hydrochloride Ph Eur 1.0% w/w; Chlorocresol Eur 0.1% w/w; and Cetylpyridinium Chloride Ph Eur 02% w/w.

PHARMACEUTICAL FORM

l for oral administration.

CLINICAL PARTICULARS

Therapeutic indications

r the temporary relief of pain caused by recurrent mouth ers, denture irritation and teething.

Posology and method of administration

ults, children and the elderly: apply a small amount to affected area with a clean fingertip. Two applications mediately will normally be sufficient to obtain pain relief. e up to four times a day. Babies teething: apply a small ount to the affected area with a clean fingertip. Use up four times a day.

Contraindications

tients with a known history of hypersensitivity or allergic e reactions to any of the constituents of the product.

Special warnings and precautions for use

e following statements appear on the packaging: (i) if nptoms persist for more than 7 days, consult your ctor or pharmacist; (ii) keep all medicines out of the ch of children.

Interaction with other medicinal products and other ms of interaction

ne known.

Pregnancy and lactation

special precautions required.

4.7 Effects on ability to drive and use machines

None known.

4.8 Undesirable effects

There have been reports of non-specific ulceration following oral cetylpyridinium chloride therapy.

4.9 Overdose

Overdose is extremely unlikely considering the small size of the tube used for sale.

5. PHARMACOLOGICAL PROPERTIES

5.1 Pharmacodynamic properties

Lidocaine: Lidocaine is a local anaesthetic of the amide type which acts by reversible inhibition of nerve impulse generation and transmission. Chlorocresol: Chlorocresol has a disinfectant action. Cetylpyridinium chloride: Cetylpyridinium chloride has a disinfectant action.

5.2 Pharmacokinetic properties

Lidocaine hydrochloride: Absorption and Fate: Lidocaine is readily absorbed from mucous membranes and through damaged skin. Lidocaine undergoes first-pass metabolism in the liver and about 90% is dealkylated to form monoethylglycinexylidide and glycinexylidide. Further metabolism occurs and the metabolites are excreted in the urine with less than 10% as unchanged lidocaine. Chlorocresol: There is no significant absorption of chlorocresol through the skin or mucous membranes. Cetylpyridinium chloride: Absorption: There is no significant absorption of cetylpyridinium chloride through the skin or mucous membranes.

5.3 Preclinical safety data

The active ingredients in Anbesol Teething Gel have a well established safety record.

6. PHARMACEUTICAL PARTICULARS

6.1 List of excipients

Alcohol 96% BP; Glycerin Ph Eur; Clove Oil BP; Sodium Saccharin BP; Hydroxypropyl Cellulose Ph Eur; Ponceau 4R (E124); Purified Water Ph Eur.

6.2 Incompatibilities

None known.

6.3 Shelf life

36 months.

6.4 Special precautions for storage

Store at a temperature not exceeding 25°C.

6.5 Nature and contents of container

Membrane sealed lacquered aluminium tubes fitted with plastic caps containing 10g gel.

6.6 Special precautions for disposal and other handling

None.

7. MARKETING AUTHORISATION HOLDER

SSL International PLC. Venus, 1 Old Park Lane, Trafford Park, Manchester, M41 7HA.

8. MARKETING AUTHORISATION NUMBER(S)

PL 17905/0072

9. DATE OF FIRST AUTHORISATION/RENEWAL OF THE AUTHORISATION

23/03/06

10. DATE OF REVISION OF THE TEXT

23/03/06

Andropatch 2.5mg

(GlaxoSmithKline UK)

1. NAME OF THE MEDICINAL PRODUCT

Andropatch 2.5 mg / 24 hours Transdermal Patch

2. QUALITATIVE AND QUANTITATIVE COMPOSITION

Each Andropatch 2.5 mg System contains 12.2 mg testosterone BP.

For full list of excipients, see section 6.1.

3. PHARMACEUTICAL FORM

Andropatch 2.5 mg is a transdermal drug delivery system consisting of a beige self-adhesive patch surrounding a central drug reservoir of testosterone dissolved in an alcohol-based gel.

Each Andropatch 2.5 mg System delivers *in vivo* approximately 2.5 mg of testosterone over 24 hours across skin of average permeability. (Active surface area 7.5 cm^2).

4. CLINICAL PARTICULARS

4.1 Therapeutic indications

Andropatch 2.5 mg is indicated for testosterone replacement therapy in conditions with a deficiency or an absence of endogenous testosterone associated with primary or secondary hypogonadism.

4.2 Posology and method of administration

Adults and Elderly

The usual dose is two Andropatch 2.5 mg Systems applied nightly (approximately 10 pm) and worn for 24 hours, providing approximately 5 mg testosterone per day. The dose can be adjusted up to the equivalent of 7.5 mg nightly or down to 2.5 mg nightly depending on the serum testosterone measured in the morning after application. Measurement of serum testosterone should be repeated taking care to ensure proper system adhesion and correct time of application before the dose is adjusted. Three systems per day may be required for men with a higher body weight >130 kg). Treatment in non-virilised patients may be initiated with one system applied nightly. The dose should be adjusted as appropriate.

The duration of treatment and frequency of testosterone measurements is determined by the physician.

The adhesive side of the Andropatch 2.5 mg System should be applied to a clean, dry area of the skin on the back, abdomen, upper arms, or thighs. Bony prominences, such as the shoulder and hip areas, and areas that may be subjected to prolonged pressure during sleeping or sitting should be avoided. Application to these sites has been associated with burn-like blister reactions (see Section 4.8). Do not apply to broken or damaged skin. Do not apply to the scrotum. The sites of application should be rotated, with an interval of seven days between applications to the same site. The area selected should not be oily, damaged or irritated.

The system should be applied immediately after opening the pouch and removing the protective release liner. The system should be pressed firmly in place, making sure there is good contact with the skin, especially around the edges.

Children

Andropatch 2.5 mg is not indicated for use in children as there has been no clinical experience of its use below the age of 15.

4.3 Contraindications

Androgens are contra-indicated in men with carcinoma of the breast or known or suspected carcinoma of the prostate, nephrotic syndrome, hypercalcaemia and known hypersensitivity to testosterone.

Andropatch 2.5 mg is contra-indicated in men with known hypersensitivity to other constituents of the patch.

Andropatch 2.5 mg has not been evaluated in women and must not be used in women. Testosterone may be harmful to the foetus.

4.4 Special warnings and precautions for use

Elderly men treated with androgens may be at an increased risk for the development of prostatic hyperplasia.

Elderly men and others with an increased risk of developing prostatic cancer, should be assessed before starting testosterone replacement therapy because testosterone may promote the growth of subclinical prostate cancer.

As in men without testosterone deficiency, patients on testosterone replacement therapy should be periodically evaluated for prostate cancer.

Care should be taken in patients with skeletal metastases due to the risk of hypercalcaemia/hypercalcuria developing from androgen therapy.

If the patient develops an application site reaction, treatment should be reviewed and discontinued if necessary.

Testosterone may cause a rise in blood pressure and Andropatch 2.5 mg should be used with caution in patients with hypertension.

Oedema, with or without congestive heart failure, may result from androgen treatment in patients with pre-existing cardiac, renal, or hepatic disease. In addition to discontinuation of the drug, diuretic therapy may be required.

Andropatch 2.5 mg should be used with caution in patients with ischaemic heart disease, epilepsy and migraine as these conditions may be aggravated.

4.5 Interaction with other medicinal products and other forms of interaction

When given simultaneously with anticoagulants the anticoagulant effect can increase. Patients receiving oral anticoagulants require close monitoring especially when androgens are started or stopped.

Concurrent administration of oxyphenbutazone and androgens may result in elevated serum levels of oxyphenbutazone.

In diabetic patients, the metabolic effects of androgens may alter blood glucose and, therefore, insulin requirements.

4.6 Pregnancy and lactation

Andropatch 2.5 mg therapy has not been evaluated in and must not be used in women under any circumstances. Testosterone may be harmful to the foetus.

4.7 Effects on ability to drive and use machines

There is no evidence that Andropatch 2.5 mg will affect the ability of a patient to drive or to use machines.

4.8 Undesirable effects

In the majority of cases, transient mild to moderate skin reactions have been observed at the site of application at some time during treatment. These include pruritus; irritation with erythema, induration or burning, rash and allergic contact dermatitis. Burn-like lesions characterised by blisters, skin necrosis, and ulceration that healed over several weeks with scarring in some cases have also been observed.

The burn-like lesions occurred sporadically, usually only at one site, (most commonly over bony prominences or areas that may have been subjected to prolonged pressure during sleeping or sitting). Such lesions should be treated as burns.

As seen with other testosterone treatments, prostate abnormalities, prostate cancer, headache, depression and gastrointestinal bleeding were also observed.

Other known undesirable effects associated with testosterone treatments include hirsuitism, male pattern baldness, seborrhoea, acne, excessive frequency and duration of penile erections, nausea, cholestatic jaundice, increased or decreased libido, anxiety, generalised paraesthaesia. Oligospermia may occur at high doses. Prolonged testosterone administration may cause electrolyte disturbances, e.g. retention of sodium, chloride, potassium, calcium, inorganic phosphates and water.

4.9 Overdose

This is not likely due to the mode of administration. Serum testosterone has a half-life of 70 minutes and therefore falls rapidly once the Andropatch 2.5 mg Systems are removed.

5. PHARMACOLOGICAL PROPERTIES

5.1 Pharmacodynamic properties

Andropatch 2.5 mg delivers physiologic amounts of testosterone producing circulating testosterone concentrations that mimic the normal circadian rhythm of healthy young men.

Testosterone, the primary androgenic hormone is responsible for the normal growth and development of the male sex organs and for maintenance of secondary sex characteristics.

Male hypogonadism results from insufficient secretion of testosterone and is characterised by low serum testosterone concentrations. Symptoms associated with male hypogonadism include the following: impotence and decreased sexual desire; fatigue and loss of energy; mood depression; regression of secondary sexual characteristics.

Androgens promote retention of nitrogen, sodium, potassium and phosphorus, decreases urinary excretion of calcium, increase protein anabolism, decrease protein catabolism, are also responsible for the growth spurt of adolescence and for the eventual termination of linear growth and stimulate the production of red blood cells by enhancing erythropoietin production.

Exogenous administration of androgens inhibits endogenous testosterone release. With large doses of exogenous androgens, spermatogenesis may be suppressed.

5.2 Pharmacokinetic properties

Following Andropatch 2.5 mg application to non-scrotal skin, testosterone is continuously absorbed during the 24-hour dosing period. Daily application of two Andropatch 2.5 mg patches at approximately 10 pm results in a serum testosterone concentration profile which mimics the normal circadian variation observed in healthy young men. Maximum concentrations occur in the early morning hours with minimum concentrations in the evening.

In hypogonadal men, application of two Andropatch 2.5 mg Systems to the back, abdomen, thighs or upper arms resulted in average testosterone absorption of 4 to 5 mg over 24 hours. Applications to the chest and shins resulted in greater inter individual variability and average 24-hour absorption of 3 to 4 mg. The serum testosterone concentration profiles during application were similar for all sites.

Normal range morning serum testosterone concentrations are reached during the first day of dosing. There is no accumulation of testosterone during continuous treatment.

Upon removal of the Andropatch 2.5 mg Systems, serum testosterone concentrations decrease with an apparent half-life of approximately 70 minutes. Hypogonadal concentrations are reached within 24 hours following system removal.

5.3 Preclinical safety data

None therapeutically relevant.

6. PHARMACEUTICAL PARTICULARS

6.1 List of excipients

Ethanol, Purified Water, Glycerol (E422), glycerol monooleate, methyl laurate, Carbomer Copolymer B, Sodium Hydroxide.

6.2 Incompatibilities

No specific incompatibilities.

6.3 Shelf life

2 years.

6.4 Special precautions for storage

Do not store above 25°C. Apply to skin immediately upon removal from the protective pouch. Store in the original package.

6.5 Nature and contents of container

Each Andropatch 2.5 mg System contains 12.2 mg testosterone BP for delivery of 2.5 mg testosterone per day. Each Andropatch 2.5 mg System is individually pouched and supplied in cartons of* 10, 30 and 60 pouches. The pouch is made from paper, low density polyethylene and aluminium foil.

*Not all pack sizes may be marketed.

<u>**Components of the patch**</u>:

Silicone-coated polyester liner,

Acrylic adhesive/silicone-coated PET laminate,

Peelable LDPE/aluminium/polyester film,

Microporous HMWPE (high molecular weight polyethylene) film.

Backing film: inner layer of EVA, Surlyn® and metallised polyethylene, outer layer: polyethylene layer, pigmented with alcohol resistant beige ink to form a beige, plastic film.

6.6 Special precautions for disposal and other handling

Andropatch 2.5 mg may be discarded with household waste in a manner that avoids accidental contact by others.

Damaged systems should not be used.

The drug reservoir may be burst by excessive heat or pressure.

Administrative Data

7. MARKETING AUTHORISATION HOLDER

SmithKline Beecham plc

980 Great West Road

Brentford

Middlesex TW8 9GS

Trading as:

GlaxoSmithKline UK

Stockley Park West

Uxbridge

Middlesex UB11 1BT

8. MARKETING AUTHORISATION NUMBER(S)

PL 10592/0069

9. DATE OF FIRST AUTHORISATION/RENEWAL OF THE AUTHORISATION

02 January 2002

10. DATE OF REVISION OF THE TEXT

12 September 2007

11. Legal Status

POM

Andropatch 5mg

(GlaxoSmithKline UK)

1. NAME OF THE MEDICINAL PRODUCT

Andropatch 5 mg / 24 hours Transdermal Patch

2. QUALITATIVE AND QUANTITATIVE COMPOSITION

Each Andropatch 5 mg System contains 24.3 mg testosterone BP.

For full list of excipients, see section 6.1.

3. PHARMACEUTICAL FORM

Andropatch is a transdermal drug delivery system consisting of a beige self-adhesive patch surrounding a central drug reservoir of testosterone dissolved in an alcohol-based gel.

Each Andropatch 5 mg System delivers *in vivo* approximately 5 mg of testosterone over 24 hours across skin of average permeability. (Active surface area 15cm^2)

4. CLINICAL PARTICULARS

4.1 Therapeutic indications

Andropatch is indicated for testosterone replacement therapy in conditions with a deficiency or an absence of endogenous testosterone associated with primary or secondary hypogonadism.

4.2 Posology and method of administration

Adults and Elderly

The usual dose is one Andropatch System applied nightly (approximately 10 pm) and worn for 24 hours, providing approximately 5 mg testosterone per day. The dose can be adjusted up to the equivalent of 7.5 mg nightly or down to 2.5 mg patch nightly depending on the serum testosterone measured in the morning after application. Measurement of serum testosterone should be repeated taking care to ensure proper system adhesion and correct time of application before the dose is adjusted. The equivalent of 7.5 mg per day may be required for men with a higher body weight (>130 kg). Treatment in non-virilised patients may be initiated with one 2.5 mg system applied nightly. The dose should be adjusted as appropriate.

The duration of treatment and frequency of testosterone measurements is determined by the physician.

The adhesive side of the Andropatch System should be applied to a clean, dry area of the skin on the back, abdomen, upper arms, or thighs. Bony prominences, such as the shoulder and hip areas, and areas that may be subjected to prolonged pressure during sleeping or sitting should be avoided. Application to these sites has been associated with burn-like blister reactions (see Section 4.8). Do not apply to broken or damaged skin. Do not apply to the scrotum. The sites of application should be rotated, with an interval of seven days between applications to the same site. The area selected should not be oily, damaged or irritated.

The system should be applied immediately after opening the pouch and removing the protective release liner. The system should be pressed firmly in place, making sure there is good contact with the skin, especially around th edges.

Children

Andropatch is not indicated for use in children as there ha been no clinical experience of its use below the age of 15

4.3 Contraindications

Androgens are contra-indicated in men with carcinoma c the breast or known or suspected carcinoma of the pros tate, nephrotic syndrome, hypercalcaemia and know hypersensitivity to testosterone.

Andropatch is contra-indicated in men with known hyper sensitivity to other constituents of the patch.

Andropatch has not been evaluated in women and mus not be used in women. Testosterone may be harmful to th foetus.

4.4 Special warnings and precautions for use

Elderly men treated with androgens may be at an increase risk for the development of prostatic hyperplasia.

Elderly men and others with an increased risk of developin prostatic cancer, should be assessed before starting tes tosterone replacement therapy because testosterone ma promote the growth of subclinical prostate cancer.

As in men without testosterone deficiency, patients c testosterone replacement therapy should be periodical evaluated for prostate cancer.

Care should be taken in patients with skeletal metastase due to the risk of hypercalcaemia/hypercalcuria develop ing from androgen therapy.

If the patient develops an application site reaction, trea ment should be reviewed and discontinued if necessary

Testosterone may cause a rise in blood pressure ar Andropatch should be used with caution in patients wi hypertension.

Oedema, with or without congestive heart failure, ma result from androgen treatment in patients with pre-exis ing cardiac, renal, or hepatic disease. In addition to di continuation of the drug, diuretic therapy may be require

Andropatch should be used with caution in patients wi ischaemic heart disease, epilepsy and migraine as thes conditions may be aggravated.

4.5 Interaction with other medicinal products and oth forms of interaction

When given simultaneously with anticoagulants the anti oagulant effect can increase. Patients receiving oral anti oagulants require close monitoring especially whe androgens are started or stopped.

Concurrent administration of oxyphenbutazone and andr gens may result in elevated serum levels of oxyphenbut zone.

In diabetic patients, the metabolic effects of androge may alter blood glucose and, therefore, insulin requir ments.

4.6 Pregnancy and lactation

Andropatch therapy has not been evaluated in and mu not be used in women under any circumstances. Testo terone may be harmful to the foetus.

4.7 Effects on ability to drive and use machines

There is no evidence that Andropatch will affect the abil of a patient to drive or to use machines.

4.8 Undesirable effects

In the majority of cases, transient mild to moderate sk reactions have been observed at the site of application some time during treatment. These include pruritus; irrit tion with erythema, induration or burning, rash and allerg contact dermatitis. Burn-like lesions characterised by bli ters, skin necrosis, and ulceration that healed over sever weeks with scarring in some cases have also be observed.

The burn-like lesions occurred sporadically, usually only one site, (most commonly over bony prominences or are that may have been subjected to prolonged pressure du ing sleeping or sitting). Such lesions should be treated burns.

As seen with other testosterone treatments, prosta abnormalities, prostate cancer, headache, depressi and gastrointestinal bleeding were also observed.

Other known undesirable effects associated with testo terone treatments include hirsuitism, male pattern bal ness, seborrhoea, acne, excessive frequency and durati of penile erections, nausea, cholestatic jaundic increased or decreased libido, anxiety, generalised par esthaesia. Oligospermia may occur at high doses. Pr longed testosterone administration may cause electroly disturbances, e.g. retention of sodium, chloride, pota sium, calcium, inorganic phosphates and water.

4.9 Overdose

This is not likely due to the mode of administration. Seru testosterone has a half-life of 70 minutes and therefore fa rapidly once the Andropatch Systems are removed.

5. PHARMACOLOGICAL PROPERTIES

5.1 Pharmacodynamic properties

Andropatch delivers physiologic amounts of testostero producing circulating testosterone concentrations th mimic the normal circadian rhythm of healthy young me

estosterone, the primary androgenic hormone is respon-
ible for the normal growth and development of the male
ex organs and for maintenance of secondary sex char-
cteristics.

1ale hypogonadism results from insufficient secretion of
estosterone and is characterised by low serum testoster-
ne concentrations. Symptoms associated with male hypo-
onadism include the following: impotence and decreased
exual desire; fatigue and loss of energy; mood depression;
egression of secondary sexual characteristics.

ndrogens promote retention of nitrogen, sodium, potas-
um and phosphorus, decreases urinary excretion of cal-
um, increase protein anabolism, decrease protein
atabolism, are also responsible for the growth spurt of
dolescence and for the eventual termination of linear
rowth and stimulate the production of red blood cells
/ enhancing erythropoietin production.

xogenous administration of androgens inhibits endogen-
us testosterone release. With large doses of exogenous
ndrogens, spermatogenesis may be suppressed.

2 Pharmacokinetic properties

ollowing Andropatch application to non-scrotal skin, tes-
sterone is continuously absorbed during the 24-hour
osing period. Daily application of two 2.5 mg or one
mg Andropatch patches at approximately 10 pm results
a serum testosterone concentration profile which mimics
e normal circadian variation observed in healthy young
en. Maximum concentrations occur in the early morning
urs with minimum concentrations in the evening.

hypogonadal men, application of two 2.5 mg or one 5 mg
ndropatch Systems to the back, abdomen, thighs or
per arms resulted in average testosterone absorption
4 to 5 mg over 24 hours. Applications to the chest and
ins resulted in greater inter individual variability and
erage 24-hour absorption of 3 to 4 mg. The serum
stosterone concentration profiles during application
ere similar for all sites.

ormal range morning serum testosterone concentrations
e reached during the first day of dosing. There is no
cumulation of testosterone during continuous treatment.

on removal of the Andropatch Systems, serum testos-
one concentrations decrease with an apparent half-life
approximately 70 minutes. Hypogonadal concentrations
e reached within 24 hours following system removal.

3 Preclinical safety data

ne therapeutically relevant.

PHARMACEUTICAL PARTICULARS

List of excipients

anol, Purified Water, Glycerol (E422), glycerol mono-
ate, methyl laurate, Carbomer Copolymer B, Sodium
droxide.

Incompatibilities

specific incompatibilities.

Shelf life

ears.

Special precautions for storage

not store above 25°C. Apply to skin immediately upon
noval from the protective pouch. Store in the original
ckage.

Nature and contents of container

ch Andropatch 5 mg System contains 24.3 mg testos-
one BP for delivery of 5 mg testosterone per day. Each
dropatch 5 mg System is individually pouched and
pplied in cartons of* 5, 15 and 30 pouches. The pouch
nade from paper, low density polyethylene and alumi-
m foil.

t all pack sizes may be marketed.

mponents of the patch:

cone-coated polyester liner,

ylic adhesive/silicone-coated PET laminate,

elable LDPE/aluminium/polyester film,

roporous HMWPE (high molecular weight polyethylene)

king film: inner layer of EVA, Surlyn® and metallised
yethylene, outer layer: polyethylene layer, pigmented
alcohol resistant beige ink to form a beige, plastic film.

Special precautions for disposal and other handling

dropatch may be discarded with household waste in a
nner that avoids accidental contact by others.

naged systems should not be used.

drug reservoir may be burst by excessive heat or
ssure.

ninistrative Data

MARKETING AUTHORISATION HOLDER

thKline Beecham plc
Great West Road
ntford
ddlesex TW8 9GS
ding as:
xoSmithKline UK
ckley Park West
ridge
ddlesex UB11 1BT

8. MARKETING AUTHORISATION NUMBER(S)

PL 10592/0106

9. DATE OF FIRST AUTHORISATION/RENEWAL OF THE AUTHORISATION

26 August 2002

10. DATE OF REVISION OF THE TEXT

12 September 2007

11. Legal Status

POM

Anectine Injection

(GlaxoSmithKline UK)

1. NAME OF THE MEDICINAL PRODUCT

Anectine Injection.

2. QUALITATIVE AND QUANTITATIVE COMPOSITION

Suxamethonium Chloride Injection BP 100mg in 2ml.

3. PHARMACEUTICAL FORM

Injection.

4. CLINICAL PARTICULARS

4.1 Therapeutic indications

Used in anaesthesia as a muscle relaxant to facilitate endotracheal intubation, mechanical ventilation and a wide range of surgical and obstetric procedures.

It is also used to reduce the intensity of muscular contractions associated with pharmacologically or electrically-induced convulsions.

4.2 Posology and method of administration

Usually by bolus intravenous injection.

Adults: The dose is dependent on body weight, the degree of muscular relaxation required, the route of administration, and the response of individual patients.

To achieve endotracheal intubation Anectine is usually administered intravenously in a dose of 1 mg/kg. This dose will usually produce muscular relaxation in about 30 to 60 seconds and has a duration of action of about 2 to 6 minutes. Larger doses will produce more prolonged muscular relaxation, but doubling the dose does not necessarily double the duration of relaxation. Supplementary doses of Anectine of 50% to 100% of the initial dose administered at 5 to 10 minute intervals will maintain muscle relaxation during short surgical procedures performed under general anaesthesia.

For prolonged surgical procedures Anectine may be given by intravenous infusion as a 0.1% to 0.2% solution, diluted in 5% glucose solution or sterile isotonic saline solution, at a rate of 2.5 to 4 mg per minute. The infusion rate should be adjusted according to the response of individual patients.

The total dose of Anectine given by repeated intravenous injection or continuous infusion should not exceed 500 mg per hour.

Children: Infants and young children are more resistant to Anectine compared with adults.

The recommended intravenous dose of Anectine for neonates and infants is 2 mg/kg. A dose of 1 mg/kg in older children is recommended.

When Anectine is given as intravenous infusion in children, the dosage is as for adults with a proportionately lower initial infusion rate based on body weight.

Anectine may be given intramuscularly to infants at doses up to 4 to 5mg/kg and in older children up to 4 mg/kg. These doses produce muscular relaxation within about 3 minutes. A total dose of 150 mg should not be exceeded.

Use in the elderly: Dosage requirements of Anectine in the elderly are comparable to those for younger adults.

The elderly may be more susceptible to cardiac arrhythmias, especially if digitalis-like drugs are also being taken. See also '*Special warnings and precautions for use*'.

Instructions to open the ampoule

Ampoules are equipped with the OPC (One Point Cut) opening system and must be opened using the following instructions:

hold with the hand the bottom part of the ampoule as indicated in picture 1

put the other hand on the top of the ampoule positioning the thumb above the coloured point and press as indicated in picture 2

Picture 1

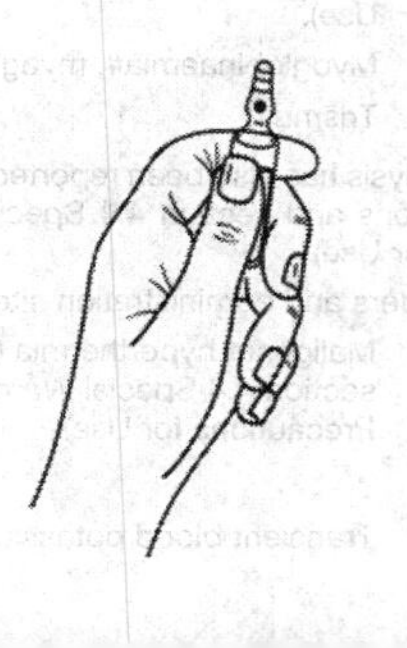

Picture 2

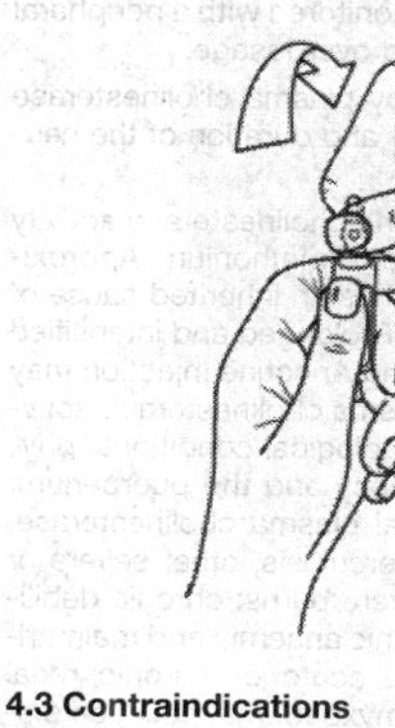

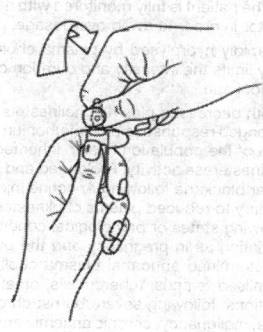

4.3 Contraindications

Anectine has no effect on the level of consciousness and should not be administered to a patient who is not fully anaesthetised.

Hypersensitivity to suxamethonium may exist in rare instances, and Anectine should not be administered to patients known to be hypersensitive to the drug.

As suxamethonium can act as a trigger of sustained myofibrillar contraction in susceptible individuals, Anectine is contra-indicated in patients with a personal or family history of malignant hyperthermia. If this condition occurs unexpectedly, all anaesthetic agents known to be associated with its development (including Anectine) must be immediately discontinued, and full supportive measures must be immediately instituted. Intravenous dantrolene sodium is the primary specific therapeutic drug and is recommended as soon as possible after the diagnosis is made.

Anectine is contra-indicated in patients known to have an inherited atypical plasma cholinesterase activity.

An acute transient rise in serum potassium often occurs following the administration of Anectine in normal individuals; the magnitude of this rise is of the order of 0.5 mmol/litre. In certain pathological states or conditions this increase in serum potassium following Anectine administration may be excessive and cause serious cardiac arrhythmias and cardiac arrest. For this reason the use of Anectine is contra-indicated in:

In patients recovering from major trauma or severe burns; the period of greatest risk of hyperkalaemia is from about 5 to 70 days after the injury and may be further prolonged if there is delayed healing due to persistent infection.

Patients with neurological deficits involving acute major muscle wasting (upper and/or lower motor neurone lesions); the potential for potassium release occurs within the first 6 months after the acute onset of the neurological deficit and correlates with the degree and extent of muscle paralysis. Patients who have been immobilised for prolonged periods of time may be at similar risk.

Patients with pre-existing hyperkalaemia. In the absence of hyperkalaemia and neuropathy, renal failure is not a contra-indication to the administration of a normal single dose of Anectine Injection, but multiple or large doses may cause clinically significant rises in serum potassium and should not be used.

Suxamethonium causes a significant transient rise in intraocular pressure, and should therefore not be used in the presence of open eye injuries or where an increase in intraocular pressure is undesirable unless the potential benefit of its use outweighs the potential risk to the eye.

Anectine should be avoided in patients with a personal or family history of congenital myotonic diseases such as myotonia congenita and dystrophia myotonica since its administration may on occasion be associated with severe myotonic spasms and rigidity.

Anectine should not be used in patients with skeletal muscle myopathies e.g. Duchenne muscular dystrophy since its administration may be associated with malignant hyperthermia, ventricular dysrhythmias and cardiac arrest secondary to acute rhabdomyolysis with hyperkalaemia.

4.4 Special warnings and precautions for use

Anectine should be administered only by or under close supervision of an anaesthetist familiar with its action, characteristics and hazards, who is skilled in the management of artificial respiration and only where there are adequate facilities for immediate endotracheal intubation with administration of oxygen by intermittent positive pressure ventilation.

High rates of cross-sensitivity (greater than 50%) between neuromuscular blocking agents have been reported. Therefore, where possible, before administering suxamethonium, hypersensitivity to other neuromuscular blocking agents should be excluded. Suxamethonium, should only be used when absolutely essential in susceptible patients. Patients who experience a hypersensitivity reaction under general anaesthesia should be tested subsequently for hypersensitivity to other neuromuscular blockers.

Anectine should not be mixed in the same syringe with any other agent, especially thiopental.

During prolonged administration of Anectine, it is recommended that the patient is fully monitored with a peripheral nerve stimulator in order to avoid overdosage.

Anectine is rapidly hydrolysed by plasma cholinesterase which thereby limits the intensity and duration of the neuromuscular blockade.

Individuals with decreased plasma cholinesterase activity exhibit a prolonged response to suxamethonium. Approximately 0.05% of the population has an inherited cause of reduced cholinesterase activity. Prolonged and intensified neuromuscular blockade following Anectine Injection may occur secondary to reduced plasma cholinesterase activity in the following states or pathological conditions: physiological variation as in pregnancy and the puerperium; genetically determined abnormal plasma cholinesterase; severe generalised tetanus, tuberculosis, other severe or chronic infections; following severe burns; chronic debilitating disease, malignancy, chronic anaemia and malnutrition; end-stage hepatic failure, acute or chronic renal failure; auto-immune diseases: myxoedema, collagen diseases; iatrogenic: following plasma exchange, plasmapheresis, cardiopulmonary bypass, and as a result of concomitant drug therapy (see *Interactions*).

If Anectine is given over a prolonged period, the characteristic depolarising neuromuscular (or Phase I) block may change to one with characteristics of a non-depolarising (or Phase II) block. Although the characteristics of a developing Phase II block resemble those of a true non-depolarising block, the former cannot always be fully or permanently reversed by anticholinesterase agents. When a Phase II block is fully established, its effects will then usually be fully reversible with standard doses of neostigmine accompanied by an anticholinergic agent.

Tachyphylaxis occurs after repeated administration of Anectine.

Muscle pains are frequently experienced after administration of suxamethonium and most commonly occur in ambulatory patients undergoing short surgical procedures under general anaesthesia. There appears to be no direct connection between the degree of visible muscle fasciculation after Anectine administration and the incidence or severity of pain. The use of small doses of non-depolarising muscle relaxants given minutes before suxamethonium administration has been advocated for the reduction of incidence and severity of suxamethonium-associated muscle pains. This technique may require the use of doses of suxamethonium in excess of 1mg/kg to achieve satisfactory conditions for endotracheal intubation.

Caution should be exercised when using suxamethonium in children, since paediatric patients are more likely to have an undiagnosed myopathy or an unknown predisposition to malignant hyperthermia and rhabdomyolysis, which places them at increased risk of serious adverse events following suxamethonium (see section 4.3 Contraindications and section 4.8 Adverse Reactions).

In patients with severe sepsis, the potential for hyperkalaemia seems to be related to the severity and duration of infection.

It is inadvisable to administer Anectine to patients with advanced myasthenia gravis. Although these patients are resistant to suxamethonium they develop a state of Phase II block which can result in delayed recovery. Patients with myasthenic Eaton-Lambert syndrome are more sensitive than normal to Anectine, necessitating dosage reduction.

In healthy adults, Anectine occasionally causes a mild transient slowing of the heart rate on initial administration. Bradycardias are more commonly observed in children and on repeated administration of suxamethonium in both children and adults. Pre-treatment with intravenous atropine or glycopyrrolate significantly reduces the incidence and severity of suxamethonium-related bradycardia.

In the absence of pre-existing or evoked hyperkalaemia, ventricular arrhythmias are rarely seen following suxamethonium administration. Patients taking digitalis-like drugs are however more susceptible to such arrhythmias. The action of suxamethonium on the heart may cause changes in cardiac rhythm including cardiac arrest.

4.5 Interaction with other medicinal products and other forms of interaction

Certain drugs or chemicals are known to reduce normal plasma cholinesterase activity and may therefore prolong the neuromuscular blocking effects of Anectine. These include: organophosphorous insecticides and metriphonate; ecothiopate eye drops; trimetaphan; specific anticholinesterase agents: neostigmine, pyridostigmine, physostigmine, edrophonium; tacrine hydrochloride; cytotoxic compounds: cyclophosphamide, mechlorethamine, triethylene-melamine, and thiotepa; psychiatric drugs: phenelzine, promazine and chlorpromazine; anaesthetic agents and drugs: ketamine, morphine and morphine antagonists, pethidine, pancuronium, propanidid.

Other drugs with potentially deleterious effects on plasma cholinesterase activity include aprotinin, diphenhydramine, promethazine, oestrogens, oxytocin, high-dose steroids, and oral contraceptives, terbutaline and metoclopramide.

Certain drugs or substances may enhance or prolong the neuromuscular effects of Anectine by mechanisms unrelated to plasma cholinesterase activity. These include: magnesium salts; lithium carbonate; azathioprine; quinine and chloroquine; antibiotics such as the aminoglycosides, clindamycin and polymyxins; antiarrhythmic drugs: quinidine, procainamide, verapamil, beta-blockers, lidocaine and procaine; volatile inhalational anaesthetic agents: halothane, enflurane, desflurane, isoflurane, diethylether and methoxyflurane have little effect on the Phase I block of Anectine injection but will accelerate the onset and enhance the intensity of a Phase II suxamethonium-induced block.

Patients receiving digitalis-like drugs are more susceptible to the effects of suxamethonium-exacerbated hyperkalaemia.

4.6 Pregnancy and lactation

No studies of the effect of suxamethonium on female fertility or pregnancy have been performed.

Suxamethonium has no direct action on the uterus or other smooth muscle structures. In normal therapeutic doses it does not cross the placental barrier in sufficient amounts to affect the respiration of the infant.

The benefits of the use of suxamethonium as part of a rapid sequence induction for general anaesthesia normally outweigh the possible risk to the foetus.

Plasma cholinesterase levels fall during the first trimester of pregnancy to about 70 to 80% of their pre-pregnancy values; a further fall to about 60 to 70% of the pre-pregnancy levels occurs within 2 to 4 days after delivery. Plasma cholinesterase levels then increase to reach normal over the next 6 weeks. Consequently, a high proportion of pregnant and puerperal patients may exhibit mildly prolonged neuromuscular blockade following Anectine injection.

It is not known whether suxamethonium or its metabolites are excreted in human milk.

4.7 Effects on ability to drive and use machines

This precaution is not relevant to the use of suxamethonium injection. Suxamethonium will always be used in combination with a general anaesthetic and therefore the usual precautions relating to performance of tasks following general anaesthesia apply.

4.8 Undesirable effects

Adverse reactions are listed below by system organ class and frequency. Estimated frequencies were determined from published data. Frequencies are defined as follows: very common ($\geq$1/10); common ($\geq$1/100 and $<$1/10), uncommon ($\geq$1/1,000 and $<$1/100); rare ($\geq$1/10,000 and $<$1/1,000); very rare ($<$1/10,000).

Immune system disorders

Very rare	Anaphylactic reactions.

Eye disorders

Common	Increased intraocular pressure.

Cardiac disorders

Common	Bradycardia, tachycardia.
Rare	Arrhythmias (including ventricular arrhythmias), cardiac arrest.

There are case reports of hyperkalaemia-related cardiac arrests following the administration of suxamethonium to patients with congenital cerebral palsy, tetanus, Duchenne muscular dystrophy, and closed head injury. Such events have also been reported rarely in children with hitherto undiagnosed muscular disorders.

Vascular disorders

Common	Skin flushing.

Hypertension and hypotension have also been reported.

Respiratory, thoracic and mediastinal disorders

Rare	Bronchospasm, prolonged respiratory depression†, apnoea.

Please refer to section 4.4 Special Warnings and Precautions for Use

Gastrointestinal disorders

Very common	Increased intragastric pressure.

Excessive salivation has also been reported

Skin and subcutaneous tissue disorders

Common	Rash.

Musculoskeletal and connective tissue disorders

Very common	Muscle fasciculation, post-operative muscle pains (Please refer to section 4.4 Special Warnings and Precautions for Use).
Common	Myoglobinaemia#, myoglobinuria#.
Rare	Trismus

Rhabdomyolysis has also been reported (see section 4.3 Contraindications and section 4.4 Special Warnings and Precautions for Use)

General disorders and administration site conditions

Very rare	Malignant hyperthermia (Please refer to section 4.4 Special Warnings and Precautions for Use).

Investigations

Common	Transient blood potassium increase.

4.9 Overdose

Apnoea and prolonged muscle paralysis are the mai serious effects of overdosage. It is essential, therefor to maintain the airway and adequate ventilation until spor taneous respiration occurs.

The decision to use neostigmine to reverse a Phase suxamethonium-induced block depends on the judgemer of the clinician in the individual case. Valuable informatic in regard to this decision will be gained by monitorir neuromuscular function. If neostigmine is used its admir istration should be accompanied by appropriate doses an anticholinergic agent such as atropine.

5. PHARMACOLOGICAL PROPERTIES

5.1 Pharmacodynamic properties

Short-acting depolarising neuromuscular blocking agen

5.2 Pharmacokinetic properties

None stated.

5.3 Preclinical safety data

Genotoxicity:-

No bacterial mutation assays have been conducted.

There are some data to suggest a weak clastogenic effe in mice, but not in patients who had received suxameth nium chloride.

Carcinogenicity:-

Carcinogenicity studies have not been performed.

Embryo-foetal Development:-

Animal reproduction studies have not been conducted w suxamethonium. It is also not known whether suxameth nium can affect reproductive capacity or cause foetal ha when administered to a pregnant woman.

6. PHARMACEUTICAL PARTICULARS

6.1 List of excipients

Water for Injections EP.

6.2 Incompatibilities

None known.

6.3 Shelf life

18 months.

6.4 Special precautions for storage

Store between 2 – 8 °C. Do not freeze. Keep in the ou carton.

6.5 Nature and contents of container

Neutral glass. 2ml ampoules.

6.6 Special precautions for disposal and other handli

For intravenous injection under medical direction.

Administrative Data

7. MARKETING AUTHORISATION HOLDER

The Wellcome Foundation Limited

Glaxo Wellcome House

Berkeley Avenue

Greenford UB6 ONN

trading as

GlaxoSmithKline UK

Stockley Park West

Uxbridge

Middlesex UB11 1BT

8. MARKETING AUTHORISATION NUMBER(S)

PL 00003/5203R

9. DATE OF FIRST AUTHORISATION/RENEWAL THE AUTHORISATION

16 May 2008

10. DATE OF REVISION OF THE TEXT

19 January 2009

11. Legal Status

POM

Anexate 500 micrograms/5ml Ampoule

(Roche Products Limit

1. NAME OF THE MEDICINAL PRODUCT

Anexate® 500 micrograms/5ml Ampoule

2. QUALITATIVE AND QUANTITATIVE COMPOSITI

Each 5ml ampoule contains 500 micrograms of fluma: (100 micrograms per ml).

For excipients, see 6.1.

3. PHARMACEUTICAL FORM

Solution for Injection or infusion.

A clear, almost colourless, sterile aqueous solution.

4. CLINICAL PARTICULARS

4.1 Therapeutic indications

Anexate is indicated for the complete or partial revers the central sedative effects of benzodiazepines. It therefore be used in anaesthesia and intensive ca the following situations:

Termination of general anaesthesia induced and/or n tained with benzodiazepines.

leversal of benzodiazepine sedation in short diagnostic nd therapeutic procedures.

'or the specific reversal of the central effects of benzodiazepines, to allow return to spontaneous respiration and onsciousness, in patients in intensive care.

.2 Posology and method of administration

\nexate is for slow intravenous injection or infusion. It hould only be administered under the supervision of an experienced physician.

Anexate may be used concurrently with other resuscitative procedures.

Adults

The recommended initial dose is 200 micrograms administered intravenously over 15 seconds. If the desired level of consciousness is not obtained within 60 seconds a further dose of 100 micrograms can be injected and repeated at 60-second intervals where necessary, up to a maximum total dose of 1mg or in intensive care situations, 2mg. The usual dose required is 300 - 600 micrograms.

f drowsiness recurs, an intravenous infusion of 100 - 400 micrograms per hour may be employed. The rate of infusion should be individually adjusted to achieve the desired evel of arousal.

The individually titrated, slow injections or infusions of Anexate should not produce withdrawal symptoms, even n patients exposed to high doses of benzodiazepines and/ or for long periods of time. If, however, unexpected signs of overstimulation occur, an individually titrated dose of diazepam (Valium) or midazolam (Hypnovel) should be given by slow intravenous injection.

f a significant improvement in consciousness or respiratory function is not obtained after repeated doses of Anexate, a non-benzodiazepine aetiology must be assumed.

Elderly

No specific data are available on the use of Anexate in the elderly, but it should be remembered that this population is more sensitive to the effects of benzodiazepines and should be treated with due caution.

Children

There are insufficient data to make dosage recommendations for Anexate in children. It should, therefore, be administered only if the potential benefits to the patient outweigh the possible risks.

Use in renal and hepatic insufficiency

o dosage adjustments are necessary in patients with enal impairment. However, since flumazenil is primarily metabolised in the liver, careful titration of dosage is recommended in patients with impaired hepatic function.

3 Contraindications

nexate is contra-indicated in patients with known hypersensitivity to flumazenil, benzodiazepines or any of the xcipients.

nexate is contra-indicated in patients who have been iven a benzodiazepine for control of a potentially lifethreatening condition (e.g. control of intracranial pressure status epilepticus).

mixed intoxications with benzodiazepines and tricyclic nd/or tetracyclic antidepressants, the toxicity of the antidepressants can be masked by protective benzodiazepine ffects. In the presence of autonomic (anticholinergic), eurological (motor abnormalities) or cardiovascular mptoms of severe intoxication with tricyclics/tetracycs, Anexate should not be used to reverse benzodiazene effects.

4 Special warnings and precautions for use

view of the short duration of action of Anexate and the ossible need for repeat doses, the patient should remain nder close observation until all possible central benzoazepine effects have subsided.

ne use of Anexate is not recommended in epileptic atients who have been receiving benzodiazepine treatment for a prolonged period. Although Anexate exerts a ght intrinsic anticonvulsant effect, its abrupt suppression the protective effect of a benzodiazepine agonist can ve rise to convulsions in epileptic patients.

nexate should be used with caution in patients with head ury as it may be capable of precipitating convulsions or tering cerebral blood flow in patients receiving benzodiapines.

enzodiazepines have a dependence potential when used ronically. Symptoms such as depression, nervousness, bound insomnia, irritability, sweating and diarrhoea may se following abrupt cessation of benzodiazepines in tients treated with high doses and/or for prolonged riods of time. Rapid injection of Anexate in such patients ay trigger these withdrawal symptoms, even in patients no stopped taking the benzodiazepine in the weeks preding Anexate administration (depending on the half-life the benzodiazepine used) and should therefore be oided. There is also a possibility of mild and transient thdrawal reactions occurring even after a short period of ministration of benzodiazepines.

nen Anexate is used with neuromuscular blocking ents, it should not be injected until the effects of neuroscular blockade have been fully reversed.

high-risk patients, the advantages of counteracting the ntral nervous system depression associated with benzodiazepines should be weighed against the drawbacks of rapid awakening.

The dosage of Anexate should be adjusted individually to the needs of patients suffering from pre-operative anxiety or having a history of chronic or episodic anxiety. In anxious patients, particularly those with coronary heart disease, it is preferable to maintain a degree of sedation throughout the early post-operative period rather than bring about complete arousal.

The pain felt by patients in the post-operative period must be taken into account. Following a major intervention, it is preferable to maintain a moderate degree of sedation.

Anexate is not recommended either as a treatment for benzodiazepine dependence or for the management of protracted benzodiazepine abstinence syndromes.

4.5 Interaction with other medicinal products and other forms of interaction

Anexate blocks the central effects of benzodiazepines by competitive interaction at the receptor level; the effects of non-benzodiazepines acting via the benzodiazepine receptor, such as zopiclone, are also blocked by Anexate. However, Anexate is ineffective when unconsciousness is due to other substances.

Interaction with other central nervous system depressants has not been observed. However, particular caution is necessary when using Anexate in cases of intentional overdosage since the toxic effects of other psychotropic drugs (especially tricyclic antidepressants) taken concurrently may increase with the subsidence of the benzodiazepine effect.

The pharmacokinetics of benzodiazepines are unaltered in the presence of Anexate and vice versa.

4.6 Pregnancy and lactation

Like other benzodiazepine compounds, Anexate is expected to cross the placenta and to enter into breast milk, although the total quantities involved would be small. There has been little human usage but animal studies have shown no teratogenic potential. The established medical principle of only administering drugs in early pregnancy when considered absolutely necessary should therefore be observed.

Emergency use of Anexate during lactation is not contra-indicated.

4.7 Effects on ability to drive and use machines

Patients who have received Anexate to reverse the effects of benzodiazepine sedation should be warned not to drive, to operate machinery or to engage in any other physically or mentally demanding activity for at least 24 hours, since the effect of the benzodiazepine may return.

4.8 Undesirable effects

Anexate is generally well tolerated. In post-operative use, nausea and/or vomiting are occasionally observed, particularly if opiates have also been employed. Flushing has also been noted. If patients are awakened too rapidly, they may become agitated, anxious or fearful.

Very rarely, seizures have been reported, particularly in patients known to suffer from epilepsy or severe hepatic impairment, particularly after long-term treatment with benzodiazepines or in cases of mixed drug overdose.

In cases of mixed-drug overdose, particularly with cyclic antidepressants, toxic effects (such as convulsions and cardiac dysrhythmias) may emerge with the reversal of benzodiazepine effects by Anexate.

Transient increases in blood pressure and heart rate may occur on awakening in intensive care patients.

Any side-effects associated with Anexate usually subside rapidly without the need for special treatment.

Excessive and/or rapidly injected doses of Anexate may induce benzodiazepine withdrawal symptoms such as anxiety attacks, tachycardia, dizziness and sweating in patients on long-term and/or high dose benzodiazepine treatment ending at any time within the weeks preceding Anexate administration (depending on the half-life of the benzodiazepine used). Such symptoms may be treated by slow intravenous injection of diazepam or midazolam (see section 4.2 Posology and method of administration). There is also a possibility of mild and transient withdrawal reactions occurring even after a short period of administration of benzodiazepines.

Anexate has been reported to provoke panic attacks in patients with a history of panic disorders.

Hypersensitivity reactions (including anaphylaxis) have occurred very rarely.

4.9 Overdose

There is very limited experience of acute overdose with Anexate.

Even when given intravenously at doses of 100mg, no symptoms of overdosage attributable to Anexate have been observed.

There is no specific antidote for overdose with Anexate. Treatment of an overdose with Anexate should consist of general supportive measures including monitoring of vital signs and observation of the clinical status of the patient.

5. PHARMACOLOGICAL PROPERTIES

5.1 Pharmacodynamic properties

Anexate, an imidazobenzodiazepine, is a specific competitive inhibitor of substances which act via the benzodiazepine receptors, specifically blocking their central effects. The hypnotic-sedative effects of the agonist are rapidly reversed by Anexate and may then reappear gradually within a few hours, depending on the half-life and dose ratio of the agonist and antagonist.

5.2 Pharmacokinetic properties

The pharmacokinetics of flumazenil are dose-proportional within and above the therapeutic range (up to 100mg).

Distribution

Flumazenil, a weak lipophilic base, is about 50% bound to plasma proteins. Albumin accounts for two thirds of plasma protein binding. Flumazenil is extensively distributed in the extravascular space. Plasma concentrations of flumazenil decrease with a half-life of 4 - 11 minutes during the distribution phase. The volume of distribution at steady state is 0.9 – 1.1 l/kg.

Metabolism

Flumazenil is extensively metabolised in the liver. The carboxylic acid metabolite is the main metabolite in plasma (free form) and urine (free form and its glucuronide). This main metabolite showed no benzodiazepine agonist or antagonist activity in pharmacological tests.

Elimination

Flumazenil is almost completely (99%) eliminated by non-renal routes. Practically no unchanged flumazenil is excreted in the urine, suggesting complete metabolic degradation of the drug. Elimination of radiolabelled drug is essentially complete within 72 hours, with 90 - 95% of the radioactivity appearing in urine and 5 - 10% in the faeces. Elimination is rapid, as shown by a short elimination half-life of 40 - 80 minutes. The total plasma clearance of flumazenil is 0.8 – 1.0 l/hr/kg and can be attributed almost entirely to hepatic clearance.

Ingestion of food during an intravenous infusion of flumazenil results in a 50% increase in clearance, most likely due to the increased hepatic blood flow that accompanies a meal.

Pharmacokinetics in special populations

In patients with impaired liver function, the elimination half-life of flumazenil is longer and the total body clearance lower than in healthy subjects. The pharmacokinetics of flumazenil are not significantly affected in the elderly, by gender, haemodialysis or renal failure.

5.3 Preclinical safety data

There are no preclinical data of relevance to the prescriber which are additional to that already included in other sections of the SPC.

6. PHARMACEUTICAL PARTICULARS

6.1 List of excipients

Disodium Edetate

Glacial Acetic Acid

Sodium Chloride

Sodium Hydroxide

Water for Injections

6.2 Incompatibilities

None stated.

6.3 Shelf life

Unopened: 5 years.

The product should be used immediately after opening.

6.4 Special precautions for storage

Do not store above 30°C.

6.5 Nature and contents of container

Clear glass 5ml ampoules. Cartons of 5 or 25.

6.6 Special precautions for disposal and other handling

Anexate ampoule solution may be diluted with Sodium Chloride Intravenous Infusion BP or Dextrose 5% Intravenous Infusion BP. Chemical and physical stability has been demonstrated for 24 hours at room temperature.

Anexate infusion should be administered within 3 hours of preparation.

No preparations other than those recommended should be added to the Anexate ampoule or mixed with the Anexate infusion solution.

For single use only. Discard any unused contents.

7. MARKETING AUTHORISATION HOLDER

Roche Products Limited, 6 Falcon Way, Shire Park, Welwyn Garden City, AL7 1TW, United Kingdom.

8. MARKETING AUTHORISATION NUMBER(S)

PL 0031/0228

9. DATE OF FIRST AUTHORISATION/RENEWAL OF THE AUTHORISATION

19 July 1999

10. DATE OF REVISION OF THE TEXT

10 November 2008

LEGAL STATUS

POM

Anexate, Hypnovel and Valium are registered trade marks

Angiox 250mg powder for concentrate for solution for injection or infusion

(The Medicines Company)

1. NAME OF THE MEDICINAL PRODUCT

Angiox ▼ 250 mg powder for concentrate for solution for injection or infusion

2. QUALITATIVE AND QUANTITATIVE COMPOSITION

Each vial contains 250 mg bivalirudin.

After reconstitution 1 ml contains 50 mg bivalirudin.

After dilution 1 ml contains 5 mg bivalirudin.

For a full list of excipients see section 6.1.

3. PHARMACEUTICAL FORM

Powder for concentrate for solution for injection or infusion.

White to off-white lyophilised powder.

4. CLINICAL PARTICULARS

4.1 Therapeutic indications

For the treatment of adult patients with acute coronary syndromes (unstable angina/non-ST segment elevation myocardial infarction (UA/NSTEMI)) planned for urgent or early intervention. Angiox should be administered with aspirin and clopidogrel.

Angiox is also indicated as an anticoagulant in patients undergoing percutaneous coronary intervention (PCI).

4.2 Posology and method of administration

Angiox should be administered by a physician experienced in either acute coronary care or in coronary intervention procedures.

Posology

Patients with acute coronary syndromes (ACS)

The recommended starting dose of Angiox for patients with ACS is an intravenous bolus of 0.1 mg/kg followed by an infusion of 0.25 mg/kg/h. Patients who are to be medically managed may continue the infusion of 0.25 mg/kg/h for up to 72 hours.

- If the patient proceeds to PCI, an additional bolus of 0.5 mg/kg of bivalirudin should be administered before the procedure and the infusion increased to 1.75 mg/kg/h for the duration of the procedure.

Following PCI, the reduced infusion dose of 0.25 mg/kg/h may be resumed for 4 to 12 hours as clinically necessary.

For patients who proceed to coronary artery bypass graft (CABG) surgery off pump, the intravenous (IV) infusion of bivalirudin should be continued until the time of surgery. Just prior to surgery, a 0.5mg/kg bolus dose should be administered followed by a 1.75mg/kg/h infusion for the duration of the surgery.

For patients who proceed to CABG surgery on pump, the IV infusion of bivalirudin should be continued until 1 hour prior to surgery after which the infusion should be discontinued and the patient treated with unfractionated heparin.

Patients undergoing PCI

The recommended dose of Angiox for patients undergoing PCI is an intravenous bolus of 0.75 mg/kg body weight followed immediately by an intravenous infusion at a rate of 1.75 mg/kg body weight/hour for at least the duration of the procedure. The infusion may be continued for up to 4 hours post-PCI as clinically warranted.

The safety and efficacy of a bolus only dose of Angiox has not been evaluated and is not recommended even if a short PCI procedure is planned.

The activated clotting time (ACT) may be used to assess bivalirudin activity.

In order to reduce the potential for low ACT values, the reconstituted and diluted product should be thoroughly mixed prior to administration and the bolus dose administered by a rapid intravenous push.

ACT values 5 minutes after bivalirudin bolus average 365 +/- 100 seconds. If the 5-minute ACT is less than 225 seconds, a second bolus dose of 0.3 mg/kg should be administered.

Once the ACT value is greater than 225 seconds, no further monitoring is required provided the 1.75mg/kg infusion dose is properly administered

The arterial sheath can be removed 2 hours after discontinuation of the bivalirudin infusion without further ACT monitoring.

Renal insufficiency

Angiox is contraindicated in patients with severe renal insufficiency (GFR<30ml/min) and also in dialysis-dependent patients (see section 4.3).

In patients with mild or moderate renal insufficiency, the ACS dose (0.1mg/kg bolus/0.25mg/kg/h infusion) should not be adjusted.

Patients with moderate renal impairment (GFR 30-59ml/min) undergoing PCI (whether being treated with bivalirudin for ACS or not) should receive a lower infusion rate of 1.4 mg/kg/h. The bolus dose should not be changed from the posology described under ACS or PCI above.

During PCI, monitoring of clotting time such as the ACT is recommended in patients with renal insufficiency. The ACT should be checked at 5 minutes post bolus dose. If the ACT is less than 225 seconds, a second bolus dose of 0.3 mg/kg should be administered and the ACT re-checked 5 minutes after the administration of the second bolus dose.

Hepatic impairment

No dose adjustment is needed. Pharmacokinetic studies indicate that hepatic metabolism of bivalirudin is limited, therefore the safety and efficacy of bivalirudin have not been specifically studied in patients with hepatic impairment.

Elderly population

Caution should be exercised in the elderly due to age-related decrease in renal function.

Paediatric patients

There is no relevant indication for use of Angiox in children less than 18 years old.

Method of administration

Angiox is intended for intravenous (IV) use.

Angiox should be initially reconstituted to give a solution of 50mg/ml bivalirudin. Reconstituted material should then be further diluted in a total volume of 50ml to give a solution of 5mg/ml bivalirudin.

Reconstituted and diluted product should be thoroughly mixed prior to administration.

Refer to section 6.6 for full instructions regarding the method of administration.

Angiox is administered as a weight based regimen consisting of an initial bolus (by rapid IV push) followed by an IV infusion.

Use with low molecular weight and unfractionated heparin

Patients can be started on Angiox 30 minutes after discontinuation of unfractionated heparin given intravenously, or 8 hours after discontinuation of low molecular weight heparin given subcutaneously.

Use with GPIIb/IIIa inhibitors

Angiox can be used in conjunction with a GPIIb/IIIa inhibitor. Refer to section 5.1 for further information regarding the use of bivalirudin with or without a GPIIb/IIIa inhibitor.

4.3 Contraindications

Angiox is contraindicated in patients with:

- a known hypersensitivity to the active substance or to any of the excipients, or to hirudins
- active bleeding or increased risk of bleeding because of haemostasis disorders and/or irreversible coagulation disorders
- severe uncontrolled hypertension
- subacute bacterial endocarditis
- severe renal impairment (GFR<30ml/min) and in dialysis-dependent patients.

4.4 Special warnings and precautions for use

Angiox is not intended for intramuscular use. Do not administer intramuscularly.

Haemorrhage

Patients must be observed carefully for symptoms and signs of bleeding during treatment particularly if bivalirudin is combined with another anticoagulant (see section 4.5). Although most bleeding associated with bivalirudin occurs at the site of arterial puncture in patients undergoing PCI, haemorrhage can occur at any site during therapy. Unexplained decreases in haematocrit, haemoglobin or blood pressure may indicate haemorrhage. Treatment should be stopped if bleeding is observed or suspected.

There is no known antidote to bivalirudin but its effect wears off quickly (T½ is 35 to 40 minutes).

Co-administration with platelet inhibitors or anti-coagulants

Combined use of anti-coagulant medicines can be expected to increase the risk of bleeding (see section 4.5). When bivalirudin is combined with a platelet inhibitor or an anti-coagulant medicine, clinical and biological parameters of haemostatsis should be regularly monitored.

In patients taking warfarin who are treated with bivalirudin, International Normalised Ratio (INR) monitoring should be considered to ensure that it returns to pre-treatment levels following discontinuation of bivalirudin treatment.

Hypersensitivity

Allergic type hypersensitivity reactions were reported uncommonly (⩾ 1/1,000 to ⩽ 1/100) in clinical trials. Necessary preparations should be made to deal with this. Patients should be informed of the early signs of hypersensitivity reactions including hives, generalised urticaria, tightness of chest, wheezing, hypotension and anaphylaxis. In the case of shock, the current medical standards for shock treatment should be applied. Anaphylaxis, including anaphylactic shock with fatal outcome has been reported very rarely (⩽ 1/10,000) in post-marketing experience (see section 4.8).

Treatment-emergent positive bivalirudin antibodies are rare and have not been associated with clinical evidence of allergic or anaphylactic reactions. Caution should be exercised in patients previously treated with lepirudin who had developed lepirudin antibodies.

Brachytherapy

Intra-procedural thrombus formation has been observe during gamma brachytherapy procedures with Angiox.

Angiox should be used with caution during beta bra chytherapy procedures.

4.5 Interaction with other medicinal products and othe forms of interaction

Interaction studies have been conducted with platelet inhi bitors, including acetylsalicylic acid, ticlopidine, clopido grel, abciximab, eptifibatide, or tirofiban. The results do no suggest pharmacodynamic interactions with these medic inal products.

From the knowledge of their mechanism of action, combined use of anti-coagulant medicinal products (heparin, warfarin, thrombolytics or antiplatelet agents) can be expected to increase the risk of bleeding.

In any case, when bivalirudin is combined with a platelet inhibitor or an anticoagulant medicine, clinical and biological parameters of haemostasis should be regularly monitored.

4.6 Pregnancy and lactation

Pregnancy

There are no or limited data from the use of bivalirudin in pregnant women. Animal studies are insufficient with respect to effects on pregnancy, embryonal/foetal development, parturition or post-natal development (see section 5.3).

Angiox should not be used during pregnancy unless the clinical condition of the woman requires treatment with bivalirudin.

Breastfeeding

It is unknown whether bivalirudin is excreted in human milk. Angiox should be administered with caution in breast-feeding mothers.

4.7 Effects on ability to drive and use machines

No studies on the effects on the ability to drive and use machines have been performed.

4.8 Undesirable effects

The ACUITY Trial (ACS)

The following adverse reaction data are based on a clinical study of bivalirudin in 13,819 patients with ACS; 4,612 were randomised to bivalirudin alone, 4,604 were randomised to bivalirudin plus GPIIb/IIIa inhibitor and 4,603 were randomised to either unfractionated heparin or enoxaparin plus GPIIb/IIIa inhibitor. Adverse reactions were more frequent in females and in patients more than 65 years of age in both the bivalirudin and the heparin-treated comparator groups compared to male or younger patients.

Approximately 23.3% of patients receiving bivalirudir experienced at least one adverse event and 2.1% experienced an adverse reaction. Adverse event reactions are listed by system organ class in Table 1.

Platelets, bleeding and clotting

In ACUITY, bleeding data were collected separately from adverse reactions.

ACUITY major bleeding was defined as any one of the following: intracranial, retroperitoneal, intraocular, access site haemorrhage requiring radiological or surgical intervention, ⩾5 cm diameter haematoma at puncture site reduction in haemoglobin concentration of ⩾4 g/dl without an overt source of bleeding, reduction in haemoglobin concentration of ⩾3 g/dl with an overt source of bleeding re-operation for bleeding or use of any blood product transfusion. Minor bleeding was defined as any observed bleeding event that did not meet the criteria as major. Minor bleeding occurred very commonly (⩾ 1/10) and major bleeding occurred commonly (⩾1/100 and <1/10).

Major bleeding rates are shown in Table 5. Both major and minor bleeds were significantly less frequent with bivalirudin alone than the heparin plus GPIIb/IIIa inhibitor and bivalirudin plus GPIIb/IIIa inhibitor groups. Similar reductions in bleeding were observed in patients who were switched to bivalirudin from heparin-based therapies (N = 2,078).

Major bleeding occurred most frequently at the sheath puncture site. Other less frequently observed bleeding sites with greater than 0.1% (uncommon) bleeding included "other" puncture site, retroperitoneal, gastrointestinal, ear, nose or throat.

Thrombocytopenia was reported in 10 bivalirudin-treated patients participating in the ACUITY study (0.1%). The majority of these patients received concomitant acetylsalicylic acid and clopidogrel, and 6 out of the 10 patients also received a GPIIb/IIIa inhibitor. Mortality among these patients was nil.

Table 1. ACUITY trial; adverse reaction data

(see Table 1 on next page)

The REPLACE-2 Trial (PCI)

The following adverse reaction data is based on a clinical study of bivalirudin in 6000 patients undergoing PCI, half of whom were treated with bivalirudin (REPLACE-2). Adverse events were more frequent in females and in patients more than 65 years of age in both the bivalirudin and the heparin treated comparator groups compared to male or younger patients.

Table 1 ACUITY trial; adverse reaction data

System organ class	Very common (⩾1/10)	Common (⩾1/100 to <1/10)	Uncommon (⩾1/1,000 to ⩽1/100)	Rare ⩾1/10,000 to ⩽1/1,000
Blood and lymphatic system disorders			INR increased, Thrombocytopenia, Anaemia.	
Immune system disorders			Hypersensitivity, including anaphylactic reaction and shock, including reports with fatal outcome[1]	
Nervous system disorders			Headache	Intracranial haemorrhage[1]
Ear and labyrinth disorders				Ear haemorrhage
Cardiac disorders				Bradycardia, Pericardial haemorrhage
Vascular disorders	Minor haemorrhage at any site	Major haemorrhage at any site including reports with fatal outcome[1], Thrombosis including reports with fatal outcome[1]	Hypotension,	Vascular pseudoaneurysm
Respiratory, thoracic and mediastinal disorders			Epistaxis	Pharyngeal haemorrhage, Haemoptysis
Gastrointestinal disorders			Gastrointestinal haemorrhage, Gingival haemorrhage, Nausea, Retroperitoneal haemorrhage, Melaena, Vomiting	Haematemesis
Skin and subcutaneous tissue disorders		Ecchymosis		Urticaria, Rash
Musculoskeletal and connective tissue disorders			Chest pain, Back pain, Groin pain	
Renal and urinary disorders			Haematuria	
General disorders and administration site conditions	Vessel puncture site haemorrhage, Vessel puncture site haematoma < 5 cm[1]		Vessel puncture site haematoma > 5 cm[1]	Injection site reactions

This reaction has also been seen in post-marketing exposure

pproximately 30% of patients receiving bivalirudin perienced at least one adverse event and 3% experi-ced an adverse reaction. Adverse reactions are listed by stem organ class in Table 2.

atelets, bleeding and clotting

REPLACE-2, bleeding data were collected separately m adverse events. Major bleeding rates for the intent to at and per protocol trial populations are shown in Table

ajor bleeding was defined as the occurrence of any of the lowing: intracranial haemorrhage, retroperitoneal hae-rrhage, blood loss leading to a transfusion of at least o units of whole blood or packed red blood cells, or eding resulting in a haemoglobin drop of more than 3 g/ or a fall in haemoglobin greater than 4 g/dl (or 12% of ematocrit) with no bleeding site identified. Minor hae-rrhage was defined as any observed bleeding event that not meet the criteria for a major haemorrhage. Minor eding occurred very commonly (⩾ 1/10) and major eding occurred commonly (⩾1/100 and <1/10).

th minor and major bleeds were significantly less fre-ent with bivalirudin than the heparin plus GPIIb/IIIa inhi-or comparator group. Major bleeding occurred most quently at the sheath puncture site. Other less frequently served bleeding sites with greater than 0.1% (uncom-n) bleeding included "other" puncture site, retroperito-al, gastrointestinal, ear, nose or throat.

ble 2. REPLACE-2 trial; adverse reaction data

e Table 2 on next page)

st-marketing experience

e following events have been reported in post-marketing perience with bivalirudin, and are described in the tables ove:

Serious bleeding, including haematoma and bleeding h a fatal outcome

ntracranial haemorrhage

hrombosis formation, including reports with a fatal out-ne

Hypersensitivity, including urticaria, anaphylactic reac-n, anaphylactic shock, and fatal shock.

Overdose

ses of overdose of up to 10 times the recommended se have been reported in clinical trials. Single bolus ses of bivalirudin up to 7.5mg/kg have also been orted. None of these cases were associated with bleed-or other adverse events.

cases of overdose, treatment with bivalirudin should be nediately discontinued and the patient monitored clo-for signs of bleeding.

he event of major bleeding, treatment with bivalirudin uld be immediately discontinued. There is no known dote to bivalirudin, however, bivalirudin is haemo-dia-ble

5. PHARMACOLOGICAL PROPERTIES

5.1 Pharmacodynamic properties

Pharmacotherapeutic group: Direct thrombin inhibitors, ATC code: B01AE06.

Angiox contains bivalirudin, a direct and specific thrombin inhibitor that binds both to the catalytic site and the anion-binding exosite of fluid-phase and clot-bound thrombin.

Thrombin plays a central role in the thrombotic process, acting to cleave fibrinogen into fibrin monomers and to activate Factor XIII to Factor XIIIa, allowing fibrin to develop a covalently cross-linked framework that stabilises the thrombus. Thrombin also activates Factors V and VIII, promoting further thrombin generation, and activates platelets, stimulating aggregation and granule release. Bivalirudin inhibits each of these thrombin effects.

The binding of bivalirudin to thrombin, and therefore its activity, is reversible as thrombin slowly cleaves the bivalirudin, Arg_3-Pro_4, bond, resulting in recovery of thrombin active site function. Thus, bivalirudin initially acts as a complete non-competitive inhibitor of thrombin, but transitions over time to become a competitive inhibitor enabling initially inhibited thrombin molecules to interact with other clotting substrates and to coagulation if required.

In vitro studies have indicated that bivalirudin inhibits both soluble (free) and clot-bound thrombin. Bivalirudin remains active and is not neutralised by products of the platelet release reaction.

In vitro studies have also shown that bivalirudin prolongs the activated partial thromboplastin time (aPTT) thrombin time (TT) and pro-thrombin time (PT) of normal human plasma in a concentration-dependent manner and that bivalirudin does not induce a platelet aggregation response against sera from patients with a history of Heparin-Induced Thrombocytopenia/Thrombosis Syndrome (HIT/HITTS).

In healthy volunteers and patients, bivalirudin exhibits dose- and concentration dependent anticoagulant activity as evidenced as prolongation of the ACT, aPTT, PT, INR and TT. Intravenous administration of bivalirudin produces measurable anticoagulation within minutes.

The pharmacodynamic effects of bivalirudin may be assessed using measures of anticoagulation including the ACT. The ACT value is positively correlated with the dose and plasma concentration of bivalirudin administered. Data from 366 patients indicates that the ACT is unaffected by concomitant treatment with a GPIIb/IIIa inhibitor.

In clinical studies bivalirudin has been shown to provide adequate anticoagulation during PCI procedures.

ACUITY Trial

The ACUITY trial was a prospective, randomised open-label, trial of bivalirudin with or without GPIIb/IIIa inhibitor (Arms B and C respectively) versus unfractionated heparin or enoxaparin with GPIIb/IIIa inhibitor (Arm A) in 13,819 high risk ACS patients.

In Arms B and C of the ACUITY trial, the recommended dose of bivalirudin was an initial post-randomisation IV bolus of 0.1mg/kg followed by a continuous IV infusion of 0.25 mg/kg/h during angiography or as clinically warranted.

For patients undergoing PCI, an additional IV bolus of 0.5mg/kg bivalirudin was administered and the rate of IV infusion increased to 1.75 mg/kg/h.

In Arm A of the ACUITY trial, UFH or enoxaparin was administered in accordance with the relevant guidelines for the management of ACS in patients with UA and NSTEMI. Patients in Arms A and B were also randomised to receive a GPIIb/IIIa inhibitor either upfront at the time of randomization (prior to angiography) or at the time of PCI. A total of 356 (7.7%) of patients randomised to Arm C also received a GPIIb/IIIa inhibitor.

High risk patient characteristics of the ACUITY population that mandated angiography within 72 hours were balanced across the three treatment arms. Approximately 77% of patients had recurrent ischaemia, approximately 70% had dynamic ECG changes or elevated cardiac biomarkers, approximately 28% had diabetes and approximately 99% of patients underwent angiography within 72 hours.

Following angiographic assessment, patients were triaged to either medical management (33%), PCI (56%) or CABG (11%). Additional anti-platelet therapy utilised in the study included aspirin and clopidogrel.

The primary analysis and results for ACUITY at 30-days and 1 year for the overall (ITT) population and for the patients that received aspirin and clopidogrel as per protocol (pre-angiography or pre-PCI) are shown in Tables 3 and 4.

Table 3. ACUITY trial; 30-day and 1-year risk differences for the composite ischaemic endpoint and its components for the overall population (ITT)

(see Table 3 on next page)

Table 4. ACUITY trial; 30-day and 1-year risk differences for the composite ischaemic endpoint and its components for patients that received aspirin and clopidogrel as per protocol*

(see Table 4 on page 99)

The incidence of both ACUITY-scale and TIMI-scale bleeding events up to day 30 is presented in Table 5 for the overall (ITT) population and for patients that received aspirin and clopidogrel as per protocol.

Table 5. ACUITY trial; bleeding events up to day 30 for the overall (ITT) population and the population of patients who received aspirin and clopidogrel as per protocol*

(see Table 5 on page 99)

Table 2 REPLACE-2 trial; adverse reaction data

System organ class	Very common (≥1/10)	Common (≥1/100 to <1/10)	Uncommon (≥1/1,000 to ≤1/100)	Rare ≥1/10,000 to ≤1/1,000
Blood and the lymphatic system disorders			Thrombocytopenia, anaemia	
Immune system disorders			Hypersensitivity, including anaphylactic reaction and shock, including reports with fatal outcome[1]	
Nervous system disorders			Headache	Intracranial haemorrhage[1]
Ear and labyrinth disorders				Ear haemorrhage
Cardiac disorders			Angina pectoris, Pericardial haemorrhage, Ventricular tachycardia, Bradycardia	
Vascular disorders	Minor haemorrhage at any site	Major haemorrhage at any site, including reports with fatal outcome[1], Thrombosis including reports with fatal outcome[1]	Hypotension, Vascular disorder, Vascular anomaly	
Respiratory, thoracic and mediastinal disorders			Epistaxis, Pharyngeal haemorrhage, Dyspnoea, Haemoptysis	
Gastrointestinal disorders			Nausea, Gingival haemorrhage Vomiting, Retroperitoneal haemmorrhage, Gastrointestinal haemorrhage	
Skin and subcutaneous tissue disorders			Rash, Urticaria	
Musculoskeletal and connective tissue disorders			Back pain	
Renal and urinary disorders			Haematuria	
General disorders and administration site conditions			Vessel puncture site haemorrhage, Injection site pain, Chest pain, Injection site haemorrhage.	

[1] This reaction has also been seen in post-marketing exposure

ACUITY major bleeding defined as any one of the following: intracranial, retroperitoneal, intraocular, access site haemorrhage requiring radiological or surgical intervention, ≥5cm diameter haematoma at puncture site, reduction in haemoglobin concentration of ≥4g/dl without an overt source of bleeding, reduction in haemaglobin concentration of ≥3g/dl with an overt source of bleeding, re-operation for bleeding, use of any blood product transfusion.

[2]TIMI major bleeding defined as intracranial bleeding or a decrease in haemoglobin concentration ≥5g/dL

The advantage of bivalirudin over UFH/enoxaparin plus GPIIb/IIIa inhibitor in terms of bleeding events was only observed in the bivalirudin monotherapy arm.

The 30-day results based on quadruple and triple endpoints from a randomized, double-blind trial of over 6,000 patients undergoing PCI (REPLACE-2), are shown in Table 6. Major bleeding in REPLACE-2 was defined by non-TIMI criteria.

Table 3 ACUITY trial; 30-day and 1-year risk differences for the composite ischaemic endpoint and its components for the overall population (ITT)

	Overall population (ITT)				
	Arm A UFH/enox +GPIIb/IIIa inhibitor (N=4603) %	Arm B bival +GPIIb/IIIa inhibitor (N=4604) %	B – A Risk diff. (95% CI)	Arm C bival alone (N=4612) %	C – A Risk diff. (95% CI)
30-day					
Composite ischaemia	7.3	7.7	0.48 (-0.60, 1.55)	7.8	0.55 (-0.53, 1.63)
Death	1.3	1.5	0.17 (-0.31, 0.66)	1.6	0.26 (-0.23, 0.75)
MI	4.9	5.0	0.04 (-0.84, 0.93)	5.4	0.45 (-0.46, 1.35)
Unplanned revasc.	2.3	2.7	0.39 (-0.24, 1.03)	2.4	0.10 (-0.51, 0.72)
1-year					
Composite ischaemia	15.3	15.9	0.65 (-0.83, 2.13)	16.0	0.71 (-0.77, 2.19)
Death	3.9	3.8	0.04 (-0.83, 0.74)	3.7	-0.18 (-0.96, 0.60)
MI	6.8	7.0	0.19 (-0.84, 1.23)	7.6	0.83 (-0.22, 1.89)
Unplanned revasc.	8.1	8.8	0.78 (-0.36, 1.92)	8.4	0.37 (-0.75, 1.50)

Table 6. REPLACE-2 study results: 30-day endpoints (intent-to-treat and per-protocol populations

(see Table 6 on next page)

Heparin-induced thrombocytopenia (HIT) and heparin-induced thrombocytopenia-thrombosis syndrome (HIT/HITTS): Clinical trials in a small number of patients have provided limited information about the use of Angiox in patients with HIT/HITTS.

5.2 Pharmacokinetic properties

The pharmacokinetic properties of bivalirudin have been evaluated and found to be linear in patients undergoing Percutaneous Coronary Intervention and in patients with ACS.

Absorption: The bioavailability of bivalirudin for intravenous use is complete and immediate. The mean steady-state concentration of bivalirudin following a constant intravenous infusion of 2.5 mg/kg/h is 12.4 μg/ml.

Distribution: Bivalirudin is rapidly distributed between plasma and extracellular fluid. The steady-state volume of distribution is 0.1 l/kg. Bivalirudin does not bind to plasma proteins (other than thrombin) or to red blood cells.

Biotransformation: As a peptide, bivalirudin is expected to undergo catabolism to its constituent amino acids, with subsequent recycling of the amino acid in the body pool. Bivalirudin is metabolized by proteases, including thrombin. The primary metabolite resulting from the cleavage of Arg_3-Pro_4 bond of the N-terminal sequence by thrombin is not active because of the loss of affinity to the catalytic active site of thrombin. About 20% of bivalirudin is excreted unchanged in the urine.

Elimination: The concentration-time profile following intravenous administration is well described by a two-compartment model. Elimination follows a first order process with a terminal half-life of 25 ± 12 minutes in patients with normal renal function. The corresponding clearance is about 3.4 ± 0.5 ml/min/kg.

Hepatic Insufficiency: The pharmacokinetics of bivalirudin have not been studied in patients with hepatic impairment but are not expected to be altered because bivalirudin is not metabolized by liver enzymes such as cytochrome P-450 isozymes.

Renal Insufficiency: The systemic clearance of bivalirudin decreases with glomerular filtration rate (GFR). The clearance of bivalirudin is similar in patients with normal renal function and those with mild renal impairment. Clearance is reduced by approximately 20% in patients with moderate or severe renal impairment, and 80% in dialysis-dependent patients (Table 7).

Table 7. Pharmacokinetic parameters for bivalirudin in patients with normal and impaired renal function

Renal function (GFR)	Clearance (ml/min/kg)	Half-life (minutes)
Normal renal function (≥ 90ml/min)	3.4	25
Mild renal impairment (60-89 ml/min)	3.4	22
Moderate renal impairment (30-59 ml/min)	2.7	34
Severe renal impairment (10-29 ml/min)	2.8	57
Dialysis dependent patients (off-dialysis)	1.0	3.5 hours

In patients with renal insufficiency, coagulation parameters such as the ACT should be monitored during Angiox therapy.

Table 4 ACUITY trial; 30-day and 1-year risk differences for the composite ischaemic endpoint and its components for patients that received aspirin and clopidogrel as per protocol*

	Patients receiving aspirin & clopidogrel as per protocol					
	Arm A UFH/enox +GPIIb/IIIa inhibitor (N=2842) %	Arm B bival +GPIIb/IIIa inhibitor (N=2924) %	B – A Risk diff. (95% CI)	Arm C bival alone (N=2911) %	C – A Risk diff. (95% CI)
30-day					
Composite ischaemia	7.4	7.4	0.03 (-1.32, 1.38)	7.0	-0.35 (-1.68, 0.99)
Death	1.4	1.4	-0.00 (-0.60, 0.60)	1.2	-0.14 (-0.72, 0.45)
MI	4.8	4.9	0.04 (-1.07, 1.14)	4.7	-0.08 (-1.18, 1.02)
Unplanned revasc.	2.6	2.8	0.23 (-0.61, 1.08)	2.2	-0.41 (-1.20, 0.39)
-year					
Composite ischaemia	16.1	16.8	0.68 (-1.24, 2.59)	15.8	-0.35 (-2.24, 1.54)
Death	3.7	3.9	0.20 (-0.78, 1.19)	3.3	-0.36 (-1.31, 0.59)
MI	6.7	7.3	0.60 (-0.71, 1.91)	6.8	0.19 (-1.11, 1.48)
Unplanned revasc.	9.4	10.0	0.59 (-0.94, 2.12)	8.9	-0.53 (-2.02, 0.96)

opidogrel pre-angiography or pre-PCI

lerly: Pharmacokinetics have been evaluated in elderly tients as part of a renal pharmacokinetic study. Dose ustments for this age group should be on the basis of al function, see section 4.2.

nder: There are no gender effects in the pharmacokitics of bivalirudin.

ight: Bivalirudin dose is body weight adjusted in mg/kg.

Preclinical safety data

n-clinical data reveal no special hazard for humans sed on conventional studies of safety, pharmacology, eated dose toxicity, genotoxicity, or toxicity to reproction.

xicity in animals upon repeated or continuous exposure day to 4 weeks at exposure levels of up to 10 times the clinical steady state plasma concentration) was limited to exaggerated pharmacological effects. Comparison of the single and repeated dose studies revealed that toxicity was related primarily to duration of exposure. All the undesirable effects, primary and secondary, resulting from excessive pharmacological activity were reversible. Undesirable effects that resulted from prolonged physiological stress in response to a non-homeostatic state of coagulation were not seen after short exposure comparable to that in clinical use, even at much higher doses.

Bivalirudin is intended for short-term administration and therefore no data on the long-term carcinogenic potential of bivalirudin are available. However, bivalirudin was not mutagenic or clastogenic in standard assays for such effects.

Table 5 ACUITY trial; bleeding events up to day 30 for the overall (ITT) population and the population of patients who received aspirin and clopidogrel as per protocol*

	Overall population (ITT)			Patients receiving aspirin & clopidogrel as per protocol		
	UFH/enox + GPIIb/IIIa inhibitor (N=4603) %	bival + GPIIb/IIIa inhibitor (N=4604) %	bival alone (N=4612) %	UFH/enox + GPIIb/IIIa inhibitor (N=2842) %	bival + GPIIb/IIIa inhibitor (N=2924) %	bival alone (N=2911) %
CUITY scale major[1]	5.7	5.3	3.0	5.9	5.4	3.1
MI scale major[2]	1.9	1.7	0.9	1.9	1.9	0.8

opidogrel pre-angiography or pre-PCI[1]

Table 6 REPLACE-2 study results: 30-day endpoints (intent-to-treat and per-protocol populations

ndpoint	Intent-to-treat		Per-protocol	
	bivalirudin (N=2994) %	heparin + GPIIb/IIIa inhibitor (N=3008) %	bivalirudin (N=2902) %	heparin + GPIIb/IIIa inhibitor (N=2882) %
uadruple endpoint	9.2	10.0	9.2	10.0
iple endpoint*	7.6	7.1	7.8	7.1
omponents:				
eath	0.2	0.4	0.2	0.4
yocardial Infarction	7.0	6.2	7.1	6.4
ajor bleeding** (based on non-MI criteria - see section 4.8)	2.4	4.1	2.2	4.0
gent revascularization	1.2	1.4	1.2	1.3

cludes major bleeding component. **p<0.001

6. PHARMACEUTICAL PARTICULARS

6.1 List of excipients

Mannitol

Sodium hydroxide solution (for pH adjustment).

6.2 Incompatibilities

The following medicinal products should not be administered in the same intravenous line as bivalirudin since they result in haze formation, micro-particulate formation or gross precipitation; alteplase, amiodarone HCl, amphotericin B, chlorpromazine HCl, diazepam, prochlorperazine edisylate, reteplase, streptokinase and vancomycin HCl.

6.3 Shelf life

4 years

Reconstituted solution: Chemical and physical in-use stability has been demonstrated for 24 hours at 2-8°C.

Diluted solution: Chemical and physical in-use stability has been demonstrated for 24 hours at 25°C.

From a microbiological point of view, the product should be used immediately. If not used immediately, in use storage times and conditions prior to use are the responsibility of the user and would normally not be longer than 24 hours at 2 – 8 °C, unless reconstitution/dilution has taken place in controlled and validated aseptic conditions.

6.4 Special precautions for storage

Lyophilised powder: Do not store above 25°C.

Reconstituted solution: Store in a refrigerator (2 – 8°C). Do not freeze.

Diluted solution: Do not store above 25°C. Do not freeze.

6.5 Nature and contents of container

Angiox is supplied as a lyophilised powder in 10 ml single use glass vials (Type 1) closed with a butyl rubber stopper and sealed with a crimped aluminum seal.

Angiox is available in packs of 2 and 10 vials.

Not all pack sizes may be marketed.

6.6 Special precautions for disposal and other handling

Instructions for preparation

Aseptic procedures should be used for the preparation and administration of Angiox.

Add 5 ml sterile water for injections to one vial of Angiox and swirl gently until completely dissolved and the solution is clear.

Withdraw 5 ml from the vial, and further dilute in a total volume of 50 ml of glucose solution for injection 5%, or sodium chloride 9 mg/ml (0.9%) solution for injection to give a final bivalirudin concentration of 5 mg/ml.

The reconstituted/diluted solution should be inspected visually for particulate matter and discolouration. Solutions containing particulate matter should not be used.

The reconstituted/diluted solution will be a clear to slightly opalescent, colourless to slightly yellow solution.

Any unused product or waste material should be disposed of in accordance with local requirements.

7. MARKETING AUTHORISATION HOLDER

The Medicines Company UK Ltd
115L Milton Park
Abingdon
Oxfordshire
OX14 4SA
UNITED KINGDOM

8. MARKETING AUTHORISATION NUMBER(S)

EU/1/04/289/001-002

9. DATE OF FIRST AUTHORISATION/RENEWAL OF THE AUTHORISATION

20.09.2004

10. DATE OF REVISION OF THE TEXT

18.06.2009

Detailed information on this product is available on the web site of the European medicines Agency (EMEA) http://www.emea.europa.eu"

Anhydrol Forte 20% w/v Cutaneous Solution

(Dermal Laboratories Limited)

1. NAME OF THE MEDICINAL PRODUCT

ANHYDROL® FORTE 20% w/v CUTANEOUS SOLUTION

2. QUALITATIVE AND QUANTITATIVE COMPOSITION

Aluminium Chloride Hexahydrate 20.0% w/v.

3. PHARMACEUTICAL FORM

Clear, colourless evaporative cutaneous solution.

4. CLINICAL PARTICULARS

4.1 Therapeutic indications

For the topical treatment of hyperhidrosis specifically involving axillae, hands or feet.

4.2 Posology and method of administration

For adults, children and the elderly: Apply to the affected sites at night, as required, and allow to dry. Wash off in the morning.

4.3 Contraindications
Not to be used in cases of sensitivity to any of the ingredients.

4.4 Special warnings and precautions for use
Care should be taken to restrict the application to the affected sites only. Keep away from the eyes. Care should be taken to avoid Anhydrol Forte coming into direct contact with clothing, polished surfaces, jewellery or metal. Replace cap tightly after use.

4.5 Interaction with other medicinal products and other forms of interaction
Do not bathe immediately before use and, if the axillae are treated, do not shave or use depilatories on this area within 12 hours before or after use.

4.6 Pregnancy and lactation
No special precautions.

4.7 Effects on ability to drive and use machines
None known.

4.8 Undesirable effects
If applied too frequently, Anhydrol Forte may cause irritation which should be treated with a mild topical hydrocortisone cream.

4.9 Overdose
See section 4.8 above (undesirable effects).

5. PHARMACOLOGICAL PROPERTIES

5.1 Pharmacodynamic properties
Aluminium chloride is believed to denature the protein content of sweat issuing from eccrine glands, and to combine with the intraductal keratin fibrils, producing a functional closure. The antibacterial action of the aluminium ion also precludes the development of miliaria. Accordingly, there is no secondary inflammation. The intraluminal pressure rises to the point where it acts as a feedback system, shutting off acinar secretion.

The formulation of Anhydrol Forte has been tested in widespread clinical practice, and has been shown to be effective when used in accordance with the recommended instructions.

5.2 Pharmacokinetic properties
As the active ingredient is applied in an alcoholic solution of low surface tension, it therefore penetrates into the terminal pores of the sweat ducts, when applied, as recommended, to dry skin. The alcohol then evaporates off, leaving the salt deposited in close contact with the lining of the duct. The use of the preparation is restricted to small areas of skin, namely the axillae, hands or feet, to ensure that there are no detrimental effects from widespread obstruction of sweating.

5.3 Preclinical safety data
No special information.

6. PHARMACEUTICAL PARTICULARS

6.1 List of excipients
Industrial Methylated Spirit.

6.2 Incompatibilities
None known.

6.3 Shelf life
36 months.

6.4 Special precautions for storage
Highly flammable. Do not store above 25°C. Store upright and away from flames.

6.5 Nature and contents of container
60 ml plastic bottle with roll-on applicator and screwcap. This is supplied as an original pack (OP).

6.6 Special precautions for disposal and other handling
Not applicable.

7. MARKETING AUTHORISATION HOLDER
Dermal Laboratories

Tatmore Place, Gosmore

Hitchin, Herts SG4 7QR, UK.

8. MARKETING AUTHORISATION NUMBER(S)
00173/0030.

9. DATE OF FIRST AUTHORISATION/RENEWAL OF THE AUTHORISATION
17 December 2006.

10. DATE OF REVISION OF THE TEXT
July 2007.

Antabuse Tablets 200mg

(Actavis UK Ltd)

1. NAME OF THE MEDICINAL PRODUCT
Antabuse® tablets 200 mg.

Disulfiram tablets 200 mg.

2. QUALITATIVE AND QUANTITATIVE COMPOSITION
Each tablet contains 200 mg disulfiram.

3. PHARMACEUTICAL FORM
Tablets.

4. CLINICAL PARTICULARS

4.1 Therapeutic indications
Alcohol deterrent compound. Disulfiram may be indicated as an adjuvant in the treatment of carefully selected and co-operative patients with drinking problems. Its use must be accompanied by appropriate supportive treatment.

4.2 Posology and method of administration
Adults and elderly patients only:

It is recommended that treatment with Disulfiram should be initiated only in a hospital or specialised clinic and by physicians experienced in its use. The patient should have adequate social and family support to avoid ingestion of alcohol. Suitable patients should not have ingested alcohol for at least 24 hours and must be warned that a Disulfiram-alcohol reaction is potentially dangerous.

On the first day of treatment, the patient should be given no more than 4 tablets of Disulfiram in one dose (800 mg). The next day the patient should take 3 tablets followed on the third day by 2 tablets and on the fourth and fifth days by 1 tablet. Subsequently, daily dosing should continue at 1 or half a tablet daily for as long as advised by the physician but no longer than six months without review.

In the routine management of the alcoholic it is not recommended to carry out an alcohol challenge test. If the clinician feels an alcohol challenge test is essential for the success of the therapy, full information of the procedure and risks of this test can be obtained from the company. As severe reactions can occur any alcohol challenge should be carried out in specialised units by physicians acquainted with the procedure. Full resuscitation facilities must be immediately available.

Children:

Not applicable.

4.3 Contraindications
Presence of cardiac failure, coronary artery disease, previous history of CVA, hypertension, severe personality disorder, suicidal risk or psychosis.

4.4 Special warnings and precautions for use
Caution should be exercised in the presence of renal failure, hepatic or respiratory disease, diabetes mellitus and epilepsy.

Before initiating treatment it is advised that appropriate examinations should be carried out to establish the suitability of the patient for treatment. Patients must not ingest alcohol during or for 1 week after ceasing Disulfiram therapy. Patients must be warned of the unpredictable and potentially severe nature of a Disulfiram-alcohol reaction as, in rare cases deaths have been reported following the drinking of alcohol by patients receiving Disulfiram. Certain foods, liquid medicines, remedies, tonics, toiletries, perfumes and aerosol sprays may contain sufficient alcohol to elicit a Disulfiram-alcohol reaction and patients should be made aware of this. Caution should also be exercised with low alcohol and "non-alcohol" or "alcohol-free" beers and wines, which may provoke a reaction when consumed in sufficient quantities. All personnel involved in the administration of Disulfiram to the patient know that Disulfiram should not be given during a drinking episode.

4.5 Interaction with other medicinal products and other forms of interaction
Disulfiram blocks the metabolism of alcohol and leads to an accumulation of acetaldehyde in the blood stream. The Disulfiram-alcohol reaction can occur within 10 minutes of ingestion of alcohol and may last several hours. It is characterised by intense flushing, dyspnoea, headache, palpitations, tachycardia, hypotension, nausea and vomiting.

Supportive therapy should be available and measures may be necessary to counteract hypotension. Severe vomiting might occur requiring administration of intravenous fluids.

Disulfiram may potentiate the toxic effects of warfarin, antipyrine, phenytoin, chlordiazepoxide and diazepam by inhibiting their metabolism. Animal studies have indicated similar inhibition of metabolism of pethidine, morphine and amphetamines. A few case reports of increase in confusion and changes in affective behaviour have been noted with the concurrent administration of metronidazole, isoniazid or paraldehyde. Potentiation of organic brain syndrome and choreoathetosis following pimozide have occurred very rarely. The intensity of the Disulfiram-alcohol reaction may be increased by amitriptyline and decreased by diazepam. Chlorpromazine while decreasing certain components of the Disulfiram-alcohol reaction may increase the overall intensity of the reaction. Disulfiram inhibits the oxidation and renal excretion of rifampicin.

4.6 Pregnancy and lactation
Pregnancy: The use of Disulfiram in the first trimester of pregnancy is not advised. The risk/benefit ratio in assessing adverse effects of alcoholism in pregnancy should be taken into account when considering the use of Disulfiram in pregnant patients.

There have been rare reports of congenital abnormalities in infants whose mothers have received Disulfiram in conjunction with other medicines.

Lactation: Should not be used. No information is available on whether Disulfiram is excreted in breast milk. Its use during breast feeding is not advised especially where there is a possibility of interaction with medicines that the baby may be taking.

4.7 Effects on ability to drive and use machines
Presumed to be safe or unlikely to produce an effect.

4.8 Undesirable effects
During initial treatment, drowsiness and fatigue may occur nausea, vomiting, halitosis and reduction in libido have been reported. If side effects are marked the dosage may be reduced. Psychotic reactions, including depression, paranoia, schizophrenia and mania occur rarely in patients receiving Disulfiram. Allergic dermatitis, peripheral neuritis and hepatic cell damage have also been reported.

4.9 Overdose
Disulfiram alone has low toxicity. Reports of the ingestion of quantities of up to 25 g refer to central and peripheral neurological symptoms which have resolved without sequel. Treatment should be symptomatic, gastric lavage and observation are recommended.

Disulfiram blocks the metabolism of alcohol and leads to an accumulation of acetaldehyde in the blood stream. The Disulfiram-alcohol reaction can occur within 10 minutes of ingestion of alcohol and may last several hours. It is characterised by intense flushing, dyspnoea and vomiting.

Supportive therapy should be available and measures may be necessary to counteract hypotension. Severe vomiting might occur requiring administration of intravenous fluids.

Symptoms: Vomiting, headache, drowsiness, fatigue, apathy, ataxia.

Treatment: Gastric lavage. Observation. Disulfiram by itself has low toxicity.

5. PHARMACOLOGICAL PROPERTIES

5.1 Pharmacodynamic properties
The effect of Disulfiram is primarily due to irreversible inactivation of liver ALDH. In the absence of this enzyme the metabolism of ethanol is blocked and the intracellular acetaldehyde concentration rises. The symptoms of the Disulfiram-alcohol reaction (DAR) are due partly to the high levels of acetaldehyde. The conversion of dopamine to noradrenaline is also inhibited and the depletion of noradrenaline in the heart and blood vessels allows acetaldehyde to act directly on these tissues to cause flushing, tachycardia and hypotension.

In addition to its affect on acetaldehyde dehydrogenase disulfiram inhibits other enzyme systems including dopamine-beta-hydroxylase (which converts dopamine and noradrenaline) and hepatic microsomal mixed function oxidases (which are responsible for the metabolism of many drugs). Disulfiram may thus potentiate the action of drugs which are metabolised by these enzymes.

5.2 Pharmacokinetic properties
Following oral administration, absorption is variable distribution is primarily to the kidney, pancreas, liver, intestines and fat. Disulfiram is rapidly metabolised to diethyldithiocarbamic acid (DDC), is conjugated with glucuronic acid, oxidised to sulphate, methylated and decomposed to diethylamine and carbon disulphide. Excretion is primarily through the kidneys.

5.3 Preclinical safety data
None.

6. PHARMACEUTICAL PARTICULARS

6.1 List of excipients
Lactose, potato starch, povidone, microcrystalline cellulose, polysorbate 20, tartaric acid, colloidal anhydrous silica, sodium bicarbonate, maize starch, magnesium stearate.

6.2 Incompatibilities
None.

6.3 Shelf life
3 years.

6.4 Special precautions for storage
Store below 25°C in a dry place and keep tightly closed. Protect from light.

6.5 Nature and contents of container
Polyethylene container with a polyethylene screw cap tamper evident closure, pack size of 50 tablets.

6.6 Special precautions for disposal and other handling
Not applicable.

7. MARKETING AUTHORISATION HOLDER
Actavis Group PTC ehf

Reykjavikuvegi 76-78

220 Hafnarfjordur

Iceland.

8. MARKETING AUTHORISATION NUMBER(S)
PL 30306/0036

9. DATE OF FIRST AUTHORISATION/RENEWAL OF THE AUTHORISATION
16 August 1994

10. DATE OF REVISION OF THE TEXT
24 September 2007

ntepsin Suspension

(Chugai Pharma UK Limited)

NAME OF THE MEDICINAL PRODUCT

ntepsin 1g/5ml Oral Suspension

QUALITATIVE AND QUANTITATIVE COMPOSITION

ach 5 mL dose contains 1 gram sucralfate.

or excipients, see section 6.1

. PHARMACEUTICAL FORM

ral Suspension

/hite to off-white viscous suspension with an odour of niseed/caramel.

. CLINICAL PARTICULARS

.1 Therapeutic indications

reatment of duodenal ulcer, gastric ulcer, chronic gastri-s, and the prophylaxis of gastrointestinal haemorrhage rom stress ulceration in seriously ill patients.

.2 Posology and method of administration

or oral administration.

Duodenal ulcer, gastric ulcer, chronic gastritis:

dults: The usual dose is 2 grams twice daily to be taken on ising and at bedtime, or 1 gram 4 times a day to be taken 1 hour before meals and at bedtime. Maximum daily dose: 8 grams.

Four to six weeks' treatment is usually needed for ulcer healing, but up to twelve weeks may be necessary in resistant cases.

Antacids may be used as required for relief of pain, but should not be taken half an hour before or after Antepsin.

Children and Elderly: see below

Prophylaxis of gastrointestinal haemorrhage from stress ulceration:

Adults: The usual dose is 1 gram six times a day. A maximum dose of 8 grams daily should not be exceeded. Antacids may be used as required for relief of pain, but should not be taken half an hour before or after Antepsin.

Elderly: There are no special dosage requirements for elderly patients but as with all medicines, the lowest effective dose should be used.

Children: Safety and effectiveness in children has not been established.

4.3 Contraindications

Contraindicated in individuals who are hypersensitive to any of the ingredients of Antepsin.

4.4 Special warnings and precautions for use

The product should only be used with caution in patients with renal dysfunction, due to the possibility of increased aluminium absorption.

In patients with severe renal impairment or on dialysis, Antepsin should be used with extreme caution and only for short-term treatment. The concomitant use of other aluminium containing medications is not recommended in view of the enhanced potential for aluminium absorption and toxicity. Antepsin may also cause allergic reactions (possibly delayed).

Bezoars (an insoluble mass formed with the gastric lumen) have been reported occasionally in patients taking Antepsin Suspension. The majority of these patients had underlying conditions that may predispose to bezoar formation such as delayed gastric emptying, or were receiving concomitant enteral feeding (see under Interactions). Bezoars have been reported after administration of Antepsin Suspension to severely ill patients in ITU, especially in premature infants in whom the use of sucralfate is not recommended.

4.5 Interaction with other medicinal products and other forms of interaction

Concomitant administration of Antepsin may reduce the bioavailability of certain drugs including tetracycline, ciprofloxacin, norfloxacin, ketoconazole, digoxin, warfarin, phenytoin, theophylline, thyroxine, quinidine and H_2 antagonists. The bioavailability of these agents may be restored by separating the administration of these agents from Antepsin by two hours. This interaction appears to be non systemic in origin presumably resulting from these agents being bound by Antepsin in the gastrointestinal tract. Because of the potential of Antepsin to alter the absorption of some drugs from the gastrointestinal tract, the separate administration of Antepsin from that of other agents should be considered when alterations in bioavailability are felt to be critical for concomitantly administered drugs.

The administration of Antepsin Suspension and enteral feeds by nasogastric tube should be separated by one hour in patients receiving Antepsin Suspension for the prophylaxis of stress ulceration. In rare cases bezoar formation has been reported when Antepsin and enteral feeds have been given too closely together.

4.6 Pregnancy and lactation

Pregnancy:

Teratogenicity studies in mice, rats and rabbits at doses up to 50 times the human dose have revealed no evidence of harm to the foetus. Safety in pregnant women has not been established and Antepsin should be used during pregnancy only if clearly needed.

Lactation:

It is not known whether this drug is excreted in human milk. Caution should be exercised when Antepsin is administered to breast-feeding women.

4.7 Effects on ability to drive and use machines

Do not drive if you feel dizzy or drowsy.

4.8 Undesirable effects

Adverse reactions to Antepsin in clinical trials were minor and only rarely led to discontinuation of the drug. Adverse events seen during use of Antepsin have included constipation, diarrhoea, nausea, vomiting, gastric discomfort, indigestion, flatulence, dry mouth, rash, back pain, dizziness, headache, vertigo, drowsiness and hypersensitivity reactions including pruritus, oedema, urticaria and shortness of breath.

4.9 Overdose

There is no experience in humans with overdose. Acute oral toxicity studies in animals, however, using doses up to 12 g/kg body weight, could not find a lethal dose. Risks associated with overdose, should, therefore, be minimal.

5. PHARMACOLOGICAL PROPERTIES

5.1 Pharmacodynamic properties

Pharmacotherapeutic group: Alimentary tract and metabolism, ATC code: A02B X02

The action of Antepsin is non-systemic as the drug is only minimally absorbed from the gastro-intestinal tract. The small amounts that are absorbed are excreted primarily in the urine. Antepsin exerts a generalised cytoprotective effect by preventing gastro-intestinal mucosal injury.

Studies in humans and animal models show that Antepsin forms an ulcer adherent complex with the proteinaceous exudate of the ulcer site. This property enables Antepsin to form a protective barrier over the ulcer lesion giving sustained protection against the penetration and action of gastric acid, pepsin and bile.

Studies both in humans and animals demonstrate that Antepsin protects the gastric mucosa against various irritants such as alcohol, acetylsalicylic acid and sodium taurocholate.

Antepsin also directly inhibits pepsin activity and absorbs bile salts. It has only weak antacid activity. It does not alter gastric emptying time, nor normal digestive function. Antepsin has no demonstrated pharmacological effect on the cardiovascular or central nervous systems.

5.2 Pharmacokinetic properties

Sucralfate is only minimally absorbed from the gastrointestinal tract. The small amounts that are absorbed are excreted primarily in the urine. Absorption of aluminium from sucralfate may be increased in patients on dialysis or with renal dysfunction (see also "other special warnings and precautions").

5.3 Preclinical safety data

There was no evidence of carcinogenesis in mice and rats receiving oral sucralfate in dosages of up to 1 g/kg daily (12 times the usual human dosage) for 2 years. In animal studies there was no effect evidence of impaired fertility. The effect of sucralfate on human fertility is not known.

6. PHARMACEUTICAL PARTICULARS

6.1 List of excipients

Saccharin sodium

Sodium dihydrogen phosphate

Purified water

Glycerol

Sodium propyl hydroxybenzoate (E217)

Sodium methyl hydroxybenzoate (E219)

Xanthan gum

Aniseed flavour

Caramel flavour

6.2 Incompatibilities

Not applicable

6.3 Shelf life

3 years

6.4 Special precautions for storage

Store below 25°C.

6.5 Nature and contents of container

Glass bottle (pack size 250 mL)

6.6 Special precautions for disposal and other handling

No special requirements.

7. MARKETING AUTHORISATION HOLDER

Chugai Pharma UK Ltd.

Mulliner House

Flanders Road

Turnham Green

London

W4 1NN

UK

8. MARKETING AUTHORISATION NUMBER(S)

PL 12185/0010

9. DATE OF FIRST AUTHORISATION/RENEWAL OF THE AUTHORISATION

29/09/2005

10. DATE OF REVISION OF THE TEXT

5 November 2007

Antepsin Tablets 1g

(Chugai Pharma UK Limited)

1. NAME OF THE MEDICINAL PRODUCT

Antepsin 1g Tablets

2. QUALITATIVE AND QUANTITATIVE COMPOSITION

Each tablet contains 1 gram of sucralfate.

For excipients, see section 6.1.

3. PHARMACEUTICAL FORM

Tablet

Biconvex, oblong, white tablets with a dividing score on one side.

4. CLINICAL PARTICULARS

4.1 Therapeutic indications

Treatment of duodenal ulcer, gastric ulcer, chronic gastritis.

4.2 Posology and method of administration

For oral administration.

Duodenal ulcer, gastric ulcer, chronic gastritis:

Adults: The usual dose is 2 grams twice daily to be taken on rising and at bedtime, or 1 gram 4 times a day to be taken 1 hour before meals and at bedtime. Maximum daily dose: 8 grams. For ease of administration, Antepsin Tablets may be dispersed in 10-15 mL of water. Four to six weeks' treatment is usually needed for ulcer healing, but up to twelve weeks may be necessary in resistant cases.

Antacids may be used as required for relief of pain, but should not be taken half an hour before or after Antepsin.

Elderly: There are no special dosage requirements for elderly patients but, as with all medicines, the lowest effective dose should be used.

Children: Safety and effectiveness in children has not been established.

4.3 Contraindications

Contraindicated in individuals who are hypersensitive to any of the ingredients of Antepsin.

4.4 Special warnings and precautions for use

The product should only be used with caution in patients with renal dysfunction, due to the possibility of increased aluminium absorption. In patients with severe renal impairment or on dialysis, Antepsin should be used with extreme caution and only for short-term treatment. The concomitant use of other aluminium containing medications is not recommended in view of the enhanced potential for aluminium absorption and toxicity.

Bezoars (an insoluble mass formed within the gastric lumen) have been reported occasionally in patients taking Antepsin Suspension. The majority of these patients had underlying conditions that may predispose to bezoar formation such as delayed gastric emptying, or were receiving concomitant enteral feeding (see under Interactions). Bezoars have been reported after administration of Antepsin Suspension to severely ill patients in ITU, especially in premature infants in whom the use of sucralfate is not recommended.

4.5 Interaction with other medicinal products and other forms of interaction

Concomitant administration of Antepsin may reduce the bioavailability of certain drugs including tetracycline, ciprofloxacin, norfloxacin, ketoconazole, digoxin, warfarin, phenytoin, theophylline, thyroxine, quinidine and H_2 antagonists. The bioavailability of these agents may be restored by separating the administration of these agents from Antepsin by two hours. This interaction appears to be non systemic in origin presumably resulting from these agents being bound by Antepsin in the gastrointestinal tract. Because of the potential of Antepsin to alter the absorption of some drugs from the gastrointestinal tract, the separate administration of Antepsin from that of other agents should be considered when alterations in bioavailability are felt to be critical for concomitantly administered drugs.

The administration of Antepsin Tablets 1 g and enteral feeds by nasogastric tube should be separated by one hour in patients receiving Antepsin Tablets 1 g for the prophylaxis of stress ulceration. In rare cases bezoar formation has been reported when Antepsin and enteral feeds have been given too closely together.

4.6 Pregnancy and lactation

Pregnancy:

Teratogenicity studies in mice, rats and rabbits at doses up to 50 times the human dose have revealed no evidence of harm to the foetus. Safety in pregnant women has not been established and Antepsin should be used during pregnancy only if clearly needed.

Lactation:

It is not known whether this drug is excreted in human milk. Caution should be exercised when Antepsin is administered to breast-feeding women.

4.7 Effects on ability to drive and use machines
Do not drive if you feel dizzy or drowsy.

4.8 Undesirable effects
Adverse reactions to Antepsin in clinical trials were minor and only rarely led to discontinuation of the drug. Adverse events seen during use of Antepsin have included constipation, diarrhoea, nausea, vomiting, gastric discomfort, indigestion, flatulence, dry mouth, rash, back pain, dizziness, headache, vertigo, drowsiness and hypersensitivity reactions including pruritus, oedema, urticaria and shortness of breath.

4.9 Overdose
There is no experience in humans with overdose. Acute oral toxicity studies in animals, however, using doses up to 12g/kg body weight, could not find a lethal dose. Risks associated with overdose, should, therefore, be minimal.

5. PHARMACOLOGICAL PROPERTIES

5.1 Pharmacodynamic properties
The action of Antepsin is non-systemic as the drug is only minimally absorbed from the gastro-intestinal tract. The small amounts that are absorbed are excreted primarily in the urine. Antepsin exerts a generalised cytoprotective effect by preventing gastro-intestinal mucosal injury.

Studies in humans and animal models show that Antepsin forms an ulcer adherent complex with the proteinaceous exudate of the ulcer site. This property enables Antepsin to form a protective barrier over the ulcer lesion giving sustained protection against the penetration and action of gastric acid, pepsin and bile.

Studies both in humans and animals demonstrate that Antepsin protects the gastric mucosa against various irritants such as alcohol, acetylsalicylic acid and sodium taurocholate.

Antepsin also directly inhibits pepsin activity and absorbs bile salts. It has only weak antacid activity. It does not alter gastric emptying time, nor normal digestive function. Antepsin has no demonstrated pharmacological effect on the cardiovascular or central nervous systems.

5.2 Pharmacokinetic properties
Sucralfate is only minimally absorbed from the gastro-intestinal tract. The small amounts that are absorbed are excreted primarily in the urine. Absorption of aluminium from sucralfate may be increased in patients on dialysis or with renal dysfunction (see also "other special warnings and precautions").

5.3 Preclinical safety data
There was no evidence of carcinogenesis in mice and rats receiving oral sucralfate in dosages of up to 1 g/kg daily (12 times the usual human dosage) for 2 years. In animal studies there was no effect evidence of impaired fertility. The effect of sucralfate on human fertility is not known.

6. PHARMACEUTICAL PARTICULARS

6.1 List of excipients
Macrogol 6000

Microcrystalline cellulose

Calcium Carmellose

Magnesium stearate.

6.2 Incompatibilities
Not applicable

6.3 Shelf life
3 years

6.4 Special precautions for storage
Store below 25°C.

6.5 Nature and contents of container
Blister packs (pack size 50 tablets).

6.6 Special precautions for disposal and other handling
No special requirements.

7. MARKETING AUTHORISATION HOLDER
Chugai Pharma UK Ltd.

Mulliner House

Flanders Road

Turnham Green

London

W4 1NN

U.K.

8. MARKETING AUTHORISATION NUMBER(S)
PL 12185/0008

9. DATE OF FIRST AUTHORISATION/RENEWAL OF THE AUTHORISATION
1 December 1998

10. DATE OF REVISION OF THE TEXT
5 November 2007

Anugesic HC Cream

(Pfizer Limited)

1. NAME OF THE MEDICINAL PRODUCT
ANUGESIC HC CREAM

2. QUALITATIVE AND QUANTITATIVE COMPOSITION
Each 100g of cream contains zinc oxide EP 12.35g, balsam peru EP 1.85g, benzyl benzoate EP 1.2g, pramocaine hydrochloride USP 1g, bismuth oxide 0.875g, hydrocortisone acetate EP 0.5g.

3. PHARMACEUTICAL FORM
A smooth, homogeneous, buff coloured cream with the characteristic odour of balsam peru.

4. CLINICAL PARTICULARS

4.1 Therapeutic indications
Anugesic HC cream provides antiseptic, astringent, emollient and decongestant properties. In addition hydrocortisone exerts an anti-inflammatory effect. Pramocaine is a rapidly acting local anaesthetic. The cream may be used to provide lubrication for suppositories.

Anugesic HC cream is indicated for the comprehensive symptomatic treatment of severe and acute discomfort or pain associated with internal and external haemorrhoids and pruritus ani.

4.2 Posology and method of administration
For topical use.

Adults:

Apply cream to the affected area at night, in the morning and after each evacuation. Thoroughly cleanse the affected area, dry and apply cream by gently smoothing onto the affected area. For internal conditions use rectal nozzle provided and clean it after each use.

Not to be taken orally.

Elderly (over 65 years):

As for adults.

Children:

Not recommended.

4.3 Contraindications
Tubercular, fungal and most viral lesions including herpes simplex, vaccinia and varicella. History of sensitivity to any of the constituents.

4.4 Special warnings and precautions for use
As with all products containing topical steroids the possibility of systemic absorption should be borne in mind.

Prolonged or excessive use may produce systemic corticosteroid effects and use for periods longer than seven days is not recommended.

Following symptomatic relief definite diagnosis should be established.

4.5 Interaction with other medicinal products and other forms of interaction
None known.

4.6 Pregnancy and lactation
There is inadequate evidence of safety in human pregnancy and there may be a very small risk of cleft palate and intrauterine growth retardation as well as suppression of the neonatal HPA axis. There is evidence of harmful effects in animals. Use in pregnancy only when there is no safer alternative and when the disease itself carries risks for the mother or child.

4.7 Effects on ability to drive and use machines
None known.

4.8 Undesirable effects
Rarely, sensitivity reactions. Patients may occasionally experience transient burning on application, especially if the anoderm is not intact.

4.9 Overdose
If swallowed, fever, nausea, vomiting, stomach cramps and diarrhoea may develop 3-12 hours after ingestion.

Pramocaine is relatively non-toxic and less sensitising than other local anaesthetics. Hydrocortisone does not normally produce toxic effects in an acute single overdose.

Treatment of a large acute overdosage should include gastric lavage, purgation with magnesium sulphate and complete bed rest. If necessary, give oxygen and general supportive measures. Methaemoglobinaemia should be treated by intravenous methylthioninium chloride

5. PHARMACOLOGICAL PROPERTIES

5.1 Pharmacodynamic properties
Pramocaine hydrochloride is a surface anaesthetic used on the skin and mucous membranes to relieve surface pain and pruritis.

Hydrocortisone acetate has the general properties of hydrocortisone and the anti-inflammatory action is of primary interest in this product.

Benzyl benzoate is used as a solubilizing agent and has mild antiseptic and preservative properties.

Bismuth oxide exerts a protective action on mucous membranes and raw surfaces. It is weakly astringent and is reported to have antiseptic properties.

Balsam peru has protective properties and a very mi[ld] antiseptic action by virtue of its content of cinnamic ar[d] benzoic acids. It is believed to promote the growth [of] epithelial cells.

Zinc oxide acts as an astringent and mild antiseptic.

5.2 Pharmacokinetic properties
It is well known that topically applied corticosteroids ca[n] be absorbed percutaneously. This appears to be mor[e] likely upon repeated or prolonged use.

The remaining active ingredients in Anugesic HC Crea[m] exert their therapeutic effect without being absorbed int[o] the systemic circulation. These observations are sup[-]ported by evidence from various studies and reviews.

5.3 Preclinical safety data
The results of the preclinical tests do not add anything o[f] further significance to the prescriber.

6. PHARMACEUTICAL PARTICULARS

6.1 List of excipients
Liquid paraffin, glyceryl monostearate, propylene glyco[l] polysorbate 60, sorbitan stearate, titanium dioxide E171 methyl hydroxybenzoate, propyl hydroxybenzoate an[d] purified water.

6.2 Incompatibilities
None known

6.3 Shelf life
2 years

6.4 Special precautions for storage
Do not store above 25°C.

6.5 Nature and contents of container
Aluminium tube externally printed and internally lacquered with plastic cap. Supplied in packs of 15, 25 and 30 g.

6.6 Special precautions for disposal and other handling
No special instructions needed.

7. MARKETING AUTHORISATION HOLDER
Pfizer Limited

Sandwich

Kent CT13 9NJ

United Kingdom

8. MARKETING AUTHORISATION NUMBER(S)
PL 00057/0520

9. DATE OF FIRST AUTHORISATION/RENEWAL OF THE AUTHORISATION
27th June 2003

10. DATE OF REVISION OF THE TEXT
June 2007

Anugesic HC Suppositories

(Pfizer Limited)

1. NAME OF THE MEDICINAL PRODUCT
Anugesic HC Suppositories.

2. QUALITATIVE AND QUANTITATIVE COMPOSITION
Each 2.8g suppository contains pramocaine hydrochloride USP 27mg, hydrocortisone acetate EP 5mg, benzyl benzoate EP 33mg, bismuth oxide 24mg, bismuth subgallate EP 59mg, balsam peru EP 49mg, zinc oxide EP 296mg.

3. PHARMACEUTICAL FORM
Buff coloured suppositories having the characteristic odour of balsam peru.

4. CLINICAL PARTICULARS

4.1 Therapeutic indications
Anugesic HC Suppositories provide antiseptic, astringent, emollient and decongestant properties. In addition hydrocortisone exerts an anti-inflammatory effect. Pramocaine is a rapidly acting local anaesthetic.

Anugesic HC Suppositories are indicated for the comprehensive symptomatic treatment of severe and acute discomfort or pain associated with internal and external haemorrhoids and pruritus ani.

4.2 Posology and method of administration
For rectal use. Not to be taken orally.

Adults:

Remove plastic cover and insert one suppository into the anus at night, in the morning and after each evacuation.

Elderly (over 65 years):

As for adults.

Children:

Not recommended.

4.3 Contraindications
Tubercular, fungal and most viral lesions including herpes simplex, vaccinia and varicella. History of sensitivity to any of the constituents.

4.4 Special warnings and precautions for use
Following symptomatic relief definitive diagnosis should be established.

5 Interaction with other medicinal products and other forms of interaction

None known.

4.6 Pregnancy and lactation

There is inadequate evidence of safety in human pregnancy and there may be a very small risk of cleft palate and intrauterine growth retardation as well as suppression of the neonatal HPA axis. There is evidence of harmful effects in animals. Use in pregnancy only when there is no safer alternative and when the disease itself carries risks for the mother or child.

4.7 Effects on ability to drive and use machines

None known.

4.8 Undesirable effects

As with all products containing topical steroids the possibility of systemic absorption should be borne in mind.

Prolonged or excessive use may produce systemic corticosteroid effects and use for periods longer than seven days is not recommended.

Rarely, sensitivity reactions.

Patients may occasionally experience transient burning on application, especially if the anoderm is not intact.

4.9 Overdose

If swallowed, fever, nausea, vomiting, stomach cramps and diarrhoea may develop 3-12 hours after ingestion.

Pramocaine is relatively non-toxic and less sensitising than other local anaesthetics. Hydrocortisone does not normally produce toxic effects in an acute single overdose.

Treatment of a large acute overdosage should include gastric lavage, purgation with magnesium sulphate and complete bed rest. If necessary, give oxygen and general supportive measures. Methaemoglobinaemia should be treated by intravenous methylthioninium chloride.

5. PHARMACOLOGICAL PROPERTIES

5.1 Pharmacodynamic properties

Pramocaine hydrochloride is a surface anaesthetic used on the skin and mucous membranes to relieve surface pain and pruritis.

Hydrocortisone acetate has the general properties of hydrocortisone and the anti-inflammatory action is of primary interest in this product.

Benzyl benzoate is used as a solubilising agent and has mild antiseptic and preservative properties.

Bismuth oxide, zinc oxide and bismuth subgallate exert a protective action on mucous membranes and raw surfaces. They are mildly astringent and are reported to have antiseptic properties.

Balsam peru has protective properties and a very mild antiseptic action by virtue of its content of cinnamic and benzoic acids. It is believed to promote the growth of epithelial cells.

5.2 Pharmacokinetic properties

It is well known that topically applied corticosteroids can be absorbed percutaneously. This appears to be more likely upon repeated or prolonged use.

The remaining active ingredients in Anugesic HC Suppositories exert their therapeutic effect without being absorbed into the systemic circulation. These observations are supported by evidence from various studies and reviews.

5.3 Preclinical safety data

The results of the preclinical tests do not add anything of further significance to the prescriber.

6. PHARMACEUTICAL PARTICULARS

6.1 List of excipients

Calcium hydrogen phosphate, hard fat "A", hard fat "C" and theobroma oil.

6.2 Incompatibilities

None known

6.3 Shelf life

2 years.

6.4 Special precautions for storage

Store below 25°C.

6.5 Nature and contents of container

Printed strip pack consisting of white opaque PVC/polyethylene laminated film. Supplied in packs of 12 and 24 suppositories.

6.6 Special precautions for disposal and other handling

No special instructions needed.

7. MARKETING AUTHORISATION HOLDER

Pfizer Limited

Sandwich

Kent CT13 9NJ

United Kingdom

8. MARKETING AUTHORISATION NUMBER(S)

PL 00057/0521

9. DATE OF FIRST AUTHORISATION/RENEWAL OF THE AUTHORISATION

1st July 2003

10. DATE OF REVISION OF THE TEXT

June 2007

Apidra 100 U/ml solution for injection in OptiClik cartridge

(sanofi-aventis)

1. NAME OF THE MEDICINAL PRODUCT

Apidra100 U/ml, solution for injection in cartridge.

2. QUALITATIVE AND QUANTITATIVE COMPOSITION

Each ml contains 100 U insulin glulisine (equivalent to 3.49 mg).

Each cartridge contains 3 ml of solution for injection, equivalent to 300 U.

Insulin glulisine is produced by recombinant DNA technology in Escherichia coli.

For excipients, see section 6.1.

3. PHARMACEUTICAL FORM

Solution for injection in cartridge for OptiClik.

Clear, colourless, aqueous solution.

4. CLINICAL PARTICULARS

4.1 Therapeutic indications

Treatment of adults, adolescents and children, 6 years or older with diabetes mellitus, where treatment with insulin is required.

4.2 Posology and method of administration

The potency of this preparation is stated in units. These units are exclusive to Apidra and are not the same as IU or the units used to express the potency of other insulin analogues. See section 5.1 (Pharmacodynamics).

Apidra should be given shortly (0-15 min) before or soon after meals.

Apidra should be used in regimens that include an intermediate or long acting insulin or basal insulin analogue and can be used with oral hypoglycaemic agents.

The dosage of Apidra should be individually adjusted.

<u>Administration</u>

Apidra should be given by subcutaneous injection or by continuous subcutaneous pump infusion.

Apidra should be administered subcutaneously in the abdominal wall, thigh or deltoid or by continuous infusion in the abdominal wall. Injection sites and infusion sites within an injection area (abdomen, thigh or deltoid) should be rotated from one injection to the next. The rate of absorption, and consequently the onset and duration of action, may be affected by the injection site, exercise and other variables. Subcutaneous injection in the abdominal wall ensures a slightly faster absorption than other injection sites (see section 5.2).

Care should be taken to ensure that a blood vessel has not been entered. After injection, the site of injection should not be massaged. Patients must be educated to use proper injection techniques.

Mixing with insulins

Apidra must not be mixed with any preparations other than NPH (Neutral Protamine Hagedorn) human insulin.

For further details on handling, see section 6.6

<u>Special populations</u>

Renal impairment

The pharmacokinetic properties of insulin glulisine are generally maintained in patients with renal impairment. However, insulin requirements may be reduced in the presence of renal impairment (see section 5.2).

Hepatic impairment

The pharmacokinetic properties of insulin glulisine have not been investigated in patients with decreased liver function. In patients with hepatic impairment, insulin requirements may be diminished due to reduced capacity for gluconeogenesis and reduced insulin metabolism.

Elderly

Limited pharmacokinetic data are available in elderly patients with diabetes mellitus. Deterioration of renal function may lead to a decrease in insulin requirements.

Children and adolescents

There is insufficient clinical information on the use of Apidra in children younger than the age of 6 years.

4.3 Contraindications

Hypersensitivity to the active substance or to any of the excipients.

Hypoglycaemia.

4.4 Special warnings and precautions for use

Transferring a patient to a new type or brand of insulin should be done under strict medical supervision. Changes in strength, brand (manufacturer), type (regular, NPH, lente, etc.), species (animal) and/or method of manufacturing may result in a change in dosage. Concomitant oral antidiabetic treatment may need to be adjusted.

The use of inadequate dosages or discontinuation of treatment, especially in insulin-dependent diabetic, may lead to hyperglycaemia and diabetic ketoacidosis; conditions which are potentially lethal.

Switching a patient to another type or brand of insulin should be done under strict medical supervision and may require change in dose.

Hypoglycaemia

The time of occurrence of hypoglycaemia depends on the action profile of the insulins used and may, therefore, change when the treatment regimen is changed.

Conditions which may make the early warning symptoms of hypoglycaemia different or less pronounced include long duration of diabetes, intensified insulin therapy, diabetic nerve disease, medicinal products such as beta blockers or after transfer from animal-source insulin to human insulin.

Adjustment of dosage may be also necessary if patients undertake increased physical activity or change their usual meal plan. Exercise taken immediately after a meal may increase the risk of hypoglycaemia.

When compared with soluble human insulin, if hypoglycaemia occurs after an injection with rapid acting analogues, it may occur earlier.

Uncorrected hypoglycaemic or hyperglycaemic reactions can cause loss of consciousness, coma, or death.

Insulin requirements may be altered during illness or emotional disturbances.

4.5 Interaction with other medicinal products and other forms of interaction

Studies on pharmacokinetic interactions have not been performed. Based on empirical knowledge from similar medicinal products, clinically relevant pharmacokinetic interactions are unlikely to occur.

A number of substances affect glucose metabolism and may require dose adjustment of insulin glulisine and particularly close monitoring.

Substances that may enhance the blood-glucose-lowering activity and increase susceptibility to hypoglycaemia include oral antidiabetic agents, angiotensin converting enzyme (ACE) inhibitors, disopyramide, fibrates, fluoxetine, monoamide oxidase inhibitors (MAOIs), pentoxifylline, propoxyphene, salicylates and sulfonamide antibiotics.

Substances that may reduce the blood-glucose-lowering activity include corticosteroids, danazol, diazoxide, diuretics, glucagon, isoniazid, phenothiazine derivatives, somatropin, sympathomimetic agents (e.g. epinephrine [adrenaline], salbutamol, terbutaline), thyroid hormones, estrogens, progestins (e.g. in oral contraceptives), protease inhibitors and atypical antipsychotic medicinal products (e.g. olanzapine and clozapine).

Beta-blockers, clonidine, lithium salts or alcohol may either potentiate or weaken the blood-glucose-lowering activity of insulin. Pentamidine may cause hypoglycaemia, which may sometimes be followed by hyperglycaemia.

In addition, under the influence of sympatholytic medicinal products such as beta-blockers, clonidine, guanethidine and reserpine, the signs of adrenergic counter-regulation may be reduced or absent.

4.6 Pregnancy and lactation

Pregnancy

There are no adequate data on the use of insulin glulisine in pregnant women.

Animal reproduction studies have not revealed any differences between insulin glulisine and human insulin regarding pregnancy, embryonal/foetal development, parturition or postnatal development (see section 5.3).

Caution should be exercised when prescribing to pregnant women. Careful monitoring of glucose control is essential.

It is essential for patients with pre-existing or gestational diabetes to maintain good metabolic control throughout pregnancy. Insulin requirements may decrease during the first trimester and generally increase during the second and third trimesters. Immediately after delivery, insulin requirements decline rapidly.

Lactation

It is unknown whether insulin glulisine is excreted in human milk, but in general insulin does not pass into breast milk and is not absorbed after oral administration.

Breast-feeding mothers may require adjustments in insulin dose and diet.

4.7 Effects on ability to drive and use machines

The patient's ability to concentrate and react may be impaired as a result of hypoglycaemia or hyperglycaemia or, for example, as a result of visual impairment. This may constitute a risk in situations where these abilities are of special importance (e.g. driving a car or operating machinery).

Patients should be advised to take precautions to avoid hypoglycaemia whilst driving. This is particularly important in those who have reduced or absent awareness of the warning symptoms of hypoglycaemia or have frequent episodes of hypoglycaemia. The advisability of driving should be considered in these circumstances.

4.8 Undesirable effects

Hypoglycaemia, the most frequent undesirable effect of insulin therapy, may occur if the insulin dose is too high in relation to the insulin requirement.

The following related adverse reactions from clinical investigations were listed below by system organ class and in order of decreasing incidence (very common: $>1/10$; common: $>1/100$, $<1/10$; uncommon: $>1/1,000$, $<1/100$; rare: $>1/10,000$, $<1/1,000$; very rare: $<1/10,000$).

Within each frequency grouping, undesirable effects are presented in order of decreasing seriousness.

Metabolism and nutrition disorders

Very common: Hypoglycaemia

Symptoms of hypoglycaemia usually occur suddenly. They may include cold sweats, cool pale skin, fatigue, nervousness or tremor, anxiousness, unusual tiredness or weakness, confusion, difficulty in concentration, drowsiness, excessive hunger, vision changes, headache, nausea and palpitation. Hypoglycaemia can become severe and may lead to unconsciousness and/or convulsions and may result in temporary or permanent impairment of brain function or even death.

Skin and subcutaneous tissue disorders

Common: injection site reactions and local hypersensitivity reactions.

Local hypersensitivity reactions (redness, swelling and itching at the injection site) may occur during treatment with insulin. These reactions are usually transitory and normally they disappear during continued treatment.

Rare: Lipodystrophy

Lipodystrophy may occur at the injection site as a consequence of failure to rotate injection sites within an area.

General disorders

Uncommon: Systemic hypersensitivity reactions

Systemic hypersensitivity reactions may include urticaria, chest tightness, dyspnea, allergic dermatitis and pruritus. Severe cases of generalized allergy, including anaphylactic reaction, may be life threatening.

4.9 Overdose

Hypoglycaemia may occur as a result of an excess of insulin activity relative to food intake and energy expenditure.

There are no specific data available concerning overdose with insulin glulisine. However, hypoglycaemia may develop over sequential stages:

Mild hypoglycaemic episodes can be treated by oral administration of glucose or sugary products. It is therefore recommended that the diabetic patient constantly carries some sugar lumps, sweets, biscuits or sugary fruit juice.

Severe hypoglycaemic episodes, where the patient has become unconscious, can be treated by glucagon (0.5 to 1 mg) given intramuscularly or subcutaneously by a person who has received appropriate instruction, or by glucose given intravenously by a medical professional. Glucose must also be given intravenously, if the patient does not respond to glucagon within 10 to 15 minutes.

Upon regaining consciousness, administration of oral carbohydrate is recommended for the patient in order to prevent relapse.

After an injection of glucagon, the patient should be monitored in a hospital in order to find the reason for this severe hypoglycaemia and prevent other similar episodes.

5. PHARMACOLOGICAL PROPERTIES

5.1 Pharmacodynamic properties

Pharmacotherapeutic group: insulin and analogues, fast-acting. ATC code: A10AB06

Insulin glulisine is a recombinant human insulin analogue that is equipotent to regular human insulin. Insulin glulisine has a more rapid onset of action and a shorter duration of action than regular human insulin.

The primary activity of insulins and insulin analogues, including insulin glulisine, is regulation of glucose metabolism. Insulins lower blood glucose levels by stimulating peripheral glucose uptake, especially by skeletal muscle and fat, and by inhibiting hepatic glucose production. Insulin inhibits lipolysis in the adipocyte, inhibits proteolysis and enhances protein synthesis.

Studies in healthy volunteers and patients with diabetes demonstrated that insulin glulisine is more rapid in onset of action and of shorter duration of action than regular human insulin when given subcutaneously. When insulin glulisine is injected subcutaneously, the glucose lowering activity will begin within 10 – 20 minutes. The glucose-lowering activities of insulin glulisine and regular human insulin are equipotent when administered by intravenous route. One unit of insulin glulisine has the same glucose-lowering activity as one unit of regular human insulin.

Dose proportionality

In a study with 18 male subjects with diabetes mellitus type 1 aged 21 to 50 years, insulin glulisine displayed dose-proportional glucose lowering effect in the therapeutic relevant dose range 0.075 to 0.15 U/kg, and less than proportional increase in glucose lowering effect with 0.3 U/kg or higher, like human insulin.

Insulin glulisine takes effect about twice as fast as regular human insulin and completes the glucose lowering effect about 2 hours earlier than regular human insulin.

A phase I study in patients with type 1 diabetes mellitus assessed the glucose lowering profiles of insulin glulisine and regular human insulin administered subcutaneously at a dose of 0.15 U/kg, at different times in relation to a 15-minute standard meal. Data indicated that insulin glulisine administered 2 minutes before the meal gives similar post-prandial glycemic control compared to regular human insulin given 30 minutes before the meal. When given 2

Figure 1

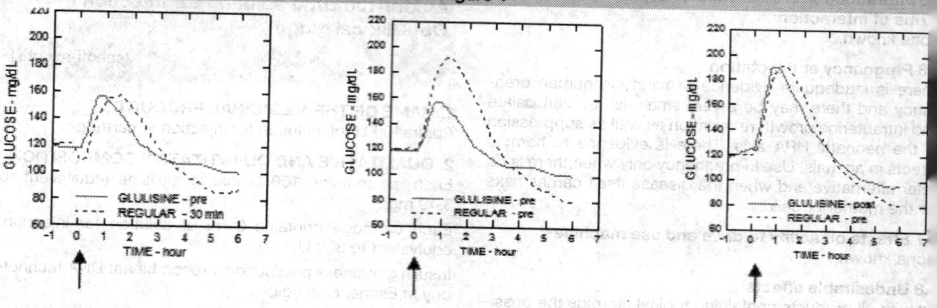

Figure 1 A Figure 1B Figure 1C

Figure 1: Average glucose-lowering effect over 6 hours in 20 patients with type 1 diabetes mellitus. Insulin glulisine given 2 minutes (GLULISINE pre) before the start of a meal compared to regular human insulin given 30 minutes (REGULAR 30 min) before the start of the meal (figure 1A) and compared to regular human insulin given 2 minutes (REGULAR pre) before a meal (figure 1B). Insulin glulisine given 15 minutes (GLULISINE post) after start of a meal compared to regular human insulin given 2 minutes (REGULAR pre) before start of the meal (figure 1C). On the x-axis, zero (arrow) is the start of a 15-minute meal.

minutes prior to meal, insulin glulisine provided better postprandial control than regular human insulin given 2 minutes before the meal. Insulin glulisine administered 15 minutes after starting the meal gives similar glycemic control as regular human insulin given 2 minutes before the meal (see figure 1).

(see Figure 1 above)

Figure 1: Average glucose-lowering effect over 6 hours in 20 patients with type 1 diabetes mellitus. Insulin glulisine given 2 minutes (GLULISINE pre) before the start of a meal compared to regular human insulin given 30 minutes (REGULAR 30 min) before the start of the meal (figure 1A) and compared to regular human insulin given 2 minutes (REGULAR pre) before a meal (figure 1B). Insulin glulisine given 15 minutes (GLULISINE post) after start of a meal compared to regular human insulin given 2 minutes (REGULAR pre) before start of the meal (figure 1C). On the x-axis, zero (arrow) is the start of a 15-minute meal.

Obesity

A phase I study carried out with insulin glulisine, lispro and regular human insulin in an obese population has demonstrated that insulin glulisine maintains its rapid-acting properties. In this study, the time to 20% of total AUC and the AUC (0-2h) representing the early glucose lowering activity were respectively of 114 minutes and 427mg.kg^{-1} for insulin glulisine, 121 minutes and 354mg.kg^{-1} for lispro, 150 minutes and 197mg.kg^{-1} for regular human insulin (see figure 2).

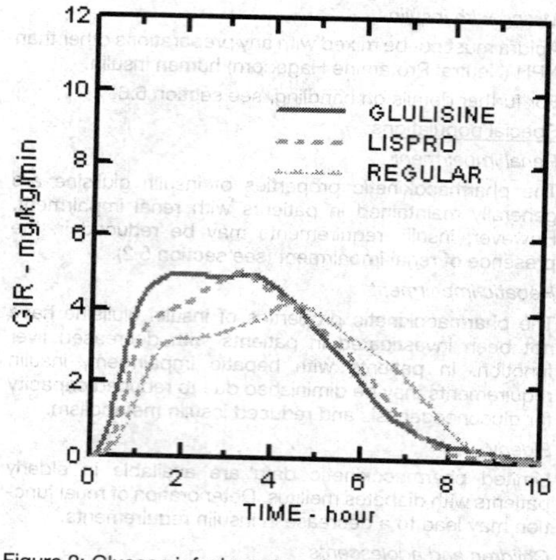

Figure 2: Glucose infusion rates after subcutaneous injection of 0.3 U/kg of insulin glulisine (GLULISINE) or insulin lispro (LISPRO) or regular human insulin (REGULAR) in an obese population.

Another phase I study with insulin glulisine and insulin lispro in a non-diabetic population in 80 subjects with a wide range of body mass indices (18-46 kg/m^2) has demonstrated that rapid action is generally maintained across a wide range of body mass indices, while total glucose lowering effect decreases with increasing obesity.

The average total GIR AUC between 0–1 hour was 102±75 mg/kg and 158±100 mg/kg with 0.2 and 0.4 U/kg insulin glulisine, respectively, and was 83.1±72.8 mg/kg and 112.3±70.8 mg/kg with 0.2 and 0.4 U/kg insulin lispro respectively.

A phase I study in 18 obese patients with type 2 diabetes mellitus (BMI between 35 and 40 kg/m2) with insulin glulisine and insulin lispro [90% CI:0.81, 0.95 (p=<0.01)]has shown that insulin glulisine effectively controls diurnal post-prandial blood glucose excursions.

Clinical studies

Type 1 diabetes mellitus-Adults

In a 26-week phase III clinical study comparing insulin glulisine with insulin lispro both injected subcutaneously shortly (0-15 minutes) before a meal in patients with type 1 diabetes mellitus using insulin glargine as basal insulin, insulin glulisine was comparable to insulin lispro for glycemic control as reflected by changes in glycated haemoglobin (expressed as HbA_{1c} equivalent) from baseline to endpoint. Comparable self-monitored blood glucose values were observed. No increase in the basal insulin dose was needed with insulin glulisine, in contrast to insulin lispro.

A 12-week phase III clinical study performed in patients with type 1 diabetes mellitus receiving insulin glargine as basal therapy indicate that the immediate postmeal administration of insulin glulisine provides efficacy that was comparable to immediate premeal insulin glulisine (0-15 minutes) or regular insulin (30-45 minutes).

In the per protocol population there was a significantly larger observed reduction in GHb in the premeal glulisine group compared with the regular insulin group.

Type 1 diabetes mellitus -Paediatric

A 26-week phase III clinical study compared insulin glulisine with insulin lispro both injected subcutaneously shortly (0-15 minutes) before a meal in children (4-5 years: n=9; 6-7 years: n=32 and 8-11 years: n=149) and adolescents (12-17 years: n=382) with type 1 diabetes mellitus using insulin glargine or NPH as basal insulin. Insulin glulisine was comparable to insulin lispro for glycaemic control as reflected by changes in glycated haemoglobin (GHb expressed as HbA_{1c} equivalent) from baseline to endpoint and by self-monitored blood glucose values.

There is insufficient clinical information on the use of Apidra in children younger than the age of 6 years.

Type 2 diabetes mellitus-Adults

A 26-week phase III clinical study followed by a 26-week extension safety study was conducted to compare insulin glulisine (0-15 minutes before a meal) with regular human insulin (30-45 minutes before a meal) injected subcutaneously in patients with type 2 diabetes mellitus also using NPH insulin as basal insulin. The average body mass index (BMI) of patients was 34.55 kg/m^2. Insulin glulisine was shown to be comparable to regular human insulin with regard to glycated haemoglobin (expressed as HbA_{1c} equivalent) changes from baseline to the 6-month endpoint (-0.46% for insulin glulisine and -0.30% for regular human insulin, p=0.0029) and from baseline to the 12-month endpoint (-0.23% for insulin glulisine and -0.13% for regular human insulin, difference not significant). In this study, the majority of patients (79%) mixed their short acting insulin with NPH insulin immediately prior to injection and 58 % of subjects used oral hypoglycemic agents at randomization and were instructed to continue to use them at the same dose.

Race and Gender

In controlled clinical trials in adults, insulin glulisine did not show differences in safety and efficacy in subgroup analyses based on race and gender.

5.2 Pharmacokinetic properties

In insulin glulisine the replacement of the human insulin amino acid asparagine in position B3 by lysine and the lysine in position B29 by glutamic acid favors more rapid absorption.

In a study with 18 male subjects with diabetes mellitus type 1 aged 21 to 50 years, insulin glulisine displays dose-proportionality for early, maximum and total exposure in the dose range 0.075 to 0.4U/kg.

Absorption and bioavailability

Pharmacokinetic profiles in healthy volunteers and diabetes patients (type 1 or 2) demonstrated that absorption of insulin glulisine was about twice as fast with a peak oncentration approximately twice as high as compared to egular human insulin.

a study in patients with type 1 diabetes mellitus after ubcutaneous administration of 0.15 U/kg, for insulin glusine the T_{max} was 55 minutes and C_{max} was 82 ± 1.3 μU/ml ompared to a T_{max} of 82 minutes and a C_{max} of 46 ± .3 μU/ml for regular human insulin. The mean residence me of insulin glulisine was shorter (98 min) than for regular uman insulin (161 min) (see figure3).

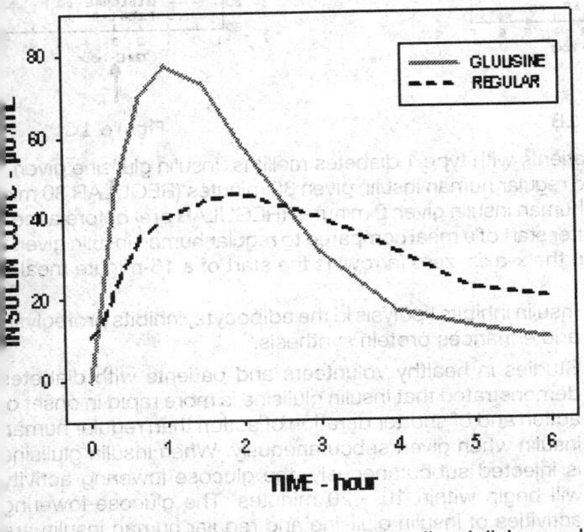

Figure 3: Pharmacokinetic profile of insulin glulisine and regular human insulin in type 1 diabetes mellitus patients after a dose of 0.15 U/kg.

In a study in patients with type 2 diabetes mellitus after subcutaneous administration of 0.2 U/kg insulin glulisine, the Cmax was 91 μU/ml with the interquartile range from 78 to 104 μU/ml.

When insulin glulisine was injected subcutaneously into abdomen, deltoid and thigh, the concentration-time profiles were similar with a slightly faster absorption when administered in the abdomen compared to the thigh. Absorption from deltoid sites was in-between (see section 4.2). The absolute bioavailability (70%) of insulin glulisine was similar between injection sites and of low intra-subject variability (11%CV).

Obesity

Another phase I study with insulin glulisine and insulin lispro in a non-diabetic population in 80 subjects with a wide range of body mass indices (18-46 kg/m^2) has demonstrated that rapid absorption and total exposure is generally maintained across a wide range of body mass indices. The time to 10% of total INS exposure was reached earlier by approximately 5–6 min with insulin glulisine.

Distribution and elimination

The distribution and elimination of insulin glulisine and regular human insulin after intravenous administration is similar with volumes of distribution of 13 l and 22 l and half-lives of 13 and 18 minutes, respectively.

After subcutaneous administration, insulin glulisine is eliminated more rapidly than regular human insulin with an apparent half-life of 42 minutes compared to 86 minutes. In an across study analysis of insulin glulisine in either healthy subjects or subjects with type 1 or type 2 diabetes mellitus the apparent half-life ranged from 37 to 75 minutes (interquartile range).

Insulin glulisine shows low plasma protein binding, similar to human insulin.

Special populations

Renal impairment

In a clinical study performed in non-diabetic subjects covering a wide range of renal function (CrCl > 80 ml/min, 30-50 ml/min, < 30 ml/min), the rapid-acting properties of insulin glulisine were generally maintained. However, insulin requirements may be reduced in the presence of renal impairment.

Hepatic impairment

The pharmacokinetic properties have not been investigated in patients with impaired liver function.

Elderly

Very limited pharmacokinetic data are available for elderly patients with diabetes mellitus.

Children and adolescents

The pharmacokinetic and pharmacodynamic properties of insulin glulisine were investigated in children (7-11 years) and adolescents (12-16 years) with type 1 diabetes mellitus. Insulin glulisine was rapidly absorbed in both age groups, with similar T_{max} and C_{max} as in adults (see section 4.2). Administered immediately before a test meal, insulin glulisine provided better postprandial control than regular human insulin, as in adults (see section 5.1). The glucose excursion (AUC_{0-6h}) was 641 mg.h.dl^{-1} for insulin glulisine and 801mg.h.dl^{-1} for regular human insulin.

5.3 Preclinical safety data

Non-clinical data did not reveal toxicity findings others than those linked to the blood glucose lowering pharmacodynamic activity (hypoglycemia), different from regular human insulin or of clinical relevance for humans.

6. PHARMACEUTICAL PARTICULARS

6.1 List of excipients

Metacresol

Sodium chloride

Trometamol

Polysorbate 20

Hydrochloric acid, concentrated

Sodium hydroxide

Water for injections

6.2 Incompatibilities

In the absence of compatibility studies, this medicinal product must not be mixed with other medicinal products except NPH human insulin.

6.3 Shelf life

2 years.

Shelf life after first use of the cartridge

The product may be stored for a maximum of 4 weeks not above 25°C away from direct heat or direct light. The pen containing the cartridge must not be stored in the refrigerator. The pen cap must be put back on the pen after each injection in order to protect from light.

6.4 Special precautions for storage

Unopened

Store in a refrigerator (2°C - 8°C).

Do not freeze.

Do not put Apidra next to the freezer compartment or a freezer pack.

Keep the cartridge in the outer carton in order to protect from light.

In use conditions:

For storage precautions, see section 6.3.

6.5 Nature and contents of container

3 ml solution in a cartridge (type I colourless glass cartridge) with a plunger (elastomeric rubber) and a flanged cap (aluminium) with a stopper (elastomeric rubber).

The glass cartridge is irreversibly integrated in a transparent container and attached to a plastic mechanism by a threaded rod at one extremity.

Packs of 5 cartridges for OptiClik are available.

6.6 Special precautions for disposal and other handling

The cartridges for OptiClik are to be used in conjunction with OptiClik only, and as recommended in the information provided by the device manufacturer.

The manufacturer's instructions for using the pen must be followed carefully for loading the cartridge, attaching the needle, and administering the insulin injection.

If OptiClik is damaged or not working properly (due to mechanical defects) it has to be discarded, and a new OptiClik has to be used.

Before insertion of the cartridge into the reusable pen, the cartridge must be stored at room temperature for 1 to 2 hours. Inspect the cartridge before use. It must only be used if the cartridge is intact and the solution is clear, colourless, with no solid particles visible.

Air bubbles must be removed from the cartridge before injection (see instruction for using pen). Empty cartridges must not be refilled.

If the pen malfunctions, (see instructions for using the pen) the solution may be drawn from the cartridge into a syringe (suitable for an insulin with 100 U/ml) and injected.

To prevent any kind of contamination, the re-usable pen should be used by a single patient only.

Mixing with insulins

When mixed with NPH human insulin, Apidra should be drawn into the syringe first. Injection should be given immediately after mixing as no data are available regarding the mixtures made up a significant time before injection.

7. MARKETING AUTHORISATION HOLDER

Sanofi-Aventis Deutschland GmbH, Brueningstrasse 50, D-65926 Frankfurt am Main, Germany.

8. MARKETING AUTHORISATION NUMBER(S)

EU/1/04/285/024

9. DATE OF FIRST AUTHORISATION/RENEWAL OF THE AUTHORISATION

27 September 2004

10. DATE OF REVISION OF THE TEXT

20th June 2008

Legal category: POM

Apidra 100 U/ml, solution for injection

(sanofi-aventis)

1. NAME OF THE MEDICINAL PRODUCT

Apidra 100 U/ml, solution for injection in a vial

Apidra 100 U/ml, solution for injection in a cartridge

Apidra 100 U/ml, solution for injection in pre-filled pen.

2. QUALITATIVE AND QUANTITATIVE COMPOSITION

Each ml contains 100 U insulin glulisine (equivalent to 3.49 mg).

Each vial contains 10 ml of solution for injection, equivalent to 1000 U.

Each cartridge contains 3 ml of solution for injection, equivalent to 300 U.

Each pen contains 3 ml of solution for injection, equivalent to 300 U.

Insulin glulisine is produced by recombinant DNA technology in Escherichia *coli*.

For a full list of excipients, see section 6.1.

3. PHARMACEUTICAL FORM

Solution for injection in a vial.

Solution for injection in a cartridge.

Solution for injection in pre-filled pen. OptiSet.

Clear, colourless, aqueous solution.

4. CLINICAL PARTICULARS

4.1 Therapeutic indications

Treatment of adults, adolescents and children, 6 years or older with diabetes mellitus, where treatment with insulin is required.

4.2 Posology and method of administration

The potency of this preparation is stated in units. These units are exclusive to Apidra and are not the same as IU or the units used to express the potency of other insulin analogues. See section 5.1 (Pharmacodynamics).

Apidra should be given shortly (0-15 min) before or soon after meals.

Apidra should be used in regimens that include an intermediate or long acting insulin or basal insulin analogue and can be used with oral hypoglycaemic agents.

The dosage of Apidra should be individually adjusted.

Administration

Apidra should be given by subcutaneous injection or by continuous subcutaneous pump infusion.

Apidra should be administered subcutaneously in the abdominal wall, thigh or deltoid or by continuous infusion in the abdominal wall. Injection sites and infusion sites within an-injection area (abdomen, thigh or deltoid) should be rotated from one injection to the next. The rate of absorption, and consequently the onset and duration of action, may be affected by the injection site, exercise and other variables. Subcutaneous injection in the abdominal wall ensures a slightly faster absorption than other injection sites (see section 5.2).

Care should be taken to ensure that a blood vessel has not been entered. After injection, the site of injection should not be massaged. Patients must be educated to use proper injection techniques.

Mixing with insulins

In the absence of compatibility studies, insulin glulisine must not be mixed with other medicinal products except NPH human insulin.

For further details on handling, see section 6.6.

Before using OptiSet, the Instructions for Use included in the Package Leaflet must be read carefully (see section 6.6).

Continuous subcutaneous infusion pump

When used with an insulin infusion pump, Apidra must not be mixed with diluents or any other insulin.

For further details on handling, see section 6.6.

Special populations

Renal impairment

The pharmacokinetic properties of insulin glulisine are generally maintained in patients with renal impairment. However, insulin requirements may be reduced in the presence of renal impairment (see section 5.2).

Hepatic impairment

The pharmacokinetic properties of insulin glulisine have not been investigated in patients with decreased liver function. In patients with hepatic impairment, insulin requirements may be diminished due to reduced capacity for gluconeogenesis and reduced insulin metabolism.

Elderly

Limited pharmacokinetic data are available in elderly patients with diabetes mellitus. Deterioration of renal function may lead to a decrease in insulin requirements.

Children and adolescents

There is insufficient clinical information on the use of Apidra in children younger than the age of 6 years.

4.3 Contraindications

Hypersensitivity to the active substance or to any of the excipients.

Hypoglycaemia.

4.4 Special warnings and precautions for use

Transferring a patient to a new type or brand of insulin should be done under strict medical supervision. Changes in strength, brand (manufacturer), type (regular, NPH, lente, etc.), species (animal) and/or method of manufacturing may result in a change in dosage. Concomitant oral antidiabetic treatment may need to be adjusted.

The use of inadequate dosages or discontinuation of treatment, especially in insulin-dependent diabetic, may lead to hyperglycaemia and diabetic ketoacidosis; conditions which are potentially lethal.

Switching a patient to another type or brand of insulin should be done under strict medical supervision and may require change in dose.

Hypoglycaemia

The time of occurrence of hypoglycaemia depends on the action profile of the insulins used and may therefore change when the treatment regimen is changed.

Conditions which may make the early warning symptoms of hypoglycaemia different or less pronounced include long duration of diabetes, intensified insulin therapy, diabetic nerve disease, medicinal products such as beta blockers or after transfer from animal-source insulin to human insulin.

Adjustment of dosage may be also necessary if patients undertake increased physical activity or change their usual meal plan. Exercise taken immediately after a meal may increase the risk of hypoglycaemia.

When compared with soluble human insulin, if hypoglycaemia occurs after an injection with rapid acting analogues, it may occur earlier.

Uncorrected hypoglycaemic or hyperglycaemic reactions can cause loss of consciousness, coma, or death.

Insulin requirements may be altered during illness or emotional disturbances.

Handling of the OptiSet pen

Before using OptiSet, the Instructions for Use included in the Package Leaflet must be read carefully. OptiSet has to be used as recommended in these Instructions for Use (see 6.6).

4.5 Interaction with other medicinal products and other forms of interaction

Studies on pharmacokinetic interactions have not been performed. Based on empirical knowledge from similar medicinal products, clinically relevant pharmacokinetic interactions are unlikely to occur.

A number of substances affect glucose metabolism and may require dose adjustment of insulin glulisine and particularly close monitoring.

Substances that may enhance the blood-glucose-lowering activity and increase susceptibility to hypoglycaemia include oral antidiabetic agents, angiotensin converting enzyme (ACE) inhibitors, disopyramide, fibrates, fluoxetine, monoamide oxidase inhibitors (MAOIs), pentoxifylline, propoxyphene, salicylates and sulfonamide antibiotics.

Substances that may reduce the blood-glucose-lowering activity include corticosteroids, danazol, diazoxide, diuretics, glucagon, isoniazid, phenothiazine derivatives, somatropin, sympathomimetic agents (e.g. epinephrine [adrenaline], salbutamol, terbutaline), thyroid hormones, estrogens, progestins (e.g. in oral contraceptives), protease inhibitors and atypical antipsychotic medicinal products (e.g. olanzapine and clozapine).

Beta-blockers, clonidine, lithium salts or alcohol may either potentiate or weaken the blood-glucose-lowering activity of insulin. Pentamidine may cause hypoglycaemia, which may sometimes be followed by hyperglycaemia.

In addition, under the influence of sympatholytic medicinal products such as beta-blockers, clonidine, guanethidine and reserpine, the signs of adrenergic counter-regulation may be reduced or absent.

4.6 Pregnancy and lactation

Pregnancy

There are no adequate data on the use of insulin glulisine in pregnant women.

Animal reproduction studies have not revealed any differences between insulin glulisine and human insulin regarding pregnancy, embryonal/foetal development, parturition or postnatal development (see section 5.3).

Caution should be exercised when prescribing to pregnant women. Careful monitoring of glucose control is essential.

It is essential for patients with pre-existing or gestational diabetes to maintain good metabolic control throughout pregnancy. Insulin requirements may decrease during the first trimester and generally increase during the second and third trimesters. Immediately after delivery, insulin requirements decline rapidly.

Lactation

It is unknown whether insulin glulisine is excreted in human milk, but in general insulin does not pass into breast milk and is not absorbed after oral administration.

Breast-feeding mothers may require adjustments in insulin dose and diet.

4.7 Effects on ability to drive and use machines

The patient's ability to concentrate and react may be impaired as a result of hypoglycaemia or hyperglycaemia or, for example, as a result of visual impairment. This may constitute a risk in situations where these abilities are of special importance (e.g. driving a car or operating machinery).

Patients should be advised to take precautions to avoid hypoglycaemia whilst driving. This is particularly important in those who have reduced or absent awareness of the warning symptoms of hypoglycaemia or have frequent episodes of hypoglycaemia. The advisability of driving should be considered in these circumstances.

Figure 1

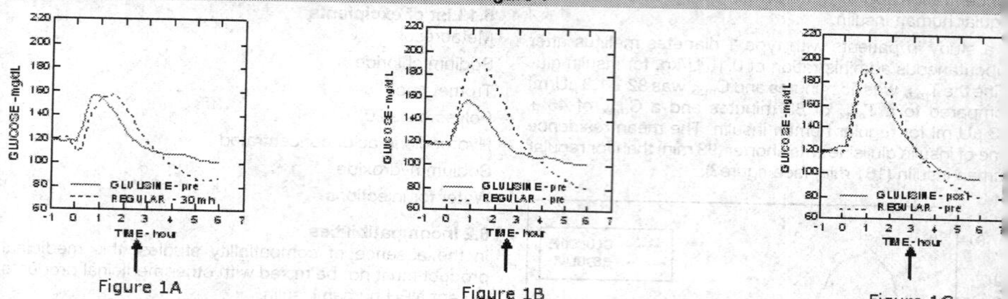

Figure 1A Figure 1B Figure 1C

Figure 1: Average glucose-lowering effect over 6 hours in 20 patients with type 1 diabetes mellitus. Insulin glulisine given 2 minutes (GLULISINE pre) before the start of a meal compared to regular human insulin given 30 minutes (REGULAR 30 min) before the start of the meal (figure 1A) and compared to regular human insulin given 2 minutes (REGULAR pre) before a meal (figure 1B). Insulin glulisine given 15 minutes (GLULISINE post) after start of a meal compared to regular human insulin given 2 minutes (REGULAR pre) before start of the meal (figure 1C). On the x-axis, zero (arrow) is the start of a 15-minute meal.

4.8 Undesirable effects

Hypoglycaemia, the most frequent undesirable effect of insulin therapy, may occur if the insulin dose is too high in relation to the insulin requirement.

The following related adverse reactions from clinical investigations were listed below by system organ class and in order of decreasing incidence (very common: > 1/10; common: > 1/100, < 1/10; uncommon: > 1/1,000, < 1/100; rare: > 1/10,000, < 1/1,000; very rare: < 1/10,000).

Within each frequency grouping, undesirable effects are presented in order of decreasing seriousness.

Metabolism and nutrition disorders

Very common: Hypoglycaemia

Symptoms of hypoglycaemia usually occur suddenly. They may include cold sweats, cool pale skin, fatigue, nervousness or tremor, anxiousness, unusual tiredness or weakness, confusion, difficulty in concentration, drowsiness, excessive hunger, vision changes, headache, nausea and palpitation. Hypoglycaemia can become severe and may lead to unconsciousness and/or convulsions and may result in temporary or permanent impairment of brain function or even death.

Skin and subcutaneous tissue disorders

Common: injection site reactions and local hypersensitivity reactions.

Local hypersensitivity reactions (redness, swelling and itching at the injection site) may occur during treatment with insulin. These reactions are usually transitory and normally they disappear during continued treatment.

Rare: Lipodystrophy

Lipodystrophy may occur at the injection site as a consequence of failure to rotate injection sites within an area.

General disorders

Uncommon: Systemic hypersensitivity reactions

Systemic hypersensitivity reactions may include urticaria, chest tightness, dyspnea, allergic dermatitis and pruritus. Severe cases of generalized allergy, including anaphylactic reaction, may be life-threatening.

4.9 Overdose

Hypoglycaemia may occur as a result of an excess of insulin activity relative to food intake and energy expenditure.

There are no specific data available concerning overdose with insulin glulisine. However, hypoglycaemia may develop over sequential stages:

Mild hypoglycaemic episodes can be treated by oral administration of glucose or sugary products. It is therefore recommended that the diabetic patient constantly carries some sugar lumps, sweets, biscuits or sugary fruit juice.

Severe hypoglycaemic episodes, where the patient has become unconscious, can be treated by glucagon (0.5 to 1 mg) given intramuscularly or subcutaneously by a person who has received appropriate instruction, or by glucose given intravenously by a medical professional.

Glucose must also be given intravenously, if the patient does not respond to glucagon within 10 to 15 minutes.

Upon regaining consciousness, administration of oral carbohydrate is recommended for the patient in order to prevent relapse.

After an injection of glucagon, the patient should be monitored in a hospital in order to find the reason for this severe hypoglycaemia and prevent other similar episodes.

5. PHARMACOLOGICAL PROPERTIES

5.1 Pharmacodynamic properties

Pharmacotherapeutic group: insulin and analogues, fast-acting. ATC code: A10AB06

Insulin glulisine is a recombinant human insulin analogue that is equipotent to regular human insulin. Insulin glulisine has a more rapid onset of action and a shorter duration of action than regular human insulin.

The primary activity of insulins and insulin analogues, including insulin glulisine, is regulation of glucose metabolism. Insulins lower blood glucose levels by stimulating peripheral glucose uptake, especially by skeletal muscle and fat, and by inhibiting hepatic glucose production. Insulin inhibits lipolysis in the adipocyte, inhibits proteolysis and enhances protein synthesis.

Studies in healthy volunteers and patients with diabetes demonstrated that insulin glulisine is more rapid in onset of action and of shorter duration of action than regular human insulin when given subcutaneously. When insulin glulisine is injected subcutaneously, the glucose lowering activity will begin within 10 – 20 minutes. The glucose-lowering activities of insulin glulisine and regular human insulin are equipotent when administered by intravenous route. One unit of insulin glulisine has the same glucose-lowering activity as one unit of regular human insulin.

Dose proportionality

In a study with 18 male subjects with diabetes mellitus type 1 aged 21 to 50 years, insulin glulisine displayed dose-proportional glucose lowering effect in the therapeutic relevant dose range 0.075 to 0.15 U/kg, and less than proportional increase in glucose lowering effect with 0.3 U/kg or higher, like human insulin.

Insulin glulisine takes effect about twice as fast as regular human insulin and completes the glucose lowering effect about 2 hours earlier than regular human insulin.

A phase I study in patients with type 1 diabetes mellitus assessed the glucose lowering profiles of insulin glulisine and regular human insulin administered subcutaneously at a dose of 0.15 U/kg, at different times in relation to a 15-minute standard meal. Data indicated that insulin glulisine administered 2 minutes before the meal gives similar postprandial glycemic control compared to regular human insulin given 30 minutes before the meal. When given 2 minutes prior to meal, insulin glulisine provided better postprandial control than regular human insulin given 2 minutes before the meal. Insulin glulisine administered 15 minutes after starting the meal gives similar glycemic control as regular human insulin given 2 minutes before the meal (see figure 1).

(see Figure 1 above)

Figure 1: Average glucose-lowering effect over 6 hours in 20 patients with type 1 diabetes mellitus. Insulin glulisine given 2 minutes (GLULISINE pre) before the start of a meal compared to regular human insulin given 30 minutes (REGULAR 30 min) before the start of the meal (figure 1A) and compared to regular human insulin given 2 minutes (REGULAR pre) before a meal (figure 1B). Insulin glulisine given 15 minutes (GLULISINE post) after start of a meal compared to regular human insulin given 2 minutes (REGULAR pre) before start of the meal (figure 1C). On the x-axis, zero (arrow) is the start of a 15-minute meal.

Obesity

A phase I study carried out with insulin glulisine, lispro and regular human insulin in an obese population has demonstrated that insulin glulisine maintains its rapid-acting properties. In this study, the time to 20% of total AUC and the AUC (0-2h) representing the early glucose lowering activity were respectively of 114 minutes and 427mg.kg^{-1} for insulin glulisine, 121 minutes and 354mg.kg^{-1} for lispro, 150 minutes and 197mg.kg^{-1} for regular human insulin (see figure 2).

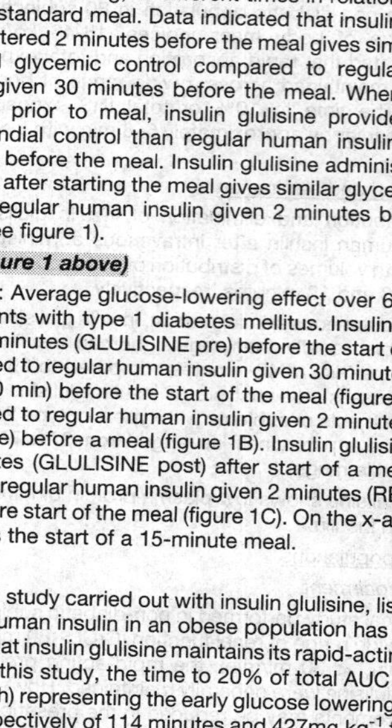

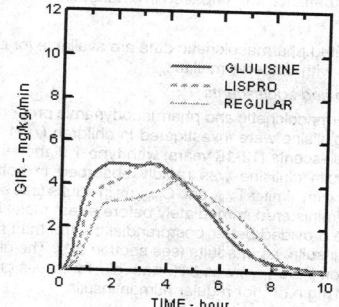

Figure 2: Glucose infusion rates after subcutaneous injection of 0.3 U/kg of insulin glulisine (GLULISINE) or insulin lispro (LISPRO) or regular human insulin (REGULAR) in an obese population.

nother phase I study with insulin glulisine and insulin pro in a non-diabetic population in 80 subjects with a de range of body mass indices (18-46 kg/m^2) s demonstrated that rapid action is generally maintained cross a wide range of body mass indices, while tal glucose lowering effect decreases with increasing besity.

he average total GIR AUC between 0–1 hour was 2±75 mg/kg and 158±100 mg/kg with 0.2 and 0.4 U/ insulin glulisine, respectively, and was 83.1±72.8 mg/kg d 112.3±70.8 mg/kg with 0.2 and 0.4 U/kg insulin lispro espectively.

phase I study in 18 obese patients with type 2 diabetes ellitus (BMI between 35 and 40 kg/m2) with insulin glusine and insulin lispro [90% CI:0.81, 0.95 (p=<0.01)]has hown that insulin glulisine effectively controls diurnal ost-prandial blood glucose excursions.

linical studies

ype 1 diabetes mellitus-Adults

 a 26-week phase III clinical study comparing insulin lulisine with insulin lispro both injected subcutaneously hortly (0-15 minutes) before a meal in patients with type 1 iabetes mellitus using insulin glargine as basal insulin, nsulin glulisine was comparable to insulin lispro for glycemic control as reflected by changes in glycated haemoglobin (expressed as HbA_{1c} equivalent) from baseline to endpoint. Comparable self-monitored blood glucose values were observed. No increase in the basal insulin dose was needed with insulin glulisine, in contrast to insulin spro.

A 12-week phase III clinical study performed in patients with type 1 diabetes mellitus receiving insulin glargine as basal therapy indicate that the immediate postmeal administration of insulin glulisine provides efficacy that was comparable to immediate premeal insulin glulisine (0-15 minutes) or regular insulin (30-45 minutes).

In the per protocol population there was a significantly larger observed reduction in GHb in the premeal glulisine group compared with the regular insulin group.

Type 1 diabetes mellitus -Paediatric

A 26-week phase III clinical study compared insulin glulisine with insulin lispro both injected subcutaneously shortly (0-15 minutes) before a meal in children (4-5 years: n=9; 6-7 years: n=32 and 8-11 years: n=149) and adolescents (12-17 years: n=382) with type 1 diabetes mellitus using insulin glargine or NPH as basal insulin. Insulin glulisine was comparable to insulin lispro for glycaemic control as reflected by changes in glycated haemoglobin (GHb expressed as HbA_{1c} equivalent) from baseline to endpoint and by self-monitored blood glucose values.

There is insufficient clinical information on the use of Apidra in children younger than the age of 6 years.

Type 2 diabetes mellitus-Adults

A 26-week phase III clinical study followed by a 26-week extension safety study was conducted to compare insulin glulisine (0-15 minutes before a meal) with regular human insulin (30-45 minutes before a meal) injected subcutaneously in patients with type 2 diabetes mellitus also using NPH insulin as basal insulin. The average body mass index (BMI) of patients was 34.55 kg/m^2. Insulin glulisine was shown to be comparable to regular human insulin with regard to glycated haemoglobin (expressed as HbA_{1c} equivalent) changes from baseline to the 6-month endpoint (-0.46% for insulin glulisine and -0.30% for regular human insulin, p=0.0029) and from baseline to the 12-month endpoint (-0.23% for insulin glulisine and -0.13% for regular human insulin, difference not significant). In this study, the majority of patients (79%) mixed their short acting insulin with NPH insulin immediately prior to injection and 58 % of subjects used oral hypoglycemic agents at randomization and were instructed to continue to use them at the same dose.

Race and Gender

In controlled clinical trials in adults, insulin glulisine did not show differences in safety and efficacy in subgroup analyses based on race and gender.

5.2 Pharmacokinetic properties

In insulin glulisine the replacement of the human insulin amino acid asparagine in position B3 by lysine and the lysine in position B29 by glutamic acid favors more rapid absorption.

In a study with 18 male subjects with diabetes mellitus type 1 aged 21 to 50 years, insulin glulisine displays dose-proportionality for early, maximum and total exposure in the dose range 0.075 to 0.4U/kg.

Absorption and bioavailability

Pharmacokinetic profiles in healthy volunteers and diabetes patients (type 1 or 2) demonstrated that absorption of insulin glulisine was about twice as fast with a peak concentration approximately twice as high as compared to regular human insulin.

In a study in patients with type 1 diabetes mellitus after subcutaneous administration of 0.15 U/kg, for insulin glulisine the T_{max} was 55 minutes and C_{max} was 82 ± 1.3 µU/ml compared to a T_{max} of 82 minutes and a C_{max} of 46 ± 1.3 µU/ml for regular human insulin. The mean residence time of insulin glulisine was shorter (98 min) than for regular human insulin (161 min) (see figure3).

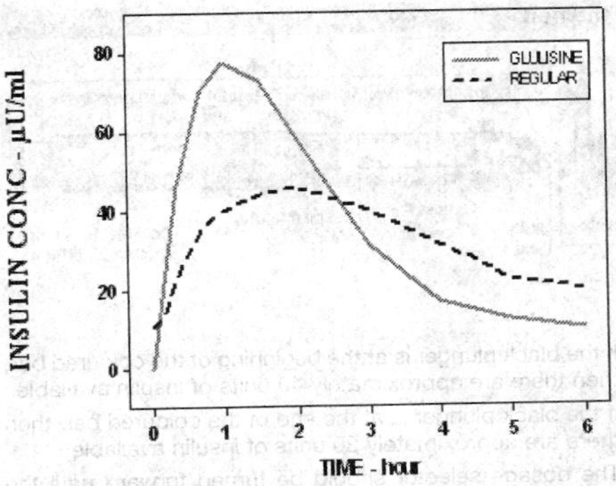

Figure 3: Pharmacokinetic profile of insulin glulisine and regular human insulin in type 1 diabetes mellitus patients after a dose of 0.15 U/kg.

In a study in patients with type 2 diabetes mellitus after subcutaneous administration of 0.2 U/kg insulin glulisine, the Cmax was 91 µU/ml with the interquartile range from 78 to 104 µU/ml.

When insulin glulisine was injected subcutaneously into abdomen, deltoid and thigh, the concentration-time profiles were similar with a slightly faster absorption when administered in the abdomen compared to the thigh. Absorption from deltoid sites was in-between (see section 4.2). The absolute bioavailability (70%) of insulin glulisine was similar between injection sites and of low intra-subject variability (11%CV).

Obesity

Another phase I study with insulin glulisine and insulin lispro in a non-diabetic population in 80 subjects with a wide range of body mass indices (18-46 kg/m^2) has demonstrated that rapid absorption and total exposure is generally maintained across a wide range of body mass indices.

The time to 10% of total INS exposure was reached earlier by approximately 5–6 min with insulin glulisine.

Distribution and elimination

The distribution and elimination of insulin glulisine and regular human insulin after intravenous administration is similar with volumes of distribution of 13l and 22l and half-lives of 13 and 18 minutes, respectively.

After subcutaneous administration, insulin glulisine is eliminated more rapidly than regular human insulin with an apparent half-life of 42 minutes compared to 86 minutes. In an across study analysis of insulin glulisine in either healthy subjects or subjects with type 1 or type 2 diabetes mellitus the apparent half-life ranged from 37 to 75 minutes (interquartile range).

Insulin glulisine shows low plasma protein binding, similar to human insulin.

Special populations

Renal impairment

In a clinical study performed in non-diabetic subjects covering a wide range of renal function (CrCl> 80 ml/min, 30-50 ml/min, < 30 ml/min), the rapid-acting properties of insulin glulisine were generally maintained. However, insulin requirements may be reduced in the presence of renal impairment.

Hepatic impairment

The pharmacokinetic properties have not been investigated in patients with impaired liver function.

Elderly

Very limited pharmacokinetic data are available for elderly patients with diabetes mellitus.

Children and adolescents

The pharmacokinetic and pharmacodynamic properties of insulin glulisine were investigated in children (7-11 years) and adolescents (12-16 years) with type 1 diabetes mellitus. Insulin glulisine was rapidly absorbed in both age groups, with similar T_{max} and C_{max} as in adults (see section 4.2). Administered immediately before a test meal, insulin glulisine provided better postprandial control than regular human insulin, as in adults (see section 5.1). The glucose excursion (AUC_{0-6h}) was 641 $mg.h.dl^{-1}$ for insulin glulisine and 801$mg.h.dl^{-1}$ for regular human insulin.

5.3 Preclinical safety data

Non-clinical data did not reveal toxicity findings others than those linked to the blood glucose lowering pharmacodynamic activity (hypoglycemia), different from regular human insulin or of clinical relevance for humans.

6. PHARMACEUTICAL PARTICULARS

6.1 List of excipients

Metacresol

Sodium chloride

Trometamol

Polysorbate 20

Hydrochloric acid, concentrated

Sodium hydroxide

Water for injections

6.2 Incompatibilities

In the absence of compatibility studies this medicinal product must not be mixed with any preparations other than NPH human insulin.

When used with an insulin infusion pump, Apidra must not be mixed with other medicinal products.

6.3 Shelf life

2 years.

Shelf life after first use:

The product may be stored for a maximum of 4 weeks not above 25°C away from direct heat or direct light.

Vials:

Keep the vial in the outer carton in order to protect from light. It is recommended that the date of the first use from the vial be noted on the label.

Cartridges or OptiSet Pens:

Pens in use must not be stored in the refrigerator. The pen cap must be put back on the pen after each injection in order to protect from light.

6.4 Special precautions for storage

Unopened

Store in a refrigerator (2°C - 8°C)

Do not freeze.

Do not put Apidra next to the freezer compartment or a freezer pack.

Keep the vial, cartridge and pre-filled pen in the outer carton in order to protect from light.

In use conditions:

For storage precautions, see section 6.3

6.5 Nature and contents of container

Vial:

10 ml solution in a vial (type I colourless glass) with a stopper (flanged aluminium overseal, elastomeric rubber) and a tear-off cap. Packs of 1 vial are available.

Cartridge:

3 ml solution in a cartridge (type I colourless glass) with a plunger (elastomeric rubber) and a flanged cap (aluminium) with a stopper (elastomeric rubber). Packs of 5 cartridges are available.

OptiSet Prefilled Pen:

3 ml solution in a cartridge (colourless glass) with a plunger (elastomeric rubber) and a flanged cap (aluminium) with a stopper (elastomeric rubber). The cartridge is sealed in a disposable pre-filled pen. Packs of 5 pens are available.

6.6 Special precautions for disposal and other handling

Vials

Apidra vials are for use with insulin syringes with the corresponding unit scale and for use with an insulin pump system (see section 4.2).

Inspect the vials, cartridges and pens before use. It must only be used if the solution is clear, colourless, with no solid particles visible. Since Apidra is a solution, it does not require resuspension before use.

Cartridges

The cartridges are to be used in conjunction with an insulin pen such as OptiPen and other pens suitable for Apidra cartridges, and as recommended in the information provided by the device manufacturer.

The manufacturer's instructions for using the pen must be followed carefully for loading the cartridge, attaching the needle, and administering the insulin injection. Inspect the cartridge before use. It must only be used if the solution is clear, colourless, with no solid particles visible. Before insertion of the cartridge into the reusable pen, the cartridge must be stored at room temperature for 1 to 2 hours. Air bubbles must be removed from the cartridge before injection (see instruction for using pen). Empty cartridges must not be refilled.

If the pen malfunctions (see instructions for using the pen), the solution may be drawn from the cartridge into a syringe (suitable for an insulin with 100 Units/ml) and injected. If the insulin pen is damaged or not working properly (due to mechanical defects) it has to be discarded, and a new insulin pen has to be used.

To prevent any kind of contamination, the re-usable pen and the pre-filled Optiset should be used by a single patient only.

OptiSet Prefilled Pen

Before first use, the pen must be stored at room temperature for 1 to 2 hours.

Inspect the cartridge before use. It must only be used if the solution is clear, colourless, with no solid particles visible, and if it is of water-like consistency. Since Apidra is a solution, it does not require resuspension before use.

Empty pens must never be used and must be properly discarded.

To prevent any kind of contamination, the use of the pre-filled pen should remain strictly for a single patient use.

Handling of the pen

The Instructions for Use included in the Package Leaflet must be read carefully before using OptiSet.

(see Handling of the pen on next page)

Handling of the pen

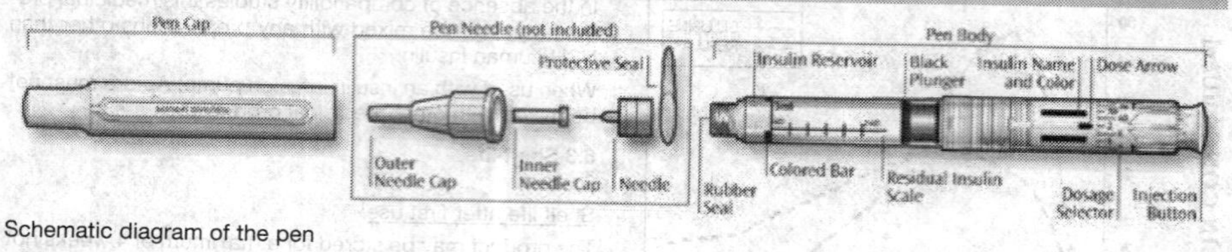

Schematic diagram of the pen

Important information for use of OptiSet:

- Always attach a new needle before each use. Only use needles that are compatible for use with OptiSet.
- Always perform the safety test before each injection.
- If a new OptiSet is used the initial safety test must be done with the 8 units preset by the manufacturer.
- The dosage selector can only be turned in one direction.
- Never turn the dosage selector (change the dose) after injection button has been pulled out.
- This pen is only for the patients use. It must not be shared with anyone else.
- If the injection is given by another person, special caution must be taken by this person to avoid accidental needle injury and transmission of infection.
- Never use OptiSet if it is damaged or if you are not sure that it is working properly.
- Always have a spare OptiSet in case your OptiSet is lost or damaged.

Storage Instructions

Please check section 6.4 of this leaflet for instructions on how to store OptiSet.

If OptiSet is in cool storage, it should be taken out 1 to 2 hours before injection to allow it to warm up. Cold insulin is more painful to inject.

The used OptiSet must be discarded as required by your local authorities.

Maintenance

OptiSet has to be protected from dust and dirt.

You can clean the outside of your OptiSet by wiping it with a damp cloth.

Do not soak, wash or lubricate the pen as this may damage it.

OptiSet is designed to work accurately and safely. It should be handled with care. Avoid situations where OptiSet might be damaged. If you are concerned that your OptiSet may be damaged, use a new one.

Step 1 Check the Insulin

After removing the pen cap, the label on the pen and the insulin reservoir should be checked to make sure it contains the correct insulin. The appearance of insulin should also be checked: the insulin solution must be clear, colourless, with no solid particles visible, and must have a water-like consistency. Do not use this OptiSet if the insulin is cloudy, coloured or has particles.

Step 2 Attach the needle

The needle should be carefully attached straight onto the pen.

Step 3 Perform a safety test

Prior to each injection a safety test has to be performed.

For a new and unused OptiSet, a dose of 8 units is already preset by the manufacturer for the first safety test.

In-use OptiSet, select a dose of 2 units by turning the dosage selector forward till the dose arrow points to 2. The dosage selector will only turn in one direction.

Pull out the injection button completely in order to load the dose. Never turn the dosage selector after injection button has been pulled out.

The outer and inner needle caps should be removed. Keep the outer cap to remove the used needle.

While holding the pen with the needle pointing upwards, the insulin reservoir should be tapped with the finger so that any air bubbles rise up towards the needle.

Then the injection button should be pressed all the way in.

If insulin has been expelled through the needle tip, then the pen and the needle are working properly.

If no insulin appears at the needle tip, step 3 should be repeated two more times until insulin appears at the needle tip. If still no insulin comes out, change the needle, as it might be blocked and try again. If no insulin comes out after changing the needle, the OptiSet may be damaged. Do not use this OptiSet.

Step 4 Select the dose

The dose can be set in steps of 2 units, from a minimum of 2 units to a maximum of 40 units. If a dose greater than 40 units is required, it should be given as two or more injections.

Check if you have enough insulin for the dose.

The residual insulin scale on the transparent insulin reservoir shows approximately how much insulin remains in the OptiSet. This scale must not be used to set the insulin dose.

If the black plunger is at the beginning of the coloured bar, then there are approximately 40 units of insulin available.

If the black plunger is at the end of the coloured bar, then there are approximately 20 units of insulin available.

The dosage selector should be turned forward until the dose arrow points to the required dose.

Step 5 Load the dose

The injection button should be pulled out as far as it will go in order to load the pen.

Check if the selected dose is fully loaded. Note that the injection button only goes out as far as the amount of insulin that is left in the reservoir.

The injection button allows checking the actual loaded dose. The injection button must be held out under tension during this check. The last thick line visible on the injection button shows the amount of insulin loaded. When the injection button is held out only the top part of this thick line can be seen.

Step 6 Inject the dose

The patient should be informed on the injection technique by his health care professional.

The needle should be inserted into the skin

The injection button should be pressed all the way in. A clicking sound can be heard, which will stop when the injection button has been pressed in completely. Then the injection button should be held down 10 seconds before withdrawing the needle from the skin. This ensures that the full dose of insulin has been delivered.

Step 7 Remove and discard the needle

The needle should be removed after each injection and discarded. This helps prevent contamination and/or infection as well as entry of air into the insulin reservoir and leakage, of the insulin, which can cause inaccurate dosing. Needles must not be reused.

The pen cap should be replaced on the pen.

Mixing with insulins

When mixed with NPH human insulin, Apidra should be drawn into the syringe first. Injection should be given immediately after mixing as no data are available regarding the mixtures made up a significant time before injection.

Continuous subcutaneous infusion pump

Apidra may be used for Continuous Subcutaneous Insulin Infusion (CSII) in pump systems suitable for insulin infusion with the appropriate catheters and reservoirs.

Patients using CSII should be comprehensively instructed on the use of the pump system. The infusion set and reservoir should be changed every 48 hours using aseptic technique.

Patients administering Apidra by CSII must have alternative insulin available in case of pump system failure.

7. MARKETING AUTHORISATION HOLDER

Sanofi-Aventis Deutschland GmbH, Brueningstrasse 50, D-65926 Frankfurt am Main, Germany.

8. MARKETING AUTHORISATION NUMBER(S)

Vial: EU/1/04/285/001

Cartridge: EU/1/04/285/008

Optiset pen: EU/1/04/285/016

9. DATE OF FIRST AUTHORISATION/RENEWAL OF THE AUTHORISATION

27 September 2004

10. DATE OF REVISION OF THE TEXT

20th June 2008

Legal category: POM

Apidra 100 Units/ml solution for injection in SoloStar pre-filled pen

(sanofi-aventis)

1. NAME OF THE MEDICINAL PRODUCT

Apidra 100 Units/ml, solution for injection in a pre-filled pen.

2. QUALITATIVE AND QUANTITATIVE COMPOSITION

Each ml contains 100 Units insulin glulisine (equivalent to 3.49 mg).

Each pen contains 3 ml of solution for injection, equivalent to 300 Units.

Insulin glulisine is produced by recombinant DNA technology in *Escherichia coli*.

For a full list of excipients, see section 6.1.

3. PHARMACEUTICAL FORM

Solution for injection in a pre-filled pen. SoloStar.

Clear, colourless, aqueous solution.

4. CLINICAL PARTICULARS

4.1 Therapeutic indications

Treatment of adults, adolescents and children, 6 years or older with diabetes mellitus, where treatment with insulin is required.

4.2 Posology and method of administration

The potency of this preparation is stated in units. These units are exclusive to Apidra and are not the same as IU or the units used to express the potency of other insulin analogues. See section 5.1 (Pharmacodynamics).

Apidra should be given shortly (0-15 min) before or soon after meals.

Apidra should be used in regimens that include an intermediate or long acting insulin or basal insulin analogue and can be used with oral hypoglycaemic agents.

The dosage of Apidra should be individually adjusted.

__Administration__

Apidra should be given by subcutaneous injection or by continuous subcutaneous pump infusion.

Apidra should be administered subcutaneously in the abdominal wall, thigh or deltoid or by continuous infusion in the abdominal wall. Injection sites and infusion sites within an injection area (abdomen, thigh or deltoid) should be rotated from one injection to the next. The rate of absorption, and consequently the onset and duration of action, may be affected by the injection site, exercise and other variables. Subcutaneous injection in the abdominal wall ensures a slightly faster absorption than other injection sites (see section 5.2).

Care should be taken to ensure that a blood vessel has not been entered. After injection, the site of injection should not be massaged. Patients must be educated to use proper injection techniques.

Mixing with insulins

In the absence of compatibility studies, insulin glulisine must not be mixed with other medicinal products except NPH human insulin.

Before using SoloStar, the Instructions for Use included in the Package Leaflet must be read carefully (see section 6.6).

__Special populations__

Renal impairment

The pharmacokinetic properties of insulin glulisine are generally maintained in patients with renal impairment. However, insulin requirements may be reduced in the presence of renal impairment (see section 5.2).

Hepatic impairment

The pharmacokinetic properties of insulin glulisine have not been investigated in patients with decreased liver function. In patients with hepatic impairment, insulin requirements may be diminished due to reduced capacity for gluconeogenesis and reduced insulin metabolism.

Elderly

Limited pharmacokinetic data are available in elderly patients with diabetes mellitus. Deterioration of renal function may lead to a decrease in insulin requirements.

Children and adolescents

There is insufficient clinical information on the use of Apidra in children younger than the age of 6 years.

4.3 Contraindications

Hypersensitivity to the active substance or to any of the excipients.

Hypoglycaemia.

4.4 Special warnings and precautions for use

Transferring a patient to a new type or brand of insulin should be done under strict medical supervision. Changes in strength, brand (manufacturer), type (regular, NPH, lente, etc.), species (animal) and/or method of manufacturing may result in a change in dosage. Concomitant oral antidiabetic treatment may need to be adjusted.

The use of inadequate dosages or discontinuation of treatment, especially in insulin-dependent diabetic, may lead to hyperglycaemia and diabetic ketoacidosis; conditions which are potentially lethal.

Switching a patient to another type or brand of insulin should be done under strict medical supervision and may require change in dose.

Hypoglycaemia

The time of occurrence of hypoglycaemia depends on the action profile of the insulins used and may, therefore, change when the treatment regimen is changed.

Conditions which may make the early warning symptoms of hypoglycaemia different or less pronounced include long duration of diabetes, intensified insulin therapy, diabetic nerve disease, medicinal products such as beta blockers or after transfer from animal-source insulin to human insulin.

Adjustment of dosage may be also necessary if patients undertake increased physical activity or change their usual meal plan. Exercise taken immediately after a meal may increase the risk of hypoglycaemia.

hen compared with soluble human insulin, if hypogly-aemia occurs after an injection with rapid acting analo-ues, it may occur earlier.

ncorrected hypoglycaemic or hyperglycaemic reactions an cause loss of consciousness, coma, or death.

sulin requirements may be altered during illness or emo-onal disturbances.

andling of the pen

efore using SoloStar, the Instructions for Use included in e Package Leaflet must be read carefully. SoloStar has to e used as recommended in these Instructions for Use (see ection 6.6).

.5 Interaction with other medicinal products and other rms of interaction

tudies on pharmacokinetic interactions have not been erformed. Based on empirical knowledge from similar edicinal products, clinically relevant pharmacokinetic teractions are unlikely to occur.

number of substances affect glucose metabolism and ay require dose adjustment of insulin glulisine and parti-ularly close monitoring.

ubstances that may enhance the blood-glucose-lowering ctivity and increase susceptibility to hypoglycaemia nclude oral antidiabetic agents, angiotensin converting nzyme (ACE) inhibitors, disopyramide, fibrates, fluoxe-ine, monoamide oxidase inhibitors (MAOIs), pentoxifylline, ropoxyphene, salicylates and sulfonamide antibiotics.

ubstances that may reduce the blood-glucose-lowering ctivity include corticosteroids, danazol, diazoxide, diure-ics, glucagon, isoniazid, phenothiazine derivatives, somatropin, sympathomimetic agents (e.g. epinephrine adrenaline], salbutamol, terbutaline), thyroid hormones, estrogens, progestins (e.g. in oral contraceptives), pro-ease inhibitors and atypical antipsychotic medicinal pro-ducts (e.g. olanzapine and clozapine).

Beta-blockers, clonidine, lithium salts or alcohol may either potentiate or weaken the blood-glucose-lowering activity of insulin. Pentamidine may cause hypoglycaemia, which may sometimes be followed by hyperglycaemia.

In addition, under the influence of sympatholytic medicinal products such as beta-blockers, clonidine, guanethidine and reserpine, the signs of adrenergic counter-regulation may be reduced or absent.

4.6 Pregnancy and lactation

Pregnancy

There are no adequate data on the use of insulin glulisine in pregnant women.

Animal reproduction studies have not revealed any differ-ences between insulin glulisine and human insulin regard-ing pregnancy, embryonal/foetal development, parturition or postnatal development (see section 5.3).

Caution should be exercised when prescribing to pregnant women. Careful monitoring of glucose control is essential.

It is essential for patients with pre-existing or gestational diabetes to maintain good metabolic control throughout pregnancy. Insulin requirements may decrease during the first trimester and generally increase during the second and third trimesters. Immediately after delivery, insulin require-ments decline rapidly.

Lactation

It is unknown whether insulin glulisine is excreted in human milk, but in general insulin does not pass into breast milk and is not absorbed after oral administration.

Breast-feeding mothers may require adjustments in insulin dose and diet.

4.7 Effects on ability to drive and use machines

The patient's ability to concentrate and react may be impaired as a result of hypoglycaemia or hyperglycaemia or, for example, as a result of visual impairment. This may constitute a risk in situations where these abilities are of special importance (e.g. driving a car or operating machin-ery).

Patients should be advised to take precautions to avoid hypoglycaemia whilst driving. This is particularly important in those who have reduced or absent awareness of the warning symptoms of hypoglycaemia or have frequent episodes of hypoglycaemia. The advisability of driving should be considered in these circumstances.

4.8 Undesirable effects

Hypoglycaemia, the most frequent undesirable effect of insulin therapy, may occur if the insulin dose is too high in relation to the insulin requirement.

The following related adverse reactions from clinical inves-tigations were listed below by system organ class and in order of decreasing incidence (very common: >1/10; com-mon: >1/100, <1/10; uncommon: > 1/1,000, < 1/100; rare: >1/10,000, <1/1,000; very rare: < 1/10,000).

Within each frequency grouping, undesirable effects are presented in order of decreasing seriousness.

Metabolism and nutrition disorders

Very common: Hypoglycaemia

Symptoms of hypoglycaemia usually occur suddenly. They may include cold sweats, cool pale skin, fatigue, nervous-ness or tremor, anxiousness, unusual tiredness or weak-ness, confusion, difficulty in concentration, drowsiness, excessive hunger, vision changes, headache, nausea

Figure 1

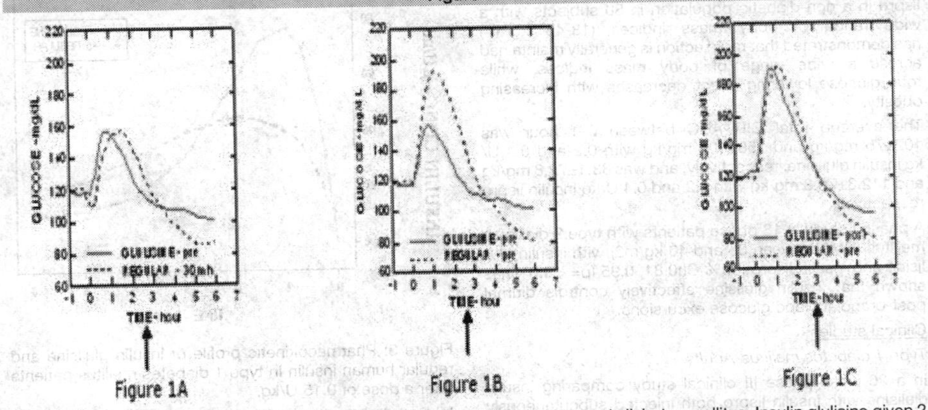

Figure 1: Average glucose-lowering effect over 6 hours in 20 patients with type 1 diabetes mellitus. Insulin glulisine given 2 minutes (GLULISINE pre) before the start of a meal compared to regular human insulin given 30 minutes (REGULAR 30 min) before the start of the meal (figure 1A) and compared to regular human insulin given 2 minutes (REGULAR pre) before a meal (figure 1B). Insulin glulisine given 15 minutes (GLULISINE post) after start of a meal compared to regular human insulin given 2 minutes (REGULAR pre) before start of the meal (figure 1C). On the x-axis, zero (arrow) is the start of a 15-minute meal.

and palpitation. Hypoglycaemia can become severe and may lead to unconsciousness and/or convulsions and may result in temporary or permanent impairment of brain func-tion or even death.

Skin and subcutaneous tissue disorders

Common: injection site reactions and local hypersensitivity reactions.

Local hypersensitivity reactions (redness, swelling and itching at the injection site) may occur during treatment with insulin. These reactions are usually transitory and normally they disappear during continued treatment.

Rare: Lipodystrophy

Lipodystrophy may occur at the injection site as a conse-quence of failure to rotate injection sites within an area.

General disorders

Uncommon: Systemic hypersensitivity reactions

Systemic hypersensitivity reactions may include urticaria, chest tightness, dyspnea, allergic dermatitis and pruritus. Severe cases of generalized allergy, including anaphylactic reaction, may be life-threatening.

4.9 Overdose

Hypoglycaemia may occur as a result of an excess of insulin activity relative to food intake and energy expendi-ture.

There are no specific data available concerning overdose with insulin glulisine. However, hypoglycaemia may develop over sequential stages:

Mild hypoglycaemic episodes can be treated by oral administration of glucose or sugary products. It is therefore recommended that the diabetic patient constantly carries some sugar lumps, sweets, biscuits or sugary fruit juice.

Severe hypoglycaemic episodes, where the patient has become unconscious, can be treated by glucagon (0.5 to 1 mg) given intramuscularly or subcutaneously by a person who has received appropriate instruction, or by glucose given intravenously by a medical professional. Glucose must also be given intravenously, if the patient does not respond to glucagon within 10 to 15 minutes.

Upon regaining consciousness, administration of oral car-bohydrate is recommended for the patient in order to prevent relapse.

After an injection of glucagon, the patient should be mon-itored in a hospital in order to find the reason for this severe hypoglycaemia and prevent other similar episodes.

5. PHARMACOLOGICAL PROPERTIES

5.1 Pharmacodynamic properties

Pharmacotherapeutic group: insulin and analogues, fast-acting. ATC code: A10AB06

Insulin glulisine is a recombinant human insulin analogue that is equipotent to regular human insulin. Insulin glulisine has a more rapid onset of action and a shorter duration of action than regular human insulin.

The primary activity of insulins and insulin analogues, including insulin glulisine, is regulation of glucose metabo-lism. Insulins lower blood glucose levels by stimulating peripheral glucose uptake, especially by skeletal muscle and fat, and by inhibiting hepatic glucose production. Insulin inhibits lipolysis in the adipocyte, inhibits proteolysis and enhances protein synthesis.

Studies in healthy volunteers and patients with diabetes demonstrated that insulin glulisine is more rapid in onset of action and of shorter duration of action than regular human insulin when given subcutaneously. When insuline glulisine is injected subcutaneously, the glucose lowering activity will begin within 10 – 20 minutes. The glucose-lowering activities of insulin glulisine and regular human insulin are equipotent when administered by intravenous route. One unit of insulin glulisine has the same glucose-lowering activity as one unit of regular human insulin.

Dose proportionality

In a study with 18 male subjects with diabetes mellitus type 1 aged 21 to 50 years, insulin glulisine displayed dose-proportional glucose lowering effect in the therapeutic relevant dose range 0.075 to 0.15 U/kg, and less than proportional increase in glucose lowering effect with 0.3 U/kg or higher, like human insulin.

Insulin glulisine takes effect about twice as fast as regular human insulin and completes the glucose lowering effect about 2 hours earlier than regular human insulin.

A phase I study in patients with type 1 diabetes mellitus assessed the glucose lowering profiles of insulin glulisine and regular human insulin administered subcutaneously at a dose of 0.15 U/kg, at different times in relation to a 15-minute standard meal. Data indicated that insulin glulisine administered 2 minutes before the meal gives similar post-prandial glycemic control compared to regular human insulin given 30 minutes before the meal. When given 2 minutes prior to meal, insulin glulisine provided better postprandial control than regular human insulin given 2 minutes before the meal. Insulin glulisine administered 15 minutes after starting the meal gives similar glycemic con-trol as regular human insulin given 2 minutes before the meal (see figure 1).

(see Figure 1 above)

Figure 1: Average glucose-lowering effect over 6 hours in 20 patients with type 1 diabetes mellitus. Insulin glulisine given 2 minutes (GLULISINE pre) before the start of a meal compared to regular human insulin given 30 minutes (REG-ULAR 30 min) before the start of the meal (figure 1A) and compared to regular human insulin given 2 minutes (REG-ULAR pre) before a meal (figure 1B). Insulin glulisine given 15 minutes (GLULISINE post) after start of a meal com-pared to regular human insulin given 2 minutes (REGULAR pre) before start of the meal (figure 1C). On the x-axis, zero (arrow) is the start of a 15-minute meal.

Obesity

A phase I study carried out with insulin glulisine, lispro and regular human insulin in an obese population has demon-strated that insulin glulisine maintains its rapid-acting prop-erties. In this study, the time to 20% of total AUC and the AUC (0-2h) representing the early glucose lowering activity were respectively of 114 minutes and 427mg.kg^{-1} for insu-lin glulisine, 121 minutes and 354mg.kg^{-1} for lispro, 150 minutes and 197mg.kg^{-1} for regular human insulin (see figure 2).

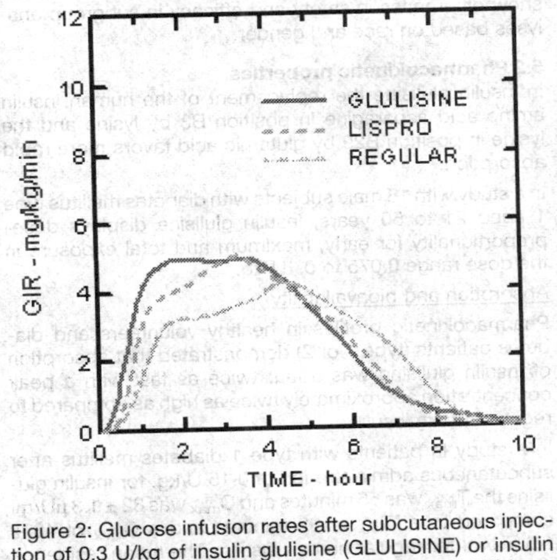

Figure 2: Glucose infusion rates after subcutaneous injec-tion of 0.3 U/kg of insulin glulisine (GLULISINE) or insulin lispro (LISPRO) or regular human insulin (REGULAR) in an obese population.

Another phase I study with insulin glulisine and insulin lispro in a non-diabetic population in 80 subjects with a wide range of body mass indices (18-46 kg/m^2) has demonstrated that rapid action is generally maintained across a wide range of body mass indices, while total glucose lowering effect decreases with increasing obesity.

The average total GIR AUC between 0–1 hour was 102±75 mg/kg and 158±100 mg/kg with 0.2 and 0.4 U/kg insulin glulisine, respectively, and was 83.1±72.8 mg/kg and 112.3±70.8 mg/kg with 0.2 and 0.4 U/kg insulin lispro respectively.

A phase I study in 18 obese patients with type 2 diabetes mellitus (BMI between 35 and 40 kg/m2) with insulin glulisine and insulin lispro [90% CI:0.81, 0.95 (p=<0.01)]has shown that insulin glulisine effectively controls diurnal post-prandial blood glucose excursions.

Clinical studies

Type 1 diabetes mellitus-Adults

In a 26-week phase III clinical study comparing insulin glulisine with insulin lispro both injected subcutaneously shortly (0-15 minutes) before a meal in patients with type 1 diabetes mellitus using insulin glargine as basal insulin, insulin glulisine was comparable to insulin lispro for glycemic control as reflected by changes in glycated haemoglobin (expressed as HbA_{1c} equivalent) from baseline to endpoint. Comparable self-monitored blood glucose values were observed. No increase in the basal insulin dose was needed with insulin glulisine, in contrast to insulin lispro.

A 12-week phase III clinical study performed in patients with type 1 diabetes mellitus receiving insulin glargine as basal therapy indicate that the immediate postmeal administration of insulin glulisine provides efficacy that was comparable to immediate premeal insulin glulisine (0-15 minutes) or regular insulin (30-45 minutes).

In the per protocol population there was a significantly larger observed reduction in GHb in the premeal glulisine group compared with the regular insulin group.

Type 1 diabetes mellitus -Paediatric

A 26-week phase III clinical study compared insulin glulisine with insulin lispro both injected subcutaneously shortly (0-15 minutes) before a meal in children (4-5 years: n=9; 6-7 years: n=32 and 8-11 years: n=149) and adolescents (12-17 years: n=382) with type 1 diabetes mellitus using insulin glargine or NPH as basal insulin. Insulin glulisine was comparable to insulin lispro for glycaemic control as reflected by changes in glycated haemoglobin (GHb expressed as HbA_{1c} equivalent) from baseline to endpoint and by self-monitored blood glucose values.

There is insufficient clinical information on the use of Apidra in children younger than the age of 6 years.

Type 2 diabetes mellitus-Adults

A 26-week phase III clinical study followed by a 26-week extension safety study was conducted to compare insulin glulisine (0-15 minutes before a meal) with regular human insulin (30-45 minutes before a meal) injected subcutaneously in patients with type 2 diabetes mellitus also using NPH insulin as basal insulin. The average body mass index (BMI) of patients was 34.55 kg/m^2. Insulin glulisine was shown to be comparable to regular human insulin with regard to glycated haemoglobin (expressed as HbA_{1c} equivalent) changes from baseline to the 6-month endpoint (-0.46% for insulin glulisine and -0.30% for regular human insulin, p=0.0029) and from baseline to the 12-month endpoint (-0.23% for insulin glulisine and -0.13% for regular human insulin, difference not significant). In this study, the majority of patients (79%) mixed their short acting insulin with NPH insulin immediately prior to injection and 58 % of subjects used oral hypoglycemic agents at randomization and were instructed to continue to use them at the same dose.

Race and Gender

In controlled clinical trials in adults, insulin glulisine did not show differences in safety and efficacy in subgroup analyses based on race and gender.

5.2 Pharmacokinetic properties

In insulin glulisine the replacement of the human insulin amino acid asparagine in position B3 by lysine and the lysine in position B29 by glutamic acid favors more rapid absorption.

In a study with 18 male subjects with diabetes mellitus type 1 aged 21 to 50 years, insulin glulisine displays dose-proportionality for early, maximum and total exposure in the dose range 0.075 to 0.4U/kg.

Absorption and bioavailability

Pharmacokinetic profiles in healthy volunteers and diabetes patients (type 1 or 2) demonstrated that absorption of insulin glulisine was about twice as fast with a peak concentration approximately twice as high as compared to regular human insulin.

In a study in patients with type 1 diabetes mellitus after subcutaneous administration of 0.15 U/kg, for insulin glulisine the T_{max} was 55 minutes and C_{max} was 82 ± 1.3 μU/ml compared to a T_{max} of 82 minutes and a C_{max} of 46 ± 1.3 μU/ml for regular human insulin. The mean residence time of insulin glulisine was shorter (98 min) than for regular human insulin (161 min) (see figure3).

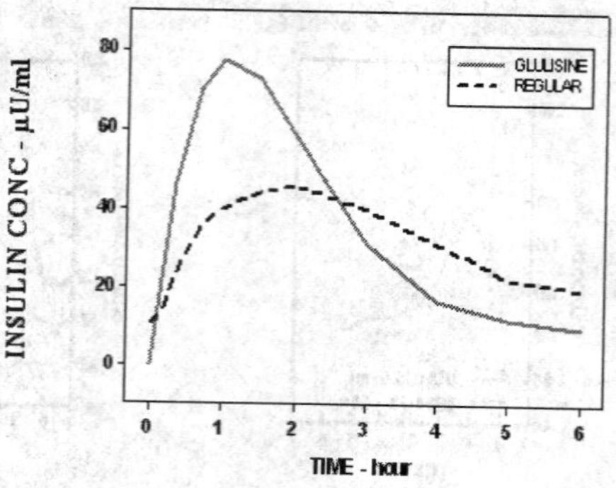

Figure 3: Pharmacokinetic profile of insulin glulisine and regular human insulin in type 1 diabetes mellitus patients after a dose of 0.15 U/kg.

In a study in patients with type 2 diabetes mellitus after subcutaneous administration of 0.2 U/kg insulin glulisine, the Cmax was 91 μU/ml with the interquartile range from 78 to 104 μU/ml.

When insulin glulisine was injected subcutaneously into abdomen, deltoid and thigh, the concentration-time profiles were similar with a slightly faster absorption when administered in the abdomen compared to the thigh. Absorption from deltoid sites was in-between (see section 4.2). The absolute bioavailability (70%) of insulin glulisine was similar between injection sites and of low intra-subject variability (11%CV).

Obesity

Another phase I study with insulin glulisine and insulin lispro in a non-diabetic population in 80 subjects with a wide range of body mass indices (18-46 kg/m^2) has demonstrated that rapid absorption and total exposure is generally maintained across a wide range of body mass indices. The time to 10% of total INS exposure was reached earlier by approximately 5–6 min with insulin glulisine.

Distribution and elimination

The distribution and elimination of insulin glulisine and regular human insulin after intravenous administration is similar with volumes of distribution of 13 l and 22 l and half-lives of 13 and 18 minutes, respectively.

After subcutaneous administration, insulin glulisine is eliminated more rapidly than regular human insulin with an apparent half-life of 42 minutes compared to 86 minutes. In an across study analysis of insulin glulisine in either healthy subjects or subjects with type 1 or type 2 diabetes mellitus the apparent half-life ranged from 37 to 75 minutes (interquartile range).

Insulin glulisine shows low plasma protein binding, similar to human insulin.

Special populations

Renal impairment

In a clinical study performed in non-diabetic subjects covering a wide range of renal function (CrCl> 80 ml/min, 30-50 ml/min, < 30 ml/min), the rapid-acting properties of insulin glulisine were generally maintained. However, insulin requirements may be reduced in the presence of renal impairment.

Hepatic impairment

The pharmacokinetic properties have not been investigated in patients with impaired liver function.

Elderly

Very limited pharmacokinetic data are available for elderly patients with diabetes mellitus.

Children and adolescents

The pharmacokinetic and pharmacodynamic properties of insulin glulisine were investigated in children (7-11 years) and adolescents (12-16 years) with type 1 diabetes mellitus. Insulin glulisine was rapidly absorbed in both age groups, with similar T_{max} and C_{max} as in adults (see section 4.2). Administered immediately before a test meal, insulin glulisine provided better postprandial control than regular human insulin, as in adults (see section 5.1). The glucose excursion (AUC_{0-6h}) was 641 mg.h.dl^{-1} for insulin glulisine and 801mg.h.dl^{-1} for regular human insulin.

5.3 Preclinical safety data

Non-clinical data did not reveal toxicity findings others than those linked to the blood glucose lowering pharmacodynamic activity (hypoglycemia), different from regular human insulin or of clinical relevance for humans.

6. PHARMACEUTICAL PARTICULARS

6.1 List of excipients

Metacresol

Sodium chloride

Trometamol

Polysorbate 20

Hydrochloric acid, concentrated

Sodium hydroxide

Water for injections

6.2 Incompatibilities

In the absence of compatibility studies, this medicinal product must not be mixed with other medicinal product except NPH human insulin.

6.3 Shelf life

2 years.

Shelf life after first use of the pen:

The product may be stored for a maximum of 4 weeks not above 25°C away from direct heat or direct light. Pens in use must not be stored in the refrigerator. The pen cap must be put back on the pen after each injection in order to protect from light.

6.4 Special precautions for storage

Not in-use pens

Store in a refrigerator (2°C - 8°C).

Do not freeze.

Do not put Apidra next to the freezer compartment or a freezer pack.

Keep the pre-filled pen in the outer carton in order to protect from light.

In use pens

For storage precautions, see section 6.3.

6.5 Nature and contents of container

3 ml solution in a cartridge (colourless glass) with a plunger (elastomeric rubber) and a flanged cap (flanged aluminium) with a stopper (elastomeric rubber). The cartridge is sealed in a disposable pre-filled pen. Packs of 5, pens are available.

6.6 Special precautions for disposal and other handling

Before first use, the pen must be stored at room temperature for 1 to 2 hours.

Inspect the cartridge before use. It must only be used if the solution is clear, colourless, with no solid particles visible, and if it is of water-like consistency. Since Apidra is a solution, it does not require resuspension before use.

Empty pens must never be used and must be properly discarded.

To prevent any kind of contamination, the use of the pre-filled pen should remain strictly for a single patient use.

Handling of the pen

The Instructions for Use included in the Package Leaflet must be read carefully before using SoloStar.

(see Handling of the pen below)

Important information for use of SoloStar:

Before each use, a new needle must always be carefully attached and a safety test must be performed. Only use needles that are compatible for use with SoloStar.

Special caution must be taken to avoid accidental needle injury and transmission of infection.

Never use SoloStar if it is damaged or if you are not sure that it is working properly.

Always have a spare SoloStar in case your SoloStar is lost or damaged.

Storage Instructions

Please check section 6.4 for instructions on how to store SoloStar.

If SoloStar is in cool storage, it should be taken out 1 to 2 hours before you inject to allow it to warm up. Cold insulin is more painful to inject.

The used SoloStar must be discarded as required by your local authorities.

Maintenance

SoloStar has to be protected from dust and dirt.

The outside of SoloStar can be cleaned by wiping it with a damp cloth.

Do not soak, wash or lubricate the pen as this may damage it.

Handling of the pen

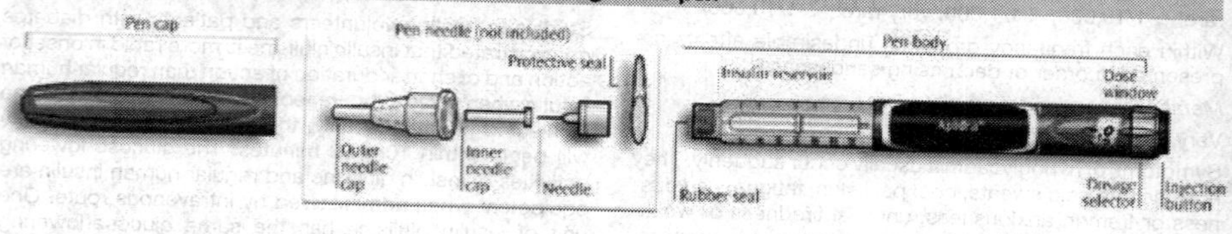

Schematic diagram of the pen

SoloStar is designed to work accurately and safely. It should be handled with care. Situations where SoloStar might be damaged must be avoided. If you are concerned that your SoloStar may be damaged, use a new one.

Step 1 Check the Insulin

The label on the pen should be checked to make sure it contains the correct insulin. The Apidra SoloStar is blue. It has a dark blue injection button with a raised ring on the top. After removing the pen cap, the appearance of insulin should also be checked: the insulin solution must be clear, colourless, with no solid particles visible, and must have a water-like consistency.

Step 2 Attach the needle

Only needles that are compatible for use with SoloStar should be used.

A new sterile needle will be always used for each injection. After removing the cap, the needle should be carefully attached straight onto the pen.

Step 3 Perform a safety test

Prior to each injection a safety test has to be performed.

Select a dose of 2.

The outer and inner needle caps should be removed.

While holding the pen with the needle pointing upwards, the insulin reservoir should be tapped gently with the finger so that any air bubbles rise up towards the needle.

Then the injection button should be pressed in completely.

If insulin has been expelled through the needle tip, then the pen and the needle are working properly.

If no insulin appears at the needle tip, step 3 should be repeated until insulin appears at the needle tip.

Step 4 Select the dose

The dose can be set in steps of 1 unit, from a minimum of 1 unit to a maximum of 80 units. If a dose greater than 80 units is required, it should be given as two or more injections.

The dose window must show "0" following the safety test. The dose can then be selected.

Step 5 Inject the dose

The patient should be informed on the injection technique by his health care professional.

The needle should be inserted into the skin.

The injection button should be pressed in completely. Then the injection button should be held down 10 seconds before withdrawing the needle. This ensures that the full dose of insulin has been injected.

Step 6 Remove and discard the needle

The needle should always be removed after each injection and discarded. This helps prevent contamination and/or infection, entry of air into the insulin reservoir and leakage of insulin. Needles must not be reused.

Special caution must be taken when removing and disposing the needle. Follow recommended safety measures for removal and disposal of needles (e.g. a one handed capping technique) in order to reduce the risk of accidental needle injury and transmission of infectious diseases.

The pen cap should be replaced on the pen.

Mixing with insulins

When mixed with NPH human insulin, Apidra should be drawn into the syringe first. Injection should be given immediately after mixing, as no data are available regarding the mixtures made up a significant time before injection.

7. MARKETING AUTHORISATION HOLDER

Sanofi-Aventis Deutschland GmbH, Brueningstrasse 50, D-65926 Frankfurt am Main, Germany.

8. MARKETING AUTHORISATION NUMBER(S)

EU/1/04/285/032

9. DATE OF FIRST AUTHORISATION/RENEWAL OF THE AUTHORISATION

Date of first authorisation: 27 September 2004

10. DATE OF REVISION OF THE TEXT

20th June 2008

Legal category

POM

APO-go ampoules 10mg/ml

(Britannia Pharmaceuticals)

1. NAME OF THE MEDICINAL PRODUCT

APO-go AMPOULES 10 mg/ml Solution for Injection

or

APO-go AMPUL 10 mg/ml Solution for Injection (Denmark)

or

APO-go 10 mg/ml Solution for Injection (Sweden)

or

APOgo 10 mg/ml Solution for Injection (France)

2. QUALITATIVE AND QUANTITATIVE COMPOSITION

Each ml contains 10mg apomorphine hydrochloride 0.5 H_2O

2ml contains 20mg apomorphine hydrochloride 0.5 H_2O

5ml contains 50mg apomorphine hydrochloride 0.5 H_2O

For a full list of excipients, see section 6.1

3. PHARMACEUTICAL FORM

Solution for Injection

Solution is clear and colourless

4. CLINICAL PARTICULARS

4.1 Therapeutic indications

The treatment of disabling motor fluctuations ("on-off" phenomena) in patients with Parkinson's disease which persist despite individually titrated treatment with levodopa (with a peripheral decarboxylase inhibitor) and/or other dopamine agonists.

4.2 Posology and method of administration

APO-go Ampoules 10 mg/ml Solution for Injection is for subcutaneous use by intermittent bolus injection. APO-go Ampoules 10 mg/ml Solution for Injection may also be administered as a continuous subcutaneous infusion by minipump and/or syringe-driver (see section 6.6).

Apomorphine must not be used via the intravenous route.

Dosage

Adults

Administration

Selection of Patients suitable for APO-go injections:

Patients selected for treatment with APO-go should be able to recognise the onset of their 'off' symptoms and be capable of injecting themselves or else have a responsible carer able to inject for them when required.

It is essential that the patient is established on domperidone, usually 20mg three times daily, for at least two days prior to initiation of therapy.

Apomorphine should be initiated in the controlled environment of a specialist clinic. The patient should be supervised by a physician experienced in the treatment of Parkinson's disease (e.g. neurologist). The patient's treatment with levodopa, with or without dopamine agonists, should be optimised before starting APO-go treatment.

Determination of the threshold dose.

The appropriate dose for each patient is established by incremental dosing schedules. The following schedule is suggested:-

1mg of apomorphine HCl (0.1ml), that is approximately 15-20 micrograms/kg, may be injected subcutaneously during a hypokinetic or 'off' period and the patient is observed over 30 minutes for a motor response.

If no response, or an inadequate response, is obtained a second dose of 2 mg of apomorphine HCl (0.2ml) is injected subcutaneously and the patient observed for an adequate response for a further 30 minutes.

The dosage may be increased by incremental injections with at least a forty minute interval between succeeding injections, until a satisfactory motor response is obtained.

Establishment of treatment.

Once the appropriate dose is determined, a single subcutaneous injection may be given into the lower abdomen or outer thigh at the first signs of an 'off' episode. It cannot be excluded that absorption may differ with different injection sites within a single individual. Accordingly, the patient should then be observed for the next hour to assess the quality of their response to treatment. Alterations in dosage may be made according to the patient's response.

The optimal dosage of apomorphine hydrochloride varies between individuals but, once established, remains relatively constant for each patient.

Precautions on continuing treatment.

The daily dose of APO-go varies widely between patients, typically within the range of 3-30 mg, given as 1-10 injections and sometimes as many as 12 separate injections per day.

It is recommended that the total daily dose of apomorphine HCl should not exceed 100 mg and that individual bolus injections should not exceed 10 mg.

In clinical studies it has usually been possible to make some reduction in the dose of levodopa; this effect varies considerably between patients and needs to be carefully managed by an experienced physician.

Once treatment has been established, domperidone therapy may be gradually reduced in some patients but successfully eliminated only in a few, without any vomiting or hypotension.

Continuous Infusion

Patients who have shown a good 'on' period response during the initiation stage, but whose overall control remains unsatisfactory using intermittent injections, or who require many and frequent injections (more than 10 per day), may be commenced on or transferred to continuous subcutaneous infusion by minipump and/or syringe-driver (see section 6.6)as follows:-

Continuous infusion is started at a rate of 1 mg apomorphine HCl (0.1 ml) per hour then increased according to the individual response. Increases in the infusion rate should not exceed 0.5 mg per hour at intervals of not less than 4 hours. Hourly infusion rates may range between 1 mg and 4 mg (0.1 ml and 0.4 ml), equivalent to 0.015 - 0.06 mg/kg/hour. Infusions should run for waking hours only. Unless the patient is experiencing severe night-time problems, 24 hour infusions are not advised. Tolerance to the therapy does not seem to occur as long as there is an overnight period without treatment of at least 4 hours. In any event, the infusion site should be changed every 12 hours.

Patients may need to supplement their continuous infusion with intermittent bolus boosts via the pump system as necessary, and as directed by their physician.

A reduction in dosage of other dopamine agonists may be considered during continuous infusion.

Children and adolescents:

APO-go Ampoules 10 mg/ml Solution for Injection is contraindicated for children and adolescents under 18 years of age (see section 4.3).

Elderly:

The elderly are well represented in the population of patients with Parkinson's disease and constitute a high proportion of those studied in clinical trials of APO-go. The management of elderly patients treated with APO-go has not differed from that of younger patients.

Renal impairment:

A dose schedule similar to that recommended for adults, and the elderly, can be followed for patients with renal impairment (see section 4.4).

4.3 Contraindications

In patients with respiratory depression, dementia, psychotic diseases or hepatic insufficiency.

Intermittent apomorphine HCl treatment is not suitable for patients who have an 'on' response to levodopa which is marred by severe dyskinesia or dystonia.

APO-go should not be administered to patients who have a known hypersensitivity to apomorphine or any excipients of the medicinal product.

APO-go is contraindicated for children and adolescents under 18 years of age.

4.4 Special warnings and precautions for use

Apomorphine HCl should be given with caution to patients with renal, pulmonary or cardiovascular disease and persons prone to nausea and vomiting.

Extra caution is recommended during initiation of therapy in elderly and/or debilitated patients.

Since apomorphine may produce hypotension, even when given with domperidone pretreatment, care should be exercised in patients with pre-existing cardiac disease or in patients taking vasoactive medicinal products such as antihypertensives, and especially in patients with pre-existing postural hypotension.

Apomorphine is associated with local subcutaneous effects. These can sometimes be reduced by the rotation of injection sites or possibly by the use of ultrasound (if available) to areas of nodularity and induration.

APO-go Ampoules 10mg/ml Solution for Injection contains sodium metabisulphite which may rarely cause severe allergic reactions and bronchospasm.

Haemolytic anaemia and thrombocytopenia have been reported in patients treated with apomorphine. Haematology tests should be undertaken at regular intervals as with levodopa, when given concomitantly with apomorphine.

Caution is advised when combining apomorphine with other medicinal products, especially those with a narrow therapeutic range (see section 4.5).

Neuropsychiatric problems co-exist in many patients with advanced Parkinson's disease. There is evidence that for some patients neuropsychiatric disturbances may be exacerbated by apomorphine. Special care should be exercised when apomorphine is used in these patients.

Apomorphine has been associated with somnolence, and other dopamine agonists can be associated with sudden sleep onset episodes, particularly in patients with Parkinson's disease. Patients must be informed of this and advised to exercise caution while driving or operating machines during treatment with apomorphine. Patients who have experienced somnolence must refrain from driving or operating machines. Furthermore, a reduction of dosage or termination of therapy may be considered.

Pathological gambling, increased libido and hypersexuality have been reported in patients treated with dopamine agonists for Parkinson's disease, including apomorphine.

4.5 Interaction with other medicinal products and other forms of interaction

Patients selected for treatment with apomorphine HCl are almost certain to be taking concomitant medications for their Parkinson's disease. In the initial stages of apomorphine HCl therapy, the patient should be monitored for unusual side-effects or signs of potentiation of effect.

Neuroleptic medicinal products may have an antagonistic effect if used with apomorphine. There is a potential interaction between clozapine and apomorphine, however clozapine may also be used to reduce the symptoms of neuropsychiatric complications.

If neuroleptic medicinal products have to be used in patients with Parkinson's disease treated by dopamine agonists, a gradual reduction in apomorphine dose may be considered when administration is by minipump and/or syringe-driver (symptoms suggestive of neuroleptic malignant syndrome have been reported rarely with abrupt withdrawal of dopaminergic therapy).

4.6 Pregnancy and lactation

There is no experience of apomorphine usage in pregnant women.

Animal reproduction studies do not indicate any teratogenic effects, but doses given to rats which are toxic to the mother can lead to failure to breathe in the newborn. The potential risk for humans is unknown. See Section 5.3.

APO-go should not be used in pregnancy unless clearly necessary.

It is not known whether apomorphine is excreted in breast milk. A decision on whether to continue/discontinue breastfeeding or to continue/discontinue therapy with APO-go should be made taking into account the benefit of breast-feeding to the child and the benefit to APO-go to the women.

4.7 Effects on ability to drive and use machines

Patients being treated with apomorphine and presenting with somnolence and/or sudden sleep episodes must be informed to refrain from driving or engaging in activities (e.g. operating machines) where impaired alertness may put themselves or others at risk of serious injury or death until such recurrent episodes and somnolence have resolved (see also section 4.4).

4.8 Undesirable effects

Very common ($\geq$1/10)

Common ($\geq$1/100 to $<$1/10)

Uncommon ($\geq$1/1,000 to $<$1/100)

Rare ($\geq$1/10,000 to $<$1/1,000)

Very rare ($<$1/10,000)

Not known (cannot be estimated from the available data)

Blood and lymphatic system disorders

Uncommon:

Haemolytic anaemia and thrombocytopenia have been reported in patients treated with apomorphine.

Rare:

Eosinophilia has rarely occurred during treatment with apomorphine HCl.

Immune system disorders

Rare:

Due to the presence of sodium metabisulphite, allergic reactions (including anaphylaxis and bronchospasm) may occur.

Psychiatric disorders

Common:

Neuropsychiatric disturbances are common in parkinsonian patients. APO-go should be used with special caution in these patients. Neuropsychiatric disturbances (including transient mild confusion and visual hallucinations) have occurred during apomorphine HCl therapy.

Not known:

Patients treated with dopamine agonists for treatment of Parkinson's disease, including apomorphine, especially at high doses, have been reported as exhibiting signs of pathological gambling, increased libido and hypersexuality; generally reversible upon reduction of the dose or treatment discontinuation.

Nervous system disorders

Common:

Transient sedation with each dose of apomorphine HCl at the start of therapy may occur; this usually resolves over the first few weeks.

Apomorphine is associated with somnolence.

Dizziness / light-headedness have also been reported.

Uncommon:

Apomorphine may induce dyskinesias during 'on' periods, which can be severe in some cases, and in a few patients may result in cessation of therapy.

Vascular disorders

Uncommon:

Postural hypotension is seen infrequently and is usually transient (See Section 4.4).

Respiratory, thoracic and mediastinal disorders

Common:

Yawning has been reported during apomorphine therapy.

Uncommon:

Breathing difficulties have been reported.

Gastrointestinal disorders

Common:

Nausea and vomiting, particularly when apomorphine treatment is first initiated, usually as a result of the omission of domperidone (See Section 4.2).

Skin and subcutaneous tissue disorders

Uncommon:

Local and generalised rashes have been reported.

General disorders and administration site conditions

Very common:

Most patients experience injection site reactions, particularly with continuous use. These may include subcutaneous nodules, induration, erythema, tenderness and panniculitis. Various other local reactions (such as irritation, itching, bruising and pain) may also occur.

Uncommon:

Injection site necrosis and ulceration have been reported.

Not Known:

Peripheral oedema has been reported.

Investigations

Uncommon:

Positive Coombs' tests have been reported for patients receiving apomorphine.

4.9 Overdose

There is little clinical experience of overdose with apomorphine by this route of administration. Symptoms of overdosemay be treated empirically as suggested below:-

Excessive emesis may be treated with domperidone.

Respiratory depression may be treated with naloxone.

Hypotension: appropriate measures should be taken, e.g. raising the foot of the bed.

Bradycardia may be treated with atropine.

5. PHARMACOLOGICAL PROPERTIES

5.1 Pharmacodynamic properties

Pharmacotherapeutic group: Dopamine agonists ATC Classification: N04B C07

Apomorphine is a direct stimulant of dopamine receptors and, while possessing both D1 and D2 receptor agonist properties, does not share transport or metabolic pathways with levodopa.

Although in intact experimental animals, administration of apomorphine suppresses the rate of firing of nigro-striatal cells and in low dose has been found to produce a reduction in locomotor activity (thought to represent pre-synaptic inhibition of endogenous dopamine release) its actions on parkinsonian motor disability are likely to be mediated at post-synaptic receptor sites. This biphasic effect is also seen in humans.

5.2 Pharmacokinetic properties

After subcutaneous injection of apomorphine its fate can be described by a two-compartment model, with a distribution half-life of 5 (±1.1) minutes and an elimination half-life of 33 (±3.9)minutes. Clinical response correlates well with levels of apomorphine in the cerebrospinal fluid; the active substance distribution being best described by a two-compartment model. Apomorphine is rapidly and completely absorbed from subcutaneous tissue, correlating with the rapid onset of clinical effects (4-12 minutes), and that the brief duration of clinical action of the active substance (about 1 hour) is explained by its rapid clearance. The metabolism of apomorphine is by glucuronidation and sulphonation to at least ten per cent of the total; other pathways have not been described.

5.3 Preclinical safety data

Repeat dose subcutaneous toxicity studies reveal no special hazard for humans, beyond the information included in other sections of the SmPC.

In vitro genotoxicity studies demonstrated mutagenic and clastogenic effects, most likely due to products formed by oxidation of apomorphine. However, apomorphine was not genotoxic in the *in vivo* studies performed.

The effect of apomorphine on reproduction has been investigated in rats. Apomorphine was not teratogenic in this species, but it was noted that doses which are toxic to the mother can cause loss of maternal care and failure to breathe in the newborn.

No carcinogenicity studies have been performed.

6. PHARMACEUTICAL PARTICULARS

6.1 List of excipients

Sodium metabisulphite (E223)

Hydrochloric acid (37%)

Sodium hydroxide (99%)

Water for injections

6.2 Incompatibilities

In the absence of compatibility studies, this medicinal product must not be mixed with other medicinal products.

6.3 Shelf life

3 years

6.4 Special precautions for storage

Do not store above 25°C.

Store in the original package in order to protect from light.

6.5 Nature and contents of container

Type I glass ampoules containing 2ml solution for injection, in packs of 5 ampoules.

Type I glass ampoules containing 5ml solution for injection, in packs of 5 ampoules.

Bundle pack of 25 and 50 ampoules are available in some territories.

The 25 ampoule bundles pack consists of 5 packs each containing 5 ampoules.

The 50 ampoule bundles pack consists of 10 packs each containing 5 ampoules.

Not all pack sizes are marketed.

6.6 Special precautions for disposal and other handlir

Do not use if the solution has turned green.

The solution should be inspected visually prior to use. On clear and colourless solutions should be used.

For single use only. Any unused solution should be di carded.

Continuous infusion and the use of a minipump and/c syringe-driver.

The choice of which minipump and/or syringe-driver t use, and the dosage settings required, will be determine by the physician in accordance with the particular needs c the patient.

7. MARKETING AUTHORISATION HOLDER

Britannia Pharmaceuticals Limited

41 - 51 Brighton Road

Redhill

Surrey

RH1 6YS

United Kingdom

8. MARKETING AUTHORISATION NUMBER(S)

PL 04483/0064

PA 356/9/2

9. DATE OF FIRST AUTHORISATION/RENEWAL OF THE AUTHORISATION

January 2000 / January 2005

10. DATE OF REVISION OF THE TEXT

July 2009

APO-go Pen 10mg/ml Solution for Injection

(Britannia Pharmaceuticals)

1. NAME OF THE MEDICINAL PRODUCT

APO-go PEN 10 mg/ml Solution for Injection*

*** Abbreviated to APO-go® Pen in the text**

2. QUALITATIVE AND QUANTITATIVE COMPOSITION

1ml contains 10mg apomorphine hydrochloride

For a full list of excipients see section 6.1

3. PHARMACEUTICAL FORM

Solution for injection.

Solution is clear and colourless.

4. CLINICAL PARTICULARS

4.1 Therapeutic indications

The treatment of disabling motor fluctuations ('on-off' phenomena) in patients with Parkinson's disease which persist despite individually titrated treatment with levodopa (with a peripheral decarboxylase inhibitor) and/or other dopamine agonists.

4.2 Posology and method of administration

APO-go Pen 10 mg/ml Solution for Injection is for subcutaneous use by intermittent bolus injection.

Dosage

Adults

Administration

Selection of patients suitable for APO-go injections:

> Patients selected for treatment with APO-go should be able to recognise the onset of their 'off' symptoms and be capable of injecting themselves or else have a responsible carer able to inject for them when required. It is essential that the patient is established on domperidone, usually 20mg three times daily for at least two days prior to initiation of therapy. Apomorphine should be initiated in the controlled environment of a specialist clinic. The treatment should be supervised by a physician experienced in the treatment of Parkinson's disease (e.g. Neurologist). The patient's treatment with levodopa, with or without dopamine agonists, should be optimised before starting APO-go treatment.

Determination of the threshold dose.

The appropriate dose for each patient is established by incremental dosing schedules. The following schedule is suggested:-

1mg of apomorphine HCl (0.1ml), that is approximately 15-20 micrograms/kg, may be injected subcutaneously during a hypokinetic, or 'off' period and the patient is observed over 30 minutes for a motor response.

If no response, or an inadequate response, is obtained a second dose of 2 mg of apomorphine HCl (0.2ml) is injected subcutaneously and the patient observed for an adequate response for a further 30 minutes.

The dosage may be increased by incremental injections with at least a forty minute interval between succeeding injections, until a satisfactory motor response is obtained.

Establishment of treatment.

Once the appropriate dose is determined, a single subcutaneous injection may be given into the lower abdomen or outer thigh at the first signs of an 'off' episode. It cannot be excluded that absorption may differ with different ection sites within a single individual. Accordingly, the atient should then be observed for the next hour to assess e quality of their response to treatment. Alterations in osage may be made according to the patient's response.

e optimal dosage of apomorphine hydrochloride varies etween individuals but, once established, remains relaely constant for each patient.

ecautions on continuing treatment.

e daily dose of APO-go varies widely between patients, pically within the range of 3-30mg, given as 1-10 injecons and sometimes as many as 12 separate injections per ay.

is recommended that the total daily dose of apomorphine Cl should not exceed 100mg and that individual bolus jections should not exceed 10mg.

clinical studies it has usually been possible to make ome reduction in the dose of levodopa; this effect varies onsiderably between patients and needs to be carefully anaged by an experienced physician.

nce treatment has been established domperidone therpy may be gradually reduced in some patients but sucessfully eliminated only in a few, without any vomiting or ypotension.

hildren and adolescents:

PO-go Pen 10mg/ml Solution for Injection is contra-indiated for children and adolescents under 18 years of age ee section 4.3).

lderly:

he elderly are well represented in the population of atients with Parkinson's disease and constitute a high roportion of those studied in clinical trials of APO-go. The anagement of elderly patients treated with APO-go has ot differed from that of younger patients.

enal impairment:

dose schedule similar to that recommended for adults, nd the elderly, can be followed for patients with renal npairment (see section 4.4).

.3 Contraindications

n patients with respiratory depression, dementia, psychoic diseases or hepatic insufficiency.

ntermittent apomorphine HCl treatment is not suitable for atients who have an 'on' response to levodopa, which is narred by severe dyskinesia or dystonia.

APO-go should not be administered to patients who have a known hypersensitivity to apomorphine or any excipients of the medicinal product.

APO-go is contra-indicated for children and adolescents under 18 years of age.

4.4 Special warnings and precautions for use

Apomorphine HCl should be given with caution to patients with renal, pulmonary or cardiovascular disease and persons prone to nausea and vomiting.

Extra caution is recommended during initiation of therapy in elderly and/or debilitated patients.

Since apomorphine may produce hypotension, even when given with domperidone pretreatment, care should be exercised in patients with pre-existing cardiac disease or in patients taking vasoactive medicinal products such as antihypertensives, especially in patients with pre-existing postural hypotension.

Apomorphine is associated with local subcutaneous effects. These can sometimes be reduced by the rotation of injection sites or possibly by the use of ultrasound (if available) to areas of nodularity and induration.

APO-go Pen 10mg/ml Solution for Injection contains sodium bisulphite which may rarely cause severe allergic reactions and bronchospasm.

Haemolytic anaemia and thrombocytopenia have been reported in patients treated with apomorphine. Haematology tests should be undertaken at regular intervals, as with levodopa, when given concomitantly with apomorphine.

Caution is advised when combining apomorphine with other medicinal products, especially those with a narrow therapeutic range (see section 4.5).

Neuropsychiatric problems co-exist in many patients with advanced Parkinson's disease. There is evidence that for some patients neuropsychiatric disturbances may be exacerbated by apomorphine.

Special care should be exercised when apomorphine is used in these patients.

Apomorphine has been associated with somnolence, and other dopamine agonists can be associated with sudden sleep onset episodes, particularly in patients with Parkinson's disease. Patients must be informed of this and advised to exercise caution while driving or operating machines during treatment with apomorphine. Patients who have experienced somnolence must refrain from driving or operating machines. Furthermore, a reduction of dosage or termination of therapy may be considered.

Pathological gambling, increased libido and hypersexuality have been reported in patients treated with dopamine agonists for Parkinson's disease, including apomorphine.

4.5 Interaction with other medicinal products and other forms of interaction

Patients selected for treatment with apomorphine HCl are almost certain to be taking concomitant medications for their Parkinson's disease. In the initial stages of apomorphine HCl therapy the patient should be monitored for unusual side-effects or signs of potentiation of effect.

Neuroleptic medicinal products may have an antagonistic effect if used with apomorphine. There is a potential interaction between clozapine and apomorphine, however clozapine may also be used to reduce the symptoms of neuropsychiatric complications.

The possible effects of apomorphine on the plasma concentrations of other drugs have not been studied. Therefore caution is advised when combining apomorphine with other medicinal products, especially those with a narrow therapeutic range.

Antihypertensive and Cardiac Active Medicinal Drugs

Even when co-administered with domperidone, apomorphine may potentiate the antihypertensive effects of these drugs. (See section 4.4).

4.6 Pregnancy and lactation

There is no experience of apomorphine usage in pregnant women.

Animal reproduction studies do not indicate any teratogenic effects, but doses given to rats which are toxic to the mother can lead to failure to breathe in the newborn. The potential risk for humans is unknown. See Section 5.3.

APO-go should not be used during pregnancy unless clearly necessary.

It is not know whether apomorphine is excreted in breast milk. A decision on whether to continue/discontinue breastfeeding or to continue/discontinue therapy with APO-go should be made taking into account the benefit of breast-feeding to the child and the benefit of APO-go to the woman.

4.7 Effects on ability to drive and use machines

Patients being treated with apomorphine and presenting with somnolence must be informed to refrain from driving or engaging in activities (e.g. operating machines) where impaired alertness may put themselves or others at risk of serious injury or death unless patients have overcome such experiences of somnolence (see also Section 4.4).

4.8 Undesirable effects

Very common (≥1/10)

Common (≥1/100 to <1/10)

Uncommon (≥1/1,000 to <1/100)

Rare (≥1/10,000 to <1/1,000)

Very rare (<1/10,000)

Not known (cannot be estimated from the available data)

Blood and lymphatic system disorders

Uncommon:

Haemolytic anaemia and thrombocytopenia have been reported in patients treated with apomorphine.

Rare:

Eosinophilia has rarely occurred during treatment with apomorphine HCl.

Immune system disorders

Rare:

Due to the presence of sodium metabisulphite, allergic reactions (including anaphylaxis and bronchospasm) may occur.

Psychiatric disorders

Common:

Neuropsychiatric disturbances are common in parkinsonian patients. APO-go should be used with special caution in these patients. Neuropsychiatric disturbances (including transient mild confusion and visual hallucinations) have occurred during apomorphine HCl therapy.

Not known:

Patients treated with dopamine agonists for treatment of Parkinson's disease, including apomorphine, especially at high doses, have been reported as exhibiting signs of pathological gambling, increased libido and hypersexuality; generally reversible upon reduction of the dose or treatment discontinuation.

Nervous system disorders

Common:

Transient sedation with each dose of apomorphine HCl at the start of therapy may occur; this usually resolves over the first few weeks.

Apomorphine is associated with somnolence.

Dizziness / light-headedness have also been reported.

Uncommon:

Apomorphine may induce dyskinesias during 'on' periods, which can be severe in some cases, and in a few patients may result in cessation of therapy.

Vascular disorders

Uncommon:

Postural hypotension is seen infrequently and is usually transient (See Section 4.4).

Respiratory, thoracic and mediastinal disorders

Common:

Yawning has been reported during apomorphine therapy.

Uncommon:

Breathing difficulties have been reported.

Gastrointestinal disorders

Common:

Nausea and vomiting, particularly when apomorphine treatment is first initiated, usually as a result of the omission of domperidone (See Section 4.2).

Skin and subcutaneous tissue disorders

Uncommon:

Local and generalised rashes have been reported.

General disorders and administration site conditions

Very common:

Most patients experience injection site reactions, particularly with continuous use. These may include subcutaneous nodules, induration, erythema, tenderness and panniculitis. Various other local reactions (such as irritation, itching, bruising and pain) may also occur.

Uncommon:

Injection site necrosis and ulceration have been reported.

Not known:

Peripheral oedema has been reported.

Investigations

Uncommon:

Positive Coombs' tests have been reported for patients receiving apomorphine.

4.9 Overdose

There is little clinical experience of overdose with apomorphine by this route of administration. Symptoms of overdose may be treated empirically as suggested below:-

Excessive emesis may be treated with domperidone.

Respiratory depression may be treated with naloxone.

Hypotension: appropriate measures should be taken, e.g. raising the foot of the bed.

Bradycardia may be treated with atropine.

5. PHARMACOLOGICAL PROPERTIES

5.1 Pharmacodynamic properties

Pharmatherapeutic group: Dopamine agonists

ATC Classification: N04B C07

Apomorphine is a direct stimulant of dopamine receptors and, while possessing both D1 and D2 receptor agonist properties, does not share transport or metabolic pathways with levodopa.

Although in intact experimental animals, administration of apomorphine suppresses the rate of firing of nigro-striatal cells and in low dose has been found to produce a reduction in locomotor activity (thought to represent pre-synaptic inhibition of endogenous dopamine release) its actions on parkinsonian motor disability are likely to be mediated at post-synaptic receptor sites. This biphasic effect is also seen in humans.

5.2 Pharmacokinetic properties

After subcutaneous injection of apomorphine its fate can be described by a two-compartment model, with a distribution half-life of 5 (± 1.1) minutes and an elimination half-life of 33 (± 3.9) minutes. Clinical response correlates well with levels of apomorphine in the cerebrospinal fluid; the drug distribution being best described by a two- compartment model. Apomorphine is rapidly and completely absorbed from subcutaneous tissue, correlating with the rapid onset of clinical effects (4-12 minutes), and that the brief duration of clinical action of the drug (about 1 hour) is explained by its rapid clearance. The metabolism of apomorphine is by glucuronidation and sulphonation to at least ten per cent of the total; other pathways have not been described.

5.3 Preclinical safety data

Repeat dose subcutaneous toxicity studies reveal no special hazard for humans, beyond the information included in other sections of the SmPC.

In vitro genotoxicity studies demonstrated mutagenic and clastogenic effects, most likely due to products formed by oxidation of apomorphine. However, apomorphine was not genotoxic in the in vivo studies performed.

The effect of apomorphine on reproduction has been investigated in rats. Apomorphine was not teratogenic in this species, but it was noted that doses which are toxic to the mother can cause loss of maternal care and failure to breathe in the newborn.

No carcinogenicity studies have been performed.

6. PHARMACEUTICAL PARTICULARS

6.1 List of excipients

Sodium bisulphite (E222)
Hydrochloric Acid (37%), concentrated (to adjust pH to 3.0 – 4.0)
Water for injection

6.2 Incompatibilities

In the absence of compatibility studies, this medicinal product must not be mixed with other medicinal products.

Figure 1 HOW TO USE YOUR APO-go PEN

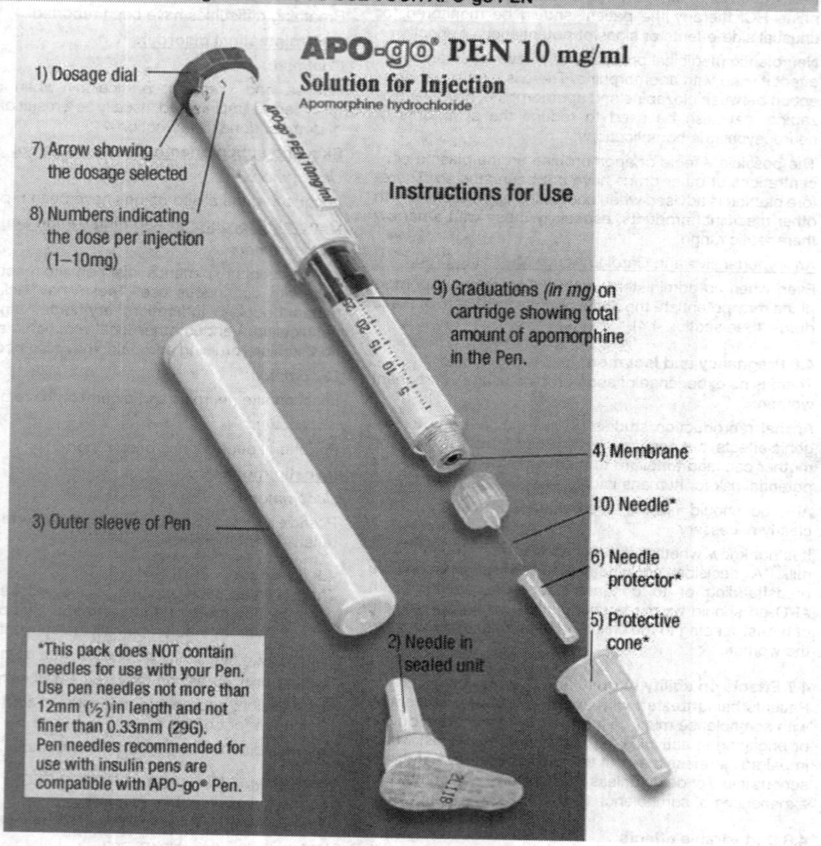

6.3 Shelf life

2 years

48 hours after first opening

6.4 Special precautions for storage

Do not store above 25°C.

Store in the original container.

6.5 Nature and contents of container

Cartridge.

APO-go Pen 10 mg/ml is a disposable multiple dose pen injector system incorporating a clear glass (type I) cartridge containing a clear solution for injection. The glass cartridge is sealed at one end with a bromobutyl rubber piston, and at the other end with a bromobutyl rubber/aluminium membrane.

APO-go Pen is available in packs containing 1, 5, or 10 × 3ml pens in a moulded plastic tray in an outer cardboard carton. Each pen contains 3ml of solution for injection. Bundle Packs containing 25 Pens are available in some territories. These bundle packs consist of 5 boxes each containing 5 pens.

Not all pack sizes are marketed.

6.6 Special precautions for disposal and other handling

APO-go PEN

Do not use if solution has turned green.

Discard each pen no later than 48 hours from first use.

(see attached diagram)

(see Figure 1 above)

HOW TO USE YOUR APO-go PEN

Read these instructions carefully

DO NOT PULL THE RED DIAL BEFORE YOU HAVE SET THE DOSAGE (See f)

(see attached diagram)

ATTACHING THE NEEDLE

(a) Before using your pen system you will need a surgical wipe and one needle in its protective cone (see 5). Take the pen out of its box and remove the outer sleeve (see 3).

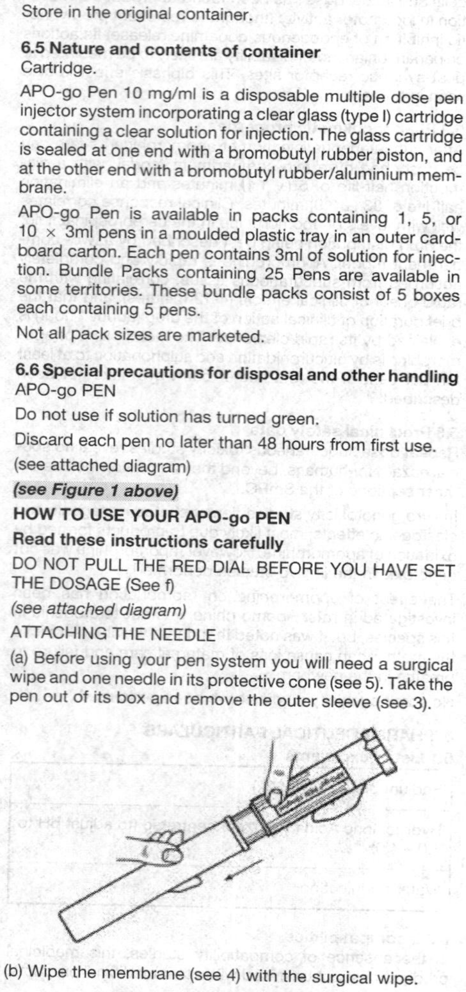

(b) Wipe the membrane (see 4) with the surgical wipe.

(c) Peel off the paper from the needle cone (see 2), and screw the cone *clockwise* onto the membrane. This will attach needle securely.

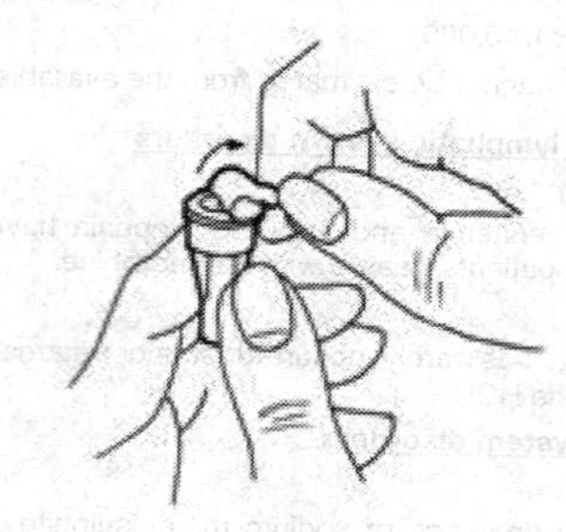

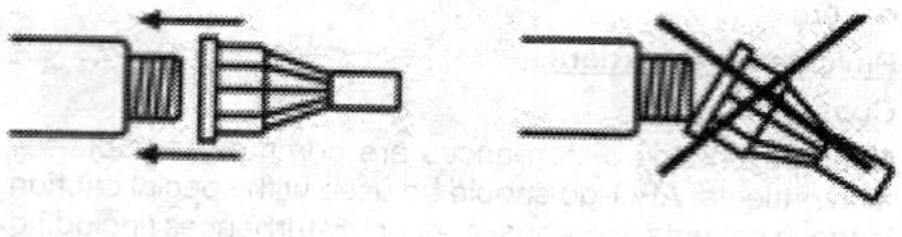

PLEASE NOTE

It is important to bring the needle to the Pen in a straight line, as shown. If the needle is presented at an angle it may cause the Pen to leak. This will attach the needle securely.

(d) Remove the protective cone, *but do not throw it away*. Do not remove the needle protector at this stage (see 6).

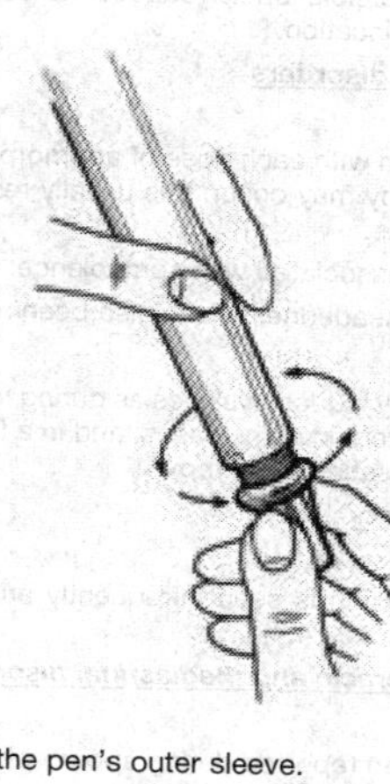

(e) Replace the pen's outer sleeve.

HOW TO SELECT YOUR CORRECT DOSAGE

(see attached diagram)

(f) Press the red dosage dial (see 1) and turn the di clockwise until the arrow points to your prescribed dosag (see 7,8). Then release downward pressure on the red di The dose is now set, and you do not need to redial f subsequent injections.

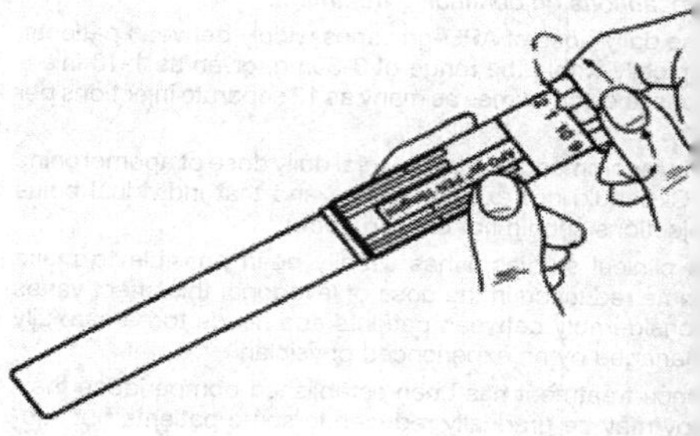

Important; If you pass your prescribed dose while turnin the dial, just continue pressing and turning in the sam direction until you arrive at it again. *Never pull and turn th red dosage dial at the same time.*

If your prescribed dose is 2mg or less, it is necessary t "prime" the pen before injecting the first dose. Do this b emptying the first 2mg dose onto a paper tissue an discard. Then, set the dose you require for injection an inject in the usual way (see below under "INJECTING"). I the first dose required is more than 2mg, then it is no necessary to "prime" the pen.

INJECTING

(see attached diagram)

(g) Pull out the red dosage dial as far as it will go. Check the white scale on the plunger and inject only if the highes number visible corresponds to the intended dose.

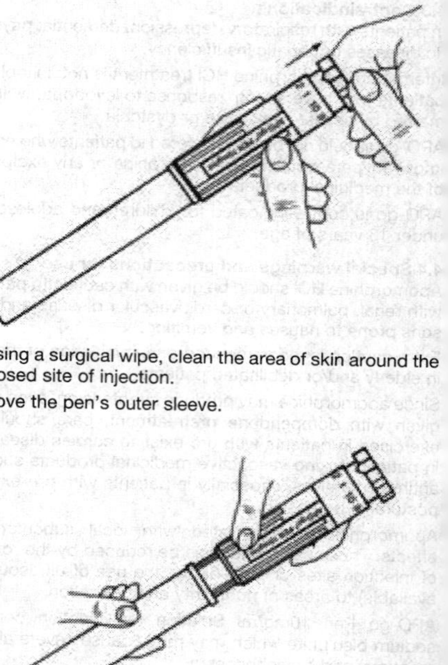

(h) Using a surgical wipe, clean the area of skin around the proposed site of injection.

Remove the pen's outer sleeve.

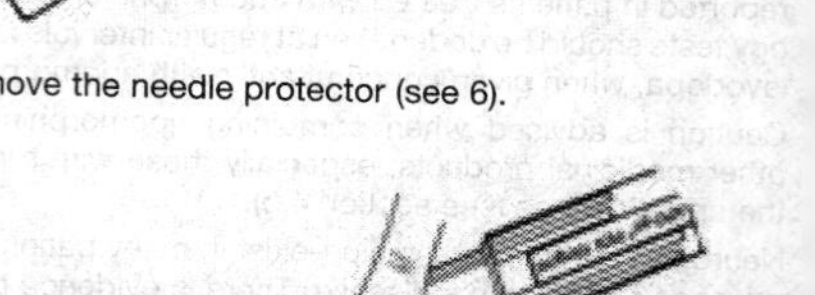

(i) Remove the needle protector (see 6).

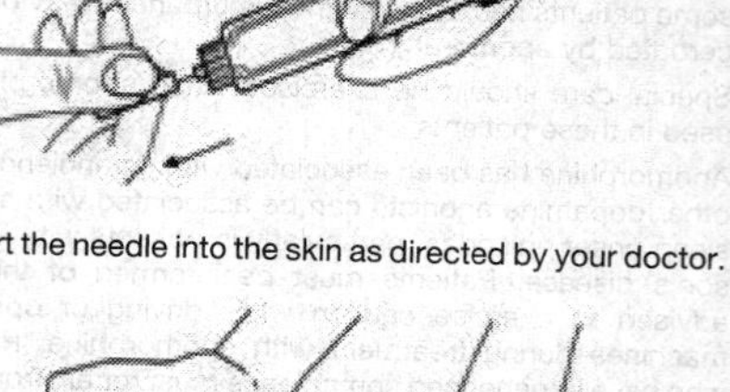

(j) Insert the needle into the skin as directed by your doctor.

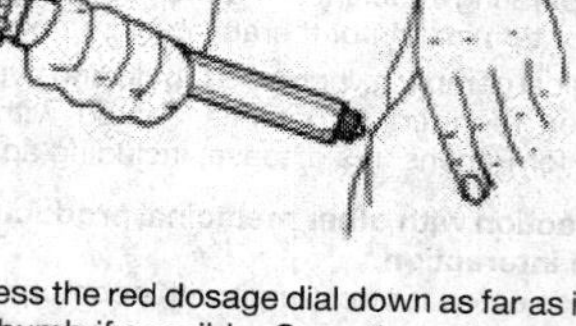

To inject, press the red dosage dial down as far as it will go, using your thumb if possible. Once the red dosage dial is lly depressed, count to three before withdrawing the needle.

Remove and discard the needle, using the protective one (see 5). This is done by replacing the protective cone nto the used needle, and pushing it gently into place. nce secure, you can unscrew the needle anti-clockwise. scard the needle in a safe place.

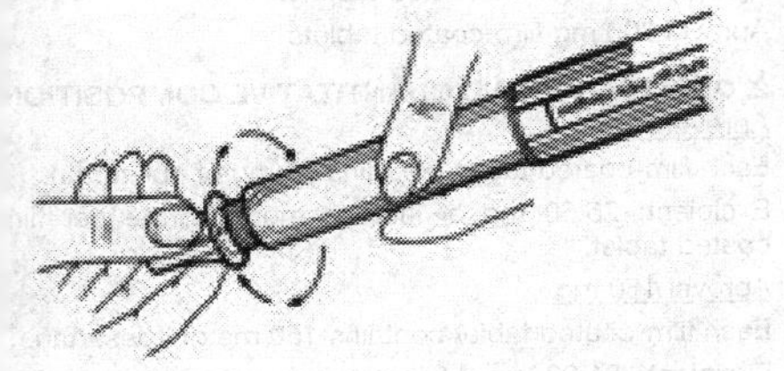

nportant: *Each needle can only be used once.*

REPARING FOR THE NEXT INJECTION:

:heck that there is enough apomorphine left in the caridge for the next injection (see 9). If there is, put a new eedle in place, following the same procedure as before. *Remember not to throw away the protective cone).*

there is not enough apomorphine left for another injecon, prepare another pen.

inally, replace the outer sleeve of the pen.

. MARKETING AUTHORISATION HOLDER

Britannia Pharmaceuticals Limited

1 - 51 Brighton Road

Redhill

Surrey

RH1 6YS

United Kingdom

. MARKETING AUTHORISATION NUMBER(S)

PL 04483/0065

PA 356/9/1

. DATE OF FIRST AUTHORISATION/RENEWAL OF THE AUTHORISATION

31 March 1999/ 1 April 2004

10. DATE OF REVISION OF THE TEXT

July 2009

APO-go PFS 5mg/ml Solution for Infusion in Pre-filled Syringe

(Britannia Pharmaceuticals)

1. NAME OF THE MEDICINAL PRODUCT

APO-go PFS 5mg/ml Solution for Infusion in Pre-filled Syringe (United Kingdom/Ireland)

APO-go 5mg/ml Infusionslösung in einer Fertigspritze (Austria/Germany)

APO-go Pumpfill 5 mg/ml infusionsvæske, opløsning i fyldt injektionssprøjte (Denmark)

APO-go PFS 5mg/ml (Greece)

APO-go 5mg/ml oplossing voor infusie in een voorgevulde spuit (the Netherlands)

APO-go Pumpfill 5 mg/ml infusionsvätska, lösning i förfylld spruta (Sweden)

2. QUALITATIVE AND QUANTITATIVE COMPOSITION

1ml contains 5mg apomorphine hydrochloride.

Each 10ml pre-filled syringe contains 50mg apomorphine hydrochloride.

Excipient:

Sodium metabisulphite 0.5 mg per ml

For a full list of excipients, see Section 6.1

3. PHARMACEUTICAL FORM

Solution for Infusion, pre-filled syringe

Solution is clear and colourless

pH 3.0-4.0

4. CLINICAL PARTICULARS

4.1 Therapeutic indications

Treatment of motor fluctuations ('on-off' phenomena) in patients with Parkinson's disease which are not sufficiently controlled by oral anti-Parkinson medication

4.2 Posology and method of administration

Selection of Patients Suitable for APO-go:

Patients selected for treatment with APO-go should be able to recognise the onset of their 'off' symptoms and be capable of injecting themselves or else have a responsible carer able to inject for them when required.

It is essential that the patient is established on domperidone, usually 20 mg three times daily for at least two days prior to initiation of therapy.

Apomorphine should be initiated in the controlled environment of a specialist clinic. The patient should be supervised by a physician experienced in the treatment of Parkinson's disease (e.g. neurologist). The patient's treatment with levodopa, with or without dopamine agonists, should be optimised before starting APO-go treatment.

Administration

APO-go PFS 5mg/ml Solution for Infusion in Pre-filled Syringe is a pre-diluted pre-filled syringe intended for use without dilution as a continuous subcutaneous infusion by minipump and / or syringe-driver. It is not intended to be used for intermittent injection.

Apomorphine must not be used via the intravenous route.

Do not use if the solution has turned green. The solution should be inspected visually prior to use. Only clear, colourless and particle free solution should be used.

Continuous Infusion

Patients who have shown a good 'on' period response during the initiation stage of apomorphine therapy, but whose overall control remains unsatisfactory using intermittent injections, or who require many and frequent injections (more than 10 per day), may be commenced on or transferred to continuous subcutaneous infusion by minipump and / or syringe driver as follows:-

The choice, of which minipump and / or syringe-driver to use, and the dosage settings required, will be determined by the physician in accordance with the particular needs of the patient.

The threshold dose for continuous infusion should be determined as follows: Continuous infusion is started at a rate of 1 mg apomorphine HCl (0.2 ml) per hour then increased according to the individual response each day. Increases in the infusion rate should not exceed 0.5 mg at intervals of not less than 4 hours. Hourly infusion rates may range between 1 mg and 4 mg (0.2 ml and 0.8 ml), equivalent to 0.014 - 0.06 mg/kg/hour. Infusions should run for waking hours only. Unless the patient is experiencing severe night-time problems, 24 hour infusions are not advised. Tolerance to the therapy does not seem to occur as long as there is an overnight period without treatment of at least 4 hours. In any event, the infusion site should be changed every 12 hours.

Patients may need to supplement their continuous infusion with intermittent bolus boosts, as necessary, and as directed by their physician.

A reduction in dosage of other dopamine agonists may be considered during continuous infusion.

Establishment of treatment.

Alterations in dosage may be made according to the patient's response.

The optimal dosage of apomorphine hydrochloride varies between individuals but, once established, remains relatively constant for each patient.

Precautions on continuing treatment

The daily dose of APO-go varies widely between patients, typically within the range of 3-30 mg.

It is recommended that the total daily dose of apomorphine HCl should not exceed 100 mg.

In clinical studies it has usually been possible to make some reduction in the dose of levodopa; this effect varies considerably between patients and needs to be carefully managed by an experienced physician.

Once treatment has been established domperidone therapy may be gradually reduced in some patients but successfully eliminated only in a few, without any vomiting or hypotension.

Children and adolescents

APO-go PFS 5mg/ml Solution for Infusion in Pre-filled Syringe is contra-indicated for children and adolescents under18 years of age (see Section 4.3).

Elderly

The elderly are well represented in the population of patients with Parkinson's disease and constitute a high proportion of those studied in clinical trials of APO-go. The management of elderly patients treated with APO-go has not differed from that of younger patients. However, extra caution is recommended during initiation of therapy in elderly patients because of the risk of postural hypotension.

Renal impairment

A dose schedule similar to that recommended for adults, and the elderly, can be followed for patients with renal impairment (see Section 4.4).

4.3 Contraindications

In patients with respiratory depression, dementia, psychotic diseases or hepatic insufficiency.

Apomorphine HCl treatment must not be administered to patients who have an 'on' response to levodopa which is marred by severe dyskinesia or dystonia.

APO-go should not be administered to patients who have a hypersensitivity to apomorphine or any excipients of the medicinal product.

APO-go is contra-indicated for children and adolescents under 18 years of age.

4.4 Special warnings and precautions for use

Apomorphine HCl should be given with caution to patients with renal, pulmonary or cardiovascular disease and persons prone to nausea and vomiting.

Extra caution is recommended during initiation of therapy in elderly and/or debilitated patients.

Since apomorphine may produce hypotension, even when given with domperidone pretreatment, care should be exercised in patients with pre-existing cardiac disease or in patients taking vasoactive medicinal products such as antihypertensives, and especially in patients with pre-existing postural hypotension.

Apomorphine is associated with local subcutaneous effects. These can sometimes be reduced by the rotation of injection sites or possibly by the use of ultrasound (if available) to areas of nodularity and induration.

Haemolytic anaemia and thrombocytopenia have been reported in patients treated with apomorphine. Haematology tests should be undertaken at regular intervals as with levodopa, when given concomitantly with apomorphine.

Caution is advised when combining apomorphine with other medicinal products, especially those with a narrow therapeutic range (see Section 4.5)

Neuropyschiatric problems co-exist in many patients with advanced Parkinson's disease. There is evidence that for some patients neuropsychiatric disturbances may be exacerbated by apomorphine. Special care should be exercised when apomorphine is used in these patients.

Apomorphine has been associated with somnolence, and other dopamine agonists can be associated with sudden sleep onset episodes, particularly in patients with Parkinson's disease. Patients must be informed of this and advised to exercise caution while driving or operating machines during treatment with apomorphine. Patients who have experienced somnolence must refrain from driving or operating machines. Furthermore a reduction of dosage or termination of therapy may be considered.

Pathological gambling, increased libido and hypersexuality have been reported in patients treated with dopamine agonists for Parkinson's disease, including apomorphine.

APO-go PFS 5mg/ml Solution for Infusion in Pre-filled Syringe contains sodium metabisulphite which may rarely cause severe allergic reactions and bronchospasm.

This medicinal product contains less than 1 mmol sodium (23 mg) per 10 ml, i.e. essentially "sodium-free".

4.5 Interaction with other medicinal products and other forms of interaction

Patients selected for treatment with apomorphine HCl are almost certain to be taking concomitant medicinal products for their Parkinson's disease. In the initial stages of apomorphine HCl therapy, the patient should be monitored for unusual undesirable effects or signs of potentiation of effect.

Neuroleptic medicinal products may have an antagonistic effect if used with apomorphine. There is a potential interaction between clozapine and apomorphine, however clozapine may also be used to reduce the symptoms of neuropsychiatric complications.

If neuroleptic medicinal products have to be used in patients with Parkinson's disease treated by dopamine agonists, a gradual reduction in apomorphine dose may be considered when administration is by minipump and / or syringe- driver (symptoms suggestive of neuroleptic malignant syndrome have been reported rarely with abrupt withdrawal of dopaminergic therapy).

The possible effects of apomorphine on the plasma concentrations of other medicinal products have not been studied. Therefore caution is advised when combining apomorphine with other medicinal products, especially those with a narrow therapeutic range.

Antihypertensive and Cardiac Active Medicinal Products

Even when co-administered with domperidone, apomorphine may potentiate the antihypertensive effects of these medicinal products (see Section 4.4).

4.6 Pregnancy and lactation

There is no experience of apomorphine usage in pregnant women.

Animal reproduction studies do not indicate any teratogenic effects, but doses given to rats which are toxic to the mother can lead to failure to breathe in the newborn. The potential risk to humans is unknown. See Section 5.3.

APO-go should not be used in pregnancy unless clearly necessary.

It is not known whether apomorphine is excreted in breast milk. A decision on whether to continue/discontinue breastfeeding or to continue/discontinue therapy with APO-go should be made taking into account the benefit of breast-feeding to the child and the benefit of APO-go to the woman.

4.7 Effects on ability to drive and use machines

Patients being treated with apomorphine and presenting with somnolence and/or sudden sleep episodes must be informed to refrain from driving or engaging in activities (e.g. operating machines) where impaired alertness may put themselves or others at risk of serious injury or death until such recurrent episodes and somnolence have resolved (see also Section 4.4).

4.8 Undesirable effects

Very common (≥1/10)

Common (≥1/100 to <1/10)

Uncommon (≥1/1,000 to <1/100)

Rare (≥1/10,000 to <1/1,000)

Very rare (<1/10,000)

Not known (cannot be estimated from the available data)

Blood and lymphatic system disorders

Uncommon:

Haemolytic anaemia and thrombocytopenia has been reported in patients treated with apomorphine.

Rare:

Eosinophilia has rarely occurred during treatment with apomorphine HCl.

Immune system disorders

Rare:

Due to the presence of sodium metabisulphite, allergic reactions (including anaphylaxis and bronchospasm) may occur.

Psychiatric disorders

Common:

Neuropsychiatric disturbances are common in parkinsonian patients. APO-go should be used with special caution in these patients. Neuropsychiatric disturbances (including transient mild confusion and visual hallucinations) have occurred during apomorphine HCl therapy.

Not known:

Patients treated with dopamine agonists for treatment of Parkinson's disease, including apomorphine, especially at high doses, have been reported as exhibiting signs of pathological gambling, increased libido and hypersexuality; generally reversible upon reduction of the dose or treatment discontinuation.

Nervous system disorders

Common:

Transient sedation with each dose of apomorphine HCl at the start of therapy may occur; this usually resolves over the first few weeks.

Apomorphine is associated with somnolence.

Dizziness / light-headedness have also been reported.

Uncommon:

Apomorphine may induce dyskinesias during 'on' periods, which can be severe in some cases, and in a few patients may result in cessation of therapy.

Vascular disorders

Uncommon:

Postural hypotension is seen infrequently and is usually transient (See Section 4.4).

Respiratory, thoracic and mediastinal disorders

Common:

Yawning has been reported during apomorphine therapy.

Uncommon:

Breathing difficulties have been reported.

Gastrointestinal disorders

Common:

Nausea and vomiting, particularly when apomorphine treatment is first initiated, usually as a result of the omission of domperidone (See Section 4.2).

Skin and subcutaneous tissue disorders

Uncommon:

Local and generalised rashes have been reported.

General disorders and administration site conditions

Very common:

Most patients experience injection site reactions, particularly with continuous use. These may include subcutaneous nodules, induration, erythema, tenderness and panniculitis. Various other local reactions (such as irritation, itching, bruising and pain) may also occur.

Uncommon:

Injection site necrosis and ulceration have been reported.

Not known:

Peripheral oedema has been reported.

Investigations

Uncommon:

Positive Coombs' tests have been reported for patients receiving apomorphine and levodopa.

4.9 Overdose

There is little clinical experience of overdosewith apomorphine by this route of administration. Symptoms of overdosemay be treated empirically as suggested below:-

Excessive emesis may be treated with domperidone.

Respiratory depression may be treated with naloxone.

Hypotension: appropriate measures should be taken, e.g. raising the foot of the bed.

Bradycardia may be treated with atropine.

5. PHARMACOLOGICAL PROPERTIES

5.1 Pharmacodynamic properties

Pharmatherapeutic group: Dopamine agonists ATC Code: N04B C07

Apomorphine is a direct stimulant of dopamine receptors and, while possessing both D1 and D2 receptor agonist properties, does not share transport or metabolic pathways with levodopa.

Although in intact experimental animals, administration of apomorphine suppresses the rate of firing of nigro-striatal cells and in low dose has been found to produce a reduction in locomotor activity (thought to represent pre-synaptic inhibition of endogenous dopamine release) its actions on parkinsonian motor disability are likely to be mediated at post-synaptic receptor sites. This biphasic effect is also seen in humans.

5.2 Pharmacokinetic properties

After subcutaneous injection of apomorphineits fate can be described by a two-compartment model, with a distribution half-life of 5 (±1.1) minutes and an elimination half-life of 33 (±3.9)minutes. Clinical response correlates well with levels of apomorphine in the cerebrospinal fluid; the active substance distribution being best described by a two-compartment model. Apomorphine is rapidly and completely absorbed from subcutaneous tissue, correlating with the rapid onset of clinical effects (4-12 minutes), and the brief duration of clinical action of the active substance (about 1 hour) is explained by its rapid clearance. The metabolism of apomorphine is by glucuronidation and sulphonation to at least ten per cent of the total; other pathways have not been described.

5.3 Preclinical safety data

Repeat dose subcutaneous toxicity studies reveal no special hazard for humans, beyond the information included in other sections of the SmPC.

In vitro genotoxicity studies demonstrated mutagenic and clastogenic effects, most likely due to products formed by oxidation of apomorphine. However, apomorphine was not genotoxic in the in vivo studies performed.

The effect of apomorphine on reproduction has been investigated in rats. Apomorphine was not teratogenic in this species, but it was noted that doses which are toxic to the mother can cause loss of maternal care and failure to breathe in the newborn.

No carcinogenicity studies have been performed.

6. PHARMACEUTICAL PARTICULARS

6.1 List of excipients

Sodium metabisulphite (E223)

Hydrochloric acid (37%), (for pH adjustment)

Water for injections

6.2 Incompatibilities

In the absence of compatibility studies, this medicinal product must not be mixed with other medicinal products.

6.3 Shelf life

2 years

Once opened the pre-filled syringe should be used immediately.

From a microbiological point of view, unless the method of opening precludes the risk of microbial contamination, the product should be used immediately.

If not used immediately in-use storage times and conditions are the responsibility of the user.

6.4 Special precautions for storage

Keep the pre-filled syringe in the outer carton in order to protect from light.

For storage of the product after opening see Section 6.3.

Do not store above 25°C.

6.5 Nature and contents of container

Clear glass (Type I) pre-filled syringe, 10 ml with a chlorobutyl rubber stopper and tip.

Packs contain 5 Pre-filled Syringes in a cardboard tray in an outer cardboard carton.

6.6 Special precautions for disposal and other handling

APO-go PFS 5mg/ml Solution for Infusion in Pre-filled Syringe is for single use only. Any unused solution should be discarded.

After single use, adaptors and syringes should be discarded and disposed of in a "Sharps" bin.

Administrative Data

7. MARKETING AUTHORISATION HOLDER

Forum Products Limited

41 - 51 Brighton Road

Redhill

Surrey

RH1 6YS

United Kingdom

8. MARKETING AUTHORISATION NUMBER(S)

PL 05928/0025

PA 454/2/3

9. DATE OF FIRST AUTHORISATION/RENEWAL OF THE AUTHORISATION

September 2004

10. DATE OF REVISION OF THE TEXT

July 2009

Aprovel Film-Coated Tablets (sanofi-aventis

(sanofi-aventis

1. NAME OF THE MEDICINAL PRODUCT

Aprovel 75 mg film-coated tablets.

Aprovel 150 mg film-coated tablets.

Aprovel 300 mg film-coated tablets

2. QUALITATIVE AND QUANTITATIVE COMPOSITION

Aprovel 75 mg

Each film-coated tablet contains 75 mg of irbesartan.

Excipient: 25.50 mg of lactose monohydrate per film-coated tablet.

Aprovel 150 mg

Each film-coated tablet contains 150 mg of irbesartan.

Excipient: 51.00 mg of lactose monohydrate per film-coated tablet.

Aprovel 300 mg

Each film-coated tablet contains 300 mg of irbesartan.

Excipient: 102.00 mg of lactose monohydrate per film-coated tablet.

For a full list of excipients, see section 6.1.

3. PHARMACEUTICAL FORM

Film-coated tablet.

Aprovel 75 mg

White to off-white, biconvex, and oval-shaped with a heart debossed on one side and the number 2871 engraved on the other side.

Aprovel 150 mg

White to off-white, biconvex, and oval-shaped with a heart debossed on one side and the number 2872 engraved on the other side.

Aprovel 300 mg

White to off-white biconvex, and oval-shaped with a heart debossed on one side and the number 2873 engraved on the other side.

4. CLINICAL PARTICULARS

4.1 Therapeutic indications

Treatment of essential hypertension.

Treatment of renal disease in patients with hypertension and type 2 diabetes mellitus as part of an antihypertensive medicinal product regimen (see section 5.1).

4.2 Posology and method of administration

The usual recommended initial and maintenance dose is 150 mg once daily, with or without food. Aprovel at a dose of 150 mg once daily generally provides a better 24 hour blood pressure control than 75 mg. However, initiation of therapy with 75 mg could be considered, particularly in haemodialysed patients and in the elderly over 75 years.

In patients insufficiently controlled with 150 mg once daily, the dose of Aprovel can be increased to 300 mg, or other anti-hypertensive agents can be added. In particular, the addition of a diuretic such as hydrochlorothiazide has been shown to have an additive effect with Aprovel (see section 4.5).

In hypertensive type 2 diabetic patients, therapy should be initiated at 150 mg irbesartan once daily and titrated up to 300 mg once daily as the preferred maintenance dose for treatment of renal disease.

The demonstration of renal benefit of Aprovel in hypertensive type 2 diabetic patients is based on studies where irbesartan was used in addition to other antihypertensive agents, as needed, to reach target blood pressure (see section 5.1).

Renal impairment: no dosage adjustment is necessary in patients with impaired renal function. A lower starting dose (75 mg) should be considered for patients undergoing haemodialysis (see section 4.4).

Hepatic impairment: no dosage adjustment is necessary in patients with mild to moderate hepatic impairment. There is no clinical experience in patients with severe hepatic impairment.

Elderly patients: although consideration should be given to initiating therapy with 75 mg in patients over 75 years of age, dosage adjustment is not usually necessary for the elderly.

Paediatric patients: irbesartan is not recommended for use in children and adolescents due to insufficient data on safety and efficacy (see sections 4.8, 5.1 and 5.2).

4.3 Contraindications

Hypersensitivity to the active substance, or to any of the excipients (see section 6.1).

Second and third trimesters of pregnancy (see sections 4.4 and 4.6).

4.4 Special warnings and precautions for use

Intravascular volume depletion: symptomatic hypotension, especially after the first dose, may occur in patients who are volume and/or sodium depleted by vigorous diuretic therapy, dietary salt restriction, diarrhoea or vomiting. Such conditions should be corrected before the administration of Aprovel.

enovascular hypertension: there is an increased risk of vere hypotension and renal insufficiency when patients th bilateral renal artery stenosis or stenosis of the artery a single functioning kidney are treated with medicinal oducts that affect the renin-angiotensin-aldosterone stem. While this is not documented with Aprovel, a nilar effect should be anticipated with angiotensin-II ceptor antagonists.

enal impairment and kidney transplantation: when Apro- l is used in patients with impaired renal function, a eriodic monitoring of potassium and creatinine serum vels is recommended. There is no experience regarding e administration of Aprovel in patients with a recent dney transplantation.

ypertensive patients with type 2 diabetes and renal dis- ase: the effects of irbesartan both on renal and cardio- ascular events were not uniform across all subgroups, in n analysis carried out in the study with patients with dvanced renal disease. In particular, they appeared less vourable in women and non-white subjects (see section .1).

lyperkalaemia: as with other medicinal products that ffect the renin-angiotensin-aldosterone system, hyperka- aemia may occur during the treatment with Aprovel, espe- ially in the presence of renal impairment, overt proteinuria lue to diabetic renal disease, and/or heart failure. Close nonitoring of serum potassium in patients at risk is recom- nended (see section 4.5).

ithium: the combination of lithium and Aprovel is not ecommended (see section 4.5).

ortic and mitral valve stenosis, obstructive hypertrophic cardiomyopathy: as with other vasodilators, special cau- ion is indicated in patients suffering from aortic or mitral stenosis, or obstructive hypertrophic cardiomyopathy.

Primary aldosteronism: patients with primary aldosteron- sm generally will not respond to anti-hypertensive medic- nal products acting through inhibition of the renin- angiotensin system. Therefore, the use of Aprovel is not recommended.

General: in patients whose vascular tone and renal function depend predominantly on the activity of the renin-angio- tensin-aldosterone system (e.g. patients with severe con- gestive heart failure or underlying renal disease, including renal artery stenosis), treatment with angiotensin convert- ing enzyme inhibitors or angiotensin-II receptor antago- nists that affect this system has been associated with acute hypotension, azotaemia, oliguria, or rarely acute renal failure. As with any anti-hypertensive agent, exces- sive blood pressure decrease in patients with ischaemic cardiopathy or ischaemic cardiovascular disease could result in a myocardial infarction or stroke.

As observed for angiotensin converting enzyme inhibitors, irbesartan and the other angiotensin antagonists are apparently less effective in lowering blood pressure in black people than in non-blacks, possibly because of higher prevalence of low-renin states in the black hyper- tensive population (see section 5.1).

Pregnancy: Angiotensin II Receptor Antagonists (AIIRAs) should not be initiated during pregnancy. Unless continued AIIRA therapy is considered essential, patients planning pregnancy should be changed to alternative anti-hyperten- sive treatments which have an established safety profile for use in pregnancy. When pregnancy is diagnosed, treat- ment with AIIRAs should be stopped immediately, and, if appropriate, alternative therapy should be started (see sections 4.3 and 4.6).

Lactose: this medicinal product contains lactose. Patients with rare hereditary problems of galactose intolerance, the Lapp lactase deficiency or glucose-galactose malabsorp- tion should not take this medicinal product.

Paediatric patients: irbesartan has been studied in paedia- tric populations aged 6 to 16 years old but the current data are insufficient to support an extension of the use in chil- dren until further data become available (see sections 4.8, 5.1 and 5.2).

4.5 Interaction with other medicinal products and other forms of interaction

Diuretics and other antihypertensive agents: other antihy- pertensive agents may increase the hypotensive effects of irbesartan; however Aprovel has been safely administered with other antihypertensive agents, such as beta-blockers, long-acting calcium channel blockers, and thiazide diure- tics. Prior treatment with high dose diuretics may result in volume depletion and a risk of hypotension when initiating therapy with Aprovel (see section 4.4).

Potassium supplements and potassium-sparing diuretics: based on experience with the use of other medicinal pro- ducts that affect the renin-angiotensin system, concomi- tant use of potassium-sparing diuretics, potassium supplements, salt substitutes containing potassium or other medicinal products that may increase serum potas- sium levels (e.g. heparin) may lead to increases in serum potassium and is, therefore, not recommended (see sec- tion 4.4).

Lithium: reversible increases in serum lithium concentra- tions and toxicity have been reported during concomitant administration of lithium with angiotensin converting enzyme inhibitors. Similar effects have been very rarely reported with irbesartan so far. Therefore, this combination is not recommended (see section 4.4). If the combination proves necessary, careful monitoring of serum lithium levels is recommended.

Non-steroidal anti-inflammatory drugs: when angiotensin II antagonists are administered simultaneously with non- steroidal anti-inflammatory drugs (i.e. selective COX-2 inhibitors, acetylsalicylic acid (> 3 g/day) and non-selec- tive NSAIDs), attenuation of the antihypertensive effect may occur.

As with ACE inhibitors, concomitant use of angiotensin II antagonists and NSAIDs may lead to an increased risk of worsening of renal function, including possible acute renal failure, and an increase in serum potassium, especially in patients with poor pre-existing renal function. The combi- nation should be administered with caution, especially in the elderly. Patients should be adequately hydrated and consideration should be given to monitoring renal function after initiation of concomitant therapy, and periodically thereafter.

Additional information on irbesartan interactions: in clinical studies, the pharmacokinetic of irbesartan is not affected by hydrochlorothiazide. Irbesartan is mainly metabolised by CYP2C9 and to a lesser extent by glucuronidation. No significant pharmacokinetic or pharmacodynamic interac- tions were observed when irbesartan was coadministered with warfarin, a medicinal product metabolised by CYP2C9. The effects of CYP2C9 inducers such as rifam- picin on the pharmacokinetic of irbesartan have not been evaluated. The pharmacokinetic of digoxin was not altered by coadministration of irbesartan.

4.6 Pregnancy and lactation

Pregnancy

The use of AIIRAs is not recommended during the first trimester of pregnancy (see section 4.4). The use of AIIRAs is contraindicated during the second and third trimesters of pregnancy (see sections 4.3 and 4.4).

Epidemiological evidence regarding the risk of teratogeni- city following exposure to ACE inhibitors during the first trimester of pregnancy has not been conclusive; however a small increase in risk cannot be excluded. Whilst there is no controlled epidemiological data on the risk with Angioten- sin II Receptor Antagonists (AIIRAs), similar risks may exist for this class of drugs. Unless continued AIIRA therapy is considered essential, patients planning pregnancy should be changed to alternative anti-hypertensive treatments which have an established safety profile for use in preg- nancy. When pregnancy is diagnosed, treatment with AIIRAs should be stopped immediately, and, if appropriate, alternative therapy should be started.

Exposure to AIIRA therapy during the second and third trimesters is known to induce human fetotoxicity (decreased renal function, oligohydramnios, skull ossifica- tion retardation) and neonatal toxicity (renal failure, hypo- tension, hyperkalaemia). (see section 5.3).

Should exposure to AIIRAs have occurred from the second trimester of pregnancy, ultrasound check of renal function and skull is recommended.

Infants whose mothers have taken AIIRAs should be clo- sely observed for hypotension (see also sections 4.3 and 4.4).

Lactation:

Because no information is available regarding the use of CoAprovel during breast-feeding, CoAprovel is not recom- mended and alternative treatments with better established safety profiles during breast-feeding are preferable, espe- cially while nursing a newborn or preterm infant.

4.7 Effects on ability to drive and use machines

No studies on the effects on the ability to drive and use machines have been performed. Based on its pharmaco- dynamic properties, irbesartan is unlikely to affect this ability. When driving vehicles or operating machines, it should be taken into account that dizziness or weariness may occur during treatment.

4.8 Undesirable effects

In placebo-controlled trials in patients with hypertension, the overall incidence of adverse events did not differ between the irbesartan (56.2%) and the placebo groups (56.5%). Discontinuation due to any clinical or laboratory adverse event was less frequent for irbesartan-treated patients (3.3%) than for placebo-treated patients (4.5%). The incidence of adverse events was not related to dose (in the recommended dose range), gender, age, race, or dura- tion of treatment.

In diabetic hypertensive patients with microalbuminuria and normal renal function, orthostatic dizziness and ortho- static hypotension were reported in 0.5% of the patients (i.e., uncommon) but in excess of placebo.

The following table presents the adverse drug reactions that were reported in placebo-controlled trials in which 1,965 hypertensive patients received irbesartan. Terms marked with a star (*) refer to the adverse reactions that were additionally reported in > 2% of diabetic hyperten- sive patients with chronic renal insufficiency and overt proteinuria and in excess of placebo.

The frequency of adverse reactions listed below is defined using the following convention:

very common (≥ 1/10); common (≥ 1/100, < 1/10); uncommon (≥ 1/1,000, < 1/100); rare (≥ 1/10,000, < 1/ 1,000); very rare (< 1/10,000). Within each frequency grouping, undesirable effects are presented in order of decreasing seriousness.

Investigations:

Very common: Hyperkalaemia* occurred more often in diabetic patients treated with irbesartan than with placebo. In diabetic hypertensive patients with microalbuminuria and normal renal function, hyperkalaemia (≥ 5.5 mEq/L) occurred in 29.4% of the patients in the irbesartan 300 mg group and 22% of the patients in the placebo group. In diabetic hypertensive patients with chronic renal insuffi- ciency and overt proteinuria, hyperkalaemia (≥ 5.5 mEq/L) occurred in 46.3% of the patients in the irbesartan group and 26.3% of the patients in the placebo group.

Common: significant increases in plasma creatine kinase were commonly observed (1.7%) in irbesartan treated subjects. None of these increases were associated with identifiable clinical musculoskeletal events.

In 1.7% of hypertensive patients with advanced diabetic renal disease treated with irbesartan, a decrease in hae- moglobin*, which was not clinically significant, has been observed.

Cardiac disorders:

Uncommon: tachycardia

Nervous system disorders:

Common: dizziness, orthostatic dizziness*

Respiratory, thoracic and mediastinal disorders:

Uncommon: cough

Gastrointestinal disorders:

Common: nausea/vomiting

Uncommon: diarrhoea, dyspepsia/heartburn

Musculoskeletal and connective tissue disorders:

Common: musculoskeletal pain*

Vascular disorders:

Common: orthostatic hypotension*

Uncommon: flushing

General disorders and administration site conditions:

Common: fatigue

Uncommon: chest pain

Reproductive system and breast disorders:

Uncommon: sexual dysfunction

The following additional adverse reactions have been reported during post-marketing experience; they are derived from spontaneous reports and therefore, the frequency of these adverse reactions is not known:

Nervous system disorders:

Headache

Ear and labyrinth disorders:

Tinnitus

Gastrointestinal disorders:

Dysgeusia

Renal and urinary disorders:

Impaired renal function including cases of renal failure in patients at risk (see section 4.4)

Skin and subcutaneous tissue disorders:

Leukocytoclastic vasculitis

Musculoskeletal and connective tissue disorders:

Arthralgia, myalgia (in some cases associated with increased plasma creatine kinase levels), muscle cramps

Metabolism and nutrition disorders:

Hyperkalaemia

Immune system disorders:

Hypersensitivity reactions such as angioedema, rash, urti- caria

Hepato-biliary disorders:

Hepatitis, abnormal liver function

Paediatric patients: in a randomised trial of 318 hyper- tensive children and adolescents aged 6 to 16 years, the following related adverse events occurred in the 3-week double-blind phase: headache (7.9%), hypotension (2.2%), dizziness (1.9%), cough (0.9%). In the 26-week open-label period of this trial the most frequent laboratory abnormalities observed were creatinine increases (6.5%) and elevated CK values in 2% of child recipients.

4.9 Overdose

Experience in adults exposed to doses of up to 900 mg/day for 8 weeks revealed no toxicity. The most likely manifesta- tions of overdose are expected to be hypotension and tachycardia; bradycardia might also occur from overdose. No specific information is available on the treatment of overdose with Aprovel. The patient should be closely mon- itored, and the treatment should be symptomatic and supportive. Suggested measures include induction of emesis and/or gastric lavage. Activated charcoal may be useful in the treatment of overdose. Irbesartan is not removed by haemodialysis.

5. PHARMACOLOGICAL PROPERTIES

5.1 Pharmacodynamic properties

Pharmacotherapeutic group: Angiotensin-II antagonists, plain.

ATC code: C09C A04.

Mechanism of action: Irbesartan is a potent, orally active, selective angiotensin-II receptor (type AT_1) antagonist. It is expected to block all actions of angiotensin-II mediated by the AT_1 receptor, regardless of the source or route of synthesis of angiotensin-II. The selective antagonism of the angiotensin-II (AT_1) receptors results in increases in plasma renin levels and angiotensin-II levels, and a decrease in plasma aldosterone concentration. Serum potassium levels are not significantly affected by irbesartan alone at the recommended doses. Irbesartan does not inhibit ACE (kininase-II), an enzyme which generates angiotensin-II and also degrades bradykinin into inactive metabolites. Irbesartan does not require metabolic activation for its activity.

Clinical efficacy:

Hypertension

Irbesartan lowers blood pressure with minimal change in heart rate. The decrease in blood pressure is dose-related for once a day doses with a tendency towards plateau at doses above 300 mg. Doses of 150-300 mg once daily lower supine or seated blood pressures at trough (i.e. 24 hours after dosing) by an average of 8-13/5-8 mm Hg (systolic/diastolic) greater than those associated with placebo.

Peak reduction of blood pressure is achieved within 3-6 hours after administration and the blood pressure lowering effect is maintained for at least 24 hours. At 24 hours the reduction of blood pressure was 60-70% of the corresponding peak diastolic and systolic responses at the recommended doses. Once daily dosing with 150 mg produced trough and mean 24 hour responses similar to twice daily dosing on the same total dose.

The blood pressure lowering effect of Aprovel is evident within 1-2 weeks, with the maximal effect occurring by 4-6 weeks after start of therapy. The antihypertensive effects are maintained during long term therapy. After withdrawal of therapy, blood pressure gradually returns toward baseline. Rebound hypertension has not been observed.

The blood pressure lowering effects of irbesartan and thiazide-type diuretics are additive. In patients not adequately controlled by irbesartan alone, the addition of a low dose of hydrochlorothiazide (12.5 mg) to irbesartan once daily results in a further placebo-adjusted blood pressure reduction at trough of 7-10/3-6 mm Hg (systolic/diastolic).

The efficacy of Aprovel is not influenced by age or gender. As is the case with other medicinal products that affect the renin-angiotensin system, black hypertensive patients have notably less response to irbesartan monotherapy. When irbesartan is administered concomitantly with a low dose of hydrochlorothiazide (e.g. 12.5 mg daily), the antihypertensive response in black patients approaches that of white patients.

There is no clinically important effect on serum uric acid or urinary uric acid secretion.

Reduction of blood pressure with 0.5 mg/kg (low), 1.5 mg/kg (medium) and 4.5 mg/kg (high) target titrated doses of irbesartan was evaluated in 318 hypertensive or at risk (diabetic, family history of hypertension) children and adolescents aged 6 to 16 years over a three week period. At the end of the three weeks the mean reduction from baseline in the primary efficacy variable, trough seated systolic blood pressure (SeSBP) was 11.7 mmHg (low dose), 9.3 mmHg (medium dose), 13.2 mmHg (high dose). No significant difference was apparent between these doses. Adjusted mean change of trough seated diastolic blood pressure (SeDBP) was as follows: 3.8 mmHg (low dose), 3.2 mmHg (medium dose), 5.6 mmHg (high dose). Over a subsequent two week period where patients were re-randomized to either active medicinal product or placebo, patients on placebo had increases of 2.4 and 2.0 mmHg in SeSBP and SeDBP compared to +0.1 and -0.3 mmHg changes respectively in those on all doses of irbesartan (see section 4.2).

Hypertension and type 2 diabetes with renal disease

The "Irbesartan Diabetic Nephropathy Trial (IDNT)" shows that irbesartan decreases the progression of renal disease in patients with chronic renal insufficiency and overt proteinuria. IDNT was a double blind, controlled, morbidity and mortality trial comparing Aprovel, amlodipine and placebo. In 1,715 hypertensive patients with type 2 diabetes, proteinuria $\geqslant$ 900 mg/day and serum creatinine ranging from 1.0-3.0 mg/dl, the long-term effects (mean 2.6 years) of Aprovel on the progression of renal disease and all-cause mortality were examined. Patients were titrated from 75 mg to a maintenance dose of 300 mg Aprovel, from 2.5 mg to 10 mg amlodipine, or placebo as tolerated. Patients in all treatment groups typically received between 2 and 4 antihypertensive agents (e.g., diuretics, beta blockers, alpha blockers) to reach a predefined blood pressure goal of $\leqslant$ 135/85 mmHg or a 10 mmHg reduction in systolic pressure if baseline was $>$ 160 mmHg. Sixty per cent (60%) of patients in the placebo group reached this target blood pressure whereas this figure was 76% and 78% in the irbesartan and amlodipine groups respectively. Irbesartan significantly reduced the relative risk in the primary combined endpoint of doubling serum creatinine, end-stage renal disease (ESRD) or all-cause mortality. Approximately 33% of patients in the irbesartan group reached the primary renal composite endpoint compared to 39% and 41% in the placebo and amlodipine groups [20% relative risk reduction versus placebo ($p = 0.024$) and 23% relative risk reduction compared to amlodipine ($p = 0.006$)]. When the individual components of the primary endpoint were analysed, no effect in all cause mortality was observed, while a positive trend in the reduction in ESRD and a significant reduction in doubling of serum creatinine were observed.

Subgroups consisting of gender, race, age, duration of diabetes, baseline blood pressure, serum creatinine, and albumin excretion rate were assessed for treatment effect. In the female and black subgroups which represented 32% and 26% of the overall study population respectively, a renal benefit was not evident, although the confidence intervals do not exclude it. As for the secondary endpoint of fatal and non-fatal cardiovascular events, there was no difference among the three groups in the overall population, although an increased incidence of non-fatal MI was seen for women and a decreased incidence of non-fatal MI was seen in males in the irbesartan group versus the placebo-based regimen. An increased incidence of non-fatal MI and stroke was seen in females in the irbesartan-based regimen versus the amlodipine-based regimen, while hospitalization due to heart failure was reduced in the overall population. However, no proper explanation for these findings in women has been identified.

The study of the "Effects of Irbesartan on Microalbuminuria in Hypertensive Patients with type 2 Diabetes Mellitus (IRMA 2)" shows that irbesartan 300 mg delays progression to overt proteinuria in patients with microalbuminuria. IRMA 2 was a placebo-controlled double blind morbidity study in 590 patients with type 2 diabetes, microalbuminuria (30-300 mg/day) and normal renal function (serum creatinine $\leqslant$ 1.5 mg/dl in males and $<$ 1.1 mg/dl in females). The study examined the long-term effects (2 years) of Aprovel on the progression to clinical (overt) proteinuria (urinary albumin excretion rate (UAER) $>$ 300 mg/day, and an increase in UAER of at least 30% from baseline). The predefined blood pressure goal was $\leqslant$ 135/85 mmHg. Additional antihypertensive agents (excluding ACE inhibitors, angiotensin II receptor antagonists and dihydropyridine calcium blockers) were added as needed to help achieve the blood pressure goal. While similar blood pressure was achieved in all treatment groups, fewer subjects in the irbesartan 300 mg group (5.2%) than in the placebo (14.9%) or in the irbesartan 150 mg group (9.7%) reached the endpoint of overt proteinuria, demonstrating a 70% relative risk reduction versus placebo ($p = 0.0004$) for the higher dose. An accompanying improvement in the glomerular filtration rate (GFR) was not observed during the first three months of treatment. The slowing in the progression to clinical proteinuria was evident as early as three months and continued over the 2 year period. Regression to normoalbuminuria ($<$ 30 mg/day) was more frequent in the Aprovel 300 mg group (34%) than in the placebo group (21%).

5.2 Pharmacokinetic properties

After oral administration, irbesartan is well absorbed: studies of absolute bioavailability gave values of approximately 60-80%. Concomitant food intake does not significantly influence the bioavailability of irbesartan. Plasma protein binding is approximately 96%, with negligible binding to cellular blood components. The volume of distribution is 53 - 93 litres. Following oral or intravenous administration of ^{14}C irbesartan, 80-85% of the circulating plasma radioactivity is attributable to unchanged irbesartan. Irbesartan is metabolised by the liver via glucuronide conjugation and oxidation. The major circulating metabolite is irbesartan glucuronide (approximately 6%). *In vitro* studies indicate that irbesartan is primarily oxidised by the cytochrome P450 enzyme CYP2C9; isoenzyme CYP3A4 has negligible effect.

Irbesartan exhibits linear and dose proportional pharmacokinetics over the dose range of 10 to 600 mg. A less than proportional increase in oral absorption at doses beyond 600 mg (twice the maximal recommended dose) was observed; the mechanism for this is unknown. Peak plasma concentrations are attained at 1.5 - 2 hours after oral administration. The total body and renal clearance are 157 - 176 and 3 - 3.5 ml/min, respectively. The terminal elimination half-life of irbesartan is 11 - 15 hours. Steady-state plasma concentrations are attained within 3 days after initiation of a once-daily dosing regimen. Limited accumulation of irbesartan ($<$ 20%) is observed in plasma upon repeated once-daily dosing. In a study, somewhat higher plasma concentrations of irbesartan were observed in female hypertensive patients. However, there was no difference in the half-life and accumulation of irbesartan. No dosage adjustment is necessary in female patients. Irbesartan AUC and Cmax values were also somewhat greater in elderly subjects ($\geqslant$ 65 years) than those of young subjects (18 - 40 years). However the terminal half-life was not significantly altered. No dosage adjustment is necessary in elderly patients.

Irbesartan and its metabolites are eliminated by both biliary and renal pathways. After either oral or IV administration of ^{14}C irbesartan, about 20% of the radioactivity is recovered in the urine, and the remainder in the faeces. Less than 2% of the dose is excreted in the urine as unchanged irbesartan.

The pharmacokinetics of irbesartan were evaluated in 23 hypertensive children after the administration of single and multiple daily doses of irbesartan (2 mg/kg) up to a maximum daily dose of 150 mg for four weeks. Of those 23 children, 21 were evaluable for comparison of pharmac kinetics with adults (twelve children over 12 years, ni children between 6 and 12 years). Results showed th Cmax, AUC and clearance rates were comparable to tho observed in adult patients receiving 150 mg irbesart daily. A limited accumulation of irbesartan (18%) in plasm was observed upon repeated once daily dosing.

Renal impairment: in patients with renal impairment those undergoing haemodialysis, the pharmacokinet parameters of irbesartan are not significantly altered. Irb sartan is not removed by haemodialysis.

Hepatic impairment: in patients with mild to modera cirrhosis, the pharmacokinetic parameters of irbesarta are not significantly altered.

Studies have not been performed in patients with seve hepatic impairment.

5.3 Preclinical safety data

There was no evidence of abnormal systemic or targe organ toxicity at clinically relevant doses. In non-clinic safety studies, high doses of irbesartan ($\geqslant$ 250 mg/kg/da in rats and $\geqslant$ 100 mg/kg/day in macaques) caused reduction of red blood cell parameters (erythrocytes, hae moglobin, haematocrit). At very high doses ($\geqslant$ 500 mg/kg day) degenerative changes in the kidney (such as inter stitial nephritis, tubular distension, basophilic tubules increased plasma concentrations of urea and creatinine were induced by irbesartan in the rat and the macaque an are considered secondary to the hypotensive effects of th medicinal product which led to decreased renal perfusior Furthermore, irbesartan induced hyperplasia/hypertroph of the juxtaglomerular cells (in rats at $\geqslant$ 90 mg/kg/day, i macaques at $\geqslant$ 10 mg/kg/day). All of these changes wer considered to be caused by the pharmacological action c irbesartan. For therapeutic doses of irbesartan in humans the hyperplasia/ hypertrophy of the renal juxtaglomerula cells does not appear to have any relevance.

There was no evidence of mutagenicity, clastogenicity o carcinogenicity.

Animal studies with irbesartan showed transient toxic effects (increased renal pelvic cavitation, hydroureter o subcutaneous oedema) in rat foetuses, which were resolved after birth. In rabbits, abortion or early resorption were noted at doses causing significant maternal toxicity including mortality. No teratogenic effects were observed in the rat or rabbit.

6. PHARMACEUTICAL PARTICULARS

6.1 List of excipients

Tablet core:

Lactose monohydrate

Microcrystalline cellulose

Croscarmellose sodium

Hypromellose

Silicon dioxide

Magnesium stearate.

Film-coating:

Lactose monohydrate

Hypromellose

Titanium dioxide

Macrogol 3000

Carnauba wax.

6.2 Incompatibilities

Not applicable.

6.3 Shelf life

3 years.

6.4 Special precautions for storage

Do not store above 30°C.

6.5 Nature and contents of container

Cartons of 28 film-coated tablets: 2 blister cards of 14 film-coated tablets in PVC/PVDC/Aluminium blisters.

6.6 Special precautions for disposal and other handling

Any unused product or waste material should be disposed of in accordance with local requirements.

7. MARKETING AUTHORISATION HOLDER

SANOFI PHARMA BRISTOL-MYERS SQUIBB SNC

174 avenue de France

F-75013 Paris - France

8. MARKETING AUTHORISATION NUMBER(S)

EU/1/97/046/017

EU/1/97/046/022

EU/1/97/046/027

9. DATE OF FIRST AUTHORISATION/RENEWAL OF THE AUTHORISATION

Date of first authorisation: 27 August 1997

Date of latest renewal: 27 August 2007

10. DATE OF REVISION OF THE TEXT

31 March 2009

Legal Category: POM

Detailed information on this product is available on the website of the European Medicines Agency (EMEA) http://www.emea.europa.eu/

ptivus 250 mg soft capsules

(Boehringer Ingelheim Limited)

NAME OF THE MEDICINAL PRODUCT

PTIVUS ▼ 250 mg soft capsules.

QUALITATIVE AND QUANTITATIVE COMPOSITION

ach soft capsule contains 250 mg tipranavir.

xcipients (per capsule): 100.0 mg Ethanol, 455.0 mg acrogolglycerol Ricinoleate and 12.6 mg Sorbitol (constituent in « Sorbitol Special-Glycerin Blend »)

or a full list of excipients, see section 6.1.

PHARMACEUTICAL FORM

oft capsule.

ach capsule is pink and is imprinted with "TPV 250".

CLINICAL PARTICULARS

.1 Therapeutic indications

PTIVUS, co-administered with low dose ritonavir, is indicated for combination antiretroviral treatment of HIV-1 nfection in highly pre-treated adults and adolescents 12 ears of age or older with virus resistant to multiple protease inhibitors. APTIVUS should only be used as part of an ctive combination antiretroviral regimen in patients with o other therapeutic options.

his indication is based on the results of two phase III tudies, performed in highly pre-treated adult patients median number of 12 prior antiretroviral agents) with virus esistant to protease inhibitors and of one phase II study nvestigating pharmacokinetics, safety and efficacy of PTIVUS in mostly treatment-experienced adolescent atients aged 12 to 18 years (see section 5.1).

n deciding to initiate treatment with APTIVUS, co-administered with low dose ritonavir, careful consideration hould be given to the treatment history of the individual atient and the patterns of mutations associated with ifferent agents. Genotypic or phenotypic testing (when vailable) and treatment history should guide the use of PTIVUS. Initiation of treatment should take into account he combinations of mutations which may negatively mpact the virological response to APTIVUS, co-administered with low dose ritonavir (see section 5.1).

.2 Posology and method of administration

APTIVUS must always be given with low dose ritonavir as a pharmacokinetic enhancer, and in combination with other antiretroviral medicinal products. The Summary of Product Characteristics of ritonavir must therefore be consulted prior to initiation of therapy with APTIVUS (especially as regards the contraindications, warnings and undesirable effects sections).

APTIVUS should be prescribed by physicians who are experienced in the treatment of HIV-1 infection.

APTIVUS soft capsules co-administered with low dose ritonavir should be taken with food (see section 5.2).

APTIVUS/ritonavir should not be used in treatment-naïve patients.

Adults and adolescents from 12 years of age

The recommended dose of APTIVUS is 500 mg, co-administered with 200 mg ritonavir (low dose ritonavir), twice daily (see section 4.4 for precautionary measures in adolescents).

Doses of ritonavir lower than 200 mg twice daily should not be used as they might alter the efficacy profile of the combination.

Since currently only limited efficacy and safety data are available for adolescents (see section 5.1) close monitoring of virologic response and tolerance is particularly warranted in this patient group.

Children under 12 years of age:

No data are available on the efficacy and safety of APTIVUS capsules in children under 12 years of age. Also, appropriate dose adjustments for children under 12 years cannot be achieved with APTIVUS capsules. APTIVUS oral solution is available for children between 2 and 12 years of age (please refer to the respective SPC for further details).

APTIVUS is not recommended for use in children under 2 years of age due to insufficient data on safety and efficacy.

Elderly

Clinical studies of APTIVUS did not include sufficient numbers of subjects aged 65 and over to determine whether they respond differently from younger subjects (see section 5.2).

Liver impairment

Tipranavir is metabolised by the hepatic system. Liver impairment could therefore result in an increase of tipranavir exposure and a worsening of its safety profile. Therefore, APTIVUS should be used with caution, and with increased monitoring frequency, in patients with mild hepatic impairment (Child-Pugh Class A). APTIVUS is contraindicated in patients with moderate or severe (Child-Pugh Class B or C) hepatic impairment (see sections 4.3, 4.4 and 5.2).

Renal impairment:

No dosage adjustment is required in patients with renal impairment (see sections 4.4 and 5.2).

4.3 Contraindications

Hypersensitivity to the active substance or to any of the excipients.

Patients with moderate or severe (Child-Pugh B or C) hepatic impairment.

Combination of rifampicin with APTIVUS with concomitant low dose ritonavir is contraindicated (see section 4.5).

Herbal preparations containing St John's wort (*Hypericum perforatum*) must not be used while taking APTIVUS due to the risk of decreased plasma concentrations and reduced clinical effects of tipranavir (see section 4.5).

Co-administration of APTIVUS with low dose ritonavir, with active substances that are highly dependent on CYP3A for clearance and for which elevated plasma concentrations are associated with serious and/or life-threatening events is contraindicated. These active substances include antiarrhythmics (amiodarone, bepridil, quinidine), antihistamines (astemizole, terfenadine), ergot derivatives (dihydroergotamine, ergonovine, ergotamine, methylergonovine), gastrointestinal motility agents (cisapride), neuroleptics (pimozide, sertindole), sedatives/hypnotics (orally administered midazolam and triazolam. For caution on parenterally administered midazolam see section 4.5) and HMG-CoA reductase inhibitors (simvastatin and lovastatin). In addition, co-administration of APTIVUS with low dose ritonavir, and medicinal products that are highly dependent on CYP2D6 for clearance, such as the antiarrhythmics flecainide, propafenone and metoprolol given in heart failure, is contraindicated (see section 4.5).

4.4 Special warnings and precautions for use

APTIVUS must be administered with low dose ritonavir to ensure its therapeutic effect (see section 4.2). Failure to correctly co-administer tipranavir with ritonavir will result in reduced plasma levels of tipranavir that may be insufficient to achieve the desired antiviral effect. Patients should be instructed accordingly.

APTIVUS is not a cure for HIV-1 infection or AIDS. Patients receiving APTIVUS or any other antiretroviral therapy may continue to develop opportunistic infections and other complications of HIV-1 infection.

Patients should be advised that current antiretroviral therapy has not been proven to prevent the risk of transmission of HIV to others through blood or sexual contact. Appropriate precautions should continue to be employed.

Switching from APTIVUS capsules to the oral solution: APTIVUS capsules are not interchangeable with the oral solution. Compared to the capsules, tipranavir exposure is higher when administering the same dose as oral solution. Also, the composition of the oral solution is different from that of the capsules, with the high vitamin E content being especially noteworthy. Both of these factors may contribute to an increased risk of adverse reactions (type, frequency and/or severity). Therefore patients should not be switched from APTIVUS capsules to APTIVUS oral solution (see sections 5.1 and 5.2).

Switching from APTIVUS oral solution to the capsules: APTIVUS oral solution is not interchangeable with the capsules. Compared to the oral solution, tipranavir exposure is lower when administering the same dose as capsules. However, children previously treated with APTIVUS oral solution and becoming 12 years of age should be switched to capsules, particularly because of the more favourable safety profile of the capsules. It has to be noted that the switch from the oral solution to the capsule formulation of APTIVUS could be associated with decreased exposure. Therefore, it is recommended that patients switching from APTIVUS oral solution to capsules at the age of 12 years are closely monitored for the virologic response of their antiretroviral regimen (see sections 5.1 and 5.2).

Elderly: In general, caution should be exercised in the administration and monitoring of APTIVUS in elderly patients reflecting the greater frequency of decreased hepatic, renal, or cardiac function, and of concomitant disease or other therapy.

Liver disease: APTIVUS is contraindicated in patients with moderate or severe (Child-Pugh Class B or C) hepatic insufficiency. Limited data are currently available for the use of APTIVUS, co-administered with low dose ritonavir, in patients co-infected with hepatitis B or C. Patients with chronic hepatitis B or C and treated with combination antiretroviral therapy are at an increased risk for severe and potentially fatal hepatic adverse events. APTIVUS should be used in this patient population only if the potential benefit outweighs the potential risk, and with increased clinical and laboratory monitoring. In the case of concomitant antiviral therapy for hepatitis B or C, please refer also to the relevant Summary of Product Characteristics for these medicinal products.

Patients with mild hepatic impairment (Child-Pugh Class A) should be closely monitored.

Patients with pre-existing liver dysfunction including chronic active hepatitis have an increased frequency of liver function abnormalities during combination therapy and should be monitored according to standard practice. APTIVUS/ritonavir should be discontinued once signs of worsening liver function occur in patients with pre-existing liver disease.

APTIVUS co-administered with low dose ritonavir, has been associated with reports of clinical hepatitis and hepatic decompensation, including some fatalities. These have generally occurred in patients with advanced HIV disease taking multiple concomitant medicinal products. Caution should be exercised when administering APTIVUS to patients with liver enzyme abnormalities or with a history of hepatitis. Increased ALAT/ASAT monitoring should be considered in these patients.

APTIVUS therapy should not be initiated in patients with pre-treatment ASAT or ALAT greater than 5 times the Upper Limit Normal (ULN) until baseline ASAT/ALAT is stabilised at less than 5X ULN, unless the potential benefit justifies the potential risk.

APTIVUS therapy should be discontinued in patients experiencing ASAT or ALAT elevations greater than 10X ULN, or developing signs or symptoms of clinical hepatitis during therapy. If another cause is identified (eg acute hepatitis A, B or C virus, gallbladder disease, other medicinal products), then rechallenge with APTIVUS may be considered when ASAT/ALAT have returned to the patient's baseline levels.

Liver monitoring

Monitoring of hepatic tests should be done prior to initiation of therapy, after two, four and then every four weeks until 24 weeks, and then every eight to twelve weeks thereafter. Increased monitoring (i.e. prior to initiation of therapy, every two weeks during the first three months of treatment, then monthly until 48 weeks, and then every eight to twelve weeks thereafter) is warranted when APTIVUS and low dose ritonavir are administered to patients with elevated ASAT and ALAT levels, mild hepatic impairment, chronic hepatitis B or C or other underlying liver disease.

Treatment-naïve patients

In a study performed in antiretroviral naïve adult patients, APTIVUS/ritonavir 500 mg/200 mg twice daily, as compared to lopinavir/ritonavir, was associated with an excess in the occurrence of significant (grade 3 and 4) transaminase elevations without any advantage in terms of efficacy (trend towards a lower efficacy). Therefore, this study was prematurely stopped after 60 weeks.

Renal impairment

Since the renal clearance of tipranavir is negligible, increased plasma concentrations are not expected in patients with renal impairment.

Haemophilia

There have been reports of increased bleeding, including spontaneous skin haematomas and haemarthrosis in patients with haemophilia type A and B treated with protease inhibitors. In some patients additional Factor VIII was given. In more than half of the reported cases, treatment with protease inhibitors was continued or reintroduced if treatment had been discontinued. A causal relationship has been evoked, although the mechanism of action had not been elucidated. Haemaophiliac patients should therefore be made aware of the possibility of increased bleeding.

Bleeding

RESIST participants receiving APTIVUS/ritonavir tended to have an increased risk of bleeding; at 24 weeks the relative risk was 1.98 (95% CI=1.03, 3.80). At 48-weeks the relative risk decreased to 1.27 (95% CI=0.76, 2.12). There was no pattern for the bleeding events and no difference between treatment groups in coagulation parameters. The significance of this finding is being further studied.

Fatal and non-fatal intracranial haemorrhages (ICH) have been reported in patients receiving APTIVUS, many of whom had other medical conditions or were receiving concomitant medicinal products that may have caused or contributed to these events. However, in some cases the role of APTIVUS cannot be excluded. No pattern of abnormal haematological or coagulation parameters has been observed in patients in general, or preceding the development of ICH. Therefore, routine measurement of coagulation parameters is not currently indicated in the management of patients on APTIVUS.

An increased risk of ICH has previously been observed in patients with advanced HIV disease/AIDS such as those treated in the APTIVUS clinical trials.

In *in vitro* experiments, tipranavir was observed to inhibit human platelet aggregation at levels consistent with exposures observed in patients receiving APTIVUS/ritonavir.

In rats, co-administration with vitamin E increased the bleeding effects of tipranavir (see section 5.3 Preclinical safety data).

APTIVUS, co-administered with low dose ritonavir, should be used with caution in patients who may be at risk of increased bleeding from trauma, surgery or other medical conditions, or who are receiving medicinal products known to increase the risk of bleeding such as antiplatelet agents and anticoagulants or who are taking supplemental vitamin E. Based on the limits of exposure available from observation in clinical trials, it is recommended not to co-administer to patients more than 1200 IU vitamin E per day.

Diabetes mellitus/hyperglycaemia

New onset of diabetes mellitus, hyperglycaemia or exacerbations of existing diabetes mellitus has been reported in patients receiving antiretroviral therapy, including protease inhibitors. In some of these the hyperglycaemia was severe and in some cases also associated with ketoacidosis. Many of the patients had confounding medical conditions, some of which required therapy with agents that have been associated with the development of diabetes mellitus or hyperglycaemia.

Lipid elevations

Treatment with APTIVUS co-administered with low dose ritonavir and other antiretroviral agents has resulted in increased plasma total triglycerides and cholesterol. Triglyceride and cholesterol testing should be performed prior to initiating tipranavir therapy and during therapy. Treatment-related lipid elevations should be managed as clinically appropriate.

Fat redistribution

Combination antiretroviral therapy has been associated with the redistribution of body fat (lipodystrophy) in HIV infected patients. The long-term consequences of these events are currently unknown. Knowledge about the mechanism is incomplete. A connection between visceral lipomatosis and protease inhibitors, and lipoatrophy and nucleoside reverse transcriptase inhibitors, has been hypothesised. A higher risk of lipodystrophy has been associated with individual factors such as older age, and with factors related to the active substance such as longer duration of antiretroviral treatment and associated metabolic disturbances. Clinical examination should include evaluation for physical signs of fat redistribution. Consideration should be given to the measurement of fasting serum lipids and blood glucose. Lipid disorders should be managed as clinically appropriate (see section 4.8).

Immune reactivation syndrome

In HIV-infected patients with severe immune deficiency at the time of institution of combination antiretroviral therapy (CART), an inflammatory reaction to asymptomatic or residual opportunistic pathogens may arise and cause serious clinical conditions, or aggravation of symptoms. Typically, such reactions have been observed within the first few weeks or months of initiation of CART. Relevant examples are cytomegalovirus retinitis, generalised and/or focal mycobacterial infections and Pneumocystis pneumonia. Any inflammatory symptoms should be evaluated and treatment instituted when necessary. In addition, reactivation of herpes simplex and herpes zoster has been observed in clinical studies with APTIVUS, co-administered with low dose ritonavir.

APTIVUS contains macrogolglycerol ricinoleate which may cause stomach upset and diarrhoea.

APTIVUS soft capsules contain small amounts of alcohol (7% ethanol, ie 100 mg per capsule or 200 mg per dose).

Rash

Mild to moderate rashes including urticarial rash, maculopapular rash, and photosensitivity have been reported in subjects receiving APTIVUS, co-administered with low dose ritonavir. At 48-weeks in Phase III trials, rash of various types was observed in 15.5% males and 20.5% females receiving APTIVUS co-administered with low dose ritonavir. Additionally, in one interaction trial, in healthy female volunteers administered a single dose of ethinyl oestradiol followed by APTIVUS co-administered with low dose ritonavir, 33% of subjects developed a rash. Rash accompanied by joint pain or stiffness, throat tightness, or generalized pruritus has been reported in both men and women receiving APTIVUS co-administered with low dose ritonavir. In the paediatric clinical trial, the frequency of rash (all grades, all causality) through 48 weeks of treatment was higher than in adult patients.

Osteonecrosis

Although the aetiology is considered to be multifactorial (including corticosteroid use, alcohol consumption, severe immunosuppression, higher body mass index), cases of osteonecrosis have been reported particularly in patients with advanced HIV-disease and/or long-term exposure to combination antiretroviral therapy (CART). Patients should be advised to seek medical advice if they experience joint aches and pain, joint stiffness or difficulty in movement.

Interactions

The interaction profile of APTIVUS, co-administered with low dose ritonavir, is complex. For a description of the mechanisms and potential mechanisms contributing to the interaction profile of APTIVUS, see section 4.5.

Abacavir and zidovudine: The concomitant use of APTIVUS, co-administered with low dose ritonavir, with zidovudine or abacavir, results in a significant decrease in plasma concentration of these nucleoside reverse transcriptase inhibitors (NRTIs). Therefore, the concomitant use of zidovudine or abacavir with APTIVUS, co-administered with low dose ritonavir, is not-recommended unless there are no other available NRTIs suitable for patient management (see section 4.5).

Protease inhibitors: Concomitant use of APTIVUS, co-administered with low dose ritonavir, with the protease inhibitors amprenavir, lopinavir or saquinavir (each co-administered with low dose ritonavir) in a dual-boosted regimen, results in significant decreases in plasma concentrations of these protease inhibitors. A significant decrease in plasma concentrations of atazanavir and a marked increase of tipranavir and ritonavir concentrations was observed when APTIVUS, associated with low dose ritonavir, was co-administered with atazanavir (see section 4.5). No data are currently available on interactions of APTIVUS, co-administered with low dose ritonavir, with protease inhibitors other than those listed above. Therefore, the co-administration of APTIVUS, co-administered with low dose ritonavir, with protease inhibitors is not recommended.

Oral contraceptives and oestrogens: Since levels of ethinyl oestradiol are decreased, the co-administration of APTIVUS co-administered with low dose ritonavir is not recommended. Alternative or additional contraceptive measures are to be used when oestrogen based oral contraceptives are co-administered with APTIVUS co-administered with low dose ritonavir (see section 4.5). Patients using oestrogens as hormone replacement therapy should be clinically monitored for signs of oestrogen deficiency. Women using oestrogens may have an increased risk of non serious rash.

Anticonvulsants: Caution should be used when prescribing carbamazepine, phenobarbital, and phenytoin. APTIVUS may be less effective due to decreased tipranavir plasma concentrations in patients taking these agents concomitantly.

Halofantrine, Lumefantrine: Due to their metabolic profile and inherent risk of inducing torsades de pointes, administration of halofantrine and lumefantrine with APTIVUS co-administered with low dose ritonavir, is not recommended.

Disulfiram/metronidazole: APTIVUS soft capsules contain alcohol (7% ethanol, ie 100 mg per capsule or up to 200 mg per dose) which can produce disulfiram-like reactions when co-administered with disulfiram or other medicinal products which produce this reaction (eg metronidazole).

Fluticasone: Concomitant use of APTIVUS, co-administered with low dose ritonavir, and fluticasone or other glucocorticoids that are metabolised by CYP3A4 is not recommended unless the potential benefit of treatment outweighs the risk of systemic corticosteroid effects, including Cushing's syndrome and adrenal suppression (see section 4.5).

Atorvastatin: APTIVUS, co-administered with low dose ritonavir, increases the plasma concentrations of atorvastatin (see section 4.5). The combination is not recommended. Other HMG-CoA reductase inhibitors should be considered such as pravastatin, fluvastatin or rosuvastatin. However, if atorvastatin is specifically required for patient management, careful monitoring is necessary.

Omeprazole: APTIVUS co-administered with low dose ritonavir decreases the plasma concentrations of omeprazole and esomeprazole (see section 4.5). Therefore, the combined use of APTIVUS/ritonavir with either omeprazole or esomeprazole is not recommended. If unavoidable, upward dose adjustments for either omeprazole or esomeprazole may be considered based on clinical response to therapy. Recommendations for maximal doses of omeprazole or esomeprazole are found in the corresponding product information.

Due to APTIVUS containing small amounts of sorbitol, patients with rare hereditary problems of fructose intolerance should not take this medicine.

4.5 Interaction with other medicinal products and other forms of interaction

The interaction profile of APTIVUS, co-administered with low dose ritonavir, is complex and requires special attention in particular in combination with other antiretroviral agents.

Interaction studies have only been performed in adults.

Metabolic profile of tipranavir:

Tipranavir is a substrate, an inducer and an inhibitor of cytochrome P450 CYP3A. When co-administered with ritonavir at the recommended dosage (see section 4.2) there is a net inhibition of P450 CYP3A. Co-administration of APTIVUS and low dose ritonavir with agents primarily metabolised by CYP3A may result in changed plasma concentrations of tipranavir or the other agents, which could alter their therapeutic and undesirable effects (see list and details of considered agents, below). Agents that are contraindicated specifically due to the expected magnitude of interaction and potential for serious adverse reactions are detailed in this section, and listed in section 4.3.

A cocktail study was conducted in 16 healthy volunteers with twice-daily APTIVUS/ritonavir 500 mg/200 mg capsule administration for 10 days to assess the net effect on the activity of hepatic CYP 1A2 (caffeine), 2C9 (warfarin), 2D6 (dextromethorphan), both intestinal/hepatic CYP 3A4 (midazolam) and P-glycoprotein (Pgp) (digoxin). At steady state, there was a significant induction of CYP 1A2 and a slight induction on CYP 2C9. Potent inhibition of CYP 2D6 and both hepatic and intestinal CYP 3A4 activities were observed. Pgp activity is significantly inhibited after the first dose, but there was a slight induction at steady state. Practical recommendations deriving from this study are displayed below.

Studies in human liver microsomes indicated tipranavir is an inhibitor of CYP 1A2, CYP 2C9, CYP 2C19 and CYP 2D6. The potential net effect of tipranavir/ritonavir on CYP 2D6 is inhibition, because ritonavir is also a CYP 2D6 inhibitor. The *in vivo* net effect of tipranavir/ritonavir on CYP 1A2, CYP 2C9 and CYP 2C19, indicates, through a preliminary study, an inducing potential of APTIVUS/ritonavir on CYP1A2 and, to a lesser extent, on CYP2C9 ar P-gp after several days of treatment. Data are not availab to indicate whether tipranavir inhibits or induces glucur nosyl transferases.

In vitro studies show that tipranavir is a substrate and als an inhibitor of Pgp.

It is difficult to predict the net effect of APTIVUS co-adm nistered with low dose ritonavir on oral bioavailability ar plasma concentrations of agents that are dual substrate of CYP3A and Pgp. The net effect will vary depending c the relative affinity of the co-administered substance fc CYP3A and Pgp, and the extent of intestinal first-pas metabolism/efflux.

Co-administration of APTIVUS and agents that induc CYP3A and/or Pgp may decrease tipranavir concentra tions and reduce its therapeutic effect (see list and detai of considered agents, below). Co-administration of APT VUS and medicinal products that inhibit Pgp may increas tipranavir plasma concentrations.

Nucleoside reverse transcriptase inhibitors: Since there no significant impact of nucleoside and nucleotide analo gues on the P450 enzyme system no dosage adjustment c APTIVUS is required when co-administered with thes agents.

Abacavir and zidovudine: APTIVUS, co-administered wit low dose ritonavir, decreases the AUC of abacavir b approximately 40% and the AUC of zidovudine by approxi mately 35%. There is no impact on glucuronidated-ZD levels. The clinical relevance of these reductions has no been established, but may decrease the efficacy of these antiretroviral agents. Therefore the concomitant use o tipranavir, co-administered with low dose ritonavir, with either abacavir or zidovudine is not recommended unless there are no other available NRTIs suitable for patien management. In such cases no dosage adjustment o abacavir or zidovudine can be recommended.

Didanosine: APTIVUS, co-administered with low dose ritonavir, causes a reduction in the AUC of didanosine. The clinical relevance of the reduction in didanosine levels has not been established. Dosing of enteric-coated didanosine and APTIVUS soft capsules, co-administered with low dose ritonavir, should be separated by at least 2 hours to avoid formulation incompatibility.

Lamivudine and stavudine: APTIVUS, co-administered with low dose ritonavir, does not cause a significant change in the AUC of lamivudine or stavudine. No dosage adjustment of lamivudine or stavudine is recommended.

Nucleotide reverse transcriptase inhibitors

Tenofovir: APTIVUS, co-administered with low dose ritonavir, did not cause a significant change in the plasma concentrations of tenofovir. No dosage adjustment of tenofovir is recommended.

Non-nucleoside reverse transcriptase inhibitors (NNRTIs)

Efavirenz: Steady-state efavirenz 600 mg once daily co-administered with steady-state APTIVUS and low-dose ritonavir (500 mg/200 mg twice daily) did not significantly alter tipranavir AUC and C_{max} and increased C_{p12h} by 19.2% which is not considered as clinically relevant. APTIVUS, co-administered with low-dose ritonavir, had no significant impact on the C_{min} of efavirenz.

Nevirapine: No specific drug-drug interaction study has been performed between APTIVUS and low-dose ritonavir (500 mg/200 mg twice daily) with nevirapine. However, the limited data available from a phase IIa study in HIV-infected patients suggest that no significant interaction is expected between nevirapine and APTIVUS co-administered with low dose ritonavir. Moreover a study with APTIVUS and low dose ritonavir and another NNRTI (efavirenz) did not show any clinically relevant interaction (see above). Therefore no dose adjustments are necessary.

Protease inhibitors

Amprenavir, lopinavir, saquinavir: In a clinical study of dual-boosted protease inhibitor combination therapy in multiple-treatment experienced HIV-positive adults, APTIVUS, co-administered with low dose ritonavir, caused a 55%, 70% and 78% reduction in the C_{min} of amprenavir, lopinavir and saquinavir, respectively. Therefore the concomitant administration of APTIVUS, co-administered with low dose ritonavir, with amprenavir/ritonavir, lopinavir/ritonavir or saquinavir/ritonavir, is not recommended, as the clinical relevance of the reduction in their levels has not been established. If the combination is nevertheless considered necessary, a monitoring of the plasma levels of these protease inhibitors is strongly encouraged.

Co-administration of Tipranavir/ritonavir and Atazanavir/ritonavir:

In a study performed in healthy volunteers co-administration of atazanavir 300 mg with TPV/r 500 mg/100 mg twice daily resulted on one hand in a marked increase of Tipranavir exposure (notably Cp12h ratio of 1.75 with 90% CI [1.39-2.20]) and ritonavir exposure (AUC ratio of 1.51 with 90% CI [1.24-1.83] and C_{max} ratio of 1.38 with 90% CI [1.13-1.67]) associated with a risk of over-toxicity and on the other hand on a marked decrease of atazanavir exposure associated with a risk of loss of efficacy (AUC_{0-24h} ratio of 0.32 with 90% CI [0.29-0.36], C_{max} ratio of 0.43 with 90% CI [0.38-0.50] and Cp24h ratio of 0.19 with 90% CI [0.15-0.24]).

›nsequently, this co-administration is not recommended. :he co-administration is nevertheless considered neces-ry, a close monitoring of the safety of tipranavir and a onitoring of plasma concentrations of atazanavir are ·ongly encouraged.

› data are currently available on interactions of APTIVUS, -administered with low dose ritonavir, with protease ıibitors other than those listed above. Hence their com-ıation with tipranavir co-administered with low dose ›navir, is not recommended (see section 4.4).

sion inhibitors

studies where tipranavir co-administered with low-dose ›navir was used with or without enfuvirtide, it has been served that the steady-state plasma tipranavir trough ncentration of patients receiving enfuvirtide were 45% gher as compared to patients not receiving enfuvirtide. information is available for the parameters AUC and ıax. A pharmacokinetic interaction is mechanistically expected and the interaction has not been confirmed a controlled interaction study. The clinical impact of the served data, especially regarding the tipranavir/ritonavir 'ety profile, remains unknown. Nevertheless, the clinical ta available from the RESIST trials did not suggest any nificant alteration of the tipranavir/ritonavir safety profile en combined with enfuvirtide as compared to patients ated with tipranavir/ritonavir without enfuvirtide.

ticonvulsants

rbamazepine, phenobarbital, and phenytoin induce 'P3A4 and should be used with caution in combination h APTIVUS/ritonavir. Concomitant use of carbamaze-e at a dose of 200mg BID resulted in decreased con-ıtrations of tipranavir (C_{min} decreased by 61% ımpared to historical controls), which may result in creased effectiveness. Higher doses of carbamazepine y result in even larger decreases in tipranavir plasma ıcentrations. The total C_{min} of carbamazepine and its ive metabolite C_{min} is increased by 23% which is not ›ected to have clinical consequences.

tifungals

conazole: APTIVUS, co-administered with low dose navir, does not substantially affect the steady-state armacokinetics of fluconazole. Fluconazole increases AUC and C_{min} of tipranavir by 56% and 104%, respec-ıly, when compared to historical data. No dosage ustments are recommended. Fluconazole doses '00 mg/day are not recommended.

conazole/ketoconazole: Based on theoretical consid-tions APTIVUS, co-administered with low dose ritona-is expected to increase itraconazole or ketoconazole centrations. Itraconazole or ketoconazole should be d with caution (doses >200 mg/day are not recom-nded).

iconazole: Due to multiple enzyme systems being olved in voriconazole metabolism, it is difficult to predict interaction.

G CoA reductase inhibitors

vastatin and lovastatin: The HMG-CoA reductase inhi-ors simvastatin and lovastatin are highly dependent on P3A for metabolism, thus concomitant use of APTIVUS administered with low dose ritonavir, with simvastatin ovastatin are contra-indicated due to an increased risk myopathy, including rhabdomyolysis (see section 4.3).

rvastatin: APTIVUS, co-administered with low dose navir, increases the plasma concentrations of single e atorvastatin by approximately 8-10 fold and reduces AUCs of its metabolites by approximately 85 %. Ator-tatin does not significantly change the AUC, C_{max} or of tipranavir. The combination is not recommended. er HMG-CoA reductase inhibitors should be consid-d such as pravastatin, fluvastatin or rosuvastatin. How-r, if atorvastatin is specifically required for patient ıagement, careful monitoring is necessary (see section).

ˀ isoenzyme inducers

mpicin: Rifampicin is a strong CYP3A4 inducer and has n shown to cause profound decreases in concentra-s of other protease inhibitors which can result in vir-gical failure and resistance development. During mpts to overcome the decreased exposure by increas-the dose of other protease inhibitors with ritonavir, a 1 frequency of liver reactions was seen. The combina-of rifampicin with APTIVUS with concomitant low-dose ıavir is contraindicated (see section 4.3).

butin: APTIVUS, co-administered with low dose rito-ir, increases plasma concentrations of rifabutin by up to ıld, and its active metabolite by up to 20 fold. Rifabutin eases the C_{min} of tipranavir by 16 %. Dosage reduc-s of rifabutin by at least 75% of the usual 300 mg/day recommended (ie 150 mg on alternate days, or three es per week). Patients receiving rifabutin with APTIVUS/ ıavir should be closely monitored for emergence of erse events associated with rifabutin therapy. Further age reduction may be necessary.

John's wort (Hypericum perforatum): Plasma levels of anavir can be reduced by concomitant use of the herbal paration St John's wort (*Hypericum perforatum*). This is to induction of drug metabolising enzymes by St n's wort. Herbal preparations containing St John's wort uld not be used concomitantly with APTIVUS. If a patient is already taking St John's wort, stop St John's wort, check viral levels and if possible tipranavir levels. Tipranavir levels may increase on stopping St John's wort, and the dose of APTIVUS may need adjusting. The inducing effect of St John's wort may persist for at least 2 weeks after cessation of treatment (see section 4.3).

CYP isoenzyme inhibitors

Clarithromycin: APTIVUS, co-administered with low dose ritonavir, increases the AUC and C_{min} of clarithromycin by 19% and 68%, respectively, and decreases the AUC of the 14-hydroxy active metabolite by over 95%. Whilst the changes in clarithromycin parameters are not considered clinically relevant, the reduction in the 14-OH metabolite AUC should be considered for the treatment of infections caused by *Haemophilus influenzae* in which the 14-OH metabolite is most active. Clarithromycin increases the C_{min} of tipranavir by more than 100%. This large increase in C_{min} may be clinically relevant. Patients using clarithromycin at doses higher than 500 mg twice daily should be carefully monitored for signs of toxicity. For patients with renal impairment the following dosage adjustments should be considered: For patients with CL_{CR} 30 to 60 ml/min the dose of clarithromycin should be reduced by 50 %. For patients with $CL_{CR} < 30$ ml/min the dose of clarithromycin should be decreased by 75 %. No dosage adjustments for patients with normal renal function are necessary.

Other agents

Co-administration of APTIVUS with low dose ritonavir, with active substances that are highly dependent on CYP3A for clearance and for which elevated plasma concentrations are associated with serious and/or life-threatening events is contraindicated. These active substances include antiarrhythmics (amiodarone, bepridil, quinidine), antihistamines (astemizole, terfenadine), ergot derivatives (dihydroergotamine, ergonovine, ergotamine, methylergonovine), gastrointestinal motility agents (cisapride), neuroleptics (pimozide, sertindole) and sedatives/hypnotics (triazolam) (see section 4.3).

In addition, co-administration of APTIVUS with low dose ritonavir, with substances that are highly dependent on CYP2D6 for clearance, such as the antiarrhythmics flecainide, propafenone and metoprolol given in heart failure, is contraindicated (see section 4.3).

Some anti-infectives are not recommended (halofantrine, lumefantrine) as well as miscellaneous agents (tolterodine) (see section 4.4).

Oral contraceptives/oestrogens

APTIVUS, co-administered with low dose ritonavir, decreases the AUC and C_{max} of ethinyl-oestradiol by 50 %, but does not significantly alter the pharmacokinetic behaviour of norethindrone. The concomitant administration with APTIVUS, co-administered with low dose ritonavir, is not recommended. Alternative or additional contraceptive measures are to be used when oestrogen based oral contraceptives are co-administered with APTIVUS and low dose ritonavir. Patients using oestrogens as hormone replacement therapy should be clinically monitored for signs of oestrogen deficiency (see section 4.4 and section 4.6).

Phosphodiesterase 5 (PDE5) inhibitors

Sildenafil and vardenafil: Particular caution should be used when prescribing the phosphodiesterase (PDE5) inhibitors sildenafil or vardenafil in patients receiving APTIVUS co-administered with low dose ritonavir. Co-administration of APTIVUS and low dose ritonavir with PDE5 inhibitors is expected to substantially increase PDE5 concentrations and may result in an increase in PDE5 inhibitor-associated adverse events including hypotension, visual changes and priapism.

Tadalafil: In a pharmacokinetic study performed in healthy male volunteers, co-administration of APTIVUS and low dose ritonavir with single dose tadalafil increased tadalafil exposure (AUC increased by 2.3 fold) at the first dose and did not change tadalafil exposure at steady-state. Therefore it is recommended to prescribe tadalafil after at least 7 days of APTIVUS/ritonavir dosing.

Narcotic analgesics (Methadone/Meperidine): Co-administration of APTIVUS and low dose ritonavir with single dose methadone was demonstrated to decrease methadone pharmacokinetic parameters (AUC_{0-24h} ratio of 0.47 with 90% CI [0.44; 0.51] and C_{max} ratio of 0.45 with 90% CI [0.41; 0.49]), in a study conducted in fasted healthy subjects. Therefore in such cases, patients should be monitored for opiate withdrawal syndrome. Dosage of methadone may need to be increased.

APTIVUS, co-administered with low dose ritonavir, is expected to decrease meperidine concentrations and increase normeperidine metabolite concentrations. Dosage increase and long-term use of meperidine with APTIVUS co-administered with low dose ritonavir are not recommended due to the increased concentrations of the metabolite normeperidine which has both analgesic activity and CNS stimulant activity (eg seizures).

(see Table 1 below)

Immunosuppressants (cyclosporin, tacrolimus, sirolimus): Concentrations of cyclosporin, tacrolimus, or sirolimus cannot be predicted when co-administered with APTIVUS co-administered with low dose ritonavir, due to conflicting effect of APTIVUS, co-administered with low dose ritonavir, on CYP 3A and Pgp. More frequent concentration monitoring of these medicinal products is recommended until blood levels have been stabilised.

Warfarin and other oral anticoagulants: Co-administration of APTIVUS with low dose ritonavir and warfarin may alter the metabolism of S-warfarin (initial inhibition and after 10 days a net induction was observed). Consequently, APTIVUS co-administered with low dose ritonavir, may be associated with changes in INR (International Normalised Ratio) values, and may affect anticoagulation (thrombogenic effect) or increase the risk of bleeding. Close clinical and biological (INR measurement) monitoring is recommended when these medicinal products are combined.

Antacids: When APTIVUS, co-administered with low dose ritonavir, was co-administered with 20 ml of aluminium- and magnesium-based liquid antacid, tipranavir AUC_{12h}, C_{max} and C_{min} were reduced by 25-29 %. Dosing of APTIVUS, co-administered with low dose ritonavir, with antacids should be separated by at least a two hours time interval.

Proton pump inhibitors

Omeprazole: In clinical pharmacokinetic studies of tipranavir/ritonavir in combination with omeprazole (40 mg once daily), no clinically important changes in tipranavir/ritonavir plasma concentrations were observed and thus no tipranavir/ritonavir dose adjustment is required. Tipranavir/ritonavir at steady state resulted in decreases in omeprazole AUC and Cmax by 71% and 73%, respectively. Similar effects were observed for the S-enantiomer, esomeprazole. Therefore, the combined use of tipranavir/ritonavir with either omeprazole or esomeprazole is not recommended (see section 4.4). If unavoidable, upward dose adjustments for either omeprazole or esomeprazole may be considered based on clinical response to therapy. There are no data available indicating that omeprazole or esomeprazole dose adjustments will overcome the observed pharmacokinetic interaction. Recommendations for maximal doses of omeprazole or esomeprazole are found in the corresponding product information.

H2-receptor antagonists: No data are available for H2-receptor antagonists in combination with tipranavir and low dose ritonavir. An increase in gastric pH that may result from H2-receptor antagonist therapy is not expected to have an impact on tipranavir plasma concentrations. Caution should be exercised when such substances are combined with tipranavir and low dose ritonavir.

Theophylline: Based on data from the cocktail study where caffeine (CYP1A2 substrate) AUC was reduced by 43%, APTIVUS/ritonavir is expected to decrease theophylline concentrations. Theophylline plasma concentrations should be monitored during the first two weeks of co-administration with APTIVUS/ritonavir and the theophylline dose should be increased as needed.

Desipramine: APTIVUS, co-administered with low dose ritonavir, is expected to increase desipramine concentrations. Dosage reduction and concentration monitoring of desipramine is recommended.

Midazolam: Concomitant use of APTIVUS/ritonavir and oral midazolam is contra-indicated (see section 4.3). Ritonavir is a potent inhibitor of CYP3A4 and therefore will affect substances metabolised by this enzyme. When co-administered with APTIVUS/ritonavir at steady-state concentrations of intravenously administered single dose midazolam were increased 2.8 fold (AUC_{0-24h}) and concentrations of orally administered midazolam were increased 10 fold. If APTIVUS/ritonavir is administered with parenteral midazolam, close clinical monitoring for respiratory depression and/or prolonged sedation should be instituted and dosage adjustment should be considered.

Digoxin: APTIVUS, co-administered with low dose ritonavir, may double the exposure of orally administered digoxin at first dose, while the net effect at steady state may rather consist in a slight decrease in digoxin exposure. Monitoring of digoxin serum concentrations is recommended until steady state has been obtained.

Trazodone: In a pharmacokinetic study performed in healthy volunteers, concomitant use of low dose ritonavir (200 mg twice daily) with a single dose of trazodone led to an increased plasma concentration of trazodone (AUC increased by 2.4 fold). Adverse events of nausea,

Table 1

Buprenorphine/ Naloxone	Buprenorphine ↔ Norbuprenorphine AUC ↓ 0.21 Norbuprenorphine Cmax ↓ 0.20 Norbuprenorphine Cmin ↓ 0.20	Due to reduction in the levels of the active metabolite norbuprenorphine, co-administration of APTIVUS, co-administered with low dose ritonavir, and buprenorphine/ naloxone may result in decreased clinical efficacy of buprenorphine. Therefore, patients should be monitored for opiate withdrawal syndrome.

dizziness, hypotension and syncope have been observed following co-administration of trazodone and ritonavir in this study. However, it is unknown whether the combination of tipranavir/ritonavir might cause a larger increase in trazodone exposure. The combination should be used with caution and a lower dose of trazodone should be considered.

Bupropion: APTIVUS co-administered with low-dose ritonavir at steady-state resulted in approximately a 50% decrease in bupropion Cmax and AUC0-12h. This effect may be due to induction of bupropion metabolism. There was no relevant change in TPV Cmin. If the co-administration with bupropion is judged unavoidable, this should be done under close clinical monitoring for bupropion efficacy, without exceeding the recommended dosage, despite the observed induction.

Loperamide: A pharmacodynamic interaction study in healthy volunteers demonstrated that administration of loperamide and APTIVUS, co-administered with low dose ritonavir does not cause any clinically relevant change in the respiratory response to carbon dioxide. The pharmacokinetic analysis showed that the AUC and C_{max} of loperamide are reduced by 51% and 61%, respectively, and the C_{min} of tipranavir by 26%. The clinical relevance of these changes is unknown.

Fluticasone propionate (interaction with ritonavir): In a clinical study where ritonavir 100 mg capsules twice daily were co-administered with 50 μg intranasal fluticasone propionate (four times daily) for 7 days in healthy subjects, the fluticasone propionate plasma levels increased significantly, whereas the intrinsic cortisol levels decreased by approximately 86% (90% confidence interval 82-89%). Greater effects may be expected when fluticasone propionate is inhaled. Systemic corticosteroid effects including Cushing's syndrome and adrenal suppression have been reported in patients receiving ritonavir and inhaled or intranasally administered fluticasone propionate; this could also occur with other corticosteroids metabolised via the P450 3A pathway e.g. budesonide. Consequently, concomitant administration of tipranavir, co-administered with low dose ritonavir, and these glucocorticoids is not recommended unless the potential benefit of treatment outweighs the risk of systemic corticosteroid effects (see section 4.4). A dose reduction of the glucocorticoid should be considered with close monitoring of local and systemic effects, or a switch to a glucocorticoid which is not a substrate for CYP3A4 (e.g. beclomethasone). Moreover, in case of withdrawal of glucocorticoids progressive dose reduction may have to be performed over a longer period. The effects of high fluticasone systemic exposure on ritonavir plasma levels are as yet unknown.

4.6 Pregnancy and lactation

There are no adequate data from the use of APTIVUS in pregnant women. Studies in animals have shown reproductive toxicity (see section 5.3). The potential risk for humans is unknown. Tipranavir should be used during pregnancy only if the potential benefit justifies the potential risk to the foetus.

APTIVUS adversely interacts with oral contraceptives. Therefore, an alternative, effective, safe method of contraception should be used during treatment.

Consistent with the recommendation that HIV-infected mothers should not breast-feed their infants under any circumstances to avoid risking postnatal transmission of HIV, mothers should discontinue breast-feeding if they are receiving APTIVUS.

4.7 Effects on ability to drive and use machines

No studies on the effects on the ability to drive and use machines have been performed.

Patients should be informed that APTIVUS soft capsules contain small amounts of alcohol (7% ethanol, ie 100 mg per capsule or 200 mg per dose).

4.8 Undesirable effects

APTIVUS co-administered with low dose ritonavir, has been associated with reports of significant liver toxicity. In Phase III RESIST trials, the frequency of transaminase elevations was significantly increased in the APTIVUS/ritonavir arm compared to the comparator arm. Close monitoring is therefore needed in patients treated with APTIVUS, co-administered with low dose ritonavir (see section 4.4). Limited data are currently available for the use of APTIVUS, co-administered with low dose ritonavir, in patients co-infected with hepatitis B or C. APTIVUS should therefore be used with caution in patients co-infected with hepatitis B or C. APTIVUS should be used in this patient population only if the potential benefit outweighs the potential risk, and with increased clinical and laboratory monitoring.

Adults

Tipranavir (as soft capsules), co-administered with low dose ritonavir has been studied in a total of 6308 HIV-positive adults as combination therapy in clinical studies, including compassionate use studies. Of these 5219 patients received the dose of 500 mg/200 mg twice daily. 909 adults in clinical trials, including 541 in the RESIST-1 and RESIST-2 Phase III pivotal trials, have been treated with 500 mg/200 mg twice daily for at least 48 weeks.

The following clinical safety features (hepatotoxicity, hyperlipidaemia, bleeding events, rash) were seen at higher frequency among APTIVUS/ritonavir treated patients when compared with the comparator arm treated patients in the RESIST trials, or have been observed with APTIVUS/ritonavir administration. The clinical significance of these observations has not been fully explored.

Hepatotoxicity: After 48 weeks of follow-up, the frequency of Grade 3 or 4 ALAT and/or ASAT abnormalities was higher in APTIVUS/ritonavir patients compared with comparator arm patients (10 % and 3.4 %, respectively). Multivariate analyses showed that baseline ALAT or ASAT above DAIDS Grade 1 and co-infection with hepatitis B or C were risk factors for these elevations. Most patients were able to continue treatment with APTIVUS/ritonavir.

Hyperlipidaemia: Grade 3 or 4 elevations of triglycerides occurred more frequently in the APTIVUS/ritonavir arm compared with the comparator arm. At 48 weeks these rates were 25.2 % of patients in the APTIVUS/ritonavir arm and 15.6 % in the comparator arm.

Bleeding: RESIST participants receiving APTIVUS/ritonavir tended to have an increased risk of bleeding; at 24 weeks the relative risk was 1.98 (95% CI=1.03, 3.80). At 48-weeks the relative risk decreased to 1.27 (95% CI=0.76, 2.12). There was no pattern for the bleeding events and no difference between treatment groups in coagulation parameters. The significance of this finding is being further studied.

Fatal and non-fatal intracranial haemorrhage (ICH) have been reported in patients receiving APTIVUS, many of whom had other medical conditions or were receiving concomitant medicinal products that may have caused or contributed to these events. However, in some cases the role of APTIVUS cannot be excluded. No pattern of abnormal haematological or coagulation parameters has been observed in patients in general, or preceding the development of ICH. Therefore, routine measurement of coagulation parameters is not currently indicated in the management of patients on APTIVUS.

An increased risk of ICH has previously been observed in patients with advanced HIV disease/AIDS such as those treated in the APTIVUS clinical trials.

Rash: An interaction study in women between APTIVUS, co-administered with low dose ritonavir, and ethinyl oestradiol/norethindrone demonstrated a high frequency of non-serious rash. In the RESIST trials, the risk of rash was similar between APTIVUS/ritonavir and comparator arms (16.3 % vs. 12.5 %, respectively; see section 4.4). No cases of Stevens-Johnson Syndrome or Toxic Epidermal Necrolysis have been reported in the clinical development programme of APTIVUS.

The most frequent adverse reactions of any intensity (Grades 1-4) reported in the Phase III clinical studies in the APTIVUS/ritonavir arms (n=749) are listed below by system organ class and frequency according to the following categories:

Very common (≥ 1/10), common (≥ 1/100 to < 1/10)

Metabolism and nutrition disorders:

Common: hypertriglyceridaemia, hyperlipidaemia, anorexia.

Nervous system disorders:

Common: headache.

Gastrointestinal disorders:

Very common: diarrhoea, nausea.

Common: vomiting, flatulence, abdominal distension, abdominal pain, loose stools, dyspepsia.

Skin and subcutaneous tissue disorders:

Common: rash, pruritus.

General disorders and administration site conditions:

Common: fatigue.

Clinically meaningful adverse reactions of moderate to severe intensity occurring in less than 1% (< 1/100) of adult patients in all Phase II and III trials treated with the 500 mg/200 mg tipranavir/ritonavir dose (n=1397) are listed below by system organ class and frequency according to the following categories:

Uncommon (≥ 1/1,000 to < 1/100), rare (≥ 1/10,000 to < 1/1,000)

Blood and lymphatic system disorders:

Uncommon: anaemia, neutropenia, thrombocytopenia.

Immune system disorders:

Uncommon: hypersensitivity.

Metabolism and nutrition disorders:

Uncommon: decreased appetite, diabetes mellitus, hyperamylasaemia, hypercholesterolaemia.

Rare: dehydration, facial wasting, hyperglycaemia.

Psychiatric disorders:

Uncommon: insomnia, sleep disorder.

Nervous system disorders:

Uncommon: dizziness, neuropathy peripheral, somnolence.

Respiratory, thoracic and mediastinal disorders:

Uncommon: dyspnoea.

Gastrointestinal disorders:

Uncommon: gastrooesophageal reflux disease, pancre titis.

Hepatobiliary disorders:

Uncommon: cytolytic hepatitis, hepatic steatosis, hepa tis, toxic hepatitis.

Rare: hepatic failure (including fatal outcome), hyperbil ubinaemia.

Skin and subcutaneous tissue disorders:

Uncommon: exanthem, lipoatrophy, lipodystrop acquired, lipohypertrophy.

Musculoskeletal and connective tissue disorders:

Uncommon: muscle cramp, myalgia.

Renal and urinary disorders:

Uncommon: renal insufficiency.

General disorders and administration site conditions:

Uncommon: influenza like illness, malaise, pyrexia.

Investigations:

Uncommon: hepatic enzymes increased (ALAT, ASA lipase increased, liver function test abnormal (ALA ASAT), weight decreased.

Laboratory abnormalities

Frequencies of marked clinical laboratory abnormaliti (Grade 3 or 4) reported in at least 2 % of patients in t APTIVUS/ritonavir arms in the phase III clinical studi (RESIST-1 and RESIST-2) after 48-weeks were increas ASAT (6.1 %), increased ALAT (9.7 %), increased amyla (6.0 %), increased cholesterol (4.2 %), increased triglyc ides (24.9 %), and decreased white blood cell cou (5.7 %).

Combination antiretroviral therapy, including regime containing a protease inhibitor, is associated with red tribution of body fat in some patients, including loss peripheral subcutaneous fat, increased intra-abdomi fat, breast hypertrophy and dorsocervical fat accumulati (buffalo hump). Protease inhibitors are also associated w metabolic abnormalities such as hypertriglyceridaem hypercholesterolaemia, insulin resistance and hyperg caemia.

Increased CPK, myalgia, myositis and, rarely, rhabdomy lysis, have been reported with protease inhibitors, partic larly in combination with nucleoside reverse transcripta inhibitors.

In HIV-infected patients with severe immune deficiency the time of initiation of combination antiretroviral thera (CART), an inflammatory reaction to asymptomatic or re dual opportunistic infections may arise (see section 4. Reactivation of herpes simplex and herpes zoster vi infections were observed in the RESIST trials.

Cases of osteonecrosis have been reported, particularly patients with generally acknowledged risk facto advanced HIV disease or long-term exposure to combi tion antiretroviral therapy (CART). The frequency of this unknown (see section 4.4).

Paediatrics

In an open-label, dose-finding study of APTIVUS p ritonavir (Trial 1182.14), 28 children who were 12 years age or above received APTIVUS capsules. In gene adverse reactions were similar to those seen in adults, w the exception of vomiting, rash and pyrexia, which w reported more frequently in children than in adults. T most frequently reported moderate or severe adve reactions in the 48 week analyses are noted below.

Most frequently reported moderate or severe adver reactions in pediatric patients aged 12 to 18 years w took Aptivus capsules (reported in 2 or more childr Trial 1182.14, week 48 analyses, Full Analysis Set).

Total patients treated (N)	28
Events [N(%)]	
Vomiting/ retching	3 (10.7)
Nausea	2 (7.1)
Abdominal pain[1]	2 (7.1)
Rash[2]	3 (10.7)
Insomnia	2 (7.1)
ALAT increased	4 (14.3)

1. Includes abdominal pain (N=1) and dyspepsia (N=1)

2. Rash consists of one or more of the preferred terms rash, drug eruption, rash macular, rash papular, erythen rash maculo-papular, rash pruitic, and urticaria

4.9 Overdose

There is no known antidote for APTIVUS overdose. Tre ment of overdose should consist of general support measures, including monitoring of vital signs and obser tion of the patient's clinical status. If indicated, eliminat of unabsorbed tipranavir should be achieved by emesis gastric lavage. Administration of activated charcoal m also be used to aid in removal of unabsorbed substan nce tipranavir is highly protein bound, dialysis is unlikely be beneficial in significant removal of this medicine.

PHARMACOLOGICAL PROPERTIES

1 Pharmacodynamic properties

harmacotherapeutic group: protease inhibitor, ATC code:)5AE09

echanism of action

he human immunodeficiency virus (HIV-1) encodes an spartyl protease that is essential for the cleavage and aturation of viral protein precursors. Tipranavir is a non-eptidic inhibitor of the HIV-1 protease that inhibits viral plication by preventing the maturation of viral particles.

ntiviral activity *in vitro*

pranavir inhibits the replication of laboratory strains of IV-1 and clinical isolates in acute models of T-cell infec-on, with 50% and 90% effective concentrations (EC_{50} and C_{90}) ranging from 0.03 to 0.07 μM (18-42 ng/ml) and 0.07 0.18 μM (42-108 ng/ml), respectively. Tipranavir demon-rates antiviral activity *in vitro* against a broad panel of IV-1 group M non-clade B isolates (A, C, D, F, G, H, RF01 AE, CRF02 AG, CRF12 BF). Group O and HIV-2 olates have reduced susceptibility *in vitro* to tipranavir ith EC_{50} values ranging from 0.164-1 μM and 0.233-.522 μM, respectively. Protein binding studies have nown that the antiviral activity of tipranavir decreases n average 3.75-fold in conditions where human serum present.

esistance

he development of resistance to tipranavir *in vitro* is slow nd complex. In one particular *in vitro* resistance experi-ent, an HIV-1 isolate that was 87-fold resistant to tipra-avir was selected after 9 months, and contained 10 utations in the protease: L10F, I13V, V32I, L33F, M36I, K45I, I54V/T, A71V, V82L, I84V as well as a mutation in the ag polyprotein CA/P2 cleavage site. Reverse genetic xperiments showed that the presence of 6 mutations in e protease (I13V, V32I, L33F, K45I, V82L, I84V) was equired to confer > 10-fold resistance to tipranavir while he full 10-mutation genotype conferred 69-fold resistance o tipranavir. *In vitro*, there is an inverse correlation etween the degree of resistance to tipranavir and the apacity of viruses to replicate. Recombinant viruses howing ≥ 3-fold resistance to tipranavir grow at less than % of the rate detected for wild type HIV-1 in the same onditions. Tipranavir resistant viruses which emerge *in vitro* from wild-type HIV-1 show decreased susceptibility to he protease inhibitors amprenavir, atazanavir, indinavir, opinavir, nelfinavir and ritonavir but remain sensitive to saquinavir.

Through a series of multiple stepwise regression analyses of baseline and on-treatment genotypes from all clinical studies, 16 amino acids have been associated with reduced tipranavir susceptibility and/or reduced 48-week viral load response: 10V, 13V, 20M/R/V, 33F, 35G, 36I, 43T, 46L, 47V, 54A/M/V, 58E, 69K, 74P, 82L/T, 83D and 84V. Clinical isolates that exhibited a ≥ 10-fold decrease in tipranavir susceptibility harboured 8 or more tipranavir-associated mutations. In Phase II and III clinical trials, 276 patients with on-treatment genotypes have demon-strated that the predominant emerging mutations with APTIVUS treatment are L33F/I/V, V82T/L and I84V. Com-bination of all three of these is usually required for reduced susceptibility. Mutations at position 82 occur via two path-ways: one from pre-existing mutation 82A selecting to 82T, the other from wild type 82V selecting to 82L.

Cross-resistance

Tipranavir maintains significant antiviral activity (< 4-fold resistance) against the majority of HIV-1 clinical isolates showing post-treatment decreased susceptibility to the currently approved protease inhibitors: amprenavir, ataza-navir, indinavir, lopinavir, ritonavir, nelfinavir and saquina-vir. Greater than 10-fold resistance to tipranavir is uncommon (< 2.5 % of tested isolates) in viruses obtained from highly treatment experienced patients who have received multiple peptidic protease inhibitors.

Clinical pharmacodynamic data

The following clinical data is derived from analyses of 48-week data from ongoing studies (RESIST-1 and RESIST-2) measuring effects on plasma HIV RNA levels and CD4 cell counts. RESIST-1 and RESIST-2 are ongoing, randomised, open-label, multicentre studies in HIV-positive, triple-class experienced patients, evaluating treatment with APTIVUS co-administered with low dose ritonavir (500 mg/200 mg twice daily) plus an optimised background regimen (OBR) individually defined for each patient based on genotypic resistance testing and patient history. The comparator regimen included a ritonavir-boosted PI (also individually defined) plus an OBR. The ritonavir-boosted PI was chosen from among saquinavir, amprenavir, indinavir or lopinavir/ritonavir.

All patients had received at least two PI-based antiretro-viral regimens and were failing a PI-based regimen at the time of study entry. At least one primary protease gene mutation from among 30N, 46I, 46L, 48V, 50V, 82A, 82F, 82L, 82T, 84V or 90M had to be present at baseline, with not more than two mutations on codons 33, 82, 84 or 90.

After Week 8, patients in the comparator arm who met the protocol defined criteria of initial lack of virologic response had the option of discontinuing treatment and switching over to APTIVUS/ritonavir in a separate roll-over study.

Table 2 Treatment response* at week 48 (pooled studies RESIST-1 and RESIST-2 in treatment-experienced patients)

RESIST study	APTIVUS/RTV		CPI/RTV**		p-value
	n (%)	N	n (%)	N	
Overall population					
FAS	255 (34.2)	746	114 (15.5)	737	<0.0001
PP	171 (37.7)	454	74 (17.1)	432	<0.0001
- with ENF (FAS)	85 (50.0)	170	28 (20.7)	135	<0.0001
- without ENF (FAS)	170 (29.5)	576	86 (14.3)	602	<0.0001
Genotypically Resistant					
LPV/rtv					
FAS	66 (28.9)	228	23 (9.5)	242	<0.0001
PP	47 (32.2)	146	13 (9.1)	143	<0.0001
APV/rtv					
FAS	50 (33.3)	150	22 (14.9)	148	<0.0001
PP	38 (39.2)	97	17 (18.3)	93	0.0010
SQV/rtv					
FAS	22 (30.6)	72	5 (7.0)	71	<0.0001
PP	11 (28.2)	39	2 (5.7)	35	0.0650
IDV/rtv					
FAS	6 (46.2)	13	1 (5.3)	19	0.0026
PP	3 (50.0)	6	1 (7.1)	14	0.0650

* Composite endpoint defined as patients with a confirmed 1 log RNA drop from baseline and without evidence of treatment failure

** Comparator PI/RTV: LPV/r 400 mg/100 mg twice daily (n=358), IDV/r 800 mg/100 mg twice daily (n=23), SQV/r 1000 mg/100 mg twice daily or 800 mg/200 mg twice daily (n=162), APV/r 600 mg/100 mg twice daily (n=194)

ENF Enfuvirtide; FAS Full Analysis Set; PP Per Protocol; APV/rtv Amprenavir/ritonavir; IDV/rtv Indinavir/ritonavir; LPV/rtv Lopinavir/ritonavir; SQV/rtv Saquinavir/ritonavir

The 1483 patients included in the primary analysis had a median age of 43 years (range 17-80), were 86 % male, 75 % white, 13 % black and 1 % Asian. In the APTIVUS and comparator arms median baseline CD4 cell counts were 158 and 166 cells/mm^3, respectively, (ranges 1-1893 and 1-1184 cells/mm^3); median baseline plasma HIV-1 RNA was 4.79 and 4.80 log_{10} copies/ml, respectively (ranges 2.34-6.52 and 2.01-6.76 log_{10} copies/ml).

Patients had prior exposure to a median of 6 NRTIs, 1 NNRTI, and 4 PIs. In both studies, a total of 67% patient viruses were resistant and 22% were possibly resistant to the pre-selected comparator PIs. A total of 10% of patients had previously used enfuvirtide. Patients had baseline HIV-1 isolates with a median of 16 HIV-1 protease gene muta-tions, including a median of 3 primary protease gene mutations D30N, L33F/I, V46I/L, G48V, I50V, V82A/F/T/L, I84V, and L90M. With respect to mutations on codons 33, 82, 84 and 90 approximately 4% had no mutations, 24% had mutations at codons 82 (less than 1% of patients had the mutation V82L) and 90, 18% had mutations at codons 84 and 90 and 53% had at least one key mutation at codon 90. One patient in the APTIVUS arm had four mutations. In addition the majority of participants had mutations asso-ciated with both NRTI and NNRTI resistance. Baseline phenotypic susceptibility was evaluated in 454 baseline patient samples. There was an average decrease in sus-ceptibility of 2-fold wild type (WT) for tipranavir, 12-fold WT for amprenavir, 55-fold WT for atazanavir, 41-fold WT for indinavir, 87-fold WT for lopinavir, 41-fold WT for nelfinavir, 195-fold WT for ritonavir, and 20-fold WT for saquinavir.

Combined 48-week treatment response (composite end-point defined as patients with a confirmed ≥1 log RNA drop from baseline and without evidence of treatment fail-ure) for both studies was 34% in the APTIVUS/ritonavir arm and 15% in the comparator arm. Treatment response is presented for the overall population (displayed by enfuvir-tide use), and detailed by PI strata for the subgroup of patients with genotypically resistant strains in the Table below.

Treatment response* at week 48 (pooled studies RESIST-1 and RESIST-2 in treatment-experienced patients)

(see Table 2 above)

Combined 48-week median time to treatment failure for both studies was 115 days in the APTIVUS/ritonavir arm and 0 days in the comparator arm (no treatment response was imputed to day 0).

Through 48 weeks of treatment, the proportion of patients in the APTIVUS/ritonavir arm compared to the comparator PI/ritonavir arm with HIV-1 RNA < 400 copies/ml was 30% and 14% respectively, and with HIV-1 RNA < 50 copies/ml was 23% and 10% respectively. Among all randomised and treated patients, the median change from baseline in

Table 3 Baseline characteristics for patients 12 – 18 years of age who took capsule

Variable		Value
Number of Patients		29
Age-Median (years)		15.1
Gender	% Male	48.3%
Race	% White	69.0%
	% Black	31.0%
	% Asian	0.0%
Baseline HIV-1 RNA (log_{10} copies/mL)	Median (Min – Max)	4.6 (3.0 – 6.8)
	% with VL > 100,000 copies/mL	27.6%
Baseline CD4+ (cells/mm^3)	Median (Min – Max)	330 (12 – 593)
	% ≤ 200	27.6%
Baseline % CD4+ cells	Median (Min – Max)	18.5% (3.1% – 37.4%)
Previous ADI*	% with Category C	29.2%
Treatment history	% with any ARV	96.6%
	Median # previous NRTIs	5
	Median # previous NNRTIs	1
	Median # previous PIs	3

* AIDS defining illness

HIV-1 RNA at the last measurement up to Week 48 was -0.64 $\log_{10}$ copies/ml in patients receiving APTIVUS/ritonavir versus -0.22 $\log_{10}$ copies/ml in the comparator PI/ritonavir arm.

Among all randomised and treated patients, the median change from baseline in CD4+ cell count at the last measurement up to Week 48 was +23 cells/mm^3 in patients receiving APTIVUS/ritonavir (N=740) versus +4 cells/mm^3 in the comparator PI/ritonavir (N=727) arm.

The superiority of APTIVUS co-administered with low dose ritonavir over the comparator protease inhibitor/ritonavir arm was observed for all efficacy parameters at week 48. It has not been shown that APTIVUS is superior to these boosted comparator protease inhibitors in patients harbouring strains susceptible to these protease inhibitors. RESIST data also demonstrate that APTIVUS co-administered with low dose ritonavir exhibits a better treatment response at 48 weeks when the OBR contains genotypically available antiretroviral agents (eg enfuvirtide).

At present there are no results from controlled trials evaluating the effect of APTIVUS on clinical progression of HIV.

Paediatric patients

HIV-positive, paediatric patients, aged 2 through 18 years, were studied in a randomized, open-label, multicenter study (trial 1182.14). Patients were required to have a baseline HIV-1 RNA concentration of at least 1500 copies/ml, were stratified by age (2 to < 6 years, 6 to < 12 years and 12 to 18 years) and randomized to receive one of two APTIVUS/ritonavir dose regimens: 375 mg/m^2/150 mg/m^2 dose, compared to the 290 mg/m^2/115 mg/m^2 dose, plus background therapy of at least two non-protease inhibitor antiretroviral medicinal products, optimized using baseline genotypic resistance testing. All patients initially received APTIVUS oral solution. Paediatric patients who were 12 years or older and received the maximum dose of 500 mg/200 mg twice daily could change to APTIVUS capsules from study day 28. The trial evaluated pharmacokinetics, safety and tolerability, as well as virologic and immunologic responses through 48 weeks.

No data are available on the efficacy and safety of APTIVUS capsules in children less than 12 years of age. Since APTIVUS capsules and oral solution are not bioequivalent, results obtained with the oral solution cannot be extrapolated to the capsules (see also section 5.2). In patients with a body surface area of less than 1.33 m^2 appropriate dose adjustments cannot be achieved with the capsule formulation.

The baseline characteristics and the key efficacy results at 48 weeks for the paediatric patients receiving APTIVUS capsules are displayed in the tables below. Data on the 29 patients who switched to capsules during the first 48 weeks are presented. Due to limitations in the study design (e.g. non-randomized switch allowed according to patient/clinician decision), any comparisons between patients taking capsules and oral solution are not meaningful.

Baseline characteristics for patients 12 – 18 years of age who took capsule

(see Table 3 on previous page)

Key efficacy results at 48 weeks for patients 12 – 18 years of age who took capsule

Endpoint	Result
Number of patients	29
Primary efficacy endpoint: % with VL < 400	31.0%
Median change from baseline in log10 HIV-1 RNA (copies/mL)	-0.79
Median change from baseline in CD4+ cell count (cells/mm3)	39
Median change from baseline in % CD4+ cells	3%

Analyses of tipranavir resistance in treatment experienced patients

APTIVUS/ritonavir response rates in the RESIST studies were assessed by baseline tipranavir genotype and phenotype. Relationships between baseline phenotypic susceptibility to tipranavir, primary PI mutations, protease mutations at codons 33, 82, 84 and 90, tipranavir resistance-associated mutations, and response to APTIVUS/ritonavir therapy were assessed.

Of note, patients in the RESIST studies had a specific mutational pattern at baseline of at least one primary protease gene mutation among codons 30N, 46I, 46L, 48V, 50V, 82A, 82F, 82L, 82T, 84V or 90M, and no more than two mutations on codons 33, 82, 84 or 90.

The following observations were made:

–Primary PI mutations:

Analyses were conducted to assess virological outcome by the number of primary PI mutations (any change at protease codons 30, 32, 36, 46, 47, 48, 50, 53, 54, 82, 84, 88 and 90) present at baseline. Response rates were higher in APTIVUS/ritonavir patients than comparator PI boosted with ritonavir in new enfuvirtide patients, or patients without new enfuvirtide. However, without new enfuvirtide some patients began to lose antiviral activity between weeks 4 and 8.

–Mutations at protease codons 33, 82, 84 and 90:

A reduced virological response was observed in patients with viral strains harbouring two or more mutations at HIV protease codons 33, 82, 84 or 90, and not receiving new enfuvirtide.

–Tipranavir resistance-associated mutations:

Virological response to APTIVUS/ritonavir therapy has been evaluated using a tipranavir-associated mutation score based on baseline genotype in RESIST-1 and RESIST-2 patients. This score (counting the 16 amino acids that have been associated with reduced tipranavir susceptibility and/or reduced viral load response: 10V, 13V, 20M/R/V, 33F, 35G, 36I, 43T, 46L, 47V, 54A/M/V, 58E, 69K, 74P, 82L/T, 83D and 84V) was applied to baseline viral protease sequences. A correlation between the tipranavir mutation score and response to APTIVUS/ritonavir therapy at week 48 has been established.

This score has been determined from the selected RESIST patient population having specific mutation inclusion criteria and therefore extrapolation to a wider population mandates caution.

At 48-weeks, a higher proportion of patients receiving APTIVUS/ ritonavir achieved a treatment response in comparison to the comparator protease inhibitor/ritonavir for nearly all of the possible combinations of genotypic resistance mutations (see table below).

Proportion of patients achieving treatment response at Week 48 (confirmed ≥1 $\log_{10}$ copies/ml decrease in viral load compared to baseline), according to tipranavir baseline mutation score and enfuvirtide use in RESIST patients

	New ENF	No New ENF*
Number of TPV Score Mutations**	TPV/r	TPV/r
0,1	73%	53%
2	61%	33%
3	75%	27%
4	59%	23%
≥ 5	47%	13%
All patients	61%	29%

* Includes patients who did not receive ENF and those who were previously treated with and continued ENF

** Mutations in HIV protease at positions L10V, I13V, K20M/R/V, L33F, E35G, M36I, K43T, M46L, I47V, I54A/M/V, 58E, H69K, T74P, V82L/T, N83D or I84V

ENF Enfuvirtide; TPV/r Tipranavir/ritonavir

Sustained HIV-1 RNA decreases up to week 48 were mainly observed in patients who received APTIVUS/ritonavir and new enfuvirtide. If patients did not receive APTIVUS/ritonavir with new enfuvirtide, diminished treatment responses at week 48 were observed, relative to new enfuvirtide use (see Table below).

Mean decrease in viral load from baseline to week 48, according to tipranavir baseline mutation score and enfuvirtide use in RESIST patients

	New ENF	No New ENF*
Number of TPV Score Mutations**	TPV/r	TPV/r
0, 1	-2.3	-1.6
2	-2.1	-1.1
3	-2.4	-0.9
4	-1.7	-0.8
≥ 5	-1.9	-0.6
All patients	-2.0	-1.0

* Includes patients who did not receive ENF and those who were previously treated with and continued ENF

** Mutations in HIV protease at positions L10V, I13V, K20M/R/V, L33F, E35G, M36I, K43T, M46L, I47V, I54A/M/V, 58E, H69K, T74P, V82L/T, N83D or I84V

ENF Enfuvirtide; TPV/r Tipranavir/ritonavir

–Tipranavir phenotypic resistance:

Increasing baseline phenotypic fold change to tipranavir in isolates is correlated to decreasing virological response. Isolates with baseline fold change of >0 to 3 are considered susceptible; isolates with >3 to 10 fold changes have decreased susceptibility; isolates with >10 fold changes are resistant.

Conclusions regarding the relevance of particular mutations or mutational patterns are subject to change with additional data, and it is recommended to always consult current interpretation systems for analysing resistance test results.

5.2 Pharmacokinetic properties

In order to achieve effective tipranavir plasma concentrations and a twice daily dosing regimen, coadministration of tipranavir with low dose ritonavir twice daily is essential (see section 4.2). Ritonavir acts by inhibiting hepatic cytochrome P450 CYP3A, the intestinal P-glycoprotein (Pgp) efflux pump and possibly intestinal cytochrome P450 CYP3A as well. As demonstrated in a dose-ranging evaluation in 113 HIV-negative healthy male and female volunteers, ritonavir increases AUC_{0-12h}, C_{max} and C_{min} and decreases the clearance of tipranavir. Tipranavir co-administered with low dose ritonavir (500 mg/200 mg twice daily) was associated with a 29-fold increase in the geometric mean morning steady-state trough plasma concentrations compared to tipranavir 500 mg twice daily without ritonavir.

Absorption

Absorption of tipranavir in humans is limited, though no absolute quantification of absorption is available. Tipranavir is a Pgp substrate, a weak Pgp inhibitor and appears to be a potent Pgp inducer as well. Data suggest that although ritonavir is a Pgp inhibitor, the net effect of APTIVUS, co-administered with low dose ritonavir, at the proposed dose regimen at steady-state, is Pgp induction. Peak plasma concentrations are reached within 1 to [illegible] hours after dose administration depending upon the dosage used. With repeated dosing, tipranavir plasma concentrations are lower than predicted from single dose data, presumably due to hepatic enzyme induction. Steady-state is attained in most subjects after 7 days of dosing. Tipranavir, co-administered with low dose ritonavir, exhibits linear pharmacokinetics at steady state.

Dosing with APTIVUS capsules 500 mg twice daily concomitant with 200 mg ritonavir twice daily for 2 to 4 weeks and without meal restriction produced a mean tipranavir peak plasma concentration (C_{max}) of 94.8 ± 22.8 μM for female patients (n=14) and 77.6 ± 16.6 μM for male patients (n=106), occurring approximately 3 hours after administration. The mean steady-state trough concentration prior to the morning dose was 41.6 ± 24.3 μM for female patients and 35.6 ± 16.7 μM for male patients. Tipranavir AUC over a 12 hour dosing interval averaged 851 ± 309 μM•h (CL=1.15 l/h) for female patients and 710 ± 207 μM•h (CL=1.27 l/h) for male patients. The mean half-life was 5.5 (females) or 6.0 hours (males).

Effects of food on oral absorption

Food improves the tolerability of tipranavir/ritonavir. Therefore APTIVUS, co-administered with low dose ritonavir, should be given with food. Data are awaited to substantiate the influence of food on oral absorption.

Absorption of tipranavir, co-administered with low dose ritonavir, is reduced in the presence of antacids (see section 4.5).

Distribution

Tipranavir is extensively bound to plasma proteins (>99.9%). From clinical samples of healthy volunteers and HIV-1 positive subjects who received tipranavir without ritonavir the mean fraction of tipranavir unbound in plasma was similar in both populations (healthy volunteers 0.015% ± 0.006%; HIV-positive subjects 0.019% ± 0.076%). Total plasma tipranavir concentrations for these samples ranged from 9 to 82 μM. The unbound fraction of tipranavir appeared to be independent of total concentration over this concentration range.

No studies have been conducted to determine the distribution of tipranavir into human cerebrospinal fluid or semen.

Metabolism

In vitro metabolism studies with human liver microsomes indicated that CYP3A4 is the predominant CYP isoform involved in tipranavir metabolism.

The oral clearance of tipranavir decreased after the addition of ritonavir which may represent diminished first-pass clearance of the substance at the gastrointestinal tract as well as the liver.

The metabolism of tipranavir in the presence of low dose ritonavir is minimal. In a ^{14}C-tipranavir human study (^{14}C-tipranavir/ritonavir, 500 mg/200 mg twice daily), unchanged tipranavir was predominant and accounted for 98.4% or greater of the total plasma radioactivity circulating at 3, 8, or 12 hours after dosing. Only a few metabolites were found in plasma, and all were at trace levels (0.2% or less of the plasma radioactivity). In faeces, unchanged tipranavir represented the majority of faecal radioactivity (79.9% of faecal radioactivity). The most abundant faecal metabolite, at 4.9% of faecal radioactivity (3.2% of dose), was a hydroxyl metabolite of tipranavir. In urine, unchanged tipranavir was found in trace amounts (0.5% of urine radioactivity). The most abundant urinary metabolite, at 11.0% of urine radioactivity (0.5% of dose) was a glucuronide conjugate of tipranavir.

Elimination

Administration of ^{14}C-tipranavir to subjects (n = 8) that received tipranavir/ritonavir 500 mg/200 mg twice daily dosed to steady-state demonstrated that most radioactivity (median 82.3%) was excreted in faeces, while only a median of 4.4% of the radioactive dose administered was recovered in urine. In addition, most radioactivity (56%) was excreted between 24 and 96 hours after dosing. The effective mean elimination half-life of tipranavir/ritonavir in healthy volunteers (n = 67) and HIV-infected adult patients (n = 120) was approximately 4.8 and 6.0 hours, respectively, at steady state following a dose of 500 mg/200 mg twice daily with a light meal.

ecial populations

hough data available at this stage are currently limited to ow a definitive analysis, they suggest that the pharma-kinetic profile is unchanged in elderly and comparable tween races. By contrast, evaluation of the steady-state asma tipranavir trough concentrations at 10-14 h after sing from the RESIST-1 and RESIST-2 studies demon-rate that females generally had higher tipranavir concen-ations than males. After four weeks of APTIVUS/ritonavir 0 mg/200 mg twice daily) the median plasma trough ncentration of tipranavir was 43.9 μM for females and .1 μM for males. This difference in concentrations does t warrant a dose adjustment.

nal dysfunction: Tipranavir pharmacokinetics have not en studied in patients with renal impairment. However, ce the renal clearance of tipranavir is negligible, a crease in total body clearance is not expected in tients with renal impairment.

patic dysfunction: In a study comparing 9 patients with ld (Child-Pugh A) hepatic impairment to 9 controls, the gle and multiple dose exposure of tipranavir and ritona- were increased in patients with hepatic impairment but l within the range observed in clinical studies. No dosing justment is required in patients with mild hepatic impair-ent but patients should be closely monitored (see sec-ns 4.2 and 4.4).

e influence of moderate (Child-Pugh B) or severe (Child-gh C) hepatic impairment on the multiple dose pharma-kinetics of either tipranavir or ritonavir has so far not en investigated. APTIVUS is contraindicated in moder- or severe hepatic impairment (see sections 4.2 and 3).

ediatrics

e oral solution has been shown to have greater bioavail-ility than the soft capsule formulation.

3 Preclinical safety data

imal toxicology studies have been conducted with tipra-vir alone, in mice, rats and dogs, and co-administered h ritonavir (3.75:1 w/w ratio) in rats and dogs. Studies h co-administration of tipranavir and ritonavir did not eal any additional toxicological effects when compared those seen in the tipranavir single agent toxicological dies.

e predominant effects of repeated administration of ranavir across all species toxicologically tested were the gastrointestinal tract (emesis, soft stool, diarrhoea) d the liver (hypertrophy). The effects were reversible with mination of treatment. Additional changes included eding in rats at high doses (rodents specific). Bleeding served in rats was associated with prolonged prothrom- time (PT), activated partial thromboplastin time (APTT) d a decrease in some vitamin K dependent factors. The -administration of tipranavir with vitamin E in the form of GS (d-alphatocopherol polyethylene glycol 1000 succi-te) from 2,322 IU/m^2 upwards in rats resulted in a sig-cant increase in effects on coagulation parameters, eding events and death. In preclinical studies of tipra-vir in dogs, an effect on coagulation parameters was not en. Co-administration of tipranavir and vitamin E has not en studied in dogs.

e majority of the effects in repeat-dose toxicity studies peared at systemic exposure levels which are equivalent or even below the human exposure levels at the recom-ended clinical dose.

in-vitro studies, Tipranavir was found to inhibit platelet gregation when using human platelets (see section 4.4) d thromboxane A2 binding in an in vitro cell model at els consistent with exposure observed in patients ceiving APTIVUS/ritonavir. The clinical implications of se findings are not known.

a study conducted in rats with tipranavir at systemic posure levels (AUC) equivalent to human exposure at the commended clinical dose, no adverse effects on mating fertility were observed. At maternal doses producing stemic exposure levels similar to or below those at the commended clinical dose, tipranavir did not produce atogenic effects. At tipranavir exposures in rats at 0.8- d human exposure at the clinical dose, foetal toxicity creased sternebrae ossification and body weights) was served. In pre- and post-natal development studies with ranavir in rats, growth inhibition of pups was observed at ternally toxic doses approximating 0.8-fold human posure.

rcinogenicity studies of tipranavir in mice and rats ealed tumourigenic potential specific for these species, ich are regarded as of no clinical relevance. Tipranavir owed no evidence of genetic toxicity in a battery of *in* o and *in vivo* tests.

PHARMACEUTICAL PARTICULARS

List of excipients

psule contents:

crogolglycerol ricinoleate

anol

ono/diglycerides of caprylic/capric acid

opylene glycol

rified water

metamol

opyl gallate.

Capsule shell:

Gelatin

Red iron oxide (E172)

Propylene glycol

Purified water

'Sorbitol special-glycerin blend' (d-sorbitol, 1,4 sorbitan, mannitol and glycerin)

Titanium dioxide (E171).

Black printing ink:

Propylene glycol

Black iron oxide (E172)

Polyvinyl acetate phthalate

Macrogol

Ammonium hydroxide.

6.2 Incompatibilities

Not applicable.

6.3 Shelf life

3 years.

In use storage: 60 days (below 25 °C), after first opening of the bottle. It is advisable that the patient writes the date of opening the bottle on the label and/or carton.

6.4 Special precautions for storage

Store in a refrigerator (2 - 8°C).

6.5 Nature and contents of container

High density polyethylene (HDPE) bottle with two-piece child-resistant closure (outer shell HDPE, inner shell polypropylene, with a pulpboard/aluminium liner). Each bottle contains 120 soft capsules.

6.6 Special precautions for disposal and other handling

No special requirements.

7. MARKETING AUTHORISATION HOLDER

Boehringer Ingelheim International GmbH

Binger Strasse 173

D-55216 Ingelheim am Rhein

Germany

8. MARKETING AUTHORISATION NUMBER(S)

EU/1/05/315/001

9. DATE OF FIRST AUTHORISATION/RENEWAL OF THE AUTHORISATION

25 October 2005

10. DATE OF REVISION OF THE TEXT

23 June 2009

LEGAL CATEGORY

POM

Detailed information on this product is available on the website of the European Medicines Agency (EMEA) http://www.emea.europa.eu/

Aquadrate 10% w/w Cream

(Alliance Pharmaceuticals)

1. NAME OF THE MEDICINAL PRODUCT

Aquadrate 10% w/w Cream

Hydromol Intensive

2. QUALITATIVE AND QUANTITATIVE COMPOSITION

Aquadrate/Hydromol Intensive contains urea Ph Eur 10% w/w.

3. PHARMACEUTICAL FORM

A smooth, unperfumed, non greasy, off white cream for topical administration.

4. CLINICAL PARTICULARS

4.1 Therapeutic indications

For the treatment of ichthyosis and hyperkeratotic skin conditions associated with atopic eczema, xeroderma, iasteatosis and other chronic dry skin conditions.

4.2 Posology and method of administration

Aquadrate/Hydromol Intensive is applied topically. Wash affected areas well, rinse off all traces of soap, dry, and apply sparingly twice daily. Occlusive dressings may be used but are usually unnecessary because of the self-occlusive nature of the cream.

4.3 Contraindications

Known hypersensitivity to the product.

4.4 Special warnings and precautions for use

Avoid application to moist or broken skin.

4.5 Interaction with other medicinal products and other forms of interaction

Aquadrate/Hydromol Intensive may increase the penetration through the skin barrier of other topically applied medicaments.

4.6 Pregnancy and lactation

Animal reproduction studies have not been conducted with Aquadrate/Hydromol Intensive. Aquadrate/Hydromol Intensive should only be used if the anticipated benefits outweigh the risks.

4.7 Effects on ability to drive and use machines

Aquadrate/Hydromol Intensive does not interfere with the ability to drive or use machines.

4.8 Undesirable effects

May produce local irritations (including erythema, burning or pruritus) and oedema when applied to sensitive, moist or fissured skin.

4.9 Overdose

Topical applications of excessive amounts of Aquadrate/Hydromol Intensive might cause skin irritation but no other effects would be expected. Ingestion of a large amount of Aquadrate/Hydromol Intensive would be expected to result in gastrointestinal irritation (nausea and vomiting). Symptomatic and supportive care should be given. Liberal oral administration of milk or water may be helpful.

5. PHARMACOLOGICAL PROPERTIES

5.1 Pharmacodynamic properties

Urea has a therapeutic effect in chronic dry skin conditions through its hydrating, keratolytic and anti-pruritic properties.

5.2 Pharmacokinetic properties

There is no information available on the pharmacokinetics of urea.

6. PHARMACEUTICAL PARTICULARS

6.1 List of excipients

The cream also contains white soft paraffin, maize starch, isopropyl myristate, syncrowax HR-C, palmitic acid, sorbitan laurate and arlatone G.

6.2 Incompatibilities

None known.

6.3 Shelf life

Two years.

6.4 Special precautions for storage

Store below 30°C.

6.5 Nature and contents of container

Aquadrate/Hydromol Intensive is available in tubes of 30g and 100g.

6.6 Special precautions for disposal and other handling

A patient leaflet is provided with details of use and handling of the product.

7. MARKETING AUTHORISATION HOLDER

Alliance Pharmaceuticals Ltd

Avonbridge House

Bath Road

Chippenham

Wiltshire

SN15 2BB

8. MARKETING AUTHORISATION NUMBER(S)

PL 16853/0061

9. DATE OF FIRST AUTHORISATION/RENEWAL OF THE AUTHORISATION

10 September 1991

10. DATE OF REVISION OF THE TEXT

5th December 2008

Arava 10, 20 and 100mg Tablets

(sanofi-aventis)

1. NAME OF THE MEDICINAL PRODUCT

Arava 10 mg film-coated tablets

Arava 20 mg film-coated tablets

Arava 100 mg film-coated tablets

2. QUALITATIVE AND QUANTITATIVE COMPOSITION

Each 10mg tablet contains 10 mg of leflunomide.

Each 20mg tablet contains 20 mg of leflunomide.

Each 100mg tablet contains 100 mg of leflunomide.

Excipient:

Each 10mg film-coated tablet contains 78 mg of lactose monohydrate.

Each 20mg film-coated tablet contains 72 mg of lactose monohydrate.

Each 100mg film-coated tablet contains 38.42 mg of lactose monohydrate.

For a full list of excipients, see section 6.1.

3. PHARMACEUTICAL FORM

Film-coated tablet.

Arava 10 mg film-coated tablets are white to almost white, round film-coated, imprinted with ZBN on one side.

Arava 20 mg film-coated tablets are yellowish to ochre and triangular film-coated tablets, imprinted with ZBO on one side.

Arava 100 mg film-coated tablets are white to almost white, round film-coated tablets with a diameter of about 1 cm, imprinted with ZBP on one side.

4. CLINICAL PARTICULARS

4.1 Therapeutic indications

Leflunomide is indicated for the treatment of adult patients with:

- active rheumatoid arthritis as a "disease-modifying antirheumatic drug" (DMARD),
- active psoriatic arthritis.

Recent or concurrent treatment with hepatotoxic or haematotoxic DMARDs (e.g. methotrexate) may result in an increased risk of serious adverse reactions; therefore, the initiation of leflunomide treatment has to be carefully considered regarding these benefit/risk aspects.

Moreover, switching from leflunomide to another DMARD without following the washout procedure (see section 4.4) may also increase the risk of serious adverse reactions even for a long time after the switching.

4.2 Posology and method of administration

The treatment should be initiated and supervised by specialists experienced in the treatment of rheumatoid arthritis and psoriatic arthritis.

Alanine aminotransferase (ALT) or serum glutamopyruvate transferase (SGPT) and a complete blood cell count, including a differential white blood cell count and a platelet count, must be checked simultaneously and with the same frequency:

- before initiation of leflunomide,
- every two weeks during the first six months of treatment, and
- every 8 weeks thereafter (see section 4.4).

Posology

Leflunomide therapy is started with a loading dose of 100 mg once daily for 3 days.

- The recommended maintenance dose for rheumatoid arthritis is leflunomide 10 mg to 20 mg once daily. Patients may be started on leflunomide 10 mg or 20 mg depending on the severity (activity) of the disease.
- The recommended maintenance dose is 20 mg for patients with psoriatic arthritis is once daily (see section 5.1).

The therapeutic effect usually starts after 4 to 6 weeks and may further improve up to 4 to 6 months.

There is no dose adjustment recommended in patients with mild renal insufficiency.

No dosage adjustment is required in patients above 65 years of age.

Paediatric population

Arava is not recommended for use in patients below 18 years since efficacy and safety in juvenile rheumatoid arthritis (JRA) have not been established (see sections 5.1 and 5.2).

Administration

Arava tablets should be swallowed whole with sufficient amounts of liquid. The extent of leflunomide absorption is not affected if it is taken with food.

4.3 Contraindications

- Hypersensitivity to the active substance (especially previous Stevens-Johnson syndrome, toxic epidermal necrolysis, erythema multiforme) or to any of the excipients.
- Patients with impairment of liver function.
- Patients with severe immunodeficiency states, e.g. AIDS.
- Patients with significantly impaired bone marrow function or significant anaemia, leucopenia, neutropenia or thrombocytopenia due to causes other than rheumatoid or psoriatic arthritis.
- Patients with serious infections (see section 4.4).
- Patients with moderate to severe renal insufficiency, because insufficient clinical experience is available in this patient group.
- Patients with severe hypoproteinaemia, e.g. in nephrotic syndrome.
- Pregnant women, or women of childbearing potential who are not using reliable contraception during treatment with leflunomide and thereafter as long as the plasma levels of the active metabolite are above 0.02 mg/l (see section 4.6). Pregnancy must be excluded before start of treatment with leflunomide.
- Breast-feeding women (see section 4.6).

4.4 Special warnings and precautions for use

Concomitant administration of hepatotoxic or haematotoxic DMARDs (e.g. methotrexate) is not advisable.

The active metabolite of leflunomide, A771726, has a long half-life, usually 1 to 4 weeks. Serious undesirable effects might occur (e.g. hepatotoxicity, haematotoxicity or allergic reactions, see below), even if the treatment with leflunomide has been stopped. Therefore, when such toxicities occur or if for any other reason A771726 needs to be cleared rapidly from the body, the washout procedure has to be followed. The procedure may be repeated as clinically necessary.

For washout procedures and other recommended actions in case of desired or unintended pregnancy see section 4.6.

Liver reactions

Rare cases of severe liver injury, including cases with fatal outcome, have been reported during treatment with leflunomide. Most of the cases occurred within the first 6 months of treatment. Co-treatment with other hepatotoxic medicinal products was frequently present. It is considered essential that monitoring recommendations are strictly adhered to.

ALT (SGPT) must be checked before initiation of leflunomide and at the same frequency as the complete blood cell count (every two weeks) during the first six months of treatment and every 8 weeks thereafter.

For ALT (SGPT) elevations between 2- and 3-fold the upper limit of normal, dose reduction from 20 mg to 10 mg may be considered and monitoring must be performed weekly. If ALT (SGPT) elevations of more than 2-fold the upper limit of normal persist or if ALT elevations of more than 3-fold the upper limit of normal are present, leflunomide must be discontinued and wash-out procedures initiated. It is recommended that monitoring of liver enzymes be maintained after discontinuation of leflunomide treatment, until liver enzyme levels have normalised.

Due to a potential for additive hepatotoxic effects, it is recommended that alcohol consumption be avoided during treatment with leflunomide.

Since the active metabolite of leflunomide, A771726, is highly protein bound and cleared via hepatic metabolism and biliary secretion, plasma levels of A771726 are expected to be increased in patients with hypoproteinaemia. Arava is contraindicated in patients with severe hypoproteinaemia or impairment of liver function (see section 4.3).

Haematological reactions

Together with ALT, a complete blood cell count, including differential white blood cell count and platelets, must be performed before start of leflunomide treatment as well as every 2 weeks for the first 6 months of treatment and every 8 weeks thereafter.

In patients with pre-existing anaemia, leucopenia, and/or thrombocytopenia as well as in patients with impaired bone marrow function or those at risk of bone marrow suppression, the risk of haematological disorders is increased. If such effects occur, a washout (see below) to reduce plasma levels of A771726 should be considered.

In case of severe haematological reactions, including pancytopenia, Arava and any concomitant myelosuppressive treatment must be discontinued and a leflunomide washout procedure initiated.

Combinations with other treatments

The use of leflunomide with antimalarials used in rheumatic diseases (e.g. chloroquine and hydroxychloroquine), intramuscular or oral gold, D-penicillamine, azathioprine and other immunosuppressive agents (with the exception of methotrexate, see section 4.5) has not been studied up to now. The risk associated with combination therapy, in particular in long-term treatment, is unknown. Since such therapy can lead to additive or even synergistic toxicity (e.g. hepato- or haematotoxicity), combination with another DMARD (e.g. methotrexate) is not advisable.

Caution is advised when leflunomide is given together with drugs, other than NSAIDs, metabolised by CYP2C9 such as phenytoin, warfarin, phenprocoumon and tolbutamide.

Switching to other treatments

As leflunomide has a long persistence in the body, a switching to another DMARD (e.g. methotrexate) without performing the washout procedure (see below) may raise the possibility of additive risks even for a long time after the switching (i.e. kinetic interaction, organ toxicity).

Similarly, recent treatment with hepatotoxic or haematotoxic medicinal products (e.g. methotrexate) may result in increased side effects; therefore, the initiation of leflunomide treatment has to carefully be considered regarding these benefit/risk aspects and closer monitoring is recommended in the initial phase after switching.

Skin reactions

In case of ulcerative stomatitis, leflunomide administration should be discontinued.

Very rare cases of Stevens Johnson syndrome or toxic epidermal necrolysis have been reported in patients treated with leflunomide. As soon as skin and/or mucosal reactions are observed which raise the suspicion of such severe reactions, Arava and any other possibly associated treatment must be discontinued, and a leflunomide washout procedure initiated immediately. A complete washout is essential in such cases. In such cases re-exposure to leflunomide is contra-indicated (see section 4.3).

Infections

It is known that medicinal products with immunosuppressive properties - like leflunomide - may cause patients to be more susceptible to infections, including opportunistic infections. Infections may be more severe in nature and may, therefore, require early and vigorous treatment. In the event that severe, uncontrolled infections occur, it may be necessary to interrupt leflunomide treatment and administer a washout procedure as described below.

Patients with tuberculin reactivity must be carefully monitored because of the risk of tuberculosis reactivation.

Respiratory reactions

Interstitial Lung disease has been reported during trea ment with leflunomide (see section 4.8). Interstitial lu disease is a potentially fatal disorder, which may occ acutely during therapy. Pulmonary symptoms, such cough and dyspnoea, may be a reason for discontinuati of the therapy and for further investigation, as appropria

Blood pressure

Blood pressure must be checked before the start of lefl nomide treatment and periodically thereafter.

Procreation (recommendations for men)

Male patients should be aware of the possible mal mediated foetal toxicity. Reliable contraception duri treatment with leflunomide should also be guaranteed.

There are no specific data on the risk of male-mediat foetal toxicity. However, animal studies to evaluate th specific risk have not been conducted. To minimise a possible risk, men wishing to father a child should consid discontinuing use of leflunomide and taking colestyrami 8 g 3 times daily for 11 days or 50 g of activated powder charcoal 4 times daily for 11 days.

In either case the A771726 plasma concentration is th measured for the first time. Thereafter, the A7717 plasma concentration must be determined again after interval of at least 14 days. If both plasma concentratio are below 0.02 mg/l, and after a waiting period of at leas months, the risk of foetal toxicity is very low.

Washout procedure

Colestyramine 8 g is administered 3 times daily. Alterr tively, 50 g of activated powdered charcoal is administer 4 times daily. Duration of a complete washout is usually days. The duration may be modified depending on clini or laboratory variables.

Lactose

Arava contains lactose. Patients with rare hereditary pr blems of galactose intolerance, the Lapp lactase de ciency or glucose-galactose malabsorption should r take this medicinal product.

4.5 Interaction with other medicinal products and oth forms of interaction

Interactions studies have only been performed in adults

Increased side effects may occur in case of recent concomitant use of hepatotoxic or haematotoxic dru or when leflunomide treatment is followed by such dru without a washout period (see also guidance concerni combination with other treatments, section 4.4). Therefo closer monitoring of liver enzymes and haematologi parameters is recommended in the initial phase af switching.

In a small (n=30) study with co-administration of leflur mide (10 to 20 mg per day) with methotrexate (10 to 25 r per week) a 2- to 3-fold elevation in liver enzymes was se on 5 of 30 patients. All elevations resolved, 2 with cc tinuation of both drugs and 3 after discontinuation leflunomide. A more than 3-fold increase was seen another 5 patients. All of these also resolved, 2 with cc tinuation of both drugs and 3 after discontinuation leflunomide.

In patients with rheumatoid arthritis, no pharmacokine interaction between the leflunomide (10 to 20 mg per d and methotrexate (10 to 25 mg per week) was demc strated.

It is recommended that patients receiving leflunomide not treated with colestyramine or activated powder charcoal because this leads to a rapid and significa decrease in plasma A771726 (the active metabolite leflunomide; see also section 5) concentration. T mechanism is thought to be by interruption of enteroh patic recycling and/or gastrointestinal dialysis of A7717

If the patient is already receiving nonsteroidal anti-infla matory drugs (NSAIDs) and/or corticosteroids, these m be continued after starting leflunomide.

The enzymes involved in the metabolism of leflunomi and its metabolites are not exactly known. An *in v* interaction study with cimetidine (non-specific cytochro P450 inhibitor) has demonstrated a lack of a significa interaction. Following concomitant administration of a s gle dose of leflunomide to subjects receiving multi doses of rifampicin (non-specific cytochrome P450 inc cer) A771726 peak levels were increased by approximat 40%, whereas the AUC was not significantly changed. T mechanism of this effect is unclear.

In vitro studies indicate that A771726 inhibits cytochror P4502C9 (CYP2C9) activity. In clinical trials no safety p blems were observed when leflunomide and NSAIDs me bolised by CYP2C9 were co-administered. Caution advised when leflunomide is given together with dru other than NSAIDs, metabolised by CYP2C9 such as ph nytoin, warfarin, phenprocoumon and tolbutamide.

In a study in which leflunomide was given concomitan with a triphasic oral contraceptive pill containing 30 ethinyloestradiol to healthy female volunteers, there w no reduction in contraceptive activity of the pill, a A771726 pharmacokinetics were within predicted rang

Vaccinations

No clinical data are available on the efficacy and safety vaccinations under leflunomide treatment. Vaccinati

:h live attenuated vaccines is, however, not recomended. The long half-life of leflunomide should be conlered when contemplating administration of a live enuated vaccine after stopping Arava.

5 Pregnancy and lactation

egnancy

e active metabolite of leflunomide, A771726 is suscted to cause serious birth defects when administered ring pregnancy.

ava is contraindicated in pregnancy (see section 4.3).

omen of childbearing potential have to use effective ntraception during and up to 2 years after treatment e "waiting period" below) or up to 11 days after treatent (see abbreviated "washout period" below).

e patient must be advised that if there is any delay in set of menses or any other reason to suspect pregncy, they must notify the physician immediately for egnancy testing, and if positive, the physician and tient must discuss the risk to the pregnancy. It is posle that rapidly lowering the blood level of the active tabolite, by instituting the drug elimination procedure scribed below, at the first delay of menses may crease the risk to the foetus from leflunomide.

women receiving leflunomide treatment and who wish become pregnant, one of the following procedures is ommended in order to ascertain that the foetus is not posed to toxic concentrations of A771726 (target conntration below 0.02 mg/l):

iting period

71726 plasma levels can be expected to be above 2 mg/l for a prolonged period. The concentration may expected to decrease below 0.02 mg/l about 2 years er stopping the treatment with leflunomide.

er a 2-year waiting period, the A771726 plasma conntration is measured for the first time.

ereafter, the A771726 plasma concentration must be ermined again after an interval of at least 14 days. If h plasma concentrations are below 0.02 mg/l no tergenic risk is to be expected.

further information on the sample testing please cont the Marketing Authorisation Holder or its local repretative (see section 7).

shout procedure

er stopping treatment with leflunomide:

olestyramine 8 g is administered 3 times daily for a iod of 11 days,

lternatively, 50 g of activated powdered charcoal is ministered 4 times daily for a period of 11 days.

wever, also following either of the washout procedures, ification by 2 separate tests at an interval of at least 14 s and a waiting period of one-and-a-half months ween the first occurrence of a plasma concentration ow 0.02 mg/l and fertilisation is required.

omen of childbearing potential should be told that a ting period of 2 years after treatment discontinuation equired before they may become pregnant. If a waiting iod of up to approximately 2 years under reliable contration is considered unpractical, prophylactic institution a washout procedure may be advisable.

h colestyramine and activated powdered charcoal may uence the absorption of oestrogens and progestogens h that reliable contraception with oral contraceptives not be guaranteed during the washout procedure with estyramine or activated powdered charcoal. Use of rnative contraceptive methods is recommended.

tation

mal studies indicate that leflunomide or its metabolites s into breast milk. Breast-feeding women must, there, not receive leflunomide.

Effects on ability to drive and use machines

he case of side effects such as dizziness the patient's lity to concentrate and to react properly may be paired. In such cases patients should refrain from driving s and using machines.

Undesirable effects

e most frequently adverse effects reported commonly /100 to <1/10) with leflunomide are: mild increase in od pressure, leucopenia, paraesthesia, headache, dizess, diarrhoea, nausea, vomiting, oral mucosal disors (e.g. aphthous stomatitis, mouth ulceration), dominal pain, increased hair loss, eczema, rash (includmaculo-papular rash), pruritus, dry skin, tenosynovitis, K increased, anorexia, weight loss (usually insignifit), asthenia, mild allergic reactions and elevation of liver ameters (transaminases (especially ALT), less often nma-GT, alkaline phosphatise, bilirubin))

ssification of expected frequencies:

y common (≥1/10); common (≥1/100 to <1/10); common (≥1/1,000 to <1/100); rare (≥1/10,000 to /1,000); very rare (<1/10,000), not known (cannot be mated from the available data).

hin each frequency grouping, undesirable effects are sented in order of decreasing seriousness.

ctions and infestations

e: severe infections, including sepsis which may be

Like other agents with immunosuppressive potential, leflunomide may increase susceptibility to infections, including opportunistic infections (see also section 4.4). Thus, the overall incidence of infections can increase (in particular of rhinitis, bronchitis and pneumonia).

Neoplasms benign, malignant and unspecified (incl. cysts and polyps)

The risk of malignancy, particularly lymphoproliferative disorders, is increased with use of some immunosuppressive agents.

Blood and lymphatic system disorders

Common: leucopenia (leucocytes >2 G/l)

Uncommon: anaemia, mild thrombocytopenia (platelets <100 G/l)

Rare: pancytopenia (probably by antiproliferative mechanism), leucopenia (leucocytes <2 G/l), eosinophilia

Very rare: agranulocytosis

Recent, concomitant or consecutive use of potentially myelotoxic agents may be associated with a higher risk of haematological effects.

Immune system disorders

Common: mild allergic reactions

Very rare: severe anaphylactic/anaphylactoid reactions, vasculitis, including cutaneous necrotizing vasculitis

Metabolism and nutrition disorders

Common: CPK increased

Uncommon: hypokalaemia, hyperlipidemia, hypophosphataemia

Rare: LDH increased

Not known: hypouricemia

Psychiatric disorders

Uncommon: anxiety

Nervous system disorders

Common: paraesthesia, headache, dizziness

Very rare: peripheral neuropathy

Cardiac disorders

Common: mild increase in blood pressure

Rare: severe increase in blood pressure

Respiratory, thoracic and mediastinal disorders

Rare: interstitial lung disease (including interstitial pneumonitis), which may be fatal

Gastrointestinal disorders

Common: diarrhoea, nausea, vomiting, oral mucosal disorders (e.g., aphthous stomatitis, mouth ulceration), abdominal pain

Uncommon: taste disturbances

Very rare: pancreatitis

Hepatobiliary disorders

Common: elevation of liver parameters (transaminases [especially ALT], less often gamma-GT, alkaline phosphatase, bilirubin)

Rare: hepatitis, jaundice/cholestasis

Very rare: severe liver injury such as hepatic failure and acute hepatic necrosis that may be fatal

Skin and subcutaneous tissue disorders

Common: increased hair loss, eczema, rash (including maculopapular rash), pruritus, dry skin

Uncommon: urticaria

Very rare: toxic epidermal necrolysis, Stevens-Johnson syndrome, erythema multiforme

Musculoskeletal and connective tissue disorders

Common: tenosynovitis

Uncommon: tendon rupture

Renal and urinary disorders

Not known: renal failure

Reproductive system and breast disorders

Not known: marginal (reversible) decreases in sperm concentration, total sperm count and rapid progressive motility

General disorders and administration site conditions

Common: anorexia, weight loss (usually insignificant), asthenia

4.9 Overdose

Symptoms

There have been reports of chronic overdose in patients taking Arava at daily doses up to five times the recommended daily dose, and reports of acute overdose in adults and children. There were no adverse events reported in the majority of case reports of overdose. Adverse events consistent with the safety profile for leflunomide were: abdominal pain, nausea, diarrhoea, elevated liver enzymes, anaemia, leucopenia, pruritus and rash.

Management

In the event of an overdose or toxicity, colestyramine or charcoal is recommended to accelerate elimination. Colestyramine given orally at a dose of 8 g three times a day for 24 hours to three healthy volunteers decreased plasma levels of A771726 by approximately 40% in 24 hours and by 49% to 65% in 48 hours.

Administration of activated charcoal (powder made into a suspension) orally or via nasogastric tube (50 g every 6 hours for 24 hours) has been shown to reduce plasma concentrations of the active metabolite A771726 by 37% in 24 hours and by 48% in 48 hours.

These washout procedures may be repeated if clinically necessary.

Studies with both hemodialysis and CAPD (chronic ambulatory peritoneal dialysis) indicate that A771726, the primary metabolite of leflunomide, is not dialysable.

5. PHARMACOLOGICAL PROPERTIES

5.1 Pharmacodynamic properties

Pharmacotherapeutic group: selective immunosuppressants, ATC code: L04AA13.

Human pharmacology

Leflunomide is a disease-modifying anti-rheumatic agent with antiproliferative properties.

Animal pharmacology

Leflunomide is effective in animal models of arthritis and of other autoimmune diseases and transplantation, mainly if administered during the sensitisation phase. It has immunomodulating/ immunosuppressive characteristics, acts as an antiproliferative agent, and displays anti-inflammatory properties. Leflunomide exhibits the best protective effects on animal models of autoimmune diseases when administered in the early phase of the disease progression. *In vivo*, it is rapidly and almost completely metabolised to A771726 which is active *in vitro*, and is presumed to be responsible for the therapeutic effect.

Mode of action

A771726, the active metabolite of leflunomide, inhibits the human enzyme dihydroorotate dehydrogenase (DHODH) and exhibits antiproliferative activity.

Rheumatoid arthritis

The efficacy of Arava in the treatment of rheumatoid arthritis was demonstrated in 4 controlled trials (1 in phase II and 3 in phase III). The phase II trial, study YU203, randomised 402 subjects with active rheumatoid arthritis to placebo (n=102), leflunomide 5 mg (n=95), 10 mg (n=101) or 25 mg/day (n=104). The treatment duration was 6 months.

All leflunomide patients in the phase III trials used an initial dose of 100 mg for 3 days.

Study MN301 randomised 358 subjects with active rheumatoid arthritis to leflunomide 20 mg/day (n=133), sulphasalazine 2 g/day (n=133), or placebo (n=92). Treatment duration was 6 months. Study MN303 was an optional 6-month blinded continuation of MN301 without the placebo arm, resulting in a 12-month comparison of leflunomide and sulphasalazine.

Study MN302 randomised 999 subjects with active rheumatoid arthritis to leflunomide 20 mg/day (n=501) or methotrexate at 7.5 mg/week increasing to 15 mg/week (n=498). Folate supplementation was optional and only used in 10% of patients. Treatment duration was 12-months.

Study US301 randomised 482 subjects with active rheumatoid arthritis to leflunomide 20 mg/day (n=182), methotrexate 7.5 mg/week increasing to 15 mg/week (n=182), or placebo (n=118). All patients received folate 1 mg bid. Treatment duration was 12 months.

Leflunomide at a daily dose of at least 10 mg (10 to 25 mg in study YU203, 20 mg in studies MN301 and US301) was statistically significantly superior to placebo in reducing the signs and symptoms of rheumatoid arthritis in all 3 placebo-controlled trials. The ACR (AmericanCollege of Rheumatology) response rates in study YU203 were 27.7% for placebo, 31.9% for 5 mg, 50.5% for 10 mg and 54.5% for 25 mg/day. In the phase III trials, the ACR response rates for leflunomide 20 mg/day vs. placebo were 54.6% vs. 28.6% (study MN301), and 49.4% vs. 26.3% (study US301). After 12 months with active treatment, the ACR response rates in leflunomide patients were 52.3% (studies MN301/303), 50.5% (study MN302) and 49.4% (study US301), compared to 53.8% (studies MN301/303) in sulphasalazine patients, 64.8% (study MN302), and 43.9% (study US301) in methotrexate patients. In study MN302 leflunomide was significantly less effective than methotrexate. However, in study US301 no significant differences were observed between leflunomide and methotrexate in the primary efficacy parameters. No difference was observed between leflunomide and sulphasalazine (study MN301). The leflunomide treatment effect was evident by 1 month, stabilised by 3 to 6 months and continued throughout the course of treatment.

A randomised, double-blind, parallel-group non-inferiority study compared the relative efficacy of two different daily maintenance doses of leflunomide, 10 mg and 20 mg. From the results it can be concluded that efficacy results of the 20 mg maintenance dose were more favourable, on the other hand, the safety results favoured the 10 mg daily maintenance dose.

Paediatrics

Leflunomide was studied in a single multicenter, randomized, double-blind, active-controlled trial in 94 patients (47 per arm) with polyarticular course juvenile rheumatoid arthritis. Patients were 3–17 years of age with active polyarticular course JRA regardless of onset type and naive to methotrexate or leflunomide. In this trial, the loading dose and maintenance dose of leflunomide was based on three weight categories: <20kg, 20-40 kg, and >40kg. After 16 weeks treatment, the difference in response rates was statistically significant in favour of methotrexate for the JRA Definition of Improvement (DOI) ≥30 % (p=0.02). In responders, this response was maintained during 48 weeks. (see section 4.2).

The pattern of adverse events of leflunomide and methotrexate seems to be similar, but the dose used in lighter subjects resulted in a relatively low exposure (see section 5.2). These data do not allow an effective and safe dose recommendation.

Psoriatic arthritis

The efficacy of Arava was demonstrated in one controlled, randomised, double blind study 3L01 in 188 patients with psoriatic arthritis, treated at 20mg/day. Treatment duration was 6 months.

Leflunomide 20mg/day was significantly superior to placebo in reducing the symptoms of arthritis in patients with psoriatic arthritis: the PsARC (Psoriatic Arthritis treatment Response Criteria) responders were 59% in the leflunomide group and 29.7% in the placebo group by 6 months (p < 0.0001). The effect of leflunomide on improvement of function and on reduction of skin lesions was modest.

5.2 Pharmacokinetic properties

Leflunomide is rapidly converted to the active metabolite, A771726, by first-pass metabolism (ring opening) in gut wall and liver. In a study with radiolabelled ^{14}C-leflunomide in three healthy volunteers, no unchanged leflunomide was detected in plasma, urine or faeces. In other studies, unchanged leflunomide levels in plasma have rarely been detected, however, at ng/ml plasma levels. The only plasma-radiolabelled metabolite detected was A771726. This metabolite is responsible for essentially all the *in vivo* activity of Arava.

Absorption

Excretion data from the ^{14}C study indicated that at least about 82 to 95% of the dose is absorbed. The time to peak plasma concentrations of A771726 is very variable; peak plasma levels can occur between 1 hour and 24 hours after single administration. Leflunomide can be administered with food, since the extent of absorption is comparable in the fed and fasting state. Due to the very long half-life of A771726 (approximately 2 weeks), a loading dose of 100 mg for 3 days was used in clinical studies to facilitate the rapid attainment of steady-state levels of A771726. Without a loading dose, it is estimated that attainment of steady-state plasma concentrations would require nearly two months of dosing. In multiple dose studies in patients with rheumatoid arthritis, the pharmacokinetic parameters of A771726 were linear over the dose range of 5 to 25 mg. In these studies, the clinical effect was closely related to the plasma concentration of A771726 and to the daily dose of leflunomide. At a dose level of 20 mg/day, average plasma concentration of A771726 at steady state is approximately 35 µg/ml. At steady state plasma levels accumulate about 33- to 35-fold compared with single dose.

Distribution

In human plasma, A771726 is extensively bound to protein (albumin). The unbound fraction of A771726 is about 0.62%. Binding of A771726 is linear in the therapeutic concentration range. Binding of A771726 appeared slightly reduced and more variable in plasma from patients with rheumatoid arthritis or chronic renal insufficiency. The extensive protein binding of A771726 could lead to displacement of other highly-bound drugs. *In vitro* plasma protein binding interaction studies with warfarin at clinically relevant concentrations, however, showed no interaction. Similar studies showed that ibuprofen and diclofenac did not displace A771726, whereas the unbound fraction of A771726 is increased 2- to 3-fold in the presence of tolbutamide. A771726 displaced ibuprofen, diclofenac and tolbutamide but the unbound fraction of these drugs is only increased by 10% to 50%. There is no indication that these effects are of clinical relevance. Consistent with extensive protein binding A771726 has a low apparent volume of distribution (approximately 11 litres). There is no preferential uptake in erythrocytes.

Metabolism

Leflunomide is metabolised to one primary (A771726) and many minor metabolites including TFMA (4-trifluoromethylaniline). The metabolic biotransformation of leflunomide to A771726 and subsequent metabolism of A771726 is not controlled by a single enzyme and has been shown to occur in microsomal and cytosolic cellular fractions. Interaction studies with cimetidine (non-specific cytochrome P450 inhibitor) and rifampicin (non-specific cytochrome P450 inducer), indicate that *in vivo* CYP enzymes are involved in the metabolism of leflunomide only to a small extent.

Elimination

Elimination of A771726 is slow and characterised by an apparent clearance of about 31 ml/hr. The elimination half-life in patients is approximately 2 weeks. After administration of a radiolabelled dose of leflunomide, radioactivity was equally excreted in faeces, probably by biliary elimination, and in urine. A771726 was still detectable in urine and faeces 36 days after a single administration. The principal urinary metabolites were glucuronide products derived from leflunomide (mainly in 0 to 24 hour samples) and an oxanilic acid derivative of A771726. The principal faecal component was A771726.

It has been shown in man that administration of an oral suspension of activated powdered charcoal or colestyramine leads to a rapid and significant increase in A771726 elimination rate and decline in plasma concentrations (see section 4.9). This is thought to be achieved by a gastrointestinal dialysis mechanism and/or by interrupting enterohepatic recycling.

Pharmacokinetics in renal failure

Leflunomide was administered as a single oral 100 mg dose to 3 haemodialysis patients and 3 patients on continuous peritoneal dialysis (CAPD). The pharmacokinetics of A771726 in CAPD subjects appeared to be similar to healthy volunteers. A more rapid elimination of A771726 was observed in haemodialysis subjects which was not due to extraction of drug in the dialysate.

Pharmacokinetics in liver failure

No data are available regarding treatment of patients with hepatic impairment. The active metabolite A771726 is extensively protein bound and cleared via hepatic metabolism and biliary secretion. These processes may be affected by hepatic dysfunction.

Pharmacokinetics in paediatrics

The pharmacokinetics of A771726 following oral administration of leflunomide have been investigated in 73 pediatric patients with polyarticular course Juvenile Rheumatoid Arthritis (JRA) who ranged in age from 3 to 17 years. The results of a population pharmacokinetic analysis of these trials have demonstrated that pediatric patients with body weights ≤40 kg have a reduced systemic exposure (measured by C_{ss}) of A771726 relative to adult rheumatoid arthritis patients (see section 4.2).

Pharmacokinetics in elderly

Pharmacokinetic data in elderly (>65 years) are limited but consistent with pharmacokinetics in younger adults.

5.3 Preclinical safety data

Leflunomide, administered orally and intraperitoneally, has been studied in acute toxicity studies in mice and rats. Repeated oral administration of leflunomide to mice for up to 3 months, to rats and dogs for up to 6 months and to monkeys for up to 1 month's duration revealed that the major target organs for toxicity were bone marrow, blood, gastrointestinal tract, skin, spleen, thymus and lymph nodes. The main effects were anaemia, leucopenia, decreased platelet counts and panmyelopathy and reflect the basic mode of action of the compound (inhibition of DNA synthesis). In rats and dogs, Heinz bodies and/or Howell-Jolly bodies were found. Other effects found on heart, liver, cornea and respiratory tract could be explained as infections due to immunosuppression. Toxicity in animals was found at doses equivalent to human therapeutic doses.

Leflunomide was not mutagenic. However, the minor metabolite TFMA (4-trifluoromethylaniline) caused clastogenicity and point mutations in vitro, whilst insufficient information was available on its potential to exert this effect *in vivo*.

In a carcinogenicity study in rats, leflunomide did not show carcinogenic potential. In a carcinogenicity study in mice an increased incidence of malignant lymphoma occurred in males of the highest dose group, considered to be due to the immunosuppressive activity of leflunomide. In female mice an increased incidence, dose-dependent, of bronchiolo-alveolar adenomas and carcinomas of the lung was noted. The relevance of the findings in mice relative to the clinical use of leflunomide is uncertain.

Leflunomide was not antigenic in animal models.

Leflunomide was embryotoxic and teratogenic in rats and rabbits at doses in the human therapeutic range and exerted adverse effects on male reproductive organs in repeated dose toxicity studies. Fertility was not reduced.

6. PHARMACEUTICAL PARTICULARS

6.1 List of excipients

Tablet core:

Arava 10 mg film-coated tablets: Maize starch, povidone (E1201), crospovidone (E1202), silica colloidal anhydrous, magnesium stearate (E470b), lactose monohydrate.

Arava 20 mg film-coated tablets: Maize starch, povidone (E1201), crospovidone (E1202), silica colloidal anhydrous, magnesium stearate (E470b), lactose monohydrate.

Arava 100 mg film-coated tablets: Maize starch, povidone (E1201), crospovidone (E1202), talc (E553b), silica colloidal anhydrous, magnesium stearate (E470b), lactose monohydrate.

Film-Coating:

Arava 10 mg film-coated tablets: Talc (E553b), hypromellose (E464), titanium dioxide (E171), macrogol 8000.

Arava 20 mg film-coated tablets: Talc (E553b), hypromellose (E464), titanium dioxide (E171), macrogol 8000, and yellow ferric oxide (E172).

Arava 100 mg film-coated tablets: Talc (E553b), hypromellose (E464), titanium dioxide (E171), macrogol 8000.

6.2 Incompatibilities

Not applicable.

6.3 Shelf life

3 years.

6.4 Special precautions for storage

Blister: Store in the original package.

Bottle: Keep the container tightly closed.

6.5 Nature and contents of container

Arava 10 mg and Arava 20 mg film-coated tablets:

Bottle: 100 ml HDPE-wide-necked bottle, with screw c[...] with integrated desiccant container, containing 30 fil[...] coated tablets

Arava 100 mg film-coated tablets:

Aluminium / Aluminium blister. Pack size: 3 film-coate[...] tablets.

6.6 Special precautions for disposal and other handlin[...]

No special requirements.

7. MARKETING AUTHORISATION HOLDER

Sanofi-Aventis Deutschland GmbH, D-65926 Frankfurt a[...] Main, Germany

8. MARKETING AUTHORISATION NUMBER(S)

Arava 10 mg film-coated tablets: EU/1/99/118/003

Arava 20 mg film-coated tablets: EU/1/99/118/007

Arava 100 mg film-coated tablets: EU/1/99/118/009

9. DATE OF FIRST AUTHORISATION/RENEWAL O[...] THE AUTHORISATION

Date of first authorisation: 02 September 1999

Date of latest renewal: 1 July 2009

10. DATE OF REVISION OF THE TEXT

July 2009

Legal category: POM

Detailed information on this medicinal product is availabl[...] on the website of the European Medicines Agency (EMEA[...] http://www.emea.europa.eu/.

Arcoxia 30mg, 60 mg, 90 mg & 120 mg Film-coated Tablets

(Merck Sharp & Dohme Limited)

1. NAME OF THE MEDICINAL PRODUCT

ARCOXIA®▼ 30 mg film-coated tablets

ARCOXIA®▼ 60 mg film-coated tablets

ARCOXIA®▼ 90 mg film-coated tablets

ARCOXIA®▼ 120 mg film-coated tablets

2. QUALITATIVE AND QUANTITATIVE COMPOSITION

Each film-coated tablet contains 30, 60, 90 or 120 mg of etoricoxib.

Excipient:

30 mg: lactose 1.4 mg

60 mg: lactose 2.8 mg

90 mg: lactose 4.2 mg

120 mg: lactose 5.6 mg

For a full list of excipients, see section 6.1.

3. PHARMACEUTICAL FORM

Film-coated tablet (tablet).

30 mg Tablets: Blue-green, apple-shaped biconvex tablets debossed '101' on one side and 'ACX 30' on the other side.

60 mg Tablets: Dark green, apple-shaped, biconvex tablets debossed '200' on one side and 'ARCOXIA 60' on the other side.

90 mg Tablets: White, apple-shaped, biconvex tablets debossed '202' on one side and 'ARCOXIA 90' on the other side.

120 mg Tablets: Pale-green, apple-shaped, biconvex tablets debossed '204' on one side and 'ARCOXIA 120' on the other side.

4. CLINICAL PARTICULARS

4.1 Therapeutic indications

For the symptomatic relief of osteoarthritis (OA), rheumatoid arthritis (RA), ankylosing spondylitis, and the pain and signs of inflammation associated with acute gouty arthritis.

The decision to prescribe a selective COX-2 inhibitor should be based on an assessment of the individual patient's overall risks (see sections 4.3, 4.4).

4.2 Posology and method of administration

ARCOXIA is administered orally and may be taken with or without food. The onset of the effect of the medicinal product may be faster when ARCOXIA is administered without food. This should be considered when rapid symptomatic relief is needed.

As the cardiovascular risks of etoricoxib may increase with dose and duration of exposure, the shortest duration possible and the lowest effective daily dose should be used. The patient's need for symptomatic relief and response to therapy should be re-evaluated periodically, especially in patients with osteoarthritis (see sections 4.3, 4.4, 4.8 and 5.1).

Osteoarthritis

The recommended dose is 30 mg once daily. In some patients with insufficient relief from symptoms, an increased dose of 60 mg once daily may increase efficacy.

the absence of an increase in therapeutic benefit, other rapeutic options should be considered.

eumatoid arthritis

e recommended dose is 90 mg once daily.

ute gouty arthritis

e recommended dose is 120 mg once daily. Etoricoxib 0 mg should be used only for the acute symptomatic riod. In clinical trials for acute gouty arthritis, etoricoxib as given for 8 days.

kylosing spondylitis

e recommended dose is 90 mg once daily.

oses greater than those recommended for each indica-on have either not demonstrated additional efficacy or ve not been studied. Therefore:

e dose for OA should not exceed 60 mg daily.

e dose for RA and ankylosing spondylitis should not ceed 90 mg daily.

ne dose for acute gout should not exceed 120 mg daily, nited to a maximum of 8 days treatment.

derly

o dosage adjustment is necessary for elderly patients. As ith other drugs, caution should be exercised in elderly atients (see section 4.4).

epatic insufficiency

egardless of indication, in patients with mild hepatic ysfunction (Child-Pugh score 5-6) a dose of 60 mg once aily should not be exceeded. In patients with moderate epatic dysfunction (Child-Pugh score 7-9), regardless of dication, the dose of 60 mg ***every other day*** should not e exceeded; administration of 30 mg once daily can also e considered.

Clinical experience is limited particularly in patients with noderate hepatic dysfunction and caution is advised. here is no clinical experience in patients with severe epatic dysfunction (Child-Pugh score ≥10); therefore, s use is contra-indicated in these patients (see sections .3, 4.4 and 5.2).

Renal insufficiency

No dosage adjustment is necessary for patients with crea-nine clearance ≥30 ml/min (see section 5.2). The use of etoricoxib in patients with creatinine clearance <30 ml/min s contra-indicated (see sections 4.3 and 4.4).

Paediatric patients

Etoricoxib is contra-indicated in children and adolescents under 16 years of age (see section 4.3).

4.3 Contraindications

Hypersensitivity to the active substance or to any of the excipients (see section 6.1).

Active peptic ulceration or active gastro-intestinal (GI) bleeding.

Patients who have experienced bronchospasm, acute rhi-nitis, nasal polyps, angioneurotic oedema, urticaria, or allergic-type reactions after taking acetylsalicylic acid or NSAIDs including COX-2 (cyclooxygenase-2) inhibitors.

Pregnancy and lactation (see sections 4.6 and 5.3).

Severe hepatic dysfunction (serum albumin <25 g/l or Child-Pugh score ≥10).

Estimated renal creatinine clearance <30 ml/min.

Children and adolescents under 16 years of age.

Inflammatory bowel disease.

Congestive heart failure (NYHA II-IV).

Patients with hypertension whose blood pressure is per-sistently elevated above 140/90mmHg and has not been adequately controlled.

Established ischaemic heart disease, peripheral arterial disease, and/or cerebrovascular disease.

4.4 Special warnings and precautions for use

Gastrointestinal effects

Upper gastrointestinal complications [perforations, ulcers or bleedings (PUBs)], some of them resulting in fatal out-come, have occurred in patients treated with etoricoxib.

Caution is advised with treatment of patients most at risk of developing a gastrointestinal complication with NSAIDs; the elderly, patients using any other NSAID or acetylsa-licylic acid concomitantly or patients with a prior history of gastrointestinal disease, such as ulceration and GI bleed-ing.

There is a further increase in the risk of gastrointestinal adverse effects (gastrointestinal ulceration or other gastro-intestinal complications) when etoricoxib is taken conco-mitantly with acetylsalicylic acid (even at low doses). A significant difference in GI safety between selective COX-2 inhibitors + acetylsalicylic acid *vs.* NSAIDs + acet-ylsalicylic acid has not been demonstrated in long-term clinical trials (see section 5.1).

Cardiovascular effects

Clinical trials suggest that the selective COX-2 inhibitor class of drugs may be associated with a risk of thrombotic events (especially myocardial infarction (MI) and stroke), relative to placebo and some NSAIDs. As the cardiovas-cular risks of etoricoxib may increase with dose and dura-tion of exposure, the shortest duration possible and the lowest effective daily dose should be used. The patient's need for symptomatic relief and response to therapy should be re-evaluated periodically, especially in patients with osteoarthritis (see sections 4.2, 4.3, 4.8 and 5.1).

Patients with significant risk factors for cardiovascular events (e.g. hypertension, hyperlipidaemia, diabetes mel-litus, smoking) should only be treated with etoricoxib after careful consideration (see section 5.1).

COX-2 selective inhibitors are not a substitute for acetyl-salicylic acid for prophylaxis of cardiovascular thrombo-embolic diseases because of their lack of antiplatelet effect. Therefore antiplatelet therapies should not be dis-continued (see sections above, 4.5 and 5.1.).

Renal effects

Renal prostaglandins may play a compensatory role in the maintenance of renal perfusion. Therefore, under condi-tions of compromised renal perfusion, administration of etoricoxib may cause a reduction in prostaglandin forma-tion and, secondarily, in renal blood flow, and thereby impair renal function. Patients at greatest risk of this response are those with pre-existing significantly impaired renal function, uncompensated heart failure, or cirrhosis. Monitoring of renal function in such patients should be considered.

Fluid retention, oedema and hypertension

As with other medicinal products known to inhibit prosta-glandin synthesis, fluid retention, oedema and hyperten-sion have been observed in patients taking etoricoxib. All Nonsteroidal Anti-inflammatory Drugs (NSAIDs), including etoricoxib, can be associated with new onset or recurrent congestive heart failure. For information regarding a dose related response for etoricoxib see section 5.1. Caution should be exercised in patients with a history of cardiac failure, left ventricular dysfunction, or hypertension and in patients with pre-existing oedema from any other reason. If there is clinical evidence of deterioration in the condition of these patients, appropriate measures including disconti-nuation of etoricoxib should be taken.

Etoricoxib may be associated with more frequent and severe hypertension than some other NSAIDs and selec-tive COX-2 inhibitors, particularly at high doses. Therefore, hypertension should be controlled before treatment with etoricoxib (see section 4.3) and special attention should be paid to blood pressure monitoring during treatment with etoricoxib. Blood pressure should be monitored within two weeks after initiation of treatment and periodically there-after. If blood pressure rises significantly, alternative treat-ment should be considered.

Hepatic effects

Elevations of alanine aminotransferase (ALT) and/or aspar-tate aminotransferase (AST) (approximately three or more times the upper limit of normal) have been reported in approximately 1% of patients in clinical trials treated for up to one year with etoricoxib 30, 60 and 90 mg daily.

Any patients with symptoms and/or signs suggesting liver dysfunction, or in whom an abnormal liver function test has occurred, should be monitored. If signs of hepatic insuffi-ciency occur, or if persistently abnormal liver function tests (three times the upper limit of normal) are detected, etor-icoxib should be discontinued.

General

If during treatment, patients deteriorate in any of the organ system functions described above, appropriate measures should be taken and discontinuation of etoricoxib therapy should be considered. Medically appropriate supervision should be maintained when using etoricoxib in the elderly and in patients with renal, hepatic, or cardiac dysfunction.

Caution should be used when initiating treatment with etoricoxib in patients with dehydration. It is advisable to rehydrate patients prior to starting therapy with etoricoxib.

Serious skin reactions, some of them fatal, including exfo-liative dermatitis, Stevens-Johnson syndrome, and toxic epidermal necrolysis, have been reported very rarely in association with the use of NSAIDs and some selective COX-2 inhibitors during post-marketing surveillance (see section 4.8). Patients appear to be at highest risk for these reactions early in the course of therapy with the onset of the reaction occurring in the majority of cases within the first month of treatment. Serious hypersensitivity reactions (such as anaphylaxis and angioedema) have been reported in patients receiving etoricoxib (see section 4.8). Some selective COX-2 inhibitors have been associated with an increased risk of skin reactions in patients with a history of any drug allergy. Etoricoxib should be discontinued at the first appearance of skin rash, mucosal lesions, or any other sign of hypersensitivity.

Etoricoxib may mask fever and other signs of inflammation.

Caution should be exercised when co-administering etor-icoxib with warfarin or other oral anticoagulants (see sec-tion 4.5).

The use of etoricoxib, as with any medicinal product known to inhibit cyclooxygenase / prostaglandin synthesis, is not recommended in women attempting to conceive (see sec-tions 4.6, 5.1, and 5.3).

ARCOXIA tablets contain lactose. Patients with rare her-editary problems of galactose intolerance, the Lapp lac-tase deficiency or glucose-galactose malabsorption should not take this medicine.

4.5 Interaction with other medicinal products and other forms of interaction

Pharmacodynamic interactions

Oral anticoagulants: In subjects stabilised on chronic war-farin therapy, the administration of etoricoxib 120 mg daily was associated with an approximate 13% increase in prothrombin time International Normalised Ratio (INR). Therefore, patients receiving oral anticoagulants should be closely monitored for their prothrombin time INR, parti-cularly in the first few days when therapy with etoricoxib is initiated or the dose of etoricoxib is changed (see section 4.4).

Diuretics, ACE inhibitors and Angiotensin II Antagonists: NSAIDs may reduce the effect of diuretics and other anti-hypertensive drugs. In some patients with compromised renal function (e.g. dehydrated patients or elderly patients with compromised renal function) the co-administration of an ACE inhibitor or Angiotensin II antagonist and agents that inhibit cyclo-oxygenase may result in further deteriora-tion of renal function, including possible acute renal failure, which is usually reversible. These interactions should be considered in patients taking etoricoxib concomitantly with ACE inhibitors or angiotensin II antagonists. Therefore, the combination should be administered with caution, espe-cially in the elderly. Patients should be adequately hydrated and consideration should be given to monitoring of renal function after initiation of concomitant therapy, and peri-odically thereafter.

Acetylsalicylic Acid: In a study in healthy subjects, at steady state, etoricoxib 120 mg once daily had no effect on the anti-platelet activity of acetylsalicylic acid (81 mg once daily). Etoricoxib can be used concomitantly with acetylsalicylic acid at doses used for cardiovascular pro-phylaxis (low-dose acetylsalicylic acid). However, conco-mitant administration of low-dose acetylsalicylic acid with etoricoxib may result in an increased rate of GI ulceration or other complications compared to use of etoricoxib alone. Concomitant administration of etoricoxib with doses of acetylsalicylic acid *above* those for cardiovascular prophy-laxis or with other NSAIDs is not recommended (see sec-tions 5.1 and 4.4.).

Ciclosporin and tacrolimus: Although this interaction has not been studied with etoricoxib, coadministration of ciclosporin or tacrolimus with any NSAID may increase the nephrotoxic effect of ciclosporin or tacrolimus. Renal function should be monitored when etoricoxib and either of these drugs is used in combination.

Pharmacokinetic interactions

The effect of etoricoxib on the pharmacokinetics of other drugs

Lithium: NSAIDs decrease lithium renal excretion and therefore increase lithium plasma levels. If necessary, monitor blood lithium closely and adjust the lithium dosage while the combination is being taken and when the NSAID is withdrawn.

Methotrexate: Two studies investigated the effects of etor-icoxib 60, 90 or 120 mg administered once daily for seven days in patients receiving once-weekly methotrexate doses of 7.5 to 20 mg for rheumatoid arthritis. Etoricoxib at 60 and 90 mg had no effect on methotrexate plasma concentrations or renal clearance. In one study, etoricoxib 120 mg had no effect, but in the other study, etoricoxib 120 mg increased methotrexate plasma concentrations by 28% and reduced renal clearance of methotrexate by 13%. Adequate monitoring for methotrexate-related toxi-city is recommended when etoricoxib and methotrexate are administered concomitantly.

Oral contraceptives: Etoricoxib 60 mg given concomitantly with an oral contraceptive containing 35 micrograms ethi-nyl estradiol (EE) and 0.5 to 1 mg norethindrone for 21 days increased the steady state $AUC_{0\text{-}24hr}$ of EE by 37%. Etor-icoxib 120 mg given with the same oral contraceptive concomitantly or separated by 12 hours, increased the steady state $AUC_{0\text{-}24hr}$ of EE by 50 to 60%. This increase in EE concentration should be considered when selecting an oral contraceptive for use with etoricoxib. An increase in EE exposure can increase the incidence of adverse events associated with oral contraceptives (e.g., venous thrombo-embolic events in women at risk).

Hormone Replacement Therapy (HRT): Administration of etoricoxib 120 mg with hormone replacement therapy consisting of conjugated estrogens (0.625 mg PREMAR-IN™) for 28 days, increased the mean steady state $AUC_{0\text{-}24hr}$ of unconjugated estrone (41%), equilin (76%), and 17-β-estradiol (22%). The effect of the recommended chronic doses of etoricoxib (30, 60, and 90 mg) has not been studied. The effects of etoricoxib 120 mg on the exposure ($AUC_{0\text{-}24hr}$) to these estrogenic components of PREMARIN were less than half of those observed when PREMARIN was administered alone and the dose was increased from 0.625 to 1.25 mg. The clinical significance of these increases is unknown, and higher doses of PREMARIN were not studied in combination with etoricoxib. These increases in estrogenic concentration should be taken into consideration when selecting post-menopausal hormone therapy for use with etoricoxib because the increase in oestrogen exposure might increase the risk of adverse events associated with HRT.

Prednisone/prednisolone: In drug-interaction studies, etor-icoxib did not have clinically important effects on the pharmacokinetics of prednisone/prednisolone.

Digoxin: Etoricoxib 120 mg administered once daily for 10 days to healthy volunteers did not alter the steady-state plasma $AUC_{0\text{-}24hr}$ or renal elimination of digoxin. There was an increase in digoxin C_{max} (approximately 33%). This increase is not generally important for most patients. However, patients at high risk of digoxin toxicity should be monitored for this when etoricoxib and digoxin are administered concomitantly.

Effect of etoricoxib on drugs metabolised by sulfotransferases

Etoricoxib is an inhibitor of human sulfotransferase activity, particularly SULT1E1, and has been shown to increase the serum concentrations of ethinyl estradiol. While knowledge about effects of multiple sulfotransferases is presently limited and the clinical consequences for many drugs are still being examined, it may be prudent to exercise care when administering etoricoxib concurrently with other drugs primarily metabolised by human sulfotransferases (e.g., oral salbutamol and minoxidil).

Effect of etoricoxib on drugs metabolised by CYP isoenzymes

Based on *in vitro* studies, etoricoxib is not expected to inhibit cytochromes P450 (CYP) 1A2, 2C9, 2C19, 2D6, 2E1 or 3A4. In a study in healthy subjects, daily administration of etoricoxib 120 mg did not alter hepatic CYP3A4 activity as assessed by the erythromycin breath test.

Effects of other drugs on the pharmacokinetics of etoricoxib

The main pathway of etoricoxib metabolism is dependent on CYP enzymes. CYP3A4 appears to contribute to the metabolism of etoricoxib *in vivo*. *In vitro* studies indicate that CYP2D6, CYP2C9, CYP1A2 and CYP2C19 also can catalyse the main metabolic pathway, but their quantitative roles have not been studied *in vivo*.

Ketoconazole: Ketoconazole, a potent inhibitor of CYP3A4, dosed at 400 mg once a day for 11 days to healthy volunteers, did not have any clinically important effect on the single-dose pharmacokinetics of 60 mg etoricoxib (43% increase in AUC).

Rifampicin: Co-administration of etoricoxib with rifampicin, a potent inducer of CYP enzymes, produced a 65% decrease in etoricoxib plasma concentrations. This interaction may result in recurrence of symptoms when etoricoxib is co-administered with rifampicin. While this information may suggest an increase in dose, doses of etoricoxib greater than those listed for each indication have not been studied in combination with rifampicin and are therefore not recommended (see section 4.2).

Antacids: Antacids do not affect the pharmacokinetics of etoricoxib to a clinically relevant extent.

4.6 Pregnancy and lactation

Pregnancy

The use of etoricoxib, as with any drug substance known to inhibit COX-2, is not recommended in women attempting to conceive.

No clinical data on exposed pregnancies are available for etoricoxib. Studies in animals have shown reproductive toxicity (see section 5.3). The potential for human risk in pregnancy is unknown. Etoricoxib, as with other medicinal products inhibiting prostaglandin synthesis, may cause uterine inertia and premature closure of the ductus arteriosus during the last trimester. Etoricoxib is contraindicated in pregnancy (see section 4.3). If a woman becomes pregnant during treatment, etoricoxib must be discontinued.

Lactation

It is not known whether etoricoxib is excreted in human milk. Etoricoxib is excreted in the milk of lactating rats. Women who use etoricoxib must not breast feed (see sections 4.3 and 5.3).

4.7 Effects on ability to drive and use machines

No studies on the effect of etoricoxib on the ability to drive or use machines have been performed. However, patients who experience dizziness, vertigo or somnolence while taking etoricoxib should refrain from driving or operating machinery.

4.8 Undesirable effects

In clinical trials, etoricoxib was evaluated for safety in 7152 individuals, including 4614 patients with OA, RA, chronic low back pain or ankylosing spondylitis (approximately 600 patients with OA or RA were treated for one year or longer).

In clinical studies, the undesirable effects profile was similar in patients with OA or RA treated with etoricoxib for one year or longer.

In a clinical study for acute gouty arthritis, patients were treated with etoricoxib 120 mg once daily for eight days. The adverse experience profile in this study was generally similar to that reported in the combined OA, RA, and chronic low back pain studies.

In a cardiovascular safety outcomes programme of pooled data from three active comparator controlled trials, 17, 412 patients with OA or RA were treated with etoricoxib (60 mg or 90 mg) for a mean duration of approximately 18 months. The safety data and details from this programme are presented in section 5.1.

The following undesirable effects were reported at an incidence greater than placebo in clinical trials in patients with OA, RA, chronic low back pain or ankylosing spondylitis treated with etoricoxib 30 mg, 60 mg or 90 mg for up to 12 weeks, or in the MEDAL Programme studies, or in post-marketing experience:

[Very Common (≥1/10) Common (≥1/100 to <1/10) Uncommon (≥1/1000 to <1/100) Rare (≥1/10,000 to <1/1,000) Very rare (<1/10,000), not known (cannot be estimated from the available data)]

Infections and infestations:

Uncommon: gastroenteritis, upper respiratory infection, urinary tract infection.

Blood and lymphatic system disorders:

Uncommon: anaemia (primarily associated with gastrointestinal bleeding), leukopenia, thrombocytopenia.

Immune system disorder:

Very rare: hypersensitivity reactions, including angioedema, anaphylactic/anaphylactoid reactions including shock.

Metabolism and nutrition disorders:

Common: oedema/fluid retention

Uncommon: appetite increase or decrease, weight gain.

Psychiatric disorders:

Uncommon: anxiety, depression, mental acuity decreased.

Very rare: confusion, hallucinations.

Nervous system disorder:

Common: dizziness, headache.

Uncommon: dysgeusia, insomnia, paresthaesia/hypaesthesia, somnolence.

Eye disorders:

Uncommon: blurred vision, conjunctivitis.

Ear and labyrinth disorders:

Uncommon: tinnitus, vertigo.

Cardiac disorders:

Common: palpitations.

Uncommon: atrial fibrillation, congestive heart failure, non-specific ECG changes, angina pectoris, myocardial infarction*.

Not known: tachycardia.

Vascular disorders:

Common: hypertension.

Uncommon: flushing, cerebrovascular accident*, transient ischaemic attack.

Very rare: hypertensive crisis.

Respiratory, thoracic and mediastinal disorders:

Uncommon: cough, dyspnoea, epistaxis.

Very rare: bronchospasm.

Gastrointestinal disorders:

Common: gastrointestinal disorders (e.g., abdominal pain, flatulence, heartburn), diarrhoea, dyspepsia, epigastric discomfort, nausea.

Uncommon: abdominal distention, acid reflux, bowel movement pattern change, constipation, dry mouth, gastroduodenal ulcer, irritable bowel syndrome, oesophagitis, oral ulcer, vomiting, gastritis.

Very rare: peptic ulcers including gastrointestinal perforation and bleeding (mainly in the elderly).

Not known: pancreatitis.

Hepatobiliary disorders:

Common: ALT increased, AST increased.

Very rare: hepatitis.

Not known: jaundice.

Skin and subcutaneous tissue disorders:

Common: ecchymosis.

Uncommon: facial oedema, pruritus, rash.

Rare: erythema.

Very rare: urticaria, Stevens-Johnson syndrome, toxic epidermal necrolysis.

Musculoskeletal, connective tissue and bone disorders:

Uncommon: muscular cramp/spasm, musculoskeletal pain/stiffness.

Renal and urinary disorders:

Uncommon: proteinuria, serum creatinine increased.

Very rare: renal insufficiency, including renal failure, usually reversible upon discontinuation of treatment (see section 4.4).

General disorders and administration site conditions:

Common: asthenia/fatigue, flu-like disease.

Uncommon: chest pain.

Investigations:

Uncommon: blood urea nitrogen increased, creatine phosphokinase increased, hyperkalaemia, uric acid increased.

Rare: blood sodium decreased.

The following serious undesirable effects have been reported in association with the use of NSAIDs and cannot be ruled out for etoricoxib: nephrotoxicity including interstitial nephritis and nephrotic syndrome; hepatotoxicity including hepatic failure.

* Based on analyses of long-term placebo and acti controlled clinical trials, selective COX-2 inhibitors ha been associated with an increased risk of serious thror botic arterial events, including myocardial infarction ar stroke. The absolute risk increase for such events is un kely to exceed 1% per year based on existing data (uncor mon).

4.9 Overdose

In clinical studies, administration of single doses of etc icoxib up to 500 mg and multiple doses up to 150 mg/d for 21 days did not result in significant toxicity. There ha been reports of acute overdosage with etoricoxib, althoug adverse experiences were not reported in the majority cases. The most frequently observed adverse experience were consistent with the safety profile for etoricoxib (e. gastrointestinal events, cardiorenal events).

In the event of overdose, it is reasonable to employ th usual supportive measures, e.g., remove unabsorbe material from the GI tract, employ clinical monitorin and institute supportive therapy, if required.

Etoricoxib is not dialysable by haemodialysis; it is nc known whether etoricoxib is dialysable by peritoneal dia lysis.

5. PHARMACOLOGICAL PROPERTIES

5.1 Pharmacodynamic properties

Pharmacotherapeutic group: Anti-inflammatory and ant rheumatic products, non-steroids, coxibs, ATC Code: MO AH05

Mechanism of Action

Etoricoxib is an oral, selective cyclo-oxygenase-2 (COX-2 inhibitor within the clinical dose range.

Across clinical pharmacology studies, ARCOXIA producec dose-dependent inhibition of COX-2 without inhibition o COX-1 at doses up to 150 mg daily. Etoricoxib did no inhibit gastric prostaglandin synthesis and had no effect or platelet function.

Cyclooxygenase is responsible for generation of prostaglandins. Two isoforms, COX-1 and COX-2, have beer identified. COX-2 is the isoform of the enzyme that has been shown to be induced by pro-inflammatory stimuli and has been postulated to be primarily responsible for the synthesis of prostanoid mediators of pain, inflammation, and fever. COX-2 is also involved in ovulation, implantation and closure of the ductus arteriosus, regulation of renal function, and central nervous system functions (fever induction, pain perception and cognitive function). It may also play a role in ulcer healing. COX-2 has been identified in tissue around gastric ulcers in man but its relevance to ulcer healing has not been established.

Efficacy

In patients with osteoarthritis (OA), etoricoxib 60 mg once daily provided significant improvements in pain and patient assessments of disease status. These beneficial effects were observed as early as the second day of therapy and maintained for up to 52 weeks. Studies with etoricoxib 30 mg once daily demonstrated efficacy superior to placebo over a 12 week treatment period (using similar assessments as the above studies). In a dose ranging study, etoricoxib 60 mg demonstrated significantly greater improvement than 30 mg for all 3 primary endpoints over 6 weeks of treatment. The 30 mg dose has not been studied in osteoarthritis of hands.

In patients with rheumatoid arthritis (RA), etoricoxib 90 mg once daily provided significant improvements in pain, inflammation, and mobility. These beneficial effects were maintained over the 12-week treatment periods.

In patients experiencing attacks of acute gouty arthritis, etoricoxib 120 mg once daily over an eight-day treatment period, relieved moderate to extreme joint pain and inflammation comparable to indomethacin 50 mg three times daily. Pain relief was observed as early as four hours after initiation of treatment.

In patients with ankylosing spondylitis, etoricoxib 90 mg once daily provided significant improvements in spine pain, inflammation, stiffness and function. The clinical benefit of etoricoxib was observed as early as the second day of therapy after initiation of treatment and was maintained throughout the 52-week treatment period.

In studies specifically designed to measure the onset of action of etoricoxib, the onset of action occurred as early as 24 minutes after dosing.

Safety

Multinational Etoricoxib and Diclofenac Arthritis Long-term (MEDAL) Programme

The MEDAL Programme was a prospectively designed Cardiovascular (CV) Safety Outcomes Programme of pooled data from three randomized, double-blind active comparator controlled trials, the MEDAL study, EDGE II and EDGE.

The MEDAL Study, was an endpoint driven CV Outcomes study in 17,804 OA and 5,700 RA patients treated with etoricoxib 60 (OA) or 90 mg (OA and RA) or diclofenac 150 mg daily for a mean period of 20.3 months (maximum of 42.3 months, median 21.3 months). In this trial, only serious adverse events and discontinuations due to any adverse events were recorded.

The EDGE and EDGE II studies compared the gastrointestinal tolerability of etoricoxib versusdiclofenac. The

Table 1 Rates of Confirmed Thrombotic CV Events (Pooled MEDAL Programme)

	Etoricoxib (N=16819) 25836 Patient-Years	Diclofenac (N=16483) 24766 Patient-Years	Between Treatment Comparison
	Rate† (95% CI)	Rate† (95% CI)	Relative Risk (95% CI)
Confirmed Thrombotic Cardiovascular Serious Adverse Events			
Per-protocol	1.24 (1.11, 1.38)	1.30 (1.17, 1.45)	0.95 (0.81, 1.11)
Intent-to-treat	1.25 (1.14, 1.36)	1.19 (1.08, 1.30)	1.05 (0.93, 1.19)
Confirmed Cardiac Events			
Per-protocol	0.71 (0.61, 0.82)	0.78 (0.68, 0.90)	0.90 (0.74, 1.10)
Intent-to-treat	0.69 (0.61, 0.78)	0.70 (0.62, 0.79)	0.99 (0.84, 1.17)
Confirmed Cerebrovascular Events			
Per-protocol	0.34 (0.28, 0.42)	0.32 (0.25, 0.40)	1.08 (0.80, 1.46)
Intent-to-treat	0.33 (0.28, 0.39)	0.29 (0.24, 0.35)	1.12 (0.87, 1.44)
Confirmed Peripheral Vascular Events			
Per-protocol	0.20 (0.15, 0.27)	0.22 (0.17, 0.29)	0.92 (0.63, 1.35)
Intent-to-treat	0.24 (0.20, 0.30)	0.23 (0.18, 0.28)	1.08 (0.81, 1.44)

†Events per 100 Patient-Years; CI=confidence interval

N=total number of patients included in Per-protocol population

Per-protocol: all events on study therapy or within 14 days of discontinuation (excluded: patients who took < 75% of their study medication or took non-study NSAIDs > 10% of the time).

Intent-to-treat: all confirmed events up to the end of the trial (included patients potentially exposed to non-study interventions following discontinuation of study medication). Total number of patients randomised, n= 17412 on etoricoxib and 17289 on diclofenac.

EDGE study included 7111 OA patients treated with a dose of etoricoxib 90 mg daily (1.5 times the dose recommended for OA) or diclofenac 150 mg daily for a mean period of 9.1 months (maximum 16.6 months, median 11.4 months). The EDGE II study included 4086 RA patients treated with etoricoxib 90 mg daily or diclofenac 150 mg daily for a mean period of 19.2 months (maximum 33.1 months, median 24 months).

In the pooled MEDAL Programme, 34,701 patients with OA or RA were treated for a mean duration of 17.9 months (maximum 42.3 months, median 16.3 months) with approximately 12,800 patients receiving treatment for more than 24 months. Patients enrolled in the Programme had a wide range of cardiovascular and gastrointestinal risk factors at baseline. Patients with a recent history of myocardial infarction, coronary artery bypass grafting or percutaneous coronary intervention within 6 months preceding enrollment were excluded. Use of gastroprotective agents and low dose aspirin were permitted in the studies.

Overall Safety:

There was no significant difference between etoricoxib and diclofenac in the rate of cardiovascular thrombotic events. Cardiorenal adverse events were observed more frequently with etoricoxib than with diclofenac, and this effect was dose-dependent (see specific results below). Gastrointestinal and hepatic adverse events were observed significantly more frequently with diclofenac than etoricoxib. The incidence of adverse experiences in EDGE and EDGE II and of adverse experiences considered serious or resulting in discontinuation in the MEDAL study was higher with etoricoxib than diclofenac.

Cardiovascular safety results:

The rate of confirmed thrombotic cardiovascular serious adverse events (consisting of cardiac, cerebrovascular, and peripheral vascular events) was comparable between etoricoxib and diclofenac, and data are summarized in the table below. There were no statistically significant differences in thrombotic event rates between etoricoxib and diclofenac across all subgroups analyzed including patient categories across a range of baseline cardiovascular risk. When considered separately, the relative risks for confirmed thrombotic cardiovascular serious adverse events with etoricoxib 60 mg or 90 mg compared with diclofenac 150mg were similar.

(see Table 1 above)

CV mortality, as well as overall mortality, was similar between the etoricoxib and diclofenac treatment groups.

Cardiorenal Events:

Approximately 50% of patients enrolled in the MEDAL study had a history of hypertension at baseline. In the study, the incidence of discontinuations due to hypertension-related adverse events was statistically significantly higher for etoricoxib than for diclofenac. The incidence of congestive heart failure adverse events (discontinuations and serious events) occurred at similar rates on etoricoxib 60 mg compared to diclofenac 150 mg but was higher for etoricoxib 90 mg compared to diclofenac 150 mg (statistically significant for 90 mg etoricoxib vs. 150 mg diclofenac in MEDAL OA cohort). The incidence of confirmed congestive heart failure adverse events (events that were serious and resulted in hospitalisation or a visit to an emergency department) was non-significantly higher with etoricoxib than diclofenac 150 mg, and this effect was dose-dependent. The incidence of discontinuations due to edema-related adverse events was higher for etoricoxib than diclofenac 150 mg, and this effect was dose-dependent (statistically significant for etoricoxib 90 mg, but not for etoricoxib 60 mg).

The cardiorenal results for EDGE and EDGE II were consistent with those described for the MEDAL Study.

In the individual MEDAL Programme studies, for etoricoxib (60 mg or 90 mg), the absolute incidence of discontinuation in any treatment group was up to 2.6% for hypertension, up to 1.9% for edema, and up to 1.1% for congestive heart failure, with higher rates of discontinuation observed with etoricoxib 90 mg than etoricoxib 60 mg.

MEDAL Programme Gastrointestinal Tolerability Results:

A significantly lower rate of discontinuations of treatment for any clinical (e.g., dyspepsia, abdominal pain, ulcer) GI adverse event was observed with etoricoxib compared with diclofenac within each of the three component studies of the MEDAL Programme. The rates of discontinuations due to adverse clinical GI events per hundred patient-years over the entire period of study were as follows: 3.23 for etoricoxib and 4.96 for diclofenac in the MEDAL Study; 9.12 with etoricoxib and 12.28 with diclofenac in the EDGE study; and 3.71 with etoricoxib and 4.81 with diclofenac in the EDGE II study.

MEDAL Programme Gastrointestinal Safety Results:

Overall upper GI events were defined as perforations, ulcers and bleeds. The subset of overall upper GI events considered complicated included perforations, obstructions, and complicated bleeding; the subset of upper GI events considered uncomplicated included uncomplicated bleeds and uncomplicated ulcers. A significantly lower rate of overall upper GI events was observed with etoricoxib compared to diclofenac. There was no significant difference between etoricoxib and diclofenac in the rate of complicated events. For the subset of upper GI hemorrhage events (complicated and uncomplicated combined), there was no significant difference between etoricoxib and diclofenac. The upper GI benefit for etoricoxib compared with diclofenac was not statistically significant in patients taking concomitant low-dose aspirin (approximately 33% of patients).

The rates per hundred patient-years of confirmed complicated and uncomplicated upper GI clinical events (perforations, ulcers and bleeds (PUBs)) were 0.67 (95% CI 0.57, 0.77) with etoricoxib and 0.97 (95% CI 0.85, 1.10) with diclofenac, yielding a relative risk of 0.69 (95% CI 0.57, 0.83).

The rate for confirmed upper GI events in elderly patients was evaluated and the largest reduction was observed in patients ≥ 75 years of age (1.35 [95% CI 0.94, 1.87] vs. 2.78 [95% CI 2.14, 3.56] events per hundred patient-years for etoricoxib and diclofenac, respectively.

The rates of confirmed lower GI clinical events (small or large bowel perforation, obstruction, or hemorrhage, (POBs)) were not significantly different between etoricoxib and diclofenac.

MEDAL Programme Hepatic Safety Results:

Etoricoxib was associated with a statistically significantly lower rate of discontinuations due to hepatic-related adverse experiences than diclofenac. In the pooled MEDAL Programme, 0.3% of patients on etoricoxib and 2.7% of patients on diclofenac discontinued due to hepatic-related adverse experiences. The rate per hundred patient-years was 0.22 on etoricoxib and 1.84 for diclofenac (p-value was <0.001 for etoricoxib vs. diclofenac). However, most hepatic adverse experiences in the MEDAL Programme were non-serious.

Additional Thrombotic Cardiovascular Safety Data

In clinical studies excluding the MEDAL Programme Studies, approximately 3100 patients were treated with etoricoxib ≥60 mg daily for 12 weeks or longer. There was no discernible difference in the rate of confirmed serious thrombotic cardiovascular events between patients receiving etoricoxib ≥60 mg, placebo, or non-naproxen NSAIDs. However, the rate of these events was higher in patients receiving etoricoxib compared with those receiving naproxen 500 mg twice daily. The difference in antiplatelet activity between some COX-1 inhibiting NSAIDs and selective COX-2 inhibitors may be of clinical significance in patients at risk of thrombo-embolic events. Selective COX-2 inhibitors reduce the formation of systemic (and therefore possibly endothelial) prostacyclin without affecting platelet thromboxane. The clinical relevance of these observations has not been established.

Additional Gastrointestinal Safety Data

In two 12-week double-blind endoscopy studies, the cumulative incidence of gastroduodenal ulceration was significantly lower in patients treated with etoricoxib 120 mg once daily than in patients treated with either naproxen 500 mg twice daily or ibuprofen 800 mg three times daily. Etoricoxib had a higher incidence of ulceration as compared to placebo.

Renal Function Study in the Elderly

A randomized, double-blind, placebo-controlled, parallel-group study evaluated the effects of 15 days of treatment of etoricoxib (90 mg), celecoxib (200 mg bid), naproxen (500 mg bid) and placebo on urinary sodium excretion, blood pressure, and other renal function parameters in subjects 60 to 85 years of age on a 200-mEq/day sodium diet. Etoricoxib, celecoxib, and naproxen had similar effects on urinary sodium excretion over the 2 weeks of treatment. All active comparators showed an increase relative to placebo with respect to systolic blood pressures; however, etoricoxib was associated with a statistically significant increase at Day 14 when compared to celecoxib and naproxen (mean change from baseline for systolic blood pressure: etoricoxib 7.7 mmHg, celecoxib 2.4 mmHg, naproxen 3.6 mmHg).

5.2 Pharmacokinetic properties

Absorption

Orally administered etoricoxib is well absorbed. The absolute bioavailability is approximately 100%. Following 120 mg once-daily dosing to steady state, the peak plasma concentration (geometric mean C_{max} = 3.6 μg/ml) was observed at approximately 1 hour (T_{max}) after administration to fasted adults. The geometric mean area under the curve (AUC_{0-24hr}) was 37.8 μg•hr/ml. The pharmacokinetics of etoricoxib are linear across the clinical dose range.

Dosing with food (a high-fat meal) had no effect on the extent of absorption of etoricoxib after administration of a 120-mg dose. The rate of absorption was affected, resulting in a 36% decrease in C_{max} and an increase in T_{max} by 2 hours. These data are not considered clinically significant. In clinical trials, etoricoxib was administered without regard to food intake.

Distribution

Etoricoxib is approximately 92% bound to human plasma protein over the range of concentrations of 0.05 to 5 μg/ml. The volume of distribution at steady state (V_{dss}) was approximately 120 l in humans.

Etoricoxib crosses the placenta in rats and rabbits, and the blood-brain barrier in rats.

Metabolism

Etoricoxib is extensively metabolised with <1% of a dose recovered in urine as the parent drug. The major route of metabolism to form the 6'-hydroxymethyl derivative is catalyzed by CYP enzymes. CYP3A4 appears to contribute to the metabolism of etoricoxib *in vivo*. *In vitro* studies indicate that CYP2D6, CYP2C9, CYP1A2 and CYP2C19 also can catalyse the main metabolic pathway, but their quantitative roles *in vivo* have not been studied.

Five metabolites have been identified in man. The principal metabolite is the 6'-carboxylic acid derivative of etoricoxib formed by further oxidation of the 6'-hydroxymethyl derivative. These principal metabolites either demonstrate no measurable activity or are only weakly active as COX-2 inhibitors. None of these metabolites inhibit COX-1.

Elimination

Following administration of a single 25-mg radiolabeled intravenous dose of etoricoxib to healthy subjects, 70% of radioactivity was recovered in urine and 20% in faeces, mostly as metabolites. Less than 2% was recovered as unchanged drug.

Elimination of etoricoxib occurs almost exclusively through metabolism followed by renal excretion. Steady state concentrations of etoricoxib are reached within seven days of once daily administration of 120 mg, with an accumulation ratio of approximately 2, corresponding to a half-life of approximately 22 hours. The plasma clearance after a 25-mg intravenous dose is estimated to be approximately 50 ml/min.

Characteristics in patients

Elderly: Pharmacokinetics in the elderly (65 years of age and older) are similar to those in the young.

Gender: The pharmacokinetics of etoricoxib are similar between men and women.

Hepatic insufficiency: Patients with mild hepatic dysfunction (Child-Pugh score 5-6) administered etoricoxib 60 mg once daily had an approximately 16% higher mean AUC as compared to healthy subjects given the same regimen. Patients with moderate hepatic dysfunction (Child-Pugh score 7-9) administered etoricoxib 60 mg ***every other day*** had similar mean AUC to the healthy subjects given etoricoxib 60 mg once daily; etoricoxib 30 mg once daily has not been studied in this population. There are no clinical or pharmacokinetic data in patients with severe hepatic dysfunction (Child-Pugh score ≥10). (See sections 4.2 and 4.3.)

Renal insufficiency: The pharmacokinetics of a single dose of etoricoxib 120 mg in patients with moderate to severe renal insufficiency and patients with end-stage renal disease on hemodialysis were not significantly different from those in healthy subjects. Hemodialysis contributed negligibly to elimination (dialysis clearance approximately 50 ml/min). (See sections 4.3 and 4.4.)

Paediatric patients: The pharmacokinetics of etoricoxib in paediatric patients (<12 years old) have not been studied.

In a pharmacokinetic study (n=16) conducted in adolescents (aged 12 to 17) the pharmacokinetics in adolescents weighing 40 to 60 kg given etoricoxib 60 mg once daily and adolescents >60 kg given etoricoxib 90 mg once daily were similar to the pharmacokinetics in adults given etoricoxib 90 mg once daily. Safety and effectiveness of etoricoxib in paediatric patients have not been established (see section 4.2).

5.3 Preclinical safety data

In preclinical studies, etoricoxib has been demonstrated not to be genotoxic. Etoricoxib was not carcinogenic in mice. Rats developed hepatocellular and thyroid follicular cell adenomas at >2-times the daily human dose [90 mg] based on systemic exposure when dosed daily for approximately two years. Hepatocellular and thyroid follicular cell adenomas observed in rats are considered to be a consequence of rat-specific mechanism related to hepatic CYP enzyme induction. Etoricoxib has not been shown to cause hepatic CYP3A enzyme induction in humans.

In the rat, gastrointestinal toxicity of etoricoxib increased with dose and exposure time. In the 14-week toxicity study etoricoxib caused gastrointestinal ulcers at exposures greater than those seen in man at the therapeutic dose. In the 53- and 106-week toxicity study, gastrointestinal ulcers were also seen at exposures comparable to those seen in man at the therapeutic dose. In dogs, renal and gastrointestinal abnormalities were seen at high exposures.

Etoricoxib was not teratogenic in reproductive toxicity studies conducted in rats at 15 mg/kg/day (this represents approximately 1.5 times the daily human dose [90 mg] based on systemic exposure). In rabbits, a treatment related increase in cardiovascular malformations was observed at exposure levels below the clinical exposure at the daily human dose (90mg). However no treatment-related external or skeletal foetal malformations were observed. In rats and rabbits, there was a dose dependent increase in post implantation loss at exposures greater than or equal to 1.5 times the human exposure (see sections 4.3 and 4.6).

Etoricoxib is excreted in the milk of lactating rats at concentrations approximately two-fold those in plasma. There was a decrease in pup body weight following exposure of pups to milk from dams administered etoricoxib during lactation.

6. PHARMACEUTICAL PARTICULARS

6.1 List of excipients

Core:

Calcium hydrogen phosphate (anhydrous)

Croscarmellose sodium

Magnesium stearate

Microcrystalline cellulose

Tablet coating:

Carnauba wax

Lactose monohydrate

Hypromellose

Titanium dioxide (E171)

Triacetin

The 30-, 60- and 120-mg tablets also contain indigo carmine lake (E132) and yellow ferric oxide (E172).

6.2 Incompatibilities

Not applicable.

6.3 Shelf life

3 years.

6.4 Special precautions for storage

Bottles: Keep the container tightly closed in order to protect from moisture.

Blisters: Store in the original package in order to protect from moisture.

6.5 Nature and contents of container

30 mg

Aluminum/aluminium blisters in packs containing 2, 7, 14, 20, 28 tablets or multi-packs containing 98 (2 packs of 49) tablets.

60, 90 and 120 mg

Aluminum/aluminium blisters in packs containing 2, 5, 7, 10, 14, 20, 28, 30, 50, 84, 100 tablets or multi-packs containing 98 (2 packs of 49) tablets.

Aluminum/aluminium blisters (unit doses) in packs of 50 or 100 tablets.

White, round, HDPE bottles with a white, polypropylene closure containing 30 tablets and two1-gram desiccant containers or 90 tablets and one 1-gram desiccant container.

Not all pack sizes may be marketed.

6.6 Special precautions for disposal and other handling

No special requirements.

7. MARKETING AUTHORISATION HOLDER

Merck Sharp & Dohme Limited

Hertford Road, Hoddesdon, Hertfordshire EN11 9BU, UK

8. MARKETING AUTHORISATION NUMBER(S)

30 mg Tablets: PL 0025/0478

60 mg Tablets PL 0025/0422

90 mg Tablets PL 0025/0423

120 mg Tablets PL 0025/0424

9. DATE OF FIRST AUTHORISATION/RENEWAL OF THE AUTHORISATION

30 mg Tablets 22/10/2007

60 mg Tablets 13/02/2002

90 mg Tablets 13/02/2002

120 mg Tablets 13/02/2002

10. DATE OF REVISION OF THE TEXT

17 September 2009

LEGAL CATEGORY

POM

® denotes registered trademark of Merck & Co., Inc., Whitehouse Station, NJ, USA.

ARCOXIA SPC.ACX.08.UK.2944.II-023

Aricept

(Eisai Ltd)

1. NAME OF THE MEDICINAL PRODUCT

ARICEPT® 5 mg film coated tablets

ARICEPT® 10 mg film coated tablets

2. QUALITATIVE AND QUANTITATIVE COMPOSITION

Each 5 mg tablet contains 5 mg donepezil hydrochloride, equivalent to 4.56 mg of donepezil free base. 87.17 mg lactose/film-coated tablet

Each 10 mg tablet contains 10 mg donepezil hydrochloride equivalent to 9.12 mg donepezil free base. 174.33 mg lactose/film-coated tablet

For full list of excipients, see section 6.1

3. PHARMACEUTICAL FORM

Film-coated tablet.

5 mg donepezil as white, round, biconvex tablets embossed 'ARICEPT' on one side and '5' on the other side.

10 mg donepezil as yellow, round, biconvex tablets embossed 'ARICEPT' on one side and '10' on the other side

4. CLINICAL PARTICULARS

4.1 Therapeutic indications

ARICEPT tablets are indicated for the symptomatic treatment of mild to moderately severe Alzheimer's dementia.

4.2 Posology and method of administration

Adults/Elderly:

Treatment is initiated at 5 mg/day (once-a-day dosing). ARICEPT should be taken orally, in the evening, just prior to retiring. The 5 mg/day dose should be maintained for at least one month in order to allow the earliest clinical responses to treatment to be assessed and to allow steady-state concentrations of donepezil hydrochloride to be achieved. Following a one-month clinical assessment of treatment at 5 mg/day, the dose of ARICEPT can be increased to 10 mg/day (once-a-day dosing). The maximum recommended daily dose is 10 mg. Doses greater than 10 mg/day have not been studied in clinical trials.

Treatment should be initiated and supervised by a physician experienced in the diagnosis and treatment of Alzheimer's dementia. Diagnosis should be made according to accepted guidelines (e.g. DSM IV, ICD 10). Therapy with donepezil should only be started if a caregiver is availab who will regularly monitor drug intake for the patier Maintenance treatment can be continued for as long as therapeutic benefit for the patient exists. Therefore, th clinical benefit of donepezil should be reassessed on regular basis. Discontinuation should be considered whe evidence of a therapeutic effect is no longer preser Individual response to donepezil cannot be predicted.

Upon discontinuation of treatment, a gradual abatement of the beneficial effects of ARICEPT is seen.

Renal and hepatic impairment:

A similar dose schedule can be followed for patients wi renal impairment, as clearance of donepezil hydrochlorio is not affected by this condition.

Due to possible increased exposure in mild to moderat hepatic impairment (see section 5.2), dose escalatio should be performed according to individual tolerabilit There are no data for patients with severe hepatic impai ment.

Children:

ARICEPT is not recommended for use in children.

4.3 Contraindications

ARICEPT is contraindicated in patients with a know hypersensitivity to donepezil hydrochloride, piperidin derivatives, or to any excipients used in the formulation.

4.4 Special warnings and precautions for use

The use of ARICEPT in patients with severe Alzheimer' dementia, other types of dementia or other types of mem ory impairment (e.g., age-related cognitive decline), ha not been investigated.

Anaesthesia: ARICEPT, as a cholinesterase inhibitor, is likely to exaggerate succinylcholine-type muscle relaxatio during anaesthesia.

Cardiovascular Conditions: Because of their pharmacological action, cholinesterase inhibitors may have vagotonic effects on heart rate (e.g., bradycardia). The potential fo this action may be particularly important to patients with "sick sinus syndrome" or other supraventricular cardiac conduction conditions, such as sinoatrial or atrioventricular block.

There have been reports of syncope and seizures. In investigating such patients the possibility of heart block or long sinusal pauses should be considered.

Gastrointestinal Conditions: Patients at increased risk for developing ulcers, e.g., those with a history of ulcer disease or those receiving concurrent nonsteroidal anti-inflammatory drugs (NSAIDs), should be monitored for symptoms. However, the clinical studies with ARICEPT showed no increase, relative to placebo, in the incidence of either peptic ulcer disease or gastrointestinal bleeding.

Genitourinary: Although not observed in clinical trials of ARICEPT, cholinomimetics may cause bladder outflow obstruction.

Neurological Conditions: Seizures: Cholinomimetics are believed to have some potential to cause generalised convulsions. However, seizure activity may also be a manifestation of Alzheimer's Disease.

Cholinomimetics may have the potential to exacerbate or induce extrapyramidal symptoms.

Pulmonary Conditions: Because of their cholinomimetic actions, cholinesterase inhibitors should be prescribed with care to patients with a history of asthma or obstructive pulmonary disease.

The administration of ARICEPT concomitantly with other inhibitors of acetylcholinesterase, agonists or antagonists of the cholinergic system should be avoided.

Severe Hepatic Impairment: There are no data for patients with severe hepatic impairment.

This medicinal product contains lactose. Patients with rare hereditary problems of galactose intolerance, the Lapp lactase deficiency or glucose-galactose malabsorption should not take this medicine.

Mortality in Vascular Dementia Clinical Trials

Three clinical trials of 6 months duration were conducted studying individuals meeting the NINDS-AIREN criteria for probable or possible vascular dementia (VaD). The NINDS-AIREN criteria are designed to identify patients whose dementia appears to be due solely to vascular causes and to exclude patients with Alzheimer's disease. In the first study, the mortality rates were 2/198 (1.0%) on donepezil hydrochloride 5 mg, 5/206 (2.4%) on donepezil hydrochloride 10 mg and 7/199 (3.5%) on placebo. In the second study, the mortality rates were 4/208 (1.9%) on donepezil hydrochloride 5 mg, 3/215 (1.4%) on donepezil hydrochloride 10 mg and 1/193 (0.5%) on placebo. In the third study, the mortality rates were 11/648 (1.7%) on donepezil hydrochloride 5 mg and 0/326 (0%) on placebo. The mortality rate for the three VaD studies combined in the donepezil hydrochloride group (1.7%) was numerically higher than in the placebo group (1.1%), however, this difference was not statistically significant. The majority of deaths in patients taking either donepezil hydrochloride or placebo appear to result from various vascular related causes, which could be expected in this elderly population with underlying vascular disease. An analysis of all serious non-fatal and fatal vascular events showed no difference in the rate of occurrence in the donepezil hydrochloride group relative to placebo.

Table 1

System Organ Class	Very Common	Common	Uncommon	Rare
Infections and infestations		Common cold		
Metabolism and nutrition disorders		Anorexia		
Psychiatric disorders		Hallucinations** Agitation** Aggressive behaviour**		
Nervous system disorders		Syncope* Dizziness Insomnia	Seizure*	Extrapyramidal symptoms
Cardiac disorders			Bradycardia	Sino-atrial block Atrioventricular block
Gastrointestinal disorders	Diarrhoea Nausea	Vomiting Abdominal disturbance	Gastrointestinal haemorrhage Gastric and duodenal ulcers	
Hepato-biliary disorders				Liver dysfunction including hepatitis***
Skin and subcutaneous tissue disorders		Rash Pruritis		
Musculoskeletal, connective tissue and bone disorders		Muscle cramps		
Renal and urinary disorders		Urinary incontinence		
General disorders and administration site conditions	Headache	Fatigue Pain		
Investigations			Minor increase in serum concentration of muscle creatine kinase	
Injury and poisoning		Accident		

* In investigating patients for syncope or seizure the possibility of heart block or long sinusal pauses should be considered (see section 4.4)

** Reports of hallucinations, agitation and aggressive behaviour have resolved on dose-reduction or discontinuation of treatment.

*** In cases of unexplained liver dysfunction, withdrawal of ARICEPT should be considered.

In pooled Alzheimer's disease studies (n=4146), and when these Alzheimer's disease studies were pooled with other dementia studies including the vascular dementia studies (total n=6888), the mortality rate in the placebo groups numerically exceeded that in the donepezil hydrochloride groups.

4.5 Interaction with other medicinal products and other forms of interaction

Donepezil hydrochloride and/or any of its metabolites do not inhibit the metabolism of theophylline, warfarin, cimetidine or digoxin in humans. The metabolism of donepezil hydrochloride is not affected by concurrent administration of digoxin or cimetidine. In vitro studies have shown that the cytochrome P450 isoenzymes 3A4 and to a minor extent 2D6 are involved in the metabolism of donepezil. Drug interaction studies performed in vitro show that ketoconazole and quinidine, inhibitors of CYP3A4 and 2D6 respectively, inhibit donepezil metabolism. Therefore these and other CYP3A4 inhibitors, such as itraconazole and erythromycin, and CYP2D6 inhibitors, such as fluoxetine could inhibit the metabolism of donepezil. In a study in healthy volunteers, ketoconazole increased mean donepezil concentrations by about 30%. Enzyme inducers, such as rifampicin, phenytoin, carbamazepine and alcohol may reduce the levels of donepezil. Since the magnitude of an inhibiting or inducing effect is unknown, such drug combinations should be used with care. Donepezil hydrochloride has the potential to interfere with medications having anticholinergic activity. There is also the potential for synergistic activity with concomitant treatment involving medications such as succinylcholine, other neuromuscular blocking agents or cholinergic agonists or beta blocking agents which have effects on cardiac conduction.

4.6 Pregnancy and lactation

Pregnancy:

There are no adequate data from the use of donepezil in pregnant women.

Studies in animals have not shown teratogenic effect but have shown peri and post natal toxicity (see section 5.3 preclinical safety data). The potential risk for humans is unknown.

Aricept should not be used during pregnancy unless clearly necessary.

Lactation:

Donepezil is excreted in the milk of rats. It is not known whether donepezil hydrochloride is excreted in human breast milk and there are no studies in lactating women. Therefore, women on donepezil should not breast feed.

4.7 Effects on ability to drive and use machines

Donepezil has minor or moderate influence on the ability to drive and use machines.

Dementia may cause impairment of driving performance or compromise the ability to use machinery. Furthermore, donepezil can induce fatigue, dizziness and muscle cramps, mainly when initiating or increasing the dose. The treating physician should routinely evaluate the ability of patients on donepezil to continue driving or operating complex machines.

4.8 Undesirable effects

The most common adverse events are diarrhoea, muscle cramps, fatigue, nausea, vomiting and insomnia.

Adverse reactions reported as more than an isolated case are listed below, by system organ class and by frequency. Frequencies are defined as: very common (≥ 1/10) common (≥ 1/100, < 1/10), uncommon (≥ 1/1,000, < 1/100), rare (≥ 1/10,000, < 1/1,000); very rare (< 1/10000) and not known (cannot be estimated from available data).

(see Table 1 above)

4.9 Overdose

The estimated median lethal dose of donepezil hydrochloride following administration of a single oral dose in mice and rats is 45 and 32 mg/kg, respectively, or approximately 225 and 160 times the maximum recommended human dose of 10 mg per day. Dose-related signs of cholinergic stimulation were observed in animals and included reduced spontaneous movement, prone position, staggering gait, lacrimation, clonic convulsions, depressed respiration, salivation, miosis, fasciculation and lower body surface temperature.

Overdosage with cholinesterase inhibitors can result in cholinergic crisis characterized by severe nausea, vomiting, salivation, sweating, bradycardia, hypotension, respiratory depression, collapse and convulsions. Increasing muscle weakness is a possibility and may result in death if respiratory muscles are involved.

As in any case of overdose, general supportive measures should be utilised. Tertiary anticholinergics such as atropine may be used as an antidote for ARICEPT overdosage. Intravenous atropine sulphate titrated to effect is recommended: an initial dose of 1.0 to 2.0 mg IV with subsequent doses based upon clinical response. Atypical responses in blood pressure and heart rate have been reported with other cholinomimetics when co-administered with quaternary anticholinergics such as glycopyrrolate. It is not known whether donepezil hydrochloride and/or its metabolites can be removed by dialysis (hemodialysis, peritoneal dialysis, or hemofiltration).

5. PHARMACOLOGICAL PROPERTIES

5.1 Pharmacodynamic properties

The pharmacotherapeutic group: anti-dementia drugs; anticholinesterase; ATC-code N06DA02.

Donepezil hydrochloride is a specific and reversible inhibitor of acetylcholinesterase, the predominant cholinesterase in the brain. Donepezil hydrochloride is *in vitro* over 1000 times more potent an inhibitor of this enzyme than of butyrylcholinesterase, an enzyme that is present mainly outside the central nervous system.

Alzheimer's Dementia

In patients with Alzheimer's Dementia participating in clinical trials, administration of single daily doses of 5 mg or 10 mg of ARICEPT produced steady-state inhibition of acetylcholinesterase activity (measured in erythrocyte membranes) of 63.6% and 77.3%, respectively when measured post dose. The inhibition of acetylcholinesterase (AChE) in red blood cells by donepezil hydrochloride has been shown to correlate to changes in ADAS-cog, a sensitive scale which examines selected aspects of cognition. The potential for donepezil hydrochloride to alter the course of the underlying neuropathology has not been studied. Thus Aricept cannot be considered to have any effect on the progress of the disease.

Efficacy of treatment with Aricept has been investigated in four placebo-controlled trials, 2 trials of 6-month duration and 2 trials of 1-year duration.

In the 6 months clinical trial, an analysis was done at the conclusion of donepezil treatment using a combination of three efficacy criteria: the ADAS-Cog (a measure of cognitive performance), the Clinician Interview Based Impression of Change with Caregiver Input (a measure of global function) and the Activities of Daily Living Subscale of the Clinical Dementia Rating Scale (a measure of capabilities in community affairs, home and hobbies and personal care).

Patients who fulfilled the criteria listed below were considered treatment responders.

Response = Improvement of ADAS-Cog of at least 4 points

No deterioration of CIBIC +

No Deterioration of Activities of Daily Living Subscale of the Clinical Dementia Rating Scale

	% Response	
	Intent to Treat Population n=365	Evaluable Population n=352
Placebo Group	10%	10%
Aricept 5-mg Group	18%*	18%*
Aricept 10-mg Group	21%*	22%**

* p<0.05

** p<0.01

Aricept produced a dose-dependent statistically significant increase in the percentage of patients who were judged treatment responders.

5.2 Pharmacokinetic properties

Absorption: Maximum plasma levels are reached approximately 3 to 4 hours after oral administration. Plasma concentrations and area under the curve rise in proportion to the dose. The terminal disposition half-life is approximately 70 hours, thus, administration of multiple single-daily doses results in gradual approach to steady-state. Approximate steady-state is achieved within 3 weeks after initiation of therapy. Once at steady-state, plasma donepezil hydrochloride concentrations and the related pharmacodynamic activity show little variability over the course of the day.

Food did not affect the absorption of donepezil hydrochloride.

Distribution: Donepezil hydrochloride is approximately 95% bound to human plasma proteins. The plasma protein binding of the active metabolite 6-O-desmethyldonepezil is not known. The distribution of donepezil hydrochloride in various body tissues has not been definitively studied. However, in a mass balance study conducted in healthy male volunteers, 240 hours after the administration of a single 5 mg dose of ^{14}C-labelled donepezil hydrochloride, approximately 28% of the label remained unrecovered. This suggests that donepezil hydrochloride and/or its metabolites may persist in the body for more than 10 days.

Metabolism/Excretion: Donepezil hydrochloride is both excreted in the urine intact and metabolised by the cytochrome P450 system to multiple metabolites, not all of which have been identified. Following administration of a single 5 mg dose of ^{14}C-labelled donepezil hydrochloride, plasma radioactivity, expressed as a percent of the administered dose, was present primarily as intact donepezil hydrochloride (30%), 6-O-desmethyl donepezil (11% - only metabolite that exhibits activity similar to donepezil hydrochloride), donepezil-cis-N-oxide (9%), 5-O-desmethyl donepezil (7%) and the glucuronide conjugate of 5-O-desmethyl donepezil (3%). Approximately 57% of the total administered radioactivity was recovered from the urine (17% as unchanged donepezil), and 14.5% was recovered from the faeces, suggesting biotransformation and urinary excretion as the primary routes of elimination. There is no evidence to suggest enterohepatic recirculation of donepezil hydrochloride and/or any of its metabolites.

Plasma donepezil concentrations decline with a half-life of approximately 70 hours.

Sex, race and smoking history have no clinically significant influence on plasma concentrations of donepezil hydrochloride. The pharmacokinetics of donepezil has not been formally studied in healthy elderly subjects or in Alzheimer's or vascular dementia patients. However mean plasma levels in patients closely agreed with those of young healthy volunteers.

Patients with mild to moderate hepatic impairment had increased donepezil steady state concentrations; mean AUC by 48% and mean C_{max} by 39% (see section 4.2).

5.3 Preclinical safety data

Extensive testing in experimental animals has demonstrated that this compound causes few effects other than the intended pharmacological effects consistent with its action as a cholinergic stimulator (see Section 4.9). Donepezil is not mutagenic in bacterial and mammalian cell mutation assays. Some clastogenic effects were observed in vitro at concentrations overtly toxic to the cells and more than 3000 times the steady-state plasma concentrations. No clastogenic or other genotoxic effects were observed in the mouse micronucleus model in vivo. There was no evidence of oncogenic potential in long term carcinogenicity studies in either rats or mice.

Donepezil hydrochloride had no effect on fertility in rats, and was not teratogenic in rats or rabbits, but had a slight effect on still births and early pup survival when administered to pregnant rats at 50 times the human dose (see Section 4.6).

6. PHARMACEUTICAL PARTICULARS

6.1 List of excipients

Lactose monohydrate

Maize starch

Microcrystalline cellulose

Hyprolose

Magnesium stearate.

Film coating:

Talc

Macrogol

Hypromellose

Titanium dioxide "E171".

Additionally the 10 mg tablet contains yellow iron oxide "E172".

6.2 Incompatibilities

Not applicable

6.3 Shelf life

3 years

6.4 Special precautions for storage

Do not store above 30°C.

6.5 Nature and contents of container

Bottles (HDPE) of 28, 30 and 100

Blister (PVC/Aluminium)

Pack sizes: 7, 14, 28, 30, 50, 56, 60, 84, 98, 112 or 120 tablets

Not all pack sizes may be marketed.

6.6 Special precautions for disposal and other handling

No special requirements

7. MARKETING AUTHORISATION HOLDER

Eisai Ltd., European Knowledge Centre, Mosquito Way, Hatfield, Herts, AL10 9SN, United Kingdom.

8. MARKETING AUTHORISATION NUMBER(S)

PL 10555/0006 (5 mg)

PL 10555/0007 (10 mg)

9. DATE OF FIRST AUTHORISATION/RENEWAL OF THE AUTHORISATION

Date of first authorisation: 14th February 1997

Date of last renewal: 10th January 2007

10. DATE OF REVISION OF THE TEXT

12th May 2009

Aricept Evess

(Eisai Ltd)

1. NAME OF THE MEDICINAL PRODUCT

Aricept Evess 5 mg orodispersible tablet

Aricept Evess 10 mg orodispersible tablet

2. QUALITATIVE AND QUANTITATIVE COMPOSITION

Each 5 mg tablet contains 5 mg donepezil hydrochloride, equivalent to 4.56 mg of donepezil free base.

Each 10 mg tablet contains 10 mg donepezil hydrochloride, equivalent to 9.12 mg of donepezil free base.

For full list of excipients, see 6.1

3. PHARMACEUTICAL FORM

Orodispersible tablet

5 mg donepezil as white tablet embossed with "5" on one side and "Aricept" on the other side.

10 mg donepezil as yellow tablet embossed with "10" on one side and "Aricept" on the other side.

4. CLINICAL PARTICULARS

4.1 Therapeutic indications

Aricept Evess tablets are indicated for the symptomatic treatment of mild to moderately severe Alzheimer's dementia.

4.2 Posology and method of administration

Adults/Elderly:

Treatment is initiated at 5 mg/day (once-a-day dosing). Aricept Evess should be taken orally, in the evening, just prior to retiring. The tablet should be placed on the tongue and allowed to disintegrate before swallowing with or without water, according to patient preference. The 5 mg/day dose should be maintained for at least one month in order to allow the earliest clinical responses to treatment to be assessed and to allow steady-state concentrations of donepezil hydrochloride to be achieved. Following a one-month clinical assessment of treatment at 5 mg/day, the dose of Aricept Evess can be increased to 10 mg/day (once-a-day dosing). The maximum recommended daily dose is 10 mg. Doses greater than 10 mg/day have not been studied in clinical trials.

Treatment should be initiated and supervised by a physician experienced in the diagnosis and treatment of Alzheimer's dementia. Diagnosis should be made according to accepted guidelines (e.g. DSM IV, ICD 10). Therapy with donepezil should only be started if a caregiver is available who will regularly monitor drug intake for the patient. Maintenance treatment can be continued for as long as a therapeutic benefit for the patient exists. Therefore, the clinical benefit of donepezil should be reassessed on a regular basis. Discontinuation should be considered when evidence of a therapeutic effect is no longer present. Individual response to donepezil cannot be predicted.

Upon discontinuation of treatment, a gradual abatement of the beneficial effects of Aricept is seen.

Renal and hepatic impairment:

A similar dose schedule can be followed for patients with renal impairment, as clearance of donepezil hydrochloride is not affected by this condition.

Due to possible increased exposure in mild to moderate hepatic impairment (see section 5.2), dose escalation should be performed according to individual tolerability. There are no data for patients with severe hepatic impairment.

Children:

Aricept is not recommended for use in children.

4.3 Contraindications

Aricept is contraindicated in patients with a known hypersensitivity to donepezil hydrochloride, piperidine derivatives, or to any excipients used in the formulation.

4.4 Special warnings and precautions for use

The use of Aricept in patients with severe dementia, other types of dementia or other types of memory impairment (e.g., age-related cognitive decline), has not been investigated.

Anaesthesia: Aricept, as a cholinesterase inhibitor, is likely to exaggerate succinylcholine-type muscle relaxation during anaesthesia.

Cardiovascular Conditions: Because of their pharmacological action, cholinesterase inhibitors may have vagotonic effects on heart rate (e.g., bradycardia). The potential for this action may be particularly important to patients with "sick sinus syndrome" or other supraventricular cardiac conduction conditions, such as sinoatrial or atrioventricular block.

There have been reports of syncope and seizures. In investigating such patients the possibility of heart block or long sinusal pauses should be considered.

Gastrointestinal Conditions: Patients at increased risk for developing ulcers, e.g., those with a history of ulcer disease or those receiving concurrent nonsteroidal anti-inflammatory drugs (NSAIDs), should be monitored for symptoms. However, the clinical studies with Aricept showed no increase, relative to placebo, in the incidence of either peptic ulcer disease or gastrointestinal bleeding.

Genitourinary: Although not observed in clinical trials of Aricept, cholinomimetics may cause bladder outflow obstruction.

Neurological Conditions: Seizures: Cholinomimetics are believed to have some potential to cause generalised convulsions. However, seizure activity may also be a manifestation of Alzheimer's Disease.

Cholinomimetics may have the potential to exacerbate or induce extrapyramidal symptoms

Pulmonary Conditions: Because of their cholinomimetic actions, cholinesterase inhibitors should be prescribed with care to patients with a history of asthma or obstructive pulmonary disease.

The administration of Aricept concomitantly with other inhibitors of acetylcholinesterase, agonists or antagonists of the cholinergic system should be avoided.

Severe Hepatic Impairment: There are no data for patients with severe hepatic impairment.

Mortality in Vascular Dementia Clinical Trials

Three clinical trials of 6 months duration were conducted studying individuals meeting the NINDS-AIREN criteria for probable or possible vascular dementia (VaD). The NINDS AIREN criteria are designed to identify patients whos dementia appears to be due solely to vascular cause and to exclude patients with Alzheimer's disease. In th first study, the mortality rates were 2/198 (1.0%) on done pezil hydrochloride 5 mg, 5/206 (2.4%) on donepezil hydro chloride 10 mg and 7/199 (3.5%) on placebo. In the secon study, the mortality rates were 4/208 (1.9%) on donepez hydrochloride 5 mg, 3/215 (1.4%) on donepezil hydrochlo ide 10 mg and 1/193 (0.5%) on placebo. In the third study the mortality rates were 11/648 (1.7%) on donepezil hydro chloride 5 mg and 0/326 (0%) on placebo. The mortalit rate for the three VaD studies combined in the donepez hydrochloride group (1.7%) was numerically higher than i the placebo group (1.1%), however, this difference was no statistically significant. The majority of deaths in patient taking either donepezil hydrochloride or placebo appear t result from various vascular related causes, which could b expected in this elderly population with underlying vascula disease. An analysis of all serious non-fatal and fatal vas cular events showed no difference in the rate of occurrence in the donepezil hydrochloride group relative to placebo.

In pooled Alzheimer's disease studies (n=4146), and wher these Alzheimer's disease studies were pooled with othe dementia studies including the vascular dementia studies (total n=6888), the mortality rate in the placebo groups numerically exceeded that in the donepezil hydrochloride groups

4.5 Interaction with other medicinal products and other forms of interaction

Donepezil hydrochloride and/or any of its metabolites do not inhibit the metabolism of theophylline, warfarin, cimetidine or digoxin in humans. The metabolism of donepezil hydrochloride is not affected by concurrent administration of digoxin or cimetidine. *In vitro* studies have shown that the cytochrome P450 isoenzymes 3A4 and to a minor extent 2D6 are involved in the metabolism of donepezil. Drug interaction studies performed *in vitro* show that ketoconazole and quinidine, inhibitors of CYP3A4 and 2D6 respectively, inhibit donepezil metabolism. Therefore these and other CYP3A4 inhibitors, such as itraconazole and erythromycin, and CYP2D6 inhibitors, such as fluoxetine, could inhibit the metabolism of donepezil. In a study in healthy volunteers, ketoconazole increased mean donepezil concentrations by about 30%. Enzyme inducers, such as rifampicin, phenytoin, carbamazepine and alcohol may reduce the levels of donepezil. Since the magnitude of an inhibiting or inducing effect is unknown, such drug combinations should be used with care. Donepezil hydrochloride has the potential to interfere with medications having anticholinergic activity. There is also the potential for synergistic activity with concomitant treatment involving medications such as succinylcholine, other neuromuscular blocking agents or cholinergic agonists or beta blocking agents that have effects on cardiac conduction.

4.6 Pregnancy and lactation

Pregnancy:

There are no adequate data from the use of donepezil in pregnant women.

Studies in animals have not shown teratogenic effect but have shown peri and post natal toxicity (see section 5.3 preclinical safety data). The potential risk for humans is unknown.

Aricept should not be used during pregnancy unless clearly necessary.

Lactation:

Donepezil is excreted in the milk of rats. It is not known whether donepezil hydrochloride is excreted in human breast milk and there are no studies in lactating women. Therefore, women on donepezil should not breast feed.

4.7 Effects on ability to drive and use machines

Donepezil has minor or moderate influence on the ability to drive and use machines.

Dementia may cause impairment of driving performance or compromise the ability to use machinery. Furthermore, donepezil can induce fatigue, dizziness and muscle cramps, mainly when initiating or increasing the dose. The treating physician should routinely evaluate the ability of patients on donepezil to continue driving or operating complex machines.

4.8 Undesirable effects

The most common adverse events are diarrhoea, muscle cramps, fatigue, nausea, vomiting and insomnia.

Adverse reactions reported as more than an isolated case are listed below, by system organ class and by frequency. Frequencies are defined as: very common (≥1/10), common (≥1/100, < 1/10), uncommon (≥1/1,000, < 1/100) rare (>1/10,000, <1/1,000); very rare (<1/10000) and not known (cannot be estimated from available data).

(see Table 1 on next page)

4.9 Overdose

The estimated median lethal dose of donepezil hydrochloride following administration of a single oral dose in mice and rats is 45 and 32 mg/kg, respectively, or approximately 225 and 160 times the maximum recommended human dose of 10 mg per day. Dose-related signs of cholinergic stimulation were observed in animals and included reduced spontaneous movement, prone position,

Table 1

System Organ Class	Very Common	Common	Uncommon	Rare
Infections and infestations		Common cold		
Metabolism and nutrition disorders		Anorexia		
Psychiatric disorders		Hallucinations** Agitation** Aggressive behaviour**		
Nervous system disorders		Syncope* Dizziness Insomnia	Seizure*	Extrapyramidal symptoms
Cardiac disorders			Bradycardia	Sino-atrial block Atrioventricular block
Gastrointestinal disorders	Diarrhoea Nausea	Vomiting Abdominal disturbance	Gastrointestinal haemorrhage Gastric and duodenal ulcers	
Hepato-biliary disorders				Liver dysfunction including hepatitis***
Skin and subcutaneous tissue disorders		Rash Pruritis		
Musculoskeletal, connective tissue and bone disorders		Muscle cramps		
Renal and urinary disorders		Urinary incontinence		
General disorders and administration site conditions	Headache	Fatigue Pain		
Investigations			Minor increase in serum concentration of muscle creatine kinase	
Injury and poisoning		Accident		

* In investigating patients for syncope or seizure the possibility of heart block or long sinusal pauses should be considered (see section 4.4)

** Reports of hallucinations, agitation and aggressive behaviour have resolved on dose-reduction or discontinuation of treatment.

*** In cases of unexplained liver dysfunction, withdrawal of ARICEPT should be considered.

staggering gait, lacrimation, clonic convulsions, depressed respiration, salivation, miosis, fasciculation and lower body surface temperature.

Overdosage with cholinesterase inhibitors can result in cholinergic crisis characterized by severe nausea, vomiting, salivation, sweating, bradycardia, hypotension, respiratory depression, collapse and convulsions. Increasing muscle weakness is a possibility and may result in death if respiratory muscles are involved.

As in any case of overdose, general supportive measures should be utilised. Tertiary anticholinergics such as atropine may be used as an antidote for Aricept overdosage. Intravenous atropine sulphate titrated to effect is recommended: an initial dose of 1.0 to 2.0 mg IV with subsequent doses based upon clinical response. Atypical responses in blood pressure and heart rate have been reported with other cholinomimetics when co-administered with quaternary anticholinergics such as glycopyrrolate. It is not known whether donepezil hydrochloride and/or its metabolites can be removed by dialysis (haemodialysis, peritoneal dialysis, or haemofiltration).

5. PHARMACOLOGICAL PROPERTIES

5.1 Pharmacodynamic properties

The pharmacotherapeutic group: anti-dementia drugs; anticholinesterases; ATC-code N06DA02.

Donepezil hydrochloride is a specific and reversible inhibitor of acetylcholinesterase, the predominant cholinesterase in the brain. Donepezil hydrochloride is *in vitro* over 1000 times more potent an inhibitor of this enzyme than of butyrylcholinesterase, an enzyme which is present mainly outside the central nervous system.

Alzheimer's Dementia

In patients with Alzheimer's Dementia participating in clinical trials, administration of single daily doses of 5 mg or 10 mg of Aricept produced steady-state inhibition of acetylcholinesterase activity (measured in erythrocyte membranes) of 63.6% and 77.3%, respectively when measured post dose. The inhibition of acetylcholinesterase (AChE) in red blood cells by donepezil hydrochloride has been shown to correlate to changes in ADAS-cog, a sensitive scale which examines selected aspects of cognition. The potential for donepezil hydrochloride to alter the course of the underlying neuropathology has not been studied. Thus Aricept cannot be considered to have any effect on the progress of the disease.

Efficacy of treatment of Alzheimer's Dementia with Aricept has been investigated in four placebo-controlled trials, 2 trials of 6-month duration and 2 trials of 1-year duration.

In the 6 months clinical trial, an analysis was done at the conclusion of donepezil treatment using a combination of three efficacy criteria: the ADAS-Cog (a measure of cognitive performance), the Clinician Interview Based Impression of Change with Caregiver Input (a measure of global function) and the Activities of Daily Living Subscale of the Clinical Dementia Rating Scale (a measure of capabilities in community affairs, home and hobbies and personal care).

Patients who fulfilled the criteria listed below were considered treatment responders.

Response = Improvement of ADAS-Cog of at least 4 points
No deterioration of CIBIC +
No Deterioration of Activities of Daily Living Subscale of the Clinical Dementia Rating Scale

	% Response	
	Intent to Treat Population n=365	Evaluable Population n=352
Placebo Group	10%	10%
Aricept 5-mg Group	18%*	18%*
Aricept 10-mg Group	21%*	22%**

* $p<0.05$

** $p<0.01$

Aricept produced a dose-dependent statistically significant increase in the percentage of patients who were judged treatment responders.

5.2 Pharmacokinetic properties

Absorption: Maximum plasma levels are reached approximately 3 to 4 hours after oral administration. Plasma concentrations and area under the curve rise in proportion to the dose. The terminal disposition half-life is approximately 70 hours, thus, administration of multiple single-daily doses results in gradual approach to steady-state. Approximate steady-state is achieved within 3 weeks after initiation of therapy. Once at steady-state, plasma donepezil hydrochloride concentrations and the related pharmacodynamic activity show little variability over the course of the day.

Food did not affect the absorption of donepezil hydrochloride.

Distribution: Donepezil hydrochloride is approximately 95% bound to human plasma proteins. The plasma protein binding of the active metabolite 6-O-desmethyldonepezil is not known. The distribution of donepezil hydrochloride in various body tissues has not been definitively studied. However, in a mass balance study conducted in healthy male volunteers, 240 hours after the administration of a single 5 mg dose of ^{14}C-labelled donepezil hydrochloride, approximately 28% of the label remained unrecovered. This suggests that donepezil hydrochloride and/or its metabolites may persist in the body for more than 10 days.

Metabolism/Excretion: Donepezil hydrochloride is both excreted in the urine intact and metabolised by the cytochrome P450 system to multiple metabolites, not all of which have been identified. Following administration of a single 5 mg dose of ^{14}C-labelled donepezil hydrochloride, plasma radioactivity, expressed as a percent of the administered dose, was present primarily as intact donepezil hydrochloride (30%), 6-O-desmethyldonepezil (11% - only metabolite that exhibits activity similar to donepezil hydrochloride), donepezil-cis-N-oxide (9%), 5-O-desmethyldonepezil (7%) and the glucuronide conjugate of 5-O-desmethyl-donepezil (3%). Approximately 57% of the total administered radioactivity was recovered from the urine (17% as unchanged donepezil), and 14.5% was recovered from the faeces, suggesting biotransformation and urinary excretion as the primary routes of elimination. There is no evidence to suggest enterohepatic recirculation of donepezil hydrochloride and/or any of its metabolites.

Plasma donepezil concentrations decline with a half-life of approximately 70 hours.

Sex, race and smoking history have no clinically significant influence on plasma concentrations of donepezil hydrochloride. The pharmacokinetics of donepezil has not been formally studied in healthy elderly subjects or in Alzheimer's or vascular dementia patients. However mean plasma levels in patients closely agreed with those of young healthy volunteers.

Patients with mild to moderate hepatic impairment had increased donepezil steady state concentrations; mean AUC by 48% and mean C_{max} by 39% (see section 4.2).

5.3 Preclinical safety data

Extensive testing in experimental animals has demonstrated that this compound causes few effects other than the intended pharmacological effects consistent with its action as a cholinergic stimulator (see section 4.9). Donepezil is not mutagenic in bacterial and mammalian cell mutation assays. Some clastogenic effects were observed *in vitro* at concentrations overtly toxic to the cells and more than 3000 times the steady-state plasma concentrations. No clastogenic or other genotoxic effects were observed in the mouse micronucleus model *in vivo*. There was no evidence of oncogenic potential in long term carcinogenicity studies in either rats or mice.

Donepezil hydrochloride had no effect on fertility in rats, and was not teratogenic in rats or rabbits, but had a slight effect on still-births and early pup survival when administered to pregnant rats at 50 times the human dose (see section 4.6).

6. PHARMACEUTICAL PARTICULARS

6.1 List of excipients

Mannitol

Colloidal anhydrous Silica

κ-Carrageenan

Polyvinyl alcohol

Additionally the 10 mg tablet contains Yellow iron oxide "E172".

6.2 Incompatibilities

Not applicable

6.3 Shelf life

3 years

6.4 Special precautions for storage

This medicinal product does not require any special storage conditions.

6.5 Nature and contents of container

5 mg and 10 mg tablets:

Blister (PVC/PVdC/PE/PVdC/PVC/Aluminium foil)

Pack sizes: 7, 28, 30, 50, 56, 60, 98 or 120 tablets

Not all pack sizes may be marketed.

6.6 Special precautions for disposal and other handling

No special requirements

7. MARKETING AUTHORISATION HOLDER

Eisai Ltd.,

Hammersmith International Centre,

3 Shortlands,

London

W6 8EE

8. MARKETING AUTHORISATION NUMBER(S)

PL 10555/0019 (5 mg)

PL 10555/0020 (10 mg)

9. DATE OF FIRST AUTHORISATION/RENEWAL OF THE AUTHORISATION

17th May 2005

10. DATE OF REVISION OF THE TEXT

9th September 2007

LEGAL CATEGORY

POM

Arimidex 1mg Film-Coated Tablet

(AstraZeneca UK Limited)

1. NAME OF THE MEDICINAL PRODUCT
Arimidex® 1 mg Film-coated Tablets

2. QUALITATIVE AND QUANTITATIVE COMPOSITION
Each tablet contains 1 mg anastrozole.

For excipients, see 6.1.

3. PHARMACEUTICAL FORM
Film-coated tablet.

White, round, biconvex tablet with logo on one side and strength on the other.

4. CLINICAL PARTICULARS
4.1 Therapeutic indications
Treatment of advanced breast cancer in postmenopausal women. Efficacy has not been demonstrated in oestrogen receptor negative patients unless they had a previous positive clinical response to tamoxifen.

Adjuvant treatment of postmenopausal women with hormone receptor positive early invasive breast cancer.

Adjuvant treatment of early breast cancer in hormone receptor positive postmenopausal women who have received 2 to 3 years of adjuvant tamoxifen.

4.2 Posology and method of administration
Adults including the elderly: One 1 mg tablet to be taken orally once a day.

Children: Not recommended for use in children (see sections 5.1 and 5.2).

Renal impairment: No dose change is recommended in patients with mild or moderate renal impairment

Hepatic impairment: No dose change is recommended in patients with mild hepatic disease.

For early disease, the recommended duration of treatment should be 5 years.

4.3 Contraindications
Arimidex is contraindicated in:

- premenopausal women.
- pregnant or lactating women.
- patients with severe renal impairment (creatinine clearance less than 20 ml/min).
- patients with moderate or severe hepatic disease.
- patients with known hypersensitivity to anastrozole or to any of the excipients as referenced in section 6.1.

Oestrogen-containing therapies should not be co-administered with Arimidex as they would negate its pharmacological action.

Concurrent tamoxifen therapy (see section 4.5).

4.4 Special warnings and precautions for use
Arimidex is not recommended for use in children as safety and efficacy have not been established in this group of patients (see sections 5.1 and 5.2).

The menopause should be defined biochemically in any patient where there is doubt about hormonal status.

There are no data to support the safe use of Arimidex in patients with moderate or severe hepatic impairment, or patients with severe impairment of renal function (creatinine clearance less than 20 ml/min).

Women with osteoporosis or at risk of osteoporosis, should have their bone mineral density formally assessed by bone densitometry e.g. DEXA scanning at the commencement of treatment and at regular intervals thereafter. Treatment or prophylaxis for osteoporosis should be initiated as appropriate and carefully monitored.

There are no data available for the use of anastrozole with LHRH analogues. This combination should not be used outside clinical trials.

As Arimidex lowers circulating oestrogen levels it may cause a reduction in bone mineral density with a possible consequent increased risk of fracture. The use of bisphosphonates may stop further bone mineral loss caused by anastrozole in postmenopausal women and could be considered.

This product contains lactose. Patients with rare hereditary problems of galactose intolerance, the Lapp lactase deficiency or glucose-galactose malabsorption should not take this medicine.

4.5 Interaction with other medicinal products and other forms of interaction
Antipyrine and cimetidine clinical interaction studies indicate that the co-administration of Arimidex with other drugs is unlikely to result in clinically significant drug interactions mediated by cytochrome P450.

A review of the clinical trial safety database did not reveal evidence of clinically significant interaction in patients treated with Arimidex who also received other commonly prescribed drugs. There were no clinically significant interactions with bisphosphonates (see section 5.1).

Oestrogen-containing therapies should not be co-administered with Arimidex as they would negate its pharmacological action.

Tamoxifen should not be co-administered with Arimidex, as this may diminish its pharmacological action (see section 4.3).

4.6 Pregnancy and lactation
Arimidex is contraindicated in pregnant or lactating women.

4.7 Effects on ability to drive and use machines
Arimidex is unlikely to impair the ability of patients to drive and operate machinery. However, asthenia and somnolence have been reported with the use of Arimidex and caution should be observed when driving or operating machinery while such symptoms persist.

4.8 Undesirable effects
Unless specified, the following frequency categories were calculated from the number of adverse events reported in a large phase III study conducted in 9366 postmenopausal women with operable breast cancer treated for five years (ATAC study).

Frequency	System Organ Class	Adverse reaction
Very common (≥ 10%)	*Vascular*	Hot flushes, mainly mild or moderate in nature
	General	Asthenia, mainly mild or moderate in nature
	Musculoskeletal, connective tissue and bone	Joint pain/stiffness, mainly mild or moderate in nature
	Nervous system	Headache, mainly mild or moderate in nature
	Gastrointestinal	Nausea, mainly mild or moderate in nature
	Skin and subcutaneous tissue	Rash, mainly mild or moderate in nature
Common (≥ 1% and < 10%)	*Skin and subcutaneous tissue*	Hair thinning (Alopecia), mainly mild or moderate in nature Allergic reactions
	Gastrointestinal	Diarrhoea, mainly mild or moderate in nature Vomiting, mainly mild or moderate in nature
	Nervous system	Somnolence, mainly mild or moderate in nature Carpal Tunnel Syndrome
	Hepatobiliary disorders	Increases in alkaline phosphatase, alanine aminotransferase and aspartate aminotransferase
	Reproductive system and breast	Vaginal dryness, mainly mild or moderate in nature Vaginal bleeding, mainly mild or moderate in nature*
	Metabolism and nutrition	Anorexia, mainly mild in nature Hypercholesterolaemia, mainly mild or moderate in nature
Uncommon (≥ 0.1% and < 1%)	*Hepatobiliary disorders*	Increases in gamma-GT and bilirubin Hepatitis
	Skin and subcutaneous tissue	Urticaria
	Musculoskeletal, connective tissue and bone	Trigger finger
Rare (≥ 0.01% and < 0.1%)	*Skin and subcutaneous tissue*	Erythema multiforme Anaphylactoid reaction
Not known	*Skin and subcutaneous tissue*	Stevens-Johnson syndrome** Angioedema**

* Vaginal bleeding has been reported commonly, mainly in patients with advanced breast cancer during the first few weeks after changing from existing hormonal therapy to treatment with Arimidex. If bleeding persists, further evaluation should be considered.

** Cannot be estimated from the available data.

As Arimidex lowers circulating oestrogen levels, it may cause a reduction in bone mineral density placing some patients at a higher risk of fracture (see section 4.4). The table below presents the frequency of pre-specified adverse events in the ATAC study, irrespective of causality, reported in patients receiving trial therapy and up to 14 days after cessation of trial therapy.

Adverse effects	Arimidex (N=3092)	Tamoxifen (N=3094)
Hot flushes	1104 (35.7%)	1264 (40.9%)
Joint pain/stiffness	1100 (35.6%)	911 (29.4%)
Mood disturbances	597 (19.3%)	554 (17.9%)
Fatigue/asthenia	575 (18.6%)	544 (17.6%)
Nausea and vomiting	393 (12.7%)	384 (12.4%)
Fractures	315 (10.2%)	209 (6.8%)
Fractures of the spine, hip, or wrist/Colles	133 (4.3%)	91 (2.9%)
Wrist/Colles fractures	67 (2.2%)	50 (1.6%)
Spine fractures	43 (1.4%)	22 (0.7%)
Hip fractures	28 (0.9%)	26 (0.8%)
Cataracts	182 (5.9%)	213 (6.9%)
Vaginal bleeding	167 (5.4%)	317 (10.2%)
Ischaemic cardiovascular disease	127 (4.1%)	104 (3.4%)
Angina pectoris	71 (2.3%)	51 (1.6%)
Myocardial infarct	37 (1.2%)	34 (1.1%)
Coronary artery disorder	25 (0.8%)	23 (0.7%)
Myocardial ischaemia	22 (0.7%)	14 (0.5%)
Vaginal discharge	109 (3.5%)	408 (13.2%)
Any venous thromboembolic event	87 (2.8%)	140 (4.5%)
Deep venous thromboembolic events including PE	48 (1.6%)	74 (2.4%)
Ischaemic cerebrovascular events	62 (2.0%)	88 (2.8%)
Endometrial cancer	4 (0.2%)	13 (0.6%)

Fracture rates of 22 per 1000 patient-years and 15 per 1000 patient-years were observed for the Arimidex and tamoxifen groups, respectively, after a median follow-up of 68 months. The observed fracture rate for Arimidex is similar to the range reported in age-matched postmenopausal populations. It has not been determined whether the rates of fracture and osteoporosis seen in ATAC in patients on anastrozole treatment reflect a protective effect of tamoxifen, a specific effect of anastrozole, or both.

The incidence of osteoporosis was 10.5% in patients treated with Arimidex and 7.3% in patients treated with tamoxifen.

4.9 Overdose
There is limited clinical experience of accidental overdosage. In animal studies, anastrozole demonstrated low acute toxicity. Clinical trials have been conducted with various dosages of Arimidex, up to 60 mg in a single dose given to healthy male volunteers and up to 10 mg daily given to postmenopausal women with advanced breast cancer; these dosages were well tolerated. A single dose of Arimidex that results in life-threatening symptoms has not been established. There is no specific antidote to overdosage and treatment must be symptomatic.

In the management of an overdose, consideration should be given to the possibility that multiple agents may have been taken. Vomiting may be induced if the patient is alert. Dialysis may be helpful because Arimidex is not highly protein bound. General supportive care, including frequent monitoring of vital signs and close observation of the patient, is indicated.

5. PHARMACOLOGICAL PROPERTIES
5.1 Pharmacodynamic properties
ATC Code: L02B G03 (Enzyme inhibitors)

Arimidex is a potent and highly selective non-steroidal aromatase inhibitor. In postmenopausal women, estradiol is produced primarily from the conversion of androstenedione to estrone through the aromatase enzyme complex in peripheral tissues. Estrone is subsequently converted to estradiol. Reducing circulating estradiol levels has been shown to produce a beneficial effect in women with breast cancer. In postmenopausal women, Arimidex at a daily dose of 1 mg produced estradiol suppression of greater than 80% using a highly sensitive assay.

Arimidex does not possess any progestogenic, androgenic or oestrogenic activity.

Daily doses of Arimidex up to 10 mg do not have any effect on cortisol or aldosterone secretion, measured before or

Table 1 ATAC endpoint summary: 5-year treatment completion analysis

Efficacy endpoints	Number of events (frequency)			
	Intention-to-treat population		Hormone-receptor-positive tumour status	
	Arimidex (N=3125)	Tamoxifen (N=3116)	Arimidex (N=2618)	Tamoxifen (N=2598)
Disease-free survival [a]	575 (18.4)	651 (20.9)	424 (16.2)	497 (19.1)
Hazard ratio	0.87		0.83	
2-sided 95% CI	0.78 to 0.97		0.73 to 0.94	
p-value	0.0127		0.0049	
Distant disease-free survival [b]	500 (16.0)	530 (17.0)	370 (14.1)	394 (15.2)
Hazard ratio	0.94		0.93	
2-sided 95% CI	0.83 to 1.06		0.80 to 1.07	
p-value	0.2850		0.2838	
Time to recurrence [c]	402 (12.9)	498 (16.0)	282 (10.8)	370 (14.2)
Hazard ratio	0.79		0.74	
2-sided 95% CI	0.70 to 0.90		0.64 to 0.87	
p-value	0.0005		0.0002	
Time to distant recurrence [d]	324 (10.4)	375 (12.0)	226 (8.6)	265 (10.2)
Hazard ratio	0.86		0.84	
2-sided 95% CI	0.74 to 0.99		0.70 to 1.00	
p-value	0.0427		0.0559	
Contralateral breast primary	35 (1.1)	59 (1.9)	26 (1.0)	54 (2.1)
Odds ratio	0.59		0.47	
2-sided 95% CI	0.39 to 0.89		0.30 to 0.76	
p-value	0.0131		0.0018	
Overall survival [e]	411 (13.2)	420 (13.5)	296 (11.3)	301 (11.6)
Hazard ratio	0.97		0.97	
2-sided 95% CI	0.85 to 1.12		0.83 to 1.14	
p-value	0.7142		0.7339	

a Disease-free survival includes all recurrence events and is defined as the first occurrence of loco-regional recurrence, contralateral new breast cancer, distant recurrence or death (for any reason).

b Distant disease-free survival is defined as the first occurrence of distant recurrence or death (for any reason).

c Time to recurrence is defined as the first occurrence of loco-regional recurrence, contralateral new breast cancer, distant recurrence or death due to breast cancer.

d Time to distant recurrence is defined as the first occurrence of distant recurrence or death due to breast cancer.

e Number (%) of patients who had died.

after standard ACTH challenge testing. Corticoid supplements are therefore not needed.

Primary adjuvant treatment of early breast cancer

In a large phase III study conducted in 9366 postmenopausal women with operable breast cancer treated for 5 years, Arimidex was shown to be statistically superior to tamoxifen in disease-free survival. A greater magnitude of benefit was observed for disease-free survival in favour of Arimidex versus tamoxifen for the prospectively defined hormone receptor positive population. Arimidex was statistically superior to tamoxifen in time to recurrence. The difference was of even greater magnitude than in disease-free survival for both the Intention To Treat (ITT) population and hormone receptor positive population. Arimidex was statistically superior to tamoxifen in terms of time to distant recurrence. The incidence of contralateral breast cancer was statistically reduced for Arimidex compared to tamoxifen. Following 5 years of therapy, anastrozole is at least as effective as tamoxifen in terms of overall survival. However, due to low death rates, additional follow-up is required to determine more precisely the long-term survival for anastrozole relative to tamoxifen. With 68 months median follow-up, patients in the ATAC study have not been followed up for sufficient time after 5 years of treatment, to enable a comparison of long-term post treatment effects of Arimidex relative to tamoxifen.

(see Table 1 above)

As with all treatment decisions, women with breast cancer and their physician should assess the relative benefits and risks of the treatment.

When Arimidex and tamoxifen were co-administered, the efficacy and safety were similar to tamoxifen when given alone, irrespective of hormone receptor status. The exact mechanism of this is not yet clear. It is not believed to be due to a reduction in the degree of estradiol suppression produced by Arimidex.

Adjuvant treatment of early breast cancer for patients being treated with adjuvant tamoxifen

In a phase III trial (ABCSG 8) conducted in 2579 postmenopausal women with hormone receptor positive early breast cancer who had received surgery with or without radiotherapy and no chemotherapy, switching to Arimidex after 2 years adjuvant treatment with tamoxifen was statistically superior in disease-free survival when compared to remaining on tamoxifen, after a median follow-up of 24 months.

Time to any recurrence, time to local or distant recurrence and time to distant recurrence confirmed a statistical advantage for Arimidex, consistent with the results of disease-free survival. The incidence of contralateral breast cancer was very low in the two treatment arms with a numerical advantage for Arimidex. Overall survival was similar for the two treatment groups.

ABCSG 8 trial endpoint and results summary

Efficacy endpoints	Number of events (frequency)	
	Arimidex (N=1297)	Tamoxifen (N=1282)
Disease-free survival	65 (5.0)	93 (7.3)
Hazard ratio	0.67	
2-sided 95% CI	0.49 to 0.92	
p-value	0.014	
Time to any recurrence	36 (2.8)	66 (5.1)
Hazard ratio	0.53	
2-sided 95% CI	0.35 to 0.79	
p-value	0.002	
Time to local or distant recurrence	29 (2.2)	51 (4.0)
Hazard ratio	0.55	
2-sided 95% CI	0.35 to 0.87	
p-value	0.011	
Time to distant recurrence	22 (1.7)	41(3.2)
Hazard ratio	0.52	
2-sided 95% CI	0.31 to 0.88	
p-value	0.015	
New contralateral breast cancer	7 (0.5)	15 (1.2)
Odds ratio	0.46	
2-sided 95% CI	0.19 to 1.13	
p-value	0.090	
Overall survival	43(3.3)	45 (3.5)
Hazard ratio	0.96	
2-sided 95% CI	0.63 to 1.46	
p-value	0.840	

Two further similar trials (GABG/ARNO 95 and ITA), in one of which patients had received surgery and chemotherapy, as well as a combined analysis of ABCSG 8 and GABG/ARNO 95, supported these results.

The Arimidex safety profile in these 3 studies was consistent with the known safety profile established in postmenopausal women with hormone receptor positive early breast cancer.

Study of anastrozole with the bisphosphonate risedronate (SABRE)

Bone Mineral Density (BMD)

In the phase III/IV SABRE study, 234 postmenopausal women with hormone receptor positive early breast cancer scheduled for treatment with Arimidex 1 mg/day were stratified to low, moderate and high risk groups according to their existing risk of fragility fracture. The primary efficacy parameter was the analysis of lumbar spine bone mass density using DEXA scanning. All patients received treatment with vitamin D and calcium. Patients in the low risk group received Arimidex alone (N=42), those in the moderate group were randomised to Arimidex plus risedronate 35 mg once a week (N=77) or Arimidex plus placebo (N=77) and those in the high risk group received Arimidex plus risedronate 35 mg once a week (N=38). The primary endpoint was change from baseline in lumbar spine bone mass density at 12 months.

The 12-month main analysis has shown that patients already at moderate to high risk of fragility fracture showed no decrease in their bone mass density (assessed by lumbar spine bone mineral density using DEXA scanning) when managed by using Arimidex 1 mg/day in combination with risedronate 35 mg once a week. In addition, a decrease in BMD which was not statistically significant was seen in the low risk group treated with Arimidex 1 mg/day alone. These findings were mirrored in the secondary efficacy variable of change from baseline in total hip BMD at 12 months.

This study provides evidence that the use of bisphosphonates should be considered in the management of possible bone mineral loss in postmenopausal women with early breast cancer scheduled to be treated with Arimidex.

Lipids

In the SABRE study there was a neutral effect on plasma lipids in those patients treated with Arimidex plus risedronate.

Paediatrics

Three clinical trials were conducted in paediatric patients (2 in pubertal boys with gynaecomastia and 1 in girls with McCune-Albright Syndrome).

Gynaecomastia studies

Trial 0006 was a randomised, double-blind, multi-centre study of 82 pubertal boys (aged 11-18 years inclusive) with gynaecomastia of greater than 12 months duration treated with Arimidex 1 mg/day or placebo daily for up to 6 months. No significant difference in the number of patients who had a 50% or greater reduction in total breast volume after 6 months of treatment was observed between the anastrozole 1 mg treated group and the placebo group.

Trial 0001 was an open-label, multiple-dose pharmacokinetic study of Arimidex 1 mg/day in 36 pubertal boys with gynaecomastia of less than 12 months duration. The secondary objectives were to evaluate the proportion of patients with reductions from baseline in the calculated volume of gynaecomastia of both breasts combined of at least 50% between day 1 and after 6 months of study treatment, and patient tolerability and safety.

A pharmacodynamic subpopulation of 25 boys was selected in this study to explore the potential benefits of anastrozole. It was noted a decrease in total breast volume of 50% or greater at 6 months was seen in 55.6% (as measured by ultrasound) and 77.8% (as measured by caliper) of the boys (observational data only, no statistical analysis conducted on these results).

McCune-Albright Syndrome study

Trial 0046 was an international, multi-centre, open-label exploratory trial of Arimidex in 28 girls (aged 2 to ≤10 years) with McCune-Albright Syndrome (MAS). The primary objective was to evaluate the safety and efficacy of anastrozole 1 mg/day in patients with MAS. The efficacy of study treatment was based on the proportion of patients fulfilling defined criteria relating to vaginal bleeding, bone age, and growth velocity.

No statistically significant change in the frequency of vaginal bleeding days on treatment was observed. There were no clinically significant changes in Tanner staging, mean ovarian volume or mean uterine volume. No statistically significant change in the rate of increase in bone age on treatment compared to the rate during baseline was observed. Growth rate (in cm/year) was significantly reduced ($p<0.05$) from pre-treatment through month 0 to month 12, and from pre-treatment to the second 6 months (month 7 to month 12). Of the patients with baseline vaginal bleeding, 28% experienced a ≥50% reduction in the frequency of bleeding days on treatment; 40% experienced a cessation over a 6-month period, and 12% experienced a cessation over a 12-month period.

The overall assessment of the adverse events in children less than 18 years of age raised no safety or tolerability concerns.

5.2 Pharmacokinetic properties

Absorption of anastrozole is rapid and maximum plasma concentrations typically occur within two hours of dosing (under fasted conditions). Anastrozole is eliminated slowly with a plasma elimination half-life of 40 to 50 hours. Food slightly decreases the rate but not the extent of absorption. The small change in the rate of absorption is not expected to result in a clinically significant effect on steady-state plasma concentrations during once daily dosing of Arimidex tablets. Approximately 90 to 95% of plasma anastrozole steady-state concentrations are attained after 7 daily doses. There is no evidence of time or dose-dependency of anastrozole pharmacokinetic parameters.

Anastrozole pharmacokinetics are independent of age in postmenopausal women.

In boys with pubertal gynaecomastia, anastrozole was rapidly absorbed, was widely distributed, and was eliminated slowly with a half-life of approximately 2 days. Clearance of anastrozole was lower in girls than in boys and exposure higher. Anastrozole in girls was widely distributed and slowly eliminated, with an estimated half-life of approximately 0.8 days.

Anastrozole is only 40% bound to plasma proteins.

Anastrozole is extensively metabolised by postmenopausal women with less than 10% of the dose excreted in the urine unchanged within 72 hours of dosing. Metabolism of anastrozole occurs by N-dealkylation, hydroxylation and glucuronidation. The metabolites are excreted primarily via the urine. Triazole, the major metabolite in plasma, does not inhibit aromatase.

The apparent oral clearance of anastrozole in volunteers with stable hepatic cirrhosis or renal impairment was in the range observed in healthy volunteers.

5.3 Preclinical safety data

Acute toxicity

In acute toxicity studies in rodents, the median lethal dose of anastrozole was greater than 100 mg/kg/day by the oral route and greater than 50 mg/kg/day by the intraperitoneal route. In an oral acute toxicity study in the dog, the median lethal dose was greater than 45 mg/kg/day.

Chronic toxicity

Multiple dose toxicity studies utilized rats and dogs. No no-effect levels were established for anastrozole in the toxicity studies, but those effects that were observed at the low doses (1 mg/kg/day) and mid doses (dog 3 mg/kg/day; rat 5 mg/kg/day) were related to either the pharmacological or enzyme-inducing properties of anastrozole and were unaccompanied by significant toxic or degenerative changes.

Mutagenicity

Genetic toxicology studies with anastrozole show that it is not a mutagen or a clastogen.

Reproductive toxicology

Oral administration of anastrozole to female rats produced a high incidence of infertility at 1 mg/kg/day and increased pre-implantation loss at 0.02 mg/kg/day. These effects occurred at clinically relevant doses. An effect in man cannot be excluded. These effects were related to the pharmacology of the compound and were completely reversed after a 5-week compound withdrawal period.

Oral administration of anastrozole to pregnant rats and rabbits caused no teratogenic effects at doses up to 1.0 and 0.2 mg/kg/day respectively. Those effects that were seen (placental enlargement in rats and pregnancy failure in rabbits) were related to the pharmacology of the compound.

The survival of litters born to rats given anastrozole at 0.02 mg/kg/day and above (from day 17 of pregnancy to day 22 post-partum) was compromised. These effects were related to the pharmacological effects of the compound on parturition. There were no adverse effects on behaviour or reproductive performance of the first generation offspring attributable to maternal treatment with anastrozole.

Carcinogenicity

A two year rat oncogenicity study resulted in an increase in incidence of hepatic neoplasms and uterine stromal polyps in females and thyroid adenomas in males at the high dose (25 mg/kg/day) only. These changes occurred at a dose which represents 100-fold greater exposure than occurs at human therapeutic doses, and are considered not to be clinically relevant to the treatment of patients with anastrozole.

A two year mouse oncogenicity study resulted in the induction of benign ovarian tumours and a disturbance in the incidence of lymphoreticular neoplasms (fewer histiocytic sarcomas in females and more deaths as a result of lymphomas). These changes are considered to be mouse-specific effects of aromatase inhibition and not clinically relevant to the treatment of patients with anastrozole.

6. PHARMACEUTICAL PARTICULARS

6.1 List of excipients

Lactose Monohydrate

Povidone

Sodium Starch Glycollate

Magnesium Stearate

Hypromellose

Macrogol 300

Titanium Dioxide

6.2 Incompatibilities

Not applicable.

6.3 Shelf life

The shelf-life of Arimidex is 5 years.

6.4 Special precautions for storage

Do not store above 30°C.

6.5 Nature and contents of container

PVC blister/aluminium foil packs of 20, 28, 30, 84, 98, 100 and 300 tablets contained in a carton. Not all pack sizes may be marketed.

6.6 Special precautions for disposal and other handling

No special requirements.

7. MARKETING AUTHORISATION HOLDER

AstraZeneca UK Limited,

600 Capability Green,

Luton, LU1 3LU, UK

8. MARKETING AUTHORISATION NUMBER(S)

PL 17901/0002

9. DATE OF FIRST AUTHORISATION/RENEWAL OF THE AUTHORISATION

18 June 2000/10 August 2005

10. DATE OF REVISION OF THE TEXT

27 March 2009

Arixtra 1.5 mg/0.3 ml solution for injection, pre-filled syringe

(GlaxoSmithKline UK)

1. NAME OF THE MEDICINAL PRODUCT

Arixtra ▼ 1.5 mg/0.3 ml solution for injection, pre-filled syringe.

2. QUALITATIVE AND QUANTITATIVE COMPOSITION

Each pre-filled syringe (0.3 ml) contains 1.5 mg of fondaparinux sodium.

Excipient(s): Contains less than 1 mmol of sodium (23 mg) per dose, and therefore is essentially sodium free.

For a full list of excipients, see section 6.1.

3. PHARMACEUTICAL FORM

Solution for injection.

The solution is a clear and colourless liquid.

4. CLINICAL PARTICULARS

4.1 Therapeutic indications

Prevention of Venous Thromboembolic Events (VTE) in patients undergoing major orthopaedic surgery of the lower limbs such as hip fracture, major knee surgery or hip replacement surgery.

Prevention of Venous Thromboembolic Events (VTE) in patients undergoing abdominal surgery who are judged to be at high risk of thromboembolic complications, such as patients undergoing abdominal cancer surgery (see section 5.1).

Prevention of Venous Thromboembolic Events (VTE) in medical patients who are judged to be at high risk for VTE and who are immobilised due to acute illness such as cardiac insufficiency and/or acute respiratory disorders, and/or acute infectious or inflammatory disease.

4.2 Posology and method of administration

Patients undergoing major orthopaedic or abdominal sur-gery

The recommended dose of fondaparinux is 2.5 mg once daily administered post-operatively by subcutaneous injection.

The initial dose should be given 6 hours following surgical closure provided that haemostasis has been established.

Treatment should be continued until the risk of venous thrombo-embolism has diminished, usually until the patient is ambulant, at least 5 to 9 days after surgery. Experience shows that in patients undergoing hip fracture surgery, the risk of VTE continues beyond 9 days after surgery. In these patients the use of prolonged prophylaxis with fondaparinux should be considered for up to an additional 24 days (see section 5.1).

Medical patients who are at high risk for thromboembolic complications based on an individual risk assessment

The recommended dose of fondaparinux is 2.5 mg once daily administered by subcutaneous injection. A treatment duration of 6-14 days has been clinically studied in medical patients (see section 5.1).

Special populations

In patients undergoing surgery, timing of the first fondaparinux injection requires strict adherence in patients ≥75 years, and/or with body weight <50 kg and/or with renal impairment with creatinine clearance ranging between 20 to 50 ml/min.

The first fondaparinux administration should be given not earlier than 6 hours following surgical closure. The injection should not be given unless haemostasis has been established (see section 4.4).

Renal impairment - Fondaparinux should not be used in patients with creatinine clearance <20 ml/min (see section 4.3). The dose should be reduced to 1.5 mg once daily in patients with creatinine clearance in the range of 20 to 50 ml/min (see sections 4.4 and 5.2). No dosage reduction is required for patients with mild renal impairment (creatinine clearance >50 ml/min).

Hepatic impairment - No dosing adjustment is necessary in patients with either mild or moderate hepatic impairment. In patients with severe hepatic impairment, fondaparinux should be used with care as this patient group has not been studied (see sections 4.4 and 5.2).

Paediatric population - Fondaparinux is not recommended for use in children below 17 years of age due to a lack of data on safety and efficacy.

Method of administration

Fondaparinux is administered by deep subcutaneous injection while the patient is lying down. Sites of administration should alternate between the left and the right anterolateral and left and right posterolateral abdominal wall. To avoid the loss of medicinal product when using the pre-filled syringe do not expel the air bubble from the syringe before the injection. The whole length of the needle should be inserted perpendicularly into a skin fold held between the thumb and the forefinger; the skin fold should be held throughout the injection.

For additional instructions for use and handling and disposal see section 6.6.

4.3 Contraindications

- hypersensitivity to the active substance or to any of the excipients
- active clinically significant bleeding
- acute bacterial endocarditis
- severe renal impairment defined by creatinine clearance < 20 ml/min.

4.4 Special warnings and precautions for use

Fondaparinux is intended for subcutaneous use only. Do not administer intramuscularly.

Haemorrhage

Fondaparinux should be used with caution in patients who have an increased risk of haemorrhage, such as those with congenital or acquired bleeding disorders (e.g. platelet count <50,000/mm^3), active ulcerative gastrointestinal disease and recent intracranial haemorrhage or shortly after brain, spinal or ophthalmic surgery and in special patient groups as outlined below.

Agents that may enhance the risk of haemorrhage should not be administered concomitantly with fondaparinux. These agents include desirudin, fibrinolytic agents, GP IIb/IIIa receptor antagonists, heparin, heparinoids, or Low Molecular Weight Heparin (LMWH). When required, concomitant therapy with vitamin K antagonist should be administered in accordance with the information of Section 4.5. Other antiplatelet medicinal products (acetylsalicylic acid, dipyridamole, sulfinpyrazone, ticlopidine or clopidogrel), and NSAIDs should be used with caution. If co-administration is essential, close monitoring is necessary.

Spinal / Epidural anaesthesia

In patients undergoing major orthopaedic surgery, epidural or spinal haematomas that may result in long-term or permanent paralysis cannot be excluded with the concurrent use of fondaparinux and spinal/epidural anaesthesia or spinal puncture. The risk of these rare events may be higher with post-operative use of indwelling epidural atheters or the concomitant use of other medicinal products affecting haemostasis.

lderly patients

he elderly population is at increased risk of bleeding. As nal function is generally decreasing with age, elderly atients may show reduced elimination and increased xposure of fondaparinux (see section 5.2). Fondaparinux hould be used with caution in elderly patients (see section 2).

ow body weight

atients with body weight <50 kg are at increased risk of eeding. Elimination of fondaparinux decreases with eight. Fondaparinux should be used with caution in these atients (see section 4.2).

enal impairment

ondaparinux is known to be mainly excreted by the kidey. Patients with creatinine clearance <50 ml/min are at creased risk of bleeding and VTE and should be treated ith caution (see sections 4.2, 4.3 and 5.2). There are mited clinical data available from patients with creatinine learance less than 30 ml/min.

evere hepatic impairment

osing adjustment of fondaparinux is not necessary. However, the use of fondaparinux should be considered with aution because of an increased risk of bleeding due to a eficiency of coagulation factors in patients with severe epatic impairment (see section 4.2).

Patients with Heparin Induced Thrombocytopenia

Fondaparinux should be used with caution in patients with a history of HIT. The efficacy and safety of fondaparinux have not been formally studied in patients with HIT type II. Fondaparinux does not bind to platelet factor 4 and does not cross-react with sera from patients with Heparin Induced Thrombocytopenia (HIT) type II. However, rare spontaneous reports of HIT in patients treated with fondaparinux have been received. To date a causal association between treatment with fondaparinux and the occurrence of HIT has not been established.

4.5 Interaction with other medicinal products and other forms of interaction

Bleeding risk is increased with concomitant administration of fondaparinux and agents that may enhance the risk of haemorrhage (see section 4.4).

Oral anticoagulants (warfarin), platelet inhibitors (acetylsalicylic acid), NSAIDs (piroxicam) and digoxin did not interact with the pharmacokinetics of fondaparinux. The fondaparinux dose (10 mg) in the interaction studies was higher than the dose recommended for the present indications. Fondaparinux neither influenced the INR activity of warfarin, nor the bleeding time under acetylsalicylic acid or piroxicam treatment, nor the pharmacokinetics of digoxin at steady state.

Follow-up therapy with another anticoagulant medicinal product

If follow-up treatment is to be initiated with heparin or LMWH, the first injection should, as a general rule, be given one day after the last fondaparinux injection.

If follow up treatment with a Vitamin K antagonist is required, treatment with fondaparinux should be continued until the target INR value has been reached.

4.6 Pregnancy and lactation

There are no adequate data from the use of fondaparinux in pregnant women. Animal studies are insufficient with respect to effects on pregnancy, embryo/foetal development, parturition and postnatal development because of limited exposure. Fondaparinux should not be prescribed to pregnant women unless clearly necessary.

Fondaparinux is excreted in rat milk but it is not known whether fondaparinux is excreted in human milk. Breast-feeding is not recommended during treatment with fondaparinux. Oral absorption by the child is however unlikely.

4.7 Effects on ability to drive and use machines

No studies on the effect on the ability to drive and to use machines have been performed.

4.8 Undesirable effects

The safety of fondaparinux 2.5 mg has been evaluated in 3,595 patients undergoing major orthopaedic surgery of the lower limbs treated up to 9 days, in 327 patients undergoing hip fracture surgery treated for 3 weeks following an initial prophylaxis of 1 week, 1,407 patients undergoing abdominal surgery treated up to 9 days, and in 425 medical patients who are at risk for thromboembolic complications treated up to 14 days.

The adverse reactions reported by the investigator as at least possibly related to fondaparinux are presented within each frequency grouping (very common ⩾ 1/10; common: ⩾1/100 to < 1/10; uncommon: ⩾ 1/1,000 to < 1/100; rare: ⩾ 1/10,000 to <1/1,000; very rare <1/10,000) and system organ class by decreasing order of seriousness; these adverse reactions should be interpreted within the surgical and medical context.

(see Table 1 below)

In other studies or in post-marketing experience, rare cases of intracranial / intracerebral and retroperitoneal bleedings have been reported.

4.9 Overdose

Fondaparinux doses above the recommended regimen may lead to an increased risk of bleeding. There is no known antidote to fondaparinux.

Overdose associated with bleeding complications should lead to treatment discontinuation and search for the primary cause. Initiation of appropriate therapy such as surgical haemostasis, blood replacements, fresh plasma transfusion, plasmapheresis should be considered.

Table 1

System organ class MedDRA	Undesirable effects in patients undergoing major orthopaedic surgery of lower limbs and/or abdominal surgery	Undesirable effects in medical patients
Infections and infestations	*Rare:* post-operative wound infection	
Blood and lymphatic system disorders	*Common:* post-operative haemorrhage, anaemia *Uncommon:* bleeding (epistaxis, gastrointestinal, haemoptysis, haematuria, haematoma) thrombocytopenia, purpura, thrombocythaemia, platelet abnormal, coagulation disorder	*Common:* bleeding (haematoma, haematuria, haemoptysis, gingival bleeding) *Uncommon:* anaemia
Immune system disorders	*Rare:* allergic reaction	
Metabolism and nutrition disorders	*Rare:* hypokalaemia	
Nervous system disorders	*Rare:* anxiety, somnolence, vertigo, dizziness, headache, confusion	
Vascular disorders	*Rare:* hypotension	
Respiratory, thoracic and mediastinal disorders	*Rare:* dyspnoea, coughing	*Uncommon:* dyspnoea
Gastrointestinal disorders	*Uncommon:* nausea, vomiting *Rare:* abdominal pain, dyspepsia, gastritis, constipation, diarrhoea	
Hepatobiliary disorders	*Uncommon:* hepatic enzymes increased, hepatic function abnormal *Rare:* bilirubinaemia	
Skin and subcutaneous tissue disorders	*Uncommon:* rash, pruritus	*Uncommon:* rash, pruritus
General disorders and administration site conditions	*Uncommon:* oedema, oedema peripheral, fever, wound secretion *Rare:* chest pain, fatigue, hot flushes, leg pain, oedema genital, flushing, syncope	*Uncommon:* chest pain

5. PHARMACOLOGICAL PROPERTIES

5.1 Pharmacodynamic properties

Pharmacotherapeutic group: antithrombotic agents.

ATC code: B01AX05

Pharmacodynamic effects

Fondaparinux is a synthetic and selective inhibitor of activated Factor X (Xa). The antithrombotic activity of fondaparinux is the result of antithrombin III (ATIII) mediated selective inhibition of Factor Xa. By binding selectively to ATIII, fondaparinux potentiates (about 300 times) the innate neutralization of Factor Xa by ATIII. Neutralisation of Factor Xa interrupts the blood coagulation cascade and inhibits both thrombin formation and thrombus development. Fondaparinux does not inactivate thrombin (activated Factor II) and has no effects on platelets.

At the 2.5 mg dose, fondaparinux does not affect routine coagulation tests such as activated partial thromboplastin time (aPTT), activated clotting time (ACT) or prothrombin time (PT)/International Normalised Ratio (INR) tests in plasma nor bleeding time or fibrinolytic activity. However, rare spontaneous reports of aPTT prolongation have been received.

Fondaparinux does not cross-react with sera from patients with heparin-induced thrombocytopaenia.

Clinical studies

Prevention of Venous Thromboembolic Events (VTE) in patients undergoing major orthopaedic surgery of the lower limbs treated up to 9 days

The fondaparinux clinical program was designed to demonstrate the efficacy of fondaparinux for the prevention of venous thromboembolic events (VTE), i.e. proximal and distal deep vein thrombosis (DVT) and pulmonary embolism (PE) in patients undergoing major orthopaedic surgery of the lower limbs such as hip fracture, major knee surgery or hip replacement surgery. Over 8,000 patients (hip fracture – 1,711, hip replacement – 5,829, major knee surgery – 1,367) were studied in controlled Phase II and III clinical studies. Fondaparinux 2.5 mg once daily started 6-8 hours postoperatively was compared with enoxaparin 40 mg once daily started 12 hours before surgery, or 30 mg twice daily started 12-24 hours after surgery.

In a pooled analysis of these studies, the recommended dose regimen of fondaparinux versus enoxaparin was associated with a significant decrease (54% [95% CI, 44 %; 63%]) in the rate of VTE evaluated up to day 11 after surgery, irrespective of the type of surgery performed. The majority of endpoint events were diagnosed by a prescheduled venography and consisted mainly of distal DVT, but the incidence of proximal DVT was also significantly reduced. The incidence of symptomatic VTE, including PE was not significantly different between treatment groups.

In studies versus enoxaparin 40 mg once daily started 12 hours before surgery, major bleeding was observed in 2.8% of fondaparinux patients treated with the recommended dose, compared to 2.6% with enoxaparin.

Prevention of Venous Thromboembolic Events (VTE) in patients undergoing hip fracture surgery treated for up to 24 days following an initial prophylaxis of 1 week

In a randomised double-blind clinical trial, 737 patients were treated with fondaparinux 2.5 mg once daily for 7 +/- 1 days following hip fracture surgery. At the end of this period, 656 patients were randomised to receive fondaparinux 2.5 mg once daily or placebo for an additional 21 +/- 2 days. Fondaparinux provided a significant reduction in the overall rate of VTE compared with placebo [3 patients (1.4%) vs 77 patients (35%), respectively]. The majority (70/80) of the recorded VTE events were venographically detected non-symptomatic cases of DVT. Fondaparinux also provided a significant reduction in the rate of symptomatic VTE (DVT, and / or PE) [1 (0.3%) vs 9 (2.7%) patients, respectively] including two fatal PE reported in the placebo group. Major bleedings, all at surgical site and none fatal, were observed in 8 patients (2.4%) treated with fondaparinux 2.5 mg compared to 2 (0.6%) with placebo.

Prevention of Venous Thromboembolic Events (VTE) in patients undergoing abdominal surgery who are judged to be at high risk of thromboembolic complications, such as patients undergoing abdominal cancer surgery

In a double-blind clinical study, 2,927 patients were randomized to receive fondaparinux 2.5mg once daily or dalteparin 5,000 IU once daily, with one 2,500 IU preoperative injection and a first 2,500 IU post-operative injection, for 7±2 days. The main sites of surgery were colonic/rectal, gastric, hepatic, cholecystectomy or other biliary. Sixty-nine percent of the patients underwent surgery for cancer. Patients under-going urological (other than kidney) or gynaecological surgery, laparoscopic surgery or vascular surgery were not included in the study.

In this study, the incidence of total VTE was 4.6% (47/1,027) with fondaparinux, versus 6.1%: (62/1,021) with dalteparin: odds ratio reduction [95%CI] = -25.8% [-49.7%, 9.5%]. The difference in total VTE rates between the treatment groups, which was not statistically significant, was mainly due to a reduction of asymptomatic distal DVT. The incidence of symptomatic DVT was similar between treatment groups: 6 patients (0.4%) in the fondaparinux group vs 5 patients (0.3%) in the dalteparin group.

In the large subgroup of patients undergoing cancer surgery (69% of the patient population), the VTE rate was 4.7% in the fondaparinux group, versus 7.7% in the dalteparin group.

Major bleeding was observed in 3.4% of the patients in the fondaparinux group and in 2.4% of the dalteparin group.

Prevention of Venous Thromboembolic Events (VTE) in medical patients who are at high risk for thromboembolic complications due to restricted mobility during acute illness

In a randomised double-blind clinical trial, 839 patients were treated with fondaparinux 2.5 mg once daily or placebo for 6 to 14 days. This study included acutely ill medical patients, aged ≥ 60 years, expected to require bed rest for at least four days, and hospitalized for congestive heart failure NYHA class III/IV and/or acute respiratory illness and/or acute infectious or inflammatory disease. Fondaparinux significantly reduced the overall rate of VTE compared to placebo [18 patients (5.6%) vs 34 patients (10.5%), respectively]. The majority of events were asymptomatic distal DVT. Fondaparinux also significantly reduced the rate of adjudicated fatal PE [0 patients (0.0%) vs 5 patients (1.2%), respectively]. Major bleedings were observed in 1 patient (0.2%) of each group.

5.2 Pharmacokinetic properties

Absorption

After subcutaneous dosing, fondaparinux is completely and rapidly absorbed (absolute bioavailability 100%). Following a single subcutaneous injection of fondaparinux 2.5 mg to young healthy subjects, peak plasma concentration (mean C_{max} = 0.34 mg/l) is obtained 2 hours post-dosing. Plasma concentrations of half the mean C_{max} values are reached 25 minutes post-dosing.

In elderly healthy subjects, pharmacokinetics of fondaparinux are linear in the range of 2 to 8 mg by subcutaneous route. Following once daily dosing, steady state of plasma levels is obtained after 3 to 4 days with a 1.3-fold increase in C_{max} and AUC.

Mean (CV%) steady state pharmacokinetic parameters estimates of fondaparinux in patients undergoing hip replacement surgery receiving fondaparinux 2.5 mg once daily are: C_{max} (mg/l) - 0.39 (31%), T_{max} (h) - 2.8 (18%) and C_{min} (mg/l) -0.14 (56%). In hip fracture patients, associated with their increased age, fondaparinux steady state plasma concentrations are: C_{max} (mg/l) - 0.50 (32%), C_{min} (mg/l) - 0.19 (58%).

Distribution

The distribution volume of fondaparinux is limited (7-11 litres). *In vitro*, fondaparinux is highly and specifically bound to antithrombin protein with a dose-dependant plasma concentration binding (98.6% to 97.0% in the concentration range from 0.5 to 2 mg/l). Fondaparinux does not bind significantly to other plasma proteins, including platelet factor 4 (PF4).

Since fondaparinux does not bind significantly to plasma proteins other than ATIII, no interaction with other medicinal products by protein binding displacement are expected.

Metabolism

Although not fully evaluated, there is no evidence of fondaparinux metabolism and in particular no evidence for the formation of active metabolites.

Fondaparinux does not inhibit CYP450s (CYP1A2, CYP2A6, CYP2C9, CYP2C19, CYP2D6, CYP2E1 or CYP3A4) *in vitro*. Thus, fondaparinux is not expected to interact with other medicinal products *in vivo* by inhibition of CYP-mediated metabolism.

Excretion/Elimination

The elimination half-life ($t_{½}$) is about 17 hours in healthy young subjects and about 21 hours in healthy elderly subjects. Fondaparinux is excreted to 64 – 77 % by the kidney as unchanged compound.

<u>*Special populations*</u>

Paediatric patients - Fondaparinux has not been investigated in this population.

Elderly patients - Renal function may decrease with age and thus, the elimination capacity for fondaparinux may be reduced in elderly. In patients >75 years undergoing orthopaedic surgery, the estimated plasma clearance was 1.2 to 1.4 times lower than in patients <65 years.

Renal impairment - Compared with patients with normal renal function (creatinine clearance > 80 ml/min), plasma clearance is 1.2 to 1.4 times lower in patients with mild renal impairment (creatinine clearance 50 to 80 ml/min) and on average 2 times lower in patients with moderate renal impairment (creatinine clearance 30 to 50 ml/min). In severe renal impairment (creatinine clearance < 30 ml/min), plasma clearance is approximately 5 times lower than in normal renal function. Associated terminal half-life values were 29 h in moderate and 72 h in patients with severe renal impairment.

Gender - No gender differences were observed after adjustment for body weight.

Race - Pharmacokinetic differences due to race have not been studied prospectively. However, studies performed in Asian (Japanese) healthy subjects did not reveal a different pharmacokinetic profile compared to Caucasian healthy subjects. Similarly, no plasma clearance differences were observed between black and Caucasian patients undergoing orthopaedic surgery.

Body weight - Plasma clearance of fondaparinux increases with body weight (9% increase per 10 kg).

Hepatic impairment - Following a single, subcutaneous dose of fondaparinux in subjects with moderate hepatic impairment (Child-Pugh Category B), total (i.e., bound and unbound) C_{max} and AUC were decreased by 22% and 39%, respectively, as compared to subjects with normal liver function. The lower plasma concentrations of fondaparinux were attributed to reduced binding to ATIII secondary to the lower ATIII plasma concentrations in subjects with hepatic impairment thereby resulting in increased renal clearance of fondaparinux. Consequently, unbound concentrations of fondaparinux are expected to be unchanged in patients with mild to moderate hepatic impairment, and therefore, no dose adjustment is necessary based on pharmacokinetics.

The pharmacokinetics of fondaparinux has not been studied in patients with severe hepatic impairment (see sections 4.2 and 4.4).

5.3 Preclinical safety data

Non-clinical data reveal no special hazard for humans based on conventional studies of safety pharmacology, repeated dose toxicity, and genotoxicity. Animal studies are insufficient with respect to effects on toxicity to reproduction because of limited exposure.

6. PHARMACEUTICAL PARTICULARS

6.1 List of excipients

Sodium chloride

Water for injections

Hydrochloric acid

Sodium hydroxide

6.2 Incompatibilities

In the absence of compatibility studies, this medicinal product must not be mixed with other medicinal products.

6.3 Shelf life

3 years.

6.4 Special precautions for storage

Do not freeze.

6.5 Nature and contents of container

Type I glass barrel (1 ml) affixed with a 27 gauge × 12.7 mm needle and stoppered with a bromobutyl or chlorobutyl elastomer plunger stopper.

Arixtra is available in pack sizes of 2, 7, 10 and 20 pre-filled syringes. There are two types of syringes:

- syringe with a yellow plunger and an automatic safety system
- syringe with yellow plunger and a manual safety system.

Not all pack sizes may be marketed.

6.6 Special precautions for disposal and other handling

The subcutaneous injection is administered in the same way as with a classical syringe.

Parenteral solutions should be inspected visually for particulate matter and discoloration prior to administration.

Instruction for self-administration is mentioned in the Package Leaflet.

The needle protection system of the Arixtra pre-filled syringes have been designed with a safety system to protect from needle stick injuries following injection.

Any unused product or waste material should be disposed of in accordance with local requirements.

7. MARKETING AUTHORISATION HOLDER

Glaxo Group Ltd

Greenford

Middlesex

UB6 0NN

United Kingdom

8. MARKETING AUTHORISATION NUMBER(S)

EU/1/02/206/005-008 and 024-026

9. DATE OF FIRST AUTHORISATION/RENEWAL OF THE AUTHORISATION

Date of first authorisation: 21 March 2002

Date of latest renewal: 21 March 2007

10. DATE OF REVISION OF THE TEXT

25 March 2009

Detailed information on this medicinal product is available on the website of the European Medicines Agency (EMEA) http://www.emea.europa.eu

Arixtra 2.5mg/0.5ml solution for injection, pre-filled syringe.

(GlaxoSmithKline UK)

1. NAME OF THE MEDICINAL PRODUCT

Arixtra ▼ 2.5 mg/0.5 ml solution for injection, pre-filled syringe.

2. QUALITATIVE AND QUANTITATIVE COMPOSITIO

Each pre-filled syringe (0.5 ml) contains 2.5 mg of fond parinux sodium.

Excipient(s): Contains less than 1 mmol of sodium (23 m per dose, and therefore is essentially sodium free.

For a full list of excipients, see section 6.1.

3. PHARMACEUTICAL FORM

Solution for injection.

The solution is a clear and colourless liquid.

4. CLINICAL PARTICULARS

4.1 Therapeutic indications

Prevention of Venous Thromboembolic Events (VTE) patients undergoing major orthopaedic surgery of th lower limbs such as hip fracture, major knee surgery c hip replacement surgery.

Prevention of Venous Thromboembolic Events (VTE) i patients undergoing abdominal surgery who are judge to be at high risk of thromboembolic complications, suc as patients undergoing abdominal cancer surgery (se section 5.1).

Prevention of Venous Thromboembolic Events (VTE) i medical patients who are judged to be at high risk fo VTE and who are immobilised due to acute illness suc as cardiac insufficiency and/or acute respiratory disorders and/or acute infectious or inflammatory disease.

Treatment of unstable angina or non-ST segment elevatio myocardial infarction (UA/NSTEMI) in patients for whon urgent (< 120 mins) invasive management (PCI) is no indicated (see sections 4.4 and 5.1).

Treatment of ST segment elevation myocardial infarctio (STEMI) in patients who are managed with thrombolytics o who initially are to receive no other form of reperfusio therapy.

4.2 Posology and method of administration

Patients undergoing major orthopaedic or abdominal surgery

The recommended dose of fondaparinux is 2.5 mg once daily administered post-operatively by subcutaneous injection.

The initial dose should be given 6 hours following surgical closure provided that haemostasis has been established.

Treatment should be continued until the risk of venous thrombo-embolism has diminished, usually until the patient is ambulant, at least 5 to 9 days after surgery. Experience shows that in patients undergoing hip fracture surgery, the risk of VTE continues beyond 9 days after surgery. In these patients the use of prolonged prophylaxis with fondaparinux should be considered for up to an additional 24 days (see section 5.1).

Medical patients who are at high risk for thromboembolic complications based on an individual risk assessment

The recommended dose of fondaparinux is 2.5 mg once daily administered by subcutaneous injection. A treatment duration of 6-14 days has been clinically studied in medical patients (see section 5.1).

Treatment of unstable angina/non- ST segment elevation myocardial infarction (UA/NSTEMI)

The recommended dose of fondaparinux is 2.5 mg once daily, administered by subcutaneous injection. Treatment should be initiated as soon as possible following diagnosis and continued for up to a maximum of 8 days or until hospital discharge if that occurs earlier.

If a patient is to undergo percutaneous coronary intervention (PCI), unfractionated heparin (UFH) as per local practice should be administered during PCI, taking into account the patient's potential risk of bleeding, including the time since the last dose of fondaparinux (see section 4.4). The timing of restarting subcutaneous fondaparinux after sheath removal should be based on clinical judgment. In the pivotal UA/NSTEMI clinical trial, treatment with fondaparinux was restarted no earlier than 2 hours after sheath removal.

Treatment of ST segment elevation myocardial infarction (STEMI)

The recommended dose of fondaparinux is 2.5 mg once daily. The first dose of fondaparinux is administered intravenously and subsequent doses are administered by subcutaneous injection. Treatment should be initiated as soon as possible following diagnosis and continued for up to a maximum of 8 days or until hospital discharge if that occurs earlier.

If a patient is to undergo non-primary PCI, unfractionated heparin (UFH) as per local practice should be administered during PCI, taking into account the patient's potential risk of bleeding, including the time since the last dose of fondaparinux (see section 4.4). The timing of restarting subcutaneous fondaparinux after sheath removal should be based on clinical judgment. In the pivotal STEMI clinical trial, treatment with fondaparinux was restarted no earlier than 3 hours after sheath removal.

In STEMI or UA/NSTEMI patients who are to undergo coronary artery bypass graft (CABG) surgery, fondaparinux where possible, should not be given during the 24 hours before surgery and may be restarted 48 hours post-operatively.

pecial populations

revention of VTE following Surgery

patients undergoing surgery, timing of the first fonda-arinux injection requires strict adherence in patients ≥75 ears, and/or with body weight <50 kg and/or with renal npairment with creatinine clearance ranging between 20 50 ml/min.

he first fondaparinux administration should be given not arlier than 6 hours following surgical closure. The injection hould not be given unless haemostasis has been estab-shed (see section 4.4).

enal impairment

Prophylaxis of VTE - Fondaparinux should not be used in atients with creatinine clearance <20 ml/min (see section .3). The dose should be reduced to 1.5 mg once daily in atients with creatinine clearance in the range of 20 to 0 ml/min (see sections 4.4 and 5.2). No dosage reduction s required for patients with mild renal impairment (creati-ine clearance >50 ml/min).

Treatment of UA/NSTEMI and STEMI - fondaparinux hould not be used in patients with creatinine clearance < 20 ml/min (see section 4.3). No dosage reduction is equired for patients with creatinine clearance > 20 ml/nin.

Hepatic impairment - No dosing adjustment is necessary in atients with either mild or moderate hepatic impairment. n patients with severe hepatic impairment, fondaparinux should be used with care as this patient group has not been studied (see sections 4.4 and 5.2).

Paediatric population - Fondaparinux is not recommended or use in children below 17 years of age due to a lack of data on safety and efficacy.

Method of administration

• *Subcutaneous administration*

Fondaparinux is administered by deep subcutaneous injection while the patient is lying down. Sites of adminis-tration should alternate between the left and the right anterolateral and left and right posterolateral abdominal wall. To avoid the loss of medicinal product when using the pre-filled syringe do not expel the air bubble from the syringe before the injection. The whole length of the needle should be inserted perpendicularly into a skin fold held between the thumb and the forefinger; the skin fold should be held throughout the injection.

• *Intravenous administration (first dose in patients with STEMI only)*

Intravenous administration should be through an existing intravenous line either directly or using a small volume (25 or 50ml) 0.9% saline minibag. To avoid the loss of medic-inal product when using the pre-filled syringe do not expel the air bubble from the syringe before the injection. The intravenous tubing should be well flushed with saline after injection to ensure that all of the medicinal product is administered. If administered via a minibag, the infusion should be given over 1 to 2 minutes.

For additional instructions for use and handling and dis-posal see section 6.6.

4.3 Contraindications

- hypersensitivity to the active substance or to any of the excipients

- active clinically significant bleeding

- acute bacterial endocarditis

- severe renal impairment defined by creatinine clearance < 20 ml/min.

4.4 Special warnings and precautions for use

Fondaparinux must not be administered intramuscularly.

Haemorrhage

Fondaparinux should be used with caution in patients who have an increased risk of haemorrhage, such as those with congenital or acquired bleeding disorders (e.g. platelet count <50,000/mm^3), active ulcerative gastrointestinal disease and recent intracranial haemorrhage or shortly after brain, spinal or ophthalmic surgery and in special patient groups as outlined below.

For prevention of VTE, agents that may enhance the risk of haemorrhage should not be administered concomitantly with fondaparinux. These agents include desirudin, fibri-nolytic agents, GP IIb/IIIa receptor antagonists, heparin, heparinoids, or Low Molecular Weight Heparin (LMWH). When required, concomitant therapy with vitamin K antagonist should be administered in accordance with the information of section 4.5. Other antiplatelet medicinal products (acetylsalicylic acid, dipyridamole, sulfinpyra-zone, ticlopidine or clopidogrel), and NSAIDs should be used with caution. If co-administration is essential, close monitoring is necessary.

For treatment of UA/NSTEMI and STEMI, fondaparinux should be used with caution in patients who are being treated concomitantly with other agents that increase the risk of haemorrhage (such as GPIIb/IIIa inhibitors or throm-bolytics).

PCI and risk of guiding catheter thrombus

In STEMI patients undergoing primary PCI, the use of fondaparinux prior to and during PCI is not recommended. Similarly, in UA/NSTEMI patients with life threatening conditions that require urgent revascularisation, the use of fondaparinux prior to and during PCI is not recommended. These are patients with refractory or recurrent angina associated with dynamic ST deviation, heart failure, life-threatening arrhythmias or haemodynamic instability.

In UA/NSTEMI and STEMI patients undergoing non-primary PCI, the use of fondaparinux as the sole anticoagu-lant during PCI is not recommended, therefore UFH should be used according to local practice (see section 4.2).

There are limited data on the use of UFH during non-primary PCI in patients treated with fondaparinux (see section 5.1). In those patients who underwent non-primary PCI 6-24 hours after the last dose of fondaparinux, the median dose of UFH was 8,000 IU and the incidence of major bleeding was 2% (2/98). In those patients who underwent non-primary PCI <6 hours after the last dose of fondaparinux, the median dose of UFH was 5,000 IU and the incidence of major bleeding was 4.1% (2/49).

Clinical trials have shown a low but increased risk of guid-ing catheter thrombus in patients treated with fondapar-inux for anticoagulation during PCI compared to control. Incidences in non-primary PCI in UA/NSTEMI were 1.0% vs 0.3% (fondaparinux vs. enoxaparin) and in primary PCI in STEMI were 1.2% vs 0% (fondaparinux vs. control).

Spinal / Epidural anaesthesia

In patients undergoing major orthopaedic surgery, epidural or spinal haematomas that may result in long-term or permanent paralysis cannot be excluded with the concur-rent use of fondaparinux and spinal/epidural anaesthesia or spinal puncture. The risk of these rare events may be higher with post-operative use of indwelling epidural catheters or the concomitant use of other medicinal pro-ducts affecting haemostasis.

Elderly patients

The elderly population is at increased risk of bleeding. As renal function is generally decreasing with age, elderly patients may show reduced elimination and increased exposure of fondaparinux (see section 5.2). Fondaparinux should be used with caution in elderly patients (see section 4.2).

Low body weight

Patients with body weight <50 kg are at increased risk of bleeding. Elimination of fondaparinux decreases with weight. Fondaparinux should be used with caution in these patients (see section 4.2).

Renal impairment

Fondaparinux is known to be mainly excreted by the kid-ney.

• *Prophylaxis of VTE* - Patients with creatinine clearance <50 ml/min are at increased risk of bleeding and VTE and should be treated with caution (see sections 4.2, 4.3 and 5.2). There are limited clinical data available from patients with creatinine clearance less than 30 ml/min.

• *Treatment of UA/NSTEMI and* STEMI - For the treatment of UA/NSTEMI and STEMI, there are limited clinical data available on the use of fondaparinux 2.5mg once daily in patients with creatinine clearance between 20 and 30 ml/min. Therefore the physician should determine if the benefit of treatment outweighs the risk (see sections 4.2 and 4.3).

Severe hepatic impairment

Dosing adjustment of fondaparinux is not necessary. How-ever, the use of fondaparinux should be considered with caution because of an increased risk of bleeding due to a deficiency of coagulation factors in patients with severe hepatic impairment (see section 4.2).

Patients with Heparin Induced Thrombocytopenia

Fondaparinux should be used with caution in patients with a history of HIT. The efficacy and safety of fondaparinux have not been formally studied in patients with HIT type II. Fondaparinux does not bind to platelet factor 4 and does not cross-react with sera from patients with Heparin Induced Thrombocytopenia (HIT) type II. However, rare spontaneous reports of HIT in patients treated with fonda-parinux have been received. To date a causal association between treatment with fondaparinux and the occurrence of HIT has not been established.

4.5 Interaction with other medicinal products and other forms of interaction

Bleeding risk is increased with concomitant administration of fondaparinux and agents that may enhance the risk of haemorrhage (see section 4.4).

Oral anticoagulants (warfarin), platelet inhibitors (acetylsa-licylic acid), NSAIDs (piroxicam) and digoxin did not inter-act with the pharmacokinetics of fondaparinux. The fondaparinux dose (10 mg) in the interaction studies was higher than the dose recommended for the present indica-tions. Fondaparinux neither influenced the INR activity of warfarin, nor the bleeding time under acetylsalicylic acid or piroxicam treatment, nor the pharmacokinetics of digoxin at steady state.

Follow-up therapy with another anticoagulant medicinal product

If follow-up treatment is to be initiated with heparin or LMWH, the first injection should, as a general rule, be given one day after the last fondaparinux injection.

If follow up treatment with a Vitamin K antagonist is required, treatment with fondaparinux should be continued until the target INR value has been reached.

4.6 Pregnancy and lactation

There are no adequate data from the use of fondaparinux in pregnant women. Animal studies are insufficient with respect to effects on pregnancy, embryo/foetal develop-ment, parturition and postnatal development because of limited exposure. Fondaparinux should not be prescribed to pregnant women unless clearly necessary.

Fondaparinux is excreted in rat milk but it is not known whether fondaparinux is excreted in human milk. Breast-feeding is not recommended during treatment with fonda-parinux. Oral absorption by the child is however unlikely.

4.7 Effects on ability to drive and use machines

No studies on the effect on the ability to drive and to use machines have been performed.

4.8 Undesirable effects

The safety of fondaparinux 2.5 mg has been evaluated in:

- 3,595 patients undergoing major orthopaedic surgery of the lower limbs treated up to 9 days

- 327 patients undergoing hip fracture surgery treated for 3 weeks following an initial prophylaxis of 1 week

- 1,407 patients undergoing abdominal surgery treated up to 9 days

- 425 medical patients who are at risk for thromboembolic complications treated up to 14 days

- 10,057 patients undergoing treatment of UA or NSTEMI ACS

- 6,036 patients undergoing treatment of STEMI ACS.

For the prevention of VTE, the adverse reactions reported by the investigator as at least possibly related to fondapar-inux are presented within each frequency grouping (very common ≥ 1/10; common: ≥1/100 to < 1/10; uncom-mon: ≥ 1/1,000 to < 1/100; rare: ≥ 1/10,000 to <1/1,000; very rare <1/10,000) and system organ class by decreas-ing order of seriousness; these adverse reactions should be interpreted within the surgical and medical context.

(see Table 1 on next page)

In other studies or in post-marketing experience, rare cases of intracranial / intracerebral and retroperitoneal bleedings have been reported.

The adverse event profile reported in the ACS program is consistent with the adverse drug reactions identified for VTE prophylaxis.

Bleeding was a commonly reported event in patients with UA/NSTEMI and STEMI. The incidence of adjudicated major bleeding was 2.1% (fondaparinux) vs. 4.1% (enox-aparin) up to and including Day 9 in the Phase III UA/NSTEMI study, and the incidence of adjudicated severe haemorrhage by modified TIMI criteria was 1.1% (fonda-parinux) vs. 1.4% (control [UFH/placebo]) up to and includ-ing Day 9 in the Phase III STEMI study.

In the Phase III UA/NSTEMI study, the most commonly reported non-bleeding adverse events (reported in at least 1% of subjects on fondaparinux) were headache, chest pain and atrial fibrillation.

In the Phase III study in STEMI patients, the most com-monly reported non-bleeding adverse events (reported in at least 1% of subjects on fondaparinux) were atrial fibrilla-tion, pyrexia, chest pain, headache, ventricular tachycar-dia, vomiting, and hypotension.

4.9 Overdose

Fondaparinux doses above the recommended regimen may lead to an increased risk of bleeding. There is no known antidote to fondaparinux.

Overdose associated with bleeding complications should lead to treatment discontinuation and search for the pri-mary cause. Initiation of appropriate therapy such as sur-gical haemostasis, blood replacements, fresh plasma transfusion, plasmapheresis should be considered.

5. PHARMACOLOGICAL PROPERTIES

5.1 Pharmacodynamic properties

Pharmacotherapeutic group: antithrombotic agents.

ATC code: B01AX05

Pharmacodynamic effects

Fondaparinux is a synthetic and selective inhibitor of acti-vated Factor X (Xa). The antithrombotic activity of fonda-parinux is the result of antithrombin III (ATIII) mediated selective inhibition of Factor Xa. By binding selectively to ATIII, fondaparinux potentiates (about 300 times) the innate neutralization of Factor Xa by ATIII. Neutralisation of Factor Xa interrupts the blood coagulation cascade and inhibits both thrombin formation and thrombus development. Fon-daparinux does not inactivate thrombin (activated Factor II) and has no effects on platelets.

At the 2.5 mg dose, fondaparinux does not affect routine coagulation tests such as activated partial thromboplastin time (aPTT), activated clotting time (ACT) or prothrombin time (PT)/International Normalised Ratio (INR) tests in plasma nor bleeding time or fibrinolytic activity. However, rare spontaneous reports of aPTT prolongation have been received.

Table 1

System organ class MedDRA	Undesirable effects in patients undergoing major orthopaedic surgery of lower limbs and/or abdominal surgery	Undesirable effects in medical patients
Infections and infestations	*Rare:* post-operative wound infection	
Blood and lymphatic system disorders	*Common:* post-operative haemorrhage, anaemia *Uncommon:* bleeding (epistaxis, gastrointestinal, haemoptysis, haematuria, haematoma) thrombocytopenia, purpura, thrombocythaemia, platelet abnormal, coagulation disorder	*Common:* bleeding (haematoma, haematuria, haemoptysis, gingival bleeding) *Uncommon:* anaemia
Immune system disorders	*Rare:* allergic reaction	
Metabolism and nutrition disorders	*Rare:* hypokalaemia	
Nervous system disorders	*Rare:* anxiety, somnolence, vertigo, dizziness, headache, confusion	
Vascular disorders	*Rare:* hypotension	
Respiratory, thoracic and mediastinal disorders	*Rare:* dyspnoea, coughing	*Uncommon:* dyspnoea
Gastrointestinal disorders	*Uncommon:* nausea, vomiting *Rare:* abdominal pain, dyspepsia, gastritis, constipation, diarrhoea	
Hepatobiliary disorders	*Uncommon:* hepatic enzymes increased, hepatic function abnormal *Rare:* bilirubinaemia	
Skin and subcutaneous tissue disorders	*Uncommon:* rash, pruritus	*Uncommon:* rash, pruritus
General disorders and administration site conditions	*Uncommon:* oedema, oedema peripheral, fever, wound secretion *Rare:* chest pain, fatigue, hot flushes, leg pain, oedema genital, flushing, syncope	*Uncommon:* chest pain

Fondaparinux does not cross-react with sera from patients with heparin-induced thrombocytopaenia.

Clinical studies

Prevention of Venous Thromboembolic Events (VTE) in patients undergoing major orthopaedic surgery of the lower limbs treated up to 9 days

The fondaparinux clinical program was designed to demonstrate the efficacy of fondaparinux for the prevention of venous thromboembolic events (VTE), i.e. proximal and distal deep vein thrombosis (DVT) and pulmonary embolism (PE) in patients undergoing major orthopaedic surgery of the lower limbs such as hip fracture, major knee surgery or hip replacement surgery. Over 8,000 patients (hip fracture – 1,711, hip replacement – 5,829, major knee surgery – 1,367) were studied in controlled Phase II and III clinical studies. Fondaparinux 2.5 mg once daily started 6-8 hours postoperatively was compared with enoxaparin 40 mg once daily started 12 hours before surgery, or 30 mg twice daily started 12-24 hours after surgery.

In a pooled analysis of these studies, the recommended dose regimen of fondaparinux versus enoxaparin was associated with a significant decrease (54% [95% CI, 44 %; 63%]) in the rate of VTE evaluated up to day 11 after surgery, irrespective of the type of surgery performed. The majority of endpoint events were diagnosed by a prescheduled venography and consisted mainly of distal DVT, but the incidence of proximal DVT was also significantly reduced. The incidence of symptomatic VTE, including PE was not significantly different between treatment groups.

In studies versus enoxaparin 40 mg once daily started 12 hours before surgery, major bleeding was observed in 2.8% of fondaparinux patients treated with the recommended dose, compared to 2.6% with enoxaparin.

Prevention of Venous Thromboembolic Events (VTE) in patients undergoing hip fracture surgery treated for up to 24 days following an initial prophylaxis of 1 week

In a randomised double-blind clinical trial, 737 patients were treated with fondaparinux 2.5 mg once daily for 7 +/- 1 days following hip fracture surgery. At the end of this period, 656 patients were randomised to receive fondaparinux 2.5 mg once daily or placebo for an additional 21 +/- 2 days. Fondaparinux provided a significant reduction in the overall rate of VTE compared with placebo [3 patients (1.4%) vs 77 patients (35%), respectively]. The majority (70/80) of the recorded VTE events were venographically detected non-symptomatic cases of DVT. Fondaparinux also provided a significant reduction in the rate of symptomatic VTE (DVT, and / or PE) [1 (0.3%) vs 9 (2.7%) patients, respectively] including two fatal PE reported in the placebo group. Major bleedings, all at surgical site and none fatal, were observed in 8 patients (2.4%) treated with fondaparinux 2.5 mg compared to 2 (0.6%) with placebo.

Prevention of Venous Thromboembolic Events (VTE) in patients undergoing abdominal surgery who are judged to be at high risk of thromboembolic complications, such as patients undergoing abdominal cancer surgery

In a double-blind clinical study, 2,927 patients were randomized to receive fondaparinux 2.5mg once daily or dalteparin 5,000 IU once daily, with one 2,500 IU preoperative injection and a first 2,500 IU post-operative injection, for 7±2 days. The main sites of surgery were colonic/rectal, gastric, hepatic, cholecystectomy or other biliary. Sixty-nine percent of the patients underwent surgery for cancer. Patients under-going urological (other than kidney) or gynaecological surgery, laparoscopic surgery or vascular surgery were not included in the study.

In this study, the incidence of total VTE was 4.6% (47/1,027) with fondaparinux, versus 6.1%: (62/1,021) with dalteparin: odds ratio reduction [95%CI] = -25.8% [-49.7%, 9.5%]. The difference in total VTE rates between the treatment groups, which was not statistically significant, was mainly due to a reduction of asymptomatic distal DVT. The incidence of symptomatic DVT was similar between treatment groups: 6 patients (0.4%) in the fondaparinux group vs 5 patients (0.3%) in the dalteparin group. In the large subgroup of patients undergoing cancer surgery (69% of the patient population), the VTE rate was 4.7% in the fondaparinux group, versus 7.7% in the dalteparin group.

Major bleeding was observed in 3.4% of the patients in the fondaparinux group and in 2.4% of the dalteparin group.

Prevention of Venous Thromboembolic Events (VTE) in medical patients who are at high risk for thromboembolic complications due to restricted mobility during acute illness

In a randomised double-blind clinical trial, 839 patients were treated with fondaparinux 2.5 mg once daily or placebo for 6 to 14 days. This study included acutely ill medical patients, aged ≥ 60 years, expected to require bed rest for at least four days, and hospitalized for congestive heart failure NYHA class III/IV and/or acute respiratory illness and/or acute infectious or inflammatory disease. Fondaparinux significantly reduced the overall rate of VTE compared to placebo [18 patients (5.6%) vs 34 patients (10.5%), respectively]. The majority of events were asymptomatic distal DVT. Fondaparinux also significantly reduced the rate of adjudicated fatal PE [0 patients (0.0%) vs 5 patients (1.2%), respectively]. Major bleedings were observed in 1 patient (0.2%) of each group.

Treatment of unstable angina or non-ST segment elevation myocardial infarction (UA/NSTEMI)

OASIS 5 was a double-blind, randomised, non-inferiority study with fondaparinux 2.5 mg subcutaneously once daily versus enoxaparin 1 mg/kg subcutaneously twice daily in approximately 20,000 patients with UA/NSTEMI. All patients received standard medical treatment for UA/NSTEMI, with 34% of patients undergoing PCI and 9% undergoing CABG. The mean treatment duration was 5. days in the fondaparinux group and 5.2 days in the enox aparin group. If PCI was performed, patients receive either intravenous fondaparinux (fondaparinux patients or weight adjusted intravenous UFH (enoxaparin patients as adjunctive therapy, dependent on the timing of the las subcutaneous dose and planned use of GP IIb/IIIa inhibito The mean age of the patients was 67 years, and approximately 60% were at least 65 years old. Approximately 40% and 17% of patients had mild (creatinine clearance ≥50 t <80 ml/min) or moderate (creatinine clearance ≥30 t <50 ml/min) renal impairment, respectively.

The primary adjudicated endpoint was a composite o death, myocardial infarction (MI) and refractory ischaemi (RI) within 9 days of randomisation. Of the patients in th fondaparinux group, 5.8% experienced an event by Day 9 compared to 5.7% for enoxaparin-treated patients (hazar ratio 1.01, 95% CI, 0.90, 1.13, one-sided non-inferiority p value = 0.003).

By Day 30, the incidence of all cause mortality was significantly reduced from 3.5% on enoxaparin to 2.9% o fondaparinux (hazard ratio 0.83, 95% CI, 0.71;0.97 p = 0.02). The effects on the incidence of MI and RI were not statistically different between the fondaparinux and enoxaparin treatment groups.

At Day 9 the incidence of major bleeding on fondaparinux and enoxaparin was 2.1% and 4.1%, respectively (hazard ratio 0.52, 95% CI, 0.44;0.61, p < 0.001).

The efficacy findings and results on major bleeding were consistent across prespecified subgroups such as elderly, renally impaired patients, type of concomitant platelet aggregation inhibitors (aspirin, thienopyridines or GP IIb/IIIa inhibitors).

In the subgroup of patients treated with fondaparinux or enoxaparin who underwent PCI, 8.8% and 8.2% of patients respectively, experience death/MI/RI within 9 days of randomisation (hazard ratio 1.08, 95% CI, 0.92;1.27). In this subgroup, the incidence of major bleeding on fondaparinux and enoxaparin at Day 9 was 2.2% and 5.0% respectively (hazard ratio 0.43, 95% CI, 0.33;0.57).

Treatment of ST segment elevation myocardial infarction (STEMI)

OASIS 6 was a double blind, randomised study assessing the safety and efficacy of fondaparinux 2.5 mg once daily, versus usual care (placebo (47%) or UFH (53%) in approximately 12,000 patients with STEMI. All patients received standard treatments for STEMI, including primary PCI (31%), thrombolytics (45%) or no reperfusion (24%). Of the patients treated with a thrombolytic, 84% were treated with a non-fibrin specific agent (primarily streptokinase). The mean treatment duration was 6.2 days on fondaparinux. The mean age of the patients was 61 years, and approximately 40% were at least 65 years old. Approximately 40% and 14% of patients had mild (creatinine clearance ≥50 to <80 ml/min) or moderate (creatinine clearance ≥30 to <50 ml/min) renal impairment, respectively.

The primary adjudicated endpoint was a composite of death and recurrent MI (re-MI) within 30 days of randomisation. The incidence of death/re-MI at Day 30 was significantly reduced from 11.1% for the control group to 9.7% for the fondaparinux group (hazard ratio 0.86, 95% CI, 0.77, 0.96, p = 0.008). In the predefined stratum comparing fondaparinux to placebo (i.e patients treated with non-fibrin specific lytics (77.3%), no reperfusion (22%), fibrin-specific lytics (0.3%), primary PCI (0.4%), the incidence of death/re-MI at Day 30 was significantly reduced from 14.0% on placebo to 11.3% (hazard ratio 0.80, 95% CI, 0.69, 0.93, p = 0.003). In the predefined stratum comparing fondaparinux to UFH (patients treated with primary PCI (58.5%), fibrin-specific lytics (13%), non-fibrin-specific lytics (2.6%) and no reperfusion (25.9%), the effects of fondaparinux and UFH on the incidence of death/re-MI at Day 30 were not statistically different: respectively, 8.3% vs 8.7% (hazard ratio 0.94, 95% CI, 0.79, 1.11 p = 0.460). However, in this stratum, in the subgroup of indicated population undergoing thrombolysis or no reperfusion (i.e patients not undergoing primary PCI), the incidence of death/re-MI at Day 30 was significantly reduced from 14.3% on UFH to 11.5% with fondaparinux (hazard ratio 0.79, 95% CI, 0.64, 0.98, p = 0.03).

The incidence of all cause mortality at Day 30 was also significantly reduced from 8.9% for the control group to 7.8% in the fondaparinux group (hazard ratio 0.87, 95% CI, 0.77;0.98, p = 0.02). The difference in mortality was statistically significant in stratum 1 (placebo comparator) but not in stratum 2 (UFH comparator). The mortality benefit shown in the fondaparinux group was maintained until the end of follow-up at Day 180.

In patients who were revascularised with a thrombolytic, fondaparinux significantly reduced the incidence of death/re-MI at Day 30 from 13.6% for the control group to 10.9% (hazard ratio 0.79, 95%CI, 0.68;0.93, p = 0.003). Among patients initially not reperfused, the incidence of death/re-MI at Day 30 was significantly reduced from 15% for the control group to 12.1% for the fondaparinux group (hazard ratio 0.79, 95% CI, 0.65;0.97, p = 0.023). In patients treated with primary PCI, the incidence of death/re-MI at Day 30 as not statistically different between the two groups .0% in fondaparinux group vs 4.8% in the control group; azard ratio 1.26, 95% CI, 0.96, 1.66].

y Day 9, 1.1% of patients treated with fondaparinux and .4% of control patients experienced a severe haemorrhage. In patients given a thrombolytic, severe haemorrhage occurred in 1.3% of the fondaparinux patients and in .0% of controls. In patients initially not reperfused, the incidence of severe haemorrhage was 1.2% for fondaparinux vs 1.5% for controls. For patients receiving primary CI, the incidence of severe haemorrhage was 1.0% for ondaparinux and 0.4% for controls.

he efficacy findings and results on severe haemorrhage were consistent across prespecified subgroups such as elderly, renally impaired patients, type of concomitant platelet aggregation inhibitors (aspirin, thienopyridines).

.2 Pharmacokinetic properties

Absorption

After subcutaneous dosing, fondaparinux is completely and rapidly absorbed (absolute bioavailability 100%). Following a single subcutaneous injection of fondaparinux 2.5 mg to young healthy subjects, peak plasma concentration (mean C_{max} = 0.34 mg/l) is obtained 2 hours post-dosing. Plasma concentrations of half the mean C_{max} values are reached 25 minutes post-dosing.

n elderly healthy subjects, pharmacokinetics of fondaparinux are linear in the range of 2 to 8 mg by subcutaneous route. Following once daily subcutaneous dosing, steady state of plasma levels is obtained after 3 to 4 days with a 1.3-fold increase in C_{max} and AUC.

Mean (CV%) steady state pharmacokinetic parameters estimates of fondaparinux in patients undergoing hip replacement surgery receiving fondaparinux 2.5 mg once daily are: C_{max} (mg/l) - 0.39 (31%), T_{max} (h) - 2.8 (18%) and C_{min} (mg/l) -0.14 (56%). In hip fracture patients, associated with their increased age, fondaparinux steady state plasma concentrations are: C_{max} (mg/l) - 0.50 (32%), C_{min} (mg/l) - 0.19 (58%).

Distribution

The distribution volume of fondaparinux is limited (7-11 litres). *In vitro*, fondaparinux is highly and specifically bound to antithrombin protein with a dose-dependant plasma concentration binding (98.6% to 97.0% in the concentration range from 0.5 to 2 mg/l). Fondaparinux does not bind significantly to other plasma proteins, including platelet factor 4 (PF4).

Since fondaparinux does not bind significantly to plasma proteins other than ATIII, no interaction with other medicinal products by protein binding displacement are expected.

Metabolism

Although not fully evaluated, there is no evidence of fondaparinux metabolism and in particular no evidence for the formation of active metabolites.

Fondaparinux does not inhibit CYP450s (CYP1A2, CYP2A6, CYP2C9, CYP2C19, CYP2D6, CYP2E1 or CYP3A4) *in vitro*. Thus, fondaparinux is not expected to interact with other medicinal products *in vivo* by inhibition of CYP-mediated metabolism.

Excretion/Elimination

The elimination half-life ($t_{½}$) is about 17 hours in healthy young subjects and about 21 hours in healthy elderly subjects. Fondaparinux is excreted to 64 – 77 % by the kidney as unchanged compound.

Special populations

Paediatric patients - Fondaparinux has not been investigated in this population.

Elderly patients - Renal function may decrease with age and thus, the elimination capacity for fondaparinux may be reduced in elderly. In patients >75 years undergoing orthopaedic surgery, the estimated plasma clearance was 1.2 to 1.4 times lower than in patients <65 years.

Renal impairment - Compared with patients with normal renal function (creatinine clearance > 80 ml/min), plasma clearance is 1.2 to 1.4 times lower in patients with mild renal impairment (creatinine clearance 50 to 80 ml/min) and on average 2 times lower in patients with moderate renal impairment (creatinine clearance 30 to 50 ml/min). In severe renal impairment (creatinine clearance < 30 ml/min), plasma clearance is approximately 5 times lower than in normal renal function. Associated terminal half-life values were 29 h in moderate and 72 h in patients with severe renal impairment.

Gender - No gender differences were observed after adjustment for body weight.

Race - Pharmacokinetic differences due to race have not been studied prospectively. However, studies performed in Asian (Japanese) healthy subjects did not reveal a different pharmacokinetic profile compared to Caucasian healthy subjects. Similarly, no plasma clearance differences were observed between black and Caucasian patients undergoing orthopaedic surgery.

Body weight - Plasma clearance of fondaparinux increases with body weight (9% increase per 10 kg).

Hepatic impairment - Following a single, subcutaneous dose of fondaparinux in subjects with moderate hepatic impairment (Child-Pugh Category B), total (i.e., bound and unbound) C_{max} and AUC were decreased by 22% and 39%, respectively, as compared to subjects with normal liver function. The lower plasma concentrations of fondaparinux were attributed to reduced binding to ATIII secondary to the lower ATIII plasma concentrations in subjects with hepatic impairment thereby resulting in increased renal clearance of fondaparinux. Consequently, unbound concentrations of fondaparinux are expected to be unchanged in patients with mild to moderate hepatic impairment, and therefore, no dose adjustment is necessary based on pharmacokinetics.

The pharmacokinetics of fondaparinux has not been studied in patients with severe hepatic impairment (see sections 4.2 and 4.4).

5.3 Preclinical safety data

Non-clinical data reveal no special hazard for humans based on conventional studies of safety pharmacology, repeated dose toxicity, and genotoxicity. Animal studies are insufficient with respect to effects on toxicity to reproduction because of limited exposure.

6. PHARMACEUTICAL PARTICULARS

6.1 List of excipients

Sodium chloride

Water for injections

Hydrochloric acid

Sodium hydroxide

6.2 Incompatibilities

In the absence of compatibility studies, this medicinal product must not be mixed with other medicinal products.

6.3 Shelf life

3 years.

If fondaparinux sodium is added to a 0.9% saline minibag it should ideally be infused immediately, but can be stored at room temperature for up to 24 hours.

6.4 Special precautions for storage

Do not freeze.

6.5 Nature and contents of container

Type I glass barrel (1 ml) affixed with a 27 gauge × 12.7 mm needle and stoppered with a bromobutyl or chlorobutyl elastomer plunger stopper.

Arixtra is available in pack sizes of 2, 7, 10 and 20 pre-filled syringes. There are two types of syringes:

- syringe with a blue plunger and an automatic safety system
- syringe with blue plunger and a manual safety system.

Not all pack sizes may be marketed.

6.6 Special precautions for disposal and other handling

The subcutaneous injection is administered in the same way as with a classical syringe. Intravenous administration should be through an existing intravenous line either directly or using a small volume (25 or 50ml) 0.9% saline minibag.

Parenteral solutions should be inspected visually for particulate matter and discoloration prior to administration.

Instruction on self-administration by subcutaneous injection is included in the Package Leaflet.

The needle protection system of the Arixtra pre-filled syringes have been designed with a safety system to protect from needle stick injuries following injection.

Any unused product or waste material should be disposed of in accordance with local requirements.

7. MARKETING AUTHORISATION HOLDER

Glaxo Group Ltd

Greenford

Middlesex

UB6 0NN

United Kingdom

8. MARKETING AUTHORISATION NUMBER(S)

EU/1/02/206/001-004 and 021-023

9. DATE OF FIRST AUTHORISATION/RENEWAL OF THE AUTHORISATION

Date of first authorisation: 21 March 2002

Date of latest renewal: 21 March 2007

10. DATE OF REVISION OF THE TEXT

25 March 2009

Detailed information on this medicinal product is available on the website of the European Medicines Agency (EMEA) http://www.emea.europa.eu

Arixtra 5mg, 7.5mg, 10mg solution for injection, pre-filled syringe

(GlaxoSmithKline UK)

1. NAME OF THE MEDICINAL PRODUCT

Arixtra ▼ 5 mg/0.4 ml solution for injection, pre-filled syringe.

Arixtra ▼ 7.5 mg/0.6 ml solution for injection, pre-filled syringe.

Arixtra ▼ 10 mg/0.8 ml solution for injection, pre-filled syringe.

2. QUALITATIVE AND QUANTITATIVE COMPOSITION

Each pre-filled syringe contains 5 mg, 7.5 mg or 10 mg of fondaparinux sodium in 0.4 ml, 0.6 ml or 10ml solution for injection.

Excipient(s): Contains less than 1 mmol of sodium (23 mg) per dose, and therefore is essentially sodium free.

For a full list of excipients, see section 6.1.

3. PHARMACEUTICAL FORM

Solution for injection.

The solution is a clear and colourless to slightly yellow liquid.

4. CLINICAL PARTICULARS

4.1 Therapeutic indications

Treatment of acute Deep Vein Thrombosis (DVT) and treatment of acute Pulmonary Embolism (PE), except in haemodynamically unstable patients or patients who require thrombolysis or pulmonary embolectomy.

4.2 Posology and method of administration

The recommended dose of fondaparinux is 7.5 mg (patients with body weight ⩾ 50, ⩽ 100kg) once daily administered by subcutaneous injection. For patients with body weight < 50 kg, the recommended dose is 5 mg. For patients with body weight > 100 kg, the recommended dose is 10 mg.

Treatment should be continued for at least 5 days and until adequate oral anticoagulation is established (International Normalised Ratio 2 to 3). Concomitant oral anticoagulation treatment should be initiated as soon as possible and usually within 72 hours. The average duration of administration in clinical trials was 7 days and the clinical experience from treatment beyond 10 days is limited.

Special populations

Elderly patients - No dosing adjustment is necessary. In patients ⩾75 years, fondaparinux should be used with care, as renal function decreases with age (see section 4.4).

Renal impairment - Fondaparinux should be used with caution in patients with moderate renal impairment (see section 4.4).

There is no experience in the subgroup of patients with *both* high body weight (>100 kg) and moderate renal impairment (creatinine clearance 30-50 ml/min). In this subgroup, after an initial 10 mg daily dose, a reduction of the daily dose to 7.5 mg may be considered, based on pharmacokinetic modelling (see section 4.4).

Fondaparinux should not be used in patients with severe renal impairment (creatinine clearance < 30 ml/min) (see section 4.3).

Hepatic impairment - No dosing adjustment is necessary in patients with either mild or moderate hepatic impairment. In patients with severe hepatic impairment, fondaparinux should be used with care as this patient group has not been studied (see sections 4.4 and 5.2).

Paediatric population - Fondaparinux is not recommended for use in children below 17 years of age due to a lack of data on safety and efficacy.

Method of administration

Fondaparinux is administered by deep subcutaneous injection while the patient is lying down. Sites of administration should alternate between the left and the right anterolateral and left and right posterolateral abdominal wall. To avoid the loss of medicinal product when using the pre-filled syringe do not expel the air bubble from the syringe before the injection. The whole length of the needle should be inserted perpendicularly into a skin fold held between the thumb and the forefinger; the skin fold should be held throughout the injection.

For additional instructions for use and handling and disposal see section 6.6.

4.3 Contraindications

- hypersensitivity to the active substance or to any of the excipients
- active clinically significant bleeding
- acute bacterial endocarditis
- severe renal impairment defined by creatinine clearance < 30 ml/min.

4.4 Special warnings and precautions for use

Fondaparinux is intended for subcutaneous use only. Do not administer intramuscularly.

There is limited experience from treatment with fondaparinux in haemodynamically unstable patients and no experience in patients requiring thrombolysis, embolectomy or insertion of a vena cava filter.

Haemorrhage

Fondaparinux should be used with caution in patients who have an increased risk of haemorrhage, such as those with congenital or acquired bleeding disorders (e.g. platelet count <50,000/mm³), active ulcerative gastrointestinal disease and recent intracranial haemorrhage or shortly after brain, spinal or ophthalmic surgery and in special patient groups as outlined below.

As for other anticoagulants, fondaparinux should be used with caution in patients who have undergone recent surgery (<3 days) and only once surgical haemostasis has been established.

Agents that may enhance the risk of haemorrhage should not be administered concomitantly with fondaparinux. These agents include desirudin, fibrinolytic agents, GP IIb/IIIa receptor antagonists, heparin, heparinoids, or Low Molecular Weight Heparin (LMWH). During treatment of VTE, concomitant therapy with vitamin K antagonist should be administered in accordance with the information of Section 4.5. Other antiplatelet medicinal products (acetylsalicylic acid, dipyridamole, sulfinpyrazone, ticlopidine or clopidogrel), and NSAIDs should be used with caution. If co-administration is essential, close monitoring is necessary.

Spinal / Epidural anaesthesia

In patients receiving fondaparinux for treatment of VTE rather than prophylaxis, spinal/epidural anaesthesia in case of surgical procedures should not be used.

Elderly patients

The elderly population is at increased risk of bleeding. As renal function generally decreases with age, elderly patients may show reduced elimination and increased exposure of fondaparinux (see section 5.2). Incidences of bleeding events in patients receiving the recommended regimen in the treatment of DVT or PE and aged <65 years, 65-75 and >75 years were 3.0 %, 4.5 % and 6.5 %, respectively. The corresponding incidences in patients receiving the recommended regimen of enoxaparin in the treatment of DVT were 2.5%, 3.6% and 8.3% respectively, while the incidences in patients receiving the recommended regimen of UFH in the treatment of PE were 5.5%, 6.6% and 7.4%, respectively. Fondaparinux should be used with caution in elderly patients (see section 4.2).

Low body weight

Clinical experience is limited in patients with body weight <50 kg. Fondaparinux should be used with caution at a daily dose of 5 mg in this population (see sections 4.2 and 5.2).

Renal impairment

The risk of bleeding increases with increasing renal impairment. Fondaparinux is known to be excreted mainly by the kidney. Incidences of bleeding events in patients receiving the recommended regimen in the treatment of DVT or PE with normal renal function, mild renal impairment, moderate renal impairment and severe renal impairment were 3.0 % (34/1,132), 4.4 % (32/733), 6.6% (21/318), and 14.5 % (8/55) respectively. The corresponding incidences in patients receiving the recommended regimen of enoxaparin in the treatment of DVT were 2.3% (13/559), 4.6% (17/368), 9.7% (14/145) and 11.1% (2/18) respectively, and in patients receiving the recommended regimen of unfractionated heparin in the treatment of PE were 6.9% (36/523), 3.1% (11/352), 11.1% (18/162) and 10.7% (3/28), respectively.

Fondaparinux is contra-indicated in severe renal impairment (creatinine clearance <30 ml/min) and should be used with caution in patients with moderate renal impairment (creatinine clearance 30-50 ml/min). The duration of treatment should not exceed that evaluated during clinical trial (mean 7 days) (see sections 4.2, 4.3 and 5.2).

There is no experience in the subgroup of patients with both high body weight (>100 kg) and moderate renal impairment (creatinine clearance 30-50 ml/min). Fondaparinux should be used with care in these patients. After an initial 10 mg daily dose, a reduction of the daily dose to 7.5 mg may be considered, based on pharmacokinetic modelling (see section 4.2).

Severe hepatic impairment

The use of fondaparinux should be considered with caution because of an increased risk of bleeding due to a deficiency of coagulation factors in patients with severe hepatic impairment (see section 4.2).

Patients with Heparin Induced Thrombocytopenia

Fondaparinux should be used with caution in patients with a history of HIT. The efficacy and safety of fondaparinux have not been formally studied in patients with HIT type II. Fondaparinux does not bind to platelet factor 4 and does not cross-react with sera from patients with Heparin Induced Thrombocytopenia (HIT) type II. However, rare spontaneous reports of HIT in patients treated with fondaparinux have been received. To date a causal association between treatment with fondaparinux and the occurrence of HIT has not been established.

4.5 Interaction with other medicinal products and other forms of interaction

Bleeding risk is increased with concomitant administration of fondaparinux and agents that may enhance the risk of haemorrhage (see section 4.4).

In clinical studies performed with fondaparinux, oral anticoagulants (warfarin) did not interact with the pharmacokinetics of fondaparinux; at the 10 mg dose used in the interaction studies, fondaparinux did not influence the anticoagulation monitoring (INR) activity of warfarin.

Platelet inhibitors (acetylsalicylic acid), NSAIDs (piroxicam) and digoxin did not interact with the pharmacokinetics of fondaparinux. At the 10 mg dose used in the interaction studies, fondaparinux did not influence the bleeding time under acetylsalicylic acid or piroxicam treatment, nor the pharmacokinetics of digoxin at steady state.

4.6 Pregnancy and lactation

No clinical data on exposed pregnancies are available. Animal studies are insufficient with respect to effects on pregnancy, embryo/foetal development, parturition and postnatal development because of limited exposure. Fondaparinux should not be prescribed to pregnant women unless clearly necessary.

Fondaparinux is excreted in rat milk but it is not known whether fondaparinux is excreted in human milk. Breast-feeding is not recommended during treatment with fondaparinux. Oral absorption by the child is however unlikely.

4.7 Effects on ability to drive and use machines

No studies on the effect on the ability to drive and to use machines have been performed.

4.8 Undesirable effects

The safety of fondaparinux has been evaluated in 2,517 patients treated for Venous Thrombo-Embolism and treated with fondaparinux for an average of 7 days. The most common adverse reactions were bleeding complications (see section 4.4).

The adverse reactions reported by the investigator as at least possibly related to fondaparinux are presented within each frequency grouping (very common ≥ 1/10; common: ≥1/100 to < 1/10; uncommon: ≥ 1/1,000 to < 1/100; rare: ≥ 1/10,000 to <1/1,000; very rare <1/10,000) and system organ class by decreasing order of seriousness.

System organ class MedDRA	Undesirable effects in patients treated for VTE[1]
Blood and lymphatic system disorders	*Common:* bleeding (gastrointestinal, haematuria, haematoma, epistaxis, haemoptysis, utero-vaginal haemorrhage, haemarthrosis, ocular, purpura, bruise) *Uncommon:* anaemia, thrombocytopaenia *Rare:* other bleeding (hepatic, retroperitoneal, intracranial/ intracerebral), thrombocythaemia
Immune system disorders	*Rare:* allergic reaction
Metabolism and nutrition disorders	*Rare:* non-protein-nitrogen (Npn) [2] increased
Nervous system disorders	*Uncommon:* headache *Rare:* dizziness
Gastrointestinal disorders	*Uncommon:* nausea, vomiting
Hepatobiliary disorders	*Uncommon:* abnormal liver function
Skin and subcutaneous tissue disorders	*Rare:* rash erythematous
General disorders and administration site conditions	*Uncommon:* pain, oedema, *Rare:* reaction at injection site

(1) Isolated AEs have not been considered except if they were medically relevant.

(2) Npn stands for non-protein-nitrogen such as urea, uric acid, amino acid, etc.

4.9 Overdose

Fondaparinux doses above the recommended regimen may lead to an increased risk of bleeding. There is no known antidote to fondaparinux.

Overdose associated with bleeding complications should lead to treatment discontinuation and search for the primary cause. Initiation of appropriate therapy such as surgical haemostasis, blood replacements, fresh plasma transfusion, plasmapheresis should be considered.

5. PHARMACOLOGICAL PROPERTIES

5.1 Pharmacodynamic properties

Pharmacotherapeutic group: antithrombotic agents.

ATC code: B01AX05

Pharmacodynamic effects

Fondaparinux is a synthetic and selective inhibitor of activated Factor X (Xa). The antithrombotic activity of fondaparinux is the result of antithrombin III (antithrombin) mediated selective inhibition of Factor Xa. By binding selectively to antithrombin, fondaparinux potentiates (about 300 times) the innate neutralization of Factor Xa by antithrombin. Neutralisation of Factor Xa interrupts the blood coagulation cascade and inhibits both thrombin formation and thrombus development. Fondaparinux does not inactivate thrombin (activated Factor II) and has no effects on platelets.

At the doses used for treatment, fondaparinux does not, to a clinically relevant extent, affect routine coagulation tests such as activated partial thromboplastin time (aPTT), activated clotting time (ACT) or prothrombin time (PT)/International Normalised Ratio (INR) tests in plasma nor bleeding time or fibrinolytic activity. However, rare spontaneous reports of aPTT prolongation have been received. At highe[r] doses, moderate changes in aPTT can occur. At the 10 m[g] dose used in interaction studies, fondaparinux did no[t] significantly influence the anticoagulation activity (INR) o[f] warfarin.

Fondaparinux does not cross-react with sera from patient[s] with heparin-induced thrombocytopaenia.

Clinical studies

The fondaparinux clinical program in treatment of Venous Thromboembolism was designed to demonstrate the effi[]cacy of fondaparinux for the treatment of deep vein throm[]bosis (DVT) and pulmonary embolism (PE). Over 4,87[4] patients were studied in controlled Phase II and III clinica[l] studies.

Treatment of Deep Venous Thrombosis

In a randomised, double-blind, clinical trial in patients with a confirmed diagnosis of acute symptomatic DVT, fondaparinux 5 mg (body weight < 50 kg), 7.5 mg (body weight ≥ 50 kg, ≤ 100 kg) or 10 mg (body weight >100 kg) SC once daily was compared to enoxaparin sodium 1 mg/kg SC twice daily. A total of 2,192 patients were treated; for both groups, patients were treated for at least 5 days and up to 26 days (mean 7 days). Both treatment groups received Vitamin K antagonist therapy usually initiated within 72 hours after the first study drug administration and continued for 90 ± 7 days, with regular dose adjustments to achieve an INR of 2-3. The primary efficacy endpoint was the composite of confirmed symptomatic recurrent non-fatal VTE and fatal VTE reported up to Day 97. Treatment with fondaparinux was demonstrated to be non-inferior to enoxaparin (VTE rates 3.9% and 4.1%, respectively).

Major bleeding during the initial treatment period was observed in 1.1% of fondaparinux patients, compared to 1.2% with enoxaparin.

Treatment of Pulmonary Embolism

A randomised, open-label, clinical trial was conducted in patients with acute symptomatic PE. The diagnosis was confirmed by objective testing (lung scan, pulmonary angiography or spiral CT scan). Patients who required thrombolysis or embolectomy or vena cava filter were excluded. Randomised patients could have been pre-treated with UFH during the screening phase but patients treated for more than 24 hours with therapeutic dose of anticoagulant or with uncontrolled hypertension were excluded. Fondaparinux 5 mg (body weight < 50 kg), 7.5 mg (body weight ≥ 50kg, ≤ 100 kg) or 10 mg (body weight >100 kg) SC once daily was compared to unfractionated heparin IV bolus (5,000 IU) followed by a continuous IV infusion adjusted to maintain 1.5–2.5 times aPTT control value. A total of 2,184 patients were treated; for both groups, patients were treated for at least 5 days and up to 22 days (mean 7 days). Both treatment groups received Vitamin K antagonist therapy usually initiated within 72 hours after the first study drug administration and continued for 90 ± 7 days, with regular dose adjustments to achieve an INR of 2-3. The primary efficacy endpoint was the composite of confirmed symptomatic recurrent non-fatal VTE and fatal VTE reported up to Day 97. Treatment with fondaparinux was demonstrated to be non-inferior to unfractionated heparin (VTE rates 3.8% and 5.0%, respectively).

Major bleeding during the initial treatment period was observed in 1.3% of fondaparinux patients, compared to 1.1% with unfractionated heparin.

5.2 Pharmacokinetic properties

The pharmacokinetics of fondaparinux sodium are derived from fondaparinux plasma concentrations quantified via anti factor Xa activity. Only fondaparinux can be used to calibrate the anti-Xa assay (the international standards of heparin or LMWH are not appropriate for this use). As a result, the concentration of fondaparinux is expressed as milligrams (mg).

Absorption

After subcutaneous dosing, fondaparinux is completely and rapidly absorbed (absolute bioavailability 100%). Following a single subcutaneous injection of fondaparinux 2.5 mg to young healthy subjects, peak plasma concentration (mean C_{max} = 0.34 mg/l) is obtained 2 hours post-dosing. Plasma concentrations of half the mean C_{max} values are reached 25 minutes post-dosing.

In elderly healthy subjects, pharmacokinetics of fondaparinux is linear in the range of 2 to 8 mg by subcutaneous route. Following once daily dosing, steady state of plasma levels is obtained after 3 to 4 days with a 1.3-fold increase in C_{max} and AUC.

Mean (CV%) steady state pharmacokinetic parameters estimates of fondaparinux in patients undergoing hip replacement surgery receiving fondaparinux 2.5 mg once daily are: C_{max} (mg/l) - 0.39 (31%), T_{max} (h) - 2.8 (18%) and C_{min} (mg/l) -0.14 (56%). In hip fracture patients, associated with their increased age, fondaparinux steady state plasma concentrations are: C_{max} (mg/l) - 0.50 (32%), C_{min} (mg/l) - 0.19 (58%).

In DVT and PE treatment, patients receiving fondaparinux 5 mg (body weight <50 kg), 7.5 mg (body weight 50-100 kg inclusive) and 10 mg (body weight >100 kg) once daily, the body weight-adjusted doses provide similar exposure across all body weight categories. The mean (CV%) steady tate pharmacokinetic parameters estimates of fondaparıux in patients with VTE receiving the fondaparinux proosed dose regimen once daily are: C_{max} (mg/l) - 1.41 23 %), T_{max} (h) – 2.4 (8%) and C_{min} (mg/l) -0.52 (45 %). he associated 5th and 95th percentiles are, respectively, .97 and 1.92 for C_{max} (mg/l), and 0.24 and 0.95 for C_{min} mg/l).

Distribution

he distribution volume of fondaparinux is limited (7-11 tres). *In vitro*, fondaparinux is highly and specifically ound to antithrombin protein with a dose-dependant lasma concentration binding (98.6% to 97.0% in the oncentration range from 0.5 to 2 mg/l). Fondaparinux loes not bind significantly to other plasma proteins, includng platelet factor 4 (PF4).

Since fondaparinux does not bind significantly to plasma roteins other than antithrombin, no interaction with other nedicinal products by protein binding displacement are xpected.

Metabolism

Although not fully evaluated, there is no evidence of fondaparinux metabolism and in particular no evidence for the ormation of active metabolites.

Fondaparinux does not inhibit CYP450s (CYP1A2, CYP2A6, CYP2C9, CYP2C19, CYP2D6, CYP2E1 or CYP3A4) *in vitro*. Thus, fondaparinux is not expected to nteract with other medicinal products *in vivo* by inhibition of CYP-mediated metabolism.

Excretion/Elimination

The elimination half-life ($t_{½}$) is about 17 hours in healthy young subjects and about 21 hours in healthy elderly subjects. Fondaparinux is excreted to 64 – 77 % by the kidney as unchanged compound.

Special populations

Paediatric patients - Fondaparinux has not been investigated in this population.

Elderly patients - Renal function may decrease with age and thus, the elimination capacity for fondaparinux may be reduced in elderly. In patients >75 years undergoing orthopaedic surgery and receiving fondaparinux 2.5 mg once daily, the estimated plasma clearance was 1.2 to 1.4 times lower than in patients <65 years. A similar pattern is observed in DVT and PE treatment patients.

Renal impairment - Compared with patients with normal renal function (creatinine clearance > 80 ml/min) undergoing orthopaedic surgery and receiving fondaparinux 2.5 mg once daily, plasma clearance is 1.2 to 1.4 times lower in patients with mild renal impairment (creatinine clearance 50 to 80 ml/min) and on average 2 times lower in patients with moderate renal impairment (creatinine clearance 30 to 50 ml/min). In severe renal impairment (creatinine clearance <30 ml/min), plasma clearance is approximately 5 times lower than in normal renal function. Associated terminal half-life values were 29 h in moderate and 72 h in patients with severe renal impairment. A similar pattern is observed in DVT and PE treatment patients.

Body weight - Plasma clearance of fondaparinux increases with body weight (9% increase per 10 kg).

Gender - No gender differences were observed after adjustment for body weight.

Race - Pharmacokinetic differences due to race have not been studied prospectively. However, studies performed in Asian (Japanese) healthy subjects did not reveal a different pharmacokinetic profile compared to Caucasian healthy subjects. Similarly, no plasma clearance differences were observed between black and Caucasian patients undergoing orthopaedic surgery.

Hepatic impairment - Following a single, subcutaneous dose of fondaparinux in subjects with moderate hepatic impairment (Child-Pugh Category B), total (i.e., bound and unbound) C_{max} and AUC were decreased by 22% and 39%, respectively, as compared to subjects with normal liver function. The lower plasma concentrations of fondaparinux were attributed to reduced binding to ATIII secondary to the lower ATIII plasma concentrations in subjects with hepatic impairment thereby resulting in increased renal clearance of fondaparinux. Consequently, unbound concentrations of fondaparinux are expected to be unchanged in patients with mild to moderate hepatic impairment, and therefore, no dose adjustment is necessary based on pharmacokinetics.

The pharmacokinetics of fondaparinux has not been studied in patients with severe hepatic impairment (see sections 4.2 and 4.4).

5.3 Preclinical safety data

Non-clinical data reveal no special hazard for humans based on conventional studies of safety pharmacology and genotoxicity. The repeated dose and reproduction toxicity studies did not reveal any special risk but did not provide adequate documentation of safety margins due to limited exposure in the animal species.

6. PHARMACEUTICAL PARTICULARS

6.1 List of excipients

Sodium chloride

Water for injections

Hydrochloric acid

Sodium hydroxide

6.2 Incompatibilities

In the absence of compatibility studies, this medicinal product must not be mixed with other medicinal products.

6.3 Shelf life

3 years

6.4 Special precautions for storage

Do not freeze.

6.5 Nature and contents of container

Type I glass barrel (1 ml) affixed with a 27 gauge × 12.7 mm needle and stoppered with a chlorobutyl elastomer plunger stopper.

Arixtra 5 mg/0.4 ml is available in pack sizes of 2, 7, 10 and 20 pre-filled syringes. There are two types of syringes:

- syringe with a orange plunger and an automatic safety system
- syringe with orange plunger and a manual safety system.

Arixtra 7.5 mg/0.6 ml is available in pack sizes of 2, 7, 10 and 20 pre-filled syringes. There are two types of syringes:

- syringe with a magenta plunger and an automatic safety system
- syringe with magenta plunger and a manual safety system.

Arixtra 10 mg/0.8 ml is available in pack sizes of 2, 7, 10 and 20 pre-filled syringes. There are two types of syringes:

- syringe with a violet plunger and an automatic safety system
- syringe with violet plunger and a manual safety system.

Not all pack sizes may be marketed.

6.6 Special precautions for disposal and other handling

The subcutaneous injection is administered in the same way as with a classical syringe.

Parenteral solutions should be inspected visually for particulate matter and discoloration prior to administration.

Instruction for self-administration is mentioned in the Package Leaflet.

The Arixtra pre-filled syringes have been designed with a needle protection system to prevent needle stick injuries following injection.

Any unused product or waste material should be disposed of in accordance with local requirements.

This medicinal product is for single use only.

7. MARKETING AUTHORISATION HOLDER

Glaxo Group Ltd

Greenford

Middlesex

UB6 0NN

United Kingdom

8. MARKETING AUTHORISATION NUMBER(S)

Arixtra 5 mg/0.4 ml EU/1/02/206/009-011, 018 and 027-028, 033

Arixtra 7.5 mg/0.6 ml EU/1/02/206/012-014, 019 and 029-030, 034

Arixtra 10 mg/0.8 ml EU/1/02/206/015-017, 020 and 031-032, 035

9. DATE OF FIRST AUTHORISATION/RENEWAL OF THE AUTHORISATION

Date of first authorisation: 21 March 2002

Date of latest renewal: 21 March 2007

10. DATE OF REVISION OF THE TEXT

22 December 2008

Detailed information on this medicinal product is available on the website of the European Medicines Agency (EMEA) http://www.emea.europa.eu

Aromasin

(Pharmacia Limited)

1. NAME OF THE MEDICINAL PRODUCT

Aromasin®25 mg coated tablets.

2. QUALITATIVE AND QUANTITATIVE COMPOSITION

Active substance: exemestane

Each coated tablet contains 25 mg exemestane.

Each tablet contains 30.2mg of sucrose and 0.003mg of methyl parahydroxybenzoate (E218). For full list of excipients, see section 6.1.

3. PHARMACEUTICAL FORM

Coated tablet

Round, biconvex, off-white coated tablet marked 7663 on one side.

4. CLINICAL PARTICULARS

4.1 Therapeutic indications

Aromasin®is indicated for the adjuvant treatment of postmenopausal women with oestrogen receptor positive invasive early breast cancer, following 2 – 3 years of initial adjuvant tamoxifen therapy.

Aromasin® is indicated for the treatment of advanced breast cancer in women with natural or induced postmenopausal status whose disease has progressed following anti-oestrogen therapy. Efficacy has not been demonstrated in patients with oestrogen receptor negative status.

4.2 Posology and method of administration

Adult and elderly patients

The recommended dose of Aromasin® is one 25 mg tablet to be taken once daily, preferably after a meal.

In patients with early breast cancer, treatment with Aromasin® should continue until completion of five years of combined sequential adjuvant hormonal therapy (tamoxifen followed by Aromasin®), or earlier if tumour relapse occurs.

In patients with advanced breast cancer, treatment with Aromasin® should continue until tumour progression is evident.

No dose adjustments are required for patients with hepatic or renal insufficiency (see 5.2).

Children

Not recommended for use in children

4.3 Contraindications

Aromasin® tablets are contraindicated in patients with a known hypersensitivity to the active substance or to any of the excipients, in pre-menopausal women and in pregnant or lactating women.

4.4 Special warnings and precautions for use

Aromasin® should not be administered to women with premenopausal endocrine status. Therefore, whenever clinically appropriate, the post-menopausal status should be ascertained by assessment of LH, FSH and oestradiol levels.

Aromasin®should be used with caution in patients with hepatic or renal impairment.

Aromasin®tablets contain sucrose and should not be administered to patients with rare hereditary problems of fructose intolerance, glucose-galactose malabsorption or sucrase-isomaltase insufficiency.

Aromasin®tablets contain methyl-p-hydroxybenzoate which may cause allergic reactions (possibly delayed).

Aromasin® is a potent oestrogen lowering agent, and a reduction in bone mineral density and an increased fracture rate-has been observed following administration (see section 5.1). During adjuvant treatment with Aromasin®, women with osteoporosis or at risk of osteoporosis should have their bone mineral density formally assessed by bone densitometry at the commencement of treatment. Although adequate data to show the effects of therapy in the treatment of the bone mineral density loss caused by Aromasin® are not available, treatment for osteoporosis should be initiated in at risk patients. Patients treated with Aromasin® should be carefully monitored.

4.5 Interaction with other medicinal products and other forms of interaction

In vitro evidence showed that the drug is metabolised through cytochrome P450 (CYP) 3A4 and aldoketoreductases (see 5.2) and does not inhibit any of the major CYP isoenzymes. In a clinical pharmacokinetic study, the specific inhibition of CYP 3A4 by ketoconazole showed no significant effects on the pharmacokinetics of exemestane.

In an interaction study with rifampicin, a potent CYP450 inducer, at a dose of 600mg daily and a single dose of exemestane 25mg, the AUC of exemestane was reduced by 54% and Cmax by 41%. Since the clinical relevance of this interaction has not been evaluated, the co-administration of drugs, such as rifampicin, anticonvulsants (e.g. phenytoin and carbamazepine) and herbal preparations containing hypericum perforatum (St John's Wort) known to induce CYP3A4 may reduce the efficacy of Aromasin®.

Aromasin® should be used cautiously with drugs that are metabolised via CYP3A4 and have a narrow therapeutic window. There is no clinical experience of the concomitant use of Aromasin® with other anticancer drugs.

Aromasin® should not be coadministered with oestrogen-containing medicines as these would negate its pharmacological action.

4.6 Pregnancy and lactation

Pregnancy

No clinical data on exposed pregnancies are available with Aromasin®. Studies on animals have shown reproductive toxicity (See section 5.3). Aromasin® is therefore contra-indicated in pregnant women.

Lactation

It is not known whether exemestane is excreted into human milk. Aromasin® should not be administered to lactating woman.

Women of perimenopausal status or child-bearing potential

The physician needs to discuss the necessity of adequate contraception with women who have the potential to become pregnant including women who are perimenopausal or who have recently become postmenopausal, until their postmenopausal status is fully established (see sections 4.3 'Contraindications' and 4.4 – 'Special warnings and precautions for use').

4.7 Effects on ability to drive and use machines

Drowsiness, somnolence, asthenia and dizziness have been reported with the use of the drug. Patients should be advised that, if these events occur, their physical and/or mental abilities required for operating machinery or driving a car may be impaired.

4.8 Undesirable effects

Aromasin® was generally well tolerated across all clinical studies conducted with Aromasin® at a standard dose of 25 mg/day, and undesirable effects were usually mild to moderate.

The withdrawal rate due to adverse events was 7.4% in patients with early breast cancer receiving adjuvant treatment with Aromasin® following initial adjuvant tamoxifen therapy. The most commonly reported adverse reactions were hot flushes (22%), arthralgia (18%) and fatigue (16%).

The withdrawal rate due to adverse events was 2.8% in the overall patient population with advanced breast cancer. The most commonly reported adverse reactions were hot flushes (14%) and nausea (12%).

Most adverse reactions can be attributed to the normal pharmacological consequences of oestrogen deprivation (e.g. hot flushes).

The reported adverse reactions are listed below by system organ class and by frequency.

Frequencies are defined as: very common (> 10%), common (> 1%, ≤ 10%), uncommon (> 0.1%, ≤ 1%), rare (> 0.01%, ≤ 0.1%).

Metabolism and nutrition disorders:	
Common	Anorexia
Psychiatric disorders:	
Very common	Insomnia
Common	Depression
Nervous system disorders:	
Very common	Headache
Common	Dizziness, carpal tunnel syndrome
Uncommon	Somnolence
Vascular disorders:	
Very common	Hot flushes
Gastrointestinal disorders:	
Very common	Nausea
Common	Abdominal pain, vomiting, constipation, dyspepsia, diarrhoea
Skin and subcutaneous tissue disorders:	
Very common	Increased sweating
Common	Rash, alopecia
Musculoskeletal and bone disorders:	
Very common	Joint and musculoskeletal pain (*)
Common	Osteoporosis, fracture
General disorders and administration site conditions:	
Very common	Fatigue
Common	Pain, peripheral oedema
Uncommon	Asthenia

(*) Includes: arthralgia, and less frequently pain in limb, osteoarthritis, back pain, arthritis, myalgia and joint stiffness

Blood and lymphatic system disorders

In patients with advanced breast cancer thrombocytopenia and leucopenia have been rarely reported. An occasional decrease in lymphocytes has been observed in approximately 20% of patients receiving Aromasin®, particularly in patients with pre-existing lymphopenia; however, mean lymphocyte values in these patients did not change significantly over time and no corresponding increase in viral infections was observed. These effects have not been observed in patients treated in early breast cancer studies.

Hepatobiliary disorders

Elevation of liver function test parameters including enzymes, bilirubin and alkaline phosphatase have been observed.

The table below presents the frequency of pre-specified adverse events and illnesses in the early breast cancer study (IES), irrespective of causality, reported in patients receiving trial therapy and up to 30 days after cessation of trial therapy.

Adverse events and illnesses	Exemestane (N = 2249)	Tamoxifen (N = 2279)
Hot flushes	491 (21.8%)	457 (20.1%)
Fatigue	367 (16.3%)	344 (15.1%)
Headache	305 (13.6%)	255 (11.2%)
Insomnia	290 (12.9%)	204 (9.0%)
Sweating increased	270 (12.0%)	242 (10.6%)
Gynaecological	235 (10.5%)	340 (14.9%)
Dizziness	224 (10.0%)	200 (8.8%)
Nausea	200 (8.9%)	208 (9.1%)
Osteoporosis	116 (5.2%)	66 (2.9%)
Vaginal haemorrhage	90 (4.0%)	121 (5.3%)
Other primary cancer	84 (3.6%)	125 (5.3%)
Vomiting	50 (2.2%)	54 (2.4%)
Visual disturbance	45 (2.0%)	53 (2.3%)
Thromboembolism	16 (0.7%)	42 (1.8%)
Osteoporotic fracture	14 (0.6%)	12 (0.5%)
Myocardial infarction	13 (0.6%)	4 (0.2%)

In the IES study, the frequency of ischemic cardiac events in the exemestane and tamoxifen treatment arms was 4.5% versus 4.2%, respectively. No significant difference was noted for any individual cardiovascular event including hypertension (9.9% versus 8.4%), myocardial infarction (0.6% versus 0.2%) and cardiac failure (1.1% versus 0.7%).

In the IES study, exemestane was associated with a greater incidence of hypercholesterolemia compared with tamoxifen (3.7% vs. 2.1%).

In a separate double blinded, randomized study of postmenopausal women with early breast cancer at low risk treated with exemestane (N=73) or placebo (N=73) for 24 months, exemestane was associated with an average 7-9% mean reduction in plasma HDL-cholesterol, versus a 1% increase on placebo. There was also a 5-6% reduction in apolipoprotein A1 in the exemestane group versus 0-2% for placebo. The effect on the other lipid parameters analysed (total cholesterol, LDL cholesterol, triglycerides, apolipoprotein-B and lipoprotein-a) was very similar in the two treatment groups. The clinical significance of these results is unclear.

In the IES study, gastric ulcer was observed at a higher frequency in the exemestane arm compared to tamoxifen (0.7% versus <0.1%). The majority of patients on exemestane with gastric ulcer received concomitant treatment with non-steroidal anti-inflammatory agents and/or had a prior history.

Adverse reactions from post-marketing experience

Hepatobiliary disorders: Hepatitis, cholestatic hepatitis

Because reactions are reported voluntarily from a population of uncertain size, it is not always possible to reliably estimate their frequency or establish a causal relationship to drug exposure.

4.9 Overdose

Clinical trials have been conducted with Aromasin® given up to 800 mg in a single dose to healthy female volunteers and up to 600 mg daily to postmenopausal women with advanced breast cancer; these dosages were well tolerated. The single dose of Aromasin® that could result in life-threatening symptoms is not known. In rats and dogs, lethality was observed after single oral doses equivalent respectively to 2000 and 4000 times the recommended human dose on a mg/m^2 basis. There is no specific antidote to overdosage and treatment must be symptomatic. General supportive care, including frequent monitoring of vital signs and close observation of the patient, is indicated.

5. PHARMACOLOGICAL PROPERTIES

5.1 Pharmacodynamic properties

Pharmacotherapeutic group: steroidal aromatase inhibitor; anti-neoplastic agent

ATC: L02BG06.

Exemestane is an irreversible, steroidal aromatase inhibitor, structurally related to the natural substrate androstenedione. In post-menopausal women, oestrogens are produced primarily from the conversion of androgens into oestrogens through the aromatase enzyme in peripheral tissues. Oestrogen deprivation through aromatase inhibition is an effective and selective treatment for hormone dependent breast cancer in postmenopausal women. In postmenopausal women, Aromasin® p.o. significantly lowered serum oestrogen concentrations starting from a 5 mg dose, reaching maximal suppression (>90%) with a dos of 10-25 mg. In postmenopausal breast cancer patient treated with the 25 mg daily dose, whole body aromatization was reduced by 98%.

Exemestane does not possess any progestogenic or oestrogenic activity. A slight androgenic activity, probably du to the 17-hydro derivative, has been observed mainly a high doses. In multiple daily doses trials, Aromasin® had n detectable effects on adrenal biosynthesis of cortisol c aldosterone, measured before or after ACTH challenge thus demonstrating its selectivity with regard to the othe enzymes involved in the steroidogenic pathway.

Glucocorticoid or mineralocorticoid replacements ar therefore not needed. A non dose-dependent sligh increase in serum LH and FSH levels has been observe even at low doses: this effect is, however, expected for th pharmacological class and is probably the result of feed back at the pituitary level due to the reduction in oestroger levels that stimulate the pituitary secretion of gonadotropins also in postmenopausal women.

Adjuvant Treatment of Early Breast Cancer

In a multicentre, randomised, double-blind study, conducted in 4724 postmenopausal patients with oestrogen-receptor-positive or unknown primary breast cancer patients who had remained disease-free after receiving adjuvant tamoxifen therapy for 2 to 3 years were randomised to receive 3 to 2 years of Aromasin® (25 mg/day) o tamoxifen (20 or 30 mg/day) to complete a total of 5 years of hormonal therapy.

After a median duration of therapy of about 30 months and a median follow-up of about 52 months, results showed that sequential treatment with Aromasin® after 2 to 3 years of adjuvant tamoxifen therapy was associated with a clinically and statistically significant improvement in disease-free survival (DFS) compared with continuation of tamoxifen therapy. Analysis showed that in the observed study period Aromasin® reduced the risk of breast cancer recurrence by 24% compared with tamoxifen (hazard ratio 0.76; p=0.00015). The beneficial effect of exemestane over tamoxifen with respect to DFS was apparent regardless of nodal status or prior chemotherapy.

Aromasin® also significantly reduced the risk of contralateral breast cancer (hazard ratio 0.57, p=0.04158).

In the whole study population, a trend for improved overall survival was observed for exemestane (222 deaths) compared to tamoxifen (262 deaths) with a hazard ratio 0.85 (log-rank test: p = 0.07362), representing a 15% reduction in the risk of death in favour of exemestane. A statistically significant 23% reduction in the risk of dying (hazard ratio for overall survival 0.77; Wald chi square test: p = 0.0069) was observed for exemestane compared to tamoxifen when adjusting for the pre-specified prognostic factors (i.e., ER status, nodal status, prior chemotherapy, use of HRT and use of bisphosphonates).

Main efficacy results in all patients (intention to treat population) and oestrogen receptor positive patients are summarised in the table below:

(see Table 1 on next page)

In the additional analysis for the subset of patients with **oestrogen** receptor positive or unknown status, the unadjusted overall survival hazard ratio was 0.83 (log-rank test: p = 0.04250), representing a clinically and statistically significant 17% reduction in the risk of dying.

Results from a bone substudy demonstrated that women treated with Aromasin® following 2 to 3 years of tamoxifen treatment experienced moderate reduction in bone mineral density. In the overall study, the treatment emergent fracture incidence evaluated during the 30 months treatment period was higher in patients treated with Aromasin® compared with tamoxifen (4.5% and 3.3% correspondingly, p=0.038).

Results from an endometrial substudy indicate that after 2 years of treatment there was a median 33% reduction of endometrial thickness in the Aromasin®-treated patients compared with no notable variation in the tamoxifen-treated patients. Endometrial thickening, reported at the start of study treatment, was reversed to normal (< 5 mm) for 54% of patients treated with Aromasin®.

Treatment of Advanced Breast Cancer

In a randomised peer reviewed controlled clinical trial, Aromasin® at the daily dose of 25 mg has demonstrated statistically significant prolongation of survival, Time to Progression (TTP), Time to Treatment Failure (TTF) as compared to a standard hormonal treatment with megestrol acetate in postmenopausal patients with advanced breast cancer that had progressed following, or during, treatment with tamoxifen either as adjuvant therapy or as first-line treatment for advanced disease.

5.2 Pharmacokinetic properties

Absorption:

After oral administration of Aromasin® tablets, exemestane is absorbed rapidly. The fraction of the dose absorbed from the gastrointestinal tract is high. The absolute bioavailability in humans is unknown, although it is anticipated to be limited by an extensive first pass effect. A similar effect resulted in an absolute bioavailability in rats and dogs of 5%. After a single dose of 25 mg, maximum plasma levels of 18 ng/ml are reached after 2 hours. Concomitant intake with food increases the bioavailability by 40%.

Table 1

Endpoint Population	Exemestane Events /N (%)	Tamoxifen Events /N (%)	Hazard Ratio (95% CI)	p-value*
Disease-free survival [a]				
All patients	**354**/2352 (15.1%)	**453**/2372 (19.1%)	0.76 (0.67-0.88)	0.00015
ER+ patients	**289**/2023 (14.3%)	**370**/2021 (18.3%)	0.75 (0.65-0.88)	0.00030
Contralateral breast cancer				
All patients	**20**/2352 (0.9%)	**35**/2372 (1.5%)	0.57 (0.33-0.99)	0.04158
ER+ patients	**18**/2023 (0.9%)	**33**/2021 (1.6%)	0.54 (0.30-0.95)	0.03048
Breast cancer free survival [b]				
All patients	**289**/2352 (12.3%)	**373**/2372 (15.7%)	0.76 (0.65-0.89)	0.00041
ER+ patients	**232**/2023 (11.5%)	**305**/2021 (15.1%)	0.73 (0.62-0.87)	0.00038
Distant recurrence free survival [c]				
All patients	**248**/2352 (10.5%)	**297**/2372 (12.5%)	0.83 (0.70-0.98)	0.02621
ER+ patients	**194**/2023 (9.6%)	**242**/2021 (12.0%)	0.78 (0.65-0.95)	0.01123
Overall survival *d*				
All patients	**222**/2352 (9.4%)	**262**/2372 (11.0%)	0.85 (0.71-1.02)	0.07362
ER+ patients	**178**/2023 (8.8%)	**211**/2021 (10.4%)	0.84 (0.68-1.02)	0.07569

* Log-rank test; ER+ patients = oestrogen receptor positive patients;
[a] Disease-free survival is defined as the first occurrence of local or distant recurrence, contralateral breast cancer, or death from any cause;
[b] Breast cancer free survival is defined as the first occurrence of local or distant recurrence, contralateral breast cancer or breast cancer death;
[c] Distant recurrence free survival is defined as the first occurrence of distant recurrence or breast cancer death;
[d] Overall survival is defined as occurrence of death from any cause.

Distribution:

The volume of distribution of exemestane, not corrected for the oral bioavailability, is ca 20000 l. The kinetics is linear and the terminal elimination half-life is 24 h. Binding to plasma proteins is 90% and is concentration independent. Exemestane and its metabolites do not bind to red blood cells.

Exemestane does not accumulate in an unexpected way after repeated dosing.

Metabolism and excretion:

Exemestane is metabolised by oxidation of the methylene moiety on the 6 position by CYP 3A4 isoenzyme and/or reduction of the 17-keto group by aldoketoreductase followed by conjugation. The clearance of exemestane is ca 500 l/h, not corrected for the oral bioavailability.

The metabolites are inactive or the inhibition of aromatase is less than the parent compound.

The amount excreted unchanged in urine is 1% of the dose. In urine and faeces equal amounts (40%) of ^{14}C-labeled exemestane were eliminated within a week.

Special populations

Age: No significant correlation between the systemic exposure of Aromasin® and the age of subjects has been observed.

Renal insufficiency:

In patients with severe renal impairment ($CL_{cr} < 30$ ml/min) the systemic exposure to exemestane was 2 times higher compared with healthy volunteers.

Given the safety profile of exemestane, no dose adjustment is considered to be necessary.

Hepatic insufficiency:

In patients with moderate or severe hepatic impairment the exposure of exemestane is 2-3 fold higher compared with healthy volunteers. Given the safety profile of exemestane, no dose adjustment is considered to be necessary.

5.3 Preclinical safety data

Toxicological studies: Findings in the repeat dose toxicology studies in rat and dog were generally attributable to the pharmacological activity of exemestane, such as effects on reproductive and accessory organs. Other toxicological effects (on liver, kidney or central nervous system) were observed only at exposures considered sufficiently in excess of the maximum human exposure indicating little relevance to clinical use.

Mutagenicity: Exemestane was not genotoxic in bacteria (Ames test), in V79 Chinese hamster cells, in rat hepatocytes or in the mouse micronucleus assay. Although exemestane was clastogenic in lymphocytes *in vitro*, it was not clastogenic in two *in vivo* studies.

Reproductive toxicology: Exemestane was embryotoxic in rats and rabbits at systemic exposure levels similar to those obtained in humans at 25 mg/day. There was no evidence of teratogenicity.

Carcinogenicity: In a two-year carcinogenicity study in female rats, no treatment-related tumors were observed. In male rats the study was terminated on week 92, because of early death by chronic nephropathy. In a two-year carcinogenicity study in mice, an increase in the incidence of hepatic neoplasms in both genders was observed at the intermediate and high doses (150 and 450 mg/kg/day). This finding is considered to be related to the induction of hepatic microsomal enzymes, an effect observed in mice but not in clinical studies. An increase in the incidence of renal tubular adenomas was also noted in male mice at the high dose (450 mg/kg/day). This change is considered to be species and gender-specific and occurred at a dose which represents 63-fold greater exposure than occurs at the human therapeutic dose. None of these observed effects is considered to be clinically relevant to the treatment of patients with exemestane.

6. PHARMACEUTICAL PARTICULARS

6.1 List of excipients

Tablet core: Silica colloidal hydrated; Crospovidone; Hypromellose; Magnesium stearate; Mannitol; Microcrystalline cellulose; Sodium starch glycolate (Type A); polysorbate

Sugar-coating: Hypromellose; Polyvinylalcohol; Simeticone; Macrogol: Sucrose; Magnesium carbonate, light; Titanium dioxide(E171); Methyl Parahydroxybenzoate (E218); Cetyl esters wax; Talc; Carnauba wax.

Printing ink: Ethyl alcohol; Shellac; Iron oxides (E172), Titanium oxide (E171)

6.2 Incompatibilities

Not applicable.

6.3 Shelf life

3 years.

6.4 Special precautions for storage

This medicinal product does not require any special storage conditions.

6.5 Nature and contents of container

30 and 90 tablets in blister packs (Aluminium-PVDC/PVC-PVDC)

6.6 Special precautions for disposal and other handling

No special requirements.

7. MARKETING AUTHORISATION HOLDER

Pharmacia Ltd.
Ramsgate Road
Sandwich
CT13 9NJ
UK

8. MARKETING AUTHORISATION NUMBER(S)

PL 0032/0236

9. DATE OF FIRST AUTHORISATION/RENEWAL OF THE AUTHORISATION

16th December 1998 / 8th August 2008

10. DATE OF REVISION OF THE TEXT

15/05/09

Legal category: POM

Company reference AM8_0

Arthrotec 50 Tablets

(Pharmacia Limited)

1. NAME OF THE MEDICINAL PRODUCT

Arthrotec 50 modified-release tablets.

2. QUALITATIVE AND QUANTITATIVE COMPOSITION

Each tablet consists of a gastro-resistant core containing 50mg diclofenac sodium surrounded by an outer mantle containing 200mcg misoprostol.

Excipient(s):

Each tablet contains 13 mg lactose monohydrate.

For a full list of excipients, see section 6.1.

3. PHARMACEUTICAL FORM

Modified-release tablet.

White, round, biconvex tablets marked on one side and 'Searle 1411' on the other side.

4. CLINICAL PARTICULARS

4.1 Therapeutic indications

Arthrotec 50 is indicated for patients who require the non-steroidal anti-inflammatory drug diclofenac together with misoprostol.

The diclofenac component of Arthrotec 50 is indicated for the symptomatic treatment of osteoarthritis and rheumatoid arthritis. The misoprostol component of Arthrotec 50 is indicated for patients with a special need for the prophylaxis of NSAID-induced gastric and duodenal ulceration

4.2 Posology and method of administration

Adults

One tablet to be taken with food, two or three times daily. Tablets should be swallowed whole, not chewed.

Elderly/Renal Impairment/Hepatic Impairment

No adjustment of dosage is necessary in the elderly or in patients with hepatic impairment or mild to moderate renal impairment as pharmacokinetics are not altered to any clinically relevant extent. Nevertheless patients with renal or hepatic impairment should be closely monitored (see section 4.4 and section 4.8).

Children

The safety and efficacy of Arthrotec 50 in children has not been established.

Undesirable effects may be minimised by using the lowest effective dose for the shortest duration necessary to control symptoms (see section 4.4).

4.3 Contraindications

Arthrotec 50 is contraindicated in:

- Patients with active peptic ulcer/haemorrhage or perforation or who have active GI bleeding or other active bleedings e.g. cerebrovascular bleedings.
- Pregnant women and in women planning a pregnancy.
- Patients with a known hypersensitivity to diclofenac, aspirin, other NSAIDs, misoprostol, other prostaglandins, or any other ingredient of the product.
- Patients in whom attacks of asthma, urticaria or acute rhinitis are precipitated by aspirin or other non-steroidal anti-inflammatory agents.
- Treatment of peri-operative pain in the setting of coronary bypass graft (CABG) surgery.
- Patients with severe renal and hepatic failure.
- Patients with severe heart failure.

4.4 Special warnings and precautions for use

Warnings

The use of diclofenac/misoprostol with concomitant NSAIDs including COX-2 inhibitors should be avoided.

Use in pre-menopausal women (see also section 4.3))

Arthrotec 50 should not be used in pre-menopausal women unless they use effective contraception and have been advised of the risks of taking the product if pregnant (see section 4.6). The label will state: 'Not for use by pre-menopausal women unless using effective contraception'.

Precautions

Undesirable effects may be minimised by using the lowest effective dose for the shortest duration necessary to control symptoms (see section 4.2, and GI and cardiovascular risks below).

- Renal/Cardiac/Hepatic

In patients with renal, cardiac or hepatic impairment caution is required since the use of NSAIDs may result in deterioration of renal function. In the following conditions Arthrotec 50 should be used only in exceptional circumstances and with close clinical monitoring: advanced cardiac failure, advanced kidney failure, advanced liver disease, severe dehydration.

Diclofenac metabolites are eliminated primarily by the kidneys (see section 5.2). The extent to which the metabolites may accumulate in patients with renal failure has not been studied. As with other NSAIDs, metabolites of which are excreted by the kidney, patients with significantly impaired renal function should be more closely monitored.

In rare cases, NSAIDs, including diclofenac/misoprostol, may cause interstitial nephritis, glomerulitis, papillary necrosis and the nephrotic syndrome. NSAIDs inhibit the synthesis of renal prostaglandin which plays a supportive role in the maintenance of renal perfusion in patients whose renal blood flow and blood volume are decreased. In these patients, administration of an NSAID may precipitate overt renal decompensation, which is typically followed by recovery to pretreatment state upon discontinuation of NSAID therapy. Patients at greatest risk of such a reaction are those with congestive heart failure, liver cirrhosis, nephrotic syndrome and overt renal disease. Such patients should be carefully monitored while receiving NSAID therapy.

Appropriate monitoring and advice are required for patients with a history of hypertension and/or mild to moderate congestive heart failure as fluid retention and oedema have been reported in association with NSAID therapy.

As with all NSAIDS, diclofenac/misoprostol can lead to the onset of new hypertension or worsening of pre-existing hypertension, either of which may contribute to the increased incidence of cardiovascular events. NSAIDs, including diclofenac/misoprostol, should be used with caution in patients with hypertension. Blood pressure should be monitored closely during the initiation of therapy with diclofenac/misoprostol and throughout the course of therapy.

Patients with uncontrolled hypertension, congestive heart failure, established ischaemic heart disease, peripheral arterial disease, and/or cerebrovascular disease should only be treated with diclofenac after careful consideration. Similar consideration should be made before initiating longer-term treatment of patients with risk factors for cardiovascular events (e.g. hypertension, hyperlipidaemia, diabetes mellitus, smoking).

Clinical trial and epidemiological data suggest that use of diclofenac, particularly at high dose (150mg daily) and in long term treatment may be associated with a small increased risk of serious arterial thrombotic events (for example myocardial infarction or stroke).

Physicians and patients should remain alert for the development of such events, even in the absence of previous cardiovascular symptoms. Patients should be informed about the signs and/or symptoms of serious cardiovascular toxicity and the steps to take if they occur (see section 4.3).

• Blood system/Gastrointestinal

NSAIDs, including diclofenac/misoprostol, can cause serious gastrointestinal (GI) adverse events including inflammation, bleeding, ulceration, and perforation of the stomach, small intestine, or large intestine, which can be fatal. When GI bleeding or ulceration occurs in patients receiving diclofenac/misoprostol, the treatment should be withdrawn. These events can occur at any time during treatment, with or without warning symptoms or in patients with a previous history of serious GI events.

Patients most at risk of developing these types of GI complications with NSAIDs are those treated at higher doses, the elderly, patients with cardiovascular disease, patients using concomitant aspirin, or patients with a prior history of, or active, gastrointestinal disease, such as ulceration, GI bleeding or inflammatory conditions.

Therefore, diclofenac/misoprostol should be used with caution in these patients and commence on treatment at the lowest dose available (see section 4.3).

Patients with a history of GI toxicity, particularly when elderly, should report any unusual abdominal symptoms (especially GI bleeding) particularly in the initial stages of treatment. Caution should be advised in patients receiving concomitant medicines which could increase the risk of ulceration or bleeding, such as oral corticosteroids, anticoagulants such as warfarin, selective serotonin-reuptake inhibitors or anti-platelet agents such as aspirin (see section 4.5).

Arthrotec 50, in common with other NSAIDs, may decrease platelet aggregation and prolong bleeding time. Extra supervision is recommended in haematopoietic disorders or in conditions with defective coagulation or in patients with a history of cerebrovascular bleeding.

Caution is required in patients suffering from ulcerative colitis or Crohn's Disease as these conditions may be exacerbated (see section 4.8).

Care should be taken in elderly patients and in patients treated with corticosteroids, other NSAIDs, or anti-coagulants (see section 4.5).

• Skin Reactions

Serious skin reactions, some of them fatal, including exfoliative dermatitis, Stevens-Johnson syndrome, and toxic epidermal necrolysis, have been reported very rarely in association with the use of NSAIDs, including diclofenac/misoprostol (see section 4.8). Patients appear to be at highest risk for these events early in the course of therapy, the onset of the event occurring in the majority of cases within the first month of treatment. Diclofenac/misoprostol should be discontinued at the first appearance of skin rash, mucosal lesions, or any other sign of hypersensitivity

• Hypersensitivity

NSAIDs may precipitate bronchospasm in patients suffering from, or with a history of, bronchial asthma or allergic disease.

• Long-term treatment

All patients who are receiving long-term treatment with NSAIDs should be monitored as a precautionary measure (e.g. renal, hepatic function and blood counts). During long-term, high dose treatment with analgesic/anti-inflammatory drugs, headaches can occur which must not be treated with higher doses of the medicinal product.

Arthrotec may mask fever and thus an underlying infection.

Patients with rare hereditary problems of galactose intolerance, the Lapp lactase deficiency or glucose-galactose malabsorption should not take this medicine.

4.5 Interaction with other medicinal products and other forms of interaction

NSAIDs may attenuate the natriuretic efficacy of diuretics due to inhibition of intrarenal synthesis of prostaglandins. Concomitant treatment with potassium-sparing diuretics may be associated with increased serum potassium levels, hence serum potassium should be monitored.

Because of their effect on renal prostaglandins, cyclo-oxygenase inhibitors such as diclofenac can increase the nephrotoxicity of ciclosporin. There is a possible increased risk of nephrotoxicity when NSAIDs are given with tacrolimus.

Steady state plasma lithium and digoxin levels may be increased and ketoconazole levels may be decreased.

Pharmacodynamic studies with diclofenac have shown no potentiation of oral hypoglycaemic and anticoagulant drugs. However as interactions have been reported with other NSAIDs, caution and adequate monitoring are, nevertheless advised (see statement on platelet aggregation in Precautions).

Because of decreased platelet aggregation caution is also advised when using Arthrotec 50 with anti-coagulants. NSAIDs may enhance the effects of anti-coagulants, such as warfarin, antiplatelet agents, such as aspirin, and serotonin re-uptake inhibitors (SSRIs) thereby increasing the risk of gastrointestinal bleeding (see section 4.4).

Cases of hypo and hyperglycaemia have been reported when diclofenac was associated with antidiabetic agents.

Caution is advised when methotrexate is administered concurrently with NSAIDs because of possible enhancement of its toxicity by the NSAID as a result of increase in methotrexate plasma levels.

Concomitant use with other NSAIDs or with corticosteroids may increase the frequency of side effects generally.

Anti-hypertensives including diuretics, angiotensin-converting enzyme (ACE) inhibitors and angiotensin II antagonists (AIIA): NSAIDs can reduce the efficacy of diuretics and other antihypertensive drugs.

In patients with impaired renal function (e.g. dehydrated patients or elderly patients with compromised renal function), the co-administration of an ACE inhibitor or an AIIA with a cyclo-oxygenase inhibitor can increase the deterioration of the renal function, including the possibility of acute renal failure, which is usually reversible. The occurrence of these interactions should be considered in patients taking diclofenac/misoprostol with an ACE inhibitor or an AIIA.

Antacids may delay the absorption of diclofenac. Magnesium-containing antacids have been shown to exacerbate misoprostol-associated diarrhoea.

Animal data indicate that NSAIDs can increase the risk of convulsions associated with quinolone antibiotics. Patients taking NSAIDs and quinolones may have an increased risk of developing convulsions.

NSAIDs should not be used for 8-12 days after mifepristone administration as NSAIDs can reduce the effect of mifepristone.

4.6 Pregnancy and lactation

Pregnancy

Arthrotec 50 is contraindicated in pregnant women and in women planning a pregnancy because misoprostol induces uterine contractions and is associated with abortion, premature birth, and foetal death. Use of misoprostol has been associated with birth defects. Also diclofenac may cause premature closure of the ductus arteriosus.

Women of childbearing potential should not be started on diclofenac/misoprostol until pregnancy is excluded, and should be fully counseled on the importance of adequate contraception while undergoing treatment. If pregnancy is suspected, use of the product should be discontinued.

Lactation

Misoprostol is rapidly metabolised in the mother to misoprostol acid, which is biologically active and is excreted in breast milk. Diclofenac is excreted in breast milk in very small quantities. In general, the potential effects on the infant from any exposure to misoprostol and its metabolites via breast feeding are unknown. However, diarrhoea is a recognised side effect of misoprostol and could occur in infants of nursing mothers. Arthrotec 50 should therefore not be administered to nursing mothers.

4.7 Effects on ability to drive and use machines

Patients who experience dizziness or other central nervous system disturbances while taking NSAIDs should refrain from driving or operating machinery.

4.8 Undesirable effects

In the table below the incidence of adverse drug reactio reported in controlled clinical studies where Arthrotec wa administered to more than 2000 patients are listed. Add tionally, adverse drug reactions reported during post-ma keting surveillance are whose frequency cannot b estimated from the available data, such as spontaneou reports, have been listed at frequency 'unknown'. Th most commonly observed adverse events are gastrointes inal in nature.

(see Table 1 on next page)

Given the lack of precise and/or reliable denominator ar numerator figures, the spontaneous adverse event repor ing system through which post marketing safety data a collected does not allow for a medically meaningful *fr quency of occurrence* of any undesirable effects.

With regard to the *relative frequency of reporting* adverse reactions during post marketing surveillance, th undesirable effects at the gastrointestinal level were thos received most frequently by the MAH (approximately 45 of all case reports in the company safety database) fo lowed by cutaneous/hypersensitivity-type reaction which is in agreement with the known side effects prof of the NSAIDs drug class.

Clinical trial and epidemiological data suggest that use diclofenac, particularly at high doses (150 mg daily) and long term treatment may be associated with a sm increased risk of arterial thrombotic events (for examp myocardial infarction or stroke) (see section 4.4).

4.9 Overdose

The toxic dose of Arthrotec 50 has not been determin and there is no experience of overdosage. Intensification the pharmacological effects may occur with overdosag Management of acute poisoning with NSAIDs essentia consists of supportive and symptomatic measures. It reasonable to take measures to reduce absorption of a recently consumed drug by forced emesis, gastric lava or activated charcoal.

5. PHARMACOLOGICAL PROPERTIES

5.1 Pharmacodynamic properties

Pharmacotherapeutic group (ATC code): M01BX

Arthrotec 50 is a non-steroidal, anti-inflammatory dr which is effective in treating the signs and symptoms arthritic conditions.

This activity is due to the presence of diclofenac which h been shown to have anti-inflammatory and analgesic pro erties.

Arthrotec 50 also contains the gastroduodenal muco protective component misoprostol which is a synthe prostaglandin E_1 analogue that enhances several of t factors that maintain gastroduodenal mucosal integrity.

5.2 Pharmacokinetic properties

The pharmacokinetic profiles of diclofenac and misopro tol administered as Arthrotec 50 are similar to the profi when the two drugs are administered as separate table and there are no pharmacokinetic interactions between t two components.

Diclofenac sodium is completely absorbed from t gastrointestinal (GI) tract after fasting oral administratio Only 50 % of the absorbed dose is systemically availa due to first pass metabolism. Peak plasma levels a achieved in 2 hours (range 1-4 hours), and the are under-the plasma-concentration curve (AUC) is dose p portional within the range of 25 mg to 150 mg. The extent diclofenac sodium absorption is not significantly affect by food intake.

The terminal half-life is approximately 2 hours. Clearan and volume of distribution are about 350 ml/min a 550 ml/kg, respectively. More than 99 % of diclofen sodium is reversibly bound to human plasma album and this has been shown not to be age dependent.

Diclofenac sodium is eliminated through metabolism a subsequent urinary and biliary excretion of the glucuroni and the sulfate conjugates of the metabolites. Appro mately 65 % of the dose is excreted in the urine and 35 % the bile. Less than 1 % of the parent drug is excret unchanged.

Misoprostol is rapidly and extensively absorbed, and undergoes rapid metabolism to its active metabolite, m oprostol acid, which is eliminated with an elimination $t_{1/2}$ about 30 minutes. No accumulation of misoprostol a was found in multiple-dose studies, and plasma stea state was achieved within 2 days. The serum protein bin ing of misoprostol acid is less than 90 %. Approximat 70 % of the administered dose is excreted in the urin mainly as biologically inactive metabolites.

5.3 Preclinical safety data

In co-administration studies in animals, the addition misoprostol did not enhance the toxic effects of diclofen The combination was also shown not to be teratogenic mutagenic. The individual components show no eviden of carcinogenic potential.

Misoprostol in multiples of the recommended therapeu dose in animals has produced gastric mucosal hyperp sia. This characteristic response to E-series prostagla dins reverts to normal on discontinuation of the compou

Table 1

Organ System	Very Common (≥ 1/10)	Common (≥ 1/100 and < 1/10)	Uncommon (≥ 1/1,000 and < 1/100)	Rare (≥ 1/10,000, and < 1/1,000)	Frequency: Unknown (Post-marketing experience)
Infections and infestations					Aseptic meningitis[1]
Blood and lymphatic system disorders			Thrombo-cytopenia		Aplastic anaemia, agranulocytosis, haemolytic anaemia, leucopenia
Immune system disorders				Anaphylactic reaction	Hypersensitivity
Metabolism and nutrition disorders					Anorexia
Psychiatric disorders		Insomnia			Psychotic reaction, disorientation, depression, anxiety, nightmares, mood change, irritability
Nervous system disorders		Headache, dizziness			Convulsions, memory disturbance, drowsiness, tremor, taste disturbance, paraesthesia
Eyes disorders					Visual disturbances, blurred vision
Ear and labyrinth disorders					Tinnitus
Cardiac disorders					Cardiac failure, palpitations
Vascular disorders					Shock, hypertension, hypotension, vasculitis
Respiratory, thoracic and mediastinal disorders					Asthma, pneumonitis, dyspnoea
Gastrointestinal disorders	Abdominal pain, diarrhoea[2], nausea, dyspepsia	Gastritis, vomiting, flatulence, eructation, constipation, peptic ulcer	Stomatitis		GI perforation [3], gastrointestinal bleeding [3], melaena, haematemesis, colitis, Crohn's disease, oesophageal disorder, mouth ulceration, glossitis, tongue odema, dry mouth
Hepato-biliary disorders		Alanine amino-transferase increased		Hepatitis, jaundice	Hepatitis fulminant, aspartate aminotransferase increased, blood bilirubin increased
Skin and subcutaneous tissue disorders		Erythema multiforme, rash, pruritus	Purpura, urticaria	Angioedema	Toxic epidermal necrolysis[4], Stevens-Johnson syndrome[4], dermatitis exfoliative[4], dermatitis bullous, Henoch Schonlein purpura, mucocutaneous rash, rash vesicular, photosensitivity reaction, alopecia, urticaria
Renal and urinary disorders					Renal failure, acute renal failure, renal papillary necrosis, nephritis interstitial, nephrotic syndrome, proteinuria, haematuria
Pregnancy, puerperium and perinatal conditions					Intra-uterine death, uterine rupture, incomplete abortion, premature baby, anaphylactoid syndrome of pregnancy, retained placenta or membranes, uterine contractions abnormal
Reproductive system and breast disorders			Menorrhagia, metrorrhagia, vaginal haemorrhage, postmenopausal haemorrhage		Uterine haemorrhage
Congenital, familial and genetic disorders					Birth defects
General disorders and administration site conditions					Oedema[5], chest pain, face oedema, fatigue, pyrexia, chills, inflammation
Investigations		Blood alkaline phosphatase increased			Decreased haemoglobin
Injury, poisoning and procedural complications					Uterine perforation

[1] Symptoms of aseptic meningitis (stiff neck, headache, nausea, vomiting, fever or impaired consciousness) have been reported during treatment with NSAIDs. Patients suffering from autoimmune disease (e.g. lupus erythematosus, mixed connective tissue disorders) seem to be more susceptible.

[2] Diarrhoea is usually mild to moderate and transient and can be minimised by taking Arthrotec 50 with food and by avoiding the use of predominantly magnesium-containing antacids.

[3] GI perforation or bleeding can sometimes be fatal, particularly in the elderly (see section 4.4).

[4] Serious skin reactions, some of them fatal, have been reported very rarely (see section 4.4).

[5] Especially in patients with hypertension or impaired renal function (see section 4.4).

6. PHARMACEUTICAL PARTICULARS

6.1 List of excipients

Arthrotec 50 tablets contain:

Core:

Lactose monohydrate

microcrystalline cellulose

maize starch

povidone K-30

magnesium stearate

Mantle/Coat:

cellulose acetate phthalate

diethyl phthalate

methylhydroxpropylcellulose

crospovidone

hydrogenated castor oil

colloidal silicon dioxide

microcrystalline cellulose

6.2 Incompatibilities

Not applicable.

6.3 Shelf life

Arthrotec 50 has a shelf-life of 3 years when stored in cold-formed blisters.

6.4 Special precautions for storage

Store in a dry place. Do not store above 25°C.

6.5 Nature and contents of container

Arthrotec 50 is presented in cold formed aluminium blisters in pack sizes of 6, 7, 56, 60, 84, 100, 120 and 140 (supplied as 14 packs of 10 tablets shrink wrapped together) tablets.

Not all pack sizes may be marketed.

6.6 Special precautions for disposal and other handling

No Special requirements.

7. MARKETING AUTHORISATION HOLDER

Pharmacia Limited

Ramsgate Road

Sandwich

Kent

CT13 9NJ

United Kingdom

8. MARKETING AUTHORISATION NUMBER(S)

PL 00032/0396

9. DATE OF FIRST AUTHORISATION/RENEWAL OF THE AUTHORISATION

Date of first authorisation: 15 April 2002

Date of last renewal: 23 January 2007

10. DATE OF REVISION OF THE TEXT

September 2009

11. LEGAL CATEGORY

POM

Ref: AE 8_0

Arthrotec 75 Tablets

(Pharmacia Limited)

1. NAME OF THE MEDICINAL PRODUCT

Arthrotec 75 modified-release tablets

2. QUALITATIVE AND QUANTITATIVE COMPOSITION

Each tablet consists of a gastro-resistant core containing 75 mg diclofenac sodium surrounded by an outer mantle containing 200 micrograms misoprostol.

Excipient(s):

Each tablet contains 19.5 mg lactose monohydrate.

For a full list of excipients, see section 6.1.

3. PHARMACEUTICAL FORM

Modified-release tablet.

White, round, biconvex tablets marked 'SEARLE' over '1421' on one side, and four times 'A' around the circumference with '75' in the centre on the reverse side.

4. CLINICAL PARTICULARS

4.1 Therapeutic indications

Arthrotec 75 is indicated for patients who require the non-steroidal anti-inflammatory drug diclofenac together with misoprostol.

The diclofenac component of Arthrotec 75 is indicated for the symptomatic treatment of osteoarthritis and rheumatoid arthritis. The misoprostol component of Arthrotec 75 is indicated for patients with a special need for the prophylaxis of NSAID-induced gastric and duodenal ulceration.

4.2 Posology and method of administration

Undesirable effects may be minimised by using the lowest effective dose for the shortest duration necessary to control symptoms (see section 4.4).

Adults

One tablet to be taken with food, two times daily. Tablets should be swallowed whole, not chewed.

Elderly/Renal, Cardiac and Hepatic Impairment

No adjustment of dosage is necessary in the elderly or in patients with hepatic impairment or mild to moderate renal impairment as pharmacokinetics are not altered to any clinically relevant extent. Nevertheless, elderly patients and patients with renal, cardiac or hepatic impairment should be closely monitored (see section 4.4 and section 4.8).

Children (under 18 years)

The safety and efficacy of Arthrotec 75 in children has not been established.

4.3 Contraindications

Arthrotec 75 is contraindicated in:

- Patients with active peptic ulcer/haemorrhage or perforation or who have active GI bleeding or other active bleedings e.g. cerebrovascular bleedings.
- Pregnant women and in women planning a pregnancy.
- Patients with a known hypersensitivity to diclofenac, aspirin, other NSAIDs, misoprostol, other prostaglandins, or any other ingredient of the product.
- Patients in whom, attacks of asthma, urticaria or acute rhinitis are precipitated by aspirin or other non-steroidal anti-inflammatory agents.
- Treatment of peri-operative pain in the setting of coronary artery bypass graft (CABG) surgery.
- Patients with severe renal and hepatic failure.
- Patients with severe heart failure.

4.4 Special warnings and precautions for use

Warnings

The use of diclofenac/misoprostol with concomitant NSAIDs including COX-2 inhibitors should be avoided.

Use in pre-menopausal women (see also section 4.3)

Arthrotec 75 should not be used in pre-menopausal women unless they use effective contraception and have been advised of the risks of taking the product if pregnant (see section 4.6).

The label will state: 'Not for use in pre-menopausal women unless using effective contraception'.

Precautions

Undesirable effects may be minimised by using the lowest effective dose for the shortest duration necessary to control symptoms (see section 4.2, and GI and cardiovascular risks below).

• Renal/Cardiac/Hepatic

In patients with renal, cardiac or hepatic impairment and in the elderly, caution is required since the use of NSAIDs may result in deterioration of renal function. In the following conditions Arthrotec 75 should be used only in exceptional circumstances and with close clinical monitoring: advanced cardiac failure, advanced kidney failure, advanced liver disease, severe dehydration.

Diclofenac metabolites are eliminated primarily by the kidneys (see section 5.2). The extent to which the metabolites may accumulate in patients with renal failure has not been studied. As with other NSAIDs, metabolites of which are excreted by the kidney, patients with significantly impaired renal function should be more closely monitored.

In rare cases, NSAIDs, including diclofenac/misoprostol, may cause interstitial nephritis, glomerulitis, papillary necrosis and the nephrotic syndrome. NSAIDs inhibit the synthesis of renal prostaglandin which plays a supportive role in the maintenance of renal perfusion in patients whose renal blood flow and blood volume are decreased. In these patients, administration of an NSAID may precipitate overt renal decompensation, which is typically followed by recovery to pre-treatment state upon discontinuation of NSAID therapy. Patients at greatest risk of such a reaction are those with congestive heart failure, liver cirrhosis, nephrotic syndrome and overt renal disease. Such patients should be carefully monitored while receiving NSAID therapy.

Appropriate monitoring and advice are required for patients with a history of hypertension and/or mild to moderate congestive heart failure as fluid retention and oedema have been reported in association with NSAID therapy.

As with all NSAIDS, diclofenac/misoprostol can lead to the onset of new hypertension or worsening of pre-existing hypertension, either of which may contribute to the increased incidence of cardiovascular events. NSAIDs, including diclofenac/misoprostol, should be used with caution in patients with hypertension. Blood pressure should be monitored closely during the initiation of therapy with diclofenac/misoprostol and throughout the course of therapy.

Patients with uncontrolled hypertension, congestive heart failure, established ischaemic heart disease, peripheral arterial disease, and/or cerebrovascular disease should only be treated with diclofenac after careful consideration. Similar consideration should be made before initiating longer-term treatment of patients with risk factors for cardiovascular events (e.g. hypertension, hyperlipidaemia, diabetes mellitus, smoking).

Clinical trial and epidemiological data suggest that use of diclofenac, particularly at high dose (150mg daily) and in long term treatment may be associated with a small increased risk of serious arterial thrombotic events (for example myocardial infarction or stroke).

Physicians and patients should remain alert for the development of such events, even in the absence of previous cardiovascular symptoms. Patients should be informed about the signs and/or symptoms of serious cardiovascular toxicity and the steps to take if they occur (see section 4.3).

• Blood system/Gastrointestinal

NSAIDs, including diclofenac/misoprostol, can cause serious gastrointestinal (GI) adverse events including inflammation, bleeding, ulceration, and perforation of the stomach, small intestine, or large intestine, which can be fatal. When GI bleeding or ulceration occurs in patients receiving diclofenac/misoprostol, the treatment should be withdrawn. These events can occur at any time during treatment, with or without warning symptoms or in patients with a previous history of serious GI events.

Patients most at risk of developing these types of GI complications with NSAIDs are those treated at higher doses, the elderly, patients with cardiovascular disease, patients using concomitant aspirin, or patients with a prior history of, or active, gastrointestinal disease, such as ulceration, GI bleeding or inflammatory conditions.

Therefore, diclofenac/misoprostol should be used with caution in these patients and commence on treatment at the lowest dose available (see section 4.3).

Patients with a history of GI toxicity, particularly when elderly, should report any unusual abdominal symptoms (especially GI bleeding) particularly in the initial stages of treatment. Caution should be advised in patients receiving concomitant medicines which could increase the risk of ulceration or bleeding, such as oral corticosteroids, anticoagulants such as warfarin, selective serotonin-reuptake inhibitors or anti-platelet agents such as aspirin (see section 4.5).

Arthrotec 75 in common with other NSAIDs, may decrease platelet aggregation and prolong bleeding time. Extra supervision is recommended in haematopoietic disorders or in conditions with defective coagulation or in patients with a history of cerebrovascular bleeding.

Caution is required in patients suffering from ulcerative colitis or Crohn's Disease as these conditions may be exacerbated (see section 4.8).

Care should be taken in elderly patients and in patients treated with corticosteroids, other NSAIDs, or anti-coagulants (see section 4.5).

• Skin Reactions

Serious skin reactions, some of them fatal, including exfoliative dermatitis, Stevens-Johnson syndrome, and toxic epidermal necrolysis, have been reported very rarely in association with the use of NSAIDs, including diclofenac/misoprostol (see section 4.8). Patients appear to be at highest risk for these events early in the course of therapy, the onset of the event occurring in the majority of cases within the first month of treatment. Diclofenac/misoprostol should be discontinued at the first appearance of skin rash, mucosal lesions, or any other sign of hypersensitivity.

• Hypersensitivity

NSAIDs may precipitate bronchospasm in patients suffering from, or with a history of bronchial asthma or allergic disease.

• Long-term treatment

All patients who are receiving long-term treatment with NSAIDs should be monitored as a precautionary measure (e.g. renal, hepatic function and blood counts). During long-term, high dose treatment with analgesic/anti-inflammatory drugs, headaches can occur which must not be treated with higher doses of the medicinal product.

• Arthrotec may mask fever and thus an underlying infection.

• Patients with rare hereditary problems of galactose intolerance, the Lapp lactase deficiency or glucose-galactose malabsorption should not take this medicine.

4.5 Interaction with other medicinal products and oth forms of interaction

NSAIDs may attenuate the natriuretic efficacy of diureti due to inhibition of intrarenal synthesis of prostaglandir Concomitant treatment with potassium-sparing diuretic may be associated with increased serum potassium level hence serum potassium should be monitored.

Because of their effect on renal prostaglandins, cycl oxygenase inhibitors such as diclofenac can increase th nephrotoxicity of ciclosporin. There is a possible increase risk of nephrotoxicity when NSAIDs are given with tacr limus.

Steady state plasma lithium and digoxin levels may b increased and ketoconazole levels may be decreased.

Pharmacodynamic studies with diclofenac have shown n potentiation of oral hypoglycaemic and anticoagular drugs. However as interactions have been reported wit other NSAIDs, caution and adequate monitoring ar nevertheless advised (see statement on platelet aggrega tion in Precautions).

Because of decreased platelet aggregation caution i advised when using Arthrotec 75 with anti-coagulants NSAIDs may enhance the effects of anti-coagulants, suc as warfarin, aniplatelet agents, such as aspirin, and ser otonin re-uptake inhibitors (SSRIs) thereby increasing th risk of gastrointestinal bleeding (see section 4.4).

Cases of hypo and hyperglycaemia have been reporte when diclofenac was associated with antidiabetic agents

Caution is advised when methotrexate is administere concurrently with NSAIDs because of possible enhance ment of its toxicity by the NSAID as a result of increase i methotrexate plasma levels.

Concomitant use with other NSAIDs or with corticosteroids may increase the frequency of gastrointestinal ulceration o bleeding and of side effects generally.

Anti-hypertensives including diuretics, angiotensin-converting enzyme (ACE) inhibitors and angiotensin II antagonists (AIIA): NSAIDs can reduce the efficacy of diuretics and other antihypertensive drugs.

In patients with impaired renal function (e.g. dehydrated patients or elderly patients with compromised renal function), the co-administration of an ACE inhibitor or an AIIA with a cyclo-oxygenase inhibitor can increase the deterioration of the renal function, including the possibility of acute renal failure, which is usually reversible. The occurrence of these interactions should be considered in patients taking diclofenac/misoprostol with an ACE inhibitor or an AIIA.

Antacids may delay the absorption of diclofenac. Magnesium-containing antacids have been shown to exacerbate misoprostol-associated diarrhoea.

Animal data indicate that NSAIDs can increase the risk of convulsions associated with quinolone antibiotics. Patients taking NSAIDs and quinolones may have an increased risk of developing convulsions.

NSAIDs should not be used for 8-12 days after mifepristone administration as NSAIDs can reduce the effect of mifepristone.

4.6 Pregnancy and lactation

Pregnancy

Arthrotec 75 is contraindicated in pregnant women and in women planning a pregnancy because misoprostol induces uterine contractions and is associated with abortion, premature birth, and foetal death. Use of misoprostol has been associated with birth defects. Also diclofenac may cause premature closure of the ductus arteriosus.

Women of childbearing potential should not be started on diclofenac/misoprostol until pregnancy is excluded, and should be fully counselled on the importance of adequate contraception while undergoing treatment. If pregnancy is suspected, use of the product should be discontinued.

Lactation

Misoprostol is rapidly metabolised in the mother to misoprostol acid, which is biologically active and is excreted in breast milk. Diclofenac is excreted in breast milk in very small quantities. In general, the potential effects on the infant from any exposure to misoprostol and its metabolites via breast feeding are unknown. However, diarrhoea is a recognised side effect of misoprostol and could occur in infants of nursing mothers. Arthrotec 75 should therefore not be administered to nursing mothers.

4.7 Effects on ability to drive and use machines

Patients who experience dizziness or other central nervous system disturbances while taking NSAIDs should refrain from driving or operating machinery.

4.8 Undesirable effects

In the table below the incidence of adverse drug reactions reported in controlled clinical studies where Arthrotec was administered to more than 2000 patients are listed. Additionally, adverse drug reactions reported during post-marketing surviellance are whose frequency cannot be estimated from the availalbe data, such as spontaneous reports, have been listed at frequency 'unknown'. The most commonly observed adverse events are gastrointestinal in nature.

(see Table 1 on next page)

Given the lack of precise and/or reliable denominator and numerator figures, the spontaneous adverse event

Table 1

Organ System	Very Common (≥ 1/10)	Common (≥1/100 and <1/10)	Uncommon (≥1/1,000 and <1/100)	Rare (≥1/10,000, and <1/1,000)	Frequency: Unknown (Post-marketing experience)
Infections and infestations					Aseptic meningitis[1]
Blood and lymphatic system disorders			Thrombo-cytopenia		Aplastic anaemia, agranulocytosis, haemolytic anaemia, leucopenia
Immune system disorders				Anaphylactic reaction	Hypersensitivity
Metabolism and nutrition disorders					Anorexia
Psychiatric disorders		Insomnia			Psychotic reaction, disorientation, depression, anxiety, nightmares, mood change, irritability
Nervous system disorders		Headache, dizziness			Convulsions, memory disturbance, drowsiness, tremor, taste disturbance, paraesthesia
Eyes disorders					Visual disturbances, blurred vision
Ear and labyrinth disorders					Tinnitus
Cardiac disorders					Cardiac failure, palpitations
Vascular disorders					Shock, hypertension, hypotension, vasculitis
Respiratory, thoracic and mediastinal disorders					Asthma, pneumonitis, dyspnoea
Gastrointestinal disorders	Abdominal pain, diarrhoea[2], nausea, dyspepsia	Gastritis, vomiting, flatulence, eructation, constipation, peptic ulcer	Stomatitis		GI perforation[3], gastrointestinal bleeding[3], melaena, haematemesis, colitis, Crohn's disease, oesophageal disorder, mouth ulceration, glossitis, tongue odema, dry mouth
Hepato-biliary disorders		Alanine amino-transferase increased		Hepatitis, jaundice	Hepatitis fulminant, aspartate aminotransferase increased, blood bilirubin increased
Skin and subcutaneous tissue disorders		Erythema multiforme, rash, pruritus	Purpura, urticaria	Angioedema	Toxic epidermal necrolysis[4], Stevens-Johnson syndrome[4], dermatitis exfoliative[4], dermatitis bullous, Henoch Schonlein purpura, mucocutaneous rash, rash vesicular, photosensitivity reaction, alopecia, urticaria
Renal and urinary disorders					Renal failure, acute renal failure, renal papillary necrosis, nephritis interstitial, nephrotic syndrome, proteinuria, haematuria
Pregnancy, puerperium and perinatal conditions					Intra-uterine death, uterine rupture, incomplete abortion, premature baby, anaphylactoid syndrome of pregnancy, retained placenta or membranes, uterine contractions abnormal
Reproductive system and breast disorders			Menorrhagia, metrorrhagia, vaginal haemorrhage, postmenopausal haemorrhage		Uterine haemorrhage
Congenital, familial and genetic disorders					Birth defects
General disorders and administration site conditions					Oedema[5], chest pain, face oedema, fatigue, pyrexia, chills, inflammation
Investigations		Blood alkaline phosphatase increased			Decreased haemoglobin
Injury, poisoning and procedural complications					Uterine perforation

[1] Symptoms of aseptic meningitis (stiff neck, headache, nausea, vomiting, fever or impaired consciousness) have been reported during treatment with NSAIDs. Patients suffering from autoimmune disease (e.g. lupus erythematosus, mixed connective tissue disorders) seem to be more susceptible.

[2] Diarrhoea is usually mild to moderate and transient and can be minimised by taking Arthrotec 75 with food and by avoiding the use of predominantly magnesium-containing antacids.

[3] GI perforation or bleeding can sometimes be fatal, particularly in the elderly (see section 4.4).

[4] Serious skin reactions, some of them fatal, have been reported very rarely (see section 4.4).

[5] Especially in patients with hypertension or impaired renal function (see section 4.4).

reporting system through which post marketing safety data are collected does not allow for a medically meaningful *frequency of occurrence* of any undesirable effects.

With regard to the *relative frequency of reporting* of adverse reactions during post marketing surveillance, the undesirable effects at the gastrointestinal level were those received most frequently by the MAH (approximately 45% of all case reports in the company safety database) followed by cutaneous/hypersensitivity-type reactions, which is in agreement with the known side effects profile of the NSAIDs drug class.

Clinical trial and epidemiological data suggest that use of diclofenac, particularly at high doses (150 mg daily) and in long term treatment may be associated with a small increased risk of arterial thrombotic events (for example myocardial infarction or stroke) (see section 4.4).

4.9 Overdose

The toxic dose of Arthrotec 75 has not been determined and there is no experience of overdosage. Intensification of the pharmacological effects may occur with overdosage. Management of acute poisoning with NSAIDs essentially consists of supportive and symptomatic measures. It is reasonable to take measures to reduce absorption of any recently consumed drug by forced emesis, gastric lavage or activated charcoal.

5. PHARMACOLOGICAL PROPERTIES

5.1 Pharmacodynamic properties

Pharmacotherapeutic group (ATC code): M01BX

Arthrotec 75 is a non-steroidal, anti-inflammatory drug, which is effective in treating the signs and symptoms of arthritic conditions.

This activity is due to the presence of diclofenac, which has been shown to have anti-inflammatory and analgesic properties.

Arthrotec 75 also contains the gastroduodenal mucosal protective component misoprostol, which is a synthetic prostaglandin E_1 analogue that enhances several of the factors that maintain gastroduodenal mucosal integrity.

Arthrotec 75 administered bd provides 200 micrograms less misoprostol than Arthrotec tds, whilst providing the same daily dose (150 mg) of diclofenac and may offer a better therapeutic ratio for certain patients.

5.2 Pharmacokinetic properties

The pharmacokinetic profiles following oral administration of a single dose or multiple doses of diclofenac sodium and misoprostol administered as Arthrotec 75 are similar to the profiles when the two drugs are administered as separate tablets. There are no pharmacokinetic interactions between the two components, apart from a slight decrease in diclofenac sodium Cmax when administered concomitantly with misoprostol.

Diclofenac sodium is completely absorbed from the gastrointestinal (GI) tract after fasting oral administration. Only 50 % of the absorbed dose is systemically available due to first pass metabolism. Peak plasma levels are achieved in 2 hours (range 1-4 hours), when given as a single dose under fasting conditions. Under fed conditions diclofenac Tmax is increased to 4 hours. The area-under-the plasma-concentration curve (AUC) is dose proportional within the range of 25 mg to 150 mg. The steady state absorption of diclofenac is reduced following the administration of Arthrotec 75 tablets with food, Cmax and AUC are reduced by approximately 40% and 20%, respectively.

The terminal half-life is approximately 2 hours. Clearance and volume of distribution are about 350 ml/min and 550 ml/kg, respectively. More than 99 % of diclofenac sodium is reversibly bound to human plasma albumin, and this has been shown not to be age dependent.

Diclofenac sodium is eliminated through metabolism and subsequent urinary and biliary excretion of the glucuronide and the sulfate conjugates of the metabolites. Approximately 65 % of the dose is excreted in the urine and 35 % in the bile. Less than 1 % of the parent drug is excreted unchanged.

Misoprostol is rapidly and extensively absorbed, and it undergoes rapid metabolism to its active metabolite, misoprostol acid, which is eliminated with an elimination $t_{½}$ of about 30 minutes. No accumulation of misoprostol acid was found in multiple-dose studies, and plasma steady state was achieved within 2 days. The serum protein binding of misoprostol acid is less than 90 %. Approximately 70 % of the administered dose is excreted in the urine, mainly as biologically inactive metabolites.

Single and multiple dose studies have been conducted comparing the pharmacokinetics of Arthrotec 75 with the diclofenac 75 mg and misoprostol 200 micrograms components administered separately. Bioequivalence between the two methods of providing diclofenac were demonstrable for AUC and absorption rate (C_{max}/AUC). In the steady state comparisons under fasted conditions bioequivalence was demonstrable in terms of AUC. Food reduced the rate and extent of absorption of diclofenac for both Arthrotec 75 and co-administered diclofenac. Despite the virtually identical mean AUCs in the fed, steady state, statistical bioequivalence was not established. This however is due to the broad co-efficients of variation in these studies due to the wide inter-individual variability in time to absorption and the extensive first-pass metabolism that occurs with diclofenac.

Bioequivalence in terms of AUC (0-24 h) was demonstrable when comparing steady state pharmacokinetics of Arthrotec 75 given bd with diclofenac 50 mg/misoprostol 200 micrograms given tds, both regimens providing a total daily dose of 150 mg diclofenac.

With respect to administration of misoprostol, bioequivalence was demonstrated after a single dose of Arthrotec 75 or misoprostol administered alone. Under steady state conditions food decreases the misoprostol C_{max} after Arthrotec 75 administration and slightly delays absorption, but the AUC is equivalent.

5.3 Preclinical safety data

In co-administration studies in animals, the addition of misoprostol did not enhance the toxic effects of diclofenac. The combination was also shown not to be teratogenic or mutagenic. The individual components show no evidence of carcinogenic potential.

Misoprostol in multiples of the recommended therapeutic dose in animals has produced gastric mucosal hyperplasia. This characteristic response to E-series prostaglandins reverts to normal on discontinuation of the compound.

6. PHARMACEUTICAL PARTICULARS

6.1 List of excipients

Arthrotec 75 tablets contain:

Core:

lactose monohydrate
microcrystalline cellulose
maize starch
povidone K-30
magnesium stearate

Mantle/Coat:

methylacrylic acid copolymer type C
sodium hydroxide
talc
triethylcitrate
hypromellose
crospovidone
hydrogenated castor oil
colloidal silicon dioxide
microcrystalline cellulose

6.2 Incompatibilities

Not applicable.

6.3 Shelf life

3 years.

6.4 Special precautions for storage

Do not store above 25 °C. Store in the original package.

6.5 Nature and contents of container

Arthrotec 75 is presented in cold-formed aluminium blisters in pack sizes of 10, 20, 30, 60, 90, 100 and 140 tablets.

Not all pack sizes may be marketed.

6.6 Special precautions for disposal and other handling

No special requirements.

7. MARKETING AUTHORISATION HOLDER

Pharmacia Limited
Ramsgate Road
Sandwich
Kent
CT13 9NJ
United Kingdom

8. MARKETING AUTHORISATION NUMBER(S)

PL 00032/0397

9. DATE OF FIRST AUTHORISATION/RENEWAL OF THE AUTHORISATION

Date of first authorisation: 13th May 1996

Date of last renewal: 23rd January 2007

10. DATE OF REVISION OF THE TEXT

8th September 2009

11. LEGAL STATUS

POM

Ref: AE11_0

Arythmol

(Abbott Laboratories Limited)

1. NAME OF THE MEDICINAL PRODUCT

Arythmol

2. QUALITATIVE AND QUANTITATIVE COMPOSITION

Each tablet contains 150 mg or 300mg propafenone HCl.

3. PHARMACEUTICAL FORM

Tablets.

4. CLINICAL PARTICULARS

4.1 Therapeutic indications

Arythmol is indicated for the prophylaxis and treatment of ventricular arrhythmias.

Arythmol is also indicated for the prophylaxis and treatment of paroxysmal supraventricular tachyarrhythmias which include paroxysmal atrial flutter/fibrillation and paroxysmal re-entrant tachycardias involving the AV node or accessory bypass tracts, when standard therapy has failed or is contra-indicated.

4.2 Posology and method of administration

It is recommended that Arythmol therapy should be initiated under hospital conditions, by a physician experienced in the treatment of arrhythmias. The individual maintenance dose should be determined under cardiological surveillance including ECG monitoring and blood pressure control. If the QRS interval is prolonged by more than 20%, the dose should be reduced or discontinued until the ECG returns to normal limits.

Adults: Initially, 150 mg three times daily increasing at a minimum of three-day intervals to 300 mg twice daily and if necessary, to a maximum of 300 mg three times daily.

The tablets should be swallowed whole and taken with a drink after food. A reduction in the total daily dose is recommended for patients below 70 kg bodyweight.

Elderly: Higher plasma concentrations of propafenone have been noted during treatment. Elderly patients may therefore respond to a lower dose.

Children: A suitable dosage form of Arythmol for children is not available.

Dosage in impaired liver function: Arythmol is extensively metabolised via a saturable hepatic oxidase pathway. In view of the increased bioavailability and elimination half-life of propafenone, a reduction in the recommended dose may be necessary.

Dosage in impaired renal function: Although the elimination of propafenone and its major metabolite is not affected by renal impairment, Arythmol should be administered cautiously.

4.3 Contraindications

Known hypersensitivity to propafenone or to any of the other ingredients.

Arythmol is contra-indicated in patients with uncontrolled congestive heart failure, cardiogenic shock (unless arrhythmia-induced), severe bradycardia, uncontrolled electrolyte disturbances, severe obstructive pulmonary disease or marked hypotension.

Arythmol may worsen myasthenia gravis.

Unless patients are adequately paced (see section 4.4, Special Warnings and Precautions for Use), Arythmol should not be used in the presence of sinus node dysfunction, atrial conduction defects, second degree or greater AV block, bundle branch block or distal block.

Minor prolongation of the PR interval and intra-ventricular conduction defects (QRS duration of less than 20%) are to be expected during treatment with Arythmol and do not warrant dose reduction or drug withdrawal.

4.4 Special warnings and precautions for use

The weak negative inotropic effect of Arythmol may assume importance in patients predisposed to cardiac failure.

In common with other anti-arrhythmic drugs, Arythmol has been shown to alter sensitivity and pacing threshold. In patients with pacemakers, appropriate adjustments may be required.

There is potential for conversion of paroxysmal atrial fibrillation to atrial flutter with accompanying 2:1 or 1:1 conduction block.

Because of the beta-blocking effect, care should be exercised in the treatment of patients with obstructive airways disease or asthma.

As with other class IC anti-arrhythmic agents, patients with structural heart disease may be predisposed to serious adverse effects.

It is essential that each patient given Arythmol be evaluated electrocardiographically and clinically prior to and during therapy to determine whether the response to Arythmol supports continued treatment.

4.5 Interaction with other medicinal products and other forms of interaction

The effects of Arythmol may be potentiated if it is given in combination with other local anaesthetic type agents or agents which depress myocardial activity.

Arythmol has been shown to increase the plasma levels of digoxin and caution should be exercised with regard to digitalis toxicity.

Arythmol has been shown to increase the plasma levels of oral anticoagulants, with an accompanying increase in prothrombin time, which may require a reduction in the dose of oral anticoagulants.

Plasma levels of propafenone may be increased by concomitant administration of cimetidine.

Increased propranolol and metoprolol plasma levels have been observed when these beta-blockers were used concurrently with Arythmol. Thus, dose reduction of these beta-blockers may be required. Details of interactions with other beta-blockers are not known.

Coadministration of propafenone hydrochloride with drugs metabolised by CYP2D6 (such as venlafaxine) might lead to increased levels of these drugs.

Drugs that inhibit CYP2D6, CYP1A2 and CYP3A4, e.g. ketoconazole, cimetidine, quinidine, tropisetron, dolasetron, mizolastine, erythromycin and grapefruit juice may lead to increased levels of propafenone hydrochloride. When propafenone hydrochloride is administered with inhibitors of these enzymes, the patients should be closely monitored and the dose adjusted accordingly.

Due to the potential for increased plasma concentrations, co-administration of 800-1200mg/day doses of ritonavir and propafenone hydrochloride is contraindicated.

Combination therapy of amiodarone and propafenone hydrochloride can affect conduction and repolarisation and lead to abnormalities that have the potential to be proarrhythmic. Dose adjustments of both compounds based on therapeutic response may be required.

No significant effects on the pharmacokinetics of propafenone or lidocaine have been seen following their concomitant use in patients. However, concomitant use of propafenone hydrochloride and intravenous lidocaine have been reported to increase the risks of central nervous system side effects of lidocaine.

Phenobarbital is a known inducer of CYP3A4. Response to propafenone hydrochloride therapy should be monitored during concomitant chronic phenobarbital use.

There has been a report of the lowering of propafenone levels by rifampicin, via the hepatic mixed oxidase system. This reduction may lead to breakthrough arrhythmias.

Cases of possible interactions with cyclosporin (levels increased with deterioration in renal function), theophylline (levels increased), desipramine (levels increased) have also been reported.

Due to the arrhythmogenic effects of tricyclic and related antidepressants and/or neuroleptics, these drugs may interact adversely when used concomitantly with anti-arrhythmic drugs including propafenone.

Concomitant administration of propafenone hydrochloride and fluoxetine in extensive metabolisers increased the S propafenone C_{max} and AUC by 39 and 50% and the R propafenone C_{max} and AUC by 71 and 50%. Elevated levels of plasma propafenone may occur when propafenone hydrochloride is used concomitantly with paroxetine. Lower doses of propafenone may be sufficient to achieve the desired therapeutic response.

4.6 Pregnancy and lactation

Animal studies have not shown any teratogenic effects but as there is no experience of the use of the drug in human pregnancy, Arythmol should not be used during pregnancy and lactation.

4.7 Effects on ability to drive and use machines

Blurred vision, dizziness, fatigue and postural hypotension may affect the patient's speed of reaction and impair the individual's ability to operate machinery or motor vehicles.

4.8 Undesirable effects

The following adverse events have been reported with this or other formulations of propafenone hydrochloride. A cause and effect relationship may not have been established.

Blood and lymphatic system disorders

Leukocytopenia and/ or granulocytopenia or thrombocytopenia; agranulocytosis.

Immune system disorders

Allergic reactions, hypersensitivity reactions (manifested by cholestasis, blood dyscrasias).

Metabolism and nutritional disorders

Anorexia

Psychiatric disorders

Anxiety, confusion

Nervous system disorders

Dizziness, headache, syncope, ataxia, restlessness, nightmares, sleep disorders, extrapyramidal symptoms, vertigo, paresthesia. Rare cases of seizures have been reported.

Eye disorders

Blurred vision

Cardiac disorders

A marked reduction in heart rate (bradycardia) or conduction disorders (i.e. sinoatrial, atrioventricular or intraventricular block) may occur. Proarrhythmic effects which anifest as an increase in heart rate (tachycardia), or ntricular fibrillation may also occur.

ascular disorders

ypotension, including postural hypotension and orthoatic hypotension

astrointestinal disorders

ausea, vomiting, constipation, dry mouth, bitter taste, odominal pain, diarrhoea, bloating and retching

epatobiliary disorders

ver abnormalities, including hepatocellular injury, cholessis, jaundice and hepatitis,

kin and subcutaneous tissue disorders

eddening of the skin, rash, pruritis, exanthema, urticaria

lusculoskeletal and connective tissue disorders

upus syndrome

eproductive system and breast disorders

 some cases a diminution of potency and a drop in sperm ount have been observed after high doses of Arythmol. his is reversible when treatment is discontinued.

eneral disorders and administration site conditions

atigue, chest pain

ivestigations

levated liver enzymes (serum transaminases and alkaline hosphatase)

9 Overdose

xperience with overdosage is limited. No specific antidote known.

rocedures to enhance drug elimination from the body by aemodialysis or haemoperfusion are unlikely to succeed ecause of the large volume of drug distribution. The ffects of propafenone hydrochloride overdose in the myoardium manifest as impulse generation and conduction isorders such as PQ prolongation, QRS widening, supression of sinus node automaticity, AV block, ventricular achycardia, ventricular flutter and ventricular fibrillation. lypotension may also occur. Convulsions, somnolence nd death may occur.

he usual emergency measures for acute cardiovascular ollapse should be applied. In severe conduction disturance associated with compromised cardiac function, tropine, isoprenaline or pacemaker therapy may be equired. If electrical stimulation is not possible, an attempt hould be made to shorten the QRS duration and increase he heart rate with high doses of isoprenaline. Bundle ranch block by itself is not an indication for isoprenaline. Hypotension may require inotropic support. Convulsions hould be treated with i.v. diazepam.

. PHARMACOLOGICAL PROPERTIES

.1 Pharmacodynamic properties

Propafenone is a class IC anti-arrhythmic agent.

t has a stabilising action on myocardial membranes, educes the fast inward current carried by sodium ions with a reduction in depolarisation rate and prolongs the mpulse conduction time in the atrium, AV node and primarily, in the His-Purkinje system.

mpulse conduction through accessory pathways, as in WPW syndrome, is either inhibited, by prolongation of the refractory period or blockade of the conduction pathway, both in anterograde but mostly retrograde direction. At the same time, spontaneous excitability is reduced by an increase of the myocardial stimulus threshold while electrical excitability of the myocardium is decreased by an increase of the ventricular fibrillation threshold.

Anti-arrhythmic effects: Slowing of upstroke velocity of the action potential, decrease of excitability, homogenisation of conduction rates, suppression of ectopic automaticity, lowered myocardial disposition to fibrillation.

Propafenone has moderate beta-sympatholytic activity without clinical relevance. However, the possibility exists that high daily doses (900 - 1200 mg) may trigger a sympatholytic (anti-adrenergic) effect.

In the ECG, propafenone causes a slight prolongation of P, PR and QRS intervals while the QTC interval remains unaffected as a rule.

In digitalised patients with an ejection fraction of 35-50%, contractility of the left ventricle is slightly decreased. In patients with acute transmural infarction and heart failure, the intravenous administration of propafenone may markedly reduce the left ventricular ejection fraction but to an essentially lesser extent in patients in the acute stages of infarction without heart failure. In both cases, pulmonary arterial pressure is minimally raised. Peripheral arterial pressure does not show any significant changes. This demonstrates that propafenone does not exert an unfavourable effect on left ventricular function which would be of clinical relevance. A clinically-relevant reduction of left ventricular function is to be expected only in patients with pre-existing poor ventricular function.

Untreated heart failure might then deteriorate possibly resulting in decompensation.

5.2 Pharmacokinetic properties

Following oral administration, propafenone is nearly completely absorbed from the gastrointestinal tract in a dose-dependent manner and distributed rapidly in the body.

After a single dose of one tablet, bioavailability is about 50%. With repeated doses, plasma concentration and bioavailability rise disproportionately due to saturation of the first pass metabolism in the liver. Steady state is reached after 3 or 4 days, when bioavailability increases to about 100%. Therapeutic plasma levels are in the range of 150 ng/ml to 1500 ng/ml. In the therapeutic concentration range, more than 95% of propafenone is bound to plasma proteins. Comparing cumulative urinary excretion over 24 hours allowed for the calculation that 1.3% of intravenous (70 mg) and 0.65% of oral (600 mg) propafenone is excreted unchanged in the urine, i.e. propafenone is almost exclusively metabolised in the liver. Even in the presence of impaired renal function, reduced elimination of propafenone is not likely, which is confirmed by case reports and single kinetic studies in patients on chronic haemodialysis. Clinical chemistry values did not differ from those of patients with uncompromised kidneys.

Terminal elimination half-life in patients is 5-7 hours (12 hours in single cases) following repeated doses. A close positive correlation between plasma level and AV conduction time was seen in the majority of both healthy volunteers and patients.

After a plasma level of 500 ng/ml, the PR interval is statistically significantly prolonged as compared to baseline values which allows for dose titration and monitoring of the patients with the help of ECG readings. The frequency of ventricular extrasystoles decreases as plasma concentrations increase. Adequate anti-arrhythmic activity has, in single cases, been observed at plasma levels as low as <500 ng/ml.

5.3 Preclinical safety data

None.

6. PHARMACEUTICAL PARTICULARS

6.1 List of excipients

Microcrystalline cellulose, maize starch, hypromellose, croscarmellose sodium, purified water, macrogol 6000, titanium dioxide, macrogol 400 and magnesium stearate.

6.2 Incompatibilities

None.

6.3 Shelf life

5 years.

6.4 Special precautions for storage

Do not store above 30°C.

6.5 Nature and contents of container

Arythmol Tablets 150 mg: PVC/aluminium blister strips containing 90 tablets.

Arythmol Tablets 300 mg: PVC/aluminium blister strips containing 60 tablets.

6.6 Special precautions for disposal and other handling

None.

7. MARKETING AUTHORISATION HOLDER

Abbott Laboratories Limited

Queenborough

Kent

ME11 5EL

United Kingdom

8. MARKETING AUTHORISATION NUMBER(S)

Arythmol 150 mg Tablets PL 00037/0331

Arythmol 300 mg Tablets PL 00037/0332

9. DATE OF FIRST AUTHORISATION/RENEWAL OF THE AUTHORISATION

5 December 2001

10. DATE OF REVISION OF THE TEXT

18 November 2008

Asacol 400mg MR Tablets

(Procter & Gamble Pharmaceuticals UK Limited)

1. NAME OF THE MEDICINAL PRODUCT

Asacol 400mg MR Tablets

2. QUALITATIVE AND QUANTITATIVE COMPOSITION

400 mg mesalazine (5-aminosalicylic acid) per tablet.

3. PHARMACEUTICAL FORM

Red-brown, oblong, modified release tablets.

4. CLINICAL PARTICULARS

4.1 Therapeutic indications

Ulcerative Colitis:

For the treatment of mild to moderate acute exacerbations.
For the maintenance of remission.

Crohn's ileo-colitis

For the maintenance of remission.

4.2 Posology and method of administration

Swallow whole with water. Do not break, crush or chew the tablets before swallowing.

ADULTS:

Oral:

Acute disease: Six tablets a day in divided doses, with concomitant corticosteroid therapy where clinically indicated.

Maintenance therapy: Three to six tablets a day in divided doses.

ELDERLY: The normal adult dosage may be used unless renal function is impaired (see section 4.4).

CHILDREN: There is no dosage recommendation.

4.3 Contraindications

A history of sensitivity to salicylates or renal sensitivity to sulphasalazine. Confirmed severe renal impairment (GFR less than 20 ml/min). Children under 2 years of age.

4.4 Special warnings and precautions for use

Use in the elderly should be cautious and subject to patients having normal renal function.

Renal disorder: Mesalazine is excreted rapidly by the kidney, mainly as its metabolite, N-acetyl-5-aminosalicylic acid. In rats, large doses of mesalazine injected intravenously produce tubular and glomerular toxicity. Asacol should be used with extreme caution in patients with confirmed mild to moderate renal impairment (see section 4.3). Patients on mesalazine should have renal function monitored, (with serum creatinine levels measured) prior to treatment start. Renal function should then be monitored periodically during treatment, for example every 3 months for the first year, then 6 monthly for the next 4 years and annually thereafter, based on individual patient history. Physicians should take into account risk factors such as prior and concomitant medications, duration and severity of disease and concurrent illnesses. Treatment with mesalazine should be discontinued if renal function deteriorates. If dehydration develops, normal electrolyte and fluid balance should be restored as soon as possible.

Serious blood dyscrasias have been reported very rarely with mesalazine. Haematological investigations should be performed if the patient develops unexplained bleeding, bruising, purpura, anaemia, fever or sore throat. Treatment should be stopped if there is suspicion or evidence of blood dyscrasia.

4.5 Interaction with other medicinal products and other forms of interaction

'Asacol' Tablets should not be given with lactulose or similar preparations, which lower stool pH and may prevent release of mesalazine.

Concurrent use of other known nephrotoxic agents, such as NSAIDs and azathioprine, may increase the risk of renal reactions (see section 4.4)

4.6 Pregnancy and lactation

No information is available with regard to teratogenicity; however, negligible quantities of mesalazine are transferred across the placenta and are excreted in breast milk following sulphasalazine therapy. Use of 'Asacol' during pregnancy should be with caution, and only if the potential benefits are greater than the possible hazards. 'Asacol' should, unless essential, be avoided by nursing mothers.

4.7 Effects on ability to drive and use machines

Not applicable.

4.8 Undesirable effects

The side effects are predominantly gastrointestinal, including nausea, diarrhoea and abdominal pain. Headache has also been reported.

There have been rare reports of leucopenia, neutropenia, agranulocytosis, aplastic anaemia and thrombocytopenia, alopecia, peripheral neuropathy, pancreatitis, abnormalities of hepatic function and hepatitis, myocarditis and pericarditis, allergic and fibrotic lung reactions, lupus erythematosus-like reactions and rash (including urticaria), drug fever, interstitial nephritis and nephrotic syndrome with oral mesalazine treatment, usually reversible on withdrawal. Renal failure has been reported. Mesalazine-induced nephrotoxicity should be suspected in patients developing renal dysfunction during treatment.

Mesalazine may very rarely be associated with an exacerbation of the symptoms of colitis, Stevens Johnson syndrome and erythema multiforme.

Other side effects observed with sulphasalazine such as depression of sperm count and function, have not been reported with 'Asacol'.

4.9 Overdose

Following tablet ingestion, gastric lavage and intravenous transfusion of electrolytes to promote diuresis. There is no specific antidote.

5. PHARMACOLOGICAL PROPERTIES

5.1 Pharmacodynamic properties

Mesalazine is one of the two components of sulphasalazine, the other being sulphapyridine. It is the latter which is responsible for the majority of the side effects associated with sulphasalazine therapy whilst mesalazine is known to be the active moiety in the treatment of ulcerative colitis.

5.2 Pharmacokinetic properties

'Asacol' Tablets contain 400 mg of available mesalazine. This is released in the terminal ileum and large bowel by the effect of pH. Above pH 7 the Eudragit S coat disintegrates and releases the active constituent. 'Asacol' Tablets contain, in a single tablet, an equivalent quantity of mesalazine to that theoretically available from the complete azo-reduction of 1g of sulphasalazine.

5.3 Preclinical safety data
There are no preclinical data of relevance to the prescriber which are additional to that already included in other sections of the SPC.

6. PHARMACEUTICAL PARTICULARS

6.1 List of excipients
Core: lactose, sodium starch glycollate, magnesium stearate, talc, polyvinylpyrrolidone.

Coating: Eudragit S, dibutylphthalate, iron oxides (E172) and polyethylene glycol.

6.2 Incompatibilities
Not applicable.

6.3 Shelf life
2 years.

6.4 Special precautions for storage
Store tablets in a dry place at a temperature not exceeding 25°C and protect from direct sunlight. Keep the bottle tightly closed

6.5 Nature and contents of container
HDPE bottle with a child-resistant closure, cotton, and silica gel desiccant pouches. Pack-sizes of 90 or 120 tablets.

6.6 Special precautions for disposal and other handling
No special requirements.

7. MARKETING AUTHORISATION HOLDER
Procter & Gamble Pharmaceuticals UK Ltd.
Rusham Park
Whitehall Lane
Egham
Surrey
TW20 9NW

8. MARKETING AUTHORISATION NUMBER(S)
PL00364/0073

9. DATE OF FIRST AUTHORISATION/RENEWAL OF THE AUTHORISATION
1.2.88 / 21.05.2002

10. DATE OF REVISION OF THE TEXT
3 September 2007

Asacol 800mg MR Tablets

(Procter & Gamble Pharmaceuticals UK Limited)

1. NAME OF THE MEDICINAL PRODUCT
Asacol 800mg MR tablets

2. QUALITATIVE AND QUANTITATIVE COMPOSITION
Each tablet contains 800 mg of mesalazine (active substance) and 152.75 mg of lactose monohydrate (excipient).
For full list of excipients, see section 6.1

3. PHARMACEUTICAL FORM
Modified ReleaseTablets
Red-brown, oblong tablets marked 'PG 800'.

4. CLINICAL PARTICULARS

4.1 Therapeutic indications
Ulcerative colitis: For the treatment of mild to moderate acute exacerbations. For the maintenance of remission.

Crohn's ileo-colitis: For the maintenance of remission.

4.2 Posology and method of administration
Swallow whole with water. Do not break, crush or chew the tablets before swallowing.

ADULTS:

Mild acute exacerbations of ulcerative colitis: Three tablets (2.4g) a day in divided doses.

Moderate acute exacerbations of ulcerative colitis: Six tablets (4.8g) a day in divided doses.

Maintenance of remission of ulcerative colitis and Crohn's ileocolitis: Up to three tablets (2.4g) a day in divided doses.

ELDERLY: The normal adult dosage may be used unless renal function is impaired (see section 4.4).

CHILDREN: Not recommended.

4.3 Contraindications
A history of sensitivity to salicylates or renal sensitivity to sulfasalazine. Confirmed severe renal impairment (GFR less than 20 ml/min). Hypersensitivity to any of the ingredients. Severe hepatic impairment. Gastric or duodenal ulcer, haemorrhagic tendency.

4.4 Special warnings and precautions for use
Geriatric Use
Use in the elderly should be cautious and subject to patients having normal renal function

Intolerance
Discontinue treatment immediately if acute symptoms of intolerance occur including vomiting, abdominal pain or rash. This medicine contains lactose. Patients with the rare hereditary problems of galactose intolerance, the Lapp lactase deficiency or glucose-galactose malabsorption should not take this medicine because of the presence of lactose monohydrate.

Mesalazine inhibits the thiopurine methyl-transferase (TPMT) activity *in vitro* and may therefore impair the metabolism of azathioprine and 6-mercaptopurine. Standard haematological indices (including the white cell count) should be monitored repeatedly in patients taking azathioprine, especially at the beginning of such combination therapy, whether or not mesalazine is prescribed.

Renal disorder
Mesalazine is excreted rapidly by the kidney, mainly as its metabolite, N-acetyl-5-aminosalicylic acid. In rats, large doses of mesalazine injected intravenously produce tubular and glomerular toxicity. Asacol should be used with extreme caution in patients with confirmed mild to moderate renal impairment (see section 4.3). Patients on mesalazine should have renal function monitored, (with serum creatinine levels measured) prior to treatment start. Renal function should then be monitored periodically during treatment, for example every 3 months for the first year, then every 6 months for the next 4 years and annually thereafter, based on individual patient history. Physicians should take into account risk factors such as prior and concomitant medications, duration and severity of disease and concurrent illnesses. Treatment with mesalazine should be discontinued if renal function deteriorates. If dehydration develops, normal electrolyte and fluid balance should be restored as soon as possible.

Blood Dyscrasias
Serious blood dyscrasias (some with fatal outcome) have been reported very rarely with mesalazine. Haematological investigations including a complete blood count may be performed prior to initiation and whilst on therapy according to the physician's judgement. Such tests should be done immediately if the patient develops unexplained bleeding, bruising, purpura, anaemia, fever or sore throat. Treatment should be stopped if there is suspicion or evidence of blood dyscrasia.

4.5 Interaction with other medicinal products and other forms of interaction
'Asacol' tablets should not be given with lactulose or similar preparations, which lower stool pH and may prevent release of mesalazine.

Concurrent use of other known nephrotoxic agents, such as NSAIDs and azathioprine, may increase the risk of renal reactions (see section 4.4).

4.6 Pregnancy and lactation
Pregnancy
Mesalazine is known to cross the placental barrier, but the limited data available on its use in pregnant women do not allow accurate assessment of possible adverse effects.

Mesalazine should therefore be used with caution during pregnancy and lactation when the potential benefit outweighs the possible hazards in the opinion of the physician.

Animal studies do not indicate direct or indirect harmful effects with respect to pregnancy, embryonal/foetal development, parturition or postnatal development (see section 5.3).

Lactation
Low concentrations of mesalazine and higher concentrations of its N-acetyl metabolite have been detected in human milk. While the clinical significance of this has not been determined, caution should be exercised when mesalazine is administered to a nursing woman. Hypersensitivity reactions like diarrhoea cannot be excluded. Therefore, if the suckling neonate develops suspected adverse reactions consideration should be given to discontinuation of breast-feeding or discontinuation of treatment of the mother.

4.7 Effects on ability to drive and use machines
No influence.

4.8 Undesirable effects
In Phase III clinical studies in patients with moderate active ulcerative colitis, treated for 6 weeks with either 2.4g/day or 4.8g/day, there was no difference in the adverse event profiles between doses. The events are presented in the table below:

Adverse Events Reported in ⩾ 2% of Patients in Either Treatment Group

Adverse Event*	Asacol 800 mg (4.8 g/day) N = 213 (%)	Mesalazine 400 mg (2.4 g/day) N = 235 (%)
Headache	16 (7.5%)	14 (6.0%)
Abdominal pain	9 (4.2%)	12 (5.1%)
Diarrhoea	8 (3.8%)	9 (3.8%)
Nausea	8 (3.8%)	4 (1.7%)
Respiratory infection	7 (3.3%)	4 (1.7%)
Exacerbation of colitis	6 (2.8%)	6 (2.6%)
Dyspepsia	6 (2.8%)	5 (2.1%)
Vomiting	6 (2.8%)	2 (0.9%)
Flatulence	5 (2.3%)	7 (3.0%)
Rectal disorder	4 (1.9%)	6 (2.6%)
Flu syndrome	3 (1.4%)	8 (3.4%)
Rash	3 (1.4%)	5 (2.1%)
Increased cough	1 (0.5%)	9 (3.8%)
Sinusitis	1 (0.5%)	5 (2.1%)
Rhinitis	0 (0.0%)	7 (3.0%)

*Adverse events are listed by decreasing frequency a observed in the 4.8 g/day treatment group

Adverse events seen with oral mesalazine products ar predominantly gastrointestinal, including nausea, vomit ing, diarrhoea, and abdominal pain. Headache and arthral gia/myalgia have also been reported.

Blood and lymphatic system disorders:

Rare (<1/1,000): leucopenia, neutropenia, agranulocyto sis, aplastic anaemia and thrombocytopenia.

Cardiac disorders:

Rare (<1/1,000): myocarditis, pericarditis

Nervous disorders:

Common (⩾ 1/100 to <1/10): headache

Rare (<1/1,000): peripheral neuropathy, vertigo

Respiratory, thoracic and mediastinal disorders:

Rare (<1/1,000): bronchospasm, eosinophilic pneumonia

Very rare (<1/10,000): interstitial pneumonitis

Gastrointestinal disorders:

Common (⩾ 1/100 to <1/10): nausea, vomiting, diarrhoea, abdominal pain

Rare (<1/1,000): pancreatitis

Very rare (<1/10,000): exacerbation of the symptoms o colitis

Hepato-biliary disorders:

Rare (<1/1,000): abnormalities of hepatic function / abnormal liver function test, hepatitis

Skin and subcutaneous tissue disorders:

Rare (<1/1,000): alopecia, lupus erythematosus-like reactions, rash (including urticaria), bullous skin reactions,

Very rare(<1/10,000): Stevens Johnson syndrome, erythema multiforme

Musculo-skeletal:

Common (⩾ 1/100 to <1/10): arthralgia/myalgia

Renal and urinary disorders

Rare (<1/1,000): interstitial nephritis and nephrotic syndrome with oral mesalazine treatment, usually reversible on withdrawal. Renal failure has been reported. Mesalazine-induced nephrotoxicity should be suspected in patients developing renal dysfunction during treatment.

General disorders and administration site conditions

Rare (<1/1,000): Drug fever

4.9 Overdose
There is no clinical experience with overdose of Asacol 800 mg. Mesalazine is not metabolized to salicylate. There is no specific antidote for mesalazine overdose and treatment is symptomatic and supportive. It may include intravenous infusion of appropriate electrolytes.

5. PHARMACOLOGICAL PROPERTIES

5.1 Pharmacodynamic properties
ATC code: A07EC02

Mesalazine is thought to have a topical anti-inflammatory effect on the intestinal mucosa, where it has been shown to inhibit prostaglandin and leukotriene synthesis, release of reactive oxygen species and other actions.

Moderately active ulcerative colitis:

Two active-controlled trials enrolled a total of 687 patients comparing Asacol 4.8 g/day (800 mg formulation) with mesalazine enteric coated tablets 2.4 g/day (400 mg formulation) in patients with mildly to moderately active ulcerative colitis. Both studies were of six weeks duration. Treatment success was defined on the basis of the Physician's Global Assessment (PGA), which took into consideration clinical assessments of rectal bleeding, stool frequency, and the patient's functional assessment and sigmoidoscopic examination. Across the two studies 4.8 g/day provided superior efficacy in patients with moderately active disease.

In the first study a total of 301 patients with mildly to moderately active UC were enrolled. Of these, 169 patients with moderately active disease were assessed for efficacy in a pre-defined subgroup analysis. In these patients, 4.8 g/day gave greater treatment success than 2.4 g/day (72% treatment success compared with 57%).

the second study a total of 386 patients with mildly moderately active ulcerative colitis were randomly ıssigned to treatment. In the 254 patients with moderately ctive disease, the pre-defined primary efficacy analysis ıowed that 4.8 g/day gave greater treatment success an 2.4 g/day (72% treatment success compared to 9%).

both studies, more patients showed improvement on 8 g/day compared to 2.4 g/day across the clinical ssessments (stool frequency, rectal bleeding, sigmoido- copy and PGA). In combined studies, 4.8 g/day showed atistically significant superiority in the sigmoidoscopy nd PGA scores.

: Week 3, more patients with moderately active disease chieved treatment success on 4.8 g/day compared with 4 g/day in each study and in the combined analysis (62% s. 53%). These differences were not statistically signifi- ant.

ı combined studies among patients with moderately ctive disease, the efficacy benefit of 4.8 g/day over .4 g/day was consistent across various subgroups includ- ıg age, gender, race, ulcerative colitis disease history, rior medication usage and extent of disease (proctitis, roctosigmoiditis, left-sided colitis and pancolitis).

.2 Pharmacokinetic properties

sacol 800mg MR tablets are coated with an acrylic-based esin. Tablets coated with this specific resin have been hown to delay release of mesalazine until it reaches the erminal ileum and beyond.

3ased on cumulative urinary recovery of 5-aminosalicylic cid and its metabolite, N-acetyl-5-aminosalicylic acid (N- c-5-ASA) from single dose studies in healthy volunteers, pproximately 20% of the orally administered mesalazine ı Asacol 800mg MR tablets is systemically absorbed, eaving the remainder available for local action and elim- ıation in the faeces. The absorbed mesalazine is rapidly cetylated in the gut mucosal wall and by the liver to N-Ac- -ASA which is excreted mainly by the kidney.

'he extent of systemic exposure to mesalazine, based on UC and Ae%, following oral administration of Asacol 00mg MR tablets, is similar in fasted and fed subjects.

'harmacokinetics studies for Asacol 800mg MR tablets ndicated that the tmax for mesalazine and its metabolite, J-Ac-5-ASA, is prolonged, reflecting the modified release characteristics, and ranged from 4 to 12 hours. Large ntersubject variability in the plasma concentrations and erminal exponential half-lives (t1/2) of mesalazine and N- Ac-5-ASA is seen following administration of Asacol 300mg MR tablets. The mean (t1/2) for mesalazine and N-Ac-5-ASA are usually about 12 hours, but may vary from 2 to 15 hours.

n patients with mildly to moderately active ulcerative colitis who participated in clinical safety and efficacy studies, the mean plasma concentrations of mesalazine and N-Ac-5- ASA following oral administration of 4.8g/day with the Asacol 800mg MR tablet for 6 weeks (N = 273) were 1931 ng/mL and 2951 ng/mL, respectively. In these studies, the mean plasma concentrations of mesalazine and N-Ac-5-ASA were 967 ng/mL and 1789 ng/mL, respectively, in patients with mildly to moderately active ulcerative colitis who were orally administered 2.4g/day with a mesalazine 400mg modified release tablet for 6 weeks (N = 275). The systemic exposure to mesalazine and N-Ac-5-ASA in patients with moderately active UC is similar to that observed in patients with mildly active UC.

5.3 Preclinical safety data

Apart from effects on the kidney (see section 4.4), preclinical data reveal no special hazard for humans based on conventional studies of safety pharmacology, repeated-dose toxicity, genotoxicity, carcinogenic potential and toxicity to reproduction. The latter was studied in rats and rabbits at oral doses up to 480 mg/kg/day and no evidence was detected for teratogenic effects or foetal toxicity due to mesalazine.

6. PHARMACEUTICAL PARTICULARS

6.1 List of excipients

Core	lactose monohydrate
	sodium starch glycolate
	talc
	povidone
	magnesium stearate
	colloidal anhydrous silica
Coating	methacrylic acid – methyl methacrylate copolymer (1:2)
	talc
	dibutyl phthalate
	ferric oxide red (E172)
	methacrylic acid – methyl methacrylate copolymer (1:1)
	ferric oxide yellow (E172)
	macrogol
Black ink containing	propylene glycol
	ferric oxide black (E172)
	ammonium hydroxide
	ethanol
	shellac glaze (bleached, de-waxed)

6.2 Incompatibilities

Not applicable.

6.3 Shelf life

3 years.

6.4 Special precautions for storage

This medicinal product does not require any special storage conditions. Keep the bottle tightly closed.

6.5 Nature and contents of container

HDPE bottle with a child-resistant closure, cotton, and silica gel desiccant pouches. Pack-sizes of 12, 36 or 180 tablets.

Not all pack sizes may be marketed.

6.6 Special precautions for disposal and other handling

No special requirements.

7. MARKETING AUTHORISATION HOLDER

Procter and Gamble Pharmaceuticals UK Ltd
Rusham Park
Whitehall Lane
Egham
Surrey
TW20 9NW

8. MARKETING AUTHORISATION NUMBER(S)

PL00364/0083

9. DATE OF FIRST AUTHORISATION/RENEWAL OF THE AUTHORISATION

14/09/2007

10. DATE OF REVISION OF THE TEXT

14/09/2007

Asacol Foam Enema

(Procter & Gamble Pharmaceuticals UK Limited)

1. NAME OF THE MEDICINAL PRODUCT

Asacol® Foam Enema.

2. QUALITATIVE AND QUANTITATIVE COMPOSITION

Mesalazine (5-aminosalicylic acid), 1g per metered dose.

3. PHARMACEUTICAL FORM

White, aerosol foam enema.

4. CLINICAL PARTICULARS

4.1 Therapeutic indications

For the treatment of mild to moderate acute exacerbations of ulcerative colitis affecting the distal colon.

4.2 Posology and method of administration

Route of administration: Rectal.

Adults: For disease affecting the rectosigmoid region, one metered dose 1g a day for 4 - 6 weeks; for disease involving the descending colon, two metered doses 2g once a day for 4 - 6 weeks.

Elderly: The normal adult dosage may be used unless renal function is impaired (see Section 4.4).

Children: There is no dosage recommendation.

4.3 Contraindications

A history of sensitivity to salicylates or renal sensitivity to sulphasalazine. Confirmed severe renal impairment (GFR less than 20 ml/min). Children under 2 years of age.

4.4 Special warnings and precautions for use

Use in the elderly should be cautious and subject to patients having a normal renal function.

Renal disorder: Mesalazine is excreted rapidly by the kidney, mainly as its metabolite, N-acetyl-5-aminosalicylic acid. In rats, large doses of mesalazine injected intravenously produce tubular and glomerular toxicity. Asacol should be used with extreme caution in patients with confirmed mild to moderate renal impairment (see section 4.3). Treatment with mesalazine should be discontinued if renal function deteriorates. If dehydration develops, normal electrolyte and fluid balance should be restored as soon as possible.

Serious blood dyscrasias have been reported very rarely with mesalazine. Haematological investigations should be performed if the patient develops unexplained bleeding, bruising, purpura, anaemia, fever or sore throat. Treatment should be stopped if there is suspicion or evidence of blood dyscrasia.

4.5 Interaction with other medicinal products and other forms of interaction

Concurrent use of other known nephrotoxic agents, such as NSAIDs and azathioprine, may increase the risk of renal reactions (see section 4.4).

4.6 Pregnancy and lactation

No information is available with regard to teratogenicity; however, negligible quantities of mesalazine are transferred across the placenta and are excreted in breast milk following sulphasalazine therapy. Use of 'Asacol' during pregnancy should be with caution, and only if the potential benefits are greater than the possible hazards. 'Asacol' should, unless essential, be avoided by nursing mothers.

4.7 Effects on ability to drive and use machines

Not applicable.

4.8 Undesirable effects

The side effects are predominantly gastrointestinal, including nausea, diarrhoea and abdominal pain. Headache has also been reported.

There have been rare reports of leucopenia, neutropenia, agranulocytosis, aplastic anaemia and thrombocytopenia, alopecia, peripheral neuropathy, pancreatitis, abnormalities of hepatic function and hepatitis, myocarditis and pericarditis, allergic and fibrotic lung reactions, lupus erythematosus-like reactions and rash (including urticaria), interstitial nephritis and nephrotic syndrome with oral mesalazine treatment, usually reversible on withdrawal. Renal failure has been reported. Mesalazine-induced nephrotoxicity should be suspected in patients developing renal dysfunction during treatment.

Mesalazine may very rarely be associated with an exacerbation of the symptoms of colitis, Stevens Johnson syndrome and erythema multiforme.

Other side effects observed with sulphasalazine such as depression of sperm count and function, have not been reported with 'Asacol'.

Rarely, local irritation may occur after administration of rectal dosage forms containing mesalazine.

4.9 Overdose

Not applicable.

5. PHARMACOLOGICAL PROPERTIES

5.1 Pharmacodynamic properties

Mesalazine is one of the two components of sulphasalazine, the other being sulphapyridine. It is the latter which is responsible for the majority of the side effects associated with sulphasalazine therapy whilst mesalazine is known to be the active moiety in the treatment of ulcerative colitis.

5.2 Pharmacokinetic properties

The foam enema is intended to deliver mesalazine directly to the proposed site of action in the colon and rectum.

5.3 Preclinical safety data

There are no preclinical data of relevance to the prescriber which are additonal to those already included in other sections of the SPC.

6. PHARMACEUTICAL PARTICULARS

6.1 List of excipients

Sorbitan mono-oleate, polysorbate 20, emulsifying wax, colloidal anhydrous silica, sodium metabisulphite, disodium edetate, methylhydroxybenzoate, propylhydroxybenzoate, sodium phosphate dodecahydrate or heptahydrate, sodium acid phosphate, glycerol, Macrogol 300, purified water, propane, iso-butane, n-butane.

6.2 Incompatibilities

Not applicable.

6.3 Shelf life

Three years.

6.4 Special precautions for storage

Store the foam enema below 30°C. This is a pressurised canister, containing a flammable propellant. It should be kept away from any flames or sparks, including cigarettes. It should be protected from direct sunlight and must not be pierced or burned even when empty.

6.5 Nature and contents of container

Cartoned aerosol cans, each carton consisting of one aerosol can containing 14 metered doses, plus 14 disposable applicators and 14 disposable plastic bags.

6.6 Special precautions for disposal and other handling

Read the instructions carefully before using 'Asacol' Foam Enema for the first time.

Mix contents by shaking the can vigorously for about five seconds.

Before using the enema for the first time, remove the safety tag from under the dome.

Push the plastic applicator firmly on to the spout of the can and align the notch beneath the dome with the spout.

Hold the can in the palm of one hand with the dome pointing downwards. This product must only be dispensed when the can is upside down, with the dome nearest to the ground. (If the can is not upside down the foam will not come out properly.)

You may find that the easiest way to use the enema is to raise one foot on to a firm surface, such as a stool or chair, and insert the applicator into the rectum as far as is comfortable. You can apply a lubricating jelly to the tip of the applicator for comfort if you wish.

To administer a dose, fully depress the dome once and release it. The foam will not come out of the can until you release the dome. To administer a second dose, press and release the dome again. Wait for 15 seconds before withdrawing the applicator.

Note: the can will only work when held with the dome pointing down.

Remove the applicator and dispose of it in one of the plastic bags provided. Do not flush it down the toilet.

7. MARKETING AUTHORISATION HOLDER
Procter & Gamble Pharmaceuticals UK Ltd.
Rusham Park
Whitehall Lane
Egham
Surrey
TW20 9NW
United Kingdom

8. MARKETING AUTHORISATION NUMBER(S)
PL 00364/0077

9. DATE OF FIRST AUTHORISATION/RENEWAL OF THE AUTHORISATION
3.6.94/21.05.2002

10. DATE OF REVISION OF THE TEXT
October 2002

11. Legal Status
POM

Asacol Suppositories 250 mg & 500 mg

(Procter & Gamble Pharmaceuticals UK Limited)

1. NAME OF THE MEDICINAL PRODUCT
Asacol® Suppositories 250 mg & 500 mg

2. QUALITATIVE AND QUANTITATIVE COMPOSITION
Asacol Suppositories contain 250 or 500 mg mesalazine per suppository.

3. PHARMACEUTICAL FORM
Opaque, beige suppositories, containing 250 mg or 500 mg mesalazine.

4. CLINICAL PARTICULARS
4.1 Therapeutic indications
For the treatment of mild to moderate acute exacerbations of ulcerative colitis.

The suppositories are particularly appropriate in patients with distal disease.

For the maintenance of remission of ulcerative colitis.

4.2 Posology and method of administration
ADULTS:

Suppositories 250 mg: Three to six suppositories a day in divided doses, with the last dose at bedtime.

Suppositories 500 mg: A maximum of three suppositories a day in divided doses, with the last dose at bedtime.

ELDERLY: The normal adult dosage may be used unless renal function is impaired (see section 4.4).

CHILDREN: There is no dosage recommendation.

4.3 Contraindications
A history of sensitivity to salicylates or renal sensitivity to sulphasalazine. Confirmed severe renal impairment (GFR <20 ml/min). Children under 2 years of age.

4.4 Special warnings and precautions for use
Use in the elderly should be cautious and subject to patients having normal renal function.

Renal disorder: Mesalazine is excreted rapidly by the kidney, mainly as its metabolite, N-acetyl-5-aminosalicylic acid. In rats, large doses of mesalazine injected intravenously produce tubular and glomerular toxicity. Asacol should be used with extreme caution in patients with confirmed mild to moderate renal impairment (see section 4.3). Treatment with mesalazine should be discontinued if renal function deteriorates. If dehydration develops, normal electrolyte and fluid balance should be restored as soon as possible.

Serious blood dyscrasias have been reported very rarely with mesalazine. Haematological investigations should be performed if the patient develops unexplained bleeding, bruising, purpura, anaemia, fever or sore throat. Treatment should be stopped if there is suspicion or evidence of blood dyscrasia.

4.5 Interaction with other medicinal products and other forms of interaction
Concurrent use of other known nephrotoxic agents, such as NSAIDs and azathioprine, may increase the risk of renal reactions (see section 4.4)

4.6 Pregnancy and lactation
No information is available with regard to teratogenicity; however, negligible quantities of mesalazine are transferred across the placenta and are excreted in breast milk following sulphasalazine therapy. Use of Asacol during pregnancy should be with caution, and only if the potential benefits are greater than the possible hazards. Asacol should, unless essential, be avoided by nursing mothers.

4.7 Effects on ability to drive and use machines
Not applicable.

4.8 Undesirable effects
The side effects are predominantly gastrointestinal, including nausea, diarrhoea and abdominal pain. Headache has also been reported.

There have been rare reports of leucopenia, neutropenia, agranulocytosis, aplastic anaemia and thrombocytopenia, alopecia, peripheral neuropathy, pancreatitis, abnormalities of hepatic function and hepatitis, myocarditis and pericarditis, allergic and fibrotic lung reactions, lupus erythematosus-like reactions and rash (including urticaria), interstitial nephritis and nephrotic syndrome with oral mesalazine treatment, usually reversible on withdrawal. Renal failure has been reported. Mesalazine-induced nephrotoxicity should be suspected in patients developing renal dysfunction during treatment.

Mesalazine may very rarely be associated with an exacerbation of the symptoms of colitis, Stevens Johnson syndrome and erythema multiforme.

Other side effects observed with sulphasalazine such as depression of sperm count and function, have not been reported with Asacol.

Rarely, local irritation may occur after administration of rectal dosage forms containing mesalazine.

4.9 Overdose
There is no specific antidote.

5. PHARMACOLOGICAL PROPERTIES
5.1 Pharmacodynamic properties
Mesalazine is one of the two components of sulphasalazine, the other being sulphapyridine. It is the latter which is responsible for the majority of the side effects associated with sulphasalazine therapy whilst mesalazine is known to be the active moiety in the treatment of ulcerative colitis. Asacol consists only of this active component which is delivered directly by the suppositories.

5.2 Pharmacokinetic properties
The suppository is designed to deliver mesalazine directly to the proposed site of action in the distal bowel.

5.3 Preclinical safety data
There are no preclinical data of relevance to the prescriber which are additional to that already included in other sections of the SPC.

6. PHARMACEUTICAL PARTICULARS
6.1 List of excipients
Witepsol W45 (Hard Fat).

6.2 Incompatibilities
Not applicable.

6.3 Shelf life
Suppositories 250 mg: 4 years.
Suppositories 500 mg: 3 years.

6.4 Special precautions for storage
Store below 25°C. Protect from light.

6.5 Nature and contents of container
Cartoned plastic moulds (OP), each containing 20 suppositories (250 mg) or 10 suppositories (500 mg).

6.6 Special precautions for disposal and other handling
For rectal administration.

7. MARKETING AUTHORISATION HOLDER
Procter & Gamble Pharmaceuticals UK Ltd.
Rusham Park
Whitehall Lane
Egham
Surrey
TW20 9NW
United Kingdom

8. MARKETING AUTHORISATION NUMBER(S)
Asacol Suppositories 250 mg 00364/0075
Asacol Suppositories 500 mg 00364/0076

9. DATE OF FIRST AUTHORISATION/RENEWAL OF THE AUTHORISATION
Asacol Suppositories 250 mg 20.4.88/21.05.2002
Asacol Suppositories 500 mg 22.3.90/21.05.2002

10. DATE OF REVISION OF THE TEXT
October 2002

11. Legal Status
POM.

Asasantin Retard

(Boehringer Ingelheim Limited)

1. NAME OF THE MEDICINAL PRODUCT
ASASANTIN® Retard

2. QUALITATIVE AND QUANTITATIVE COMPOSITION
Each capsule contains dipyridamole 200 mg and aspirin 25 mg.

3. PHARMACEUTICAL FORM
Capsule containing aspirin in standard release form and dipyridamole in modified release form.

Capsules consisting of a red cap and an ivory body imprinted with the company logo and the figures "01A".

4. CLINICAL PARTICULARS
4.1 Therapeutic indications
Secondary prevention of ischaemic stroke and transie ischaemic attacks.

4.2 Posology and method of administration
For oral administration.

Adults, including the elderly

The recommended dose is one capsule twice daily, usual one in the morning and one in the evening preferably wi meals.

The capsules should be swallowed whole without chewin together with a glass of water.

Children

ASASANTIN Retard is not indicated for use in children an young people. Do not give to children aged under 16 years unless specifically indicated (e.g. for Kawasaki's disease

Alternative regimen in case of intolerable headaches

In the event of intolerable headaches during treatmer initiation, switch to one capsule at bedtime and low-dos acetylsalicylic acid (ASA) in the morning. Because there ar no outcome data with this regimen and headache become less of a problem as treatment continues, patient should return to the usual regimen as soon as possible usually within one week.

4.3 Contraindications
Hypersensitivity to any component of the product or sali cylates.

Patients with active gastric or duodenal ulcers or with bleeding disorders.

Patients in the last trimester of pregnancy.

In case of rare hereditary conditions that may be incompatible with an excipient of the product (please refer to "special warnings and precautions") the use of the produc is contraindicated.

4.4 Special warnings and precautions for use
Due to the risk of bleeding, as with other antiplatelet agents, ASASANTIN should be used with caution in patients at increased bleeding risk and patients should be followed carefully for any signs of bleeding, including occult bleeding.

Caution should be advised in patients receiving concomitant medication which may increase the risk of bleeding, such as anti-platelet agents (e.g. clopidogrel, ticlopidine) or selective serotonin reuptake inhibitors (SSRIs), please see section 4.5.

Headache or migraine-like headache which may occur especially at the beginning of ASASANTIN therapy should not be treated with analgesic doses of acetylsalicylic acid.

Among other properties dipyridamole acts as a vasodilator. It should be used with caution in patients with severe coronary artery disease, including unstable angina and/or recent myocardial infarction, left ventricular outflow obstruction, or haemodynamic instability (e.g. decompensated heart failure).

Patients being treated with regular oral doses of ASASANTIN Retard should not receive additional intravenous dipyridamole. Clinical experience suggests that patients being treated with oral dipyridamole who also require pharmacological stress testing with intravenous dipyridamole, should discontinue drugs containing oral dipyridamole twenty-four hours prior to stress testing.

In patients with myasthenia gravis readjustment of therapy may be necessary after changes in dipyridamole dosage (see Interactions).

Due to the aspirin component, ASASANTIN Retard should be used in caution in patients with asthma, allergic rhinitis, nasal polyps, chronic or recurring gastric or duodenal complaints, impaired renal (avoid if severe) or hepatic function or glucose-6-phosphate dehydrogenase deficiency.

In addition, caution is advised in patients hypersensitive to other non-steroidal anti-inflammatory drugs.

ASASANTIN Retard is not indicated for use in children and young people. There is a possible association between aspirin and Reye's syndrome when given to children. Reye's syndrome is a very rare disease, which affects the brain and liver, and can be fatal. For this reason aspirin should not be given to children aged under 16 years unless specifically indicated (e.g. for Kawasaki's disease).

The dose of aspirin in ASASANTIN Retard has not been studied in secondary prevention of myocardial infarction.

The product contains 106 mg of lactose and 22.64 mg sucrose per maximum recommended daily dose. Patients with rare hereditary problems of fructose intolerance, galactose intolerance, the Lapp lactase deficiency, glucose-galactose malabsorption or sucrase-isomaltase insufficiency should not take this medicine.

4.5 Interaction with other medicinal products and other forms of interaction
When dipyridamole is used in combination with aspirin or with warfarin, the statements regarding precautions, warnings and tolerance for these preparations must be observed.

Aspirin has been shown to enhance the effect of anticoagulants (e.g. coumarin derivatives and heparin), antiplatelet drugs (e.g. clopidogrel, ticlopidine) and selective erotonin reuptake inhibitors (SSRIs) and may increase the sk of bleeding.

spirin may enhance the effect of valproic acid and pheytoin with possible increased risk of side effects.

astrointestinal side effects may increase when aspirin is dministered concomitantly with NSAIDs, corticosteroids chronic alcohol use. The addition of dipyridamole to spirin does not increase the incidence of bleeding events. Vhen dipyridamole was administered concomitantly with arfarin, bleeding was no greater in frequency or severity han that observed when warfarin was administered alone.

ipyridamole increases the plasma levels and cardiovasular effects of adenosine. Adjustment of adenosine osage should therefore be considered if use with dipyridamole is unavoidable.

Dipyridamole may increase the hypotensive effect of blood ressure lowering drugs and may counteract the anticolinesterase effect of cholinesterase inhibitors thereby otentially aggravating myasthenia gravis.

he effect of hypoglycaemic agents and the toxicity of nethotrexate may be increased by the concomitant dministration of aspirin.

spirin may decrease the natriuretic effect of spironolacone and inhibit the effect of uricosuric agents (e.g. probeecid, sulphinpyrazone).

There is some experimental evidence that ibuprofen intereres with aspirin induced inhibition of platelet cyclooxygenase. This interaction could reduce the beneficial ardiovascular effects of aspirin, however the evidence or this is not conclusive. Further, in view of the known ncreased risk of gastrointestinal toxicity associated with NSAID and aspirin co-medication, this combination should be avoided wherever possible. When such a combination s necessary the balance of gastrointestinal and cardiovascular risks should be considered.

4.6 Pregnancy and lactation

There is inadequate evidence of the safety in human pregnancy regarding dipyridamole and aspirin at low dose.

Animal studies performed with the drug combination revealed no increased teratogenic risk over the individual components alone. Fertility studies and studies covering the peri-postnatal period have not been performed with the combination.

ASASANTIN Retard should only be used with caution in the first and second trimester if considered essential by the physician in terms of benefit and risk. Asasantin Retard should be completely avoided in the third trimester.

Dipyridamole and salicylates are excreted in breast milk. Therefore ASASANTIN Retard should only be administered to nursing mothers if clearly needed.

4.7 Effects on ability to drive and use machines

None stated.

4.8 Undesirable effects

Two large scale trials (ESPS-2, PRoFESS) enrolling a total of 26,934 patients, thereof 11,831 patients treated with ASASANTIN, were used to define the side effects profile of ASASANTIN. In addition, from spontaneous reporting also those events where facts and evidence qualified these as side effects have been included.

Due to the granularity of the coding system, bleeding events are distributed over several System Organ Classes (SOC); therefore, a summary description of **bleeding** is given in Table 1 below.

Table 1 Bleeding events broken down to any bleeding, major bleeding, haemorrhage intracranial and gastrointestinal haemorrhage

	ESPS-2		PRoFESS
	ASASANTIN	Placebo	ASASANTIN
Patients treated (N (%))	1,650 (100)	1,649 (100)	10,055 (100)
Mean exposure (years)	1.4		1.9
Any Bleeding (%)	8.7	4.5	5.3
Major bleeding (%)	1.6	0.4	3.3
Haemorrhage intracranial (%)	0.6	0.4	1.2*
Gastrointestinal haemorrhage (%)	4.3	2.6	1.9

* PRoFESS: intracranial haemorrhage (1.0%) and intraocular haemorrhage (0.2%)

Side effects of ASASANTIN broken down to System Organ Classes:

Frequency: Very common (≥ 1/10); Common (≥ 1/100 to < 1/10); Uncommon (≥ 1/1,000 to < 1/100); Rare (≥ 1/10,000 to < 1/1,000); and Very rare (< 1/10,000) including isolated reports.

System Organ Class: MedDRA Term	Frequency
Blood and lymphatic system disorders:	
Anaemia	Common
Thrombocytopenia (reduction of platelet count)	Rare
Iron deficiency anaemia due to occult gastrointestinal bleeding	Rare
Immune system disorders:	
Hypersensitivity reactions	Common
rash	
urticaria	
severe bronchospasm	
angioedema	
Nervous system disorders:	
Haemorrhage intracranial	Common
Headache	Very Common
Migraine-like headache	Common
Dizziness	Very Common
Eye disorders:	
Eye haemorrhage (intraocular haemorrhage)	Uncommon
Cardiac disorders:	
Tachycardia	Uncommon
Worsening of symptoms of coronary heart disease	Common
(coronary artery disease)	
Syncope	Common
Vascular disorders:	
Hypotension	Uncommon
Hot flush	Uncommon
Respiratory, thoracic and mediastinal disorders:	
Epistaxis	Common
Gastrointestinal disorders:	
Dyspepsia (epigastric distress)	Very Common
Vomiting	Common
Diarrhoea	Very Common
Nausea	Very Common
Gastritis erosive	Rare
Gastric ulcer, Duodenal ulcer	Uncommon
(severe) Gastrointestinal haemorrhage	Common
Abdominal pain	Very Common
Skin and subcutaneous tissue disorders:	
Skin haemorrhage	Not known*
contusion	
ecchymosis	
haematoma	
Musculoskeletal, connective tissue and bone disorders:	
Myalgia	Common
Investigations:	
Bleeding time prolonged	Not known*
Injury, poisoning and procedural complications:	
Post procedural haemorrhage	Not known*
Operative haemorrhage	Not known*

* These ADRs were not reported in clinical trials, therefore a frequency could not be calculated.

In addition to those side effects listed for ASASANTIN, for the relevant monocompounds also the below listed side effects are established; however, have not been reported for ASASANTIN yet.

Dipyridamole:

Additional side effects reported with dipyridamole monotherapy were as follows:

Dipyridamole has been shown to be incorporated into gallstones.

Acetylsalicylic acid:

Additional side effects reported with acetylsalicylic acid monotherapy were as follows:

Blood and lymphatic system disorders

Disseminated intravascular coagulation, coagulopathy

Immune system disorders

Anaphylactic reactions (especially in patients with asthma)

Metabolism and nutrition disorders

Hypoglycaemia (children), hyperglycaemia, thirst, dehydration, hyperkaleamia, metabolic acidosis, respiratory alkalosis

Psychiatric disorders

Confusional state

Nervous system disorders

Agitation, brain oedema, lethargy, convulsion

Ear and labyrinth disorders

Tinnitus, deafness

Cardiac disorders

Arrhythmia

Respiratory, thoracic and mediastinal disorders

Dyspnoea, gingival bleeding, laryngeal oedema, hyperventilation, pulmonary oedema, tachypnoea

Gastrointestinal disorders

Gastric ulcer perforation, duodenal ulcer perforation, melaena, haematemesis, pancreatitis

Hepatobiliary disorders

Hepatitis, Reye's syndrome

Skin and subcutaneous tissue disorders

Erythema exsudativum multiforme

Musculoskeletal, connective tissue and bone disorders

Rhabdomyolysis

Renal and urinary disorders

Renal failure, nephritis interstitial, renal papillary necrosis, proteinuria

Pregnancy, puerperium and perinatal conditions

Prolonged pregnancy, prolonged labour, small for dates baby, stillbirth, antepartum haemorrhage, postpartum haemorrhage

General disorders and administration site conditions

Pyrexia, hypothermia

Investigations

Liver function test abnormal, blood uric acid increased (may lead to gout attacks), prothrombin time prolonged

4.9 Overdose

Symptoms

Because of the dose ratio of dipyridamole to aspirin, overdosage is likely to be dominated by signs and symptoms of dipyridamole overdose.

Due to the low number of observations, experience with dipyridamole overdose is limited.

Symptoms such as a warm feeling, flushes, sweating, accelerated pulse, restlessness, feeling of weakness, dizziness, drop in blood pressure and anginal complaints can be expected.

Salicylate poisoning is usually associated with plasma concentrations >350 mg/L (2.5 mmol/L). Most adult deaths occur in patients whose concentrations exceed 700 mg/L (5.1 mmol/L). Single doses less than 100 mg/kg are unlikely to cause serious poisoning.

Symptoms of salicylate overdose commonly include vomiting, dehydration, tinnitus, vertigo, deafness, sweating, warm extremities with bounding pulses, increased respiratory rate and hyperventilation. Some degree of acid-base disturbance is present in most cases.

A mixed respiratory alkalosis and metabolic acidosis with normal or high arterial pH (normal or reduced hydrogen ion concentration) is usual in adults and children over the age of four years. In children aged four years or less, a dominant metabolic acidosis with low arterial pH (raised hydrogen ion concentration) is common. Acidosis may increase salicylate transfer across the blood brain barrier.

Uncommon features of salicylate poisoning include haematemesis, hyperpyrexia, hypoglycaemia, hypokalaemia, thrombocytopaenia, increased INR/PTR, intravascular coagulation, renal failure and non-cardiac pulmonary oedema. Central nervous system features including confusion, disorientation, coma and convulsions are less common in adults than in children.

Therapy

Administration of xanthine derivatives (e.g. aminophylline) may reverse the haemodynamic effects of dipyridamole overdose. Due to its wide distribution to tissues and its predominantly hepatic elimination, dipyridamole is not likely to be accessible to enhanced removal procedures.

In the case of salicylate poisoning activated charcoal should be given to adults who present within one hour of ingestion of more than 250 mg/kg. the plasma salicylate concentration should be measured, although the severity of poisoning cannot be determined from this alone and the clinical and biochemical features must be taken into account. Elimination is increased by urinary alkalinisation, which is achieved by the administration of 1.26% sodium bicarbonate. The urine pH should be monitored. Correct metabolic acidosis with intravenous 8.4% sodium bicarbonate (first check serum potassium). Forced diuresis should not be used since it does not enhance salicylate excretion and may cause pulmonary oedema.

Haemodialysis is the treatment of choice for severe poisoning and should be considered in patients with plasma salicylate concentrations > 700 mg/L (5.1 mmol/L), or lower concentrations associated with severe clinical or metabolic features. Patients under ten years or over 70 have increased risk of salicylate toxicity and may require dialysis at an earlier stage.

5. PHARMACOLOGICAL PROPERTIES

5.1 Pharmacodynamic properties

The antithrombotic action of the Acetylsalicylic acid (aspirin)/dipyridamole combination is based on the different biochemical mechanisms involved. Acetylsalicylic acid (aspirin) inactivates irreversibly the enzyme cyclo-oxygenase in platelets thus preventing the production of thromboxane A2, a powerful inducer of platelet aggregation and vasoconstriction.

Dipyridamole inhibits the uptake of adenosine into erythrocytes, platelets and endothelial cells in vitro and in vivo; the inhibition amounts to approximately 80% at maximum and occurs dose-dependently at therapeutic concentrations (0.5 – 2 mcg/ml). Consequently, there is an increased concentration of adenosine locally to act on the platelet A_2-receptor, stimulating platelet adenylate cyclase, thereby increasing platelet cAMP levels.

Reduced platelet aggregation reduces platelet consumption towards normal levels. In addition, adenosine has a vasodilator effect and this is one of the mechanisms by which dipyridamole produces vasodilation.

Dipyridamole has also been shown in stroke patients to reduce the density of prothrombotic surface proteins (PAR-1: Thrombin receptor) on platelets as well as to reduce levels of c-reactive protein (CRP) and von Willebrand Factor (vWF). In-vitro investigations have shown that dipyridamole selectively inhibits inflammatory cytokines (MCP-1 and MMP-9) arising from platelet-monocyte interaction. Dipyridamole inhibits phosphodiesterase (PDE) in various tissues.

Whilst the inhibition of cAMP-PDE is weak, therapeutic levels of dipyridamole inhibit cGMP-PDE, thereby augmenting the increase in cGMP produced by EDRF (endothelium-derived relaxing factor, identified as nitric oxide (NO)).

Dipyridamole increases the release of t-PA from microvascular endothelial cells and was shown to amplify the antithrombotic properties of endothelial cells on thrombus formation on adjacent subendothelial matrix in a dose dependent manner. Dipyridamole is a potent radical scavenger for oxy- and peroxy-radicals.

Dipyridamole also stimulates the biosynthesis and release of prostacyclin by the endothelium and reduces the thrombogenicity of subendothelial structures by increasing the concentration of the protective mediator 13-HODE (13-hydroxyoctadecadienic acid).

Whereas acetylsalicylic acid (aspirin) inhibits only platelet aggregation, dipyridamole in addition inhibits platelet activation and adhesion. Therefore an additional benefit from combining both drugs can be expected

Clinical Trials:

ASASANTIN Retard® was studied in a double-blind, placebo-controlled, 24-month study (**E**uropean **S**troke **P**revention **S**tudy **2**, **ESPS2**) in which 6602 patients had an ischemic stroke or transient ischemic attack (TIA) within three months prior to entry. Patients were randomized to one of four treatment groups: ASASANTIN Retard (ASA / extended-release dipyridamole) 25 mg/200 mg; extended-release dipyridamole (ER-DP) 200 mg alone; ASA 25 mg alone; or placebo. Patients received one capsule twice daily (morning and evening). Efficacy assessments included analyses of stroke (fatal or nonfatal) and death (from all causes) as confirmed by a blinded morbidity and mortality assessment group. In ESPS-2 ASASANTIN Retard reduced the risk of stroke by 22.1% compared to ASA.

50 mg/day alone (p =0.008) and reduced the risk of stroke by 24.4% compared to extended-release dipyridamole 400 mg/day alone (p = 0.002). ASASANTIN Retard reduced the risk of stroke by 36.8% compared to placebo (p <0.001).

The results of the ESPS-2 study are supported by the **E**uropean/**A**ustralasian **S**troke **P**revention in **R**eversible **I**schaemia **T**rial **(ESPRIT)** study [112] which studied a combination treatment of diypridamole 400 mg daily (83% of patients treated with the extended-release dipyridamole formulation) and ASA 30-325 mg daily. A total of 2739 patients after ischaemic stroke of arterial origin were enrolled in the ASA-alone (n = 1376) and combination ASA plus dipyridamole (n = 1363) arm. The primary outcome event was the composite of death from all vascular causes, non-fatal stroke, non-fatal myocardial infarction (MI), or major bleeding complications. Patients in the ASA plus dipyridamole group showed a 20% risk reduction (p<0.05) for the primary composite endpoint compared with those in the ASA alone group (12.7% vs. 15.7%; hazard ratio [HR] 0.80, 95% CI 0.66–0.98).

The PRoFESS (**PR**evention Regimen **F**or **E**ffectively avoiding **S**econd **S**trokes) study was a randomized, parallel group, international, double-blind, double-dummy, active and placebo controlled, 2x2 factorial study to compare ASASANTIN with clopidogrel, and telmisartan with matching placebo in the prevention of stroke in patients who had already experienced an ischaemic stroke of noncardioembolic origin. Individuals who were ≥ 55 years of age and who had had an ischemic stroke within 90 days of entry to the study were included. A total of 20,332 patients were randomized to ASASANTIN (n = 10,181) or clopidogrel (n = 10,151), both given on a background of standard treatment. The primary endpoint was the time to first recurrent stroke of any type.

The incidence of the primary endpoint was similar in both treatment groups (9.0% for ASASANTIN vs. 8.8% for clopidogrel; HR 1.01, 95 % CI 0.92-1.11). No significant difference between the ASASANTIN and clopidogrel treatment groups were detected for several other important pre-specified endpoints, including the composite of recurrent stroke, myocardial infarction, or death due to vascular causes (13.1% in both treatment groups; HR 0.99, 95 % CI 0.92-1.07) and the composite of recurrent stroke or major haemorrhagic event (11.7% for ASASANTIN vs. 11.4% for clopidogrel; HR 1.03, 95 % CI 0.95-1.11). The functional neurological outcome 3 months post recurrent stroke was assessed by the Modified Rankin Scale (MRS) and no significant difference in the distribution of the MRS between ASASANTIN and clopidogrel was observed (p = 0.3073 by Cochran-Armitage test for linear trend).

More patients randomised to ASA+ER-DP (4.1%) than to clopidogrel (3.6%) experienced a major haemorrhagic event (HR = 1.15; 95% CI 1.00, 1.32; p = 0.0571). The difference between the treatment groups was mainly due to the higher incidence of non-life threatening major haemorrhagic events in the ASA+ER-DP group (2.9%) than in the clopidogrel group (2.5%) while the incidences of life threatening haemorrhagic events were similar in both groups (128 patients vs. 116 patients). The overall incidence of intracranial haemorrhage was higher in the ASA+ER-DP group (1.4%) than in the clopidogrel group (1.0%) resulting in a HR of 1.42 (95% CI 1.11, 1.83) with a p-value of 0.0062. The difference between the treatment groups resulted mainly from the higher incidence of haemorrhagic strokes in the ASA+ER-DP group (0.9% vs. clopidogrel 0.5%).

5.2 Pharmacokinetic properties

There is no noteworthy pharmacokinetic interaction between the extended release pellets of dipyridamole and aetylsalicylic acid (aspirin). Therefore pharmacokinetics of ASASANTIN Retard is reflected by the pharmacokinetics of the individual components.

Dipyridamole

(Most pharmacokinetic data refer to healthy volunteers.)

With dipyridamole, there is dose linearity for all doses used in therapy.

For long-term treatment dipyridamole modified release capsules, formulated as pellets were developed. The pH dependent solubility of dipyridamole which prevents dissolution in the lower parts of the gastro-intestinal tract (where sustained release preparations must still release the active principle) was overcome by combination with tartaric acid. Retardation is achieved by a diffusion membrane, which is sprayed onto the pellets.

Various kinetic studies at steady state showed, that all pharmacokinetic parameters which are appropriate to characterise the pharmacokinetic properties of modified release preparations are either equivalent or somewhat improved with dipyridamole modified release capsules given b.i.d. compared to dipyridamole tablets administered t.d.s./q.d.s.: Bioavailability is slightly greater, peak concentrations are similar, trough concentrations are considerably higher and peak trough fluctuation is reduced.

Absorption

The absolute bioavailability is about 70%. As first pass removes approx. 1/3 of the dose administered, near to complete absorption of dipyridamole following administration of acetylsalicylic acid (aspirin) modified release capsules can be assumed.

Peak plasma concentrations of dipyridamole following a daily dose of 400 mg acetylsalicylic acid (aspirin) (given as 200 mg b.i.d) are reached about 2 - 3 hours after administration. There is no relevant effect of food on the pharmacokinetics of dipyridamole in acetylsalicylic acid (aspirin) modified release capsules.

Distribution

The apparent volume of distribution of the central compartment (Vc) is about 5 l (similar to plasma volume). The apparent volume of distribution at steady state is about 100 l, reflecting distribution to various compartments.

The drug does not cross the blood-brain barrier to a significant extent.

The protein binding of Dipyridamole is about 97-99%, primarily it is bound to alpha 1-acid glycoprotein and albumin.

Metabolism

Metabolism of dipyridamole occurs in the liver. Dipyridamole is metabolized primarily by conjugation with glucuronic acid to form mainly a monoglucuronide and only small amounts of diglucuronide. In plasma about 80% of the total amount is present as parent compound, and 20% of the total amount as monoglucuronide. The pharmacodynamic activity of dipyridamole glucuronides is considerably lower than of dipyridamole.

Elimination

The dominant half-life with oral administration is about 40 minutes as it is the case with i.v. administration.

Renal excretion of parent compound is negligible (< 0.5%). Urinary excretion of the glucuronide metabolite is low (5%), the metabolites are mostly (about 95%) excreted via the bile into the faeces, with some evidence of entero-hepatic recirculation.

Total clearance is approximately 250 ml/min and mean residence time is about 11 hours (resulting from an intrinsic MRT of about 6.4 h and a mean time of absorption of 4.6 h).

As with i.v. administration a prolonged terminal elimination half-life of approximately 13 hours is observed.

This terminal elimination phase is of relatively minor importance in that it represents a small proportion of the total AUC, as evidenced by the fact that steady state is achieve within 2 days with b.i.d. regimens of modified releas capsules. There is no significant accumulation of the dru with repeated dosing.

Kinetics in elderly

Dipyridamole plasma concentrations (determined as AUC in elderly subjects (> 65 years) were about 50% higher f tablet treatment and about 30% higher with intake c ASASANTIN Retard modified release capsules than i young (<55 years) subjects. The difference is cause mainly by reduced clearance; absorption appears to b similar.

Similar increases in plasma concentrations in elder patients were observed in the ESPS2 study for PERSAN TIN® modified release capsules as well as for ASASANTI Retard.

Kinetics in patients with renal impairment

Since renal excretion is very low (5%), no change in phar macokinetics is to be expected in cases of renal insuffi ciency. In the ESPS2 trial, in patients with creatinin clearances ranging from about 15 mL/min to >100 mL min, no changes were observed in the pharmacokinetics c dipyridamole or its glucuronide metabolite if data wer corrected for differences in age.

Kinetics in patients with hepatic impairment

Patients with hepatic insufficiency show no change i plasma concentrations of dipyridamole, but an increase of (pharmacodynamically low active) glucuronides. It is suggested to dose dipyridamole without restriction as lon as there is no clinical evidence of liver failure.

Acetylsalicylic acid (aspirin)

Absorption

After oral administration acetylsalicylic acid (aspirin) is rapidly and completely absorbed in the stomach and intestine. Approximately 30% of the dose of acetylsalicylic acid (aspirin) is hydrolyzed presystemically to salicylic acid. Maximum plasma concentrations after a daily dose of 50 mg acetylsalicylic acid from ASASANTIN Retard (given as 25 mg twice daily) are attained after 30 minutes of each dose, and peak plasma concentration at steady state amounted to approximately 360 ng/mL for acetylsalicylic acid (aspirin); maximum plasma concentrations of salicylic acid are achieved after 60-90 minutes and amount to approximately 1100 ng/ml. There is no relevant effect of food on the pharmacodynamics of acetylsalicylic acid in ASASANTIN Retard.

Distribution

Acetylsalicylic acid (aspirin) is rapidly converted to salicylate but is the predominant form of the drug in the plasma during the first 20 minutes following oral administration.

Plasma acetylsalicylic acid (aspirin) concentrations decline rapidly with a half-life of approx. 15 minutes. Its major metabolite, salicylic acid, is highly bound to plasma proteins, and its binding is concentration-dependent (nonlinear). At low concentrations (<100 μg/mL), approximately 90% of salicylic acid is bound to albumin. Salicylates are widely distributed to all tissues and fluids in the body, including the central nervous system, breast milk, and fetal tissues.

Metabolism

Acetylsalicylic acid (aspirin) is metabolised rapidly by non-specific esterases to salicylic acid. Salicylic acid is metabolised to salicyluric acid, salicyl phenolic glucuronide, salicylic acyl glucuronide, and to a minor extent to gentisic acid and gentisuric acid. The formation of the major metabolites salicyluric acid and salicylic phenolic glucuronide is easily saturated and follows Michaelis-Menten kinetics; the other metabolic routes are first-order processes.

Elimination

Acetylsalicylic acid (aspirin) has an elimination half-life of elimination of 15-20 minutes in plasma; the major metabolite salicylic acid has a half-life of elimination of 2-3 hours at low doses (e.g. 325 mg), which may rise to 30 hours at higher doses because of nonlinearity in metabolism and plasma protein binding.

More than 90% of acetylsalicylic acid (aspirin) is excreted as metabolites via the kidneys. The fraction of salicylic acid excreted unchanged in the urine increases with increasing dose and the renal clearance of total salicylate also increases with increasing urinary pH.

Kinetics in patients with renal impairment

Renal dysfunction: acetylsalicylic acid (aspirin) is to be avoided in patients with severe renal failure (glomerular filtration rate less than 10 mL/min). An increase in total plasma concentrations and in the unbound fraction of salicylic acid has been reported.

Kinetics in patients with hepatic impairment

Hepatic dysfunction: acetylsalicylic acid is to be avoided in patients with severe hepatic insufficiency. An increase in the unbound fraction of salicylic acid has been reported.

5.3 Preclinical safety data

Dipyridamole and aspirin separately have been extensively investigated in animal models and no clinically significant findings have been observed at doses equivalent to therapeutic doses in humans. Toxicokinetic evaluations were not included in these studies.

studies with the drug combination dipyridamole/aspirin in a ratio of 1:4 revealed additive, but no potentiating toxic effects. A single dose study in rats using dipyridamole/aspirin in a ratio of 1:0.125 gave comparable results to studies with the 1:4 combination.

6. PHARMACEUTICAL PARTICULARS

6.1 List of excipients

Tartaric acid

Povidone

Methacrylic acid-methyl methacrylate copolymer (1:2)

Talc

Acacia

Hypromellose phthalate

Hypromellose

Triacetin

Dimethicone 350

Stearic acid

Lactose

Aluminium stearate

Colloidal silica

Maize starch

Microcrystalline cellulose

Sucrose

Titanium dioxide; E171

Capsule Shells:

Gelatin

Titanium dioxide; E171

Red and yellow iron oxides; E172

Printing Ink:

Shellac

Ethyl alcohol

Isopropyl alcohol

Propylene glycol

N-butyl alcohol

Ammonium hydroxide

Potassium hydroxide

Purified water

Red iron oxide; E172

6.2 Incompatibilities

None stated.

6.3 Shelf life

30 months

6.4 Special precautions for storage

Store below 25°C

Discard any capsules remaining 6 weeks after first opening.

6.5 Nature and contents of container

White polypropylene tubes with low-density polyethylene Air-sec stoppers filled with desiccating agent (90% white silicon gel/10% molecular sieves). Packs contain 60 capsules.

6.6 Special precautions for disposal and other handling

None stated.

7. MARKETING AUTHORISATION HOLDER

Boehringer Ingelheim limited

Ellesfield Avenue

Bracknell

Berkshire

RG12 8YS

England

8. MARKETING AUTHORISATION NUMBER(S)

PL 00015/0224

9. DATE OF FIRST AUTHORISATION/RENEWAL OF THE AUTHORISATION

12 May 1998 / 22 December 2003

10. DATE OF REVISION OF THE TEXT

May 2009

Legal category

Prescription only medicine

Ashton & Parsons Infants' Powders

(SSL International plc)

1. NAME OF THE MEDICINAL PRODUCT

Ashton & Parsons Infants' Powders.

2. QUALITATIVE AND QUANTITATIVE COMPOSITION

Tincture of Matricaria 0.002ml.

3. PHARMACEUTICAL FORM

Powder containing Tincture of Matricaria 0.002ml.

4. CLINICAL PARTICULARS

4.1 Therapeutic indications

This is a herbal product traditionally used in infants for the symptomatic relief of the pain and gastric upset associated with teething.

4.2 Posology and method of administration

Route of administration: Oral. This product is only intended for use in teething infants. *Children aged over 6 months:* One powder, dry on the tongue, night and morning. *Children aged 6 months and under:* Half a powder, taken as above. If the child is very restless, the dose may be repeated every 1, 2, or 3 hours if necessary until improvement occurs.

4.3 Contraindications

There are no known contraindications to matricaria tincture. The product is contraindicated in cases of established lactose intolerance.

4.4 Special warnings and precautions for use

Label Warnings: If symptoms persist for more than 5 days, consult your doctor. Keep out of the reach of children.

4.5 Interaction with other medicinal products and other forms of interaction

None stated.

4.6 Pregnancy and lactation

None stated.

4.7 Effects on ability to drive and use machines

None stated.

4.8 Undesirable effects

None stated.

4.9 Overdose

Overdosage with this product would cause diarrhoea due to excessive lactose intake. Treatment: Treatment would be withdrawal of the product and supportive measures such as oral rehydration therapy.

5. PHARMACOLOGICAL PROPERTIES

5.1 Pharmacodynamic properties

Matricaria Chamomilla is monographed in the Homeopathic Pharmacopoeia and is recommended for complaints of the newly born and during dentition. It is listed in Martindale-The Extra Pharmacopoeia as a domestic remedy for indigestion and as a carminative. It is traditionally used for pain relief during teething and has been shown to have anti-inflammatory activity. Tincture of matricaria is an alcoholic decoction of Matricaria Chamomilla and is therefore credited with the same activity.

5.2 Pharmacokinetic properties

None stated.

5.3 Preclinical safety data

None stated.

6. PHARMACEUTICAL PARTICULARS

6.1 List of excipients

Lactose Ph Eur.

6.2 Incompatibilities

None stated.

6.3 Shelf life

36 months.

6.4 Special precautions for storage

None.

6.5 Nature and contents of container

The powder is contained in a wrapper made of glazed paper. 20 wrappers are packed in a boxboard outer.

6.6 Special precautions for disposal and other handling

Not applicable

7. MARKETING AUTHORISATION HOLDER

SSL International PLC. Venus, 1 Old Park Lane, Trafford Park, Manchester, M41 7HA.

8. MARKETING AUTHORISATION NUMBER(S)

PL 17905/0070

9. DATE OF FIRST AUTHORISATION/RENEWAL OF THE AUTHORISATION

23/03/06

10. DATE OF REVISION OF THE TEXT

23/03/06

Asmabec Clickhaler 50, 100, 250

(UCB Pharma Limited)

1. NAME OF THE MEDICINAL PRODUCT

Asmabec Clickhaler 50 micrograms. Inhalation powder

Asmabec Clickhaler 100micrograms. Inhalation powder

Asmabec Clickhaler 250micrograms. Inhalation powder

2. QUALITATIVE AND QUANTITATIVE COMPOSITION

Each metered actuation of 1.3mg contains 50 micrograms of beclometasone dipropionate and delivers 45 micrograms of beclometasone dipropionate.

Each metered actuation of 2.6mg contains 100 micrograms of beclometasone dipropionate and delivers 90 micrograms of beclometasone dipropionate.

Each metered actuation of 6.6mg contains 250 micrograms of beclometasone dipropionate and delivers 225 micrograms of beclometasone dipropionate.

For excipients see 6.1.

3. PHARMACEUTICAL FORM

Inhalation powder

White free-flowing powder.

4. CLINICAL PARTICULARS

4.1 Therapeutic indications

Beclometasone Dipropionate is indicated for the control of persistent asthma.

4.2 Posology and method of administration

The product is intended for oral inhalation only. For optimum results Asmabec Clickhaler should be used regularly.

The initial dose should be appropriate to the severity of the disease and the maintenance dose titrated to the lowest dose at which effective control of asthma is achieved.

Adults:

The initial dose for patients with mild asthma is 200 to 400 micrograms per day; this may be increased to 800 micrograms per day if required.

For patients with moderate asthma and severe asthma the initial dose can be 800 to 1600 micrograms per day, increased to 2000 micrograms in severe cases. The normal maximum daily dose for adults is 2000 micrograms.

The maintenance dose is normally 200 to 400 micrograms twice daily. If necessary the dose may be increased to 1600 to 2000 micrograms per day divided into two to four doses and be reduced later when asthma is stabilised.

Children aged 6 - 12 years:

Up to 100 micrograms 2 to 4 times daily according to the clinical response.

Normally the maximum daily dose in children is 400μg. However some cases of severe asthma may not be controlled and higher doses may be required in line with international guidelines. Once the asthma is controlled, the dose of Asmabec Clickhaler should be reduced to the minimum to maintain control.

When transferring a patient to Asmabec Clickhaler from other devices, treatment should be individualised taking into consideration the active ingredient and method of administration.

4.3 Contraindications

Asmabec Clickhaler is contra-indicated in patients with hypersensitivity (allergy) to beclometasone dipropionate or to the excipient (see 6.1 List of Excipients).

4.4 Special warnings and precautions for use

Patients should be instructed in the proper use of the inhaler. They should also be made aware of the prophylactic nature of therapy with Asmabec Clickhaler and that they should use it regularly, every day, even when they are asymptomatic. Beclometasone dipropionate is not suitable for the treatment of an acute asthma attack.

Increasing use of bronchodilators, in particular short-acting inhaled β_2-agonists, to relieve symptoms indicates deterioration of asthma control. If patients find that short-acting relief bronchodilator treatment becomes less effective, or they need more inhalations than usual, medical attention must be sought. In this situation patients should be reassessed and consideration given to the need for increased anti-inflammatory therapy (e.g. higher doses of inhaled corticosteroids or a course of oral corticosteroids). Severe exacerbations of asthma must be treated in the normal way.

Systemic effects of inhaled corticosteroids may occur, particularly at high doses prescribed for prolonged periods. Possible systemic effects include adrenal suppression, growth retardation in children and adolescents, decrease in bone mineral density, cataract and glaucoma. It is important therefore that the dose of inhaled steroids is titrated to the lowest dose at which effective control of symptoms is achieved.

It is recommended that the height of children receiving prolonged treatment with inhaled steroids is regularly monitored. If growth is slowed, therapy should be reviewed with the aim of reducing the dose of inhaled corticosteroid if possible, to the lowest dose at which effective control of symptoms is achieved.

Doses in excess of 1500 micrograms per day may induce adrenal suppression. In such patients the risks of developing adrenal suppression should be balanced against the therapeutic advantages, and precautions should be taken to provide systemic steroid cover in situations of stress or elective surgery.

The transfer to inhaled beclometasone dipropionate of patients who have been treated with systemic steroids for long periods of time, or at high dose, needs special care and subsequent management as recovery from impaired adrenocortical function is slow. With these patients adrenocortical function should be monitored regularly and their dose of systemic steroid reduced cautiously. Gradual withdrawal of the systemic steroid should commence after about one week. Reductions in dosage, appropriate to the level of maintenance systemic steroid, should be introduced at not less than weekly intervals.

Some patients may feel unwell in a non-specific way during withdrawal of the systemic steroid. They should be encouraged to persevere with the inhaled beclometasone dipropionate, unless there are objective signs of adrenal insufficiency.

Patients who have been transferred from oral steroids whose adrenocortical function is impaired should carry a steroid warning card indicating that they may need supplementary systemic steroids during periods of stress, eg. worsening asthma attacks, chest infections, major intercurrent illness, surgery, trauma etc.

Replacement of systemic steroid treatment with inhaled therapy sometimes unmasks allergies such as allergic rhinitis or eczema previously controlled by the systemic drug.

In the case of massive mucus secretion in the respiratory tract, de-obstruction and a short course of oral steroids may be necessary to ensure efficacy of the inhaled beclometasone.

Special care is necessary in patients with active or quiescent pulmonary tuberculosis and in patients with viral, bacterial and fungal infections of the eye, mouth or respiratory tract. In the case of bacterial infection of the respiratory tract adequate antibiotic co-medication may be required.

Treatment with Asmabec Clickhaler especially at high doses should not be stopped abruptly.

The presence of lactose may trigger hypersensitivity reactions, including bronchospasm, in patients with a known hypersensitivity to milk proteins.

4.5 Interaction with other medicinal products and other forms of interaction

Due to the very low plasma concentration achieved after inhaled dosing, clinically significant drug interactions are in general unlikely. Care should be taken when co-administering known strong CYP 3A4 inhibitors (e.g. ketoconazole, itraconazole, nelfinavir, ritonavir) as there is a potential for increased systemic exposure to beclomethasone.

4.6 Pregnancy and lactation

Pregnancy: There are insufficient data regarding the safety of beclometasone dipropionate during human pregnancy. Systemic administration of relatively high doses of corticosteroids to pregnant animals can cause abnormalities of foetal development including cleft palate and intra-uterine growth retardation. There may therefore be a very small risk of such effects in the human foetus. Because beclometasone dipropionate is delivered directly to the lungs by the inhaled route it avoids the high level of exposure that occurs when corticosteroids are given by systemic routes.

The use of beclometasone dipropionate in pregnancy requires that the possible benefits of the drug be weighed against the possible hazards. It should be noted that the drug has been in widespread use for many years without apparent ill consequence.

Lactation It is reasonable to assume that beclometasone dipropionate is secreted in milk, but at the dosages used for direct inhalation there is low potential for significant levels in breast milk.

The use of beclometasone dipropionate in mothers breast feeding their babies requires that the therapeutic benefits of the drug be weighed against the potential hazards to the mother and baby.

4.7 Effects on ability to drive and use machines

None known

4.8 Undesirable effects

Infections and infestations: candidiasis of the mouth and throat. This may be treated whilst still continuing with Asmabec Clickhaler.

Immune system disorders: easy bruising of the skin, very rarely hypersensitivity including rash and angioedema may occur.

Endocrine disorders: decrease in bone mineral density, adrenal suppression, growth retardation in children and adolescents

Psychiatric disorders: anxiety, sleep disorders, behavioural changes, including hyperactivity and irritability (predominately seen in children)

Eye disorders: cataract and glaucoma

Respiratory, thoracic and mediastinal disorders: hoarseness, paradoxical bronchospasm. If bronchospasm occurs the preparation should be discontinued immediately and if necessary alternative therapy instituted.

It is recommended to rinse out the mouth thoroughly with water immediately after inhalation in order to reduce the risks of candidiasis and hoarseness.

Systemic effects of inhaled corticosteroids may occur, particularly at high doses prescribed for prolonged periods (see also section 4.4).

4.9 Overdose

Acute Inhalation of a large amount of the drug over a short period may lead to temporary suppression of adrenal function. No emergency action is required. Treatment with beclometasone dipropionate by inhalation should be continued at a dose sufficient to control asthma; adrenal function recovers in a few days and can be verified by measuring plasma cortisol.

Chronic Use of excessive doses of inhaled beclometasone dipropionate over a prolonged period may cause adrenal suppression and a degree of atrophy of the adrenal cortex. Transfer to a maintenance dose of a systemic steroid may be required until the condition is stabilised. Treatment with inhaled beclometasone dipropionate should then be continued at a dose sufficient to control asthma.

If higher than approved doses are continued over prolonged periods, significant adrenal suppression and adrenal crisis are possible. Presenting symptoms of adrenal crisis may initially be non-specific and include anorexia, abdominal pain, weight loss, tiredness, headache, nausea, vomiting. Hypoglycaemia with decreased consciousness and/or convulsions is a typical symptom. Situations which could potentially trigger acute adrenal crisis include exposure to trauma, surgery, infection or any rapid reduction in dosage.

5. PHARMACOLOGICAL PROPERTIES

5.1 Pharmacodynamic properties

ATC code: R03B A01. Other anti-asthmatics, inhalants, glucocorticoids.

Beclometasone dipropionate given by inhalation has a glucocorticoid anti-inflammatory action within the lungs.

The exact mechanism responsible for this anti-inflammatory effect is unknown.

5.2 Pharmacokinetic properties

Absorption from the gastrointestinal tract is slow and bioavailability is low, suggesting that most of the absorbed drug is metabolised during its first passage through the liver. Since the dose of oral beclometasone dipropionate needed to suppress plasma cortisol is greater than that required by inhalation, this suggests that the portion absorbed from the lungs is mainly responsible for any systemic effects.

5.3 Preclinical safety data

Studies in a number of animal species, including rats, rabbits and dogs, have shown no unusual toxicity during acute experiments. The effects of beclometasone dipropionate in producing signs of glucocorticoid excess during chronic administration by various routes are dose related. Teratogenicity testing has shown cleft palate in mice, as with other glucocorticoids. Beclometasone dipropionate is non-genotoxic and demonstrates no oncogenic potential in lifetime studies with rats.

6. PHARMACEUTICAL PARTICULARS

6.1 List of excipients

Lactose monohydrate (which contains milk proteins).

6.2 Incompatibilities

None known

6.3 Shelf life

3 years.

6 months when removed from the foil pouch.

6.4 Special precautions for storage

Do not store above 30°C. Store in a dry place.

6.5 Nature and contents of container

A plastic inhaler device incorporating a metering pump and a mouthpiece enclosed within a polyester/ aluminium / polyethylene heat-sealed sachet.

Each 50 microgram inhaler contains 200 actuations.

Each 100 microgram inhaler contains 200 actuations.

Each 250 microgram inhaler contains 100 actuations.

6.6 Special precautions for disposal and other handling

1. Remove mouthpiece cover from the inhaler

2. Shake the inhaler well

3. Hold the inhaler upright with thumb on the base and finger on the push button.

Press the dosing button down firmly - once only.

4. Breathe out as far as is comfortable.

Note: do not blow into the device at any time.

5. Place mouthpiece in your mouth. Close lips firmly around it (do not bite it).

6. Breathe in through your mouth steadily and deeply, to draw the medicine into your lungs.

7. Hold your breath, take the inhaler from your mouth and continue holding your breath for about 5 seconds.

8. For the second puff, keep the inhaler upright and repeat steps 2-7.

9. Replace the mouthpiece cover.

7. MARKETING AUTHORISATION HOLDER

UCB Pharma Limited

208 Bath Road

Slough

Berkshire,

SL1 3WE

8. MARKETING AUTHORISATION NUMBER(S)

PL 00039/0501 Asmabec Clickhaler 50microgram

PL 00039/0502 Asmabec Clickhaler 100microgram

PL 00039/0503 Asmabec Clickhaler 250microgram

9. DATE OF FIRST AUTHORISATION/RENEWAL OF THE AUTHORISATION

30 October 1998

10. DATE OF REVISION OF THE TEXT

Approved: April 2008

POM

Asmasal Clickhaler

(UCB Pharma Limited)

1. NAME OF THE MEDICINAL PRODUCT

Asmasal Clickhaler inhalation powder, 95 micrograms/inhalation

2. QUALITATIVE AND QUANTITATIVE COMPOSITION

Each metered actuation of 3 mg of inhalation powder contains 114 micrograms of salbutamol sulphate (95 micrograms salbutamol base) and delivers 110 micrograms of salbutamol sulphate (90 micrograms of salbutamol base).

Excipient: Lactose Monohydrate 2.886 mg per actuation.

For a full list of excipients see section 6.1.

3. PHARMACEUTICAL FORM

Inhalation powder

A plastic inhalation device incorporating an actuating and metering mechanism enclosed within an aluminium foil heat sealed bag.

4. CLINICAL PARTICULARS

4.1 Therapeutic indications

Asmasal Clickhaler is indicated for the symptomatic treatment of bronchospasm in bronchial asthma and other conditions with associated reversible airways obstruction. Appropriate anti-inflammatory therapy should be considered in line with current practice.

Asmasal Clickhaler may be used when necessary to relieve attacks of acute dyspnoea due to bronchoconstriction.

Asmasal Clickhaler may also be used before exertion to prevent exercise-induced bronchospasm or before exposure to a known unavoidable allergen challenge.

4.2 Posology and method of administration

Adults: For the relief of acute bronchospasm and for managing intermittent episodes of asthma, one inhalation may be administered as a single dose; this may be increased to two inhalations if necessary. If the response is inadequate, higher doses than two inhalations can be used. The maximum recommended dose is two inhalations three or four times a day.

To prevent exercise-induced bronchospasm one or two inhalations should be taken 15 minutes before exertion.

One or two inhalations may also be taken before foreseeable contact with allergens.

Elderly: as for adults

Children: One inhalation is the recommended dose for the relief of acute bronchospasm, in the management of episodic asthma or before exercise. If the response is inadequate, higher doses than one inhalation can be used.

On demand use should not exceed four times daily. The bronchodilator effect of each administration of inhaled salbutamol lasts for at least four hours except in patients whose asthma is becoming worse. Such patients should be warned not to increase their usage of the inhaler, but should seek medical advice since treatment with, or an increased dose of an inhaled and/or systemic glucocorticosteroid is indicated.

As there may be adverse effects associated with excessive dosing, the dosage or frequency of administration should only be increased on medical advice.

The following instructions for use are included in the Patient Information Leaflet:

1. Remove mouthpiece cover from the inhaler

2. Shake the inhaler well

3. Hold the inhaler upright with thumb on the base and finger on the push button. Press the dosing button down firmly - once only

4. Breathe out as far as is comfortable.

Note: do not blow into the device at any time.

5. Place mouthpiece in your mouth. Close lips firmly around it (do not bite it)

6. Breathe in through your mouth steadily and deeply, to draw the medicine into your lungs.

7. Hold your breath, take the inhaler from your mouth and continue holding your breath for about 5 seconds.

8. For the second puff, keep the inhaler upright and repeat steps 2-7.

9. Replace the mouthpiece cover.

.3 Contraindications
smasal Clickhaler is contra-indicated in patients with tolerance or hypersensitivity to the active ingredient or ie excipient.

.4 Special warnings and precautions for use
ronchodilators should not be the only or main treatment in atients with moderate to severe or unstable asthma. evere asthma requires regular medical assessment cluding lung function testing as patients are at risk of evere attacks and even death. Physicians should consider using the maximum recommended dose of inhaled orticosteroid and/or oral corticosteroid therapy in these atients. Increasing use of bronchodilators, in particular hort-acting inhaled beta-2-agonists to relieve symptoms, dicates deterioration of asthma control. If patients find at short-acting bronchodilator treatment becomes less fective or they need more inhalations than usual, they hould be warned by the prescriber of the need for consulting immediately. In this situation, patients should be assessed and consideration given to the need for creased anti-inflammatory therapy (eg. higher doses of haled corticosteroids or a course of oral corticosteroids).

albutamol should be administered cautiously, especially ith systemic therapy, to patients suffering from thyrotoxosis, myocardial insufficiency, hypertension, known neurysms, decreased glucose tolerance, manifest diaetes, phaeochromocytoma and concomitant use of carac glycosides. Caution should also be applied in patients ith myocardial ischemia, tachyarrythmias and hyperophic obstructive cardiomyopathy.

ardiovascular effects may be seen with sympathomietic drugs, including salbutamol. There is some evidence om post-marketing data and published literature of rare ccurrences of myocardial ischemia associated with salutamol. Patients with underlying severe heart disease .g. ischemic heart disease, arrhythmia or severe heart ilure) who are receiving salbutamol should be warned to eek medical advice if they experience chest pain or other mptoms of worsening heart disease. Attention should be aid to assessment of symptoms such as dyspnoea and nest pain, as they may be of either respiratory or cardiac rigin.

albutamol and non-selective beta-blocking drugs, such s propranolol, should not usually be prescribed together.

otentially serious hypokalaemia has resulted from sysmic β_2-agonist therapy. Particular caution is advised in cute severe asthma as this effect may be potentiated by oncomitant treatment with xanthine derivatives, steroids, uretics and by hypoxia. It is recommended that serum otassium levels are monitored in such situations.

atients with rare hereditary problems of galactose intolance, the Lapp lactase deficiency or glucose-galactose alabsorption should not take this medicine.

5 Interaction with other medicinal products and other rms of interaction
albutamol and non-selective beta-blocking drugs, such s propranolol, should not usually be prescribed together. aution is also advised in patients using cardiac glycodes.

otentially serious hypokalaemia has resulted from sysmic β_2-agonist therapy. Particular caution is advised in cute severe asthma as this effect may be potentiated by oncomitant treatment with xanthine derivatives, steroids, uretics and by hypoxia.

atients should be instructed to discontinue salbutamol at ast 6 hours before intended anaesthesia with halogeated anaesthetics, wherever possible.

.6 Pregnancy and lactation
regnancy: Administration of salbutamol during pregnancy hould only be considered if the expected benefit to the other is greater than any possible risk to the fetus. As with e majority of drugs there is little published evidence of its afety in the early stages of pregnancy, but in animal tudies, there was evidence of some harmful effects in e fetus at very high dose levels.

actation: Salbutamol may be secreted in breast milk. It is ot known whether salbutamol has a harmful effect on the eonate and so its use should be restricted to situations here it is felt that the expected benefit to the mother is kely to outweigh any potential risk to the neonate.

.7 Effects on ability to drive and use machines
ndividual reactions, especially at higher doses, may be uch that patients' ability to drive or use machines may be ffected, particularly so at the beginning of treatment and conjunction with alcohol.

he possible side effects of salbutamol such as transient nuscle cramps and tremor may necessitate caution when sing machines.

.8 Undesirable effects
he side effects are dose dependent and due to the direct nechanism of β_2-agonists.

ypersensitivity reactions include angioedema and urtiaria, bronchospasm, hypotension and collapse and have een reported very rarely.

lood and the lymphatic system disorders: potentially serous hypokalaemia may result from systemic β_2-agonist nerapy. Special precautions should be taken in patients sing β_2 -agonists with hypokalaemia because of the increased risk of tachycardia and arrhythmias. Hypokalaemia may be potentiated by concomitant therapy with corticosteroids, diuretics and xanthines.

Psychiatric disorders: nervousness, feeling of tenseness. As with other β_2 agonists, hyperactivity in children has been reported rarely.

Nervous system disorders: mild tremor, headache, dizziness.

Cardiac disorders: tachycardia, angioedema, hypotension, cardiac arrhythmias (including atrial fibrillation, supraventricular tachycardia and extrasystoles) and myocardial ischaemia (see Section 4.4) have been reported in association with β_2 agonists, usually in susceptible patients.

Respiratory, thoracic and mediastinal disorders: as with other inhalation therapy, the potential for paradoxical bronchospasm should be kept in mind. If it occurs, the preparation should be discontinued immediately and alternative therapy instituted.

Gastrointestinal disorders: nausea

Skin and subcutaneous tissue disorders: urticaria.

Musculoskeletal, connective tissue and bone disorders: there have been rare reports of transient muscle cramps

General disorders and administration site conditions: oral and pharyngeal irritation can occur.

4.9 Overdose
An overdose should be treated symptomatically.

The preferred antidote for overdosage with salbutamol is a cardioselective beta-blocking agent but beta-blocking drugs should be used with caution in patients with a history of bronchospasm.

If hypokalaemia occurs potassium replacement via the oral route should be given. In patients with severe hypokalaemia intravenous replacement may be necessary.

Increased serum lactate levels, and rarely, lactic acidosis, have been reported following therapy with salbutamol, particularly after high dose administration. Symptoms include deep, rapid breathing, cold and blue coloured fingers and toes, inability to concentrate and general malaise.

5. PHARMACOLOGICAL PROPERTIES

5.1 Pharmacodynamic properties
ATC Code: R03A C02

Salbutamol is a beta-adrenergic stimulant which has a selective action on bronchial β_2-adrenoceptors at therapeutic doses. Following inhalation, salbutamol exerts a stimulating action on β_2 receptors on bronchial smooth muscles, and thus ensures rapid bronchodilation which becomes significant within a few minutes and persists for 4 to 6 hours.

The drug also causes vasodilation leading to a reflex chronotropic effect and widespread metabolic effects, including hypokalaemia.

5.2 Pharmacokinetic properties
Following treatment with salbutamol by inhalation, only approximately 10% or less of the drug is deposited in the airways and the remainder is swallowed. Pre-systemic metabolism of salbutamol is considerable and occurs primarily in the gastrointestinal tract and by conjugation to form an inactive sulphate ester. The systemic clearance for salbutamol is 30 l/hr. Salbutamol is eliminated both through excretion of unchanged drug in urine and through metabolism mainly via sulphate conjugation. The elimination half-life varies between 3 and 7 hours. Salbutamol is well absorbed from the gastrointestinal tract.

5.3 Preclinical safety data
Preclinical data reveal no special hazard for humans based on conventional studies of safety pharmacology, repeated dose toxicity and genotoxicity. Findings concerning teratogenicity in rabbits at high systemic exposure and the induction of benign mesovarian leiomyomas in rats are not considered of clinical concern.

6. PHARMACEUTICAL PARTICULARS

6.1 List of excipients
Lactose monohydrate (which contains milk protein)

6.2 Incompatibilities
Not applicable

6.3 Shelf life
3 years in unopened foil pouch. 6 months when removed from foil pouch.

6.4 Special precautions for storage
Do not store above 30°C. Store in a dry place.

6.5 Nature and contents of container
A plastic inhaler device incorporating an actuating and metering mechanism enclosed within an aluminium foil heat sealed bag. Each device contains 750mg of powder - sufficient for 200 actuations.

6.6 Special precautions for disposal and other handling
Instructions for use are included in the patient information leaflet. These are also included in Section 4.2.

7. MARKETING AUTHORISATION HOLDER
UCB Pharma Limited
208 Bath Road
Slough, Berkshire
SL1 3WE
UK

8. MARKETING AUTHORISATION NUMBER(S)
PL 00039/0497

9. DATE OF FIRST AUTHORISATION/RENEWAL OF THE AUTHORISATION
9 May 1997

10. DATE OF REVISION OF THE TEXT
Approved September 2009.

AT10
(Intrapharm Laboratories Ltd)

1. NAME OF THE MEDICINAL PRODUCT
AT10

2. QUALITATIVE AND QUANTITATIVE COMPOSITION
Dihydrotachysterol BP 0.025% w/v

3. PHARMACEUTICAL FORM
Oily solution

4. CLINICAL PARTICULARS

4.1 Therapeutic indications
AT10 is recommended for use in acute, chronic and latent forms of hypocalcaemic tetany due to hypoparathyroidism where its action is to increase the rate of absorption and utilisation of calcium.

4.2 Posology and method of administration
Adults (and the elderly):
In acute cases 3-5ml may be given on each of the first three days of treatment, followed two to three days later by blood and urinary calcium estimations. The maintenance dose of AT10 is usually within the range of 1-7ml each week, but the precise amount depends on the results of serum and urinary calcium determinations. In chronic cases an initial dose of 2ml of AT10 daily, or on alternate days, may be sufficient to maintain normocalcaemia in moderate cases. The dose of AT10 usually has to be increased during menstruation and periods of unusual activity.

Children
No specific dosage recommendations.

Route of Administration
Oral.

4.3 Contraindications
Hypersensitivity to dihydrotachysterol.
Hypercalcaemia.
Hypervitaminosis D.
Allergy to nuts (including peanuts).

4.4 Special warnings and precautions for use
AT10 contains Arachis oil (peanut oil) and should not be taken by patients known to be allergic to peanut. As there is a possible relationship between allergy to peanut and allergy to Soya, patients with Soya allergy should also avoid AT10.

As with calciferol, uncontrolled prolonged administration of AT10 can result in hypercalcaemia which may lead to nephrocalcinosis. Therefore accurate blood calcium determinations must be made at the beginning of treatment and then periodically until the required maintenance dose has been established. The serum calcium level should subsequently be kept between 2.25-2.5mmol/litre. Serum phosphate, magnesium, and alkaline phosphatase should also be measured periodically to monitor progress.

If nausea and vomiting are present, serum calcium level should be checked.

Monitoring of calciuria is a convenient supplement to blood calcium determinations, but it should not be regarded as a substitute because in hypoparathyroid patients treated with AT10 hypercalciuria can occur in the presence of hypocalcaemia.

Certain individuals, particularly those suffering from sarcoidosis, are very sensitive to the effect of Vitamin D and it is advisable to consult a physician in cases of doubt.

4.5 Interaction with other medicinal products and other forms of interaction
Several classes of medicine interact with Vitamin D analogues calling for adjustment in the dosage of AT10. Thyroid replacement therapy may increase clearance of dihydrotachysterol; cholestyramine may impair its absorption; thiazide diuretics may enhance the calcaemic response leading to hypercalcaemia; barbiturates, anticonvulsants, rifampicin and isoniazid may reduce the effectiveness of AT10. Hypercalcaemia induced by excessive dosaging of AT10 may enhance the toxic effects of cardiac glycosides.

4.6 Pregnancy and lactation
The safety of dihydrotachysterol in pregnancy is not established. Since there is some evidence that use during pregnancy could lead to foetal damage and hypercalcaemia in

the newborn, treatment with AT10 is only justified if potential benefits outweigh possible risks. Dihydrotachysterol is excreted in breast milk and may cause hypercalcaemia in the suckling infant. AT10 is contraindicated in breast feeding mothers.

4.7 Effects on ability to drive and use machines
None stated.

4.8 Undesirable effects
Side effects are most likely to be due to hypercalcaemia, the first signs of which are loss of appetite, listlessness and nausea.

More severe manifestations include vomiting, urgency of micturition, polyuria, dehydration, thirst, vertigo, stupor, headache, abdominal cramps and paralysis.

The calcium and phosphorus concentrations of serum and urine are increased.

With chronic overdosage, calcium may be deposited in many tissues, including arteries and the kidneys, leading to hypertension and renal failure. Plasma cholesterol may also be increased.

4.9 Overdose
Treatment

The symptoms of hypercalcaemia in chronic overdosage will usually respond to withdrawal of medication, bed rest, liberal fluid intake and the use of laxatives.

In acute overdosage, consideration should be given to recovery of AT10 by emesis or gastric lavage if ingestion is recent. Serum calcium estimations should be helpful in determining management.

In massive overdosage of Vitamin D, corticosteroids have been found useful and also neutral phosphate in resistant cases. Several months management may be needed in such cases.

5. PHARMACOLOGICAL PROPERTIES

5.1 Pharmacodynamic properties
Dihydrotachysterol is a synthetic analogue of Vitamin D and is used in the treatment of hypoparathyroidism. However, it is not useful in the treatment of rickets since its antirachitic activity is considerably weaker than that of Vitamin D.

The actions of dihydrotachysterol resemble those of calciferol and Vitamin D_3. It promotes the absorption of calcium from the intestine and the mobilisation of calcium from bone as effectively as calciferol. Dihydrotachysterol acts more rapidly and is more rapidly eliminated than calciferol and its action is therefore more readily controlled; in practice, calciferol is generally used for the treatment of Vitamin D deficiency and dihydrotachysterol for other conditions.

5.2 Pharmacokinetic properties
Vitamin D substances are well absorbed from the gastro-intestinal tract. The presence of bile is essential for adequate intestinal absorption; absorption may be decreased in patients with decreased fat absorption.

Vitamin D compounds and their metabolites are excreted mainly in the bile and faeces with only small amounts appearing in urine.

5.3 Preclinical safety data
There are no preclinical data of relevance to the prescriber which are additional to that already included in other sections of the SPC.

6. PHARMACEUTICAL PARTICULARS

6.1 List of excipients
Arachis oil, Sodium sulphate anhydrous.

6.2 Incompatibilities
None.

6.3 Shelf life
48 months.

6.4 Special precautions for storage
Store in well-closed containers protected from heat and light.

6.5 Nature and contents of container
15ml bottles with a 1ml dropper.

Pack size: 15ml.

6.6 Special precautions for disposal and other handling
None.

Administrative Data

7. MARKETING AUTHORISATION HOLDER
Intrapharm Laboratories Limited
Maidstone
Kent
ME15 9QS

8. MARKETING AUTHORISATION NUMBER(S)
PL 17509/0004

9. DATE OF FIRST AUTHORISATION/RENEWAL OF THE AUTHORISATION
30 April 1999

10. DATE OF REVISION OF THE TEXT
May 2003

11. Legal category
P

ATARAX 10mg

(Alliance Pharmaceuticals)

1. NAME OF THE MEDICINAL PRODUCT
Atarax™

2. QUALITATIVE AND QUANTITATIVE COMPOSITION
Hydroxyzine hydrochloride 10mg

3. PHARMACEUTICAL FORM
10mg film coated tablets, coloured orange and coded on one side with 'AX'.

4. CLINICAL PARTICULARS

4.1 Therapeutic indications
Atarax is indicated to assist in the management of anxiety in adults.

Atarax is indicated for the management of pruritus associated with acute and chronic urticaria, including cholinergic and physical types, and atopic and contact dermatitis in adults and children.

4.2 Posology and method of administration
Method of administration: oral.

Dosage:

Anxiety

Adults 50-100mg four times daily.

Pruritus

Adults Starting dose of 25mg at night increasing as necessary to 25mg three or four times daily.

Use in the elderly Atarax may be used in elderly patients with no special precautions other than the care always necessary in this age group. The lowest effective maintenance dose and careful observation for side-effects are important.

Use in children From 6 months to 6 years 5-15mg rising to 50mg daily in divided doses and for children over 6 years, 15-25mg rising to 50-100mg daily in divided doses.

As with all medications, the dosage should be adjusted according to the patient's response to therapy.

Renal impairment The total daily dosage should be reduced by half (see 'Special Warnings and Precautions for Use').

4.3 Contraindications
Atarax is contra-indicated in patients who have shown previous hypersensitivity to it.

4.4 Special warnings and precautions for use
Atarax should be used with caution in patients with impaired renal function (see 'Posology and Method of Administration'). It is uncertain whether the drug may accumulate or have other adverse effects in such patients. Atarax is completely metabolised and one of the metabolites is the active metabolite cetirizine. Cetirizine is renally excreted and clearance is reduced in patients with moderate renal impairment and on dialysis compared to normal volunteers.

Because of its potential anticholinergic effects, Atarax should be used with caution in patients with bladder outflow obstruction.

4.5 Interaction with other medicinal products and other forms of interaction
Patients should be warned that Atarax may enhance their response to alcohol, barbiturates and other CNS depressants.

4.6 Pregnancy and lactation
Atarax is contra-indicated in early pregnancy. Hydroxyzine, when administered to the pregnant mouse, rat and rabbit, induced foetal abnormalities at doses substantially above the human therapeutic range. Clinical data in humans are inadequate to establish safety in early pregnancy. There is inadequate evidence of safety in the later stages of pregnancy. Use in pregnancy only when there is no safe alternative or when the disease itself carries risks for the mother or child.

Use in nursing mothers It is not known whether Atarax is excreted in human milk. Since many drugs are so excreted, Atarax should not be given to nursing mothers.

4.7 Effects on ability to drive and use machines
Patients should be warned that Atarax may impair their ability to perform activities requiring mental alertness or physical co-ordination such as operating machinery or driving a vehicle.

4.8 Undesirable effects
Therapeutic doses of Atarax seldom produce marked impairment of mental alertness. Drowsiness may occur; if so, it is usually transitory and may disappear after a few days of continued therapy or upon reduction of the dose. Dryness of the mouth may be encountered at higher doses. Dizziness, weakness, headache and confusion, and urinary retention have been reported.

Extensive clinical use has substantiated the absence of toxic effects on the liver or bone marrow when administered for over four years of uninterrupted therapy. The absence of side-effects has been further demonstrated in experimental studies in which excessively high doses were administered.

Involuntary motor activity, including rare instances of tre mor and convulsions, have been reported, usually wit doses considerably higher than those recommended. Con tinuous therapy with over 1g/day has been employed i some patients without these effects having been encoun tered.

4.9 Overdose
The most common manifestation of Atarax overdosage i hypersedation. As in the management of overdosage wit any drug, it should be borne in mind that multiple agent may have been taken. If vomiting has not occurred spon taneously in conscious patients it should be induce Immediate gastric lavage is also recommended. Genera supportive care, including frequent monitoring of the vit signs and close observation of the patient is indicate Hypotension, though unlikely, may be controlled with intra venous fluids and noradrenaline, or metaraminol. Adrena line should not be used in this situation as Atara counteracts its pressor action.

There is no specific antidote. It is doubtful whether hae modialysis has any value in the treatment of overdosag with Atarax. However, if other agents such as barbiturate have been ingested concomitantly, haemodialysis may b indicated.

5. PHARMACOLOGICAL PROPERTIES

5.1 Pharmacodynamic properties
Atarax is unrelated chemically to phenothiazine, reserpin and meprobamate.

Atarax has been shown clinically to be a rapid-actin anxiolytic with a wide margin of safety. It induces a calmin effect in anxious tense adults. It is not a cortical depres sant, but its action may be due to a suppression of activit in certain key regions of the subcortical area of the centr nervous system.

Antihistamine effects have been demonstrated experimen tally and confirmed clinically; it is highly effective in alle viating pruritus.

5.2 Pharmacokinetic properties
Atarax is rapidly absorbed from the gastro-intestinal trac and effects are usually noted within 15 to 30 minutes afte oral administration.

5.3 Preclinical safety data
None stated.

6. PHARMACEUTICAL PARTICULARS

6.1 List of excipients
Tablet core:

- Lactose (anhydrous)
- Calcium Hydrogen Phosphate Anhydrous
- Starch, Pregelatinised.
- Magnesium Stearate
- Sodium Laurilsulphate
- Silica, colloidal anhydrous.

Tablet coating:

Opadry II Orange 85G23730 (10mg only) -contains:

- Poly (vinyl alcohol)
- Talc
- Macrogol 3350
- Sunset yellow (E110)
- Titanium dioxide (E171)
- Iron oxide yellow (E172)
- Quinoline yellow (E104)
- Lecithin (E322).

6.2 Incompatibilities
None stated.

6.3 Shelf life
24 Months.

6.4 Special precautions for storage
Do not store above 25°C.

6.5 Nature and contents of container
White opaque 250/51 micron PVC/PCTFE (Aclar) - 2 micron aluminium foil blister strips containin 84 × 10mg tablets, (6 blister strips per carton)

6.6 Special precautions for disposal and other handlin
No special requirements.

7. MARKETING AUTHORISATION HOLDER
Alliance Pharmaceuticals Limited
Avonbridge House
Chippenham
Wiltshire
SN15 2BB
United Kingdom

8. MARKETING AUTHORISATION NUMBER(S)
Atarax 10mg Tablets PL 16853/0094

9. DATE OF FIRST AUTHORISATION/RENEWAL O THE AUTHORISATION
Atarax 10mg Tablets 27 April 1987/30 July 1997

10. DATE OF REVISION OF THE TEXT
October 2008

ATARAX 25mg Tablets

(Alliance Pharmaceuticals)

. NAME OF THE MEDICINAL PRODUCT
TARAX™

. QUALITATIVE AND QUANTITATIVE COMPOSITION
Hydroxyzine hydrochloride 25mg

. PHARMACEUTICAL FORM
25mg film coated tablets, coloured green and coded on one side with 'AX'.

. CLINICAL PARTICULARS

4.1 Therapeutic indications
Atarax is indicated to assist in the management of anxiety in adults.

Atarax is indicated for the management of pruritus associated with acute and chronic urticaria, including cholinergic and physical types, and atopic and contact dermatitis in adults and children.

4.2 Posology and method of administration
Method of administration: oral.

Dosage:

Anxiety

Adults 50-100mg four times daily.

Pruritus

Adults Starting dose of 25mg at night increasing as necessary to 25mg three or four times daily.

Use in the elderly Atarax may be used in elderly patients with no special precautions other than the care always necessary in this age group. The lowest effective maintenance dose and careful observation for side-effects are important.

Use in children From 6 months to 6 years 5-15mg rising to 50mg daily in divided doses and for children over 6 years, 15-25mg rising to 50-100mg daily in divided doses.

As with all medications, the dosage should be adjusted according to the patient's response to therapy.

Renal impairment The total daily dosage should be reduced by half (see 'Special Warnings and Precautions for Use').

4.3 Contraindications
Atarax is contra-indicated in patients who have shown previous hypersensitivity to it.

4.4 Special warnings and precautions for use
Atarax should be used with caution in patients with impaired renal function (see 'Posology and Method of Administration'). It is uncertain whether the drug may accumulate or have other adverse effects in such patients. Atarax is completely metabolised and one of the metabolites is the active metabolite cetirizine. Cetirizine is renally excreted and clearance is reduced in patients with moderate renal impairment and on dialysis compared to normal volunteers.

Because of its potential anticholinergic effects, Atarax should be used with caution in patients with bladder outflow obstruction.

4.5 Interaction with other medicinal products and other forms of interaction
Patients should be warned that Atarax may enhance their response to alcohol, barbiturates and other CNS depressants.

4.6 Pregnancy and lactation
Atarax is contra-indicated in early pregnancy. Hydroxyzine, when administered to the pregnant mouse, rat and rabbit, induced foetal abnormalities at doses substantially above the human therapeutic range. Clinical data in humans are inadequate to establish safety in early pregnancy. There is inadequate evidence of safety in the later stages of pregnancy. Use in pregnancy only when there is no safe alternative or when the disease itself carries risks for the mother or child.

Use in nursing mothers It is not known whether Atarax is excreted in human milk. Since many drugs are so excreted, Atarax should not be given to nursing mothers.

4.7 Effects on ability to drive and use machines
Patients should be warned that Atarax may impair their ability to perform activities requiring mental alertness or physical co-ordination such as operating machinery or driving a vehicle.

4.8 Undesirable effects
Therapeutic doses of Atarax seldom produce marked impairment of mental alertness. Drowsiness may occur; if so, it is usually transitory and may disappear after a few days of continued therapy or upon reduction of the dose. Dryness of the mouth may be encountered at higher doses. Dizziness, weakness, headache and confusion, and urinary retention have been reported.

Extensive clinical use has substantiated the absence of toxic effects on the liver or bone marrow when administered for over four years of uninterrupted therapy. The absence of side-effects has been further demonstrated in experimental studies in which excessively high doses were administered.

Involuntary motor activity, including rare instances of tremor and convulsions, have been reported, usually with doses considerably higher than those recommended. Continuous therapy with over 1g/day has been employed in some patients without these effects having been encountered.

4.9 Overdose
The most common manifestation of Atarax overdosage is hypersedation. As in the management of overdosage with any drug, it should be borne in mind that multiple agents may have been taken. If vomiting has not occurred spontaneously in conscious patients it should be induced. Immediate gastric lavage is also recommended. General supportive care, including frequent monitoring of the vital signs and close observation of the patient is indicated. Hypotension, though unlikely, may be controlled with intravenous fluids and noradrenaline, or metaraminol. Adrenaline should not be used in this situation as Atarax counteracts its pressor action.

There is no specific antidote. It is doubtful whether haemodialysis has any value in the treatment of overdosage with Atarax. However, if other agents such as barbiturates have been ingested concomitantly, haemodialysis may be indicated.

5. PHARMACOLOGICAL PROPERTIES

5.1 Pharmacodynamic properties
Atarax is unrelated chemically to phenothiazine, reserpine and meprobamate.

Atarax has been shown clinically to be a rapid-acting anxiolytic with a wide margin of safety. It induces a calming effect in anxious tense adults. It is not a cortical depressant, but its action may be due to a suppression of activity in certain key regions of the subcortical area of the central nervous system.

Antihistamine effects have been demonstrated experimentally and confirmed clinically; it is highly effective in alleviating pruritus.

5.2 Pharmacokinetic properties
Atarax is rapidly absorbed from the gastro-intestinal tract and effects are usually noted within 15 to 30 minutes after oral administration.

5.3 Preclinical safety data
None stated.

6. PHARMACEUTICAL PARTICULARS

6.1 List of excipients
Tablet core:

- Lactose (anhydrous)
- Calcium Hydrogen Phosphate Anhydrous
- Starch, Pregelatinised.
- Magnesium Stearate
- Sodium Laurilsulphate
- Silica, colloidal anhydrous.

Tablet coating:
Opadry II Green 85G24674 (25mg only) -contains:

- Poly (vinyl alcohol)
- Talc
- Macrogol 3350
- Quinoline yellow (E104)
- Titanium dioxide (E171)
- Brilliant blue (E1331)
- Indigo carmine (E132)
- Lecithin (E322).

6.2 Incompatibilities
None stated.

6.3 Shelf life
24 Months.

6.4 Special precautions for storage
Do not store above 25°C.

6.5 Nature and contents of container
White opaque 250/5/120 micron PVC/TE/PVdC - 20 micron aluminium foil blister strips containing 28 × 25mg tablets (2 blister strips per carton).

6.6 Special precautions for disposal and other handling
No special requirements.

7. MARKETING AUTHORISATION HOLDER
Alliance Pharmaceuticals Limited
Avonbridge House
Chippenham
Wiltshire
SN15 2BB
United Kingdom

8. MARKETING AUTHORISATION NUMBER(S)
Atarax 25mg Tablets PL 16853/0095

9. DATE OF FIRST AUTHORISATION/RENEWAL OF THE AUTHORISATION
Atarax 25mg Tablets 24 July 1985/24 July 2002

10. DATE OF REVISION OF THE TEXT
October 2008

Ativan Injection

(Wyeth Pharmaceuticals)

1. NAME OF THE MEDICINAL PRODUCT
Ativan® Injection

2. QUALITATIVE AND QUANTITATIVE COMPOSITION
Ativan Injection contains the active ingredient lorazepam at a concentration of 4 mg/ml.

Lorazepam (INN, BAN) is chemically defined as 7-chloro-5-(o-chlorphenyl)-1,3-dihydro-3-hydroxy-2H-1,4-benzodiazepin-2-one.

3. PHARMACEUTICAL FORM
Solution for injection

Clear, colourless solution supplied in clear glass ampoules containing 4 mg lorazepam in 1 ml of solution.

4. CLINICAL PARTICULARS

4.1 Therapeutic indications
Pre-operative medication or premedication for uncomfortable or prolonged investigations, e.g. bronchoscopy, arteriography, endoscopy.

The treatment of acute anxiety states, acute excitement or acute mania.

The control of status epilepticus.

4.2 Posology and method of administration
Dosage and duration of therapy should be individualised. The lowest effective dose should be prescribed for the shortest time possible.

Treatment in all patients should be withdrawn gradually to minimise possible withdrawal symptoms (See Special Warnings and Special Precautions for Use).

Route of administration
Ativan Injection can be given intravenously or intramuscularly. However, the intravenous route is to be preferred. Care should be taken to avoid injection into small veins and intra-arterial injection.

Absorption from the injection site is considerably slower if the intramuscular route is used and as rapid an effect may be obtained by oral administration of Ativan tablets.

Ativan should not be used for long-term chronic treatment.

Preparation of the injection
Ativan Injection is slightly viscid when cool. To facilitate injection it may be diluted 1:1 with normal Saline or Water for Injection BP immediately before administration. If given intramuscularly it should always be diluted.

Ativan Injection is presented as a 1ml solution in a 2ml ampoule to facilitate dilution.

Ativan Injection should not be mixed with other drugs in the same syringe.

Dosage:

1. Premedication:
Adults: 0.05mg/kg (3.5mg for an average 70kg man). By the intravenous route the injection should be given 30-45 minutes before surgery when sedation will be evident after 5-10 minutes and maximal loss of recall will occur after 30-45 minutes.

By the intramuscular route the injection should be given 1-$1^1/_2$ hours before surgery when sedation will be evident after 30-45 minutes and maximal loss of recall will occur after 60-90 minutes.

Children: Ativan Injection is not recommended in children under 12.

2. Acute Anxiety
Adults: 0.025-0.03mg/kg (1.75-2.1mg for an average 70kg man). Repeat 6 hourly.

Children: Ativan Injection is not recommended in children under 12.

3. Status epilepticus
Adults: 4mg intravenously

Children: 2mg intravenously

Elderly: The elderly may respond to lower doses and half the normal adult dose may be sufficient.

Patients with Renal or Hepatic impairment:
Lower doses may be sufficient in these patients *(See Special Warnings and Precautions for Use)*. Use in patients with severe hepatic insufficiency is contraindicated.

4.3 Contraindications

- Acute pulmonary insufficiency.
- Hypersensitivity to benzodiazepines, including Ativan Injection or any of the vehicle constituents (polyethylene glycol, propylene glycol, benzyl alcohol).
- Sleep apnoea syndrome
- Myasthenia gravis
- Severe hepatic insufficiency
- Ativan Injection contains benzyl alcohol and is contra-indicated in infants or young children, up to 3 years old.

Ativan Injection is not recommended for out-patient use unless the patient is accompanied.

4.4 Special warnings and precautions for use
Prior to use, Ativan Injection may be diluted with equal amounts of compatible diluent *(see Posology and Method*

of Administration). Intravenous injection should be made slowly except in the control of status epilepticus where rapid injection is required.

The possibility that respiratory arrest may occur or that the patient may have partial airway obstruction should be considered. Therefore, equipment necessary to maintain a patent airway and to support respiration/ventilation should be available and used where necessary.

The use of benzodiazepines, including lorazepam, may lead to physical and psychological dependence.

Severe anaphylactic/anaphylactoid reactions have been reported with the use of benzodiazepines. Cases of angioedema involving the tongue, glottis or larynx have been reported in patients after taking the first or subsequent doses of benzodiazepines. Some patients taking benzodiazepines have had additional symptoms such as dyspnoea, throat closing, or nausea and vomiting. Some patients have required medical therapy in the emergency department. If angioedema involves the tongue, glottis or larynx, airway obstruction may occur and be fatal. Patients who develop angioedema after treatment with a benzodiazepine should not be rechallenged with the drug.

It is recommended that patients receiving Ativan Injection should remain under observation for at least eight hours and preferably overnight. When Ativan Injection is used for short procedures on an outpatient basis, the patient should be accompanied when discharged.

Patients should be advised that their tolerance for alcohol and other CNS depressants will be diminished in the presence of Ativan Injection. Alcoholic beverages should not be consumed for at least 24 to 48 hours after receiving Ativan Injection.

Use of benzodiazepines, including lorazepam, may lead to potentially fatal respiratory depression. Extreme care must be taken in administering Ativan Injection to elderly or very ill patients and to those with limited pulmonary reserve or compromised respiratory function (eg, chronic obstructive pulmonary disease [COPD], sleep apnoea syndrome), because of the possibility that apnoea and/or cardiac arrest may occur. Care should also be exercised when administering Ativan Injection to a patient with status epilepticus, especially when the patient has received other central nervous system depressants.

There is no evidence to support the use of Ativan Injection in coma or shock.

Ativan is not intended for the primary treatment of psychotic illness or depressive disorders, and should not be used alone to treat depressed patients. The use of benzodiazepines may have a disinhibiting effect and may release suicidal tendencies in depressed patients.

Pre-existing depression may emerge during benzodiazepine use.

There are no clinical data available for Ativan Injection with regard to abuse or dependence. However, based upon experience with oral benzodiazepines, doctors should be aware that repeated doses of Ativan Injection over a prolonged period of time may lead to physical and psychological dependence. The risk of dependence on Ativan is low when used at the recommended dose and duration, but increases with higher doses and longer term use. The risk of dependence is further increased in patients with a history of alcoholism or drug abuse, or in patients with significant personality disorders. Therefore, use in individuals with a history of alcoholism or drug abuse should be avoided.

Dependence may lead to withdrawal symptoms, especially if treatment is discontinued abruptly. Therefore, **the drug should always be discontinued gradually** - using the oral preparation if necessary.

Symptoms reported following discontinuation of oral benzodiazepines include headaches, muscle pain, anxiety, tension, depression, insomnia, restlessness, confusion, irritability, sweating, and the occurrence of "rebound" phenomena whereby the symptoms that led to treatment with benzodiazepines recur in an enhanced form. These symptoms may be difficult to distinguish from the original symptoms for which the drug was prescribed.

In severe cases the following symptoms may occur: derealisation; depersonalisation; hyperacusis; tinnitus; numbness and tingling of the extremities; hypersensitivity to light, noise, and physical contact; involuntary movements; vomiting; hallucinations; convulsions. Convulsions may be more common in patients with pre-existing seizure disorders or who are taking other drugs that lower the convulsive threshold, such as antidepressants.

It may be useful to inform the patient that treatment will be of limited duration and that it will be discontinued gradually. The patient should also be made aware of the possibility of "rebound" phenomena to minimise anxiety should they occur.

Withdrawal symptoms (eg, rebound insomnia) can appear following cessation of recommended doses after as little as one week of therapy.

There are indications that, in the case of benzodiazepines with a short duration of action, withdrawal phenomena can become manifest within the dosage interval, especially when the dosage is high.

When benzodiazepines with a long duration of action are being used, it is important to warn against changing to a benzodiazepine with a short duration of action, as withdrawal symptoms may develop.

Abuse of benzodiazepines has been reported.

Anxiety or insomnia may be a symptom of several other disorders. The possibility should be considered that the complaint may be related to an underlying physical or psychiatric disorder for which there is more specific treatment.

Caution should be used in the treatment of patients with acute narrow-angle glaucoma.

As with all benzodiazepines, the use of lorazepam may worsen hepatic encephalopathy.

Patients with impaired renal or hepatic function should be monitored frequently and have their dosage adjusted carefully according to patient response. Lower doses may be sufficient in these patients. The same precautions apply to elderly or debilitated patients and patients with chronic respiratory insufficiency.

As with all CNS-depressants, the use of benzodiazepines may precipitate encephalopathy in patients with severe hepatic insufficiency. Therefore, use in these patients is contraindicated.

Some patients taking benzodiazepines have developed a blood dyscrasia, and some have had elevations in liver enzymes. Periodic haematologic and liver-function assessments are recommended where repeated courses of treatment are considered clinically necessary.

Transient anterograde amnesia or memory impairment has been reported in association with the use of benzodiazepines. This effect may be advantageous when Ativan is used as a premedicant.

Paradoxical reactions have been occasionally reported during benzodiazepine use (see Undesirable effects). Such reactions may be more likely to occur in children and the elderly. Should these occur, use of the drug should be discontinued.

Although hypotension has occurred only rarely, benzodiazepines should be administered with caution to patients in whom a drop in blood pressure might lead to cardiovascular or cerebrovascular complications. This is particularly important in elderly patients.

Ativan Injection contains the excipients polyethylene glycol and propylene glycol. There have been rare reports of propylene glycol toxicity (e.g. lactic acidosis, hyperosmolality, hypotension) and polyethylene glycol toxicity (e.g. acute tubular necrosis) during administration of Ativan Injection at higher than recommended doses. Central nervous system toxicity, including seizures, as well as unresponsiveness, tachypnoea, tachycardia and diaphoresis have also been associated with propylene glycol toxicity. Symptoms may be more likely to develop in patients with renal or hepatic impairment and in paediatric patients.

4.5 Interaction with other medicinal products and other forms of interaction

Not recommended: Concomitant intake with alcohol

The sedative effects may be enhanced when the product is used in combination with alcohol. This affects the ability to drive or use machines.

The benzodiazepines, including Ativan Injection, produce additive CNS depressant effects when co-administered with other medications which themselves produce CNS depression, e.g. barbiturates, antipsychotics, sedatives/hypnotics, anxiolytics, antidepressants, narcotic analgesics, sedative antihistamines, anticonvulsants and anaesthetics.

Concurrent administration of lorazepam with valproate may result in increased plasma concentrations and reduced clearance of lorazepam. Lorazepam dosage should be reduced to approximately 50% when co-administered with valproate.

Concurrent administration of lorazepam with probenecid may result in a more rapid onset or prolonged effect of lorazepam due to increased half-life and decreased total clearance. Lorazepam dosage needs to be reduced by approximately 50% when co-administered with probenecid.

An enhancement of the euphoria induced by narcotic analgesics may occur with benzodiazepine use, leading to an increase in psychic dependence.

Compounds which inhibit certain hepatic enzymes (particularly cytochrome P450) may enhance the activity of benzodiazepines. To a lesser degree this also applies to benzodiazepines which are metabolised only by conjugation.

The addition of scopolamine to Ativan Injection is not recommended, since their combination has been observed to cause an increased incidence of sedation, hallucination and irrational behaviour.

Concomitant use of clozapine and lorazepam may produce marked sedation, excessive salivation, and ataxia.

Administration of theophylline or aminophylline may reduce the sedative effects of benzodiazepines, including lorazepam.

There have been reports of apnoea, coma, bradycardia, heart arrest and death with the concomitant use of lorazepam injection solution and haloperidol.

4.6 Pregnancy and lactation

Ativan Injection should not be used during pregnanc[y], especially during the first and last trimesters, unless [in] the judgement of the physician such administration [is] clinically justifiable. Benzodiazepines may cause foet[al] damage when administered to pregnant women.

If the drug is prescribed to a woman of childbearing poten[tial], she should be warned to contact her physician abou[t] stopping the drug if she intends to become, or suspect[s] that she is, pregnant.

Use of Ativan Injection during the late phase of pregnanc[y] may require ventilation of the infant at birth.

If, for compelling medical reasons, the product is adminis[tered] during the late phase of pregnancy, or during labou[r] at high doses, effects on the neonate, such as hypother[mia], hypotonia and moderate respiratory depression, ca[n] be expected, due to the pharmacological action of th[e] compound.

Infants of mothers who ingested benzodiazepines for several weeks or more preceding delivery have been reporte[d] to have withdrawal symptoms during the postnatal period.

Symptoms such as hypotonia, hypothermia, respiratory depression, apnoea, feeding problems, and impaired metabolic response to cold stress have been reported in neonates born of mothers who have received benzodiazepines during the late phase of pregnancy or at delivery.

There are insufficient data regarding obstetrical safety of parenteral Ativan, including use in cesarean section. Such use, therefore, is not recommended.

Since benzodiazepines are found in breast milk, Ativan Injection should not be given to breast feeding mothers unless the expected benefit to the woman outweighs the potential risk to the infant.

4.7 Effects on ability to drive and use machines

Sedation, amnesia, impaired concentration and impaired muscular function may adversely affect the ability to drive or use machines. Therefore, patients should not drive or operate machinery within 24-48 hours of administration of Ativan Injection and should be advised not to take alcohol *(see also Interactions).*

4.8 Undesirable effects

Lorazepam is well tolerated and imbalance or ataxia are signs of excessive dosage. Drowsiness may occur. Occasional confusion, hangover, headache on waking, dizziness, blurred vision, nausea, vomiting, restlessness, depression, crying, sobbing, hallucinations, diplopia have been reported. In addition, blood dyscrasias and increased liver enzymes have occasionally been reported. On rare occasions visual disturbances, hypotension, hypertension, gastrointestinal disturbances and mild transient skin rashes have been reported. Convulsion/seizure has been reported during or following treatment with lorazepam but causality has not been established.

Tolerance at the injection site is generally good although, rarely, pain and redness have been reported after Ativan Injection.

Transient anterograde amnesia or memory impairment may occur using therapeutic doses, the risk increasing at higher doses *(see Special Warnings and Special Precautions for Use).*

Paradoxical reactions, such as restlessness, agitation, irritability, aggressiveness, delusion, rage, nightmares, hallucinations, psychoses and inappropriate behaviour, have been occasionally reported during benzodiazepine use. Such reactions may be more likely to occur in children and the elderly *(see Special Warnings and Special Precautions for Use).*

4.9 Overdose

In the management of overdosage with any drug, it should be borne in mind that multiple agents may have been taken.

Overdosage of benzodiazepines is usually manifested by degrees of central nervous system depression ranging from drowsiness to coma. In mild cases, symptoms include drowsiness, mental confusion and lethargy. In more serious cases, and especially when other CNS-depressant drugs or alcohol are ingested, symptoms may include ataxia, hypotension, hypotonia, respiratory depression, cardiovascular depression, coma and, very rarely, death.

Rarely, propylene glycol toxicity and polyethylene glycol toxicity have been reported following higher than recommended doses of Ativan Injection *(See Section 4.4 Special warnings and precautions for use).*

Treatment of overdosage is mainly supportive including monitoring of vital signs and close observation of the patient. An adequate airway should be maintained and assisted respiration used as needed. Hypotension, though unlikely, may be controlled with noradrenaline. Lorazepam is poorly dialysable.

The benzodiazepine antagonist, flumazenil, may be useful in hospitalised patients for the management of benzodiazepine overdosage. Flumazenil product information should be consulted prior to use. The physician should be aware of a risk of seizure in association with flumazenil treatment, particularly in long-term benzodiazepine users and in tricyclic antidepressant overdose.

. PHARMACOLOGICAL PROPERTIES

.1 Pharmacodynamic properties

tivan is a benzodiazepine with anxiolytic, sedative, hypnotic, anticonvulsant and muscle relaxant properties.

.2 Pharmacokinetic properties

tivan Injection is readily absorbed when given intramuscularly. Peak plasma concentrations occur approximately 0-90 minutes following intramuscular administration.

tivan is metabolised by a simple one-step process to a harmacologically inactive glucuronide. There is minimal sk of accumulation after repeated doses, giving a wide nargin of safety.

There are no major active metabolites. The elimination halffe is about 12-16 hours when given intramuscularly or ntravenously.

.3 Preclinical safety data

Nothing of relevance to the prescriber.

. PHARMACEUTICAL PARTICULARS

.1 List of excipients

Polyethylene glycol 400

Benzyl alcohol

Propylene glycol

6.2 Incompatibilities

None known

6.3 Shelf life

18 months

6.4 Special precautions for storage

Store and transport refrigerated (2°C to 8°C).

Keep ampoule in the outer carton.

6.5 Nature and contents of container

10 × 1ml solution (in 2ml ampoules) per pack.

6.6 Special precautions for disposal and other handling

None.

7. MARKETING AUTHORISATION HOLDER

John Wyeth and Brother Limited
trading as: Wyeth Laboratories
Huntercombe Lane South
Taplow
Maidenhead
Berkshire SL6 OPH

8. MARKETING AUTHORISATION NUMBER(S)

Ativan Injection: PL 0011/0051

9. DATE OF FIRST AUTHORISATION/RENEWAL OF THE AUTHORISATION

First Authorisation: 25 March 1988

Last Renewal: 9 February 1999

10. DATE OF REVISION OF THE TEXT

04 August 2009

Atriance 5 mg/ml solution for infusion

(GlaxoSmithKline UK)

1. NAME OF THE MEDICINAL PRODUCT

Atriance▼ 5 mg/ml solution for infusion

2. QUALITATIVE AND QUANTITATIVE COMPOSITION

Each ml contains 5 mg of nelarabine.

Each vial contains 250 mg of nelarabine.

Excipients:

Each ml contains 1.725 mg (75 micromols) of sodium.

For a full list of excipients, see section 6.1.

3. PHARMACEUTICAL FORM

Solution for infusion.

Clear, colourless solution.

4. CLINICAL PARTICULARS

4.1 Therapeutic indications

Nelarabine is indicated for the treatment of patients with T-cell acute lymphoblastic leukaemia (T-ALL) and T-cell lymphoblastic lymphoma (T-LBL) whose disease has not responded to or has relapsed following treatment with at least two chemotherapy regimens.

Due to the small patient populations in these disease settings, the information to support these indications is based on limited data.

4.2 Posology and method of administration

Nelarabine is for intravenous use only and must only be administered under the supervision of a physician experienced in the use of cytotoxic agents. Nelarabine is not diluted prior to administration. The appropriate dose of nelarabine is transferred into polyvinylchloride (PVC) or ethyl vinyl acetate (EVA) infusion bags or glass containers and administered as a two-hour infusion in adult patients and as a one-hour infusion in paediatric patients.

Complete blood counts including platelets must be monitored regularly (see sections 4.4 and 4.8).

Patients receiving nelarabine are recommended to receive intravenous hydration according to standard medical practice for the management of hyperuricemia in patients at risk for tumour lysis syndrome. For patients at risk of hyperuricemia, the use of allopurinol should be considered (see section 4.4).

Adults and adolescents (aged 16 years and older)

The recommended dose of nelarabine for adults is 1,500 mg/m^2 administered intravenously over two hours on days 1, 3 and 5 and repeated every 21 days.

Children and adolescents (aged 21 years and younger)

The recommended dose of nelarabine for children is 650 mg/m^2 administered intravenously over one hour daily for 5 consecutive days, repeated every 21 days.

In clinical studies, the 650 mg/m^2 and 1,500 mg/m^2 dose have both been used in patients in the age range 16 to 21 years. Efficacy and safety were similar for both regimens. The prescribing physician should consider which regimen is appropriate when treating patients in this age range.

Limited clinical pharmacology data are available for patients below the age of 4 years.

Dose modification

Nelarabine must be discontinued at the first sign of neurological events of National Cancer Institute Common Terminology Criteria Adverse Event (NCI CTCAE) grade 2 or greater. Delaying subsequent dosing is an option for other toxicities, including haematological toxicity.

Elderly

Insufficient numbers of patients aged 65 years of age and older have been treated with nelarabine to determine whether they respond differently than younger patients (see sections 4.4 and 5.2).

Renal Impairment

Nelarabine has not been studied in individuals with renal impairment. Nelarabine and 9-β-D-arabinofuranosylguanine (ara-G) are partially renally excreted (see section 5.2 — Renal impairment). There are insufficient data to support a dose adjustment recommendation for patients with a renal clearance of creatinin Cl_{cr} less than 50 ml/min. Patients with renal impairment must be closely monitored for toxicities when treated with nelarabine.

Hepatic Impairment

Nelarabine has not been studied in patients with hepatic impairment. These patients should be treated with caution.

4.3 Contraindications

Hypersensitivity to the active substance or to any of the excipients.

4.4 Special warnings and precautions for use

NEUROLOGICAL ADVERSE EVENTS

Severe neurological events have been reported with the use of nelarabine. These events have included altered mental states including severe somnolence, central nervous system effects including convulsions, and peripheral neuropathy ranging from numbness and paresthesias to motor weakness and paralysis. There have also been reports of events associated with demyelination, and ascending peripheral neuropathies similar in appearance to Guillain-Barré Syndrome.

Full recovery from these events has not always occurred with cessation of nelarabine. Therefore, close monitoring for neurological events is strongly recommended, and nelarabine must be discontinued at the first sign of neurological events of NCI CTCAE Grade 2 or greater.

Neurotoxicity is the dose-limiting toxicity of nelarabine. It is advised that patients undergoing therapy with nelarabine be closely observed for signs and symptoms of neurological toxicity.

Common signs and symptoms of nelarabine-related neurotoxicity include somnolence, confusion, convulsions, ataxia, paraesthesias, and hypoesthesia. Severe neurological toxicity can manifest as coma, status epilepticus, demyelination, or ascending neuropathy similar in appearance to Guillain-Barré syndrome (see section 4.8).

Patients treated previously or concurrently with intrathecal chemotherapy or previously with craniospinal irradiation are potentially at increased risk for neurological adverse events (see section 4.2 - dose modification) and therefore concomitant intrathecal therapy and/or craniospinal irradiation is not recommended.

Immunisation using a live organism vaccine has the potential to cause infection in immunocompromised hosts. Therefore, immunisations with live organism vaccines are not recommended.

Leukopenia, thrombocytopenia, anaemia, and neutropenia, (including febrile neutropenia) have been associated with nelarabine therapy. Complete blood counts including platelets must be monitored regularly (see sections 4.2 and 4.8).

Patients receiving nelarabine are recommended to receive intravenous hydration according to standard medical practice for the management of hyperuricemia in patients at risk of tumour lysis syndrome. For patients at risk of hyperuricemia, the use of allopurinol should be considered.

Elderly

Clinical studies of nelarabine did not include sufficient numbers of patients aged 65 and over to determine whether they respond differently from younger patients. In an exploratory analysis, increasing age, especially aged 65 years and older, appeared to be associated with increased rates of neurological adverse events.

Carcinogenicity and mutagenicity

Carcinogenicity testing of nelarabine has not been performed. Nelarabine however, is known to be genotoxic to mammalian cells (see section 5.3).

Sodium warning

This medicinal product contains 1.725 mg/ml (75 micromols) of sodium. To be taken into consideration by patients on a controlled sodium diet.

4.5 Interaction with other medicinal products and other forms of interaction

Nelarabine and ara-G did not significantly inhibit the activities of the major hepatic cytochrome P450 (CYP) isoenzymes CYP1A2, CYP2A6, CYP2B6, CYP2C8, CYP2C9, CYP2C19, CYP2D6, or CYP3A4 *in vitro*.

Concomitant administration of nelarabine in combination with adenosine deaminase inhibitors, such as pentostatin is not recommended. Concomitant administration may reduce the efficacy of nelarabine and/or change the adverse event profile of either active substance.

4.6 Pregnancy and lactation

There are no adequate data from the use of nelarabine in pregnant women.

Studies in animals have shown reproductive toxicity including malformations (see section 5.3). The potential risk in humans is unknown, however, exposure during pregnancy will likely lead to anomalies and malformations of the foetus.

Nelarabine should not be used during pregnancy unless clearly necessary. If a patient becomes pregnant during treatment with nelarabine, they should be informed of the possible risk to the foetus.

Both sexually active men and women should use effective methods of contraception during treatment and for at least three months following cessation of treatment.

The effect of nelarabine on fertility in humans is unknown. Based on the pharmacological action of the compound, undesirable effects on fertility are possible. Family planning should be discussed with patients as appropriate.

It is unknown whether nelarabine or its metabolites are excreted in human breast milk. The excretion of nelarabine in milk has not been studied in animals. However, because of the potential for serious adverse reactions in infants, breastfeeding should be discontinued.

4.7 Effects on ability to drive and use machines

No studies on the effects on the ability to drive and use machines have been performed.

Patients treated with nelarabine are potentially at risk of suffering from somnolence during and for several days after treatment. Patients must be cautioned that somnolence can affect performance of skilled tasks, such as driving.

4.8 Undesirable effects

Clinical trial data

Pivotal clinical trial data

The safety profile from pivotal clinical trials at the recommended doses of nelarabine in adults (1,500 mg/m^2) and children (650 mg/m^2) is based on data from 103 adults and 84 paediatric patients respectively. The most frequently occurring adverse events were fatigue; gastrointestinal disorders; haematological disorders; respiratory disorders; nervous system disorders; and pyrexia. Neurotoxicity is the dose limiting toxicity associated with nelarabine therapy (see section 4.4).

The following convention has been utilised for the classification of frequency: Very common ($\geq$1/10), Common ($\geq$1/100 to $<$1/10), Uncommon ($\geq$1/1,000 to $<$1/100), Rare ($\geq$1/10,000 to $<$1/1,000) and Very rare ($<$1/10,000), not known (cannot be estimated from the available data)

(see Table 1 on next page)

Data from NCI studies/compassionate use programme and phase I studies

In addition to the adverse reactions seen in the pivotal clinical trials, there are also data from 875 patients from NCI studies/compassionate use programme (694 patients) and Phase I (181 patients) studies of nelarabine. The following additional adverse reactions were seen:

Neoplasms benign and malignant (including cysts and polyps)

Tumour lysis syndrome – 7 cases (see sections 4.2 and 4.4)

4.9 Overdose

No case of overdose has been reported.

Nelarabine has been administered in clinical trials up to a dose of 75 mg/kg (approximately 2,250 mg/m^2) daily for 5 days to a paediatric patient, up to a dose of 60 mg/kg (approximately 2,400 mg/m^2) daily for 5 days to 5 adult patients and up to 2,900 mg/m^2 in a further 2 adults on days 1, 3 and 5.

Symptoms and signs

It is likely that nelarabine overdose would result in severe neurotoxicity (possibly including paralysis, coma), myelosuppression and potentially death. At a dose of 2200 mg/m^2 given on days 1, 3 and 5 every 21 days, 2 patients developed a significant grade 3 ascending sensory

Table 1

MedDRA Preferred Term(s)	Adults (1,500 mg/m²) N=103 (%)	Children (650 mg/m²) N=84 (%)
Infections and infestations		
Infection (including but not limited to; sepsis, bacteraemia, pneumonia, fungal infection)	Very common: 40 (39)	Very common: 13 (15)
There was a single additional report of biopsy confirmed progressive multifocal leukoencephalopathy in the adult population. There have been reports of sometimes fatal opportunistic infections in patients receiving nelarabine therapy.		
Neoplasms benign and malignant (including cysts and polyps)		
Tumour lysis syndrome (see also Data from compassionate use programme and non-pivotal studies)	Common: 1 (1)	N/A
Blood and lymphatic system disorders		
Febrile neutropenia	Very common: 12 (12)	Common: 1 (1)
Neutropenia	Very common: 83 (81)	Very common: 79 (94)
Leukopenia	Common: 3 (3)	Very common: 32 (38)
Thrombocytopenia	Very common: 89 (86)	Very common: 74 (88)
Anaemia	Very common: 102 (99)	Very common: 80 (95)
Metabolism and nutrition disorders		
Hypoglycaemia	N/A	Common: 5 (6)
Hypocalcaemia	Common: 3 (3)	Common: 7 (8)
Hypomagnesaemia	Common: 4 (4)	Common: 5 (6)
Hypokalaemia	Common: 4 (4)	Very common: 9 (11)
Anorexia	Common: 9 (9)	N/A
Psychiatric disorders		
Confusional state	Common: 8 (8)	Common: 2 (2)
Nervous system disorders		
Seizures (including convulsions, grand mal convulsions, status epilepticus)	Common: 1 (1)	Common: 5 (6)
Amnesia	Common: 3 (3)	N/A
Somnolence	Very common: 24 (23)	Common: 6 (7)
Peripheral neurological disorders (sensory and motor)	Very common: 22 (21)	Very common: 10 (12)
Hypoesthesia	Very common: 18 (17)	Common: 5 (6)
Paresthesia	Very common: 15 (15)	Common: 3 (4)
Ataxia	Common: 9 (9)	Common: 2 (2)
Balance disorder	Common: 2 (2)	N/A
Tremor	Common: 5 (5)	Common: 3 (4)
Dizziness	Very common: 22 (21)	N/A
Headache	Very common: 15 (15)	Very common: 14 (17)
Dysgeusia	Common: 3 (3)	N/A
There have also been reports of events associated with demyelination and ascending peripheral neuropathies similar in appearance to Guillain-Barré syndrome. One subject in the paediatric group had a fatal neurological event of status epilepticus.		
Eye disorders		
Blurred vision	Common: 4 (4)	N/A
Vascular disorders		
Hypotension	Common: 8 (8)	N/A
Respiratory, thoracic, and mediastinal disorders		
Pleural effusion	Common: 10 (10)	N/A
Wheezing	Common: 5 (5)	N/A
Dyspnea	Very common: 21 (20)	N/A
Cough	Very common: 26 (25)	N/A
Gastrointestinal disorders		
Diarrhoea	Very common: 23 (22)	Common: 2 (2)
Stomatitis	Common: 8 (8)	Common: 1 (1)
Vomiting	Very common: 23 (22)	Common: 8 (10)
Abdominal pain	Common: 9 (9)	N/A
Constipation	Very common: 22 (21)	Common: 1 (1)
Nausea	Very common: 42 (41)	Common: 2 (2)
Hepatobiliary disorders		
Hyperbilirubinaemia	Common: 3 (3)	Common: 8 (10)
Transaminases increased	N/A	Very common: 10 (12)
Aspartate aminotransferase increased	Common: 6 (6)	N/A
Musculoskeletal and connective tissue disorders		
Muscle weakness	Common: 8 (8)	N/A
Myalgia	Very common: 13 (13)	N/A
Arthralgia	Common: 9 (9)	Common: 1 (1)
Back pain	Common: 8 (8)	N/A
Pain in extremity	Common: 7 (7)	Common: 2 (2)
Renal and urinary disorders		
Blood creatinine increased	Common: 2 (2)	Common: 5 (6)
General disorders and administrative site conditions		
Oedema	Very common: 11 (11)	N/A
Gait abnormal	Common: 6 (6)	N/A
Oedema peripheral	Very common: 15 (15)	N/A
Pyrexia	Very common: 24 (23)	Common: 2 (2)
Pain	Very common: 11 (11)	N/A
Fatigue	Very common: 51 (50)	Common: 1 (1)
Asthenia	Very common: 18 (17)	Common: 5 (6)

neuropathy. MRI evaluations of the 2 patients demo strated findings consistent with a demyelinating proces in the cervical spine.

Treatment

There is no known antidote for nelarabine overdose. Sup portive care consistent with good clinical practice shoul be provided.

5. PHARMACOLOGICAL PROPERTIES

5.1 Pharmacodynamic properties

Pharmacotherapeutic group: Antineoplastic agents, anti metabolites, purine analogues, ATC code: L01B B 07.

Nelarabine is a pro-drug of the deoxyguanosine analogu ara-G. Nelarabine is rapidly demethylated by adenosin deaminase (ADA) to ara-G and then phosphorylated intra cellularly by deoxyguanosine kinase and deoxycytidin kinase to its 5'-monophosphate metabolite. The monopho sphate metabolite is subsequently converted to the active 5'-triphosphate form, ara-GTP. Accumulation of ara-GTF in leukaemic blasts allows for preferential incorporation o ara-GTP into deoxyribonucleic acid (DNA) leading to inhi bition of DNA synthesis. This results in cell death. Othe mechanisms may contribute to the cytotoxic effects o nelarabine. *In vitro*, T-cells are more sensitive than B-cells to the cytotoxic effects of nelarabine.

Clinical studies

Adult studies

In an open-label study carried out by the Cancer and Leukaemia Group B and the Southwest Oncology Group, the safety and efficacy of nelarabine were evaluated in 39 adults with T-cell acute lymphoblastic leukaemia (T-ALL) or lymphoblastic lymphoma (T-LBL). Twenty-eight of the 39 adults had relapsed or were refractory to at least two prior induction regimens and aged between 16 to 65 years of age (mean 34 years). Nelarabine at a dose of 1500 mg/m²/day was administered intravenously over two hours on days 1, 3 and 5 of a 21 day cycle. Five of the 28 patients (18%) [95% CI: 6%—37%] treated with nelarabine achieved a complete response (bone marrow blast counts ≤ 5%, no other evidence of disease, and full recovery of peripheral blood counts). A total of 6 patients (21%) [95% CI: 8%–41%] achieved a complete response with or without haematological recovery. Time to complete response in both classifications of response ranged from 2.9 to 11.7 weeks. Duration of response (in both classifications of response (n=5) ranged between 15 and 195+ weeks. Median overall survival was 20.6 weeks [95% CI: 10.4–36.4]. Survival at one year was 29% [95% CI: 12%–45%].

Paediatric studies

In an open-label, multicenter study carried out by Childrens Oncology Group, nelarabine was administered intravenously over 1 hour for 5 days to 151 patients ≤ 21 years of age, 149 of whom had relapsed or refractory T-cell acute lymphoblastic leukaemia (T-ALL) or T-cell lymphoblastic lymphoma (T-LBL). Eighty-four (84) patients, 39 of whom had received two or more prior induction regimens and 31 whom had received one prior induction regimen, were treated with 650 mg/m²/day of nelarabine administered intravenously over 1 hour daily for 5 consecutive days repeated every 21 days.

Of the 39 patients who had received two or more prior induction regimens, 5 (13%) [95% CI: 4%-27%] achieved a complete response (bone marrow blast counts ≤ 5%, no other evidence of disease, and full recovery of peripheral blood counts) and 9 (23%) [95% CI: 11%–39%] achieved complete responses with or without full haematological recovery. Duration of response in both classifications of response ranged between 4.7 and 36.4 weeks and median overall survival was 13.1 weeks [95% CI: 8.7–17.4] and survival at one year was 14% [95% CI: 3%–26%].

Thirteen (42%) of the 31 patients treated with one prior induction regimen achieved a complete response overall. Nine of these 31 patients failed to respond to prior induction (refractory patients). Four (44%) of the nine refractory patients experienced a complete response to nelarabine.

This medicinal product has been authorised under "Exceptional Circumstances". This means that due to the rarity of the disease it has not been possible to obtain complete information on this medicinal product. The European Medicines Agency (EMEA) will review any new information which may become available every year and this SPC will be updated as necessary.

5.2 Pharmacokinetic properties

Nelarabine is a pro-drug of the deoxyguanosine analogue ara-G. Nelarabine is rapidly demethylated by adenosine deaminase (ADA) to ara-G and then phosphorylated intracellularly by deoxyguanosine kinase and deoxycytidine kinase to its 5'-monophosphate metabolite. The monophosphate metabolite is subsequently converted to the active 5'-triphosphate from, ara-GTP. Accumulation of ara-GTP in leukaemic blasts allows for preferential incorporation of ara-GTP into deoxyribonucleic acid (DNA) leading to inhibition of DNA synthesis. This results in cell death. Other mechanisms may contribute to the cytotoxic effects of nelarabine. *In vitro*, T-cells are more sensitive than B-cells to the cytotoxic effects of nelarabine.

In a cross-study analysis using data from four Phase I studies, the pharmacokinetics of nelarabine and ara-G were characterized in patients aged less than 18 years and adult patients with refractory leukaemia or lymphoma *bsorption*

dults

lasma ara-G C_{max} values generally occurred at the end of ie nelarabine infusion and were generally higher than elarabine C_{max} values, suggesting rapid and extensive onversion of nelarabine to ara-G. After infusion of ,500 mg/m^2 nelarabine over two hours in adult patients, iean (%CV) plasma nelarabine C_{max} and AUC_{inf} values vere 13.9 μM (81%) and 13.5 μM.h (56%) respectively. Mean plasma ara-G C_{max} and AUC_{inf} values were 115 μM 16%) and 571 μM.h (30%), respectively.

ntracellular C_{max} for ara-GTP appeared within 3 to 25 iours on day 1. Mean (%CV) intracellular ara-GTP C_{max} nd AUC values were 95.6 μM (139%) and 2214 μM.h 263%) at this dose.

Paediatric patients

After infusion of 400 or 650 mg/m^2 nelarabine over one iour in 6 paediatric patients, mean (%CV) plasma nelarabine C_{max} and AUC_{inf} values, adjusted to a 650 mg/m^2 dose, were 45.0 μM (40%) and 38.0 μM.h (39%), respectively. Mean plasma ara-G C_{max} and AUC_{inf} values were 60.1 μM (17%) and 212 μM.h (18%), respectively.

Distribution

Nelarabine and ara-G are extensively distributed throughout the body based on combined Phase I pharmacokinetic data at nelarabine doses of 104 to 2,900 mg/m^2. Specifically, for nelarabine, mean (%CV) V_{SS} values were 115 l/m^2 (159%) and 89.4 l/m^2 (278%) in adult and paediatric patients, respectively. For ara-G, mean V_{SS}/F values were 44.8 l/m^2 (32%) and 32.1 l/m^2 (25%) in adult and paediatric patients, respectively.

Nelarabine and ara-G are not substantially bound to human plasma proteins (less than 25%) *in vitro*, and binding is independent of nelarabine or ara-G concentrations up to 600 μM.

No accumulation of nelarabine or ara-G was observed in plasma after nelarabine administration on either a daily or a day 1, 3, 5 schedule.

Intracellular ara-GTP concentrations in leukaemic blasts were quantifiable for a prolonged period after nelarabine administration. Intracellular ara-GTP accumulated with repeated administration of nelarabine. On the day 1, 3, and 5 schedule, C_{max} and $AUC_{(0-t)}$ values on day 3 were approximately 50% and 30%, respectively, greater than C_{max} and $AUC_{(0-t)}$ values on day 1.

Metabolism

The principal route of metabolism for nelarabine is O-demethylation by adenosine deaminase to form ara-G, which undergoes hydrolysis to form guanine. In addition, some nelarabine is hydrolysed to form methylguanine, which is O-demethylated to form guanine. Guanine is N-deaminated to form xanthine, which is further oxidized to yield uric acid.

Elimination

Nelarabine and ara-G are rapidly eliminated from plasma with a half-life of approximately 30 minutes and 3 hours, respectively. These findings were demonstrated in patients with refractory leukaemia or lymphoma given a dose of 1,500 mg/m^2 nelarabine (adults) or a 650 mg/m^2 (paediatrics).

Combined Phase 1 pharmacokinetic data at nelarabine doses of 104 to 2,900 mg/m^2 indicate that mean (%CV) clearance (Cl) values for nelarabine are 138 l/h/m^2 (104%) and 125 l/h/m^2 (214%) in adult and paediatric patients, respectively, on day 1 (n = 65 adults, n = 21 paediatric patients). The apparent clearance of ara-G (Cl/F) is comparable between the two groups [9.5 l/h/m^2 (35%) in adult patients and 10.8 l/h/m^2 (36%) in paediatric patients] on day 1.

Nelarabine and ara-G are partially eliminated by the kidneys. In 28 adult patients, 24 hours after nelarabine infusion on day 1, mean urinary excretion of nelarabine and ara-G was 5.3% and 23.2% of the administered dose, respectively. Renal clearance averaged 9.0 l/h/m^2 (151%) for nelarabine and 2.6 l/h/m^2 (83%) for ara-G in 21 adult patients.

Because the timecourse of intracellular ara-GTP was prolonged, its elimination half-life could not be accurately estimated.

Children

Limited clinical pharmacology data are available for patients below the age of 4 years.

Combined Phase 1 pharmacokinetic data at nelarabine doses of 104 to 2,900 mg/m^2 indicate that the clearance (Cl) and V_{ss} values for nelarabine and ara-G are comparable between the two groups. Further data with respect to nelarabine and ara-G pharmacokinetics in the paediatric population are provided in other subsections.

Gender

Gender has no effect on nelarabine or ara-G plasma pharmacokinetics. Intracellular ara-GTP C_{max} and $AUC_{(0-t)}$ values at the same dose level were 2– to 3– fold greater on average in adult female than in adult male patients.

Race

The effect of race on nelarabine and ara-G pharmacokinetics has not been specifically studied. In a pharmacokinetic/pharmacodynamic cross study analysis, race had no apparent effect on nelarabine, ara-G, or intracellular ara-GTP pharmacokinetics.

Renal Impairment

The pharmacokinetics of nelarabine and ara-G have not been specifically studied in renally impaired or haemodialysed patients. Nelarabine is excreted by the kidney to a small extent (5 to 10% of the administered dose). Ara-G is excreted by the kidney to a greater extent (20 to 30% of the administered nelarabine dose). Adults and children in clinical studies were categorized into the three groups according to renal impairment: normal with Cl_{cr} greater than 80 ml/min (n = 56), mild with Cl_{cr} equalling 50 to 80 ml/min (n = 12), and moderate with Cl_{cr} less than 50 ml/min (n = 2). The mean apparent clearance (Cl/F) of ara-G was about 7% lower in patients with mild renal impairment than in patients with normal renal function (see section 4.2). No data are available to provide a dose advice for patients with Cl_{cr} less than 50 ml/min.

Elderly

Age has no effect on the pharmacokinetics of nelarabine or ara-G. Decreased renal function, which is more common in the elderly, may reduce ara-G clearance (see section 4.2).

5.3 Preclinical safety data

Adverse reactions not observed in clinical studies, but seen in animals at exposure levels similar to clinical exposure levels and with possible relevance to clinical use were as follows: nelarabine caused histopathological changes to the central nervous system (white matter) vacuolation and degenerative changes in cerebrum, cerebellum and spinal cord of monkeys after treatment with nelarabine daily during 23 days, at exposures below the human therapeutic exposure. Nelarabine showed *in vitro* cytotoxicity to monocytes and macrophages.

Carcinogenicity

Carcinogenicity testing of nelarabine has not been performed.

Mutagenicity

Nelarabine was mutagenic to L5178Y/TK mouse lymphoma cells with and without metabolic activation.

Reproduction toxicity

Compared to controls, nelarabine caused increased incidences of fetal malformations, anomalies, and variations in rabbits when given at doses approximately 24% of the adult human dose on a mg/m^2 basis during the period of organogenesis. Cleft palate was seen in rabbits given a dose approximately 2-fold the adult human dose, absent pollices in rabbits given a dose approximately 79% of the adult human dose while absent gall bladder, accessory lung lobes, fused or extra sternebrae and delayed ossification was seen at all doses. Maternal body weight gain and fetal body weights were reduced in rabbits given a dose approximately 2-fold the adult human dose.

Fertility

No studies have been conducted in animals to assess the effects of nelarabine on fertility. However, no undesirable effects were seen in the testes or ovaries of monkeys given nelarabine intravenously at doses up to approximately 32% of the adult human dose on a mg/m^2 basis for 30 consecutive days.

6. PHARMACEUTICAL PARTICULARS

6.1 List of excipients

Sodium chloride

Water for injections

Hydrochloric acid (to adjust the pH)

Sodium hydroxide (to adjust the pH)

6.2 Incompatibilities

Not applicable.

6.3 Shelf life

3 years

Atriance is stable for up to 8 hours at up to 30°C once the vial is opened.

6.4 Special precautions for storage

This medicinal product does not require any special storage conditions.

6.5 Nature and contents of container

Clear glass (Type I) vials with a non-latex bromobutyl rubber stopper, sealed with an aluminium cap.

Each vial contains 50 ml. Atriance is supplied in packs of 6 vials.

6.6 Special precautions for disposal and other handling

The normal procedures for proper handling and disposal of anti-tumour medicinal products should be adopted, namely:

- Staff should be trained in how to handle and transfer the medicinal product.

- Pregnant staff should be excluded from working with this medicinal product.

- Personnel handling this medicinal product during handling/transfer should wear protective clothing including mask, goggles and gloves.

- All items for administration or cleaning, including gloves, should be placed in high-risk, waste disposal bags for high-temperature incineration. Liquid waste may be flushed with large amounts of water.

- Accidental contact with the skin or eyes should be treated immediately with copious amounts of water.

Any unused product or waste material should be disposed of in accordance with local requirements.

7. MARKETING AUTHORISATION HOLDER

Glaxo Group Limited, Berkeley Avenue, Greenford, Middlesex UB6 0NN, United Kingdom

8. MARKETING AUTHORISATION NUMBER(S)

EU/1/07/403/001

9. DATE OF FIRST AUTHORISATION/RENEWAL OF THE AUTHORISATION

22 August 2007

10. DATE OF REVISION OF THE TEXT

19 November 2008

Detailed information on this medicinal product is available on the website of the European Medicines Agency (EMEA) http://www.emea.europa.eu/.

Atripla 600 mg/200 mg/245 mg film-coated tablets

(Gilead Sciences Ltd)

1. NAME OF THE MEDICINAL PRODUCT

Atripla 600 mg/200 mg/245 mg film-coated tablets

2. QUALITATIVE AND QUANTITATIVE COMPOSITION

Each film-coated tablet contains 600 mg of efavirenz, 200 mg of emtricitabine and 245 mg of tenofovir disoproxil (as fumarate).

Excipient(s):

Each film-coated tablet contains 1 mmol (23.6 mg) of sodium.

For a full list of excipients, see section 6.1.

3. PHARMACEUTICAL FORM

Film-coated tablet.

Pink, capsule shaped, film-coated tablet, debossed with "123" on one side, plain on the other side.

4. CLINICAL PARTICULARS

4.1 Therapeutic indications

Atripla is a fixed-dose combination of efavirenz, emtricitabine and tenofovir disoproxil fumarate. It is indicated for the treatment of human immunodeficiency virus-1 (HIV-1) infection in adults with virologic suppression to HIV-1 RNA levels of < 50 copies/ml on their current combination antiretroviral therapy for more than three months. Patients must not have experienced virological failure on any prior antiretroviral therapy and must be known not to have harboured virus strains with mutations conferring significant resistance to any of the three components contained in Atripla prior to initiation of their first antiretroviral treatment regimen (see sections 4.4 and 5.1).

The demonstration of the benefit of Atripla is primarily based on 48-week data from a clinical study in which patients with stable virologic suppression on a combination antiretroviral therapy changed to Atripla (see section 5.1). No data are currently available from clinical studies with Atripla in treatment-naïve or in heavily pretreated patients.

No data are available to support the combination of Atripla and other antiretroviral agents.

4.2 Posology and method of administration

Therapy should be initiated by a physician experienced in the management of human immunodeficiency virus (HIV) infection.

Posology

Adults: the recommended dose of Atripla is one tablet taken orally once daily.

Method of administration

It is recommended that Atripla be swallowed whole with water.

It is recommended that Atripla be taken on an empty stomach since food may increase efavirenz exposure and may lead to an increase in the frequency of adverse reactions (see sections 4.4 and 4.8). In order to improve the tolerability to efavirenz with respect to undesirable effects on the nervous system, bedtime dosing is recommended (see section 4.8).

It is anticipated that tenofovir exposure will be approximately 35% lower following administration of Atripla on an empty stomach as compared to the individual component tenofovir disoproxil fumarate when taken with food (see section 5.2). In virologically suppressed patients, the clinical relevance of this reduction can be expected to be limited (see section 5.1). Further data on the clinical translation of the decrease in pharmacokinetic exposure is awaited.

Children and adolescents: Atripla is not recommended for use in children below 18 years of age due to lack of data on safety and efficacy.

Elderly: insufficient numbers of elderly patients have been evaluated in clinical studies of the components of Atripla to determine whether they respond differently than younger patients. Caution should be exercised when prescribing Atripla to the elderly, keeping in mind the greater frequency of decreased hepatic or renal function in these patients.

Dose adjustment: if Atripla is co-administered with rifampicin, an additional 200 mg/day (800 mg total) of efavirenz is recommended (see section 4.5).

Renal insufficiency: Atripla is not recommended for patients with moderate or severe renal impairment (creatinine clearance (CrCl) < 50 ml/min). Patients with moderate or severe renal impairment require dose interval adjustment of emtricitabine and tenofovir disoproxil fumarate that cannot be achieved with the combination tablet (see sections 4.4 and 5.2).

Hepatic impairment: the pharmacokinetics of Atripla have not been studied in patients with hepatic impairment. Patients with mild-to-moderate liver disease (Child-Pugh-Turcotte (CPT), Grade A or B) may be treated with the normal recommended dose of Atripla (see sections 4.3, 4.4 and 5.2). Patients should be monitored carefully for adverse reactions, especially nervous system symptoms related to efavirenz (see sections 4.3 and 4.4).

If Atripla is discontinued in patients co-infected with HIV and HBV, these patients should be closely monitored for evidence of exacerbation of hepatitis (see section 4.4).

It is important to take Atripla on a regular dosing schedule to avoid missing doses. Patients should be told that if they forget to take Atripla, they should take the missed dose right away, unless it is less than 12 hours until the next day's dose. In this case, patients should be told not to take the missed dose and to take their next dose at the usual time.

Where discontinuation of therapy with one of the components of Atripla is indicated or where dose modification is necessary, separate preparations of efavirenz, emtricitabine and tenofovir disoproxil fumarate are available. Please refer to the Summary of Product Characteristics for these medicinal products.

If therapy with Atripla is discontinued, consideration should be given to the long half-life of efavirenz (see section 5.2) and long intracellular half-lives of tenofovir and emtricitabine. Because of interpatient variability in these parameters and concerns regarding development of resistance, HIV treatment guidelines should be consulted, also taking into consideration the reason for discontinuation.

4.3 Contraindications

Hypersensitivity to the active substances or to any of the excipients.

Atripla must not be used in patients with severe hepatic impairment (CPT Grade C) (see section 5.2).

Atripla must not be administered concurrently with terfenadine, astemizole, cisapride, midazolam, triazolam, pimozide, bepridil, or ergot alkaloids (for example, ergotamine, dihydroergotamine, ergonovine, and methylergonovine), because competition for cytochrome P450 (CYP) 3A4 by efavirenz could result in inhibition of metabolism and create the potential for serious and/or life-threatening undesirable effects (for example, cardiac arrhythmias, prolonged sedation or respiratory depression) (see section 4.5).

Herbal preparations containing St. John's wort (*Hypericum perforatum*) must not be used while taking Atripla due to the risk of decreased plasma concentrations and reduced clinical effects of efavirenz (see section 4.5).

Efavirenz significantly decreases voriconazole plasma concentrations while voriconazole also significantly increases efavirenz plasma concentrations. Since Atripla is a fixed-dose combination product, the dose of efavirenz cannot be altered; therefore, voriconazole and Atripla must not be co-administered (see section 4.5).

4.4 Special warnings and precautions for use

General: as a fixed combination, Atripla should not be administered concomitantly with other medicinal products containing any of the same active components, efavirenz, emtricitabine or tenofovir disoproxil fumarate. Due to similarities with emtricitabine, Atripla should not be administered concomitantly with other cytidine analogues, such as lamivudine (see section 4.5). Atripla should not be administered concomitantly with adefovir dipivoxil.

Currently available data indicate a trend that in patients on a PI-based antiretroviral regimen the switch to Atripla may lead to a reduction of the response to the therapy (see section 5.1). These patients should be carefully monitored for rises in viral load and, since the safety profile of efavirenz differs from that of protease inhibitors, for adverse reactions.

Lactic acidosis: lactic acidosis, usually associated with hepatic steatosis, has been reported with the use of nucleoside analogues. Early symptoms (symptomatic hyperlactataemia) include benign digestive symptoms (nausea, vomiting and abdominal pain), non-specific malaise, loss of appetite, weight loss, respiratory symptoms (rapid and/or deep breathing) or neurological symptoms (including motor weakness). Lactic acidosis has a high mortality and may be associated with pancreatitis, liver failure or renal failure. Lactic acidosis generally occurred after a few or several months of treatment.
Treatment with nucleoside analogues must be discontinued in the setting of symptomatic hyperlactataemia and metabolic/lactic acidosis, progressive hepatomegaly, or rapidly elevating aminotransferase levels.
Caution should be exercised when administering nucleoside analogues to any patient (particularly obese women) with hepatomegaly, hepatitis or other known risk factors for liver disease and hepatic steatosis (including certain medicinal products and alcohol). Co-infection with hepatitis C and treatment with alpha interferon and ribavirin may constitute a special risk.
Patients at increased risk must be followed closely.

Opportunistic infections: patients receiving Atripla or any other antiretroviral therapy may continue to develop opportunistic infections and other complications of HIV infection, and therefore should remain under close clinical observation by physicians experienced in the treatment of patients with HIV associated diseases.

Transmission of HIV: patients must be advised that antiretroviral therapies, including Atripla, have not been proven to prevent the risk of transmission of HIV to others through sexual contact or contamination with blood. Appropriate precautions must continue to be used.

Liver disease: the pharmacokinetics, safety and efficacy of Atripla have not been established in patients with significant underlying liver disorders (see section 5.2). Atripla is contraindicated in patients with severe hepatic impairment (see section 4.3). Since efavirenz is principally metabolised by the cytochrome P450 (CYP450) system, caution should be exercised in administering Atripla to patients with mild-to-moderate liver disease. These patients should be carefully monitored for efavirenz adverse reactions, especially nervous system symptoms. Laboratory tests should be performed to evaluate their liver disease at periodic intervals (see section 4.2).

Patients with pre-existing liver dysfunction including chronic active hepatitis have an increased frequency of liver function abnormalities during combination antiretroviral therapy and should be monitored according to standard practice. If there is evidence of worsening liver disease or persistent elevations of serum transaminases to greater than 5 times the upper limit of the normal range, the benefit of continued therapy with Atripla needs to be weighed against the potential risks of significant liver toxicity. In such patients, interruption or discontinuation of treatment must be considered (see section 4.8).

In patients treated with other medicinal products associated with liver toxicity, monitoring of liver enzymes is also recommended.

Patients with HIV and hepatitis B (HBV) or C virus (HCV) co-infection: patients with chronic hepatitis B or C and treated with combination antiretroviral therapy are at an increased risk for severe and potentially fatal hepatic adverse reactions.

Physicians should refer to current HIV treatment guidelines for the optimal management of HIV infection in patients co-infected with HBV.

In case of concomitant antiviral therapy for hepatitis B or C, please refer also to the relevant Summary of Product Characteristics for these medicinal products.

The safety and efficacy of Atripla have not been studied for the treatment of chronic HBV infection. Emtricitabine and tenofovir individually and in combination have shown activity against HBV in pharmacodynamic studies (see section 5.1). Limited clinical experience suggests that emtricitabine and tenofovir disoproxil fumarate have an anti-HBV activity when used in antiretroviral combination therapy to control HIV infection. Discontinuation of Atripla therapy in patients co-infected with HIV and HBV may be associated with severe acute exacerbations of hepatitis. Patients co-infected with HIV and HBV who discontinue Atripla must be closely monitored with both clinical and laboratory follow-up for at least four months after stopping treatment with Atripla. If appropriate, resumption of anti-hepatitis B therapy may be warranted. In patients with advanced liver disease or cirrhosis, treatment discontinuation is not recommended since post-treatment exacerbation of hepatitis may lead to hepatic decompensation.

Psychiatric symptoms: psychiatric adverse reactions have been reported in patients treated with efavirenz. Patients with a prior history of psychiatric disorders appear to be at greater risk of these serious psychiatric adverse reactions. In particular, severe depression was more common in those with a history of depression. There have also been post-marketing reports of severe depression, death by suicide, delusions and psychosis-like behaviour. Patients should be advised that if they experience symptoms such as severe depression, psychosis or suicidal ideation, they should contact their doctor immediately to assess the possibility that the symptoms may be related to the use of efavirenz, and if so, to determine whether the risk of continued therapy outweighs the benefits (see section 4.8).

Nervous system symptoms: symptoms including, but not limited to, dizziness, insomnia, somnolence, impaired concentration and abnormal dreaming are frequently reported undesirable effects in patients receiving efavirenz 600 mg daily in clinical studies. Dizziness was also seen in clinical studies with emtricitabine and tenofovir disoproxil fumarate. Headache has been reported in clinical studies with emtricitabine (see section 4.8). Nervous system symptoms associated with efavirenz usually begin during the first one or two days of therapy and generally resolve after the first two to four weeks. Patients should be informed that if they do occur, these common symptoms are likely to improve with continued therapy and are not predictive of subsequent onset of any of the less frequent psychiatric symptoms.

Seizures: convulsions have been observed in patients receiving efavirenz, generally in the presence of a known medical history of seizures. Patients who are receiving concomitant anticonvulsant medicinal products primarily metabolised by the liver, such as phenytoin, carbamazepine and phenobarbital, may require periodic monitoring of plasma levels. In a drug interaction study, carbamazepir plasma concentrations were decreased when carbamaze pine was co-administered with efavirenz (see section 4.5 Caution must be taken in any patient with a history of seizures.

Renal impairment: Atripla is not recommended for patient with moderate or severe renal impairment. Patients wit moderate or severe renal impairment require a dos adjustment of emtricitabine and tenofovir disoproxil fuma rate that cannot be achieved with the combination table (see sections 4.2 and 5.2). Use of Atripla should be avoide with concurrent or recent use of a nephrotoxic medicina product. If concomitant use of Atripla and nephrotoxi agents (e.g. aminoglycosides, amphotericin B, foscarnet ganciclovir, pentamidine, vancomycin, cidofovir, interleu kin-2) is unavoidable, renal function must be monitore weekly (see section 4.5).

Renal failure, renal impairment, elevated creatinine, hypo phosphataemia and proximal tubulopathy (including Fanconi syndrome) have been reported with the use o tenofovir disoproxil fumarate in clinical practice (see section 4.8).

It is recommended that creatinine clearance is calculated in all patients prior to initiating therapy with Atripla and rena function (creatinine clearance and serum phosphate) is also monitored every four weeks during the first year and then every three months. In patients with a history of renal dysfunction or in patients who are at risk for renal dysfunction, consideration must be given to more frequent monitoring of renal function.

If serum phosphate is < 1.5 mg/dl (0.48 mmol/l) or creatinine clearance is decreased to < 50 ml/min in any patient receiving Atripla, renal function must be re-evaluated within one week, including measurements of blood glucose, blood potassium and urine glucose concentrations (see section 4.8, proximal tubulopathy). Since Atripla is a combination product and the dosing interval of the individual components cannot be altered, treatment with Atripla must be interrupted in patients with confirmed creatinine clearance < 50 ml/min or decreases in serum phosphate to < 1.0 mg/dl (0.32 mmol/l). Where discontinuation of therapy with one of the components of Atripla is indicated or where dose modification is necessary, separate preparations of efavirenz, emtricitabine and tenofovir disoproxil fumarate are available.

Skin reactions: mild-to-moderate rash has been reported with the individual components of Atripla. The rash associated with the efavirenz component usually resolves with continued therapy. Appropriate antihistamines and/or corticosteroids may improve tolerability and hasten the resolution of rash. Severe rash associated with blistering, moist desquamation or ulceration has been reported in less than 1% of patients treated with efavirenz (see section 4.8). The incidence of erythema multiforme or Stevens-Johnson syndrome was approximately 0.1%. Atripla must be discontinued in patients developing severe rash associated with blistering, desquamation, mucosal involvement or fever. Patients who discontinued treatment with other non-nucleoside reverse transcriptase inhibitors due to rash may be at higher risk of developing rash during treatment with Atripla.

Lipodystrophy and metabolic abnormalities: combination antiretroviral therapy has been associated with the redistribution of body fat (lipodystrophy) in HIV patients. The long-term consequences of these events are currently unknown. Knowledge about the mechanism is incomplete. A connection between visceral lipomatosis and protease inhibitors (PI) and lipoatrophy and nucleoside reverse transcriptase inhibitors (NRTIs) has been hypothesised. A higher risk of lipodystrophy has been associated with individual factors such as older age, and with drug-related factors such as longer duration of antiretroviral treatment and associated metabolic disturbances. Clinical examination should include evaluation for physical signs of fat redistribution. Consideration should be given to the measurement of fasting serum lipids and blood glucose. Lipid disorders should be managed as clinically appropriate (see section 4.8).

Effect of food: the administration of Atripla with food may increase efavirenz exposure (see section 5.2) and may lead to an increase in frequency of adverse reactions (see section 4.8). It is recommended that Atripla be taken on an empty stomach, preferably at bedtime.

Mitochondrial dysfunction: nucleoside and nucleotide analogues have been demonstrated *in vitro* and *in vivo* to cause a variable degree of mitochondrial damage. There have been reports of mitochondrial dysfunction in HIV negative infants exposed *in utero* and/or postnatally to nucleoside analogues. The main adverse events reported are haematological disorders (anaemia, neutropenia), metabolic disorders (hyperlactataemia, hyperlipasaemia). These events are often transitory. Some late-onset neurological disorders have been reported (hypertonia, convulsion, abnormal behaviour). Whether the neurological disorders are transient or permanent is currently unknown. Any child exposed *in utero* to nucleoside and nucleotide analogues, even HIV negative children, should have clinical and laboratory follow-up and should be fully investigated for possible mitochondrial dysfunction in case of relevant signs or symptoms. These findings do not affect current national recommendations to use antiretroviral therapy in pregnant women to prevent vertical transmission of HIV.

mmune Reactivation Syndrome: in HIV infected patients vith severe immune deficiency at the time of institution of ombination antiretroviral therapy (CART), an inflammatory eaction to asymptomatic or residual opportunistic pathogens may arise and cause serious clinical conditions, or ggravation of symptoms. Typically, such reactions have been observed within the first few weeks or months of nitiation of CART. Relevant examples are cytomegalovirus etinitis, generalised and/or focal mycobacterial infections, and pneumonia caused by *Pneumocystis jiroveci* (formerly known as *Pneumocystis carinii*). Any inflammatory symptoms should be evaluated and treatment instituted when necessary.

Osteonecrosis: although the etiology is considered to be multifactorial (including corticosteroid use, alcohol consumption, severe immunosuppression, higher body mass index), cases of osteonecrosis have been reported particularly in patients with advanced HIV disease and/or long term exposure to combination antiretroviral therapy (CART). Patients should be advised to seek medical advice if they experience joint aches and pain, joint stiffness or difficulty in movement.

Bone: in a 144-week controlled clinical study that compared tenofovir disoproxil fumarate with stavudine in combination with lamivudine and efavirenz in antiretroviral-naïve patients, small decreases in bone mineral density of the hip and spine were observed in both treatment groups. Decreases in bone mineral density of spine and changes in bone biomarkers from baseline were significantly greater in the tenofovir disoproxil fumarate treatment group at 144 weeks. Decreases in bone mineral density of the hip were significantly greater in this group until 96 weeks. However, there was no increased risk of fractures or evidence for clinically relevant bone abnormalities over 144 weeks.

Bone abnormalities (infrequently contributing to fractures) may be associated with proximal renal tubulopathy (see section 4.8). If bone abnormalities are suspected then appropriate consultation should be obtained.

Other antiretroviral agents: no data are available on the safety and efficacy of Atripla in combination with other antiretroviral agents.

Didanosine: co-administration of Atripla and didanosine is not recommended since exposure to didanosine is significantly increased following co-administration with tenofovir disoproxil fumarate (see section 4.5).

Patients with HIV-1 harbouring mutations: Atripla should be avoided in patients with HIV-1 harbouring the K65R, M184V/I or K103N mutation (see sections 4.1 and 5.1).

Excipients: this medicinal product contains 1 mmol (23.6 mg) of sodium per dose which should be taken into consideration by patients on a controlled sodium diet.

4.5 Interaction with other medicinal products and other forms of interaction

No drug interaction studies have been conducted using Atripla. As Atripla contains efavirenz, emtricitabine and tenofovir disoproxil fumarate, any interactions that have been identified with these agents individually may occur with Atripla. Interaction studies with these agents have only been performed in adults.

As a fixed combination, Atripla should not be administered concomitantly with other medicinal products containing any of the components, efavirenz, emtricitabine or tenofovir disoproxil as fumarate. Due to similarities with emtricitabine, Atripla should not be administered concomitantly with other cytidine analogues, such as lamivudine. Atripla should not be administered concomitantly with adefovir dipivoxil.

Efavirenz is an inducer of CYP3A4 and an inhibitor of some CYP450 isoenzymes including CYP3A4 (see section 5.2). Other compounds that are substrates of CYP3A4 may have decreased plasma concentrations when co-administered with efavirenz. Efavirenz exposure may also be altered when given with medicinal products or food (for example, grapefruit juice) which affect CYP3A4 activity. *In vitro* and clinical pharmacokinetic interaction studies have shown the potential for CYP450-mediated interactions involving emtricitabine and tenofovir disoproxil fumarate with other medicinal products is low.

Contraindications of concomitant use

Atripla must not be administered concurrently with terfenadine, astemizole, cisapride, midazolam, triazolam, pimozide, bepridil, or ergot alkaloids (for example, ergotamine, dihydroergotamine, ergonovine, and methylergonovine), since inhibition of their metabolism may lead to serious, life-threatening events (see section 4.3).

Voriconazole: co-administration of standard doses of efavirenz and voriconazole is contraindicated. Since Atripla is a fixed-dose combination product, the dose of efavirenz cannot be altered; therefore, voriconazole and Atripla must not be co-administered (see section 4.3 and Table 1).

St. John's wort (Hypericum perforatum): co-administration of Atripla and St. John's wort or herbal preparations containing St. John's wort is contraindicated (see section 4.3).

Concomitant use not recommended

Atazanavir/ritonavir: insufficient data are available to make a dosing recommendation for atazanavir/ritonavir in combination with Atripla. Therefore co-administration of atazanavir/ritonavir and Atripla is not recommended (see Table 1).

Didanosine: co-administration of Atripla and didanosine is not recommended (see section 4.4 and Table 1).

Renally eliminated medicinal products: since emtricitabine and tenofovir are primarily eliminated by the kidneys, co-administration of Atripla with medicinal products that reduce renal function or compete for active tubular secretion (e.g. cidofovir) may increase serum concentrations of emtricitabine, tenofovir and/or the co-administered medicinal products.

Use of Atripla should be avoided with concurrent or recent use of a nephrotoxic medicinal product. Some examples include, but are not limited to, aminoglycosides, amphotericin B, foscarnet, ganciclovir, pentamidine, vancomycin, cidofovir or interleukin-2 (see section 4.4).

Other interactions

Interactions between the components of Atripla and protease inhibitors, antiretroviral agents other than protease inhibitors and other non-antiretroviral medicinal products are listed in Table 1 below (increase is indicated as "↑", decrease as "↓", no change as "↔", twice daily as "b.i.d.", once daily as "q.d." and once every 8 hours as "q8h"). If available, 90% confidence intervals are shown in parentheses.

Table 1: Interactions between the individual components of Atripla and other medicinal products

(see Table 1 on next page)

Studies conducted with other medicinal products: there were no clinically significant pharmacokinetic interactions when efavirenz was administered with azithromycin, cetirizine, lorazepam, nelfinavir, zidovudine, aluminium/magnesium hydroxide antacids, famotidine or fluconazole. The potential for interactions with efavirenz and other imidazole antifungals, such as ketoconazole, has not been studied.

There were no clinically significant pharmacokinetic interactions when emtricitabine was administered with stavudine, zidovudine or famciclovir. There were no clinically significant pharmacokinetic interactions when tenofovir disoproxil fumarate was co-administered with adefovir dipivoxil, emtricitabine, nelfinavir or ribavirin.

4.6 Pregnancy and lactation

Atripla should not be used during pregnancy unless clearly necessary (there are no other appropriate treatment options).

Women of child bearing potential: pregnancy should be avoided in women receiving Atripla. Barrier contraception should always be used in combination with other methods of contraception (for example, oral or other hormonal contraceptives) while on therapy with Atripla. Because of the long half-life of efavirenz, use of adequate contraceptive measures for 12 weeks after discontinuation of Atripla is recommended. Women of childbearing potential should undergo pregnancy testing before initiation of Atripla.

Pregnancy: there are no adequate or well-controlled studies of Atripla or its components in pregnant women. In post-marketing experience through an antiretroviral pregnancy registry, more than 200 pregnancies with first-trimester exposure to efavirenz as part of a combination antiretroviral regimen have been reported with no specific malformation pattern. Retrospectively in this registry, a small number of cases of neural tube defects, including meningomyelocele, have been reported but causality has not been established. Studies of efavirenz in animals have shown reproductive toxicity including marked teratogenic effects (see section 5.3).

Lactation: studies in rats have demonstrated that efavirenz and tenofovir are excreted in milk; concentrations of efavirenz were much higher than those in maternal plasma. It is not known whether efavirenz, emtricitabine or tenofovir are excreted in human milk. Because of the potential for both HIV transmission and the potential for serious undesirable effects in breast-feeding infants, mothers should be instructed not to breast-feed if they are receiving Atripla.

4.7 Effects on ability to drive and use machines

No studies on the effects on the ability to drive and use machines have been performed. However, dizziness has been reported during treatment with efavirenz, emtricitabine and tenofovir disoproxil fumarate. Efavirenz may also cause impaired concentration and/or somnolence. Patients should be instructed that if they experience these symptoms they should avoid potentially hazardous tasks such as driving and operating machinery.

4.8 Undesirable effects

Assessment of adverse reactions for the fixed combination Atripla is based on experience from:

- a 48-week clinical study of Atripla (see Table 2)
- a clinical study in which efavirenz, emtricitabine and tenofovir disoproxil fumarate were co-administered (see Table 3)
- clinical study and post-marketing experience with the individual components of Atripla (see Table 4).

In Tables 2, 3 and 4 undesirable effects are presented in order of decreasing seriousness within each frequency grouping. Frequencies are defined as very common (⩾ 1/10), common (⩾ 1/100, < 1/10) or uncommon (⩾ 1/1,000, < 1/100).

Adverse reactions from clinical study experience with Atripla

In a 48-week open-label randomised clinical study in HIV infected patients with successful virological suppression on their current antiretroviral regimen, patients either changed to Atripla (n=203) or continued on their original antiretroviral treatment regimen (n=97). Treatment-emergent adverse reactions considered possibly or probably related to study drugs reported in patients who received Atripla in study AI266073 are listed by body system organ class and frequency in Table 2.

Table 2: All treatment-emergent adverse reactions considered possibly or probably related to Atripla reported in study AI266073 (over 48 weeks)

	Atripla (n=203)
Metabolism and nutrition disorders:	
Common	anorexia
Uncommon	fat redistribution, hypertriglyceridaemia, weight decreased, increased appetite
Psychiatric disorders:	
Common	nightmare, depression, depressed mood, anxiety, insomnia, mood altered, abnormal dreams, sleep disorder
Uncommon	confusional state, disorientation, personality change, mood swings, libido decreased
Nervous system disorders:	
Very common	dizziness
Common	somnolence, headache
Uncommon	incoherent speech
Eye disorders:	
Uncommon	vision blurred, altered visual depth perception
Ear and labyrinth disorders:	
Uncommon	vertigo
Vascular disorders:	
Common	hot flush
Gastrointestinal disorders:	
Common	diarrhoea, nausea
Uncommon	pancreatitis acute, vomiting, paraesthesia oral, hypoaesthesia oral, flatulence, dry mouth
Hepatobiliary disorders:	
Uncommon	hepatitis acute
Skin and subcutaneous tissue disorders:	
Common	rash, night sweats
Uncommon	pruritus
Musculoskeletal and connective tissue disorders:	
Uncommon	myalgia
Renal and urinary disorders:	
Common	blood creatinine increased
Reproductive system and breast disorders:	
Uncommon	breast enlargement
General disorders and administration site conditions:	
Common	fatigue, energy increased
Uncommon	feeling abnormal, feeling jittery, chills

Adverse reactions from clinical study experience with efavirenz + emtricitabine + tenofovir disoproxil fumarate

The following data are derived from a clinical study (GS-01-934) in which efavirenz, emtricitabine and tenofovir disoproxil fumarate were co-administered without regard to food as individual formulations or as a dual fixed combination of emtricitabine and tenofovir disoproxil fumarate with efavirenz.

Selected treatment-emergent adverse reactions considered possibly or probably related to study drugs from this

Table 1 Interactions between the individual components of Atripla and other medicinal products

Medicinal product by therapeutic areas (dose in mg)	Effects on drug levels Mean percent change in AUC, C_{max}, C_{min} with 90% confidence intervals if available (mechanism)	Recommendation concerning co-administration with Atripla (efavirenz 600 mg, emtricitabine 200 mg, tenofovir disoproxil fumarate 300 mg)
ANTI-INFECTIVES		
Antiretrovirals		
Protease inhibitors		
Amprenavir/Efavirenz (1,200 b.i.d./600 q.d.)	Amprenavir: AUC: ~↓ 40% C_{max}: ~↓ 40% C_{min}: ~↓ 40% (CYP3A4 induction, the effect of efavirenz is compensated by the pharmacokinetic booster effect of ritonavir) For co-administration of efavirenz with low-dose ritonavir in combination with a protease inhibitor, see section on ritonavir below.	Co-administration of amprenavir/ritonavir and Atripla is not recommended.
Amprenavir/Emtricitabine	Interaction not studied.	
Amprenavir/Tenofovir disoproxil fumarate	Interaction not studied.	
Atazanavir/Ritonavir/Tenofovir disoproxil fumarate (300 q.d./100 q.d./300 q.d.)	Atazanavir: AUC: ↓ 25% (↓ 42 to ↓ 3) C_{max}: ↓ 28% (↓ 50 to ↑ 5) C_{min}: ↓ 26% (↓ 46 to ↑ 10) Co-administration of atazanavir/ritonavir with tenofovir resulted in increased exposure to tenofovir. Higher tenofovir concentrations could potentiate tenofovir-associated adverse events, including renal disorders.	Co-administration of atazanavir/ritonavir and Atripla is not recommended.
Atazanavir/Ritonavir/Efavirenz	Co-administration of efavirenz with atazanavir in combination with low-dose ritonavir resulted in substantial decreases in atazanavir exposure due to CYP3A4 induction, necessitating dosage adjustment of atazanavir (refer to the Summary of Product Characteristics for the medicinal product containing atazanavir). Co-administration of efavirenz and atazanavir in combination with ritonavir may lead to increases in efavirenz exposure which may worsen the tolerability profile of efavirenz.	
Atazanavir/Ritonavir/Emtricitabine	Interaction not studied.	
Indinavir/Efavirenz (800 q8h/200 q.d.) Indinavir/Efavirenz (1,000 q8h/600 q.d.)	Efavirenz: AUC: ↔ C_{max}: ↔ C_{min}: ↔ Indinavir: Morning AUC: ↓ 33%* (↓ 26 to ↓ 39) Afternoon AUC: ↓ 37%* (↓ 26 to ↓ 46) Evening AUC: ↓ 46%* (↓ 37 to ↓ 54) Morning C_{max}: ↔* Afternoon C_{max}: ↔* Evening C_{max}: ↓ 29%* (↓ 11 to ↓ 43) Morning C_{min}: ↓ 39%* (↓ 24 to ↓ 51) Afternoon C_{min}: ↓ 52%* (↓ 47 to ↓ 57) Evening C_{min}: ↓ 57%* (↓ 50 to ↓ 63) * when compared to indinavir 800 q8h alone (CYP3A4 induction) For co-administration of efavirenz with low-dose ritonavir in combination with a protease inhibitor, see section on ritonavir below.	Insufficient data are available to make a dosing recommendation for indinavir when dosed with Atripla. While the clinical significance of decreased indinavir concentrations has not been established, the magnitude of the observed pharmacokinetic interaction should be taken into consideration when choosing a regimen containing both efavirenz, a component of Atripla, and indinavir.
Indinavir/Emtricitabine (800 q8h/200 q.d.)	Indinavir: AUC: ↔ C_{max}: ↔ Emtricitabine: AUC: ↔ C_{max}: ↔	
Indinavir/Tenofovir disoproxil fumarate (800 q8h/300 q.d.)	Indinavir: AUC: ↔ C_{max}: ↔ Tenofovir: AUC: ↔ C_{max}: ↔	
Lopinavir/Ritonavir/Tenofovir disoproxil fumarate (400 b.i.d./100 b.i.d./300 q.d.)	Lopinavir/Ritonavir: AUC: ↔ C_{max}: ↔ C_{min}: ↔ Tenofovir: AUC: ↑ 32% (↑ 25 to ↑ 38) C_{max}: ↔ C_{min}: ↑ 51% (↑ 37 to ↑ 66) Higher tenofovir concentrations could potentiate tenofovir-associated adverse events, including renal disorders.	Insufficient data are available to make a dosing recommendation for lopinavir/ritonavir when dosed with Atripla. Co-administration of lopinavir/ritonavir and Atripla is not recommended.
Lopinavir/Ritonavir/Efavirenz	Co-administration of lopinavir/ritonavir with efavirenz resulted in a substantial decrease in lopinavir exposure, necessitating dosage adjustment of lopinavir/ritonavir. When used in combination with efavirenz and two NRTIs, 533/133 mg lopinavir/ritonavir (soft capsules) twice daily yielded similar lopinavir plasma concentrations as compared to lopinavir/ritonavir (soft capsules) 400/100 mg twice daily without efavirenz (historical data). Refer to the Summary of Product Characteristics for lopinavir/ritonavir tablets for pharmacokinetic data when this formulation was administered with efavirenz. For co-administration of efavirenz with low-dose ritonavir in combination with a protease inhibitor, see section on ritonavir below.	
Lopinavir/Ritonavir/Emtricitabine	Interaction not studied.	
Ritonavir/Efavirenz (500 b.i.d./600 q.d.)	Ritonavir: Morning AUC: ↑ 18% (↑ 6 to ↑ 33) Evening AUC: ↔ Morning C_{max}: ↑ 24% (↑ 12 to ↑ 38) Evening C_{max}: ↔ Morning C_{min}: ↑ 42% (↑ 9 to ↑ 86) Evening C_{min}: ↑ 24% (↑ 3 to ↑ 50) Efavirenz: AUC: ↑ 21% (↑ 10 to ↑ 34) C_{max}: ↑ 14% (↑ 4 to ↑ 26) C_{min}: ↑ 25% (↑ 7 to ↑ 46) (inhibition of CYP-mediated oxidative metabolism) When efavirenz was given with ritonavir 500 mg or 600 mg twice daily, the combination was not well tolerated (for example, dizziness, nausea, paraesthesia and elevated liver enzymes occurred). Sufficient data on the tolerability of efavirenz with low-dose ritonavir (100 mg, once or twice daily) are not available.	Co-administration of ritonavir at doses of 600 mg and Atripla is not recommended. When using Atripla in a regimen including low-dose ritonavir, the possibility of an increase in the incidence of efavirenz-associated adverse events should be considered, due to possible pharmacodynamic interaction.
Ritonavir/Emtricitabine (600 b.i.d./600 q.d.)	Interaction not studied.	
Ritonavir/Tenofovir disoproxil fumarate (600 b.i.d./600 q.d.)	Interaction not studied.	

Medicinal product by therapeutic areas (dose in mg)	Effects on drug levels Mean percent change in AUC, C_{max}, C_{min} with 90% confidence intervals if available (mechanism)	Recommendation concerning co-administration with Atripla (efavirenz 600 mg, emtricitabine 200 mg, tenofovir disoproxil fumarate 300 mg)
Saquinavir/Efavirenz (1,200 soft capsule formulation q8h/600 q.d.)	Saquinavir: AUC: ↓ 62% (↓ 45 to ↓ 74) C_{max}: ↓ 50% (↓ 28 to ↓ 66) C_{min}: ↓ 56% (↓ 16 to ↓ 77) (decrease in saquinavir concentrations: CYP3A4 induction) Efavirenz: AUC: ↓ 12% (↓ 4 to ↓ 19) C_{max}: ↓ 13% (↓ 5 to ↓ 20) C_{min}: ↓ 14% (↓ 2 to ↓ 24)	Use of Atripla in combination with saquinavir as the sole protease inhibitor is not recommended.
Saquinavir/Tenofovir disoproxil fumarate (1,000 q.d./300 q.d.)	Saquinavir: AUC: ↔ C_{max}: ↔ Tenofovir: AUC: ↔ C_{max}: ↔ Co-administration of tenofovir disoproxil fumarate with ritonavir boosted saquinavir also resulted in no pharmacokinetic interaction.	
Saquinavir/Emtricitabine	Interaction not studied.	
Saquinavir/Ritonavir/Efavirenz	No data are available on the potential interactions of efavirenz with the combination of saquinavir and ritonavir. For co-administration of efavirenz with low-dose ritonavir in combination with a protease inhibitor, see section on ritonavir above.	Insufficient data are available to make a dosing recommendation for saquinavir/ritonavir when dosed with Atripla. Co-administration of saquinavir/ritonavir and Atripla is not recommended.
NRTIs and NNRTIs		
NRTIs/Efavirenz	Specific interaction studies have not been performed with efavirenz and NRTIs other than lamivudine (see section 4.4), zidovudine and tenofovir disoproxil fumarate. Clinically significant interactions would not be expected since the NRTIs are metabolised via a different route than efavirenz and would be unlikely to compete for the same metabolic enzymes and elimination pathways.	
NNRTIs/Efavirenz	Interaction not studied. The potential for pharmacokinetic or pharmacodynamic interactions is unknown.	Since use of two NNRTIs proved not beneficial in terms of efficacy and safety, co-administration of Atripla and another NNRTI is not recommended.
Didanosine/Tenofovir disoproxil fumarate	Co-administration of tenofovir disoproxil fumarate and didanosine results in a 40-60% increase in systemic exposure to didanosine that may increase the risk for didanosine-related adverse events. Rare cases of pancreatitis and lactic acidosis, sometimes fatal, have been reported. Co-administration of tenofovir disoproxil fumarate and didanosine at a dose of 400 mg daily has been associated with a significant decrease in CD4 cell count, possibly due to an intracellular interaction increasing phosphorylated (i.e. active) didanosine. A decreased dosage of 250 mg didanosine co-administered with tenofovir disoproxil fumarate therapy has been associated with reports of high rates of virologic failure within several tested combinations.	Co-administration of Atripla and didanosine is not recommended (see section 4.4).
Didanosine/Efavirenz	Interaction not studied.	
Didanosine/Emtricitabine	Interaction not studied.	
Antibiotics		
Clarithromycin/Efavirenz (500 b.i.d./400 q.d.)	Clarithromycin: AUC: ↓ 39% (↓ 30 to ↓ 46) C_{max}: ↓ 26% (↓ 15 to ↓ 35) Clarithromycin 14-hydroxymetabolite: AUC: ↑ 34% (↑ 18 to ↑ 53) C_{max}: ↑ 49% (↑ 32 to ↑ 69) Efavirenz: AUC: ↔ C_{max}: ↑ 11% (↑ 3 to ↑ 19) (CYP3A4 induction) Rash developed in 46% of uninfected volunteers receiving efavirenz and clarithromycin.	The clinical significance of these changes in clarithromycin plasma levels is not known. Alternatives to clarithromycin (e.g. azithromycin) may be considered. Other macrolide antibiotics, such as erythromycin, have not been studied in combination with Atripla.
Clarithromycin/Emtricitabine	Interaction not studied.	
Clarithromycin/Tenofovir disoproxil fumarate	Interaction not studied.	
Antimycobacterials		
Rifabutin/Efavirenz (300 q.d./600 q.d.)	Rifabutin: AUC: ↓ 38% (↓ 28 to ↓ 47) C_{max}: ↓ 32% (↓ 15 to ↓ 46) C_{min}: ↓ 45% (↓ 31 to ↓ 56) Efavirenz: AUC: ↔ C_{max}: ↔ C_{min}: ↓ 12% (↓ 24 to ↑ 1) (CYP3A4 induction)	The daily dose of rifabutin should be increased by 50% when given with Atripla. Consider doubling the rifabutin dose in regimens where rifabutin is given 2 or 3 times a week in combination with Atripla.
Rifabutin/Emtricitabine	Interaction not studied.	
Rifabutin/Tenofovir disoproxil fumarate	Interaction not studied.	
Rifampicin/Efavirenz (600 q.d./600 q.d.)	Efavirenz: AUC: ↓ 26% (↓ 15 to ↓ 36) C_{max}: ↓ 20% (↓ 11 to ↓ 28) C_{min}: ↓ 32% (↓ 15 to ↓ 46) (CYP3A4 and CYP2B6 induction)	An additional 200 mg/day (800 mg total) of efavirenz is recommended when rifampicin is co-administered with Atripla. No dose adjustment of rifampicin is recommended when given with Atripla.
Rifampicin/Tenofovir disoproxil fumarate (600 q.d./300 q.d.)	Rifampicin: AUC: ↔ C_{max}: ↔ Tenofovir: AUC: ↔ C_{max}: ↔	
Rifampicin/Emtricitabine	Interaction not studied.	
Antifungals		
Itraconazole/Efavirenz (200 b.i.d./600 q.d.)	Itraconazole: AUC: ↓ 39% (↓ 21 to ↓ 53) C_{max}: ↓ 37% (↓ 20 to ↓ 51) C_{min}: ↓ 44% (↓ 27 to ↓ 58) (decrease in itraconazole concentrations: CYP3A4 induction) Hydroxyitraconazole: AUC: ↓ 37% (↓ 14 to ↓ 55) C_{max}: ↓ 35% (↓ 12 to ↓ 52) C_{min}: ↓ 43% (↓ 18 to ↓ 60) Efavirenz: AUC: ↔ C_{max}: ↔ C_{min}: ↔	No dose recommendations can be made for the use of Atripla in combination with itraconazole. An alternative antifungal treatment should be considered.
Itraconazole/Emtricitabine	Interaction not studied.	
Itraconazole/Tenofovir disoproxil fumarate	Interaction not studied.	

Medicinal product by therapeutic areas (dose in mg)	Effects on drug levels Mean percent change in AUC, C_{max}, C_{min} with 90% confidence intervals if available (mechanism)	Recommendation concerning co-administration with Atripla (efavirenz 600 mg, emtricitabine 200 mg, tenofovir disoproxil fumarate 300 mg)
Voriconazole/Efavirenz (200 b.i.d./400 q.d.)	Voriconazole: AUC: ↓ 77% C_{max}: ↓ 61% Efavirenz: AUC: ↑ 44% C_{max}: ↑ 38% (competitive inhibition of oxidative metabolism) Co-administration of standard doses of efavirenz and voriconazole is contraindicated (see section 4.3).	Since Atripla is a fixed-dose combination product, the dose of efavirenz cannot be altered; therefore, voriconazole and Atripla must not be co-administered.
Voriconazole/Emtricitabine	Interaction not studied.	
Voriconazole/Tenofovir disoproxil fumarate	Interaction not studied.	
ANTICONVULSANTS		
Carbamazepine/Efavirenz (400 q.d./600 q.d.)	Carbamazepine: AUC: ↓ 27% (↓ 20 to ↓ 33) C_{max}: ↓ 20% (↓ 15 to ↓ 24) C_{min}: ↓ 35% (↓ 24 to ↓ 44) Efavirenz: AUC: ↓ 36% (↓ 32 to ↓ 40) C_{max}: ↓ 21% (↓ 15 to ↓ 26) C_{min}: ↓ 47% (↓ 41 to ↓ 53) (decrease in carbamazepine concentrations: CYP3A4 induction; decrease in efavirenz concentrations: CYP3A4 and CYP2B6 induction) Co-administration of higher doses of either efavirenz or carbamazepine has not been studied.	No dose recommendation can be made for the use of Atripla with carbamazepine. An alternative anticonvulsant should be considered. Carbamazepine plasma levels should be monitored periodically.
Carbamazepine/Emtricitabine	Interaction not studied.	
Carbamazepine/Tenofovir disoproxil fumarate	Interaction not studied.	
Phenytoin, Phenobarbital, and other anticonvulsants that are substrates of CYP450 isoenzymes	Interaction not studied with efavirenz, emtricitabine, or tenofovir disoproxil fumarate. There is a potential for reduction or increase in the plasma concentrations of phenytoin, phenobarbital and other anticonvulsants that are substrates of CYP450 isoenzymes with efavirenz.	When Atripla is co-administered with an anticonvulsant that is a substrate of CYP450 isoenzymes, periodic monitoring of anticonvulsant levels should be conducted.
Vigabatrin/Efavirenz Gabapentin/Efavirenz	Interaction not studied. Clinically significant interactions are not expected since vigabatrin and gabapentin are exclusively eliminated unchanged in the urine and are unlikely to compete for the same metabolic enzymes and elimination pathways as efavirenz.	Atripla and vigabatrin or gabapentin can be co-administered without dose adjustment.
Vigabatrin/Emtricitabine Gabapentin/Emtricitabine	Interaction not studied.	
Vigabatrin/Tenofovir disoproxil fumarate Gabapentin/Tenofovir disoproxil fumarate	Interaction not studied.	
ANTIDEPRESSANTS		
Selective Serotonin Reuptake Inhibitors (SSRIs)		
Sertraline/Efavirenz (50 q.d./600 q.d.)	Sertraline: AUC: ↓ 39% (↓ 27 to ↓ 50) C_{max}: ↓ 29% (↓ 15 to ↓ 40) C_{min}: ↓ 46% (↓ 31 to ↓ 58) Efavirenz: AUC: ↔ C_{max}: ↑ 11% (↑ 6 to ↑ 16) C_{min}: ↔ (CYP3A4 induction)	When co-administered with Atripla, sertraline dose increases should be guided by clinical response.
Sertraline/Emtricitabine	Interaction not studied.	
Sertraline/Tenofovir disoproxil fumarate	Interaction not studied.	
Paroxetine/Efavirenz (20 q.d./600 q.d.)	Paroxetine: AUC: ↔ C_{max}: ↔ C_{min}: ↔ Efavirenz: AUC: ↔ C_{max}: ↔ C_{min}: ↔	Atripla and paroxetine can be co-administered without dose adjustment.
Paroxetine/Emtricitabine	Interaction not studied.	
Paroxetine/Tenofovir disoproxil fumarate	Interaction not studied.	
Fluoxetine/Efavirenz	Interaction not studied. Since fluoxetine shares a similar metabolic profile with paroxetine, i.e. a strong CYP2D6 inhibitory effect, a similar lack of interaction would be expected for fluoxetine.	Atripla and fluoxetine can be co-administered without dose adjustment.
Fluoxetine/Emtricitabine	Interaction not studied.	
Fluoxetine/Tenofovir disoproxil fumarate	Interaction not studied.	
CARDIOVASCULAR AGENTS		
Calcium Channel Blockers		
Diltiazem/Efavirenz (240 q.d./600 q.d.)	Diltiazem: AUC: ↓ 69% (↓ 55 to ↓ 79) C_{max}: ↓ 60% (↓ 50 to ↓ 68) C_{min}: ↓ 63% (↓ 44 to ↓ 75) Desacetyl diltiazem: AUC: ↓ 75% (↓ 59 to ↓ 84) C_{max}: ↓ 64% (↓ 57 to ↓ 69) C_{min}: ↓ 62% (↓ 44 to ↓ 75) N-monodesmethyl diltiazem: AUC: ↓ 37% (↓ 17 to ↓ 52) C_{max}: ↓ 28% (↓ 7 to ↓ 44) C_{min}: ↓ 37% (↓ 17 to ↓ 52) Efavirenz: AUC: ↑ 11% (↑ 5 to ↑ 18) C_{max}: ↑ 16% (↑ 6 to ↑ 26) C_{min}: ↑ 13% (↑ 1 to ↑ 26) (CYP3A4 induction) The increase in efavirenz pharmacokinetic parameters is not considered clinically significant.	Dose adjustments of diltiazem when co-administered with Atripla should be guided by clinical response (refer to the Summary of Product Characteristics for diltiazem).
Diltiazem/Emtricitabine	Interaction not studied.	
Diltiazem/Tenofovir disoproxil fumarate	Interaction not studied.	
Verapamil, Felodipine, Nifedipine and Nicardipine	Interaction not studied with efavirenz, emtricitabine, or tenofovir disoproxil fumarate. When efavirenz is co-administered with a calcium channel blocker that is a substrate of the CYP3A4 enzyme, there is a potential for reduction in the plasma concentrations of the calcium channel blocker.	Dose adjustments of calcium channel blockers when co-administered with Atripla should be guided by clinical response (refer to the Summary of Product Characteristics for the calcium channel blocker).

Medicinal product by therapeutic areas (dose in mg)	Effects on drug levels Mean percent change in AUC, C_{max}, C_{min} with 90% confidence intervals if available (mechanism)	Recommendation concerning co-administration with Atripla (efavirenz 600 mg, emtricitabine 200 mg, tenofovir disoproxil fumarate 300 mg)
LIPID LOWERING MEDICINAL PRODUCTS		
HMG Co-A Reductase Inhibitors		
Atorvastatin/Efavirenz (10 q.d./600 q.d.)	Atorvastatin: AUC: ↓ 43% (↓ 34 to ↓ 50) C_{max}: ↓ 12% (↓ 1 to ↓ 26) 2-hydroxy atorvastatin: AUC: ↓ 35% (↓ 13 to ↓ 40) C_{max}: ↓ 13% (↓ 0 to ↓ 23) 4-hydroxy atorvastatin: AUC: ↓ 4% (↓ 0 to ↓ 31) C_{max}: ↓ 47% (↓ 9 to ↓ 51) Total active HMG Co-A reductase inhibitors: AUC: ↓ 34% (↓ 21 to ↓ 41) C_{max}: ↓ 20% (↓ 2 to ↓ 26)	Cholesterol levels should be periodically monitored when atorvastatin, pravastatin, or simvastatin is co-administered with Atripla. Dosage adjustments of statins may be required (refer to the Summary of Product Characteristics for the statin).
Atorvastatin/Emtricitabine	Interaction not studied.	
Atorvastatin/Tenofovir disoproxil fumarate	Interaction not studied.	
Pravastatin/Efavirenz (40 q.d./600 q.d.)	Pravastatin: AUC: ↓ 40% (↓ 26 to ↓ 57) C_{max}: ↓ 18% (↓ 59 to ↑ 12)	
Pravastatin/Emtricitabine	Interaction not studied.	
Pravastatin/Tenofovir disoproxil fumarate	Interaction not studied.	
Simvastatin/Efavirenz (40 q.d./600 q.d.)	Simvastatin: AUC: ↓ 69% (↓ 62 to ↓ 73) C_{max}: ↓ 76% (↓ 63 to ↓ 79) Simvastatin acid: AUC: ↓ 58% (↓ 39 to ↓ 68) C_{max}: ↓ 51% (↓ 32 to ↓ 58) Total active HMG Co-A reductase inhibitors: AUC: ↓ 60% (↓ 52 to ↓ 68) C_{max}: ↓ 62% (↓ 55 to ↓ 78) Total HMG Co-A reductase inhibitors: AUC: ↓ 60% (↓ 54 to ↓ 74) C_{max}: ↓ 70% (↓ 58 to ↓ 85) (CYP3A4 induction) Co-administration of efavirenz with atorvastatin, pravastatin, or simvastatin did not affect efavirenz AUC or C_{max} values.	
Simvastatin/Emtricitabine	Interaction not studied.	
Simvastatin/Tenofovir disoproxil fumarate	Interaction not studied.	
HORMONAL CONTRACEPTIVES		
Ethinyloestradiol/Efavirenz (50 µg single dose/400 q.d.)	Ethinyloestradiol: AUC: ↑ 37% (↑ 25 to ↑ 51) C_{max}: ↔ Efavirenz: AUC: ↔ C_{max}: ↔ (mechanism unknown) The clinical significance of the effect on ethinyloestradiol AUC is not known.	Because the potential interaction of efavirenz, a component of Atripla, with oral contraceptives has not been fully characterised, a reliable method of barrier contraception must be used in addition to oral contraceptives (see section 4.6).
Ethinyloestradiol/Tenofovir disoproxil fumarate (-/300 q.d.)	Ethinyloestradiol: AUC: ↔ C_{max}: ↔ Tenofovir: AUC: ↔ C_{max}: ↔	
Norgestimate/Ethinyloestradiol/ Emtricitabine	Interaction not studied.	
IMMUNOSUPPRESSANTS		
Tacrolimus/Efavirenz	Interaction not studied. ↓ exposure of tacrolimus may be expected (CYP3A4 induction). Tacrolimus is not anticipated to impact exposure of efavirenz.	Dose adjustments of tacrolimus may be required. Close monitoring of tacrolimus concentrations for at least two weeks (until stable concentrations are reached) is recommended when starting or stopping treatment with Atripla.
Tacrolimus/Emtricitabine/Tenofovir disoproxil fumarate (0.1 mg/kg q.d./200 mg/300 mg q.d.)	Tacrolimus: AUC: ↔ C_{max}: ↔ C_{24}: ↔ Emtricitabine: AUC: ↔ C_{max}: ↔ C_{24}: ↔ Tenofovir disoproxil fumarate: AUC: ↔ C_{max}: ↔ C_{24}: ↔	
OPIOIDS		
Methadone/Efavirenz (35-100 q.d./600 q.d.)	Methadone: AUC: ↓ 52% (↓ 33 to ↓ 66) C_{max}: ↓ 45% (↓ 25 to ↓ 59) (CYP3A4 induction) In a study of HIV infected intravenous drug users, co-administration of efavirenz with methadone resulted in decreased plasma levels of methadone and signs of opiate withdrawal. The methadone dose was increased by a mean of 22% to alleviate withdrawal symptoms.	Patients receiving methadone and Atripla concomitantly should be monitored for signs of withdrawal and their methadone dose increased as required to alleviate withdrawal symptoms.
Methadone/Tenofovir disoproxil fumarate (40-110 q.d./300 q.d.)	Methadone: AUC: ↔ C_{max}: ↔ C_{min}: ↔ Tenofovir: AUC: ↔ C_{max}: ↔ C_{min}: ↔	
Methadone/Emtricitabine	Interaction not studied.	
HERBAL PRODUCTS		
St. John's wort (*Hypericum perforatum*)/Efavirenz	Plasma levels of efavirenz can be reduced by concomitant use of St. John's wort due to induction of drug metabolising enzymes and/or transport proteins by St. John's wort.	Co-administration of Atripla and St. John's wort is contraindicated. If a patient is already taking St. John's wort, stop St. John's wort, check viral levels and if possible efavirenz levels. Efavirenz levels may increase on stopping St. John's wort. The inducing effect of St. John's wort may persist for at least 2 weeks after cessation of treatment.
St. John's wort (*Hypericum perforatum*)/Emtricitabine	Interaction not studied.	
St. John's wort (*Hypericum perforatum*)/Tenofovir disoproxil fumarate	Interaction not studied.	

study reported in patients after 144 weeks of treatment are listed by body system organ class and frequency in Table 3.

Table 3: Selected treatment-emergent adverse reactions considered possibly or probably related to study drugs (efavirenz, emtricitabine and tenofovir disoproxil fumarate) in clinical study GS-01-934 over 144 weeks

	Efavirenz+emtricitabine+tenofovir disoproxil fumarate (n=257)
Blood and lymphatic system disorders:	
Uncommon	neutropenia
Nervous system disorders:	
Very common	dizziness
Common	somnolence, stupor, lethargy, headache, disturbance of attention
Uncommon	amnesia, ataxia, balance disorder, dysgeusia
Eye disorders:	
Uncommon	vision blurred
Ear and labyrinth disorders:	
Common	vertigo
Respiratory, thoracic and mediastinal disorders:	
Uncommon	dyspnoea
Gastrointestinal disorders:	
Very common	nausea
Common	diarrhoea, vomiting, abdominal pain, flatulence, abdominal distension, dry mouth
Uncommon	dyspepsia
Skin and subcutaneous tissue disorders:	
Very common	rash
Common	pruritus, skin hyperpigmentation, dermatitis
Uncommon	urticaria, dry skin, eczema
Metabolism and nutrition disorders:	
Common	decreased appetite, increased appetite
Uncommon	hypertriglyceridaemia, anorexia
Vascular disorders:	
Common	hot flush
General disorders and administration site conditions:	
Common	fatigue, fever
Uncommon	asthenia, feeling drunk
Psychiatric disorders:	
Very common	abnormal dreams
Common	nightmares, depression, insomnia, sleep disorder, euphoric mood
Uncommon	paranoia, psychomotor agitation, delusion, confusional state, anxiety, aggression, nervousness, disorientation

Laboratory test abnormalities: Liver enzymes: in a 144-week clinical study (GS-01-934), elevations of aspartate aminotransferase (AST> 5 times ULN (upper limit of normal)) and of alanine aminotransferase (ALT> 5 times ULN) were reported in 3% and 2% of patients treated with efavirenz, emtricitabine, and tenofovir disoproxil fumarate (n=257) and 3% and 3% of patients treated with efavirenz and fixed-dose zidovudine/lamivudine (n=254), respectively.

Adverse reactions associated with the individual components of Atripla

The adverse reactions from clinical study and post-marketing experience with the individual components of Atripla in antiretroviral combination therapy are listed in Table 4 below by body system organ class and frequency.

The most notable adverse reactions that have been reported in clinical studies with efavirenz are rash and nervous system symptoms. The administration of efavirenz

Table 4 Adverse reactions associated with the individual components of Atripla based on clinical study and post-marketing safety experience

	Efavirenz	Emtricitabine	Tenofovir disoproxil fumarate
Blood and lymphatic system disorders:			
Common		neutropenia	
Uncommon		anaemia	
Nervous system disorders:			
Very common		headache	dizziness
Common	somnolence, headache, disturbance in attention, dizziness	dizziness	
Uncommon	convulsions, amnesia, thinking abnormal, ataxia, coordination abnormal, agitation		
Not known*	cerebellar coordination and balance disturbances		
Eye disorders:			
Uncommon	vision blurred		
Ear and labyrinth disorders:			
Uncommon	vertigo		
Respiratory, thoracic and mediastinal disorders:			
Not known*			dyspnoea
Gastrointestinal disorders:			
Very common		diarrhoea, nausea	diarrhoea, vomiting, nausea
Common	diarrhoea, vomiting, abdominal pain, nausea	elevated amylase including elevated pancreatic amylase, elevated serum lipase, vomiting, abdominal pain, dyspepsia	flatulence
Uncommon	pancreatitis acute		
Not known*			pancreatitis
Renal and urinary disorders:			
Not known*			renal failure (acute and chronic), acute tubular necrosis, proximal renal tubulopathy including Fanconi syndrome, nephritis, acute interstitial nephritis, nephrogenic diabetes insipidus, increased creatinine, proteinuria
Skin and subcutaneous tissue disorders:			
Very common	rash (all grades, 18%)		
Common	pruritus	allergic reaction, vesiculobullous rash, pustular rash, maculopapular rash, rash, pruritus, urticaria, skin discolouration (increased pigmentation)	
Uncommon	Stevens-Johnson syndrome, erythema multiforme, severe rash (< 1%)		
Not known*	photoallergic dermatitis		rash
Musculoskeletal and connective tissue disorders:			
Very common		elevated creatine kinase	
Not known*			rhabdomyolysis, osteomalacia (manifested as bone pain and infrequently contributing to fractures), muscular weakness, myopathy
Metabolism and nutrition disorders:			
Very common			hypophosphataemia
Common		hyperglycaemia, hypertriglyceridaemia	
Not known*			lactic acidosis, hypokalaemia
General disorders and administration site conditions:			
Common	fatigue	pain, asthenia	
Not known*			asthenia
Immune system disorders:			
Uncommon	hypersensitivity		
Hepatobiliary disorders:			
Common		elevated serum aspartate aminotransferase (AST) and/or elevated serum alanine aminotransferase (ALT), hyperbilirubinaemia	
Uncommon	hepatitis acute		
Not known*	hepatic failure		hepatitis, increased transaminases, hepatic steatosis
Reproductive system and breast disorders:			
Uncommon	gynaecomastia		
Psychiatric disorders:			
Common	depression (severe in 1.6%), anxiety, abnormal dreams, insomnia	abnormal dreams, insomnia	
Uncommon	suicide attempt, suicide ideation, mania, paranoia, hallucination, euphoric mood, affect lability, confusional state, aggression		
Not known*	completed suicide, psychosis, delusion, neurosis		

* These adverse reactions have been identified through post-marketing safety surveillance and the frequency is not known.

th food may increase efavirenz exposure and may lead to increase in the frequency of adverse reactions (see ction 4.4). There have been post-marketing reports in sociation with tenofovir disoproxil fumarate of renal and inary disorders including renal failure, proximal tubulopathy (including Fanconi syndrome), acute tubular necros and nephrogenic diabetes insipidus.

able 4: Adverse reactions associated with the individual components of Atripla based on clinical study and ost-marketing safety experience

ee Table 4 on previous page)

he following adverse reactions, listed under the body ystem headings above, may occur as a consequence of roximal renal tubulopathy: rhabdomyolysis, osteomalacia nanifested as bone pain and infrequently contributing to actures), hypokalaemia, muscular weakness, myopathy nd hypophosphataemia. These events are not considered be causally associated with tenofovir disoproxil fumaate therapy in the absence of proximal renal tubulopathy.

Rash with efavirenz: rashes are usually mild-to-moderate naculopapular skin eruptions that occur within the first two veeks of initiating therapy with efavirenz. In most patients ash resolves with continuing therapy with efavirenz within ne month. In clinical studies, 1.7% of patients treated with favirenz discontinued therapy because of rash. Efavirenz can be reinitiated in patients interrupting therapy because of rash. Use of appropriate antihistamines and/or corticosteroids is recommended when efavirenz is restarted.

Experience with efavirenz in patients who discontinued other antiretroviral agents of the non-nucleoside reverse transcriptase inhibitor (NNRTI) class is limited. Nineteen patients who discontinued nevirapine because of rash have been treated with efavirenz. Nine of these patients developed mild-to-moderate rash while receiving therapy with efavirenz, and two discontinued because of rash.

Psychiatric symptoms with efavirenz: patients with a history of psychiatric disorders appear to be at greater risk of serious psychiatric adverse reactions listed in the efavirenz column of Table 4 with the frequency of events ranging from 0.3% for manic reactions to 2.0% for both severe depression and suicidal ideation.

Nervous system symptoms with efavirenz: in clinical controlled studies, nervous system symptoms of moderate-to-severe intensity were experienced by 19.4% of patients compared to 9.0% of patients receiving control regimens. These symptoms were severe in 2.0% of patients receiving efavirenz 600 mg daily and in 1.3% of patients receiving control regimens. In clinical studies 2.1% of patients treated with 600 mg of efavirenz discontinued therapy because of nervous system symptoms.

Nervous system symptoms usually begin during the first one or two days of therapy and generally resolve after the first two to four weeks. Nervous system symptoms may occur more frequently when efavirenz is taken concomitantly with meals possibly due to increased efavirenz plasma levels (see section 5.2). Dosing at bedtime seems to improve the tolerability of these symptoms (see section 4.2).

Analysis of long-term data from a clinical study (median follow-up 180 weeks, 102 weeks and 76 weeks for patients treated with efavirenz + zidovudine + lamivudine, efavirenz + indinavir, and indinavir + zidovudine + lamivudine, respectively) showed that, beyond 24 weeks of therapy, the incidences of new-onset nervous system symptoms among efavirenz-treated patients were generally similar to those in the control arm.

Lactic acidosis: lactic acidosis, usually associated with hepatic steatosis, has been reported with the use of nucleoside analogues (see section 4.4).

HIV/HBV or HCV co-infected patients: Only a limited number of patients were co-infected with HBV (n=13) or HCV (n=26) in study GS-01-934. The adverse reaction profile of efavirenz, emtricitabine and tenofovir disoproxil fumarate in patients co-infected with HIV/HBV or HIV/HCV was similar to that observed in patients infected with HIV without co-infection. However, as would be expected in this patient population, elevations in AST and ALT occurred more frequently than in the general HIV infected population.

Amylase: in clinical studies, asymptomatic increases in serum amylase levels > 1.5 times the ULN were seen in 10% of patients treated with efavirenz and 6% of patients treated with control regimens. The clinical significance of asymptomatic increases in serum amylase is unknown.

Lipids, lipodystrophy and metabolic abnormalities: combination antiretroviral therapy has been associated with metabolic abnormalities such as hypertriglyceridaemia, hypercholesterolaemia, insulin-resistance, hyperglycaemia and hyperlactataemia (see section 4.4).

Combination antiretroviral therapy has been associated with redistribution of body fat (lipodystrophy) in HIV patients including the loss of peripheral and facial subcutaneous fat, increased intra-abdominal and visceral fat, breast hypertrophy and dorsocervical fat accumulation (buffalo hump) (see section 4.4).

Immune Reactivation Syndrome: in HIV infected patients with severe immune deficiency at the time of initiation of CART, an inflammatory reaction to asymptomatic or residual opportunistic infections may arise (see section 4.4).

Cannabinoid test interaction: efavirenz does not bind to cannabinoid receptors. False positive urine cannabinoid test results have been reported in uninfected volunteers who received efavirenz. False positive test results have only been observed with the CEDIA DAU Multi-Level THC assay, which is used for screening, and have not been observed with other cannabinoid assays tested including tests used for confirmation of positive results.

Osteonecrosis: cases of osteonecrosis have been reported, particularly in patients with generally acknowledged risk factors, advanced HIV disease or long-term exposure to combination antiretroviral therapy (CART). The frequency of this is unknown (see section 4.4).

4.9 Overdose

Some patients accidentally taking 600 mg efavirenz twice daily have reported increased nervous system symptoms. One patient experienced involuntary muscle contractions.

If overdose occurs, the patient must be monitored for evidence of toxicity (see section 4.8), and standard supportive treatment applied as necessary.

Administration of activated charcoal may be used to aid removal of unabsorbed efavirenz. There is no specific antidote for overdose with efavirenz. Since efavirenz is highly protein bound, dialysis is unlikely to remove significant quantities of it from blood.

Up to 30% of the emtricitabine dose and approximately 10% of the tenofovir dose can be removed by haemodialysis. It is not known whether emtricitabine or tenofovir can be removed by peritoneal dialysis.

5. PHARMACOLOGICAL PROPERTIES

5.1 Pharmacodynamic properties

Pharmacotherapeutic group: Antivirals for treatment of HIV infections, combinations, ATC code: J05AR06

Mechanism of action: efavirenz is an NNRTI of HIV-1. Efavirenz non-competitively inhibits HIV-1 reverse transcriptase (RT) and does not significantly inhibit human immunodeficiency virus-2 (HIV-2) RT or cellular deoxyribonucleic acid (DNA) polymerases (α, β, γ, and δ). Emtricitabine is a nucleoside analogue of cytidine. Tenofovir disoproxil fumarate is converted *in vivo* to tenofovir, a nucleoside monophosphate (nucleotide) analogue of adenosine monophosphate.

Emtricitabine and tenofovir are phosphorylated by cellular enzymes to form emtricitabine triphosphate and tenofovir diphosphate, respectively. *In vitro* studies have shown that both emtricitabine and tenofovir can be fully phosphorylated when combined together in cells. Emtricitabine triphosphate and tenofovir diphosphate competitively inhibit HIV-1 reverse transcriptase, resulting in DNA chain termination.

Both emtricitabine triphosphate and tenofovir diphosphate are weak inhibitors of mammalian DNA polymerases and there was no evidence of toxicity to mitochondria *in vitro* and *in vivo*.

Antiviral activity in vitro: efavirenz demonstrated antiviral activity against most non-clade B isolates (subtypes A, AE, AG, C, D, F, G, J, and N) but had reduced antiviral activity against group O viruses. Emtricitabine displayed antiviral activity against HIV-1 clades A, B, C, D, E, F, and G. Tenofovir displayed antiviral activity against HIV-1 clades A, B, C, D, E, F, G, and O. Both emtricitabine and tenofovir showed strain specific activity against HIV-2 and antiviral activity against HBV.

In combination studies evaluating the *in vitro* antiviral activity of efavirenz and emtricitabine together, efavirenz and tenofovir together, and emtricitabine and tenofovir together, additive to synergistic antiviral effects were observed.

Resistance: resistance to efavirenz can be selected *in vitro* and resulted in single or multiple amino acid substitutions in HIV-1 RT, including L100I, V108I, V179D, and Y181C. K103N was the most frequently observed RT substitution in viral isolates from patients who experienced rebound in viral load during clinical studies of efavirenz. Substitutions at RT positions 98, 100, 101, 108, 138, 188, 190 or 225 were also observed, but at lower frequencies, and often only in combination with K103N. Cross-resistance profiles for efavirenz, nevirapine and delavirdine *in vitro* demonstrated that the K103N substitution confers loss of susceptibility to all three NNRTIs.

The potential for cross-resistance between efavirenz and NRTIs is low because of the different binding sites on the target and mechanism of action. The potential for cross-resistance between efavirenz and PIs is low because of the different enzyme targets involved.

Resistance to emtricitabine or tenofovir has been seen *in vitro* and in some HIV-1 infected patients due to the development of an M184V or M184I substitution in RT with emtricitabine or a K65R substitution in RT with tenofovir. No other pathways of resistance to emtricitabine or tenofovir have been identified. Emtricitabine-resistant viruses with the M184V/I mutation were cross-resistant to lamivudine, but retained sensitivity to didanosine, stavudine, tenofovir and zidovudine. The K65R mutation can also be selected by abacavir or didanosine and results in reduced susceptibility to these agents plus lamivudine, emtricitabine and tenofovir. Tenofovir disoproxil fumarate should be avoided in patients with HIV-1 harbouring the K65R mutation. Both the K65R and M184V/I mutation remain fully susceptible to efavirenz.

Patients with HIV-1 expressing three or more thymidine analogue associated mutations (TAMs) that included either an M41L or an L210W substitution in RT showed reduced susceptibility to tenofovir disoproxil fumarate.

In vivo resistance (antiretroviral-naïve patients): extremely limited resistance data from patients treated with Atripla are currently available. However, in a 144-week open-label randomised clinical study (GS-01-934) in antiretroviral-naïve patients, where efavirenz, emtricitabine and tenofovir disoproxil fumarate were used as individual formulations (or as efavirenz and the fixed combination of emtricitabine and tenofovir disoproxil fumarate (Truvada) from week 96 to 144), genotyping was performed on plasma HIV-1 isolates from all patients with confirmed HIV RNA> 400 copies/ml at week 144 or early study drug discontinuation (see section on *Clinical experience*). As of week 144:

- The M184V/I mutation developed in 2/19 (10.5%) isolates analysed from patients in the efavirenz + emtricitabine + tenofovir disoproxil fumarate group and in 10/29 (34.5%) isolates analysed from the efavirenz + lamivudine/zidovudine group (p-value < 0.05, Fisher's Exact test comparing the emtricitabine + tenofovir disoproxil fumarate group to the lamivudine/zidovudine group among all subjects).
- No virus analysed contained the K65R mutation.
- Genotypic resistance to efavirenz, predominantly the K103N mutation, developed in virus from 13/19 (68%) patients in the efavirenz + emtricitabine + tenofovir disoproxil fumarate group and in virus from 21/29 (72%) patients in the efavirenz + lamivudine/zidovudine group. A summary of resistance mutation development is shown in Table 5.

Table 5: Development of resistance in study GS-01-934 through week 144

(see Table 5 on next page)

Please refer to the Summary of Product Characteristics for the individual components for additional information regarding *in vivo* resistance with these medicinal products.

Clinical experience

In a 144-week open-label randomised clinical study (GS-01-934) antiretroviral treatment-naïve HIV-1 infected patients received either a once-daily regimen of efavirenz, emtricitabine and tenofovir disoproxil fumarate or a fixed combination of lamivudine and zidovudine (Combivir) administered twice daily and efavirenz once daily (please refer to the Summary of Product Characteristics for Truvada). Patients who completed 144 weeks of treatment with either treatment arm in study GS-01-934 were given the option to continue in an open-label extended phase of the study with Atripla on an empty stomach. Preliminary 24-week data are available from a total of 286 patients who changed to Atripla: 160 had previously received efavirenz, emtricitabine and tenofovir disoproxil fumarate, and 126 had previously received Combivir and efavirenz. The majority of patients from both initial treatment groups maintained virologic suppression after changing to Atripla. In 91% of the patients the HIV-1 RNA plasma concentrations remained < 50 copies/ml and in 97% < 400 copies/ml, after 24 weeks of Atripla treatment (intention to treat analysis (ITT), missing=failure).

Study AI266073 was a 48-week open-label randomised clinical study in HIV infected patients comparing the efficacy of Atripla to antiretroviral therapy consisting of at least two nucleoside or nucleotide reverse transcriptase inhibitors (NRTIs) with a protease inhibitor or non-nucleoside reverse transcriptase inhibitor; however not a regimen containing all Atripla components (efavirenz, emtricitabine and tenofovir disoproxil fumarate). Atripla was administered on an empty stomach (see section 4.2). Patients had never experienced virological failure on a previous antiretroviral therapy, had no known HIV-1 mutations that confer resistance to any of the three components within Atripla, and had been virologically suppressed for at least three months at baseline. Patients either changed to Atripla (N=203) or continued on their original antiretroviral treatment regimen (N=97). Forty-eight week data showed that high levels of virologic suppression, comparable to the original treatment regimen, were maintained in patients who were randomised to change to Atripla (see Table 6).

Table 6: 48-week efficacy data from study AI266073 in which Atripla was administered to virologically suppressed patients on combination antiretroviral therapy

(see Table 6 on next page)

When the two strata were analysed separately, response rates in the stratum with prior PI-treatment were numerically lower for patients switched to Atripla [92.4% versus 94.0% for the PVR (sensitivity analysis) for Atripla and SBR patients respectively; a difference (95%CI) of -1.6% (-10.0%, 6.7%)]. In the prior-NNRTI stratum, response rates were 98.9% vs 97.4% for Atripla and SBR patients respectively; a difference (95%CI) of 1.4% (-4.0%, 6.9%).

No data are currently available from clinical studies with Atripla in treatment-naïve patients or in heavily pretreated patients. There is no clinical experience with Atripla in patients who are experiencing virological failure in a first-line antiretroviral treatment regimen or in combination with other antiretroviral agents.

Table 5 Development of resistance in study GS-01-934 through week 144

	Efavirenz+emtricitabine+ tenofovir disoproxil fumarate (N=244)		Efavirenz +lamivudine/zidovudine (N=243)	
Resistance analysis by week 144	19		31	
On-therapy genotypes	19	(100%)	29	(100%)
Efavirenz resistance[1]	13	(68%)	21	(72%)
K103N	8	(42%)	18*	(62%)
K101E	3	(16%)	3	(10%)
G190A/S	2	(10.5%)	4	(14%)
Y188C/H	1	(5%)	2	(7%)
V108I	1	(5%)	1	(3%)
P225H	0		2	(7%)
M184V/I	2	(10.5%)	10*	(34.5%)
K65R	0		0	
TAMs[2]	0		2	(7%)

* p-value < 0.05, Fisher's Exact test comparing efavirenz + emtricitabine + tenofovir disoproxil fumarate group to efavirenz + lamivudine/zidovudine group among all patients.

[1] Other efavirenz resistance mutations included A98G (n=1), K103E (n=1), V179D (n=1), and M230L (n=1).

[2] Thymidine analogue associated mutations included D67N (n=1) and K70R (n=1).

Table 6 48-week efficacy data from study AI266073 in which Atripla was administered to virologically suppressed patients on combination antiretroviral therapy

	Treatment group		
Endpoint	Atripla (N=203) **n/N (%)**	Stayed on original treatment regimen (N=97) **n/N (%)**	Difference between Atripla and original treatment regimen (95%CI)
	patients with HIV-1 RNA < 50 copies/ml		
PVR (KM)	94.5%	85.5%	8.9% (-7.7% to 25.6%)
M=Excluded	179/181 (98.9%)	85/87 (97.7%)	1.2% (-2.3% to 6.7%)
M=Failure	179/203 (88.2%)	85/97 (87.6%)	0.5% (-7.0% to 9.3%)
Modified LOCF	190/203 (93.6%)	94/97 (96.9%)	-3.3% (-8.3% to 2.7%)
	patients with HIV-1 RNA < 200 copies/ml		
PVR (KM)	98.4%	98.9%	-0.5% (-3.2% to 2.2%)
M=Excluded	181/181 (100%)	87/87 (100%)	0% (-2.4% to 4.2%)
M=Failure	181/203 (89.2%)	87/97 (89.7%)	-0.5% (-7.6% to 7.9%)

PVR (KM): Pure virologic response assessed using the Kaplan Meier (KM) method

M: Missing

Modified LOCF: Post-hoc analysis where patients who failed virologically or discontinued for adverse events were treated as failures; for other drop-outs, the LOCF (last observation carried forward) method was applied

Patients coinfected with HIV and HBV: limited clinical experience in patients co-infected with HIV and HBV suggests that treatment with emtricitabine or tenofovir disoproxil fumarate in antiretroviral combination therapy to control HIV infection also results in a reduction in HBV DNA (3 $\log_{10}$ reduction or 4 to 5 $\log_{10}$ reduction, respectively) (see section 4.4).

5.2 Pharmacokinetic properties

The separate pharmaceutical forms of efavirenz, emtricitabine and tenofovir disoproxil fumarate were used to determine the pharmacokinetics of efavirenz, emtricitabine and tenofovir disoproxil fumarate, administered separately in HIV infected patients. The bioequivalence of one Atripla film-coated tablet with one efavirenz 600 mg film-coated tablet plus one emtricitabine 200 mg hard capsule plus one tenofovir disoproxil 245 mg film-coated tablet (equivalent to 300 mg tenofovir disoproxil fumarate) administered together, was established following single dose administration to fasting healthy subjects in study GS-US-177-0105 (see Table 7).

Table 7: Summary of pharmacokinetic data from stu
GS-US-177-0105

(see Table 7 below)

Absorption: in HIV infected patients, peak efavirenz plasm concentrations were attained by 5 hours and steady-sta concentrations reached in 6 to 7 days. In 35 patien receiving efavirenz 600 mg once daily, steady-state pea concentration (C_{max}) was 12.9 ± 3.7 μM (29%) [mean standard deviation (S.D.) (coefficient of variation (%CV) steady-state C_{min} was 5.6 ± 3.2 μM (57%), and AUC wa 184 ± 73 μM•h (40%).

Emtricitabine is rapidly absorbed with peak plasma co centrations occurring at 1 to 2 hours post-dose. Followir multiple dose oral administration of emtricitabine to 20 H infected patients, steady-state C_{max} was 1.8 ± 0.7 μg/ (mean ± S.D.) (39%CV), steady-state C_{min} was 0.09 0.07 μg/ml (80%) and the AUC was 10.0 ± 3.1 μg•h/ (31%) over a 24 hour dosing interval.

Following oral administration of a single 300 mg dose tenofovir disoproxil fumarate to HIV-1 infected patients the fasted state, maximum tenofovir concentrations we achieved within one hour and the C_{max} and AUC (mean S.D.) (%CV) values were 296 ± 90 ng/ml (30%) and 2,287 685 ng•h/ml (30%), respectively. The oral bioavailability tenofovir from tenofovir disoproxil fumarate in faste patients was approximately 25%.

Effect of food: Atripla has not been evaluated in the pr sence of food.

Administration of efavirenz capsules with a high fat me increased the mean AUC and C_{max} of efavirenz by 28 and 79%, respectively, compared to administration in fasted state. Compared to fasted administration, dosing tenofovir disoproxil fumarate and emtricitabine in comb nation with either a high fat meal or a light meal increase the mean AUC and C_{max} of tenofovir by 35% and 15% respectively without affecting emtricitabine exposures.

Atripla is recommended for administration on an emp stomach since food may increase efavirenz exposure ar may lead to an increase in the frequency of adverse rea tions (see sections 4.4 and 4.8). It is anticipated th tenofovir exposure will be approximately 35% lower fo lowing administration of Atripla on an empty stomach compared to the individual component tenofovir disopro fumarate when taken with food. Forty-eight week data fro a clinical study (AI266073) showed maintenance of virol gic suppression for patients who had stable virologic su pression on combination antiretroviral therapy ar subsequently changed to Atripla with a recommendatio for administration of Atripla on an empty stomach.

Distribution: efavirenz is highly bound (> 99%) to huma plasma proteins, predominantly albumin.

In vitro binding of emtricitabine to human plasma protei is (< 4% and independent of concentrations over th range of 0.02 to 200 μg/ml. Following intravenous admi istration the volume of distribution of emtricitabine wa approximately 1.4 l/kg. After oral administration, emtric tabine is widely distributed throughout the body. The mea plasma to blood concentration ratio was approximately 1 and the mean semen to plasma concentration ratio wa approximately 4.0.

In vitro binding of tenofovir to human plasma or seru protein is < 0.7% and 7.2%, respectively over the tend fovir concentration range 0.01 to 25 μg/ml. Following intr venous administration the volume of distribution tenofovir was approximately 800 ml/kg. After oral admi istration, tenofovir is widely distributed throughout th body.

Biotransformation: studies in humans and *in vitro* studie using human liver microsomes have demonstrated th efavirenz is principally metabolised by the cytochrom P450 system to hydroxylated metabolites with subseque glucuronidation of these hydroxylated metabolites. Thes metabolites are essentially inactive against HIV-1. The *vitro* studies suggest that CYP3A4 and CYP2B6 are th major isoenzymes responsible for efavirenz metabolis

Table 7 Summary of pharmacokinetic data from study GS-US-177-0105

	Efavirenz (n=45)			Emtricitabine (n=45)			Tenofovir disoproxil fumarate (n=45)		
Parameters	**Test**	**Reference**	**GMR (%) (90%CI)**	**Test**	**Reference**	**GMR (%) (90%CI)**	**Test**	**Reference**	**GMR (%) (90%CI)**
C_{max} (ng/ml)	2,264.3 (26.8)	2,308.6 (30.3)	98.79 (92.28, 105.76)	2,130.6 (25.3)	2,384.4 (20.4)	88.84 (84.02, 93.94)	325.1 (34.2)	352.9 (29.6)	91.46 (84.64, 98.83)
AUC_{0-last} (ng•h/ml)	125,623.6 (25.7)	132,795.7 (27.0)	95.84 (90.73, 101.23)	10,682.6 (18.1)	10,874.4 (14.9)	97.98 (94.90, 101.16)	1,948.8 (32.9)	1,969.0 (32.8)	99.29 (91.02, 108.32)
AUC_{inf} (ng•h/ml)	146,074.9 (33.1)	155,518.6 (34.6)	95.87 (89.63, 102.55)	10,854.9 (17.9)	11,054.3 (14.9)	97.96 (94.86, 101.16)	2,314.0 (29.2)	2,319.4 (30.3)	100.45 (93.22, 108.23)
$T_{1/2}$ (h)	180.6 (45.3)	182.5 (38.3)		14.5 (53.8)	14.6 (47.8)		18.9 (20.8)	17.8 (22.6)	

Test: single fixed-dose combination tablet taken under fasted conditions.

Reference: single dose of a 600 mg efavirenz tablet, 200 mg emtricitabine capsule and 300 mg tenofovir disoproxil fumarate tablet taken under fasted conditions.

Values for Test and Reference are mean (% coefficient of variation).

GMR=geometric least-squares mean ratio, CI=confidence interval d that it inhibits P450 isoenzymes 2C9, 2C19, and 3A4. in vitro studies efavirenz did not inhibit CYP2E1 and hibited CYP2D6 and CYP1A2 only at concentrations well ove those achieved clinically.

avirenz plasma exposure may be increased in patients th homozygous G516T genetic variant of the CYP2B6 oenzyme. The clinical implications of such an association e unknown; however, the potential for an increased equency and severity of efavirenz-associated adverse vents cannot be excluded.

favirenz has been shown to induce P450 enzymes, result-g in the induction of its own metabolism. In uninfected lunteers, multiple doses of 200 to 400 mg per day for 10 ays resulted in a lower than predicted extent of accumu-(22 to 42% lower) and a shorter terminal half-life of 40 55 hours (single dose half-life 52 to 76 hours).

here is limited metabolism of emtricitabine. The biotrans-rmation of emtricitabine includes oxidation of the thiol oiety to form the 3'-sulphoxide diastereomers (approxi-ately 9% of dose) and conjugation with glucuronic acid to rm 2'-O-glucuronide (approximately 4% of dose). *In vitro* udies have determined that neither tenofovir disoproxil marate nor tenofovir are substrates for the CYP450 nzymes. Neither emtricitabine nor tenofovir inhibited *in tro* drug metabolism mediated by any of the major human YP450 isoforms involved in drug biotransformation. Also, mtricitabine did not inhibit uridine 5'-diphosphoglucuro-yl transferase, the enzyme responsible for glucuronida-on.

limination: efavirenz has a relatively long terminal half-life f at least 52 hours after single doses (see also data from ioequivalence study described above) and 40 to 55 hours fter multiple doses. Approximately 14 to 34% of a radi-labelled dose of efavirenz was recovered in the urine and ess than 1% of the dose was excreted in urine as nchanged efavirenz.

ollowing oral administration, the elimination half-life of mtricitabine is approximately 10 hours. Emtricitabine is rimarily excreted by the kidneys with complete recovery f the dose achieved in urine (approximately 86%) and aeces (approximately 14%). Thirteen percent of the emtri-citabine dose was recovered in urine as three metabolites. he systemic clearance of emtricitabine averaged 307 ml/ min.

Following oral administration, the elimination half-life of enofovir is approximately 12 to 18 hours. Tenofovir is primarily excreted by the kidney by both filtration and an active tubular transport system with approximately 70 to 30% of the dose excreted unchanged in urine following ntravenous administration. The apparent clearance of enofovir averaged approximately 307 ml/min. Renal clear-ance has been estimated to be approximately 210 ml/min, which is in excess of the glomerular filtration rate. This indicates that active tubular secretion is an important part of the elimination of tenofovir.

Age, gender and ethnicity: the pharmacokinetics of emtri-citabine and tenofovir are similar in male and female patients. Although limited data suggest that females as well as Asian and Pacific Island patients may have higher exposure to efavirenz, they do not appear to be less tolerant of efavirenz.

Pharmacokinetic studies have not been performed with efavirenz, emtricitabine or tenofovir in the elderly (over 65 years).

Pharmacokinetic studies with Atripla have not been per-formed in infants and children (see section 4.2).

Renal impairment: the pharmacokinetics of efavirenz, emtricitabine and tenofovir disoproxil fumarate after co-administration of the separate pharmaceutical forms or as Atripla have not been studied in HIV infected patients with renal impairment.

Pharmacokinetic parameters were determined following administration of single doses of the individual prepara-tions of emtricitabine 200 mg or tenofovir disoproxil 245 mg to non-HIV infected patients with varying degrees of renal impairment. The degree of renal impairment was defined according to baseline creatinine clearance (normal renal function when creatinine clearance > 80 ml/min; mild impairment with creatinine clearance=50 to 79 ml/min; moderate impairment with creatinine clearance=30 to 49 ml/min and severe impairment with creatinine clear-ance=10 to 29 ml/min).

The mean (%CV) emtricitabine exposure increased from 12 μg•h/ml (25%) in subjects with normal renal function to 20 μg•h/ml (6%), 25 μg•h/ml (23%) and 34 μg•h/ml (6%) in patients with mild, moderate and severe renal impairment, respectively.

The mean (%CV) tenofovir exposure increased from 2,185 ng•h/ml (12%) in patients with normal renal function, to 3,064 ng•h/ml (30%), 6,009 ng•h/ml (42%) and 15,985 ng•h/ml (45%) in patients with mild, moderate and severe renal impairment, respectively.

In patients with end-stage renal disease (ESRD) requiring haemodialysis, between dialysis drug exposures substan-tially increased over 72 hours to 53 μg•h/ml (19%) of emtricitabine, and over 48 hours to 42,857 ng•h/ml (29%) of tenofovir.

The pharmacokinetics of efavirenz have not been studied in patients with renal impairment. However, less than 1% of an efavirenz dose is excreted unchanged in the urine, so the impact of renal impairment on exposure to efavirenz is likely to be minimal.

Atripla is not recommended for patients with moderate or severe renal impairment (creatinine clearance < 50 ml/ min). Patients with moderate or severe renal impairment require dose interval adjustment of emtricitabine and teno-fovir disoproxil fumarate that cannot be achieved with the combination tablet (see sections 4.2 and 4.4).

Hepatic impairment: the pharmacokinetics of Atripla have not been studied in HIV infected patients with hepatic impairment. Atripla should be administered with caution to patients with mild-to-moderate liver disease (see sec-tions 4.3 and 4.4).

Atripla must not be used in patients with severe hepatic impairment (see section 4.3).

In the single patient studied with severe hepatic impair-ment (CPT, Grade C), half-life of efavirenz was doubled indicating a potential for a much greater degree of accu-mulation.

The pharmacokinetics of emtricitabine have not been stu-died in non-HBV infected patients with varying degrees of hepatic insufficiency. In general, emtricitabine pharmaco-kinetics in HBV infected patients were similar to those in healthy subjects and in HIV infected patients.

A single 300 mg dose of tenofovir disoproxil fumarate was administered to non-HIV infected patients with varying degrees of hepatic impairment defined according to CPT classification. Tenofovir pharmacokinetics were not sub-stantially altered in subjects with hepatic impairment sug-gesting that no dose adjustment of tenofovir disoproxil fumarate is required in these subjects.

5.3 Preclinical safety data

Malformations were observed in 3 of 20 foetuses/new-borns from efavirenz-treated cynomolgus monkeys given doses resulting in plasma efavirenz concentrations similar to those seen in humans. Anencephaly and unilateral anophthalmia with secondary enlargement of the tongue were observed in one foetus, micro-ophthalmia was observed in another foetus, and cleft palate was observed in a third foetus. Efavirenz induced foetal resorptions in rats. No malformations were observed in foetuses from efavirenz-treated rats and rabbits.

Conventional reproductive/developmental toxicity studies with emtricitabine and tenofovir disoproxil fumarate revealed no special hazard for humans.

Carcinogenicity studies using efavirenz showed an increased incidence of hepatic and pulmonary tumours in female mice, but not in male mice. The mechanism of tumour formation and the potential relevance for humans are not known. Carcinogenicity studies using efavirenz in male mice and in male and female rats were negative. While the carcinogenic potential in humans is unknown, these data suggest that the clinical benefit of efavirenz outweighs the potential carcinogenic risk to humans.

Tenofovir disoproxil fumarate did not show any carcino-genic potential in a long-term oral carcinogenicity study in rats. A long-term oral carcinogenicity study in mice showed a low incidence of duodenal tumours, considered likely related to high local concentrations in the gastrointestinal tract at a dose of 600 mg/kg/day. While the mechanism of tumour formation is uncertain, the findings are unlikely to be of relevance to humans.

Emtricitabine did not show any carcinogenic potential in long-term studies in rats and mice.

Efavirenz and emtricitabine were negative in conventional genotoxic assays. Tenofovir disoproxil fumarate was posi-tive in two out of three *in vitro* genotoxicity studies but negative in the *in vivo* micronucleus assay. The combina-tion of emtricitabine and tenofovir disoproxil fumarate was positive in the *in vitro* mouse lymphoma assay, with com-parable results to those obtained for tenofovir disoproxil fumarate alone. The combination of emtricitabine and tenofovir disoproxil fumarate was negative in the bacterial reverse mutation assay (Ames assay).

Biliary hyperplasia was observed in cynomolgus monkeys given efavirenz for ⩾ 1 year at a dose resulting in mean AUC values approximately 2-fold greater than those in humans given the recommended dose. The biliary hyper-plasia regressed upon cessation of dosing. Biliary fibrosis has been observed in rats. Non-sustained convulsions were observed in some monkeys receiving efavirenz for ⩾ 1 year, at doses yielding plasma AUC values 4- to 13-fold greater than those in humans given the recommended dose (see sections 4.4 and 4.8).

Preclinical studies of tenofovir disoproxil fumarate con-ducted in rats, dogs and monkeys revealed effects on bone and a decrease in serum phosphate concentration. Bone toxicity was diagnosed as osteomalacia (monkeys) and reduced bone mineral density (rats and dogs). Findings in the rat and monkey studies indicated that there was a substance-related decrease in intestinal absorption of phosphate with potential secondary reduction in bone mineral density. The mechanisms of these toxicities are not completely understood.

A one month dog study using the combination of emtrici-tabine and tenofovir disoproxil fumarate found no exacer-bation of toxicological effects compared to the separate components.

6. PHARMACEUTICAL PARTICULARS

6.1 List of excipients

Tablet core:

Croscarmellose sodium

Hydroxypropylcellulose

Magnesium stearate

Microcrystalline cellulose

Sodium laurilsulfate

Film-coating:

Iron oxide black

Iron oxide red

Macrogol 3350

Poly(vinyl alcohol)

Talc

Titanium dioxide

6.2 Incompatibilities

Not applicable.

6.3 Shelf life

3 years.

6.4 Special precautions for storage

Store in the original package in order to protect from moisture. Keep the bottle tightly closed.

6.5 Nature and contents of container

High density polyethylene (HDPE) bottle with a polypropy-lene child-resistant closure containing 30 film-coated tablets and silica gel desiccant.

The following pack sizes are available: outer cartons con-taining 1 × 30 film-coated tablet and 3 × 30 film-coated tablet bottles. Not all pack sizes may be marketed.

6.6 Special precautions for disposal and other handling

Any unused product or waste material should be disposed of in accordance with local requirements.

7. MARKETING AUTHORISATION HOLDER

Bristol-Myers Squibb and Gilead Sciences Limited

Unit 13, Stillorgan Industrial Park

Blackrock

Co. Dublin

Ireland

8. MARKETING AUTHORISATION NUMBER(S)

EU/1/07/430/001

EU/1/07/430/002

9. DATE OF FIRST AUTHORISATION/RENEWAL OF THE AUTHORISATION

13 December 2007

10. DATE OF REVISION OF THE TEXT

03/2009

Detailed information on this medicinal product is available on the website of the European Medicines Agency (EMEA) http://www.emea.europa.eu/.

Atropine Injection BP Minijet

(International Medication Systems (UK) Ltd)

1. NAME OF THE MEDICINAL PRODUCT

Atropine Injection BP Minijet

2. QUALITATIVE AND QUANTITATIVE COMPOSITION

Atropine Sulphate 0.1 mg/ml

3. PHARMACEUTICAL FORM

Sterile aqueous solution for parenteral administration to humans.

4. CLINICAL PARTICULARS

4.1 Therapeutic indications

Acute myocardial infarction with AV conduction block due to excess vagal tone (Wenkebach Type I, second-degree AV block) and sinus bradycardia, with associated hypoten-sion and increased ventricular irritability.

Atropine can also be used in cardiopulmonary resuscita-tion for the treatment of sinus bradycardia accompanied by hypotension, hypoperfusion or ectopic arrhythmias.

Parenteral atropine is indicated as an antisialogogue in anaesthetic premedication to prevent or reduce secretions of the respiratory tract.

During anaesthesia, atropine may be used to prevent reflex bradycardia and restore cardiac rate and arterial pressure resulting from increased vagal activity associated with laryngoscopy, tracheal intubation and intra-abdominal manipulation. It may also be administered to block mus-carinic effects when neostigmine is used to counteract muscle relaxants such as tubocurarine.

Parenteral atropine is an antidote for cardiovascular col-lapse following overdose of anticholinesterases; in the treatment of poisoning from organophosphorous insecti-cides or from chemical warfare 'nerve' gases and in the treatment of mushroom poisoning.

4.2 Posology and method of administration
Adults, children over 12 and the elderly:

Bradyarrhythmias: intramuscular or intravenous, 300 to 600 mcg (0.3 to 0.6 mg) every four to six hours to a total dose of 2 mg.

In cardiac resuscitation, intravenous 500 mcg (0.5 mg) repeated at 5 minute intervals until the desired heart rate is achieved. In asystole, 3 mg may be given intravenously as a once only single dose. If atropine cannot be administered intravenously during resuscitation, 2-3 times the intravenous dose may be administered via an endotracheal tube.

Premedication before anaesthesia: intramuscular or subcutaneous, 300 to 600 mcg (0.3 to 0.6 mg) 30-60 minutes before surgery or the same dose intravenously immediately before surgery.

To control muscarinic side effects of neostigmine: intravenous, 600 to 1200 mcg (0.6 - 1.2 mg).

Anticholinesterase poisoning: intramuscular or intravenous, 1 to 2 mg repeated every 5 to 60 minutes until signs and symptoms disappear, up to a maximum of 100 mg in the first 24 hours.

Children up to the age of 12 years:

The usual intramuscular, intravenous or subcutaneous dose in children is 10 mcg/kg (0.01 mg/kg), but generally not exceeding 400 mcg (0.4 mg). If necessary, these doses may be repeated every 4-6 hours.

Cardiac: for advanced cardiac life support: intravenous, 20mcg/kg (0.02 mg/kg) with a minimum dose of 10 mcg (0.01 mg) repeated at 5 minute intervals, to a maximum dose of 100 mcg (0.1 mg).

Premedication before anaesthesia: intramuscular or subcutaneous; 30-60 minutes before surgery.

Up to 3 kg - 100 mcg (0.1mg)

7 - 9 kg - 200 mcg (0.2mg)

12 - 16 kg - 300 mcg (0.3mg)

Over 20 kg - as for adults.

To control the muscarinic side effects of neostigmine: intravenous; neonates, infants and children - 20 mcg/kg (0.02 mg/kg). Maximum dosage 600 mcg.

Anticholinesterase poisoning: intramuscular or intravenous, 50 mcg/kg (0.05 mg/kg) every 10-30 minutes until muscarinic signs and symptoms disappear.

4.3 Contraindications

Contra-indications are not applicable to the use of atropine in life-threatening emergencies (eg. asystole).

Atropine is contraindicated in patients with known hypersensitivity to the drug, obstruction of the bladder neck eg due to prostatic hypertrophy, reflux oesophagitis, closed angle glaucoma, myasthenia gravis (unless used to treat the adverse effects of an anticholinesterase agent), paralytic ileus, severe ulcerative colitis and obstructive disease of the gastrointestinal tract.

4.4 Special warnings and precautions for use

Antimuscarinic agents should be used with caution in the elderly and children since these patients may be more susceptible to adverse effects. Atropine should also be used with caution in patients with hyperthyroidism, hepatic or renal disease or hypertension. Use with caution in febrile patients or when ambient temperature is high since antimuscarinics may cause an increase in temperature. Antimuscarinics block vagal inhibition of the SA nodal pacemaker and should thus be used with caution in patients with tachyarrhythmias, congestive heart failure or coronary heart disease. Parenterally administered atropine should be used cautiously in patients with chronic pulmonary disease since a reduction in bronchial secretions may lead to formation of bronchial plugs. Antimuscarinics should be used with extreme caution in patients with autonomic neuropathy.

Antimuscarinics decrease gastric motility, relax the lower oesophageal sphincter and may delay gastric emptying; they should therefore be used with caution in patients with gastric ulcer, oesophageal reflux or hiatus hernia associated with reflux oesophagitis, diarrhoea or GI infection.

4.5 Interaction with other medicinal products and other forms of interaction

The effects of atropine may be enhanced by the concomitant administration of other drugs with anticholinergic activity eg. tricyclic antidepressants, antispasmodics, anti-parkinsonian drugs, some antihistamines, phenothiazines, disopyramide and quinidine. By delaying gastric emptying, atropine may alter the absorption of other drugs.

4.6 Pregnancy and lactation

Atropine crosses the placenta. Studies in humans have not been done and only limited information is available from animal studies. Intravenous administration of atropine during pregnancy or at term may cause tachycardia in the foetus. Atropine should only be administered to pregnant women if the benefits outweigh the risks to the foetus. Trace amounts of atropine appear in the breast milk and may cause antimuscarinic effects in the infant; lactation may be inhibited.

4.7 Effects on ability to drive and use machines

Not applicable; this preparation is intended for use only in emergencies.

4.8 Undesirable effects

Adverse effects are dose-related and usually reversible when therapy is discontinued. In relatively small doses, atropine reduces salivary, bronchial and sweat secretions; dry mouth and anhidrosis may develop, these effects being intensified as the dosage is increased. Reduced bronchial secretion may cause dehydration of residual secretion and consequent formation of thick bronchial plugs that are difficult to eject from the respiratory tract.

Larger doses dilate the pupil and inhibit accommodation of the eye, and block vagal impulses with consequent increase in heart rate with possible atrial arrhythmias, A-V dissociation and multiple ventricular ectopics; parasympathetic control of the urinary bladder and gastrointestinal tract is inhibited, causing urinary retention and constipation. Further increase in dosage inhibits gastric secretion. Anaphylaxis, urticaria and rash occasionally progressing to exfoliation may develop in some patients. Other effects include hallucinations, increased ocular tension, loss of taste, headache, nervousness, drowsiness, weakness, dizziness, flushing, insomnia, nausea, vomiting and bloated feeling. Mental confusion and/or excitement may occur especially in the elderly.

4.9 Overdose

Symptoms: marked dryness of the mouth accompanied by a burning sensation, difficulty in swallowing, pronounced photophobia, flushing and dryness of the skin, raised body temperature, rash, nausea, vomiting, tachycardia and hypertension. Restlessness, tremor, confusion, excitement, hallucinations and delirium may result from CNS stimulation; this is followed by increasing drowsiness, stupor and general central depression terminating in death from circulatory and respiratory failure.

Treatment: In severe cases, physostigmine, 1 to 4 mg, should be administered intravenously, intramuscularly or subcutaneously, the dose may be repeated if necessary since it is rapidly eliminated from the body. Diazepam may be administered for sedation of the delirious patient but the risk of central depression occurring late in the course of atropine poisoning contraindicates large doses of sedative. An adequate airway should be maintained and respiratory failure may be treated with oxygen and carbon dioxide inhalation. Fever is reduced by the application of cold packs or sponging with tepid water. Adequate fluid intake is important. Urethral catheterisation may be necessary. If photophobia is present or likely, the patient should be nursed in a darkened room.

5. PHARMACOLOGICAL PROPERTIES

5.1 Pharmacodynamic properties

Atropine is an antimuscarinic agent which competitively antagonizes acetylcholine at postganglionic nerve endings, thus affecting receptors of the exocrine glands, smooth muscle, cardiac muscle and the central nervous system.

Peripheral effects include tachycardia, decreased production of saliva, sweat, bronchial, nasal, lachrymal and gastric secretions, decreased intestinal motility and inhibition of micturition.

Atropine increases sinus rate and sinoatrial and AV conduction. Usually heart rate is increased but there may be an initial bradycardia.

Atropine inhibits secretions throughout the respiratory tract and relaxes bronchial smooth muscle producing bronchodilatation.

5.2 Pharmacokinetic properties

Following intravenous administration, the peak increase in heart rate occurs within 2 to 4 minutes. Peak plasma concentrations of atropine after intramuscular administration are reached within 30 minutes, although peak effects on the heart, sweating and salivation may occur nearer one hour after intramuscular administration.

Plasma levels after intramuscular and intravenous injection are comparable at one hour. Atropine is distributed widely throughout the body and crosses the blood brain barrier. The elimination half life is about 2 to 5 hours. Up to 50% of the dose is protein bound. It disappears rapidly from the circulation.

Atropine is metabolised in the liver by oxidation and conjugation to give inactive metabolites.

About 50% of the dose is excreted within 4 hours and 90% in 24 hours in the urine, about 30 to 50% as unchanged drug.

5.3 Preclinical safety data

Not applicable since atropine has been used in clinical practice for many years and its effects in man are well known.

6. PHARMACEUTICAL PARTICULARS

6.1 List of excipients

Sodium Citrate Dihydrate USP

Citric Acid Monohydrate USP

Sodium Chloride USP

Water for Injection USP

6.2 Incompatibilities

None known.

6.3 Shelf life

36 months

6.4 Special precautions for storage

Store below 25°C. Protect from light.

6.5 Nature and contents of container

The solution is contained in a USP type I glass vial with a elastomeric closure which meets all the relevant US specifications. The product is available either as 5, 10 or 30ml.

6.6 Special precautions for disposal and other handling

The container is specially designed for use with the IMS Minijet injector.

7. MARKETING AUTHORISATION HOLDER

International Medication Systems (UK) Ltd

208 Bath Road

Slough

Berkshire

SL1 3WE

UK

8. MARKETING AUTHORISATION NUMBER(S)

PL 03265/0013R

9. DATE OF FIRST AUTHORISATION/RENEWAL OF THE AUTHORISATION

Date first granted: 20.03.91

Date renewed: 17 March 1997/16 March 2002

10. DATE OF REVISION OF THE TEXT

August 2005

11. LEGAL CATEGORY

POM

Atrovent Inhaler CFC-Free

(Boehringer Ingelheim Limited)

1. NAME OF THE MEDICINAL PRODUCT

ATROVENT Inhaler ▼ CFC-Free 20 micrograms/actuation pressurised inhalation solution.

2. QUALITATIVE AND QUANTITATIVE COMPOSITION

One metered dose (ex-valve) contains 20 micrograms ipratropium bromide (as the monohydrate).

For excipients, see 6.1.

3. PHARMACEUTICAL FORM

Pressurised inhalation, solution.

Each container is filled with 10 ml of a clear, colourless liquid, free from suspended particles.

ATROVENT Inhaler CFC-Free contains a new propellant, HFA-134a, and does not contain any chlorofluorocarbons (CFCs).

4. CLINICAL PARTICULARS

4.1 Therapeutic indications

ATROVENT Inhaler CFC-Free is indicated for the regular treatment of reversible bronchospasm associated with chronic obstructive pulmonary disease (COPD) and chronic asthma.

4.2 Posology and method of administration

For inhalation use.

Adults (including the elderly):

Usually 1 or 2 puffs three or four times daily, although some patients may need up to 4 puffs at a time to obtain maximum benefit during early treatment.

Children:

6-12 years: Usually 1 or 2 puffs three times daily.

Under 6 years: Usually 1 puff three times daily.

In order to ensure that the inhaler is used correctly, administration should be supervised by an adult.

The recommended dose should not be exceeded.

If therapy does not produce a significant improvement, if the patient's condition gets worse or if a reduced response to treatment becomes apparent, medical advice must be sought. In the case of acute or rapidly worsening dyspnoea (difficulty in breathing) a doctor should be consulted immediately.

Administration

The correct administration of ipratropium bromide from the inhaler is essential for successful therapy. For detailed information on instructions for use please refer to the Patient Information Leaflet.

The canister should be pressed twice to release two metered doses into the air before the inhaler is used for the first time, or when the inhaler has not been used for 3 days or more, to ensure that the inhaler is working properly and that it is ready for use.

Before each occasion on which the inhaler is used the following should be observed:

1. Remove protective cap.

2. Hold the inhaler upright (the arrow on the base of the container should be pointing upwards), breathe out gently and then close the lips over the mouthpiece

3. Breathe in slowly and deeply, pressing the base of the canister firmly at the same time; this releases one metered dose. Hold the breath for 10 seconds or as long as is

omfortable, then remove the mouthpiece from the mouth nd breathe out slowly.

. If a second inhalation is required you should wait at least ne minute and then repeat Points 2 and 3 above.

. Replace the protective cap after use.

he inhaler can be used with the Aerochamber Plus^{TM} pacer device. This may be useful for patients, e.g. chilren, who find it difficult to synchronise breathing in and haler actuation.

he canister is not transparent. It is therefore not possible o see when it is empty. The inhaler will deliver 200 actuaons. When these have all been used (usually after 3 – 4 veeks of regular use) the inhaler may still appear to contain small amount of fluid. However the inhaler should be eplaced in order to ensure that each metered dose conains the correct amount of medicine.

VARNING:

he plastic mouthpiece has been specially designed for se with ATROVENT Inhaler CFC-Free to ensure that each netered dose contains the correct amount of medicine. he mouthpiece must never be used with any other netered dose inhaler nor must ATROVENT Inhaler CFC-ree be used with any mouthpiece other than the one supplied with the product.

The mouthpiece should always be kept clean. To clean the nouthpiece, the canister and dustcap must be removed. The mouthpiece should then be washed in warm soapy water, rinsed and dried. Care should be taken to ensure that the small hole in the mouthpiece is flushed through thoroughly. The canister and dustcap should be replaced once the mouthpiece is dry.

4.3 Contraindications

ATROVENT Inhaler CFC-Free should not be taken by patients with known hypersensitivity to atropine or its derivatives, or to ipratropium bromide or to any other component of the product.

4.4 Special warnings and precautions for use

When using ATROVENT Inhaler CFC-Free for the first time, some patients may notice that the taste is slightly different from that of the CFC-containing formulation. Patients should be made aware of this when changing from one formulation to the other. They should also be told that the formulations have been shown to be interchangeable for all practical purposes and that the difference in taste has no consequences in terms of the safety or the efficacy of the new formulation.

Caution is advocated in the use of anticholinergic agents in patients predisposed to or with narrow-angle glaucoma, or with prostatic hyperplasia or bladder-outflow obstruction.

As patients with cystic fibrosis may be prone to gastro-intestinal motility disturbances, ipratropium bromide, as with other anticholinergics, should be used with caution in these patients.

Hypersensitivity reactions following the use of ipratropium bromide have been seen and have presented as urticaria, angioedema, rash, bronchospasm, oropharyngeal oedema and anaphylaxis.

There have been isolated reports of ocular complications (i.e. mydriasis, increased intraocular pressure, narrow-angle glaucoma, eye pain) when aerosolised ipratropium bromide, either alone or in combination with an adrenergic beta$_2$-agonist, has come into contact with the eyes. Thus patients must be instructed in the correct administration of ATROVENT Inhaler CFC-Free and warned against the accidental release of the contents into the eye. Antiglaucoma therapy is effective in the prevention of acute narrow-angle glaucoma in susceptible individuals and patients who may be susceptible to glaucoma should be warned specifically on the need for ocular protection.

Eye pain or discomfort, blurred vision, visual halos or coloured images in association with red eyes from conjunctival congestion and corneal oedema may be signs of acute narrow-angle glaucoma. Should any combination of these symptoms develop, treatment with miotic drops should be initiated and specialist advice sought immediately.

Patients should be informed when starting treatment that the onset of action of ipratropium bromide is slower than that of inhaled sympathomimetic bronchodilators.

4.5 Interaction with other medicinal products and other forms of interaction

There is evidence that the administration of ipratropium bromide with beta-adrenergic drugs and xanthine preparations may produce an additive bronchodilatory effect.

4.6 Pregnancy and lactation

There is no experience of the use of this product in pregnancy and lactation in humans. It should not be used in pregnancy or lactation unless the expected benefits to the mother are thought to outweigh any potential risks to the fetus or neonate.

The safety of ipratropium bromide during human pregnancy has not been established. The benefits of using ipratropium bromide during a confirmed or suspected pregnancy must be weighed against the possible hazards to the unborn child. Preclinical studies have shown no embryotoxic or teratogenic effects following inhalation or intranasal application at doses considerably higher than those recommended in man.

It is not known whether ipratropium bromide is excreted into breast milk. It is unlikely that ipratropium bromide would reach the infant to an important extent, however caution should be exercised when ipratropium bromide is administered to nursing mothers.

Studies of HFA-134a administered to pregnant and lactating rats and rabbits have not revealed any special hazard.

4.7 Effects on ability to drive and use machines

On the basis of the pharmacodynamic profile and reported adverse drug reactions it is not likely that ipratropium bromide has an effect on ability to drive and use machines.

4.8 Undesirable effects

The following side effects have been reported. The frequencies given below are based on clinical trials involving 3250 patients who have been treated with ATROVENT (ipratropium bromide).

Frequencies

Very common: ⩾ 1/10

Common: ⩾ 1/100 < 1/10

Uncommon: ⩾ 1/1,000 < 1/100

Rare: ⩾ 1/10,000 < 1/1,000

Very rare: < 1/10,000

Immune system disorders

Urticaria (1): Uncommon

Anaphylactic reaction: Rare

Angio-oedema of tongue, lips, face: Rare

Nervous system disorders

Headache: Common

Dizziness: Common

Eye disorders

Ocular accommodation disturbances: Uncommon

Angle closure glaucoma(2): Uncommon

Intraocular pressure increased (2): Rare

Eye pain (2): Rare

Mydriasis(2): Rare

Cardiac Disorders

Tachycardia: Uncommon

Palpitations: Rare

Supraventricular tachycardia: Rare

Atrial fibrillation: Rare

Respiratory, Thoracic and Mediastinal Disorders

Cough: Common

Local irritation: Common

Inhalation induced bronchoconstriction(3): Common

Laryngospasm: Rare

Gastro-intestinal Disorders

Dryness of mouth: Common

Vomiting: Common

Gastro-intestinal motility disorder (4): Common

Nausea: Rare

Skin and Subcutaneous Disorders

Skin rash: Uncommon

Pruritus: Uncommon

Renal and Urinary Disorders

Urinary retention (5): Rare

When using ATROVENT Inhaler CFC-Free for the first time some patients may notice that the taste is slightly different from that of the CFC-containing formulation. Some patients have described the taste as unpleasant.

(1) including giant urticaria

(2) ocular complications have been reported when aerosolised ipratropium bromide, either alone or in combination with an adrenergic beta$_2$-agonist, has come into contact with the eyes – see section 4.4.

(3) as with other inhalation therapy, inhalation induced bronchoconstriction may occur with an immediate increase in wheezing after dosing. This should be treated straight away with a fast acting inhaled bronchodilator. ATROVENT Inhaler CFC-Free should be discontinued immediately, the patient assessed and, if necessary, alternative treatment instituted.

(4) e.g. constipation, diarrhoea

(5) the risk of urinary retention may be increased in patients with pre-existing urinary outflow tract obstruction.

4.9 Overdose

No symptoms specific to overdosage have been encountered. In view of the wide therapeutic window and topical administration of ipratropium bromide, no serious anticholinergic symptoms are to be expected. As with other anticholinergics, dry mouth, visual accommodation disturbances and tachycardia would be the expected symptoms and signs of overdose.

5. PHARMACOLOGICAL PROPERTIES

5.1 Pharmacodynamic properties

ATC Code: R03B B01

Trials with a treatment duration of up to three months involving adult asthmatics and COPD patients, and asthmatic children, in which the HFA formulation and the CFC formulation have been compared have shown the two formulations to be therapeutically equivalent.

Ipratropium bromide is a quaternary ammonium compound with anticholinergic (parasympatholytic) properties. In preclinical studies, it appears to inhibit vagally mediated reflexes by antagonising the action of acetylcholine, the transmitter agent released from the vagus nerve. Anticholinergics prevent the increase in intracellular concentration of cyclic guanosine monophosphate (cyclic GMP) caused by interaction of acetylcholine with the muscarinic receptor on bronchial smooth muscle.

The bronchodilation following inhalation of ipratropium bromide is induced by local drug concentrations sufficient for anticholinergic efficacy at the bronchial smooth muscle and not by systemic drug concentrations.

In clinical trials using metered dose inhalers in patients with reversible bronchospasm associated with asthma or chronic obstructive pulmonary disease significant improvements in pulmonary function (FEV_1 increases of 15% or more) occurred within 15 minutes, reached a peak in 1-2 hours, and persisted for approximately 4 hours.

Preclinical and clinical evidence suggest no deleterious effect of ipratropium bromide on airway mucous secretion, mucociliary clearance or gas exchange.

5.2 Pharmacokinetic properties

The therapeutic effect of ipratropium bromide is produced by a local action in the airways. Therefore time courses of bronchodilation and systemic pharmacokinetics do not run in parallel.

Following inhalation, dose portions from 10 to 30%, depending on the formulation, device and inhalation technique, are generally deposited in the lungs. The major part of the dose is swallowed and passes through the gastro-intestinal tract.

Due to the negligible gastrointestinal absorption of ipratropium bromide the bioavailability of the swallowed dose portion is only approximately 2%. This fraction of the dose does not make a relevant contribution to the plasma concentrations of the active ingredient. The portion of the dose deposited in the lungs reaches the circulation rapidly (within minutes).

Limited data on total systemic bioavailability (pulmonary and gastrointestinal portions), based on renal excretion (0 – 24 hours) of ipratropium bromide, suggests a range of 7 to 28% when delivery is via a nebuliser or a MDI product. It is assumed that this is also a valid range for inhalation from the powder preparation. This is also a valid range for inhalation from the metered aerosol with HFA 134a propellant because the kinetic results (renal excretion, AUC and Cmax) from the HFA formulation and the conventional CFC formulation are closely comparable.

Kinetic parameters describing the distribution of ipratropium bromide were calculated from plasma concentrations after i.v. administration.

A rapid biphasic decline in plasma concentrations is observed. The volume of distribution (V_β) is 338 L (≙ 4.6 L/kg). The drug is minimally (less then 20%) bound to plasma proteins. The ipratropium ion does not cross the blood-brain barrier, consistent with the ammonium structure of the molecule.

The half-life of the terminal elimination phase is about 1.6 hours.

The mean total clearance of the drug is determined to be 2.3 L/min. The major portion of approximately 60% of the systemic available dose is eliminated by metabolic degradation, probably in the liver. The main urinary metabolites bind poorly to the muscarinic receptor and have to be regarded as ineffective.

A portion of approximately 40% of the systemic available dose is cleared via urinary excretion corresponding to an experimental renal clearance of 0.9 L/min. A study with radiolabelled material showed that approximately 10% of orally administered ipratropium bromide was absorbed from the gastrointestinal tract and metabolised. Less than 1% of an oral dose is renally excreted as parent compound.

In excretion balance studies after intravenous administration of a radioactive dose, less than 10% of the drug-related radioactivity (including parent compound and all metabolites) is excreted via the biliary-faecal route. The dominant excretion of drug-related radioactivity occurs via the kidneys.

5.3 Preclinical safety data

Preclinical data reveal no special hazard for humans based on conventional studies of safety pharmacology, repeated dose toxicity, genotoxicity, carcinogenic potential and toxicity to reproduction.

6. PHARMACEUTICAL PARTICULARS

6.1 List of excipients

1,1,1,2 – Tetrafluoroethane (HFA-134a)

Ethanol anhydrous

Purified water

Citric acid anhydrous.

6.2 Incompatibilities

Not applicable.

6.3 Shelf life

36 months.

6.4 Special precautions for storage

Do not store above 25°C. Protect from direct sunlight, heat and frost.

The canister contains a pressurised liquid. Do not expose to temperatures higher than 50°C. Do not pierce the canister.

6.5 Nature and contents of container

17 ml stainless steel pressurised container with a 50 µl metering valve and oral adaptor. Each canister contains 200 actuations.

6.6 Special precautions for disposal and other handling

None.

7. MARKETING AUTHORISATION HOLDER

Boehringer Ingelheim Limited
Ellesfield Avenue
Bracknell
Berkshire
RG12 8YS
United Kingdom

8. MARKETING AUTHORISATION NUMBER(S)

PL 00015/0266

9. DATE OF FIRST AUTHORISATION/RENEWAL OF THE AUTHORISATION

1 March 2004

10. DATE OF REVISION OF THE TEXT

September 2006

11. LEGAL CATEGORY

POM

A9e/UK/SPC/4

Atrovent UDVs

(Boehringer Ingelheim Limited)

1. NAME OF THE MEDICINAL PRODUCT

Atrovent® 250 UDVs®, 1 ml

Atrovent® UDVs®, 2 ml

2. QUALITATIVE AND QUANTITATIVE COMPOSITION

Each single dose unit contains 0.025 % w/v ipratropium bromide i.e. 250 micrograms in 1 ml and 500 micrograms in 2 ml.

For excipients, see 6.1.

3. PHARMACEUTICAL FORM

Nebuliser solution.

4. CLINICAL PARTICULARS

4.1 Therapeutic indications

ATROVENT UDVs are indicated for treatment of reversible bronchospasm associated with chronic obstructive pulmonary disease (COPD).

ATROVENT UDVs are indicated, when used concomitantly with inhaled beta$_2$-agonists, for treatment of reversible airways obstruction as in acute and chronic asthma.

4.2 Posology and method of administration

The dosage should be adapted to the individual needs of the patient. In children aged 12 years and under, only ATROVENT 250 UDVs, 1 ml should be used. The following doses are recommended:

Adults (including the elderly) and children over 12 years of age:

250 - 500 micrograms (i.e. one vial of 250 micrograms in 1 ml or 1 vial of 500 micrograms in 2 ml) 3 to 4 times daily.

For treatment of acute bronchospasm, 500 micrograms.

Repeated doses can be administered until the patient is stable. The time interval between the doses may be determined by the physician.

It is advisable not to exceed the recommended daily dose during either acute or maintenance treatment. Daily doses exceeding 2 mg in adults and children over 12 years of age should only be given under medical supervision.

Children 6 - 12 years of age:

250 micrograms (i.e. one vial of 250 micrograms in 1ml) up to a total daily dose of 1mg (4 vials).

The time interval between doses may be determined by the physician.

Children 0 – 5 years of age (for treatment of acute asthma only):

125 – 250 micrograms (i.e. half to one vial of 250 micrograms in 1 ml) up to a total daily dose of 1 mg (4 vials).

Ipratropium bromide should be administered no more frequently than 6 hourly in children under 5 years of age.

For acute bronchospasm, repeated doses may be administered until the patient is stable.

If therapy does not produce a significant improvement or if the patient's condition gets worse, medical advice must be sought. In the case of acute or rapidly worsening dyspnoea (difficulty in breathing) a doctor should be consulted immediately.

ATROVENT UDVs may be combined with a short-acting beta$_2$-agonist in the same nebuliser chamber, for simultaneous administration where co-administration is required. The solution should be used as soon as possible after mixing and any unused solution should be discarded.

ATROVENT UDVs can be administered using a range of commercially available nebulising devices. The dose of nebuliser solution may need to be diluted in order to obtain a final volume suitable for the particular nebuliser being used (usually 2 – 4 ml); if dilution is necessary use only sterile sodium chloride 0.9% solution.

ATROVENT UDVs and disodium cromoglycate inhalation solutions that contain the preservative benzalkonium chloride should not be administered simultaneously in the same nebuliser as precipitation may occur.

The unit dose vials are intended only for inhalation with suitable nebulising devices and should not be taken orally or administered parenterally.

Please refer to the patient information leaflet for instructions on use with a nebuliser.

4.3 Contraindications

Known hypersensitivity to atropine or its derivatives, or to any other component of the product.

4.4 Special warnings and precautions for use

Use of the nebuliser solution should be subject to close medical supervision during initial dosing.

Caution is advocated in the use of anticholinergic agents in patients predisposed to or with narrow-angle glaucoma, or with prostatic hyperplasia or bladder-outflow obstruction.

As patients with cystic fibrosis may be prone to gastro-intestinal motility disturbances, ATROVENT, as with other anticholinergics, should be used with caution in these patients.

Immediate hypersensitivity reactions following the use of ATROVENT have been demonstrated by rare cases of urticaria, angioedema, rash, bronchospasm, oropharyngeal oedema and anaphylaxis.

There have been isolated reports of ocular complications (i.e. mydriasis, increased intra-ocular pressure, narrow-angle glaucoma, eye pain) when aerosolised ipratropium bromide, either alone or in combination with an adrenergic beta$_2$-agonist, has come into contact with the eyes during nebuliser therapy.

Eye pain or discomfort, blurred vision, visual halos or coloured images in association with red eyes from conjunctival congestion and corneal oedema may be signs of acute narrow-angle glaucoma. Should any combination of these symptoms develop, treatment with miotic drops should be initiated and specialist advice sought immediately.

Patients must be instructed in the correct administration of ATROVENT UDVs. Care must be taken not to allow the solution or mist to enter the eyes. It is recommended that the nebulised solution is administered via a mouthpiece. If this is not available and a nebuliser mask is used, it must fit properly. Patients who may be predisposed to glaucoma should be warned specifically to protect their eyes.

4.5 Interaction with other medicinal products and other forms of interaction

There is evidence that the administration of ATROVENT with beta-adrenergic drugs and xanthine preparations may produce an additive bronchodilatory effect.

The risk of acute glaucoma in patients with a history of narrow-angle glaucoma (see Special Warnings and Precautions for Use) may be increased when nebulised ipratropium bromide and beta$_2$-agonists are administered simultaneously.

4.6 Pregnancy and lactation

The safety of ATROVENT during human pregnancy has not been established. The benefits of using ATROVENT during a confirmed or suspected pregnancy must be weighed against the possible hazards to the unborn child. Preclinical studies have shown no embryotoxic or teratogenic effects following inhalation or intranasal application at doses considerably higher than those recommended in man.

It is not known whether ipratropium bromide is excreted into breast milk. It is unlikely that ipratropium bromide would reach the infant to an important extent, however caution should be exercised when ATROVENT is administered to nursing mothers.

4.7 Effects on ability to drive and use machines

None stated.

4.8 Undesirable effects

The following side effects have been reported. The frequencies given below are based on clinical trials involving 3250 patients who have been treated with ATROVENT (ipratropium bromide).

Frequencies

Very common	≥ 1/10
Common	≥ 1/100 < 1/10
Uncommon	≥ 1/1,000 < 1/100
Rare	≥ 1/10,000 < 1/1,000
Very rare	< 1/10,000

Immune system disorders	
Urticaria[1]	Uncommon
Anaphylactic reaction	Rare
Angio-oedema of tongue, lips, face	Rare
Nervous system disorders	
Headache	Common
Dizziness	Common
Eye disorders	
Ocular accommodation disturbances	Uncommon
Angle closure glaucoma[2]	Uncommon
Intraocular pressure increased [2]	Rare
Eye pain[2]	Rare
Mydriasis[2]	Rare
Cardiac Disorders	
Tachycardia	Uncommon
Palpitations	Rare
Supraventricular tachycardia	Rare
Atrial fibrillation	Rare
Respiratory, Thoracic and Mediastinal Disorders	
Cough	Common
Local irritation	Common
Inhalation induced bronchospasm	Common
Laryngospasm	Rare
Gastro-intestinal Disorders	
Dryness of mouth	Common
Vomiting	Common
Gastro-intestinal motility disorder [3]	Common
Nausea	Rare
Skin and Subcutaneous Disorders	
Skin rash	Uncommon
Pruritus	Uncommon
Renal and Urinary Disorders	
Urinary retention [4]	Rare

[1] including giant urticaria

[2] ocular complications have been reported when aerolised ipratropium bromide, either alone or in combination with an adrenergic beta$_2$-agonist, has come into contact with the eyes during nebuliser therapy– see section 4.4.

[3] e.g. constipation, diarrhoea

[4] the risk of urinary retention may be increased in patients with pre-existing urinary outflow tract obstruction.

4.9 Overdose

No symptoms specific to overdosage have been encountered. In view of the wide therapeutic window and topical administration of ATROVENT, no serious anticholinergic symptoms are to be expected. As with other anticholinergics, dry mouth, visual accommodation disturbances and tachycardia would be the expected symptoms and signs of overdose.

5. PHARMACOLOGICAL PROPERTIES

5.1 Pharmacodynamic properties

ATROVENT is a quaternary ammonium compound with anticholinergic (parasympatholytic) properties. In preclinical studies, it appears to inhibit vagally mediated reflexes by antagonising the action of acetylcholine, the transmitter agent released from the vagus nerve. Anticholinergics prevent the increase in intracellular concentration of cyclic guanosine monophosphate (cyclic GMP) caused by interaction of acetylcholine with the muscarinic receptor on bronchial smooth muscle.

The bronchodilation following inhalation of ATROVENT is induced by local drug concentrations sufficient for anticholinergic efficacy at the bronchial smooth muscle and not by systemic drug concentrations.

In clinical trials using metered dose inhalers in patients with reversible bronchospasm associated with chronic obstructive pulmonary disease significant improvements in pulmonary function (FEV$_1$ increases of 15% or more) occurred within 15 minutes, reached a peak in 1-2 hours, and persisted for approximately 4 hours.

Preclinical and clinical evidence suggest no deleterious effect of ATROVENT on airway mucous secretion, mucociliary clearance or gas exchange.

The bronchodilator effect of ATROVENT in the treatment of acute bronchospasm associated with asthma has been shown in studies in adults and children over 6 years of age. In most of these studies ATROVENT was administered in combination with an inhaled beta$_2$-agonist.

5.2 Pharmacokinetic properties

The therapeutic effect of ATROVENT is produced by a local action in the airways. Therefore time courses of bronchodilation and systemic pharmacokinetics do not run in parallel.

Following inhalation, dose portions from 10 to 30%, depending on the formulation, device and inhalation technique, are generally deposited in the lungs. The major part of the dose is swallowed and passes through the gastro-intestinal tract.

Due to the negligible gastro-intestinal absorption of ipratropium bromide the bioavailability of the swallowed dose portion is only approximately 2%. This fraction of the dose does not make a relevant contribution to the plasma oncentrations of the active ingredient. The portion of the ose deposited in the lungs reaches the circulation rapidly within minutes).

imited data on total systemic bioavailability (pulmonary nd gastro-intestinal portions), based on renal excretion) – 24 hours) of ipratropium bromide, suggests a range of 7 28% when delivery is via a nebuliser or a MDI product. It is ssumed that this is also a valid range for inhalation from ne powder preparation.

Kinetic parameters describing the distribution of ipratro- ium bromide were calculated from plasma concentrations fter i.v. administration.

A rapid biphasic decline in plasma concentrations is observed. The volume of distribution (V_β) is 338 L (≙ 4.6 L/kg). The drug is minimally (less then 20%) bound to plasma proteins. The ipratropium ion does not cross the blood-brain barrier, consistent with the ammonium structure of the molecule.

The half-life of the terminal elimination phase is about 1.6 hours.

The mean total clearance of the drug is determined to be 2.3 L/min. The major portion of approximately 60% of the systemic available dose is eliminated by metabolic degradation, probably in the liver. The main urinary metabolites bind poorly to the muscarinic receptor and have to be regarded as ineffective.

A portion of approximately 40% of the systemic available dose is cleared via urinary excretion corresponding to an experimental renal clearance of 0.9 L/min. A study with radiolabelled material showed that approximately 10% of orally administered ipratropium bromide was absorbed from the gastro-intestinal tract and metabolised. Less than 1% of an oral dose is renally excreted as parent compound.

In excretion balance studies after intravenous administration of a radioactive dose, less than 10% of the drug-related radioactivity (including parent compound and all metabolites) is excreted via the biliary-faecal route. The dominant excretion of drug-related radioactivity occurs via the kidneys.

5.3 Preclinical safety data

There are no pre-clinical data of relevance to the prescriber which are additional to that already included in other sections of the SPC.

6. PHARMACEUTICAL PARTICULARS

6.1 List of excipients

Sodium Chloride

1N Hydrochloric Acid

Purified Water

6.2 Incompatibilities

Not applicable.

6.3 Shelf life

24 months (unopened).

As the product contains no preservative, a fresh vial should be used for each dose and the vial should be opened immediately before administration. Any solution left in the vial should be discarded.

6.4 Special precautions for storage

Do not store above 25°C. Keep vials in the outer carton.

6.5 Nature and contents of container

Polyethylene unit dose vials containing either 1 ml or 2 ml of solution

Pack sizes of 10, 20, 30, 50, 60, 80, 100, 120, 150, 200, 300, 500 and 1000.

Not all pack sizes may be marketed

6.6 Special precautions for disposal and other handling

None.

7. MARKETING AUTHORISATION HOLDER

Boehringer Ingelheim Limited

Ellesfield Avenue

Bracknell

Berkshire

RG12 8YS

8. MARKETING AUTHORISATION NUMBER(S)

PL 0015/0108

9. DATE OF FIRST AUTHORISATION/RENEWAL OF THE AUTHORISATION

27 August 1986 / 23 December 2005

10. DATE OF REVISION OF THE TEXT

June 2009

11. Legal Category

Prescription Only Medicine

Augmentin 125/31 SF Suspension

(GlaxoSmithKline UK)

1. NAME OF THE MEDICINAL PRODUCT

Augmentin® 125/31 SF Suspension

2. QUALITATIVE AND QUANTITATIVE COMPOSITION

Augmentin 125/31 SF Suspension: When reconstituted each 5 ml contains co-amoxiclav 125/31.

The amoxicillin is present as amoxicillin trihydrate and the clavulanic acid is present as potassium clavulanate.

3. PHARMACEUTICAL FORM

Augmentin 125/31 SF Suspension: Dry powder for reconstitution in water, at time of dispensing, to form an oral sugar-free suspension.

4. CLINICAL PARTICULARS

4.1 Therapeutic indications

Augmentin is an antibiotic agent with a notably broad spectrum of activity against the commonly occurring bacterial pathogens in general practice and hospital. The β-lactamase inhibitory action of clavulanate extends the spectrum of amoxicillin to embrace a wider range of organisms, including many resistant to other β-lactam antibiotics.

Augmentin oral preparations are indicated for short term treatment of bacterial infections at the following sites when amoxicillin resistant beta-lactamase producing strains are suspected as the cause. In other situations, amoxicillin alone should be considered.

- *Upper Respiratory Tract Infections (including ENT)* in particular sinusitis, otitis media, recurrent tonsillitis. These infections are often caused by *Streptococcus pneumoniae, Haemophilus influenzae**, *Moraxella catarrhalis** and *Streptococcus pyogenes*.

- *Lower Respiratory Tract Infections* in particular acute exacerbations of chronic bronchitis (especially if considered severe), bronchopneumonia. These infections are often caused by *Streptococcus pneumoniae, Haemophilus influenzae** and *Moraxella catarrhalis**.

- *Genito-urinary Tract and Abdominal Infections* in particular cystitis (especially when recurrent or complicated - excluding prostatitis), septic abortion, pelvic or puerperal sepsis and intra-abdominal sepsis. These infections are often caused by *Enterobacteriaceae** (mainly *Escherichia coli**), *Staphylococcus saprophyticus, Enterococcus* species.*

- *Skin and Soft Tissue Infections* in particular cellulitis, animal bites and severe dental abscess with spreading cellulitis. These infections are often caused by *Staphylococcus aureus**, *Streptococcus pyogenes* and *Bacteroides species**.

- A comprehensive list of sensitive organisms is provided in Section 5.

* Some members of these species of bacteria produce beta-lactamase, rendering them insensitive to amoxicillin alone.

Mixed infections caused by amoxicillin-susceptible organisms in conjunction with Augmentin-susceptible beta-lactamase-producing organisms may be treated with Augmentin. These infections should not require the addition of another antibiotic resistant to beta-lactamases.

4.2 Posology and method of administration

Usual dosages for the treatment of infection

Adults and children over 12 years of age:	This formulation is not applicable to this age group
Children under 12 years of age:	The usual recommended daily dosage is 25 mg/kg/day* in divided doses every eight hours. The table below presents guidance for children.

Augmentin Suspension	
Under 1 year	25 mg/kg/day*, for example a 7.5 kg child would require 2 ml Augmentin 125/31 SF Suspension t.d.s.
1- 6 years (10-18 kg)	5ml Augmentin 125/31 SF Suspension t.d.s.
Over 6 years (18-40 kg)	5ml Augmentin 250/62 SF Suspension t.d.s.

In more serious infections the dosage may be increased up to 50 mg/kg/day in divided doses every eight hours.

* Each 25 mg Augmentin provides co-amoxiclav 20/5.

Dosage in renal impairment

Mild impairment (creatinine clearance >30 ml/min): no change in dosage.

Moderate to severe impairment (creatinine clearance <30 ml/min): A reduction in dosage should be made in proportion to the recommendation for adults.

Dosage in hepatic impairment

Dose with caution; monitor hepatic function at regular intervals.

There are, as yet, insufficient data on which to base a dosage recommendation.

Administration

Oral: Suspensions. To minimise potential gastrointestinal intolerance, administer at the start of a meal. The absorption of Augmentin is optimised when taken at the start of a meal.

Duration of therapy should be appropriate to the indication and should not exceed 14 days without review.

4.3 Contraindications

Penicillin hypersensitivity. Attention should be paid to possible cross-sensitivity with other β-lactam antibiotics, e.g. cephalosporins.

A previous history of Augmentin- or penicillin-associated jaundice/hepatic dysfunction.

4.4 Special warnings and precautions for use

Changes in liver function tests have been observed in some patients receiving Augmentin. The clinical significance of these changes is uncertain but Augmentin should be used with caution in patients with evidence of hepatic dysfunction.

Cholestatic jaundice, which may be severe, but is usually reversible, has been reported rarely. Signs and symptoms may not become apparent for several weeks after treatment has ceased.

In patients with renal impairment, dosage should be adjusted according to the degree of impairment (see Section 4.2).

In patients with reduced urine output, crystalluria has been observed very rarely, predominantly with parenteral therapy. During the administration of high doses of amoxicillin, it is advisable to maintain adequate fluid intake and urinary output in order to reduce the possibility of amoxicillin crystalluria (See Section 4.9 Overdose).

Serious and occasionally fatal hypersensitivity (anaphylactoid) reactions have been reported in patients on penicillin therapy. These reactions are more likely to occur in individuals with a history of penicillin hypersensitivity (see 4.3).

Erythematous rashes have been associated with glandular fever in patients receiving amoxicillin.

Prolonged use may also occasionally result in overgrowth of non-susceptible organisms.

Augmentin Suspensions contain 12.5 mg aspartame per 5 ml dose and therefore care should be taken in phenylketonuria.

4.5 Interaction with other medicinal products and other forms of interaction

Prolongation of bleeding time and prothrombin time have been reported in some patients receiving Augmentin. Augmentin should be used with care in patients on anti-coagulation therapy. In common with other broad-spectrum antibiotics, Augmentin may reduce the efficacy of oral contraceptives and patients should be warned accordingly.

Concomitant use of allopurinol during treatment with amoxicillin can increase the likelihood of allergic skin reactions. There are no data on the concomitant use of Augmentin and allopurinol.

4.6 Pregnancy and lactation

Reproduction studies in animals (mice and rats) with orally and parenterally administered Augmentin have shown no teratogenic effects. In a single study in women with preterm, premature rupture of the foetal membrane (pPROM), it was reported that prophylactic treatment with Augmentin may be associated with an increased risk of necrotising enterocolitis in neonates. As with all medicines, use should be avoided in pregnancy, especially during the first trimester, unless considered essential by the physician.

Augmentin may be administered during the period of lactation. With the exception of the risk of sensitisation, associated with the excretion of trace quantities in breast milk, there are no known detrimental effects for the breast-fed infant.

4.7 Effects on ability to drive and use machines

None known.

4.8 Undesirable effects

Side effects are uncommon and mainly of a mild and transitory nature.

Gastrointestinal reactions:

Diarrhoea, indigestion, nausea, vomiting, and mucocutaneous candidiasis have been reported. Antibiotic-associated colitis (including pseudomembranous colitis and haemorrhagic colitis) has been reported rarely. Nausea, although uncommon, is more often associated with higher oral dosages. If gastrointestinal side effects occur with oral therapy they may be reduced by taking Augmentin at the start of meals.

As with other antibiotics the incidence of gastrointestinal side effects may be raised in children under 2 years. In clinical trials, however, only 4% of children under 2 years were withdrawn from treatment.

Superficial tooth discolouration has been reported rarely, mostly with the suspension. It can usually be removed by brushing.

Renal and urinary tract disorders:

Crystalluria has been reported very rarely (See Section 4.9 Overdose).

Genito-urinary effects:

Vaginal itching, soreness and discharge may occur.

Hepatic effects:

Moderate and asymptomatic rises in AST and/or ALT and alkaline phosphatases have been reported occasionally. Hepatitis and cholestatic jaundice have been reported rarely. These hepatic reactions have been reported more commonly with Augmentin than with other penicillins.

After Augmentin hepatic reactions have been reported more frequently in males and elderly patients, particularly those over 65 years. The risk increases with duration of treatment longer than 14 days. These reactions have been very rarely reported in children.

Signs and symptoms usually occur during or shortly after treatment but in some cases may not occur until several weeks after treatment has ended. Hepatic reactions are usually reversible but they may be severe and, very rarely, deaths have been reported.

Hypersensitivity reactions:

Urticarial and erythematous skin rashes sometimes occur. Rarely erythema multiforme, Stevens-Johnson syndrome, toxic epidermal necrolysis, bullous exfoliative dermatitis, acute generalised exanthematous pustulosis (AGEP), serum sickness-like syndrome and hypersensitivity vasculitis have been reported. Treatment should be discontinued if one of these disorders occurs. In common with other β-lactam antibiotics angioedema and anaphylaxis have been reported. Interstitial nephritis can occur rarely.

Haematological effects:

As with other β-lactams transient leucopenia (including neutropenia and agranulocytosis), thrombocytopenia and haemolytic anaemia have been reported rarely. Prolongation of bleeding time and prothrombin time has also been reported rarely (see 4.5).

CNS effects:

CNS effects have been seen very rarely. These include reversible hyperactivity, dizziness, headache and convulsions. Convulsions may occur with impaired renal function or in those receiving high doses.

4.9 Overdose

Gastrointestinal symptoms and disturbance of the fluid and electrolyte balances may be evident. They may be treated symptomatically with attention to the water electrolyte balance. Augmentin may be removed from the circulation by haemodialysis.

Amoxicillin crystalluria, in some cases leading to renal failure, has been observed (see Section 4.4 Special Warnings and Special Precautions for Use)

5. PHARMACOLOGICAL PROPERTIES

5.1 Pharmacodynamic properties

Resistance to many antibiotics is caused by bacterial enzymes which destroy the antibiotic before it can act on the pathogen. The clavulanate in Augmentin anticipates this defence mechanism by blocking the β-lactamase enzymes, thus rendering the organisms sensitive to amoxicillin's rapid bactericidal effect at concentrations readily attainable in the body.

Clavulanate by itself has little antibacterial activity; however, in association with amoxicillin as Augmentin, it produces an antibiotic agent of broad spectrum with wide application in hospital and general practice.

Augmentin is bactericidal to a wide range of organisms including:

Gram-positive

Aerobes: *Enterococcus faecalis**, *Enterococcus faecium**, *Streptococcus pneumoniae*, *Streptococcus pyogenes*, *Streptococcus viridans*, *Staphylococcus aureus**, *Coagulase negative staphylococci** (including *Staphylococcus epidermidis**), *Corynebacterium* species, *Bacillus anthracis**, *Listeria monocytogenes*.

Anaerobes: *Clostridium* species, *Peptococcus* species, *Peptostreptococcus*.

Gram-negative

Aerobes: *Haemophilus influenzae**, *Moraxella catarrhalis** *(Branhamella catarrhalis)*, *Escherichia coli**, *Proteus mirabilis**, *Proteus vulgaris**, *Klebsiella* species*, *Salmonella* species*, *Shigella* species*, *Bordetella pertussis*, *Brucella* species, *Neisseria gonorrhoeae**, *Neisseria meningitidis**, *Vibrio cholerae*, *Pasteurella multocida*.

Anaerobes: *Bacteroides* species* including *B. fragilis*.

* Some members of these species of bacteria produce beta-lactamase, rendering them insensitive to amoxicillin alone.

5.2 Pharmacokinetic properties

The pharmacokinetics of the two components of Augmentin are closely matched. Peak serum levels of both occur about 1 hour after oral administration. Absorption of Augmentin is optimised at the start of a meal. Both clavulanate and amoxicillin have low levels of serum binding; about 70% remains free in the serum.

Doubling the dosage of Augmentin approximately doubles the serum levels achieved.

5.3 Preclinical safety data

Not relevant

6. PHARMACEUTICAL PARTICULARS

6.1 List of excipients

Augmentin 125/31 SF Suspension

The powder contains xanthan gum, hydroxypropyl methylcellulose, aspartame, silicon dioxide, colloidal silica, succinic acid, raspberry, orange and golden syrup dry flavours.

6.2 Incompatibilities

None

6.3 Shelf life

Augmentin 125/31 SF Suspension Dry powder: 24 months

Reconstituted suspensions: 7 days

6.4 Special precautions for storage

Augmentin 125/31 SF Suspension: the dry powder should be stored in a dry place. Reconstituted suspensions should be kept in a refrigerator (but not frozen) for up to 7 days.

6.5 Nature and contents of container

Augmentin 125/31 SF Suspension: Clear glass bottles containing powder for reconstitution to 100 ml.

6.6 Special precautions for disposal and other handling

Augmentin 125/31 SF Suspension: At time of dispensing, the dry powder should be reconstituted to form an oral suspension as detailed below:

Strength	Volume of water to be added to reconstitute	Nominal bottle size	Final volume of reconstituted oral suspension
125/31	92 ml	150 ml	100 ml

Administrative Data

7. MARKETING AUTHORISATION HOLDER

Beecham Group plc

980 Great West Road

Brentford, Middlesex TW8 9GS

Trading as

GlaxoSmithKline UK

Stockley Park West

Uxbridge

Middlesex UB11 1BT

8. MARKETING AUTHORISATION NUMBER(S)

PL 00038/0298

9. DATE OF FIRST AUTHORISATION/RENEWAL OF THE AUTHORISATION

8 December 2003

10. DATE OF REVISION OF THE TEXT

15 August 2007

11. Legal Status

POM

Augmentin 250/62 SF Suspension

(GlaxoSmithKline UK)

1. NAME OF THE MEDICINAL PRODUCT

Augmentin® 250/62 SF Suspension

2. QUALITATIVE AND QUANTITATIVE COMPOSITION

Augmentin *250/62 SF* Suspension*:* When reconstituted each 5 ml contains co-amoxiclav 250/62.

The amoxicillin is present as amoxicillin trihydrate and the clavulanic acid is present as potassium clavulanate.

3. PHARMACEUTICAL FORM

Augmentin 250/62 SF: Dry powder for reconstitution in water, at time of dispensing, to form an oral sugar-free suspension.

4. CLINICAL PARTICULARS

4.1 Therapeutic indications

Augmentin is an antibiotic agent with a notably broad spectrum of activity against the commonly occurring bacterial pathogens in general practice and hospital. The β-lactamase inhibitory action of clavulanate extends the spectrum of amoxicillin to embrace a wider range of organisms, including many resistant to other β-lactam antibiotics.

Augmentin oral preparations are indicated for short term treatment of bacterial infections at the following sites when amoxicillin resistant beta-lactamase producing strains are suspected as the cause. In other situations, amoxicillin alone should be considered.

- *Upper Respiratory Tract Infections (including ENT)* in particular sinusitis, otitis media, recurrent tonsillitis. These infections are often caused by *Streptococcus pneumoniae*, *Haemophilus influenzae**, *Moraxella catarrhalis** and *Streptococcus pyogenes*.

- *Lower Respiratory Tract Infections* in particular acute exacerbations of chronic bronchitis (especially if considered severe), bronchopneumonia. These infections are often caused by *Streptococcus pneumoniae*, *Haemophilus influenzae** and *Moraxella catarrhalis**.

- *Genito-urinary Tract and Abdominal Infections* in particular cystitis (especially when recurrent or complicated - excluding prostatitis), septic abortion, pelvic or puerperal sepsis and intra-abdominal sepsis. These infections are often caused by *Enterobacteriaceae** (mainly *Escherichia coli**), *Staphylococcus saprophyticus*, *Enterococcus* species.*

- *Skin and Soft Tissue Infections* in particular cellulitis, animal bites and severe dental abscess with spreading cellulitis. These infections are often caused by *Staphylococcus aureus**, *Streptococcus pyogenes* and *Bacteroides species**.

- A comprehensive list of sensitive organisms is provided i Section 5.

* Some members of these species of bacteria produc beta-lactamase, rendering them insensitive to amoxicilli alone.

Mixed infections caused by amoxicillin-susceptible organ isms in conjunction with Augmentin-susceptible beta lactamase-producing organisms may be treated with Aug mentin. These infections should not require the addition c another antibiotic resistant to beta-lactamases.

4.2 Posology and method of administration

Usual dosages for the treatment of infection

Adults and children over 12 years of age:	This formulation is not applicabl to this age group
Children under 12 years of age:	The usual recommended daily dosage is 25 mg/kg/day* in divided doses every eight hours The table below presents guidance for children.
Augmentin Suspension	
Under 1 year	25 mg/kg/day*, for example a 7.5 kg child would require 2 ml Augmentin 125/31 SF Suspension t.d.s.
1-6 years (10-18 kg)	5ml Augmentin 125/31 SF Suspension t.d.s.
Over 6 years (18-40 kg)	5ml Augmentin 250/62 SF Suspension t.d.s.

Alternatively, children weighing under 15 kg may be given 25 mg/kg/day using Augmentin 250/62 SF Suspension, administered with the syringe dosing device. For example a 7.5 kg child would require 1 ml Augmentin 250/62 SF Suspension t.d.s. #

In more serious infections the dosage may be increased up to 50 mg/kg/day in divided doses every eight hours.

* Each 25 mg Augmentin provides co-amoxiclav 20/5.

 # This section will only be inserted on the printed SPC if the pack is available in the market

Dosage in renal impairment

Mild impairment (creatinine clearance >30 ml/min): no change in dosage.

Moderate to severe impairment (creatinine clearance <30 ml/min): A reduction in dosage should be made in proportion to the recommendation for adults.

Dosage in hepatic impairment

Dose with caution; monitor hepatic function at regular intervals.

There are, as yet, insufficient data on which to base a dosage recommendation.

Administration

Oral: SuspensionTo minimise potential gastrointestinal intolerance, administer at the start of a meal. The absorption of Augmentin is optimised when taken at the start of a meal.

Duration of therapy should be appropriate to the indication and should not exceed 14 days without review.

4.3 Contraindications

Penicillin hypersensitivity. Attention should be paid to possible cross-sensitivity with other β-lactam antibiotics, e.g. cephalosporins.

A previous history of Augmentin- or penicillin-associated jaundice/hepatic dysfunction.

4.4 Special warnings and precautions for use

Changes in liver function tests have been observed in some patients receiving Augmentin. The clinical significance of these changes is uncertain but Augmentin should be used with caution in patients with evidence of hepatic dysfunction.

Cholestatic jaundice, which may be severe, but is usually reversible, has been reported rarely. Signs and symptoms may not become apparent for several weeks after treatment has ceased.

In patients with renal impairment, dosage should be adjusted according to the degree of impairment (see Section 4.2).

In patients with reduced urine output, crystalluria has been observed very rarely, predominantly with parenteral therapy. During the administration of high doses of amoxicillin, it is advisable to maintain adequate fluid intake and urinary output in order to reduce the possibility of amoxicillin crystalluria (see Section 4.9 Overdose).

Serious and occasionally fatal hypersensitivity (anaphylactoid) reactions have been reported in patients on penicillin therapy. These reactions are more likely to occur in individuals with a history of penicillin hypersensitivity (see 4.3).

Erythematous rashes have been associated with glandular fever in patients receiving amoxicillin.

Prolonged use may also occasionally result in overgrowth of non-susceptible organisms.

Augmentin Suspensions contain 12.5 mg aspartame per 5 ml dose and therefore care should be taken in phenylketonuria.

.5 Interaction with other medicinal products and other orms of interaction

'rolongation of bleeding time and prothrombin time have een reported in some patients receiving Augmentin. Augmentin should be used with care in patients on anti-coaulation therapy. In common with other broad-spectrum ntibiotics, Augmentin may reduce the efficacy of oral ontraceptives and patients should be warned accordngly.

Concomitant use of allopurinol during treatment with moxicillin can increase the likelihood of allergic skin reacons. There are no data on the concomitant use of Augnentin and allopurinol.

.6 Pregnancy and lactation

Reproduction studies in animals (mice and rats) with orally nd parenterally administered Augmentin have shown no eratogenic effects. In a single study in women with preerm, premature rupture of the foetal membrane (pPROM), t was reported that prophylactic treatment with Augmentin nay be associated with an increased risk of necrotising enterocolitis in neonatesAs with all medicines, use should oe avoided in pregnancy, especially during the first trimester, unless considered essential by the physician.

Augmentin may be administered during the period of lacation. With the exception of the risk of sensitisation, assoiated with the excretion of trace quantities in breast milk, here are no known detrimental effects for the breast-fed nfant.

4.7 Effects on ability to drive and use machines

None known.

4.8 Undesirable effects

Side effects are uncommon and mainly of a mild and transitory nature.

Gastrointestinal reactions:

Diarrhoea, indigestion, nausea, vomiting, and mucocutaneous candidiasis have been reported. Antibiotic-associated colitis (including pseudomembranous colitis and haemorrhagic colitis) has been reported rarely. Nausea, although uncommon, is more often associated with higher oral dosages. If gastrointestinal side effects occur with oral therapy they may be reduced by taking Augmentin at the start of meals.

As with other antibiotics the incidence of gastrointestinal side effects may be raised in children under 2 years. In clinical trials, however, only 4% of children under 2 years were withdrawn from treatment.

Superficial tooth discolouration has been reported rarely, mostly with the suspension. It can usually be removed by brushing.

Renal and urinary tract disorders:

Crystalluria has been reported very rarely (See Section 4.9 Overdose).

Genito-urinary effects:

Vaginal itching, soreness and discharge may occur.

Hepatic effects:

Moderate and asymptomatic rises in AST and/or ALT and alkaline phosphatases have been reported occasionally. Hepatitis and cholestatic jaundice have been reported rarely. These hepatic reactions have been reported more commonly with Augmentin than with other penicillins.

After Augmentin hepatic reactions have been reported more frequently in males and elderly patients, particularly those over 65 years. The risk increases with duration of treatment longer than 14 days. These reactions have been very rarely reported in children.

Signs and symptoms usually occur during or shortly after treatment but in some cases may not occur until several weeks after treatment has ended. Hepatic reactions are usually reversible but they may be severe and, very rarely, deaths have been reported.

Hypersensitivity reactions:

Urticarial and erythematous skin rashes sometimes occur. Rarely erythema multiforme, Stevens-Johnson syndrome, toxic epidermal necrolysis, bullous exfoliative dermatitis, acute generalised exanthematous pustulosis (AGEP), serum sickness-like syndrome and hypersensitivity vasculitis have been reported. Treatment should be discontinued if one of these disorders occurs. In common with other β-lactam antibiotics angioedema and anaphylaxis have been reported. Interstitial nephritis can occur rarely.

Haematological effects:

As with other β-lactams transient leucopenia (including neutropenia and agranulocytosis), thrombocytopenia and haemolytic anaemia have been reported rarely. Prolongation of bleeding time and prothrombin time has also been reported rarely (see 4.5).

CNS effects:

CNS effects have been seen very rarely. These include reversible hyperactivity, dizziness, headache and convulsions. Convulsions may occur with impaired renal function or in those receiving high doses.

4.9 Overdose

Gastrointestinal symptoms and disturbance of the fluid and electrolyte balances may be evident. They may be treated symptomatically with attention to the water electrolyte balance. Augmentin may be removed from the circulation by haemodialysis.

Amoxicillin crystalluria, in some cases leading to renal failure, has been observed (see Section 4.4 Special Warnings and Special Precautions for Use)

5. PHARMACOLOGICAL PROPERTIES

5.1 Pharmacodynamic properties

Resistance to many antibiotics is caused by bacterial enzymes which destroy the antibiotic before it can act on the pathogen. The clavulanate in Augmentin anticipates this defence mechanism by blocking the β-lactamase enzymes, thus rendering the organisms sensitive to amoxicillin's rapid bactericidal effect at concentrations readily attainable in the body.

Clavulanate by itself has little antibacterial activity; however, in association with amoxicillin as Augmentin, it produces an antibiotic agent of broad spectrum with wide application in hospital and general practice.

Augmentin is bactericidal to a wide range of organisms including:

Gram-positive

Aerobes: *Enterococcus faecalis*, Enterococcus faecium*, Streptococcus pneumoniae, Streptococcus pyogenes, Streptococcus viridans, Staphylococcus aureus*, Coagulase negative staphylococci** (including *Staphylococcus epidermidis*), Corynebacterium* species, *Bacillus anthracis*, Listeria monocytogenes.*

Anaerobes: *Clostridium* species, *Peptococcus* species, *Peptostreptococcus.*

Gram-negative

Aerobes: *Haemophilus influenzae*, Moraxella catarrhalis* (Branhamella catarrhalis), Escherichia coli*, Proteus mirabilis*, Proteus vulgaris*, Klebsiella* species*, *Salmonella* species*, *Shigella* species*, *Bordetella pertussis, Brucella* species, *Neisseria gonorrhoeae*, Neisseria meningitidis*, Vibrio cholerae, Pasteurella multocida.*

Anaerobes: *Bacteroides* species* including *B. fragilis*.

* Some members of these species of bacteria produce beta-lactamase, rendering them insensitive to amoxicillin alone.

5.2 Pharmacokinetic properties

The pharmacokinetics of the two components of Augmentin are closely matched. Peak serum levels of both occur about 1 hour after oral administration. Absorption of Augmentin is optimised at the start of a meal. Both clavulanate and amoxicillin have low levels of serum binding; about 70% remains free in the serum.

Doubling the dosage of Augmentin approximately doubles the serum levels achieved.

5.3 Preclinical safety data

Not relevant

6. PHARMACEUTICAL PARTICULARS

6.1 List of excipients

Augmentin 250/62 SF Suspension

The powder contains xanthan gum, hydroxypropyl methylcellulose, aspartame, silicon dioxide, colloidal silica, succinic acid, raspberry, orange and golden syrup dry flavours.

6.2 Incompatibilities

None

6.3 Shelf life

Augmentin 250/62 SF Suspension	Dry powder: 24 months Reconstituted suspensions: 7 days

6.4 Special precautions for storage

Augmentin 250/62 SF Suspensions: the dry powder should be stored in a dry place. Reconstituted suspensions should be kept in a refrigerator (but not frozen) for up to 7 days.

6.5 Nature and contents of container

Augmentin 250/62 SF Suspensions: Clear glass bottles containing powder for reconstitution to 60 or 100 ml or 20 ml (with a plastic dosing syringe).

6.6 Special precautions for disposal and other handling

Augmentin 250/62 SF Suspensions: At time of dispensing, the dry powder should be reconstituted to form an oral suspension as detailed below:

Strength	Volume of water to be added to reconstitute	Nominal bottle size	Final volume of reconstituted oral suspension
250/62	90 ml	150 ml	100 ml

Administrative Data

7. MARKETING AUTHORISATION HOLDER

Beecham Group plc
980 Great West Road
Brentford, Middlesex TW8 9GS
Trading as:
GlaxoSmithKline UK
Stockley Park West
Uxbridge
Middlesex UB11 1BT

8. MARKETING AUTHORISATION NUMBER(S)

Augmentin 250/62 SF Suspension PL 00038/0337

9. DATE OF FIRST AUTHORISATION/RENEWAL OF THE AUTHORISATION

Augmentin 250/62 SF Suspension 11 October 2005

10. DATE OF REVISION OF THE TEXT

20 August 2007

11. Legal Status

POM

Augmentin 375mg Dispersible Tablets

(GlaxoSmithKline UK)

1. NAME OF THE MEDICINAL PRODUCT

Augmentin® Dispersible Tablets 375 mg

2. QUALITATIVE AND QUANTITATIVE COMPOSITION

Augmentin Dispersible Tablets 375 mg: Each tablet contains co-amoxiclav 250/125.

The amoxicillin is present as amoxicillin trihydrate and the clavulanic acid is present as potassium clavulanate.

3. PHARMACEUTICAL FORM

Augmentin Dispersible Tablets 375 mg: White round tablets engraved Augmentin

4. CLINICAL PARTICULARS

4.1 Therapeutic indications

Augmentin is an antibiotic agent with a notably broad spectrum of activity against the commonly occurring bacterial pathogens in general practice and hospital. The β-lactamase inhibitory action of clavulanate extends the spectrum of amoxicillin to embrace a wider range of organisms, including many resistant to other β-lactam antibiotics.

Augmentin oral preparations are indicated for short term treatment of bacterial infections at the following sites when amoxicillin resistant beta-lactamase producing strains are suspected as the cause. In other situations, amoxicillin alone should be considered.

- Upper Respiratory Tract Infections (including ENT) in particular sinusitis, otitis media, recurrent tonsillitis. These infections are often caused by Streptococcus pneumoniae, Haemophilus influenzae*, Moraxella catarrhalis* and Streptococcus pyogenes.

- Lower Respiratory Tract Infections in particular acute exacerbations of chronic bronchitis (especially if considered severe), bronchopneumonia. These infections are often caused by Streptococcus pneumoniae, Haemophilus influenzae* and Moraxella catarrhalis*.

- Genito-urinary Tract and Abdominal Infections in particular cystitis (especially when recurrent or complicated - excluding prostatitis), septic abortion, pelvic or puerperal sepsis and intra-abdominal sepsis. These infections are often caused by *Enterobacteriaceae** (mainly *Escherichia coli*), Staphylococcus saprophyticus, Enterococcus* species.*

- *Skin and Soft Tissue Infections* in particular cellulitis, animal bites and severe dental abscess with spreading cellulitis. These infections are often caused by *Staphylococcus aureus*, Streptococcus pyogenes* and *Bacteroides species*.*

- A comprehensive list of sensitive organisms is provided in Section 5.

* Some members of these species of bacteria produce beta-lactamase, rendering them insensitive to amoxicillin alone.

Mixed infections caused by amoxicillin-susceptible organisms in conjunction with Augmentin-susceptible beta-lactamase-producing organisms may be treated with Augmentin. These infections should not require the addition of another antibiotic resistant to beta-lactamases.

4.2 Posology and method of administration

Usual dosages for the treatment of infection

Adults and children over 12 years	One Augmentin 375 mg Tablet or Dispersible Tablet three times a day. (In severe infections one Augmentin 625 mg Tablet three times a day.) Therapy can be started parenterally and continued with an oral preparation.

Not recommended in children of 12 years and under.

Dosage in dental infections (e.g. dentoalveolar abscess)

Adults and children over 12 years: one Augmentin Tablet 375 mg three times a day for five days.

Dosage in renal impairment

Adults:

Mild impairment (Creatinine clearance >30 ml/min)	Moderate impairment (Creatinine clearance 10-30 ml/min)	Severe impairment (Creatinine clearance <10 ml/min)
No change in dosage	One 375 mg tablet 12 hourly	Not more than one 375 mg tablet 12 hourly.

Dosage in hepatic impairment

Dose with caution; monitor hepatic function at regular intervals.

There are, as yet, insufficient data on which to base a dosage recommendation.

Administration

Oral: Dispersible tablets. To minimise potential gastrointestinal intolerance, administer at the start of a meal. The absorption of Augmentin is optimised when taken at the start of a meal. Dispersible tablets should be stirred into a little water before taking.

Duration of therapy should be appropriate to the indication and should not exceed 14 days without review.

4.3 Contraindications

Penicillin hypersensitivity. Attention should be paid to possible cross-sensitivity with other -lactam antibiotics, e.g. cephalosporins.

A previous history of Augmentin- or penicillin-associated jaundice/hepatic dysfunction.

4.4 Special warnings and precautions for use

Changes in liver function tests have been observed in some patients receiving Augmentin. The clinical significance of these changes is uncertain but Augmentin should be used with caution in patients with evidence of hepatic dysfunction.

Cholestatic jaundice, which may be severe, but is usually reversible, has been reported rarely. Signs and symptoms may not become apparent for several weeks after treatment has ceased.

In patients with renal impairment, dosage should be adjusted according to the degree of impairment (see Section 4.2).

In patients with reduced urine output, crystalluria has been observed very rarely, predominantly with parenteral therapy. During the administration of high doses of amoxicillin, it is advisable to maintain adequate fluid intake and urinary output in order to reduce the possibility of amoxicillin crystalluria (See Section 4.9 Overdose).

Serious and occasionally fatal hypersensitivity (anaphylactoid) reactions have been reported in patients on penicillin therapy. These reactions are more likely to occur in individuals with a history of penicillin hypersensitivity (see 4.3).

Erythematous rashes have been associated with glandular fever in patients receiving amoxicillin.

Prolonged use may also occasionally result in overgrowth of non-susceptible organisms.

4.5 Interaction with other medicinal products and other forms of interaction

Prolongation of bleeding time and prothrombin time have been reported in some patients receiving Augmentin. Augmentin should be used with care in patients on anti-coagulation therapy. In common with other broad-spectrum antibiotics, Augmentin may reduce the efficacy of oral contraceptives and patients should be warned accordingly.

Concomitant use of allopurinol during treatment with amoxicillin can increase the likelihood of allergic skin reactions. There are no data on the concomitant use of Augmentin and allopurinol.

4.6 Pregnancy and lactation

Reproduction studies in animals (mice and rats) with orally and parenterally administered Augmentin have shown no teratogenic effects. In a single study in women with preterm, premature rupture of foetal membrane (pPROM), it was reported that prophylactic treatment with Augmentin may be associated with an increased risk of necrotising enterocolitis in neonates. As with all medicines, use should be avoided in pregnancy, especially during the first trimester, unless considered essential by the physician.

Augmentin may be administered during the period of lactation. With the exception of the risk of sensitisation, associated with the excretion of trace quantities in breast milk, there are no known detrimental effects for the breast-fed infant.

4.7 Effects on ability to drive and use machines

None known.

4.8 Undesirable effects

Side effects are uncommon and mainly of a mild and transitory nature.

Gastrointestinal reactions:

Diarrhoea, indigestion, nausea, vomiting, and mucocutaneous candidiasis have been reported. Antibiotic-associated colitis (including pseudomembranous colitis and haemorrhagic colitis) has been reported rarely. Nausea, although uncommon, is more often associated with higher oral dosages. If gastrointestinal side effects occur with oral therapy they may be reduced by taking Augmentin at the start of meals.

Superficial tooth discolouration has been reported rarely, mostly with the suspension. It can usually be removed by brushing.

Renal and urinary tract disorders:

Crystalluria has been reported very rarely (see Section 4.9 Overdose).

Genito-urinary effects:

Vaginal itching, soreness and discharge may occur.

Hepatic effects:

Moderate and asymptomatic rises in AST and/or ALT and alkaline phosphatases have been reported occasionally. Hepatitis and cholestatic jaundice have been reported rarely. These hepatic reactions have been reported more commonly with Augmentin than with other penicillins.

After Augmentin hepatic reactions have been reported more frequently in males and elderly patients, particularly those over 65 years. The risk increases with duration of treatment longer than 14 days.

Signs and symptoms usually occur during or shortly after treatment but in some cases may not occur until several weeks after treatment has ended. Hepatic reactions are usually reversible but they may be severe and, very rarely, deaths have been reported.

Hypersensitivity reactions:

Urticarial and erythematous skin rashes sometimes occur. Rarely erythema multiforme, Stevens-Johnson syndrome, toxic epidermal necrolysis, bullous exfoliative dermatitis, acute generalised exanthematous pustulosis (AGEP), serum sickness-like syndrome and hypersensitivity vasculitis have been reported. Treatment should be discontinued if one of these disorders occurs. In common with other -lactam antibiotics angioedema and anaphylaxis have been reported. Interstitial nephritis can occur rarely.

Haematological effects:

As with other -lactams transient leucopenia (including neutropenia and agranulocytosis), thrombocytopenia and haemolytic anaemia have been reported rarely. Prolongation of bleeding time and prothrombin time has also been reported rarely (see 4.5).

CNS effects:

CNS effects have been seen very rarely. These include reversible hyperactivity, dizziness, headache and convulsions. Convulsions may occur with impaired renal function or in those receiving high doses.

4.9 Overdose

Gastrointestinal symptoms and disturbance of the fluid and electrolyte balances may be evident. They may be treated symptomatically with attention to the water electrolyte balance. Augmentin may be removed from the circulation by haemodialysis.

Amoxicillin crystalluria, in some cases leading to renal failure, has been observed (see Section 4.4 Special Warnings and Special Precautions for Use)

5. PHARMACOLOGICAL PROPERTIES

5.1 Pharmacodynamic properties

Resistance to many antibiotics is caused by bacterial enzymes which destroy the antibiotic before it can act on the pathogen. The clavulanate in Augmentin anticipates this defence mechanism by blocking the β-lactamase enzymes, thus rendering the organisms sensitive to amoxicillin's rapid bactericidal effect at concentrations readily attainable in the body.

Clavulanate by itself has little antibacterial activity; however, in association with amoxicillin as Augmentin, it produces an antibiotic agent of broad spectrum with wide application in hospital and general practice.

Augmentin is bactericidal to a wide range of organisms including:

Gram-positive

Aerobes: *Enterococcus faecalis**, *Enterococcus faecium**, *Streptococcus pneumoniae, Streptococcus pyogenes, Streptococcus viridans, Staphylococcus aureus**, *Coagulase negative staphylococci** (including *Staphylococcus epidermidis**), *Corynebacterium* species, *Bacillus anthracis**, *Listeria monocytogenes.*

Anaerobes: *Clostridium* species, *Peptococcus* species, *Peptostreptococcus.*

Gram-negative

Aerobes: *Haemophilus influenzae**, *Moraxella catarrhalis** *(Branhamella catarrhalis), Escherichia coli**, *Proteus mirabilis**, *Proteus vulgaris**, *Klebsiella* species*, *Salmonella* species*, *Shigella* species*, *Bordetella pertussis, Brucella* species, *Neisseria gonorrhoeae**, *Neisseria meningitidis**, *Vibrio cholerae, Pasteurella multocida.*

Anaerobes: *Bacteroides* species* including *B. fragilis.*

* Some members of these species of bacteria produce beta-lactamase, rendering them insensitive to amoxicillin alone.

5.2 Pharmacokinetic properties

The pharmacokinetics of the two components of Augmentin are closely matched. Peak serum levels of both occur about 1 hour after oral administration. Absorption of Augmentin is optimised at the start of a meal. Both clavulanate and amoxicillin have low levels of serum binding; about 70% remains free in the serum.

Doubling the dosage of Augmentin approximately doubles the serum levels achieved.

5.3 Preclinical safety data

Not relevant

6. PHARMACEUTICAL PARTICULARS

6.1 List of excipients

Each tablet contains polyvinylpyrrolidone (cross-linked) silica gel, saccharin sodium, pineapple, strawberry and blood orange dry flavours, magnesium stearate and microcrystalline cellulose.

6.2 Incompatibilities

None

6.3 Shelf life

Augmentin Dispersible Tablets 375 mg 24M

6.4 Special precautions for storage

Augmentin Dispersible Tablets 375 mg should be stored in a dry place.

6.5 Nature and contents of container

Blister Pack of 6, 21, 30, 90, 100, or 500 in a carton.

Bottles of 6, 21, 30, 90, 100, or 500 with either a molecular sieve or silica gel dessicant.

6.6 Special precautions for disposal and other handling

The dispersible tablets should be stirred with a little water before taking.

Administrative Data

7. MARKETING AUTHORISATION HOLDER

Beecham Group plc

980 Great West Road

Brentford, Middlesex TW8 9GS

Trading as:

GlaxoSmithKline UK

Stockley Park West

Uxbridge

Middlesex UB11 1BT

8. MARKETING AUTHORISATION NUMBER(S)

PL 00038/0272

9. DATE OF FIRST AUTHORISATION/RENEWAL OF THE AUTHORISATION

27 July 2002

10. DATE OF REVISION OF THE TEXT

11 January 2005

11. Legal Status

POM

Augmentin 375mg Tablets

(GlaxoSmithKline UK)

1. NAME OF THE MEDICINAL PRODUCT

Augmentin® 375 mg Tablets

2. QUALITATIVE AND QUANTITATIVE COMPOSITION

Augmentin 375 mg Tablets: Each tablet contains co-amoxiclav 250/125.

The amoxicillin is present as amoxicillin trihydrate and the clavulanic acid is present as potassium clavulanate.

3. PHARMACEUTICAL FORM

Augmentin 375 mg Tablets: White to off-white, oval film-coated tablets engraved Augmentin on one side.

4. CLINICAL PARTICULARS

4.1 Therapeutic indications

Augmentin is an antibiotic agent with a notably broad spectrum of activity against the commonly occurring bacterial pathogens in general practice and hospital. The β-lactamase inhibitory action of clavulanate extends the spectrum of amoxicillin to embrace a wider range of organisms, including many resistant to other β-lactam antibiotics.

Augmentin oral preparations are indicated for short term treatment of bacterial infections at the following sites when amoxicillin resistant beta-lactamase producing strains are suspected as the cause. In other situations, amoxicillin alone should be considered.

- *Upper Respiratory Tract Infections (including ENT)* in particular sinusitis, otitis media, recurrent tonsillitis. These infections are often caused by *Streptococcus pneumoniae, Haemophilus influenzae**, *Moraxella catarrhalis** and *Streptococcus pyogenes.*

- *Lower Respiratory Tract Infections* in particular acute exacerbations of chronic bronchitis (especially if considered severe), bronchopneumonia. These infections are often caused by *Streptococcus pneumoniae, Haemophilus influenzae** and *Moraxella catarrhalis**.

- *Genito-urinary Tract and Abdominal Infections* in particular cystitis (especially when recurrent or complicated - excluding prostatitis), septic abortion, pelvic or puerperal sepsis and intra-abdominal sepsis. These infections are often caused by *Enterobacteriaceae** (mainly *Escherichia coli**), *Staphylococcus saprophyticus, Enterococcus* species.*- *Skin and Soft Tissue Infections* in particular cellulitis, animal bites and severe dental abscess with spreading cellulitis. These infections are often caused by *Staphylococcus aureus**, *Streptococcus pyogenes* and *Bacteroides* species*.

A comprehensive list of sensitive organisms is provided in ection 5.

Some members of these species of bacteria produce eta-lactamase, rendering them insensitive to amoxicillin one.

ixed infections caused by amoxicillin-susceptible organ-ms in conjunction with Augmentin-susceptible beta-ctamase-producing organisms may be treated with Aug-entin. These infections should not require the addition of nother antibiotic resistant to beta-lactamases.

.2 Posology and method of administration

sual dosages for the treatment of infection

dults and children ver 12 years	One Augmentin 375 mg Tablet three times a day. *In severe infections this may be increased to two tablets (375 mg) three times a day**. Therapy can be started parenterally and continued with an oral preparation.

ugmentin 375 mg Tablets are not recommended in chil-ren of 12 years and under.

)osage in dental infections (e.g. dentoalveolar abscess)

dults and children over 12 years: one Augmentin Tablet 75 mg three times a day for five days.

)osage in renal impairment

Adults:

Mild impairment Creatine clearance >30 ml/min)	Moderate impairment (Creatinine clearance 10-30 ml/min)	Severe impairment (Creatinine clearance <10 ml/min)
No change in dosage	One 375 mg tablet or one 625 mg tablet 12 hourly	Not more than one 375 mg tablet 12 hourly; 625 mg tablets are not recommended.

Children:

Similar reductions in dosage should be made for children.

**This dosage regimen is not promoted and will not appear on the printed SPC.*

Dosage in hepatic impairment

Dose with caution; monitor hepatic function at regular intervals.

There are, as yet, insufficient data on which to base a dosage recommendation.

Each 375 mg tablet of Augmentin contains 0.63 mmol (25 mg) of potassium.

Administration

Oral: Tablets. To minimise potential gastrointestinal intolerance, administer at the start of a meal. The absorption of Augmentin is optimised when taken at the start of a meal.

Duration of therapy should be appropriate to the indication and should not exceed 14 days without review.

4.3 Contraindications

Penicillin hypersensitivity. Attention should be paid to possible cross-sensitivity with other -lactam antibiotics, e.g. cephalosporins.

A previous history of Augmentin- or penicillin-associated jaundice/hepatic dysfunction.

4.4 Special warnings and precautions for use

Changes in liver function tests have been observed in some patients receiving Augmentin. The clinical significance of these changes is uncertain but Augmentin should be used with caution in patients with evidence of hepatic dysfunction.

Cholestatic jaundice, which may be severe, but is usually reversible, has been reported rarely. Signs and symptoms may not become apparent for several weeks after treatment has ceased.

In patients with renal impairment, dosage should be adjusted according to the degree of impairment (see Section 4.2).

In patients with reduced urine output, crystalluria has been observed very rarely, predominantly with parenteral therapy. During the administration of high doses of amoxicillin, it is advisable to maintain adequate fluid intake and urinary output in order to reduce the possibility of amoxicillin crystalluria (see Section 4.9 Overdose).

Serious and occasionally fatal hypersensitivity (anaphylactoid) reactions have been reported in patients on penicillin therapy. These reactions are more likely to occur in individuals with a history of penicillin hypersensitivity (see 4.3).

Erythematous rashes have been associated with glandular fever in patients receiving amoxicillin.

Prolonged use may also occasionally result in overgrowth of non-susceptible organisms.

4.5 Interaction with other medicinal products and other forms of interaction

Prolongation of bleeding time and prothrombin time have been reported in some patients receiving Augmentin. Augmentin should be used with care in patients on anti-coagulation therapy. In common with other broad-spectrum antibiotics, Augmentin may reduce the efficacy of oral contraceptives and patients should be warned accordingly.

Concomitant use of allopurinol during treatment with amoxicillin can increase the likelihood of allergic skin reactions. There are no data on the concomitant use of Augmentin and allopurinol.

4.6 Pregnancy and lactation

Reproduction studies in animals (mice and rats) with orally and parenterally administered Augmentin have shown no teratogenic effects. In a single study in women with preterm, premature rupture of the foetal membrane (pPROM), it was reported that prophylactic treatment with Augmentin may be associated with an increased risk of necrotising enterocolitis in neonates. As with all medicines, use should be avoided in pregnancy, especially during the first trimester, unless considered essential by the physician.

Augmentin may be administered during the period of lactation. With the exception of the risk of sensitisation, associated with the excretion of trace quantities in breast milk, there are no known detrimental effects for the breast-fed infant.

4.7 Effects on ability to drive and use machines

None known.

4.8 Undesirable effects

Side effects are uncommon and mainly of a mild and transitory nature.

Gastrointestinal reactions:

Diarrhoea, indigestion, nausea, vomiting, and mucocutaneous candidiasis have been reported. Antibiotic-associated colitis (including pseudomembranous colitis and haemorrhagic colitis) has been reported rarely. Nausea, although uncommon, is more often associated with higher oral dosages. If gastrointestinal side effects occur with oral therapy they may be reduced by taking Augmentin at the start of meals.

Superficial tooth discolouration has been reported rarely, mostly with the suspension. It can usually be removed by brushing.

Renal and urinary tract disorders:

Crystalluria has been reported very rarely (see Section 4.9 Overdose).

Genito-urinary effects:

Vaginal itching, soreness and discharge may occur.

Hepatic effects:

Moderate and asymptomatic rises in AST and/or ALT and alkaline phosphatases have been reported occasionally. Hepatitis and cholestatic jaundice have been reported rarely. These hepatic reactions have been reported more commonly with Augmentin than with other penicillins.

After Augmentin hepatic reactions have been reported more frequently in males and elderly patients, particularly those over 65 years. The risk increases with duration of treatment longer than 14 days.

Signs and symptoms usually occur during or shortly after treatment but in some cases may not occur until several weeks after treatment has ended. Hepatic reactions are usually reversible but they may be severe and, very rarely, deaths have been reported.

Hypersensitivity reactions:

Urticarial and erythematous skin rashes sometimes occur. Rarely erythema multiforme, Stevens-Johnson syndrome, toxic epidermal necrolysis, bullous exfoliative dermatitis, acute generalised exanthematous pustulosis (AGEP), serum sickness-like syndrome and hypersensitivity vasculitis have been reported. Treatment should be discontinued if one of these disorders occurs. In common with other -lactam antibiotics angioedema and anaphylaxis have been reported. Interstitial nephritis can occur rarely.

Haematological effects:

As with other -lactams transient leucopenia (including neutropenia and agranulocytosis), thrombocytopenia and haemolytic anaemia have been reported rarely. Prolongation of bleeding time and prothrombin time has also been reported rarely (see 4.5).

CNS effects:

CNS effects have been seen very rarely. These include reversible hyperactivity, dizziness, headache and convulsions. Convulsions may occur with impaired renal function or in those receiving high doses.

4.9 Overdose

Gastrointestinal symptoms and disturbance of the fluid and electrolyte balances may be evident. They may be treated symptomatically with attention to the water electrolyte balance. Augmentin may be removed from the circulation by haemodialysis.

Amoxicillin crystalluria, in some cases leading to renal failure, has been observed (see Section 4.4 Special Warnings and Special Precautions for Use)

5. PHARMACOLOGICAL PROPERTIES

5.1 Pharmacodynamic properties

Resistance to many antibiotics is caused by bacterial enzymes which destroy the antibiotic before it can act on the pathogen. The clavulanate in Augmentin anticipates this defence mechanism by blocking the β-lactamase enzymes, thus rendering the organisms sensitive to amoxicillin's rapid bactericidal effect at concentrations readily attainable in the body.

Clavulanate by itself has little antibacterial activity; however, in association with amoxicillin as Augmentin, it produces an antibiotic agent of broad spectrum with wide application in hospital and general practice.

Augmentin is bactericidal to a wide range of organisms including:

Gram-positive

Aerobes: *Enterococcus faecalis**, *Enterococcus faecium**, *Streptococcus pneumoniae*, *Streptococcus pyogenes*, *Streptococcus viridans*, *Staphylococcus aureus**, *Coagulase negative staphylococci** (including *Staphylococcus epidermidis**), *Corynebacterium* species, *Bacillus anthracis**, *Listeria monocytogenes*.

Anaerobes: *Clostridium* species, *Peptococcus* species, *Peptostreptococcus*.

Gram-negative

Aerobes: *Haemophilus influenzae**, *Moraxella catarrhalis** *(Branhamella catarrhalis)*, *Escherichia coli**, *Proteus mirabilis**, *Proteus vulgaris**, *Klebsiella* species*, *Salmonella* species*, *Shigella* species*, *Bordetella pertussis*, *Brucella* species, *Neisseria gonorrhoeae**, *Neisseria meningitidis**, *Vibrio cholerae*, *Pasteurella multocida*.

Anaerobes: *Bacteroides* species* including *B. fragilis*.

* Some members of these species of bacteria produce beta-lactamase, rendering them insensitive to amoxicillin alone.

5.2 Pharmacokinetic properties

The pharmacokinetics of the two components of Augmentin are closely matched. Peak serum levels of both occur about 1 hour after oral administration. Absorption of Augmentin is optimised at the start of a meal. Both clavulanate and amoxicillin have low levels of serum binding; about 70% remains free in the serum.

Doubling the dosage of Augmentin approximately doubles the serum levels achieved.

5.3 Preclinical safety data

Not relevant

6. PHARMACEUTICAL PARTICULARS

6.1 List of excipients

Augmentin 375 mg tablets:

Each tablet contains magnesium stearate, sodium starch glycollate, colloidal silica, microcrystalline cellulose, titanium dioxide (E171), hydroxypropyl methylcellulose, polyethylene glycol and silicone oil.

6.2 Incompatibilities

None

6.3 Shelf life

Augmentin 375 mg Tablets Blister enclosed in pouch 24M, Glass Bottles 24M

6.4 Special precautions for storage

Augmentin 375 mg Tablets should be stored in a dry place at 25°C or below.

6.5 Nature and contents of container

Augmentin 375 mg Tablets: Aluminium PVC/PVdC blister enlcosed within an aluminium laminate pouch containing a desiccant sachet. Each pouch contains a plaque of 7 tablets. 3 pouches are enclosed within a carton to provide a pack of 21 tablets. Tablets are also supplied in amber glass bottles of 50 and 100*.

6.6 Special precautions for disposal and other handling

None

Administrative Data

7. MARKETING AUTHORISATION HOLDER

Beecham Group plc

980 Great West Road

Brentford

Middlesex TW8 9GS

Trading as:

GlaxoSmithKline UK

Stockley Park West

Uxbridge

Middlesex UB11 1BT

8. MARKETING AUTHORISATION NUMBER(S)

PL 00038/0270

9. DATE OF FIRST AUTHORISATION/RENEWAL OF THE AUTHORISATION

27 July 2002

10. DATE OF REVISION OF THE TEXT

11th January 2005

11. Legal Status

POM

Augmentin 625mg Tablets

(GlaxoSmithKline UK)

1. NAME OF THE MEDICINAL PRODUCT

Augmentin® 625 mg Tablets

2. QUALITATIVE AND QUANTITATIVE COMPOSITION

Augmentin 625 mg Tablets: Each tablet contains co-amoxiclav 500/125.

The amoxicillin is present as amoxicillin trihydrate and the clavulanic acid is present as potassium clavulanate.

3. PHARMACEUTICAL FORM

Augmentin 625 mg Tablets:

Film-coated tablet

White to off-white, oval film-coated tablets debossed with 'AC' and a score line one side and plain on the other side.

4. CLINICAL PARTICULARS

4.1 Therapeutic indications

Augmentin is an antibiotic agent with a notably broad spectrum of activity against the commonly occurring bacterial pathogens in general practice and hospital. The β-lactamase inhibitory action of clavulanate extends the spectrum of amoxicillin to embrace a wider range of organisms, including many resistant to other β-lactam antibiotics.

Augmentin oral preparations are indicated for short term treatment of bacterial infections at the following sites when amoxicillin resistant beta-lactamase producing strains are suspected as the cause. In other situations, amoxicillin alone should be considered.

- *Upper Respiratory Tract Infections (including ENT)* in particular sinusitis, otitis media, recurrent tonsillitis. These infections are often caused by *Streptococcus pneumoniae, Haemophilus influenzae**, *Moraxella catarrhalis** and *Streptococcus pyogenes.*

- *Lower Respiratory Tract Infections* in particular acute exacerbations of chronic bronchitis (especially if considered severe), bronchopneumonia. These infections are often caused by *Streptococcus pneumoniae, Haemophilus influenzae** and *Moraxella catarrhalis**.

- *Genito-urinary Tract and Abdominal Infections* in particular cystitis (especially when recurrent or complicated - excluding prostatitis), septic abortion, pelvic or puerperal sepsis and intra-abdominal sepsis. These infections are often caused by *Enterobacteriaceae** (mainly *Escherichia coli**), *Staphylococcus saprophyticus, Enterococcus* species.*

- *Skin and Soft Tissue Infections* in particular cellulitis, animal bites and severe dental abscess with spreading cellulitis. These infections are often caused by *Staphylococcus aureus**, *Streptococcus pyogenes* and *Bacteroides species**.

- A comprehensive list of sensitive organisms is provided in Section 5.

* Some members of these species of bacteria produce beta-lactamase, rendering them insensitive to amoxicillin alone.

Mixed infections caused by amoxicillin-susceptible organisms in conjunction with Augmentin-susceptible beta-lactamase-producing organisms may be treated with Augmentin. These infections should not require the addition of another antibiotic resistant to beta-lactamases.

4.2 Posology and method of administration

Usual dosages for the treatment of infection

Adults and children over 12 years	In severe infections one Augmentin 625 mg Tablet three times a day. Therapy can be started parenterally and continued with an oral preparation.

Not recommended in children of 12 years and under.

Dosage in renal impairment

Adults:

Mild impairment (Creatinine clearance >30 ml/min)	Moderate impairment (Creatinine clearance 10-30 ml/min)	Severe impairment (Creatinine clearance <10 ml/min)
No change in dosage	One 625 mg tablet 12 hourly	Not recommended.

Dosage in hepatic impairment

Dose with caution; monitor hepatic function at regular intervals.

There are, as yet, insufficient data on which to base a dosage recommendation.

Administration

Oral: Tablets To minimise potential gastrointestinal intolerance, administer at the start of a meal. The absorption of Augmentin is optimised when taken at the start of a meal.

Duration of therapy should be appropriate to the indication and should not exceed 14 days without review.

4.3 Contraindications

Penicillin hypersensitivity. Attention should be paid to possible cross-sensitivity with other β-lactam antibiotics, e.g. cephalosporins.

A previous history of Augmentin- or penicillin-associated jaundice/hepatic dysfunction.

4.4 Special warnings and precautions for use

Changes in liver function tests have been observed in some patients receiving Augmentin. The clinical significance of these changes is uncertain but Augmentin should be used with caution in patients with evidence of hepatic dysfunction.

Cholestatic jaundice, which may be severe, but is usually reversible, has been reported rarely. Signs and symptoms may not become apparent for several weeks after treatment has ceased.

In patients with renal impairment, dosage should be adjusted according to the degree of impairment (see Section 4.2).

In patients with reduced urine output, crystalluria has been observed very rarely, predominantly with parenteral therapy. During the administration of high doses of amoxicillin, it is advisable to maintain adequate fluid intake and urinary output in order to reduce the possibility of amoxicillin crystalluria (see Section 4.9 Overdose).

Serious and occasionally fatal hypersensitivity (anaphylactoid) reactions have been reported in patients on penicillin therapy. These reactions are more likely to occur in individuals with a history of penicillin hypersensitivity (see 4.3).

Erythematous rashes have been associated with glandular fever in patients receiving amoxicillin.

Prolonged use may also occasionally result in overgrowth of non-susceptible organisms.

4.5 Interaction with other medicinal products and other forms of interaction

Prolongation of bleeding time and prothrombin time have been reported in some patients receiving Augmentin. Augmentin should be used with care in patients on anti-coagulation therapy.

In common with other broad-spectrum antibiotics, Augmentin may reduce the efficacy of oral contraceptives and patients should be warned accordingly.

Concomitant use of allopurinol during treatment with amoxicillin can increase the likelihood of allergic skin reactions. There are no data on the concomitant use of Augmentin and allopurinol.

4.6 Pregnancy and lactation

Reproduction studies in animals (mice and rats) with orally and parenterally administered Augmentin have shown no teratogenic effects. In a single study in women with preterm, premature rupture of the foetal membrane (pPROM), it was reported that prophylactic treatment with Augmentin may be associated with an increased risk of necrotising enterocolitis in neonates. As with all medicines, use should be avoided in pregnancy, especially during the first trimester, unless considered essential by the physician.

Augmentin may be administered during the period of lactation. With the exception of the risk of sensitisation, associated with the excretion of trace quantities in breast milk, there are no known detrimental effects for the breast-fed infant.

4.7 Effects on ability to drive and use machines

None known.

4.8 Undesirable effects

Side effects are uncommon and mainly of a mild and transitory nature.

Gastrointestinal reactions:

Diarrhoea, indigestion, nausea, vomiting, and mucocutaneous candidiasis have been reported. Antibiotic-associated colitis (including pseudomembranous colitis and haemorrhagic colitis) has been reported rarely. Nausea, although uncommon, is more often associated with higher oral dosages. If gastrointestinal side effects occur with oral therapy they may be reduced by taking Augmentin at the start of meals.

Superficial tooth discolouration has been reported rarely, mostly with the suspension. It can usually be removed by brushing.

Renal and urinary tract disorders:

Crystalluria has been reported very rarely (see Section 4.9 Overdose).

Genito-urinary effects:

Vaginal itching, soreness and discharge may occur.

Hepatic effects:

Moderate and asymptomatic rises in AST and/or ALT and alkaline phosphatases have been reported occasionally. Hepatitis and cholestatic jaundice have been reported rarely. These hepatic reactions have been reported more commonly with Augmentin than with other penicillins.

After Augmentin hepatic reactions have been reported more frequently in males and elderly patients, particularly those over 65 years. The risk increases with duration of treatment longer than 14 days.

Signs and symptoms usually occur during or shortly after treatment but in some cases may not occur until several weeks after treatment has ended. Hepatic reactions are usually reversible but they may be severe and, very rarely, deaths have been reported.

Hypersensitivity reactions:

Urticarial and erythematous skin rashes sometimes occur. Rarely erythema multiforme, Stevens-Johnson syndrome, toxic epidermal necrolysis, bullous exfoliative dermatitis, acute generalised exanthematous pustulosis (AGEF serum sickness-like syndrome and hypersensitivity vasc litis have been reported. Treatment should be discontinue if one of these disorders occurs. In common with other β lactam antibiotics angioedema and anaphylaxis have bee reported. Interstitial nephritis can occur rarely.

Haematological effects:

As with other β-lactams transient leucopenia (includin neutropenia and agranulocytosis), thrombocytopenia ar haemolytic anaemia have been reported rarely. Prolonga tion of bleeding time and prothrombin time has also bee reported rarely (see 4.5).

CNS effects:

CNS effects have been seen very rarely. These incluc reversible hyperactivity, dizziness, headache and convu sions. Convulsions may occur with impaired renal functic or in those receiving high doses.

4.9 Overdose

Gastrointestinal symptoms and disturbance of the fluid ar electrolyte balances may be evident. They may be treate symptomatically with attention to the water electroly balance. Augmentin may be removed from the circulatic by haemodialysis.

Amoxicillin crystalluria, in some cases leading to ren failure, has been observed (see Section 4.4 Special War ings and Precautions for Use).

5. PHARMACOLOGICAL PROPERTIES

5.1 Pharmacodynamic properties

Resistance to many antibiotics is caused by bacter enzymes which destroy the antibiotic before it can act c the pathogen. The clavulanate in Augmentin anticipat this defence mechanism by blocking the β-lactama enzymes, thus rendering the organisms sensitive to amo icillin's rapid bactericidal effect at concentrations read attainable in the body.

Clavulanate by itself has little antibacterial activity; hov ever, in association with amoxicillin as Augmentin, it pr duces an antibiotic agent of broad spectrum with wi application in hospital and general practice.

Augmentin is bactericidal to a wide range of organisn including:

Gram-positive

Aerobes: *Enterococcus faecalis**, *Enterococcus faeciun Streptococcus pneumoniae, Streptococcus pyogene Streptococcus viridans, Staphylococcus aureus**, *Coag lase negative staphylococci** (including *Staphylococc epidermidis**), *Corynebacterium* species, *Bacillus anth cis**, *Listeria monocytogenes.*

Anaerobes: *Clostridium* species, *Peptococcus* specie *Peptostreptococcus.*

Gram-negative

Aerobes: *Haemophilus influenzae**, *Moraxella catarrhal (Branhamella catarrhalis), Escherichia coli**, *Proteus m abilis**, *Proteus vulgaris**, *Klebsiella* species*, *Salmone* species*, *Shigella* species*, *Bordetella pertussis, Bruce* species, *Neisseria gonorrhoeae**, *Neisseria meningitidi Vibrio cholerae, Pasteurella multocida.*

Anaerobes: *Bacteroides* species* including *B. fragilis.*

* Some members of these species of bacteria produ beta-lactamase, rendering them insensitive to amoxici alone.

5.2 Pharmacokinetic properties

The pharmacokinetics of the two components of Augme tin are closely matched. Peak serum levels of both occ about one hour after oral administration. Absorption Augmentin is optimised at the start of a meal. Both clav lanate and amoxicillin have low levels of serum bindir about 70% remains free in the serum.

Doubling the dosage of Augmentin approximately doub the serum levels achieved.

5.3 Preclinical safety data

Not relevant.

6. PHARMACEUTICAL PARTICULARS

6.1 List of excipients

Augmentin 625 mg tablets:

Each tablet contains

Magnesium stearate,

Sodium starch glycollate

Colloidal silica

Microcrystalline cellulose

Titanium dioxide (E171)

Hydroxypropyl methylcellulose

Polyethylene glycol

Silicone oil

6.2 Incompatibilities

None

6.3 Shelf life

Augmentin 625 mg Tablets	Blister enclosed in pouch 24 months, Glass Bottles 36 months

.4 Special precautions for storage
ugmentin 625 mg Tablets should be stored in a dry place t 25°C or below.

.5 Nature and contents of container
ugmentin 625 mg Tablets: Aluminium PVC/PVdC blister nclosed within an aluminium laminate pouch containing a esiccant sachet. Each pouch contains a plaque of 7 ablets. 3 pouches are enclosed within a carton to provide pack of 21 tablets. Tablets are also supplied amber glass ottles of 30, 50 100 or 500.

.6 Special precautions for disposal and other handling
ugmentin 625 mg Tablets: None.

dministrative Data

. MARKETING AUTHORISATION HOLDER
eecham Group plc
80 Great West Road
rentford
Aiddlesex
W8 9GS
rading as:
ilaxoSmithKline UK
tockley Park West
Jxbridge
Aiddlesex UB11 1BT

. MARKETING AUTHORISATION NUMBER(S)
L 00038/0362

. DATE OF FIRST AUTHORISATION/RENEWAL OF THE AUTHORISATION
16 November 2005

10. DATE OF REVISION OF THE TEXT
21 September 2007

11. Legal Status
POM

Augmentin Intravenous

(GlaxoSmithKline UK)

1. NAME OF THE MEDICINAL PRODUCT
Augmentin® Intravenous

2. QUALITATIVE AND QUANTITATIVE COMPOSITION
Vials of sterile powder providing co-amoxiclav 500/100 (600 mg Augmentin) or co-amoxiclav 1000/200 (1.2 g Augmentin). For reconstitution as an intravenous injection or infusion.

The amoxicillin is present as amoxicillin sodium and the clavulanic acid is present as potassium clavulanate.

3. PHARMACEUTICAL FORM
Powder for solution for injection or infusion.

4. CLINICAL PARTICULARS

4.1 Therapeutic indications
Augmentin is an antibiotic agent with a notably broad spectrum of activity against the commonly occurring bacterial pathogens in general practice and hospital. The β-lactamase inhibitory action of clavulanate extends the spectrum of amoxicillin to embrace a wider range of organisms, including many resistant to other β-lactam antibiotics.

Augmentin Intravenous is indicated for short-term treatment of bacterial infections at the following sites when amoxicillin-resistant β-lactamase-producing strains are suspected as the cause. In other situations, amoxicillin alone should be considered.

- *Upper Respiratory Tract Infections (including ENT)* in particular sinusitis, otitis media, recurrent tonsillitis. These infections are often caused by *Streptococcus pneumoniae, Haemophilus influenzae**, *Moraxella catarrhalis** and *Streptococcus pyogenes*.

- *Lower Respiratory Tract Infections* in particular acute exacerbations of chronic bronchitis (especially if considered severe), bronchopneumonia. These infections are often caused by *Streptococcus pneumoniae, Haemophilus influenzae** and *Moraxella catarrhalis**.

- *Genito-urinary Tract and Abdominal Infections* in particular cystitis (especially when recurrent or complicated - excluding prostatitis), septic abortion, pelvic or puerperal sepsis and intra-abdominal sepsis. These infections are often caused by *Enterobacteriaceae** (mainly *Escherichia coli**), *Staphylococcus saprophyticus, Enterococcus* species.*

- *Skin and Soft Tissue Infections* in particular cellulitis, animal bites and severe dental abscess with spreading cellulitis. These infections are often caused by *Staphylococcus aureus**, *Streptococcus pyogenes* and *Bacteroides* species*.

- *Prophylaxis of wound infection associated with surgical procedures* in particular gastrointestinal, pelvic, major head and neck surgery and after limb amputation for infection.

- A comprehensive list of sensitive organisms is provided in Section 5.

* Some members of these species of bacteria produce β-lactamase, rendering them insensitive to amoxicillin alone.

Mixed infections caused by amoxicillin-susceptible organisms in conjunction with Augmentin-susceptible β-lactamase-producing organisms may be treated with Augmentin. These infections should not require the addition of another antibiotic resistant to β-lactamases.

4.2 Posology and method of administration
Dosages for the treatment of infection

Adults and children over 12 years: Usually 1.2 g eight hourly. In more serious infections, increase frequency to six-hourly intervals.

Children 3 months-12 years: Usually 30 mg/kg * Augmentin eight hourly. In more serious infections, increase frequency to six-hourly intervals.

Children 0-3 months: 30 mg/kg* Augmentin every 12 hours in premature infants and in full-term infants during the perinatal period, increasing to eight hours thereafter.

*Each 30 mg Augmentin provides co-amoxiclav 25/5.

Adult dosage for surgical prophylaxis

The usual dose is 1.2 g Augmentin Intravenous given at the induction of anaesthesia. Operations where there is a high risk of infection, e.g. colorectal surgery, may require three, and up to four, doses of 1.2 g Augmentin Intravenous in a 24-hour period. These doses are usually given at 0, 8, 16 (and 24) hours. This regimen can be continued for several days if the procedure has a significantly increased risk of infection.

Clear clinical signs of infection at operation will require a normal course of intravenous or oral Augmentin therapy post-operatively.

Dosage in renal impairment

Adults

Mild impairment (creatinine clearance >30 ml/min)	Moderate impairment (creatinine clearance 10-30 ml/min)	Severe impairment (creatinine clearance <10 ml/min)
No change in dosage.	1.2 g IV stat., followed by 600 mg IV 12 hourly.	1.2 g IV stat., followed by 600 mg IV 24 hourly. Dialysis decreases serum concentrations of Augmentin and an additional 600 mg IV dose may need to be given during dialysis and at the end of dialysis.

Children

Similar reductions in dosage should be made for children.

Dosage in hepatic impairment

Dose with caution; monitor hepatic function at regular intervals.

There are, as yet, insufficient data on which to base a dosage recommendation.

Each 1.2 g vial of Augmentin contains 1.0 mmol of potassium and 2.7 mmol of sodium (approx).

Administration

Augmentin Intravenous may be administered either by intravenous injection or by intermittent infusion (see Section 6.6). It is not suitable for intramuscular administration.

Duration of therapy should be appropriate to the indication and should not exceed 14 days without review.

4.3 Contraindications
Penicillin hypersensitivity. Attention should be paid to possible cross-sensitivity with other β-lactam antibiotics, e.g. cephalosporins.

A previous history of Augmentin- or penicillin-associated jaundice/hepatic dysfunction.

4.4 Special warnings and precautions for use
Changes in liver function tests have been observed in some patients receiving Augmentin. The clinical significance of these changes is uncertain but Augmentin should be used with caution in patients with evidence of hepatic dysfunction.

Cholestatic jaundice, which may be severe, but is usually reversible, has been reported rarely. Signs and symptoms may not become apparent for several weeks after treatment has ceased.

In patients with renal impairment, dosage should be adjusted according to the degree of impairment (see Section 4.2).

The presence of clavulanic acid in Augmentin may cause a non-specific binding of IgG and albumin by red cell membranes leading to a false positive Coombs test.

If the parenteral administration of high doses is necessary, the sodium content must be taken into account in patients on a sodium restricted diet.

In patients with reduced urine output crystalluria has been observed very rarely, predominantly with parenteral therapy. During administration of high doses of amoxicillin it is advisable to maintain adequate fluid intake and urinary output in order to reduce the possibility of amoxicillin crystalluria (see Section 4.9 Overdose). Amoxicillin has been reported to precipitate in bladder catheters after intravenous administration of large doses. A regular check of patency should be maintained.

Serious and occasionally fatal hypersensitivity (anaphylactoid) reactions have been reported in patients on penicillin therapy. These reactions are more likely to occur in individuals with a history of penicillin hypersensitivity (see Section 4.3).

Erythematous rashes have been associated with glandular fever in patients receiving amoxicillin.

Prolonged use may also occasionally result in overgrowth of non-susceptible organisms.

4.5 Interaction with other medicinal products and other forms of interaction
Probenecid decreases the renal tubular secretion of amoxicillin. Concurrent use with Augmentin may result in increased and prolonged blood levels of amoxicillin, but not of clavulanic acid.

Prolongation of bleeding time and prothrombin time have been reported in some patients receiving Augmentin. Augmentin should be used with care in patients on anti-coagulation therapy.

In common with other antibiotics, Augmentin may affect the gut flora, leading to lower oestrogen reabsorption and reduced efficacy of combined oral contraceptives. Therefore, alternative non-hormonal methods of contraception are recommended.

Penicillins reduce the excretion of methotrexate (potential increase in toxicity).

Concomitant use of allopurinol during treatment with amoxicillin can increase the likelihood of allergic skin reactions. There are no data on the concomitant use of Augmentin and allopurinol.

The presence of clavulanic acid in Augmentin may cause a non-specific binding of IgG and albumin by red cell membranes leading to a false positive Coombs test.

4.6 Pregnancy and lactation
Reproduction studies in animals (mice and rats) with orally and parenterally administered Augmentin have shown no teratogenic effects. In a single study in women with preterm, premature rupture of the foetal membrane (pPROM), it was reported that prophylactic treatment with Augmentin may be associated with an increased risk of necrotising enterocolitis in neonates. As with all medicines, use should be avoided in pregnancy, especially during the first trimester, unless considered essential by the physician.

Augmentin may be administered during the period of lactation. With the exception of the risk of sensitisation, associated with the excretion of trace quantities in breast milk, there are no known detrimental effects for the breast-fed infant.

4.7 Effects on ability to drive and use machines
None known.

4.8 Undesirable effects
The following convention has been utilised for the classification of undesirable effects: -

Very common (>1/10), common (>1/100, <1/10), uncommon (>1/1000, <1/100), rare (>1/10,000, <1/1000), very rare (<1/10,000)

The majority of side effects listed below are not unique to Augmentin and may occur when using other penicillins.

Infections and infestations

Common: Mucocutaneous candidiasis

Blood and lymphatic system disorders

Rare: Reversible leucopenia (including neutropenia) and thrombocytopenia

Very rare: Reversible agranulocytosis and haemolytic anaemia.

Prolongation of bleeding time and prothrombin time (see section 4.5)

Immune system disorders

Very rare: As with other antibiotics, severe allergic reactions, including angioneurotic oedema, anaphylaxis, serum sickness-like syndrome and hypersensitivity vasculitis.

If hypersensitivity reaction is reported, the treatment must be discontinued.

Nervous system disorders

Uncommon: Dizziness, headache

Very rare: Convulsions may occur in patients with impaired renal function or in those receiving high doses.

Vascular disorders

Rare: Thrombophlebitis at the site of injection

Gastrointestinal disorders

Common: Diarrhoea

Uncommon: Nausea, vomiting, indigestion

Very rare: Antibiotic associated colitis (including pseudomembraneous colitis and haemorrhagic colitis), less likely to occur after parenteral administration.

Hepato-biliary disorders

Uncommon: Moderate rise in AST and/or ALT, the significance is unknown.

Very rare: Hepatitis and cholestatic jaundice

Hepatic events have been reported predominately in males and elderly patients and may be associated with prolonged treatment

Signs and symptoms usually occur during or shortly after treatment but in some cases may not become apparent until several weeks after treatment has ceased. These are usually reversible. Hepatic events may be severe and in extremely rare circumstances, deaths have been reported.

Skin and subcutaneous tissue disorders

Uncommon: Skin rash, pruritus, urticaria

Rare: Erythema multiforme

Very rare: Stevens-Johnson syndrome, toxic epidermal necrolysis, Bullous exfoliative-dermatitis, acute generalised exanthemous pustulosis (AGEP)

If any hypersensitivity dermatitis reaction is reported, the treatment must be discontinued.

Renal and urinary disorders

Very rare: Interstitial nephritis, Crystalluria (see Section 4.4 and 4.9)

4.9 Overdose

Gastrointestinal symptoms and disturbance of the fluid and electrolyte balances may be evident. They may be treated symptomatically with attention to the water electrolyte balance. Augmentin may be removed from the circulation by haemodialysis.

Amoxicillin crystalluria, in some cases leading to renal failure, has been observed (see Section 4.4 Special Warnings and Special Precautions for Use)

5. PHARMACOLOGICAL PROPERTIES

5.1 Pharmacodynamic properties

Resistance to many antibiotics is caused by bacterial enzymes which destroy the antibiotic before it can act on the pathogen. The clavulanate in Augmentin anticipates this defence mechanism by blocking the β-lactamase enzymes, thus rendering the organisms sensitive to amoxicillin's rapid bactericidal effect at concentrations readily attainable in the body.

Clavulanate by itself has little antibacterial activity; however, in association with amoxicillin as Augmentin, it produces an antibiotic agent of broad spectrum with wide application in hospital and general practice.

Augmentin is bactericidal to a wide range of organisms including:

Gram-positive

Aerobes: *Enterococcus faecalis**, *Enterococcus faecium**, *Streptococcus pneumoniae, Streptococcus pyogenes, Streptococcus viridans, Staphylococcus aureus**, Coagulase negative *staphylococci** (including *Staphylococcus epidermidis**), *Corynebacterium* species, *Bacillus anthracis**, *Listeria monocytogenes.*

Anaerobes: *Clostridium* species, *Peptococcus* species, *Peptostreptococcus.*

Gram-negative

Aerobes: *Haemophilus influenzae**, *Moraxella catarrhalis** *(Branhamella catarrhalis), Escherichia coli**, *Proteus mirabilis**, *Proteus vulgaris**, *Klebsiella* species*, *Salmonella* species*, *Shigella* species*, *Bordetella pertussis, Brucella* species, *Neisseria gonorrhoeae**, *Neisseria meningitidis**, *Vibrio cholerae, Pasteurella multocida.*

Anaerobes: *Bacteroides* species* including *B. fragilis.*

* Some members of these species of bacteria produce β-lactamase, rendering them insensitive to amoxicillin alone.

5.2 Pharmacokinetic properties

The pharmacokinetics of the two components of Augmentin are closely matched. Both clavulanate and amoxicillin have low levels of serum binding; about 70% remains free in the serum.

Doubling the dosage of Augmentin approximately doubles the serum levels achieved.

5.3 Preclinical safety data

Not relevant

6. PHARMACEUTICAL PARTICULARS

6.1 List of excipients

None

6.2 Incompatibilities

Augmentin Intravenous should not be mixed with blood products, other proteinaceous fluids such as protein hydrolysates or with intravenous lipid emulsions.

If Augmentin is prescribed concurrently with an aminoglycoside, the antibiotics should not be mixed in the syringe, intravenous fluid container or giving set because loss of activity of the aminoglycoside can occur under these conditions.

6.3 Shelf life

Two years

6.4 Special precautions for storage

Augmentin vials should be stored in a dry place. Do not store above 25°C.

6.5 Nature and contents of container

Clear glass vials (Ph.Eur. Type I or Ph.Eur. Type III, moulded or tubular), of 10 ml or 25 ml nominal volume, fitted with chlorobutyl rubber bungs and aluminium overseals or chlorobutyl rubber bungs, aluminium overseals and flip-top lids.

6.6 Special precautions for disposal and other handling

600 mg vial: To reconstitute dissolve in 10 ml Water for Injections BP.

(Final volume 10.5 ml.)

1.2 g vial: To reconstitute dissolve in 20 ml Water for Injections BP.

(Final volume 20.9 ml.)

Augmentin Intravenous should be given by slow intravenous injection over a period of three to four minutes and used within 20 minutes of reconstitution. It may be injected directly into a vein or via a drip tube.

Alternatively, Augmentin Intravenous may be infused in Water for Injections BP or Sodium Chloride Intravenous Injection BP (0.9% w/v). Add, without delay, 600 mg reconstituted solution to 50 ml infusion fluid or 1.2 g reconstituted solution to 100 ml infusion fluid (e.g. using a minibag or in-line burette). Infuse over 30-40 minutes and complete within four hours of reconstitution. For other appropriate infusion fluids, see Package Enclosure Leaflet.

Any residual antibiotic solutions should be discarded.

Augmentin Intravenous is less stable in infusions containing glucose, dextran or bicarbonate. Reconstituted solution should, therefore, not be added to such infusions but may be injected into the drip tubing over a period of three to four minutes.

Administrative Data

7. MARKETING AUTHORISATION HOLDER

Beecham Group plc

980 Great West Road

Brentford

Middlesex TW8 9GS

Trading as:

GlaxoSmithKline UK

Stockley Park West

Uxbridge

Middlesex UB11 1BT

8. MARKETING AUTHORISATION NUMBER(S)

PL 00038/0320

9. DATE OF FIRST AUTHORISATION/RENEWAL OF THE AUTHORISATION

2 August 2002

10. DATE OF REVISION OF THE TEXT

10 July 2007

11. Legal Status

POM

Augmentin-Duo 400/57

(GlaxoSmithKline UK)

1. NAME OF THE MEDICINAL PRODUCT

Augmentin®-Duo 400/57.

2. QUALITATIVE AND QUANTITATIVE COMPOSITION

Augmentin-Duo 400/57 contains 400 mg amoxicillin and 57 mg clavulanic acid per 5ml (co-amoxiclav 400/57).

The amoxicillin is present as amoxicillin trihydrate and the clavulanic acid is present as potassium clavulanate.

3. PHARMACEUTICAL FORM

Dry powder for reconstitution in water, at time of dispensing, to form an oral sugar-free suspension.

4. CLINICAL PARTICULARS

4.1 Therapeutic indications

Augmentin-Duo 400/57 is an antibiotic agent with a notably broad spectrum of activity against the commonly occurring bacterial pathogens in general practice and hospital. The β-lactamase inhibitory action of clavulanate extends the spectrum of amoxicillin to embrace a wider range of organisms, including many resistant to other β-lactam antibiotics.

Augmentin-Duo 400/57, for twice-daily (b.i.d) oral dosing, is indicated for short-term treatment of bacterial infections at the following sites when amoxicillin resistant β-lactamase-producing strains are suspected as the cause. In other situations, amoxicillin alone should be considered.

- *Upper Respiratory Tract Infections (including ENT)* in particular sinusitis, otitis media, recurrent tonsillitis. These infections are often caused by *Streptococcus pneumoniae, Haemophilus influenzae**, *Moraxella catarrhalis** and *Streptococcus pyogenes.*

- *Lower Respiratory Tract Infections* in particular acute exacerbations of chronic bronchitis (especially if considered severe), bronchopneumonia. These infections are often caused by *Streptococcus pneumoniae, Haemophilus influenzae** and *Moraxella catarrhalis**.

- *Urinary Tract Infections* in particular cystitis (especially when recurrent or complicated - excluding prostatitis). These infections are often caused by *Enterobacteriaceae** (mainly *Escherichia coli**), *Staphylococcus saprophyticus, Enterococcus* species.*

- *Skin and Soft Tissue Infections* in particular cellulitis, animal bites and severe dental abscess with spreading cellulitis. These infections are often caused by *Staphylc coccus aureus**, *Streptococcus pyogenes* and *Bacteroide* species*.

- A comprehensive list of sensitive organisms is provided ; Section 5.

* Some members of these species of bacteria produce β lactamase, rendering them insensitive to amoxicillin alone

Mixed infections caused by amoxicillin-susceptible organ isms in conjunction with Augmentin-Duo 400/57-suscep tible β-lactamase-producing organisms may be treate with Augmentin-Duo 400/57. These infections should no require the addition of another antibiotic resistant to β lactamases.

4.2 Posology and method of administration

The usual recommended daily dosage is:

25/3.6 mg/kg/day in mild to moderate infections (uppe respiratory tract infections, e.g. recurrent tonsillitis, lowe respiratory infections and skin and soft tissue infections)

45/6.4 mg/kg/day for the treatment of more serious infec tions (upper respiratory tract infections, e.g. otitis media and sinusitis, lower respiratory tract infections, e.g bronchopneumonia and urinary tract infections)

The tables below give guidance for children.

Children over 2 years

25/3.6 mg/kg/day	2 - 6 years (13 - 21 kg)	2.5 ml Augmentin-Duo 400/57 Suspension b.i.d.
	7 - 12 years (22 - 40 kg)	5.0 ml Augmentin-Duo 400/57 Suspension b.i.d.
45/6.4 mg/kg/day	2 - 6 years (13 - 21 kg)	5.0 ml Augmentin-Duo 400/57 Suspension b.i.d.
	7 - 12 years (22 - 40 kg)	10.0 ml Augmentin-Duo 400/57 Suspension b.i.d.

Children aged 2 months to 2 years

Children under 2 years should be dosed according to body weight

Weight (kg)	25/3.6 mg/kg/day) (ml/b.i.d.*)	45/6.4 mg/kg/day (ml/b.i.d.*)
2	0.3	0.6
3	0.5	0.8
4	0.6	1.1
5	0.8	1.4
6	0.9	1.7
7	1.1	2.0
8	1.3	2.3
9	1.4	2.5
10	1.6	2.8
11	1.7	3.1
12	1.9	3.4
13	2.0	3.7
14	2.2	3.9
15	2.3	4.2

* The 35 ml presentation is supplied with a syringe dosing device - See Sections 6.5 and 6.6

There is insufficient experience with Augmentin-Duo' to make dosage recommendations for children under 2 months old.

Infants with immature kidney function

For children with immature renal function Augmentin-Duo 400/57 is not recommended.

Renal impairment

For children with a GFR of >30 ml/min no adjustment in dosage is required. For children with a GFR of <30 ml/min Augmentin-Duo 400/57 is not recommended.

Hepatic impairment

Dose with caution; monitor hepatic function at regular intervals. There is, as yet, insufficient evidence on which to base a dosage recommendation.

Method of administration

To minimise potential gastrointestinal intolerance, administer at the start of a meal. The absorption of co-amoxiclav is optimised when taken at the start of a meal. Duration of therapy should be appropriate to the indication and should not exceed 14 days without review. Therapy can be started parenterally and continued with an oral preparation.

4.3 Contraindications

Penicillin hypersensitivity.

Attention should be paid to possible cross-sensitivity with other β-lactam antibiotics, e.g. cephalosporins.

A previous history of co-amoxiclav- or penicillin-associated jaundice/hepatic dysfunction.

4.4 Special warnings and precautions for use

Changes in liver function tests have been observed in some patients receiving co-amoxiclav. The clinical significance of these changes is uncertain but co-amoxiclav should be used with caution in patients with evidence of hepatic dysfunction.

Cholestatic jaundice, which may be severe, but is usually reversible, has been reported rarely. Signs and symptoms ay not become apparent for several weeks after treatment has ceased.

patients with renal impairment, dosage should be djusted according to the degree of impairment (see Section 4.2). In patients with moderate or severe renal impairment Augmentin-Duo 400/57 is not recommended.

n patients with reduced urine output, crystalluria has been bserved very rarely, predominantly with parenteral therpy. During the administration of high doses of amoxicillin, is advisable to maintain adequate fluid intake and urinary utput in order to reduce the possibility of amoxicillin rystalluria (see Section 4.9 Overdose).

Serious and occasionally fatal hypersensitivity (anaphylacoid) reactions have been reported in patients on penicillin herapy. These reactions are more likely to occur in individuals with a history of penicillin hypersensitivity (see Section 4.3).

Erythematous rashes have been associated with glandular ever in patients receiving amoxicillin.

Prolonged use may also occasionally result in overgrowth of non-susceptible organisms.

Augmentin-Duo 400/57 contains 16.64 mg aspartame per 5 ml dose and therefore care should be taken in phenylketonuria.

4.5 Interaction with other medicinal products and other forms of interaction

Probenecid decreases the renal tubular secretion of amoxicillin. Concurrent use with co-amoxiclav may result in increased and prolonged blood levels of amoxicillin, but not of clavulanic acid.

Prolongation of bleeding time and prothrombin time have been reported in some patients receiving co-amoxiclav. Co-amoxiclav should be used with care in patients on anticoagulation therapy.

In common with other antibiotics, co-amoxiclav may affect the gut flora, leading to lower oestrogen reabsorption and reduced efficacy of combined oral contraceptives. See local/national guidelines or BNF for specific advice.

Concomitant use of allopurinol during treatment with amoxicillin can increase the likelihood of allergic skin reactions. There are no data on the concomitant use of co-amoxiclav and allopurinol.

Penicillins reduce the excretion of methotrexate (potential increase in toxicity).

4.6 Pregnancy and lactation

Use in pregnancy

Reproduction studies in animals (mice and rats) with orally and parenterally administered co-amoxiclav have shown no teratogenic effects In a single study in women with preterm, premature rupture of the foetal membrane (pPROM), it was reported that prophylactic treatment with Augmentin may be associated with an increased risk of necrotising enterocolitis in neonates. As with all medicines, use should be avoided in pregnancy, especially during the first trimester, unless considered essential by the physician.

Use in lactation

Co-amoxiclav may be administered during the period of lactation. With the exception of the risk of sensitisation, associated with the excretion of trace quantities in breast milk, there are no known detrimental effects for the breast-fed infant.

4.7 Effects on ability to drive and use machines

Adverse effects on the ability to drive or operate machinery have not been observed.

4.8 Undesirable effects

The following convention has been utilised for the classification of undesirable effects: -

Very common >1/10), common >1/100, <1/10), uncommon >1/1000, <1/100), rare >1/10,000, <1/1000), very rare (<1/10,000)

The majority of side effects listed below are not unique to co-amoxiclav and may occur when using other penicillins.

Infections and infestations

Common: Mucocutaneous candidiasis

Blood and lymphatic system disorders

Rare: Reversible leucopenia (including neutropenia) and thrombocytopenia

Very rare: Reversible agranulocytosis and haemolytic anaemia.

Prolongation of bleeding time and prothrombin time (see section 4.5)

Immune system disorders

Very rare: As with other antibiotics, severe allergic reactions, including angioneurotic oedema, anaphylaxis, serum sickness-like syndrome and hypersensitivity vasculitis.

If hypersensitivity reaction is reported, the treatment must be discontinued.

Nervous system disorders

Uncommon: Dizziness, headache

Very rare: Convulsions may occur in patients with impaired renal function or in those receiving high doses.

Gastrointestinal disorders

Adults

Very Common: Diarrhoea

Common: Nausea, vomiting

Children

Common: Diarrhoea, nausea, vomiting

All populations

Nausea is more often associated with higher oral dosages. If gastrointestinal side effects are evident, they may be reduce by taking co-amoxiclav at the start of a meal

Uncommon: Indigestion

Very rare: Antibiotic associated colitis (including pseudomembraneous colitis and haemorrhagic colitis)

Black hairy tongue

Superficial tooth discolouration has been reported in children. Good oral hygiene may help prevent tooth discolouration as it can usually be removed by brushing

Hepato-biliary disorders

Uncommon: Moderate rise in AST and/or ALT, the significance is unknown.

Very rare: Hepatitis and cholestatic jaundice

Hepatic events have been reported predominately in males and elderly patients and may be associated with prolonged treatment.

These events have been rarely reported in children.

Signs and symptoms usually occur during or shortly after treatment but in some cases may not become apparent until several weeks after treatment has ceased. These are usually reversible. Hepatic events may be severe and in extremely rare circumstances, deaths have been reported.

Skin and subcutaneous tissue disorders

Uncommon: Skin rash, pruritus, urticaria

Rare: Erythema multiforme

Very rare: Stevens-Johnson syndrome, toxic epidermal necrolysis, Bullous exfoliative-dermatitis, acute generalised exanthemous pustulosis (AGEP)

If any hypersensitivity dermatitis reaction is reported, the treatment must be discontinued.

Renal and urinary disorders

Very rare: Interstitial nephritis, Crystalluria (see Section 4.4 and 4.9)

4.9 Overdose

Overdosage

Gastrointestinal symptoms and disturbance of the fluid and electrolyte balances may be evident. They may be treated symptomatically, with attention to the water/electrolyte balance. Co-amoxiclav may be removed from the circulation by haemodialysis.

Amoxicillin crystalluria, in some cases leading to renal failure, has been observed (see Section 4.4 Special warnings and special precautions for use)

Drug abuse and dependence

Drug dependency, addiction and recreational abuse have not been reported as a problem with this compound.

5. PHARMACOLOGICAL PROPERTIES

Augmentin-Duo 400/57 contains a combination of amoxicillin and clavulanic acid, co-amoxiclav 400/57.

5.1 Pharmacodynamic properties

Microbiology

Amoxicillin is a semi-synthetic antibiotic with a broad spectrum of antibacterial activity against many Gram-positive and Gram-negative micro-organisms. Amoxicillin is, however, susceptible to degradation by β-lactamases and therefore the spectrum of activity of amoxicillin alone does not include organisms which produce these enzymes.

Clavulanic acid is a β-lactam, structurally related to the penicillins, which possesses the ability to inactivate a wide range of β-lactamase enzymes commonly found in micro-organisms resistant to penicillins and cephalosporins. In particular, it has good activity against the clinically important plasmid mediated beta-lactamases frequently responsible for transferred drug resistance. It is generally less effective against chromosomally-mediated type 1 β-lactamases.

The presence of clavulanic acid in Augmentin-Duo 400/57 protects amoxicillin from degradation by β-lactamase enzymes and effectively extends the antibacterial spectrum of amoxicillin to include many bacteria normally resistant to amoxicillin and other penicillins and cephalosporins. Thus Augmentin-Duo 400/57 possesses the distinctive properties of a broad spectrum antibiotic and a β-lactamase inhibitor. Augmentin-Duo 400/57 is bactericidal to a wide range of organisms including:

Gram-positive

Aerobes: *Enterococcus faecalis**, *Enterococcus faecium**, *Streptococcus pneumoniae*, *Streptococcus pyogenes*, *Streptococcus viridans*, *Staphylococcus aureus**, Coagulase negative *staphylococci** (including *Staphylococcus epidermidis**), *Corynebacterium* species, *Bacillus anthracis**, *Listeria monocytogenes*.

Anaerobes: *Clostridium* species, *Peptococcus* species, *Peptostreptococcus*.

Gram-negative

Aerobes: *Haemophilus influenzae**, *Moraxella catarrhalis** *(Branhamella catarrhalis)*, *Escherichia coli**, *Proteus mirabilis**, *Proteus vulgaris**, *Klebsiella* species*, *Salmonella* species*, *Shigella* species*, *Bordetella pertussis*, *Brucella* species, *Neisseria gonorrhoeae**, *Neisseria meningitidis**, *Vibrio cholerae*, *Pasteurella multocida*.

Anaerobes: *Bacteroides* species* including *B. fragilis*.

* Some members of these species of bacteria produce β-lactamase, rendering them insensitive to amoxicillin alone.

5.2 Pharmacokinetic properties

a. Absorption:

The two components of Augmentin-Duo 400/57, amoxicillin and clavulanic acid, are each fully dissociated in aqueous solution at physiological pH. Both components are rapidly and well absorbed by the oral route of administration. Absorption of co-amoxiclav is optimised when taken at the start of a meal.

b. Pharmacokinetics

Pharmacokinetic studies have been performed in children, including one study [25000/382] which has compared co-amoxiclav t.i.d and b.i.d. All of these data indicate that the elimination pharmacokinetics seen in adults also apply to children with mature kidney function.

The mean AUC values for amoxicillin are essentially the same following twice-a-day dosing with the 875/125 mg tablet or three-times-a-day dosing with the 500/125 mg tablet, in adults. No differences between the 875 mg bid and 500mg t.i.d dosing regimes are seen when comparing the amoxicillin $T_{½}$, or C_{max} after normalisation for the different doses of amoxicillin administered. Similarly, no differences are seen for the clavulanate $T_{½}$, C_{max} or AUC values after appropriate dose normalisation [Study 360].

The time of dosing of co-amoxiclav relative to the start of a meal has no marked effects on the pharmacokinetics of amoxicillin in adults. In a study of the 875/125 mg tablet [Study 362], the time of dosing relative to ingestion of a meal had a marked effect on the pharmacokinetics of clavulanate. For clavulanate AUC and C_{max}, the highest mean values and smallest inter-subject variabilities were achieved by administering co-amoxiclav at the start of a meal, compared to the fasting state or 30 or 150 minutes after the start of a meal.

The mean C_{max}, T_{max}, $T_{½}$ and AUC values for amoxicillin and clavulanic acid are given below for an 875 mg/125 mg dose of co-amoxiclav administered at the start of a meal [Study 362].

Mean Pharmacokinetic Parameters

(see Table 1 below)

Amoxicillin serum concentrations achieved with co-amoxiclav are similar to those produced by the oral administration of equivalent doses of amoxicillin alone.

c. Distribution:

Following intravenous administration therapeutic concentrations of both amoxicillin and clavulanic acid may be detected in the tissues and interstitial fluid. Therapeutic concentrations of both drugs have been found in gall bladder, abdominal tissue, skin, fat, and muscle tissues; fluids found to have therapeutic levels include synovial and peritoneal fluids, bile and pus.

Neither amoxicillin nor clavulanic acid is highly protein bound, studies show that about 25% for clavulanic acid and 18% for amoxicillin of total plasma drug content is bound to protein. From animal studies there is no evidence to suggest that either component accumulates in any organ.

Amoxicillin, like most penicillins, can be detected in breast milk. There are no data available on the passage of clavulanic acid into breast milk.

Reproduction studies in animals have shown that both amoxicillin and clavulanic acid penetrate the placental barrier. However, no evidence of impaired fertility or harm to the foetus was detected.

Table 1 Mean Pharmacokinetic Parameters

Drug Administration	Dose (mg)	C_{max} (mg/L)	T_{max}* (hours)	AUC (mg.h/L)	$T_{½}$ (hours)
AUGMENTIN 1 g					
Amoxicillin	875 mg	12.4	1.5	29.9	1.36
Clavulanic acid	125 mg	3.3	1.3	6.88	0.92

* Median values

Table 2

Fill Weight	Volume of water to be added to reconstitute	Nominal bottle size	Final volume of reconstituted oral suspension
6.3 g	32 ml	107 ml	35 ml
12.6 g	64 ml	147 ml	70 ml
25.2 g	127 ml	200 ml	140 ml

d. Elimination:

As with other penicillins, the major route of elimination for amoxicillin is via the kidney, whereas for clavulanate elimination is by both non-renal and renal mechanisms. Approximately 60-70% of the amoxicillin and approximately 40-65% of the clavulanic acid are excreted unchanged in urine during the first 6 hours after administration of a single 375 or 625 mg tablet.

Amoxicillin is also partly excreted in the urine as the inactive penicilloic acid in quantities equivalent to 10-25% of the initial dose. Clavulanic acid is extensively metabolised in man to 2,5-dihydro-4-(2- hydroxyethyl)-5-oxo-1H-pyrrole-3-carboxylic acid and 1-amino-4-hydroxy- butan-2-one and eliminated in urine and faeces and as carbon dioxide in expired air.

5.3 Preclinical safety data

No further information of relevance.

6. PHARMACEUTICAL PARTICULARS

6.1 List of excipients

Xantham gum, aspartame, colloidal silica, silicon dioxide, crospovidone, carmellose sodium, magnesium stearate, sodium benzoate, strawberry flavour.

6.2 Incompatibilities

None known.

6.3 Shelf life

Glass Bottles

Dry powder: 24 months when stored at temperatures at or below 25°C.

Reconstituted suspensions: seven days when stored in a refrigerator (2-8°C).

Sachets

18 months when stored at temperatures at or below 25°C.

6.4 Special precautions for storage

The dry powder should be stored in well-sealed containers in a dry place.

6.5 Nature and contents of container

Clear, glass bottles containing an off-white dry powder. The 35 ml presentation is supplied in a carton with a polystyrene syringe dosing device.

or

Single-dose sachets. Four sachets are supplied in a carton.

When reconstituted, an off-white suspension is formed

6.6 Special precautions for disposal and other handling

Glass bottles:

At time of dispensing, the dry powder should be reconstituted to form an oral suspension, as detailed below:

(see Table 2 above)

The 35 ml presentation is provided with a syringe dosing device which should be used in place of the cap following reconstitution. This device is used to dose patients under 2 years according to the schedule in Section 4.2.

Sachets:

Single-dose sachets contain powder for a 2.5 ml dose.

Directions for use: Check that the sachet is intact before use

1. Cut sachet along dotted line
2. Empty contents into a glass
3. Half fill sachet with water
4. Pour into the glass, stir well and drink immediately

If two or four sachets have to be taken at once then they can be mixed in the same glass.

Administrative Data

7. MARKETING AUTHORISATION HOLDER

SmithKline Beecham plc

980 Great West Road

Brentford

Middlesex TW8 9GS

Trading as:

GlaxoSmithKline UK

Stockley Park West

Uxbridge

Middlesex, UB11 1BT

8. MARKETING AUTHORISATION NUMBER(S)

PL 10592/0070

9. DATE OF FIRST AUTHORISATION/RENEWAL OF THE AUTHORISATION

2 January 2002

10. DATE OF REVISION OF THE TEXT

9 July 2007

11. Legal Status

POM

Avamys

(GlaxoSmithKline UK)

1. NAME OF THE MEDICINAL PRODUCT

AVAMYS▼ 27.5 micrograms/spray

nasal spray suspension

2. QUALITATIVE AND QUANTITATIVE COMPOSITION

Each spray actuation delivers 27.5 micrograms of fluticasone furoate.

For a full list of excipients, see section 6.1.

3. PHARMACEUTICAL FORM

Nasal spray, suspension.

White suspension.

4. CLINICAL PARTICULARS

4.1 Therapeutic indications

Adults, adolescents (12 years and over) and children (6 – 11 years)

Avamys is indicated for the treatment of:

- the symptoms of allergic rhinitis

4.2 Posology and method of administration

Avamys nasal spray is for administration by the intranasal route only.

For full therapeutic benefit regular, scheduled usage is recommended. Onset of action has been observed as early as 8 hours after initial administration. However, it may take several days of treatment to achieve maximum benefit, and the patient should be informed that their symptoms will improve with continuous regular use (see section 5.1). The duration of treatment should be restricted to the period that corresponds to allergenic exposure.

Adults and Adolescents (12 years and over)

The recommended starting dose is two spray actuations (27.5 micrograms of fluticasone furoate per spray actuation) in each nostril once daily (total daily dose, 110 micrograms).

Once adequate control of symptoms is achieved, dose reduction to one spray actuation in each nostril (total daily dose 55 micrograms) may be effective for maintenance.

The dose should be titrated to the lowest dose at which effective control of symptoms is maintained.

Children (6 to 11 years of age)

The recommended starting dose is one spray actuation (27.5 micrograms of fluticasone furoate per spray actuation) in each nostril once daily (total daily dose, 55 micrograms).

Patients not adequately responding to one spray actuation in each nostril once daily (total daily dose, 55 micrograms) may use two spray actuations in each nostril once daily (total daily dose, 110 micrograms).

Once adequate control of symptoms is achieved, dose reduction to one spray actuation in each nostril once daily (total daily dose, 55 micrograms) is recommended.

Children under 6 years of age: The experience in children under the age of 6 years is limited (see section 5.1 and 5.2). Safety and efficacy in this group has not been well established.

Elderly Patients: No dose adjustment is required in this population (see section 5.2).

Renal Impaired Patients: No dose adjustment is required in this population (see section 5.2).

Hepatic Impaired Patients: No dose adjustment is required in mild to moderate hepatic impairment. There are no data in patients with severe hepatic impairment (see section 4.4 and 5.2).

The intranasal device should be shaken before use. The device is primed by pressing the mist release button for at least six spray actuations (until a fine mist is seen), whilst holding the device upright. Re-priming (approximately 6 sprays until a fine mist is seen) is only necessary if the cap is left off for 5 days or the intranasal device has not been used for 30 days or more.

The device should be cleaned after each use and the cap replaced.

4.3 Contraindications

Hypersensitivity to the active substance or to any of the excipients of Avamys.

4.4 Special warnings and precautions for use

Avamys undergoes extensive first-pass metabolism, therefore the systemic exposure of intranasal fluticasone furoate in patients with severe liver disease is likely to increased. This may result in a higher frequency of systemic adverse events (see section 4.2 and 5.2). Caution advised when treating these patients.

Ritonavir

Concomitant administration with ritonavir is not recommended because of the risk of increased systemic exposure of fluticasone furoate (see section 4.5).

Systemic effects of nasal corticosteroid may occur, particularly at high doses prescribed for prolonged periods. These effects vary between patients and different corticosteroids (see section 5.2).

Treatment with higher than recommended doses of nasal corticosteroids may result in clinically significant adrenal suppression. If there is evidence for higher than recommended doses being used, then additional systemic corticosteroid cover should be considered during periods of stress or elective surgery. Fluticasone furoate 110 micrograms once daily was not associated with hypothalamic pituitary-adrenal (HPA) axis suppression in adult, adolescent or paediatric subjects. However the dose of intranasal fluticasone furoate should be reduced to the lowest dose at which effective control of the symptoms of rhinitis is maintained. As with all intranasal corticosteroids, the total systemic burden of corticosteroids should be considered whenever other forms of corticosteroid treatment are prescribed concurrently.

Growth retardation has been reported in children receiving some nasal corticosteroids at licensed doses. It is recommended that the height of children receiving prolonged treatment with nasal corticosteroids is regularly monitored. If growth is slowed, therapy should be reviewed with the aim of reducing the dose of nasal corticosteroid if possible, to the lowest dose at which effective control of symptoms is maintained. In addition, consideration should be given to referring the patient to a paediatric specialist (see section 5.1).

If there is any reason to believe that adrenal function is impaired, care must be taken when transferring patients from systemic steroid treatment to fluticasone furoate.

Nasal and inhaled corticosteroids may result in the development of glaucoma and/or cataracts. Therefore close monitoring is warranted in patients with a change in vision or with a history of increased intraocular pressure, glaucoma and/or cataracts.

Avamys contains benzalkonium chloride. It may cause irritation of the nasal mucosa.

4.5 Interaction with other medicinal products and other forms of interaction

Fluticasone furoate is rapidly cleared by extensive first pass metabolism mediated by the cytochrome P450 3A4.

Based on data with another glucocorticoid (fluticasone propionate), that is metabolised by CYP3A4, coadministration with ritonavir is not recommended because of the risk of increased systemic exposure of fluticasone furoate.

Caution is recommended when co-administering fluticasone furoate with potent CYP3A4 inhibitors as an increase in systemic exposure cannot be ruled out. In a drug interaction study of intranasal fluticasone furoate with the potent CYP3A4 inhibitor ketoconazole there were more subjects with measurable fluticasone furoate concentrations in the ketoconazole group (6 of the 20 subjects) compared to placebo (1 out of 20 subjects). This small increase in exposure did not result in a statistically significant difference in 24 hour serum cortisol levels between the two groups (see section 4.4).

The enzyme induction and inhibition data suggest that there is no theoretical basis for anticipating metabolic interactions between fluticasone furoate and the cytochrome P450 mediated metabolism of other compounds at clinically relevant intranasal doses. Therefore, no clinical studies have been conducted to investigate interactions of fluticasone furoate on other drugs.

4.6 Pregnancy and lactation

There are no adequate data from the use of fluticasone furoate in pregnant women. In animal studies glucocorticoids have been shown to induce malformations including cleft palate and intra-uterine growth retardation. This is not likely to be relevant for humans given recommended nasal doses which results in minimal systemic exposure (see section 5.2). Fluticasone furoate should be used in pregnancy only if the benefits to the mother outweigh the potential risks to the foetus or child.

It is unknown whether nasal administered fluticasone furoate is excreted in human breast milk.

Administration of fluticasone furoate to women who are breastfeeding should only be considered if the expected benefit to the mother is greater than any possible risk to the child.

4.7 Effects on ability to drive and use machines

No studies on the effects on the ability to drive and use machines have been performed as fluticasone furoate is not expected to affect this ability.

4.8 Undesirable effects

Data from large clinical trials were used to determine the frequency of adverse reactions.

The following convention has been used for the classification of frequencies: Very common ≥1/10; Common ≥1/

00 to < 1/10; Uncommon ⩾ 1/1000 to < 1/100; Rare ⩾ 1/ 0,000 to < 1/1000; Very rare < 1/10,000.

Respiratory, thoracic and mediastinal disorders	
Very common	Epistaxis
Common	Nasal ulceration

Epistaxis was generally mild to moderate in intensity. In adults and adolescents, the incidence of epistaxis was higher in longer-term use (more than 6 weeks) than in short-term use (up to 6 weeks). In paediatric clinical studies of up to 12 weeks duration the incidence of epistaxis was similar between patients receiving fluticasone furoate and patients receiving placebo.

Systemic effects of nasal corticosteroids may occur, particularly when prescribed at high doses for prolonged periods.

4.9 Overdose

In a bioavailability study, intranasal doses of up to 2640 micrograms per day were administered over three days with no adverse systemic effects observed (see section 5.2).

Acute overdose is unlikely to require any therapy other than observation.

5. PHARMACOLOGICAL PROPERTIES

5.1 Pharmacodynamic properties

Pharmacotherapeutic group: Corticosteroids. ATC code: R01AD12

Fluticasone furoate is a synthetic trifluorinated corticosteroid that possesses a very high affinity for the glucocorticoid receptor and has a potent anti-inflammatory action.

Clinical experience:

Seasonal Allergic Rhinitis in adults and adolescents

Compared with placebo, fluticasone furoate nasal spray 110 micrograms once daily significantly improved nasal symptoms (comprising rhinorrhoea, nasal congestion, sneezing and nasal itching) and ocular symptoms (comprising itching/burning, tearing/watering and redness of the eyes) in all 4 studies. Efficacy was maintained over the full 24-hours dosing period with once daily administration.

Onset of therapeutic benefit was observed as early as 8 hours after initial administration, with further improvement observed for several days afterwards.

Fluticasone furoate nasal spray significantly improved the patients' perception of overall response to therapy, and the patients' disease-related quality of life (Rhinoconjunctivitis Quality of Life Questionnaire – RQLQ), in all 4 studies.

Perennial Allergic Rhinitis in adults and adolescents:

Fluticasone furoate nasal spray 110 micrograms once daily significantly improved nasal symptoms as well as patients' perception of overall response to therapy compared to placebo in both studies.

Fluticasone furoate nasal spray 110 micrograms once daily significantly improved ocular symptoms as well as improving patients' disease-related quality of life (RQLQ) compared to placebo in one study.

Efficacy was maintained over the full 24-hour dosing period with once daily administration.

Seasonal and perennial allergic rhinitis in children:

The paediatric posology is based on assessment of the efficacy data across the allergic rhinitis population in children.

In seasonal allergic rhinitis, fluticasone furoate nasal spray 110 micrograms once daily was effective but no significant differences were observed between fluticasone furoate nasal spray 55 micrograms once daily and placebo on any endpoint.

In perennial allergic rhinitis, fluticasone furoate nasal spray 55 micrograms once daily exhibited a more consistent efficacy profile than fluticasone furoate nasal spray 110 micrograms once daily over 4 weeks' treatment. Post-hoc analysis over 6 and 12 weeks in the same study, as well as 6-week HPA axis safety study, supported the efficacy of fluticasone furoate nasal spray 110 micrograms once daily.

A 6-week study that assessed the effect of fluticasone furoate nasal spray 110 micrograms once daily on adrenal function in children aged 2 to 11 years showed that there was no significant effect on 24-hour serum cortisol profiles, compared with placebo.

Results from a placebo-controlled knemometry study of fluticasone furoate nasal spray 110 micrograms once daily revealed no clinically relevant effects on short-term lower leg growth rate in children (6 to 11 years).

Seasonal and perennial allergic rhinitis in children (under 6 years):

Safety and efficacy studies were performed in a total of 271 patients from 2 to 5 years of age in both seasonal and perennial allergic rhinitis, of whom 176 were exposed to fluticasone furoate.

Safety and efficacy in this group has not been well established.

5.2 Pharmacokinetic properties

Absorption: Fluticasone furoate undergoes incomplete absorption and extensive first-pass metabolism in the liver and gut resulting in negligible systemic exposure. The intranasal dosing of 110 micrograms once daily does not typically result in measurable plasma concentrations (< 10 pg/ml). The absolute bioavailability for intranasal fluticasone furoate is 0.50 %, such that less than 1 microgram of fluticasone furoate would be systemically available after administration of 110 micrograms (see section 4.9).

Distribution: The plasma protein binding of fluticasone furoate is greater than 99 %. Fluticasone furoate is widely distributed with volume of distribution at steady-state of, on average, 608 l.

Metabolism: Fluticasone furoate is rapidly cleared (total plasma clearance of 58.7 l/h) from systemic circulation principally by hepatic metabolism to an inactive 17β-carboxylic metabolite (GW694301X), by the cytochrome P450 enzyme CYP3A4. The principal route of metabolism was hydrolysis of the Sfluoromethyl carbothioate function to form the 17β-carboxylic acid metabolite. In vivo studies have revealed no evidence of cleavage of the furoate moiety to form fluticasone.

Elimination: Elimination was primarily via the faecal route following oral and intravenous administration indicative of excretion of fluticasone furoate and its metabolites via the bile. Following intravenous administration, the elimination phase half-life averaged 15.1 hours. Urinary excretion accounted for approximately 1 % and 2 % of the orally and intravenously administered dose, respectively.

Children:

In the majority of patients fluticasone furoate is not quantifiable (< 10 pg/ml) following intranasal dosing of 110 micrograms once daily. Quantifiable levels were observed in 15.1 % of paediatric patients following intranasal dosing of 110 micrograms once daily and only 6.8 % of paediatric patients following 55 micrograms once daily. There was no evidence for higher quantifiable levels of fluticasone furoate in younger children (less than 6 years of age). Median fluticasone furoate concentrations in those subjects with quantifiable levels at 55 micrograms were 18.4 pg/ml and 18.9 pg/ml for 2-5 yrs and 6-11 yrs, respectively.

At 110 micrograms, median concentrations in those subjects with quantifiable levels were 14.3 pg/ml and 14.4 pg/ml for 2-5 yrs and 6-11 yrs, respectively. The values are similar to those seen in adults (12+) where median concentrations in those subjects with quantifiable levels were 15.4 pg/ml and 21.8 pg/ml at 55 micrograms and 110 micrograms, respectively.

Elderly:

Only a small number of elderly patients (⩾65 years, n=23/872; 2.6 %) provided pharmacokinetic data. There was no evidence for a higher incidence of patients with quantifiable fluticasone furoate concentrations in the elderly, when compared with the younger patients.

Renal Impairment:

Fluticasone furoate is not detectable in urine from healthy volunteers after intranasal dosing. Less than 1 % of dose-related material is excreted in urine and therefore renal impairment would not be expected to affect the pharmacokinetics of fluticasone furoate.

Hepatic Impairment:

There are no data with intranasal fluticasone furoate in patients with hepatic impairment. A study of a single 400 microgram dose of orally inhaled fluticasone furoate in patients with moderate hepatic impairment resulted in increased Cmax (42 %) and AUC(0-∞) (172 %) and a modest (on average 23 %) decrease in cortisol levels in patients compared to healthy subjects. From this study the average predicted exposure of 110 micrograms of intranasal fluticasone furoate in patients with moderate hepatic impairment would not be expected to result in suppression of cortisol. Therefore moderate hepatic impairment is not predicted to result in a clinically relevant effect for the normal adult dose. There are no data in patients with severe hepatic impairment. The exposure of fluticasone furoate is likely to be further increased in such patients.

5.3 Preclinical safety data

Findings in general toxicology studies were similar to those observed with other glucocorticoids and are associated with exaggerated pharmacological activity. These findings are not likely to be relevant for humans given recommended nasal doses which results in minimal systemic exposure. No genotoxic effects of fluticasone furoate have been observed in conventional genotoxicity tests. Further, there were no treatment-related increases in the incidence of tumours in two year inhalation studies in rats and mice.

6. PHARMACEUTICAL PARTICULARS

6.1 List of excipients

Glucose anhydrous

Dispersible cellulose

Polysorbate 80

Benzalkonium chloride

Disodium edetate

Purified water

6.2 Incompatibilities

Not applicable.

6.3 Shelf life

3 years

In-use shelf life: 2 months

6.4 Special precautions for storage

Do not refrigerate or freeze.

6.5 Nature and contents of container

Avamys nasal spray is a predominantly off-white plastic device with a dose indicator window, light blue side actuated lever and lid which contains a stopper. The plastic device contains the nasal spray suspension within a Type I amber bottle (glass) fitted with a metering spray pump.

The medicinal product is available in three pack sizes: 30, 60 and 120 sprays.

Not all pack sizes may be marketed.

6.6 Special precautions for disposal and other handling

No special requirements.

7. MARKETING AUTHORISATION HOLDER

Glaxo Group Ltd

Greenford, Middlesex, UB6 0NN

United Kingdom

8. MARKETING AUTHORISATION NUMBER(S)

EU/1/07/434/001 - 003

9. DATE OF FIRST AUTHORISATION/RENEWAL OF THE AUTHORISATION

11 January 2008

10. DATE OF REVISION OF THE TEXT

02 June 2009

Detailed information on this medicine is available on the European Medicines Agency (EMEA) website:

http://www.emea.europa.eu/

Avandamet Film-Coated Tablets

(GlaxoSmithKline UK)

1. NAME OF THE MEDICINAL PRODUCT

Avandamet 2 mg/500 mg film-coated tablets ▼.

Avandamet 2 mg/1000 mg film-coated tablets ▼.

Avandamet 4 mg/1000 mg film-coated tablets ▼.

2. QUALITATIVE AND QUANTITATIVE COMPOSITION

Each tablet contains rosiglitazone maleate corresponding to 2 or 4mg rosiglitazone in combination with metformin hydrochloride 500 mg or 1000 mg (corresponding to metformin free base 390 mg or 780 mg respectively).

Excipient

AVANDAMET 2 mg/500 mg and AVANDAMET 2 mg/1000 mg – Each tablet contains lactose (approximately 11 mg)

AVANDAMET 4 mg/1000 mg - Contains lactose (approximately 23 mg)

For a full list of excipients, see section 6.1.

3. PHARMACEUTICAL FORM

Film-coated tablet.

AVANDAMET 2 mg/500 mg - Pale pink film-coated tablets marked "gsk" on one side and "2/500" on the other.

AVANDAMET 2 mg/1000 mg - Yellow film-coated tablets marked "gsk" on one side and "2/1000" on the other.

AVANDAMET 4 mg/1000 mg - Pink film-coated tablets marked "gsk" on one side and "4/1000" on the other.

4. CLINICAL PARTICULARS

4.1 Therapeutic indications

AVANDAMET is indicated in the treatment of type 2 diabetes mellitus patients, particularly overweight patients:

- who are unable to achieve sufficient glycaemic control at their maximally tolerated dose of oral metformin alone.

- in triple oral therapy with sulphonylurea in patients with insufficient glycaemic control despite dual oral therapy with their maximally tolerated dose of metformin and a sulphonylurea (see section 4.4).

4.2 Posology and method of administration

For the different dosage regimens, AVANDAMET is available in appropriate strengths.

The usual starting dose of AVANDAMET is 4 mg/day rosiglitazone plus 2000 mg/day metformin hydrochloride.

Rosiglitazone can be increased to 8 mg/day after 8 weeks if greater glycaemic control is required. The maximum recommended daily dose of AVANDAMET is 8 mg rosiglitazone plus 2000 mg metformin hydrochloride.

The total daily dose of AVANDAMET should be given in two divided doses.

Dose titration with rosiglitazone (added to the optimal dose of metformin) may be considered before the patient is switched to AVANDAMET.

When clinically appropriate, direct change from metformin monotherapy to AVANDAMET may be considered.

Taking AVANDAMET with or just after food may reduce gastrointestinal symptoms associated with metformin.

Triple oral therapy (rosiglitazone, metformin and sulphonylurea) (see section 4.4)

- Patients on metformin and sulphonylurea: when appropriate AVANDAMET may be initiated at 4 mg/day rosiglitazone with the dose of metformin substituting that already being taken. An increase in the rosiglitazone component to 8 mg/day should be undertaken cautiously following appropriate clinical evaluation to assess the patient's risk of developing adverse reactions relating to fluid retention (see sections 4.4 and 4.8).

- Patients established on triple oral therapy: when appropriate, AVANDAMET may substitute rosiglitazone and metformin doses already being taken.

Where appropriate, AVANDAMET may be used to substitute concomitant rosiglitazone and metformin in existing dual or triple oral therapy to simplify treatment.

Elderly

As metformin is excreted via the kidney, and elderly patients have a tendency to decreased renal function, elderly patients taking AVANDAMET should have their renal function monitored regularly (see sections 4.3 and 4.4).

Patients with renal impairment

AVANDAMET should not be used in patients with renal failure or renal dysfunction e.g. serum creatinine levels > 135 μmol/l in males and > 110 μmol/l in females and/or creatinine clearance < 70 ml/min (see sections 4.3 and 4.4).

Children and adolescents

AVANDAMET is not recommended for use in children and adolescents below 18 years of age as there are no data available on its safety and efficacy in this age group (see sections 5.1 and 5.2).

4.3 Contraindications

AVANDAMET is contraindicated in patients with:

- hypersensitivity to rosiglitazone, metformin hydrochloride or to any of the excipients
- cardiac failure or history of cardiac failure (New York Heart Association (NYHA) stages I to IV)
- an Acute Coronary Syndrome (unstable angina, NSTEMI and STEMI) (see section 4.4)
- acute or chronic disease which may cause tissue hypoxia such as:
  - cardiac or respiratory failure
  - recent myocardial infarction
  - shock
- hepatic impairment
- acute alcohol intoxication, alcoholism (see section 4.4)
- diabetic ketoacidosis or diabetic pre-coma
- renal failure or renal dysfunction e.g. serum creatinine levels > 135 μmol/l in males and > 110 μmol/l in females and/or creatinine clearance < 70 ml/min (see section 4.4)
- acute conditions with the potential to alter renal function such as:
  - dehydration
  - severe infection
  - shock
  - intravascular administration of iodinated contrast agents (see section 4.4)
- lactation.

4.4 Special warnings and precautions for use

Lactic acidosis

Lactic acidosis is a very rare, but serious, metabolic complication that can occur due to metformin accumulation. Reported cases of lactic acidosis in patients on metformin have occurred primarily in diabetic patients with significant renal failure. The incidence of lactic acidosis can and should be reduced by also assessing other associated risk factors such as poorly controlled diabetes, ketosis, prolonged fasting, excessive alcohol intake, hepatic insufficiency and any conditions associated with hypoxia.

Diagnosis:

Lactic acidosis is characterised by acidotic dyspnoea, abdominal pain and hypothermia followed by coma. Diagnostic laboratory findings are decreased blood pH, plasma lactate levels above 5 mmol/l and an increased anion gap and lactate/pyruvate ratio. If metabolic acidosis is suspected, treatment with the medicinal product should be discontinued and the patient hospitalised immediately (see section 4.9).

Renal function

As metformin is excreted by the kidney, serum creatinine concentrations should be determined regularly:

- at least once a year in patients with normal renal function
- at least two to four times a year in patients with serum creatinine levels at the upper limit of normal and in elderly patients.

Decreased renal function in elderly patients is frequent and asymptomatic. Special caution should be exercised in situations where renal function may become impaired, for example when initiating antihypertensive or diuretic therapy or when starting treatment with an NSAID.

Fluid retention and cardiac failure

Thiazolidinediones can cause fluid retention which may exacerbate or precipitate signs or symptoms of congestive heart failure. Rosiglitazone can cause dose-dependent fluid retention. The possible contribution of fluid retention to weight gain should be individually assessed as rapid and excessive weight gain has been reported very rarely as a sign of fluid retention. All patients, particularly those receiving concurrent insulin but also sulphonylurea therapy, those at risk for heart failure, and those with reduced cardiac reserve, should be monitored for signs and symptoms of adverse reactions relating to fluid retention, including weight gain and heart failure. AVANDAMET must be discontinued if any deterioration in cardiac status occurs.

The use of AVANDAMET in combination with a sulphonylurea or insulin may be associated with increased risks of fluid retention and heart failure (see section 4.8). The decision to initiate AVANDAMET in combination with a sulphonylurea should include consideration of alternative therapies. Increased monitoring of the patient is recommended if AVANDAMET is used in combination particularly with insulin but also with a sulphonylurea.

Heart failure was also reported more frequently in patients with a history of heart failure, oedema and heart failure was also reported more frequently in elderly patients and in patients with mild or moderate renal failure. Caution should be exercised in patients over 75 years because of the limited experience in this patient group. Since NSAIDs, insulin and rosiglitazone are all associated with fluid retention, concomitant administration may increase the risk of oedema.

Combination with insulin

An increased incidence of cardiac failure has been observed in clinical trials when rosiglitazone is used in combination with insulin. Insulin and rosiglitazone are both associated with fluid retention, concomitant administration may increase the risk of oedema and could increase the risk of ischaemic heart disease. Insulin should only be added to established rosiglitazone therapy in exceptional cases and under close supervision.

Myocardial Ischaemia

The available data indicate that treatment with rosiglitazone may be associated with an increased risk of myocardial ischaemic events (see section 4.8). There are limited clinical trial data in patients with ischaemic heart disease and/or peripheral arterial disease. Therefore, as a precaution, the use of rosiglitazone is not recommended in these patients, particularly those with myocardial ischaemic symptoms.

Acute Coronary Syndrome (ACS)

Patients experiencing an ACS have not been studied in rosiglitazone controlled clinical trials. In view of the potential for development of heart failure in these patients, rosiglitazone should therefore not be initiated in patients having an acute coronary event and it should be discontinued during the acute phase (see section 4.3).

Monitoring of liver function

There have been rare reports of hepatocellular dysfunction during post-marketing experience with rosiglitazone (see section 4.8). There is limited experience with rosiglitazone in patients with elevated liver enzymes (ALT> 2.5 times the upper limit of normal). Therefore, liver enzymes should be checked prior to the initiation of therapy with AVANDAMET in all patients and periodically thereafter based on clinical judgement. Therapy with AVANDAMET should not be initiated in patients with increased baseline liver enzyme levels (ALT> 2.5 times the upper limit of normal) or with any other evidence of liver disease. If ALT levels are increased to > 3 times the upper limit of normal during AVANDAMET therapy, liver enzyme levels should be reassessed as soon as possible. If ALT levels remain > 3 times the upper limit of normal, therapy should be discontinued. If any patient develops symptoms suggesting hepatic dysfunction, which may include unexplained nausea, vomiting, abdominal pain, fatigue, anorexia and/or dark urine, liver enzymes should be checked. The decision whether to continue the patient on therapy with AVANDAMET should be guided by clinical judgement pending laboratory evaluations. If jaundice is observed, therapy should be discontinued.

Eye disorders

Post-marketing reports of new-onset or worsening diabetic macular oedema with decreased visual acuity have been reported with thiazolidinediones, including rosiglitazone. Many of these patients reported concurrent peripheral oedema. It is unclear whether or not there is a direct association between rosiglitazone and macular oedema but prescribers should be alert to the possibility of macular oedema if patients report disturbances in visual acuity and appropriate ophthalmologic referral should be considered.

Weight gain

In clinical trials with rosiglitazone there was evidence of dose-related weight gain, which was greater when used in combination with insulin. Therefore weight should be closely monitored, given that it may be attributable to fluid retention, which may be associated with cardiac failure.

Anaemia

Rosiglitazone treatment is associated with a dose-related reduction of haemoglobin levels. In patients with low haemoglobin levels before initiating therapy, there is an increased risk of anaemia during treatment with AVANDAMET.

Hypoglycaemia

Patients receiving AVANDAMET in combination with a sulphonylurea or insulin may be at risk for dose-related hypoglycaemia. Increased monitoring of the patient and a reduction in the dose of the concomitant agent may be necessary.

Surgery

As AVANDAMET contains metformin hydrochloride, the treatment should be discontinued 48 hours before elective surgery with general anaesthesia and should not usually be resumed earlier than 48 hours afterwards.

Administration of iodinated contrast agent

The intravascular administration of iodinated contrast agents in radiological studies can lead to renal failure. Therefore, due to the metformin active substance, AVANDAMET should be discontinued prior to, or at the time of the test and not reinstituted until 48 hours afterwards, and only after renal function has been re-evaluated and found to be normal (see section 4.5).

Bone disorders

In a long-term study an increased incidence of bone fractures (foot, hand and arm) was observed in female patients taking rosiglitazone as monotherapy (see section 4.8). This increased incidence was noted after the first year of treatment and remained during the course of the study. The risk of fracture should be considered in the care of patients, especially female patients, treated with rosiglitazone.

Other precautions

Premenopausal women have received rosiglitazone during clinical studies. Although hormonal imbalance has been seen in preclinical studies (see section 5.3), no significant undesirable effects associated with menstrual disorders have been observed. As a consequence of improving insulin sensitivity, resumption of ovulation may occur in patients who are anovulatory due to insulin resistance. Patients should be aware of the risk of pregnancy (see section 4.6).

AVANDAMET should be used with caution during concomitant administration of CYP2C8 inhibitors (e.g. gemfibrozil) or inducers (e.g. rifampicin), due to the effect on rosiglitazone pharmacokinetics (see section 4.5). Furthermore, AVANDAMET should be used with caution during concomitant administration of cationic medicinal productsthat are eliminated by renal tubular secretion (e.g. cimetidine) due to the effect on metformin pharmacokinetics (see section 4.5). Glycaemic control should be monitored closely. AVANDAMET dose adjustment within the recommended posology or changes in diabetic treatment should be considered.

All patients should continue their diet with regular distribution of carbohydrate intake during the day. Overweight patients should continue their energy-restricted diet.

The usual laboratory tests for diabetes monitoring should be performed regularly.

AVANDAMET tablets contain lactose and therefore should not be administered to patients with rare hereditary problems of galactose intolerance, the Lapp lactase deficiency or glucose-galactose malabsorption.

4.5 Interaction with other medicinal products and other forms of interaction

There have been no formal interaction studies for AVANDAMET, however the concomitant use of the active substances in patients in clinical studies and in widespread clinical use has not resulted in any unexpected interactions. The following statements reflect the information available on the individual active substances (rosiglitazone and metformin).

There is increased risk of lactic acidosis in acute alcohol intoxication (particularly in the case of fasting, malnutrition or hepatic insufficiency) due to the metformin active substance of AVANDAMET (see section 4.4). Avoid consumption of alcohol and medicinal products containing alcohol.

Cationic medicinal products that are eliminated by renal tubular secretion (e.g. cimetidine) may interact with metformin by competing for common renal tubular transport systems. A study conducted in seven normal healthy volunteers showed that cimetidine, administered as 400 mg twice daily, increased metformin systemic exposure (AUC) by 50% and C_{max} by 81%. Therefore, close monitoring of glycaemic control, dose adjustment within the recommended posology and changes in diabetic treatment should be considered when cationic medicinal productsthat are eliminated by renal tubular secretion are co-administered (see section 4.4).

In vitro studies demonstrate that rosiglitazone is predominantly metabolised by CYP2C8, with CYP2C9 as only a minor pathway.

Co-administration of rosiglitazone with gemfibrozil (an inhibitor of CYP2C8) resulted in a twofold increase in rosiglitazone plasma concentrations. Since there is a potential for an increase in the risk of dose-related adverse reactions, a decrease in rosiglitazone dose may be needed. Close monitoring of glycaemic control should be considered (see section 4.4).

Co-administration of rosiglitazone with rifampicin (an inducer of CYP2C8) resulted in a 66% decrease in rosiglitazone plasma concentrations. It cannot be excluded that other inducers (e.g. phenytoin, carbamazepine, phenobarbital, St John's wort) may also affect rosiglitazone exposure. The rosiglitazone dose may need to be increased. Close monitoring of glycaemic control should be considered (see section 4.4).

Clinically significant interactions with CYP2C9 substrates or inhibitors are not anticipated.

Concomitant administration of rosiglitazone with the oral antihyperglycaemic agents glibenclamide and acarbose did not result in any clinically relevant pharmacokinetic interactions.

No clinically relevant interactions with digoxin, the CYP2C9 substrate warfarin, the CYP3A4 substrates nifedipine, ethinylestradiol or norethindrone were observed after co-administration with rosiglitazone.

Intravascular administration of iodinated contrast agents may lead to renal failure, resulting in metformin accumulation and a risk of lactic acidosis. Metformin should be discontinued prior to, or at the time of the test and not reinstituted until 48 hours afterwards and only after renal function has been re-evaluated and found to be normal.

Combination requiring precautions for use

Glucocorticoids (given by systemic and local routes) beta-2-agonists, and diuretics have intrinsic hyperglycaemic activity. The patient should be informed and more frequent blood glucose monitoring performed, especially at the beginning of treatment. If necessary, the dosage of the antihyperglycaemic medicinal product should be adjusted during therapy with the other medicinal product and on its discontinuation.

ACE-inhibitors may decrease the blood glucose levels. If necessary, the dosage of the antihyperglycaemic medicinal product should be adjusted during therapy with the other medicinal product and on its discontinuation.

4.6 Pregnancy and lactation

Rosiglitazone has been reported to cross the human placenta and to be detected in foetal tissues. For AVANDAMET no preclinical or clinical data on exposed pregnancies or lactation are available.

There are no adequate data from the use of rosiglitazone in pregnant women. Studies in animals have shown reproductive toxicity (see section 5.3). The potential risk for humans is unknown.

Therefore, AVANDAMET should not be used during pregnancy. If a patient wishes to become pregnant or if pregnancy occurs, treatment with AVANDAMET should be discontinued unless the expected benefit to the mother outweighs the potential risk to the foetus.

Both rosiglitazone and metformin have been detected in the milk of experimental animals. It is not known whether breast-feeding will lead to exposure of the infant to the medicinal product. AVANDAMET must therefore not be used in women who are breast-feeding (see section 4.3).

4.7 Effects on ability to drive and use machines

AVANDAMET has no or negligible influence on the ability to drive and use machines.

4.8 Undesirable effects

Adverse reactions are presented below for each of the component parts of AVANDAMET. An adverse reaction is only presented for the fixed dose combination if it has not been seen in one of the component parts of AVANDAMET or if it occurred at a higher frequency than that listed for a component part.

Adverse reactions for each treatment regimen are presented below by system organ class and absolute frequency. For dose-related adverse reactions the frequency category reflects the higher dose of rosiglitazone. Frequency categories do not account for other factors including varying study duration, pre-existing conditions and baseline patient characteristics. Adverse reaction frequency categories assigned based on clinical trial experience may not reflect the frequency of adverse events occurring during normal clinical practice. Frequencies are defined as: very common (≥1/10), common (≥1/100 to <1/10), uncommon (≥1/1,000 to <1/100), rare (≥1/10,000 to <1/1000) and very rare (<1/10,000 including isolated reports).

AVANDAMET

Data from double-blind studies confirm that the safety profile of concomitant rosiglitazone and metformin is similar to that of the combined adverse reaction profile for the twomedicinal products. Data with AVANDAMET is also consistent with this combined adverse reaction profile.

Clinical trial data (addition of insulin to established AVANDAMET therapy)

In a single study (n=322) where insulin was added to patients established on AVANDAMET, no new adverse events were observed in excess of those already defined for either AVANDAMET or rosiglitazone combination therapies.

However, the risk of both fluid related adverse events and hypoglycaemia are increased when AVANDAMET is used in combination with insulin.

Rosiglitazone

Clinical trial data

Adverse reactions for each treatment regimen are presented below by system organ class and absolute frequency. For dose-related adverse reactions the frequency category reflects the higher dose of rosiglitazone. Frequency categories do not account for other factors including varying study duration, pre-existing conditions and baseline patient characteristics.

Table 1 lists adverse reactions identified from an integrated clinical trial population of over 5,000 rosiglitazone-treated patients. Within each system organ class, adverse reactions are presented in the table by decreasing frequency for the rosiglitazone monotherapy treatment regimen. Within each frequency grouping, adverse reactions are presented in order of decreasing seriousness.

Table 1. The frequency of adverse reactions identified from clinical trial data with rosiglitazone

(see Table 1 opposite)

In double-blind clinical trials with rosiglitazone the incidence of elevations of ALT greater than three times the upper limit of normal was equal to placebo (0.2%) and less than that of the active comparators (0.5% metformin/sulphonylureas). The incidence of all adverse events relating to liver and biliary systems was <1.5% in any treatment group and similar to placebo.

Post-marketing data

In addition to the adverse reactions identified from clinical trial data, the adverse reactions presented in Table 2 have been identified in post approval use of rosiglitazone.

Table 1 The frequency of adverse reactions identified from clinical trial data with rosiglitazone

Adverse reaction	Frequency of adverse reaction by treatment regimen		
	Rosiglitazone monotherapy	**Rosiglitazone with metformin**	**Rosiglitazone with metformin and sulphonylurea**
Blood and the lymphatic system disorders			
anaemia	Common	Common	Common
granulocytopaenia			Common
Metabolism and nutrition disorders			
hypercholesterolaemia[1]	Common	Common	Common
hypertriglyceridaemia	Common		
hyperlipaemia	Common	Common	Common
weight increase	Common	Common	Common
increased appetite	Common		
hypoglycaemia		Common	Very common
Nervous system disorders			
dizziness*		Common	
headache*			Common
Cardiac disorders			
cardiac failure[2]			Common
cardiac ischaemia[3]*	Common	Common	Common
Gastrointestinal disorders			
constipation	Common	Common	Common
Musculoskeletal and connective tissue disorders			
bone fractures[4]	Common		
myalgia*			Common
General disorders and administration site conditions			
oedema	Common	Common	Very common

*The frequency category for the background incidence of these events, as taken from placebo group data from clinical trials, is 'common'.

[1] Hypercholesterolaemia was reported in up to 5.3% of patients treated with rosiglitazone (monotherapy, dual or triple oral therapy). The elevated total cholesterol levels were associated with an increase in both LDLc and HDLc, but the ratio of total cholesterol: HDLc was unchanged or improved in long term studies. Overall, these increases were generally mild to moderate and usually did not require discontinuation of treatment.

[2] An increased incidence of heart failure has been observed when rosiglitazone was added to treatment regimens with a sulphonylurea (either as dual or triple therapy), and appeared higher with 8 mg rosiglitazone compared to 4 mg rosiglitazone (total daily dose). The incidence of heart failure on triple oral therapy was 1.4% in the main double blind study, compared to 0.4% for metformin plus sulphonylurea dual therapy. The incidence of heart failure in combination with insulin (rosiglitazone added to established insulin therapy) was 2.4%, compared to insulin alone, 1.1%.

[3] In a retrospective analysis of data from 42 pooled short-term clinical studies, the overall incidence of events typically associated with cardiac ischaemia was higher for rosiglitazone containing regimens, 2.00% versus combined active and placebo comparators, 1.53% [Hazard ratio 1.30 (95% confidence interval 1.004 - 1.69)]. This risk was increased when rosiglitazone was added to established insulin and in patients receiving nitrates for known ischaemic heart disease. In a large observational study where patients were well-matched at baseline, the incidence of the composite endpoint myocardial infarction and coronary revascularization was 17.46 events per 1000 person years for rosiglitazone containing regimens and 17.57 events per 1000 person years for other anti-diabetic agents [Hazard ratio 0.93 (95% confidence interval 0.80 - 1.10)]. Three large long-term prospective randomised controlled clinical trials (mean duration 41 months; 14,067 patients), comparing rosiglitazone to some other approved oral antidiabetic agents or placebo, have not confirmed or excluded this risk. In their entirety, the available data on the risk of myocardial ischaemia are inconclusive.

[4] In a long-term randomised (4 to 6 year) monotherapy study in recently diagnosed patients with type 2 diabetes mellitus, an increased incidence of bone fractures was noted after the first year of treatment in female patients taking rosiglitazone (9.3%, 2.7 patients per 100 patient years) vs metformin (5.1%, 1.5 patients per 100 patient years) or glyburide/glibenclamide (3.5%, 1.3 patients per 100 patient years). This increased risk remained during the course of the study. The majority of the fractures in the females who received rosiglitazone were reported in the foot, hand and arm.

Table 2. The frequency of adverse reactions identified from post-marketing data with rosiglitazone

Adverse reaction	Frequency
Metabolism and nutrition disorders	
rapid and excessive weight gain	Very rare
Immune system disorders (see Skin and subcutaneous tissue disorders)	
anaphylactic reaction	Very rare
Eye disorders	
macular oedema	Rare
Cardiac disorders	

congestive heart failure/pulmonary oedema	Rare
Hepatobiliary disorders	
hepatic dysfunction, primarily evidenced by elevated hepatic enzymes[5]	Rare
Skin and subcutaneous tissue disorders (see Immune system disorders)	
angioedema	Very rare
skin reactions (e.g. urticaria, pruritis, rash)	Very rare

[5]Rare cases of elevated liver enzymes and hepatocellular dysfunction have been reported. In very rare cases, a fatal outcome has been reported.

Metformin

Clinical Trial Data and Post-marketing data

Table 3 presents adverse reactions by system organ class and by frequency category. Frequency categories are based on information available from metformin Summary of Product Characteristics available in the EU.

Table 3. The frequency of metformin adverse reactions identified from clinical trial and post-marketing data

Adverse reaction	Frequency
Gastrointestinal disorders	
gastrointestinal symptoms[6]	Very common
Metabolism and nutrition disorders	
lactic acidosis	Very rare
vitamin B12 deficiency[7]	Very rare
Nervous system disorders	
metallic taste	Common
Hepatobiliary disorders	
liver function disorders	Very rare
hepatitis	Very rare
Skin and subcutaneous disorders	
urticaria	Very rare
erythema	Very rare
pruritis	Very rare

[6] Gastrointestinal symptoms such as nausea, vomiting, diarrhoea, abdominal pain and loss of appetite occur most frequently during initiation of therapy and resolve spontaneously in most cases.

[7] Long-term treatment with metformin has been associated with a decrease in vitamin B12 absorption which may very rarely result in clinically significant vitamin B12 deficiency (e.g. megaloblastic anaemia).

4.9 Overdose

No data are available with regard to overdose of AVANDAMET.

Limited data are available with regard to overdose of rosiglitazone in humans. In clinical studies in volunteers rosiglitazone has been administered at single oral doses of up to 20 mg and was well tolerated.

A large overdose of metformin (or coexisting risks of lactic acidosis) may lead to lactic acidosis which is a medical emergency and must be treated in hospital.

In the event of an overdose, it is recommended that appropriate supportive treatment is initiated as dictated by the patient's clinical status. The most effective method to remove lactate and metformin is haemodialysis, however rosiglitazone is highly protein bound and is not cleared by haemodialysis.

5. PHARMACOLOGICAL PROPERTIES

5.1 Pharmacodynamic properties

Pharmacotherapeutic group: Combinations of oral blood glucose loweringmedicinal products, ATC code: A10BD03

AVANDAMET combines two antihyperglycaemic agents with complimentary mechanisms of action to improve glycaemic control in patients with type 2 diabetes: rosiglitazone maleate, a member of the thiazolidinedione class and metformin hydrochloride, a member of the biguanide class. Thiazolidinediones act primarily by reducing insulin resistance and biguanides act primarily by decreasing endogenous hepatic glucose production.

Rosiglitazone

Rosiglitazone is a selective agonist at the PPARγ (peroxisome proliferator activated receptor gamma) nuclear receptor and is a member of the thiazolidinedione class of antihyperglycaemic agents. It reduces glycaemia by reducing insulin resistance at adipose tissue, skeletal muscle and liver.

The antihyperglycaemic activity of rosiglitazone has been demonstrated in a number of animal models of type 2 diabetes. In addition, rosiglitazone preserved β-cell function as shown by increased pancreatic islet mass and insulin content and prevented the development of overt hyperglycaemia in animal models of type 2 diabetes. Rosiglitazone did not stimulate pancreatic insulin secretion or induce hypoglycaemia in rats and mice. The major metabolite (a para-hydroxy-sulphate) with high affinity to the soluble human PPARγ, exhibited relatively high potency in a glucose tolerance assay in obese mice. The clinical relevance of this observation has not been fully elucidated.

In clinical trials, the glucose lowering effects observed with rosiglitazone are gradual in onset with near maximal reductions in fasting plasma glucose (FPG) evident following approximately 8 weeks of therapy. The improved glycaemic control is associated with reductions in both fasting and post-prandial glucose.

Rosiglitazone was associated with increases in weight. In mechanistic studies, the weight increase was predominantly shown to be due to increased subcutaneous fat with decreased visceral and intra-hepatic fat.

Consistent with the mechanism of action, rosiglitazone in combination with metformin reduced insulin resistance and improved pancreatic β-cell function. Improved glycaemic control was also associated with significant decreases in free fatty acids. As a consequence of different but complementary mechanisms of action, combination therapy of rosiglitazone with metformin resulted in additive effects on glycaemic control in type 2 diabetic patients.

In studies with a maximal duration of three years, rosiglitazone given once or twice daily in dual oral therapy with metformin produced a sustained improvement in glycaemic control (FPG and HbA1c). A more pronounced glucose-lowering effect was observed in obese patients. An outcome study has not been completed with rosiglitazone, therefore the long-term benefits associated with improved glycaemic control of rosiglitazone have not been demonstrated.

At 18 months, in an ongoing long term comparator study, rosiglitazone in dual oral therapy with metformin was non-inferior to the combination of sulphonylurea plus metformin for lowering HbA1c.

An active controlled clinical trial (rosiglitazone up to 8 mg daily or metformin up to 2,000 mg daily) of 24 weeks duration was performed in 197 children (10-17 years of age) with type 2 diabetes. Improvement in HbA1c from baseline achieved statistical significance only in the metformin group. Rosiglitazone failed to demonstrate non-inferiority to metformin. Following rosiglitazone treatment, there were no new safety concerns noted in children compared to adult patients with type 2 diabetes mellitus. No long-term efficacy and safety data are available in paediatric patients.

ADOPT (A Diabetes Outcome Progression Trial) was a multicentre, double-blind, controlled trial with a treatment duration of 4-6 years (median duration of 4 years), in which rosiglitazone at doses of 4 to 8 mg/day was compared to metformin (500 mg to 2000 mg/day) and glibenclamide (2.5 to 15 mg/day) in 4351 drug naive subjects recently diagnosed ($\leq$3 years) with type 2 diabetes. Rosiglitazone treatment significantly reduced the risk of reaching monotherapy failure (FPG $>$10.0 mmol/L) by 63% relative to glibenclamide (HR 0.37, CI 0.30-0.45) and by 32% relative to metformin (HR 0.68, CI 0.55-0.85) during the course of the study (up to 72 months of treatment). This translates to a cumulative incidence of treatment failure of 10.3% for rosiglitazone, 14.8% for metformin and 23.3% for glibenclamide treated patients. Overall, 43%, 47% and 42% of subjects in the rosiglitazone, glibenclamide and metformin groups respectively withdrew due to reasons other than monotherapy failure. The impact of these findings on disease progression or on microvascular or macrovascular outcomes has not been determined (see section 4.8). In this study, the adverse events observed were consistent with the known adverse event profile for each of the treatments, including continuing weight gain with rosiglitazone. An additional observation of an increased incidence of bone fractures was seen in women with rosiglitazone (see sections 4.4 and 4.8).

There are no studies completed assessing long-term cardiovascular outcome in patients receiving rosiglitazone in combination with metformin.

Metformin

Metformin is a biguanide with antihyperglycaemic effects, lowering both basal and postprandial plasma glucose. It does not stimulate insulin secretion and therefore does not produce hypoglycaemia.

Metformin may act via three mechanisms:

- by reduction of hepatic glucose production by inhibiting gluconeogenesis and glycogenolysis
- in muscle, by modestly increasing insulin sensitivity, improving peripheral glucose uptake and utilisation
- by delaying intestinal glucose absorption.

Metformin stimulates intracellular glycogen synthesis by acting on glycogen synthase.

Metformin increases the transport capacity of specific types of membrane glucose transporters (GLUT-1 and GLUT-4).

In humans, independently of its action on glycaemia, metformin has favourable effects on lipid metabolism. This has been shown at therapeutic doses in controlled, medium-term or long-term clinical studies: metformin reduces total cholesterol, LDLc and triglyceride levels.

The prospective randomised (UKPDS) study has established the long-term benefit of intensive blood glucose control in type 2 diabetes. Analysis of the results for overweight patients treated with metformin after failure of diet alone showed:

- a significant reduction of the absolute risk of any diabetes-related complication in the metformin group (29.8 events/1,000 patient-years) versus diet alone (43.3 events/1,000 patient-years), p=0.0023, and versus the combined sulphonylurea and insulin monotherapy groups (40.1 events/1,000 patient-years), p=0.0034
- a significant reduction of the absolute risk of diabetes-related mortality: metformin 7.5 events/1,000 patient-years, diet alone 12.7 events/1,000 patient-years, p=0.017
- a significant reduction of the absolute risk of overall mortality: metformin 13.5 events/1,000 patient-years versus diet alone 20.6 events/1,000 patient-years (p=0.011), and versus the combined sulphonylurea and insulin monotherapy groups 18.9 events/1,000 patient-years (p=0.021)
- a significant reduction in the absolute risk of myocardial infarction: metformin 11 events/1,000 patient-years, diet alone 18 events/1,000 patient-years (p=0.01).

5.2 Pharmacokinetic properties

AVANDAMET

Absorption

No statistically significant difference was observed between the absorption characteristics of rosiglitazone and metformin from the AVANDAMET tablet and those obtained from rosiglitazone maleate and metformin hydrochloride tablets, respectively.

Food had no effect on the AUC of rosiglitazone or metformin when AVANDAMET was administered to healthy volunteers. In the fed state, C_{max} was lower (22% rosiglitazone and 15% metformin) and t_{max} delayed (by approximately 1.5 h rosiglitazone and 0.5 h metformin). This food-effect is not considered clinically significant.

The following statements reflect the pharmacokinetic properties of the individual active substances of AVANDAMET.

Rosiglitazone

Absorption

Absolute bioavailability of rosiglitazone following both a 4 and an 8 mg oral dose is approximately 99%. Rosiglitazone plasma concentrations peak at around 1 h after dosing. Plasma concentrations are approximately dose proportional over the therapeutic dose range.

Administration of rosiglitazone with food resulted in no change in overall exposure (AUC), although a small decrease in C_{max} (approximately 20-28%) and a delay in t_{max} (approximately 1.75 h) were observed compared to dosing in the fasting state. These small changes are not clinically significant and, therefore, it is not necessary to administer rosiglitazone at any particular time in relation to meals. The absorption of rosiglitazone is not affected by increases in gastric pH.

Distribution

The volume of distribution of rosiglitazone is approximately 14 l in healthy volunteers. Plasma protein binding of rosiglitazone is high (approximately 99.8%) and is not influenced by concentration or age. The protein binding of the major metabolite (a para-hydroxy-sulphate) is very high ($>$ 99.99%).

Metabolism

Metabolism of rosiglitazone is extensive with no parent compound being excreted unchanged. The major routes of metabolism are N-demethylation and hydroxylation, followed by conjugation with sulphate and glucuronic acid. The contribution of the major metabolite (a para-hydroxy-sulphate) to the overall antihyperglycaemic activity of rosiglitazone has not been fully elucidated in man and it cannot be ruled out that the metabolite may contribute to the activity. However, this raises no safety concern regarding target or special populations as hepatic impairment is contraindicated and the phase III clinical studies included a considerable number of elderly patients and patients with mild to moderate renal impairment.

In vitro studies demonstrate that rosiglitazone is predominantly metabolised by CYP2C8, with a minor contribution by CYP2C9.

Since there is no significant *in vitro* inhibition of CYP1A2, 2A6, 2C19, 2D6, 2E1, 3A or 4A with rosiglitazone, there is a low probability of significant metabolism-based interactions with substances metabolised by these P450 enzymes. Rosiglitazone showed moderate inhibition of CYP2C8 (IC_{50} 18 μM) and low inhibition of CYP2C9 (IC_{50} 50 μM) *in vitro* (see section 4.5). An *in vivo* interaction study with warfarin indicated that rosiglitazone does not interact with CYP2C9 substrates *in vivo*.

Elimination

Total plasma clearance of rosiglitazone is around 3 l/h and the terminal elimination half-life of rosiglitazone is approximately 3-4 h. There is no evidence for unexpected ccumulation of rosiglitazone after once or twice daily dosing. The major route of excretion is the urine with approximately two-thirds of the dose being eliminated by this route, whereas faecal elimination accounts for approximately 25% of dose. No intact active substance is excreted in urine or faeces. The terminal half-life for radioactivity was about 130 h indicating that elimination of metabolites is very slow. Accumulation of the metabolites in plasma is expected upon repeated dosing, especially that of the major metabolite (a para-hydroxy-sulphate) for which an 8-fold accumulation is anticipated.

Special populations

Gender: In the pooled population pharmacokinetic analysis, there were no marked differences in the pharmacokinetics of rosiglitazone between males and females.

Elderly: In the pooled population pharmacokinetic analysis, age was not found to influence the pharmacokinetics of rosiglitazone to any significant extent.

Children and adolescents: Population pharmacokinetic analysis including 96 paediatric patients aged 10 to 18 years and weighing 35 to 178 kg suggested similar mean CL/F in children and adults. Individual CL/F in the paediatric population was in the same range as individual adult data. CL/F seemed to be independent of age, but increased with weight in the paediatric population.

Hepatic impairment: In cirrhotic patients with moderate (Child-Pugh B) hepatic impairment, unbound C_{max} and AUC were 2- and 3-fold higher than in normal subjects. The inter-subject variability was large, with a 7-fold difference in unbound AUC between patients.

Renal insufficiency: There are no clinically significant differences in the pharmacokinetics of rosiglitazone in patients with renal impairment or end stage renal disease on chronic dialysis.

Metformin

Absorption

After an oral dose of metformin, t_{max} is reached in 2.5 h. Absolute bioavailability of a 500 mg metformin tablet is approximately 50-60% in healthy subjects. After an oral dose, the non-absorbed fraction recovered in faeces was 20-30%.

After oral administration, metformin absorption is saturable and incomplete. It is assumed that the pharmacokinetics of metformin absorption is non-linear. At the usual metformin doses and dosing schedules, steady state plasma concentrations are reached within 24-48 h and are generally less than 1 μg/ml. In controlled clinical trials, maximum metformin plasma levels (C_{max}) did not exceed 4 μg/ml, even at maximum doses.

Food decreases the extent and slightly delays the absorption of metformin. Following administration of a dose of 850 mg, a 40% lower plasma peak concentration, a 25% decrease in AUC and a 35 min prolongation of time to peak plasma concentration was observed. The clinical relevance of this decrease is unknown.

Distribution

Plasma protein binding is negligible. Metformin partitions into erythrocytes. The blood peak is lower than the plasma peak and appears at approximately the same time. The red blood cells most likely represent a secondary compartment of distribution. The mean V_d ranged between 63 – 276 l.

Metabolism

Metformin is excreted unchanged in the urine. No metabolites have been identified in humans.

Elimination

Renal clearance of metformin is > 400 ml/min, indicating that metformin is eliminated by glomerular filtration and tubular secretion. Following an oral dose, the apparent terminal elimination half-life is approximately 6.5 h. When renal function is impaired, renal clearance is decreased in proportion to that of creatinine and thus the elimination half-life is prolonged, leading to increased levels of metformin in plasma.

5.3 Preclinical safety data

No animal studies have been conducted with the combined products in AVANDAMET. The following data are findings in studies performed with rosiglitazone or metformin individually.

Rosiglitazone

Undesirable effects observed in animal studies with possible relevance to clinical use were as follows: An increase in plasma volume accompanied by decrease in red cell parameters and increase in heart weight. Increases in liver weight, plasma ALT (dog only) and fat tissue were also observed. Similar effects have been seen with other thiazolidinediones.

In reproductive toxicity studies, administration of rosiglitazone to rats during mid-late gestation was associated with foetal death and retarded foetal development. In addition, rosiglitazone inhibited ovarian oestradiol and progesterone synthesis and lowered plasma levels of these hormones resulting in effects on oestrus/menstrual cycles and fertility (see section 4.4).

In an animal model for familial adenomatous polyposis (FAP), treatment with rosiglitazone at 200 times the pharmacologically active dose increased tumour multiplicity in the colon. The relevance of this finding is unknown. However, rosiglitazone promoted differentiation and reversal of mutagenic changes in human colon cancer cells *in vitro*. In addition, rosiglitazone was not genotoxic in a battery of *in vivo* and *in vitro* genotoxicity studies and there was no evidence of colon tumours in lifetime studies of rosiglitazone in two rodent species.

Metformin

Non-clinical data for metformin reveal no special hazard for humans based on conventional studies of safety pharmacology, repeated dose toxicity, genotoxicity, carcinogenic potential, toxicity to reproduction.

6. PHARMACEUTICAL PARTICULARS

6.1 List of excipients

Tablet-core:

Sodium starch glycollate, hypromellose (E464), microcrystalline cellulose (E460), lactose monohydrate, povidone (E1201), magnesium stearate.

Avandamet 2 mg/1000 mg film-coating:

Hypromellose (E464), titanium dioxide (E171), macrogol, iron oxide yellow (E172).

Avandamet 2 mg/500 mg and Avandamet 4 mg/1000 mg film-coating:

Hypromellose (E464), titanium dioxide (E171), macrogol, iron oxide red (E172).

6.2 Incompatibilities

Not applicable.

6.3 Shelf life

3 years.

6.4 Special precautions for storage

This medicinal product does not require any special storage conditions.

6.5 Nature and contents of container

Avandamet 2 mg/500 mg tablets:

Opaque blisters (PVC/PVdC/aluminium). Packs of 112 tablets.

Avandamet 2 mg/1000 mg and 4 mg/1000 mg tablets:

Opaque blisters (PVC/PVdC/aluminium). Packs of 56 tablets.

6.6 Special precautions for disposal and other handling

Any unused product should be disposed of in accordance with local requirements.

7. MARKETING AUTHORISATION HOLDER

SmithKline Beecham plc

980 Great West Road

Brentford, Middlesex

TW8 9GS

United Kingdom

8. MARKETING AUTHORISATION NUMBER(S)

EU/1/03/258/006 – Avandamet 2 mg/500 mg – 112 film-coated tablets.

EU/1/03/258/009 – Avandamet 2 mg/1000 mg – 56 film coated tablets

EU/1/03/258/012 – Avandamet 4 mg/1000 mg – 56 film-coated tablets

9. DATE OF FIRST AUTHORISATION/RENEWAL OF THE AUTHORISATION

Date of First Authorisation:

20 October 2003 - Avandamet 2 mg/500 mg

02 September 2004 – Avandamet 2 mg/1000 mg

02 September 2004 – Avandamet 4 mg/1000 mg

Date of latest renewal: 08 August 2008 (all presentations)

10. DATE OF REVISION OF THE TEXT

25 August 2009

Avandia 4mg & 8mg film-coated Tablets

(GlaxoSmithKline UK)

1. NAME OF THE MEDICINAL PRODUCT

AVANDIA 4 mg film-coated tablets.

AVANDIA 8 mg film-coated tablets.

2. QUALITATIVE AND QUANTITATIVE COMPOSITION

Each tablet contains rosiglitazone maleate corresponding to 4 or 8 mg rosiglitazone.

Excipient

AVANDIA 4 mg – contains lactose (approximately 105 mg).

AVANDIA 8 mg – contains lactose (approximately 209 mg).

For a full list of excipients, see section 6.1.

3. PHARMACEUTICAL FORM

Film-coated tablet.

AVANDIA 4 mg – orange film-coated tablets debossed with "GSK" on one side and "4" on the other side.

AVANDIA 8 mg – Red-brown film-coated tablets debossed with "GSK" on one side and "8" on the other side.

4. CLINICAL PARTICULARS

4.1 Therapeutic indications

Rosiglitazone is indicated in the treatment of type 2 diabetes mellitus:

as **monotherapy**

– in patients (particularly overweight patients) inadequately controlled by diet and exercise for whom metformin is inappropriate because of contraindications or intolerance

as **dual oral therapy** in combination with

– metformin, in patients (particularly overweight patients) with insufficient glycaemic control despite maximal tolerated dose of monotherapy with metformin

– a sulphonylurea, only in patients who show intolerance to metformin or for whom metformin is contraindicated, with insufficient glycaemic control despite monotherapy with a sulphonylurea

as **triple oral therapy** in combination with

– metformin and a sulphonylurea, in patients (particularly overweight patients) with insufficient glycaemic control despite dual oral therapy (see section 4.4).

4.2 Posology and method of administration

Rosiglitazone therapy is usually initiated at 4 mg/day. This dose can be increased to 8 mg/day after eight weeks if greater glycaemic control is required. In patients administered rosiglitazone in combination with a sulphonylurea, an increase in rosiglitazone to 8 mg/day should be undertaken cautiously following appropriate clinical evaluation to assess the patient's risk of developing adverse reactions relating to fluid retention (see 4.4 and 4.8).

Rosiglitazone may be given once or twice a day.

Rosiglitazone may be taken with or without food.

Elderly (see section 4.4 Fluid retention and cardiac failure)

No dose adjustment is required in the elderly.

Patients with renal impairment (see section 4.4 Fluid retention and cardiac failure)

No dose adjustment is required in patients with mild and moderate renal insufficiency. Limited data are available in patients with severe renal insufficiency (creatinine clearance < 30 ml/min) and therefore rosiglitazone should be used with caution in these patients.

Patients with hepatic impairment

Rosiglitazone should not be used in patients with hepatic impairment.

Children and adolescents

There are no data available on the use of rosiglitazone in patients under 10 years of age. For children aged 10 to 17 years, there are limited data on rosiglitazone as monotherapy (see sections 5.1 and 5.2). The available data do not support efficacy in the paediatric population and therefore such use is not recommended.

4.3 Contraindications

Use of rosiglitazone is contraindicated in patients with:

– known hypersensitivity to rosiglitazone or to any of the excipients

– cardiac failure or history of cardiac failure (NYHA class I to IV)

– an Acute Coronary Syndrome (unstable angina, NSTEMI and STEMI) (see section 4.4)

– hepatic impairment.

– diabetic ketoacidosis and diabetic pre-coma.

4.4 Special warnings and precautions for use

Fluid retention and cardiac failure

Thiazolidinediones can cause fluid retention which may exacerbate or precipitate signs or symptoms of congestive heart failure. Rosiglitazone can cause dose-dependent fluid retention. The possible contribution of fluid retention to weight gain should be individually assessed as rapid and excessive weight gain has been reported very rarely as a sign of fluid retention. All patients, particularly those receiving concurrent insulin or sulphonylurea therapy, those at risk for heart failure, and those with reduced cardiac reserve, should be monitored for signs and symptoms of adverse reactions relating to fluid retention, including weight gain and heart failure. Increased monitoring of the patient is recommended if rosiglitazone is used in combination with metformin and insulin. Rosiglitazone should be discontinued if any deterioration in cardiac status occurs. Heart failure was also reported more frequently in patients with a history of heart failure; oedema and heart failure was also reported more frequently in elderly patients and in patients with mild or moderate renal failure. Caution should be exercised in patients over 75 years because of the limited experience in this patient group. Since NSAIDs and rosiglitazone are associated with fluid retention, concomitant administration may increase the risk of oedema.

Combination with insulin

An increased incidence of cardiac failure has been observed in clinical trials when rosiglitazone is used in combination with insulin. Insulin and rosiglitazone are both associated with fluid retention, concomitant administration may increase the risk of oedema and could increase the risk of ischaemic heart disease. Insulin should only be added to established rosiglitazone therapy in exceptional cases and under close supervision.

Myocardial Ischaemia

The available data indicate that treatment with rosiglitazone may be associated with an increased risk of myocardial ischaemic events (see section 4.8). There are limited clinical trial data in patients with ischaemic heart disease and/or peripheral arterial disease. Therefore, as a precaution, the use of rosiglitazone is not recommended in these patients, particularly those with myocardial ischaemic symptoms.

Acute Coronary Syndrome (ACS)

Patients experiencing an ACS have not been studied in rosiglitazone controlled clinical trials. In view of the potential for development of heart failure in these patients, rosiglitazone should therefore not be initiated in patients having an acute coronary event and it should be discontinued during the acute phase (see section 4.3).

Monitoring of liver function

There have been rare reports of hepatocellular dysfunction during post-marketing experience (see section 4.8). There is limited experience with rosiglitazone in patients with elevated liver enzymes (ALT > 2.5X upper limit of normal). Therefore, liver enzymes should be checked prior to the initiation of therapy with rosiglitazone in all patients and periodically thereafter based on clinical judgement. Therapy with rosiglitazone should not be initiated in patients with increased baseline liver enzyme levels (ALT > 2.5X upper limit of normal) or with any other evidence of liver disease. If ALT levels are increased to > 3X upper limit of normal during rosiglitazone therapy, liver enzyme levels should be reassessed as soon as possible. If ALT levels remain > 3X the upper limit of normal, therapy should be discontinued. If any patient develops symptoms suggesting hepatic dysfunction, which may include unexplained nausea, vomiting, abdominal pain, fatigue, anorexia and/or dark urine, liver enzymes should be checked. The decision whether to continue the patient on therapy with rosiglitazone should be guided by clinical judgement pending laboratory evaluations. If jaundice is observed, drug therapy should be discontinued.

Eye disorders

Post-marketing reports of new-onset or worsening diabetic macular oedema with decreased visual acuity have been reported with thiazolidinediones, including rosiglitazone. Many of these patients reported concurrent peripheral oedema. It is unclear whether or not there is a direct association between rosiglitazone and macular oedema but prescribers should be alert to the possibility of macular oedema if patients report disturbances in visual acuity and appropriate ophthalmologic referral should be considered.

Weight gain

In clinical trials with rosiglitazone there was evidence of dose-related weight gain, which was greater when used in combination with insulin. Therefore weight should be closely monitored, given that it may be attributable to fluid retention, which may be associated with cardiac failure.

Anaemia

Rosiglitazone treatment is associated with a dose-related reduction of haemoglobin levels. In patients with low haemoglobin levels before initiating therapy, there is an increased risk of anaemia during treatment with rosiglitazone.

Hypoglycaemia

Patients receiving rosiglitazone in combination therapy with a sulphonylurea or with insulin may be at risk for dose-related hypoglycaemia. Increased monitoring of the patient and a reduction in the dose of the concomitant agent may be necessary.

Triple oral therapy

The use of rosiglitazone in triple oral therapy, in combination with metformin and a sulphonylurea, may be associated with increased risks for fluid retention and heart failure, as well as hypoglycaemia (see section 4.8). Increased monitoring of the patient is recommended and adjustment of the dose of sulphonylurea may be necessary. The decision to initiate triple oral therapy should include consideration of the alternative to switch the patient to insulin.

Bone disorders

In a long-term study an increased incidence of bone fractures (foot, hand and arm) was observed in female patients taking rosiglitazone as monotherapy (see section 4.8). This increased incidence was noted after the first year of treatment and remained during the course of the study. The risk of fracture should be considered in the care of patients, especially female patients, treated with rosiglitazone.

Others

Premenopausal women have received rosiglitazone during clinical studies. Although hormonal imbalance has been seen in preclinical studies (see section 5.3), no significant undesirable effects associated with menstrual disorders have been observed. As a consequence of improving insulin sensitivity, resumption of ovulation may occur in patients who are anovulatory due to insulin resistance. Patients should be aware of the risk of pregnancy and if a patient wishes to become pregnant or if pregnancy occurs the treatment should be discontinued (see section 4.6).

Rosiglitazone should be used with caution in patients with severe renal insufficiency (creatinine clearance < 30 ml/min).

Rosiglitazone should be used with caution during concomitant administration of CYP2C8 inhibitors (e.g. gemfibrozil) or inducers (e.g. rifampicin). Glycaemic control should be monitored closely. Rosiglitazone dose adjustment within the recommended posology or changes in diabetic treatment should be considered (see section 4.5).

AVANDIA tablets contain lactose and therefore should not be administered to patients with rare hereditary problems of galactose intolerance, the Lapp lactase deficiency or glucose-galactose malabsorption.

4.5 Interaction with other medicinal products and other forms of interaction

In vitro studies demonstrate that rosiglitazone is predominantly metabolised by CYP2C8, with CYP2C9 as only a minor pathway.

Co-administration of rosiglitazone with gemfibrozil (an inhibitor of CYP2C8) resulted in a twofold increase in rosiglitazone plasma concentrations. Since there is a potential for an increase in the risk of dose-related adverse reactions, a decrease in rosiglitazone dose may be needed. Close monitoring of glycaemic control should be considered (see section 4.4).

Co-administration of rosiglitazone with rifampicin (an inducer of CYP2C8) resulted in a 66% decrease in rosiglitazone plasma concentrations. It cannot be excluded that other inducers (e.g. phenytoin, carbamazepine, phenobarbital, St John's wort) may also affect rosiglitazone exposure. The rosiglitazone dose may need to be increased. Close monitoring of glycaemic control should be considered (see section 4.4).

Clinically significant interactions with CYP2C9 substrates or inhibitors are not anticipated.

Concomitant administration with the oral anti-diabetic agents metformin, glibenclamide and acarbose did not result in any clinically relevant pharmacokinetic interactions with rosiglitazone. Moderate ingestion of alcohol with rosiglitazone has no effect on glycaemic control.

Table 1 The frequency of adverse reactions identified from clinical trial data

Adverse reaction	Frequency of adverse reaction by treatment regimen			
	RSG	RSG + MET	RSG + SU	RSG +MET +SU
Blood and the lymphatic system disorders				
anaemia	Common	Common	Common	Common
leucopaenia			Common	
thrombocytopaenia			Common	
granulocytopaenia				Common
Metabolism and nutrition disorders				
hypercholesterolaemia[1]	Common	Common	Common	Common
hypertriglyceridaemia	Common		Common	
hyperlipaemia	Common	Common	Common	Common
weight increase	Common	Common	Common	Common
increased appetite	Common		Uncommon	
hypoglycaemia		Common	Very common	Very common
Nervous system disorders				
dizziness*		Common	Common	
headache*				Common
Cardiac disorders				
cardiac failure[2]			Common	Common
cardiac ischaemia[3]*	Common	Common	Common	Common
Gastrointestinal disorders				
constipation	Common	Common	Common	Common
Musculoskeletal and connective tissue disorders				
bone fractures[4]	Common			
myalgia*				Common
General disorders and administration site conditions				
oedema	Common	Common	Very common	Very common

RSG - Rosiglitazone monotherapy; RSG + MET - Rosiglitazone with metformin; RSG + SU - Rosiglitazone with sulphonylurea; RSG + MET + SU - Rosiglitazone with metformin and sulphonylurea

*The frequency category for the background incidence of these events, as taken from placebo group data from clinical trials, is 'common'.

[1] Hypercholesterolaemia was reported in up to 5.3% of patients treated with rosiglitazone (monotherapy, dual or triple oral therapy). The elevated total cholesterol levels were associated with increase in both LDLc and HDLc, but the ratio of total cholesterol: HDLc was unchanged or improved in long term studies. Overall, these increases were generally mild to moderate and usually did not require discontinuation of treatment.

[2] An increased incidence of heart failure has been observed when rosiglitazone was added to treatment regimens with a sulphonylurea (either as dual or triple therapy), and appeared higher with 8 mg rosiglitazone compared to 4 mg rosiglitazone (total daily dose). The incidence of heart failure on triple oral therapy was 1.4% in the main double blind study, compared to 0.4% for metformin plus sulphonylurea dual therapy. The incidence of heart failure in combination with insulin (rosiglitazone added to established insulin therapy) was 2.4%, compared to insulin alone, 1.1%. Moreover in patients with congestive heart failure NYHA class I-II, a placebo-controlled one-year trial demonstrated worsening or possible worsening of heart failure in 6.4% of patients treated with rosiglitazone, compared with 3.5% on placebo.

[3] In a retrospective analysis of data from 42 pooled short-term clinical studies, the overall incidence of events typically associated with cardiac ischaemia was higher for rosiglitazone containing regimens, 2.00% versus combined active and placebo comparators, 1.53% [Hazard ratio 1.30 (95% confidence interval 1.004 - 1.69)]. This risk was increased when rosiglitazone was added to established insulin and in patients receiving nitrates for known ischaemic heart disease. In a large observational study where patients were well-matched at baseline, the incidence of the composite endpoint myocardial infarction and coronary revascularization was 17.46 events per 1000 person years for rosiglitazone containing regimens and 17.57 events per 1000 person years for other anti-diabetic agents [Hazard ratio 0.93 (95% confidence interval 0.80 - 1.10)]. Three large long-term prospective randomised controlled clinical trials (mean duration 41 months; 14,067 patients), comparing rosiglitazone to some other approved oral antidiabetic agents or placebo, have not confirmed or excluded this risk. In their entirety, the available data on the risk of myocardial ischaemia are inconclusive.

[4] In a long-term randomised (4 to 6 year) monotherapy study in recently diagnosed patients with type 2 diabetes mellitus, an increased incidence of bone fractures was noted after the first year of treatment in female patients taking rosiglitazone (9.3%, 2.7 patients per 100 patient years) vs metformin (5.1%, 1.5 patients per 100 patient years) or glyburide/glibenclamide (3.5%, 1.3 patients per 100 patient years). This increased risk remained during the course of the study. The majority of the fractures in the females who received rosiglitazone were reported in the foot, hand and arm.

No clinically relevant interactions with digoxin, the CYP2C9 substrate warfarin, the CYP3A4 substrates nifedipine, ethinylestradiol or norethindrone were observed after co-administration with rosiglitazone.

4.6 Pregnancy and lactation

Rosiglitazone has been reported to cross the human placenta and to be detectable in the foetal tissues. There are no adequate data from the use of rosiglitazone in pregnant women. Studies in animals have shown reproductive toxicity (see section 5.3). The potential risk for humans is unknown. Rosiglitazone should not be used during pregnancy.

Rosiglitazone has been detected in the milk of experimental animals. It is not known whether breast-feeding will lead to exposure of the infant to drug. Rosiglitazone should therefore not be used in women who are breast-feeding.

4.7 Effects on ability to drive and use machines

AVANDIA has no or negligible influence on the ability to drive and use machines.

4.8 Undesirable effects

Clinical trial data

Adverse reactions for each treatment regimen are presented below by system organ class and absolute frequency. For dose-related adverse reactions the frequency category reflects the higher dose of rosiglitazone. Frequency categories do not account for other factors including varying study duration, pre-existing conditions and baseline patient characteristics. Adverse reaction frequency categories assigned based on clinical trial experience may not reflect the frequency of adverse events occurring during normal clinical practice. Frequencies are defined as: very common $\geqslant$ 1/10; common $\geqslant$ 1/100, < 1/10; and uncommon $\geqslant$ 1/1000, < 1/100.

Table 1 lists adverse reactions identified from an integrated clinical trial population of over 5,000 rosiglitazone-treated patients. Within each system organ class, adverse reactions are presented in the table by decreasing frequency for the rosiglitazone monotherapy treatment regimen. Within each frequency grouping, adverse reactions are presented in order of decreasing seriousness.

Table 1. The frequency of adverse reactions identified from clinical trial data

(see Table 1 on previous page)

In double-blind clinical trials with rosiglitazone the incidence of elevations of ALT greater than three times the upper limit of normal was equal to placebo (0.2%) and less than that of the active comparators (0.5% metformin/sulphonylureas). The incidence of all adverse events relating to liver and biliary systems was < 1.5% in any treatment group and similar to placebo.

Post-marketing data

In addition to the adverse reactions identified from clinical trial data, the adverse reactions presented in Table 2 have been identified in post approval use of rosiglitazone. Frequencies are defined as: rare $\geqslant$1/10,000, <1/1000 and very rare <1/10,000 including isolated reports.

Table 2. The frequency of adverse reactions identified from post-marketing data

Adverse reaction	Frequency
Metabolism and nutrition disorders	
rapid and excessive weight gain	Very rare
Immune system disorders (see Skin and subcutaneous tissue disorders)	
anaphylactic reaction	Very rare
Eye disorders	
macular oedema	Rare
Cardiac disorders	
congestive heart failure/pulmonary oedema	Rare
Hepatobiliary disorders	
hepatic dysfunction, primarily evidenced by elevated hepatic enzymes[5]	Rare
Skin and subcutaneous tissue disorders (see Immune system disorders)	
angioedema	Very rare
skin reactions (e.g. urticaria, pruritus, rash)	Very rare

[5] Rare cases of elevated liver enzymes and hepatocellular dysfunction have been reported. In very rare cases a fatal outcome has been reported.

4.9 Overdose

Limited data are available with regard to overdose in humans. In clinical studies in volunteers rosiglitazone has been administered at single oral doses of up to 20 mg and was well tolerated.

In the event of an overdose, it is recommended that appropriate supportive treatment should be initiated, as dictated by the patient's clinical status. Rosiglitazone is highly protein bound and is not cleared by haemodialysis.

5. PHARMACOLOGICAL PROPERTIES

5.1 Pharmacodynamic properties

Pharmacotherapeutic group: oral blood glucose lowering drugs, thiazolidinediones, ATC code: A10 BG 02

Rosiglitazone is a selective agonist at the PPARγ (peroxisomal proliferator activated receptor gamma) nuclear receptor and is a member of the thiazolidinedione class of anti-diabetic agents. It reduces glycaemia by reducing insulin resistance at adipose tissue, skeletal muscle and liver.

Preclinical data

The antihyperglycaemic activity of rosiglitazone has been demonstrated in a number of animal models of type 2 diabetes. In addition, rosiglitazone preserved β-cell function as shown by increased pancreatic islet mass and insulin content and prevented the development of overt hyperglycaemia in animal models of type 2 diabetes. Rosiglitazone did not stimulate pancreatic insulin secretion or induce hypoglycaemia in rats and mice. The major metabolite (para-hydroxy-sulphate) with high affinity to the soluble human PPARγ, exhibited relatively high potency in a glucose tolerance assay in obese mouse. The clinical relevance of this observation has not been fully elucidated.

Clinical trials data

The glucose lowering effects observed with rosiglitazone are gradual in onset with near maximal reductions in fasting plasma glucose (FPG) evident following approximately 8 weeks of therapy. The improved glycaemic control is associated with reductions in both fasting and post-prandial glucose.

Rosiglitazone was associated with increases in weight. In mechanistic studies, the weight increase was predominantly shown to be due to increased subcutaneous fat with decreased visceral and intra-hepatic fat.

Consistent with the mechanism of action, rosiglitazone reduced insulin resistance and improved pancreatic β-cell function. Improved glycaemic control was also associated with significant decreases in free fatty acids. As a consequence of different but complementary mechanisms of action, dual oral therapy of rosiglitazone with a sulphonylurea or metformin resulted in additive effects on glycaemic control in type 2 diabetic patients.

In studies with a maximal duration of three years, rosiglitazone given once or twice daily produced a sustained improvement in glycaemic control (FPG and HbA1c). A more pronounced glucose-lowering effect was observed in obese patients. An outcome study has not been completed with rosiglitazone, therefore the long-term benefits associated with improved glycaemic control have not been demonstrated.

At 18 months, in an ongoing long term comparator study, rosiglitazone in dual oral therapy with metformin or a sulphonylurea was non-inferior to the combination of sulphonylurea plus metformin for lowering HbA1c.

An active controlled clinical trial (rosiglitazone up to 8 mg daily or metformin up to 2,000 mg daily) of 24 weeks duration was performed in 197 children (10-17 years of age) with type 2 diabetes. Improvement in HbA1c from baseline achieved statistical significance only in the metformin group. Rosiglitazone failed to demonstrate non-inferiority to metformin. Following rosiglitazone treatment, there were no new safety concerns noted in children compared to adult patients with type 2 diabetes mellitus. No long-term efficacy and safety data are available in paediatric patients.

ADOPT (A Diabetes Outcome Progression Trial) was a multicentre, double-blind, controlled trial with a treatment duration of 4-6 years (median duration of 4 years), in which rosiglitazone at doses of 4 to 8 mg/day was compared to metformin (500 mg to 2000 mg/day) and glibenclamide (2.5 to 15 mg/day) in 4351 drug naive subjects recently diagnosed ($\leqslant$3 years) with type 2 diabetes. Rosiglitazone treatment significantly reduced the risk of reaching monotherapy failure (FPG >10.0 mmol/L) by 63% relative to glibenclamide (HR 0.37, CI 0.30-0.45) and by 32% relative to metformin (HR 0.68, CI 0.55-0.85) during the course of the study (up to 72 months of treatment). This translates to a cumulative incidence of treatment failure of 10.3% for rosiglitazone, 14.8% for metformin and 23.3% for glibenclamide treated patients. Overall, 43%, 47% and 42% of subjects in the rosiglitazone, glibenclamide and metformin groups respectively withdrew due to reasons other than monotherapy failure. The impact of these findings on disease progression or on microvascular or macrovascular outcomes has not been determined (see section 4.8). In this study, the adverse events observed were consistent with the known adverse event profile for each of the treatments, including continuing weight gain with rosiglitazone. An additional observation of an increased incidence of bone fractures was seen in women with rosiglitazone (see sections 4.4 and 4.8).

There are no studies completed assessing long-term cardiovascular outcome in patients receiving rosiglitazone.

5.2 Pharmacokinetic properties

Absorption

Absolute bioavailability of rosiglitazone following both a 4 and an 8 mg oral dose is approximately 99%. Rosiglitazone plasma concentrations peak at around 1 hour after dosing. Plasma concentrations are approximately dose proportional over the therapeutic dose range.

Administration of rosiglitazone with food resulted in no change in overall exposure (AUC), although a small decrease in C_{max} (approximately 20% to 28%) and a delay in t_{max} (ca.1.75 h) were observed compared to dosing in the fasting state. These small changes are not clinically significant and, therefore, it is not necessary to administer rosiglitazone at any particular time in relation to meals. The absorption of rosiglitazone is not affected by increases in gastric pH.

Distribution

The volume of distribution of rosiglitazone is approximately 14 litres in healthy volunteers. Plasma protein binding of rosiglitazone is high (approximately 99.8%) and is not influenced by concentration or age. The protein binding of the major metabolite (para-hydroxy-sulphate) is very high (>99.99%).

Metabolism

Metabolism of rosiglitazone is extensive with no parent compound being excreted unchanged. The major routes of metabolism are N-demethylation and hydroxylation, followed by conjugation with sulphate and glucuronic acid. The contribution of the major metabolite (para-hydroxy-sulphate) to the overall anti-diabetic activity of rosiglitazone has not been fully elucidated in man and it cannot be ruled out that the metabolite may contribute to the activity. However, this raises no safety concern regarding target or special populations as hepatic impairment is contraindicated and the phase III clinical studies included a considerable number of elderly patients and patients with mild to moderate renal impairment.

In vitro studies demonstrate that rosiglitazone is predominantly metabolised by CYP2C8, with a minor contribution by CYP2C9.

Since there is no significant *in vitro* inhibition of CYP1A2, 2A6, 2C19, 2D6, 2E1, 3A or 4A with rosiglitazone, there is a low probability of significant metabolism-based interactions with substances metabolised by these P450 enzymes. Rosiglitazone showed moderate inhibition of CYP2C8 (IC_{50} 18 μM) and low inhibition of CYP2C9 (IC_{50} 50 μM) *in vitro* (see section 4.5). An *in vivo* interaction study with warfarin indicated that rosiglitazone does not interact with CYP2C9 substrates *in vivo*.

Elimination

Total plasma clearance of rosiglitazone is around 3 l/h and the terminal elimination half-life of rosiglitazone is approximately 3 to 4 hours. There is no evidence for unexpected accumulation of rosiglitazone after once or twice daily dosing. The major route of excretion is the urine with approximately two-thirds of the dose being eliminated by this route, whereas faecal elimination accounts for approximately 25% of dose. No intact drug is excreted in urine or faeces. The terminal half-life for radioactivity was about 130 hours indicating that elimination of metabolites is very slow. Accumulation of the metabolites in plasma is expected upon repeated dosing, especially that of the major metabolite (para-hydroxy-sulphate) for which an 8-fold accumulation is anticipated.

Special populations

Gender: In the pooled population pharmacokinetic analysis, there were no marked differences in the pharmacokinetics of rosiglitazone between males and females.

Elderly: In the pooled population pharmacokinetic analysis, age was not found to influence the pharmacokinetics of rosiglitazone to any significant extent.

Children and adolescents: Population pharmacokinetic analysis including 96 paediatric patients aged 10 to 18 years and weighing 35 to 178 kg suggested similar mean CL/F in children and adults. Individual CL/F in the paediatric population was in the same range as individual adult data. CL/F seemed to be independent of age, but increased with weight in the paediatric population.

Hepatic impairment: In cirrhotic patients with moderate (Child-Pugh B) hepatic impairment, unbound C_{max} and AUC were 2- and 3-fold higher than in normal subjects. The inter-subject variability was large, with a 7-fold difference in unbound AUC between patients.

Renal insufficiency: There are no clinically significant differences in the pharmacokinetics of rosiglitazone in patients with renal impairment or end stage renal disease on chronic dialysis.

5.3 Preclinical safety data

Adverse effects observed in animal studies with possible relevance to clinical use were as follows: An increase in plasma volume accompanied by decrease in red cell parameters and increase in heart weight. Increases in liver weight, plasma ALT (dog only) and fat tissue were also observed. Similar effects have been seen with other thiazolidinediones.

In reproductive toxicity studies, administration of rosiglitazone to rats during mid-late gestation was associated with foetal death and retarded foetal development. In addition, rosiglitazone inhibited ovarian oestradiol and progesterone synthesis and lowered plasma levels of these hormones resulting in effects on oestrus/menstrual cycles and fertility (see section 4.4).

In an animal model for familial adenomatous polyposis (FAP), treatment with rosiglitazone at 200 times the pharmacologically active dose increased tumour multiplicity in the colon. The relevance of this finding is unknown. However, rosiglitazone promoted differentiation and reversal of mutagenic changes in human colon cancer cells *in vitro*. In addition, rosiglitazone was not genotoxic in a battery of *in vivo* and *in vitro* genotoxicity studies and there was no evidence of colon tumours in lifetime studies of rosiglitazone in two rodent species.

6. PHARMACEUTICAL PARTICULARS

6.1 List of excipients

4 and 8 mg Tablet core:

Sodium starch glycollate (Type A), hypromellose, microcrystalline cellulose, lactose monohydrate, magnesium stearate.

4 mg Film coating:

Opadry orange OY-L-23028 (hypromellose 6cP, titanium dioxide E171, macrogol 3000, purified talc, lactose monohydrate, glycerol triacetate, iron oxide red E172, iron oxide yellow E172).

8 mg Film coating:

Opadry pink OY-L-24803 (hypromellose 6cP, titanium dioxide E171, macrogol 3000, lactose monohydrate, glycerol triacetate, iron oxide red E172).

6.2 Incompatibilities

Not applicable.

6.3 Shelf life

2 years.

6.4 Special precautions for storage

This medicinal product does not require any special storage conditions.

6.5 Nature and contents of container

Opaque blister packs (PVC/ aluminium).

4 mg - 28 and 56 film-coated tablets.

8 mg - 28 film-coated tablets

6.6 Special precautions for disposal and other handling

Any unused product should be disposed of in accordance with local requirements.

7. MARKETING AUTHORISATION HOLDER

SmithKline Beecham plc

980 Great West Road

Brentford

Middlesex

TW8 9GS

United Kingdom

8. MARKETING AUTHORISATION NUMBER(S)

EU/1/00/137/006 - Avandia 4 mg - 28 Film-coated tablets

EU/1/00/137/007 - Avandia 4 mg - 56 Film-coated tablets

EU/1/00/137/011 - Avandia 8 mg - 28 Film-coated tablets

9. DATE OF FIRST AUTHORISATION/RENEWAL OF THE AUTHORISATION

Date of first authorisation: 11 July 2000.

Date of renewal: 18 July 2005.

10. DATE OF REVISION OF THE TEXT

28 May 2009

Avastin 25mg/ml concentrate for solution for infusion

(Roche Products Limited)

1. NAME OF THE MEDICINAL PRODUCT

Avastin▼ 25 mg/ml concentrate for solution for infusion.

2. QUALITATIVE AND QUANTITATIVE COMPOSITION

Bevacizumab 25 mg per ml. Each vial contains 100 mg of bevacizumab in 4 ml and 400 mg in 16 ml respectively.

Bevacizumab is a recombinant humanised monoclonal antibody produced by DNA technology in Chinese Hamster ovary cells.

For a full list of excipients, see section 6.1.

3. PHARMACEUTICAL FORM

Concentrate for solution for infusion.

Clear to slightly opalescent, colourless to pale brown liquid.

4. CLINICAL PARTICULARS

4.1 Therapeutic indications

Avastin (bevacizumab) in combination with fluoropyrimidine-based chemotherapy is indicated for treatment of patients with metastatic carcinoma of the colon or rectum.

Avastin in combination with paclitaxel or docetaxel is indicated for first-line treatment of patients with metastatic breast cancer. For further information as to HER2 status, please refer to section 5.1.

Avastin, in addition to platinum-based chemotherapy, is indicated for first-line treatment of patients with unresectable advanced, metastatic or recurrent non-small cell lung cancer other than predominantly squamous cell histology.

Avastin in combination with interferon alfa-2a is indicated for first line treatment of patients with advanced and/or metastatic renal cell cancer.

4.2 Posology and method of administration

General

Avastin must be administered under the supervision of a physician experienced in the use of antineoplastic medicinal products.

It is recommended that treatment be continued until progression of the underlying disease.

The initial dose should be delivered over 90 minutes as an intravenous infusion. If the first infusion is well tolerated, the second infusion may be administered over 60 minutes. If the 60-minute infusion is well tolerated, all subsequent infusions may be administered over 30 minutes.

Do not administer as an intravenous push or bolus.

Instructions for the preparation of Avastin infusions are described in section 6.6. Avastin infusions should not be administered or mixed with glucose solutions (see section 6.2).

Dose reduction for adverse events is not recommended. If indicated, therapy should either be permanently discontinued or temporarily suspended as described in section 4.4.

Metastatic carcinoma of the colon or rectum (mCRC)

The recommended dose of Avastin, administered as an intravenous infusion, is either 5 mg/kg or 10 mg/kg of body weight given once every 2 weeks or 7.5 mg/kg or 15 mg/kg of body weight given once every 3 weeks.

Metastatic breast cancer (mBC)

The recommended dose of Avastin is 10 mg/kg of body weight given once every 2 weeks or 15 mg/kg of body weight given once every 3 weeks as an intravenous infusion.

Non-small cell lung cancer (NSCLC)

Avastin is administered in addition to platinum-based chemotherapy for up to 6 cycles of treatment followed by Avastin as a single agent until disease progression.

The recommended dose of Avastin is 7.5 mg/kg or 15 mg/kg of body weight given once every 3 weeks as an intravenous infusion.

Clinical benefit in NSCLC patients has been demonstrated with both 7.5 mg/kg and 15 mg/kg doses. For details refer to section 5.1 *Pharmacodynamic Properties, Non-small cell lung cancer (NSCLC)*.

Advanced and/or metastatic Renal Cell Cancer (mRCC)

The recommended dose of Avastin is 10 mg/kg of body weight given once every 2 weeks as an intravenous infusion.

Special populations

Children and Adolescents: The safety and efficacy in children and adolescents have not been established. Avastin is not recommended for use in children and adolescents due to a lack of data on safety and efficacy (see section 5.3).

Elderly: No dose adjustment is required in the elderly.

Renal impairment: The safety and efficacy have not been studied in patients with renal impairment.

Hepatic impairment: The safety and efficacy have not been studied in patients with hepatic impairment.

4.3 Contraindications

- Hypersensitivity to the active substance or to any of the excipients.
- Hypersensitivity to Chinese hamster ovary (CHO) cell products or other recombinant human or humanised antibodies.
- Pregnancy (see section 4.6).

4.4 Special warnings and precautions for use

Gastrointestinal perforations (see section 4.8)

Patients may be at an increased risk for the development of gastrointestinal perforation when treated with Avastin. Intra-abdominal inflammatory process may be a risk factor for gastrointestinal perforations in patients with metastatic carcinoma of the colon or rectum, therefore, caution should be exercised when treating these patients. Therapy should be permanently discontinued in patients who develop gastrointestinal perforation.

Fistulae (see section 4.8)

Patients may be at increased risk for the development of fistulae when treated with Avastin.

Permanently discontinue Avastin in patients with TE (tracheoesophageal) fistula or any grade 4 fistula. Limited information is available on the continued use of Avastin in patients with other fistulae.

In cases of internal fistula not arising in the GI tract, discontinuation of Avastin should be considered

Wound Healing Complications (see section 4.8)

Avastin may adversely affect the wound healing process. Therapy should not be initiated for at least 28 days following major surgery or until the surgical wound is fully healed. In patients who experienced wound healing complications during therapy, treatment should be withheld until the wound is fully healed. Therapy should be withheld for elective surgery.

Hypertension (see section 4.8)

An increased incidence of hypertension was observed in Avastin-treated patients. Clinical safety data suggest that the incidence of hypertension is likely to be dose-dependent. Pre existing hypertension should be adequately controlled before starting Avastin treatment. There is no information on the effect of Avastin in patients with uncontrolled hypertension at the time of initiating therapy. Monitoring of blood pressure is generally recommended during therapy.

In most cases hypertension was controlled adequately using standard antihypertensive treatment appropriate for the individual situation of the affected patient. The use of diuretics to manage hypertension is not advised in patients who receive a cisplatin-based chemotherapy regimen. Avastin should be permanently discontinued, if medically significant hypertension cannot be adequately controlled with antihypertensive therapy, or if the patient develops hypertensive crisis or hypertensive encephalopathy.

Reversible Posterior Leukoencephalopathy Syndrome (RPLS) (see section 4.8)

There have been rare reports of Avastin-treated patients developing signs and symptoms that are consistent with Reversible Posterior Leukoencephalopathy Syndrome (RPLS), a rare neurologic disorder, which can present with the following signs and symptoms among others: seizures, headache, altered mental status, visual disturbance, or cortical blindness, with or without associated hypertension. A diagnosis of RPLS requires confirmation by brain imaging. In patients developing RPLS, treatment of specific symptoms including control of hypertension is recommended along with discontinuation of Avastin. The safety of reinitiating Avastin therapy in patients previously experiencing RPLS is not known.

Proteinuria (see section 4.8)

Patients with a history of hypertension may be at increased risk for the development of proteinuria when treated with Avastin. There is evidence suggesting that Grade 1 [US National Cancer Institute-Common Toxicity Criteria (NCI-CTC) version 2.0] proteinuria may be related to the dose. Monitoring of proteinuria by dipstick urinalysis is recommended prior to starting and during therapy. Therapy should be permanently discontinued in patients who develop Grade 4 proteinuria (nephrotic syndrome).

Arterial Thromboembolism (see section 4.8)

In five randomised clinical trials, the incidence of arterial thromboembolic events including cerebrovascular accidents (CVAs), transient ischaemic attacks (TIAs) and myocardial infarctions (MIs) was higher in patients receiving Avastin in combination with chemotherapy compared to those who received chemotherapy alone.

Patients, receiving Avastin plus chemotherapy, with a history of arterial thromboembolism or age greater than 65 years have an increased risk of developing arterial thromboembolic events during therapy. Caution should be taken when treating these patients with Avastin.

Therapy should be permanently discontinued in patients who develop arterial thromboembolic events.

Venous Thromboembolism (see section 4.8)

Patients may be at risk of developing venous thromboembolic events, including pulmonary embolism under Avastin treatment. Avastin should be discontinued in patients with life-threatening (Grade 4) pulmonary embolism, patients with ≤Grade 3 need to be closely monitored.

Haemorrhage

Patients treated with Avastin have an increased risk of haemorrhage, especially tumour-associated haemorrhage. Avastin should be discontinued permanently in patients who experience Grade 3 or 4 bleeding during Avastin therapy (see section 4.8).

Patients with untreated CNS metastases were routinely excluded from clinical trials with Avastin, based on imaging procedures or signs and symptoms. Therefore, the risk of CNS haemorrhage in such patients has not been prospectively evaluated in randomised clinical studies (see section 4.8). Patients should be monitored for signs and symptoms of CNS bleeding, and Avastin treatment discontinued in case of intracranial bleeding.

There is no information on the safety profile of Avastin in patients with congenital bleeding diathesis, acquired coagulopathy or in patients receiving full dose of anticoagulants for the treatment of thromboembolism prior to starting Avastin treatment, as such patients were excluded from clinical trials. Therefore, caution should be exercised before initiating therapy in these patients. However, patients who developed venous thrombosis while receiving therapy did not appear to have an increased rate of grade 3 or above bleeding when treated with a full dose of warfarin and Avastin concomitantly.

Pulmonary Haemorrhage/Haemoptysis

Patients with non-small cell lung cancer treated with Avastin may be at risk of serious, and in some cases fatal, pulmonary haemorrhage/haemoptysis. Patients with recent pulmonary haemorrhage/ haemoptysis (> 2.5 ml of red blood) should not be treated with Avastin.

Congestive Heart Failure (CHF) (see section 4.8)

events consistent with CHF were reported in clinical trials. The symptoms ranged from asymptomatic declines in left ventricular ejection fraction to symptomatic CHF, requiring treatment or hospitalisation. Most of the patients who experienced CHF had metastatic breast cancer and had received previous treatment with anthracyclines, prior radiotherapy to the left chest wall or other risk factors for CHF, such as pre-existing coronary heart disease or concomitant cardiotoxic therapy.

Caution should be exercised when treating patients with clinically significant cardiovascular disease or pre-existing congestive heart failure with Avastin.

Neutropenia (see section 4.8)

Increased rates of severe neutropenia, febrile neutropenia, or infection with severe neutropenia (including some fatalities) have been observed in patients treated with some myelotoxic chemotherapy regimens plus Avastin in comparison to chemotherapy alone.

4.5 Interaction with other medicinal products and other forms of interaction

Effect of antineoplastic agents on bevacizumab pharmacokinetics

No clinically relevant pharmacokinetic interaction of co-administered chemotherapy on Avastin pharmacokinetics has been observed based on the results of a population PK analysis. There was neither statistical significance nor clinically relevant difference in clearance of Avastin in patients receiving Avastin monotherapy compared to patients receiving Avastin in combination with Interferon alpha 2a or other chemotherapies (IFL, 5-FU/LV, carboplatin-paclitaxel, capecitabine doxorubicin or cisplatin/gemcitabine).

Effect of bevacizumab on the pharmacokinetics of other antineoplastic agents

Results from a dedicated drug-drug interaction study, demonstrated no significant effect of bevacizumab on the pharmacokinetics of irinotecan and its active metabolite SN38.

Results from one study in metastatic colorectal cancer patients demonstrated no significant effect of bevacizumab on the pharmacokinetic of capecitabine and its metabolites, and on the pharmacokinetics of oxaliplatin, as determined by measurement of free and total platinum.

Results from one study in renal cancer patients demonstrated no significant effect of bevacizumab on the pharmacokinetics of interferon alfa-2a.

The potential effect of bevacizumab on the pharmacokinetics of cisplatin and gemcitabine was investigated in non-squamous NSCLC patients. Study results demonstrated no significant effect of bevacizumab on the pharmacokinetics of cisplatin. Due to high inter-patient variability and limited sampling, the results from that study do not allow firm conclusions to be drawn on the impact of bevacizumab on gemcitabine pharmacokinetics.

Combination of bevacizumab and sunitinib malate

In two clinical studies of metastatic renal cell carcinoma, microangiopathic haemolytic anaemia (MAHA) was reported in 7 of 19 patients treated with bevacizumab (10 mg/kg every two weeks) and sunitinib malate (50 mg daily) combination.

MAHA is a haemolytic disorder which can present with red cell fragmentation, anaemia, and thrombocytopenia. In addition, hypertension (including hypertensive crisis), elevated creatinine, and neurological symptoms were observed in some of these patients. All of these findings were reversible upon discontinuation of bevacizumab and sunitinib malate (see Hypertension, Proteinuria, RPLS in section 4.4 Special warnings and precautions for use).

Radiotherapy

The safety and efficacy of concomitant administration of radiotherapy and Avastin has not been established.

4.6 Pregnancy and lactation

Pregnancy

There are no data on the use of Avastin in pregnant women. Studies in animals have shown reproductive toxicity including malformations (see section 5.3). IgGs are known to cross the placenta, and Avastin is anticipated to inhibit angiogenesis in the foetus, and thus is suspected to cause serious birth defects when administered during pregnancy. Avastin is contraindicated (see section 4.3) in pregnancy. Women of childbearing potential have to use effective contraception during (and up to 6 months after) treatment.

Lactation

It is not known whether bevacizumab is excreted in human milk. As maternal IgG is excreted in milk and bevacizumab could harm infant growth and development (see section 5.3), women must discontinue breast-feeding during therapy and not breast feed for at least six months following the last dose of Avastin.

4.7 Effects on ability to drive and use machines

No studies on the effects on the ability to drive and use machines have been performed. However, there is no evidence that Avastin treatment results in an increase in adverse events that might lead to impairment of the ability to drive or operate machinery or impairment of mental ability.

4.8 Undesirable effects

The overall safety profile of Avastin is based on data from over 3,500 patients with various malignancies, predominantly treated with Avastin in combination with chemotherapy in clinical trials.

The most serious adverse drug reactions were:

- Gastrointestinal perforations (see section 4.4).
- Haemorrhage, including pulmonary haemorrhage/haemoptysis, which is more common in non-small cell lung cancer patients (see section 4.4).
- Arterial thromboembolism (see section 4.4).

The most frequently observed adverse drug reactions across clinical trials in patients receiving Avastin were hypertension, fatigue or asthenia, diarrhoea and abdominal pain.

Analyses of the clinical safety data suggest that the occurrence of hypertension and proteinuria with Avastin therapy are likely to be dose-dependent.

Table 1 lists adverse drug reactions associated with the use of Avastin in combination with different chemotherapy regimens in multiple indications. These reactions had occurred either with at least a 2% difference compared to the control arm (NCI-CTC grade 3-5 reactions) or with at least a 10% difference compared to the control arm (NCI-CTC grade 1-5 reactions), in at least one of the major clinical trials.

The adverse drug reactions listed in this table fall into the following categories: Very Common (⩾ 10%) and Common (⩾ 1% - < 10%). Adverse drug reactions are added to the appropriate category in the table below according to the highest incidence seen in any of the major clinical trials.

Within each frequency grouping adverse drug reactions are presented in the order of decreasing seriousness. Some of the adverse drug reactions are reactions commonly seen with chemotherapy, (e.g. palmar-plantar erythrodysaesthesia syndrome with capecitabine and peripheral sensory neuropathy with paclitaxel or oxaliplatin); however, an exacerbation by Avastin therapy can not be excluded.

Table 1: Very Common and Common Adverse Drug Reactions

(see Table 1 below)

Further information on selected serious adverse drug reactions:

Gastrointestinal perforations (see section 4.4):

Avastin has been associated with serious cases of gastrointestinal perforation or fistulae (see also under heading *Fistulae*).

Gastrointestinal perforation have been reported in clinical trials with an incidence of less than 1% in patients with metastatic breast cancer or non-squamous non-small cell lung cancer, and in up to 2.0% in metastatic colorectal cancer patients. Fatal outcome was reported in approximately a third of serious cases of gastrointestinal perforations, which represents between 0.2%-1% of all Avastin treated patients.

The presentation of these events varied in type and severity, ranging from free air seen on the plain abdominal X-ray, which resolved without treatment, to intestinal perforation with abdominal abscess and fatal outcome. In some cases underlying intra-abdominal inflammation was present, either from gastric ulcer disease, tumour necrosis, diverticulitis, or chemotherapy-associated colitis.

Fistulae (see section 4.4):

Avastin use has been associated with serious cases of fistulae including events resulting in death.

In clinical trials, gastrointestinal fistulae have been reported with an incidence of up to 2% in patients with metastatic colorectal cancer, but were also reported less commonly in patients with other types of cancers. Uncommon (⩾ 0.1% to < 1%) reports of other types of fistulae that involve

Table 1 Very Common and Common Adverse Drug Reactions

System Organ Class (SOC)	**NCI-CTC Grade 3-5 Reactions (⩾ 2% difference between the study arms in at least one clinical trial)**		**All Grade Reactions (⩾ 10% difference between the study arms in at least one clinical trial)**
	Very common	**Common**	**Very Common**
Infections and infestations		Sepsis Abscess Infection	
Blood and the lymphatic systems disorders	Febrile neutropenia Leucopenia Thrombocytopenia Neutropenia	Anaemia	
Metabolism and nutrition disorders		Dehydration	Anorexia
Nervous system disorders	Peripheral sensory neuropathy	Cerebrovascular accident Syncope Somnolence Headache	Dysgeusia Headache
Eye disorders			Eye disorder Lacrimation increased
Cardiac disorders		Cardiac failure congestive Supraventricular tachycardia	
Vascular disorders	Hypertension	Thromboembolism (arterial)* Deep vein thrombosis Haemorrhage	Hypertension
Respiratory, thoracic and mediastinal disorders		Pulmonary embolism Dyspnoea Hypoxia Epistaxis	Dyspnoea Epistaxis Rhinitis
Gastrointestinal disorders	Diarrhoea Nausea Vomiting	Intestinal Perforation Ileus Intestinal obstruction Abdominal pain Gastrointestinal disorder Stomatitis	Constipation Stomatitis Rectal haemorrhage
Skin and subcutaneous tissue disorders		Palmar-plantar erythrodysaesthesia syndrome	Exfoliative dermatitis Dry skin Skin discolouration
Musculoskeletal, connective tissue and bone disorders		Muscular weakness Myalgia	Arthralgia
Renal and urinary disorders		Proteinuria Urinary Tract Infection	Proteinuria
General disorders and administration site conditions	Asthenia Fatigue	Pain Lethargy Mucosal inflammation	Pyrexia Asthenia Pain Mucosal inflammation

** Pooled arterial thromboembolic events including cerebrovascular accident, myocardial infarction, transient ischaemic attack and other arterial thromboembolic events.*

Data are unadjusted for the differential time on treatment.

areas of the body other than the gastrointestinal tract (e.g. bronchopleural, urogenital and biliary fistulae) were observed across various indications. Fistulae have also been reported in post-marketing experience.

Events were reported at various time points during treatment ranging from one week to greater than 1 year from initiation of Avastin, with most events occurring within the first 6 months of therapy.

Wound healing (see section 4.4):

As Avastin may adversely impact wound healing, patients who had major surgery within the last 28 days were excluded from participation in phase III clinical trials.

In clinical trials of metastatic carcinoma of the colon or rectum, there was no increased risk of post-operative bleeding or wound healing complications observed in patients who underwent major surgery 28-60 days prior to starting Avastin. An increased incidence of post-operative bleeding or wound healing complication occurring within 60 days of major surgery was observed if the patient was being treated with Avastin at the time of surgery. The incidence varied between 10% (4/40) and 20% (3/15).

In locally recurrent and metastatic breast cancer trials, Grade 3-5 wound healing complications were observed in up to 1.1% of patients receiving Avastin compared with up to 0.9% of patients in the control arms.

Hypertension (see section 4.4):

An increased incidence of hypertension (all grades) of up to 34% has been observed in Avastin-treated patients in clinical trials compared with up to 14% in those treated with comparator. Grade 3 and 4 hypertension (requiring oral anti-hypertensive medication) in patients receiving Avastin ranged from 0.4% to 17.9%. Grade 4 hypertension (hypertensive crisis) occurred in up to 1.0% of patients treated with Avastin and chemotherapy compared to up to 0.2% of patients treated with the same chemotherapy alone.

Hypertension was generally adequately controlled with oral anti-hypertensives such as angiotensin-converting enzyme inhibitors, diuretics and calcium-channel blockers. It rarely resulted in discontinuation of Avastin treatment or hospitalisation.

Very rare cases of hypertensive encephalopathy have been reported, some of which were fatal.

The risk of Avastin-associated hypertension did not correlate with the patients' baseline characteristics, underlying disease or concomitant therapy.

Proteinuria (see section 4.4):

In clinical trials, proteinuria has been reported within the range of 0.7% to 38% of patients receiving Avastin.

Proteinuria ranged in severity from clinically asymptomatic, transient, trace proteinuria to nephrotic syndrome, with the great majority as Grade 1 proteinuria. Grade 3 proteinuria was reported in < 3% of treated patients: however, in patients treated for advanced and/or metastatic renal cell carcinoma this was up to 7%. Grade 4 proteinuria (nephrotic syndrome) was seen in up to 1.4% of treated patients. The proteinuria seen in clinical trials was not associated with renal dysfunction and rarely required permanent discontinuation of therapy. Testing for proteinuria is recommended prior to start of Avastin therapy. In most clinical studies urine protein levels of ⩾ 2g/24 hrs led to the holding of Avastin until recovery to < 2g/24 hrs.

Haemorrhage (see section 4.4):

In clinical trials across all indications the overall incidence of NCI-CTC Grade 3-5 bleeding events ranged from 0.4% to 5% in Avastin treated patients, compared with up to 2.9% of patients in chemotherapy control group.

The haemorrhagic events that have been observed in clinical studies were predominantly tumour-associated haemorrhage (see below) and minor mucocutaneous haemorrhage (e.g. epistaxis).

Tumour-associated haemorrhage (see section 4.4).

Major or massive pulmonary haemorrhage/haemoptysis has been observed primarily in studies in patients with non-small cell lung cancer (NSCLC). Possible risk factors include squamous cell histology, treatment with antirheumatic/anti-inflammatory drugs, treatment with anticoagulants, prior radiotherapy, Avastin therapy, previous medical history of atherosclerosis, central tumour location and cavitation of tumours prior to or during therapy. The only variables that showed statistically significant correlations with bleeding were Avastin therapy and squamous cell histology. Patients with NSCLC of known squamous cell histology or mixed cell type with predominant squamous cell histology were excluded from subsequent phase III studies, while patients with unknown tumour histology were included.

In patients with NSCLC excluding predominant squamous histology, all grade events were seen with a frequency of up to 9% when treated with Avastin plus chemotherapy compared with 5% in the patients treated with chemotherapy alone. Grade 3-5 events have been observed in up to 2.3% of patients treated with Avastin plus chemotherapy as compared with < 1% with chemotherapy alone. Major or massive pulmonary haemorrhage/haemoptysis can occur suddenly and up to two thirds of the serious pulmonary haemorrhages resulted in a fatal outcome.

Gastrointestinal haemorrhages, including rectal bleeding and melaena have been reported in colorectal cancer patients, and have been assessed as tumour-associated haemorrhages.

Tumour-associated haemorrhage was also seen rarely in other tumour types and locations, including cases of central nervous system (CNS) bleeding in patients with CNS metastases (see section 4.4).

The incidence of CNS bleeding in patients with untreated CNS metastases receiving bevacizumab has not been prospectively evaluated in randomised clinical studies. In an exploratory retrospective analysis of data from 13 completed randomised trials in patients with various tumour types, 3 patients out of 91 (3.3%) with brain metastases experienced CNS bleeding (all Grade 4) when treated with bevacizumab, compared to 1 case (Grade 5) out of 96 patients (1%) that were not exposed to bevacizumab. In two ongoing studies in patients with treated brain metastases, one case of Grade 2 CNS haemorrhage was reported in 83 subjects treated with bevacizumab (1.2%) at the time of interim safety analysis.

Across all clinical trials, mucocutaneous haemorrhage has been seen in up to 50% of Avastin-treated patients. These were most commonly NCI-CTC Grade 1 epistaxis that lasted less than 5 minutes, resolved without medical intervention and did not require any changes in the Avastin treatment regimen. Clinical safety data suggest that the incidence of minor mucocutaneous haemorrhage (e.g. epistaxis) may be dose-dependent.

There have also been less common events of minor mucocutaneous haemorrhage in other locations, such as gingival bleeding or vaginal bleeding.

Thromboembolism (see section 4.4):

Arterial thromboembolism:

An increased incidence of arterial thromboembolic events was observed in patients treated with Avastin across indications, including cerebrovascular accidents, myocardial infarction, transient ischemic attacks, and other arterial thromboembolic events.

In clinical trials, the overall incidence of arterial thromboembolic events ranged up to 3.8% in the Avastin containing arms compared with up to 1.7% in the chemotherapy control arms. Fatal outcome was reported in 0.8% of patients receiving Avastin compared to 0.5% in patients receiving chemotherapy alone. Cerebrovascular accidents (including transient ischemic attacks) were reported in up to 2.3% of patients treated with Avastin in combination with chemotherapy compared to 0.5% of patients treated with chemotherapy alone. Myocardial infarction was reported in 1.4% of patients treated with Avastin in combination with chemotherapy compared to 0.7% of patients treated with chemotherapy alone.

In one clinical trial, AVF2192g, patients with metastatic colorectal cancer who were not candidates for treatment with irinotecan were included. In this trial arterial thromboembolic events were observed in 11% (11/100) of patients compared to 5.8% (6/104) in the chemotherapy control group.

Venous thromboembolism:

The incidence of venous thromboembolic events in clinical trials was similar in patients receiving Avastin in combination with chemotherapy compared to those receiving the control chemotherapy alone. Venous thromboembolic events include deep venous thrombosis, pulmonary embolism and thrombophlebitis.

In clinical trials across indications, the overall incidence of venous thromboembolic events ranged from 2.8% to 17.3% of Avastin-treated patients compared with 3.2% to 15.6% in the control arms.

Grade 3-5 venous thromboembolic events have been reported in up to 7.8% of patients treated with chemotherapy plus bevacizumab compared with up to 4.9% in patients treated with chemotherapy alone.

Patients who have experienced a venous thromboembolic event may be at higher risk for a recurrence if they receive Avastin in combination with chemotherapy versus chemotherapy alone.

Congestive Heart Failure (CHF)

In clinical trials with Avastin, congestive heart failure (CHF) was observed in all cancer indications studied to date, but occurred predominantly in patients with metastatic breast cancer. In two phase III studies (AVF2119g and E2100) in patients with metastatic breast cancer an increase of CHF Grade 3 or more with Avastin was seen. CHF was reported in up to 3.5% of patients treated with Avastin compared with up to 0.9% in the control arms. Most of these patients showed improved symptoms and/or left ventricular function following appropriate medical therapy.

In most clinical trials of Avastin, patients with pre-existing CHF of NYHA (New York Heart Association (NYHA) II-IV were excluded, therefore, no information is available on the risk of CHF in this population.

Prior anthracyclines exposure and/or prior radiation to the chest wall may be possible risk factors for the development of CHF.

Elderly Patients

In randomised clinical trials, age > 65 years was associated with an increased risk of developing arterial thromboembolic events, including cerebrovascular accidents (CVAs), transient ischaemic attacks (TIAs) and myocardial infarctions (MIs). Other reactions with a higher frequency seen in patients over 65 were grade 3-4 leucopenia and thrombocytopenia; and all grade neutropenia, diarrhoea, nausea, headache and fatigue as compared to those aged ⩽ 65 years when treated with Avastin (see sections 4.4 and 4.8 under *Thromboembolism*).

No increase in the incidence of other reactions, including gastrointestinal perforation, wound healing complications, hypertension, proteinuria, congestive heart failure, and haemorrhage was observed in elderly patients (> 65 years) receiving Avastin as compared to those aged ⩽ 65 years treated with Avastin.

Laboratory Abnormalities:

Decreased neutrophil count, decreased white blood cell count and presence of urine protein may be associated with Avastin treatment.

Across clinical trials, the following Grade 3 and 4 laboratory abnormalities occurred in patients treated with Avastin with at least a 2% difference compared to the corresponding control groups: hyperglycaemia, decreased haemoglobin, hypokalaemia, hyponatraemia, decreased white blood cell count, increased international normalised ratio (INR).

Post-marketing experience:

Table 2: Adverse reactions reported in post-marketing setting

System Organ Class (SOC)	***Reactions (frequency*)***
Nervous system disorders	Hypertensive encephalopathy (very rare) (see also section 4.4 Special warnings and precautions for use, and *Hypertension* in section 4.8 Undesirable Effects) Reversible Posterior Leukoencephalopathy Syndrome (rare) (see also section 4.4 Special warnings and precautions for use)
Vascular Disorders	Renal Thrombotic Microangiopathy, clinically manifested as proteinuria (frequency not known). For further information on proteinuria see section 4.4 Special warnings and precautions for use, and *Proteinuria* in section 4.8 Undesirable Effects.
Respiratory, thoracic and mediastinal disorders	Nasal septum perforation (not known) Pulmonary hypertension (not known) Dysphonia (common)

* if specified, the frequency has been derived from clinical trial data

4.9 Overdose

The highest dose tested in humans (20 mg/kg of body weight, intravenous every 2 weeks) was associated with severe migraine in several patients.

5. PHARMACOLOGICAL PROPERTIES

5.1 Pharmacodynamic properties

Pharmacotherapeutic group: Antineoplastic agents, monoclonal antibody, ATC code: L01X C07

Mechanism of action

Bevacizumab binds to vascular endothelial growth factor (VEGF), the key driver of vasculogenesis and angiogenesis, and thereby inhibits the binding of VEGF to its receptors, Flt-1 (VEGFR-1) and KDR (VEGFR-2), on the surface of endothelial cells. Neutralising the biological activity of VEGF regresses the vascularisation of tumours, normalises remaining tumour vasculature, and inhibits the formation of new tumour vasculature, thereby inhibiting tumour growth.

Pharmacodynamic effects

Administration of bevacizumab or its parental murine antibody to xenotransplant models of cancer in nude mice resulted in extensive anti-tumour activity in human cancers, including colon, breast, pancreas and prostate. Metastatic disease progression was inhibited and microvascular permeability was reduced.

Clinical efficacy

Metastatic carcinoma of the colon or rectum (mCRC)

The safety and efficacy of the recommended dose (5 mg/kg of body weight every two weeks) in metastatic carcinoma of the colon or rectum were studied in three randomised, active-controlled clinical trials in combination with fluoropyrimidine-based first-line chemotherapy. Avastin was combined with two chemotherapy regimens:

- **AVF2107g**: A weekly schedule of irinotecan/bolus 5-fluorouracil/folinic acid (IFL) for a total of 4 weeks of each 6 week-cycle (Saltz regimen).
- **AVF0780g**: In combination with bolus 5-fluorouracil/folinic acid (5-FU/FA) for a total of 6 weeks of each 8 week-cycle (Roswell Park regimen).
- **AVF2192g**: In combination with bolus 5-FU/FA for a total of 6 weeks of each 8 week-cycle (Roswell Park regimen) in patients who were not optimal candidates for first-line irinotecan treatment.

Two additional studies were conducted in first (NO16966) and second line (E3200) treatment of metastatic carcinoma of the colon or rectum, with Avastin administered in the following dosing regimens, in combination with FOLFOX-4

5FU/LV/Oxaliplatin) and XELOX (Capecitabine/Oxaliplatin):

NO16966: Avastin 7.5 mg/kg of body weight every 3 weeks in combination with oral capecitabine and intravenous oxaliplatin (XELOX) or Avastin 5 mg/kg every 2 weeks in combination with leucovorin plus 5-fluorouracil bolus, followed by 5-fluorouracil infusion, with intravenous oxaliplatin (FOLFOX-4).

- E3200: Avastin 10 mg/kg of body weight every 2 weeks in combination with leucovorin and 5-fluorouracil bolus, followed by 5-fluorouracil infusion, with intravenous oxaliplatin (FOLFOX-4).

AVF2107g: This was a phase III randomised, double-blind, active-controlled clinical trial evaluating Avastin in combination with IFL as first-line treatment for metastatic carcinoma of the colon or rectum. Eight hundred and thirteen patients were randomised to receive IFL + placebo (Arm 1) or IFL + Avastin (5 mg/kg every 2 weeks, Arm 2). A third group of 110 patients received bolus 5-FU/FA+Avastin (Arm 3). Enrolment in Arm 3 was discontinued, as pre-specified, once safety of Avastin with the IFL regimen was established and considered acceptable. All treatments were continued until disease progression. The overall mean age was 59.4 years; 56.6% of patients had an ECOG performance status of 0, 43% had a value of 1 and 0.4% had a value of 2. 15.5% had received prior radiotherapy and 28.4% prior chemotherapy.

The primary efficacy variable of the trial was overall survival. The addition of Avastin to IFL resulted in statistically significant increases in overall survival, progression-free survival and overall response rate (see Table 3). The clinical benefit, as measured by overall survival, was seen in all pre-specified patient subgroups, including those defined by age, sex, performance status, location of primary tumour, number of organs involved and duration of metastatic disease.

The efficacy results of Avastin in combination with IFL-chemotherapy are displayed in Table 3.

Table 3 Efficacy results for study AVF2107g

	AVF2107g	
	Arm 1 IFL + Placebo	Arm 2 IFL + Avastin[a]
Number of Patients	411	402
Overall survival		
Median time (months)	15.6	20.3
95% Confidence Interval	14.29 – 16.99	18.46 – 24.18
Hazard ratio[b]	0.660 (p-value = 0.00004)	
Progression-free survival		
Median time (months)	6.2	10.6
Hazard ratio	0.54 (p-value < 0.0001)	
Overall response rate		
Rate (%)	34.8	44.8
	(p-value = 0.0036)	

[a] 5 mg/kg every 2 weeks.

[b] Relative to control arm.

Among the 110 patients randomised to Arm 3 (5-FU/FA + Avastin) prior to discontinuation of this arm, the median overall survival was 18.3 months and the median progression free survival was 8.8 months.

AVF2192g: This was a phase II randomised, double-blind, active-controlled clinical trial evaluating the efficacy and safety of Avastin in combination with 5-FU/FA as first-line treatment for metastatic colorectal cancer in patients who were not optimal candidates for first-line irinotecan treatment. One hundred and five patients were randomised to 5-FU/FA + placebo arm and 104 patients to 5-FU/FA + Avastin (5 mg/kg every 2 weeks) arm. All treatments were continued until disease progression. The addition of Avastin 5 mg/kg every two weeks to 5-FU/FA resulted in higher objective response rates, significantly longer progression-free survival, and a trend in longer survival as compared to 5-FU/FA chemotherapy alone.

AVF0780g: This was a phase II randomised, active-controlled, open-labelled clinical trial investigating Avastin in combination with 5-FU/FA as first-line treatment of metastatic colorectal cancer. The median age was 64 years. 19% of the patients had received prior chemotherapy and 14% prior radiotherapy. Seventy-one patients were randomised to receive bolus 5-FU/FA or 5-FU/FA + Avastin (5 mg/kg every 2 weeks). A third group of 33 patients received bolus 5-FU/FA + Avastin (10 mg/kg every 2 weeks). Patients were treated until disease progression. The primary endpoints of the trial were objective response rate and progression-free survival. The addition of Avastin 5 mg/kg every two weeks to 5-FU/FA resulted in higher objective response rates, longer progression-free survival, and a trend in longer survival, compared with 5-FU/FA

Table 4 Efficacy results for studies AVF0780g and AVF2192g

	AVF0780g			AVF2192g	
	5-FU/FA	5-FU/FA + Avastin[a]	5-FU/FA + Avastin[b]	5-FU/FA + placebo	5-FU/FA + Avastin
Number of Patients	36	35	33	105	104
Overall survival					
Median time (months)	13.6	17.7	15.2	12.9	16.6
95% Confidence Interval				10.35 - 16.95	13.63 – 19.32
Hazard ratio[c]	-	0.52	1.01		0.79
p-value		0.073	0.978		0.16
Progression-free survival					
Median time (months)	5.2	9.0	7.2	5.5	9.2
Hazard ratio		0.44	0.69		0.5
p-value	-	0.0049	0.217		0.0002
Overall response rate					
Rate (percent)	16.7	40.0	24.2	15.2	26
95% CI	7.0 – 33.5	24.4 – 57.8	11.7 – 42.6	9.2 - 23.9	18.1 - 35.6
p-value		0.029	0.43		0.055
Duration of response					
Median time (months)	NR	9.3	5.0	6.8	9.2
25–75 percentile (months)	5.5 – NR	6.1 – NR	3.8 – 7.8	5.59 - 9.17	5.88 - 13.01

[a] 5 mg/kg every 2 weeks.

[b] 10 mg/kg every 2 weeks.

[c] Relative to control arm.

NR = Not reached.

chemotherapy alone (see Table 4). These efficacy data are consistent with the results from study AVF2107g.

The efficacy data from studies AVF0780g and AVF2192g investigating Avastin in combination with 5-FU/FA-chemotherapy are summarised in Table 4.

Table 4: Efficacy results for studies AVF0780g and AVF2192g

(see Table 4 above)

NO16966

This was a phase III randomised, double-blind (for bevacizumab), clinical trial investigating Avastin 7.5 mg/kg in combination with oral capecitabine and IV oxaliplatin (XELOX), administered on a 3-weekly schedule; or Avastin 5 mg/kg in combination with leucovorin with 5-fluorouracil bolus, followed by 5-fluorouracil infusional, with IV oxaliplatin (FOLFOX-4), administered on a 2-weekly schedule. The study contained two parts: an initial unblinded 2-arm part (Part I) in which patients were randomised to two different treatment groups (XELOX and FOLFOX-4) and a subsequent 2 × 2 factorial 4-arm part (Part II) in which patients were randomised to four treatment groups (XELOX + placebo, FOLFOX-4 + placebo, XELOX + Avastin, FOLFOX-4 + Avastin). In Part II, treatment assignment was double-blind with respect to Avastin.

Approximately 350 patients were randomised into each of the 4 study arms in the Part II of the trial.

Table 5 Treatment Regimens in Study N016966 (mCRC)

(see Table 5 below)

The primary efficacy parameter of the trial was the duration of progression-free survival. In this study, there were two primary objectives: to show that XELOX was non-inferior to FOLFOX-4 and to show that Avastin in combination with FOLFOX-4 or XELOX chemotherapy was superior to chemotherapy alone. Both co-primary objectives were met:

i) Non-inferiority of the XELOX-containing arms compared with the FOLFOX-4-containing arms in the overall comparison was demonstrated in terms of progression-free survival and overall survival in the eligible per-protocol population.

ii) Superiority of the Avastin-containing arms versus the chemotherapy alone arms in the overall comparison was demonstrated in terms of progression-free survival in the ITT population (Table 6)

Secondary PFS analyses, based on 'on-treatment'-based response assessments, confirmed the significantly superior clinical benefit for patients treated with Avastin (analyses shown in Table 6), consistent with the statistically significant benefit observed in the pooled analysis.

Table 6 Key efficacy results for the superiority analysis (ITT population, Study NO16966)

(see Table 6 on next page)

In the FOLFOX treatment subgroup, the median PFS was 8.6 months in placebo and 9.4 months in bevacizumab treated patients, HR = 0.89, 97.5% CI = [0.73; 1.08]; p-value = 0.1871, the corresponding results in the XELOX treatment subgroup being 7.4 vs. 9.3 months, HR = 0.77, 97.5% CI = [0.63; 0.94]; p-value = 0.0026.

The median overall survival was 20.3 months in placebo and 21.2 months in bevacizumab treated patients in the FOLFOX treatment subgroup, HR=0.94, 97.5% CI = [0.75; 1.16]; p-value = 0.4937, the corresponding results in the XELOX, treatment subgroup being 19.2 vs. 21.4 months, HR = 0.84, 97.5% CI = [0.68; 1.04]; p-value = 0.0698.

Table 5 Treatment Regimens in Study N016966 (mCRC)

	Treatment	Starting Dose	Schedule
FOLFOX-4 or FOLFOX-4 + Avastin	Oxaliplatin	85 mg/m² IV 2 h	Oxaliplatin on Day 1 Leucovorin on Day 1 and 2 5-fluorouracil IV bolus/infusion, each on Days 1 and 2
	Leucovorin	200 mg/m² IV 2 h	
	5-Fluorouracil	400 mg/m² IV bolus, 600 mg/ m² IV 22 h	
	Placebo or Avastin	5 mg/kg IV 30-90 min	Day 1, prior to FOLFOX-4, every 2 weeks
XELOX or XELOX+ Avastin	Oxaliplatin	130 mg/m² IV 2 h	Oxaliplatin on Day 1 Capecitabine oral bid for 2 weeks (followed by 1 week off treatment)
	Capecitabine	1000 mg/m² oral bid	
	Placebo or Avastin	7.5 mg/kg IV 30-90 min	Day 1, prior to XELOX, q 3 weeks

5-Fluorouracil: IV bolus injection immediately after leucovorin

Table 6 Key efficacy results for the superiority analysis (ITT population, Study NO16966)

Endpoint (months)	FOLFOX-4 or XELOX + Placebo (n=701)	FOLFOX-4 or XELOX + Bevacizumab (n=699)	P Value
Primary endpoint			
Median PFS**	8.0	9.4	0.0023
Hazard ratio (97.5% CI)a	0.83 (0.72–0.95)		
Secondary endpoints			
Median PFS (on treatment)**	7.9	10.4	<0.0001
Hazard ratio (97.5% CI)	0.63 (0.52-0.75)		
Overall response rate (Invest. Assessment)**	49.2%,	46.5%	
Median overall survival*	19.9	21.2	0.0769
Hazard ratio (97.5% CI)	0.89 (0.76-1.03)		

* Overall survival analysis at clinical cut-off 31 January 2007

** Primary analysis at clinical cut-off 31 January 2006

[a] relative to control arm

ECOG E3200

This was a phase III randomised, active-controlled, open-label study investigating Avastin 10 mg/kg in combination with leucovorin with 5-fluorouracil bolus and then 5-fluorouracil infusional, with IV oxaliplatin (FOLFOX-4), administered on a 2-weekly schedule in previously-treated patients (second line) with advanced colorectal cancer. In the chemotherapy arms, the FOLFOX-4 regimen used the same doses and schedule as shown in Table 5 for Study NO16966.

The primary efficacy parameter of the trial was overall survival, defined as the time from randomization to death from any cause. Eight hundred and twenty-nine patients were randomised (292 FOLFOX-4, 293 Avastin + FOLFOX-4 and 244 Avastin monotherapy). The addition of Avastin to FOLFOX-4 resulted in a statistically significant prolongation of survival. Statistically significant improvements in progression-free survival and objective response rate were also observed (see Table 7).

Table 7 Efficacy Results for Study E3200

	E3200	
	FOLFOX-4	FOLFOX-4 + Avastin[a]
Number of Patients	292	293
Overall Survival		
Median (months)	10.8	13.0
95% confidence interval	10.12 – 11.86	12.09 – 14.03
Hazard ratio[b]	0.751 (p-value = 0.0012)	
Progression-Free Survival		
Median (months)	4.5	7.5
Hazard ratio	0.518 (p-value < 0.0001)	
Objective Response Rate		
Rate	8.6%	22.2%
	(p-value <0.0001)	

a 10 mg/kg every 2 weeks

b Relative to control arm

No significant difference was observed in the duration of overall survival between patients who received Avastin monotherapy compared to patients treated with FOLFOX-4. Progression-free survival and objective response rate were inferior in the Avastin monotherapy arm compared to the FOLFOX-4 arm.

The benefit of Avastin re-treatment in metastatic colorectal cancer patients who were exposed to Avastin in previous therapies has not been addressed in randomized clinical trials.

Metastatic breast cancer (mBC)

ECOG E2100

Study E2100 was an open-label, randomised, active controlled, multicentre clinical trial evaluating Avastin in combination with paclitaxel for locally recurrent or metastatic breast cancer in patients who had not previously received chemotherapy for locally recurrent and metastatic disease. Patients were randomised to paclitaxel alone (90 mg/m^2 IV over 1 hour once weekly for three out of four weeks) or in combination with Avastin (10 mg/kg IV infusion every two weeks). Prior hormonal therapy for the treatment of metastatic disease was allowed. Adjuvant taxane therapy was allowed only if it was completed at least 12 months prior to study entry. Of the 722 patients in the study, the majority of patients had HER2-negative disease (90%), with a small number of patients with unknown (8%) or confirmed HER2-positive status (2%), who had previously been treated with or were considered unsuitable for trastuzumab therapy. Furthermore, 65% of patients had received adjuvant chemotherapy including 19% prior taxanes and 49% prior anthracyclines. Patients with central nervous system metastasis, including previously treated or resected brain lesions, were excluded.

In Study E2100, patients were treated until disease progression. In situations where early discontinuation of chemotherapy was required, treatment with Avastin as a single agent continued until disease progression. The patient characteristics were similar across the study arms. The primary endpoint of this trial was progression free survival (PFS), based on study investigators' assessment of disease progression. In addition, an independent review of the primary endpoint was also conducted. The results of this study are presented in Table 8.

Table 8 Study E2100 Efficacy Results:
(see Table 8 below)

Overall Survival		
	Paclitaxel (n=354)	Paclitaxel/Avastin (n=368)
Median OS (months)	24.8	26.5
HR (95% CI)	0.869 (0.722; 1.046)	
p-value	0.1374	

The clinical benefit of Avastin as measured by PFS was seen in all pre-specified subgroups tested (including disease-free interval, number of metastatic sites, prior receip of adjuvant chemotherapy and estrogen receptor (ER status).

BO17708

Study BO17708 was a randomised, double-blind, placebo controlled, multicentre (phase III) trial to evaluate the effi cacy and safety of Avastin in combination with docetaxe compared with docetaxel plus placebo, as first-line treatment for patients with HER2-negative metastatic or locally recurrent breast cancer who have not received prior chemotherapy for their metastatic disease.

Patients were randomised in a 1:1:1 ratio to treatment with either

- placebo + docetaxel 100 mg/m2 every 3 weeks
- Avastin 7.5 mg/kg + docetaxel 100 mg/m2 every 3 weeks
- Avastin 15 mg/kg + docetaxel 100 mg/m2 every 3 weeks.

Docetaxel, Avastin or placebo treatment was continued until disease progression/death or unacceptable toxicity. Docetaxel treatment was limited to a maximum of 9 cycles. The patient and disease characteristics were similar across the three arms.

On documented disease progression, patients from all three treatment arms could enter into a post-study treatment phase during which they received open-label Avastin together with a wide-range of subsequent lines of therapies. (The percentage of patients in each arm who received open-label Avastin were: placebo + doc: 42%, Avastin 7.5 + doc: 37% and Avastin 15 + doc: 26%).

The primary endpoint was progression free survival (PFS), as assessed by investigators. For the efficacy endpoints two comparisons were performed:

- Avastin 7.5 mg/kg + docetaxel 100 mg/m2 every 3 weeks versus placebo + docetaxel 100 mg/m2 every 3 weeks
- Avastin 15 mg/kg + docetaxel 100 mg/m2 every 3 weeks vs placebo + docetaxel 100 mg/m2 every 3 weeks.

The results of this study are presented in Table 9. For progression free survival and response rates this includes results from the pre-specified final analysis and results from an exploratory (updated) analysis carried out at the same time as the pre-specified final OS analysis which included an additional 18 months of follow-up. Overall survival results presented are those from the pre-specified final analysis for OS. At this point approximately 45% of patients across all treatment arms had died.

Table 9 Efficacy results for study BO17708

(see Table 9 on next page)

Non-small cell lung cancer (NSCLC)

The safety and efficacy of Avastin, in addition to platinum-based chemotherapy, in the first-line treatment of patients with non-squamous non-small cell lung cancer (NSCLC), was investigated in studies E4599 and BO17704. An overall survival benefit has been demonstrated in study E4599 with a 15 mg/kg/q3wk dose of bevacizumab. Study BO17704 has demonstrated that both 7.5 mg/kg/q3wk and 15 mg/kg/q3wk bevacizumab doses increase progression free survival and response rate.

E4599

E4599 was an open-label, randomised, active-controlled, multicentre clinical trial evaluating Avastin as first-line treatment of patients with locally advanced (stage IIIb with malignant pleural effusion), metastatic or recurrent NSCLC other than predominantly squamous cell histology.

Patients were randomized to platinum-based chemotherapy (paclitaxel 200 mg/m2 and carboplatin AUC = 6.0, both by IV infusion) (PC) on day 1 of every 3-week cycle for up to 6 cycles or PC in combination with Avastin at a dose of

Table 8 Study E2100 Efficacy Results

Progression-free survival	Investigator Assessment*		IRF Assessment	
	Paclitaxel (n=354)	Paclitaxel/Avastin (n=368)	Paclitaxel (n=354)	Paclitaxel/Avastin (n=368)
Median PFS (months)	5.8	11.4	5.8	11.3
HR (95% CI)	0.421 (0.343; 0.516)		0.483 (0.385; 0.607)	
p-value	<0.0001		<0.0001	

Response rates (for patients with measurable disease)	Investigator Assessment		IRF Assessment	
	Paclitaxel (n=273)	Paclitaxel/Avastin (n=252)	Paclitaxel (n=243)	Paclitaxel/Avastin (n=229)
% pts with objective response	23.4	48.0	22.2	49.8
p-value	<0.0001		<0.0001	

* primary analysis

Table 9 Efficacy results for study BO17708

Progression-free survival			
	Docetaxel + Placebo q 3 weeks (n=241)	Docetaxel + Avastin 7.5 mg/kg q 3 weeks (n=248)	Docetaxel + Avastin 15 mg/kg q 3 weeks (n=247)
Median PFS (months) *[updated analysis]*	8.0 *[8.2]*	8.7 *[9.0]*	8.8 *[10.1]*
Hazard ratio vs placebo arm (95% CI) *[updated analysis]*		0.79 (0.63; 0.98) *[0.86]* *[(0.72; 1.04)]*	0.72 (0.57; 0.90) *[0.77]* *[(0.64; 0.93)]*
P value (log rank test) vs placebo arm *[exploratory p value from updated analysis]*		0.0318 *[0.1163]*	0.0099 *[0.0061]*
Progression-free survival (sensitivity analysis)*			
	Docetaxel + Placebo q 3 weeks (n=241)	Docetaxel + Avastin 7.5 mg/kg q 3 weeks (n=248)	Docetaxel + Avastin 15 mg/kg q 3 weeks (n=247)
Median PFS (months) *[updated analysis]*	8.0 *[8.1]*	8.7 *[9.0]*	8.8 *[10.0]*
Hazard ratio vs placebo arm (95% CI) *[updated analysis]*		0.69 (0.54; 0.89) *[0.80]* *[(0.65; 1.00)]*	0.61 (0.48; 0.78) *[0.67]* *[(0.54; 0.83)]*
P value (log rank test) vs placebo arm *[exploratory p value from updated analysis]*		0.0035 *[0.0450]*	0.0001 *[0.0002]*
Response rates (for patients with measurable disease)			
	Docetaxel + Placebo q 3 weeks (n=207)	Docetaxel + Avastin 7.5 mg/kg q 3 weeks (n=201)	Docetaxel + Avastin 15 mg/kg q 3 weeks (n=206)
% pts with objective response *[updated analysis]*	44.4 *[46.4]*	55.2 *[55.2]*	63.1 *[64.1]*
p-value vs placebo arm *[exploratory p value from updated analysis]*		0.0295 *[0.0739]*	0.0001 *[0.0003]*
Overall Survival			
HR (95% CI)		1.05 (0.81; 1.36)	1.03 (0.79; 1.33)
p-value		0.7198	0.8528

* Stratified analysis which included all progression and death events except those where non-protocol therapy (NPT) was initiated prior to documented progression - those patients were censored at the last tumor assessment prior to the start of NPT.

15 mg/kg IV infusion day 1 of every 3-week cycle. After completion of six cycles of carboplatin-paclitaxel chemotherapy or upon premature discontinuation of chemotherapy, patients on the Avastin + carboplatin-paclitaxel arm continued to receive Avastin as a single agent every 3 weeks until disease progression. 878 patients were randomised to the two arms.

During the study, of the patients who received trial treatment, 32.2% (136/422) of patients received 7-12 administrations of Avastin and 21.1% (89/422) of patients received 13 or more administrations of Avastin.

The primary endpoint was duration of survival. Results are presented in Table 10.

Table 10 Efficacy results for study E4599

	Arm 1 **Carboplatin/ Paclitaxel**	**Arm 2 Carboplatin/ Paclitaxel + Avastin 15 mg/kg q 3 weeks**
Number of Patients	444	434
Overall Survival		
Median (months)	10.3	12.3
Hazard ratio	0.80 (p=0.003) 95% CI (0.69, 0.93)	
Progression-Free Survival		
Median (months)	4.8	6.4
Hazard ratio	0.65 (p<0.0001) 95% CI (0.56, 0.76)	
Overall Response Rate		
Rate (percent)	12.9	29.0 (p<0.0001)

In an exploratory analysis, the extent of Avastin benefit on overall survival was less pronounced in the subgroup of patients who did not have adenocarcinoma histology.

BO17704

Study BO17704 was a randomised, double-blind phase III study of Avastin in addition to cisplatin and gemcitabine versus placebo, cisplatin and gemcitabine in patients with locally advanced (stage IIIb with supraclavicular lymph node metastases or with malignant pleural or pericardial effusion), metastatic or recurrent non-squamous NSCLC, who had not received prior chemotherapy. The primary endpoint was progression free survival, secondary endpoints for the study included the duration of overall survival.

Patients were randomised to platinum-based chemotherapy, cisplatin 80 mg/m2 i.v. infusion on day 1 and gemcitabine 1250 mg/m2 i.v. infusion on days 1 and 8 of every 3-week cycle for up to 6 cycles (CG) with placebo or CG with Avastin at a dose of 7.5 or 15 mg/kg IV infusion day 1 of every 3-week cycle. In the Avastin-containing arms, patients could receive Avastin as a single-agent every 3 weeks until disease progression or unacceptable toxicity. Study results show that 94% (277 / 296) of eligible patients went on to receive single agent bevacizumab at cycle 7. A high proportion of patients (approximately 62%) went on to receive a variety of non-protocol specified anti-cancer therapies, which may have impacted the analysis of overall survival.

The efficacy results are presented in Table 11.

Table 11 Efficacy results for study BO17704

(see Table 11 on next page)

Overall Survival			
Median (months)	13.1	13.6 (p = 0.4203)	13.4 (p = 0.7613)
Hazard ratio		0.93 [0.78; 1.11]	1.03 [0.86, 1.23]

Advanced and/or metastatic Renal Cell Cancer (mRCC)

Avastin in Combination with Interferon alfa-2a for the First-Line Treatment of Advance and/ or Metastatic Renal Cell Cancer (BO17705)

This was a phase III randomised double-blind trial conducted to evaluate the efficacy and safety of Avastin in combination with interferon (IFN) alfa-2a (Roferon®) versus IFN alfa-2a alone as first-line treatment in mRCC. The 649 randomized patients (641 treated) had Karnofsky Performance Status (KPS) of ⩾ 70%, no CNS metastases and adequate organ function. Patients were nephrectomised for primary renal cell carcinoma. Avastin 10 mg/kg was given every 2 weeks until disease progression. IFN alfa-2a was given up to 52 weeks or until disease progression at a recommend starting dose of 9 MIU three times a week, allowing a dose reduction to 3 MIU three times a week in 2 steps. Patients were stratified according to country and Motzer score and the treatment arms were shown to be well balanced for the prognostic factors.

The primary endpoint was overall survival, with secondary endpoints for the study including progression-free survival. The addition of Avastin to IFN-alpha-2a significantly increased PFS and objective tumour response rate. These results have been confirmed through an independent radiological review. However, the increase in the primary endpoint of overall survival by 2 months was not significant (HR= 0.91). A high proportion of patients (approximately 63% IFN/placebo; 55% Avastin/IFN) received a variety of non-specified post-study anti-cancer therapies, including antineoplastic agents, which may have impacted the analysis of overall survival.

The efficacy results are presented in Table 12

Table 12 Efficacy Results for Study BO17705

	BO17705	
	Placebo+ IFN[a]	Bv[b] + IFN[a]
Number of Patients	322	327
Progression-Free Survival		
Median (months)	5.4	10.2
Hazard ratio 95% CI	0.63 0.52, 0.75 (p-value < 0.0001)	
Objective Response Rate (%) in Patients with Measurable Disease n	289	306
Response rate	12.8%	31.4%
	(p-value <0.0001)	

[a] Interferon alfa-2a 9 MIU 3x/week

[b] Bevacizumab 10 mg/kg q 2 wk

Overall Survival		
Median (months)	21.3	23.3
Hazard ratio 95% CI	0.91 0.76, 1.10 (p-value 0.3360)	

An exploratory multivariate Cox regression model using backward selection indicated that the following baseline prognostic factors were strongly associated with survival independent of treatment: gender, white blood cell count, platelets, body weight loss in the 6 months prior to study entry, number of metastatic sites, sum of longest diameter of target lesions, Motzer score. Adjustment for these baseline factors resulted in a treatment hazard ratio of 0.78 (95% CI [0.63;0.96], p = 0.0219), indicating a 22% reduction in the risk of death for patients in the Avastin+ IFN alfa-2a arm compared to IFN alfa-2a arm.

Ninety seven (97) patients in the IFN alfa-2a arm and 131 patients in the Avastin arm reduced the dose of IFN alfa-2a from 9 MIU to either 6 or 3 MIU three times a week as pre-specified in the protocol. Dose-reduction of IFN alfa-2a did not appear to affect the efficacy of the combination of Avastin and IFN alfa-2a based on PFS event free rates over time, as shown by a sub-group analysis. The 131 patients in the Avastin + IFN alfa-2a arm who reduced and maintained the IFN alfa-2a dose at 6 or 3 MIU during the study, exhibited at 6, 12 and 18 months PFS event free rates of 73, 52 and 21% respectively, as compared to 61, 43 and 17% in the total population of patients receiving Avastin + IFN alfa-2a.

AVF2938

This was a randomised, double-blind, phase II clinical study investigating Avastin 10 mg/kg in a 2 weekly schedule with the same dose of Avastin in combination with 150 mg daily erlotinib, in patients with metastatic clear cell RCC. A total of 104 patients were randomised to treatment in this study, 53 to Avastin 10 mg/kg every 2 weeks plus

Table 11 Efficacy results for study BO17704

	Cisplatin/Gemcitabine + placebo	Cisplatin/Gemcitabine + Avastin 7.5 mg/kg q 3 weeks	Cisplatin/Gemcitabine + Avastin 15 mg/kg q 3 weeks
Number of Patients	347	345	351
Progression-Free Survival			
Median (months)	6.1	6.7 (p = 0.0026)	6.5 (p = 0.0301)
Hazard ratio		0.75 [0.62;0.91]	0.82 [0.68;0.98]
Best Overall Response Rate [a]	20.1%	34.1% (p< 0.0001)	30.4% (p=0.0023)

a patients with measurable disease at baseline

placebo and 51 to Avastin 10 mg/kg every 2 weeks plus erlotinib 150 mg daily. The analysis of the primary endpoint showed no difference between the Avastin + Placebo arm and the Avastin + Erlotinib arm (median PFS 8.5 versus 9.9 months). Seven patients in each arm had an objective response. The addition of erlotinib to bevacizumab did not result in an improvement in OS (HR = 1.764; p=0.1789), duration of objective response (6.7 vs 9.1 months) or time to symptom progression (HR = 1.172; p = 0.5076).

AVF0890

This was a randomised phase II trial conducted to compare the efficacy and safety of bevacizumab versus placebo. A total of 116 patients were randomized to receive bevacizumab 3 mg/kg every 2 weeks (n=39), 10 mg/kg every 2 weeks; (n=37), or placebo (n=40). An interim analysis showed there was a significant prolongation of the time to progression of disease in the 10 mg/kg group as compared with the placebo group (hazard ratio, 2.55; p<0.001). There was a small difference, of borderline significance, between the time to progression of disease in the 3 mg/kg group and that in the placebo group (hazard ratio, 1.26; p=0.053). Four patients had objective (partial) response, and all of these had received the 10 mg/kg dose bevacizumab; the ORR for the 10 mg/kg dose was 10%.

5.2 Pharmacokinetic properties

The pharmacokinetic data for bevacizumab are available from ten clinical trials in patients with solid tumours. In all clinical trials, bevacizumab was administered as an IV infusion. The rate of infusion was based on tolerability, with an initial infusion duration of 90 minutes. The pharmacokinetics of bevacizumab was linear at doses ranging from 1 to 10 mg/kg.

Absorption

Not applicable.

Distribution

The typical value for central volume (V_c) was 2.73 L and 3.28 L for female and male patients respectively, which is in the range that has been described for IgGs and other monoclonal antibodies. The typical value for peripheral volume (V_p) was 1.69 L and 2.35 L for female and male patients respectively, when bevacizumab is coadministered with anti-neoplastic agents. After correcting for body weight, male patients had a larger Vc (+ 20%) than female patients.

Metabolism

Assessment of bevacizumab metabolism in rabbits following a single IV dose of ^{125}I-bevacizumab indicated that its metabolic profile was similar to that expected for a native IgG molecule which does not bind VEGF. The metabolism and elimination of bevacizumab is similar to endogenous IgG i.e. primarily via proteolytic catabolism throughout the body, including endothelial cells, and does not rely primarily on elimination through the kidneys and liver. Binding of the IgG to the FcRn receptor result in protection from cellular metabolism and the long terminal half-life.

Elimination

The value for clearance is, on average, equal to 0.188 and 0.220 L/day for female and male patients, respectively. After correcting for body weight, male patients had a higher bevacizumab clearance (+ 17%) than females. According to the two-compartmental model, the elimination half-life is 18 days for a typical female patient and 20 days for a typical male patient.

Low albumin and high tumour burden are generally indicative of disease severity. Bevacizumab clearance was approximately 30% faster in patients with low levels of serum albumin and 7% faster in subjects with higher tumour burden when compared with a typical patient with median values of albumin and tumour burden.

Pharmacokinetics in Special Populations

The population pharmacokinetics were analysed to evaluate the effects of demographic characteristics. The results showed no significant difference in the pharmacokinetics of bevacizumab in relation to age.

Children and adolescents: The pharmacokinetics of bevacizumab have been studied in a limited number of paediatric patients. The resulting pharmacokinetic data suggest that the volume of distribution and clearance of bevacizumab were comparable to that in adults with solid tumours.

Renal impairment: No studies have been conducted to investigate the pharmacokinetics of bevacizumab in renally impaired patients since the kidneys are not a major organ for bevacizumab metabolism or excretion.

Hepatic impairment: No studies have been conducted to investigate the pharmacokinetics of bevacizumab in patients with hepatic impairment since the liver is not a major organ for bevacizumab metabolism or excretion.

5.3 Preclinical safety data

In studies of up to 26 weeks duration in cynomolgus monkeys, physeal dysplasia was observed in young animals with open growth plates, at bevacizumab average serum concentrations below the expected human therapeutic average serum concentrations. In rabbits, bevacizumab was shown to inhibit wound healing at doses below the proposed clinical dose. Effects on wound healing were shown to be fully reversible.

Studies to evaluate the mutagenic and carcinogenic potential of bevacizumab have not been performed.

No specific studies in animals have been conducted to evaluate the effect on fertility. An adverse effect on female fertility can however be expected as repeat dose toxicity studies in animals have shown inhibition of the maturation of ovarian follicles and a decrease/absence of corpora lutea and associated decrease in ovarian and uterus weight as well as a decrease in the number of menstrual cycles.

Bevacizumab has been shown to be embryotoxic and teratogenic when administered to rabbits. Observed effects included decreases in maternal and foetal body weights, an increased number of foetal resorptions and an increased incidence of specific gross and skeletal foetal malformations. Adverse foetal outcomes were observed at all tested doses, of which the lowest dose resulted in average serum concentrations approximately 3 times larger than in humans receiving 5 mg/kg every 2 weeks.

6. PHARMACEUTICAL PARTICULARS

6.1 List of excipients

Trehalose dihydrate

Sodium phosphate

Polysorbate 20

Water for injections

6.2 Incompatibilities

A concentration dependent degradation profile of bevacizumab was observed when diluted with glucose solutions (5%).

6.3 Shelf life

2 years.

Chemical and physical in-use stability has been demonstrated for 48 hours at 2°C to 30°C in sodium chloride 9 mg/ml (0.9%) solution for injection. From a microbiological point of view, the product should be used immediately. If not used immediately, in-use storage times and conditions are the responsibility of the user and would normally not be longer than 24 hours at 2°C to 8°C, unless dilution has taken place in controlled and validated aseptic conditions.

6.4 Special precautions for storage

Store in a refrigerator (2°C-8°C).

Do not freeze.

Keep the vial in the outer carton in order to protect from light.

For storage conditions of the diluted medicinal product, see section 6.3.

6.5 Nature and contents of container

Single-use vial (Type I glass) with a butyl rubber stopper containing 100 mg of bevacizumab in 4 ml of concentrate for solution for infusion.

Single-use vial (Type I glass) with a butyl rubber stopper containing 400 mg of bevacizumab in 16 ml of concentrate for solution for infusion.

Pack of 1 vial containing 4 ml.

Pack of 1 vial containing 16 ml.

6.6 Special precautions for disposal and other handling

Avastin does not contain any antimicrobial preservative; therefore, care must be taken to ensure the sterility of the prepared solution.

Avastin should be prepared by a healthcare professional using aseptic technique. Withdraw the necessary amount of bevacizumab and dilute to the required administration volume with 0.9% sodium chloride solution for injection. The concentration of the final bevacizumab solution should be kept within the range of 1.4-16.5 mg/ml.

Discard any unused portion left in a vial, as the product contains no preservatives. Parenteral medicinal products should be inspected visually for particulate matter and discolouration prior to administration.

No incompatibilities between Avastin and polyvinyl chloride or polyolefine bags or infusion sets have been observed.

7. MARKETING AUTHORISATION HOLDER

Roche Registration Limited

6 Falcon Way

Shire Park

Welwyn Garden City

AL7 1TW

United Kingdom

8. MARKETING AUTHORISATION NUMBER(S)

EU/1/04/300/001 – 100 mg/4 ml vial

EU/1/04/300/002 – 400 mg/16 ml vial

9. DATE OF FIRST AUTHORISATION/RENEWAL OF THE AUTHORISATION

12 January 2005

10. DATE OF REVISION OF THE TEXT

23 July 2009

LEGAL STATUS

POM

Avloclor Tablets

(AstraZeneca UK Limited)

1. NAME OF THE MEDICINAL PRODUCT

Avloclor Tablets

2. QUALITATIVE AND QUANTITATIVE COMPOSITION

Tablets containing 250mg chloroquine phosphate Ph. Eur. which is equivalent to 155mg chloroquine base.

3. PHARMACEUTICAL FORM

Tablets.

4. CLINICAL PARTICULARS

4.1 Therapeutic indications

a) Treatment of malaria.

b) Prophylaxis and suppression of malaria.

c) Treatment of amoebic hepatitis and abscess.

d) Treatment of discoid and systemic lupus erythematosus.

e) Treatment of rheumatoid arthritis.

4.2 Posology and method of administration

The dose should be taken after food.

a) Treatment of malaria

i) P. falciparum and P. malariae infections

Adults: A single dose of four tablets, followed by two tablets six hours later and then two tablets a day for two days.

Children: A single dose of 10mg base/kg, followed by 5mg base/kg six hours later and then 5mg base/kg a day for two days.

(see Table 1 on next page)

ii) P. vivax and P. ovale infections

Adults: A single dose of four tablets, followed by two tablets six hours later and then two tablets a day for two days. Follow with a course of treatment with primaquine if a radical cure is required.

Children: A single dose of 10mg base/kg, followed by 5mg base/kg six hours later and then 5mg base/kg a day for two days. Follow with a course of treatment with primaquine if a radical cure is required.

Elderly Patients: There are no special dosage recommendations for the elderly, but it may be advisable to monitor elderly patients so that optimum dosage can be individually determined.

Hepatic or Renally Impaired Patients: Caution is necessary when giving Avloclor to patients with renal disease or hepatic disease.

b) Prophylaxis and suppression of malaria

Adults: Two tablets taken once a week, on the same day each week. Start one week before exposure to risk and continue until four weeks after leaving the malarious area.

Children: A single dose of 5mg chloroquine base/kg per week on the same day each week. Start one week before exposure to risk and continue until four weeks after leaving the malarious area.

For practical purposes, children aged over 14 years may be treated as adults. The dose given to infants and children should be calculated on their body weight and must not exceed the adult dose regardless of weight.

Table 1

Age (years)	Initial dose	Second dose 6 hours after first	Dose on each of the two subsequent days
1 – 4	1 Tablet	½ Tablet	½ Tablet
5 – 8	2 Tablets	1 Tablet	1 Tablet
9 -14	3 Tablets	1 ½ Tablets	1 ½ Tablets

- 4 years ½ tablet
5 - 8 years 1 tablet
9 - 15 years 1 ½ tablets

Elderly Patients: There are no special dosage recommendations for the elderly, but it may be advisable to monitor elderly patients so that optimum dosage can be individually determined.

Hepatic or Renally Impaired Patients: Caution is necessary when giving Avloclor to patients with renal disease or hepatic disease.

c) Amoebic hepatitis

Adults: Four tablets daily for two days followed by one tablet twice daily for two or three weeks.

Elderly Patients: There are no special dosage recommendations for the elderly, but it may be advisable to monitor elderly patients so that optimum dosage can be individually determined.

Hepatic or Renally Impaired Patients: Caution is necessary when giving Avloclor to patients with renal disease or hepatic disease.

d) Lupus erythematosus

Adults: One tablet twice daily for one to two weeks followed by a maintenance dosage of one tablet daily.

Elderly Patients: There are no special dosage recommendations for the elderly, but it may be advisable to monitor elderly patients so that optimum dosage can be individually determined.

Hepatic or Renally Impaired Patients: Caution is necessary when giving Avloclor to patients with renal disease or hepatic disease.

e) Rheumatoid arthritis

Adults: The usual dosage is one tablet daily.

Elderly Patients: There are no special dosage recommendations for the elderly, but it may be advisable to monitor elderly patients so that optimum dosage can be individually determined.

Hepatic or Renally Impaired Patients: Caution is necessary when giving Avloclor to patients with renal disease or hepatic disease.

4.3 Contraindications

Known hypersensitivity to chloroquine or any other ingredients of the formulation.

Concomitant use with amiodarone. (See section 4.5)

4.4 Special warnings and precautions for use

When used as malaria prophylaxis official guidelines and local information on prevalence of resistance to anti-malarial drugs should be taken into consideration.

Caution is necessary when giving Avloclor to patients with impaired hepatic function, particularly when associated with cirrhosis.

Caution is also necessary in patients with porphyria. Avloclor may precipitate severe constitutional symptoms and an increase in the amount of porphyrins excreted in the urine. This reaction is especially apparent in patients with high alcohol intake.

Caution is necessary when giving Avloclor to patients with renal disease.

Avloclor should be used with care in patients with a history of epilepsy. Potential risks and benefits should be carefully evaluated before use in subjects on anticonvulsant therapy or with a history of epilepsy as rare cases of convulsions have been reported in association with chloroquine.

Considerable caution is needed in the use of Avloclor for long-term high dosage therapy and such use should only be considered when no other drug is available. Patients on long-term therapy should also be monitored for cardiomyopathy.

Irreversible retinal damage and corneal changes may develop during long term therapy and after the drug has been discontinued. Ophthalmic examination prior to and at 3 – 6 monthly intervals during use is required if patients are receiving chloroquine

- at continuous high doses for longer than 12 months
- as weekly treatment for longer than 3 years
- when total consumption exceeds 1.6g/kg (cumulative dose 100g)

Full blood counts should be carried out regularly during extended treatment as bone marrow suppression may occur rarely. Caution is required if drugs known to induce blood disorders are used concurrently.

The use of Avloclor in patients with psoriasis may precipitate a severe attack.

Caution is advised in patients with glucose-6-phosphate dehydrogenase deficiency, as there may be a risk of haemolysis.

4.5 Interaction with other medicinal products and other forms of interaction

If the patient is taking amiodarone then chloroquine and hydroxychloroquine may increase the risk of cardiac arrhythmias including ventricular arrhythmias, bradycardias and cardiac conduction defect. Concurrent use is contraindicated.

Antacids (aluminium, calcium and magnesium salts) and adsorbents (e.g. kaolin) may reduce the absorption of chloroquine, so should be taken well separated from Avloclor (at least four hours apart).

If the patient is taking ciclosporin then chloroquine may cause an increase in ciclosporin levels.

Pre-exposure intradermal human diploid-cell rabies vaccine should not be administered to patients taking chloroquine as this may suppress the antibody response. When vaccinated against rabies, that vaccine should precede the start of the antimalarial dosing, otherwise the effectiveness of the vaccine might be reduced.

Chloroquine significantly reduces levels of praziquantel. Caution is therefore advised during co-administration. Prescribers may consider increasing the dose of praziquantel if the patient does not respond to the initial dose.

Other antimalarials: increased risk of convulsion with mefloquine.

Cardiac glycosides: hydroxychloroquine and possibly chloroquine increase plasma concentration of digoxin.

Parasympathomimetics: chloroquine and hydroxychloroquine have potential to increase symptoms of myasthenia gravis and thus diminish effect of neostigmine and pyridostigmine.

Ulcer healing drugs: cimetidine inhibits metabolism of chloroquine (increased plasma concentration).

4.6 Pregnancy and lactation

Pregnancy

Avloclor should not be used during pregnancy unless, in the judgement of the physician, potential benefit outweighs the risk.

Short-term malaria prophylaxis:

Malaria in pregnant women increases the risk of maternal death, miscarriage, still-birth and low birth weight with the associated risk of neonatal death. Travel to malarious areas should be avoided during pregnancy but, if this is not possible, women should receive effective prophylaxis.

Long-term high dose:

There is evidence to suggest that Avloclor given to women in high doses throughout pregnancy can give rise to foetal abnormalities including visual loss, ototoxicity and cochlear-vestibular dysfunction.

Lactation

Although Avloclor is excreted in breast milk, the amount is too small to be harmful when used for malaria prophylaxis but as a consequence is insufficient to confer any benefit on the infant. Separate chemoprophylaxis for the infant is required. However, when long-term high doses are used for rheumatoid disease, breast feeding is not recommended.

4.7 Effects on ability to drive and use machines

Defects in visual accommodation may occur on first taking Avloclor and patients should be warned regarding driving or operating machinery.

4.8 Undesirable effects

The adverse reactions which may occur at doses used in the prophylaxis or treatment of malaria are generally not of a serious nature. Where prolonged high dosage is required, i.e. in the treatment of rheumatoid arthritis, adverse reactions can be of a more serious nature.

Cardiovascular: hypotension and ECG changes (at high doses) cardiomyopathy.

Central nervous system: convulsions and psychotic reactions including hallucinations (rare), anxiety, personality changes.

Eye disorders: retinal degeneration, macular defects of colour vision, pigmentation, optic atrophy scotomas, field defects, blindness, corneal opacities and pigmented deposits, blurring of vision, difficulty in accommodation, diplopia.

Gastro-intestinal: gastro-intestinal disturbances, nausea, vomiting, diarrhoea, abdominal cramps.

General: headache.

Haematological: bone marrow depression, aplastic anaemia, agranulocytosis, thrombocytopenia, neutropenia.

Hepatic: Changes in liver function, including hepatitis and abnormal liver function tests, have been reported rarely.

Hypersensitivity: allergic and anaphylactic reactions, including urticaria, angioedema and vasculitis.

Hearing disorders: tinnitus, reduced hearing, nerve deafness.

Muscular: neuromyopathy and myopathy.

Skin: macular, urticarial and purpuric skin eruptions, occasional depigmentation or loss of hair, erythema multiforme, Stevens-Johnson syndrome, toxic epidermal necrolysis, precipitation of psoriasis, pruritus, photosensitivity, lichen-planus type reaction, pigmentation of the skin and mucous membranes (long term use).

4.9 Overdose

Chloroquine is highly toxic in overdose and children are particularly susceptible. The chief symptoms of overdosage include circulatory collapse due to a potent cardiotoxic effect, respiratory arrest and coma. Symptoms may progress rapidly after initial nausea and vomiting. Cardiac complications may occur without progressively deepening coma.

Death may result from circulatory or respiratory failure or cardiac arrhythmia. If there is no demonstrable cardiac output due to arrhythmias, asystole or electromechanical dissociation, external chest compression should be persisted with for as long as necessary, or until adrenaline and diazepam can be given (see below).

Gastric lavage should be carried out urgently, first protecting the airway and instituting artificial ventilation where necessary. There is a risk of cardiac arrest following aspiration of gastric contents in more serious cases. Activated charcoal left in the stomach may reduce absorption of any remaining chloroquine from the gut. Circulatory status (with central venous pressure measurement), respiration, plasma electrolytes and blood gases should be monitored, with correction of hypokalaemia and acidosis if indicated. Cardiac arrhythmias should not be treated unless life threatening; drugs with quinidine-like effects should be avoided. Intravenous sodium bicarbonate 1-2mmol/kg over 15 minutes may be effective in conduction disturbances, and DC shock is indicated for ventricular tachycardia and ventricular fibrillation.

Early administration of the following has been shown to improve survival in cases of serious poisoning:

1. Adrenaline infusion 0.25micrograms/kg/min initially, with increments of 0.25micrograms/kg/min until adequate systolic blood pressure (more than 100mg/Hg) is restored; adrenaline reduces the effects of chloroquine on the heart through its inotropic and vasoconstrictor effects.

2. Diazepam infusion (2mg/kg over 30 minutes as a loading dose, followed by 1-2mg/kg/day for up to 2-4 days). Diazepam may minimise cardiotoxicity.

Acidification of the urine, haemodialysis, peritoneal dialysis or exchange transfusion have not been shown to be of value in treating chloroquine poisoning. Chloroquine is excreted very slowly, therefore cases of overdosage require observation for several days.

5. PHARMACOLOGICAL PROPERTIES

5.1 Pharmacodynamic properties

The mode of action of chloroquine on plasmodia has not been fully elucidated. Chloroquine binds to and alters the properties of DNA. Chloroquine also binds to ferriprotoporphyrin IX and this leads to lysis of the plasmodial membrane.

In suppressive treatment, chloroquine inhibits the erythrocytic stage of development of plasmodia. In acute attacks of malaria, it interrupts erythrocytic schizogony of the parasite. Its ability to concentrate in parasitised erythrocytes may account for the selective toxicity against the erythrocytic stages of plasmodial infection.

5.2 Pharmacokinetic properties

Studies in volunteers using single doses of chloroquine phosphate equivalent to 300mg base have found peak plasma levels to be achieved within one to six hours. These levels are in the region of 54 - 102microgram/litre, the concentration in whole blood being some 4 to 10 times higher. Following a single dose, chloroquine may be detected in plasma for more than four weeks. Mean bioavailability from tablets of chloroquine phosphate is 89%. Chloroquine is widely distributed in body tissues such as the eyes, kidneys, liver, and lungs where retention is prolonged. The elimination of chloroquine is slow, with a multi exponential decline in plasma concentration. The initial distribution phase has a half-life of 2-6 days while the terminal elimination phase is 10-60 days. Approximately 50-70% of chloroquine in plasma is bound to the plasma proteins.

The principal metabolite is monodesethylchloroquine, which reaches a peak concentration of 10-20 microgram/litre within a few hours. Mean urinary recovery, within 3-13 weeks, is approximately 50% of the administered dose, most being unchanged drug and the remainder as metabolite. Chloroquine may be detected in urine for several months.

5.3 Preclinical safety data

Avloclor has been widely used for many years in clinical practice. There is no animal data which adds significant information relevant to the prescriber, to that covered elsewhere in this document.

6. PHARMACEUTICAL PARTICULARS

6.1 List of excipients

Magnesium stearate Ph. Eur.

Maize starch Ph. Eur.

6.2 Incompatibilities

None have been reported or are known.

6.3 Shelf life

5 years.

6.4 Special precautions for storage

Do not store above 30°C. Protect from light and moisture.

6.5 Nature and contents of container

HDPE bottle of 100's and PVC/Aluminium Foil Blister Pack of 20's

6.6 Special precautions for disposal and other handling

No special instructions.

7. MARKETING AUTHORISATION HOLDER

AstraZeneca UK Limited
600 Capability Green,
Luton, LU1 3LU, UK

8. MARKETING AUTHORISATION NUMBER(S)

PL 17901/0003

9. DATE OF FIRST AUTHORISATION/RENEWAL OF THE AUTHORISATION

18th June 2000/4th June 2005

10. DATE OF REVISION OF THE TEXT

28th July 2009

Avodart 0.5mg soft capsules

(GlaxoSmithKline UK)

1. NAME OF THE MEDICINAL PRODUCT

Avodart® 0.5 mg soft capsules.

2. QUALITATIVE AND QUANTITATIVE COMPOSITION

Each capsule contains 0.5 mg dutasteride.

For a full list of excipients, see section 6.1.

3. PHARMACEUTICAL FORM

Capsules, soft.

The capsules are opaque, yellow, oblong soft gelatin capsules imprinted with GX CE2 on one side in red ink.

4. CLINICAL PARTICULARS

4.1 Therapeutic indications

Treatment of moderate to severe symptoms of benign prostatic hyperplasia (BPH).

Reduction in the risk of acute urinary retention (AUR) and surgery in patients with moderate to severe symptoms of BPH.

For information on effects of treatment and patient populations studied in clinical trials please see section 5.1.

4.2 Posology and method of administration

Avodart can be administered alone or in combination with the alpha-blocker tamsulosin (0.4mg) (see sections 4.4, 4.8 and 5.1).

Adults (including elderly):

The recommended dose of Avodart is one capsule (0.5 mg) taken orally once a day. The capsules should be swallowed whole and not chewed or opened as contact with the capsule contents may result in irritation of the oropharyngeal mucosa. The capsules may be taken with or without food. Although an improvement may be observed at an early stage, it can take up to 6 months before a response to the treatment can be achieved. No dose adjustment is necessary in the elderly.

Renal impairment

The effect of renal impairment on dutasteride pharmacokinetics has not been studied. No adjustment in dosage is anticipated for patients with renal impairment (see section 5.2).

Hepatic impairment

The effect of hepatic impairment on dutasteride pharmacokinetics has not been studied so caution should be used in patients with mild to moderate hepatic impairment (see section 4.4 and section 5.2). In patients with severe hepatic impairment, the use of dutasteride is contraindicated (see section 4.3).

4.3 Contraindications

Avodart is contraindicated in:

- women and children and adolescents (see section 4.6).
- patients with hypersensitivity to dutasteride, other 5-alpha reductase inhibitors, or any of the excipients.
- patients with severe hepatic impairment.

4.4 Special warnings and precautions for use

Combination therapy should be prescribed after careful benefit risk assessment due to the potential increased risk of adverse events and after consideration of alternative treatment options including monotherapies (see section 4.2).

Digital rectal examination, as well as other evaluations for prostate cancer, must be performed on patients with BPH prior to initiating therapy with Avodart and periodically thereafter.

Dutasteride is absorbed through the skin, therefore, women, children and adolescents must avoid contact with leaking capsules (see section 4.6). If contact is made with leaking capsules, the contact area should be washed immediately with soap and water.

Dutasteride was not studied in patients with liver disease. Caution should be used in the administration of dutasteride to patients with mild to moderate hepatic impairment (see section 4.2, section 4.3 and section 5.2).

Serum prostate-specific antigen (PSA) concentration is an important component in the detection of prostate cancer. Generally, a total serum PSA concentration greater than 4 ng/mL (Hybritech) requires further evaluation and consideration of prostate biopsy. Physicians should be aware that a baseline PSA less than 4 ng/mL in patients taking Avodart does not exclude a diagnosis of prostate cancer. Avodart causes a decrease in serum PSA levels by approximately 50%, after 6 months, in patients with BPH, even in the presence of prostate cancer. Although there may be individual variation, the reduction in PSA by approximately 50% is predictable as it was observed over the entire range of baseline PSA values (1.5 to 10 ng/mL). Therefore to interpret an isolated PSA value in a man treated with Avodart for six months or more, PSA values should be doubled for comparison with normal ranges in untreated men. This adjustment preserves the sensitivity and specificity of the PSA assay and maintains its ability to detect prostate cancer. Any sustained increases in PSA levels while on Avodart should be carefully evaluated, including consideration of noncompliance to therapy with Avodart.

Total serum PSA levels return to baseline within 6 months of discontinuing treatment. The ratio of free to total PSA remains constant even under the influence of Avodart. If clinicians elect to use percent free PSA as an aid in the detection of prostate cancer in men undergoing Avodart therapy, no adjustment to its value appears necessary.

4.5 Interaction with other medicinal products and other forms of interaction

For information on the decrease of serum PSA levels during treatment with dutasteride and guidance concerning prostate cancer detection, please see section 4.4.

Effects of other drugs on the pharmacokinetics of dutasteride

Use together with CYP3A4 and/or P-glycoprotein-inhibitors:

Dutasteride is mainly eliminated via metabolism. *In vitro* studies indicate that this metabolism is catalysed by CYP3A4 and CYP3A5. No formal interaction studies have been performed with potent CYP3A4 inhibitors. However, in a population pharmacokinetic study, dutasteride serum concentrations were on average 1.6 to 1.8 times greater, respectively, in a small number of patients treated concurrently with verapamil or diltiazem (moderate inhibitors of CYP3A4 and inhibitors of P-glycoprotein) than in other patients.

Long-term combination of dutasteride with drugs that are potent inhibitors of the enzyme CYP3A4 (e.g. ritonavir, indinavir, nefazodone, itraconazole, ketoconazole administered orally) may increase serum concentrations of dutasteride. Further inhibition of 5-alpha reductase at increased dutasteride exposure, is not likely. However, a reduction of the dutasteride dosing frequency can be considered if side effects are noted. It should be noted that in the case of enzyme inhibition, the long half-life may be further prolonged and it can take more than 6 months of concurrent therapy before a new steady state is reached.

Administration of 12g colestyramine one hour before a 5mg single dose of dutasteride did not affect the pharmacokinetics of dutasteride.

Effects of dutasteride on the pharmacokinetics of other drugs

Dutasteride has no effect on the pharmacokinetics of warfarin or digoxin. This indicates that dutasteride does not inhibit/induce CYP2C9 or the transporter P-glycoprotein. *In vitro* interaction studies indicate that dutasteride does not inhibit the enzymes CYP1A2, CYP2D6, CYP2C9, CYP2C19 or CYP3A4.

In a small study (N=24) of two weeks duration in healthy men, dutasteride (0.5 mg daily) had no effect on the pharmacokinetics of tamsulosin or terazosin. There was also no indication of a pharmacodynamic interaction in this study.

4.6 Pregnancy and lactation

Avodart is contraindicated for use by women.

Fertility

Dutasteride has been reported to affect semen characteristics (reduction in sperm count, semen volume, and sperm motility) in healthy men (see section 5.1). The possibility of reduced male fertility cannot be excluded.

Pregnancy

As with other 5 alpha reductase inhibitors, dutasteride inhibits the conversion of testosterone to dihydrotestosterone and may, if administered to a woman carrying a male foetus, inhibit the development of the external genitalia c the foetus (see section 4.4). Small amounts of dutasterid have been recovered from the semen in subjects receivin Avodart 0.5 mg day. Based on studies in animals, it i unlikely that a male foetus will be adversely affected his mother is exposed to the semen of a patient bein treated with Avodart (the risk of which is greatest during th first 16 weeks of pregnancy). However, as with all 5 alph reductase inhibitors, when the patient's partner is or ma potentially be pregnant it is recommended that the patien avoids exposure of his partner to semen by use of a condom.

Lactation

It is not known whether dutasteride is excreted in humar milk.

4.7 Effects on ability to drive and use machines

Based on the pharmacodynamic properties of dutasteride, treatment with dutasteride would not be expected to interfere with the ability to drive or operate machinery.

4.8 Undesirable effects

AVODART AS MONOTHERAPY

Approximately 19% of the 2167 patients who received dutasteride in the 2 year Phase III placebo-controlled trials developed adverse reactions during the first year of treatment. The majority of events were mild to moderate and occurred in the reproductive system. No change to the adverse event profile was apparent over a further 2 years in open-label extension studies.

The following table shows adverse reactions from controlled clinical trials and post-marketing experience. The listed adverse events from clinical trials are investigator-judged drug-related events (with incidence more than or equal to 1%) reported with a higher incidence in patients treated with dutasteride compared with placebo during the first year of treatment. Adverse events from post-marketing experience were identified from spontaneous post-marketing reports; therefore the true incidence is unknown:

(see Table 1 on next page)

AVODART IN COMBINATION WITH THE ALPHA-BLOCKER TAMSULOSIN

Year 2 data from the CombAT Study, comparing dutasteride 0.5mg (n=1623) and tamsulosin 0.4mg (n=1611) once daily alone and in combination (n=1610) have shown that the incidence of any investigator-judged drug-related adverse event during the first and second years of treatment respectively was 22% and 5% for dutasteride/tamsulosin combination therapy, 14% and 5% for dutasteride monotherapy and 13% and 4% for tamsulosin monotherapy. The higher incidence of adverse events in the combination therapy group in the first year of treatment was due to a higher incidence of reproductive disorders, specifically ejaculation disorders, observed in this group.

The following investigator-judged drug-related adverse events have been reported with an incidence of greater than or equal to 1% during the first year of treatment in the Year 2 analysis of the CombAT Study; the incidence of these events during the first and second year of treatment is shown in the table below:

(see Table 2 on next page)

4.9 Overdose

In volunteer studies of Avodart, single daily doses of dutasteride up to 40 mg/day (80 times the therapeutic dose) have been administered for 7 days without significant safety concerns. In clinical studies, doses of 5mg daily have been administered to subjects for 6 months with no additional adverse effects to those seen at therapeutic doses of 0.5 mg. There is no specific antidote for Avodart, therefore, in suspected overdosage symptomatic and supportive treatment should be given as appropriate.

5. PHARMACOLOGICAL PROPERTIES

5.1 Pharmacodynamic properties

Pharmacotherapeutic group: testosterone-5-alpha-reductase inhibitors.

ATC code: G04C B02.

Dutasteride reduces circulating levels of dihydrotestosterone (DHT) by inhibiting both type 1 and type 2, 5α-reductase isoenzymes which are responsible for the conversion of testosterone to 5α-DHT.

AVODART AS MONOTHERAPY

Effects on DHT/Testosterone:

Effect of daily doses of Avodart on the reduction on DHT is dose dependant and is observed within 1-2 weeks (85% and 90% reduction, respectively).

In patients with BPH treated with dutasteride 0.5 mg/day, the median decrease in serum DHT was 94% at 1 year and 93% at 2 years and the median increase in serum testosterone was 19% at both 1 and 2 years.

Effect on Prostate Volume:

Significant reductions in prostate volume have been detected as early as one month after initiation of treatment and reductions continued through Month 24 ($p<0.001$). Avodart led to a mean reduction of total prostate volume of 23.6% (from 54.9 ml at baseline to 42.1 ml) at Month 12 compared with a mean reduction of 0.5% (from 54.0 ml to 53.7 ml) in the placebo group. Significant ($p<0.001$) reductions also occurred in prostate transitional zone volume as early as one month continuing through Month 24, with a

Table 1

Organ system	Adverse reaction	Incidence from clinical trial data	
		Incidence during year 1 of treatment (n=2167)	Incidence during year 2 of treatment (n=1744)
Reproductive system and breast disorders	Impotence	6.0%	1.7%
	Altered (decreased) libido	3.7%	0.6%
	Ejaculation disorders	1.8%	0.5%
	Breast disorders (includes breast enlargement and/or breast tenderness)	1.3%	1.3%
Immune system disorders	Allergic reactions including rash, pruritus, urticaria, localised oedema, and angioedema	Incidence estimated from post-marketing data	
		Unknown	

Table 2

System Organ Class	Adverse reaction	Incidence during year 1 of treatment			Incidence during year 2 of treatment		
		Dutasteride + Tamsulosin (n=1610)	Dutasteride (n=1623)	Tamsulosin (n=1611)	Dutasteride + Tamsulosin (n=1424)	Dutasteride (n=1457)	Tamsulosin (n=1468)
Reproductive system and breast disorders, Psychiatric disorders and Investigations	Impotence	6.5%	4.9%	3.3%	1.1%	1.3%	0.7%
	Altered (decreased) libido	5.2%	3.8%	2.5%	0.4%	0.9%	0.6%
	Ejaculation disorders	8.9%	1.6%	2.7%	0.5%	0.3%	0.5%
	Breast disorders (includes breast enlargement and/or breast tenderness)	2.0%	1.8%	0.8%	0.9%	1.2%	0.3%
Nervous system disorders	Dizziness	1.4%	0.6%	1.3%	0.2%	0.1%	0.4%

nean reduction in prostate transitional zone volume of 7.8% (from 26.8 ml at baseline to 21.4 ml) in the Avodart roup compared to a mean increase of 7.9% (from 26.8ml 27.5 ml) in the placebo group at Month 12. The reduction f the prostate volume seen during the first 2 years of ouble-blind treatment was maintained during an additional 2 years of open-label extension studies. Reduction f the size of prostate leads to improvement of symptoms nd a decreased risk for AUR and BPH-related surgery.

CLINICAL STUDIES

Avodart 0.5 mg/day or placebo was evaluated in 4325 male subjects with moderate to severe symptoms of BPH who ad prostates ⩾30 ml and a PSA value within the range 1.5 10 ng/mL in three primary efficacy 2-year multicenter, multinational, placebo-controlled, double-blind studies. The studies then continued with an open-label extension o 4 years with all patients remaining in the study receiving utasteride at the same 0.5mg dose. 37% of initially placebo-randomized patients and 40% of dutasteride-randomized patients remained in the study at 4 years. The majority (71%) of the 2,340 subjects in the open-label extensions completed the 2 additional years of open-label treatment.

The most important clinical efficacy parameters were American Urological Association Symptom Index (AUA-SI), maximum urinary flow (Qmax) and the incidence of acute urinary retention and BPH-related surgery.

AUA-SI is a seven-item questionnaire about BPH-related symptoms with a maximum score of 35. At baseline the average score was approx. 17. After six months, one and two years treatment the placebo group had an average improvement of 2.5, 2.5 and 2.3 points respectively while the Avodart group improved 3.2, 3.8 and 4.5 points respectively. The differences between the groups were statistically significant. The improvement in AUA-SI seen during the first 2 years of double-blind treatment was maintained during an additional 2 years of open-label extension studies.

Qmax (maximum urine flow):

Mean baseline Qmax for the studies was approx 10 ml/sec (normal Qmax ⩾15 ml/sec). After one and two years treatment the flow in the placebo group had improved by 0.8 and 0.9 ml/sec respectively and 1.7 and 2.0 ml/sec respectively in the Avodart group. The difference between the groups was statistically significant from Month 1 to Month 24. The increase in maximum urine flow rate seen during the first 2 years of double blind treatment continued throughout an additional 2 years of open-label extension studies.

Acute Urinary Retention and Surgical Intervention

After two years of treatment, the incidence of AUR was 4.2% in the placebo group against 1.8% in the Avodart group (57% risk reduction). This difference is statistically significant and means that 42 patients (95% CI 30-73) need to be treated for two years to avoid one case of AUR.

The incidence of BPH-related surgery after two years was 4.1% in the placebo group and 2.2% in the Avodart group (48% risk reduction). This difference is statistically significant and means that 51 patients (95% CI 33-109) need to be treated for two years to avoid one surgical intervention.

Hair distribution

The effect of dutasteride on hair distribution was not formally studied during the phase III programme, however, 5 alpha-reductase inhibitors could reduce hair loss and may induce hair growth in subjects with male pattern hair loss (male androgenetic alopecia).

Thyroid function:

Thyroid function was evaluated in a one year study in healthy men. Free thyroxine levels were stable on dutasteride treatment but TSH levels were mildly increased (by 0.4 MCIU/mL) compared to placebo at the end of one year's treatment. However, as TSH levels were variable, median TSH ranges (1.4 - 1.9 MCIU/mL) remained within normal limits (0.5 - 5/6 MCIU/mL), free thyroxine levels were stable within the normal range and similar for both placebo and dutasteride treatment, the changes in TSH were not considered clinically significant. In all the clinical studies, there has been no evidence that dutasteride adversely affects thyroid function.

Breast neoplasia:

In the 2 year clinical trials, providing 3374 patient years of exposure to dutasteride, and at the time of registration in the 2 year open label extension, there were 2 cases of breast cancer reported in dutasteride-treated patients and 1 case in a patient who received placebo.

However, the relationship between breast cancer and dutasteride is not clear.

Effects on male fertility

The effects of dutasteride 0.5mg/day on semen characteristics were evaluated in healthy volunteers aged 18 to 52 (n=27 dutasteride, n=23 placebo) throughout 52 weeks of treatment and 24 weeks of post-treatment follow-up. At 52 weeks, the mean percent reduction from baseline in total sperm count, semen volume and sperm motility were 23%, 26% and 18%, respectively, in the dutasteride group when adjusted for changes from baseline in the placebo group. Sperm concentration and sperm morphology were unaffected. After 24 weeks of follow-up, the mean percent change in total sperm count in the dutasteride group remained 23% lower than baseline. While mean values for all parameters at all time points remained within the normal ranges and did not meet the predefined criteria for a clinically significant change (30%), two subjects in the dutasteride group had decreases in sperm count of greater than 90% from baseline at 52 weeks, with partial recovery at the 24 week follow-up. The possibility of reduced male fertility cannot be excluded.

AVODART IN COMBINATION WITH THE ALPHA-BLOCKER TAMSULOSIN

Avodart 0.5 mg/day (n = 1,623), tamsulosin 0.4 mg/day (n = 1,611) or the combination of Avodart 0.5 mg plus tamsulosin 0.4 mg (n = 1,610) were evaluated in male subjects with moderate to severe symptoms of BPH who had prostates ⩾30 ml and a PSA value within the range 1.5 - 10 ng/mL in a multicentre, multinational, randomized double-blind, parallel group study. Approximately 52% of subjects had previous exposure to 5-alpha reductase inhibitor or alpha-blocker treatment. Efficacy endpoints during the first 2 years of treatment were change in International Prostate Symptom Score (IPSS), maximum urine flow rate (Qmax) and prostate volume. IPSS is an 8-item instrument based on AUA-SI with an additional question on quality of life.

Results following 2 years of treatment are presented below:

(see Table 3 below)

5.2 Pharmacokinetic properties

Absorption

Following oral administration of a single 0.5 mg dutasteride dose, the time to peak serum concentrations of dutasteride is 1 to 3 hours. The absolute bioavailability is approximately 60%. The bioavailability of dutasteride is not affected by food.

Distribution

Dutasteride has a large volume of distribution (300 to 500 L) and is highly bound to plasma proteins >99.5%). Following daily dosing, dutasteride serum concentrations achieve 65% of steady state concentration after 1 month and approximately 90% after 3 months.

Steady state serum concentrations (C_{ss}) of approximately 40 ng/mL are achieved after 6 months of dosing 0.5mg once a day. Dutasteride partitioning from serum into semen averaged 11.5%.

Elimination

Dutasteride is extensively metabolized *in vivo*. *In vitro*, dutasteride is metabolized by the cytochrome P450 3A4 and 3A5 to three monohydroxylated metabolites and one dihydroxylated metabolite.

Following oral dosing of dutasteride 0.5 mg/day to steady state, 1.0% to 15.4% (mean of 5.4%) of the administered

Table 3

Parameter	Time-point	Combination	Avodart	Tamsulosin
IPSS (units)	[Baseline] Month 24 (Change from Baseline)	[16.6] -6.2	[16.4] -4.9a	[16.4] -4.3b
Qmax (mL/sec)	[Baseline] Month 24 (Change from Baseline)	[10.9] 2.4	[10.6] 1.9c*	[10.7] 0.9d*
Prostate Volume	[Baseline] (ml) Month 24 (% Change from Baseline)	[54.7] -26.9	[54.6] -28.0	[55.8] 0.0*
Prostate Transition Zone Volume	[Baseline] (ml) Month 24 (% Change from Baseline)	[27.7] -23.4	[30.3] -22.8	[30.5] 8.8*
BPH Impact Index (BII) (units)	[Baseline] Month 24 (Change from Baseline)	[5.3] -2.1	[5.3] -1.7*	[5.3] -1.5*
IPSS Question 8 (BPH-related Health Status)	[Baseline] Month 24 (Change from Baseline)	[3.6] -1.4	[3.6] -1.1*	[3.6] -1.1*

a. Combination achieved significance ($p<0.001$) vs. Avodart from Month 3
b. Combination achieved significance ($p<0.001$) vs. tamsulosin from Month 9
c. Combination achieved significance ($p<=0.006$) vs. Avodart from Month 6
d. Combination achieved significance ($p<0.001$) vs. tamsulosin from Month 6
* $p<0.01$

dose is excreted as unchanged dutasteride in the faeces. The remainder is excreted in the faeces as 4 major metabolites comprising 39%, 21%, 7%, and 7% each of drug-related material and 6 minor metabolites (less than 5% each). Only trace amounts of unchanged dutasteride (less than 0.1% of the dose) are detected in human urine.

The elimination of dutasteride is dose dependent and the process appears to be described by two elimination pathways in parallel, one that is saturable at clinically relevant concentrations and one that is non saturable.

At low serum concentrations (less than 3ng/mL), dutasteride is cleared rapidly by both the concentration dependent and concentration independent elimination pathways. Single doses of 5 mg or less showed evidence of rapid clearance and a short half-life of 3 to 9 days.

At therapeutic concentrations, following repeat dosing of 0.5 mg/day, the slower, linear elimination pathway is dominating and the half-life is approx. 3-5 weeks.

Elderly

Dutasteride pharmacokinetics were evaluated in 36 healthy male subjects between the ages of 24 and 87 years following administration of a single 5mg dose of dutasteride. No significant influence of age was seen on the exposure of dutasteride but the half-life was shorter in men under 50 years of age. Half-life was not statistically different when comparing the 50-69 year old group to the greater than 70 years old.

Renal impairment

The effect of renal impairment on dutasteride pharmacokinetics has not been studied. However, less than 0.1% of a steady-state 0.5 mg dose of dutasteride is recovered in human urine, so no clinically significant increase of the dutasteride plasma concentrations is anticipated for patients with renal impairment (see section 4.2).

Hepatic impairment

The effect on the pharmacokinetics of dutasteride in hepatic impairment has not been studied (see section 4.3). Because dutasteride is eliminated mainly through metabolism the plasma levels of dutasteride are expected to be elevated in these patients and the half-life of dutasteride be prolonged (see section 4.2 and section 4.4).

5.3 Preclinical safety data

Current studies of general toxicity, genotoxicity and carcinogenicity did not show any particular risk to humans.

Reproduction toxicity studies in male rats have shown a decreased weight of the prostate and seminal vesicles, decreased secretion from accessory genital glands and a reduction in fertility indices (caused by the pharmacological effect of dutasteride). The clinical relevance of these findings is unknown.

As with other 5 alpha reductase inhibitors, feminisation of male foetuses in rats and rabbits has been noted when dutasteride was administered during gestation. Dutasteride has been found in blood from female rats after mating with dutasteride treated males. When dutasteride was administered during gestation to primates, no feminisation of male foetuses was seen at blood exposures sufficiently in excess of those likely to occur via human semen. It is unlikely that a male foetus will be adversely affected following seminal transfer of dutasteride.

6. PHARMACEUTICAL PARTICULARS

6.1 List of excipients

Capsule contents:

mono- and diglycerides of caprylic/capric acid

butylhydroxytoluene (E321).

Capsule shell:

gelatin

glycerol

titanium dioxide (E171)

iron oxide yellow (E172)

triglycerides, medium chain

lecithin.

Red printing ink containing iron oxide red (E172) as the colourant, polyvinyl acetate phthalate, propylene glycol and Macrogol 400.

6.2 Incompatibilities

Not applicable.

6.3 Shelf life

4 years.

6.4 Special precautions for storage

Do not store above 30°C.

6.5 Nature and contents of container

Blisters of opaque PVC/PVDC film containing 10 soft gelatin capsules packed into containers of 10, 30, 60 and 90 capsules. Not all pack sizes may be marketed.

6.6 Special precautions for disposal and other handling

Dutasteride is absorbed through the skin, therefore contact with leaking capsules must be avoided. If contact is made with leaking capsules, the contact area should be washed immediately with soap and water (see section 4.4).

Any unused product or waste material should be disposed of in accordance with local requirements.

Administrative Data

7. MARKETING AUTHORISATION HOLDER

GlaxoSmithKline UK Limited
980 Great West Road
Brentford
Middlesex
TW8 9GS
United Kingdom
Trading as:
GlaxoSmithKline UK Ltd
Stockley Park West
Uxbridge
Middlesex,
UB11 1BT

8. MARKETING AUTHORISATION NUMBER(S)

19494/0006

9. DATE OF FIRST AUTHORISATION/RENEWAL OF THE AUTHORISATION

17 January 2003/ 13 February 2008

10. DATE OF REVISION OF THE TEXT

14 August 2008

Avomine Tablets 25mg

(Manx Healthcare)

1. NAME OF THE MEDICINAL PRODUCT

Avomine Tablets 25mg

2. QUALITATIVE AND QUANTITATIVE COMPOSITION

Promethazine teoclate 25mg

3. PHARMACEUTICAL FORM

Tablet

4. CLINICAL PARTICULARS

4.1 Therapeutic indications

Avomine is a long acting anti-emetic, indicated for:

- prevention and treatment of nausea and vomiting, including motion sickness and post operative vomiting;

- vertigo due to Meniere's syndrome, labyrinitis and other causes

4.2 Posology and method of administration

Motion sickness

Adults

For the prevention on long journeys: one 25mg tablet each evening at bedtime, starting the day before setting out. The duration of action is such that a second dose in 24 hours is not often necessary.

For the prevention of motion sickness on short journeys: one 25mg tablet one or two hours before travelling or as soon after as possible.

Treatment of motion sickness: one 25mg tablet as soon as possible and repeated the same evening followed by a third tablet the following evening.

Nausea and vomiting due to other causes

Adults

One 25mg tablet at night is often sufficient, but two or three tablets are sometimes necessary. Alternatively, more frequent administration such as 25mg two or three times a day may be required for some patients. It is often not necessary to give more than four of the 25mg Avomine Tablets in 24 hours.

Children

In the above indications children over 10 years of age may be given the lower adult doses described above. Children between 5 and 10 years may be given half the adult dose. Tablets are not suitable for administration to children aged between 2 and 5 years. An oral liquid preparation is recommended in this age group. Not for use in children under 2 years of age (see section 4.3).

Elderly

No specific dosage recommendations.

Administration: Oral.

4.3 Contraindications

Avomine should not be used in patients with:

- Hypersensitivity to promethazine or any of the excipients
- Hypersensitivity to other phenothiazines
- Coma or CNS depression of any cause

Avomine should not be used in children less than two years of age because of the potential for fatal respiratory depression.

Avomine should not be administered to patients who have been taking monoamine oxidase inhibitors within the previous 14 days.

4.4 Special warnings and precautions for use

Avomine may thicken or dry lung secretions and impair expectoration, it should therefore be used with caution in patients with asthma, bronchitis or bronchiectasis.

Use with care in patients with severe coronary artery disease, narrow angle glaucoma, epilepsy or hepatic and renal insufficiency.

Caution should be exercised in patients with bladder, neck or pyloro-duodenal obstruction.

Promethazine may mask the warnings signs of ototoxicity caused by ototoxic drugs e.g salicylates.

Promethazine may also delay the early diagnosis of intestinal obstruction or raised intracranial pressure through suppression of vomiting.

The use of promethazine should be avoided in children and adolescents with signs and symptoms suggestive of Reye's syndrome.

Avomine should not be used for longer than seven days without seeking medical advice.

Contains lactose. Patients with rare hereditary problems of galactose intolerance, the Lapp lactase deficiency or glucose-galactose malabsorption should not take this medicine.

4.5 Interaction with other medicinal products and other forms of interaction

Avomine may enhance the action of any anticholinergic agent, tricyclic antidepressant, sedative or hypnotic. Alcohol should be avoided during treatment.

Avomine may interfere with immunologic urine pregnancy tests to produce false-positive and false-negative results.

Avomine should be discontinued at least 72 hours before any skin tests using allergen extracts as it may inhibit the cutaneous histamine response thus producing false-negative results.

4.6 Pregnancy and lactation

Use in pregnancy: It should be not used in pregnancy unless the physician considers it essential. The use of Avomine Tablets is not recommended in the two weeks prior to delivery in view of the risk of irritability and excitement in the neonate.

Use in lactation: Available evidence suggests that the amount excreted in milk is insignificant. However, there are risks of neonate irritability and excitement.

4.7 Effects on ability to drive and use machines

Ambulant patients receiving Avomine for the first time should not be in control of vehicles or machinery for the first few days until it is established that they are not hypersensitive to the central nervous effects of the drug and do not suffer from disorientation, confusion or dizziness.

4.8 Undesirable effects

Side effects may be seen in a few patients: drowsiness, dizziness, restlessness, headaches, nightmare, tiredness and disorientation. Anticholinergic side effects such as blurred vision, dry mouth and urinary retention occur occasionally. Newborn and premature infants are susceptible to the anticholinergic effects of promethazine, while other children may display paradoxical hyperexcitability. The elderly are particularly susceptible to the anticholinergic effects and confusion may occur.

Other side effects include anorexia, gastric irritation, palpitations, hypotension, arrhythmias, extrapyramidal effects, muscle spasms and tic-like movements of the head and face. Anaphylaxis, jaundice and blood dyscrasias including haemolytic anaemia rarely occur. Photosensitive skin reactions have been reported; strong sunlight should be avoided during treatment.

4.9 Overdose

Symptoms

Common features may include nausea, vomiting, dilated pupils, dry mouth and tongue, hot dry skin, fever, drowsiness and delirium. Symptoms of severe overdosage are variable. They are characterised in children by various combinations of excitement, ataxia, inco-ordination, athetosis and hallucinations, while adults may become drowsy and lapse into coma. Convulsions may occur in both adults and children; coma and excitement may precede their occurrence. Cardiac conduction abnormalities and dysrhythmias may occur; cardiorespiratory depression is uncommon. Patients who have been unconscious may be hypothermic.

Treatment

Consider use of activated charcoal only if the patient presents within one hour of ingestion. Treatment is otherwise supportive with attention to maintenance of adequate respiratory and circulatory status. Convulsions should be treated with intravenous diazepam and delirium treated with oral diazepam or other suitable anticonvulsant. Arrhythmias may be treated by correction of hypoxia, acidosis and other biochemical abnormalities. The use of antiarrhythmic drugs to treat dysrhythmias should be avoided. Procyclidine injection may be effective in the treatment of dystonic reactions.

5. PHARMACOLOGICAL PROPERTIES

5.1 Pharmacodynamic properties

Promethazine teoclate is a long acting antihistamine with anti-emetic, central sedative and anticholinergic properties.

Promethazine is metabolised in the liver (the major metabolite being the sulphoxide) and slowly excreted in the urine. The drug is highly bound to plasma proteins.

2 Pharmacokinetic properties

romethazine is well absorbed after oral administration, eak plasma concentrations occurring in 2-3 hours. It is idely distributed in the body. It enters the brain and rosses the placenta. Phenothiazines pass into the milk : low concentrations.

.3 Preclinical safety data

one stated

PHARMACEUTICAL PARTICULARS

.1 List of excipients

actose

odium metabisulphite

otato starch

extrin

ellulose

tearic acid

lagnesium stearate

.2 Incompatibilities

lone

.3 Shelf life

ive (5) years

.4 Special precautions for storage

store in the original container

.5 Nature and contents of container

Blister pack of 10 × 25mg tablets

Blister pack of 28 × 25mg tablets

Blister pack of 30 × 25mg tablets

Securitainer of 60 × 25mg tablets

Securitainer or polyethylene bottle of 250 × 25mg tablets

6.6 Special precautions for disposal and other handling

Not applicable

7. MARKETING AUTHORISATION HOLDER

Manx Pharma Ltd

Taylor Group House

Wedgnock Lane

Warwick

CV34 5YA

United Kingdom

8. MARKETING AUTHORISATION NUMBER(S)

PL 15833/0003

9. DATE OF FIRST AUTHORISATION/RENEWAL OF THE AUTHORISATION

September 1997

10. DATE OF REVISION OF THE TEXT

September 2009

AVONEX 30 micrograms powder and solvent for solution for injection

(Biogen Idec Ltd)

1. NAME OF THE MEDICINAL PRODUCT

AVONEX 30 micrograms powder and solvent for solution for injection

2. QUALITATIVE AND QUANTITATIVE COMPOSITION

Each BIO-SET vial contains 30 micrograms (6 million IU) of interferon beta-1a.

Following reconstitution with the solvent (water for injections) the vial contains 1.0 ml of solution. The concentration is 30 micrograms per ml.

Using the World Health Organisation (WHO) International Standard for Interferon, 30 micrograms of AVONEX contains 6 million IU of antiviral activity. The activity against other standards is not known.

For a full list of excipients, see section 6.1.

3. PHARMACEUTICAL FORM

Powder and solvent for solution for injection.

The vial contains a white to off-white cake.

4. CLINICAL PARTICULARS

4.1 Therapeutic indications

AVONEX is indicated for the treatment of

- Patients diagnosed with relapsing multiple sclerosis (MS). In clinical trials, this was characterised by two or more acute exacerbations (relapses) in the previous three years without evidence of continuous progression between relapses; AVONEX slows the progression of disability and decreases the frequency of relapses.
- Patients with a single demyelinating event with an active inflammatory process, if it is severe enough to warrant treatment with intravenous corticosteroids, if alternative diagnoses have been excluded, and if they are determined to be at high risk of developing clinically definite multiple sclerosis (see section 5.1).

AVONEX should be discontinued in patients who develop progressive MS.

4.2 Posology and method of administration

Treatment should be initiated under supervision of a physician experienced in the treatment of the disease.

Adults: The recommended dosage for the treatment of relapsing MS is 30 micrograms (1 ml solution), administered by intramuscular (IM) injection once a week (see section 6.6). No additional benefit has been shown by administering a higher dose (60 micrograms) once a week.

Children and adolescents: No formal clinical trials or pharmacokinetic studies have been conducted in children or adolescents. However, limited published data suggest that the safety profile in adolescents from 12 to 16 years of age receiving AVONEX 30 micrograms IM once per week is similar to that seen in adults. There is no information on the use of AVONEX in children under 12 years of age and therefore AVONEX should not be used in this population.

Elderly: Clinical studies did not include a sufficient number of patients aged 65 and over to determine whether they respond differently than younger patients. However, based on the mode of clearance of the active substance there are no theoretical reasons for any requirement for dose adjustments in the elderly.

The intramuscular injection site should be varied each week (see section 5.3).

Doctors may prescribe a 25 mm, 25 gauge needle to patients for whom such a needle is appropriate to administer an intramuscular injection.

Prior to injection and for an additional 24 hours after each injection, an antipyretic analgesic is advised to decrease flu-like symptoms associated with AVONEX administration. These symptoms are usually present during the first few months of treatment.

At the present time, it is not known for how long patients should be treated. Patients should be clinically evaluated after two years of treatment and longer-term treatment should be decided on an individual basis by the treating physician. Treatment should be discontinued if the patient develops chronic progressive MS.

4.3 Contraindications

- Initiation of treatment in pregnancy (see section 4.6).

- Patients with a history of hypersensitivity to natural or recombinant interferon -β, human albumin or to any excipients.

- Patients with current severe depression and/or suicidal ideation (see sections 4.4 and 4.8).

4.4 Special warnings and precautions for use

AVONEX should be administered with caution to patients with previous or current depressive disorders, in particular to those with antecedents of suicidal ideation (see section 4.3). Depression and suicidal ideation are known to occur in increased frequency in the multiple sclerosis population and in association with interferon use. Patients should be advised to immediately report any symptoms of depression and/or suicidal ideation to their prescribing physician.

Patients exhibiting depression should be monitored closely during therapy and treated appropriately. Cessation of therapy with AVONEX should be considered (see also sections 4.3 and 4.8).

AVONEX should be administered with caution to patients with a history of seizures, to those receiving treatment with anti-epileptics, particularly if their epilepsy is not adequately controlled with anti-epileptics (see sections 4.5 and 4.8).

Caution should be used and close monitoring considered when administering AVONEX to patients with severe renal and hepatic failure and to patients with severe myelosuppression.

Hepatic injury including elevated serum hepatic enzyme levels, hepatitis, autoimmune hepatitis and hepatic failure has been reported with interferon beta in post-marketing (see section 4.8). In some cases, these reactions have occurred in the presence of other medicinal products that have been associated with hepatic injury. The potential of additive effects from multiple medicinal products or other hepatotoxic agents (e.g. alcohol) has not been determined. Patients should be monitored for signs of hepatic injury and caution exercised when interferons are used concomitantly with other medicinal products associated with hepatic injury.

Patients with cardiac disease, such as angina, congestive heart failure or arrhythmia, should be closely monitored for worsening of their clinical condition during treatment with AVONEX. Flu-like symptoms associated with AVONEX therapy may prove stressful to patients with underlying cardiac conditions.

Laboratory abnormalities are associated with the use of interferons. Therefore, in addition to those laboratory tests normally required for monitoring patients with MS, complete and differential white blood cell counts, platelet counts, and blood chemistry, including liver function tests, are recommended during AVONEX therapy. Patients with myelosuppression may require more intensive monitoring of complete blood cell counts, with differential and platelet counts.

Patients may develop antibodies to AVONEX. The antibodies of some of those patients reduce the activity of interferon beta-1a *in vitro* (neutralising antibodies). Neutralising antibodies are associated with a reduction in the *in vivo* biological effects of AVONEX and may potentially be associated with a reduction of clinical efficacy. It is estimated that the plateau for the incidence of neutralising antibody formation is reached after 12 months of treatment. Data from patients treated up to two years with AVONEX suggests that approximately 8% develop neutralising antibodies.

The use of various assays to detect serum antibodies to interferons limits the ability to compare antigenicity among different products.

4.5 Interaction with other medicinal products and other forms of interaction

No formal interaction studies have been performed in humans.

The interaction of AVONEX with corticosteroids or adrenocorticotropic hormone (ACTH) has not been studied systematically. The clinical studies indicate that MS patients can receive AVONEX and corticosteroids or ACTH during relapses.

Interferons have been reported to reduce the activity of hepatic cytochrome P450-dependent enzymes in humans and animals. The effect of high-dose AVONEX administration on P450-dependent metabolism in monkeys was evaluated and no changes in liver metabolising capabilities were observed. Caution should be exercised when AVONEX is administered in combination with medicinal products that have a narrow therapeutic index and are largely dependent on the hepatic cytochrome P450 system for clearance, e.g. antiepileptics and some classes of antidepressants.

4.6 Pregnancy and lactation

Pregnancy

There is limited information on the use of AVONEX in pregnancy. Available data indicates that there may be an increased risk of spontaneous abortion. Initiation of treatment is contraindicated during pregnancy (see section 4.3).

Women of child-bearing potential

Women of child-bearing potential have to take appropriate contraceptive measures. If the patient becomes pregnant or plans to become pregnant while taking AVONEX she should be informed of the potential hazards and discontinuation of therapy should be considered (see section 5.3). In patients with a high relapse rate before treatment started, the risk of a severe relapse following discontinuation of AVONEX in the event of pregnancy should be weighed against a possible increased risk of spontaneous abortion.

Lactation

It is not known whether AVONEX is excreted in human milk. Because of the potential for serious adverse reactions in nursing infants, a decision should be made either to discontinue breast-feeding or AVONEX therapy.

4.7 Effects on ability to drive and use machines

No studies on the effects of AVONEX on the ability to drive and use machines have been performed. Central nervous system-related adverse reactions may have a minor influence on the ability to drive and use machines in susceptible patients (see section 4.8).

4.8 Undesirable effects

The highest incidence of adverse reactions associated with AVONEX therapy is related to flu-like symptoms. The most commonly reported flu-like symptoms are myalgia, fever, chills, sweating, asthenia, headache and nausea. Flu-like symptoms tend to be most prominent at the initiation of therapy and decrease in frequency with continued treatment.

Transient neurological symptoms that may mimic MS exacerbations may occur following injections. Transient episodes of hypertonia and/or severe muscular weakness that prevent voluntary movements may occur at any time during treatment. These episodes are of limited duration, temporally related to the injections and may recur after subsequent injections. In some cases these symptoms are associated with flu-like symptoms.

The frequencies of adverse reactions are expressed in patient-years, according to the following categories:

Very common (≥1/10 patient-years);

Common (≥1/100 to <1/10 patient-years);

Uncommon (≥1/1, 000 to <1/100 patient-years);

Rare (≥1/10, 000 to <1/1,000 patient-years);

Very rare (<1/10,000 patient-years);

Not known (cannot be estimated from the available data).

Patient-time is the sum of individual units of time that the patient in the study has been exposed to AVONEX before experiencing the adverse reaction. For example, 100 person-years could be observed in 100 patients who were on treatment for one year or in 200 patients who were on treatment for half a year.

Adverse reactions identified from studies (clinical trials and observational studies, with a period of follow-up ranging from two years to six years) and other adverse reactions identified through spontaneous reporting from the market, with unknown frequency, are provided in the table below.

Within each frequency grouping, undesirable effects are presented in order of decreasing seriousness.

Investigations	
common	lymphocyte count decreased, white blood cell count decreased, neutrophil count decreased, hematocrit decreased, blood potassium increased, blood urea nitrogen increased
uncommon	platelet count decreased
not known	weight decreased, weight increased, liver function tests abnormal
Cardiac disorders	
not known	cardiomyopathy, congestive heart failure (see section 4.4), palpitations, arrhythmia, tachycardia
Blood and lymphatic system disorders	
not known	pancytopenia, thrombocytopenia
Nervous system disorders	
very common	headache[2]
common	muscle spasticity, hypoesthesia
not known	neurological symptoms, syncope[3], hypertonia, dizziness, paraesthesia, seizures, migraine
Respiratory, thoracic and mediastinal disorders	
common	rhinorrhoea
rare	dyspnoea
Gastrointestinal disorders	
common	vomiting, diarrhoea, nausea[2]
Skin and subcutaneous tissue disorders	
common	rash, sweating increased, contusion
uncommon	alopecia
not known	angioneurotic oedema, pruritus, rash vesicular, urticaria, aggravation of psoriasis
Musculoskeletal and connective tissue disorders	
common	muscle cramp, neck pain, myalgia[2], arthralgia, pain in extremity, back pain, muscle stiffness, musculoskeletal stiffness
not known	systemic lupus erythematosus, muscle weakness, arthritis
Endocrine disorders	
not known	hypothyroidism, hyperthyroidism
Metabolism and nutrition disorders	
common	anorexia
Infections and infestations	
not known	injection site abscess[1]
Vascular disorders	
common	flushing
not known	vasodilatation
General disorders and administration site conditions	
very common	flu-like symptoms, pyrexia[2], chills[2], sweating[2]
common	injection site pain, injection site erythema, injection site bruising, asthenia[2], pain, fatigue[2], malaise, night sweats
uncommon	injection site burning
Not known	injection site reaction, injection site inflammation, injection site cellulitis[1], injection site necrosis, injection site bleeding, chest pain
Immune system disorders	
not known	anaphylactic reaction, anaphylactic shock, hypersensitivity reactions (angioedema, dyspnoea, urticaria, rash, pruritic rash)
Hepatobiliary disorders	
not known	hepatic failure (see section 4.4), hepatitis, autoimmune hepatitis
Reproductive system and breast disorders	
uncommon	metrorrhagia, menorrhagia
Psychiatric disorders	
common	depression (see section 4.4), insomnia
not known	suicide, psychosis, anxiety, confusion, emotional lability

[1]Injection site reactions including pain, inflammation and very rare cases of abscess or cellulitis that may require surgical intervention have been reported.

[2]The frequency of occurrence is higher at the beginning of treatment.

[3]A syncope episode may occur after AVONEX injection, it is normally a single episode that usually appears at the beginning of the treatment and does not recur with subsequent injections.

4.9 Overdose

No case of overdose has been reported. However, in case of overdose, patients should be hospitalised for observation and appropriate supportive treatment given.

5. PHARMACOLOGICAL PROPERTIES

5.1 Pharmacodynamic properties

Pharmacotherapeutic Group: Interferons, ATC code: L03 AB07.

Interferons are a family of naturally occurring proteins that are produced by eukaryotic cells in response to viral infection and other biological inducers. Interferons are cytokines that mediate antiviral, antiproliferative and immunomodulatory activities. Three major forms of interferons have been distinguished: alpha, beta and gamma. Interferons alpha and beta are classified as Type I interferons and interferon gamma is a Type II interferon. These interferons have overlapping but clearly distinguishable biological activities. They can also differ with respect to their cellular sites of synthesis.

Interferon beta is produced by various cell types including fibroblasts and macrophages. Natural interferon beta and AVONEX (interferon beta-1a) are glycosylated and have a single N-linked complex carbohydrate moiety. Glycosylation of other proteins is known to affect their stability, activity, biodistribution, and half-life in blood. However, the effects of interferon beta that are dependent on glycosylation are not fully defined.

AVONEX exerts its biological effects by binding to specific receptors on the surface of human cells. This binding initiates a complex cascade of intracellular events that leads to the expression of numerous interferon-induced gene products and markers. These include MHC Class I, Mx protein, 2′/5′-oligoadenylate synthetase, β_2-microglobulin, and neopterin. Some of these products have been measured in the serum and cellular fractions of blood collected from patients treated with AVONEX. After a single intramuscular dose of AVONEX, serum levels of these products remain elevated for at least four days and up to one week.

Whether the mechanism of action of AVONEX in MS mediated by the same pathway as the biological effect described above is not known because the pathophysic ogy of MS is not well established.

The effects of lyophilised AVONEX in the treatment of M were demonstrated in a placebo-controlled study of 30 patients (AVONEX n=158, placebo n=143) with relapsin MS characterised by at least 2 exacerbations in the pre vious 3 years or at least one exacerbation per year prior t entry when the duration of the disease was less than years. Patients with an EDSS of 1.0 to 3.5 at entry wer included in the clinical trial. Due to the design of the study patients were followed for variable lengths of time. 15 AVONEX-treated patients completed one year on stud and 85 completed two years on study. In the study, th cumulative percentage of patients who developed dis ability progression (by Kaplan-Meier life table analysis) b the end of two years was 35% for placebo-treate patients and 22% for AVONEX-treated patients. Disabilit progression was measured as an increase in th Expanded Disability Status Scale (EDSS) of 1.0 point sustained for at least six months. It was also shown tha there was a one-third reduction in annual relapse rate This latter clinical effect was observed after more than one year of treatment.

A double-blind randomised dose comparison study of 80 relapsing MS patients (AVONEX 30 micrograms n=402 AVONEX 60 micrograms n=400) has shown no statistically significant differences or trends between the 30 micrograms and the 60 micrograms doses of AVONEX in clinica and general MRI parameters.

The effects of AVONEX in the treatment of MS were also demonstrated in a randomised double-blind study performed with 383 patients (AVONEX n=193, placebo n=190) with a single demyelinating event associated with at least two compatible brain MRI lesions. A reduction of the risk of experiencing a second event was noted in the AVONEX treatment group. An effect on MRI parameters was also seen. The estimated risk of a second event was 50% in three years and 39% in two years in the placebo group and 35% (three years) and 21% (two years) in the AVONEX group. In a post-hoc analysis, those patients with a baseline MRI with at least one Gd-enhancing lesion and nine T2 lesions had a two-year risk of suffering a second event of 56% in the placebo group and 21% in the AVONEX treatment group. However, the impact of early treatment with AVONEX is unknown even in this high-risk subgroup as the study was mainly designed to assess the time to the second event rather than the long term evolution of the disease. Furthermore, for the time-being there is no well established definition of a high risk patient although a more conservative approach is to accept at least nine T2 hyperintense lesions on the initial scan and at least one new T2 or one new Gd-enhancing lesion on a follow-up scan taken at least three months after the initial scan. In any case, treatment should only be considered for patients classified at high risk.

5.2 Pharmacokinetic properties

The pharmacokinetic profile of AVONEX has been investigated indirectly with an assay that measures interferon antiviral activity. This assay is limited in that it is sensitive for interferon but lacks specificity for interferon beta. Alternative assay techniques are not sufficiently sensitive.

Following intramuscular administration of AVONEX, serum antiviral activity levels peak between 5 and 15 hours post-dose and decline with a half-life of approximately 10 hours. With appropriate adjustment for the rate of absorption from the injection site, the calculated bioavailability is approximately 40%. The calculated bioavailability is greater without such adjustments. Intramuscular bioavailability is three-fold higher than subcutaneous bioavailability. Subcutaneous administration cannot be substituted for intramuscular administration.

5.3 Preclinical safety data

Carcinogenesis: No carcinogenicity data for interferon beta-1a are available in animals or humans.

Chronic Toxicity: In a 26-week, repeated-dose toxicity study in rhesus monkeys by intramuscular route once per week, administered in combination with another immunomodulating agent, an anti CD40 ligand monoclonal antibody, no immune response toward interferon beta-1a and no signs of toxicity were demonstrated.

Local Tolerance: Intramuscular irritation has not been evaluated in animals following repeated administration to the same injection site.

Mutagenesis: Limited but relevant mutagenesis tests have been carried out. The results have been negative.

Impairment of Fertility: Fertility and developmental studies in rhesus monkeys have been carried out with a related form of interferon beta-1a. At very high doses, anovulatory and abortifacient effects in test animals were observed. Similar reproductive dose-related effects have also been observed with other forms of alpha and beta interferons. No teratogenic effects or effects on foetal development have been observed, but the available information on the effects of interferon beta-1a in the peri- and postnatal periods is limited.

No information is available on the effects of interferon beta-1a on male fertility.

PHARMACEUTICAL PARTICULARS

.1 List of excipients

luman serum albumin,

ibasic sodium phosphate,

Monobasic sodium phosphate,

odium chloride.

.2 Incompatibilities

lot applicable.

.3 Shelf life

years.

VONEX should be administered as soon as possible after reconstitution. However, the reconstituted solution can be stored at 2 °C-8 °C for up to six hours, prior to injection.

.4 Special precautions for storage

Store below 25 °C.

DO NOT FREEZE the powder or the reconstituted product.

For storage conditions of the reconstituted medicinal product see section 6.3.

.5 Nature and contents of container

AVONEX is available as a package of four individual doses. Each dose is supplied in a 3 ml clear glass vial with BIO-SET device and a 13 mm bromobutyl rubber stopper. It is provided with a 1 ml pre-filled glass syringe of solvent for reconstitution (water for injections) and one needle.

6.6 Special precautions for disposal and other handling

Use the supplied pre-filled syringe of solvent to reconstitute AVONEX for injection. Do not use any other solvent. Inject the content of the syringe into the vial of AVONEX by connecting the pre-filled syringe to the BIO-SET device. Gently swirl the contents in the vial until all materials are dissolved; DO NOT SHAKE. Inspect the reconstituted product: If it contains particulate matter or is other than colourless to slightly yellow in colour, the vial must not be used. After reconstitution, draw all the liquid (1 ml) from the vial back into the syringe for the administration of 30 micrograms AVONEX. The needle for intramuscular injection is provided. The formulation does not contain a preservative. Each vial of AVONEX contains a single dose only. Discard the unused portion of any vial.

Any unused product or waste material should be disposed of in accordance with local requirements.

7. MARKETING AUTHORISATION HOLDER

BIOGEN IDEC LIMITED
Innovation House
70 Norden Road
Maidenhead
Berkshire
SL6 4AY
United Kingdom

8. MARKETING AUTHORISATION NUMBER(S)

EU/1/97/033/002

9. DATE OF FIRST AUTHORISATION/RENEWAL OF THE AUTHORISATION

Date of first authorisation: 13 March 1997

Date of latest renewal: 13 March 2007

10. DATE OF REVISION OF THE TEXT

06/2008

Detailed information on this medicinal product is available on the website of the European Medicines Agency (EMEA) http://www.emea.europa.eu

AVONEX 30 micrograms/0.5 ml solution for injection.

(Biogen Idec Ltd)

1. NAME OF THE MEDICINAL PRODUCT

AVONEX 30 micrograms/0.5 ml solution for injection.

2. QUALITATIVE AND QUANTITATIVE COMPOSITION

Each 0.5 ml pre-filled syringe contains 30 micrograms (6 million IU) of interferon beta-1a.

The concentration is 30 micrograms per 0.5 ml.

Using the World Health Organisation (WHO) International Standard for Interferon, 30 micrograms of AVONEX contains 6 million IU of antiviral activity. The activity against other standards is not known.

For a full list of excipients, see section 6.1.

3. PHARMACEUTICAL FORM

Solution for injection.

Clear and colourless solution.

4. CLINICAL PARTICULARS

4.1 Therapeutic indications

AVONEX is indicated for the treatment of

• Patients diagnosed with relapsing multiple sclerosis (MS). In clinical trials, this was characterised by two or more acute exacerbations (relapses) in the previous three-years without evidence of continuous progression between relapses; AVONEX slows the progression of disability and decreases the frequency of relapses.

• Patients with a single demyelinating event with an active inflammatory process, if it is severe enough to warrant treatment with intravenous corticosteroids, if alternative diagnoses have been excluded, and if they are determined to be at high risk of developing clinically definite multiple sclerosis (see section 5.1).

AVONEX should be discontinued in patients who develop progressive MS.

4.2 Posology and method of administration

Treatment should be initiated under supervision of a physician experienced in the treatment of the disease.

Adults: The recommended dosage for the treatment of relapsing MS is 30 micrograms (0.5 ml solution), administered by intramuscular (IM) injection once a week (see section 6.6).

At the initiation of treatment, patients may either be started on a full dose of 30 micrograms (0.5 ml solution) or on approximately half the dose once a week to help them to adjust to treatment and thereafter increased to the full dose of 30 micrograms (0.5 ml solution). In order to obtain adequate efficacy, a dose of 30 micrograms (0.5 ml solution) once a week should be reached and maintained after the initial titration period. A manual titration device to enable delivery of approximately half the dose is available for patients initiating AVONEX treatment.

No additional benefit has been shown by administering a higher dose (60 micrograms) once a week.

Children and adolescents: No formal clinical trials or pharmacokinetic studies have been conducted in children or adolescents. However, limited published data suggest that the safety profile in adolescents from 12 to 16 years of age receiving AVONEX 30 micrograms IM once per week is similar to that seen in adults. There is no information on the use of AVONEX in children under 12 years of age and therefore AVONEX should not be used in this population.

Elderly: Clinical studies did not include a sufficient number of patients aged 65 and over to determine whether they respond differently than younger patients. However, based on the mode of clearance of the active substance there are no theoretical reasons for any requirement for dose adjustments in the elderly.

The intramuscular injection site should be varied each week (see section 5.3).

Doctors may prescribe a 25 mm, 25 gauge needle to patients for whom such a needle is appropriate to administer an intramuscular injection.

Prior to injection and for an additional 24 hours after each injection, an antipyretic analgesic is advised to decrease flu-like symptoms associated with AVONEX administration. These symptoms are usually present during the first few months of treatment.

At the present time, it is not known for how long patients should be treated. Patients should be clinically evaluated after two years of treatment and longer-term treatment should be decided on an individual basis by the treating physician. Treatment should be discontinued if the patient develops chronic progressive MS.

4.3 Contraindications

- Initiation of treatment in pregnancy (see section 4.6).

- Patients with a history of hypersensitivity to natural or recombinant interferon-β or to any excipients.

- Patients with current severe depression and/or suicidal ideation (see sections 4.4 and 4.8).

4.4 Special warnings and precautions for use

AVONEX should be administered with caution to patients with previous or current depressive disorders, in particular to those with antecedents of suicidal ideation (see section 4.3). Depression and suicidal ideation are known to occur in increased frequency in the multiple sclerosis population and in association with interferon use. Patients should be advised to immediately report any symptoms of depression and/or suicidal ideation to their prescribing physician.

Patients exhibiting depression should be monitored closely during therapy and treated appropriately. Cessation of therapy with AVONEX should be considered (see also sections 4.3 and 4.8).

AVONEX should be administered with caution to patients with a history of seizures, to those receiving treatment with anti-epileptics, particularly if their epilepsy is not adequately controlled with anti-epileptics (see sections 4.5 and 4.8).

Caution should be used and close monitoring considered when administering AVONEX to patients with severe renal and hepatic failure and to patients with severe myelosuppression.

Hepatic injury including elevated serum hepatic enzyme levels, hepatitis, autoimmune hepatitis and hepatic failure has been reported with interferon beta in post-marketing (see section 4.8). In some cases, these reactions have occurred in the presence of other medicinal products that have been associated with hepatic injury. The potential of additive effects from multiple medicinal products or other hepatotoxic agents (e.g. alcohol) has not been determined. Patients should be monitored for signs of hepatic injury and caution exercised when interferons are used concomitantly with other medicinal products associated with hepatic injury.

Patients with cardiac disease, such as angina, congestive heart failure or arrhythmia, should be closely monitored for worsening of their clinical condition during treatment with AVONEX. Flu-like symptoms associated with AVONEX therapy may prove stressful to patients with underlying cardiac conditions.

Laboratory abnormalities are associated with the use of interferons. Therefore, in addition to those laboratory tests normally required for monitoring patients with MS, complete and differential white blood cell counts, platelet counts, and blood chemistry, including liver function tests, are recommended during AVONEX therapy. Patients with myelosuppression may require more intensive monitoring of complete blood cell counts, with differential and platelet counts.

Patients may develop antibodies to AVONEX. The antibodies of some of those patients reduce the activity of interferon beta-1a *in vitro* (neutralising antibodies). Neutralising antibodies are associated with a reduction in the *in vivo* biological effects of AVONEX and may potentially be associated with a reduction of clinical efficacy. It is estimated that the plateau for the incidence of neutralising antibody formation is reached after 12 months of treatment. Recent clinical studies with patients treated up to three years with AVONEX suggest that approximately 5% to 8% develop neutralising antibodies.

The use of various assays to detect serum antibodies to interferons limits the ability to compare antigenicity among different products.

4.5 Interaction with other medicinal products and other forms of interaction

No formal interaction studies have been performed in humans.

The interaction of AVONEX with corticosteroids or adrenocorticotropic hormone (ACTH) has not been studied systematically. The clinical studies indicate that MS patients can receive AVONEX and corticosteroids or ACTH during relapses.

Interferons have been reported to reduce the activity of hepatic cytochrome P450-dependent enzymes in humans and animals. The effect of high-dose AVONEX administration on P450-dependent metabolism in monkeys was evaluated and no changes in liver metabolising capabilities were observed. Caution should be exercised when AVONEX is administered in combination with medicinal products that have a narrow therapeutic index and are largely dependent on the hepatic cytochrome P450 system for clearance, e.g. antiepileptics and some classes of antidepressants.

4.6 Pregnancy and lactation

Pregnancy

There is limited information on the use of AVONEX in pregnancy. Available data indicates that there may be an increased risk of spontaneous abortion. Initiation of treatment is contraindicated during pregnancy (see section 4.3).

Women of child-bearing potential

Women of child-bearing potential have to take appropriate contraceptive measures. If the patient becomes pregnant or plans to become pregnant while taking AVONEX she should be informed of the potential hazards and discontinuation of therapy should be considered (see section 5.3). In patients with a high relapse rate before treatment started, the risk of a severe relapse following discontinuation of AVONEX in the event of pregnancy should be weighed against a possible increased risk of spontaneous abortion.

Lactation

It is not known whether AVONEX is excreted in human milk. Because of the potential for serious adverse reactions in nursing infants, a decision should be made either to discontinue breast-feeding or AVONEX therapy.

4.7 Effects on ability to drive and use machines

No studies of the effects of AVONEX on the ability to drive and use machines have been performed. Central nervous system-related adverse reactions may have a minor influence on the ability to drive and use machines in susceptible patients (see section 4.8).

4.8 Undesirable effects

The highest incidence of adverse reactions associated with AVONEX therapy is related to flu-like symptoms. The most commonly reported flu-like symptoms are myalgia, fever, chills, sweating, asthenia, headache and nausea. Flu-like symptoms tend to be most prominent at the initiation of therapy and decrease in frequency with continued treatment.

Transient neurological symptoms that may mimic MS exacerbations may occur following injections. Transient episodes of hypertonia and/or severe muscular weakness that prevent voluntary movements may occur at any time during treatment. These episodes are of limited duration, temporally related to the injections and may recur after subsequent injections. In some cases these symptoms are associated with flu-like symptoms.

The frequencies of adverse reactions are expressed in patient-years, according to the following categories:

Very common ($\geq$1/10 patient-years);

Common ($\geq$1/100 to $<$1/10 patient-years);

Uncommon (≥1/1, 000 to <1/100 patient-years);

Rare (≥1/10, 000 to <1/1,000 patient-years);

Very rare (<1/10,000 patient-years);

Not known (cannot be estimated from the available data).

Patient-time is the sum of individual units of time that the patient in the study has been exposed to AVONEX before experiencing the adverse reaction. For example, 100 person-years could be observed in 100 patients who were on treatment for one year or in 200 patients who were on treatment for half a year.

Adverse reactions identified from studies (clinical trials and observational studies, with a period of follow-up ranging from two years to six years) and other adverse reactions identified through spontaneous reporting from the market, with unknown frequency, are provided in the table below.

Within each frequency grouping, undesirable effects are presented in order of decreasing seriousness.

Investigations	
common	lymphocyte count decreased, white blood cell count decreased, neutrophil count decreased, hematocrit decreased, blood potassium increased, blood urea nitrogen increased
uncommon	platelet count decreased
not known	weight decreased, weight increased, liver function tests abnormal
Cardiac disorders	
not known	cardiomyopathy, congestive heart failure (see section 4.4), palpitations, arrhythmia, tachycardia
Blood and lymphatic system disorders	
not known	pancytopenia, thrombocytopenia
Nervous system disorders	
very common	headache[2]
common	muscle spasticity, hypoesthesia
not known	neurological symptoms, syncope[3], hypertonia, dizziness, paraesthesia, seizures, migraine
Respiratory, thoracic and mediastinal disorders	
common	rhinorrhoea
rare	dyspnoea
Gastrointestinal disorders	
common	vomiting, diarrhoea, nausea[2]
Skin and subcutaneous tissue disorders	
common	rash, sweating increased, contusion
uncommon	alopecia
not known	angioneurotic oedema, pruritus, rash vesicular, urticaria, aggravation of psoriasis
Musculoskeletal and connective tissue disorders	
common	muscle cramp, neck pain, myalgia[2], arthralgia, pain in extremity, back pain, muscle stiffness, musculoskeletal stiffness
not known	systemic lupus erythematosus, muscle weakness, arthritis
Endocrine disorders	
not known	hypothyroidism, hyperthyroidism
Metabolism and nutrition disorders	
common	anorexia
Infections and infestations	
not known	injection site abscess[1]
Vascular disorders	
common	flushing
not known	vasodilatation
General disorders and administration site conditions	
very common	flu-like symptoms, pyrexia[2], chills[2], sweating[2]
common	injection site pain, injection site erythema, injection site bruising, asthenia[2], pain, fatigue[2], malaise, night sweats
uncommon	injection site burning
not known	injection site reaction, injection site inflammation, injection site cellulitis[1], injection site necrosis, injection site bleeding, chest pain
Immune system disorders	
not known	anaphylactic reaction, anaphylactic shock, hypersensitivity reactions (angioedema, dyspnoea, urticaria, rash, pruritic rash)
Hepatobiliary disorders	
not known	hepatic failure (see section 4.4), hepatitis, autoimmune hepatitis
Reproductive system and breast disorders	
uncommon	metrorrhagia, menorrhagia
Psychiatric disorders	
common	depression (see section 4.4), insomnia
not known	suicide, psychosis, anxiety, confusion, emotional lability

[1]Injection site reactions including pain, inflammation and very rare cases of abscess or cellulitis that may require surgical intervention have been reported.

[2]The frequency of occurrence is higher at the beginning of treatment.

[3]A syncope episode may occur after AVONEX injection, it is normally a single episode that usually appears at the beginning of the treatment and does not recur with subsequent injections.

4.9 Overdose

No case of overdose has been reported. However, in case of overdose, patients should be hospitalised for observation and appropriate supportive treatment given.

5. PHARMACOLOGICAL PROPERTIES

5.1 Pharmacodynamic properties

Pharmacotherapeutic Group: Interferons, ATC code: L03 AB07.

Interferons are a family of naturally occurring proteins that are produced by eukaryotic cells in response to viral infection and other biological inducers. Interferons are cytokines that mediate antiviral, antiproliferative, and immunomodulatory activities. Three major forms of interferons have been distinguished: alpha, beta, and gamma. Interferons alpha and beta are classified as Type I interferons, and interferon gamma is a Type II interferon. These interferons have overlapping but clearly distinguishable biological activities. They can also differ with respect to their cellular sites of synthesis.

Interferon beta is produced by various cell types including fibroblasts and macrophages. Natural interferon beta and AVONEX (interferon beta-1a) are glycosylated and have a single N-linked complex carbohydrate moiety. Glycosylation of other proteins is known to affect their stability, activity, biodistribution, and half-life in blood. However, the effects of interferon beta that are dependent on glycosylation are not fully defined.

AVONEX exerts its biological effects by binding to specific receptors on the surface of human cells. This binding initiates a complex cascade of intracellular events that leads to the expression of numerous interferon-induced gene products and markers. These include MHC Class I, Mx protein, 2' / 5'-oligoadenylate synthetase, β_2-microglobulin, and neopterin. Some of these products have been measured in the serum and cellular fractions of blood collected from patients treated with AVONEX. After a single intramuscular dose of AVONEX, serum levels of these products remain elevated for at least four days and up to one week.

Whether the mechanism of action of AVONEX in MS is mediated by the same pathway as the biological effects described above is not known because the pathophysiology of MS is not well established.

The effects of lyophilised AVONEX in the treatment of MS were demonstrated in a placebo-controlled study of 301 patients (AVONEX n=158, placebo n=143) with relapsing MS characterised by at least 2 exacerbations in the previous 3 years or at least one exacerbation per year prior to entry when the duration of the disease was less than 3 years. Patients with an EDSS of 1.0 to 3.5 at entry were included in the clinical trial. Due to the design of the study, patients were followed for variable lengths of time. 150 AVONEX-treated patients completed one year on study and 85 completed two years on study. In the study, the cumulative percentage of patients who developed disability progression (by Kaplan-Meier life table analysis) by the end of two years was 35% for placebo-treated patients and 22% for AVONEX-treated patients. Disability progression was measured as an increase in the Expanded Disability Status Scale (EDSS) of 1.0 point, sustained for at least six months. It was also shown that there was a one third reduction in annual relapse rate. This latter clinical effect was observed after more than one year of treatment.

A double-blind randomised dose comparison study of 802 relapsing MS patients (AVONEX 30 micrograms n=402, AVONEX 60 micrograms n=400) has shown no statistically significant differences or trends between the 30 micrograms and the 60 micrograms doses of AVONEX in clinical and general MRI parameters.

The effects of AVONEX in the treatment of MS were also demonstrated in a randomised double-blind study performed with 383 patients (AVONEX n=193, placebo n=190) with a single demyelinating event associated with at least two compatible brain MRI lesions. A reduction of the risk of experiencing a second event was noted in the AVONEX treatment group. An effect on MRI parameters was also seen. The estimated risk of a second event was 50% in three years and 39% in two years in the placebo group and 35% (three years) and 21% (two years) in the AVONEX group. In a post-hoc analysis, those patients with a baseline MRI with at least one Gd-enhancing lesion and nine T2 lesions had a two-year risk of suffering a second event of 56% in the placebo group and 21% in the AVONEX treatment group. However, the impact of early treatment with AVONEX is unknown even in this high-risk subgroup as the study was mainly designed to assess the time to the second event rather than the long-term evolution of the disease. Furthermore, for the time-being there is no well established definition of a high risk patient although a more conservative approach is to accept at least nine T2 hyperintense lesions on the initial scan and at least one new T2 or one new Gd-enhancing lesion on a follow-up scan taken at least three months after the initial scan. In any case, treatment should only be considered for patients classified at high risk.

5.2 Pharmacokinetic properties

The pharmacokinetic profile of AVONEX has been investigated indirectly with an assay that measures interferon antiviral activity. This assay is limited in that it is sensitive for interferon but lacks specificity for interferon beta. Alternative assay techniques are not sufficiently sensitive.

Following intramuscular administration of AVONEX, serum antiviral activity levels peak between 5 and 15 hours post-dose and decline with a half-life of approximately 10 hours. With appropriate adjustment for the rate of absorption from the injection site, the calculated bioavailability is approximately 40%. The calculated bioavailability is greater without such adjustments. Intramuscular bioavailability is three-fold higher than subcutaneous bioavailability. Subcutaneous administration cannot be substituted for intramuscular administration.

5.3 Preclinical safety data

Carcinogenesis: No carcinogenicity data for interferon beta-1a are available in animals or humans.

Chronic Toxicity: In a 26-week repeated dose toxicity study in rhesus monkeys by intramuscular route once per week, administered in combination with another immunomodulating agent, an anti CD40 ligand monoclonal antibody, no immune response toward interferon beta-1a and no signs of toxicity were demonstrated.

Local Tolerance: Intramuscular irritation has not been evaluated in animals following repeated administration to the same injection site.

Mutagenesis: Limited but relevant mutagenesis tests have been carried out. The results have been negative.

Impairment of Fertility: Fertility and developmental studies in rhesus monkeys have been carried out with a related form of interferon beta-1a. At very high doses, anovulatory and abortifacient effects in test animals were observed. Similar reproductive dose-related effects have also been observed with other forms of alpha and beta interferons. No teratogenic effects or effects on foetal development have been observed, but the available information on the effects of Interferon beta-1a in the peri- and postnatal periods is limited.

No information is available on the effects of interferon beta-1a on male fertility.

6. PHARMACEUTICAL PARTICULARS

6.1 List of excipients

Sodium acetate trihydrate,

Acetic acid, glacial,

Arginine hydrochloride,

Polysorbate 20,

Water for injections.

6.2 Incompatibilities

Not applicable.

6.3 Shelf life

2 years.

6.4 Special precautions for storage

Store in a refrigerator (2 °C -8 °C).

DO NOT FREEZE.

AVONEX can be stored at room temperature (between 15 °C and 30 °C) for up to one week.

tore in the original package (sealed plastic tray) in order to rotect from light (see section 6.5).

.5 Nature and contents of container

ml pre-filled syringe made of glass (Type I) with a tamper vident cap and plunger stopper (bromobutyl) containing .5 ml of solution.

ack size: box of four or twelve pre-filled syringes of 0.5 ml. ach syringe is packed in a sealed plastic tray, which also ontains one injection needle for intramuscular use.

Not all pack sizes may be marketed.

.6 Special precautions for disposal and other handling

AVONEX is provided as ready to use solution for injection in pre-filled syringe.

Once removed from the refrigerator, AVONEX in a pre-filled yringe should be allowed to warm to room temperature 15 °C -30 °C) for about 30 minutes.

Do not use external heat sources such as hot water to warm AVONEX 30 micrograms solution for injection.

f the solution for injection contains particulate matter or if it s any colour other than clear colourless, the pre-filled syringe must not be used. The injection needle for intramuscular injection is provided. The formulation does not contain a preservative. Each pre-filled syringe of AVONEX contains a single dose only. Discard the unused portion of any pre-filled syringe.

Any unused product or waste material should be disposed of in accordance with local requirements.

7. MARKETING AUTHORISATION HOLDER

BIOGEN IDEC LIMITED
Innovation House
70 Norden Road
Maidenhead
Berkshire
SL6 4AY
United Kingdom

8. MARKETING AUTHORISATION NUMBER(S)

EU/1/97/033/003
EU/1/97/033/004

9. DATE OF FIRST AUTHORISATION/RENEWAL OF THE AUTHORISATION

Date of first authorisation: 13 March 1997

Date of latest renewal: 13 March 2007

10. DATE OF REVISION OF THE TEXT

12/2008

Detailed information on this medicinal product is available on the website of the European Medicines Agency (EMEA) http://www.emea.europa.eu

Axsain

(Cephalon Limited)

1. NAME OF THE MEDICINAL PRODUCT

Axsain Cream

2. QUALITATIVE AND QUANTITATIVE COMPOSITION

Capsaicin 0.075% w/w

3. PHARMACEUTICAL FORM

Cream for topical application.

4. CLINICAL PARTICULARS

4.1 Therapeutic indications

1. For the symptomatic relief of neuralgia associated with and following Herpes Zoster infections (post-herpetic neuralgia) after open skin lesions have healed.

2. For the symptomatic management of painful diabetic peripheral polyneuropathy.

4.2 Posology and method of administration

Adults and the elderly:

For topical administration to unbroken skin. Apply only a small amount of cream (pea size) to the affected area 3 or 4 times daily. These applications should be evenly spaced throughout the waking hours and not more often than every 4 hours. The cream should be gently rubbed in, there should be no residue left on the surface. Hands should be washed immediately after application of Axsain with the fingers. Do not apply near the eyes.

Patients using Axsain for the treatment of painful diabetic peripheral polyneuropathy should only do so under the direct supervision of a hospital consultant who has access to specialist resources. The recommended duration of use in the first instance is 8 weeks, since there is no clinical trial evidence of efficacy for treatment of more than 8 weeks duration. After this time, it is recommended that the patient's condition should be fully clinically assessed prior to continuation of treatment, and regularly re-evaluated thereafter, by the supervising consultant.

Not suitable for use in children.

4.3 Contraindications

Axsain cream is contra-indicated for use on broken or irritated skin.

Axsain Cream is contra-indicated in patients with known hypersensitivity to capsaicin or any of the excipients used in this product.

4.4 Special warnings and precautions for use

Keep away from the eyes.

After applying Axsain cream with the fingers, hands should be washed immediately. Patients should avoid taking a hot bath or shower just before or after applying Axsain, as it can enhance the burning sensation.

Patients and carers should avoid inhalation of vapours from the cream, as transient irritation of the mucous membranes of the eyes and respiratory tract (including exacerbation of asthma) has been reported.

If the condition worsens, seek medical advice.

4.5 Interaction with other medicinal products and other forms of interaction

Not applicable.

4.6 Pregnancy and lactation

The safety of Axsain during pregnancy or lactation has not been established in either humans or animals. However, in the small amounts absorbed transdermally from Axsain Cream, it is considered unlikely that capsaicin will cause any adverse effects in humans.

4.7 Effects on ability to drive and use machines

Not applicable.

4.8 Undesirable effects

Axsain may cause transient burning on application. This burning is observed more frequently when application schedules of less than 3-4 times daily are utilised. The burning can be enhanced if too much cream is used and if it is applied just before or after a bath or shower.

Irritation of the mucous membranes of the eyes and respiratory tract (such as coughing, sneezing, and runny eyes) on application of Axsain cream has been reported rarely. These events are usually mild and self-limiting. There have been a few reports of dyspnoea, wheezing and exacerbation of asthma.

4.9 Overdose

Not applicable.

5. PHARMACOLOGICAL PROPERTIES

5.1 Pharmacodynamic properties

Although the precise mechanism of action of capsaicin is not fully understood, current evidence suggests that capsaicin renders skin insensitive to pain by depleting and preventing re-accumulation of substance P in peripheral sensory neurons. Substance P is thought to be the principal chemo-mediator of pain impulses from the periphery to the Central Nervous System.

5.2 Pharmacokinetic properties

Absorption after topical application is unknown. Average consumption of dietary spice from capsicum fruit has been estimated as 2.5g/person/day in India and 5.0g/person/day in Thailand. Capsaicin content in capsicum fruit is approximately 1% therefore daily dietary intake of capsaicin may range from 0.5 - 1mg/kg/day for a 50kg person. Application of two tubes of Axsain Cream 0.075% (90g) each week results in a 9.6mg/day topical exposure. Assuming 100% absorption in a 50kg person, daily exposure would be 0.192mg/kg which is approximately one third to one quarter of the above mentioned dietary intake.

5.3 Preclinical safety data

The available animal toxicity data relating to capsicum, capsicum extracts and capsaicin do not suggest that, in usual doses, they pose any significant toxicity hazard to man. Thus, in both single and repeat dosing studies which have been reported, capsicum extracts and capsaicin are generally well tolerated at many times even the highest estimated human intakes. The safety of Axsain for use in human pregnancy has not been established since no formal reproduction studies have been performed on either animals or man. However, there is no reason to suspect from human or animal studies currently available that any adverse effects in humans are likely.

Studies reported in the published literature, which relate to potential genotoxic and carcinogenic action of capsaicin have produced inconclusive and conflicting data. However, it is unlikely that capsaicin, in the quantities absorbed transdermally from Axsain Cream, will pose any significant hazard to humans.

6. PHARMACEUTICAL PARTICULARS

6.1 List of excipients

Purified water
Sorbitol solution
Isopropyl myristate
Cetyl alcohol
White Soft Paraffin
Glyceryl stearate and PEG-100 stearate (Arlacel 165)
Benzyl alcohol

6.2 Incompatibilities

Not applicable.

6.3 Shelf life

3 years

6.4 Special precautions for storage

Store below 25°C.

6.5 Nature and contents of container

Aluminium tubes with epoxyphenolic lining and polypropylene spiked cap containing 45g Axsain Cream, or 7.5g for use as professional sample.

6.6 Special precautions for disposal and other handling

Not applicable.

Administrative Data

7. MARKETING AUTHORISATION HOLDER

Cephalon Limited
1 Albany Place
Hyde Way
WelwynGarden City
Hertfordshire
AL7 3BT

8. MARKETING AUTHORISATION NUMBER(S)

PL 21799/0002

9. DATE OF FIRST AUTHORISATION/RENEWAL OF THE AUTHORISATION

30th January 2006

10. DATE OF REVISION OF THE TEXT

October 2007

11. Legal Category

POM

Azzalure

(Galderma (U.K) Ltd)

1. NAME OF THE MEDICINAL PRODUCT

Azzalure, 10 Speywood units/0.05ml, powder for solution for injection

2. QUALITATIVE AND QUANTITATIVE COMPOSITION

Botulinum toxin type A * 10 Speywood units **/0.05ml of reconstituted solution

Vial of 125 units

*Clostridium botulinum toxin A haemagglutinin complex

**One Speywood unit (U) is defined as the median lethal peritoneal dose in mice (LD50).

The Speywood units of Azzalure are specific to the preparation and are not interchangeable with other preparations of botulinum toxin

For a full list of excipients see Section 6.1.

3. PHARMACEUTICAL FORM

Powder for solution for injection.

The powder is white.

4. CLINICAL PARTICULARS

4.1 Therapeutic indications

Azzalure is indicated for the temporary improvement in the appearance of moderate to severe glabellar lines (vertical lines between the eyebrows) seen at frown, in adult patients under 65 years, when the severity of these lines has an important psychological impact on the patient.

4.2 Posology and method of administration

Botulinum toxin units are different depending on the medicinal products. The Speywood units of Azzalure are specific to the preparation and are not interchangeable with other preparations of botulinum toxin.

Azzalure should only be administered by physicians with appropriate qualifications and expertise in this treatment and having the required equipment.

Once reconstituted, Azzalure should only be used to treat a single patient, during a single session.

Prior to injection, the product should be reconstituted, instructions for which are given in Section 6.6.

Remove any make-up and disinfect the skin with a local antiseptic.

Intramuscular injections should be performed at right angles to the skin using a sterile 29-30 gauge needle.

The recommended dose is 50 Speywood units (0.25 ml of reconstituted solution) of Azzalure to be divided into 5 injection sites, 10 Speywood units (0.05 ml of reconstituted solution) are to be administered intramuscularly into each of the 5 sites: 2 injections into each *corrugator* muscle and one into the *procerus* muscle near the nasofrontal angle as shown below:

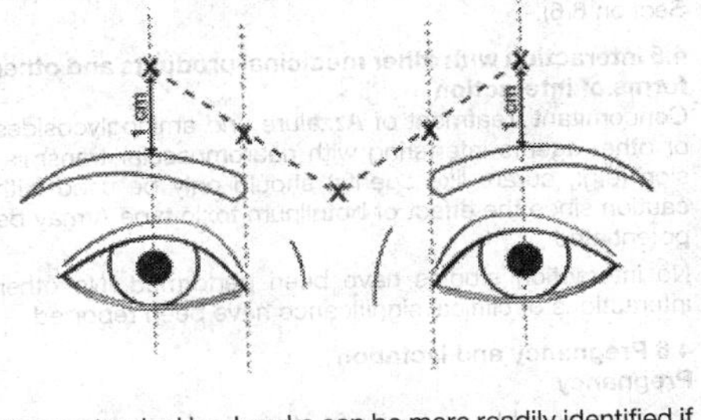

The anatomical landmarks can be more readily identified if observed and palpated at maximal frown. Before injection, place the thumb or index finger firmly below the orbital rim in order to prevent extravasation below the orbital rim. The needle should be pointed upward and medially during the injection. In order to reduce the risk of ptosis, avoid injections near the *levator palpebrae superioris* muscle, particularly in patients with larger brow-depressor complexes (*depressor supercilii*). Injections in the corrugator muscle must be made into the central part of that muscle, at least 1 cm above the orbital rim.

The treatment interval depends on the individual patient's response after assessment. In clinical studies, an optimal effect was demonstrated for up to 4 months after injection. Some patients were still responders at 5 months (see section 5.1). Treatment interval should not be more frequent than every three months.

In the event of treatment failure or diminished effect following repeat injections, alternative treatment methods should be employed. In case of treatment failure after the first treatment session, the following approaches may be considered:

• Analysis of the causes of failure, e.g. incorrect muscles injected, injection technique, and formation of toxin-neutralising antibodies;

• Re-evaluation of the relevance of treatment with botulinum toxin A

Use in children

The safety and effectiveness of Azzalure in individuals under 18 years of age have not been demonstrated.

4.3 Contraindications

Azzalure is contraindicated,

- In individuals with a known hypersensitivity to botulinum toxin A or to any of the excipients of the formulation;

- In the presence of infection at the proposed injection sites;

- In the presence of myasthenia gravis, Eaton Lambert Syndrome or Amyotrophic lateral sclerosis.

4.4 Special warnings and precautions for use

Azzalure should be used with caution in patients with a risk of, or clinical evidence of, marked defective neuro-muscular transmission. Such patients may have an increased sensitivity to agents such as Azzalure, which may result in excessive muscle weakness.

Adverse reactions possibly related to the distribution of the effects of the toxin to sites remote from the site of administration have been reported very rarely with botulinum toxin. Patients treated with therapeutic doses may experience exaggerated muscle weakness.

Injection of Azzalure is not recommended in patients with a history of dysphagia and aspiration.

Patients or care-givers should be advised to seek immediate medical care if swallowing, speech or respiratory difficulties arise.

The recommended dose and frequency of administration for Azzalure must not be exceeded.

It is essential to study the patient's facial anatomy prior to administering Azzalure. Facial asymmetry, ptosis, excessive dermatochalasis, scarring and any alterations to this anatomy, as a result of previous surgical interventions should be taken into consideration.

Caution should be taken when Azzalure is used in the presence of inflammation at the proposed injection site(s) or when the targeted muscle shows excessive weakness or atrophy.

As with all intramuscular injections, Azzalure treatment is not recommended in patients who have a prolonged bleeding time.

Injections at more frequent intervals or at higher doses can increase the risk of antibody formation to botulinum toxin. Clinically, the formation of neutralising antibodies may reduce the effectiveness of subsequent treatment.

The effect of administering different botulinum neurotoxins during the course of treatment with Azzalure is unknown and must be avoided.

This product contains a small amount of human albumin. The risk of transmission of an infection cannot be excluded with absolute certainty following the use of blood products.

It is mandatory that Azzalure is used for one single patient treatment only during a single session. The excess of unused product must be disposed of as detailed in section 6.6. Particular precautions should be taken for product preparation and administration as well as for the inactivation and disposal of the remaining unused solution (see Section 6.6).

4.5 Interaction with other medicinal products and other forms of interaction

Concomitant treatment of Azzalure and aminoglycosides or other agents interfering with neuromuscular transmission (e.g., curare-like agents) should only be used with caution since the effect of botulinum toxin type A may be potentiated.

No interaction studies have been performed. No other interactions of clinical significance have been reported.

4.6 Pregnancy and lactation

Pregnancy

Azzalure should not be used during pregnancy unless clearly necessary. There are no adequate data from the use of botulinum toxin type A in pregnant women. Studies in animals have shown reproductive toxicity at high doses (see Section 5.3). The potential risk for humans is unknown.

Lactation

There is no information on whether Azzalure is excreted in human milk. The use of Azzalure during lactation cannot be recommended.

4.7 Effects on ability to drive and use machines

There is a potential risk of localised muscle weakness or visual disturbances linked with the use of this medicinal product which may temporarily impair the ability to drive or operate machinery.

4.8 Undesirable effects

More than 1900 patients were exposed to Azzalure in the different clinical trials.

In pivotal clinical studies, over 1500 patients with moderate to severe glabellar lines have been treated at the recommended dose of 50 Units in double-blind placebo-controlled and long-term open-label studies.

In pivotal double-blind placebo-controlled single dose studies, 22.3% of patients treated at the recommended Azzalure dose (50U) and 16.6% of patients treated with placebo, experienced a reaction that was related to treatment, injection technique or both. In the long-term open-label dose Phase III study in which patients received multiple injection cycles, 26% of patients experienced at least one related reaction after the first injection. The incidence of treatment/injection technique related reactions decreased over repeat cycles.

The most frequently occurring related reactions are headache and injection site reactions. In general, treatment/injection technique related reactions occur within the first week following injection and are transient. Most of these reactions reported were of mild to moderate severity and were reversible.

The frequency of undesirable effects is classified as follows:

Very common (≥ 1/10); common (≥ 1/100 to < 1/10); uncommon (≥ 1/1,000 to <1/100); rare (≥ 1/10,000 to < 1/1,000); very rare (< 1/10,000); not known (cannot be estimated from the available data).

Nervous system disorders	Very Common Headache Common Facial paresis (predominantly describes brow paresis) Uncommon Dizziness
Eye disorders	Common Asthenopia, Ptosis, Eyelid oedema, Lacrimation increase, Dry eye, Muscle twitching (twitching of muscles around the eyes) Uncommon Visual disturbances, Vision blurred, Diplopia Rare Eye movement disorder
Skin and subcutaneous tissue disorders	Uncommon Pruritus, Rash Rare Urticaria
General disorders and administration site conditions	Very Common Injection site reactions (e.g. erythema, oedema, irritation, rash, pruritus, paraesthesia, pain, discomfort, stinging and bruising)
Immune system disorders	Uncommon Hypersensitivity

4.9 Overdose

There were no cases of overdose during clinical studies.

Excessive doses of botulinum toxin may be expected to produce neuromuscular weakness with a variety of symptoms. Respiratory support may be required where excessive doses cause paralysis of respiratory muscles. In the event of overdose the patient should be medically monitored for symptoms of excessive muscle weakness or muscle paralysis. Symptomatic treatment should be instigated if necessary.

Symptoms of overdose may not present immediately following injection.

Admission to hospital should be considered in patients presenting symptoms of botulinum toxin A poisoning (e.g. a combination of muscle weakness, ptosis, diplopia, swallowing and speech disorders, or paresis of the respiratory muscles).

5. PHARMACOLOGICAL PROPERTIES

5.1 Pharmacodynamic properties

Pharmacotherapeutic group: Other muscle relaxants, peripherally acting agents

ATC code: M03AX01

The primary pharmacodynamic effect of *Clostridium botulinum* toxin type A is due to chemical denervation of the treated muscle resulting in a measurable decrease of th compound muscle action potential, causing a localiz reduction of, or paralysis in, muscle activity.

Clinical data

During the clinical development of Azzalure, more tha 2600 patients were included in the different clinical trials

In clinical studies, 1907 patients with moderate to sever glabellar lines have been treated at the recommende dose of 50 Speywood Units. Of these, 305 were treate with 50U in two pivotal Phase III double-blind placebo controlled studies and 1200 treated with 50U in a long-tern open-label repeated dose Phase III study. The remainin patients were treated in supportive and dose-ranging stu dies.

The median time to onset of response was 2 to 3 day following treatment, with the maximum effect observed a day thirty. In both pivotal placebo-controlled phase I studies, Azzalure injections significantly reduced the severity of glabellar lines for up to 4 months. The effec was still significant after 5 months in one of the two pivota studies.

Thirty days following injection, the assessment of the investigators showed that 90% (273/305) of patients hac responded to treatment (exhibited no or mild glabellar lines at maximum frown), compared to 3% (4/153) placebo-treated patients. Five months after injection, 17% (32/ 190) of patients treated with Azzalure were still responding to treatment compared to 1% (1/92) of placebo treated patients in the concerned study. The patients own assessment at maximum frown after thirty days gave a response rate of 82% (251/305) for those treated with Azzalure and 6% (9/153) for those treated with placebo. The proportion of patients exhibiting a two-grade improvement according to the investigator assessment at maximum frown, was 77% (79/103) in the one pivotal Phase III study where this was assessed.

A subset of 177 patients had moderate or severe glabellar lines at rest prior to treatment. Assessment by investigators of this population, thirty days after treatment, showed that 71% (125/177) of Azzalure-treated patients were considered responders versus 10% (8/78) of placebo-treated patients.

The long-term repeat dose open label study showed that the median time to onset of response of 3 days was maintained across repeated dose cycles. The responder rate at maximum frown as determined by the investigator at day 30 was maintained over repeated cycles (ranging between 80% and 91% over the 5 cycles). The responder rate at rest over repeated dose cycles was also consistent with the single dose studies, with 56% to 74% of Azzalure-treated patients considered by investigators to be responders thirty days after treatment.

None of the clinical endpoints included an objective evaluation of the psychological impact.

5.2 Pharmacokinetic properties

Azzalure is not expected to be present in the peripheral blood at measurable levels following IM injection at the recommended dose. Therefore pharmacokinetic studies have not been performed with Azzalure.

5.3 Preclinical safety data

In reproductive studies in rats and rabbits, severe maternal toxicity associated with implantation loses was observed at high doses. At doses corresponding to 60 to 100 times the human recommended dose (50U) in rabbits and rats respectively, no embryofetal toxicity was observed. No teratogenic effects were observed in these species. In rats, fertility of the males and females was decreased due to reduced mating secondary to muscle paralysis at high doses.

In a chronic toxicity study performed in rats, there was no indication of systemic toxicity at doses corresponding to 75 times the human recommended dose (50U) divided equally between the right and left gluteus muscles.

Studies on acute toxicity, chronic toxicity and local tolerance at the injection site did not show unusual adverse local or systemic effects at clinically relevant dose levels.

6. PHARMACEUTICAL PARTICULARS

6.1 List of excipients

Human Albumin 200g/L.

Lactose Monohydrate.

6.2 Incompatibilities

This medicinal product must not be mixed with other medicinal products except those mentioned in section 6.6.

6.3 Shelf life

2 years.

Reconstituted solution:

From a microbiological point of view, the product should be used immediately. However, chemical and physical in-use stability has been demonstrated for 4 hours at between 2°C and 8°C.

6.4 Special precautions for storage

Store in a refrigerator (2°C - 8°C).

Do not freeze.

For storage of the reconstituted medicinal product see Section 6.3.

.5 Nature and contents of container
25 Speywood Units in a powder in a vial (Type I glass), ith a stopper (halobutyl) and seal (aluminium).

ack size of 1 or 2 vial(s).

lot all pack sizes may be marketed.

.6 Special precautions for disposal and other handling
he instructions for use, handling and disposal should be trictly followed.

econstitution should be performed in accordance with ood practice rules, particularly in the respect of asepsis.

zzalure should be reconstituted using 0.63 ml of sodium hloride 9 mg/ml (0.9%) solution for injection. This will rovide a clear solution containing 125 Speywood Units f active substance at a concentration of 10U per 0.05ml of econstituted solution.

The accurate measurement of 0.63ml can be achieved sing 1ml insulin type syringes. These are graduated to 1 ml in 0.1 ml and 0.01 ml increments.

RECOMMENDATIONS FOR THE DISPOSAL OF CONTAMINATED MATERIALS

mmediately after use and prior to disposal, unused reconstituted Azzalure (in the vial or in the syringe) should be inactivated with 2ml of dilute sodium hypochlorite solution at 0.55 or 1% (Dakin's solution).

Used vials, syringes and materials should not be emptied and must be discarded into appropriate containers and disposed of in accordance with local requirements.

RECOMMENDATIONS SHOULD ANY INCIDENT OCCUR DURING THE HANDLING OF BOTULINUM TOXIN

- Any spills of the product must be wiped up: either using absorbent material impregnated with a solution of sodium hypochlorite (bleach) in case of the powder, or with dry, absorbent material in case of reconstituted product.
- The contaminated surfaces should be cleaned using absorbent material impregnated with a solution of sodium hypochlorite (bleach), then dried.
- If a vial is broken, proceed as mentioned above by carefully collecting the pieces of broken glass and wiping up the product, avoiding any cuts to the skin.
- If the product comes into contact with the skin, wash the affected area with a solution of sodium hypochlorite (bleach) then rinse abundantly with water.
- If product enters into contact with the eyes, rinse thoroughly with plenty of water or with an ophthalmic eyewash solution.
- If product enters into contact with a wound, cut or broken skin, rinse thoroughly with plenty of water and take the appropriate medical steps according to the dose injected.

These instructions for use handling and disposal should be strictly followed.

7. MARKETING AUTHORISATION HOLDER
Ipsen Limited
190 Bath Road
Slough SL1 3XE
United Kingdom

8. MARKETING AUTHORISATION NUMBER(S)
PL 06958/0031

9. DATE OF FIRST AUTHORISATION/RENEWAL OF THE AUTHORISATION
26/02/2009

10. DATE OF REVISION OF THE TEXT
26/02/2009

Bacteriostatic Saline for Injection

(Pharmacia Limited)

1. NAME OF THE MEDICINAL PRODUCT
Bacteriostatic Saline for Injection

2. QUALITATIVE AND QUANTITATIVE COMPOSITION
Sodium Chloride, EP 0.9% w/v.

3. PHARMACEUTICAL FORM
Solution

4. CLINICAL PARTICULARS

4.1 Therapeutic indications
To be used to reconstitute certain medicinal products.

4.2 Posology and method of administration
Extra-amniotic only.

4.3 Contraindications
Not applicable.

4.4 Special warnings and precautions for use
Not applicable.

4.5 Interaction with other medicinal products and other forms of interaction
Not applicable.

4.6 Pregnancy and lactation
Not applicable.

4.7 Effects on ability to drive and use machines
Not applicable.

4.8 Undesirable effects
Benzyl alcohol is contained in the diluent and has been reported to be associated with a fatal "gasping syndrome" in premature infants.

4.9 Overdose
Not applicable.

5. PHARMACOLOGICAL PROPERTIES

5.1 Pharmacodynamic properties
Not applicable.

5.2 Pharmacokinetic properties
Not applicable.

6. PHARMACEUTICAL PARTICULARS

6.1 List of excipients
Benzyl alcohol and water for injection.

6.2 Incompatibilities
Not applicable.

6.3 Shelf life
60 months.

6.4 Special precautions for storage
Store below 25°. Discard any remaining solution after use.

6.5 Nature and contents of container
Type I flint glass vials and rubber closures (EP) which are sealed with a flip-top aluminium cap. Vials contain 18.5 ml or 50 ml.

6.6 Special precautions for disposal and other handling
No special requirements.

7. MARKETING AUTHORISATION HOLDER
Pharmacia Limited

Davy Avenue

Milton Keynes

MK5 8PH

UK

8. MARKETING AUTHORISATION NUMBER(S)
PL 0032/0149

9. DATE OF FIRST AUTHORISATION/RENEWAL OF THE AUTHORISATION
Date of first authorisation: 15 February 1990

Date of renewal of authorisation: 23 May 2003

10. DATE OF REVISION OF THE TEXT
April 2001

Ref: BA1_0

Legal category: POM

Bacteriostatic Water for Injection

(Pharmacia Limited)

1. NAME OF THE MEDICINAL PRODUCT
Bacteriostatic Water for Injections

2. QUALITATIVE AND QUANTITATIVE COMPOSITION
Not applicable

3. PHARMACEUTICAL FORM
Sterile solution.

4. CLINICAL PARTICULARS

4.1 Therapeutic indications
None. The product is intended as a diluent for Caverject Powder for Injection (PL 00032/0188, 0203, 0214, 0227).

4.2 Posology and method of administration
Intracavernosal injection

4.3 Contraindications
Hypersensitivity to benzyl alcohol.

4.4 Special warnings and precautions for use
None stated.

4.5 Interaction with other medicinal products and other forms of interaction
None stated.

4.6 Pregnancy and lactation
None stated.

4.7 Effects on ability to drive and use machines
None stated.

4.8 Undesirable effects
None stated.

4.9 Overdose
None stated.

5. PHARMACOLOGICAL PROPERTIES

5.1 Pharmacodynamic properties
None stated.

5.2 Pharmacokinetic properties
None stated.

5.3 Preclinical safety data
There are no pre-clinical data of relevance to the prescriber which are additional to that already included in other sections of this Summary of Product Characteristics.

6. PHARMACEUTICAL PARTICULARS

6.1 List of excipients
Benzyl alcohol Ph.Eur

Water for injection Ph.Eur

6.2 Incompatibilities
None stated

6.3 Shelf life
36 months

6.4 Special precautions for storage
Store below 25°C.

6.5 Nature and contents of container
1 ml pre-filled syringe with butyl rubber plunger stopper and tip cap containing 1 ml of solution.

Or

1 ml pre-filled syringe with butyl rubber plunger stopper, syringe tip cap, tamper evident seal and locking device containing 1 ml of solution.

6.6 Special precautions for disposal and other handling
No special requirements.

Administrative Data

7. MARKETING AUTHORISATION HOLDER
Pharmacia Limited

Davy Avenue

Milton Keynes

MK5 8PH

UK

8. MARKETING AUTHORISATION NUMBER(S)
PL 00032/0193

9. DATE OF FIRST AUTHORISATION/RENEWAL OF THE AUTHORISATION
15 March 1994 / 16 March 1999

10. DATE OF REVISION OF THE TEXT
December 2003

Legal Category: **POM**

Ref: 1_0

Bactroban Cream

(GlaxoSmithKline UK)

1. NAME OF THE MEDICINAL PRODUCT
Bactroban® Cream.

2. QUALITATIVE AND QUANTITATIVE COMPOSITION
1g Cream contains: 21.5mg Mupirocin calcium equivalent to 20.0mg mupirocin.

For excipients, see Section 6.1.

3. PHARMACEUTICAL FORM
Cream.

Bactroban Cream is presented as a white cream of homogeneous appearance.

4. CLINICAL PARTICULARS

4.1 Therapeutic indications
Bactroban Cream is indicated for the topical treatment of secondarily infected traumatic lesions such as small lacerations, sutured wounds or abrasions (up to 10cm in length or $100cm^2$ in area), due to susceptible strains of *Staphylococcus aureus* and *Streptococcus pyogenes*.

4.2 Posology and method of administration

Dosage

Adults/children/elderly

Three times a day for up to 10 days, depending on the response.

Patients not showing a clinical response within 3 to 5 days should be re-evaluated.

The duration of treatment should not exceed 10 days.

Hepatic impairment: No dosage adjustment is necessary.

Renal impairment: No dosage adjustment is necessary.

Method of administration

A thin layer of cream should be applied to the affected area with a piece of clean cotton wool or gauze swab.

The treated area may be covered by a dressing.

Do not mix with other preparations, as there is a risk of dilution, resulting in a reduction in the antibacterial activity and potential loss of stability of the mupirocin in the cream.

4.3 Contraindications
Hypersensitivity to mupirocin or any of the excipients (see section 6.1).

4.4 Special warnings and precautions for use
Avoid contact with the eyes.

Should a possible sensitisation reaction or severe local irritation occur with the use of Bactroban Cream, treatment should be discontinued, the product should be washed off and appropriate alternative therapy for the infection instituted.

As with other antibacterial products, prolonged use may result in overgrowth of non-susceptible organisms.

Bactroban Cream has not been studied in infants under 1 year old and therefore it should not be used in these patients until further data become available.

Bactroban Cream contains cetyl alcohol and stearyl alcohol. These inactive ingredients may cause local skin reactions (e.g. contact dermatitis).

4.5 Interaction with other medicinal products and other forms of interaction
No drug interactions have been identified.

4.6 Pregnancy and lactation

Use in pregnancy:

Reproduction studies on mupirocin in animals have revealed no evidence of harm to the foetus. As there is no clinical experience on its use during pregnancy, mupirocin should only be used in pregnancy when the potential benefits outweigh the possible risks of treatment.

Use in lactation:

There is no information on the excretion of mupirocin in milk. If a cracked nipple is to be treated, it should be thoroughly washed prior to breast feeding.

4.7 Effects on ability to drive and use machines
No adverse effects on the ability to drive or operate machinery have been identified.

4.8 Undesirable effects
Data from clinical trials was used to determine the frequency of very common to rare undesirable effects.

The following convention has been used for the classification of frequency:-

very common $\geq$1/10, common $\geq$1/100 and <1/10, uncommon $\geq$1/1000 and <1/100, rare $\geq$1/10,000 and <1/1000, very rare <1/10,000.

Skin and subcutaneous tissue disorders:

Common: Application site hypersensitivity reactions including urticaria, pruritus, erythema, burning sensation, contact dermatitis, rash

Skin dryness and erythema have been reported in irritancy studies in volunteers.

4.9 Overdose
The toxicity of mupirocin is very low. In the event of accidental ingestion of the cream symptomatic treatment should be given.

5. PHARMACOLOGICAL PROPERTIES

5.1 Pharmacodynamic properties

ATC classification

Properties

ATC-code: D06A X09, Antibiotics and chemotherapeutics for dermatological use.

Mode of Action

Mupirocin is an antibiotic produced through fermentation by *Pseudomonas fluorescens*. Mupirocin inhibits isoleucyl transfer-RNA synthetase, thereby arresting bacterial protein synthesis. Due to this particular mode of action and its unique chemical structure, mupirocin does not show any cross-resistance with other clinically available antibiotics.

Mupirocin has bacteriostatic properties at minimum inhibitory concentrations and bactericidal properties at the higher concentrations reached when applied locally.

Activity

Mupirocin is a topical antibacterial agent showing *in vivo* activity against *Staphylococcus aureus* (including methicillin-resistant strains), *S. epidermidis* and beta-haemolytic *Streptococcus* species.

The *in-vitro* spectrum of activity includes but is not limited to the following bacteria which are most often implicated in skin infections:

- *Staphylococcus aureus* (including beta-lactamase-producing strains and methicillin resistant strains).
- *Staphylococcus epidermidis* (including beta-lactamase-producing strains and methicillin-resistant strains).
- Other coagulase-negative staphylococci (including methicillin-resistant strains).
- *Streptococcus* species.

5.2 Pharmacokinetic properties

Absorption

Systemic absorption of mupirocin through intact human skin is low although it may occur through broken/diseased skin. However, clinical trials have shown that when given systemically, it is metabolised to the microbiologically inactive metabolite monic acid and rapidly excreted.

Excretion

Mupirocin is rapidly eliminated from the body by metabolism to its inactive metabolite monic acid which is rapidly excreted by the kidney.

5.3 Preclinical safety data

Pre-clinical effects were seen only at exposures which give no cause for concern for man under normal conditions of clinical use. Mutagenicity studies revealed no risks to man.

6. PHARMACEUTICAL PARTICULARS

6.1 List of excipients

Xanthan gum, liquid paraffin, cetomacrogol 1000, stearyl alcohol, cetyl alcohol, phenoxyethanol, benzyl alcohol, purified water.

6.2 Incompatibilities

None known

6.3 Shelf life

18 months

6.4 Special precautions for storage

Do not store above 25°C. Do not freeze.

6.5 Nature and contents of container

Squeezable aluminium tubes with a screw cap containing 15 g of white cream.

6.6 Special precautions for disposal and other handling

Any product remaining at the end of treatment should be discarded.

Administrative Data

7. MARKETING AUTHORISATION HOLDER

Beecham Group plc

980 Great West Road, Brentford

Middlesex TW8 9GS

Trading as:

GlaxoSmithKline UK

Stockley Park West,

Uxbridge,

Middlesex, UB11 1BT

8. MARKETING AUTHORISATION NUMBER(S)

PL 00038/0372

9. DATE OF FIRST AUTHORISATION/RENEWAL OF THE AUTHORISATION

28 October 1998

10. DATE OF REVISION OF THE TEXT

28 October 2008

11. Legal category

POM

Bactroban Nasal Ointment

(GlaxoSmithKline UK)

1. NAME OF THE MEDICINAL PRODUCT

Bactroban® Nasal Ointment

2. QUALITATIVE AND QUANTITATIVE COMPOSITION

Mupirocin 2.0% w/w as mupirocin calcium.

3. PHARMACEUTICAL FORM

White soft paraffin based ointment containing a glycerin ester.

4. CLINICAL PARTICULARS

4.1 Therapeutic indications

The elimination of nasal carriage of staphylococci, including methicillin resistant *Staphylococcus aureus* (MRSA).

4.2 Posology and method of administration

Dosage: Adults (including the elderly) and children:

Bactroban Nasal Ointment should be applied to the anterior nares two to three times a day as follows:

A small amount of the ointment about the size of a match head is placed on the little finger and applied to the inside of each nostril. The nostrils are closed by pressing the sides of the nose together; this will spread the ointment throughout the nares. A cotton bud may be used instead of the little finger for the application in particular to infants or patients who are very ill.

Nasal carriage should normally clear within 5-7 days of commencing treatment.

Administration: Topical.

4.3 Contraindications

Bactroban Nasal Ointment should not be given to patients with a history of hypersensitivity to any of the constituents.

4.4 Special warnings and precautions for use

As with all topical preparations care should be taken to avoid the eyes.

In the rare event of a possible sensitisation reaction or severe local irritation occuring with the use of Bactroban Nasal Ointment, treatment should be discontinued, the product should be wiped off and appropriate alternative therapy for the infection instituted.

4.5 Interaction with other medicinal products and other forms of interaction

The product is not known to interact with other medicaments.

4.6 Pregnancy and lactation

This product should not be used during pregnancy and lactation unless considered essential by the physician.

Pregnancy: Adequate human data on use during pregnancy are not available. However animal studies have not identified any risk to pregnancy or embryo-foetal development.

Lactation: Adequate human and animal data on use during lactation are not available.

4.7 Effects on ability to drive and use machines

None known.

4.8 Undesirable effects

Adverse reactions are listed below by system organ class and frequency. Frequencies are defined as: very common (≥1/10), common (≥1/100, <1/10), uncommon (≥1/1000, <1/100), rare (≥1/10,000, <1/1000), very rare (<1/10,000), including isolated reports. Uncommon adverse reactions were determined from pooled safety data from a clinical trial population of 422 treated patients encompassing 12 clinical studies. Very rare adverse reactions were primarily determined from post-marketing experience data and therefore refer to reporting rate rather than true frequency.

Immune system disorders

Very rare: Cutaneous hypersensitivity reactions.

Respiratory, thoracic and mediastinal disorders

Uncommon: Nasal mucosa reactions.

4.9 Overdose

The toxicity of mupirocin is very low. In the event of overdose, symptomatic treatment should be given.

5. PHARMACOLOGICAL PROPERTIES

5.1 Pharmacodynamic properties

Mupirocin is a novel antibiotic formulated for topical application only. Its spectrum of *in-vitro* antibacterial activity includes *Staphylococcus aureus* (including methicillin resistant strains), *Staphylococcus epidermidis*, *Streptococcus* species and certain Gram-negative bacteria, particularly *Haemophilus influenzae* and *Escherichia coli*. Other Gram-negative bacteria are less susceptible and Pseudomonas aeruginosa is resistant.

Mupirocin is the major antibacterial compound of a group of structurally related metabolites produced by submerged fermentation of Ps. Fluorescens. Mupirocin has a novel mode of action, inhibiting bacterial iso-leucyl transfer-RNA synthetase and thus cross-resistance with other antibiotics is not experienced.

5.2 Pharmacokinetic properties

Studies have shown that following topical application of mupirocin there is very little systemic absorption of drug-related material. To mimic possible enhanced systemic penetration of mupirocin by application to damaged skin or a vascular site such as the mucous membrane, intravenous studies have been performed. Mupirocin was rapidly eliminated from the plasma by metabolism to monic acid, which in turn was excreted mainly in the urine.

5.3 Preclinical safety data

No further information of relevance.

6. PHARMACEUTICAL PARTICULARS

6.1 List of excipients

White soft paraffin and Softisan 649.

6.2 Incompatibilities

None known.

6.3 Shelf life

Bactroban Nasal Ointment has a shelf-life of three years.

6.4 Special precautions for storage

Store at room temperature (below 25°C).

6.5 Nature and contents of container

Lacquered aluminium tube fitted with a nozzle and screw cap - 3 g ointment.

6.6 Special precautions for disposal and other handling

None stated.

Administrative Data

7. MARKETING AUTHORISATION HOLDER

Beecham Group plc

980 Great West Road

Brentford

Middlesex TW8 9GS

trading as:

GlaxoSmithKline UK,

Stockley Park West,

Uxbridge,

Middlesex, UB11 1BT

8. MARKETING AUTHORISATION NUMBER(S)

PL 00038/0347

9. DATE OF FIRST AUTHORISATION/RENEWAL OF THE AUTHORISATION

21 May 2008

10. DATE OF REVISION OF THE TEXT

21 May 2008

11. Legal Status

POM

Bactroban Ointment

(GlaxoSmithKline UK)

1. NAME OF THE MEDICINAL PRODUCT

Bactroban® Ointment

2. QUALITATIVE AND QUANTITATIVE COMPOSITION

Mupirocin 2.0% w/w

3. PHARMACEUTICAL FORM

Ointment in a white, translucent, water-soluble, polyethylene glycol base. For topical administration.

4. CLINICAL PARTICULARS

4.1 Therapeutic indications

Bactroban is a topical antibacterial agent, active against those organisms responsible for the majority of skin infections, e.g. *Staphylococcus aureus*, including methicillin-resistant strains, other staphylococci, streptococci. It is also active against Gram-negative organisms such as *Escherichia coli* and *Haemophilus influenzae*. Bactroban Ointment is used for skin infections, e.g. impetigo, folliculitis, furunculosis.

4.2 Posology and method of administration

Dosage:

Adults (including elderly) and children:

Bactroban Ointment should be applied to the affected area up to three times a day for up to 10 days.

The area may be covered with a dressing or occluded if desired.

Administration:

Topical.

Do not mix with other preparations as there is a risk of dilution, resulting in a reduction of the antibacterial activity and potential loss of stability of the mupirocin in the ointment.

4.3 Contraindications

Bactroban ointment should not be given to patients with a history of hypersensitivity to any of its constituents.

This Bactroban Ointment formulation is not suitable for ophthalmic or intranasal use.

4.4 Special warnings and precautions for use

When Bactroban Ointment is used on the face, care should be taken to avoid the eyes.

Polyethylene glycol can be absorbed from open wounds and damaged skin and is excreted by the kidneys. In common with other polyethylene glycol-based ointments, Bactroban Ointment should be used with caution if there is evidence of moderate or severe renal impairment.

In the rare event of a possible sensitisation reaction or severe local irritation occurring with the use of Bactroban ointment, treatment should be discontinued, the product hould be rinsed off and appropriate alternative therapy for ne infection instituted.

.5 Interaction with other medicinal products and other orms of interaction
one stated.

.6 Pregnancy and lactation
his product should not be used during pregnancy and actation unless considered essential by the physician.

regnancy: Adequate human data on use during pregnancy are not available. However animal studies have not dentified any risk to pregnancy or embryo-foetal development.

actation: Adequate human and animal data on use during actation are not available.

.7 Effects on ability to drive and use machines
one stated.

.8 Undesirable effects
dverse reactions are listed below by system organ class nd frequency. Frequencies are defined as: very common ≥1/10), common (≥1/100, <1/10), uncommon (≥1/ 000, <1/100), rare (≥1/10,000, <1/1000), very rare <1/10,000), including isolated reports. Common and ncommon adverse reactions were determined from ooled safety data from a clinical trial population of 1573 reated patients encompassing 12 clinical studies. Very are adverse reactions were primarily determined from ost-marketing experience data and therefore refer to eporting rate rather than true frequency.

mmune system disorders:

ery rare: Systemic allergic reactions have been reported with Bactroban Ointment.

Skin and subcutaneous tissue disorders:

Common: Burning localised to the area of application.

Uncommon: Itching, erythema, stinging and dryness localised to the area of application.

Uncommon: Cutaneous sensitisation reactions to mupirocin or the ointment base.

4.9 Overdose
The toxicity of mupirocin is very low. In the event of overdose, symptomatic treatment should be given.

5. PHARMACOLOGICAL PROPERTIES

5.1 Pharmacodynamic properties
Bactroban (mupirocin) potently inhibits bacterial protein and RNA synthesis by inhibition of isoleucyl-transfer RNA synthetase.

5.2 Pharmacokinetic properties
After topical application of Bactroban Ointment, mupirocin is only very minimally absorbed systemically and that which is absorbed is rapidly metabolised to the antimicrobially inactive metabolite, monic acid. Penetration of mupirocin into the deeper epidermal and dermal layers of the skin is enhanced in traumatised skin and under occlusive dressings.

5.3 Preclinical safety data
None stated.

6. PHARMACEUTICAL PARTICULARS

6.1 List of excipients
Polyethylene Glycol 400 USNF

Polyethylene Glycol 3350 USNF

6.2 Incompatibilities
None stated.

6.3 Shelf life
Bactroban Ointment has a shelf-life of two years.

6.4 Special precautions for storage
Store at room temperature (below 25°C).

6.5 Nature and contents of container
Original pack of 5 and 15 g* (sealed tube in a carton) with Patient Information Leaflet.

6.6 Special precautions for disposal and other handling
No special instructions.

Administrative Data

7. MARKETING AUTHORISATION HOLDER
Beecham Group plc

980 Great West Road,

Brentford,

Middlesex TW8 9GS

Trading as:

GlaxoSmithKine UK,

Stockley Park West,

Uxbridge,

Middlesex UB11 1BT

8. MARKETING AUTHORISATION NUMBER(S)
PL 00038/0319

9. DATE OF FIRST AUTHORISATION/RENEWAL OF THE AUTHORISATION
21 May 2008

10. DATE OF REVISION OF THE TEXT
21 May 2008

11. Legal Status
POM

* At time of printing only the details relevant to marketed packs will be included.

Bambec Tablets 10mg

(AstraZeneca UK Limited)

1. NAME OF THE MEDICINAL PRODUCT
Bambec Tablets 10 mg

2. QUALITATIVE AND QUANTITATIVE COMPOSITION
Each tablet contains 10 mg Bambuterol hydrochloride

For excipients, see Section 6.1

3. PHARMACEUTICAL FORM
Tablet

4. CLINICAL PARTICULARS

4.1 Therapeutic indications
Management of asthma, bronchospasm and/or reversible airways obstruction.

4.2 Posology and method of administration
Bambec is formulated as a tablet and should be taken once daily, shortly before bedtime. The dose should be individualised.

Adults: The recommended starting doses are 10 mg–20 mg. The 10 mg dose may be increased to 20 mg if necessary after 1–2 weeks, depending on the clinical effect.

In patients who have previously tolerated β_2-agonists well, the recommended starting dose, as well as maintenance dose, is 20 mg.

Children: Until the clinical documentation has been completed, Bambec should not be used in children.

Elderly: Dose adjustment is not required in the elderly.

Significant hepatic dysfunction: Not recommended because of unpredictable conversion to terbutaline.

Moderate to severely impaired renal function (GFR < 50ml/min): It is recommended that the starting dose of Bambec should be halved in these patients.

4.3 Contraindications
Bambec tablets are contraindicated in patients with a history of hypersensitivity to any of their ingredients. Bambec is presently not recommended for children due to limited clinical data in this age group.

4.4 Special warnings and precautions for use
As terbutaline is excreted mainly via the kidneys, the dose of Bambec should be halved in patients with moderately to severely impaired renal function (GFR ≤ 50 mL/min).

Care should be taken with patients suffering from thyrotoxicosis.

Cardiovascular effects may be seen with sympathomimetic drugs, including Bambec. There is some evidence from post-marketing data and published literature of rare occurrences of myocardial ischaemia associated with beta agonists. Patients with underlying severe heart disease (e.g. ischaemic heart disease, arrhythmia or severe heart failure) who are receiving Bambec should be warned to seek medical advice if they experience chest pain or other symptoms of worsening heart disease. Attention should be paid to assessment of symptoms such as dyspnoea and chest pain, as they may be of either respiratory or cardiac origin.

Due to the hyperglycaemic effects of β_2-stimulants, additional blood glucose measurements are recommended initially when Bambec therapy is commenced in diabetic patients.

Due to the positive inotropic effects of β_2-agonists these drugs should not be used in patients with hypertrophic cardiomyopathy.

β_2-agonists may be arrhythmogenic and this must be considered in the treatment of the individual patient.

Unpredictable inter-individual variation in the metabolism of bambuterol to terbutaline has been shown in subjects with liver cirrhosis. The use of an alternative β_2-agonist is recommended in patients with cirrhosis and other forms of severely impaired liver function.

Potentially serious hypokalaemia may result from β_2-agonist therapy mainly from parenteral or nebulised administration. Particular caution is advised in acute severe asthma as this effect may be augmented by hypoxia. The hypokalaemic effect may be potentiated by concomitant treatment with xanthine derivatives, corticosteroids and/or diuretics. It is recommended that serum potassium levels are monitored in such situations.

If a previously effective dosage regimen no longer gives the same symptomatic relief, the patient should urgently seek further medical advice. Consideration should be given to the requirements for additional therapy (including increased dosages of anti-inflammatory medication). Severe exacerbations of asthma should be treated as an emergency in the usual manner.

Patients with rare hereditary problems of galactose intolerance, the Lapp lactase deficiency or glucose galactose malabsorption should not take this medicine.

4.5 Interaction with other medicinal products and other forms of interaction
Bambuterol may interact with suxamethonium (succinylcholine). A prolongation of the muscle-relaxing effect of suxamethonium of up to 2-fold has been observed in some patients after taking Bambec 20 mg on the evening prior to surgery. The interaction is dose-dependent. It is due to the fact that plasma cholinesterase, which inactivates suxamethonium, is partly, but fully reversibly, inhibited by bambuterol. In extreme situations, the interaction may result in a prolonged apnoea time which may be of clinical importance.

Bambuterol may also interact with other muscle relaxants metabolised by plasma cholinesterase.

Beta-receptor blocking agents including eyedrops, especially non-selective ones, may partly or totally inhibit the effect of beta-stimulants. Therefore, Bambec tablets and non-selective β-blockers should not normally be administered concurrently. Bambec should be used with caution in patients receiving other sympathomimetics.

Hypokalemia may result from β_2-agonist therapy and may be potentiated by concomitant treatment with xanthine derivatives, corticosteroids and diuretics (see Section 4.4, Warnings and Precautions).

4.6 Pregnancy and lactation
Unless there are compelling reasons, avoid in pregnancy, lactation and women of child-bearing potential who are not taking adequate contraceptive precautions. Although no teratogenic effects have been observed in animals after administration of bambuterol, there is no experience of use in human pregnancy. Terbutaline, the active metabolite of bambuterol, has been in widespread clinical use for many years and may be considered in such patients. Terbutaline should be used with caution in the first trimester of pregnancy. Maternal β_2-agonist treatment may result in transient hypoglycaemia in pre-term newborn infants.

It is not known whether bambuterol or intermediary metabolites pass into breast milk. Terbutaline does pass into breast milk, but an effect on the infant is unlikely at therapeutic doses.

4.7 Effects on ability to drive and use machines
None stated.

4.8 Undesirable effects
Adverse events are listed below by system organ class and frequency. Frequencies are defined as: very common (≥1/10), common (≥1/100 to <1/10), uncommon (≥1/1000 to < 1/100), rare (≥1/10,000 to < 1/1000), very rare (<1/10,000) and unknown (cannot be estimated from available data).

Most of the adverse reactions are characteristic of sympathomimetic amines. The intensity of the adverse reactions is dose-dependent. Tolerance to the effects has usually developed within 1-2 weeks.

(see Table 1 on next page)

4.9 Overdose
Overdosing may result in high levels of terbutaline.

Symptoms

The signs and symptoms described here have been recorded after terbutaline overdose.

Possible signs and symptoms: Headache, anxiety, tremor, nausea, cramps, palpitations, tachycardia, cardiac arrhythmias. A fall in blood pressure sometimes occurs.

Laboratory findings: Hypokalaemia, hyperglycaemia and lactic acidosis sometimes occur.

Overdose of Bambec is also likely to cause a prolonged inhibition of plasma cholinesterase.

Management

Mild and moderate cases: Reduce the dose.

Severe cases: Administration of activated charcoal if ingestion is recent. Determination of acid-base balance, blood sugar and electrolytes. Monitoring of heart rate and rhythm and blood pressure.

Metabolic changes should be corrected. A cardioselective β-blocker (e.g. metoprolol) is recommended for the treatment of haemodynamically significant cardiac arrhythmias. The β-blocker should be used with care because of the possibility of inducing bronchoconstriction. Serum potassium levels should be monitored. If the β_2-mediated vasodilation contributes significantly to the fall in blood pressure, a volume expander should be given.

5. PHARMACOLOGICAL PROPERTIES

5.1 Pharmacodynamic properties
Pharmacotherapeutic group: selective β_2-agonists, bambuterol, ATC code: R03C C12.

Bambuterol is an active precursor of the selective β_2-adrenergic agonist terbutaline. Bambuterol is the bis-dimethylcarbamate of terbutaline, and is present in the formulation as a 1:1 racemate.

Pharmacodynamic studies have shown that after oral administration of bambuterol to guinea pigs, a sustained protective effect was achieved against histamine-induced bronchoconstriction. At equipotent doses, the duration of the relaxing activity was more prolonged than after plain

Table 1

System Organ Class (SOC)	Frequency Classification	Adverse Drug Reaction
Immune system disorders	Unknown	Hypersensitivity reactions including angioedema, urticaria, exanthema, bronchospasm, hypotension and collapse.
Metabolism and nutrition disorders	Unknown	Hypokalemia
Psychiatric disorders	Very Common	Restlessness
	Common	Sleep disturbances
	Uncommon	Agitation
	Unknown	Hyperactivity
Nervous system disorders	Very common	Tremor, headache
Cardiac disorders	Common	Palpitations
	Uncommon	Tachycardia Cardiac arrhythmias, e.g. atrial fibrillation, supraventricular tachycardia and extrasystoles
	Unknown	Myocardial ischemia (see section 4.4)
Respiratory, thoracic and mediastinal disorders	Unknown	Paradoxical bronchospasm
Gastrointestinal disorders	Unknown	Nausea
Musculoskeletal, connective tissue and bone disorders	Common	Muscle cramps

terbutaline. Bambuterol, or the monocarbamate ester, did not exert any smooth muscle relaxing properties. The bronchoprotective effects seen after oral administration of bambuterol are related to the generation of terbutaline, as were the secondary effects (effects on other organs).

Pharmacodynamic studies have been conducted in asthmatics and healthy volunteers. The effects observed were bronchodilation, tremor and increases in heart rate. The metabolic effects included a small increase in blood glucose, while the effect on serum potassium was negligible. In short-term studies on lipoprotein metabolism, an increase in HDL cholesterol has been observed. In conclusion, all pharmacodynamic effects observed can be ascribed to the active metabolite terbutaline.

5.2 Pharmacokinetic properties

On average, 17.5% of an oral dose is absorbed. Approximately 70–90% of the absorption occurs in the first 24 hours.

Bambuterol is metabolised in the liver and terbutaline is formed by both hydrolysis and oxidation. After absorption from the gut, about 2/3 of terbutaline is first-pass metabolised, bambuterol escapes this first-pass metabolism. Of the absorbed amount, about 65% reaches the circulation. Bambuterol therefore has a bioavailability of about 10%.

Protein binding of bambuterol is low, 40–50% at therapeutic concentrations.

The terminal half-life of bambuterol after an oral dose is 9–17 hours.

Studies on the effects on plasma cholinesterase showed that bambuterol inhibited activity, but that this was reversible.

All categories of subjects studied were able to form terbutaline in a predictive way except for liver cirrhotics.

5.3 Preclinical safety data

Bambuterol has not revealed any adverse effects which pose a risk to man at therapeutic dosages in the toxicity studies.

Bambuterol is given as a racemate: (-)-bambuterol is responsible for the pharmacodynamic effects via generation of (-)-terbutaline. (+)-bambuterol generates the pharmacodynamic inactive (+)-terbutaline. Both (+) and (-)-bambuterol are equally active as plasma cholinesterase inhibitors. This inhibition is reversible.

The toxicity studies showed that bambuterol has β_2-stimulatory effects, expressed as cardiotoxicity in dogs, and at high doses, observed in the acute toxicity studies, cholinergic effects.

There is no evidence from the preclinical safety data to indicate that bambuterol cannot be used in man for the intended indications with sufficient safety.

6. PHARMACEUTICAL PARTICULARS

6.1 List of excipients

Lactose monohydrate; maize starch; povidone; microcrystalline cellulose; magnesium stearate; water, purified.

6.2 Incompatibilities

Not applicable.

6.3 Shelf life

3 years.

6.4 Special precautions for storage

Do not store above 30°C.

6.5 Nature and contents of container

Amber glass bottle with LD-polyethene cap: 7, 14, 28, 30, 56 or 100 tablets.

HDPE container with LD-polyethene cap: 7, 14, 28, 30, 56 or 100 tablets.

HDPE container with polypropylene cap: 7, 14, 28, 30, 56 or 100 tablets.

PVC blisters: 7, 14, 28, 30, 56 or 100 tablets.

6.6 Special precautions for disposal and other handling

None.

7. MARKETING AUTHORISATION HOLDER

AstraZeneca UK Ltd.,

600 Capability Green,

Luton, LU1 3LU, UK.

8. MARKETING AUTHORISATION NUMBER(S)

PL 17901/0103

9. DATE OF FIRST AUTHORISATION/RENEWAL OF THE AUTHORISATION

21st May 2002

10. DATE OF REVISION OF THE TEXT

26th June 2009

Bambec Tablets 20mg

(AstraZeneca UK Limited)

1. NAME OF THE MEDICINAL PRODUCT

Bambec Tablets 20 mg

2. QUALITATIVE AND QUANTITATIVE COMPOSITION

Each tablet contains 20 mg Bambuterol hydrochloride

For excipients, see Section 6.1

3. PHARMACEUTICAL FORM

Tablet

4. CLINICAL PARTICULARS

4.1 Therapeutic indications

Management of asthma, bronchospasm and/or reversible airways obstruction.

4.2 Posology and method of administration

Bambec is formulated as a tablet and should be taken once daily, shortly before bedtime. The dose should be individualised.

Adults: The recommended starting doses are 10 mg–20 mg. The 10 mg dose may be increased to 20 mg if necessary after 1–2 weeks, depending on the clinical effect.

In patients who have previously tolerated β_2-agonists well, the recommended starting dose, as well as maintenance dose, is 20 mg.

Children: Until the clinical documentation has been completed, Bambec should not be used in children.

Elderly: Dose adjustment is not required in the elderly.

Significant hepatic dysfunction: Not recommende because of unpredictable conversion to terbutaline.

Moderate to severely impaired renal function (GF < 50ml/min): It is recommended that the starting dos of Bambec should be halved in these patients.

4.3 Contraindications

Bambec tablets are contraindicated in patients with history of hypersensitivity to any of their ingredients. Bambec is presently not recommended for children due t limited clinical data in this age group.

4.4 Special warnings and precautions for use

As terbutaline is excreted mainly via the kidneys, the dose of Bambec should be halved in patients with moderately t severely impaired renal function (GFR ≤ 50 mL/min).

Care should be taken with patients suffering from thyro toxicosis.

Cardiovascular effects may be seen with sympathomi metic drugs, including Bambec. There is some evidence from post-marketing data and published literature of rare occurrences of myocardial ischaemia associated with beta agonists. Patients with underlying severe heart disease (e.g. ischaemic heart disease, arrhythmia or severe heart failure) who are receiving Bambec should be warned t seek medical advice if they experience chest pain or other symptoms of worsening heart disease. Attention should be paid to assessment of symptoms such as dyspnoea and chest pain, as they may be of either respiratory or cardiac origin.

Due to the hyperglycaemic effects of β_2-stimulants, additional blood glucose measurements are recommended initially when Bambec therapy is commenced in diabetic patients.

Due to the positive inotropic effects of β_2-agonists these drugs should not be used in patients with hypertrophic cardiomyopathy.

β_2-agonists may be arrhythmogenic and this must be considered in the treatment of the individual patient.

Unpredictable inter-individual variation in the metabolism of bambuterol to terbutaline has been shown in subjects with liver cirrhosis. The use of an alternative β_2-agonist is recommended in patients with cirrhosis and other forms of severely impaired liver function.

Potentially serious hypokalaemia may result from β_2-agonist therapy mainly from parenteral or nebulised administration. Particular caution is advised in acute severe asthma as this effect may be augmented by hypoxia. The hypokalaemic effect may be potentiated by concomitant treatment with xanthine derivatives, corticosteroids and/or diuretics. It is recommended that serum potassium levels are monitored in such situations.

If a previously effective dosage regimen no longer gives the same symptomatic relief, the patient should urgently seek further medical advice. Consideration should be given to the requirements for additional therapy (including increased dosages of anti-inflammatory medication). Severe exacerbations of asthma should be treated as an emergency in the usual manner.

Patients with rare hereditary problems of galactose intolerance, the Lapp lactase deficiency or glucose galactose malabsorption should not take this medicine.

4.5 Interaction with other medicinal products and other forms of interaction

Bambuterol may interact with suxamethonium (succinylcholine). A prolongation of the muscle-relaxing effect of suxamethonium of up to 2-fold has been observed in some patients after taking Bambec 20 mg on the evening prior to surgery. The interaction is dose-dependent. It is due to the fact that plasma cholinesterase, which inactivates suxamethonium, is partly, but fully reversibly, inhibited by bambuterol. In extreme situations, the interaction may result in a prolonged apnoea time which may be of clinical importance.

Bambuterol may also interact with other muscle relaxants metabolised by plasma cholinesterase.

Beta-receptor blocking agents including eyedrops, especially non-selective ones, may partly or totally inhibit the effect of beta-stimulants. Therefore, Bambec tablets and non-selective β-blockers should not normally be administered concurrently. Bambec should be used with caution in patients receiving other sympathomimetics.

Hypokalemia may result from β_2-agonist therapy and may be potentiated by concomitant treatment with xanthine derivatives, corticosteroids and diuretics (see Section 4.4, Warnings and Precautions).

4.6 Pregnancy and lactation

Unless there are compelling reasons, avoid in pregnancy, lactation and women of child-bearing potential who are not taking adequate contraceptive precautions. Although no teratogenic effects have been observed in animals after administration of bambuterol, there is no experience of use in human pregnancy. Terbutaline, the active metabolite of bambuterol, has been in widespread clinical use for many years and may be considered in such patients. Terbutaline should be used with caution in the first trimester of pregnancy. Maternal β_2-agonist treatment may result in transient hypoglycaemia in pre-term newborn infants.

It is not known whether bambuterol or intermediary metabolites pass into breast milk. Terbutaline does pass into breast milk, but an effect on the infant is unlikely at therapeutic doses.

4.7 Effects on ability to drive and use machines
None stated.

4.8 Undesirable effects
Adverse events are listed below by system organ class and frequency. Frequencies are defined as: very common (≥1/10), common (≥1/100 to <1/10), uncommon (≥1/1000 to < 1/100), rare (≥1/10,000 to < 1/1000), very rare (<1/10,000) and unknown (cannot be estimated from available data).

Most of the adverse reactions are characteristic of sympathomimetic amines. The intensity of the adverse reactions is dose-dependent. Tolerance to the effects has usually developed within 1-2 weeks.

(see Table 1 below)

4.9 Overdose
Overdosing may result in high levels of terbutaline.

Symptoms

The signs and symptoms described here have been recorded after terbutaline overdose.

Possible signs and symptoms: Headache, anxiety, tremor, nausea, cramps, palpitations, tachycardia, cardiac arrhythmias. A fall in blood pressure sometimes occurs.

Laboratory findings: Hypokalaemia, hyperglycaemia and lactic acidosis sometimes occur.

Overdose of Bambec is also likely to cause a prolonged inhibition of plasma cholinesterase.

Management

Mild and moderate cases: Reduce the dose.

Severe cases: Administration of activated charcoal if ingestion is recent. Determination of acid-base balance, blood sugar and electrolytes. Monitoring of heart rate and rhythm and blood pressure.

Metabolic changes should be corrected. A cardioselective β-blocker (e.g. metoprolol) is recommended for the treatment of haemodynamically significant cardiac arrhythmias. The β-blocker should be used with care because of the possibility of inducing bronchoconstriction. Serum potassium levels should be monitored. If the β_2-mediated vasodilation contributes significantly to the fall in blood pressure, a volume expander should be given.

5. PHARMACOLOGICAL PROPERTIES

5.1 Pharmacodynamic properties
Pharmacotherapeutic group: selective β_2-agonists, bambuterol, ATC code: R03C C12.

Bambuterol is an active precursor of the selective β_2-adrenergic agonist terbutaline. Bambuterol is the bis-dimethylcarbamate of terbutaline, and is present in the formulation as a 1:1 racemate.

Pharmacodynamic studies have shown that after oral administration of bambuterol to guinea pigs, a sustained protective effect was achieved against histamine-induced bronchoconstriction. At equipotent doses, the duration of the relaxing activity was more prolonged than after plain terbutaline. Bambuterol, or the monocarbamate ester, did not exert any smooth muscle relaxing properties. The bronchoprotective effects seen after oral administration of bambuterol are related to the generation of terbutaline, as were the secondary effects (effects on other organs).

Pharmacodynamic studies have been conducted in asthmatics and healthy volunteers. The effects observed were bronchodilation, tremor and increases in heart rate. The metabolic effects included a small increase in blood glucose, while the effect on serum potassium was negligible. In short-term studies on lipoprotein metabolism, an increase in HDL cholesterol, has been observed. In conclusion, all pharmacodynamic effects observed can be ascribed to the active metabolite terbutaline.

5.2 Pharmacokinetic properties
On average, 17.5% of an oral dose is absorbed. Approximately 70–90% of the absorption occurs in the first 24 hours.

Bambuterol is metabolised in the liver and terbutaline is formed by both hydrolysis and oxidation. After absorption from the gut, about 2/3 of terbutaline is first-pass metabolised, bambuterol escapes this first-pass metabolism. Of the absorbed amount, about 65% reaches the circulation. Bambuterol therefore has a bioavailability of about 10%.

Protein binding of bambuterol is low, 40–50% at therapeutic concentrations.

The terminal half-life of bambuterol after an oral dose is 9–17 hours.

Studies on the effects on plasma cholinesterase showed that bambuterol inhibited activity, but that this was reversible.

All categories of subjects studied were able to form terbutaline in a predictive way except for liver cirrhotics.

5.3 Preclinical safety data
Bambuterol has not revealed any adverse effects which pose a risk to man at therapeutic dosages in the toxicity studies.

Bambuterol is given as a racemate: (-)-bambuterol is responsible for the pharmacodynamic effects via generation of (-)-terbutaline. (+)-bambuterol generates the pharmacodynamic inactive (+)-terbutaline. Both (+) and (-)-bambuterol are equally active as plasma cholinesterase inhibitors. This inhibition is reversible.

The toxicity studies showed that bambuterol has β_2-stimulatory effects, expressed as cardiotoxicity in dogs, and at high doses, observed in the acute toxicity studies, cholinergic effects.

There is no evidence from the preclinical safety data to indicate that bambuterol cannot be used in man for the intended indications with sufficient safety.

6. PHARMACEUTICAL PARTICULARS

6.1 List of excipients
Lactose monohydrate; maize starch; povidone; microcrystalline cellulose; magnesium stearate; water, purified.

6.2 Incompatibilities
Not applicable.

6.3 Shelf life
3 years.

6.4 Special precautions for storage
Do not store above 30°C.

6.5 Nature and contents of container
Amber glass bottle with LD-polyethene cap: 7, 14, 28, 30, 56 or 100 tablets.
HDPE container with LD-polyethene cap: 7, 14, 28, 30, 56 or 100 tablets.
HDPE container with polypropylene cap: 7, 14, 28, 30, 56 or 100 tablets.
PVC blisters: 7, 14, 28, 30, 56 or 100 tablets.

6.6 Special precautions for disposal and other handling
None.

7. MARKETING AUTHORISATION HOLDER
AstraZeneca UK Ltd.,
600 Capability Green,
Luton, LU1 3LU, UK.

8. MARKETING AUTHORISATION NUMBER(S)
PL 17901/0104

9. DATE OF FIRST AUTHORISATION/RENEWAL OF THE AUTHORISATION
21st May 2002

10. DATE OF REVISION OF THE TEXT
26th June 2009

Table 1

System Organ Class (SOC)	Frequency Classification	Adverse Drug Reaction
Immune system disorders	Unknown	Hypersensitivity reactions including angioedema, urticaria, exanthema, bronchospasm, hypotension and collapse.
Metabolism and nutrition disorders	Unknown	Hypokalemia
Psychiatric disorders	Very Common	Restlessness
	Common	Sleep disturbances
	Uncommon	Agitation
	Unknown	Hyperactivity
Nervous system disorders	Very common	Tremor, headache
Cardiac disorders	Common	Palpitations
	Uncommon	Tachycardia Cardiac arrhythmias, e.g. atrial fibrillation, supraventricular tachycardia and extrasystoles
	Unknown	Myocardial ischemia (see section 4.4)
Respiratory, thoracic and mediastinal disorders	Unknown	Paradoxical bronchospasm
Gastrointestinal disorders	Unknown	Nausea
Musculoskeletal, connective tissue and bone disorders	Common	Muscle cramps

Becodisks 100mcg

(Allen & Hanburys)

1. NAME OF THE MEDICINAL PRODUCT
Becodisks 100 Micrograms

2. QUALITATIVE AND QUANTITATIVE COMPOSITION
Beclometasone Dipropionate 100 micrograms

3. PHARMACEUTICAL FORM
Dry Powder for Inhalation via Diskhaler Device

4. CLINICAL PARTICULARS

4.1 Therapeutic indications
Clinical Indications

Beclometasone dipropionate provides effective anti-inflammatory action in the lungs, with a lower incidence and severity of adverse effects than those observed when corticosteroids are administered systemically. It also offers preventive treatment of asthma.

Becodisks are indicated for the following:

Adults

Prophylactic management in:

Mild asthma (PEF values greater than 80% predicted at baseline with less than 20% variability):

Patients requiring intermittent symptomatic bronchodilator asthma medication on more than an occasional basis.

Moderate asthma (PEF values 60-80% predicted at baseline with 20-30% variability):

Patients requiring regular asthma medication and patients with unstable or worsening asthma on other prophylactic therapy or bronchodilator alone.

Severe asthma (PEF values less than 60% predicted at baseline with greater than 30% variability):

Patients with severe chronic asthma. On transfer to high dose inhaled beclometasone dipropionate, many patients who are dependent on systemic corticosteroids for adequate control of symptoms may be able to reduce significantly or eliminate their requirement for oral corticosteroids.

4.2 Posology and method of administration
Becodisks are for administration by the inhalation route only using a Diskhaler device.

Patients should be made aware of the prophylactic nature of therapy with inhaled beclometasone dipropionate and that it should be taken regularly everyday even when they are asymptomatic.

Patients should be given a starting dose of inhaled beclometasone dipropionate which is appropriate for severity of their disease. The dose may then be adjusted until control is achieved and should be titrated to the lowest dose at which effective control of asthma is maintained.

Adults

400 microgram twice daily is the usual starting dose. One 400 microgram blister or two 200 micrograms blisters twice daily is the usual maintenance dose. Alternatively, 200 micrograms may be administered three or four times daily.

Children

100 micrograms two, three or four times a day, according to the response. Alternatively, the usual starting dose of 200 micrograms twice daily may be administered.

Special Patient Groups

There is no need to adjust the dose in elderly patients or in those with hepatic or renal impairment.

4.3 Contraindications
Hypersensitivity to Becodisks or any of its compnents is a contraindication. (See Pharmaceutical Particulars – List of Excipients).

Special care is necessary in patients with active or quiescent pulmonary tuberculosis.

4.4 Special warnings and precautions for use

Patients should be instructed in the proper use of the Diskhaler to ensure that the drug reaches the target areas within the lungs. They should be made aware that Becodisks have to be used regularly everyday for optimum benefit. Patients should be made aware of the prophylactic nature of therapy with Becodisks and that they should be used regularly, even when they are asymptomatic.

Becodisks are not designed to relieve acute asthmatic symptoms for which an inhaled short-acting bronchodilator is required. Patients should be advised to have such rescue medication available.

Severe asthma requires regular medical assessment including lung function testing as patients are at risk of severe attacks and even death.

Increasing use of bronchodilators, in particular short-acting inhaled $beta_2$ agonists to relieve symptoms indicates deterioration of asthma control. If patients find that short acting relief bronchodilator treatment becomes less effective or they need more inhalations than usual, medical attention must be sought.

In this situation patients should be reassessed and consideration given to the need for increased anti-inflammatory therapy (e.g. Higher doses of inhaled corticosteroids or a course of oral corticosteroids). Severe exacerbations of asthma must be treated in the normal way.

Systemic effects of inhaled corticosteroids may occur, particularly at high doses prescribed for prolonged periods. These effects are much less likely to occur than with oral corticosteroids. Possible systemic effects include Cushing's syndrome, Cushingoid features, adrenal suppression, growth retardation in children and adolescents, decrease in bone mineral density, cataract and glaucoma. It is important therefore that the dose of inhaled corticosteroid is titrated to the lowest dose at which effective control of asthma is maintained.

It is recommended that the height of children receiving prolonged treatment with inhaled corticosteroids is regularly monitored. If growth is slowed, therapy should be reviewed with the aim of reducing the dose of inhaled corticosteroid, if possible, to the lowest dose at which effective control of asthma is maintained. In addition, consideration should be given to referring the patient to a paediatric respiratory specialist.

Prolonged treatment with high doses of inhaled corticosteroids, particularly higher than recommended doses, may result in clinically significant adrenal suppression. Additional systemic corticosteroid cover should be considered during periods of stress or elective surgery.

Lack of response or severe exacerbations of asthma should be treated by increasing the dose of inhaled beclometasone dipropionate and, if necessary, by giving a systemic steroid and/or antibiotic if there is an infection, and by use of beta-agonist therapy.

For the transfer of patients being treated with oral corticosteroids:

The transfer of oral steroid-dependent patients to Becodisks and their subsequent management needs special care as recovery from impaired adrenocortical function, caused by prolonged systemic steroid therapy, may take a considerable time.

Patients who have been treated with systemic steroids for long periods of time or at a high dose may have adrenocortical suppression. With these patients adrenocortical function should be monitored regularly and their dose of systemic steroid reduced cautiously.

After approximately a week, gradual withdrawal of the systemic steroid is commenced. Decrements in dosages should be appropriate to the level of maintenance systemic steroid, and introduced at not less than weekly intervals. For maintenance doses of prednisolone (or equivalent) of 10mg daily or less, the decrements in dose should not be greater than 1mg per day, at not less than weekly intervals. For maintenance doses of prednisolone in excess of 10mg daily, it may be appropriate to employ cautiously, larger decrements in dose at weekly intervals.

Some patients feel unwell in a non-specific way during the withdrawal phase despite maintenance or even improvement of the respiratory function. They should be encouraged to persevere with the Diskhaler and withdrawal of systemic steroid continued, unless there are objective signs of adrenal insufficiency.

Patients weaned off oral steroids whose adrenocortical function is impaired should carry a steroid warning card indicating that they may need supplementary systemic steroid during periods of stress, e.g. Worsening asthma attacks, chest infections, major intercurrent illness, surgery, trauma, etc.

Replacement of systemic steroid treatment with inhaled therapy sometimes unmasks allergies such as allergic rhinitis or eczema previously controlled by the systemic drug. These allergies should be symptomatically treated with antihistamine and/or topical preparations, including topical steroids.

Treatment with Becodisks should not be stopped abruptly.

As with all inhaled corticosteroids, special care is necessary in patients with active or quiescent pulmonary tuberculosis

4.5 Interaction with other medicinal products and other forms of interaction

No interactions have been reported.

4.6 Pregnancy and lactation

There is inadequate evidence of safety in human pregnancy. Administration of corticosteroids to pregnant animals can cause abnormalities of foetal development including cleft palate and intra-uterine growth retardation. There may therefore be a very small risk of such effects in the human foetus. It should be noted, however, that the foetal changes in animals occur after relatively high systemic exposure. Because beclometasone dipropionate is delivered directly to the lungs by the inhaled route it avoids the high level of exposure that occurs when corticosteroids are given by systemic routes.

The use of beclometasone dipropionate in pregnancy requires that the possible benefits of the drug be weighed against the possible hazards. It should be noted that the drug has been in widespread use for many years without apparent ill consequence.

No specific studies examining the transference of beclometasone dipropionate into the milk of lactating animals have been performed. It is reasonable to assume that beclometasone dipropionate is secreted in milk but at the dosages used for direct inhalation, there is low potential for significant levels in breast milk. The use of beclometasone dipropionate in mothers breast feeding their babies requires that the therapeutic benefits of the drug be weighed against the potential hazards to the mother and baby.

4.7 Effects on ability to drive and use machines

No adverse effect has been reported.

4.8 Undesirable effects

Adverse events are listed below by system organ class and frequency. Frequencies are defined as: very common (≥1/10), common (≥1/100 and <1/10), uncommon (≥1/1000 and <1/100), rare (≥1/10,000 and <1/1000) and very rare (<1/10,000) including isolated reports. Very common, common and uncommon events were generally determined from clinical trial data. The incidence in placebo and comparator group has not been taken into account in estimation of these frequencies. Rare and very rare events were generally determined from spontaneous data.

System Organ Class	Adverse Event	Frequency
Infections & Infestations	Candidiasis of the mouth and throat.	Very Common
Immune System Disorders	Hypersensitivity reactions with the following manifestations:	
	Rashes, urticaria, pruritis, erythema.	Uncommon
	Oedema of the eyes, face, lips and throat	Very Rare
	Respiratory symptoms (dyspnoea and/or bronchospasm)	Very Rare
	Anaphylactoid/ anaphylactic reactions	Very Rare
Endocrine Disorders	Cushing's syndrome, Cushingoid features, adrenal suppression, growth retardation in children and adolescents, decrease in bone mineral density, cataract, glaucoma	Very Rare
Psychiatric Disorders	Anxiety, sleep disorders, behavioural changes, including hyperactivity and irritability (predominantly in children)	Very Rare
Respiratory, Thoracic & Mediastinal Disorders	Hoarseness/throat irritation	Common
	Paradoxical bronchospasm	Very Rare

Candidiasis of the mouth and throat (thrush) occurs in some patients, the incidence of which is increased with doses greater than 400 micrograms beclometasone dipropionate per day. Patients with high blood levels of *Candida precipitins*, indicating a previous infection, are most likely to develop this complication. Patients may find it helpful to rinse out their mouth with water after using the Diskhaler. Symptomatic candidiasis can be treated with topical anti-fungal therapy whilst still continuing with beclometasone dipropionate treatment.

Systemic effects of inhaled corticosteroids may occur, particularly at high doses prescribed for prolonged periods. Possible systemic effects include Cushing's syndrome, Cushingoid features, adrenal suppression, growth retardation in children and adolescents, decrease in bone mineral density, cataract, glaucoma (see 4.4 Special Warnings and Precautions for Use).

In some patients inhaled beclometasone dipropionate may cause hoarseness or throat irritation. It may be helpful to rinse out the mouth with water immediately after inhalation.

As with other inhalation therapy, paradoxical bronchospasm may occur with an immediate increase in wheezing after dosing. This should be treated immediately with a fast-acting inhaled bronchodilator. The beclometasone dipropionate preparation should be discontinued immediately, the patient assessed, and if necessary alternative therapy instituted.

4.9 Overdose

Acute - inhalation of the drug in doses in excess of those recommended may lead to temporary suppression of adrenal function. This does not necessitate emergency action being taken. In these patients treatment with beclometasone dipropionate by inhalation should be continued at a dose sufficient to control asthma; adrenal function recovers in a few days and can be verified by measuring plasma cortisol.

Chronic - use of inhaled beclometasone dipropionate in daily doses in excess of 1500 micrograms over prolonged periods may lead to adrenal suppression. Monitoring of adrenal reserve may be indicated. Treatment with inhaled beclometasone dipropionate should be continued at a dose sufficient to control asthma.

5. PHARMACOLOGICAL PROPERTIES

5.1 Pharmacodynamic properties

BDP is a pro-drug with weak glucocorticoid receptor binding activity. It is hydrolysed via esterase enzymes to the active metabolite beclometasone-17-monopropionate (B-17-MP), which has high topical anti-inflammatory activity.

5.2 Pharmacokinetic properties

Absorption

When administered via inhalation (via metered dose inhaler) there is extensive conversion of BDP to the active metabolite B-17-MP within the lungs prior to systemic absorption. The systemic absorption of B-17-MP arises from both lung deposition and oral absorption of the swallowed dose. When administered orally, in healthy male volunteers, the bioavailability of BDP is negligible but pre-systemic conversion to B-17-MP results in 41% (95% CI 27 - 62 %) of the dose being available as B-17-MP.

Metabolism

BDP is cleared very rapidly from the systemic circulation, owing to extensive first pass metabolism. The main product of metabolism is the active metabolite (B-17-MP). Minor inactive metabolites, beclometasone-21-monopropionate (B-21-MP) and beclometasone (BOH), are also formed but these contribute little to systemic exposure.

Distribution

The tissue distribution at steady state for BDP is moderate (20L) but more extensive for B-17-MP (424L). Plasma protein binding is moderately high (87%).

Elimination

The elimination of BDP and B-17-MP are characterised by high plasma clearance (150 and 120L/h) with corresponding terminal elimination half lives of 0.5h and 2.7h. Following oral administration of tritiated BDP, approximately 60% of the dose was excreted in the faeces within 96 hours mainly as free and conjugated polar metabolites. Approximately 12% of the dose was excreted as free and conjugated polar metabolites in the urine.

5.3 Preclinical safety data

No clinically relevant findings were observed in preclinical studies.

6. PHARMACEUTICAL PARTICULARS

6.1 List of excipients

Lactose (which contains milk protein)

6.2 Incompatibilities

No incompatibilities have been reported.

6.3 Shelf life

36 months

6.4 Special precautions for storage

Do not store above 30°C

6.5 Nature and contents of container

Circular double foil blister pack consisting of:

A) Lidding material (i) polyester over-lacquer/hard tempered aluminium foil/heat seal lacquer of total thickness = 39.4 - 48.6microns or (ii) nitrocellulose over-lacquer/hard tempered aluminium foil/heat seal lacquer of total thickness = 37.0 - 42.0microns.

Blister material - pvc film/aluminium foil/orientated polyamide. Becodisks are supplied as 8 blisters per Becodisk as follows:

Carton containing 14 disks plus a Diskhaler

Carton containing 15 disks plus a Diskhaler

Carton containing 5 disks plus a Diskhaler (Hospital pack)

Refill packs of 14 disks

Refill packs of 15 disks

Not all pack sizes may be marketed

6.6 Special precautions for disposal and other handling
See Patient Information Leaflet

Administrative Data

7. MARKETING AUTHORISATION HOLDER

Glaxo Wellcome UK Ltd.
Trading as Allen & Hanburys,
Stockley Park West,
Uxbridge
Middlesex, UB11 1BT

8. MARKETING AUTHORISATION NUMBER(S)
PL 10949/0055

9. DATE OF FIRST AUTHORISATION/RENEWAL OF THE AUTHORISATION
7 October 1993/11 December 1997

10. DATE OF REVISION OF THE TEXT
26 January 2006

11. Legal Status
POM

Becodisks 200mcg

(Allen & Hanburys)

1. NAME OF THE MEDICINAL PRODUCT
Becodisks 200 Micrograms

2. QUALITATIVE AND QUANTITATIVE COMPOSITION
Beclometasone Dipropionate 200micrograms

3. PHARMACEUTICAL FORM
Dry Powder for Inhalation via Diskhaler Device

4. CLINICAL PARTICULARS

4.1 Therapeutic indications

Clinical Indications

Beclometasone dipropionate provides effective anti-inflammatory action in the lungs, with a lower incidence and severity of adverse effects than those observed when corticosteroids are administered systemically. It also offers preventive treatment of asthma.

Becodisks are indicated for the following:

Adults

Prophylactic management in:

Mild asthma (PEF values greater than 80% predicted at baseline with less than 20% variability):

Patients requiring intermittent symptomatic bronchodilator asthma medication on more than an occasional basis.

Moderate asthma (PEF values 60-80% predicted at baseline with 20-30% variability):

Patients requiring regular asthma medication and patients with unstable or worsening asthma on other prophylactic therapy or bronchodilator alone.

Severe asthma (PEF values less than 60% predicted at baseline with greater than 30% variability):

Patients with severe chronic asthma. On transfer to high dose inhaled beclometasone dipropionate, many patients who are dependent on systemic corticosteroids for adequate control of symptoms may be able to reduce significantly or eliminate their requirement for oral corticosteroids.

4.2 Posology and method of administration

Becodisks are for administration by the inhalation route only using a Diskhaler device.

Patients should be made aware of the prophylactic nature of therapy with inhaled beclometasone dipropionate and that it should be taken regularly everyday even when they are asymptomatic.

Patients should be given a starting dose of inhaled beclometasone dipropionate which is appropriate for severity of their disease. The dose may then be adjusted until control is achieved and should be titrated to the lowest dose at which effective control of asthma is maintained.

Adults

400 microgram twice daily is the usual starting dose. One 400 microgram blister or two 200 micrograms blisters twice daily is the usual maintenance dose. Alternatively, 200 micrograms may be administered three or four times daily.

Children

100 micrograms two, three or four times a day, according to the response. Alternatively, the usual starting dose of 200 micrograms twice daily may be administered.

Special Patient Groups

There is no need to adjust the dose in elderly patients or in those with hepatic or renal impairment.

4.3 Contraindications

Hypersensitivity to Becodisks or any of its compnents is a contraindication. (See Pharmaceutical Particulars – List of Excipients).

Special care is necessary in patients with active or quiescent pulmonary tuberculosis.

4.4 Special warnings and precautions for use

Patients should be instructed in the proper use of the Diskhaler to ensure that the drug reaches the target areas within the lungs. They should be made aware that Becodisks have to be used regularly everyday for optimum benefit. Patients should be made aware of the prophylactic nature of therapy with Becodisks and that they should be used regularly, even when they are asymptomatic.

Becodisks are not designed to relieve acute asthmatic symptoms for which an inhaled short-acting bronchodilator is required. Patients should be advised to have such rescue medication available.

Severe asthma requires regular medical assessment including lung function testing as patients are at risk of severe attacks and even death.

Increasing use of bronchodilators, in particular short-acting inhaled beta$_2$ agonists to relieve symptoms indicates deterioration of asthma control. If patients find that short acting relief bronchodilator treatment becomes less effective or they need more inhalations than usual, medical attention must be sought.

In this situation patients should be reassessed and consideration given to the need for increased anti-inflammatory therapy (e.g. Higher doses of inhaled corticosteroids or a course of oral corticosteroids). Severe exacerbations of asthma must be treated in the normal way.

Systemic effects of inhaled corticosteroids may occur, particularly at high doses prescribed for prolonged periods. These effects are much less likely to occur than with oral corticosteroids. Possible systemic effects include Cushing's syndrome, Cushingoid features, adrenal suppression, growth retardation in children and adolescents, decrease in bone mineral density, cataract and glaucoma. It is important therefore that the dose of inhaled corticosteroid is titrated to the lowest dose at which effective control of asthma is maintained.

It is recommended that the height of children receiving prolonged treatment with inhaled corticosteroids is regularly monitored. If growth is slowed, therapy should be reviewed with the aim of reducing the dose of inhaled corticosteroid, if possible, to the lowest dose at which effective control of asthma is maintained. In addition, consideration should be given to referring the patient to a paediatric respiratory specialist.

Prolonged treatment with high doses of inhaled corticosteroids, particularly higher than recommended doses, may result in clinically significant adrenal suppression. Additional systemic corticosteroid cover should be considered during periods of stress or elective surgery.

Lack of response or severe exacerbations of asthma should be treated by increasing the dose of inhaled beclometasone dipropionate and, if necessary, by giving a systemic steroid and/or antibiotic if there is an infection, and by use of beta-agonist therapy.

For the transfer of patients being treated with oral corticosteroids:

The transfer of oral steroid-dependent patients to Becodisks and their subsequent management needs special care as recovery from impaired adrenocortical function, caused by prolonged systemic steroid therapy, may take a considerable time.

Patients who have been treated with systemic steroids for long periods of time or at a high dose may have adrenocortical suppression. With these patients adrenocortical function should be monitored regularly and their dose of systemic steroid reduced cautiously.

After approximately a week, gradual withdrawal of the systemic steroid is commenced. Decrements in dosages should be appropriate to the level of maintenance systemic steroid, and introduced at not less than weekly intervals. For maintenance doses of prednisolone (or equivalent) of 10mg daily or less, the decrements in dose should not be greater than 1mg per day, at not less than weekly intervals. For maintenance doses of prednisolone in excess of 10mg daily, it may be appropriate to employ cautiously, larger decrements in dose at weekly intervals.

Some patients feel unwell in a non-specific way during the withdrawal phase despite maintenance or even improvement of the respiratory function. They should be encouraged to persevere with the Diskhaler and withdrawal of systemic steroid continued, unless there are objective signs of adrenal insufficiency.

Patients weaned off oral steroids whose adrenocortical function is impaired should carry a steroid warning card indicating that they may need supplementary systemic steroid during periods of stress, e.g. Worsening asthma attacks, chest infections, major intercurrent illness, surgery, trauma, etc.

Replacement of systemic steroid treatment with inhaled therapy sometimes unmasks allergies such as allergic rhinitis or eczema previously controlled by the systemic drug. These allergies should be symptomatically treated with antihistamine and/or topical preparations, including topical steroids.

Treatment with Becodisks should not be stopped abruptly.

As with all inhaled corticosteroids, special care is necessary in patients with active or quiescent pulmonary tuberculosis

4.5 Interaction with other medicinal products and other forms of interaction

No interactions have been reported

4.6 Pregnancy and lactation

There is inadequate evidence of safety in human pregnancy. Administration of corticosteroids to pregnant animals can cause abnormalities of foetal development including cleft palate and intra-uterine growth retardation. There may therefore be a very small risk of such effects in the human foetus. It should be noted, however, that the foetal changes in animals occur after relatively high systemic exposure. Because beclometasone dipropionate is delivered directly to the lungs by the inhaled route it avoids the high level of exposure that occurs when corticosteroids are given by systemic routes.

The use of beclometasone dipropionate in pregnancy requires that the possible benefits of the drug be weighed against the possible hazards. It should be noted that the drug has been in widespread use for many years without apparent ill consequence.

No specific studies examining the transference of beclometasone dipropionate into the milk of lactating animals have been performed. It is reasonable to assume that beclometasone dipropionate is secreted in milk but at the dosages used for direct inhalation, there is low potential for significant levels in breast milk. The use of beclometasone dipropionate in mothers breast feeding their babies requires that the therapeutic benefits of the drug be weighed against the potential hazards to the mother and baby.

4.7 Effects on ability to drive and use machines

No adverse effect has been reported.

4.8 Undesirable effects

Adverse events are listed below by system organ class and frequency. Frequencies are defined as: very common (≥1/10), common (≥1/100 and <1/10), uncommon (≥1/1000 and <1/100), rare (≥1/10,000 and <1/1000) and very rare (<1/10,000) including isolated reports. Very common, common and uncommon events were generally determined from clinical trial data. The incidence in placebo and comparator group has not been taken into account in estimation of these frequencies. Rare and very rare events were generally determined from spontaneous data.

System Organ Class	Adverse Event	Frequency
Infections & Infestations	Candidiasis of the mouth and throat.	Very Common
Immune System Disorders	Hypersensitivity reactions with the following manifestations:	
	Rashes, urticaria, pruritis, erythema.	Uncommon
	Oedema of the eyes, face, lips and throat	Very Rare
	Respiratory symptoms (dyspnoea and/or bronchospasm)	Very Rare
	Anaphylactoid/anaphylactic reactions	Very Rare
Endocrine Disorders	Cushing's syndrome, Cushingoid features, adrenal suppression, growth retardation in children and adolescents, decrease in bone mineral density, cataract, glaucoma	Very Rare
Psychiatric Disorders	Anxiety, sleep disorders, behavioural changes, including hyperactivity and irritability (predominantly in children)	Very Rare
Respiratory, Thoracic & Mediastinal Disorders	Hoarseness/throat irritation	Common
	Paradoxical bronchospasm	Very Rare

Candidiasis of the mouth and throat (thrush) occurs in some patients, the incidence of which is increased with doses greater than 400 micrograms beclometasone dipropionate per day. Patients with high blood levels of *Candida precipitins*, indicating a previous infection, are most likely to develop this complication. Patients may find it helpful to rinse out their mouth with water after using the Diskhaler. Symptomatic candidiasis can be treated with topical anti-fungal therapy whilst still continuing with beclometasone dipropionate treatment.

Systemic effects of inhaled corticosteroids may occur, particularly at high doses prescribed for prolonged periods. Possible systemic effects include Cushing's syndrome, Cushingoid features, adrenal suppression, growth retardation in children and adolescents, decrease in bone mineral density, cataract, glaucoma (see 4.4 Special Warnings and Precautions for Use).

In some patients inhaled beclometasone dipropionate may cause hoarseness or throat irritation. It may be helpful to rinse out the mouth with water immediately after inhalation.

As with other inhalation therapy, paradoxical bronchospasm may occur with an immediate increase in wheezing after dosing. This should be treated immediately with a fast-acting inhaled bronchodilator. The beclometasone dipropionate preparation should be discontinued immediately, the patient assessed, and if necessary alternative therapy instituted.

4.9 Overdose

Acute - inhalation of the drug in doses in excess of those recommended may lead to temporary suppression of adrenal function. This does not necessitate emergency action being taken. In these patients treatment with beclometasone dipropionate by inhalation should be continued at a dose sufficient to control asthma; adrenal function recovers in a few days and can be verified by measuring plasma cortisol.

Chronic - use of inhaled beclometasone dipropionate in daily doses in excess of 1500 micrograms over prolonged periods may lead to adrenal suppression. Monitoring of adrenal reserve may be indicated. Treatment with inhaled beclometasone dipropionate should be continued at a dose sufficient to control asthma.

5. PHARMACOLOGICAL PROPERTIES

5.1 Pharmacodynamic properties

BDP is a pro-drug with weak glucocorticoid receptor binding activity. It is hydrolysed via esterase enzymes to the active metabolite beclometasone-17-monopropionate (B-17-MP), which has high topical anti-inflammatory activity.

5.2 Pharmacokinetic properties

Absorption

When administered via inhalation (via metered dose inhaler) there is extensive conversion of BDP to the active metabolite B-17-MP within the lungs prior to systemic absorption. The systemic absorption of B-17-MP arises from both lung deposition and oral absorption of the swallowed dose. When administered orally, in healthy male volunteers, the bioavailability of BDP is negligible but pre-systemic conversion to B-17-MP results in 41% (95% CI 27- 62 %) of the dose being available as B-17-MP.

Metabolism

BDP is cleared very rapidly from the systemic circulation, owing to extensive first pass metabolism. The main product of metabolism is the active metabolite (B-17-MP). Minor inactive metabolites, beclometasone-21-monopropionate (B-21-MP) and beclometasone (BOH), are also formed but these contribute little to systemic exposure.

Distribution

The tissue distribution at steady state for BDP is moderate (20L) but more extensive for B-17-MP (424L). Plasma protein binding is moderately high (87%).

Elimination

The elimination of BDP and B-17-MP are characterised by high plasma clearance (150 and 120L/h) with corresponding terminal elimination half lives of 0.5h and 2.7h. Following oral administration of tritiated BDP, approximately 60% of the dose was excreted in the faeces within 96 hours mainly as free and conjugated polar metabolites. Approximately 12% of the dose was excreted as free and conjugated polar metabolites in the urine.

5.3 Preclinical safety data

No clinically relevant findings were observed in preclinical studies.

6. PHARMACEUTICAL PARTICULARS

6.1 List of excipients

Lactose (which contains milk protein)

6.2 Incompatibilities

No incompatibilities have been reported.

6.3 Shelf life

36 months

6.4 Special precautions for storage

Do not store above 30°C.

6.5 Nature and contents of container

Circular double foil blister pack consisting of:

A) Lidding material (i) polyester over-lacquer/hard tempered aluminium foil/heat seal lacquer of total thickness = 39.4 - 48.6microns or (ii) nitrocellulose over-lacquer/hard tempered aluminium foil/heat seal lacquer of total thickness = 37.0 - 42.0microns.

B) Blister material - pvc film/aluminium foil/orientated polyamide.

Becodisks are supplied as 8 blisters per Becodisk as follows:

- Carton containing 14 disks plus a Diskhaler
- Carton containing 15 disks plus a Diskhaler
- Carton containing 5 disks plus a Diskhaler (Hospital pack)
- Refill packs of 14 disks
- Refill packs of 15 disks

Not all pack sizes may be marketed

6.6 Special precautions for disposal and other handling

See Patient Information Leaflet

Administrative Data

7. MARKETING AUTHORISATION HOLDER

Glaxo Wellcome UK Ltd.

Trading as Allen & Hanburys,

Stockley Park West,

Uxbridge

Middlesex,

UB11 1BT

8. MARKETING AUTHORISATION NUMBER(S)

PL 10949/0056

9. DATE OF FIRST AUTHORISATION/RENEWAL OF THE AUTHORISATION

27 September 1993/11 December 1997

10. DATE OF REVISION OF THE TEXT

26 January 2006

11. Legal Status

POM

Becodisks 400mcg

(Allen & Hanburys)

1. NAME OF THE MEDICINAL PRODUCT

Becodisks 400 Micrograms

2. QUALITATIVE AND QUANTITATIVE COMPOSITION

Beclometasone Dipropionate Monohydrate (Micronised) 414μg equivalent to 400μg Beclometasone Dipropionate

3. PHARMACEUTICAL FORM

Dry Powder for Inhalation via Diskhaler Device

4. CLINICAL PARTICULARS

4.1 Therapeutic indications

Clinical Indications

Beclometasone dipropionate provides effective anti-inflammatory action in the lungs, with a lower incidence and severity of adverse effects than those observed when corticosteroids are administered systemically. It also offers preventive treatment of asthma.

Becodisks are indicated for the following:

Adults

Prophylactic management in:

Mild asthma (PEF values greater than 80% predicted at baseline with less than 20% variability):

Patients requiring intermittent symptomatic bronchodilator asthma medication on more than an occasional basis.

Moderate asthma (PEF values 60-80% predicted at baseline with 20-30% variability):

Patients requiring regular asthma medication and patients with unstable or worsening asthma on other prophylactic therapy or bronchodilator alone.

Severe asthma (PEF values less than 60% predicted at baseline with greater than 30% variability):

Patients with severe chronic asthma. On transfer to high dose inhaled beclometasone dipropionate, many patients who are dependent on systemic corticosteroids for adequate control of symptoms may be able to reduce significantly or eliminate their requirement for oral corticosteroids.

4.2 Posology and method of administration

Becodisks are for administration by the inhalation route only using a Diskhaler device.

Patients should be made aware of the prophylactic nature of therapy with inhaled beclometasone dipropionate and that it should be taken regularly everyday even when they are asymptomatic.

Patients should be given a starting dose of inhaled beclometasone dipropionate which is appropriate for the severity of their disease. The dose may then be adjusted until control is achieved and should be titrated to the lowest dose at which effective control of asthma is maintained.

Adults

The contents of one blister (400 micrograms) twice daily is the usual maintenance dose. This may be increased to two blisters (800 micrograms) twice daily in patients for whom there is a clinical need.

Children

Not recommended in children.

Special Patient Groups

There is no need to adjust the dose in elderly patients or in those with hepatic or renal impairment.

4.3 Contraindications

Hypersensitivity to Becodisks or any of its components is a contraindication. (See Pharmaceutical Particulars – List of Excipients).

Special care is necessary in patients with active or quiescent pulmonary tuberculosis

4.4 Special warnings and precautions for use

Patients should be instructed in the proper use of the Diskhaler to ensure that the drug reaches the target areas within the lungs. They should be made aware that Beco disks have to be used regularly everyday for optimum benefit. Patients should be made aware of the prophylactic nature of therapy with Becodisks and that they should be used regularly, even when they are asymptomatic.

Becodisks are not designed to relieve acute asthmatic symptoms for which an inhaled short-acting bronchodilator is required. Patients should be advised to have such rescue medication available.

Severe asthma requires regular medical assessmen including lung function testing as patients are at risk o severe attacks and even death.

Increasing use of bronchodilators, in particular short-act ing inhaled beta$_2$ agonists to relieve symptoms indicate deterioration of asthma control. If patients find that shor acting relief bronchodilator treatment becomes less effec tive or they need more inhalations than usual, medica attention must be sought.

In this situation patients should be reassessed and con sideration given to the need or increased anti-inflammator therapy (e.g. Higher doses of inhaled corticosteroids or course of oral corticosteroids). Severe exacerbations c asthma must be treated in the normal way.

Systemic effects of inhaled corticosteroids may occu particularly at high doses prescribed for prolonged per ods. These effects are much less likely to occur than wit oral corticosteroids. Possible systemic effects includ Cushing's syndrome, Cushingoid features, adrenal sup pression, growth retardation in children and adolescent decrease in bone mineral density, cataract and glaucoma It is important therefore that the dose of inhaled corticos teroid is titrated to the lowest dose at which effectiv control of asthma is maintained.

It is recommended that the height of children receivin prolonged treatment with inhaled corticosteroids is regu larly monitored. If growth is slowed, therapy should b reviewed with the aim of reducing the dose of inhale corticosteroid, if possible, to the lowest dose at whic effective control of asthma is maintained. In addition, co sideration should be given to referring the patient to paediatric respiratory specialist.

Prolonged treatment with high doses of inhaled cortico teroids, particularly higher than recommended doses, ma result in clinically significant adrenal suppression. Add tional systemic corticosteroid cover should be considere during periods of stress or elective surgery.

Lack of response or severe exacerbations of asthm should be treated by increasing the dose of inhaled becl metasonedipropionate and, if necessary, by giving a sy temic steroid and/or antibiotic if there is an infection, ar by use of beta-agonist therapy.

For the transfer of patients being treated with oral cor costeroids:

The transfer of oral steroid-dependent patients to Bec disks and their subsequent management needs spec care as recovery from impaired adrenocortical functio caused by prolonged systemic steroid therapy, may take considerable time.

Patients who have been treated with systemic steroids f long periods of time or at a high dose may have adren cortical suppression. With these patients adrenocortic function should be monitored regularly and their dose systemic steroid reduced cautiously.

After approximately a week, gradual withdrawal of th systemic steroid is commenced. Decrements in dosag should be appropriate to the level of maintenance system steroid, and introduced at not less than weekly interval For maintenance doses of prednisolone (or equivalent) 10mg daily or less, the decrements in dose should not b greater than 1mg per day, at not less than weekly interva For maintenance doses of prednisolone in excess of 10n daily, it may be appropriate to employ cautiously, larg decrements in dose at weekly intervals.

Some patients feel unwell in a non-specific way during t withdrawal phase despite maintenance or even improv ment of the respiratory function. They should be encou aged to persevere with the Diskhaler and withdrawal systemic steroid continued, unless there are objecti signs of adrenal insufficiency.

Patients weaned off oral steroids whose adrenocortic function is impaired should carry a steroid warning ca indicating that they may need supplementary systen steroid during periods of stress, e.g. Worsening asthn attacks, chest infections, major intercurrent illness, su gery, trauma, etc.

Replacement of systemic steroid treatment with inhal therapy sometimes unmasks allergies such as allerg rhinitis or eczema previously controlled by the systen drug. These allergies should be symptomatically treat with antihistamine and/or topical preparations, includi topical steroids.

Treatment with Becodisks should not be stopped abrupt

As with all inhaled corticosteroids, special care is nece sary in patients with active or quiescent pulmonary tub culosis.

4.5 Interaction with other medicinal products and oth forms of interaction

No interactions have been reported

4.6 Pregnancy and lactation

There is inadequate evidence of safety in human pregnancy. Administration of corticosteroids to pregnant animals can cause abnormalities of foetal development including cleft palate and intra-uterine growth retardation. There may therefore be a very small risk of such effects in the human foetus. It should be noted, however, that the foetal changes in animals occur after relatively high systemic exposure. Because beclometasone dipropionate is delivered directly to the lungs by the inhaled route it avoids the high level of exposure that occurs when corticosteroids are given by systemic routes.

The use of beclometasone dipropionate in pregnancy requires that the possible benefits of the drug be weighed against the possible hazards. It should be noted that the drug has been in widespread use for many years without apparent ill consequence.

No specific studies examining the transference of beclometasone dipropionate into the milk of lactating animals have been performed. It is reasonable to assume that beclometasone dipropionate is secreted in milk but at the dosages used for direct inhalation, there is low potential for significant levels in breast milk. The use of beclometasone dipropionate in mothers breast feeding their babies requires that the therapeutic benefits of the drug be weighed against the potential hazards to the mother and baby.

4.7 Effects on ability to drive and use machines

No adverse effect has been reported.

4.8 Undesirable effects

Adverse events are listed below by system organ class and frequency. Frequencies are defined as: very common (≥1/10), common (≥1/100 and <1/10), uncommon (≥1/1000 and <1/100), rare (≥1/10,000 and <1/1000) and very rare (<1/10,000) including isolated reports. Very common, common and uncommon events were generally determined from clinical trial data. The incidence in placebo and comparator group has not been taken into account in estimation of these frequencies. Rare and very rare events were generally determined from spontaneous data.

System Organ Class	Adverse Event	Frequency
Infections & Infestations	Candidiasis of the mouth and throat.	Very Common
Immune System Disorders	Hypersensitivity reactions with the following manifestations:	
	Rashes, urticaria, pruritis, erythema.	Uncommon
	Oedema of the eyes, face, lips and throat	Very Rare
	Respiratory symptoms (dyspnoea and/or bronchospasm)	Very Rare
	Anaphylactoid/ anaphylactic reactions	Very Rare
Endocrine Disorders	Cushing's syndrome, Cushingoid features, adrenal suppression, growth retardation in children and adolescents, decrease in bone mineral density, cataract, glaucoma	Very Rare
Psychiatric Disorders	Anxiety, sleep disorders, behavioural changes, including hyperactivity and irritability (predominantly in children)	Very Rare
Respiratory, Thoracic & Mediastinal Disorders	Hoarseness/throat irritation	Common
	Paradoxical bronchospasm	Very Rare

Candidiasis of the mouth and throat (thrush) occurs in some patients, the incidence of which is increased with doses greater than 400 micrograms beclometasone dipropionate per day. Patients with high blood levels of *Candida precipitins*, indicating a previous infection, are most likely to develop this complication. Patients may find it helpful to rinse out their mouth with water after using the Diskhaler. Symptomatic candidiasis can be treated with topical anti-fungal therapy whilst still continuing with beclometasone dipropionate treatment.

Systemic effects of inhaled corticosteroids may occur, particularly at high doses prescribed for prolonged periods. Possible systemic effects include Cushing's syndrome, Cushingoid features, adrenal suppression, growth retardation in children and adolescents, decrease in bone mineral density, cataract, glaucoma (see 4.4 Special Warnings and Precautions for Use).

In some patients inhaled beclometasone dipropionate may cause hoarseness or throat irritation. It may be helpful to rinse out the mouth with water immediately after inhalation.

As with other inhalation therapy, paradoxical bronchospasm may occur with an immediate increase in wheezing after dosing. This should be treated immediately with a fast-acting inhaled bronchodilator. The beclometasone dipropionate preparation should be discontinued immediately, the patient assessed, and if necessary alternative therapy instituted.

4.9 Overdose

Acute - inhalation of the drug in doses in excess of those recommended may lead to temporary suppression of adrenal function. This does not necessitate emergency action being taken. In these patients treatment with beclometasone dipropionate by inhalation should be continued at a dose sufficient to control asthma; adrenal function recovers in a few days and can be verified by measuring plasma cortisol.

Chronic - use of inhaled beclometasone dipropionate in daily doses in excess of 1500 micrograms over prolonged periods may lead to adrenal suppression. Monitoring of adrenal reserve may be indicated. Treatment with inhaled beclometasone dipropionate should be continued at a dose sufficient to control asthma.

5. PHARMACOLOGICAL PROPERTIES

5.1 Pharmacodynamic properties

BDP is a pro-drug with weak glucocorticoid receptor binding activity. It is hydrolysed via esterase enzymes to the active metabolite beclometasone -17-monopropionate (B-17-MP), which has high topical anti-inflammatory activity.

5.2 Pharmacokinetic properties

Absorption

When administered via inhalation (via metered dose inhaler) there is extensive conversion of BDP to the active metabolite B-17-MP within the lungs prior to systemic absorption. The systemic absorption of B-17-MP arises from both lung deposition and oral absorption of the swallowed dose. When administered orally, in healthy male volunteers, the bioavailability of BDP is negligible but pre-systemic conversion to B-17-MP results in 41% (95% CI 27- 62 %) of the dose being available as B-17-MP.

Metabolism

BDP is cleared very rapidly from the systemic circulation, owing to extensive first pass metabolism. The main product of metabolism is the active metabolite (B-17-MP). Minor inactive metabolites, beclometasone-21-monopropionate (B-21-MP) and beclometasone (BOH), are also formed but these contribute little to systemic exposure.

Distribution

The tissue distribution at steady state for BDP is moderate (20L) but more extensive for B-17-MP (424L). Plasma protein binding is moderately high (87%).

Elimination

The elimination of BDP and B-17-MP are characterised by high plasma clearance (150 and 120L/h) with corresponding terminal elimination half lives of 0.5h and 2.7h. Following oral administration of titrated BDP, approximately 60% of the dose was excreted in the faeces within 96 hours mainly as free and conjugated polar metabolites. Approximately 12% of the dose was excreted as free and conjugated polar metabolites in the urine.

5.3 Preclinical safety data

No clinically relevant findings were observed in preclinical studies.

6. PHARMACEUTICAL PARTICULARS

6.1 List of excipients

Lactose (which contains milk protein)

6.2 Incompatibilities

No incompatibilities have been reported.

6.3 Shelf life

36 months

6.4 Special precautions for storage

Do not store above 30°C

6.5 Nature and contents of container

Circular double foil blister pack consisting of:

A) Lidding material (i) polyester over-lacquer/hard tempered aluminium foil/heat seal lacquer of total thickness = 39.4 - 48.6μ or (ii) nitrocellulose over-lacquer/hard tempered aluminium foil/heat seal lacquer of total thickness = 37.0 - 42.0μ.

B) Blister material - pvc film/aluminium foil/orientated polyamide.

Becodisks are supplied as 8 blisters per Becodisk as follows:

- Carton containing 7 disks plus a Diskhaler
- Carton containing 15 disks plus a Diskhaler
- Carton containing 2 disks plus a Diskhaler
- Refill pack of 7 disks
- Refill pack of 15 disks
- A starter pack consisting of a Diskhaler pre-load with one disk

Not all pack sizes may be marketed

6.6 Special precautions for disposal and other handling

See Patient Information Leaflet

Administrative Data

7. MARKETING AUTHORISATION HOLDER

Glaxo Wellcome UK Ltd.
Trading as Allen & Hanburys,
Stockley Park West,
Uxbridge
Middlesex,
UB11 1BT

8. MARKETING AUTHORISATION NUMBER(S)

PL10949/0057

9. DATE OF FIRST AUTHORISATION/RENEWAL OF THE AUTHORISATION

1 October 1993/27 September 1999

10. DATE OF REVISION OF THE TEXT

26 January 2006

11. Legal Status

POM

Beconase Aqueous Nasal Spray

(Allen & Hanburys)

1. NAME OF THE MEDICINAL PRODUCT

Beconase Aqueous Nasal Spray

2. QUALITATIVE AND QUANTITATIVE COMPOSITION

Beclometasone Dipropionate 50μg (as monohydrate, micronised)

3. PHARMACEUTICAL FORM

Aqueous suspension for intranasal inhalation via metered dose atomising pump.

4. CLINICAL PARTICULARS

4.1 Therapeutic indications

Beconase Aqueous Nasal Spray is indicated for the prophylaxis and treatment of perennial and seasonal allergic rhinitis including hayfever, and vasomotor rhinitis. Beclometasone dipropionate has a potent anti-inflammatory effect within the respiratory tract, with a lower incidence and severity of adverse events than those observed when corticosteroids are administered systemically.

4.2 Posology and method of administration

Beconase Aqueous Nasal Spray is for administration by the intranasal route only.

Adults and children over six years of age:

The recommended dosage is two sprays into each nostril twice daily (400 micrograms/day). Once control has been established it may be possible to maintain control with fewer sprays. A dosage regimen of one spray into each nostril morning and evening has been shown to be efficacious in some patients. However, should symptoms recur, patients should revert to the recommended dosage of two sprays into each nostril morning and evening. The minimum dose should be used at which effective control of symptoms is maintained. Total daily administration should not normally exceed eight sprays.

For full therapeutic benefit regular usage is essential. The co-operation of the patient should be sought to comply with the regular dosage schedule and it should be explained that maximum relief may not be obtained within the first few applications.

For children under six years old, there are insufficient clinical data to recommend use.

4.3 Contraindications

Beconase Aqueous Nasal Spray is contra-indicated in patients with a history of hypersensitivity to any of its components.

4.4 Special warnings and precautions for use

Systemic effects of nasal corticosteroids may occur, particularly at high doses prescribed for prolonged periods. Growth retardation has been reported in children receiving nasal corticosteroids at licensed doses.

It is recommended that the height of children receiving prolonged treatment with nasal corticosteroids is regularly monitored. If growth is slowed, therapy should be reviewed with the aim of reducing the dose of nasal corticosteroid, if possible to the lowest dose at which effective control of symptoms is maintained. In addition, consideration should be given to referring the patient to a paediatric specialist.

Treatment with higher than recommended doses may result in clinically significant adrenal suppression. If there is evidence for higher than recommended doses being used then additional systemic corticosteroid cover should be considered during periods of stress or elective surgery.

Care must be taken while transferring patients from systemic steroid treatment to Beconase Aqueous Nasal Spray if there is any reason to suppose that their adrenal function is impaired.

Infections of the nasal passages and paranasal sinuses should be appropriately treated but do not constitute a specific contra-indication to treatment with Beconase Aqueous Nasal Spray.

Although Beconase Aqueous Nasal Spray will control seasonal allergic rhinitis in most cases, an abnormally heavy challenge of summer allergens may in certain instances necessitate appropriate additional therapy particularly to control eye symptoms.

4.5 Interaction with other medicinal products and other forms of interaction
Not applicable

4.6 Pregnancy and lactation
There is inadequate evidence of safety in human pregnancy. Administration of corticosteroids to pregnant animals can cause abnormalities of foetal development including cleft palate and intra-uterine growth retardation. There may therefore be a very small risk of such effects in the human foetus. It should be noted, however, that the foetal changes in animals occur after relatively high systemic exposure. Beconase Aqueous Nasal Spray delivers beclometasone dipropionate directly to the nasal mucosa and so minimises systemic exposure.

The use of beclometasone dipropionate should be avoided during pregnancy unless thought essential by the doctor.

No specific studies examining the transference of beclometasone dipropionate into the milk of lactating animals have been performed. It is reasonable to assume that beclometasone dipropionate is secreted in milk but at the dosages used for direct intranasal administration there is low potential for significant levels in breast milk. The use of beclometasone dipropionate in mothers breast feeding their babies requires that the therapeutic benefits of the drug be weighed against the potential hazards to the mother and baby.

4.7 Effects on ability to drive and use machines
Not applicable

4.8 Undesirable effects
Adverse events are listed below by system organ class and frequency. Frequencies are defined as: very common (≥1/10), common (≥1/100 and <1/10), uncommon (≥1/1000 and <1/100), rare (≥1/10,000 and <1/1000) and very rare (<1/10,000) including isolated reports. Very common, common and uncommon events were generally determined from clinical trial data. Rare and very rare events were generally determined from spontaneous data. In assigning adverse event frequencies, the background rates in placebogroups were not taken into account, since these rates were generally comparable to those in the active treatment group.

System Organ Class	Adverse Event	Frequency
Immune system disorders	Hypersensitivity reactions including:	
	Rashes, urticaria, pruritis, erythema.	Common
	Oedema of the eyes, face, lips and throat	Very rare
	Dyspnoea and/or bronchospasm	Very rare
	Anaphylactoid/ anaphylactic reactions	Very rare
Nervous system disorders	Unpleasant taste, unpleasant smell.	Common
Eye disorders	Glaucoma, raised intraocular pressure, cataract.	Very rare
Respiratory, Thoracic & Mediastinal disorders	Epistaxis, nasal dryness, nasal irritation, throat dryness, throat irritation.	Common
	Nasal septum perforation.	Very rare

As with other nasal sprays, dryness and irritation of the nose and throat, and epistaxis have been reported. Nasal septal perforation has also been reported following the use of intranasal corticosteroids.

Systemic effects of nasal corticosteroids may occur particularly when used at high doses for prolonged periods.

4.9 Overdose
The only harmful effect that follows inhalation of large amounts of the drug over a short time period is suppression of Hypothalamic-Pituitary-Adrenal (HPA) function. No special emergency action need be taken. Treatment with Beconase Aqueous Nasal Spray should be continued at the recommended dose. HPA function recovers in a day or two.

5. PHARMACOLOGICAL PROPERTIES

5.1 Pharmacodynamic properties
Following topical administration beclometasone 17,21-dipropionate (BDP) produces potent anti-inflammatory and vasoconstrictor effects.

BDP is a pro-drug with weak corticosteroid receptor binding affinity. It is hydrolysed via esterase enzymes to the highly active metabolite beclometasone-17-monopropionate (B-17-MP), which has high topical anti-inflammatory activity.

Beclometasone dipropionate offers a preventative background treatment for hayfever when taken prior to allergen challenge. After which with regular use, BDP can continue to prevent allergy symptoms from reappearing.

5.2 Pharmacokinetic properties
Absorption
Following intranasal administration of BDP in healthy males, the systemic absorption was assessed by measuring the plasma concentrations of its active metabolite B-17-MP, for which the absolute bioavailability following intranasal administration is 44% (95% CI 28%, 70%). After intranasal administration, <1% of the dose is absorbed by the nasal mucosa. The remainder after being cleared from the nose, either by drainage or mucociliary clearance, is available for absorption from the gastrointestinal tract. Plasma B-17-MP is almost entirely due to conversion of BDP absorbed from the swallowed dose.

Following oral administration of BDP in healthy males, the systemic absorption was also assessed by measuring the plasma concentrations of its active metabolite B-17-MP, for which the absolute bioavailability following oral administration is 41% (95% CI 27%, 62%).

Following an oral dose, B-17-MP is absorbed slowly with peak plasma levels reached 3-5 hours after dosing.

Metabolism
BDP is cleared very rapidly from the circulation and plasma concentrations are undetectable (< 50pg/ml) following oral or intranasal dosing. There is rapid metabolism of the majority of the swallowed portion of BDP during its first passage through the liver. The main product of metabolism is the active metabolite (B-17-MP). Minor inactive metabolites, beclometasone-21-monopropionate (B-21-MP) and beclometasone (BOH), are also formed but these contribute little to systemic exposure.

Distribution
The tissue distribution at steady-state for BDP is moderate (20l) but more extensive for B-17-MP (424l). Plasma protein binding of BDP is moderately high (87%).

Elimination
The elimination of BDP and B-17-MP are characterised by high plasma clearance (150 and 120l/h) with corresponding terminal elimination half-lives of 0.5h and 2.7h. Following oral administration of tritiated BDP, approximately 60% of the dose was excreted in the faeces within 96 hours mainly as free and conjugated polar metabolites. Approximately 12% of the dose was excreted as free and conjugated polar metabolites in the urine.

5.3 Preclinical safety data
No clinically relevant findings were observed in preclinical studies.

6. PHARMACEUTICAL PARTICULARS

6.1 List of excipients
Avicel RC 591 (Microcrystalline Cellulose And Carboxymethylcellulose Sodium) US NF
Anhydrous Dextrose BP
Benzalkonium Chloride BP
Phenylethyl Alcohol USP
Polysorbate 80 BP
Purified Water BP

6.2 Incompatibilities
Not applicable

6.3 Shelf life
24 months when not stored above 30°C

6.4 Special precautions for storage
Beconase Aqueous Nasal Spray should not be stored above 30°C. Keepcontainer in the outer carton. Do not refrigerate.

6.5 Nature and contents of container
A 25ml amber neutral glass bottle fitted with a metering atomising pump, or a 30ml polypropylene bottle fitted with a tamper-resistant metering atomising pump. The pumps are manufactured by: Valois S.A. Le Prieure BPG, 27110 Le Neubourg, France.

Pack size: 200 Metered Spray.

6.6 Special precautions for disposal and other handling
Refer to Patient Information Leaflet.

Administrative Data

7. MARKETING AUTHORISATION HOLDER
Glaxo Wellcome UK Ltd.
Trading as Allen and Hanburys,
Stockley Park West,
Uxbridge
Middlesex, UB11 1BT

8. MARKETING AUTHORISATION NUMBER(S)
PL 10949/0104

9. DATE OF FIRST AUTHORISATION/RENEWAL OF THE AUTHORISATION
12th April 2003

10. DATE OF REVISION OF THE TEXT
26 January 2006

11. Legal Status
POM

Begrivac 2009/2010 suspension for injection in pre-filled syringe

(Novartis Vaccines)

1. NAME OF THE MEDICINAL PRODUCT
Begrivac® 2009/2010 / suspension for injection in pre-filled syringe
Influenza vaccine (split virion, inactivated)

2. QUALITATIVE AND QUANTITATIVE COMPOSITION
Split influenza virus, inactivated containing antigens equivalent to*:

A/Brisbane/59/2007 (H1N1) like strain used (A/Brisbane/59/2007, Reass. IVR-148) 15 micrograms HA**

A/Brisbane/10/2007 (H3N2) like strain used (A/Uruguay/716/2007, Reass. NYMC X-175C) 15 micrograms HA**

B/Brisbane/60/2008 like strain used (B/Brisbane/60/2008) 15 micrograms HA**

per 0.5 ml dose

* propagated in fertilised hen's eggs from healthy chicken flocks.

** haemagglutinin

This vaccine complies with the WHO recommendation (northern hemisphere) and EU decision for the 2009/2010 season.

For a full list of excipients see section 6.1.

3. PHARMACEUTICAL FORM
Suspension for injection in pre-filled syringe.
Slightly opalescent.

4. CLINICAL PARTICULARS

4.1 Therapeutic indications
Prophylaxis of influenza, especially in those who run an increased risk of associated complications.

The use of Begrivac 2009/2010 should be based on official recommendations.

4.2 Posology and method of administration
Adults and children from 36 months: 0.5 ml.

Children from 6 months to 35 months: Clinical data are limited. Dosages of 0.25 ml or 0.5 ml have been used.

For children who have not previously been vaccinated, a second dose should be given after an interval of at least 4 weeks.

Immunisation should be carried out by intramuscular or deep subcutaneous injection.

For instructions for preparation, see section 6.6.

4.3 Contraindications
Hypersensitivity to the active substances, to any of the excipients and to eggs, chicken protein, formaldehyde, diethyleter or polysorbate 80.

Begrivac 2009/2010 does not contain more than 1.0 μg ovalbumin per dose. The vaccine may contain residues of polymyxin B.

Immunisation shall be postponed in patients with febrile illness or acute infection.

4.4 Special warnings and precautions for use
As with all injectable vaccines, appropriate medical treatment and supervision should always be readily available in case of an anaphylactic event following the administration of the vaccine.

Begrivac 2009/2010 should under no circumstances be administered intravascularly.

Antibody response in patients with endogenous or iatrogenic immunosuppression may be insufficient.

4.5 Interaction with other medicinal products and other forms of interaction
Begrivac 2009/2010 may be given at the same time as other vaccines. Immunisation should be carried out on separate limbs. It should be noted that the adverse reactions may be intensified.

The immunological response may be diminished if the patient is undergoing immuno-suppressant treatment.

Following influenza vaccination, false positive results in serology tests using the ELISA method to detect antibodies against HIV1, Hepatitis C and especially HTLV1 have been observed. The Western Blot technique disproves the false-positive ELISA test results. The transient false positive reactions could be due to the IgM response by the vaccine.

4.6 Pregnancy and lactation
The limited data from vaccinations in pregnant women do not indicate that adverse fetal and maternal outcomes were attributable to the vaccine. The use of this vaccine may be considered from the second trimester of pregnancy. For pregnant women with medical conditions that increase their risk of complications from influenza, administration of the vaccine is recommended, irrespective of their stage of pregnancy.

Begrivac 2009/2010 may be used during lactation.

4.7 Effects on ability to drive and use machines
The vaccine is unlikely to produce an effect on the ability to drive and use machines.

4.8 Undesirable effects

Adverse reactions observed from clinical trials

The safety of trivalent inactivated influenza vaccines is assessed in open label, uncontrolled clinical trials performed as annual update requirement, including at least 50 adults aged 18 – 60 years of age and at least 50 elderly aged 61 years or older. Safety evaluation is performed during the first 3 days following vaccination.

The following undesirable effects have been observed during clinical trials with the following frequencies:

Very common (>1/10); common (≥1/100, <1/10); uncommon (≥1/1,000, <1/100); rare (≥1/10,000, <1/1,000); very rare (<1/10,000), including isolated reports.

Nervous system disorders

Common:

Headache*

Skin and subcutaneous tissue disorders

Common:

Sweating*

Musculoskeletal and connective tissue disorders

Common:

Myalgia, arthralgia*

General disorders and administration site conditions

Common:

Fever, malaise, shivering, fatigue. Local reactions: redness, swelling, pain, ecchymosis, induration.*

* These reactions usually disappear within 1-2 days without treatment.

Adverse reactions reported from post-marketing surveillance

Adverse reactions reported from post-marketing surveillance are, next to the reactions which have also been observed during the clinical trials, the following:

Blood and lymphatic system disorders:

Transient thrombocytopenia, transient lymphadenopathy

Immune system disorders:

Allergic reactions, in rare cases leading to shock, angioedema

Nervous system disorders:

Neuralgia, paraesthesia, febrile convulsions, neurological disorders, such as encephalomyelitis, neuritis and Guillain Barré syndrome

Vacsular disorders:

Vasculitis associated in very rare cases with transient renal involvement.

Skin and subcutaneous tissue disorders:

Generalised skin reactions including pruritus, urticaria or non-specific rash.

4.9 Overdose

Overdosage is unlikely to have any untoward effect.

5. PHARMACOLOGICAL PROPERTIES

5.1 Pharmacodynamic properties

Pharmacotherapeutic group: Influenza vaccine

ATC-Code: J07BB02

Seroprotection is generally obtained within 2 to 3 weeks. The duration of postvaccinal immunity to homologous strains or to strains closely related to the vaccine strains varies but is usually 6-12 months.

5.2 Pharmacokinetic properties

Not applicable

5.3 Preclinical safety data

Not applicable

6. PHARMACEUTICAL PARTICULARS

6.1 List of excipients

Sucrose, buffer solution (pH = 7.2) containing: sodium chloride, potassium chloride, magnesium chloride hexahydrate, disodium phosphate dihydrate, potassium dihydrogen phosphate and water for injections.

6.2 Incompatibilities

In the absence of compatibility studies, this medicinal product must not be mixed with other medicinal products.

6.3 Shelf life

1 year

6.4 Special precautions for storage

Store in a refrigerator (2 °C – 8 °C). Do not freeze. Keep the syringe in the outer carton in order to protect from light.

6.5 Nature and contents of container

0.5 ml suspension in pre-filled syringe (Type I glass) with plunger stopper (bromobutyl rubber) with or without needle – in pack sizes of 1, 10 or 20 (2 × 10)

Not all pack sizes may be marketed.

6.6 Special precautions for disposal and other handling

Unused vaccine and other waste material should be disposed of in compliance with local rules for the disposal of product of this nature.

The vaccine should be allowed to reach room temperature before use.

Shake before use.

For children, when a dose of 0.25 ml is indicated, the following procedure is recommended:

Syringe without mark for the 0.25 ml dose:

The pre-filled syringe should be held in the upright position and half of the volume should be eliminated. The remaining volume should be injected.

Syringe with a mark for the 0.25 ml dose:

Discard half the contained volume up to the mark (little black line indicated on the syringe barrel below the label), before injection.

7. MARKETING AUTHORISATION HOLDER

Novartis Vaccines and Diagnostics GmbH & Co. KG
P.O. Box 1630
D-35006 Marburg

8. MARKETING AUTHORISATION NUMBER(S)

national:

MRP: DE/H/125/01

9. DATE OF FIRST AUTHORISATION/RENEWAL OF THE AUTHORISATION

Date of first authorization (national): 8. August 1996

Renewal of the authorization: 30 December 2002

10. DATE OF REVISION OF THE TEXT

May 2009

BeneFIX

(Wyeth Pharmaceuticals)

1. NAME OF THE MEDICINAL PRODUCT

BeneFIX 250 IU, BeneFIX 500 IU, BeneFIX 1000 IU, BenеFIX 2000 IU powder and solvent for solution for injection.

2. QUALITATIVE AND QUANTITATIVE COMPOSITION

BeneFIX 250 IU powder and solvent for solution for injection contains nominally 250 IU nonacog alfa (recombinant coagulation factor IX). After reconstitution with the accompanying 5 ml (0.234%) sodium chloride solution for injection, each ml of the solution contains approximately 50 IU nonacog alfa.

BeneFIX 500 IU powder and solvent for solution for injection contains nominally 500 IU nonacog alfa (recombinant coagulation factor IX). After reconstitution with the accompanying 5 ml (0.234%) sodium chloride solution for injection, each ml of the solution contains approximately 100 IU nonacog alfa

BeneFIX 1000 IU powder and solvent for solution for injection contains nominally 1000 IU nonacog alfa (recombinant coagulation factor IX). After reconstitution with the accompanying 5 ml (0.234%) sodium chloride solution for injection, each ml of the solution contains approximately 200 IU nonacog alfa

BeneFIX 2000 IU powder and solvent for solution for injection contains nominally 2000 IU nonacog alfa (recombinant coagulation factor IX). After reconstitution with the accompanying 5 ml (0.234%) sodium chloride solution for injection, each ml of the solution contains approximately 400 IU nonacog alfa.

The potency (IU) is determined using the European Pharmacopoeia one-stage clotting assay. The specific activity of BeneFIX is not less than 200 IU/mg protein.

BeneFIX contains recombinant coagulation factor IX, (INN = nonacog alfa). Nonacog alfa is a purified protein that has 415 amino acids in a single chain. It has a primary amino acid sequence that is comparable to the Ala^{148} allelic form of plasma-derived factor IX, and some post-translational modifications of the recombinant molecule are different from those of the plasma-derived molecule. Recombinant coagulation factor IX is a glycoprotein that is secreted by genetically engineered mammalian cells derived from a Chinese hamster ovary (CHO) cell line.

Excipients:

Each vial contains 40 mg sucrose.

For a full list of excipients, see section 6.1.

3. PHARMACEUTICAL FORM

White/almost white powder and clear and colourless solvent for solution for injection.

4. CLINICAL PARTICULARS

4.1 Therapeutic indications

Treatment and prophylaxis of bleeding in patients with haemophilia B (congenital factor IX deficiency).

4.2 Posology and method of administration

Treatment should be initiated under the supervision of a physician experienced in the treatment of haemophilia.

Posology

The dosage and duration of the substitution therapy depends on the severity of the factor IX deficiency, the location and extent of bleeding, and the patient's clinical condition. Dosing of BeneFIX may differ from that of plasma-derived factor IX products.

To ensure that the desired factor IX activity level has been achieved, precise monitoring using the factor IX activity assay is advised and doses should be calculated taking the factor IX activity, pharmacokinetic parameters such as half-life and recovery, as well as the clinical situation into consideration in order to adjust the dose as appropriate.

The amount to be administered and the frequency of administration should always be oriented to the clinical effectiveness in the individual case. Factor IX products rarely require to be administered more than once daily.

The number of units of factor IX administered is expressed in International Units (IU), which are related to the current WHO standard for factor IX products. Factor IX activity in plasma is expressed either as a percentage (relative to normal human plasma) or in International Units (relative to an international standard for factor IX in plasma).

One International Unit (IU) of factor IX activity is equivalent to that quantity of factor IX in one ml of normal human plasma. Estimation of the required dose of BeneFIX can be based on the finding that one unit of factor IX activity per kg body weight is expected to increase the circulating level of factor IX, an average of 0.8 IU/dl (range from 0.4 to 1.4 IU/dl) in adult patients (≥ 15 years). Pharmacokinetics have to be assessed regularly in each patient and posology has to be adjusted accordingly.

The required dosage is determined using the following formula:

(see Table 1 below)

For a recovery 0.8 IU/dl (average increase of factor IX), then:

(see Table 2 below)

In the case of the following haemorrhagic events, the factor IX activity should not fall below the given plasma activity levels (in % of normal or in IU/dl) in the corresponding period. The following table can be used to guide dosing in bleeding episodes and surgery:

(see Table 3 on next page)

During the course of treatment, appropriate determination of factor IX levels is advised to guide the dose to be administered and the frequency of repeated infusions. In the case of major surgical interventions in particular, precise monitoring of the substitution therapy by means of coagulation analysis (plasma factor IX activity) is indispensable. Individual patients may vary in their response to factor IX, achieving different levels of in vivo recovery and demonstrating different half-lives.

For long term prophylaxis against bleeding in patients with severe haemophilia B, BeneFIX may be administered. In a clinical study for routine secondary prophylaxis the average dose for previously treated patients (PTP) was 40IU/kg (range 13 to 78 IU/kg) at intervals of 3 to 4 days. In younger patients, shorter dosage intervals or higher doses may be necessary.

Paediatric patients

There are insufficient data to recommend the use of BeneFIX in children less than 6 years of age. In clinical studies, 57% of the paediatric patients increased their doses due to lower than expected recovery or to obtain sufficient therapeutic response or both, some to an average dose of >50 IU/kg. Therefore, close monitoring of factor IX plasma activity should be performed, as well as calculation of pharmacokinetic parameters such as recovery and half-life, as clinically indicated, in order to adjust doses as appropriate. If doses >100 IU/kg have been repeatedly needed during routine prophylaxis or treatment, a switch to another FIX product should be considered.

Patients should be monitored for the development of factor IX inhibitors. If the expected factor IX activity plasma levels are not attained, or if bleeding is not controlled with an appropriate dose, biological testing should be performed to determine if a factor IX inhibitor is present.

In patients with high levels of inhibitor factor IX therapy may not be effective and other therapeutic options must be considered. Management of such patients should be directed by physicians with experience in the care of patients with haemophilia. See also section 4.4.

Table 1

Number of factor IX IU required	=	body weight (in kg)	X	desired factor IX increase (%) or (IU/dl)	X	reciprocal of observed recovery

Table 2

Number of factor IX IU required	=	body weight (in kg)	X	desired factor IX increase (%) or (IU/dl)	X	1.3 IU/kg

Table 3

Degree of haemorrhage/Type of surgical procedure	Factor IX level required (%) or (IU/dl)	Frequency of doses (hours)/Duration of Therapy (days)
Haemorrhage		
Early haemarthrosis, muscle bleeding or oral bleeding	20-40	Repeat every 24 hours. At least 1 day, until the bleeding episode as indicated by pain is resolved or healing is achieved.
More extensive haemarthrosis, muscle bleeding or haematoma	30-60	Repeat infusion every 24 hours for 3-4 days or more until pain and acute disability are resolved.
Life-threatening haemorrhages	60-100	Repeat infusion every 8 to 24 hours until threat is resolved.
Surgery		
Minor: Including tooth extraction	30-60	Every 24 hours, at least 1 day, until healing is achieved.
Major	80-100 (pre- and postoperative)	Repeat infusion every 8-24 hours until adequate wound healing, then therapy for at least another 7 days to maintain a factor IX activity of 30% to 60% (IU/dl)

Method of administration

BeneFIX is administered by intravenous infusion after reconstitution of the lyophilised powder for solution for injection with sterile 0.234% sodium chloride solution (see section 6.6).

BeneFIX should be administered at a slow infusion rate. In most of the cases, an infusion rate of up to 4 ml per minute has been used. The rate of administration should be determined by the patient's comfort level.

Administration by continuous infusion has not been approved and is not recommended (see also sections 4.4, 4.8 and 6.6).

4.3 Contraindications

Hypersensitivity to the active substance or to any of the excipients.

Known allergic reaction to hamster proteins.

4.4 Special warnings and precautions for use

Activity-neutralizing antibodies (inhibitors) are an uncommon event in previously treated patients (PTPs) receiving factor IX-containing products. Since during clinical studies one PTP treated with BeneFIX developed a clinically relevant low responding inhibitor and experience on antigenicity with recombinant factor IX is still limited, patients treated with BeneFIX should be carefully monitored for the development of factor IX inhibitors that should be titrated in Bethesda Units using appropriate biological testing.

Sufficient data have not been obtained from ongoing clinical studies on the treatment of previously untreated patients (PUPs), with BeneFIX. Additional safety and efficacy studies in paediatric patients are ongoing in previously treated, minimally treated, and previously untreated paediatric patients. Clinical studies of BeneFIX did not include sufficient numbers of subjects aged 65 and over to determine whether they respond differently from younger subjects. As with any patient receiving BeneFIX, dose selection for an elderly patient should be individualised.

As with any intravenous protein product, allergic-type hypersensitivity reactions are possible. The product contains traces of hamster proteins. Potentially life-threatening anaphylactic/anaphylactoid reactions have occurred with factor IX products, including BeneFIX. Patients should be informed of early signs of hypersensitivity reactions including difficult breathing, shortness of breath, swelling, hives, itching, tightness of the chest, bronchospasm, laryngospasm, wheezing, hypotension, and anaphylaxis.

If allergic or anaphylactic-type reactions occur, the administration of BeneFIX has to be discontinued immediately and an appropriate treatment has to be initiated. In some cases, these reactions have progressed to severe anaphylaxis. In the case of shock, the current medical standards for treatment of shock should be observed. In case of severe allergic reactions, alternative haemostatic measures should be considered.

There have been reports in the literature showing a correlation between the occurrence of a factor IX inhibitor and allergic reactions. Therefore, patients experiencing allergic reactions should be evaluated for the presence of an inhibitor. It should be noted that patients with factor IX inhibitors may be at an increased risk of anaphylaxis with subsequent challenge with factor IX. Preliminary information suggests a relationship may exist between the presence of major deletion mutations in a patient's factor IX gene and an increased risk of inhibitor formation and of acute hypersensitivity reactions. Patients known to have major deletion mutations of the factor IX gene should be observed closely for signs and symptoms of acute hypersensitivity reactions, particularly during the early phases of initial exposure to product.

Because of the risk of allergic reactions with factor IX concentrates, the initial administrations of factor IX should, according to the treating physician's judgement, be performed under medical observation where proper medical care for allergic reactions could be provided.

Posology has to be adjusted according to the pharmacokinetics of each patient.

Although BeneFIX contains only factor IX, the risk of thrombosis and disseminated intravascular coagulation (DIC) should be recognised. Since the use of factor IX complex concentrates has historically been associated with the development of thromboembolic complications, the use of factor IX-containing products may be potentially hazardous in patients with signs of fibrinolysis and in patients with disseminated intravascular coagulation (DIC). Because of the potential risk of thrombotic complications, clinical surveillance for early signs of thrombotic and consumptive coagulopathy should be initiated with appropriate biological testing when administering this product to patients with liver disease, to patients post-operatively, to neonates, or to patients at risk of thrombotic phenomena or DIC. In each of these situations, the benefit of treatment with BeneFIX should be weighed against the risk of these complications.

The safety and efficacy of BeneFIX administration by continuous infusion have not been established (see also sections 4.2 and 4.8). There have been post-marketing reports of thrombotic events, including life-threatening superior vena cava (SVC) syndrome in critically ill neonates, while receiving continuous-infusion BeneFIX through a central venous catheter (see also section 4.8).

There have been reports of agglutination of red blood cells in the tube/syringe with the administration of BeneFIX. So far, no clinical sequelae have been reported in association with this observation. To minimize the possibility of agglutination, it is important to limit the amount of blood entering the tubing. Blood should not enter the syringe. If agglutination of red blood cells in the tubing/syringe is observed, discard all this material (tubing, syringe and BeneFIX solution) and resume administration with a new package.

Nephrotic syndrome has been reported following attempted immune tolerance induction in haemophilia B patients with Factor IX inhibitors and a history of allergic reaction. The safety and efficacy of using BeneFIX for immune tolerance induction has not been established.

In the interest of patients, it is recommended that, whenever possible, every time that BeneFIX is administered to them, the name and batch number of the product is registered.

4.5 Interaction with other medicinal products and other forms of interaction

No interaction studies have been performed.

4.6 Pregnancy and lactation

Animal reproduction studies have not been conducted with factor IX. Based on the rare occurrence of haemophilia B in women, experience regarding the use of factor IX during pregnancy and breastfeeding is not available. Therefore, factor IX should be used during pregnancy and breastfeeding only if clearly indicated.

4.7 Effects on ability to drive and use machines

No studies on the effects on the ability to drive and use machines have been performed.

4.8 Undesirable effects

To date, no adverse reactions reported in association with BeneFIX occurred with a frequency of ≥1/100 to <1/10 (common). The frequency of adverse reactions reported in association with BeneFIX would be categorized as uncommon (≥1/1,000 to ≤1/100) or rare (≥1/10,000 to ≤1/1,000). Of these the most significant include: anaphylaxis, cellulitis, phlebitis, and neutralising antibodies.

Adverse reactions based on experience from clinical trials and postmarketing experience are presented below by system organ class and frequency of occurrence. Within each frequency grouping, undesirable effects are presented in order of decreasing seriousness. These frequencies have been estimated on a per-infusion basis and are described using the following categories: uncommon (≥1/1,000 to ≤1/100); rare (≥1/10,000 to ≤1/1,000).

Nervous system disorders

Uncommon: Dizziness, headache, altered taste, lightheadedness

Gastrointestinal disorders

Uncommon: Nausea

Rare: Vomiting

General disorders and administration site conditions

Uncommon: Cellulitis, phlebitis, injection site reaction (including burning infusion site and injection site stinging) injection site discomfort

Rare: Pyrexia

Immune system disorders

Uncommon: Neutralising antibodies (factor IX inhibition)*

Rare: Hypersensitivity/allergic reactions; such reactions may include anaphylaxis*, bronchospasm/respiratory distress, (dyspnoea), hypotension, angioedema, tachycardia, chest tightness, urticaria, hives, rash, burning sensation in jaw and skull, chills (rigors), tingling, flushing, lethargy, restlessness, dry cough/sneezing

* See additional information below.

Hypersensitivity/allergic reactions

Hypersensitivity or allergic reactions have been infrequently observed in patients treated with factor IX containing products, including BeneFIX. In some cases, these reactions have progressed to severe anaphylaxis. Allergic reactions have occurred in close temporal association with development of factor IX inhibitor (see also section 4.4).

The aetiology of the allergic reactions to BeneFIX has not yet been elucidated. These reactions are potentially life threatening. If allergic/anaphylactic reactions occur, the administration of BeneFIX should be discontinued at once. In case of severe allergic reactions, alternative haemostatic measures should be considered. The treatment required depends on the nature and severity of side-effects (see also section 4.4). Due to the production process BeneFIX contains trace amounts of hamster cell proteins. Hypersensitivity responses can occur.

Inhibitor development

Patients with haemophilia B may develop neutralising antibodies (inhibitors) to factor IX. If such inhibitors occur, the condition may manifest itself as an insufficient clinical response. In such cases, it is recommended that a specialised haemophilia centre be contacted. A clinically relevant, low responding inhibitor was detected in 1 out of 65 BeneFIX patients (including 9 patients participating only in the surgery study) who had previously received plasma derived products. This patient was able to continue treatment with BeneFIX with no anamnestic rise in inhibitor or anaphylaxis. There are insufficient data to provide information on inhibitor incidence in PUPs.

Nephrotic syndrome has been reported following high doses of plasma-derived Factor IX to induce immune tolerance in haemophilia B patients with factor IX inhibitors and a history of allergic reactions.

Renal

In a clinical trial, twelve days after a dose of BeneFIX for a bleeding episode, one hepatitis C antibody positive patient developed a renal infarct. The relationship of the infarct to prior administration of BeneFIX is uncertain. The patient continued to be treated with BeneFIX.

Thrombotic events

There have been post-marketing reports of thrombotic events, including life-threatening SVC syndrome in critically ill neonates, while receiving continuous-infusion BeneFIX through a central venous catheter. Cases of peripheral thrombophlebitis and deep venous thrombosis have also been reported; in most of these cases, BeneFIX was administered via continuous infusion, which is not an approved method of administration (see also sections 4.2 and 4.4).

Inadequate therapeutic response and inadequate factor IX recovery

Inadequate therapeutic response and inadequate factor IX recovery have been reported during the post-marketing use of BeneFIX (see also section 4.2).

If any adverse reaction takes place that is thought to be related to the administration of BeneFIX, the rate of infusion should be decreased or the infusion stopped.

4.9 Overdose

No case of overdose has been reported.

5. PHARMACOLOGICAL PROPERTIES

5.1 Pharmacodynamic properties

Pharmacotherapeutic group: antihaemorrhagic Blood Coagulation Factor IX; ATC code: B02BD09

BeneFIX contains recombinant coagulation factor IX, (nonacog alfa). Recombinant coagulation factor IX is a single chain glycoprotein with an approximate molecular mass of 55,000 Daltons that is a member of the serine protease family of vitamin K-dependent coagulation factors. Recombinant coagulation factor IX is a recombinant

DNA-based protein therapeutic which has structural and functional characteristics comparable to endogenous factor IX. Factor IX is activated by factor VII/tissue factor complex in the extrinsic pathway as well as factor XIa in the intrinsic coagulation pathway. Activated factor IX, in combination with activated factor VIII, activates factor X. This results ultimately in the conversion of prothrombin to thrombin. Thrombin then converts fibrinogen into fibrin and a clot can be formed. Factor IX activity is absent or greatly reduced in patients with haemophilia B and substitution therapy may be required.

Haemophilia B is a sex-linked hereditary disorder of blood coagulation due to decreased levels of factor IX and results in profuse bleeding into joints, muscles or internal organs, either spontaneously or as a result of accidental or surgical trauma. By replacement therapy the plasma levels of factor IX is increased, thereby enabling a temporary correction of the factor deficiency and correction of the bleeding tendencies.

There are insufficient data to recommend the use of BeneFIX in children less than 6 years of age.

The medicinal product has been authorised under "Exceptional Circumstances".

This means that due to the rarity of the disease it has not been possible to obtain complete information on this medicinal product.

The European Medicines Agency (EMEA) will review any new information which may become available every year and this SPC will be updated as necessary.

5.2 Pharmacokinetic properties

Infusion of BeneFIX into 56 PTP patients (baseline data) with haemophilia B has shown an *in vivo* recovery ranging from 15 to 62% (mean 33.7 ± 10.3%). One International Unit of BeneFIX showed a mean 0.75 IU/dl (range 0.3 to 1.4 IU/dl) increase in the circulating level of factor IX. The biologic half-life ranged from 11 to 36 hours (mean of 19.3 ± 5.0 hours).

For a subset of the 56 patients, data are available from baseline to 24 months. The pharmacokinetic data for these patients at various time points are shown in the following table:

(see Table 4 below)

A 28% lower recovery of BeneFIX in comparison to plasma-derived Factor IX was shown. Pharmacokinetic parameters of BeneFIX have also been determined after single and multiple intravenous doses in different species. The pharmacokinetic parameters obtained in studies comparing BeneFIX to plasma-derived Factor IX were similar to those obtained in human studies. Structural differences of BeneFIX compared with plasma-derived Factor IX appear to contribute to the different recovery compared to plasma-derived Factor IX.

5.3 Preclinical safety data

Non-clinical data reveal no special hazard for humans based on conventional studies of genotoxicity.

No investigations on carcinogenicity, fertility impairment and foetal development have been conducted.

6. PHARMACEUTICAL PARTICULARS

6.1 List of excipients

Powder

Sucrose

Glycine

L-Histidine

Polysorbate 80

Solvent

Sodium chloride solution

6.2 Incompatibilities

In the absence of compatibility studies, this medicinal product must not be mixed with other medicinal products. Only the provided infusion set should be used. Treatment failure can occur as a consequence of human coagulation factor IX adsorption to the internal surfaces of some infusion equipment.

6.3 Shelf life

3 years

The reconstituted product should be used immediately, but no longer than 3 hours after reconstitution. Chemical and physical in-use stability has been demonstrated for 3 hours at temperatures up to 25°C.

6.4 Special precautions for storage

Store and transport refrigerated (2°C - 8°C). Do not freeze, in order to prevent damage to the prefilled syringe.

For the purpose of ambulatory use the product may be removed from refrigerated storage for one single period of maximum 1 month at room temperature (up to 25 °C). At the end of this period, the product should not be put back in the refrigerator, but should be used or discarded.

Table 4 Summary of BeneFIX Pharmacokinetic Parameters for Activity Data by Month in Previously Treated Patients

Parameter	Month	n	Mean	Median	SD	Range	95% CI
Recovery (%)	0	56	33.7	31.5	10.31	15.3–62.2	30.9, 36.4
	6	53	31.8	31.0	9.04	15.3–56.7	29.4, 34.3
	12	50	31.3	30.5	8.75	16.2–53.1	28.8, 33.7
	18	47	30.7	28.9	9.24	12.6–62.1	28.0, 33.5
	24	47	31.0	30.6	8.80	16.2–59.4	28.4, 33.6
FIX increase (IU/dl per IU/kg)	0	56	0.75	0.70	0.23	0.34–1.38	0.69, 0.81
	6	53	0.71	0.69	0.20	0.34–1.26	0.65, 0.76
	12	50	0.70	0.68	0.19	0.36–1.18	0.64, 0.75
	18	47	0.68	0.64	0.21	0.28–1.38	0.62, 0.74
	24	47	0.69	0.68	0.20	0.36–1.32	0.63, 0.75
Elimination half-life (h)	0	56	19.3	19.1	4.97	11.1–36.4	18.0, 20.7
	6	53	19.8	18.2	6.26	9.6–38.2	18.1, 21.6
	12	49	18.5	16.6	5.89	10.6–33.7	16.8, 20.2
	18	46	18.9	16.3	7.02	10.7–38.3	16.8, 21.0
	24	45	18.9	17.3	6.84	10.9–42.2	16.8, 20.9
$AUC_{0-\infty}$ (IU × h/dl)	0	56	619.8	605.2	155.7	366.5–1072.6	578.1, 661.5
	6	53	579.8	562.2	146.1	330.9–900.1	539.5, 620.1
	12	49	575.7	566.0	151.0	290.3–1080.8	532.4, 619.1
	18	46	561.8	560.9	155.6	254.5–940.8	515.7, 608.0
	24	45	577.6	551.7	154.7	284.1–1045.4	531.1, 624.1
Half-life Initial Phase (h)	0	54	2.0	1.5	1.60	0.07–5.73	1.6,2.5
	6	52	2.3	1.0	2.62	0.12–9.98	1.5,3.0
	12	48	2.2	1.2	2.70	0.13–14.34	1.5,3.0
	18	44	2.0	1.3	1.94	0.13–6.21	1.4,2.6
	24	43	1.8	0.78	2.07	0.11–7.43	1.1,2.4
Clearance (ml/h/kg)	0	56	8.4	8.2	2.01	4.66–13.64	7.86,8.94
	6	53	9.2	8.9	2.48	5.55–15.11	8.53,9.89
	12	49	9.3	8.8	2.53	4.63–17.22	8.56,10.01
	18	46	9.6	8.9	2.85	5.31–19.65	8.78,10.47
	24	45	9.2	9.1	2.40	4.78–17.60	8.52,9.96
MRT (h)	0	56	26.0	25.8	6.07	15.81–46.09	24.35,27.60
	6	53	25.6	25.3	5.68	13.44–42.26	24.01,27.15
	12	49	24.6	22.2	6.47	14.83–38.75	22.75,26.47
	18	46	24.7	22.7	7.40	15.30–50.75	22.55,26.94
	24	45	25.1	23.9	6.94	15.65–47.52	23.00,27.17

Data exclude those collected from one patient after evidence of inhibitor development was observed at 9 months.

$AUC_{0-\infty}$= Area Under the Curve

MRT = Mean Residence Time

SD = Standard Deviation

CI = Confidence Interval

6.5 Nature and contents of container

BeneFIX 250 IU powder and solvent for solution for injection: 250 IU of powder in a 10 ml vial (type 1 glass) with a stopper (chlorobutyl) and a flip-off seal (aluminium) and 5 ml of solvent in a prefilled syringe (type 1 glass) with a plunger stopper (bromobutyl), a tip-cap (bromobutyl) and a sterile vial adapter reconstitution device, a sterile infusion set, two alcohol swabs, a plaster, and a gauze pad.

BeneFIX 500 IU powder and solvent for solution for injection: 500 IU of powder in a 10 ml vial (type 1 glass) with a stopper (chlorobutyl) and a flip-off seal (aluminium) and 5 ml of solvent in a prefilled syringe (type 1 glass) with a plunger stopper (bromobutyl), a tip-cap (bromobutyl) and a sterile vial adapter reconstitution device, a sterile infusion set, two alcohol swabs, a plaster, and a gauze pad.

BeneFIX 1000 IU powder and solvent for solution for injection: 1000 IU of powder in a 10 ml vial (type 1 glass) with a stopper (chlorobutyl) and a flip-off seal (aluminium) and 5 ml of solvent in a prefilled syringe (type 1 glass) with a plunger stopper (bromobutyl), a tip-cap (bromobutyl) and a sterile vial adapter reconstitution device, a sterile infusion set, two alcohol swabs, a plaster, and a gauze pad.

BeneFIX 2000 IU powder and solvent for solution for injection: 2000 IU of powder in a 10 ml vial (type 1 glass) with a stopper (chlorobutyl) and a flip-off seal (aluminium) and 5 ml of solvent in a prefilled syringe (type 1 glass) with a plunger stopper (bromobutyl), a tip-cap (bromobutyl) and a sterile vial adapter reconstitution device, a sterile infusion set, two alcohol swabs, a plaster, and a gauze pad.

6.6 Special precautions for disposal and other handling

BeneFIX is administered by intravenous (IV) injection after reconstitution of the lyophilised powder for injection with the supplied solvent (0.234% w/v sodium chloride solution) in the pre-filled syringe.

BeneFIX, when reconstituted, contains polysorbate-80, which is known to increase the rate of di-(2-ethylhexyl)phthalate (DEHP) extraction from polyvinyl chloride (PVC). This should be considered during the preparation and administration of BeneFIX. It is important that the recommendations in section 4.2 be followed closely.

Any unused product or waste material should be disposed of in accordance with local requirements.

The product does not contain a preservative, and the reconstituted solution should be used immediately or within 3 hours after reconstitution.

Because the use of BeneFIX by continuous infusion has not been evaluated, BeneFIX should not be mixed with infusion solutions or be given in a drip.

7. MARKETING AUTHORISATION HOLDER

Wyeth Europa Ltd.

Huntercombe Lane South

Taplow, Maidenhead

Berkshire, SL6 0PH

United Kingdom

8. MARKETING AUTHORISATION NUMBER(S)

BeneFIX 250 IU powder and solvent for solution for injection: EU/1/97/047/004

BeneFIX 500 IU powder and solvent for solution for injection: EU/1/97/047/005

BeneFIX 1000 IU powder and solvent for solution for injection: EU/1/97/047/006

BeneFIX 2000 IU powder and solvent for solution for injection: EU/1/97/047/007

9. DATE OF FIRST AUTHORISATION/RENEWAL OF THE AUTHORISATION

Date of first authorisation: 27 August 1997

Date of last renewal: 27 August 2007

10. DATE OF REVISION OF THE TEXT

22 April 2009

Detailed information on this medicinal product is available on the website of the European Medicines Agency (EMEA) http://www.emea.europa.eu.

Berinert SPC

(CSL Behring UK Limited)

1. NAME OF THE MEDICINAL PRODUCT

Berinert®▼

500 units

Powder and solvent for solution for injection / infusion.

2. QUALITATIVE AND QUANTITATIVE COMPOSITION

Active substance: C1-esterase inhibitor, human

Berinert contains 500 units C1-esterase inhibitor per injection vial. 1 U is equivalent to the C1-esterase inhibitor activity in 1 ml of fresh citrated plasma of healthy donors, 1 U is equivalent to 6 Levy-Lepow units.

The product contains 50 U/ml C1-esterase inhibitor after reconstitution with 10 ml water for injections.

The total protein content of the reconstituted solution is 6.5 mg/ml.

Excipients recognized to have a known effect:

Sodium up to 486 mg (approximately 21 mmol) per 100 ml solution.

For a full list of excipients, see section 6.1.

3. PHARMACEUTICAL FORM

Powder (white lyophilisate) and solvent for solution for injection / infusion.

4. CLINICAL PARTICULARS

4.1 Therapeutic indications

Hereditary angioedema type I and II (HAE)

Treatment of acute episodes

4.2 Posology and method of administration

Treatment should be initiated under the supervision of a physician experienced in the treatment of C1-esterase inhibitor deficiency.

Posology

20 units per kilogram body weight (20 U/kg b.w.)

Dosage for neonates, infants and children

The dose for children is 20 units per kilogram body weight (20 U/kg b.w.).

Method of administration

Berinert is to be reconstituted according to section 6.6. The reconstituted solution is to be administered by slow i.v. injection or infusion.

4.3 Contraindications

Known hypersensitivity to any of the components of the product.

4.4 Special warnings and precautions for use

In patients with known tendency towards allergies, antihistamines and corticosteroids should be administered prophylactically.

If allergic or anaphylactic-type reactions occur, the administration of Berinert has to be stopped immediately (e.g. discontinue injection/infusion) and an appropriate treatment has to be initiated. Therapeutic measures depend on the kind and severity of the undesirable effect. The current medical standards for shock treatment are to be observed.

Patients with laryngeal oedema require particularly careful monitoring with emergency treatment in stand-by.

Unlicenced use or treatment of Capillary Leak Syndrome (CLS) with Berinert (see also section "4.8 Undesirable effects") is not advised.

Berinert contains up to 486 mg sodium (approximately 21 mmol) per 100 ml solution. To be taken into consideration by patients on a controlled sodium diet.

Virus safety

Standard measures to prevent infections resulting from the use of medicinal products prepared from human blood or plasma include selection of donors, screening of individual donations and plasma pools for specific markers of infection and the inclusion of effective manufacturing steps for the inactivation/removal of viruses. Despite this, when medicinal products prepared from human blood or plasma are administered, the possibility of transmitting infective agents cannot be totally excluded. This also applies to unknown or emerging viruses and other pathogens.

The measures taken are considered effective for enveloped viruses such as HIV, HBV and HCV and for the non-enveloped virus HAV.

The measures taken may be of limited value against non-enveloped viruses such as parvovirus B19.

Parvovirus B19 infection may be serious for pregnant women (foetal infection) and for individuals with immunodeficiency or increased erythropoiesis (e.g. haemolytic anaemia).

Appropriate vaccination (hepatitis A and B) should be generally considered for patients in regular/repeated receipt of human plasma-derived products.

It is strongly recommended that every time Berinert is administered to a patient, the name and batch number of the product are recorded in order to maintain a link between the patient and the batch of the product.

4.5 Interaction with other medicinal products and other forms of interaction

No interaction studies have been performed.

4.6 Pregnancy and lactation

Pregnancy

There are limited amount of data that indicate no increased risk from the use of Berinert in pregnant women. Berinert is a physiological component of human plasma. Therefore, no studies on reproduction and developmental toxicity have been performed in animals and no adverse effects on fertility, pre- and postnatal development are expected in humans.

Therefore, Berinert should be given to a pregnant woman only if clearly needed.

Lactation

It is unknown whether Berinert is excreted in human milk, but due to its high molecular weight, the transfer of Berinert into breast milk seems unlikely. However, breastfeeding is questionable in women suffering from hereditary angioedema. A decision must be made whether to discontinue breastfeeding or to discontinue the Berinert therapy taking into account the benefit of breastfeeding for the child and the benefit of therapy for the woman.

Table 1

Organ class	Very common	Common	Uncommon	Rare	Very rare
Vascular disorders				Development of thrombosis*	
General disorders and administration site conditions				Rise in temperature, reactions at the injection side	
Immune system disorders				Allergic or anaphylactic-type reactions (e.g. tachycardia, hyper- or hypotension, flushing, hives, dyspnoea, headache, dizziness, nausea)	Shock

* In treatment attempts with high doses of Berinert for prophylaxis or therapy of Capillary Leak Syndrome (CLS) before, during or aft cardiac surgery under extracorporal circulation (unlicensed indication and dose), in single cases with fatal outcome.

4.7 Effects on ability to drive and use machines

No studies on the effects on the ability to drive and use machines have been performed.

4.8 Undesirable effects

The following adverse reactions are based on post marketing experience as well as scientific literature. The following standard categories of frequency are used:

Very common: ⩾ 1/10

Common: ⩾ 1/100 and < 1/10

Uncommon: ⩾ 1/1,000 and < 1/100

Rare: ⩾ 1/10,000 and < 1/1,000

Very rare: < 1/10,000 (including reported single cases)

Undesired reactions with Berinert are rare.

(see Table 1 above)

For safety with respect to transmissible agents, see section 4.4.

4.9 Overdose

No case of overdose has been reported.

5. PHARMACOLOGICAL PROPERTIES

5.1 Pharmacodynamic properties

Pharmacotherapeutic group: C1-inhibitor

ATC code: B02A B03

C1-esterase inhibitor is a plasma glycoprotein with a molecular weight of 105 kD and a carbohydrate moiety of 40 %. Its concentration in human plasma ranges around 240 mg/l. Besides its occurrence in human plasma, also the placenta, the liver cells, monocytes and platelets contain C1-esterase inhibitor.

C1-esterase inhibitor belongs to the serine-protease-inhibitor-(serpin)-system of human plasma as do also other proteins like antithrombin III, alpha-2-antiplasmin, alpha-1-antitrypsin and others.

Under physiological conditions C1-esterase inhibitor blocks the classical pathway of the complement system by inactivating the enzymatic active components C1s and C1r. The active enzyme forms a complex with the inhibitor in a stoichiometry of 1:1.

Furthermore, C1-esterase inhibitor represents the most important inhibitor of the contact activation of coagulation by inhibiting factor XIIa and its fragments. In addition, it serves, besides alpha-2-macroglobulin, as the main inhibitor of plasma kallikrein.

The therapeutic effect of Berinert in hereditary angioedema is induced by the substitution of the deficient C1-esterase inhibitor activity.

5.2 Pharmacokinetic properties

The product is to be administered intravenously and is immediately available in the plasma with a plasma concentration corresponding to the administered dose.

Pharmacokinetic properties have been investigated in 40 patients (6 patients < 18 years) with hereditary angioedema. These included 15 patients under prophylactic treatment (with frequent/severe attacks), as well as 25 patients with less frequent/mild attacks and "on demand" treatment. The data were generated in an attack-free interval.

The median *in-vivo* recovery (IVR) was 86.7 % (range: 54.0 – 254.1 %). The IVR for children was slightly higher (98.2 %, range: 69.2 – 106.8 %)) than for adults (82.5 %, range: 54.0 – 254.1 %). Patients with severe attacks had a higher IVR (101.4 %) compared to patients with mild attacks (75.8 %, range: 57.2 – 195.9 %).

The median increase in activity was 2.3%/U/kg b.w. (range: 1.4 – 6.9 %/U/kg b.w.). No significant differences were seen between adults and children. Patients with severe attacks showed a slightly higher increase in activity than patients with mild attacks (2.9, range: 1.4 – 6.9 vs. 2.1, range: 1.5 – 5.1 %/U/kg b.w.).

The maximum concentration of C1-esterase inhibitor activity in plasma was reached within 0.8 hours after administration of Berinert without significant differences between the patient groups.

The median half-life was 36.1 hours. It was slightly shorte in children than in adults (32.9 vs. 36.1 hours) and patients with severe attacks than in patients with mi attacks (30.9 vs. 37.0).

5.3 Preclinical safety data

Berinert contains as active ingredient C1-esteras inhibitor. It is derived from human plasma and ac like an endogenous constituent of plasma. Single-dos application of Berinert in rats and mice and repeate dose applications in rats did not show any evidence toxicity.

Preclinical studies with repeated-dose application investigate carcinogenicity and reproductive toxicity hav not been conducted because they cannot be reasonab performed in conventional animal models due to the deve opment of antibodies following the application of heter logous human proteins.

The *in-vitro* Ouchterlony test and the *in-vivo* PCA mod in guinea pigs did not show any evidence of new arising antigenic determinants in Berinert followir pasteurisation.

6. PHARMACEUTICAL PARTICULARS

6.1 List of excipients

Powder:

Glycine

Sodium chloride

Sodium citrate

Solvent:

Water for injections

6.2 Incompatibilities

Berinert should not be mixed with other medicinal produc and diluents in the syringe/infusion set.

6.3 Shelf life

30 months

After reconstitution, from a microbiological point of vie and as Berinert contains no preservative, the reconstitute product should be used immediately. The physico-chem cal stability has been demonstrated for 48 hours at roo temperature (max. 25°C). However, if it is not administere immediately, storage shall not exceed 8 hours at roo temperature.

6.4 Special precautions for storage

Do not store above 25 °C.

Do not freeze.

Keep the vial in the outer carton in order to protect fro light.

6.5 Nature and contents of container

Powder: Injection vial of colourless glass Type II, seale with bromobutyl rubber infusion stopper Type I, aluminiu seal and plastic flip-off cap.

Solvent: 10 ml water for injections in an injection vial colourless glass Type I, sealed with chlorobutyl rubb infusion stopper Type I, aluminium seal and plastic fli off cap.

Administration set: 1 filter transfer device 20/20, 1 disp sable 10 ml syringe, 1 venipuncture set, 2 alcohol swabs, plaster

6.6 Special precautions for disposal and other handli

Any unused product or waste material should be dispos of in accordance with local requirements.

Method of administration

General instructions

- The solution should be clear or slightly opalescent. Aft filtering/withdrawal (see below) reconstituted produ should be inspected visually for particulate matter a discoloration prior to administration.

- Do not use solutions that are cloudy or have deposits

- Reconstitution and withdrawal must be carried out und aseptic conditions.

Reconstitution

Bring the solvent to room temperature. Ensure product a solvent vial flip caps are removed and the stoppers a treated with an aseptic solution and allowed to dry prior opening the Mix2Vial package.

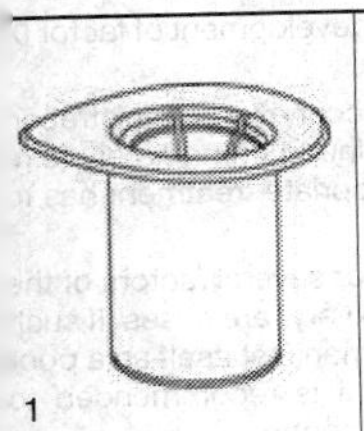
1

1. Open the Mix2Vial package by peeling off the lid. Do **not** remove the Mix2Vial from the blister package!

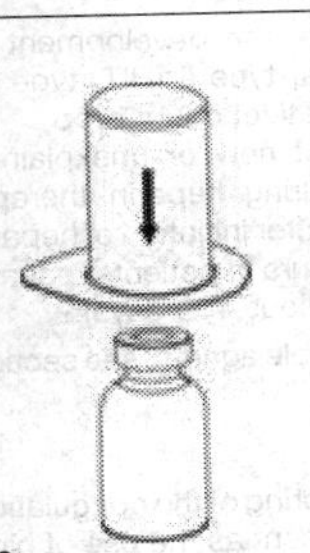
2

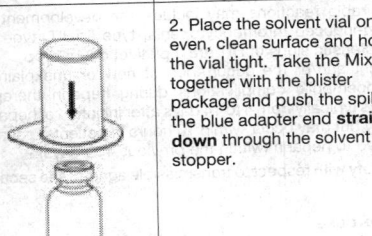

2. Place the solvent vial on an even, clean surface and hold the vial tight. Take the Mix2Vial together with the blister package and push the spike of the blue adapter end **straight down** through the solvent vial stopper.

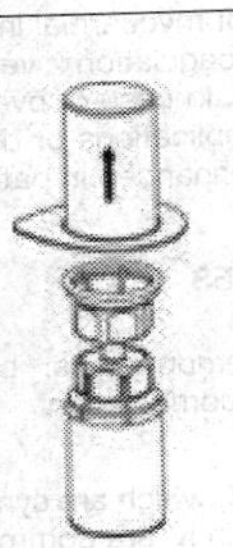
3

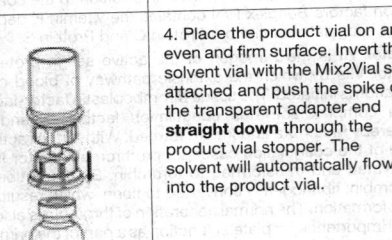

3. Carefully remove the blister package from the Mix2Vial set by holding at the rim, and pulling **vertically** upwards. Make sure that you only pull away the blister package and not the Mix2Vial set.

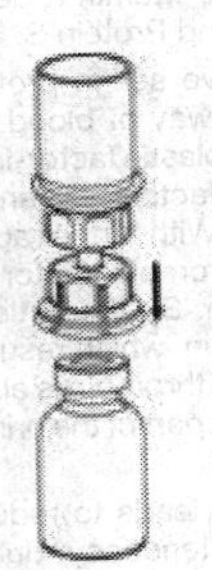
4

4. Place the product vial on an even and firm surface. Invert the solvent vial with the Mix2Vial set attached and push the spike of the transparent adapter end **straight down** through the product vial stopper. The solvent will automatically flow into the product vial.

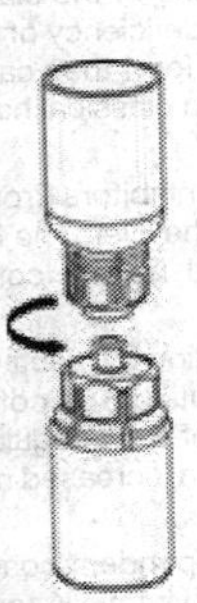
5

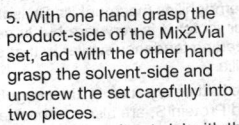

5. With one hand grasp the product-side of the Mix2Vial set, and with the other hand grasp the solvent-side and unscrew the set carefully into two pieces.
Discard the solvent vial with the blue Mix2Vial adapter attached.

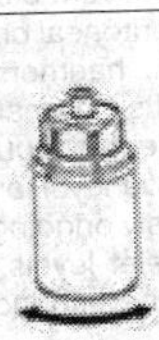
6

6. Gently swirl the product vial with the transparent adapter attached until the substance is fully dissolved. Do not shake.

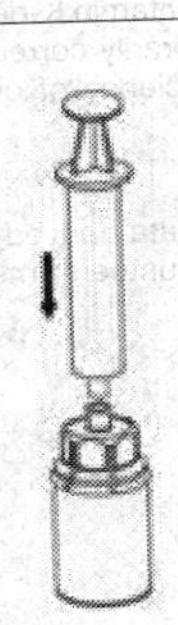
7

7. Draw air into an empty, sterile syringe. While the product vial is upright, connect the syringe to the Mix2Vial's Luer Lock fitting. Inject air into the product vial.

Withdrawal and application

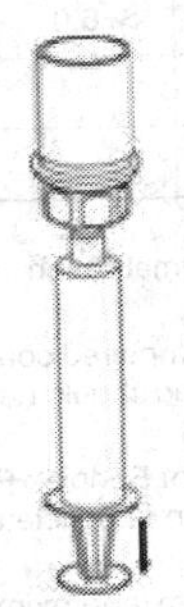
8

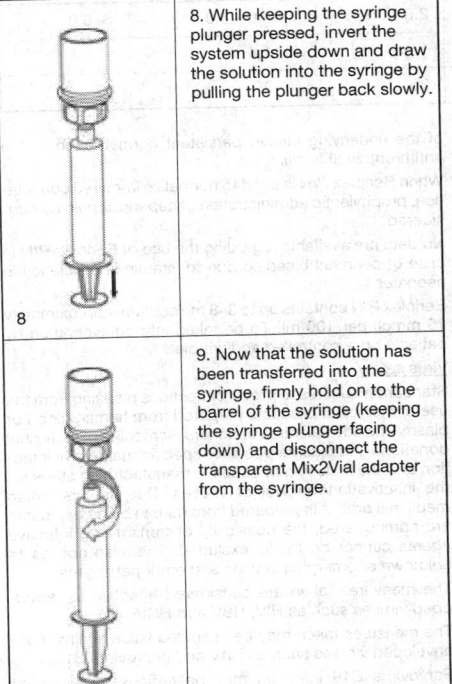

8. While keeping the syringe plunger pressed, invert the system upside down and draw the solution into the syringe by pulling the plunger back slowly.

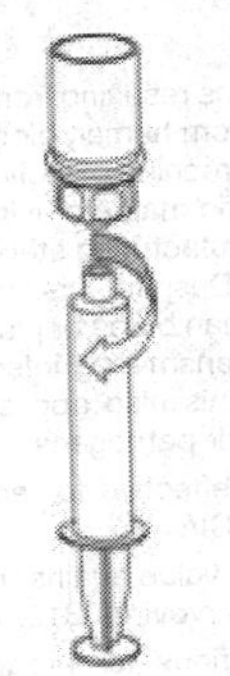
9

9. Now that the solution has been transferred into the syringe, firmly hold on to the barrel of the syringe (keeping the syringe plunger facing down) and disconnect the transparent Mix2Vial adapter from the syringe.

7. MARKETING AUTHORISATION HOLDER
CSL Behring GmbH
Emil-von-Behring-Strasse 76
35041 Marburg
Germany

8. MARKETING AUTHORISATION NUMBER(S)
PL 15036/0030

9. DATE OF FIRST AUTHORISATION/RENEWAL OF THE AUTHORISATION
29 January 2009

10. DATE OF REVISION OF THE TEXT
29 January 2009

Beriplex P/N
(CSL Behring UK Limited)

1. NAME OF THE MEDICINAL PRODUCT
Beriplex P/N 250 & 500, powder and solvent for solution for injection ▼

2. QUALITATIVE AND QUANTITATIVE COMPOSITION
Beriplex P/N is presented as powder and solvent for solution for injection containing human prothrombin complex. The product nominally contains the following IU of the human coagulation factors tabled below:

(see Table 1 below)

The total protein content is 6 – 14 mg/ml of reconstituted solution.

The specific activity of factor IX is 2.5 IU per mg total protein.

The activities of all coagulation factors as well as Protein C and S (antigen) have been tested according to the current valid international WHO-Standards.

For a full list of excipients, see section 6.1.

3. PHARMACEUTICAL FORM
Powder and solvent for solution for injection.

4. CLINICAL PARTICULARS
4.1 Therapeutic indications
- Treatment and perioperative prophylaxis of bleedings in acquired deficiency of the prothrombin complex coagulation factors, such as deficiency caused by treatment with vitamin K antagonists, or in case of overdose of vitamin K antagonists, when rapid correction of the deficiency is required.

- Treatment and perioperative prophylaxis of bleedings in congenital deficiency of any of the vitamin K dependent coagulation factors when purified specific coagulation factor products are not available.

4.2 Posology and method of administration
Posology

Only general dosage guidelines are given below. Treatment should be initiated under the supervision of a physician experienced in the treatment of coagulation disorders. The dosage and duration of the substitution therapy depend on the severity of the disorder, on the location and extent of bleeding and on the patient's clinical condition.

The amount and the frequency of administration should be calculated on an individual patient basis. Dosage intervals must be adapted to the different circulating half-lives of the respective coagulation factors in the prothrombin complex (see section 5.2). Individual dosage requirements can only be identified on the basis of regular determinations of the individual plasma levels of the coagulation factors of interest, or on global tests of the prothrombin complex levels (INR, Quick's test), and a continuous monitoring of the clinical condition of the patient.

In case of major surgical interventions, precise monitoring of the substitution therapy by means of coagulation assays is essential (specific coagulation factor assays and/or global tests for prothrombin complex levels).

The posology and method of administration in elderly people (> 65 years) is equivalent to the general recommendations.

There is no experience in children (see section 4.4 and 5.2).

• Treatment and perioperative prophylaxis of bleedings during vitamin K antagonist treatment.

The dose will depend on the INR before treatment and the targeted INR. In the following table approximate doses (ml/kg body weight of the reconstituted product and IU FIX/kg b.w.) required for normalisation of INR (e.g. $\leq$ 1.3) at different initial INR levels are given.

(see Table 2 on next page)

It is recommended that the maximum single dose should not exceed 5000 IU FIX.

The correction of the vitamin K antagonist-induced impairment of haemostasis is reached at the latest 30 minutes after the injection and will persist for approximately 6 – 8 hours. However, the effect of vitamin K, if administered simultaneously, is usually achieved within 4 – 6 hours. Thus, repeated treatment with human prothrombin complex is not usually required when vitamin K has been administered.

These recommendations are based on data from clinical studies with a limited number of subjects. Recovery and the duration of effect may vary, therefore monitoring of INR during treatment is mandatory.

• Bleedings and perioperative prophylaxis in congenital deficiency of any of the vitamin K dependent coagulation factors when specific coagulation factor products are not available.

The calculation of the required dosage of prothrombin complex concentrate is based on data from clinical studies:

- 1 IU of factor IX per kg body weight can be expected to raise the plasma factor IX activity by 1.3 % (0.013 IU/ml) of normal
- 1 IU of factor VII per kg body weight raises the plasma factor VII activity by 1.7 % (0.017 IU/ml) of normal
- 1 IU of factor II per kg body weight raises the plasma factor II activity by 1.9 % (0.019 IU/ml) of normal
- 1 IU of factor X per kg body weight raises the plasma factor X activity by 1.8 % (0.018 IU/ml) of normal.

Table 1

Name of the ingredients	Content after reconstitution (IU/ml)	Beriplex P/N 250 content per vial (IU)	Beriplex P/N 500 content per vial (IU)
Active Ingredients			
Human coagulation factor II	20 – 48	200 – 480	400 – 960
Human coagulation factor VII	10 – 25	100 – 250	200 – 500
Human coagulation factor IX	20 – 31	200 – 310	400 – 620
Human coagulation factor X	22 – 60	220 – 600	440 – 1200
Further active ingredients			
Protein C	15 – 45	150 – 450	300 – 900
Protein S	12 - 38	120 - 380	240 - 760

Table 2

Initial INR	2.0 – 3.9	4.0 – 6.0	> 6.0
Approximate dose ml/kg body weight	1	1.4	2
Approximate dose IU (Factor IX)/kg body weight	25	35	50

The dose of a specific factor administered is expressed in International Units (IU), which are related to the current WHO standard for each factor. The activity in the plasma of a specific coagulation factor is expressed either as a percentage (relative to normal plasma) or in International Units (relative to the international standard for the specific coagulation factor).

One International Unit (IU) of a coagulation factor activity is equivalent to the quantity in one ml of the normal human plasma.

For example, the calculation of the required dosage of factor X is based on the finding that 1 International Unit (IU) of factor X per kg body weight raises the plasma factor X activity by 0.018 IU/ml.

The required dosage is determined using the following formula:

Required units = body weight [kg] × desired factor X rise [IU/ml] × 56

where 56 (ml/kg) is the reciprocal of the estimated recovery.

If the individual recovery is known, that value should be used for calculation.

Method of administration

Beriplex P/N should be reconstituted according to section 6.6. The reconstituted solution should be administered intravenously (not more than 3 IU/kg/min, max. 210 IU/min, approximately 8 ml/min).

4.3 Contraindications

Known hypersensitivity to any of the components of the product.

Risk of thrombosis, angina pectoris, recent myocardial infarction (exception: life-threatening haemorrhages following overdosage of oral anticoagulants, and before induction of a fibrinolytic therapy).

In the case of disseminated intravascular coagulation, prothrombin complex-preparations may only be applied after termination of the consumptive state.

Known history of heparin-induced thrombocytopenia.

4.4 Special warnings and precautions for use

The advice of a specialist experienced in the management of coagulation disorders should be sought.

In patients with acquired deficiency of the vitamin K-dependent coagulation factors (e.g. as induced by treatment of vitamin K antagonists), Beriplex P/N should only be used when rapid correction of the prothrombin complex levels is necessary, such as major bleedings or emergency surgery. In other cases, reduction of the dose of the vitamin K antagonist and/or administration of vitamin K is usually sufficient.

Patients receiving a vitamin K antagonist may have an underlying hypercoaguable state and infusion of human prothrombin complex may exacerbate this.

In congenital deficiency of any of the vitamin K-dependent factors, specific coagulation factor products should be used when available.

If allergic or anaphylactic-type reactions occur, the administration of Beriplex P/N has to be stopped immediately (e.g. discontinue injection) and an appropriate treatment has to be initiated. Therapeutic measures depend on the kind and severity of the undesirable effect. The current medical standards for shock treatment are to be observed.

There is a risk of thrombosis or disseminated intravascular coagulation when patients, with either congenital or acquired deficiency, are treated with human prothrombin complex particularly with repeated dosing. The risk may be higher in treatment of isolated factor VII deficiency, since the other vitamin K-dependent coagulation factors, with longer half-lives, may accumulate to levels considerably higher than normal. Patients given human prothombin complex should be observed closely for signs or symptoms of disseminated intravascular coagulation or thrombosis.

Because of the risk of thromboembolic complications, close monitoring should be exercised when administering Beriplex P/N to patients with a history of coronary heart disease or myocardial infarction, to patients with liver disease, to patients postoperatively, to neonates or to patients at risk of thromboembolic phenomena or disseminated intravascular coagulation or simultaneous inhibitor deficiency. In each of these situations, the potential benefit of treatment with Beriplex P/N should be weighed against the potential risk of such complications. In patients with DIC and sepsis antithrombin III substitution should be considered prior to treatment with Beriplex P/N.

In patients with disseminated intravascular coagulation, it may, under certain circumstances, be necessary to substitute the coagulation factors of the prothrombin complex. This substitution may, however, only be carried out after termination of the consumptive state (e.g. by treatment of the underlying cause, persistent normalization of the antithrombin III level).

When Beriplex P/N is used to normalize impaired coagulation, prophylactic administration of heparin should be considered.

No data are available regarding the use of Beriplex P/N in case of perinatal bleeding due to vitamin K deficiency in neonates.

Beriplex P/N contains up to 343 mg sodium (approximately 15 mmol) per 100 ml. To be taken into consideration by patients on a controlled sodium diet.

Virus safety

Standard measures to prevent infections resulting from the use of medicinal products prepared from human blood or plasma include selection of donors, screening of individual donations and plasma pools for specific markers of infection and the inclusion of effective manufacturing steps for the inactivation/removal of viruses. Despite this, when medicinal products prepared from human blood or plasma are administered, the possibility of transmitting infective agents cannot be totally excluded. This also applies to unknown or emerging viruses and other pathogens.

The measures taken are considered effective for enveloped viruses such as HIV, HBV and HCV.

The measures taken may be of limited value against non-enveloped viruses such as HAV and parvovirus B19.

Parvovirus B19 infection may be serious for pregnant women (fetal infection) and for individuals with immunodeficiency or increased erythropoiesis (e.g. haemolytic anaemia).

Appropriate vaccination (hepatits A and B) should be generally considered for patients in regular/repeated receipt of human plasma-derived products.

It is strongly recommended that every time that Beriplex P/N is administered to a patient, the name and batch number of the product are recorded in order to maintain a link between the patient and the batch of the product.

4.5 Interaction with other medicinal products and other forms of interaction

Human prothrombin complex products neutralise the effect of vitamin K antagonist treatment, but no interactions with other medicinal products are known.

When performing clotting tests which are sensitive to heparin in patients receiving high doses of human prothrombin complex, the heparin as a constituent of the administered product must be taken into account.

4.6 Pregnancy and lactation

The safety of Beriplex P/N for use in human pregnancy and during lactation has not been established. Animal studies are not suitable to assess the safety with respect to pregnancy, embryonal/foetal development, parturition or postnatal development.

Therefore, Beriplex P/N should be used during pregnancy and lactation only if clearly indicated.

4.7 Effects on ability to drive and use machines

No studies on the effects on the ability to drive and use machines have been performed.

4.8 Undesirable effects

The following adverse reactions are based on post marketing experience as well as scientific literature. The following standard categories of frequency are used:

Very common: ≥ 1/10

Common: ≥ 1/100 and < 1/10

Uncommon: ≥ 1/1,000 and < 1/100

Rare: ≥ 1/10,000 and < 1/1,000

Very rare: < 1/10,000 (including reported single cases)

Renal and urinary disorders:

Nephrotic syndrome has been reported in single cases following attempted immune tolerance induction in haemophilia B patients with factor IX inhibitors and a history of allergic reaction.

Vascular disorders:

There is a risk of thromboembolic episodes following the administration of human prothrombin complex (see section 4.4).

General disorders and administration site conditions:

Increase in body temperature is observed in very rare cases.

Immune system disorders:

Hypersensitivity or allergic reactions (which may include angioedema, burning and stinging at the injection site, chills, flushing, generalized urticaria, headache, hives, hypotension, lethargy, nausea, restlessness, tachycardia, angina pectoris, tingling, vomiting or wheezing) have been observed very rarely in patients treated with factor IX containing products. In some cases, these reactions have progressed to severe anaphylaxis, and they have occurred in close temporal association with development of factor IX inhibitors (see section 4.4).

If allergic-anaphylactic reactions occur, the administration of Beriplex P/N has to be discontinued immediately (e.g. discontinue injection) and an appropriate treatment has to be initiated (see section 4.4).

Development of antibodies to one or several factors of the prothrombin complex may occur in very rare cases. If such inhibitors occur, the condition will manifest itself as a poor clinical response. In such cases, it is recommended to contact a specialised haemophilia centre.

Undesirable reactions may include the development of heparin-induced thrombocytopenia, type II (HIT, type II). Characteristic signs of HIT are a platelet count drop > 50 per cent and/or the occurrence of new or unexplained thromboembolic complications during heparin therapy. Onset is typically from 4 to 14 days after initiation of heparin therapy but may occur within 10 hours in patients recently exposed to heparin (within the previous 100 days).

For safety with respect to transmissible agents, see section 4.4.

4.9 Overdose

To avoid overdosage, regular monitoring of the coagulation status is indicated during the treatment as the use of high doses of prothrombin complex concentrate (overdosage) has been associated with instances of myocardial infarction, disseminated intravascular coagulation, venous thrombosis and pulmonary embolism. In case of overdosage the risk of thromboembolic complications or disseminated intravascular coagulation is enhanced in patients at risk of these complications.

5. PHARMACOLOGICAL PROPERTIES

5.1 Pharmacodynamic properties

Pharmacotherapeutic group: antihaemorrhagics, blood coagulation factors II, VII, IX and X in combination

ATC code: B02B D01

The coagulation factors II, VII, IX and X, which are synthesised in the liver with the help of vitamin K, are commonly called the prothrombin complex. In addition to the coagulation factors Beriplex P/N contains the vitamin K dependent coagulation inhibitors Protein C and Protein S.

Factor VII is the zymogen of the active serine protease factor VIIa by which the extrinsic pathway of blood coagulation is initiated. The tissue thromboplastin factor-factor VIIa complex activates coagulation factors IX and X, whereby factor IXa and Xa are formed. With further activation of the coagulation cascade, prothrombin (factor II) is activated and transformed to thrombin. By the action of thrombin, fibrinogen is converted to fibrin, which results in clot formation. The normal generation of thrombin is also of vital importance for platelet function as a part of the primary haemostasis.

Isolated severe deficiency of factor VII leads to reduced thrombin formation and a bleeding tendency due to impaired fibrin formation and impaired primary haemostasis. Isolated deficiency of factor IX is one of the classical haemophilias (haemophilia B). Isolated deficiency of factor II or factor X is very rare but in severe form they cause a bleeding tendency similar to that seen in classical haemophilia.

The further ingredients, the coagulation inhibitors Protein C and Protein S, are also synthesized in the liver. The biological activity of Protein C is enforced by the cofactor Protein S.

Activated Protein C inhibits the coagulation by inactivating the coagulation factors Va and VIIIa. Protein S as cofactor of Protein C supports the inactivation of the coagulation. Protein C deficiency is associated with an increased risk of thrombosis.

Acquired deficiency of the vitamin K-dependent coagulation factors occurs during treatment with vitamin K antagonists. If the deficiency becomes severe, a severe bleeding tendency results, characterised by retroperitoneal or cerebral bleeds rather than muscle and joint haemorrhage. Severe hepatic insufficiency also results in markedly reduced levels of the vitamin K-dependent coagulation factors and a clinical relevant bleeding tendency. However this is often complex due to a simultaneously ongoing low-grade intravascular coagulation, low platelet levels, deficiency of coagulation inhibitors and disturbed fibrinolysis.

The administration of human prothrombin complex provides an increase in plasma levels of the vitamin K-dependent coagulation factors, and can temporarily correct the coagulation defect of patients with deficiency of one or several of these factors.

5.2 Pharmacokinetic properties

Plasma half-life is indicated as follows (data derived from a clinical study including 15 healthy volunteers; median values, range):

Factor II:	60	(25 – 135)	hours
Factor VII:	4	(2 – 9)	hours
Factor IX:	17	(10 – 127)	hours*
Factor X:	31	(17 – 44)	hours
Protein C:	47	(9 – 122)	hours*
Protein S:	49	(33 – 83)	hours*

*terminal half-life; two-compartment-model

Beriplex P/N is distributed and metabolized in the organism in the same way as the endogenous coagulation factors II, VII, IX and X.

Intravenous administration means that the preparation is available immediately; bioavailability is proportional to the dose administered.

5.3 Preclinical safety data

Beriplex P/N contains as active ingredients the factors of the prothrombin complex (factors II, VII, IX and X). They are derived from human plasma and act like endogenous constituents of plasma.

Single dose toxicity studies with the predecessing pasteurized but not nanofiltrated product showed moderate toxicity in mice after the administration of 200 IU/kg, the highest dose tested. Preclinical studies with repeated dose applications (chronic toxicity, cancerogenicity and reproductive toxicity) cannot be reasonably performed in conventional animal models due to the development of antibodies following the application of heterologous human proteins.

The local tolerance after intravenous administration of Beriplex P/N was shown in rabbits. A neoantigenicity study with rabbits has shown no indication of generation of a neoepitop due to the pasteurization process.

6. PHARMACEUTICAL PARTICULARS

6.1 List of excipients

Powder:

Heparin

Human albumin

Human antithrombin III

Sodium chloride

Sodium citrate

HCl or NaOH (in small amounts for pH adjustment)

Solvent:

Water for injections

6.2 Incompatibilities

Beriplex P/N must not be mixed with other medicinal products, diluents or solvents.

6.3 Shelf life

3 years

After reconstitution, from a microbiological point of view and as Beriplex P/N contains no preservative, the reconstituted product should be used immediately. The physicochemical stability has been demonstrated for 24 hours at room temperature (max. 25°C). However, if it is not administered immediately, storage shall not exceed 8 hours at room temperature.

6.4 Special precautions for storage

Do not store above 25°C. Do not freeze.

Keep the vial in the outer carton, in order to protect from light.

6.5 Nature and contents of container

Beriplex P/N 250:

Powder: Injection vial of colourless glass (Type I), sealed with rubber infusion stopper, aluminium seal and plastic flip-off cap.

Solvent: 10 ml Water for injections in an injection vial of colourless glass (Type I), sealed with rubber infusion stopper, aluminium seal and plastic flip-off cap.

Injection device: 1 filter transfer device 20/20

Beriplex P/N 500:

Powder: Injection vial of colourless glass (Type II), sealed with rubber infusion stopper, aluminium seal and plastic flip-off cap.

Solvent: 20 ml Water for injections in an injection vial of colourless glass (Type I), sealed with rubber infusion stopper, aluminium seal and plastic flip-off cap.

Injection device: 1 filter transfer device 20/20

Not all pack sizes may be marketed.

6.6 Special precautions for disposal and other handling

Any unused product or waste material should be disposed of in accordance with local requirements.

Method of administration

General instructions

- The solution should be clear or slightly opalescent. After filtering/withdrawal (see below) reconstituted product should be inspected visually for particulate matter and discoloration prior to administration. Do not use solutions that are cloudy or have deposits.

- Reconstitution and withdrawal must be carried out under aseptic conditions.

Reconstitution

Bring the solvent to room temperature. Ensure that product and diluent vial flip caps are removed and the stoppers are treated with an aseptic solution and allowed to dry prior to opening the Mix2Vial package.

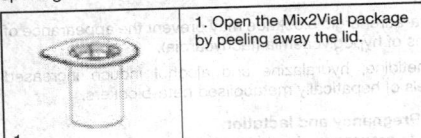

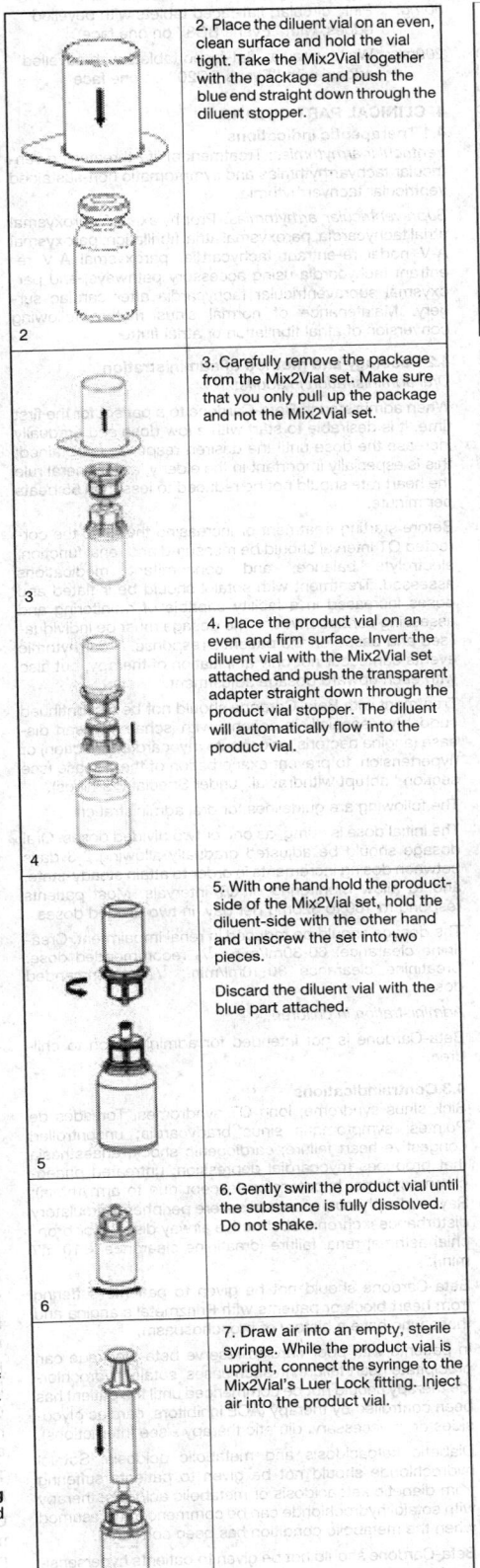

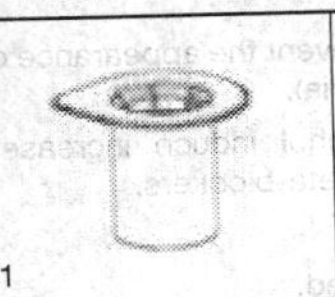 1	1. Open the Mix2Vial package by peeling away the lid.
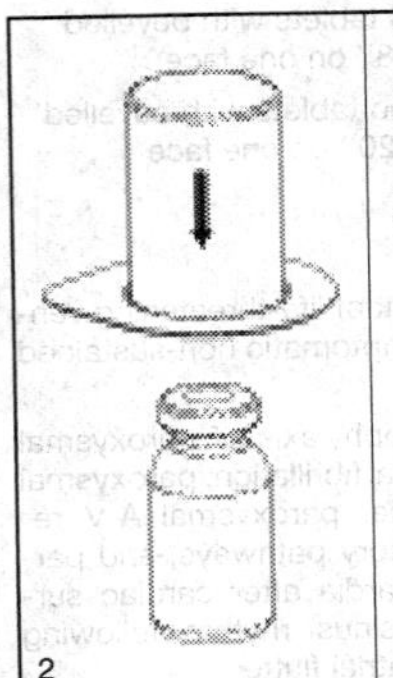 2	2. Place the diluent vial on an even, clean surface and hold the vial tight. Take the Mix2Vial together with the package and push the blue end straight down through the diluent stopper.
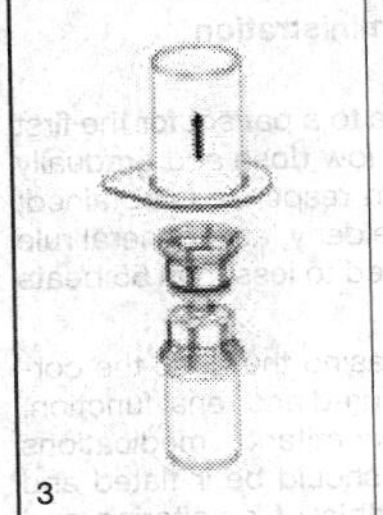 3	3. Carefully remove the package from the Mix2Vial set. Make sure that you only pull up the package and not the Mix2Vial set.
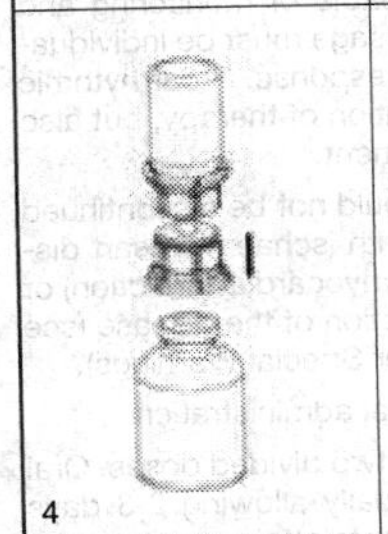 4	4. Place the product vial on an even and firm surface. Invert the diluent vial with the Mix2Vial set attached and push the transparent adapter straight down through the product vial stopper. The diluent will automatically flow into the product vial.
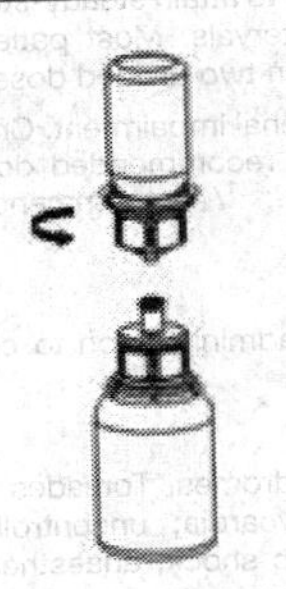 5	5. With one hand hold the product-side of the Mix2Vial set, hold the diluent-side with the other hand and unscrew the set into two pieces. Discard the diluent vial with the blue part attached.
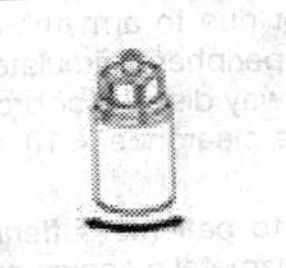 6	6. Gently swirl the product vial until the substance is fully dissolved. Do not shake.
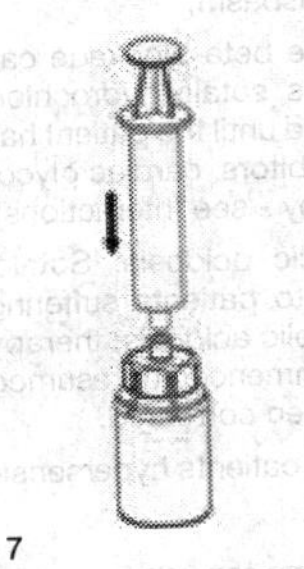 7	7. Draw air into an empty, sterile syringe. While the product vial is upright, connect the syringe to the Mix2Vial's Luer Lock fitting. Inject air into the product vial.

Withdrawal and application

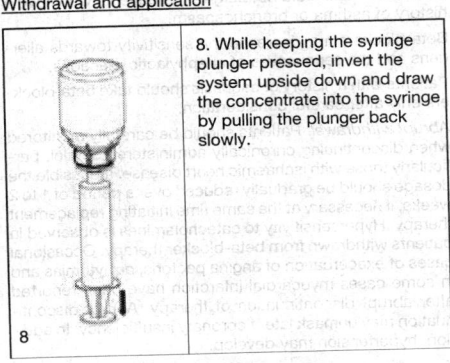

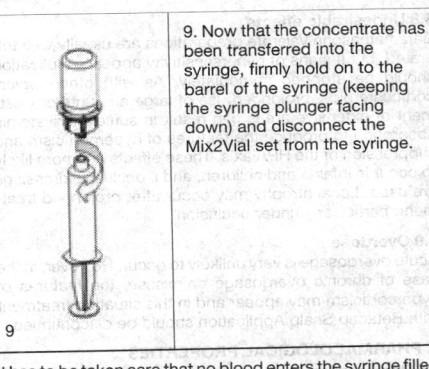

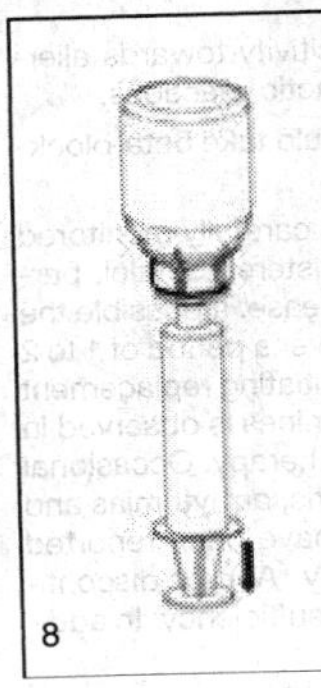 8	8. While keeping the syringe plunger pressed, invert the system upside down and draw the concentrate into the syringe by pulling the plunger back slowly.
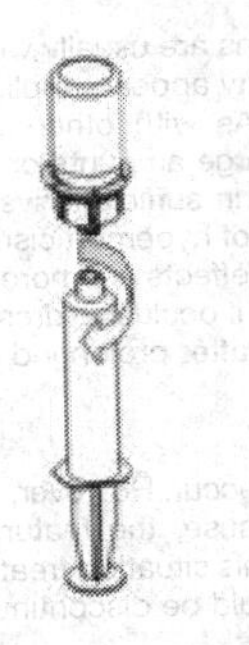 9	9. Now that the concentrate has been transferred into the syringe, firmly hold on to the barrel of the syringe (keeping the syringe plunger facing down) and disconnect the Mix2Vial set from the syringe.

It has to be taken care that no blood enters the syringe filled with product, as there is a risk that the blood could coagulate in the syringe and fibrin clots would therefore be administered to the patient.

The reconstituted solution should be administered by a separate infusion line.

7. MARKETING AUTHORISATION HOLDER

CSL Behring GmbH

Emil-von-Behring-Strasse 76

35041 Marburg

Germany

8. MARKETING AUTHORISATION NUMBER(S)

Beriplex P/N 250: PL 15036/0028

Beriplex P/N 500: PL 15036/0029

9. DATE OF FIRST AUTHORISATION/RENEWAL OF THE AUTHORISATION

11 January 2008

10. DATE OF REVISION OF THE TEXT

August 2008

Betacap Scalp Application

(Dermal Laboratories Limited)

1. NAME OF THE MEDICINAL PRODUCT

BETACAP™ SCALP APPLICATION

2. QUALITATIVE AND QUANTITATIVE COMPOSITION

Betamethasone (as valerate) 0.1% w/w.

3. PHARMACEUTICAL FORM

Cutaneous solution.

Transparent, slightly gelled, emollient, scalp application.

4. CLINICAL PARTICULARS

4.1 Therapeutic indications

For the topical treatment of dermatoses of the scalp, such as psoriasis and seborrhoeic dermatitis, which are unresponsive to less potent corticosteroids.

4.2 Posology and method of administration

For adults, including the elderly, and children over the age of one year: Betacap Scalp Application should be applied sparingly to the scalp night and morning until improvement is noticeable. It may then be possible to sustain improvement by applying once a day, or less frequently.

For the treatment of seborrhoeic dermatitis in children, the product should not be used for longer than 5 to 7 days.

4.3 Contraindications

Not to be used where there is bacterial, fungal or viral infection of the scalp. Not to be used in cases of sensitivity to any of the ingredients. Not to be used in children under the age of one year.

4.4 Special warnings and precautions for use

Keep away from the eyes. Betacap is highly flammable. Do not use near a fire or naked flame. Allow the treated scalp to dry naturally. Long-term continuous topical therapy should be avoided where possible, particularly in infants and children, as adrenal suppression can occur even without occlusion. Complications sometimes associated with the use of topical corticosteroids in psoriasis include the possibility of rebound relapses, development of tolerance, risk of generalised pustular psoriasis and development of local or systemic toxicity due to impaired barrier function of the skin. If used in psoriasis, careful patient supervision is important. For external use only.

4.5 Interaction with other medicinal products and other forms of interaction

None known.

4.6 Pregnancy and lactation

There is inadequate evidence of safety in human pregnancy. Topical administration of corticosteroids to pregnant animals can cause abnormalities of foetal development including cleft palate and intra-uterine growth retardation. There may therefore be a very small risk of such effects in the human foetus.

4.7 Effects on ability to drive and use machines

None known.

4.8 Undesirable effects
Betamethasone valerate preparations are usually well tolerated, but if signs of hypersensitivity appear, application should be stopped immediately. As with other topical corticosteroids, prolonged use of large amounts or treatment of extensive areas can result in sufficient systemic absorption to produce the features of hypercorticism and suppression of the HPA axis. These effects are more likely to occur in infants and children, and if occlusive dressings are used. Local atrophy may occur after prolonged treatment, particularly under occlusion.

4.9 Overdose
Acute overdosage is very unlikely to occur. However, in the case of chronic overdosage or misuse, the features of hypercorticism may appear and in this situation treatment with Betacap Scalp Application should be discontinued.

5. PHARMACOLOGICAL PROPERTIES
5.1 Pharmacodynamic properties
Betamethasone (as valerate) is a well-established example of a corticosteroid which is used in dermatological therapy in pharmacological doses for its anti-inflammatory and immuno-suppressive glucocorticoid properties. It suppresses the clinical manifestations of a wide range of inflammatory dermatoses and is frequently used at the concentration of 0.1% (as valerate). Betacap Scalp Application complies with the specification given in the monograph for Betamethasone Valerate Scalp Application BP. Betacap Scalp Application includes a coconut-oil related emollient ingredient to reduce the drying effect that a standard alcoholic vehicle may otherwise have on the scalp. The vehicle also contains isopropyl alcohol, which has antiseptic activity.

5.2 Pharmacokinetic properties
For clinical usage, the betamethasone valerate is presented as a slightly thickened evaporative solution which allows drug availability over the affected area, whilst reducing the propensity to spread onto uninvolved skin. In addition, after rapidly drying, the drug substance is thus deposited uniformly in a micronised crystalline form for efficient absorption into the skin. The lipid characteristics of the drug substance ensure that these micro-fine crystals rapidly dissolve in skin lipids to enhance molecular diffusion through the outer epidermal tissue and to encourage permeation into the deeper layers where it reverses the pathological processes responsible for the inflammation.

5.3 Preclinical safety data
No relevant information additional to that contained elsewhere in this SPC.

6. PHARMACEUTICAL PARTICULARS
6.1 List of excipients
Macrogol 7 Glyceryl Cocoate (a water dispersible derivative of coconut oil); Isopropyl Alcohol; Carbomer; Sodium Hydroxide; Purified Water.

6.2 Incompatibilities
None known.

6.3 Shelf life
36 months.

6.4 Special precautions for storage
Do not store above 25°C. Protect from light. Return bottle to carton between use.

6.5 Nature and contents of container
100 ml plastic squeeze bottle with integral nozzle applicator for convenient direct application to the scalp through the hair, and tamper-evident replaceable cap.

6.6 Special precautions for disposal and other handling
Not applicable.

7. MARKETING AUTHORISATION HOLDER
Dermal Laboratories

Tatmore Place, Gosmore

Hitchin, Herts SG4 7QR, UK.

8. MARKETING AUTHORISATION NUMBER(S)
00173/0149.

9. DATE OF FIRST AUTHORISATION/RENEWAL OF THE AUTHORISATION
22 May 2008.

10. DATE OF REVISION OF THE TEXT
June 2008.

Beta-Cardone Tablets 40, 80, 200mg

(UCB Pharma Limited)

1. NAME OF THE MEDICINAL PRODUCT
Beta-Cardone Tablets 40mg, 80mg or 200mg

2. QUALITATIVE AND QUANTITATIVE COMPOSITION
Sotalol Hydrochloride 40mg, 80mg or 200mg

For excipients see 6.1.

3. PHARMACEUTICAL FORM
Tablet

40mg: Green, circular, flat-faced tablets with bevelled edges, with "Evans/BC4" on one face.

80mg: Pink, circular, flat-faced tablets with bevelled edges, with "Evans/BC8" on one face.

200mg: White, circular, flat-faced tablets with bevelled edges, with "Evans/BC20" on one face

4. CLINICAL PARTICULARS
4.1 Therapeutic indications
Ventricular arrhythmias: Treatment of life-threatening ventricular tachyarrhythmias and symptomatic non-sustained ventricular tachyarrhythmias.

Supraventricular arrhythmias: Prophylaxis of paroxysmal atrial tachycardia, paroxysmal atrial fibrillation, paroxysmal A-V nodal re-entrant tachycardia, paroxysmal A-V re-entrant tachycardia using accessory pathways, and paroxysmal supraventricular tachycardia after cardiac surgery. Maintenance of normal sinus rhythm following conversion of atrial fibrillation or atrial flutter.

4.2 Posology and method of administration
Oral administration in adults:

When administering Beta-Cardone to a patient for the first time, it is desirable to start with a low dose and gradually increase the dose until the desired response is obtained; this is especially important in the elderly, as a general rule the heart rate should not be reduced to less than 55 beats per minute.

Before starting treatment or increasing the dose the corrected QT interval should be measured and renal function, electrolyte balance, and concomitant medications assessed. Treatment with sotalol should be initiated and doses increased in a facility capable of monitoring and assessing cardiac rhythm. The dosage must be individualised and based on the patient's response. Proarrhythmic events can occur not only at initiation of therapy, but also with each upward dosage adjustment.

Treatment with Beta-Cardone should not be discontinued suddenly, especially in patients with ischaemic heart disease (angina pectoris, prior acute myocardial infarction) or hypertension, to prevent exacerbation of the disease (see section "abrupt withdrawal" under Special Warnings).

The following are guidelines for oral administration.

The initial dose is 80mg, as one or two divided doses. Oral dosage should be adjusted gradually allowing 2-3 days between dosing increments in order to attain steady-state, and to allow monitoring of QT intervals. Most patients respond to 160 to 320mg per day, in two divided doses.

The dosage should be reduced in renal impairment. Creatinine clearance: 60-30ml/min.: $^1/_2$ recommended dose. Creatinine clearance 30-10ml/min.: $^1/_4$ recommended dose.

Administration in children:

Beta-Cardone is not intended for administration to children.

4.3 Contraindications
Sick sinus syndrome; long QT syndromes, Torsades de Pointes; symptomatic sinus bradycardia; uncontrolled congestive heart failure; cardiogenic shock; anaesthesia that produces myocardial depression; untreated phaeochromocytoma; hypotension (except due to arrhythmia); Raynaud's phenomenon and severe peripheral circulatory disturbances; chronic obstructive airway disease or bronchial asthma; renal failure (creatinine clearance <10 ml/min.).

Beta-Cardone should not be given to patients suffering from heart block or patients with Prinzmetal's angina and those who have a history of bronchospasm,

In patients with poor cardiac reserve beta-blockade can precipitate heart failure; in such cases, sotalol hydrochloride therapy should not be commenced until the patient has been controlled by therapy (ACE inhibitors, cardiac glycosides or, if necessary, diuretic therapy - see Interactions).

Diabetic ketoacidosis and metabolic acidosis: Sotalol hydrochloride should not be given to patients suffering from diabetic ketoacidosis or metabolic acidosis; therapy with sotalol hydrochloride can be commenced or resumed when the metabolic condition has been corrected.

Beta-Cardone should not be given to patients hypersensitive to sotalol.

4.4 Special warnings and precautions for use
Beta-Cardone should not be given to patients who have a history of asthma or bronchospasm.

Beta-blockers may increase the sensitivity towards allergens and the seriousness of anaphylactic reactions.

Patients with a history of psoriasis should take beta-blockers only after careful consideration.

Abrupt withdrawal: Patients should be carefully monitored when discontinuing chronically administered sotalol, particularly those with ischaemic heart disease. If possible the dosage should be gradually reduced over a period of 1 to 2 weeks, if necessary at the same time initiating replacement therapy. Hypersensitivity to catecholamines is observed in patients withdrawn from beta-blocker therapy. Occasional cases of exacerbation of angina pectoris, arrhythmias and in some cases myocardial infarction have been reported after abrupt discontinuation of therapy. Abrupt discontinuation may unmask latent coronary insufficiency. In addition, hypertension may develop.

Proarrhythmias: Rarely, Beta-Cardone causes aggravation of pre-existing arrhythmias or the provocation of new arrhythmias.

Risk factors for Torsades de Pointes include prolongation of the QT interval, bradycardia, reduction in serum potassium and magnesium, and history of cardiomegaly or congestive heart failure, sustained ventricular tachycardia.

Proarrhythmic events can occur on initiating therapy and with every upward dose adjustment. The incidence of Torsades de Pointes is dose dependent.

Caution should be used if the QT_C exceeds 500 msec whilst on therapy. It is advisable to reduce dose or discontinue therapy when the QT_C interval exceeds 550 msec.

Electrolyte disturbances: Sotalol should not be used in patients with hypokalaemia or hypomagnesaemia. Potassium levels should be monitored. In conditions likely to provoke hypokalaemia/hypomagnesaemia, such as persistent diarrhoea, appropriate corrective clinical measures should be taken.

Heart failure: Beta-blockade may precipitate heart failure. Following myocardial infarction careful monitoring and dose titration are critical during initiation and follow-up of therapy. Sotalol should be avoided in patients with left ventricular ejection fractions ≤40% without serious ventricular arrhythmias.

Thyrotoxicosis: Beta-blockade may mask certain clinical signs of hyperthyroidism.

Treated diabetes: Beta-Cardone, like other beta-blocking agents, may reduce or mask the usual pre-hypoglycaemic warning signs. It may be necessary to adjust the dose of anti-diabetic therapy.

General anaesthesia: If desired, Beta-Cardone may be stopped four days prior to surgery. However, where sudden withdrawal might expose the patient to severe angina or arrhythmias, anaesthesia can proceed provided that the following precautions are taken.

1. Vagal dominance is counteracted by premedication with atropine sulphate (0.25 to 2.0mg) administered intravenously.

2. Anaesthetic agents such as ether, chloroform, cyclopropane, trichlorethylene, methoxyflurane and enflurane are not used.

Alcoholism: Beta-adrenoceptor blocking drugs may precipitate cardiac failure in alcoholic patients.

Upper respiratory infections: In these conditions patients without a history of airways obstruction may suffer bronchospasm from beta-blockade.

The product labelling will bear a statement warning against use in patients with a history of wheezing or asthma.

Patients with rare hereditary problems of galactose intolerance, the Lapp-lactose deficiency, or glucose-galactose malabsorption should not take this medicine.

4.5 Interaction with other medicinal products and other forms of interaction
In combined therapy, clonidine should not be discontinued until several days after withdrawal of Beta-Cardone.

Use with great caution with drugs that also prolong QT interval, e.g. disopyramide, amiodarone, class I antiarrhythmic agents, calcium antagonists of the verapamil type or tricyclic antidepressants.

Concomitant potassium-depleting diuretics may increase the potential for Torsade de Pointes.

Proarrhythmic events are more common in patients also receiving digitalis glycosides.

Phenothiazines, terfenadine, astemizole, diltiazem and halofantrine.

Concomitant use of reserpine, guanethidine, or alpha methyldopa: Closely monitor for evidence of hypotension and/or marked bradycardia, syncope.

Tubocurarine: Neuromuscular blockade is prolonged by beta-blocking agents.

Calcium antagonists: Dihydropyridine derivatives such as nifedipine. The risk of hypotension may be increased. In patients with latent cardiac insufficiency, concomitant treatment with beta-blockers may lead to cardiac failure.

Prostaglandin synthetase inhibiting drugs may decrease the hypotensive effects of beta-blockers.

Sympathicomimetic agents: may counteract the effect of beta-adrenergic agents.

Concomitant administration of tricyclic antidepressants, barbiturates and phenothiazines as well as other antihypertensive agents may increase the blood pressure lowering effect.

Precautions for use:

Insulin and oral antidiabetic drugs, may intensify the blood sugar lowering effect (especially non-selective beta-blockers).

Beta-adrenergic blockade may prevent the appearance of signs of hypoglycaemia (tachycardia).

Cimetidine, hydralazine and alcohol induce increased levels of hepatically metabolised beta-blockers.

4.6 Pregnancy and lactation
Use in pregnancy should be avoided.

Pregnancy: Animal studies with sotalol hydrochloride have shown no evidence of teratogenicity or other harmful effects on the foetus. Nevertheless its use throughout pregnancy should be avoided unless it is absolutely necessary as it crosses the placenta and may cause foetal bradycardia.

Beta-blockers reduce placental perfusion which may result in intrauterine foetal death, immature and premature deliveries. In addition, adverse effects (especially hypoglycaemia and bradycardia) may occur in the foetus and neonate. There is an increased risk of cardiac and pulmonary complications in the neonate in the postnatal period. Most beta-blockers, particularly lipophilic compounds, will pass into breast milk although to a variable extent.

Lactation: Infants should not be fed with breast milk from mothers being treated with Beta-Cardone.

Newborns exposed near delivery should be closely observed for the first 24-48 hours for signs and symptoms of beta-blockade.

4.7 Effects on ability to drive and use machines
Side-effects such as dizziness and fatigue should be taken into account.

4.8 Undesirable effects
The most significant adverse effects are those due to proarrhythmia, including Torsades de Pointes. There is an increased risk of Torsades de Pointes in women.

Also bradycardia, dyspnoea, chest pain, palpitations, oedema, ECG abnormalities, hypotension, proarrhythmia, syncope, heart failure, presyncope. Nausea/vomiting, diarrhoea, dyspepsia, abdominal pain, flatulence, cramps, fatigue, dizziness, asthenia, lightheadedness, headache, sleep disturbances, depression, paraesthesia, mood changes, anxiety, sexual dysfunction, visual disturbances, taste abnormalities, hearing disturbances, fever, slowed AV-conduction or increase of an existing AV-block, cold and cyanotic extremities, Raynaud's phenomenon, increase of intermittent claudication.

Beta-blockers, even those with apparent cardioselectivity should not be used in patients with asthma or a history of obstructive airways disease unless no alternative treatment is available. In such cases, the risk of inducing bronchospasm should be appreciated and appropriate precautions taken. If bronchospasm should occur after the use of Beta-Cardone it can be treated with a $beta_2$-agonist by inhalation e.g. salbutamol (the dose of which may need to be greater than the usual dose in asthma) and, if necessary, intravenous atropine 1mg.

There have been reports of skin rashes and especially exacerbation of psoriasis disorders of lacrimation including dry eyes and conjunctivitis. In most cases the symptoms have cleared when the treatment was withdrawn. Discontinuance of the drug should be considered if any such reaction is not otherwise explicable. Cessation of therapy with a beta-blocker should be gradual.

An increase in Anti Nuclear Antibodies has been seen; its clinical relevance is not clear.

4.9 Overdose
Symptoms of overdose are: bradycardia, hypotension, bronchospasm and acute cardiac insufficiency.

After ingestion of an overdose or in the case of hypersensitivity, the patient should be kept under close supervision and treated in an intensive care ward. Absorption of any drug material still present in the gastro-intestinal tract can be prevented by gastric lavage, administration of activated charcoal and a laxative. Artificial respiration may be required. Bradycardia or extensive vagal reactions should be treated by administering atropine or methylatropine. Hypotension and shock should be treated with plasma/ plasma substitutes and if necessary, catecholamines. The beta-blocking effect can be counteracted by slow intravenous administration of isoprenaline hydrochloride, starting with a dose of approximately 5 micrograms/minute, or dobutamine, starting with a dose of 2.5 micrograms/minute, until the required effect has been obtained.

In refractory cases isoprenaline can be combined with dopamine. If this does not produce the desired effect either, Intravenous administration of 8-10 mg of glucagon may be considered. If required the injection should be repeated within one hour, to be followed - if required - by an i.v. infusion of glucagon at an administration rate of 1-3 mg/hour. Administration of calcium ions, or the use of a cardiac pacemaker may also be considered. In patients intoxicated with hydrophylic beta-blocking agents hemodialysis or hemoperfusion may be considered.

Prolongation of the QT_c interval has been reported. Transvenous pacing may be required.

5. PHARMACOLOGICAL PROPERTIES

5.1 Pharmacodynamic properties
Sotalol has both beta-adrenoreceptor blocking (Vaughan Williams Class II) and cardiac action potential duration prolongation (Vaughan Williams Class III) antiarrhythmic properties. The d- and l-isomers of sotalol have similar Class III antiarrhythmic effects while the l-isomer is responsible for virtually all of the beta-blocking activity.

5.2 Pharmacokinetic properties
Sotalol is completely absorbed from the gastrointestinal tract and peak plasma concentrations are obtained about 2 or 3 hours after a dose. It is excreted unchanged in the urine. After oral administration the plasma half-life has been shown to be 17 hours. It is not bound to plasma proteins. The lipid solubility is very low.

5.3 Preclinical safety data
None stated.

6. PHARMACEUTICAL PARTICULARS

6.1 List of excipients
Lactose
Maize Starch
Pregelatinised Starch
Talc
Magnesium Stearate
Dispersed Blue 11076 and Quinoline Yellow Lake 19248 (40mg only)
Dispersed Red 11652 (80mg only)

6.2 Incompatibilities
None known.

6.3 Shelf life
36 months

6.4 Special precautions for storage
Beta-Cardone Tablets should be protected from light.

6.5 Nature and contents of container
Polypropylene securitainers containing 30 tablets (200mg only); 100 or 500 tablets (40mg, 80mg or 200mg).

PVC, PVdC and foil blister pack containing 56 tablets (40mg and 80mg only)

Polypropylene TraCeR pack containing 28 tablets (200mg only)

6.6 Special precautions for disposal and other handling
None stated.

7. MARKETING AUTHORISATION HOLDER
UCB Pharma Ltd
208 Bath Road
Slough
Berkshire
SL1 3WE
UK

8. MARKETING AUTHORISATION NUMBER(S)
40mg: PL 00039/0414
80mg: PL 00039/0415
200mg: PL00039/0416

9. DATE OF FIRST AUTHORISATION/RENEWAL OF THE AUTHORISATION
12 January 1993/11 May 2000

10. DATE OF REVISION OF THE TEXT
June 2005

11. Legal Category
POM

Betagan

(Allergan Ltd)

1. NAME OF THE MEDICINAL PRODUCT
Betagan®
Betagan® Eye Drops 0.5% w/v

2. QUALITATIVE AND QUANTITATIVE COMPOSITION
Levobunolol hydrochloride 0.5% w/v (equivalent to levobunolol 0.445% w/v)

3. PHARMACEUTICAL FORM
Eye Drops, Solution

4. CLINICAL PARTICULARS

4.1 Therapeutic indications
Reduction of intraocular pressure in chronic open-angle glaucoma and ocular hypertension.

4.2 Posology and method of administration
Adults (including the elderly)

The usual dose is one drop instilled in the affected eye(s) once or twice daily. In common with other topical ophthalmic beta-adrenergic blocking agents, full clinical response may take several weeks to occur. Intraocular pressure should therefore be measured approximately four weeks after starting treatment. Because of diurnal variations in intraocular pressure, satisfactory response is best determined by measuring the intraocular pressure at different times of the day.

Use in Children

Betagan is not currently recommended for use in children.

Concomitant administration

If the patient's intraocular pressure is not satisfactory on this regimen, concomitant therapy with dipivefrin or adrenaline and/or pilocarpine and other miotics, and/or systemically administered carbonic anhydrase inhibitors can be instituted.

4.3 Contraindications
Bronchial asthma; history of bronchial asthma; chronic obstructive pulmonary disease; sinus bradycardia; second and third degree atrioventricular block; cardiac failure; cardiogenic shock; hypersensitivity to any component; sick sinus syndrome (including sino-atrial block); Prinzmetal's angina; untreated phaeochromocytoma; metabolic acidosis; hypotension.

4.4 Special warnings and precautions for use
As with other topically applied ophthalmic drugs, Betagan may be absorbed systemically and adverse reactions typical of oral beta-adrenoceptor agents may occur.

Respiratory and cardiac reactions have been reported including, rarely, death due to bronchospasm or associated with cardiac failure.

Congestive heart failure should be adequately controlled before commencing therapy with Betagan. In patients with a history of cardiac disease pulse rates should be monitored.

Diabetic control should be monitored during Betagan therapy in patients with labile diabetes. Beta-blockers may mask the symptoms of thyrotoxicosis.

Betagan has little or no effect on pupil size and if administered in angle-closure glaucoma, for reduction of intraocular pressure, must only be given in combination with a miotic.

Betagan contains benzalkonium chloride and should not be used in patients continuing to wear hydrophilic (soft) lenses.

Diminished response after prolonged therapy has been reported in some patients. If necessary, concomitant therapy with dipivefrin/ adrenaline, pilocarpine and/ or carbonic anhydrase inhibitors can be instituted.

In patients with peripheral circulatory disorders (Raynaud's disease or syndrome, intermittent claudication), beta-blockers should be used with great caution as aggravation of these disorders may occur.

Beta-blockers may induce bradycardia. If the pulse rate decreases to less than 50-55 beats per minute at rest and the patient experiences symptoms related to the bradycardia, review of intraocular pressure lowering therapy may be required.

Due to its negative effect on conduction time, beta-blockers should only be given with caution to patients with first degree heart block.

Beta-blockers may increase both the sensitivity towards allergens and the seriousness of anaphylactic reactions.

4.5 Interaction with other medicinal products and other forms of interaction
Caution should be exercised when used concomitantly with oral beta-adrenergic blocking agents, because of the potential for additive effects on systemic blockade.

4.6 Pregnancy and lactation
Betagan has not been studied in human pregnancy. It is recommended that Betagan be avoided in pregnancy. If treatment with Betagan during lactation is considered necessary for the benefit of the mother, consideration should be given to the cessation of breast feeding.

4.7 Effects on ability to drive and use machines
There are no studies on the effect of this medicine on the ability to drive. When driving vehicles or operating machines it should be taken into account that occasionally dizziness or fatigue may occur.

4.8 Undesirable effects
Ocular: Transient burning and stinging on installation, conjunctival hyperaemia, eyelid oedema, impaired vision, blepharoconjunctivitis and iridocyclitis have been reported occasionally. Dry eye has been rarely reported. The pharmacological and physical properties of levobunolol indicate a potential for post-installation reduction in corneal sensitivity: this potential has not been confirmed in clinical studies with Betagan.

Cardiovascular: Bradycardia, hypotension, heart block and paraesthesia have been reported.

Respiratory: There have been reports of dyspnoea and asthma.

CNS: Headache, transient ataxia and dizziness, hallucinations, confusion, impotence, sleep disturbances, depression and lethargy have been reported occasionally.

Gastrointestinal: Nausea, vomiting, and diarrhoea have been reported occasionally.

Dermatological: Urticaria and pruritis have been rarely reported.

Immunological: Post-marketing reports of ocular and systemic hypersensitivity / allergic reactions have been received rarely.

4.9 Overdose
There are no data available on human overdosage with Betagan, which is unlikely to occur via the ocular route. Should accidental overdosage occur, flush the eye(s) with water or normal saline. If accidentally ingested, systemic symptoms of bradycardia, hypotension, bronchospasm and acute cardiac insufficiency may occur.

5. PHARMACOLOGICAL PROPERTIES

5.1 Pharmacodynamic properties
Levobunolol hydrochloride is a non-cardioselective beta-adrenoceptor blocking agent, equipotent at both beta-1 and beta-2 receptors. Levobunolol does not have

significant local anaesthetic (membrane-stabilizing) or intrinsic sympathomimetic activity.

Because of levobunolol's affinity for beta-1 receptors there exists the theoretical possibility of a negative inotropic effect.

The primary mechanism of the ocular hypotensive activity of levobunolol hydrochloride is likely to be a decrease in aqueous humour production. There is little effect on pupil size or accommodation.

5.2 Pharmacokinetic properties
The onset of action of one drop of Betagan can be detected one hour after installation with the maximum effect seen between 2 and 6 hours. The half lives of orally ingested levobunolol and of its active metabolite dihydrolevobunolol are between 6 and 7 hours.

5.3 Preclinical safety data
Not applicable.

6. PHARMACEUTICAL PARTICULARS

6.1 List of excipients
Benzalkonium chloride Ph. Eur.

Disodium edetate Ph. Eur.

Polyvinyl alcohol USP

Sodium chloride Ph. Eur.

Sodium phosphate, dibasic, heptahydrate USP

Potassium phosphate, monobasic NF

Sodium metabisulphite BP

Sodium hydroxide or hydrochloric acid to adjust pH Ph. Eur.

Purified water Ph. Eur.

6.2 Incompatibilities
None known.

6.3 Shelf life
24 months unopened.

Discard 28 days after first opening.

6.4 Special precautions for storage
Do not store above 25°C.

Protect from light.

6.5 Nature and contents of container
10 ml white bottle and dropper tip made of low density polyethylene. The cap is either a "traditional" green, medium impact, polystyrene cap or a white medium impact polystyrene cap or a white, medium impact, polystyrene compliance cap (C-Cap®) with an external rotating sleeve indicating daily dosage status. Each have a safety seal to ensure integrity. The bottle is filled with either 5 or 10 ml of Betagan.

6.6 Special precautions for disposal and other handling
No special instructions.

7. MARKETING AUTHORISATION HOLDER
Allergan Ltd

Marlow International

The Parkway

Marlow

Bucks

SL7 1YL

UK

8. MARKETING AUTHORISATION NUMBER(S)
PL 00426/0060

9. DATE OF FIRST AUTHORISATION/RENEWAL OF THE AUTHORISATION
23rd March 1989/14th July 2005

10. DATE OF REVISION OF THE TEXT
20th December 2007

Betagan Unit Dose

(Allergan Ltd)

1. NAME OF THE MEDICINAL PRODUCT
Betagan Unit Dose

2. QUALITATIVE AND QUANTITATIVE COMPOSITION
Levobunolol hydrochloride 0.5% USP

3. PHARMACEUTICAL FORM
Eye drops, solution.

Clear, greenish-yellow to light greenish-yellow solution.

Sterile aqueous ophthalmic solution.

4. CLINICAL PARTICULARS

4.1 Therapeutic indications
Reduction of intraocular pressure in chronic open-angle glaucoma and ocular hypertension.

4.2 Posology and method of administration
Adults (including the elderly)

The recommended adult dose is one drop of Betagan Unit Dose once or twice daily in the affected eye(s). Discard product after use.

Children

Use in children is not currently recommended.

4.3 Contraindications
Bronchial asthma; history of bronchial asthma; chronic obstructive pulmonary disease; sinus bradycardia; second and third degree atrioventricular block; cardiac failure; cardiogenic shock; hypersensitivity to any component.

4.4 Special warnings and precautions for use
As with other topically applied ophthalmic drugs, Betagan may be absorbed systemically.

4.5 Interaction with other medicinal products and other forms of interaction
Betagan may have additive effects in patients taking systemic antihypertensive drugs. These possible additive effects may include hypotension, including orthostatic hypotension, bradycardia, dizziness, and/ or syncope. Conversely, systemic beta-adrenoceptor blocking agents may potentiate the ocular hypotensive effect of Betagan.

Betagan may potentially add to the effects of oral calcium antagonists, rauwolfia alkaloids or beta blockers to induce hypotension and/ or marked bradycardia.

4.6 Pregnancy and lactation
There are no adequate and well-controlled studies in pregnant women. Levobunolol should be used during pregnancy only if the potential benefit justifies the potential risk to the foetus.

It is not known whether this drug is excreted in human milk. Systemic beta-blockers and topical Timolol maleate are known to be excreted in human milk. Because similar drugs are excreted in human milk, caution should be exercised when Betagan is administered to a nursing woman.

4.7 Effects on ability to drive and use machines
None known.

4.8 Undesirable effects
Blepharoconjunctivitis, transient ocular burning, stinging, and decreases in heart rate and blood pressure have been reported occasionally with the use of Betagan. Urticaria has been reported rarely with the use of Betagan.

The following adverse effects have been reported rarely and a definite relationship with the use of Betagan has not been established: change in heart rhythm, iridocyclitis, browache, transient ataxia, lethargy, urticaria, elevated liver enzymes, eructation, dizziness and itching.

The following additional adverse reactions have been reported with ophthalmic use of $beta_1$ and $beta_2$ non selective blocking agents:

Special senses: conjunctivitis, blepharitis, keratitis and decreased corneal sensitivity, visual disturbances, including refractory changes, diplopia and ptosis.

Cardiovascular: bradycardia, hypotension, syncope, heartblock, cerebrovascular accident, cerebral ischaemia, congestive heart failure, palpitation and cardiac arrest.

Respiratory: bronchospasm, respiratory failure and dyspenea.

Body as a whole: asthenia, nausea and depression.

4.9 Overdose
There are no data available on human overdosage with Betagan which is unlikely to occur via the ocular route. Should accidental ocular overdosage occur, flush the eye(s) with water or normal saline. If accidentally ingested, efforts to decrease further absorption may be appropriate.

5. PHARMACOLOGICAL PROPERTIES

5.1 Pharmacodynamic properties
Levobunolol is a non-cardioselective beta-adrenoceptor blocking agent, equipotent at both $beta_1$ and $beta_2$ receptors. Levobunolol is greater than 60 times more potent than its dextro isomer in its beta-blocking activity. In order to obtain the highest degree of beta-blocking potential without increasing the potential for direct myocardial depression, the levo isomer, levobunolol, is used. Levobunolol does not have significant local anaesthetic (membrane-stabilising) or intrinsic sympathomimetic activity. Betagan has shown to be as effective as Timolol in lowering intraocular pressure.

Betagan when instilled in the eye will lower elevated intraocular pressure as well as normal intraocular pressure, whether or not accompanied by glaucoma. Elevated intraocular pressure presents a major risk factor in the pathogenesis of glaucomatous field loss. The higher the level of intraocular pressure, the likelihood of optic nerve damage and visual field loss.

The primary mechanism of action of levobunolol in reducing intraocular pressure is most likely a decrease in aqueous humor production. Betagan reduces intraocular pressure with little or no effect on pupil size in contrast to the miosis which cholinergic agents are known to produce.

The blurred vision and night blindness often associated with miotics would not be expected with the use of Betagan. Patients with cateracts avoid the inability to see around lenticular opacities caused by pupil constriction.

5.2 Pharmacokinetic properties
The onset of action with one drop of Betagan can be detected within one hour of treatment, with maximum effect seen between two and six hours. A significant decrease can be maintained for up to 24 hours following a single dose.

5.3 Preclinical safety data
Not applicable

6. PHARMACEUTICAL PARTICULARS

6.1 List of excipients
Polyvinyl alcohol USP

Sodium chloride EP

Disodium edetate EP

Sodium phosphate dibasic, heptahydrate USP

Potassium phosphate monobasic NF

Sodium hydroxide or hydrochloric acid (to adjust pH) EP

Purified water EP

6.2 Incompatibilities
No major incompatibilities have been reported from topical use of levobunolol.

6.3 Shelf life
24 months.

6.4 Special precautions for storage
Store at or below 25°.

Protect from light.

Discard after use.

6.5 Nature and contents of container
Low density polyethylene (LDPE) blow-fill-seal unit dose container (0.9 ml volume) filled with 0.4 ml solution.

Unit dose containers are packaged into a foil covered pouch (5 containers per pouch).

Pouches are packaged into cartons such that each carton contains 30 or 60 unit dose containers.

6.6 Special precautions for disposal and other handling
None.

7. MARKETING AUTHORISATION HOLDER
Allergan Limited

Marlow International

The Parkway

Marlow

Bucks

SL7 1YL

UK

8. MARKETING AUTHORISATION NUMBER(S)
PL 00426/0072

9. DATE OF FIRST AUTHORISATION/RENEWAL OF THE AUTHORISATION
20th April 1993 / 26th July 2003

10. DATE OF REVISION OF THE TEXT
24th April 2008

Betaloc I.V. Injection

(AstraZeneca UK Limited)

1. NAME OF THE MEDICINAL PRODUCT
Betaloc I.V. Injection

2. QUALITATIVE AND QUANTITATIVE COMPOSITION
Each ampoule of 5 ml contains 5 mg Metoprolol tartrate Ph. Eur.

3. PHARMACEUTICAL FORM
Solution for Injection

4. CLINICAL PARTICULARS

4.1 Therapeutic indications
Control of tachyarrhythmias, especially supraventricular tachyarrhythmias.

Early intervention with Betaloc in acute myocardial infarction reduces infarct size and the incidence of ventricular fibrillation. Pain relief may also decrease the need for opiate analgesics.

Betaloc has been shown to reduce mortality when administered to patients with acute myocardial infarction.

4.2 Posology and method of administration
The dose must always be adjusted to the individual requirements of the patient. The following are guidelines:

Cardiac arrhythmias:

Initially up to 5 mg injected intravenously at a rate of 1-2 mg per minute. The injection can be repeated at 5 minute intervals until a satisfactory response has been obtained. A total dose of 10-15 mg generally proves sufficient.

Because of the risk of a pronounced drop of blood pressure, the I.V. administration of Betaloc to patients with a systolic blood pressure below 100 mmHg should only be given with special care.

During Anaesthesia:

2-4 mg injected slowly I.V. at induction is usually sufficient to prevent the development of arrhythmias during anaesthesia. The same dosage can also be used to control arrhythmias developing during anaesthesia. Further injections of 2 mg may be given as required to a maximum overall dose of 10 mg.

Myocardial infarction:

Intravenous Betaloc should be initiated in a coronary care or similar unit when the patient's haemodynamic condition has stabilised. Therapy should commence with 5 mg I.V. every 2 minutes to a maximum of 15 mg total as determined by blood pressure and heart rate. The second or third dose should not be given if the systolic blood pressure is <90 mmHg, the heart rate is <40 beats/min and the P-Q time is >0.26 seconds, or if there is any aggravation of dyspnoea or cold sweating. Oral therapy should commence 15 minutes after the last injection with 50 mg every 6 hours for 48 hours. Patients who fail to tolerate the full intravenous dose should be given half the suggested oral dose.

Impaired Renal Function:

Dose adjustment is generally not needed in patients with impaired renal function.

Impaired Hepatic Function:

Dose adjustment is normally not needed in patients suffering from liver cirrhosis because metoprolol has a low protein binding (5 - 10 %). However, in patients with severe hepatic dysfunction a reduction in dosage may be necessary.

Elderly:

Several studies indicate that age related physiological changes have negligible effects on the pharmacokinetics of metoprolol. Dose adjustment is not needed in the elderly, but careful dose titration is important in all patients.

Children:

The safety and efficacy of metoprolol in children has not been established.

4.3 Contraindications

Betaloc Injection, as with other beta blockers, should not be used in patients with any of the following:

- Hypotension,
- AV block of second- or third-degree,
- Decompensated cardiac failure (pulmonary oedema, hypoperfusion or hypotension),
- Continuous or intermittent inotropic therapy acting through beta-receptor agonism,
- Bradycardia (<45 bpm),
- Sick sinus syndrome,
- Cardiogenic shock,
- Severe peripheral arterial circulatory disorder
- Untreated phaeochromocytoma,
- Metabolic acidosis.

Known hypersensitivity to any component of Betaloc Injection or other beta-blockers.

Betaloc Injection is also contra-indicated when suspected acute myocardial infarction is complicated by bradycardia (<45 bpm), first-degree heart block or systolic blood pressure <100 mmHg and/or severe heart failure.

4.4 Special warnings and precautions for use

When treating patients with suspected or definite myocardial infarction the haemodynamic status of the patient should be carefully monitored after each of the three 5 mg intravenous doses. The second or third dose should not be given if the heart rate is <40 beats/min, the systolic blood pressure is <90 mmHg and the P-Q time is >0.26 sec, or if there is any aggravation of dyspnoea or cold sweating.

Betaloc, as with other beta blockers:

- should not be withdrawn abruptly during oral treatment. When possible, Betaloc should be withdrawn gradually over a period of 10 - 14 days, in diminishing doses to 25 mg daily for the last 6 days. During its withdrawal patients should be kept under close surveillance, especially those with known ischaemic heart disease. The risk for coronary events, including sudden death, may increase during the withdrawal of beta-blockade.
- must be reported to the anaesthetist prior to general anaesthesia. It is not generally recommended to stop Betaloc treatment in patients undergoing surgery. If withdrawal of metoprolol is considered desirable, this should, if possible, be completed at least 48 hours before general anaesthesia. However, in some patients it may be desirable to employ a beta-blocker as premedication. By shielding the heart against the effects of stress, the beta-blocker may prevent excessive sympathetic stimulation provoking cardiac arrhythmias or acute coronary insufficiency. If a beta-blocker is given for this purpose, an anaesthetic with little negative inotropic activity should be selected to minimise the risk of myocardial depression.
- although contra-indicated in severe peripheral arterial circulatory disturbances (see Section 4.3), may also aggravate less severe peripheral arterial circulatory disorders.
- may be administered when heart failure has been controlled. Digitalisation and/or diuretic therapy should also be considered for patients with a history of heart failure, or patients known to have a poor cardiac reserve. Betaloc should be used with caution in patients where cardiac reserve is poor.
- may cause patients to develop increasing bradycardia, in such cases the Betaloc Injection dosage should be reduced or gradually withdrawn.
- due to the negative effect on conduction time, should only be given with caution to patients with first-degree heart block.
- may increase the number and duration of angina attacks in patients with Prinzmetal's angina, due to unopposed alpha-receptor mediated coronary artery vasoconstriction. Betaloc Injection is a $beta_1$-selective beta-blocker; consequently, its use may be considered although utmost caution must be exercised.
- may mask the early signs of acute hypoglycaemia, in particular tachycardia. During treatment with Betaloc Injection, the risk of interfering with carbohydrate metabolism or masking hypoglycaemia is less than with non-selective beta-blockers.
- may mask the symptoms of thyrotoxicosis.
- may increase both the sensitivity towards allergens and the seriousness of anaphylactic reactions.

Although cardioselective beta-blockers may have less effect on lung function than non-selective beta-blockers, as with all beta-blockers, these should be avoided in patients with reversible obstructive airways disease unless there are compelling clinical reasons for their use. When administration is necessary, these patients should be kept under close surveillance. The use of a $beta_2$-bronchodilator (e.g. terbutaline) may be advisable in some patients. The dosage of the $beta_2$-agonist may require an increase when treatment with Betaloc Injection is commenced.

The label shall state - "Use with caution in patients who have a history of wheezing, asthma or any other breathing difficulties, see enclosed user leaflet."

Like all beta-blockers, careful consideration should be given to patients with psoriasis before Betaloc i.v. is administered.

In patients with a phaeochromocytoma, an alpha-blocker should be given concomitantly.

In labile and insulin-dependent diabetes it may be necessary to adjust the hypoglycaemic therapy.

Intravenous administration of calcium antagonists of the verapamil type should not be given to patients treated with beta-blockers.

4.5 Interaction with other medicinal products and other forms of interaction

Metoprolol is a metabolic substrate for the Cytochrome P450 isoenzyme CYP2D6. Drugs that act as enzyme-inducing and enzyme-inhibiting substances may exert an influence on the plasma level of metoprolol. Enzyme inducing agents (e.g. rifampicin) may reduce plasma concentrations of Betaloc whereas enzyme inhibitors (e.g. cimetidine, alcohol and hydralazine) may increase plasma concentrations.

Patients receiving concomitant treatment with sympathetic ganglion blocking agents, other beta blockers (i.e. eye drops), or Mono Amine Oxidase (MAO) inhibitors should be kept under close surveillance.

If concomitant treatment with clonidine is to be discontinued, Betaloc Injection should be withdrawn several days before clonidine.

Increased negative inotropic and chronotropic effects may occur when metoprolol is given together with calcium antagonists of the verapamil and diltiazem type. In patients treated with beta-blockers intravenous administration of calcium antagonists of the verapamil-type should not be given.

Beta-blockers may enhance the negative inotropic and negative dromotropic effect of antiarrhythmic agents (of the quinidine type and amiodarone).

Digitalis glycosides, in association with beta-blockers, may increase atrioventricular conduction time and may induce bradycardia.

In patients receiving beta-blocker therapy, inhalation anaesthetics enhance the cardiodepressant effect.

Concomitant treatment with indometacin and other prostaglandin synthetase inhibiting drugs may reduce the antihypertensive effect of beta-blockers.

The administration of adrenaline (epinephrine) to patients undergoing beta-blockade can result in an increase in blood pressure and bradycardia although this is less likely to occur with $beta_1$-selective drugs.

Betaloc Injection will antagonise the $beta_1$-effects of sympathomimetic agents but should have little influence on the bronchodilator effects of $beta_2$-agonists at normal therapeutic doses.

Metoprolol may impair the elimination of lidocaine.

As with other beta-blockers, concomitant therapy with dihydropyridines e.g. nifedipine, may increase the risk of hypotension, and cardiac failure may occur in patients with latent cardiac insufficiency.

The dosages of oral antidiabetic agents and also of insulin may have to be readjusted in patients receiving beta-blockers.

As beta-blockers may affect the peripheral circulation, care should be exercised when drugs with similar activity e.g. ergotamine are given concurrently.

The effects of Betaloc Injection and other drugs with an antihypertensive effect on blood pressure are usually additive. Care should be taken when combining with other antihypertensive drugs or drugs that might reduce blood pressure such as tricyclic antidepressants, barbiturates and phenothiazines. However, combinations of antihypertensive drugs may often be used with benefit to improve control of hypertension.

4.6 Pregnancy and lactation

Pregnancy

Betaloc should not be used in pregnancy or nursing mothers unless the physician considers that the benefit outweighs the possible hazard to the foetus/infant. Beta-blockers reduce placental perfusion, which may result in intrauterine foetal death, immature and premature deliveries. As with all beta-blockers, Betaloc Injection may cause side-effects especially bradycardia and hypoglycaemia in the foetus, and in the newborn and breastfed infant. There is an increased risk of cardiac and pulmonary complications in the neonate. Betaloc Injection has, however, been used in pregnancy-associated hypertension under close supervision, after 20 weeks gestation. Although Betaloc crosses the placental barrier and is present in cord blood, no evidence of foetal abnormalities has been reported.

Lactation

Breast feeding is not recommended. The amount of metoprolol ingested via breast milk should not produce significant beta-blocking effects in the neonate if the mother is treated with normal therapeutic doses.

4.7 Effects on ability to drive and use machines

When driving vehicles or operating machines, it should be taken into account that occasionally dizziness or fatigue may occur.

4.8 Undesirable effects

The following events have been reported as adverse events in clinical trials or reported from routine use.

The following definitions of frequencies are used:

Very common (≥10%), common (1-9.9%), uncommon (0.1-0.9%), rare (0.01-0.09%) and very rare (<0.01%).

Infections and infestations

Very rare: Gangrene in patients with pre existing severe peripheral circulatory disorders.

Blood and lymphatic system disorders

Very rare: Thrombocytopenia.

Psychiatric disorders

Uncommon: Depression, insomnia, nightmares.

Rare: Nervousness, anxiety.

Very rare: Confusion, hallucinations.

Nervous system disorders

Common: Dizziness, headache.

Uncommon: Concentration impairment, somnolence, paraesthesiae.

Very rare: Amnesia/memory impairment, taste disturbances.

Eye disorders

Rare: Disturbances of vision, dry and/or irritated eyes, conjunctivitis.

Ear and labyrinth disorders

Very rare: Tinnitus.

Cardiac disorders

Common: Bradycardia, palpitations.

Uncommon: Deterioration of heart failure symptoms, cardiogenic shock in patients with acute myocardial infarction*, first degree heart block.

Rare: Disturbances of cardiac conduction, cardiac arrhythmias, increased existing AV block.

* Excess frequency of 0.4 % compared with placebo in a study of 46,000 patients with acute myocardial infarction where the frequency of cardiogenic shock was 2.3 % in the metoprolol group and 1.9 % in the placebo group in the subset of patients with low shock risk index. The corresponding excess frequency for patients in Killip class I was 0.7% (metoprolol 3.5% and placebo 2.8%). The shock risk index was based on the absolute risk of shock in each individual patient derived from age, sex, time delay, Killip class, blood pressure, heart rate, ECG abnormality, and prior history of hypertension. The patient group with low shock risk index corresponds to the patients in which metoprolol is indicated for use in acute myocardial infarction.

Vascular disorders

Common: Postural disorders (very rarely with syncope).

Rare: Raynauds phenomenon.

Very rare: Increase of pre-existing intermittent claudication.

Respiratory, thoracic and mediastinal disorders

Common: Dyspnoea on exertion.

Uncommon: Bronchospasm.

Rare: Rhinitis.

Gastrointestinal disorders

Common: Nausea, abdominal pain, diarrhoea, constipation.

Uncommon: Vomiting.

Rare: Dry mouth.

Hepato-biliary disorders

Very rare: Hepatitis.

Skin and subcutaneous tissue disorders

Uncommon: Rash (in the form of psoriasiform urticaria and dystrophic skin lesions), increased sweating.

Rare: Loss of hair.

Very rare: Photosensitivity reactions, aggravated psoriasis.

Musculoskeletal and connective tissue disorders

Very rare: Arthralgia.

Uncommon: Muscle cramps.

Reproductive system and breast disorders

Rare: Impotence/sexual dysfunction.

General disorders and administration site disorders

Very common: Fatigue.

Common: Cold hands and feet.

Uncommon: Precordial pain, oedema.

Investigations

Uncommon: Weight gain.

Rare: Liver function test abnormalities, positive anti-nuclear antibodies (not associated with SLE).

4.9 Overdose

The symptoms of overdose may include bradycardia, hypotension, acute cardiac insufficiency and bronchospasm.

General treatment should include:

Close supervision, treatment in an intensive care ward and the use of plasma or plasma substitutes to treat hypotension and shock.

Excessive bradycardia can be countered with atropine 1-2 mg intravenously and/or a cardiac pacemaker. If necessary, this may be followed by a bolus dose of glucagon 10 mg intravenously. If required, this may be repeated or followed by an intravenous infusion of glucagon 1-10 mg/hour depending on response. If no response to glucagon occurs or if glucagon is unavailable, a beta adrenoceptor stimulant such as dobutamine 2.5 to 10 micrograms/kg/minute by intravenous infusion may be given.

Dobutamine, because of its positive inotropic effect could also be used to treat hypotension and acute cardiac insufficiency. It is likely that these doses would be inadequate to reverse the cardiac effects of beta blockade if a large overdose has been taken. The dose of dobutamine should therefore be increased if necessary to achieve the required response according to the clinical condition of the patient.

Administration of calcium ions may also be considered. Bronchospasm can usually be reversed by bronchodilators.

5. PHARMACOLOGICAL PROPERTIES

5.1 Pharmacodynamic properties

Pharmacotherapeutic group: Beta blocking agents, selective

ATC code: C07AB02

Metoprolol is a competitive beta-adrenoceptor antagonist. It acts preferentially to inhibit beta-adrenoceptors (conferring some cardioselectivity), is devoid of intrinsic sympathomimetic activity (partial agonist activity) and possesses beta-adrenoceptor blocking activity comparable in potency with propranolol.

A negative chronotrophic effect on the heart is a consistent feature of metoprolol administration. Thus, cardiac output and systolic blood pressure rapidly decrease following acute administration.

The intention to treat trial COMMIT included 45,852 patients admitted to hospital within 24 hours of the onset of symptoms of suspected acute myocardial infarction with supporting ECG abnormalities (i.e. ST elevation, ST depression or left bundle-branch block). Patients were randomly allocated to metoprolol (up to 15 mg intravenous then 200 mg oral) or placebo and treated until discharge or up to 4 weeks in hospital. The two co-primary outcomes were: (1) composite of death, reinfarction or cardiac arrest; and (2) death from any cause during the scheduled treatment period. Neither of the co-primary outcomes was significantly reduced by metoprolol. However, metoprolol treatment was associated with fewer people having reinfarction and ventricular fibrillation but an increased rate of cardiogenic shock during the first day after admission. There was substantial net hazard in haemodynamically unstable patients. There was moderate net benefit in those who were stable, particularly after days 0-1.

5.2 Pharmacokinetic properties

Metoprolol is eliminated mainly by hepatic metabolism, the average elimination half-life is 3.5 hours (range 1-9 hours). Rates of metabolism vary between individuals, with poor metabolisers (approximately 10%) showing higher plasma concentrations and slower elimination than extensive metabolisers. Within individuals, however, plasma concentrations are stable and reproducible.

Metoprolol undergoes oxidative metabolism in the liver primarily by the CYP2D6 isoenzyme.

5.3 Preclinical safety data

Pre-clinical information has not been included because the safety profile of metoprolol tartrate has been established after many years of clinical use. Please refer to section 4.

6. PHARMACEUTICAL PARTICULARS

6.1 List of excipients

Sodium chloride and water for injections.

6.2 Incompatibilities

None known.

6.3 Shelf life

4 years.

6.4 Special precautions for storage

Protect from light. Store below 25°C.

6.5 Nature and contents of container

5 ml glass ampoule.

6.6 Special precautions for disposal and other handling

None

7. MARKETING AUTHORISATION HOLDER

AstraZeneca UK Ltd.,

600 Capability Green,

Luton, LU1 3LU, UK.

8. MARKETING AUTHORISATION NUMBER(S)

PL 17901/0106

9. DATE OF FIRST AUTHORISATION/RENEWAL OF THE AUTHORISATION

Date of first authorisation: 28th May 2002

Date of renewal of authorisation: 16th July 2005

10. DATE OF REVISION OF THE TEXT

17th September 2008

Betaloc SA

(AstraZeneca UK Limited)

1. NAME OF THE MEDICINAL PRODUCT

Betaloc SA

2. QUALITATIVE AND QUANTITATIVE COMPOSITION

Metoprolol tartrate Ph. Eur. 200mg

3. PHARMACEUTICAL FORM

Extended release formulation (Durules®)

4. CLINICAL PARTICULARS

4.1 Therapeutic indications

In the management of angina pectoris and hypertension. Prophylaxis of migraine.

4.2 Posology and method of administration

Betaloc SA should be swallowed with liquid. Betaloc SA should not be chewed or crushed.

The dose of metoprolol must always be titrated and adjusted to the individual requirements of the patient using other suitable formulations and doses. The following are guidelines:

Hypertension

The recommended maintenance dosage in patients with hypertension is 100 – 200 mg daily. If needed, other antihypertensive agents may be added.

Angina Pectoris

The recommended maintenance dosage is 100 – 200 mg daily. If needed, other anti-anginal agents may be added.

Migraine Prophylaxis

The recommended dosage is 100 – 200 mg daily.

Impaired Renal Function

Dose adjustment is generally not needed in patients with impaired renal function.

Impaired Hepatic Function

Dose adjustment is normally not needed in patients suffering from liver cirrhosis because metoprolol has a low protein binding (5 – 10%). However, in patients with severe hepatic dysfunction a reduction in dosage may be necessary.

Elderly

Several studies indicate that age–related physiological changes have negligible effects on the pharmacokinetics of metoprolol. Dose adjustment is not needed in the elderly, but careful dose titration is important in all patients.

Children

The safety and efficacy of metoprolol in children has not been established.

4.3 Contraindications

Betaloc SA, as with other beta–blockers, should not be used in patients with any of the following:

- Hypotension,
- AV block of second- or third-degree,
- Decompensated cardiac failure (pulmonary oedema, hypoperfusion or hypotension),
- Continuous or intermittent inotropic therapy acting through beta–receptor agonism,
- Bradycardia (<45bpm),
- Sick-sinus syndrome,
- Cardiogenic shock,
- Severe peripheral arterial circulatory disorder,
- Untreated phaeochromocytoma,
- Metabolic acidosis.

Known hypersensitivity to any component of Betaloc SA o other beta–blockers.

Betaloc SA is also contra-indicated when suspected acute myocardial infarction is complicated by bradycardi (<45bpm), first-degree heart block or systolic blood pres sure <100mmHg and/or severe heart failure.

4.4 Special warnings and precautions for use

Betaloc SA as with other beta–blockers:

- should not be withdrawn abruptly. When possible, Betaloc should be withdrawn gradually over a period of 10-14 days, in diminishing doses to 25 mg daily for the last 6 days. During its withdrawal patients should be kept under close surveillance, especially those with known ischaemic heart disease. The risk for coronary events, including sudden death, may increase during the withdrawal of beta-blockade.
- must be reported to the anaesthetist prior to general anaesthesia. It is not generally recommended to stop Betaloc treatment in patients undergoing surgery. If withdrawal of metoprolol is considered desirable, this should, if possible, be completed at least 48 hours before general anaesthesia. However, in some patients it may be desirable to employ a beta-blocker as premedication. By shielding the heart against the effects of stress, the beta-blocker may prevent excessive sympathetic stimulation provoking cardiac arrhythmias or acute coronary insufficiency. If a beta-blocker is given for this purpose, an anaesthetic with little negative inotropic activity should be selected to minimise the risk of myocardial depression.
- although contra–indicated in severe peripheral arterial circulatory disturbances (see Section 4.3), may also aggravate less severe peripheral arterial circulatory disorders.
- may be administered when heart failure has been controlled. Digitalisation and/or diuretic therapy should also be considered for patients with a history of heart failure, or patients known to have a poor cardiac reserve. Betaloc should be used with caution in patients where cardiac reserve is poor.
- may cause patients to develop increasing bradycardia, in such cases the Betaloc SA dosage should be reduced or gradually withdrawn.
- due to the negative effect on conduction time, should only be given with caution to patients with first-degree heart block.
- may increase the number and duration of angina attacks in patients with Prinzmetal's angina, due to unopposed alpha–receptor mediated coronary artery vasoconstriction. Betaloc SA is a beta$_1$–selective beta–blocker; consequently, its use may be considered although utmost caution must be exercised.
- may mask the early signs of acute hypoglycaemia, in particular tachycardia. During treatment with Betaloc SA, the risk of interfering with carbohydrate metabolism or masking hypoglycaemia is less than with non–selective beta–blockers.
- may mask the symptoms of thyrotoxicosis.
- may increase both the sensitivity towards allergens and the seriousness of anaphylactic reactions.

Although cardioselective beta-blockers may have less effect on lung function than non-selective beta-blockers, as with all beta-blockers these should be avoided in patients with reversible obstructive airways disease unless there are compelling clinical reasons for their use. When administration is necessary, these patients should be kept under close surveillance. The use of a beta$_2$-bronchodilator (e.g. terbutaline) may be advisable in some patients. The dosage of the beta$_2$ agonist may require an increase when treatment with Betaloc SA is commenced.

The label shall state - "If you have a history of wheezing, asthma or any other breathing difficulties, you must tell your doctor before you take this medicine."

Like all beta-blockers, careful consideration should be given to patients with psoriasis before Betaloc SA is administered.

In the presence of liver cirrhosis the bioavailability of Betaloc SA may be increased

In patients with a phaeochromocytoma, an alpha-blocker should be given concomitantly.

In labile and insulin-dependent diabetes it may be necessary to adjust the hypoglycaemic therapy.

Intravenous administration of calcium antagonists of the verapamil type should not be given to patients treated with beta-blockers.

4.5 Interaction with other medicinal products and other forms of interaction

Metoprolol is a metabolic substrate for the Cytochrome P450 isoenzyme CYP2D6. Drugs that act as enzyme–inducing and enzyme–inhibiting substances may exert an influence on the plasma level of metoprolol. Enzyme–inducing agents (e.g. rifampicin) may reduce plasma concentrations of Betaloc, whereas enzyme inhibitors (e.g. cimetidine, alcohol and hydralazine) may increase plasma concentrations.

Patients receiving concomitant treatment with sympathetic ganglion blocking agents, other beta-blockers (i.e. eye rops), or Mono Amine Oxidase (MAO) inhibitors should be ept under close surveillance.

concomitant treatment with clonidine is to be discontin-ed, Betaloc SA should be withdrawn several days before onidine.

ıcreased negative inotropic and chronotropic effects may ccur when metoprolol is given together with calcium ntagonists of the verapamil and diltiazem type. In patients eated with beta-blockers, intravenous administration of alcium antagonists of the verapamil-type should not be iven.

3eta-blockers may enhance the negative inotropic and egative dromotropic effect of antiarrhythmic agents (of he quinidine type and amiodarone).

)igitalis glycosides, in association with beta-blockers, may ıcrease atrioventricular conduction time and may induce oradycardia.

n patients receiving beta-blocker therapy, inhalation ınaesthetics enhance the cardiodepressant effect.

Concomitant treatment with indometacin and other pros-taglandin synthetase inhibiting drugs may reduce the anti-hypertensive effect of beta-blockers.

The administration of adrenaline (epinephrine) to patients undergoing beta-blockade can result in an increase in blood pressure and bradycardia although this is less likely to occur with $beta_1$-selective drugs.

Betaloc SA will antagonise the $beta_1$-effects of sympatho-mimetic agents but should have little influence on the bronchodilator effects of $beta_2$-agonists at normal thera-peutic doses.

Metoprolol may impair the elimination of lidocaine.

As with other beta-blockers, concomitant therapy with dihydropyridines e.g. nifedipine, may increase the risk of hypotension, and cardiac failure may occur in patients with latent cardiac insufficiency.

The dosages of oral antidiabetic agents and also of insulin may have to be readjusted in patients receiving beta-blockers.

As beta-blockers may affect the peripheral circulation, care should be exercised when drugs with similar activity e.g. ergotamine are given concurrently.

The effects of Betaloc SA and other drugs with an anti-hypertensive effect on blood pressure are usually additive. Care should be taken when combining with other antihy-pertensive drugs or drugs that might reduce blood pres-sure such as tricyclic antidepressants, barbiturates and phenothiazines. However, combinations of antihyperten-sive drugs may often be used with benefit to improve control of hypertension.

4.6 Pregnancy and lactation

Pregnancy

Betaloc SA should not be used in pregnancy or nursing mothers unless the physician considers that the benefit outweighs the possible hazard to the foetus/infant. Beta blockers reduce placental perfusion, which may result in intrauterine foetal death, immature and premature deliv-eries. As with all beta-blockers, Betaloc SA may cause side-effects, especially bradycardia and hypoglycaemia in the foetus, and in the newborn and breastfed infant. There is an increased risk of cardiac and pulmonary complica-tions in the neonate. Betaloc SA has, however, been used in pregnancy-associated hypertension under close super-vision, after 20 weeks gestation. Although Betaloc SA crosses the placental barrier and is present in cord blood, no evidence of foetal abnormalities has been reported.

Lactation

Breast feeding is not recommended. The amount of meto-prolol ingested via breast milk should not produce signifi-cant beta-blocking effects in the neonate if the mother is treated with normal therapeutic doses.

4.7 Effects on ability to drive and use machines

When driving vehicles or operating machines, it should be taken into account that occasionally dizziness or fatigue may occur.

4.8 Undesirable effects

The following events have been reported as adverse events in clinical trials or reported from routine use.

The following definitions of frequencies are used:

Very common ($\geqslant$10%), common (1 – 9.9 %), uncommon (0.1 – 0.9%), rare (0.01 – 0.09%) and very rare (<0.01%).

Infections and infestations

Very rare: Gangrene in patients with pre existing severe peripheral circulatory disorders.

Blood and lymphatic system disorders

Very rare: Thrombocytopenia.

Psychiatric disorders

Uncommon: Depression, insomnia, nightmares.

Rare: Nervousness, anxiety.

Very rare: Confusion, hallucinations.

Nervous system disorders

Common: Dizziness, headache.

Uncommon: Concentration impairment, somnolence, paraesthesiae.

Very rare: Amnesia/memory impairment, taste distur-bances.

Eye disorders

Rare: Disturbances of vision, dry and/or irritated eyes, conjunctivitis.

Ear and labyrinth disorders

Very rare: Tinnitus.

Cardiac disorders

Common: Bradycardia, palpitations.

Uncommon: Deterioration of heart failure symptoms, first degree heart block.

Rare: Disturbances of cardiac conduction, cardiac arrhyth-mias, increased existing AV block.

Vascular disorders

Common: Postural disorders (very rarely with syncope).

Rare: Raynauds phenomenon.

Very rare: Increase of pre-existing intermittent claudica-tion.

Respiratory, thoracic and mediastinal disorders

Common: Dyspnoea on exertion.

Uncommon: Bronchospasm.

Rare: Rhinitis.

Gastrointestinal disorders

Common: Nausea, abdominal pain, diarrhoea, constipa-tion.

Uncommon: Vomiting.

Rare: Dry mouth.

Hepato-biliary disorders

Very rare: Hepatitis.

Skin and subcutaneous tissue disorders

Uncommon: Rash (in the form of psoriasiform urticaria and dystrophic skin lesions), increased sweating.

Rare: Loss of hair.

Very rare: Photosensitivity reactions, aggravated psoriasis.

Musculoskeletal and connective tissue disorders

Very rare: Arthralgia.

Uncommon: Muscle cramps.

Reproductive system and breast disorders

Rare: Impotence/sexual dysfunction.

General disorders and administration site disorders

Very common: Fatigue.

Common: Cold hands and feet.

Uncommon: Precordial pain, oedema.

Investigations

Uncommon: Weight gain.

Rare: Liver function test abnormalities, positive anti-nuclear antibodies (not associated with SLE).

4.9 Overdose

The symptoms of overdose may include bradycardia, hypotension, acute cardiac insufficiency and bronchos-pasm.

General treatment should include:

Close supervision, treatment in an intensive care ward, the use of gastric lavage, activated charcoal and a laxative to prevent absorption of any drug still present in the gastro-intestinal tract, the use of plasma or plasma substitutes to treat hypotension and shock.

Excessive bradycardia can be countered with atropine 1-2 mg intravenously and/or a cardiac pacemaker. If neces-sary, this may be followed by a bolus dose of glucagon 10 mg intravenously. If required, this may be repeated or followed by an intravenous infusion of glucagon 1-10 mg/hour depending on response. If no response to glucagon occurs or if glucagon is unavailable, a beta adrenoceptor stimulant such as dobutamine 2.5 to 10 micrograms/kg/minute by intravenous infusion may be given.

Dobutamine, because of its positive inotropic effect could also be used to treat hypotension and acute cardiac insuf-ficiency. It is likely that these doses would be inadequate to reverse the cardiac effects of beta blockade if a large overdose has been taken. The dose of dobutamine should therefore be increased if necessary to achieve the required response according to the clinical condition of the patient.

Administration of calcium ions may also be considered. Bronchospasm can usually be reversed by bronchodila-tors.

5. PHARMACOLOGICAL PROPERTIES

5.1 Pharmacodynamic properties

Metoprolol is a competitive beta-adrenoceptor antagonist. It acts preferentially to inhibit $beta_1$-adrenoceptors (con-ferring some cardioselectivity), is devoid of intrinsic sym-pathomimetic activity (partial agonist activity) and possesses beta-adrenoceptor blocking activity compar-able in potency with propranolol.

A negative chronotropic effect on the heart is a consistent feature of metoprolol administration. Thus cardiac output and systolic blood pressure rapidly decrease following acute administration.

5.2 Pharmacokinetic properties

Metoprolol is almost completely absorbed over a large part of the gastrointestinal tract, but bioavailability after oral administration is 40-50% of that after i.v. injection, because of hepatic first pass metabolism. The bioavail-ability of metoprolol after CR tablet administration is about 70% of that after plain tablets.

The steady state V_D of metoprolol is 3.2 L/kg and protein binding is about 12%.

Metoprolol undergoes oxidative metabolism in the liver primarily by the CYP2D6 isoenzyme.

Elimination half life of metoprolol is usually between about 3 and 5 hours. Elimination is by liver metabolism and metabolites are largely inactive. With metoprolol CR T_{max} is prolonged to about 8 hours. Mean C_{max} after Betaloc SA was 519 nmol/L, achieved after 4 hours. Plasma levels at 24 hours were about 85 nmol/L after Betaloc SA.

Initial absorption of metoprolol CR was more rapid and AUC increased when given together with food.

Urine recovery of unchanged drug was about 4% after metoprolol CR and metoprolol plain tablets. The pharma-cokinetics and beta-blocking effect of metoprolol are not significantly altered in patients with renal failure.

In healthy elderly volunteers there was no significant dif-ference in the volume of distribution, elimination half life, total body clearance or bioavailability of metoprolol com-pared with young volunteers.

In patients with cirrhosis of the liver the bioavailability of metoprolol was increased and total body clearance reduced.

5.3 Preclinical safety data

There is no toxicity data that would indicate that metoprolol tartrate is unsafe for use in the indications given. Signs in rats and dogs indicate that metoprolol can exert a cardi-opressive action at high plasma levels.

6. PHARMACEUTICAL PARTICULARS

6.1 List of excipients

Sodium aluminium silicate, paraffin, magnesium stearate, ethylcellulose, ethanol (used during manufacture), hydro-xypropyl methylcellulose, polyethylene glycol, titanium dioxide (E171), hydrogen peroxide (30%) and water pur-ified.

6.2 Incompatibilities

None known

6.3 Shelf life

5 years.

6.4 Special precautions for storage

Store below 25°C.

6.5 Nature and contents of container

Blister strips (press through packs of thermoformed PVC) 7 tablets per strip - pack size 28.

Securitainers of 300 tablets.

6.6 Special precautions for disposal and other handling

Not applicable

7. MARKETING AUTHORISATION HOLDER

AstraZeneca UK Ltd.,
600 Capability Green,
Luton, LU1 3LU, UK.

8. MARKETING AUTHORISATION NUMBER(S)

PL 17901/0107

9. DATE OF FIRST AUTHORISATION/RENEWAL OF THE AUTHORISATION

28th May 2002 / 16th July 2005

10. DATE OF REVISION OF THE TEXT

12th August 2008

Betesil 2.250mg Medicated Plaster

(Genus Pharmaceuticals)

1. NAME OF THE MEDICINAL PRODUCT

BETESIL 2.250 mg medicated plaster.

2. QUALITATIVE AND QUANTITATIVE COMPOSITION

Each 7.5 cm × 10 cm medicated plaster contains:

2.250 mg of betamethasone valerate (corresponding to 1.845 mg of betamethasone).

For a full list of excipients, see section 6.1.

3. PHARMACEUTICAL FORM

Medicated plaster.

Colourless plaster.

4. CLINICAL PARTICULARS

4.1 Therapeutic indications

Treatment of inflammatory skin disorders which do not respond to treatment with less potent corticosteroids, such as eczema, lichenification, lichen planus, granuloma annu-lare, palmoplantar pustulosis and mycosis fungoides.

Due to its particular pharmaceutical form, BETESIL is suitable for chronic plaque psoriasis localized in difficult to treat areas (e.g. knees, elbows and anterior face of the tibia on an area not greater than 5% of the body surface).

4.2 Posology and method of administration

Posology

Adults

Apply the medicated plaster to the skin area to be treated once a day. Do not exceed the maximum daily dose of six medicated plasters and the maximum treatment period of 30 days.

A new medicated plaster must be applied every 24 hours. It is also advisable to wait at least 30 minutes between one application and the next.

Once an appreciable improvement has been obtained, you can discontinue the application and possibly continue the treatment with a less potent corticosteroid.

Children

The safety and efficacy of this medicinal product have not been shown in children; until sufficient data has been acquired, limit use of BETESIL to adults.

Method of administration

Cleanse and carefully dry the area to be treated before each application so that the medicated plaster adheres well to the skin.

Open the sachet containing the medicated plaster and cut the plaster, if necessary, so that it fits the area to be treated. Peel off the protective film and apply the adhesive medicated part to the area concerned.

Any unused part of the plaster should be put back into the sachet so that it keeps and can be used at the next application (see section 6.3).

The medicated plaster must not be removed and reused.

Once the medicated plaster has been applied, the skin must not come in contact with water. It is advisable to take a bath or have a shower between applications.

Furthermore, if the medicated plaster is applied to particularly mobile parts (e.g. an elbow or knee) and its edges start to lift, it is advisable to apply a small adhesive tape to the detached part only.

Never cover the medicated plaster completely with occlusive material or dressing.

4.3 Contraindications

Hypersensitivity to the active substance or to any of the excipients.

Cutaneous tuberculosis and viral skin infections (including vaccinia pustules, herpes zoster and herpes simplex). Exudative lesions and primary skin infections caused by fungi or bacteria. Acne, acne rosacea, perioral dermatitis, skin ulcers, burns and frostbite.

Do not apply to face.

Do not use on patients under 18 years of age.

4.4 Special warnings and precautions for use

In general, use of topical corticosteroids on large areas of the body and for prolonged periods, as well as the use of occlusive dressing can cause a temporary suppression of the hypothalamus-pituitary-adrenal axis, leading to secondary hypoadrenalism and adrenal hypercorticism, including the Cushing's syndrome. In these situations, treatment should be discontinued gradually and under strict control of a doctor due to the risk of acute adrenal insufficiency.

Sudden withdrawal of the treatment in psoriatic patients, may also lead to symptoms exacerbation or generalized pustular psoriasis.

Prolonged use of BETESIL in diffuse psoriasis (except for the treatment of isolated plaques) or diffuse eczema or application on lesions located in skin folds is not recommended, as these conditions may increase systemic absorption. The use of occlusive bandages, especially with plastic material, may increase this effect. The symptoms of this are: facial redness, weight changes (fat increase in body and face and loss in legs and arms), reddish streaks on stomach, headache, menstrual alterations, or an increase in unwanted face and body hair. In this regard, it is known that certain skin areas (face, eyelids, armpits, scalp and scrotum) absorb more easily than others (skin on the knees, elbows, palms of the hands and feet on soles).

Application of topical medicinal products, especially if prolonged, may give rise to hypersensitivity reaction. Skin atrophy has also been reported after three-week treatment periods.

In case of drug intolerance, for example if skin irritation or contact dermatitis occur during treatment, it is necessary to stop the medicated plaster application and start suitable treatment (see section 4.8 "Undesirable effects").

Corticosteroids may affect the results of the nitroblue tetrazolium test (NBT) for diagnosing bacterial infections by producing false negatives.

Medicinal products containing corticosteroids must be used with caution in patients with impaired immune system function (T-lymphocytes) or in those being treated with immunosuppressive therapy.

The product contains methyl parahydroxybenzoate and propyl parahydroxybenzoate, which may cause hypersensitivity reactions (possibly delayed).

4.5 Interaction with other medicinal products and other forms of interaction

At recommended doses, Betamethasone valerate for topical use is not known to cause medically significant drug interactions. BETESIL did not show significant systemic absorption of betamethasone valerate.

4.6 Pregnancy and lactation

Pregnancy

Topical administration of corticosteroids to pregnant laboratory animals may cause impairment of foetal maturation. The importance of this preclinical data has not been evaluated in humans: however, topical steroids must not be used in pregnant women on large areas of skin and specifically, in large quantities or for long period of time. Therefore, this medicinal product must only be used in case of need and under direct medical control, after having assessed the real benefits for the mother against the possible risks for the foetus and having evaluated the treatment period and the size of the skin area to be treated.

Lactation

Systemic corticosteroids are excreted in human breast milk. It is unknown whether topical corticosteroids are excreted in human breast milk.

Therefore topical corticosteroids should be used with caution also in nursing women and should not be applied to the breast.

4.7 Effects on ability to drive and use machines

There are neither assumptions, nor evidences that the drug may affect attentiveness or reaction times.

4.8 Undesirable effects

The commonly reported adverse reactions are skin and subcutaneous tissue disorders, occurring in about 15% of patients treated. These undesirable effects are mainly due to the pharmacological effects of the medicinal product. They are local effects on the skin in the plaster application area. No systemic effects have been observed.

The following list of adverse reactions has been observed during controlled clinical trials.

Reported adverse reactions have been classified according to their frequency of observation using the following convention: very common ($\geq$1/10); common ($\geq$1/100, $\leq$1/10), uncommon ($\geq$1/1,000, $\leq$1/100); rare ($\geq$1/10,000, $\leq$1/1,000); very rare ($\leq$1/10,000), including isolated cases.

All cases reported were found to be common. Within each frequency grouping, adverse reactions are presented in order of decreasing seriousness.

Skin and subcutaneous tissue disorders	Common	Skin atrophy Telangiectasia Pustules Papules Furuncle Erythema Pruritus Skin erosion

Other undesirable reactions not observed with BETESIL, but reported with topical corticosteroids are: contact dermatitis, hypersensitivity, oedema, purpura, striae atrophicae, dry skin, skin exfoliation, capillary fragility, skin irritation, hypertrichosis, hyperaesthesia, perioral dermatitis, burning or stretching sensation, folliculitis and skin hypopigmentation.

The use of topical corticosteroids on large areas of the body and for long periods, as well as the use of occlusive dressing can cause temporary suppression of the hypothalamus-pituitary-adrenal axis, leading to secondary hypoadrenalism and adrenal hypercorticism, including the Cushing's syndrome. In these situations, treatment should be discontinued gradually and under strict control of a doctor due to the risk of acute adrenal insufficiency.

Sudden withdrawal of the treatment in psoriatic patients, may also lead to symptoms exacerbation or generalized pustular psoriasis (see section 4.4 "Special warnings and precautions for use").

Hypersensitivity reactions to occlusive plastic material have been observed rarely.

4.9 Overdose

No case of overdose has been reported.

Due to the product characteristics and the route of administration, the occurrence of symptoms and signs of corticosteroid overdose is unlikely.

However, prolonged use of topical corticosteroids may cause the temporary suppression of the hypothalamus-pituitary-adrenal axis, leading to secondary hypoadrenalism. Adrenal hypercorticism symptoms spontaneously reverse and their treatment is symptomatic. If necessary, act to restore the hydroelectrolytic balance. In the event of chronic toxicity, remove the corticosteroid from the organism slowly.

5. PHARMACOLOGICAL PROPERTIES

5.1 Pharmacodynamic properties

Pharmacotherapeutic group: Corticosteroids, dermatological products: active corticosteroids (group III). ATC code: D07AC01.

Betamethasone valerate for topical application is active in the treatment of dermatosis, which responds to corticosteroids, due to its anti-inflammatory, antipruriginous and vasoconstrictor action.

5.2 Pharmacokinetic properties

Corticosteroids applied to the skin are mainly held back b[y] the stratum corneum, and only a small part reaches th[e] dermis where they can be absorbed. Several factors ma[y] however favour greater absorption: the location and area o[f] the skin to be treated, the type of lesion, the treatmen[t] duration and any occlusive dressing.

Betamethasone valerate is mainly metabolized in the liver where it is inactivated. It is then conjugated in the liver an[d] kidneys with sulphate or glycuronic acid and excreted i[n] urine.

5.3 Preclinical safety data

There are no significant data from preclinical trials, which may be relevant to physicians other than those already reported in other sections of the Summary of Product Characteristics.

6. PHARMACEUTICAL PARTICULARS

6.1 List of excipients

Plaster: unwoven cloth (polypropylene/polyethylene and rayon fibres) laminated with an ethylene-methyl methacrylate copolymer film.

Adhesive layer: sodium hyaluronate, 1,3-butylene glycol, glycerol, disodium edetate, tartaric acid, aluminium glycinate, polyacrylic acid, sodium polyacrylate, hydroxypropylcellulose, carmellose sodium, methyl parahydroxybenzoate, propyl parahydroxybenzoate, purified water.

Protective film: polyethylene terephthalate film.

6.2 Incompatibilities

Not applicable.

6.3 Shelf life

3 years.

After opening the sachet: 1 month.

6.4 Special precautions for storage

Do not store above 25 °C.

Store the medicated plaster in its original sachet in order to preserve its integrity.

6.5 Nature and contents of container

Boxes: 4 medicated plasters / 8 medicated plasters / 16 medicated plasters

Each medicated plaster is packed individually in a paper/ polyethylene/ aluminium/ ethylene-methacrylic acid copolymer sachet.

Not all pack sizes may be marketed

6.6 Special precautions for disposal and other handling

No special requirements

Used medicated plasters must not be flushed down toilets. Plasters should be disposed of in accordance with local requirements.

7. MARKETING AUTHORISATION HOLDER

IBSA FARMACEUTICI ITALIA S.r.l. – Via Martiri di Cefalonia, 2 – 26900 Lodi (ITALY)

8. MARKETING AUTHORISATION NUMBER(S)

PL 21039 / 0009

9. DATE OF FIRST AUTHORISATION/RENEWAL OF THE AUTHORISATION

12/03/2007 (first authorisation) – 09/10/2011 (renewal)

10. DATE OF REVISION OF THE TEXT

6 March 2009

Betnovate Cream

(GlaxoSmithKline UK)

1. NAME OF THE MEDICINAL PRODUCT

Betnovate Cream

2. QUALITATIVE AND QUANTITATIVE COMPOSITION

Betamethasone Valerate BP 0.122% $^{W}/_{w}$

3. PHARMACEUTICAL FORM

Aqueous Cream

4. CLINICAL PARTICULARS

4.1 Therapeutic indications

Betamethasone valerate is an active topical corticosteroid which produces a rapid response in those inflammatory dermatoses that are normally responsive to topical corticosteroid therapy, and is often effective in the less responsive conditions such as psoriasis.

Betnovate preparations are indicated for the treatment of eczema in children and adults, including atopic and discoid eczemas, prurigo nodularis, psoriasis (excluding widespread plaque psoriasis); neurodermatoses, including lichen simplex, lichen planus; seborrhoeic dermatitis; contact sensitivity reactions; discoid lupus erythematosus and they may be used as an adjunct to systemic steroid therapy in generalised erythroderma.

4.2 Posology and method of administration

A small quantity of Betnovate should be applied gently to the affected area two or three times daily until improvement occurs. It may then be possible to maintain improvement by applying once a day, or even less often, or by using the appropriate ready-diluted (1 in 4) preparation Betnovate

.D. If no improvement is seen within two to four weeks, eassessment of the diagnosis, or referral, may be necessary.

etnovate and Betnovate R.D. creams are especially ppropriate for dry, lichenified or scaly lesions, but this is ot invariably so.

n the more recent resistant lesions, such as the thickened laques of psoriasis on elbows and knees, the effect of etnovate can be enhanced, if necessary, by occluding the reatment area with polythene film. Overnight occlusion nly is usually adequate to bring about a satisfactory esponse in such lesions; thereafter improvement can sually be maintained by regular application without occluion.

hildren

ourses should be limited to five days. Occlusion should ot be used.

or topical administration.

.3 Contraindications

Rosacea, acne and perioral dermatitis. Primary cutaneous iral infections (e.g. herpes simplex, chickenpox). Hypersensitivity to any component of the preparation.

he use of Betnovate skin preparations is not indicated in he treatment of primarily infected skin lesions caused by nfections with fungi (e.g. candidiasis, tinea); or bacteria e.g. impetigo); primary or secondary infections due to easts; peri-anal and genital pruritus; dermatoses in children under 1 year of age, including dermatitis and napkin eruptions.

.4 Special warnings and precautions for use

ong-term continuous topical therapy should be avoided where possible, particularly in infants and children, as adrenal suppression, with or without clinical features of Cushing's syndrome, can occur even without occlusion. In this situation, topical steroids should be discontinued gradually under medical supervision because of the risk of adrenal insufficiency (see section 4.8 Undesirable Effects and Section 4.9 Overdose).

The face, more than other areas of the body, may exhibit atrophic changes after prolonged treatment with potent topical corticosteroids. This must be borne in mind when treating such conditions as psoriasis, discoid lupus erythematosus and severe eczema. If applied to the eyelids, care is needed to ensure that the preparation does not enter the eye, as glaucoma might result.

If used in childhood, or on the face, courses should be limited to five days and occlusion should not be used.

Topical corticosteroids may be hazardous in psoriasis for a number of reasons including rebound relapses, development of tolerance, risk of generalised pustular psoriasis and development of local or systemic toxicity due to impaired barrier function of the skin. If used in psoriasis careful patient supervision is important.

Appropriate antimicrobial therapy should be used whenever treating inflammatory lesions which have become infected. Any spread of infection requires withdrawal of topical corticosteroid therapy and systemic administration of antimicrobial agents. Bacterial infection is encouraged by the warm, moist conditions induced by occlusive dressings, and so the skin should be cleansed before a fresh dressing is applied.

Further Information

The least potent corticosteroid which will control the disease should be selected. None of these preparations contain lanolin. Betnovate Cream and Ointment and the corresponding RD preparations do not contain parabens. Betnovate Lotion contains parabens.

4.5 Interaction with other medicinal products and other forms of interaction

None known.

4.6 Pregnancy and lactation

There is inadequate evidence of safety in human pregnancy. Topical administration of corticosteroids to pregnant animals can cause abnormalities of foetal development including cleft palate and intra-uterine growth retardation. There may therefore be a very small risk of such effects in the human foetus.

4.7 Effects on ability to drive and use machines

None known

4.8 Undesirable effects

Adverse events are listed below by system organ class and frequency. Frequencies are defined as: very common (≥1/10), common (≥1/100 and <1/10), uncommon (≥1/1000 and <1/100), rare (≥1/10,000 and <1/1000) and very rare (<1/10,000) including isolated reports. Very common, common and uncommon events were generally determined from clinical trial data. The background rates in placebo and comparator groups were not taken into account when assigning frequency categories to adverse events derived from clinical trial data, since these rates were generally comparable to those in the active treatment group. Rare and very rare events were generally determined from spontaneous data.

Immune system disorders

Very rare: Hypersensitivity.

If signs of hypersensitivity appear, application should stop immediately.

Endocrine disorders

Very rare: Features of Cushing's syndrome

As with other topical corticosteroids, prolonged use of large amounts or treatment of extensive areas can result in sufficient systemic absorption to produce suppression of the HPA axis and the clinical features of Cushing's syndrome (see Section 4.4 Special Warnings and Precautions for use). These effects are more likely to occur in infants and children, and if occlusive dressings are used. In infants the napkin may act as an occlusive dressing.

Skin and subcutaneous tissue disorders

Common: Local skin burning and pruritus.

Very rare: Local atrophic changes in the skin such as thinning, striae and dilatation of the superficial blood vessels may be caused by prolonged and intensive treatment with highly active corticosteroid preparations, particularly when occlusive dressings are used or when skin folds are involved.

Pigmentation changes, hypertrichosis, allergic contact dermatitis, exacerbation of symptoms, pustular psoriasis (due to treatment of psoriasis with corticosteroids or its withdrawal: see Section 4.4. Special Warnings and Precautions for use)

4.9 Overdose

Acute overdosage is very unlikely to occur. However, in the case of chronic overdosage or misuse the features of Cushing's syndrome may appear and in this situation topical steroids should be discontinued gradually under medical supervision (see Section 4.4 Special Warnings and Precautions for use).

5. PHARMACOLOGICAL PROPERTIES

5.1 Pharmacodynamic properties

Betamethasone valerate is an active corticosteroid with topical anti-inflammatory activity.

5.2 Pharmacokinetic properties

The extent of percutaneous absorption of topical corticosteroids is determined by many factors including the vehicle, the integrity of the epidermal barrier, and the use of occlusive dressings.

Topical corticosteroids can be absorbed from normal intact skin. Inflammation and/or other disease processes in the skin increase percutaneous absorption. Occlusive dressings on the skin increase percutaneous absorption. Occlusive dressings substantially increase the percutaneous absorption of topical corticosteroids.

Once absorbed through the skin, topical corticosteroids are handled through pharmacokinetic pathways similar to systematically administered corticosteroids. Corticosteroids are bound to plasma proteins in varying degrees. Corticosteroids are metabolised primarily by the liver and are then excreted by the kidneys.

5.3 Preclinical safety data

There are no preclinical data of relevance to the prescriber which are additional to that in other sections of the SmPC.

6. PHARMACEUTICAL PARTICULARS

6.1 List of excipients

Chlorocresol	BP
Cetomacrogol 1000	BP
Cetostearyl Alcohol	BP
White Soft Paraffin	BP
Liquid Paraffin	BP
Sodium Acid Phosphate	BP
Phosphoric Acid	BP
Sodium Hydroxide	BP
Purified Water	BP

6.2 Incompatibilities

None known.

6.3 Shelf life

Tubes	36 Months
500gm pots	18 months

6.4 Special precautions for storage

Store below 25°C.

6.5 Nature and contents of container

15gm, 30gm and 100gm collapsible aluminium tubes internally coated with an epoxy resin based lacquer and closed with a cap.

500mg opaque high density polythene pots with black urea formaldehyde screw caps having a steran faced wad.

Not all pack sizes may be marketed

6.6 Special precautions for disposal and other handling

No special instructions.

Administrative Data

7. MARKETING AUTHORISATION HOLDER

Glaxo Wellcome UK Ltd.,

T/A GlaxoSmithKline UK

Stockley Park West,

Uxbridge,

Middlesex UB11 1BT

8. MARKETING AUTHORISATION NUMBER(S)

PL10949/0014

9. DATE OF FIRST AUTHORISATION/RENEWAL OF THE AUTHORISATION

24 October 1997

10. DATE OF REVISION OF THE TEXT

25th January 2005

Betnovate Lotion

(GlaxoSmithKline UK)

1. NAME OF THE MEDICINAL PRODUCT

Betnovate Lotion

2. QUALITATIVE AND QUANTITATIVE COMPOSITION

Betamethasone Valerate 0.122% w/w

3. PHARMACEUTICAL FORM

Lotion

4. CLINICAL PARTICULARS

4.1 Therapeutic indications

Betamethasone valerate is an active topical corticosteroid, which produces a rapid response in those inflammatory dermatoses that are normally responsive to topical corticosteroid therapy, and is often effective in the less responsive conditions such as psoriasis.

Betnovate preparations are indicated in the treatment of: eczema in children and adults; including atopic and discoid eczemas, prurigo nodularis; psoriasis (excluding widespread plaque psoriasis); neurodermatoses, including lichen simplex, lichen planus, seborrhoeic dermatitis; contact sensitivity reactions; discoid lupus erythematosus and they may be used as an adjunct to systemic steroid therapy in generalised erythroderma.

4.2 Posology and method of administration

A small quantity of Betnovate should be applied to the affected area two or three times daily until improvement occurs. It may then be possible to maintain improvement by applying once a day, or even less often. If no improvement is seen within two to four weeks, reassessment of the diagnosis or referral, may be necessary.

Betnovate lotion is particularly suitable when a minimal application to a large area is required.

In the more resistant lesions, such as the thickened plaques of psoriasis on elbows and knees, the effect of Betnovate can be enhanced, if necessary, by occluding the treatment area with polythene film. Overnight occlusion only is usually adequate to bring about a satisfactory response in such lesions. Thereafter improvement can usually be maintained by regular application without occlusion.

Children

Courses should be limited to five days if possible. Occlusion should not be used.

4.3 Contraindications

Rosacea, acne vulgaris and perioral dermatitis. Primary cutaneous viral infections (e.g. herpes simplex, chickenpox). Hypersensitivity to the preparation.

The use of Betnovate skin preparations is not indicated in the treatment of primarily infected skin lesions caused by infection with fungi (e.g. candidiasis, tinea); or bacteria (e.g. impetigo); primary or secondary infections due to yeast; perianal and genital pruritus; dermatoses in children under 1 year of age, including dermatitis and napkin eruptions.

4.4 Special warnings and precautions for use

Long-term continuous topical therapy should be avoided where possible, particularly in infants and children, as adrenal suppression, with or without clinical features of Cushing's syndrome, can occur even without occlusion. In this situation, topical steroids should be discontinued gradually under medical supervision because of the risk of adrenal insufficiency (see section 4.8 Undesirable Effects and Secion 4.9 Overdose).

The face, more than other areas of the body, may exhibit atrophic changes after prolonged treatment with potent topical corticosteroids. This must be borne in mind when treating such conditions as psoriasis, discoid lupus erythematosus and severe eczema. If applied to the eyelids, care is needed to ensure that the preparation does not enter the eye, as glaucoma might result.

If used in childhood, or on the face, courses should be limited to five days and occlusion should not be used.

Topical corticosteroids may be hazardous in psoriasis for a number of reasons including rebound relapses, development of tolerance, risk of generalised pustular psoriasis and development of local or systemic toxicity due to impaired barrier function of the skin. If used in psoriasis careful patient supervision is important.

Appropriate antimicrobial therapy should be used whenever treating inflammatory lesions, which have become infected. Any spread of infection requires withdrawal of topical corticosteroid therapy and systemic administration of antimicrobial agents.

Bacterial infection is encouraged by the warm moist conditions induced by occlusive dressings and so the skin should be cleansed before a fresh dressing is applied.

Further information:

The least potent corticosteroid, which will control the disease, should be selected. None of these preparations contain lanolin. Betnovate cream and ointment and the corresponding RD preparations do not contain parabens. Betnovate lotion contains parabens.

4.5 Interaction with other medicinal products and other forms of interaction

None known.

4.6 Pregnancy and lactation

There is inadequate evidence of safety in human pregnancy. Topical administration of corticosteroids to pregnant animals can cause abnormalities of foetal development including cleft palate and intrauterine growth retardation. There may therefore be a very small risk of such effects in the human foetus.

4.7 Effects on ability to drive and use machines

None known.

4.8 Undesirable effects

Adverse events are listed below by system organ class and frequency. Frequencies are defined as: very common (≥1/10), common (≥1/100 and <1/10), uncommon (≥1/1000 and <1/100), rare (≥1/10,000 and <1/1000) and very rare (<1/10,000) including isolated reports. Very common, common and uncommon events were generally determined from clinical trial data. The background rates in placebo and comparator groups were not taken into account when assigning frequency categories to adverse events derived from clinical trial data, since these rates were generally comparable to those in the active treatment group. Rare and very rare events were generally determined from spontaneous data.

Immune system disorders

Very rare: Hypersensitivity.

If signs of hypersensitivity appear, application should stop immediately.

Endocrine disorders

Very rare: Features of Cushing's syndrome

As with other topical corticosteroids, prolonged use of large amounts or treatment of extensive areas can result in sufficient systemic absorption to produce suppression of the HPA axis and the clinical features of Cushing's syndrome (see Section 4.4 Special Warnings and Precautions for use). These effects are more likely to occur in infants and children, and if occlusive dressings are used. In infants the napkin may act as an occlusive dressing.

Skin and subcutaneous tissue disorders

Common: Local skin burning and pruritus.

Very rare: Local atrophic changes in the skin such as thinning, striae and dilatation of the superficial blood vessels may be caused by prolonged and intensive treatment with highly active corticosteroid preparations, particularly when occlusive dressings are used or when skin folds are involved.

Pigmentation changes, hypertrichosis, allergic contact dermatitis, exacerbation of symptoms, pustular psoriasis (due to treatment of psoriasis with corticosteroids or its withdrawal: see Section 4.4. Special Warnings and Precautions for use)

4.9 Overdose

Acute overdosage is very unlikely to occur. However, in the case of chronic overdosage or misuse the features of Cushing's syndrome may appear and in this situation topical steroids should be discontinued gradually under medical supervision (see Section 4.4 Special Warnings and Precautions for use).

5. PHARMACOLOGICAL PROPERTIES

5.1 Pharmacodynamic properties

Betamethasone valerate is an active corticosteroid with topical anti-inflammatory activity.

5.2 Pharmacokinetic properties

The extent of percutaneous absorption of topical corticosteroid is determined by many factors including the vehicle, the integrity of the epidermal barrier, and the use of occlusive dressings.

Topical corticosteroids can be absorbed from normal intact skin. Inflammation and/or other disease processes in the skin increase percutaneous absorption. Occlusive dressings substantially increase the percutaneous absorption of topical corticosteroids.

Once absorbed through the skin, topical corticosteroids are handled through pharmacokinetic pathways similar to systemically administered corticosteroids. Corticosteroids are bound to plasma proteins in varying degrees. Corticosteroids are metabolised primarily by the liver and are then excreted by the kidneys.

5.3 Preclinical safety data

There are no preclinical data of relevance to the prescriber which are additional to that in other sections of the SmPC.

6. PHARMACEUTICAL PARTICULARS

6.1 List of excipients

Methyl Hydroxybenzoate BP

Xanthan Gum USP

Cetostearyl Alcohol BP

Liquid Paraffin BP

Isopropyl Alcohol BP

Glycerol BP

Cetomacrogol 1000 BP

Sodium citrate BP

Citric Acid Monohydrate BP

Purified Water BP

6.2 Incompatibilities

None known

6.3 Shelf life

36 months

6.4 Special precautions for storage

Store below 25°C

6.5 Nature and contents of container

Polyethylene squeeze bottle with a polyethylene nozzle and a polystyrene or polyethylene cap or

White High Density Polyethylene (HDPE) Hostalen GF4750 and Remafin white CEG 020 container with a polyethylene nozzle and a polystyrene or polyethylene cap.

Pack size: 20 ml; 100 ml

Not all pack sizes may be marketed.

6.6 Special precautions for disposal and other handling

No special instructions

7. MARKETING AUTHORISATION HOLDER

Glaxo Wellcome UK Limited

T/A Glaxo Laboratories and/or GlaxoSmithKline UK

Stockley Park West

Uxbridge

Middlesex

UB11 1BT

8. MARKETING AUTHORISATION NUMBER(S)

PL 10949/0044

9. DATE OF FIRST AUTHORISATION/RENEWAL OF THE AUTHORISATION

Date of first authorisation: 1 February 1993

Date of latest renewal: 26 September 2007

10. DATE OF REVISION OF THE TEXT

26 September 2007

Betnovate Ointment

(GlaxoSmithKline UK)

1. NAME OF THE MEDICINAL PRODUCT

Betnovate Ointment

2. QUALITATIVE AND QUANTITATIVE COMPOSITION

Betamethasone Valerate B.P. 0.122% w/w

3. PHARMACEUTICAL FORM

Ointment

4. CLINICAL PARTICULARS

4.1 Therapeutic indications

Betamethasone valerate is an active topical corticosteroid which provides a rapid response in those inflammatory dermatoses that are often effective in the less responsive conditions such as psoriasis.

Betnovate preparations are indicated for the treatment of: eczema in children and adults; including atopic and discoid eczemas, prurigo nodularis; psoriasis (excluding widespread plaque psoriasis); neurodermatoses, including lichen simplex, lichen planus; seborrhoeic dermatitis; contact sensitivity reactions; discoid lupus erythematosus and they may be used as an adjunct to systemic steroid therapy in generalised erythroderma.

4.2 Posology and method of administration

A small quantity of Betnovate should be applied to the affected area two or three times daily until improvement occurs. It may then be possible to maintain improvement by applying once a day, or even less often, or by using the appropriate ready diluted (1 in 4) preparation, Betnovate RD. If no improvement is seen within two to four weeks, reassessment of the diagnosis, or referral, may be necessary.

Betnovate and Betnovate RD ointments are especially appropriate for dry, lichenified or scaly lesions, but this is not invariably so.

In the more resistant lesions, such as the thickened plaques of psoriasis on elbows and knees, the effect of Betnovate can be enhanced, if necessary, by occluding the treatment area with polythene film. Overnight occlusion only is usually adequate to bring about a satisfactory response in such lesions; thereafter improvement can usually be maintained by regular application without occlusion.

Children

Courses should be limited to five days. Occlusion should not be used.

For topical administration.

4.3 Contraindications

Rosacea, acne vulgaris, perioral dermatitis, primary cutaneous viral infections (e.g. herpes simplex, chickenpox). Hypersensitivity to any component of the preparation.

The use of Betnovate skin preparations is not indicated in the treatment of primarily infected skin lesions caused by infections with fungi (e.g. candidiasis, tinea); or bacteria (e.g. impetigo); primary or secondary infections due to yeast; peri-anal and genital pruritus; dermatoses in children under 1 year of age, including dermatitis and napkin eruptions.

4.4 Special warnings and precautions for use

Long-term continuous topical therapy should be avoided where possible, particularly in infants and children, as adrenal suppression, with or without clinical features of Cushing's syndrome, can occur even without occlusion. In this situation, topical steroids should be discontinued gradually under medical supervision because of the risk of adrenal insufficiency (see section 4.8 Undesirable Effects and Section 4.9 Overdose).

The face, more than other areas of the body, may exhibit atrophic changes after prolonged treatment with potent topical corticosteroids. This must be borne in mind when treating such conditions as psoriasis, discoid lupus erythematosus and severe eczema. If applied to the eyelids, care is needed to ensure that the preparation does not enter the eye, as glaucoma might result.

If used in childhood, or on the face, courses should be limited to five days and occlusion should not be used.

Topical corticosteroids may be hazardous in psoriasis for a number of reasons including rebound relapses, development of tolerance, risk of generalised pustular psoriasis and development of local or systemic toxicity due to impaired barrier function of the skin. If used in psoriasis careful patient supervision is important.

Appropriate antimicrobial therapy should be used whenever treating inflammatory lesions which have become infected. Any spread of infection requires withdrawal of topical corticosteroid therapy and systemic administration of antimicrobial agents. Bacterial infection is encouraged by the warm, moist conditions induced by occlusive dressings, and so the skin should be cleansed before a fresh dressing is applied.

Further information:

The least potent corticosteroid, which will control the disease, should be selected. None of these preparations contain lanolin. Betnovate ointment and cream and the corresponding RD preparations do not contain parabens.

4.5 Interaction with other medicinal products and other forms of interaction

None known.

4.6 Pregnancy and lactation

There is inadequate evidence of safety in human pregnancy. Topical administration of corticosteroids to pregnant animals can cause abnormalities of foetal development including cleft palate and intrauterine growth retardation. There may therefore be a very small risk of such effects in the human foetus.

4.7 Effects on ability to drive and use machines

None known.

4.8 Undesirable effects

Adverse events are listed below by system organ class and frequency. Frequencies are defined as: very common (≥1/10), common (≥1/100 and <1/10), uncommon (≥1/1000 and <1/100), rare (≥1/10,000 and <1/1000) and very rare (<1/10,000) including isolated reports. Very common, common and uncommon events were generally determined from clinical trial data. The background rates in placebo and comparator groups were not taken into account when assigning frequency categories to adverse events derived from clinical trial data, since these rates were generally comparable to those in the active treatment group. Rare and very rare events were generally determined from spontaneous data.

Immune system disorders

Very rare: Hypersensitivity.

If signs of hypersensitivity appear, application should stop immediately.

Endocrine disorders

Very rare: Features of Cushing's syndrome.

As with other topical corticosteroids, prolonged use of large amounts or treatment of extensive areas can result in sufficient systemic absorption to produce suppression of the HPA axis and the clinical features of Cushing's syndrome (see Section 4.4 Special Warnings and Precautions for use). These effects are more likely to occur in infants and children, and if occlusive dressings are used. In infants the napkin may act as an occlusive dressing.

Skin and subcutaneous tissue disorders

Common: Local skin burning and pruritus.

Very rare: Local atrophic changes in the skin such as thinning, striae and dilatation of the superficial blood essels may be caused by prolonged and intensive treatment with highly active corticosteroid preparations, particularly when occlusive dressings are used or when skin folds are involved.

Pigmentation changes, hypertrichosis, allergic contact dermatitis, exacerbation of symptoms, pustular psoriasis (due to treatment of psoriasis with corticosteroids or its withdrawal: see Section 4.4. Special Warnings and Precautions for use)

4.9 Overdose
Acute overdosage is very unlikely to occur. However, in the case of chronic overdosage or misuse the features of Cushing's syndrome may appear and in this situation topical steroids should be discontinued gradually under medical supervision (see Section 4.4 Special Warnings and Precautions for use).

5. PHARMACOLOGICAL PROPERTIES

5.1 Pharmacodynamic properties
Bethamethasone valerate is an active corticosteroid with topical anti-inflammatory activity.

5.2 Pharmacokinetic properties
The extent of percutaneous absorption of topical corticosteroid is determined by many factors including the vehicle, the integrity of the epidermal barrier, and the use of occlusive dressings.

Topical corticosteroids can be absorbed from normal intact skin. Inflammation and/or other disease processes in the skin increase percutaneous absorption. Occlusive dressings substantially increase the percutaneous absorption of topical corticosteroids.

Once absorbed through the skin, topical corticosteroids are handled through pharmacokinetic pathways similar to systematically administered corticosteroids. Corticosteroids are bound to plasma proteins in varying degrees. Corticosteroids are metabolised primarily by the liver and are then excreted by the kidneys.

5.3 Preclinical safety data
There are no preclinical data of relevance to the prescriber which are additional to that in other sections of the SmPC.

6. PHARMACEUTICAL PARTICULARS

6.1 List of excipients
Liquid Paraffin BP
White Soft Paraffin BP

6.2 Incompatibilities
None known

6.3 Shelf life
Tubes 36 months
Pump Dispenser 24 months

6.4 Special precautions for storage
Tubes Store below 30°C
Pump Dispenser Store below 25°C

6.5 Nature and contents of container
30 gm and 100 gm collapsible aluminium tubes internally coated with an epoxy resin based lacquer and closed with a polypropylene cap.

100 gm polypropylene/polyethylene pump dispenser with natural (translucent) polypropylene body. The nozzle is sealed with a polyethylene acetyl tab. The pump is closed with an opaque polypropylene overcap and overwrapped with an opaque shrink-wrap.

Not all pack sizes may be marketed

6.6 Special precautions for disposal and other handling
No special instructions

7. MARKETING AUTHORISATION HOLDER
Glaxo Wellcome UK Limited
T/A Glaxo Laboratories and/or GlaxoSmithKline UK
Stockley Park West
Uxbridge
Middlesex
UB11 1BT

8. MARKETING AUTHORISATION NUMBER(S)
PL 10949/0020

9. DATE OF FIRST AUTHORISATION/RENEWAL OF THE AUTHORISATION
Date of first authorisation: 24 February 1995
Date of latest renewal: 26 September 2007

10. DATE OF REVISION OF THE TEXT
26 September 2007

Betnovate RD Cream

(GlaxoSmithKline UK)

1. NAME OF THE MEDICINAL PRODUCT
Betnovate RD Cream

2. QUALITATIVE AND QUANTITATIVE COMPOSITION
Betamethasone Valerate B.P. Equivalent to Betamethasone 0.025%.

3. PHARMACEUTICAL FORM
Cream

4. CLINICAL PARTICULARS

4.1 Therapeutic indications
Betamethasone valerate is an active topical corticosteroid which produces a rapid response in those inflammatory dermatoses that are normally responsive to topical corticosteroid therapy, and is often effective in the less responsive conditions such as psoriasis.

Betnovate preparations are indicated for the treatment of: eczema in children and adults; including atopic and discoid eczemas; prurigo nodularis; psoriasis (excluding widespread plaque psoriasis); neurodermatoses, including lichen simplex, lichen planus; seborrhoeic dermatitis; contact sensitivity reactions; discoid lupus erythematosus and they may be used as an adjunct to systemic steroid therapy in generalised erythroderma.

Betnovate RD preparations are indicated for maintenance treatment when control has been achieved with Betnovate.

4.2 Posology and method of administration
A small quantity of Betnovate should be applied to the affected area two or three times daily until improvement occurs. It may then be possible to maintain improvement by applying once a day, or even less often, or by using the appropriate ready-diluted (1 in 4) preparation Betnovate RD. If no improvement is seen within two or four weeks, reassessment of the diagnosis, or referral, may be necessary.

Betnovate and Betnovate RD Creams are especially appropriate for moist or weeping surfaces but this is not invariably so.

In the more resistant lesions, such as the thickened plaques of psoriasis on elbows and knees, the effect of Betnovate can be enhanced, if necessary, by occluding the treatment area with polythene film. Overnight occlusion only is usually adequate to bring about a satisfactory response in such lesions; thereafter improvement can usually be maintained by regular application without occlusion.

Children
Courses should be limited to five days if possible. Occlusion should not be used.

4.3 Contraindications
Rosacea, acne vulgaris and peri-oral dermatitis. Primary cutaneous viral infections (e.g. herpes simplex, chickenpox). Hypersensitivity to the preparation.

The use of Betnovate skin preparations is not indicated in the treatment of primarily infected skin lesions caused by infection with fungi (e.g. candidiasis, tinea), or bacteria (e.g. impetigo); primary or secondary infections due to yeast; peri-anal and genital pruritus; dermatoses in children under 1 year of age, including dermatitis and napkin eruptions.

4.4 Special warnings and precautions for use
Long-term continuous topical therapy should be avoided where possible, particularly in infants and children, as adrenal suppression, with or without clinical features of Cushing's syndrome, can occur even without occlusion. In this situation, topical steroids should be discontinued gradually under medical supervision because of the risk of adrenal insufficiency (see section 4.8 Undesirable Effects and Section 4.9 Overdose).

The face, more than other areas of the body, may exhibit atrophic changes after prolonged treatment with potent topical corticosteroids. This must be borne in mind when treating such conditions as psoriasis, discoid lupus erythematosus and severe eczema. If applied to the eyelids, care is needed to ensure that the preparation does not enter the eye, as glaucoma might result.

If used in childhood or on the face, courses should be limited if possible to five days and occlusion should not be used.

Topical corticosteroids may be hazardous in psoriasis for a number of reasons including rebound relapses, development of tolerance, risk of generalised pustular psoriasis and development of local or systemic toxicity due to impaired barrier function of the skin. If used in psoriasis careful patient supervision is important.

Appropriate antimicrobial therapy should be used whenever treating inflammatory lesions which have become infected. Any spread of infection requires withdrawal of topical corticosteroid therapy and systemic administration of antimicrobial agents. Bacterial infection is encouraged by the warm, moist conditions induced by occlusive dressings, and so the skin should be cleansed before a fresh dressing is applied.

In rare instances, treatment of psoriasis with corticosteroids (or its withdrawal) is thought to have provoked the pustular form of the disease. Betnovate RD is usually well tolerated but if signs of hypersensitivity appear, application should stop immediately.

4.5 Interaction with other medicinal products and other forms of interaction
None known.

4.6 Pregnancy and lactation
Avoid extensive use in pregnancy. There is inadequate evidence of safety. Topical administration of corticosteroids to pregnant animals can cause abnormalities of foetal development including cleft palate and intrauterine growth retardation. There may therefore be a very small risk of such effects in the human foetus.

4.7 Effects on ability to drive and use machines
None known.

4.8 Undesirable effects
Adverse events are listed below by system organ class and frequency. Frequencies are defined as: very common (≥1/10), common (≥1/100 and <1/10), uncommon (≥1/1000 and <1/100), rare (≥1/10,000 and <1/1000) and very rare (<1/10,000) including isolated reports. Very common, common and uncommon events were generally determined from clinical trial data. The background rates in placebo and comparator groups were not taken into account when assigning frequency categories to adverse events derived from clinical trial data, since these rates were generally comparable to those in the active treatment group. Rare and very rare events were generally determined from spontaneous data.

Immune system disorders
Very rare: Hypersensitivity.

If signs of hypersensitivity appear, application should stop immediately.

Endocrine disorders
Very rare: Features of Cushing's syndrome

As with other topical corticosteroids, prolonged use of large amounts or treatment of extensive areas can result in sufficient systemic absorption to produce suppression of the HPA axis and the clinical features of Cushing's syndrome (see Section 4.4 Special Warnings and Precautions for Use). These effects are more likely to occur in infants and children, and if occlusive dressings are used. In infants the napkin may act as an occlusive dressing.

Skin and subcutaneous tissue disorders
Common: Local skin burning and pruritus.

Very rare: Local atrophic changes in the skin such as thinning, striae and dilatation of the superficial blood vessels may be caused by prolonged and intensive treatment with highly active corticosteroid preparations, particularly when occlusive dressings are used or when skin folds are involved.

Pigmentation changes, hypertrichosis, allergic contact dermatitis, exacerbation of symptoms, pustular psoriasis (due to treatment of psoriasis with corticosteroids or its withdrawal: see Section 4.4. Special Warnings and Precautions for use)

4.9 Overdose
Acute overdosage is very unlikely to occur. However, in the case of chronic overdosage or misuse the features of Cushing's syndromemay appear and in this situation topical steroids should be discontinued gradually under medical supervision (see Section 4.4 Special Warnings and Precautions for use).

5. PHARMACOLOGICAL PROPERTIES

5.1 Pharmacodynamic properties
Betamethasone is a corticosteroid with topical anti-inflammatory activity.

5.2 Pharmacokinetic properties
The extent of percutaneous absorption of topical corticosteroid is determined by many factors including the vehicle, the integrity of the epidermal barrier, and the use of occlusive dressings.

Topical corticosteroids can be absorbed from normal intact skin. Inflammation and/or other disease processes in the skin increase percutaneous absorption of topical corticosteroids.

Once absorbed through the skin, topical corticosteroids are handled through pharmacokinetic pathways similar to systematically administered corticosteroids. Corticosteroids are metabolised primarily by the liver and are then excreted by the kidneys.

5.3 Preclinical safety data
No additional data of relevance.

6. PHARMACEUTICAL PARTICULARS

6.1 List of excipients
Cetostearyl Alcohol B.P.
Cetomacrogol 1000 B.P.
White Soft Paraffin B.P.
Liquid Paraffin B.P.
Chlorocresol B.P.
Disodium Hydrogen Phosphate, Anhydrous
Citric Acid Monohydrate B.P.
Purified Water B.P.

6.2 Incompatibilities
None known.

6.3 Shelf life
36 months.

6.4 Special precautions for storage
Store below 25°C.

6.5 Nature and contents of container
100gm lacquered aluminium tubes with polypropylene screw caps.

6.6 Special precautions for disposal and other handling
No special instructions.

Administrative Data

7. MARKETING AUTHORISATION HOLDER
Glaxo Wellcome UK Ltd, trading as GlaxoSmithKline UK
Stockley Park West,
Uxbridge,
Middlesex UB11 1BT.

8. MARKETING AUTHORISATION NUMBER(S)
PL 10949/0021

9. DATE OF FIRST AUTHORISATION/RENEWAL OF THE AUTHORISATION
14 October 1996

10. DATE OF REVISION OF THE TEXT
25th January 2005

Betnovate RD Ointment

(GlaxoSmithKline UK)

1. NAME OF THE MEDICINAL PRODUCT
Betnovate RD Ointment

2. QUALITATIVE AND QUANTITATIVE COMPOSITION
Betamethasone Valerate B.P. 0.0305%. Equivalent to Betamethasone 0.025%.

3. PHARMACEUTICAL FORM
Ointment

4. CLINICAL PARTICULARS

4.1 Therapeutic indications
Betamethasone valerate is an active topical corticosteroid, which produces a rapid response in those inflammatory dermatoses that are normally responsive to topical corticosteroid therapy, and is often effective in the less responsive conditions such as psoriasis.

Betnovate preparations are indicated for the treatment of: eczema in children and adults; including atopic and discoid eczemas; prurigo nodularis; psoriasis (excluding widespread plaque psoriasis); neurodermatoses, including lichen simplex, lichen planus; seborrhoeic dermatitis; contact sensitivity reactions; discoid lupus erythematosus and they may be used as an adjunct to systemic steroid therapy in generalised erythroderma.

Betnovate RD preparations are indicated for maintenance treatment when control has been achieved with Betnovate.

4.2 Posology and method of administration
A small quantity of Betnovate should be applied to the affected area two or three times daily until improvement occurs. It may then be possible to maintain improvement by applying once a day, or even less often, or by using the appropriate ready-diluted (1 in 4) preparation Betnovate RD. If no improvement is seen within two or four weeks, reassessment of the diagnosis, or referral, may be necessary.

Betnovate and Betnovate RD ointments are especially appropriate for dry, lichenified or scaly lesions, but this is not invariably so.

In the more resistant lesions, such as the thickened plaques of psoriasis on elbows and knees, the effect of Betnovate can be enhanced, if necessary, by occluding the treatment area with polythene film. Overnight occlusion only is usually adequate to bring about a satisfactory response in such lesions; thereafter improvement can usually be maintained by regular application without occlusion.

Children

Courses should be limited to five days if possible. Occlusion should not be used.

4.3 Contraindications
Rosacea, acne vulgaris and peri-oral dermatitis. Primary cutaneous viral infections (e.g. herpes simplex, chickenpox). Hypersensitivity to the preparation.

The use of Betnovate skin preparations is not indicated in the treatment of primarily infected skin lesions caused by infection with fungi (e.g. candidiasis, tinea), or bacteria (e.g. impetigo); primary or secondary infections due to yeast; peri-anal and genital pruritus; dermatoses in children under 1 year of age, including dermatitis and napkin eruptions.

4.4 Special warnings and precautions for use
Long-term continuous topical therapy should be avoided where possible, particularly in infants and children, as adrenal suppression, with or without clinical features of Cushing's syndrome, can occur even without occlusion. In this situation, topical steroids should be discontinued gradually under medical supervision because of the risk of adrenal insufficiency (see section 4.8 Undesirable Effects and Secion 4.9 Overdose).

The face, more than other areas of the body, may exhibit atrophic changes after prolonged treatment with potent topical corticosteroids. This must be borne in mind when treating such conditions as psoriasis, discoid lupus erythematosus and severe eczema. If applied to the eyelids, care is needed to ensure that the preparation does not enter the eye, as glaucoma might result.

If used in childhood or on the face, courses should be limited if possible to five days and occlusion should not be used.

Topical corticosteroids may be hazardous in psoriasis for a number of reasons including rebound relapses, development of tolerance, risk of generalised pustular psoriasis and development of local or systemic toxicity due to impaired barrier function of the skin. If used in psoriasis careful patient supervision is important.

Appropriate antimicrobial therapy should be used whenever treating inflammatory lesions, which have become infected. Any spread of infection requires withdrawal of topical corticosteroid therapy and systemic administration of antimicrobial agents. Bacterial infection is encouraged by the warm, moist conditions induced by occlusive dressings, and so the skin should be cleansed before a fresh dressing is applied.

In rare instances, treatment of psoriasis with corticosteroids (or its withdrawal) is thought to have provoked the pustular form of the disease. Betnovate RD is usually well tolerated but if signs of hypersensitivity appear, application should stop immediately.

4.5 Interaction with other medicinal products and other forms of interaction
None known.

4.6 Pregnancy and lactation
Avoid extensive use in pregnancy. There is inadequate evidence of safety. Topical administration of corticosteroids to pregnant animals can cause abnormalities of foetal development including cleft palate and intrauterine growth retardation. There may therefore be a very small risk of such effects in the human foetus.

4.7 Effects on ability to drive and use machines
None known.

4.8 Undesirable effects
Adverse events are listed below by system organ class and frequency. Frequencies are defined as: very common ($\geq$1/10), common ($\geq$1/100 and <1/10), uncommon ($\geq$1/1000 and <1/100), rare ($\geq$1/10,000 and <1/1000) and very rare (<1/10,000) including isolated reports. Very common, common and uncommon events were generally determined from clinical trial data. The background rates in placebo and comparator groups were not taken into account when assigning frequency categories to adverse events derived from clinical trial data, since these rates were generally comparable to those in the active treatment group. Rare and very rare events were generally determined from spontaneous data.

Immune system disorders
Very rare: Hypersensitivity.

If signs of hypersensitivity appear, application should stop immediately.

Endocrine disorders
Very rare: Features of Cushing's syndrome

As with other topical corticosteroids, prolonged use of large amounts or treatment of extensive areas can result in sufficient systemic absorption to produce suppression of the HPA axis and the clinical features of Cushing's syndrome (see Section 4.4 Special Warnings and Precautions for use). These effects are more likely to occur in infants and children, and if occlusive dressings are used. In infants the napkin may act as an occlusive dressing.

Skin and subcutaneous tissue disorders
Common: Local skin burning and pruritus.

Very rare: Local atrophic changes in the skin such as thinning, striae and dilatation of the superficial blood vessels may be caused by prolonged and intensive treatment with highly active corticosteroid preparations, particularly when occlusive dressings are used or when skin folds are involved.

Pigmentation changes, hypertrichosis, allergic contact dermatitis, exacerbation of symptoms, pustular psoriasis (due to treatment of psoriasis with corticosteroids or its withdrawal: see Section 4.4. Special Warnings and Precautions for use).

4.9 Overdose
Acute overdosage is very unlikely to occur. However, in the case of chronic overdosage or misuse the features of Cushing's syndrome may appear and in this situation topical steroids should be discontinued gradually under medical supervision (see Section 4.4 Special Warnings and Precautions for use).

5. PHARMACOLOGICAL PROPERTIES

5.1 Pharmacodynamic properties
Betamethasone is a corticosteroid with topical anti-inflammatory activity.

5.2 Pharmacokinetic properties
The extent of percutaneous absorption of topical corticosteroid is determined by many factors including the vehicle, the integrity of the epidermal barrier, and the use of occlusive dressings.

Topical corticosteroids can be absorbed from normal intact skin. Inflammation and/or other disease processes in the skin increase percutaneous absorption of topica corticosteroids.

Once absorbed through the skin, topical corticosteroid are handled through pharmacokinetic pathways similar t systemically administered corticosteroids. Corticoster oids are metabolised primarily by the liver and are the excreted by the kidneys.

5.3 Preclinical safety data
No additional data of relevance.

6. PHARMACEUTICAL PARTICULARS

6.1 List of excipients
White Soft Paraffin B.P.
Liquid Paraffin B.P.

6.2 Incompatibilities
None known.

6.3 Shelf life
36 months.

6.4 Special precautions for storage
Store below 30°C.

6.5 Nature and contents of container
100gm lacquered aluminium tubes with polypropylene screw caps.

6.6 Special precautions for disposal and other handling
No special instructions.

Administrative Data

7. MARKETING AUTHORISATION HOLDER
Glaxo Wellcome UK Ltd,
trading as GlaxoSmithKline UK
Stockley Park West,
Uxbridge,
Middlesex
UB11 1BT.

8. MARKETING AUTHORISATION NUMBER(S)
PL 10949/0022

9. DATE OF FIRST AUTHORISATION/RENEWAL OF THE AUTHORISATION
28 May 2008

10. DATE OF REVISION OF THE TEXT
28 May 2008

11. Legal Category
POM

Betnovate Scalp Application

(GlaxoSmithKline UK)

1. NAME OF THE MEDICINAL PRODUCT
Betnovate Scalp Application.

2. QUALITATIVE AND QUANTITATIVE COMPOSITION
Betamethasone Valerate BP 0.122% $^{w}/_{w}$.

3. PHARMACEUTICAL FORM
Aqueous Suspension.

4. CLINICAL PARTICULARS

4.1 Therapeutic indications
Steroid responsive dermatoses of the scalp, such as psoriasis and seborrhoeic dermatitis.

4.2 Posology and method of administration
A small quantity of Betnovate Scalp Application should be applied to the scalp night and morning until improvement is noticeable. It may then be possible to sustain improvement by applying once a day, or less frequently.

For topical application.

4.3 Contraindications
Infections of the scalp. Hypersensitivity to the preparation. Dermatoses in children under one year of age, including dermatitis.

4.4 Special warnings and precautions for use
Care must be taken to keep the preparation away from the eyes. Does not use near a naked flame.

Long-term continuous topical therapy should be avoided where possible, particularly in infants and children, as adrenal suppression, with or without clinical features of Cushing's syndrome, can occur even without occlusion. In this situation, topical steroids should be discontinued gradually under medical supervision because of the risk of adrenal insufficiency (see section 4.8 Undesirable Effects and Section 4.9 Overdose).

Topical corticosteroids may be hazardous in psoriasis for a number of reasons including rebound relapses, development of tolerance, risk of generalised pustular psoriasis and development of local or systemic toxicity due to impaired barrier function of the skin. If used in psoriasis careful patient supervision is important.

Development of secondary infection requires withdrawal of topical corticosteroid therapy and commencement of appropriate systemic antimicrobial therapy.

The least potent corticosteroid which will control the disease should be selected. The viscosity of the scalp application has been adjusted so that the preparation spreads easily without being too fluid. The specially-designed bottle and nozzle allow easy application direct to the scalp through the hair.

4.5 Interaction with other medicinal products and other forms of interaction
None known.

4.6 Pregnancy and lactation
There is inadequate evidence of safety in human pregnancy. Topical administration of corticosteroids to pregnant animals can cause abnormalities of fetal development including cleft palate and intrauterine growth retardation. There may therefore be a very small risk of such effects in the human foetus.

4.7 Effects on ability to drive and use machines
None known.

4.8 Undesirable effects
Adverse events are listed below by system organ class and frequency. Frequencies are defined as: very common (≥1/10), common (≥1/100 and <1/10), uncommon (≥1/1000 and <1/100), rare (≥1/10,000 and <1/1000) and very rare (<1/10,000) including isolated reports. Very common, common and uncommon events were generally determined from clinical trial data. The background rates in placebo and comparator groups were not taken into account when assigning frequency categories to adverse events derived from clinical trial data, since these rates were generally comparable to those in the active treatment group. Rare and very rare events were generally determined from spontaneous data.

Immune system disorders
Very rare: Hypersensitivity.

If signs of hypersensitivity appear, application should be stopped immediately.

Endocrine disorders
Very rare: Features of Cushing's syndrome

As with other topical corticosteroids, prolonged use of large amounts or treatment of extensive areas can result in sufficient systemic absorption to produce suppression of the HPA axis and the clinical features of Cushing's syndrome (see Section 4.4 Special Warnings and Precautions for use). These effects are more likely to occur in infants and children, and if occlusive dressings are used.

Skin and subcutaneous tissue disorders
Common: Local skin burning and pruritus.

Very rare: Local atrophic changes in the skin such as thinning, striae and dilatation of the superficial blood vessels may be caused by prolonged and intensive treatment with highly active corticosteroid preparations, particularly when occlusive dressings are used or when skin folds are involved.

Pigmentation changes, hypertrichosis, allergic contact dermatitis, exacerbation of symptoms, pustular psoriasis (due to treatment of psoriasis with corticosteroids or its withdrawal: see Section 4.4. Special Warnings and Precautions for use)

4.9 Overdose
Acute overdosage is very unlikely to occur. However, in the case of chronic overdosage or misuse the features of Cushing's syndrome may appear and in this situation topical steroids should be discontinued gradually under medical supervision (see Section 4.4 Special Warnings and Precautions for use).

5. PHARMACOLOGICAL PROPERTIES

5.1 Pharmacodynamic properties
Betamethasone valerate is an active corticosteroid with topical anti-inflammatory activity.

5.2 Pharmacokinetic properties
The extent of percutaneous absorption of topical corticosteroids is determined by many factors including the vehicle, the integrity of the epidermal barrier, and the use of occlusive dressings.

Topical corticosteroids can be absorbed from normal intact skin. Inflammation and/or other disease processes in the skin increase percutaneous absorption.

Occlusive dressings substantially increase the percutaneous absorption of topical corticosteroids.

Once absorbed through the skin, topical corticosteroids are handled through pharmacokinetic pathways similar to systemically administered corticosteroids. Corticosteroids are bound to plasma proteins in varying degrees. Corticosteroids are metabolised primarily by the liver and are then excreted by the kidneys.

5.3 Preclinical safety data
There are no preclinical data of relevance to the prescriber which are additional to that in other sections of the SPC.

6. PHARMACEUTICAL PARTICULARS

6.1 List of excipients
Carbomer

Isopropyl Alcohol

Sodium Hydroxide

Purified Water

6.2 Incompatibilities
None known.

6.3 Shelf life
24 months.

6.4 Special precautions for storage
Store below 25°C

6.5 Nature and contents of container
Polyethylene squeeze bottle with a polyethylene nozzle and a polystyrene or polyethylene cap or

white High Density Polyethylene (HDPE) Hostalen GF4750 and Remafin white CEG 020 container with a polyethylene nozzle and a polystyrene or polyethylene cap.

Pack size: 30ml; 100ml

Not all pack sizes may be marketed

6.6 Special precautions for disposal and other handling
No special instructions.

Administrative Data

7. MARKETING AUTHORISATION HOLDER
Glaxo Wellcome UK Limited

trading as GlaxoSmithKline UK

Stockley Park West

Uxbridge

Middlesex

UB11 1BT

8. MARKETING AUTHORISATION NUMBER(S)
PL 10949/0045.

9. DATE OF FIRST AUTHORISATION/RENEWAL OF THE AUTHORISATION
9 December 1997

10. DATE OF REVISION OF THE TEXT
25th January 2005

11. Legal Status
POM

Bezalip 200mg tablets

(Actavis UK Ltd)

1. NAME OF THE MEDICINAL PRODUCT
Bezalip

2. QUALITATIVE AND QUANTITATIVE COMPOSITION
Bezafibrate 200mg

3. PHARMACEUTICAL FORM
Tablet for oral use.

Bezalip is a round film-coated tablet with a white core and is imprinted G6.

4. CLINICAL PARTICULARS

4.1 Therapeutic indications
Bezalip is indicated for use in hyperlipidaemias of Type IIa, IIb, III, IV and V (Fredrickson classification).

Bezalip should be employed only in patients with a fully defined and diagnosed lipid abnormality which is inadequately controlled by dietary means, or by other changes in life-style such as physical exercise and weight reduction, and in whom the long-term risks associated with the condition warrant treatment.

The rationale for the use of Bezalip is to control abnormalities of serum lipids and lipoproteins to reduce or prevent the long term effects which have been shown by many epidemiological studies to be positively and strongly correlated with such hyperlipidaemias.

4.2 Posology and method of administration

Adults
The recommended dosage for Bezalip tablets is three tablets daily, equivalent to 600mg bezafibrate. The tablets should be swallowed whole with a little fluid after each meal.

Elderly
No specific dosage reduction is necessary in elderly patients.

Children
At present there is inadequate information regarding an appropriate dosage in children.

Renal impairment
In patients with renal insufficiency the dose should be adjusted according to serum creatinine levels or creatinine clearance as shown in the following table;

Serum creatinine (μ mol/l)	Creatinine clearance (ml/min)	Dosage (tablets/day)
Up to 135	Over 60	3
136 – 225	60 – 40	2
226 – 530	40 – 15	1 every 1 or 2 days
Over 530	Less than 15	Contra-indicated

In dialysis patients the dosage must be further reduced. As a general rule a dosage of one Bezalip tablet every third day is recommended, to avoid overdosage. The patient should be carefully monitored.

The response to therapy is normally rapid, although a progressive improvement may occur over a number of weeks. Treatment should be withdrawn if an adequate response has not been achieved within 3 to 4 months.

4.3 Contraindications
Significant hepatic disease (other than fatty infiltration of the liver associated with raised triglyceride values), severe renal insufficiency (serum creatinine > 530μmol/l; creatinine clearance <15ml/min), gall bladder disease with or without cholelithiasis, nephrotic syndrome, known photo-allergic or phototoxic reactions to fibrates and hypersensitivity to bezafibrate or any component of the product or to other fibrates.

4.4 Special warnings and precautions for use
See *Preclinical safety data*.

Bezafibrate could cause cholelithiasis, although there is no evidence of an increased frequency of gallstones in patients treated with Bezalip. Appropriate diagnostic procedures should be performed if cholelithic symptoms and signs occur (see section *4.8 Undesirable effects).*

Muscle effects: Bezafibrate and other fibrates may cause myopathy, manifested as muscle weakness or pain, often accompanied by a considerable increase in creatine kinase (CPK). In isolated cases severe muscle damage (rhabdomyolysis) may occur. The risk of rhabdomyolysis may be increased in patients with predisposing factors for myopathy, (including renal impairment, hypothyroidism, severe infection, trauma, surgery, disturbances of hormone or electrolyte imbalance and a high alcohol intake).

Bezafibrate should be used with caution in combination with HMG CoA reductase inhibitors as the combination of HMG CoA inhibitors and fibrates has been shown to increase the incidence and severity of myopathy. Patients should be monitored for signs of myopathy and increased CPK activity and combination therapy discontinued if signs of myopathy develop. Combination therapy should not be used in patients with predisposing factors for myopathy (see section *4.5 Interaction with other medicaments and other forms of interaction).*

4.5 Interaction with other medicinal products and other forms of interaction
Care is required in administering Bezalip to patients taking coumarin-type anti-coagulants, the action of which may be potentiated. The dosage of anti-coagulant should be reduced by up to 50% and readjusted by monitoring blood coagulation.

As bezafibrate improves glucose utilisation the action of antidiabetic medication, including insulin, may be potentiated. Hypoglycaemia has not been observed although increased monitoring of the glycaemic status may be warranted for a brief period after introduction of Bezalip.

In isolated cases, a pronounced though reversible impairment of renal function (accompanied by a corresponding increase in serum creatinine level) has been reported in organ transplant patients receiving cyclosporin therapy and concomitant bezafibrate. Accordingly, renal function should be closely monitored in these patients and, in the event of relevant significant changes in laboratory parameters, bezafibrate, should if necessary, be discontinued. Should combined therapy with an ion-exchange resin be considered necessary, there should be an interval of 2 hours between the intake of the resin and Bezalip as the absorption of bezafibrate otherwise may be impaired.

Concomitant therapy with HMG CoA reductase inhibitors and fibrates has been reported to increase the risk of myopathy (see section *4.4 Special warnings and precautions*). The underlying mechanism for this remains unclear; the available data do not suggest a pharmacokinetic interaction between bezafibrate and HMG CoA reductase inhibitors.

MAO-inhibitors (with hepatotoxic potential) should not be administered together with bezafibrate.

Since oestrogens may lead to a rise in lipid levels, the necessity for treatment with Bezalip in patients receiving oestrogens or oestrogen containing preparations should be considered on an individual basis.

4.6 Pregnancy and lactation
Although the drug substance has not been shown in animal studies to have any adverse effects on the foetus, it is recommended that Bezalip should not be administered to either pregnant women or to those who are breast feeding.

4.7 Effects on ability to drive and use machines
None known.

4.8 Undesirable effects

Gastro-intestinal system:

– occasionally gastro-intestinal symptoms such as loss of appetite, feelings of fullness in the stomach and nausea may occur. These side-effects are usually transient and generally do not require withdrawal of the drug. In susceptible patients a slowly increasing dosage over 5 to 7 days may help to avoid such symptoms.

Hepato-biliary system:

– in isolated cases, increase of transaminases, cholestasis and gallstones (see section *4.4 Special warnings and special precautions for use*).

Hypersensitivity:

– occasionally allergic skin reactions such as pruritus or urticaria.

– in isolated cases, photosensitivity or generalised hypersensitivity reactions may occur.

Haematology:

Isolated cases of:

– decreases in haemoglobin and leucocytes.

– thrombocytopenia, which may cause bleeding (e.g. purpura).

– pancytopenia.

Renal system:

– frequently slight increases in serum creatinine. In patients with existing impairment of renal function, if dosage recommendations are not followed, myopathy may develop (in extreme cases rhabdomyolysis).

Muscular system:

– Muscular weakness, myalgia and muscle cramps, often accompanied by a considerable increase in creatine kinase may occur. In isolated cases, severe muscular damage (rhabdomyolysis) has been observed. In cases of rhabdomyolysis, bezafibrate must be stopped immediately and renal function closely monitored.

Others:

– in rare cases, headache and dizziness, alopecia.

– isolated cases of potency disorders have been reported.

In general, most of the adverse drug reactions disappear after withdrawal of Bezalip.

4.9 Overdose

No specific effects of acute overdose are known. Rhabdomyolysis has occurred. In cases of rhabdomyolysis, bezafibrate must be stopped immediately and renal function carefully monitored.

5. PHARMACOLOGICAL PROPERTIES

5.1 Pharmacodynamic properties

Bezafibrate lowers elevated levels of serum cholesterol and triglycerides (i.e. lowers elevated low density lipoprotein and very low density lipoprotein levels, and raises lowered high density lipoprotein levels) by stimulating lipoprotein lipase and hepatic lipase, and by suppressing the activity of 3 HMGCo-A reductase resulting in stimulation of low density lipoprotein receptors on the cell surface.

Studies have shown bezafibrate to be effective in treating hyperlipidaemia in patients with diabetes mellitus. Some cases showed a beneficial reduction in fasting blood glucose.

Significant reductions in serum fibrinogen levels have been observed in hyperfibrinogenaemic patients treated with bezafibrate.

5.2 Pharmacokinetic properties

Maximum concentrations of bezafibrate appear around 2 hours after ingestion of Bezalip tablets. The protein-binding of bezafibrate in serum is approximately 95%. The elimination half-life is in the order of 2.1 hours although elimination is markedly slowed in the presence of limited renal function. Elimination may be increased in forced diuresis. The drug substance is non-dialysable (cuprophane filter).

5.3 Preclinical safety data

The chronic administration of a high dose of bezafibrate to rats was associated with hepatic tumour formation in females. This dosage was in the order of 30 to 40 times the human dosage. No such effect was apparent at reduced intake levels approximating more closely to the lipid-lowering dosage in humans.

6. PHARMACEUTICAL PARTICULARS

6.1 List of excipients

Table core:

maize starch,

microcrystalline cellulose,

colloidal silicon dioxide,

sodium starch glycollate,

magnesium stearate.

Film-coating:

polyvinyl alcohol,

titanium dioxide (E171),

macrogol,

talc.

6.2 Incompatibilities

Not applicable.

6.3 Shelf life

5 years.

6.4 Special precautions for storage

Do not store above 25 °C.

6.5 Nature and contents of container

Packs of 84 or 100 tablets in PVC/Aluminium blister strips.

6.6 Special precautions for disposal and other handling

Not applicable.

7. MARKETING AUTHORISATION HOLDER

Actavis Group PTC ehf

Reykjavikurvegi 76-78

220 Hafnarfjordur

Iceland.

8. MARKETING AUTHORISATION NUMBER(S)

PL 30306/0125

9. DATE OF FIRST AUTHORISATION/RENEWAL OF THE AUTHORISATION

1 April 1999

10. DATE OF REVISION OF THE TEXT

06/07/09

Bezalip Mono (Actavis UK)

(Actavis UK Ltd)

1. NAME OF THE MEDICINAL PRODUCT

Bezalip Mono

2. QUALITATIVE AND QUANTITATIVE COMPOSITION

Bezafibrate 400mg.

For excipients see section 6.1.

3. PHARMACEUTICAL FORM

Modified release tablet for oral use.

Bezalip Mono is a round film-coated tablet with a white core and is imprinted D9.

4. CLINICAL PARTICULARS

4.1 Therapeutic indications

Bezalip Mono is indicated for use in hyperlipidaemias of Type IIa, IIb, III, IV and V (Fredrickson classification).

Bezalip Mono should be employed only in patients with a fully defined and diagnosed lipid abnormality which is inadequately controlled by dietary means, or by other changes in life-style such as physical exercise and weight reduction, and in whom the long-term risks associated with the condition warrant treatment.

The rationale for the use of Bezalip Mono is to control abnormalities of serum lipids and lipoproteins to reduce or prevent the long term effects which have been shown by many epidemiological studies to be positively and strongly correlated with such hyperlipidaemias.

4.2 Posology and method of administration

Adults

The dosage for Bezalip Mono is one tablet daily, equivalent to 400mg bezafibrate. The tablets should be swallowed whole with sufficient fluid after a meal either at night or in the morning.

Elderly

Bezalip Mono should not be used in elderly patients if the creatinine clearance is below 60 ml/min (see Renal impairment below).

Children

At present there is inadequate information regarding an appropriate dosage in children.

Renal impairment

In dialysis patients the use of bezafibrate is contraindicated.

Bezalip Mono is contra-indicated in patients with renal impairment with serum creatinine > 135 micromol/l or creatinine clearance < 60ml/min. Such patients may be treated with conventional Bezalip tablets (200mg bezafibrate) using an appropriately reduced daily dosage.

The response to therapy is normally rapid, although a progressive improvement may occur over a number of weeks. Treatment should be withdrawn if an adequate response has not been achieved within 3 to 4 months.

4.3 Contraindications

Significant hepatic disease (other than fatty infiltration of the liver associated with raised triglyceride values), gall bladder disease with or without cholelithiasis, nephrotic syndrome or renal impairment (serum creatinine > 135 micromol/l or creatinine clearance < 60ml/min.) Patients undergoing dialysis, known photoallergic or phototoxic reactions to fibrates. Hypersensitivity to bezafibrate or any component of the product or to other fibrates. Concomitant use of HMG CoA reductase inhibitors (statins) in patients with predisposing factors for myopathy (see sections 4.4 and 4.5).

4.4 Special warnings and precautions for use

Patients with impaired renal function should be monitored regularly. In these patients acute renal failure may develop if dosage recommendations according to the presenting serum creatinine or creatinine clearance are not strictly followed.

Bezafibrate and other fibrates may cause myopathy, manifested as muscle weakness or pain, often accompanied by a considerable increase in creatine kinase (CPK). In isolated cases severe muscle damage (rhabdomyolysis) has been observed. The risk of rhabdomyolysis may be increased when higher than recommended doses of bezafibrate are used, most frequently in the presence of impaired renal function and in patients with predisposing factors for myopathy, (including renal impairment hypothyroidism, severe infection, trauma, surgery, disturbances of hormone or electrolyte imbalance and a high alcohol intake).

Because of the risk of rhabdomyolysis, bezafibrate should be used in combination with HMG CoA reductase inhibitors only in exceptional cases when strictly indicated. Patients should be informed of and monitored for signs of myopathy and increased CPK activity and combination therapy discontinued immediately if signs of myopathy develop.

Bezafibrate alters the composition of bile. There have been isolated reports of the development of gallstones.

As bezafibrate could cause cholelithiasis appropriate diagnostic procedures should be performed if cholelithic symptoms and signs occur (see section *4.8 Undesirable effects).*

When Bezalip Mono is given in combination with anion-exchange resins (e.g. cholestyramine) the two drugs should always be taken at least 2 hours apart.

4.5 Interaction with other medicinal products and other forms of interaction

Care is required in administering Bezalip Mono to patients taking coumarin-type anti-coagulants, the action of which may be potentiated. The dosage of anti-coagulant should be reduced by up to 50% and readjusted by monitoring blood coagulation.

As bezafibrate improves glucose utilisation the action of antidiabetic medication, including insulin, may be potentiated. Hypoglycaemia has not been observed although increased monitoring of the glycaemic status may be warranted for a brief period after introduction of Bezalip Mono.

In isolated cases, a pronounced though reversible impairment of renal function (accompanied by a corresponding increase in serum creatinine level) has been reported in organ transplant patients receiving cyclosporin therapy and concomitant bezafibrate. Accordingly, renal function should be closely monitored in these patients and, in the event of relevant significant changes in laboratory parameters, bezafibrate, should if necessary, be discontinued.

Should combined therapy with an ion-exchange resin be considered necessary, there should be an interval of 2 hours between the intake of the resin and Bezalip Mono as the absorption of bezafibrate otherwise may be impaired.

Interaction between HMG CoA reductase inhibitors and fibrates may vary in nature and intensity depending on the combination of the administered drugs. A pharmacodynamic interaction between these two classes of drugs may, in some cases, also contribute to an increase in the risk of myopathy (see section *4.3 Contraindications*). For specific dose restrictions of statins refer to the SPC of the relevant product.

MAO-inhibitors (with hepatotoxic potential) should not be administered together with bezafibrate.

Since oestrogens may lead to a rise in lipid levels, the necessity for treatment with Bezalip Mono in patients receiving oestrogens or oestrogen containing preparations should be considered on an individual basis.

4.6 Pregnancy and lactation

Animal studies are insuffcient with respect to effects on pregnancy, embryonal/foetal development, parturition or postnatal development. The potential risk for humans is unknown.

There is insufficient information on the excretion of bezafibrate or its metabolites into breast milk.

Bezalip Mono should not be used during pregnancy or lacation unless clearly indicated.

4.7 Effects on ability to drive and use machines

Bezalip has been shown to cause dizziness and can have a minor to moderate effect on the ability to drive or use machines. Patients should not drive or use machines if they are affected.

4.8 Undesirable effects

The overall safety profile of bezafibrate is based on a combination of clinical data from Boehringer Mannheim and post-marketing experience.

The frequency of adverse drug reactions according to MedDRA System Organ Class is displayed below:

Frequency of reporting:	Common (>1/100)
	Uncommon (≥1/1,000 and <1/100)
	Very rare (<1/10,000)

Blood and Lymphatic System

Very rare:	Pancytopenia Thrombocytopenia purpura Haemoglobin decreased Platelet increased White blood cell count decreased

Immune System

Uncommon:	Hypersensitivity reactions

Metabolism and Nutrition System

Common:	Decreased appetite

Nervous System

Uncommon:	Dizziness Headache

Gastro-intestinal Disorders

Uncommon:	Abdominal distensionNausea

Hepato-biliary Disorders:

Uncommon:	Cholestasis Blood alkaline phosphatase increased Decreased gamma-glutamyl transferase and in parallel decreased alkaline phosphatase
Very rare:	Cholelithiasis (see section 4.4 Special warnings and special precautions for use) Gamma-glutyl transferase increased Transaminase increased

Skin and Appendages Disorders

Uncommon:	Pruritis Urticaria Photosensitivity reactions
Very rare:	Erythema multiforme Stevens-Johnson Syndrome Toxic epidermal necrolysis Alopecia

Musculoskeletal and Connective Tissue Disorders

Uncommon:	Muscular weakness Myalgia Muscle cramps
Very rare:	Rhabdomyolysis

Renal and Urinary Disorders

Uncommon:	Acute renal failure Blood creatinine increased

Reproductive System and Breast Disorders

Uncommon:	Erectile dysfunction Nos

Investigations

Uncommon:	Increased blood creatinine phosphokinase

4.9 Overdose

No specific effects of acute overdose are known (apart from rhabdomyolysis). There is no specific antidote. Thus appropriate symptomatic therapy is recommended in case of overdose. In cases of rhabdomyolysis bezafibrate must be stopped immediately and renal function carefully monitored.

5. PHARMACOLOGICAL PROPERTIES

5.1 Pharmacodynamic properties

ATC Code: C10AB02

Bezafibrate lowers elevated levels of serum cholesterol and triglycerides (i.e. lowers elevated low density lipoprotein and very low density lipoprotein levels, and raises lowered high density lipoprotein levels) by stimulating lipoprotein lipase and hepatic lipase, and by suppressing the activity of 3 HMGCo-A reductase resulting in stimulation of low density lipoprotein receptors on the cell surface.

Studies have shown bezafibrate to be effective in treating hyperlipidaemia in patients with diabetes mellitus. Some cases showed a beneficial reduction in fasting blood glucose.

Significant reductions in serum fibrinogen levels have been observed in hyperfibrinogenaemic patients treated with bezafibrate.

5.2 Pharmacokinetic properties

Absorption

With 400 mg Bezalip Mono, a peak concentration of about 8 mg is reached after about 4 hours. The relative bioavailability of bezafibrate retard compared to the standard form is about 70%.

Distribution

The protein-binding of bezafibrate in serum is approximately 95% and the apparent volume of distribution is 17 litres.

Metabolism

50% of the administered bezafibrate dose is recovered in the urine as unchanged drug and 20% in the form of glucuronides.

Elimination

Elimination is rapid with excretion almost exclusively renal. 95% of the activity of 14C-labelled drug is recovered in the urine and 3% in the faeces within 48 hours. The rate of clearance ranges from 3.4 to 6.0 l/h. The elimination half-life is in the order of 1-2 hours although elimination is markedly slowed in the presence of limited renal function.

5.3 Preclinical safety data

The chronic administration of a high dose of bezafibrate to rats was associated with hepatic tumour formation. The dosage was in the order of 30 to 40 times the human dosage. No such effect was apparent at reduced intake levels approximating more closely to the lipid-lowering dosage in humans.

6. PHARMACEUTICAL PARTICULARS

6.1 List of excipients

Lactose
Povidone
Sodium laurilsulfate
Hypromellose
Silica, colloidal hydrated
Magnesium stearate (E572)
Polymethacrylic acid esters
Macrogol 10,000
Talc (E553b)
Titanium dioxide (E171)
Polysorbate 80
Sodium citrate (E331).

6.2 Incompatibilities

Not applicable.

6.3 Shelf life

5 years.

6.4 Special precautions for storage

Bezalip Mono requires no special storage conditions.

6.5 Nature and contents of container

Packs of 28 or 30 tablets in PVC/Aluminium blister strips. HDPE containers of 28 tablets.

6.6 Special precautions for disposal and other handling

Not applicable.

7. MARKETING AUTHORISATION HOLDER

Actavis Group PTC ehf
Reykjavíkurvegi 76-78
220 Hafnarfjordur
Iceland.

8. MARKETING AUTHORISATION NUMBER(S)

PL 30306/0126

9. DATE OF FIRST AUTHORISATION/RENEWAL OF THE AUTHORISATION

1 April 1999

10. DATE OF REVISION OF THE TEXT

03/04/09

Bicalutamide 150mg (AstraZeneca UK Ltd)

(AstraZeneca UK Limited)

1. NAME OF THE MEDICINAL PRODUCT

Bicalutamide 150 mg Film-coated Tablets.

2. QUALITATIVE AND QUANTITATIVE COMPOSITION

Each tablet contains 150 mg bicalutamide (INN)

For excipients, see Section 6.1.

3. PHARMACEUTICAL FORM

Film-coated tablet.

White, round, biconvex film-coated tablet with 'BCL' impressed on one side and '150' impressed on the other side.

4. CLINICAL PARTICULARS

4.1 Therapeutic indications

Bicalutamide 150 mg is indicated either alone or as adjuvant to radical prostatectomy or radiotherapy in patients with locally advanced prostate cancer at high risk for disease progression (see section 5.1).

Bicalutamide 150 mg is also indicated for the management of patients with locally advanced, non-metastatic prostate cancer for whom surgical castration or other medical intervention is not considered appropriate or acceptable.

4.2 Posology and method of administration

Adult males including the elderly: The dosage is one 150 mg tablet to be taken orally once a day.

Bicalutamide 150 mg should be taken continuously for at least 2 years or until disease progression.

Renal Impairment: No dosage adjustment is necessary for patients with renal impairment.

Hepatic Impairment: No dosage adjustment is necessary for patients with mild hepatic impairment. Increased accumulation may occur in patients with moderate to severe hepatic impairment (see section 4.4).

4.3 Contraindications

Bicalutamide 150 mg is contraindicated in females and children.

Bicalutamide 150 mg must not be given to any patient who has shown a hypersensitivity to the active substance or any of the excipients.

Co-administration of terfenadine, astemizole or cisapride with Bicalutamide is contraindicated (see section 4.5).

4.4 Special warnings and precautions for use

Bicalutamide is extensively metabolised in the liver. Data suggest that its elimination may be slower in subjects with severe hepatic impairment and this could lead to increased accumulation of bicalutamide. Therefore, Bicalutamide 150 mg should be used with caution in patients with moderate to severe hepatic impairment.

Periodic liver function testing should be considered due to the possibility of hepatic changes. The majority of cases are expected to occur within the first 6 months of Bicalutamide therapy.

Severe hepatic changes and hepatic failure have been observed rarely with Bicalutamide 150 mg (see section 4.8). Bicalutamide 150 mg therapy should be discontinued if changes are severe.

For patients who have an objective progression of disease together with elevated PSA, cessation of Bicalutamide therapy should be considered.

Bicalutamide has been shown to inhibit cytochrome P450 (CYP 3A4), as such, caution should be exercised when co-administered with drugs metabolised predominantly by CYP 3A4, see sections 4.3 and 4.5.

Patients with rare hereditary problems of galactose intolerance, the Lapp lactase deficiency or glucose-galactose malabsorption should not take this medicine.

4.5 Interaction with other medicinal products and other forms of interaction

In vitro studies have shown that R- bicalutamide is an inhibitor of CYP 3A4, with lesser inhibitory effects on CYP 2C9, 2C19 and 2D6 activity. Although clinical studies using antipyrine as a marker of cytochrome P450 (CYP) activity showed no evidence of a drug interaction potential with Bicalutamide, mean midazolam exposure (AUC) was increased by up to 80%, after co-administration of Bicalutamide for 28 days. For drugs with a narrow therapeutic index such an increase could be of relevance. As such, concomitant use of terfenadine, astemizole and cisapride is contraindicated and caution should be exercised with the co-administration of Bicalutamide with compounds such as ciclosporin and calcium channel blockers. Dosage reduction may be required for these drugs particularly if there is evidence of enhanced or adverse drug effect. For ciclosporin, it is recommended that plasma concentrations and clinical condition are closely monitored following initiation or cessation of Bicalutamide therapy.

Caution should be exercised when prescribing Bicalutamide with other drugs which may inhibit drug oxidation e.g. cimetidine and ketoconazole. In theory, this could result in increased plasma concentrations of bicalutamide which theoretically could lead to an increase in side effects.

In vitro studies have shown that bicalutamide can displace the coumarin anticoagulant, warfarin, from its protein binding sites. It is therefore recommended that if Bicalutamide 150 mg is started in patients who are already receiving coumarin anticoagulants, prothrombin time should be closely monitored.

4.6 Pregnancy and lactation

Bicalutamide is contraindicated in females and must not be given to pregnant women or nursing mothers.

4.7 Effects on ability to drive and use machines

No effects on ability to drive and use machines have been observed during treatment with Bicalutamide 150 mg.

4.8 Undesirable effects

The frequencies of adverse events are ranked according to the following: Very common ($\geqslant$10%); Common ($\geqslant$1% and <10%); Uncommon ($\geqslant$0.1% and <1%); Rare ($\geqslant$0.01% and <0.1%).

Frequency of Adverse Reactions

(see Table 1 on next page)

4.9 Overdose

There is no human experience of overdosage. There is no specific antidote; treatment should be symptomatic. Dialysis may not be helpful, since bicalutamide is highly protein bound and is not recovered unchanged in the urine. General supportive care, including frequent monitoring of vital signs, is indicated.

5. PHARMACOLOGICAL PROPERTIES

5.1 Pharmacodynamic properties

Antiandrogen, ATC code L02 B B03

Bicalutamide is a non-steroidal antiandrogen, devoid of other endocrine activity. It binds to the wild type or normal androgen receptor without activating gene expression, and thus inhibits the androgen stimulus. Regression of prostatic tumours results from this inhibition. Clinically, discontinuation of Bicalutamide can result in the 'antiandrogen withdrawal syndrome' in a subset of patients.

Bicalutamide 150 mg was studied as a treatment for patients with localised (T1-T2, N0 or NX, M0) or locally advanced (T3-T4, any N, M0; T1-T2, N+, M0) non-metastatic prostate cancer in a combined analysis of three placebo controlled, double-blind studies in 8113 patients, where Bicalutamide was given as immediate hormonal therapy or as adjuvant to radical prostatectomy or radiotherapy (primarily external beam radiation). At 7.4 years median follow up, 27.4% and 30.7% of all Bicalutamide and placebo-treated patients, respectively, had experienced objective disease progression.

A reduction in risk of objective disease progression was seen across most patients groups but was most evident in those at highest risk of disease progression. Therefore, clinicians may decide that the optimum medical strategy for a patient at low risk of disease progression, particularly in the adjuvant setting following radical prostatectomy, may be to defer hormonal therapy until signs that the disease is progressing.

No overall survival difference was seen at 7.4 years median follow up with 22.9% mortality (HR=0.99; 95% CI 0.91 to 1.09). However, some trends were apparent in exploratory subgroup analyses.

Progression-free survival and overall survival data for patients with locally advanced disease are summarised in the following tables:

Table 2 Progression-free survival in locally advanced disease by therapy sub-group

(see Table 2 on next page)

Table 3 Overall survival in locally advanced disease by therapy sub-group

(see Table 3 on next page)

Table 1 Frequency of Adverse Reactions

System Organ Class	Frequency	Event
Blood and the lymphatic system disorders	Common	Anaemia
	Uncommon	Thrombocytopenia
Immune system disorders	Uncommon	Hypersensitivity reactions, including angioneurotic oedema and urticaria
Psychiatric disorders	Common	Decreased libido
	Uncommon	Depression
Vascular disorders	Common	Hot flushes
Respiratory, thoracic and mediastinal disorders	Uncommon	Interstitial lung disease
Gastrointestinal disorders	Common	Nausea
	Uncommon	Abdominal pain Dyspepsia
Hepato-biliary disorders	Common	Hepatic changes (elevated levels of transaminases, cholestasis and jaundice)[1]
	Rare	Hepatic failure
Skin and subcutaneous tissue disorders	Common	Alopecia Hair regrowth Dry skin Pruritis
Renal and urinary disorders	Uncommon	Haematuria
Reproductive system and breast disorders	Very common	Gynaecomastia[2] Breast tenderness[2]
	Common	Impotence
General disorders and administration site conditions	Common	Asthenia
Investigations	Common	Weight gain

1. Hepatic changes are rarely severe and were frequently transient, resolving or improving with continued therapy or following cessation of therapy (see section 4.4).

2. The majority of patients receiving Bicalutamide 150 mg as monotherapy experience gynaecomastia and/or breast pain. In studies these symptoms were considered to be severe in up to 5% of the patients. Gynaecomastia may not resolve spontaneously following cessation of therapy, particularly after prolonged treatment.

Table 2 Progression-free survival in locally advanced disease by therapy sub-group

Analysis population	Events (%) in Bicalutamide patients	Events (%) in placebo patients	Hazard ratio (95% CI)
Watchful waiting	193/335 (57.6)	222/322 (68.9)	0.60 (0.49 to 0.73)
Radiotherapy	66/161 (41.0)	86/144 (59.7)	0.56 (0.40 to 0.78)
Radical prostatectomy	179/870 (20.6)	213/849 (25.1)	0.75 (0.61 to 0.91)

Table 2 Overall survival in locally advanced disease by therapy sub-group

Analysis population	Deaths (%) in Bicalutamide patients	Deaths (%) in placebo patients	Hazard ratio (95% CI)
Watchful waiting	164/335 (49.0)	183/322 (56.8)	0.81 (0.66 to 1.01)
Radiotherapy	49/161 (30.4)	61/144 (42.4)	0.65 (0.44 to 0.95)
Radical prostatectomy	137/870 (15.7)	122/849 (14.4)	1.09 (0.85 to 1.39)

For patients with localised disease receiving Bicalutamide alone, there was no significant difference in progression free survival. In these patients there was also a trend toward decreased survival compared with placebo patients (HR=1.16; 95% CI 0.99 to 1.37). In view of this, the benefit-risk profile for the use of Bicalutamide is not considered favourable in this group of patients.

In a separate programme, the efficacy of Bicalutamide 150 mg for the treatment of patients with locally advanced non-metastatic prostate cancer for whom immediate castration was indicated, was demonstrated in a combined analysis of 2 studies with 480 previously untreated patients with non-metastatic (M0) prostate cancer. At 56% mortality and a median follow-up of 6.3 years, there was no significant difference between Bicalutamide and castration in survival (hazard ratio = 1.05 [CI 0.81 to 1.36]); however, equivalence of the two treatments could not be concluded statistically.

In a combined analysis of 2 studies with 805 previously untreated patients with metastatic (M1) disease at 43% mortality, Bicalutamide 150 mg was demonstrated to be less effective than castration in survival time (hazard ratio = 1.30 [CI 1.04 to 1.65]), with a numerical difference in estimated time to death of 42 days (6 weeks) over a median survival time of 2 years.

Bicalutamide is a racemate with its antiandrogen activity being almost exclusively in the R-enantiomer.

5.2 Pharmacokinetic properties

Bicalutamide is well absorbed following oral administration. There is no evidence of any clinically relevant effect of food on bioavailability.

The (S)-enantiomer is rapidly cleared relative to (R)-enantiomer, the latter having a plasma elimination half-life of about 1 week.

On daily administration of Bicalutamide 150 mg, the (R)-enantiomer accumulates about 10-fold in plasma as a consequence of its long half-life.

Steady state plasma concentrations of the (R)-enantiomer, of approximately 22 microgram/ml are observed during daily administration of Bicalutamide 150 mg. At steady state, the predominantly active (R)-enantiomer accounts for 99% of the total circulating enantiomers.

The pharmacokinetics of the (R)-enantiomer are unaffected by age, renal impairment or mild to moderate hepatic impairment. There is evidence that for subjects with severe hepatic impairment, the (R)-enantiomer is more slowly eliminated from plasma.

Bicalutamide is highly protein bound (racemate 96%, (R) enantiomer > 99%) and extensively metabolised (oxidation and glucuronidation); its metabolites are eliminated via the kidneys and bile in approximately equal proportions.

In a clinical study the mean concentration of R-bicalutamide in semen of men receiving Bicalutamide 150 mg was 4.9 microgram/ml. The amount of bicalutamide potentially delivered to a female partner during intercourse is low and equates to approximately 0.3 microgram/kg. This is below that required to induce changes in offspring of laboratory animals.

5.3 Preclinical safety data

Bicalutamide is a potent antiandrogen and a mixed function oxidase enzyme inducer in animals. Target organ changes, including tumour induction (Leydig cells, thyroid, liver) in animals, are related to these activities. Enzyme induction has not been observed in man and none of these findings is considered to have relevance to the treatment of patients with prostate cancer. Atrophy of seminiferous tubules is a predicted class effect with antiandrogens and has been observed for all species examined. Full reversal of testicular atrophy was 24 weeks after a 12-month repeated dose toxicity study in rats, although functional reversal was evident in reproduction studies 7 weeks after the end of an 11 week dosing period. A period of subfertility or infertility should be assumed in man.

6. PHARMACEUTICAL PARTICULARS

6.1 List of excipients

Bicalutamide 150 mg includes the following excipients:

Tablet core: Lactose Monohydrate, Magnesium Stearate, Povidone, Sodium Starch Glycolate

Film-coating material: Hypromellose, Macrogol 300, Titanium Dioxide.

6.2 Incompatibilities

Not applicable.

6.3 Shelf life

4 years.

6.4 Special precautions for storage

Do not store above 30°C.

6.5 Nature and contents of container

PVC/Aluminium foil blister pack comprising strips of 5, 10 and 14 tablets to give pack sizes of 10, 20, 30, 40, 50, 80, 90, 100, 200 or 14, 28, 56, 84, 140 and 280 tablets.

Not all pack sizes may be marketed.

6.6 Special precautions for disposal and other handling

No special requirements.

7. MARKETING AUTHORISATION HOLDER

AstraZeneca UK Ltd

600 Capability Green,

Luton, LU1 3LU, UK.

8. MARKETING AUTHORISATION NUMBER(S)

PL 17901/0190

9. DATE OF FIRST AUTHORISATION/RENEWAL OF THE AUTHORISATION

15th May 2002/03rd August 2007

10. DATE OF REVISION OF THE TEXT

18th June 2008

Binocrit Solution for Injection in a pre-filled syringe

(Sandoz Limited)

1. NAME OF THE MEDICINAL PRODUCT

Binocrit 1000 ▼ IU/0.5 ml solution for injection in a pre-filled syringe

Binocrit 2000 ▼ IU/1 ml solution for injection in a pre-filled syringe

Binocrit 3000 ▼ IU/0.3 ml solution for injection in a pre-filled syringe

Binocrit 4000 ▼ IU/0.4 ml solution for injection in a pre-filled syringe

Binocrit 5000 ▼ IU/0.5 ml solution for injection in a pre-filled syringe

Binocrit 6000 ▼ IU/0.6 ml solution for injection in a pre-filled syringe

Binocrit 7000 ▼ IU/0.7 ml solution for injection in a pre-filled syringe

Binocrit 8000 ▼ IU/0.8 ml solution for injection in a pre-filled syringe

Binocrit 9000 ▼ IU/0.9 ml solution for injection in a pre-filled syringe

Binocrit 10 000 ▼ IU/1 ml solution for injection in a pre-filled syringe

. QUALITATIVE AND QUANTITATIVE COMPOSITION

000 IU/0.5 ml: Each ml of solution contains 2000 IU of •poetin alfa* corresponding to 16.8 micrograms per ml. 1 •re-filled syringe of 0.5 ml contains 1000 international units U) corresponding to 8.4 micrograms epoetin alfa.

'000 IU/1 ml: Each ml of solution contains 2000 IU of epoetin alfa* corresponding to 16.8 micrograms per ml. 1 ore-filled syringe of 1 ml contains 2000 international units IU) corresponding to 16.8 micrograms epoetin alfa.

3000 IU/0.3 ml: Each ml of solution contains 10 000 IU of epoetin alfa* corresponding to 84.0 micrograms per ml. 1 •re-filled syringe of 0.3 ml contains 3000 international units IU) corresponding to 25.2 micrograms epoetin alfa.

4000 IU/0.4 ml: Each ml of solution contains 10 000 IU of epoetin alfa* corresponding to 84.0 micrograms per ml. 1 ore-filled syringe of 0.4 ml contains 4000 international units IU) corresponding to 33.6 micrograms epoetin alfa.

5000 IU/0.5 ml: Each ml of solution contains 10 000 IU of epoetin alfa* corresponding to 84.0 micrograms per ml. 1 ore-filled syringe of 0.5 ml contains 5000 international units (IU) corresponding to 42.0 micrograms epoetin alfa.

6000 IU/0.6 ml: >Each ml of solution contains 10 000 IU of epoetin alfa* corresponding to 84.0 micrograms per ml. 1 pre-filled syringe of 0.6 ml contains 6000 international units (IU) corresponding to 50.4 micrograms epoetin alfa.

7000 IU/0.7 ml: Each ml of solution contains 10 000 IU of epoetin alfa* corresponding to 84.0 micrograms per ml. 1 pre-filled syringe of 0.7 ml contains 7000 international units (IU) corresponding to 58.8 micrograms epoetin alfa.

8000 IU/0.8 ml: >Each ml of solution contains 10 000 IU of epoetin alfa* corresponding to 84.0 micrograms per ml. 1 pre-filled syringe of 0.8 ml contains 8000 international units (IU) corresponding to 67.2 micrograms epoetin alfa.

9000 IU/0.9 ml: Each ml of solution contains 10 000 IU of epoetin alfa* corresponding to 84.0 micrograms per ml. 1 pre-filled syringe of 0.9 ml contains 9000 international units (IU) corresponding to 75.6 micrograms epoetin alfa.

Binocrit 10 000 IU/1 ml: Each ml of solution contains 10 000 IU of epoetin alfa* corresponding to 84.0 micrograms per ml. 1 pre-filled syringe of 1 ml contains 10 000 international units (IU) corresponding to 84.0 micrograms epoetin alfa.

* Produced in CHO cell line by recombinant DNA technology

For a full list of excipients, see section 6.1.

3. PHARMACEUTICAL FORM

Solution for injection in a pre-filled syringe (injection)

Clear colourless solution

4. CLINICAL PARTICULARS

4.1 Therapeutic indications

Treatment of symptomatic anaemia associated with chronic renal failure (CRF) in adult and paediatric patients:

- Treatment of anaemia associated with chronic renal failure in paediatric and adult patients on haemodialysis and adult patients on peritoneal dialysis (See section 4.4).

- Treatment of severe anaemia of renal origin accompanied by clinical symptoms in adult patients with renal insufficiency not yet undergoing dialysis (See section 4.4).

Treatment of anaemia and reduction of transfusion requirements in adult patients receiving chemotherapy for solid tumours, malignant lymphoma or multiple myeloma, and at risk of transfusion as assessed by the patient's general status (e.g. cardiovascular status, pre-existing anaemia at the start of chemotherapy).

Binocrit can be used to increase the yield of autologous blood from patients in a predonation programme. Its use in this indication must be balanced against the reported risk of thromboembolic events. Treatment should only be given to patients with moderate anaemia (haemoglobin (Hb) 10 – 13 g/dl [6.2 – 8.1 mmol/l], no iron deficiency), if blood saving procedures are not available or insufficient when the scheduled major elective surgery requires a large volume of blood (4 or more units of blood for females or 5 or more units for males).

Binocrit can be used to reduce exposure to allogeneic blood transfusions in adult non-iron deficient patients prior to major elective orthopaedic surgery, having a high perceived risk for transfusion complications. Use should be restricted to patients with moderate anaemia (e.g. Hb 10 - 13 g/dl) who do not have an autologous predonation programme available and with an expected blood loss of 900 to 1800 ml.

4.2 Posology and method of administration

Treatment with Binocrit has to be initiated under the supervision of physicians experienced in the management of patients with the above indications.

Posology

Treatment of symptomatic anaemia in adult and paediatric chronic renal failure patients:

In patients with chronic renal failure the medicinal product has to be administered intravenously (see section 4.4).

The haemoglobin concentration aimed for is between 10 and 12 g/dl (6.2 - 7.5 mmol/l), except in paediatric patients in whom the haemoglobin concentration should be between 9.5 and 11 g/dl (5.9 - 6.8 mmol/l).

Anaemia symptoms and sequelae may vary with age, gender, and overall burden of disease; a physician's evaluation of the individual patient's clinical course and condition is necessary. Binocrit should be administered intravenously in order to increase haemoglobin to not greater than 12 g/dl (7.5 mmol/l). A rise in haemoglobin of greater than 2 g/dl (1.25 mmol/l) over a four week period should be avoided. If it occurs, appropriate dose adjustments should be made as provided. Due to intra-patient variability, occasional individual haemoglobin values for a patient above and below the desired haemoglobin level may be observed. Haemoglobin variability should be addressed through dose management, with consideration for the haemoglobin target range of 10 g/dl (6.2 mmol/l) to 12 g/dl (7.5 mmol/l).

In paediatric patients the recommended target haemoglobin range is between 9.5 and 11 g/dl (5.9 - 6.8 mmol/l).

A sustained haemoglobin level of greater than 12 g/dl (7.5 mmol/l) should be avoided. If the haemoglobin is rising by more than 2 g/dl (1.25 mmol/l) per month, or if the sustained haemoglobin exceeds 12 g/dl (7.5 mmol/l) reduce the epoetin alfa dose by 25%. If the haemoglobin exceeds 13 g/dl (8.1 mmol/l), discontinue therapy until it falls below 12 g/dl (7.5 mmol/l) and then reinstitute epoetin alfa therapy at a dose 25% below the previous level.

Patients should be monitored closely to ensure that the lowest approved dose of Epoetin alfa is used to provide adequate control of anaemia and of the symptoms of anaemia.

Iron status should be evaluated prior to and during treatment and iron supplementation administered if necessary. In addition, other causes of anaemia, such as vitamin B_{12} or folate deficiency, should be excluded before instituting therapy with epoetin alfa. Non response to epoetin alfa therapy may have the following causes: iron, folate, or vitamin B_{12} deficiency; aluminium intoxication; intercurrent infections; inflammatory or traumatic episodes; occult blood loss; haemolysis, and bone marrow fibrosis of any origin.

Adult haemodialysis patients:

The treatment is divided into two stages:

Correction phase:

50 IU/kg 3 times per week by the intravenous route. When a dose adjustment is necessary, this should be done in steps of at least four weeks. At each step, the increase or reduction in dose should be of 25 IU/kg 3 times per week.

Maintenance phase:

Dose adjustment in order to maintain haemoglobin values at the desired level: Hb between 10 and 12 g/dl (6.2 - 7.5 mmol/l).

The recommended total weekly dose is between 75 and 300 IU/kg given by the intravenous route.

The clinical data available suggest that those patients whose initial haemoglobin is very low (< 6 g/dl or < 3.75 mmol/l) may require higher maintenance doses than those whose initial anaemia is less severe (Hb > 8 g/dl or > 5 mmol/l).

Paediatric haemodialysis patients:

The treatment is divided into two stages:

Correction phase:

50 IU/kg 3 times per week by the intravenous route. When a dose adjustment is necessary, this should be done in steps of 25 IU/kg 3 times per week at intervals of at least 4 weeks until the desired goal is achieved.

Maintenance phase:

Dose adjustment in order to maintain haemoglobin values at the desired level: Hb between 9.5 and 11 g/dl (5.9 - 6.8 mmol/l).

Generally, children under 30 kg require higher maintenance doses than children over 30 kg and adults.

The following maintenance doses were observed in clinical trials after 6 months of treatment:

	Dose (IU/kg given 3x /week)	
Weight (kg)	Median	Usual maintenance dose
< 10	100	75 - 150
10 - 30	75	60 - 150
> 30	33	30 - 100

The clinical data available suggest that those patients whose initial haemoglobin is very low (< 6.8 g/dl or < 4.25 mmol/l) may require higher maintenance doses than those whose initial anaemia is less severe (Hb > 6.8 g/dl or > 4.25 mmol/l).

Adult peritoneal dialysis patients:

The treatment is divided into two stages:

Correction phase:

Starting dose of 50 IU/kg 2 times per week by the intravenous route.

Maintenance phase:

Dose adjustment in order to maintain haemoglobin values at the desired level: Hb between 10 and 12 g/dl (6.2 - 7.5 mmol/l). Maintenance dose between 25 and 50 IU/kg 2 times per week into 2 equal injections.

Adult patients with renal insufficiency not yet undergoing dialysis:

The treatment is divided into two stages:

Correction phase:

Starting dose of 50 IU/kg 3 times per week by the intravenous route, followed if necessary by a dose increase with 25 IU/kg increments (3 times per week) until the desired goal is achieved (this should be done in steps of at least four weeks).

Maintenance phase:

Dose adjustment in order to maintain haemoglobin values at the desired level: Hb between 10 and 12 g/dl (6.2 - 7.5 mmol/l). Maintenance dose between 17 and 33 IU/kg 3 times per week by the intravenous route.

The maximum dose should not exceed 200 IU/kg 3 times per week.

Treatment of patients with chemotherapy induced anaemia:

Epoetin alfa should be administered by the subcutaneous route to patients with anaemia (e.g. haemoglobin concentration ⩽ 10 g/dl (6.2 mmol/l)). Anaemia symptoms and sequelae may vary with age, gender, and overall burden of disease; a physician's evaluation of the individual patient's clinical course and condition is necessary.

Due to intra-patient variability, occasional individual haemoglobin values for a patient above and below the desired haemoglobin level may be observed. Haemoglobin variability should be addressed through dose management with consideration for the haemoglobin target range of 10 g/dl (6.2 mmol/l) to 12 g/dl (7.5 mmol/l). A sustained haemoglobin level of greater than 12 g/dl (7.5 mmol/l) should be avoided; guidance for appropriate dose adjustment for when haemoglobin values exceeding 12 g/dl (7.5 mmol/l) are observed are described below.

Patients should be monitored closely to ensure that the lowest approved dose of Epoetin alfa is used to provide adequate control of the symptoms of anaemia.

Epoetin alfa therapy should continue until one month after the end of chemotherapy.

The initial dose is 150 IU/kg given subcutaneously 3 times per week. Alternatively, epoetin alfa can be administered at an initial dose of 450 IU/kg subcutaneously once weekly. If haemoglobin has increased by at least 1 g/dl (0.62 mmol/l) or the reticulocyte count has increased ⩾ 40,000 cells/µl above baseline after 4 weeks of treatment, the dose should remain at 150 IU/kg 3 times a week or 450 IU/kg once weekly. If the haemoglobin increase is < 1 g/dl (< 0.62 mmol/l) and the reticulocyte count has increased < 40,000 cells/µl above baseline, increase the dose to 300 IU/kg 3 times per week. If after an additional 4 weeks of therapy at 300 IU/kg 3 times per week, the haemoglobin has increased ⩾ 1 g/dl (⩾ 0.62 mmol/l) or the reticulocyte count has increased ⩾ 40,000 cells/µl the dose should remain at 300 IU/kg 3 times per week. However, if the haemoglobin has increased < 1 g/dl (< 0.62 mmol/l) and the reticulocyte count has increased < 40,000 cells/µl above baseline, response to epoetin alfa therapy is unlikely and treatment should be discontinued.

The recommended dosing regimen is described in the following diagram:

(see Figure 1 on next page)

Dosage adjustment to maintain haemoglobin concentration between 10 g/dl - 12 g/dl:

If the haemoglobin is rising by more than 2 g/dl (1.25 mmol/l) per month, or if the haemoglobin exceeds 12 g/dl (7.5 mmol/l), the dose should be reduced by approximately 25 to 50%. If the haemoglobin exceeds 13 g/dl (8.1 mmol/l), discontinue therapy until it falls below 12 g/dl (7.5 mmol/l) and than reinstitute epoetin alfa therapy at a dose 25% below the previous dose.

Adult surgery patients in an autologous predonation programme:

Binocrit should be given by the intravenous route.

At the time of donating blood, Binocrit should be administered after the completion of the blood donation procedure.

Mildly anaemic patients (haematocrit of 33 - 39%) requiring predeposit of ⩾ 4 units of blood should be treated with Binocrit at a dose of 600 IU/kg body weight 2 times weekly for 3 weeks prior to surgery.

All patients being treated with Binocrit should receive adequate iron supplementation (e.g. 200 mg oral elemental iron daily) throughout the course of treatment. Iron supplementation should be started as soon as possible, even several weeks prior to initiating the autologous predeposit, in order to achieve high iron stores prior to starting Binocrit therapy.

Treatment of adult patients scheduled for major elective orthopaedic surgery:

The subcutaneous route of administration should be used.

The recommended dose is 600 IU/kg epoetin alfa, given weekly for three weeks (days 21, 14 and 7) prior to surgery and on the day of surgery (day 0). In cases where there is a medical need to shorten the lead time before surgery to less than three weeks, 300 IU/kg epoetin alfa should be

Figure 1

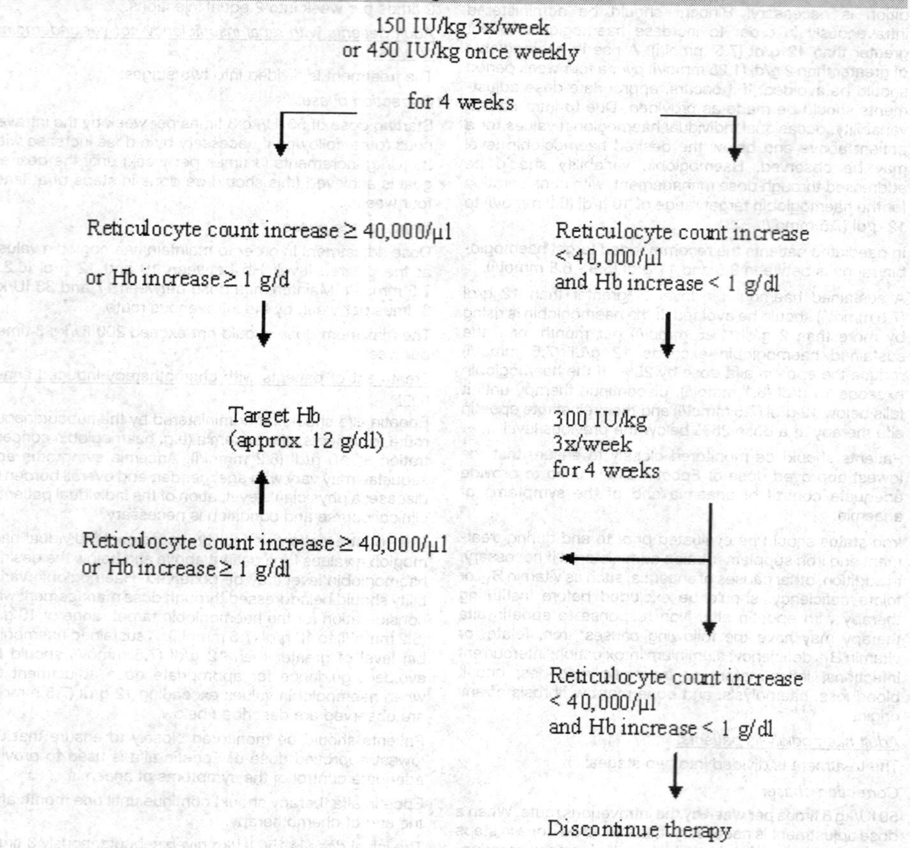

given daily for 10 consecutive days prior to surgery, on the day of surgery and for four days immediately thereafter. When performing haematologic assessments during the preoperative period, if the haemoglobin level reaches 15 g/dl, or higher, administration of epoetin alfa should be stopped and further doses should not be given.

Care should be taken to ensure that at the outset of the treatment patients are not iron deficient.

All patients being treated with epoetin alfa should receive adequate iron supplementation (e.g. oral iron substitution of 200 mg Fe^{2+} daily) throughout the course of epoetin alfa treatment. Iron supplementation should be started prior to epoetin alfa therapy, to achieve adequate iron stores.

Method of administration

Binocrit is a sterile but unpreserved product and is for single use only. Administer the amount required. This medicinal product must not be administered by intravenous infusion, or mixed with other medicinal products.

1. Intravenous injection: over at least one to five minutes, depending on the total dose. In haemodialysed patients, a bolus injection may be given during the dialysis session through a suitable venous port in the dialysis line. Alternatively, the injection can be given at the end of the dialysis session via the fistula needle tubing, followed by 10 ml of isotonic saline to rinse the tubing and ensure satisfactory injection of the product into the circulation.

A slower injection is preferable in patients who react to the treatment with "flu-like" symptoms.

2. Subcutaneous injection: a maximum volume of 1 ml at one injection site should generally not be exceeded. In case of larger volumes, more than one site should be chosen for the injection.

The injections are given in the thighs or the anterior abdominal wall.

In chronic renal failure patients Binocrit has not to be administered subcutaneously! The intravenous route has to be used (please see section 4.4 - chronic renal failure patients).

4.3 Contraindications

Hypersensitivity to the active substance or to any of the excipients.

Patients who develop Pure Red Cell Aplasia (PRCA) following treatment with any erythropoietin should not receive Binocrit or any other erythropoietin (see section 4.4 - Pure Red Cell Aplasia).

Uncontrolled hypertension.

In the indication "increasing the yield of autologous blood": myocardial infarction or stroke in the month preceding treatment, unstable angina pectoris, increased risk of deep venous thrombosis such as history of venous thromboembolic disease.

Patients who for any reason cannot receive adequate antithrombotic prophylaxis.

The use of epoetin alfa in patients scheduled for major elective orthopaedic surgery and not participating in an autologous blood predonation programme is contraindicated in patients with severe coronary, peripheral arterial, carotid or cerebral vascular disease, including patients with recent myocardial infarction or cerebral vascular accident.

4.4 Special warnings and precautions for use

General

In all patients receiving epoetin alfa, blood pressure should be closely monitored and controlled as necessary. Epoetin alfa should be used with caution in the presence of untreated, inadequately treated or poorly controllable hypertension. It may be necessary to add or increase antihypertensive treatment. If blood pressure cannot be controlled, epoetin alfa treatment should be discontinued.

Epoetin alfa should be used with caution in the presence of epilepsy and chronic liver failure.

There may be a moderate dose-dependent rise in the platelet count within the normal range during treatment with epoetin alfa. This regresses during the course of continued therapy. It is recommended that the platelet count is regularly monitored during the first 8 weeks of therapy.

All other causes of anaemia (iron deficiency, haemolysis, blood loss, vitamin B_{12} or folate deficiencies) should be considered and treated prior to initiating therapy with epoetin alfa. In most cases, the ferritin values in the serum fall simultaneously with the rise in packed cell volume. In order to ensure optimum response to epoetin alfa, adequate iron stores should be assured:

- iron supplementation, e.g. 200 - 300 mg Fe^{2+}/day orally (100 - 200 mg Fe^{2+}/day for paediatric patients) is recommended for chronic renal failure patients whose serum ferritin levels are below 100 ng/ml

- oral iron substitution of 200 - 300 mg Fe^{2+}/day is recommended for all cancer patients whose transferrin saturation is below 20%.

All of these additive factors of anaemia should also be carefully considered when deciding to increase the dose of epoetin alfa in cancer patients.

Good blood management practices should always be used in the perisurgical setting

Pure Red Cell Aplasia (PRCA)

Antibody-mediated PRCA has been very rarely reported after months to years of subcutaneous erythropoietin treatment. In patients developing sudden lack of efficacy defined by a decrease in haemoglobin (1 to 2 g/dl per month) with increased need for transfusions, a reticulocyte count should be obtained and typical causes of non-response (e.g. iron, folate or, vitamin B_{12} deficiency, aluminium intoxication, infection or inflammation, blood loss and haemolysis) should be investigated.

If the reticulocyte count corrected for anaemia (i.e., the reticulocyte "index") is low (< 20,000/mm³ or < 20,000 microlitre or < 0.5%), platelet and white blood cell count are normal, and if no other cause of loss of effect has been found, anti-erythropoietin antibodies should be determined and bone marrow examination should be considered for diagnosis of PRCA.

If anti-erythropoietin, antibody-mediated PRCA is suspected, therapy with Binocrit should be discontinued immediately. No other erythropoietic therapy should be commenced because of the risk of cross-reaction. Appropriate therapy such as blood transfusions may be given to patients when indicated.

Chronic renal failure patients

Immunogenicity data for subcutaneous use of Binocrit in patients at risk for antibody-induced PRCA, i.e. patients with renal anaemia, are not sufficient. Therefore, in patients with renal anaemia the medicinal product has to be administered intravenously.

In patients with chronic renal failure, maintenance haemoglobin concentration should not exceed the upper limit of the target haemoglobin concentration recommended in section 4.2. In clinical trials, an increased risk of death and serious cardiovascular events was observed when erythropoiesis stimulating agents (ESAs) were administered to target a haemoglobin of greater than 12 g/dl (7.5 mmol/l).

Controlled clinical trials have not shown significant benefits attributable to the administration of epoetins when haemoglobin concentration is increased beyond the level necessary to control symptoms of anaemia and to avoid blood transfusion.

Haemoglobin levels should be measured on a regular basis until a stable level is achieved and periodically thereafter. The rate of increase in haemoglobin should be approximately 1 g/dl (0.62 mmol/l) per month and should not exceed 2 g/dl (1.25 mmol/l) per month to minimise risks of an increase in hypertension.

Hyperkalaemia has been observed in isolated cases. Correction for anaemia may lead to increased appetite, and potassium and protein intake. Dialysis prescriptions may have to be adjusted periodically to maintain urea, creatinine and potassium in the desired range. Serum electrolytes should be monitored in chronic renal failure patients. If an elevated (or rising) serum potassium level is detected then consideration should be given to ceasing epoetin alfa administration until hyperkalaemia has been corrected.

An increase in heparin dose during haemodialysis is frequently required during the course of therapy with epoetin alfa as a result of the increased packed cell volume. Occlusion of the dialysis system is possible if heparinisation is not optimum.

In patients with chronic renal failure and clinically evident ischaemic heart disease or congestive heart failure, maintenance haemoglobin concentration should not exceed the upper limit of the target haemoglobin concentration as recommended under section 4.2.

Based on information available to date, correction of anaemia with epoetin alfa in adult patients with renal insufficiency not yet undergoing dialysis does not accelerate the rate of progression of renal insufficiency.

Adult cancer patients with symptomatic anaemia receiving chemotherapy

In cancer patients receiving chemotherapy, the 2 - 3 week delay between epoetin alfa administration and the appearance of erythropoietin-induced red cells should be taken into account when assessing if epoetin alfa therapy is appropriate (patient at risk of being transfused).

Haemoglobin levels should be measured on a regular basis until a stable level is achieved and periodically thereafter. If the rate of increase in haemoglobin exceeds 2 g/dl (1.25 mmol/l) per month or the haemoglobin level exceeds 13 g/dl (8.1 mmol/l)m, the dose adaptation detailed in section 4.2 should be thoroughly performed to minimise the risk for thrombotic events (see section 4.2 Treatment of patients with chemotherapy induced anaemia - Dosage adjustment to maintain haemoglobin concentration between 10 g/dl - 12 g/dl).

As an increased incidence of thrombotic vascular events (TVEs) has been observed in cancer patients receiving erythropoiesis-stimulating agents (see section 4.8), this risk should be carefully weighed against the benefit to be derived from treatment (with epoetin alfa) particularly in cancer patients with an increased risk of thrombotic vascular events, such as obesity and patients with a prior history of TVEs (e.g. deep vein thrombosis or pulmonary embolism). An investigational study (BEST study) in women with metastatic breast cancer was designed to determine whether epoetin alfa treatment that extended beyond the correction of anaemia could improve treatment outcomes. In that study the incidence of fatal thromboembolic events was higher in patients receiving epoetin alfa than in those receiving placebo (see section 5.1).

In view of the above, in some clinical situations blood transfusions should be the preferred treatment for the management of anaemia in patients with cancer. The decision to administer recombinant erythropoietins should be based on a benefit-risk assessment with the participation of the individual patient, which should also take into account the specific clinical context. Factors that should be considered in this assessment should include the type of tumour and its stage; the degree of anaemia; life-expectancy; the environment in which the patient is being treated; and patient preference (see section 5.1).

Adult surgery patients in an autologous predonation programme

All special warnings and precautions associated with autologous predonation programmes, especially routine volume replacement, should be respected.

Patients scheduled for major elective orthopaedic surgery

In patients scheduled for major elective orthopaedic surgery the cause of anaemia should be established and treated, if possible, before the start of epoetin alfa treatment. Thrombotic events can be a risk in this population and this possibility should be carefully weighed against the benefit to be derived from the treatment in this patient group.

Patients scheduled for major elective orthopaedic surgery should receive adequate antithrombotic prophylaxis, as thrombotic and vascular events may occur in surgical patients, especially in those with underlying cardiovascular disease. In addition, special precaution should be taken in patients with predisposition for development of deep vein thrombosis (DVTs). Moreover, in patients with a baseline haemoglobin of > 13 g/dl, the possibility that epoetin alfa treatment may be associated with an increased risk of postoperative thrombotic/vascular events cannot be excluded. Therefore, it should not be used in patients with baseline haemoglobin > 13 g/dl.

Tumour growth potential

Erythropoietins are growth factors that primarily stimulate red blood cell production. Erythropoietin receptors may be expressed on the surface of a variety of tumour cells. As with all growth factors, there is a concern that epoetins could stimulate the growth of tumours. In several controlled studies, epoetins have not been shown to improve overall survival or decrease the risk of tumour progression in patients with anaemia associated with cancer.

In controlled clinical studies, use of Epoetin alfa and other erythropoiesis-stimulating agents (ESAs) have shown:

- decreased locoregional control in patients with advanced head and neck cancer receiving radiation therapy when administered to target a haemoglobin of greater than 14 g/dl (8.7 mmol/l),

- shortened overall survival and increased deaths attributed to disease progression at 4 months in patients with metastatic breast cancer receiving chemotherapy when administered to target a haemoglobin of 12 - 14 g/dl (7.5 – 8.7 mmol/l),

- increased risk of death when administered to target a haemoglobin of 12 g/dl (7.5 mmol/l) in patients with active malignant disease receiving neither chemotherapy nor radiation therapy. ESAs are not indicated for use in this patient population.

Excipients

This medicinal product contains less than 1 mmol sodium (23 mg) per dose, i.e. essentially "sodium-free".

4.5 Interaction with other medicinal products and other forms of interaction

No evidence exists that indicates that treatment with epoetin alfa alters the metabolism of other medicinal products. However, since cyclosporin is bound by red blood cells there is potential for an interaction. If epoetin alfa is given concomitantly with cyclosporin, blood levels of cyclosporin should be monitored and the dose of cyclosporin adjusted as the haematocrit rises.

No evidence exists that indicates an interaction between epoetin alfa and G-CSF or GM-CSF with regard to haematological differentiation or proliferation of tumour biopsy specimens *in vitro*.

4.6 Pregnancy and lactation

There are no adequate and well-controlled studies in pregnant women. Studies in animals have shown reproduction toxicity (see section 5.3).

Consequently:

- In chronic renal failure patients, epoetin alfa should be used in pregnancy only if the potential benefit outweighs the potential risk to the foetus.

- In pregnant or lactating surgical patients participating in an autologous blood predonation programme, the use of epoetin alfa is not recommended.

4.7 Effects on ability to drive and use machines

Binocrit has no influence on the ability to drive and use machines.

4.8 Undesirable effects

The most frequent adverse reaction is an increase in blood pressure or aggravation of existing hypertension. Hypertensive crisis with encephalopathy-like symptoms can occur. Attention should be paid to sudden stabbing migraine-like headaches as a possible warning signal.

General

Non-specific skin rashes have been described in association with epoetin alfa.

"Flu-like" symptoms such as headaches, joint pains, feelings of weakness, dizziness, and tiredness may occur, especially at the start of treatment.

Thrombocytosis has been observed but its occurrence is very rare (see section 4.4).

Thrombotic/vascular events, such as myocardial ischaemia, myocardial infarction, cerebrovascular accidents (cerebral haemorrhage and cerebral infarction), transient ischaemic attacks, deep vein thrombosis, arterial thrombosis, pulmonary emboli, aneurysms, retinal thrombosis, and clotting of an artificial kidney have been reported in patients receiving erythropoietic agents, including patients receiving epoetin alfa.

Hypersensitivity reactions have been rarely reported with epoetin alfa including isolated cases of angioedema and anaphylactic reaction.

Antibody-mediated erythroblastopenia (PRCA) has been reported after months to years of treatment with epoetin alfa. In most of these patients, antibodies to erythropoietins have been observed (see sections 4.3 and 4.4 – *Pure Red Cell Aplasia*)

Adult and paediatric haemodialysis patients, adult peritoneal dialysis patients and adult patients with renal insufficiency not yet undergoing dialysis

The most frequent adverse reaction during treatment with epoetin alfa is a dose-dependent increase in blood pressure or aggravation of existing hypertension. These increases in blood pressure can be treated with medicinal products. Moreover, monitoring of the blood pressure is recommended particularly at the start of therapy. The following reactions have also occurred in isolated patients with normal or low blood pressure: hypertensive crisis with encephalopathy-like symptoms (e.g. headaches and confused state) and generalised tonoclonal seizures, requiring the immediate attention of a physician and intensive medical care. Particular attention should be paid to sudden stabbing migraine-like headaches as a possible warning signal.

Shunt thromboses may occur, especially in patients who have a tendency to hypotension or whose arteriovenous fistulae exhibit complications (e.g. stenoses, aneurysms, etc.). Early shunt revision and thrombosis prophylaxis by administration of acetylsalicylic acid, for example, is recommended in these patients.

Adult cancer patients with symptomatic anaemia receiving chemotherapy

Hypertension may occur in epoetin alfa treated patients. Consequently, haemoglobin and blood pressure should be closely monitored.

An increased incidence of thrombotic vascular events (see section 4.4 and section 4.8 - General) has been observed in patients receiving erythropoietic agents.

Surgery patients in autologous predonation programmes

Independent of erythropoietin treatment, thrombotic and vascular events may occur in surgical patients with underlying cardiovascular disease following repeated phlebotomy. Therefore, routine volume replacement should be performed in such patients.

Patients scheduled for major elective orthopaedic surgery

In patients scheduled for major elective orthopaedic surgery, with a baseline haemoglobin of 10 to 13 g/dl, the incidence of thrombotic/vascular events (most of which were DVTs), in the overall patient population of the clinical trials, appeared to be similar across the different epoetin alfa dosing groups and placebo group, although the clinical experience is limited.

Moreover, in patients with a baseline haemoglobin of > 13 g/dl, the possibility that epoetin alfa treatment may be associated with an increased risk of postoperative thrombotic/vascular events cannot be excluded.

4.9 Overdose

The therapeutic margin of epoetin alfa is very wide. Overdose of epoetin alfa may produce effects that are extensions of the pharmacological effects of the hormone. Phlebotomy may be performed if excessively high haemoglobin levels occur. Additional supportive care should be provided as necessary.

5. PHARMACOLOGICAL PROPERTIES

5.1 Pharmacodynamic properties

Pharmacotherapeutic group: antianaemic, ATC code: B03XA01

Erythropoietin is a glycoprotein that stimulates, as a mitosis-stimulating factor and differentiating hormone, the formation of erythrocytes from precursors of the stem cell compartment.

The apparent molecular weight of erythropoietin is 32,000 to 40,000 dalton. The protein fraction of the molecule contributes about 58% and consists of 165 amino acids. The four carbohydrate chains are attached via three N-glycosidic bonds and one O-glycosidic bond to the protein. Epoetin alfa obtained by gene technology is glycosylated and is identical in its amino acid and carbohydrate composition to endogenous human erythropoietin that has been isolated from the urine of anaemic patients.

Binocrit has the highest possible purity according to the present state of the art. In particular, no residues of the cell line used for the production are detectable at the concentrations of the active ingredient that are used in humans.

The biological efficacy of epoetin alfa has been demonstrated in various animal models *in vivo* (normal and anaemic rats, polycythaemic mice). After administration of epoetin alfa, the number of erythrocytes, the Hb values and reticulocyte counts increase as well as the ^{59}Fe-incorporation rate.

An increased ^{3}H-thymidine incorporation in the erythroid nucleated spleen cells has been found *in vitro* (mouse spleen cell culture) after incubation with epoetin alfa.

It could be shown with the aid of cell cultures of human bone marrow cells that epoetin alfa stimulates erythropoiesis specifically and does not affect leucopoiesis. Cytotoxic actions of epoetin alfa on bone marrow cells could not be detected.

721 cancer patients receiving non-platinum chemotherapy were included in three placebo-controlled studies, 389 patients with haematological malignancies (221 multiple myeloma, 144 non-Hodgkin's lymphoma, and 24 other haematological malignancies) and 332 with solid tumours (172 breast, 64 gynaecological, 23 lung, 22 prostate, 21 gastro-intestinal, and 30 other tumour types). In two large, open-label studies, 2697 cancer patients receiving non-platinum chemotherapy were included, 1895 with solid tumours (683 breast, 260 lung, 174 gynaecological, 300 gastro-intestinal, and 478 other tumour types) and 802 with haematological malignancies.

In a prospective, randomised, double-blind, placebo-controlled trial conducted in 375 anaemic patients with various non-myeloid malignancies receiving non-platinum chemotherapy, there was a significant reduction of anaemia-related sequelae (e.g. fatigue, decreased energy, and activity reduction), as measured by the following instruments and scales: Functional Assessment of Cancer Therapy-Anaemia (FACT-An) general scale, FACT-An fatigue scale, and Cancer Linear Analogue Scale (CLAS). Two other smaller, randomised, placebo-controlled trials failed to show a significant improvement in quality of life parameters on the EORTC-QLQ-C30 scale or CLAS, respectively.

Erythropoietin is a growth factor that primarily stimulates red cell production. Erythropoietin receptors may be expressed on the surface of a variety of tumour cells.

Survival and tumour progression have been examined in five large controlled studies involving a total of 2833 patients, of which four were double-blind placebo-controlled studies and one was an open-label study. The studies either recruited patients who were being treated with chemotherapy (two studies) or used patient populations in which erythropoiesis stimulating agents are not indicated: anaemia in patients with cancer not receiving chemotherapy, and head and neck cancer patients receiving radiotherapy. The target haemoglobin concentration in two studies was > 13 g/dl; in the remaining three studies it was 12 - 14 g/dl. In the open-label study there was no difference in overall survival between patients treated with recombinant human erythropoietin and controls. In the four placebo-controlled studies the hazard ratios for overall survival ranged between 1.25 and 2.47 in favour of controls. These studies have shown an consistent unexplained statistically significant excess mortality in patients who have anaemia associated with various common cancers who received recombinant human erythropoietin compared to controls. Overall survival outcome in the trials could not be satisfactorily explained by differences in the incidence of thrombosis and related complications between those given recombinant human erythropoietin and those in the control group.

A systematic review has also been performed involving more than 9000 cancer patients participating in 57 clinical trials. Meta-analysis of overall survival data produced a hazard ratio point estimate of 1.08 in favour of controls (95% CI: 0.99, 1,18; 42 trials and 8167 patients). An increased relative risk of thromboembolic events (RR 1.67, 95% CI: 1.35, 2.06, 35 trials and 6769 patients) was observed in patients treated with recombinant human erythropoietin. There is an increased risk for thromboembolic events in patients with cancer treated with recombinant human erythropoietin and a negative impact on overall survival cannot be excluded. The extent to which these outcomes might apply to the administration of recombinant human erythropoietin to patients with cancer, treated with chemotherapy to achieve haemoglobin concentrations less than 13 g/dl, is unclear because few patients with these characteristics were included in the data reviewed.

5.2 Pharmacokinetic properties

Intravenous route

Measurement of epoetin alfa following multiple dose intravenous administration revealed a half-life of approximately 4 hours in normal volunteers and a somewhat more prolonged half-life in renal failure patients, approximately 5 hours. A half-life of approximately 6 hours has been reported in children.

Subcutaneous route

Following subcutaneous injection, serum levels of epoetin alfa are much lower than the levels achieved following intravenous injection, the levels increase slowly and reach a peak between 12 and 18 hours postdose. The peak is always well below the peak achieved using the intravenous route (approximately 1/20th of the value).

There is no accumulation: the levels remain the same, whether they are determined 24 hours after the first injection or 24 hours after the last injection.

The half-life is difficult to evaluate for the subcutaneous route and is estimated about 24 hours.

The bioavailability of subcutaneous injectable epoetin alfa is much lower than that of the intravenous medicinal product: approximately 20%.

5.3 Preclinical safety data

In some preclinical toxicological studies in dogs and rats, but not in monkeys, epoetin alfa therapy was associated with subclinical bone marrow fibrosis (bone marrow fibrosis is a known complication of chronic renal failure in humans and may be related to secondary hyperparathyroidism or unknown factors. The incidence of bone marrow fibrosis was not increased in a study of haemodialysis patients who were treated with epoetin alfa for 3 years compared to a matched control group of dialysis patients who had not been treated with epoetin alfa.).

In animal studies, epoetin alfa has been shown to decrease foetal body weight, delay ossification and increase foetal mortality when given in weekly doses of approximately 20 times the recommended human weekly dose. These changes are interpreted as being secondary to decreased maternal body weight gain.

Epoetin alfa did not show any changes in bacterial and mammalian cell culture mutagenicity tests and an *in vivo* micronucleus test in mice.

Long-term carcinogenicity studies have not been carried out. There are conflicting reports in the literature regarding whether erythropoietins may play a major role as tumour proliferators. These reports are based on *in vitro* findings from human tumour samples, but are of uncertain significance in the clinical situation.

6. PHARMACEUTICAL PARTICULARS

6.1 List of excipients

Sodium dihydrogen phosphate dihydrate

Disodium phosphate dihydrate

Sodium chloride

Glycine

Polysorbate 80

Water for injections

Hydrochloric acid (for pH-adjustment)

Sodium hydroxide (for pH-adjustment)

6.2 Incompatibilities

In the absence of compatibility studies, this medicinal product must not be mixed with other medicinal products.

6.3 Shelf life

2 years

6.4 Special precautions for storage

Store and transport refrigerated (2°C - 8°C).

Do not freeze.

Keep the pre-filled syringe in the outer carton in order to protect from light.

For the purpose of ambulatory use, the patient may remove Binocrit from the refrigerator and store it not above 25°C for one single period of up to 3 days.

6.5 Nature and contents of container

Pre-filled syringes (glass type I) with plunger (Teflon-faced rubber) sealed in a blister.

1000 IU/0.5 ml:	The syringes contain 0.5 ml (1000 IU) of solution.
2000 IU/1 ml:	The syringes contain 1 ml (2000 IU) of solution.
3000 IU/0.3 ml:	The syringes contain 0.3 ml (3000 IU) of solution.
4000 IU/0.4 ml:	The syringes contain 0.4 ml (4000 IU) of solution.
5000 IU/0.5 ml:	The syringes contain 0.5 ml (5000 IU) of solution.
6000 IU/0.6 ml:	The syringes contain 0.6 ml (6000 IU) of solution.
7000 IU/0.7 ml:	The syringes contain 0.7 ml (7000 IU) of solution.
8000 IU/0.8 ml:	The syringes contain 0.8 ml (8000 IU) of solution.
9000 IU/0.9 ml:	The syringes contain 0.9 ml (9000 IU) of solution.
10 000 IU/1 ml:	The syringes contain 1 ml (10 000 IU) of solution.

Syringes are embossed with graduation rings and the filling volume is indicated by a stick-on label in order to enable partial use if required.

Pack of 1 or 6 syringes. Not all pack sizes may be marketed.

6.6 Special precautions for disposal and other handling

Binocrit must not be used

- if the solution is cloudy or there are particles in it.
- if the seal is broken.
- if the solution has been accidentally frozen.

The pre-filled syringes are ready to use (see section 4.2 – Method of administration). After injection of the necessary amount of the solution from the pre-filled syringe, discard any remaining contents. The pre-filled syringe should not be shaken.

Any unused product or waste material should be disposed of in accordance with local requirements.

7. MARKETING AUTHORISATION HOLDER

Sandoz GmbH
Biochemiestr. 10
A-6250 Kundl
Austria

8. MARKETING AUTHORISATION NUMBER(S)

1000IU/0.5ml:	EU/1/07/410/001 – 1 pre-filled syringe EU/1/07/410/002 – 6 pre-filled syringes
2000IU/1ml:	EU/1/07/410/003 – 1 pre-filled syringe EU/1/07/410/004 - 6 pre-filled syringes
3000IU/0.3ml:	EU/1/07/410/005 – 1 pre-filled syringe EU/1/07/410/006 – 6 pre-filled syringes
4000IU/0.4ml:	EU/1/07/410/007 – 1 pre-filled syringe EU/1/07/410/008 – 6 pre-filled syringes
5000IU/0.5ml:	EU/1/07/410/009 – 1 pre-filled syringe EU/1/07/410/010 – 6 pre-filled syringes
6000IU/0.6ml:	EU/1/07/410/011 – 1 pre-filled syringe EU/1/07/410/012 – 6 pre-filled syringes
7000IU/0.7ml:	EU/1/07/410/017 – 1 pre-filled syringe EU/1/07/410/018 – 6 pre-filled syringes
8000IU/0.8ml:	EU/1/07/410/013 – 1 pre-filled syringe EU/1/07/410/014 – 6 pre-filled syringes
9000IU/0.9ml:	EU/1/07/410/019 – 1 pre-filled syringe EU/1/07/410/020 – 6 pre-filled syringes
10000IU/1ml:	EU/1/07/410/015 – 1 pre-filled syringe EU/1/07/410/016 – 6 pre-filled syringes

9. DATE OF FIRST AUTHORISATION/RENEWAL OF THE AUTHORISATION

28 August 2007

10. DATE OF REVISION OF THE TEXT

21 November 2008

Binovum Oral Contraceptive Tablets.

(Janssen-Cilag Ltd)

1. NAME OF THE MEDICINAL PRODUCT

BINOVUM® Oral Contraceptive Tablets.

2. QUALITATIVE AND QUANTITATIVE COMPOSITION

White Tablets

Norethisterone	EP	0.5 mg
Ethinylestradiol	EP	0.035 mg

Peach Tablets

Norethisterone	EP	1.0 mg
Ethinylestradiol	EP	0.035 mg

For a full list of excipients, see section 6.1.

3. PHARMACEUTICAL FORM

Tablets.

4. CLINICAL PARTICULARS

4.1 Therapeutic indications

Contraception and the recognised indications for such oestrogen/progestogen combinations.

4.2 Posology and method of administration

Adults

It is preferable that tablet intake from the first pack is started on the first day of menstruation in which case no extra contraceptive precautions are necessary.

If menstruation has already begun (that is 2, 3 or 4 days previously), tablet taking should commence on day 5 of the menstrual period. In this case, additional contraceptive precautions must be taken for the first 7 days of tablet taking.

If menstruation began more than 5 days previously then the patient should be advised to wait until her next menstrual period before starting to take Binovum.

How to take Binovum:

One tablet is taken daily at the same time (preferably in the evening) without interruption for 21 days, followed by a break of 7 tablet-free days. (A white tablet is taken every day for 7 days, then a peach coloured tablet is taken every day for 14 days, then 7 tablet-free days). Each subsequent pack is started after the 7 tablet-free days have elapsed. Additional contraceptive precautions are not then required.

Elderly:

Not applicable.

Children:

Not recommended.

4.3 Contraindications

Absolute contra-indications

– Pregnancy or suspected pregnancy (that cannot yet be excluded).

– Circulatory disorders (cardiovascular or cerebrovascular) such as thrombophlebitis and thrombo-embolic processes, or a history of these conditions (including history of confirmed venous thrombo-embolism (VTE), family history of idiopathic VTE and other known risk factors for VTE), moderate to severe hypertension, hyperlipoproteinaemia. In addition, the presence of more than one of the risk factors for arterial disease.

– Severe liver disease, cholestatic jaundice or hepatitis (viral or non-viral) or a history of these conditions if the results of liver function tests have failed to return to normal, and for 3 months after liver function tests have been found to be normal; a history of jaundice of pregnancy or jaundice due to the use of steroids, Rotor syndrome and Dubin-Johnson syndrome, hepatic cell tumours and porphyria.

– Cholelithiasis.

– Known or suspected oestrogen-dependent tumours; endometrial hyperplasia; undiagnosed vaginal bleeding.

– Systemic lupus erythematosus or a history of this condition.

– A history during pregnancy or previous use of steroids of:

- severe pruritus
- herpes gestationis
- a manifestation or deterioration of otosclerosis

Relative contra-indications:

If any relative contra-indication listed below are present, the benefits of oestrogen/progestogen containing preparations must be weighed against the possible risk for each individual case and the patient kept under close supervision. In case of aggravation or appearance of any of these conditions whilst the patient is taking the pill, its use should be discontinued.

– Conditions implicating an increasing risk of developing venous thrombo-embolic complications, eg severe varicose veins or prolonged immobilisation or major surgery.

– Disorders of coagulation.

– Presence of any risk factor for arterial disease e.g. smoking, hyperlipidaemia or hypertension.

– Other conditions associated with an increased risk of circulatory disease such as latent or overt cardiac failure, renal dysfunction, or a history of these conditions.

– Epilepsy or a history of this condition.

– Migraine or a history of this condition.

– A history of cholelithiasis.

– Presence of any risk factor for oestrogen-dependent tumours; oestrogen-sensitive gynaecological disorders such as uterine fibromyomata and endometriosis.

– Diabetes mellitus.

– Severe depression or a history of this condition. If this is accompanied by a disturbance in tryptophan metabolism, administration of vitamin B6 might be of therapeutic value.

– Sickle cell haemoglobinopathy, since under certain circumstances, e.g. during infections or anoxia, oestrogen containing preparations may induce thrombo-embolic process in patients with this condition.

– If the results of liver function tests become abnormal, use should be discontinued.

4.4 Special warnings and precautions for use

Post partum administration

Following a vaginal delivery, oral contraceptive administration to non-breast-feeding mothers can be started 21 days post-partum provided the patient is fully ambulant and there are no puerperal complications. No additional contraceptive precautions are required. If post partum administration begins more than 21 days after delivery, additional contraceptive precautions are required for the first 7 days of pill-taking.

If intercourse has taken place post-partum, oral contraceptive use should be delayed until the first day of the first menstrual period.

After miscarriage or abortion, administration should start immediately, in which case no additional contraceptive precautions are required.

Changing from a 21 day pill or 22 day pill to Binovum

All tablets in the old pack should be finished. The first Binovum tablet is taken the next day i.e. no gap is left between taking tablets nor does the patient need to wait for her period to begin. Tablets should be taken as instructed in 'How to take Binovum' (see 4.2). Additional contraceptive precautions are not required. The patient will not have a period until the end of the first Binovum pack, but this is not harmful, nor does it matter if she experiences some bleeding on tablet-taking days.

Changing from a combined every day pill (28 day tablet) to Binovum

Binovum should be started after taking the last active tablet from the 'Every day Pill' pack (ie after taking 21 or 22 tablets). The first Binovum tablet is taken the next day, ie no gap is left between taking tablets nor does the patient need to wait for her period to begin. Tablets should be taken as instructed in 'How to take Binovum' (see 4.2).

dditional contraceptive precautions are not required. emaining tablets from the every day (ED) pack should e discarded.

he patient will not have a period until the end of the first inovum pack, but this is not harmful, nor does it matter if he experiences some bleeding on tablet-taking days.

hanging from a progestogen-only pill (POP or mini pill) to inovum

he first Binovum tablet should be taken on the first day of e period, even if the patient has already taken a mini pill n that day. Tablets should be taken as instructed in 'How take Binovum' (see 4.2). Additional contraceptive pre-autions are not required. All the remaining progestogen-nly pills in the mini pill pack should be discarded.

the patient is taking a mini pill, then she may not always ave a period, especially when she is breast-feeding. The rst Binovum tablet should be taken on the day after opping the mini pill. All remaining pills in the mini pill acket must be discarded. Additional contraceptive pre-autions must be taken for the first 7 days.

o skip a period

o skip a period, a new pack of Binovum should be started n the day after finishing the current pack (the patient skips e tablet-free days). Tablet-taking should be continued in e usual way.

uring the use of the second pack, she may experience ight spotting or break-through bleeding but contracep-ve protection will not be diminished provided there are no blet omissions.

he next pack of Binovum is started after the usual 7 tablet-ee days, regardless of whether the period has completely nished or not.

educed reliability

/hen Binovum is taken according to the directions for use e occurrence of pregnancy is highly unlikely. However e reliability of oral contraceptives may be reduced under e following circumstances:

Forgotten tablets

the patient forgets to take a tablet, she should take it as oon as she remembers and take the next one at the ormal time. This may mean that two tablets are taken in e day. Provided she is less than 12 hours late in taking er tablet, Binovum will still give contraceptive protection uring this cycle and the rest of the pack should be taken s usual.

she is more than 12 hours late in taking one or more blets, then she should take the last missed pill as soon as e remembers but leave the other missed pills in the pack. he should continue to take the rest of the pack as usual ut must use extra precautions (e.g. sheath, diaphragm, us spermicide) and follow the '7-day rule' (see Further formation for the '7 day rule').

there are 7 or more pills left in the pack after the missed nd delayed pills then the usual 7-day break can be left efore starting the next pack. If there are less than 7 pills ft in the pack after the missed and delayed pills then when e pack is finished the next pack should be started the ext day. If withdrawal bleeding does not occur at the end the second pack then a pregnancy test should be erformed.

Vomiting or diarrhoea

after tablet intake, vomiting or diarrhoea occurs, a tablet ay not be absorbed properly by the body. If the symp-oms disappear within 12 hours of tablet-taking, the patient hould take an extra tablet from a spare pack and continue ith the rest of the pack as usual.

owever, if the symptoms continue beyond those 12 ours, additional contraceptive precautions are necessary r any sexual intercourse during the stomach or bowel oset and for the following 7 days (the patient must be dvised to follow the '7-day rule').

) Change in bleeding pattern

after taking Binovum for several months there is a sudden ccurrence of spotting or breakthrough bleeding (not bserved in previous cycles) or the absence of withdrawal eeding, contraceptive effectiveness may be reduced. If ithdrawal bleeding fails to occur and none of the above entioned events has taken place, pregnancy is highly nlikely and oral contraceptive use can be continued until e end of the next pack. (If withdrawal bleeding fails to ccur at the end of the second cycle, tablet intake should e discontinued and pregnancy excluded before oral con-aceptive use can be resumed.) However, if withdrawal eeding is absent and any of the above mentioned events as occurred, tablet intake should be discontinued and regnancy excluded before oral contraceptive use can be sumed.

edical examination/consultation

ssessment of women prior to starting oral contraceptives nd at regular intervals thereafter) should include a perso-al and family medical history of each woman. Physical xamination should be guided by this and by the contra-dications (Section 4.3) and warnings (Section 4.4) for this roduct. The frequency and nature of these assessments hould be based upon relevant guidelines and should be dapted to the individual woman, but should include mea-urement of blood pressure and, if judged appropriate by the clinician, breast, abdominal and pelvic examination including cervical cytology.

Caution should be observed when prescribing oral contraceptives to young women whose cycles are not yet stabilised.

Venous thrombo-embolic disease

An increased risk of venous thrombo-embolic disease (VTE) associated with the use of oral contraceptives is well established but is smaller than that associated with pregnancy, which has been estimated at 60 cases per 100,000 pregnancies. Some epidemiological studies have reported a greater risk of VTE for women using combined oral contraceptives containing desogestrel or gestodene (the so-called 'third generation' pills) than for women using pills containing levonorgestrel or norethisterone (the so-called 'second generation' pills).

The spontaneous incidence of VTE in healthy non-pregnant women (not taking any oral contraceptive) is about 5 cases per 100,000 per year. The incidence in users of second generation pills is about 15 per 100,000 women per year of use. The incidence in users of third generation pills is about 25 cases per 100,000 women per year of use; this excess incidence has not been satisfactorily explained by bias or confounding. The level of all of these risks of VTE increases with age and is likely to be further increased in women with other known risk factors for VTE such as obesity. The excess risk of VTE is highest during the first year a woman ever uses a combined oral contraceptive.

Surgery, varicose veins or immobilisation

In patients using oestrogen-containing preparations, the risk of deep vein thrombosis may be temporarily increased when undergoing a major operation (eg abdominal, orthopaedic), and surgery to the legs, medical treatment for varicose veins or prolonged immobilisation. Therefore, it is advisable to discontinue oral contraceptive use at least 4 to 6 weeks prior to these procedures if performed electively and to (re)start not less than 2 weeks after full ambulation. The latter is also valid with regard to immobilisation after an accident or emergency surgery. In case of emergency surgery, thrombotic prophylaxis is usually indicated, eg with subcutaneous heparin.

Chloasma

Chloasma may occasionally occur, especially in women with a history of chloasma gravidarum. Women with a tendency to chloasma should avoid exposure to the sun or ultraviolet radiation whilst taking this preparation. Chloasma is often not fully reversible.

Laboratory tests

The use of steroids may influence the results of certain laboratory tests. In the literature, at least a hundred different parameters have been reported to possibly be influenced by oral contraceptive use, predominantly by the oestrogenic component. Among these are: biochemical parameters of the liver, thyroid, adrenal and renal function, plasma levels of (carrier) proteins and lipid/lipoprotein fractions and parameters of coagulation and fibrinolysis.

Further information

Additional contraceptive precautions

When additional contraceptive precautions are required, the patient should be advised either not to have sex, or to use a cap plus spermicide or for her partner to use a condom. Rhythm methods should not be advised as the pill disrupts the usual cyclical changes associated with the natural menstrual cycle, eg changes in temperature and cervical mucus.

The 7-day rule

If any one tablet is forgotten for more than 12 hours.

If the patient has vomiting or diarrhoea for more than 12 hours.

If the patient is taking any of the drugs listed under 'Interactions'.

The patient should continue to take her tablets as usual and:

– Additional contraceptive precautions must be taken for the next 7 days.

But - if these 7 days run beyond the end of the current pack, the next pack must be started as soon as the current one is finished, ie no gap should be left between packs. (This prevents an extended break in tablet taking which may increase the risk of the ovaries releasing an egg and thus reducing contraceptive protection.) The patient will not have a period until the end of 2 packs but this is not harmful nor does it matter if she experiences some bleeding on tablet taking days.

4.5 Interaction with other medicinal products and other forms of interaction

Irregular cycles and reduced reliability of oral contraceptives may occur when these preparations are used concomitantly with drugs such as anticonvulsants, barbiturates, antibiotics (eg tetracyclines, ampicillin, rifampicin, etc), griseofulvin, activated charcoal and certain laxatives. Special consideration should be given to patients being treated with antibiotics for acne. They should be advised to use a non-hormonal method of contraception, or to use an oral contraceptive containing a progestogen showing minimal androgenicity, which have been reported as helping to improve acne without using an antibiotic. Oral contraceptives may diminish glucose tolerance and increase the need for insulin or other antidiabetic drugs in diabetics.

The herbal remedy St John's Wort *(Hypericum perforatum)* should not be taken concomitantly with this medicine as this could potentially lead to a loss of contraceptive effect.

4.6 Pregnancy and lactation

Binovum is contra-indicated for use during pregnancy or suspected pregnancy, since it has been suggested that combined oral contraceptives, in common with many other substances, might be capable of affecting the normal development of the child in the early stages of pregnancy. It can be concluded, however, that, if a risk of abnormality exists at all, it must be very small.

Mothers who are breast-feeding should be advised not to use the combined pill since this may reduce the amount of breast milk, but may be advised instead to use a progestogen-only pill (POP).

4.7 Effects on ability to drive and use machines

Not applicable.

4.8 Undesirable effects

Various adverse reactions have been associated with oral contraceptive use. The first appearance of symptoms indicative of any one of these reactions necessitates immediate cessation of oral contraceptive use while appropriate diagnostic and therapeutic measures are undertaken.

Serious Adverse Reactions

– There is a general opinion, based on statistical evidence that users of combined oral contraceptives experience more often than non-users, various disorders of the coagulation. How often these disorders occur in users of modern low-oestrogen oral contraceptives is unknown, but there are reasons for suggesting that they may occur less often than with the older types of pill which contain more oestrogen.

Various reports have associated oral contraceptive use with the occurrence of deep venous thrombosis, pulmonary embolism and other embolisms. Other investigations of these oral contraceptives have suggested an increased risk of oestrogen and/or progestogen dose-dependent coronary and cerebrovascular accidents, predominantly in heavy smokers. Thrombosis has very rarely been reported to occur in other veins or arteries, eg hepatic, mesenteric, renal or retinal.

It should be noted that there is no consensus about often contradictory findings obtained in early studies. The physician should bear in mind the possibility of vascular accidents occurring and that there may not be full recovery from such disorders and they may be fatal. The physician should take into account the presence of risk factors for arterial disease and deep venous thrombosis when prescribing oral contraceptives. Risk factors for arterial disease include smoking, the presence of hyperlipidaemia, hypertension or diabetes.

Signs and symptoms of a thrombotic event may include: sudden severe pain in the chest, whether or not reaching to the left arm; sudden breathlessness; and unusual severe, prolonged headache, especially if it occurs for the first time or gets progressively worse, or is associated with any of the following symptoms: sudden partial or complete loss of vision or diplopia, aphasia, vertigo, a bad fainting attack or collapse with or without focal epilepsy, weakness or very marked numbness suddenly affecting one side or one part of the body, motor disturbances; severe pain in the calf of one leg; acute abdomen.

Cigarette smoking increases the risk of serious cardiovascular adverse reactions to oral contraceptive use. The risk increases with age and with heavy smoking and is more marked in women over 35 years of age. Women who use oral contraceptives should be strongly advised not to smoke.

– The use of oestrogen-containing oral contraceptives may promote growth of existing sex steroid dependent tumours. For this reason, the use of these oral contraceptives in patients with such tumours is contra-indicated. Numerous epidemiological studies have been reported on the risk of ovarian, endometrial, cervical and breast cancer in women using combined oral contraceptives.

The evidence is clear that combined oral contraceptives offer substantial protection against both ovarian and endometrial cancer. An increased risk of cervical cancer in long term users of combined oral contraceptives has been reported in some studies, but there continues to be controversy about the extent to which this is attributable to the confounding effects of sexual behaviour and other factors.

A meta-analysis from 54 epidemiological studies reported that there is a slightly increased relative risk (RR = 1.24) of having breast cancer diagnosed in women who are currently using combined oral contraceptives (COCs). The observed pattern of increased risk may be due to an earlier diagnosis of breast cancer in COC users, the biological effects of COCs or a combination of both. The additional breast cancers diagnosed in current users of COCs or in women who have used COCs in the last 10 years are more likely to be localised to the breast than those in women who never used COCs.

Breast cancer is rare among women under 40 years of age whether or not they take COCs. Whilst this background risk increases with age, the excess number of breast cancer

Figure 1

Estimated number of breast cancers found in 10,000 women who took the Pill for 5 years then stopped, or who never took the Pill

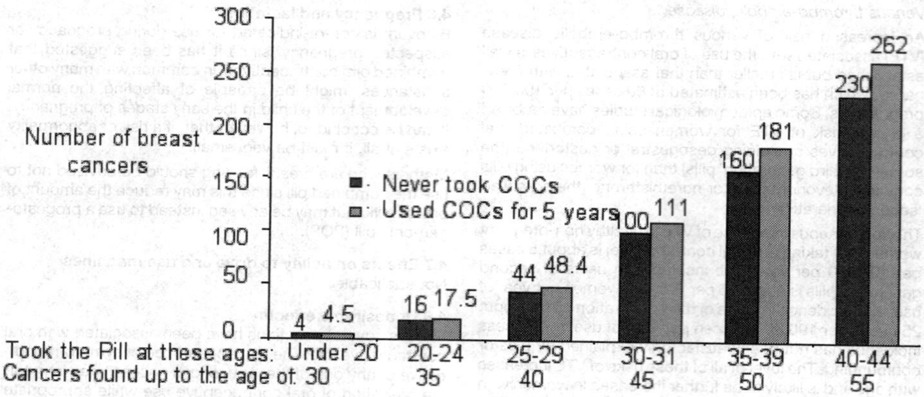

diagnoses in current and recent COC users is small in relation to the overall risk of breast cancer (see bar chart). The most important risk factor for breast cancer in COC users is the age women discontinue the COC; the older the age at stopping, the more breast cancers are diagnosed. Duration of use is less important and the excess risk gradually disappears during the course of the 10 years after stopping COC use such that by 10 years there appears to be no excess.

The possible increase in risk of breast cancer should be discussed with the user and weighed against the benefits of COCs taking into account the evidence that they offer substantial protection against the risk of developing certain other cancers (eg ovarian and endometrial cancer).

(see Figure 1 above)

– Malignant hepatic tumours have been reported on rare occasions in long-term users of oral contraceptives. Benign hepatic tumours have also been associated with oral contraceptive usage. A hepatic tumour should be considered in the differential diagnosis when upper abdominal pain, enlarged liver or signs of intra-abdominal haemorrhage occur.

– The use of oral contraceptives may sometimes lead to the development of cholestatic jaundice or cholelithiasis.

– On rare occasions the use of oral contraceptives may trigger or reactivate systemic lupus erythematosus.

– A further rare complication of oral contraceptive use is the occurrence of chorea which can be reversed by discontinuing the pill. The majority of cases of oral contraceptive-induced chorea show a pre-existing predisposition which often relates to acute rheumatism.

Other Adverse Reactions

–Cardiovascular System

Rise of blood pressure. If hypertension develops, treatment should be discontinued.

–Genital Tract

Intermenstrual bleeding, post-medication amenorrhoea, changes in cervical secretion, increase in size of uterine fibromyomata, aggravation of endometriosis, certain vaginal infections, eg candidosis.

–Breast

Tenderness, pain, enlargement, secretion.

–Gastro-intestinal Tract

Nausea, vomiting, cholelithiasis, cholestatic jaundice.

–Skin

Erythema nodosum, rash, chloasma, erythema multiforme, hirsutism, loss of scalp hair.

–Eyes

Discomfort of the cornea if contact lenses are used.

–CNS

Headache, migraine, mood changes, depression.

–Metabolic

Fluid retention, change in body weight, reduced glucose tolerance.

–Other

Changes in libido, leg cramp, premenstrual-like syndrome.

4.9 Overdose

There have been no reports of serious ill-health from overdosage even when a considerable number of tablets has been taken by a small child. In general, it is therefore unnecessary to treat overdosage. However, if overdosage is discovered within two or three hours and is large, then gastric lavage can be safely used. There are no antidotes and further treatment should be symptomatic.

5. PHARMACOLOGICAL PROPERTIES

5.1 Pharmacodynamic properties

Binovum Oral Contraceptive Tablets act through the mechanism of gonadotrophin suppression by the oestrogenic and progestational actions of the ethinylestradiol and norethisterone. The primary mechanism of action is inhibition of ovulation, but alterations to the cervical mucus and to the endometrium may also contribute to the efficacy of the product.

5.2 Pharmacokinetic properties

Norethisterone and ethinylestradiol are absorbed from the gastro-intestinal tract and metabolised in the liver. To obtain maximal contraceptive effectiveness, the tablets should be taken as directed and at approximately the same time each day.

Because the active ingredients are metabolised in the liver, reduced contraceptive efficacy has been associated with concomitant use of oral contraceptives and rifampicin. A similar association has been suggested with oral contraceptives and barbiturates, phenytoin sodium, phenylbutazone, griseofulvin and ampicillin.

5.3 Preclinical safety data

The toxicology of norethisterone and ethinylestradiol has been extensively investigated in animal studies and through long term clinical experience with widespread use in contraceptives.

6. PHARMACEUTICAL PARTICULARS

6.1 List of excipients

White Tablets:

Magnesium Stearate

Pregelatinised Starch

Lactose

Methanol

Peach Coloured Tablets:

Magnesium Stearate

Pregelatinised Starch

Lactose

FD & C Yellow No.6

Methanol

Purified water

6.2 Incompatibilities

Not applicable.

6.3 Shelf life

Two years

6.4 Special precautions for storage

Do not store above 30°C. Protect from light.

6.5 Nature and contents of container

Clear, uncoloured PVC/foil blister strips in a cardboard carton.

Cartons containing 1 (starter pack)*, 3, and 50* PVC/foil blister strips of 21 tablets each.

*Non-marketed pack sizes.

6.6 Special precautions for disposal and other handling

Not applicable.

7. MARKETING AUTHORISATION HOLDER

Janssen-Cilag Limited

50-100 Holmers Farm Way

High Wycombe

Buckinghamshire

HP12 4EG

UK

8. MARKETING AUTHORISATION NUMBER(S)

PL 0242/0208

9. DATE OF FIRST AUTHORISATION/RENEWAL OF THE AUTHORISATION

23 February 2009

10. DATE OF REVISION OF THE TEXT

23 February 2009

Biorphen

(Alliance Pharmaceuticals)

1. NAME OF THE MEDICINAL PRODUCT

Biorphen

2. QUALITATIVE AND QUANTITATIVE COMPOSITION

Orphenadrine Hydrochloride BP 25 mg/5mL

3. PHARMACEUTICAL FORM

An anise scented and flavoured clear colourless aqueous liquid.

4. CLINICAL PARTICULARS

4.1 Therapeutic indications

Parkinsonism, particularly with apathy and depression, and drug induced extrapyramidal syndrome.

4.2 Posology and method of administration

Oral dose

Adult and Elderly:

150 mg daily in divided doses. Maximum dose 400mg daily. Optimal dose range 150 to 300 mg; this is usually achieved by raising the dose to 50 mg every two to three days.

Children:

Not recommended.

4.3 Contraindications

Hypersensitivity to orphenadrine, or to any of the excipients.

Glaucoma, prostatic hypertrophy, urinary retention, porphyria.

4.4 Special warnings and precautions for use

Caution in renal and hepatic disease.

Antimuscarinic agents, including orphenadrine, should be used with caution in patients with pre-existing tachycardia, (e.g. in heart failure, thyrotoxicosis) as they may cause further acceleration of the heart rate.

Anti-muscarinic agents such as orphenadrine are not effective in the treatment of tardive dyskinesia which may be made worse, and should not be used in patients with this condition.

Avoid abrupt discontinuation of treatment.

Contains sorbitol. Patients with rare hereditary problems of fructose intolerance should not take this medicine.

4.5 Interaction with other medicinal products and other forms of interaction

May additionally increase anticholinergic activity.

As with other similar agents, the antimuscarinic effects of orphenadrine may be enhanced by the concomitant administration of other medications with antimuscarinic properties, such as antihistamines, antispasmodics, tricyclic antidepressants, phenothiazines, dopaminergic anti-parkinsonian drugs including amantadine, and anti-arrhythmics such as disopyramide. Although the additive effect may be minor, there is the potential for development of severe constipation and ileus, atropine-like psychoses and heat stroke.

Due to the anti-muscarinic effects of orphenadrine on the gastrointestinal tract, a reduction in gastric motility may occur which may affect the absorption of other orally administered drugs.

4.6 Pregnancy and lactation

No studies with Biorphen have been carried out, therefore the drug should only be used in pregnancy if there is no safer alternative.

It is not known whether orphenadrine passes into the breast milk, therefore mothers should refrain from breast feeding whilst taking Biorphen.

4.7 Effects on ability to drive and use machines

Patients should be warned of the potential hazards of driving or operating machinery if they experience blurred vision.

4.8 Undesirable effects

Occasionally dry mouth, disturbances of visual accommodation, gastro-intestinal disturbances, dizziness and micturition difficulties may occur; these usually disappear spontaneously or may be controlled by a slight reduction in dosage. Less commonly, tachycardia, hypersensitivity, nervousness, euphoria, hallucinations, confusion and co-ordination disturbances and insomnia may be seen.

4.9 Overdose

Effects seen on overdose are anti-cholinergic in nature and include agitation, confusion, hallucinations, incoordination, delirium, tachycardia and occasionally convulsions. Fatalities have been reported. Gastric lavage, emetic and high enema is recommended. Cholinergics may be useful.

5. PHARMACOLOGICAL PROPERTIES

5.1 Pharmacodynamic properties

Orphenadrine is a tertiary amine antimuscarinic agent.

5.2 Pharmacokinetic properties

Orphenadrine is readily absorbed from the gastro-intestinal tract and is almost completely metabolised, to at least 8 metabolites. It is mainly excreted in the urine.

5.3 Preclinical safety data
No formal preclinical studies have been undertaken with Biorphen, as its active ingredient is a well established pharmaceutical.

6. PHARMACEUTICAL PARTICULARS

6.1 List of excipients
Sorbitol, glycerol, anise water condensed, saccharin sodium, Tween 20, benzoic acid solution, water.

6.2 Incompatibilities
None known.

6.3 Shelf life
24 months.

6.4 Special precautions for storage
None.

6.5 Nature and contents of container
200 ml and 1000 ml amber glass bottles with polycone lined closures.

6.6 Special precautions for disposal and other handling
None stated.

7. MARKETING AUTHORISATION HOLDER
Alliance Pharmaceuticals Ltd
Avonbridge House
Bath Road
Chippenham
Wiltshire
SN15 2BB

8. MARKETING AUTHORISATION NUMBER(S)
PL16853/0022

9. DATE OF FIRST AUTHORISATION/RENEWAL OF THE AUTHORISATION
04 April 2002

10. DATE OF REVISION OF THE TEXT
28th May 2008

Alliance, Alliance Pharmaceuticals and associated devices are registered Trademarks of Alliance Pharmaceuticals Ltd.

Bisodol Extra Strong Mint Tablets
(Forest Laboratories UK Limited)

1. NAME OF THE MEDICINAL PRODUCT
Bisodol Extra Strong Mint Tablets

2. QUALITATIVE AND QUANTITATIVE COMPOSITION
Active ingredients per tablet:

Calcium Carbonate Ph.Eur.	522mg
Magnesium Carbonate Light Ph.Eur.	68mg
Sodium Bicarbonate Ph.Eur.	64mg

3. PHARMACEUTICAL FORM
Chewable tablet

4. CLINICAL PARTICULARS

4.1 Therapeutic indications
For relief from indigestion, dyspepsia, heartburn, acidity and flatulence.

4.2 Posology and method of administration
Adults, elderly and children over 12 years:
Take one or two tablets as required. Suck slowly or chew as preferred.
Children below 12 years:
Not recommended.

4.3 Contraindications
Hypophosphataemia, and avoid in patients with heart or renal failure.

4.4 Special warnings and precautions for use
The label will contain the following statements:

1. If symptoms persist, consult your doctor.
2. Keep all medicines out of the reach of children.
3. Not to be taken during the first three months of pregnancy.

4.5 Interaction with other medicinal products and other forms of interaction
Antacids are known to reduce the absorption of certain medicines including tetracyclines and iron salts.

4.6 Pregnancy and lactation
No clinical data on exposed pregnancies are available.

Animal studies do not indicate direct or indirect harmful effects with respect to pregnancy, embryonal/foetal development, parturition or postnatal development (see section 5.3).

Caution should be exercised when prescribing to pregnant women.

4.7 Effects on ability to drive and use machines
None stated

4.8 Undesirable effects
Calcium salts can have a constipating effect and magnesium salts can have a laxative effect. The mixture of antacids is intended to avoid the lower gastrointestinal effects seen with single antacid preparations. No side effects associated with sodium bicarbonate except when taken in excess. Rebound hyperacidity may occur with prolonged dosage.

4.9 Overdose
Hypermagnesaemia – intravenous administration of calcium salts.

Hypernatraemia – give plenty of salt free liquids.

Hypercalcaemia – remove source of calcium.

5. PHARMACOLOGICAL PROPERTIES

5.1 Pharmacodynamic properties
Sodium bicarbonate, calcium carbonate and magnesium carbonate are antacids. They act by neutralising the hydrochloric acid produced by the stomach and thus reducing gastric and duodenal irritation.

Sodium Bicarbonate

Sodium bicarbonate is a rapid onset, short acting antacid which neutralises acid secretions in the gastrointestinal tract by reacting with hydrochloric acid to produce sodium chloride. During neutralisation carbon dioxide is released, facilitating erucation which provides a sense of relief.

Calcium Carbonate

Calcium carbonate is an antacid with a more prolonged effect than sodium bicarbonate. It rapidly reacts with gastric acid to produce calcium chloride.

Magnesium Carbonate

Magnesium carbonate reacts with gastric acid to form soluble magnesium chloride and carbon dioxide. Because of its crystalline structure it reacts less rapidly than sodium bicarbonate giving it a slower onset of action, and providing longer lasting relief.

5.2 Pharmacokinetic properties
Sodium Bicarbonate

Administration of sodium bicarbonate by mouth causes neutralisation of gastric acid with the production of carbon dioxide. Bicarbonate not involved in that reaction is absorbed and in the absence of a deficit of bicarbonate in the plasma, bicarbonate ions are excreted in the urine that is rendered alkaline with an accompanying diuresis.

Calcium Carbonate

Calcium carbonate is converted to calcium chloride by gastric acid. Some of the calcium is absorbed from the intestines but about 85% is reconverted to insoluble calcium salts, such as the carbonate and is excreted in the faeces.

Magnesium Carbonate

Magnesium carbonate reacts with gastric acid to form soluble magnesium chloride and carbon dioxide in the stomach. Some magnesium is absorbed but is usually excreted rapidly in the urine.

5.3 Preclinical safety data
The active ingredients in Bisodol Tablets have a well-established safety record.

6. PHARMACEUTICAL PARTICULARS

6.1 List of excipients
Saccharin Soluble
Starch
Sucrose
Calcium Stearate
Peppermint Essential Oil

6.2 Incompatibilities
None known

6.3 Shelf life
60 months

6.4 Special precautions for storage
Store at a temperature not exceeding 25°C.

6.5 Nature and contents of container
Tablets in a polypropylene container with polypropylene lid.

Pack size: 30

Carton of 5 rolls of 20 tablets in wax laminated foil with paper label.

Pack size: 100

6.6 Special precautions for disposal and other handling
None

7. MARKETING AUTHORISATION HOLDER
Forest Laboratories UK Limited
Bourne Road
Bexley
Kent DA5 1NX

8. MARKETING AUTHORISATION NUMBER(S)
PL 0108/0125

9. DATE OF FIRST AUTHORISATION/RENEWAL OF THE AUTHORISATION
22nd November 1993/26th May 2004

10. DATE OF REVISION OF THE TEXT
September 2004

11. Legal Category
GSL

Bisodol Indigestion Relief Tablets
(Forest Laboratories UK Limited)

1. NAME OF THE MEDICINAL PRODUCT
Bisodol Indigestion Relief Tablets

2. QUALITATIVE AND QUANTITATIVE COMPOSITION
Active ingredients:

Sodium Bicarbonate Ph.Eur.	64mg/tablet
Calcium Carbonate Ph.Eur.	522mg/tablet
Magnesium Carbonate Light Ph.Eur.	68mg/tablet

3. PHARMACEUTICAL FORM
Chewable tablet for oral administration

4. CLINICAL PARTICULARS

4.1 Therapeutic indications
For relief of the symptoms of gastric hyperacidity, variously called indigestion, heartburn, dyspepsia and flatulence.

4.2 Posology and method of administration
Adults, elderly and children over 12 years:
Suck slowly or chew one or two tablets as required.
Children under 12 years:
Not recommended.

4.3 Contraindications
Hypophosphataemia, and avoid in patients with heart failure or renal failure.

4.4 Special warnings and precautions for use
If symptoms persist, consult your doctor.

Keep all medicines out of the reach of children.

Not to be taken during the first three months of pregnancy.

4.5 Interaction with other medicinal products and other forms of interaction
Antacids are known to reduce the absorption of certain medicines including tetracyclines and iron salts.

4.6 Pregnancy and lactation
Animal studies are insufficient with respect to effects on pregnancy/embryonal/foetal development/parturition and postnatal development.

Caution should be exercised when prescribing to pregnant women.

4.7 Effects on ability to drive and use machines
None stated

4.8 Undesirable effects
Calcium salts can have a constipating effect and magnesium salts can have a laxative effect. The specific mixture of antacids is intended to avoid the lower gastrointestinal effects seen with single antacid preparations. No side effects associated with sodium bicarbonate except when taken in excess.

Rebound hyperacidity may occur with prolonged dosage.

4.9 Overdose
Hypermagnesaemia – intravenous administration of calcium salts.

Hypernatraemia – give plenty of salt free fluids.

Hypercalcaemia – remove source of calcium.

5. PHARMACOLOGICAL PROPERTIES

5.1 Pharmacodynamic properties
Sodium bicarbonate, calcium carbonate and magnesium carbonate are antacids. They act by neutralising the hydrochloric acid produced by the stomach and thus reducing gastric and duodenal irritation.

5.2 Pharmacokinetic properties
Calcium Carbonate

Calcium carbonate is converted to calcium chloride by gastric acid. Some of the calcium is absorbed from the intestines but about 85% is reconverted to insoluble calcium salts, such as the carbonate and is excreted in the faeces.

Magnesium Carbonate

Magnesium carbonate reacts with gastric acid to form soluble magnesium chloride and carbon dioxide in the stomach. Some magnesium is absorbed but is usually excreted rapidly in the urine.

Sodium Bicarbonate

Administration of sodium bicarbonate by mouth causes neutralisation of gastric acid with the production of carbon dioxide. Bicarbonate not involved in that reaction is absorbed and in the absence of a deficit of bicarbonate in the plasma, bicarbonate ions are excreted in the urine that is rendered alkaline with an accompanying diuresis.

5.3 Preclinical safety data
The active ingredients in Bisodol Indigestion Relief Tablets have a well documented safety record.

6. PHARMACEUTICAL PARTICULARS

6.1 List of excipients

Saccharin Soluble

Maize Starch

Sugar

Calcium Stearate

Peppermint Essential Oil Hanningtons White Diamond (374611E)

6.2 Incompatibilities

None stated

6.3 Shelf life

Polypropylene packs: 36 months

Other packs: 60 months

6.4 Special precautions for storage

Store at a temperature not exceeding 25°C.

6.5 Nature and contents of container

Cellulose over wrapped shell and slide cardboard cartons.

Pack sizes: 12, 30.

250 micron UPVC /20 micron coated aluminium blister packs in cardboard cartons.

Pack sizes: 24, 48.

Cellophane overwrapped carton of 5 rolls of 20 tablets in wax laminated foil with paper labels.

Pack size: 100.

Polypropylene roll holder with a polypropylene cap attached by a banding strip to the 100 tablet carton.

Amber glass bottle with black plastic cap.

Pack size: 250.

Rolls of 20 tablets in wax laminated foil with paper label.

Pack size: 20.

Polypropylene container and polypropylene lid.

Pack sizes: 30, 50.

Two rolls of 20 tablets in wax laminated foil packed together in cardboard carton.

Pack size: 40

Three rolls of 20 tablets in wax laminated foil packed together in cardboard carton.

Pack size: 60

Not all pack sizes may be marketed.

6.6 Special precautions for disposal and other handling

None

7. MARKETING AUTHORISATION HOLDER

Forest Laboratories UK Limited

Bourne Road

Bexley

Kent DA5 1NX

8. MARKETING AUTHORISATION NUMBER(S)

PL 0108/0123

9. DATE OF FIRST AUTHORISATION/RENEWAL OF THE AUTHORISATION

29th January 1987 / 20th January 2004

10. DATE OF REVISION OF THE TEXT

December 2005

11. Legal Category

GSL

Bleo-Kyowa

(Kyowa Hakko Kirin UK Ltd)

1. NAME OF THE MEDICINAL PRODUCT

Bleo-Kyowa

2. QUALITATIVE AND QUANTITATIVE COMPOSITION

Bleomycin Sulphate equivalent to 15,000 IU (15 × 10^3 IU)

3. PHARMACEUTICAL FORM

Powder for solution for injection

White to light yellowish, freeze-dried substance

4. CLINICAL PARTICULARS

4.1 Therapeutic indications

a. Squamous cell carcinoma affecting the mouth, nasopharynx and paranasal sinuses, larynx, oesophagus, external genitalia, cervix or skin. Well differentiated tumours usually respond better than anaplastic ones.

b. Hodgkin's disease and other malignant lymphomas, including mycosis fungoides.

c. Testicular teratoma

d. Malignant effusions of serous cavities.

e. Secondary indications in which Bleomycin has been shown to be of some value (alone or in combination with other drugs) include metastatic malignant melanoma, carcinoma of the thyroid, lung and bladder.

4.2 Posology and method of administration

Adults

Routes of administration

Bleomycin is usually administered intramuscularly but may be given intravenously (bolus or drip), intra-arterially, intrapleurally or intraperitoneally as a solution in physiological saline.

Local injection directly into the tumour may occasionally be indicated.

Recommended dose and dosage schedules

Squamous cell carcinoma and testicular teratoma:

Used alone the normal dosage is 15 × 10^3 IU (1 vial) three times a week or 30 × 10^3 IU (2 vials) twice a week, either intramuscularly or intravenously. Treatment may continue on consecutive weeks, or more usually at intervals of 3-4 weeks, up to a total cumulative dose of 500 × 10^3 IU although young men with testicular tumours have frequently tolerated twice this amount. Continuous intravenous infusion at a rate of 15 × 10^3 IU (1 vial) per 24 hours for up to 10 days, or 30 × 10^3 IU (2 vials) per 24 hours for up to 5 days may produce a therapeutic effect more rapidly. The development of stomatitis is the most useful guide to the determination of individual tolerance of maximum therapeutic response. The dose may need to be adjusted when bleomycin is used in combination chemotherapy. Use in elderly or children – see below.

Malignant lymphomas:

Used alone the recommended dosage regime is 15 × 10^3 IU (1 vial) once or twice a week, intramuscularly, to a total dose of 225 × 10^3 IU (15 vials). Dosage should be reduced in the elderly. The dose may need to be adjusted when bleomycin is used in combination chemotherapy. Use in elderly or children – see below.

Malignant effusions:

After drainage of the affected serous cavity 60 × 10^3 IU (4 vials) bleomycin dissolved in 100 ml physiological saline is introduced via the drainage needle or cannula. After instillation, the drainage needle or cannula may be withdrawn. Administration may be repeated if necessary subject to a total cumulative dose of 500 × 10^3 IU (about 33 vials). Use in the elderly or children – see below.

Combination therapy:

Bleomycin is commonly used in conjunction with radiotherapy, particularly in treatment of cancer of the head and neck region. Such a combination may enhance mucosal reactions if full doses of both forms of treatment are used and bleomycin dosage may require reduction, e.g. to 5 × 10^3 IU at the time of each radiotherapy fraction five days a week. Bleomycin is frequently used as one of the drugs in multiple chemotherapy regimes (e.g. squamous cell carcinoma, testicular teratoma, lymphoma). The mucosal toxicity of bleomycin should be borne in mind in the selection and dosage of drugs with similar toxic potential used in such combinations.

Elderly Patients:

The total dose of bleomycin used in the treatment of squamous cell carcinoma, testicular teratoma or malignant effusions should be reduced as indicated below

Age in years	Total Dose (IU)	Dose per week (IU)
80 and over	100 × 10^3	15 × 10^3
70 – 79	150 – 200 × 10^3	30 × 10^3
60 – 69	200 – 300 × 10^3	30 – 60 × 10^3
Under 60	500 × 10^3	30 – 60 × 10^3

Children

Until further data are available, administration of bleomycin to children should take place only under exceptional circumstances and in special centres. The dosage should be based on that recommended for adults and adjusted to body surface area or body weight.

Reduced kidney function

With serum creatinine values of 2-4 mg%, it is recommended to half the above dosages. With serum cretinine above 4 mg%, a further reduction in dose is indicated.

Preparation of solution

For intramuscular injections the required dose is dissolved in up to 5 ml of suitable solvents such as physiological saline. If pain occurs at the site of injection a 1% solution of lignocaine may be used as a solvent.

For intravenous injections the dose required is dissolved in 5-200 ml of physiological saline and injected slowly or added to the reservoir of a running intravenous infusion. For intra-arterial administration a slow infusion in physiological saline is used. For intra-cavity injection 60 × 10^3 IU is dissolved in 100ml of normal saline.

For local injections bleomycin is dissolved in physiological saline to make a 1-3 × 10^3 IU/ml solution

4.3 Contraindications

Bleomycin is contra-indicated in patients with acute pulmonary infection or greatly reduced lung function

Patients who have previously had a hypersensitivity or idiosyncratic reaction to bleomycin.

4.4 Special warnings and precautions for use

Patients undergoing treatment with bleomycin should have chest X-rays weekly. These should continue to be taken for up to 4 weeks after completion of the course. If breathlessness or infiltrates appear, not obviously attributable to tumour or to co-existent lung disease, administration of the drug must be stopped immediately and patients should be treated with a corticosteriod and a broad spectrum antibiotic. High oxygen concentrations should be used with caution in these cases.

Lung function tests which use 100% oxygen should not be used in patients who have been treated with Bleomycin. Lung function tests using less than 21% oxygen are recommended as an alternative.

When Bleomycin has been administered pre-operatively, reduced oxygen concentrations should be used during operation and post operatively.

Patients treated previously or concurrently with radiation to the chest may develop more frequent or severe toxicity.

Bleomycin should be used with caution in patients with significant renal impairment as clearance may be reduced and toxicity increased (see Section 4.2 "Posology and Method of Administration")

Bleomycin should be used with caution in patients with severe heart disease.

4.5 Interaction with other medicinal products and other forms of interaction

When bleomycin is used as one of the drugs in multiple chemotherapy regimes the toxicity of bleomycin should be borne in mind in the selection and dosage of drugs with similar toxic potential. The addition of other cytotoxic drugs can necessitate changes and dose alterations. Increased pulmonary toxicity has been noted when bleomycin is given with cisplatin.

Previous or concurrent radiotherapy to the chest is an important factor in increasing the incidence and severity of lung toxicity.

Because of bleomycin's sensitisation of lung tissue, patients who have received bleomycin pre-operatively are at greater risk of developing pulmonary toxicity when oxygen is administered at surgery and a reduction in inspired oxygen concentration during operation and post-operatively is recommended (See Section 4.4).

In patients treated for testicular cancer with a combination of bleomycin and vinca alkaloids a syndrome has been reported corresponding to morbus Raynaud, ischaemia which can lead to necrosis of peripheral parts of the body (fingers, toes, nose tip).

The following clinical incompatibilities have been noted:- Cytotoxics possibly reduce the absorption of phenytoin. Concommitant use of bleomycin with clozapine should be avoided due to an increased risk of agranulocytosis

4.6 Pregnancy and lactation

Bleomycin should not normally be administered to patients who are pregnant or to mothers who are breast-feeding.

Animal experiences have revealed that bleomycin, like most cytotoxics, may have teratogenic and carcinogenic potential.

4.7 Effects on ability to drive and use machines

This depends on the patient's condition and should be considered in co-operation with the doctor.

4.8 Undesirable effects

The most frequently observed adverse reactions in 1613 patients receiving bleomycin were pulmonary manifestations such as interstitial pneumonia or pulmonary fibrosis (10.2%), sclerosis of skin, pigmentation (40.6%), fever and rigors (39.8%), alopecia (29.5%), anorexia and weight decrease (28.7%), general malaise (16.0%), nausea and vomiting (14.6%), stomatitis (13.3%) and nail changes (11.2%).

Haematologic:	
Common	Haemorrhage
Uncommon	Leukopenia
Nervous:	
Common	Headache
Uncommon	Dizziness
Respiratory:	
Very common	Interstitial pneumonia and pulmonary fibrosis
Gastrointestinal:	
Very common	Anorexia, weight decrease, nausea and vomiting and stomatitis
Common	Angular stomatitis
Uncommon	Diarrhoea
Hepatic:	
Uncommon	Hepatic disturbances

Skin:	
Very common	Hypertrophy of the skin, pigmentation, alopecia and deformation and discolouration of the nail
Common	Rash, urticaria and erythroderma assocated with fever
Renal and Urinary:	
Uncommon	Oligurea, micturition pain, polyuria and feeling of residual urine
General Disorders and Adminsitration Site Conditions:	
Very common	Fever, rigors and malaise
Uncommon	Pain at the tumour site
	Hypertrophy of the venous wall and narrowing of the venous lumen when given by intravenous injection
	Induration when given by intramuscular or local injection

Like most cytotoxic agents bleomycin can give rise to both immediate and to delayed toxic effects. The most immediate effect is fever on the day of injection. Anorexia, tiredness or nausea also may occur. Pain at the injection site or in the region of the tumour has occasionally been reported, and other rare adverse effects are hypotension and local thrombophlebitis after intravenous administration.

The majority of patients who receive a full course of bleomycin develop lesions of the skin or oral mucosa. Induration, hyperkeratotis, reddening, tenderness and swelling of the tips of the fingers, ridging of the nails, bulla formation over pressure points such as elbows, loss of hair and stomatitis are rarely serious and usually disappear soon after completion of the course.

The most serious delayed effect is interstitial pneumonia, which may develop during, or occasionally after, a course of treatment. This condition may sometimes develop into fatal pulmonary fibrosis, although such an occurrence is rare at recommended doses. Previous or concurrent radiotherapy to the chest is an important factor in increasing the incidence and severity of lung toxicity.

A few cases of acute fulminant reactions with hyperpyrexia and cardiorespiratory collapse have been observed after intravenous injections of doses higher than those recommended. Hypotension, hyperpyrexia and drug-related deaths have been reported rarely following intra-cavitary instillation of bleomycin.

During postmarketing surveillance the following events have been reported: sepsis, pancytopenia, thrombocytopenia, anaemia, neutropenia, chest pain, myocardial infarction, Raynaud's syndrome, embolism, thrombosis and digital ischaemia.

4.9 Overdose

The acute reaction to an overdosage of bleomycin would probably include hypotension, fever, rapid pulse and general symptoms of shock.

Treatment is purely symptomatic. In the event of respiratory complications the patient should be treated with a corticosteroid and a broad-spectrum antibiotic. There is no specific antidote to bleomycin.

5. PHARMACOLOGICAL PROPERTIES

5.1 Pharmacodynamic properties

ATC code: LO1D C01, other cytotoxic antibiotics

Bleomycin is a basic, water-soluble glycopeptide with cytotoxic activity. The mechanism of action of bleomycin is believed to involve single-strand scission of DNA, leading to inhibition of cell division, of growth and of DNA synthesis in tumour cells.

Apart from its antibacterial and antitumour properties, bleomycin is relatively free from biological activity. When injected intravenously it may have a histamine-like effect on blood pressure and may cause a rise in body temperature.

5.2 Pharmacokinetic properties

Bleomycin is administered parenterally. After intravenous (IV) administration of a bolus dose of 15×10^3 IU/m^2 body surface, peak concentrations of 1 to 10 IU are achieved in plasma. Following the intramuscular (IM) injection of 15×10^3 IU peak plasma concentrations of about 1 IU/ml have been reported. The peak plasma concentration is reached 30 minutes after an IM injection. Continuous infusion of bleomycin 30×10^3 IU daily, for 4 to 5 days, resulted in an average steady state plasma concentration of 100-300 milli IU/ml. After IV injections of bleomycin in a dose of 15×10^3 IU/m^2 body surface, the area under the serum concentration curve is, on average, 300 milli IU $\times$ min $\times$ ml^{-1}.

Bleomycin is only bound to plasma proteins to a slight extent. Bleomycin is rapidly distributed in body tissues, with the highest concentrations in skin, lungs, peritoneum and lymph. Low concentrations are seen in the bone marrow. Bleomycin could not be detected in cerebrospinal fluid after intravenous injection. Bleomycin appears to cross the placental barrier.

The mechanism for bio-transformation is not yet fully known. Inactivation takes place during enzymatic breakdown by bleomycin hydrolase, primarily in plasma, liver and other organs and, to a much lesser degree, in skin and lungs. When bleomycin was administered as an IV bolus injection in a dose of 15×10^3 IU/m^2 body surface, initial and terminal half-lives were 0.5 and 4 hours respectively. Given as a continuous intravenous infusion in a dose of 30×10^3 IU daily for 4 to 5 days bleomycin disappears from plasma with initial and terminal half-lives of about 1.3 hours and 9 hours, respectively. About two thirds of the administered drug is excreted unchanged in the urine, probably by glomerular filtration. Approximately 50% is recovered in the urine in the 24 hours following an IV or IM injection. The rate of excretion, therefore, is highly influenced by renal function; concentrations in plasma are greatly elevated if usual doses are given to patients with renal impairment with only up to 20% excreted in 24 hours. Observations indicate that it is difficult to eliminate bleomycin from the body by dialysis.

5.3 Preclinical safety data

There are no preclinical data of relevance to the prescriber which are additional to that already included in other sections of the Summary of Product Characteristics.

6. PHARMACEUTICAL PARTICULARS

6.1 List of excipients

None

6.2 Incompatibilities

Bleomycin solution should not be mixed with solutions of essential amino acids, riboflavine, ascorbic acid, dexamethasone, aminophylline or frusemide.

6.3 Shelf life

3 years

6.4 Special precautions for storage

Protect from light. Store at 2°C -8°C.

6.5 Nature and contents of container

5 ml colourless glass vials with rubber closure and aluminium cap containing freeze dried bleomycin sulphate equivalent to 15,000 IU. Ten vials per carton.

6.6 Special precautions for disposal and other handling

Bleomycin should be handled with care. Precautions should be taken to avoid bleomycin coming into contact with skin, mucous membranes or eyes, but in the event of contamination the effected part should be washed with water

7. MARKETING AUTHORISATION HOLDER

Kyowa Hakko Kirin UK Ltd
258 Bath Road
Slough
Berkshire SL1 4DX
UK

8. MARKETING AUTHORISATION NUMBER(S)

PL 12196/0005

9. DATE OF FIRST AUTHORISATION/RENEWAL OF THE AUTHORISATION

03/07/2006

10. DATE OF REVISION OF THE TEXT

15/01/2009

BLISTEX RELIEF CREAM

(DDD Limited)

1. NAME OF THE MEDICINAL PRODUCT

BLISTEX RELIEF CREAM

2. QUALITATIVE AND QUANTITATIVE COMPOSITION

Strong ammonia solution 0.100% w/w

Aromatic ammonia solution 6.040% w/w

Liquefied phenol 0.494% w/w

For excipients, see 6.1.

3. PHARMACEUTICAL FORM

Cream.

Off white smooth cream.

4. CLINICAL PARTICULARS

4.1 Therapeutic indications

For quick relief of occasional cold sores, cracked lips or chapped lips.

4.2 Posology and method of administration

At first symptoms apply every hour. By topical application to the lips.

4.3 Contraindications

Hypersensitivity to the active substances or to any of the excipients.

4.4 Special warnings and precautions for use

If you suffer from recurrent cold sores consult your doctor.

4.5 Interaction with other medicinal products and other forms of interaction

None known.

4.6 Pregnancy and lactation

Not contraindicated.

4.7 Effects on ability to drive and use machines

None.

4.8 Undesirable effects

None known.

4.9 Overdose

No known problems associated with overdosage.

5. PHARMACOLOGICAL PROPERTIES

Pharmacotherapeutic group: Other dermatologicals ATC code: D11 AX

5.1 Pharmacodynamic properties

The product was developed for topical use and is for the relief of occasional cold sores, cracked lips and chapped lips.

Ammonia is incorporated into the formulation for its rubefacient properties. Phenol is present in the formulation for its disinfectant properties. Phenol is bacteriostatic in concentrations of about 0.02% to 1% bactericidal to some organisms in concentrations as low as 0.4%. Phenol is also reported to be active against certain viruses.

These two actives are present in an emollient emulsion base, comprising largely of lanolin 25.4% w/w and White Soft Paraffin 33% w/w. These oleaginous substances, also known as occlusive agents and humectants, are employed as protectives and as agents for softening the skin and rendering it more pliable, but chiefly as vehicles for the more active drugs above.

Emollients soften the skin by forming an occlusive oil film on the stratum corneum, thus preventing drying from evaporation of the water that diffuses to the surface from the underlying layers of skin.

In this way, Blistex Relief Cream provides an effective treatment for the relief of occasional cold sores, cracked lips and chapped lips.

(References abstracted from Goodman & Gillman and Martindale).

5.2 Pharmacokinetic properties

Approximately 80mg of Blistex Relief Cream is applied to the lips at any one time. Blistex Relief Cream is a topical treatment with locally acting agents.

Any trace quantities of ammonia entering the blood system via Blistex Relief Cream would be so small compared to normal background concentrations of ammonia as to be inconsequential.

Ammonia in the body represents that which is liberated from the deamination of amino acids and the deamination of amides. Portal venous blood contains a high concentration of ammonia. Normally about 20% of the urea produced in the body diffuses into the gut, where it is converted by bacteria to ammonia and carbon dioxide. Intestinal bacteria also produce ammonia from dietary proteins. The ammonia is absorbed and converted back to urea in the liver, by way of the ornithine cycle. Another significant role of ammonia is in the synthesis of glutamine.

Renal excretion – Normal renal venous blood contains a high concentration of ammonia synthesised from glutamine and other amino acids in the kidney. The ammonia that is formed by the kidney is excreted when the urine is acidic, but is largely returned to the systemic circulation if the urine is alkaline. In an acidic urine, NH_3 accepts a proton and exists almost entirely as NH_4^+. Under normal states of metabolism about 70mEq of non-volatile acid is generated per day: about one half of this is excreted in the urine in conjunction with NH_4^+, and the remainder is excreted as titratable acid. Renal production of ammonia is stimulated by acidosis: ammonia buffers urinary acid and allows further secretion of protons into the tabular fluid. Potassium depletion also results in a primary increase in the alkalinization of the urine (Tannen, 1977). This may increase the amount of ammonia that is returned to the circulation via the renal vein and have a deleterious effect when potassium depletion coexists with hepatic failure.

Normal physiological mechanisms are designed to keep the concentration of ammonia in the blood as low as possible. Thus, ammonia added to the venous circulation by the kidney or gastrointestinal tract is converted to urea by the liver.

Phenol – A paper published by JAMA in 1953 showed that phenol readily penetrates the human skin and that detoxification by conjugation is initiated immediately.

The pharmaceutical form of Blistex Relief Cream is similar to the aromatised liquid petrolatum of Camphor phenique. This being so, we would expect that after local application the amount of phenol in blood attributable to Blistex Relief Cream would be of the order of 0.0003 mg/100ml of blood.

According to the Journal of Clinical Pathology 12:129, 1942 the residual phenol content of blood in normal human beings varies from 0.0 to 0.08 mg/100ml free phenol and 0.0 to 0.08 mg/100ml conjugated phenol.

This suggests that residual phenol in normal humans can be anything up to 250 times greater than that which is likely to come from Blistex Relief Cream.

The results of the 1953 paper indicate that phenol from Blistex Relief Cream is rapidly absorbed through the skin and is rapidly detoxified due to its extremely low concentrations.

5.3 Preclinical safety data
N/A

6. PHARMACEUTICAL PARTICULARS

6.1 List of excipients
White soft paraffin
Purified water
Modified lanolin
Sorbitan palmitate
Peppermint oil
Polysorbate 40
Ethanol 96%
Cineole
Racemic camphor
Saccharin sodium

6.2 Incompatibilities
Not applicable

6.3 Shelf life
3 years

6.4 Special precautions for storage
Do not store above 25°C.

Keep all medicines out of the reach of children.

6.5 Nature and contents of container
Collapsible printed aluminium tube with elongated nozzle and plastic screw-on cap, containing 3.5 g or 5 g of cream.

Not all pack sizes may be marketed.

6.6 Special precautions for disposal and other handling
No special requirements

Administrative Data

7. MARKETING AUTHORISATION HOLDER
DDD limited
94 Rickmansworth Road
Watford
Hertfordshire
United Kingdom. WD18 7JJ

8. MARKETING AUTHORISATION NUMBER(S)
PL 0133/5007

9. DATE OF FIRST AUTHORISATION/RENEWAL OF THE AUTHORISATION
29.07.99

10. DATE OF REVISION OF THE TEXT
February 2004

Bondronat Concentrate for Solution for Infusion

(Roche Products Limited)

1. NAME OF THE MEDICINAL PRODUCT
***Bondronat 2 mg*▼**
***Bondronat 6 mg*▼**
Concentrate for solution for infusion

2. QUALITATIVE AND QUANTITATIVE COMPOSITION
Bondronat 2 mg
One vial with 2 ml concentrate for solution for infusion contains 2 mg ibandronic acid (as 2.25 mg ibandronic acid, monosodium salt, monohydrate).

Bondronat 6 mg
One vial with 6 ml concentrate for solution for infusion contains 6 mg ibandronic acid (as 6.75 mg ibandronic acid, monosodium salt, monohydrate)

Excipients:

For a full list of excipients, see section 6.1.

3. PHARMACEUTICAL FORM
Concentrate for solution for infusion.

Clear, colourless solution

4. CLINICAL PARTICULARS

4.1 Therapeutic indications
Bondronat is indicated for:

- Prevention of skeletal events (pathological fractures, bone complications requiring radiotherapy or surgery) in patients with breast cancer and bone metastases.
- Treatment of tumour-induced hypercalcaemia with or without metastases.

4.2 Posology and method of administration
Bondronat therapy should only be initiated by physicians experienced in the treatment of cancer.

For intravenous administration.

For single use only. Only clear solution without particles should be used.

Prevention of Skeletal Events in Patients with Breast Cancer and Bone Metastases

The recommended dose for prevention of skeletal events in patients with breast cancer and bone metastases is 6 mg intravenous injection given every 3-4 weeks. The dose should be infused over at least 15 minutes. For infusion, the contents of the vials(s) should only be added to 100 ml isotonic sodium chloride solution or 100 ml 5% glucose solution.

A shorter (i.e. 15 min) infusion time should only be used for patients with normal renal function or mild renal impairment. There are no data available characterising the use of a shorter infusion time in patients with creatinine clearance below 50 ml/min. Prescribers should consult the section *Patients with Renal Impairment* (Section 4.2) for recommendations on dosing and administration in this patient group.

Treatment of Tumour-Induced Hypercalcaemia

Prior to treatment with Bondronat the patient should be adequately rehydrated with 9 mg/ml (0.9%) sodium chloride. Consideration should be given to the severity of the hypercalcaemia as well as the tumour type. In general patients with osteolytic bone metastases require lower doses than patients with the humoral type of hypercalcaemia. In most patients with severe hypercalcaemia (albumin-corrected serum calcium* ⩾ 3 mmol/l or ⩾ 12 mg/dl) 4 mg is an adequate single dosage. In patients with moderate hypercalcaemia (albumin-corrected serum calcium < 3 mmol/l or < 12 mg/dl) 2 mg is an effective dose. The highest dose used in clinical trials was 6 mg but this dose does not add any further benefit in terms of efficacy.

*Note albumin-corrected serum calcium concentrations are calculated as follows:

Albumin-corrected serum calcium (mmol/l) = serum calcium (mmol/l) - [0.02 × albumin (g/l)] + 0.8

Or

Albumin-corrected serum calcium (mg/dl) = serum calcium (mg/dl) + 0.8 × [4 - albumin (g/dl)]

To convert the albumin-corrected serum calcium in mmol/l value to mg/dl, multiply by 4.

In most cases a raised serum calcium level can be reduced to the normal range within 7 days. The median time to relapse (return of albumin-corrected serum calcium to levels above 3 mmol/l) was 18 - 19 days for the 2 mg and 4 mg doses. The median time to relapse was 26 days with a dose of 6 mg.

A limited number of patients (50 patients) have received a second infusion for hypercalcaemia. Repeated treatment may be considered in case of recurrent hypercalcaemia or insufficient efficacy.

Bondronat concentrate for solution for infusion should be administered as an intravenous infusion. For this purpose, the contents of the vials are to be added to 500 ml isotonic sodium chloride solution (or 500 ml 5% dextrose solution) and infused over two hours.

As the inadvertent intra-arterial administration of preparations not expressly recommended for this purpose as well as paravenous administration can lead to tissue damage, care must be taken to ensure that Bondronat concentrate for solution for infusion is administered intravenously.

Patients with hepatic impairment

No dosage adjustment is required (see section 5.2).

Patients with renal impairment

There is no evidence of a reduction in tolerability associated with an increase in exposure to ibandronate in patients with various degrees of renal impairment. However, for the prevention of skeletal events in patients with breast cancer and bone metastases the following recommendations should be followed:

Creatinine Clearance (ml/min)	Dosage / Infusion time [1]	Infusion Volume [2]
⩾ 50	6mg / 15 minutes	100ml
30 ⩽ CLcr < 50	6mg / 1 hour	500ml
<30	2mg / 1 hour	500ml

[1] Administration every 3 to 4 week

[2] 0.9% sodium chloride solution or 5% glucose solution

A 15 minute infusion time has not been studied in cancer patients with CLCr < 50 mL/min.

Elderly

No dose adjustment is required.

Children and adolescents

Bondronat is not recommended for patients below age 18 years due to insufficient data on safety and efficacy.

4.3 Contraindications
Hypersensitivity to the active substance or to any of the excipients.

Caution is to be taken in patients with known hypersensitivity to other bisphosphonates.

Bondronat should not be used in children.

4.4 Special warnings and precautions for use
Clinical studies have not shown any evidence of deterioration in renal function with long term Bondronat therapy. Nevertheless, according to clinical assessment of the individual patient, it is recommended that renal function serum calcium, phosphate and magnesium should be monitored in patients treated with Bondronat.

As no clinical data are available, dosage recommendations cannot be given for patients with severe hepatic insufficiency.

Overhydration should be avoided in patients at risk of cardiac failure.

Hypocalcaemia and other disturbances of bone and mineral metabolism should be effectively treated before starting Bondronat therapy for metastatic bone disease.

Adequate intake of calcium and vitamin D is important in all patients. Patients should receive supplemental calcium and/or vitamin D if dietary intake is inadequate.

Osteonecrosis of the jaw, generally associated with tooth extraction and/or local infection (including osteomyelitis) has been reported in patients with cancer receiving treatment regimens including primarily intravenously administered bisphosphonates. Many of these patients were also receiving chemotherapy and corticosteroids. Osteonecrosis of the jaw has also been reported in patients with osteoporosis receiving oral bisphosphonates.

A dental examination with appropriate preventive dentistry should be considered prior to treatment with bisphosphonates in patients with concomitant risk factors (e.g. cancer, chemotherapy, radiotherapy, corticosteroids, poor oral hygiene).

While on treatment, these patients should avoid invasive dental procedures if possible. For patients who develop osteonecrosis of the jaw while on bisphosphonate therapy, dental surgery may exacerbate the condition. For patients requiring dental procedures, there are no data available to suggest whether discontinuation of bisphosphonate treatment reduces the risk of osteonecrosis of the jaw. Clinical judgement of the treating physician should guide the management plan of each patient based on individual benefit/risk assessment.

4.5 Interaction with other medicinal products and other forms of interaction
Bondronat should not be mixed with calcium containing solutions.

No interaction was observed when co-administered with melphalan/prednisolone in patients with multiple myeloma.

Other interaction studies in postmenopausal women have demonstrated the absence of any interaction potential with tamoxifen or hormone replacement therapy (oestrogen).

In relation to disposition, no drug interactions of clinical significance are likely. Ibandronic acid is eliminated by renal secretion only and does not undergo any biotransformation. The secretory pathway does not appear to include known acidic or basic transport systems involved in the excretion of other active substances. In addition, ibandronic acid does not inhibit the major human hepatic P450 isoenzymes and does not induce the hepatic cytochrome P450 system in rats. Plasma protein binding is low at therapeutic concentrations and ibandronic acid is therefore unlikely to displace other active substances.

Caution is advised when bisphosphonates are administered with aminoglycosides, since both agents can lower serum calcium levels for prolonged periods. Attention should also be paid to the possible existence of simultaneous hypomagnesaemia.

In clinical studies, Bondronat has been administered concomitantly with commonly used anticancer agents, diuretics, antibiotics and analgesics without clinically apparent interactions occurring.

Interaction studies have only been performed in adults.

4.6 Pregnancy and lactation
There are no adequate data from the use of ibandronic acid in pregnant women. Studies in rats have shown reproductive toxicity (see section 5.3). The potential risk for humans is unknown. Therefore, Bondronat should not be used during pregnancy.

It is not known whether ibandronic acid is excreted in human milk. Studies in lactating rats have demonstrated the presence of low levels of ibandronic acid in the milk following intravenous administration. Bondronat should not be used during lactation.

4.7 Effects on ability to drive and use machines
No studies on the effects on the ability to drive and use machines have been performed.

4.8 Undesirable effects
Adverse reactions are ranked under heading of frequency, the most frequent first, using the following convention: very common (⩾ 10%), common (⩾ 1% and <10%), uncommon (⩾ 0.1% and <1%), rare (⩾ 0.01% and <0.1%), and very rare (⩽ 0.01%).

Treatment of Tumour Induced Hypercalcaemia

The safety profile for Bondronat in tumour-induced hypercalcaemia is derived from controlled clinical trials in this indication and after the intravenous administration of Bondronat at the recommended doses. Treatment was most commonly associated with a rise in body temperature. Occasionally, a flu-like syndrome consisting of fever, chills, bone and/or muscle ache-like pain was reported. In most cases no specific treatment was required and the symptoms subsided after a couple of hours/days.

Table 1 lists adverse reactions recorded in the trials (events were recorded irrespective of a determination of causality).

Table 1. Number (percentage) of Patients Reporting Adverse Reactions in Controlled Clinical Trials in Tumour-Induced Hypercalcaemia after treatment with Bondronat

System Organ Class / Adverse Reaction	Frequency Number (%) (n=352)
Metabolism and nutrition disorders	
Common: Hypocalcaemia	10 (2.8)
Musculoskeletal and connective tissue disorders:	
Common: Bone Pain	6 (1.7)
Uncommon: Myalgia	1 (0.3)
General disorders and administration site conditions:	
Very common: Pyrexia	39 (11.1)
Uncommon: Influenza-like illness	2 (0.6)
Rigors	1 (0.3)

Note: Data for both the 2 mg and 4 mg doses of ibandronic acid are pooled. Events were recorded irrespective of a determination of causality.

Frequently, decreased renal calcium excretion is accompanied by a fall in serum phosphate levels not requiring therapeutic measures. The serum calcium level may fall to hypocalcaemic values.

Other reactions reported at lower frequency are as follows:

Immune system disorders:

Very rare: Hypersensitivity.

Skin and subcutaneous tissue disorders:

Very rare: Angioneurotic oedema

Respiratory, thoracic and mediastinal disorders:

Very rare: Bronchospasm.

Administration of other bisphosphonates has been associated with broncho-constriction in acetylsalicylic acid-sensitive asthmatic patients.

Prevention of Skeletal Events in Patients with Breast Cancer and Bone Metastases

The safety profile of intravenous Bondronat in patients with breast cancer and bone metastases is derived from a controlled clinical trial in this indication and after the intravenous administration of Bondronat at the recommended dose.

Table 2 lists adverse reactions from the pivotal phase III study (152 patients treated with Bondronat 6 mg), i.e. adverse events with remote, possible, or probable relationship to study medication, occurring commonly and more frequently in the active treatment group than in placebo.

Table 2 Adverse Reactions Occurring Commonly and Greater than Placebo in Patients with Metastatic Bone Disease due to Breast Cancer Treated with Bondronat 6 mg administered intravenously.

Adverse Reaction	Placebo (n = 157) No. (%)	Bondronat 6 mg (n = 152) No. (%)
Infections and Infestations:		
Infection	1 (0.6)	2 (1.3)
Endocrine disorders:		
Parathyroid disorder	1 (0.6)	2 (1.3)
Nervous System disorders:		
Headache	4 (2.5)	9 (5.9)
Dizziness	2 (1.3)	4 (2.6)
Dysgeusia (taste perversion)	0 (0.0)	2 (1.3)
Eye disorders:		
Cataract	1 (0.6)	2 (1.3)
Cardiac disorders:		
Bundle branch block	1 (0.6)	2 (1.3)
Respiratory, thoracic and mediastinal disorders:		
Pharyngitis	0 (0.0)	3 (2.0)
Gastrointestinal disorders:		
Diarrhoea	1 (0.6)	8 (5.3)
Dyspepsia	5 (3.2)	6 (3.9)
Vomiting	2 (1.3)	5 (3.3)
Gastrointestinal pain	2 (1.3)	4 (2.6)
Tooth disorder	0 (0.0)	3 (2.0)
Skin and subcutaneous tissue disorders:		
Skin disorder	0 (0.0)	2 (1.3)
Ecchymosis	0 (0.0)	2 (1.3)
Musculoskeletal and connective tissue disorders:		
Myalgia	6 (3.8)	8 (5.3)
Arthralgia	1 (0.6)	2 (1.3)
Joint disorder	0 (0.0)	2 (1.3)
Osteoarthritis	0 (0.0)	2 (1.3)
General disorders:		
Asthenia	8 (5.1)	10 (6.6)
Influenza-like illness	2 (1.3)	8 (5.3)
Oedema Peripheral	2 (1.3)	3 (2.0)
Thirst	0 (0.0)	2 (1.3)
Investigations:		
Gamma-GT increased	1 (0.6)	4 (2.6)
Creatinine increased	1 (0.6)	3 (2.0)

Other adverse reactions reported at a lower frequency are as follows:

Uncommon:

Infection and infestation: cystitis, vaginitis, oral candidiasis

Neoplasms benign and malignant (including cysts and polyps): benign skin neoplasm

Blood and lymphatic system: anaemia, blood dyscrasia

Metabolism and nutrition disorders: hypophosphataemia

Psychiatric disorders: sleep disorder, anxiety, affection lability

Nervous system disorders: cerbrovascular disorder, nerve root lesion, amnesia, migraine, neuralgia, hypertonia, hyperaestesia, paraesthesia circumoral, parosmia.

Ear and labyrinth disorders: deafness

Cardiac disorders: myocardial ischaemia, cardiovascular disorder, palpitations

Vascular disorders: hypertension, lymphoedema, varicose veins

Respiratory, thoracic and mediastinal disorders: lung oedema, stridor

Gastrointestinal disorders: gastroenteritis, dysphagia, gastritis, mouth ulceration, cheilitis

Hepato-biliary disorders: cholelithiasis

Skin and subcutaneous tissue disorders: rash, alopecia

Renal and urinary disorders: urinary retention, renal cyst

Reproductive system and breast disorders: pelvic pain

General disorders and administration site conditions: hypothermia

Investigations: blood alkaline phosphatase increase, weight decrease

Injury, poisoning and procedural complications: injury, injection site pain

Osteonecrosis of the jaw has been reported in patients treated by bisphosphonates. The majority of the reports refer to cancer patients, but such cases have also been reported in patients treated for osteoporosis. Osteonecrosis of the jaw is generally associated with tooth extraction and / or local infection (including osteomyelitis). Diagnosis of cancer, chemotherapy, radiotherapy, corticosteroids and poor oral hygiene are also deemed as risk factors (see section 4.4).

4.9 Overdose

Up to now there is no experience of acute poisoning with Bondronat concentrate for solution for infusion. Since both the kidney and the liver were found to be target organs for toxicity in preclinical studies with high doses, kidney and liver function should be monitored. Clinically relevant hypocalcaemia should be corrected by intravenous administration of calcium gluconate.

5. PHARMACOLOGICAL PROPERTIES

5.1 Pharmacodynamic properties

Pharmaco-therapeutic group: Bisphosphonate, ATC Code: M05B A 06

Ibandronic acid belongs to the bisphosphonate group of compounds which act specifically on bone. Their selective action on bone tissue is based on the high affinity of bisphosphonates for bone mineral. Bisphosphonates act by inhibiting osteoclast activity, although the precise mechanism is still not clear.

In vivo, ibandronic acid prevents experimentally-induced bone destruction caused by cessation of gonadal function, retinoids, tumours or tumour extracts. The inhibition of endogenous bone resorption has also been documented by ^{45}Ca kinetic studies and by the release of radioactive tetracycline previously incorporated into the skeleton.

At doses that were considerably higher than the pharmacologically effective doses, ibandronic acid did not have any effect on bone mineralisation.

Bone resorption due to malignant disease is characterised by excessive bone resorption that is not balanced with appropriate bone formation. Ibandronic acid selectively inhibits osteoclast activity, reducing bone resorption and thereby reducing skeletal complications of the malignant disease.

Clinical Studies in the Treatment of Tumour-Induced Hypercalcaemia

Clinical studies in hypercalcaemia of malignancy demonstrated that the inhibitory effect of ibandronic acid on tumour-induced osteolysis, and specifically on tumour-induced hypercalcaemia, is characterised by a decrease in serum calcium and urinary calcium excretion.

In the dose range recommended for treatment, the following response rates with the respective confidence intervals have been shown in clinical trials for patients with baseline albumin-corrected serum calcium ⩾ 3.0 mmol/l after adequate rehydration.

(see Figure 1 on next page)

For these patients and dosages, the median time to achieve normocalcaemia was 4 to 7 days. The median time to relapse (return of albumin-corrected serum calcium above 3.0 mmol/l) was 18 to 26 days.

Clinical Studies in the Prevention of Skeletal Events in Patients with Breast Cancer and Bone Metastases

Clinical studies in patients with breast cancer and bone metastases have shown that there is a dose dependent inhibitory effect on bone osteolysis, expressed by markers of bone resorption, and a dose dependent effect on skeletal events.

Prevention of skeletal events in patients with breast cancer and bone metastases with Bondronat 6 mg administered intravenously was assessed in one randomised placebo controlled phase III trial with duration of 96 weeks. Female patients with breast cancer and radiologically confirmed bone metastases were randomised to receive placebo (158 patients) or 6 mg Bondronat (154 patients). The results from this trial are summarised below.

Primary Efficacy Endpoints

The primary endpoint of the trial was the skeletal morbidity period rate (SMPR). This was a composite endpoint which had the following skeletal related events (SREs) as subcomponents:

- radiotherapy to bone for treatment of fractures/impending fractures
- surgery to bone for treatment of fractures
- vertebral fractures
- non-vertebral fractures.

The analysis of the SMPR was time-adjusted and considered that one or more events occurring in a single 12 week period could be potentially related. Multiple events were therefore counted only once for the purposes of the analysis. Data from this study demonstrated a significant advantage for intravenous Bondronat 6 mg over placebo in the reduction in SREs measured by the time-adjusted SMPR (p=0.004). The number of SREs was also significantly reduced with Bondronat 6 mg and there was a 40% reduction in the risk of a SRE over placebo (relative risk 0.6, p = 0.003). Efficacy results are summarised in Table 3.

Table 3 Efficacy Results (Breast Cancer Patients with Metastatic Bone Disease)

	All Skeletal Related Events (SREs)		
	Placebo n=158	Bondronat 6 mg n=154	p-value
SMPR (per patient year)	1.48	1.19	p=0.004
Number of events (per patient)	3.64	2.65	p=0.025
SRE relative risk	-	0.60	p=0.003

Secondary Efficacy Endpoints

A statistically significant improvement in bone pain score was shown for intravenous Bondronat 6 mg compared to placebo. The pain reduction was consistently below baseline throughout the entire study and accompanied by a significantly reduced use of analgesics. The deterioration in Quality of Life was significantly less in Bondronat treated patients compared with placebo. A tabular summary of these secondary efficacy results is presented in Table 4.

Table 4 Secondary Efficacy Results (Breast cancer Patients with Metastatic Bone Disease)

	Placebo n=158	Bondronat 6 mg n=154	p-value
Bone pain *	0.21	-0.28	p< 0.001
Analgesic use *	0.90	0.51	p=0.083
Quality of Life *	-45.4	-10.3	p=0.004

* Mean change from baseline to last assessment.

There was a marked depression of urinary markers of bone resorption (pyridinoline and deoxypyridinoline) in patients treated with Bondronat that was statistically significant compared to placebo.

In a study in 130 patients with metastatic breast cancer the safety of Bondronat infused over 1 hour or 15 minutes was compared. No difference was observed in the indicators of renal function. The overall adverse event profile of ibandronic acid following the 15 minute infusion was consistent with the known safety profile over longer infusion times and no new safety concerns were identified relating to the use of a 15 minute infusion time.

A 15 minute infusion time has not been studied in cancer patients with a creatinine clearance of < 50ml/min.

Figure 1

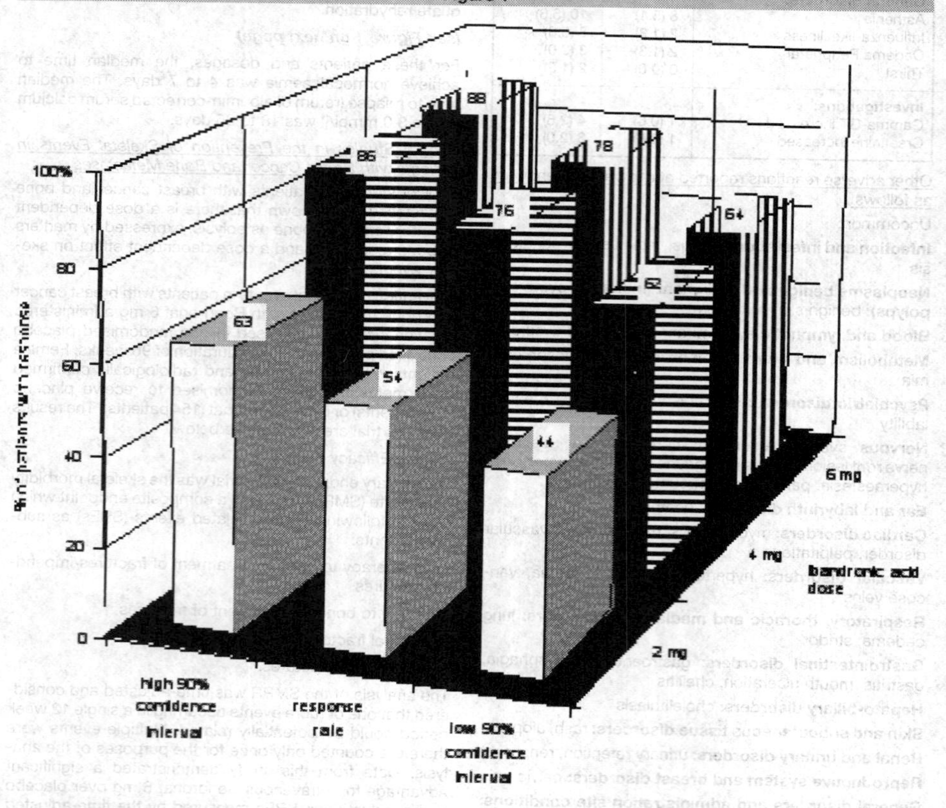

5.2 Pharmacokinetic properties

After a 2 hour infusion of 2, 4 and 6 mg ibandronic acid pharmacokinetic parameters are dose proportional.

Distribution

After initial systemic exposure, ibandronic acid rapidly binds to bone or is excreted into urine. In humans, the apparent terminal volume of distribution is at least 90 l and the amount of dose reaching the bone is estimated to be 40 - 50% of the circulating dose. Protein binding in human plasma is approximately 87% at therapeutic concentrations, and thus drug-drug interaction due to displacement is unlikely.

Metabolism

There is no evidence that ibandronic acid is metabolised in animals or humans.

Elimination

The range of observed apparent half-lives is broad and dependent on dose and assay sensitivity, but the apparent terminal half-life is generally in the range of 10 - 60 hours. However, early plasma levels fall quickly, reaching 10% of peak values within 3 and 8 hours after intravenous or oral administration respectively. No systemic accumulation was observed when ibandronic acid was administered intravenously once every 4 weeks for 48 weeks to patients with metastatic bone disease.

Total clearance of ibandronic acid is low with average values in the range 84 – 160 ml/min. Renal clearance (about 60 ml/min in healthy postmenopausal females) accounts for 50 - 60% of total clearance and is related to creatinine clearance. The difference between the apparent total and renal clearances is considered to reflect the uptake by bone.

Pharmacokinetics in Special Populations

Gender

Bioavailability and pharmacokinetics of ibandronic acid are similar in both men and women.

Race

There is no evidence for clinically relevant interethnic differences between Asians and Caucasians in ibandronic acid disposition. There are only very few data available on patients with African origin.

Patients with renal impairment

Exposure to ibandronic acid in patients with various degrees of renal impairment is related to creatinine clearance (CLcr). In clinical pharmacology trial WP18551, after a single dose intravenous administration of 6 mg (15 minutes infusion), mean AUC_{0-24} increased by 14% and 86%, respectively, in subjects with mild (mean estimated CLcr=68.1 mL/min) and moderate (mean estimated CLcr=41.2 mL/min) renal impairment compared to healthy volunteers (mean estimated CLcr=120 mL/min). Mean C_{max} was not increased in patients with mild renal impairment and increased by 12% in patients with moderate renal impairment. There is no evidence of a reduction in tolerability associated with an increase in exposure. However, an adjustment in the dose or infusion time is recommended in patients being treated for the prevention of skeletal events in patients with breast cancer and bone metastases (see section 4.2).

Patients with hepatic impairment

There are no pharmacokinetic data for ibandronic acid in patients who have hepatic impairment. The liver has no significant role in the clearance of ibandronic acid since it is not metabolised but is cleared by renal excretion and by uptake into bone. Therefore dosage adjustment is not necessary in patients with hepatic impairment. Further, as protein binding of ibandronic acid is approximately 87% at therapeutic concentrations, hypoproteinaemia in severe liver disease is unlikely to lead to clinically significant increases in free plasma concentration.

Elderly

In a multivariate analysis, age was not found to be an independent factor of any of the pharmacokinetic parameters studied. As renal function decreases with age, this is the only factor that should be considered (see renal impairment section).

Children and adolescents

There are no data on the use of Bondronat in patients less than 18 years old.

5.3 Preclinical safety data

Effects in non-clinical studies were observed only at exposures sufficiently in excess of the maximum human exposure indicating little relevance to clinical use. As with other bisphosphonates, the kidney was identified to be the primary target organ of systemic toxicity.

Mutagenicity/Carcinogenicity:

No indication of carcinogenic potential was observed. Tests for genotoxicity revealed no evidence of effects on genetic activity for ibandronic acid.

Reproductive toxicity:

No evidence of direct foetal toxicity or teratogenic effects were observed for ibandronic acid in intravenously treated rats and rabbits. Adverse effects of ibandronic acid in reproductive toxicity studies in the rat were those expected for this class of drug (bisphosphonates). They include a decreased number of implantation sites, interference with natural delivery (dystocia), an increase in visceral variations (renal pelvis ureter syndrome) and teeth abnormalities in F1 offspring in rats.

6. PHARMACEUTICAL PARTICULARS

6.1 List of excipients

Sodium chloride

Acetic acid (99%)

Sodium acetate

Water for injections

6.2 Incompatibilities

To avoid potential incompatibilities Bondronat concentrate for solution for infusion should only be diluted with isotonic sodium chloride solution or 5% glucose solution.

Bondronat should not be mixed with calcium containing solutions.

6.3 Shelf life

5 years.

After reconstitution: 24 hours.

6.4 Special precautions for storage

No special precautions for storage prior to reconstitution.

After reconstitution: Store at 2°C - 8°C (in a refrigerator).

From a microbiological point of view, the product should be used immediately. If not used immediately, in-use storage times and conditions prior to use are the responsibility of the user and would normally not be longer than 24 hours at 2 to 8°C, unless reconstitution has taken place in controlled and validated aseptic conditions.

6.5 Nature and contents of container

Bondronat 2 mg is supplied as packs containing 1 vial (2 ml type 1 glass vial).

Bondronat 6 mg is supplied as packs containing 1, 5 and 10 vials (6 ml type 1 glass vials). The vials are closed with rubber stoppers complying with Ph.Eur. Not all pack sizes may be marketed.

6.6 Special precautions for disposal and other handling

Any unused product or waste material should be disposed of in accordance with local requirements.

7. MARKETING AUTHORISATION HOLDER

Roche Registration Limited
6 Falcon Way
Shire Park
Welwyn Garden City
AL7 1TW
United Kingdom

8. MARKETING AUTHORISATION NUMBER(S)

Bondronat 2 mg

EU/1/96/012/004 - Packs of 1 vial

Bondronat 6 mg

EU/1/96/012/011 - Packs of 1 vial
EU/1/96/012/012 - Packs of 5 vials
EU/1/96/012/013 - Packs of 10 vials

9. DATE OF FIRST AUTHORISATION/RENEWAL OF THE AUTHORISATION

Bondronat 2 mg

Date of First Authorisation: 25 June 1996

Date of last renewal: 25 June 2006

Bondronat 6 mg

Date of first Authorisation: 25 June 1996

Date of last renewal: 25 June 2006

10. DATE OF REVISION OF THE TEXT

March 2007

LEGAL STATUS

POM

Detailed information on this medicinal product is available on the website of the European Medicines Agency (EMEA) http://www.emea.europa.eu/.

Bondronat is a registered trade mark

Bondronat 50mg Film-coated Tablets

(Roche Products Limited)

1. NAME OF THE MEDICINAL PRODUCT

Bondronat ▼ 50 mg Film Coated Tablets

2. QUALITATIVE AND QUANTITATIVE COMPOSITION

Each film-coated tablet contains 50 mg of ibandronic acid (as ibandronic sodium monohydrate).

Excipients:

For a full list of excipients, see section 6.1.

Bondronat tablets contain lactose and should not be administered to patients with rare hereditary problems of galactose intolerance, Lapp lactase deficiency or glucose-galactose malabsorption.

3. PHARMACEUTICAL FORM

Film-coated tablets.

White to off-white film-coated tablets, of oblong shape engraved "L2" on one side and "IT" on the other side.

4. CLINICAL PARTICULARS

4.1 Therapeutic indications

Bondronat is indicated for the prevention of skeletal events (pathological fractures, bone complications requiring radiotherapy or surgery) in patients with breast cancer and bone metastases.

4.2 Posology and method of administration

Bondronat therapy should only be initiated by physicians experienced in the treatment of cancer.

For oral use.

The recommended dose is one 50 mg film-coated tablet daily.

Bondronat tablets should be taken after an overnight fast (at least 6 hours) and before the first food or drink of the day. Medicinal products and supplements (including calcium) should similarly be avoided prior to taking Bondronat tablets. Fasting should be continued for at least 30 minutes after taking the tablet. Plain water may be taken at any time during the course of Bondronat treatment.

- The tablets should be swallowed whole with a full glass of plain water (180 to 240 ml) while the patient is standing or sitting in an upright position.
- Patients should not lie down for 60 minutes after taking Bondronat.
- Patients should not chew or suck the tablet because of a potential for oropharyngeal ulceration.
- Plain water is the only drink that should be taken with Bondronat. Please note that some mineral waters may have a higher concentration of calcium and therefore should not be used.

Patients with hepatic impairment

No dosage adjustment is required (see section 5.2).

Patients with renal impairment

No dosage adjustment is necessary for patients with mild or moderate renal impairment where creatinine clearance is equal to or greater than 30 ml/min.

Below 30 ml/min creatinine clearance, the recommended dose is 50 mg once weekly. See dosing instructions, above.

Elderly

No dose adjustment is necessary.

Children and adolescents

Bondronat is not recommended for patients below age 18 years due to insufficient data on safety and efficacy.

4.3 Contraindications

Hypersensitivity to ibandronic acid or to any of the excipients.

Bondronat should not be used in children.

4.4 Special warnings and precautions for use

Caution is indicated in patients with known hypersensitivity to other bisphosphonates.

Hypocalcaemia and other disturbances of bone and mineral metabolism should be effectively treated before starting Bondronat therapy. Adequate intake of calcium and vitamin D is important in all patients. Patients should receive supplemental calcium and/or vitamin D if dietary intake is inadequate.

Oral bisphosphonates have been associated with dysphagia, oesophagitis and oesophageal or gastric ulcers. Therefore, patients should pay particular attention to the dosing instructions (see section 4.2).

Physicians should be alert to signs or symptoms signalling a possible oesophageal reaction during therapy, and patients should be instructed to discontinue Bondronat and seek medical attention if they develop symptoms of oesophageal irritation such as new or worsening dysphagia, pain on swallowing, retrosternal pain, or heartburn.

Since NSAIDS are associated with gastrointestinal irritation, caution should be taken during concomitant oral medication with Bondronat.

Clinical studies have not shown any evidence of deterioration in renal function with long term Bondronat therapy. Nevertheless, according to clinical assessment of the individual patient, it is recommended that renal function, serum calcium, phosphate and magnesium should be monitored in patients treated with Bondronat.

Bondronat tablets contain lactose and should not be administered to patients with rare hereditary problems of galactose intolerance, Lapp lactase deficiency or glucose-galactose malabsorption.

Osteonecrosis of the jaw, generally associated with tooth extraction and/or local infection (including osteomyelitis) has been reported in patients with cancer receiving treatment regimens including primarily intravenously administered bisphosphonates. Many of these patients were also receiving chemotherapy and corticosteroids. Osteonecrosis of the jaw has also been reported in patients with osteoporosis receiving oral bisphosphonates.

A dental examination with appropriate preventive dentistry should be considered prior to treatment with bisphosphonates in patients with concomitant risk factors (e.g. cancer, chemotherapy, radiotherapy, corticosteroids, poor oral hygiene).

While on treatment, these patients should avoid invasive dental procedures if possible. For patients who develop osteonecrosis of the jaw while on bisphosphonate therapy, dental surgery may exacerbate the condition. For patients requiring dental procedures, there are no data available to suggest whether discontinuation of bisphosphonate treatment reduces the risk of osteonecrosis of the jaw. Clinical judgement of the treating physician should guide the management plan of each patient based on individual benefit/risk assessment.

4.5 Interaction with other medicinal products and other forms of interaction

Interaction studies have only been performed in adults.

Drug-Food Interactions

Products containing calcium and other multivalent cations (such as aluminium, magnesium, iron), including milk and food, are likely to interfere with absorption of Bondronat tablets. Therefore, with such products, including food, intake must be delayed at least 30 minutes following oral administration.

Bioavailability was reduced by approximately 75% when Bondronat tablets were administered 2 hours after a standard meal. Therefore, it is recommended that the tablets should be taken after an overnight fast (at least 6 hours) and fasting should continue for at least 30 minutes after the dose has been taken (see section 4.2).

Drug-Drug Interactions

When co-administered with melphalan/prednisolone in patients with multiple myeloma, no interaction was observed.

Other interaction studies in postmenopausal women have demonstrated the absence of any interaction potential with tamoxifen or hormone replacement therapy (oestrogen).

In healthy male volunteers and postmenopausal women, intravenous ranitidine caused an increase in ibandronic acid bioavailability of about 20% (which is within the normal variability of the bioavailability of ibandronic acid), probably as a result of reduced gastric acidity. However, no dosage adjustment is required when Bondronat is administered with H_2-antagonists or other drugs that increase gastric pH.

In relation to disposition, no drug interactions of clinical significance are likely. Ibandronic acid is eliminated by renal secretion only and does not undergo any biotransformation. The secretory pathway does not appear to include known acidic or basic transport systems involved in the excretion of other active substances. In addition, ibandronic acid does not inhibit the major human hepatic P450 isoenzymes and does not induce the hepatic cytochrome P450 system in rats. Plasma protein binding is low at therapeutic concentrations and ibandronic acid is therefore unlikely to displace other active substances.

Caution is advised when bisphosphonates are administered with aminoglycosides, since both agents can lower serum calcium levels for prolonged periods. Attention should also be paid to the possible existence of simultaneous hypomagnesaemia.

In clinical studies, Bondronat has been administered concomitantly with commonly used anticancer agents, diuretics, antibiotics and analgesics without clinically apparent interactions occurring.

4.6 Pregnancy and lactation

There are no adequate data from the use of ibandronic acid in pregnant women. Studies in rats have shown reproductive toxicity (see section 5.3). The potential risk for humans is unknown. Therefore, Bondronat should not be used during pregnancy.

It is not known whether ibandronic acid is excreted in human milk. Studies in lactating rats have demonstrated the presence of low levels of ibandronic acid in the milk following intravenous administration. Bondronat should not be used during lactation.

4.7 Effects on ability to drive and use machines

No studies on the effects on the ability to drive and use machines have been performed.

4.8 Undesirable effects

The safety profile of Bondronat is derived from controlled clinical trials in the approved indication and after the oral administration of Bondronat at the recommended dose.

In the pooled database from the 2 pivotal phase III trials (286 patients treated with Bondronat 50 mg), the proportion of patients who experienced an adverse reaction with a possible or probable relationship to Bondronat was 27%.

Adverse reactions are ranked under heading of frequency, the most frequent first, using the following convention: very common (≥10%), common (≥1% and <10%), uncommon (≥0.1% and <1%), rare (≥0.01% and <0.1%), very rare (≤0.01%).

Table 1 lists common adverse reactions from the pooled phase III trials. Adverse reactions that are equally frequent in both active and placebo or more frequent in placebo-treated patients are excluded.

Table 1 Adverse ReactionsReported Commonly and Greater than Placebo

Adverse Reaction	Placebo p. o. daily (n=277 patients) No. (%)	Bondronat 50 mg p.o. daily (n=286 patients) No. (%)
Metabolism and Nutrition Disorders		
Hypocalcaemia	14 (5.1)	27 (9.4)
Gastrointestinal Disorders		
Dyspepsia	13 (4.7)	20 (7.0)
Nausea	4 (1.4)	10 (3.5)
Abdominal Pain	2 (0.7)	6 (2.1)
Oesophagitis	2 (0.7)	6 (2.1)
General Disorders		
Asthenia	2 (0.7)	4 (1.4)

Adverse drug reactions occurring at a frequency <1%:

The following list provides information on adverse drug reactions reported in study MF 4414 and MF 4434 occurring more frequently with Bondronat 50 mg than with placebo:

Uncommon:

Blood and Lymphatic System Disorders	anaemia
Nervous System Disorders	paraesthesia, dysgeusia (taste perversion)
Gastrointestinal Disorders	haemorrhage, duodenal ulcer, gastritis, dysphagia, abdominal pain, dry mouth
Skin and Subcutaneous Tissue Disorders	pruritus
Renal and Urinary Disorders	azotaemia (uraemia)
General Disorders:	chest pain, influenza-like illness, malaise, pain
Investigations	Blood parathyroid hormone increased

Osteonecrosis of the jaw has been reported in patients treated by bisphosphonates. The majority of the reports refer to cancer patients, but such cases have also been reported in patients treated for osteoporosis. Osteonecrosis of the jaw is generally associated with tooth extraction and / or local infection (including osteomyelitis). Diagnosis of cancer, chemotherapy, radiotherapy, corticosteroids and poor oral hygiene are also deemed as risk factors (see section 4.4).

4.9 Overdose

No case of overdose has been reported.

No specific information is available on the treatment of overdosage with Bondronat. However, oral overdosage may result in upper gastrointestinal events, such as upset stomach, heartburn, oesophagitis, gastritis or ulcer. Milk or antacids should be given to bind Bondronat. Owing to the risk of oesophageal irritation, vomiting should not be induced and the patient should remain fully upright.

5. PHARMACOLOGICAL PROPERTIES

5.1 Pharmacodynamic properties

Pharmaco-therapeutic group: Bisphosphonate, ATC Code: M05B A 06

Ibandronic acid belongs to the bisphosphonate group of compounds which act specifically on bone. Their selective action on bone tissue is based on the high affinity of bisphosphonates for bone mineral. Bisphosphonates act by inhibiting osteoclast activity, although the precise mechanism is still not clear.

In vivo, ibandronic acid prevents experimentally-induced bone destruction caused by cessation of gonadal function, retinoids, tumours or tumour extracts. The inhibition of endogenous bone resorption has also been documented by ^{45}Ca kinetic studies and by the release of radioactive tetracycline previously incorporated into the skeleton.

At doses that were considerably higher than the pharmacologically effective doses, ibandronic acid did not have any effect on bone mineralisation.

Bone resorption due to malignant disease is characterized by excessive bone resorption that is not balanced with appropriate bone formation. Ibandronic acid selectively inhibits osteoclast activity, reducing bone resorption and thereby reducing skeletal complications of the malignant disease.

Clinical studies in patients with breast cancer and bone metastases have shown that there is a dose dependent inhibitory effect on bone osteolysis, expressed by markers of bone resorption, and a dose dependent effect on skeletal events.

Prevention of skeletal events in patients with breast cancer and bone metastases with Bondronat 50 mg tablets was assessed in two randomized placebo controlled phase III trials with duration of 96 weeks. Female patients with breast cancer and radiologically confirmed bone metastases were randomised to receive placebo (277 patients) or 50 mg Bondronat (287 patients). The results from these trials are summarised below.

Primary Efficacy Endpoints

The primary endpoint of the trials was the skeletal morbidity period rate (SMPR). This was a composite endpoint which had the following skeletal related events (SREs) as sub-components:

- radiotherapy to bone for treatment of fractures/impending fractures
- surgery to bone for treatment of fractures
- vertebral fractures
- non-vertebral fractures

The analysis of the SMPR was time-adjusted and considered that one or more events occurring in a single 12 week period could be potentially related. Multiple events were therefore, counted only once in any given 12 week period for the purposes of the analysis. Pooled data from these studies demonstrated a significant advantage for Bondronat 50 mg p.o. over placebo in the reduction in SREs measured by the SMPR (p=0.041). There was also a

38% reduction in the risk of developing an SRE for Bondronat treated patients when compared with placebo (relative risk 0.62, p=0.003). Efficacy results are summarised in Table 2.

Table 2 Efficacy Results (Breast Cancer Patients with Metastatic Bone Disease)

	All Skeletal Related Events (SREs)		
	Placebo n=277	Bondronat 50 mg n=287	p-value
SMPR (per patient year)	1.15	0.99	p=0.041
SRE relative risk	-	0.62	p=0.003

Secondary Efficacy Endpoints

A statistically significant improvement in bone pain score was shown for Bondronat 50 mg compared to placebo. The pain reduction was consistently below baseline throughout the entire study and accompanied by a significantly reduced use of analgesics compared to placebo. The deterioration in Quality of Life and WHO performance status was significantly less in Bondronat treated patients compared with placebo. Urinary concentrations of the bone resorption marker CTx (C-terminal telopeptide released from Type I collagen) were significantly reduced in the Bondronat group compared to placebo. This reduction in urinary CTx levels was significantly correlated with the primary efficacy endpoint SMPR (Kendall-tau-b ($p<0.001$)). A tabular summary of the secondary efficacy results is presented in Table 3.

Table 3 Secondary Efficacy Results (Breast Cancer Patients with Metastatic Bone Disease)

	Placebo n=277	Bondronat 50 mg n=287	p-value
Bone pain *	0.20	-0.10	p=0.001
Analgesic use *	0.85	0.60	p=0.019
Quality of Life *	-26.8	-8.3	p=0.032
WHO performance score *	0.54	0.33	p=0.008
Urinary CTx **	10.95	-77.32	p=0.001

* Mean change from baseline to last assessment.

** Median change from baseline to last assessment

5.2 Pharmacokinetic properties

Absorption

The absorption of ibandronic acid in the upper gastrointestinal tract is rapid after oral administration. Maximum observed plasma concentrations were reached within 0.5 to 2 hours (median 1 hour) in the fasted state and absolute bioavailability was about 0.6%. The extent of absorption is impaired when taken together with food or beverages (other than plain water). Bioavailability is reduced by about 90% when ibandronic acid is administered with a standard breakfast in comparison with bioavailability seen in fasted subjects. When taken 30 minutes before a meal, the reduction in bioavailability is approximately 30%. There is no meaningful reduction in bioavailability provided ibandronic acid is taken 60 minutes before a meal.

Bioavailability was reduced by approximately 75% when Bondronat tablets were administered 2 hours after a standard meal. Therefore, it is recommended that the tablets should be taken after an overnight fast (minimum 6 hours) and fasting should continue for at least 30 minutes after the dose has been taken (see Section 4.2).

Distribution

After initial systemic exposure, ibandronic acid rapidly binds to bone or is excreted into urine. In humans, the apparent terminal volume of distribution is at least 90 l and the amount of dose reaching the bone is estimated to be 40-50% of the circulating dose. Protein binding in human plasma is approximately 87% at therapeutic concentrations, and thus drug-drug interaction due to displacement is unlikely.

Metabolism

There is no evidence that ibandronic acid is metabolized in animals or humans.

Elimination

The absorbed fraction of ibandronic acid is removed from the circulation via bone absorption (estimated to be 40-50%) and the remainder is eliminated unchanged by the kidney. The unabsorbed fraction of ibandronic acid is eliminated unchanged in the faeces.

The range of observed apparent half-lives is broad and dependent on dose and assay sensitivity, but the apparent terminal half-life is generally in the range of 10-60 hours. However, early plasma levels fall quickly, reaching 10% of peak values within 3 and 8 hours after intravenous or oral administration respectively.

Total clearance of ibandronic acid is low with average values in the range 84-160 ml/min. Renal clearance (about 60 ml/min in healthy postmenopausal females) accounts for 50-60% of total clearance and is related to creatinine clearance. The difference between the apparent total and renal clearances is considered to reflect the uptake by bone.

Pharmacokinetics in Special Populations

Gender

Bioavailability and pharmacokinetics of ibandronic acid are similar in both men and women.

Race

There is no evidence for clinically relevant interethnic differences between Asians and Caucasians in ibandronic acid disposition. There are only very few data available on patients with African origin.

Patients with renal impairment

Renal clearance of ibandronic acid in patients with various degrees of renal impairment is linearly related to creatinine clearance (CLcr). No dosage adjustment is necessary for patients with mild or moderate renal impairment (CLcr ≥30 ml/min). Subjects with severe renal impairment (CLcr ≤ 30 ml/min) receiving oral administration of 10 mg ibandronic acid daily for 21 days, had 2-3 fold higher plasma concentrations than subjects with normal renal function. Total clearance of ibandronic acid was reduced to 44 ml/min in the subjects with severe renal impairment. After intravenous administration of 0.5 mg, total, renal, and non-renal clearances decreased by 67%, 77% and 50%, respectively, in subjects with severe renal impairment. However, there was no reduction in tolerability associated with the increase in exposure. Reduction of the oral dose to one 50 mg tablet once weekly is recommended in patients with severe renal impairment (CLcr <30 ml/min) (see Section 4.2).

Patients with hepatic impairment

There are no pharmacokinetic data for ibandronic acid in patients who have hepatic impairment. The liver has no significant role in the clearance of ibandronic acid since it is not metabolized but is cleared by renal excretion and by uptake into bone. Therefore dosage adjustment is not necessary in patients with hepatic impairment. Further, as protein binding of ibandronic acid is approximately 87% at therapeutic concentrations, hypoproteinaemia in severe liver disease is unlikely to lead to clinically significant increases in free plasma concentration.

Elderly

In a multivariate analysis, age was not found to be an independent factor of any of the pharmacokinetic parameters studied. As renal function decreases with age, this is the only factor to take into consideration (see renal impairment section).

Children and adolescents

There are no data on the use of Bondronat in patients less than 18 years old.

5.3 Preclinical safety data

Effects in non-clinical studies were observed only at exposures sufficiently in excess of the maximum human exposure indicating little relevance to clinical use. As with other bisphosphonates, the kidney was identified to be the primary target organ of systemic toxicity.

Mutagenicity/Carcinogenicity:

No indication of carcinogenic potential was observed. Tests for genotoxicity revealed no evidence of genetic activity for ibandronic acid.

Reproductive toxicity:

No evidence of direct foetal toxicity or teratogenic effects was observed for ibandronic acid in intravenously or orally treated rats and rabbits. Adverse effects of ibandronic acid in reproductive toxicity studies in the rat were those expected for this class of drugs (bisphosphonates). They include a decreased number of implantation sites, interference with natural delivery (dystocia), an increase in visceral variations (renal pelvis ureter syndrome) and teeth abnormalities in F1 offspring in rats.

6. PHARMACEUTICAL PARTICULARS

6.1 List of excipients

Tablet core:

Lactose monohydrate

Povidone

Cellulose, microcrystalline

Crospovidone

Stearic acid

Silica, anhydrous colloidal

Tablet coat:

Hypromellose

Titanium dioxide E171

Talc

Macrogol 6000

6.2 Incompatibilities

Not applicable.

6.3 Shelf life

5 years.

6.4 Special precautions for storage

Store in the original package in order to protect from moisture.

6.5 Nature and contents of container

Bondronat 50 mg film coated tablets are supplied in blisters (aluminium) containing 7 tablets, which are presented as packs containing 28 or 84 tablets. Not all pack sizes may be marketed.

6.6 Special precautions for disposal and other handling

No special requirements.

7. MARKETING AUTHORISATION HOLDER

Roche Registration Limited

6 Falcon Way

Shire Park

Welwyn Garden City

AL7 1TW

United Kingdom

8. MARKETING AUTHORISATION NUMBER(S)

EU/1/96/012/009

EU/1/96/012/010

9. DATE OF FIRST AUTHORISATION/RENEWAL OF THE AUTHORISATION

Date of first Authorisation: 25 June 1996

Date of last renewal: 25 June 2006

10. DATE OF REVISION OF THE TEXT

10 March 2009

Detailed information on this medicinal product is available on the website of the European Medicines Agency (EMEA) http://www.emea.europa.eu/.

Bonviva 150mg Film-Coated Tablets

(Roche Products Limited)

1. NAME OF THE MEDICINAL PRODUCT

Bonviva ▼150 mg film-coated tablets

2. QUALITATIVE AND QUANTITATIVE COMPOSITION

Each film-coated tablet contains 150 mg ibandronic acid (as ibandronic sodium monohydrate).

Excipients

Each film-coated tablet contains 162.75 mg lactose monohydrate. For a full list of excipients, see section 6.1.

3. PHARMACEUTICAL FORM

Film-coated tablet

White to off white film-coated tablets, of oblong shape marked "BNVA" on one side, and "150" on the other side.

4. CLINICAL PARTICULARS

4.1 Therapeutic indications

Treatment of osteoporosis in postmenopausal women at increased risk of fracture (see section 5.1).

A reduction in the risk of vertebral fractures has been demonstrated, efficacy on femoral neck fractures has not been established.

4.2 Posology and method of administration

Posology:

The recommended dose is one 150 mg film-coated tablet once a month. The tablet should preferably be taken on the same date each month.

Bonviva should be taken after an overnight fast (at least 6 hours) and 1 hour before the first food or drink (other than water) of the day (see section 4.5) or any other oral medicinal products or supplementation (including calcium).

In case a dose is missed, patients should be instructed to take one Bonviva 150 mg tablet the morning after the tablet is remembered, unless the time to the next scheduled dose is within 7 days. Patients should then return to taking their dose once a month on their originally scheduled date.

If the next scheduled dose is within 7 days, patients should wait until their next dose and then continue taking one tablet once a month as originally scheduled.

Patients should not take two tablets within the same week.

Patients should receive supplemental calcium and / or vitamin D if dietary intake is inadequate (see section 4.4 and section 4.5).

Special Populations

Patients with renal impairment

No dose adjustment is necessary for patients with mild or moderate renal impairment where creatinine clearance is equal or greater than 30 ml/min.

Bonviva is not recommended for patients with a creatinine clearance below 30 ml/min due to limited clinical experience (see section 4.4 and section 5.2).

Patients with hepatic impairment

No dose adjustment is required (see section 5.2).

Elderly Population

No dose adjustment is required (see section 5.2).

Paediatric Population

There is no relevant use of Bonviva in children, and Bonviva was not studied in the paediatric population.

Method of Administration:

For oral use.

Tablets should be swallowed whole with a glass of plain water (180 to 240 ml) while the patient is sitting or standing in an upright position. Patients should not lie down for 1 hour after taking Bonviva.

Plain water is the only drink that should be taken with Bonviva. Please note that some mineral waters may have a higher concentration of calcium and therefore, should not be used.

Patients should not chew or suck the tablet, because of a potential for oropharyngeal ulceration.

4.3 Contraindications

- Hypocalcaemia (see section 4.4)
- Hypersensitivity to ibandronic acid or to any of the excipients.

4.4 Special warnings and precautions for use

Gastrointestinal Disorders

Bisphosphonates have been associated with dysphagia, oesophagitis and oesophageal or gastric ulcers. Therefore patients, especially those with a history of prolonged oesophageal transit time, should pay particular attention to and be able to comply with the dosing instructions (see section 4.2).

Physicians should be alert to signs or symptoms signalling a possible oesophageal reaction during therapy, and patients should be instructed to discontinue Bonviva and seek medical attention if they develop symptoms of oesophageal irritation such as new or worsening dysphagia, pain on swallowing, retrosternal pain, or heartburn.

Since Nonsteroidal Anti-Inflammatory Drugs and bisphosphonates are both associated with gastrointestinal irritation, caution should be taken during concomitant administration.

Hypocalcaemia

Existing hypocalcaemia must be corrected before starting Bonviva therapy. Other disturbances of bone and mineral metabolism should also be effectively treated. Adequate intake of calcium and vitamin D is important in all patients.

Renal impairment

Due to limited clinical experience, Bonviva is not recommended for patients with a creatinine clearance below 30 ml/min (see section 5.2).

Osteonecrosis of the Jaw

Osteonecrosis of the jaw, generally associated with tooth extraction and/or local infection (including osteomyelitis) has been reported in patients with cancer receiving treatment regimens including primarily intravenously administered bisphosphonates. Many of these patients were also receiving chemotherapy and corticosteroids. Osteonecrosis of the jaw has also been reported in patients with osteoporosis receiving oral bisphosphonates.

A dental examination with appropriate preventive dentistry should be considered prior to treatment with bisphosphonates in patients with concomitant risk factors (e.g. cancer, chemotherapy, radiotherapy, corticosteroids, poor oral hygiene).

While on treatment, these patients should avoid invasive dental procedures if possible. For patients who develop osteonecrosis of the jaw while on bisphosphonate therapy, dental surgery may exacerbate the condition. For patients requiring dental procedures, there are no data available to suggest whether discontinuation of bisphosphonate treatment reduces the risk of osteonecrosis of the jaw. Clinical judgement of the treating physician should guide the management plan of each patient based on individual benefit/risk assessment.

Galactose intolerance

Patients with rare hereditary problems of galactose intolerance, the Lapp lactase deficiency or glucose-galactose malabsorption should not take this medicinal product.

4.5 Interaction with other medicinal products and other forms of interaction

Oral bioavailability of ibandronic acid is generally reduced in the presence of food. In particular, products containing calcium and other multivalent cations (such as aluminium, magnesium, iron), including milk, are likely to interfere with absorption of Bonviva, which is consistent with findings in animal studies. Therefore, patients should fast overnight (at least 6 hours) before taking Bonviva and continue fasting for 1 hour following intake of Bonviva (see section 4.2).

Calcium supplements, antacids and some oral medicinal products containing multivalent cations (such as aluminium, magnesium, iron) are likely to interfere with the absorption of Bonviva. Therefore, patients should not take other oral medicinal products for at least 6 hours before taking Bonviva and for 1 hour following intake of Bonviva.

Metabolic interactions are not considered likely, since ibandronic acid does not inhibit the major human hepatic P450 isoenzymes and has been shown not to induce the hepatic cytochrome P450 system in rats. Furthermore, plasma protein binding is approximately 85 % - 87 % (determined *in vitro* at therapeutic concentrations), and thus there is a low potential for interaction with other medicinal products due to displacement. Ibandronic acid is eliminated by renal excretion only and does not undergo any biotransformation. The secretory pathway appears not to include known acidic or basic transport systems involved in the excretion of other active substances.

In a two-year study in postmenopausal women with osteoporosis (BM 16549), the incidence of upper gastrointestinal events in patients concomitantly taking aspirin or NSAIDs was similar in patients taking ibandronic acid 2.5 mg daily or 150 mg once monthly after one and two years.

Of over 1500 patients enrolled in study BM 16549 comparing monthly with daily dosing regimens of ibandronic acid, 14 % and 18 % of patients used histamine (H2) blockers or proton pump inhibitors after one and two years, respectively. Among these patients, the incidence of upper gastrointestinal events in the patients treated with Bonviva 150 mg once monthly was similar to that in patients treated with ibandronic acid 2.5 mg daily.

In healthy male volunteers and postmenopausal women, intravenous administration of ranitidine caused an increase in ibandronic acid bioavailability of about 20 %, probably as a result of reduced gastric acidity. However, since this increase is within the normal variability of the bioavailability of ibandronic acid, no dose adjustment is considered necessary when Bonviva is administered with H2-antagonists or other active substances which increase gastric pH.

Pharmacokinetic interaction studies in postmenopausal women have demonstrated the absence of any interaction potential with tamoxifen or hormone replacement therapy (oestrogen).

No interaction was observed when co-administered with melphalan/prednisolone in patients with multiple myeloma.

4.6 Pregnancy and lactation

Pregnancy

There are no adequate data from the use of ibandronic acid in pregnant women. Studies in rats have shown some reproductive toxicity (see section 5.3). The potential risk for humans is unknown.

Bonviva should not be used during pregnancy.

Lactation

It is not known whether ibandronic acid is excreted in human milk. Studies in lactating rats have demonstrated the presence of low levels of ibandronic acid in the milk following intravenous administration.

Bonviva should not be used during lactation.

4.7 Effects on ability to drive and use machines

No studies on the effects on the ability to drive and use machines have been performed.

4.8 Undesirable effects

The safety of oral treatment with ibandronic acid 2.5 mg daily was evaluated in 1251 patients treated in 4 placebo-controlled clinical studies, with the large majority of patients coming from the pivotal three year fracture study (MF4411). The overall safety profile of ibandronic acid 2.5 mg daily in all these studies was similar to that of placebo.

In a two-year study in postmenopausal women with osteoporosis (BM 16549) the overall safety of Bonviva 150 mg once monthly and ibandronic acid 2.5 mg daily was similar. The overall proportion of patients who experienced an adverse reaction, was 22.7 % and 25.0 % for Bonviva 150 mg once monthly after one and two years, respectively. The majority of adverse reactions were mild to moderate in intensity. Most cases did not lead to cessation of therapy.

The most commonly reported adverse reaction was arthralgia.

Adverse reactions considered by investigators to be causally related to Bonviva are listed below by System Organ Class.

Frequencies are defined as common (≥ 1/100 to < 1/10), uncommon (≥ 1/1,000 to < 1/100), and rare (≥ 1/10,000 to < 1/1,000). Within each frequency grouping, adverse reactions are presented in order of decreasing seriousness.

Table 1: Adverse reactions occurring in postmenopausal women receiving Bonviva 150mg once monthly or ibandronic acid 2.5mg daily in the phase III studies BM16549 and MF4411.

(see Table 1 below)

Patients with a previous history of gastrointestinal disease including patients with peptic ulcer without recent bleeding or hospitalisation, and patients with dyspepsia or reflux controlled by medication were included in the once monthly treatment study. For these patients, there was no difference in the incidence of upper gastrointestinal adverse events with the 150 mg once monthly regimen compared to the 2.5 mg daily regimen.

Laboratory test findings

In the pivotal three-year study with ibandronic acid 2.5 mg daily (MF 4411) there was no difference compared with placebo for laboratory abnormalities indicative of hepatic or renal dysfunction, an impaired haematologic system, hypocalcaemia or hypophosphataemia. Similarly, no differences were noted between the groups in study BM 16549 after one and two years.

Post-marketing Experience

Osteonecrosis of the jaw has been reported in patients treated by bisphosphonates. The majority of the reports refer to cancer patients, but such cases have also been reported in patients treated for osteoporosis. Osteonecrosis of the jaw is generally associated with tooth extraction and / or local infection (including osteomyelitis). Diagnosis of cancer, chemotherapy, radiotherapy, corticosteroids and poor oral hygiene are also deemed as risk factors (see section 4.4).

4.9 Overdose

No specific information is available on the treatment of overdosage with Bonviva.

However, based on a knowledge of this class of compounds, oral over-dosage may result in upper gastrointestinal adverse reactions (such as upset stomach, dyspepsia, oesophagitis, gastritis, or ulcer) or hypocalcaemia. Milk or antacids should be given to bind Bonviva, and any adverse reactions treated symptomatically. Owing to the risk of oesophageal irritation, vomiting should not be induced and the patient should remain fully upright.

5. PHARMACOLOGICAL PROPERTIES

5.1 Pharmacodynamic properties

Pharmacotherapeutic group: Bisphosphonates, ATC code: M05B A06

Table 1 Adverse reactions occurring in postmenopausal women receiving Bonviva 150mg once monthly or ibandronic acid 2.5mg daily in the phase III studies BM16549 and MF4411.

System Organ Class	Frequency	Adverse reactions
Immune system disorders	Rare	Hypersensitivity reaction
Nervous system disorders	Common	Headache
	Uncommon	Dizziness
Gastrointestinal disorders	Common	Oesophagitis, Gastritis, Gastro oesophageal reflux disease, Dyspepsia, Diarrhoea, Abdominal pain, Nausea
	Uncommon	Oesophagitis including oesophageal ulcerations or strictures and dysphagia, Vomiting, Flatulence
	Rare	Duodenitis
Skin and subcutaneous tissues disorders	Common	Rash
	Rare	Angioedema, Face oedema, Urticaria
Musculoskeletal, connective tissue and bone disorders	Common	Arthralgia, Myalgia, Musculoskeletal pain, Muscle cramp, Musculoskeletal stiffness
	Uncommon	Back pain
General disorders and administration site conditions	Common	Influenza like illness*
	Uncommon	Fatigue

MedDRA version 7.1

* Transient, influenza-like symptoms have been reported with Bonviva 150 mg once monthly, typically in association with the first dose. Such symptoms were generally of short duration, mild or moderate in intensity, and resolved during continuing treatment without requiring remedial measures. Influenza-like illness includes events reported as acute phase reaction or symptoms including myalgia, arthralgia, fever, chills, fatigue, nausea, loss of appetite, or bone pain.

Table 2 Mean relative change from baseline of lumbar spine, total hip, femoral neck and trochanter BMD after one year (primary analysis) and two years of treatment (Per-Protocol Population) in study BM 16549.

	One year data in study BM 16549		Two year data in study BM 16549	
Mean relative changes from baseline % [95% CI]	ibandronic acid 2.5 mg daily (N=318)	Bonviva 150 mg once monthly (N=320)	ibandronic acid 2.5 mg daily (N=294)	Bonviva 150 mg once monthly (N=291)
Lumbar spine L2-L4 BMD	3.9 [3.4, 4.3]	4.9 [4.4, 5.3]	5.0 [4.4, 5.5]	6.6 [6.0, 7.1]
Total hip BMD	2.0 [1.7, 2.3]	3.1 [2.8, 3.4]	2.5 [2.1, 2.9]	4.2 [3.8, 4.5]
Femoral neck BMD	1.7 [1.3, 2.1]	2.2 [1.9, 2.6]	1.9 [1.4, 2.4]	3.1 [2.7, 3.6]
Trochanter BMD	3.2 [2.8, 3.7]	4.6 [4.2, 5.1]	4.0 [3.5, 4.5]	6.2 [5.7, 6.7]

Mechanism of action

Ibandronic acid is a highly potent bisphosphonate belonging to the nitrogen-containing group of bisphosphonates, which act selectively on bone tissue and specifically inhibit osteoclast activity without directly affecting bone formation. It does not interfere with osteoclast recruitment. Ibandronic acid leads to progressive net gains in bone mass and a decreased incidence of fractures through the reduction of elevated bone turnover towards premenopausal levels in postmenopausal women.

Pharmacodynamic effects

The pharmacodynamic action of ibandronic acid is inhibition of bone resorption. *In vivo*, ibandronic acid prevents experimentally induced bone destruction caused by cessation of gonadal function, retinoids, tumours or tumour extracts. In young (fast growing) rats, the endogenous bone resorption is also inhibited, leading to increased normal bone mass compared with untreated animals.

Animal models confirm that ibandronic acid is a highly potent inhibitor of osteoclastic activity. In growing rats, there was no evidence of impaired mineralization even at doses greater than 5,000 times the dose required for osteoporosis treatment.

Both daily and intermittent (with prolonged dose-free intervals) long-term administration in rats, dogs and monkeys was associated with formation of new bone of normal quality and maintained or increased mechanical strength even at doses in the toxic range. In humans, the efficacy of both daily and intermittent administration with a dose-free interval of 9-10 weeks of ibandronic acid was confirmed in a clinical trial (MF 4411), in which ibandronic acid demonstrated anti-fracture efficacy.

In animal models ibandronic acid produced biochemical changes indicative of dose-dependent inhibition of bone resorption, including suppression of urinary biochemical markers of bone collagen degradation (such as deoxypyridinoline, and cross-linked N-telopeptides of type I collagen (NTX)).

In a Phase 1 bioequivalence study conducted in 72 postmenopausal women receiving 150 mg orally every 28 days for a total of four doses, inhibition in serum CTX following the first dose was seen as early as 24 hours post-dose (median inhibition 28 %), with median maximal inhibition (69 %) seen 6 days later. Following the third and fourth dose, the median maximum inhibition 6 days post dose was 74 % with reduction to a median inhibition of 56 % seen 28 days following the fourth dose. With no further dosing, there is a loss of suppression of biochemical markers of bone resorption.

Clinical efficacy

Independent risk factors, for example, low BMD, age, the existence of previous fractures, a family history of fractures, high bone turnover and low body mass index should be considered in order to identify women at increased risk of osteoporotic fractures.

Bonviva 150 mg once monthly

Bone mineral density (BMD)

Bonviva 150 mg once monthly was shown to be at least as effective as ibandronic acid 2.5 mg daily at increasing BMD in a two year, double-blind, multicentre study (BM 16549) of postmenopausal women with osteoporosis (lumbar spine BMD T score below -2.5 SD at baseline). This was demonstrated in both the primary analysis at one year and in the confirmatory analysis at two years endpoint (Table 2).

Table 2: Mean relative change from baseline of lumbar spine, total hip, femoral neck and trochanter BMD after one year (primary analysis) and two years of treatment (Per-Protocol Population) in study BM 16549.

(*see Table 2 above*)

Furthermore, Bonviva 150 mg once monthly was proven superior to ibandronic acid 2.5 mg daily for increases in lumbar spine BMD in a prospectively planned analysis at one year, p=0.002, and at two years, p<0.001.

At one year (primary analysis), 91.3 % (p=0.005) of patients receiving Bonviva 150 mg once monthly had a lumbar spine BMD increase above or equal to baseline (BMD responders), compared with 84.0 % of patients receiving ibandronic acid 2.5 mg daily. At two years, 93.5 % (p=0.004) and 86.4 % of patients receiving Bonviva 150 mg once monthly or ibandronic acid 2.5 mg daily, respectively, were responders.

For total hip BMD, 90.0 % (p<0.001) of patients receiving Bonviva 150 mg once monthly and 76.7 % of patients receiving ibandronic acid 2.5 mg daily had total hip BMD increases above or equal to baseline at one year. At two years 93.4 % (p<0.001) of patients receiving Bonviva 150 mg once monthly and 78.4 %, of patients receiving ibandronic acid 2.5 mg daily had total hip BMD increases above or equal to baseline.

When a more stringent criterion is considered, which combines both lumbar spine and total hip BMD, 83.9 % (p<0.001) and 65.7 % of patients receiving Bonviva 150 mg once monthly or ibandronic acid 2.5 mg daily, respectively, were responders at one year. At two years, 87.1 % (p<0.001) and 70.5 %, of patients met this criterion in the 150 mg monthly and 2.5 mg daily arms respectively.

Biochemical markers of bone turn-over

Clinically meaningful reductions in serum CTX levels were observed at all time points measured, i.e. months 3, 6, 12 and 24. After one year (primary analysis) the median relative change from baseline was -76 % for Bonviva 150 mg once monthly and -67 % for ibandronic acid 2.5 mg daily. At two years the median relative change was -68 % and -62 %, in the 150 mg monthly and 2.5 mg daily arms respectively.

At one year, 83.5 % (p= 0.006) of patients receiving Bonviva 150 mg once monthly and 73.9 % of patients receiving ibandronic acid 2.5 mg daily were identified as responders (defined as a decrease ≥50 % from baseline). At two years 78.7 % (p=0.002) and 65.6 % of patients were identified as responders in the 150 mg monthly and 2.5 mg daily arms respectively.

Based on the results of study BM 16549, Bonviva 150 mg once monthly is expected to be at least as effective in preventing fractures as ibandronic acid 2.5 mg daily.

Ibandronic acid 2.5 mg daily

In the initial three-year, randomised, double-blind, placebo-controlled, fracture study (MF 4411), a statistically significant and medically relevant decrease in the incidence of new radiographic morphometric and clinical vertebral fractures was demonstrated (table 3). In this study, ibandronic acid was evaluated at oral doses of 2.5 mg daily and 20 mg intermittently as an exploratory regimen. Ibandronic acid was taken 60 minutes before the first food or drink of the day (post-dose fasting period). The study enrolled women aged 55 to 80 years, who were at least 5 years postmenopausal, who had a BMD at lumbar spine of 2 to 5 SD below the premenopausal mean (T-score) in at least one vertebra [L1-L4], and who had one to four prevalent vertebral fractures. All patients received 500 mg calcium and 400 IU vitamin D daily. Efficacy was evaluated in 2,928 patients. ibandronic acid 2.5 mg administered daily, showed a statistically significant and medically relevant reduction in the incidence of new vertebral fractures. This regimen reduced the occurrence of new radiographic vertebral fractures by 62 % (p=0.0001) over the three year duration of the study. A relative risk reduction of 61 % was observed after 2 years (p=0.0006). No statistically significant difference was attained after 1 year of treatment (p=0.056). The anti-fracture effect was consistent over the duration of the study. There was no indication of a waning of the effect over time.

The incidence of clinical vertebral fractures was also significantly reduced by 49 % (p=0.011). The strong effect on vertebral fractures was furthermore reflected by a statistically significant reduction of height loss compared to placebo (p<0.0001).

Table 3: Results from 3 years fracture study MF 4411 (%, 95 % CI)

	Placebo (N=974)	ibandronic acid 2.5 mg daily (N=977)
Relative Risk Reduction New morphometric vertebral fractures		62 % (40.9, 75.1)
Incidence of new morphometric vertebral fractures	9.56 % (7.5, 11.7)	4.68 % (3.2,6.2)
Relative risk reduction of clinical vertebral fracture		49 % (14.03, 69.49)
Incidence of clinical vertebral fracture	5.33 % (3.73, 6.92)	2.75 % (1.61, 3.89)
BMD – mean change relative to baseline lumbar spine at year 3	1.26 % (0.8, 1.7)	6.54 % (6.1, 7.0)
BMD – mean change relative to baseline total hip at year 3	-0.69 % (-1.0, -0.4)	3.36 % (3.0, 3.7)

The treatment effect of ibandronic acid was further assessed in an analysis of the subpopulation of patients who at baseline had a lumbar spine BMD T-score below -2.5. The vertebral fracture risk reduction was very consistent with that seen in the overall population.

Table 4: Results from 3 years fracture study MF 4411 (%, 95 % CI) for patients with lumbar spine BMD T-score below -2.5 at baseline

	Placebo (N=587)	ibandronic acid 2.5 mg daily (N=575)
Relative Risk Reduction New morphometric vertebral fractures		59 % (34.5, 74.3)
Incidence of new morphometric vertebral fractures	12.54 % (9.53, 15.55)	5.36 % (3.31, 7.41)
Relative risk reduction of clinical vertebral fracture		50 % (9.49, 71.91)
Incidence of clinical vertebral fracture	6.97 % (4.67, 9.27)	3.57 % (1.89, 5.24)
BMD – mean change relative to baseline lumbar spine at year 3	1.13 % (0.6, 1.7)	7.01 % (6.5, 7.6)
BMD – mean change relative to baseline total hip at year 3	-0.70 % (-1.1, -0.2)	3.59 % (3.1, 4.1)

In the overall patient population of the study MF4411, no reduction was observed for non-vertebral fractures, however daily ibandronate appeared to be effective in a high-risk subpopulation (femoral neck BMD T-score < -3.0), where a non-vertebral fracture risk reduction of 69% was observed.

Daily treatment with 2.5 mg resulted in progressive increases in BMD at vertebral and nonvertebral sites of the skeleton.

Three-year lumbar spine BMD increase compared to placebo was 5.3 % and 6.5 % compared to baseline. Increases at the hip compared to baseline were 2.8 % at the femoral neck, 3.4 % at the total hip, and 5.5 % at the trochanter.

Biochemical markers of bone turnover (such as urinary CTX and serum Osteocalcin) showed the expected pattern of suppression to premenopausal levels and reached maximum suppression within a period of 3-6 months.

A clinically meaningful reduction of 50 % of biochemical markers of bone resorption was observed as early as one month after start of treatment with ibandronic acid 2.5 mg.

Following treatment discontinuation, there is a reversion to the pathological pre-treatment rates of elevated bone resorption associated with postmenopausal osteoporosis.

The histological analysis of bone biopsies after two and three years of treatment of postmenopausal women showed bone of normal quality and no indication of a mineralization defect.

5.2 Pharmacokinetic properties

The primary pharmacological effects of ibandronic acid on bone are not directly related to actual plasma concentrations, as demonstrated by various studies in animals and humans.

Absorption

The absorption of ibandronic acid in the upper gastrointestinal tract is rapid after oral administration and plasma concentrations increase in a dose-proportional manner up to 50 mg oral intake, with greater than dose-proportional increases seen above this dose. Maximum observed plasma concentrations were reached within 0.5 to 2 hours (median 1 hour) in the fasted state and absolute bioavailability was about 0.6 %. The extent of absorption is impaired when taken together with food or beverages (other than plain water). Bioavailability is reduced by about 90 % when ibandronic acid is administered with a standard breakfast in comparison with bioavailability seen in fasted subjects. There is no meaningful reduction in bioavailability provided ibandronic acid is taken 60 minutes before the first food of the day. Both bioavailability and BMD gains are reduced when food or beverage is taken less than 60 minutes after ibandronic acid is ingested.

Distribution

After initial systemic exposure, ibandronic acid rapidly binds to bone or is excreted into urine. In humans, the apparent terminal volume of distribution is at least 90 l and the amount of dose reaching the bone is estimated to be 40-50 % of the circulating dose. Protein binding in human plasma is approximately 85 % - 87 % (determined *in vitro* at therapeutic concentrations), and thus there is a low potential for interaction with other medicinal products due to displacement.

Metabolism

There is no evidence that ibandronic acid is metabolised in animals or humans.

Elimination

The absorbed fraction of ibandronic acid is removed from the circulation via bone absorption (estimated to be 40-50 % in postmenopausal women) and the remainder is eliminated unchanged by the kidney. The unabsorbed fraction of ibandronic acid is eliminated unchanged in the faeces.

The range of observed apparent half-lives is broad, the apparent terminal half-life is generally in the range of 10-72 hours. As the values calculated are largely a function of the duration of study, the dose used, and assay sensitivity, the true terminal half-life is likely to be substantially longer, in common with other bisphosphonates. Early plasma levels fall quickly reaching 10 % of peak values within 3 and 8 hours after intravenous or oral administration respectively.

Total clearance of ibandronic acid is low with average values in the range 84-160 ml/min. Renal clearance (about 60 mL/min in healthy postmenopausal females) accounts for 50-60 % of total clearance and is related to creatinine clearance. The difference between the apparent total and renal clearances is considered to reflect the uptake by bone.

Pharmacokinetics in special clinical situations

Gender

Bioavailability and pharmacokinetics of ibandronic acid are similar in men and women.

Race

There is no evidence for any clinically relevant inter-ethnic differences between Asians and Caucasians in ibandronic acid disposition. There are few data available on patients of African origin.

Patients with renal impairment

Renal clearance of ibandronic acid in patients with various degrees of renal impairment is linearly related to creatinine clearance.

No dose adjustment is necessary for patients with mild or moderate renal impairment (CLcr equal or greater than 30 ml/min), as shown in study BM 16549 where the majority of patients had mild to moderate renal impairment.

Subjects with severe renal failure (CLcr less than 30 ml/min) receiving daily oral administration of 10 mg ibandronic acid for 21 days, had 2-3 fold higher plasma concentrations than subjects with normal renal function and total clearance of ibandronic acid was 44 ml/min. After intravenous administration of 0.5 mg, total, renal, and non-renal clearances decreased by 67 %, 77 % and 50 %, respectively, in subjects with severe renal failure but there was no reduction in tolerability associated with the increase in exposure. Due to the limited clinical experience, Bonviva is not recommended in patients with severe renal impairment (see section 4.2 and section 4.4). The pharmacokinetics of ibandronic acid was not assessed in patients with end-stage renal disease managed by other than haemodialysis. The pharmacokinetics of ibandronic acid in these patients is unknown, and ibandronic acid should not be used under these circumstances.

Patients with hepatic impairment

There are no pharmacokinetic data for ibandronic acid in patients who have hepatic impairment. The liver has no significant role in the clearance of ibandronic acid which is not metabolised but is cleared by renal excretion and by uptake into bone. Therefore dose adjustment is not necessary in patients with hepatic impairment.

Elderly Population

In a multivariate analysis, age was not found to be an independent factor of any of the pharmacokinetic parameters studied. As renal function decreases with age this is the only factor to take into consideration (see renal impairment section).

Paediatric Population

There are no data on the use of Bonviva in these age groups.

5.3 Preclinical safety data

Toxic effects, e.g signs of renal damage, were observed in dogs only at exposures considered sufficiently in excess of the maximum human exposure indicating little relevance to clinical use.

Mutagenicity/Carcinogenicity:

No indication of carcinogenic potential was observed. Tests for genotoxicity revealed no evidence of genetic activity for ibandronic acid.

Reproductive toxicity:

There was no evidence for a direct foetal toxic or teratogenic effect of ibandronic acid in orally treated rats and rabbits and there were no adverse effects on the development in F_1 offspring in rats at an extrapolated exposure of at least 35 times above human exposure. Adverse effects of ibandronic acid in reproductive toxicity studies in the rat were those observed with bisphosphonates as a class. They include a decreased number of implantation sites, interference with natural delivery (dystocia), and an increase in visceral variations (renal pelvis ureter syndrome).

6. PHARMACEUTICAL PARTICULARS

6.1 List of excipients

Tablet core

Lactose monohydrate

Povidone

Cellulose, microcrystalline

Crospovidone

Stearic acid

Silica, colloidal anhydrous

Tablet coat

Hypromellose

Titanium dioxide E171

Talc

Macrogol 6,000

6.2 Incompatibilities

Not applicable.

6.3 Shelf life

3 years.

6.4 Special precautions for storage

This medicinal product does not require any special storage conditions.

6.5 Nature and contents of container

Bonviva 150 mg film-coated tablets are supplied in blisters (PVC/PVDC) containing 1 or 3 tablets.

Not all pack sizes may be marketed.

6.6 Special precautions for disposal and other handling

No special requirements.

7. MARKETING AUTHORISATION HOLDER

Roche Registration Limited

6 Falcon Way

Shire Park

Welwyn Garden City

AL7 1TW

United Kingdom

8. MARKETING AUTHORISATION NUMBER(S)

EU/1/03/265/003

EU/1/03/265/004

9. DATE OF FIRST AUTHORISATION/RENEWAL OF THE AUTHORISATION

23.02.2004/23.02.2009

10. DATE OF REVISION OF THE TEXT

2 July 2009

Detailed information on this medicinal product is available on the website of the European Medicines Agency (EMEA) http://www.emea.europa.eu/

Bonviva 3mg/3ml solution for injection in pre-filled syringe

(Roche Products Limited)

1. NAME OF THE MEDICINAL PRODUCT

Bonviva ▼ 3 mg solution for injection

2. QUALITATIVE AND QUANTITATIVE COMPOSITION

One pre-filled syringe of 3 ml solution contains 3 mg ibandronic acid (as 3.375 mg ibandronic acid, monosodium salt, monohydrate).

The concentration of ibandronic acid in the solution for injection is 1mg per ml.

For a full list of excipients, see section 6.1.

3. PHARMACEUTICAL FORM

Solution for injection.

Clear, colourless solution.

4. CLINICAL PARTICULARS

4.1 Therapeutic indications

Treatment of osteoporosis in postmenopausal women at increased risk of fracture (see section 5.1).

A reduction in the risk of vertebral fractures has been demonstrated, efficacy on femoral neck fractures has not been established.

4.2 Posology and method of administration

Posology:

The recommended dose of ibandronic acid is 3 mg, administered as an intravenous injection over 15 - 30 seconds, every three months.

Patients must receive supplemental calcium and vitamin D (see section 4.4 and section 4.5)

If a dose is missed, the injection should be administered as soon as convenient. Thereafter, injections should be scheduled every 3 months from the date of the last injection.

Special Populations

Patients with renal impairment

No dose adjustment is necessary for patients with mild or moderate renal impairment where serum creatinine is equal or below 200 μmol/l (2.3 mg/dl) or where creatinine clearance (measured or estimated) is equal or greater than 30 ml/min.

Bonviva injection is not recommended for use in patients who have a serum creatinine above 200 μmol/l (2.3 mg/dl) or who have a creatinine clearance (measured or estimated) below 30 ml/min, because of limited clinical data available from studies including such patients (see section 4.4 and section 5.2)

Patients with hepatic impairment

No dose adjustment is required (see section 5.2).

Elderly Population

No dose adjustment is required (see section 5.2).

Paediatric Population

There is no relevant use of Bonviva in children, and Bonviva was not studied in the paediatric population.

Method of Administration:

For intravenous use.

Strict adherence to the intravenous administration route is required (see section 4.4).

4.3 Contraindications

- Hypocalcaemia (see section 4.4)

- Hypersensitivity to ibandronic acid or to any of the excipients.

4.4 Special warnings and precautions for use

Administration failures

Strict adherence to the intravenous route of administration is required. Care must be taken not to administer Bonviva injection via intra-arterial or paravenous administration as this could lead to tissue damage.

Hypocalcaemia

Bonviva, like other bisphosphonates administered intravenously, may cause a transient decrease in serum calcium values.

Existing hypocalcaemia must be corrected before starting Bonviva injection therapy. Other disturbances of bone and mineral metabolism should also be effectively treated before starting Bonviva injection therapy.

All patients must receive adequate supplemental calcium and vitamin D.

Renal impairment

Patients with concomitant diseases, or who use medicinal products which have potential for undesirable effects on the kidney, should be reviewed regularly in line with good medical practice during treatment.

Due to limited clinical experience, Bonviva injection is not recommended for patients with a serum creatinine above 200 μmol/l (2.3 mg/dl) or with a creatinine clearance below 30 ml/min (see section 4.2 and section 5.2).

Osteonecrosis of the jaw

Osteonecrosis of the jaw, generally associated with tooth extraction and/or local infection (including osteomyelitis) has been reported in patients with cancer receiving treatment regimens including primarily intravenously administered bisphosphonates. Many of these patients were also receiving chemotherapy and corticosteroids. Osteonecrosis of the jaw has also been reported in patients with osteoporosis receiving oral bisphosphonates.

A dental examination with appropriate preventive dentistry should be considered prior to treatment with bisphosphonates in patients with concomitant risk factors (e.g. cancer, chemotherapy, radiotherapy, corticosteroids, poor oral hygiene).

While on treatment, these patients should avoid invasive dental procedures if possible. For patients who develop osteonecrosis of the jaw while on bisphosphonate therapy, dental surgery may exacerbate the condition. For patients requiring dental procedures, there are no data available to suggest whether discontinuation of bisphosphonate treatment reduces the risk of osteonecrosis of the jaw. Clinical judgement of the treating physician should guide the management plan of each patient based on individual benefit/risk assessment.

4.5 Interaction with other medicinal products and other forms of interaction

Metabolic interactions are not considered likely, since ibandronic acid does not inhibit the major human hepatic P450 isoenzymes and has been shown not to induce the hepatic cytochrome P450 system in rats. Furthermore, plasma protein binding is approximately 85 % - 87 % (determined *in vitro* at therapeutic ibandronic acid concentrations), and thus there is a low potential for interaction with other medicinal products due to displacement. Ibandronic acid is eliminated by renal excretion only and does not undergo any biotransformation. The secretory pathway appears not to include known acidic or basic transport systems involved in the excretion of other active substances.

Pharmacokinetic interaction studies in postmenopausal women have demonstrated the absence of any interaction potential with tamoxifen or hormone replacement therapy (oestrogen).

No interaction was observed when co-administered with melphalan/prednisolone in patients with multiple myeloma.

4.6 Pregnancy and lactation

Pregnancy

There are no adequate data from the use of ibandronic acid in pregnant women. Studies in rats have shown some reproductive toxicity (see section 5.3). The potential risk for humans is unknown. Bonviva should not be used during pregnancy.

Lactation

It is not known whether ibandronic acid is excreted in human milk. Studies in lactating rats have demonstrated the presence of low levels of ibandronic acid in the milk following intravenous administration. Bonviva should not be used during lactation.

4.7 Effects on ability to drive and use machines

No studies on the effects on the ability to drive and use machines have been performed.

4.8 Undesirable effects

The safety of oral treatment with ibandronic acid 2.5 mg daily was evaluated in 1251 patients treated in 4 placebo-controlled clinical studies, with the large majority of patients coming from the pivotal three-year fracture study (MF 4411). The overall safety profile of ibandronic acid 2.5 mg daily in all these studies was similar to that of placebo.

In the pivotal two-year study in postmenopausal women with osteoporosis (BM16550), the overall safety of intravenous injection of Bonviva 3 mg every 3 months and oral ibandronic acid 2.5 mg daily were shown to be similar. The overall proportion of patients who experienced an adverse reaction was 26.0 % and 28.6 % for Bonviva 3 mg injection every 3 months after one year and two years, respectively. The majority of adverse reactions were mild to moderate in intensity. Most cases of adverse reactions did not lead to cessation of therapy.

The most commonly reported adverse reaction was influenza like illness.

Adverse reactions considered by investigators to be causally related to Bonviva are listed below by System Organ Class.

Frequencies are defined as common (≥ 1/100 to < 1/10), uncommon (≥ 1/1,000 to < 1/100), and rare (≥ 1/10,000 to < 1/1,000). Within each frequency grouping, adverse reactions are presented in order of decreasing seriousness.

Table 1: Adverse reactions occurring in postmenopausal women receiving Bonviva 3mg injection every 3 months or ibandronic acid 2.5mg daily in the phase III studies BM16550 and MF 4411.

System Organ Class	Frequency	Adverse reactions
Immune system disorders	Rare	Hypersensitivity reaction
Nervous system disorders	Common	Headache
Vascular disorders	Uncommon	Phlebitis/ thrombophlebitis
Gastrointestinal disorders	Common	Gastritis, Dyspepsia, Diarrhoea, Abdominal pain, Nausea, Constipation
Skin and subcutaneous tissues disorders	Common	Rash
	Rare	Angioedema, Facial swelling/oedema, Urticaria
Musculoskeletal, connective tissue and bone disorders	Common	Arthralgia, Myalgia, Musculoskeletal pain, Back pain
	Uncommon	Bone pain
General disorders and administration site conditions	Common	Influenza like illness*, Fatigue
	Uncommon	Injection site reactions, Asthenia

MedDRA version 8.0

* Transient, influenza-like symptoms have been reported in patients receiving intravenous injection of Bonviva 3 mg every 3 months, typically in association with the first dose. Influenza-like illness includes events reported as acute phase reaction or symptoms, including myalgia, arthralgia, fever, chills, fatigue, nausea, loss of appetite, and bone pain. Such symptoms were generally of short duration, mild or moderate in intensity, and resolved during continuing treatment without requiring remedial measures.

Laboratory test findings

In the pivotal three-year study with oral ibandronic acid 2.5 mg daily (MF 4411) there was no difference compared with placebo for laboratory abnormalities indicative of hepatic or renal dysfunction, impaired haematologic system, hypocalcaemia or hypophosphataemia. Similarly, no differences were noted between the groups in the pivotal study with Bonviva 3 mg injection every 3 months (BM 16550).

Post-marketing Experience

Osteonecrosis of the jaw has been reported in patients treated by bisphosphonates. The majority of the reports refer to cancer patients, but such cases have also been reported in patients treated for osteoporosis. Osteonecrosis of the jaw is generally associated with tooth extraction and / or local infection (including osteomyelitis). Diagnosis of cancer, chemotherapy, radiotherapy, corticosteroids and poor oral hygiene are also deemed as risk factors (see section 4.4).

4.9 Overdose

No specific information is available on the treatment of overdosage with Bonviva.

Based on knowledge of this class of compounds, intravenous overdosage may result in hypocalcaemia, hypophosphataemia, and hypomagnesaemia. Clinically relevant reductions in serum levels of calcium, phosphorus, and magnesium should be corrected by intravenous administration of calcium gluconate, potassium or sodium phosphate, and magnesium sulfate, respectively.

5. PHARMACOLOGICAL PROPERTIES

5.1 Pharmacodynamic properties

Pharmacotherapeutic group: Bisphosphonates, ATC code: M05B A06

Mechanism of action

Ibandronic acid is a highly potent bisphosphonate belonging to the nitrogen-containing group of bisphosphonates, which act selectively on bone tissue and specifically inhibit osteoclast activity without directly affecting bone formation. It does not interfere with osteoclast recruitment. Ibandronic acid leads to progressive net gains in bone mass and a decreased incidence of fractures through the reduction of elevated bone turnover towards premenopausal levels in postmenopausal women.

Pharmacodynamic effects

The pharmacodynamic action of ibandronic acid is inhibition of bone resorption. *In vivo*, ibandronic acid prevents bone destruction experimentally induced by cessation of gonadal function, retinoids, tumours or tumour extracts. In young (fast growing) rats, the endogenous bone resorption is also inhibited, leading to increased normal bone mass compared with untreated animals.

Animal models confirm that ibandronic acid is a highly potent inhibitor of osteoclastic activity. In growing rats, there was no evidence of impaired mineralisation even at doses greater than 5,000 times the dose required for osteoporosis treatment.

Both daily and intermittent (with prolonged dose-free intervals) long-term administration in rats, dogs and monkeys was associated with formation of new bone of normal quality and maintained or increased mechanical strength even at doses in the toxic range. In humans, the efficacy of both daily and intermittent administration with a dose-free interval of 9 - 10 weeks of ibandronic acid was confirmed in a clinical trial (MF 4411), in which ibandronic acid demonstrated anti-fracture efficacy.

In animal models ibandronic acid produced biochemical changes indicative of dose-dependent inhibition of bone resorption, including suppression of urinary biochemical markers of bone collagen degradation (such as deoxypyridinoline, and cross-linked N-telopeptides of type I collagen (NTX)).

Both daily, intermittent (with a dose-free interval of 9 - 10 weeks per quarter) oral doses as well as intravenous doses of ibandronic acid in postmenopausal women produced biochemical changes indicative of dose-dependent inhibition of bone resorption.

Bonviva intravenous injection decreased levels of serum C telopeptide of the alpha chain of Type I collagen (CTX) within 3 - 7 days of starting treatment and decreased levels of osteocalcin within 3 months.

Following treatment discontinuation, there is a reversion to the pathological pre-treatment rates of elevated bone resorption associated with postmenopausal osteoporosis.

The histological analysis of bone biopsies after two and three years of treatment of postmenopausal women with doses of oral ibandronic acid 2.5 mg daily and intermittent intravenous doses of up to 1 mg every 3 months showed bone of normal quality and no indication of a mineralisation defect. An expected decrease in bone turnover, normal quality of bone and absence of defects in mineralization were also seen after two years of treatment with Bonviva 3 mg injection.

Clinical efficacy

Independent risk factors, for example, low BMD, age, the existence of previous fractures, a family history of fractures, high bone turnover and low body mass index should be considered in order to identify women at increased risk of osteoporotic fractures.

Bonviva 3 mg injection every 3 months

Bone mineral density (BMD)

Bonviva 3 mg intravenous injection, administered every 3 months, was shown to be at least as effective as oral ibandronic acid 2.5 mg daily in a 2-year, randomised, double-blind, multicentre, non-inferiority study (BM16550) of postmenopausal women (1386 women aged 55 - 80) with osteoporosis (lumbar spine BMD T-score below -2.5 SD at baseline). This was demonstrated in both the primary analysis at one year and in the confirmatory analysis at two years endpoint (Table 2).

The primary analysis of data from study BM16550 at one year and the confirmatory analysis at 2 years demonstrated the non-inferiority of 3 mg every 3 months injection dosing regimen compared to 2.5 mg oral daily dosing regimen, in terms of mean increases in BMD at lumbar spine, total hip, femoral neck and trochanter (Table 2).

Table 2: Mean relative change from baseline of lumbar spine, total hip, femoral neck and trochanter BMD after one year (primary analysis) and two years of treatment (Per-Protocol Population) in study BM 16550.

(see Table 2 below)

Furthermore, Bonviva 3 mg injection every 3 months was proven superior to oral ibandronic acid 2.5 mg daily for increases in lumbar spine BMD in a prospectively planned analysis at one year, $p<0.001$, and at two years, $p<0.001$.

For lumbar spine BMD, 92.1 % of patients receiving 3 mg injection every 3 months increased or maintained their BMD after 1 year of treatment (i.e. were responders) compared with 84.9 % of patients receiving oral 2.5 mg daily ($p=0.002$). After 2 years of treatment, 92.8 % of patients receiving 3 mg injections and 84.7 % of patient receiving 2.5 mg oral therapy had increased or maintained lumbar spine BMD ($p=0.001$).

For total hip BMD, 82.3 % of patients receiving 3 mg injection every 3 months were responders at one year, compared with 75.1 % of patients receiving 2.5 mg daily orally ($p=0.02$). After 2 years of treatment, 85.6 % of patients receiving 3 mg injections and 77.0 % of patient receiving 2.5 mg oral therapy had increased or maintained total hip BMD ($p=0.004$).

The proportion of patients who increased or maintained their BMD at one year at both lumbar spine and total hip was 76.2 % in the 3 mg injection every 3 months arm and 67.2 % in the 2.5 mg daily orally arm ($p=0.007$). At two years, 80.1 % and 68.8 % of patients met this criterion in the 3 mg every 3 months injection arm and the 2.5 mg daily arm ($p=0.001$).

Biochemical markers of bone turn-over

Clinically meaningful reductions in serum CTX levels were observed at all time points measured. At 12 months median relative changes from baseline were −58.6 % for the intravenous injection of 3 mg every 3 months regimen and −62.6 % for oral 2.5 mg daily regimen. In addition, 64.8 % of patients receiving 3 mg every 3 months injection were identified as responders (defined as a decrease ≥50 % from baseline), compared with 64.9 % of patients receiving

Table 2 Mean relative change from baseline of lumbar spine, total hip, femoral neck and trochanter BMD after one year (primary analysis) and two years of treatment (Per-Protocol Population) in study BM 16550.

	One year data in study BM 16550		Two year data in study BM 16550	
Mean relative changes from baseline % [95% CI]	ibandronic acid 2.5 mg daily (N=377)	Bonviva 3 mg injection every 3 months (N=365)	ibandronic acid 2.5 mg daily (N=334)	Bonviva 3 mg injection every 3 months (N=334)
Lumbar spine L2-L4 BMD	3.8 [3.4, 4.2]	4.8 [4.5, 5.2]	4.8 [4.3, 5.4]	6.3 [5.7, 6.8]
Total hip BMD	1.8 [1.5, 2.1]	2.4 [2.0, 2.7]	2.2 [1.8, 2.6]	3.1 [2.6, 3.6]
Femoral neck BMD	1.6 [1.2, 2.0]	2.3 [1.9, 2.7]	2.2 [1.8, 2.7]	2.8 [2.3, 3.3]
Trochanter BMD	3.0 [2.6, 3.4]	3.8 [3.2, 4.4]	3.5 [3.0, 4.0]	4.9 [4.1, 5.7]

2.5 mg daily orally. Serum CTX reduction was maintained over the 2 years, with more than half of the patients identified as responders in both treatment groups.

Based on the results of study BM 16550, Bonviva 3 mg intravenous injection, administered every 3 months is expected to be at least as effective in preventing fractures as the oral regimen of ibandronic acid 2.5 mg daily.

Ibandronic acid 2.5 mg daily tablets

In the initial three-year, randomised, double-blind, placebo-controlled, fracture study (MF 4411), a statistically significant and medically relevant decrease in the incidence of new radiographic morphometric and clinical vertebral fractures was demonstrated (table 3). In this study, ibandronic acid was evaluated at oral doses of 2.5 mg daily and 20 mg intermittently as an exploratory regimen. Ibandronic acid was taken 60 minutes before the first food or drink of the day (post-dose fasting period). The study enrolled women aged 55 to 80 years, who were at least 5 years postmenopausal, who had a BMD at the lumbar spine of -2 to -5 SD below the premenopausal mean (T-score) in at least one vertebra [L1-L4], and who had one to four prevalent vertebral fractures. All patients received 500 mg calcium and 400 IU vitamin D daily. Efficacy was evaluated in 2,928 patients. Ibandronic acid 2.5 mg administered daily, showed a statistically significant and medically relevant reduction in the incidence of new vertebral fractures. This regimen reduced the occurrence of new radiographic vertebral fractures by 62 % (p=0.0001) over the three year duration of the study. A relative risk reduction of 61 % was observed after 2 years (p=0.0006). No statistically significant difference was attained after 1 year of treatment (p=0.056). The anti-fracture effect was consistent over the duration of the study. There was no indication of a waning of the effect over time.

The incidence of clinical vertebral fractures was also significantly reduced by 49 % after 3 years (p=0.011). The strong effect on vertebral fractures was furthermore reflected by a statistically significant reduction of height loss compared to placebo (p<0.0001).

Table 3: Results from 3 years fracture study MF 4411 (%, 95 % CI)

	Placebo (N=974)	ibandronic acid 2.5 mg daily (N=977)
Relative risk reduction New morphometric vertebral fractures		62% (40.9, 75.1)
Incidence of new morphometric vertebral fractures	9.56% (7.5, 11.7)	4.68% (3.2, 6.2)
Relative risk reduction of clinical vertebral fracture		49% (14.03, 69.49)
Incidence of clinical vertebral fracture	5.33% (3.73, 6.92)	2.75% (1.61, 3.89)
BMD – mean change relative to baseline lumbar spine at year 3	1.26% (0.8, 1.7)	6.54% (6.1, 7.0)
BMD – mean change relative to baseline total hip at year 3	-0.69% (-1.0, -0.4)	3.36% (3.0, 3.7)

The treatment effect of ibandronic acid was further assessed in an analysis of the subpopulation of patients who, at baseline, had a lumbar spine BMD T-score below –2.5 (table 4). The vertebral fracture risk reduction was very consistent with that seen in the overall population.

Table 4: Results from 3 years fracture study MF 4411 (%, 95 % CI) for patients with lumbar spine BMD T-score below –2.5 at baseline

	Placebo (N=587)	ibandronic acid 2.5 mg daily (N=575)
Relative Risk Reduction New morphometric vertebral fractures		59% (34.5, 74.3)
Incidence of new morphometric vertebral fractures	12.54% (9.53, 15.55)	5.36% (3.31, 7.41)
Relative risk reduction of clinical vertebral fracture		50% (9.49, 71.91)
Incidence of clinical vertebral fracture	6.97% (4.67, 9.27)	3.57% (1.89, 5.24)
BMD – mean change relative to baseline lumbar spine at year 3	1.13% (0.6, 1.7)	7.01% (6.5, 7.6)
BMD – mean change relative to baseline total hip at year 3	-0.70% (-1.1, -0.2)	3.59% (3.1, 4.1)

In the overall patient population of the study MF4411, no reduction was observed for non-vertebral fractures, however daily ibandronate appeared to be effective in a high-risk subpopulation (femoral neck BMD T-score < -3.0), where a non-vertebral fracture risk reduction of 69% was observed.

Daily oral treatment with ibandronic acid 2.5 mg tablets resulted in progressive increases in BMD at vertebral and nonvertebral sites of the skeleton.

Three-year lumbar spine BMD increase compared to placebo was 5.3 % and 6.5 % compared to baseline. Increases at the hip compared to baseline were 2.8 % at the femoral neck, 3.4 % at the total hip, and 5.5 % at the trochanter.

Biochemical markers of bone turnover (such as urinary CTX and serum Osteocalcin) showed the expected pattern of suppression to premenopausal levels and reached maximum suppression within a period of 3 - 6 months of using 2.5 mg ibandronic acid daily.

A clinically meaningful reduction of 50 % of biochemical markers of bone resorption was observed as early as one month after starting treatment with ibandronic acid 2.5 mg.

5.2 Pharmacokinetic properties

The primary pharmacological effects of ibandronic acid on bone are not directly related to actual plasma concentrations, as demonstrated by various studies in animals and humans.

Plasma concentrations of ibandronic acid increase in a dose-proportional manner after intravenous administration of 0.5 mg to 6 mg.

Absorption

Not applicable

Distribution

After initial systemic exposure, ibandronic acid rapidly binds to bone or is excreted into urine. In humans, the apparent terminal volume of distribution is at least 90 l and the amount of dose reaching the bone is estimated to be 40 – 50 % of the circulating dose. Protein binding in human plasma is approximately 85 % - 87 % (determined *in vitro* at therapeutic ibandronic acid concentrations), and thus there is a low potential for interaction with other medicinal products due to displacement.

Metabolism

There is no evidence that ibandronic acid is metabolised in animals or humans.

Elimination

Ibandronic acid is removed from the circulation via bone absorption (estimated to be 40 – 50 % in postmenopausal women) and the remainder is eliminated unchanged by the kidney.

The range of observed apparent half-lives is broad, the apparent terminal half-life is generally in the range of 10 - 72 hours. As the values calculated are largely a function of the duration of study, the dose used, and assay sensitivity, the true terminal half-life is likely to be substantially longer, in common with other bisphosphonates. Early plasma levels fall quickly, reaching 10 % of the peak values within 3 and 8 hours after intravenous or oral administration, respectively.

Total clearance of ibandronic acid is low with average values in the range 84 - 160 ml/min. Renal clearance (about 60 ml/min in healthy postmenopausal females) accounts for 50 – 60 % of total clearance, and is related to creatinine clearance. The difference between the apparent total and renal clearances is considered to reflect the uptake by bone.

Pharmacokinetics in special clinical situations

Gender

Pharmacokinetics of ibandronic acid are similar in men and women.

Race

There is no evidence for any clinically relevant inter-ethnic differences between Asians and Caucasians in ibandronic acid disposition. There is limited data available on patients of African origin.

Patients with renal impairment

Renal clearance of ibandronic acid in patients with various degrees of renal impairment is linearly related to creatinine clearance (CLcr).

No dose adjustment is necessary for patients with mild or moderate renal impairment (CLcr equal or above 30 ml/min).

Subjects with severe renal impairment (CLcr less than 30 ml/min) receiving daily oral administration of 10 mg ibandronic acid for 21 days, had 2 - 3 fold higher plasma concentrations than subjects with normal renal function and total clearance of ibandronic acid was 44 ml/min. After intravenous administration of 0.5 mg of ibandronic acid, total, renal, and non-renal clearances decreased by 67 %, 77 % and 50 %, respectively, in subjects with severe renal failure, but there was no reduction in tolerability associated with the increase in exposure. Due to the limited clinical experience, Bonviva is not recommended in patients with severe renal impairment (see section 4.2 and section 4.4). The pharmacokinetics of ibandronic acid in patients with end-stage renal disease was only assessed in a small number of patients managed by haemodialysis, therefore, the pharmacokinetics of ibandronic acid in the patients not undergoing haemodialysis is unknown. Due to the limited data available, ibandronic acid should not be used in all patients with end-stage renal disease.

Patients with hepatic impairment

There are no pharmacokinetic data for ibandronic acid in patients who have hepatic impairment. The liver has no significant role in the clearance of ibandronic acid, which is not metabolised but is cleared by renal excretion and by uptake into bone. Therefore dose adjustment is not necessary in patients with hepatic impairment.

Elderly Population

In a multivariate analysis, age was not found to be an independent factor of any of the pharmacokinetic parameters studied. As renal function decreases with age, renal function is the only factor to take into consideration (see renal impairment section).

Paediatric Population

There are no data on the use of Bonviva in these age groups.

5.3 Preclinical safety data

Toxic effects, e.g. signs of renal damage, were observed in dogs only at exposures considered sufficiently in excess of the maximum human exposure, indicating little relevance to clinical use.

Mutagenicity/Carcinogenicity:

No indication of carcinogenic potential was observed. Tests for genotoxicity revealed no evidence of genetic activity for ibandronic acid.

Reproductive toxicity:

Specific studies for the 3-monthly dosing regimen have not been performed. In studies with daily i.v. dosing regimen, there was no evidence for a direct foetal toxic or teratogenic effect of ibandronic acid in rats and rabbits. Body weight gain was decreased in F_1 offspring in rats. Other adverse reactions to ibandronic acid in reproductive toxicity studies in the rat were those observed with bisphosphonates as a class. They include a decreased number of implantation sites, interference with natural delivery (dystocia), and an increase in visceral variations (renal pelvis ureter syndrome).

6. PHARMACEUTICAL PARTICULARS

6.1 List of excipients

Sodium chloride

Glacial acetic acid

Sodium acetate trihydrate

Water for injections

6.2 Incompatibilities

Bonviva solution for injection must not be mixed with calcium-containing solutions or other intravenously administered medicinal products.

6.3 Shelf life

2 years.

6.4 Special precautions for storage

This medicinal product does not require any special storage conditions.

6.5 Nature and contents of container

Pre-filled syringes (5 ml) made of colourless type I glass, the grey rubber plunger stopper and tip cap are made of fluororesin-laminated butyl rubber, containing 3 ml of solution for injection.

Packs of 1 pre-filled syringe and 1 injection needle or 4 pre-filled syringes and 4 injection needles.

Not all pack sizes may be marketed.

6.6 Special precautions for disposal and other handling

Where the product is administered into an existing intravenous infusion line, the infusate should be restricted to either isotonic saline or 50 mg/ml (5 %) glucose solution. This also applies to solutions used to flush butterfly and other devices.

Any unused solution for injection, syringe and injection needle should be disposed of in accordance with local requirements.

7. MARKETING AUTHORISATION HOLDER

Roche Registration Limited

6 Falcon Way

Shire Park

Welwyn Garden City

AL7 1TW

United Kingdom

8. MARKETING AUTHORISATION NUMBER(S)

EU/1/03/265/005

EU/1/03/265/006

9. DATE OF FIRST AUTHORISATION/RENEWAL OF THE AUTHORISATION

23.02.2004/23.02.2009

10. DATE OF REVISION OF THE TEXT

2 July 2009

Detailed information on this medicinal product is available on the website of the European Medicines Agency (EMEA) http://www.emea.europa.eu/

BOTOX® 100 Units

(Allergan Ltd)

1. NAME OF THE MEDICINAL PRODUCT

BOTOX

100 Allergan units

Powder for solution for injection

2. QUALITATIVE AND QUANTITATIVE COMPOSITION

Botulinum toxin* type A, 100 Allergan Units/vial.

* from *Clostridium botulinum*

Botulinum toxin units are not interchangeable from one product to another.

For a full list of excipients, see section 6.1.

3. PHARMACEUTICAL FORM

Powder for solution for injection.

4. CLINICAL PARTICULARS

4.1 Therapeutic indications

BOTOX is indicated for the symptomatic relief of blepharospasm, hemifacial spasm and idiopathic cervical dystonia (spasmodic torticollis). It is indicated for the management of severe hyperhidrosis of the axillae, which does not respond to topical treatment with antiperspirants or antihidrotics.

BOTOX is also indicated for focal spasticity, including the treatment of

- dynamic equinus foot deformity due to spasticity in ambulant paediatric cerebral palsy patients, two years of age or older and

- wrist and hand disability due to upper limb spasticity associated with stroke in adults

The injections should be administered by appropriately trained personnel in hospital specialist centres.

The safety and effectiveness of BOTOX in the treatment of blepharospasm, hemifacial spasm, or idiopathic cervical dystonia, or focal hyperhidrosis in children have not been demonstrated.

4.2 Posology and method of administration

Doses recommended for BOTOX are not interchangeable with other preparations of botulinum toxin.

Adequate studies on geriatric dosing have not been performed. Dose selection should be the same; however, the lowest effective dose is recommended.

Blepharospasm

After reconstitution, BOTOX is injected using a sterile, 27-30 gauge needle. Electromyographic guidance is not necessary. The initial recommended dose is 1.25-2.5 Units (0.05-0.1 ml volume at each site) injected into the medial and lateral orbicularis oculi of the upper lid and the lateral orbicularis oculi of the lower lid. Additional sites in the brow area, the lateral orbicularis and in the upper facial area may also be injected if spasms here interfere with vision. In general, the initial effect of the injections is seen within three days and reaches a peak at one to two weeks post-treatment. Each treatment lasts approximately three months, following which the procedure can be repeated indefinitely. At repeat treatment sessions, the dose may be increased up to two-fold if the response from the initial treatment is considered insufficient - usually defined as an effect that does not last longer than two months. However, there appears to be little benefit obtainable from injecting more than 5 Units per site. The initial dose should not exceed 25 Units per eye. Normally no additional benefit is conferred by treating more frequently than every three months. It is rare for the effect to be permanent.

In the management of blepharospasm total dosing should not exceed 100 Units every 12 weeks.

Hemifacial spasm

Patients with hemifacial spasm or VIIth nerve disorders should be treated as for unilateral blepharospasm, with other affected facial muscles being injected as needed. Electromyographic control may be necessary to identify affected small circumoral muscles.

Cervical dystonia

Several dosing regimens have been used in clinical trials for treatment of cervical dystonia with BOTOX. Dosing must be tailored to the individual patient based on the patient's head and neck position, location of pain, muscle hypertrophy, patient's body weight, and patient response.

In practice, the maximum total dose is not usually more than 200 Units. No more than 50 Units should be given at any one injection site. The dilutions suggested are indicated in the following table:

Diluent added	Resulting dose in units per 0.1 ml
0.5 ml	20 Units
1 ml	10 Units
2 ml	5 Units
4 ml	2.5 Units
8 ml	1.25 Units

The following doses are recommended:

Type I Head **rotated** toward side of shoulder elevation	Sternomastoid Levator scapulae Scalene Splenius capitis Trapezius	50 - 100 Units; at least 2 sites 50 Units; 1 - 2 sites 25 - 50 Units; 1 - 2 sites 25 - 75 Units; 1 - 3 sites 25 - 100 Units; 1 - 8 sites
Type II Head rotation only	Sternomastoid	25 - 100 Units; at least 2 sites if >25 Units given
Type III Head **tilted** toward side of shoulder elevation	Sternomastoid Levator scapulae Scalene Trapezius	25 - 100 Units at posterior border; at least 2 sites if >25 Units given 25 - 100 Units; at least 2 sites 25 - 75 Units; at least 2 sites 25 - 100 Units; 1 - 8 sites
Type IV Bilateral posterior cervical muscle spasm with elevation of the face	Splenius capitis and cervicis	50 - 200 Units; 2 - 8 sites, treat bilaterally (This is the total dose and not the dose for each side of the neck)

The treatment of cervical dystonia typically may include injection of BOTOX into the sternocleidomastoid, levator scapulae, scalene, splenius capitis, and/or the trapezius muscle(s). The muscle mass and the degree of hypertrophy are factors to be taken into consideration when selecting the appropriate dose.

The sternocleidomastoid muscle should not be injected bilaterally as there is an increased risk of adverse effects (in particular dysphagia) when bilateral injections or doses in excess of 100 Units are administered to this muscle.

A 25, 27 or 30 gauge needle may be used for superficial muscles, and a 22 gauge needle may be used for deeper musculature. For cervical dystonia, localisation of the involved muscles with electromyographic guidance may be useful.

Multiple injection sites allow BOTOX to have more uniform contact with the innervation areas of the dystonic muscle and are especially useful in larger muscles. The optimal number of injection sites is dependent upon the size of the muscle to be chemically denervated.

Hyperhidrosis of the axillae

The recommended injection volume for intradermal injection in axillary hyperhidrosis is 0.1-0.2 ml. Reconstituted BOTOX (100 Units/4 mL) is injected using a 30 gauge needle. 50 Units of BOTOX is injected intradermally to each axilla, evenly distributed in multiple sites approximately 1-2 cm apart. The hyperhidrotic area to be injected may be defined by using standard staining techniques, e.g. Minor's iodine-starch test.

Clinical improvement generally occurs within the first week after injection. Repeat injections of axillary hyperhidrosis should be administered when effects from previous injections subside. Treatment response has been reported to persist for 4-7 months.

Paediatric cerebral palsy

Diluted BOTOX is injected using a sterile 23-26 gauge needle. It is administered into each of two sites in the medial and lateral heads of the affected gastrocnemius muscle. The recommended total dose is 4 Units/kg body weight. When both lower limbs are to be injected on the same occasion this dose should be divided between the two limbs.

Clinical improvement generally occurs within the first two weeks after injection. Repeat doses should be administered when the clinical effect of a previous injection diminishes but not more frequently than every two months.

Focal spasticity associated with stroke

Reconstituted BOTOX is injected using a sterile 25, 27 or 30 gauge needle for superficial muscles, and a longer needle for deeper musculature. Localisation of the involved muscles with electromyographic guidance or nerve stimulation techniques may be useful. Multiple injection sites may allow BOTOX to have more uniform contact with the innervation areas of the muscle and are especially useful in larger muscles.

The exact dosage and number of injection sites may be tailored to the individual based on the size, number and location of muscles involved, the severity of spasticity, and the presence of local muscle weakness.

In the controlled Phase 3 clinical trial the following doses were administered:

Muscle	Total Dose
Flexor digitorum profundus	50 Units
Flexor digitorum sublimis	50 Units
Flexor carpi radialis	50 Units
Flexor carpi ulnaris	50 Units
Adductor Pollicis	20 Units
Flexor Pollicis Longus	20 Units

In all clinical trials, the doses did not exceed 360 Units divided among selected muscles at any treatment session.

Clinical improvement in muscle tone generally occurs within two weeks following treatment and the peak effect is generally seen within four to six weeks following treatment. Data on the repeated and long-term treatment are limited.

4.3 Contraindications

BOTOX is contraindicated:

- in individuals with a known hypersensitivity to botulinum toxin type A or to any of the excipients;

- in the presence of infection at the proposed injection site(s).

4.4 Special warnings and precautions for use

The relevant anatomy, and any alterations to the anatomy due to prior surgical procedures, must be understood prior to administering BOTOX. The recommended dosages and frequencies of administration of BOTOX should not be exceeded.

Serious and/or immediate hypersensitivity reactions have been rarely reported including anaphylaxis, serum sickness, urticaria, soft tissue oedema, and dyspnoea. Some of these reactions have been reported following the use of BOTOX either alone or in conjunction with other products associated with similar reactions. If such a reaction occurs further injection of BOTOX should be discontinued and appropriate medical therapy, such as epinephrine, immediately instituted. Please see section 4.8c) for further information.

Side effects related to spread of toxin distant from the site of administration have been reported (See section 4.8), sometimes resulting in death, which in some cases was associated with dysphagia, pneumonia and/or significant debility.

Patients treated with therapeutic doses may experience exaggerated muscle weakness. Patients with underlying neurological disorders including swallowing difficulties are at increased risk of these side effects. The botulinum toxin product should be used under specialist supervision in these patients and should only be used if the benefit of treatment is considered to outweigh the risk. Patients with a history of dysphagia and aspiration should be treated with extreme caution.

Patients or caregivers should be advised to seek immediate medical care if swallowing, speech or respiratory disorders arise.

Dysphagia has also been reported following injection to sites other than the cervical musculature (see section 4.4 'Cervical Dystonia' for further information).

Clinical fluctuations during the repeated use of BOTOX (as with all botulinum toxins) may be a result of different vial reconstitution procedures, injection intervals, muscles injected and slightly differing potency values given by the biological test method used.

Formation of neutralizing antibodies to botulinum toxin type A may reduce the effectiveness of BOTOX treatment by inactivating the biological activity of the toxin. Results from some studies suggest that BOTOX injections at more frequent intervals or at higher doses may lead to greater incidence of antibody formation.

As with any treatment with the potential to allow previously-sedentary patients to resume activities, the sedentary patient should be cautioned to resume activity gradually.

Caution should be used when BOTOX is used in the presence of inflammation at the proposed injection site(s) or when excessive weakness or atrophy is present in the target muscle. Caution should also be exercised when BOTOX is used for treatment of patients with peripheral motor neuropathic diseases (e.g., amyotrophic lateral sclerosis or motor neuropathy).

BOTOX should only be used with extreme caution and under close supervision in patients with subclinical or clinical evidence of defective neuromuscular transmission e.g. myasthenia gravis or Eaton Lambert Syndrome; such patients may have an increased sensitivity to agents such as BOTOX, which may result in excessive muscle weakness. Patients with neuromuscular disorders may be at an increased risk of clinically significant systemic effects including severe dysphagia and respiratory compromise from typical doses of BOTOX.

BOTOX contains human serum albumin. When medicinal products derived from human blood or plasma are administered, the possibility of transmitting infectious agents cannot be totally excluded. To reduce the risk of transmission of infective agents, stringent controls are applied to the selection of blood donors and donations. In addition, virus inactivation procedures are included in the production process.

As with any injection, procedure-related injury could occur. An injection could result in localized infection, pain, inflammation, paraesthesia, hypoaesthesia, tenderness, swelling, erythema, and/or bleeding/bruising. Needle-related pain and/or anxiety may result in vasovagal responses e.g. syncope, hypotension, etc. Care should be taken when injecting near vulnerable anatomic structures.

Blepharospasm

Reduced blinking following botulinum toxin injection into the orbicularis muscle can lead to corneal pathology. Careful testing of corneal sensation in eyes previously operated upon, avoidance of injection into the lower lid area to avoid ectropion, and vigorous treatment of any epithelial defect should be employed. This may require protective drops, ointment, therapeutic soft contact lenses, or closure of the eye by patching or other means.

Ecchymosis occurs easily in the soft eyelid tissues. This can be minimised by applying gentle pressure at the injection site immediately after injection.

Because of the anticholinergic activity of botulinum toxin, caution should be exercised when treating patients at risk for angle closure glaucoma.

Cervical dystonia

Patients with cervical dystonia should be informed of the possibility of experiencing dysphagia which may be very mild, but could be severe. Dysphagia may persist for two to three weeks after injection, but has been reported to last up to five months post-injection. Consequent to the dysphagia there is the potential for aspiration, dyspnoea and occasionally the need for tube feeding. In rare cases dysphagia followed by aspiration pneumonia and death has been reported.

Limiting the dose injected into the sternocleidomastoid muscle to less than 100 Units may decrease the occurrence of dysphagia. Patients with smaller neck muscle mass, or patients who receive bilateral injections into the sternocleidomastoid muscle, have been reported to be at greater risk of dysphagia. Dysphagia is attributable to the spread of the toxin to the oesophageal musculature. Injections into the levator scapulae may be associated with an increased risk of upper respiratory infection and dysphagia.

Dysphagia may contribute to decreased food and water intake resulting in weight loss and dehydration. Patients with subclinical dysphagia may be at increased risk of experiencing more severe dysphagia following a BOTOX injection.

Hyperhidrosis of the axillae

Medical history and physical examination, along with specific additional investigations as required, should be performed to exclude potential causes of secondary hyperhidrosis (e.g. hyperthyroidism, phaeochromocytoma). This will avoid symptomatic treatment of hyperhidrosis without the diagnosis and/or treatment of underlying disease.

Focal spasticity associated with paediatric cerebral palsy and spasticity of the hand and wrist in adult post-stroke patients

BOTOX is a treatment of focal spasticity that has only been studied in association with usual standard of care regimens, and is not intended as a replacement for these treatment modalities. BOTOX is not likely to be effective in improving range of motion at a joint affected by a fixed contracture.

4.5 Interaction with other medicinal products and other forms of interaction

Theoretically, the effect of botulinum toxin may be potentiated by aminoglycoside antibiotics or spectinomycin, or other medicinal products that interfere with neuromuscular transmission (e.g. tubocurarine-type muscle relaxants).

The effect of administering different botulinum neurotoxin serotypes at the same time or within several months of each other is unknown. Excessive neuromuscular weakness may be exacerbated by administration of another botulinum toxin prior to the resolution of the effects of a previously administered botulinum toxin.

No interaction studies have been performed. No interactions of clinical significance have been reported.

4.6 Pregnancy and lactation

Pregnancy

There are no adequate data from the use of botulinum toxin type A in pregnant women. Studies in animals have shown reproductive toxicity (see Section 5.3). The potential risk for humans is unknown. BOTOX should not be used during pregnancy unless clearly necessary.

Lactation

There is no information on whether BOTOX is excreted in human milk. The use of BOTOX during lactation cannot be recommended.

4.7 Effects on ability to drive and use machines

The effects of BOTOX on the ability to drive or to use machines can only be assessed after treatment.

4.8 Undesirable effects

a) General

Based on controlled clinical trial data patients would be expected to experience an adverse reaction after treatment with BOTOX at the rates of 35% for blepharospasm, 28% for cervical dystonia, 17% for paediatric cerebral palsy and 11% for primary hyperhidrosis of the axillae. Sixteen percent (16%) of participants in clinical trials treated with BOTOX for focal spasticity of the upper limb associated with stroke experienced an adverse reaction.

In general, adverse reactions occur within the first few days following injection and are transient.

In rare cases, adverse reactions may have a duration of several months or longer.

Local muscle weakness represents the expected pharmacological action of botulinum toxin in muscle tissue.

As is expected for any injection procedure, localised pain, tenderness and/or bruising may be associated with the injection. Fever and flu syndrome have also been reported after injections of botulinum toxin.

b) Adverse reactions - frequency by indication

For each indication the frequency of adverse reactions arising from clinical experience is given. The frequency is defined as follows:

Very Common (> 1/10); Common (>1/100, <1/10); Uncommon (>1/1,000, <1/100); Rare (>1/10,000, <1/1,000); Very Rare (<1/10,000).

Blepharospasm/hemifacial spasm	
Nervous system disorders	
Uncommon:	Dizziness, facial paresis and facial palsy.
Eye Disorders:	
Very common:	Eyelid ptosis.
Common:	Punctate keratitis, lagophthalmos, dry eye, photophobia and lacrimation increase.
Uncommon:	Keratitis, ectropion, diplopia, entropion, visual disturbance and vision blurred.
Rare:	Eyelid oedema.
Very rare:	Corneal ulceration.
Skin and subcutaneous tissue disorders	
Uncommon:	Rash/dermatitis.
General disorders and administration site conditions	
Common:	Irritation and face oedema.
Uncommon:	Fatigue.
Cervical dystonia	
Infections and infestations	
Common:	Rhinitis and upper respiratory infection.
Nervous system disorders	
Common:	Dizziness, hypertonia, hypoaesthesia, somnolence and headache.
Eye Disorders:	
Uncommon:	Diplopia and eyelid ptosis.
Respiratory, thoracic and mediastinal disorders	
Uncommon:	Dyspnoea and dysphonia.
Gastrointestinal disorders	
Very common:	Dysphagia (see section c. below).
Common:	Dry mouth and nausea.
Musculoskeletal and connective tissue disorders	
Very common:	Muscular weakness.
Common:	Musculoskeletal stiffness and soreness.
General disorders and administration site conditions	
Very common:	Pain.
Common:	Asthenia, influenza like illness and malaise.
Uncommon:	Pyrexia.
Paediatric cerebral palsy	
Infections and infestations	
Very common:	Viral infection and ear infection.
Nervous system disorders	
Common:	Somnolence and paraesthesia.
Skin and subcutaneous tissue disorders	
Common:	Rash.
Musculoskeletal and connective tissue disorders	
Common:	Myalgia and muscular weakness.
Renal and urinary disorders	
Common:	Urinary incontinence.
General disorders and administration site conditions	
Common:	Gait disturbance and malaise.
Focal upper limb spasticity associated with stroke	
Psychiatric disorders	
Uncommon:	Depression and insomnia.
Nervous system disorders	
Common:	Hypertonia
Uncommon:	Hypoaesthesia, headache, paraesthesia, incoordination and amnesia.
Ear and labyrinth disorders	
Uncommon:	Vertigo.
Vascular disorders	
Uncommon:	Orthostatic hypotension.
Gastrointestinal disorders	
Uncommon:	Nausea and paraesthesia oral.
Skin and subcutaneous tissue disorders	
Common:	Ecchymosis and purpura.
Uncommon:	Dermatitis, pruritus and rash.
Musculoskeletal and connective tissue disorders	
Common:	Pain in extremity and muscle weakness.
Uncommon:	Arthralgia and bursitis.
General disorders and administration site conditions	
Common:	Injection site hemorrhage and injection site irritation.
Uncommon:	Asthenia, pain, injection site hypersensitivity, malaise and oedema peripheral.
Some of the uncommon events may be disease related.	
Primary hyperhidrosis of the axillae	
Nervous system disorders	
Common:	Headache
Vascular disorders	
Common:	Hot flushes.
Gastrointestinal disorders	
Uncommon:	Nausea
Skin and subcutaneous tissue disorders	
Common:	Hyperhidrosis (non-axillary sweating).
Uncommon:	Pruritus.
Musculoskeletal and connective tissue disorders	
Uncommon:	Muscular weakness, myalgia, arthropathy and pain in extremity.
General disorders and administration site conditions	
Common:	Injection site reactions and pain.
Uncommon:	Asthenia, injection site oedema and injection site pain

In the management of primary axillary hyperhidrosis, increase in non axillary sweating was reported in 4.5% of patients within 1 month after injection and showed no pattern with respect to anatomical sites affected. Resolution was seen in approximately 30% of the patients within four months.

Weakness of the arm has been also reported uncommonly (0.7%) and was mild, transient, did not require treatment and recovered without sequelae. This adverse event may be related to treatment, injection technique, or both. In the uncommon event of muscle weakness being reported a neurological examination may be considered. In addition, a re-evaluation of injection technique prior to subsequent injection is advisable to ensure intradermal placement of injections.

c) Additional information

Dysphagia ranges in severity from mild to severe, with potential for aspiration, which occasionally may require medical intervention. See Section 4.4.

Side effects related to spread of toxin distant from the site of administration have been reported very rarely (exaggerated muscle weakness, dysphagia, aspiration/aspiration pneumonia, with fatal outcome in some cases). (See section 4.4).

The following other adverse events have been reported since the drug has been marketed: dysarthria; abdominal pain; vision blurred; pyrexia; focal facial paralysis; hypoaesthesia; malaise; myalgia; pruritus; hyperhidrosis; diarrhoea; anorexia; hypoacusis; tinnitus; radiculopathy; syncope; myasthenia gravis; erythema multiforme; dermatitis psoriasiform; vomiting and brachial plexopathy.

There have also been rare reports of adverse events involving the cardiovascular system, including arrhythmia and myocardial infarction, some with fatal outcomes. Some of these patients had risk factors including cardiovascular disease.

Serious and/or immediate hypersensitivity reactions have been rarely reported, including anaphylaxis, serum sickness, urticaria, soft tissue oedema, and dyspnoea. Some of these reactions have been reported following the use of BOTOX either alone or in conjunction with other agents known to cause similar reactions.

A case of peripheral neuropathy has been reported in a large adult male after receiving four sets of BOTOX injections, totalling 1800 Units (for neck and back spasm, and severe pain) over an 11 week period.

Angle closure glaucoma has been reported very rarely following botulinum toxin treatment for blepharospasm.

New onset or recurrent seizures have been reported, typically in patients, who are predisposed to experiencing these events. The exact relationship of these events to the botulinum toxin injection has not been established. The reports in children were reports predominantly from cerebral palsy patients treated for spasticity.

Needle-related pain and/or anxiety may result in vasovagal responses, e.g. syncope, hypotension, etc.

4.9 Overdose

No cases of systemic toxicity resulting from accidental injection of BOTOX have been observed. No cases of ingestion of BOTOX have been reported. Signs of overdose are not apparent immediately post-injection. Should accidental injection or ingestion occur, the patient should be medically supervised for several days for signs and symptoms of systemic weakness or muscle paralysis.

Patients presenting with the symptoms of botulinum toxin type A poisoning (generalised weakness, ptosis, diplopia, swallowing and speech disorders, or paresis of the respiratory muscles) should be considered for admission to hospital.

With increasing dosage, generalised and profound muscular paralysis occurs. When the musculature of the oropharynx and oesophagus are affected, aspiration may occur which may lead to development of aspiration pneumonia. If the respiratory muscles become paralysed, intubation and assisted respiration will be required until recovery takes place.

5. PHARMACOLOGICAL PROPERTIES

5.1 Pharmacodynamic properties

ATC class M03A X01 and ATC class D11AX

The active constituent in BOTOX is a protein complex derived from *Clostridium botulinum*. The protein consists of type A neurotoxin and several other proteins. Under physiological conditions it is presumed that the complex dissociates and releases the pure neurotoxin.

Clostridium botulinum toxin type A neurotoxin complex blocks peripheral acetyl choline release at presynaptic cholinergic nerve terminals.

Intramuscular injection of the neurotoxin complex blocks cholinergic transport at the neuromuscular junction by preventing the release of acetylcholine. The nerve endings of the neuromuscular junction no longer respond to nerve impulses and secretion of the chemotransmitter is prevented (chemical denervation). Re-establishment of impulse transmission is by newly formed nerve endings and motor end plates. Recovery after intramuscular injection takes place normally within 12 weeks of injection as nerve terminals sprout and reconnect with the endplates.

After intradermal injection, where the target is the eccrine sweat glands, the effect lasted for about 4-7 months in patients treated with 50 Units per axilla.

5.2 Pharmacokinetic properties

a) General characteristics of the active substance:

Classical absorption, distribution, biotransformation and elimination studies on the active substance have not been performed due to the extreme toxicity of botulinum toxin type A.

b) Characteristics in patients:

Human ADME studies have not been performed due to the nature of the product. It is believed that little systemic distribution of therapeutic doses of BOTOX occurs. BOTOX is probably metabolised by proteases and the molecular components recycled through normal metabolic pathways.

5.3 Preclinical safety data

Acute toxicity

In monkeys receiving a single intramuscular (i.m.) injection of BOTOX, the No Observed Effect Level (NOEL) ranged from 4 to 24 Units/kg. The i.m. LD_{50} was reported to be 39 Units/kg.

Toxicity on repeated injection

In three different studies (six months in rats; 20 weeks in juvenile monkeys; 1 year in monkeys) where the animals received i.m. injections, the NOEL was at the following respective BOTOX dosage levels: < 4 Units/kg, 8 Units/kg and 4 Units/kg. The main systemic effect was a transient decrease in body weight gain.

There was no indication of a cumulative effect in the animal studies when BOTOX was given at dosage intervals of 1 month or greater.

Local toxicity

BOTOX was shown not to cause ocular or dermal irritation, or give rise to toxicity when injected into the vitreous body in rabbits.

Allergic or inflammatory reactions in the area of the injection sites are rarely observed after BOTOX administration. However, formation of haematoma may occur.

Reproduction toxicology

Teratogenic effects

When pregnant mice and rats were injected intramuscularly during the period of organogenesis, the developmental NOEL of BOTOX was at 4 Units/kg. Reductions in ossification were observed at 8 and 16 Units/kg (mice) and reduced ossification of the hyoid bone at 16 Units/kg (rats). Reduced foetal body weights were observed at 8 and 16 Units/kg (rats).

In a range-finding study in rabbits, daily injections at dosages of 0.5 Units/kg/day (days 6 to 18 of gestation), and 4 and 6 Units/kg (administered on days 6 and 13 of gestation), caused death and abortions among surviving dams. External malformations were observed in one foetus each in the 0.125 Units/kg/day and the 2 Units/kg dosage groups. The rabbit appears to be a very sensitive species to BOTOX treatment.

Impairment of fertility and reproduction

The reproductive NOEL following i.m. injection of BOTOX was 4 Units/kg in male rats and 8 Units/kg in female rats. Higher dosages were associated with dose-dependent reductions in fertility. Provided impregnation occurred, there were no adverse effects on the numbers or viability of the embryos sired or conceived by treated male or female rats.

Pre- and post-natal developmental effects

In female rats, the reproductive NOEL was 16 Units/kg. The developmental NOEL was 4 Units/kg.

Mutagenicity

BOTOX has been evaluated and shown to be non-mutagenic in a number of *in vitro* and *in vivo* systems including the Ames test, the AS52/XPRT Mammalian Cell Forward Gene Mutation assay and the CHO test, and non-clastogenic in the mouse PCE test.

Carcinogenicity

No animal studies have been conducted.

Antigenicity

BOTOX showed antigenicity in mice only in the presence of adjuvant. BOTOX was found to be slightly antigenic in the guinea pig.

Blood compatibility

No haemolysis was detected up to 100 Units/ml of BOTOX in normal human blood.

6. PHARMACEUTICAL PARTICULARS

6.1 List of excipients

Human albumin

Sodium chloride

6.2 Incompatibilities

In the absence of compatibility studies, this medicinal product should not be mixed with other medicinal products.

6.3 Shelf life

3 years.

After reconstitution, stability has been demonstrated for 24 hours at 2°C – 8°C.

From a microbiological point of view, the product should be used immediately. If not used immediately, in-use storage times and conditions prior to use are the responsibility of the user and would normally not be longer than 24 hours at 2°C to 8°C (see also section 6.6).

6.4 Special precautions for storage

Store in a refrigerator (2°C-8°C), or store in a freezer (at or below -5°C).

For storage conditions of the reconstituted medicinal product see section 6.3.

6.5 Nature and contents of container

Clear glass vial, with rubber stopper and tamper-proof aluminium seal, containing white powder for solution for injection.

Pack size:

- Carton comprising one 100 Allergan Unit vial and package leaflet.
- Packs containing two, three or six cartons.

Not all pack sizes may be marketed.

6.6 Special precautions for disposal and other handling

BOTOX is reconstituted prior to use with sterile unpreserved normal saline (0.9% sodium chloride for injection). It is good practice to perform vial reconstitution and syringe preparation over plastic-lined paper towels to catch any spillage. An appropriate amount of diluent (see dilution table below) is drawn up into a syringe. The exposed portion of the rubber septum of the vial is cleaned with alcohol (70%) prior to insertion of the needle. Since BOTOX is denatured by bubbling or similar violent agitation, the diluent should be injected gently into the vial. Discard the vial if a vacuum does not pull the diluent into the vial. Reconstituted BOTOX is a clear colourless to slightly yellow solution free of particulate matter. When reconstituted, BOTOX may be stored in a refrigerator (2-8°C) for up to 24 hours prior to use. After this period used or unused vials should be discarded.

Each vial is for single use only.

Dilution table: Diluent added	Resulting dose in units per 0.1 ml
0.5 ml	20 Units
1 ml	10 Units
2 ml	5 Units
4 ml	2.5 Units
8 ml	1.25 Units

The 'unit' by which the potency of preparations of BOTOX is measured should be used to calculate dosages of BOTOX only and is not transferable to other preparations of botulinum toxin.

An injection volume of approximately 0.1 ml is recommended. A decrease or increase in the BOTOX dose is possible by administering a smaller or larger injection volume. The smaller the injection volume the less discomfort and less spread of toxin in the injected muscle occurs. This is of benefit in reducing effects on nearby muscles when small muscle groups are being injected.

For safe disposal, unused vials should be reconstituted with a small amount of water then autoclaved. Any used vials, syringes, and spillages etc. should be autoclaved, or the residual BOTOX inactivated using dilute hypochlorite solution (0.5%).

Any unused product or waste material should be disposed of in accordance with local requirements.

7. MARKETING AUTHORISATION HOLDER

Allergan Ltd.,

Marlow International,

The Parkway, Marlow,

Bucks, SL7 1YL, UK

8. MARKETING AUTHORISATION NUMBER(S)

PL 00426/0074

9. DATE OF FIRST AUTHORISATION/RENEWAL OF THE AUTHORISATION

17 May 1994

10. DATE OF REVISION OF THE TEXT

22nd May 2009

BOTOX® 50 Units

(Allergan Ltd)

1. NAME OF THE MEDICINAL PRODUCT

BOTOX

50 Allergan Units

Powder for solution for injection

2. QUALITATIVE AND QUANTITATIVE COMPOSITION

Botulinum toxin* type A, 50 Allergan units/vial.

* from *Clostridium botulinum*

Botulinum toxin units are not interchangeable from one product to another.

For full list of excipients, see section 6.1

3. PHARMACEUTICAL FORM

Powder for solution for injection.

4. CLINICAL PARTICULARS

4.1 Therapeutic indications

BOTOX is indicated for the symptomatic relief of blepharospasm, hemifacial spasm and idiopathic cervical dystonia (spasmodic torticollis). It is indicated for the management of severe hyperhidrosis of the axillae, which does not respond to topical treatment with antiperspirants or antihidrotics.

BOTOX is also indicated for focal spasticity, including the treatment of

- dynamic equinus foot deformity due to spasticity in ambulant paediatric cerebral palsy patients, two years of age or older

and

- wrist and hand disability due to upper limb spasticity associated with stroke in adults

The injections should be administered by appropriately trained personnel in hospital specialist centres.

The safety and effectiveness of BOTOX in the treatment of blepharospasm, hemifacial spasm, or idiopathic cervical dystonia, or focal hyperhidrosis in children have not been demonstrated.

4.2 Posology and method of administration

Doses recommended for BOTOX are not interchangeable with other preparations of botulinum toxin.

Adequate studies on geriatric dosing have not been performed. Dose selection should be the same; however, the lowest effective dose is recommended.

Blepharospasm

After reconstitution, BOTOX is injected using a sterile, 27-30 gauge needle. Electromyographic guidance is not necessary. The initial recommended dose is 1.25-2.5 Units (0.05-0.1 ml volume at each site) injected into the medial and lateral orbicularis oculi of the upper lid and the lateral orbicularis oculi of the lower lid. Additional sites in the brow area, the lateral orbicularis and in the upper facial area may also be injected if spasms here interfere with vision. In general, the initial effect of the injections is seen within three days and reaches a peak at one to two weeks post-treatment. Each treatment lasts approximately three months, following which the procedure can be repeated indefinitely. At repeat treatment sessions, the dose may be increased up to two-fold if the response from the initial treatment is considered insufficient - usually defined as an effect that does not last longer than two months. However, there appears to be little benefit obtainable from injecting more than 5 Units per site. The initial dose should not exceed 25 Units per eye. Normally no additional benefit is conferred by treating more frequently than every three months. It is rare for the effect to be permanent.

In the management of blepharospasm total dosing should not exceed 100 Units every 12 weeks.

Hemifacial spasm

Patients with hemifacial spasm or VIIth nerve disorders should be treated as for unilateral blepharospasm, with other affected facial muscles being injected as needed. Electromyographic control may be necessary to identify affected small circumoral muscles.

Cervical dystonia

Several dosing regimens have been used in clinical trials for treatment of cervical dystonia with BOTOX. Dosing must be tailored to the individual patient based on the patient's head and neck position, location of pain, muscle hypertrophy, patient's body weight, and patient response.

In practice, the maximum total dose is not usually more than 200 Units. No more than 50 Units should be given at any one injection site. The dilutions suggested are indicated in the following table:

Diluent added	Resulting dose in units per 0.1 ml
0.5 ml	10.0 Units
1 ml	5.0 Units
2 ml	2.50 Units
4 ml	1.25 Units

The following doses are recommended:

Type I Head **rotated** toward side of shoulder elevation	Sternomastoid	50 - 100 Units; at least 2 sites
	Levator scapulae	50 Units; 1 - 2 sites
	Scalene	25 - 50 Units; 1 - 2 sites
	Splenius capitis	25 - 75 Units; 1 - 3 sites
	Trapezius	25 - 100 Units; 1 - 8 sites
Type II Head rotation only	Sternomastoid	25 - 100 Units; at least 2 sites if >25 Units given
Type III Head **tilted** toward side of shoulder elevation	Sternomastoid	25 - 100 Units at posterior border; at least 2 sites if >25 Units given
	Levator scapulae	25 - 100 Units; at least 2 sites
	Scalene	25 - 75 Units; at least 2 sites
	Trapezius	25 - 100 Units; 1 - 8 sites
Type IV Bilateral posterior cervical muscle spasm with elevation of the face	Splenius capitis and cervicis	50 - 200 Units; 2 - 8 sites, treat bilaterally (This is the total dose and not the dose for each side of the neck)

The treatment of cervical dystonia typically may include injection of BOTOX into the sternocleidomastoid, levator scapulae, scalene, splenius capitis, and/or the trapezius muscle(s). The muscle mass and the degree of hypertrophy are factors to be taken into consideration when selecting the appropriate dose.

The sternocleidomastoid muscle should not be injected bilaterally as there is an increased risk of adverse effects (in particular dysphagia) when bilateral injections or doses in excess of 100 Units are administered to this muscle.

A 25, 27 or 30 gauge needle may be used for superficial muscles, and a 22 gauge needle may be used for deeper musculature. For cervical dystonia, localisation of the involved muscles with electromyographic guidance may be useful.

Multiple injection sites allow BOTOX to have more uniform contact with the innervation areas of the dystonic muscle and are especially useful in larger muscles. The optimal number of injection sites is dependent upon the size of the muscle to be chemically denervated.

Hyperhidrosis of the axillae

The recommended injection volume for intradermal injection in axillary hyperhidrosis is 0.1-0.2 ml. Reconstituted BOTOX (100 Units/4 mL) is injected using a 30 gauge needle. 50 Units of BOTOX is injected intradermally to each axilla, evenly distributed in multiple sites approximately 1-2 cm apart. The hyperhidrotic area to be injected may be defined by using standard staining techniques, e.g. Minor's iodine-starch test.

Clinical improvement generally occurs within the first week after injection. Repeat injections of axillary hyperhidrosis should be administered when effects from previous injections subside. Treatment response has been reported to persist for 4-7 months.

Paediatric cerebral palsy

Diluted BOTOX is injected using a sterile 23-26 gauge needle. It is administered into each of two sites in the medial and lateral heads of the affected gastrocnemius muscle. The recommended total dose is 4 Units/kg body weight. When both lower limbs are to be injected on the same occasion this dose should be divided between the two limbs.

Clinical improvement generally occurs within the first two weeks after injection. Repeat doses should be administered when the clinical effect of a previous injection diminishes but not more frequently than every two months.

Focal spasticity associated with stroke

Reconstituted BOTOX is injected using a sterile 25, 27 or 30 gauge needle for superficial muscles, and a longer needle for deeper musculature. Localisation of the involved muscles with electromyographic guidance or nerve stimulation techniques may be useful. Multiple injection sites may allow BOTOX to have more uniform contact with the innervation areas of the muscle and are especially useful in larger muscles.

The exact dosage and number of injection sites may be tailored to the individual based on the size, number and location of muscles involved, the severity of spasticity, and the presence of local muscle weakness.

In the controlled Phase 3 clinical trial the following doses were administered:

Muscle	Total Dose
Flexor digitorum profundus	50 Units
Flexor digitorum sublimis	50 Units
Flexor carpi radialis	50 Units
Flexor carpi ulnaris	50 Units
Adductor Pollicis	20 Units
Flexor Pollicis Longus	20 Units

In all clinical trials, the doses did not exceed 360 Units divided among selected muscles at any treatment session.

Clinical improvement in muscle tone generally occurs within two weeks following treatment and the peak effect is generally seen within four to six weeks following treatment. Data on the repeated and long-term treatment are limited.

4.3 Contraindications

BOTOX is contraindicated:

- in individuals with a known hypersensitivity to botulinum toxin type A or to any of the excipients;

- in the presence of infection at the proposed injection site(s).

4.4 Special warnings and precautions for use

The relevant anatomy, and any alterations to the anatomy due to prior surgical procedures, must be understood prior to administering BOTOX. The recommended dosages and frequencies of administration of BOTOX should not be exceeded.

Serious and/or immediate hypersensitivity reactions have been rarely reported including anaphylaxis, serum sickness, urticaria, soft tissue oedema, and dyspnoea. Some of these reactions have been reported following the use of BOTOX either alone or in conjunction with other products associated with similar reactions. If such a reaction occurs further injection of BOTOX should be discontinued and appropriate medical therapy, such as epinephrine, immediately instituted. Please see section 4.8c) for further information.

Side effects related to spread of toxin distant from the site of administration have been reported (See section 4.8), sometimes resulting in death, which in some cases was associated with dysphagia, pneumonia and/or significant debility.

Patients treated with therapeutic doses may experience exaggerated muscle weakness. Patients with underlying neurological disorders including swallowing difficulties are at increased risk of these side effects. The botulinum toxin product should be used under specialist supervision in these patients and should only be used if the benefit of treatment is considered to outweigh the risk. Patients with a history of dysphagia and aspiration should be treated with extreme caution.

Patients or caregivers should be advised to seek immediate medical care if swallowing, speech or respiratory disorders arise.

Dysphagia has also been reported following injection to sites other than the cervical musculature (see section 4.4 'Cervical Dystonia' for further information).

Clinical fluctuations during the repeated use of BOTOX (as with all botulinum toxins) may be a result of different vial reconstitution procedures, injection intervals, muscles injected and slightly differing potency values given by the biological test method used.

Formation of neutralizing antibodies to botulinum toxin type A may reduce the effectiveness of BOTOX treatment by inactivating the biological activity of the toxin. Results from some studies suggest that BOTOX injections at more frequent intervals or at higher doses may lead to greater incidence of antibody formation.

As with any treatment with the potential to allow previously-sedentary patients to resume activities, the sedentary patient should be cautioned to resume activity gradually.

Caution should be used when BOTOX is used in the presence of inflammation at the proposed injection site(s) or when excessive weakness or atrophy is present in the target muscle. Caution should also be exercised when BOTOX is used for treatment of patients with peripheral motor neuropathic diseases (e.g., amyotrophic lateral sclerosis or motor neuropathy).

BOTOX should only be used with extreme caution and under close supervision in patients with subclinical or clinical evidence of defective neuromuscular transmission e.g. myasthenia gravis or Eaton Lambert Syndrome; such patients may have an increased sensitivity to agents such as BOTOX, which may result in excessive muscle weakness. Patients with neuromuscular disorders may be at an increased risk of clinically significant systemic effects including severe dysphagia and respiratory compromise from typical doses of BOTOX.

BOTOX contains human albumin. When medicinal products derived from human blood or plasma are administered, the possibility of transmitting infectious agents cannot be totally excluded. To reduce the risk of transmission of infective agents, stringent controls are applied to the selection of blood donors and donations. In addition, virus inactivation procedures are included in the production process.

As with any injection, procedure-related injury could occur. An injection could result in localized infection, pain, inflammation, paraesthesia, hypoaesthesia, tenderness, swelling, erythema, and/or bleeding/bruising. Needle-related pain and/or anxiety may result in vasovagal responses, e.g. syncope, hypotension, etc. Care should be taken when injecting near vulnerable anatomic structures.

Blepharospasm

Reduced blinking following botulinum toxin injection into the orbicularis muscle can lead to corneal pathology. Careful testing of corneal sensation in eyes previously operated upon, avoidance of injection into the lower lid area to avoid ectropion, and vigorous treatment of any epithelial defect should be employed. This may require protective drops, ointment, therapeutic soft contact lenses, or closure of the eye by patching or other means.

Ecchymosis occurs easily in the soft eyelid tissues. This can be minimised by applying gentle pressure at the injection site immediately after injection.

Because of the anticholinergic activity of botulinum toxin, caution should be exercised when treating patients at risk for angle closure glaucoma.

Cervical dystonia

Patients with cervical dystonia should be informed of the possibility of experiencing dysphagia which may be very mild, but could be severe. Dysphagia may persist for two to three weeks after injection, but has been reported to last up to five months post-injection. Consequent to the dysphagia there is the potential for aspiration, dyspnoea and occasionally the need for tube feeding. In rare cases dysphagia followed by aspiration pneumonia and death has been reported.

Limiting the dose injected into the sternocleidomastoid muscle to less than 100 Units may decrease the occurrence of dysphagia. Patients with smaller neck muscle mass, or patients who receive bilateral injections into the sternocleidomastoid muscle, have been reported to be at greater risk of dysphagia. Dysphagia is attributable to the spread of the toxin to the oesophageal musculature. Injections into the levator scapulae may be associated with an increased risk of upper respiratory infection and dysphagia.

Dysphagia may contribute to decreased food and water intake resulting in weight loss and dehydration. Patients with subclinical dysphagia may be at increased risk of experiencing more severe dysphagia following a BOTOX injection.

Hyperhidrosis of the axillae

Medical history and physical examination, along with specific additional investigations as required, should be performed to exclude potential causes of secondary hyperhidrosis (e.g. hyperthyroidism, phaeochromocytoma). This will avoid symptomatic treatment of hyperhidrosis without the diagnosis and/or treatment of underlying disease.

Focal spasticity associated with paediatric cerebral palsy and spasticity of the hand and wrist in adult post-stroke patients

BOTOX is a treatment of focal spasticity that has only been studied in association with usual standard of care regimens, and is not intended as a replacement for these treatment modalities. BOTOX is not likely to be effective in improving range of motion at a joint affected by a fixed contracture.

4.5 Interaction with other medicinal products and other forms of interaction

Theoretically, the effect of botulinum toxin may be potentiated by aminoglycoside antibiotics or spectinomycin, or other medicinal products that interfere with neuromuscular transmission (e.g. tubocurarine-type muscle relaxants).

The effect of administering different botulinum neurotoxin serotypes at the same time or within several months of each other is unknown. Excessive neuromuscular weakness may be exacerbated by administration of another botulinum toxin prior to the resolution of the effects of a previously administered botulinum toxin.

No interaction studies have been performed. No interactions of clinical significance have been reported.

4.6 Pregnancy and lactation

Pregnancy

There are no adequate data from the use of botulinum toxin type A in pregnant women. Studies in animals have shown reproductive toxicity (see Section 5.3). The potential risk for humans is unknown. BOTOX should not be used during pregnancy unless clearly necessary.

Lactation

There is no information on whether BOTOX is excreted in human milk. The use of BOTOX during lactation cannot be recommended.

4.7 Effects on ability to drive and use machines

The effects of BOTOX on the ability to drive or to use machines can only be assessed after treatment.

4.8 Undesirable effects

a) General

Based on controlled clinical trial data patients would be expected to experience an adverse reaction after treatment with BOTOX at the rates of 35% for blepharospasm, 28% for cervical dystonia, 17% for paediatric cerebral palsy and 11% for primary hyperhidrosis of the axillae. Sixteen percent (16%) of participants in clinical trials treated with BOTOX for focal spasticity of the upper limb associated with stroke experienced an adverse reaction.

In general, adverse reactions occur within the first few days following injection and are transient.

In rare cases, adverse reactions may have a duration of several months or longer.

Local muscle weakness represents the expected pharmacological action of botulinum toxin in muscle tissue.

As is expected for any injection procedure, localised pain, tenderness and/or bruising may be associated with the injection. Fever and flu syndrome have also been reported after injections of botulinum toxin.

b) Adverse reactions - frequency by indication

For each indication the frequency of adverse reactions arising from clinical experience is given. The frequency is defined as follows:

Very Common (> 1/10); Common (>1/100, <1/10); Uncommon (>1/1,000, <1/100); Rare (>1/10,000, <1/1,000); Very Rare (<1/10,000).

Blepharospasm/hemifacial spasm

Nervous system disorders

Uncommon: Dizziness, facial paresis and facial palsy.

Eye Disorders

Very common: Eyelid ptosis.

Common: Punctate keratitis, lagophthalmos, dry eye, photophobia and lacrimation increase.

Uncommon: Keratitis, ectropion, diplopia, entropion, visual disturbance and vision blurred.

Rare: Eyelid oedema.

Very rare: Corneal ulceration.

Skin and subcutaneous tissue disorders

Uncommon: Rash/dermatitis.

General disorders and administration site conditions

Common: Irritation and face oedema.

Uncommon: Fatigue.

Cervical dystonia

Infections and infestations

Common: Rhinitis and upper respiratory infection.

Nervous system disorders

Common: Dizziness, hypertonia, hypoaesthesia, somnolence and headache.

Eye Disorders

Uncommon: Diplopia and eyelid ptosis.

Respiratory, thoracic and mediastinal disorders

Uncommon: Dyspnoea and dysphonia.

Gastrointestinal disorders

Very common: Dysphagia (see section c. below).

Common: Dry mouth and nausea.

Musculoskeletal and connective tissue disorders

Very common: Muscular weakness.

Common: Musculoskeletal stiffness and soreness.

General disorders and administration site conditions

Very common: Pain.

Common: Asthenia, influenza like illness and malaise.

Uncommon: Pyrexia.

Paediatric cerebral palsy

Infections and infestations

Very common: Viral infection and ear infection.

Nervous system disorders

Common: Somnolence and paraesthesia.

Skin and subcutaneous tissue disorders

Common: Rash.

Musculoskeletal and connective tissue disorders

Common: Myalgia and muscular weakness.

Renal and urinary disorders

Common: Urinary incontinence.

General disorders and administration site conditions

Common: Gait disturbance and malaise.

Focal upper limb spasticity associated with stroke

Psychiatric disorders

Uncommon: Depression and insomnia.

Nervous system disorders

Common: Hypertonia

Uncommon: Hypoaesthesia, headache, paraesthesia, incoordination and amnesia.

Ear and labyrinth disorders

Uncommon: Vertigo.

Vascular disorders

Uncommon: Orthostatic hypotension.

Gastrointestinal disorders

Uncommon: Nausea and paraesthesia oral.

Skin and subcutaneous tissue disorders

Common: Ecchymosis and purpura.

Uncommon: Dermatitis, pruritus and rash.

Musculoskeletal and connective tissue disorders

Common: Pain in extremity and muscle weakness.

Uncommon: Arthralgia and bursitis.

General disorders and administration site conditions

Common: Injection site hemorrhage and injection site irritation.

Uncommon: Asthenia, pain, injection site hypersensitivity, malaise and oedema peripheral.

Some of the uncommon events may be disease related.

Primary hyperhidrosis of the axillae

Nervous system disorders

Common: Headache

Vascular disorders

Common: Hot flushes.

Gastrointestinal disorders

Uncommon: Nausea

Skin and subcutaneous tissue disorders

Common: Hyperhidrosis (non-axillary sweating).

Uncommon: Pruritus.

Musculoskeletal and connective tissue disorders

Uncommon: Muscular weakness, myalgia, arthropathy and pain in extremity.

General disorders and administration site conditions

Common: Injection site reactions and pain.

Uncommon: Asthenia, injection site oedema and injection site pain

In the management of primary axillary hyperhidrosis, increase in non axillary sweating was reported in 4.5% of patients within 1 month after injection and showed no pattern with respect to anatomical sites affected. Resolution was seen in approximately 30% of the patients within four months.

Weakness of the arm has been also reported uncommonly (0.7%) and was mild, transient, did not require treatment and recovered without sequelae. This adverse event may be related to treatment, injection technique, or both. In the uncommon event of muscle weakness being reported a neurological examination may be considered. In addition, a re-evaluation of injection technique prior to subsequent injection is advisable to ensure intradermal placement of injections.

c) Additional information

Dysphagia ranges in severity from mild to severe, with potential for aspiration, which occasionally may require medical intervention. See Section 4.4.

Side effects related to spread of toxin distant from the site of administration have been reported very rarely (exaggerated muscle weakness, dysphagia, aspiration/aspiration pneumonia, with fatal outcome in some cases). (See section 4.4).

The following other adverse events have been reported since the drug has been marketed: dysarthria; abdominal pain; vision blurred; pyrexia; focal facial paralysis; hypoaesthesia; malaise; myalgia; pruritus; hyperhidrosis; diarrhoea; anorexia; hypoacusis; tinnitus; radiculopathy; syncope; myasthenia gravis; erythema multiforme; dermatitis psoriasiform; vomiting and brachial plexopathy.

There have also been rare reports of adverse events involving the cardiovascular system, including arrhythmia and myocardial infarction, some with fatal outcomes. Some of these patients had risk factors including cardiovascular disease.

Serious and/or immediate hypersensitivity reactions have been rarely reported, including anaphylaxis, serum sickness, urticaria, soft tissue oedema, and dyspnoea. Some of these reactions have been reported following the use of BOTOX either alone or in conjunction with other agents known to cause similar reactions.

A case of peripheral neuropathy has been reported in a large adult male after receiving four sets of BOTOX injections, totalling 1800 Units (for neck and back spasm, and severe pain) over an 11 week period.

Angle closure glaucoma has been reported very rarely following botulinum toxin treatment for blepharospasm.

New onset or recurrent seizures have been reported, typically in patients, who are predisposed to experiencing these events. The exact relationship of these events to the botulinum toxin injection has not been established. The reports in children were reports predominantly from cerebral palsy patients treated for spasticity.

Needle-related pain and/or anxiety may result in vasovagal responses, e.g. syncope, hypotension, etc.

4.9 Overdose

No cases of systemic toxicity resulting from accidental injection of BOTOX have been observed. No cases of ingestion of BOTOX have been reported. Signs of overdose are not apparent immediately post-injection. Should accidental injection or ingestion occur, the patient should be medically supervised for several days for signs and symptoms of systemic weakness or muscle paralysis.

Patients presenting with the symptoms of botulinum toxin type A poisoning (generalised weakness, ptosis, diplopia, swallowing and speech disorders, or paresis of the respiratory muscles) should be considered for admission to hospital.

With increasing dosage, generalised and profound muscular paralysis occurs. When the musculature of the oropharynx and oesophagus are affected, aspiration may occur which may lead to development of aspiration pneumonia. If the respiratory muscles become paralysed, intubation and assisted respiration will be required until recovery takes place.

5. PHARMACOLOGICAL PROPERTIES

5.1 Pharmacodynamic properties

ATC class M03A X01 and ATC class D11AX.

The active constituent in BOTOX is a protein complex derived from *Clostridium botulinum*. The protein consists of type A neurotoxin and several other proteins. Under physiological conditions it is presumed that the complex dissociates and releases the pure neurotoxin.

Clostridium botulinum toxin type A neurotoxin complex blocks peripheral acetyl choline release at presynaptic cholinergic nerve terminals.

Intramuscular injection of the neurotoxin complex blocks cholinergic transport at the neuromuscular junction by preventing the release of acetylcholine. The nerve endings of the neuromuscular junction no longer respond to nerve impulses and secretion of the chemotransmitter is prevented (chemical denervation). Re-establishment of impulse transmission is by newly formed nerve endings and motor end plates. Recovery after intramuscular injection takes place normally within 12 weeks of injection as nerve terminals sprout and reconnect with the endplates.

After intradermal injection, where the target is the eccrine sweat glands, the effect lasted for about 4-7 months in patients treated with 50 Units per axilla.

5.2 Pharmacokinetic properties

a) General characteristics of the active substance:

Classical absorption, distribution, biotransformation and elimination studies on the active substance have not been performed due to the extreme toxicity of botulinum toxin type A.

5.2) Characteristics in patients:

Human ADME studies have not been performed due to the nature of the product. It is believed that little systemic distribution of therapeutic doses of BOTOX occurs.

BOTOX is probably metabolised by proteases and the molecular components recycled through normal metabolic pathways.

5.3 Preclinical safety data

Acute toxicity

In monkeys receiving a single intramuscular (i.m.) injection of BOTOX, the No Observed Effect Level (NOEL) ranged from 4 to 24 Units/kg. The i.m. LD_{50} was reported to be 39 Units/kg.

Toxicity on repeated injection

In three different studies (six months in rats; 20 weeks in juvenile monkeys; 1 year in monkeys) where the animals received i.m. injections, the NOEL was at the following respective BOTOX dosage levels: < 4 Units/kg, 8 Units/kg and 4 Units/kg. The main systemic effect was a transient decrease in body weight gain.

There was no indication of a cumulative effect in the animal studies when BOTOX was given at dosage intervals of 1 month or greater.

Local toxicity

BOTOX was shown not to cause ocular or dermal irritation, or give rise to toxicity when injected into the vitreous body in rabbits.

Allergic or inflammatory reactions in the area of the injection sites are rarely observed after BOTOX administration. However, formation of haematoma may occur.

Reproduction toxicology

Teratogenic effects

When pregnant mice and rats were injected intramuscularly during the period of organogenesis, the developmental NOEL of BOTOX was at 4 Units/kg. Reductions in ossification were observed at 8 and 16 Units/kg (mice) and reduced ossification of the hyoid bone at 16 Units/kg (rats). Reduced foetal body weights were observed at 8 and 16 Units/kg (rats).

In a range-finding study in rabbits, daily injections at dosages of 0.5 Units/kg/day (days 6 to 18 of gestation), and 4 and 6 Units/kg (administered on days 6 and 13 of gestation), caused death and abortions among surviving dams. External malformations were observed in one foetus each in the 0.125 Units/kg/day and the 2 Units/kg dosage groups. The rabbit appears to be a very sensitive species to BOTOX treatment.

Impairment of fertility and reproduction

The reproductive NOEL following i.m. injection of BOTOX was 4 Units/kg in male rats and 8 Units/kg in female rats. Higher dosages were associated with dose-dependent reductions in fertility. Provided impregnation occurred, there were no adverse effects on the numbers or viability of the embryos sired or conceived by treated male or female rats.

Pre- and post-natal developmental effects

In female rats, the reproductive NOEL was 16 Units/kg. The developmental NOEL was 4 Units/kg.

Mutagenicity

BOTOX has been evaluated and shown to be non-mutagenic in a number of *in vitro* and *in vivo* systems including the Ames test, the AS52/XPRT Mammalian Cell Forward Gene Mutation assay and the CHO test, and non-clastogenic in the mouse PCE test.

Carcinogenicity

No animal studies have been conducted.

Antigenicity

BOTOX showed antigenicity in mice only in the presence of adjuvant. BOTOX was found to be slightly antigenic in the guinea pig.

Blood compatibility

No haemolysis was detected up to 100 Units/ml of BOTOX in normal human blood.

6. PHARMACEUTICAL PARTICULARS

6.1 List of excipients

Human albumin

Sodium chloride

6.2 Incompatibilities

In the absence of compatibility studies, this medicinal product should not be mixed with other medicinal products.

6.3 Shelf life

3 years.

After reconstitution, stability has been demonstrated for 24 hours at 2°C – 8°C.

6.4 Special precautions for storage

Store in a refrigerator (2°C-8°C), or store in a freezer (at or below -5°C).

For storage conditions of the reconstituted medicinal product see section 6.3.

From a microbiological point of view, the product should be used immediately. If not used immediately, in-use storage times and conditions prior to use are the responsibility of the user and would normally not be longer than 24 hours at 2°C to 8°C (see also section 6.6).

6.5 Nature and contents of container

Clear glass vial, with rubber stopper and tamper-proof aluminium seal, containing white powder for solution for injection.

Pack size:

- Carton comprising one 50 Allergan Unit vial and package leaflet.
- Packs containing one, two, three or six cartons.

Not all pack sizes may be marketed.

6.6 Special precautions for disposal and other handling

BOTOX is reconstituted prior to use with sterile unpreserved normal saline (0.9% sodium chloride for injection). It is good practice to perform vial reconstitution and syringe preparation over plastic-lined paper towels to catch any spillage. An appropriate amount of diluent (see dilution table below) is drawn up into a syringe. The exposed portion of the rubber septum of the vial is cleaned with alcohol (70%) prior to insertion of the needle. Since BOTOX is denatured by bubbling or similar violent agitation, the diluent should be injected gently into the vial. Discard the vial if a vacuum does not pull the diluent into the vial. Reconstituted BOTOX is a clear colourless to slightly yellow solution free of particulate matter. When reconstituted, BOTOX may be stored in a refrigerator (2-8°C) for up to 24 hours prior to use. After this period used or unused vials should be discarded.

Each vial is for single use only.

Dilution table: Diluent added	Resulting dose in units per 0.1 ml
0.5 ml	10 Units
1 ml	5 Units
2 ml	2.5 Units
4 ml	1.25 Units

The 'unit' by which the potency of preparations of BOTOX is measured should be used to calculate dosages of BOTOX only and is not transferable to other preparations of botulinum toxin.

An injection volume of approximately 0.1 ml is recommended. A decrease or increase in the BOTOX dose is possible by administering a smaller or larger injection volume. The smaller the injection volume the less discomfort and less spread of toxin in the injected muscle occurs. This is of benefit in reducing effects on nearby muscles when small muscle groups are being injected.

For safe disposal, unused vials should be reconstituted with a small amount of water then autoclaved. Any used vials, syringes, and spillages etc. should be autoclaved, or the residual BOTOX inactivated using dilute hypochlorite solution (0.5%).

Any unused product or waste material should be disposed of in accordance with local requirements.

7. MARKETING AUTHORISATION HOLDER

Allergan Ltd.,
Marlow International,
The Parkway, Marlow,
Bucks, SL7 1YL, UK

8. MARKETING AUTHORISATION NUMBER(S)

PL 00426/0118

9. DATE OF FIRST AUTHORISATION/RENEWAL OF THE AUTHORISATION

21/09/2007

10. DATE OF REVISION OF THE TEXT

21/09/2007

Brevinor Tablets

(Pharmacia Limited)

1. NAME OF THE MEDICINAL PRODUCT

Brevinor.

2. QUALITATIVE AND QUANTITATIVE COMPOSITION

Each tablet contains 0.5 milligrams norethisterone and 35 micrograms ethinylestradiol.

3. PHARMACEUTICAL FORM

Blue, flat, circular, bevel-edged tablet inscribed 'SEARLE' on one side and 'BX' on the other side.

4. CLINICAL PARTICULARS

4.1 Therapeutic indications

Brevinor is indicated for oral contraception, with the benefit of a low intake of oestrogen.

4.2 Posology and method of administration

Oral Administration: The dosage of Brevinor for the initial cycle of therapy is 1 tablet taken at the same time each day from the first day of the menstrual cycle. For subsequent cycles, no tablets are taken for 7 days, then a new course is started of 1 tablet daily for the next 21 days. This sequence of 21 days on treatment, seven days off treatment is repeated for as long as contraception is required.

Patients unable to start taking Brevinor tablets on the first day of the menstrual cycle may start treatment on any day up to and including the 5th day of the menstrual cycle.

Patients starting on day 1 of their period will be protected at once. Those patients delaying therapy up to day 5 may not be protected immediately and it is recommended that another method of contraception is used for the first 7 days of tablet-taking. Suitable methods are condoms, caps plus spermicides and intra-uterine devices. The rhythm, temperature and cervical-mucus methods should not be relied upon.

Tablet omissions

Tablets must be taken daily in order to maintain adequate hormone levels and contraceptive efficacy.

If a tablet is missed within 12 hours of the correct dosage time then the missed tablet should be taken as soon as possible, even if this means taking 2 tablets on the same day, this will ensure that contraceptive protection is maintained. If one or more tablets are missed for more than 12 hours from the correct dosage time it is recommended that the patient takes the last missed tablet as soon as possible and then continues to take the rest of the tablets in the normal manner. In addition, it is recommended that extra contraceptive protection, such as a condom, is used for the next 7 days.

Patients who have missed one or more of the last 7 tablets in a pack should be advised to start the next pack of tablets as soon as the present one has finished (i.e. without the normal seven day gap between treatments). This reduces the risk of contraceptive failure resulting from tablets being missed close to a 7 day tablet free period.

Changing from another oral contraceptive

In order to ensure that contraception is maintained it is advised that the first dose of Brevinor tablets is taken on the day immediately after the patient has finished the previous pack of tablets.

Use after childbirth, miscarriage or abortion

Providing the patient is not breast feeding the first dose of Brevinor tablets should be taken on the 21st day after childbirth. This will ensure the patient is protected immediately. If there is any delay in taking the first dose, contraception may not be established until 7 days after the first tablet has been taken. In these circumstances patients should be advised that extra contraceptive methods will be necessary.

After a miscarriage or abortion patients can take the first dose of Brevinor tablets on the next day; in this way they will be protected immediately.

4.3 Contraindications

As with all combined progestogen/oestrogen oral contraceptives, the following conditions should be regarded as contra-indications:

i. History of confirmed venous thromboembolic disease (VTE), family history of idiopathic VTE and other known risk factors of VTE

ii. Thrombophlebitis, cerebrovascular disorders, coronary artery disease, myocardial infarction, angina, hyperlipidaemia or a history of these conditions.

iii. Acute or severe chronic liver disease, including liver tumours, Dubin-Johnson or Rotor syndrome.

iv. History during pregnancy of idiopathic jaundice, severe pruritus or pemphigoid gestationis.

v. Known or suspected breast or genital cancer.

vi. Known or suspected oestrogen-dependent neoplasia.

vii. Undiagnosed abnormal vaginal bleeding.

viii. A history of migraines classified as classical focal or crescendo.

ix. Pregnancy.

4.4 Special warnings and precautions for use

Assessment of women prior to starting oral contraceptives (and at regular intervals thereafter) should include a personal and family medical history of each woman. Physical examination should be guided by this and by the contraindications (section 4.3) and warnings (section 4.4) for this product. The frequency and nature of these assessments should be based upon relevant guidelines and should be adapted to the individual woman, but should include measurement of blood pressure and, if judged appropriate by the clinician, breast, abdominal and pelvic examination including cervical cytology.

Women taking oral contraceptives require careful observation if they have or have had any of the following conditions: breast nodules; fibrocystic disease of the breast or an abnormal mammogram; uterine fibroids; a history of severe depressive states; varicose veins; sickle-cell anaemia; diabetes; hypertension; cardiovascular disease; migraine; epilepsy; asthma; otosclerosis; multiple sclerosis; porphyria; tetany; disturbed liver functions; gallstones; kidney disease; chloasma; any condition that is likely to worsen during pregnancy. The worsening or first appearance of any of these conditions may indicate that the oral contraceptive should be stopped. Discontinue treatment if there is a gradual or sudden, partial or complete loss of vision or any evidence of ocular changes, onset or aggravation of migraine or development of headache of a new kind, which is recurrent, persistent or severe.

Gastro-intestinal upsets, such as vomiting and diarrhoea, may interfere with the absorption of the tablets leading to a reduction in contraceptive efficacy. Patients should continue to take Brevinor, but they should also be encouraged to use another contraceptive method during the period of gastro-intestinal upset and for the next 7 days.

Progestogen oestrogen preparations should be used with caution in patients with a history of hepatic dysfunction or hypertension.

An increased risk of venous thromboembolic disease (VTE) associated with the use of oral contraceptives is well established but is smaller than that associated with pregnancy, which has been estimated at 60 cases per 100,000 pregnancies. Some epidemiological studies have reported a greater risk of VTE for women using combined oral contraceptives containing desogestrel or gestodene (the so-called 'third generation' pills) than for women using pills containing levonorgestrel or norethisterone (the so-called 'second generation' pills

The spontaneous incidence of VTE in healthy non-pregnant women (not taking any oral contraceptive) is about 5 cases per 100,000 per year. The incidence in users of second generation pills is about 15 per 100,000 women per year of use. The incidence in users of third generation pills is about 25 cases per 100,000 women per year of use; this excess incidence has not been satisfactorily explained by bias or confounding. The level of all of these risks of VTE increases with age and is likely to be further increased in women with other known risk factors for VTE such as obesity. The excess risk of VTE is highest during the first year a woman ever uses a combined oral contraceptive.

Patients receiving oral contraceptives should be kept under regular surveillance, in view of the possibility of development of conditions such as thromboembolism.

The risk of coronary artery disease in women taking oral contraceptives is increased by the presence of other predisposing factors such as cigarette smoking, hypercholesterolaemia, obesity, diabetes, history of pre-eclamptic toxaemia and increasing age. After the age of thirty-five years, the patient and physician should carefully re-assess the risk/benefit ratio of using combined oral contraceptives as opposed to alternative methods of contraception.

Brevinor should be discontinued at least four weeks before, and for two weeks following, elective operations and during immobilisation. Patients undergoing injection treatment for varicose veins should not resume taking Brevinor until 3 months after the last injection.

Benign and malignant liver tumours have been associated with oral contraceptive use. The relationship between occurrence of liver tumours and use of female sex hormones is not known at present. These tumours may rupture causing intra-abdominal bleeding. If the patient presents with a mass or tenderness in the right upper quadrant or an acute abdomen, the possible presence of a tumour should be considered.

An increased risk of congenital abnormalities, including heart defects and limb defects, has been reported following the use of sex hormones, including oral contraceptives, in pregnancy. If the patient does not adhere to the prescribed schedule, the possibility of pregnancy should be considered at the time of the first missed period and further use of oral contraceptives should be withheld until pregnancy has been ruled out. It is recommended that for any patient who has missed two consecutive periods, pregnancy should be ruled out before continuing the contraceptive regimen. If pregnancy is confirmed the patient should be advised of the potential risks to the foetus and the advisability of continuing the pregnancy should be discussed in the light of these risks. It is advisable to discontinue Brevinor three months before a planned pregnancy.

The risk of arterial thrombosis associated with combined oral contraceptives increases with age, and this risk is aggravated by cigarette smoking. The use of combined oral contraceptives by women in the older age group, especially those who are cigarette smokers, should therefore be discouraged and alternative methods advised.

The use of this product in patients suffering from epilepsy, migraine, asthma or cardiac dysfunction may result in exacerbation of these disorders because of fluid retention. Caution should also be observed in patients who wear contact lenses.

Decreased glucose tolerance may occur in diabetic patients on this treatment, and their control must be carefully supervised.

The use of oral contraceptives has also been associated with a possible increased incidence of gall bladder disease.

Women with a history of oligomenorrhoea or secondary amenorrhoea or young women without regular cycles may have a tendency to remain anovulatory or to become amenorrhoeic after discontinuation of oral contraceptives. Women with these pre-existing problems should be advised of this possibility and encouraged to use other contraceptive methods.

Numerous epidemiological studies have been reported on the risks of ovarian, endometrial, cervical and breast cancer in women using combined oral contraceptives. The evidence is clear that combined oral contraceptives offer substantial protection against both ovarian and endometrial cancer.

Figure 1

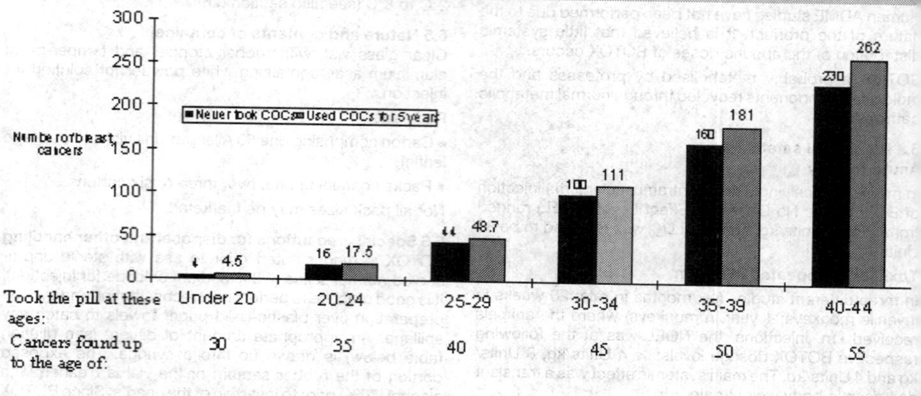

An increased risk of cervical cancer in long-term users of combined oral contraceptives has been reported in some studies, but there continues to be controversy about the extent to which this is attributable to the confounding effects of sexual behaviour and other factors.

A meta-analysis from 54 epidemiological studies reported that there is a slightly increased relative risk (RR = 1.24) of having breast cancer diagnosed in women who are currently using combined oral contraceptives (COCs). The observed pattern of increased risk may be due to an earlier diagnosis of breast cancer in COC users, the biological effects of COCs or a combination of both. The additional breast cancers diagnosed in current users of COCs or in women who have used COCs in the last ten years are more likely to be localised to the breast than those in women who never used COCs.

Breast cancer is rare among women under 40 years of age whether or not they take COCs. Whilst this background risk increases with age, the excess number of breast cancer diagnoses in current and recent COC users is small in relation to the overall risk of breast cancer (see bar chart).

The most important risk factor for breast cancer in COC users is the age women discontinue the COC; the older the age at stopping, the more breast cancers are diagnosed. Duration of use is less important and the excess risk gradually disappears during the course of the 10 years after stopping COC use such that by 10 years there appears to be no excess.

The possible increase in risk of breast cancer should be discussed with the user and weighed against the benefits of COCs taking into account the evidence that they offer substantial protection against the risk of developing certain other cancers (e.g. ovarian and endometrial cancer).

Estimated cumulative numbers of breast cancers per 10,000 women diagnosed in 5 years of use and up to 10 years after stopping COCs, compared with numbers of breast cancers diagnosed in 10,000 women who had never used COCs.

(see Figure 1 above)

4.5 Interaction with other medicinal products and other forms of interaction

The herbal remedy St John's wort (*Hypericum perforatum*) should not be taken concomitantly with this medicine as this could potentially lead to a loss of contraceptive effect.

Some drugs may modify the metabolism of Brevinor reducing its effectiveness; these include certain sedatives, antibiotics, anti-epileptic and anti-arthritic drugs. During the time such agents are used concurrently, it is advised that mechanical contraceptives also be used.

The results of a large number of laboratory tests have been shown to be influenced by the use of oestrogen containing oral contraceptives, which may limit their diagnostic value. Among these are: biochemical markers of thyroid and liver function; plasma levels of carrier proteins, triglycerides, coagulation and fibrinolysis factors.

4.6 Pregnancy and lactation

Contra-indicated in pregnancy.

Patients who are fully breast-feeding should not take Brevinor tablets since, in common with other combined oral contraceptives, the oestrogen component may reduce the amount of milk produced. In addition, active ingredients or their metabolites have been detected in the milk of mothers taking oral contraceptives. The effect of Brevinor on breast-fed infants has not been determined.

4.7 Effects on ability to drive and use machines

None.

4.8 Undesirable effects

As with all oral contraceptives, there may be slight nausea at first, weight gain or breast discomfort, which soon disappear.

Other side-effects known or suspected to occur with oral contraceptives include gastro-intestinal symptoms, changes in libido and appetite, headache, exacerbation of existing uterine fibroid disease, depression, and changes in carbohydrate, lipid and vitamin metabolism.

Spotting or bleeding may occur during the first few cycles. Usually menstrual bleeding becomes light and occasionally there may be no bleeding during the tablet-free days.

Hypertension, which is usually reversible on discontinuing treatment, has occurred in a small percentage of women taking oral contraceptives.

4.9 Overdose

Overdosage may be manifested by nausea, vomiting, breast enlargement and vaginal bleeding. There is no specific antidote and treatment should be symptomatic. Gastric lavage may be employed if the overdose is large and the patient is seen sufficiently early (within four hours).

5. PHARMACOLOGICAL PROPERTIES

5.1 Pharmacodynamic properties

The mode of action of Brevinor is similar to that of other progestogen/oestrogen oral contraceptives and includes the inhibition of ovulation, the thickening of cervical mucus so as to constitute a barrier to sperm and the rendering of the endometrium unreceptive to implantation. Such activity is exerted through a combined effect on one or more of the following: hypothalamus, anterior pituitary, ovary, endometrium and cervical mucus.

5.2 Pharmacokinetic properties

Norethisterone is rapidly and completely absorbed after oral administration, peak plasma concentrations occurring in the majority of subjects between 1 and 3 hours. Due to first-pass metabolism, blood levels after oral administration are 60% of those after i.v. administration. The half life of elimination varies from 5 to 12 hours, with a mean of 7.6 hours. Norethisterone is metabolised mainly in the liver. Approximately 60% of the administered dose is excreted as metabolites in urine and faeces.

Ethinylestradiol is rapidly and well absorbed from the gastro-intestinal tract but is subject to some first-pass metabolism in the gut-wall. Compared to many other oestrogens it is only slowly metabolised in the liver. Excretion is via the kidneys with some appearing also in the faeces.

5.3 Preclinical safety data

The toxicity of norethisterone is very low. Reports of teratogenic effects in animals are uncommon. No carcinogenic effects have been found even in long-term studies.

Long-term continuous administration of oestrogens in some animals increases the frequency of carcinoma of the breast, cervix, vagina and liver.

6. PHARMACEUTICAL PARTICULARS

6.1 List of excipients

Brevinor tablets contain:

Maize starch, polyvidone, magnesium stearate, lactose and E132.

6.2 Incompatibilities

None stated.

6.3 Shelf life

The shelf life of Brevinor tablets is 5 years.

6.4 Special precautions for storage

Store in a dry place, below 25°C, away from direct sunlight.

6.5 Nature and contents of container

Brevinor tablets are supplied in pvc/foil blister packs of 21 and 63 tablets.

6.6 Special precautions for disposal and other handling

None.

7. MARKETING AUTHORISATION HOLDER

Pharmacia Limited

Ramsgate Road

Sandwich

Kent CT13 9NJ, UK

8. MARKETING AUTHORISATION NUMBER(S)

PL 00032/0398

9. DATE OF FIRST AUTHORISATION/RENEWAL OF THE AUTHORISATION
27 June 2002

10. DATE OF REVISION OF THE TEXT
June 2007

Brevoxyl 4% Cream

(Stiefel Laboratories (UK) Limited)

1. NAME OF THE MEDICINAL PRODUCT
Brevoxyl 4% Cream

2. QUALITATIVE AND QUANTITATIVE COMPOSITION
Benzoyl peroxide 4%w/w as hydrous benzoyl peroxide Ph Eur

100g cream contains 4g benzoyl peroxide.

For excipients, see section 6.1

3. PHARMACEUTICAL FORM
Cream

A white to off white cream.

4. CLINICAL PARTICULARS
4.1 Therapeutic indications
Brevoxyl is indicated for the treatment of moderate acne vulgaris.

4.2 Posology and method of administration
Adolescents and Adults:

Apply to the whole of the affected area once or twice daily. Wash with soap and water prior to application.

Paediatric use:

The safety and efficacy of Brevoxyl has not been established in children since acne vulgaris rarely presents in this age group.

Initial application of the product may be varied at the physicians instructions to reflect the patients skin type and to avoid undesirable effects.

Improvement can generally be seen after 4-6 weeks of treatment. However, longer use may be necessary.

4.3 Contraindications
Patients with known hypersensitivity to any of the ingredients should not use the product.

4.4 Special warnings and precautions for use
Avoid contact with the eyes, mouth and other mucous membranes. Care should be taken when applying the product to the neck and other sensitive areas. Propylene glycol alginate may cause skin irritation. Stearyl alcohol and cetyl alcohol may cause local skin reaction (e.g. contact dermatitis).

It is recommended that exposure to sun or sunlamps should be minimised.

Simultaneous use of other keratolytics such as salicylates or sulphur may increase occurrence of skin irritation.

During the first weeks of treatment, a sudden increase in peeling and reddening will occur in most patients; this is not harmful and will normally subside in a day or two if treatment is temporarily discontinued.

The product may bleach hair and coloured or dyed fabrics.

4.5 Interaction with other medicinal products and other forms of interaction
Simultaneous application of Brevoxyl and topical acne preparations containing vitamin A derivatives should be avoided.

4.6 Pregnancy and lactation
The safety of Brevoxyl in human pregnancy is not established. During pregnancy and lactation Brevoxyl should be used only with special caution and after the physician's assessment of benefit and risk. In the last month of pregnancy Brevoxyl should not be used.

There is no knowledge about the excretion of Brevoxyl in breast milk.

4.7 Effects on ability to drive and use machines
Not relevant.

4.8 Undesirable effects
In normal use, a mild burning sensation will probably be felt on first application and a moderate reddening and peeling of the skin will occur within a few days. During the first few weeks of treatment, a sudden increase in peeling and reddening will occur in most patients; this is not harmful and will normally subside in a day or two if treatment is temporarily discontinued. The patient may also experience temporary pruritus, facial oedema, dermatitis or rash. As for other benzoyl peroxide preparations allergic contact dermatitis could occasionally occur.

4.9 Overdose
Not applicable.

5. PHARMACOLOGICAL PROPERTIES
5.1 Pharmacodynamic properties
ATC Code: D10A E01

Benzoyl peroxide is keratolytic and is an oxidising agent with antibacterial activity against Propionibacterium acnes, the organism implicated in acne vulgaris. It has keratolytic activity and is sebostatic, counteracting the hyperkeratinisation and excessive sebum production associated with acne.

5.2 Pharmacokinetic properties
After topical application, benzoyl peroxide is absorbed in varying quantities through the skin of man and animals.

Radio-labelled studies have shown that absorption of benzoyl peroxide through the skin can only occur following its conversion to benzoic acid. Benzoic acid is mostly conjugated to form hippuric acid which is excreted via the kidneys.

5.3 Preclinical safety data
Animal toxicity studies of benzoyl peroxide have shown that the compound is non-toxic when applied topically.

Benzoic acid, to which benzoyl peroxide is converted prior to absorption, has a wide margin of safety. Benzoic acid is an approved food additive.

Benzoyl peroxide is a free radical generating compound. The release of oxygen during its conversion to benzoic acid may be implicated in a tumour promoting effect seen in mouse skin.

Benzoyl peroxide at high doses (>20 times the normal human dose) has been shown to increase tumour growth initiated by dimethyl benzanthracene (DMBA) in mice. DMBA is a powerful chemical carcinogen to which patients are unlikely to be exposed. The relevance of these results to man is limited. Studies in mice have also shown that benzoyl peroxide does not increase the growth of tumours initiated by ultra violet light.

No reproductive toxicology studies have been performed. Up to date there are no indications that the topical use of Brevoxyl causes damage to the unborn child.

6. PHARMACEUTICAL PARTICULARS
6.1 List of excipients
Cetyl alcohol

Promulgen G (Stearyl alcohol and Macrogol cetostearyl ether)

Simethicone emulsion

Propylene glycol alginate

Dimethyl isosorbide

Fragrance X-23304

Purified water

6.2 Incompatibilities
Not applicable

6.3 Shelf life
2 years

6.4 Special precautions for storage
Do not store above 25°C.

6.5 Nature and contents of container
Lacquered aluminium or laminated (aluminium/plastic) tubes with white polypropylene screw caps.

Licensed pack sizes: 6g, 40g and 50g.

6.6 Special precautions for disposal and other handling
No special requirements.

7. MARKETING AUTHORISATION HOLDER
Stiefel Laboratories (UK) Ltd

Holtspur Lane

Wooburn Green

High Wycombe

Bucks HP10 0AU

8. MARKETING AUTHORISATION NUMBER(S)
PL 00174/0193

9. DATE OF FIRST AUTHORISATION/RENEWAL OF THE AUTHORISATION
29 May 1996/ 28 May 2006

10. DATE OF REVISION OF THE TEXT
28/05/06

Bricanyl Injection, 0.5 mg/ml, solution for injection or infusion

(AstraZeneca UK Limited)

1. NAME OF THE MEDICINAL PRODUCT
Bricanyl® Injection, 0.5 mg/ml, solution for injection or infusion.

2. QUALITATIVE AND QUANTITATIVE COMPOSITION
Terbutaline sulphate 0.5 mg/ml.

For excipients see Section 6.1.

3. PHARMACEUTICAL FORM
Solution for injection or infusion.

A clear aqueous solution.

4. CLINICAL PARTICULARS
4.1 Therapeutic indications
Bronchodilation

Terbutaline is a selective β_2-adrenergic agonist recommended for the relief of bronchospasm in bronchial asthma and other bronchopulmonary disorders in which bronchospasm is a complicating factor.

For the management of uncomplicated premature labour

To arrest labour between 24 and 33 weeks of gestation in patients with no medical or obstetric contraindication to tocolytic therapy. The main effect of tocolytic therapy is a delay in delivery of up to 48 hours; no statistically significant effect on perinatal mortality or morbidity has as yet been observed in randomised, controlled trials. The greatest benefit from tocolytic therapy is gained by using the delay in delivery to administer glucocorticoids or to implement other measures known to improve perinatal health.

4.2 Posology and method of administration
Routes of administration

Parenteral - subcutaneous, intramuscular, intravenous.

The dosage should be individualised.

For bronchodilation

When a rapid therapeutic response is required, Bricanyl can be administered by any of the three standard parenteral routes: subcutaneous, intramuscular, or i.v. bolus. The preferred routes will usually be subcutaneous or intramuscular. When given as an i.v. bolus the injection must be made slowly noting patient response.

Adults:0.5 - 1 ml (0.25 - 0.5 mg) up to four times a day.

Children 2 - 15 years: 0.01 mg/kg body weight to a maximum of 0.3 mg total.

Age	Average weight		mg	ml
	kg	(lb)	terbutaline	volume
<3	10	(22)	0.1	0.2
3	15	(33)	0.15	0.3
6	20	(44)	0.2	0.4
8	25	(55)	0.25	0.5
10+	30+	(66+)	0.3	0.6

By infusion: 3 - 5 ml (1.5 - 2.5 mg) in 500 ml 5% dextrose, saline or dextrose/saline given by continuous intravenous infusion at a rate of 10 - 20 drops (0.5 - 1 ml) per minute for 8 to 10 hours. A corresponding reduction in dosage should be made for children.

Elderly: Dosage as for adults.

For the management of premature labour

Procedure: To be administered as early as possible after the diagnosis of premature labour, and after evaluation of the patient to rule out contraindications to the use of terbutaline (*see Section 4.3, Contraindications*).

Initially, 5 mcg/min should be infused during the first 20 minutes increasing by 2.5 mcg/min at 20 minute intervals until the contractions stop. More than 10 mcg/min should seldom be given, 20 mcg/min should not be exceeded.

The infusion should be stopped if labour progresses despite treatment at the maximum dose.

If successful, the infusion should continue for 1 hour at the chosen rate and then be decreased by 2.5 mcg/min every 20 minutes to the lowest dose that produces suppression of contractions. Keep the infusion at this rate for 12 hours and then continue with oral maintenance therapy.

As an alternative, subcutaneous injections of 250 mcg should be given four times a day for a few days before oral treatment is commenced. Oral treatment may be continued for as long as the physician considers it desirable to prolong pregnancy.

Special cautions for infusion: The dose must be individually titrated with reference to suppression of contractions, increase in pulse rate and changes in blood pressure, which are limiting factors. These parameters should be carefully monitored during treatment. A maternal heart rate of more than 135 beats/min should be avoided.

Careful control of the level of hydration is essential to avoid the risk of maternal pulmonary oedema (*see Section 4.8, Undesirable effects*). The volume of fluid in which the drug is administered should thus be kept to a minimum. A controlled infusion device should be used, preferably a syringe pump.

Dilution:

The recommended infusion fluid is 5% dextrose. If a syringe pump is available, the concentration of the drug infused should be 0.1 mg/ml (10 ml Bricanyl Injection should be added to 40 ml of 5% dextrose).

At this dilution:

5 mcg/min ≡ 0.05 ml/min and

10 mcg/min ≡ 0.1 ml/min

If no syringe pump is available, the concentration of the drug should be 0.01 mg/ml (10 ml Bricanyl Injection should be added to 490 ml of 5% dextrose).

At this dilution:

5 mcg/min ≡ 0.5 ml/min and

10 mcg/min ≡ 1 ml/min.

4.3 Contraindications
Bricanyl solution for injection should not be used as a tocolytic agent in patients with pre-existing ischaemic

heart disease or those patients with significant risk factors for ischaemic heart disease.

Although Bricanyl solution for injection is used in the management of uncomplicated premature labour, use in the following conditions is contra-indicated:

- any condition of the mother or foetus in which prolongation of the pregnancy is hazardous, e.g. severe toxaemia, anti-partum haemorrhage, intra-uterine infection, intrauterine infection, severe preeclampsia, abruptio placentae, threatened abortion during the 1st and 2nd trimester, or cord compression.

Bricanyl solution for injection should not be used in patients with a history of hypersensitivity to any of the ingredients.

4.4 Special warnings and precautions for use

As for all beta$_2$-agonists caution should be observed in patients with thyrotoxicosis.

Cardiovascular effects may be seen with sympathomimetic drugs, including Bricanyl. There is some evidence from post-marketing data and published literature of myocardial ischaemia associated with beta agonists.

Due to the positive inotropic effect of the beta$_2$-agonists, these drugs should not be used in patients with hypertrophic cardiomyopathy.

Tocolysis

Bricanyl should be used with caution in tocolysis and supervision of cardiorespiratory function, including ECG monitoring, should be considered. Treatment should be discontinued if signs of myocardial ischaemia (such as chest pain or ECG changes) develop. Bricanyl should not be used as a tocolytic agent in patients with significant risk factors for or pre-existing heart disease (see section 4.3, Contraindications).

In premature labour in a patient with known or suspected cardiac disease, a physician experienced in cardiology should assess the suitability of treatment before intravenous infusion with Bricanyl.

In order to minimise the risk of hypotension associated with tocolytic therapy, special care should be taken to avoid caval compression by keeping the patient in the left or right lateral positions throughout the infusion.

In treatment of premature labour, hyperglycaemia and ketoacidosis have been found in pregnant women with diabetes after treatment with beta$_2$-agonists. It may therefore be necessary to adjust the insulin dose when beta$_2$-agonists are used in the treatment.

Increased tendency to uterine bleeding has been reported in connection with Caesarian section. However, this can be effectively stopped by propranolol 1-2 mg injected intravenously.

Respiratory indications

Patients with underlying severe heart disease (e.g. ischaemic heart disease, arrhythmia or severe heart failure) who are receiving Bricanyl should be warned to seek medical advice if they experience chest pain or other symptoms of worsening heart disease.

Attention should be paid to assessment of symptoms such as dyspnoea and chest pain, as they may be of either respiratory or cardiac origin.

Due to the hyperglycaemic effects of beta$_2$-agonists, additional blood glucose controls are recommended initially in diabetic patients.

Potentially serious hypokalaemia may result from beta$_2$-agonist therapy. Particular caution is recommended in acute severe asthma as the associated risk may be augmented by hypoxia. The hypokalaemic effect may be potentiated by concomitant treatments (see section 4.5, Interactions). It is recommended that serum potassium levels are monitored in such situations.

If a previously effective dosage regimen no longer gives the same symptomatic relief, the patient should urgently seek further medical advice. Consideration should be given to the requirements for additional therapy (including increased dosages of anti-inflammatory medication). Severe exacerbations of asthma should be treated as an emergency in the usual manner.

4.5 Interaction with other medicinal products and other forms of interaction

Beta-blocking agents (including eye drops), especially the non-selective ones such as propranolol, may partially or totally inhibit the effect of beta-stimulants. Therefore, Bricanyl preparations and non-selective beta-blockers should not normally be administered concurrently. Bricanyl should be used with caution in patients receiving other sympathomimetics.

Hypokalaemia may result from beta$_2$-agonist therapy and may be potentiated by concomitant treatment with xanthine derivatives, corticosteroids and diuretics (*see Section 4.4, Special Warnings and Precautions for use*).

4.6 Pregnancy and lactation

Although no teratogenic effects have been observed in animals or in patients, Bricanyl should only be administered with caution in patients during the first trimester of pregnancy.

Terbutaline is secreted into breast milk, but any effects on the infant are unlikely at therapeutic doses.

Transient hypoglycaemia has been reported in newborn preterm infants after maternal beta$_2$-agonist treatment.

Table 1 Bronchial asthma. Chronic bronchitis, emphysema and other lung diseases where bronchospasm is a complicating factor.

Frequency Classification	Adverse Drug Reaction System Organ Class (SOC)	Preferred term (PT)
Very Common (>1/10)	Nervous System Disorders	Tremor Headache
Common (>1/100, <1/10)	Cardiac Disorders	Tachycardia Palpitations
	Musculoskeletal and Connective Tissue Disorders #	Muscle spasms
	Metabolism and Nutrition Disorders	Hypokalaemia (see section 4.4)
Not Known ^	Cardiac Disorders	Arrhythmias, e.g. atrial fibrillation, supraventricular tachycardia and extrasystoles Myocardial ischaemia (see section 4.4)
	Vascular Disorders	Peripheral vasodilation
	Immune System Disorders	Hypersensitivity reactions including angioedema, bronchospasm, hypotension and collapse
	Gastrointestinal Disorders	Nausea Mouth and throat irritation
	Psychiatric Disorders	Sleep disorder and Behavioural disturbances, such as agitation and restlessness
	Respiratory, Thoracic and Mediastinal Disorders	Paradoxical bronchospasm*
	Skin and Subcutaneous Tissue Disorders	Urticaria Rash

A few patients feel tense; this is also due to the effects on skeletal muscle and not to direct CNS stimulation.

^ Reported spontaneously in post-marketing data and therefore frequency regarded as unknown

* In rare cases, through unspecified mechanisms, paradoxical bronchospasm may occur, with wheezing immediately after inhalation. This should be immediately treated with a rapid-onset bronchodilator. Bricanyl therapy should be discontinued and after assessment, an alternative therapy initiated.

4.7 Effects on ability to drive and use machines

Bricanyl does not affect the ability to drive or use machines.

4.8 Undesirable effects

The intensity of the adverse reactions depends on dosage and route of administration. An initial dose titration will often reduce the adverse reactions. Most of the adverse reactions are characteristic of sympathomimetic amines. The majority of these effects have reversed spontaneously within the first 1-2 weeks of treatment.

The frequency of side effects is low at the recommended doses.

Adverse events are listed below by system organ class and frequency. Frequencies are defined as: very common (>1/10), common (>1/100 and <1/10), uncommon (>1/1,000 and <1/100), rare (>1/10,000 and <1/1,000), very rare (<1/10,000) and not known (cannot be estimated from the available data).

Bronchial asthma. Chronic bronchitis, emphysema and other lung diseases where bronchospasm is a complicating factor.

(see Table 1 above)

Preterm labour

(see Table 2 on next page)

During treatment of preterm labour, when high doses of Bricanyl are used, diabetic mothers may develop hyperglycaemia and lactacidosis. In these patients glucose and acid-base balance should be carefully monitored. High doses of beta$_2$-stimulants may cause hypokalaemia as a result of redistribution of potassium. Symptoms of pulmonary oedema have also been reported following treatment of preterm labour, in some cases this has proved fatal. Predisposing factors include fluid overload, multiple pregnancy, pre-existing cardiac disease and maternal infection. Close monitoring of the patient's state of hydration is essential. If signs of pulmonary oedema develop (e.g. cough, shortness of breath), treatment should be discontinued immediately and diuretic therapy instituted.

An increased tendency to bleeding has been described in connection with caesarean section (give propranolol, 1-2 mg i.v.) in patients treated with Bricanyl for preterm labour

4.9 Overdose

i) Possible symptoms and signs: Headache, anxiety, tremor, nausea, tonic cramp, palpitations, tachycardia and arrhythmia. A fall in blood pressure sometimes occurs. Laboratory findings: hypokalaemia, hyperglycaemia and lactic acidosis sometimes occur.

ii) Treatment:

Mild and moderate cases: Reduce the dose.

Severe cases: Determination of acid-base balance, blood sugar and electrolytes, particularly serum potassium levels. Monitoring of heart rate and rhythm and blood pressure. Metabolic changes should be corrected. A cardioselective beta-blocker (e.g. metoprolol) is recommended for the treatment of arrhythmias causing haemodynamic deterioration. The beta-blocker should be used with care because of the possibility of inducing bronchoconstriction: use with caution in patients with a history of bronchospasm. If the beta$_2$-mediated reduction in peripheral vascular resistance significantly contributes to the fall in blood pressure, a volume expander should be given.

In preterm labour:

Pulmonary oedema: discontinue administration of Bricanyl. A normal dose of loop diuretic (e.g. frusemide) should be given intravenously.

Increased bleeding in connection with Caesarean section: propranolol, 1 - 2 mg intravenously.

5. PHARMACOLOGICAL PROPERTIES

5.1 Pharmacodynamic properties

Pharmaco-therapeutic group: selective beta$_2$-agonist, terbutaline, ATC code: R03C C03.

Terbutaline is a selective beta$_2$-adrenergic stimulant, having the following pharmacological effects:

i) In the lung: bronchodilation; increase in mucociliary clearance; suppression of oedema and anti-allergic effects.

ii) In skeletal muscle: stimulates Na^+/K^+ transport and also causes depression of subtetanic contractions in slow-contracting muscle.

iii) In uterine muscle: inhibition of uterine contractions.

iv) In the CNS: low penetration into the blood-brain barrier at therapeutic doses, due to the highly hydrophilic nature of the molecule.

v) In the CVS: administration of terbutaline results in cardiovascular effects mediated through β_2-receptors in the peripheral arteries and in the heart e.g. in healthy subjects, 0.25 - 0.5 mg injected s.c is associated with an increase in cardiac output (up to 85% over controls) due to an increase in heart rate and a larger stroke volume. The increase in heart rate is probably due to a combination of a reflex tachycardia, via a fall in peripheral resistance and a direct positive chronotropic effect of the drug.

5.2 Pharmacokinetic properties

Basic parameters have been evaluated in man after i.v. and oral administration of therapeutic doses, e.g.

i.v. single dose

Volume of distribution (VSS) -	114 L
Total body clearance (CL) -	213 ml/min
Mean residence time (MRT) -	9.0 h
Renal clearance (CLR) -	149 ml/min (males)

Table 2 Preterm labour

Frequency Classification	Adverse Drug Reaction System Organ Class (SOC)	Preferred term (PT)
Very Common (>1/10)	Cardiac Disorders	Tachycardia
	Nervous System Disorders	Tremor Headache
	Gastrointestinal Disorders	Nausea
Common (>1/100, <1/10)	Cardiac Disorders	Palpitations
	Metabolism and Nutrition Disorders	Hypokalaemia (see section 4.4)
Not Known ^	Blood and Lymphatic System Disorders	An increased tendency to bleeding in connection with caesarean section
	Vascular Disorders	Peripheral vasodilation
	Immune System Disorders	Hypersensitivity reactions including angioedema, bronchospasm, hypotension and collapse
	Cardiac Disorders	Arrhythmias, e.g. atrial fibrillation, supraventricular tachycardia and extrasystoles Myocardial ischaemia (see section 4.4)
	Respiratory, Thoracic and Mediastinal Disorders	Symptoms of pulmonary oedema Paradoxical bronchospasm*
	Gastrointestinal Disorders	Mouth and throat irritation
	Psychiatric Disorders	Sleep disorder and Behavioural disturbances, such as agitation and restlessness
	Nervous System Disorders	Hyperactivity
	Metabolism and Nutrition Disorders	Hyperglycaemia Hyperlactacidaemia
	Skin and Subcutaneous Tissue Disorders	Urticaria Rash
	Musculoskeletal and Connective Tissue Disorders #	Muscle spasms

A few patients feel tense; this is also due to the effects on skeletal muscle and not to direct CNS stimulation.

^ Reported spontaneously in post-marketing data and therefore frequency regarded as unknown

* In rare cases, through unspecified mechanisms, paradoxical bronchospasm may occur, with wheezing immediately after inhalation. This should be immediately treated with a rapid-onset bronchodilator. Bricanyl therapy should be discontinued and after assessment, an alternative therapy initiated.

Oral dose

Renal clearance (CLR) - 1.925 ml/min (males)

Renal clearance (CLR) - 2.32 ml/min (females)

The plasma concentration/time curve after i.v. administration is characterised by a fast distribution phase, an intermediate elimination phase and a late elimination phase.

Terminal half-life ($t_{1/2}$) has been determined after single and multiple dosing (mean values varied between 16 - 20 h).

Bioavailability

Food reduces bioavailability following oral dosing (10% on average); fasting values of 14 - 15% have been obtained.

Metabolism

The main metabolite after oral dosing is the sulphate conjugate and also some glucuronide conjugate can be found in the urine.

5.3 Preclinical safety data

The major toxic effect of terbutaline, observed in toxicological studies in rats and dogs at exposures in excess of maximum human exposure, is focal myocardial necrosis. This type of cardiotoxicity is a well known pharmacological manifestation seen after the administration of high doses of $beta_2$-agonists.

In rats, an increase in the incidence of benign uterine leiomyomas has been observed. This effect is looked upon as a class-effect observed in rodents after long term exposure to high doses of $beta_2$-agonists

6. PHARMACEUTICAL PARTICULARS

6.1 List of excipients

Sodium chloride, hydrochloric acid and water for injection.

6.2 Incompatibilities

Bricanyl solution for injection should not be mixed with alkaline solutions, i.e. solutions with a pH higher than 7.0.

6.3 Shelf life

24 months

6.4 Special precautions for storage

Do not store above 25°C. Keep in the outer carton.

6.5 Nature and contents of container

Packs of 5 × 1ml glass ampoules

Packs of 10 × 5ml glass ampoules

6.6 Special precautions for disposal and other handling

Bronchodilation: the recommended diluent is 5% dextrose, saline or dextrose/saline.

In the management of premature labour, the recommended infusion fluid is 5% dextrose. Saline should be avoided due to the risk of pulmonary oedema. If saline is used, the patient should be carefully monitored.

7. MARKETING AUTHORISATION HOLDER

AstraZeneca UK Ltd.,

600 Capability Green,

Luton, LU1 3LU, UK.

8. MARKETING AUTHORISATION NUMBER(S)

PL 17901/0112

9. DATE OF FIRST AUTHORISATION/RENEWAL OF THE AUTHORISATION

7th May 2002 / 12th May 2007

10. DATE OF REVISION OF THE TEXT

30th March 2009

Bricanyl Respules

(AstraZeneca UK Limited)

1. NAME OF THE MEDICINAL PRODUCT

Bricanyl® Respules®

2. QUALITATIVE AND QUANTITATIVE COMPOSITION

Terbutaline sulphate 2.5mg/ml.

Each single dose respule contains 2ml (5mg).

For excipients see Section 6.1.

3. PHARMACEUTICAL FORM

Nebuliser Solution.

A clear, aqueous, isotonic solution.

4. CLINICAL PARTICULARS

4.1 Therapeutic indications

Terbutaline is a selective $beta_2$-adrenergic agonist recommended for the relief of severe bronchospasm in bronchial asthma and in chronic bronchitis and other bronchopulmonary disorders in which bronchospasm is a complicating factor.

4.2 Posology and method of administration

In most patients, the use of terbutaline sulphate, based on the doses below, given 2-4 times daily will be sufficient to relieve bronchospasm. In acute, severe asthma, additional doses may be necessary.

Bricanyl Respules:

Adults: 1 or 2 Respules (5 or 10mg)

Children: (>25kg) 1 Respule (5mg)

Children: (<25kg) use multidose bottles.

Multidose Bottles:

Adults: 0.5 to 1 ml (5 to 10mg) diluted to required nebuliser volume with sterile physiological saline.

Children: 0.2 to 0.5ml (2 to 5mg), see table, diluted to required nebuliser volume with sterile physiological saline.

Table illustrating ml undiluted solution from multidose bottle required for administration to children

Age	Average kg	weight lb	mg terbutaline	ml undiluted solution
<3	10	22	2.0	0.2
3	15	33	3.0	0.3
6	20	44	4.0	0.4
8+	25+	55+	5.0	0.5

Elderly: Dosage as for adults.

Instructions for use and cleaning are provided in the Patient Information Leaflet which can be found in each pack.

4.3 Contraindications

Bricanyl preparations are contra-indicated in patients with a history of hypersensitivity to any of their constituents.

4.4 Special warnings and precautions for use

Patients should be instructed in proper use and their inhalation technique checked regularly.

If a previously effective dosage regimen no longer gives the same symptomatic relief, the patient should urgently seek further medical advice. Consideration should be given to the requirements for additional therapy (including increased dosages of anti-inflammatory medication). Severe exacerbations of asthma should be treated as an emergency in the usual manner.

As for all $beta_2$-agonists caution should be observed in patients with thyrotoxicosis.

Due to the positive inotropic effect of the $beta_2$-agonists, these drugs should not be used in patients with hypertrophic cardiomyopathy.

Cardiovascular effects may be seen with sympathomimetic drugs, including Bricanyl. There is some evidence from post-marketing data and published literature of rare occurrences of myocardial ischaemia associated with beta agonists. Patients with underlying severe heart disease (e.g. ischaemic heart disease, arrhythmia or severe heart failure) who are receiving Bricanyl should be warned to seek medical advice if they experience chest pain or other symptoms of worsening heart disease. Attention should be paid to assessment of symptoms such as dyspnoea and chest pain, as they may be of either respiratory or cardiac origin.

Due to the hyperglycaemic effects of $beta_2$-agonists, additional blood glucose controls are recommended initially in diabetic patients.

Potentially serious hypokalaemia may result from $beta_2$-agonist therapy. Particular caution is recommended in acute severe asthma as the associated risk may be augmented by hypoxia. The hypokalaemic effect may be potentiated by concomitant treatments (see section 4.5, Interactions). It is recommended that serum potassium levels are monitored in such situations.

4.5 Interaction with other medicinal products and other forms of interaction

Beta-blocking agents (including eye drops), especially the non-selective ones such as propranolol, may partially or totally inhibit the effect of beta-stimulants. Therefore, Bricanyl preparations and non-selective beta-blockers should not normally be administered concurrently. Bricanyl should be used with caution in patients receiving other sympathomimetics.

Hypokalaemia may result from $beta_2$-agonist therapy and may be potentiated by concomitant treatment with xanthine derivatives, corticosteroids and diuretics (see *Section 4.4, Special Warnings and Precautions for use*).

4.6 Pregnancy and lactation

Although no teratogenic effects have been observed in animals or in patients, Bricanyl should only be administered with caution during the first trimester of pregnancy.

Table 1

Frequency Classification	Adverse Drug Reaction	
	System Organ Class (SOC)	**Preferred term (PT)**
Very Common (>1/10)	Nervous System Disorders	Tremor Headache
Common (>1/100, <1/10)	Cardiac Disorders	Tachycardia Palpitations
	Musculoskeletal and Connective Tissue Disorders #	Muscle spasms
	Metabolism and Nutrition Disorders	Hypokalaemia (See section 4.4)
Not Known ^	Cardiac Disorders	Arrhythmias, e.g. atrial fibrillation, supraventricular tachycardia and extrasystoles Myocardial ischaemia (See section 4.4)
	Vascular Disorders	Peripheral vasodilation
	Immune System Disorders	Hypersensitivity reactions including angioedema, bronchospasm, hypotension and collapse
	Gastrointestinal Disorders	Nausea Mouth and throat irritation
	Psychiatric Disorders	Sleep disorder and Behavioural disturbances, such as agitation and restlessness
	Respiratory, Thoracic and Mediastinal Disorders	Paradoxical bronchospasm *
	Skin and Subcutaneous Tissue Disorders	Urticaria Rash

A few patients feel tense; this is also due to the effects on skeletal muscle and not to direct CNS stimulation.

^ Reported spontaneously in post-marketing data and therefore frequency regarded as unknown

* In rare cases, through unspecified mechanisms, paradoxical bronchospasm may occur, with wheezing immediately after inhalation. This should be immediately treated with a rapid-onset bronchodilator. Bricanyl therapy should be discontinued and after assessment, an alternative therapy initiated.

Terbutaline is secreted via breast milk, but effect on the infant is unlikely at therapeutic doses.

4.7 Effects on ability to drive and use machines
None Known

4.8 Undesirable effects
The frequency of adverse reactions is low at the recommended dose. Terbutaline given by inhalation is unlikely to produce significant systemic effects when given in recommended doses. Most of the adverse reactions are characteristic of sympathomimetic amines. The majority of these effects have reversed spontaneously within the first 1-2 weeks of treatment.

The frequency of side-effects is low at the recommended doses.

Adverse events are listed below by system organ class and frequency. Frequencies are defined as: very common (>1/10), common (>1/100 and <1/10), uncommon (>1/1,000 and <1/100), rare (>1/10,000 and <1/1,000), very rare (<1/10,000) and not known (cannot be estimated from the available data).

(see Table 1 above)

4.9 Overdose
i) Possible symptoms and signs
Headache, anxiety, tremor, nausea, tonic cramp, palpitations, tachycardia and arrhythmia. A fall in blood pressure sometimes occurs. Laboratory findings; hypokalaemia, hyperglycaemia and metabolic acidosis sometimes occur.

ii) Treatment
Mild and moderate cases: Reduce the dose.

Severe cases: Gastric lavage, administration of activated charcoal, (where suspected that significant amounts have been swallowed). Determination of acid-base balance, blood sugar and electrolytes, particularly serum potassium levels. Monitoring of heart rate and rhythm and blood pressure. Metabolic changes should be corrected. A cardioselective beta-blocker (e.g. metoprolol) is recommended for the treatment of arrhythmias causing haemodynamic deterioration. The beta-blocker should be used with care because of the possibility of inducing bronchoconstriction: use with caution in patients with a history of bronchospasm. If the beta-mediated reduction in peripheral vascular resistance significantly contributes to the fall in blood pressure, a volume expander should be given.

5. PHARMACOLOGICAL PROPERTIES

5.1 Pharmacodynamic properties
Pharmaco-therapeutic group: selective beta$_2$-agonist, terbutaline, ATC code: R03A C03.

Terbutaline is a selective beta$_2$-adrenergic stimulant, having the following pharmacological effects:-

i) In the lung: bronchodilation; increase in mucociliary clearance; suppression of oedema and anti-allergic effects.

ii) In skeletal muscle: stimulates Na^+/K^+ transport and also causes depression of subtetanic contractions in slow-contracting muscle.

iii) In uterine muscle: Inhibition of uterine contractions.

iv) In the C.N.S: Low penetration into the blood-brain barrier at therapeutic doses, due to the highly hydrophilic nature of the molecule.

v) In the C.V.S.: Administration of terbutaline results in cardiovascular effects mediated through beta$_2$-receptors in the peripheral arteries and in the heart e.g. in healthy subjects, 0.25 - 0.5 mg injected s.c., is associated with an increase in cardiac output (up to 85% over controls) due to an increase in heart rate and a larger stroke volume. The increase in heart rate is probably due to a combination of a reflex tachycardia, via a fall in peripheral resistance, and a direct positive chronotropic effect of the drug.

5.2 Pharmacokinetic properties
Basic parameters have been evaluated in man after i.v. and oral administration of therapeutic doses, e.g.

I.V. single dose
Volume distribution (VSS) - 114L

Total body clearance (CL) - 213 ml/min.

Mean residence time (MRT) - 9.0 h.

Renal clearance (CLR) - 149 ml/min.(males)

Oral dose
Renal clearance (CLR) - 1.925 ml/min. (males)

Renal clearance (CLR) - 2.32 ml/min. (females)

The plasma concentration/time curve after i.v. administration is characterised by a fast distribution phase, an intermediate elimination phase and a late elimination phase.

Terminal half-life $t_{½}$ has been determined after single and multiple dosing (mean values varied between 16-20 h.).

Bioavailability
Food reduces bioavailability following oral dosing (10% on average) fasting values of 14-15% have been obtained.

Metabolism
The main metabolite after oral dosing is the sulphate conjugate and also some glucoronide conjugate can be found in the urine.

5.3 Preclinical safety data
The major toxic effect of terbutaline, observed in toxicological studies in rats and dogs at exposures in excess of maximum human exposure, is focal myocardial necrosis. This type of cardiotoxicity is a well known pharmacological manifestation seen after the administration of high doses of beta$_2$-agonists.

In rats, an increase in the incidence of benign uterine leiomyomas has been observed. This effect is looked upon as a class-effect observed in rodents after long term exposure to high doses of beta$_2$-agonists

6. PHARMACEUTICAL PARTICULARS

6.1 List of excipients
Sodium chloride, disodium edetate, hydrochloric acid water for injections.

6.2 Incompatibilities
None known.

6.3 Shelf life
36 months

Single dose units in an opened foil envelope should be used within 3 months.

6.4 Special precautions for storage
Do not store above 30°C.

Store in the original container.

6.5 Nature and contents of container
Single dose, plastic units (Respules) in cartons of 20 Respules, as 4 strips of 5 units, each wrapped in a foil envelope.

6.6 Special precautions for disposal and other handling
Bricanyl Respules will not normally require dilution at recommended doses. The pH of Bricanyl Respules is 3-4.5.

If dilution is required use sterile normal saline.

7. MARKETING AUTHORISATION HOLDER
AstraZeneca UK Limited
600 Capability Green
Luton
LU1 3LU
United Kingdom

8. MARKETING AUTHORISATION NUMBER(S)
PL 17901/0114

9. DATE OF FIRST AUTHORISATION/RENEWAL OF THE AUTHORISATION
7th May 2002 / 12th May 2007

10. DATE OF REVISION OF THE TEXT
30th March 2009

Bricanyl Syrup

(AstraZeneca UK Limited)

1. NAME OF THE MEDICINAL PRODUCT
Bricanyl Syrup

2. QUALITATIVE AND QUANTITATIVE COMPOSITION
Terbutaline sulphate 0.3mg/ml.

For excipients see Section 6.1.

3. PHARMACEUTICAL FORM
Oral Solution.

Bricanyl syrup is a clear colourless raspberry flavoured oral solution.

4. CLINICAL PARTICULARS

4.1 Therapeutic indications
For bronchodilation

Terbutaline is a selective beta$_2$-adrenergic agonist recommended for the relief and prevention of bronchospasm in bronchial asthma and other bronchopulmonary disorders in which bronchospasm is a complicating factor.

For the management of uncomplicated premature labour.

4.2 Posology and method of administration
Use in bronchospasm

Bricanyl Syrup has a duration of action of 7 to 8 hours. The minimum recommended dosage interval is therefore 7 hours.

Adults: The starting dose should be 2 × 5ml spoonfuls 3 times in 24 hours. The dose may then be increased to 3 × 5ml spoonfuls 3 times in 24 hours if necessary to achieve adequate bronchodilation.

Elderly: Dosage as for Adults.

Children: The following dosage is recommended - 0.075mg (0.25ml)/kg body weight 3 times in a 24 hour period.

e.g.

Body weight (kg)	Dosage
14	3.5 ml × 3
16	4 ml × 3
18	4.5 ml × 3
20	5 ml × 3
24	6 ml × 3
28	7 ml × 3
32	8 ml × 3
36	9 ml × 3
40	10 ml × 3

Use in the management of premature labour.

Oral treatment should not be used initially in an attempt to arrest premature labour. After uterine contractions have been controlled by intravenous infusion of Bricanyl Injection, (see Bricanyl Injection Summary of Product Characteristics) or subcutaneous injections (0.25mg, 4 times in a 24 hour period for a few days) maintenance therapy can be continued with oral treatment (5mg, 3 times in a 24 hour period). Oral treatment may be continued for as long as the physician considers it desirable to prolong pregnancy.

4.3 Contraindications

Bricanyl Syrup should not be used as a tocolytic agent in patients with pre-existing ischaemic heart disease or those patients with significant risk factors for ischaemic heart disease.

Although Bricanyl Syrup is used in the management of uncomplicated premature labour, use in the following conditions is contra-indicated: -

- any condition of the mother or foetus in which prolongation of the pregnancy is hazardous, e.g. severe toxaemia, anti-partum haemorrhage, intra-uterine infection, severe pre-eclampsia, abruptio placentae, threatened abortion during the 1st and 2nd trimester, or cord compression.

Bricanyl Syrup should not be used in patients with a history of hypersensitivity to any of the ingredients.

4.4 Special warnings and precautions for use

As for all beta$_2$-agonists caution should be observed in patients with thyrotoxicosis.

Cardiovascular effects may be seen with sympathomimetic drugs, including Bricanyl. There is some evidence from post-marketing data and published literature of myocardial ischaemia associated with beta agonists.

Due to the positive inotropic effect of beta$_2$-agonists, these drugs should not be used in patients with hypertrophic cardiomyopathy.

Tocolysis

Bricanyl should be used with caution in tocolysis and supervision of cardiorespiratory function, including ECG monitoring, should be considered. Treatment should be discontinued if signs of myocardial ischaemia (such as chest pain or ECG changes) develop. Bricanyl should not be used as a tocolytic agent in patients with significant risk factors for or pre-existing heart disease (see section 4.3, Contraindications).

During infusion treatment in pregnant women with beta$_2$-stimulants in combination with corticosteroids a rare complication with a pathological picture resembling pulmonary oedema, has been reported.

Increased tendency to uterine bleeding has been reported in connection with Caesarean section. However, this can be effectively stopped by propranolol 1-2 mg injected intravenously.

Respiratory indications

Patients with underlying severe heart disease (e.g. ischaemic heart disease, arrhythmia or severe heart failure) who are receiving Bricanyl should be warned to seek medical advice if they experience chest pain or other symptoms of worsening heart disease.

Attention should be paid to assessment of symptoms such as dyspnoea and chest pain, as they may be of either respiratory or cardiac origin.

Due to the hyperglycaemic effects of beta$_2$-agonists, additional blood glucose controls are recommended initially in diabetic patients.

Potentially serious hypokalaemia may result from beta$_2$-agonist therapy. Particular caution is recommended in acute severe asthma as the associated risk may be augmented by hypoxia. The hypokalaemic effect may be potentiated by concomitant treatments (see section 4.5, Interactions). It is recommended that serum potassium levels are monitored in such situations.

If a previously effective dosage regimen no longer gives the same symptomatic relief, the patient should urgently seek further medical advice. Consideration should be given to the requirements for additional therapy (including increased dosages of anti-inflammatory medication). Severe exacerbations of asthma should be treated as an emergency in the usual manner.

4.5 Interaction with other medicinal products and other forms of interaction

Beta-blocking agents (including eye drops), especially the non-selective ones such as propranolol, may partially or totally inhibit the effect of beta-stimulants. Therefore Bricanyl preparations and non-selective beta-blockers should not normally be administered concurrently. Bricanyl should be used with caution in patients receiving other sympathomimetics.

Hypokalaemia may result from beta$_2$-agonist therapy and may be potentiated by concomitant treatment with xanthine derivatives, corticosteroids and diuretics (*see Section 4.4, Special Warnings and Precautions for use*).

4.6 Pregnancy and lactation

Although no teratogenic effects have been observed in animals or in patients, Bricanyl should only be administered with caution during the first trimester of pregnancy.

Terbutaline is secreted in breast milk, but effect on the infant is unlikely at therapeutic doses.

Table 1

Frequency Classification	Adverse Drug Reaction	
	System Organ Class (SOC)	Preferred term (PT)
Very Common (>1/10)	Nervous System Disorders	Tremor Headache
Common (>1/100, <1/10)	Cardiac Disorders	Tachycardia Palpitations
	Musculoskeletal and Connective Tissue Disorders #	Muscle spasms
	Metabolism and Nutrition Disorders	Hypokalaemia (See section 4.4)
Not Known ^	Cardiac Disorders	Arrhythmias, e.g. atrial fibrillation, supraventricular tachycardia and extrasystoles Myocardial ischaemia (See section 4.4)
	Vascular Disorders	Peripheral vasodilation
	Immune System Disorders	Hypersensitivity reactions including angioedema, bronchospasm, hypotension and collapse
	Gastrointestinal Disorders	Nausea Mouth and throat irritation
	Psychiatric Disorders	Sleep disorder and Behavioural disturbances, such as agitation and restlessness
	Respiratory, Thoracic and Mediastinal Disorders	Paradoxical bronchospasm *
	Skin and Subcutaneous Tissue Disorders	Urticaria Rash

A few patients feel tense; this is also due to the effects on skeletal muscle and not to direct CNS stimulation.

^ Reported spontaneously in post-marketing data and therefore frequency regarded as unknown

* In rare cases, through unspecified mechanisms, paradoxical bronchospasm may occur, with wheezing immediately after inhalation. This should be immediately treated with a rapid-onset bronchodilator. Bricanyl therapy should be discontinued and after assessment, an alternative therapy initiated.

Transient hypoglycaemia has been reported in newborn preterm infants after maternal beta$_2$-agonist treatment.

4.7 Effects on ability to drive and use machines

None Known.

4.8 Undesirable effects

The intensity of the adverse reactions depends on dosage and route of administration. Most of the adverse reactions are characteristic of sympathomimetic amines. The majority of these effects have reversed spontaneously within the first 1-2 weeks of treatment.

The frequency of side-effects is low at the recommended doses.

Adverse events are listed below by system organ class and frequency. Frequencies are defined as: very common (>1/10), common (>1/100 and <1/10), uncommon (>1/1,000 and <1/100), rare (>1/10,000 and <1/1,000), very rare (<1/10,000) and not known (cannot be estimated from the available data).

(see Table 1 above)

4.9 Overdose

Possible symptoms and signs

Headache, anxiety, tremor, nausea, tonic cramp, palpitations, tachycardia, arrhythmia. A fall in blood pressure sometimes occurs.

Laboratory findings; hypokalaemia, hyperglycaemia and lactic acidosis sometimes occur.

Treatment

Mild and moderate cases: Reduce the dose.

Severe cases: Gastric lavage, administration of activated charcoal. Determination of acid-base balance, blood sugar and electrolytes, particularly serum potassium levels. Monitoring of the heart rate and rhythm and blood pressure. Metabolic changes should be corrected.

A cardioselective beta-blocker (e.g. metoprolol) is recommended for the treatment of arrhythmias causing haemodynamic deterioration. The beta-blocker should be used with care because of the possibility of inducing bronchoconstriction: use with caution in patients with a history of bronchospasm. If the beta$_2$-mediated reduction in the peripheral vascular resistance significantly contributes to the fall in blood pressure, a volume expander should be given.

Preterm labour: Pulmonary oedema: discontinue administration of Bricanyl. A normal dose of loop diuretic (e.g. frusemide) should be given intravenously.

Increased bleeding in connection with Caesarian section: propranolol, 1-2mg intravenously.

5. PHARMACOLOGICAL PROPERTIES

5.1 Pharmacodynamic properties

Pharmaco-therapeutic group: selective beta$_2$-agonist, terbutaline ATC code:R03C C03.

Terbutaline is a selective beta$_2$ -adrenergic stimulant having the following pharmacological effects:-

i) *In the lung*: bronchodilation; increase in mucociliary clearance; suppression of oedema and anti-allergic effects.

ii) *In skeletal muscle*: stimulates Na^+/K^+transport and also causes depression of subtetanic contractions in slow-contracting muscle.

iii) *In uterine muscle*: inhibition of uterine contractions.

iv) *In the CNS*: low penetration into the blood-brain barrier at therapeutic doses, due to the highly hydrophilic nature of the molecule.

v) *In the CVS*: administration of terbutaline results in cardiovascular effects mediated through beta$_2$ -receptors in the peripheral arteries and in the heart e.g. in healthy subjects, 0.25 - 0.5mg injected s.c., is associated with an increase in cardiac output (up to 85% over controls) due to an increase in heart rate and a larger stroke volume. The increase in heart rate is probably due to a combination of a reflex tachycardia via a fall in peripheral resistance and a direct positive chronotropic effect of the drug.

5.2 Pharmacokinetic properties

Basic parameters have been evaluated in man after i.v and oral administration of therapeutic doses, e.g.

i.v. single dose.

Volume distribution (VSS): 114 L

Total body clearance (CL): 213 ml/min

Mean residence time (MRT): 9.0 h

Renal clearance (CLR): 149 ml/min (males)

Oral dose

renal clearance (CLR): 1.925/ml/min (males)

renal clearance (CLR): 2.32ml/min (females)

The plasma concentration/time curve after iv administration is characterised by a fast distribution phase, an intermediate elimination phase and a late elimination phase.

Terminal half-life T½ has been determined after single and multiple dosing (mean values varied between 16-20 h)

Bioavailability

Food reduces bioavailability following oral dosing (10% on average).

Fasting values of 14-15% have been obtained.

Metabolism

The main metabolite after oral dosing is the sulphate conjugate and also some glucoronide conjugate can be found in the urine.

5.3 Preclinical safety data

The major toxic effect of terbutaline, observed in toxicological studies in rats and dogs at exposures in excess of maximum human exposure, is focal myocardial necrosis. This type of cardiotoxicity is a well known pharmacological manifestation seen after the administration of high doses of $beta_2$-agonists.

In rats, an increase in the incidence of benign uterine leiomyomas has been observed. This effect is looked upon as a class-effect observed in rodents after long term exposure to high doses of $beta_2$-agonists

6. PHARMACEUTICAL PARTICULARS

6.1 List of excipients

Citric Acid, disodium edetate, ethanol, glycerol, sodium hydroxide, sorbitol, sodium benzoate, essence of raspberry, water.

6.2 Incompatibilities

None known.

6.3 Shelf life

4 years.

6.4 Special precautions for storage

Do not store above 25°C.

6.5 Nature and contents of container

Bottles of 100ml, 300ml and 1 litre.

6.6 Special precautions for disposal and other handling

Not applicable.

7. MARKETING AUTHORISATION HOLDER

AstraZeneca UK Ltd

600 Capability Green

Luton

LU1 3LU

United Kingdom

8. MARKETING AUTHORISATION NUMBER(S)

PL17901/0111

9. DATE OF FIRST AUTHORISATION/RENEWAL OF THE AUTHORISATION

7 May 2002 / 12 May 2007

10. DATE OF REVISION OF THE TEXT

30th March 2009

Bricanyl Tablets 5mg

(AstraZeneca UK Limited)

1. NAME OF THE MEDICINAL PRODUCT

Bricanyl® Tablets 5mg

2. QUALITATIVE AND QUANTITATIVE COMPOSITION

Each tablet contains 5mg terbutaline sulphate.

For excipients see Section 6.1.

3. PHARMACEUTICAL FORM

Tablet.

Off white, circular, biconvex tablet, engraved A/BT and scored on one side, symbol '5' on the reverse.

4. CLINICAL PARTICULARS

4.1 Therapeutic indications

For bronchodilation: Terbutaline is a selective $beta_2$-adrenergic agonist recommended for the relief and prevention of bronchospasm in bronchial asthma and other broncho-pulmonary disorders in which bronchospasm is a complicating factor.

For the management of uncomplicated premature labour.

4.2 Posology and method of administration

Use in bronchospasm: Bricanyl Tablets have a duration of action of 7 to 8 hours. The minimum recommended dosage interval is therefore 7 hours.

Adults: During the first 1 - 2 weeks, 2.5mg (half a tablet) 3 times in a 24-hour period is recommended. The dose may then be increased to 5mg (1 tablet) 3 times in a 24-hour period to achieve adequate bronchodilation.

Elderly: Dosage as for Adults.

Children 7 - 15 years: The starting dose should normally be 2.5mg (half a tablet) 2 times in 24 hours. However, in some patients, the dose may need to be increased to 2.5mg 3 times in 24 hours.

Use in the management of premature labour: Oral treatment should not be used initially in an attempt to arrest premature labour. After uterine contractions have been controlled by intravenous infusion of Bricanyl Injection, (see Bricanyl Injection Summary of Product Characteristics) or subcutaneous injections (0.25mg, 4 times in a 24-hour period for a few days) maintenance therapy can be continued with oral treatment (5mg, 3 times in a 24-hour period). Oral treatment may be continued for as long as the physician considers it desirable to prolong pregnancy.

4.3 Contraindications

Bricanyl Tablets should not be used as a tocolytic agent in patients with pre-existing ischaemic heart disease or those patients with significant risk factors for ischaemic heart disease.

Although Bricanyl Tablets are used in the management of uncomplicated premature labour, their use in the following conditions is contraindicated:

- any condition of the mother or foetus in which prolongation of the pregnancy is hazardous, e.g. severe toxaemia, ante-partum haemorrhage, intra-uterine infection, severe pre-eclampsia, abruptio placentae, threatened abortion during the 1st and 2nd trimesters, or cord compression.

Bricanyl Tablets should not be used in patients with a history of hypersensitivity to any of the ingredients.

4.4 Special warnings and precautions for use

As for all $beta_2$-agonists caution should be observed in patients with thyrotoxicosis.

Cardiovascular effects may be seen with sympathomimetic drugs, including Bricanyl. There is some evidence from post-marketing data and published literature of myocardial ischaemia associated with beta agonists.

Due to the positive inotropic effect of $beta_2$-agonists, these drugs should not be used in patients with hypertrophic cardiomyopathy.

Tocolysis

Bricanyl should be used with caution in tocolysis and supervision of cardiorespiratory function, including ECG monitoring, should be considered. Treatment should be discontinued if signs of myocardial ischaemia (such as chest pain or ECG changes) develop. Bricanyl should not be used as a tocolytic agent in patients with significant risk factors for or pre-existing heart disease (see section 4.3, Contraindications).

During infusion treatment in pregnant women with $beta_2$-stimulants in combination with corticosteroids, a rare complication with a pathological picture resembling pulmonary oedema has been reported.

Increased tendency to uterine bleeding has been reported in connection with Caesarean section. However, this can be effectively stopped by propranolol 1-2 mg injected intravenously.

Respiratory indications

Patients with underlying severe heart disease (e.g. ischaemic heart disease, arrhythmia or severe heart failure) who are receiving Bricanyl should be warned to seek medical advice if they experience chest pain or other symptoms of worsening heart disease.

Attention should be paid to assessment of symptoms such as dyspnoea and chest pain, as they may be of either respiratory or cardiac origin.

Due to the hyperglycaemic effects of $beta_2$-agonists, additional blood glucose controls are recommended initially in diabetic patients.

Potentially serious hypokalaemia may result from $beta_2$-agonist therapy. Particular caution is recommended in acute severe asthma as the associated risk may be augmented by hypoxia. The hypokalaemic effect may be potentiated by concomitant treatments (see section 4.5, Interactions). It is recommended that serum potassium levels are monitored in such situations.

If a previously effective dosage regimen no longer gives the same symptomatic relief, the patient should urgently seek further medical advice. Consideration should be given to the requirements for additional therapy (including increased dosages of anti-inflammatory medication). Severe exacerbations of asthma should be treated as an emergency in the usual manner.

4.5 Interaction with other medicinal products and other forms of interaction

Beta-blocking agents (including eye drops), especially the non selective ones such as propranolol, may partially or totally inhibit the effect of beta-stimulants. Therefore, Bricanyl preparations and non-selective beta-blockers should not normally be administered concurrently. Bricanyl should be used with caution in patients receiving other sympathomimetics.

Hypokalaemia may result from $beta_2$-agonist therapy and may be potentiated by concomitant treatment with xanthine derivatives, corticosteroids and diuretics (*see Section 4.4, Special Warnings and Precautions for use*).

4.6 Pregnancy and lactation

Although no teratogenic effects have been observed in animals or in patients, Bricanyl should only be administered with caution during the first trimester of pregnancy.

Terbutaline is secreted into breast milk, but any effect on the infant is unlikely at therapeutic doses.

Transient hypoglycaemia has been reported in newborn preterm infants after maternal $beta_2$-agonist treatment.

4.7 Effects on ability to drive and use machines

None

4.8 Undesirable effects

The intensity of the adverse reactions depends on dosage and route of administration. Most of the adverse reactions are characteristic of sympathomimetic amines. The majority of these effects have reversed spontaneously within the first 1-2 weeks of treatment.

The frequency of side-effects is low at the recommended doses.

Adverse events are listed below by system organ class and frequency. Frequencies are defined as: very common (>1/10), common (>1/100 and <1/10), uncommon (>1/1,000 and <1/100), rare (>1/10,000 and <1/1,000), very rare (<1/10,000) and not known (cannot be estimated from the available data).

(see Table 1 below)

4.9 Overdose

Possible symptoms and signs: Headache, anxiety, tremor, nausea, tonic cramp, palpitations, tachycardia, arrhythmia. A fall in blood pressure sometimes occurs. Laboratory findings: hypokalaemia, hyperglycaemia and lactic acidosis sometimes occur.

Table 1

Frequency Classification	Adverse Drug Reaction System Organ Class (SOC)	Preferred term (PT)
Very Common (>1/10)	Nervous System Disorders	Tremor Headache
Common (>1/100, <1/10)	Cardiac Disorders	Tachycardia Palpitations
	Musculoskeletal and Connective Tissue Disorders #	Muscle spasms
	Metabolism and Nutrition Disorders	Hypokalaemia (See section 4.4)
Not Known ^	Cardiac Disorders	Arrhythmias, e.g. atrial fibrillation, supraventricular tachycardia and extrasystoles Myocardial ischaemia (See section 4.4)
	Vascular Disorders	Peripheral vasodilation
	Immune System Disorders	Hypersensitivity reactions including angioedema, bronchospasm, hypotension and collapse
	Gastrointestinal Disorders	Nausea Mouth and throat irritation
	Psychiatric Disorders	Sleep disorder and Behavioural disturbances, such as agitation and restlessness
	Respiratory, Thoracic and Mediastinal Disorders	Paradoxical bronchospasm *
	Skin and Subcutaneous Tissue Disorders	Urticaria Rash

A few patients feel tense; this is also due to the effects on skeletal muscle and not to direct CNS stimulation.

^ Reported spontaneously in post-marketing data and therefore frequency regarded as unknown

* In rare cases, through unspecified mechanisms, paradoxical bronchospasm may occur, with wheezing immediately after inhalation. This should be immediately treated with a rapid-onset bronchodilator. Bricanyl therapy should be discontinued and after assessment, an alternative therapy initiated.

Treatment:

Mild and moderate cases: Reduce the dose.

Severe cases: Gastric lavage, administration of activated charcoal. Determination of acid-base balance, blood sugar and electrolytes, particularly serum potassium levels. Monitoring of the heart rate and rhythm and blood pressure. Metabolic changes should be corrected. A cardioselective β-blocker (e.g. metoprolol) is recommended for the treatment of arrhythmias causing haemodynamic deterioration. The β-blocker should be used with care because of the possibility of inducing bronchoconstriction: use with caution in patients with a history of bronchospasm. If the beta$_2$-mediated reduction in the peripheral vascular resistance significantly contributes to the fall in blood pressure, a volume expander should be given.

Preterm labour: Pulmonary oedema: discontinue administration of Bricanyl. A normal dose of loop diuretic (e.g. frusemide) should be given intravenously.

Increased bleeding in connection with Caesarian section: propranolol, 1 - 2mg intravenously.

5. PHARMACOLOGICAL PROPERTIES

5.1 Pharmacodynamic properties

Pharmaco-therapeutic group: selective beta$_2$-agonist, terbutaline, ATC code: R03C C03.

Terbutaline is a selective beta$_2$-adrenergic stimulant having the following pharmacological effects:-

i) In the lung - bronchodilation; increased mucociliary clearance; suppression of oedema and anti-allergic effects.

ii) In skeletal muscle - stimulates Na^+/K^+ transport and also causes depression of subtetanic contractions in slow-contracting muscle.

iii) In uterine muscle - inhibition of uterine contractions.

iv) In the CNS - low penetration of the blood-brain barrier at therapeutic doses, due to the highly hydrophilic nature of the molecule.

v) In the CVS - administration of terbutaline results in cardiovascular effects mediated through beta$_2$-receptors in the peripheral arteries and in the heart e.g. in healthy subjects, 0.25 - 0.5mg injected s.c. is associated with an increase in cardiac output (up to 85% over controls) due to an increase in heart rate and a larger stroke volume. The increase in heart rate is probably due to a combination of a reflex tachycardia via a fall in peripheral resistance and a direct positive chronotropic effect of the drug.

5.2 Pharmacokinetic properties

Basic parameters have been evaluated in man after i.v and oral administration of therapeutic doses, e.g.

i.v single dose

Volume distribution (vss): 114 L

Total body clearance (cl): 213 ml/min

Mean residence time (mrt): 9.0 h

Renal clearance (clr): 149 ml/min (males)

Oral dose

Renal clearance (clr): 1.925 ml/min (males)

Renal clearance (clr): 2.32 ml/min (females)

The plasma concentration/time curve after iv administration is characterised by a fast distribution phase, an intermediate elimination phase and a late elimination phase. Terminal half-life ($t_{½}$) has been determined after single and multiple dosing (mean values varied between 16 - 20 h).

Bioavailability

Food reduces bioavailability following oral dosing (10% on average).

Fasting values of 14 - 15% have been obtained.

Metabolism

The main metabolite after oral dosing is the sulphate conjugate and also some glucuronide conjugate can be found in the urine.

5.3 Preclinical safety data

The major toxic effect of terbutaline, observed in toxicological studies in rats and dogs at exposures in excess of maximum human exposure, is focal myocardial necrosis. This type of cardiotoxicity is a well known pharmacological manifestation seen after the administration of high doses of beta$_2$-agonists.

In rats, an increase in the incidence of benign uterine leiomyomas has been observed. This effect is looked upon as a class-effect observed in rodents after long term exposure to high doses of beta$_2$-agonists

6. PHARMACEUTICAL PARTICULARS

6.1 List of excipients

Lactose monohydrate, maize starch, povidone, microcrystalline cellulose and magnesium stearate.

6.2 Incompatibilities

None known.

6.3 Shelf life

4 years.

6.4 Special precautions for storage

Do not store above 25°C.

6.5 Nature and contents of container

Glass bottles and Securitainers of 100 and 500 tablets.

6.6 Special precautions for disposal and other handling

Not applicable

7. MARKETING AUTHORISATION HOLDER

AstraZeneca UK Ltd.,

600 Capability Green,

Luton, LU1 3LU, UK.

8. MARKETING AUTHORISATION NUMBER(S)

PL 17901/0116

9. DATE OF FIRST AUTHORISATION/RENEWAL OF THE AUTHORISATION

28th May 2002 / 15th May 2007

10. DATE OF REVISION OF THE TEXT

30th March 2009

Bricanyl Turbohaler, 0.5mg/dose, inhalation powder

(AstraZeneca UK Limited)

1. NAME OF THE MEDICINAL PRODUCT

Bricanyl® Turbohaler®, 0.5mg/dose, inhalation powder

2. QUALITATIVE AND QUANTITATIVE COMPOSITION

Terbutaline Sulphate 0.5mg/dose.

For excipients see Section 6.1.

3. PHARMACEUTICAL FORM

Inhalation powder.

Breath-actuated metered dose powder inhaler.

4. CLINICAL PARTICULARS

4.1 Therapeutic indications

Terbutaline is a selective beta$_2$-adrenergic agonist recommended for the relief and prevention of bronchospasm in bronchial asthma and other bronchopulmonary disorders in which bronchospasm or reversible airways obstruction is a complicating factor.

4.2 Posology and method of administration

Adults and Children: One inhalation (0.5mg) as required. Not more than 4 inhalations should be required in any 24-hour period.

The duration of action of a single dose is up to 6 hours.

Elderly: Dosage as for adults.

Instructions for use and cleaning are provided in the Patient Information Leaflet, which can be found in each pack.

4.3 Contraindications

Bricanyl preparations are contraindicated in patients with a history of sensitivity to terbutaline sulphate.

4.4 Special warnings and precautions for use

Patients should be instructed in proper use and their inhalation technique checked regularly.

If a previously effective dosage regimen no longer gives the same symptomatic relief, the patient should urgently seek further medical advice. Consideration should be given to the requirements for additional therapy (including increased dosages of anti-inflammatory medication). Severe exacerbations of asthma should be treated as an emergency in the usual manner.

As for all beta$_2$-agonists caution should be observed in patients with thyrotoxicosis.

Due to the positive inotropic effect of beta$_2$-agonists, these drugs should not be used in patients with hypertrophic cardiomyopathy.

Cardiovascular effects may be seen with sympathomimetic drugs, including Bricanyl. There is some evidence from post-marketing data and published literature of rare occurrences of myocardial ischaemia associated with beta agonists. Patients with underlying severe heart disease (e.g. ischaemic heart disease, arrhythmia or severe heart failure) who are receiving Bricanyl should be warned to seek medical advice if they experience chest pain or other symptoms of worsening heart disease. Attention should be paid to assessment of symptoms such as dyspnoea and chest pain, as they may be of either respiratory or cardiac origin.

Due to the hyperglycaemic effects of beta$_2$-agonists, additional blood glucose controls are recommended initially in diabetic patients.

Potentially serious hypokalaemia may result from beta$_2$-agonist therapy. Particular caution is recommended in acute severe asthma as the associated risk may be augmented by hypoxia. The hypokalaemic effect may be potentiated by concomitant treatments (see section 4.5, Interactions). It is recommended that serum potassium levels are monitored in such situations.

4.5 Interaction with other medicinal products and other forms of interaction

Beta-blocking agents (including eye drops), especially the non-selective ones such as propranolol, may partially or totally inhibit the effect of beta-stimulants. Therefore, Bricanyl preparations and non-selective beta-blockers should not normally be administered concurrently. Bricanyl should be used with caution in patients receiving other sympathomimetics.

Hypokalaemia may result from beta$_2$-agonist therapy and may be potentiated by concomitant treatment with xanthine derivatives, corticosteroids and diuretics (*see Section 4.4, Special Warnings and Precautions for use*).

4.6 Pregnancy and lactation

Although no teratogenic effects have been observed in animals or in patients, Bricanyl should only be administered with caution during the first trimester of pregnancy.

Terbutaline is secreted via breast milk but any effect on the infant is unlikely at therapeutic doses.

4.7 Effects on ability to drive and use machines

None.

4.8 Undesirable effects

The frequency of adverse reactions is low at the recommended dose. Terbutaline given by inhalation is unlikely to produce significant systemic effects when given in recommended doses. Most of the adverse reactions are characteristic of sympathomimetic amines. The majority of these effects have reversed spontaneously within the first 1-2 weeks of treatment.

The frequency of side-effects is low at the recommended doses.

Adverse events are listed below by system organ class and frequency. Frequencies are defined as: very common (>1/10), common (>1/100 and <1/10), uncommon (>1/1,000 and <1/100), rare (>1/10,000 and <1/1,000), very rare (<1/10,000) and not known (cannot be estimated from the available data).

(see Table 1 on next page)

4.9 Overdose

i) Possible symptoms and signs:

Headache, anxiety, tremor, nausea, tonic cramp, palpitations, tachycardia and arrhythmia. A fall in blood pressure sometimes occurs. Laboratory findings: Hypokalaemia, hyperglycaemia and metabolic acidosis sometimes occur.

ii) Treatment:

Mild and moderate cases: Reduce the dose.

Severe cases: Gastric lavage, administration of activated charcoal (where suspected that significant amounts have been swallowed). Determination of acid-base balance, blood sugar and electrolytes, particularly serum potassium levels. Monitoring of heart rate and rhythm and blood pressure. Metabolic changes should be corrected. A cardioselective beta-blocker (e.g. metoprolol) is recommended for the treatment of arrhythmias causing haemodynamic deterioration. The beta-blocker should be used with care because of the possibility of inducing bronchoconstriction: use with caution in patients with a history of bronchospasm. If the beta$_2$-mediated reduction in peripheral vascular resistance significantly contributes to the fall in blood pressure, a volume expander should be given.

5. PHARMACOLOGICAL PROPERTIES

5.1 Pharmacodynamic properties

Pharmaco-therapeutic group: selective beta$_2$-agonist, terbutaline, ATC code: R03A C03.

Terbutaline sulphate is a selective beta$_2$-adrenoceptor agonist, thus producing relaxation of bronchial smooth muscle, inhibition of the release of endogenous spasmogens, inhibitions of oedema caused by endogenous mediators, increased mucociliary clearance and relaxation of the uterine muscle.

5.2 Pharmacokinetic properties

Pharmacokinetic data from terbutaline inhaled from a pressurised aerosol reveal that less than 10% of the dose is absorbed from the airways. The remaining 90% is swallowed but is largely prevented from entering the systemic circulation due to extensive first pass metabolism.

Data suggest that inhaled terbutaline acts topically in the airways.

5.3 Preclinical safety data

The major toxic effect of terbutaline, observed in toxicological studies in rats and dogs at exposures in excess of maximum human exposure, is focal myocardial necrosis. This type of cardiotoxicity is a well known pharmacological manifestation seen after the administration of high doses of beta$_2$-agonists.

In rats, an increase in the incidence of benign uterine leiomyomas has been observed. This effect is looked upon as a class-effect observed in rodents after long term exposure to high doses of beta$_2$-agonists.

6. PHARMACEUTICAL PARTICULARS

6.1 List of excipients

None

6.2 Incompatibilities

None known.

6.3 Shelf life

24 months

6.4 Special precautions for storage

Do not store above 30°C.

6.5 Nature and contents of container

Bricanyl Turbohaler consists of a number of assembled plastic details, the main parts being the dosing mechanism, the drug substance store, the desiccant store and the

Table 1

Frequency Classification	Adverse Drug Reaction	
	System Organ Class (SOC)	**Preferred term (PT)**
Very Common (>1/10)	Nervous System Disorders	Tremor Headache
Common (>1/100, <1/10)	Cardiac Disorders	Tachycardia Palpitations
	Musculoskeletal and Connective Tissue Disorders #	Muscle spasms
	Metabolism and Nutrition Disorders	Hypokalaemia (See section 4.4)
Not Known ^	Cardiac Disorders	Arrhythmias, e.g. atrial fibrillation, supraventricular tachycardia and extrasystoles Myocardial ischaemia (See section 4.4)
	Vascular Disorders	Peripheral vasodilation
	Immune System Disorders	Hypersensitivity reactions including angioedema, bronchospasm, hypotension and collapse
	Gastrointestinal Disorders	Nausea Mouth and throat irritation
	Psychiatric Disorders	Sleep disorder and Behavioural disturbances, such as agitation and restlessness
	Respiratory, Thoracic and Mediastinal Disorders	Paradoxical bronchospasm *
	Skin and Subcutaneous Tissue Disorders	Urticaria Rash

A few patients feel tense; this is also due to the effects on skeletal muscle and not to direct CNS stimulation.

^ Reported spontaneously in post-marketing data and therefore frequency regarded as unknown

* In rare cases, through unspecified mechanisms, paradoxical bronchospasm may occur, with wheezing immediately after inhalation. This should be immediately treated with a rapid-onset bronchodilator. Bricanyl therapy should be discontinued and after assessment, an alternative therapy initiated.

mouthpiece. The inhaler is protected by an outer tubular cover screwed onto a bottom plate.

Each inhaler contains 100 doses.

6.6 Special precautions for disposal and other handling

None.

7. MARKETING AUTHORISATION HOLDER

AstraZeneca UK Ltd.,
600 Capability Green,
Luton, LU1 3LU, UK.

8. MARKETING AUTHORISATION NUMBER(S)

PL 17901/0117

9. DATE OF FIRST AUTHORISATION/RENEWAL OF THE AUTHORISATION

4th June 2002 / 12th May 2007

10. DATE OF REVISION OF THE TEXT

30th March 2009

BritLofex Tablets 0.2mg

(Britannia Pharmaceuticals)

1. NAME OF THE MEDICINAL PRODUCT

BritLofex Tablets 0.2mg

2. QUALITATIVE AND QUANTITATIVE COMPOSITION

Lofexidine hydrochloride 0.2mg

3. PHARMACEUTICAL FORM

Film-coated tablet.

Peach coloured, round tablet.

4. CLINICAL PARTICULARS

4.1 Therapeutic indications

To relieve symptoms in patients undergoing opiate detoxification.

4.2 Posology and method of administration

The recommended route of administration is by mouth.

ADULTS

The dosage of lofexidine should be titrated according to the patient's response. Initial dosage should be 0.8mg per day in divided doses. The dosage may be increased by increments of 0.4 to 0.8mg per day up to a maximum of 2.4mg daily. Maximum single dose should not exceed 4 × 0.2mg tablets (0.8mg). Each patient should be assessed on an individual basis; those undergoing acute detoxification will usually require the highest recommended dose and dosage increments to provide optimum relief at the time of expected peak withdrawal symptoms.

In cases where no opiate use occurs during detoxification, a duration of treatment of 7-10 days is recommended. In some cases the physician may consider longer treatment is warranted.

CHILDREN:

Safety and effectiveness in children has not been established.

ELDERLY:

There is no experience of dosing in the elderly from clinical studies. Should use in the elderly be necessary it is advised that special caution is observed in the presence of heart disease or anti-hypertensive therapy.

4.3 Contraindications

BritLofex tablets are contraindicated in patients who are allergic to lofexidine or to other imidazoline derivatives or to any excipients of BritLofex.

4.4 Special warnings and precautions for use

As with other hypotensive agents, therapy with lofexidine should not be discontinued abruptly. Dosage should be reduced gradually over a period of 2-4 days or longer, to minimise blood pressure elevation and associated signs and symptoms. Lofexidine should be used with caution in patients with severe coronary insufficiency, recent myocardial infarction, cerebrovascular disease or chronic renal failure and in patients with bradycardia or hypotension. Blood pressure and pulse rate should be assessed frequently. Patients with a history of depression should be carefully observed during long-term therapy with lofexidine.

There have been reports of QT prolongation during lofexidine treatment. Whilst the nature of the relationship between lofexidine and these ECG changes is not yet clear, it would be prudent to avoid the use of lofexidine in patients at risk of QT prolongation i.e. those with known QT problems, metabolic disturbances, pre-existing cardiovascular disease, relevant family history or those taking other drugs known to prolong the QT interval.

This medicine contains lactose. Patients with rare hereditary problems of galactose intolerance, the Lapp lactase deficiency or glucose-galactose malabsorption should not take this medicine.

Allergic reactions may occur due to the presence of E110 (Sunset Yellow).

4.5 Interaction with other medicinal products and other forms of interaction

Lofexidine may enhance the CNS depressive effects of alcohol, barbiturates and other sedatives.

Lofexidine may enhance the effects of anti-hypertensive drug therapy.

Concomitant use of tricyclic antidepressants may reduc the efficacy of lofexidine.

Concomitant use of drug which prolong the QT interval c cause electrolyte imbalance should be avoided.

4.6 Pregnancy and lactation

Pregnancy:

The safety of lofexidine in pregnant women has not bee established. High doses of lofexidine given to pregna dogs and rabbits caused a reduction in foetal weight ar increased abortions. Lofexidine should only be adminis tered during pregnancy if the benefit outweighs the pote tial risk to mother and foetus.

Lactation:

It is not known whether this drug is excreted in human mi and caution should be exercised when it is administered a nursing woman.

4.7 Effects on ability to drive and use machines

Lofexidine may have a sedative effect. If affected, patien should be advised not to drive or operate machines.

4.8 Undesirable effects

The adverse effects of the drug are primarily related to central alpha-adrenergic agonist effects:

Very common (≥1/10)
Common (≥1/100 to <1/10)
Uncommon (≥1/1,000 to <1/100)
Rare (≥1/10,000 to <1/1,000)
Very rare (<1/10,000)
Not known (cannot be estimated from the available dat

Immune system disorders:

Not known:

Allergic reactions may occur due to the presence of E1 (Sunset Yellow).

Nervous system disorders:

Very common:

Dizziness has been reported following treatment w lofexidine.

Drowsiness and related symptoms including sedation a somnolence have been reported.

Cardiac disorders:

Very common:

Bradycardia has been reported.

Not known:

There have been reports of QT prolongation during lof idine treatment.

Vascular disorders:

Very common:

Hypotension has been reported

General disorders and administration site conditio

Very common:

Dryness of mucous membranes especially the mo throat and nose has been reported.

4.9 Overdose

Overdosage may cause hypotension, bradycardia a sedation. Gastric lavage should be carried out wh appropriate. In most cases, all that is required are gen supportive measures.

5. PHARMACOLOGICAL PROPERTIES

5.1 Pharmacodynamic properties

Pharmacotherapeutic Group: Drugs used in opioid dep dence

ATC Classification: N07BC04

Lofexidine hydrochloride is an orally active imidazo adrenergic alpha-2-receptor agonist; and is believed have a high affinity for 2A receptor subtypes resultin less anti-hypertensive activity than clonidine, a non-se tive alpha-2-receptor agonist. Hypotension may occu susceptible subjects, accompanied by a decrease in h rate.

Abrupt discontinuation of lofexidine has been, in s cases, associated with a transient increase in blood p sure to higher than pre-treatment levels.

5.2 Pharmacokinetic properties

Lofexidine is extensively absorbed and achieves p plasma concentration at 3 hours after administration single dose. The elimination half-life is 11 hours with ac mulation occurring up to four days with repeat dos Lofexidine undergoes extensive metabolism in the and excretion is mainly by the kidney.

5.3 Preclinical safety data

Animal toxicology. Lofexidine was tolerated at high dos in singe dose toxicity studies in animals, the LD_{50} b >77 mg/kg. With repeat dosing in mice, rats and c symptoms related to the pharmacology of the drug (ata sedation, tremor, unkempt appearance and exhaus appeared.

Studies of mutagenicity are incomplete but lofexidine not display mutagenicity in the Ames test. Long-term dies in rats showed no evidence of carcinogenicity.

High doses of lofexidine given to pregnant rats and rabbits caused a reduction in the foetal weight and increased abortions. No teratogenic effects were found.

6. PHARMACEUTICAL PARTICULARS

6.1 List of excipients

Lactose (monohydrate)

Citric acid

Povidone

Microcrystalline cellulose

Calcium stearate

Sodium lauryl sulphate

Purified water

Film Coat:

Opadry OY-S-9480 Brown

containing

Hydroxypropylmethyl cellulose

Titanium dioxide

Propylene glycol

Indigo Carmine (E132)

Sunset Yellow (E110)

6.2 Incompatibilities

None known

6.3 Shelf life

36 months

6.4 Special precautions for storage

Store below 25°C. Store in original package.

6.5 Nature and contents of container

Aluminium foil/aluminium foil blister strips

Aluminium foil/PVC blister strips

6.6 Special precautions for disposal and other handling

No special instructions.

7. MARKETING AUTHORISATION HOLDER

Britannia Pharmaceuticals Limited

41 - 51 Brighton Road

Redhill

Surrey

RH1 6YS

United Kingdom

8. MARKETING AUTHORISATION NUMBER(S)

PL 04483/0036

9. DATE OF FIRST AUTHORISATION/RENEWAL OF THE AUTHORISATION

October 1990

10. DATE OF REVISION OF THE TEXT

7 May 2009

Broflex Syrup 5mg/5ml

(Alliance Pharmaceuticals)

1. NAME OF THE MEDICINAL PRODUCT

Broflex syrup (5mg/5mL).

2. QUALITATIVE AND QUANTITATIVE COMPOSITION

Trihexyphenidyl hydrochloride BP 5mg/5mL.

3. PHARMACEUTICAL FORM

A blackcurrant scented and flavoured clear pink syrup.

4. CLINICAL PARTICULARS

4.1 Therapeutic indications

Parkinsonism and drug induced extrapyramidal syndrome.

4.2 Posology and method of administration

Adults and Elderly:

Initial dose 2mg. Subsequent doses up to 20mg as recommended by a physician.

Children:

Not recommended.

4.3 Contraindications

Hypersensitivity to trihexyphenidyl or any of the other ingredients.

Incipient glaucoma may be precipitated. The following are not absolute contra-indications, nevertheless caution must be observed in patients with: hypertension, cardiac, liver or kidney dysfunction, glaucoma, obstructive disease of the gastro-intestinal or genito-urinary tracts and in males with a prostatic hypertrophy.

4.4 Special warnings and precautions for use

Anticholinergic medications, including trihexyphenidyl, should not be withdrawn abruptly in patients on long-term therapy, to avoid recurrence of the original symptoms and possible anticholinergic rebound. Prescribers should be aware that trihexyphenidyl may be the subject of abuse due to its euphoric or hallucinogenic properties.

Since atropine-like drugs may cause psychiatric symptoms such as confusion, delusion and hallucinations, trihexyphenidyl should be used with extreme caution in elderly patients.

As trihexyphenidyl may provoke or exacerbate tardive dyskinesia, it is not recommended for use in patients with this condition.

Since trihexyphenidyl has been associated with clinical worsening of myasthenia gravis, the drug should be avoided or used with great caution in patients with myasthenia gravis.

Patients with rare hereditary problems of fructose intolerance, glucose-galactose malabsoprtion or sucrase-maltase insufficiency should not take this medicine.

4.5 Interaction with other medicinal products and other forms of interaction

Monoamine oxidase inhibitors (MAOI's), antihistamines, disopyramide, phenothiazines and tricyclic antidepressants increase the side effects of blurred vision and dry mouth, constipation, urinary retention. MAOI's, amantidine and some tricyclic antidepressents may also cause excitation, confusion and hallucination.

4.6 Pregnancy and lactation

Pregnancy

There is inadequate information regarding the use of trihexyphenidyl in pregnancy. Animal studies are insufficient with regard to effects on pregnancy, embryonal/foetal development, parturition and postnatal development. The potential risk for humans is unknown. Trihexyphenidyl should not be used during pregnancy unless clearly necessary.

Lactation

It is unknown whether trihexyphenidyl is excreted in human breast milk. The excretion of trihexyphenidyl in milk has not been studied in animals. Infants may be very sensitive to the effects of antimuscarinic medications. Trihexyphenidyl should not be used during breast feeding.

4.7 Effects on ability to drive and use machines

Patients should be warned of the potential hazards of driving or operating machinery if they experience blurred vision or a reduction in alertness.

4.8 Undesirable effects

Dry mouth, constipation and blurred vision may occur. This is more frequent in the elderly but reduces with tolerance. Psychiatric symptoms such as agitation, confusion, hallucinations, euphoria, insomnia, restlessness and very occasionally paranoid delusions have been reported. These are more likely to occur in patients receiving higher than recommended doses. There have been reports of abuse of trihexyphenidyl due to its euphoric and hallucinogenic properties.

Impairment of immediate and short-term memory functions has also been reported.

4.9 Overdose

Symptoms

Symptoms of overdose with antimuscarinic agents include flushing and dryness of the skin, dilated pupils, dry mouth and tongue, tachycardia, rapid respiration, hyperpyrexia, hypertension, nausea, vomiting. A rash may appear on the face or upper trunk. Symptoms of CNS stimulation include restlessness, confusion, hallucinations, paranoid and psychotic reactions, incoordination, delirium and occasionally convulsions. In severe overdose, CNS depression may occur with coma, circulatory and respiratory failure and death.

Treatment

Treatment should always be supportive. An adequate airway should be maintained. Diazepam may be administered to control excitement and convulsions but the risk of central nervous system depression should be considered. Hypoxia and acidosis should be corrected. Antiarrhythmic drugs are not recommended if dysrhythmias occur.

5. PHARMACOLOGICAL PROPERTIES

5.1 Pharmacodynamic properties

Trihexyphenidyl is a tertiary amine antimuscarinic. It also has a direct antispasmodic action on smooth muscle.

5.2 Pharmacokinetic properties

Trihexyphenidyl is well absorbed from the gastro-intestinal tract.

5.3 Preclinical safety data

No formal preclinical studies have been undertaken with Broflex, as its active ingredient is a well established pharmaceutical.

6. PHARMACEUTICAL PARTICULARS

6.1 List of excipients

Anhydrous citric acid, benzoic acid, propylene glycol, amaranth E123, glycerol, chloroform spirit, blackcurrant flavour A402, syrup, purified water.

6.2 Incompatibilities

None known.

6.3 Shelf life

24 months.

6.4 Special precautions for storage

None.

6.5 Nature and contents of container

200 mL pack size in amber glass bottle with polycone lined enclosure.

6.6 Special precautions for disposal and other handling

None stated.

7. MARKETING AUTHORISATION HOLDER

Alliance Pharmaceuticals Ltd

Avonbridge House

Bath Road

Chippenham

Wiltshire

SN15 2BB

8. MARKETING AUTHORISATION NUMBER(S)

PL16853/0023

9. DATE OF FIRST AUTHORISATION/RENEWAL OF THE AUTHORISATION

30 June 1999

10. DATE OF REVISION OF THE TEXT

25th July 2007.

Alliance, Alliance Pharmaceuticals and associated devices are registered Trademarks of Alliance Pharmaceuticals Ltd.

Brufen 200 mg Tablets

(Abbott Laboratories Limited)

1. NAME OF THE MEDICINAL PRODUCT

Brufen Tablets 200 mg

2. QUALITATIVE AND QUANTITATIVE COMPOSITION

Active ingredient	Quantity
Ibuprofen	200 mg

3. PHARMACEUTICAL FORM

A white, pillow-shaped, film-coated tablet with 'Brufen' printed in black on one face

4. CLINICAL PARTICULARS

4.1 Therapeutic indications

Brufen is indicated for its analgesic and anti-inflammatory effects in the treatment of rheumatoid arthritis (including juvenile rheumatoid arthritis or Still's disease), ankylosing spondylitis, osteoarthritis and other non-rheumatoid (seronegative) arthropathies.

In the treatment of non-articular rheumatic conditions, Brufen is indicated in periarticular conditions such as frozen shoulder (capsulitis), bursitis, tendonitis, tenosynovitis and low back pain; Brufen can also be used in soft tissue injuries such as sprains and strains.

Brufen is also indicated for its analgesic effect in the relief of mild to moderate pain such as dysmenorrhoea, dental and post-operative pain and for symptomatic relief of headache, including migraine headache.

4.2 Posology and method of administration

Undesirable effects may be minimised by using the lowest effective dose for the shortest duration necessary to control symptoms (see section 4.4).

Adults: The recommended dosage of Brufen is 1200-1800 mg daily in divided doses. Some patients can be maintained on 600-1200 mg daily. In severe or acute conditions, it can be advantageous to increase the dosage until the acute phase is brought under control, provided that the total daily dose does not exceed 2400 mg in divided doses.

Children: The daily dosage of Brufen is 20 mg/kg of body weight in divided doses.

In Juvenile Rheumatoid Arthritis, up to 40 mg/kg of body weight daily in divided doses may be taken.

Not recommended for children weighing less than 7 kg.

Elderly: The elderly are at increased risk of serious consequences of adverse reactions. If an NSAID is considered necessary, the lowest effective dose should be used and for the shortest possible duration. The patient should be monitored regularly for GI bleeding during NSAID therapy. If renal or hepatic function is impaired, dosage should be assessed individually.

For oral administration. To be taken preferably with or after food.

4.3 Contraindications

Brufen is contraindicated in patients with hypersensitivity to the active substance or to any of the excipients.

Brufen should not be used in patients who have previously shown hypersensitivity reactions (e.g. asthma, urticaria, angioedema or rhinitis) after taking ibuprofen, aspirin or other NSAIDs.

Brufen is also contraindicated in patients with a history of gastrointestinal bleeding or perforation, related to previous NSAID therapy. Brufen should not be used in patients with active, or history of, recurrent peptic ulcer or gastrointestinal haemorrhage (two or more distinct episodes of proven ulceration or bleeding).

Brufen is contraindicated in patients with severe heart failure, hepatic failure and renal failure (see section 4.4).

Brufen is contraindicated during the last trimester of pregnancy (see section 4.6).

4.4 Special warnings and precautions for use

Undesirable effects may be minimised by using the lowest effective dose for the shortest duration necessary to control symptoms (see section 4.2, and GI and cardiovascular risks below).

Patients with rare hereditary problems of galactose intolerance, the Lapp lactose deficiency or glucose-galactose malabsorption should not take this medication.

As with other NSAIDs, ibuprofen may mask the signs of infection.

The use of Brufen with concomitant NSAIDs, including cyclooxygenase-2 selective inhibitors, should be avoided due to the potential for additive effects (see section 4.5).

Elderly

The elderly have an increased frequency of adverse reactions to NSAIDs, especially gastrointestinal bleeding and perforation, which may be fatal (see section 4.2).

Gastrointestinal bleeding, ulceration and perforation

GI bleeding, ulceration or perforation, which can be fatal, has been reported with all NSAIDs at anytime during treatment, with or without warning symptoms or a previous history of serious GI events.

The risk of GI bleeding, ulceration or perforation is higher with increasing NSAID doses, in patients with a history of ulcer, particularly if complicated with haemorrhage or perforation (see section 4.3), and in the elderly. These patients should commence treatment on the lowest dose available. Combination therapy with protective agents (e.g. misoprostol or proton pump inhibitors) should be considered for these patients, and also for patients requiring concomitant low dose aspirin, or other drugs likely to increase gastrointestinal risk (see below and section 4.5).

Patients with a history of gastrointestinal disease, particularly when elderly, should report any unusual abdominal symptoms (especially gastrointestinal bleeding) particularly in the initial stages of treatment.

Caution should be advised in patients receiving concomitant medications which could increase the risk of ulceration or bleeding, such as oral corticosteroids, anticoagulants such as warfarin, selective serotonin-reuptake inhibitors or anti-platelet agents such as aspirin (see section 4.5).

When GI bleeding or ulceration occurs in patients receiving Brufen, the treatment should be withdrawn.

NSAIDs should be given with care to patients with a history of ulcerative colitis or Crohn's disease as these conditions may be exacerbated (see section 4.8).

Respiratory disorders

Caution is required if Brufen is administered to patients suffering from, or with a previous history of, bronchial asthma since NSAIDs have been reported to precipitate bronchospasm in such patients.

Cardiovascular, renal and hepatic impairment

The administration of an NSAID may cause a dose dependent reduction in prostaglandin formation and precipitate renal failure. Patients at greatest risk of this reaction are those with impaired renal function, cardiac impairment, liver dysfunction, those taking diuretics and the elderly. Renal function should be monitored in these patients (see also section 4.3).

Brufen should be given with care to patients with a history of heart failure or hypertension since oedema has been reported in association with ibuprofen administration.

Cardiovascular and cerebrovascular effects

Appropriate monitoring and advice are required for patients with a history of hypertension and/or mild to moderate congestive heart failure as fluid retention and oedema have been reported in association with NSAID therapy.

Epidemiological data suggest that use of ibuprofen, particularly at a high dose (2400 mg/ daily) and in long term treatment, may be associated with a small increased risk of arterial thrombotic events such as myocardial infarction or stroke. Overall, epidemiological studies do not suggest that low dose ibuprofen (e.g. ⩽ 1200mg daily) is associated with an increased risk of arterial thrombotic events, particularly myocardial infarction.

Patients with uncontrolled hypertension, congestive heart failure, established ischaemic heart disease, peripheral arterial disease, and/or cerebrovascular disease should only be treated with ibuprofen after careful consideration. Similar consideration should be made before initiating longer-term treatment of patients with risk factors for cardiovascular events (e.g. hypertension, hyperlipidaemia, diabetes mellitus, smoking).

Renal effects

Caution should be used when initiating treatment with ibuprofen in patients with considerable dehydration.

As with other NSAIDs, long-term administration of ibuprofen has resulted in renal papillary necrosis and other renal pathologic changes. Renal toxicity has also been seen in patients in whom renal prostaglandins have a compensatory role in the maintenance of renal perfusion. In these patients, administration of an NSAID may cause a dose-dependant reduction in prostaglandin formation and, secondarily, in renal blood flow, which may precipitate overt renal decompensation. Patients at greatest risk of this reaction are those with impaired renal function, heart failure, liver dysfunction, those taking diuretics and ACE inhibitors and the elderly. Discontinuation of NSAID therapy is usually followed by recovery to the pre-treatment state.

SLE and mixed connective tissue disease

In patients with systemic lupus erythematosus (SLE) and mixed connective tissue disorders there may be an increased risk of aseptic meningitis (see below and section 4.8).

Dermatological effects

Serious skin reactions, some of them fatal, including exfoliative dermatitis, Stevens-Johnson syndrome, and toxic epidermal necrolysis, have been reported very rarely in association with the use of NSAIDs (see section 4.8). Patients appear to be at highest risk of these reactions early in the course of therapy, the onset of the reaction occurring within the first month of treatment in the majority of cases. Brufen should be discontinued at the first appearance of skin rash, mucosal lesions, or any other sign of hypersensitivity.

Haematological effects

Ibuprofen, like other NSAIDs, can interfere with platelet aggregation and has been shown to prolong bleeding time in normal subjects.

Aseptic meningitis

Aseptic meningitis has been observed on rare occasions in patients on ibuprofen therapy. Although it is probably more likely to occur in patients with systematic lupus erythematosus and related connective tissue diseases, it has been reported in patients who do not have an underlying chronic disease.

Impaired female fertility

The use of Brufen may impair female fertility and is not recommended in women attempting to conceive. In women who have difficulties conceiving or who are undergoing investigation of infertility, withdrawal of Brufen should be considered.

4.5 Interaction with other medicinal products and other forms of interaction

Care should be taken in patients treated with any of the following drugs as interactions have been reported in some patients.

Antihypertensives: Reduced antihypertensive effect.

Diuretics: Reduced diuretic effect. Diuretics can increase the risk of nephrotoxicity of NSAIDs.

Cardiac glycosides: NSAIDs may exacerbate cardiac failure, reduce GFR and increase plasma cardiac glycoside levels.

Lithium: Decreased elimination of lithium.

Methotrexate: Decreased elimination of methotrexate.

Ciclosporin: Increased risk of nephrotoxicity.

Mifepristone: NSAIDs should not be used for 8-12 days after mifepristone administration as NSAIDs can reduce the effects of mifepristone.

Other analgesics and cyclooxygenase-2 selective inhibitors: Avoid concomitant use of two or more NSAIDs, including Cox-2 inhibitors, as this may increase the risk of adverse effects (see section 4.4).

Aspirin: As with other products containing NSAIDs, concomitant administration of ibuprofen and aspirin is not generally recommended because of the potential of increased adverse effects.

Experimental data suggest that ibuprofen may inhibit the effect of low dose aspirin on platelet aggregation when they are dosed concomitantly. However, the limitations of these data and the uncertainties regarding extrapolation of ex vivo data to the clinical situation imply that no firm conclusions can be made for regular ibuprofen use, and no clinically relevant effect is considered to be likely for occasional use (see section 5.1).

Corticosteroids: Increased risk of gastrointestinal ulceration or bleeding with NSAIDs (see section 4.4).

Anticoagulants: NSAIDs may enhance the effects of anticoagulants, such as warfarin (see section 4.4).

Quinolone antibiotics: Animal data indicate that NSAIDs can increase the risk of convulsions associated with quinolone antibiotics. Patients taking NSAIDs and quinolones may have an increased risk of developing convulsions.

Anti-platelet agents and selective serotonin reuptake inhibitors (SSRIs): Increased risk of gastrointestinal bleeding with NSAIDs (see section 4.4).

Tacrolimus: Possible increased risk of nephrotoxicity when NSAIDs are given with tacrolimus.

Zidovudine: Increased risk of haematological toxicity when NSAIDs are given with zidovudine. There is evidence of an increased risk of haemarthroses and haematoma in HIV(+) haemophiliacs receiving concurrent treatment with zidovudine and ibuprofen.

Aminoglycosides: NSAIDs may decrease the excretion of aminoglycosides.

Herbal extracts: Ginkgo biloba may potentiate the risk of bleeding with NSAIDs.

4.6 Pregnancy and lactation

Pregnancy

Congenital abnormalities have been reported in association with NSAID administration in man; however, these are low in frequency and do not appear to follow any discernible pattern. In view of the known effects of NSAIDs on the foetal cardiovascular system (risk of closure of the ductus arteriosus), use in the last trimester of pregnancy is contraindicated. The onset of labour may be delayed and the duration increased with an increased bleeding tendency in both mother and child (see section 4.3). NSAIDs should not be used during the first two trimesters of pregnancy or labour unless the potential benefit to the patient outweighs the potential risk to the foetus.

Lactation

In the limited studies so far available, NSAIDs can appear in the breast milk in very low concentrations. NSAIDs should, if possible, be avoided when breastfeeding.

See section 4.4 Special warnings and precautions for use, regarding female fertility.

4.7 Effects on ability to drive and use machines

Undesirable effects such as dizziness, drowsiness, fatigue and visual disturbances are possible after taking NSAIDs. If affected, patients should not drive or operate machinery.

4.8 Undesirable effects

Gastrointestinal disorders: The most commonly observed adverse events are gastrointestinal in nature. Peptic ulcers, perforation or GI bleeding, sometimes fatal, particularly in the elderly, may occur (see section 4.4). Nausea, vomiting, diarrhoea, flatulence, constipation, dyspepsia, abdominal pain, melaena, haematemesis, ulcerative stomatitis, exacerbation of colitis and Crohn's disease (see section 4.4) have been reported following ibuprofen administration. Less frequently, gastritis has been observed. Pancreatitis has been reported very rarely.

Immune system disorders: Hypersensitivity reactions have been reported following treatment withNSAIDs. These may consist of (a) non-specific allergic reaction and anaphylaxis, (b) respiratory tract reactivity comprising asthma, aggravated asthma, bronchospasm or dyspnoea, or (c) assorted skin disorders, including rashes of various types, pruritus, urticaria, purpura, angioedema and, more rarely, exfoliative and bullous dermatoses (including Stevens-Johnson syndrome, toxic epidermal necrolysis and erythema multiforme).

Cardiac disorders and vascular disorders: Oedema, hypertension and cardiac failure have been reported in association with NSAID treatment. Epidemiological data suggest that use of ibuprofen, particularly at high dose (2400 mg/ daily), and in long term treatment, may be associated with a small increased risk of arterial thrombotic events such as myocardial infarction or stroke (see section 4.4).

Other adverse events reported less commonly and for which causality has not necessarily been established include:

Blood and lymphatic system disorders: Thrombocytopenia, neutropenia, agranulocytosis, aplastic anaemia and haemolytic anaemia.

Psychiatric disorders: Depression, confusional state, hallucination

Nervous system disorders: Optic neuritis, headache, paraesthesia, dizziness, somnolence

Aseptic meningitis (especially in patients with existing autoimmune disorders, such as systemic lupus erythematosus and mixed connective tissue disease) with symptoms of stiff neck, headache, nausea, vomiting, fever or disorientation (see section 4.4).

Eye disorders: Visual disturbance

Ear and labyrinth disorders: Tinnitus, vertigo

Hepatobiliary disorders: Abnormal liver function, hepatic failure, hepatitis and jaundice.

Skin and subcutaneous tissue disorders: Bullous reactions, including Stevens-Johnson syndrome and toxic epidermal necrolysis (very rare), and photosensitivity reaction.

Renal and urinary disorders: Impaired renal function and toxic nephropathy in various forms, including interstitial nephritis, nephrotic syndrome and renal failure.

General disorders and administration site conditions: Malaise, fatigue

4.9 Overdose

Symptoms

Symptoms include headache, nausea, vomiting, epigastric pain, gastrointestinal bleeding, rarely diarrhoea, disorientation, excitation, drowsiness, dizziness, tinnitus, fainting, depression of the CNS and respiratory system, coma, occasionally convulsions and rarely, loss of consciousness. In cases of significant poisoning, acute renal failure and liver damage are possible.

Therapeutic measures

Patients should be treated symptomatically as required. Within one hour of ingestion of a potentially toxic amount, activated charcoal should be considered. Alternatively, in adults, gastric lavage should be considered within one hour of ingestion of a potentially life-threatening overdose.

Good urine output should be ensured.

Renal and liver function should be closely monitored.

Patients should be observed for at least four hours after ingestion of potentially toxic amounts.

Frequent or prolonged convulsions should be treated with intravenous diazepam. Other measures may be indicated by the patient's clinical condition.

5. PHARMACOLOGICAL PROPERTIES

5.1 Pharmacodynamic properties

Ibuprofen is a propionic acid derivative with analgesic, anti-inflammatory and anti-pyretic activity. The drug's therapeutic effects as an NSAID are thought to result from its inhibitory effect on the enzyme cyclo-oxygenase, which results in a marked reduction in prostaglandin synthesis.

Experimental data suggest that ibuprofen may inhibit the effect of low dose aspirin on platelet aggregation when they are dosed concomitantly. In one study, when a single dose of ibuprofen 400mg was taken within 8 hours before or within 30 minutes after immediate release aspirin dosing (81mg), a decreased effect of aspirin on the formation of thromboxane or platelet aggregation occurred. However, the limitations of these data and the uncertainties regarding extrapolation of ex vivo data to the clinical situation imply that no firm conclusions can be made for regular ibuprofen use, and no clinically relevant effect is considered to be likely for occasional ibuprofen use.

5.2 Pharmacokinetic properties

Ibuprofen is rapidly absorbed from the gastrointestinal tract, peak serum concentrations occurring 1-2 hours after administration. The elimination half-life is approximately 2 hours.

Ibuprofen is metabolised in the liver to two inactive metabolites and these, together with unchanged ibuprofen, are excreted by the kidney either as such or as conjugates. Excretion by the kidney is both rapid and complete.

Ibuprofen is extensively bound to plasma proteins.

5.3 Preclinical safety data

Not applicable.

6. PHARMACEUTICAL PARTICULARS

6.1 List of excipients

Microcrystalline cellulose

Croscarmellose sodium

Lactose monohydrate

Colloidal anhydrous silica

Sodium lauryl sulphate

Magnesium stearate

Opadry white

or

Hydroxypropylmethylcellulose

plus

Talc

plus

Opaspray white M-1-7111B

Opacode S-1-8152HV black

Butanol

or

Industrial methylated spirit

Purified water

6.2 Incompatibilities

None known.

6.3 Shelf life

HDPE bottles: 36 months

PVC or PVC/PVDC blister packs: 36 months

6.4 Special precautions for storage

HDPE bottles: Do not store above 30°C

PVC or PVC/PVDC blister packs: Do not store above 25°C, store in the original pack.

6.5 Nature and contents of container

White high-density polyethylene bottle with a white polypropylene screw cap fitted with a waxed aluminium-faced pulpboard liner - pack size 9, 12, 100, 250 or 500 tablets.

Blister pack comprising of transparent polyvinyl chloride (PVC) with aluminium foil backing – pack size 60 tablets.

Blister pack comprising of transparent polyvinyl chloride (PVC) film coated on one face with polyvinylidene chloride (PVDC) with aluminium foil backing – pack size 60 tablets.

Not all pack sizes are marketed.

6.6 Special precautions for disposal and other handling

No special instructions.

Administrative Data

7. MARKETING AUTHORISATION HOLDER

Abbott Laboratories Limited

Queenborough

Kent

ME11 5EL

United Kingdom

8. MARKETING AUTHORISATION NUMBER(S)

PL 00037/0333

9. DATE OF FIRST AUTHORISATION/RENEWAL OF THE AUTHORISATION

25 February 2009

10. DATE OF REVISION OF THE TEXT

03 March 2009

Brufen 400 mg Tablets

(Abbott Laboratories Limited)

1. NAME OF THE MEDICINAL PRODUCT

Brufen Tablets 400mg

2. QUALITATIVE AND QUANTITATIVE COMPOSITION

Each Brufen tablet contains 400 mg Ibuprofen.

3. PHARMACEUTICAL FORM

A white, pillow-shaped, film-coated tablet with 'Brufen 400' printed in black on one face

4. CLINICAL PARTICULARS

4.1 Therapeutic indications

Brufen is indicated for its analgesic and anti-inflammatory effects in the treatment of rheumatoid arthritis (including juvenile rheumatoid arthritis or Still's disease), ankylosing spondylitis, osteoarthritis and other non-rheumatoid (seronegative) arthropathies.

In the treatment of non-articular rheumatic conditions, Brufen is indicated in periarticular conditions such as frozen shoulder (capsulitis), bursitis, tendonitis, tenosynovitis and low back pain; Brufen can also be used in soft tissue injuries such as sprains and strains.

Brufen is also indicated for its analgesic effect in the relief of mild to moderate pain such as dysmenorrhoea, dental and post-operative pain and for symptomatic relief of headache, including migraine headache.

4.2 Posology and method of administration

Undesirable effects may be minimised by using the lowest effective dose for the shortest duration necessary to control symptoms (see section 4.4).

Adults: The recommended dosage of Brufen is 1200-1800 mg daily in divided doses. Some patients can be maintained on 600-1200 mg daily. In severe or acute conditions, it can be advantageous to increase the dosage until the acute phase is brought under control, provided that the total daily dose does not exceed 2400 mg in divided doses.

Children: The daily dosage of Brufen is 20 mg/kg of body weight in divided doses.

In Juvenile Rheumatoid Arthritis, up to 40 mg/kg of body weight daily in divided doses may be taken.

Not recommended for children weighing less than 7 kg.

Elderly: The elderly are at increased risk of serious consequences of adverse reactions. If an NSAID is considered necessary, the lowest effective dose should be used and for the shortest possible duration. The patient should be monitored regularly for GI bleeding during NSAID therapy. If renal or hepatic function is impaired, dosage should be assessed individually.

For oral administration. To be taken preferably with or after food.

4.3 Contraindications

Brufen is contraindicated in patients with hypersensitivity to the active substance or to any of the excipients.

Brufen should not be used in patients who have previously shown hypersensitivity reactions (e.g. asthma, urticaria, angioedema or rhinitis) after taking ibuprofen, aspirin or other NSAIDs.

Brufen is also contraindicated in patients with a history of gastrointestinal bleeding or perforation, related to previous NSAID therapy. Brufen should not be used in patients with active, or history of, recurrent peptic ulcer or gastrointestinal haemorrhage (two or more distinct episodes of proven ulceration or bleeding).

Brufen is contraindicated in patients with severe heart failure, hepatic failure and renal failure (see section 4.4).

Brufen is contraindicated during the last trimester of pregnancy (see section 4.6).

4.4 Special warnings and precautions for use

Undesirable effects may be minimised by using the lowest effective dose for the shortest duration necessary to control symptoms (see section 4.2, and GI and cardiovascular risks below).

Patients with rare hereditary problems of galactose intolerance, the Lapp lactose deficiency or glucose-galactose malabsorption should not take this medication.

As with other NSAIDs, ibuprofen may mask the signs of infection.

The use of Brufen with concomitant NSAIDs, including cyclooxygenase-2 selective inhibitors, should be avoided due to the potential for additive effects (see section 4.5).

Elderly

The elderly have an increased frequency of adverse reactions to NSAIDs, especially gastrointestinal bleeding and perforation, which may be fatal (see section 4.2).

Gastrointestinal bleeding, ulceration and perforation

GI bleeding, ulceration or perforation, which can be fatal, has been reported with all NSAIDs at anytime during treatment, with or without warning symptoms or a previous history of serious GI events.

The risk of GI bleeding, ulceration or perforation is higher with increasing NSAID doses, in patients with a history of ulcer, particularly if complicated with haemorrhage or perforation (see section 4.3), and in the elderly. These patients should commence treatment on the lowest dose available. Combination therapy with protective agents (e.g. misoprostol or proton pump inhibitors) should be considered for these patients, and also for patients requiring concomitant low dose aspirin, or other drugs likely to increase gastrointestinal risk (see below and section 4.5).

Patients with a history of gastrointestinal disease, particularly when elderly, should report any unusual abdominal symptoms (especially gastrointestinal bleeding) particularly in the initial stages of treatment.

Caution should be advised in patients receiving concomitant medications which could increase the risk of ulceration or bleeding, such as oral corticosteroids, anticoagulants such as warfarin, selective serotonin-reuptake inhibitors or anti-platelet agents such as aspirin (see section 4.5).

When GI bleeding or ulceration occurs in patients receiving Brufen, the treatment should be withdrawn.

NSAIDs should be given with care to patients with a history of ulcerative colitis or Crohn's disease as these conditions may be exacerbated (see section 4.8).

Respiratory disorders

Caution is required if Brufen is administered to patients suffering from, or with a previous history of, bronchial asthma since NSAIDs have been reported to precipitate bronchospasm in such patients.

Cardiovascular, renal and hepatic impairment

The administration of an NSAID may cause a dose dependent reduction in prostaglandin formation and precipitate renal failure. Patients at greatest risk of this reaction are those with impaired renal function, cardiac impairment, liver dysfunction, those taking diuretics and the elderly. Renal function should be monitored in these patients (see also section 4.3).

Brufen should be given with care to patients with a history of heart failure or hypertension since oedema has been reported in association with ibuprofen administration.

Cardiovascular and cerebrovascular effects

Appropriate monitoring and advice are required for patients with a history of hypertension and/or mild to moderate congestive heart failure as fluid retention and oedema have been reported in association with NSAID therapy.

Epidemiological data suggest that use of ibuprofen, particularly at a high dose (2400 mg/ daily) and in long term treatment, may be associated with a small increased risk of arterial thrombotic events such as myocardial infarction or stroke. Overall, epidemiological studies do not suggest that low dose ibuprofen (e.g. ⩽ 1200mg daily) is associated with an increased risk of arterial thrombotic events, particularly myocardial infarction.

Patients with uncontrolled hypertension, congestive heart failure, established ischaemic heart disease, peripheral arterial disease, and/or cerebrovascular disease should only be treated with ibuprofen after careful consideration. Similar consideration should be made before initiating longer-term treatment of patients with risk factors for cardiovascular events (e.g. hypertension, hyperlipidaemia, diabetes mellitus, smoking).

Renal effects

Caution should be used when initiating treatment with ibuprofen in patients with considerable dehydration.

As with other NSAIDs, long-term administration of ibuprofen has resulted in renal papillary necrosis and other renal pathologic changes. Renal toxicity has also been seen in patients in whom renal prostaglandins have a compensatory role in the maintenance of renal perfusion. In these patients, administration of an NSAID may cause a dose-dependant reduction in prostaglandin formation and, secondarily, in renal blood flow, which may precipitate overt renal decompensation. Patients at greatest risk of this reaction are those with impaired renal function, heart failure, liver dysfunction, those taking diuretics and ACE inhibitors and the elderly. Discontinuation of NSAID therapy is usually followed by recovery to the pre-treatment state.

SLE and mixed connective tissue disease

In patients with systemic lupus erythematosus (SLE) and mixed connective tissue disorders there may be an increased risk of aseptic meningitis (see below and section 4.8).

Dermatological effects

Serious skin reactions, some of them fatal, including exfoliative dermatitis, Stevens-Johnson syndrome, and toxic epidermal necrolysis, have been reported very rarely in association with the use of NSAIDs (see section 4.8). Patients appear to be at highest risk of these reactions early in the course of therapy, the onset of the reaction occurring within the first month of treatment in the majority of cases. Brufen should be discontinued at the first appearance of skin rash, mucosal lesions, or any other sign of hypersensitivity.

Haematological effects

Ibuprofen, like other NSAIDs, can interfere with platelet aggregation and has been shown to prolong bleeding time in normal subjects.

Aseptic meningitis

Aseptic meningitis has been observed on rare occasions in patients on ibuprofen therapy. Although it is probably more likely to occur in patients with systematic lupus erythematosus and related connective tissue diseases, it has been reported in patients who do not have an underlying chronic disease.

Impaired female fertility

The use of Brufen may impair female fertility and is not recommended in women attempting to conceive. In women who have difficulties conceiving or who are undergoing investigation of infertility, withdrawal of Brufen should be considered.

4.5 Interaction with other medicinal products and other forms of interaction

Care should be taken in patients treated with any of the following drugs as interactions have been reported in some patients.

Antihypertensives: Reduced antihypertensive effect.

Diuretics: Reduced diuretic effect. Diuretics can increase the risk of nephrotoxicity of NSAIDs.

Cardiac glycosides: NSAIDs may exacerbate cardiac failure, reduce GFR and increase plasma cardiac glycoside levels.

Lithium: Decreased elimination of lithium.

Methotrexate: Decreased elimination of methotrexate.

Ciclosporin: Increased risk of nephrotoxicity.

Mifepristone: NSAIDs should not be used for 8-12 days after mifepristone administration as NSAIDs can reduce the effects of mifepristone.

Other analgesics and cyclooxygenase-2 selective inhibitors: Avoid concomitant use of two or more NSAIDs, including Cox-2 inhibitors, as this may increase the risk of adverse effects (see section 4.4).

Aspirin: As with other products containing NSAIDs, concomitant administration of ibuprofen and aspirin is not generally recommended because of the potential of increased adverse effects.

Experimental data suggest that ibuprofen may inhibit the effect of low dose aspirin on platelet aggregation when they are dosed concomitantly. However, the limitations of these data and the uncertainties regarding extrapolation of ex vivo data to the clinical situation imply that no firm conclusions can be made for regular ibuprofen use, and no clinically relevant effect is considered to be likely for occasional use (see section 5.1).

Corticosteroids: Increased risk of gastrointestinal ulceration or bleeding with NSAIDs (see section 4.4).

Anticoagulants: NSAIDs may enhance the effects of anticoagulants, such as warfarin (see section 4.4).

Quinolone antibiotics: Animal data indicate that NSAIDs can increase the risk of convulsions associated with quinolone antibiotics. Patients taking NSAIDs and quinolones may have an increased risk of developing convulsions.

Anti-platelet agents and selective serotonin reuptake inhibitors (SSRIs): Increased risk of gastrointestinal bleeding with NSAIDs (see section 4.4).

Tacrolimus: Possible increased risk of nephrotoxicity when NSAIDs are given with tacrolimus.

Zidovudine: Increased risk of haematological toxicity when NSAIDs are given with zidovudine. There is evidence of an increased risk of haemarthroses and haematoma in HIV(+) haemophiliacs receiving concurrent treatment with zidovudine and ibuprofen.

Aminoglycosides: NSAIDs may decrease the excretion of aminoglycosides.

Herbal extracts: Ginkgo biloba may potentiate the risk of bleeding with NSAIDs.

4.6 Pregnancy and lactation

Pregnancy

Congenital abnormalities have been reported in association with NSAID administration in man; however, these are low in frequency and do not appear to follow any discernible pattern. In view of the known effects of NSAIDs on the foetal cardiovascular system (risk of closure of the ductus arteriosus), use in the last trimester of pregnancy is contraindicated. The onset of labour may be delayed and the duration increased with an increased bleeding tendency in both mother and child (see section 4.3). NSAIDs should not be used during the first two trimesters of pregnancy or labour unless the potential benefit to the patient outweighs the potential risk to the foetus.

Lactation

In the limited studies so far available, NSAIDs can appear in the breast milk in very low concentrations. NSAIDs should, if possible, be avoided when breastfeeding.

See section 4.4 Special warnings and precautions for use, regarding female fertility.

4.7 Effects on ability to drive and use machines

Undesirable effects such as dizziness, drowsiness, fatigue and visual disturbances are possible after taking NSAIDs. If affected, patients should not drive or operate machinery.

4.8 Undesirable effects

Gastrointestinal disorders: The most commonly observed adverse events are gastrointestinal in nature. Peptic ulcers, perforation or GI bleeding, sometimes fatal, particularly in the elderly, may occur (see section 4.4). Nausea, vomiting, diarrhoea, flatulence, constipation, dyspepsia, abdominal pain, melaena, haematemesis, ulcerative stomatitis, exacerbation of colitis and Crohn's disease (see section 4.4) have been reported following ibuprofen administration. Less frequently, gastritis has been observed. Pancreatitis has been reported very rarely.

Immune system disorders: Hypersensitivity reactions have been reported following treatment withNSAIDs. These may consist of (a) non-specific allergic reaction and anaphylaxis, (b) respiratory tract reactivity comprising asthma, aggravated asthma, bronchospasm or dyspnoea, or (c) assorted skin disorders, including rashes of various types, pruritus, urticaria, purpura, angioedema and, more rarely, exfoliative and bullous dermatoses (including Stevens-Johnson syndrome, toxic epidermal necrolysis and erythema multiforme).

Cardiac disorders and vascular disorders: Oedema, hypertension and cardiac failure have been reported in association with NSAID treatment. Epidemiological data suggest that use of ibuprofen, particularly at high dose (2400 mg/daily), and in long term treatment, may be associated with a small increased risk of arterial thrombotic events such as myocardial infarction or stroke (see section 4.4).

Other adverse events reported less commonly and for which causality has not necessarily been established include:

Blood and lymphatic system disorders: Thrombocytopenia, neutropenia, agranulocytosis, aplastic anaemia and haemolytic anaemia.

Psychiatric disorders: Depression, confusional state, hallucination

Nervous system disorders: Optic neuritis, headache, paraesthesia, dizziness, somnolence

Aseptic meningitis (especially in patients with existing autoimmune disorders, such as systemic lupus erythematosus and mixed connective tissue disease) with symptoms of stiff neck, headache, nausea, vomiting, fever or disorientation (see section 4.4).

Eye disorders: Visual disturbance

Ear and labyrinth disorders: Tinnitus, vertigo

Hepatobiliary disorders: Abnormal liver function, hepatic failure, hepatitis and jaundice.

Skin and subcutaneous tissue disorders: Bullous reactions, including Stevens-Johnson syndrome and toxic epidermal necrolysis (very rare), and photosensitivity reaction.

Renal and urinary disorders: Impaired renal function and toxic nephropathy in various forms, including interstitial nephritis, nephrotic syndrome and renal failure.

General disorders and administration site conditions: Malaise, fatigue

4.9 Overdose

Symptoms

Symptoms include headache, nausea, vomiting, epigastric pain, gastrointestinal bleeding, rarely diarrhoea, disorientation, excitation, drowsiness, dizziness, tinnitus, fainting, depression of the CNS and respiratory system, coma, occasionally convulsions and rarely, loss of consciousness. In cases of significant poisoning, acute renal failure and liver damage are possible.

Therapeutic measures

Patients should be treated symptomatically as required. Within one hour of ingestion of a potentially toxic amount, activated charcoal should be considered. Alternatively, in adults, gastric lavage should be considered within one hour of ingestion of a potentially life-threatening overdose.

Good urine output should be ensured.

Renal and liver function should be closely monitored.

Patients should be observed for at least four hours after ingestion of potentially toxic amounts.

Frequent or prolonged convulsions should be treated with intravenous diazepam. Other measures may be indicated by the patient's clinical condition.

5. PHARMACOLOGICAL PROPERTIES

5.1 Pharmacodynamic properties

Ibuprofen is a propionic acid derivative with analgesic, anti-inflammatory and anti-pyretic activity. The drug's therapeutic effects as an NSAID are thought to result from its inhibitory effect on the enzyme cyclo-oxygenase, which results in a marked reduction in prostaglandin synthesis.

Experimental data suggest that ibuprofen may inhibit the effect of low dose aspirin on platelet aggregation when they are dosed concomitantly. In one study, when a single dose of ibuprofen 400mg was taken within 8 hours before or within 30 minutes after immediate release aspirin dosing (81mg), a decreased effect of aspirin on the formation of thromboxane or platelet aggregation occurred. However, the limitations of these data and the uncertainties regarding extrapolation of ex vivo data to the clinical situation imply that no firm conclusions can be made for regular ibuprofen use, and no clinically relevant effect is considered to be likely for occasional ibuprofen use.

5.2 Pharmacokinetic properties

Ibuprofen is rapidly absorbed from the gastrointestinal tract, peak serum concentrations occurring 1-2 hours after administration. The elimination half-life is approximately 2 hours.

Ibuprofen is metabolised in the liver to two inactive metabolites and these, together with unchanged ibuprofen, are excreted by the kidney either as such or as conjugates. Excretion by the kidney is both rapid and complete.

Ibuprofen is extensively bound to plasma proteins.

5.3 Preclinical safety data

Not applicable.

6. PHARMACEUTICAL PARTICULARS

6.1 List of excipients

Microcrystalline cellulose

Croscarmellose sodium

Lactose monohydrate

Colloidal anhydrous silica

Sodium lauryl sulphate

Magnesium stearate

Opadry white

or

Hydroxypropylmethylcellulose

plus

Talc

plus

Opaspray white M-1-7111B

Opacode S-1-8152HV black

Butanol

or

Industrial methylated spirit

Purified water

6.2 Incompatibilities

Not applicable.

6.3 Shelf life

HDPE bottles: 36 months

PVC or PVC/PVDC blister packs: 36 months

6.4 Special precautions for storage

HDPE bottles: Do not store above 30°C.

PVC or PVC/PVDC blister packs: Do not store above 25°C, store in the original pack.

6.5 Nature and contents of container

White high-density polyethylene bottle with a white polypropylene screw cap fitted with a waxed aluminium-faced pulpboard liner - pack size 9, 12, 100, 250 or 500 tablets.

Blister pack comprising of transparent polyvinyl chloride (PVC) with aluminium foil backing – pack size 60 tablets.

Blister pack comprising of transparent polyvinyl chloride (PVC) film coated on one face with polyvinylidene chloride (PVDC) with aluminium foil backing – pack size 60 tablets.

Not all pack sizes are marketed.

6.6 Special precautions for disposal and other handling

None.

7. MARKETING AUTHORISATION HOLDER

Abbott Laboratories Limited

Queenborough

Kent

ME11 5EL

United Kingdom

8. MARKETING AUTHORISATION NUMBER(S)

PL 00037/0334

9. DATE OF FIRST AUTHORISATION/RENEWAL OF THE AUTHORISATION

04 March 2009

10. DATE OF REVISION OF THE TEXT

04 March 2009

Brufen 600 mg Tablets

(Abbott Laboratories Limited)

1. NAME OF THE MEDICINAL PRODUCT

Brufen Tablets 600 mg

2. QUALITATIVE AND QUANTITATIVE COMPOSITION

Each Brufen Tablet contains 600 mg Ibuprofen.

3. PHARMACEUTICAL FORM

A white, pillow-shaped, film-coated tablet with 'Brufen 600' printed in black on one face.

4. CLINICAL PARTICULARS

4.1 Therapeutic indications

Brufen is indicated for its analgesic and anti-inflammatory effects in the treatment of rheumatoid arthritis (including juvenile rheumatoid arthritis or Still's disease), ankylosing spondylitis, osteoarthritis and other non-rheumatoid (seronegative) arthropathies.

In the treatment of non-articular rheumatic conditions, Brufen is indicated in periarticular conditions such as frozen shoulder (capsulitis), bursitis, tendinitis, tenosynovitis and low back pain; Brufen can also be used in soft tissue injuries such as sprains and strains.

rufen is also indicated for its analgesic effect in the relief f mild to moderate pain such as dysmenorrhoea, dental nd post-operative pain and for symptomatic relief of eadache, including migraine headache.

2 Posology and method of administration

ndesirable effects may be minimised by using the lowest ffective dose for the shortest duration necessary to con-ol symptoms (see section 4.4).

dults: The recommended dosage of Brufen is 1200-300 mg daily in divided doses. Some patients can be aintained on 600-1200 mg daily. In severe or acute con-tions, it can be advantageous to increase the dosage until e acute phase is brought under control, provided that the tal daily dose does not exceed 2400 mg in divided doses.

hildren: The daily dosage of Brufen is 20 mg/kg of body eight in divided doses.

Juvenile Rheumatoid Arthritis, up to 40 mg/kg of body eight daily in divided doses may be taken.

ot recommended for children weighing less than 7 kg.

derly: The elderly are at increased risk of serious con-quences of adverse reactions. If an NSAID is considered cessary, the lowest effective dose should be used and the shortest possible duration. The patient should be onitored regularly for GI bleeding during NSAID therapy. renal or hepatic function is impaired, dosage should be sessed individually.

r oral administration. To be taken preferably with or after od.

3 Contraindications

ufen is contraindicated in patients with hypersensitivity the active substance or to any of the excipients.

ufen should not be used in patients who have previously own hypersensitivity reactions (e.g. asthma, urticaria, gioedema or rhinitis) after taking ibuprofen, aspirin or ner NSAIDs.

ufen is also contraindicated in patients with a history of strointestinal bleeding or perforation, related to previous SAID therapy. Brufen should not be used in patients with tive, or history of, recurrent peptic ulcer or gastrointest-l haemorrhage (two or more distinct episodes of proven eration or bleeding).

ufen is contraindicated in patients with severe heart ure, hepatic failure and renal failure (see section 4.4).

ufen is contraindicated during the last trimester of preg-ncy (see section 4.6).

Special warnings and precautions for use

desirable effects may be minimised by using the lowest ective dose for the shortest duration necessary to con-symptoms (see section 4.2, and GI and cardiovascular ks below).

tients with rare hereditary problems of galactose intol-nce, the Lapp lactose deficiency or glucose-galactose labsorption should not take this medication.

with other NSAIDs, ibuprofen may mask the signs of ection.

e use of Brufen with concomitant NSAIDs, including looxygenase-2 selective inhibitors, should be avoided e to the potential for additive effects (see section 4.5).

erly

elderly have an increased frequency of adverse reac-ns to NSAIDs, especially gastrointestinal bleeding and foration, which may be fatal (see section 4.2).

strointestinal bleeding, ulceration and perforation

bleeding, ulceration or perforation, which can be fatal, been reported with all NSAIDs at anytime during treat-nt, with or without warning symptoms or a previous ory of serious GI events.

risk of GI bleeding, ulceration or perforation is higher n increasing NSAID doses, in patients with a history of er, particularly if complicated with haemorrhage or per-tion (see section 4.3), and in the elderly. These patients uld commence treatment on the lowest dose available. mbination therapy with protective agents (e.g. miso-stol or proton pump inhibitors) should be considered these patients, and also for patients requiring conco-ant low dose aspirin, or other drugs likely to increase trointestinal risk (see below and section 4.5).

ents with a history of gastrointestinal disease, particu-when elderly, should report any unusual abdominal ptoms (especially gastrointestinal bleeding) particu-in the initial stages of treatment.

tion should be advised in patients receiving concomi-medications which could increase the risk of ulceration bleeding, such as oral corticosteroids, anticoagulants h as warfarin, selective serotonin-reuptake inhibitors or -platelet agents such as aspirin (see section 4.5).

en GI bleeding or ulceration occurs in patients receiving fen, the treatment should be withdrawn.

AIDs should be given with care to patients with a history lcerative colitis or Crohn's disease as these conditions be exacerbated (see section 4.8).

piratory disorders

tion is required if Brufen is administered to patients ering from, or with a previous history of, bronchial ma since NSAIDs have been reported to precipitate nchospasm in such patients.

Cardiovascular, renal and hepatic impairment

The administration of an NSAID may cause a dose dependent reduction in prostaglandin formation and precipitate renal failure. Patients at greatest risk of this reaction are those with impaired renal function, cardiac impairment, liver dysfunction, those taking diuretics and the elderly. Renal function should be monitored in these patients (see also section 4.3).

Brufen should be given with care to patients with a history of heart failure or hypertension since oedema has been reported in association with ibuprofen administration.

Cardiovascular and cerebrovascular effects

Appropriate monitoring and advice are required for patients with a history of hypertension and/or mild to moderate congestive heart failure as fluid retention and oedema have been reported in association with NSAID therapy.

Epidemiological data suggest that use of ibuprofen, particularly at a high dose (2400 mg/ daily) and in long term treatment, may be associated with a small increased risk of arterial thrombotic events such as myocardial infarction or stroke. Overall, epidemiological studies do not suggest that low dose ibuprofen (e.g. ≤ 1200mg daily) is associated with an increased risk of arterial thrombotic events, particularly myocardial infarction.

Patients with uncontrolled hypertension, congestive heart failure, established ischaemic heart disease, peripheral arterial disease, and/or cerebrovascular disease should only be treated with ibuprofen after careful consideration. Similar consideration should be made before initiating longer-term treatment of patients with risk factors for cardiovascular events (e.g. hypertension, hyperlipidaemia, diabetes mellitus, smoking).

Renal effects

Caution should be used when initiating treatment with ibuprofen in patients with considerable dehydration.

As with other NSAIDs, long-term administration of ibuprofen has resulted in renal papillary necrosis and other renal pathologic changes. Renal toxicity has also been seen in patients in whom renal prostaglandins have a compensatory role in the maintenance of renal perfusion. In these patients, administration of an NSAID may cause a dose-dependant reduction in prostaglandin formation and, secondarily, in renal blood flow, which may precipitate overt renal decompensation. Patients at greatest risk of this reaction are those with impaired renal function, heart failure, liver dysfunction, those taking diuretics and ACE inhibitors and the elderly. Discontinuation of NSAID therapy is usually followed by recovery to the pre-treatment state.

SLE and mixed connective tissue disease

In patients with systemic lupus erythematosus (SLE) and mixed connective tissue disorders there may be an increased risk of aseptic meningitis (see below and section 4.8).

Dermatological effects

Serious skin reactions, some of them fatal, including exfoliative dermatitis, Stevens-Johnson syndrome, and toxic epidermal necrolysis, have been reported very rarely in association with the use of NSAIDs (see section 4.8). Patients appear to be at highest risk of these reactions early in the course of therapy, the onset of the reaction occurring within the first month of treatment in the majority of cases. Brufen should be discontinued at the first appearance of skin rash, mucosal lesions, or any other sign of hypersensitivity.

Haematological effects

Ibuprofen, like other NSAIDs, can interfere with platelet aggregation and has been shown to prolong bleeding time in normal subjects.

Aseptic meningitis

Aseptic meningitis has been observed on rare occasions in patients on ibuprofen therapy. Although it is probably more likely to occur in patients with systematic lupus erythematosus and related connective tissue diseases, it has been reported in patients who do not have an underlying chronic disease.

Impaired female fertility

The use of Brufen may impair female fertility and is not recommended in women attempting to conceive. In women who have difficulties conceiving or who are undergoing investigation of infertility, withdrawal of Brufen should be considered.

4.5 Interaction with other medicinal products and other forms of interaction

Care should be taken in patients treated with any of the following drugs as interactions have been reported in some patients.

Antihypertensives: Reduced antihypertensive effect.

Diuretics: Reduced diuretic effect. Diuretics can increase the risk of nephrotoxicity of NSAIDs.

Cardiac glycosides: NSAIDs may exacerbate cardiac failure, reduce GFR and increase plasma cardiac glycoside levels.

Lithium: Decreased elimination of lithium.

Methotrexate: Decreased elimination of methotrexate.

Ciclosporin: Increased risk of nephrotoxicity.

Mifepristone: NSAIDs should not be used for 8-12 days after mifepristone administration as NSAIDs can reduce the effects of mifepristone.

Other analgesics and cyclooxygenase-2 selective inhibitors: Avoid concomitant use of two or more NSAIDs, including Cox-2 inhibitors, as this may increase the risk of adverse effects (see section 4.4).

Aspirin: As with other products containing NSAIDs, concomitant administration of ibuprofen and aspirin is not generally recommended because of the potential of increased adverse effects.

Experimental data suggest that ibuprofen may inhibit the effect of low dose aspirin on platelet aggregation when they are dosed concomitantly. However, the limitations of these data and the uncertainties regarding extrapolation of ex vivo data to the clinical situation imply that no firm conclusions can be made for regular ibuprofen use, and no clinically relevant effect is considered to be likely for occasional use (see section 5.1).

Corticosteroids: Increased risk of gastrointestinal ulceration or bleeding with NSAIDs (see section 4.4).

Anticoagulants: NSAIDs may enhance the effects of anticoagulants, such as warfarin (see section 4.4).

Quinolone antibiotics: Animal data indicate that NSAIDs can increase the risk of convulsions associated with quinolone antibiotics. Patients taking NSAIDs and quinolones may have an increased risk of developing convulsions.

Anti-platelet agents and selective serotonin reuptake inhibitors (SSRIs): Increased risk of gastrointestinal bleeding with NSAIDs (see section 4.4).

Tacrolimus: Possible increased risk of nephrotoxicity when NSAIDs are given with tacrolimus.

Zidovudine: Increased risk of haematological toxicity when NSAIDs are given with zidovudine. There is evidence of an increased risk of haemarthroses and haematoma in HIV(+) haemophiliacs receiving concurrent treatment with zidovudine and ibuprofen.

Aminoglycosides: NSAIDs may decrease the excretion of aminoglycosides.

Herbal extracts: Ginkgo biloba may potentiate the risk of bleeding with NSAIDs.

4.6 Pregnancy and lactation

Pregnancy

Congenital abnormalities have been reported in association with NSAID administration in man; however, these are low in frequency and do not appear to follow any discernible pattern. In view of the known effects of NSAIDs on the foetal cardiovascular system (risk of closure of the ductus arteriosus), use in the last trimester of pregnancy is contraindicated. The onset of labour may be delayed and the duration increased with an increased bleeding tendency in both mother and child (see section 4.3). NSAIDs should not be used during the first two trimesters of pregnancy or labour unless the potential benefit to the patient outweighs the potential risk to the foetus.

Lactation

In the limited studies so far available, NSAIDs can appear in the breast milk in very low concentrations. NSAIDs should, if possible, be avoided when breastfeeding.

See section 4.4 Special warnings and precautions for use, regarding female fertility.

4.7 Effects on ability to drive and use machines

Undesirable effects such as dizziness, drowsiness, fatigue and visual disturbances are possible after taking NSAIDs. If affected, patients should not drive or operate machinery.

4.8 Undesirable effects

Gastrointestinal disorders: The most commonly observed adverse events are gastrointestinal in nature. Peptic ulcers, perforation or GI bleeding, sometimes fatal, particularly in the elderly, may occur (see section 4.4). Nausea, vomiting, diarrhoea, flatulence, constipation, dyspepsia, abdominal pain, melaena, haematemesis, ulcerative stomatitis, exacerbation of colitis and Crohn's disease (see section 4.4) have been reported following ibuprofen administration. Less frequently, gastritis has been observed. Pancreatitis has been reported very rarely.

Immune system disorders: Hypersensitivity reactions have been reported following treatment withNSAIDs. These may consist of (a) non-specific allergic reaction and anaphylaxis, (b) respiratory tract reactivity comprising asthma, aggravated asthma, bronchospasm or dyspnoea, or (c) assorted skin disorders, including rashes of various types, pruritus, urticaria, purpura, angioedema and, more rarely, exfoliative and bullous dermatoses (including Stevens-Johnson syndrome, toxic epidermal necrolysis and erythema multiforme).

Cardiac disorders and vascular disorders: Oedema, hypertension and cardiac failure have been reported in association with NSAID treatment. Epidemiological data suggest that use of ibuprofen, particularly at high dose (2400 mg/ daily), and in long term treatment, may be associated with a small increased risk of arterial thrombotic events such as myocardial infarction or stroke (see section 4.4).

Other adverse events reported less commonly and for which causality has not necessarily been established include:

Blood and lymphatic system disorders: Thrombocytopenia, neutropenia, agranulocytosis, aplastic anaemia and haemolytic anaemia.

Psychiatric disorders: Depression, confusional state, hallucination

Nervous system disorders: Optic neuritis, headache, paraesthesia, dizziness, somnolence

Aseptic meningitis (especially in patients with existing autoimmune disorders, such as systemic lupus erythematosus and mixed connective tissue disease) with symptoms of stiff neck, headache, nausea, vomiting, fever or disorientation (see section 4.4).

Eye disorders: Visual disturbance

Ear and labyrinth disorders: Tinnitus, vertigo

Hepatobiliary disorders: Abnormal liver function, hepatic failure, hepatitis and jaundice.

Skin and subcutaneous tissue disorders: Bullous reactions, including Stevens-Johnson syndrome and toxic epidermal necrolysis (very rare), and photosensitivity reaction.

Renal and urinary disorders: Impaired renal function and toxic nephropathy in various forms, including interstitial nephritis, nephrotic syndrome and renal failure.

General disorders and administration site conditions: Malaise, fatigue

4.9 Overdose

Symptoms

Symptoms include headache, nausea, vomiting, epigastric pain, gastrointestinal bleeding, rarely diarrhoea, disorientation, excitation, drowsiness, dizziness, tinnitus, fainting, depression of the CNS and respiratory system, coma, occasionally convulsions and rarely, loss of consciousness. In cases of significant poisoning, acute renal failure and liver damage are possible.

Therapeutic measures

Patients should be treated symptomatically as required. Within one hour of ingestion of a potentially toxic amount, activated charcoal should be considered. Alternatively, in adults, gastric lavage should be considered within one hour of ingestion of a potentially life-threatening overdose.

Good urine output should be ensured.

Renal and liver function should be closely monitored.

Patients should be observed for at least four hours after ingestion of potentially toxic amounts.

Frequent or prolonged convulsions should be treated with intravenous diazepam. Other measures may be indicated by the patient's clinical condition.

5. PHARMACOLOGICAL PROPERTIES

5.1 Pharmacodynamic properties

Ibuprofen is a propionic acid derivative with analgesic, anti-inflammatory and anti-pyretic activity. The drug's therapeutic effects as an NSAID are thought to result from its inhibitory effect on the enzyme cyclo-oxygenase, which results in a marked reduction in prostaglandin synthesis.

Experimental data suggest that ibuprofen may inhibit the effect of low dose aspirin on platelet aggregation when they are dosed concomitantly. In one study, when a single dose of ibuprofen 400mg was taken within 8 hours before or within 30 minutes after immediate release aspirin dosing (81mg), a decreased effect of aspirin on the formation of thromboxane or platelet aggregation occurred. However, the limitations of these data and the uncertainties regarding extrapolation of ex vivo data to the clinical situation imply that no firm conclusions can be made for regular ibuprofen use, and no clinically relevant effect is considered to be likely for occasional ibuprofen use.

5.2 Pharmacokinetic properties

Ibuprofen is rapidly absorbed from the gastrointestinal tract, peak serum concentrations occurring 1-2 hours after administration. The elimination half-life is approximately 2 hours.

Ibuprofen is metabolised in the liver to two inactive metabolites and these, together with unchanged ibuprofen, are excreted by the kidney either as such or as conjugates. Excretion by the kidney is both rapid and complete.

Ibuprofen is extensively bound to plasma proteins.

5.3 Preclinical safety data

Not applicable.

6. PHARMACEUTICAL PARTICULARS

6.1 List of excipients

Microcrystalline cellulose

Croscarmellose sodium

Lactose monohydrate

Colloidal anhydrous silica

Sodium lauryl sulphate

Magnesium stearate

Opadry white

or

Hydroxypropylmethylcellulose

plus

Talc

plus

Opaspray white M-1-7111B

Opacode S-1-8152HV black

Butanol

or

Industrial methylated spirit

Purified water

6.2 Incompatibilities

None.

6.3 Shelf life

HDPE bottles: 36 months.

PVC or PVC/PVDC blister packs: 36 months

6.4 Special precautions for storage

HDPE bottles: Do not store above 30°C

PVC or PVC/PVDC blister packs: Do not store above 25°C, store in the original pack.

6.5 Nature and contents of container

White high-density polyethylene bottle with a white polypropylene screw cap fitted with a waxed aluminium-faced pulpboard liner - pack size 12, 30, 100 tablets.

Blister pack comprising of transparent polyvinyl chloride (PVC) with aluminium foil backing – pack size 60 tablets.

Blister pack comprising of transparent polyvinyl chloride (PVC) film coated on one face with polyvinylidene chloride (PVDC) with aluminium foil backing – pack size 60 tablets.

Not all pack sizes are marketed.

6.6 Special precautions for disposal and other handling

None.

7. MARKETING AUTHORISATION HOLDER

Abbott Laboratories Limited

Queenborough

Kent

ME11 5EL

United Kingdom

8. MARKETING AUTHORISATION NUMBER(S)

PL 00037/0335

9. DATE OF FIRST AUTHORISATION/RENEWAL OF THE AUTHORISATION

25 February 2009

10. DATE OF REVISION OF THE TEXT

03 March 2009

Brufen Granules

(Abbott Laboratories Limited)

1. NAME OF THE MEDICINAL PRODUCT

Brufen Granules

2. QUALITATIVE AND QUANTITATIVE COMPOSITION

Ibuprofen BP 600 mg

3. PHARMACEUTICAL FORM

Effervescent granules

4. CLINICAL PARTICULARS

4.1 Therapeutic indications

Brufen Granules are indicated for their analgesic and anti-inflammatory effects in the treatment of rheumatoid arthritis, ankylosing spondylitis, osteoarthritis and other non-rheumatoid (seronegative) arthropathies.

In the treatment of non-articular rheumatic conditions, Brufen Granules are indicated in peri-articular conditions such as frozen shoulder (capsulitis), bursitis, tendinitis, tenosynovitis and low back pain; Brufen Granules can also be used in soft-tissue injuries such as sprains and strains.

Brufen Granules are also indicated for their analgesic effect in the relief of mild to moderate pain such as dysmenorrhoea, dental and post-operative pain and for symptomatic relief of headache including migraine headache.

4.2 Posology and method of administration

Undesirable effects may be minimised by using the lowest effective dose for the shortest duration necessary to control symptoms (see section 4.4).

Adults: The recommended dosage of Brufen is 1200-1800 mg daily in divided doses. Some patients can be maintained on 600-1200 mg daily. Total daily dose should not exceed 2400 mg.

Children: Brufen Granules are not suitable for use in children.

Elderly: The elderly are at increased risk of serious consequences of adverse reactions. If an NSAID is considered necessary, the lowest effective dose should be used and for the shortest possible duration. The patient should be monitored regularly for GI bleeding during NSAID therapy. If renal or hepatic function is impaired, dosage should be assessed individually.

For oral administration. To be taken preferably with or after food.

4.3 Contraindications

Brufen is contraindicated in patients with hypersensitivity to the active substance or to any of the excipients.

Brufen should not be used in patients who have previously shown hypersensitivity reactions (e.g. asthma, urticaria angioedema or rhinitis) after taking ibuprofen, aspirin or other NSAIDs.

Brufen is also contraindicated in patients with a history of gastrointestinal bleeding or perforation, related to previous NSAID therapy. Brufen should not be used in patients with active, or history of, recurrent peptic ulcer or gastrointestinal haemorrhage (two or more distinct episodes of proven ulceration or bleeding).

Brufen is contraindicated in patients with severe heart failure, hepatic failure and renal failure (see section 4.4).

Brufen is contraindicated during the last trimester of pregnancy (see section 4.6).

4.4 Special warnings and precautions for use

Undesirable effects may be minimised by using the lowest effective dose for the shortest duration necessary to control symptoms (see section 4.2, and GI and cardiovascular risks below).

Patients with rare hereditary problems of fructose intolerance, glucose-galactose malaabsorption or sucrase-isomaltase insufficiency should not take this medicine.

As with other NSAIDs, ibuprofen may mask the signs of infection.

Each Brufen Granules sachet contains 197mg (approximately 9 mEq) sodium. This should be considered in patients whose overall intake of sodium must be markedly restricted.

The use of Brufen with concomitant NSAIDs, including cyclooxygenase-2 selective inhibitors, should be avoided due to the potential for additive effects (see section 4.5).

Elderly

The elderly have an increased frequency of adverse reactions to NSAIDs, especially gastrointestinal bleeding and perforation, which may be fatal (see section 4.2).

Gastrointestinal bleeding, ulceration and perforation

GI bleeding, ulceration or perforation, which can be fatal, has been reported with all NSAIDs at anytime during treatment, with or without warning symptoms or a previous history of serious GI events.

The risk of GI bleeding, ulceration or perforation is higher with increasing NSAID doses, in patients with a history of ulcer, particularly if complicated with haemorrhage or perforation (see section 4.3), and in the elderly. These patients should commence treatment on the lowest dose available. Combination therapy with protective agents (e.g. misoprostol or proton pump inhibitors) should be considered for these patients, and also for patients requiring concomitant low dose aspirin, or other drugs likely to increase gastrointestinal risk (see below and section 4.5).

Patients with a history of gastrointestinal disease, particularly when elderly, should report any unusual abdominal symptoms (especially gastrointestinal bleeding) particularly in the initial stages of treatment.

Caution should be advised in patients receiving concomitant medications which could increase the risk of ulceration or bleeding, such as oral corticosteroids, anticoagulants such as warfarin, selective serotonin-reuptake inhibitors or anti-platelet agents such as aspirin (see section 4.5).

When GI bleeding or ulceration occurs in patients receiving Brufen, the treatment should be withdrawn.

NSAIDs should be given with care to patients with a history of ulcerative colitis or Crohn's disease as these conditions may be exacerbated (see section 4.8).

Respiratory disorders

Caution is required if Brufen is administered to patients suffering from, or with a previous history of, bronchial asthma since NSAIDs have been reported to precipitate bronchospasm in such patients.

Cardiovascular, renal and hepatic impairment

The administration of an NSAID may cause a dose dependent reduction in prostaglandin formation and precipitate renal failure. Patients at greatest risk of this reaction are those with impaired renal function, cardiac impairment, liver dysfunction, those taking diuretics and the elderly. Renal function should be monitored in these patients (see also section 4.3).

Brufen should be given with care to patients with a history of heart failure or hypertension since oedema has been reported in association with ibuprofen administration.

Cardiovascular and cerebrovascular effects

Appropriate monitoring and advice are required for patients with a history of hypertension and/or mild to moderate congestive heart failure as fluid retention and oedema have been reported in association with NSAID therapy.

Epidemiological data suggest that use of ibuprofen, particularly at a high dose (2400 mg/ daily) and in long term treatment, may be associated with a small increased risk of arterial thrombotic events such as myocardial infarction or stroke. Overall, epidemiological studies do not suggest that low dose ibuprofen (e.g. ≤ 1200mg daily) is associated with an increased risk of arterial thrombotic events, particularly myocardial infarction.

Patients with uncontrolled hypertension, congestive heart failure, established ischaemic heart disease, peripheral arterial disease, and/or cerebrovascular disease should only be treated with ibuprofen after careful consideration. Similar consideration should be made before initiating longer-term treatment of patients with risk factors for cardiovascular events (e.g. hypertension, hyperlipidaemia, diabetes mellitus, smoking).

Renal effects

Caution should be used when initiating treatment with ibuprofen in patients with considerable dehydration.

As with other NSAIDs, long-term administration of ibuprofen has resulted in renal papillary necrosis and other renal pathologic changes. Renal toxicity has also been seen in patients in whom renal prostaglandins have a compensatory role in the maintenance of renal perfusion. In these patients, administration of an NSAID may cause a dose-dependant reduction in prostaglandin formation and, secondarily, in renal blood flow, which may precipitate overt renal decompensation. Patients at greatest risk of this reaction are those with impaired renal function, heart failure, liver dysfunction, those taking diuretics and ACE inhibitors and the elderly. Discontinuation of NSAID therapy is usually followed by recovery to the pre-treatment state.

SLE and mixed connective tissue disease

In patients with systemic lupus erythematosus (SLE) and mixed connective tissue disorders there may be an increased risk of aseptic meningitis (see below and section 4.8).

Dermatological effects

Serious skin reactions, some of them fatal, including exfoliative dermatitis, Stevens-Johnson syndrome, and toxic epidermal necrolysis, have been reported very rarely in association with the use of NSAIDs (see section 4.8). Patients appear to be at highest risk of these reactions early in the course of therapy, the onset of the reaction occurring within the first month of treatment in the majority of cases. Brufen should be discontinued at the first appearance of skin rash, mucosal lesions, or any other sign of hypersensitivity.

Haematological effects

Ibuprofen, like other NSAIDs, can interfere with platelet aggregation and has been shown to prolong bleeding time in normal subjects.

Aseptic meningitis

Aseptic meningitis has been observed on rare occasions in patients on ibuprofen therapy. Although it is probably more likely to occur in patients with systematic lupus erythematosus and related connective tissue diseases, it has been reported in patients who do not have an underlying chronic disease.

Impaired female fertility

The use of Brufen may impair female fertility and is not recommended in women attempting to conceive. In women who have difficulties conceiving or who are undergoing investigation of infertility, withdrawal of Brufen should be considered.

4.5 Interaction with other medicinal products and other forms of interaction

Care should be taken in patients treated with any of the following drugs as interactions have been reported in some patients.

Antihypertensives: Reduced antihypertensive effect.

Diuretics: Reduced diuretic effect. Diuretics can increase the risk of nephrotoxicity of NSAIDs.

Cardiac glycosides: NSAIDs may exacerbate cardiac failure, reduce GFR and increase plasma cardiac glycoside levels.

Lithium: Decreased elimination of lithium.

Methotrexate: Decreased elimination of methotrexate.

Ciclosporin: Increased risk of nephrotoxicity.

Mifepristone: NSAIDs should not be used for 8-12 days after mifepristone administration as NSAIDs can reduce the effects of mifepristone.

Other analgesics and cyclooxygenase-2 selective inhibitors: Avoid concomitant use of two or more NSAIDs, including Cox-2 inhibitors, as this may increase the risk of adverse effects (see section 4.4).

Aspirin: As with other products containing NSAIDs, concomitant administration of ibuprofen and aspirin is not generally recommended because of the potential of increased adverse effects.

Experimental data suggest that ibuprofen may inhibit the effect of low dose aspirin on platelet aggregation when they are dosed concomitantly. However, the limitations of these data and the uncertainties regarding extrapolation of ex vivo data to the clinical situation imply that no firm conclusions can be made for regular ibuprofen use, and no clinically relevant effect is considered to be likely for occasional use (see section 5.1).

Corticosteroids: Increased risk of gastrointestinal ulceration or bleeding with NSAIDs (see section 4.4).

Anticoagulants: NSAIDs may enhance the effects of anticoagulants, such as warfarin (see section 4.4).

Quinolone antibiotics: Animal data indicate that NSAIDs can increase the risk of convulsions associated with quinolone antibiotics. Patients taking NSAIDs and quinolones may have an increased risk of developing convulsions.

Anti-platelet agents and selective serotonin reuptake inhibitors (SSRIs): Increased risk of gastrointestinal bleeding with NSAIDs (see section 4.4).

Tacrolimus: Possible increased risk of nephrotoxicity when NSAIDs are given with tacrolimus.

Zidovudine: Increased risk of haematological toxicity when NSAIDs are given with zidovudine. There is evidence of an increased risk of haemarthroses and haematoma in HIV(+) haemophiliacs receiving concurrent treatment with zidovudine and ibuprofen.

Aminoglycosides: NSAIDs may decrease the excretion of aminoglycosides.

Herbal extracts: Ginkgo biloba may potentiate the risk of bleeding with NSAIDs.

4.6 Pregnancy and lactation

Pregnancy

Congenital abnormalities have been reported in association with NSAID administration in man; however, these are low in frequency and do not appear to follow any discernible pattern. In view of the known effects of NSAIDs on the foetal cardiovascular system (risk of closure of the ductus arteriosus), use in the last trimester of pregnancy is contraindicated. The onset of labour may be delayed and the duration increased with an increased bleeding tendency in both mother and child (see section 4.3). NSAIDs should not be used during the first two trimesters of pregnancy or labour unless the potential benefit to the patient outweighs the potential risk to the foetus.

Lactation

In the limited studies so far available, NSAIDs can appear in the breast milk in very low concentrations. NSAIDs should, if possible, be avoided when breastfeeding.

See section 4.4 Special warnings and precautions for use, regarding female fertility.

4.7 Effects on ability to drive and use machines

Undesirable effects such as dizziness, drowsiness, fatigue and visual disturbances are possible after taking NSAIDs. If affected, patients should not drive or operate machinery.

4.8 Undesirable effects

Gastrointestinal disorders: The most commonly observed adverse events are gastrointestinal in nature. Peptic ulcers, perforation or GI bleeding, sometimes fatal, particularly in the elderly, may occur (see section 4.4). Nausea, vomiting, diarrhoea, flatulence, constipation, dyspepsia, abdominal pain, melaena, haematemesis, ulcerative stomatitis, exacerbation of colitis and Crohn's disease (see section 4.4) have been reported following ibuprofen administration. Less frequently, gastritis has been observed. Pancreatitis has been reported very rarely.

Immune system disorders: Hypersensitivity reactions have been reported following treatment with NSAIDs. These may consist of (a) non-specific allergic reaction and anaphylaxis, (b) respiratory tract reactivity comprising asthma, aggravated asthma, bronchospasm or dyspnoea, or (c) assorted skin disorders, including rashes of various types, pruritus, urticaria, purpura, angioedema and, more rarely, exfoliative and bullous dermatoses (including Stevens-Johnson syndrome, toxic epidermal necrolysis and erythema multiforme).

Cardiac disorders and vascular disorders: Oedema, hypertension and cardiac failure have been reported in association with NSAID treatment. Epidemiological data suggest that use of ibuprofen, particularly at high dose (2400 mg/daily), and in long term treatment, may be associated with a small increased risk of arterial thrombotic events such as myocardial infarction or stroke (see section 4.4).

Other adverse events reported less commonly and for which causality has not necessarily been established include:

Blood and lymphatic system disorders: Thrombocytopenia, neutropenia, agranulocytosis, aplastic anaemia and haemolytic anaemia.

Psychiatric disorders: Depression, confusional state, hallucination

Nervous system disorders: Optic neuritis, headache, paraesthesia, dizziness, somnolence

Aseptic meningitis (especially in patients with existing autoimmune disorders, such as systemic lupus erythematosus and mixed connective tissue disease) with symptoms of stiff neck, headache, nausea, vomiting, fever or disorientation (see section 4.4).

Eye disorders: Visual disturbance

Ear and labyrinth disorders: Tinnitus, vertigo

Hepatobiliary disorders: Abnormal liver function, hepatic failure, hepatitis and jaundice.

Skin and subcutaneous tissue disorders: Bullous reactions, including Stevens-Johnson syndrome and toxic epidermal necrolysis (very rare), and photosensitivity reaction.

Renal and urinary disorders: Impaired renal function and toxic nephropathy in various forms, including interstitial nephritis, nephrotic syndrome and renal failure.

General disorders and administration site conditions: Malaise, fatigue

4.9 Overdose

Symptoms

Symptoms include headache, nausea, vomiting, epigastric pain, gastrointestinal bleeding, rarely diarrhoea, disorientation, excitation, drowsiness, dizziness, tinnitus, fainting, depression of the CNS and respiratory system, coma, occasionally convulsions and rarely, loss of consciousness. In cases of significant poisoning, acute renal failure and liver damage are possible.

Therapeutic measures

Patients should be treated symptomatically as required. Within one hour of ingestion of a potentially toxic amount, activated charcoal should be considered. Alternatively, in adults, gastric lavage should be considered within one hour of ingestion of a potentially life-threatening overdose.

Good urine output should be ensured.

Renal and liver function should be closely monitored.

Patients should be observed for at least four hours after ingestion of potentially toxic amounts.

Frequent or prolonged convulsions should be treated with intravenous diazepam. Other measures may be indicated by the patient's clinical condition.

5. PHARMACOLOGICAL PROPERTIES

5.1 Pharmacodynamic properties

Ibuprofen is a propionic acid derivative with analgesic, anti-inflammatory and anti-pyretic activity. The drug's therapeutic effects as an NSAID are thought to result from its inhibitory effect on the enzyme cyclo-oxygenase, which results in a marked reduction in prostaglandin synthesis.

Experimental data suggest that ibuprofen may inhibit the effect of low dose aspirin on platelet aggregation when they are dosed concomitantly. In one study, when a single dose of ibuprofen 400mg was taken within 8 hours before or within 30 minutes after immediate release aspirin dosing (81mg), a decreased effect of aspirin on the formation of thromboxane or platelet aggregation occurred. However, the limitations of these data and the uncertainties regarding extrapolation of ex vivo data to the clinical situation imply that no firm conclusions can be made for regular ibuprofen use, and no clinically relevant effect is considered to be likely for occasional ibuprofen use.

5.2 Pharmacokinetic properties

Ibuprofen is rapidly absorbed from the gastrointestinal tract, peak serum concentrations occurring 1-2 hours after administration. The elimination half-life is approximately 2 hours.

Ibuprofen is metabolised in the liver to two inactive metabolites and these, together with unchanged ibuprofen, are excreted by the kidney either as such or as conjugates. Excretion by the kidney is both rapid and complete.

Ibuprofen is extensively bound to plasma proteins.

5.3 Preclinical safety data

Not applicable.

6. PHARMACEUTICAL PARTICULARS

6.1 List of excipients

Anhydrous sodium carbonate

Microcrystalline cellulose

Croscarmellose sodium

Malic acid

Sodium saccharin (76% saccharin)

Pulverised sugar

Povidone (K29-32)

Sodium bicarbonate

Orange flavour 57.403/TP05.51 firme

Sodium lauryl sulphate

Isopropyl alcohol

6.2 Incompatibilities

Not applicable.

6.3 Shelf life

3 years.

6.4 Special precautions for storage

Store below 25°C.

6.5 Nature and contents of container

A heat-sealed sachet consisting of a paper/polythene/aluminium foil/polythene laminate.

Pack sizes: 2, 3, 20, 21, 50, 100.

6.6 Special precautions for disposal and other handling

None stated.

Administrative Data

7. MARKETING AUTHORISATION HOLDER

Abbott Laboratories Limited

Queenborough

Kent

ME11 5EL

United Kingdom

8. MARKETING AUTHORISATION NUMBER(S)

PL 00037/0337

9. DATE OF FIRST AUTHORISATION/RENEWAL OF THE AUTHORISATION

25 February 2009

10. DATE OF REVISION OF THE TEXT
03 March 2009

Brufen Retard

(Abbott Laboratories Limited)

1. NAME OF THE MEDICINAL PRODUCT
Brufen Retard

2. QUALITATIVE AND QUANTITATIVE COMPOSITION
Active Ingredient: Ibuprofen BP (800 mg)

3. PHARMACEUTICAL FORM
Sustained-release tablets.

4. CLINICAL PARTICULARS

4.1 Therapeutic indications
Brufen Retard is indicated for its analgesic and anti-inflammatory effects in the treatment of rheumatoid arthritis (including juvenile rheumatoid arthritis or Still's disease), ankylosing spondylitis, osteoarthritis and other non-rheumatoid (seronegative) arthropathies.

In the treatment of non-articular rheumatic conditions, Brufen Retard is indicated in periarticular conditions such as frozen shoulder (capsulitis), bursitis, tendinitis, tenosynovitis and low back pain; Brufen Retard can also be used in soft-tissue injuries such as sprains and strains.

Brufen Retard is also indicated for its analgesic effect in the relief of mild to moderate pain such as dysmenorrhoea, dental and post-operative pain and for symptomatic relief of headache including migraine headache.

4.2 Posology and method of administration
Undesirable effects may be minimised by using the lowest effective dose for the shortest duration necessary to control symptoms (see section 4.4).

Adults: Two tablets taken as a single daily dose, preferably in the early evening well before retiring to bed. The tablets should be swallowed whole with plenty of fluid. In severe or acute conditions, total daily dosage may be increased to three tablets in two divided doses.

Children: Not recommended for children under 12 years.

Elderly: The elderly are at increased risk of serious consequences of adverse reactions. If an NSAID is considered necessary, the lowest effective dose should be used and for the shortest possible duration. The patient should be monitored regularly for GI bleeding during NSAID therapy. If renal or hepatic function is impaired, dosage should be assessed individually.

For oral administration. To be taken preferably with or after food.

4.3 Contraindications
Brufen is contraindicated in patients with hypersensitivity to the active substance or to any of the excipients.

Brufen should not be used in patients who have previously shown hypersensitivity reactions (e.g. asthma, urticaria, angioedema or rhinitis) after taking ibuprofen, aspirin or other NSAIDs.

Brufen is also contraindicated in patients with a history of gastrointestinal bleeding or perforation, related to previous NSAID therapy. Brufen should not be used in patients with active, or history of, recurrent peptic ulcer or gastrointestinal haemorrhage (two or more distinct episodes of proven ulceration or bleeding).

Brufen is contraindicated in patients with severe heart failure, hepatic failure and renal failure (see section 4.4).

Brufen is contraindicated during the last trimester of pregnancy (see section 4.6).

4.4 Special warnings and precautions for use
Undesirable effects may be minimised by using the lowest effective dose for the shortest duration necessary to control symptoms (see section 4.2, and GI and cardiovascular risks below). As with other NSAIDs, ibuprofen may mask the signs of infection.

The use of Brufen with concomitant NSAIDs, including cyclooxygenase-2 selective inhibitors, should be avoided due to the potential for additive effects (see section 4.5).

Elderly

The elderly have an increased frequency of adverse reactions to NSAIDs, especially gastrointestinal bleeding and perforation, which may be fatal (see section 4.2).

Gastrointestinal bleeding, ulceration and perforation

GI bleeding, ulceration or perforation, which can be fatal, has been reported with all NSAIDs at anytime during treatment, with or without warning symptoms or a previous history of serious GI events.

The risk of GI bleeding, ulceration or perforation is higher with increasing NSAID doses, in patients with a history of ulcer, particularly if complicated with haemorrhage or perforation (see section 4.3), and in the elderly. These patients should commence treatment on the lowest dose available. Combination therapy with protective agents (e.g. misoprostol or proton pump inhibitors) should be considered for these patients, and also for patients requiring concomitant low dose aspirin, or other drugs likely to increase gastrointestinal risk (see below and section 4.5).

Patients with a history of gastrointestinal disease, particularly when elderly, should report any unusual abdominal symptoms (especially gastrointestinal bleeding) particularly in the initial stages of treatment.

Caution should be advised in patients receiving concomitant medications which could increase the risk of ulceration or bleeding, such as oral corticosteroids, anticoagulants such as warfarin, selective serotonin-reuptake inhibitors or anti-platelet agents such as aspirin (see section 4.5).

When GI bleeding or ulceration occurs in patients receiving Brufen, the treatment should be withdrawn.

NSAIDs should be given with care to patients with a history of ulcerative colitis or Crohn's disease as these conditions may be exacerbated (see section 4.8).

Respiratory disorders

Caution is required if Brufen is administered to patients suffering from, or with a previous history of, bronchial asthma since NSAIDs have been reported to precipitate bronchospasm in such patients.

Cardiovascular, renal and hepatic impairment

The administration of an NSAID may cause a dose dependent reduction in prostaglandin formation and precipitate renal failure. Patients at greatest risk of this reaction are those with impaired renal function, cardiac impairment, liver dysfunction, those taking diuretics and the elderly. Renal function should be monitored in these patients (see also section 4.3).

Brufen should be given with care to patients with a history of heart failure or hypertension since oedema has been reported in association with ibuprofen administration.

Cardiovascular and cerebrovascular effects

Appropriate monitoring and advice are required for patients with a history of hypertension and/or mild to moderate congestive heart failure as fluid retention and oedema have been reported in association with NSAID therapy.

Epidemiological data suggest that use of ibuprofen, particularly at a high dose (2400 mg/ daily) and in long term treatment, may be associated with a small increased risk of arterial thrombotic events such as myocardial infarction or stroke. Overall, epidemiological studies do not suggest that low dose ibuprofen (e.g. ≤ 1200mg daily) is associated with an increased risk of arterial thrombotic events, particularly myocardial infarction.

Patients with uncontrolled hypertension, congestive heart failure, established ischaemic heart disease, peripheral arterial disease, and/or cerebrovascular disease should only be treated with ibuprofen after careful consideration. Similar consideration should be made before initiating longer-term treatment of patients with risk factors for cardiovascular events (e.g. hypertension, hyperlipidaemia, diabetes mellitus, smoking).

Renal effects

Caution should be used when initiating treatment with ibuprofen in patients with considerable dehydration.

As with other NSAIDs, long-term administration of ibuprofen has resulted in renal papillary necrosis and other renal pathologic changes. Renal toxicity has also been seen in patients in whom renal prostaglandins have a compensatory role in the maintenance of renal perfusion. In these patients, administration of an NSAID may cause a dose-dependant reduction in prostaglandin formation and, secondarily, in renal blood flow, which may precipitate overt renal decompensation. Patients at greatest risk of this reaction are those with impaired renal function, heart failure, liver dysfunction, those taking diuretics and ACE inhibitors and the elderly. Discontinuation of NSAID therapy is usually followed by recovery to the pre-treatment state.

SLE and mixed connective tissue disease

In patients with systemic lupus erythematosus (SLE) and mixed connective tissue disorders there may be an increased risk of aseptic meningitis (see below and section 4.8).

Dermatological effects

Serious skin reactions, some of them fatal, including exfoliative dermatitis, Stevens-Johnson syndrome, and toxic epidermal necrolysis, have been reported very rarely in association with the use of NSAIDs (see section 4.8). Patients appear to be at highest risk of these reactions early in the course of therapy, the onset of the reaction occurring within the first month of treatment in the majority of cases. Brufen should be discontinued at the first appearance of skin rash, mucosal lesions, or any other sign of hypersensitivity.

Haematological effects

Ibuprofen, like other NSAIDs, can interfere with platelet aggregation and has been shown to prolong bleeding time in normal subjects.

Aseptic meningitis

Aseptic meningitis has been observed on rare occasions in patients on ibuprofen therapy. Although it is probably more likely to occur in patients with systematic lupus erythematosus and related connective tissue diseases, it has been reported in patients who do not have an underlying chronic disease.

Impaired female fertility

The use of Brufen may impair female fertility and is not recommended in women attempting to conceive. In women who have difficulties conceiving or who are undergoing investigation of infertility, withdrawal of Brufen should be considered.

4.5 Interaction with other medicinal products and other forms of interaction
Care should be taken in patients treated with any of the following drugs as interactions have been reported in some patients.

Antihypertensives: Reduced antihypertensive effect.

Diuretics: Reduced diuretic effect. Diuretics can increase the risk of nephrotoxicity of NSAIDs.

Cardiac glycosides: NSAIDs may exacerbate cardiac failure, reduce GFR and increase plasma cardiac glycoside levels.

Lithium: Decreased elimination of lithium.

Methotrexate: Decreased elimination of methotrexate.

Ciclosporin: Increased risk of nephrotoxicity.

Mifepristone: NSAIDs should not be used for 8-12 days after mifepristone administration as NSAIDs can reduce the effects of mifepristone.

Other analgesics and cyclooxygenase-2 selective inhibitors: Avoid concomitant use of two or more NSAIDs, including Cox-2 inhibitors, as this may increase the risk of adverse effects (see section 4.4).

Aspirin: As with other products containing NSAIDs, concomitant administration of ibuprofen and aspirin is not generally recommended because of the potential of increased adverse effects.

Experimental data suggest that ibuprofen may inhibit the effect of low dose aspirin on platelet aggregation when they are dosed concomitantly. However, the limitations of these data and the uncertainties regarding extrapolation of ex vivo data to the clinical situation imply that no firm conclusions can be made for regular ibuprofen use, and no clinically relevant effect is considered to be likely for occasional use (see section 5.1).

Corticosteroids: Increased risk of gastrointestinal ulceration or bleeding with NSAIDs (see section 4.4).

Anticoagulants: NSAIDs may enhance the effects of anticoagulants, such as warfarin (see section 4.4).

Quinolone antibiotics: Animal data indicate that NSAIDs can increase the risk of convulsions associated with quinolone antibiotics. Patients taking NSAIDs and quinolones may have an increased risk of developing convulsions.

Anti-platelet agents and selective serotonin reuptake inhibitors (SSRIs): Increased risk of gastrointestinal bleeding with NSAIDs (see section 4.4).

Tacrolimus: Possible increased risk of nephrotoxicity when NSAIDs are given with tacrolimus.

Zidovudine: Increased risk of haematological toxicity when NSAIDs are given with zidovudine. There is evidence of an increased risk of haemarthroses and haematoma in HIV(+) haemophiliacs receiving concurrent treatment with zidovudine and ibuprofen.

Aminoglycosides: NSAIDs may decrease the excretion of aminoglycosides.

Herbal extracts: Ginkgo biloba may potentiate the risk of bleeding with NSAIDs.

4.6 Pregnancy and lactation

Pregnancy

Congenital abnormalities have been reported in association with NSAID administration in man; however, these are low in frequency and do not appear to follow any discernible pattern. In view of the known effects of NSAIDs on the foetal cardiovascular system (risk of closure of the ductus arteriosus), use in the last trimester of pregnancy is contraindicated. The onset of labour may be delayed and the duration increased with an increased bleeding tendency in both mother and child (see section 4.3). NSAIDs should not be used during the first two trimesters of pregnancy or labour unless the potential benefit to the patient outweighs the potential risk to the foetus.

Lactation

In the limited studies so far available, NSAIDs can appear in the breast milk in very low concentrations. NSAIDs should, if possible, be avoided when breastfeeding.

See section 4.4 Special warnings and precautions for use, regarding female fertility.

4.7 Effects on ability to drive and use machines
Undesirable effects such as dizziness, drowsiness, fatigue and visual disturbances are possible after taking NSAIDs. If affected, patients should not drive or operate machinery.

4.8 Undesirable effects
Gastrointestinal disorders: The most commonly observed adverse events are gastrointestinal in nature. Peptic ulcers, perforation or GI bleeding, sometimes fatal, particularly in the elderly, may occur (see section 4.4). Nausea, vomiting, diarrhoea, flatulence, constipation, dyspepsia, abdominal pain, melaena, haematemesis, ulcerative stomatitis, exacerbation of colitis and Crohn's disease (see section 4.4) have been reported following ibuprofen

administration. Less frequently, gastritis has been observed. Pancreatitis has been reported very rarely.

Immune system disorders: Hypersensitivity reactions have been reported following treatment withNSAIDs. These may consist of (a) non-specific allergic reaction and anaphylaxis, (b) respiratory tract reactivity comprising asthma, aggravated asthma, bronchospasm or dyspnoea, or (c) assorted skin disorders, including rashes of various types, pruritus, urticaria, purpura, angioedema and, more rarely, exfoliative and bullous dermatoses (including Stevens-Johnson syndrome, toxic epidermal necrolysis and erythema multiforme).

Cardiac disorders and vascular disorders: Oedema, hypertension and cardiac failure have been reported in association with NSAID treatment. Epidemiological data suggest that use of ibuprofen, particularly at high dose (2400 mg/daily), and in long term treatment, may be associated with a small increased risk of arterial thrombotic events such as myocardial infarction or stroke (see section 4.4).

Other adverse events reported less commonly and for which causality has not necessarily been established include:

Blood and lymphatic system disorders: Thrombocytopenia, neutropenia, agranulocytosis, aplastic anaemia and haemolytic anaemia.

Psychiatric disorders: Depression, confusional state, hallucination

Nervous system disorders: Optic neuritis, headache, paraesthesia, dizziness, somnolence

Aseptic meningitis (especially in patients with existing autoimmune disorders, such as systemic lupus erythematosus and mixed connective tissue disease) with symptoms of stiff neck, headache, nausea, vomiting, fever or disorientation (see section 4.4).

Eye disorders: Visual disturbance

Ear and labyrinth disorders: Tinnitus, vertigo

Hepatobiliary disorders: Abnormal liver function, hepatic failure, hepatitis and jaundice.

Skin and subcutaneous tissue disorders: Bullous reactions, including Stevens-Johnson syndrome and toxic epidermal necrolysis (very rare), and photosensitivity reaction.

Renal and urinary disorders: Impaired renal function and toxic nephropathy in various forms, including interstitial nephritis, nephrotic syndrome and renal failure.

General disorders and administration site conditions: Malaise, fatigue

4.9 Overdose

Symptoms

Symptoms include headache, nausea, vomiting, epigastric pain, gastrointestinal bleeding, rarely diarrhoea, disorientation, excitation, drowsiness, dizziness, tinnitus, fainting, depression of the CNS and respiratory system, coma, occasionally convulsions and rarely, loss of consciousness. In cases of significant poisoning, acute renal failure and liver damage are possible.

Therapeutic measures

Patients should be treated symptomatically as required. Within one hour of ingestion of a potentially toxic amount, activated charcoal should be considered. Alternatively, in adults, gastric lavage should be considered within one hour of ingestion of a potentially life-threatening overdose.

Good urine output should be ensured.

Renal and liver function should be closely monitored.

Patients should be observed for at least four hours after ingestion of potentially toxic amounts.

Frequent or prolonged convulsions should be treated with intravenous diazepam. Other measures may be indicated by the patient's clinical condition.

5. PHARMACOLOGICAL PROPERTIES

5.1 Pharmacodynamic properties

Ibuprofen is a propionic acid derivative with analgesic, anti-inflammatory and antipyretic activity. The drug's therapeutic effect as an NSAID are thought to result from its inhibitory effect on the enzyme cyclo-oxygenase, which results in a marked reduction in prostaglandin synthesis.

Experimental data suggest that ibuprofen may inhibit the effect of low dose aspirin on platelet aggregation when they are dosed concomitantly. In one study, when a single dose of ibuprofen 400mg was taken within 8 hours before or within 30 minutes after immediate release aspirin dosing (81mg), a decreased effect of aspirin on the formation of thromboxane or platelet aggregation occurred. However, the limitations of these data and the uncertainties regarding extrapolation of ex vivo data to the clinical situation imply that no firm conclusions can be made for regular ibuprofen use, and no clinically relevant effect is considered to be likely for occasional ibuprofen use.

5.2 Pharmacokinetic properties

The pharmacokinetic profile of Brufen Retard compared with that of conventional-release 400mg tablets showed that the sustained-release formulation reduced the peaks and troughs characteristic of the conventional-release tablets and gave higher levels at 5, 10, 15 and 24 hours. Compared with conventional-release tablets, the area under the plasma concentration time curve for sustained-release tablets was almost identical.

Both mean plasma profiles and the pre-dose plasma levels showed no major differences between the young and elderly age groups. In several studies, Brufen Retard produced a double peak plasma profile when taken under fasting conditions. The elimination half-life of ibuprofen is approximately 2 hours. Ibuprofen is metabolised in the liver to two inactive metabolites and these, together with unchanged ibuprofen, are excreted by the kidney either as such or as conjugates. Excretion by the kidney is both rapid and complete. Ibuprofen is extensively bound to plasma proteins.

5.3 Preclinical safety data

None stated.

6. PHARMACEUTICAL PARTICULARS

6.1 List of excipients

Colloidal Silicon Dioxide NF, Isopropyl Alcohol BP, Povidone BP, Stearic Acid BPC PDR BPC, Xanthan Gum NF.

French Chalk for tablets (Talc EP) EP, Hydroxypropylmethylcellulose USP, Purified Water EP, Opaspray White M-1-7111B (Solids), Opacode S-1-9005 HV Red (Solids), Industrial Methylated Spirit BP.

6.2 Incompatibilities

None.

6.3 Shelf life

All packs: 36 months.

6.4 Special precautions for storage

HDPE bottle and nylon/aluminium/PVC blister: store cool, dry, below 25°C.

PVC/PVDC blister: store cool, dry, below 25°C.

6.5 Nature and contents of container

1. White pigmented HDPE bottle with a white polypropylene screw cap with a waxed aluminium pulp-board liner. Pack size: 60.

2. A blister consisting of 250 μm opaque PVC/40 gsm PVDC bonded to 20 μm aluminium foil. The blisters are packed in a cardboard carton.

Pack size: 8 or 56.

3. A blister consisting of 25 μm polyamide/40 μm aluminium/60 μm PVC bonded to 20 μm aluminium foil. The blisters are packed in a cardboard carton. Pack size: 8 or 56.

6.6 Special precautions for disposal and other handling

None.

Administrative Data

7. MARKETING AUTHORISATION HOLDER

Abbott Laboratories Limited

Queenborough

Kent

ME11 5EL

United Kingdom

8. MARKETING AUTHORISATION NUMBER(S)

PL 00037/0338

9. DATE OF FIRST AUTHORISATION/RENEWAL OF THE AUTHORISATION

25 February 2009

10. DATE OF REVISION OF THE TEXT

03 March 2009

Brufen Syrup

(Abbott Laboratories Limited)

1. NAME OF THE MEDICINAL PRODUCT

Brufen Syrup

2. QUALITATIVE AND QUANTITATIVE COMPOSITION

Ibuprofen BP 100 mg/5 ml

3. PHARMACEUTICAL FORM

An orange-coloured, orange-flavoured, syrupy suspension.

4. CLINICAL PARTICULARS

4.1 Therapeutic indications

Brufen Syrup is indicated for its analgesic and anti-inflammatory effects in the treatment of rheumatoid arthritis (including juvenile rheumatoid arthritis or Still's disease), ankylosing spondylitis, osteoarthritis and other non-rheumatoid (seronegative) arthropathies.

In the treatment of non-articular rheumatic conditions, Brufen Syrup is indicated in peri-articular conditions such as frozen shoulder (capsulitis), bursitis, tendinitis, tenosynovitis and low back pain; Brufen Syrup can also be used in soft-tissue injuries such as sprains and strains.

Brufen Syrup is also indicated for its analgesic effect in the relief of mild to moderate pain such as dysmenorrhoea, dental and post-operative pain and for symptomatic relief of headache including migraine headache.

Brufen Syrup is indicated in short-term use for the treatment of pyrexia in children over one year of age.

4.2 Posology and method of administration

Undesirable effects may be minimised by using the lowest effective dose for the shortest duration necessary to control symptoms (see section 4.4).

Adults: The recommended dosage of Brufen is 1200-1800 mg daily in divided doses. Some patients can be maintained on 600-1200 mg daily. Total daily dose should not exceed 2400 mg.

Children: The daily dosage of Brufen is 20 mg/kg of bodyweight in divided doses. This can be achieved as follows:

1-2 years: One 2.5 ml spoonful (50 mg) three to four times a day.

3-7 years: One 5 ml spoonful (100 mg) three to four times a day.

8-12 years: Two 5 ml spoonfuls (200 mg) three to four times a day.

Not recommended for children weighing less than 7 kg.

In juvenile rheumatoid arthritis, up to 40 mg/kg of bodyweight daily in divided doses may be taken.

Elderly: The elderly are at increased risk of serious consequences of adverse reactions. If an NSAID is considered necessary, the lowest effective dose should be used and for the shortest possible duration. The patient should be monitored regularly for GI bleeding during NSAID therapy. If renal or hepatic function is impaired, dosage should be assessed individually.

For oral administration. To be taken preferably with or after food.

4.3 Contraindications

Brufen is contraindicated in patients with hypersensitivity to the active substance or to any of the excipients.

Brufen should not be used in patients who have previously shown hypersensitivity reactions (e.g. asthma, urticaria, angioedema or rhinitis) after taking ibuprofen, aspirin or other NSAIDs.

Brufen is also contraindicated in patients with a history of gastrointestinal bleeding or perforation, related to previous NSAID therapy. Brufen should not be used in patients with active, or history of, recurrent peptic ulcer or gastrointestinal haemorrhage (two or more distinct episodes of proven ulceration or bleeding).

Brufen is contraindicated in patients with severe heart failure, hepatic failure and renal failure (see section 4.4).

Brufen is contraindicated during the last trimester of pregnancy (see section 4.6).

4.4 Special warnings and precautions for use

Undesirable effects may be minimised by using the lowest effective dose for the shortest duration necessary to control symptoms (see section 4.2, and GI and cardiovascular risks below).

Patients with rare hereditary problems of fructose intolerance, glucose-galactose malaabsorption or sucrase-isomaltase insufficiency should not take this medicine.

As with other NSAIDs, ibuprofen may mask the signs of infection.

The use of Brufen with concomitant NSAIDs, including cyclooxygenase-2 selective inhibitors, should be avoided due to the potential for additive effects (see section 4.5).

Elderly

The elderly have an increased frequency of adverse reactions to NSAIDs, especially gastrointestinal bleeding and perforation, which may be fatal (see section 4.2).

Gastrointestinal bleeding, ulceration and perforation

GI bleeding, ulceration or perforation, which can be fatal, has been reported with all NSAIDs at anytime during treatment, with or without warning symptoms or a previous history of serious GI events.

The risk of GI bleeding, ulceration or perforation is higher with increasing NSAID doses, in patients with a history of ulcer, particularly if complicated with haemorrhage or perforation (see section 4.3), and in the elderly. These patients should commence treatment on the lowest dose available. Combination therapy with protective agents (e.g. misoprostol or proton pump inhibitors) should be considered for these patients, and also for patients requiring concomitant low dose aspirin, or other drugs likely to increase gastrointestinal risk (see below and section 4.5).

Patients with a history of gastrointestinal disease, particularly when elderly, should report any unusual abdominal symptoms (especially gastrointestinal bleeding) particularly in the initial stages of treatment.

Caution should be advised in patients receiving concomitant medications which could increase the risk of ulceration or bleeding, such as oral corticosteroids, anticoagulants such as warfarin, selective serotonin-reuptake inhibitors or anti-platelet agents such as aspirin (see section 4.5).

When GI bleeding or ulceration occurs in patients receiving Brufen, the treatment should be withdrawn.

NSAIDs should be given with care to patients with a history of ulcerative colitis or Crohn's disease as these conditions may be exacerbated (see section 4.8).

Respiratory disorders

Caution is required if Brufen is administered to patients suffering from, or with a previous history of, bronchial asthma since NSAIDs have been reported to precipitate bronchospasm in such patients.

Cardiovascular, renal and hepatic impairment

The administration of an NSAID may cause a dose dependent reduction in prostaglandin formation and precipitate renal failure. Patients at greatest risk of this reaction are those with impaired renal function, cardiac impairment, liver dysfunction, those taking diuretics and the elderly. Renal function should be monitored in these patients (see also section 4.3).

Brufen should be given with care to patients with a history of heart failure or hypertension since oedema has been reported in association with ibuprofen administration.

Cardiovascular and cerebrovascular effects

Appropriate monitoring and advice are required for patients with a history of hypertension and/or mild to moderate congestive heart failure as fluid retention and oedema have been reported in association with NSAID therapy.

Epidemiological data suggest that use of ibuprofen, particularly at a high dose (2400 mg/ daily) and in long term treatment, may be associated with a small increased risk of arterial thrombotic events such as myocardial infarction or stroke. Overall, epidemiological studies do not suggest that low dose ibuprofen (e.g. ≤ 1200mg daily) is associated with an increased risk of arterial thrombotic events, particularly myocardial infarction.

Patients with uncontrolled hypertension, congestive heart failure, established ischaemic heart disease, peripheral arterial disease, and/or cerebrovascular disease should only be treated with ibuprofen after careful consideration. Similar consideration should be made before initiating longer-term treatment of patients with risk factors for cardiovascular events (e.g. hypertension, hyperlipidaemia, diabetes mellitus, smoking).

Renal effects

Caution should be used when initiating treatment with ibuprofen in patients with considerable dehydration.

As with other NSAIDs, long-term administration of ibuprofen has resulted in renal papillary necrosis and other renal pathologic changes. Renal toxicity has also been seen in patients in whom renal prostaglandins have a compensatory role in the maintenance of renal perfusion. In these patients, administration of an NSAID may cause a dose-dependant reduction in prostaglandin formation and, secondarily, in renal blood flow, which may precipitate overt renal decompensation. Patients at greatest risk of this reaction are those with impaired renal function, heart failure, liver dysfunction, those taking diuretics and ACE inhibitors and the elderly. Discontinuation of NSAID therapy is usually followed by recovery to the pre-treatment state.

SLE and mixed connective tissue disease

In patients with systemic lupus erythematosus (SLE) and mixed connective tissue disorders there may be an increased risk of aseptic meningitis (see below and section 4.8).

Dermatological effects

Serious skin reactions, some of them fatal, including exfoliative dermatitis, Stevens-Johnson syndrome, and toxic epidermal necrolysis, have been reported very rarely in association with the use of NSAIDs (see section 4.8). Patients appear to be at highest risk of these reactions early in the course of therapy, the onset of the reaction occurring within the first month of treatment in the majority of cases. Brufen should be discontinued at the first appearance of skin rash, mucosal lesions, or any other sign of hypersensitivity.

Haematological effects

Ibuprofen, like other NSAIDs, can interfere with platelet aggregation and has been shown to prolong bleeding time in normal subjects.

Asceptic meningitis

Aseptic meningitis has been observed on rare occasions in patients on ibuprofen therapy. Although it is probably more likely to occur in patients with systematic lupus erythematosus and related connective tissue diseases, it has been reported in patients who do not have an underlying chronic disease.

Impaired female fertility

The use of Brufen may impair female fertility and is not recommended in women attempting to conceive. In women who have difficulties conceiving or who are undergoing investigation of infertility, withdrawal of Brufen should be considered.

4.5 Interaction with other medicinal products and other forms of interaction

Care should be taken in patients treated with any of the following drugs as interactions have been reported in some patients.

Antihypertensives: Reduced antihypertensive effect.

Diuretics: Reduced diuretic effect. Diuretics can increase the risk of nephrotoxicity of NSAIDs.

Cardiac glycosides: NSAIDs may exacerbate cardiac failure, reduce GFR and increase plasma cardiac glycoside levels.

Lithium: Decreased elimination of lithium.

Methotrexate: Decreased elimination of methotrexate.

Ciclosporin: Increased risk of nephrotoxicity.

Mifepristone: NSAIDs should not be used for 8-12 days after mifepristone administration as NSAIDs can reduce the effects of mifepristone.

Other analgesics and cyclooxygenase-2 selective inhibitors: Avoid concomitant use of two or more NSAIDs, including Cox-2 inhibitors, as this may increase the risk of adverse effects (see section 4.4).

Aspirin: As with other products containing NSAIDs, concomitant administration of ibuprofen and aspirin is not generally recommended because of the potential of increased adverse effects.

Experimental data suggest that ibuprofen may inhibit the effect of low dose aspirin on platelet aggregation when they are dosed concomitantly. However, the limitations of these data and the uncertainties regarding extrapolation of ex vivo data to the clinical situation imply that no firm conclusions can be made for regular ibuprofen use, and no clinically relevant effect is considered to be likely for occasional use (see section 5.1).

Corticosteroids: Increased risk of gastrointestinal ulceration or bleeding with NSAIDs (see section 4.4).

Anticoagulants: NSAIDs may enhance the effects of anticoagulants, such as warfarin (see section 4.4).

Quinolone antibiotics: Animal data indicate that NSAIDs can increase the risk of convulsions associated with quinolone antibiotics. Patients taking NSAIDs and quinolones may have an increased risk of developing convulsions.

Anti-platelet agents and selective serotonin reuptake inhibitors (SSRIs): Increased risk of gastrointestinal bleeding with NSAIDs (see section 4.4).

Tacrolimus: Possible increased risk of nephrotoxicity when NSAIDs are given with tacrolimus.

Zidovudine: Increased risk of haematological toxicity when NSAIDs are given with zidovudine. There is evidence of an increased risk of haemarthroses and haematoma in HIV(+) haemophiliacs receiving concurrent treatment with zidovudine and ibuprofen.

Aminoglycosides: NSAIDs may decrease the excretion of aminoglycosides.

Herbal extracts: Ginkgo biloba may potentiate the risk of bleeding with NSAIDs.

4.6 Pregnancy and lactation

Pregnancy

Congenital abnormalities have been reported in association with NSAID administration in man; however, these are low in frequency and do not appear to follow any discernible pattern. In view of the known effects of NSAIDs on the foetal cardiovascular system (risk of closure of the ductus arteriosus), use in the last trimester of pregnancy is contraindicated. The onset of labour may be delayed and the duration increased with an increased bleeding tendency in both mother and child (see section 4.3). NSAIDs should not be used during the first two trimesters of pregnancy or labour unless the potential benefit to the patient outweighs the potential risk to the foetus.

Lactation

In the limited studies so far available, NSAIDs can appear in the breast milk in very low concentrations. NSAIDs should, if possible, be avoided when breastfeeding.

See section 4.4 Special warnings and precautions for use, regarding female fertility.

4.7 Effects on ability to drive and use machines

Undesirable effects such as dizziness, drowsiness, fatigue and visual disturbances are possible after taking NSAIDs. If affected, patients should not drive or operate machinery.

4.8 Undesirable effects

Gastrointestinal disorders: The most commonly observed adverse events are gastrointestinal in nature. Peptic ulcers, perforation or GI bleeding, sometimes fatal, particularly in the elderly, may occur (see section 4.4). Nausea, vomiting, diarrhoea, flatulence, constipation, dyspepsia, abdominal pain, melaena, haematemesis, ulcerative stomatitis, exacerbation of colitis and Crohn's disease (see section 4.4) have been reported following ibuprofen administration. Less frequently, gastritis has been observed. Pancreatitis has been reported very rarely.

Immune system disorders: Hypersensitivity reactions have been reported following treatment withNSAIDs. These may consist of (a) non-specific allergic reaction and anaphylaxis, (b) respiratory tract reactivity comprising asthma, aggravated asthma, bronchospasm or dyspnoea, or (c) assorted skin disorders, including rashes of various types, pruritus, urticaria, purpura, angioedema and, more rarely, exfoliative and bullous dermatoses (including Stevens-Johnson syndrome, toxic epidermal necrolysis and erythema multiforme).

Cardiac disorders and vascular disorders: Oedema, hypertension and cardiac failure have been reported in association with NSAID treatment. Epidemiological data suggest that use of ibuprofen, particularly at high dose (2400 mg/ daily), and in long term treatment, may be associated with a small increased risk of arterial thrombotic events such as myocardial infarction or stroke (see section 4.4).

Other adverse events reported less commonly and for which causality has not necessarily been established include:

Blood and lymphatic system disorders: Thrombocytopenia, neutropenia, agranulocytosis, aplastic anaemia and haemolytic anaemia.

Psychiatric disorders: Depression, confusional state, hallucination

Nervous system disorders: Optic neuritis, headache, paraesthesia, dizziness, somnolence

Aseptic meningitis (especially in patients with existing autoimmune disorders, such as systemic lupus erythematosus and mixed connective tissue disease) with symptoms of stiff neck, headache, nausea, vomiting, fever or disorientation (see section 4.4).

Eye disorders: Visual disturbance

Ear and labyrinth disorders: Tinnitus, vertigo

Hepatobiliary disorders: Abnormal liver function, hepatic failure, hepatitis and jaundice.

Skin and subcutaneous tissue disorders: Bullous reactions, including Stevens-Johnson syndrome and toxic epidermal necrolysis (very rare), and photosensitivity reaction.

Renal and urinary disorders: Impaired renal function and toxic nephropathy in various forms, including interstitial nephritis, nephrotic syndrome and renal failure.

General disorders and administration site conditions: Malaise, fatigue

4.9 Overdose

Symptoms

Symptoms include headache, nausea, vomiting, epigastric pain, gastrointestinal bleeding, rarely diarrhoea, disorientation, excitation, drowsiness, dizziness, tinnitus, fainting, depression of the CNS and respiratory system, coma, occasionally convulsions and rarely, loss of consciousness. In cases of significant poisoning, acute renal failure and liver damage are possible.

Therapeutic measures

Patients should be treated symptomatically as required. Within one hour of ingestion of a potentially toxic amount, activated charcoal should be considered. Alternatively, in adults, gastric lavage should be considered within one hour of ingestion of a potentially life-threatening overdose.

Good urine output should be ensured.

Renal and liver function should be closely monitored.

Patients should be observed for at least four hours after ingestion of potentially toxic amounts.

Frequent or prolonged convulsions should be treated with intravenous diazepam. Other measures may be indicated by the patient's clinical condition.

5. PHARMACOLOGICAL PROPERTIES

5.1 Pharmacodynamic properties

Ibuprofen is a propionic acid derivative with analgesic, anti-inflammatory and anti-pyretic activity. The drug's therapeutic effects as an NSAID are thought to result from its inhibitory effect on the enzyme cyclo-oxygenase, which results in a marked reduction in prostaglandin synthesis.

Experimental data suggest that ibuprofen may inhibit the effect of low dose aspirin on platelet aggregation when they are dosed concomitantly. In one study, when a single dose of ibuprofen 400mg was taken within 8 hours before or within 30 minutes after immediate release aspirin dosing (81mg), a decreased effect of aspirin on the formation of thromboxane or platelet aggregation occurred. However, the limitations of these data and the uncertainties regarding extrapolation of ex vivo data to the clinical situation imply that no firm conclusions can be made for regular ibuprofen use, and no clinically relevant effect is considered to be likely for occasional ibuprofen use.

5.2 Pharmacokinetic properties

Ibuprofen is rapidly absorbed from the gastrointestinal tract, peak serum concentrations occurring 1-2 hours after administration. The elimination half-life is approximately 2 hours.

Ibuprofen is metabolised in the liver to two inactive metabolites and these, together with unchanged ibuprofen, are excreted by the kidney either as such or as conjugates. Excretion by the kidney is both rapid and complete.

Ibuprofen is extensively bound to plasma proteins.

5.3 Preclinical safety data

Not applicable.

6. PHARMACEUTICAL PARTICULARS

6.1 List of excipients

Methyl hydroxybenzoate

Propyl hydroxybenzoate

Refined sugar

Citric acid monohydrate granular

Sodium benzoate

Agar powder

Glycerin

Sorbitol solution 70% (non-crystallising)

Irradiated light kaolin

Polysorbate 80

Sunset yellow

Orange flavour D717

Purified water

.2 Incompatibilities
lone known.

.3 Shelf life
6 months.

.4 Special precautions for storage
tore below 25°C and protect from light.

.5 Nature and contents of container
n amber glass bottle with either a wadless polypropylene ap or a thermoset cap with an expanded polythene liner.

r

mber-coloured polyethylene terephthalate bottle with a ilfer-proof neck finish, with a thermoplastic or a thermoset crew cap fitted with a low density polythene cone liner.

r

n amber-coloured polyethylene terephthalate (PET) bottle ith an aluminium roll-on pilfer-proof cap fitted with an xpanded polyethylene liner lined with a film of low-density olyethylene.

ack sizes of 150, 200, 500 or 1000 ml for each of the ontainers.

.6 Special precautions for disposal and other handling
lone stated.

dministrative Data

. MARKETING AUTHORISATION HOLDER
bbott Laboratories Limited
ueenborough
ent
IE11 5EL
nited Kingdom

. MARKETING AUTHORISATION NUMBER(S)
L 00037/0339

. DATE OF FIRST AUTHORISATION/RENEWAL OF HE AUTHORISATION
5 February 2009

0. DATE OF REVISION OF THE TEXT
3 March 2009

Brulidine Cream

(Manx Healthcare)

. NAME OF THE MEDICINAL PRODUCT
rulidine Cream
oyds Antiseptic Cream

. QUALITATIVE AND QUANTITATIVE COMPOSITION
ibrompropamidine isethionate 0.15%w/w

. PHARMACEUTICAL FORM
ream

. CLINICAL PARTICULARS

.1 Therapeutic indications
dications

) First aid dressing for minor burns, scalds, abrasions and ther open injuries and their routine treatment

) For the treatment of surface infections due to suscep-ble organisms, particularly in cases with penicillin resis-nt Staphylococci or certain Gram-negative bacilli

) Treatment of ringworm of the scalp (Microsporum canis) nd other superficial fungal infections

) Treatment of pyodermias, including impetigo and syco-s barbae

) Treatment of otitis externa

Treatment of nappy rash

2 Posology and method of administration
dults: apply to the affected area, either directly or on a ght dressing, two or three times a day.

derly and children: no specific recommendations.

3 Contraindications
rulidine Cream should not be used in patients with known ypersensitivity to dibrompropamidine or any of the other gredients.

4 Special warnings and precautions for use
rolonged use may interfere with healing and cause skin ecrosis in infants.

5 Interaction with other medicinal products and other rms of interaction
one known

6 Pregnancy and lactation
here is no evidence of the drug's safety in human use nor there any evidence from animal work that it is free from azard. Avoid unless considered essential.

7 Effects on ability to drive and use machines
one

8 Undesirable effects
here is always the possibility, although rare, of a sensiti-ation reaction or contact dermatitis occurring: in such an vent, treatment should be discontinued immediately.

4.9 Overdose
The 25g tube of Brulidine Cream contains 37.5mg of dibrompropamidine and the 30g contains 45mg.

No toxic effects are likely to occur even if the contents of a full tube are accidentally ingested. Similarly, the ingredients of the base are unlikely to have toxic effects in the quantities present.

5. PHARMACOLOGICAL PROPERTIES

5.1 Pharmacodynamic properties
Dibrompropamidine isethionate is an antibacterial agent active against pathogenic Streptococci and Staphylococci, including penicillin resistant strains, and has some activity against a number of Gram negative bacilli. Its antibacterial action in not inhibited by pus, blood or p-aminobenzoic acid. In addition, it has useful activity against certain species of pathogenic fungi. Brulidine Cream is well tolerated and rarely gives rise to sensitisation reactions or contact dermatitis.

5.2 Pharmacokinetic properties
No data available

5.3 Preclinical safety data
No relevant data

6. PHARMACEUTICAL PARTICULARS

6.1 List of excipients
Caster oil, virgin
Cetostearyl alcohol
Polyethylene glycol 600 monostearate
Methyl parahydroxybenzoate
Silicone MS antifoam A
Purified water

6.2 Incompatibilities
Not applicable

6.3 Shelf life
36 months

6.4 Special precautions for storage
Store below 25°C

6.5 Nature and contents of container
Collapsible aluminium internally lacquered tube with extended nozzle containing 25g or 30g cream

Polythene plug seal cap

6.6 Special precautions for disposal and other handling
Not applicable

7. MARKETING AUTHORISATION HOLDER
Manx Pharma Ltd
Taylor Group House
Wedgnock Lane
Warwick
CV34 5YA
United Kingdom

8. MARKETING AUTHORISATION NUMBER(S)
PL 15833/0002

9. DATE OF FIRST AUTHORISATION/RENEWAL OF THE AUTHORISATION
1 September 1997 / 30 May 2002

10. DATE OF REVISION OF THE TEXT
February 2009

Budenofalk 2mg/dose rectal foam

(Dr. Falk Pharma UK Ltd)

1. NAME OF THE MEDICINAL PRODUCT
Budenofalk® 2mg/dose rectal foam

2. QUALITATIVE AND QUANTITATIVE COMPOSITION
Each dose of 1.2 g foam contains 2 mg of budesonide

Excipients: cetyl alcohol, propylene glycol

For a full list of excipients, see section 6.1.

3. PHARMACEUTICAL FORM
Rectal foam, pressurised container

White to pale white, creamy firm foam

4. CLINICAL PARTICULARS

4.1 Therapeutic indications
For the treatment of active ulcerative colitis that is limited to the rectum and the sigmoid colon

4.2 Posology and method of administration

Posology:

Adults aged > 18 years:

One actuation of 2 mg budesonide daily.

Children and adolescents:

Budenofalk® 2mg rectal foam should not be taken by children due to insufficient experience in this age group.

Method of Administration:

Budenofalk® 2mg rectal foam can be applied in the morning or evening.

The canister is first fitted with an applicator and then shaken for about 15 seconds before the applicator is inserted into the rectum as far as comfortable. Note that the dose is only sufficiently accurate when the pump dome is held downwards as vertically as possible. To administer a dose of Budenofalk® 2mg rectal foam, the pump dome is fully pushed down and very slowly released. Following the activation the applicator should be held in position for 10-15 seconds before being withdrawn from the rectum.

The best results are obtained when the intestine is evacuated prior to administration of Budenofalk® 2mg rectal foam.

The attending physician determines the duration of use. An acute episode generally subsides after 6 to 8 weeks. Budenofalk® 2mg rectal foam should not be used after this time.

4.3 Contraindications
Budenofalk® 2mg rectal foam must not be used in:

- hypersensitivity to budesonide or any of the ingredients
- hepatic cirrhosis with signs of portal hypertension, e.g. late-stage primary biliary cirrhosis

4.4 Special warnings and precautions for use
Treatment with Budenofalk® 2mg rectal foam results in lower systemic steroid levels than oral therapy with systemically acting corticoids. If a patient is transferred from systemic corticoids to Budenofalk, the theoretical risk of recurrence of symptoms due to differences in the pharmacokinetics has to be taken into account.

Caution is required in patients with tuberculosis, hypertension, diabetes mellitus, osteoporosis, peptic ulcer, glaucoma, cataracts, family history of diabetes, family history of glaucoma.

Infection:

Suppression of the inflammatory response and immune function increases the susceptibility to infections and their severity. The risk of deterioration of bacterial, fungal, amoebic, and viral infections during glucocorticoid treatment should be carefully considered. The clinical presentation may often be atypical and serious infections such as septicaemia and tuberculosis may be masked and may reach an advanced stage before being recognised.

Chickenpox: Chickenpox is of particular concern since this normally minor illness may be fatal in immunosuppressed patients. Patients without a definite history of chickenpox should be advised to avoid close personal contact with chickenpox or herpes zoster and if exposed they should seek urgent medical attention. If the patient is a child, parents must be given the above advice. Passive immunisation with varicella-zoster immunoglobulin (VZIG) is needed by exposed non-immune patients who are receiving systemic corticosteroids or who have used them within the previous 3 months; this should be given within 10 days of exposure to chickenpox. If a diagnosis of chickenpox is confirmed, the illness warrants specialist care and urgent treatment. In some cases corticosteroids should not be stopped and the dose may need to be increased.

Measles: Patients with compromised immunity who have come into contact with measles should, wherever possible, receive normal immunoglobulin as soon as possible after exposure.

Live vaccines: Live vaccines should not be given to individuals with impaired immune responsiveness. The antibody response to other vaccines may be diminished.

In patients with severe liver function disorders, the elimination of glucocorticoids including Budenofalk® 2mg rectal foam will be reduced, and their systemic bioavailability will be increased.

Caution should be exercised in patients with slight to moderate hepatic impairment.

Corticosteroids may cause suppression of the HPA axis and reduce the stress response. Where patients are subject to surgery or other stresses, supplementary systemic glucocorticoid treatment is recommended.

Concomitant treatment with ketoconazole or other CYP3A4 inhibitors should be avoided (see section 4.5).

4.5 Interaction with other medicinal products and other forms of interaction

Pharmacodynamic interactions

Cardiac glycosides:

The action of the glycoside can be potentiated by potassium deficiency.

Saluretics:

Potassium excretion can be enhanced.

Pharmacokinetic interactions

Cytochrome P450:

- CYP3A4 inhibitors:

Ketoconazole 200 mg once daily p.o. increased the plasma concentrations of budesonide (3 mg single dose) approximately 6-fold during concomitant administration. When ketoconazole was administered 12 hours after budesonide, the concentrations increased approximately 3-fold. As there are not enough data to give dose recommendations, the combination should be avoided.

Other potent inhibitors of CYP3A4 such as ritonavir, itraconazole, and clarithromycin are also likely to give a marked increase of the plasma concentrations of budesonide. In addition, concomitant intake of grapefruit juice should be avoided.

- CYP3A4 inducers:

Compounds or drugs such as carbamazepine and rifampicin, which induce CYP3A4, might reduce the systemic but also the local exposure of budesonide at the gut mucosa. An adjustment of the budesonide dose might be necessary.

- CYP3A4 substrates:

Compounds or drugs which are metabolized by CYP3A4 might be in competition with budesonide. This might lead to an increased budesonide plasma concentration if the competing substance has a stronger affinity to CYP3A4, or - if budesonide binds stronger to CYP3A4 - the competing substance might be increased in plasma and a dose-adaptation/reduction of this drug might be required.

Elevated plasma concentrations and enhanced effects of corticosteroids have been reported in women also receiving oestrogens or oral contraceptives, but this has not been observed with oral low dose combination contraceptives.

4.6 Pregnancy and lactation

Administration during pregnancy should be avoided unless there are compelling reasons for Budenofalk® 2mg rectal foam therapy. In pregnant animals, budesonide, like other glucocorticosteroids, has been shown to cause abnormalities of foetal development. The relevance of this to man has not been established.

It is not known if budesonide passes into breastmilk. A decision on whether to continue/discontinue breast-feeding or to continue/discontinue therapy with Budenofalk 2mg rectal foam should be made taking into account the benefit of breast-feeding to the child and the benefit of the therapy to the woman.

4.7 Effects on ability to drive and use machines

No effects are known.

4.8 Undesirable effects

The assessment of undesirable effects is based on the following frequencies.

Very common: (⩾ 1/10)

Common: (⩾ 1/100 to < 1/10)

Uncommon: (⩾ 1/1000 to < 1/100)

Rare: (⩾ 1/10,000 to < 1/1000)

Very rare: (< 1/10,000), not known (cannot be estimated from the available data)

Undesirable effects were reported in 8% of patients in clinical trials with Budenofalk rectal foam. Burning in the rectum or pain were common and nausea, headache, increase in liver enzymes were uncommon.

The details of the side effects observed during clinical trials are as follows:

Infections and parasitic diseases

Uncommon: urinary tract infections

Blood and lymphatic system disorders

Uncommon: anaemia, increase in erythrocyte sedimentation rate, leukocytosis

Metabolism and nutrition disorders

Uncommon: increased appetite

Psychiatric disorders

Uncommon: insomnia

Nervous system disorders

Uncommon: headache, dizziness, disturbances of smell

Vascular disorders

Uncommon: hypertension

Gastrointestinal disorders

Uncommon: nausea, abdominal pain, dyspepsia, flatulence, paraesthesias in the abdominal region, anal fissure, aphthous stomatitis, frequent urge to defecate, haemorrhoids, rectal bleeding

Hepatobiliary disorders

Uncommon: increase in transaminases (GOT, GPT), increase in parameters of cholestasis (GGT, AP)

Skin and subcutaneous tissue disorders

Uncommon: acne, increased sweating

Investigations

Uncommon: increase in amylase, change in cortisol

General disorders and administration site conditions

Common: burning in the rectum and pain

Uncommon: asthenia, increase in body weight

Occasionally side effects may occur which are typical for systemically acting glucocorticosteroids. The side effects listed below depend on the dosage, the period of treatment, concomitant or previous treatment with other glucocorticosteroids and the individual sensitivity.

Immune system disorders:

Interference with the immune response (e.g. increase in risk of infections).

An exacerbation or the reappearance of extraintestinal manifestations (especially affecting skin and joints) can occur on switching a patient from the systemically acting glucocorticosteroids to the locally acting budesonide.

Metabolism and nutrition disorders:

Cushing's syndrome: moon-face, truncal obesity, reduced glucose tolerance, diabetes mellitus, sodium retention with oedema formation, increased excretion of potassium, inactivity or atrophy of the adrenal cortex, growth retardation in children, disturbance of sex hormone secretion (e.g. amenorrhoea, hirsutism, impotence)

Nervous system disorders:

depression, irritability, euphoria

in isolated cases (< 1/10,000): pseudotumor cerebri (including papilloedema) in adolescents.

Eye disorders:

glaucoma, cataract

Vascular disorders:

hypertension, increased risk of thrombosis, vasculitis (withdrawal syndrome after long-term therapy)

Gastro intestinal disorders:

stomach complaints, duodenal ulcer, pancreatitis, constipation

Skin and subcutaneous tissue disorders:

allergic exanthema, red striae, petechiae, ecchymoses, steroid acne, delayed wound healing.

Due to the cetyl alcohol and propylene glycol content local skin reactions may occur, e.g. contact dermatitis.

Musculoskeletal, connective tissue and bone disorders:

aseptic necrosis of bone (femur and head of the humerus), diffuse muscle pain and weakness, osteoporosis.

General disorders:

Tiredness, malaise.

Some of the undesired effects were reported after long-term use of orally administered budesonide.

Due to its local action, the risk of unwanted effects of Budenofalk® 2mg rectal foam is generally lower than when taking systemically acting glucocorticoids.

4.9 Overdose

To date, no cases of overdosage with budesonide are known. In view of the properties of budesonide contained in Budenofalk® 2mg rectal foam, an overdose resulting in toxic damage is extremely unlikely.

5. PHARMACOLOGICAL PROPERTIES

5.1 Pharmacodynamic properties

Pharmacotherapeutic group: Corticosteroids acting locally

ATC code: A07EA06

The exact mechanism of action of budesonide in the treatment of ulcerative colitis/procto-sigmoiditis is not fully understood. Data from clinical pharmacology studies and controlled clinical trials strongly indicate that the mode of action of budesonide is predominantly based on a local action in the gut. Budesonide is a glucocorticosteroid with a high local anti-inflammatory effect. At a dosage of 2 mg budesonide, applied rectally, budesonide leads to practically no suppression of the hypothalamus-hypophysis-adrenal cortex axis.

Budenofalk® 2mg rectal foam investigated up to the daily dosage of 4 mg budesonide showed virtually no influence on the plasma cortisol level.

5.2 Pharmacokinetic properties

Absorption:

After oral application the systemic availability of budesonide is about 10%. After rectal administration the areas under the concentration time curves are about 1.5-fold higher than in historical controls considering the identical oral budesonide dose. Peak levels are obtained after an average of 2-3 hours after administering Budenofalk® 2mg rectal foam.

Distribution:

Budesonide has a high volume of distribution (about 3 l/kg). Plasma protein binding averages 85 -90%.

Biotransformation:

Budesonide undergoes extensive biotransformation in the liver (approximately 90 %) to metabolites of low glucocorticosteroid activity. The glucocorticosteroid activity of the major metabolites, 6β-hydroxybudesonide and 16α-hydroxyprednisolone, is less than 1 % of that of budesonide.

Elimination:

The average elimination half-life is about 3 - 4 hours. The mean clearance rate is about 10 -15 l/min for budesonide, determined by HPLC-based methods.

Spread:

A scintigraphic investigation with technetium-marked Budenofalk® 2mg rectal foam on patients with ulcerative colitis showed that the foam spreads out over the entire sigmoid.

Specific patient populations (liver diseases):

Dependent on the type and severity of liver diseases the metabolism of budesonide might be decreased.

5.3 Preclinical safety data

Preclinical investigations on dogs have shown that Budenofalk® 2mg rectal foam is well tolerated locally.

Preclinical data in acute, subchronic and chronic toxicological studies with budesonide showed atrophies of the thymus gland and adrenal cortex and a reduction especially of lymphocytes. These effects were less pronounced or at the same magnitude as observed with other glucocorticosteroids. These steroid effects might also be of relevance in man.

Budesonide had no mutagenic effects in a number of *in vitro* and *in vivo* tests.

A slightly increased number of basophilic hepatic foci were observed in chronic rat studies with budesonide, and in carcinogenicity studies there was an increased incidence of primary hepatocellular neoplasms, astrocytomas (in male rats) and mammary tumours (female rats) observed. These tumours are probably due to the specific steroid receptor action, increased metabolic burden on the liver and anabolic effects, effects which are also known from other glucocorticosteroids in rat studies and therefore represent a class effect. No similar effects have ever been observed in man for budesonide, neither in clinical trials nor from spontaneous reports.

In general, preclinical data reveal no special hazard for humans based on conventional studies of safety pharmacology, repeated dose toxicity, genotoxicity, carcinogenic potential.

In pregnant animals, budesonide, like other glucocorticosteroids, has been shown to cause abnormalities of foetal development, but the relevance to man has not been established (see also section 4.6).

6. PHARMACEUTICAL PARTICULARS

6.1 List of excipients

Cetyl alcohol

Citric acid monohydrate

Disodium edetate

Emulsifying wax

Macrogol stearyl ether

Propylene glycol

Purified water

Propellant:

n-Butane

Isobutane

Propane

6.2 Incompatibilities

Not applicable.

6.3 Shelf life

2 years

After first opening: 4 weeks.

6.4 Special precautions for storage

Do not store above 25 °C.

Do not refrigerate or freeze.

This is a pressurised container, containing of inflammable propellant.

Do not expose to temperature higher than 50°C, protect from direct sunlight. Do not pierce or burn even when empty.

6.5 Nature and contents of container

Aluminium pressurised container with metering valve together with 14 PVC applicators coated with white soft paraffin and liquid paraffin for administration of the foam and 14 plastic bags for hygienic disposal of the applicators.

Pack sizes:

Original pack with 1 pressurised container, contains at least 14 doses of 1.2 g rectal foam each.

Original pack with 2 pressurised containers, contains at least 2 × 14 doses of 1.2 g rectal foam each.

Hospital pack with 1 pressurised container, contains at least 14 doses of 1.2 g rectal foam each.

Not all pack sizes may be marketed.

6.6 Special precautions for disposal and other handling

No special requirements

7. MARKETING AUTHORISATION HOLDER

Dr. Falk Pharma GmbH

Leinenweberstr. 5

Postfach 6529

D-79041 Freiburg

Germany

8. MARKETING AUTHORISATION NUMBER(S)

PL 08637/0011

9. DATE OF FIRST AUTHORISATION/RENEWAL OF THE AUTHORISATION

15/06/2006

10. DATE OF REVISION OF THE TEXT

July 2009.

Budenofalk 3mg gastro-resistant capsules

(Dr. Falk Pharma UK Ltd)

1. NAME OF THE MEDICINAL PRODUCT

Budenofalk 3 mg gastro-resistant capsules

2. QUALITATIVE AND QUANTITATIVE COMPOSITION

Each capsule contains 3 mg budesonide

Excipients: Each capsule contains 240mg Sucrose and 12mg Lactose Monohydrate.

For a full list of excipients, see 6.1.

3. PHARMACEUTICAL FORM

Gastro-resistant capsules, hard (gastro-resistant capsules)

Capsule, hard, pink containing white gastro-resistant granules

4. CLINICAL PARTICULARS

4.1 Therapeutic indications

– Induction of remission in patients with mild to moderate active Crohn's disease affecting the ileum and/or the ascending colon

– Symptomatic relief of chronic diarrhoea due to collagenous colitis

Please note:

Treatment with Budenofalk 3 mg does not appear useful in patients with Crohn's disease affecting the upper gastro-intestinal tract. Extraintestinal symptoms, e.g. involving the skin, eyes or joints, are unlikely to respond to Budenofalk 3 mg because of its local action.

4.2 Posology and method of administration

Posology:

Adults aged > 18 years:

The recommended daily dose is one capsule (containing 3 mg budesonide) three times daily (morning, midday and evening) about a half hour before meals.

Children:

Budenofalk 3 mg should not be taken by children due to insufficient experience in this age group.

Method of Administration:

The capsules containing the gastro-resistant granules should be taken before meals, swallowed whole with plenty of fluid (e.g. a glass of water).

The duration of treatment in active Crohn's Disease and in collagenous colitis should be limited to 8 weeks.

The treatment with Budenofalk 3 mg should not be stopped abruptly, but withdrawn gradually (tapering doses). In the first week, the dosage should be reduced to two capsules daily, one in the morning, one in the evening. In the second week, only one capsule should be taken in the morning. Afterwards treatment can be stopped.

4.3 Contraindications

Budenofalk 3 mg must not be used in:

– hypersensitivity to budesonide or any of the ingredients

– hepatic cirrhosis with signs of portal hypertension, e.g. late-stage primary biliary cirrhosis

4.4 Special warnings and precautions for use

Treatment with Budenofalk 3 mg results in lower systemic steroid levels than conventional oral steroid therapy. Transfer from other steroid therapy may result in symptoms relating to the change in systemic steroid levels. Caution is required in patients with tuberculosis, hypertension, diabetes mellitus, osteoporosis, peptic ulcer, glaucoma, cataracts, family history of diabetes, family history of glaucoma.

Systemic effects of corticosteroids may occur, particularly when prescribed at high doses and for prolonged periods. Such effects may include Cushing's syndrome, adrenal suppression, growth retardation, decreased bone mineral density, cataract, glaucoma and very rarely a wide range of psychiatric/behavioural effects (see section 4.8.)

Infection:

Suppression of the inflammatory response and immune function increases the susceptibility to infections and their severity. The risk of deterioration of bacterial, fungal, amoebic and viral infections during glucocorticoid treatment should be carefully considered. The clinical presentation may often be atypical and serious infections such as septicaemia and tuberculosis may be masked, and therefore may reach an advanced stage before being recognised.

Chickenpox: Chickenpox is of particular concern since this normally minor illness may be fatal in immunosuppressed patients. Patients without a definite history of chickenpox should be advised to avoid close personal contact with chickenpox or herpes zoster and if exposed they should seek urgent medical attention. If the patient is a child, parents must be given the above advice. Passive immunisation with varicella zoster immunoglobulin (VZIG) is needed by exposed non-immune patients who are receiving systemic corticosteroids or who have used them within the previous 3 months; this should be given within 10 days of exposure to chickenpox. If a diagnosis of chickenpox is confirmed, the illness warrants specialist care and urgent treatment. Corticosteroids should not be stopped and the dose may need to be increased.

Measles: Patients with compromised immunity who have come into contact with measles should, wherever possible, receive normal immunglobulin as soon as possible after exposure.

Live vaccines: Live vaccines should not be given to individuals with impaired immune responsiveness. The antibody response to other vaccines may be diminished.

In patients with severe liver function disorders, the elimination of glucocorticosteroids including Budenofalk will be reduced, and their systemic bioavailability will be increased.

Corticosteroids may cause suppression of the HPA axis and reduce the stress response. Where patients are subject to surgery or other stresses, supplementary systemic glucocorticoid treatment is recommended.

Concomitant treatment with ketoconazole or other CYP3A4 inhibitors should be avoided (see section 4.5.)

Budenofalk 3mg capsules contain lactose and sucrose. Patients with rare hereditary problems of galactose or fructose intolerance, glucose-galactose malabsorption, sucrase-isomaltase insufficiency, the Lapp lactase deficiency or the congenital lactase deficiency should not take this medicine.

4.5 Interaction with other medicinal products and other forms of interaction

Pharmacodynamic interactions

Cardiac glycosides:

The action of the glycoside can be potentiated by potassium deficiency.

Saluretics:

Potassium excretion can be enhanced.

Pharmacokinetic interactions

Cytochrome P450:

– CYP3A4 inhibitors:

Ketoconazole 200 mg once daily p.o. increased the plasma concentrations of budesonide (3 mg single dose) approximately 6-fold during concomitant administration. When ketoconazole was administered 12 hours after budesonide, the concentrations increased approximately 3-fold. As there are not enough data to give dose recommendations, the combination should be avoided.

Other potent inhibitors of CYP3A4 such as ritonavir, itraconazole, and clarithromycin are also likely to give a marked increase of the plasma concentrations of budesonide. In addition, concomitant intake of grapefruit juice should be avoided.

–CYP3A4 inducers:

Compounds or drugs such as carbamazepine and rifampicin, which induce CYP3A4, might reduce the systemic but also the local exposure of budesonide at the gut mucosa. An adjustment of the budesonide dose might be necessary.

–CYP3A4 substrates:

Compounds or drugs which are metabolized by CYP3A4 might be in competition with budesonide. This might lead to an increased budesonide plasma concentration if the competing substance has a stronger affinity to CYP3A4, or – if budesonide binds stronger to CYP3A4 – the competing substance might be increased in plasma and a dose-adaption/reduction of this drug might be required.

Elevated plasma concentrations and enhanced effects of corticosteroids have been reported in women also receiving oestrogens or oral contraceptives, but this has not been observed with oral low dose combination contraceptives.

Cimetidine at recommended doses in combination with budesonide has a small but insignificant effect on pharmacokinetics of budesonide. Omeprazole has no effect on the pharmacokinetics of budesonide.

Steroid-binding compounds:

In theory, potential interactions with steroid-binding synthetic resins such as cholestyramine, and with antacids cannot be ruled out. If given at the same time as Budenofalk 3 mg, such interactions could result in a reduction in the effect of budesonide. Therefore these preparations should not be taken simultaneously, but at least two hours apart.

4.6 Pregnancy and lactation

Administration during pregnancy should be avoided unless there are compelling reasons for Budenofalk 3 mg therapy. In pregnant animals, budesonide, like other glucocorticosteroids, has been shown to cause abnormalities of foetal development. The relevance of this to man has not been established.

Since it is not known if budesonide passes into breast milk, the infant should not be breast-fed during treatment with Budenofalk 3 mg.

4.7 Effects on ability to drive and use machines

No effects are known.

4.8 Undesirable effects

The following undesirable effects and frequencies of Budenofalk 3 mg have been spontaneously reported:

Very rare (< 1/10,000), including isolated reports:

•*Metabolism and nutritional disorders:* oedema of legs, Cushing's syndrome

•*Nervous system disorders:* Pseudotumor cerebri (including papilloedema) in adolescents

•*Gastrointestinal disorders:* Constipation

•*Musculoskeletal, connective tissue and bone disorders:* diffuse muscle pain and weakness, osteoporosis

•*General disorders:* tiredness, malaise

Some of the undesired effects were reported after long-term use.

Occasionally side effects may occur which are typical for systemic glucocorticosteroids. These side effects depend on the dosage, the period of treatment, concomitant or previous treatment with other glucocorticosteroids and the individual sensitivity.

Clinical studies showed that the frequency of glucocorticosteroid associated side effects is lower with Budenofalk 3 mg (approx. by half) than with oral treatment of equivalent dosages of prednisolone.

Immune system disorders:

Interference with the immune response (e.g. increase in risk of infections).

An exacerbation or the reappearance of extraintestinal manifestations (especially affecting skin and joints) can occur on switching a patient from the systemically acting glucocorticosteroids to the locally acting budesonide.

Metabolism and nutrition disorders:

Cushing's syndrome: moon-face, truncal obesity, reduced glucose tolerance, diabetes mellitus, sodium retention with oedema formation, increased excretion of potassium, inactivity or atrophy of the adrenal cortex, growth retardation in children, disturbance of sex hormone secretion (e.g. amenorrhoea, hirsutism, impotence)

Psychiatric disorders:

Depression, irritability, euphoria

In addition very rarely a wide range of psychiatric/behavioural effects may occur.

Eyes disorders:

Glaucoma, cataract

Vascular disorders:

Hypertension, increased risk of thrombosis, vasculitis (withdrawal syndrome after long-term therapy)

Gastrointestinal disorders:

Stomach complaints, gastroduodenal ulcer, pancreatitis

Skin and subcutaneous tissue disorders:

Allergic exanthema, red striae, petechiae, ecchymosis, steroid acne, delayed wound healing, contact dermatitis

Musculoskeletal, connective tissue and bone disorders:

Aseptic necrosis of bone (femur and head of the humerus)

4.9 Overdose

To date, no cases of overdosage with budesonide are known. In view of the properties of budesonide contained in Budenofalk 3 mg, an overdose resulting in toxic damage is extremely unlikely.

5. PHARMACOLOGICAL PROPERTIES

5.1 Pharmacodynamic properties

Pharmacotherapeutic group: Glucocorticosteroid ATC code: A07EA06

The exact mechanism of budesonide in the treatment of Crohn's disease is not fully understood. Data from clinical pharmacology studies and controlled clinical trials strongly indicate that the mode of action of Budenofalk 3 mg capsules is predominantly based on a local action in the gut. Budesonide is a glucocorticosteroid with a high local anti-inflammatory effect. At doses clinically equivalent to systemically acting glucocorticosteroids, budesonide gives significantly less HPA axis suppression and has a lower impact on inflammatory markers.

Budenofalk 3 mg capsules show a dose-dependent influence on cortisol plasma levels which is at the recommended dose of 3 × 3 mg budesonide/day significantly smaller than that of clinically equivalent effective doses of systemic glucocorticosteroids.

5.2 Pharmacokinetic properties

Absorption:

Budenofalk 3 mg capsules, which contain gastric juice resistant granules, have – due to the specific coating of the granules – a lag phase of 2–3 hours. In healthy volunteers, as well as in patients with Crohn's disease, mean maximal budesonide plasma concentrations of 1-2 ng/ml were seen at about 5 hours following an oral dose of Budenofalk 3 mg capsules at a single dose of 3 mg, taken before meals. The maximal release therefore occurs in the terminal ileum and caecum, the main area of inflammation in Crohn's disease.

In ileostomy patients release of budesonide from Budenofalk 3 mg is comparable to healthy subjects or Crohn's disease patients. In ileostomy patients it was demonstrated that about 30–40 % of released budesonide is still found in the ileostomy bag, indicating that a substantial amount of budesonide from Budenofalk 3 mg will be transferred normally into the colon.

Concomitant intake of food may delay release of granules from stomach by 2–3 hours, prolonging the lag phase to about 4–6 hours, without change in absorption rates.

Distribution:

Budesonide has a high volume of distribution (about 3 l/kg). Plasma protein binding averages 85–90 %.

Biotransformation:

Budesonide undergoes extensive biotransformation in the liver (approximately 90 %) to metabolites of low glucocorticosteroid activity. The glucocorticosteroid activity of the major metabolites, 6β-hydroxybudesonide and 16α-hydroxyprednisolone, is less than 1 % of that of budesonide.

Elimination:

The average elimination half-life is about 3–4 hours. The systemic availability in healthy volunteers as well as in fasting patients with Crohn's disease is about 9–13 %. The clearance rate is about 10–15 l/min for budesonide, determined by HPLC-based methods.

Specific patient populations (liver diseases):

Dependent on the type and severity of liver diseases and due to the fact that budesonide is metabolised by CYP3A4, the metabolization of budesonide might be decreased. Therefore, the systemic exposure of budesonide might be increased in patients with impaired hepatic functions, as has been shown for patients with autoimmune hepatitis (AIH). With improving the liver function and disease, metabolization of budesonide will normalize.

The bioavailability of budesonide has been found to be significantly higher in patients in the late stage of primary biliary cirrhosis (PBC Stage IV) than in patients in the early stages of primary biliary cirrhosis (PBC Stage I/II); on average, the areas under the plasma concentration-time curves were threefold greater in patients with late-stage PBC, following repeated administration of budesonide 3 × 3 mg daily, than in patients with early-stage PBC.

5.3 Preclinical safety data

Preclinical data in acute, subchronic and chronic toxicological studies with budesonide showed atrophies of the thymus gland and adrenal cortex and a reduction especially of lymphocytes. These effects were less pronounced or at the same magnitude as observed with other glucocorticosteroids. Like with other glucocorticosteroids, and in dependence of the dose and duration and in dependence of the diseases these steroid effects might also be of relevance in man.

Budesonide had no mutagenic effects in a number of *in vitro* and *in vivo* tests.

A slightly increased number of basophilic hepatic foci were observed in chronic rat studies with budesonide, and in carcinogenicity studies was an increased incidence of primary hepatocellular neoplasms, astrocytomas (in male rats) and mammary tumors (female rats) observed. These tumors are probably due to the specific steroid receptor action, increased metabolic burden on the liver and anabolic effects, effects which are also known from other glucocorticosteroids in rat studies and therefore represent a class effect. No similar effects have ever been observed in man for budesonide, neither in clinical trials nor from spontaneous reports.

In general, preclinical data reveal no special hazard for humans based on conventional studies of safety pharmacology, repeated dose toxicity, genotoxicity, carcinogenic potential.

In pregnant animals, budesonide, like other glucocorticosteroids, has been shown to cause abnormalities of foetal development. But the relevance to man has not been established (see also section 4.6.)

6. PHARMACEUTICAL PARTICULARS

6.1 List of excipients

Capsules contents:

Lactose monohydrate

Maize starch

Methacrylic acid, methylmethacrylate copolymer (1:1) (Eudragit L 100)

Methacrylic acid, methylmethacrylate copolymer (1:2) (Eudragit S 100)

Poly(ethylacrylate, methylmethacrylate, trimethylammonium ethylmethacrylate chloride) (1:2:0.2) (solution with 12.5 percent Eudragit RL 12.5)

Poly(ethylacrylic acid, methylmethacrylate, trimethylammonium ethylmethacrylate chloride) (1:2:0.1) (dispersion with 12.5 percent Eudragit RS 12.5)

Povidone K25

Purified water*

Sucrose

Talc

Triethyl citrate

* intermediate excipient

Capsule shell:

Black iron oxide (E 172)

Erythrosine (E 127)

Gelatin

Purified water

Red iron oxide (E 172)

Sodium Laurilsulphate

Titanium dioxide (E 171)

6.2 Incompatibilities

Not applicable

6.3 Shelf life

3 years.

6.4 Special precautions for storage

Do not store above 25 °C.

6.5 Nature and contents of container

Al/PVC/PVDC blister strips.

Pack sizes: 10, 50, 90, 100 or 120 capsules. Not all pack sizes may be marketed.

6.6 Special precautions for disposal and other handling

No special requirements.

7. MARKETING AUTHORISATION HOLDER

Dr. Falk Pharma GmbH

Leinenweberstr. 5

79108 Freiburg

Postfach 6529

79041 Freiburg

8. MARKETING AUTHORISATION NUMBER(S)

PL08637/0002

9. DATE OF FIRST AUTHORISATION/RENEWAL OF THE AUTHORISATION

January 4, 1999

10. DATE OF REVISION OF THE TEXT

April 2009

Bumetanide Injection 0.5mg/ml, solution for injection (Leo Laboratories Ltd)

(Leo Laboratories Limited)

1. NAME OF THE MEDICINAL PRODUCT

Bumetanide Injection 0.5 mg/ml, solution for injection.

2. QUALITATIVE AND QUANTITATIVE COMPOSITION

Bumetanide Ph Eur 0.5 mg/ml.

3. PHARMACEUTICAL FORM

Solution for injection.

4. CLINICAL PARTICULARS

4.1 Therapeutic indications

Bumetanide is indicated whenever diuretic therapy is required in the treatment of oedema, e.g. that associated with congestive heart failure, cirrhosis of the liver and renal disease including the nephrotic syndrome.

For those oedematous conditions where a prompt diuresis is required, Bumetanide Injection 0.5 mg/ml may be used, e.g. acute pulmonary oedema, acute and chronic renal failure. Bumetanide Injection 0.5 mg/ml can be given intravenously or intramuscularly to those patients who are unable to take Burinex Tablets or who fail to respond satisfactorily to oral therapy.

4.2 Posology and method of administration

Route of administration: parenteral.

Pulmonary oedema: Initially 1 - 2 mg by intravenous injection. This can be repeated, if necessary, 20 minutes later.

In those conditions in which an infusion is appropriate, 2 - 5 mg may be given in 500 ml infusion fluid over 30 - 60 minutes. (See Section 4.4, special warnings and precautions for use).

When intramuscular administration is considered appropriate, a dose of 1 mg should be given initially and the dose then adjusted according to diuretic response.

Children: not recommended for children under 12 years of age.

Dosage in the elderly: adjust dosage according to response. A dose of 0.5 mg bumetanide per day may be sufficient in some elderly patients.

4.3 Contraindications

Although bumetanide can be used to induce diuresis in renal insufficiency, any marked increase in blood urea or the development of oliguria or anuria during treatment of severe progressing renal disease are indications for stopping treatment with bumetanide.

Hypersensitivity to any of the ingredients. Bumetanide is contra-indicated in hepatic coma and care should be taken in states of severe electrolyte depletion.

As with other diuretics, bumetanide should not be administered concurrently with lithium salts. Diuretics can reduce lithium clearance resulting in high serum levels of lithium.

4.4 Special warnings and precautions for use

Excessively rapid mobilisation of oedema, particularly in elderly patients, may give rise to sudden changes in cardiovascular pressure-flow relationships with circulatory collapse. This should be borne in mind when bumetanide is given in high doses intravenously or orally. Electrolyte disturbances may occur, particularly in those patients taking a low salt diet. Regular checks of serum electrolytes, in particular sodium, potassium, chloride and bicarbonate should be performed and replacement therapy instituted where indicated.

Like other diuretics, bumetanide shows a tendency to increase the excretion of potassium which can lead to an increase in the sensitivity of the myocardium to the toxic effects of digitalis. Thus the dose may need adjustment when given in conjunction with cardiac glycosides.

Bumetanide may potentiate the effects of antihypertensive drugs. Therefore, the dose of the latter may need adjustment when bumetanide is used to treat oedema in hypertensive patients.

As with other diuretics, bumetanide may cause an increase in blood uric acid. Periodic checks on urine and blood glucose should be made in diabetics and patients suspected of latent diabetes.

Patients with chronic renal failure on high doses of bumetanide should remain under constant hospital supervision.

Pharmaceutical precautions

Bumetanide Injection 0.5 mg/ml is presented in amber glass containers to protect against deterioration due to exposure to light.

When an intravenous infusion is required, Bumetanide Injection 0.5 mg/ml may be added to Dextrose Injection BP, Sodium Chloride Injection BP or Sodium Chloride and Dextrose Injection BP.

When 25 mg bumetanide (as Bumetanide Injection 0.5 mg/ml) was added to 1 litre of these infusion fluids, no evidence of precipitation was observed over a period of 72 hours. Higher concentrations of bumetanide in these infusion fluids may cause precipitation. It is good practice to inspect all infusion fluids containing bumetanide from time to time. Should cloudiness appear, the infusion should be discarded.

4.5 Interaction with other medicinal products and other forms of interaction

See Section 4.4 above.

4.6 Pregnancy and lactation

Although tests in four animal species have shown no teratogenic effects, the ordinary precaution of avoiding use of bumetanide in the first trimester of pregnancy should at present be observed. Since it is not known whether bumetanide is distributed into breast milk, a nursing mother should either stop breast feeding or observe the infant for any adverse effects if the drug is absolutely necessary for the mother.

4.7 Effects on ability to drive and use machines

None known.

4.8 Undesirable effects

Reported reactions include skin rashes and muscular cramps in the legs, abdominal discomfort, thrombocytopenia and gynaecomastia. Bone marrow depression associated with the use of bumetanide has been reported rarely, but it has not been proven definitely to be attributed to the drug. Hearing disturbance after administration of bumetanide is rare and reversible. The possibility of hearing disturbance must be considered, particularly when bumetanide is injected too quickly and in high doses.

High Dose Therapy

In patients with severe chronic renal failure given high doses of bumetanide, there have been reports of severe, generalised, musculoskeletal pain sometimes associated with muscle spasm, occurring one to two hours after administration and lasting up to 12 hours. The lowest reported dose causing this type of adverse reaction was 5 mg by intravenous injection and the highest was 75 mg orally in a single dose. All patients recovered fully and there was no deterioration in their renal function.

The cause of this pain is uncertain but it may be a result of varying electrolyte gradients at the cell membrane level.

Experience suggests that the incidence of such reactions is reduced by initiating treatment at 5-10 mg daily and titrating upwards using a twice daily dosage regimen at doses of 20 mg per day or more.

4.9 Overdose

Symptoms would be those caused by excessive diuresis. General measures should be taken to restore blood volume, maintain blood pressure and correct electrolyte disturbance.

5. PHARMACOLOGICAL PROPERTIES

5.1 Pharmacodynamic properties

Mode of action: bumetanide is a potent high ceiling diuretic with a rapid onset and a short duration of action.

5.2 Pharmacokinetic properties

After intravenous injection, diuresis usually starts within a few minutes and ceases in about two hours.

In most patients, 1mg of bumetanide produces a similar diuretic effect to 40 mg furosemide. Bumetanide excretion in the urine shows a good correlation with the diuretic response. In patients with chronic renal failure, the liver takes more importance as an excretory pathway although the duration of action in such patients is not markedly prolonged.

5.3 Preclinical safety data

There are no pre-clinical data of relevance to the prescriber which are additional to that already included in other sections of the SPC.

6. PHARMACEUTICAL PARTICULARS

6.1 List of excipients

Xylitol, disodium hydrogen phosphate dihydrate, sodium dihydrogen phosphate dihydrate and water for injections.

6.2 Incompatibilities

None known.

6.3 Shelf life

3 years.

6.4 Special precautions for storage

Do not store above 25°C.

6.5 Nature and contents of container
5 × 4 ml amber glass ampoules (OP), each ampoule containing 2mg bumetanide.

6.6 Special precautions for disposal and other handling
None.

7. MARKETING AUTHORISATION HOLDER
Leo Laboratories Limited
Longwick Road
Princes Risborough
Bucks HP27 9RR
UK

8. MARKETING AUTHORISATION NUMBER(S)
PL 0043/0060

9. DATE OF FIRST AUTHORISATION/RENEWAL OF THE AUTHORISATION
24 November 1978/13 January 1995.

10. DATE OF REVISION OF THE TEXT
November 2005

LEGAL CATEGORY
POM

Burinex 1mg Tablets

(Leo Laboratories Limited)

1. NAME OF THE MEDICINAL PRODUCT
Burinex® 1 mg Tablets.

2. QUALITATIVE AND QUANTITATIVE COMPOSITION
Bumetanide Ph Eur 1 mg.

3. PHARMACEUTICAL FORM
Tablet.

4. CLINICAL PARTICULARS

4.1 Therapeutic indications
Burinex is indicated whenever diuretic therapy is required in the treatment of oedema, e.g. that associated with congestive heart failure, cirrhosis of the liver and renal disease including the nephrotic syndrome.

In oedema of cardiac or renal origin where high doses of a potent short acting diuretic are required, Burinex 5 mg tablets may be used.

4.2 Posology and method of administration
For oral administration.

Most patients require a daily dose of 1 mg which can be given as a single morning or early evening dose. Depending on the patient's response, a second dose can be given six to eight hours later. In refractory cases, the dose can be increased until a satisfactory diuretic response is obtained, or infusions of Burinex can be given.

Children: not recommended for children under 12 years of age.

Dosage in the elderly: adjust dosage according to response. A dose of 0.5 mg bumetanide per day may be sufficient in some elderly patients.

4.3 Contraindications
Although Burinex can be used to induce diuresis in renal insufficiency, any marked increase in blood urea or the development of oliguria or anuria during treatment of severe progressing renal disease are indications for stopping treatment with Burinex.

Hypersensitivity to Burinex. Burinex is contra-indicated in hepatic coma and care should be taken in states of severe electrolyte depletion.

As with other diuretics, Burinex should not be administered concurrently with lithium salts. Diuretics can reduce lithium clearance resulting in high serum levels of lithium.

4.4 Special warnings and precautions for use
Excessively rapid mobilisation of oedema, particularly in elderly patients, may give rise to sudden changes in cardiovascular pressure-flow relationships with circulatory collapse. This should be borne in mind when Burinex is given in high doses intravenously or orally. Electrolyte disturbances may occur, particularly in those patients taking a low salt diet. Regular checks of serum electrolytes, in particular sodium, potassium, chloride and bicarbonate, should be performed and replacement therapy instituted where indicated.

Encephalopathy may be precipitated in patients with pre-existing hepatic impairment.

Burinex should be used with caution in patients already receiving nephrotoxic or ototoxic drugs.

4.5 Interaction with other medicinal products and other forms of interaction
Like other diuretics, Burinex shows a tendency to increase the excretion of potassium which can lead to an increase in the sensitivity of the myocardium to the toxic effects of digitalis. Thus the dose may need adjustment when given in conjunction with cardiac glycosides.

Burinex may potentiate the effects of antihypertensive drugs. Therefore, the dose of the latter may need adjustment when Burinex is used to treat oedema in hypertensive patients.

As with other diuretics, Burinex may cause an increase in blood uric acid. Periodic checks on urine and blood glucose should be made in diabetics and patients suspected of latent diabetes.

Patients with chronic renal failure on high doses of Burinex should remain under constant hospital supervision.

Certain non-steroidal anti-inflammatory drugs have been shown to antagonise the action of diuretics.

4.6 Pregnancy and lactation
Although tests in four animal species have shown no teratogenic effects, the ordinary precaution of avoiding use of Burinex in the first trimester of pregnancy should at present be observed. Since it is not known whether bumetanide is distributed into breast milk, a nursing mother should either stop breast feeding or observe the infant for any adverse effects if the drug is absolutely necessary for the mother.

4.7 Effects on ability to drive and use machines
None known.

4.8 Undesirable effects
Reported reactions include abdominal pain, vomiting, dyspepsia, diarrhoea, stomach and muscle cramps, arthralgia, dizziness, fatigue, hypotension, headache, nausea, encephalopathy (in patients with pre-existing hepatic disease), fluid and electrolyte depletion, dehydration, hyperuricaemia, raised blood urea and serum creatinine, hyperglycaemia, abnormalities of serum levels of hepatic enzymes, skin rashes, pruritus, urticaria, thrombocytopenia, gynaecomastia and painful breasts. Bone marrow depression associated with the use of Burinex has been reported rarely but it has not been proven definitely to be attributed to the drug. Hearing disturbance after administration of Burinex is rare and reversible.

High dose therapy:

In patients with severe chronic renal failure given high doses of Burinex, there have been reports of severe, generalised musculoskeletal pain sometimes associated with muscle spasm, occurring one to two hours after administration and lasting up to 12 hours. The lowest reported dose causing this type of adverse reaction was 5 mg by intravenous injection and the highest was 75 mg orally in a single dose. All patients recovered fully and there was no deterioration in their renal function. The cause of this pain is uncertain but it may be a result of varying electrolyte gradients at the cell membrane level.

Experience suggests that the incidence of such reactions is reduced by initiating treatment at 5-10 mg daily and titrating upwards using a twice daily dosage regimen at doses of 20 mg per day or more.

4.9 Overdose
Symptoms would be those caused by excessive diuresis. Empty stomach by gastric lavage or emesis. General measures should be taken to restore blood volume, maintain blood pressure and correct electrolyte disturbance.

5. PHARMACOLOGICAL PROPERTIES

5.1 Pharmacodynamic properties
Burinex is a potent, high ceiling loop diuretic with a rapid onset and a short duration of action. The primary site of action is the ascending limb of the Loop of Henlé where it exerts inhibiting effects on electrolyte reabsorption causing the diuretic and natriuretic action observed.

After oral administration of 1 mg Burinex, diuresis begins within 30 minutes with a peak effect between one and two hours. The diuretic effect is virtually complete in three hours after a 1 mg dose.

5.2 Pharmacokinetic properties
Burinex is well absorbed after oral administration with the bioavailability reaching between 80 and 95%. The elimination half life ranges from between 0.75 to 2.6 hours. No active metabolites are known. Renal excretion accounts for approximately half the clearance with hepatic excretion responsible for the other half. There is an increase in half-life and a reduced plasma clearance in the presence of renal or hepatic disease. In patients with chronic renal failure the liver takes more importance as an excretory pathway although the duration of action is not markedly prolonged.

5.3 Preclinical safety data
There are no pre-clinical data of relevance to the prescriber which are additional to that already included in other sections of the SPC.

6. PHARMACEUTICAL PARTICULARS

6.1 List of excipients
Maize starch, lactose, colloidal anhydrous silica, povidone, polysorbate 80, agar powder, talc and magnesium stearate.

6.2 Incompatibilities
None known

6.3 Shelf life
5 years.

6.4 Special pre
None.

6.5 Nature a
Blister pack

6.6 Special precautions for disposal and other handling
None.

7. MARKETING AUTHORISATION HOLDER
LEO Laboratories Limited
Longwick Road
Princes Risborough
Bucks HP27 9RR
UK

8. MARKETING AUTHORISATION NUMBER(S)
PL 0043/0021R

9. DATE OF FIRST AUTHORISATION/RENEWAL OF THE AUTHORISATION
27 June 1996.

10. DATE OF REVISION OF THE TEXT
December 2005

LEGAL CATEGORY
POM

Burinex 5mg Tablets

(Leo Laboratories Limited)

1. NAME OF THE MEDICINAL PRODUCT
Burinex® 5 mg Tablets.

2. QUALITATIVE AND QUANTITATIVE COMPOSITION
Bumetanide Ph Eur 5 mg.

3. PHARMACEUTICAL FORM
Tablet.

4. CLINICAL PARTICULARS

4.1 Therapeutic indications
Burinex is indicated whenever diuretic therapy is required in the treatment of oedema, e.g. that associated with congestive heart failure, cirrhosis of the liver and renal disease including the nephrotic syndrome.

In oedema of cardiac or renal origin where high doses of a potent short acting diuretic are required, Burinex 5 mg tablets may be used.

4.2 Posology and method of administration
For oral administration.

The dose should be carefully titrated in each patient according to the patient's response and the required therapeutic activity. As a general rule, in patients not controlled on lower doses, dosage should be started at 5 mg daily and then increased by 5 mg increments every 12-24 hours until the required response is obtained or side-effects appear.

Consideration should be given to a twice daily dosage rather than once daily. Direct substitution of Burinex for furosemide in a 1:40 ratio at high doses should be avoided. Treatment should be initiated at a lower equivalent dose and gradually increased in 5 mg increments.

Children: not recommended for children under 12 years of age.

Dosage in the elderly: adjust dosage according to response. A dose of 0.5 mg bumetanide per day may be sufficient in some elderly patients.

4.3 Contraindications
Although Burinex can be used to induce diuresis in renal insufficiency, any marked increase in blood urea or the development of oliguria or anuria during treatment of severe progressing renal disease are indications for stopping treatment with Burinex.

Hypersensitivity to Burinex. Burinex is contra-indicated in hepatic coma and care should be taken in states of severe electrolyte depletion.

As with other diuretics, Burinex should not be administered concurrently with lithium salts. Diuretics can reduce lithium clearance resulting in high serum levels of lithium.

4.4 Special warnings and precautions for use
Excessively rapid mobilisation of oedema, particularly in elderly patients, may give rise to sudden changes in cardiovascular pressure-flow relationships with circulatory collapse. This should be borne in mind when Burinex is given in high doses intravenously or orally. Electrolyte disturbances may occur, particularly in those patients taking a low salt diet. Regular checks of serum electrolytes, in particular sodium, potassium, chloride and bicarbonate, should be performed and replacement therapy instituted where indicated.

Encephalopathy may be precipitated in patients with pre-existing hepatic impairment.

Burinex should be used with caution in patients already receiving nephrotoxic or ototoxic drugs.

4.5 Interaction with other medicinal products and other forms of interaction
Like other diuretics, Burinex shows a tendency to increase the excretion of potassium which can lead to an increase in the sensitivity of the myocardium to the toxic effects of digitalis. Thus the dose may need adjustment when given in conjunction with cardiac glycosides.

Burinex may potentiate the effects of antihypertensive drugs. Therefore, the dose of the latter may need adjustment when Burinex is used to treat oedema in hypertensive patients.

As with other diuretics, Burinex may cause an increase in blood uric acid. Periodic checks on urine and blood glucose should be made in diabetics and patients suspected of latent diabetes.

Patients with chronic renal failure on high doses of Burinex should remain under constant hospital supervision.

Certain non-steroidal anti-inflammatory drugs have been shown to antagonise the action of diuretics.

4.6 Pregnancy and lactation

Although tests in four animal species have shown no teratogenic effects, the ordinary precaution of avoiding use of Burinex in the first trimester of pregnancy should at present be observed. Since it is not known whether bumetanide is distributed into breast milk, a nursing mother should either stop breast feeding or observe the infant for any adverse effects if the drug is absolutely necessary for the mother.

4.7 Effects on ability to drive and use machines

None known.

4.8 Undesirable effects

Reported reactions include abdominal pain, vomiting, dyspepsia, diarrhoea, stomach and muscle cramps, arthralgia, dizziness, fatigue, hypotension, headache, nausea, encephalopathy (in patients with pre-existing hepatic disease), fluid and electrolyte depletion, dehydration, hyperuricaemia, raised blood urea and serum creatinine, hyperglycaemia, abnormalities of serum levels of hepatic enzymes, skin rashes, pruritus, urticaria, thrombocytopenia, gynaecomastia and painful breasts. Bone marrow depression associated with the use of Burinex has been reported rarely but it has not been proven definitely to be attributed to the drug. Hearing disturbance after administration of Burinex is rare and reversible.

High dose therapy:

In patients with severe chronic renal failure given high doses of Burinex, there have been reports of severe, generalised musculoskeletal pain sometimes associated with muscle spasm, occurring one to two hours after administration and lasting up to 12 hours. The lowest reported dose causing this type of adverse reaction was 5 mg by intravenous injection and the highest was 75 mg orally in a single dose. All patients recovered fully and there was no deterioration in their renal function. The cause of this pain is uncertain but it may be a result of varying electrolyte gradients at the cell membrane level.

Experience suggests that the incidence of such reactions is reduced by initiating treatment at 5-10 mg daily and titrating upwards using a twice daily dosage regimen at doses of 20 mg per day or more.

4.9 Overdose

Symptoms would be those caused by excessive diuresis. Empty stomach by gastric lavage or emesis. General measures should be taken to restore blood volume, maintain blood pressure and correct electrolyte disturbance.

5. PHARMACOLOGICAL PROPERTIES

5.1 Pharmacodynamic properties

Burinex is a potent, high ceiling loop diuretic with a rapid onset and a short duration of action. The primary site of action is the ascending limb of the Loop of Henlé where it exerts inhibiting effects on electrolyte reabsorption causing the diuretic and natriuretic action observed.

After oral administration of 1 mg Burinex, diuresis begins within 30 minutes with a peak effect between one and two hours. The diuretic effect is virtually complete in three hours after a 1 mg dose.

5.2 Pharmacokinetic properties

Burinex is well absorbed after oral administration with the bioavailability reaching between 80 and 95%. The elimination half life ranges from between 0.75 to 2.6 hours. No active metabolites are known. Renal excretion accounts for approximately half the clearance with hepatic excretion responsible for the other half. There is an increase in half-life and a reduced plasma clearance in the presence of renal or hepatic disease. In patients with chronic renal failure the liver takes more importance as an excretory pathway although the duration of action is not markedly prolonged.

5.3 Preclinical safety data

There are no pre-clinical data of relevance to the prescriber which are additional to that already included in other sections of the SPC.

6. PHARMACEUTICAL PARTICULARS

6.1 List of excipients

Maize starch, lactose, colloidal anhydrous silica, povidone, polysorbate 80, agar powder, talc and magnesium stearate.

6.2 Incompatibilities

None known

6.3 Shelf life

5 years.

6.4 Special precautions for storage

None.

6.5 Nature and contents of container

Blister packs of 28 tablets (OP).

6.6 Special precautions for disposal and other handling

None.

7. MARKETING AUTHORISATION HOLDER

Leo Laboratories Limited
Longwick Road
Princes Risborough
Bucks HP27 9RR
UK

8. MARKETING AUTHORISATION NUMBER(S)

PL 0043/0043R

9. DATE OF FIRST AUTHORISATION/RENEWAL OF THE AUTHORISATION

27 June 1996.

10. DATE OF REVISION OF THE TEXT

December 2005

LEGAL CATEGORY

POM

Buscopan Ampoules

(Boehringer Ingelheim Limited)

1. NAME OF THE MEDICINAL PRODUCT

Buscopan Ampoules 20mg/ml solution for injection.

2. QUALITATIVE AND QUANTITATIVE COMPOSITION

Each 1ml ampoule contains 20 mg hyoscine butylbromide.

For excipients, see 6.1.

3. PHARMACEUTICAL FORM

Solution for injection

A colourless or almost colourless, clear solution

4. CLINICAL PARTICULARS

4.1 Therapeutic indications

Buscopan Ampoules are indicated in acute spasm, as in renal or biliary colic, in radiology for differential diagnosis of obstruction and to reduce spasm and pain in pyelography, and in other diagnostic procedures where spasm may be a problem, e.g. gastro-duodenal endoscopy.

4.2 Posology and method of administration

Not recommended for children.

<u>Adults</u>:

One ampoule (20 mg) intramuscularly or intravenously, repeated after half an hour if necessary. Intravenous injection should be performed 'slowly' (in rare cases a marked drop in blood pressure and even shock may be produced by Buscopan). When used in endoscopy this dose may need to be repeated more frequently.

Maximum daily dose of 100mg.

<u>Diluent</u>:

Buscopan injection solution may be diluted with dextrose or with sodium chloride 0.9% injection solutions.

No specific information on the use of this product in the elderly is available. Clinical trials have included patients over 65 years and no adverse reactions specific to this age group have been reported.

4.3 Contraindications

Buscopan Ampoules should not be administered to patients with myasthenia gravis, megacolon, narrow angle glaucoma, tachycardia, prostatic enlargement with urinary retention, mechanical stenoses in the region of the gastro-intestinal tract or paralytic ileus.

Buscopan should not be used in patients who have demonstrated prior hypersensitivity to hyoscine butylbromide or any other component of the product.

BUSCOPAN ampoules should not be given by intramuscular injection to patients being treated with anticoagulant drugs since intramuscular haematoma may occur.

4.4 Special warnings and precautions for use

Buscopan Ampoules should be used with caution in conditions characterised by tachycardia such as thyrotoxicosis, cardiac insufficiency or failure and in cardiac surgery where it may further accelerate the heart rate.

Because of the possibility that anticholinergics may reduce sweating, Buscopan should be administered with caution to patients with pyrexia.

Elevation of intraocular pressure may be produced by the administration of anticholinergic agents such as Buscopan in patients with undiagnosed and therefore untreated narrow angle glaucoma. Therefore, patients should seek urgent ophthalmological advice in case they should develop a painful, red eye with loss of vision after the injection of Buscopan.

After parenteral administration of Buscopan, cases of anaphylaxis including episodes of shock have been observed. As with all drugs causing such reactions, patients receiving Buscopan by injection should be kept under observation.

4.5 Interaction with other medicinal products and other forms of interaction

The anticholinergic effect of drugs ... tricyclic antidepressants, antihistamines, quini... ...ntadine, phenothiazines, butyrophenones, di... and other

anticholinergics (e.g. tiotropium, ipratropium) may be intensified by Buscopan.

The tachycardic effects of beta-adrenergic agents may be enhanced by Buscopan.

Concomitant treatment with dopamine antagonists such as metoclopramide may result in diminution of the effects of both drugs on the gastrointestinal tract.

4.6 Pregnancy and lactation

Although Buscopan has been in wide general use for many years, there is no definitive evidence of ill-consequence during human pregnancy; animal studies have shown no hazard. Nevertheless, medicines should not be used in pregnancy, especially the first trimester, unless the expected benefit is thought to outweigh any possible risk to the foetus.

Safety during lactation has not yet been established.

4.7 Effects on ability to drive and use machines

Because of visual accommodation disturbances patients should not drive or operate machinery after parenteral administration of Buscopan until vision has normalised.

4.8 Undesirable effects

Many of the listed undesirable effects can be assigned to the anticholinergic properties of BUSCOPAN.

<u>Immune system disorders</u>

Anaphylactic shock including cases with fatal outcome, anaphylactic reactions, dyspnoea, skin reactions and other hypersensitivity.

<u>Eye disorders</u>

Accommodation disorders

<u>Cardiac disorders</u>

Tachycardia

<u>Vascular disorders</u>

Blood pressure decreased, dizziness, flushing

<u>Gastrointestinal disorders</u>

Dry mouth, constipation

<u>Skin and subcutaneous tissue disorders</u>

Dyshidrosis

<u>Renal and urinary disorders</u>

Urinary retention

Injection site pain, particularly after intramuscular use, occurs.

Hyoscine butylbromide, the active ingredient of Buscopan, due to its chemical structure as a quaternary ammonium derivate, is not expected to enter the central nervous system. Hyoscine butylbromide does not readily pass the blood-brain barrier. However, it cannot totally be ruled out that under certain circumstances psychiatric disorders (e.g. confusion) may also occur after administration of Buscopan.

4.9 Overdose

Symptoms

Serious signs of poisoning following acute overdosage have not been observed in man. In the case of overdosage, anticholinergic symptoms such as urinary retention, dry mouth, reddening of the skin, tachycardia, inhibition of gastrointestinal motility and transient visual disturbances may occur, and Cheynes-Stokes respiration has been reported.

Therapy

Symptoms of Buscopan overdosage respond to parasympathomimetics. For patients with glaucoma, pilocarpine should be given locally. Cardiovascular complications should be treated according to usual therapeutic principles. In case of respiratory paralysis, intubation and artificial respiration. Catheterisation may be required for urinary retention.

In addition, appropriate supportive measures should be used as required.

5. PHARMACOLOGICAL PROPERTIES

5.1 Pharmacodynamic properties

Buscopan is an antispasmodic agent which relaxes smooth muscle of the organs of the abdominal and pelvic cavities. It is believed to act predominantly on the intramural parasympathetic ganglia of these organs.

5.2 Pharmacokinetic properties

After intravenous administration hyoscine butylbromide is rapidly distributed into the tissues. The volume of distribution (Vss) is 128 l. The half-life of the terminal elimination phase ($t_{1/2}\gamma$) is approximately 5 hours. The total clearance is 1.2 l/min, approximately half of the clearance is renal.

In rat, highest concentrations of hyoscine butylbromide are found in the tissue of the gastrointestinal tract, liver and kidneys. Plasma protein binding of hyoscine butylbromide is low.

Hyoscine butylbromide does not readily pass the blood-brain barrier.

5.3 Preclinical safety data

None stated

6. PHARMACEUTICAL PARTICULARS

6.1 List of excipients

Sodium Chloride

Water for injections

6.2 Incompatibilities
None known

6.3 Shelf life
Unopened: 5 years

Once opened, use immediately and discard any unused contents

6.4 Special precautions for storage
Store below 30°C.

Store in the outer carton.

6.5 Nature and contents of container
1ml colourless glass (Ph. Eur. Type I) ampoules marketed in cartons containing 10 ampoules.

6.6 Special precautions for disposal and other handling
For single use only. Any unused solution should be discarded.

7. MARKETING AUTHORISATION HOLDER
Boehringer Ingelheim Limited

Ellesfield Avenue

Bracknell

Berkshire

RG12 8YS

United Kingdom

8. MARKETING AUTHORISATION NUMBER(S)
PL 00015/5005R

9. DATE OF FIRST AUTHORISATION/RENEWAL OF THE AUTHORISATION
23/06/2006

10. DATE OF REVISION OF THE TEXT
July 2008

Legal Category
POM

Busilvex

(Pierre Fabre Limited)

1. NAME OF THE MEDICINAL PRODUCT
Busilvex ▼ 6 mg/ml concentrate for solution for infusion

2. QUALITATIVE AND QUANTITATIVE COMPOSITION
One ml of concentrate contains 6 mg of busulfan (60 mg in 10 ml).

After dilution: 1 ml of solution contains 0.5 mg of busulfan

For a full list of excipients see section 6.1

3. PHARMACEUTICAL FORM
Concentrate for solution for infusion (sterile concentrate).

Clear, colourless solution.

4. CLINICAL PARTICULARS

4.1 Therapeutic indications
Busilvex followed by cyclophosphamide (BuCy2) is indicated as conditioning treatment prior to conventional haematopoietic progenitor cell transplantation (HPCT) in adult patients when the combination is considered the best available option.

Busilvex followed by cyclophosphamide (BuCy4) or melphalan (BuMel) is indicated as conditioning treatment prior to conventional haematopoietic progenitor cell transplantation in paediatric patients.

4.2 Posology and method of administration
Busilvex administration should be supervised by a physician experienced in conditioning treatment prior to haematopoietic progenitor cell transplantation.

Busilvex is administered prior the conventional haematopoietic progenitor cell transplantation (HPCT).

Dosage in adults

The recommended dosage and schedule of administration is:

- 0.8 mg/kg body weight (BW) of busulfan as a two-hour infusion every 6 hours over 4 consecutive days for a total of 16 doses,

- followed by cyclophosphamide at 60 mg/kg/day over 2 days initiated for a least 24 hours following the 16th dose of Busilvex (see section 4.5).

Dosage in paediatric patients (0 to 17 years)

The recommended dose of Busilvex is as follows:

Actual body weight (kg)	Busulfex dose (mg/kg)
< 9	1.0
9 to < 16	1.2
16 to 23	1.1
> 23 to 34	0.95
> 34	0.8

followed by:

- 4 cycles of 50 mg/kg body weight (BW) cyclophosphamide (BuCy4) or

- one administration of 140 mg/m² melphalan (BuMel)

initiated for a least 24 hours following the 16th dose of Busilvex.(see section 4.5).

Busilvex is administered as a two-hour infusion every 6 hours over 4 consecutive days for a total of 16 doses prior to cyclophosphamide or melphalan and conventional haematopoietic progenitor cell transplantation (HPCT)

Administration

Busilvex must be diluted prior to administration (see section 6.6). A final concentration of approximately 0.5 mg/ml busulfan should be achieved. Busilvex should be administered by intravenous infusion via central venous catheter.

Busilvex should not be given by rapid intravenous, *bolus* or peripheral injection.

All patients should be pre-medicated with anticonvulsant medicinal products to prevent seizures reported with the use of high dose busulfan.

It is recommended to administer anticonvulsants 12 h prior to Busilvex to 24 h after the last dose of Busilvex.

In adults all studied patients received phenytoin. There is no experience with other anticonvulsant agents such as benzodiazepines (see sections 4.4 and 4.5).

In children studied patients received either phenytoin or benzodiazepines.

Antiemetics should be administered prior to the first dose of Busilvex and continued on a fixed schedule according to local practice through its administration.

Obese patients

In adults

For obese patients, dosing based on adjusted ideal body weight (AIBW) should be considered.

Ideal body weight (IBW) is calculated as follows:

IBW men (kg)=50 + 0.91x (height in cm-152);

IBW women (kg)= 45 + 0.91x (height in cm-152).

Adjusted ideal body weight (AIBW) is calculated as follows:

AIBW= IBW+0.25x (actual body weight - IBW).

In paediatric patients

The medicinal product is not recommended in obese children and adolescents with body mass index Weight (kg)/(m)² > 30 kg/m² until further data become available.

Renally impaired patient:

Studies in renally impaired patients have not been conducted, however, as busulfan is moderately excreted in the urine, dose modification is not recommended in these patients.

However, caution is recommended (see sections 4.8 and 5.2).

Hepatically impaired patient:

Busilvex as well as busulfan has not been studied in patients with hepatic impairment.

Caution is recommended, particularly in those patients with severe hepatic impairment (see section 4.4).

Elderly patient:

Patients older than 50 years of age (n=23) have been successfully treated with Busilvex without dose-adjustment. However, for the safe use of Busilvex in patients older than 60 years only limited information is available. Same dose (see section 5.2) for elderly as for adults (< 50 years old) should be used.

4.3 Contraindications
Hypersensitivity to the active substance or to any of the excipients

Pregnancy (see section 4.6)

4.4 Special warnings and precautions for use
The consequence of treatment with Busilvex at the recommended dose and schedule is profound myelosuppression, occurring in all patients. Severe granulocytopenia, thrombocytopenia, anaemia, or any combination thereof may develop. Frequent complete blood counts, including differential white blood cell counts, and platelet counts should be monitored during the treatment and until recovery is achieved.

Prophylactic or empiric use of anti-infectives (bacterial, fungal, viral) should be considered for the prevention and management of infections during the neutropenic period. Platelet and red blood cell support, as well as the use of growth factors such as granulocyte colony stimulating agent (G-CSF), should be employed as medically indicated.

In adults, absolute neutrophil counts < $0.5x10^9$/l at a median of 4 days post transplant occurred in 100% of patients and recovered at median day 10 and 13 days following autologous and allogeneic transplant respectively (median neutropenic period of 6 and 9 days respectively). Thrombocytopenia (< $25x10^9$/l or requiring platelet transfusion) occurred at a median of 5-6 days in 98% of patients. Anaemia (haemoglobin < 8.0 g/dl) occurred in 69% of patients.

In paediatric patients, absolute neutrophil counts < $0.5x10^9$/l at a median of 3 days post transplant occurred in 100% of patients and lasted 5 and 18.5 days in autologous and allogeneic transplant respectively. In children, thrombocytopenia (< $25x10^9$/l or requiring platelet transfusion) occurred in 100% of patients. Anaemia (haemoglobin < 8.0 g/dl) occurred in 100% of patients.

The Fanconi anaemia cells have hypersensitivity to cross-linking agents. There is limited clinical experience of the use of busulfan as a component of a conditioning regimen prior to HSCT in children with Fanconi's anaemia. Therefore Busilvex should be used with caution in this type of patients.

Busilvex as well as busulfan has not been studied in patients with hepatic impairment. Since busulfan is mainly metabolized through the liver, caution should be observed when Busilvex is used in patients with pre-existing impairment of liver function, especially in those with severe hepatic impairment. It is recommended when treating these patients that serum transaminase, alkaline phosphatase, and bilirubin should be monitored regularly 28 days following transplant for early detection of hepatotoxicity.

Hepatic veno-occlusive disease is a major complication that can occur during treatment with Busilvex. Patients who have received prior radiation therapy, greater than or equal to three cycles of chemotherapy, or prior progenitor cell transplant may be at an increased risk (see section 4.8).

Caution should be exercised when using paracetamol prior to (less than 72 hours) or concurrently with Busilvex due to a possible decrease in the metabolism of busulfan (See section 4.5).

As documented in clinical studies, no treated patients experienced cardiac tamponade or other specific cardiac toxicities related to Busilvex. However cardiac function should be monitored regularly in patients receiving Busilvex (see section 4.8).

Occurrence of acute respiratory distress syndrome with subsequent respiratory failure associated with interstitial pulmonary fibrosis was reported in Busilvex studies in one patient who died, although, no clear aetiology was identified. In addition, busulfan might induce pulmonary toxicity that may be additive to the effects produced by other cytotoxic agents. Therefore, attention should be paid to this pulmonary issue in patients with prior history of mediastinal or pulmonary radiation (see section 4.8).

Periodic monitoring of renal function should be considered during therapy with Busilvex (see section 4.8).

Seizures have been reported with high dose busulfan treatment. Special caution should be exercised when administering the recommended dose of Busilvex to patients with a history of seizures. Patients should receive adequate anti-convulsant prophylaxis. In adults, all data with Busilvex were obtained using phenytoin. There are no data available on the use of other anticonvulsant agents such as benzodiazepines. Thus, the effect of anticonvulsant agents (other than phenytoin) on busulfan pharmacokinetics is not known. (see sections 4.2 and 4.5).

In paediatric patients, data with Busilvex were obtained using benzodiazepines or phenytoin.

The increased risk of a second malignancy should be explained to the patient. On the basis of human data, busulfan has been classified by the International Agency for Research on Cancer (IARC) as a human carcinogen. The World Health Association has concluded that there is a causal relationship between busulfan exposure and cancer. Leukaemia patients treated with busulfan developed many different cytological abnormalities, and some developed carcinomas. Busulfan is thought to be leukemogenic.

Fertility: busulfan can impair fertility. Therefore, men treated with Busilvex are advised not to father a child during and up to 6 months after treatment and to seek advice on cryo-conservation of sperm prior to treatment because of the possibility of irreversible infertility due to therapy with Busilvex. Ovarian suppression and amenorrhoea with menopausal symptoms commonly occur in pre-menopausal patients. Busulfan treatment in a pre-adolescent girl prevented the onset of puberty due to ovarian failure. Impotence, sterility, azoospermia, and testicular atrophy have been reported in male patients. The solvent dimethylacetamide (DMA) may also impair fertility. DMA decreases fertility in male and female rodents (see sections 4.6 and 5.3)

4.5 Interaction with other medicinal products and other forms of interaction
No specific clinical trial was carried out to assess drug-drug interaction between intravenous busulfan and itraconazole. From published studies, in adults administration of itraconazole to patients receiving high-dose busulfan may result in reduced busulfan clearance. Patients should be monitored for signs of busulfan toxicity when itraconazole is used as an antifungal prophylaxis with intravenous busulfan.

Published studies in adults described that ketobemidone (analgesic) might be associated with high levels of plasma busulfan. Therefore special care is recommended when combining these two compounds.

In adults, for the BuCy2 regimen it has been reported that the time interval between the last oral busulfan administration and the first cyclophosphamide administration may influence the development of toxicities. A reduced incidence of Hepatic Veino Occlusive Disease (HVOD) and other regimen-related toxicity have been observed in patients when the lag time between the last dose of oral busulfan and the first dose of cyclophosphamide is > 24hours.

In paediatric patients, for the BuMel regimen it has been reported that the administration of melphalan less than 24 hours after the last oral busulfan administration may influence the development of toxicities.

Paracetamol is described to decrease glutathione levels in blood and tissues, and may therefore decrease busulfan clearance when used in combination (see section 4.4).

Phenytoin or benzodiazepines were administered for seizure prophylaxis in all patients in the clinical trials conducted with intravenous busulfan. The concomitant systemic administration of phenytoin to patients receiving high-dose busulfan has been reported to increase busulfan clearance, due to induction of glutathion-S-transferase. However no evidence of this effect has been seen in intravenous data.(see section 4.4)

No interaction has been reported when benzodiazepines such as diazepam, clonazepam or lorazepam have been used to prevent seizures with high-dose busulfan (see sections 4.2 and 4.4).

No interaction was observed when busulfan was combined with fluconazole (antifungal agent) or 5 HT_3 antiemetics such as ondansetron or granisetron.

4.6 Pregnancy and lactation

Pregnancy

HPCT is contraindicated in pregnant women; therefore, Busilvex is contraindicated during pregnancy. Busulfan has caused embryofoetal lethality and malformations in pre-clinical studies.(see section 5.3)

There are no adequate data from the use of either busulfan or DMA in pregnant woman. A few cases of congenital abnormalities have been reported with low-dose oral busulfan, not necessarily attributable to the active substance, and third trimester exposure may be associated with impaired intrauterine growth.

Women of childbearing potential have to use effective contraception during and up to 6 months after treatment.

Lactation

It is not known whether busulfan and DMA are excreted in human milk. Because of the potential for tumorigenicity shown for busulfan in human and animal studies, breast-feeding should be discontinued at the start of therapy.

Fertility

Busulfan and DMA can impair fertility in man or woman. Therefore it is advised not to father child during the treatment and up to 6 months after treatment and to seek advice on cryo-conservation of sperm prior to treatment because of the possibility of irreversible infertility (see section 4.4).

4.7 Effects on ability to drive and use machines

Not relevant

4.8 Undesirable effects

Averse events in adults

Adverse events information is derived from two clinical trials (n=103) of Busilvex.

Serious toxicities involving the haematologic, hepatic and respiratory systems were considered as expected consequences of the conditioning regimen and transplant process. These include infection and Graft-versus host disease (GVHD) which although not directly related, were the major causes of morbidity and mortality, especially in allogeneic HPCT.

Blood and the lymphatic system disorders:

Myelo-suppression and immuno-suppression were the desired therapeutic effects of the conditioning regimen. Therefore all patients experienced profound cytopenia: leukopenia 96%, thrombocytopenia 94%, and anemia 88%. The median time to neutropenia was 4 days for both autologous and allogeneic patients. The median duration of neutropenia was 6 days and 9 days for autologous and allogeneic patients.

Immune system disorders:

The incidence of acute graft versus host disease (a-GVHD) data was collected in OMC-BUS-4 study(allogeneic)(n=61). A total of 11 patients (18%) experienced a-GVHD. The incidence of a-GVHD grades I-II was 13% (8/61), while the incidence of grade III-IV was 5% (3/61). Acute GVHD was rated as serious in 3 patients. Chronic GVHD (c-GVHD) was reported if serious or the cause of death, and was reported as the cause of death in 3 patients.

Infections and infestations:

39% of patients (40/103) experienced one or more episodes of infection, of which 83% (33/40) were rated as mild or moderate. Pneumonia was fatal in 1% (1/103) and life-threatening in 3% of patients. Other infections were considered severe in 3% of patients. Fever was reported in 87% of patients and graded as mild/moderate in 84% and severe in 3%. 47% of patients experienced chills which were mild/moderate in 46% and severe in 1%.

Hepato-biliary disorders:

15% of SAEs involved liver toxicity. HVOD is a recognized potential complication of conditioning therapy post-transplant. Six of 103 patients (6%) experienced HVOD. HVOD occurred in: 8.2% (5/61) allogeneic patients (fatal in 2 patients) and 2.5% (1/42) of autologous patients. Elevated bilirubine (n=3) and elevated AST (n=1) were also observed. Two of the above four patients with serious serum hepatotoxicity were among patients with diagnosed HVOD.

Respiratory, thoracic and mediastinal disorders:

One patient experienced a fatal case of acute respiratory distress syndrome with subsequent respiratory failure associated with interstitial pulmonary fibrosis in the Busilvex studies.

In addition the literature review reports alterations of cornea and lens of the eye with oral busulfan.

Adverse events in paediatric patients

Adverse events information are derived from the clinical study in paediatrics (n=55). Serious toxicities involving the hepatic and respiratory systems were considered as expected consequences of the conditioning regimen and transplant process.

Immune system disorders:

The incidence of acute graft versus host disease (a-GVHD) data was collected in allogeneic patients (n=28). A total of 14 patients (50%) experienced a-GVHD. The incidence of a-GVHD grades I-II was 46.4% (13/28), while the incidence of grade III-IV was 3.6% (1/28). Chronic GVHD was reported only if it is the cause of death: one patient died 13 months post-transplant.

Infections and infestations:

Infections (documented and non documented febrile neutropenia) were experienced in 89% of patients (49/55). Mild/moderate fever was reported in 76% of patients.

Hepato-biliary disorders:

Grade 3 elevated transaminases were reported in 24% of patients.

Veino occlusive disease (VOD) was reported in 15% (4/27) and 7% (2/28) of the autologous and allogenic transplant respectively. VOD observed were neither fatal nor severe and resolved in all cases.

Adverse reactions reported both in adults and paediatric patients as more than an isolated case are listed below, by system organ class and by frequency. Within each frequency grouping, adverse events are presented in order of decreasing seriousness. Frequencies are defined as: very common (⩾ 1/10), common (⩾ 1/100, < 1/10), uncommon (⩾ 1/1,000, < 1/100).

(see Table 1 on next page)

4.9 Overdose

The principal toxic effect is profound myeloablation and pancytopenia but the central nervous system, liver, lungs, and gastrointestinal tract may also be affected.

There is no known antidote to Busilvex other than haematopoietic progenitor cell transplantation. In the absence of haematopoietic progenitor cell transplantation, the recommended dosage of Busilvex would constitute an overdose of busulfan. The haematologic status should be closely monitored and vigorous supportive measures instituted as medically indicated.

There have been two reports that busulfan is dialyzable, thus dialysis should be considered in the case of an overdose. Since, busulfan is metabolized through conjugation with glutathione, administration of glutathione might be considered.

It must be considered that overdose of Busilvex will also increase exposure to DMA. In human the principal toxic effects were hepatotoxicity and central nervous system (CNS) effects. CNS changes precede any of the more severe side effects. No specific antidote for DMA overdose is known. In case of overdose, management would include general supportive care.

5. PHARMACOLOGICAL PROPERTIES

5.1 Pharmacodynamic properties

Pharmacotherapeutic group: Alkyl sulfonates, ATC code: L01AB01.

Busulfan is a potent cytotoxic agent and a bifunctional alkylating agent. In aqueous media, release of the methanesulphonate groups produces carbonium ions which can alkylate DNA, thought to be an important biological mechanism for its cytotoxic effect.

Clinical trials in adults

Documentation of the safety and efficacy of Busilvex in combination with cyclophosphamide in the BuCy2 regimen prior to conventional allogeneic and/or autologous HPCT derive from two clinical trials (OMC-BUS-4 and OMC-BUS-3).

Two prospective, single arm, open-label, uncontrolled phase II studies were conducted in patients with haematological disease, the majority of whom had advanced disease.

Diseases included were acute leukemia past first remission, in first or subsequent relapse, in first remission (high risk), or induction failures; chronic melogenous leukemia in chronic or advanced phase; primary refractory or resistant relapsed Hodgkin's disease or non-Hodgkin's lymphoma, and myelodysplastic syndrome.

Patients received doses of 0.8 mg/kg busulfan every 6 hours infusion for a total 16 doses followed by cyclophosphamide at 60 mg/kg once per day for two days (BuCy2 regimen).

The primary efficacy parameters in these studies were myeloablation, engraftment, relapse, and survival.

In both studies, all patients received a 16/16 dose regimen of Busilvex. No patients were discontinued from treatment due to adverse reactions related to Busilvex.

All patients experienced a profound myelosuppression. The time to Absolute Neutrophil Count (ANC) greater than $0.5x10^9$ /l was 13 days (range 9-29 days) in allogenic patients (OMC-BUS 4), and 10 days (range 8-19 days) in autologous patients (OMC-BUS 3). All evaluable patients engrafted. There is no primary nor secondary graft rejection. Overall mortality and non- relapse mortality at more than 100 days post-transplant was (8/61) 13% and (6/61) 10% in allotransplanted patients, respectively. During the same period there was no death in autologous recipients.

Clinical trials in paediatric patients

Documentation of the safety and efficacy of Busilvex in combination with cyclophosphamide in the BuCy4 or with melphalan in the BuMel regimen prior to conventional allogeneic and/or autologous HPCT derives from clinical trial F60002 IN 101 G0.

The patients received the dosing mentioned in section 4.2.

All patients experienced a profound myelosuppression. The time to Absolute Neutrophil Count (ANC) greater than $0.5x10^9$/l was 21 days (range 12-47 days) in allogenic patients, and 11 days (range 10-15 days) in autologous patients. All children engrafted. There is no primary or secondary graft rejection. 93% of allogeneic patients showed complete chimerism. There was no regimen-related death through the first 100-day post-transplant and up to one year post-transplant.

5.2 Pharmacokinetic properties

The pharmacokinetics of Busilvex has been investigated. The information presented on metabolism and elimination is based on oral busulfan.

Pharmacokinetics in adults

Absorption

The pharmacokinetics of intravenous busulfan was studied in 124 evaluable patients following a 2-hour intravenous infusion for a total of 16 doses over four days. Immediate and complete availability of the dose is obtained after intravenous infusion of busulfan. Similar blood exposure was observed when comparing plasma concentrations in adult patients receiving oral and intravenous busulfan at 1 mg/kg and 0.8 mg/kg respectively. Low inter (CV=21%) and intra (CV=12%) patient variability on busulfan exposure was demonstrated through a population pharmacokinetic analysis, performed on 102 patients.

Distribution

Terminal volume of distribution V_z ranged between 0.62 and 0.85 l/kg.

Busulfan concentrations in the cerebrospinal fluid are comparable to those in plasma although these concentrations are probably insufficient for anti-neoplastic activity.

Reversible binding to plasma proteins was around 7% while irreversible binding, primarily to albumin, was about 32%.

Metabolism

Busulfan is metabolised mainly through conjugation with glutathione (spontaneous and glutathione-S-transferase mediated). The glutathione conjugate is then further metabolised in the liver by oxidation. None of the metabolites is thought to contribute significantly to either efficacy or toxicity.

Elimination

Total clearance in plasma ranged 2.25 - 2.74 ml/minute/kg. The terminal half-life ranged from 2.8 to 3.9 hours.

Approximately 30% of the administered dose is excreted into the urine over 48 hours with 1% as unchanged busulfan. Elimination in faeces is negligible. Irreversible protein binding may explain the incomplete recovery. Contribution of long-lasting metabolites is not excluded.

Pharmacokinetic linearity

The dose proportional increase of busulfan exposure was demonstrated following intravenous busulfan up to 1 mg/kg.

Pharmacokinetic/pharmacodynamic relationships

The literature on busulfan suggests a therapeutic window between 900 and 1500 μMol.minute for AUC. During clinical trials with intravenous busulfan, 90% of patients AUCs were below the upper AUC limit (1500 μMol.minute) and at least 80% were within the targeted therapeutic window (900-1500 μMol.minute).

Special populations

The effects of renal dysfunction on intravenous. busulfan disposition have not been assessed.

The effects of hepatic dysfunction on intravenous busulfan disposition have not been assessed. Nevertheless the risk of liver toxicity may be increased in this population.

No age effect on busulfan clearance was evidenced from available intravenous busulfan data in patients over 60 years.

Table 1

System organ class	Very common	Common	Uncommon
Infections and infestations	Rhinitis Pharyngitis		
Blood and lymphatic system disorders	Neutropenia Thrombocytopenia Febrile neutropenia Anaemia Pancytopenia		
Immune system disorders	Allergic reaction		
Metabolism and nutrition disorders	Anorexia Hyperglycaemia Hypocalcaemia Hypokalaemia Hypomagnesaemia Hypophosphatemia	Hyponatraemia	
Psychiatric disorders	Anxiety Depression Insomnia	Confusion	Delirium Nervousness Hallucination Agitation
Nervous system disorders	Headache Dizziness		Seizure Encephalopathy Cerebral haemorrhage
Cardiac disorders	Tachycardia	Arrhythmia Atrial fibrillation Cardiomegaly Pericardial effusion Pericarditis	Ventricular extrasystoles Bradycardia
Vascular disorders	Hypertension Hypotension Thrombosis Vasodilatation		Femoral artery thrombosis Capillary leak syndrome
Respiratory thoracic and mediastinal disorders	Dyspnoea Epistaxis Cough Hiccup	Hyperventilation Respiratory failure Alveolar haemorrhages Asthma Atelectasis Pleural effusion	Hypoxia
Gastrointestinal disorders	Stomatitis Diarrhoea Abdominal pain Nausea Vomiting Dyspepsia Ascites Constipation Anus discomfort	Haematemesis Ileus Oesophagitis	Gastrointestinal haemorrhage
Hepato-biliary disorders	Hepatomegaly Jaundice		
Skin and subcutaneous tissue disorders	Rash Pruritis Alopecia	Skin desquamation Erythema Pigmentation disorder	
Musculoskeletal and connective tissue disorders	Myalgia Back pain Arthralgia		
Renal and urinary disorders	Dysuria Oliguria	Haematuria Moderate renal insufficiency	
General disorders and administration site conditions	Asthenia Chills Fever Chest pain Oedema Oedema general Pain Pain or inflammation at injection site Mucositis		
Investigations	Transaminases increased Bilirubin increased GGT increased Alkaline phosphatases increased Weight increased Abnormal breath sounds Creatinine elevated	Bun increase Decrease ejection fraction	

Pharmacokinetics in paediatric patients

A continuous variation of clearance ranging from 2.49 to 3.92 ml/minute/kg has been established in children from < 6 months up to 17 years old. The terminal half life ranged from 2.26 to 2.52 h.

The dosing recommended in section 4.2. allows to achieve a similar AUC whatever the children's age, the targeted range of AUCs being the one used for adults. Inter and intra patient variabilities in plasma exposure were lower than 20% and 10%, respectively.

Pharmacokinetic/pharmacodynamic relationships:

The successful engraftment achieved in all patients during phase II trials suggests the appropriateness of the targeted AUCs. Occurrence of VOD was not related to overexposure. PK/PD relationship was observed between stomatitis and AUCs in autologous patients and between bilirubin increase and AUCs in a combined autologous and allogeneic patient analysis.

5.3 Preclinical safety data

Busulfan is mutagenic and clastogenic. Busulfan was mutagenic in *Salmonella typhimurium, Drosophila melanogaster* and barley. Busulfan induced chromosomal aberrations *in vitro* (rodent and human cell) and *in vivo* (rodents and humans). Various chromosome aberrations have been observed in cells from patients receiving oral busulfan.

Busulfan belongs to a class of substances which are potentially carcinogenic based on their mechanism of action. On the basis of human data, busulfan has been classified by the IARC as a human carcinogen. WHO has concluded that there is a causal relationship between busulfan exposure and cancer. The available data in animals support the carcinogenic potential of busulfan. Intravenous administration of busulfan to mice significantly increased the incidences of thymic and ovarian tumours.

Busulfan is teratogen in rats, mice and rabbits. Malformations and anomalies included significant alterations in the musculoskeletal system, body weight gain, and size. In pregnant rats, busulfan produced sterility in both male and female offspring due to the absence of germinal cells in testes and ovaries. Busulfan was shown to cause sterility in rodents. Busulfan depleted oocytes of female rats, and induced sterility in male rats and hamster.

Repeated doses of DMA produced signs of liver toxicity, the first being increases in serum clinical enzymes followed by histopatological changes in the hepatocytes. Higher doses can produce hepatic necrosis and liver damage can be seen following single high exposures.

DMA is teratogenic in rats. Doses of 400 mg/kg/day DMA administered during organogenesis caused significant developmental anomalies. The malformations included serious heart and/or major vessels anomalies: a common truncus arteriosis and no ductus arteriosis, coarctation of the pulmonary trunk and the pulmonary arteries, intraventricular defects of the heart. Other frequent anomalies included cleft palate, anasarca and skeletal anomalies of the vertebrae and ribs. DMA decreases fertility in male and female rodents. A single s.c. dose of 2.2 g/kg administered on gestation day 4 terminated pregnancy in 100% of tested hamster. In rats, a DMA daily dose of 450 mg/kg given to rats for nine days caused inactive spermatogenesis.

6. PHARMACEUTICAL PARTICULARS

6.1 List of excipients

Dimethylacetamide

Macrogol 400.

6.2 Incompatibilities

In the absence of compatibility studies, this medicinal product must not be mixed with other medicinal products except those mentioned in section 6.6.

Do not use polycarbonate syringes with Busilvex.

6.3 Shelf life

Vials: 2 years

Diluted solution

Chemical and physical in-use stability after dilution in glucose 5% or sodium chloride 9 mg/ml (0.9%) solution for injection has been demonstrated for:

- 8 hours (including infusion time) after dilution when stored at 20 °C ± 5 °C

- 12 hours after dilution when stored at 2 °C-8 °C followed by 3 hours stored at 20 °C ± 5 °C (including infusion time).

From a microbiological point of view, the product should be used immediately after dilution. If not used immediately, in-use storage times and conditions prior to use are the responsibility of the user and would normally not be longer than the above mentioned conditions when dilution has taken place in controlled and validated aseptic conditions.

6.4 Special precautions for storage

Store in a refrigerator (2°C- 8°C).

Do not freeze the diluted solution.

For storage conditions of the diluted medicinal product see section 6.3

6.5 Nature and contents of container

10 ml of concentrate for solution for infusion in clear glass vials (type I) with a butyl rubber stopper covered by a purple flip-off aluminium seal cap.

Pack size: 8 vials per box

6.6 Special precautions for disposal and other handling

Preparation of Busilvex

Procedures for proper handling and disposal of anticancer medicinal products should be considered.

All transfer procedures require strict adherence to aseptic techniques, preferably employing a vertical laminar flow safety hood

As with other cytotoxic compounds, caution should be exercised in handling and preparing the Busilvex solution:

- The use of gloves and protective clothing is recommended.

- If Busilvex or diluted Busilvex solution contacts the skin or mucosa, wash them thoroughly with water immediately.

Calculation of the quantity of Busilvex to be diluted and of the diluent

Busilvex must be diluted prior to use with either sodium chloride 9 mg/ml (0.9%) solution for injection or glucose solution for injection 5%.

The quantity of the diluent must be 10 times the volume of Busilvex ensuring the final concentration of busulfan remains at approximately 0.5 mg/ml. By example:

The amount of Busilvex and diluent to be administered would be calculated as follows:

for a patient with a Y kg body weight:

- Quantity of Busilvex:

$$\frac{Y\ (kg) \times D\ (mg/kg)}{6\ (mg/ml)} = A \text{ ml of Busilvex to be diluted}$$

Y: body weight of the patient in kg

D: dose of Busilvex (see section 4.2)

• Quantity of diluent:

(A ml Busilvex) × (10) = B ml of diluent

To prepare the final solution for infusion, add (A) ml of Busilvex to (B) ml of diluent (sodium chloride 9 mg/ml (0.9%) solution for injection or glucose solution for injection 5%)

Preparation of the solution for infusion

• Busilvex must be prepared by a healthcare professional using sterile transfer techniques. Using a non polycarbonate syringe fitted with a needle:

- the calculated volume of Busilvex must be removed from the vial.

- the contents of the syringe must be dispensed into an intravenous bag (or syringe) which already contains the calculated amount of the selected diluent. Busilvex must always be added to the diluent, not the diluent to Busilvex. Busilvex must not be put into an intravenous bag that does not contain sodium chloride 9 mg/ml (0.9%) solution for injection or glucose solution for injection 5%.

• The diluted solution must be mixed thoroughly by inverting several times

After dilution, 1 ml of solution for infusion contains 0.5 mg of busulfan

Diluted Busilvex is a clear colourless solution

Instructions for use

Prior to and following each infusion, flush the indwelling catheter line with approximately 5 ml of sodium chloride 9 mg/ml (0.9%) solution for injection or glucose (5%) solution for injection.

The residual medicinal product must not be flushed in the administration tubing as rapid infusion of Busilvex has not been tested and is not recommended.

The entire prescribed Busilvex dose should be delivered over two hours.

Small volumes may be administered over 2 hours using electric syringes. In this case infusion sets with minimal priming space should be used (i.e 0.3-0.6 ml), primed with medicinal product solution prior to beginning the actual Busilvex infusion and then flushed with sodium chloride 9 mg/ml (0.9%) solution for injection or glucose (5%) solution for injection.

Busilvex must not be infused concomitantly with another intravenous solution.

Polycarbonate syringes must not be used with Busilvex.

For single use only. Only a clear solution without any particles should be used.

Any unused product or waste material should be disposed of in accordance with local requirements for cytotoxic medicinal products.

7. MARKETING AUTHORISATION HOLDER

Pierre Fabre Médicament

45, Place Abel Gance

F-92654 Boulogne Billancourt Cedex

France

8. MARKETING AUTHORISATION NUMBER(S)

EU/1/03/254/002

9. DATE OF FIRST AUTHORISATION/RENEWAL OF THE AUTHORISATION

Date of first authorisation: 09 July, 2003

Date of latest renewal: 09 July 2008

10. DATE OF REVISION OF THE TEXT

09 July 2008

BuTrans 5, 10 and 20ug/h Transdermal Patch

(Napp Pharmaceuticals Limited)

1. NAME OF THE MEDICINAL PRODUCT

BuTrans 5 µg/h, 10 µg/h and 20 µg/h transdermal patch

2. QUALITATIVE AND QUANTITATIVE COMPOSITION

5 µg/h transdermal patch contains:

5 mg buprenorphine.

Area containing active substance: 6.25 cm^2.

Nominal release rate: 5 micrograms of buprenorphine per hour (over a period of 7 days).

10 µg/h transdermal patch contains:

10 mg buprenorphine.

Area containing active substance: 12.5 cm^2.

Nominal release rate: 10 micrograms of buprenorphine per hour (over a period of 7 days).

20 µg/h transdermal patch contains:

20 mg buprenorphine.

Area containing active substance: 25 cm^2.

Nominal release rate: 20 micrograms of buprenorphine per hour (over a period of 7 days).

For a full list of excipients, see section 6.1.

3. PHARMACEUTICAL FORM

Transdermal patch.

Beige coloured patch with rounded corners

Square patch marked ***BuTrans*** 5 µg/h

Rectangular patch marked ***BuTrans***, 10 µg/h

Square patch marked: ***BuTrans*** 20 µg/h

4. CLINICAL PARTICULARS

4.1 Therapeutic indications

Treatment of non-malignant pain of moderate intensity when an opioid is necessary for obtaining adequate analgesia.

BuTrans is not suitable for the treatment of acute pain.

4.2 Posology and method of administration

BuTrans should be administered every 7th day.

Patients aged 18 years and over:

The lowest ***BuTrans*** dose (***BuTrans*** 5 µg/h transdermal patch) should be used as the initial dose. Consideration should be given to the previous opioid history of the patient (see section 4.5) as well as to the current general condition and medical status of the patient.

Titration:

During initiation and titration with ***BuTrans***, patients should use the usual recommended doses of short-acting supplemental analgesics (see section 4.5) as needed until analgesic efficacy with ***BuTrans*** is attained.

The dose should not be increased before 3 days, when the maximum effect of a given dose is established. Subsequent dosage increases may then be titrated based on the need for supplemental pain relief and the patient's analgesic response to the patch.

To increase the dose, a larger patch should replace the patch that is currently being worn, or a combination of patches should be applied in different places to achieve the desired dose. It is recommended that no more than two patches are applied at the same time, regardless of the patch strength. A new patch should not be applied to the same skin site for the subsequent 3-4 weeks (see section 5.2). Patients should be carefully and regularly monitored to assess the optimum dose and duration of treatment.

Conversion from opioids:

BuTrans can be used as an alternative to treatment with other opioids. Such patients should be started on the lowest available dose (***BuTrans*** 5 µg/h transdermal patch) and continue taking short-acting supplemental analgesics (see section 4.5) during titration, as required.

Patients under 18 years of age:

As ***BuTrans*** has not been studied in patients under 18 years of age the use of ***BuTrans*** in patients below this age is not recommended.

Elderly:

No dosage adjustment of ***BuTrans*** is required in elderly patients.

Renal impairment:

No special dose adjustment of ***BuTrans*** is necessary in patients with renal impairment.

Hepatic impairment:

Buprenorphine is metabolised in the liver. The intensity and duration of its action may be affected in patients with impaired liver function. Therefore patients with hepatic insufficiency should be carefully monitored during treatment with ***BuTrans***.

Patients with severe hepatic impairment may accumulate buprenorphine during ***BuTrans*** treatment. Consideration of alternate therapy should be considered, and ***BuTrans*** should be used with caution, if at all, in such patients.

Patch application:

BuTrans should be applied to non-irritated, intact skin of the upper outer arm, upper chest, upper back or the side of the chest, but not to any parts of the skin with large scars. ***BuTrans*** should be applied to a relatively hairless or nearly hairless skin site. If none are available, the hair at the site should be cut with scissors, not shaven.

If the application site must be cleaned, it should be done with clean water only. Soaps, alcohol, oils, lotions or abrasive devices must not be used. The skin must be dry before the patch is applied. ***BuTrans*** should be applied immediately after removal from the sealed sachet. Following removal of the protective layer, the transdermal patch should be pressed firmly in place with the palm of the hand for approximately 30 seconds, making sure the contact is complete, especially around the edges. If the edges of the patch begin to peel off, the edges may be taped down with suitable skin tape.

The patch should be worn continuously for 7 days.

Bathing, showering, or swimming should not affect the patch. If a patch falls off, a new one should be applied.

Duration of administration:

BuTrans should under no circumstances be administered for longer than absolutely necessary. If long-term pain treatment with ***BuTrans*** is necessary in view of the nature and severity of the illness, then careful and regular monitoring should be carried out (if necessary with breaks in treatment) to establish whether and to what extent further treatment is necessary.

Discontinuation:

After removal of the patch, buprenorphine serum concentrations decrease gradually and thus the analgesic effect is maintained for a certain amount of time. This should be considered when therapy with ***BuTrans*** is to be followed by other opioids. As a general rule, a subsequent opioid should not be administered within 24 hours after removal of the patch. At present, only limited information is available on the starting dose of other opioids administered after discontinuation of the transdermal patch (see section 4.5).

Patients with fever or exposed to external heat:

While wearing the patch, patients should be advised to avoid exposing the application site to external heat sources, such as heating pads, electric blankets, heat lamps, sauna, hot tubs, and heated water beds, etc., as an increase in absorption of buprenorphine may occur. When treating febrile patients, one should be aware that fever may also increase absorption resulting in increased plasma concentrations of buprenorphine and thereby increased risk of opioid reactions.

4.3 Contraindications

BuTrans is contra-indicated in:

- patients with known hypersensitivity to the active substance buprenorphine or to any of the excipients (see section 6.1)

- opioid dependent patients and for narcotic withdrawal treatment

- conditions in which the respiratory centre and function are severely impaired or may become so

- patients who are receiving MAO inhibitors or have taken them within the last two weeks (see section 4.5)

- patients suffering from myasthenia gravis

- patients suffering from delirium tremens.

4.4 Special warnings and precautions for use

BuTrans should be used with particular caution in patients with convulsive disorders, head injury, shock, a reduced level of consciousness of uncertain origin, intracranial lesions or increased intracranial pressure, or in patients with severe hepatic impairment (see section 4.2).

Significant respiratory depression has been associated with buprenorphine, particularly by the intravenous route. A number of overdose deaths have occurred when addicts have intravenously abused buprenorphine, usually with benzodiazepines concomitantly. Additional overdose deaths due to ethanol and benzodiazepines in combination with buprenorphine have been reported.

BuTrans is not recommended for analgesia in the immediate post-operative period or in other situations characterised by a narrow therapeutic index or a rapidly varying analgesic requirement.

Controlled human and animal studies indicate that buprenorphine has a lower dependence liability than pure agonist analgesics. In humans limited euphorigenic effects have been observed with buprenorphine. This may result in some abuse of the product and caution should be exercised when prescribing to patients known to have, or suspected of having, a history of drug abuse.

As with all opioids, chronic use of buprenorphine can result in the development of physical dependence. Withdrawal (abstinence syndrome), when it occurs, is generally mild, begins after 2 days and may last up to 2 weeks. Withdrawal symptoms include agitation, anxiety, nervousness, insomnia, hyperkinesia, tremor and gastrointestinal disorders.

4.5 Interaction with other medicinal products and other forms of interaction

BuTrans must not be used concomitantly with MAOIs or in patients who have received MAOIs within the previous two weeks (see section 4.3).

Effect of other active substances on the pharmacokinetics of buprenorphine:

Buprenorphine is primarily metabolised by glucuronidation and to a lesser extent (about 30%) by CYP3A4. Concomitant treatment with CYP3A4 inhibitors may lead to elevated plasma concentrations with intensified efficacy of buprenorphine.

A drug interaction study with the CYP3A4 inhibitor ketoconazole did not produce clinically relevant increases in mean maximum (Cmax) or total (AUC) buprenorphine exposure following ***BuTrans*** with ketoconazole as compared to ***BuTrans*** alone.

The interaction between buprenorphine and CYP3A4 enzyme inducers has not been studied.

Co-administration of ***BuTrans*** and enzyme inducers (e.g. phenobarbital, carbamazepine, phenytoin and rifampicin) could lead to increased clearance which might result in reduced efficacy.

Reductions in hepatic blood flow induced by some general anaesthetics (e.g. halothane) and other medicinal products may result in a decreased rate of hepatic elimination of buprenorphine.

Pharmacodynamic interactions:

BuTrans should be used cautiously with:

Benzodiazepines: This combination can potentiate respiratory depression of central origin, with risk of death (see section 4.4).

Other central nervous system depressants: other opioid derivatives (analgesics and antitussives containing e.g. morphine, dextropropoxyphene, codeine, dextromethorphan or noscapine). Certain antidepressants, sedative

H1-receptor antagonists, alcohol, anxiolytics, neuroleptics, clonidine and related substances. These combinations increase the CNS depressant activity.

Buprenorphine is a partial mu-receptor agonist but it is described to function as a pure mu receptor agonist at typical analgesic doses. These doses produce buprenorphine exposures comparable to or greater than those produced by ***BuTrans*** 5, 10, and 20 μg/h transdermal patches. In ***BuTrans*** clinical studies, where subjects receiving full mu agonist opioids (up to 90 mg oral morphine or oral morphine equivalents per day) were transferred to ***BuTrans***, there were no reports of abstinence syndrome or opioid withdrawal during conversion from entry opioid to ***BuTrans*** (see section 4.4).

4.6 Pregnancy and lactation

Pregnancy

There are no data from the use of ***BuTrans*** in pregnant women. Studies in animals have shown reproductive toxicity (see Section 5.3). The potential risk for humans is unknown.

Towards the end of pregnancy high doses of buprenorphine may induce respiratory depression in the neonate even after a short period of administration. Long-term administration of buprenorphine during the last three months of pregnancy may cause a withdrawal syndrome in the neonate.

Therefore ***BuTrans*** should not be used during pregnancy and in women of childbearing potential who are not using effective contraception.

Lactation

Studies in rats have shown that buprenorphine may inhibit lactation. Excretion of buprenorphine into the milk in rats has been observed. Data on excretion into human milk are not available. Therefore the use of ***BuTrans*** during lactation should be avoided.

4.7 Effects on ability to drive and use machines

BuTrans has a major influence on the ability to drive and use machines. Even when used according to instructions, ***BuTrans*** may affect the patient's reactions to such an extent that road safety and the ability to operate machinery may be impaired. This applies particularly in the beginning of treatment and in conjunction with other centrally acting substances including alcohol, tranquillisers, sedatives and hypnotics. An individual recommendation should be given by the physician. A general restriction is not necessary in cases where a stable dose is used.

In patients who are affected, such as during treatment initiation or titration to a higher dose, these patients should not drive or use machines, nor for at least 24 hours after the patch has been removed.

4.8 Undesirable effects

Serious adverse reactions that may be associated with ***BuTrans*** therapy in clinical use are similar to those observed with other opioid analgesics, including respiratory depression (especially when used with other CNS depressants) and hypotension (see section 4.4).

The following undesirable effects have occurred:

Very common (≥1/10), common (≥1/100, <1/10), uncommon (≥1/1000, <1/100), rare (≥1/10,000, <1/1000), very rare (<1/10,000), not known (cannot be estimated from the available data).

Immune system disorders

Uncommon	hypersensitivity
Very rare:	anaphylactic reaction, anaphylactoid reaction

Metabolism and nutrition disorders

Common:	anorexia
Uncommon:	dehydration

Psychiatric disorders

Common:	confusion, depression, insomnia, nervousness,
Uncommon:	sleep disorder, restlessness, agitation, depersonalisation, euphoric mood, affect lability, anxiety, hallucinations, nightmares
Rare:	psychotic disorder, decreased libido
Very rare:	drug dependence, mood swings

Nervous system disorders

Very common:	headache, dizziness, somnolence
Common:	paraesthesia
Uncommon:	sedation, dysgeusia, dysarthria, hypoaesthesia, memory impairment, migraine, syncope, tremor, abnormal co-ordination, disturbance in attention
Rare:	balance disorder, speech disorder,
Very rare:	involuntary muscle contractions

Eye disorders

Uncommon:	dry eye, blurred vision
Rare:	visual disturbance, eyelid oedema, miosis

Ear and labyrinth disorders

Uncommon:	tinnitus, vertigo
Very rare:	ear pain

Cardiac/disorders

Uncommon:	angina pectoris, palpitations, tachycardia,

Vascular disorders

Common:	vasodilatation
Uncommon:	hypotension, circulatory collapse, hypertension, flushing

Respiratory, thoracic and mediastinal disorders

Common:	dyspnoea
Uncommon:	asthma aggravated, cough, hypoxia, rhinitis, wheezing, hyperventilation, hiccups
Rare:	respiratory depression, respiratory failure

Gastrointestinal disorders

Very common:	constipation, dry mouth, nausea, vomiting
Common:	abdominal pain, diarrhoea, dyspepsia
Uncommon:	flatulence
Rare:	diverticulitis, dysphagia, ileus

Hepatobiliary disorders

Rare:	biliary colic

Skin and subcutaneous tissue disorders

Very common:	pruritus, erythema
Common:	rash, sweating, exanthema
Uncommon:	dry skin, face oedema, urticaria
Very rare:	pustules, vesicles

Musculoskeletal and connective tissue disorders

Uncommon:	muscle cramp, myalgia, muscular weakness, muscle spasms

Renal and urinary disorders

Uncommon:	urinary retention, micturition disorder

Reproductive system and breast disorders

Rare:	erectile dysfunction, sexual dysfunction

General disorders and administration site conditions

Very common:	application site pruritus, application site reaction
Common:	tiredness, asthenia, pain, peripheral oedema, application site erythema, application site rash, chest pain
Uncommon:	fatigue, influenza like illness, pyrexia, rigors, malaise, oedema, drug withdrawal syndrome
Rare:	application site inflammation*

Investigations

Uncommon:	alanine aminotransferase increased, weight decreased

Injury, poisoning and procedural complications

Uncommon:	accidental injury, fall

* In some cases delayed local allergic reactions occurred with marked signs of inflammation. In such cases treatment with ***BuTrans*** should be terminated.

Buprenorphine has a low risk of physical dependence. After discontinuation of ***BuTrans***, withdrawal symptoms are unlikely. This may be due to the very slow dissociation of buprenorphine from the opioid receptors and to the gradual decrease of buprenorphine plasma concentrations (usually over a period of 30 hours after removal of the last patch). However, after long-term use of ***BuTrans***, withdrawal symptoms similar to those occurring during opioid withdrawal, cannot be entirely excluded. These symptoms include agitation, anxiety, nervousness, insomnia, hyperkinesia, tremor and gastrointestinal disorders.

4.9 Overdose

Symptoms: Symptoms similar to those of other centrally acting analgesics are to be expected. These include respiratory depression, sedation, drowsiness, nausea, vomiting, cardiovascular collapse and marked miosis.

Treatment: Remove any patches from the patient's skin. Establish and maintain a patent airway, assist or control respiration as indicated and maintain adequate body temperature and fluid balance. Oxygen, intravenous fluids, vasopressors and other supportive measures should be employed as indicated.

A specific opioid antagonist such as naloxone may reverse the effects of buprenorphine. The dose of naloxone may be in the range 5 to 12 mg intravenously. The onset of the naloxone effect may be delayed by 30 minutes or more. Maintenance of adequate ventilation is more important than treatment with naloxone.

5. PHARMACOLOGICAL PROPERTIES

5.1 Pharmacodynamic properties

Pharmacotherapeutic group: Analgesics, opioids; ATC code: N02 AE01

Buprenorphine is a partial agonist opioid, acting at the mu opioid receptor. It also has antagonistic activity at the kappa opioid receptor.

Efficacy has been demonstrated in five pivotal phase III studies of up to 12 weeks duration in patients with non-malignant pain of various aetiologies. These included patients with moderate and severe OA and back pain. ***BuTrans*** demonstrated clinically significant reductions in pain scores (approximately 3 points on the BS-11 scale) and significantly greater pain control compared with placebo.

A long term, open-label extension study (n=384) has also been performed in patients with non-malignant pain. With chronic dosing, 63% of patients were maintained in pain control for 6 months, 39% of patients for 12 months, 13% of patients for 18 months and 6% for 21 months. Approximately 17% were stabilised on the 5 mg dose, 35% on the 10 mg dose and 48% on the 20 mg dose.

5.2 Pharmacokinetic properties

There is evidence of enterohepatic recirculation.

Studies in non-pregnant and pregnant rats have shown that buprenorphine passes the blood-brain and placental barriers. Concentrations in the brain (which contained only unchanged buprenorphine) after parenteral administration were 2-3 times higher than after oral administration. After intramuscular or oral administration buprenorphine apparently accumulates in the foetal gastrointestinal lumen – presumably due to biliary excretion, as enterohepatic circulation has not fully developed.

Each patch provides a steady delivery of buprenorphine for up to seven days. Steady state is achieved during the first application. After removal of ***BuTrans***, buprenorphine concentrations decline, decreasing approximately 50% in 12 hours (range 10–24 h).

Absorption:

Following ***BuTrans*** application, buprenorphine diffuses from the patch through the skin. In clinical pharmacology studies, the median time for "***BuTrans*** 10 μg/h" to deliver detectable buprenorphine concentrations (25 picograms/ml) was approximately 17 hours. Analysis of residual buprenorphine in patches after 7-day use shows 15% of the original load delivered. A study of bioavailability, relative to intravenous administration, confirms that this amount is systemically absorbed. Buprenorphine concentrations remain relatively constant during the 7-day patch application.

Application site:

A study in healthy subjects demonstrated that the pharmacokinetic profile of buprenorphine delivered by ***BuTrans*** is similar when applied to upper outer arm, upper chest, upper back or the side of the chest (midaxillary line, 5th intercostal space). The absorption varies to some extent depending on the application site and the exposure is at the most approximately 26 % higher when applied to the upper back compared to the side of the chest.

In a study of healthy subjects receiving ***BuTrans*** repeatedly to the same site, an almost doubled exposure was seen with a 14 day rest period. For this reason, rotation of application sites is recommended, and a new patch should not be applied to the same skin site for 3-4 weeks.

In a study of healthy subjects, application of a heating pad directly on the transdermal patch caused a transient 26 - 55% increase in blood concentrations of buprenorphine. Concentrations returned to normal within 5 hours after the heat was removed. For this reason, applying direct heat sources such as hot water bottles, heat pads or electric blankets directly to the patch is not recommended. A heating pad applied to a ***BuTrans*** site immediately after patch removal did not alter absorption from the skin depot.

Distribution:

Buprenorphine is approximately 96% bound to plasma proteins.

Studies of intravenous buprenorphine have shown a large volume of distribution, implying extensive distribution of buprenorphine. In a study of intravenous buprenorphine in healthy subjects, the volume of distribution at steady state was 430 l, reflecting the large volume of distribution and lipophilicity of the active substance.

Following intravenous administration, buprenorphine and its metabolites are secreted into bile, and within several minutes, distributed into the cerebrospinal fluid. Buprenorphine concentrations in the cerebrospinal fluid appear to be approximately 15% to 25% of concurrent plasma concentrations.

Biotransformation and elimination:

Buprenorphine metabolism in the skin following ***BuTrans*** application is negligible. Following transdermal application, buprenorphine is eliminated via hepatic metabolism, with subsequent biliary excretion and renal excretion of soluble metabolites. Hepatic metabolism, through CYP3A4 and UGT1A1/1A3 enzymes, results in two primary metabolites, norbuprenorphine and buprenorphine 3-O-glucuronide, respectively. Norbuprenorphine is glucuronidated before elimination. Buprenorphine is also eliminated in the faeces. In a study in post-operative patients, the total elimination of buprenorphine was shown to be approximately 55l/h.

Norbuprenorphine is the only known active metabolite of buprenorphine.

Effect of buprenorphine on the pharmacokinetics of other active substances:

Based on *in vitro* studies in human microsomes and hepatocytes, buprenorphine does not have the potential to inhibit metabolism catalysed by the CYP450 enzymes CYP1A2, CYP2A6 and CYP3A4 at concentrations obtained with use of ***BuTrans*** 20μg/h transdermal patch.

The effect on metabolism catalysed by CYP2C8, CYP2C9 and CYP2C19 has not been studied.

5.3 Preclinical safety data

In single- and repeat-dose toxicity studies in rats, rabbits, guinea pigs, dogs and minipigs, ***BuTrans*** caused minimal or no adverse systemic events, whereas skin irritation was observed in all species examined. No teratogenic effects were observed in rats or rabbits. However, perinatal mortality was reported in the literature for rats treated with buprenorphine.

A standard battery of genotoxicity tests indicated that buprenorphine is non-genotoxic.

In long-term studies in rats and mice there was no evidence of any carcinogenic potential relevant for humans.

Toxicological data available did not indicate a sensitising potential of the additives of the transdermal patches.

6. PHARMACEUTICAL PARTICULARS

6.1 List of excipients

Adhesive matrix (containing buprenorphine):

[(Z)-octadec-9-en-1-yl] (Oleyl oleate),

Povidone K90,

4-oxopentanic acid, (Levulinic Acid)

Poly[acrylic acid-co-butylacrylate-co-(2-ethylhexyl)acrylate-co-vinylacetate] (5:15:75:5), cross-linked (DuroTak 387-2054)

Adhesive matrix (without buprenorphine):

Poly[acrylic acid-co-butylacrylate-co-(2-ethylhexyl) acrylate-co-vinylacetate] (5:15:75:5), not cross-linked (DuroTak 387-2051).

Separating foil between the adhesive matrices with and without buprenorphine: Poly(Ethyleneterephthalate) – foil.

Backing layer:

Poly(Ethyleneterephthalate) – tissue.

Release liner (on the front covering the adhesive matrix containing buprenorphine) (to be removed before applying the patch):

Poly(Ethyleneterephthalate) – foil, siliconised, coated on one side with aluminium.

6.2 Incompatibilities

Not applicable

6.3 Shelf life

2 years

6.4 Special precautions for storage

Do not store above 25°C.

6.5 Nature and contents of container

Sealed sachet, composed of identical top and bottom layers of heat-sealable laminate, comprising (from outside to inside) paper, LDPE, aluminium and poly(acrylic acid-co-ethylene).

Pack Sizes:

BuTrans 5 μg/h: 2 transdermal patches

BuTrans 10 μg/h and 20 μg/h: 4 transdermal patches

Not all pack sizes may be marketed.

6.6 Special precautions for disposal and other handling

The patch should not be used if the seal is broken.

Disposal after use:

When changing the patch, the used patch should be removed, the adhesive layer folded inwards on itself, and the patch disposed of safely and out of sight and reach of children.

7. MARKETING AUTHORISATION HOLDER

Napp Pharmaceuticals Limited

Cambridge Science Park

Milton Road

Cambridge

CB4 0GW

UK

8. MARKETING AUTHORISATION NUMBER(S)

PL 16950/0136-0138

9. DATE OF FIRST AUTHORISATION/RENEWAL OF THE AUTHORISATION

Date of first authorisation 10th June 2005

Date of last renewal 27th November 2008

10. DATE OF REVISION OF THE TEXT

November 2008

Byetta 5 micrograms solution for injection, prefilled pen. Byetta 10 micrograms solution for injection, prefilled pen.

(Eli Lilly and Company Limited)

1. NAME OF THE MEDICINAL PRODUCT

BYETTA*▼ 5 micrograms solution for injection, pre-filled pen.

BYETTA 10 micrograms solution for injection, pre-filled pen.

2. QUALITATIVE AND QUANTITATIVE COMPOSITION

Each dose contains 5 micrograms (μg) synthetic exenatide in 20 microlitres (μl), (0.25mg exenatide per ml).

Excipients: Each dose contains 44μg metacresol.

Each dose contains 10 micrograms (μg) synthetic exenatide in 40 microlitres (μl), (0.25mg exenatide per ml).

Excipients: Each dose contains 88μg metacresol.

This medicinal product contains less than 1mmol sodium per dose, i.e., essentially 'sodium-free'.

For a full list of excipients, see section 6.1.

3. PHARMACEUTICAL FORM

Solution for injection, pre-filled pen.

Clear, colourless solution.

4. CLINICAL PARTICULARS

4.1 Therapeutic indications

BYETTA is indicated for treatment of Type 2 diabetes mellitus in combination with metformin and/or sulphonylureas in patients who have not achieved adequate glycaemic control on maximally tolerated doses of these oral therapies.

4.2 Posology and method of administration

BYETTA therapy should be initiated at 5μg exenatide per dose, administered twice daily (BID), for at least one month in order to improve tolerability. The dose of exenatide can then be increased to 10μg BID to further improve glycaemic control. Doses higher than 10μg BID are not recommended.

BYETTA is available as either a 5μg or a 10μg exenatide per dose pre-filled pen.

BYETTA can be administered at any time within the 60-minute period before the morning and evening meal (or two main meals of the day, approximately 6 hours or more apart). BYETTA **should not** be administered after a meal. If an injection is missed, the treatment should be continued with the next scheduled dose.

Each dose should be administered as a subcutaneous injection in the thigh, abdomen, or upper arm.

BYETTA is recommended for use in patients with Type 2 diabetes mellitus who are already receiving metformin and/or a sulphonylurea. When BYETTA is added to existing metformin therapy, the current dose of metformin can be continued, as no increased risk of hypoglycaemia is anticipated compared to metformin alone. When BYETTA is added to sulphonylurea therapy, a reduction in the dose of sulphonylurea should be considered to reduce the risk of hypoglycaemia (see section 4.4).

The dose of BYETTA does not need to be adjusted on a day-by-day basis depending on self-monitored glycaemia. However, blood glucose self-monitoring may become necessary to adjust the dose of sulphonylureas.

Limited experience exists concerning the combination of BYETTA with thiazolidinediones (see section 5.1).

Specific Patient Groups

Elderly: BYETTA should be used with caution and dose escalation from 5μg to 10μg should proceed conservatively in patients >70 years. The clinical experience in patients >75 years is very limited.

Patients with renal impairment: No dosage adjustment of BYETTA is necessary in patients with mild renal impairment (creatinine clearance 50-80ml/min).

In patients with moderate renal impairment (creatinine clearance 30-50ml/min), dose escalation from 5μg to 10μg should proceed conservatively (see section 5.2).

BYETTA is not recommended for use in patients with end-stage renal disease or severe renal impairment (creatinine clearance <30ml/min) (see section 4.4).

Patients with hepatic impairment: No dosage adjustment of BYETTA is necessary in patients with hepatic impairment (see section 5.2).

Children and adolescents: The safety and effectiveness of exenatide have not been established in patients under 18 years of age (see section 5.2).

4.3 Contraindications

Hypersensitivity to the active substance or to any of the excipients.

4.4 Special warnings and precautions for use

BYETTA should not be used in patients with Type 1 diabetes mellitus or for the treatment of diabetic ketoacidosis.

BYETTA should not be used in Type 2 diabetes patients who require insulin therapy due to beta-cell failure.

Intravenous or intramuscular injection of BYETTA is not recommended.

In patients with end-stage renal disease receiving dialysis, single doses of BYETTA 5μg increased frequency and severity of undesirable gastrointestinal effects. BYETTA is not recommended for use in patients with end-stage renal disease or severe renal impairment (creatinine clearance <30ml/min). The clinical experience in patients with moderate renal impairment is very limited.

There have been rare, spontaneously reported events of altered renal function, including increased serum creatinine, renal impairment, worsened chronic renal failure and acute renal failure, sometimes requiring haemodialysis. Some of these events occurred in patients experiencing events that may affect hydration, including nausea, vomiting, and/or diarrhoea, and/or receiving pharmacological agents known to affect renal function/hydration status. Concomitant agents included angiotensin converting enzymes inhibitors, angiotensin-II antagonists, nonsteroidal anti-inflammatory medicinal products and diuretics. Reversibility of altered renal function has been observed with supportive treatment and discontinuation of potentially causative agents, including BYETTA.

BYETTA has not been studied in patients with severe gastrointestinal disease, including gastroparesis. Its use is commonly associated with gastrointestinal adverse reactions, including nausea, vomiting, and diarrhoea. Therefore, the use of BYETTA is not recommended in patients with severe gastrointestinal disease.

There have been rare, spontaneously reported events of acute pancreatitis. Patients should be informed of the characteristic symptom of acute pancreatitis: persistent, severe abdominal pain. Resolution of pancreatitis has been observed with supportive treatment, but very rare cases of necrotizing or haemorrhagic pancreatitis and/or death have been reported. If pancreatitis is suspected, BYETTA and other potentially suspect medicinal products should be discontinued. Treatment with BYETTA should not be resumed after pancreatitis has been diagnosed.

The concurrent use of BYETTA with insulin, D-phenylalanine derivatives (meglitinides), or alpha-glucosidase inhibitors has not been studied and cannot be recommended.

The experience in patients with BMI ≤25 is limited.

This medicinal product contains metacresol, which may cause allergic reactions.

Hypoglycaemia

When BYETTA was used in combination with a sulphonylurea, the incidence of hypoglycaemia was increased over that of placebo in combination with a sulphonylurea. In the clinical studies, patients on a sulphonylurea combination, with mild renal impairment, had an increased incidence of hypoglycaemia compared to patients with normal renal function. To reduce the risk of hypoglycaemia associated with the use of a sulphonylurea, reduction in the dose of sulphonylurea should be considered.

Interactions

The effect of BYETTA to slow gastric emptying may reduce the extent and rate of absorption of orally administered medicinal products. BYETTA should be used with caution in patients receiving oral medicinal products that require rapid gastrointestinal absorption and medicinal products with a narrow therapeutic ratio. Specific recommendations regarding intake of such medicinal products in relation to BYETTA is given in section 4.5.

4.5 Interaction with other medicinal products and other forms of interaction

The effect of BYETTA to slow gastric emptying may reduce the extent and rate of absorption of orally administered medicinal products. Patients receiving medicinal products of either a narrow therapeutic ratio or medicinal products that require careful clinical monitoring should be followed closely. These medicinal products should be taken in a standardised way in relation to BYETTA injection. If such medicinal products are to be administered with food, patients should be advised to, if possible, take them with a meal when BYETTA is not administered.

For oral medicinal products that are particularly dependent on threshold concentrations for efficacy, such as antibiotics, patients should be advised to take those medicinal products at least 1 hour before BYETTA injection.

BYETTA is not expected to have any clinically relevant effects on the pharmacokinetics of metformin or sulphonylureas. Hence, no restriction in timing of intake of these medicinal products in relation to BYETTA injection are needed.

Gastro-resistant formulations containing substances sensitive for degradation in the stomach, such as proton pump inhibitors, should be taken at least 1 hour before or more than 4 hours after BYETTA injection.

Paracetamol

Paracetamol was used as a model medicinal product to evaluate the effect of exenatide on gastric emptying. When 1,000mg paracetamol was given with 10μg BYETTA (0 h) and 1 h, 2 h, and 4 h after BYETTA injection, paracetamol AUCs were decreased by 21%, 23%, 24%, and 14%, respectively; C_{max} was decreased by 37%, 56%, 54%, and 41%, respectively; T_{max} was increased from 0.6 h in the control period to 0.9 h, 4.2 h, 3.3 h, and 1.6 h, respectively. Paracetamol AUC, C_{max}, and T_{max} were not significantly changed when paracetamol was given 1 hour before BYETTA injection. No adjustment to paracetamol dosing is required based on these study results.

HMG CoA Reductase Inhibitors

Lovastatin AUC and C_{max} were decreased approximately 40% and 28%, respectively, and T_{max} was delayed about 4 h when BYETTA (10μg BID) was administered concomitantly with a single dose of lovastatin (40mg) compared with lovastatin administered alone. In the 30-week placebo-controlled clinical trials, concomitant use of BYETTA and HMG CoA reductase inhibitors was not associated with consistent changes in lipid profiles (see section 5.1). Although no predetermined dose adjustment is required, one should be aware of possible changes in LDL-C or total cholesterol. Lipid profiles should be monitored regularly.

Digoxin, Lisinopril and Warfarin

A delay in T_{max} of about 2 h was observed when digoxin, lisinopril, or warfarin was administered 30 minutes after exenatide. No clinically relevant effects on C_{max} or AUC were observed. However, since market introduction, increased INR has been reported during concomitant use of warfarin and BYETTA. INR should be closely monitored during initiation and dose increase of BYETTA therapy in patients on warfarin and/or cumarol derivatives (see section 4.8).

Ethinyl Oestradiol and Levonorgestrel

Administration of a combination oral contraceptive (30μg ethinyl oestradiol plus 150μg levonorgestrel) one hour before BYETTA (10 μg BID) did not alter the AUC, C_{max} or C_{min} of either ethinyl oestradiol or levonorgestrel. Administration of the oral contraceptive 30 minutes after BYETTA did not affect AUC but resulted in a reduction of the C_{max} of ethinyl oestradiol by 45%, and C_{max} of levonorgestrel by 27-41%, and a delay in T_{max} by 2-4 h due to delayed gastric emptying. The reduction in C_{max} is of limited clinical relevance and no adjustment of dosing of oral contraceptives is required.

4.6 Pregnancy and lactation

There are no adequate data from the use of BYETTA in pregnant women. Studies in animals have shown reproductive toxicity (see section 5.3). The potential risk for humans is unknown. BYETTA should not be used during pregnancy, and the use of insulin is recommended. If a patient wishes to become pregnant, or pregnancy occurs, treatment with BYETTA should be discontinued.

It is unknown whether exenatide is excreted in human milk. BYETTA should not be used if breast-feeding.

4.7 Effects on ability to drive and use machines

No studies on the effects on the ability to drive and use machines have been performed. When BYETTA is used in combination with a sulphonylurea, patients should be advised to take precautions to avoid hypoglycaemia while driving and using machines.

4.8 Undesirable effects

Table 1 lists adverse reactions reported from Phase 3 studies. The table presents adverse reactions that occurred with an incidence ≥5% and more frequently among BYETTA-treated patients than insulin- or placebo-treated patients. The table also includes adverse reactions that occurred with an incidence ≥1% and with a statistically significantly higher and/or ≥2X incidence among BYETTA-treated patients than insulin- or placebo-treated patients.

The reactions are listed below as MedDRA preferred term by system organ class and absolute frequency. Patient frequencies are defined as: very common (≥1/10), common (≥1/100, <1/10) and uncommon (≥1/1,000 to <1/100).

Table 1 **Adverse Reactions Reported in Long-Term Phase 3 Controlled Studies**

(see Table 1 below)

Hypoglycaemia

In studies in patients treated with BYETTA and a sulphonylurea (with or without metformin), the incidence of hypoglycaemia was increased compared to placebo (23.5% and 25.2% versus 12.6% and 3.3%) and appeared to be dependent on the doses of both BYETTA and the sulphonylurea. Most episodes of hypoglycaemia were mild to moderate in intensity, and all resolved with oral administration of carbohydrate.

Nausea

The most frequently reported adverse reaction was nausea. In patients treated with 5μg or 10μg BYETTA, generally 40-50% reported at least one episode of nausea. Most episodes of nausea were mild to moderate and occurred in a dose-dependent fashion. With continued therapy, the frequency and severity decreased in most patients who initially experienced nausea.

The incidence of withdrawal due to adverse events was 8% for BYETTA-treated patients, 3% for placebo-treated and 1% for insulin-treated patients in the long-term controlled trials (16 weeks or longer). The most common adverse events leading to withdrawal for BYETTA-treated patients were nausea (4% of patients) and vomiting (1%). For placebo-treated or insulin-treated patients, <1% withdrew due to nausea or vomiting.

BYETTA-treated patients in the open-label extension studies at 82 weeks experienced similar types of adverse events observed in the controlled trials.

Injection Site Reactions

Injection site reactions have been reported in approximately 5.1% of subjects receiving BYETTA in long-term (16 weeks or longer) controlled trials. These reactions have usually been mild and usually did not result in discontinuation of BYETTA.

Immunogenicity

Consistent with the potentially immunogenic properties of protein and peptide pharmaceuticals, patients may develop anti-exenatide antibodies following treatment with BYETTA. In most patients who develop antibodies, antibody titres diminish over time and remain low through 82 weeks.

Overall, the percentage of antibody positive patients was consistent across clinical trials. Patients who developed anti-exenatide antibodies had similar rates and types of adverse events as those with no anti-exenatide antibodies. In the three placebo-controlled trials (n = 963), 38% of patients had low titre anti-exenatide antibodies at 30 weeks. For this group, the level of glycaemic control (HbA_{1c}) was generally comparable to that observed in those without antibody titres. An additional 6% of patients had higher titre antibodies at 30 weeks. About half of this 6% (3% of the total patients given BYETTA in the controlled studies) had no apparent glycaemic response to BYETTA. In two insulin-comparator controlled trials (n = 475), comparable efficacy and adverse events were observed in BYETTA-treated patients regardless of antibody titre.

Examination of antibody-positive specimens from one long-term uncontrolled study revealed no significant cross-reactivity with similar endogenous peptides (glucagon or GLP-1).

Spontaneous Reports

Since market introduction of BYETTA, the following additional adverse reactions have been reported:

Immune system disorders: Anaphylactic reaction, very rarely.

Metabolism and nutritional disorders: Dehydration, generally associated with nausea, vomiting and/or diarrhoea.

Nervous system disorders: Dysgeusia, somnolence.

Gastrointestinal disorders: Eructation, constipation, flatulence.

Renal and urinary disorders: Altered renal function, including acute renal failure, worsened chronic renal failure, renal impairment, increased serum creatinine (see section 4.4).

Skin and subcutaneous tissue disorders: Macular rash, papular rash, pruritus, urticaria, angioneurotic oedema.

Investigations: International normalised ratio increased with concomitant warfarin, some reports associated with bleeding (see section 4.5).

4.9 Overdose

Signs and symptoms of overdose may include severe nausea, severe vomiting and rapidly declining blood glucose concentrations. In the event of overdose, appropriate supportive treatment (possibly given parenterally) should be initiated according to the patient's clinical signs and symptoms.

5. PHARMACOLOGICAL PROPERTIES

5.1 Pharmacodynamic properties

Pharmacotherapeutic group: Other blood glucose lowering drugs, excl. insulins. *ATC code:* A10BX04.

Mechanism of Action

Exenatide is an incretin mimetic that exhibits several antihyperglycaemic actions of glucagon-like peptide-1 (GLP-1). The amino acid sequence of exenatide partially overlaps that of human GLP-1. Exenatide has been shown to bind to and activate the known human GLP-1 receptor *in vitro*, its mechanism of action mediated by cyclic AMP and/or other intracellular signalling pathways.

Exenatide increases, on a glucose-dependent basis, the secretion of insulin from pancreatic beta cells. As blood glucose concentrations decrease, insulin secretion subsides. When exenatide was used in combination with metformin alone, no increase in the incidence of hypoglycaemia was observed over that of placebo in combination with metformin, which may be due to this glucose-dependent insulinotropic mechanism (see section 4.4).

Exenatide suppresses glucagon secretion which is known to be inappropriately elevated in Type 2 diabetes. Lower glucagon concentrations lead to decreased hepatic glucose output. However, exenatide does not impair the normal glucagon response and other hormone responses to hypoglycaemia.

Exenatide slows gastric emptying, thereby reducing the rate at which meal-derived glucose appears in the circulation.

Pharmacodynamic Effects

BYETTA improves glycaemic control through the immediate and sustained effects of lowering both postprandial and fasting glucose concentrations in patients with Type 2 diabetes.

Clinical Efficacy

The clinical studies comprised 3,945 subjects (2,997 treated with exenatide), 56% men and 44% women; 319 subjects (230 treated with exenatide) were ≥70 years of age and 34 subjects (27 treated with exenatide) were ≥75 years of age.

BYETTA reduced HbA_{1c} and body weight in patients treated for 30 weeks in three placebo-controlled studies, whether the BYETTA was added to metformin, a

Table 1 Adverse Reactions Reported in Long-Term Phase 3 Controlled Studies[1]

Body system/adverse reaction terms	Frequency of occurrence		
Reactions	Very common	Common	Uncommon
Metabolism and nutrition disorders			
Hypoglycaemia (with metformin and a sulphonylurea) [2]	X		
Hypoglycaemia (with a sulphonylurea)	X		
Decreased appetite		X	
Nervous system disorders			
Headache [2]		X	
Dizziness		X	
Gastrointestinal disorders			
Nausea	X		
Vomiting	X		
Diarrhoea	X		
Dyspepsia		X	
Abdominal pain		X	
Gastro-oesophageal reflux disease		X	
Abdominal distension		X	
Acute pancreatitis			X[3]
Skin and subcutaneous tissue disorders			
Hyperhidrosis [2]		X	
General disorders and administrative site conditions			
Feeling jittery		X	
Asthenia [2]		X	

n = 1,788 BYETTA-treated intent-to-treat (ITT) patients.

[1] Data from Phase 3 comparator-controlled studies versus placebo, insulin glargine or 30% soluble insulin aspart/70% insulin aspart protamine crystals (biphasic insulin aspart) in which patients also received metformin, thiazolidinediones or sulphonylurea in addition to BYETTA or comparator.

[2] In insulin-comparator controlled studies in which metformin and a sulphonylurea were concomitant medicinal products, the incidence for these adverse reactions was similar for insulin- and BYETTA-treated patients.

[3] Does not conform to criteria previously cited; acute pancreatitis events were uncommon in all treatment groups.

Table 2 Combined Results of the 30-Week Placebo-Controlled Studies (Intent to Treat Patients)

	Placebo	BYETTA 5μg BID	BYETTA 10μg BID
n	483	480	483
Base line HbA_{1c} (%)	8.48	8.42	8.45
HbA_{1c} (%) change from base line	0.08	-0.59	-0.89
Proportion of patients (%) achieving $HbA_{1c} \leq 7\%$	7.9	25.3	33.6
Proportion of patients (%) achieving $HbA_{1c} \leq 7\%$ (patients completing studies)	10.0	29.6	38.5
Base line weight (kg)	99.26	97.10	98.11
Change of weight from base line (kg)	-0.65	-1.41	-1.91

sulphonylurea or a combination of both. These reductions in HbA_{1c} were generally observed at 12 weeks after initiation of treatment. See *Table 2*. The reduction in HbA_{1c} was sustained, and the weight loss continued for at least 82 weeks in the subset of 10μg BID patients completing both the placebo-controlled studies and the uncontrolled study extensions (n = 137).

Table 2 **Combined Results of the 30-Week Placebo-Controlled Studies (Intent to Treat Patients)**

(see Table 2 above)

In a placebo-controlled study of 16 weeks duration, BYETTA (n = 121) or placebo (n = 112) was added to existing thiazolidinedione treatment, with or without metformin. BYETTA (5μg BID for 4 weeks, followed by 10μg BID) resulted in statistically significant reductions from base line HbA_{1c} compared to placebo (-0.8% versus +0.1%), as well as significant reductions in body weight (-1.5 versus -0.2 kg). When BYETTA was used in combination with a thiazolidinedione, the incidence of hypoglycaemia was similar to that of placebo in combination with a thiazolidinedione. The experience in patients >65 years and in patients with impaired renal function is limited.

In insulin-comparator studies, BYETTA (5μg BID for 4 weeks, followed by 10μg BID), in combination with metformin and sulphonylurea, significantly (statistically and clinically) improved glycaemic control, as measured by decrease in HbA_{1c}. This treatment effect was comparable to that of insulin glargine in a 26-week study (mean insulin dose 24.9 IU/day, range 4-95 IU/day, at the end of study) and biphasic insulin aspart in a 52-week study (mean insulin dose 24.4 IU/day, range 3-78 IU/day, at the end of study). BYETTA lowered HbA_{1c} from 8.21 (n = 228) and 8.6% (n = 222) by 1.13 and 1.01%, while insulin glargine lowered from 8.24 (n = 227) by 1.10% and biphasic insulin aspart from 8.67 (n = 224) by 0.86%. Weight loss of 2.3 kg (2.6%) was achieved with BYETTA in the 26-week study and a loss of 2.5 kg (2.7%) in a 52-week study, whereas treatment with insulin was associated with weight gain. Treatment differences (BYETTA minus comparator) were -4.1 kg in the 26-week study and -5.4 kg in the 52-week study. Seven-point self-monitored blood glucose profiles (before and after meals and at 3 am) demonstrated significantly reduced glucose values compared to insulin in the postprandial periods after BYETTA injection. Premeal blood glucose concentrations were generally lower in patients taking insulin compared to BYETTA. Mean daily blood glucose values were similar between BYETTA and insulin. In these studies, the incidence of hypoglycaemia was similar for BYETTA and insulin treatment.

BYETTA has shown no adverse effects on lipid parameters. A trend for a decrease in triglycerides has been observed with weight loss.

Clinical studies with BYETTA have indicated improved beta-cell function, using measures such as the homeostasis model assessment for beta-cell function (HOMA-B) and the proinsulin to insulin ratio. A pharmacodynamic study demonstrated, in patients with Type 2 diabetes (n = 13), a restoration of first-phase insulin secretion and improved second-phase insulin secretion in response to an intravenous bolus of glucose.

A reduction in body weight was seen in patients treated with BYETTA irrespective of the occurrence of nausea, although the reduction was larger in the group with nausea (mean reduction 2.4 kg versus 1.7 kg) in the long-term controlled studies of up to 52 weeks.

Administration of exenatide has been shown to reduce food intake, due to decreased appetite and increased satiety.

5.2 Pharmacokinetic properties

Absorption

Following subcutaneous administration to patients with Type 2 diabetes, exenatide reaches median peak plasma concentrations in 2 h. Mean peak exenatide concentration (C_{max}) was 211pg/ml and overall mean area under the curve (AUC_{0-inf}) was 1036pg •h/ml following subcutaneous administration of a 10μg dose of exenatide. Exenatide exposure increased proportionally over the therapeutic dose range of 5μg to 10μg. Similar exposure is achieved with subcutaneous administration of exenatide in the abdomen, thigh, or arm.

Distribution

The mean apparent volume of distribution of exenatide following subcutaneous administration of a single dose of exenatide is 28 l.

Metabolism and Elimination

Non-clinical studies have shown that exenatide is predominantly eliminated by glomerular filtration, with subsequent proteolytic degradation. In clinical studies, the mean apparent clearance of exenatide is 9 l/h and the mean terminal half-life is 2.4 h. These pharmacokinetic characteristics of exenatide are independent of the dose.

Special Populations

Patients with renal impairment: In patients with mild (creatinine clearance 50 to 80ml/min) or moderate renal impairment (creatinine clearance 30 to 50ml/min), exenatide clearance was mildly reduced compared to clearance in individuals with normal renal function (13% reduction in mild and 36% reduction in moderate renal impairment). Clearance was significantly reduced by 84% in patients with end-stage renal disease receiving dialysis (see section 4.2).

Patients with hepatic insufficiency: No pharmacokinetic study has been performed in patients with hepatic insufficiency. Exenatide is cleared primarily by the kidney; therefore, hepatic dysfunction is not expected to affect blood concentrations of exenatide.

Gender and race: Gender and race have no clinically relevant influence on exenatide pharmacokinetics.

Elderly: Data in elderly are limited, but suggest no marked changes in exenatide exposure with increased age up to about 75 years old. There are no pharmacokinetic data in patients >75 years.

Children and adolescents: In a single-dose pharmacokinetic study in 13 patients with Type 2 diabetes and between the ages of 12 and 16 years, administration of exenatide (5μg) resulted in slightly lower mean AUC (16% lower) and C_{max} (25% lower) compared to those observed in adults.

5.3 Preclinical safety data

Non-clinical data reveal no special hazards for humans based on conventional studies of safety pharmacology, repeat-dose toxicity, or genotoxicity.

In female rats given exenatide for 2 years, an increased incidence of benign thyroid C−cell adenomas was observed at the highest dose, 250μg/kg/day, a dose that produced an exenatide plasma exposure 130-fold the human clinical exposure. This incidence was not statistically significant when adjusted for survival. There was no tumorigenic response in male rats or either sex of mice.

Animal studies did not indicate direct harmful effects with respect to fertility or pregnancy. High doses of exenatide during mid-gestation caused skeletal effects and reduced foetal growth in mice and reduced foetal growth in rabbits. Neonatal growth was reduced in mice exposed to high doses during late gestation and lactation.

6. PHARMACEUTICAL PARTICULARS

6.1 List of excipients

Metacresol

Mannitol

Glacial acetic acid

Sodium acetate trihydrate

Water for injections

6.2 Incompatibilities

This medicinal product must not be mixed with other medicinal products.

6.3 Shelf life

2 years.

Shelf-life for pen in use: 30 days.

6.4 Special precautions for storage

Store in a refrigerator (2°C-8°C).

Do not freeze.

In use: Store below 25°C.

The pen should not be stored with the needle attached.

Replace cap on pen in order to protect from light.

6.5 Nature and contents of container

Type I glass cartridge with a (bromobutyl) rubber plunger, rubber disc, and aluminium seal. Each cartridge is assembled into a disposable pen-injector (pen).

Each pre-filled pen contains 60 doses of sterile preserved solution (approximately 1.2ml [5μg] or 2.4ml [10μg]).

Pack size of 1 and 3 pens. Not all pack sizes may be marketed.

Injection needles are not included. The following are examples of disposable needles that can be used with the BYETTA pen: 29, 30, or 31 gauge (diameter 0.25-0.33mm) and 12.7, 8, or 5mm length.

6.6 Special precautions for disposal and other handling

The patient should be instructed to discard the needle after each injection.

Any unused medicinal product or waste material should be disposed of in accordance with local requirements.

Instructions for Use

BYETTA is for use by one person only.

The instructions for using the pen, included with the leaflet, must be followed carefully.

The pen is stored without needle.

BYETTA should not be used if particles appear or if the solution is cloudy and/or coloured.

BYETTA that has been frozen must not be used.

7. MARKETING AUTHORISATION HOLDER

Eli Lilly Nederland BV, Grootslag 1-5, NL-3991 RA Houten, The Netherlands.

8. MARKETING AUTHORISATION NUMBER(S)

EU/1/06/362/001:	5μg (1 pen)
EU/1/06/362/002:	5μg (3 pens)
EU/1/06/362/003:	10μg (1 pen)
EU/1/06/362/004:	10μg (3 pens)

9. DATE OF FIRST AUTHORISATION/RENEWAL OF THE AUTHORISATION

20 November 2006

10. DATE OF REVISION OF THE TEXT

06 March 2009

LEGAL CATEGORY

POM

*BYETTA (exenatide) is a trademark of Amylin Pharmaceuticals, Inc.

BY6M

Cabaser 1 mg & 2 mg Tablets

(Pharmacia Limited)

1. NAME OF THE MEDICINAL PRODUCT

Cabaser® Tablets 1 mg

Cabaser® Tablets 2 mg

2. QUALITATIVE AND QUANTITATIVE COMPOSITION

Cabergoline INN 1 mg, 2 mg,

For excipients, see 6.1

3. PHARMACEUTICAL FORM

Tablet

Cabaser 1 mg tablets are white, oval, 3.8 × 7.4mm and concave with one side scored and engraved '7' on the left and '01' on the right

Cabaser 2 mg tablets are white, oval, 5.1 × 10mm and concave with one side scored and engraved '7' on the left and '02' on the right

4. CLINICAL PARTICULARS

4.1 Therapeutic indications

Treatment of Parkinson's disease

If treatment with a dopamine agonist is being considered, cabergoline is indicated as second line therapy in patients who are intolerant or fail treatment with a non-ergot compound, as monotherapy, or as adjunctive treatment to levodopa plus dopa-decarboxylase inhibitor, in the management of the signs and symptoms of Parkinson's disease.

Treatment should be initiated under specialist supervision. The benefit of continued treatment should be regularly reassessed taking into account the risk of fibrotic reactions and valvulopathy (see sections 4.3, 4.4 & 4.8)

4.2 Posology and method of administration

The tablets are for oral administration.

Since the tolerability of dopaminergic agents is improved when administered with food, it is recommended that Cabaser be taken with meals.

Cabaser is intended for chronic, long term treatment.

Adults and elderly patients

As expected for dopamine agonists, dose response for both efficacy and side effects appears to be linked to individual sensitivity. Optimization of dose should be obtained through slow initial dose titration, from starting doses of 1 mg daily. The dosage of concurrent levodopa may be gradually decreased, while the dosage of Cabaser is increased, until the optimum balance is determined. In view of the long half-life of the compound, increments of the daily dose of 0.5-1 mg should be done at weekly (initial weeks) or bi-weekly intervals, up to optimal doses.

The recommended therapeutic dosage is 2 to 3 mg/day for patients with signs and symptoms of Parkinson's disease. Cabaser should be given as a single daily dose.

Use in children

The safety and efficacy of Cabaser have not been investigated in children as Parkinson's disease does not affect this population.

4.3 Contraindications

Hypersensitivity to cabergoline, other ergot alkaloids or to any of the excipients.

History of pulmonary, pericardial and retroperitoneal fibrotic disorders.

For long-term treatment: Evidence of cardiac valvulopathy as determined by pre-treatment echocardiography.

4.4 Special warnings and precautions for use

Fibrosis and Cardiac Valvulopathy and Possibly Related Clinical Phenomena

Fibrotic and serosal inflammatory disorders such as pleuritis, pleural effusion, pleural fibrosis, pulmonary fibrosis, pericarditis, pericardial effusion, cardiac valvulopathy involving one or more valves (aortic, mitral and tricuspid) or retroperitoneal fibrosis have occurred after prolonged usage of ergot derivatives with agonist activity at the serotonin $5HT_{2B}$ receptor, such as cabergoline. In some cases, symptoms or manifestations of cardiac valvulopathy improved after discontinuation of cabergoline. Erythrocyte sedimentation rate (ESR) has been found to be abnormally increased in association with pleural effusion/fibrosis. Chest x-ray examination is recommended in cases of unexplained ESR increases to abnormal values.

Serum creatine measurements can also be used to help in the diagnosis of fibrotic disorder.

Valvulopathy has been associated with cumulative doses, therefore patients should be treated with thelowest effective dose. At each visit, the risk benefit profile of cabergoline treatment for the patient should be reassessed to determine the suitability of continued treatment with cabergoline.

Before initiating long-term treatment:

All patients must undergo a cardiovascular evaluation, including echocardiogram, to assess the potential presence of asymptomatic valvular disease. It is also appropriate to perform baseline investigations of ESR or other inflammatory markers, lung function/chest x-ray and renal function prior to initiation of therapy.

In patients with valvular regurgitation, it is not known whether cabergoline treatment might worsen the underlying disease. If fibrotic valvular disease is detected, the patient should not be treated with cabergoline (See Section 4.3).

During long-term treatment:

Fibrotic disorders can have an insidious onset and patients should be regularly monitored for possible manifestations of progressive fibrosis. Therefore during treatment, attention should be paid to the signs and symptoms of:

- Pleuropulmonary disease, such as dyspnoea, shortness of breath, persistent cough, or chest pain.
- Renal insufficiency or ureteral/abdominal vascular obstruction that may occur with pain in the loin/flank, and lower limb oedema, as well as any possible abdominal masses or tenderness that may indicate retroperitoneal fibrosis.
- Cardiac failure: cases of valvular and pericardial fibrosis have often manifested as cardiac failure. Therefore, valvular fibrosis (and constrictive pericarditis) should be excluded if such symptoms occur.

Clinical diagnostic monitoring for development of valvular disease or fibrosis, as appropriate, is essential. Following treatment initiation, the first echocardiogram should occur within 3-6 months, thereafter, the frequency of echocardiographic monitoring should be determined by appropriate individual clinical assessment with particular emphasis on the above-mentioned signs and symptoms, but must occur at least every 6 to 12 months.

Cabergoline should be discontinued if an echocardiogram reveals new or worsened valvular regurgitation, valvular restriction or valve leaflet thickening. (See Section 4.3) The need for other clinical monitoring (e.g., physical examination including, cardiac auscultation, X-ray, CT scan) should be determined on an individual basis. Additional appropriate investigations such as erythrocyte sedimentation rate, and serum creatinine measurements should be performed if necessary to support a diagnosis of a fibrotic disorder.

While renal insufficiency has been shown not to modify cabergoline kinetics, hepatic insufficiency of severe degree (> 10 Child-Pugh score, maximum score 12) has been shown to be associated with an increase of AUC, thus indicating that dose regimens in Parkinsonian patients with severe hepatic insufficiency should be modified accordingly.

In addition, by analogy with other ergot derivatives, Cabaser should be given with caution to patients suffering from severe cardiovascular disease, Raynaud's syndrome, peptic ulcer, gastrointestinal bleeding or a history of serious, particularly psychotic mental disease. Symptomatic hypotension can occur following adminstration of Cabaser: particular attention should be paid when administering Cabaser concomitantly with other drugs known to lower blood pressure.

Cabergoline has been associated with somnolence and episodes of sudden sleep onset, particularly in Patients with Parkinson's disease. Sudden onset of sleep during activities, in some cases without awareness or warning signs, has been reported uncommonly. Patients must be informed of this and advised to exercise caution while driving or operating machines during treatment with cabergoline. Patients who have experienced somnolence and/or an episode of sudden sleep onset must refrain from driving or operating machines. Furthermore a reduction of dosage or termination of therapy may be considered.

The effects of alcohol on overall tolerability of Cabaser are currently unknown.

Pathological gambling, increased libido and hypersexuality have been reported in patients treated with dopamine agonists for Parkinson's disease, including Cabergoline/Cabaser.

4.5 Interaction with other medicinal products and other forms of interaction

No pharmacokinetic interaction with L-Dopa or selegiline was observed in the studies carried out in parkinsonian patients. The concomitant use of other drugs, particularly other antiparkinsonian non-dopamine-agonist agents, was not associated with detectable interactions modifying the efficacy and safety of Cabaser.

No other information is available about possible interaction between Cabaser and other ergot alkaloids: therefore the concomitant use of these medications during long term treatment with Cabaser is not recommended.

Since Cabaser exerts its therapeutic effect by direct stimulation of dopamine receptors, it should not be concurrently administered with drugs which have dopamine antagonist activity (such as phenothiazines, butyrophenones, thioxanthenes, metoclopramide) since these might reduce the therapeutic effect of Cabaser.

By analogy with other ergot derivatives, Cabaser should not be used in association with macrolide antibiotics (e.g erythromycin) since the systemic bioavailability of Cabaser and adverse effects could increase.

4.6 Pregnancy and lactation

Cabaser has been shown to cross the placenta in rats: it is unknown whether this occurs also in humans.

Animal studies in rats and mice have not demonstrated any teratogenic effect or any effect of the compound on global reproductive performance. In clinical studies there have been over 100 pregnancies in women treated with cabergoline for hyperprolactinemic disorders. The compound was generally taken during the first 8 weeks after conception. Among the pregnancies evaluable so far, there were approximately 85% live births and about 10% spontaneous abortions. Three cases of congenital abnormalities (Down's syndrome, hydrocephalus, malformation of lower limbs) which led to therapeutic abortion and three cases of minor abnormalities in live births were observed.

These incidence rates are comparable with those quoted for normal populations and for women exposed to other ovulation-inducing drugs. Based on the above data, the use of the product does not appear to be associated with an increased risk of abortion, premature delivery, multiple pregnancy or congenital abnormalities.

Because clinical experience is still limited and the drug has a long half-life, as a precautionary measure it is recommended that women seeking pregnancy discontinue Cabaser one month before intended conception, in order to prevent possible foetal exposure to the drug. If conception occurs during therapy, treatment is to be discontinued as soon as pregnancy is confirmed, to limit foetal exposure to the drug.

In rats cabergoline and/or its metabolites are excreted in milk. Lactation is expected to be inhibited/suppressed by Cabaser, in view of its dopamine-agonist properties. Therefore, while no information on the excretion of cabergoline in maternal milk in humans is available, puerperal women should be advised not to breast-feed in case of failed lactation inhibition/suppression by the product.

4.7 Effects on ability to drive and use machines

Patients being treated with cabergoline and presenting with somnolence and/or sudden sleep onset episodes must be informed to refrain from driving or engaging in activities where impaired alertness may put themselves or others at risk of serious injury or death (e.g. operating machines) until such episodes and somnolence have resolved (see also Section 4.4).

4.8 Undesirable effects

About 1070 parkinsonian patients have received Cabaser as adjuvant therapy to L-dopa in clinical studies; of these 74% had at least one adverse event, mainly of mild to moderate severity and transient in nature, and requiring discontinuation in a small proportion of cases.

In the majority of cases (51%), events were related to the nervous system: most frequently reported events were dyskinesia, hyperkinesia, hallucinations or confusion. The gastrointestinal system was involved in 33% of cases: events most frequently reported were nausea, vomiting, dyspepsia and gastritis. The cardiovascular system was involved in 27% of cases, most frequently reported events being dizziness and hypotension.

There have been reports of fibrotic and serosal inflammatory conditions, such as pleuritis, pleural effusion, pleural fibrosis, pulmonary fibrosis, pericarditis, pericardial effusion, cardiac valvulopathy and retroperitoneal fibrosis, in patients taking cabergoline (see 'Special warnings and special precautions for use'). The incidence of cardiac valvulopathy (including regurgitation) and related disorders (pericarditis and pericardial effusion) is considered to be very common.

There is limited information available on the reversibility of these reactions.

Other adverse events expected for the pharmacological class, in view of the vasoconstrictive properties, include angina (reported in about 1% of the patients on cabergoline) and erythromelalgia (observed in 0.4% of the patients). Similarly expected for the pharmacological class, peripheral oedema occurred in 6% of patients.

Gastric upset was more frequent in female than in male patients, while CNS events were more frequent in the elderly.

A blood pressure decrease of clinical relevance was observed mainly on standing in a minority of patients. The effect was mainly evident in the first weeks of therapy. Neither modification of heart rate nor consistent changes of ECG tracing were observed during Cabaser treatment.

Cabergoline is associated with somnolence and has been associated uncommonly with excessive daytime somnolence and sudden sleep onset episodes.

Alterations in standard laboratory tests are uncommon during long term therapy with Cabaser.

Patients treated with dopamine agonists for treatment of Parkinson's disease, including Cabergoline/Cabaser, especially at high doses, have been reported as exhibiting signs of pathological gambling, increased libido and hypersexuality, generally reversible upon reduction of the dose or treatment discontinuation.

4.9 Overdose

The acute toxicity studies carried out in animals indicate very low toxicity, with a wide safety margin with respect to pharmacologically active doses. Clinical signs and cause of death, if any, were related to CNS stimulation.

There is no experience in humans of overdosage with Cabaser in the proposed indication: it is likely to lead to symptoms due to over-stimulation of dopamine receptors. These might include nausea, vomiting, gastric complaints, hypotension, confusion/psychosis or hallucinations. The vomiting stimulating properties of dopamine agonists are expected to favour removal of unabsorbed drug. Supportive measures should be directed to maintain blood pressure, if necessary. In addition, in case of pronounced central nervous system effects (hallucinations) the administration of dopamine antagonist drugs may be advisable.

5. PHARMACOLOGICAL PROPERTIES

5.1 Pharmacodynamic properties

Cabaser is a dopaminergic ergoline derivative endowed with potent and long-lasting dopamine D2 receptor agonist properties. In rats the compound, acting at D2 dopamine receptors on pituitary lactotrophic cells, decreases PRL secretion at oral doses of 3-25 mcg/kg, and in vitro at a concentration of 45 pg/ml. In addition, Cabaser exerts a central dopaminergic effect via D2 receptor stimulation at doses higher than those effective in lowering serum PRL levels. Improvement of motor deficit in animal models of parkinson's disease was present at oral daily doses of 1-2.5 mg/kg in rats and at s.c. doses of 0.5-1 mg/kg in monkeys.

In healthy volunteers the administration of Cabaser at single oral doses of 0.3-2.5 mg was associated with a significant decrease in serum PRL levels. The effect is prompt (within 3 hours of administration) and persistent (up to 7-28 days). The PRL-lowering effect is dose-related both in terms of degree of effect and duration of action.

The pharmacodynamic actions of Cabaser not linked to the therapeutic effect relate only to blood pressure decrease. The maximal hypotensive effect of Cabaser as a single dose usually occurs during the first 6 hours after drug intake and is dose-dependent both in terms of maximal decrease and frequency.

5.2 Pharmacokinetic properties

The pharmacokinetic and metabolic profiles of Cabaser have been studied in healthy volunteers of both sexes, in female hyperprolactinemic patients and in parkinsonian patients. After oral administration of the labelled compound, radioactivity was rapidly absorbed from the gastrointestinal tract as the peak of radioactivity in plasma was between 0.5 and 4 hours. Ten days after administration about 18/20% and 55/72% of the radioactive dose (^{3}H-cabergoline/^{14}C-cabergoline) was recovered in urine and faeces, respectively. Unchanged drug in urine accounted for 2-3% of the dose.

In urine, the main metabolite identified was 6-allyl-8b-carboxy-ergoline, which accounted for 4-6% of the dose. Three additional metabolites were identified in urine, which accounted overall for less than 3% of the dose. The metabolites have been found to be much less potent than Cabaser as D_2 dopamine receptor agonists "in vitro".

The low urinary excretion of unchanged Cabaser has been confirmed also in studies with non-radioactive product. The elimination half-life of Cabaser, estimated from urinary excretion rates, is long (63-68 hours in healthy volunteers, 79-115 hours in hyperprolactinemic patients).

The pharmacokinetics of Cabaser seem to be dose-independent both in healthy volunteers (doses of 0.5-1.5 mg) and parkinsonian patients (steady state of daily doses up to 7 mg/day).

On the basis of the elimination half-life, steady state conditions should be achieved after 4 weeks, as confirmed by the mean peak plasma levels of Cabaser obtained after a single dose (37$\pm$8 pg/ml) and after a 4 week multiple-regimen (101$\pm$43 pg/ml). "In vitro" experiments showed that the drug at concentrations of 0.1-10 ng/ml is 41-42% bound to plasma proteins.

Food does not appear to affect absorption and disposition of Cabaser.

While renal insufficiency has been shown not to modify cabergoline kinetics, hepatic insufficiency of severe degree (> 10 Child-Pugh score, maximum score 12) has been shown to be associated with an increase of AUC.

5.3 Preclinical safety data

Almost all the findings noted throughout the series of preclinical safety studies are a consequence of the central dopaminergic effects or the long-lasting inhibition of PRL in rodents with a specific hormonal physiology different to man.

Preclinical safety studies of Cabaser indicate a consistent safety margin for this compound in rodents and in monkeys, as well as a lack of teratogenic, genotoxic or carcinogenic potential.

6. PHARMACEUTICAL PARTICULARS

6.1 List of excipients

Lactose anhydrous NF, USP

Leucine Ph Eur

6.2 Incompatibilities

Not applicable

6.3 Shelf life

24 months at room temperature (25°C).

6.4 Special precautions for storage

There are no special precautions for storage.

6.5 Nature and contents of container

The tablets are contained in Type I amber glass bottles with tamper resistant screw caps which contain silica gel desiccant.

Each bottle contains 20 or 30 tablets and is enclosed in an outer cardboard carton.

6.6 Special precautions for disposal and other handling

Bottles of Cabaser are supplied with desiccant in the caps. This desiccant must not be removed.

Administrative Data

7. MARKETING AUTHORISATION HOLDER

Pharmacia Laboratories Limited

Ramsgate Road

Sandwich

Kent

CT13 9NJ

United Kingdom

8. MARKETING AUTHORISATION NUMBER(S)

1mg: PL 00022/0169

2mg: PL 00022/0170

9. DATE OF FIRST AUTHORISATION/RENEWAL OF THE AUTHORISATION

14 February 1996

10. DATE OF REVISION OF THE TEXT

December 2008

Company Ref: CA9_2

Cacit D3 Effervescent Granules 500 mg/440 IU

(Procter & Gamble Pharmaceuticals UK Limited)

1. NAME OF THE MEDICINAL PRODUCT

CACIT VITAMIN D3 500 mg/440 IU, effervescent granules for oral solution in sachet

2. QUALITATIVE AND QUANTITATIVE COMPOSITION

One sachet of 4 g contains:

Calcium carbonate 1250 mg (equivalent to calcium element 500 mg or 12.5 mmol)

Colecalciferol concentrate (powder form) 440 IU (equivalent to colecalciferol (Vitamin D_3) 11µg)

For excipients, see 6.1.

3. PHARMACEUTICAL FORM

Effervescent white granules for oral solution.

4. CLINICAL PARTICULARS

4.1 Therapeutic indications

- Correction of vitamin D and calcium combined deficiency in elderly people.

- Vitamin D and calcium supplementation as an adjunct to specific therapy for osteoporosis treatment in patients with established, or at high risk of vitamin D and calcium combined deficiencies.

4.2 Posology and method of administration

- Posology:

One or two sachets per day.

- Method of administration:

Oral.

Pour the contents of the sachet into a glass, add a large quantity of water, then drink immediately.

4.3 Contraindications

- Diseases and/or conditions resulting in hypercalcaemia and/or hypercalciuria
- Nephrolithiasis
- Hypervitaminosis D
- Hypersensitivity to the active substances or to any of the excipients (in particular soya oil).

4.4 Special warnings and precautions for use

During long-term treatment, serum calcium levels should be followed and renal function should be monitored through measurements of serum creatinine. Monitoring is especially important in elderly patients on concomitant treatment with cardiac glycosides or diuretics (see section 4.5) and in patients with a high tendency to calculus formation. In case of hypercalcaemia or signs of impaired renal function the dose should be reduced or the treatment discontinued.

Vitamin D3 should be used with caution in patients with impairment of renal function and the effect on calcium and phosphate levels should be monitored. The risk of soft tissue calcification should be taken into account. In patients with severe renal insufficiency, vitamin D in the form of cholecalciferol is not metabolised normally and other forms of vitamin D should be used (see section 4.3 contraindications)

Cacit Vitamin D3 sachets should be prescribed with caution to patients suffering from sarcoidosis, due to the risk of increased metabolism of vitamin D into its active form. These patients, should be monitored with regard to the calcium content in serum and urine.

Calcium/vitamin D3 sachets should be used with caution in immobilised patients with osteoporosis due to the increased risk of hypercalcaemia.

The contentof vitamin D3 (440 IU) in Cacit Vitamin D3 sachets should be considered when prescribing other medicinal products containing vitamin D. Additional doses of calcium or vitamin D should be taken under close medical supervision. In such cases it is necessary to monitor serum calcium levels and urinary calcium excretion frequently.

Cacit Vitamin D3 sachets are not intended for use in children.

- Special warnings:

Cacit Vitamin D3 sachets contain sucrose.

Patients with rare hereditary problems of fructose intolerance, glucose-galactose malabsorption or sucrose-isomaltase insufficiency should not take this medicine.

4.5 Interaction with other medicinal products and other forms of interaction

Concomitant use requiring precautions:

- Digitalis and other cardiac glycosides: the oral administration of calcium combined with vitamin D increases the toxicity of digitalis (risk of dysrythmia). Strict medical supervision, and if necessary, monitoring ECG and calcaemia are necessary.

- Bisphosphonate, sodium fluoride: it is advisable to allow a minimum period of two hours before taking the calcium (risk of reduction of the gastrointestinal absorption of bisphosphonate and sodium fluoride).

- Thiazide diuretics: reduce urinary elimination of calcium therefore supervision of calcaemia is recommended.

- Phenytoin or barbiturates: can decrease the effect of vitamin D because of metabolic inactivation.

- Glucocorticosteroid: can decrease the effect of vitamin D

- Tetracyclines by oral route: it is advisable to delay taking the calcium by at least three hours (calcium salts reduce the absorption of tetracyclines).

- Possible interactions with food (e.g. containing oxalic acid, phosphate or phytinic acid).

4.6 Pregnancy and lactation

The product may be used during pregnancy and lactation. However, the daily intake should not exceed

1500 mg calcium and 600 IU vitamin D3.

In pregnancy overdoses of colecalciferol must be avoided

- Overdoses of vitamin D have shown teratogenic effects in pregnant animals.

- In humans overdoses of colecalciferol must be avoided as permanent hypercalcaemia can lead to physical and mental retardation, supravalvular aortic stenosis and retinopathy in the child.

There are however several case reports of administration of very high doses in hypoparathyroidism in the mother where normal children were born.

Vitamin D and its metabolites pass into the breast milk.

4.7 Effects on ability to drive and use machines

No remarkable findings. No effect expected.

4.8 Undesirable effects

Adverse reactions are listed below, by system organ class and frequency. Frequencies are defined as: uncommon (>1/1,000, <1/100) or rare (>1/10,000 <1/1,000).

Metabolism and nutrition disorders

Uncommon: Hypercalcaemia and hypercalciuria.

Gastrointestinal disorders

Rare: Constipation, flatulence, nausea, abdominal pain and diarrhoea.

Skin and subcutaneous disorders

Rare: Pruritus, rash and urticaria.

4.9 Overdose

Consequence of overdose are hypercalciuria and hypercalcaemia. Symptoms include:

nausea, vomiting, thirst, polydipsia, polyuria, constipation.

Chronic overdoses can lead to vascular and organ calcifications as a result of hypercalcaemia.

Treatment:

Stop all intake of calcium and vitamin D, rehydration.

5. PHARMACOLOGICAL PROPERTIES

5.1 Pharmacodynamic properties

Vitamin D corrects an insufficient intake of vitamin D and increases intestinal absorption of calcium.

Calcium intake corrects a lack of calcium in the diet.

The commonly accepted requirement of calcium in the elderly is 1500 mg/day.

The optimal amount of vitamin D in the elderly is 500 - 1000 IU/day.

Vitamin D and calcium correct secondary senile hyperparathyroidism.

In a double blind placebo controlled study of 18 months, including 3270 women aged 84 ± 6 years with a low intake of calcium and living in nursing homes, had their diet supplemented with colecalciferol (800 UI/day) + Calcium (1.2 g/day). A significant decrease in PTH secretion has been observed.

After 18 months, results of the intend to treat analysis showed 80 hip fractures (5.7%) in the Calcium Vitamin D group and 110 hip fractures (7.9%) in the placebo group ($p = 0.004$). Therefore, in these study conditions, the treatment of 1387 women prevented 30 hip fractures. After 36 months of follow up, 137 women presented at least one hip fracture (11.6%) in the Calcium Vitamin D group ($n = 1176$) and 178 (15.8%) in the placebo group ($n = 1127$) ($p \leqslant 0.02$).

5.2 Pharmacokinetic properties

During dissolution the calcium salt contained in CACIT VITAMIN D3 is transformed into calcium citrate.

Calcium citrate is well absorbed, approximately 30% to 40% of the ingested dose.

Calcium is eliminated in the urine and faeces and secreted in the sweat.

Vitamin D is absorbed in the intestine and transported by protein binding in the blood to the liver (first hydroxylation) then to the kidney (second hydroxylation).

The non-hydroxylated vitamin D is stored in reserve compartments such as adipose and muscle tissue. Its plasma half-life is several days; it is eliminated in the faeces and the urine.

5.3 Preclinical safety data

No remarkable findings.

6. PHARMACEUTICAL PARTICULARS

6.1 List of excipients

Citric acid anhydrous, Malic acid, Gluconolactone, Maltodextrin, Sodium cyclamate, Saccharin sodium, Lemon flavouring (containing: Sorbitol, Mannitol, D-gluconolactone, Dextrin, Gum arabic, Lemon oil), Rice starch, Potassium carbonate, -Tocopherol, Soya-bean oil hydrogenated, Gelatin, Sucrose, Corn starch.

Quantity of sodium per sachet: 5 mg or 0.22 mmol

6.2 Incompatibilities

Not applicable.

6.3 Shelf life

3 years.

6.4 Special precautions for storage

Do not store above 25°C.

6.5 Nature and contents of container

4 g sachets (paper/aluminium/polyethylene); boxes of 20, 28, 30, 46, 50, 56, 60 or 100 sachets and sample pack of 10 sachets.

Not all pack sizes may be marketed.

6.6 Special precautions for disposal and other handling

No special requirements

7. MARKETING AUTHORISATION HOLDER

Procter & Gamble Pharmaceuticals UK Limited.

Rusham Park,

Whitehall Lane,

Egham,

Surrey.

TW20 9NW, UK.

8. MARKETING AUTHORISATION NUMBER(S)

PL 0364/0060

9. DATE OF FIRST AUTHORISATION/RENEWAL OF THE AUTHORISATION

03 March 2001 (Renewal)

10. DATE OF REVISION OF THE TEXT

February 2006

Cacit Effervescent Tablets 500mg

(Procter & Gamble Pharmaceuticals UK Limited)

1. NAME OF THE MEDICINAL PRODUCT

Cacit Effervescent Tablets 500mg

2. QUALITATIVE AND QUANTITATIVE COMPOSITION

Each tablet contains 1.25g Calcium Carbonate Ph Eur which when dissolved in water provides 500mg of calcium as calcium citrate.

3. PHARMACEUTICAL FORM

Effervescent tablet

4. CLINICAL PARTICULARS

4.1 Therapeutic indications

1. Treatment of calcium deficiency states including osteomalacia, rickets and malabsorption syndromes affecting the upper gastrointestinal tract.

2. An adjunct to conventional therapy in the arrest or slowing down of bone demineralisation in osteoporosis.

3. In the arrest or slowing down of bone demineralisation in osteoporosis, where other effective treatment is contra-indicated.

4. As a therapeutic supplement during times when intake may be inadequate, particularly those associated with the increased demand of childhood, old age, pregnancy and lactation.

4.2 Posology and method of administration

The tablets must be dissolved in a glass of water and the solution should then be drunk immediately after complete dissolution of the tablets.

Adults and the Elderly

For calcium deficiency states including malabsorption, the dosage should be tailored to the individual patient's needs. A dose of 1.0 g to 2.5g per day is recommended.

For the treatment of osteoporosis a dose of up to 1.5g per day is normally required. In patients with adequate dietary calcium intake, 500mg daily may be sufficient.

Up to 1.5g of calcium per day is the recommended dosage for therapeutic supplementation.

Children

For calcium deficiency states including malabsorption and rickets, the dosage recommendation under adult dosage should be followed.

For therapeutic supplementation, a dose of up to 1.0g per day is recommended.

4.3 Contraindications

Hypercalcaemia (eg. due to hyperparathyroidism, hypervitaminosis D, decalcifying tumours, severe renal failure, bone metastases), severe hypercalciuria calci-lithiasis and renal calculi. Long term immobilisation accompanied by hypercalciuria and/or hypercalcaemia. Hypersensitivity to any of the ingredients.

4.4 Special warnings and precautions for use

In mild hypercalciuria (exceeding 7.5 mmol/24 hours in adults or 0.12-0.15 mmol/kg/24 hours in children) or renal failure, or where there is evidence of stone formation in the urinary tract; adequate checks must be kept on urinary calcium excretion. If necessary the dosage should be reduced or calcium therapy discontinued. The product should be administered with caution in patients with sarcoidosis because of possible increased metabolism of vitamin D to its active form. These patients should be monitored for serum and urinary calcium.

4.5 Interaction with other medicinal products and other forms of interaction

Concomitant administration with vitamin D causes an increase in calcium absorption and plasma levels may continue to rise after stopping vitamin D therapy.

The effects of digoxin and other cardiac glycosides may be accentuated by calcium and toxicity may be produced, especially in combination with vitamin D.

Calcium salts reduce the absorption of some drugs, in particular tetracyclines It is therefore recommended that administration of Cacit tablets be separated from these products by at least 3 hours.

Thiazide diuretics increase renal absorption of calcium, so the risk of hypercalcaemia should be considered.

Bisphosphonate, sodium fluoride: it is advisable to allow a two hour minimum period before taking Cacit (risk of reduction of the gastrointestinal absorption of bisphosphonate and sodium fluoride).

4.6 Pregnancy and lactation

Calcium supplements have been in wide use for many years without apparent ill consequence.

4.7 Effects on ability to drive and use machines

None

4.8 Undesirable effects

Mild gastrointestinal disturbances have occurred rarely (eg. nausea, abdominal pain, diarrhoea, constipation, flatulence and eructation). Hypercalciuria and, in rare cases, hypercalcaemia in cases of long-term treatment with high doses.

Skin reactions, such as pruritis, rash, and urticaria (especially urticaria in patients with a past history of allergy) have been reported. The colouring agent E110 can cause allergic type reactions including asthma. Allergy is more common in those people who are allergic to aspirin

4.9 Overdose

The amount of calcium absorbed will depend on the individuals calcium status. Deliberate overdosage is unlikely with effervescent preparations and acute overdosage has not been reported. It might cause gastrointestinal disturbance but would not be expected to cause hypercalcaemia, except in patients treated with excessive doses of vitamin D. Symptoms of overdose may include nausea, vomiting, polydipsia, polyuria and constipation. Treatment should be aimed at lowering serum calcium levels, eg. administration of oral phosphates and rehydration.

Chronic overdoses can lead to vascular and organ calcifications as a result of hypercalcaemia.

5. PHARMACOLOGICAL PROPERTIES

5.1 Pharmacodynamic properties

Calcium is an essential element of tissues and plasma.

5.2 Pharmacokinetic properties

When the tablets are added to water, insoluble calcium carbonate is converted into absorbable calcium citrate.

5.3 Preclinical safety data

Not Applicable

6. PHARMACEUTICAL PARTICULARS

6.1 List of excipients

Citric acid

Sodium saccharin

Sodium cyclamate

Sunset Yellow FCF (E110) and flavour.

Cacit tablets contain no sugar and have a low sodium content.

6.2 Incompatibilities

None

6.3 Shelf life

Three years.

6.4 Special precautions for storage

Store in a dry place.

6.5 Nature and contents of container

Supplied in boxes of 76 tablets (4 polypropylene tubes with polyethylene stoppers each containing 19 tablets).

6.6 Special precautions for disposal and other handling

To be dissolved in water before administration as described in Section 4.2

7. MARKETING AUTHORISATION HOLDER

Procter & Gamble Pharmaceuticals UK Limited

Rusham Park

Whitehall Lane

Egham

Surrey

TW20 9NW

UK

8. MARKETING AUTHORISATION NUMBER(S)

PL 0364/0045

9. DATE OF FIRST AUTHORISATION/RENEWAL OF THE AUTHORISATION

2 October 1989/28 october 2005

10. DATE OF REVISION OF THE TEXT

28/10/2005

Cafergot Suppositories 2mg

(Alliance Pharmaceuticals)

1. NAME OF THE MEDICINAL PRODUCT

Cafergot® Suppositories 2mg.

2. QUALITATIVE AND QUANTITATIVE COMPOSITION

Ergotamine tartrate PhEur 2mg and caffeine PhEur 100mg.

3. PHARMACEUTICAL FORM

2mg off-white suppositories, 3cm in length, 1cm in diameter.

4. CLINICAL PARTICULARS

4.1 Therapeutic indications

Acute attacks of migraine and migraine variants unresponsive to simple analgesics.

4.2 Posology and method of administration

Adults:

There is considerable inter-individual variation in the sensitivity of patients to ergotamine. Care should therefore be exercised in selecting the optimum therapeutic dose for an individual patient which will not give rise to unwanted effects, either acutely or chronically. The maximum recommended dosages should not be exceeded and ergotamine treatment should not be administered at intervals of less than 4 days.

For maximum efficacy, the optimal dose (in the preferred presentation) should be administered immediately prodromal symptoms are experienced.

One suppository should be administered at the first warning of an attack. This dose is normally sufficient, although some individuals may require higher dosages which should never exceed 2 suppositories (4mg ergotamine) in 24 hours. It is essential to use the minimum effective dose.

The maximum recommended weekly dosage of 4 suppositories (8mg ergotamine) should never be exceeded.

Children under 12 years: Not recommended.

Elderly: Whilst there is no evidence to suggest that the elderly require different dosages of Cafergot, the contraindications of this drug are common in the elderly, eg. coronary heart disease, renal impairment, hepatic impairment and severe hypertension. Caution should therefore be exercised when prescribing for this age group.

4.3 Contraindications

Known hypersensitivity to ergot alkaloids, caffeine, or any other components of the formulation.

Patients with impaired peripheral circulation, obliterative vascular disease, coronary heart disease, inadequately controlled hypertension, septic conditions or shock. Impaired hepatic or renal function, temporal arteritis and patients with hemiplegic or basilar migraine are also contraindicated.

Pregnancy or nursing mothers.

Concomitant treatment with macrolide antibiotics, HIV-protease or reverse-transcriptase inhibitors, azole antifungals (see 4.5 Interactions with other medicinal products and other forms of interaction).

Concomitant treatment with vasoconstrictive agents (including ergot alkaloids, sumatriptan and other $5HT_1$-receptor agonists (see 4.5 Interactions with other medicinal products and other forms of interaction).

4.4 Special warnings and precautions for use

Cafergot is only indicated for the treatment of acute migraine attacks and not for prevention.

Continued daily use of Cafergot or use in excess of the recommended doses must be avoided since this may cause vasospasm.

Owing to its vasoconstrictor properties, ergotamine may cause myocardial ischaemia or, in rare cases, infarction, even in patients with no known history of coronary heart disease.

Patients who are being treated with Cafergot should be informed of the maximum doses allowed and of the first symptoms of over dosage: hypoaesthesia, paraesthesia (eg numbness, tingling) in the fingers and toes, non-migraine-related nausea and vomiting, and symptoms of myocardial ischaemia (e.g. precordial pain). If symptoms such as tingling in the fingers or toes occur, the drug should be discontinued at once and the physician consulted.

If contrary to recommendations ergotamine-containing drugs are used excessively over years, they may induce fibrotic changes, in particular of the pleura and retroperitoneum. There have also been rare reports of fibrotic changes of the cardiac valves.

The occurrence of drug-induced headaches has been reported during prolonged and uninterrupted treatment with Cafergot.

Rare cases of solitary rectal or anal ulcer have occurred from abuse of ergotamine containing suppositories, usually at higher than recommended doses or with continuous use at the recommended dose for many years.

4.5 Interaction with other medicinal products and other forms of interaction

Ergotism (increased peripheral vasoconstriction)

Several drugs increase the risk of ergotism (vasoconstriction, convulsions, other CNS and GI effects) and concomitant use of the following with Cafergot should be avoided (see section 4.3): -

Antibacterials

- Macrolides (eg erythromycin, azithromycin, clarithromycin, spiramycin) or telithromycin
- quinupristin/dalfopristin
- tetracycline

Antifungals

- Imidazoles (eg ketaconazole, miconazole)
- Triazoles (eg itraconazole, posaconazole, voriconazole)
- Antivirals (eg amprenavir, indinavir, nelfinavir, ritonavir, saquinavir. atazinavir, efavirenz)

$5HT_1$ agonists

- Avoid Cafergot for 6 hours after almotriptan, rizatriptan, sumatriptan or zolmitriptan. Avoid almotriptan, rizatriptan, sumatriptan or zolmitriptan for 24 hours after Cafergot.
- Avoid Cafergot for 24 hours after eletriptan or frovatriptan. Avoid eletriptan or frovatriptan for 24 hours after Cafergot.

Cimetidine

Sympathomimetic agents

Beta-blockers

Other vasoconstrictors - excessive nicotine may enhance vasoconstriction

Other

Anaesthetics

- Halothane reduces the effect of ergometrine on the parturient uterus

Antidepressants

- Reboxetine - possible increase in hypertension in association with ergot

4.6 Pregnancy and lactation

Ergotamine-containing products are contraindicated in pregnancy due to oxytocic and vasoconstrictor effects on the placenta and umbilical cord.

Ergotamine is excreted in breast milk and may cause symptoms of vomiting, diarrhoea, weak pulse and unstable blood pressure in infants. Thus, Cafergot are contraindicated in nursing mothers.

4.7 Effects on ability to drive and use machines

Dizziness and feelings of anxiety (trembling, sweating etc) have been reported with Cafergot. If a patient is affected they should not drive, operate machinery or take part in activities where these reactions may put themselves or others at risk.

4.8 Undesirable effects

The caffeine component of Cafergot may give rise to unwanted stimulant effects.

Side effects of Cafergot are related in the main to the ergotamine component.

The most common of all side-effects are nausea and vomiting. Depending on the dose of ergotamine, signs and symptoms of vasoconstriction may occur.

Adverse reactions (Table 1) are ranked under heading of frequency, the most frequent first, using the following convention: very common (greater than or equal to 1 in 10); common (less than or equal to 1 in 100, less than 1 in 10); uncommon (greater than or equal to 1 in 1,000, less than 1 in 100); rare (greater than or less than 1 in 10,000, less than 1 in 1,000) very rare (less than 1 in 10,000), including isolated reports.

Table 1

Immune system disorders
Rare: Hypersensitivity reactions[1]
Nervous system disorders
Common: Dizziness
Uncommon: Paraesthesia (e.g. tingling), hypoaesthesia (e.g numbness)
Ear and labyrinth disorders
Rare: Vertigo
Cardiac disorders
Uncommon: Cyanosis
Rare: Bradycardia, tachycardia
Very rare: Myocardial ischaemia, myocardial infarction
Vascular disorders
Uncommon: Peripheral vasoconstriction
Rare: Increase in blood pressure
Very rare: Gangrene
Respiratory, thoracic and mediastinal disorders
Rare: Dyspnoea
Gastrointestinal disorders
Common: Nausea and vomiting (not migraine related), abdominal pain
Uncommon: Diarrhoea
Skin and subcutaneous tissue disorders
Uncommon: Pain in extremities
Rare: Myalgia
General disorders and administration site conditions
Uncommon: Weakness in extremities
Investigations
Rare: Absence of pulse
Injury, poisoning and procedural complications
Rare: Ergotism[2]

1. Hypersensitivity reactions such as skin rash, face oedema, urticaria and dyspnoea.

2. Ergotism is defined as an intense arterial vasoconstriction, producing signs and symptoms of vascular ischemia of the extremities and other tissues (such as renal or cerebral vasospasm)

Rare cases of intestinal ischaemia have been associated with chronic use and overuse of ergotamine-containing preparations. Rarely, headache may be provoked either by chronic overdosage or by rapid withdrawal of the product.

Excessive use of ergotamine-containing products for prolonged periods may result in fibrotic changes, in particular of the pleura and retroperitoneum. Rare cases of fibrosis of cardiac valves have also been reported.

The occurrence of drug induced headaches has been reported during prolonged and uninterrupted treatment with Cafergot (see 4.4 Special Warnings and Precautions).

Rectal and anal ulcers may occur after long term use or use at doses higher than recommended dose of ergotamine containing suppositories (see 4.4 Special Warnings and Precautions).

4.9 Overdose

Symptoms: Nausea, vomiting, drowsiness, confusion, tachycardia, dizziness, respiratory depression, hypotension, convulsion, shock, coma and symptoms and complications of ergotism.

Ergotism is defined as an intense arterial vasoconstriction, producing signs and symptoms of vascular ischemia of the extremities such as tingling, numbness and pain in the extremities, cyanosis, absence of pulse and if the condition is allowed to progress untreated, gangrene may result. Furthermore ergotism can also involve signs and symptoms of vascular ischaemia of other tissues such as renal and cerebral vasospasm. Most cases of ergotism are associated with chronic intoxication and/or overdose.

Treatment: should be directed to the elimination of ingested material by aspiration and gastric lavage.

Treatment should be symptomatic. In the event of severe vasospastic reactions, i.v. administration of a peripheral vasodilator such as nitroprusside, phentolamine or dihydralazine, local application of warmth to the affected area and nursing care to prevent tissue damage are recommended. In the event of coronary constriction, appropriate treatment such as nitroglycerin should be initiated.

5. PHARMACOLOGICAL PROPERTIES

5.1 Pharmacodynamic properties

Ergotamine is a highly vasoactive ergot alkaloid having characteristically complex pharmacological actions. It is a partial tryptaminic agonist in certain blood vessels and both a partial agonist and antagonist of α-adrenergic receptors of blood vessels.

Although its exact mode of action in migraine is not known, its therapeutic effects have been attributed to its ability to cause vasoconstriction, thereby eliminating the painful dilation/pulsation of branches of the external carotid artery.

5.2 Pharmacokinetic properties

There is great interindividual variation in the absorption of ergotamine in patients and volunteers. Bioavailability is of the order of 5% or less by oral or rectal administration. After im or iv administration, plasma concentrations decay in a bi-exponential fashion. The elimination half life is 2 to 2.5 hours and clearance is about 0.68L/h/kg. Metabolism occurs in the liver. The major enzyme involved in the metabolism of ergotamine is Cytochrome P450 (CYP) 3A4. The primary route of excretion is biliary.

5.3 Preclinical safety data

There are no pre-clinical data of relevance to the prescriber which are additional to those already included in other sections of the Summary of Product Characteristics.

6. PHARMACEUTICAL PARTICULARS

6.1 List of excipients

Tartaric acid, lactose, Suppocire AM.

6.2 Incompatibilities

None

6.3 Shelf life

3 years.

6.4 Special precautions for storage

Store below 25°C.

6.5 Nature and contents of container

Carton of 30 suppositories in an aluminium blister pack.

6.6 Special precautions for disposal and other handling

None.

7. MARKETING AUTHORISATION HOLDER

Alliance Pharmaceuticals Ltd

Avonbridge House

Bath Road

Chippenham

Wiltshire

SN15 2BB

8. MARKETING AUTHORISATION NUMBER(S)

PL16853/0003

9. DATE OF FIRST AUTHORISATION/RENEWAL OF THE AUTHORISATION

25 June 1998

10. DATE OF REVISION OF THE TEXT

30 March 2009

Cafergot Tablets

(Alliance Pharmaceuticals)

1. NAME OF THE MEDICINAL PRODUCT

Cafergot® tablets 1mg

2. QUALITATIVE AND QUANTITATIVE COMPOSITION

Ergotamine tartrate PhEur 1.0mg and caffeine PhEur 100mg.

3. PHARMACEUTICAL FORM

White, round, sugar coated tablets

4. CLINICAL PARTICULARS

4.1 Therapeutic indications

Acute attacks of migraine and migraine variants unresponsive to simple analgesics.

4.2 Posology and method of administration

Adults:

There is considerable inter-individual variation in the sensitivity of patients to ergotamine. Care should therefore be exercised in selecting the optimum therapeutic dose for an individual patient which will not give rise to unwanted effects, either acutely or chronically. The maximum recommended dosages should not be exceeded and ergotamine treatment should not be administered at intervals of less than 4 days.

For maximum efficacy, the optimal dose (in the preferred presentation) should be administered immediately prodromal symptoms are experienced.

One or two tablets taken at the first warning of an attack are normally sufficient to obtain migraine relief. Some individuals may require higher dosages which should never exceed 4 tablets (4mg ergotamine) in 24 hours. It is essential to use the minimum effective dose.

The maximum recommended weekly dose of 8 tablets (8mg ergotamine) should not be exceeded.

Children under 12 years: *Not recommended.*

Elderly: Whilst there is no evidence to suggest that the elderly require different dosages of Cafergot, the contra-indications of this drug are common in the elderly, e.g. coronary heart disease, renal impairment, hepatic impairment and severe hypertension. Caution should therefore be exercised when prescribing for this age group.

4.3 Contraindications

Known hypersensitivity to ergot alkaloids, caffeine, or any other components of the formulation.

Patients with impaired peripheral circulation, obliterative vascular disease, coronary heart disease, inadequately controlled hypertension, septic conditions or shock. Impaired hepatic or renal function, temporal arteritis and patients with hemiplegic or basilar migraine are also contraindicated.

Pregnancy or nursing mothers.

Concomitant treatment with macrolide antibiotics, HIV-protease or reverse-transcriptase inhibitors, azole antifungals (see 4.5 Interactions with other medicinal products and other forms of interaction).

Concomitant treatment with vasoconstrictive agents (including ergot alkaloids, sumatriptan and other $5HT_1$-receptor agonists (see 4.5 Interactions with other medicinal products and other forms of interaction).

4.4 Special warnings and precautions for use

Cafergot is only indicated for the treatment of acute migraine attacks and not for prevention.

Continued daily use of Cafergot or use in excess of the recommended doses must be avoided since this may cause vasospasm.

Owing to its vasoconstrictor properties, ergotamine may cause myocardial ischaemia or, in rare cases, infarction, even in patients with no known history of coronary heart disease.

Patients who are being treated with Cafergot should be informed of the maximum doses allowed and of the first symptoms of over dosage: hypoaesthesia, paraesthesia (eg numbness, tingling) in the fingers and toes, non-migraine-related nausea and vomiting, and symptoms of myocardial ischaemia (e.g. precordial pain). If symptoms such as tingling in the fingers or toes occur, the drug should be discontinued at once and the physician consulted.

If contrary to recommendations ergotamine-containing drugs are used excessively over years, they may induce fibrotic changes, in particular of the pleura and retroperitoneum. There have also been rare reports of fibrotic changes of the cardiac valves.

The occurrence of drug-induced headaches has been reported during prolonged and uninterrupted treatment with Cafergot.

4.5 Interaction with other medicinal products and other forms of interaction

Ergotism (increased peripheral vasoconstriction)

Several drugs increase the risk of ergotism (vasoconstriction, convulsions, other CNS and GI effects) and concomitant use of the following with Cafergot should be avoided (see section 4.3): -

Antibacterials

- Macrolides (eg erythromycin, azithromycin, clarithromycin, spiramycin) or telithromycin
- quinupristin/dalfopristin
- tetracycline

Antifungals

- Imidazoles (eg ketaconazole, miconazole)
- Triazoles (eg itraconazole, posaconazole, voriconazole)
- Antivirals (eg amprenavir, indinavir, nelfinavir, ritonavir, saquinavir. atazinavir, efavirenz)

$5HT_1$ agonists

- Avoid Cafergot for 6 hours after almotriptan, rizatriptan, sumatriptan or zolmitriptan. Avoid almotriptan, rizatriptan, sumatriptan or zolmitriptan for 24 hours after Cafergot.
- Avoid Cafergot for 24 hours after eletriptan or frovatriptan. Avoid eletriptan or frovatriptan for 24 hours after Cafergot.

Cimetidine

Sympathomimetic agents

Beta-blockers

Other vasoconstrictors - excessive nicotine may enhance vasoconstriction

Other

Anaesthetics

- Halothane reduces the effect of ergometrine on the parturient uterus

Antidepressants

- Reboxetine - possible increase in hypertension in association with ergot

4.6 Pregnancy and lactation

Ergotamine-containing products are contraindicated in pregnancy due to oxytocic and vasoconstrictor effects on the placenta and umbilical cord.

Ergotamine is excreted in breast milk and may cause symptoms of vomiting, diarrhoea, weak pulse and unstable blood pressure in infants. Thus, Cafergot are contraindicated in nursing mothers.

4.7 Effects on ability to drive and use machines

Dizziness and feelings of anxiety (trembling, sweating etc) have been reported with Cafergot. If a patient is affected they should not drive, operate machinery or take part in activities where these reactions may put themselves or others at risk.

4.8 Undesirable effects

The caffeine component of Cafergot may give rise to unwanted stimulant effects.

Side effects of Cafergot are related in the main to the ergotamine component.

The most common of all side-effects are nausea and vomiting. Depending on the dose of ergotamine, signs and symptoms of vasoconstriction may occur.

Adverse reactions (Table 1) are ranked under heading of frequency, the most frequent first, using the following convention: very common (greater than or equal to 1 in 10); common (less than or equal to 1 in 100, less than 1 in 10); uncommon (greater than or equal to 1 in 1,000, less than 1 in 100); rare (greater than or less than 1 in 10,000, less than 1 in 1,000) very rare (less than 1 in 10,000), including isolated reports.

Table 1

Immune system disorders
Rare: Hypersensitivity reactions[1]
Nervous system disorders
Common: Dizziness
Uncommon: Paraesthesia (e.g. tingling), hypoaesthesia (e.g numbness)
Ear and labyrinth disorders
Rare: Vertigo
Cardiac disorders
Uncommon: Cyanosis
Rare: Bradycardia, tachycardia
Very rare: Myocardial ischaemia, myocardial infarction
Vascular disorders
Uncommon: Peripheral vasoconstriction
Rare: Increase in blood pressure
Very rare: Gangrene
Respiratory, thoracic and mediastinal disorders
Rare: Dyspnoea
Gastrointestinal disorders
Common: Nausea and vomiting (not migraine related), abdominal pain
Uncommon: Diarrhoea
Skin and subcutaneous tissue disorders
Uncommon: Pain in extremities
Rare: Myalgia
General disorders and administration site conditions
Uncommon: Weakness in extremities
Investigations
Rare: Absence of pulse
Injury, poisoning and procedural complications
Rare: Ergotism[2]

1. Hypersensitivity reactions such as skin rash, face oedema, urticaria and dyspnoea.

2. Ergotism is defined as an intense arterial vasoconstriction, producing signs and symptoms of vascular ischemia of the extremities and other tissues (such as renal or cerebral vasospasm)

Rare cases of intestinal ischaemia have been associated with chronic use and overuse of ergotamine-containing preparations. Rarely, headache may be provoked either by chronic overdosage or by rapid withdrawal of the product.

Excessive use of ergotamine-containing products for prolonged periods may result in fibrotic changes, in particular of the pleura and retroperitoneum. Rare cases of fibrosis of cardiac valves have also been reported.

The occurrence of drug induced headaches has been reported during prolonged and uninterrupted treatment with Cafergot (see 4.4 Special Warnings and Precautions).

4.9 Overdose

Symptoms: Nausea, vomiting, drowsiness, confusion, tachycardia, dizziness, respiratory depression, hypotension, convulsion, shock, coma and symptoms and complications of ergotism.

Ergotism is defined as an intense arterial vasoconstriction, producing signs and symptoms of vascular ischemia of the extremities such as tingling, numbness and pain in the extremities, cyanosis, absence of pulse and if the condition is allowed to progress untreated, gangrene may result. Furthermore ergotism can also involve signs and symptoms of vascular ischemia of other tissues such as renal or cerebral vasospasm. Most cases of ergotism are associated with chronic intoxication and/or overdose.

Treatment: should be directed to the elimination of ingested material by aspiration and gastric lavage. Treatment should be symptomatic. In the event of severe vasospastic reactions, i.v. administration of a peripheral vasodilator such as nitroprusside, phentolamine or dihydralazine, local application of warmth to the affected area and nursing care to prevent tissue damage are recommended. In the event of coronary constriction, appropriate treatment such as nitroglycerin should be initiated.

5. PHARMACOLOGICAL PROPERTIES

5.1 Pharmacodynamic properties

Ergotamine is a highly vasoactive ergot alkaloid having characteristically complex pharmacological actions. It is a partial tryptaminic agonist in certain blood vessels and both a partial agonist and antagonist of α-adrenergic receptors of blood vessels.

Although its exact mode of action in migraine is not known, its therapeutic effects have been attributed to its ability to cause vasoconstriction, thereby eliminating the painful dilation/pulsation of branches of the external carotid artery.

5.2 Pharmacokinetic properties

There is great interindividual variation in the absorption of ergotamine in patients and volunteers. Bioavailability is of the order of 5% or less by oral or rectal administration. After im or iv administration, plasma concentrations decay in a bi-exponential fashion. The elimination half life is 2 to 2.5 hours and clearance is about 0.68L/h/kg. Metabolism occurs in the liver. The major enzyme involved in the metabolism of ergotamine is Cytochrome P450 (CYP) 3A4. The primary route of excretion is biliary.

5.3 Preclinical safety data

There are no pre-clinical data of relevance to the prescriber which are additional to those already included in other sections of the Summary of Product Characteristics.

6. PHARMACEUTICAL PARTICULARS

6.1 List of excipients

Tartaric acid, gelatin, stearic acid, lactose, starch, talc, gum acacia, sugar, and carnauba wax.

6.2 Incompatibilities

None

6.3 Shelf life

2 years

6.4 Special precautions for storage

None

6.5 Nature and contents of container

Cartons of 30 tablets in opaque aluminium/PVdC blister packs.

6.6 Special precautions for disposal and other handling

None

7. MARKETING AUTHORISATION HOLDER

Alliance Pharmaceuticals Ltd

Avonbridge House

Bath Road

Chippenham

Wiltshire

SN15 2BB

8. MARKETING AUTHORISATION NUMBER(S)

PL 16853/0004

9. DATE OF FIRST AUTHORISATION/RENEWAL OF THE AUTHORISATION

25 June 1998

10. DATE OF REVISION OF THE TEXT

30 March 2009

Calceos

(Galen Limited)

1. NAME OF THE MEDICINAL PRODUCT

CALCEOS Chewable Tablets.

2. QUALITATIVE AND QUANTITATIVE COMPOSITION

Calcium Carbonate 1250mg (i.e. 500mg or 12.5mmol of elemental calcium).

Colecalciferol (INN) (Vitamin D_3) 10μg (corresponding to 400IU of Vitamin D_3).

For a full list of excipients, see section 6.1.

3. PHARMACEUTICAL FORM

Chewable tablets, for oral administration.

4. CLINICAL PARTICULARS

4.1 Therapeutic indications

Vitamin D and calcium deficiency correction in the elderly. Vitamin and calcium supplement as an adjunct to specific therapy for osteoporosis.

4.2 Posology and method of administration

Oral use. For adults only. One tablet, twice per day. Chew the tablets and drink a glass of water.

4.3 Contraindications

Hypersensitivity to one of the constituents. Hypercalcaemia as a result of hyperparathyroidism (primary or secondary), hypercalciuria, calcium lithiasis, tissue calcification (nephrocalcinosis). Vitamin D overdose. Myeloma and bone metastases. Renal insufficiency (creatinine clearance less than 20ml/min). Calceos tablets are also contra-indicated in patients where prolonged immobilisation is accompanied by hypercalcaemia and/or hypercalciuria. In these cases, treatments should only be resumed when the patient becomes mobile.

This product contains partially hydrogenated soybean oil. Patients should not take this medicinal product if they are allergic to peanut or soya.

4.4 Special warnings and precautions for use

Calculate the total Vitamin D intake in case of treatment with another drug containing this vitamin.

The following may be important in patient monitoring: plasma calcium and urinary calcium determinations.

Precautions:

Plasma and urinary calcium levels should be monitored regularly.

In the elderly, renal function must be monitored regularly.

In patients with renal failure, dosage has to be adapted according to the creatinine clearance.

In case of long term treatment, the urinary calcium excretion must be monitored and treatment must be reduced or momentarily suspended if urinary calcium exceeds 7.5 to 9mmol/24h (300 to 360mg/24h).

This product contains sorbitol (E420) and sucrose. Patients with rare hereditary problems of fructose intolerance, glucose-galactose malabsorption or sucrase-isomaltase insufficiency should not take this medicine.

The sucrose in this product may be harmful to teeth if taken chronically, e.g. for two weeks or more.

4.5 Interaction with other medicinal products and other forms of interaction

In case of treatment with digitalis glycosides: risk of cardiac arrhythmias. Clinical surveillance is required and possibly electrocardiographic and plasma calcium monitoring are recommended.

Associations to be taken into account in the case of treatment with thiazide diuretics: risk of hypercalcaemia by decreasing urinary calcium excretion.

Calcium may impair the absorption of tetracyclines, etidronate, fluoride and iron. At least 3 hours should intervene between taking Calceos and these agents.

4.6 Pregnancy and lactation

Normal requirements for calcium and vitamin D are raised during pregnancy and lactation. If supplementation is necessary, it should be given at a different time to iron supplements. Calcium is excreted in breast milk but not sufficiently to produce an adverse effect in the infant.

4.7 Effects on ability to drive and use machines

None known.

4.8 Undesirable effects

- Hypercalciuria in cases of prolonged treatment at high doses, exceptionally hypercalcaemia.
- Hypophosphataemia
- Nausea
- Mild gastro-intestinal disturbances such as constipation can occur but are infrequent.
- This product contains sucrose. May be harmful to teeth if taken chronically, e.g. for two weeks or more.

4.9 Overdose

Clinical signs: Anorexia, intense thirst, nausea, vomiting, polyuria, polydipsia, dehydration, hypertension, vasomotor disorders, constipation.

Laboratory signs: Hypercalcaemia, hypercalciuria, impaired renal function tests.

Emergency treatment:

- Stop all calcium and vitamin D supplements.
- Rehydration and, according to the severity of the intoxication, isolated or combined use of diuretics, corticosteroids, calcitonin, peritoneal dialysis.

5. PHARMACOLOGICAL PROPERTIES

5.1 Pharmacodynamic properties

Calceos is a fixed combination of calcium and vitamin D. The high calcium and vitamin D concentration in each dose unit facilitates absorption of a sufficient quantity of calcium with a limited number of doses. Vitamin D is involved in calcium-phosphorus metabolism. It allows active absorption of calcium and phosphorus from the intestine and their uptake by bone.

5.2 Pharmacokinetic properties

Calcium Carbonate:

Absorption:

In the stomach, calcium carbonate releases calcium ion as a function of pH. Calcium is essentially absorbed in the proximal part of the small intestine. The rate of absorption of calcium in the gastrointestinal tract is of the order of 30% of the dose ingested.

Elimination:

Calcium is eliminated in sweat and gastrointestinal secretions. The urinary calcium excretion depends on the glomerular filtration and rate of tubular resorption of calcium.

Vitamin D_3:

Vitamin D_3 is absorbed from the intestine and transported by protein binding in the blood to the liver (first hydroxylation) and to the kidney (second hydroxylation).

Non-hydroxylated Vitamin D_3 is stored in reserve compartments such as muscle and adipose tissues. Its plasma half-life is of the order of several days; it is eliminated in faeces and urine.

5.3 Preclinical safety data

None stated.

6. PHARMACEUTICAL PARTICULARS

6.1 List of excipients

Xylitol

Sorbitol (E420)

Povidone

Lemon flavouring*

Magnesium stearate

* Composition of the lemon flavouring: essential oils of lemon, orange and litsea cubeba, maltodextrin, acacia gum and sodium citrate.

The colecalciferol is present as a concentrate powder that also contains:

DL-alpha-Tocopherol

Partially hydrogenated soybean oil

Gelatin

Sucrose

Corn starch

6.2 Incompatibilities

None known.

6.3 Shelf life

36 months.

6.4 Special precautions for storage

None.

6.5 Nature and contents of container

Polypropylene tube and polyethylene stopper with silica gel desiccant containing 10, 15, 30, 60 and 100 tablets. Packs of 1, 2, 4 or 10 tubes in card outers.

6.6 Special precautions for disposal and other handling

None.

7. MARKETING AUTHORISATION HOLDER

Laboratoire Innotech International

22 avenue Aristide Briand

94110 Arcueil

France

8. MARKETING AUTHORISATION NUMBER(S)

PL 19152/0001

9. DATE OF FIRST AUTHORISATION/RENEWAL OF THE AUTHORISATION

31 October 2001

10. DATE OF REVISION OF THE TEXT

12 March 2009

Calcichew 500mg Chewable Tablets

(Shire Pharmaceuticals Limited)

1. NAME OF THE MEDICINAL PRODUCT

Calcichew 500mg Chewable Tablets

2. QUALITATIVE AND QUANTITATIVE COMPOSITION

Per tablet: Calcium carbonate 1250mg equivalent to 500mg of elemental calcium.

Contains sorbitol, 390mg; isomalt, 62mg; and aspartame, 1mg.

For a full list of excipients see Section 6.1.

3. PHARMACEUTICAL FORM

Chewable tablet.

Round, white, uncoated and convex tablets. May have small specks.

4. CLINICAL PARTICULARS

4.1 Therapeutic indications

Calcichew 500mg Chewable Tablets are to be chewed as a supplemental source of calcium in the correction of dietary deficiencies or when normal requirements are high.

Calcichew 500mg Chewable Tablets may be used as an adjunct to conventional therapy in the prevention and treatment of osteoporosis. They may be used as a phosphate binding agent in the management of renal failure in patients on renal dialysis.

4.2 Posology and method of administration

Oral.

Adults and elderly:

Adjunct to osteoporosis therapy 2 to 3 tablets daily.

Dietary deficiency 2 to 3 tablets daily.

Osteomalacia 2 to 6 tablets daily.

Children:

Dietary deficiency 2 to 3 tablets daily.

Phosphate Binder:

Adults, children and elderly Dose as required by the individual patient depending on serum phosphate level.

The tablets should be taken just before, during or just after each meal. Tablets may be chewed or sucked.

4.3 Contraindications

- Severe hypercalcaemia and hypercalciuria, for example in hyperparathyroidism, vitamin D overdosage, decalcifying tumours such as plasmocytoma and skeletal metastases, in severe renal failure untreated by renal dialysis and in osteoporosis due to immobilisation.
- Nephrolithiasis
- Hypersensitivity to the active substance or to any of the excipients.

4.4 Special warnings and precautions for use

Calcichew 500mg chewable tablets contain aspartame (a source of phenylalanine) and should be avoided by patients with phenylketonuria.

Calcichew 500 mg Chewable Tablets contain sorbitol (E420) and isomalt (E953). Patients with rare hereditary problems of fructose intolerance, glucose-galactose malabsorption or sucrase-isomaltase insufficiency should not take this medicine.

In renal insufficiency the tablets should be given only under controlled conditions for hyperphosphataemia. Caution should be exercised in patients with a history of renal calculi.

During high dose therapy and especially during concomitant treatment with vitamin D, there is a risk of hypercalcaemia with subsequent kidney function impairment. In these patients, serum calcium levels should be followed and renal function should be monitored.

4.5 Interaction with other medicinal products and other forms of interaction

Thiazide diuretics reduce the urinary excretion of calcium. Due to increased risk of hypercalcaemia, serum calcium should be regularly monitored during concomitant use of thiazide diuretics.

Systemic corticosteroids reduce calcium absorption. During concomitant use, it may be necessary to increase the dose of Calcichew 500mg Chewable Tablets.

Calcium carbonate may interfere with the absorption of concomitantly administered tetracycline preparations. For this reason, tetracycline preparations should be administered at least two hours before, or four to six hours after, oral intake of calcium.

Hypercalcaemia may increase the toxicity of cardiac glycosides during treatment with calcium. Patients should be monitored with regard to electrocardiogram (ECG) and serum calcium levels.

If a bisphosphonate or sodium fluoride is used concomitantly, this preparation should be administered at least three hours before the intake of Calcichew 500mg Chewable Tablets since gastrointestinal absorption may be reduced.

Oxalic acid (found in spinach and rhubarb) and phytic acid (found in whole cereals) may inhibit calcium absorption through formation of insoluble calcium salts. The patient should not take calcium products within two hours of eating foods high in oxalic acid and phytic acid.

4.6 Pregnancy and lactation

The adequate daily intake (including food and supplementation) for normal pregnant and lactating women is 1000-1300 mg calcium. During pregnancy, the daily intake of calcium should not exceed 1500 mg. Significant amounts of calcium are secreted in milk during lactation. Calcichew 500mg Chewable Tablets can be used during pregnancy in case of a calcium deficiency.

4.7 Effects on ability to drive and use machines

There are no data about the effect of this product on driving capacity. An effect is, however, unlikely.

4.8 Undesirable effects

Adverse reactions are listed below, by system organ class and frequency. Frequencies are defined as: uncommon (>1/1,000, <1/100) or rare (>1/10,000, <1/1,000).

Metabolism and nutrition disorders

Uncommon: Hypercalcaemia and hypercalciuria.

Gastrointestinal disorders

Rare: Constipation, flatulence, nausea, abdominal pain and diarrhoea.

Skin and subcutaneous disorders

Rare: Pruritus, rash and urticaria.

4.9 Overdose

Overdose can lead to hypercalcaemia. Symptoms of hypercalcaemia may include anorexia, thirst, nausea, vomiting, constipation, abdominal pain, muscle weakness, fatigue, mental disturbances, polydipsia, polyuria, bone pain, nephrocalcinosis, nephrolithiasis and in severe cases, cardiac arrhythmias. Extreme hypercalcaemia may result in coma and death. Persistently high calcium levels may lead to irreversible renal damage and soft tissue calcification.

Treatment of hypercalcaemia: The treatment with calcium must be discontinued. Treatment with thiazide diuretics, lithium, vitamin A, vitamin D and cardiac glycosides must so be discontinued. Treatment: rehydration, and, according to severity of hypercalcaemia, isolated or combined treatment with loop diuretics, bisphosphonates, calcitonin and corticosteroids should be considered. Serum electrolytes, renal function and diuresis must be monitored. In severe cases, ECG and CVP should be followed.

5. PHARMACOLOGICAL PROPERTIES

5.1 Pharmacodynamic properties

Pharmacotherapeutic group: Calcium

ATC-code: A12A A04

An adequate intake of calcium is of importance during growth, pregnancy and breastfeeding.

5.2 Pharmacokinetic properties

Absorption: The amount of calcium absorbed through the gastrointestinal tract is approximately 30% of the swallowed dose.

Distribution and metabolism: 99% of the calcium in the body is concentrated in the hard structure of bones and teeth. The remaining 1% is present in the intra- and extracellular fluids. About 50% of the total blood-calcium content is in the physiologically active ionised form with approximately 10% being complexed to citrate, phosphate or other anions, the remaining 40% being bound to proteins, principally albumin.

Elimination: Calcium is eliminated through faeces, urine and sweat. Renal excretion depends on glomerular filtration and calcium tubular reabsorption.

5.3 Preclinical safety data

There is no information of relevance to the safety assessment in addition to what is stated in other parts of the SmPC.

6. PHARMACEUTICAL PARTICULARS

6.1 List of excipients

Sorbitol (E420)

Povidone

Magnesium stearate

Aspartame (E951)

Orange flavour:

Isomalt (E953)

Flavouring (orange)

Mono, di-fatty acid glycerides

6.2 Incompatibilities

Not applicable.

6.3 Shelf life

3 years.

6.4 Special precautions for storage

Do not store above 30°C.

Keep the container tightly closed.

6.5 Nature and contents of container

Securitainer containing 100 tablets.

6.6 Special precautions for disposal and other handling

No special requirements.

7. MARKETING AUTHORISATION HOLDER

Shire Pharmaceuticals Ltd.

Hampshire International Business Park

Chineham

Basingstoke

Hampshire RG24 8EP

United Kingdom

8. MARKETING AUTHORISATION NUMBER(S)

PL 08557/0003

9. DATE OF FIRST AUTHORISATION/RENEWAL OF THE AUTHORISATION

27 November 1987/27 November 1997

10. DATE OF REVISION OF THE TEXT

18 July 2007

Calcichew D3 Chewable Tablets

(Shire Pharmaceuticals Limited)

1. NAME OF THE MEDICINAL PRODUCT

Calcichew-D_3 Chewable Tablets

2. QUALITATIVE AND QUANTITATIVE COMPOSITION

Per tablet:	Calcium carbonate (equivalent to 500mg of elemental calcium)	1250mg
	Colecalciferol (equivalent to 5 micrograms vitamin D_3)	200iu

Contains sorbitol, 390mg; isomalt, 62mg; aspartame, 1mg; sucrose 0.76mg and soya bean oil, hydrogenated, 0.15mg.

For a full list of excipients see section 6.1.

3. PHARMACEUTICAL FORM

Chewable tablet.

Round, white, uncoated and convex tablets. May have small specks.

4. CLINICAL PARTICULARS

4.1 Therapeutic indications

Calcichew-D_3 Chewable Tablets should be used only as a therapeutic and not as a food supplement when the diet is deficient or when normal requirement of both components is increased.

Calcichew-D_3 Chewable Tablets may be used as an adjunct to specific therapy for osteoporosis or as a therapeutic supplement in established osteomalacia, pregnant patients at high risk of needing such a therapeutic supplementation or malnutrition when dietary intake is less than that required.

4.2 Posology and method of administration

Oral.

Adjunctive therapy in osteoporosis:

One chewable tablet 2-3 times per day

Calcium and vitamin D deficiency:

Adults One chewable tablet 2-3 times per day

Children One chewable tablet 1-2 times per day.

The tablet may be chewed or sucked.

Dosage in hepatic impairment:

No dose adjustment is required.

Dosage in renal impairment:

Calcichew-D_3 chewable tablets should not be used in patients with severe renal impairment.

4.3 Contraindications

- Diseases and/or conditions resulting in hypercalcaemia and/or hypercalciuria
- Nephrolithiasis
- Hypervitaminosis D
- Hypersensitivity to soya or peanut
- Hypersensitivity to the active substances or to any of the excipients

4.4 Special warnings and precautions for use

During long-term treatment, serum calcium levels should be followed and renal function should be monitored through measurement of serum creatinine. Monitoring is especially important in elderly patients on concomitant treatment with cardiac glycosides or diuretics (see section 4.5) and in patients with a high tendency to calculus formation. In case of hypercalcaemia or signs of impaired renal function, the dose should be reduced or the treatment discontinued.

Vitamin D should be used with caution in patients with impairment of renal function and the effect on calcium and phosphate levels should be monitored. The risk of soft tissue calcification should be taken into account. In patients with severe renal insufficiency, vitamin D in the form of colecalciferol is not metabolised normally and other forms of vitamin D should be used (see section 4.3, contraindications).

Calcichew-D_3 chewable tablets should be prescribed with caution to patients suffering from sarcoidosis because of the risk of increased metabolism of vitamin D to its active form. These patients should be monitored with regard to the calcium content in serum and urine.

Calcichew-D_3 Chewable Tablets should be used with caution in immobilised patients with osteoporosis due to the increased risk of hypercalcaemia.

The content of colecalciferol (200 IU) in Calcichew-D_3 Chewable Tablets should be considered when prescribing other medicinal products containing vitamin D. Additional doses of calcium or vitamin D should be taken under close medical supervision. In such cases it is necessary to monitor serum calcium levels and urinary calcium excretion frequently.

Calcichew-D_3 Chewable Tablets contain aspartame (a source of phenylalanine) which may be harmful for people with phenylketonuria.

Calcichew-D_3 Chewable Tablets contain sorbitol (E420), isomalt and sucrose. Patients with rare hereditary problems of fructose intolerance, glucose-galactose malabsorption or sucrase-isomaltase insufficiency should not take this medicine.

4.5 Interaction with other medicinal products and other forms of interaction

Thiazide diuretics reduce the urinary excretion of calcium. Due to increased risk of hypercalcaemia, serum calcium should be regularly monitored during concomitant use of thiazide diuretics.

Systemic corticosteroids reduce calcium absorption. During concomitant use, it may be necessary to increase the dose of Calcichew-D_3 Chewable Tablets.

Simultaneous treatment with ion exchange resins such as cholestyramine or laxatives such as paraffin oil may reduce the gastrointestinal absorption of vitamin D.

Calcium carbonate may interfere with the absorption of concomitantly administered tetracycline preparations. For this reason, tetracycline preparations should be administered at least two hours before, or four to six hours after, oral intake of calcium.

Hypercalcaemia may increase the toxicity of cardiac glycosides during treatment with calcium and vitamin D. Patients should be monitored with regard to electrocardiogram (ECG) and serum calcium levels.

If a bisphosphonate or sodium fluoride is used concomitantly, this preparation should be administered at least three hours before the intake of Calcichew-D_3 Chewable Tablets since gastrointestinal absorption may be reduced.

Oxalic acid (found in spinach and rhubarb) and phytic acid (found in whole cereals) may inhibit calcium absorption through formation of insoluble calcium salts. The patient should not take calcium products within two hours of eating foods high in oxalic acid and phytic acid.

4.6 Pregnancy and lactation

Pregnancy

During pregnancy the daily intake should not exceed 1500 mg calcium and 600 IU vitamin D). Studies in animals have shown reproductive toxicity with high doses of vitamin D. In pregnant women, overdoses of calcium and vitamin D should be avoided as permanent hypercalcaemia has been related to adverse effects on the developing foetus. There are no indications that vitamin D at therapeutic doses is teratogenic in humans. Calcichew-D_3 Chewable Tablets can be used during pregnancy, in case of a calcium and vitamin D deficiency.

Lactation

Calcichew-D_3 Chewable Tablets can be used during breast-feeding. Calcium and vitamin D_3 pass into breast milk. This should be considered when giving additional vitamin D to the child.

4.7 Effects on ability to drive and use machines

There are no data about the effect of this product on driving capacity. An effect is, however, unlikely.

4.8 Undesirable effects

Adverse reactions are listed below, by system organ class and frequency. Frequencies are defined as: uncommon ($>1/1{,}000$, $<1/100$) or rare ($>1/10{,}000$, $<1/1{,}000$).

Metabolism and nutrition disorders

Uncommon: Hypercalcaemia and hypercalciuria.

Gastrointestinal disorders

Rare: Constipation, flatulence, nausea, abdominal pain and diarrhoea.

Skin and subcutaneous disorders

Rare: Pruritus, rash and urticaria.

4.9 Overdose

Overdose can lead to hypervitaminosis D and hypercalcaemia. Symptoms of hypercalcaemia may include anorexia, thirst, nausea, vomiting, constipation, abdominal pain, muscle weakness, fatigue, mental disturbances, polydipsia, polyuria, bone pain, nephrocalcinosis, nephrolithiasis and in severe cases, cardiac arrhythmias. Extreme hypercalcaemia may result in coma and death. Persistently high calcium levels may lead to irreversible renal damage and soft tissue calcification.

Treatment of hypercalcaemia: The treatment with calcium and vitamin D must be discontinued. Treatment with thiazide diuretics, lithium, vitamin A and cardiac glycosides must also be discontinued. Teatment is rehydration, and, according to severity of hypercalcaemia, isolated or combined treatment with loop diuretics, bisphosphonates, calcitonin and corticosteroids should be considered. Serum electrolytes, renal function and diuresis must be monitored. In severe cases, ECG and CVP should be followed.

5. PHARMACOLOGICAL PROPERTIES

5.1 Pharmacodynamic properties

Pharmacotherapeutic group: Mineral supplements

ATC code: A12AX

Vitamin D increases the intestinal absorption of calcium.

Administration of calcium and vitamin D_3 counteracts the increase of parathyroid hormone (PTH) which is caused by calcium deficiency and which causes increased bone resorption.

A clinical study of institutionalised patients suffering from vitamin D deficiency indicated that a daily intake of two tablets of calcium 500mg/vitamin D 400 IU for six months normalised the value of the 25-hydroxylated metabolite of vitamin D_3 and reduced secondary hyperparathyroidism and alkaline phosphatases.

5.2 Pharmacokinetic properties

Calcium

Absorption: The amount of calcium absorbed through the gastrointestinal tract is approximately 30% of the swallowed dose.

Distribution and metabolism: 99% of the calcium in the body is concentrated in the hard structure of bones and teeth. The remaining 1% is present in the intra- and extracellular fluids. About 50% of the total blood-calcium content is in the physiologically active ionised form with approximately 10% being complexed to citrate, phosphate or other anions, the remaining 40% being bound to proteins, principally albumin.

Elimination: Calcium is eliminated through faeces, urine and sweat. Renal excretion depends on glomerular filtration and calcium tubular reabsorption.

Vitamin D

Absorption: Vitamin D is easily absorbed in the small intestine.

Distribution and metabolism: Colecalciferol and its metabolites circulate in the blood bound to a specific globulin.

Colecalciferol is converted in the liver by hydroxylation to the active form 25-hydroxycolecalciferol. It is then further converted in the kidneys to 1,25-hydroxycolecalciferol; 1,25-hydroxycolecalciferol is the metabolite responsible for increasing calcium absorption. Vitamin D which is not metabolised is stored in adipose and muscle tissues.

Elimination: Vitamin D is excreted in faeces and urine.

5.3 Preclinical safety data
At doses far higher than the human therapeutic range teratogenicity has been observed in animal studies. There is no further information of relevance to the safety assessment in addition to what is stated in other parts of the SmPC.

6. PHARMACEUTICAL PARTICULARS

6.1 List of excipients
Sorbitol (E420)

Povidone

Isomalt (E953)

Flavour (orange)

Magnesium stearate

Aspartame (E951)

Mono, di-fatty acid glycerides

Sucrose

Gelatin

Soya-bean oil, hydrogenated

Tocopherol

Maize starch

6.2 Incompatibilities
Not applicable.

6.3 Shelf life
3 years.

6.4 Special precautions for storage
Do not store above 30°C. Keep the container tightly closed.

6.5 Nature and contents of container
White HD Polyethylene containers with a primary tamper-evident seal and secondary re-sealable closure containing 60 and 100 tablets.

Not all pack sizes may be marketed.

6.6 Special precautions for disposal and other handling
No special requirements.

7. MARKETING AUTHORISATION HOLDER
Shire Pharmaceuticals Ltd.

Hampshire International Business Park

Chineham

Basingstoke

Hampshire RG24 8EP

United Kingdom

8. MARKETING AUTHORISATION NUMBER(S)
PL 08557/0021

9. DATE OF FIRST AUTHORISATION/RENEWAL OF THE AUTHORISATION
26 November 1991

10. DATE OF REVISION OF THE TEXT
April 2007

Calcichew D3 Forte Chewable Tablets

(Shire Pharmaceuticals Limited)

1. NAME OF THE MEDICINAL PRODUCT
Calcichew-D_3 Forte Chewable Tablets

2. QUALITATIVE AND QUANTITATIVE COMPOSITION
Per tablet: Calcium carbonate 1250 mg

(equivalent to 500 mg of elemental calcium)

Colecalciferol 400 IU

(equivalent to 10 micrograms vitamin D_3)

Contains sorbitol, 390mg; isomalt, 49.90mg; aspartame, 1mg; sucrose, 1.52mg; and soya bean oil, hydrogenated, 0.30mg. For a full list of excipients, see Section 6.1.

3. PHARMACEUTICAL FORM
Chewable tablet.

Round, white, uncoated and convex tablets. May have small specks.

4. CLINICAL PARTICULARS

4.1 Therapeutic indications
The treatment and prevention of vitamin D/calcium deficiency (characterised by raised serum alkaline phosphatase levels associated with increased bone loss, raised levels of serum PTH and lowered 25-hydroxyvitamin D) particularly in the housebound and institutionalised elderly subjects.

The supplementation of vitamin D and calcium as an adjunct to specific therapy for osteoporosis, in pregnancy, in established vitamin D dependent osteomalacia, and in other situations requiring therapeutic supplementation of malnutrition.

4.2 Posology and method of administration
Oral.

Adults and elderly:

2 chewable tablets per day, preferably one tablet morning and evening.

The tablet may be chewed or sucked.

Dosage in hepatic impairment:

No dose adjustment is required.

Dosage in renal impairment:

Calcichew-D_3 Forte Chewable Tablets should not be used in patients with severe renal impairment.

4.3 Contraindications

- Diseases and/or conditions resulting in hypercalcaemia and/or hypercalciuria
- Nephrolithiasis
- Hypervitaminosis D
- Hypersensitivity to soya or peanut
- Hypersensitivity to the active substances or to any of the excipients

4.4 Special warnings and precautions for use
During long-term treatment, serum calcium levels should be followed and renal function should be monitored through measurements of serum creatinine. Monitoring is especially important in elderly patients on concomitant treatment with cardiac glycosides or diuretics (see section 4.5) and in patients with a high tendency to calculus formation. In case of hypercalcaemia or signs of impaired renal function the dose should be reduced or the treatment discontinued.

Vitamin D should be used with caution in patients with impairment of renal function and the effect on calcium and phosphate levels should be monitored. The risk of soft tissue calcification should be taken into account. In patients with severe renal insufficiency, vitamin D in the form of colecalciferol is not metabolised normally and other forms of vitamin D should be used (see section 4.3, contra-indications).

Calcichew-D_3 Forte Chewable Tablets should be prescribed with caution to patients suffering from sarcoidosis because of the risk of increased metabolism of vitamin D to its active form. These patients should be monitored with regard to the calcium content in serum and urine.

Calcichew-D_3 Forte Chewable Tablets should be used with caution in immobilised patients with osteoporosis due to the increased risk of hypercalcaemia.

The content of colecalciferol (400 IU) in Calcichew-D_3 Forte Chewable Tablets should be considered when prescribing other medicinal products containing vitamin D. Additional doses of calcium or vitamin D should be taken under close medical supervision. In such cases it is necessary to monitor serum calcium levels and urinary calcium excretion frequently.

Calcichew-D_3 ForteChewable Tablets contain aspartame (a source of phenylalanine) which may be harmful for people with phenylketonuria.

Calcichew-D_3 ForteChewable Tablets contain sorbitol (E420), isomalt and sucrose. Patients with rare hereditary problems of fructose intolerance, glucose-galactose malabsorption or sucrase-isomaltase insufficiency should not take this medicine.

Calcichew-D_3 ForteChewable Tablets are not intended for use in children.

4.5 Interaction with other medicinal products and other forms of interaction
Thiazide diuretics reduce the urinary excretion of calcium. Due to increased risk of hypercalcaemia, serum calcium should be regularly monitored during concomitant use of thiazide diuretics.

Systemic corticosteroids reduce calcium absorption. During concomitant use, it may be necessary to increase the dose of Calcichew-D_3 Forte Chewable Tablets.

Simultaneous treatment with ion exchange resins such as cholestyramine or laxatives such as paraffin oil may reduce the gastrointestinal absorption of vitamin D.

Calcium carbonate may interfere with the absorption of concomitantly administered tetracycline preparations. For this reason, tetracycline preparations should be administered at least two hours before, or four to six hours after, oral intake of calcium.

Hypercalcaemia may increase the toxicity of cardiac glycosides during treatment with calcium and vitamin D. Patients should be monitored with regard to electrocardiogram (ECG) and serum calcium levels.

If a bisphosphonate or sodium fluoride is used concomitantly, this preparation should be administered at least three hours before the intake of Calcichew-D_3 Forte Chewable Tablets since gastrointestinal absorption may be reduced.

Oxalic acid (found in spinach and rhubarb) and phytic acid (found in whole cereals) may inhibit calcium absorption through formation of insoluble calcium salts. The patient should not take calcium products within two hours of eating foods high in oxalic acid and phytic acid.

4.6 Pregnancy and lactation

Pregnancy

During pregnancy the daily intake should not exceed 1500 mg calcium and 600 IU colecalciferol (15μg vitamin D). Studies in animals have shown reproductive toxicity with high doses of vitamin D. In pregnant women, overdoses of calcium and vitamin D should be avoided as permanent hypercalcaemia has been related to adverse effects on the developing foetus. There are no indications that vitamin D at therapeutic doses is teratogenic in humans. Calcichew-D_3 Forte Chewable Tablets can be used during pregnancy, in case of a calcium and vitamin D deficiency.

Lactation

Calcichew-D_3 Forte Chewable Tablets can be used during breast-feeding. Calcium and vitamin D_3 pass into breast milk. This should be considered when giving additional vitamin D to the child.

4.7 Effects on ability to drive and use machines
There are no data about the effect of this product on driving capacity. An effect is, however, unlikely.

4.8 Undesirable effects
Adverse reactions are listed below, by system organ class and frequency. Frequencies are defined as: uncommon $>1/1,000$, $<1/100$) or rare $>1/10,000$, $<1/1,000$).

Metabolism and nutrition disorders

Uncommon: Hypercalcaemia and hypercalciuria.

Gastrointestinal disorders

Rare: Constipation, flatulence, nausea, abdominal pain and diarrhoea.

Skin and subcutaneous disorders

Rare: Pruritus, rash and urticaria.

4.9 Overdose
Overdose can lead to hypercalcaemia. Symptoms of hypercalcaemia may include anorexia, thirst, nausea, vomiting, constipation, abdominal pain, muscle weakness, fatigue, mental disturbances, polydipsia, polyuria, bone pain, nephrocalcinosis, nephrolithiasis and in severe cases, cardiac arrhythmias. Extreme hypercalcaemia may result in coma and death. Persistently high calcium levels may lead to irreversible renal damage and soft tissue calcification.

Treatment of hypercalcaemia: The treatment with calcium must be discontinued. Treatment with thiazide diuretics, lithium, vitamin A, vitamin D and cardiac glycosides must also be discontinued. Treatment: rehydration, and, according to severity of hypercalcaemia, isolated or combined treatment with loop diuretics, bisphosphonates, calcitonin and corticosteroids should be considered. Serum electrolytes, renal function and diuresis must be monitored. In severe cases, ECG and CVP should be followed.

5. PHARMACOLOGICAL PROPERTIES

5.1 Pharmacodynamic properties
Pharmacotherapeutic group: Mineral supplements

ATC code: A12AX

Vitamin D increases the intestinal absorption of calcium.

Administration of calcium and vitamin D_3 counteracts the increase of parathyroid hormone (PTH), which is caused by calcium deficiency and which causes increased bone resorption.

A clinical study of institutionalised patients suffering from vitamin D deficiency indicated that a daily intake of two tablets of Calcichew-D_3 Forte chewable tablets for six months normalised the value of the 25-hydroxylated metabolite of vitamin D_3 and reduced secondary hyperparathyroidism and alkaline phosphatases.

An 18 month double-blind, placebo controlled study including 3270 institutionalised women aged 84+/- 6 years who received supplementation of vitamin D (800 IU/day) and calcium phosphate (corresponding to 1200 mg/day of elemental calcium), showed a significant decrease of PTH secretion. After 18 months, an "intent-to treat" analysis showed 80 hip fractures in the calcium-vitamin D group and 110 hip fractures in the placebo group (p=0.004). A follow-up study after 36 months showed 137 women with at least one hip fracture in the calcium-vitamin D group (n=1176) and 178 in the placebo group (n=1127) ($p \leqslant 0.02$).

5.2 Pharmacokinetic properties

Calcium

Absorption: The amount of calcium absorbed through the gastrointestinal tract is approximately 30% of the swallowed dose.

Distribution and metabolism: 99% of the calcium in the body is concentrated in the hard structure of bones and teeth. The remaining 1% is present in the intra- and extracellular fluids. About 50% of the total blood-calcium content is in the physiologically active ionised form with approximately 10% being complexed to citrate, phosphate or other anions, the remaining 40% being bound to proteins, principally albumin.

Elimination: Calcium is eliminated through faeces, urine and sweat. Renal excretion depends on glomerular filtration and calcium tubular reabsorption.

Vitamin D

Absorption: Vitamin D is easily absorbed in the small intestine.

Distribution and metabolism: Colecalciferol and its metabolites circulate in the blood bound to a specific globulin. Colecalciferol is converted in the liver by hydroxylation to the active form 25-hydroxycholecalciferol. It is then further converted in the kidneys to 1,25-hydroxycholecalciferol; 1,25-hydroxycholecalciferol is the metabolite responsible for increasing calcium absorption. Vitamin D, which is not metabolised, is stored in adipose and muscle tissues.

Elimination: Vitamin D is excreted in faeces and urine.

5.3 Preclinical safety data

At doses far higher than the human therapeutic range teratogenicity has been observed in animal studies. There is no further information of relevance to the safety assessment in addition to what is stated in other parts of the SmPC.

6. PHARMACEUTICAL PARTICULARS

6.1 List of excipients

Sorbitol E420

Povidone

Isomalt (E953)

Flavouring (lemon)

Fatty acid mono- and diglycerides

Aspartame (E951)

Magnesium stearate

Sucrose

Gelatin

Soya bean oil, hydrogenated

Tocopherol

Maize starch

6.2 Incompatibilities

Not applicable.

6.3 Shelf life

3 years.

6.4 Special precautions for storage

Do not store above 30°C. Keep the container tightly closed.

6.5 Nature and contents of container

White, high density polyethylene bottles containing 20, 30, 60, 90 or 100 tablets with tamper-evident seal.

Not all pack sizes may be marketed.

6.6 Special precautions for disposal and other handling

No special requirements.

7. MARKETING AUTHORISATION HOLDER

Shire Pharmaceuticals Limited

Hampshire International Business Park

Chineham

Basingstoke

Hampshire RG24 8EP

United Kingdom

8. MARKETING AUTHORISATION NUMBER(S)

PL 08557/0029

9. DATE OF FIRST AUTHORISATION/RENEWAL OF THE AUTHORISATION

26 March 1996

10. DATE OF REVISION OF THE TEXT

April 2007

Calcichew Forte Chewable Tablets

(Shire Pharmaceuticals Limited)

1. NAME OF THE MEDICINAL PRODUCT

Calcichew Forte Chewable Tablets

2. QUALITATIVE AND QUANTITATIVE COMPOSITION

Per tablet: Calcium carbonate 2500mg equivalent to 1g of elemental calcium.

Contains sorbitol, 780mg; isomalt, 124mg; and aspartame, 2mg.

For a full list of excipients see Section 6.1.

3. PHARMACEUTICAL FORM

Chewable tablet.

Round, white, uncoated and convex tablets. May have small specks.

4. CLINICAL PARTICULARS

4.1 Therapeutic indications

Calcichew Forte Chewable Tablets are to be chewed as a supplemental source of calcium in the correction of dietary deficiencies or when normal requirements are high.

Calcichew Forte Chewable Tablets may be used as an adjunct to conventional therapy in the prevention and treatment of osteoporosis. They may be used as a phosphate binding agent in the management of renal failure in patients on renal dialysis.

4.2 Posology and method of administration

Oral.

Adults and elderly:

Adjunct to osteoporosis therapy One tablet to be chewed daily.

Dietary deficiency One tablet to be chewed daily.

Osteomalacia 1-3 tablets daily is recommended.

Children:

Dietary deficiency One tablet to be chewed daily.

Phosphate Binder:

Adults, children and elderly: Dose as required by the individual patient depending on serum phosphate level.

The tablets should be taken just before, during or just after each meal.

The tablets may be chewed or sucked.

4.3 Contraindications

- Severe hypercalcaemia and hypercalciuria, for example in hyperparathyroidism, vitamin D overdosage, decalcifying tumours such as plasmocytoma and skeletal metastases, in severe renal failure untreated by renal dialysis and in osteoporosis due to immobilisation.
- Nephrolithiasis
- Hypersensitivity to the active substance or to any of the excipients.

4.4 Special warnings and precautions for use

Calcichew Forte chewable tablets contain aspartame (a source of phenylalanine) and should be avoided by patients with phenylketonuria.

Calcichew 500 mg Chewable Tablets contain sorbitol (E420) and isomalt (E953). Patients with rare hereditary problems of fructose intolerance, glucose-galactose malabsorption or sucrase-isomaltase insufficiency should not take this medicine.

In renal insufficiency the tablets should be given only under controlled conditions for hyperphosphataemia. Caution should be exercised in patients with a history of renal calculi.

During high dose therapy and especially during concomitant treatment with vitamin D, there is a risk of hypercalcaemia with subsequent kidney function impairment. In these patients, serum calcium levels should be followed and renal function should be monitored.

4.5 Interaction with other medicinal products and other forms of interaction

Thiazide diuretics reduce the urinary excretion of calcium. Due to increased risk of hypercalcaemia, serum calcium should be regularly monitored during concomitant use of thiazide diuretics.

Systemic corticosteroids reduce calcium absorption. During concomitant use, it may be necessary to increase the dose of Calcichew Forte Chewable Tablets.

Calcium carbonate may interfere with the absorption of concomitantly administered tetracycline preparations. For this reason, tetracycline preparations should be administered at least two hours before, or four to six hours after, oral intake of calcium.

Hypercalcaemia may increase the toxicity of cardiac glycosides during treatment with calcium. Patients should be monitored with regard to electrocardiogram (ECG) and serum calcium levels.

If a bisphosphonate or sodium fluoride is used concomitantly, this preparation should be administered at least three hours before the intake of Calcichew Forte Chewable Tablets since gastrointestinal absorption may be reduced.

Oxalic acid (found in spinach and rhubarb) and phytic acid (found in whole cereals) may inhibit calcium absorption through formation of insoluble calcium salts. The patient should not take calcium products within two hours of eating foods high in oxalic acid and phytic acid.

4.6 Pregnancy and lactation

The adequate daily intake (including food and supplementation) for normal pregnant and lactating women is 1000-1300 mg calcium. During pregnancy, the daily intake of calcium should not exceed 1500 mg. Significant amounts of calcium are secreted in milk during lactation. Calcichew Forte Chewable Tablets can be used during pregnancy in case of a calcium deficiency.

4.7 Effects on ability to drive and use machines

There are no data about the effect of this product on driving capacity. An effect is, however, unlikely.

4.8 Undesirable effects

Adverse reactions are listed below, by system organ class and frequency. Frequencies are defined as: uncommon (>1/1,000, <1/100) or rare (>1/10,000, <1/1,000).

Metabolism and nutrition disorders

Uncommon: Hypercalcaemia and hypercalciuria.

Gastrointestinal disorders

Rare: Constipation, flatulence, nausea, abdominal pain and diarrhoea.

Skin and subcutaneous disorders

Rare: Pruritus, rash and urticaria.

4.9 Overdose

Overdose can lead to hypercalcaemia. Symptoms of hypercalcaemia may include anorexia, thirst, nausea, vomiting, constipation, abdominal pain, muscle weakness, fatigue, mental disturbances, polydipsia, polyuria, bone pain, nephrocalcinosis, nephrolithiasis and in severe cases, cardiac arrhythmias. Extreme hypercalcaemia may result in coma and death. Persistently high calcium levels may lead to irreversible renal damage and soft tissue calcification.

Treatment of hypercalcaemia: The treatment with calcium must be discontinued. Treatment with thiazide diuretics, lithium, vitamin A, vitamin D and cardiac glycosides must also be discontinued. Treatment: rehydration, and, according to severity of hypercalcaemia, isolated or combined treatment with loop diuretics, bisphosphonates, calcitonin and corticosteroids should be considered. Serum electrolytes, renal function and diuresis must be monitored. In severe cases, ECG and CVP should be followed.

5. PHARMACOLOGICAL PROPERTIES

5.1 Pharmacodynamic properties

Pharmacotherapeutic group: Calcium

ATC-code: A12A A04

An adequate intake of calcium is of importance during growth, pregnancy and breastfeeding.

5.2 Pharmacokinetic properties

Absorption: The amount of calcium absorbed through the gastrointestinal tract is approximately 30% of the swallowed dose.

Distribution and metabolism: 99% of the calcium in the body is concentrated in the hard structure of bones and teeth. The remaining 1% is present in the intra- and extracellular fluids. About 50% of the total blood-calcium content is in the physiologically active ionised form with approximately 10% being complexed to citrate, phosphate or other anions, the remaining 40% being bound to proteins, principally albumin.

Elimination: Calcium is eliminated through faeces, urine and sweat. Renal excretion depends on glomerular filtration and calcium tubular reabsorption.

5.3 Preclinical safety data

There is no information of relevance to the safety assessment in addition to what is stated in other parts of the SmPC.

6. PHARMACEUTICAL PARTICULARS

6.1 List of excipients

Sorbitol (E420)

Povidone

Magnesium stearate

Aspartame (E951)

Orange flavour:

Isomalt (E953)

Flavouring (orange)

Mono, di-fatty acid glycerides

6.2 Incompatibilities

Not applicable.

6.3 Shelf life

3 years.

6.4 Special precautions for storage

Do not store above 30°C.

Keep the container tightly closed.

6.5 Nature and contents of container

WiMo Box of 28, 30, 56, 60, 90 and 100 tablets. Not all pack sizes may be marketed.

It is a high density polyethylene cylindrical bottle with high density polyethylene screw cap and medium density polyethylene tamper-evident liner.

6.6 Special precautions for disposal and other handling

No special requirements.

7. MARKETING AUTHORISATION HOLDER

Shire Pharmaceuticals Limited

Hampshire International Business Park

Chineham

Basingstoke

Hampshire RG24 8EP

United Kingdom

8. MARKETING AUTHORISATION NUMBER(S)

PL 08557/0022

9. DATE OF FIRST AUTHORISATION/RENEWAL OF THE AUTHORISATION

2 January 1992

10. DATE OF REVISION OF THE TEXT

17 July 2007

Calcium Chloride BP Sterile Solution (UCB Pharma Ltd)

(UCB Pharma Limited)

1. NAME OF THE MEDICINAL PRODUCT

Calcium Chloride BP Sterile Solution

2. QUALITATIVE AND QUANTITATIVE COMPOSITION
Calcium Chloride Dihydrate BP 13.4% w/v
'For excipients, see 6.1'

3. PHARMACEUTICAL FORM
Sterile solution for slow intravenous injection.

4. CLINICAL PARTICULARS
4.1 Therapeutic indications
Calcium Chloride Sterile Solution is indicated for the treatment of acute hypocalcaemia where there is a requirement for the rapid replacement of calcium, e.g. severe hypocalcaemic tetany or hypoparathyroidism, or where the oral route is inappropriate due to malabsorption.

4.2 Posology and method of administration
Route of Administration: Slow intravenous injection.

Adults
A typical dose is 2.25 to 4.5 mmol of calcium given by slow intravenous injection not exceeding 1 ml per minute and repeated as necessary.

Children
The cause of the hypocalcaemia must be fully assessed before starting therapy including dietary review, measurement of vitamin D and PTH, together with regular serum calcium and phosphate levels. For children with hypocalcaemic tetany a dosage of 0.25 to 0.35 mmol/kg of calcium given by slow intravenous injection may be given, repeated every six to eight hours until a response is seen. For other hypocalcaemia conditions initial doses of 0.5 to 3.5 mmol of calcium may be given to elevate serum calcium concentrations.

Infants
Calcium chloride has been given to infants at doses of under 0.5 mmol of calcium, but calcium gluconate is usually preferred due to the irritancy of calcium chloride.

4.3 Contraindications
Parenteral calcium therapy is contraindicated in patients receiving cardiac glycosides. Unsuitable for the treatment of hypocalcaemia caused by renal insufficiencies.

Must not be given intramuscularly and subcutaneously as severe necrosis and sloughing may occur.

4.4 Special warnings and precautions for use
Calcium chloride can cause gastro-intestinal irritation due to the stimulatory effects of calcium on gastric acid production. However, the effect would be most likely with oral administration.

Close monitoring of serum calcium levels is essential following IV administration of calcium.

Calcium salts should be used with caution in patients with impaired renal function, cardiac disease or sarcoidosis.

Because it is acidifying, calcium chloride should be used cautiously in patients with respiratory acidosis or respiratory failure.

4.5 Interaction with other medicinal products and other forms of interaction
Calcium salts reduce the absorption of a number of drugs such as bisphosphonates, fluoride, some fluoroquinolones and tetracyclines; administration should be separated by at least 3 hours.

Calcium chloride infusion reduces the cardiotonic effects of dobutamine.

The effects of digitalis can be increased by increases in blood calcium levels, and the administration of intravenous calcium may result in the development of potentially life-threatening digitalis induced heart arrhythmias.

Thiazide diuretics decrease urinary calcium excretion, and caution is required if such drugs are administered with both calcium chloride and other calcium-containing preparations.

4.6 Pregnancy and lactation
Calcium chloride has no known effects on the foetus or infant, but as with all drugs it should not be administered during pregnancy or breast feeding unless considered essential.

4.7 Effects on ability to drive and use machines
None stated.

4.8 Undesirable effects
Rapid intravenous injection may cause vasodilation, decreased blood pressure, bradycardia and arrhythmias.

The patient may complain of tingling sensations, a chalky 'calcium' taste and a sense of oppression or 'heat wave'.

Irritation can occur after intravenous injection. Extravasation can cause burning, necrosis and sloughing of tissue, cellulitis and soft tissue calcification.

4.9 Overdose
Excessive administration of calcium salts leads to hypercalcaemia. Too rapid injection of calcium salts may also lead to many of the symptoms of hypercalcaemia as well as chalky taste, hot flushes and peripheral vasodilation. Treatment of hypercalcaemia is by the administration of sodium chloride by intravenous infusion.

5. PHARMACOLOGICAL PROPERTIES
5.1 Pharmacodynamic properties
ATC code:A12 A07

Calcium is an essential electrolyte involved in the function of nervous, muscular and skeletal systems, cell membrane and capillary permeability. The cation is also an important activator in many enzymatic reactions and plays a regulatory role in the release and storage of neurotransmitters and hormones.

5.2 Pharmacokinetic properties
Intravenously administered calcium will be absorbed directly into the blood system. Serum calcium levels will increase immediately and may return to normal values in thirty minutes to two hours depending on the rate of renal clearance.

5.3 Preclinical safety data
None stated.

6. PHARMACEUTICAL PARTICULARS
6.1 List of excipients
Sodium hydroxide

Hydrochloric acid

Water for injections

6.2 Incompatibilities
Calcium salts are incompatible with oxidising agents, citrates, soluble carbonates, bicarbonates, phosphates, tartrates and sulphates.

6.3 Shelf life
36 months.

6.4 Special precautions for storage
Store below 25°C.

6.5 Nature and contents of container
10ml neutral Type 1 glass ampoules in packs of 10.

6.6 Special precautions for disposal and other handling
None stated.

7. MARKETING AUTHORISATION HOLDER
UCB Pharma Limited
208 Bath Road
Slough
Berkshire
SL1 3 WE
UK

8. MARKETING AUTHORISATION NUMBER(S)
PL 00039/5888R

9. DATE OF FIRST AUTHORISATION/RENEWAL OF THE AUTHORISATION
18 February 1993, 17 February 2003

10. DATE OF REVISION OF THE TEXT
June 2005

11. Legal Category
POM

Calcium Chloride Injection
(International Medication Systems (UK) Ltd)

1. NAME OF THE MEDICINAL PRODUCT
Calcium Chloride Injection Minijet 10% w/v.

2. QUALITATIVE AND QUANTITATIVE COMPOSITION
Calcium Chloride Dihydrate USP 100mg in 1ml (0.68mmol/ml).

3. PHARMACEUTICAL FORM
Sterile aqueous solution for intracardiac or slow intravenous administration.

4. CLINICAL PARTICULARS
4.1 Therapeutic indications
Calcium Chloride Injection 10% w/v is indicated in the immediate treatment of hypocalcaemic tetany. Other therapy, such as parathyroid hormone and/or vitamin D, may be indicated according to the etiology of the tetany. It is also important to institute oral calcium therapy as soon as practicable.

In cardiac resuscitation, particularly after open heart surgery, calcium chloride has been used when adrenaline has failed to improve weak or ineffective myocardial contractions.

Calcium salts have been used as adjunctive therapy in a number of conditions, including the following:

1. In severe hyperkalaemia, calcium may be injected slowly while the ECG is monitoring the heart.

2. As an aid in the treatment of depression due to overdosage of magnesium sulphate (calcium is the antagonist of magnesium toxicity).

Routes of administration:

For intracardiac or slow intravenous use only.

4.2 Posology and method of administration
Intracardiac use:

In cardiac resuscitation, injection may be made into the ventricular cavity. Do not inject into the myocardium.

Adult dosage: 200-400mg (2-4ml)

Paediatric dosage: 0.2ml/kg of bodyweight.

Intravenous use:

Hypocalcaemic disorders

Adult dosage: 500mg to 1g (5-10ml) at intervals of 1 to 3 days, depending on response of the patient or serum calcium determinations. Repeated injection may be required.

Paediatric dosage: 0.2ml/kg of bodyweight. Maximum 1-10ml/day.

Magnesium Intoxication

Adult dosage: 500mg (5ml) administered promptly. Observe patient for signs of recovery before further doses are given.

Hyperkalaemic ECG disturbances of cardiac function

Adult dosage: Adjust dosage by constant monitoring of ECG changes during administration.

Geriatric patient dosage is the same as an adult.

4.3 Contraindications
In cardiac resuscitation, the use of calcium is contraindicated in the presence of ventricular fibrillation. Calcium chloride injection is contraindicated for injection into tissue (subcutaneous or intramuscular) as it may cause necrosis and sloughing.

Calcium chloride is also contraindicated in those patients with conditions associated with hypercalcaemia and hypercalcuria (e.g. some forms of malignant disease) or in those with conditions associated with elevated vitamin D levels (e.g. sarcoidosis) or in those with renal calculi or a history of calcium renal calculi.

4.4 Special warnings and precautions for use
A moderate fall in blood pressure due to vasodilation may attend the injection. Since calcium chloride is an acidifying salt, it is usually undesirable in the treatment of hypocalcaemia of renal insufficiency.

Calcium chloride injection, 10% w/v is for intracardiac or slow intravenous injection only. Care should be taken not to infiltrate the perivascular tissue due to possible necrosis. Solutions should be warmed to body temperature. Injections should be made slowly through a small needle into a large vein to minimize venous irritation and avoid undesirable reactions.

It is particularly important to prevent a high concentration of calcium from reaching the heart because of danger of cardiac syncope. If injected into the ventricular cavity in cardiac resuscitation care must be taken to avoid injection into the myocardial tissue. Calcium chloride injection should never be given to infants orally because of severe irritation to the gastrointestinal tract. Infant injections should not be given through the scalp.

The use of calcium chloride is undesirable in patients with respiratory acidosis or respiratory failure due to the acidifying nature of the salt.

4.5 Interaction with other medicinal products and other forms of interaction
Because of the danger involved in the simultaneous use of calcium salts and drugs of the digitalis group, a digitalized patient should not receive an intravenous injection of a calcium compound unless the indications are clearly defined. Calcium salts should not generally be mixed with carbonates, phosphates, sulphates or tartrate in parenteral mixtures.

Biphosphonates may interact with calcium chloride causing reduced absorption of biphosphates. Thiazide diuretics may increase the risk of hypercalcaemia.

4.6 Pregnancy and lactation
Studies on the effects of calcium chloride on pregnant women have not been carried out and problems have not been documented. Calcium crosses the placenta. The benefits of administration must outweigh any potential risk.

Calcium is excreted in breast milk but there are no data on the effects, if any, on the infant.

4.7 Effects on ability to drive and use machines
Not applicable.

4.8 Undesirable effects
Rapid intravenous injections may cause the patient to complain of tingling sensations, a calcium taste, a sense of oppression or "heat wave". Injections of calcium chloride are accompanied by peripheral vasodilation as well as a local burning sensation and there may be a moderate fall in blood pressure.

Necrosis and sloughing with subcutaneous or intramuscular administration or if extravasation occurs have been reported. Soft tissue calcification, bradycardia or arrhythmias have also been reported.

4.9 Overdose
Symptoms: anorexia, nausea, vomiting, constipation, abdominal pain, muscle weakness, mental disturbances, polydipsia, polyuria, bone pain, nephrocalcinosis, renal calculi and, in severe cases, cardiac arrhythmias and coma.

Treatment: withholding calcium administration will usually resolve mild hypercalcaemia in asymptomatic patients, provided renal function is adequate.

When serum calcium concentrations are greater than 12mg per 100ml, immediate measures may be required such as hydration, loop diuretics, chelating agents, calcitonin and corticosteroids. Serum calcium concentration should be determined at frequent intervals to guide therapy adjustments.

5. PHARMACOLOGICAL PROPERTIES

5.1 Pharmacodynamic properties

Calcium is essential for the functional integrity of the nervous and muscular systems. It is necessary for normal cardiac function. It is also one of the factors involved in the mechanism of blood coagulation.

Calcium ions increase the force of myocardial contraction. In response to electrical stimulation of muscle, calcium ions enter the sarcoplasm from the extracellular space. Calcium ions contained in the sarcoplasmic reticulum are rapidly transferred to the sites of interaction between the actin and myosin filaments of the sarcomere to initiate myofibril shortening. Thus, calcium increases myocardial function. Calcium's positive inotropic effects are modulated by its action on systemic vascular resistance. Calcium may either increase or decrease systemic vascular resistance. In the normal heart, calcium's positive inotropic and vasoconstricting effect produces a predictable rise in systemic arterial pressure.

5.2 Pharmacokinetic properties

The precise mechanism of action of calcium is not known.

Excretion is renal and varies directly with serum calcium ion concentration.

5.3 Preclinical safety data

Not applicable since calcium chloride has been used in clinical practice for many years and its effects in man are well known.

6. PHARMACEUTICAL PARTICULARS

6.1 List of excipients

Calcium Hydroxide

Hydrochloric Acid

Water for Injections

6.2 Incompatibilities

Calcium salts should not be mixed with carbonates, phosphates, sulphates, tartrates or tetracycline antibiotics in parenteral mixtures.

6.3 Shelf life

36 months.

6.4 Special precautions for storage

Store below 25°C.

6.5 Nature and contents of container

The solution is contained in a USP type I glass vial with an elastomeric closure which meets all the relevant USP specifications. The product is available as 10ml.

6.6 Special precautions for disposal and other handling

The container is specially designed for use with the IMS Minijet injector.

7. MARKETING AUTHORISATION HOLDER

International Medication Systems (UK) Limited

208 Bath Road

Slough

Berkshire

SL1 3WE

UK

8. MARKETING AUTHORISATION NUMBER(S)

PL 03265/0018

9. DATE OF FIRST AUTHORISATION/RENEWAL OF THE AUTHORISATION

Date first granted: PL 10 December 1976

Date renewed: PL 10 December 1996

10. DATE OF REVISION OF THE TEXT

April 2002

POM

Calcium Resonium

(sanofi-aventis)

1. NAME OF THE MEDICINAL PRODUCT

Calcium Resonium

2. QUALITATIVE AND QUANTITATIVE COMPOSITION

Contains Calcium Polystyrene Sulphonate 99.934% w/w

3. PHARMACEUTICAL FORM

An ion-exchange resin presented as a powder.

4. CLINICAL PARTICULARS

4.1 Therapeutic indications

Calcium Resonium is an ion-exchange resin that is recommended for the treatment of hyperkalaemia associated with anuria or severe oliguria. It is also used to treat hyperkalaemia in patients requiring dialysis and in patients on regular haemodialysis or on prolonged peritoneal dialysis.

4.2 Posology and method of administration

Calcium Resonium is to be taken either orally or rectally.

The dosage recommendations detailed below are a guide only; the precise requirements should be decided on the basis of regular serum electrolyte determinations.

Adults, including the elderly:

Oral

Usual dose 15g, three to four times a day. The resin is given by mouth in a little water, or it may be made into a paste with some sweetened vehicle.

Rectal

In cases where vomiting may make oral administration difficult, the resin may be given rectally as a suspension of 30g resin in 100ml 2% methylcellulose (medium viscosity) and 100ml water, as a daily retention enema. In the initial stages administration by this route as well as orally may help to achieve a rapid lowering of the serum potassium level.

The enema should if possible be retained for a least nine hours, then the colon should be irrigated to remove the resin. If both routes are used initially it is probably unnecessary to continue rectal administration once the oral resin has reached the rectum.

Children:

Oral

1g/kg body weight daily in divided doses in acute hyperkalaemia. Dosage may be reduced to 0.5g/kg body weight daily in divided doses for maintenance therapy.

The resin is given orally, preferably with a drink (not a fruit squash because of the high potassium content) or a little jam or honey.

Rectal

When refused by mouth it should be given rectally using a dose at least as great as that which would have been given orally, diluted in the same ratio as described for adults. Following retention of the enema, the colon should be irrigated to ensure adequate removal of the resin.

Neonates:

Calcium Resonium should not be given by the oral route. With rectal administration, the minimum effective dosage within the range 0.5g/kg to 1g/kg should be employed, diluted as for adults with adequate irrigation to ensure recovery of the resin.

4.3 Contraindications

- In patients with plasma potassium levels below 5mmol/litre.
- Conditions associated with hypercalcaemia (e.g. hyperparathyroidism, multiple myeloma, sarcoidosis or metastatic carcinoma).
- History of hypersensitivity to polystyrene sulphonate resins.
- Obstructive bowel disease.
- Calcium Resonium should not be administered orally to neonates and is contraindicated in neonates with reduced gut motility (post-operatively or drug-induced).

4.4 Special warnings and precautions for use

Hypokalaemia: The possibility of severe potassium depletion should be considered and adequate clinical and biochemical control is essential during treatment, especially in patients on digitalis. Administration of the resin should be stopped when the serum potassium falls to 5mmol/litre.

Other electrolyte disturbances: Like all cation-exchange resins, calcium polystyrene sulphonate is not totally selective for potassium. Hypomagnesemia and/or hypercalcemia may occur. Accordingly, patients should be monitored for all applicable electrolyte disturbances. Serum calcium levels should be estimated at weekly intervals to detect the early development of hypercalcaemia, and the dose of resin adjusted to levels at which hypercalcaemia and hypokalaemia are prevented.

Other risks: In the event of clinically significant constipation, treatment should be discontinued until normal bowel movement has resumed. Magnesium-containing laxatives should not be used (see section 4.5 Interactions).

The patient should be positioned carefully when ingesting the resin, to avoid aspiration, which may lead to bronchopulmonary complications.

Children and neonates: In neonates, calcium polystyrene sulphonate should not be given by the oral route. In children and neonates, particular care is needed with rectal administration as excessive dosage or inadequate dilution could result in impaction of the resin. Due to the risk of digestive haemorrhage or colonic necrosis, particular care should be observed in premature infants or low birth weight infants.

4.5 Interaction with other medicinal products and other forms of interaction

Concomitant use not recommended

Sorbitol (oral or rectal): Concomitant use of sorbitol with sodium polystyrene sulphonate may cause colonic necrosis. Therefore concomitant administration of sorbitol with calcium polystyrene sulphonate is not recommended.

To be used with caution

Cation-donating agents: may reduce the potassium binding effectiveness of Calcium Resonium.

Non-absorbable cation-donating antacids and laxatives: There have been reports of systemic alkalosis following concurrent administration of cation-exchange resins and non-absorbable cation-donating antacids and laxatives such as magnesium hydroxide and aluminium carbonate.

Aluminium hydroxide: Intestinal obstruction due to concretions of aluminium hydroxide has been reported when aluminium hydroxide has been combined with the resin (sodium form).

Digitalis-like drugs: The toxic effects of digitalis on the heart, especially various ventricular arrhythmias and A-V nodal dissociation, are likely to be exaggerated if hypokalaemia and/or hypercalcaemia are allowed to develop (see 4.4 Special warnings and special precautions for use).

Lithium: Possible decrease of lithium absorption.

Levothyroxine: Possible decrease of levothyroxine absorption.

4.6 Pregnancy and lactation

No data are available regarding the use of polystyrene sulphonate resins in pregnancy and lactation. The administration of Calcium Resonium in pregnancy and during breast feeding therefore, is not advised unless, in the opinion of the physician, the potential benefits outweigh any potential risks.

4.7 Effects on ability to drive and use machines

There are no specific warnings.

4.8 Undesirable effects

In accordance with its pharmacological actions, the resin may give rise to hypokalaemia and hypercalcaemia and their related clinical manifestations (see Warnings and Precautions and Overdosage).

Hypercalcaemia has been reported in well dialysed patients receiving calcium resin, and in the occasional patient with chronic renal failure. Many patients in chronic renal failure have low serum calcium and high serum phosphate, but some, who cannot be screened out beforehand, show a sudden rise in serum calcium to high levels after therapy. The risk emphasises the need for adequate biochemical control.

- **Gastrointestinal disorders**

Gastric irritation, anorexia, nausea, vomiting, constipation and occasionally diarrhoea may occur. Faecal impaction following rectal administration particularly in children and gastrointestinal concretions (bezoars) following oral administration have been reported. Intestinal obstruction has also been reported although this has been extremely rare and, possibly, a reflection of co-existing pathology or inadequate dilution of resin.

Gastro-intestinal tract ulceration or necrosis which could lead to intestinal perforation have been reported following administration of sodium polystyrene sulphonate.

- **Respiratory disorders**

Some cases of acute bronchitis and/or bronchopneumonia associated with inhalation of particles of calcium polystyrene sulphonate have been described.

4.9 Overdose

Biochemical disturbances from overdosage may give rise to clinical signs of symptoms of hypokalaemia, including irritability, confusion, delayed thought processes, muscle weakness, hyporeflexia and eventual paralysis. Apnoea may be a serious consequence of this progression. Electrocardiographic changes may be consistent with hypokalaemia or hypercalcaemia; cardiac arrhythmia may occur. Appropriate measures should be taken to correct serum electrolytes and the resin should be removed from the alimentary tract by appropriate use of laxatives or enemas.

5. PHARMACOLOGICAL PROPERTIES

5.1 Pharmacodynamic properties

Ion-exchange resin

5.2 Pharmacokinetic properties

Not applicable as this product is not absorbed.

5.3 Preclinical safety data

There are no pre-clinical data of relevance to the prescriber which are additional to that already included in other sections of the SPC.

6. PHARMACEUTICAL PARTICULARS

6.1 List of excipients

Calcium Resonium also contains Vanillin and Saccharin.

6.2 Incompatibilities

There are no specific incompatibilities.

6.3 Shelf life

The shelf-life of Calcium Resonium is 5 years.

6.4 Special precautions for storage

Store in a dry place

6.5 Nature and contents of container

HDPE containers of 300g.

6.6 Special precautions for disposal and other handling

None

7. MARKETING AUTHORISATION HOLDER
sanofi-aventis
One Onslow Street
Guildford
Surrey
GU1 4YS
UK

8. MARKETING AUTHORISATION NUMBER(S)
PL 11723/0010

9. DATE OF FIRST AUTHORISATION/RENEWAL OF THE AUTHORISATION
2 April 2003

10. DATE OF REVISION OF THE TEXT
27th April 2009

Legal category: P

Calcium-Sandoz Syrup

(Alliance Pharmaceuticals)

1. NAME OF THE MEDICINAL PRODUCT
Calcium-Sandoz® Syrup

2. QUALITATIVE AND QUANTITATIVE COMPOSITION
Calcium glubionate 1.09g and calcium lactobionate USP 0.727g per 5ml.

3. PHARMACEUTICAL FORM
Colourless to pale straw coloured, fruit flavoured syrup.

4. CLINICAL PARTICULARS

4.1 Therapeutic indications
1. An adjunct to conventional therapy in the arrest or slowing down of bone demineralisation in osteoporosis.
2. In the arrest or slowing down of bone demineralisation in osteoporosis where other effective treatment is contra-indicated.
3. A supplemental source of calcium in the correction of dietary deficiencies or when normal requirements are high.
4. Neonatal hypocalcaemia.

4.2 Posology and method of administration
Treatment or therapeutic supplementation should aim to restore or maintain normal levels of calcium (2.25 to 2.75mmol/L or 4.5 to 5.5mEq/L).

Calcium Sandoz Syrup should be taken by mouth either as provided or after dilution with syrup BP.

Indication	Daily Dose Syrup (5ml spoonfuls)
Adults	
Osteoporosis	11-15
Therapeutic supplement (dose dependent upon severity)	3-15
Children	
Calcium deficiency	6-9
Dietary supplementation	2-6

Neonatal hypocalcaemia: Calcium-Sandoz Syrup may be given at a dose of 1mmol calcium/kg/24 hours in divided doses. Serum calcium levels should be monitored and the dosage adjusted if necessary. Doses may be mixed with the first (small) part of milk feeds. Note: 1mmol of calcium is equivalent to 1.85ml Calcium-Sandoz Syrup.

Elderly: No evidence exists that tolerance of Calcium-Sandoz is directly affected by advanced age; however, elderly patients should be supervised as factors sometimes associated with ageing, such as poor diet or impaired renal function, may indirectly affect tolerance and may require dosage reduction.

4.3 Contraindications
Hypercalcaemia (e.g., in hyperparathyroidism, vitamin D overdosage, decalcifying tumours such as plasmocytoma, severe renal failure, bone metastases), severe hypercalciuria, and renal calculi.

Due to its galactose component Calcium-Sandoz Syrup should not be given to patients with galactosaemia.

4.4 Special warnings and precautions for use
In mild hypercalciuria (exceeding 300mg (7.5mmol)/24 hours) or renal failure, or where there is evidence of stone formation in the urinary tract, adequate checks must be kept on urinary calcium excretion; if necessary the dosage should be reduced or calcium therapy discontinued.

The sugar content of Calcium-Sandoz Syrup should be taken into account in diabetic patients.

4.5 Interaction with other medicinal products and other forms of interaction
High vitamin D intake should be avoided during calcium therapy, unless especially indicated (see also Section 4.9, "Overdose").

Thiazide diuretics reduce urinary calcium excretion, so the risk of hypercalcaemia should be considered.

Oral calcium supplementation is aimed at restoring normal serum levels. Although it is extremely unlikely that high enough levels will be achieved to adversely affect digitalised patients, this theoretical possibility should be considered.

Oral calcium administration may reduce the absorption of oral tetracycline or fluoride preparations. An interval of 3 hours should be observed if the two are to be given.

4.6 Pregnancy and lactation
The likelihood of hypercalcaemia is increased in pregnant women in whom calcium and vitamin D are co-administered. Epidemiological studies with calcium have shown no increase in the teratogenic hazard to the foetus if used in the doses recommended. Although supplemental calcium may be excreted in breast milk, the concentration is unlikely to be sufficient to produce any adverse effect on the neonate.

4.7 Effects on ability to drive and use machines
None known.

4.8 Undesirable effects
Mild gastrointestinal disturbances (e.g., constipation, diarrhoea) have occurred rarely. Although hypercalcaemia would not be expected in patients unless their renal function were impaired, the following symptoms could indicate the possibility of hypercalcaemia: nausea, vomiting, anorexia, constipation, abdominal pain, bone pain, thirst, polyuria, muscle weakness, drowsiness or confusion.

4.9 Overdose
The amount of calcium absorbed following overdosage with Calcium-Sandoz Syrup will depend on the individual's calcium status. Deliberate overdosage is unlikely and acute overdosage has not been reported. It might cause gastrointestinal disturbances but would not be expected to cause hypercalcaemia except in patients treated with excessive doses of vitamin D. Treatment should be aimed at lowering serum calcium levels, e.g., administration of oral phosphates.

5. PHARMACOLOGICAL PROPERTIES

5.1 Pharmacodynamic properties
Calcium is an endogenous ion of the body essential for the maintenance of a number of physiologic processes. It participates as an integral factor in the maintenance of the functional integrity of the nervous system, in the contractile mechanisms of muscle tissue, in the clotting of blood, and in the formulation of the major structural material of the skeleton.

A dynamic equilibrium occurs between blood calcium and skeletal calcium, homeostasis being mainly regulated by the parathyroid hormone, by calcitonin and by vitamin D. Variations in the concentration of ionised calcium are responsible for the symptoms of hyper/hypocalcaemia. Soluble calcium salts are commonly used in the treatment of calcium deficiency and may be given by mouth or injection.

5.2 Pharmacokinetic properties
Concentrations of plasma calcium are determined chiefly by gastrointestinal absorption, bone metabolism and renal excretion, and levels are closely regulated within the normal limits of 4.5 – 5.5mEq/l (2.25-2.75mmol/L) of which 50-60% is present in ionized form. Up to 10% is present as diffusible complexes with organic acids; the remainder is present as non-diffusible complexes with proteins. More than 99% of the body calcium is deposited in bone as hydroxyapatite crystals, which are available for exchange with calcium in the extracellular fluids. In bone as a whole, about 1% of calcium is in a readily exchangeable pool. Bone therefore functions as the main reservoir of these ions from which they may be readily mobilised if the plasma concentration falls, or in which they may be deposited if the plasma level rises.

5.3 Preclinical safety data
There are no pre-clinical data of relevance to the prescriber which are additional to those already included in other sections of the Summary of Product Characteristics.

6. PHARMACEUTICAL PARTICULARS

6.1 List of excipients
Orange natural flavour, tamaris flavour, benzoic acid, formic acid, sugar and water.

6.2 Incompatibilities
None known.

6.3 Shelf life
Three years unopened. Up to 1 year once the bottle has been opened.

6.4 Special precautions for storage
None.

6.5 Nature and contents of container
Amber glass bottles of 300ml with a polythene closure (polythene wad faced with PP, PVDC or PET lining).

6.6 Special precautions for disposal and other handling
Calcium-Sandoz Syrup may be diluted with Syrup BP; the diluted syrup should be used within 14 days.

Administrative Data

7. MARKETING AUTHORISATION HOLDER
Alliance Pharmaceuticals Ltd
Avonbridge House
Bath Road
Chippenham
Wiltshire
SN15 2BB

8. MARKETING AUTHORISATION NUMBER(S)
PL16853/0005

9. DATE OF FIRST AUTHORISATION/RENEWAL OF THE AUTHORISATION
25 June 1998

10. DATE OF REVISION OF THE TEXT
March 1999

11. Legal status
Pharmacy

Alliance, Alliance Pharmaceuticals and associated devices are registered Trademarks of Alliance Pharmaceuticals Ltd.

Calcort 6mg Tablets

(sanofi-aventis)

1. NAME OF THE MEDICINAL PRODUCT
Calcort 6mg

2. QUALITATIVE AND QUANTITATIVE COMPOSITION
Active ingredient: deflazacort 6mg

3. PHARMACEUTICAL FORM
Round, white, uncoated tablets, marked with a cross on one face and a 6 on the other face.

4. CLINICAL PARTICULARS

4.1 Therapeutic indications
A wide range of conditions may sometimes need treatment with glucocorticoids. The indications include:

Anaphylaxis, asthma, severe hypersensitivity reactions

Rheumatoid arthritis, juvenile chronic arthritis, polymyalgia rheumatica

Systemic lupus erythematosus, dermatomyositis, mixed connective tissue disease (other than systemic sclerosis), polyarteritis nodosa, sarcoidosis

Pemphigus, bullous pemphigoid, pyoderma gangrenosum

Minimal change nephrotic syndrome, acute interstitial nephritis

Rheumatic carditis

Ulcerative colitis, Crohn's disease

Uveitis, optic neuritis

Autoimmune haemolytic anaemia, idiopathic thrombocytopenic purpura

Acute and lymphatic leukaemia, malignant lymphoma, multiple myeloma

Immune suppression in transplantation

4.2 Posology and method of administration
Deflazacort is a glucocorticoid derived from prednisolone and 6mg of deflazacort has approximately the same anti-inflammatory potency as 5mg prednisolone or prednisone.

Doses vary widely in different diseases and different patients. In more serious and life-threatening conditions, high doses of deflazacort may need to be given. When deflazacort is used long term in relatively benign chronic diseases, the maintenance dose should be kept as low as possible. Dosage may need to be increased during periods of stress or in exacerbation of illness.

The dosage should be individually titrated according to diagnosis, severity of disease and patient response and tolerance. The lowest dose that will produce an acceptable response should be used (see Warnings and Precautions).

Adults

For acute disorders, up to 120 mg/day deflazacort may need to be given initially. Maintenance doses in most conditions are within the range 3 - 18 mg/day. The following regimens are for guidance only.

Rheumatoid arthritis: The maintenance dose is usually within the range 3 - 18 mg/day. The smallest effective dose should be used and increased if necessary.

Bronchial asthma: In the treatment of an acute attack, high doses of 48-72 mg/day may be needed depending on severity and gradually reduced once the attack has been controlled. For maintenance in chronic asthma, doses should be titrated to the lowest dose that controls symptoms.

Other conditions: The dose of deflazacort depends on clinical need titrated to the lowest effective dose for maintenance. Starting doses may be estimated on the basis of ratio of 5mg prednisone or prednisolone to 6mg deflazacort.

Hepatic Impairment

In patients with hepatic impairment, blood levels of deflazacort may be increased. Therefore the dose of deflazacort should be carefully monitored and adjusted to the minimum effective dose.

Renal Impairment

In renally impaired patients, no special precautions other than those usually adopted in patients receiving glucocorticoid therapy are necessary.

Elderly

In elderly patients, no special precautions other than those usually adopted in patients receiving glucocorticoid therapy are necessary. The common adverse effects of systemic corticosteroids may be associated with more serious consequences in old age (see Warnings and Precautions).

Children

There has been limited exposure of children to deflazacort in clinical trials.

In children, the indications for glucocorticoids are the same as for adults, but it is important that the lowest effective dosage is used. Alternate day administration may be appropriate (see Warnings and Precautions).

Doses of deflazacort usually lie in the range 0.25 - 1.5 mg/kg/day. The following ranges provide general guidance:

Juvenile chronic arthritis: The usual maintenance dose is between 0.25 - 1.0 mg/kg/day.

Nephrotic syndrome: Initial dose of usually 1.5 mg/kg/day followed by down titration according to clinical need.

Bronchial asthma: On the basis of the potency ratio, the initial dose should be between 0.25 - 1.0 mg/kg deflazacort on alternate days.

Deflazacort withdrawal

In patients who have received more than physiological doses of systemic corticosteroids (approximately 9mg per day or equivalent) for greater than 3 weeks, withdrawal should not be abrupt. How dose reduction should be carried out depends largely on whether the disease is likely to relapse as the dose of systemic corticosteroids is reduced. Clinical assessment of disease activity may be needed during withdrawal. If the disease is unlikely to relapse on withdrawal of systemic corticosteroids but there is uncertainty about HPA suppression, the dose of systemic corticosteroids may be reduced rapidly to physiological doses. Once a daily dose equivalent to 9mg deflazacort is reached, dose reduction should be slower to allow the HPA-axis to recover.

Abrupt withdrawal of systemic corticosteroid treatment, which has continued up to 3 weeks is appropriate if it is considered that the disease is unlikely to relapse. Abrupt withdrawal of doses up to 48 mg daily of deflazacort, or equivalent for 3 weeks is unlikely to lead to clinically relevant HPA-axis suppression, in the majority of patients. In the following patient groups, gradual withdrawal of systemic corticosteroid therapy should be *considered* even after courses lasting 3 weeks or less:

- Patients who have had repeated courses of systemic corticosteroids, particularly if taken for greater than 3 weeks.
- When a short course has been prescribed within one year of cessation of long-term therapy (months or years).
- Patients who may have reasons for adrenocortical insufficiency other than exogenous corticosteroid therapy.
- Patients receiving doses of systemic corticosteroid greater than 48 mg daily of deflazacort (or equivalent),
- Patients repeatedly taking doses in the evening.

4.3 Contraindications

Systemic infection unless specific anti-infective therapy is employed.

Hypersensitivity to deflazacort or any of the ingredients. Patients receiving live virus immunisation.

4.4 Special warnings and precautions for use

A patient information leaflet should be supplied with this product.

Patients with rare hereditary problems of galactose intolerance, the Lapp lactose deficiency or glucose-galactose malabsorption should not take this medicine.

Undesirable effects may be minimised by using the lowest effective dose for the minimum period, and by administering the daily requirement as a single morning dose or whenever possible as a single morning dose on alternate days. Frequent patient review is required to appropriately titrate the dose against disease activity (see Dosage section).

Adrenal suppression

Adrenal cortical atrophy develops during prolonged therapy and may persist for years after stopping treatment. Withdrawal of corticosteroids after prolonged therapy must therefore always be gradual to avoid acute adrenal insufficiency, being tapered off over weeks or months according to the dose and duration of treatment. During prolonged therapy, any intercurrent illness, trauma or surgical procedure will require a temporary increase in dosage; if corticosteroids have been stopped following prolonged therapy, they may need to be temporarily re-introduced.

Patients should carry 'Steroid treatment' cards which give clear guidance on the precautions to be taken to minimise risk and which provide details of prescriber, drug, dosage and the duration of treatment.

Anti-inflammatory/immunosuppressive effects and infection

Suppression of the inflammatory response and immune function increases the susceptibility to infections and their severity. The clinical presentation may often be atypical and serious infections such as septicaemia and tuberculosis may be masked and may reach an advanced stage before being recognised.

Chickenpox is of particular concern since this normally minor illness may be fatal in immunosuppressed patients. Patients (or parents of children) without a definite history of chicken pox should be advised to avoid close personal contact with chickenpox or herpes zoster and, if exposed, they should seek urgent medical attention. Passive immunisation with varicella zoster immunoglobulin (VZIG) is needed by exposed non-immune patients who are receiving systemic corticosteroids or who have used them within the previous 3 months; this should be given within 10 days of exposure to chickenpox. If a diagnosis of chickenpox is confirmed, the illness warrants specialist care and urgent treatment. Corticosteroids should not be stopped and the dose may need to be increased.

Patients should be advised to take particular care to avoid exposure to measles and to seek immediate medical advice if exposure occurs. Prophylaxis with intramuscular normal immunoglobulin may be needed.

Live vaccines should not be given to individuals with impaired responsiveness. The antibody response to other vaccines may be diminished.

Prolonged use of glucocorticoids may produce posterior subcapsular cataracts, glaucoma with possible damage to the optic nerves and may enhance the establishment of secondary ocular infections due to fungi or viruses.

Use in active tuberculosis should be restricted to those cases of fulminating and disseminated tuberculosis in which deflazacort is used for management with appropriate antituberculosis regimen. If glucocorticoids are indicated in patients with latent tuberculosis or tuberculin reactivity, close observation is necessary as reactivation of the disease may occur. During prolonged glucocorticoid therapy, these patients should receive chemoprophylaxis.

Special precautions

The following clinical conditions require special caution and frequent patient monitoring is necessary:-

- Cardiac disease or congestive heart failure (except in the presence of active rheumatic carditis), hypertension, thromboembolic disorders. Glucocorticoids can cause salt and water retention and increased excretion of potassium. Dietary salt restriction and potassium supplementation may be necessary.
- Gastritis or oesophagitis, diverticulitis, ulcerative colitis if there is probability of impending perforation, abscess or pyogenic infections, fresh intestinal anastomosis, active or latent peptic ulcer.
- Diabetes mellitus or a family history, osteoporosis, myasthenia gravis, renal insufficiency.
- Emotional instability or psychotic tendency, epilepsy.
- Previous corticosteroid-induced myopathy.
- Liver failure.
- Hypothyroidism and cirrhosis, which may increase glucocorticoid effect.
- Ocular herpes simplex because of possible corneal perforation.

Patients/and or carers should be warned that potentially severe psychiatric adverse reactions may occur with systemic steroids (see section 4.8). Symptoms typically emerge within a few days or weeks of starting the treatment. Risks may be higher with high doses/systemic exposure (see also section 4.5 pharmacokinetic interactions that can increase the risk of side effects). although dose levels do not allow prediction of the onset. type, severity or duration of reactions. Most reactions recover after either dose reduction or withdrawal, although specific treatment may be necessary. Patients/carers should be encouraged to seek medical advice if worrying psychological symptoms develop, especially if depressed mood or suicidal ideation is suspected. Patients/carers should also be alert to possible psychiatric disturbances that may occur either during or immediately after dose tapering/withdrawal of systemic steroids, although such reactions have been reported infrequently.

Particular care is required when considering the use of systemic corticosteroids in patients with existing or previous history of severe affective disorders in themselves or in their first degree relatives. These would include depressive or manic-depressive illness and previous steroid psychosis.

Use in Children

Corticosteroids cause dose-related growth retardation in infancy, childhood and adolescence which may be irreversible.

Use in Elderly

The common adverse effects of systemic corticosteroids may be associated with more serious consequences in old age, especially osteoporosis, hypertension, hypokalaemia, diabetes, susceptibility to infection and thinning of the skin. Close clinical supervision is required to avoid life-threatening reactions.

Since complications of glucocorticoid therapy are dependent on dose and duration of therapy, the lowest possible dose must be given and a risk/benefit decision must be made as to whether intermittent therapy should be used.

4.5 Interaction with other medicinal products and other forms of interaction

The same precautions should be exercised as for other glucocorticoids. Deflazacort is metabolised in the liver. It is recommended to increase the maintenance dose of deflazacort if drugs which are liver enzyme inducers are co-administered, e.g. rifampicin, rifabutin, carbamazepine, phenobarbitone, phenytoin, primidone and aminoglutethimide. For drugs which inhibit liver enzymes, e.g. ketoconazole it may be possible to reduce the maintenance dose of deflazacort.

In patients taking estrogens, corticosteroid requirements may be reduced.

The desired effects of hypoglycaemic agents (including insulin), anti-hypertensives and diuretics are antagonised by corticosteroids and the hypokalaemic effects of acetazolamide, loop diuretics, thiazide diuretics and carbenoxolone are enhanced.

The efficacy of coumarin anticoagulants may be enhanced by concurrent corticosteroid therapy and close monitoring of the INR or prothrombin time is required to avoid spontaneous bleeding.

In patients treated with systemic corticosteroids, use of non-depolarising muscle relaxants can result in prolonged relaxation and acute myopathy. Risk factors for this include prolonged and high dose corticosteroid treatment, and prolonged duration of muscle paralysis. This interaction is more likely following prolonged ventilation (such as in the ITU setting).

The renal clearance of salicylates is increased by corticosteroids and steroid withdrawal may result in salicylate intoxication.

As glucocorticoids can suppress the normal responses of the body to attack by micro-organisms, it is important to ensure that any anti-infective therapy is effective and it is recommended to monitor patients closely. Concurrent use of glucocorticoids and oral contraceptives should be closely monitored as plasma levels of glucocorticoids may be increased. This effect may be due to a change in metabolism or binding to serum proteins. Antacids may reduce bioavailability; leave at least 2 hours between administration of deflazacort and antacids.

4.6 Pregnancy and lactation

Pregnancy

The ability of corticosteroids to cross the placenta varies between individual drugs, however, deflazacort does cross the placenta.

Administration of corticosteroids to pregnant animals can cause abnormalities of foetal development including cleft palate, intra-uterine growth retardation and effects on brain growth and development. There is no evidence that corticosteroids result in an increased incidence of congenital abnormalities, such as cleft palate/lip in man. However, when administered for prolonged periods or repeatedly during pregnancy, corticosteroids may increase the risk of intra-uterine growth retardation. Hypoadrenalism may, in theory, occur in the neonate following prenatal exposure to corticosteroids but usually resolves spontaneously following birth and is rarely clinically important. As with all drugs, corticosteroids should only be prescribed when the benefits to the mother and child outweigh the risks. When corticosteroids are essential however, patients with normal pregnancies may be treated as though they were in the non-gravid state.

Lactation

Corticosteroids are excreted in breast milk, although no data are available for deflazacort. Doses of up to 50 mg daily of deflazacort are unlikely to cause systemic effects in the infant. Infants of mothers taking higher doses than this may have a degree of adrenal suppression but the benefits of breast feeding are likely to outweigh any theoretical risk.

4.7 Effects on ability to drive and use machines

On the basis of the pharmacodynamic profile and reported adverse events, it is unlikely that deflazacort will produce an effect on the ability to drive and use machines.

4.8 Undesirable effects

The incidence of predictable undesirable effects, including hypothalamic-pituitary-adrenal suppression correlates with the relative potency of the drug, dosage, timing of administration and the duration of treatment (see Warnings and Precautions).

Endocrine/metabolic

Suppression of the hypothalamic-pituitary-adrenal axis, growth suppression in infancy, childhood and adolescence, menstrual irregularity and amenorrhoea. Cushingoid facies, hirsutism, weight gain, impaired carbohydrate tolerance with increased requirement for anti-diabetic therapy. Negative protein and calcium balance. Increased appetite.

Anti-inflammatory and immunosuppressive effects

Increased susceptibility and severity of infections with suppression of clinical symptoms and signs, opportunistic infections, recurrence of dormant tuberculosis (see Warnings and Precautions).

Musculoskeletal

Osteoporosis, vertebral and long bone fractures, avascular osteonecrosis, tendon rupture. Muscle wasting or myopathy (acute myopathy may be precipitated by non-depolarising muscle relaxants – see section 4.5), negative nitrogen balance.

Fluid and electrolyte disturbance

Sodium and water retention with hypertension, oedema and heart failure, potassium loss, hypokalaemic alkalosis.

Neuropsychiatric

Headache, vertigo, psychological dependence, hypomania or depression, restlessness. Increased intra-cranial pressure with papilloedema in children (pseudotumour cerebri), usually after treatment withdrawal. Aggravation of epilepsy.

A wide range of psychiatric reactions including affective disorders (such as irritable, euphoric, depressed and labile mood, and suicidal thoughts), psychotic reactions (including mania, delusions, hallucinations, and aggravation of schizophrenia), behavioural disturbances, irritability, anxiety, sleep disturbances, and cognitive dysfunction including confusion and amnesia have been reported. Reactions are common and may occur in both adults and children. In adults, the frequency of severe reactions has been estimated to be 5-6%. Psychological effects have been reported on withdrawal of corticosteroids; the frequency is unknown.

Ophthalmic

Increased intra-ocular pressure, glaucoma, papilloedema, posterior subcapsular cataracts especially in children, corneal or scleral thinning, exacerbation of ophthalmic viral or fungal diseases.

Gastrointestinal

Dyspepsia, peptic ulceration with perforation and haemorrhage, acute pancreatitis (especially in children), candidiasis. Nausea.

Dermatological

Impaired healing, skin atrophy, bruising, telangiectasia, striae, acne.

General

Hypersensitivity including anaphylaxis has been reported. Leucocytosis. Thromboembolism. Rare incidence of benign intracranial hypertension.

Withdrawal symptoms and signs

Too rapid a reduction of corticosteroid dosage following prolonged treatment can lead to acute adrenal insufficiency, hypotension and death (see Warnings and Precautions).

A 'withdrawal syndrome' may also occur including fever, myalgia, arthralgia, rhinitis, conjunctivitis, painful itchy skin nodules and loss of weight. This may occur in patients even without evidence of adrenal insufficiency.

4.9 Overdose

It is unlikely that treatment is needed in cases of acute overdosage. The LD_{50} for the oral dose is greater than 4000 mg/kg in laboratory animals.

5. PHARMACOLOGICAL PROPERTIES

5.1 Pharmacodynamic properties

Deflazacort is a glucocorticoid. Its anti-inflammatory and immunosuppressive effects are used in treating a variety of diseases and are comparable to other anti-inflammatory steroids. Clinical studies have indicated that the average potency ratio of deflazacort to prednisolone is 0.69-0.89.

5.2 Pharmacokinetic properties

Orally administered deflazacort appears to be well absorbed and is immediately converted by plasma esterases to the pharmacologically active metabolite (D 21-OH) which achieves peak plasma concentrations in 1.5 to 2 hours. It is 40% protein-bound and has no affinity for corticosteroid-binding-globulin (transcortin). Its elimination plasma half-life is 1.1 to 1.9 hours. Elimination takes place primarily through the kidneys; 70% of the administered dose is excreted in the urine. The remaining 30% is eliminated in the faeces. Metabolism of D 21-OH is extensive; only 18% of urinary excretion represents D 21-OH. The metabolite of D 21-OH, deflazacort 6-beta-OH, represents one third of the urinary elimination.

5.3 Preclinical safety data

Safety studies have been carried out in the rat, dog, mouse and monkey. The findings are consistent with other glucocorticoids at comparable doses. Teratogenic effects demonstrated in rodents and rabbits are typical of those caused by other glucocorticoids. Deflazacort was not found to be carcinogenic in the mouse, but studies in the rat produced carcinogenic findings consistent with the findings with other glucocorticoids.

6. PHARMACEUTICAL PARTICULARS

6.1 List of excipients

Microcrystalline cellulose, lactose, maize starch and magnesium stearate.

6.2 Incompatibilities

None reported.

6.3 Shelf life

5 years.

6.4 Special precautions for storage

Store in the original package. Do not store above 25°C.

6.5 Nature and contents of container

Deflazacort is packed in blister packs of polyvinylchloride and aluminium foil presented in cardboard cartons. Each pack contains 60 tablets.

6.6 Special precautions for disposal and other handling

No special instructions for use or handling are required.

7. MARKETING AUTHORISATION HOLDER

Sanofi-aventis
One Onslow Street
Guildford
Surrey, GU1 4YS, UK

8. MARKETING AUTHORISATION NUMBER(S)

PL 04425/0629

9. DATE OF FIRST AUTHORISATION/RENEWAL OF THE AUTHORISATION

06 August 2008

10. DATE OF REVISION OF THE TEXT

22 July 2009

Legal category: POM

Calfovit D3

(A. Menarini Pharma U.K. S.R.L.)

1. NAME OF THE MEDICINAL PRODUCT

CALFOVIT D3 powder for oral suspension

2. QUALITATIVE AND QUANTITATIVE COMPOSITION

Each sachet contains:

Colecalciferol (Vitamin D3) 20 micrograms (equivalent to 800 I.U.)

Calcium phosphate 3100 mg

(equivalent to 1200 mg or 30 mmol of elemental calcium per sachet)

For excipients see 6.1.

3. PHARMACEUTICAL FORM

Powder for oral suspension.

White or slightly orange, granular powder.

4. CLINICAL PARTICULARS

4.1 Therapeutic indications

Correction of calcium and Vitamin D deficiency in the elderly.

CALFOVIT D3 may be used as an adjunct to specific therapy for osteoporosis, in patients with either established vitamin D and calcium combined deficiencies or in those patients at high risk of needing such therapeutic supplements.

4.2 Posology and method of administration

Adults and elderly: 1 sachet/day for oral use

Pour the contents of the sachet into a glass of non-carbonated water. Stir with a spoon to obtain a pleasant-tasting suspension. Drink immediately.

It is advisable to take the preparation during the evening meal.

Children: The safe or effective use of CALFOVIT D3 in children has not been established. Therefore, it should not be used in children.

Patients with hepatic dysfunction: No dosage adjustment is required.

Patients with renal dysfunction: CALFOVIT D3 should not be used in patients with severe renal dysfunction.

4.3 Contraindications

Hypersensitivity to active substances or to excipients.

Hypercalcaemia (>10.5 mg/dl), hypercalciuria (300 mg or 7.5 mmol/24 hours), severe renal insufficiency, kidney stones, calcium lithiasis, calcification of tissues, prolonged immobilisation accompanied by hypercalciurea and/or hypercalcaemia.

Hypervitaminosis D.

CALFOVIT D3 is not indicated in children, pregnancy and lactation.

4.4 Special warnings and precautions for use

CALFOVIT D3 must be used with caution in patients with renal insufficiency or when there is an evident tendency for the formation of urinary calculi. Calcaemia and calciuria must be adequately monitored in these patients to prevent the onset of hypercalcaemia. If calciuria levels exceed 7.5 mmol/24 hours (300 mg/24 hours), treatment should be temporarily interrupted.

Special caution is also required in the treatment of patients with cardiovascular disease. The effect of cardiac glycosides may be accentuated with the oral administration of calcium combined with Vitamin D. Strict medical supervision, and if necessary, monitoring ECG and calcaemia are necessary.

All other Vitamin D compounds and their derivatives, including food-stuffs which may be fortified with Vitamin D, should be withheld during treatment with CALFOVIT D3.

The product should be prescribed with caution to patients with sarcoidosis because of possible increased metabolism of Vitamin D to its active form. These patients should be monitored for serum and urinary calcium.

CALFOVIT D3 contains the colouring agent E110 which can cause allergic-type reactions including asthma. Allergy is more common in those people who are allergic to aspirin.

Patients with rare hereditary problems of fructose intolerance, glucose-galactose malabsorption or sucrase-isomaltase insufficiency should not take CALFOVIT D3.

4.5 Interaction with other medicinal products and other forms of interaction

Absorption of orally administered tetracyclines can be reduced by the simultaneous oral administration of calcium. These two drugs should be taken at least 3 hours apart.

Some diuretics (furosemide, ethacrynic acid), antacids containing aluminium salts and thyroid hormones can inhibit calcium absorption and increase renal and faecal excretion. Thiazide diuretics can reduce urinary excretion of calcium and can induce hypercalcaemia, some antibiotics such as penicillin, neomycin and chloramphenicol can increase its absorption. Monitoring of the serum calcium levels during prolonged treatment is recommended.

Colestyramine, corticosteroids and mineral oils interfere with and reduce Vitamin D absorption, while phenytoin and barbiturates favour its inactivation.

The calcium/digitalis synergism on the heart may cause severe disorders of cardiac function (see section 4.4).

In case of concomitant treatment with bisphosphonate or with sodium fluoride, it is advisable to allow a minimum period of two hours before taking CALFOVIT D3 (risk of reduction of the gastrointestinal absorption of bisphosphonate and sodium fluoride).

Possible interactions may occur with food (e.g. foods containing phosphate, oxalic or phytinic acid) with a reduction of calcium absorption.

4.6 Pregnancy and lactation

Due to its high vitamin D content, CALFOVIT D3 is not indicated for use during pregnancy and lactation as the daily dose of Vitamin D should not exceed 600 I.U. Animal studies have shown that vitamin D overdose during pregnancy leads to teratogenic effects and there are no studies on this medicinal product in human pregnancy and lactation. Vitamin D and its metabolites pass into breast milk. Therefore CALFOVIT D3 should not be used during pregnancy and breast-feeding.

4.7 Effects on ability to drive and use machines

None

4.8 Undesirable effects

There have been rare reports of mild gastrointestinal disorders (nausea, constipation, diarrhoea, epigastric pain) and hypersensitivity reactions (anaphylaxis, urticaria and allergic rashes). Although hypercalcaemia should not develop in patients with good renal function, the following symptoms may be indicative of hypercalcaemia: anorexia, nausea, vomiting, headache, weakness, apathy and drowsiness. More severe symptoms may include: thirst, dehydration, polyuria, nocturia, abdominal pain, paralytic ileus and cardiac arrhythmia.

4.9 Overdose

An acute or long-term overdose may cause hypervitaminosis D and hypercalcaemia.

Symptoms of an overdose are nausea, vomiting, thirst, polyuria and constipation; a chronic overdose may lead to vascular and organ calcification.

Treatment of an overdose: all treatments with calcium and vitamin D must be discontinued. Rehydration should be carried out.

5. PHARMACOLOGICAL PROPERTIES

5.1 Pharmacodynamic properties

Calcium, combinations with other drugs. ATC code: A12AX

CALFOVIT D3 is a preparation for oral use, in which calcium phosphate is associated with colecaliferol (Vitamin D3).

Calcium and Vitamin D have a fundamental effect on "bone rebuilding" processes and it is for this reason that they are used in those conditions of the elderly patient characterised by a negative calcium balance with low levels of circulating Vitamin D and elevated serum levels of parathormone. This secondary hyperparathyroidism is effectively corrected by the combined effect of tribasic calcium phosphate and Vitamin D3, the active ingredients in CALFOVIT D3.

Vitamin D3 regulates calcium and phosphate metabolism, guaranteeing calcium absorption by the intestinal mucosa.

5.2 Pharmacokinetic properties

Approximately 30% of administered calcium is absorbed in the proximal part of the small intestine. Vitamin D is also quickly absorbed in the intestines after oral administration. The role of bile salts in facilitating absorption is well known. Approximately 40% of plasma calcium is bound to proteins, especially albumin, approximately 1/10 is diffusable, but bound to anions (phosphates); the remaining fraction is diffusable ionic calcium which has a physiological effect.

Vitamin D has a half-life of 19 to 25 hours, and circulates in the plasma bound to a specific protein, an alpha-globulin, and it is accumulated in the body for long periods. In the liver Vitamin D is converted into the derivative 25-hydroxylate (calcidiol) which is put back into the circulation where it binds with a specific alpha-globulin and undergoes further hydroxylation in the kidneys into 1-25 hydroxyderivative (calcitriol). Vitamin D is excreted mainly in the bile. Only a small portion of the administered dose is found in the urine.

Calcium is secreted into the gastro-intestinal tract via the saliva, bile and pancreatic secretion. Calcium from these sources, along with the calcium that is not absorbed comprises the portion excreted in the faeces. Of the portion of calcium excreted via the renal system, approximately 2/3 of the filtered calcium is reabsorbed.

Parathormone stimulates calcium reabsorption in the convoluted distal tubules, while Vitamin D increments proximal reabsorption. Part of the calcium is also excreted in perspiration

5.3 Preclinical safety data

Chronic safety evaluation studies in animals show that Vitamin D and Calcium combination is generally well tolerated.

Preclinical data revealed no specific hazard for humans, except for toxicity to reproduction (see section 4.6).

6. PHARMACEUTICAL PARTICULARS

6.1 List of excipients

Propylene glycol

Sunset yellow FCF (E110)

Lemon flavouring (containing: natural flavourings, maltodextrin, gum arabic)

Saccharin sodium

Anhydrous citric acid

Microcrystalline cellulose and carmellose sodium

Monopalmitate sucrose

Silica colloidal anhydrous

Mannitol

α-tocopherol

Edible fats

Gelatin

Sucrose

Maize starch.

6.2 Incompatibilities

Not applicable

6.3 Shelf life

2 years.

Shelf life after reconstitution: use immediately.

6.4 Special precautions for storage

Do not store above 25°C.

6.5 Nature and contents of container

Single, paper-aluminium-polythene bonded, sealed sachets.

The sachets are packaged in cardboard boxes containing 2, 30 or 60 sachets.

Not all pack sizes may be marketed.

6.6 Special precautions for disposal and other handling

No special requirements

7. MARKETING AUTHORISATION HOLDER

Menarini International Operations Luxembourg S.A.

1, Avenue de la Gare

L-1611

Luxembourg

8. MARKETING AUTHORISATION NUMBER(S)

PL 16239/0027

9. DATE OF FIRST AUTHORISATION/RENEWAL OF THE AUTHORISATION

1st January 2007

10. DATE OF REVISION OF THE TEXT

May 2008

Legal category

P

Calmurid Cream

(Galderma (U.K) Ltd)

1. NAME OF THE MEDICINAL PRODUCT

Calmurid Cream

2. QUALITATIVE AND QUANTITATIVE COMPOSITION

A white cream containing Urea Ph.Eur 10.0 % w/w and Lactic Acid Ph.Eur 5.0% w/w in a stabilising emulsified base.

3. PHARMACEUTICAL FORM

Cream for topical (cutaneous) use.

4. CLINICAL PARTICULARS

4.1 Therapeutic indications

To be applied topically for the correction of hyperkeratosis and dryness in ichthyosis and allied conditions characterised by dry, rough, scaly skin.

4.2 Posology and method of administration

For external use only.

Dosage and administration:

Adults, elderly and children:

A thick layer of Calmurid is applied twice daily after washing the affected area. The cream is left on the skin for 3-5 minutes and then rubbed lightly in. Excess cream should be wiped off the skin with a tissue, not washed off. Frequency of application can be reduced as the patient progresses. In hyperkeratosis of the feet apply Calmurid as above after soaking the feet in warm water for 15 minutes and drying with a rough towel.

4.3 Contraindications

Hypersensitivity to any constituent of the product.

4.4 Special warnings and precautions for use

Calmurid is acidic and hypertonic and can cause smarting if applied to raw areas, fissures or mucous membranes. Where this is a barrier to therapy the use of Calmurid diluted 50% with aqueous cream B.P. for one week should result in freedom from smarting upon use of Calmurid.

4.5 Interaction with other medicinal products and other forms of interaction

Low pH of cream might affect stability of other drugs.

4.6 Pregnancy and lactation

There is no specific data available regarding the use in pregnant women and during lactation.

4.7 Effects on ability to drive and use machines

None known.

4.8 Undesirable effects

Calmurid is acidic and hypertonic and can cause smarting if applied to raw areas, fissures or mucous membranes.

4.9 Overdose

Unlikely. In the case of smarting, wash the cream off.

5. PHARMACOLOGICAL PROPERTIES

5.1 Pharmacodynamic properties

Urea at a concentration of 10% has keratolytic, anti microbial, anti pruritic and hydrating effects on the skin. Lactic acid has keratolytic, hydrating and anti microbial properties also. Treatment of ichthyotic patients shows a parallel between clinical improvement and increase in the otherwise depressed binding capacity of the horny layer.

5.2 Pharmacokinetic properties

Not applicable.

5.3 Preclinical safety data

Urea and lactic acid are long established materials, whose pre-clinical profile is known.

6. PHARMACEUTICAL PARTICULARS

6.1 List of excipients

Glyceryl Monostearate Ph.Eur.

Betaine Monohydrate

Diethanolamine Cetylphosphate ("Amphisol")

Adeps Solidus (Hard Fat) Ph.Eur

Cholesterol USNF

Sodium chloride Ph.Eur

Purified water Ph.Eur.

6.2 Incompatibilities

The low pH due to lactic acid means care in choice of other packages or other drugs admixed.

6.3 Shelf life

30 months.

6.4 Special precautions for storage

Store below 25°C. Do not freeze. Do not put in alloy containers.

6.5 Nature and contents of container

White low density polyethylene tubes fitted with white polypropylene screw caps

Package sizes: 15, 20, 30, 50, 100 g.

Pump dispenser: White polypropylene bottle fitted with a white polyethylene closure and a natural polyethylene follower plate.

Package sizes: 400, 500 g.

Not all pack sizes may be marketed.

6.6 Special precautions for disposal and other handling

Not relevant.

7. MARKETING AUTHORISATION HOLDER

Galderma (UK) Limited

Meridien House

69-71 Clarendon Road

Watford

Herts.

WD17 1DS

UK

8. MARKETING AUTHORISATION NUMBER(S)

PL 10590/0009

9. DATE OF FIRST AUTHORISATION/RENEWAL OF THE AUTHORISATION

9 February 1993

10. DATE OF REVISION OF THE TEXT

July 2007

11 Legal category

P

Calmurid HC Cream

(Galderma (U.K) Ltd)

1. NAME OF THE MEDICINAL PRODUCT

Calmurid HC Cream

2. QUALITATIVE AND QUANTITATIVE COMPOSITION

Urea Ph. Eur. 10.0% w/w

Lactic Acid Ph. Eur. 5.0% w/w

Hydrocortisone Ph. Eur. 1.0% w/w

3. PHARMACEUTICAL FORM

Cream for topical (cutaneous) use.

4. CLINICAL PARTICULARS

4.1 Therapeutic indications

To be used topically for the treatment of atopic eczema, Besniers prurigo, acute and chronic allergic eczema, neurodermatitis and other hyperkeratotic skin conditions with accompanying inflammation.

4.2 Posology and method of administration

For external use only.

Adults, elderly and children:

Apply twice daily to the affected area after bathing or washing. Moist lesions should be treated as to dry them before using Calmurid HC.

4.3 Contraindications

Skin tuberculosis, viral infections accompanied by dermal manifestations e.g. herpes simplex, vaccinia, chicken pox and measles. Syphilitic skin lesions. In concurrent mycotic infections, the cream should be complemented with antimycotic treatment. Hypersensitivity to any constituent of the product.

4.4 Special warnings and precautions for use

In infants, high surface area in relation to mass raises the likelihood of uptake of excessive amounts of steroid from the cream, even without occlusion, thus adrenal suppression is more likely. In infants, long term continuous topical therapy should be avoided.

4.5 Interaction with other medicinal products and other forms of interaction

None known.

4.6 Pregnancy and lactation

There is no specific data available regarding the use in pregnant women and during lactation.

Pregnancy:

Evidence from animal studies suggests that prolonged intensive therapy with steroids during pregnancy should be avoided.

Lactation:

Given the slow uptake of hydrocortisone from the skin and the rapid destruction of hydrocortisone by the body, there would seem to be little risk of significant transfer at lactation.

4.7 Effects on ability to drive and use machines

None known.

4.8 Undesirable effects

If applied to open wounds or mucous membranes the hypertonic and acidic nature of the preparation may produce smarting. In such cases wash off with water. Where smarting is a barrier to therapy, dilute with an equal quantity of aqueous cream: after a week of treatment with this material, the normal strength should be tolerated.

4.9 Overdose

The barrier function in the skin to steroid uptake, the low toxicity of hydrocortisone and the nature mechanism for its rapid inactivation make overdose unlikely.

5. PHARMACOLOGICAL PROPERTIES

5.1 Pharmacodynamic properties

Urea at a concentration of 10% has keratolytic, anti microbial, anti pruritic and hydrating effects on the skin, properties also attributable to Lactic acid. Hydrocortisone 1% is the normal concentration of the drug used as a dermatological anti-inflammatory agent. In some patients with eczema, Calmurid HC cream may be as effective as fluorinated steroid creams.

5.2 Pharmacokinetic properties

Not applicable.

5.3 Preclinical safety data

Urea, lactic acid and hydrocortisone are long established materials, whose pre-clinical profile is known.

6. PHARMACEUTICAL PARTICULARS

6.1 List of excipients

Glyceryl Monostearate Ph. Eur.

Betaine Monohydrate

Diethanolamine Cetylphosphate ("Amphisol")

Adeps Solidus (Hard Fat) Ph. Eur.

Cholesterol USNF

Soduim Chloride Ph. Eur.

Purified Water Ph. Eur.

6.2 Incompatibilities

Do not mix with other preparations, as the effect on the stability of each is unknown. Do not pack in alloy containers as they may react with the lactic acid.

6.3 Shelf life

24 months

6.4 Special precautions for storage

Store below 25°C.

6.5 Nature and contents of container

Polypropylene tubes.

Package sizes: 15, 30, 50g 100 g.

6.6 Special precautions for disposal and other handling

Not relevant.

7. MARKETING AUTHORISATION HOLDER

Galderma (UK) Limited,

Meridien House

69-71 Clarendon Road

Watford

Herts.

WD17 1DS

UK

8. MARKETING AUTHORISATION NUMBER(S)

PL 10590/0010

9. DATE OF FIRST AUTHORISATION/RENEWAL OF THE AUTHORISATION

23rd February 2006

10. DATE OF REVISION OF THE TEXT

October 2006

CAMCOLIT 250

(Norgine Limited)

1. NAME OF THE MEDICINAL PRODUCT

CAMCOLIT 250 mg, Lithium Carbonate

2. QUALITATIVE AND QUANTITATIVE COMPOSITION

The active ingredient is Lithium Carbonate; 250mg/tablet

3. PHARMACEUTICAL FORM

White film coated tablets engraved "CAMCOLIT" around one face and having a breakline on the reverse. For oral administration.

4. CLINICAL PARTICULARS

4.1 Therapeutic indications

The treatment and prophylaxis of mania, manic depressive illness and recurrent depression, and the treatment of aggressive or self mutilating behaviour.

4.2 Posology and method of administration

Regular monitoring of plasma lithium concentration is always obligatory when Lithium is used; lithium therapy should not be initiated unless adequate facilities for routine monitoring of plasma concentrations are available. On initiation of plasma therapy concentrations should be measured weekly until stabilisation is achieved, then weekly for one month and at monthly intervals thereafter.

Additional measurements should be made if signs of lithium toxicity occur, on dosage alteration, development of significant intercurrent disease, signs of manic depressions or depressive relapse and if significant change in sodium or fluid intake occurs. More frequent monitoring is required if patients are receiving any drug treatment that affects renal clearance of lithium e.g. diuretics and NSAID. As bioavailability may vary between formulations, should a change of preparations be made, blood levels should be monitored weekly until restabilisation is achieved.

Acute mania:

Adults: Treatment should be initiated in hospital where regular monitoring of plasma lithium levels can be conducted. The dosage of Camcolit should be adjusted to produce a plasma lithium level between 0.6 and 1.0 mmol/l 12 hours after the last dose. The required plasma lithium level may be achieved in one of two ways but, whichever is adopted, regular estimations must be carried out to ensure maintenance of levels within the therapeutic range. For consistent results it is essential that the blood samples for plasma lithium estimations are taken 12 hours after the last dose of lithium.

1. 1,000-1,500 mg of lithium carbonate are administered daily for the first five days. A blood sample for plasma lithium estimation is taken 12 hours after the last dose on the fifth day, and the dosage of Camcolit is adjusted to keep the plasma lithium level within the therapeutic range. Subsequently, regular plasma lithium estimations must be carried out and, where necessary, the dosage of Camcolit adjusted accordingly. The precise initial dose of lithium should be decided in the light of the age and weight of the patient; young patients often require a dose higher than average and older patients a lower dose.

2. A lithium clearance test is carried out and the initial dosage calculated from the results. Even when the initial dosage is calculated in this way, it is still desirable that plasma lithium levels should be determined at weekly intervals during the first three weeks of treatment, and any necessary adjustments to dosage made as a result of the levels actually obtained.

Most of the above applies in the treatment of hypomania as well as mania, but the patient (if not too ill) can be started on treatment as an outpatient provided that facilities for regular plasma lithium monitoring are available, and assays are initiated within one week.

Prophylaxis of recurrent affective disorders:

Adults: (Including unipolar mania & unipolar depressions and bipolar manic-depressive illness): A low dose of 300-400 mg of lithium carbonate can be administered daily for the first seven days. A blood sample for plasma lithium estimation is then taken 12 hours after the last dose, and the dosage of Camcolit is adjusted to keep the plasma lithium level within the range of 0.4-0.8 mmol/l. Toxic symptoms are usually associated with concentrations exceeding 1.5 mmol/l.

Elderly: As for prophylaxis above, but 12 hour lithium levels should be kept in the range of 0.4-0.7 mmol/l as toxic symptoms are likely with plasma concentrations above 1.0 mmol/l.

Use in children: Not recommended

4.3 Contraindications

Patients with renal disease, cardiovascular Addison's disease or those breast feeding.

4.4 Special warnings and precautions for use

Pre-treatment and periodic routine clinical monitoring is essential. This should include assessment of renal function, urine analysis, assessment of thyroid function and cardiac function, especially in patients with cardiovascular disease.

Patients should be euthyroid before initiation of lithium therapy.

Clear instructions regarding the symptoms of impending toxicity should be given by the doctor to all patients receiving long-term lithium therapy. Patients should also be warned to report if polyuria or polydipsia develop. Episodes of nausea and vomiting or other conditions leading to salt/water depletion (including severe dieting) should also be reported. Patients should be advised to maintain their usual salt and fluid intake.

Elderly patients are particularly liable to lithium toxicity.

Caution is advised in patients with cardiovascular disease or family history of QT prolongation.

Concomitant administration of antipsychotics should be avoided.

4.5 Interaction with other medicinal products and other forms of interaction

Lower doses of lithium may be required during diuretic therapy as lithium clearance is reduced.

Serum lithium concentrations may increase during concomitant therapy with non-steroidal anti-inflammatory drugs, or tetracycline, possibly resulting in lithium toxicity. Serum lithium concentrations therefore should be monitored more frequently if NSAID or tetracycline therapy is initiated or discontinued.

Raised plasma levels of ADH may occur during treatment.

Symptoms of nephrogenic diabetes insipidus are particularly prevalent in patients receiving concurrent treatment with tricyclic or tetracyclic antidepressants.

Use with concomitant QT prolonging drugs (e.g. Class IA and III antiarrhythmics, arsenic trioxide, dolasetron mesylate, mefloquine, IV erythromycin) is not recommended.

Use with drugs causing electrolyte imbalance is not recommended.

4.6 Pregnancy and lactation

Pregnancy: There is epidemiological evidence to suggest that the drug may be harmful during human pregnancy, and therefore Camcolit should not be used during pregnancy.

Lactation: Infants of mothers on lithium should be bottle fed as lithium is present in the breast milk.

4.7 Effects on ability to drive and use machines

As lithium may cause disturbances of the CNS, patients should be warned of the possible hazards when driving or operating machinery.

4.8 Undesirable effects

Long term treatment with lithium may result in permanent changes in the kidney and impairment of renal function. High serum concentrations of lithium, including episodes of acute lithium toxicity may enhance these changes. The minimum clinically effective dose of lithium should always be used. Patients should only be maintained on lithium after 3-5 years if, on assessment, benefit persists.

Renal function should be routinely monitored in patients with polyuria and polydipsia.

Side effects are usually related to serum lithium concentrations and are infrequent at levels below 1.0 mmol/l.

Mild gastro-intestinal effects, nausea, vertigo, muscle weakness and a dazed feeling may occur, but frequently disappear after stabilisation. Fine hand tremors, polyuria and mild thirst may persist. Some studies suggest that the tremor can be controlled by relatively small doses of propranolol.

Long term treatment with lithium is frequently associated with disturbances of thyroid function including goitre and hypothyroidism. These can be controlled by administration of small doses of thyroxine (0.05-0.2 mg daily) concomitantly with lithium. Thyrotoxicosis has also been reported.

Mild cognitive impairment may occur during long term use.

Hypercalcaemia, hypermagnesaemia, hyperparathyroidism and an increase in antinuclear antibodies have also been reported.

Exacerbation of psoriasis may occur.

Cardiovascular effects of lithium are rare and often benign. Reported effects are arrhythmia, oedema and sinus node dysfunction. QT interval prolongation, ventricular arrhythmias – ventricular fibrillation, ventricular tachycardia (rare), sudden unexplained death, cardiac arrest and Torsade de pointes have been reported, Any signs of cardiac disturbance e.g. syncope, heart rhythm or rate disturbances should be investigated further.

Oedema with weight gain can occur and may lead to an increased risk of lithium toxicity if treated incautiously with diuretic drugs.

4.9 Overdose

Symptoms, emergency procedures, antidotes

Appearance or aggravation of gastro-intestinal symptoms, muscle weakness, lack of coordination, drowsiness or lethargy may be early signs of intoxication. With increasing toxicity, ataxia, giddiness, tinnitus, blurred vision, coarse tremor, muscle twitching and a large output of dilute urine may be seen. At blood levels above 2 – 3 mmol/l, increasing disorientation, seizures, coma and death may occur.

There is no antidote to lithium poisoning. In the event, lithium treatment should be stopped immediately and serum levels estimated every 6 hours. When ingestion is recent, gastric lavage should be carried out, together with general supportive measures. Special attention must be given to the maintenance of fluid and electrolyte balance, and also adequate renal function. Sodium-depleting diuretics should not be used in any circumstances. Forced alkaline diuresis may be used. If the serum lithium level is above 4.0 mmol/l, or if there is a deterioration in the patient's condition, or if the serum concentration is not falling at a rate equivalent to a half-life of less than 30 hours, peritoneal dialysis or haemodialysis should be instituted promptly. This should be continued until the serum and dialysis fluid are free of lithium. Serum lithium levels should be monitored for at least another 7 days thereafter, as a rebound rise is possible due to delayed diffusion form the tissues.

5. PHARMACOLOGICAL PROPERTIES

5.1 Pharmacodynamic properties

The precise mechanism of action of lithium as a mood-stabilising agent remains unknown, although many cellular actions of lithium have been characterised.

5.2 Pharmacokinetic properties

The pharmacokinetics of lithium are extremely well documented. A single oral dose of CAMCOLIT 250 gives a peak plasma level approximately 2-3 hours later, with the level at 24 hours being approximately 40% of peak levels.

5.3 Preclinical safety data

There is no preclinical data of relevance to the prescriber.

6. PHARMACEUTICAL PARTICULARS

6.1 List of excipients

Maize Starch

Magnesium Stearate

Pregelatinised Maize Starch

Hypromellose

Macrogol 400

6.2 Incompatibilities

Not applicable.

6.3 Shelf life

The shelf life is 5 years.

6.4 Special precautions for storage

Do not store above 25°C. Keep the container tightly closed.

6.5 Nature and contents of container

Polypropylene tablet container, containing 100 or 1000 tablets. Not all pack sizes maybe included.

6.6 Special precautions for disposal and other handling

No special requirements.

7. MARKETING AUTHORISATION HOLDER
Norgine Limited
Chaplin House
Widewater Place
Moorhall Road
Harefield
Uxbridge
Middlesex UB9 6NS
United Kingdom

8. MARKETING AUTHORISATION NUMBER(S)
PL 00322/5900R

9. DATE OF FIRST AUTHORISATION/RENEWAL OF THE AUTHORISATION
12 June 2002

10. DATE OF REVISION OF THE TEXT
January 2009

CAMCOLIT 400

(Norgine Limited)

1. NAME OF THE MEDICINAL PRODUCT
CAMCOLIT 400 mg, controlled release Lithium Carbonate.

This product may also be sold as LITHONATE.

2. QUALITATIVE AND QUANTITATIVE COMPOSITION
The active ingredient is Lithium Carbonate; 400mg/tablet.

3. PHARMACEUTICAL FORM
White film coated tablet engraved "CAMCOLIT-S" around one face and having a breakline on the reverse. The tablet is a controlled release formulation. If sold as LITHONATE the tablet is engraved on one side "LIT 400"

For oral administration.

4. CLINICAL PARTICULARS
4.1 Therapeutic indications
The treatment and prophylaxis of mania, manic-depressive illness and recurrent depression, and the treatment of aggressive or self mutilating behaviour.

4.2 Posology and method of administration
Regular monitoring of plasma lithium concentration is always obligatory when lithium is used; lithium therapy should not be initiated unless adequate facilities for routine monitoring of plasma concentrations are available. On initiation of plasma therapy concentrations should be measured weekly until stabilisation is achieved, then weekly for one month and at monthly intervals thereafter.

Additional measurements should be made if signs of lithium toxicity occur, on dosage alteration, development of significant intercurrent disease, signs of manic or depressive relapse and if significant change in sodium or fluid intake occurs. More frequent monitoring is required if patients are receiving any drug treatment that affects renal clearance of lithium e.g. diuretics and NSAID. As bioavailability may vary between formulations, should a change of preparations be made, blood levels should be monitored weekly until restabilisation is achieved.

Acute mania:

Treatment should be initiated in hospital where regular monitoring of plasma lithium levels can be conducted. The dosage of Camcolit should be adjusted to produce a plasma lithium level between 0.6 and 1.0 mmol/l 12 hours after the last dose. The required plasma lithium level may be achieved in one of two ways but, whichever is adopted, regular estimations must be carried out to ensure maintenance of levels within the therapeutic range. For consistent results it is essential that the blood samples for plasma lithium estimations are taken 12 hours after the last dose of lithium.

1. 1,000-1,500 mg of lithium carbonate are administered daily for the first five days. A blood sample for plasma lithium estimation is taken 12 hours after the last dose on the fifth day, and the dosage of Camcolit is adjusted to keep the plasma lithium level within the therapeutic range. Subsequently, regular plasma lithium estimations must be carried out and, where necessary, the dosage of Camcolit adjusted accordingly. The precise initial dose of lithium should be decided in the light of the age and weight of the patient; young patients often require a dose higher than average and older patients a lower dose.

2. A lithium clearance test is carried out and the initial dosage calculated from the results. Even when the initial dosage is calculated in this way, it is still desirable that plasma lithium levels should be determined at weekly intervals during the first three weeks of treatment, and any necessary adjustments to dosage made as a result of the levels actually obtained.

Most of the above applies in the treatment of hypomania as well as mania, but the patient (if not too ill) can be started on treatment as an outpatient provided that facilities for regular plasma lithium monitoring are available, and assays are initiated within one week.

Prophylaxis of recurrent affective disorders:

(Including unipolar mania & unipolar depressions and bipolar manic-depressive illness): A low dose of 300-400 mg of lithium carbonate can be administered daily for the first seven days. A blood sample for plasma lithium estimation is then taken 12 hours after the last dose, and the dosage of Camcolit is adjusted to keep the plasma lithium level within the range of 0.4-0.8 mmol/l. Toxic symptoms are usually associated with concentrations exceeding 1.5 mmol/l.

Use in Elderly: As for prophylaxis above, but 12 hour lithium levels should be kept in the range of 0.4-0.7 mmol/l as toxic symptoms are likely with plasma concentrations above 1.0 mmol/l.

Use in children: Not recommended

4.3 Contraindications
Patients with renal disease, untreated hypothyroidism, cardiac disease, Addison's disease or those breast feeding.

4.4 Special warnings and precautions for use
Pre-treatment and periodic routine clinical monitoring is essential. This should include assessment of renal function, urine analysis, assessment of thyroid function and cardiac function, especially in patients with cardiovascular disease.

Patients should be euthyroid before initiation of lithium therapy.

Clear instructions regarding the symptoms of impending toxicity should be given by the doctor to all patients receiving long-term lithium therapy. Patients should also be warned to report if polyuria or polydipsia develop. Episodes of nausea and vomiting or other conditions leading to salt/water depletion (including severe dieting) should also be reported. Patients should be advised to maintain their usual salt and fluid intake.

Elderly patients are particularly liable to lithium toxicity.

Caution is advised in patients with cardiovascular disease or family history of QT prolongation.

Concomitant administration of antipsychotics should be avoided.

4.5 Interaction with other medicinal products and other forms of interaction
Lower doses of lithium may be required during diuretic therapy as lithium clearance is reduced.

Serum lithium concentrations may increase during concomitant therapy with non-steroidal anti-inflammatory drugs, or tetracycline, possibly resulting in lithium toxicity. Serum lithium concentrations therefore should be monitored more frequently if NSAID or tetracycline therapy is initiated or discontinued.

Raised plasma levels of ADH may occur during treatment.

Symptoms of nephrogenic diabetes insipidus are particularly prevalent in patients receiving concurrent treatment with tricyclic or tetracyclic anti-depressants.

Use with concomitant QT prolonging drugs (e.g. Class IA and III antiarrhythmics, arsenic trioxide, dolasetron mesylate, mefloquine, IV erythromycin) is not recommended.

Use with drugs causing electrolyte imbalance is not recommended.

4.6 Pregnancy and lactation
Pregnancy: There is epidemiological evidence to suggest that the drug may be harmful during human pregnancy. Should the use of lithium be unavoidable, close monitoring of serum concentrations should be made throughout pregnancy and parturition.

Lactation: Infants of mothers on lithium should be bottle fed as lithium is present in the breast milk.

4.7 Effects on ability to drive and use machines
As lithium may cause disturbances of the CNS, patients should be warned of the possible hazards when driving or operating machinery.

4.8 Undesirable effects
Long term treatment with lithium may result in permanent changes in the kidney and impairment of renal function. High serum concentrations of lithium, including episodes of acute lithium toxicity may enhance these changes. The minimum clinically effective dose of lithium should always be used. Patients should only be maintained on lithium after 3 – 5 years if, on assessment, benefit persists.

Renal function should be routinely monitored in patients with polyuria and polydipsia. Side effects are usually related to serum lithium concentrations and infrequent at levels below 1.0 mmol/l.

Mild gastro-intestinal effects, nausea, vertigo, muscle weakness and a dazed feeling may occur, but frequently disappear after stabilisation. Fine hand tremors, polyuria and mild thirst may persist. Some studies suggest that the tremor can be controlled by relatively small doses of propranolol.

Long term treatment with lithium is frequently associated with disturbances of thyroid function including goitre and hypothyroidism. These can be controlled by administration of small doses of thyroxine (0.05-0.2 mg daily) concomitantly with lithium. Thyrotoxicosis has also been reported.

Mild cognitive impairment may occur during long term use.

Hypercalcaemia, hypermagnesaemia, hyperparathyroidism and an increase in antinuclear antibodies have also been reported.

Exacerbation of psoriasis may occur.

Cardiovascular effects of lithium are rare and often benign. Reported effects are arrhythmia, oedema and sinus node dysfunction. QT interval prolongation, ventricular arrhythmias – ventricular fibrillation, ventricular tachycardia (rare), sudden unexplained death, cardiac arrest and Torsade de pointes have been reported, Any signs of cardiac disturbance e.g. syncope, heart rhythm or rate disturbances should be investigated further.

Oedema with weight gain can occur and may lead to an increased risk of lithium toxicity if treated incautiously with diuretic drugs.

4.9 Overdose
Symptoms, emergency procedures, antidotes
Appearance or aggravation of gastro-intestinal symptoms, muscle weakness, lack of coordination, drowsiness or lethargy may be early signs of intoxication. With increasing toxicity, ataxia, giddiness, tinnitus, blurred vision, coarse tremor, muscle twitching and a large output of dilute urine may be seen. At blood levels above 2 – 3 mmol/l, increasing disorientation, seizures, coma and death may occur.

There is no antidote to lithium poisoning. In the event, lithium treatment should be stopped immediately and serum levels estimated every 6 hours. When ingestion is recent, gastric lavage should be carried out, together with general supportive measures. Special attention must be given to the maintenance of fluid and electrolyte balance, and also adequate renal function. Sodium-depleting diuretics should not be used in any circumstances. Forced alkaline diuresis may be used. If the serum lithium level is above 4.0 mmol/l, or if there is a deterioration in the patient's condition, or if the serum concentration is not falling at a rate equivalent to a half-life of less than 30 hours, peritoneal dialysis or haemodialysis should be instituted promptly. This should be continued until the serum and dialysis fluid are free of lithium. Serum lithium levels should be monitored for at least another 7 days thereafter, as a rebound rise is possible due to delayed diffusion form the tissues.

5. PHARMACOLOGICAL PROPERTIES
5.1 Pharmacodynamic properties
The precise mechanism of action of lithium as a mood-stabilising agent remains unknown, although many cellular actions of lithium have been characterised.

5.2 Pharmacokinetic properties
The pharmacokinetics of lithium are extremely well documented. A single oral dose of CAMCOLIT 400 gives a peak plasma level approximately 3-4 hours later, with the level at 24 hours being approximately 40% of peak levels.

5.3 Preclinical safety data
There is no preclinical data of relevance to the prescriber.

6. PHARMACEUTICAL PARTICULARS
6.1 List of excipients
Maize Starch
Acacia
Magnesium Stearate
Sodium Lauryl Sulphate
Hypromellose
Macrogol 400
Opasrpay M-1-7111B

6.2 Incompatibilities
See 4.5 and 4.8 above.

6.3 Shelf life
The shelf life is 3 years.

6.4 Special precautions for storage
Do not store above 25°C. Keep the container tightly closed. Keep out of the reach and sight of children.

6.5 Nature and contents of container
Polypropylene containers of 100 or 500 tablet capacity, and for hospital use only, screw cap-amber glass bottles of 50 or 100 tablet capacity.

6.6 Special precautions for disposal and other handling
None.

7. MARKETING AUTHORISATION HOLDER
Norgine Limited
Chaplin House
Widewater Place
Moorhall Road
Harefield
Uxbridge
Middlesex UB9 6NS
United Kingdom

8. MARKETING AUTHORISATION NUMBER(S)
PL 00322/0015

9. DATE OF FIRST AUTHORISATION/RENEWAL OF THE AUTHORISATION
12 June 2002

10. DATE OF REVISION OF THE TEXT
Date approved: January 2009

Legal Category: POM

Campral EC

(Merck Serono)

1. NAME OF THE MEDICINAL PRODUCT
Campral EC

2. QUALITATIVE AND QUANTITATIVE COMPOSITION
Each tablet contains acamprosate (I.N.N.) calcium 333.0 mg as the active ingredient.

3. PHARMACEUTICAL FORM
Enterocoated tablets.

4. CLINICAL PARTICULARS

4.1 Therapeutic indications
Acamprosate is indicated as therapy to maintain abstinence in alcohol-dependent patients. It should be combined with counselling.

4.2 Posology and method of administration
Adults within the age range 18-65 years:

- 2 tablets three times daily with meals (2 tablets morning, noon and night) in subjects weighing 60kg or more.

- In subjects weighing less than 60kg, 4 tablets divided into three daily doses with meals (2 tablets in the morning, 1 at noon and 1 at night).

Children and the Elderly:

Acamprosate should not be administered to children and the elderly.

The recommended treatment period is one year. Treatment with acamprosate should be initiated as soon as possible after the withdrawal period and should be maintained if the patient relapses.

4.3 Contraindications
Acamprosate is contraindicated:

– in patients with a known hypersensitivity to the drug

– in pregnant women and lactating women

– in cases of renal insufficiency (serum creatinine >120 micromol/L)

– in cases with severe hepatic failure (Childs- Pugh Classification C)

4.4 Special warnings and precautions for use
Acamprosate does not constitute treatment for the withdrawal period.

Acamprosate does not prevent the harmful effects of continuous alcohol abuse. Continued alcohol abuse negates the therapeutic benefit, therefore acamprosate treatment should only be initiated after weaning therapy, once the patient is abstinent from alcohol.

Because the interrelationship between alcohol dependence, depression and suicidality is well-recognised and complex, it is recommended that alcohol-dependent patients, including those treated with acamprosate, be monitored for such symptoms.

4.5 Interaction with other medicinal products and other forms of interaction
The concomitant intake of alcohol and acamprosate does not affect the pharmacokinetics of either alcohol or acamprosate. Administering acamprosate with food diminishes the bioavailability of the drug compared with its administration in the fasting state. Pharmacokinetic studies have been completed and show no interaction between acamprosate and diazepam, disulfiram or imipramine. There is no information available on the concomitant administration of acamprosate with diuretics.

4.6 Pregnancy and lactation
Although animal studies have not shown any evidence of foetotoxicity or teratogenicity, the safety of acamprosate has not been established in pregnant women. Acamprosate should not be administered to pregnant women.

Acamprosate is excreted in the milk of lactating animals. Safe use of acamprosate has not been demonstrated in lactating women. Acamprosate should not be administered to breast feeding women.

4.7 Effects on ability to drive and use machines
Acamprosate should not impair the patient's ability to drive or operate machinery.

4.8 Undesirable effects
The following definitions apply to the frequency terminology used hereafter: very common (≥ 1/10), common (≥ 1/100, < 1/10), uncommon (≥ 1/1,000, < 1/100), rare (≥ 1/10,000, < 1/1,000), very rare (< 1/10,000, including isolated cases), frequency not known (cannot be estimated from the available data)

Within each frequency grouping, undesirable effects are presented in order of decreasing seriousness.

Gastrointestinal disorders:

Very common: Diarrhoea

Common: Abdominal pain, nausea, vomiting

Skin and subcutaneous tissue disorders:

Common: Pruritus, maculo-papular rash

Rare: Bullous skin reactions

Immune system disorders:

Very rare: Hypersensitivity reactions including urticaria, angio-oedema or anaphylactic reactions.

Reproductive system and breast disorders:

Common: Frigidity or impotence.

Psychiatric disorders:

Common: Decreased libido

Uncommon: Increased libido

4.9 Overdose
Five cases of overdose associated with acamprosate therapy have been reported in humans, including one patient who ingested 43g of acamprosate. After gastric lavage all patients had an uneventful recovery. Diarrhoea was observed in two cases. No case of hypercalcaemia was reported in the course of these overdoses. However, should this occur, the patients should be treated for acute hypercalcaemia.

5. PHARMACOLOGICAL PROPERTIES

5.1 Pharmacodynamic properties
Acamprosate (calcium acetylhomotaurinate) has a chemical structure similar to that of amino acid neuromediators, such as taurine or gamma-amino-butyric acid (GABA), including an acetylation to permit passage across the blood brain barrier. Acamprosate may act by stimulating GABAergic inhibitory neurotransmission and antagonising excitatory amino-acids, particularly glutamate. Animal experimental studies have demonstrated that acamprosate affects alcohol dependence in rats, decreasing the voluntary intake of alcohol without affecting food and total fluid intake.

5.2 Pharmacokinetic properties
Acamprosate absorption across the gastrointestinal tract is moderate, slow and sustained and varies substantially from person to person. Food reduces the oral absorption of acamprosate. Steady state levels of acamprosate are achieved by the seventh day of dosing. Acamprosate is not protein bound.

Oral absorption shows considerable variability and is usually less than 10% of the ingested drug in the first 24 hours. The drug is excreted in the urine and is not metabolised significantly. There is a linear relationship between creatinine clearance values and total apparent plasma clearance, renal clearance and plasma half-life of acamprosate.

The kinetics of acamprosate are not modified in group A or B of the Child-Pugh classification of impaired liver function, a population which is likely to be part of the target population for acamprosate. This is in accordance with the absence of hepatic metabolism of the drug.

5.3 Preclinical safety data
In the preclinical studies, signs of toxicity are related to the excessive intake of calcium and not to acetylhomotaurine. Disorders of phosphorus/calcium metabolism have been observed including diarrhoea, soft tissue calcification, renal and cardiac lesions. Acamprosate had no mutagenic or carcinogenic effect, nor any teratogenic or adverse effects on the male or female reproductive systems of animals. Detailed *in vitro* and *in vivo* research on acamprosate to detect genetic and chromosomal mutations has not produced any evidence of potential genetic toxicity.

6. PHARMACEUTICAL PARTICULARS

6.1 List of excipients
Crospovidone (KOLLIDON CL)

Microcrystalline cellulose (AVICEL PH 101)

Magnesium silicate (COMPRESSIL)

Sodium starch glycolate (EXPLOTAB)

Anhydrous colloidal silica (AEROSIL 200)

Magnesium stearate

Anionic copolymer of methacrylic and acrylic acid ethyl ester (EUDRAGIT L30 D)

Talc

Propylene glycol

6.2 Incompatibilities
None known

6.3 Shelf life
3 years

6.4 Special precautions for storage
None

6.5 Nature and contents of container
Aluminium/PVC sheets of blisters presented in cartons of 168 tablets.

6.6 Special precautions for disposal and other handling
Not applicable.

7. MARKETING AUTHORISATION HOLDER
Merck Santé s.a.s

37 rue Saint Romain

69379 Lyon Cedex 08

France

8. MARKETING AUTHORISATION NUMBER(S)
MA 13466/0001

9. DATE OF FIRST AUTHORISATION/RENEWAL OF THE AUTHORISATION
18 December 1995 (first authorization)

10. DATE OF REVISION OF THE TEXT
16 November 2007

LEGAL CATEGORY
POM

Campto 40mg/2ml and 100mg/5ml concentrate for solution for infusion

(Pfizer Limited)

1. NAME OF THE MEDICINAL PRODUCT
CAMPTO 20 mg/ml, concentrate for solution for infusion.

2. QUALITATIVE AND QUANTITATIVE COMPOSITION
The concentrate contains 20 mg/ml irinotecan hydrochloride, trihydrate (equivalent to 17.33 mg/ml irinotecan). Vials of CAMPTO contain 40 mg, 100 mg or 300 mg of irinotecan hydrochloride, trihydrate. For excipients, see section 6.1, 'List of excipients'.

3. PHARMACEUTICAL FORM
Concentrate for solution for infusion.

4. CLINICAL PARTICULARS

4.1 Therapeutic indications
CAMPTO is indicated for the treatment of patients with advanced colorectal cancer:

- in combination with 5-fluorouracil and folinic acid in patients without prior chemotherapy for advanced disease,
- as a single agent in patients who have failed an established 5-fluorouracil containing treatment regimen.

CAMPTO in combination with cetuximab is indicated for the treatment of patients with epidermal growth factor receptor (EGFR)-expressing, KRAS wild-type metastatic colorectal cancer, who had not received prior treatment for metastatic disease or after failure of irinotecan-including cytotoxic therapy (please see 5.1).

CAMPTO in combination with 5-fluorouracil, folinic acid and bevacizumab is indicated for first-line treatment of patients with metastatic carcinoma of the colon or rectum.

Campto in combination with capecitabine with or without bevacizumab is indicated for first-line treatment of patients with metastatic colorectal carcinoma.

4.2 Posology and method of administration
For adults only. CAMPTO solution for infusion should be infused into a peripheral or central vein.

Recommended dosage:

In monotherapy (for previously treated patient):

The recommended dosage of CAMPTO is 350 mg/m^2 administered as an intravenous infusion over a 30- to 90-minute period every three weeks (see «Instructions for Use/Handling» and «Special Warnings and Special Precautions for Use» sections).

In combination therapy (for previously untreated patient):

Safety and efficacy of CAMPTO in combination with 5-fluorouracil (5FU) and folinic acid (FA) have been assessed with the following schedule (see « Pharmacodynamic properties »):

- CAMPTO plus 5FU/FA in every 2 weeks schedule

The recommended dose of CAMPTO is 180 mg/m^2 administered once every 2 weeks as an intravenous infusion over a 30- to 90-minute period, followed by infusion with folinic acid and 5-fluorouracil.

For the posology and method of administration of concomitant cetuximab, refer to the product information for this medicinal product.

Normally, the same dose of irinotecan is used as administered in the last cycles of the prior irinotecan-containing regimen. Irinotecan must not be administered earlier than 1 hour after the end of the cetuximab infusion

For the posology and method of administration of bevacizumab, refer to the bevacizumab summary product of characteristics.

For the posology and method of administration of capecitabine combination, please see section 5.1 and refer to the appropriate sections in the capecitabine summary of product characteristics.

Dosage adjustments:

CAMPTO should be administered after appropriate recovery of all adverse events to grade 0 or 1 NCI-CTC grading (National Cancer Institute Common Toxicity Criteria) and when treatment-related diarrhoea is fully resolved.

At the start of a subsequent infusion of therapy, the dose of CAMPTO, and 5FU when applicable, should be decreased according to the worst grade of adverse events observed in the prior infusion. Treatment should be delayed by 1 to 2 weeks to allow recovery from treatment-related adverse events.

With the following adverse events a dose reduction of 15 to 20 % should be applied for CAMPTO and/or 5FU when applicable:

- haematological toxicity (neutropenia grade 4, febrile neutropenia (neutropenia grade 3-4 and fever grade 2-4), thrombocytopenia and leukopenia (grade 4)),
- non haematological toxicity (grade 3-4).

Recommendations for dose modifications of cetuximab when administered in combination with irinotecan must be followed according to the product information for this medicinal product.

Refer to the bevacizumab summary product of characteristics for dose modifications of bevacizumab when administered in combination with CAMPTO/5FU/FA.

In combination with capecitabine for patients 65 years of age or more, a reduction of the starting dose of capecitabine to 800 mg/m2 twice daily is recommended according to the summary of product characteristics for capecitabine. Refer also to the recommendations for dose modifications in combination regimen given in the summary of product characteristics for capecitabine.

Treatment Duration:

Treatment with CAMPTO should be continued until there is an objective progression of the disease or an unacceptable toxicity.

Special populations:

Patients with Impaired Hepatic Function: In monotherapy: Blood bilirubin levels (up to 3 times the upper limit of the normal range (UNL)) in patients with performance status $\leqslant 2$, should determine the starting dose of Campto. In these patients with hyperbilirubinemia and prothrombin time greater than 50%, the clearance of irinotecan is decreased (see "Pharmacokinetic properties" section) and therefore the risk of hematotoxicity is increased. Thus, weekly monitoring of complete blood counts should be conducted in this patient population.

- In patients with bilirubin up to 1.5 times the upper limit of the normal range (ULN), the recommended dosage of CAMPTO is 350 mg/m^2,
- In patients with bilirubin ranging from 1.5 to 3 times the ULN, the recommended dosage of CAMPTO is 200 mg/m^2,
- Patients with bilirubin beyond to 3 times the ULN should not be treated with CAMPTO (see « Contraindications » and « Special Warnings and Special Precautions for Use » sections).

No data are available in patients with hepatic impairment treated by CAMPTO in combination.

Patients with Impaired Renal Function: CAMPTO is not recommended for use in patients with impaired renal function, as studies in this population have not been conducted. (See « Special Warnings and Special Precautions for Use » and « Pharmacokinetic Properties »).

Elderly: No specific pharmacokinetic studies have been performed in elderly. However, the dose should be chosen carefully in this population due to their greater frequency of decreased biological functions. This population should require more intense surveillance (see « Special Warnings and Special Precautions for Use »).

4.3 Contraindications

- Chronic inflammatory bowel disease and/or bowel obstruction (see « Special Warnings and Special Precautions for Use »).
- History of severe hypersensitivity reactions to irinotecan hydrochloride trihydrate or to one of the excipients of CAMPTO.
- Pregnancy and lactation (see « Pregnancy and Lactation » and « Special Warnings and Special Precautions for Use » sections).
- Bilirubin > 3 times the upper limit of the normal range (see « Special warnings and Special Precautions for Use » section).
- Severe bone marrow failure.
- WHO performance status > 2.
- Concomitant use with St John's Wort (see section 4.5).

For additional contraindications of cetuximab or bevacizumab or capecitabine, refer to the product information for these medicinal products.

4.4 Special warnings and precautions for use

The use of CAMPTO should be confined to units specialised in the administration of cytotoxic chemotherapy and it should only be administered under the supervision of a physician qualified in the use of anticancer chemotherapy.

Given the nature and incidence of adverse events, CAMPTO will only be prescribed in the following cases after the expected benefits have been weighted against the possible therapeutic risks:

- in patients presenting a risk factor, particularly those with a WHO performance status = 2.
- in the few rare instances where patients are deemed unlikely to observe recommendations regarding management of adverse events (need for immediate and prolonged antidiarrhoeal treatment combined with high fluid intake at onset of delayed diarrhoea). Strict hospital supervision is recommended for such patients.

When CAMPTO is used in monotherapy, it is usually prescribed with the every-3-week-dosage schedule. However, the weekly-dosage schedule (see « Pharmacological properties ») may be considered in patients who may need a closer follow-up or who are at particular risk of severe neutropenia.

Delayed diarrhoea

Patients should be made aware of the risk of delayed diarrhoea occurring more than 24 hours after the administration of CAMPTO and at any time before the next cycle. In monotherapy, the median time of onset of the first liquid stool was on day 5 after the infusion of CAMPTO®. Patients should quickly inform their physician of its occurrence and start appropriate therapy immediately.

Patients with an increased risk of diarrhoea are those who had a previous abdominal/pelvic radiotherapy, those with baseline hyperleucocytosis, those with performance status $\geqslant 2$ and women. If not properly treated, diarrhoea can be life-threatening, especially if the patient is concomitantly neutropenic.

As soon as the first liquid stool occurs, the patient should start drinking large volumes of beverages containing electrolytes and an appropriate antidiarrhoeal therapy must be initiated immediately. This antidiarrhoeal treatment will be prescribed by the department where CAMPTO has been administered. After discharge from the hospital, the patients should obtain the prescribed drugs so that they can treat the diarrhoea as soon as it occurs. In addition, they must inform their physician or the department administering CAMPTO when/if diarrhoea is occurring.

The currently recommended antidiarrhoeal treatment consists of high doses of loperamide (4 mg for the first intake and then 2 mg every 2 hours). This therapy should continue for 12 hours after the last liquid stool and should not be modified. In no instance should loperamide be administered for more than 48 consecutive hours at these doses, because of the risk of paralytic ileus, nor for less than 12 hours.

In addition to the anti-diarrhoeal treatment, a prophylactic broad spectrum antibiotic should be given, when diarrhoea is associated with severe neutropenia (neutrophil count < 500 cells/mm^3).

In addition to the antibiotic treatment, hospitalisation is recommended for management of the diarrhoea, in the following cases:

- Diarrhoea associated with fever,
- Severe diarrhoea (requiring intravenous hydration),
- Diarrhoea persisting beyond 48 hours following the initiation of high-dose loperamide therapy.

Loperamide should not be given prophylactically, even in patients who experienced delayed diarrhoea at previous cycles.

In patients who experienced severe diarrhoea, a reduction in dose is recommended for subsequent cycles (see « Posology and Method of Administration » section).

Haematology

Weekly monitoring of complete blood cell counts is recommended during CAMPTO treatment. Patients should be aware of the risk of neutropenia and the significance of fever. Febrile neutropenia (temperature > 38°C and neutrophil count $\leqslant$ 1,000 cells/mm^3) should be urgently treated in the hospital with broad-spectrum intravenous antibiotics.

In patients who experienced severe haematological events, a dose reduction is recommended for subsequent administration (see « Posology and Method of Administration » section).

There is an increased risk of infections and haematological toxicity in patients with severe diarrhoea. In patients with severe diarrhoea, complete blood cell counts should be performed.

Liver impairment

Liver function tests should be performed at baseline and before each cycle.

Weekly monitoring of complete blood counts should be conducted in patients with bilirubin ranging from 1.5 to 3 times ULN, due to decrease of the clearance of irinotecan (see "Pharmacokinetic properties" section) and thus increasing the risk of hematotoxicity in this population. For patients with a bilirubin > 3 times ULN (see « Contraindications » section).

NAUSEA AND VOMITING

A prophylactic treatment with antiemetics is recommended before each treatment with CAMPTO. Nausea and vomiting have been frequently reported. Patients with vomiting associated with delayed diarrhoea should be hospitalised as soon as possible for treatment.

Acute cholinergic syndrome

If acute cholinergic syndrome appears (defined as early diarrhoea and various other symptoms such as sweating, abdominal cramping, lacrimation, myosis and salivation), atropine sulphate (0.25 mg subcutaneously) should be administered unless clinically contraindicated (see « Undesirable Effects » section). Caution should be exercised in patients with asthma. In patients who experienced an acute and severe cholinergic syndrome, the use of prophylactic atropine sulphate is recommended with subsequent doses of CAMPTO.

RESPIRATORY DISORDERS

Interstitial pulmonary disease presenting as pulmonary infiltrates is uncommon during irinotecan therapy. Interstitial pulmonary disease can be fatal. Risk factors possibly associated with the development of interstitial pulmonary disease include the use of pneumotoxic drugs, radiation therapy and colony stimulating factors. Patients with risk factors should be closely monitored for respiratory symptoms before and during irinotecan therapy.

ELDERLY

Due to the greater frequency of decreased biological functions, in particular hepatic function, in elderly patients, dose selection with CAMPTO should be cautious in this population (see « Posology and Method of Administration » section).

Patients with bowel obstruction

Patients must not be treated with CAMPTO until resolution of the bowel obstruction (see « Contraindications »).

Patients with Impaired Renal Function

Studies in this population have not been conducted. (see « Posology and Method of Administration » and « Pharmacokinetic Properties »).

Others

Since this medicinal contains sorbitol, it is unsuitable in hereditary fructose intolerance. Infrequent cases of renal insufficiency, hypotension or circulatory failure have been observed in patients who experienced episodes of dehydration associated with diarrhoea and/or vomiting, or sepsis. Contraceptive measures must be taken during and for at least three months after cessation of therapy.

Concomitant administration of irinotecan with a strong inhibitor (e.g. ketoconazole) or inducer (e.g. rifampicin, carbamazepine, phenobarbital, phenytoin, St John's Wort) of CYP3A4 may alter the metabolism of irinotecan and should be avoided (see section 4.5).

4.5 Interaction with other medicinal products and other forms of interaction

Interaction between irinotecan and neuromuscular blocking agents cannot be ruled out. Since CAMPTO has anticholinesterase activity, drugs with anticholinesterase activity may prolong the neuromuscular blocking effects of suxamethonium and the neuromuscular blockade of non-depolarising drugs may be antagonised.

Several studies have shown that concomitant administration of CYP3A-inducing anticonvulsant drugs (e.g., carbamazepine, phenobarbital or phenytoin) leads to reduced exposure to irinotecan, SN-38 and SN-38 glucuronide and reduced pharmacodynamic effects. The effects of such anticonvulsant drugs was reflected by a decrease in AUC of SN-38 and SN-38G by 50% or more. In addition to induction of cytochrome P450 3A enzymes, enhanced glucuronidation and enhanced biliary excretion may play a role in reducing exposure to irinotecan and its metabolites.

A study has shown that the co-administration of ketoconazole resulted in a decrease in the AUC of APC of 87% and in an increase in the AUC of SN-38 of 109% in comparison to irinotecan given alone.

Caution should be exercised in patients concurrently taking drugs known to inhibit (e.g., ketoconazole) or induce (e.g., rifampicin, carbamazepine, phenobarbital or phenytoin) drug metabolism by cytochrome P450 3A4. Concurrent administration of irinotecan with an inhibitor/inducer of this metabolic pathway may alter the metabolism of irinotecan and should be avoided (see section 4.4).

In a small pharmacokinetic study (n=5), in which irinotecan 350 mg/m2 was co-administered with St. John's Wort (Hypericum perforatum) 900 mg, a 42% decrease in the active metabolite of irinotecan, SN-38, plasma concentrations was observed.

St. John's Wort decreases SN-38 plasma levels. As a result, St. John's Wort should not be administered with irinotecan (see section 4.3).

Coadministration of 5-fluorouracil/folinic acid in the combination regimen does not change the pharmacokinetics of irinotecan.

There is no evidence that the safety profile of irinotecan is influenced by cetuximab or *vice versa*.

In one study, irinotecan concentrations were similar in patients receiving CAMPTO/5FU/FA alone and in combination with bevacizumab. Concentrations of SN-38, the active metabolite of irinotecan, were analyzed in a subset of patients (approximately 30 per treatment arm). Concentrations of SN-38 were on average 33% higher in patients receiving CAMPTO/5FU/FA in combination with bevacizumab compared with CAMPTO/5FU/FA alone. Due to high inter-patient variability and limited sampling, it is uncertain if the increase in SN-38 levels observed was due to bevacizumab. There was a small increase in diarrhoea and leukopenia adverse events. More dose reductions of irinotecan were reported for patients receiving CAMPTO/5FU/FA in combination with bevacizumab.

Patients who develop severe diarrhoea, leukopenia, or neutropenia with the bevacizumab and irinotecan combination should have irinotecan dose modifications as specified in section 4.2 Posology and method of administration.

4.6 Pregnancy and lactation

Pregnancy:

There is no information on the use of CAMPTO in pregnant women.

CAMPTO has been shown to be embryotoxic, foetotoxic and teratogenic in rabbits and rats. Therefore, CAMPTO must not be used during pregnancy (see « Contraindications » and « Special Warnings and Special Precautions for Use »).

Women of child-bearing potential:

Women of child-bearing age receiving CAMPTO should be advised to avoid becoming pregnant, and to inform the treating physician immediately should this occur (see « Contraindications » and « Special Warnings and Special Precautions for Use »).

Lactation:

In lactating rats, ^{14}C-irinotecan was detected in milk. It is not known whether irinotecan is excreted in human milk. Consequently, because of the potential for adverse reactions in nursing infants, breast-feeding must be discontinued for the duration of CAMPTO therapy (see « Contraindications »).

4.7 Effects on ability to drive and use machines

Patients should be warned about the potential for dizziness or visual disturbances which may occur within 24 hours following the administration of CAMPTO, and advised not to drive or operate machinery if these symptoms occur.

4.8 Undesirable effects

Undesirable effects detailed in this section refer to irinotecan. There is no evidence that the safety profile of irinotecan is influenced by cetuximab or *vice versa*. In combination with cetuximab, additional reported undesirable effects were those expected with cetuximab (such as acneform rash 88%). For information on adverse reactions on irinotecan in combination with cetuximab, only refer to the summary of product characteristics.

For information on adverse reactions in combination with bevacizumab, refer to the bevacizumab summary of product characteristics.

Adverse drug reactions reported in patients treated with capecitabine in combination with irinotecan in addition to those seen with capecitabine monotherapy or seen at a higher frequency grouping compared to capecitabine monotherapy include: *Very common, all grade adverse drug reactions:* thrombosis/embolism; *Common, all grade adverse drug reactions:* hypersensitivity reaction, cardiac ischemia/infarction; *Common, grade 3 and grade 4 adverse drug reactions*: febrile neutropenia. For complete information on adverse reactions of capecitabine, refer to the capecitabine summary product of characteristics.

Grade 3 and Grade 4 adverse drug reactions reported in patients treated with capecitabine in combination with irinotecan and bevacizumab in addition to those seen with capecitabine monotherapy or seen at a higher frequency grouping compared to capecitabine monotherapy include: *Common, grade 3 and grade 4 adverse drug reactions:* neutropenia, thrombosis/embolism, hypertension, and cardiac ischemia/infarction. For complete information on adverse reactions of capecitabine and bevacizumab, refer to the respective capecitabine and bevacizumab summary of product characteristics.

The following adverse reactions considered to be possibly or probably related to the administration of CAMPTO have been reported from 765 patients at the recommended dose of 350 mg/m^2 in monotherapy, and from 145 patients treated by CAMPTO in combination therapy with 5FU/FA in every 2 weeks schedule at the recommended dose of 180 mg/m^2.

Gastrointestinal disorders

Delayed diarrhoea

Diarrhoea (occurring more than 24 hours after administration) is a dose-limiting toxicity of CAMPTO.

<u>In monotherapy:</u>

Severe diarrhoea was observed in 20 % of patients who follow recommendations for the management of diarrhoea. Of the evaluable cycles, 14 % have a severe diarrhoea. The median time of onset of the first liquid stool was on day 5 after the infusion of CAMPTO.

<u>In combination therapy:</u>

Severe diarrhoea was observed in 13.1 % of patients who follow recommendations for the management of diarrhoea. Of the evaluable cycles, 3.9 % have a severe diarrhoea.

Uncommon cases of pseudo-membranous colitis have been reported, one of which has been documented bacteriologically (*Clostridium difficile*).

Nausea and vomiting

<u>In monotherapy:</u>

Nausea and vomiting were severe in approximately 10 % of patients treated with antiemetics.

<u>In combination therapy:</u>

A lower incidence of severe nausea and vomiting was observed (2.1 % and 2.8 % of patients respectively).

Dehydration

Episodes of dehydration commonly associated with diarrhoea and/or vomiting have been reported.

Infrequent cases of renal insufficiency, hypotension or cardio-circulatory failure have been observed in patients who experienced episodes of dehydration associated with diarrhoea and/or vomiting.

Other gastrointestinal disorders

Constipation relative to CAMPTO and/or loperamide has been observed, shared between:

- in monotherapy: in less than 10 % of patients
- in combination therapy: 3.4 % of patients.

Infrequent cases of intestinal obstruction, ileus, or gastrointestinal haemorrhage and rare cases of colitis, including typhlitis, ischemic and ulcerative colitis, were reported. Rare cases of intestinal perforation were reported. Other mild effects include anorexia, abdominal pain and mucositis.

Rare cases of symptomatic or asymptomatic pancreatitis have been associated with irinotecan therapy.

BLOOD DISORDERS

Neutropenia is a dose-limiting toxic effect. Neutropenia was reversible and not cumulative; the median day to nadir was 8 days whatever the use in monotherapy or in combination therapy.

<u>In monotherapy:</u>

Neutropenia was observed in 78.7 % of patients and was severe (neutrophil count < 500 cells/mm3) in 22.6 % of patients. Of the evaluable cycles, 18 % had a neutrophil count below 1,000 cells/mm^3 including 7.6 % with a neutrophil count < 500 cells/mm^3.

Total recovery was usually reached by day 22.

Fever with severe neutropenia was reported in 6.2 % of patients and in 1.7 % of cycles.

Infectious episodes occurred in about 10.3 % of patients (2.5 % of cycles) and were associated with severe neutropenia in about 5.3 % of patients (1.1 % of cycles), and resulted in death in 2 cases.

Anaemia was reported in about 58.7 % of patients (8 % with haemoglobin < 8 g/dl and 0.9 % with haemoglobin < 6.5 g/dl).

Thrombocytopenia (< 100,000 cells/mm^3) was observed in 7.4 % of patients and 1.8 % of cycles with 0.9 % with platelets count ⩽ 50,000 cells/mm3 and 0.2 % of cycles.

Nearly all the patients showed a recovery by day 22.

<u>In combination therapy:</u>

Neutropenia was observed in 82.5 % of patients and was severe (neutrophil count < 500 cells/mm3) in 9.8 % of patients.

Of the evaluable cycles, 67.3 % had a neutrophil count below 1,000 cells/mm^3 including 2.7 % with a neutrophil count < 500 cells/mm^3.

Total recovery was usually reached within 7-8 days.

Fever with severe neutropenia was reported in 3.4 % of patients and in 0.9 % of cycles.

Infectious episodes occurred in about 2 % of patients (0.5 % of cycles) and were associated with severe neutropenia in about 2.1 % of patients (0.5 % of cycles), and resulted in death in 1 case.

Anaemia was reported in 97.2 % of patients (2.1 % with haemoglobin < 8 g/dl).

Thrombocytopenia (< 100,000 cells/mm^3) was observed in 32.6 % of patients and 21.8 % of cycles. No severe thrombocytopenia (< 50,000 cells/mm^3) has been observed.

One case of peripheral thrombocytopenia with antiplatelet antibodies has been reported in the post-marketing experience.

INFECTION AND INFESTATION

Infrequent cases of renal insufficiency, hypotension or cardio-circulatory failure have been observed in patients who experienced sepsis.

GENERAL DISORDERS AND INFUSION SITE REACTIONS

Acute cholinergic syndrome

Severe transient acute cholinergic syndrome was observed in 9 % of patients treated in monotherapy and in 1.4 % of patients treated in combination therapy. The main symptoms were defined as early diarrhoea and various other symptoms such as abdominal pain, conjunctivitis, rhinitis, hypotension, vasodilatation, sweating, chills, malaise, dizziness, visual disturbances, myosis, lachrimation and increased salivation occurring during or within the first 24 hours after the infusion of CAMPTO. These symptoms disappear after atropine administration (see « Special Warning and Special Precautions for Use »).

Asthenia was severe in less than 10 % of patients treated in monotherapy and in 6.2 % of patients treated in combination therapy. The causal relationship to CAMPTO has not been clearly established. Fever in the absence of infection and without concomitant severe neutropenia, occurred in 12 % of patients treated in monotherapy and in 6.2 % of patients treated in combination therapy.

Mild infusion site reactions have been reported although uncommonly.

CARDIAC DISORDER

Rare cases of hypertension during or following the infusion have been reported.

RESPIRATORY DISORDERS

Interstitial pulmonary disease presenting as pulmonary infiltrates is uncommon during irinotecan therapy. Early effects such as dyspnoea have been reported (see section 4.4).

SKIN AND SUBCUTANEOUS TISSUE DISORDERS

Alopecia was very common and reversible. Mild cutaneous reactions have been reported although uncommonly.

IMMUNE SYSTEM DISORDERS

Uncommon mild allergy reactions and rare cases of anaphylactic/anaphylactoid reactions have been reported.

Musculoskeletal disorders

Early effects such as muscular contraction or cramps and paresthesia have been reported.

Laboratory tests

In monotherapy, transient and mild to moderate increases in serum levels of either transaminases, alkaline phosphatase or bilirubin were observed in 9.2 %, 8.1 % and 1.8 % of the patients, respectively, in the absence of progressive liver metastasis.

Transient and mild to moderate increases of serum levels of creatinine have been observed in 7.3 % of the patients.

In combination therapy transient serum levels (grades 1 and 2) of either SGPT, SGOT, alkaline phosphatase or bilirubin were observed in 15 %, 11 %, 11 % and 10 % of the patients, respectively, in the absence of progressive liver metastasis. Transient grade 3 were observed in 0 %, 0%, 0 % and 1 % of the patients, respectively. No grade 4 was observed.

Increases of amylase and/or lipase have been very rarely reported.

Rare cases of hypokalemia and hyponatremia mostly related with diarrhea and vomiting have been reported.

NERVOUS SYSTEM DISORDERS

There have been very rare postmarketing reports of transient speech disorders associated with CAMPTO infusions.

4.9 Overdose

There have been reports of overdosage at doses up to approximately twice the recommended therapeutic dose, which may be fatal. The most significant adverse reactions reported were severe neutropenia and severe diarrhoea. There is no known antidote for CAMPTO. Maximum supportive care should be instituted to prevent dehydration due to diarrhoea and to treat any infectious complications.

5. PHARMACOLOGICAL PROPERTIES

5.1 Pharmacodynamic properties

Cytostatic topoisomerase I inhibitor. ATC Code: L01XX19

Experimental data

Irinotecan is a semi-synthetic derivative of camptothecin. It is an antineoplastic agent which acts as a specific inhibitor of DNA topoisomerase I. It is metabolised by carboxylesterase in most tissues to SN-38, which was found to be more active than irinotecan in purified topoisomerase I and more cytotoxic than irinotecan against several murine and human tumour cell lines. The inhibition of DNA topoisomerase I by irinotecan or SN-38 induces single-strand DNA lesions which blocks the DNA replication fork and are responsible for the cytotoxicity. This cytotoxic activity was found time-dependent and was specific to the S phase.

In vitro, irinotecan and SN-38 were not found to be significantly recognised by the P -glycoprotein MDR, and displays cytotoxic activities against doxorubicin and vinblastine resistant cell lines.

Furthermore, irinotecan has a broad antitumor activity *in vivo* against murine tumour models (P03 pancreatic ductal adenocarcinoma, MA16/C mammary adenocarcinoma, C38 and C51 colon adenocarcinomas) and against human xenografts (Co-4 colon adenocarcinoma, Mx-1 mammary adenocarcinoma, ST-15 and SC-16 gastric adenocarcinomas). Irinotecan is also active against tumors expressing the P-glycoprotein MDR (vincristine- and doxorubicin-resistant P388 leukaemia's).

Beside the antitumor activity of CAMPTO, the most relevant pharmacological effect of irinotecan is the inhibition of acetylcholinesterase.

Clinical data

<u>In combination therapy for the first-line treatment of metastatic colorectal carcinoma</u>

In combination therapy with Folinic Acid and 5-Fluorouracil

A phase III study was performed in 385 previously untreated metastatic colorectal cancer patients treated with either every 2 weeks schedule (see « Posology and method of administration ») or weekly schedule regimens. In the every 2 weeks schedule, on day 1, the administration of CAMPTO at 180 mg/m^2 once every 2 weeks is followed by infusion with folinic acid (200 mg/m^2 over a 2-hour intravenous infusion) and 5-fluorouracil (400 mg/m^2 as an intravenous bolus, followed by 600 mg/m^2 over a 22-hour intravenous infusion). On day 2, folinic acid and 5-fluorouracil are administered at the same doses and schedules. In the weekly schedule, the administration of CAMPTO at 80 mg/m^2 is followed by infusion with folinic acid (500 mg/m^2 over a 2-hour intravenous infusion) and then by 5-fluorouracil (2300 mg/m^2 over a 24-hour intravenous infusion) over 6 weeks.

In the combination therapy trial with the 2 regimens described above, the efficacy of CAMPTO was evaluated in 198 treated patients:

(see Table 1 opposite)

In the weekly schedule, the incidence of severe diarrhoea was 44.4% in patients treated by CAMPTO in combination with 5FU/FA and 25.6% in patients treated by 5FU/FA alone. The incidence of severe neutropenia (neutrophil count < 500 cells/mm^3) was 5.8% in patients treated by CAMPTO in combination with 5FU/FA and in 2.4% in patients treated by 5FU/FA alone.

Additionally, median time to definitive performance status deterioration was significantly longer in CAMPTO combination group than in 5FU/FA alone group (p=0.046).

Quality of life was assessed in this phase III study using the EORTC QLQ-C30 questionnaire. Time to definitive deterioration constantly occurred later in the CAMPTO groups. The evolution of the Global Health Status/Quality of life was slightly better in CAMPTO combination group although not significant, showing that efficacy of CAMPTO in combination could be reached without affecting the quality of life.

In combination therapy with bevazicumab

A phase III randomised, double-blind, active-controlled clinical trial evaluated bevacizumab in combination with CAMPTO/5FU/FA as first-line treatment for metastatic carcinoma of the colon or rectum (Study AVF2107g). The addition of bevacizumab to the combination of CAMPTO/5FU/FA resulted in a statistically significant increase in overall survival. The clinical benefit, as measured by overall survival, was seen in all pre-specified patient subgroups, including those defined by age, sex, performance status, location of primary tumour, number of organs involved, and duration of metastatic disease. Refer also to the bevacizumab summary of product characteristics. The efficacy results of Study AVF2107g are summarized in the table below.

	AVF2107g	
	Arm 1 CAMPTO/ 5FU/FA + Placebo	Arm 2 CAMPTO/ 5FU/FA + Avastin[a]
Number of Patients	411	402
Overall survival		
Median time (months)	15.6	20.3
95% Confidence Interval	14.29 – 16.99	18.46 – 24.18
Hazard ratio [b]		0.660
p-value		0.00004
Progression-free survival		
Median time (months)	6.2	10.6
Hazard ratio		0.54
p-value		< 0.0001
Overall response rate		
Rate (%)	34.8	44.8
95% CI	30.2 – 39.6	39.9 – 49.8
p-value		0.0036
Duration of response		
Median time (months)	7.1	10.4
25–75 percentile (months)	4.7 – 11.8	6.7 – 15.0

[a] 5 mg/kg every 2 weeks.
[b] Relative to control arm.

In combination therapy with cetuximab

EMR 62 202-013: This randomised study in patients with metastatic colorectal cancer who had not received prior treatment for metastatic disease compared the combination of cetuximab and irinotecan plus infusional 5-fluorouracil/folinic acid (5-FU/FA) (599 patients) to the same chemotherapy alone (599 patients). The proportion of patients with KRAS wild-type tumours from the patient population evaluable for KRAS status comprised 64%.

The efficacy data generated in this study are summarised in the table below:

(see Table 2 opposite)

In combination therapy with capecitabine

Data from a randomised, controlled phase III study (CAIRO) support the use of capecitabine at a starting dose of 1000 mg/m2 for 2 weeks every 3 weeks in combination with irinotecan for the first-line treatment of patients with metastatic colorectal cancer. 820 Patients were randomized to receive either sequential treatment (n=410) or combination treatment (n=410). Sequential treatment consisted of first-line treatment with capecitabine (1250 mg/m2 twice daily for 14 days), second-line irinotecan (350 mg/m2 on day 1), and third-line combination of capecitabine (1000 mg/m2 twice daily for 14 days) with oxaliplatin (130 mg/m2 on day 1). Combination treatment consisted of first-line treatment of capecitabine (1000 mg/m2 twice daily for 14 days) combined with irinotecan (250 mg /m2 on day 1) (XELIRI) and second-line capecitabine (1000 mg/m2 twice daily for 14 days) plus oxaliplatin (130 mg/m2 on day 1). All treatment cycles were administered at intervals of 3 weeks. In first-line treatment the median progression-free survival in the intent-to-treat population was 5.8 months (95%CI, 5.1 -6.2 months) for capecitabine monotherapy and 7.8 months (95%CI, 7.0-8.3 months) for XELIRI (p=0.0002).

Data from an interim analysis of a multicentre, randomised, controlled phase II study (AIO KRK 0604) support the use of capecitabine at a starting dose of 800 mg/m2 for 2 weeks every 3 weeks in combination with irinotecan and bevacizumab for the first-line treatment of patients with metastatic colorectal cancer. 115 patients were randomised to treatment with capecitabine combined with irinotecan (XELIRI) and bevacizumab: capecitabine (800 mg/m2 twice daily for two weeks followed by a 7-day rest period), irinotecan (200 mg/m2 as a 30 minute infusion on day 1 every 3 weeks), and bevacizumab (7.5 mg/kg as a 30 to 90 minute infusion on day 1 every 3 weeks); a total of 118 patients were randomised to treatment with capecitabine combined with oxaliplatin plus bevacizumab: capecitabine (1000 mg/m2 twice daily for two weeks followed by a 7-day rest period), oxaliplatin (130 mg/m2 as a 2 hour infusion on day 1 every 3 weeks), and bevacizumab (7.5 mg/kg as a 30 to 90 minute infusion on day 1 every 3 weeks). Progression-free survival at 6 months in the intent-to-treat population was 80% (XELIRI plus bevacizumab) versus 74 % (XELOX plus bevacizumab). Overall response rate (complete response plus partial response) was 45 % (XELOX plus bevacizumab) versus 47 % (XELIRI plus bevacizumab).

In monotherapy for the second-line treatment of metastatic colorectal carcinoma:

Clinical phase II/III studies were performed in more than 980 patients in the every 3 week dosage schedule with metastatic colorectal cancer who failed a previous 5-FU regimen. The efficacy of CAMPTO was evaluated in 765 patients with documented progression on 5-FU at study entry.

(see Table 3 on next page)

In phase II studies, performed on 455 patients in the every 3-week dosage schedule, the progression free survival at 6 months was 30 % and the median survival was 9 months. The median time to progression was 18 weeks.

Additionally, non-comparative phase II studies were performed in 304 patients treated with a weekly schedule regimen, at a dose of 125 mg/m^2 administered as an intravenous infusion over 90 minutes for 4 consecutive weeks followed by 2 weeks rest. In these studies, the median time to progression was 17 weeks and median survival was 10 months. A similar safety profile has been observed in the weekly-dosage schedule in 193 patients at the starting dose of 125 mg/m^2, compared to the every 3-week-dosage schedule. The median time of onset of the first liquid stool was on day 11.

In combination with cetuximab after failure of irinotecan-including cytotoxic therapy

The efficacy of the combination of cetuximab with irinotecan was investigated in two clinical studies. A total of 356 patients with EGFR-expressing metastatic colorectal cancer who had recently failed irinotecan-including cytotoxic therapy and who had a minimum Karnofsky performance status of 60, but the majority of whom had a Karnofsky performance status of ⩾ 80 received the combination treatment.

EMR 62 202-007: This randomised study compared the combination of cetuximab and irinotecan (218 patients) with cetuximab monotherapy (111 patients).

IMCL CP02-9923: This single arm open-label study investigated the combination therapy in 138 patients.

The efficacy data from these studies are summarised in the table below:

(see Table 4 on next page)

The efficacy of the combination of cetuximab with irinotecan was superior to that of cetuximab monotherapy, in terms of objective response rate (ORR), disease control

Table 1

	Combined regimens (n=198)		Weekly schedule (n=50)		Every 2 weeks schedule (n=148)	
	CAMPTO +5FU/FA	5FU/FA	CAMPTO +5FU/FA	5FU/FA	CAMPTO +5FU/FA	5FU/FA
Response rate (%)	40.8 *	23.1 *	51.2 *	28.6 *	37.5 *	21.6 *
p value	p<0.001		p=0.045		p=0.005	
Median time to progression (months)	6.7	4.4	7.2	6.5	6.5	3.7
p value	p<0.001		NS		p=0.001	
Median duration of response (months)	9.3	8.8	8.9	6.7	9.3	9.5
p value	NS		p=0.043		NS	
Median duration of response and stabilisation (months)	8.6	6.2	8.3	6.7	8.5	5.6
p value	p<0.001		NS		p=0.003	
Median time to treatment failure (months)	5.3	3.8	5.4	5.0	5.1	3.0
p value	p=0.0014		NS		p<0.001	
Median survival (months)	16.8	14.0	19.2	14.1	15.6	13.0
p value	p=0.028		NS		p=0.041	

5FU: 5-fluorouracil
FA: folinic acid
NS: Non Significant
*: As per protocol population analysis

Table 2

Variable/statistic	Overall population		KRAS wild-type population	
	Cetuximab plus FOLFIRI (N=599)	FOLFIRI (N=599)	Cetuximab plus FOLFIRI (N=172)	FOLFIRI (N=176)
ORR				
% (95%CI)	46.9 (42.9, 51.0)	38.7 (34.8, 42.8)	59.3 (51.6, 66.7)	43.2 (35.8, 50.9)
p-value	0.0038		0.0025	
PFS				
Hazard Ratio (95% CI)	0.85 (0.726, 0.998)		0.68 (0.501, 0.934)	
p-value	0.0479		0.0167	

CI = confidence interval, FOLFIRI = irinotecan plus infusional 5-FU/FA, ORR = objective response rate (patients with complete response or partial response), PFS = progression-free survival time

Table 3

	Phases III					
	CAMPTO versus supportive care			CAMPTO versus 5FU		
	CAMPTO n=183	Supportive care n=90	p values	CAMPTO n=127	5FU n=129	p values
Progression Free Survival at 6 months (%)	NA	NA		33.5 *	26.7	p=0.03
Survival at 12 months (%)	36.2 *	13.8	p=0.0001	44.8 *	32.4	p=0.0351
Median survival (months)	9.2*	6.5	p=0.0001	10.8*	8.5	p=0.0351

NA: Non Applicable
*: Statistically significant difference

Table 4

Study	N	ORR		DCR		PFS (months)		OS (months)	
		n (%)	95% CI	n (%)	95% CI	Median	95% CI	Median	95% CI
Cetuximab+irinotecan									
EMR 62 202-007	218	50 (22.9)	17.5, 29.1	121 (55.5)	48.6, 62.2	4.1	2.8, 4.3	8.6	7.6, 9.6
IMCLCP02-9923	138	21 (15.2)	9.7, 22.3	84 (60.9)	52.2, 69.1	2.9	2.6, 4.1	8.4	7.2, 10.3
Cetuximab									
EMR 62 202-007	111	12 (10.8)	5.7, 18.1	36 (32.4)	23.9, 42.0	1.5	1.4, 2.0	6.9	5.6, 9.1

CI= confidence interval, DCR= disease control rate (patients with complete response, partial response, or stable disease for at least 6 weeks), ORR= objective response rate (patients with complete response or partial response), OS= overall survival time, PFS= progression-free survival

rate (DCR) and progression-free survival (PFS). In the randomised trial, no effects on overall survival were demonstrated (hazard ratio 0.91, p=0.48).

Pharmacokinetic/Pharmacodynamic data

The intensity of the major toxicities encountered with CAMPTO (e.g., leukoneutropenia and diarrhoea) are related to the exposure (AUC) to parent drug and metabolite SN-38. Significant correlations were observed between haematological toxicity (decrease in white blood cells and neutrophils at nadir) or diarrhoea intensity and both irinotecan and metabolite SN-38 AUC values in monotherapy.

5.2 Pharmacokinetic properties

In a phase I study in 60 patients with a dosage regimen of a 30-minute intravenous infusion of 100 to 750 mg/m^2 every three weeks, irinotecan showed a biphasic or triphasic elimination profile. The mean plasma clearance was 15 L/h/m^2 and the volume of distribution at steady state (Vss): 157 L/m^2. The mean plasma half-life of the first phase of the triphasic model was 12 minutes, of the second phase 2.5 hours, and the terminal phase half-life was 14.2 hours. SN-38 showed a biphasic elimination profile with a mean terminal elimination half-life of 13.8 hours. At the end of the infusion, at the recommended dose of 350 mg/m^2, the mean peak plasma concentrations of irinotecan and SN-38 were 7.7 μg/ml and 56 ng/ml, respectively, and the mean area under the curve (AUC) values were 34 μg.h/ml and 451 ng.h/ml, respectively. A large interindividual variability in pharmacokinetic parameters is generally observed for SN-38.

A population pharmacokinetic analysis of irinotecan has been performed in 148 patients with metastatic colorectal cancer, treated with various schedules and at different doses in phase II trials. Pharmacokinetic parameters estimated with a three compartment model were similar to those observed in phase I studies. All studies have shown that irinotecan (CPT-11) and SN-38 exposure increase proportionally with CPT-11 administered dose; their pharmacokinetics are independent of the number of previous cycles and of the administration schedule.

In vitro, plasma protein binding for irinotecan and SN-38 was approximately 65 % and 95 % respectively.

Mass balance and metabolism studies with 14 C-labelled drug have shown that more than 50% of an intravenously administered dose of irinotecan is excreted as unchanged drug, with 33% in the faeces mainly via the bile and 22% in urine.

Two metabolic pathways account each for at least 12% of the dose:

• Hydrolysis by carboxylesterase into active metabolite SN-38,SN-38 is mainly eliminated by glucuronidation, and further by biliary and renal excretion (less than 0.5% of the irinotecan dose) The SN-38 glucuronite is subsequently probably hydrolysed in the intestine.

• Cytochrome P450 3A enzymes-dependent oxidations resulting in opening of the outer piperidine ring with formation of APC (aminopentanoic acid derivate) and NPC (primary amine derivate) (see section 4.5).

Unchanged irinotecan is the major entity in plasma, followed by APC, SN-38 glucuronide and SN-38. Only SN-38 has significant cytotoxic activity.

Irinotecan clearance is decreased by about 40% in patients with bilirubinemia between 1.5 and 3 times the upper normal limit. In these patients a 200 mg/m^2 irinotecan dose leads to plasma drug exposure comparable to that observed at 350 mg/m^2 in cancer patients with normal liver parameters.

5.3 Preclinical safety data

Irinotecan and SN-38 have been shown to be mutagenic *in vitro* in the chromosomal aberration test on CHO-cells as well as in the *in vivo* micronucleus test in mice.

However, they have been shown to be devoid of any mutagenic potential in the Ames test.

In rats treated once a week during 13 weeks at the maximum dose of 150 mg/m^2 (which is less than half the human recommended dose), no treatment related tumours were reported 91 weeks after the end of treatment.

Single- and repeated-dose toxicity studies with CAMPTO have been carried out in mice, rats and dogs. The main toxic effects were seen in the haematopoietic and lymphatic systems. In dogs, delayed diarrhoea associated with atrophy and focal necrosis of the intestinal mucosa was reported. Alopecia was also observed in the dog.

The severity of these effects was dose-related and reversible.

6. PHARMACEUTICAL PARTICULARS

6.1 List of excipients

Sorbitol,

lactic acid,

sodium hydroxide (to adjust to pH 3.5),

hydrochloric acid (for pH adjustment) used for the product in polypropylene vials,

and water for injections.

6.2 Incompatibilities

None known.

Do not admix with other medications.

6.3 Shelf life

The shelf-life of unopened vials is 36 months.

The CAMPTO solution should be used immediately after reconstitution as it contains no antibacterial preservative. If reconstitution and dilution are performed under strict aseptic conditions (e.g. on Laminar Air Flow bench) CAMPTO solution should be used (infusion completed) within 12 hours at room temperature or 24 hours if stored 2°-8°C after the first breakage.

The following conditions apply to the product in plastic vials. CAMPTO solution is compatible with infusion solutions (0.9% (w/v) sodium chloride solution and 5% (w/v) glucose solution) for up to 28 days when stored in LDPE or PVC containers at 5°C or at 30°C/ambient humidity and protected from light. When exposed to light, compatibility is indicated for up to 3 days.

It is recommended, however, that in order to reduce microbiological hazard, the infusion solutions should be prepared immediately prior to use and infusion commenced as soon as practicable after preparation. If not used immediately, in-use storage times and conditions prior to use are the responsibility of the user and would normally not be longer than 24 hours at 2 to 8°C, unless reconstitution / dilution (etc) has taken place in controlled and validated aseptic conditions.

6.4 Special precautions for storage

Product in glass vials and **polypropylene vials:**

Vials of CAMPTO concentrate for solution for infusion should be stored below 25°C and protected from light.

6.5 Nature and contents of container

Single brown glass vials of 2ml (40 mg) and 5 ml (100 mg), with a halobutyl rubber closure coated with teflon on the inner side.

Single amber-coloured medical-grade polypropylene vials of 2 ml (40 mg), 5 ml (100 mg) and 20 ml (300 mg), closed with halobutyl rubber stopper.

6.6 Special precautions for disposal and other handling

As with other antineoplastic agents, CAMPTO must be prepared and handled with caution. The use of glasses, mask and gloves is required.

If CAMPTO solution or infusion solution should come into contact with the skin, wash immediately and thoroughly with soap and water. If CAMPTO solution or infusion solution should come into contact with the mucous membranes, wash immediately with water.

Preparation for the intravenous infusion administration:

As with any other injectable drugs, THE CAMPTO SOLUTION MUST BE PREPARED ASEPTICALLY (see « Shelf-life »).

If any precipitate is observed in the vials or after reconstitution, the product should be discarded according to standard procedures for cytotoxic agents.

Aseptically withdraw the required amount of CAMPTO solution from the vial with a calibrated syringe and inject into a 250 ml infusion bag or bottle containing either 0.9 % sodium chloride solution or 5 % glucose solution. The infusion should then be thoroughly mixed by manual rotation.

Disposal:

All materials used for dilution and administration should be disposed of according to hospital standard procedures applicable to cytotoxic agents.

7. MARKETING AUTHORISATION HOLDER

Pfizer Limited

Ramsgate Road

Sandwich

Kent

CT13 9NJ

8. MARKETING AUTHORISATION NUMBER(S)

Campto 20 mg/ ml Concentrate for Soution for Infusion PL 00057/0626 (40mg/2ml pack size)

Campto 20 mg/ ml Concentrate for Solution for Infusion PL 00057/0627 (100mg/5ml & 300mg/15ml pack size)

9. DATE OF FIRST AUTHORISATION/RENEWAL OF THE AUTHORISATION

September 1995

10. DATE OF REVISION OF THE TEXT

4th May 2009

Ref: 6_0

CANCIDAS (formerly Caspofungin MSD)

(Merck Sharp & Dohme Limited)

1. NAME OF THE MEDICINAL PRODUCT

CANCIDAS®▼* 50 mg powder for concentrate for solution for infusion

CANCIDAS®▼* 70 mg powder for concentrate for solution for infusion

* *Intensive monitoring is requested only when used for the recently-licensed indication extension to paediatric patients.*

2. QUALITATIVE AND QUANTITATIVE COMPOSITION

CANCIDAS 50 mg powder for concentrate for solution for infusion: Each vial contains 50 mg caspofungin (as acetate).

Each 50 mg vial contains 35.7 mg of sucrose.

CANCIDAS 70 mg powder for concentrate for solution for infusion: Each vial contains 70 mg caspofungin (as acetate).

Each 70 mg vial contains 50.0 mg of sucrose.

For a full list of excipients, see section 6.1.

3. PHARMACEUTICAL FORM

Powder for concentrate for solution for infusion.

White to off-white compact, lyophilised powder.

4. CLINICAL PARTICULARS

4.1 Therapeutic indications

• Treatment of invasive candidiasis in adult or paediatric patients.

• Treatment of invasive aspergillosis in adult or paediatric patients who are refractory to or intolerant of amphotericin

B, lipid formulations of amphotericin B and/or itraconazole. Refractoriness is defined as progression of infection or failure to improve after a minimum of 7 days of prior therapeutic doses of effective antifungal therapy.

• Empirical therapy for presumed fungal infections (such as *Candida* or *Aspergillus*) in febrile, neutropaenic adult or paediatric patients.

4.2 Posology and method of administration

CANCIDAS should be initiated by a physician experienced in the management of invasive fungal infections.

After reconstitution and dilution, the solution should be administered by slow intravenous infusion over approximately 1 hour. Do not mix or co-infuse CANCIDAS with other medicines, as there are no data available on the compatibility of CANCIDAS with other intravenous substances, additives, or medicinal products. DO NOT USE DILUENTS CONTAINING GLUCOSE, as CANCIDAS is not stable in diluents containing glucose. For reconstitution directions see section 6.6.

Both 70 mg and 50 mg vials are available.

CANCIDAS should be given as a single daily infusion.

Dosage in adult patients

A single 70 mg loading dose should be administered on Day-1, followed by 50 mg daily thereafter. In patients weighing more than 80 kg, after the initial 70 mg loading dose, CANCIDAS 70 mg daily is recommended (see section 5.2). No dosage adjustment is necessary based on gender or race (see section 5.2).

Dosage in paediatric patients (12 months to 17 years)

In paediatric patients (12 months to 17 years of age), dosing should be based on the patient's body surface area (see Instructions for Use in Paediatric Patients, Mosteller[1] Formula). For all indications, a single 70 mg/m^2 loading dose (not to exceed an actual dose of 70 mg) should be administered on Day 1, followed by 50 mg/m^2 daily thereafter (not to exceed an actual dose of 70 mg daily). If the 50-mg/m^2 daily dose is well tolerated but does not provide an adequate clinical response, the daily dose can be increased to 70 mg/m^2 daily (not to exceed an actual daily dose of 70 mg).

The efficacy and safety of CANCIDAS have not been sufficiently studied in clinical trials involving neonates and infants below 12 months of age. Caution is advised when treating this age group. Limited data suggest that CANCIDAS at 25 mg/m^2 daily in neonates and infants (less than 3 months of age) and 50 mg/m^2 daily in young children (3 to 11 months of age) can be considered (see section 5.2).

Duration of treatment

Duration of empirical therapy should be based on the patient's clinical response. Therapy should be continued until up to 72 hours after resolution of neutropaenia (ANC ≥ 500). Patients found to have a fungal infection should be treated for a minimum of 14 days and treatment should continue for at least 7 days after both neutropaenia and clinical symptoms are resolved.

Duration of treatment of invasive candidiasis should be based upon the patient's clinical and microbiological response. After signs and symptoms of invasive candidiasis have improved and cultures have become negative, a switch to oral antifungal therapy may be considered. In general, antifungal therapy should continue for at least 14 days after the last positive culture.

Duration of treatment of invasive aspergillosis is determined on a case by case basis and should be based upon the severity of the patient's underlying disease, recovery from immunosuppression, and clinical response. In general, treatment should continue for at least 7 days after resolution of symptoms.

Dosage in elderly patients

In elderly patients (65 years of age or more), the area under the curve (AUC) is increased by approximately 30 %. However, no systematic dosage adjustment is required. There is limited treatment experience in patients 65 years of age and older.

Dosage in patients with renal impairment

No dosage adjustment is necessary based on renal impairment (see section 5.2).

Dosage in patients with hepatic insufficiency

For adult patients with mild hepatic insufficiency (Child-Pugh score 5 to 6), no dosage adjustment is needed. For adult patients with moderate hepatic insufficiency (Child-Pugh score 7 to 9), CANCIDAS 35 mg daily is recommended based upon pharmacokinetic data. An initial 70 mg loading dose should be administered on Day-1. There is no clinical experience in adult patients with severe hepatic insufficiency (Child-Pugh score greater than 9) and in paediatric patients with any degree of hepatic insufficiency (see section 4.4).

Co-administration with inducers of metabolic enzymes

Limited data suggest that an increase in the daily dose of CANCIDAS to 70 mg, following the 70 mg loading dose, should be considered when co-administering CANCIDAS in adult patients with certain inducers of metabolic enzymes (see section 4.5). When CANCIDAS is co-administered to paediatric patients (12 months to 17 years of age) with these same inducers of metabolic enzymes (see section 4.5), a CANCIDAS dose of 70 mg/m^2 daily (not to exceed an actual daily dose of 70 mg) should be considered.

[1] Mosteller RD: Simplified Calculation of Body Surface Area. *N Engl J Med* 1987 Oct 22;317(17):1098 (letter)

4.3 Contraindications

Hypersensitivity to the active substance or to any of the excipients.

4.4 Special warnings and precautions for use

Limited data suggest that less common non-*Candida* yeasts and non-*Aspergillus* moulds are not covered by caspofungin. The efficacy of caspofungin against these fungal pathogens has not been established.

Concomitant use of CANCIDAS with ciclosporin has been evaluated in healthy adult volunteers and in adult patients. Some healthy adult volunteers who received two 3 mg/kg doses of ciclosporin with caspofungin showed transient increases in alanine transaminase (ALT) and aspartate transaminase (AST) of less than or equal to 3-fold the upper limit of normal (ULN) that resolved with discontinuation of the treatment. In a retrospective study of 40 patients treated during marketed use with CANCIDAS and ciclosporin for 1 to 290 days (median 17.5 days), no serious hepatic adverse events were noted. These data suggest that CANCIDAS can be used in patients receiving ciclosporin when the potential benefit outweighs the potential risk. Close monitoring of liver enzymes should be considered if CANCIDAS and ciclosporin are used concomitantly.

In adult patients with mild and moderate hepatic impairment, the AUC is increased about 20 and 75 %, respectively. A reduction of the daily dose to 35 mg is recommended for adults with moderate hepatic impairment. There is no clinical experience in adults with severe hepatic insufficiency or in paediatric patients with any degree of hepatic insufficiency. A higher exposure than in moderate hepatic insufficiency is expected and CANCIDAS should be used with caution in these patients (see sections 4.2 and 5.2).

The safety information on treatment durations longer than 4 weeks is limited.

This medicinal product contains sucrose. Patients with rare hereditary problems of fructose intolerance or sucrase-isomaltase insufficiency should not take this medicinal product.

4.5 Interaction with other medicinal products and other forms of interaction

Studies *in vitro* show that caspofungin acetate is not an inhibitor of any enzyme in the cytochrome P450 (CYP) system. In clinical studies, caspofungin did not induce the CYP3A4 metabolism of other substances. Caspofungin is not a substrate for P-glycoprotein and is a poor substrate for cytochrome P450 enzymes. However, caspofungin has been shown to interact with other medicinal products in pharmacological and clinical studies (see below).

In two clinical studies performed in healthy adult subjects, ciclosporin A (one 4 mg/kg dose or two 3 mg/kg doses 12 hours apart) increased the AUC of caspofungin by approximately 35 %. These AUC increases are probably due to reduced uptake of caspofungin by the liver. CANCIDAS did not increase the plasma levels of ciclosporin. There were transient increases in liver ALT and AST of less than or equal to 3-fold the upper limit of normal (ULN) when CANCIDAS and ciclosporin were co-administered, that resolved with discontinuation of the medicinal products. In a retrospective study of 40 patients treated during marketed use with CANCIDAS and ciclosporin for 1 to 290 days (median 17.5 days), no serious hepatic adverse events were noted (see section 4.4). Close monitoring of liver enzymes should be considered if the two medicinal products are used concomitantly.

CANCIDAS reduced the trough concentration of tacrolimus by 26 % in healthy adult volunteers. For patients receiving both therapies, standard monitoring of tacrolimus blood concentrations and appropriate tacrolimus dosage adjustments are mandatory.

Clinical studies in healthy adult volunteers show that the pharmacokinetics of CANCIDAS are not altered to a clinically relevant extent by itraconazole, amphotericin B, mycophenolate, nelfinavir, or tacrolimus. Caspofungin did not influence the pharmacokinetics of amphotericin B, itraconazole, rifampicin or mycophenolate mofetil. Although safety data are limited it appears that no special precautions are needed when amphotericin B, itraconazole, nelfinavir or mycophenolate mofetil are co-administered with caspofungin.

Rifampicin caused a 60 % increase in AUC and 170 % increase in trough concentration of caspofungin on the first day of co-administration when both medicinal products were initiated together in healthy adult volunteers. Caspofungin trough levels gradually decreased upon repeated administration. After two weeks' administration rifampicin had limited effect on AUC, but trough levels were 30 % lower than in adult subjects who received caspofungin alone. The mechanism of interaction could possibly be due to an initial inhibition and subsequent induction of transport proteins. A similar effect could be expected for other medicinal products that induce metabolic enzymes. Limited data from population pharmacokinetics studies indicate that concomitant use of CANCIDAS with the inducers efavirenz, nevirapine, rifampicin, dexamethasone, phenytoin, or carbamazepine may result in a decrease in caspofungin AUC. When co-administering inducers of metabolic enzymes, an increase in the daily dose of CANCIDAS to 70 mg, following the 70 mg loading dose, should be considered in adult patients (see section 4.2).

All adult drug-drug interaction studies described above were conducted at a 50 or 70 mg daily caspofungin dose. The interaction of higher doses of caspofungin with other medications has not been formally studied.

In paediatric patients, results from regression analyses of pharmacokinetic data suggest that co-administration of dexamethasone with CANCIDAS may result in clinically meaningful reductions in caspofungin trough concentrations. This finding may indicate that paediatric patients will have similar reductions with inducers as seen in adults. When CANCIDAS is co-administered to paediatric patients (12 months to 17 years of age) with inducers of drug clearance, such as rifampicin, efavirenz, nevirapine, phenytoin, dexamethasone, or carbamazepine, a CANCIDAS dose of 70 mg/m^2 daily (not to exceed an actual daily dose of 70 mg) should be considered.

4.6 Pregnancy and lactation

For CANCIDAS, no clinical data on exposed pregnancies are available. Caspofungin should not be used during pregnancy unless clearly necessary. There are no adequate data from the use of caspofungin in pregnant women. Developmental studies in animals have shown adverse effects (see section 5.3). Caspofungin has been shown to cross the placental barrier in animal studies. The potential risk to the human foetus is unknown.

Caspofungin is excreted in milk of lactating animals. It is not known whether it is excreted in human milk. Women receiving caspofungin should not breast-feed.

4.7 Effects on ability to drive and use machines

No studies on the effects on the ability to drive and use machines have been performed.

4.8 Undesirable effects

Adult Patients

In clinical studies, 1,865 adult individuals received single or multiple doses of CANCIDAS: 564 febrile neutropaenic patients (empirical therapy study), 382 patients with invasive candidiasis, 228 patients with invasive aspergillosis, 297 patients with localised *Candida* infections, and 394 individuals enrolled in Phase I studies. In the empirical therapy study patients had received chemotherapy for malignancy or had undergone haematopoietic stem-cell transplantation (including 39 allogeneic transplantations). In the studies involving patients with documented *Candida* infections, the majority of the patients with invasive *Candida* infections had serious underlying medical conditions (e.g., haematologic or other malignancy, recent major surgery, HIV) requiring multiple concomitant medications. Patients in the non-comparative *Aspergillus* study often had serious predisposing medical conditions (e.g., bone marrow or peripheral stem cell transplants, haematologic malignancy, solid tumours or organ transplants) requiring multiple concomitant medications.

Phlebitis was a commonly reported local injection-site adverse reaction in all patient populations. Other local reactions included erythema, pain/tenderness, itching, discharge, and a burning sensation.

Reported clinical and laboratory abnormalities among all adults treated with CANCIDAS (total 1,780) were typically mild and rarely led to discontinuation.

The following adverse reactions were reported:

[Very common (≥ 1/10), Common (≥ 1/100, < 1/10), Uncommon (> 1/1,000, < 1/100)]

Blood and lymphatic system disorders:

Common: haemoglobin decreased, haematocrit decreased, white blood cell count decreased

Uncommon: anaemia, thrombocytopaenia, coagulopathy, leukopaenia, eosinophil count increased, platelet count decreased, platelet count increased, lymphocyte count decreased, white blood cell count increased, neutrophil count decreased

Metabolism and nutrition disorders:

Common: hypokalemia

Uncommon: fluid overload, hypomagnesaemia, anorexia, electrolyte imbalance, hyperglycaemia, hypocalcaemia, metabolic acidosis

Psychiatric disorders

Uncommon: anxiety, disorientation, insomnia

Nervous system disorders:

Common: headache

Uncommon: dizziness, dysgeusia, paraesthesia, somnolence, tremor, hypoaesthesia

Eye disorders:

Uncommon: ocular icterus, vision blurred, eyelid oedema, lacrimation increased

Cardiac disorders:

Uncommon: palpitations, tachycardia, arrhythmia, atrial fibrillation, cardiac failure congestive

Vascular disorders:

Common: phlebitis

Uncommon: thrombophlebitis, flushing, hot flush, hypertension, hypotension

Respiratory, thoracic and mediastinal disorders:

Common: dyspnoea

Uncommon: nasal congestion, pharyngolaryngeal pain, tachypnoea, bronchospasm, cough, dyspnoea paroxysmal nocturnal, hypoxia, rales, wheezing

Gastrointestinal disorders:

Common: nausea, diarrhoea, vomiting

Uncommon: abdominal pain, abdominal pain upper, dry mouth, dyspepsia, stomach discomfort, abdominal distension, ascites, constipation, dysphagia, flatulence

Hepatobiliary disorders:

Common: elevated liver values (alanine aminotransferase, aspartate aminotranserase, blood alkaline phosphatase, bilirubin conjugated, blood bilirubin)

Unommon: cholestasis, hepatomegaly, hyperbilirubinaemia, jaundice, hepatic function abnormal, hepatotoxicity, liver disorder

Skin and subcutaneous tissue disorders:

Common: rash, pruritus, erythema, hyperhidrosis

Uncommon: erythema multiforme, rash macular, rash maculo-papular, rash pruritic, urticaria, dermatitis allergic, pruritus generalised, rash erythematous, rash generalised, rash morbilliform, skin lesion

Musculoskeletal and connective tissue disorders

Common: arthralgia

Uncommon: back pain, pain in extremity, bone pain, muscular weakness, myalgia

Renal and urinary disorders

Uncommon: renal failure, renal failure acute

General disorders and administration site conditions:

Common: pyrexia, chills, infusion-site pruritus

Uncommon: pain, catheter site pain, fatigue, feeling cold, feeling hot, infusion site erythema, infusion site induration, infusion site pain, infusion site swelling, injection site phlebitis, oedema peripheral, tenderness, chest discomfort, chest pain, face oedema, feeling of body temperature change, induration, infusion site extravasation, infusion site irritation, infusion site phlebitis, infusion site rash, infusion site urticaria, injection site erythema, injection site oedema, injection site pain, injection site swelling, malaise, oedema

Investigations:

Common: blood potassium decreased, blood albumin decreased

Uncommon: blood creatinine increased, red blood cells urine positive, protein total decreased, protein urine present, prothrombin time prolonged, prothrombin time shortened, blood sodium decreased, blood sodium increased, blood calcium decreased, blood calcium increased, blood chloride decreased, blood glucose increased, blood magnesium decreased, blood phosphorus decreased, blood phosphorus increased, blood urea increased, gamma-glutamyltransferase increased, activated partial thromboplastin time prolonged, blood bicarbonate decreased, blood chloride increased, blood potassium increased, blood pressure increased, blood uric acid decreased, blood urine present, breath sounds abnormal, carbon dioxide decreased, immunosuppressant drug level increased, international normalised ratio increased, urinary casts, white blood cells urine positive, and pH urine increased.

Possible histamine-mediated symptoms have been reported including reports of rash, facial swelling, pruritus, sensation of warmth, or bronchospasm. Anaphylaxis has been reported during administration of CANCIDAS.

Also reported in patients with invasive aspergillosis were pulmonary oedema, adult respiratory distress syndrome (ARDS), and radiographic infiltrates.

CANCIDAS has also been evaluated at 150 mg daily (for up to 51 days) in 100 adult patients (see section 5.1). The study compared CANCIDAS at 50 mg daily (following a 70-mg loading dose on Day 1) versus 150 mg daily in the treatment of invasive candidiasis. In this group of patients, the safety of CANCIDAS at this higher dose appeared generally similar to patients receiving the 50-mg daily dose of CANCIDAS. The proportion of patients with a serious drug-related adverse reaction or a drug-related adverse reaction leading to caspofungin discontinuation was comparable in the 2 treatment groups.

Paediatric Patients

In clinical studies, 171 paediatric patients received single or multiple doses of CANCIDAS: 104 febrile, neutropenic patients; 56 patients with invasive candidiasis; 1 patient with esophageal candidiasis; and 10 patients with invasive aspergillosis. The overall safety profile of CANCIDAS in paediatric patients is generally comparable to that in adult patients.

The following adverse reactions were reported:

[Very common (≥ 1/10), Common (≥ 1/100, < 1/10)]

Blood and lymphatic system disorders:

Common: eosinophil count increased

Nervous system disorders:

Common: headache

Cardiac disorders:

Common: tachycardia

Vascular disorders:

Common: flushing, hypotension

Hepatobiliary disorders:

Common: elevated liver enzyme levels (AST, ALT)

Skin and subcutaneous tissue disorders:

Common: rash, pruritus

General disorders and administration site conditions:

Very Common: fever

Common: chills, catheter site pain

Investigations:

Common: decreased potassium, hypomagnesaemia, increased glucose, decreased phosphorus, and increased phosphorus

As in adult patients, similar histamine-mediated symptoms have also been reported in paediatric patients.

Post-Marketing experience:

The following post-marketing adverse events have been reported:

Hepatobiliary disorders:

Hepatic dysfunction

General disorders and administration site conditions:

Swelling and peripheral oedema

Investigations:

Hypercalcaemia

4.9 Overdose

Inadvertent administration of up to 400 mg of caspofungin in one day has been reported. These occurrences did not result in clinically important adverse experiences. Caspofungin is not dialysable.

5. PHARMACOLOGICAL PROPERTIES

5.1 Pharmacodynamic properties

Pharmacotherapeutic group: antimycotics for systemic use, ATC Code: J02AX04

Caspofungin acetate is a semi-synthetic lipopeptide (echinocandin) compound synthesised from a fermentation product of *Glarea lozoyensis*. Caspofungin acetate inhibits the synthesis of beta (1,3)-D-glucan, an essential component of the cell wall of many filamentous fungi and yeast. Beta (1,3)-D-glucan is not present in mammalian cells.

Fungicidal activity with caspofungin has been demonstrated against *Candida* yeasts. Studies *in vitro* and *in vivo* demonstrate that exposure of *Aspergillus* to caspofungin results in lysis and death of hyphal apical tips and branch points where cell growth and division occur.

Caspofungin has *in vitro* activity against *Aspergillus* species (*Aspergillus fumigatus* [N = 75], *Aspergillus flavus* [N = 111], *Aspergillus niger*[N = 31], *Aspergillus nidulans* [N = 8], *Aspergillus terreus* [N = 52], and *Aspergillus candidus* [N = 3]). Caspofungin also has *in vitro* activity against *Candida* species (*Candida albicans* [N = 1,032], *Candida dubliniensis* [N = 100], *Candida glabrata* [N = 151], *Candida guilliermondii* [N = 67], *Candida kefyr* [N = 62], *Candida krusei* [N = 147], *Candida lipolytica* [N = 20], *Candida lusitaniae* [N = 80], *Candida parapsilosis* [N = 215], *Candida rugosa* [N = 1], and *Candida tropicalis* [N = 258]), including isolates with multiple resistance transport mutations and those with acquired or intrinsic resistance to fluconazole, amphotericin B, and 5-flucytosine. Susceptibility testing was performed according to a modification of both the Clinical and Laboratory Standards Institute (CLSI, formerly known as the National Committee for Clinical Laboratory Standards [NCCLS]) method M38-A (for *Aspergillus* species) and method M27-A (for *Candida* species). Mutants of *Candida* with reduced susceptibility to caspofungin have been identified in some patients during treatment. However, standardised techniques for susceptibility testing for antifungal agents, including beta (1,3)-D-glucan synthesis inhibitors, have not been established. MIC values for caspofungin should not be used to predict clinical outcome, since a correlation between MIC values and clinical outcome has not been established. Development of *in vitro* resistance to caspofungin by *Aspergillus* species has not been identified. In limited clinical experience, resistance to caspofungin in patients with invasive aspergillosis has not been observed. The incidence of resistance to caspofungin by various clinical isolates of *Candida* and *Aspergillus* is unknown.

Invasive Candidiasis in Adult Patients: Two hundred thirty-nine patients were enrolled in an initial study to compare caspofungin and amphotericin B for the treatment of invasive candidiasis. Twenty-four patients had neutropaenia. The most frequent diagnoses were bloodstream infections (candidaemia) (77 %, n=186) and *Candida* peritonitis (8 %, n=19); patients with *Candida* endocarditis, osteomyelitis, or meningitis were excluded from this study. Caspofungin 50 mg once daily was administered following a 70 mg loading dose, while amphotericin B was administered at 0.6 to 0.7 mg/kg/day to non-neutropaenic patients or 0.7 to 1.0 mg/kg/day to neutropaenic patients. The mean duration of intravenous therapy was 11.9 days, with a range of 1 to 28 days. A favourable response required both symptom resolution and microbiological clearance of the *Candida* infection. Two hundred twenty-four patients were included in the primary efficacy analysis (MITT analysis) of response at the end of IV study therapy; favourable response rates for the treatment of invasive candidiasis were comparable for caspofungin (73 % [80/109]) and amphotericin B (62 % [71/115]) [% difference 12.7 (95.6 % CI -0.7, 26.0)]. Among patients with candidaemia, favourable response rates at the end of IV study therapy were comparable for caspofungin (72 % [66/92]) and amphotericin B (63 % [59/94]) in the primary efficacy analysis (MITT analysis) [% difference 10.0 (95.0 % CI -4.5, 24.5)]. Data in patients with non-blood sites of infection were more limited. Favourable response rates in neutropaenic patients were 7/14 (50 %) in the caspofungin group and 4/10 (40 %) in the amphotericin B group. These limited data are supported by the outcome of the empirical therapy study.

In a second study, patients with invasive candidiasis received daily doses of caspofungin at 50 mg/day (following a 70-mg loading dose on Day 1) or caspofungin at 150 mg/day (see section 4.8). In this study, the caspofungin dose was administered over 2 hours (instead of the routine 1-hour administration). The study excluded patients with suspected *Candida* endocarditis, meningitis, or osteomyelitis. As this was a primary therapy study, patients who were refractory to prior antifungal agents were also excluded. The number of neutropenic patients enrolled in this study was also limited (8.0 %). Efficacy was a secondary endpoint in this study. Patients who met the entry criteria and received one or more doses of caspofungin study therapy were included in the efficacy analysis. The favorable overall response rates at the end of caspofungin therapy were similar in the 2 treatment groups: 72 % (73/102) and 78 % (74/95) for the caspofungin 50-mg and 150-mg treatment groups, respectively (difference 6.3 % [95 % CI -5.9, 18.4]).

Invasive Aspergillosis in Adult Patients: Sixty-nine adult patients (age 18-80) with invasive aspergillosis were enrolled in an open-label, non-comparative study to evaluate the safety, tolerability, and efficacy of caspofungin. Patients had to be either refractory to (disease progression or failure to improve with other antifungal therapies given for at least 7 days) (84 % of the enrolled patients) or intolerant of (16 % of enrolled patients) other standard antifungal therapies. Most patients had underlying conditions (haematologic malignancy [N = 24], allogeneic bone marrow transplant or stem cell transplant [N = 18], organ transplant [N = 8], solid tumour [N = 3], or other conditions [N = 10]). Stringent definitions, modelled after the Mycoses Study Group Criteria, were used for diagnosis of invasive aspergillosis and for response to therapy (favourable response required clinically significant improvement in radiographs as well as in signs and symptoms). The mean duration of therapy was 33.7 days, with a range of 1 to 162 days. An independent expert panel determined that 41 % (26/63) of patients receiving at least one dose of caspofungin had a favourable response. For those patients who received more than 7 days of therapy with caspofungin, 50 % (26/52) had a favourable response. The favourable response rates for patients who were either refractory to or intolerant of previous therapies were 36 % (19/53) and 70 % (7/10), respectively. Although the doses of prior antifungal therapies in 5 patients enrolled as refractory were lower than those often administered for invasive aspergillosis, the favourable response rate during therapy with caspofungin was similar in these patients to that seen in the remaining refractory patients (2/5 versus 17/48, respectively). The response rates among patients with pulmonary disease and extrapulmonary disease were 47 % (21/45) and 28 % (5/18), respectively. Among patients with extrapulmonary disease, 2 of 8 patients who also had definite, probable, or possible CNS involvement had a favourable response.

Empirical Therapy in Febrile, Neutropaenic Adult Patients: A total of 1,111 patients with persistent fever and neutropaenia were enrolled in a clinical study and treated with either caspofungin 50 mg once daily following a 70 mg loading dose or liposomal amphotericin B 3.0 mg/kg/day. Eligible patients had received chemotherapy for malignancy or had undergone hematopoietic stem-cell transplantation, and presented with neutropaenia (<500 cells/mm^3 for 96 hours) and fever (>38.0°C) not responding to ≥ 96 hours of parenteral antibacterial therapy. Patients were to be treated until up to 72 hours after resolution of neutropaenia, with a maximum duration of 28 days. However, patients found to have a documented fungal infection could be treated longer. If the drug was well tolerated but the patient's fever persisted and clinical condition deteriorated after 5 days of therapy, the dosage of study drug could be increased to 70 mg/day of caspofungin (13.3 % of patients treated) or to 5.0 mg/kg/day of liposomal amphotericin B (14.3 % of patients treated). There were 1,095 patients included in the primary Modified Intention-To-Treat (MITT) efficacy analysis of overall favourable response; caspofungin (33.9 %) was as effective as liposomal amphotericin B (33.7 %) [% difference 0.2 (95.2 % CI –5.6, 6.0)]. An overall favourable response required meeting each of 5 criteria: (1) successful treatment of any baseline fungal infection (caspofungin 51.9 % [14/27], liposomal amphotericin B 25.9 % [7/27]), (2) no breakthrough fungal infections during administration of study drug or within 7 days after completion of treatment (caspofungin 94.8 % [527/556], liposomal amphotericin B 95.5 % [515/539]), (3) survival for 7 days after completion of study therapy (caspofungin 92.6 % [515/556], liposomal amphotericin B 89.2 % [481/539]), (4) no discontinuation from the study drug because of drug-related toxicity or lack of efficacy (caspofungin 89.7 % [499/556], liposomal amphotericin B

35.5 % [461/539]), and (5) resolution of fever during the period of neutropaenia (caspofungin 41.2 % [229/556], liposomal amphotericin B 41.4 % [223/539]). Response rates to caspofungin and liposomal amphotericin B for baseline infections caused by *Aspergillus* species were, respectively, 41.7 % (5/12) and 8.3 % (1/12), and by *Candida* species were 66.7 % (8/12) and 41.7 % (5/12). Patients in the caspofungin group experienced breakthrough infections due to the following uncommon yeasts and moulds: *Trichosporon* species (1), *Fusarium* species (1), *Mucor* species (1), and *Rhizopus* species (1).

Paediatric Patients

The safety and efficacy of CANCIDAS was evaluated in paediatric patients 3 months to 17 years of age in two prospective, multicenter clinical trials. The study design, diagnostic criteria, and criteria for efficacy assessment were similar to the corresponding studies in adult patients (see section 5.1).

The first study, which enrolled 82 patients between 2 to 17 years of age, was a randomized, double-blind study comparing CANCIDAS (50 mg/m^2 IV once daily following a 70 mg/m^2 loading dose on Day 1 [not to exceed 70 mg daily]) to liposomal amphotericin B (3 mg/kg IV daily) in a 2:1 treatment fashion (56 on caspofungin, 26 on liposomal amphotericin B) as empirical therapy in paediatric patients with persistent fever and neutropenia. The overall success rates in the MITT analysis results, adjusted by risk strata, were as follows: 46.6 % (26/56) for CANCIDAS and 32.2 % (8/25) for liposomal amphotericin B.

The second study was a prospective, open-label, non-comparative study estimating the safety and efficacy of caspofungin in paediatric patients (ages 6 months to 17 years) with invasive candidiasis, esophageal candidiasis, and invasive aspergillosis (as salvage therapy). Forty-nine patients were enrolled and received CANCIDAS at 50 mg/m^2 IV once daily following a 70 mg/m^2 loading dose on Day 1 (not to exceed 70 mg daily), of whom 48 were included in the MITT analysis. Of these, 37 had invasive candidiasis, 10 had invasive aspergillosis, and 1 patient had esophageal candidiasis. The favorable response rate, by indication, at the end of caspofungin therapy was as follows in the MITT analysis: 81 % (30/37) in invasive candidiasis, 50 % (5/10) in invasive aspergillosis, and 100 % (1/1) in esophageal candidiasis.

5.2 Pharmacokinetic properties

Distribution

Caspofungin is extensively bound to albumin. The unbound fraction of caspofungin in plasma varies from 3.5 % in healthy volunteers to 7.6 % in patients with invasive candidiasis. Distribution plays the prominent role in caspofungin plasma pharmacokinetics and is the rate-controlling step in both the alpha- and beta-disposition phases. The distribution into tissues peaked at 1.5 to 2 days after dosing when 92 % of the dose was distributed into tissues. It is likely that only a small fraction of the caspofungin taken up into tissues later returns to plasma as parent compound. Therefore, elimination occurs in the absence of a distribution equilibrium, and a true estimate of the volume of distribution of caspofungin is currently impossible to obtain.

Metabolism

Caspofungin undergoes spontaneous degradation to an open ring compound. Further metabolism involves peptide hydrolysis and N-acetylation. Two intermediate products, formed during the degradation of caspofungin to this open ring compound, form covalent adducts to plasma proteins resulting in a low-level, irreversible binding to plasma proteins.

In vitro studies show that caspofungin is not an inhibitor of cytochrome P450 enzymes 1A2, 2A6, 2C9, 2C19, 2D6 or 3A4. In clinical studies, caspofungin did not induce or inhibit the CYP3A4 metabolism of other medicinal products. Caspofungin is not a substrate for P-glycoprotein and is a poor substrate for cytochrome P450 enzymes.

Elimination and excretion

The elimination of caspofungin from plasma is slow with a clearance of 10-12 ml/min. Plasma concentrations of caspofungin decline in a polyphasic manner following single 1-hour intravenous infusions. A short alpha-phase occurs immediately post-infusion, followed by a beta-phase with a half-life of 9 to 11 hours. An additional gamma-phase also occurs with a half-life of 45 hours. Distribution, rather than excretion or biotransformation, is the dominant mechanism influencing plasma clearance.

Approximately 75 % of a radioactive dose was recovered during 27 days: 41 % in urine and 34 % in faeces. There is little excretion or biotransformation of caspofungin during the first 30 hours after administration. Excretion is slow and the terminal half-life of radioactivity was 12 to 15 days. A small amount of caspofungin is excreted unchanged in urine (approximately 1.4 % of dose).

Caspofungin displays moderate non-linear pharmacokinetics with increased accumulation as the dose is increased, and a dose dependency in the time to reach steady state upon multiple-dose administration.

Special populations

Increased caspofungin exposure was seen in adult patients with renal impairment and mild liver impairment, in female subjects, and in the elderly. Generally the increase was modest and not large enough to warrant dosage adjustment. In adult patients with moderate liver impairment or in higher weight patients, a dosage adjustment may be necessary (see below).

Weight: Weight was found to influence caspofungin pharmacokinetics in the population pharmacokinetic analysis in adult candidiasis patients. The plasma concentrations decrease with increasing weight. The average exposure in an adult patient weighing 80 kg was predicted to be about 23 % lower than in an adult patient weighing 60 kg (see section 4.2).

Hepatic impairment: In adult patients with mild and moderate hepatic impairment, the AUC is increased about 20 and 75 %, respectively. There is no clinical experience in adult patients with severe hepatic insufficiency and in paediatric patients with any degree of hepatic insufficiency. In a multiple-dose study, a dose reduction of the daily dose to 35 mg in adult patients with moderate hepatic impairment has been shown to provide an AUC similar to that obtained in adult subjects with normal hepatic function receiving the standard regimen (see section 4.2).

Renal impairment: In a clinical study of single 70 mg doses, caspofungin pharmacokinetics were similar in adult volunteers with mild renal insufficiency (creatinine clearance 50 to 80 ml/min) and control subjects. Moderate (creatinine clearance 31 to 49 ml/min), advanced (creatinine clearance 5 to 30 ml/min), and end-stage (creatinine clearance <10 ml/min and dialysis dependent) renal insufficiency moderately increased caspofungin plasma concentrations after single-dose administration (range: 30 to 49 % for AUC). However, in adult patients with invasive candidiasis, oesophageal candidiasis, or invasive aspergillosis who received multiple daily doses of CANCIDAS 50 mg, there was no significant effect of mild to advanced renal impairment on caspofungin concentrations. No dosage adjustment is necessary for patients with renal insufficiency. Caspofungin is not dialysable, thus supplementary dosing is not required following haemodialysis.

Gender: Caspofungin plasma concentrations were on average 17-38 % higher in women than in men.

Elderly: A modest increase in AUC (28 %) and C_{24h} (32 %) was observed in elderly male subjects compared with young male subjects. In patients who were treated empirically or who had invasive candidiasis, a similar modest effect of age was seen in older patients relative to younger patients.

Race: Patient pharmacokinetic data indicated that no clinically significant differences in the pharmacokinetics of caspofungin were seen among Caucasians, Blacks, Hispanics, and Mestizos.

Paediatric Patients:

In adolescents (ages 12 to 17 years) receiving caspofungin at 50 mg/m^2 daily (maximum 70 mg daily), the caspofungin plasma $AUC_{0\text{-}24hr}$ was generally comparable to that seen in adults receiving caspofungin at 50 mg daily. All adolescents received doses >50 mg daily, and, in fact, 6 of 8 received the maximum dose of 70 mg/day. The caspofungin plasma concentrations in these adolescents were reduced relative to adults receiving 70 mg daily, the dose most often administered to adolescents.

In children (ages 2 to 11 years) receiving caspofungin at 50 mg/m^2 daily (maximum 70 mg daily), the caspofungin plasma $AUC_{0\text{-}24hr}$ after multiple doses was comparable to that seen in adults receiving caspofungin at 50 mg/day.

In young children and toddlers (ages 12 to 23 months) receiving caspofungin at 50 mg/m^2 daily (maximum 70 mg daily), the caspofungin plasma $AUC_{0\text{-}24hr}$ after multiple doses was comparable to that seen in adults receiving caspofungin at 50 mg daily and to that in older children (2 to 11 years of age) receiving the 50 mg/m^2 daily dose.

Overall, the available pharmacokinetic, efficacy, and safety data are limited in patients 3 to 10 months of age. Pharmacokinetic data from one 10-month old child receiving the 50 mg/m^2 daily dose indicated an $AUC_{0\text{-}24hr}$ within the same range as that observed in older children and adults at the 50 mg/m^2 and the 50 mg dose, respectively, while in one 6-month old child receiving the 50 mg/m^2 dose, the $AUC_{0\text{-}24hr}$ was somewhat higher.

In neonates and infants (<3 months) receiving caspofungin at 25 mg/m^2 daily (corresponding mean daily dose of 2.1 mg/kg), caspofungin peak concentration ($C_{1\ hr}$) and caspofungin trough concentration ($C_{24\ hr}$) after multiple doses were comparable to that seen in adults receiving caspofungin at 50 mg daily. On Day 1, $C_{1\ hr}$ was comparable and $C_{24\ hr}$ modestly elevated (36 %) in these neonates and infants relative to adults. However, variability was seen in both $C_{1\ hr}$ (Day 4 geometric mean 11.73 µg/ml, range 2.63 to 22.05 µg/ml) and $C_{24\ hr}$ (Day 4 geometric mean 3.55 µg/ml, range 0.13 to 7.17 µg/ml). $AUC_{0\text{-}24hr}$ measurements were not performed in this study due to the sparse plasma sampling. Of note, the efficacy and safety of CANCIDAS have not been adequately studied in prospective clinical trials involving neonates and infants under 3 months of age.

5.3 Preclinical safety data

Repeated dose toxicity studies in rats and monkeys using doses up to 7-8 mg/kg given intravenously showed injection site reactions in rats and monkeys, signs of histamine release in rats, and evidence of adverse effects directed at the liver in monkeys. Developmental toxicity studies in rats showed that caspofungin caused decreases in foetal body weights and an increase in the incidence of incomplete ossification of vertebra, sternebra, and skull bone at doses of 5 mg/kg that were coupled to adverse maternal effects such as signs of histamine release in pregnant rats. An increase in the incidence of cervical ribs was also noted. Caspofungin was negative in *in vitro* assays for potential genotoxicity as well as in the *in vivo* mouse bone marrow chromosomal test. No long-term studies in animals have been performed to evaluate the carcinogenic potential.

6. PHARMACEUTICAL PARTICULARS

6.1 List of excipients

Sucrose

Mannitol

Glacial acetic acid

Sodium hydroxide (to adjust the pH)

6.2 Incompatibilities

Do not mix with diluents containing glucose, as CANCIDAS is not stable in diluents containing glucose. Do not mix or co-infuse CANCIDAS with other medicinal products, as there are no data available on the compatibility of CANCIDAS with other intravenous substances, additives, or medicinal products.

6.3 Shelf life

2 years

Reconstituted concentrate: should be used immediately. Stability data have shown that the concentrate for solution for infusion can be stored for up to 24 hours when the vial is stored at 25°C or less and reconstituted with water for injections.

Dilute patient infusion solution: should be used immediately. Stability data have shown that the product can be used within 24 hours when stored at 25°C or less, or within 48 hours when the intravenous infusion bag (bottle) is stored refrigerated (2 to 8°C) and diluted with sodium chloride solution 9 mg/ml (0.9 %), 4.5 mg/ml (0.45 %), or 2.25 mg/ml (0.225 %) for infusion, or lactated Ringer's solution.

CANCIDAS contains no preservatives. From a microbiological point of view, the product should be used immediately. If not used immediately, in use storage times and conditions prior to use are the responsibility of the user and would normally not be longer than 24 hours at 2 to 8°C, unless reconstitution and dilution have taken place in controlled validated aseptic conditions.

6.4 Special precautions for storage

Unopened vials: store in a refrigerator (2°C to 8°C).

For storage conditions of the reconstituted and diluted medicinal product, see section 6.3.

6.5 Nature and contents of container

CANCIDAS 50 mg powder for concentrate for solution for infusion: 10 ml Type I glass vials with a grey butyl stopper and a plastic cap with a red aluminium band for single use only.

CANCIDAS 70 mg powder for concentrate for solution for infusion: 10 ml Type I glass vials with a grey butyl stopper and a plastic cap with a yellow/orange aluminium band for single use only.

Supplied in packs of 1 vial.

6.6 Special precautions for disposal and other handling

No special requirements.

Reconstitution of CANCIDAS

DO NOT USE ANY DILUENTS CONTAINING GLUCOSE, as CANCIDAS is not stable in diluents containing glucose. DO NOT MIX OR CO-INFUSE CANCIDAS WITH ANY OTHER MEDICINES, as there are no data available on the compatibility of CANCIDAS with other intravenous substances, additives, or medicinal products. Visually inspect the infusion solution for particulate matter or discolouration.

INSTRUCTIONS FOR USE IN ADULT PATIENTS

Step 1 Reconstitution of conventional vials

To reconstitute the powder, bring the vial to room temperature and aseptically add 10.5 ml of water for injections. The concentrations of the reconstituted vials will be 5.2 mg/ml (50 mg vial) or 7.2 mg/ml (70 mg vial).

The white to off-white compact lyophilised powder will dissolve completely. Mix gently until a clear solution is obtained. Reconstituted solutions should be visually inspected for particulate matter or discolouration. This reconstituted solution may be stored for up to 24 hours at or below 25°C.

Step 2 Addition of Reconstituted CANCIDAS to patient infusion solution

Diluents for the final solution for infusion are: sodium chloride solution for injection, or lactated Ringer's solution. The solution for infusion is prepared by aseptically adding the appropriate amount of reconstituted concentrate (as shown in the table below) to a 250 ml infusion bag or bottle. Reduced volume infusions in 100 ml may be used, when medically necessary, for 50 mg or 35 mg daily doses. Do not use if the solution is cloudy or has precipitated. This infusion solution must be used within 24 hours if stored at or below 25°C, or within 48 hours if stored refrigerated at 2 to 8°C. Chemical and physical in-use stability of the diluted solution in sterile lactated Ringer's solution and sodium chloride solution 9 mg/ml (0.9 %), 4.5 mg/ml (0.45 %), and

Table 1 PREPARATION OF THE SOLUTION FOR INFUSION IN ADULTS

DOSE*	Volume of reconstituted CANCIDAS for transfer to intravenous bag or bottle	Standard preparation (reconstituted CANCIDAS added to 250 ml) final concentration	Reduced volume infusion (reconstituted CANCIDAS added to 100 ml) final concentration
50 mg	10 ml	0.19 mg/ml	-
50 mg at reduced volume	10 ml	-	0.45 mg/ml
35 mg for moderate hepatic insufficiency (from one 50 mg vial)	7 ml	0.14 mg/ml	-
35 mg for moderate hepatic insufficiency (from one 50 mg vial) at reduced volume	7 ml	-	0.33 mg/ml
70 mg	10 ml	0.27 mg/ml	Not Recommended
70 mg (from two 50 mg vials)**	14 ml	0.27 mg/ml	Not Recommended
35 mg for moderate hepatic insufficiency (from one 70-mg vial)	5 ml	0.14 mg/ml	0.33 mg/ml

* 10.5 ml should be used for reconstitution of all vials.

** If 70 mg vial is not available, the 70 mg dose can be prepared from two 50 mg vials

2.25 mg/ml (0.225 %) for infusion has been demonstrated for 24 hours at 25°C and for 48 hours at 2 to 8°C. From a microbiological point of view, the solution must be used immediately. If not used immediately, in-use storage times and conditions prior to use are the responsibility of the user and would normally not be longer than 24 hours at 2 to 8°C, unless reconstitution and dilution has taken place in controlled and validated aseptic conditions.

PREPARATION OF THE SOLUTION FOR INFUSION IN ADULTS

(see Table 1 above)

INSTRUCTIONS FOR USE IN PAEDIATRIC PATIENTS

Calculation of Body Surface Area (BSA) for paediatric dosing

Before preparation of infusion, calculate the body surface area (BSA) of the patient using the following formula: (Mosteller Formula)

$$BSA\ (m^2) = \sqrt{\frac{\text{Height (cm)} \times \text{Weight (kg)}}{3600}}$$

Preparation of the 70 mg/m² infusion for paediatric patients >3 months of age (using a 50-mg vial or a 70-mg vial)

1. Determine the actual loading dose to be used in the paediatric patient by using the patient's BSA (as calculated above) and the following equation:

$BSA\ (m^2) \times 70\ mg/m^2$ = Loading Dose

The maximum loading dose on Day 1 should not exceed 70 mg regardless of the patient's calculated dose.

2. Equilibrate the refrigerated vial of CANCIDAS to room temperature.

3. Aseptically add 10.5 ml of 0.9 % Sodium Chloride Injection, Sterile Water for Injection or Bacteriostatic Water for Injection with methylparaben and propylparaben.[a] This reconstituted solution may be stored for up to one hour at ⩽ 25°C (⩽ 77°F).[b] This will give a final caspofungin concentration in the vial of 5.2 mg/ml (if using a 50-mg vial) or 7.2 mg/ml (if using a 70-mg vial).

4. Remove the volume of drug equal to the calculated loading dose (Step 1) from the vial. Aseptically transfer this volume (ml)[c] of reconstituted CANCIDAS to an IV bag (or bottle) containing 250 ml of 0.9%, 0.45%, or 0.225% Sodium Chloride Injection, or Lactated Ringers Injection. Alternatively, the volume (ml)[c] of reconstituted CANCIDAS can be added to a reduced volume of 0.9%, 0.45%, or 0.225% Sodium Chloride Injection or Lactated Ringers Injection, not to exceed a final concentration of 0.5 mg/ml. This infusion solution must be used within 24 hours if stored at ⩽ 25°C (⩽ 77°F) or within 48 hours if stored refrigerated at 2 to 8°C (36 to 46°F).

Preparation of the 50 mg/m² infusion for paediatric patients >3 months of age (using a 50-mg vial or a 70-mg vial)

1. Determine the actual daily maintenance dose to be used in the paediatric patient by using the patient's BSA (as calculated above) and the following equation:

$BSA\ (m^2) \times 50\ mg/m^2$ = Daily Maintenance Dose

The daily maintenance dose should not exceed 70 mg regardless of the patient's calculated dose.

2. Equilibrate the refrigerated vial of CANCIDAS to room temperature.

3. Aseptically add 10.5 ml of 0.9% Sodium Chloride Injection, Sterile Water for Injection or Bacteriostatic Water for Injection with methylparaben and propylparaben.[a] This reconstituted solution may be stored for up to one hour at ⩽ 25°C (⩽ 77°F).[b] This will give a final caspofungin concentration in the vial of 5.2 mg/ml (if using a 50-mg vial) or 7.2 mg/ml (if using a 70-mg vial).

4. Remove the volume of drug equal to the calculated daily maintenance dose (Step 1) from the vial. Aseptically transfer this volume (ml)[c] of reconstituted CANCIDAS to an IV bag (or bottle) containing 250 ml of 0.9%, 0.45%, or 0.225% Sodium Chloride Injection, or Lactated Ringers Injection. Alternatively, the volume (ml)[c] of reconstituted CANCIDAS can be added to a reduced volume of 0.9%, 0.45%, or 0.225% Sodium Chloride Injection or Lactated Ringers Injection, not to exceed a final concentration of 0.5 mg/ml. This infusion solution must be used within 24 hours if stored at ⩽ 25°C (⩽ 77°F) or within 48 hours if stored refrigerated at 2 to 8°C (36 to 46°F).

Preparation notes:

a. The white to off-white cake will dissolve completely. Mix gently until a clear solution is obtained.

b. Visually inspect the reconstituted solution for particulate matter or discolouration during reconstitution and prior to infusion. Do not use if the solution is cloudy or has precipitated.

c. CANCIDAS is formulated to provide the full labeled vial dose (50 mg or 70 mg) when 10 ml is withdrawn from the vial.

7. MARKETING AUTHORISATION HOLDER

Merck Sharp & Dohme Ltd

Hertford Road, Hoddesdon

Hertfordshire EN11 9BU

United Kingdom

8. MARKETING AUTHORISATION NUMBER(S)

CANCIDAS 50 mg Powder for concentrate for solution for infusion: EU/1/01/196/001

CANCIDAS 70 mg Powder for concentrate for solution for infusion: EU/1/01/196/003

9. DATE OF FIRST AUTHORISATION/RENEWAL OF THE AUTHORISATION

Date of first authorisation: 24 October 2001

Date of last renewal: 29 September 2006

10. DATE OF REVISION OF THE TEXT

July 2009

® denotes registered trademark of Merck & Co., Inc., Whitehouse Station, NJ, USA.

SPC.CANC.08.UK2991 (II-035; II-037)

Capasal Therapeutic Shampoo

(Dermal Laboratories Limited)

1. NAME OF THE MEDICINAL PRODUCT

CAPASAL™ THERAPEUTIC SHAMPOO

2. QUALITATIVE AND QUANTITATIVE COMPOSITION

Salicylic Acid 0.5% w/w; Coconut Oil 1.0% w/w; Distilled Coal Tar 1.0% w/w.

3. PHARMACEUTICAL FORM

Viscous, golden brown shampoo.

4. CLINICAL PARTICULARS

4.1 Therapeutic indications

For use as a shampoo in the treatment of dry, scaly scalp conditions such as seborrhoeic eczema, seborrhoeic dermatitis, pityriasis capitis, psoriasis, and cradle cap in children. It may also be used to remove previous scalp applications.

4.2 Posology and method of administration

For adults, children and the elderly: Use as a shampoo, daily if necessary. Wet the hair thoroughly. Massage a small amount of the shampoo into the scalp, leaving on for a few minutes before washing out. Repeat, producing a rich lather. Rinse hair well and dry.

4.3 Contraindications

Not to be used in cases of sensitivity to any of the ingredients.

4.4 Special warnings and precautions for use

Keep away from the eyes. Keep out of the reach of children. For external use only. In case of irritation, discontinue treatment.

4.5 Interaction with other medicinal products and other forms of interaction

None known.

4.6 Pregnancy and lactation

No known side-effects.

4.7 Effects on ability to drive and use machines

None known.

4.8 Undesirable effects

None known.

4.9 Overdose

There are no known toxic effects resulting from excessive use of Capasal.

5. PHARMACOLOGICAL PROPERTIES

5.1 Pharmacodynamic properties

The preparation has been designed as an aid in the treatment of dry, scaly scalp conditions by incorporating into a shampoo formulation three well known ingredients which have been established as safe and effective for use in this indication. They are as follows:

0.5% salicylic acid - mild keratolytic

1.0% coconut oil - emollient, softening agent and lubricant

1.0% distilled coal tar - anti-pruritic, keratoplastic

The preparation may also be used conveniently to remove any previous topical application.

5.2 Pharmacokinetic properties

The active ingredients of the formulation are readily available for intimate contact with the skin, as the shampoo is massaged into the scalp and left on for a few minutes before washing out. This is then repeated in order to produce a rich lather. The detergent effect of the shampoo will also remove any previous application to the scalp.

5.3 Preclinical safety data

No relevant information additional to that contained elsewhere in the SPC.

6. PHARMACEUTICAL PARTICULARS

6.1 List of excipients

Lauric Acid Diethanolamide; Coco Amido Propyl Dimethyl Betaine; Triethanolamine Lauryl Sulphate; Phenoxyethanol.

6.2 Incompatibilities

None known.

6.3 Shelf life

36 months.

6.4 Special precautions for storage

Do not store above 25°C. Keep away from direct sunlight.

6.5 Nature and contents of container

Plastic 'flip top' bottle containing 250 ml. This is supplied as an original pack (OP).

6.6 Special precautions for disposal and other handling

Not applicable.

7. MARKETING AUTHORISATION HOLDER

Dermal Laboratories

Tatmore Place, Gosmore

Hitchin, Herts SG4 7QR, UK.

8. MARKETING AUTHORISATION NUMBER(S)

00173/0048.

9. DATE OF FIRST AUTHORISATION/RENEWAL OF THE AUTHORISATION

29 January 2006.

10. DATE OF REVISION OF THE TEXT

July 2006.

Capreomycin Injection

(King Pharmaceuticals Ltd)

1. NAME OF THE MEDICINAL PRODUCT

CAPREOMYCIN Injection

2. QUALITATIVE AND QUANTITATIVE COMPOSITION

Each vial contains Capreomycin Sulphate, approximately equivalent to 1g Capreomycin base.

3. PHARMACEUTICAL FORM

Powder for injection

4. CLINICAL PARTICULARS

4.1 Therapeutic indications

Actions: Capreomycin is active against human strains of Mycobacterium tuberculosis.

Frequent cross-resistance occurs between capreomycin and viomycin. Varying degrees of cross-resistance between capreomycin and kanamycin and neomycin have been reported. No cross-resistance has been observed between capreomycin and isoniazid, aminosalicylic acid, cycloserine, streptomycin, ethionamide or ethambutol.

Indications: Capreomycin should be used concomitantly with other appropriate antituberculous agents for the treatment of pulmonary infections caused by capreomycin-susceptible strains of *Mycobacterium tuberculosis* when the primary agents (isoniazid, rifampicin, streptomycinand ethambutol) have been ineffective or cannot be used because of toxicity or the presence of resistant tubercle bacilli.

4.2 Posology and method of administration

The usual dose is 1g daily (but 20mg/kg/day should not be exceeded) given by deep intramuscular injection only for 60 to 120 days, followed by 1g intramuscularly two or three times a week. Capreomycin is always administered in combination with at least one other antituberculous agent to which the patient's strain of tubercle bacillus is susceptible.

Capreomycin should be dissolved in 2ml of 0.9% Sodium Chloride Intravenous Infusion BP or Water for Injections PhEur. Two to three minutes should be allowed for complete solution.

For administration of a 1g dose, the entire contents of the vial should be given. For dosages of less than 1g the following dilution table may be used:

Diluent to be added (ml)	Appropriate volume of Capreomycin solution (ml)	Approximate average concentration (mg/ml) in terms of mg of capreomycin activity
2.15	2.85	370
2.63	3.33	315
3.3	4.0	260
4.3	5.0	210

The elderly: As for adults. Reduce dosage if renal function is impaired.

Patients with reduced renal function: A reduced dosage should be given based on creatinine clearance using the guidance given in the following table. These dosages are designed to achieve a mean steady-state capreomycin level of 10 micrograms/ml, at various levels of renal function:

(see Table 1 below)

Infants and children: Not for paediatric use since the safety of capreomycin for use in infants and children has not been established.

4.3 Contraindications

Hypersensitivity to capreomycin

4.4 Special warnings and precautions for use

Warnings

The use of capreomycin in patients with renal insufficiency or pre-existing auditory impairment must be undertaken with great caution, and the risk of additional eighth cranial nerve impairment or renal injury should be weighed against the benefits to be derived from treatment.

Capreomycin must be used only in conjunction with adequate doses of other antituberculous drugs. The use of Capreomycin alone allows the rapid development of strains resistant to it.

Precautions

As capreomycin is potentially ototoxic, audiometry and assessment of vestibular function should be performed before starting treatment and at regular intervals during treatment.

Regular tests of renal function should be made throughout the period of treatment, and reduced dosage should be used in patients known, or suspected, renal impairment (see "Dosage and Administration").

Since hypokalaemia may occur during capreomycin therapy, serum potassium levels should be determined frequently.

A partial neuromuscular block can occur after large doses of capreomycin.

Capreomycin should be administered cautiously to patients with a history of allergy, particularly to drugs.

4.5 Interaction with other medicinal products and other forms of interaction

Simultaneous administration of other antituberculous drugs which also have ototoxic and nephrotoxic potential (e.g. streptomycin, viomycin) is not recommended. Also, use with other drugs that are not given for the treatment of tuberculosis but have ototoxic or nephrotoxic potential (e.g. polymyxin, colistin sulphate, amikacin, gentamicin, tobramycin, vancomycin, kanamycin and neomycin) should also be undertaken only with great caution.

4.6 Pregnancy and lactation

Pregnancy: The safety of capreomycin for use during pregnancy has not been established. Capreomycin has been shown to be teratogenic in rats when given at 3.5 times the human dose. There are no adequate and well controlled studies in pregnant women. Capreomycin should be used during pregnancy only if the potential benefit justifies the potential risk to the fetus.

Studies have not been performed to determine potential for carcinogenicity, mutagenicity, or impairment of fertility.

Nursing mothers: It is not known whether capreomycin is excreted in human milk. Caution should be exercised when administering to a nursing woman.

4.7 Effects on ability to drive and use machines

Not applicable

4.8 Undesirable effects

Renal: Elevation of serum creatinine or blood urea and abnormal urine sediment have been observed. Toxic nephritis was reported in one patient with tuberculosis and portal cirrhosis who was treated with capreomycin (1g) and aminosalicylic acid daily for one month. This patient developed renal insufficiency and oliguria and died. The post-mortem showed subsiding acute tubular necrosis.

Electrolyte disturbances resembling Bartter's syndrome have been reported in one patient.

Hepatic: A decrease in bromsulphthalein excretion without change in serum enzymes has been noted in the presence of pre-existing liver disease. Abnormal results in liver function tests have occurred in many patients receiving capreomycin in combination with other antituberculous agents which are also known to cause changes in hepatic function. Periodic determinations of liver function are recommended.

Haematological: Leucocytosis and leucopenia have been observed. Rare cases of thrombocytopenia have been reported. Most patients receiving daily capreomycin have had eosinophilia exceeding 5%, but this has subsided with the reduction of capreomycin dosage to two or three times weekly.

Hypersensitivity: Urticaria and maculopapular rashes associated in some cases with febrile reactions have been reported when capreomycin and other antituberculous drugs were given concomitantly.

Otic: Clinical and subclinical auditory loss has been noted. Some audiometric changes have proved reversible and others, with permanent loss have not been progressive following withdrawal of capreomycin. Tinnitus and vertigo have occurred.

Injection site reactions: Pain and induration at injection sites have been observed. Excessive bleeding and sterile abscesses have also been reported at these sites.

4.9 Overdose

Signs and symptoms: Hypokalaemia, hypocalcaemia, hypomagnesaemia and an electrolyte disturbance resembling Bartter's syndrome have been reported to occur in patients with capreomycin toxicity. Nephrotoxicity, including acute tubular necrosis; and ototoxicity, including dizziness, tinnitus, vertigo and loss of high-tone acuity (see 'Warnings' and 'Precautions'). Neuromuscular blockage or respiratory paralysis may occur following rapid intravenous administration.

If capreomycin is ingested, toxicity is unlikely because less than 1% is absorbed from an intact gastro-intestinal system.

Treatment: Symptomatic and supportive therapy is recommended. Activated charcoal may be more effective than emesis or lavage in reducing absorption.

Table 1

Creatinine Clearance	Capreomycin clearance	Half life	Dose for these dosing intervals (mg/kg)		
(ml/min)	(l/kg/h × 10^2)	(hours)	24h	48h	72h
0	0.54	55.5	1.29	2.58	3.87
10	1.01	29.4	2.43	4.87	7.30
20	1.49	20.0	3.58	7.16	10.70
30	1.97	15.1	4.72	9.45	14.20
40	2.45	12.2	5.87	11.70	
50	2.92	10.2	7.01	14.00	
60	3.40	8.8	8.16		
80	4.35	6.8	10.40		
100	5.31	5.6	12.70		
110	5.78	5.2	13.90		

Patients who have received an overdose of capreomycin and have normal renal function should be hydrated to maintain a urine output of 3-5ml/kg/hr. Fluid balance electrolytes and creatinine clearance should be monitored.

Haemodialysis is effective in patients with significant renal disease.

5. PHARMACOLOGICAL PROPERTIES

5.1 Pharmacodynamic properties

Capreomycin is active against human strains of Mycobacterium tuberculosis.

5.2 Pharmacokinetic properties

Capreomycin sulphate is not significantly absorbed from the gastrointestinal tract, and must be administered parenterally.

Following intramuscular injection of 1g of capreomycin in human subjects, peak serum concentrations in the range of 20-50µg/ml are achieved after 1-2 hours. Serum concentrations are low at 24 hours and daily injections of 1g for 30 days produced no significant accumulation in subjects with normal renal function.

Capreomycin is excreted in the urine, essentially unaltered, and approximately 50% of a 1g intramuscular dose is excreted within 12 hours.

5.3 Preclinical safety data

There are no preclinical data of relevance to the prescriber in addition to those summarised in other sections of the Summary of Product Characteristics.

6. PHARMACEUTICAL PARTICULARS

6.1 List of excipients

Not applicable

6.2 Incompatibilities

Not applicable.

6.3 Shelf life

Two years.

Reconstituted product should be used within 24 hours.

6.4 Special precautions for storage

Store below 25°C

6.5 Nature and contents of container

Rubber stoppered, clear glass vial, with aluminium or plastic seal, containing 1g capreomycin base, approximately, as sterile white powder.

6.6 Special precautions for disposal and other handling

Reconstituted solutions of Capreomycin may be stored below 25°C for 24 hours. Discard unused portion.

The solution may acquire a pale straw colour and darken with time, but this is not associated with loss of potency or the development of toxicity.

7. MARKETING AUTHORISATION HOLDER

King Pharmaceuticals Ltd
Donegal Street
Ballybofey
County Donegal
Ireland

8. MARKETING AUTHORISATION NUMBER(S)

PL 14385/0006

9. DATE OF FIRST AUTHORISATION/RENEWAL OF THE AUTHORISATION

19th November 1997

10. DATE OF REVISION OF THE TEXT

November 2007

Carace 10 Plus and Carace 20 Plus Tablets

(Merck Sharp & Dohme Limited)

1. NAME OF THE MEDICINAL PRODUCT

Carace® 10 Plus

Carace® 20 Plus

2. QUALITATIVE AND QUANTITATIVE COMPOSITION

'Carace' 10 Plus: Each tablet contains 10 mg lisinopril and 12.5 mg hydrochlorothiazide.

'Carace' 20 Plus: Each tablet contains 20 mg lisinopril and 12.5 mg hydrochlorothiazide.

3. PHARMACEUTICAL FORM

Tablets

'Carace' 10 Plus: Blue, hexagonal, biconvex tablet with the product code '145' on one side.

'Carace' 20 Plus: Yellow, hexagonal scored tablet with the product code 'MSD 140' on one side.

4. CLINICAL PARTICULARS

4.1 Therapeutic indications

For the management of mild to moderate hypertension in patients who have been stabilised on the individual components given in the same proportions.

4.2 Posology and method of administration

Route of administration: Oral

Adults

Essential hypertension: The usual dosage of 'Carace' Plus is 1 tablet, administered once daily. If necessary, the dosage may be increased to 2 tablets, administered once daily.

Dosage in renal insufficiency: Thiazides may not be appropriate diuretics for use in patients with renal impairment and are ineffective at creatinine clearance values of 30 ml/min or below (i.e. moderate or severe renal insufficiency). 'Carace' Plus is not to be used as initial therapy in any patient with renal insufficiency.

In patients with creatinine clearance of >30 and <80 ml/min, 'Carace' Plus may be used, but only after titration of the individual components.

Prior diuretic therapy:

Symptomatic hypotension may occur following the initial dose of 'Carace' Plus: this is more likely in patients who are volume and/or salt depleted as a result of prior diuretic therapy. If possible, the diuretic therapy should be discontinued for 2-3 days prior to initiation of therapy with lisinopril alone, in a 2.5 mg dose.

Use in the elderly

Lisinopril was equally effective in elderly (65 years or older) and non-elderly hypertensive patients. In elderly hypertensive patients, monotherapy with lisinopril was as effective in reducing diastolic blood pressure as monotherapy with either hydrochlorothiazide or atenolol. In clinical studies, age did not affect the tolerability of lisinopril.

In clinical studies the efficacy and tolerability of lisinopril and hydrochlorothiazide, administered concomitantly, were similar in both elderly and younger hypertensive patients.

Paediatric Use

Safety and effectiveness in children have not been established.

4.3 Contraindications

'Carace' Plus is contraindicated in patients with anuria or aortic stenosis or hyperkalaemia.

'Carace' Plus is contraindicated in patients who are hypersensitive to any component of the product.

'Carace' Plus is contraindicated in patients with a history of angioneurotic oedema relating to previous treatment with an angiotensin-converting enzyme inhibitor and in patients with hereditary or idiopathic angioedema.

'Carace' Plus is contraindicated in patients who are hypersensitive to other sulphonamide-derived drugs.

The use of 'Carace' Plus during pregnancy is not recommended. When pregnancy is detected 'Carace' Plus should be discontinued as soon as possible, unless it is considered life-saving for the mother.

'Carace' Plus is contraindicated in lactating women who are breast-feeding infants. It is not known whether lisinopril is excreted in human milk. Thiazides do appear in human milk. See also 'Breast-feeding mothers' under 'Pregnancy and Lactation'.

4.4 Special warnings and precautions for use

Hypotension and electrolyte/fluid imbalance: As with all antihypertensive therapy, symptomatic hypotension may occur in some patients. This was rarely seen in uncomplicated hypertensive patients but is more likely in the presence of fluid or electrolyte imbalance, e.g. volume depletion, hyponatraemia, hypochloraemic alkalosis, hypomagnesaemia or hypokalaemia which may occur from prior diuretic therapy, dietary salt restriction, dialysis, or during intercurrent diarrhoea or vomiting. Periodic determination of serum electrolytes should be performed at appropriate intervals in such patients.

Particular consideration should be given when therapy is administered to patients with ischaemic heart or cerebrovascular disease, because an excessive fall in blood pressure could result in a myocardial infarction or cerebrovascular accident.

If hypotension occurs, the patient should be placed in the supine position and, if necessary, should receive an intravenous infusion of normal saline. A transient hypotensive response is not a contraindication to further doses. Following restoration of effective blood volume and pressure, reinstitution of therapy at reduced dosage may be possible; or either of the components may be used appropriately alone.

Aortic stenosis/Hypertrophic cardiomyopathy: As with all vasodilators, ACE inhibitors should be given with caution to patients with obstruction in the outflow tract of the left ventricle.

Renal function impairment: Thiazides may not be appropriate diuretics for use in patients with renal impairment and are ineffective at creatinine clearance values of 30 ml/min or below (i.e. moderate or severe renal insufficiency). 'Carace' Plus should not be administered to patients with renal insufficiency (creatinine clearance <80 ml/min) until titration of the individual components has shown the need for the doses present in the combination tablet.

Some hypertensive patients, with no apparent pre-existing renal disease, have developed usually minor and transient increases in blood urea and serum creatinine when lisinopril has been given concomitantly with a diuretic. If this occurs during therapy with 'Carace' Plus, the combination should be discontinued. Reinstitution of therapy at reduced dosage may be possible, or either of the components may be used appropriately alone.

In some patients, with bilateral renal artery stenosis or stenosis of the single artery to a solitary kidney, increases in blood urea and serum creatinine, usually reversible upon discontinuation of therapy, have been seen with angiotensin-converting enzyme (ACE) inhibitors.

Haemodialysis patients: The use of 'Carace' Plus is not indicated in patients requiring dialysis for renal failure. A high incidence of anaphylactoid reactions has been reported in patients dialysed with high-flux membranes (e.g. AN 69) and treated concomitantly with an ACE inhibitor. In these patients consideration should be given to using a different type of dialysis membrane or a different class of antihypertensive agent.

Anaphylactoid reactions during LDL apheresis: Rarely, patients receiving ACE inhibitors during low-density lipoprotein (LDL) apheresis with dextran sulphate have experienced life-threatening anaphylactoid reactions. These reactions were avoided by temporarily withholding ACE inhibitor therapy prior to each apheresis.

Hepatic disease: Thiazides should be used with caution in patients with impaired hepatic function or progressive liver disease, since minor alterations of fluid and electrolyte balance may precipitate hepatic coma.

Surgery/anaesthesia: In patients undergoing major surgery or during anaesthesia with agents that produce hypotension, lisinopril may block angiotensin II formation secondary to compensatory renin release. If hypotension occurs and is considered to be due to this mechanism, it can be corrected by volume expansion.

Metabolic and endocrine effects: Thiazide therapy may impair glucose tolerance. Dosage adjustment of antidiabetic agents, including insulin, may be required.

Thiazides may decrease urinary calcium excretion and may cause intermittent and slight elevation of serum calcium. Marked hypercalcaemia may be evidence of hidden hyperparathyroidism. Thiazides should be discontinued before carrying out tests for parathyroid function.

Increases in cholesterol and triglyceride levels may be associated with thiazide diuretic therapy.

Thiazide therapy may precipitate hyperuricaemia and/or gout in certain patients. However, lisinopril may increase urinary uric acid and thus may attenuate the hyperuricaemic effect of hydrochlorothiazide.

Hypersensitivity/angioneurotic oedema: Angioneurotic oedema of the face, extremities, lips, tongue, glottis and/or larynx has been reported rarely in patients treated with angiotensin-converting enzyme inhibitors, including lisinopril. This may occur at anytime during treatment. In such cases, 'Carace' Plus should be discontinued promptly, and appropriate monitoring should be instituted to ensure complete resolution of symptoms prior to dismissing the patient.

In those instances where swelling has been confined to the face and lips, the condition generally resolved without treatment, although antihistamines have been useful in relieving symptoms. Angioneurotic oedema associated with laryngeal oedema may be fatal. Where there is involvement of the tongue, glottis or larynx, likely to cause airway obstruction, appropriate therapy (which may include subcutaneous ephinephrine (adrenaline) solution 1:1,000 (0.3 ml to 0.5 ml) and/or measures to ensure a patent airway) should be administered promptly.

Intestinal angioedema has also been reported very rarely in patients treated with ACE inhibitors and should be included in the differential diagnosis of patients on ACE inhibitors presenting with abdominal pain.

Black patients receiving ACE inhibitors have been reported to have a higher incidence of angioedema compared to non-blacks.

Patients with a history of angioedema unrelated to ACE-inhibitor therapy may be at increased risk of angioedema while receiving an ACE inhibitor. (See also 'Contraindications').

In patients receiving thiazides, sensitivity reactions may occur with or without a history of allergy or bronchial asthma. Exacerbation or activation of systemic lupus erythematosus has been reported with the use of thiazides.

Anaphylactoid Reactions during Hymenoptera Desensitisation: Rarely, patients receiving ACE inhibitors during desensitisation with hymenoptera venom (e.g. Bee or Wasp venom) have experienced life-threatening anaphylactoid reactions. These reactions were avoided by temporarily withholding ACE inhibitor therapy prior to each desensitisation.

Cough: Cough has been reported with the use of ACE inhibitors. Characteristically, the cough is non-productive, persistent, and resolves after discontinuation of therapy. ACE inhibitor-induced cough should be considered as part of the differential diagnosis of cough.

4.5 Interaction with other medicinal products and other forms of interaction

Serum potassium: The potassium-losing effect of thiazide diuretics is usually attenuated by the potassium-conserving effect of lisinopril.

The use of potassium supplements, potassium-sparing agents or potassium-containing salt substitutes, particularly in patients with impaired renal function, may lead to a significant increase in serum potassium. If concomitant use of 'Carace' Plus and any of these agents is deemed appropriate, they should be used with caution and with frequent monitoring of serum potassium.

Antidiabetic drugs: Epidemiological studies have suggested that concomitant administration of ACE-inhibitors and antidiabetic medicines (insulins, oral hypoglycaemic agents) may cause an increased blood-glucose-lowering effect with risk of hypoglycaemia. This phenomenon appeared to be more likely to occur during the first weeks of combined treatment and in patients with renal impairment. Long term controlled clinical trials with lisinopril have not confirmed these findings and do not preclude the use of lisinopril in diabetic patients. It is advised, however that these patients be monitored. (See below for information regarding antidiabetic drugs and thiazide diuretics.)

Lithium: Diuretic agents and ACE inhibitors reduce the renal clearance of lithium and add a high risk of lithium toxicity; concomitant use is not recommended. Refer to prescribing information for lithium preparations before use of such preparations.

Narcotic drugs/antipsychotics: Postural hypotension may occur with ACE inhibitors.

Alcohol: Alcohol may enhance the hypotensive effect of any antihypertensive.

Other agents: Indometacin may diminish the antihypertensive effect of concomitantly administered 'Carace' Plus. In some patients with compromised renal function who are being treated with non-steroidal anti-inflammatory drugs the co-administration of ACE inhibitors may result in further deterioration of renal function. These effects are usually reversible. The antihypertensive effect of 'Carace' Plus may be potentiated when given concomitantly with other agents likely to cause postural hypotension.

Non-depolarising muscle relaxants: Thiazides may increase the responsiveness to tubocurarine.

Allopurinol, cytostatic or immunosuppressive agents, systemic corticosteroids, or procainamide: Concomitant administration with ACE inhibitors may lead to an increased risk of leucopenia.

Antacids: Induce decreased bioavailability of ACE inhibitors.

Sympathomimetics: May reduce the antihypertensive effects of ACE inhibitors; patients should be carefully monitored to confirm that the desired effect is being obtained.

Ciclosporin: Increase the risk of hyperkalaemia with ACE inhibitors.

When administered concurrently, the following drugs may interact with thiazide diuretics:

Barbiturates or narcotics: Potentiation of orthostatic hypotension may occur.

Antidiabetic drugs (oral agents and insulin): Dosage adjustment of the antidiabetic drug may be required. (See above for information regarding antidiabetic drugs and lisinopril).

Colestyramine and colestipol resins: Absorption of hydrochlorothiazide is impaired in the presence of anionic exchange resins. Single doses of either colestyramine or colestipol resins bind the hydrochlorothiazide and reduce its absorption from the gastrointestinal tract by up to 85 and 43 percent, respectively.

Corticosteroids, ACTH: Intensified electrolyte depletion, particularly hypokalaemia.

Pressor amines (e.g. epinephrine (adrenaline)): Possible decreased response to pressor amines but not sufficient to preclude their use.

Non-steroidal anti-inflammatory drugs: In some patients, the administration of a non-steroidal anti-inflammatory agent can reduce the diuretic, natriuretic, and antihypertensive effects of diuretics.

4.6 Pregnancy and lactation

Pregnancy

The use of 'Carace' Plus during pregnancy is not recommended. When pregnancy is detected 'Carace' Plus should be discontinued as soon as possible, unless it is considered life-saving for the mother.

ACE inhibitors can cause foetal and neonatal morbidity and mortality when administered to pregnant women during the second and third trimesters. Use of ACE inhibitors during this period has been associated with foetal and neonatal injury including hypotension, renal failure, hyperkalaemia, and/or skull hypoplasia in the newborn. Maternal oligohydramnios, presumably representing decreased foetal renal function, has occurred and may result in limb contractures, craniofacial deformations and hypoplastic lung development.

These adverse effects to the embryo and foetus do not appear to have resulted from intrauterine ACE inhibitor exposure limited to the first trimester.

The routine use of diuretics in otherwise healthy pregnant women is not recommended and exposes mother and foetus to unnecessary hazard including foetal or neonatal jaundice, thrombocytopenia and possibly other adverse reactions which have occurred in the adult.

If 'Carace' Plus is used during pregnancy, the patient should be apprised of the potential hazard to the foetus. In those rare cases where use during pregnancy is deemed essential, serial ultrasound examinations should be performed to assess the intraamniotic environment. If oligohydramnios is detected, 'Carace' Plus should be discontinued unless it is considered life-saving for the mother. Patients and physicians should be aware, however, that oligohydramnios may not appear until after the foetus has sustained irreversible injury.

Infants whose mothers have taken 'Carace' Plus should be closely observed for hypotension, oliguria and hyperkalaemia. Lisinopril, which crosses the placenta, has been removed from the neonatal circulation by peritoneal dialysis with some clinical benefit, and theoretically may be removed by exchange transfusion. There is no experience with the removal of hydrochlorothiazide, which also crosses the placenta, from the neonatal circulation.

Lactation

Breast-feeding mothers: It is not known whether lisinopril is secreted in human milk; however, thiazides do appear in human milk. Because of the potential for serious reactions in nursing infants, a decision should be made whether to discontinue breast-feeding or to discontinue 'Carace' Plus, taking into account the importance of the drug to the mother.

4.7 Effects on ability to drive and use machines

Usually 'Carace' Plus does not interfere with the ability to drive and to operate machinery. Patients should be instructed to first determine how they respond to 'Carace' Plus before performing hazardous tasks.

4.8 Undesirable effects

'Carace' Plus is usually well tolerated. In clinical studies, side effects have usually been mild and transient, and in most instances have not required interruption of therapy. The side effects that have been observed have been limited to those reported previously with lisinopril or hydrochlorothiazide.

One of the most common clinical side effects was dizziness, which generally responded to dosage reduction and seldom required discontinuation of therapy. Other, less frequent, side effects were headache, dry cough, fatigue, and hypotension including orthostatic hypotension.

Still less common were diarrhoea, nausea, vomiting, pancreatitis, dry mouth, rash, gout, palpitation, chest discomfort, muscle cramps and weakness, paraesthesia, asthenia, and impotence.

Hypersensitivity/angioneurotic oedema: Angioneurotic oedema of the face, extremities, lips, tongue, glottis and/or larynx has been reported rarely. Intestinal angioedema has also been reported very rarely in patients treated with ACE inhibitors. (see 'Precautions').

A symptom complex has been reported which may include some or all of the following: fever, vasculitis, myalgia, arthralgia/arthritis, a positive ANA, elevated ESR, eosinophilia, and leucocytosis. Rash, photosensitivity, or other dermatological manifestations may occur.

Laboratory test findings: Laboratory side effects have rarely been of clinical importance. Occasional hyperglycaemia, hyperuricaemia and hyperkalaemia or hypokalaemia have been noted. Usually minor and transient increases in blood urea nitrogen and serum creatinine have been seen in patients without evidence of pre-existing renal impairment. If such increases persist, they are usually reversible upon discontinuation of 'Carace' Plus. Small decreases in haemoglobin and haematocrit have been reported frequently in hypertensive patients treated with 'Carace' Plus but were rarely of clinical importance unless another cause of anaemia co-existed. Rarely, elevation of liver enzymes and/or serum bilirubin have occurred, but a causal relationship to 'Carace' Plus has not been established.

Other side effects reported with the individual components alone, and which may be potential side effects with 'Carace' Plus, are:

Lisinopril: Myocardial infarction or cerebrovascular accident possibly secondary to excessive hypotension in high-risk patients (see 'Precautions'), tachycardia, abdominal pain, hepatitis - either hepatocellular or cholestatic jaundice, mood alterations, mental confusion, bronchospasm, urticaria, pruritis, diaphoresis, alopecia, uraemia, oliguria/anuria, renal dysfunction, acute renal failure, bone marrow depression manifest as anaemia and/or thrombocytopenia and/or leucopenia, hyponatraemia. Rare cases of neutropenia have been reported, although no causal relationship has been established. There have been reports of haemolytic anaemia in patients taking lisinopril, although no causal relationship has been established.

Hydrochlorothiazide: Anorexia, gastric irritation, constipation, jaundice (intrahepatic cholestatic jaundice), sialoadenitis, vertigo, xanthopsia, leucopenia, agranulocytosis, thrombocytopenia, aplastic anaemia, haemolytic anaemia, purpura, photosensitivity, urticaria, necrotising angiitis (vasculitis, cutaneous vasculitis), fever, respiratory distress including pneumonitis and pulmonary oedema, anaphylactic reactions, toxic epidermal necrolysis, hyperglycaemia, glycosuria, hyperuricaemia, electrolyte imbalance including hyponatraemia, muscle spasm, restlessness, transient blurred vision, renal failure, renal dysfunction, and interstitial nephritis.

4.9 Overdose

No specific information is available on the treatment of overdosage with 'Carace' Plus. Treatment is symptomatic and supportive. Therapy with 'Carace' Plus should be discontinued and the patient observed closely. Suggested measures include induction of emesis and/or gastric lavage, if ingestion is recent, and correction of dehydration, electrolyte imbalance and hypotension by established procedures.

Lisinopril: The most likely features of overdosage would be hypotension, for which the usual treatment would be intravenous infusion of normal saline solution, if available angiotensin II may be beneficial.

Lisinopril may be removed from the general circulation by haemodialysis. (See 'Special Warnings and Precautions, Haemodialysis Patients').

Hydrochlorothiazide: The most common signs and symptoms observed are those caused by electrolyte depletion (hypokalaemia, hypochloraemia, hyponatraemia) and dehydration resulting from excessive diuresis. If digitalis has also been administered, hypokalaemia may accentuate cardiac arrhythmias.

5. PHARMACOLOGICAL PROPERTIES

5.1 Pharmacodynamic properties

'Carace' Plus contains antihypertensive and diuretic activity. Lisinopril and hydrochlorothiazide have been used alone and concurrently for the treatment of hypertension where their effects are approximately additive.

Lisinopril is an inhibitor of the angiotensin-converting enzyme (ACE). Inhibition of the formation of angiotensin II results in vasodilation and a fall in blood pressure.

Hydrochlorothiazide is a diuretic and antihypertensive agent. Use of this agent alone results in increased renin secretion. Although lisinopril alone is antihypertensive, even in patients with low renin hypertension, concomitant administration with hydrochlorothiazide results in a greater reduction in blood pressure. Lisinopril attenuates the potassium loss associated with hydrochlorothiazide.

5.2 Pharmacokinetic properties

In clinical studies, peak serum concentrations of lisinopril occurred within about 6 to 8 hours following oral administration. Declining serum concentrations exhibited a prolonged terminal phase which did not contribute to drug accumulation. This terminal phase probably represents saturable binding to ACE and was not proportional to dose. Lisinopril did not appear to be bound to other plasma proteins.

Lisinopril does not undergo significant metabolism and is excreted unchanged predominantly in the urine. Based on urinary recovery in clinical studies, the extent of absorption of lisinopril was approximately 25%. Lisinopril absorption was not influenced by the presence of food in the gastro-intestinal tract.

On multiple dosing, lisinopril exhibited an effective accumulation half-life of 12 hours.

In patients with renal insufficiency, disposition of lisinopril was similar to that in patients with normal renal function until glomerular filtration rate reached 30 ml/min or less; peak and trough lisinopril levels, and time to peak then increased and time to steady state was sometimes prolonged. Animal studies indicate lisinopril crosses the blood-brain barrier poorly. No clinically significant pharmacokinetic interactions occurred when lisinopril was used concomitantly with propranolol, digoxin or hydrochlorothiazide.

When plasma levels of hydrochlorothiazide have been followed for at least 24 hours the plasma half-life has been observed to vary between 5.6 and 14.8 hours. Hydrochlorothiazide is not metabolised but is eliminated rapidly by the kidney. At least 61% of the oral dose is eliminated unchanged within 24 hours. Hydrochlorothiazide crosses the placental but not the blood-brain barrier.

Concomitant multiple doses of lisinopril and hydrochlorothiazide have little or no effect on the bioavailability of these drugs. The combination tablet is bioequivalent to concomitant administration of the separate entities.

5.3 Preclinical safety data

Lisinopril and hydrochlorothiazide are well established in medical use. Preclinical data is broadly consistent with clinical experience. For reproduction toxicity, see section 4.6.

6. PHARMACEUTICAL PARTICULARS

6.1 List of excipients

Mannitol BP

Calcium Hydrogen Phosphate BP

Blue FD & C Aluminium Lake (E132) ('Carace' 10 Plus)

Yellow Ferric Oxide (E172) ('Carace' 20 Plus)

Maize Starch BP

Pregelatinised Starch BP

Magnesium Stearate EP

6.2 Incompatibilities

Not applicable.

6.3 Shelf life

30 months - Bottles

36 months - Blisters

6.4 Special precautions for storage

Store in a dry place below 25°C.

6.5 Nature and contents of container

HDPE bottles of 30, 56 or 100 tablets.

Blister packs of 2, 28, 30, 56, 84 or 100 tablets.

6.6 Special precautions for disposal and other handling

Not applicable.

7. MARKETING AUTHORISATION HOLDER

Merck Sharp & Dohme Limited

Hertford Road

Hoddesdon

Hertfordshire

EN11 9BU

8. MARKETING AUTHORISATION NUMBER(S)

Carace 10 Plus PL 00025/0534

Carace 20 Plus PL 00025/0535

9. DATE OF FIRST AUTHORISATION/RENEWAL OF THE AUTHORISATION

11 February 2009

10. DATE OF REVISION OF THE TEXT

08 May 2009

LEGAL CATEGORY

POM

®denotes registered trademark of Merck & Co., Inc., Whitehouse Station, New Jersey, USA.

SPC.CAR-PLUS.09.UK.3026

Carbomix (activated charcoal) 50g

(Beacon Pharmaceuticals)

1. NAME OF THE MEDICINAL PRODUCT

Carbomix

2. QUALITATIVE AND QUANTITATIVE COMPOSITION

Charcoal Activated Ph. Eur. 81.3% w/w

3. PHARMACEUTICAL FORM

Granules for oral suspension

4. CLINICAL PARTICULARS

4.1 Therapeutic indications

Emergency treatment of acute oral poisoning or drug overdose. Carbomix adsorbs toxic substances and reduces or prevents systemic absorption. The shorter the time interval between ingestion of the toxicant and the administration of Carbomix, the greater is the benefit for the patient. However, as the absorption of massive drug overdoses is often retarded in acute conditions of intoxication. Even the delayed administration of Carbomix may be beneficial. In severe intoxication, repeated administration of Carbomix is recommended to prevent adsorbed drug being released (in an unbound state) in the lower intestinal tract or to expedite the elimination and prevent the re-absorption of any drug undergoing enterohepatic circulation.

4.2 Posology and method of administration

Adults (including the Elderly)

50g activated charcoal (one standard treatment pack), repeated if necessary.

Children under 12 years

25g activated charcoal (one small treatment pack or half the contents of the standard pack), repeated if necessary.

If a large quantity of toxicant has been ingested, and where there is a risk to life, a dose of 50g is recommended.

Carbomix should be given as soon as possible after the ingestion of the potential poison.

The contents of the bottle are made up to the red band with water and shaken thoroughly.

The suspension is then taken orally or given by intragastric tube using the applicator provided. Carbomix may be administered after emesis or gastric lavage and may be used concurrently with parenteral antidotes such as acetylcysteine.

4.3 Contraindications

There are no contraindications to the use of Carbomix but see under (4.4).

4.4 Special warnings and precautions for use

The value of Carbomix in the treatment of poisoning by strong acids, alkalis and other corrosive substances is limited. It should also be borne in mind that the presence of charcoal will render difficult any immediate endoscopy that may be required. Carbomix is poor at binding cyanide, iron salts and some solvents including methanol, ethanol and ethylene glycol. In cases where the toxicant has diuretic properties or has been ingested with alcohol. Plenty of fluid should be given after the administration of Carbomix. Carbomix should not be used concurrently with systemically active oral emetics or oral antidotes such as methionine since such agents would be adsorbed by the charcoal.

4.5 Interaction with other medicinal products and other forms of interaction

The purpose of the product is to interact with other medicaments and toxicants taken in overdose. There are no systemic interactions because the product is not absorbed from the gut.

4.6 Pregnancy and lactation
There is no evidence to suggest that Carbomix should not be used during pregnancy or lactation. The product is not systemically absorbed.

4.7 Effects on ability to drive and use machines
None (the product is not systemically absorbed).

4.8 Undesirable effects
In general, Carbomix is well tolerated. Some patients may however experience constipation or diarrhoea. Faecal impaction has been reported in a patient treated for an overdose of a diuretic with alcohol.

4.9 Overdose
Not applicable. In theory severe constipation would result from excessive use and this could be treated with laxatives.

5. PHARMACOLOGICAL PROPERTIES

5.1 Pharmacodynamic properties
Activated charcoal has well documented adsorptive properties and is effective in reducing the absorption of a wide range of toxicants, including drugs taken in overdose, from the gut. In addition, there is evidence that the administration of activated charcoal can enhance the elimination of some compounds by creating an effective concentration gradient from the circulation to the gut.

5.2 Pharmacokinetic properties
Activated charcoal is not systemically absorbed.

5.3 Preclinical safety data
No findings have been reported which add to the prescribing information given in other sections.

6. PHARMACEUTICAL PARTICULARS

6.1 List of excipients
Citric Acid, Acacia, Glycerol.

6.2 Incompatibilities
Carbomix should not be used concurrently with systemically active oral emetics or oral antidotes such as methionine since such agents would be adsorbed by the charcoal.

6.3 Shelf life
As package for sale – 5 years.

After reconstitution – 24 hours.

6.4 Special precautions for storage
Store below 25°C.

6.5 Nature and contents of container
HDPE bottle and cap 25g and 50g.

6.6 Special precautions for disposal and other handling
Carbomix granules should be mixed with water and swallowed as a suspension. The contents of the bottle are made up to the red band with water, shaken thoroughly and taken by mouth. Under medical supervision only. It may be given by intragastric tube and the cap is fitted with a universal applicator for this purpose.

Administration Details

7. MARKETING AUTHORISATION HOLDER
Beacon Pharmaceuticals Ltd, 85, High Street, Tunbridge Wells, TN1 1YG. United Kingdom

8. MARKETING AUTHORISATION NUMBER(S)
PL 18157/0020

9. DATE OF FIRST AUTHORISATION/RENEWAL OF THE AUTHORISATION
22/05/2006

10. DATE OF REVISION OF THE TEXT
22/05/2006

Cardene 20 and 30mg

(Astellas Pharma Ltd)

1. NAME OF THE MEDICINAL PRODUCT
Cardene 20 mg

Cardene 30 mg

2. QUALITATIVE AND QUANTITATIVE COMPOSITION
Nicardipine hydrochloride 20 mg

Nicardipine hydrochloride 30 mg

3. PHARMACEUTICAL FORM
Capsules

4. CLINICAL PARTICULARS

4.1 Therapeutic indications
Cardene is indicated for the prophylaxis of patients with chronic stable angina. For the treatment of hypertension considered to be mild to moderate in severity.

4.2 Posology and method of administration
Nicardipine should be taken with a little water.

Prophylaxis of chronic stable angina:

Starting dose: 20 mg every 8 hours titrating upwards as required.

Usual effective dose: 30 mg every 8 hours (range of total dose 60 mg - 120 mg per day).

Allow at least 3 days before increasing the dose of Cardene to ensure steady state plasma levels have been achieved.

Hypertension:

Starting dose: 20 mg every 8 hours titrating upwards as required.

Usual effective dose: 30 mg every 8 hours (range of total dose 60 mg - 120 mg per day).

Use in elderly:

Starting dose is 20 mg 3 times a day. Titrate upwards with care as nicardipine may lower systolic pressure more than diastolic pressure in these patients.

Children:

Cardene is not recommended in patients under the age of 18.

Cardene capsules are for oral administration.

4.3 Contraindications
(1) Pregnancy and lactation.

(2) Hypersensitivity to nicardipine hydrochloride or other dihydropyridines because of the theoretical risk of cross reactivity.

(3) Because part of the effect of nicardipine is secondary to reduced afterload, the drug should not be given to patients with advanced aortic stenosis. Reduction of diastolic pressure in these patients may worsen rather than improve myocardial infarction.

(4) Cardene should not be used in cardiogenic shock, clinically significant aortic stenosis, unstable angina, and during or within one month of a myocardial infarction.

(5) Cardene should not be used for acute attacks of angina.

(6) Cardene should not be used for secondary prevention of myocardial infarction.

4.4 Special warnings and precautions for use
If used in combination with diuretics or beta-blockers, careful titration of Cardene is advised to avoid excessive reduction in blood pressure.

If switching from beta-blockers to Cardene, gradually reduce the beta-blocker dose (preferably over 8 - 10 days) since nicardipine gives no protection against the dangers of abrupt beta-blocker withdrawal.

Stop Cardene in patients experiencing ischaemic pain within 30 minutes of starting therapy or after increasing the dose.

Use in patients with congestive heart failure or poor cardiac reserve:

Haemodynamic studies in patients with heart failure have shown that nicardipine reduces afterload and improves overall haemodynamics. In one study, intravenous nicardipine reduced myocardial contractility in patients with severe heart failure despite increases in cardiac index and ejection fraction noted in the same patients.

Since nicardipine has not been extensively studied in patients with severe left ventricular dysfunction and cardiac failure one must consider that worsening of cardiac failure may occur.

Use in patients with impaired hepatic or renal function:

Since Cardene is subject to first-pass metabolism, use with caution in patients with impaired liver function or reduced hepatic blood flow. Patients with severe liver disease showed elevated blood levels and the half-life of nicardipine was prolonged. Cardene blood levels may also be elevated in some renally impaired patients. Therefore the lowest starting dose and extending the dosing interval should be individually considered in these patients.

Use in patients following a stroke (infarction or haemorrhage):

Avoid inducing systemic hypotension when administering Cardene to these patients.

Laboratory tests:

Transient elevations of alkaline phosphatase, serum bilirubin, SGPT, SGOT and glucose, have been observed. BUN and creatinine may also become elevated. While out-of-range values were seen in T_3, T_4 and TSH, the lack of consistent alterations suggest that any changes were not drug-related.

Treatment with short acting nicardipine may induce an exaggerated fall in blood pressure and reflex tachycardia which can cause cardiovascular complications such as myocardial and cerebrovascular ischaemia.

There has been some concern about increased mortality and morbidity in the treatment of ischaemic heart disease using higher than recommended doses of some other short-acting dihydropyridines.

4.5 Interaction with other medicinal products and other forms of interaction

Digoxin

Careful monitoring of serum digoxin levels is advised in patients also receiving Cardene as levels may be increased.

Propanolol, Dipyridamole, Warfarin, Quinidine, Naproxen:

Therapeutic concentrations of these drugs does not change the *in vitro* plasma protein binding of nicardipine.

Cimetidine:

Cimetidine increases nicardipine plasma levels. Carefully monitor patients receiving both drugs.

Fentanyl Anaesthesia:

Severe hypotension has been reported during fentanyl anaesthesia with concomitant use of a beta-blocker and calcium blockade. Even though such interactions have not been seen in clinical trials, such hypotensive episodes should be vigorously treated with conventional therapy such as intravenous fluids.

Cyclosporin:

Monitor cyclosporin plasma levels and reduce dosage accordingly in patients concomitantly receiving nicardipine as elevated cyclosporin levels have been reported.

Rifampicin:

Rifampicin can interact with other dihydropyridines to substantially reduce their plasma levels and so rifampicin and nicardipine should be used together with caution.

As with other dihydropyridines, nicardipine should not be taken with grapefruit juice because bioavailability may be increased.

Cardene may be used in combination with beta-blocking and other anti-hypertensive drugs but the possibility of an additive effect resulting in postural hypotension should be considered.

4.6 Pregnancy and lactation
See contra-indications.

4.7 Effects on ability to drive and use machines
None known.

4.8 Undesirable effects
Majority are not serious and are expected consequences of the vasodilator effects of Cardene.

The most frequent side-effects reported are headache, pedal oedema, heat sensation and/or flushing, palpitations, nausea and dizziness.

Other side-effects noted in clinical trials include the following:

Cardiovascular System: As with the use of other short-acting dihydropyridines in patients with ischaemic heart disease, exacerbation of angina pectoris may occur frequently at the start of treatment with nicardipine capsules. The occurrence of myocardial infarction has been reported although it is not possible to distinguish such an event from the natural course of ischaemic heart disease.

Central nervous system: Drowsiness, insomnia, tinnitus, paraesthesia, functional disorders.

Skin: Itching, rashes.

Hepato-Renal: Impairment, frequency of micturition.

Dyspnoea, gastro-intestinal upset and, rarely, depression, impotence and thrombocytopenia, have also been reported.

4.9 Overdose
Symptoms may include marked hypotension, bradycardia, palpitations, flushing, drowsiness, confusion and slurred speech. In laboratory animals, overdosage also resulted in reversible hepatic function abnormalities, sporadic focal hepatic necrosis and progressive atrioventricular conduction block.

For treatment of overdose, standard measures including monitoring of cardiac and respiratory functions should be implemented. The patient should be positioned so as to avoid cerebral anoxia. Frequent blood pressure determinations are essential. Vasopressors are clinically indicated for patients exhibiting profound hypotension. Intravenous calcium gluconate may help reverse the effects of calcium entry blockade.

5. PHARMACOLOGICAL PROPERTIES

5.1 Pharmacodynamic properties
Cardene is a potent calcium antagonist. Pharmacological studies demonstrate its preferential high selectivity for the peripheral vasculature over the myocardium which accounts for its minimal negative inotropic effects. Cardene produces smooth muscle relaxation and marked peripheral vasodilatation.

In man Cardene produces a significant decrease in systemic vascular resistance, the degree of vasodilatation being more predominant in hypertensive patients than in normotensive subjects. Haemodynamic studies in patients with coronary artery disease and normal left ventricular function have shown significant increases in cardiac index and coronary blood flow, with little if any increase in left ventricular end-diastolic pressure.

Electrophysiologic effects: Electrophysiological studies in man show that Cardene does not depress sinus node function or atrial or ventricular conduction in patients with either normal or decreased electrical conduction systems. Refractory periods of the His-Purkinje system were actually shortened slightly by nicardipine and SA conduction time was improved.

5.2 Pharmacokinetic properties
Pharmacokinetics and metabolism: Nicardipine is rapidly and completely absorbed with plasma levels detectable 20 minutes following an oral dose. Maximal plasma levels are observed within 30 minutes to two hours (mean T_{max} = 1 hour). When given with a high fat meal peak plasma levels are reduced by 30%. Nicardipine is subject to saturable first-pass metabolism and the bioavailability is about 35% following a 30 mg oral dose at steady state.

The pharmacokinetics of Cardene are non-linear due to saturable hepatic first pass metabolism.

Steady state plasma levels are achieved after about 3 days of dosing at 20 and 30 mg tds and remain relatively constant over 28 days of dosing at 30 mg tds. Considerable intersubject variability in plasma levels is observed. Following dosing to steady state using doses of 30 and 40 mg (tds), the terminal plasma half-life of nicardipine averaged 8.6 hours. Nicardipine is highly protein-bound (>99%) in human plasma over a wide concentration range.

Nicardipine does not induce its own metabolism and does not induce hepatic microsomal enzymes.

5.3 Preclinical safety data
Please refer to section 4.6 Pregnancy and Lactation.

6. PHARMACEUTICAL PARTICULARS
6.1 List of excipients
Starch, Pregelatinised

Magnesium Stearate

Cardene 20mg

Capsule shell body

Titanium Dioxide E171

Gelatin

Cardene 30mg

Capsule shell body

Indigotine E132

Titanium Dioxide E171

Gelatin

Cardene 20mg and 30mg

Capsule shell cap

Indigotine E132

Titanium Dioxide E171

Gelatin

6.2 Incompatibilities
None known.

6.3 Shelf life
Cardene 20mg

Securitainer: 60 months.

Blister packs of 21, 100 and 200 capsules: 60 months.

Blister packs of 56 and 84 capsules: 36 months.

Cardene 30mg

Securitainer: 60 months

Blister packs of 21, 56, 60, 100 and 200 capsules: 60 months.

Blister packs of 84 capsules: 36 months.

6.4 Special precautions for storage
Do not store above 25°C.

6.5 Nature and contents of container
Cardene 20mg

Securitainer packs of 50 and 100.

PVC/aluminium foil blister strips of 21, 56, 84,100 and 200 capsules.

Cardene 30mg

Securitainer packs of 50 and 100.

PVC/aluminium foil blister strips of 21, 56, 60, 84,100 and 200 capsules.

6.6 Special precautions for disposal and other handling
Not applicable.

Administrative Data
7. MARKETING AUTHORISATION HOLDER
Astellas Pharma Limited

Lovett House

Lovett Road

Staines

TW18 3AZ

United Kingdom

8. MARKETING AUTHORISATION NUMBER(S)
Cardene 20mg - PL 00166/0181

Cardene 30mg - PL 00166/0182

9. DATE OF FIRST AUTHORISATION/RENEWAL OF THE AUTHORISATION
15 May 1998/ 15 July 2002

10. DATE OF REVISION OF THE TEXT
4 November 2005

11. Legal category
POM

Cardene SR 30 and 45mg

(Astellas Pharma Ltd)

1. NAME OF THE MEDICINAL PRODUCT
Cardene SR 30

Cardene SR 45

2. QUALITATIVE AND QUANTITATIVE COMPOSITION
Nicardipine hydrochloride 30 mg

Nicardipine hydrochloride 45 mg

3. PHARMACEUTICAL FORM
Sustained release capsules

4. CLINICAL PARTICULARS
4.1 Therapeutic indications
Treatment of mild to moderate hypertension.

4.2 Posology and method of administration
Adults

Starting dose: 30 mg every 12 hours titrating upwards as required.

Usual effective dose: 45 mg every 12 hours (range 30 mg to 60 mg every 12 hours).

Individually adjust the dose for each patient. Where appropriate Cardene SR may also be used in combination with beta-blockers and/or diuretics.

Use in the elderly:

Starting dose: 30 mg every 12 hours. Titrate upwards with care as nicardipine may lower systolic pressure more than diastolic pressure in these patients.

Children:

Cardene SR is not recommended for use in patients under the age of 18.

4.3 Contraindications
i) Use in pregnancy and lactation.

ii) Hypersensitivity to nicardipine hydrochloride or other dihydropyridines because of the theoretical risk of cross reactivity.

iii) As part of the effect of nicardipine is secondary to reduced afterload, the drug should not be given to patients with advanced aortic stenosis. Reduction in diastolic pressure in these patients may worsen rather than improve myocardial oxygen balance.

iv) Cardene should not be used in cardiogenic shock, clinically significant aortic stenosis and during or within one month of a myocardial infarction.

v) Cardene should not be used for secondary prevention of myocardial infarction.

4.4 Special warnings and precautions for use
If used in combination with diuretics or beta-blockers, careful titration of Cardene SR is advised to avoid excessive reduction in blood pressure.

If switching from beta-blockers to Cardene SR, gradually reduce the beta-blocker dose (preferably over 8 – 10 days) since nicardipine gives no protection against the dangers of abrupt beta-blocker withdrawal.

Stop Cardene SR in patients experiencing ischaemic pain within 30 minutes of starting therapy or after increasing the dose.

Use in patients with congestive heart failure or poor cardiac reserve:

Haemodynamic studies in patients with heart failure have shown that nicardipine reduces afterload and improves overall haemodynamics. In one study, intravenous nicardipine reduced myocardial contractility in patients with severe heart failure despite increases in cardiac index and ejection fraction noted in the same patients.

Since nicardipine has not been extensively studied in patients with severe left ventricular dysfunction and cardiac failure, one must consider that worsening of cardiac failure may occur.

Use in patients with impaired hepatic or renal function:

Since Cardene is subject to first-pass metabolism, use with caution in patients with impaired liver function or reduced hepatic blood flow. Patients with severe liver disease showed elevated blood levels and the half-life of nicardipine was prolonged. Cardene blood levels may also be elevated in some renally impaired patients. Therefore the lowest starting dose and extending the dosing interval should be individually considered in these patients.

Use in patients following a stroke (infarction or haemorrhage):

Avoid inducing systemic hypotension when administering Cardene SR to these patients.

Laboratory tests:

Transient elevations of alkaline phosphatase, serum bilirubin, SGPT, SGOT and glucose, have been observed. BUN and creatinine may also become elevated. While out-of-range values were seen in T_3, T_4 and TSH, the lack of consistent alterations suggest that any changes were not drug-related.

Treatment with short acting nicardipine may induce an exaggerated fall in blood pressure and reflex tachycardia which can cause cardiovascular complications such as myocardial and cerebrovascular ischaemia.

There has been some concern about increased mortality and morbidity in the treatment of ischaemic heart disease using higher than recommended doses of some other short-acting dihydropyridines.

Patients with rare hereditary problems of galactose intolerance, the Lapp lactase deficiency or glucose-galactose malabsorption should not take this medicine.

4.5 Interaction with other medicinal products and other forms of interaction
Digoxin

Careful monitoring of serum digoxin levels is advised in patients also receiving Cardene as levels may be increased.

Propranolol, Dipyridamole, Warfarin, Quinidine, Naproxen:

Therapeutic concentrations of these drugs does not change the *in vitro* plasma protein binding of nicardipine.

Cimetidine:

Cimetidine increases nicardipine plasma levels. Carefully monitor patients receiving both drugs.

Fentanyl Anaesthesia:

Severe hypotension has been reported during fentanyl anaesthesia with concomitant use of a beta-blocker and calcium blockade. Even though such interactions have not been seen in clinical trials, such hypotensive episodes should be vigorously treated with conventional therapy such as intravenous fluids.

Ciclosporin:

Monitor ciclosporin plasma levels and reduce dosage accordingly in patients concomitantly receiving nicardipine as elevated cyclosporin levels have been reported.

Rifampicin:

Rifampicin can interact with other dihydropyridines to substantially reduce their plasma levels and so rifampicin and nicardipine should be used together with caution.

As with other dihydropyridines, nicardipine should not be taken with grapefruit juice because bioavailability may be increased.

Cardene may be used in combination with beta-blocking and other anti-hypertensive drugs but the possibility of an additive effect resulting in postural hypotension should be considered.

4.6 Pregnancy and lactation
See contra-indications.

4.7 Effects on ability to drive and use machines
None known.

4.8 Undesirable effects
Most are expected consequences of the vasodilator effects of Cardene SR.

The most frequent side-effects reported are headache, pedal oedema, heat sensation and/or flushing, palpitations, nausea and dizziness.

Other side-effects noted in clinical trials include the following:

Cardiovascular System: As with the use of other sustained release dihydropyridines in patients with ischaemic heart disease, exacerbation of angina pectoris may occur rarely at the start of treatment with Cardene SR. The occurrence of myocardial infarction has been reported although it is not possible to distinguish such an event from the natural course of ischaemic heart disease.

Central Nervous System: Drowsiness, insomnia, tinnitus, paraesthesia, functional disorders.

Skin: Itching, rashes.

Hepato-Renal: Impairment, frequency.

Dyspnoea, gastro-intestinal upset and, rarely, depression, impotence and thrombocytopenia, have also been reported.

4.9 Overdose
Symptoms may include marked hypotension, bradycardia, palpitations, flushing, drowsiness, confusion and slurred speech. In laboratory animals, overdosage also resulted in reversible hepatic function abnormalities, sporadic focal hepatic necrosis and progressive atrioventricular conduction block.

Use routine measures (eg gastric lavage) including monitoring of cardiac and respiratory functions. Position the patient to avoid cerebral anoxia. Frequent blood pressure determinations are essential. Vasopressors are clinically indicated for patients exhibiting the effects of calcium entry blockade.

5. PHARMACOLOGICAL PROPERTIES
5.1 Pharmacodynamic properties
Mode of action

Cardene is a potent calcium channel blocker. Pharmacological studies suggest it is highly selective for the peripheral vasculature over the myocardium accounting for its minimal negative inotropic effects and marked peripheral vasodilatation when used clinically.

In mild to moderate hypertensive patients Cardene SR has been shown to reduce blood pressure and maintain control over 24 hours, only if the doses are regularly administered exactly 12 hours apart.

Electrophysiologic effects:

Electrophysiological studies in man show that Cardene does not depress sinus node function or atrial or ventricular conduction in patients with either normal or decreased electrical conduction systems. Refractory periods of the His-Purkinje system were actually shortened slightly by nicardipine and SA conduction time was improved.

5.2 Pharmacokinetic properties

Cardene Capsules are completely absorbed with plasma levels detectable 20 minutes following an oral dose. Maximal plasma levels are generally achieved between one and four hours. Cardene SR is subject to saturable first pass metabolism with somewhat lower bioavailability than the standard capsule formulation of nicardipine (about 35% following a 30mg oral standard capsule at steady state) except at the 60mg dose. Minimum plasma levels produced by equivalent daily doses are similar. Cardene SR thus exhibits significantly reduced fluctuation in plasma levels in comparison to standard nicardipine capsules.

When Cardene SR is taken with a high fat meal, fluctuation in plasma levels are reduced.

Cardene is extensively metabolised by the liver; none of the metabolites possess significant biological activity.

5.3 Preclinical safety data

Please refer to section 4.6 Pregnancy and Lactation.

6. PHARMACEUTICAL PARTICULARS

6.1 List of excipients

Starch, Pregelatinised

Magnesium Stearate

Microcrystalline cellulose

Starch

Lactose

Methacrylic acid co-polymer

Cardene SR 30mg

Capsule shell body

Titanium Dioxide E171

Gelatin

Cardene SR 45mg

Capsule shell body

Titanium Dioxide E171

Gelatin

Indigotine E132

Cardene SR 30mg

Capsule shell cap

Titanium Dioxide E171

Gelatin

Cardene SR 45mg

Capsule shell cap

Titanium Dioxide E171

Gelatin

Indigotine E132

6.2 Incompatibilities

None known.

6.3 Shelf life

60 months.

6.4 Special precautions for storage

Protect from light and excessive humidity. Do not store above 25°C.

6.5 Nature and contents of container

Blister packs of 56

Blister packs of 14

Securitainers of 100

6.6 Special precautions for disposal and other handling

No special instructions required.

Administrative Data

7. MARKETING AUTHORISATION HOLDER

Astellas Pharma Limited

Lovett House

Lovett Road

Staines

TW18 3AZ

United Kingdom

8. MARKETING AUTHORISATION NUMBER(S)

Cardene SR 30mg - PL 00166/0183

Cardene SR 45mg - PL 00166/0184

9. DATE OF FIRST AUTHORISATION/RENEWAL OF THE AUTHORISATION

1 July 1998/ 15 July 2002

10. DATE OF REVISION OF THE TEXT

6 June 2006.

11. LEGAL CATEGORY

POM

Cardicor 1.25mg, 2.5mg, 3.75mg, 5mg, 7.5mg, 10mg Film Coated Tablets

(Merck Serono)

1. NAME OF THE MEDICINAL PRODUCT

Cardicor 1.25 mg film-coated tablets

Cardicor 2.5 mg film-coated tablets

Cardicor 3.75 mg film-coated tablets

Cardicor 5 mg film-coated tablets

Cardicor 7.5 mg film-coated tablets

Cardicor 10 mg film-coated tablets

2. QUALITATIVE AND QUANTITATIVE COMPOSITION

Each tablet contains 1.25, 2.5, 3.75, 5, 7.5 or 10 mg bisoprolol hemifumarate

For excipients, see section 6.1.

3. PHARMACEUTICAL FORM

Film-coated tablet.

1.25mg: white, round film-coated tablets

2.5mg: white, heart shaped, scored and film-coated tablets

3.75mg: off-white, heart shaped, scored and film coated tablets

5mg: yellowish white, heart shaped, scored and film-coated tablets

7.5mg: pale yellow, heart shaped, scored and film-coated tablets

10mg: pale orange-light orange, heart shaped, scored and film-coated tablets

4. CLINICAL PARTICULARS

4.1 Therapeutic indications

Treatment of stable chronic moderate to severe heart failure with reduced systolic ventricular function (ejection fraction $\leq$35%, based on echocardiography) in addition to ACE inhibitors, and diuretics, and optionally cardiac glycosides (for additional information see section 5.1).

4.2 Posology and method of administration

The patients should have stable chronic heart failure without acute failure during the past six weeks and a mainly unchanged basic therapy during the past two weeks. They should be treated at optimal dose with an ACE inhibitor (or other vasodilator in case of intolerance to ACE inhibitors) and a diuretic, and optionally cardiac glycosides, prior to the administration of bisoprolol.

It is recommended that the treating physician should be experienced in the management of chronic heart failure.

Warning: The treatment of stable chronic heart failure with bisoprolol has to be initiated with a titration phase as given in the description below.

The treatment with bisoprolol is to be started with a gradual uptitration according to the following steps:

- 1.25 mg once daily for 1 week, if well tolerated increase to
- 2.5 mg once daily for a further week, if well tolerated increase to
- 3.75 mg once daily for a further week, if well tolerated increase to
- 5 mg once daily for the 4 following weeks, if well tolerated increase to
- 7.5 mg once daily for the 4 following weeks, if well tolerated increase to
- 10 mg once daily for the maintenance therapy.

After initiation of treatment with 1.25 mg, the patients should be observed over a period of approximately 4 hours (especially as regards blood pressure, heart rate, conduction disturbances, signs of worsening of heart failure).

The maximum recommended dose is 10 mg once daily.

Occurrence of adverse events may prevent all patients being treated with the maximum recommended dose. If necessary, the dose reached can also be decreased step by step. The treatment may be interrupted if necessary and reintroduced as appropriate. During the titration phase, in case of worsening of the heart failure or intolerance, it is recommended first to reduce the dose of bisoprolol, or to stop immediately if necessary (in case of severe hypotension, worsening of heart failure with acute pulmonary oedema, cardiogenic shock, symptomatic bradycardia or AV block).

Treatment of stable chronic heart failure with bisoprolol is generally a long-term treatment.

The treatment with bisoprolol is not recommended to be stopped abruptly since this might lead to a transitory worsening of heart failure. If discontinuation is necessary, the dose should be gradually decreased divided into halves weekly.

Bisoprolol tablets should be taken in the morning and can be taken with food. They should be swallowed with liquid and should not be chewed.

Renal or liver insufficiency

There is no information regarding pharmacokinetics of bisoprolol in patients with chronic heart failure and with impaired liver or renal function. Uptitration of the dose in these populations should therefore be made with additional caution.

Elderly

No dosage adjustment is required.

Children

There is no paediatric experience with bisoprolol, therefore its use cannot be recommended for children.

4.3 Contraindications

Bisoprolol is contraindicated in chronic heart failure patients with:

- acute heart failure or during episodes of heart failure decompensation requiring i.v. inotropic therapy
- cardiogenic shock
- AV block of second or third degree (without a pacemaker)
- sick sinus syndrome
- sinoatrial block
- bradycardia with less than 60 beats/min before the start of therapy
- hypotension (systolic blood pressure less than 100 mm Hg)
- severe bronchial asthma or severe chronic obstructive pulmonary disease
- late stages of peripheral arterial occlusive disease and Raynaud's syndrome
- untreated phaeochromocytoma (see 4.4)
- metabolic acidosis
- hypersensitivity to bisoprolol or to any of the excipients

4.4 Special warnings and precautions for use

Bisoprolol must be used with caution in:

- bronchospasm (bronchial asthma, obstructive airways diseases)
- diabetes mellitus with large fluctuations in blood glucose values; symptoms of hypoglycaemia can be masked
- strict fasting
- ongoing desensitisation therapy
- AV block of first degree
- Prinzmetal's angina
- peripheral arterial occlusive disease (intensification of complaints might happen especially during the start of therapy)
- General anaesthesia

In patients undergoing general anaesthesia beta-blockade reduces the incidence of arrhythmias and myocardial ischemia during induction and intubation, and the post-operative period. It is currently recommended that maintenance beta-blockade be continued peri-operatively. The anaesthetist must be aware of beta-blockade because of the potential for interactions with other drugs, resulting in bradyarrhythmias, attenuation of the reflex tachycardia and the decreased reflex ability to compensate for blood loss. If it is thought necessary to withdraw beta-blocker therapy before surgery, this should be done gradually and completed about 48 hours before anaesthesia.

There is no therapeutic experience of bisoprolol treatment of heart failure in patients with the following diseases and conditions:

- NYHA class II heart failure
- insulin dependent diabetes mellitus (type I)
- impaired renal function (serum creatinine $\geq$300 micro-mol/l)
- impaired liver function
- patients older than 80 years
- restrictive cardiomyopathy
- congenital heart disease
- haemodynamically significant organic valvular disease
- myocardial infarction within 3 months

Combination of bisoprolol with calcium antagonists of the verapamil and diltiazem type, with Class I antiarrhythmic drugs and with centrally acting antihypertensive drugs is generally not recommended, for details please refer to section 4.5.

In bronchial asthma or other chronic obstructive lung diseases, which may cause symptoms, bronchodilating therapy should be given concomitantly. Occasionally an increase of the airway resistance may occur in patients with asthma, therefore the dose of $beta_2$-stimulants may have to be increased.

As with other beta-blockers, bisoprolol may increase both the sensitivity towards allergens and the severity of anaphylactic reactions. Adrenaline treatment does not always give the expected therapeutic effect.

Patients with psoriasis or with a history of psoriasis should only be given beta-blockers (e.g. bisoprolol) after carefully balancing the benefits against the risks.

In patients with phaeochromocytoma bisoprolol must not be administered until after alpha-receptor blockade.

Under treatment with bisoprolol the symptoms of a thyreotoxicosis may be masked.

The initiation of treatment with bisoprolol necessitates regular monitoring. For the posology and method of administration please refer to section 4.2.

The cessation of therapy with bisoprolol should not be done abruptly unless clearly indicated. For further information please refer to section 4.2.

4.5 Interaction with other medicinal products and other forms of interaction

Combinations not recommended

Calcium antagonists of the verapamil type and to a lesser extent of the diltiazem type: Negative influence on contractility and atrio-ventricular conduction. Intravenous administration of verapamil in patients on β-blocker treatment may lead to profound hypotension and atrioventricular block.

Class I antiarrhythmic drugs (e.g. quinidine, disopyramide; lidocaine, phenytoin; flecainide, propafenone): Effect on atrio-ventricular conduction time may be potentiated and negative inotropic effect increased.

Centrally acting antihypertensive drugs such as clonidine and others (e.g. methyldopa, moxonodine, rilmenidine): Concomitant use of centrally acting antihypertensive drugs may worsen heart failure by a decrease in the central sympathetic tonus (reduction of heart rate and cardiac output, vasodilation). Abrupt withdrawal, particularly if prior to beta-blocker discontinuation, may increase risk of "rebound hypertension".

Combinations to be used with caution

Calcium antagonists of the dihydropyridine type such as felodipine and amlodipine: Concomitant use may increase the risk of hypotension, and an increase in the risk of a further deterioration of the ventricular pump function in patients with heart failure cannot be excluded.

Class-III antiarrhythmic drugs (e.g. amiodarone): Effect on atrio-ventricular conduction time may be potentiated.

Topical beta-blockers (e.g. eye drops for glaucoma treatment) may add to the systemic effects of bisoprolol.

Parasympathomimetic drugs: Concomitant use may increase atrio-ventricular conduction time and the risk of bradycardia.

Insulin and oral antidiabetic drugs: Intensification of blood sugar lowering effect. Blockade of beta-adrenoreceptors may mask symptoms of hypoglycaemia.

Anaesthetic agents: Attenuation of the reflex tachycardia and increase of the risk of hypotension (for further information on general anaesthesia see also section 4.4.).

Digitalis glycosides: Reduction of heart rate, increase of atrio-ventricular conduction time.

Non-steroidal anti-inflammatory drugs (NSAIDs): NSAIDs may reduce the hypotensive effect of bisoprolol.

β-Sympathomimetic agents (e.g. isoprenaline, dobutamine): Combination with bisoprolol may reduce the effect of both agents.

Sympathomimetics that activate both β- and α-adrenoceptors (e.g. noradrenaline, adrenaline): Combination with bisoprolol may unmask the α-adrenoceptor-mediated vasoconstrictor effects of these agents leading to blood pressure increase and exacerbated intermittent claudication. Such interactions are considered to be more likely with nonselective β-blockers.

Concomitant use with antihypertensive agents as well as with other drugs with blood pressure lowering potential (e.g. tricyclic antidepressants, barbiturates, phenothiazines) may increase the risk of hypotension.

Combinations to be considered

Mefloquine: increased risk of bradycardia

Monoamine oxidase inhibitors (except MAO-B inhibitors): Enhanced hypotensive effect of the beta-blockers but also risk for hypertensive crisis.

4.6 Pregnancy and lactation

Pregnancy:

Bisoprolol has pharmacological effects that may cause harmful effects on pregnancy and/or the fetus/newborn. In general, beta-adrenoceptor blockers reduce placental perfusion, which has been associated with growth retardation, intrauterine death, abortion or early labour. Adverse effects (e.g. hypoglycaemia and bradycardia) may occur in the fetus and newborn infant. If treatment with beta-adrenoceptor blockers is necessary, beta$_1$-selective adrenoceptor blockers are preferable.

Bisoprolol should not be used during pregnancy unless clearly necessary. If treatment with bisoprolol is considered necessary, the uteroplacental blood flow and the fetal growth should be monitored. In case of harmful effects on pregnancy or the fetus alternative treatment should be considered. The newborn infant must be closely monitored. Symptoms of hypoglycaemia and bradycardia are generally to be expected within the first 3 days.

Lactation:

It is not known whether this drug is excreted in human milk. Therefore, breastfeeding is not recommended during administration of bisoprolol.

4.7 Effects on ability to drive and use machines

In a study with coronary heart disease patients bisoprolol did not impair driving performance. However, due to individual variations in reactions to the drug, the ability to drive a vehicle or to operate machinery may be impaired. This should be considered particularly at start of treatment and upon change of medication as well as in conjunction with alcohol.

4.8 Undesirable effects

Clinical trial data

The table below shows incidences of adverse events reported from both the placebo and the bisoprolol cohort of the CIBIS II trial. Regardless of causal relationship all adverse events are included. Each patient is only counted once for each adverse event occurring in at least 5% of the study population.

(see Table 1 below)

Post-marketing data

The following data results from post-marketing experience with bisoprolol:

Common (≥1% and <10%), uncommon (≥0.1% and <1%), rare (≥0.01% and <0.1%), very rare (<0.01%), single cases.

Cardiac disorders:

Uncommon: bradycardia, AV-stimulus disturbances, worsening of heart failure.

Ear and labyrinth disorders:

Rare: hearing impairment.

Eye disorders:

Rare: reduced tear flow (to be considered if the patient uses lenses).

Very rare: conjunctivitis.

Gastrointestinal disorders:

Common: Nausea, vomiting, diarrhoea, constipation.

General disorders:

Uncommon: Muscular weakness and cramps.

Hepatobiliary disorders:

Rare: increased liver enzymes (ALAT, ASAT), hepatitis.

Metabolism and nutrition disorders:

Rare: Increased triglycerides.

Nervous system disorders:

Common: Tiredness*, exhaustion*, dizziness*, headache*.

Uncommon: Sleep disturbances, depression.

Rare: Nightmares, hallucinations, syncope

Reproductive system and breast disorders:

Rare: Potency disorders.

Respiratory, thoracic and mediastinal disorders:

Uncommon: Bronchospasm in patients with bronchial asthma or a history of obstructive airways disease.

Rare: allergic rhinitis.

Skin and subcutaneous tissue disorders:

Rare: hypersensitivity reactions (itching, flush, rash).

Very rare: beta-blockers may provoke or worsen psoriasis or induce psoriasis-like rash, alopecia.

Vascular disorders:

Common: Feeling of coldness or numbness in the extremities.

Uncommon: orthostatic hypotension.

* These symptoms especially occur at the beginning of the therapy. They are generally mild and usually disappear within 1-2 weeks.

4.9 Overdose

With overdose (e.g. daily dose of 15 mg instead of 7.5 mg) third degree AV-block, bradycardia, and dizziness have been reported. In general the most common signs expected with overdosage of a beta-blocker are bradycardia, hypotension, bronchospasm, acute cardiac insufficiency and hypoglycaemia. To date a few cases of overdose (maximum: 2000 mg) with bisoprolol have been reported in patients suffering from hypertension and/or coronary heart disease showing bradycardia and/or hypotension; all patients recovered. There is a wide interindividual variation in sensitivity to one single high dose of bisoprolol and patients with heart failure are probably very sensitive. Therefore it is mandatory to initiate the treatment of these patients with a gradual uptitration according to the scheme given in section 4.2.

If overdose occurs, bisoprolol treatment should be stopped and supportive and symptomatic treatment should be provided. Limited data suggest that bisoprolol is hardly dialysable. Based on the expected pharmacologic actions and recommendations for other beta-blockers, the following general measures should be considered when clinically warranted.

Bradycardia: Administer intravenous atropine. If the response is inadequate, isoprenaline or another agent with positive chronotropic properties may be given cautiously. Under some circumstances, transvenous pacemaker insertion may be necessary.

Hypotension: Intravenous fluids and vasopressors should be administered. Intravenous glucagon may be useful.

AV block (second or third degree): Patients should be carefully monitored and treated with isoprenaline infusion or transvenous cardiac pacemaker insertion.

Acute worsening of heart failure: Administer i.v. diuretics, inotropic agents, vasodilating agents.

Bronchospasm: Administer bronchodilator therapy such as isoprenaline, beta$_2$-sympathomimetic drugs and/or aminophylline.

Hypoglycaemia: Administer i.v. glucose.

5. PHARMACOLOGICAL PROPERTIES

5.1 Pharmacodynamic properties

Pharmacotherapeutic group: Beta blocking agents, selective

ATC Code: C07AB07

Bisoprolol is a highly beta$_1$-selective-adrenoceptor blocking agent, lacking intrinsic stimulating and relevant membrane stabilising activity. It only shows low affinity to the beta$_2$-receptor of the smooth muscles of bronchi and vessels as well as to the beta$_2$-receptors concerned with metabolic regulation. Therefore, bisoprolol is generally not to be expected to influence the airway resistance and beta$_2$-mediated metabolic effects. Its beta$_1$-selectivity extends beyond the therapeutic dose range.

In total 2647 patients were included in the CIBIS II trial. 83% (n = 2202) were in NYHA class III and 17% (n = 445) were in NYHA class IV. They had stable symptomatic systolic heart failure (ejection fraction ≤35%, based on echocardiography). Total mortality was reduced from 17.3% to 11.8% (relative reduction 34%). A decrease in sudden death (3.6% vs 6.3%, relative reduction 44%) and a reduced number of heart failure episodes requiring hospital admission (12% vs 17.6%, relative reduction 36%) was observed. Finally, a significant improvement of the functional status according to NYHA classification has been shown. During the initiation and titration of bisoprolol hospital admission due to bradycardia (0.53%), hypotension (0.23%), and acute decompensation (4.97%) were observed, but they were not more frequent than in the placebo-group (0%, 0.3% and 6.74%). The numbers of fatal and disabling strokes during the total study period were 20 in the bisoprolol group and 15 in the placebo group.

Bisoprolol is already used for the treatment of hypertension and angina.

In acute administration in patients with coronary heart disease without chronic heart failure bisoprolol reduces the heart rate and stroke volume and thus the cardiac output and oxygen consumption. In chronic administration the initially elevated peripheral resistance decreases.

5.2 Pharmacokinetic properties

Bisoprolol is absorbed and has a biological availability of about 90% after oral administration. The plasma protein binding of bisoprolol is about 30%. The distribution volume is 3.5 l/kg. Total clearance is approximately 15 l/h. The half-life in plasma of 10-12 hours gives a 24 hour effect after dosing once daily.

Bisoprolol is excreted from the body by two routes. 50% is metabolised by the liver to inactive metabolites which are then excreted by the kidneys. The remaining 50% is excreted by the kidneys in an unmetabolised form. Since the elimination takes place in the kidneys and the liver to

Table 1

Preferred Term WHO	Placebo (n=1321)		Bisoprolol (n=1328)	
	Pat. with AE	% Pat. with AE	Pat. with AE	% Pat. with AE
Cardiac failure	301	22.8	244	18.4
Dyspnoea	224	17.0	183	13.8
Dizziness	126	9.5	177	13.3
Cardiomyopathy	132	10.0	141	10.6
Bradycardia	60	4.5	202	15.2
Hypotension	96	7.3	152	11.4
Tachycardia	144	10.9	79	5.9
Fatigue	94	7.1	123	9.3
Viral infection	75	5.7	86	6.5
Pneumonia	69	5.2	65	4.9

AE = Adverse Events

the same extent a dosage adjustment is not required for patients with impaired liver function or renal insufficiency. The pharmacokinetics in patients with stable chronic heart failure and with impaired liver or renal function has not been studied.

The kinetics of bisoprolol are linear and independent of age.

In patients with chronic heart failure (NYHA stage III) the plasma levels of bisoprolol are higher and the half-life is prolonged compared to healthy volunteers. Maximum plasma concentration at steady state is 64±21 ng/ml at a daily dose of 10 mg and the half-life is 17±5 hours.

5.3 Preclinical safety data
Preclinical data reveal no special hazard for humans based on conventional studies of safety pharmacology, repeated dose toxicity, genotoxicity or carcinogenicity. Like other beta-blockers, bisoprolol caused maternal (decreased food intake and decreased body weight) and embryo/fetal toxicity (increased incidence of resorptions, reduced birth weight of the offspring, retarded physical development) at high doses but was not teratogenic.

6. PHARMACEUTICAL PARTICULARS
6.1 List of excipients
Cardicor 1.25 mg
Tablet core: Silica, colloidal anhydrous; magnesium stearate, crospovidone, pregelatinised maize starch, maize starch, microcrystalline cellulose, calcium hydrogen phosphate, anhydrous.

Film coating: Dimeticone, talc, macrogol 400, titanium dioxide (E171), hypromellose.

Cardicor 2.5 mg
Tablet core: Silica, colloidal anhydrous; magnesium stearate, crospovidone, microcrystalline cellulose, maize starch, calcium hydrogen phosphate, anhydrous.

Film coating: Dimeticone, macrogol 400, titanium dioxide (E171), hypromellose.

Cardicor 3.75 mg
Tablet core: Silica, colloidal anhydrous; magnesium stearate, crospovidone, microcrystalline cellulose, maize starch, calcium hydrogen phosphate, anhydrous.

Film coating: Iron oxide yellow (E172), dimeticone, macrogol 400, titanium dioxide (E171), hypromellose.

Cardicor 5 mg
Tablet core: Silica, colloidal anhydrous; magnesium stearate, crospovidone, microcrystalline cellulose, maize starch, calcium hydrogen phosphate, anhydrous.

Film coating: Iron oxide yellow (E172), dimeticone, macrogol 400, titanium dioxide (E171), hypromellose.

Cardicor 7.5 mg
Tablet core: Silica, colloidal anhydrous; magnesium stearate, crospovidone, microcrystalline cellulose, maize starch, calcium hydrogen phosphate, anhydrous.

Film coating: Iron oxide yellow (E172), dimeticone, macrogol 400, titanium dioxide (E171), hypromellose.

Cardicor 10 mg
Tablet core: Silica, colloidal anhydrous; magnesium stearate, crospovidone, microcrystalline cellulose, maize starch, calcium hydrogen phosphate, anhydrous.

Film coating: Iron oxide red (E172), iron oxide yellow (E172), dimeticone, macrogol 400, titanium dioxide (E171), hypromellose.

6.2 Incompatibilities
Not applicable.

6.3 Shelf life
3 years.

6.4 Special precautions for storage
Do not store above 25°C.

6.5 Nature and contents of container
The container is a blister, which is made of a polyvinylchloride base film and an aluminium cover foil.

Pack sizes: 20, 28, 30, 50, 56, 60, 90 and 100 tablets.

Not all pack sizes may be marketed.

6.6 Special precautions for disposal and other handling
No special requirements.

7. MARKETING AUTHORISATION HOLDER
E Merck Ltd
Bedfont Cross
Stanwell Road
Feltham
Middlesex
TW14 8NX
UK

8. MARKETING AUTHORISATION NUMBER(S)
PL 0493/0179-0184

9. DATE OF FIRST AUTHORISATION/RENEWAL OF THE AUTHORISATION
4 June 2004

10. DATE OF REVISION OF THE TEXT
July 2009

Cardura XL
(Pfizer Limited)

1. NAME OF THE MEDICINAL PRODUCT
CARDURA™ XL 4mg CARDURA™ XL 8mg

2. QUALITATIVE AND QUANTITATIVE COMPOSITION
Doxazosin mesilate:

4.85mg equivalent to 4mg doxazosin.

9.70mg equivalent to 8mg doxazosin.

For excipients, see 6.1.

3. PHARMACEUTICAL FORM
Modified release tablet

Cardura XL 4mg and 8mg tablets are white, round, biconvex shaped tablets with a hole in one side, marked CXL4 and CXL8.

4. CLINICAL PARTICULARS
4.1 Therapeutic indications
Hypertension: Cardura XL is indicated for the treatment of hypertension and can be used as the sole agent to control blood pressure in the majority of patients. In patients inadequately controlled on single antihypertensive therapy, Cardura XL may be used in combination with a thiazide diuretic, beta-adrenoceptor blocking agent, calcium antagonist or an angiotensin-converting enzyme inhibitor.

Benign prostatic hyperplasia: Cardura XL is indicated for the treatment of urinary outflow obstruction and symptoms associated with benign prostatic hyperplasia (BPH).

Cardura XL may be used in BPH patients who are either hypertensive or normotensive. While the blood pressure changes in normotensive patients with BPH are not usually clinically significant, patients with hypertension and BPH have had both conditions effectively treated with doxazosin monotherapy.

4.2 Posology and method of administration
Hypertension and benign prostatic hyperplasia: The initial dose of Cardura XL is 4mg once daily. Over 50% of patients with mild to moderate severity hypertension will be controlled on Cardura XL 4mg once daily. Optimal effect of Cardura XL may take up to 4 weeks. If necessary, the dosage may be increased following this period to 8mg once daily according to patient response.

The maximum recommended dose of Cardura XL is 8mg once daily.

Cardura XL can be taken with or without food.

The tablets should be swallowed whole with a sufficient amount of liquid.

Children: The safety and efficacy of Cardura XL in children have not been established.

Elderly: Normal adult dosage.

Patients with renal impairment: Since there is no change in pharmacokinetics in patients with impaired renal function the usual adult dose of Cardura XL is recommended. Doxazosin is not dialysable.

Patients with hepatic impairment: As with any drug wholly metabolised by the liver, Cardura XL should be administered with caution to patients with evidence of impaired hepatic function (see section 4.4 and section 5.2).

4.3 Contraindications
Cardura XL is contraindicated in:

1) Patients with a known hypersensitivity to quinazolines, (e.g. doxazosin, prazosin, terazosin), or any of the excipients.

2) Patients with a history of orthostatic hypotension

3) Patients with benign prostatic hyperplasia and concomitant congestion of the upper urinary tract, chronic urinary tract infection or bladder stones.

4) Patients with a history of gastro-intestinal obstruction, oesophageal obstruction, or any degree of decreased lumen diameter of the gastro-intestinal tract.

5) During lactation (see section 4.6)

6) Patients with hypotension (for benign prostatic hyperplasia indication only)

Doxazosin is contraindicated as monotherapy in patients with either overflow bladder or anuria with or without progressive renal insufficiency.

4.4 Special warnings and precautions for use
Information to be given to the Patient: Patients should be informed that Cardura XL tablets should be swallowed whole. Patients should not chew, divide or crush the tablets.

In Cardura XL, the active compound is surrounded by an inert, non-absorbable shell that has been specially designed to control the release of the drug over a prolonged period. After transit through the gastrointestinal tract the empty tablet shell is excreted. Patients should be advised that they should not be concerned if they occasionally observe remains in their stools that look like a tablet.

Abnormally short transit times through the gastrointestinal tract (e.g. following surgical resection) could result in incomplete absorption. In view of the long half life of doxazosin the clinical significance of this is unclear.

Postural hypotension / syncope:
Initiation of therapy - As with all alpha-blockers, a very small percentage of patients have experienced postural hypotension evidenced by dizziness and weakness, or rarely loss of consciousness (syncope), particularly with the commencement of therapy. Therefore, it is prudent medical practice to monitor blood pressure on initiation of therapy to minimise the potential for postural effects.

When instituting therapy with any effective alpha-blocker, the patient should be advised how to avoid symptoms resulting from postural hypotension and what measures to take should they develop. The patient should be cautioned to avoid situations where injury could result should dizziness or weakness occur during the initiation of Cardura XL therapy.

Use in patients with Acute Cardiac Conditions:
As with any other vasodilatory anti-hypertensive agent it is prudent medical practice to advise caution when administering doxazosin to patients with the following acute cardiac conditions:

- pulmonary oedema due to aortic or mitral stenosis
- high-output cardiac failure
- right-sided heart failure due to pulmonary embolism or pericardial effusion
- left ventricular heart failure with low filling pressure.

Use in Hepatically Impaired Patients:
As with any drug wholly metabolised by the liver, Cardura XL should be administered with particular caution to patients with evidence of impaired hepatic function (see section 4.2 and section 5.2). Since there is no clinical experience in patients with severe hepatic impairment use in these patients is not recommended.

Use with PDE-5 Inhibitors: Concomitant administration of doxazosin with phosphodiesterase-5-inhibitors (eg sildenafil, tadalafil, and vardenafil) should be done with caution as both drugs have vasodilating effects and may lead to symptomatic hypotension in some patients. To reduce the risk of orthostatic hypotension it is recommended to initiate the treatment with phosphodiesterase-5-inhibitors only if the patient is hemodynamically stabilized on alpha-blocker therapy. Furthermore, it is recommended to initiate phosphodiesterase-5-inhibitor treatment with the lowest possible dose and to respect a 6-hour time interval from intake of doxazosin. No studies have been conducted with doxazosin prolonged release formulations.

Use in patients undergoing cataract surgery: The 'Intraoperative Floppy Iris Syndrome' (IFIS, a variant of small pupil syndrome) has been observed during cataract surgery in some patients on or previously treated with tamsulosin. Isolated reports have also been received with other alpha-1 blockers and the possibility of a class effect cannot be excluded. As IFIS may lead to increased procedural complications during the cataract operation current or past use of alpha-1 blockers should be made known to the ophthalmic surgeon in advance of surgery.

4.5 Interaction with other medicinal products and other forms of interaction
Phosphodiesterase-5-inhibitors (eg. sildenafil, tadalafil, vardenafil)

Concomitant administration of doxazosin with a PDE-5 inhibitor may lead to symptomatic hypotension in some patients (see section 4.4). No studies have been conducted with doxazosin prolonged-release formulations.

Doxazosin is highly bound to plasma proteins (98%). *In vitro* data in human plasma indicates that doxazosin has no effect on protein binding of the drugs tested (digoxin, phenytoin, warfarin or indomethacin).

Conventional doxazosin has been administered without any adverse drug interactions in clinical experience with thiazide diuretics, frusemide, beta-blocking agents, non-steroidal anti-inflammatory drugs, antibiotics, oral hypoglycaemic drugs, uricosuric agents, or anticoagulants. However, data from formal drug/drug interaction studies are not present.

Doxazosin potentiates the blood pressure lowering activity of other alpha-blockers and other antihypertensives.

In an open-label, randomized, placebo-controlled trial in 22 healthy male volunteers, the administration of a single 1 mg dose of doxazosin on day 1 of a four-day regimen of oral cimetidine (400 mg twice daily) resulted in a 10% increase in mean AUC of doxazosin, and no statistically significant changes in mean Cmax and mean half-life of doxazosin. The 10% increase in the mean AUC for doxazosin with cimetidine is within intersubject variation (27%) of the mean AUC for doxazosin with placebo.

4.6 Pregnancy and lactation
For the hypertension indication:

Use during pregnancy: As there are no adequate and well-controlled studies in pregnant women, the safety of Cardura XL during pregnancy has not yet been established. Accordingly, Cardura XL should be used only when, in the opinion of the physician, the potential benefit outweighs the potential risk.

Although no teratogenic effects were seen in animal testing, reduced foetal survival was observed in animals at extremely high doses (see section 5.3). These doses were approximately 300 times the maximum recommended human dose.

Jse during lactation: Doxazosin is contraindicated during actation as animal studies have shown that doxazosin accumulates in milk of lactating rats, and there is no nformation about the excretion of the drug into the milk of lactating women.

Alternatively, mothers should stop breast-feeding when reatment with doxazosin is necessary (Please see section 5.3).

For the benign prostatic hyperplasia indication: The secion is not applicable

.7 Effects on ability to drive and use machines

The ability to drive or use machinery may be impaired, specially when initiating therapy.

.8 Undesirable effects

n clinical trials, the most common reactions associated vith Cardura XL therapy were of a postural type (rarely ssociated with fainting) or non-specific.

requencies used are as follows: Very common ≥ 1/10, Common ≥ 1/100 and < 1/10, Uncommon ≥ 1/1,000 and < 1/100, Rare ≥ 1/10,000 and < 1/1,000, Very rare < 1/0,000, Unknown (cannot be estimated from the existing ata).

see Table 1 opposite)

The adverse events for Cardura XL are similar to those with nmediate release doxazosin tablets.

.9 Overdose

Should overdosage lead to hypotension, the patient should e immediately placed in a supine, head down position. Other supportive measures should be performed if thought ppropriate in individual cases. Since doxazosin is highly rotein bound, dialysis is not indicated.

. PHARMACOLOGICAL PROPERTIES

.1 Pharmacodynamic properties

Doxazosin is a potent and selective post-junctional alpha--adrenoceptor antagonist.

dministration of Cardura XL to hypertensive patients auses a clinically significant reduction in blood pressure s a result of a reduction in systemic vascular resistance. This effect is thought to result from selective blockade of e alpha-1-adrenoreceptors located in the vasculature. Vith once daily dosing, clinically significant reductions in lood pressure are present throughout the day and at 24 ours post dose. The majority of patients are controlled on e initial dose. In patients with hypertension, the decrease blood pressure during treatment with Cardura XL was milar in both the sitting and standing position.

ubjects treated with immediate release doxazosin tablets an be transferred to Cardura XL 4mg and the dose titrated pwards as needed.

oxazosin has been shown to be free of adverse metabolic ffects and is suitable for use in patients with coexistent iabetes mellitus, gout and insulin resistance.

oxazosin is suitable for use in patients with co-existent sthma, left ventricular hypertrophy and in elderly patients. reatment with doxazosin has been shown to result in egression of left ventricular hypertrophy, inhibition of plaelet aggregation and enhanced activity of tissue plasmiogen activator. Additionally, doxazosin improves insulin ensitivity in patients with impairment.

oxazosin, in addition to its antihypertensive effect, has in ng term studies produced a modest reduction in plasma tal cholesterol, LDL-cholesterol and triglyceride concenations and therefore may be of particular benefit to ypertensive patients with concomitant hyperlipidaemia.

dministration of Cardura XL to patients with symptomatic PH results in a significant improvement in urodynamics nd symptoms. The effect in BPH is thought to result from elective blockade of the alpha-adrenoceptors located in e prostatic muscular stroma, capsule and bladder neck.

.2 Pharmacokinetic properties

bsorption: After oral administration of therapeutic doses, ardura XL is well absorbed with peak blood levels graually reached at 8 to 9 hours after dosing. Peak plasma vels are approximately one third of those of the same ose of immediate release doxazosin tablets. Trough vels at 24 hours are, however, similar.

eak/trough ratio of Cardura XL is less than half that of nmediate release doxazosin tablets.

t steady-state, the relative bioavailability of doxazosin om Cardura XL compared to immediate release form as 54% at the 4mg dose and 59% at the 8mg dose.

harmacokinetic studies with Cardura XL in the elderly ave shown no significant alterations compared to younger atients.

iotransformation/elimination: The plasma elimination biphasic with the terminal elimination half-life being 22 ours and hence this provides the basic for once daily osing. Doxazosin is extensively metabolised with <5% xcreted as unchanged drug.

harmacokinetic studies with doxazosin in patients with enal impairment also showed no significant alterations ompared to patients with normal renal function.

here are only limited data in patients with liver impairment nd on the effects of drugs known to influence hepatic etabolism (e.g. cimetidine). In a clinical study in 12 subcts with moderate hepatic impairment, single dose

Table 1

MedDRA System Organ Class	Frequency	Undesirable Effects
Infections and infestations	Common	Respiratory tract infection, urinary tract infection
Blood and lymphatic system disorders	Very Rare	Leukopenia, thrombocytopenia
Immune System Disorders	Uncommon	Allergic drug reaction
Metabolism and Nutrition Disorders	Uncommon	Anorexia, gout, increased appetite
Psychiatric Disorders	Uncommon	Anxiety, depression, insomnia
	Very Rare	Agitation, nervousness
Nervous System Disorders	Common	Dizziness, headache, somnolence
	Uncommon	Cerebrovascular accident, hypoesthesia, syncope, tremor
	Very Rare	Postural dizziness, paresthesia
Eye Disorders	Very Rare	Blurred vision
	Unknown	Intropertive floppy iris syndrome (see Section 4.4)
Ear and Labyrinth Disorders	Common	Vertigo
	Uncommon	Tinnitus
Cardiac Disorders	Common	Palpitation, tachycardia
	Uncommon	Angina pectoris, myocardial infarction
	Very Rare	Bradycardia, cardiac arrhythmias
Vascular Disorders	Common	Hypotension, postural hypotension
	Very Rare	Flush
Respiratory, Thoracic and Mediastinal Disorders	Common	Bronchitis, cough, dyspnea, rhinitis
	Uncommon	Epistaxis
	Very Rare	Bronchospasm
Gastrointestinal Disorders	Common	Abdominal pain, dyspepsia, dry mouth, nausea
	Uncommon	Constipation, diarrhoea, flatulence, vomiting, gastroenteritis
Hepatobiliary Disorders	Uncommon	Abnormal liver function tests
	Very Rare	Cholestasis, hepatitis, jaundice
Skin and Subcutaneous Tissue Disorders	Common	Pruritus
	Uncommon	Skin rash
	Very Rare	Alopecia, purpura, urticaria
Musculoskeletal and Connective Tissue Disorders	Common	Back pain, myalgia
	Uncommon	Arthralgia
	Very Rare	Muscle cramps, muscle weakness
Renal and Urinary Disorders	Common	Cystitis, urinary incontinence
	Uncommon	Dysuria, hematuria, micturition frequency
	Very Rare	Micturition disorder, nocturia, polyuria, increased diuresis
Reproductive System and Breast Disorders	Uncommon	Impotence
	Very Rare	Gynecomastia, priapism
	Unknown	Retrograde ejaculation
General Disorders and Administration Site Conditions	Common	Asthenia, chest pain, influenza-like symptoms, peripheral oedema
	Uncommon	Pain, facial oedema
	Very Rare	Fatigue, malaise,
Investigations	Uncommon	Weight increase

administration of doxazosin resulted in an increase in AUC of 43% and a decrease in apparent oral clearance of 40%.

Approximately 98% of doxazosin is protein-bound in plasma.

Doxazosin is primarily metabolised by O-demethylation and hydroxylation.

5.3 Preclinical safety data

Preclinical data reveal no special hazard for humans based on conventional animal studies in safety pharmacology, repeated dose toxicity, genotoxicity and carcinogenicity. For further information see section 4.6.

6. PHARMACEUTICAL PARTICULARS

6.1 List of excipients

Polyethylene oxide, sodium chloride, hypromellose, red ferric oxide (E172), titanium dioxide (E171), magnesium stearate, cellulose acetate, Macrogol, pharmaceutical glaze, black iron oxide (E172), ammonium hydroxide and propylene glycol.

6.2 Incompatibilities

None stated.

6.3 Shelf life

2 years.

6.4 Special precautions for storage

Do not store above 30°C.

Store in the original package.

6.5 Nature and contents of container

Blister strips of aluminium foil/aluminium foil of 7 tablets in pack size of 28 tablets.

6.6 Special precautions for disposal and other handling

No special requirements.

7. MARKETING AUTHORISATION HOLDER

Pfizer Limited

Ramsgate Road

Sandwich

Kent CT13 9NJ

United Kingdom

8. MARKETING AUTHORISATION NUMBER(S)

Cardura XL 4mg PL 00057/0417

Cardura XL 8mg PL 00057/0418

9. DATE OF FIRST AUTHORISATION/RENEWAL OF THE AUTHORISATION
6th November 2006

10. DATE OF REVISION OF THE TEXT
September 2009

11. LEGAL CATEGORY
POM
Ref: CX8_2 UK

CARDURA™ TABLETS 1mg; CARDURA™ TABLETS 2mg

(Pfizer Limited)

1. NAME OF THE MEDICINAL PRODUCT
CARDURA™

2. QUALITATIVE AND QUANTITATIVE COMPOSITION
Doxazosin mesilate:

1.213mg equivalent to 1mg doxazosin

2.43mg equivalent to 2mg doxazosin

For excipients, see 6.1.

3. PHARMACEUTICAL FORM
Tablets for oral administration.

1mg round tablets marked CN1 on one side and 'PFIZER' on the other.

2mg oblong tablets marked CN2 on one side and 'PFIZER' on the other.

4. CLINICAL PARTICULARS
4.1 Therapeutic indications
Hypertension: Cardura is indicated for the treatment of hypertension and can be used as the sole agent to control blood pressure in the majority of patients. In patients inadequately controlled on single antihypertensive therapy, Cardura may be used in combination with a thiazide diuretic, beta-adrenoceptor blocking agent, calcium antagonist or an angiotensin-converting enzyme inhibitor.

Benign prostatic hyperplasia: Cardura is indicated for the treatment of urinary outflow obstruction and symptoms associated with benign prostatic hyperplasia (BPH). Cardura may be used in BPH patients who are either hypertensive or normotensive.

4.2 Posology and method of administration
Cardura may be administered in the morning or the evening.

Hypertension: Cardura is used in a once daily regimen: the initial dose is 1mg, to minimise the potential for postural hypotension and/or syncope (see section 4.4). Dosage may then be increased to 2mg after an additional one or two weeks of therapy and thereafter, if necessary to 4mg. The majority of patients who respond to Cardura will do so at a dose of 4mg or less. Dosage can be further increased if necessary to 8mg or the maximum recommended dose of 16mg.

Benign prostatic hyperplasia: The recommended initial dosage of Cardura is 1mg given once daily to minimise the potential for postural hypotension and/or syncope (see section 4.4). Depending on the individual patient's urodynamics and BPH symptomatology dosage may then be increased to 2mg and thereafter to 4mg and up to the maximum recommended dose of 8mg. The recommended titration interval is 1-2 weeks. The usual recommended dose is 2-4mg daily.

Children: The safety and efficacy of Cardura in children have not been established.

Elderly: Normal adult dosage.

Patients with renal impairment: Since there is no change in pharmacokinetics in patients with impaired renal function, the usual adult dose of Cardura is recommended.

Cardura is not dialysable.

Patients with hepatic impairment: There are only limited data in patients with liver impairment and on the effect of drugs known to influence hepatic metabolism (e.g. cimetidine). As with any drug wholly metabolised by the liver, Cardura should be administered with caution to patients with evidence of impaired liver function (see section 4.4 and section 5.2).

4.3 Contraindications
Doxazosin is contraindicated in:

1) Patients with a known hypersensitivity to quinazolines (e.g. prazosin, terazosin, doxazosin), or any of the excipients

2) Patients with a history of orthostatic hypotension

3) Patients with benign prostatic hyperplasia and concomitant congestion of the upper urinary tract, chronic urinary tract infection or bladder stones.

4) During lactation (please see section 4.6)

5) Patients with hypotension (for benign prostatic hyperplasia indication only)

Doxazosin is contraindicated as monotherapy in patients with either overflow bladder or anuria with or without progressive renal insufficiency.

4.4 Special warnings and precautions for use
Postural Hypotension/Syncope:

Initiation of Therapy - As with all alpha-blockers, a very small percentage of patients have experienced postural hypotension evidenced by dizziness and weakness, or rarely loss of consciousness (syncope), particularly with the commencement of therapy (see section 4.2). Therefore, it is prudent medical practice to monitor blood pressure on initiation of therapy to minimise the potential for postural effects.

When instituting therapy with any effective alpha-blocker, the patient should be advised how to avoid symptoms resulting from postural hypotension and what measures to take should they develop. The patient should be cautioned to avoid situations where injury could result, should dizziness or weakness occur during the initiation of Cardura therapy.

Use in patients with Acute Cardiac Conditions:

As with any other vasodilatory anti-hypertensive agent it is prudent medical practice to advise caution when administering doxazosin to patients with the following acute cardiac conditions:

- pulmonary oedema due to aortic or mitral stenosis
- high-output cardiac failure
- right-sided heart failure due to pulmonary embolism or pericardial effusion
- left ventricular heart failure with low filling pressure.

Use in Hepatically Impaired patients:

As with any drug wholly metabolised by the liver, Cardura should be administered with particular caution to patients with evidence of impaired hepatic function (see section 4.2). Since there is no clinical experience in patients with severe hepatic impairment use in these patients is not recommended.

Use with PDE-5 Inhibitors:

Concomitant administration of doxazosin with phosphodiesterase-5-inhibitors (eg sildenafil, tadalafil, and vardenafil) should be done with caution as both drugs have vasodilating effects and may lead to symptomatic hypotension in some patients. To reduce the risk of orthostatic hypotension it is recommended to initiate the treatment with phosphodiesterase-5-inhibitors only if the patient is hemodynamically stabilized on alpha-blocker therapy. Furthermore, it is recommended to initiate phosphodiesterase-5-inhibitor treatment with the lowest possible dose and to respect a 6-hour time interval from intake of doxazosin. No studies have been conducted with doxazosin prolonged release formulations.

Use in patients undergoing cataract surgery:

The 'Intraoperative Floppy Iris Syndrome' (IFIS, a variant of small pupil syndrome) has been observed during cataract surgery in some patients on or previously treated with tamsulosin. Isolated reports have also been received with other alpha-1 blockers and the possibility of a class effect cannot be excluded. As IFIS may lead to increased procedural complications during the cataract operation current or past use of alpha-1 blockers should be made known to the ophthalmic surgeon in advance of surgery.

Patients with rare hereditary problems of galactose intolerance, the Lapp lactase deficiency or glucose-galactose malabsorption should not take this medicine.

4.5 Interaction with other medicinal products and other forms of interaction
Phosphodiesterase-5-inhibitors (eg. sildenafil, tadalafil, vardenafil)

Concomitant administration of doxazosin with a PDE-5 inhibitor may lead to symptomatic hypotension in some patients (see section 4.4). No studies have been conducted with doxazosin prolonged release formulations.

Doxazosin is highly bound to plasma proteins (98%). *In vitro* data in human plasma indicates that doxazosin has no effect on protein binding of the drugs tested (digoxin, phenytoin, warfarin or indometacin).

Conventional doxazosin has been administered without any adverse drug interaction in clinical experience with thiazide diuretics, furosemide, beta-blocking agents, non-steroidal anti-inflammatory drugs, antibiotics, oral hypoglycaemic drugs, uricosuric agents, or anticoagulants. However, data from formal drug/drug interaction studies are not present.

Doxazosin potentiates the blood pressure lowering activity of other alpha-blockers and other antihypertensives.

In an open-label, randomized, placebo-controlled trial in 22 healthy male volunteers, the administration of a single 1 mg dose of doxazosin on day 1 of a four-day regimen of oral cimetidine (400 mg twice daily) resulted in a 10% increase in mean AUC of doxazosin, and no statistically significant changes in mean Cmax and mean half-life of doxazosin. The 10% increase in the mean AUC for doxazosin with cimetidine is within intersubject variation (27%) of the mean AUC for doxazosin with placebo.

4.6 Pregnancy and lactation
For the hypertension indication:

Use during pregnancy: As there are no adequate and well-controlled studies in pregnant women, the safety of Cardura during pregnancy has not yet been established. Accordingly, Cardura should be used only when, in the opinion of the physician, the potential benefit outweighs the potential risk. Although no teratogenic effects were seen in animal testing, reduced foetal survival was observed in animals at extremely high doses (see Section 5.3). These doses were approximately 300 times the maximum recommended human dose.

Use during lactation:

Doxazosin is contraindicated during lactation as anima[l] studies have shown that doxazosin accumulates in milk of lactating rats, and there is no information about the excretion of the drug into the milk of lactating women. The clinical safety of Cardura during lactation has not been established, consequently Cardura is contra-indicated in nursing mothers.

Alternatively, mothers should stop breast-feeding when treatment with doxazosin is necessary (Please see section 5.3).

For the benign prostatic hyperplasia indication: This section is not applicable

4.7 Effects on ability to drive and use machines
The ability to drive or use machinery may be impaired especially when initiating therapy.

4.8 Undesirable effects
Hypertension: In clinical trials involving patients with hypertension, the most common reactions associated with Cardura therapy were of a postural type (rarely associated with fainting) or non-specific.

Benign prostatic hyperplasia: Experience in controlled clinical trials in BPH indicates a similar adverse event profile to that seen in hypertension.

Frequencies used are as follows: Very common ≥ 1/10, Common ≥ 1/100 and < 1/10, Uncommon ≥ 1/1,000 and < 1/100, Rare ≥ 1/10,000 and < 1/1,000, Very rare < 1/10,000, Unknown (cannot be estimated from the available data).

(see Table 1 on next page)

4.9 Overdose
Should overdosage lead to hypotension, the patient should be immediately placed in a supine, head down position. Other supportive measures may be appropriate in individual cases.

If this measure is inadequate, shock should first be treated with volume expanders. If necessary, vasopressor should then be used. Renal function should be monitored and supported as needed.

Since Cardura is highly protein bound, dialysis is not indicated.

5. PHARMACOLOGICAL PROPERTIES
5.1 Pharmacodynamic properties
Doxazosin is a potent and selective post-junctional alpha-1-adrenoceptor antagonist. This action results in a decrease in systemic blood pressure. Cardura is appropriate for oral administration in a once daily regimen in patients with essential hypertension.

Cardura has been shown to be free of adverse metabolic effects and is suitable for use in patients with coexistent diabetes mellitus, gout and insulin resistance.

Cardura is suitable for use in patients with co-existent asthma, left ventricular hypertrophy and in elderly patients. Treatment with Cardura has been shown to result in regression of left ventricular hypertrophy, inhibition of platelet aggregation and enhanced activity of tissue plasminogen activator. Additionally, Cardura improves insulin sensitivity in patients with impairment.

Cardura, in addition to its antihypertensive effect, has in long term studies produced a modest reduction in plasma total cholesterol, LDL-cholesterol and triglyceride concentrations and therefore may be of particular benefit to hypertensive patients with concomitant hyperlipidaemia.

Administration of Cardura to patients with symptomatic BPH results in a significant improvement in urodynamics and symptoms. The effect in BPH is thought to result from selective blockade of the alpha-adrenoceptors located in the muscular stroma and capsule of the prostate, and in the bladder neck.

5.2 Pharmacokinetic properties
Absorption: Following oral administration in humans (young male adults or the elderly of either sex), doxazosin is well absorbed and approximately two thirds of the dose is bioavailable.

Biotransformation/Elimination: Approximately 98% of doxazosin is protein-bound in plasma.

Doxazosin is extensively metabolised in man and in the animal species tested, with the faeces being the predominant route of excretion.

The mean plasma elimination half-life is 22 hours thus making the drug suitable for once daily administration.

After oral administration of Cardura the plasma concentrations of the metabolites are low. The most active (6' hydroxy) metabolite is present in man at one fortieth of the plasma concentration of the parent compound, which suggests that the antihypertensive activity is in the main due to doxazosin.

There are only limited data in patients with liver impairment and on the effects of drugs known to influence hepatic metabolism (e.g. cimetidine). In a clinical study in 12

Table 1

MedDRA System Organ Class	Frequency	Undesirable Effects
Infections and infestations	Common	Respiratory tract infection, urinary tract infection
Blood and lymphatic system disorders	Very Rare	Leukopenia, thrombocytopenia
Immune System Disorders	Uncommon	Allergic drug reaction
Metabolism and Nutrition Disorders	Uncommon	Gout, increased appetite, anorexia
Psychiatric Disorders	Uncommon	Agitation, depression, anxiety, insomnia, nervousness
Nervous System Disorders	Common	Somnolence, dizziness, headache
	Uncommon	Cerebrovascular accident, hypoesthesia, syncope, tremor
	Very Rare	Postural dizziness, paresthesia,
Eye Disorders	Very Rare	Blurred vision
	Unknown	Introperative floppy iris syndrome (see Section 4.4)
Ear and Labyrinth Disorders	Common	Vertigo
	Uncommon	Tinnitus
Cardiac Disorders	Common	Palpitation, tachycardia
	Uncommon	Angina pectoris, myocardial infarction,
	Very Rare	Bradycardia, cardiac arrhythmias
Vascular Disorders	Common	Hypotension, postural hypotension
	Very Rare	Hot flushes
Respiratory, Thoracic and Mediastinal Disorders	Common	Bronchitis, cough, dyspnea, rhinitis
	Uncommon	Epistaxis
	Very Rare	Aggravated bronchospasm
Gastrointestinal Disorders	Common	Abdominal pain, dyspepsia, dry mouth, nausea,
	Uncommon	Constipation, flatulence, vomiting, gastroenteritis diarrhoea
Hepatobiliary Disorders	Uncommon	Abnormal liver function tests
	Very Rare	Cholestasis, hepatitis, jaundice
Skin and Subcutaneous Tissue Disorders	Common	Pruritus
	Uncommon	Skin rash
	Very Rare	Urticaria, alopecia, purpura
Musculoskeletal and Connective Tissue Disorders	Common	Back pain, myalgia
	Uncommon	Arthralgia,
	Rare	Muscle cramps, muscle weakness
Renal and Urinary Disorders	Common	Cystitis, urinary incontinence
	Uncommon	Dysuria, micturition frequency, hematuria
	Rare	polyuria
	Very Rare	Increased diuresis, micturition disorder, nocturia
Reproductive System and Breast Disorders	Uncommon	Impotence
	Very Rare	Gynecomastia, priapism
	Unknown	Retrograde ejaculation
General Disorders and Administration Site Conditions	Common	Asthenia, chest pain, influenza-like symptoms, peripheral oedema,
	Uncommon	Pain, facial oedema
	Very Rare	Fatigue, malaise
Investigations	Uncommon	Weight increase

subjects with moderate hepatic impairment, single dose administration of doxazosin resulted in an increase in AUC of 43% and a decrease in apparent oral clearance of 40%. As with any drug wholly metabolised by the liver, Cardura should be administered with caution to patients with impaired liver function (see section 4.4).

5.3 Preclinical safety data

Preclinical data reveal no special hazard for humans based on conventional animal studies in safety pharmacology, repeated dose toxicity, genotoxicity and carcinogenicity. For further information see section 4.6.

6. PHARMACEUTICAL PARTICULARS

6.1 List of excipients

Lactose, magnesium stearate, microcrystalline cellulose, sodium lauril sulfate and sodium starch glycollate.

6.2 Incompatibilities

Not applicable.

6.3 Shelf life

5 years.

6.4 Special precautions for storage

Do not store above 30°C.

6.5 Nature and contents of container

Cardura 1mg and 2mg Tablets are available as calendar packs of 28 tablets. Aluminium/PVC/PVdC blister strips, 14 tablets/strip, 2 strips in a carton box.

6.6 Special precautions for disposal and other handling

No special requirements.

7. MARKETING AUTHORISATION HOLDER

Pfizer Limited
Ramsgate Road
Sandwich
Kent, CT13 9NJ
United Kingdom

8. MARKETING AUTHORISATION NUMBER(S)

Cardura 1mg PL 00057/0276
Cardura 2mg PL 00057/0277

9. DATE OF FIRST AUTHORISATION/RENEWAL OF THE AUTHORISATION

11 October 2006

10. DATE OF REVISION OF THE TEXT

August 2009

11. LEGAL CATEGORY

POM

Ref: CR10_3 UK

Carnitor 1 g Solution for Injection

(sigma-tau Pharma Limited UK)

1. NAME OF THE MEDICINAL PRODUCT

Carnitor 1 g Solution for Injection

2. QUALITATIVE AND QUANTITATIVE COMPOSITION

L-carnitine inner salt 1 g

3. PHARMACEUTICAL FORM

A clear, colourless or light straw- coloured solution

4. CLINICAL PARTICULARS

4.1 Therapeutic indications

Indicated for the treatment of primary and secondary carnitine deficiency in adults, children, infants and neonates.

Secondary carnitine deficiency in haemodialysis patients.

Secondary carnitine deficiency should be suspected in long-term haemodialysis patients who have the following conditions:

1. Severe and persistent muscle cramps and/or hypotensive episodes during dialysis.
2. Lack of energy causing a significant negative effect on the quality of life.
3. Skeletal muscle weakness and/or myopathy.
4. Cardiomyopathy.
5. Anaemia of uraemia unresponsive to or requiring large doses of erythropoietin.
6. Muscle mass loss caused by malnutrition.

4.2 Posology and method of administration

For slow intravenous administration over 2-3 minutes

Adults, Children, infants and neonates

It is advisable to monitor therapy by measuring free and acyl carnitine levels in both plasma and urine.

The management of inborn errors of metabolism:

The dosage required depends upon the specific inborn error of metabolism concerned and the severity of presentation at the time of treatment. However, the following can be considered as a general guide.

In acute decompensation, dosages of up to 100 mg/kg/day in 3-4 divided doses are recommended. Higher doses have been used although an increase in adverse events, primarily diarrhoea, may occur.

Secondary carnitine deficiency in haemodialysis patients:

It is strongly recommended that, before initiating therapy with Carnitor, plasma carnitine is measured. Secondary carnitine deficiency is suggested by a plasma ratio of acyl to free carnitine of greater than 0.4 and/or when free carnitine concentrations are lower than 20 μmol/litre.

A dose of 20mg per kg should be administered as an intravenous bolus at the end of each dialysis session (assuming three sessions per week). The duration of intravenous treatment should be at least three months, which is the time usually required to restore normal muscle levels of free carnitine. The overall response should be assessed by monitoring plasma acyl to free carnitine levels and by evaluating the patient's symptoms. When carnitine supplementation has been stopped there will be a progressive decline in carnitine levels. The need for a repeat course of therapy can be assessed by plasma carnitine assays at regular intervals and by monitoring the patient's symptoms.

Haemodialysis - maintenance therapy:

If significant clinical benefit has been gained by the first course of intravenous Carnitor then maintenance therapy can be considered using 1 g per day of Carnitor orally. On the day of the dialysis, oral Carnitor has to be administered at the end of the session.

4.3 Contraindications

Hypersensitivity to any of the constituents of the product.

4.4 Special warnings and precautions for use

While improving glucose utilisation, the administration of L-carnitine to diabetic patients receiving either insulin or hypoglycaemic oral treatment may result in hypoglycaemia. Plasma glucose levels in these subjects must be monitored regularly in order to adjust the hypoglycaemic treatment immediately, if required.

The safety and efficacy of oral L-carnitine has not been evaluated in patients with renal insufficiency. Chronic administration of high doses of oral L-carnitine in patients with severely compromised renal function or in end stage renal disease (ESRD) patients on dialysis may result in an accumulation of the potentially toxic metabolites, trimethylamine (TMA) and trimethylamine-N-oxide (TMAO), since these metabolites are usually excreted in the urine. This situation has not been observed following intravenous administration of L-carnitine.

4.5 Interaction with other medicinal products and other forms of interaction
There are no known interactions.

4.6 Pregnancy and lactation
Reproductive studies were performed in rats and rabbits. There was no evidence of a teratogenic effect in either species. In the rabbit but not in the rat, there was a statistically insignificant greater number of post implantation losses at the highest dose tested (600 mg/kg daily) as compared with control animals. The significance of these findings for man is unknown. There is no experience of use in pregnant patients with primary systemic carnitine deficiency.

Taking into account the serious consequences to a pregnant woman who has primary systemic carnitine deficiency stopping treatment, the risk to the mother of discontinuing treatment seems greater than the theoretical risk to the foetus if treatment is continued.

Levocarnitine is a normal component of human milk. Use of levocarnitine supplementation in nursing mothers has not been studied.

4.7 Effects on ability to drive and use machines
None known.

4.8 Undesirable effects
Various mild gastro-intestinal complaints have been reported during the long-term administration of oral levocarnitine, these include transient nausea and vomiting, abdominal cramps and diarrhoea.

Decreasing the dosage often diminishes or eliminates drug-related patient body odour or gastro-intestinal symptoms when present. Tolerance should be monitored very closely during the first week of administration and after any dosage increase.

4.9 Overdose
There have been no reports of toxicity from levocarnitine overdosage. Overdosage should be treated with supportive care.

5. PHARMACOLOGICAL PROPERTIES

5.1 Pharmacodynamic properties
ATC Code: A16AA01 (Amino acids and derivatives)

L-Carnitine is present as a natural constituent in animal tissues, micro-organisms and plants. In man the physiological metabolic requirements are met both by the consumption of food containing carnitine and the endogenous synthesis in the liver and kidneys from lysine with methionine serving as the methyl donor. Only the L-isomer is biologically active, playing an essential role in lipid metabolism as well as in the metabolism of ketone bodies as branched chain-amino-acids. L-Carnitine as a factor is necessary in the transport of long-chain fatty acids into the mitochondria – facilitating the oxidation of fatty acids rather than their incorporation into triglycerides. By releasing CoA from its thioesters, through the action of CoA; carnitine acetyl transferase, L-carnitine also enhances the metabolic flux in the Kreb's cycle; with the same mechanism it stimulates the activity of pyruvate dehydrogenase and in skeletal muscle, the oxidation of branched-chain amino acids. L-Carnitine is thus involved, directly or indirectly in several pathways so that its availability should be an important factor controlling not only the oxidative utilisation of fatty acids and ketone bodies but also that of glucose and some amino acids.

5.2 Pharmacokinetic properties
The absorbed L-carnitine is transported to various organ systems via the blood. The presence of membrane-bound proteins in several tissues including red blood cells that bind carnitine, suggest that a transport system in the blood and a cellular system for the collective uptake is present in several tissues. Tissue and serum carnitine concentration depends on several metabolic processes, carnitine biosynthesis and dietary contributions, transport into and out of tissues, degradation and excretion may all affect tissue carnitine concentrations.

Absorption
L-Carnitine is absorbed by the mucosal cells of the small intestine and enters the blood stream relatively slowly; the absorption is probably associated with an active transluminal mechanism.

The apparent systemic availability after oral administration is limited (<10%) and variable.

Distribution
Absorbed L-carnitine is transported to various organ systems via the blood; it is thought that a transport system in the blood and a cellular system for selective uptake is involved.

Excretion
L-Carnitine is excreted mainly in the urine and is variable. The excretion is directly proportional to the blood levels.

Metabolism
L-Carnitine is metabolised to a very limited extent.

5.3 Preclinical safety data
L-Carnitine is a naturally occurring body substance in human beings, plants and animals. Carnitor products are used to bring the level of L-carnitine in the body up to those found naturally. Appropriate pre-clinical studies have been undertaken and show no signs of toxicity at normal therapeutic doses.

6. PHARMACEUTICAL PARTICULARS

6.1 List of excipients
Hydrochloric acid 10%
Water for injection

6.2 Incompatibilities
None known.

6.3 Shelf life
5 years.

6.4 Special precautions for storage
Store below 25°C.
Store in the original carton in order to protect from light.

6.5 Nature and contents of container
Ph.Eur. Type 1 clear glass ampoules of 5 ml capacity.
The ampoules are packed in cardboard outer cartons containing 5 ampoules.

6.6 Special precautions for disposal and other handling
None.

7. MARKETING AUTHORISATION HOLDER
Sigma-Tau Industrie Farmaceutiche Riunite SpA,
Viale Shakespeare 47-00144,
Rome, Italy.

8. MARKETING AUTHORISATION NUMBER(S)
PL 08381/0003

9. DATE OF FIRST AUTHORISATION/RENEWAL OF THE AUTHORISATION
30 November 1999

10. DATE OF REVISION OF THE TEXT
November 2008

Carnitor 30% Paediatric Oral Solution
(sigma-tau Pharma Limited UK)

1. NAME OF THE MEDICINAL PRODUCT
Carnitor 30% Paediatric Oral Solution

2. QUALITATIVE AND QUANTITATIVE COMPOSITION
L-Carnitine inner salt 30% w/v

3. PHARMACEUTICAL FORM
Colourless or slightly yellow solution

4. CLINICAL PARTICULARS

4.1 Therapeutic indications
Indicated for the treatment of primary and secondary carnitine deficiency in children of under 12 years, infants and newborns.

4.2 Posology and method of administration
For oral administration only. The Paediatric Solution can be drunk directly or diluted further in water or fruit juices.

Children under 12 years, infants and newborns:

It is advisable to monitor therapy by measuring free and acyl carnitine levels in both plasma and urine.

The management of inborn errors of metabolism

The dosage required depends upon the specific inborn error of metabolism concerned and the severity of presentation at the time of treatment. However, the following can be considered as a general guide.

An oral dosage of up to 200mg/kg/day in divided doses (2 to 4) is recommended for chronic use in some disorders, with lower doses sufficing in other conditions. If clinical and biochemical symptoms do not improve, the dose may be increased on a short-term basis. Higher doses of up to 400mg/kg/day may be necessary in acute metabolic decompensation or the i.v. route may be required.

Haemodialysis - maintenance therapy

If significant clinical benefit has been gained by a first course of intravenous Carnitor then maintenance therapy can be considered using 1g per day of Carnitor orally. On the day of the dialysis oral Carnitor has to be administered at the end of the session.

4.3 Contraindications
Hypersensitivity to any of the constituents of the product.

4.4 Special warnings and precautions for use
While improving glucose utilisation, the administration of L-carnitine to diabetic patients receiving either insulin or hypoglycaemic oral treatment may result in hypoglycaemia. Plasma glucose levels in these subjects must be monitored regularly in order to adjust the hypoglycaemic treatment immediately, if required.

The 30% oral solution contains sucrose. This must be considered when treating diabetics or patients who are following diets to reduce calorie intake.

The safety and efficacy of oral L-carnitine has not been evaluated in patients with renal insufficiency. Chronic administration of high doses of oral L-carnitine in patients with severely compromised renal function or in end stage renal disease (ESRD) patients on dialysis may result in an accumulation of the potentially toxic metabolites, trimethylamine (TMA) and trimethylamine-N-oxide (TMAO), since these metabolites are usually excreted in the urine. This situation has not been observed following intravenous administration of L-carnitine.

4.5 Interaction with other medicinal products and other forms of interaction
There are no known interactions.

4.6 Pregnancy and lactation
Reproductive studies were performed in rats and rabbits. There was no evidence of a teratogenic effect in either species. In the rabbit but not in the rat there was a statistically insignificant greater number of post implantation losses at the highest dose tested (600mg/kg daily) as compared with control animals. The significance of these findings in man is unknown. There is no experience of use in pregnant patients with primary systemic carnitine deficiency.

Taking into account the serious consequences in a pregnant woman who has primary systemic carnitine deficiency stopping treatment, the risk to the mother of discontinuing treatment seems greater than the theoretical risk to the foetus if treatment is continued.

Levocarnitine is a normal component of human milk. Use of levocarnitine supplementation in nursing mothers has not been studied.

4.7 Effects on ability to drive and use machines
None known.

4.8 Undesirable effects
Various mild gastro-intestinal complaints have been reported during the long term administration of oral levocarnitine, these include transient nausea and vomiting, abdominal cramps and diarrhoea.

Decreasing the dosage often diminishes or eliminates drug related patient body odour or gastro-intestinal symptoms when present. Tolerance should be monitored very closely during the first week of administration and after any dosage increase.

4.9 Overdose
There have been no reports of toxicity from levocarnitine overdosage. Overdosage should be treated with supportive care.

5. PHARMACOLOGICAL PROPERTIES

5.1 Pharmacodynamic properties
ATC Code: A16AA01 (Amino acids and derivatives)

L-Carnitine is present as a natural constituent in animal tissues, micro-organisms and plants. In man the physiological metabolic requirements are met both by the consumption of food containing carnitine and the endogenous synthesis in the liver and kidneys from lysine with methionine serving as the methyl donor. Only the L-isomer is biologically active, playing an essential role in lipid metabolism as well as in the metabolism of ketone bodies as branched chain-amino-acids. L-Carnitine as a factor is necessary in the transport of long-chain fatty acids into the mitochondria - facilitating the oxidation of fatty acids rather than their incorporation into triglycerides. By releasing CoA from its thioesters, through the action of CoA; carnitine acetyl transferase, L-carnitine also enhances the metabolic flux in the Kreb's cycle; with the same mechanism it stimulates the activity of pyruvate dehydrogenase and in skeletal muscle, the oxidation of branched-chain amino acids. L-Carnitine is thus involved, directly or indirectly in several pathways so that its availability should be an important factor controlling not only the oxidative utilisation of fatty acids and ketone bodies but also that of glucose and some amino acids.

5.2 Pharmacokinetic properties
The absorbed L-carnitine is transported to various organ systems via the blood. The presence of membrane-bound proteins in several tissues including red blood cells that bind carnitine, suggest that a transport system in the blood and a cellular system for the collective uptake is present in several tissues. Tissue and serum carnitine concentration depend on several metabolic processes, carnitine biosynthesis and dietary contributions, transport into and out of tissues, degradation and excretion may all affect tissue carnitine concentrations.

It has been demonstrated that pharmacokinetic parameters increase significantly with dosage. Apparent bioavailability in healthy volunteers is about 10-16%. The data suggests a relationship between maximal plasma concentration/dosage, dosage, plasma AUC, dosage/urinary accumulation. Maximum concentration is reached about four hours after ingestion.

5.3 Preclinical safety data
L-Carnitine is a naturally occurring body substance in human beings, plants and animals. Carnitor products are used to bring the level of L-carnitine in the body up to those found naturally. Appropriate pre-clinical studies have been undertaken and show no signs of toxicity at normal therapeutic doses.

6. PHARMACEUTICAL PARTICULARS

6.1 List of excipients
Sorbitol solution (70%) (E420), tartaric acid (E334), sodium propyl hydroxybenzoate (E217), sodium methyl hydroxybenzoate (E219), colourless cherry flavour, colourless sour black cherry flavour, saccharose and purified water.

6.2 Incompatibilities
None known.

.3 Shelf life
3 years.

.4 Special precautions for storage
Store below 25°C.
Store in the original carton in order to protect from light and moisture.

.5 Nature and contents of container
0 ml amber glass bottles with a polyethylene lined, polypropylene child proof cap.

.6 Special precautions for disposal and other handling
None

. MARKETING AUTHORISATION HOLDER
Sigma-Tau Industrie Farmaceutiche Riunite SpA,
Viale Shakespeare 47-00144,
Rome, Italy.

. MARKETING AUTHORISATION NUMBER(S)
PL 08381/0005

. DATE OF FIRST AUTHORISATION/RENEWAL OF THE AUTHORISATION
0 November 1998

0. DATE OF REVISION OF THE TEXT
November 2008

Carnitor Oral Single Dose 1g

(sigma-tau Pharma Limited UK)

. NAME OF THE MEDICINAL PRODUCT
Carnitor 1 g Oral Solution

. QUALITATIVE AND QUANTITATIVE COMPOSITION
-Carnitine inner salt 1.0g

. PHARMACEUTICAL FORM
Clear, colourless or light straw- coloured solution.

. CLINICAL PARTICULARS

.1 Therapeutic indications
ndicated for the treatment of primary and secondary carnitine deficiency in adults and children over 12 years of age.

.2 Posology and method of administration
or oral administration only. The Oral Solution can be drunk directly or diluted further in water or fruit juices.

dults and children over 12 years of age
is advisable to monitor therapy by measuring free and cyl carnitine levels in both plasma and urine.

he management of inborn errors of metabolism
he dosage required depends upon the specific inborn rror of metabolism concerned and the severity of presentation at the time of treatment. However, the following can e considered as a general guide.

n oral dosage of up to 200mg/kg/day in divided doses (2 to 4) is recommended for chronic use in some disorders, with lower doses sufficing in other conditions. If clinical and biochemical symptoms do not improve, the dose may be increased on a short-term basis. Higher doses of up to 00mg/kg/day may be necessary in acute metabolic decompensation or the i.v. route may be required.

aemodialysis - maintenance therapy
significant clinical benefit has been gained by a first course of intravenous Carnitor then maintenance therapy can be considered using 1g per day of Carnitor orally. On the day of the dialysis oral Carnitor has to be administered t the end of the session.

.3 Contraindications
ypersensitivity to any of the constituents of the product.

.4 Special warnings and precautions for use
While improving glucose utilisation, the administration of L-carnitine to diabetic patients receiving either insulin or hypoglycaemic oral treatment may result in hypoglycaemia. Plasma glucose levels in these subjects must be monitored regularly in order to adjust the hypoglycaemic treatment immediately, if required.

he safety and efficacy of oral L-carnitine has not been evaluated in patients with renal insufficiency. Chronic administration of high doses of oral L-carnitine in patients with severely compromised renal function or in end stage renal disease (ESRD) patients on dialysis may result in an accumulation of the potentially toxic metabolites, trimethylamine (TMA) and trimethylamine-N-oxide (TMAO), since these metabolites are usually excreted in the urine. This situation has not been observed following intravenous administration of L-carnitine.

.5 Interaction with other medicinal products and other forms of interaction
here are no known interactions.

6 Pregnancy and lactation
eproductive studies were performed in rats and rabbits. There was no evidence of a teratogenic effect in either species. In the rabbit but not in the rat, there was a statistically insignificant greater number of post-implantation losses at the highest dose tested (600mg/kg daily) as compared with control animals. The significance of these findings in man is unknown. There is no experience of use in pregnant patients with primary systemic carnitine deficiency.

Taking into account the serious consequences in a pregnant woman who has primary systemic carnitine deficiency stopping treatment, the risk to the mother of discontinuing treatment seems greater than the theoretical risk to the foetus if treatment is continued.

Levocarnitine is a normal component of human milk. Use of levocarnitine supplementation in nursing mothers has not been studied.

4.7 Effects on ability to drive and use machines
None known.

4.8 Undesirable effects
Various mild gastro-intestinal complaints have been reported during the long-term administration of oral levocarnitine, these include transient nausea and vomiting, abdominal cramps and diarrhoea.
Decreasing the dosage often diminishes or eliminates drug related patient body odour or gastro-intestinal symptoms when present. Tolerance should be monitored very closely during the first week of administration and after any dosage increase.

4.9 Overdose
There have been no reports of toxicity from levocarnitine overdosage. Overdosage should be treated with supportive care.

5. PHARMACOLOGICAL PROPERTIES

5.1 Pharmacodynamic properties
ATC Code: A16AA01 (Amino acids and derivatives)
L-Carnitine is present as a natural constituent in animal tissues, micro-organisms and plants. In man the physiological metabolic requirements are met both by the consumption of food containing carnitine and the endogenous synthesis in the liver and kidneys from lysine with methionine serving as the methyl donor. Only the L-isomer is biologically active, playing an essential role in lipid metabolism as well as in the metabolism of ketone bodies as branched-chain amino acids. L-Carnitine as a factor is necessary in the transport of long-chain fatty acids into the mitochondria - facilitating the oxidation of fatty acids rather than their incorporation into triglycerides. By releasing CoA from its thioesters, through the action of CoA; carnitine acetyl transferase, L-carnitine also enhances the metabolic flux in the Kreb's cycle; with the same mechanism it stimulates the activity of pyruvate dehydrogenase and in skeletal muscle, the oxidation of branched-chain amino acids. L-Carnitine is thus involved, directly or indirectly in several pathways so that its availability should be an important factor controlling not only the oxidative utilisation of fatty acids and ketone bodies but also that of glucose and some amino acids.

5.2 Pharmacokinetic properties
The absorbed L-carnitine is transported to various organ systems via the blood. The presence of membrane-bound proteins in several tissues including red blood cells that bind carnitine, suggest that a transport system in the blood and a cellular system for the collective uptake is present in several tissues. Tissue and serum carnitine concentration depend on several metabolic processes, carnitine biosynthesis and dietary contributions, transport into and out of tissues, degradation and excretion may all affect tissue carnitine concentrations.

It has been demonstrated that pharmacokinetic parameters increase significantly with dosage. Apparent bioavailability in healthy volunteers is about 10-16%. The data suggests a relationship between maximal plasma concentration/dosage, dosage, plasma AUC, dosage/urinary accumulation. Maximum concentration is reached about four hours after ingestion.

5.3 Preclinical safety data
L-Carnitine is a naturally occurring body substance in human beings, plants and animals. Carnitor products are used to bring the level of L-carnitine in the body up to those found naturally. Appropriate pre-clinical studies have been undertaken and show no signs of toxicity at normal therapeutic doses.

6. PHARMACEUTICAL PARTICULARS

6.1 List of excipients
Malic acid (E296), saccharin sodium (E954), sodium methyl hydroxybenzoate (E219), sodium propyl hydroxybenzoate (E217) and purified water.

6.2 Incompatibilities
None known.

6.3 Shelf life
4 years.

6.4 Special precautions for storage
Store below 25°C.
Store in the original carton in order to protect from light.

6.5 Nature and contents of container
10 ml amber glass bottles with a fully removable low density polyethylene cap.

6.6 Special precautions for disposal and other handling
None.

7. MARKETING AUTHORISATION HOLDER
Sigma-Tau Industrie Farmaceutiche Riunite SpA,
Viale Shakespeare 47-00144,
Rome, Italy.

8. MARKETING AUTHORISATION NUMBER(S)
PL 08381/0004

9. DATE OF FIRST AUTHORISATION/RENEWAL OF THE AUTHORISATION
16 October 1998

10. DATE OF REVISION OF THE TEXT
September 2008

Casodex 150 mg Film-coated Tablets.

(AstraZeneca UK Limited)

1. NAME OF THE MEDICINAL PRODUCT
Casodex® 150 mg Film-coated Tablets

2. QUALITATIVE AND QUANTITATIVE COMPOSITION
Each tablet contains 150 mg bicalutamide (INN).
For excipients, see section 6.1.

3. PHARMACEUTICAL FORM
Film-coated tablet.
White.

4. CLINICAL PARTICULARS

4.1 Therapeutic indications
Casodex 150 mg is indicated either alone or as adjuvant to radical prostatectomy or radiotherapy in patients with locally advanced prostate cancer at high risk for disease progression (see section 5.1).

Casodex 150 mg is also indicated for the management of patients with locally advanced, non-metastatic prostate cancer for whom surgical castration or other medical intervention is not considered appropriate or acceptable.

4.2 Posology and method of administration
Adult males including the elderly: The dosage is one 150 mg tablet to be taken orally once a day.

Casodex 150 mg should be taken continuously for at least 2 years or until disease progression.

Renal impairment: No dosage adjustment is necessary for patients with renal impairment.

Hepatic impairment: No dosage adjustment is necessary for patients with mild hepatic impairment. Increased accumulation may occur in patients with moderate to severe hepatic impairment (see section 4.4).

4.3 Contraindications
Casodex 150 mg is contraindicated in females and children.

Casodex 150 mg must not be given to any patient who has shown a hypersensitivity reaction to its use.

Co-administration of terfenadine, astemizole or cisapride with Casodex is contraindicated (see section 4.5).

4.4 Special warnings and precautions for use
Initiation of treatment should be under the direct supervision of a specialist.

Bicalutamide is extensively metabolised in the liver. Data suggest that its elimination may be slower in subjects with severe hepatic impairment and this could lead to increased accumulation of bicalutamide. Therefore, Casodex 150 mg should be used with caution in patients with moderate to severe hepatic impairment.

Periodic liver function testing should be considered due to the possibility of hepatic changes. The majority of changes are expected to occur within the first 6 months of Casodex therapy.

Severe hepatic changes and hepatic failure have been observed rarely with Casodex 150 mg (see section 4.8). Casodex 150 mg therapy should be discontinued if changes are severe.

For patients who have an objective progression of disease together with elevated PSA, cessation of Casodex therapy should be considered.

Bicalutamide has been shown to inhibit cytochrome P450 (CYP 3A4), as such, caution should be exercised when co-administered with drugs metabolised predominantly by CYP 3A4 (see sections 4.3 and 4.5).

Patients with rare hereditary problems of galactose intolerance, the Lapp lactase deficiency or glucose-galactose malabsorption should not take this medicine.

4.5 Interaction with other medicinal products and other forms of interaction
In vitro studies have shown that R-bicalutamide is an inhibitor of CYP 3A4, with lesser inhibitory effects on CYP 2C9, 2C19 and 2D6 activity. Although clinical studies using antipyrine as a marker of cytochrome P450 (CYP) activity showed no evidence of a drug interaction potential with Casodex, mean midazolam exposure (AUC) was increased by up to 80%, after co-administration of Casodex for 28 days. For drugs with a narrow therapeutic index such an increase could be of relevance. As such, concomitant use of terfenadine, astemizole and cisapride is

contraindicated (see section 4.3) and caution should be exercised with the co-administration of Casodex with compounds such as ciclosporin and calcium channel blockers. Dosage reduction may be required for these drugs particularly if there is evidence of enhanced or adverse drug effect. For ciclosporin, it is recommended that plasma concentrations and clinical condition are closely monitored following initiation or cessation of Casodex therapy.

Caution should be exercised when prescribing Casodex with other drugs which may inhibit drug oxidation e.g. cimetidine and ketoconazole. In theory, this could result in increased plasma concentrations of bicalutamide which theoretically could lead to an increase in side effects.

In vitro studies have shown that bicalutamide can displace the coumarin anticoagulant, warfarin, from its protein binding sites. It is therefore recommended that if Casodex 150 mg is started in patients who are already receiving coumarin anticoagulants, prothrombin time should be closely monitored.

4.6 Pregnancy and lactation

Bicalutamide is contraindicated in females and must not be given to pregnant women or nursing mothers.

4.7 Effects on ability to drive and use machines

Casodex is unlikely to impair the ability of patients to drive or operate machinery. However, it should be noted that occasionally somnolence may occur. Any affected patients should exercise caution.

4.8 Undesirable effects

In this section, undesirable effects are defined as follows: Very common (⩾1/10); common (⩾1/100 to <1/10); uncommon (⩾1/1,000 to ⩽1/100); rare (⩾1/10,000 to ⩽1/1,000); very rare (⩽1/10,000); not known (cannot be estimated from the available data).

Table 1 Frequency of Adverse Reactions

System Organ Class	Frequency	Event
Blood and the lymphatic system disorders	Common	Anaemia
Immune system disorders	Uncommon	Hypersensitivity reactions (including angioneurotic oedema and urticaria)
Metabolism and nutrition disorders	Common	Anorexia
Psychiatric disorders	Common	Decreased libido Depression
Nervous system disorders	Common	Dizziness Somnolence
Vascular disorders	Common	Hot flush
Respiratory, thoracic and mediastinal disorders	Uncommon	Interstitial lung disease
Gastrointestinal disorders	Common	Abdominal pain Constipation Dyspepsia Flatulence Nausea
Hepato-biliary disorders	Common	Hepatic changes (including elevated levels of transaminases, jaundice)/hepato-biliary disorders[a]
	Rare	Hepatic failure[b]
Skin and subcutaneous tissue disorders	Very common	Rash
	Common	Alopecia Hirsuitism/hair regrowth Dry skin Pruritis
Renal and urinary disorders	Common	Haematuria
Reproductive system and breast disorders	Very common	Gynaecomastia and breast tenderness[c]
	Common	Impotence
General disorders and administration site conditions	Very common	Asthenia
	Common	Chest pain Oedema
Investigations	Common	Weight gain

a. Hepatic changes are rarely severe and were frequently transient, resolving or improving with continued therapy or following cessation of therapy.

b. Hepatic failure has occurred rarely in patients treated with bicalutamide, but a causal relationship has not been established with certainty. Periodic liver function testing should be considered (see also section 4.4).

c. The majority of patients receiving Casodex 150 mg as monotherapy experience gynaecomastia and/or breast pain. In studies these symptoms were considered to be severe in up to 5% of the patients. Gynaecomastia may not resolve spontaneously following cessation of therapy, particularly after prolonged treatment (⩽1/10,000), not known (cannot be estimated from the available data).

In addition, cardiac failure was reported in clinical trials (as a possible adverse drug reaction in the opinion of investigating clinicians, with a frequency of >1%) during treatment with bicalutamide plus an LHRH analogue. There is no evidence of a causal relationship with drug treatment.

4.9 Overdose

There is no human experience of overdosage. There is no specific antidote; treatment should be symptomatic. Dialysis may not be helpful, since bicalutamide is highly protein bound and is not recovered unchanged in the urine. General supportive care, including frequent monitoring of vital signs, is indicated.

5. PHARMACOLOGICAL PROPERTIES

5.1 Pharmacodynamic properties

Antiandrogen, ATC code L02 B B03

Bicalutamide is a non-steroidal antiandrogen, devoid of other endocrine activity. It binds to the wild type or normal androgen receptor without activating gene expression, and thus inhibits the androgen stimulus. Regression of prostatic tumours results from this inhibition. Clinically, discontinuation of Casodex can result in the 'antiandrogen withdrawal syndrome' in a subset of patients.

Casodex 150 mg was studied as a treatment for patients with localised (T1-T2, N0 or NX, M0) or locally advanced (T3-T4, any N, M0; T1-T2, N+, M0) non-metastatic prostate cancer in a combined analysis of three placebo controlled, double-blind studies in 8113 patients, where Casodex was given as immediate hormonal therapy or as adjuvant to radical prostatectomy or radiotherapy, (primarily external beam radiation). At 7.4 years median follow up, 27.4% and 30.7% of all Casodex and placebo-treated patients, respectively, had experienced objective disease progression.

A reduction in risk of objective disease progression was seen across most patient groups but was most evident in those at highest risk of disease progression. Therefore, clinicians may decide that the optimum medical strategy for a patient at low risk of disease progression, particularly in the adjuvant setting following radical prostatectomy, may be to defer hormonal therapy until signs that the disease is progressing.

No overall survival difference was seen at 7.4 years median follow up with 22.9% mortality (HR= 0.99; 95% CI 0.91 to1.09). However, some trends were apparent in exploratory subgroup analyses.

Progression-free survival and overall survival data for patients with locally advanced disease are summarised in the following tables:

Table 1 Progression-free survival in locally advanced disease by therapy sub-group

(see Table 1 below)

Table 2 Overall survival in locally advanced disease by therapy sub-group

(see Table 2 below)

For patients with localised disease receiving Casodex alone, there was no significant difference in progression free survival. In these patients there was also a trend toward decreased survival compared with placebo patients (HR=1.16; 95% CI 0.99 to 1.37). In view of this, the benefit-risk profile for the use of Casodex is not considered favourable in this group of patients.

In a separate programme, the efficacy of Casodex 150 mg for the treatment of patients with locally advanced non-metastatic prostate cancer for whom immediate castration was indicated, was demonstrated in a combined analysis of 2 studies with 480 previously untreated patients with non-metastatic (M0) prostate cancer. At 56% mortality and a median follow-up of 6.3 years, there was no significant difference between Casodex and castration in survival (hazard ratio = 1.05 [CI 0.81 to 1.36]); however, equivalence of the two treatments could not be concluded statistically.

In a combined analysis of 2 studies with 805 previously untreated patients with metastatic (M1) disease at 43% mortality, Casodex 150 mg was demonstrated to be less effective than castration in survival time (hazard ratio = 1.30 [CI 1.04 to 1.65]), with a numerical difference in estimated time to death of 42 days (6 weeks) over a median survival time of 2 years.

Bicalutamide is a racemate with its antiandrogen activity being almost exclusively in the R-enantiomer.

5.2 Pharmacokinetic properties

Bicalutamide is well absorbed following oral administration. There is no evidence of any clinically relevant effect of food on bioavailability.

The (S)-enantiomer is rapidly cleared relative to (R)-enantiomer, the latter having a plasma elimination half-life of about 1 week.

On daily administration of Casodex 150 mg, the (R)-enantiomer accumulates about 10-fold in plasma as a consequence of its long half-life.

Steady state plasma concentrations of the (R)-enantiomer of approximately 22 microgram/ml are observed during daily administration of Casodex 150 mg. At steady state the predominantly active (R)-enantiomer accounts for 99% of the total circulating enantiomers.

The pharmacokinetics of the (R)-enantiomer are unaffected by age, renal impairment or mild to moderate hepatic impairment. There is evidence that for subjects with severe hepatic impairment, the (R)-enantiomer is more slowly eliminated from plasma.

Bicalutamide is highly protein bound (racemate 96%, (R) enantiomer >99%) and extensively metabolised (oxidation and glucuronidation); its metabolites are eliminated via the kidneys and bile in approximately equal proportions.

In a clinical study the mean concentration of R-bicalutamide in semen of men receiving Casodex 150 mg was 4.9 microgram/ml. The amount of bicalutamide potentially delivered to a female partner during intercourse is low and equates to approximately 0.3 microgram/kg. This is below that required to induce changes in offspring of laboratory animals.

5.3 Preclinical safety data

Bicalutamide is a potent antiandrogen and a mixed function oxidase enzyme inducer in animals. Target organ changes, including tumour induction (Leydig cells, thyroid, liver) in animals, are related to these activities. Enzyme induction has not been observed in man and none of these findings is considered to have relevance to the treatment of patients with prostate cancer. Atrophy of seminiferous tubules is a predicted class effect with antiandrogens and has been observed for all species examined. Full reversal of testicular atrophy was 2[illegible] weeks after a 12-month repeated dose toxicity study in rats, although functional reversal was evident in reproduction studies 7 weeks after the end of an 11 week dosing period. A period of subfertility or infertility should be assumed in man.

6. PHARMACEUTICAL PARTICULARS

6.1 List of excipients

Casodex 150 mg includes the following excipients:

Tablet core: Lactose Monohydrate, Magnesium Stearate, Povidone, Carboxymethyl amidon sodium.

Film-coating material: Hypromellose, Macrogol 300, Titanium Dioxide.

6.2 Incompatibilities

Not applicable.

Table 1 Progression-free survival in locally advanced disease by therapy sub-group

Analysis population	Events (%) in CASODEX patients	Events (%) in placebo patients	Hazard ratio (95% CI)
Watchful waiting	193/335 (57.6)	222/322 (68.9)	0.60 (0.49 to 0.73)
Radiotherapy	66/161 (41.0)	86/144 (59.7)	0.56 (0.40 to 0.78)
Radical prostatectomy	179/870 (20.6)	213/849 (25.1)	0.75 (0.61 to 0.91)

Table 2 Overall survival in locally advanced disease by therapy sub-group

Analysis population	Deaths (%) in CASODEX patients	Deaths (%) in placebo patients	Hazard ratio (95% CI)
Watchful waiting	164/335 (49.0)	183/322 (56.8)	0.81 (0.66 to 1.01)
Radiotherapy	49/161 (30.4)	61/144 (42.4)	0.65 (0.44 to 0.95)
Radical prostatectomy	137/870 (15.7)	122/849 (14.4)	1.09 (0.85 to 1.39)

6.3 Shelf life
4 years.

6.4 Special precautions for storage
Do not store above 30°C.

6.5 Nature and contents of container
PVC/Aluminium foil blister pack comprising strips of 5, 10 and 14 tablets to give pack sizes of 10, 20, 30, 40, 50, 80, 90, 100, 200 or 14, 28, 56, 84, 140 and 280 tablets.

Not all pack sizes may be marketed.

6.6 Special precautions for disposal and other handling
No special requirements.

7. MARKETING AUTHORISATION HOLDER
AstraZeneca UK Ltd.,
600 Capability Green,
Luton, LU1 3LU, UK.

8. MARKETING AUTHORISATION NUMBER(S)
PL 17901/0006

9. DATE OF FIRST AUTHORISATION/RENEWAL OF THE AUTHORISATION
18th June 2000/16th June 2004

10. DATE OF REVISION OF THE TEXT
22nd April 2009

Casodex Tablets 50mg

(AstraZeneca UK Limited)

1. NAME OF THE MEDICINAL PRODUCT
Casodex Tablets 50 mg

2. QUALITATIVE AND QUANTITATIVE COMPOSITION
Each tablet contains 50 mg bicalutamide (INN)

3. PHARMACEUTICAL FORM
White film-coated tablet.

4. CLINICAL PARTICULARS

4.1 Therapeutic indications
Treatment of advanced prostate cancer in combination with LHRH analogue therapy or surgical castration.

4.2 Posology and method of administration
Adult males including the elderly: one tablet (50 mg) once a day.

Treatment with Casodex should be started at least 3 days before commencing treatment with an LHRH analogue, or at the same time as surgical castration.

Children: Casodex is contraindicated in children.

Renal impairment: no dosage adjustment is necessary for patients with renal impairment.

Hepatic impairment: no dosage adjustment is necessary for patients with mild hepatic impairment. Increased accumulation may occur in patients with moderate to severe hepatic impairment (see section 4.4).

4.3 Contraindications
Casodex is contraindicated in females and children.

Casodex must not be given to any patient who has shown a hypersensitivity reaction to its use.

Co-administration of terfenadine, astemizole or cisapride with Casodex is contraindicated (see section 4.5).

4.4 Special warnings and precautions for use
Initiation of treatment should be under the direct supervision of a specialist.

Casodex is extensively metabolised in the liver. Data suggests that its elimination may be slower in subjects with severe hepatic impairment and this could lead to increased accumulation of Casodex. Therefore, Casodex should be used with caution in patients with moderate to severe hepatic impairment.

Periodic liver function testing should be considered due to the possibility of hepatic changes. The majority of changes are expected to occur within the first 6 months of Casodex therapy.

Severe hepatic changes and hepatic failure have been observed rarely with Casodex (see section 4.8). Casodex therapy should be discontinued if changes are severe.

A reduction in glucose tolerance has been observed in males receiving LHRH agonists. This may manifest as diabetes or loss of glycaemic control in those with pre-existing diabetes. Consideration should therefore be given to monitoring blood glucose in patients receiving Casodex in combination with LHRH agonists.

Casodex has been shown to inhibit cytochrome P450 (CYP 3A4), as such caution should be exercised when co-administered with drugs metabolised predominantly by CYP 3A4 (see sections 4.3 and 4.5).

Patients with rare hereditary problems of galactose intolerance, the Lapp lactase deficiency or glucose-galactose malabsorption should not take this medicine.

4.5 Interaction with other medicinal products and other forms of interaction
There is no evidence of any pharmacodynamic or pharmacokinetic interactions between Casodex and LHRH analogues.

In vitro studies have shown that R-bicalutamide is an inhibitor of CYP 3A4, with lesser inhibitory effects on CYP 2C9, 2C19 and 2D6 activity.

Although clinical studies using antipyrine as a marker of cytochrome P450 (CYP) activity showed no evidence of a drug interaction potential with Casodex, mean midazolam exposure (AUC) was increased by up to 80%, after co-administration of Casodex for 28 days. For drugs with a narrow therapeutic index such an increase could be of relevance. As such, concomitant use of terfenadine, astemizole and cisapride is contraindicated (see section 4.3) and caution should be exercised with the co-administration of Casodex with compounds such as ciclosporin and calcium channel blockers. Dosage reduction may be required for these drugs particularly if there is evidence of enhanced or adverse drug effect. For ciclosporin, it is recommended that plasma concentrations and clinical condition are closely monitored following initiation or cessation of Casodex therapy.

Caution should be exercised when prescribing Casodex with other drugs which may inhibit drug oxidation e.g. cimetidine and ketoconazole. In theory, this could result in increased plasma concentrations of Casodex which theoretically could lead to an increase in side effects.

In vitro studies have shown that Casodex can displace the coumarin anticoagulant, warfarin, from its protein binding sites. It is therefore recommended that if Casodex is started in patients who are already receiving coumarin anticoagulants, prothrombin time should be closely monitored.

4.6 Pregnancy and lactation
Casodex is contraindicated in females and must not be given to pregnant women or nursing mothers.

4.7 Effects on ability to drive and use machines
Casodex is unlikely to impair the ability of patients to drive or operate machinery. However, it should be noted that occasionally somnolence may occur. Any affected patients should exercise caution.

4.8 Undesirable effects
In this section, undesirable effects are defined as follows: Very common (≥1/10); common (≥1/100 to <1/10); uncommon (≥1/1,000 to ≤1/100); rare (≥1/10,000 to ≤1/1,000); very rare (≤1/10,000); not known (cannot be estimated from the available data).

Table 1 Frequency of Adverse Reactions

System Organ Class	Frequency	Event
Blood and lymphatic system disorders	Common	Anaemia
Immune system disorders	Uncommon	Hypersensitivity reactions (including angioneurotic oedema and urticaria)
Metabolism and nutrition disorders	Common	Anorexia
Psychiatric disorders	Common	Decreased libido Depression
Nervous system disorders	Very common	Dizziness
	Common	Somnolence
Vascular disorders	Very common	Hot flush
Respiratory, thoracic and mediastinal disorders	Uncommon	Interstitial lung disease
Gastrointestinal disorders	Very common	Abdominal pain Constipation Nausea
	Common	Dyspepsia Flatulence
Hepato-biliary disorders	Common	Hepatic changes (including elevated levels of transaminases, jaundice)/hepato-biliary disorders[1]
	Rare	Hepatic failure[2]
Skin and subcutaneous tissue disorders	Common	Alopecia Hirsutism/hair re-growth Dry skin Pruritis Rash
Renal and urinary disorders	Very common	Haematuria
Reproductive system and breast disorders	Very common	Gynaecomastia and breast tenderness[3]
	Common	Impotence
General disorders and administration site conditions	Very common	Asthenia Chest pain Oedema
Investigations	Common	Weight gain

1. Hepatic changes are rarely severe and were frequently transient, resolving or improving with continued therapy or following cessation of therapy.

2. Hepatic failure has occurred rarely in patients treated with Casodex, but a causal relationship has not been established with certainty. Periodic liver function testing should be considered (see also section 4.4).

3. May be reduced by concomitant castration.

In addition, cardiac failure was reported in clinical trials (as a possible adverse drug reaction in the opinion of investigating clinicians, with a frequency of > 1%) during treatment with Casodex plus an LHRH analogue. There is no evidence of a causal relationship with drug treatment.

4.9 Overdose
There is no human experience of overdosage. There is no specific antidote; treatment should be symptomatic. Dialysis may not be helpful, since Casodex is highly protein bound and is not recovered unchanged in the urine. General supportive care, including frequent monitoring of vital signs, is indicated.

5. PHARMACOLOGICAL PROPERTIES

5.1 Pharmacodynamic properties
Casodex is a non-steroidal antiandrogen, devoid of other endocrine activity. It binds to androgen receptors without activating gene expression, and thus inhibits the androgen stimulus. Regression of prostatic tumours results from this inhibition. Clinically, discontinuation of Casodex can result in antiandrogen withdrawal syndrome in a subset of patients.

Casodex is a racemate with its antiandrogenic activity being almost exclusively in the (R)-enantiomer.

5.2 Pharmacokinetic properties
Casodex is well absorbed following oral administration. There is no evidence of any clinically relevant effect of food on bioavailability.

The (S)-enantiomer is rapidly cleared relative to the (R)-enantiomer, the latter having a plasma elimination half-life of about 1 week.

On daily administration of Casodex, the (R)-enantiomer accumulates about 10 fold in plasma as a consequence of its long half-life.

Steady state plasma concentrations of the (R)-enantiomer of approximately 9 microgram/ml are observed during daily administration of 50 mg doses of Casodex. At steady state the predominantly active (R)-enantiomer accounts for 99% of the total circulating enantiomers.

The pharmacokinetics of the (R)-enantiomer are unaffected by age, renal impairment or mild to moderate hepatic impairment. There is evidence that for subjects with severe hepatic impairment, the (R)-enantiomer is more slowly eliminated from plasma.

Casodex is highly protein bound (racemate 96%, R-bicalutamide 99.6%) and extensively metabolised (via oxidation and glucuronidation): Its metabolites are eliminated via the kidneys and bile in approximately equal proportions.

In a clinical study the mean concentration of R-bicalutamide in semen of men receiving Casodex 150 mg was 4.9 microgram/ml. The amount of bicalutamide potentially delivered to a female partner during intercourse is low and by extrapolation possibly equates to approximately 0.3 microgram/kg. This is below that required to induce changes in offspring of laboratory animals.

5.3 Preclinical safety data
Casodex is a potent antiandrogen and a mixed function oxidase enzyme inducer in animals. Target organ changes, including tumour induction, in animals, are related to these activities. None of the findings in the preclinical testing is considered to have relevance to the treatment of advanced prostate cancer patients.

6. PHARMACEUTICAL PARTICULARS

6.1 List of excipients
Casodex includes the following excipients:

Lactose Monohydrate
Magnesium Stearate
Hypromellose
Macrogol 300
Povidone
Sodium Starch Glycolate
Titanium Dioxide (E171).

6.2 Incompatibilities
None known.

6.3 Shelf life
5 years.

6.4 Special precautions for storage
Do not store above 30°C.

6.5 Nature and contents of container
PVC blister/aluminium foil packs.

6.6 Special precautions for disposal and other handling
No special precautions required.

7. MARKETING AUTHORISATION HOLDER
AstraZeneca UK Limited,
600 Capability Green,
Luton, LU1 3LU, UK.

8. MARKETING AUTHORISATION NUMBER(S)
17901/0005

9. DATE OF FIRST AUTHORISATION/RENEWAL OF THE AUTHORISATION
18th June 2000/19th January 2006

10. DATE OF REVISION OF THE TEXT
26th February 2009

Caverject Dual Chamber 10 micrograms & Caverject Dual Chamber 20 micrograms

(Pharmacia Limited)

1. NAME OF THE MEDICINAL PRODUCT
Caverject® Dual Chamber 10 or 20 micrograms, Powder and solvent for solution for injection

2. QUALITATIVE AND QUANTITATIVE COMPOSITION
Each 0.5ml cartridge delivers a maximum dose of 10 or 20 micrograms of alprostadil.

For excipients see 6.1

3. PHARMACEUTICAL FORM
Powder and solvent for solution for injection

Dual chamber glass cartridge containing a white lyophilised powder and diluent for reconstitution.

4. CLINICAL PARTICULARS

4.1 Therapeutic indications
Caverject Dual Chamber is indicated for the symptomatic treatment of erectile dysfunction in adult males due to neurogenic, vasculogenic, psychogenic, or mixed etiology.

Caverject Dual Chamber may be a useful adjunct to other diagnostic tests in the diagnosis of erectile dysfunction.

4.2 Posology and method of administration
No formal studies with Caverject have been performed in patients younger than 18 years and older than 75 years.

General Information

Caverject Dual Chamber should be administered by direct intracavernosal injection using the 1/2-inch 29 gauge needle provided. The usual site of injection is along the dorsolateral aspect of the proximal third of the penis. Visible veins should be avoided. Both the side of the penis and the site of injection must be altered between injections.

The initial injections of Caverject Dual Chamber must be administered by medically trained personnel and after proper training, alprostadil may be injected at home. It is recommended that patients are regularly monitored (e.g. every 3 months) particularly in the initial stages of self injection therapy when dose adjustments may be needed.

The dose of Caverject Dual Chamber should be individualized for each patient by careful titration under a physician's supervision. The lowest, effective dose should be used that provides the patient with an erection that is satisfactory for sexual intercourse. It is recommended that the dose administered produces a duration of the erection not exceeding one hour. If the duration is longer, the dose should be reduced. The majority of patients achieve a satisfactory response with doses in the range of 5 to 20 micrograms.

The delivery device is designed to deliver a single dose which can be set at 25% increments of the nominal dose. Doses greater than 40 micrograms of alprostadil are not routinely justified. The following doses can be given using Caverject Dual Chamber:

Presentation	Dose Available
Caverject Dual Chamber 10 micrograms	2.5, 5, 7.5, 10 micrograms
Caverject Dual Chamber 20 micrograms	5, 10, 15, 20 micrograms

A Treatment

The initial dose of alprostadil for erectile dysfunction of vasculogenic, psychogenic, or mixed aetiology is 2.5 micrograms. The second dose should be 5 micrograms if there is a partial response, and 7.5 micrograms if there is no response. Subsequent incremental increases of 5 - 10 micrograms should be given until an optimal dose is identified. If there is no response to the administered dose, then the next higher dose may be given within one hour. If there is a response, there should be a one day interval before the next dose is given.

For patients with erectile dysfunction of neurogenic origin requiring doses less than 2.5 micrograms, it should be considered to dose titrate with Caverject Powder for Injection. Starting with a dose of 1.25 micrograms, if this produces no response, the second dose should be 2.5 micrograms. Apart from the starting dose, it is possible to dose titrate with either Caverject Dual Chamber or Caverject Powder for Injection with similar increments to the treatment of non-neurogenic erectile dysfunction.

The maximum recommended frequency of injection is no more than once daily and no more than three times weekly.

B Adjunct to aetiologic diagnosis.

Subjects without evidence of neurological dysfunction: 10-20 micrograms alprostadil to be injected into the corpus cavernosum and massaged through the penis. Over 80% of subjects may be expected to respond to a single 20 micrograms dose of alprostadil.

Subjects with evidence of neurological dysfunction: These patients can be expected to respond to lower doses of alprostadil. In subjects with erectile dysfunction caused by neurologic disease/trauma the dose for diagnostic testing must not exceed 10 micrograms and an initial dose of 5 micrograms is likely to be appropriate.

Should an ensuing erection persist for more than one hour, detumescent therapy should be employed prior to the subject leaving the clinic to prevent a risk of priapism (please refer to Section 4.9 - Overdose). At the time of discharge from the clinic, the erection should have subsided entirely and the penis must be in a completely flaccid state.

In case of lack of erectile response during the titration phase, patients should be monitored for systemic adverse effects.

4.3 Contraindications
Caverject Dual Chamber should not be used in patients who have a known hypersensitivity to any of the constituents of the product; in patients who have conditions that might predispose them to priapism, such as sickle cell anaemia or trait, multiple myeloma, or leukaemia; or in patients with anatomical deformation of the penis, such as angulation, cavernosal fibrosis, or Peyronie's disease. Patients with penile implants should not be treated with Caverject Dual Chamber.

Caverject Dual Chamber should not be used in men for whom sexual activity is inadvisable or contraindicated (e.g. patients suffering from severe heart disease).

4.4 Special warnings and precautions for use
Prolonged erection and/or priapism may occur. Patients should be instructed to report to a physician any erection lasting for a prolonged time period, such as 4 hours or longer. Treatment of priapism should not be delayed more than 6 hours (please refer to Section 4.9 - Overdose).

Painful erection is more likely to occur in patients with anatomical deformations of the penis, such as angulation, phimosis, cavernosal fibrosis, Peyronie's disease or plaques. Penile fibrosis, including angulation, fibrotic nodules and Peyronie's disease may occur following the intracavernosal administration of Caverject Dual Chamber. The occurrence of fibrosis may increase with increased duration of use. Regular follow-up of patients, with careful examination of the penis, is strongly recommended to detect signs of penile fibrosis or Peyronie's disease. Treatment with Caverject Dual Chamber should be discontinued in patients who develop penile angulation, cavernosal fibrosis, or Peyronie's disease.

Patients on anticoagulants such as warfarin or heparin may have increased propensity for bleeding after the intracavernous injection. In some patients, injection of Caverject Dual Chamber can induce a small amount of bleeding at the site of injection. In patients infected with blood-born diseases, this could increase the transmission of such diseases to their partner.

Caverject should be used with care in patients who have experienced transient ischaemic attacks or those with unstable cardiovascular disorders.

Caverject Dual Chamber is not intended for co-administration with any other agent for the treatment of erectile dysfunction (see also 4.5).

The potential for abuse of caverject should be considered in patients with a history of psychiatric disorder or addiction.

Sexual stimulation and intercourse can lead to cardiac and pulmonary events in patients with coronary heart disease, congestive heart failure or pulmonary disease. Caverject should be used with care in these patients.

Reconstituted solutions of Caverject Dual Chamber are intended for single use only. Any unused contents of the syringe should be discarded.

4.5 Interaction with other medicinal products and other forms of interaction
No known interactions.

Sympathomimetics may reduce the effect of alprostadil. Alprostadil may enhance the effects of antihypertensives, vasodilative agents, anticoagulants and platelet aggregation inhibitors.

The effects of combinations of alprostadil with other treatments for erectile dysfunction (e.g. sildenafil) or other drugs inducing erection (e.g. papaverine) have not been formally studied. Such agents should not be used in combination with Caverject due to the potential for inducing prolonged erections.

4.6 Pregnancy and lactation
Not applicable.

4.7 Effects on ability to drive and use machines
Not applicable.

4.8 Undesirable effects
The most frequent adverse effects following an intracavernous injection was pain in the penis. Thirty percent of patients reported pain at least once. Pain was associated with 11% of the injections administered. In most cases pain was assessed as mild or moderate. Three per cent of patients discontinued treatment because of pain.

Penile fibrosis, including angulation, fibrotic nodules, and Peyronie's disease, was reported in 3% of clinical trial patients overall. In one self-injection study in which the duration of use was up to 18 months, the incidence of penile fibrosis was higher, approximately 8%.

Haematoma and ecchymosis at the injection site, which is related with the injection technique rather than the effect of alprostadil, was reported by 3% and 2% of patients, respectively.

Prolonged erection (an erection for 4 - 6 h) developed in 4% of patients. Priapism (a painful erection for more than 6 hours) occurred in 0.4%. In most cases it disappeared spontaneously.

Adverse drug reactions reported during clinical trials and post marketing experience are presented in the following table:

Cardiac disorders *Uncommon*: Supraventricular extrasystole
Eye disorders *Uncommon*: Mydriasis
Gastrointestinal disorders *Uncommon* Nausea; dry mouth
General disorders and administration site conditions *Common*: Haematoma; ecchymosis *Uncommon:* Haemorrhage; inflammation; irritation; swelling; oedema; injection site numbness; injection site tenderness; injection site warmth; asthenia.
Investigations *Uncommon*: Blood pressure decreased; haematuria; heart rate increased; blood creatinine increased
Musculoskeletal, connective tissue and bone disorders *Common*: Leg cramps
Infections and infestations *Uncommon:* Fungal infection; common cold.
Nervous system disorders *Uncommon*: Vasovagal reactions; hypoaesthesia
Renal and urinary disorders *Uncommon*: Dysuria; pollakiuria, micturition urgency, urethral haemorrhage
Reproductive system and breast disorders *Very Common*: Penile Pain *Common*: Prolonged erection; Peyronie's disease; penile disorders (angulation, fibrotic nodules *Uncommon*: Balanitis; priapism; phimosis; painful erection; ejaculation disorder; testicular pain; scrotal pain; pelvic pain; testicle oedema; scrotal oedema; spermatocele; testicular disorder
Skin and subcutaneous tissue disorders *Uncommon:* Rash; pruritus; scrotum erythema; diaphoresis
Vascular disorders *Uncommon:* Hypotension; vasodilation; peripheral vascular disorder, venous bleeding

Very Common (≥1/10)	Common (≥1/100, <1/10)	Uncommon (≥1/1000, < 1/100)

Benzyl alcohol may cause hypersensitivity reactions.

4.9 Overdose
Overdosage was not observed in clinical trials with alprostadil. If intracavernous overdose of Caverject Dual Chamber occurs, the patient should be placed under medical supervision until any systemic effects have resolved and/or until penile detumescence has occurred. Symptomatic treatment of any systemic symptoms would be appropriate.

The treatment of priapism (prolonged erection) should not be delayed more than 6 hours. Initial therapy should be by penile aspiration. Using aseptic technique, insert a 19-21 gauge butterfly needle into the corpus cavernosum and aspirate 20-50 ml of blood. This may detumesce the penis. If necessary, the procedure may be repeated on the opposite side of the penis until a total of up to 100 ml blood has been aspirated. If still unsuccessful, intracavernous injection of alpha-adrenergic medication is recommended. Although the usual contra-indication to intrapenile administration of a vasoconstrictor does not apply in the treatment of priapism, caution is advised when this option is exercised. Blood pressure and pulse should be continuously monitored during the procedure. Extreme caution is required in patients with coronary heart disease, uncontrolled hypertension, cerebral ischaemia, and in subjects taking monoamine oxidase inhibitors. In the latter case, facilities should be available to manage a hypertensive crisis. A 200 microgram/ml solution of phenylephrine should be prepared, and 0.5 to 1.0 ml of the solution injected every 5 to 10 minutes. Alternatively, a 20 microgram/ml solution of epinephrine should be used. If necessary, this may be followed by further aspiration of blood through the same butterfly needle. The maximum dose of phenylephrine should be 1 mg, or epinephrine 100 micrograms (5 ml of the solution). As an alternative metaraminol may be used, but it should be noted that fatal hypertensive crises have been reported. If this still fails to resolve the priapism, urgent surgical referral for further management, which may include a shunt procedure is required.

5. PHARMACOLOGICAL PROPERTIES

5.1 Pharmacodynamic properties

Pharmacotherapeutic group: Drugs used in erectile dysfunction ATC code: G04B E01

Alprostadil is the naturally occurring form of prostaglandin E_1 (PGE_1). Alprostadil has a wide variety of pharmacological actions; vasodilation and inhibition of platelet aggregation are among the most notable of these effects. In most animal species tested, alprostadil relaxed retractor penis and corpus cavernosum urethrae in vitro. Alprostadil also relaxed isolated preparations of human corpus cavernosum and spongiosum, as well as cavernous arterial segments contracted by either phenylephrine or $PGF_{2\alpha}$ in vitro. In pigtail monkeys (Macaca nemestrina), alprostadil increased cavernous arterial blood flow in vivo. The degree and duration of cavernous smooth muscle relaxation in this animal model was dose-dependent.

Alprostadil induces erection by relaxation of trabecular smooth muscle and by dilation of cavernosal arteries. This leads to expansion of lacunar spaces and entrapment of blood by compressing the venules against the tunica albuginea, a process referred to as the corporal veno-occlusive mechanism. Erection usually occurs 5 to 15 minutes after injection. Its duration is dose dependent.

5.2 Pharmacokinetic properties

Caverject Dual Chamber contains alprostadil as the active ingredient in a complex with alfadex. At reconstitution, the complex is immediately dissociated into alprostadil and alfadex. The pharmacokinetics of alprostadil is therefore unchanged in Caverject Dual Chamber in comparison with Caverject Powder for Injection.

ADME

Absorption: For the treatment of erectile dysfunction, alprostadil is administered by injection into the corpora cavernosa.

Distribution: Following intracavernosal injection of 20 micrograms alprostadil, mean plasma concentrations of alprostadil increased 22 fold from the baseline endogenous levels approximately 5 minutes post-injection. Alprostadil concentrations then returned to endogenous levels within 2 hours after injection. Alprostadil is bound in plasma primarily to albumin (81% bound) and to a lesser extent α-globulin IV-4 fraction (55% bound). No significant binding to erythrocytes or white blood cells was observed.

Metabolism: Alprostadil is rapidly converted to compounds that are further metabolized prior to excretion. Following intravenous administration, approximately 80% of circulating alprostadil is metabolized in one pass through the lungs, primarily by beta- and omega-oxidation. Hence, any alprostadil entering the systemic circulation following intracavernosal injection is rapidly metabolized. The primary metabolites of alprostadil are 15-keto-PGE_1, 15-keto-13,14-dihydro-PGE_1, and 13,14-dihydro-PGE_1. In contrast to 15-keto-PGE_1 and 15-keto-13,14-dihydro-PGE_1, which lack almost completely biological activity, 13,14-dihydro-PGE_1 has been shown to lower blood pressure and inhibit platelet aggregation. Plasma concentrations of the major circulating metabolite (15-keto-13,14-dihydro-PGE_1) increased 34 fold from the baseline endogenous levels 10 minutes after the injection and returned to baseline levels 2 hours post-injection. Plasma concentrations of 13,14-dihydro-PGE_1 increased 7 fold, 20 minutes after injection.

Elimination: The metabolites of alprostadil are excreted primarily by the kidney, with almost 90% of an administered intravenous dose excreted in urine within 24 hours. The remainder of the dose is excreted in the faeces. There is no evidence of tissue retention of alprostadil or its metabolites following intravenous administration. In healthy volunteers, 70% to 90% of alprostadil is extensively extracted and metabolized in a single pass through the lungs, resulting in a short elimination half-life of less than one minute.

Pharmacokinetics in sub-populations

Effect of renal or hepatic impairment: Pulmonary first-pass metabolism is the primary factor influencing the systemic clearance of alprostadil. Although the pharmacokinetics of alprostadil have not been formally examined in patients with renal or hepatic insufficiency, alterations in renal or hepatic function would not be expected to have a major influence on the pharmacokinetics of alprostadil.

5.3 Preclinical safety data

Preclinical effects were observed only at exposures considered sufficiently in excess of the maximum human exposure indicating little relevance to clinical use.

Alprostadil at subcutaneous doses of up to 0.2 mg/kg/day had no adverse effect on the reproductive function in male rats

A standard battery of genotoxicity studies revealed no mutagenic potential of alprostadil or alprostadil/alfadex.

Pharmaceutical Particulars

6. PHARMACEUTICAL PARTICULARS

6.1 List of excipients

Caverject Dual Chamber powder:	Lactose Monohydrate
	Sodium citrate
	Alfadex
	Hydrochloric acid
	Sodium hydroxide
Diluent:	Benzyl alcohol
	Water for injections

6.2 Incompatibilities

Not applicable.

6.3 Shelf life

Shelf life of the medicinal product as packaged for sale

36 months.

Shelf life of the medicinal product after reconstitution

Chemical and physical in-use stability has been demonstrated for 24 hours at 25°C

6.4 Special precautions for storage

No special precautions for storage.

6.5 Nature and contents of container

Two or ten*, Type I, Ph. Eur, clear, borosilicate glass cartridges divided into two compartments and sealed with a bromobutyl rubber plunger. The cartridge is sealed with an aluminium cap containing a bromobutyl rubber disc.

Two or ten* 29 G injection needles.

Four or twenty*, pouches containing isopropyl cleansing tissues.

*Not all pack sizes may be marketed.

6.6 Special precautions for disposal and other handling

Instructions for use

To perform the reconstitution, attach the needle to the device by pressing the needle onto the tip of the device and turning clockwise until it stops. Remove the outer protective cap of the needle. Turn the white plunger rod clockwise until it stops to reconstitute the alprostadil powder. Invert the device twice in order to make sure the solution is evenly mixed. The solution should be clear. Carefully remove the inner protective cap from the needle. Holding the device upright, press the plunger rod as far as it will go. A few drops will appear at the needle tip. Turn the end of the plunger rod clockwise to select the desired dose.

The package insert provides full instructions on reconstitution, cleansing of the injection site, and also how to perform the injection.

Administrative Data

7. MARKETING AUTHORISATION HOLDER

Pharmacia Limited

Ramsgate Road

Sandwich

Kent

CT13 9NJ

United Kingdom

8. MARKETING AUTHORISATION NUMBER(S)

Caverject Dual Chamber 10 micrograms: PL 00032/0263

Caverject Dual Chamber 20 micrograms: PL 0032/0264

9. DATE OF FIRST AUTHORISATION/RENEWAL OF THE AUTHORISATION

13 July 2000

10. DATE OF REVISION OF THE TEXT

14th July 2005

Ref: CJ3_0 UK

Caverject Powder for Injection 5, 10, 20, 40 Micrograms

(Pharmacia Limited)

1. NAME OF THE MEDICINAL PRODUCT

Caverject 5, 10, 20 or 40 microgramspowder for solution for injection

2. QUALITATIVE AND QUANTITATIVE COMPOSITION

Alprostadil 5, 10, 20 or 40 micrograms.

When reconstituted, each 1ml delivers a dose of 5, 10, 20 or 40 micrograms of alprostadil.

For excipients, see section 6.1.

3. PHARMACEUTICAL FORM

Powder for Solution for Injection

Powder: A white to off-white powder.

4. CLINICAL PARTICULARS

4.1 Therapeutic indications

Caverject is indicated for the treatment of erectile dysfunction in adult males due to neurogenic, vasculogenic, psychogenic or mixed aetiology.

Caverject may be a useful adjunct to other diagnostic tests in the diagnosis of erectile dysfunction.

4.2 Posology and method of administration

Caverject is administered by direct intracavernous injection. A half inch, 27 to 30 gauge needle is generally recommended. The dose of Caverject should be individualised for each patient by careful titration under supervision by a physician.

The intracavernosal injection must be done under sterile conditions. The site of injection is usually along the dorsolateral aspect of the proximal third of the penis. Visible veins should be avoided. Both the side of the penis that is injected and the site of injection must be alternated; prior to the injection, the injection site must be cleansed with an alcohol swab.

To reconstitute Caverject using the prefilled diluent syringe: flip off the plastic cap from the vial, and use one of the swabs to wipe the rubber cap. Fit the 22 gauge needle to the syringe.

Inject the 1 ml of diluent into the vial, and shake to dissolve the powder entirely. Withdraw slightly more than the required dose of Caverject solution, remove the 22 gauge needle, and fit the 30 gauge needle. Adjust volume to the required dose for injection. Following administration, any unused contents of the vial or syringe should be discarded.

A. As an aid to aetiologic diagnosis.

i) Subjects without evidence of neurological dysfunction; 20 micrograms alprostadil to be injected into the corpus cavernosum and massaged through the penis. Should an ensuing erection persist for more than one hour detumescent therapy (please refer to Section 4.9 - Overdose) should be employed prior to the subject leaving the clinic to prevent a risk of priapism.

Over 80% of subjects may be expected to respond to a single 20 micrograms dose of alprostadil. At the time of discharge from the clinic, the erection should have subsided entirely and the penis must be in a completely flaccid state.

ii) Subjects with evidence of neurological dysfunction; these patients can be expected to respond to lower doses of alprostadil. In subjects with erectile dysfunction caused by neurologic disease/trauma the dose for diagnostic testing must not exceed 10 micrograms and an initial dose of 5 micrograms is likely to be appropriate. Should an ensuing erection persist for more than one hour detumescent therapy (please refer to Section 4.9 - Overdose) should be employed prior to the subject leaving the clinic to prevent a risk of priapism. At the time of discharge from the clinic, the erection should have subsided entirely and the penis must be in a completely flaccid state.

B. Treatment

The initial dose of alprostadil in patients with erectile dysfunction of neurogenic origin secondary to spinal cord injury is 1.25 micrograms, with a second dose of 2.5 micrograms, a third of 5 micrograms, and subsequent incremental increases of 5 micrograms until an optimal dose is achieved. For erectile dysfunction of vasculogenic, psychogenic, or mixed aetiology, the initial dose is 2.5 micrograms. The second dose should be 5 micrograms if there is a partial response, and 7.5 micrograms if there is no response. Subsequent incremental increases of 5-10 micrograms should be given until an optimal dose is achieved. If there is no response to the administered dose, then the next higher dose may be given within 1 hour. If there is a response, there should be at least a 1-day interval before the next dose is given. The usual maximum recommended frequency of injection is no more than once daily and no more than three times weekly.

The first injections of alprostadil must be done by medically trained personnel. After proper training and instruction, alprostadil may be injected at home. If self-administration is planned, the physician should make an assessment of the patient's skill and competence with the procedure. It is recommended that patients are regularly monitored (e.g. every 3 months) particularly in the initial stages of self injection therapy when dose adjustments may be needed.

The dose that is selected for self-injection treatment should provide the patient with an erection that is satisfactory for sexual intercourse. It is recommended that the dose administered produces a duration of the erection not exceeding one hour. If the duration is longer, the dose should be reduced. The majority of patients achieve a satisfactory response with doses in the range of 5 to 20 micrograms. Doses of greater than 60 micrograms of alprostadil are not recommended. The lowest effective dose should be used.

4.3 Contraindications

Caverject should not be used in patients who have a known hypersensitivity to any of the constituents of the product; in patients who have conditions that might predispose them to priapism, such as sickle cell anaemia or trait, multiple myeloma, or leukaemia; or in patients with anatomical deformation of the penis, such as angulation, cavernosal fibrosis, or Peyronie's disease. Patients with penile implants should not be treated with Caverject.

Caverject should not be used in men for whom sexual activity is inadvisable or contraindicated.

4.4 Special warnings and precautions for use

Prolonged erection and/or priapism may occur. Patients should be instructed to report to a physician any erection lasting for a prolonged time period, such as 4 hours or longer. Treatment of priapism should not be delayed more than 6 hours (please refer to Section 4.9 - Overdose).

Painful erection is more likely to occur in patients with anatomical deformations of the penis, such as angulation, phimosis, cavernosal fibrosis, Peyronie's disease or plaques. Penile fibrosis, including angulation, fibrotic nodules and Peyronie's disease may occur following the intracavernosal administration of Caverject. The occurrence of fibrosis may increase with increased duration of use. Regular follow-up of patients, with careful examination of the penis, is strongly recommended to detect signs of penile fibrosis or Peyronie's disease. Treatment with Caverject should be discontinued in patients who develop penile angulation, cavernosal fibrosis, or Peyronie's disease.

Patients on anticoagulants such as warfarin or heparin may have increased propensity for bleeding after the intracavernous injection.

Underlying treatable medical causes of erectile dysfunction should be diagnosed and treated prior to initiation of therapy with Caverject.

Use of intracavernosal alprostadil offers no protection from the transmission of sexually transmitted diseases. Individuals who use alprostadil should be counselled about the protective measures that are necessary to guard against the spread of sexually transmitted diseases, including the human immunodeficiency virus (HIV). In some patients, injection of Caverject can induce a small amount of bleeding at the site of injection. In patients infected with blood-born diseases, this could increase the transmission of such diseases to their partner.

Reconstituted solutions of Caverject are intended for single use only, they should be used immediately and not stored.

4.5 Interaction with other medicinal products and other forms of interaction

No known interactions. Caverject is not intended for co-administration with any other agent for the treatment of erectile dysfunction.

4.6 Pregnancy and lactation

Not applicable.

(High doses of alprostadil (0.5 to 2.0 mg/kg subcutaneously) had an adverse effect on the reproductive potential of male rats, although this was not seen with lower doses (0.05 to 0.2 mg/kg). Alprostadil did not affect rat spermatogenesis at doses 200 times greater than the proposed human intrapenile dose.

4.7 Effects on ability to drive and use machines

Not applicable.

4.8 Undesirable effects

The most frequent adverse reaction after intracavernosal injection of Caverject is penile pain. In studies, 37% of the patients reported penile pain at least once; however, this event was associated with only 11% of the administered injections. In the majority of the cases, penile pain was rated mild or moderate in intensity. 3% of patients discontinued treatment because of penile pain.

Prolonged erection (defined as an erection that lasts for 4 to 6 hours) after intracavernosal administration of Caverject was reported in 4% of patients. The frequency of priapism (defined as an erection that lasts 6 hours or longer) was 0.4%. (Please refer to Section 4.4 - Special warnings and precautions for use). In the majority of cases, spontaneous detumescence occurred.

Penile fibrosis, including angulation, fibrotic nodules and Peyronie's disease was reported in 3% of clinical trial patients overall, however, in one self-injection study in which the duration of use was up to 18 months, the incidence of penile fibrosis was 7.8% (please refer to Section 4.4).

Haematoma and ecchymosis at the site of injection, which is related to the injection technique rather than to the effects of alprostadil, occurred in 3% and 2% of patients, respectively. Penile oedema or rash was reported by 1% of alprostadil treated patients.

The following local adverse reactions were reported by fewer than 1% of patients in clinical studies following intracavernosal injection of Caverject: balanitis, injection site haemorrhage, injection site inflammation, injection site itching, injection site swelling, injection site oedema, urethral bleeding and penile warmth, numbness, yeast infection, irritation, sensitivity, phimosis, pruritus, erythema, venous leak, painful erection and abnormal ejaculation.

In terms of systemic events, 2 to 4% of alprostadil-treated patients reported headache, hypertension, upper respiratory infection, flu-like syndrome, prostatic disorder, localised pain (buttocks pain, leg pain, genital pain, abdominal pain), trauma, and sinusitis. One percent of patients reported each of the following: dizziness, back pain, nasal congestion and cough. The following were reported for less than 1% of patients in clinical trials and were judged to be possibly related to Caverject use: testicular pain, scrotal disorder (redness, pain, spermatocele), scrotal oedema, haematuria, testicular disorder (warmth, swelling, mass, thickening), impaired urination, urinary frequency, urinary urgency, pelvic pain, hypotension, vasodilatation, peripheral vascular disorder, supraventricular extrasystoles, vasovagal reactions, hypaesthesia, non-generalised weakness, diaphoresis, rash, non-application site pruritus, skin neoplasm, nausea, dry mouth, increased serum creatinine, leg cramps and mydriasis.

Haemodynamic changes, manifested as decreases in blood pressure and increases in pulse rate, were observed during clinical studies, principally at doses above 20 micrograms and above 30 micrograms of Caverject, respectively and appeared to be dose-dependent. However, these changes were usually clinically unimportant; only three patients (0.2%) discontinued the treatment because of symptomatic hypotension.

Caverject had no clinically important effect on serum or urine laboratory tests.

4.9 Overdose

The pharmacotoxic signs of alprostadil are similar in all animal species and include depression, soft stools or diarrhoea and rapid breathing. In animals, the lowest acute LD_{50} was 12 mg/kg which is 12,000 times greater than the maximum recommended human dose of 60 micrograms.

In man, prolonged erection and/or priapism are known to occur following intracavernous administration of vasoactive substances, including alprostadil. Patients should be instructed to report to a physician any erection lasting for a prolonged time period, such as 4 hours or longer.

The treatment of priapism (prolonged erection) should not be delayed more than 6 hours. Initial therapy should be by penile aspiration. Using aseptic technique, insert a 19-21 gauge butterfly needle into the corpus cavernosum and aspirate 20-50 ml of blood. This may detumesce the penis. If necessary, the procedure may be repeated on the opposite side of the penis until a total of up to 100 ml blood has been aspirated. If still unsuccessful, intracavernous injection of alpha-adrenergic medication is recommended. Although the usual contra-indication to intrapenile administration of a vasoconstrictor does not apply in the treatment of priapism, caution is advised when this option is exercised. Blood pressure and pulse should be continuously monitored during the procedure. Extreme caution is required in patients with coronary heart disease, uncontrolled hypertension, cerebral ischaemia, and in subjects taking monoamine oxidase inhibitors. In the latter case, facilities should be available to manage a hypertensive crisis. A 200 microgram/ml solution of phenylephrine should be prepared, and 0.5 to 1.0 ml of the solution injected every 5 to 10 minutes. Alternatively, a 20 microgram/ml solution of adrenaline should be used. If necessary, this may be followed by further aspiration of blood through the same butterfly needle. The maximum dose of phenylephrine should be 1 mg, or adrenaline 100 micrograms (5 ml of the solution). As an alternative metaraminol may be used, but it should be noted that fatal hypertensive crises have been reported. If this still fails to resolve the priapism, urgent surgical referral for further management, which may include a shunt procedure, is required.

5. PHARMACOLOGICAL PROPERTIES

5.1 Pharmacodynamic properties

Alprostadil is present in various mammalian tissues and fluids. It has a diverse pharmacologic profile, among which some of its more important effects are vasodilation, inhibition of platelet aggregation, inhibition of gastric secretion, and stimulation of intestinal and uterine smooth muscle. The pharmacologic effect of alprostadil in the treatment of erectile dysfunction is presumed to be mediated by inhibition of $alpha_1$-adrenergic activity in penile tissue and by its relaxing effect on cavernosal smooth muscle.

5.2 Pharmacokinetic properties

Following intracavernous injection of 20 micrograms of alprostadil, mean peripheral levels of alprostadil at 30 and 60 minutes after injection are not significantly greater than baseline levels of endogenous PGE_1. Peripheral levels of the major circulating metabolite, 15-oxo-13,14-dihydro-PGE_1, increase to reach a peak 30 minutes after injection and return to pre-dose levels by 60 minutes after injection. Any alprostadil entering the systemic circulation from the corpus cavernosum will be rapidly metabolized. Following intravenous administration, approximately 80% of the circulating alprostadil is metabolized in one pass through the lungs, primarily by beta- and omega-oxidation. The metabolites are excreted primarily by the kidney and excretion is essentially complete within 24 hours. There is no evidence of tissue retention of alprostadil or its metabolites following intravenous administration.

5.3 Preclinical safety data

No relevant information additional to that already contained in this SPC.

6. PHARMACEUTICAL PARTICULARS

6.1 List of excipients

Lactose, sodium citrate, hydrochloric acid, sodium hydroxide

6.2 Incompatibilities

Caverject is not intended to be mixed or coadministered with any other products.

6.3 Shelf life

24 months. Reconstituted solutions should be used immediately and not stored.

40 micrograms only: 24 months under refrigerated conditions (2-8°C). After dispensing, 3 months at room temperature (do not store above 25°C), included in 24 months shelf life. After reconstitution, the product may be stored for 6 hours below 25°C.

6.4 Special precautions for storage

Do not store above 25°C. Reconstituted solutions are intended for single use only, they should be used immediately and not stored.

40 micrograms only: Store at 2-8°C until dispensed. After dispensing, may be stored at room temperature (do not store above 25°C) for up to 3 months. After reconstitution, the product may be stored for 6 hours below 25°C. Do not refrigerate or freeze.

6.5 Nature and contents of container

Single pack containing a vial of Caverject 5, 10, 20 or 40 micrograms powder

Packs also each contain a syringe of solvent, a sterile 22G and a 30G needle plus pre-injection swab.

6.6 Special precautions for disposal and other handling

The presence of benzyl alcohol in the reconstitution vehicle decreases the degree of binding to package surfaces. Therefore, a more consistent product delivery is produced when Bacteriostatic Water for Injection containing benzyl alcohol is used.

5,10 & 20 micrograms only: Use immediately after reconstitution.

7. MARKETING AUTHORISATION HOLDER

Pharmacia Limited

Ramsgate Road

Sandwich

Kent, CT13 9NJ

United Kingdom

8. MARKETING AUTHORISATION NUMBER(S)

PL 00032/0214

PL 00032/0203

PL 00032/0188

PL 00032/0227

9. DATE OF FIRST AUTHORISATION/RENEWAL OF THE AUTHORISATION

25 March 1997 / 03 April 2003

08 February 1996 / 03 April 2003

15 March 1994 / 16 March 1999

23 June 1998 / 22 June 2003

10. DATE OF REVISION OF THE TEXT

February 2004

11. LEGAL CATEGORY

POM

Ref: CJ1_0UK

Cedocard Retard 20 Tablets

(Pharmacia Limited)

1. NAME OF THE MEDICINAL PRODUCT

Cedocard Retard 20 Tablets

2. QUALITATIVE AND QUANTITATIVE COMPOSITION

Isosorbide Dinitrate BP 20.0 mg

3. PHARMACEUTICAL FORM

Uncoated sustained release tablets for oral administration.

4. CLINICAL PARTICULARS

4.1 Therapeutic indications

For the prophylaxis of angina pectoris.

4.2 Posology and method of administration

By oral administration, the tablets should be swallowed, with a little water without chewing.

Children:

There is no recommended dose for children.

Adults:

One tablet in the morning and one before retiring to sleep.

Elderly:

The dosage of nitrates in cardiovascular disease is usually determined by patient response and stabilisation. Clinical experience has not necessitated alternative advice for use in elderly patients. The pharmacokinetics of isosorbide dinitrate in patients with severe renal failure and liver cirrhosis are similar to those in normal subjects.

The onset of action is 20-30 minutes.

The duration of action is 10-12 minutes.

4.3 Contraindications
A history of sensitivity to the drug.

4.4 Special warnings and precautions for use
Tolerance and cross-tolerance to other nitrates may occur.

4.5 Interaction with other medicinal products and other forms of interaction
Alcohol may potentiate the effect of isosorbide dinitrate.

4.6 Pregnancy and lactation
No data have been reported which would indicate the possibility of adverse effects resulting from the use of isosorbide dinitrate in pregnancy. Safety in pregnancy however, has not been established. Isosorbide dinitrate should only be used in pregnancy if, in the opinion of the physician, the possible benefits of treatment outweigh the possible hazards. Lactation – there are no data available on the transfer of isosorbide dinitrate in breast milk or its effect on breast-fed children.

4.7 Effects on ability to drive and use machines
Side effects include throbbing headache and dizziness. Patients are advised not to drive or operate machinery is so affected.

4.8 Undesirable effects
Headaches may occur (common), these are usually temporary. Less frequent, cutaneous vasodilation with flushing. Transient episodes of dizziness and weakness and other signs of cerebral ischaemia may occur with postural hypotension.

4.9 Overdose
In rare cases of overdosage, gastric lavage is indicated. Passive exercise of the extremities of the recumbent patient will promote venous return.

5. PHARMACOLOGICAL PROPERTIES

5.1 Pharmacodynamic properties
Vasodilator.

5.2 Pharmacokinetic properties
After administration of one tablet of Cedocard Retard 20 at least two peak concentration of ISDN occurred in the plasma. The initial peak (mean 1.9 ng/ml, range 1.0-3.4 mg/ml) occurred during 0.5 to 2 hours, and then mean plasma concentrations declined to 1.3 ng/ml at 3 hours. The concentration then increased again to reach a major peak level (mean 6.2 ng/ml, range 1.6-12.3 ng/ml) during 4-6 hours after dosing.

Plasma concentrations of ISDN have been measured after administration of increasing doses in the range 20-100 mg (as Cedocard Retard 20 tablets).

Means of peak concentrations of 4.2 ng/ml, 13.1 ng/ml, 20.7 ng/ml, 36.8 ng/ml and 34.9 ng/ml were measured after doses of 20 mg, 40 mg, 60 mg, 80 mg and 100 mg respectively.

5.3 Preclinical safety data
There are no preclinical data of relevance to the prescriber which are additional to that already included in other sections of the SPC.

6. PHARMACEUTICAL PARTICULARS

6.1 List of excipients
Lactose
Talc
Magnesium Stearate
Polyvinyl Acetate
Quinoline Yellow (E104)
Yellow Orange S (E110)
Methylene Chloride
Water

6.2 Incompatibilities
None known.

6.3 Shelf life
60 months.

6.4 Special precautions for storage
Protect from heat and moisture.

6.5 Nature and contents of container
PVC/Aluminium foil blister strip.
Pack size: 60 tablets

6.6 Special precautions for disposal and other handling
There are no special instructions for handling.

Administrative Data

7. MARKETING AUTHORISATION HOLDER
Pharmacia Limited
Ramsgate Road
Sandwich
Kent
CT13 9NJ

8. MARKETING AUTHORISATION NUMBER(S)
PL 00032/0331

9. DATE OF FIRST AUTHORISATION/RENEWAL OF THE AUTHORISATION
30 September 2002

10. DATE OF REVISION OF THE TEXT
August 2007

Company Ref: CD1_0

Cedocard Retard 40 Tablets
(Pharmacia Limited)

1. NAME OF THE MEDICINAL PRODUCT
Cedocard Retard 40

2. QUALITATIVE AND QUANTITATIVE COMPOSITION
Isosorbide Dinitrate BP 40.0 mg

3. PHARMACEUTICAL FORM
Uncoated sustained release tablets for oral administration.

4. CLINICAL PARTICULARS

4.1 Therapeutic indications
Cedocard Retard is indicated for prophylactic treatment of angina pectoris.

4.2 Posology and method of administration
Children:
There is no recommended dose for children.
Adults:
One or two tablets to be taken twice daily.
Elderly:
Dosage as for other adults.

4.3 Contraindications
Isosorbide dinitrate is contra-indicated in patients with a history of sensitivity to the drug. Sildenafil has been shown to potentiate the hypotensive effects of nitrates, and its co-administration with nitrates, or nitric oxide donors is therefore contra-indicated.

4.4 Special warnings and precautions for use
Tolerance and cross-tolerance to other nitrates and nitrites may occur.

4.5 Interaction with other medicinal products and other forms of interaction
Tolerance and cross-tolerance to other nitrates and nitrites may occur. The hypotensive effects of nitrates are potentiated by concurrent administration of sildenafil.

4.6 Pregnancy and lactation
No data have been reported which would indicate the possibility of adverse effects resulting from the use of isosorbide dinitrate in pregnancy. Safety in pregnancy however, has not been established. Isosorbide dinitrate should only be used in pregnancy if, in the opinion of the physician, the possible benefits of treatment outweigh the possible hazards. Lactation - there are no data available on the transfer of isosorbide dinitrate in breast milk or its effect on breast fed children.

4.7 Effects on ability to drive and use machines
Side effects include throbbing headache and dizziness. Patients are advised not to drive or operate machinery if so affected.

4.8 Undesirable effects
Side effects include throbbing headache and dizziness. Patients are advised not to drive or operate machinery if so affected.

4.9 Overdose
No available data.

5. PHARMACOLOGICAL PROPERTIES

5.1 Pharmacodynamic properties
Isosorbide dinitrate is a vasodilator. It relaxes vascular smooth muscle and produces coronary vasodilation, reduction in peripheral resistance and venous return, alteration of myocardial metabolism and reduction of the myocardial oxygen demand.

5.2 Pharmacokinetic properties
The mean plasma concentrations of ISDN at the end of each 12 hour dosage interval (Cmin) during the period of administration of 40 mg as the sustained release tablets were 0.6 ng/ml, 0.6 ng/ml, 0.9 ng/ml and 0.6 ng/ml after the first, second, third and fourth doses respectively and was 0.9 ng/ml at 12 hours after the last dose. At 1, 4 and 8 hours after the first dose the mean plasma levels of ISDN were 1.3 ng/ml, 4.0 ng/ml and 2.2 ng/ml respectively. At 1, 4 and 8 hours after the 3rd dose the mean plasma levels of ISDN were 2.1 ng/ml, 4.0 ng/ml and 2.0 ng/ml respectively and after the last dose, the peak plasma concentrations of ISDN of 12.7 ng/ml occurred at 5 hours and thereafter mean concentrations of ISDN declined to 0.4 ng/ml at 14 hours after the last dose.

5.3 Preclinical safety data
Due to the age and well established safety nature of this product, preclinical data has not been included.

6. PHARMACEUTICAL PARTICULARS

6.1 List of excipients

Lactose	Ph. Eur
Talc	Ph. Eur
Magnesium stearate	Ph. Eur
Polyvinyl acetate	
Red (E124)	
Yellow-orange S (E110)	
Potato starch	Ph. Eur
Methylene chloride	USP
Water	
Sodium chloride	
Sodium sulphate	

6.2 Incompatibilities
None known.

6.3 Shelf life
60 months.

6.4 Special precautions for storage
Protect from heat and moisture.

6.5 Nature and contents of container
PVC/Aluminium blisters in packs of 60 or 1000 tablets.

6.6 Special precautions for disposal and other handling
There are no special instructions for handling.

7. MARKETING AUTHORISATION HOLDER
Pharmacia Limited
Ramsgate Road
Sandwich
Kent
CT13 9NJ

8. MARKETING AUTHORISATION NUMBER(S)
PL 00032/0332

9. DATE OF FIRST AUTHORISATION/RENEWAL OF THE AUTHORISATION
12 December 2002

10. DATE OF REVISION OF THE TEXT
August 2007

Company Ref: CD1_0

Celebrex 100mg & 200mg Capsules
(Pharmacia Limited)

1. NAME OF THE MEDICINAL PRODUCT
Celebrex 100 mg capsule, hard.
Celebrex 200 mg capsule, hard.

2. QUALITATIVE AND QUANTITATIVE COMPOSITION
Each capsule contains 100 mg or 200 mg celecoxib.
Excipients:
Each 100 mg capsule contains 149.7 mg lactose monohydrate (see section 4.4).
Each 200 mg capsule contains 49.8 mg lactose monohydrate (see section 4.4).
For a full list of excipients, see section 6.1.

3. PHARMACEUTICAL FORM
Capsule, hard.
Opaque, white with two blue bands marked 7767 and 100 (Celebrex 100 mg).
Opaque, white with two gold bands marked 7767 and 200 (Celebrex 200 mg).

4. CLINICAL PARTICULARS

4.1 Therapeutic indications
Symptomatic relief in the treatment of osteoarthritis, rheumatoid arthritis and ankylosing spondylitis.

The decision to prescribe a selective COX-2 inhibitor should be based on an assessment of the individual patient's overall risks (see sections 4.3, 4.4).

4.2 Posology and method of administration
As the cardiovascular risks of celecoxib may increase with dose and duration of exposure, the shortest duration possible and the lowest effective daily dose should be used. The patient's need for symptomatic relief and response to therapy should be re-evaluated periodically, especially in patients with osteoarthritis (4.3, 4.4, 4.8 and 5.1).

Osteoarthritis: The usual recommended daily dose is 200 mg taken once daily or in two divided doses. In some patients, with insufficient relief from symptoms, an increased dose of 200 mg twice daily may increase efficacy. In the absence of an increase in therapeutic benefit after two weeks, other therapeutic options should be considered.

Rheumatoid arthritis: The initial recommended daily dose is 200 mg taken in two divided doses. The dose may, if needed, later be increased to 200 mg twice daily. In the absence of an increase in therapeutic benefit after two weeks, other therapeutic options should be considered.

Ankylosing spondylitis: The recommended daily dose is 200 mg taken once daily or in two divided doses. In a few patients, with insufficient relief from symptoms, an increased dose of 400mg once daily or in two divided doses may increase efficacy. In the absence of an increase in therapeutic benefit after two weeks, other therapeutic options should be considered.

The maximum recommended daily dose is 400 mg for all indications.

Celebrex may be taken with or without food.

Elderly: (>65 years) As in younger adults, 200 mg per day should be used initially. The dose may, if needed, later be increased to 200 mg twice daily. Particular caution should be exercised in elderly with a body weight less than 50 kg (see 4.4 and 5.2).

Hepatic impairment: Treatment should be initiated at half the recommended dose in patients with established moderate liver impairment with a serum albumin of 25-35 g/l. Experience in such patients is limited to cirrhotic patients (see 4.3, 4.4 and 5.2).

Renal impairment: Experience with celecoxib in patients with mild or moderate renal impairment is limited; therefore such patients should be treated with caution. (see 4.3, 4.4 and 5.2).

Children: Celecoxib is not indicated for use in children.

CYP2C9 Poor Metabolisers: Patients who are known, or suspected to be CYP2C9 poor metabolisers based on genotyping or previous history/experience with other CYP2C9 substrates should be administered celecoxib with caution as the risk of dose-dependent adverse effects is increased. Consider reducing the dose to half the lowest recommended dose. (See 5.2).

4.3 Contraindications

History of hypersensitivity to the active substance or to any of the excipients (see 6.1).

Known hypersensitivity to sulphonamides.

Active peptic ulceration or gastrointestinal (GI) bleeding.

Patients who have experienced asthma, acute rhinitis, nasal polyps, angioneurotic oedema, urticaria or other allergic-type reactions after taking acetylsalicylic acid or NSAIDs including COX-2 (cyclooxygenase-2) inhibitors.

In pregnancy and in women of childbearing potential unless using an effective method of contraception (See 4.5). Celecoxib has been shown to cause malformations in the two animal species studied (See 4.6 and 5.3). The potential for human risk in pregnancy is unknown, but cannot be excluded.

Breast feeding (See 4.6 and 5.3).

Severe hepatic dysfunction (serum albumin <25 g/l or Child-Pugh score ≥10).

Patients with estimated creatinine clearance <30 ml/min.

Inflammatory bowel disease.

Congestive heart failure (NYHA II-IV).

Established ischaemic heart disease, peripheral arterial disease and/or cerebrovascular disease.

4.4 Special warnings and precautions for use

Upper gastrointestinal complications [perforations, ulcers or bleedings (PUBs)], some of them resulting in fatal outcome, have occurred in patients treated with celecoxib. Caution is advised with treatment of patients most at risk of developing a gastrointestinal complication with NSAIDs; the elderly, patients using any other NSAID or acetylsalicylic acid concomitantly or patients with a prior history of gastrointestinal disease, such as ulceration and GI bleeding.

There is further increase in the risk of gastrointestinal adverse effects for celecoxib (gastrointestinal ulceration or other gastrointestinal complications), when celecoxib is taken concomitantly with acetylsalicylic acid (even at low doses). A significant difference in GI safety between selective COX-2 inhibitors + acetylsalicylic acid vs. NSAIDs + acetylsalicylic acid has not been demonstrated in long-term clinical trials (see 5.1).

The concomitant use of celecoxib and a non-aspirin NSAID should be avoided.

Increased number of serious cardiovascular events, mainly myocardial infarction, has been found in a long-term placebo-controlled study in subjects with sporadic adenomatous polyps treated with celecoxib at doses of 200mg BID and 400mg BID compared to placebo (see 5.1).

As the cardiovascular risks of celecoxib may increase with dose and duration of exposure, the shortest duration possible and the lowest effective daily dose should be used. The patient's need for symptomatic relief and response to therapy should be re-evaluated periodically, especially in patients with osteoarthritis (4.2, 4.3, 4.8 and 5.1).

Patients with significant risk factors for cardiovascular events (e.g. hypertension, hyperlipidaemia, diabetes mellitus, smoking) should only be treated with celecoxib after careful consideration (see 5.1). COX-2 selective inhibitors are not a substitute for acetylsalicylic acid for prophylaxis of cardiovascular thrombo-embolic diseases because of their lack of antiplatelet effects. Therefore, antiplatelet therapies should not be discontinued (see section 5.1).

As with other drugs known to inhibit prostaglandin synthesis, fluid retention and oedema have been observed in patients taking celecoxib. Therefore, celecoxib should be used with caution in patients with history of cardiac failure, left ventricular dysfunction or hypertension, and in patients with pre-existing oedema from any other reason, since prostaglandin inhibition may result in deterioration of renal function and fluid retention. Caution is also required in patients taking diuretic treatment or otherwise at risk of hypovolaemia.

As with all NSAIDS, celecoxib can lead to the onset of new hypertension or worsening of pre-existing hypertension, either of which may contribute to the increased incidence of cardiovascular events. Therefore blood pressure should be monitored closely during the initiation of therapy with celecoxib and throughout the course of therapy.

Compromised renal or hepatic function and especially cardiac dysfunction are more likely in the elderly and therefore medically appropriate supervision should be maintained.

NSAIDs, including celecoxib, may cause renal toxicity. Clinical trials with celecoxib have shown renal effects similar to those observed with comparator NSAIDs. Patients at greatest risk for renal toxicity are those with impaired renal function, heart failure, liver dysfunction, and the elderly. Such patients should be carefully monitored while receiving treatment with celecoxib.

Some cases of severe hepatic reactions, including fulminant hepatitis (some with fatal outcome), liver necrosis and, hepatic failure (some with fatal outcome or requiring liver transplant), have been reported with celecoxib. Among the cases that reported time to onset, most of the severe adverse hepatic events developed within one month after initiation of celecoxib treatment (see 4.8).

If during treatment, patients deteriorate in any of the organ system functions described above, appropriate measures should be taken and discontinuation of celecoxib therapy should be considered.

Celecoxib inhibits CYP2D6. Although it is not a strong inhibitor of this enzyme, a dose reduction may be necessary for individually dose-titrated drugs that are metabolised by CYP2D6 (See 4.5).

Patients known to be CYP2C9 poor metabolisers should be treated with caution (see 5.2.).

Serious skin reactions, some of them fatal, including exfoliative dermatitis, Stevens-Johnson syndrome, and toxic epidermal necrolysis, have been reported very rarely in association with the use of celecoxib (see 4.8). Patients appear to be at highest risk for these reactions early in the course of therapy: the onset of the reaction occurring in the majority of cases within the first month of treatment. Serious hypersensitivity reactions (anaphylaxis and angioedema) have been reported in patients receiving celecoxib (see 4.8). Patients with a history of sulphonamide allergy or any drug allergy may be at greater risk of serious skin reactions or hypersensitivity reactions (see 4.3). Celecoxib should be discontinued at the first appearance of skin rash, mucosal lesions, or any other sign of hypersensitivity.

Celecoxib may mask fever and other signs of inflammation.

In patients on concurrent therapy with warfarin, serious bleeding events have occurred.

Caution should be exercised when combining celecoxib with warfarin and other oral anticoagulants (See 4.5).

Celebrex 100 mg and 200 mg capsules contain lactose (149.7 mg and 49.8 mg, respectively). Patients with rare hereditary problems of galactose intolerance, the Lapp lactase deficiency or glucose-galactose malabsorption should not take this medicine.

4.5 Interaction with other medicinal products and other forms of interaction

Pharmacodynamic interactions

Anticoagulant activity should be monitored particularly in the first few days after initiating or changing the dose of celecoxib in patients receiving warfarin or other anticoagulants since these patients have an increased risk of bleeding complications. Therefore, patients receiving oral anticoagulants should be closely monitored for their prothrombin time INR, particularly in the first few days when therapy with celecoxib is initiated or the dose of celecoxib is changed. (see 4.4). Bleeding events in association with increases in prothrombin time have been reported, predominantly in the elderly, in patients receiving celecoxib concurrently with warfarin, some of them fatal.

NSAIDs may reduce the effect of diuretics and antihypertensive medicinal products. As for NSAIDs, the risk of acute renal insufficiency, which is usually reversible, may be increased in some patients with compromised renal function (e.g. dehydrated patients or elderly patients) when ACE inhibitors or angiotensin II receptor antagonists are combined with NSAIDs, including celecoxib. Therefore, the combination should be administered with caution, especially in the elderly. Patients should be adequately hydrated and consideration should be given to monitoring of renal function after initiation of concomitant therapy, and periodically thereafter.

In a 28-day clinical study in patients with lisinopril-controlled Stage I and II hypertension, administration of celecoxib 200 mg BID resulted in no clinically significant increases, when compared to placebo treatment, in mean daily systolic or diastolic blood pressure as determined using 24-hour ambulatory blood pressure monitoring. Among patients treated with celecoxib 200 mg BID, 48% were considered unresponsive to lisinopril at the final clinic visit (defined as either cuff diastolic blood pressure >90 mmHg or cuff diastolic blood pressure increased >10% compared to baseline), compared to 27% of patients treated with placebo; this difference was statistically significant.

Co-administration of NSAIDs and ciclosporin or tacrolimus have been suggested to increase the nephrotoxic effect of ciclosporin and tacrolimus. Renal function should be monitored when celecoxib and any of these drugs are combined.

Celecoxib can be used with low dose acetylsalicylic acid but is not a substitute for acetylsalicylic acid for cardiovascular prophylaxis. In the submitted studies, as with other NSAIDs, an increased risk of gastrointestinal ulceration or other gastrointestinal complications compared to use of celecoxib alone was shown for concomitant administration of low-dose acetylsalicylic acid. (see 5.1)

Pharmacokinetic interactions

Effects of celecoxib on other drugs

Celecoxib is an inhibitor of CYP2D6. During celecoxib treatment, the plasma concentrations of the CYP2D6 substrate dextromethorphan were increased by 136%. The plasma concentrations of drugs that are substrates of this enzyme may be increased when celecoxib is used concomitantly. Examples of drugs which are metabolised by CYP2D6 are antidepressants (tricyclics and SSRIs), neuroleptics, anti-arrhythmic drugs, etc. The dose of individually dose-titrated CYP2D6 substrates may need to be reduced when treatment with celecoxib is initiated or increased if treatment with celecoxib is terminated.

In vitro studies have shown some potential for celecoxib to inhibit CYP2C19 catalysed metabolism. The clinical significance of this in vitro finding is unknown. Examples of drugs which are metabolised by CYP2C19 are diazepam, citalopram and imipramine.

In an interaction study, celecoxib had no clinically relevant effects on the pharmacokinetics of oral contraceptives (1 mg norethisterone /35 microg ethinylestradiol).

Celecoxib does not affect the pharmacokinetics of tolbutamide (CYP2C9 substrate), or glibenclamide to a clinically relevant extent.

In patients with rheumatoid arthritis celecoxib had no statistically significant effect on the pharmacokinetics (plasma or renal clearance) of methotrexate (in rheumatologic doses). However, adequate monitoring for methotrexate-related toxicity should be considered when combining these two drugs.

In healthy subjects, co-administration of celecoxib 200 mg twice daily with 450 mg twice daily of lithium resulted in a mean increase in Cmax of 16% and in AUC of 18% of lithium. Therefore, patients on lithium treatment should be closely monitored when celecoxib is introduced or withdrawn.

Effects of other drugs on celecoxib

In individuals who are CYP2C9 poor metabolisers and demonstrate increased systemic exposure to celecoxib, concomitant treatment with CYP2C9 inhibitors could result in further increases in celecoxib exposure. Such combinations should be avoided in known CYP2C9 poor metabolisers (see sections 4.2 and 5.2).

Since celecoxib is predominantly metabolised by CYP2C9 it should be used at half the recommended dose in patients receiving fluconazole. Concomitant use of 200 mg single dose of celecoxib and 200 mg once daily of fluconazole, a potent CYP2C9 inhibitor, resulted in a mean increase in celecoxib Cmax of 60% and in AUC of 130%. Concomitant use of inducers of CYP2C9 such as rifampicin, carbamazepine and barbiturates may reduce plasma concentrations of celecoxib.

Ketoconazole or antacids have not been observed to affect the pharmacokinetics of celecoxib.

4.6 Pregnancy and lactation

No clinical data on exposed pregnancies are available for celecoxib. Studies in animals (rats and rabbits) have shown reproductive toxicity; including malformations (see 4.3 and 5.3). The potential for human risk in pregnancy is unknown, but cannot be excluded. Celecoxib, as with other drugs inhibiting prostaglandin synthesis, may cause uterine inertia and premature closure of the ductus arteriosus during the last trimester. Celecoxib is contraindicated in pregnancy and in women who can become pregnant (see 4.3 and 4.4). If a woman becomes pregnant during treatment, celecoxib should be discontinued.

Celecoxib is excreted in the milk of lactating rats at concentrations similar to those in plasma. Administration of celecoxib to a limited number of lactating women has shown a very low transfer of celecoxib into breast milk. Women who take celecoxib should not breastfeed.

4.7 Effects on ability to drive and use machines

Patients who experience dizziness, vertigo or somnolence while taking celecoxib should refrain from driving or operating machinery.

4.8 Undesirable effects

Adverse reactions are listed by system organ class and ranked by frequency in **Table 1**, reflecting data from the following sources:

• Adverse reactions reported in osteoarthritis patients and rheumatoid arthritis patients at incidence rates greater than 0.01% and greater than those reported for placebo during 12 placebo- and/or active-controlled clinical trials of duration up to 12 weeks at celecoxib daily doses from

100 mg up to 800 mg. In additional studies using non-selective NSAID comparators, approximately 7400 arthritis patients have been treated with celecoxib at daily doses up to 800 mg, including approximately 2300 patients treated for 1 year or longer. The adverse reactions observed with celecoxib in these additional studies were consistent with those for osteoarthritis and rheumatoid arthritis patients listed in **Table 1**.

- Adverse reactions reported at incidence rates greater than placebo for subjects treated with celecoxib 400 mg daily in long-term polyp prevention trials of duration up to 3 years (the APC and PreSAP trials; see Section 5.1, Pharmacodynamic properties: Cardiovascular Safety – Long-Term Studies Involving Patients With Sporadic Adenomatous Polyps).
- Adverse drug reactions from post-marketing surveillance as spontaneously reported during a period in which an estimated >70 million patients were treated with celecoxib (various doses, durations, and indications). Because not all adverse drug reactions are reported to the MAH and included in the safety database, the frequencies of these reactions cannot be reliably determined.

Table 1. Adverse Drug Reactions in Celecoxib Clinical Trials and Surveillance Experience (MedDRA Preferred Terms)[1,2]

(see Table 1 on next page)

In final data (adjudicated) from the APC and PreSAP trials in patients treated with celecoxib 400 mg daily for up to 3 years (pooled data from both trials; see Section 5.1 for results from individual trials), the excess rate over placebo for myocardial infarction was 7.6 events per 1000 patients (uncommon) and there was no excess rate for stroke (types not differentiated) over placebo.

4.9 Overdose

There is no clinical experience of overdose. Single doses up to 1200 mg and multiple doses up to 1200 mg twice daily have been administered to healthy subjects for nine days without clinically significant adverse effects. In the event of suspected overdose, appropriate supportive medical care should be provided e.g. by eliminating the gastric contents, clinical supervision and, if necessary, the institution of symptomatic treatment. Dialysis is unlikely to be an efficient method of drug removal due to high protein binding.

5. PHARMACOLOGICAL PROPERTIES

5.1 Pharmacodynamic properties

Pharmacotherapeutic group: Non-steroidal anti-inflammatory and antirheumatic drugs, NSAIDs, Coxibs. ATC code: M01AH01.

Celecoxib is an oral, selective, cyclooxygenase-2 (COX-2) inhibitor within the clinical dose range (200-400 mg daily). No statistically significant inhibition of COX-1 (assessed as *ex vivo* inhibition of thromboxane B2 [TxB2] formation) was observed in this dose range in healthy volunteers.

Cyclooxygenase is responsible for generation of prostaglandins. Two isoforms, COX-1 and COX-2, have been identified. COX-2 is the isoform of the enzyme that has been shown to be induced by pro-inflammatory stimuli and has been postulated to be primarily responsible for the synthesis of prostanoid mediators of pain, inflammation, and fever. COX-2 is also involved in ovulation, implantation and closure of the ductus arteriosus, regulation of renal function, and central nervous system functions (fever induction, pain perception and cognitive function). It may also play a role in ulcer healing. COX-2 has been identified in tissue around gastric ulcers in man but its relevance to ulcer healing has not been established.

The difference in antiplatelet activity between some COX 1 inhibiting NSAIDs and COX 2 selective inhibitors may be of clinical significance in patients at risk of thrombo-embolic reactions. COX-2 selective inhibitors reduce the formation of systemic (and therefore possibly endothelial) prostacyclin without affecting platelet thromboxane.

Celecoxib is a diaryl-substituted pyrazole, chemically similar to other non-arylamine sulfonamides (e.g. thiazides, furosemide) but differs from arylamine sulfonamides (e.g. sulfamethoxizole and other sulfonamide antibiotics).

A dose dependent effect on TxB2 formation has been observed after high doses of celecoxib. However, in healthy subjects, in small multiple dose studies with 600 mg BID (three times the highest recommended dose) celecoxib had no effect on platelet aggregation and bleeding time compared to placebo.

Several clinical studies have been performed confirming efficacy and safety in osteoarthritis, rheumatoid arthritis and ankylosing spondylitis. Celecoxib was evaluated for the treatment of the inflammation and pain of OA of the knee and hip in approximately 4200 patients in placebo and active controlled trials of up to 12 weeks duration. It was also evaluated for treatment of the inflammation and pain of RA in approximately 2100 patients in placebo and active controlled trials of up to 24 weeks duration. Celecoxib at daily doses of 200 mg - 400 mg provided pain relief within 24 hours of dosing. Celecoxib was evaluated for the symptomatic treatment of ankylosing spondylitis in 896 patients in placebo and active controlled trials of up to 12 weeks duration. Celecoxib at doses of 100mg BID, 200mg QD, 200mg BID and 400mg QD in these studies demonstrated significant improvement in pain, global disease activity and function in ankylosing spondylitis.

Five randomised double-blind controlled studies have been conducted including scheduled upper gastrointestinal endoscopy in approximately 4500 patients free from initial ulceration (celecoxib doses from 50 mg - 400 mg BID). In twelve week endoscopy studies celecoxib (100 - 800 mg per day) was associated with a significantly lower risk of gastroduodenal ulcers compared with naproxen (1000 mg per day) and ibuprofen (2400 mg per day). The data were inconsistent in comparison with diclofenac (150 mg per day). In two of the 12-week studies the percentage of patients with endoscopic gastroduodenal ulceration were not significantly different between placebo and celecoxib 200 mg BID and 400 mg BID.

In a prospective long-term safety outcome study (6 to 15 month duration, CLASS study), 5,800 OA and 2, 200 RA patients received celecoxib 400 mg BID (4-fold and 2-fold the recommended OA and RA doses, respectively), ibuprofen 800 mg TID or diclofenac 75 mg BID (both at therapeutic doses). Twenty-two percent of enrolled patients took concomitant low-dose acetylsalicylic acid (≤325 mg/day), primarily for cardiovascular prophylaxis. For the primary endpoint complicated ulcers (defined as gastrointestinal bleeding, perforation or obstruction) celecoxib was not significantly different than either ibuprofen or diclofenac individually. Also for the combined NSAID group there was no statistically significant difference for complicated ulcers (relative risk 0.77, 95 % CI 0.41-1.46, based on entire study duration). For the combined endpoint, complicated and symptomatic ulcers, the incidence was significantly lower in the celecoxib group compared to the NSAID group, relative risk 0.66, 95% CI 0.45-0.97 but not between celecoxib and diclofenac. Those patients on celecoxib and concomitant low-dose acetylsalicylic acid experienced 4 fold higher rates of complicated ulcers as compared to those on celecoxib alone. The incidence of clinically significant decreases in haemoglobin (>2 g/dL), confirmed by repeat testing, was significantly lower in patients on celecoxib compared to the NSAID group, relative risk 0.29, 95% CI 0.17- 0.48. The significantly lower incidence of this event with celecoxib was maintained with or without acetylsalicylic acid use.

Cardiovascular Safety – Long-Term Studies Involving Subjects With Sporadic Adenomatous Polyps

Two studies involving subjects with sporadic adenomatous polyps were conducted with celecoxib i.e., the APC trial (Adenoma Prevention with Celecoxib) and the PreSAP trial (Prevention of Spontaneous Adenomatous Polyps). In the APC trial, there was a dose-related increase in the composite endpoint of cardiovascular death, myocardial infarction, or stroke (adjudicated) with celecoxib compared to placebo over 3 years of treatment. The PreSAP trial did not demonstrate a statistically significant increased risk for the same composite endpoint.

In the APC trial, the relative risks compared to placebo for a composite endpoint (adjudicated) of cardiovascular death, myocardial infarction, or stroke were 3.4 (95% CI 1.4 - 8.5) with celecoxib 400 mg twice daily and 2.8 (95% CI 1.1 - 7.2) with celecoxib 200 mg twice daily. Cumulative rates for this composite endpoint over 3 years were 3.0% (20/671 subjects) and 2.5% (17/685 subjects) respectively, compared to 0.9% (6/679 subjects) for placebo. The increases for both celecoxib dose groups versus placebo were mainly due to an increased incidence of myocardial infarction.

In the PreSAP trial, the relative risk compared to placebo for this same composite endpoint (adjudicated) was 1.2 (95% CI 0.6 - 2.4) with celecoxib 400 mg once daily compared to placebo. Cumulative rates for this composite endpoint over 3 years were 2.3% (21/933 subjects) and 1.9% (12/628 subjects), respectively. The incidence of myocardial infarction (adjudicated) was 1.0% (9/933 subjects) with celecoxib 400 mg once daily and 0.6% (4/628 subjects) with placebo.

Data from a third long-term study, ADAPT (The Alzheimer's Disease Anti-inflammatory Prevention Trial), did not show a significantly increased cardiovascular risk with celecoxib 200mg BID compared to placebo. The relative risk compared to placebo for a similar composite endpoint (CV death, MI, stroke) was 1.14 (95% CI 0.61 - 2.12) with celecoxib 200 mg twice daily. The incidence of myocardial infarction was 1.1% (8/717 patients) with celecoxib 200 mg twice daily and 1.2% (13/1070 patients) with placebo.

5.2 Pharmacokinetic properties

Celecoxib is well absorbed reaching peak plasma concentrations after approximately 2-3 hours. Dosing with food (high fat meal) delays absorption by about 1 hour.

Celecoxib is mainly eliminated by metabolism. Less than 1% of the dose is excreted unchanged in urine. The inter-subject variability in the exposure of celecoxib is about 10-fold. Celecoxib exhibits dose- and time-independent pharmacokinetics in the therapeutic dose range. Plasma protein binding is about 97% at therapeutic plasma concentrations and the drug is not preferentially bound to erythrocytes. Elimination half-life is 8-12 hours. Steady state plasma concentrations are reached within 5 days of treatment. Pharmacological activity resides in the parent drug. The main metabolites found in the circulation have no detectable COX-1 or COX-2 activity.

Celecoxib metabolism is primarily mediated via cytochrome P450 2C9. Three metabolites, inactive as COX-1 or COX-2 inhibitors, have been identified in human plasma i.e., a primary alcohol, the corresponding carboxylic acid and its glucuronide conjugate.

Cytochrome P450 2C9 activity is reduced in individuals with genetic polymorphisms that lead to reduced enzyme activity, such as those homozygous for the CYP2C9*3 polymorphism.

In a pharmacokinetic study of celecoxib 200 mg administered once daily in healthy volunteers, genotyped as either CYP2C9*1/*1, CYP2C9*1/*3, or CYP2C9*3/*3, the median Cmax and AUC 0-24 of celecoxib on day 7 were approximately 4-fold and 7-fold, respectively, in subjects genotyped as CYP2C9*3/*3 compared to other genotypes. In three separate single dose studies, involving a total of 5 subjects genotyped as CYP2C9*3/*3, single-dose AUC 0-24 increased by approximately 3-fold compared to normal metabolizers. It is estimated that the frequency of the homozygous *3/*3 genotype is 0.3-1.0% among different ethnic groups.

Patients who are known, or suspected to be CYP2C9 poor metabolizers based on previous history/experience with other CYP2C9 substrates should be administered celecoxib with caution (see section 4.2).

No clinically significant differences were found in PK parameters of celecoxib between elderly African-Americans and Caucasians.

The plasma concentration of celecoxib is approximately 100% increased in elderly women (>65 years).

Compared to subjects with normal hepatic function, patients with mild hepatic impairment had a mean increase in C_{max} of 53% and in AUC of 26% of celecoxib. The corresponding values in patients with moderate hepatic impairment were 41% and 146% respectively. The metabolic capacity in patients with mild to moderate impairment was best correlated to their albumin values. Treatment should be initiated at half the recommended dose in patients with moderate liver impairment (with serum albumin 25-35g/L). Patients with severe hepatic impairment (serum albumin <25 g/l) have not been studied and celecoxib is contraindicated in this patient group.

There is little experience of celecoxib in renal impairment. The pharmacokinetics of celecoxib has not been studied in patients with renal impairment but is unlikely to be markedly changed in these patients. Thus caution is advised when treating patients with renal impairment. Severe renal impairment is contraindicated.

5.3 Preclinical safety data

Conventional embryo-foetal toxicity studies resulted in dose dependent occurrences of diaphragmatic hernia in rat foetuses and of cardiovascular malformations in rabbit foetuses at systemic exposures to free drug approximately 5X (rat) and 3X (rabbit) higher than those achieved at the maximum recommended daily human dose (400 mg). Diaphragmatic hernia was also seen in a peri-post natal toxicity study in rats, which included exposure during the organogenetic period. In the latter study, at the lowest systemic exposure where this anomaly occurred in a single animal, the estimated margin relative to the maximum recommended daily human dose was 3X.

In animals, exposure to celecoxib during early embryonic development resulted in pre-implantation and post-implantation losses. These effects are expected following inhibition of prostaglandin synthesis.

Celecoxib was excreted in rat milk. In a peri-post natal study in rats, pup toxicity was observed.

Based on conventional studies, genotoxicity or carcinogenicity, no special hazard for humans was observed, beyond those addressed in other sections of the SmPC. In a two-year toxicity study an increase in nonadrenal thrombosis was observed in male rat at high doses.

6. PHARMACEUTICAL PARTICULARS

6.1 List of excipients

Capsules 100 mg contain:

lactose monohydrate

sodium lauryl sulphate

povidone K30

croscarmellose sodium

magnesium stearate

Capsule shells contain:

gelatin

titanium dioxide E171

ink contains indigotine E132

Capsules 200 mg contain:

lactose monohydrate

sodium lauryl sulphate

povidone K30

croscarmellose sodium

magnesium stearate

Capsule shells contain:

gelatin

titanium dioxide E171

ink contains iron oxide E172

6.2 Incompatibilities

Not applicable.

Table 1 Adverse Drug Reactions in Celecoxib Clinical Trials and Surveillance Experience (MedDRA Preferred Terms)[1,2]

	Adverse Drug Reaction Frequency			
Very Common (≥1/10)	**Common** (≥1/100 to <1/10)	**Uncommon** (≥1/1000 to <1/100)	**Rare** (≥1/10,000 to <1/1000)	**Frequency Not Known** (Post-marketing experience)[3]
Infections and infestations				
	Sinusitis, upper respiratory tract infection, urinary tract infection			
Blood and lymphatic system disorders				
		Anemia	Leucopenia, thrombocytopenia	Pancytopenia
Immune system disorders				
	Allergy aggravated			Serious allergic reactions, anaphylactic shock, anaphylaxis
Psychiatric disorders				
	Insomnia	Anxiety, depression, tiredness	Confusion	Hallucinations
Metabolism and nutrition disorders				
		Hyperkaelemia		
Nervous system disorders				
	Dizziness, hypertonia	Paraesthesia, somnolence, cerebral infarction[1]	Ataxia, taste alteration	Headache, aggravated epilepsy, meningitis aseptic, ageusia, anosmia, fatal intracranial haemorrhage
Eye disorders				
		Blurred vision		Conjunctivitis, ocular haemorrhage, retinal artery or vein occlusion
Ear and labyrinth disorders				
		Tinnitus, hypoacusis[1]		
Cardiac disorders				
	Myocardial infarction[1]	Heart failure, palpitations, tachycardia		Arrhythmia
Vascular disorders				
Hypertension[1]		Hypertension aggravated		Flushing, vasculitis
Respiratory, thoracic, and mediastinal disorders				
	Pharyngitis, rhinitis, cough, dyspnoea[1]			Bronchospasm
Gastrointestinal disorders				
	Abdominal pain, diarrhoea, dyspepsia, flatulence, vomiting[1], dysphagia[1]	Constipation, eructation, gastritis, stomatitis, aggravation of gastrointestinal inflammation	Duodenal, gastric, oesophageal, intestinal, and colonic ulceration, intestinal perforation, oesophagitis, melaena, pancreatitis	Nausea, gastrointestinal haemorrhage, colitis/colitis aggravated
Hepatobiliary disorders				
		Abnormal hepatic function, increased SGOT and SGPT,	Elevation of hepatic enzymes	Hepatic failure (sometimes fatal or requiring liver transplant), fulminant hepatitis (some with fatal outcome), liver necrosis, hepatitis, jaundice
Skin and subcutaneous tissue disorders				
	Rash, pruritus	Urticaria	Alopecia, photosensitivity	Ecchymosis, bullous eruption, exfoliative dermatitis, erythema multiforme, Stevens-Johnson syndrome, toxic epidermal necrolysis, angioedema, acute generalised exanthematous pustulosis
Musculoskeletal and connective tissue disorders				
		Leg cramps		Arthralgia, myositis
Renal and urinary disorders				
		Increased creatinine, BUN increased		Acute renal failure, interstitial nephritis, hyponatraemia
Reproductive system and breast disorders				
				Menstrual disorder NOS
General disorders and administrative site conditions				
	Flu-like symptoms, peripheral oedema/ fluid retention			

[1] Adverse drug reactions that occurred in polyp prevention trials, representing subjects treated with celecoxib 400 mg daily in 2 clinical trials of duration up to 3 years (the APC and PreSAP trials). The adverse drug reactions listed above for the polyp prevention trials are only those that have been previously recognized in the post-marketing surveillance experience, or have occurred more frequently than in the arthritis trials.

[2] Furthermore, the following *previously unknown* adverse reactions occurred in polyp prevention trials, representing subjects treated with celecoxib 400 mg daily in 2 clinical trials of duration up to 3 years (the APC and PreSAP trials):

Common: angina pectoris, irritable bowel syndrome, nephrolithiasis, blood creatinine increased, benign prostatic hyperplasia, weight increased.

Uncommon: helicobacter infection, herpes zoster, erysipelas, bronchopneumonia, labyrinthitis, gingival infection, lipoma, vitreous floaters, conjunctival haemorrhage, deep vein thrombosis, dysphonia, haemorrhoidal haemorrhage, frequent bowel movements, mouth ulceration, allergic dermatitis, ganglion, nocturia, vaginal haemorrhage, breast tenderness, lower limb fracture, blood sodium increased.

[3] Adverse drug reactions spontaneously reported to the safety surveillance database over a period in which an estimated >70 million patients were treated with celecoxib (various doses, durations, and indications). As a result, the frequencies of these adverse drug reactions cannot be reliably determined. Adverse drug reactions listed for the post-marketing population are only those that are not already listed for the arthritis trials or the polyp prevention trials.

6.3 Shelf life
3 years.

6.4 Special precautions for storage
Do not store above 30°C.

6.5 Nature and contents of container
Clear or opaque PVC blisters or aluminium cold-formed blisters. Pack of 2, 5, 6, 10, 20, 30, 40, 50, 60, 100, 10x10, 10x30, 10x50, 1x50 unit dose, 1x100 unit dose, 5x(10x10).

6.6 Special precautions for disposal and other handling
No special requirements.

7. MARKETING AUTHORISATION HOLDER
Pharmacia Limited
Ramsgate Road
Sandwich
Kent
CT13 9NJ
United Kingdom

8. MARKETING AUTHORISATION NUMBER(S)
Celebrex 100 mg: PL 00032/0399
Celebrex 200 mg: PL 00032/0400

9. DATE OF FIRST AUTHORISATION/RENEWAL OF THE AUTHORISATION
Date of first authorisation: 1st September 2002
Date of last renewal: 3rd December 2004

10. DATE OF REVISION OF THE TEXT
9th June 2009

11 LEGAL CATEGORY
POM
FOR FURTHER INFORMATION PLEASE CONTACT
Pfizer Limited
Walton Oaks
Dorking Road
Tadworth
Surrey KT20 7NS
Company Ref: CB 13_1

CellCept 1g/5ml powder for oral suspension

(Roche Products Limited)

1. NAME OF THE MEDICINAL PRODUCT
CellCept 1 g/5 ml powder for oral suspension.

2. QUALITATIVE AND QUANTITATIVE COMPOSITION
Each bottle contains 35 g mycophenolate mofetil in 110 g powder for oral suspension. 5 ml of the reconstituted suspension contains 1 g of mycophenolate mofetil.

For a full list of excipients, see section 6.1.

3. PHARMACEUTICAL FORM
Powder for oral suspension.

4. CLINICAL PARTICULARS
4.1 Therapeutic indications
CellCept 1 g/5 ml powder for oral suspension is indicated in combination with ciclosporin and corticosteroids for the prophylaxis of acute transplant rejection in patients receiving allogeneic renal, cardiac or hepatic transplants.

4.2 Posology and method of administration
Treatment with CellCept should be initiated and maintained by appropriately qualified transplant specialists.

Use in renal transplant:

Adults: oral CellCept 1 g/5 ml powder for oral suspension should be initiated within 72 hours following transplantation. The recommended dose in renal transplant patients is 1 g administered twice daily (2 g daily dose), i.e. 5 ml oral suspension twice daily.

Children and adolescents (aged 2 to 18 years): the recommended dose of CellCept 1 g/5 ml powder for oral suspension is 600 mg/m^2 administered twice daily (up to a maximum of 2 g/10 ml oral suspension daily). As some adverse reactions occur with greater frequency in this age group (see section 4.8) compared with adults, temporary dose reduction or interruption may be required; these will need to take into account relevant clinical factors including severity of reaction.

Children (< 2 years): there are limited safety and efficacy data in children below the age of 2 years. These are insufficient to make dosage recommendations, and therefore use in this age group is not recommended.

Use in cardiac transplant:

Adults: oral CellCept should be initiated within 5 days following transplantation. The recommended dose in cardiac transplant patients is 1.5 g administered twice daily (3 g daily dose).

Children: no data are available for paediatric cardiac transplant patients.

Use in hepatic transplant:

Adults: IV CellCept should be administered for the first 4 days following hepatic transplant, with oral CellCept initiated as soon after this as it can be tolerated. The recommended oral dose in hepatic transplant patients is 1.5 g administered twice daily (3 g daily dose).

Children: no data are available for paediatric hepatic transplant patients.

Use in elderly (≥ 65 years): the recommended dose of 1 g administered twice a day for renal transplant patients and 1.5 g twice a day for cardiac or hepatic transplant patients is appropriate for the elderly.

Use in renal impairment: in renal transplant patients with severe chronic renal impairment (glomerular filtration rate < 25 ml•min^{-1}•1.73 m^{-2}), outside the immediate post-transplant period, doses greater than 1 g administered twice a day should be avoided. These patients should also be carefully observed. No dose adjustments are needed in patients experiencing delayed renal graft function post-operatively. (see section 5.2). No data are available for cardiac or hepatic transplant patients with severe chronic renal impairment.

Use in severe hepatic impairment: no dose adjustments are needed for renal transplant patients with severe hepatic parenchymal disease. No data are available for cardiac transplant patients with severe hepatic parenchymal disease.

Treatment during rejection episodes: MPA (mycophenolic acid) is the active metabolite of mycophenolate mofetil. Renal transplant rejection does not lead to changes in MPA pharmacokinetics; dosage reduction or interruption of CellCept is not required. There is no basis for CellCept dose adjustment following cardiac transplant rejection. No pharmacokinetic data are available during hepatic transplant rejection.

Note

If required, CellCept 1 g/5 ml powder for oral suspension can be administered via a nasogastric tube with a minimum size of 8 French (minimum 1.7 mm interior diameter).

4.3 Contraindications
Hypersensitivity reactions to CellCept have been observed (see section 4.8). Therefore, CellCept is contraindicated in patients with a hypersensitivity to mycophenolate mofetil or mycophenolic acid.

CellCept is contraindicated in women who are breastfeeding (see section 4.6).

For information on use in pregnancy and contraceptive requirements, see section 4.6.

4.4 Special warnings and precautions for use
Patients receiving immunosuppressive regimens involving combinations of medicinal products, including CellCept, are at increased risk of developing lymphomas and other malignancies, particularly of the skin (see section 4.8). The risk appears to be related to the intensity and duration of immunosuppression rather than to the use of any specific agent. As general advice to minimise the risk for skin cancer, exposure to sunlight and UV light should be limited by wearing protective clothing and using a sunscreen with a high protection factor.

Patients receiving CellCept should be instructed to report immediately any evidence of infection, unexpected bruising, bleeding or any other manifestation of bone marrow depression.

Patients treated with immunosuppressants, including CellCept, are at increased risk for opportunistic infections (bacterial, fungal, viral and protozoal), fatal infections and sepsis (see section 4.8). Among the opportunistic infections are BK virus associated nephropathy and JC virus associated progressive multifocal leukoencephalopathy (PML). These infections are often related to a high total immunosuppressive burden and may lead to serious or fatal conditions that physicians should consider in the differential diagnosis in immunosuppressed patients with deteriorating renal function or neurological symptoms.

Patients receiving CellCept should be monitored for neutropenia, which may be related to CellCept itself, concomitant medications, viral infections, or some combination of these causes. Patients taking CellCept should have complete blood counts weekly during the first month, twice monthly for the second and third months of treatment, then monthly through the first year. If neutropenia develops (absolute neutrophil count < 1.3 × 10^3/μl), it may be appropriate to interrupt or discontinue CellCept.

Cases of pure red cell aplasia (PRCA) have been reported in patients treated with CellCept in combination with other immunosuppressants. The mechanism for mycophenolate mofetil induced PRCA is unknown. PRCA may resolve with dose reduction or cessation of CellCept therapy. Changes to CellCept therapy should only be undertaken under appropriate supervision in transplant recipients in order to minimise the risk of graft rejection (see section 4.8).

Patients should be advised that during treatment with CellCept, vaccinations may be less effective, and the use of live attenuated vaccines should be avoided (see section 4.5). Influenza vaccination may be of value. Prescribers should refer to national guidelines for influenza vaccination.

Because CellCept has been associated with an increased incidence of digestive system adverse events, including infrequent cases of gastrointestinal tract ulceration, haemorrhage and perforation, CellCept should be administered with caution in patients with active serious digestive system disease.

CellCept is an IMPDH (inosine monophosphate dehydrogenase) inhibitor. On theoretical grounds, therefore, it should be avoided in patients with rare hereditary deficiency of hypoxanthine-guanine phosphoribosyl-transferase (HGPRT) such as Lesch-Nyhan and Kelley-Seegmiller syndrome.

It is recommended that CellCept should not be administered concomitantly with azathioprine because such concomitant administration has not been studied.

In view of the significant reduction in the AUC of MPA by cholestyramine, caution should be used in the concomitant administration of CellCept with medicinal products that interfere with enterohepatic recirculation because of the potential to reduce the efficacy of CellCept.

CellCept 1 g/5 ml powder for oral suspension contains aspartame. Therefore, care should be taken if CellCept 1 g/5 ml powder for oral suspension is administered to patients with phenylketonuria (see section 6.1)

The risk: benefit of mycophenolate mofetil in combination with tacrolimus or sirolimus has not been established (see also section 4.5).

This medicinal product contains sorbitol. Patients with rare hereditary problems of fructose intolerance should not take this medicine.

4.5 Interaction with other medicinal products and other forms of interaction
Interaction studies have only been performed in adults.

Aciclovir: higher aciclovir plasma concentrations were observed when mycophenolate mofetil was administered with aciclovir in comparison to the administration of aciclovir alone. The changes in MPAG (the phenolic glucuronide of MPA) pharmacokinetics (MPAG increased by 8 %) were minimal and are not considered clinically significant. Because MPAG plasma concentrations are increased in the presence of renal impairment, as are aciclovir concentrations, the potential exists for mycophenolate mofetil and aciclovir, or its prodrugs, e.g. valaciclovir, to compete for tubular secretion and further increases in concentrations of both substances may occur.

Antacids with magnesium and aluminium hydroxides: absorption of mycophenolate mofetil was decreased when administered with antacids.

Cholestyramine: following single dose administration of 1.5 g of mycophenolate mofetil to normal healthy subjects pre-treated with 4 g TID of cholestyramine for 4 days, there was a 40 % reduction in the AUC of MPA. (see section 4.4, and section 5.2). Caution should be used during concomitant administration because of the potential to reduce efficacy of CellCept.

Medicinal products that interfere with enterohepatic circulation: caution should be used with medicinal products that interfere with enterohepatic circulation because of their potential to reduce the efficacy of CellCept.

Ciclosporin A: ciclosporin A (CsA) pharmacokinetics are unaffected by mycophenolate mofetil.

In contrast, if concomitant ciclosporin treatment is stopped, an increase in MPA AUC of around 30% should be expected.

Ganciclovir: based on the results of a single dose administration study of recommended doses of oral mycophenolate and IV ganciclovir and the known effects of renal impairment on the pharmacokinetics of CellCept (see section 4.2) and ganciclovir, it is anticipated that co-administration of these agents (which compete for mechanisms of renal tubular secretion) will result in increases in MPAG and ganciclovir concentration. No substantial alteration of MPA pharmacokinetics is anticipated and CellCept dose adjustment is not required. In patients with renal impairment in which CellCept and ganciclovir or its prodrugs, e.g. valganciclovir, are co-administered, the dose recommendations for ganciclovir should be observed and patients should be monitored carefully.

Oral contraceptives: the pharmacokinetics and pharmacodynamics of oral contraceptives were unaffected by coadministration of CellCept (see also section 5.2).

Rifampicin: in patients not also taking ciclosporin, concomitant administration of CellCept and rifampicin resulted in a decrease in MPA exposure (AUC0-12h) of 18% to 70%. It is recommended to monitor MPA exposure levels and to adjust CellCept doses accordingly to maintain clinical efficacy when rifampicin is administered concomitantly.

Sirolimus: in renal transplant patients, concomitant administration of CellCept and CsA resulted in reduced MPA exposures by 30-50% compared with patients receiving the combination of sirolimus and similar doses of CellCept (see also section 4.4).

Sevelamer: decrease in MPA C_{max} and AUC0-12 by 30% and 25%, respectively, were observed when CellCept was concomitantly administered with sevelamer without any clinical consequences (i.e. graft rejection). It is recommended, however, to administer CellCept at least one hour before or three hours after sevelamer intake to minimise the impact on the absorption of MPA. There is no data on CellCept with phosphate binders other than sevelamer.

Trimethoprim/sulfamethoxazole: no effect on the bioavailability of MPA was observed.

Norfloxacin and metronidazole: in healthy volunteers, no significant interaction was observed when CellCept was concomitantly administered with norfloxacin and metronidazole separately. However, norfloxacin and metronidazole combined reduced the MPA exposure by approximately 30 % following a single dose of CellCept.

Ciprofloxacin and amoxicillin plus clavulanic acid: Reductions in pre-dose (trough) MPA concentrations of about 50% have been reported in renal transplant recipients in the days immediately following commencement of oral ciprofloxacin or amoxicillin plus clavulanic acid. This effect tended to diminish with continued antibiotic use and to cease within a few days of their discontinuation. The change in predose level may not accurately represent changes in overall MPA exposure. Therefore, a change in the dose of CellCept should not normally be necessary in the absence of clinical evidence of graft dysfunction. However, close clinical monitoring should be performed during the combination and shortly after antibiotic treatment.

Tacrolimus: in hepatic transplant patients initiated on CellCept and tacrolimus, the AUC and C_{max} of MPA, the active metabolite of CellCept, were not significantly affected by coadministration with tacrolimus. In contrast, there was an increase of approximately 20 % in tacrolimus AUC when multiple doses of CellCept (1.5 g BID) were administered to patients taking tacrolimus. However, in renal transplant patients, tacrolimus concentration did not appear to be altered by CellCept (see also section 4.4).

Other interactions: co-administration of probenecid with mycophenolate mofetil in monkeys raises plasma AUC of MPAG by 3-fold. Thus, other substances known to undergo renal tubular secretion may compete with MPAG, and thereby raise plasma concentrations of MPAG or the other substance undergoing tubular secretion.

Live vaccines: live vaccines should not be given to patients with an impaired immune response. The antibody response to other vaccines may be diminished (see also section 4.4).

4.6 Pregnancy and lactation

It is recommended that CellCept therapy should not be initiated until a negative pregnancy test has been obtained. Effective contraception must be used before beginning CellCept therapy, during therapy, and for six weeks following discontinuation of therapy (see section 4.5). Patients should be instructed to consult their physician immediately should pregnancy occur.

The use of CellCept is not recommended during pregnancy and should be reserved for cases where no more suitable alternative treatment is available. CellCept should be used in pregnant women only if the potential benefit outweighs the potential risk to the foetus. There is limited data from the use of CellCept in pregnant women. However, congenital malformations including ear malformations, i.e. abnormally formed or absent external/middle ear, have been reported in children of patients exposed to CellCept in combination with other immunosuppressants during pregnancy. Cases of spontaneous abortions have been reported in patients exposed to CellCept. Studies in animals have shown reproductive toxicity (see section 5.3).

Mycophenolate mofetil has been shown to be excreted in the milk of lactating rats. It is not known whether this substance is excreted in human milk. Because of the potential for serious adverse reactions to mycophenolate mofetil in breast-fed infants, CellCept is contraindicated in nursing mothers (see section 4.3).

4.7 Effects on ability to drive and use machines

No studies on the effects on the ability to drive and use machines have been performed. The pharmacodynamic profile and the reported adverse reactions indicate that an effect is unlikely.

4.8 Undesirable effects

The following undesirable effects cover adverse reactions from clinical trials:

The principal adverse reactions associated with the administration of CellCept in combination with ciclosporin and corticosteroids include diarrhoea, leucopenia, sepsis and vomiting, and there is evidence of a higher frequency of certain types of infections (see section 4.4).

Malignancies:

Patients receiving immunosuppressive regimens involving combinations of medicinal products, including CellCept, are at increased risk of developing lymphomas and other malignancies, particularly of the skin (see section 4.4). Lymphoproliferative disease or lymphoma developed in 0.6 % of patients receiving CellCept (2 g or 3 g daily) in combination with other immunosuppressants in controlled clinical trials of renal (2 g data), cardiac and hepatic transplant patients followed for at least 1 year. Non-melanoma skin carcinomas occurred in 3.6 % of patients; other types of malignancy occurred in 1.1 % of patients. Three-year safety data in renal and cardiac transplant patients did not reveal any unexpected changes in incidence of malignancy compared to the 1-year data. Hepatic transplant patients were followed for at least 1 year, but less than 3 years.

Opportunistic infections:

All transplant patients are at increased risk of opportunistic infections; the risk increased with total immunosuppressive load (see section 4.4). The most common opportunistic infections in patients receiving CellCept (2 g or 3 g daily) with other immunosuppressants in controlled clinical trials of renal (2 g data), cardiac and hepatic transplant patients followed for at least 1 year were candida mucocutaneous, CMV viraemia/syndrome and Herpes simplex. The proportion of patients with CMV viraemia/syndrome was 13.5 %.

Children and adolescents (aged 2 to 18 years):

The type and frequency of adverse reactions in a clinical study, which recruited 92 paediatric patients aged 2 to 18 years who were given 600 mg/m² mycophenolate mofetil orally twice daily, were generally similar to those observed in adult patients given 1 g CellCept twice daily. However, the following treatment-related adverse events were more frequent in the paediatric population, particularly in children under 6 years of age, when compared to adults: diarrhoea, sepsis, leucopenia, anaemia and infection.

Elderly patients (⩾ 65 years):

Elderly patients (⩾ 65 years) may generally be at increased risk of adverse reactions due to immunosuppression. Elderly patients receiving CellCept as part of a combination immunosuppressive regimen may be at increased risk of certain infections (including cytomegalovirus tissue invasive disease) and possibly gastrointestinal haemorrhage and pulmonary oedema, compared to younger individuals.

Other adverse reactions:

Adverse reactions, probably or possibly related to CellCept, reported in ⩾1/10 and in ⩾1/100 to <1/10 of patients treated with CellCept in the controlled clinical trials of renal (2 g data), cardiac and hepatic transplant patients are listed in the following table.

Adverse Reactions, Probably or Possibly Related to CellCept, Reported in Patients Treated with CellCept in Renal, Cardiac and Hepatic Clinical Trials when Used in Combination with Ciclosporin and Corticosteroids

Within the system organ classes, undesirable effects are listed under headings of frequency, using the following categories: very common (⩾1/10); common (⩾1/100 to <1/10); uncommon (⩾1/1,000 to <1/100); rare (⩾1/10,000 to <1/1,000); very rare (<1/10,000), not known (cannot be estimated form the available data). Within each frequency grouping, undesirable effects are presented in order of decreasing seriousness.

System organ class		Adverse drug reactions
Infections and infestations	Very common	Sepsis, gastrointestinal candidiasis, urinary tract infection, herpes simplex, herpes zoster
	Common	Pneumonia, influenza, respiratory tract infection, respiratory moniliasis, gastrointestinal infection, candidiasis, gastroenteritis, infection, bronchitis, pharyngitis, sinusitis, fungal skin infection, skin candida, vaginal candidiasis, rhinitis
Neoplasms benign, malignant and unspecified (incl cysts and polyps)	Very common	-
	Common	Skin cancer, benign neoplasm of skin
Blood and lymphatic system disorders	Very common	Leucopenia, thrombocytopenia, anaemia
	Common	Pancytopenia, leucocytosis
Metabolism and nutrition disorders	Very common	-
	Common	Acidosis, hyperkalaemia, hypokalaemia, hyperglycaemia, hypomagnesaemia, hypocalcaemia, hypercholesterolaemia, hyperlipidaemia, hypophosphataemia, hyperuricaemia, gout, anorexia
Psychiatric disorders	Very common	-
	Common	Agitation, confusional state, depression, anxiety, thinking abnormal, insomnia
Nervous system disorders	Very common	-
	Common	Convulsion, hypertonia, tremor, somnolence, myasthenic syndrome, dizziness, headache, paraesthesia, dysgeusia
Cardiac disorders	Very common	-
	Common	Tachycardia
Vascular disorders	Very common	-
	Common	Hypotension, hypertension, vasodilatation
Respiratory, thoracic and mediastinal disorders	Very common	-
	Common	Pleural effusion, dyspnoea, cough
Gastrointestinal disorders	Very common	Vomiting, abdominal pain, diarrhoea, nausea
	Common	Gastrointestinal haemorrhage, peritonitis, ileus, colitis, gastric ulcer, duodenal ulcer, gastritis, oesophagitis, stomatitis, constipation, dyspepsia, flatulence, eructation
Hepatobiliary disorders	Very common	-
	Common	Hepatitis, jaundice, hyperbilirubinaemia
Skin and subcutaneous tissue disorders	Very common	-
	Common	Skin hypertrophy, rash, acne, alopecia,
Musculoskeletal and connective Tissue disorders	Very common	-
	Common	Arthralgia
Renal and urinary disorders	Very common	-
	Common	Renal impairment
General disorders and administration site conditions	Very common	-
	Common	Oedema, pyrexia, chills, pain, malaise, asthenia,
Investigations	Very common	-
	Common	Hepatic enzyme increased, blood creatinine increased, blood lactate dehydrogenase increased, blood urea increased, blood alkaline phosphatase increased, weight decreased

Note: 501 (2 g CellCept daily), 289 (3 g CellCept daily) and 277 (2 g IV / 3 g oral CellCept daily) patients were treated in Phase III studies for the prevention of rejection in renal, cardiac and hepatic transplantation, respectively.

The following undesirable effects cover adverse reactions from post-marketing experience:

The types of adverse reactions reported during post-marketing with CellCept are similar to those seen in the controlled renal, cardiac and hepatic transplant studies. Additional adverse reactions reported during post-marketing are described below with the frequencies reported within brackets if known.

Gastrointestinal: gingival hyperplasia (⩾1/100 to <1/10), colitis including cytomegaloviruscolitis, (⩾1/100 to <1/10), pancreatitis (⩾1/100 to <1/10) and intestinal villous atrophy.

Disorders related to immunosuppression: serious life-threatening infections including meningitis, endocarditis, tuberculosis and atypical mycobacterial infection. Cases of BK virus associated nephropathy, as well as cases of JC virus associated progressive multifocal leucoencephalopathy (PML), have been reported in patients treated with immunosuppressants, including CellCept.

Agranulocytosis (⩾1/1000 to <1/100) and neutropenia have been reported; therefore regular monitoring of patients taking CellCept is advised (see section 4.4). There have been reports of aplastic anaemia and bone marrow depression in patients treated with CellCept, some of which have been fatal.

Blood and lymphatic system disorder:

Cases of pure red cell aplasia (PRCA) have been reported in patients treated with CellCept (see section 4.4).

Isolated cases of abnormal neutrophil morphology, including the acquired Pelger-Huet anomaly, have been observed in patients treated with CellCept. These changes are not associated with impaired neutrophil function. These changes may suggest a 'left shift' in the maturity of neutrophils in haematological investigations, which may be mistakenly interpreted as a sign of infection in immunosuppressed patients such as those that receive CellCept.

Hypersensitivity: Hypersensitivity reactions, including angioneurotic oedema and anaphylactic reaction have been reported.

Congenital disorders: see further details in section 4.6.

4.9 Overdose

Reports of overdoses with mycophenolate mofetil have been received from clinical trials and during post-marketing experience. In many of these cases, no adverse events were reported. In those overdose cases in which adverse events were reported, the events fall within the known safety profile of the medicinal product.

It is expected that an overdose of mycophenolate mofetil could possibly result in oversuppression of the immune system and increase susceptibility to infections and bone marrow suppression (see section 4.4). If neutropenia develops, dosing with CellCept should be interrupted or the dose reduced (see section 4.4).

Haemodialysis would not be expected to remove clinically significant amounts of MPA or MPAG. Bile acid sequestrants, such as cholestyramine, can remove MPA by decreasing the enterohepatic re-circulation of the drug (see section 5.2).

5. PHARMACOLOGICAL PROPERTIES

5.1 Pharmacodynamic properties

Pharmacotherapeutic group: immunosuppressive agents ATC code L04AA06

Mycophenolate mofetil is the 2-morpholinoethyl ester of MPA. MPA is a potent, selective, uncompetitive and reversible inhibitor of inosine monophosphate dehydrogenase, and therefore inhibits the *de novo* pathway of guano sine nucleotide synthesis without incorporation into DNA. Because T- and B-lymphocytes are critically dependent for their proliferation on *de novo* synthesis of pureness whereas other cell types can utilise salvage pathways, MPA has more potent gyrostatic effects on lymphocytes than on other cells.

5.2 Pharmacokinetic properties

Following oral administration, mycophenolate mofetil undergoes rapid and extensive absorption and complete presystemic metabolism to the active metabolite, MPA. As evidenced by suppression of acute rejection following renal transplantation, the immunosuppressant activity of CellCept is correlated with MPA concentration. The mean bioavailability of oral mycophenolate mofetil, based on MPA AUC, is 94 % relative to IV mycophenolate mofetil. Food had no effect on the extent of absorption (MPA AUC) of mycophenolate mofetil when administered at doses of 1.5 g BID to renal transplant patients. However, MPA C_{max} was decreased by 40 % in the presence of food. Mycophenolate mofetil is not measurable systemically in plasma following oral administration. MPA at clinically relevant concentrations is 97 % bound to plasma albumin.

As a result of enterohepatic recirculation, secondary increases in plasma MPA concentration are usually observed at approximately 6 – 12 hours post-dose. A reduction in the AUC of MPA of approximately 40 % is associated with the co-administration of cholestyramine (4 g TID), indicating that there is a significant amount of enterohepatic recirculation.

MPA is metabolised principally by glucuronyl transferase to form the phenolic glucuronide of MPA (MPAG), which is not pharmacologically active.

A negligible amount of substance is excreted as MPA (< 1 % of dose) in the urine. Orally administered radiolabelled mycophenolate mofetil results in complete recovery of the administered dose, with 93 % of the administered dose recovered in the urine and 6 % recovered in the faeces. Most (about 87 %) of the administered dose is excreted in the urine as MPAG.

At clinically encountered concentrations, MPA and MPAG are not removed by haemodialysis. However, at high MPAG plasma concentrations (>100μg/ml), small amounts of MPAG are removed.

In the early post-transplant period (< 40 days post-transplant), renal, cardiac and hepatic transplant patients had mean MPA AUCs approximately 30 % lower and C_{max} approximately 40 % lower compared to the late post-transplant period (3 – 6 months post-transplant).

Renal impairment:

In a single dose study (6 subjects/group), mean plasma MPA AUC observed in subjects with severe chronic renal impairment (glomerular filtration rate < $25 ml \bullet min^{-1} \bullet 1.73 m^{-2}$) were 28 – 75 % higher relative to the means observed in normal healthy subjects or subjects with lesser degrees of renal impairment. However, the mean single dose MPAG AUC was 3 – 6-fold higher in subjects with severe renal impairment than in subjects with mild renal impairment or normal healthy subjects, consistent with the known renal elimination of MPAG. Multiple dosing of mycophenolate mofetil in patients with severe chronic renal impairment has not been studied. No data are available for cardiac or hepatic transplant patients with severe chronic renal impairment.

Delayed renal graft function:

In patients with delayed renal graft function post-transplant, mean MPA AUC (0–12h) was comparable to that seen in post-transplant patients without delayed graft function. Mean plasma MPAG AUC (0-12h) was 2 – 3-fold higher than in post-transplant patients without delayed graft function. There may be a transient increase in the free fraction and concentration of plasma MPA in patients with delayed renal graft function. Dose adjustment of CellCept does not appear to be necessary.

Hepatic impairment:

In volunteers with alcoholic cirrhosis, hepatic MPA glucuronidation processes were relatively unaffected by hepatic parenchymal disease. Effects of hepatic disease on this process probably depend on the particular disease. However, hepatic disease with predominantly biliary damage, such as primary biliary cirrhosis, may show a different effect.

Children and adolescents (aged 2 to 18 years):

Pharmacokinetic parameters were evaluated in 49 paediatric renal transplant patients given 600 mg/m^2 mycophenolate mofetil orally twice daily. This dose achieved MPA AUC values similar to those seen in adult renal transplant patients receiving CellCept at a dose of 1 g bid in the early and late post-transplant period. MPA AUC values across age groups were similar in the early and late post-transplant period.

Elderly patients (⩾ 65 years):

Pharmacokinetic behaviour of CellCept in the elderly has not been formally evaluated.

Oral contraceptives:

The pharmacokinetics of oral contraceptives were unaffected by coadministration of CellCept (see also section 4.5). A study of the coadministration of CellCept (1 g bid) and combined oral contraceptives containing ethinylestradiol (0.02 mg to 0.04 mg) and levonorgestrel (0.05 mg to 0.15 mg), desogestrel (0.15 mg) or gestodene (0.05 mg to 0.10 mg) conducted in 18 non-transplant women (not taking other immunosuppressants) over 3 consecutive menstrual cycles showed no clinically relevant influence of CellCept on the ovulation suppressing action of the oral contraceptives. Serum levels of LH, FSH and progesterone were not significantly affected.

5.3 Preclinical safety data

In experimental models, mycophenolate mofetil was not tumourigenic. The highest dose tested in the animal carcinogenicity studies resulted in approximately 2 – 3 times the systemic exposure (AUC or C_{max}) observed in renal transplant patients at the recommended clinical dose of 2 g/day and 1.3 – 2 times the systemic exposure (AUC or C_{max}) observed in cardiac transplant patients at the recommended clinical dose of 3 g/day.

Two genotoxicity assays (*in vitro* mouse lymphoma assay and *in vivo* mouse bone marrow micronucleus test) showed a potential of mycophenolate mofetil to cause chromosomal aberrations. These effects can be related to the pharmacodynamic mode of action, i.e. inhibition of nucleotide synthesis in sensitive cells. Other *in vitro* tests for detection of gene mutation did not demonstrate genotoxic activity.

Mycophenolate mofetil had no effect on fertility of male rats at oral doses up to 20 $mg \bullet kg^{-1} \bullet day^{-1}$. The systemic exposure at this dose represents 2 – 3 times the clinical exposure at the recommended clinical dose of 2 g/day in renal transplant patients and 1.3 – 2 times the clinical exposure at the recommended clinical dose of 3 g/day in cardiac transplant patients. In a female fertility and reproduction study conducted in rats, oral doses of 4.5 $mg \bullet kg^{-1} \bullet day^{-1}$ caused malformations (including anophthalmia, agnathia, and hydrocephaly) in the first generation offspring in the absence of maternal toxicity. The systemic exposure at this dose was approximately 0.5 times the clinical exposure at the recommended clinical dose of 2 g/day for renal transplant patients and approximately 0.3 times the clinical exposure at the recommended clinical dose of 3 g/day for cardiac transplant patients. No effects on fertility or reproductive parameters were evident in the dams or in the subsequent generation.

In teratology studies in rats and rabbits, foetal resorptions and malformations occurred in rats at 6 $mg \bullet kg^{-1} \bullet day^{-1}$ (including anophthalmia, agnathia, and hydrocephaly) and in rabbits at 90 $mg \bullet kg^{1} \bullet day^{-1}$ (including cardiovascular and renal anomalies, such as ectopia cordis and ectopic kidneys, and diaphragmatic and umbilical hernia), in the absence of maternal toxicity. The systemic exposure at these levels is approximately equivalent to or less than 0.5 times the clinical exposure at the recommended clinical dose of 2 g/day for renal transplant patients and approximately 0.3 times the clinical exposure at the recommended clinical dose of 3 g/day for cardiac transplant patients.

Refer to section 4.6.

The haematopoietic and lymphoid systems were the primary organs affected in toxicology studies conducted with mycophenolate mofetil in the rat, mouse, dog and monkey. These effects occurred at systemic exposure levels that are equivalent to or less than the clinical exposure at the recommended dose of 2 g/day for renal transplant recipients. Gastrointestinal effects were observed in the dog at systemic exposure levels equivalent to or less than the clinical exposure at the recommended dose. Gastrointestinal and renal effects consistent with dehydration were also observed in the monkey at the highest dose (systemic exposure levels equivalent to or greater than clinical exposure). The nonclinical toxicity profile of mycophenolate mofetil appears to be consistent with adverse events observed in human clinical trials which now provide safety data of more relevance to the patient population (see section 4.8).

6. PHARMACEUTICAL PARTICULARS

6.1 List of excipients

CellCept 1 g/5 ml powder for oral suspension:

sorbitol

silica, colloidal anhydrous

sodium citrate

soybean lecithin

mixed fruit flavour

xanthan gum

aspartame* (E951)

methyl parahydroxybenzoate (E218)

citric acid anhydrous

* contains phenylalanine equivalent to 2.78 mg/5 ml of suspension.

6.2 Incompatibilities

This medicinal product must not be mixed with other medicinal products except those mentioned in section 6.6.

6.3 Shelf life

The shelf-life of the powder for oral suspension is 2 years.

The shelf-life of the reconstituted suspension is 2 months.

6.4 Special precautions for storage

Powder for oral suspension and reconstituted suspension: Do not store above 30 °C.

6.5 Nature and contents of container

Each bottle contains 110 g of powder for oral suspension. When reconstituted, the volume of the suspension is 175 ml, providing a usable volume of 160 – 165 ml.

A bottle adapter and 2 oral dispensers are also provided.

6.6 Special precautions for disposal and other handling

Because mycophenolate mofetil has demonstrated teratogenic effects in rats and rabbits, avoid inhalation or direct contact with skin or mucous membranes of the dry powder as well as direct contact of the reconstituted suspension with the skin. If such contact occurs, wash thoroughly with soap and water; rinse eyes with plain water.

It is recommended that CellCept 1 g/5 ml powder for oral suspension be reconstituted by the pharmacist prior to dispensing to the patient.

Preparation of suspension

1. Tap the closed bottle several times to loosen the powder.

2. Measure 94 ml of purified water in a graduated cylinder.

3. Add approximately half of the total amount of purified water to the bottle and shake the closed bottle well for about 1 minute.

4. Add the remainder of water and shake the closed bottle well for about 1 minute.

5. Remove child-resistant cap and push bottle adapter into neck of bottle.

6. Close bottle with child-resistant cap tightly. This will assure the proper seating of the bottle adapter in the bottle and child-resistant status of the cap.

7. Write the date of expiration of the reconstituted suspension on the bottle label. (The shelf-life of the reconstituted suspension is two months.)

Any unused product or waste material should be disposed of in accordance with local requirements.

7. MARKETING AUTHORISATION HOLDER

Roche Registration Limited

6 Falcon Way

Shire Park

Welwyn Garden City

AL7 1TW

United Kingdom

8. MARKETING AUTHORISATION NUMBER(S)

EU/1/96/005/006 CellCept (1 bottle 110g)

9. DATE OF FIRST AUTHORISATION/RENEWAL OF THE AUTHORISATION

Date of first authorisation: 14 February 1996

Date of latest renewal: 14 February 2006

10. DATE OF REVISION OF THE TEXT

29 May 2009

LEGAL STATUS

POM

Detailed information on this medicinal product is available on the website of the European Medicines Agency (EMEA) http://www.emea.europa.eu/

Cellcept 250mg Capsules

(Roche Products Limited)

1. NAME OF THE MEDICINAL PRODUCT

CellCept 250 mg capsules.

2. QUALITATIVE AND QUANTITATIVE COMPOSITION

Each capsule contains 250 mg mycophenolate mofetil.

For a full list of excipients, see section 6.1.

3. PHARMACEUTICAL FORM

Capsules, hard.

CellCept capsules: oblong, blue/brown, branded with black "CellCept 250" on the capsule cap and "Company logo" on the capsule body.

4. CLINICAL PARTICULARS

4.1 Therapeutic indications

CellCept is indicated in combination with ciclosporin and corticosteroids for the prophylaxis of acute transplant rejection in patients receiving allogeneic renal, cardiac or hepatic transplants.

4.2 Posology and method of administration

Treatment with CellCept should be initiated and maintained by appropriately qualified transplant specialists.

Use in renal transplant:

Adults: oral CellCept should be initiated within 72 hours following transplantation. The recommended dose in renal transplant patients is 1 g administered twice daily (2 g daily dose).

Children and adolescents (aged 2 to 18 years): the recommended dose of mycophenolate mofetil is 600 mg/m^2 administered orally twice daily (up to a maximum of 2 g daily). CellCept capsules should only be prescribed to patients with a body surface area of at least 1.25 m^2. Patients with a body surface area of 1.25 to 1.5 m^2 may be prescribed CellCept capsules at a dose of 750 mg twice daily (1.5 g daily dose). Patients with a body surface area greater than 1.5 m^2 may be prescribed CellCept capsules at a dose of 1 g twice daily (2 g daily dose). As some adverse reactions occur with greater frequency in this age group (see section 4.8) compared with adults, temporary dose reduction or interruption may be required; these will need to take into account relevant clinical factors including severity of reaction.

Children (< 2 years): there are limited safety and efficacy data in children below the age of 2 years. These are insufficient to make dosage recommendations and therefore use in this age group is not recommended.

Use in cardiac transplant:

Adults: oral CellCept should be initiated within 5 days following transplantation. The recommended dose in cardiac transplant patients is 1.5 g administered twice daily (3 g daily dose).

Children: no data are available for paediatric cardiac transplant patients.

Use in hepatic transplant:

Adults: IV CellCept should be administered for the first 4 days following hepatic transplant, with oral CellCept initiated as soon after this as it can be tolerated. The recommended oral dose in hepatic transplant patients is 1.5 g administered twice daily (3 g daily dose).

Children: no data are available for paediatric hepatic transplant patients.

Use in elderly (≥ 65 years): the recommended dose of 1 g administered twice a day for renal transplant patients and 1.5 g twice a day for cardiac or hepatic transplant patients is appropriate for the elderly.

Use in renal impairment: in renal transplant patients with severe chronic renal impairment (glomerular filtration rate < 25 ml•min^{-1}•1.73 m^{-2}), outside the immediate post-transplant period, doses greater than 1 g administered twice a day should be avoided. These patients should also be carefully observed. No dose adjustments are needed in patients experiencing delayed renal graft function post-operatively (see section 5.2). No data are available for cardiac or hepatic transplant patients with severe chronic renal impairment.

Use in severe hepatic impairment: no dose adjustments are needed for renal transplant patients with severe hepatic parenchymal disease. No data are available for cardiac transplant patients with severe hepatic parenchymal disease.

Treatment during rejection episodes: MPA (mycophenolic acid) is the active metabolite of mycophenolate mofetil. Renal transplant rejection does not lead to changes in MPA pharmacokinetics; dosage reduction or interruption of CellCept is not required. There is no basis for CellCept dose adjustment following cardiac transplant rejection. No pharmacokinetic data are available during hepatic transplant rejection.

4.3 Contraindications

Hypersensitivity reactions to CellCept have been observed (see section 4.8). Therefore, CellCept is contraindicated in patients with a hypersensitivity to mycophenolate mofetil or mycophenolic acid.

CellCept is contraindicated in women who are breastfeeding (see section 4.6).

For information on use in pregnancy and contraceptive requirements see section 4.6.

4.4 Special warnings and precautions for use

Patients receiving immunosuppressive regimens involving combinations of medicinal products, including CellCept, are at increased risk of developing lymphomas and other malignancies, particularly of the skin (see section 4.8). The risk appears to be related to the intensity and duration of immunosuppression rather than to the use of any specific agent. As general advice to minimise the risk for skin cancer, exposure to sunlight and UV light should be limited by wearing protective clothing and using a sunscreen with a high protection factor.

Patients receiving CellCept should be instructed to report immediately any evidence of infection, unexpected bruising, bleeding or any other manifestation of bone marrow depression.

Patients treated with immunosuppressants, including CellCept, are at increased risk for opportunistic infections (bacterial, fungal, viral and protozoal), fatal infections and sepsis (see section 4.8). Among the opportunistic infections are BK virus associated nephropathy and JC virus associated progressive multifocal leukoencephalopathy (PML). These infections are often related to a high total immunosuppressive burden and may lead to serious or fatal conditions that physicians should consider in the differential diagnosis in immunosuppressed patients with deteriorating renal function or neurological symptoms.

Patients receiving CellCept should be monitored for neutropenia, which may be related to CellCept itself, concomitant medications, viral infections, or some combination of these causes. Patients taking CellCept should have complete blood counts weekly during the first month, twice monthly for the second and third months of treatment, then monthly through the first year. If neutropenia develops (absolute neutrophil count < 1.3 × 10^3/µl), it may be appropriate to interrupt or discontinue CellCept.

Cases of pure red cell aplasia (PRCA) have been reported in patients treated with CellCept in combination with other immunosuppressants. The mechanism for mycophenolate mofetil induced PRCA is unknown. PRCA may resolve with dose reduction or cessation of CellCept therapy. Changes to CellCept therapy should only be undertaken under appropriate supervision in transplant recipients in order to minimise the risk of graft rejection (see section 4.8).

Patients should be advised that during treatment with CellCept, vaccinations may be less effective and the use of live attenuated vaccines should be avoided (see section 4.5). Influenza vaccination may be of value. Prescribers should refer to national guidelines for influenza vaccination.

Because CellCept has been associated with an increased incidence of digestive system adverse events, including infrequent cases of gastrointestinal tract ulceration, haemorrhage and perforation, CellCept should be administered with caution in patients with active serious digestive system disease.

CellCept is an IMPDH (inosine monophosphate dehydrogenase) inhibitor. On theoretical grounds, therefore, it should be avoided in patients with rare hereditary deficiency of hypoxanthine-guanine phosphoribosyl-transferase (HGPRT) such as Lesch-Nyhan and Kelley-Seegmiller syndrome.

It is recommended that CellCept should not be administered concomitantly with azathioprine because such concomitant administration has not been studied.

In view of the significant reduction in the AUC of MPA by cholestyramine, caution should be used in the concomitant administration of CellCept with medicinal products that interfere with enterohepatic recirculation because of the potential to reduce the efficacy of CellCept.

The risk: benefit of mycophenolate mofetil in combination with tacrolimus or sirolimus has not been established (see also section 4.5).

4.5 Interaction with other medicinal products and other forms of interaction

Interaction studies have only been performed in adults.

Aciclovir: higher aciclovir plasma concentrations were observed when mycophenolate mofetil was administered with aciclovir in comparison to the administration of aciclovir alone. The changes in MPAG (the phenolic glucuronide of MPA) pharmacokinetics (MPAG increased by 8 %) were minimal and are not considered clinically significant. Because MPAG plasma concentrations are increased in the presence of renal impairment, as are aciclovir concentrations, the potential exists for mycophenolate mofetil and aciclovir, or its prodrugs, e.g. valaciclovir, to compete for tubular secretion and further increases in concentrations of both substances may occur.

Antacids with magnesium and aluminium hydroxides: absorption of mycophenolate mofetil was decreased when administered with antacids.

Cholestyramine: following single dose administration of 1.5 g of mycophenolate mofetil to normal healthy subjects pre-treated with 4 g TID of cholestyramine for 4 days, there was a 40 % reduction in the AUC of MPA (see section 4.4 and section 5.2). Caution should be used during concomitant administration because of the potential to reduce efficacy of CellCept.

Medicinal products that interfere with enterohepatic circulation: caution should be used with medicinal products that interfere with enterohepatic circulation because of their potential to reduce the efficacy of CellCept.

Ciclosporin A: ciclosporin A (CsA) pharmacokinetics are unaffected by mycophenolate mofetil. In contrast, if concomitant ciclosporin treatment is stopped, an increase in MPA AUC of around 30% should be expected.

Ganciclovir: based on the results of a single dose administration study of recommended doses of oral mycophenolate and IV ganciclovir and the known effects of renal impairment on the pharmacokinetics of CellCept (see section 4.2) and ganciclovir, it is anticipated that co-administration of these agents (which compete for mechanisms of renal tubular secretion) will result in increases in MPAG and ganciclovir concentration. No substantial alteration of MPA pharmacokinetics is anticipated and CellCept dose adjustment is not required. In patients with renal impairment in which CellCept and ganciclovir or its prodrugs, e.g. valganciclovir, are co-administered, the dose recommendations for ganciclovir should be observed and patients should be monitored carefully.

Oral contraceptives: the pharmacokinetics and pharmacodynamics of oral contraceptives were unaffected by coadministration of CellCept (see also section 5.2).

Rifampicin: in patients not also taking ciclosporin, concomitant administration of CellCept and rifampicin resulted in a decrease in MPA exposure (AUC0-12h) of 18% to 70%. It is recommended to monitor MPA exposure levels and to adjust CellCept doses accordingly to maintain clinical efficacy when rifampicin is administered concomitantly.

Sirolimus: in renal transplant patients, concomitant administration of CellCept and CsA resulted in reduced MPA exposures by 30-50% compared with patients receiving the combination of sirolimus and similar doses of CellCept (see also section 4.4).

Sevelamer: decrease in MPA C_{max} and AUC0-12 by 30% and 25%, respectively, were observed when CellCept was concomitantly administered with sevelamer without any clinical consequences (i.e. graft rejection). It is recommended, however, to administer CellCept at least one hour before or three hours after sevelamer intake to minimise the impact on the absorption of MPA. There is no data on CellCept with phosphate binders other than sevelamer.

Trimethoprim/sulfamethoxazole: no effect on the bioavailability of MPA was observed.

Norfloxacin and metronidazole: in healthy volunteers, no significant interaction was observed when CellCept was concomitantly administered with norfloxacin and metronidazole separately. However, norfloxacin and metronidazole combined reduced the MPA exposure by approximately 30 % following a single dose of CellCept.

Ciprofloxacin and amoxicillin plus clavulanic acid: Reductions in pre-dose (trough) MPA concentrations of about 50% have been reported in renal transplant recipients in the days immediately following commencement of oral ciprofloxacin or amoxicillin plus clavulanic acid. This effect tended to diminish with continued antibiotic use and to cease within a few days of their discontinuation. The change in predose level may not accurately represent changes in overall MPA exposure. Therefore, a change in the dose of CellCept should not normally be necessary in the absence of clinical evidence of graft dysfunction. However, close clinical monitoring should be performed during the combination and shortly after antibiotic treatment.

Tacrolimus: in hepatic transplant patients initiated on CellCept and tacrolimus, the AUC and C_{max} of MPA, the active metabolite of CellCept, were not significantly affected by coadministration with tacrolimus. In, contrast, there was an increase of approximately 20 % in tacrolimus AUC when multiple doses of CellCept (1.5 g BID) were administered to patients taking tacrolimus. However, in renal transplant patients, tacrolimus concentration did not appear to be altered by CellCept (see also section 4.4).

Other interactions: co-administration of probenecid with mycophenolate mofetil in monkeys raises plasma AUC of MPAG by 3-fold. Thus, other substances known to undergo renal tubular secretion may compete with MPAG, and thereby raise plasma concentrations of MPAG or the other substance undergoing tubular secretion.

Live vaccines: live vaccines should not be given to patients with an impaired immune response. The antibody response to other vaccines may be diminished (see also section 4.4).

4.6 Pregnancy and lactation

It is recommended that CellCept therapy should not be initiated until a negative pregnancy test has been obtained. Effective contraception must be used before beginning CellCept therapy, during therapy, and for six weeks following discontinuation of therapy (see section 4.5). Patients should be instructed to consult their physician immediately should pregnancy occur.

The use of CellCept is not recommended during pregnancy and should be reserved for cases where no more suitable alternative treatment is available. CellCept should be used in pregnant women only if the potential benefit outweighs the potential risk to the foetus. There is limited data from the use of CellCept in pregnant women. However, congenital malformations including ear malformations, i.e. abnormally formed or absent external/middle ear, have been reported in children of patients exposed to CellCept in combination with other immunosuppressants during pregnancy. Cases of spontaneous abortions have been reported in patients exposed to CellCept. Studies in animals have shown reproductive toxicity (see section 5.3).

Mycophenolate mofetil has been shown to be excreted in the milk of lactating rats. It is not known whether this substance is excreted in human milk. Because of the potential for serious adverse reactions to mycophenolate mofetil in breast-fed infants, CellCept is contraindicated in nursing mothers (see section 4.3).

4.7 Effects on ability to drive and use machines

No studies on the effects on the ability to drive and use machines have been performed. The pharmacodynamic profile and the reported adverse reactions indicate that an effect is unlikely.

4.8 Undesirable effects

The following undesirable effects cover adverse reactions from clinical trials:

The principal adverse reactions associated with the administration of CellCept in combination with ciclosporin and corticosteroids include diarrhoea, leucopenia, sepsis and vomiting, and there is evidence of a higher frequency of certain types of infections (see section 4.4).

Malignancies:

Patients receiving immunosuppressive regimens involving combinations of medicinal products, including CellCept, are at increased risk of developing lymphomas and other malignancies, particularly of the skin (see section 4.4). Lymphoproliferative disease or lymphoma developed in 0.6 % of patients receiving CellCept (2 g or 3 g daily) in combination with other immunosuppressants in controlled clinical trials of renal (2 g data), cardiac and hepatic transplant patients followed for at least 1 year. Non-melanoma skin carcinomas occurred in 3.6 % of patients; other types of malignancy occurred in 1.1 % of patients. Three-year safety data in renal and cardiac transplant patients did not reveal any unexpected changes in incidence of malignancy compared to the 1-year data. Hepatic transplant patients were followed for at least 1 year, but less than 3 years.

Opportunistic infections:

All transplant patients are at increased risk of opportunistic infections; the risk increased with total immunosuppressive load (see section 4.4). The most common opportunistic infections in patients receiving CellCept (2 g or 3 g daily) with other immunosuppressants in controlled clinical trials of renal (2 g data), cardiac and hepatic transplant patients followed for at least 1 year were candida mucocutaneous, CMV viraemia/syndrome and Herpes simplex. The proportion of patients with CMV viraemia/syndrome was 13.5 %.

Children and adolescents (aged 2 to 18 years):

The type and frequency of adverse reactions in a clinical study, which recruited 92 paediatric patients aged 2 to 18 years who were given 600 mg/m^2 mycophenolate mofetil orally twice daily, were generally similar to those observed in adult patients given 1 g CellCept twice daily. However, the following treatment-related adverse events were more frequent in the paediatric population, particularly in children under 6 years of age, when compared to adults: diarrhoea, sepsis, leucopenia, anaemia and infection.

Elderly patients (≥ 65 years):

Elderly patients (≥ 65 years) may generally be at increased risk of adverse reactions due to immunosuppression. Elderly patients receiving CellCept as part of a combination immunosuppressive regimen, may be at increased risk of certain infections (including cytomegalovirus tissue invasive disease) and possibly gastrointestinal haemorrhage and pulmonary oedema, compared to younger individuals.

Other adverse reactions:

Adverse reactions, probably or possibly related to CellCept, reported in ≥1/10 and in ≥1/100 to <1/10 of patients treated with CellCept in the controlled clinical trials of renal (2 g data), cardiac and hepatic transplant patients are listed in the following table.

Adverse Reactions, Probably or Possibly Related to CellCept, Reported in Patients Treated with CellCept in Renal, Cardiac and Hepatic Clinical Trials when Used in Combination with Ciclosporin and Corticosteroids

Within the system organ classes, undesirable effects are listed under headings of frequency, using the following categories: very common (≥1/10); common (≥1/100 to <1/10); uncommon (≥1/1,000 to <1/100); rare (≥1/10,000 to <1/1,000); very rare (<1/10,000), not known (cannot be estimated form the available data). Within each frequency grouping, undesirable effects are presented in order of decreasing seriousness.

System organ class		Adverse drug reactions
Infections and infestations	Very common	Sepsis, gastrointestinal candidiasis, urinary tract infection, herpes simplex, herpes zoster
	Common	Pneumonia, influenza, respiratory tract infection, respiratory moniliasis, gastrointestinal infection, candidiasis, gastroenteritis, infection, bronchitis, pharyngitis, sinusitis, fungal skin infection, skin candida, vaginal candidiasis, rhinitis
Neoplasms benign, malignant and unspecified (incl cysts and polyps)	Very common	-
	Common	Skin cancer, benign neoplasm of skin
Blood and lymphatic system disorders	Very common	Leucopenia, thrombocytopenia, anaemia
	Common	Pancytopenia, leucocytosis
Metabolism and nutrition disorders	Very common	-
	Common	Acidosis, hyperkalaemia, hypokalaemia, hyperglycaemia, hypomagnesaemia, hypocalcaemia, hypercholesterolaemia, hyperlipidaemia, hypophosphataemia, hyperuricaemia, gout, anorexia
Psychiatric disorders	Very common	-
	Common	Agitation, confusional state, depression, anxiety, thinking abnormal, insomnia
Nervous system disorders	Very common	-
	Common	Convulsion, hypertonia, tremor, somnolence, myasthenic syndrome, dizziness, headache, paraesthesia, dysgeusia
Cardiac disorders	Very common	-
	Common	Tachycardia
Vascular disorders	Very common	-
	Common	Hypotension, hypertension, vasodilatation
Respiratory, thoracic and mediastinal disorders	Very common	-
	Common	Pleural effusion, dyspnoea, cough
Gastrointestinal disorders	Very common	Vomiting, abdominal pain, diarrhoea, nausea
	Common	Gastrointestinal haemorrhage, peritonitis, ileus, colitis, gastric ulcer, duodenal ulcer, gastritis, oesophagitis, stomatitis, constipation, dyspepsia, flatulence, eructation
Hepatobiliary disorders	Very common	-
	Common	Hepatitis, jaundice, hyperbilirubinaemia
Skin and subcutaneous tissue disorders	Very common	-
	Common	Skin hypertrophy, rash, acne, alopecia,
Musculoskeletal and connective Tissue disorders	Very common	-
	Common	Arthralgia
Renal and urinary disorders	Very common	-
	Common	Renal impairment
General disorders and administration site conditions	Very common	-
	Common	Oedema, pyrexia, chills, pain, malaise, asthenia,
Investigations	Very common	-
	Common	Hepatic enzyme increased, blood creatinine increased, blood lactate dehydrogenase increased, blood urea increased, blood alkaline phosphatase increased, weight decreased

Note: 501 (2 g CellCept daily), 289 (3 g CellCept daily) and 277 (2 g IV / 3 g oral CellCept daily) patients were treated in Phase III studies for the prevention of rejection in renal, cardiac and hepatic transplantation, respectively.

The following undesirable effects cover adverse reactions from post-marketing experience:

The types of adverse reactions reported during post-marketing with CellCept are similar to those seen in the controlled renal, cardiac and hepatic transplant studies. Additional adverse reactions reported during post-marketing are described below with the frequencies reported within brackets if known.

Gastrointestinal: gingival hyperplasia (≥1/100 to <1/10), colitis including cytomegalovirus colitis, (≥1/100 to <1/10), pancreatitis, (≥1/100 to <1/10) and intestinal villous atrophy.

Disorders related to immunosuppression: serious life-threatening infections including meningitis, endocarditis, tuberculosis and atypical mycobacterial infection. Cases of BK virus associated nephropathy, as well as cases of JC virus associated progressive multifocal leucoencephalopathy (PML), have been reported in patients treated with immunosuppressants, including CellCept.

Agranulocytosis (≥1/1000 to <1/100) and neutropenia have been reported; therefore, regular monitoring of patients taking CellCept is advised (see section 4.4). There have been reports of aplastic anaemia and bone marrow depression in patients treated with CellCept, some of which have been fatal.

Blood and lymphatic system disorder:

Cases of pure red cell aplasia (PRCA) have been reported in patients treated with CellCept (see section 4.4).

Isolated cases of abnormal neutrophil morphology, including the acquired Pelger-Huet anomaly, have been observed in patients treated with CellCept. These changes are not associated with impaired neutrophil function. These changes may suggest a 'left shift' in the maturity of neutrophils in haematological investigations, which may be mistakenly interpreted as a sign of infection in immunosuppressed patients such as those that receive CellCept.

Hypersensitivity: Hypersensitivity reactions, including angioneurotic oedema and anaphylactic reaction, have been reported.

Congenital disorders: see further details in section 4.6.

4.9 Overdose

Reports of overdoses with mycophenolate mofetil have been received from clinical trials and during post-marketing experience. In many of these cases, no adverse events were reported. In those overdose cases in which adverse events were reported, the events fall within the known safety profile of the medicinal product.

It is expected that an overdose of mycophenolate mofetil could possibly result in oversuppression of the immune system and increase susceptibility to infections and bone marrow suppression (see section 4.4). If neutropenia develops, dosing with CellCept should be interrupted or the dose reduced (see section 4.4).

Haemodialysis would not be expected to remove clinically significant amounts of MPA or MPAG. Bile acid sequestrants, such as cholestyramine, can remove MPA by decreasing the enterohepatic re-circulation of the drug (see section 5.2).

5. PHARMACOLOGICAL PROPERTIES

5.1 Pharmacodynamic properties

Pharmacotherapeutic group: immunosuppressive agents ATC code L04AA06

Mycophenolate mofetil is the 2-morpholinoethyl ester of MPA. MPA is a potent, selective, uncompetitive and reversible inhibitor of inosine monophosphate dehydrogenase, and therefore inhibits the *de novo* pathway of guanosine nucleotide synthesis without incorporation into DNA. Because T- and B-lymphocytes are critically dependent for their proliferation on *de novo* synthesis of purines whereas other cell types can utilise salvage pathways, MPA has more potent cytostatic effects on lymphocytes than on other cells.

5.2 Pharmacokinetic properties

Following oral administration, mycophenolate mofetil undergoes rapid and extensive absorption and complete presystemic metabolism to the active metabolite, MPA. As evidenced by suppression of acute rejection following renal transplantation, the immunosuppressant activity of CellCept is correlated with MPA concentration. The mean bioavailability of oral mycophenolate mofetil, based on MPA AUC, is 94 % relative to IV mycophenolate mofetil. Food had no effect on the extent of absorption (MPA AUC) of mycophenolate mofetil when administered at doses of 1.5 g BID to renal transplant patients. However, MPA C_{max} was decreased by 40 % in the presence of food. Mycophenolate mofetil is not measurable systemically in plasma following oral administration. MPA at clinically relevant concentrations is 97 % bound to plasma albumin.

As a result of enterohepatic recirculation, secondary increases in plasma MPA concentration are usually observed at approximately 6 – 12 hours post-dose. A reduction in the AUC of MPA of approximately 40 % is associated with the co-administration of cholestyramine (4 g TID), indicating that there is a significant amount of enterohepatic recirculation.

MPA is metabolised principally by glucuronyl transferase to form the phenolic glucuronide of MPA (MPAG), which is not pharmacologically active.

A negligible amount of substance is excreted as MPA (< 1 % of dose) in the urine. Orally administered radiolabelled mycophenolate mofetil results in complete recovery of the administered dose with 93 % of the administered dose recovered in the urine and 6 % recovered in the faeces. Most (about 87 %) of the administered dose is excreted in the urine as MPAG.

At clinically encountered concentrations, MPA and MPAG are not removed by haemodialysis. However, at high MPAG plasma concentrations (>100μg/ml), small amounts of MPAG are removed.

In the early post-transplant period (< 40 days post-transplant), renal, cardiac and hepatic transplant patients had mean MPA AUCs approximately 30 % lower and C_{max} approximately 40 % lower compared to the late post-transplant period (3 – 6 months post-transplant).

Renal impairment:

In a single dose study (6 subjects/group), mean plasma MPA AUC observed in subjects with severe chronic renal impairment (glomerular filtration rate < 25 ml•min^{-1}•1.73 m^{-2}) were 28 – 75 % higher relative to the means observed in normal healthy subjects or subjects with lesser degrees of renal impairment. However, the mean single dose MPAG AUC was 3 – 6-fold higher in subjects with severe renal impairment than in subjects with mild renal impairment or normal healthy subjects, consistent with the known renal elimination of MPAG. Multiple dosing of mycophenolate mofetil in patients with severe chronic renal impairment has not been studied. No data are available for cardiac or hepatic transplant patients with severe chronic renal impairment.

Delayed renal graft function:

In patients with delayed renal graft function post-transplant, mean MPA AUC (0–12h) was comparable to that seen in post-transplant patients without delayed graft function. Mean plasma MPAG AUC (0-12h) was 2 – 3-fold higher than in post-transplant patients without delayed graft function. There may be a transient increase in the free fraction and concentration of plasma MPA in patients with delayed renal graft function. Dose adjustment of CellCept does not appear to be necessary.

Hepatic impairment:

In volunteers with alcoholic cirrhosis, hepatic MPA glucuronidation processes were relatively unaffected by hepatic parenchymal disease. Effects of hepatic disease on this process probably depend on the particular disease. However, hepatic disease with predominantly biliary damage, such as primary biliary cirrhosis, may show a different effect.

Children and adolescents (aged 2 to 18 years):

Pharmacokinetic parameters were evaluated in 49 paediatric renal transplant patients given 600 mg/m^2 mycophenolate mofetil orally twice daily. This dose achieved MPA AUC values similar to those seen in adult renal transplant patients receiving CellCept at a dose of 1 g bid in the early and late post-transplant period. MPA AUC values across age groups were similar in the early and late post-transplant period.

Elderly patients (≥ 65 years):

Pharmacokinetic behaviour of CellCept in the elderly has not been formally evaluated.

Oral contraceptives:

The pharmacokinetics of oral contraceptives were unaffected by coadministration of CellCept (see also section 4.5). A study of the coadministration of CellCept (1 g bid) and combined oral contraceptives containing ethinylestradiol (0.02 mg to 0.04 mg) and levonorgestrel (0.05 mg to 0.15 mg), desogestrel (0.15 mg) or gestodene (0.05 mg to 0.10 mg) conducted in 18 non-transplant women (not taking other immunosuppressants) over 3 consecutive menstrual cycles showed no clinically relevant influence of CellCept on the ovulation suppressing action of the oral contraceptives. Serum levels of LH, FSH and progesterone were not significantly affected.

5.3 Preclinical safety data

In experimental models, mycophenolate mofetil was not tumourigenic. The highest dose tested in the animal carcinogenicity studies resulted in approximately 2 – 3 times the systemic exposure (AUC or C_{max}) observed in renal transplant patients at the recommended clinical dose of 2 g/day and 1.3 – 2 times the systemic exposure (AUC or C_{max}) observed in cardiac transplant patients at the recommended clinical dose of 3 g/day.

Two genotoxicity assays (*in vitro* mouse lymphoma assay and *in vivo* mouse bone marrow micronucleus test) showed a potential of mycophenolate mofetil to cause chromosomal aberrations. These effects can be related to the pharmacodynamic mode of action, i.e. inhibition of nucleotide synthesis in sensitive cells. Other *in vitro* tests for detection of gene mutation did not demonstrate genotoxic activity.

Mycophenolate mofetil had no effect on fertility of male rats at oral doses up to 20 mg•kg^{-1}•day^{-1}. The systemic exposure at this dose represents 2 – 3 times the clinical exposure at the recommended clinical dose of 2 g/day in renal transplant patients and 1.3 – 2 times the clinical exposure at the recommended clinical dose of 3 g/day in cardiac transplant patients. In a female fertility and reproduction study conducted in rats, oral doses of 4.5 mg•kg^{-1}•day^{-1} caused malformations (including anophthalmia, agnathia, and hydrocephaly) in the first generation offspring in the absence of maternal toxicity. The systemic exposure at this dose was approximately 0.5 times the clinical exposure at the recommended clinical dose of 2 g/day for renal transplant patients and approximately 0.3 times the clinical exposure at the recommended clinical dose of 3 g/day for cardiac transplant patients. No effects on fertility or reproductive parameters were evident in the dams or in the subsequent generation.

In teratology studies in rats and rabbits, foetal resorptions and malformations occurred in rats at 6 mg•kg^{-1}•day^{-1} (including anophthalmia, agnathia, and hydrocephaly) and in rabbits at 90 mg•kg^{-1}•day^{-1} (including cardiovascular and renal anomalies, such as ectopia cordis and ectopic kidneys, and diaphragmatic and umbilical hernia), in the absence of maternal toxicity. The systemic exposure at these levels is approximately equivalent to or less than 0.5 times the clinical exposure at the recommended clinical dose of 2 g/day for renal transplant patients and approximately 0.3 times the clinical exposure at the recommended clinical dose of 3 g/day for cardiac transplant patients.

Refer to section 4.6.

The haematopoietic and lymphoid systems were the primary organs affected in toxicology studies conducted with mycophenolate mofetil in the rat, mouse, dog and monkey. These effects occurred at systemic exposure levels that are equivalent to or less than the clinical exposure at the recommended dose of 2 g/day for renal transplant recipients. Gastrointestinal effects were observed in the dog at systemic exposure levels equivalent to or less than the clinical exposure at the recommended dose. Gastrointestinal and renal effects consistent with dehydration were also observed in the monkey at the highest dose (systemic exposure levels equivalent to or greater than clinical exposure). The nonclinical toxicity profile of mycophenolate mofetil appears to be consistent with adverse events observed in human clinical trials which now provide safety data of more relevance to the patient population (see section 4.8).

6. PHARMACEUTICAL PARTICULARS

6.1 List of excipients

CellCept capsules:

pregelatinised maize starch

croscarmellose sodium

polyvidone (K-90)

magnesium stearate

Capsule shells:

gelatin

indigo carmine (E132)

yellow iron oxide (E172)

red iron oxide (E172)

titanium dioxide (E171)

black iron oxide (E172)

potassium hydroxide

shellac.

6.2 Incompatibilities

Not applicable.

6.3 Shelf life

3 years.

6.4 Special precautions for storage

Do not store above 30°C. Store in the original package in order to protect from moisture.

6.5 Nature and contents of container

CellCept 250 mg capsules:	1 carton contains 100 capsules (in blister packs of 10)
	1 carton contains 300 capsules (in blister packs of 10)

6.6 Special precautions for disposal and other handling

Because mycophenolate mofetil has demonstrated teratogenic effects in rats and rabbits, CellCept capsules should not be opened or crushed. Avoid inhalation or direct contact with skin or mucous membranes of the powder contained in CellCept capsules. If such contact occurs, wash thoroughly with soap and water; rinse eyes with plain water.

Any unused product or waste material should be disposed of in accordance with local requirements.

7. MARKETING AUTHORISATION HOLDER

Roche Registration Limited

6 Falcon Way

Shire Park

Welwyn Garden City

AL7 1TW

United Kingdom

8. MARKETING AUTHORISATION NUMBER(S)

EU/1/96/005/001 CellCept (100 capsules)

EU/1/96/005/003 CellCept (300 capsules)

9. DATE OF FIRST AUTHORISATION/RENEWAL OF THE AUTHORISATION

Date of first authorisation: 14 February 1996

Date of latest renewal: 14 February 2006

10. DATE OF REVISION OF THE TEXT

29 May 2009

LEGAL STATUS

POM

Detailed information on this medicinal product is available on the website of the European Medicines Agency (EMEA) http://www.emea.europa.eu/

Cellcept 500mg Powder

(Roche Products Limited)

1. NAME OF THE MEDICINAL PRODUCT

CellCept 500 mg powder for concentrate for solution for infusion.

2. QUALITATIVE AND QUANTITATIVE COMPOSITION

Each vial contains the equivalent of 500 mg mycophenolate mofetil (as hydrochloride salt).

For a full list of excipients, see section 6.1.

3. PHARMACEUTICAL FORM

Powder for concentrate for solution for infusion.

CellCept 500 mg powder for concentrate for solution for infusion must be reconstituted and further diluted with glucose intravenous infusion 5 % prior to administration to the patient (see section 6.6).

4. CLINICAL PARTICULARS

4.1 Therapeutic indications

CellCept 500 mg powder for concentrate for solution for infusion is indicated in combination with ciclosporin and corticosteroids for the prophylaxis of acute transplant rejection in patients receiving allogeneic renal or hepatic transplants.

4.2 Posology and method of administration

Treatment with CellCept should be initiated and maintained by appropriately qualified transplant specialists.

CAUTION: CELLCEPT I.V. SOLUTION SHOULD NEVER BE ADMINISTERED BY RAPID OR BOLUS INTRAVENOUS INJECTION.

CellCept 500 mg powder for concentrate for solution for infusion is an alternative dosage form to CellCept oral forms (capsules, tablets and powder for oral suspension) that may be administered for up to 14 days. The initial dose of CellCept 500 mg powder for concentrate for solution for infusion should be given within 24 hours following transplantation.

Following reconstitution to a concentration of 6 mg/ml, CellCept 500 mg powder for concentrate for solution for infusion must be administered by slow intravenous infusion over a period of 2 hours by either a peripheral or a central vein (see section 6.6).

Use in renal transplant: the recommended dose in renal transplant patients is 1 g administered twice daily (2 g daily dose).

Use in hepatic transplant: the recommended dose of CellCept for infusion in hepatic transplant patients is 1 g administered twice daily (2 g daily dose). IV CellCept should continue for the first 4 days following hepatic transplant, with oral CellCept initiated as soon after this as it can be tolerated. The recommended dose of oral CellCept in hepatic transplant patients is 1.5 g administered twice daily (3 g daily dose).

Use in children: safety and efficacy of CellCept for infusion in paediatric patients have not been established. No pharmacokinetic data with CellCept for infusion are available for paediatric renal transplant patients. No pharmacokinetic data are available for paediatric patients following hepatic transplants.

Use in elderly (≥ 65 years): the recommended dose of 1 g administered twice a day for renal or hepatic transplant patients is appropriate for the elderly.

Use in renal impairment: in renal transplant patients with severe chronic renal impairment (glomerular filtration rate < 25 ml•min^{-1}•1.73 m^{-2}), outside the immediate post-transplant period, doses greater than 1 g administered twice a day should be avoided. These patients should also be carefully observed. No dose adjustments are needed in patients experiencing delayed renal graft function post-operatively (see section 5.2). No data are available for hepatic transplant patients with severe chronic renal impairment.

Use in severe hepatic impairment: no dose adjustments are needed for renal transplant patients with severe hepatic parenchymal disease.

Treatment during rejection episodes: MPA (mycophenolic acid) is the active metabolite of mycophenolate mofetil. Renal transplant rejection does not lead to changes in MPA pharmacokinetics; dosage reduction or interruption of CellCept is not required. No pharmacokinetic data are available during hepatic transplant rejection.

4.3 Contraindications

Hypersensitivity reactions to CellCept have been observed (see section 4.8). Therefore, CellCept is contraindicated in patients with a hypersensitivity to mycophenolate mofetil or mycophenolic acid. CellCept 500 mg powder for concentrate for solution for infusion is contraindicated in patients who are allergic to polysorbate 80.

CellCept is contraindicated in women who are breastfeeding (see section 4.6).

For information on use in pregnancy and contraceptive requirements, see section 4.6.

4.4 Special warnings and precautions for use

Patients receiving immunosuppressive regimens involving combinations of medicinal products, including CellCept, are at increased risk of developing lymphomas and other malignancies, particularly of the skin (see section 4.8). The risk appears to be related to the intensity and duration of immunosuppression rather than to the use of any specific agent. As general advice to minimise the risk for skin cancer, exposure to sunlight and UV light should be limited by wearing protective clothing and using a sunscreen with a high protection factor.

Patients receiving CellCept should be instructed to report immediately any evidence of infection, unexpected bruising, bleeding or any other manifestation of bone marrow depression.

Patients treated with immunosuppressants, including CellCept, are at increased risk for opportunistic infections (bacterial, fungal, viral and protozoal), fatal infections and sepsis (see section 4.8). Among the opportunistic infections are BK virus associated nephropathy and JC virus associated progressive multifocal leukoencephalopathy (PML). These infections are often related to a high total immunosuppressive burden and may lead to serious or fatal conditions that physicians should consider in the differential diagnosis in immunosuppressed patients with deteriorating renal function or neurological symptoms.

Patients receiving CellCept should be monitored for neutropenia, which may be related to CellCept itself, concomitant medications, viral infections, or some combination of these causes. Patients taking CellCept should have complete blood counts weekly during the first month, twice monthly for the second and third months of treatment, then monthly through the first year. If neutropenia develops (absolute neutrophil count $< 1.3 \times 10^3/\mu l$) it may be appropriate to interrupt or discontinue CellCept.

Cases of pure red cell aplasia (PRCA) have been reported in patients treated with CellCept in combination with other immunosuppressants. The mechanism for mycophenolate mofetil induced PRCA is unknown. PRCA may resolve with dose reduction or cessation of CellCept therapy. Changes to CellCept therapy should only be undertaken under appropriate supervision in transplant recipients in order to minimise the risk of graft rejection (see section 4.8).

Patients should be advised that during treatment with CellCept, vaccinations may be less effective, and the use of live attenuated vaccines should be avoided (see section 4.5). Influenza vaccination may be of value. Prescribers should refer to national guidelines for influenza vaccination.

Because CellCept has been associated with an increased incidence of digestive system adverse events, including infrequent cases of gastrointestinal tract ulceration, haemorrhage and perforation, CellCept should be administered with caution in patients with active serious digestive system disease.

CellCept is an IMPDH (inosine monophosphate dehydrogenase) inhibitor. On theoretical grounds, therefore, it should be avoided in patients with rare hereditary deficiency of hypoxanthine-guanine phosphoribosyl transferase (HGPRT) such as Lesch-Nyhan and Kelley-Seegmiller syndrome.

It is recommended that CellCept should not be administered concomitantly with azathioprine because such concomitant administration has not been studied.

In view of the significant reduction in the AUC of MPA by cholestyramine, caution should be used in the concomitant administration of CellCept with medicinal products that interfere with enterohepatic recirculation because of the potential to reduce the efficacy of CellCept. Some degree of enterohepatic recirculation is anticipated following intravenous administration of CellCept.

The risk: benefit of mycophenolate mofetil in combination with tacrolimus or sirolimus has not been established (see also section 4.5).

4.5 Interaction with other medicinal products and other forms of interaction

Interaction studies have only been performed in adults.

Aciclovir: higher aciclovir plasma concentrations were observed when mycophenolate mofetil was administered with aciclovir in comparison to the administration of aciclovir alone. The changes in MPAG (the phenolic glucuronide of MPA) pharmacokinetics (MPAG increased by 8 %) were minimal and are not considered clinically significant. Because MPAG plasma concentrations are increased in the presence of renal impairment, as are aciclovir concentrations, the potential exists for mycophenolate mofetil and aciclovir, or its prodrugs, e.g. valaciclovir, to compete for tubular secretion, and further increases in concentrations of both substances may occur.

Cholestyramine: following single dose, oral administration of 1.5 g of mycophenolate mofetil to normal healthy subjects pre-treated with 4 g TID of cholestyramine for 4 days, there was a 40 % reduction in the AUC of MPA. (see section 4.4, and section 5.2). Caution should be used during concomitant administration because of the potential to reduce efficacy of CellCept.

Medicinal products that interfere with enterohepatic circulation: caution should be used with medicinal products that interfere with enterohepatic circulation because of their potential to reduce the efficacy of CellCept.

Ciclosporin A: ciclosporin A (CsA) pharmacokinetics are unaffected by mycophenolate mofetil.

In contrast, if concomitant ciclosporin treatment is stopped, an increase in MPA AUC of around 30% should be expected.

Ganciclovir: based on the results of a single dose administration study of recommended doses of oral mycophenolate and IV ganciclovir and the known effects of renal impairment on the pharmacokinetics of CellCept (see section 4.2) and ganciclovir, it is anticipated that co-administration of these agents (which compete for mechanisms of renal tubular secretion) will result in increases in MPAG and ganciclovir concentration. No substantial alteration of MPA pharmacokinetics is anticipated and CellCept dose adjustment is not required. In patients with renal impairment in which CellCept and ganciclovir or its prodrugs, e.g. valganciclovir, are co-administered, the dose recommendations for ganciclovir should be observed and patients should be monitored carefully.

Oral contraceptives: the pharmacokinetics and pharmacodynamics of oral contraceptives were unaffected by coadministration of CellCept (see also section 5.2).

Rifampicin: in patients not also taking ciclosporin, concomitant administration of CellCept and rifampicin resulted in a decrease in MPA exposure (AUC0-12h) of 18% to 70%. It is recommended to monitor MPA exposure levels and to adjust CellCept doses accordingly to maintain clinical efficacy when rifampicin is administered concomitantly.

Sirolimus: in renal transplant patients, concomitant administration of CellCept and CsA resulted in reduced MPA exposures by 30-50% compared with patients receiving the combination of sirolimus and similar doses of CellCept (see also section 4.4).

Sevelamer: decrease in MPA Cmax and AUC0-12 by 30% and 25%, respectively, were observed when CellCept was concomitantly administered with sevelamer without any clinical consequences (i.e. graft rejection). It is recommended, however, to administer CellCept at least one hour before or three hours after sevelamer intake to minimise the impact on the absorption of MPA. There is no data on CellCept with phosphate binders other than sevelamer.

Trimethoprim/sulfamethoxazole: no effect on the bioavailability of MPA was observed.

Norfloxacin and metronidazole: in healthy volunteers, no significant interaction was observed when CellCept was concomitantly administered with norfloxacin and metronidazole separately. However, norfloxacin and metronidazole combined reduced the MPA exposure by approximately 30 % following a single dose of CellCept.

Ciprofloxacin and amoxicillin plus clavulanic acid: Reductions in pre-dose (trough) MPA concentrations of about 50% have been reported in renal transplant recipients in the days immediately following commencement of oral ciprofloxacin or amoxicillin plus clavulanic acid. This effect tended to diminish with continued antibiotic use and to cease within a few days of their discontinuation. The change in predose level may not accurately represent changes in overall MPA exposure. Therefore, a change in the dose of CellCept should not normally be necessary in the absence of clinical evidence of graft dysfunction. However, close clinical monitoring should be performed during the combination and shortly after antibiotic treatment.

Tacrolimus: in hepatic transplant patients initiated on CellCept and tacrolimus, the AUC and C_{max} of MPA, the active metabolite of CellCept, were not significantly affected by coadministration with tacrolimus. In contrast, there was an increase of approximately 20 % in tacrolimus AUC when multiple doses of CellCept (1.5 g BID) were administered to patients taking tacrolimus. However, in renal transplant patients, tacrolimus concentration did not appear to be altered by CellCept (see also section 4.4).

Other interactions: co-administration of probenecid with mycophenolate mofetil in monkeys raises plasma AUC of MPAG by 3-fold. Thus, other substances known to undergo renal tubular secretion may compete with MPAG, and thereby raise plasma concentrations of MPAG or the other substance undergoing tubular secretion.

Live vaccines: live vaccines should not be given to patients with an impaired immune response. The antibody response to other vaccines may be diminished (see also section 4.4).

4.6 Pregnancy and lactation

It is recommended that CellCept therapy should not be initiated until a negative pregnancy test has been obtained. Effective contraception must be used before beginning CellCept therapy, during therapy, and for six weeks following discontinuation of therapy (see section 4.5). Patients should be instructed to consult their physician immediately should pregnancy occur.

The use of CellCept is not recommended during pregnancy and should be reserved for cases where no more suitable alternative treatment is available. CellCept should be used in pregnant women only if the potential benefit outweighs the potential risk to the foetus. There is limited data from the use of CellCept in pregnant women. However, congenital malformations including ear malformations, i.e. abnormally formed or absent external/middle ear, have been reported in children of patients exposed to CellCept in combination with other immunosuppressants during pregnancy. Cases of spontaneous abortions have been reported in patients exposed to CellCept. Studies in animals have shown reproductive toxicity (see section 5.3).

Mycophenolate mofetil has been shown to be excreted in the milk of lactating rats. It is not known whether this substance is excreted in human milk. Because of the potential for serious adverse reactions to mycophenolate mofetil in breast-fed infants, CellCept is contraindicated in nursing mothers (see section 4.3).

4.7 Effects on ability to drive and use machines

No studies on the effects on the ability to drive and use machines have been performed. The pharmacodynamic profile and the reported adverse reactions indicate that an effect is unlikely.

4.8 Undesirable effects

The following undesirable effects cover adverse reactions from clinical trials:

The principal adverse reactions associated with the administration of CellCept in combination with ciclosporin and corticosteroids include diarrhoea, leucopenia, sepsis and vomiting, and there is evidence of a higher frequency of certain types of infections (see section 4.4). The adverse reaction profile associated with the administration of CellCept 500 mg powder for concentrate for solution for infusion has been shown to be similar to that observed after oral administration.

Malignancies:

Patients receiving immunosuppressive regimens involving combinations of medicinal products, including CellCept, are at increased risk of developing lymphomas and other malignancies, particularly of the skin (see section 4.4). Lymphoproliferative disease or lymphoma developed in 0.6 % of patients receiving CellCept (2 g or 3 g daily) in combination with other immunosuppressants in controlled clinical trials of renal (2 g data), cardiac and hepatic transplant patients followed for at least 1 year. Non-melanoma skin carcinomas occurred in 3.6 % of patients; other types of malignancy occurred in 1.1 % of patients. Three-year safety data in renal and cardiac transplant patients did not reveal any unexpected changes in incidence of malignancy compared to the 1-year data. Hepatic transplant patients were followed for at least 1 year, but less than 3 years.

Opportunistic infections:

All transplant patients are at increased risk of opportunistic infections; the risk increased with total immunosuppressive load (see section 4.4). The most common opportunistic infections in patients receiving CellCept (2 g or 3 g daily) with other immunosuppressants in controlled clinical trials of renal (2 g data), cardiac and hepatic transplant patients followed for at least 1 year were candida mucocutaneous, CMV viraemia/syndrome and Herpes simplex. The proportion of patients with CMV viraemia/syndrome was 13.5 %.

Elderly patients (⩾ 65 years):

Elderly patients (⩾ 65 years) may generally be at increased risk of adverse reactions due to immunosuppression. Elderly patients receiving CellCept as part of a combination immunosuppressive regimen, may be at increased risk of certain infections (including cytomegalovirus tissue invasive disease) and possibly gastrointestinal haemorrhage and pulmonary oedema, compared to younger individuals.

Other adverse reactions:

The following data refer to the safety experience of oral CellCept in renal transplant patients. Data in hepatic transplant patients are based on i.v. dosing of CellCept for up to 14 days followed by oral dosing. Adverse reactions, probably or possibly related to CellCept, reported in ⩾1/10 and in ⩾1/100 to <1/10 of patients treated with CellCept in the controlled clinical trials of renal (2 g data) and hepatic transplant patients are listed in the following table.

Adverse Reactions, Probably or Possibly Related to CellCept, Reported in Patients Treated with CellCept in Renal and Hepatic Clinical Trials when Used in Combination with Ciclosporin and Corticosteroids

Within the system organ classes, undesirable effects are listed under headings of frequency, using the following categories: very common (⩾1/10); common (⩾1/100 to <1/10); uncommon (⩾1/1,000 to <1/100); rare (⩾1/10,000 to <1/1,000); very rare (<1/10,000), not known (cannot be estimated form the available data). Within each frequency grouping, undesirable effects are presented in order of decreasing seriousness.

System organ class		Adverse drug reactions
Infections and infestations	Very common	Sepsis, gastrointestinal candidiasis, urinary tract infection, herpes simplex, herpes zoster
	Common	Pneumonia, influenza, respiratory tract infection, respiratory moniliasis, gastrointestinal infection, candidiasis, gastroenteritis, infection, bronchitis, pharyngitis, sinusitis, fungal skin infection, skin candida, vaginal candidiasis, rhinitis
Neoplasms benign, malignant and unspecified (incl cysts and polyps)	Very common	-
	Common	Skin cancer, benign neoplasm of skin
Blood and lymphatic system disorders	Very common	Leucopenia, thrombocytopenia, anaemia
	Common	Pancytopenia, leucocytosis
Metabolism and nutrition disorders	Very common	-
	Common	Acidosis, hyperkalaemia, hypokalaemia, hyperglycaemia, hypomagnesaemia, hypocalcaemia, hypercholesterolaemia, hyperlipidaemia, hypophosphataemia, anorexia
Psychiatric disorders	Very common	-
	Common	Depression, thinking abnormal, insomnia
Nervous system disorders	Very common	-
	Common	Convulsion, hypertonia, tremor, somnolence, headache, paraesthesia
Cardiac disorders	Very common	-
	Common	Tachycardia
Vascular disorders	Very common	-
	Common	Hypotension, hypertension
Respiratory, thoracic and mediastinal disorders	Very common	-
	Common	Pleural effusion, dyspnoea, cough
Gastrointestinal disorders	Very common	Vomiting, abdominal pain, diarrhoea, nausea
	Common	Gastrointestinal haemorrhage, peritonitis, ileus, colitis, gastric ulcer, duodenal ulcer, gastritis, oesophagitis, stomatitis, constipation, dyspepsia, flatulence
Hepatobiliary disorders	Very common	-
	Common	Hepatitis
Skin and subcutaneous tissue disorders	Very common	-
	Common	Rash, acne, alopecia,
Musculoskeletal and connective Tissue disorders	Very common	-
	Common	Arthralgia
Renal and urinary disorders	Very common	-
	Common	Renal impairment
General disorders and administration site conditions	Very common	-
	Common	Oedema, pyrexia, chills, pain, malaise, asthenia,
Investigations	Very common	-
	Common	Hepatic enzyme increased, blood creatinine increased, blood lactate dehydrogenase increased, blood alkaline phosphatase increased, weight decreased

Note: 501 (2 g CellCept daily) and 277 (2 g IV / 3 g oral CellCept daily) patients were treated in Phase III studies for the prevention of rejection in renal and hepatic transplantation, respectively.

Adverse reactions attributable to peripheral venous infusion were phlebitis and thrombosis, both observed at 4 % in patients treated with CellCept 500 mg powder for concentrate for solution for infusion.

The following undesirable effects cover adverse reactions from post-marketing experience:

Adverse reactions reported during post-marketing with CellCept are similar to those seen in the controlled renal and hepatic transplant studies. Additional adverse reactions reported during post-marketing experience with CellCept are described below with the frequencies reported within brackets if known.

Gastrointestinal: gingival hyperplasia ($\geqslant$1/100 to $<$1/10), colitis including cytomegalovirus colitis, ($\geqslant$1/100 to $<$1/10), pancreatitis ($\geqslant$1/100 to $<$1/10) and intestinal villous atrophy.

Disorders related to immunosuppression: serious life-threatening infections including meningitis, endocarditis tuberculosis and atypical mycobacterial infection. Cases of BK virus associated nephropathy, as well as cases of JC virus associated progressive multifocal leucoencephalopathy (PML), have been reported in patients treated with immunosuppressants, including CellCept.

Agranulocytosis ($\geqslant$1/1000 to $<$1/100) and neutropenia have been reported; therefore regular monitoring of patients taking CellCept is advised (see section 4.4). There have been reports of aplastic anaemia and bone marrow depression in patients treated with CellCept, some of which have been fatal.

Blood and lymphatic system disorder:

Cases of pure red cell aplasia (PRCA) have been reported in patients treated with CellCept (see section 4.4).

Isolated cases of abnormal neutrophil morphology, including the acquired Pelger-Huet anomaly, have been observed in patients treated with CellCept. These changes are not associated with impaired neutrophil function. These changes may suggest a 'left shift' in the maturity of neutrophils in haematological investigations, which may be mistakenly interpreted as a sign of infection in immunosuppressed patients such as those that receive CellCept.

Hypersensitivity: Hypersensitivity reactions, including angioneurotic oedema and anaphylactic reaction, have been reported.

Congenital disorders: see further details in section 4.6.

4.9 Overdose

Reports of overdoses with mycophenolate mofetil have been received from clinical trials and during post-marketing experience. In many of these cases, no adverse events were reported. In those overdose cases in which adverse events were reported, the events fall within the known safety profile of the medicinal product.

It is expected that an overdose of mycophenolate mofetil could possibly result in oversuppression of the immune system and increase susceptibility to infections and bone marrow suppression (see section 4.4). If neutropenia develops, dosing with CellCept should be interrupted or the dose reduced (see section 4.4).

Haemodialysis would not be expected to remove clinically significant amounts of MPA or MPAG. Bile acid sequestrants, such as cholestyramine, can remove MPA by decreasing the enterohepatic re-circulation of the drug (see section 5.2).

5. PHARMACOLOGICAL PROPERTIES

5.1 Pharmacodynamic properties

Pharmacotherapeutic group: immunosuppressive agents ATC code L04AA06

Mycophenolate mofetil is the 2-morpholinoethyl ester of MPA. MPA is a potent, selective, uncompetitive and reversible inhibitor of inosine monophosphate dehydrogenase, and therefore inhibits the *de novo* pathway of guanosine nucleotide synthesis without incorporation into DNA. Because T- and B-lymphocytes are critically dependent for their proliferation on *de novo* synthesis of purines whereas other cell types can utilise salvage pathways, MPA has more potent cytostatic effects on lymphocytes than on other cells.

5.2 Pharmacokinetic properties

Following intravenous administration, mycophenolate mofetil undergoes rapid and complete metabolism to the active metabolite, MPA. MPA at clinically relevant concentrations is 97 % bound to plasma albumin. The parent substance mycophenolate mofetil can be measured systemically during intravenous infusion; however, after oral administration it is below the limit of quantitation (0.4 μg/ml).

As a result of enterohepatic recirculation, secondary increases in plasma MPA concentration are usually observed at approximately 6 – 12 hours post-dose. A reduction in the AUC of MPA of approximately 40 % is associated with the co-administration of cholestyramine (4 g TID), indicating that there is a significant amount of enterohepatic recirculation.

MPA is metabolised principally by glucuronyl transferase to form the phenolic glucuronide of MPA (MPAG), which is not pharmacologically active.

A negligible amount of substance is excreted as MPA ($<$ 1 % of dose) in the urine. Orally administered radiolabelled mycophenolate mofetil results in complete recovery of the administered dose, with 93 % of the administered dose recovered in the urine and 6 % recovered in faeces. Most (about 87 %) of the administered dose is excreted in the urine as MPAG.

At clinically encountered concentrations, MPA and MPAG are not removed by haemodialysis. However, at high MPAG plasma concentrations ($>$ 100μg/ml), small amounts of MPAG are removed.

In the early post-transplant period ($<$ 40 days post-transplant), renal, cardiac and hepatic transplant patients had mean MPA AUCs approximately 30 % lower and C_{max} approximately 40 % lower compared to the late post-transplant period (3 – 6 months post-transplant). MPA AUC values obtained following administration of 1 g BID intravenous CellCept to renal transplant patients in the early post-transplant phase are comparable to those observed following 1 g BID oral CellCept. In hepatic transplant patients, administration of 1 g BID intravenous CellCept followed by 1.5 g BID oral CellCept resulted in MPA AUC values similar to those found in renal transplant patients administered 1 g CellCept BID.

Renal impairment:

In a single dose study (6 subjects/group), mean plasma MPA AUC observed in subjects with severe chronic renal impairment (glomerular filtration rate $<$ 25 ml•min^{-1}•1.73 m^{-2}) were 28 – 75 % higher relative to the means observed in normal healthy subjects or subjects with lesser degrees of renal impairment. However, the mean single dose MPAG AUC was 3 – 6 fold higher in subjects with severe renal impairment than in subjects with mild renal impairment or normal healthy subjects, consistent with the known renal elimination of MPAG. Multiple dosing of mycophenolate mofetil in patients with severe chronic renal impairment has not been studied. No data are available for hepatic transplant patients with severe chronic renal impairment.

Delayed renal graft function:

In patients with delayed renal graft function post-transplant, mean MPA AUC (0–12h) was comparable to that seen in post-transplant patients without delayed graft function. Mean plasma MPAG AUC (0-12h) was 2 – 3-fold higher than in post-transplant patients without delayed graft function. There may be a transient increase in the free fraction and concentration of plasma MPA in patients with delayed renal graft function. Dose adjustment of CellCept does not appear to be necessary.

Hepatic impairment:

In volunteers with alcoholic cirrhosis, hepatic MPA glucuronidation processes were relatively unaffected by hepatic parenchymal disease. Effects of hepatic disease on this process probably depend on the particular disease. However, hepatic disease with predominantly biliary damage, such as primary biliary cirrhosis, may show a different effect.

Elderly patients ($\geqslant$ 65 years):

Pharmacokinetic behaviour of CellCept in the elderly has not been formally evaluated.

Oral contraceptives:

The pharmacokinetics of oral contraceptives were unaffected by coadministration of CellCept (see also section 4.5). A study of the coadministration of CellCept (1 g bid) and combined oral contraceptives containing ethinylestradiol (0.02 mg to 0.04 mg) and levonorgestrel (0.05 mg to 0.15 mg), desogestrel (0.15 mg) or gestodene (0.05 mg to 0.10 mg) conducted in 18 non-transplant women (not taking other immunosuppressants) over 3 consecutive menstrual cycles showed no clinically relevant influence of CellCept on the ovulation suppressing action of the oral contraceptives. Serum levels of LH, FSH and progesterone were not significantly affected.

5.3 Preclinical safety data

In experimental models, mycophenolate mofetil was not tumourigenic. The highest dose tested in the animal carcinogenicity studies resulted in approximately 2 – 3 times the systemic exposure (AUC or C_{max}) observed in renal transplant patients at the recommended clinical dose of 2 g/day.

Two genotoxicity assays (*in vitro* mouse lymphoma assay and *in vivo* mouse bone marrow micronucleus test) showed a potential of mycophenolate mofetil to cause chromosomal aberrations. These effects can be related to the pharmacodynamic mode of action, i.e. inhibition of nucleotide synthesis in sensitive cells. Other *in vitro* tests for detection of gene mutation did not demonstrate genotoxic activity.

Mycophenolate mofetil had no effect on fertility of male rats at oral doses up to 20 mg•kg^{-1}•day^{-1}. The systemic exposure at this dose represents 2 – 3 times the clinical exposure at the recommended clinical dose of 2 g/day. In a female fertility and reproduction study conducted in rats, oral doses of 4.5 mg•kg^{-1}•day^{-1} caused malformations (including anophthalmia, agnathia, and hydrocephaly) in the first generation offspring in the absence of maternal toxicity. The systemic exposure at this dose was approximately 0.5 times the clinical exposure at the recommended clinical dose of 2 g/day. No effects on fertility or reproductive parameters were evident in the dams or in the subsequent generation.

In teratology studies in rats and rabbits, foetal resorptions and malformations occurred in rats at 6 mg•kg^{-1}•day^{-1} (including anophthalmia, agnathia, and hydrocephaly) and in rabbits at 90 mg•kg^{-1}•day^{-1} (including cardiovascular and renal anomalies, such as ectopia cordis and ectopic kidneys, and diaphragmatic and umbilical hernia), in the absence of maternal toxicity. The systemic exposure at these levels is approximately equivalent to or less than 0.5 times the clinical exposure at the recommended clinical dose of 2 g/day.

Refer to section 4.6.

The haematopoietic and lymphoid systems were the primary organs affected in toxicology studies conducted with mycophenolate mofetil in the rat, mouse, dog and monkey. These effects occurred at systemic exposure levels that are equivalent to or less than the clinical exposure at the recommended dose of 2 g/day. Gastrointestinal effects were observed in the dog at systemic exposure levels equivalent to or less than the clinical exposure at the recommended dose. Gastrointestinal and renal effects consistent with dehydration were also observed in the monkey at the highest dose (systemic exposure levels equivalent to or greater than clinical exposure). The non-clinical toxicity profile of mycophenolate mofetil appears to be consistent with adverse events observed in human clinical trials which now provide safety data of more relevance to the patient population (see section 4.8).

6. PHARMACEUTICAL PARTICULARS

6.1 List of excipients

CellCept 500 mg powder for concentrate for solution for infusion:

polysorbate 80

citric acid

hydrochloric acid

sodium chloride.

6.2 Incompatibilities

CellCept 500 mg powder for concentrate for solution for infusion solution should not be mixed or administered concurrently via the same catheter with other intravenous medicinal products or infusion admixtures.

This medicinal product must not be mixed with other medicinal products except those mentioned in section 6.6.

6.3 Shelf life

Powder for concentrate for solution for infusion: 3 years.

Reconstituted solution and infusion solution: If the infusion solution is not prepared immediately prior to administration, the commencement of administration of the infusion solution should be within 3 hours from reconstitution and dilution of the medicinal product.

6.4 Special precautions for storage

Powder for concentrate for solution for infusion: Do not store above 30°C.

Reconstituted solution and infusion solution: Store at 15 – 30°C.

6.5 Nature and contents of container

20 ml type I clear glass vials with grey butyl rubber stopper and aluminium seals with plastic flip-off caps. CellCept 500 mg powder for concentrate for solution for infusion is available in packs containing 4 vials.

6.6 Special precautions for disposal and other handling

Preparation of Infusion Solution (6 mg/ml)

CellCept 500 mg powder for concentrate for solution for infusion does not contain an antibacterial preservative; therefore, reconstitution and dilution of the product must be performed under aseptic conditions.

CellCept 500 mg powder for concentrate for solution for infusion must be prepared in two steps: the first step is a reconstitution step with glucose intravenous infusion 5 % and the second step is a dilution step with glucose intravenous infusion 5 %. A detailed description of the preparation is given below:

Step 1

a. Two vials of CellCept 500 mg powder for concentrate for solution for infusion are used for preparing each 1 g dose. Reconstitute the content of each vial by injecting 14 ml of glucose intravenous infusion 5 %.

b. Gently shake the vial to dissolve the medicinal product yielding a slightly yellow solution.

c. Inspect the resulting solution for particulate matter and discoloration prior to further dilution. Discard the vial if particulate matter or discoloration is observed.

Step 2

a. Further dilute the content of the two reconstituted vials (approx. 2 × 15 ml) into 140 ml of glucose intravenous infusion 5 %. The final concentration of the solution is 6 mg/ml mycophenolate mofetil.

b. Inspect the infusion solution for particulate matter or discoloration. Discard the infusion solution if particulate matter or discoloration is observed.

If the infusion solution is not prepared immediately prior to administration, the commencement of administration of the infusion solution should be within 3 hours from reconstitution and dilution of the medicinal product. Keep solutions at 15 – 30° C.

Because mycophenolate mofetil has demonstrated teratogenic effects in rats and rabbits, avoid direct contact of prepared solutions of CellCept 500 mg powder for concentrate for solution for infusion with skin or mucous membranes. If such contact occurs, wash thoroughly with soap and water; rinse eyes with plain water.

Any unused product or waste material should be disposed of in accordance with local requirements.

7. MARKETING AUTHORISATION HOLDER

Roche Registration Limited

6 Falcon Way

Shire Park

Welwyn Garden City

AL7 1TW

United Kingdom

8. MARKETING AUTHORISATION NUMBER(S)

EU/1/96/005/005 CellCept (4 vials)

9. DATE OF FIRST AUTHORISATION/RENEWAL OF THE AUTHORISATION

Date of first authorisation: 14 February 1996

Date of latest renewal: 14 February 2006

10. DATE OF REVISION OF THE TEXT

29 May 2009

LEGAL STATUS

POM

Detailed information on this medicinal product is available on the website of the European Medicines Agency (EMEA) http://www.emea.europa.eu/

Cellcept 500mg Tablets

(Roche Products Limited)

1. NAME OF THE MEDICINAL PRODUCT

CellCept 500 mg tablets.

2. QUALITATIVE AND QUANTITATIVE COMPOSITION

Each tablet contains 500 mg mycophenolate mofetil.

For a full list of excipients, see section 6.1.

3. PHARMACEUTICAL FORM

Film coated tablets.

CellCept tablets: lavender coloured caplet-shaped tablet, engraved with "CellCept 500" on one side and "Company logo" on the other.

4. CLINICAL PARTICULARS

4.1 Therapeutic indications

CellCept is indicated in combination with ciclosporin and corticosteroids for the prophylaxis of acute transplant rejection in patients receiving allogeneic renal, cardiac or hepatic transplants.

4.2 Posology and method of administration

Treatment with CellCept should be initiated and maintained by appropriately qualified transplant specialists.

Use in renal transplant:

Adults: oral CellCept should be initiated within 72 hours following transplantation. The recommended dose in renal transplant patients is 1 g administered twice daily (2 g daily dose).

Children and adolescents (aged 2 to 18 years): the recommended dose of mycophenolate mofetil is 600 mg/m^2 administered orally twice daily (up to a maximum of 2 g daily). CellCept tablets should only be prescribed to patients with a body surface area greater than 1.5 m^2, at a dose of 1 g twice daily (2 g daily dose). As some adverse reactions occur with greater frequency in this age group (see section 4.8) compared with adults, temporary dose reduction or interruption may be required; these will need to take into account relevant clinical factors including severity of reaction.

Children (< 2 years): there are limited safety and efficacy data in children below the age of 2 years. These are insufficient to make dosage recommendations and therefore use in this age group is not recommended.

Use in cardiac transplant:

Adults: oral CellCept should be initiated within 5 days following transplantation. The recommended dose in cardiac transplant patients is 1.5 g administered twice daily (3 g daily dose).

Children: no data are available for paediatric cardiac transplant patients.

Use in hepatic transplant:

Adults: IV CellCept should be administered for the first 4 days following hepatic transplant, with oral CellCept initiated as soon after this as it can be tolerated. The recommended oral dose in hepatic transplant patients is 1.5 g administered twice daily (3 g daily dose).

Children: no data are available for paediatric hepatic transplant patients.

Use in elderly (≥ 65 years): the recommended dose of 1 g administered twice a day for renal transplant patients and 1.5 g twice a day for cardiac or hepatic transplant patients is appropriate for the elderly.

Use in renal impairment: in renal transplant patients with severe chronic renal impairment (glomerular filtration rate < 25 ml•min^{-1}•1.73 m^{-2}), outside the immediate post-transplant period, doses greater than 1 g administered twice a day should be avoided. These patients should also be carefully observed. No dose adjustments are needed in patients experiencing delayed renal graft function post-operatively (see section 5.2). No data are available for cardiac or hepatic transplant patients with severe chronic renal impairment.

Use in severe hepatic impairment: no dose adjustments are needed for renal transplant patients with severe hepatic parenchymal disease. No data are available for cardiac transplant patients with severe hepatic parenchymal disease.

Treatment during rejection episodes: MPA (mycophenolic acid) is the active metabolite of mycophenolate mofetil. Renal transplant rejection does not lead to changes in MPA pharmacokinetics; dosage reduction or interruption of CellCept is not required. There is no basis for CellCept dose adjustment following cardiac transplant rejection. No pharmacokinetic data are available during hepatic transplant rejection.

4.3 Contraindications

Hypersensitivity reactions to CellCept have been observed (see section 4.8). Therefore, CellCept is contraindicated in patients with a hypersensitivity to mycophenolate mofetil or mycophenolic acid.

CellCept is contraindicated in women who are breastfeeding (see section 4.6).

For information on use in pregnancy and contraceptive requirements see section 4.6.

4.4 Special warnings and precautions for use

Patients receiving immunosuppressive regimens involving combinations of medicinal products, including CellCept, are at increased risk of developing lymphomas and other malignancies, particularly of the skin (see section 4.8). The risk appears to be related to the intensity and duration of immunosuppression rather than to the use of any specific agent. As general advice to minimise the risk for skin cancer, exposure to sunlight and UV light should be limited by wearing protective clothing and using a sunscreen with a high protection factor.

Patients receiving CellCept should be instructed to report immediately any evidence of infection, unexpected bruising, bleeding or any other manifestation of bone marrow depression.

Patients treated with immunosuppressants, including CellCept, are at increased risk for opportunistic infections (bacterial, fungal, viral and protozoal), fatal infections and sepsis (see section 4.8). Among the opportunistic infections are BK virus associated nephropathy and JC virus associated progressive multifocal leukoencephalopathy (PML). These infections are often related to a high total immunosuppressive burden and may lead to serious or fatal conditions that physicians should consider in the differential diagnosis in immunosuppressed patients with deteriorating renal function or neurological symptoms.

Patients receiving CellCept should be monitored for neutropenia, which may be related to CellCept itself, concomitant medications, viral infections, or some combination of these causes. Patients taking CellCept should have complete blood counts weekly during the first month, twice monthly for the second and third months of treatment, then monthly through the first year. If neutropenia develops (absolute neutrophil count < 1.3 × 10^3/µl), it may be appropriate to interrupt or discontinue CellCept.

Cases of pure red cell aplasia (PRCA) have been reported in patients treated with CellCept in combination with other immunosuppressants. The mechanism for mycophenolate mofetil induced PRCA is unknown. PRCA may resolve with dose reduction or cessation of CellCept therapy. Changes to CellCept therapy should only be undertaken under appropriate supervision in transplant recipients in order to minimise the risk of graft rejection (see section 4.8).

Patients should be advised that during treatment with CellCept, vaccinations may be less effective, and the use of live attenuated vaccines should be avoided (see section 4.5). Influenza vaccination may be of value. Prescribers should refer to national guidelines for influenza vaccination.

Because CellCept has been associated with an increased incidence of digestive system adverse events, including infrequent cases of gastrointestinal tract ulceration, haemorrhage and perforation, CellCept should be administered with caution in patients with active serious digestive system disease.

CellCept is an IMPDH (inosine monophosphate dehydrogenase) inhibitor. On theoretical grounds, therefore, it should be avoided in patients with rare hereditary deficiency of hypoxanthine-guanine phosphoribosyl-transferase (HGPRT) such as Lesch-Nyhan and Kelley-Seegmiller syndrome.

It is recommended that CellCept should not be administered concomitantly with azathioprine because such concomitant administration has not been studied.

In view of the significant reduction in the AUC of MPA by cholestyramine, caution should be used in the concomitant administration of CellCept with medicinal products that interfere with enterohepatic recirculation because of the potential to reduce the efficacy of CellCept.

The risk: benefit of mycophenolate mofetil in combination with tacrolimus or sirolimus has not been established (see also section 4.5).

4.5 Interaction with other medicinal products and other forms of interaction

Interaction studies have only been performed in adults.

Aciclovir: higher aciclovir plasma concentrations were observed when mycophenolate mofetil was administered with aciclovir in comparison to the administration of aciclovir alone. The changes in MPAG (the phenolic glucuronide of MPA) pharmacokinetics (MPAG increased by 8 %) were minimal and are not considered clinically significant. Because MPAG plasma concentrations are increased in the presence of renal impairment, as are aciclovir concentrations, the potential exists for mycophenolate mofetil and aciclovir, or its prodrugs, e.g. valaciclovir, to compete for tubular secretion and further increases in concentrations of both substances may occur.

Antacids with magnesium and aluminium hydroxides: absorption of mycophenolate mofetil was decreased when administered with antacids.

Cholestyramine: following single dose administration of 1.5 g of mycophenolate mofetil to normal healthy subjects pre-treated with 4 g TID of cholestyramine for 4 days, there was a 40 % reduction in the AUC of MPA. (see section 4.4 and section 5.2). Caution should be used during concomitant administration because of the potential to reduce efficacy of CellCept.

Medicinal products that interfere with enterohepatic circulation: caution should be used with medicinal products that interfere with enterohepatic circulation because of their potential to reduce the efficacy of CellCept.

Ciclosporin A: ciclosporin A (CsA) pharmacokinetics are unaffected by mycophenolate mofetil.

In contrast, if concomitant ciclosporin treatment is stopped, an increase in MPA AUC of around 30% should be expected.

Ganciclovir: based on the results of a single dose administration study of recommended doses of oral mycophenolate and IV ganciclovir and the known effects of renal impairment on the pharmacokinetics of CellCept (see section 4.2) and ganciclovir, it is anticipated that co-administration of these agents (which compete for mechanisms of renal tubular secretion) will result in increases in MPAG and ganciclovir concentration. No substantial alteration of MPA pharmacokinetics is anticipated and CellCept dose adjustment is not required. In patients with renal impairment in which CellCept and ganciclovir or its prodrugs, e.g. valganciclovir, are co-administered, the dose recommendations for ganciclovir should be observed and patients should be monitored carefully.

Oral contraceptives: the pharmacokinetics and pharmacodynamics of oral contraceptives were unaffected by coadministration of CellCept (see also section 5.2).

Rifampicin: in patients not also taking ciclosporin, concomitant administration of CellCept and rifampicin resulted in a decrease in MPA exposure (AUC0-12h) of 18% to 70%. It is recommended to monitor MPA exposure levels and to adjust CellCept doses accordingly to maintain clinical efficacy when rifampicin is administered concomitantly.

Sirolimus: in renal transplant patients, concomitant administration of CellCept and CsA resulted in reduced MPA exposures by 30-50% compared with patients receiving the combination of sirolimus and similar doses of CellCept (see also section 4.4).

Sevelamer: decrease in MPA C_{max} and AUC0-12 by 30% and 25%, respectively, were observed when CellCept was concomitantly administered with sevelamer without any clinical consequences (i.e. graft rejection). It is recommended, however, to administer CellCept at least one hour before or three hours after sevelamer intake to minimise the impact on the absorption of MPA. There is no data on CellCept with phosphate binders other than sevelamer.

Trimethoprim/sulfamethoxazole: no effect on the bioavailability of MPA was observed.

Norfloxacin and metronidazole: in healthy volunteers, no significant interaction was observed when CellCept was concomitantly administered with norfloxacin and metronidazole separately. However, norfloxacin and metronidazole combined reduced the MPA exposure by approximately 30 % following a single dose of CellCept.

Ciprofloxacin and amoxicillin plus clavulanic acid: Reductions in pre-dose (trough) MPA concentrations of about 50% have been reported in renal transplant recipients in the days immediately following commencement of oral ciprofloxacin or amoxicillin plus clavulanic acid. This effect tended to diminish with continued antibiotic use and to cease within a few days of their discontinuation. The change in predose level may not accurately represent changes in overall MPA exposure. Therefore, a change in the dose of CellCept should not normally be necessary in the absence of clinical evidence of graft dysfunction. However, close clinical monitoring should be performed during the combination and shortly after antibiotic treatment.

Tacrolimus: in hepatic transplant patients initiated on CellCept and tacrolimus, the AUC and C_{max} of MPA, the active metabolite of CellCept, were not significantly affected by coadministration with tacrolimus. In contrast, there was an increase of approximately 20 % in tacrolimus AUC when multiple doses of CellCept (1.5 g BID) were administered to patients taking tacrolimus. However, in renal transplant patients, tacrolimus concentration did not appear to be altered by CellCept (see also section 4.4).

Other interactions: co-administration of probenecid with mycophenolate mofetil in monkeys raises plasma AUC of MPAG by 3-fold. Thus, other substances known to undergo renal tubular secretion may compete with MPAG, and thereby raise plasma concentrations of MPAG or the other substance undergoing tubular secretion.

Live vaccines: live vaccines should not be given to patients with an impaired immune response. The antibody response to other vaccines may be diminished (see also 4.4).

4.6 Pregnancy and lactation

It is recommended that CellCept therapy should not be initiated until a negative pregnancy test has been obtained. Effective contraception must be used before beginning CellCept therapy, during therapy, and for six weeks following discontinuation of therapy (see section 4.5). Patients should be instructed to consult their physician immediately should pregnancy occur.

The use of CellCept is not recommended during pregnancy and should be reserved for cases where no more suitable alternative treatment is available. CellCept should be used in pregnant women only if the potential benefit outweighs the potential risk to the foetus. There is limited data from the use of CellCept in pregnant women. However, congenital malformations including ear malformations, i.e. abnormally formed or absent external/middle ear, have been reported in children of patients exposed to CellCept in combination with other immunosuppressants during pregnancy. Cases of spontaneous abortions have been reported in patients exposed to CellCept. Studies in animals have shown reproductive toxicity (see section 5.3).

Mycophenolate mofetil has been shown to be excreted in the milk of lactating rats. It is not known whether this substance is excreted in human milk. Because of the potential for serious adverse reactions to mycophenolate mofetil in breast-fed infants, CellCept is contraindicated in nursing mothers (see section 4.3).

4.7 Effects on ability to drive and use machines

No studies on the effects on the ability to drive and use machines have been performed. The pharmacodynamic profile and the reported adverse reactions indicate that an effect is unlikely.

4.8 Undesirable effects

The following undesirable effects cover adverse reactions from clinical trials:

The principal adverse reactions associated with the administration of CellCept in combination with ciclosporin and corticosteroids include diarrhoea, leucopenia, sepsis and vomiting, and there is evidence of a higher frequency of certain types of infections (see section 4.4).

Malignancies:

Patients receiving immunosuppressive regimens involving combinations of medicinal products, including CellCept, are at increased risk of developing lymphomas and other malignancies, particularly of the skin (see section 4.4). Lymphoproliferative disease or lymphoma developed in 0.6 % of patients receiving CellCept (2 g or 3 g daily) in combination with other immunosuppressants in controlled clinical trials of renal (2 g data), cardiac and hepatic transplant patients followed for at least 1 year. Non-melanoma skin carcinomas occurred in 3.6 % of patients; other types of malignancy occurred in 1.1 % of patients. Three-year safety data in renal and cardiac transplant patients did not reveal any unexpected changes in incidence of malignancy compared to the 1-year data. Hepatic transplant patients were followed for at least 1 year, but less than 3 years.

Opportunistic infections:

All transplant patients are at increased risk of opportunistic infections; the risk increased with total immunosuppressive load (see section 4.4) The most common opportunistic infections in patients receiving CellCept (2 g or 3 g daily) with other immunosuppressants in controlled clinical trials of renal (2 g data), cardiac and hepatic transplant patients followed for at least 1 year were candida mucocutaneous, CMV viraemia/syndrome and Herpes simplex. The proportion of patients with CMV viraemia/syndrome was 13.5 %.

Children and adolescents (aged 2 to 18 years):

The type and frequency of adverse reactions in a clinical study, which recruited 92 paediatric patients aged 2 to 18 years who were given 600 mg/m^2 mycophenolate mofetil orally twice daily, were generally similar to those observed in adult patients given 1 g CellCept twice daily. However, the following treatment-related adverse events were more frequent in the paediatric population, particularly in children under 6 years of age, when compared to adults: diarrhoea, sepsis, leucopenia, anaemia and infection.

Elderly patients (≥ 65 years):

Elderly patients (≥ 65 years) may generally be at increased risk of adverse reactions due to immunosuppression. Elderly patients receiving CellCept as part of a combination immunosuppressive regimen, may be at increased risk of certain infections (including cytomegalovirus tissue invasive disease) and possibly gastrointestinal haemorrhage and pulmonary oedema, compared to younger individuals.

Other adverse reactions:

Adverse reactions, probably or possibly related to CellCept, reported in ≥1/10 and in ≥1/100 to <1/10 of patients treated with CellCept in the controlled clinical trials of renal (2 g data), cardiac and hepatic transplant patients are listed in the following table.

Adverse Reactions, Probably or Possibly Related to CellCept, Reported in Patients Treated with CellCept in Renal, Cardiac and Hepatic Clinical Trials when Used in Combination with Ciclosporin and Corticosteroids

Within the system organ classes, undesirable effects are listed under headings of frequency, using the following categories: very common (≥1/10); common (≥1/100 to <1/10); uncommon (≥1/1,000 to <1/100); rare (≥1/10,000 to <1/1,000); very rare (<1/10,000), not known (cannot be estimated form the available data). Within each frequency grouping, undesirable effects are presented in order of decreasing seriousness.

System organ class		Adverse drug reactions
Infections and infestations	Very common	Sepsis, gastrointestinal candidiasis, urinary tract infection, herpes simplex, herpes zoster
	Common	Pneumonia, influenza, respiratory tract infection, respiratory moniliasis, gastrointestinal infection, candidiasis, gastroenteritis, infection, bronchitis, pharyngitis, sinusitis, fungal skin infection, skin candida, vaginal candidiasis, rhinitis
Neoplasms benign, malignant and unspecified (incl cysts and polyps)	Very common	-
	Common	Skin cancer, benign neoplasm of skin
Blood and lymphatic system disorders	Very common	Leucopenia, thrombocytopenia, anaemia
	Common	Pancytopenia, leucocytosis
Metabolism and nutrition disorders	Very common	-
	Common	Acidosis, hyperkalaemia, hypokalaemia, hyperglycaemia, hypomagnesaemia, hypocalcaemia, hypercholesterolaemia, hyperlipidaemia, hypophosphataemia, hyperuricaemia, gout, anorexia
Psychiatric disorders	Very common	-
	Common	Agitation, confusional state, depression, anxiety, thinking abnormal, insomnia
Nervous system disorders	Very common	-
	Common	Convulsion, hypertonia, tremor, somnolence, myasthenic syndrome, dizziness, headache, paraesthesia, dysgeusia
Cardiac disorders	Very common	-
	Common	Tachycardia
Vascular disorders	Very common	-
	Common	Hypotension, hypertension, vasodilatation
Respiratory, thoracic and mediastinal disorders	Very common	-
	Common	Pleural effusion, dyspnoea, cough
Gastrointestinal disorders	Very common	Vomiting, abdominal pain, diarrhoea, nausea
	Common	Gastrointestinal haemorrhage, peritonitis, ileus, colitis, gastric ulcer, duodenal ulcer, gastritis, oesophagitis, stomatitis, constipation, dyspepsia, flatulence, eructation
Hepatobiliary disorders	Very common	-
	Common	Hepatitis, jaundice, hyperbilirubinaemia
Skin and subcutaneous tissue disorders	Very common	-
	Common	Skin hypertrophy, rash, acne, alopecia,
Musculoskeletal and connective Tissue disorders	Very common	-
	Common	Arthralgia
Renal and urinary disorders	Very common	-
	Common	Renal impairment

General disorders and administration site conditions	Very common	-
	Common	Oedema, pyrexia, chills, pain, malaise, asthenia,
Investigations	Very common	-
	Common	Hepatic enzyme increased, blood creatinine increased, blood lactate dehydrogenase increased, blood urea increased, blood alkaline phosphatase increased, weight decreased

Note: 501 (2 g CellCept daily), 289 (3 g CellCept daily) and 277 (2 g IV / 3 g oral CellCept daily) patients were treated in Phase III studies for the prevention of rejection in renal, cardiac and hepatic transplantation, respectively.

The following undesirable effects cover adverse reactions from post-marketing experience:

The types of adverse reactions reported during post-marketing with CellCept are similar to those seen in the controlled renal, cardiac and hepatic transplant studies. Additional adverse reactions reported during post-marketing are described below with the frequencies reported within brackets if known.

Gastrointestinal: gingival hyperplasia (≥1/100 to <1/10), colitis including cytomegalovirus colitis, (≥1/100 to <1/10), pancreatitis (≥1/100 to <1/10) and intestinal villous atrophy.

Disorders related to immunosuppression: serious life-threatening infections including meningitis, endocarditis, tuberculosis and atypical mycobacterial infection. Cases of BK virus associated nephropathy, as well as cases of JC virus associated progressive multifocal leucoencephalopathy (PML), have been reported in patients treated with immunosuppressants, including CellCept.

Agranulocytosis (≥1/1000 to <1/100) and neutropenia have been reported; therefore, regular monitoring of patients taking CellCept is advised (see section 4.4). There have been reports of aplastic anaemia and bone marrow depression in patients treated with CellCept, some of which have been fatal.

Blood and lymphatic system disorder:

Cases of pure red cell aplasia (PRCA) have been reported in patients treated with CellCept (see section 4.4).

Isolated cases of abnormal neutrophil morphology, including the acquired Pelger-Huet anomaly, have been observed in patients treated with CellCept. These changes are not associated with impaired neutrophil function. These changes may suggest a 'left shift' in the maturity of neutrophils in haematological investigations, which may be mistakenly interpreted as a sign of infection in immunosuppressed patients such as those that receive CellCept.

Hypersensitivity: Hypersensitivity reactions, including angioneurotic oedema and anaphylactic reaction have been reported.

Congenital disorders: see further details in section 4.6.

4.9 Overdose

Reports of overdoses with mycophenolate mofetil have been received from clinical trials and during post-marketing experience. In many of these cases, no adverse events were reported. In those overdose cases in which adverse events were reported, the events fall within the known safety profile of the medicinal product.

It is expected that an overdose of mycophenolate mofetil could possibly result in oversuppression of the immune system and increase susceptibility to infections and bone marrow suppression (see section 4.4). If neutropenia develops, dosing with CellCept should be interrupted or the dose reduced (see section 4.4).

Haemodialysis would not be expected to remove clinically significant amounts of MPA or MPAG. Bile acid sequestrants, such as cholestyramine, can remove MPA by decreasing the enterohepatic re-circulation of the drug (see section 5.2).

5. PHARMACOLOGICAL PROPERTIES

5.1 Pharmacodynamic properties

Pharmacotherapeutic group: immunosuppressive agents ATC code L04AA06

Mycophenolate mofetil is the 2-morpholinoethyl ester of MPA. MPA is a potent, selective, uncompetitive and reversible inhibitor of inosine monophosphate dehydrogenase, and therefore inhibits the *de novo* pathway of guanosine nucleotide synthesis without incorporation into DNA. Because T- and B-lymphocytes are critically dependent for their proliferation on *de novo* synthesis of purines whereas other cell types can utilise salvage pathways, MPA has more potent cytostatic effects on lymphocytes than on other cells.

5.2 Pharmacokinetic properties

Following oral administration, mycophenolate mofetil undergoes rapid and extensive absorption and complete presystemic metabolism to the active metabolite, MPA. As evidenced by suppression of acute rejection following renal transplantation, the immunosuppressant activity of CellCept is correlated with MPA concentration. The mean bioavailability of oral mycophenolate mofetil, based on MPA AUC, is 94 % relative to IV mycophenolate mofetil. Food had no effect on the extent of absorption (MPA AUC) of mycophenolate mofetil when administered at doses of 1.5 g BID to renal transplant patients. However, MPA C_{max} was decreased by 40 % in the presence of food. Mycophenolate mofetil is not measurable systemically in plasma following oral administration. MPA at clinically relevant concentrations, is 97 % bound to plasma albumin.

As a result of enterohepatic recirculation, secondary increases in plasma MPA concentration are usually observed at approximately 6 – 12 hours post-dose. A reduction in the AUC of MPA of approximately 40 % is associated with the co-administration of cholestyramine (4 g TID), indicating that there is a significant amount of enterohepatic recirculation.

MPA is metabolised principally by glucuronyl transferase to form the phenolic glucuronide of MPA (MPAG), which is not pharmacologically active.

A negligible amount of substance is excreted as MPA (< 1 % of dose) in the urine. Orally administered radiolabelled mycophenolate mofetil results in complete recovery of the administered dose with 93 % of the administered dose recovered in the urine and 6 % recovered in the faeces. Most (about 87 %) of the administered dose is excreted in the urine as MPAG.

At clinically encountered concentrations, MPA and MPAG are not removed by haemodialysis. However, at high MPAG plasma concentrations (>100µg/ml), small amounts of MPAG are removed.

In the early post-transplant period (< 40 days post-transplant), renal, cardiac and hepatic transplant patients had mean MPA AUCs approximately 30 % lower and C_{max} approximately 40 % lower compared to the late post-transplant period (3 – 6 months post-transplant).

Renal impairment:

In a single dose study (6 subjects/group), mean plasma MPA AUC observed in subjects with severe chronic renal impairment (glomerular filtration rate < 25 ml•min^{-1}•1.73 m^{-2}) were 28 – 75 % higher relative to the means observed in normal healthy subjects or subjects with lesser degrees of renal impairment. However, the mean single dose MPAG AUC was 3 – 6-fold higher in subjects with severe renal impairment than in subjects with mild renal impairment or normal healthy subjects, consistent with the known renal elimination of MPAG. Multiple dosing of mycophenolate mofetil in patients with severe chronic renal impairment has not been studied. No data are available for cardiac or hepatic transplant patients with severe chronic renal impairment.

Delayed renal graft function:

In patients with delayed renal graft function post-transplant, mean MPA AUC (0–12h) was comparable to that seen in post-transplant patients without delayed graft function. Mean plasma MPAG AUC (0-12h) was 2 – 3-fold higher than in post-transplant patients without delayed graft function. There may be a transient increase in the free fraction and concentration of plasma MPA in patients with delayed renal graft function. Dose adjustment of CellCept does not appear to be necessary.

Hepatic impairment:

In volunteers with alcoholic cirrhosis, hepatic MPA glucuronidation processes were relatively unaffected by hepatic parenchymal disease. Effects of hepatic disease on this process probably depend on the particular disease. However, hepatic disease with predominantly biliary damage, such as primary biliary cirrhosis, may show a different effect.

Children and adolescents (aged 2 to 18 years):

Pharmacokinetic parameters were evaluated in 49 paediatric renal transplant patients given 600 mg/m^2 mycophenolate mofetil orally twice daily. This dose achieved MPA AUC values similar to those seen in adult renal transplant patients receiving CellCept at a dose of 1 g bid in the early and late post-transplant period. MPA AUC values across age groups were similar in the early and late post-transplant period.

Elderly patients (≥ 65 years):

Pharmacokinetic behaviour of CellCept in the elderly has not been formally evaluated.

Oral contraceptives:

The pharmacokinetics of oral contraceptives were unaffected by coadministration of CellCept (see also section 4.5). A study of the coadministration of CellCept (1 g bid) and combined oral contraceptives containing ethinylestradiol (0.02 mg to 0.04 mg) and levonorgestrel (0.05 mg to 0.15 mg), desogestrel (0.15 mg) or gestodene (0.05 mg to 0.10 mg) conducted in 18 non-transplant women (not taking other immunosuppressants) over 3 consecutive menstrual cycles showed no clinically relevant influence of CellCept on the ovulation suppressing action of the oral contraceptives. Serum levels of LH, FSH and progesterone were not significantly affected.

5.3 Preclinical safety data

In experimental models, mycophenolate mofetil was not tumourigenic. The highest dose tested in the animal carcinogenicity studies resulted in approximately 2 – 3 times the systemic exposure (AUC or C_{max}) observed in renal transplant patients at the recommended clinical dose of 2 g/day and 1.3 – 2 times the systemic exposure (AUC or C_{max}) observed in cardiac transplant patients at the recommended clinical dose of 3 g/day.

Two genotoxicity assays (*in vitro* mouse lymphoma assay and *in vivo* mouse bone marrow micronucleus test) showed a potential of mycophenolate mofetil to cause chromosomal aberrations. These effects can be related to the pharmacodynamic mode of action, i.e. inhibition of nucleotide synthesis in sensitive cells. Other *in vitro* tests for detection of gene mutation did not demonstrate genotoxic activity.

Mycophenolate mofetil had no effect on fertility of male rats at oral doses up to 20 mg•kg^{-1}•day^{-1}. The systemic exposure at this dose represents 2 – 3 times the clinical exposure at the recommended clinical dose of 2 g/day in renal transplant patients and 1.3 – 2 times the clinical exposure at the recommended clinical dose of 3 g/day in cardiac transplant patients. In a female fertility and reproduction study conducted in rats, oral doses of 4.5 mg•kg^{-1}•day^{-1} caused malformations (including anophthalmia, agnathia, and hydrocephaly) in the first generation offspring in the absence of maternal toxicity. The systemic exposure at this dose was approximately 0.5 times the clinical exposure at the recommended clinical dose of 2 g/day for renal transplant patients and approximately 0.3 times the clinical exposure at the recommended clinical dose of 3 g/day for cardiac transplant patients. No effects on fertility or reproductive parameters were evident in the dams or in the subsequent generation.

In teratology studies in rats and rabbits, foetal resorptions and malformations occurred in rats at

6 mg•kg^{-1}•day^{-1} (including anophthalmia, agnathia, and hydrocephaly) and in rabbits at 90 mg•kg^{-1}•day^{-1} (including cardiovascular and renal anomalies, such as ectopia cordis and ectopic kidneys, and diaphragmatic and umbilical hernia), in the absence of maternal toxicity. The systemic exposure at these levels is approximately equivalent to or less than 0.5 times the clinical exposure at the recommended clinical dose of 2 g/day for renal transplant patients and approximately 0.3 times the clinical exposure at the recommended clinical dose of 3 g/day for cardiac transplant patients.

Refer to section 4.6.

The haematopoietic and lymphoid systems were the primary organs affected in toxicology studies conducted with mycophenolate mofetil in the rat, mouse, dog and monkey. These effects occurred at systemic exposure levels that are equivalent to or less than the clinical exposure at the recommended dose of 2 g/day for renal transplant recipients. Gastrointestinal effects were observed in the dog at systemic exposure levels equivalent to or less than the clinical exposure at the recommended dose. Gastrointestinal and renal effects consistent with dehydration were also observed in the monkey at the highest dose (systemic exposure levels equivalent to or greater than clinical exposure). The nonclinical toxicity profile of mycophenolate mofetil appears to be consistent with adverse events observed in human clinical trials which now provide safety data of more relevance to the patient population (see section 4.8).

6. PHARMACEUTICAL PARTICULARS

6.1 List of excipients

CellCept tablets:

microcrystalline cellulose

polyvidone (K-90)

croscarmellose sodium

magnesium stearate

Tablet coating:

hydroxypropyl methylcellulose

hydroxypropyl cellulose

titanium dioxide (E171)

polyethylene glycol 400

indigo carmine aluminium lake (E132)

red iron oxide (E172)

6.2 Incompatibilities

Not applicable.

6.3 Shelf life

3 years.

6.4 Special precautions for storage

Do not store above 30°C. Keep the blister in the outer carton in order to protect from light.

6.5 Nature and contents of container

CellCept 500 mg tablets: 1 carton contains 50 tablets (in blister packs of 10)

1 carton contains 150 tablets (in blister packs of 10)

6.6 Special precautions for disposal and other handling

Because mycophenolate mofetil has demonstrated teratogenic effects in rats and rabbits, CellCept tablets should not be crushed.

Any unused product or waste material should be disposed of in accordance with local requirements.

7. MARKETING AUTHORISATION HOLDER

Roche Registration Limited
6 Falcon Way
Shire Park
Welwyn Garden City
AL7 1TW
United Kingdom

8. MARKETING AUTHORISATION NUMBER(S)

EU/1/96/005/002 CellCept (50 tablets)
EU/1/96/005/004 CellCept (150 tablets)

9. DATE OF FIRST AUTHORISATION/RENEWAL OF THE AUTHORISATION

Date of first authorisation: 14 February 1996

Date of latest renewal: 14 February 2006

10. DATE OF REVISION OF THE TEXT

29 May 2009

LEGAL STATUS

POM

Detailed information on this medicinal product is available on the website of the European Medicines Agency (EMEA) http://www.emea.europa.eu/

Celluvisc 0.5% w/v, eye drops, solution

(Allergan Ltd)

1. NAME OF THE MEDICINAL PRODUCT

Celluvisc® 0.5% w/v, eye drops, solution, unit dose

2. QUALITATIVE AND QUANTITATIVE COMPOSITION

1 ml contains 5mg carmellose sodium

For excipients, see section 6.1.

3. PHARMACEUTICAL FORM

Eye drops, solution in single-dose container.

Clear, colourless to slightly yellow solution.

4. CLINICAL PARTICULARS

4.1 Therapeutic indications

Tear substitute. Treatment of the symptoms of dry eye.

4.2 Posology and method of administration

Instil 1-2 drops in the affected eye/s 4 times a day or as needed.

Ensure that the single-dose container is intact before use. The eye drop solution should be used immediately after opening.

To avoid contamination do not touch the tip to the eye or any other surface.

If Celluvisc is concomitantly used with other ocular eye medications there must be an interval of at least 15 minutes between the two medications (as displacement of a medication may occur).

The eye drops may be used with contact lenses.

4.3 Contraindications

Hypersensitivity to carmellose sodium or to any of the excipients.

4.4 Special warnings and precautions for use

If irritation, pain, redness or changes in vision occur or if the patient's condition is worsened treatment discontinuation should be considered and a new assessment made.

4.5 Interaction with other medicinal products and other forms of interaction

None known.

For the use of concomitant ocular products, see section 4.2.

4.6 Pregnancy and lactation

Due to the negligible systemic exposure and the lack of pharmacological activity Celluvisc can be used during pregnancy and lactation.

4.7 Effects on ability to drive and use machines

Celluvisc is not expected to cause blurred vision. If individual patients experience transient blurred vision they should be advised not to drive or operate machinery until vision has cleared.

4.8 Undesirable effects

Temporary burning may occur.

4.9 Overdose

Accidental overdose will present no hazard.

5. PHARMACOLOGICAL PROPERTIES

5.1 Pharmacodynamic properties

Pharmacotherapeutic group: Other ophthalmologicals

ATC code: S01XA20

Carmellose sodium has no pharmacological effect. Carmellose sodium has a high viscosity resulting in an increased retention time on the eye.

The excipients in Celluvisc were chosen to mimic the electrolyte constitution of tears.

5.2 Pharmacokinetic properties

Due to the high molecular weight (approx. 90,000 Daltons) carmellose sodium is unlikely to penetrate the cornea.

5.3 Preclinical safety data

There are no preclinical data considered relevant to clinical safety beyond data included in other sections of the SPC.

6. PHARMACEUTICAL PARTICULARS

6.1 List of excipients

Sodium chloride
Sodium lactate
Potassium chloride
Calcium chloride dihydrate
Magnesium chloride hexahydrate
Sodium hydroxide or hydrochloric acid to adjust pH
Purified water

6.2 Incompatibilities

Not applicable.

6.3 Shelf life

18 months.

After first opening: Use immediately.

6.4 Special precautions for storage

Do not store above 25°C.

6.5 Nature and contents of container

0.4 ml in LDPE single-dose container.

Pack sizes: 5, 30 or 90 single-dose containers.

Not all pack sizes may be marketed.

6.6 Special precautions for disposal and other handling

Discard any unused solution in opened container i.e. do not re-use container for subsequent doses.

7. MARKETING AUTHORISATION HOLDER

Allergan Pharmaceuticals Ireland
Castlebar Road
Westport
County Mayo
Ireland

8. MARKETING AUTHORISATION NUMBER(S)

PL 05179/0011

9. DATE OF FIRST AUTHORISATION/RENEWAL OF THE AUTHORISATION

2nd October 2006

10. DATE OF REVISION OF THE TEXT

-

Celluvisc 1.0% w/v, Eye drops, solution

(Allergan Ltd)

1. NAME OF THE MEDICINAL PRODUCT

Celluvisc 1.0% w/v Eye drops, solution, unit dose

2. QUALITATIVE AND QUANTITATIVE COMPOSITION

1 ml contains 10 mg carmellose sodium.

One drop ($\approx$ 0.05 ml) contains 0.5 mg of carmellose sodium.

For a full list of excipients, see section 6.1.

3. PHARMACEUTICAL FORM

Eye drops, solution

A clear, colourless to slightly yellow viscous solution.

4. CLINICAL PARTICULARS

4.1 Therapeutic indications

Treatment of the symptoms of dry eye.

4.2 Posology and method of administration

Instil one or two drops in the affected eye/s as needed.

Ensure that the single-dose container is intact before use. The eye drop solution should be used immediately after opening.

To avoid contamination do not touch the tip to the eye or any other surface.

4.3 Contraindications

Hypersensitivity to the active substance or to any of the excipients.

4.4 Special warnings and precautions for use

If irritation, pain, redness and changes in vision occur or worsen, treatment should be discontinued and a new assessment considered.

Contact lenses should be removed before each application and may be inserted after 15 minutes.

Concomitant ocular medication should be administered 15 minutes prior to the instillation of Celluvisc.

To avoid contamination, do not touch the tip to the eye or any surface. Discard open single dose container after use.

4.5 Interaction with other medicinal products and other forms of interaction

No interaction studies have been performed.

1. No interactions have been observed with Celluvisc. Given the formulation of Celluvisc, no interactions are anticipated.

2. If this product is used concomitantly with other topical eye medications there must be an interval of at least 15 minutes between the two medications.

4.6 Pregnancy and lactation

The constituents of Celluvisc have been used as pharmaceutical agents for many years with no untoward effects. No special precautions are necessary for the use of Celluvisc in pregnancy and lactation.

4.7 Effects on ability to drive and use machines

Celluvisc has minor or moderate influence on the ability to drive and use machines as it may cause transient blurring of vision. Do not drive or use machinery unless vision is clear.

4.8 Undesirable effects

The frequency of undesirable effects is defined as follows:

- Very Common ($\geqslant$ 1/10)
- Common ($\geqslant$1/100, $<$1/10)
- Uncommon ($\geqslant$1/1,000, $<$1/100)
- Rare ($\geqslant$1/10,000, $<$1/1,000)
- Very Rare ($<$1/10,000), not known (cannot be estimated from the available data).

Eye disorders:

Not known: eye irritation, eye pain, vision blurred, lacrimation increased.

4.9 Overdose

Accidental overdose will present no hazard.

5. PHARMACOLOGICAL PROPERTIES

5.1 Pharmacodynamic properties

Pharmacotherapeutic group: Other ophthalmologicals

ATC code: S01XA20

Carmellose sodium has no pharmacological effect. Carmellose sodium has a high viscosity resulting in an increased retention time on the eye.

5.2 Pharmacokinetic properties

Due to the high molecular weight (approx. 90,000 Daltons) carmellose sodium is unlikely to penetrate the cornea.

5.3 Preclinical safety data

No additional information of relevance for the doctor has been obtained from the preclinical testing.

6. PHARMACEUTICAL PARTICULARS

6.1 List of excipients

Sodium chloride
Sodium lactate
Potassium chloride
Calcium chloride
Purified Water

6.2 Incompatibilities

Not applicable.

6.3 Shelf life

2 years.

The eye drop solution should be used immediately after opening. Any unused solution should be discarded.

6.4 Special precautions for storage

Do not store above 25°C.

6.5 Nature and contents of container

Clear, single-dose containers made from low density polyethylene formed with a twist-off tab.

Each unit is filled with 0.4 ml of solution.

Pack sizes: 5, 10, 20, 30, 40, 60 or 90 single-dose containers.

Not all pack sizes may be marketed.

6.6 Special precautions for disposal and other handling

Ensure that the single dose container is intact before use. Discard any unused solution (i.e. once opened do not re-use container for subsequent doses).

7. MARKETING AUTHORISATION HOLDER

Allergan Pharmaceuticals Ireland
Castlebar Road
Westport
County Mayo
IRELAND

8. MARKETING AUTHORISATION NUMBER(S)

PL 05179/0001

9. DATE OF FIRST AUTHORISATION/RENEWAL OF THE AUTHORISATION

Date of first authorisation: 29th January 2001

Date of last renewal: 29th September 2003

10. DATE OF REVISION OF THE TEXT

17th March 2008

Celsentri 150mg and 300mg film-coated tablets

(Pfizer Limited)

1. NAME OF THE MEDICINAL PRODUCT

CELSENTRI▼ 150 mg film-coated tablets.

CELSENTRI▼ 300 mg film-coated tablets.

2. QUALITATIVE AND QUANTITATIVE COMPOSITION

Each film-coated tablet contains 150 mg of maraviroc. Each film-coated tablet contains 300 mg of maraviroc.

Excipients

Each 150mg film-coated tablet contains 0.84 mg of soya lecithin.

Each 300mg film-coated tablet contains 1.68 mg of soya lecithin.

For a full list of excipients, see section 6.1.

3. PHARMACEUTICAL FORM

Film-coated tablet.

Blue, biconvex, oval film-coated tablets debossed with "Pfizer" on one side and "MVC 150" on the other.

Blue, biconvex, oval film-coated tablets debossed with "Pfizer" on one side and "MVC 300" on the other.

4. CLINICAL PARTICULARS

4.1 Therapeutic indications

CELSENTRI, in combination with other antiretroviral medicinal products, is indicated for treatment-experienced adult patients infected with only CCR5-tropic HIV-1 detectable (see section 4.2).

This indication is based on safety and efficacy data from two double-blind, placebo-controlled trials in treatment-experienced patients (see section 5.1).

4.2 Posology and method of administration

Therapy should be initiated by a physician experienced in the management of HIV infection.

Before taking CELSENTRI it has to be confirmed that only CCR5-tropic HIV-1 is detectable (i.e. CXCR4 or dual/mixed tropic virus not detected) using an adequately validated and sensitive detection method on a newly drawn blood sample. The Monogram Trofile assay was used in the clinical studies of CELSENTRI (see sections 4.4 and 5.1). Other phenotypic and genotypic assays are currently being evaluated. The viral tropism cannot be safely predicted by treatment history and assessment of stored samples.

There are currently no data regarding the reuse of CELSENTRI in patients that currently have only CCR5-tropic HIV-1 detectable, but have a history of failure on CELSENTRI (or other CCR5 antagonists) with a CXCR4 or dual/mixed tropic virus. There are no data regarding the switch from a medicinal product of a different antiretroviral class to CELSENTRI in virologically suppressed patients. Alternative treatment options should be considered.

Adults: the recommended dose of CELSENTRI is 150 mg, 300 mg or 600 mg twice daily depending on interactions with co-administered antiretroviral therapy and other medicinal products (see Table 2 in Section 4.5). CELSENTRI can be taken with or without food.

Children: CELSENTRI is not recommended for use in children due to lack of data on safety, efficacy and pharmacokinetics (see section 5.2).

Elderly: there is limited experience in patients >65 years of age (see section 5.2), therefore CELSENTRI should be used with caution in this population.

Renal impairment: dosage adjustment is only recommended in patients with renal impairment who are receiving potent CYP3A4 inhibitors such as:

- protease inhibitors (except tipranavir/ritonavir)
- ketoconazole, itraconazole, clarithromycin, telithromycin.

CELSENTRI should be used with caution in patients with renal impairment (CLcr < 80ml/min) who are taking potent CYP3A4 inhibitors (see sections 4.4 and 5.2). Table 1 below provides dose interval adjustment guidelines based on simulations of increasing renal impairment in patients being coadministered potent CYP3A4 inhibitors. The safety and efficacy of these dose interval adjustments have not been clinically evaluated. Therefore, clinical response to treatment should be closely monitored in these patients.

Table 1. Dose interval adjustments based on simulations of increasing renal impairment (for dose recommendations, see Section 4.5 Table 2)

(see Table 1 below)

Hepatic impairment: limited data are available in patients with hepatic impairment, therefore CELSENTRI should be used with caution in this population (see sections 4.4 and 5.2).

4.3 Contraindications

Hypersensitivity to the active substance or to peanut or soya or to any of the excipients.

4.4 Special warnings and precautions for use

CELSENTRI should be taken as part of an antiretroviral combination regimen. CELSENTRI should optimally be combined with other antiretrovirals to which the patient's virus is sensitive (see section 5.1).

CELSENTRI should only be used when only CCR5-tropic HIV-1 is detectable (i.e. CXCR4 or dual/mixed tropic virus not detected) as determined by an adequately validated and sensitive detection method (see sections 4.1, 4.2 and 5.1). The Monogram Trofile assay was used in the clinical studies of CELSENTRI. Other phenotypic and genotypic assays are currently being evaluated. The viral tropism cannot be predicted by treatment history or assessment of stored samples.

Changes in viral tropism occur over time in HIV-1 infected patients. Therefore there is a need to start therapy shortly after a tropism test.

Background resistance to other classes of antiretrovirals have been shown to be similar in previously undetected CXCR4-tropic virus of the minor viral population, as that found in CCR5-tropic virus.

Dose adjustment: physicians should ensure that appropriate dose adjustment of CELSENTRI is made when CELSENTRI is co-administered with CYP3A4 inhibitors and/or inducers since maraviroc concentrations and its therapeutic effects may be affected (see sections 4.2 and 4.5). Please also refer to the respective Summary of Product Characteristics of the other antiretroviral medicinal products used in the combination.

Information for patients: patients should be advised that antiretroviral therapies including CELSENTRI have not been shown to prevent the risk of transmission of HIV to others through sexual contact or contamination with blood. They should continue to use appropriate precautions. Patients should also be informed that CELSENTRI is not a cure for HIV-1 infection.

Postural hypotension: when CELSENTRI was administered in studies with healthy volunteers at doses higher than the recommended dose, cases of symptomatic postural hypotension were seen at a greater frequency than with placebo. However, when CELSENTRI was given at the recommended dose in HIV infected patients in Phase 3 studies, postural hypotension was seen at a similar rate compared to placebo (approximately 0.5%). Caution should be used when administering CELSENTRI in patients with a history of postural hypotension or on concomitant medicinal products known to lower blood pressure.

Potential effect on immunity: CCR5 antagonists could potentially impair the immune response to certain infections. This should be taken into consideration when treating infections such as active tuberculosis and invasive fungal infections. The incidence of AIDS-defining infections was similar between CELSENTRI and placebo arms in the pivotal studies.

Cardiovascular safety: limited data exist with the use of CELSENTRI in patients with severe cardiovascular disease, therefore special caution should be exercised when treating these patients with CELSENTRI.

Immune reconstitution syndrome: in HIV infected patients with severe immune deficiency at the time of institution of combination antiretroviral therapy (CART), an inflammatory reaction to asymptomatic or residual opportunistic pathogens may arise and cause serious clinical conditions, or aggravation of symptoms. Typically, such reactions have been observed within the first few weeks or months of initiation of CART. Relevant examples are cytomegalovirus retinitis, generalised and/or focal mycobacterial infections, and pneumonia caused by *Pneumocystis jiroveci* (formerly known as *Pneumocystis carinii*). Any inflammatory symptoms should be evaluated and treatment initiated when necessary.

Osteonecrosis: although the etiology is considered to be multifactorial (including corticosteroid use, alcohol consumption, severe immunosuppression, higher body mass index), cases of osteonecrosis have been reported particularly in patients with advanced HIV-disease and/or long-term exposure to combination antiretroviral therapy (CART). Patients should be advised to seek medical advice if they experience joint aches and pain, joint stiffness or difficulty in movement.

Hepatic safety: the safety and efficacy of CELSENTRI have not been specifically studied in patients with significant underlying liver disorders.

A case of possible CELSENTRI-induced hepatotoxicity with allergic features has been reported in a study in healthy volunteers. In addition, an increase in hepatic adverse reactions with CELSENTRI was observed during studies of treatment-experienced subjects with HIV infection, although there was no overall increase in ACTG Grade 3/4 liver function test abnormalities (see section 4.8). Patients with pre-existing liver dysfunction, including chronic active hepatitis, can have an increased frequency of liver function abnormalities during combination antiretroviral therapy and should be monitored according to standard practice.

Discontinuation of CELSENTRI should be considered in any patient with signs or symptoms of acute hepatitis, in particular if drug-related hypersensitivity is suspected or with increased liver transaminases combined with rash or other systemic symptoms of potential hypersensitivity (e.g. pruritic rash, eosinophila or elevated IgE).

Since there are very limited data in patients with hepatitis B/C co-infection, special caution should be exercised when treating these patients with CELSENTRI. In case of concomitant antiviral therapy for hepatitis B and/or C, please refer also to the relevant product information for these medicinal products.

There is limited experience in patients with reduced hepatic function, therefore CELSENTRI should be used with caution in this population (see sections 4.2 and 5.2).

Renal impairment: the safety and efficacy of CELSENTRI have not been specifically studied in patients with renal impairment, therefore CELSENTRI should be used with caution in this population.

In the absence of metabolic inhibitors, renal clearance accounts for less than 25% of total clearance of maraviroc and hence renal impairment is not expected to significantly alter maraviroc exposures.

In the presence of metabolic inhibitors, renal clearance may account for up to 70% of total clearance of maraviroc, hence renal impairment may result in increased maraviroc exposures in this case. Therefore, CELSENTRI should be used with caution in patients with renal impairment (CLcr < 80 ml/min) who are also taking potent CYP3A4 inhibitors. Table 1 provides dose interval adjustment guidelines based on simulations of increasing renal impairment in patients being coadministered potent CYP3A4 inhibitors. The safety and efficacy of these dose interval adjustments have not been clinically evaluated. Therefore, clinical response to treatment should be closely monitored in these patients (see sections 4.2 and 5.2).

Soya lecithin: CELSENTRI contains soya lecithin. If a patient is hypersensitive to peanut or soya, CELSENTRI should not be used.

4.5 Interaction with other medicinal products and other forms of interaction

Maraviroc is a substrate of cytochrome P450 CYP3A4. Co-administration of CELSENTRI with medicinal products that induce CYP3A4 may decrease maraviroc concentrations and reduce its therapeutic effects. Co-administration of CELSENTRI with medicinal products that inhibit CYP3A4 may increase maraviroc plasma concentrations. Dose adjustment of CELSENTRI is recommended when CELSENTRI is co-administered with CYP3A4 inhibitors and/or inducers. Further details for concomitantly administered medicinal products are provided below (see Table 2).

Studies in human liver microsomes and recombinant enzyme systems have shown that maraviroc does not inhibit any of the major P450 enzymes at clinically relevant concentrations (CYP1A2, CYP2B6, CYP2C8, CYP2C9, CYP2C19, CYP2D6 and CYP3A4). Maraviroc had no clinically relevant effect on the pharmacokinetics of midazolam, the oral contraceptives ethinylestradiol and levonorgestrel, or urinary 6β-hydroxycortisol/cortisol ratio, suggesting no inhibition or induction of CYP3A4 *in vivo*. At higher exposure of maraviroc a potential inhibition of CYP2D6 cannot be excluded. Based on the *in vitro* and clinical data, the potential for maraviroc to affect the pharmacokinetics of coadministered medicinal products is low.

Renal clearance accounts for approximately 23% of total clearance of maraviroc when maraviroc is administered without CYP3A4 inhibitors. As both passive and active processes are involved, there is the potential for competition for elimination with other renally eliminated active substances. However, co-administration of CELSENTRI with tenofovir (substrate for renal elimination) and Cotrimoxazole (contains trimethoprim, a renal cation transport inhibitor), showed no effect on the pharmacokinetics of

Table 1 Dose interval adjustments based on simulations of increasing renal impairment (for dose recommendations, see Section 4.5 Table 2)

Recommended CELSENTRI dose interval	Creatinine clearance (CLcr) (ml/min)		
	50- 80 ml/min	<50 – 30 ml/min	<30 ml/min
Without potent CYP3A4 inhibitors or co-administered with tipranavir/ritonavir	No dose interval adjustment required		
If coadministered with potent CYP3A4 inhibitors, e.g. lopinavir/ritonavir, darunavir/ritonavir, atazanavir/ritonavir, ketoconazole (see also section 4.5)	Every 24 hours		
If coadministered with saquinavir/ritonavir	Every 24 hours	Every 48 hours	Every 72 hours

maraviroc. In addition, co-administration of CELSENTRI with lamivudine/zidovudine showed no effect of maraviroc on lamivudine (primarily renally cleared) or zidovudine (non-P450 metabolism and renal clearance) pharmacokinetics. In vitro results indicate that maraviroc could inhibit P-glycoprotein in the gut and may thus affect bioavailability of certain drugs.

Table 2. Interactions and dose recommendations with other medical products

(see Table 2 opposite)

4.6 Pregnancy and lactation

No meaningful clinical data on exposure during pregnancy are available. Studies in rats and rabbits showed reproductive toxicity at high exposures. Primary pharmacological activity (CCR5 receptor affinity) was limited in these species (see section 5.3). CELSENTRI should be used during pregnancy only if the potential benefit justifies the potential risk to the foetus.

Studies in lactating rats indicate that maraviroc is extensively secreted into rat milk. Primary pharmacological activity (CCR5 receptor affinity) was limited in these species. It is not known whether maraviroc is secreted into human milk. Mothers should be instructed not to breast-feed if they are receiving CELSENTRI because of the potential for HIV transmission as well as any possible undesirable effects in breast-fed infants.

4.7 Effects on ability to drive and use machines

No studies on the effects on the ability to drive and use machines have been performed. CELSENTRI may cause dizziness. Patients should be instructed that if they experience dizziness they should avoid potentially hazardous tasks such as driving or operating machinery.

4.8 Undesirable effects

The safety profile of CELSENTRI is based on 1349 HIV-1 infected patients who received at least one dose of CELSENTRI during clinical studies. This includes 427 patients who received the recommended dose 300 mg twice daily and a further 401 patients who received 300 mg once daily for at least 24 weeks. Assessment of treatment related adverse reactions is based on pooled data at the recommended dose from two Phase 3 studies (MOTIVATE 1 and MOTIVATE 2) in CCR5-tropic HIV-1 infected patients.

The most frequently reported adverse reactions occurring in the Phase 3 studies at the recommended dose regardless of the incidence compared to OBT alone were diarrhoea, nausea and headache. These adverse reactions were common (≥ 1/100 to < 1/10). The reported frequencies for these events as well as the rates of discontinuation due to any adverse reactions were similar in patients receiving CELSENTRI 300 mg twice daily + OBT (Optimised Background Therapy) compared to those receiving OBT alone.

The adverse reactions are listed by system organ class (SOC) and frequency. Within each frequency grouping, undesirable effects are presented in order of decreasing seriousness. Frequencies are defined as very common (≥ 1/10), common (≥ 1/100 to < 1/10) and uncommon (≥1/1000 to <1/100). The adverse reactions and laboratory abnormalities presented below are not exposure adjusted.

The following table presents adverse reactions occurring at a numerically higher rate among patients receiving CELSENTRI 300 mg twice daily + OBT than patients on OBT alone with an incidence of ≥1%.

Table 3. Adverse reactions occurring at a numerically higher rate among patients receiving CELSENTRI 300 mg twice daily + OBT than patients on OBT alone with an incidence of ≥1%

System Organ Class	Adverse Reaction	Frequency
Investigations	alanine aminotransferase increased, aspartate aminotransferase increased, gamma-glutamyltransferase increased, weight decreased	common
Nervous system disorders	dizziness, paraesthesia, dysgeusia, somnolence	common
Respiratory, thoracic and mediastinal disorders	Cough	common
Gastrointestinal disorders	nausea	very common
	vomiting, abdominal pain, abdominal distension, dyspepsia, constipation	common
Skin and subcutaneous tissue disorders	rash, pruritus	common
Musculoskeletal and connective tissue disorders	muscle spasms, back pain	common
General disorders and administration site conditions	Asthenia	common
Psychiatric disorders	Insomnia	common

Table 2 Interactions and dose recommendations with other medical products

Medicinal product by therapeutic areas (dose of CELSENTRI used in study)	Effects on drug levels Geometric mean change if not stated otherwise	Recommendations concerning co-administration
ANTI-INFECTIVES		
Antiretrovirals		
NRTIs		
Lamivudine 150 mg BID (maraviroc 300 mg BID)	Lamivudine AUC_{12}: ↔ 1.13 Lamivudine C_{max}: ↔ 1.16 Maraviroc concentrations not measured, no effect is expected.	No significant interaction seen/expected. **CELSENTRI 300 mg twice daily and NRTIs can be co-administered without dose adjustment.**
Tenofovir 300 mg QD (maraviroc 300 mg BID)	Maraviroc AUC_{12}: ↔ 1.03 Maraviroc C_{max}: ↔ 1.03 Tenofovir concentrations not measured, no effect is expected.	
Zidovudine 300 mg BID (maraviroc 300 mg BID)	Zidovudine AUC_{12}: ↔ 0.98 Zidovudine C_{max}: ↔ 0.92 Maraviroc concentrations not measured, no effect is expected.	
Integrase Inhibitors		
Raltegravir 400 mg BID (maraviroc 300 mg BID)	Maraviroc AUC_{12}: ↓ 0.86 Maraviroc C_{max}: ↓ 0.79 Raltegravir AUC_{12}: ↓ 0.63 Raltegravir C_{max}: ↓ 0.67 Raltegravir C_{12}: ↓ 0.72	No clinically significant interaction seen. **CELSENTRI 300 mg twice daily and raltegravir can be co-administered without dose adjustment.**
NNRTIs		
Efavirenz 600 mg QD (maraviroc 100 mg BID)	Maraviroc AUC_{12}: ↓ 0.55 Maraviroc C_{max}: ↓ 0.49 Efavirenz concentrations not measured, no effect is expected.	**CELSENTRI dose should be increased to 600 mg twice daily when co-administered with efavirenz in the <u>absence</u> of a PI (except tipranavir/ritonavir) or other potent CYP3A4 inhibitor.** For combination with efavirenz + PI, see below.
Etravirine 200 mg BID (maraviroc 300 mg BID)	Maraviroc AUC_{12}: ↓ 0.47 Maraviroc C_{max}: ↓ 0.40 Etravirine AUC_{12}: ↔ 1.06 Etravirine C_{max}: ↔ 1.05 Etravirine C_{12}: ↔ 1.08	**Etravirine is only approved for use with boosted protease inhibitors.** For combination with etravirine + PI, see below.
Nevirapine 200 mg BID (maraviroc 300 mg Single Dose)	Maraviroc AUC_{12}: ↔ compared to historical controls Maraviroc C_{max}: ↑ compared to historical controls Nevirapine concentrations not measured, no effect is expected.	Comparison to exposure in historical controls suggests that **CELSENTRI 300 mg twice daily and nevirapine can be co-administered without dose adjustment.**
PIs		
Atazanavir 400 mg QD (maraviroc 300 mg BID)	Maraviroc AUC_{12} ↑ 3.57 Maraviroc C_{max}: ↑ 2.09 Atazanavir concentrations not measured, no effect is expected.	**CELSENTRI dose should be decreased to 150 mg twice daily when co-administered with a PI; <u>except in combination with tipranavir/ritonavir or fosamprenavir/ritonavir</u> where the dose should be 300 mg BID.** Maraviroc does not significantly affect PI drug levels.
Atazanavir/ritonavir 300 mg/100 mg QD (maraviroc 300 mg BID)	Maraviroc AUC_{12} ↑ 4.88 Maraviroc C_{max}: ↑ 2.67 Atazanavir/ritonavir concentrations not measured, no effect is expected.	
Lopinavir/ritonavir 400 mg/100 mg BID (maraviroc 300 mg BID)	Maraviroc AUC_{12} ↑ 3.95 Maraviroc C_{max}: ↑ 1.97 Lopinavir/ritonavir concentrations not measured, no effect is expected.	
Saquinavir/ritonavir 1000 mg/100 mg BID (maraviroc 100 mg BID)	Maraviroc AUC_{12} ↑ 9.77 Maraviroc C_{max}: 4.78 Saquinavir/ritonavir concentrations not measured, no effect is expected.	
Darunavir/ritonavir 600 mg/100 mg BID (maraviroc 150 mg BID)	Maraviroc AUC_{12} ↑ 4.05 Maraviroc C_{max}: ↑ 2.29 Darunavir/ritonavir concentrations were consistent with historical data.	
Nelfinavir	Limited data are available for co-administration with nelfinavir. Nelfinavir is a potent CYP3A4 inhibitor and would be expected to increase maraviroc concentrations.	
Indinavir	Limited data are available for co-administration with indinavir. Indinavir is a potent CYP3A4 inhibitor. Population PK analysis in phase 3 studies suggests dose reduction of maraviroc when coadministered with indinavir gives appropriate maraviroc exposure.	
Fosamprenavir/ritonavir	Fosamprenavir is considered to be a moderate CYP3A4 inhibitor. Population PK studies suggest that a dose adjustment of maraviroc is not required.	**CELSENTRI 300 mg twice daily and tipranavir/ritonavir or fosamprenavir/ritonavir can be co-administered without dose adjustment.**
Tipranavir/ritonavir 500 mg/200 mg BID (maraviroc 150 mg BID)	Maraviroc AUC_{12} ↔ 1.02 Maraviroc C_{max}: ↔ 0.86 Tipranavir/ritonavir concentrations were consistent with historical data.	
NNRTI + PI		
Efavirenz 600 mg QD + lopinavir/ritonavir 400mg/100 mg BID (maraviroc 300 mg BID)	Maraviroc AUC_{12}: ↑ 2.53 Maraviroc C_{max}: ↑ 1.25 Efavirenz, lopinavir/ritonavir concentrations not measured, no effect expected.	**CELSENTRI dose should be decreased to 150 mg twice daily when co-administered with efavirenz in the <u>presence</u> of a PI (except fosamprenavir/ritonavir where the dose should be 300 mg twice daily and tipranavir/ritonavir where the dose should be 600 mg twice daily).**
Efavirenz 600 mg QD + saquinavir/ritonavir 1000 mg/100 mg BID (maraviroc 100 mg BID)	Maraviroc AUC_{12}: ↑ 5.00 (3.04, 6.31) Maraviroc C_{max}: ↑ 2.26 (0.68, 4.09) Efavirenz, saquinavir/ritonavir concentrations not measured, no effect expected.	
Efavirenz and atazanavir/ritonavir or darunavir/ritonavir	Not studied. Based on the extent of inhibition by atazanavir/ritonavir or darunavir/ritonavir in the absence of efavirenz, an increased exposure is expected.	

Medicinal product by therapeutic areas (dose of CELSENTRI used in study)	Effects on drug levels Geometric mean change if not stated otherwise	Recommendations concerning co-administration
Etravirine and darunavir/ ritonavir (maraviroc 150 mg BID)	Maraviroc AUC_{12}: ↑ 3.10 Maraviroc C_{max}: ↑ 1.77 Etravirine AUC_{12}: ↔ 1.00 Etravirine C_{max}: ↔ 1.08 Etravirine C_{12}: ↓ 0.81 Darunavir AUC_{12}: ↓ 0.86 Darunavir C_{max}: ↔ 0.96 Darunavir C_{12}: ↓ 0.77 Ritonavir AUC_{12}: ↔ 0.93 Ritonavir C_{max}: ↔ 1.02 Ritonavir C_{12}: ↓ 0.74	**CELSENTRI dose should be decreased to 150 mg twice daily when co-administered etravirine in the presence of a PI (except fosamprenavir/ritonavir where the dose should be 300 mg twice daily).**
Etravirine and lopinavir/ritonavir, saquinavir/ritonavir or atazanavir/ritonavir	Not studied. Based on the extent of inhibition by lopinavir/ritonavir, saquinavir/ritonavir or atazanavir/ ritonavir in the absence of etravirine, an increased exposure is expected.	
Antibiotics		
Sulphamethoxazole/ Trimethoprim 800 mg/160 mg BID (maraviroc 300 mg BID)	Maraviroc AUC_{12}: ↔ 1.11 Maraviroc C_{max}: ↔ 1.19 Sulphamethoxazole/trimethoprim concentrations not measured, no effect expected.	**CELSENTRI 300 mg twice daily and sulphamethoxazole/trimethoprim can be co-administered without dose adjustment.**
Rifampicin 600 mg QD (maraviroc 100 mg BID)	Maraviroc AUC.↓ 0.37 Maraviroc C_{max}: ↓ 0.34 Rifampicin concentrations not measured, no effect expected.	**CELSENTRI dose should be increased to 600 mg twice daily when co-administered with rifampicin in the absence of a potent CYP3A4 inhibitor.** This dose adjustment has not been studied in HIV patients. See also section 4.4.
Rifampicin + efavirenz	Combination with two inducers has not been studied. There may be a risk of suboptimal levels with risk of loss of virologic response and resistance development.	**Concomitant use of CELSENTRI and rifampicin + efavirenz is not recommended.**
Rifabutin + PI	Not studied. Rifabutin is considered to be a weaker inducer than rifampicin. When combining rifabutin with protease inhibitors that are potent inhibitors of CYP3A4 a net inhibitory effect on maraviroc is expected.	**CELSENTRI dose should be decreased to 150 mg twice daily when co-administered with rifabutin in the presence of a PI (except tipranavir/ritonavir or fosamprenavir/ritonavir where the dose should be 300 mg twice daily).** See also section 4.4.
Clarithromycin, Telithromycin	Not studied, but both are potent CYP3A4 inhibitors and would be expected to increase maraviroc concentrations.	**CELSENTRI dose should be decreased to 150 mg twice daily when co-administered with clarithromycin and telithromycin.**
Antifungals		
Ketoconazole 400 mg QD (maraviroc 100 mg BID)	Maraviroc AUC_{tau}: ↑ 5.00 Maraviroc C_{max}: ↑ 3.38 Ketoconazole concentrations not measured, no effect is expected.	**CELSENTRI dose should be decreased to 150 mg twice daily when co-administered with ketoconazole.**
Itraconazole	Not studied. Itraconazole, is a potent CYP3A4 inhibitor and would be expected to increase the exposure of maraviroc.	**CELSENTRI dose should be decreased to 150 mg twice daily when co-administered with itraconazole.**
Fluconazole	Fluconazole is considered to be a moderate CYP3A4 inhibitor. Population PK studies suggest that a dose adjustment of maraviroc is not required.	**CELSENTRI 300 mg twice daily should be administered with caution when coadministered with fluconazole.**
Antivirals		
HCV agents	Pegylated interferon and ribavirin have not been studied, no interaction is expected.	**CELSENTRI 300 mg twice daily and pegylated interferon or ribavirin can be coadministered without dose adjustment.**
DRUG ABUSE		
Methadone	Not studied, no interaction expected.	**CELSENTRI 300 mg twice daily and methadone can be coadministered without dose adjustment.**
Buprenorphine	Not studied, no interaction expected.	**CELSENTRI 300 mg twice daily and buprenorphine can be coadministered without dose adjustment.**
LIPID LOWERING MEDICINAL PRODUCTS		
Statins	Not studied, no interaction expected.	**CELSENTRI 300 mg twice daily and statins can be coadministered without dose adjustment.**
ORAL CONTRACEPTIVES		
Ethinylestradiol 30 mcg QD (maraviroc 100 mg BID)	Ethinylestradiol. AUC_{t}: ↔ 1.00 Ethinylestradiol. C_{max}: ↔ 0.99 Maraviroc concentrations not measured, no interaction expected.	**CELSENTRI 300 mg twice daily. and ethinylestradiol can be co-administered without dose adjustment.**
Levonorgestrel 150mcg QD (maraviroc 100 mg BID)	Levonorgestrel. AUC_{12}: ↔ 0.98 Levonorgestrel. C_{max}: ↔ 1.01 Maraviroc concentrations not measured, no interaction expected.	**CELSENTRI 300 mg twice daily and levonorgestrel can be co-administered without dose adjustment.**
SEDATIVES		
Benzodiazepines		
Midazolam 7.5 mg Single Dose (maraviroc 300 mg BID)	Midazolam. AUC: ↔ 1.18 Midazolam. C_{max}: ↔ 1.21 Maraviroc concentrations not measured, no interaction expected.	**CELSENTRI 300 mg twice daily and midazolam can be co-administered without dose adjustment.**
HERBAL PRODUCTS		
St John's Wort	Coadministration of maraviroc with St. John's wort is expected to substantially decrease maraviroc concentrations and may result in suboptimal levels and lead to loss of virologic response and possible resistance to maraviroc.	**Concomitant use of maraviroc and St. John's wort (Hypericum Perforatum) or products containing St. John's wort is not recommended.**

Clinically important adverse reactions occurring in less than 1% of adult patients receiving CELSENTRI in Phase 3 studies are presented below.

Table 4. Clinically important adverse reactions occurring in less than 1% of adult patients receiving CELSENTRI in Phase 3 studies

System Organ Class	Adverse Reaction	Frequency
Cardiac disorders	myocardial infarction, myocardial ischaemia	uncommon
Blood and lymphatic system disorders	pancytopenia, neutropenia, lymphadenopathy	uncommon
Nervous system disorders	loss of consciousness, epilepsy, petit mal epilepsy, convulsion, facial palsy, polyneuropathy, areflexia	uncommon
Respiratory, thoracic and Mediastinal disorders	respiratory distress, bronchospasm	uncommon
Gastrointestinal disorders	pancreatitis, rectal haemorrhage	uncommon
Renal and urinary disorders	renal failure, polyuria	uncommon
Musculoskeletal and connective tissue disorders	Myositis	uncommon
Infections and infestations	Pneumonia	uncommon
Hepatobiliary disorders	hepatic cirrhosis	uncommon
Psychiatric disorders	Hallucination	uncommon

In HIV infected patients with severe immune deficiency at the time of initiation of combination antiretroviral therapy (CART), an inflammatory reaction to asymptomatic or residual opportunistic infections may arise (see section 4.4).

Laboratory abnormalities

Table 5 shows the incidence ⩾1% of Grade 3-4 Abnormalities (ACTG Criteria) based on the maximum shift in laboratory test values without regard to baseline values.

Table 5: Incidence ⩾1% of grade 3-4 abnormalities (ACTG criteria) based on maximum shift in laboratory test values without regard to baseline studies MOTIVATE 1 and MOTIVATE 2 (pooled analysis, up to 48 weeks)

(see Table 5 on next page)

Cases of osteonecrosis have been reported, particularly in patients with generally acknowledged risk factors, advanced HIV disease or long-term exposure to combination antiretroviral therapy (CART). The frequency of this is unknown (see section 4.4).

4.9 Overdose

The highest dose administered in clinical studies was 1200 mg. The dose limiting adverse reaction was postural hypotension.

Prolongation of the QT interval was seen in dogs and monkeys at plasma concentrations 6 and 12 times, respectively, those expected in humans at the maximum recommended dose of 300 mg twice daily. However, no clinically significant QT prolongation compared to OBT alone was seen in the Phase 3 clinical studies using the recommended dose of maraviroc or in a specific pharmacokinetic study to evaluate the potential of CELSENTRI to prolong the QT interval.

There is no specific antidote for overdose with CELSENTRI. Treatment of overdose should consist of general supportive measures including keeping the patient in a supine position, careful assessment of patient vital signs, blood pressure and ECG.

If indicated, elimination of unabsorbed active maraviroc should be achieved by emesis or gastric lavage. Administration of activated charcoal may also be used to aid in removal of unabsorbed active substance. Since maraviroc is moderately protein bound, dialysis may be beneficial in removal of this medicine.

5. PHARMACOLOGICAL PROPERTIES

5.1 Pharmacodynamic properties

Pharmacotherapeutic group: Antivirals for systemic use, Other Antivirals ATC code: J05AX09

Mechanism of action:

Maraviroc is a member of a therapeutic class called CCR5 antagonists. Maraviroc selectively binds to the human chemokine receptor CCR5, preventing CCR5-tropic HIV-1 from entering cells.

Antiviral activity *in vitro:*

Maraviroc has no antiviral activity in vitro against viruses which can use CXCR4 as their entry co-receptor (dual-tropic or CXCR4-tropic viruses, collectively termed 'CXCR4-using' virus below). The serum adjusted EC90 value in 43 primary HIV-1 clinical isolates was 0.57 (0.06

Table 5 Incidence ≥1% of grade 3-4 abnormalities (ACTG criteria) based on maximum shift in laboratory test values without regard to baseline studies MOTIVATE 1 and MOTIVATE 2 (pooled analysis, up to 48 weeks)

Laboratory parameter	Limit	Celsentri 300 mg twice daily + OBT N =421* (%)	OBT alone N =207* (%)
Aspartate aminotransferase	>5.0x ULN	4.5	2.9
Alanine aminotransferase	>5.0x ULN	2.4	3.4
Total bilirubin	>5.0x ULN	5.7	5.3
Amylase	>2.0x ULN	5.5	5.8
Lipase	>2.0x ULN	4.9	6.3
Absolute neutrophil count	<750/mm^3	3.8	1.9

ULN: Upper Limit of Normal

* Percentages based on total patients evaluated for each laboratory parameter

– 10.7) ng/mL without significant changes between different subtypes tested. The antiviral activity of maraviroc against HIV-2 has not been evaluated. For details please refer to http://www.emea.europa.eu/htms/human/epar/eparintro.

When used with other antiretroviral medicinal products in cell culture, the combination of maraviroc was not antagonistic with a range of NRTIs, NNRTIs, PIs or the HIV fusion inhibitor enfuvirtide.

Resistance:

Viral escape from maraviroc can occur via 2 routes: the selection of virus which can use CXCR4 as its entry co-receptor (CXCR4-using virus) or the selection of virus that continues to use exclusively CCR5 (CCR5-tropic virus).

In vitro:

HIV-1 variants with reduced susceptibility to maraviroc have been selected *in vitro*, following serial passage of two CCR5-tropic viruses (0 laboratory strains, 2 clinical isolates). The maraviroc-resistant viruses remained CCR5-tropic and there was no conversion from a CCR5-tropic virus to a CXCR4-using virus.

Phenotypic resistance: concentration response curves for the maraviroc-resistant viruses were characterized phenotypically by curves that did not reach 100% inhibition in assays using serial dilutions of maraviroc. Traditional IC_{50}/IC_{90} fold-change was not a useful parameter to measure phenotypic resistance, as those values were sometimes unchanged despite significantly reduced sensitivity.

Genotypic resistance: mutations were found to accumulate in the gp120 envelope glycoprotein (the viral protein that binds to the CCR5 co-receptor). The position of these mutations was not consistent between different isolates. Hence, the relevance of these mutations to maraviroc susceptibility in other viruses is not known.

Cross-resistance *in vitro*:

HIV-1 clinical isolates resistant to nucleoside analogue reverse transcriptase inhibitors (NRTI), non-nucleoside analogue reverse transcriptase inhibitors (NNRTI), protease inhibitors (PI) and enfuvirtide were all susceptible to maraviroc in cell culture. Maraviroc-resistant viruses that emerged *in vitro* remained sensitive to the fusion inhibitor enfuvirtide and the protease inhibitor saquinavir.

In vivo:

Treatment naïve patients

The resistance profile in treatment-naïve patients has not been characterized.

Treatment experienced patients

In the pivotal studies (MOTIVATE 1 and MOTIVATE 2), 7.6% of patients had a change in tropism result from CCR5-tropic to CXCR4-tropic or dual/mixed-tropic between screening and baseline (a period of 4-6 weeks).

Failure with CXCR4-using virus:

CXCR4-using virus was detected at failure in approximately 60% of subjects who failed treatment on CELSENTRI, as compared to 6% of subjects who experienced treatment failure in the OBT alone arm. To investigate the likely origin of the on-treatment CXCR4-using virus, a detailed clonal analysis was conducted on virus from 20 representative subjects (16 subjects from the CELSENTRI arms and 4 subjects from the OBT alone arm) in whom CXCR4-using virus was detected at treatment failure. This analysis indicated that CXCR4-virus emerged from a pre-existing CXCR4-using reservoir not detected at baseline, rather than from mutation of CCR5-tropic virus present at baseline. An analysis of tropism following failure of CELSENTRI therapy with CXCR4-using virus in patients with CCR5 virus at baseline, demonstrated that the virus population reverted back to CCR5 tropism in 33 of 36 patients with more than 35 days of follow-up.

At time of failure with CXCR4-using virus, the resistance pattern to other antiretrovirals appears similar to that of the CCR5-tropic population at baseline, based on available data. Hence, in the selection of a treatment regimen, it should be assumed that viruses forming part of the previously undetected CXCR4 -using population (i.e. minor viral population) harbours the same resistance pattern as the CCR5-tropic population.

Failure with CCR5-tropic virus:

Phenotypic resistance: in patients with CCR5-tropic virus at time of treatment failure with CELSENTRI, 22 out of 58 patients had virus with reduced sensitivity to maraviroc. In the remaining 36 patients, there was no evidence of virus with reduced sensitivity as identified by exploratory virology analyses on a representative group. The latter group had markers correlating to low compliance (low and variable drug levels and often a calculated high residual sensitivity score of the OBT). In patients failing therapy with R5-virus only, maraviroc might be considered still active if the maximal percentage inhibition (MPI) value is ≥95% (Phenosense Entry assay). Residual activity in vivo for viruses with MPI-values <95% has not been determined.

Genotypic resistance: Key mutations (V3-loop) can presently not be suggested due to the high variability of the V3-sequence, and the low number of samples analysed.

Clinical Results

Studies in CCR5-tropic Treatment-Experienced Patients:

The clinical efficacy of CELSENTRI (in combination with other antiretroviral medicinal products) on plasma HIV RNA levels and CD4+ cell counts have been investigated in two pivotal ongoing, randomized, double blind, multicentre studies (MOTIVATE 1 and MOTIVATE 2, n=1076) in patients infected with CCR5 tropic HIV-1 as determined by the Monogram Trofile Assay.

Patients who were eligible for these studies had prior exposure to at least 3 antiretroviral medicinal product classes [≥1 nucleoside reverse transcriptase inhibitors (NRTI), ≥1 non-nucleoside reverse transcriptase inhibitors (NNRTI), ≥2 protease inhibitors (PI), and/or enfurvirtide] or documented resistance to at least one member of each class. Patients were randomised in a 2:2:1 ratio to CELSENTRI 300 mg (dose equivalence) once daily, twice daily or placebo in combination with an optimized background consisting of 3 to 6 antiretroviral medicinal products (excluding low-dose ritonavir). The OBT was selected on the basis of the subject's prior treatment history and baseline genotypic and phenotypic viral resistance measurements.

Table 6: Demographic and baseline characteristics of patients in studies MOTIVATE 1 and MOTIVATE 2 (Pooled Analysis)

Demographic and Baseline Characteristics	CELSENTRI 300 mg twice daily + OBT N = 426	OBT alone N = 209
Age (years) (Range, years)	46.3 21-73	45.7 29-72
Male Sex	89.7%	88.5%
Race (White/Black/Other)	85.2% / 12% / 2.8%	85.2% / 12.4% / 2.4%
Mean Baseline HIV-1 RNA (log_{10} copies/mL)	4.85	4.86
Median Baseline CD4+ Cell Count (cells/mm^3) (range, cells/mm^3)	166.8 (2.0-820.0)	171.3 (1.0-675.0)
Screening Viral Load ≥ 100,000 copies/mL	179 (42.0%)	84 (40.2%)
Baseline CD4+ Cell Count ≤200 cells/mm^3	250 (58.7%)	118 (56.5%)

Number (Percentage) of patients with GSS score:		
0	102 (23.9%)	51 (24.4%)
1	138 (32.4%)	53 (25.4%)
2	80 (18.8%)	41 (19.6%)
≥3	104 (24.4%)	59 (28.2%)

GeneSeq resistance assay

Limited numbers of patients from ethnicities other than Caucasian were included in the pivotal clinical studies, therefore very limited data are available in these patient populations.

The mean increase in CD4+ cell count from baseline in patients who failed with a change in tropism result to dual/mixed tropic or CXCR4, in the CELSENTRI 300 mg twice daily + OBT (+56 cells/mm^3) group was greater than that seen in patients failing OBT alone (+13.8 cells/mm^3) regardless of tropism.

Table 7. Outcomes of randomised treatment at week 48 (pooled studies MOTIVATE 1 and MOTIVATE 2)

(see Table 7 on next page)

CELSENTRI 300 mg twice daily + OBT was superior to OBT alone across all subgroups of patients analysed (see Table 8). Patients with very low CD4+ count at baseline (i.e. <50 cells/uL) had a less favourable outcome. This subgroup had a high degree of bad prognostic markers, i.e. extensive resistance and high baseline viral loads. However, a significant treatment benefit for CELSENTRI compared to OBT alone was still demonstrated (see Table 8).

Table 8. Proportion of patients achieving <50 copies/ml at Week 48 by subgroup (pooled Studies MOTIVATE 1 and MOTIVATE 2, ITT)

Subgroups	HIV-1 RNA <50 copies/ml	
	CELSENTRI 300 mg twice daily + OBT N=426	OBT alone N=209
Baseline HIV-1 RNA:		
<5.0 log_{10} copies/ml	58.4%	26.0%
≥5.0 log_{10} copies/ml	34.7%	9.5%
Baseline CD4+ (cells/uL):		
<50	16.5	2.6
50-100	36.4	12.0
101-200	56.7	21.8
201-350	57.8	21.0
≥ 350	72.9	38.5
Number of active ARVs in OBT[1,2]:		
0	32.7%	2.0%
1	44.5%	7.4%
2	58.2%	31.7%
≥3	62%	38.6%

[1]Discontinuations or virological failures considered as failures.
[2]Based on GSS.

Studies in Non-CCR5-tropic Treatment-Experienced Patients:

Study A4001029 was an exploratory study in patients infected with dual/mixed or CXCR4 tropic HIV-1 with a similar design as the studies MOTIVATE 1 and MOTIVATE 2. In this study, neither superiority nor non-inferiority to OBT alone were demonstrated although there was no adverse outcome on viral load or CD4+ cell count

5.2 Pharmacokinetic properties

Absorption: the absorption of maraviroc is variable with multiple peaks. Median peak maraviroc plasma concentrations is attained at 2 hours (range 0.5-4 hours) following single oral doses of 300 mg commercial tablet administered to healthy volunteers. The pharmacokinetics of oral maraviroc are not dose proportional over the dose range. The absolute bioavailability of a 100 mg dose is 23% and is predicted to be 33% at 300 mg. Maraviroc is a substrate for the efflux transporter P-glycoprotein.

Coadministration of a 300 mg tablet with a high fat breakfast reduced maraviroc C_{max} and AUC by 33% in healthy volunteers. There were no food restrictions in the studies that demonstrated the efficacy and safety of CELSENTRI (see section 5.1). Therefore, CELSENTRI can be taken with or without food at the recommended doses (see section 4.2).

Distribution: maraviroc is bound (approximately 76%) to human plasma proteins, and shows moderate affinity for albumin and alpha-1 acid glycoprotein. The volume of distribution of maraviroc is approximately 194 L.

Metabolism: studies in humans and *in vitro* studies using human liver microsomes and expressed enzymes have demonstrated that maraviroc is principally metabolized by the cytochrome P450 system to metabolites that are essentially inactive against HIV-1. *In vitro* studies indicate that CYP3A4 is the major enzyme responsible for maraviroc metabolism. *In vitro* studies also indicate that polymorphic enzymes CYP2C9, CYP2D6 and CYP2C19 do not contribute significantly to the metabolism of maraviroc.

Maraviroc is the major circulating component (approximately 42% radioactivity) following a single oral dose of 300 mg. The most significant circulating metabolite in

Table 7 Outcomes of randomised treatment at week 48 (pooled studies MOTIVATE 1 and MOTIVATE 2)

Outcomes	CELSENTRI 300 mg twice daily + OBT N=426	OBT alone N=209	Treatment Difference[1] (Confidence Interval[2])
HIV-1 RNA Change from baseline (log_{10} copies/mL)	-1.84	-0.78	-1.05 (-1.33, -0.78)
Proportion of patients with HIV RNA <400 copies/ml	56.1%	22.5%	Odds ratio: 4.76 (3.24, 7.00)
Proportion of patients with HIV RNA <50 copies/ml	45.5%	16.7%	Odds ratio: 4.49 (2.96, 6.83)
CD4+ cell count Change from baseline (cells/mm^3)	124.07	60.93	63.13 (44.28, 81.99)

[1]p-values < 0.0001
[2] For all efficacy endpoints the confidence intervals were 95%, except for HIV-1 RNA Change from baseline which was 97.5%

humans is a secondary amine (approximately 22% radioactivity) formed by N-dealkylation. This polar metabolite has no significant pharmacological activity. Other metabolites are products of mono-oxidation and are only minor components of plasma radioactivity.

Elimination: a mass balance/excretion study was conducted using a single 300 mg dose of ^{14}C-labeled maraviroc. Approximately 20% of the radiolabel was recovered in the urine and 76% was recovered in the faeces over 168 hours. Maraviroc was the major component present in urine (mean of 8% dose) and faeces (mean of 25% dose). The remainder was excreted as metabolites. After intravenous administration (30 mg), the half-life of maraviroc was 13.2 h, 22% of the dose was excreted unchanged in the urine and the values of total clearance and renal clearance were 44.0 L/h and 10.17 L/h respectively.

Children: the pharmacokinetics of maraviroc in paediatric patients have not been established (see section 4.2).

Elderly: population analysis of the Phase 1/2a and Phase 3 studies (16-65 years of age) has been conducted and no effect of age has been observed (see section 4.2).

Renal impairment: the pharmacokinetics of maraviroc have not been studied in patients with renal impairment. However, renal clearance contributes less than 25% of maraviroc total clearance in the absence of CYP3A4 inhibitors, therefore the impact of renal impairment on maraviroc elimination should be minimal. In the presence of metabolic inhibitors, renal clearance may account for up to 70% of total clearance of maraviroc and hence renal impairment may result in increased maraviroc exposures in this case (see sections 4.2 and 4.4).

Hepatic impairment: maraviroc is primarily metabolized and eliminated by the liver. A study compared the pharmacokinetics of a single 300 mg dose of CELSENTRI in patients with mild (Child-Pugh Class A, n=8), and moderate (Child-Pugh Class B, n=8) hepatic impairment compared to healthy subjects (n=8). Geometric mean ratios for Cmax and AUC_{last} were 11% and 25% higher respectively for subjects with mild hepatic impairment, and 32% and 46% higher respectively for subjects with moderate hepatic impairment compared to subjects with normal hepatic function. The effects of moderate hepatic impairment may be underestimated due to limited data in patients with decreased metabolic capacity and higher renal clearance in these subjects. The results should therefore be interpreted with caution. The pharmacokinetics of maraviroc have not been studied in subjects with severe hepatic impairment (see sections 4.2 and 4.4).

Race: no relevant difference between Caucasian, Asian and Black subjects has been observed. The pharmacokinetics in other races has not been evaluated.

Gender: no relevant differences in pharmacokinetics have been observed.

5.3 Preclinical safety data

Primary pharmacological activity (CCR5 receptor affinity) was present in the monkey (100% receptor occupancy) and limited in the mouse, rat, rabbit and dog. In mice and human beings that lack CCR5 receptors through genetic deletion, no significant adverse consequences have been reported.

In vitro and in vivo studies showed that maraviroc has a potential to increase QTc interval at supratherapeutic doses with no evidence of arrhythmia.

Repeated dose toxicity studies in rats identified the liver as the primary target organ for toxicity (increases in transaminases, bile duct hyperplasia, necrosis).

Maraviroc was evaluated for carcinogenic potential by a 6 month transgenic mouse study and a 24 month study in rats. In mice, no statistically significant increase in the incidence of tumors was reported at systemic exposures from 7 to 39-times the human exposure (unbound AUC 0-24h measurement) at a dose of 300 mg twice daily. In rats, administration of maraviroc at a systemic exposure 21-times the expected human exposure produced thyroid adenomas associated with adaptive liver changes. These findings are considered of low human relevance. In addition, cholangiocarcinomas (2/60 males at 900 mg/kg) and cholangioma (1/60 females at 500 mg/kg) were reported in the rat study at a systemic exposure at least 15-times the expected free human exposure.

Maraviroc was not mutagenic or genotoxic in a battery of in vitro and in vivo assays including bacterial reverse mutation, chromosome aberrations in human lymphocytes and rat bone marrow micronucleus.

Maraviroc did not impair mating or fertility of male or female rats, and did not affect sperm of treated male rats up to 1000 mg/kg. The exposure at this dose level corresponded to 39-fold the estimated free clinical AUC for a 300 mg twice daily dose.

Embryofoetal development studies were conducted in rats and rabbits at doses up to 39- and 34-fold the estimated free clinical AUC for a 300 mg twice daily dose. In rabbit, 7 foetuses had external anomalies at maternally toxic doses and 1 foetus at the mid dose of 75 mg/kg.

Pre- and post-natal developmental studies were performed in rats at doses up to 27-fold the estimated free clinical AUC for a 300 mg twice daily dose. A slight increase in motor activity in high-dose male rats at both weaning and as adults was noted, while no effects were seen in females. Other developmental parameters of these offspring, including fertility and reproductive performance, were not affected by the maternal administration of maraviroc.

6. PHARMACEUTICAL PARTICULARS

6.1 List of excipients

Tablet core:

Cellulose, microcrystalline

Calcium hydrogen phosphate, anhydrous

Sodium starch glycolate

Magnesium stearate

Film-coat:

Poly (vinyl alcohol)

Titanium dioxide

Macrogol 3350

Talc

Soya Lecithin

Indigo carmine aluminium lake (E132)

6.2 Incompatibilities

Not applicable.

6.3 Shelf life

3 years.

6.4 Special precautions for storage

This medicinal product does not require any special storage condition.

6.5 Nature and contents of container

High density polyethylene bottles (HDPE) with polypropylene child resistant (CR) closures and an aluminium foil/polyethylene heat induction seal containing 180 film-coated tablets.

Polyvinyl chloride (PVC) blisters with aluminium foil backing in a carton containing 30, 60, 90 film-coated tablets and multipacks containing 180 (2 packs of 90) film-coated tablets.

Not all pack sizes may be marketed.

6.6 Special precautions for disposal and other handling

No special requirements.

7. MARKETING AUTHORISATION HOLDER

Pfizer Limited

Ramsgate Road

Sandwich

Kent

CT13 9NJ

United Kingdom

8. MARKETING AUTHORISATION NUMBER(S)

EU/1/07/418/001 – 010

9. DATE OF FIRST AUTHORISATION/RENEWAL OF THE AUTHORISATION

Date of first authorisation: 18/09/07

Date of last renewal:

10. DATE OF REVISION OF THE TEXT

07 August 2009

11. LEGAL CATEGORY

POM

Detailed information on this medicinal product is available on the website of the European Medicines Agency (EMEA) http://www.emea.europa.eu

Cervarix

(GlaxoSmithKline UK)

1. NAME OF THE MEDICINAL PRODUCT

Cervarix ▼ suspension for injection in pre-filled syringe

Human Papillomavirus vaccine [Types 16, 18] (Recombinant, adjuvanted, adsorbed)

2. QUALITATIVE AND QUANTITATIVE COMPOSITION

1 dose (0.5 ml) contains:

Human Papillomavirus[1] type 16 L1 protein[2,3,4] 20 micrograms

Human Papillomavirus[1] type 18 L1 protein[2,3,4] 20 micrograms

[1]Human Papillomavirus = HPV

[2]adjuvanted by AS04 containing:

3-*O*-desacyl-4'- monophosphoryl lipid A (MPL)[3] 50 micrograms

[3]adsorbed on aluminium hydroxide, hydrated ($Al(OH)_3$) 0.5 milligrams Al^{3+} in total

[4]L1 protein in the form of non-infectious virus-like particles (VLPs) produced by recombinant DNA technology using a Baculovirus expression system which uses Hi-5 Rix4446 cells derived from *Trichoplusia ni*.

For a full list of excipients, see section 6.1.

3. PHARMACEUTICAL FORM

Suspension for injection in pre-filled syringe.

Turbid white suspension. Upon storage, a fine white deposit with a clear colourless supernatant may be observed.

4. CLINICAL PARTICULARS

4.1 Therapeutic indications

Cervarix is a vaccine for the prevention of premalignant cervical lesions and cervical cancer causally related to Human Papillomavirus (HPV) types 16 and 18 (see section 5.1).

The indication is based on the demonstration of efficacy in women aged 15-25 years following vaccination with Cervarix and on the immunogenicity of the vaccine in girls and women aged 10-25 years.

See section 5.1 for information on the evidence that supports the efficacy of Cervarix in prevention of premalignant cervical lesions associated with HPV-16 and/or HPV-18.

The use of Cervarix should be in accordance with official recommendations.

4.2 Posology and method of administration

The recommended vaccination schedule is 0, 1, 6 months.

The need for a booster dose has not been established (see section 5.1).

It is recommended that subjects who receive a first dose of Cervarix complete the 3-dose vaccination course with Cervarix (see section 4.4).

Girls aged less than 10 years: Cervarix is not recommended for use in girls below 10 years of age due to lack of data on safety and immunogenicity in this age-group.

Cervarix is for intramuscular injection in the deltoid region (see also sections 4.4 and 4.5).

4.3 Contraindications

Hypersensitivity to the active substances or to any of the excipients.

Administration of Cervarix should be postponed in subjects suffering from an acute severe febrile illness. However, the presence of a minor infection, such as a cold, is not a contraindication for immunisation.

4.4 Special warnings and precautions for use

As with all injectable vaccines, appropriate medical treatment and supervision should always be readily available in case of a rare anaphylactic event following the administration of the vaccine.

Cervarix should under no circumstances be administered intravascularly or intradermally.

No data are available on subcutaneous administration of Cervarix.

As with other vaccines administered intramuscularly, Cervarix should be given with caution to individuals with thrombocytopenia or any coagulation disorder since bleeding may occur following an intramuscular administration to these subjects.

Vaccination is not a substitute for regular cervical screening or for precautions against exposure to HPV and sexually transmitted diseases.

As with any vaccine, a protective immune response may not be elicited in all vaccinees.

Cervarix protects against disease caused by HPV types 16 and 18. Other oncogenic HPV types can also cause cervical cancer and therefore routine cervical screening remains critically important and should follow local recommendations.

Cervarix has not been shown to have a therapeutic effect. The vaccine is therefore not indicated for treatment of cervical cancer, cervical intraepithelial neoplasia (CIN) or any other established HPV-related lesions.

Cervarix does not prevent HPV-related lesions in women who are infected with HPV-16 or HPV-18 at the time of vaccination.

Duration of protection has not fully been established. Timing and need of booster dose(s) has not been investigated.

There are no data on the use of Cervarix in subjects with impaired immune responsiveness such as HIV infected patients or patients receiving immunosuppressive treatment. As with other vaccines, an adequate immune response may not be elicited in these individuals.

There are no safety, immunogenicity or efficacy data to support interchangeability of Cervarix with other HPV vaccines.

4.5 Interaction with other medicinal products and other forms of interaction

In all clinical trials individuals who had received immunoglobulin or blood products within 3 months prior to the first vaccine dose were excluded.

Use with other vaccines

Cervarix may be administered concomitantly with a combined booster vaccine containing diphtheria (d), tetanus (T) and pertussis [acellular] (pa) with or without inactivated poliomyelitis (IPV), (dTpa, dTpa-IPV vaccines), with no clinically relevant interference with antibody response to any of the components of either vaccine. The sequential administration of combined dTpa-IPV followed by Cervarix one month later tended to elicit lower anti-HPV-16 and anti-HPV-18 GMTs as compared to Cervarix alone. The clinical significance of this observation is not known.

If Cervarix is to be given at the same time as another injectable vaccine, the vaccines should always be administered at different injection sites.

Use with hormonal contraceptive

In clinical efficacy studies, approximately 60% of women who received Cervarix used hormonal contraceptives. There is no evidence that the use of hormonal contraceptives has an impact on the efficacy of Cervarix.

Use with systemic immunosuppressive medicinal products

As with other vaccines it may be expected that, in patients receiving immunosuppressive treatment, an adequate response may not be elicited.

4.6 Pregnancy and lactation

Specific studies of the vaccine in pregnant women were not conducted. During the pre-licensure clinical development program, a total of 1,737 pregnancies were reported including 870 in women who had received Cervarix. Overall, the proportions of pregnant subjects who experienced specific outcomes (e.g., normal infant, abnormal infants including congenital anomalies, premature birth, and spontaneous abortion) were similar between treatment groups.

Animal studies do not indicate direct or indirect harmful effects with respect to fertility, pregnancy, embryonal/foetal development, parturition or post-natal development (see section 5.3).

These data are insufficient to recommend use of Cervarix during pregnancy.

Vaccination should, therefore, be postponed until after completion of pregnancy.

The effect on breast-fed infants of the administration of Cervarix to their mothers has not been evaluated in clinical studies.

Cervarix should only be used during breast-feeding when the possible advantages outweigh the possible risks.

4.7 Effects on ability to drive and use machines

No studies on the effects on the ability to drive or use machines have been performed.

4.8 Undesirable effects

In clinical studies that enrolled girls and women aged from 10 up to 72 years (of which 79.2% were aged 10-25 years at the time of enrolment), Cervarix was administered to 16,142 subjects whilst 13,811 subjects received control. These subjects were followed for serious adverse events over the entire study period. In a pre-defined subset of subjects (Cervarix = 8,130 versus control = 5,786), adverse events were followed for 30 days after each injection.

The most common adverse reaction observed after vaccine administration was injection site pain which occurred after 78% of all doses. The majority of these reactions were of mild to moderate severity and were not long lasting.

Adverse reactions considered as being at least possibly related to vaccination have been categorised by frequency.

Frequencies are reported as:

Very common (≥1/10)

Common (≥1/100 to <1/10)

Uncommon (≥1/1,000 to <1/100)

Nervous system disorders:

Very common: headache

Uncommon: dizziness

Gastrointestinal disorders:

Common: gastrointestinal symptoms including nausea, vomiting, diarrhoea and abdominal pain

Skin and subcutaneous tissue disorders:

Common: itching/pruritus, rash, urticaria

Musculoskeletal and connective tissue disorders:

Very common: myalgia

Common: arthralgia

Infections and infestations:

Uncommon: upper respiratory tract infection

General disorders and administration site conditions:

Very common: injection site reactions including pain, redness, swelling; fatigue

Common: fever (≥38°C)

Uncommon: other injection site reactions such as induration, local paraesthesia

A similar safety profile has been observed in subjects with prior or current HPV infection as compared to subjects negative for oncogenic HPV DNA or seronegative for HPV-16 and HPV-18 antibodies.

4.9 Overdose

No case of overdose has been reported.

5. PHARMACOLOGICAL PROPERTIES

5.1 Pharmacodynamic properties

Pharmaco-therapeutic group: Papillomavirus vaccines, ATC code: J07BM02

Mechanism of action

Cervarix is a non-infectious recombinant vaccine prepared from the highly purified virus-like particles (VLPs) of the major capsid L1 protein of oncogenic HPV types 16 and 18. Since the VLPs contain no viral DNA, they cannot infect cells, reproduce or cause disease. Animal studies have shown that the efficacy of L1 VLP vaccines is largely mediated by the development of a humoral immune response.

HPV-16 and HPV-18 are responsible for approximately 70% of cervical cancers across all regions worldwide.

Clinical studies

The efficacy of Cervarix was assessed in two controlled, double-blind, randomised Phase II and III clinical trials that included a total of 19,778 women aged 15 to 25 years.

The phase II trial (study 001/007) enrolled only women who:

- Were tested negative for oncogenic HPV DNA of types 16, 18, 31, 33, 35, 39, 45, 51, 52, 56, 58, 59, 66 and 68
- Were seronegative for HPV-16 and HPV-18 and
- Had normal cytology

The primary efficacy endpoint was incident infection with HPV-16 and/or HPV-18. Twelve-month persistent infection was evaluated as additional efficacy endpoint.

The phase III trial (study 008) enrolled women without pre-screening for the presence of HPV infection, i.e. regardless of baseline cytology and HPV serological and DNA status.

The primary efficacy endpoint was CIN2+ associated with HPV-16 and/or HPV-18. The secondary endpoints included 12-month persistent infection.

Cervical Intraepithelial Neoplasia (CIN) grade 2 and 3 was used in the clinical trials as a surrogate marker for cervical cancer.

The term "premalignant cervical lesions" in section 4.1 corresponds to high-grade Cervical Intraepithelial Neoplasia (CIN 2/3).

Prophylactic efficacy against HPV-16/18 infection in a population naïve to oncogenic HPV types

Women (N=1,113) were vaccinated in study 001 and evaluated for efficacy up to month 27. A subset of women (N=776) vaccinated in study 001 was followed in study 007 up to 6.4 years (approximately 77 months) after the first dose (mean follow-up of 5.9 years). There were five cases of 12-month persistent HPV-16/18 infection (4 HPV-16; 1 HPV-18) in the control group and one HPV-16 case in the vaccine group in study 001. In study 007 the efficacy of Cervarix against 12-month persistent HPV-16/18 infection was 100% (95% CI: 80.5; 100). There were sixteen cases of persistent HPV-16 infection, and five cases of persistent HPV-18 infection, all in the control group.

Prophylactic efficacy in women naïve to HPV-16 and/or HPV-18

In study 008 the primary analyses of efficacy were conducted in the total vaccinated cohort (TVC-1). This cohort included only women who were HPV DNA negative and seronegative to the relevant HPV type (HPV-16 or HPV-18) at study entry and had received at least one dose of Cervarix or the control. Women with high-grade or missing cytology (0.5%) were excluded from the efficacy analysis. Overall, 74.0% of women enrolled were naïve to both HPV-16 and HPV-18 at study entry.

The efficacy of Cervarix in the prevention of CIN2+ associated with HPV-16 and/or HPV-18 as assessed up to 15 months after the last dose of vaccine or control and the rates of 12-month persistent infection in the TVC-1 cohort are presented in the table below:

(see Table 1 below)

All endpoints reached statistical significance for HPV-16. For HPV-18, the difference between the vaccine and control groups was not statistically significant for CIN2+ and 12 month persistent infection (TVC-1 cohort). However, in a pre-specified analysis (TVC-2) that was identical to the TVC-1 analysis except that it excluded women with abnormal cytology at study entry, the 12 month persistent infection endpoint for HPV-18 reached statistical significance with vaccine efficacy of 89.9% (97.9% CI: 11.3; 99.9). One case was observed in the vaccine group versus 10 cases in the control group.

Several of the CIN2+ lesions contained multiple oncogenic types (including non-vaccine HPV types). An additional analysis was conducted to determine vaccine efficacy against lesions likely to be causally associated with HPV-16 and/or HPV-18. This post-hoc analysis (clinical case assignment) assigned causal association of an HPV type with the lesion based on the presence of the HPV type in cytology samples prior to detection of the lesion. Based on this case assignment, the analysis excluded 3 CIN2+ cases (2 in the vaccine group and 1 in the control group) which were not considered to be causally associated with HPV-16 or HPV-18 infections acquired during the trial. Based on this analysis there were no cases in the vaccine group and 20 cases in the control group (Efficacy 100%; 97.9% CI: 74.2; 100).

Prophylactic efficacy in women with current or prior infection

There was no evidence of protection from disease caused by the HPV types for which subjects were HPV DNA positive at study entry. However, individuals already infected with one of the vaccine-related HPV types prior to vaccination were protected from clinical disease caused by the remaining HPV type.

In study 008, approximately 26% of women had evidence of current and/or prior infection. Twenty percent of women

Table 1

Study 008	Cervarix		Control		Efficacy (97.9% CI)
	N	n	N	n	
CIN2+ (primary endpoint)					
HPV-16 and/or 18*	7788	2	7838	21	90.4 (53.4; 99.3)
HPV-16	6701	1	6717	15	93.3 (47.0; 99.9)
HPV-18	7221	1	7258	6	83.3 (<0.0; 99.9)
12-month persistent infection (secondary endpoint)					
HPV-16 and/or 18*	3386	11	3437	46	75.9 (47.7; 90.2)
HPV-16	2945	7	2972	35	79.9 (48.3; 93.8)
HPV-18	3143	4	3190	12	66.2 (<0.0; 94.0)

N = number of subjects included in each group of TVC-1 cohort

n = number of cases

*protocol-specified endpoints

had evidence of prior infection (i.e. HPV-16 and/or HPV-18 seropositive). Seven percent of women were infected at time of vaccination (i.e. HPV-16 and/or HPV-18 DNA positive) of which only 0.5% were DNA positive for both types.

Immunogenicity

No minimal antibody level associated with protection against CIN of grade 2 or 3 or against persistent infection associated with vaccine HPV types has been identified for HPV vaccines.

The antibody response to HPV-16 and HPV-18 was measured using a type-specific ELISA which was shown to correlate with the pseudovirion-based neutralisation assay.

The immunogenicity induced by three doses of Cervarix has been evaluated in 5,303 female subjects from 10 to 55 years of age.

In clinical trials, 99.9% of initially seronegative subjects had seroconverted to both HPV types 16 and 18 one month after the third dose. Vaccine-induced IgG Geometric Mean Titres (GMT) were well above titres observed in women previously infected but who cleared HPV infection (natural infection). Initially seropositive and seronegative subjects reached similar titres after vaccination.

Study 001/007, which included women from 15 to 25 years of age at the time of vaccination, evaluated the immune response against HPV-16 and HPV-18 up to 76 months post dose 1.

Vaccine-induced IgG Geometric Mean Titres (GMT) for both HPV-16 and HPV-18 peaked at month 7 and then declined to reach a plateau from month 18 up to the end of the follow-up (month 76). At the end of the follow-up period, GMTs for both HPV-16 and HPV-18 were still at least 11-fold higher than titres observed in women previously infected but who cleared HPV infection and >98% of the women were still seropositive for both antigens. In study 008, immunogenicity at month 7 was similar to the response observed in study 001.

In another clinical trial (study 014) performed in women aged 15 to 55 years, all subjects seroconverted to both HPV types 16 and 18 after the third dose (at month 7). The GMTs were, however, lower in women above 25 years. Nevertheless, all subjects remained seropositive for both types throughout the follow-up phase (up to month 18) maintaining antibody levels at an order of magnitude above those encountered after natural infection.

Bridging the efficacy of Cervarix from young adult women to adolescents

In two clinical trials performed in girls and adolescents aged 10 to 14 years, all subjects seroconverted to both HPV types 16 and 18 after the third dose (at month 7) with GMTs at least 2-fold higher as compared to women aged 15 to 25 years. On the basis of these immunogenicity data, the efficacy of Cervarix is inferred from 10 to 14 years of age.

5.2 Pharmacokinetic properties

Evaluation of pharmacokinetic properties is not required for vaccines.

5.3 Preclinical safety data

Non-clinical data reveal no special hazard for humans based on conventional studies of safety pharmacology, acute and repeated dose toxicity, local tolerance, fertility, embryo-foetal and postnatal toxicity (up to the end of the lactation period).

Serological data suggest a transfer of anti-HPV-16 and anti-HPV-18 antibodies via the milk during the lactation period in rats. However, it is unknown whether vaccine-induced antibodies are excreted in human breast milk.

6. PHARMACEUTICAL PARTICULARS

6.1 List of excipients

Sodium chloride (NaCl)

Sodium dihydrogen phosphate dihydrate ($NaH_2PO_4.2H_2O$)

Water for injections

For adjuvants, see section 2.

6.2 Incompatibilities

In the absence of compatibility studies, this medicinal product must not be mixed with other medicinal products.

6.3 Shelf life

4 years.

Cervarix should be administered as soon as possible after being removed from the refrigerator. However, stability data generated indicate that Cervarix presented in monodose containers remains stable and can be administered in case it has been stored outside the refrigerator up to three days at temperatures between 8°C and 25°C or up to one day at temperatures between 25°C and 37°C.

6.4 Special precautions for storage

Store in a refrigerator (2°C – 8°C).

Do not freeze.

Store in the original package in order to protect from light.

6.5 Nature and contents of container

0.5 ml of suspension in a pre-filled syringe (type I glass) with a plunger stopper (rubber butyl) with or without needles in pack sizes of 1 and 10.

Not all pack sizes may be marketed.

6.6 Special precautions for disposal and other handling

A fine white deposit with a clear colourless supernatant may be observed upon storage of the syringe. This does not constitute a sign of deterioration.

The content of the syringe should be inspected visually both before and after shaking for any foreign particulate matter and/or abnormal physical appearance prior to administration.

In the event of either being observed, discard the vaccine.

The vaccine should be well shaken before use.

Any unused product or waste material should be disposed of in accordance with local requirements.

7. MARKETING AUTHORISATION HOLDER

GlaxoSmithKline Biologicals s.a.

Rue de l'Institut 89

B-1330 Rixensart, Belgium

8. MARKETING AUTHORISATION NUMBER(S)

EU/1/07/419/004

EU/1/07/419/005

EU/1/07/419/006

EU/1/07/419/007

EU/1/07/419/008

EU/1/07/419/009

9. DATE OF FIRST AUTHORISATION/RENEWAL OF THE AUTHORISATION

Date of first authorisation: 20 September 2007.

10. DATE OF REVISION OF THE TEXT

24 July 2009

11. LEGAL STATUS

POM

Detailed information on this medicinal product is available on the website of the European Medicines Agency (EMEA) http://www.emea.europa.eu/.

Cetraben Emollient Bath Additive

(Genus Pharmaceuticals)

1. NAME OF THE MEDICINAL PRODUCT

Cetraben Emollient Bath Additive

2. QUALITATIVE AND QUANTITATIVE COMPOSITION

Light Liquid Paraffin 82.8% w/w

For excipients see section 6.1.

3. PHARMACEUTICAL FORM

Bath Additive

Cetraben Emollient Bath Additive is a clear liquid with a faint odour.

4. CLINICAL PARTICULARS

4.1 Therapeutic indications

Cetraben Emollient Bath Additive is an emollient, moisturising and protective oil for the symptomatic relief of red, inflamed, damaged, dry or chapped skin, especially when associated with endogenous or exogenous eczema.

4.2 Posology and method of administration

Cetraben Emollient Bath Additive should be added to a warm water bath or applied to wet skin before showering.

Bath: Adults: Add one/two capfuls to a warm water bath

Children: Add half/one capful to a warm water bath

Shower: Apply lightly using a wet sponge

4.3 Contraindications

Hypersensitivity to any of the ingredients.

4.4 Special warnings and precautions for use

Allergy to any of the ingredients.

Care when entering or leaving the bath.

Avoid contact with eyes.

4.5 Interaction with other medicinal products and other forms of interaction

None known.

4.6 Pregnancy and lactation

No special precautions required.

4.7 Effects on ability to drive and use machines

None.

4.8 Undesirable effects

Very rarely, mild skin reactions have been seen.

4.9 Overdose

No cases of overdose have been reported. Patients should be advised that if they accidentally swallow Cetraben Emollient Bath Additive, they should talk to their doctor or pharmacist at once.

5. PHARMACOLOGICAL PROPERTIES

5.1 Pharmacodynamic properties

ATC Code: D02AX (Other Emollients and Protectives)

The ingredients of Cetraben Emollient Bath Additive have emollient, moisturising and protective properties.

5.2 Pharmacokinetic properties

Cetraben Emollient Bath Additive acts only on the skin.

5.3 Preclinical safety data

Not applicable.

6. PHARMACEUTICAL PARTICULARS

6.1 List of excipients

C-12-13-Pareth-3

Medium chain triglycerides

6.2 Incompatibilities

Not applicable.

6.3 Shelf life

48 months.

6.4 Special precautions for storage

Do not store above 25°C.

6.5 Nature and contents of container

Polyethylene jars containing 40ml and 500ml, with polypropylene screw caps.

6.6 Special precautions for disposal and other handling

Not applicable.

7. MARKETING AUTHORISATION HOLDER

Pharma Health Care Ltd

Russell Bedford House

City Forum

250 City Road

London

EC1V 2QQ

United Kingdom

8. MARKETING AUTHORISATION NUMBER(S)

PL 17320/0002

9. DATE OF FIRST AUTHORISATION/RENEWAL OF THE AUTHORISATION

10 August 2001

10. DATE OF REVISION OF THE TEXT

22 March 2007

Cetraben Emollient Cream

(Genus Pharmaceuticals)

1. NAME OF THE MEDICINAL PRODUCT

Cetraben Emollient Cream

2. QUALITATIVE AND QUANTITATIVE COMPOSITION

White Soft Paraffin 13.2% w/w

Light Liquid Paraffin 10.5% w/w

For excipients see section 6.1.

3. PHARMACEUTICAL FORM

Cream.

A thick white cream with the characteristic odour of paraffin oil.

4. CLINICAL PARTICULARS

4.1 Therapeutic indications

Cetraben Emollient Cream is an emollient, moisturising and protective cream for the symptomatic relief of red, inflamed, damaged, dry or chapped skin, especially when associated with endogenous or exogenous eczema.

4.2 Posology and method of administration

Cetraben Cream should be applied to the dry skin areas as often as required and rubbed in.

4.3 Contraindications

Hypersensitivity to any of the ingredients.

4.4 Special warnings and precautions for use

None known.

4.5 Interaction with other medicinal products and other forms of interaction

None known.

4.6 Pregnancy and lactation

No special precautions are required.

4.7 Effects on ability to drive and use machines

None.

4.8 Undesirable effects

Very rarely, mild allergic skin reactions including rash and erythema have been observed, in which case use of the product should be discontinued.

4.9 Overdose

None reported.

5. PHARMACOLOGICAL PROPERTIES

5.1 Pharmacodynamic properties

ATC Code: D02A X (Other Emollients and Protectives)

The ingredients of Cetraben Cream have an emollient, moisturising and protective properties.

5.2 Pharmacokinetic properties

Cetraben cream acts only on the skin.

5.3 Preclinical safety data

Not applicable.

6. PHARMACEUTICAL PARTICULARS

6.1 List of excipients

Emulsifying wax

Cetyl stearyl Alcohol

Glycerin

Butylparaben

Methylparaben

Ethylparaben

Propylparaben

Phenoxetol

Citric Acid

Purified water

6.2 Incompatibilities

None known.

6.3 Shelf life

Three years

6.4 Special precautions for storage

Do not store above 25°C.

6.5 Nature and contents of container

Polypropylene jars with a pump dispenser of 1050g, 500g, 150g and 50g, polyethylene screw capped jars* or tubes of 125g, polyethylene tubes of 50g and polyethylene tubes of 20g.

* not currently marketed.

6.6 Special precautions for disposal and other handling

Not applicable.

7. MARKETING AUTHORISATION HOLDER

Pharma Health Care Ltd

Russell Bedford House

City Forum

250 City Road

London EC1V 2QQ

United Kingdom

8. MARKETING AUTHORISATION NUMBER(S)

PL 17320/0001

9. DATE OF FIRST AUTHORISATION/RENEWAL OF THE AUTHORISATION

21/09/2006

10. DATE OF REVISION OF THE TEXT

25/09/07

Cetrotide 0.25 mg

(Merck Serono)

1. NAME OF THE MEDICINAL PRODUCT

Cetrotide 0.25 mg powder and solvent for solution for injection

2. QUALITATIVE AND QUANTITATIVE COMPOSITION

Each vial contains 0.25 mg cetrorelix (as acetate).

After reconstitution with the solvent provided, each ml of the solution contains 0.25 mg cetrorelix.

For a full list of excipients, see section 6.1.

3. PHARMACEUTICAL FORM

Powder and solvent for solution for injection.

Appearance of the powder: white lyophilisate

Appearance of the solvent: clear and colourless solution

The pH of the reconstituted solution is 4.0 – 6.0

4. CLINICAL PARTICULARS

4.1 Therapeutic indications

Prevention of premature ovulation in patients undergoing a controlled ovarian stimulation, followed by oocyte pick-up and assisted reproductive techniques.

In clinical trials Cetrotide was used with human menopausal gonadotropin (HMG), however, limited experience with recombinant follicle-stimulating hormone (FSH) suggested similar efficacy.

4.2 Posology and method of administration

Cetrotide should only be prescribed by a specialist experienced in this field.

The first administration of Cetrotide should be performed under the supervision of a physician and under conditions where treatment of possible allergic/pseudo-allergic reactions (including life-threatening anaphylaxis) is immediately available. The following injections may be self-administered as long as the patient is made aware of the signs and symptoms that may indicate hypersensitivity, the consequences of such a reaction and the need for immediate medical intervention.

The contents of 1 vial (0.25 mg cetrorelix) are to be administered once daily, at 24 h intervals, either in the morning or in the evening. Following the first administration, it is advised that the patient be kept under medical supervision for 30 minutes to ensure there is no allergic/pseudo-allergic reaction to the injection.

Cetrotide is for subcutaneous injection into the lower abdominal wall.

The injection site reactions may be minimised by rotating the injection sites, delaying injection at the same site and injecting the product in a slow rate to facilitate the progressive absorption of the product.

Administration in the morning: Treatment with Cetrotide should commence on day 5 or 6 of ovarian stimulation (approximately 96 to 120 hours after start of ovarian stimulation) with urinary or recombinant gonadotropins and is to be continued throughout the gonadotropin treatment period including the day of ovulation induction.

Administration in the evening: Treatment with Cetrotide should commence on day 5 of ovarian stimulation (approximately 96 to 108 hours after start of ovarian stimulation) with urinary or recombinant gonadotropins and is to be continued throughout the gonadotropin treatment period until the evening prior to the day of ovulation induction.

Additional information on special populations:

There is no relevant indication for the use of Cetrotide in children or geriatric populations.

For instructions for preparation, see section 6.6.

4.3 Contraindications

- Hypersensitivity to the active substance or any structural analogues of gonadotropin-releasing hormone (GnRH), extrinsic peptide hormones or to any of the excipients.
- Pregnancy and lactation.
- Postmenopausal women.
- Patients with moderate and severe renal and hepatic impairment.

4.4 Special warnings and precautions for use

Special care should be taken in women with signs and symptoms of active allergic conditions or known history of allergic predisposition. Treatment with Cetrotide is not advised in women with severe allergic conditions.

During or following ovarian stimulation an ovarian hyperstimulation syndrome can occur. This event must be considered as an intrinsic risk of the stimulation procedure with gonadotropins.

An ovarian hyperstimulation syndrome should be treated symptomatically, e.g. with rest, intravenous electrolytes/colloids and heparin therapy.

Luteal phase support should be given according to the reproductive medical centre's practice.

There is limited experience up to now with the administration of Cetrotide during a repeated ovarian stimulation procedure. Therefore Cetrotide should be used in repeated cycles only after a careful risk/benefit evaluation.

4.5 Interaction with other medicinal products and other forms of interaction

In vitro investigations have shown that interactions are unlikely with medicinal products that are metabolised by cytochrome P450 or glucuronised or conjugated in some other way. However, though there has been no evidence of drug-interactions, especially with commonly used medicinal products, gonadotropins or products that may induce histamine release in susceptible individuals, the possibility of an interaction cannot be totally excluded.

4.6 Pregnancy and lactation

Cetrotide is not intended to be used during pregnancy and lactation (see section 4.3).

Studies in animals have indicated that cetrorelix exerts a dose related influence on fertility, reproductive performance and pregnancy. No teratogenic effects occurred when the medicinal product was administered during the sensitive phase of gestation.

4.7 Effects on ability to drive and use machines

Cetrotide has no or negligible influence on the ability to drive or use machines.

4.8 Undesirable effects

The most commonly reported side effects are local injection site reactions such as erythema, swelling and pruritus that are usually transient in nature and mild in intensity. In clinical trials, these effects were observed with a frequency of 9.4% following multiple injections of *Cetrotide* 0.25 mg.

Mild to moderate ovarian hyperstimulation syndrome (OHSS) (WHO grade I or II) have been commonly reported and should be considered as an intrinsic risk of the stimulation procedure. Inversely, severe OHSS remains uncommon.

Uncommonly, cases of hypersensitivity reactions including pseudo-allergic/anaphylactoid reactions have been reported.

The adverse reactions reported below are classified according to frequency of occurrence as follows:

Very Common	≥ 1/10
Common	≥ 1/100 to < 1/10
Uncommon	≥ 1/1,000 to < 1/100
Rare	≥ 1/10,000 to < 1/1,000
Very rare	< 1/10,000

Within each frequency grouping, undesirable effects are presented in order of decreasing seriousness.

Immune system disorders	Uncommon	Systemic allergic/pseudo-allergic reactions including life-threatening anaphylaxis.
Nervous system disorders	Uncommon	Headache
Gastrointestinal disorders	Uncommon	Nausea
Reproductive system and breast disorders	Common	Mild to moderate ovarian hyperstimulation syndrome (WHO grade I or II) can occur which is an intrinsic risk of the stimulation procedure (see section 4.4).
	Uncommon	Severe ovarian hyperstimulation syndrome (WHO grade III)
General disorders and administration site conditions	Common	Local reactions at the injection site (e.g. erythema, swelling and pruritus) have been reported. Usually they were transient in nature and of mild intensity. The frequency as reported in clinical trials was 9.4% following multiple injections of 0.25 mg cetrorelix.

4.9 Overdose

Overdosage in humans may result in a prolonged duration of action but is unlikely to be associated with acute toxic effects.

In acute toxicity studies in rodents non-specific toxic symptoms were observed after intraperitoneal administration of cetrorelix doses more than 200 times higher than the pharmacologically effective dose after subcutaneous administration.

5. PHARMACOLOGICAL PROPERTIES

5.1 Pharmacodynamic properties

Pharmacotherapeutic group: anti-gonadotropin-releasing hormones, ATC code: H01CC02.

Cetrorelix is a luteinising hormone releasing hormone (LHRH) antagonist. LHRH binds to membrane receptors on pituitary cells. Cetrorelix competes with the binding of endogenous LHRH to these receptors. Due to this mode of action, cetrorelix controls the secretion of gonadotropins (LH and FSH).

Cetrorelix dose-dependently inhibits the secretion of LH and FSH from the pituitary gland. The onset of suppression is virtually immediate and is maintained by continuous treatment, without initial stimulatory effect.

In females, cetrorelix delays the LH surge and consequently ovulation. In women undergoing ovarian stimulation the duration of action of cetrorelix is dose dependent. Following a single dose of 3 mg of cetrorelix a duration of action of at least 4 days has been evaluated. On day 4 the suppression was approximately 70%. At a dose of 0.25 mg per injection repeated injections every 24 hours will maintain the effect of cetrorelix.

In animals as well as in humans, the antagonistic hormonal effects of cetrorelix were fully reversible after termination of treatment.

5.2 Pharmacokinetic properties

The absolute bioavailability of cetrorelix after subcutaneous administration is about 85%.

The total plasma clearance and the renal clearance are 1.2 $ml \times min^{-1} \times kg^{-1}$ and 0.1 $ml \times min^{-1} \times kg^{-1}$, respectively. The volume of distribution (V_d) is 1.1 $l \times kg^{-1}$. The mean terminal half-lives following intravenous and subcutaneous administration are about 12 h and 30 h, respectively, demonstrating the effect of absorption processes at the injection site. The subcutaneous administration of single doses (0.25 mg to 3 mg cetrorelix) and also daily dosing over 14 days show linear kinetics.

5.3 Preclinical safety data

Non-clinical data reveal no special hazard for humans based on conventional studies of safety pharmacology, repeated dose toxicity, genotoxicity, carcinogenic potential, toxicity to reproduction.

No target organ toxicity could be observed from acute, subacute and chronic toxicity studies in rats and dogs following subcutaneous administration of cetrorelix. No signs of medicinal product-related local irritation or incompatibility were noted in dogs after intravenous, intra-arterial and paravenous injection when cetrorelix was administered in doses clearly above the intended clinical use in man.

Cetrorelix showed no mutagenic or clastogenic potential in gene and chromosome mutation assays.

6. PHARMACEUTICAL PARTICULARS

6.1 List of excipients

Powder:

Mannitol

Solvent:

Water for injections

6.2 Incompatibilities
This medicinal product must not be mixed with other medicinal products except those mentioned in section 6.6.

6.3 Shelf life
2 years.

The solution should be used immediately after preparation.

6.4 Special precautions for storage
Do not store above 25°C. Keep the vial(s) in the outer carton in order to protect from light.

6.5 Nature and contents of container
Packs with 1 or 7 Type I glass vials sealed with a rubber stopper.

Additionally for each vial the packs contain:

1 pre-filled syringe (Type I glass cartridge closed with rubber stoppers) with 1 ml solvent for parenteral use

1 injection needle (20 gauge)

1 hypodermic injection needle (27 gauge)

2 alcohol swabs.

Not all pack sizes may be marketed.

6.6 Special precautions for disposal and other handling
Cetrotide should only be reconstituted with the solvent provided, using a gentle, swirling motion. Vigorous shaking with bubble formation should be avoided.

The reconstituted solution is without particles and clear. Do not use if the solution contains particles or if the solution is not clear.

Withdraw the entire contents of the vial. This ensures a delivery to the patient of a dose of at least 0.23 mg cetrorelix.

The solution should be used immediately after reconstitution.

7. MARKETING AUTHORISATION HOLDER
Merck Serono Europe Limited

56 Marsh Wall

London E14 9TP

United Kingdom

8. MARKETING AUTHORISATION NUMBER(S)
EU/1/99/100/001

EU/1/99/100/002

9. DATE OF FIRST AUTHORISATION/RENEWAL OF THE AUTHORISATION
Date of first authorisation: 13 April 1999

Date of first renewal: 15 April 2004

Date of latest renewal: March 2009

10. DATE OF REVISION OF THE TEXT
July 2009

Cetrotide 3 mg

(Merck Serono)

1. NAME OF THE MEDICINAL PRODUCT
Cetrotide 3 mg powder and solvent for solution for injection

2. QUALITATIVE AND QUANTITATIVE COMPOSITION
Each vial contains 3 mg cetrorelix (as acetate).

After reconstitution with the solvent provided, each ml of the solution contains 1 mg cetrorelix.

For a full list of excipients, see section 6.1.

3. PHARMACEUTICAL FORM
Powder and solvent for solution for injection.

Appearance of the powder: white lyophilisate

Appearance of the solvent: clear and colourless solution

The pH of the reconstituted solution is 4.0 – 6.0

4. CLINICAL PARTICULARS
4.1 Therapeutic indications
Prevention of premature ovulation in patients undergoing a controlled ovarian stimulation, followed by oocyte pick-up and assisted reproductive techniques.

In clinical trials Cetrotide was used with human menopausal gonadotropin (HMG), however, limited experience with recombinant follicule-stimulating hormone (FSH) suggested similar efficacy.

4.2 Posology and method of administration
Cetrotide should only be prescribed by a specialist experienced in this field.

The first administration of Cetrotide should be performed under the supervision of a physician and under conditions where treatment of possible allergic/pseudo-allergic reactions (including life-threatening anaphylaxis) is immediately available. The following injections may be self-administered as long as the patient is made aware of the signs and symptoms that may indicate hypersensitivity, the consequences of such a reaction and the need for immediate medical intervention.

The contents of 1 vial (3 mg cetrorelix) are to be administered on day 7 of ovarian stimulation (approximately 132 to 144 hours after start of ovarian stimulation) with urinary or recombinant gonadotropins. Following the first administration, it is advised that the patient be kept under medical supervision for 30 minutes to ensure there is no allergic/pseudo-allergic reaction to the injection.

If the follicle growth does not allow ovulation induction on the fifth day after injection of Cetrotide 3 mg, additionally 0.25 mg cetrorelix (Cetrotide 0.25 mg) should be administered once daily beginning 96 hours after the injection of Cetrotide 3 mg until the day of ovulation induction.

Cetrotide is for subcutaneous injection into the lower abdominal wall.

The injection site reactions may be minimised by injecting the product in a slow rate to facilitate the progressive absorption of the product.

Additional information on special populations:

There is no relevant indication for the use of Cetrotide in children or geriatric populations.

For instructions for preparation, see section 6.6.

4.3 Contraindications
- Hypersensitivity to the active substance or any structural analogues of gonadotropin-releasing hormone (GnRH), extrinsic peptide hormones or to any of the excipients.
- Pregnancy and lactation.
- Postmenopausal women.
- Patients with moderate and severe renal and hepatic impairment.

4.4 Special warnings and precautions for use
Special care should be taken in women with signs and symptoms of active allergic conditions or known history of allergic predisposition. Treatment with Cetrotide is not advised in women with severe allergic conditions.

During or following ovarian stimulation an ovarian hyperstimulation syndrome can occur. This event must be considered as an intrinsic risk of the stimulation procedure with gonadotropins.

An ovarian hyperstimulation syndrome should be treated symptomatically, e.g. with rest, intravenous electrolytes/colloids and heparin therapy.

Luteal phase support should be given according to the reproductive medical centre's practice.

There is limited experience up to now with the administration of Cetrotide during a repeated ovarian stimulation procedure. Therefore Cetrotide should be used in repeated cycles only after a careful risk/benefit evaluation.

4.5 Interaction with other medicinal products and other forms of interaction
In vitro investigations have shown that interactions are unlikely with medicinal products that are metabolised by cytochrome P450 or glucuronised or conjugated in some other way. However, though there has been no evidence of drug-interactions, especially with commonly used medicinal products, gonadotropins or products that may induce histamine release in susceptible individuals, the possibility of an interaction cannot be totally excluded.

4.6 Pregnancy and lactation
Cetrotide is not intended to be used during pregnancy and lactation (see section 4.3).

Studies in animals have indicated that cetrorelix exerts a dose related influence on fertility, reproductive performance and pregnancy. No teratogenic effects occurred when the medicinal product was administered during the sensitive phase of gestation.

4.7 Effects on ability to drive and use machines
Cetrotide has no or negligible influence on the ability to drive or use machines.

4.8 Undesirable effects
The most commonly reported side effects are local injection site reactions such as erythema, swelling and pruritus that are usually transient in nature and mild in intensity.

Mild to moderate ovarian hyperstimulation syndrome (OHSS) (WHO grade I or II) have been commonly reported and should be considered as an intrinsic risk of the stimulation procedure. Inversely, severe OHSS remains uncommon.

Uncommonly, cases of hypersensitivity reactions including pseudo-allergic/anaphylactoid reactions have been reported.

The adverse reactions reported below are classified according to frequency of occurrence as follows:

Very Common	⩾ 1/10
Common	⩾ 1/100 to < 1/10
Uncommon	⩾ 1/1,000 to < 1/100
Rare	⩾ 1/10,000 to < 1/1,000
Very rare	< 1/10,000

Within each frequency grouping, undesirable effects are presented in order of decreasing seriousness.

Immune system disorders	Uncommon	Systemic allergic/pseudo-allergic reactions including life-threatening anaphylaxis.
Nervous system disorders	Uncommon	Headache
Gastrointestinal disorders	Uncommon	Nausea
Reproductive system and breast disorders	Common	Mild to moderate ovarian hyperstimulation syndrome (WHO grade I or II) can occur which is an intrinsic risk of the stimulation procedure (see section 4.4).
	Uncommon	Severe ovarian hyperstimulation syndrome (WHO grade III)
General disorders and administration site conditions	Common	Local reactions at the injection site (e.g. erythema, swelling and pruritus) have been reported. Usually they were transient in nature and of mild intensity. The frequency as reported in clinical trials was 8.0%.

4.9 Overdose
Overdosage in humans may result in a prolonged duration of action but is unlikely to be associated with acute toxic effects.

In acute toxicity studies in rodents non-specific toxic symptoms were observed after intraperitoneal administration of cetrorelix doses more than 200 times higher than the pharmacologically effective dose after subcutaneous administration.

5. PHARMACOLOGICAL PROPERTIES
5.1 Pharmacodynamic properties
Pharmacotherapeutic group: anti-gonadotropin-releasing hormones, ATC code: H01CC02.

Cetrorelix is a luteinising hormone releasing hormone (LHRH) antagonist. LHRH binds to membrane receptors on pituitary cells. Cetrorelix competes with the binding of endogenous LHRH to these receptors. Due to this mode of action, cetrorelix controls the secretion of gonadotropins (LH and FSH).

Cetrorelix dose-dependently inhibits the secretion of LH and FSH from the pituitary gland. The onset of suppression is virtually immediate and is maintained by continuous treatment, without initial stimulatory effect.

In females, cetrorelix delays the LH surge and consequently ovulation. In women undergoing ovarian stimulation the duration of action of cetrorelix is dose dependent. Following a single dose of 3 mg of cetrorelix a duration of action of at least 4 days has been evaluated. On day 4 the suppression was approximately 70%. At a dose of 0.25 mg per injection repeated injections every 24 hours will maintain the effect of cetrorelix.

In animals as well as in humans, the antagonistic hormonal effects of cetrorelix were fully reversible after termination of treatment.

5.2 Pharmacokinetic properties
The absolute bioavailability of cetrorelix after subcutaneous administration is about 85%.

The total plasma clearance and the renal clearance are 1.2 $ml \times min^{-1} \times kg^{-1}$ and 0.1 $ml \times min^{-1} \times kg^{-1}$, respectively. The volume of distribution (V_d) is 1.1 $l \times kg^{-1}$. The mean terminal half-lives following intravenous and subcutaneous administration are about 12 h and 30 h, respectively, demonstrating the effect of absorption processes at the injection site. The subcutaneous administration of single doses (0.25 mg to 3 mg cetrorelix) and also daily dosing over 14 days show linear kinetics.

5.3 Preclinical safety data
Non-clinical data reveal no special hazard for humans based on conventional studies of safety pharmacology, repeated dose toxicity, genotoxicity, carcinogenic potential, toxicity to reproduction.

No target organ toxicity could be observed from acute, subacute and chronic toxicity studies in rats and dogs following subcutaneous administration of cetrorelix. No signs of medicinal product-related local irritation or incompatibility were noted in dogs after intravenous, intra-arterial and paravenous injection when cetrorelix was administered in doses clearly above the intended clinical use in man.

Cetrorelix showed no mutagenic or clastogenic potential in gene and chromosome mutation assays.

6. PHARMACEUTICAL PARTICULARS
6.1 List of excipients
Powder:

Mannitol

Solvent:

Water for injections

6.2 Incompatibilities
This medicinal product must not be mixed with other medicinal products except those mentioned in section 6.6.

6.3 Shelf life
2 years.

The solution should be used immediately after preparation.

6.4 Special precautions for storage
Do not store above 25°C. Keep the vial in the outer carton in order to protect from light.

6.5 Nature and contents of container
Pack with 1 Type I glass vial sealed with a rubber stopper.

Additionally the pack contains:

1 pre-filled syringe (Type I glass cartridge closed with rubber stoppers) with 3 ml solvent for parenteral use

1 injection needle (20 gauge)

1 hypodermic injection needle (27 gauge)

2 alcohol swabs.

6.6 Special precautions for disposal and other handling
Cetrotide should only be reconstituted with the solvent provided, using a gentle, swirling motion. Vigorous shaking with bubble formation should be avoided.

The reconstituted solution is without particles and clear. Do not use if the solution contains particles or if the solution is not clear.

Withdraw the entire contents of the vial. This ensures a delivery to the patient of a dose of at least 2.82 mg cetrorelix.

The solution should be used immediately after reconstitution.

7. MARKETING AUTHORISATION HOLDER
Merck Serono Europe Limited
56 Marsh Wall
London E14 9TP
United Kingdom

8. MARKETING AUTHORISATION NUMBER(S)
EU/1/99/100/003

9. DATE OF FIRST AUTHORISATION/RENEWAL OF THE AUTHORISATION
Date of first authorisation: 13 April 1999
Date of first renewal: 15 April 2004
Date of latest renewal: March 2009

10. DATE OF REVISION OF THE TEXT
July 2009

CHAMPIX 0.5 mg film-coated tablets; CHAMPIX 1 mg film-coated tablets

(Pfizer Limited)

1. NAME OF THE MEDICINAL PRODUCT
CHAMPIX ®▼ 0.5 mg film-coated tablets
CHAMPIX ®▼ 1 mg film-coated tablets

2. QUALITATIVE AND QUANTITATIVE COMPOSITION
Each film-coated tablet contains 0.5 mg of varenicline (as tartrate).

Each film-coated tablet contains 1 mg of varenicline (as tartrate).

For a full list of excipients, see section 6.1.

3. PHARMACEUTICAL FORM
Film-coated tablet

0.5 mg film-coated tablets: White, capsular-shaped, biconvex tablets debossed with "*Pfizer*" on one side and "CHX 0.5" on the other side.

1 mg film-coated tablets: Light blue, capsular-shaped, biconvex tablets debossed with "*Pfizer*" on one side and "CHX 1.0" on the other side.

4. CLINICAL PARTICULARS

4.1 Therapeutic indications
CHAMPIX is indicated for smoking cessation in adults.

4.2 Posology and method of administration
Smoking cessation therapies are more likely to succeed for patients who are motivated to stop smoking and who are provided with additional advice and support.

CHAMPIX is for oral use. The recommended dose is 1 mg varenicline twice daily following a 1-week titration as follows:

Days 1 – 3:	0.5 mg once daily
Days 4 – 7:	0.5 mg twice daily
Day 8 – End of treatment:	1 mg twice daily

The patient should set a date to stop smoking. CHAMPIX dosing should start 1-2 weeks before this date.

Patients who cannot tolerate adverse effects of CHAMPIX may have the dose lowered temporarily or permanently to 0.5 mg twice daily.

CHAMPIX tablets should be swallowed whole with water. CHAMPIX can be taken with or without food.

Patients should be treated with CHAMPIX for 12 weeks.

For patients who have successfully stopped smoking at the end of 12 weeks, an additional course of 12 weeks treatment with CHAMPIX at 1 mg twice daily may be considered (see section 5.1).

No data are available on the efficacy of an additional 12 weeks course of treatment for patients who do not succeed in stopping smoking during initial therapy or who relapse after treatment.

In smoking cessation therapy, risk for relapse to smoking is elevated in the period immediately following the end of treatment. In patients with a high risk of relapse, dose tapering may be considered (see section 4.4).

Patients with renal insufficiency

No dosage adjustment is necessary for patients with mild (estimated creatinine clearance > 50 ml/min and ≤ 80 ml/min) to moderate (estimated creatinine clearance ≥ 30 ml/min and ≤ 50 ml/min) renal impairment.

For patients with moderate renal impairment who experience adverse events that are not tolerable, dosing may be reduced to 1 mg once daily.

For patients with severe renal impairment (estimated creatinine clearance < 30 ml/min), the recommended dose of CHAMPIX is 1 mg once daily. Dosing should begin at 0.5 mg once daily for the first 3 days then increased to 1 mg once daily. Based on insufficient clinical experience with CHAMPIX in patients with end stage renal disease, treatment is not recommended in this patient population (see section 5.2).

Patients with hepatic impairment

No dosage adjustment is necessary for patients with hepatic impairment (see section 5.2).

Dosing in elderly patients

No dosage adjustment is necessary for elderly patients (see section 5.2). Because elderly patients are more likely to have decreased renal function, prescribers should consider the renal status of an elderly patient.

Paediatric patients

CHAMPIX is not recommended for use in children or adolescents below 18 years of age due to insufficient data on safety and efficacy (see section 5.2).

4.3 Contraindications
Hypersensitivity to the active substance or to any of the excipients.

4.4 Special warnings and precautions for use
Effect of smoking cessation: Physiological changes resulting from smoking cessation, with or without treatment with CHAMPIX, may alter the pharmacokinetics or pharmacodynamics of some medicinal products, for which dosage adjustment may be necessary (examples include theophylline, warfarin and insulin). As smoking induces CYP1A2, smoking cessation may result in an increase of plasma levels of CYP1A2 substrates.

Depression, suicidal ideation and behaviour and suicide attempts have been reported in patients attempting to quit smoking with Champix in the post-marketing experience. Not all patients had stopped smoking at the time of onset of symptoms and not all patients had known pre-existing psychiatric illness. Clinicians should be aware of the possible emergence of significant depressive symptomatology in patients undergoing a smoking cessation attempt, and should advise patients accordingly. Champix should be discontinued immediately if agitation, depressed mood or changes in behaviour that are of concern for the doctor, the patient, family or caregivers are observed, or if the patient develops suicidal ideation or suicidal behaviour.

Depressed mood, rarely including suicidal ideation and suicide attempt, may be a symptom of nicotine withdrawal. In addition, smoking cessation, with or without pharmacotherapy, has been associated with exacerbation of underlying psychiatric illness (e.g. depression).

The safety and efficacy of Champix in patients with serious psychiatric illness such as schizophrenia, bipolar disorder and major depressive disorder has not been established. Care should be taken with patients with a history of psychiatric illness and patients should be advised accordingly.

There is no clinical experience with CHAMPIX in patients with epilepsy.

At the end of treatment, discontinuation of CHAMPIX was associated with an increase in irritability, urge to smoke, depression, and/or insomnia in up to 3% of patients. The prescriber should inform the patient accordingly and discuss or consider the need for dose tapering.

4.5 Interaction with other medicinal products and other forms of interaction
Based on varenicline characteristics and clinical experience to date, CHAMPIX has no clinically meaningful drug interactions. No dosage adjustment of CHAMPIX or co-administered medicinal products listed below is recommended.

In vitro studies indicate that varenicline is unlikely to alter the pharmacokinetics of compounds that are primarily metabolised by cytochrome P450 enzymes.

Furthermore since metabolism of varenicline represents less than 10% of its clearance, active substances known to affect the cytochrome P450 system are unlikely to alter the pharmacokinetics of varenicline (see section 5.2) and therefore a dose adjustment of CHAMPIX would not be required.

In vitro studies demonstrate that varenicline does not inhibit human renal transport proteins at therapeutic concentrations. Therefore, active substances that are cleared by renal secretion (e.g. metformin - see below) are unlikely to be affected by varenicline.

Metformin: Varenicline did not affect the pharmacokinetics of metformin. Metformin had no effect on varenicline pharmacokinetics.

Cimetidine: Co-administration of cimetidine, with varenicline increased the systemic exposure of varenicline by 29% due to a reduction in varenicline renal clearance. No dosage adjustment is recommended based on concomitant cimetidine administration in subjects with normal renal function or in patients with mild to moderate renal impairment. In patients with severe renal impairment, the concomitant use of cimetidine and varenicline should be avoided.

Digoxin: Varenicline did not alter the steady-state pharmacokinetics of digoxin.

Warfarin: Varenicline did not alter the pharmacokinetics of warfarin. Prothrombin time (INR) was not affected by varenicline. Smoking cessation itself may result in changes to warfarin pharmacokinetics (see section 4.4).

Alcohol: There is limited clinical data on any potential interaction between alcohol and varenicline

Use with other therapies for smoking cessation:

Bupropion: Varenicline did not alter the steady-state pharmacokinetics of bupropion.

Nicotine replacement therapy (NRT): When varenicline and transdermal NRT were co-administered to smokers for 12 days, there was a statistically significant decrease in average systolic blood pressure (mean 2.6 mmHg) measured on the final day of the study. In this study, the incidence of nausea, headache, vomiting, dizziness, dyspepsia, and fatigue was greater for the combination than for NRT alone.

Safety and efficacy of CHAMPIX in combination with other smoking cessation therapies have not been studied.

4.6 Pregnancy and lactation
There are no adequate data from the use of CHAMPIX in pregnant women. Studies in animals have shown reproductive toxicity (see section 5.3). The potential risk for humans is unknown. CHAMPIX should not be used during pregnancy.

It is unknown whether varenicline is excreted in human breast milk. Animal studies suggest that varenicline is excreted in breast milk. A decision on whether to continue/discontinue breast-feeding or to continue/discontinue therapy with CHAMPIX should be made taking into account the benefit of breast-feeding to the child and the benefit of CHAMPIX therapy to the woman.

4.7 Effects on ability to drive and use machines
CHAMPIX may have minor or moderate influence on the ability to drive and use machines. CHAMPIX may cause dizziness and somnolence and therefore may influence the ability to drive and use machines. Patients are advised not to drive, operate complex machinery or engage in other potentially hazardous activities until it is known whether this medicinal product affects their ability to perform these activities.

4.8 Undesirable effects
Smoking cessation with or without treatment is associated with various symptoms. For example, dysphoric or depressed mood; insomnia, irritability, frustration or anger; anxiety; difficulty concentrating; restlessness; decreased heart rate; increased appetite or weight gain have been reported in patients attempting to stop smoking. No attempt has been made in either the design or the analysis of the CHAMPIX studies to distinguish between adverse events associated with study drug treatment or those possibly associated with nicotine withdrawal.

Clinical trials included approximately 4,000 patients treated with CHAMPIX for up to 1 year (average exposure 84 days). In general, when adverse reactions occurred, onset was in the first week of therapy; severity was generally mild to moderate and there were no differences by age, race or gender with regard to the incidence of adverse reactions.

In patients treated with the recommended dose of 1mg BID following an initial titration period the adverse event most commonly reported was nausea (28.6%). In the majority of cases nausea occurred early in the treatment period, was mild to moderate in severity and seldom resulted in discontinuation.

The treatment discontinuation rate due to adverse events was 11.4% for varenicline compared with 9.7% for placebo. In this group, the discontinuation rates for the most common adverse events in varenicline treated patients were as follows: nausea (2.7% vs. 0.6% for placebo), headache (0.6% vs. 1.0% for placebo), insomnia (1.3% vs. 1.2% for placebo), and abnormal dreams (0.2% vs. 0.2% for placebo).

In the table below all adverse reactions, which occurred at an incidence greater than placebo are listed by system organ class and frequency (very common (≥1/10), common (≥1/100 to <1/10), uncommon (≥1/1,000 to <1/100) and rare (≥1/10,000 to <1/1,000)). Within each frequency grouping, undesirable effects are presented in order of decreasing seriousness.

System Organ Class	Adverse Drug Reactions
Infections and Infestations	
Uncommon	Bronchitis, nasopharyngitis, sinusitis, fungal infection, viral infection.
Metabolism and nutrition disorders	
Common	Increased appetite
Uncommon	Anorexia, decreased appetite, polydipsia
Psychiatric disorders	
Very common	Abnormal dreams, insomnia
Uncommon	Panic reaction, bradyphrenia, thinking abnormal, mood swings
Nervous system disorders	
Very common	Headache
Common	Somnolence, dizziness, dysgeusia
Uncommon	Tremor, coordination abnormal, dysarthria, hypertonia, restlessness, dysphoria, hypoaesthesia, hypogeusia, lethargy, libido increased, libido decreased
Cardiac disorders	
Uncommon	Atrial fibrillation, palpitations
Eye disorders	
Uncommon	Scotoma, scleral discolouration, eye pain, mydriasis, photophobia, myopia, lacrimation increased
Ear and labyrinth disorders	
Uncommon	Tinnitus
Respiratory, thoracic and mediastinal disorders	
Uncommon	Dyspnoea, cough, hoarseness, pharyngolaryngeal pain, throat irritation, respiratory tract congestion, sinus congestion, post nasal drip, rhinorrhoea, snoring
Gastrointestinal disorders	
Very common	Nausea
Common	Vomiting, constipation, diarrhoea, abdominal distension, stomach discomfort, dyspepsia, flatulence, dry mouth
Uncommon	Haematemesis, haematochezia, gastritis, gastroesophageal reflux disease, abdominal pain, change of bowel habit, abnormal faeces, eructation, aphthous stomatitis, gingival pain, tongue coated
Skin and subcutaneous tissue disorders	
Uncommon	Rash generalised, erythema, pruritus, acne, hyperhidrosis, night sweats
Musculoskeletal and connective tissue disorders	
Uncommon	Joint stiffness, muscle spasms, chest wall pain, costochondritis
Renal and urinary disorders	
Uncommon	Glycosuria, nocturia, polyuria
Reproductive system and breast disorders	
Uncommon	Menorrhagia, vaginal discharge, sexual dysfunction
General disorders and administration site conditions	
Common	Fatigue
Uncommon	Chest discomfort, chest pain, pyrexia, feeling cold, asthenia, circadian rhythm sleep disorder, malaise, cyst
Investigations	
Uncommon	Blood pressure increased, electrocardiogram ST segment depression, electrocardiogram T wave amplitude decreased, heart rate increased, liver function test abnormal, platelet count decreased, weight increased, semen abnormal, C-reactive protein increased, blood calcium decreased

Post-marketing cases of depression, suicidal ideation and changes in behaviour (such as aggression and irrational behaviour) have been reported in patients taking varenicline (see section 4.4). There have also been reports of myocardial infarction, hallucinations and hypersensitivity reactions, such as angioedema and facial swelling.

4.9 Overdose

No cases of overdose were reported in pre-marketing clinical trials.

In case of overdose, standard supportive measures should be instituted as required.

Varenicline has been shown to be dialyzed in patients with end stage renal disease (see section 5.2), however, there is no experience in dialysis following overdose.

5. PHARMACOLOGICAL PROPERTIES

5.1 Pharmacodynamic properties

Pharmacotherapeutic group: Active substances used in nicotine dependence, ATC code: N07BA03

Varenicline binds with high affinity and selectivity at the $\alpha4\beta2$ neuronal nicotinic acetylcholine receptors, where it acts as a partial agonist - a compound that has both agonist activity, with lower intrinsic efficacy than nicotine, and antagonist activities in the presence of nicotine.

Electrophysiology studies *in vitro* and neurochemical studies in vivo have shown that varenicline binds to the $\alpha4\beta2$ neuronal nicotinic acetylcholine receptors and stimulates receptor-mediated activity, but at a significantly lower level than nicotine. Nicotine competes for the same human $\alpha4\beta2$ nAChR binding site for which varenicline has higher affinity. Therefore, varenicline can effectively block nicotine's ability to fully activate $\alpha4\beta2$ receptors and the mesolimbic dopamine system, the neuronal mechanism underlying reinforcement and reward experienced upon smoking. Varenicline is highly selective and binds more potently to the $\alpha4\beta2$ receptor subtype (Ki=0.15 nM) than to other common nicotinic receptors ($\alpha3\beta4$ Ki=84 nM, $\alpha7$ Ki= 620 nM, $\alpha1\beta\gamma\delta$ Ki= 3,400 nM), or to non-nicotinic receptors and transporters (Ki$>$ 1μM, except to 5-HT3 receptors: Ki=350 nM).

The efficacy of CHAMPIX in smoking cessation is a result of varenicline's partial agonist activity at the $\alpha4\beta2$ nicotinic receptor where its binding produces an effect sufficient to alleviate symptoms of craving and withdrawal (agonist activity), while simultaneously resulting in a reduction of the rewarding and reinforcing effects of smoking by preventing nicotine binding to $\alpha4\beta2$ receptors (antagonist activity).

Clinical Efficacy

The efficacy of CHAMPIX in smoking cessation was demonstrated in 3 clinical trials involving chronic cigarette smokers ($\geqslant$10 cigarettes per day). 2619 patients received CHAMPIX 1mg BID (titrated during the first week), 669 patients received bupropion 150 mg BID (also titrated) and 684 patients received placebo.

Comparative Clinical Studies

Two identical double-blind clinical trials prospectively compared the efficacy of CHAMPIX (1 mg twice daily), sustained release bupropion (150 mg twice daily) and placebo in smoking cessation. In these 52-week duration studies, patients received treatment for 12 weeks, followed by a 40-week non-treatment phase.

The primary endpoint of the two studies was the carbon monoxide (CO) confirmed, 4-week continuous quit rate (4W-CQR) from week 9 through week 12. The primary endpoint for CHAMPIX demonstrated statistical superiority to bupropion and placebo.

After the 40 week non-treatment phase, a key secondary endpoint for both studies was the Continuous Abstinence Rate (CA) at week 52. CA was defined as the proportion of all subjects treated who did not smoke (not even a puff of a cigarette) from Week 9 through Week 52 and did not have an exhaled CO measurement of $>$ 10 ppm. The 4W-CQR (weeks 9 through 12) and CA rate (weeks 9 through 52) from studies 1 and 2 are included in the following table:

(see Table 1 below)

Patient reported craving, withdrawal and reinforcing effects of smoking

Across both Studies 1 and 2 during active treatment, craving and withdrawal were significantly reduced in patients randomized to CHAMPIX in comparison with placebo. CHAMPIX also significantly reduced reinforcing effects of smoking that can perpetuate smoking behaviour in patients who smoke during treatment compared with placebo. The effect of varenicline on craving, withdrawal and reinforcing effects of smoking were not measured during the non-treatment long-term follow-up phase.

Maintenance of Abstinence Study

The third study assessed the benefit of an additional 12 weeks of CHAMPIX therapy on the maintenance of abstinence. Patients in this study (n=1,927) received open-label CHAMPIX 1 mg twice daily for 12 weeks. Patients who stopped smoking by Week 12 were then randomized to receive either CHAMPIX (1 mg twice daily) or placebo for an additional 12 weeks for a total study duration of 52 weeks.

The primary study endpoint was the CO-confirmed continuous abstinence rate from week 13 through week 24 in the double-blind treatment phase. A key secondary endpoint was the continuous abstinence (CA) rate for week 13 through week 52.

This study showed the benefit of an additional 12-week treatment with CHAMPIX 1 mg twice daily for the maintenance of smoking cessation compared to placebo. The odds of maintaining abstinence at week 24, following an additional 12 weeks of treatment with CHAMPIX, were 2.47 times those for placebo ($p<0.0001$). Superiority to placebo for CA was maintained through week 52 (Odds Ratio=1.35, $p=0.0126$).

The key results are summarised in the following table:

(see Table 2 below)

There is currently limited clinical experience with the use of CHAMPIX among black people to determine clinical efficacy.

5.2 Pharmacokinetic properties

Absorption: Maximum plasma concentrations of varenicline occur typically within 3-4 hours after oral administration. Following administration of multiple oral doses to healthy volunteers, steady-state conditions were reached within 4 days. Absorption is virtually complete after oral administration and systemic availability is high. Oral bioavailability of varenicline is unaffected by food or time-of-day dosing.

Distribution: Varenicline distributes into tissues, including the brain. Apparent volume of distribution averaged 415 litres (%CV= 50) at steady-state. Plasma protein binding of varenicline is low ($\leq$ 20%) and independent of both age and renal function. In rodents, varenicline is transferred through the placenta and excreted in milk.

Biotransformation: Varenicline undergoes minimal metabolism with 92% excreted unchanged in the urine and less than 10% excreted as metabolites. Minor metabolites in urine include varenicline N-carbamoylglucuronide and hydroxyvarenicline. In circulation, varenicline comprises 91% of drug-related material. Minor circulating metabolites include varenicline N-carbamoylglucuronide and N-glucosylvarenicline.

Elimination: The elimination half-life of varenicline is approximately 24 hours. Renal elimination of varenicline is primarily through glomerular filtration along with active

Table 1

	Study 1 (n=1022)		Study 2 (n=1023)	
	4W CQR	CA Wk 9-52	4W CQR	CA Wk 9-52
CHAMPIX	44.4%	22.1%	44.0%	23.0%
Bupropion	29.5%	16.4%	30.0%	15.0%
Placebo	17.7%	8.4%	17.7%	10.3%
Odds ratio CHAMPIX vs placebo	3.91 $p<0.0001$	3.13 $p<0.0001$	3.85 $p<0.0001$	2.66 $p<0.0001$
Odds ratio CHAMPIX vs bupropion	1.96 $p<0.0001$	1.45 p=0.0640	1.89 $p<0.0001$	1.72 p=0.0062

Table 2

	CHAMPIX n=602	Placebo n=604	Difference (95% CI)	Odds ratio (95% CI)
CA wk 13-24	70.6%	49.8%	20.8% (15.4%, 26.2%)	2.47 (1.95, 3.15)
CA wk 13-52	44.0%	37.1%	6.9% (1.4%,12.5%)	1.35 (1.07, 1.70)

tubular secretion via the organic cationic transporter, OCT2. (See section 4.5).

Linearity/Non linearity: Varenicline exhibits linear kinetics when given as single (0.1 to 3 mg) or repeated (1 to 3 mg/ day) doses.

Pharmacokinetics in special patient populations: There are no clinically meaningful differences in varenicline pharmacokinetics due to age, race, gender, smoking status, or use of concomitant medications, as demonstrated in specific pharmacokinetic studies and in population pharmacokinetic analyses.

Patients with hepatic impairment: Due to the absence of significant hepatic metabolism, varenicline pharmacokinetics should be unaffected in patients with hepatic impairment. (See section 4.2).

Renal Insufficiency: Varenicline pharmacokinetics were unchanged in subjects with mild renal impairment (estimated creatinine clearance > 50 ml/min and ≤ 80 ml/min). In patients with moderate renal impairment (estimated creatinine clearance ≥ 30 ml/min and ≤ 50 ml/min), varenicline exposure increased 1.5-fold compared with subjects with normal renal function (estimated creatinine clearance > 80 ml/min). In subjects with severe renal impairment (estimated creatinine clearance < 30 ml/ min), varenicline exposure was increased 2.1-fold. In subjects with end-stage-renal disease (ESRD), varenicline was efficiently removed by haemodialysis (see section 4.2).

Elderly: The pharmacokinetics of varenicline in elderly patients with normal renal function (aged 65-75 years) is similar to that of younger adult subjects (see section 4.2). For elderly patients with reduced renal function please refer to section 4.2.

Adolescents: When 22 adolescents aged 12 to 17 years (inclusive) received a single 0.5 mg and 1 mg dose of varenicline the pharmacokinetics of varenicline was approximately dose proportional between the 0.5 mg and 1 mg doses. Systemic exposure, as assessed by AUC (0-inf), and renal clearance of varenicline were comparable to adults. An increase of 30% in C_{max} and a shorter elimination half-life (10.9 hr) were observed in adolescents compared with adults (see section 4.2).

In vitro studies demonstrate that varenicline does not inhibit cytochrome P450 enzymes (IC50 > 6,400 ng/ml). The P450 enzymes tested for inhibition were: 1A2, 2A6, 2B6, 2C8, 2C9, 2C19, 2D6, 2E1, and 3A4/5. Also, in human hepatocytes in vitro, varenicline was shown to not induce the activity of cytochrome P450 enzymes 1A2 and 3A4. Therefore, varenicline is unlikely to alter the pharmacokinetics of compounds that are primarily metabolised by cytochrome P450 enzymes.

5.3 Preclinical safety data

Non-clinical data reveal no special hazard for humans based on conventional studies of safety pharmacology, repeated dose toxicity, genotoxicity, fertility and embryo-foetal development. In male rats dosed for 2 years with varenicline, there was a dose-related increase in the incidence of hibernoma (tumour of the brown fat). In the off-spring of pregnant rats treated with varenicline there were decreases in fertility and increases in the auditory startle response (see section 4.6). These effects were observed only at exposures considered sufficiently in excess of the maximum human exposure indicating little relevance to clinical use. Nonclinical data indicate varenicline has reinforcing properties albeit with lower potency than nicotine. In clinical studies in humans, varenicline showed low abuse potential.

6. PHARMACEUTICAL PARTICULARS

6.1 List of excipients

Core Tablet

Cellulose, Microcrystalline

Calcium Hydrogen Phosphate Anhydrous

Croscarmellose Sodium

Silica, Colloidal Anhydrous

Magnesium Stearate

Film Coating

Hypromellose

Titanium Dioxide (E171)

Macrogols

Triacetin

6.2 Incompatibilities

Not applicable.

6.3 Shelf life

2 years

6.4 Special precautions for storage

This medicinal product does not require any special storage conditions

6.5 Nature and contents of container

Treatment initiation packs

Aclar / PVC blisters with aluminium foil backing containing one clear blister of 11 × 0.5 mg film-coated tablets and a second clear blister of 14 × 1 mg film-coated tablets in secondary heat sealed card packaging.

Aclar / PVC blisters with aluminium foil backing containing one clear blister of 11 × 0.5 mg film-coated tablets and a second clear blister containing 14 × 1 mg film-coated tablets in a carton.

Aclar / PVC / blisters with aluminium foil backing containing one clear blister of 11 × 0.5 mg and 14 × 1 mg film-coated tablets and a second clear blister of 28 × 1 mg film-coated tablets in secondary heat sealed card packaging.

Maintenance packs

Aclar / PVC blisters with aluminium foil backing in a pack containing 28 × 0.5 mg film-coated tablets in secondary heat sealed card packaging.

Aclar / PVC blisters with aluminium foil backing in a pack containing 56 × 0.5 mg film-coated tablets in secondary heat sealed card packaging.

High-density polyethylene (HDPE) blue white tablet container with polypropylene child resistant closure and an aluminium foil / polyethylene induction seal containing 56 × 0.5 mg film-coated tablets

Aclar / PVC blisters with aluminium foil backing in a pack containing 28 × 1 mg film-coated tablets in secondary heat sealed card packaging.

Aclar / PVC blisters with aluminium foil backing in a pack containing 56 × 1 mg film-coated tablets in secondary heat sealed card packaging.

Aclar / PVC blisters with aluminium foil backing in a pack containing 28 × 1 mg film-coated tablets in a carton.

Aclar / PVC blisters with aluminium foil backing in a pack containing 56 × 1 mg film-coated tablets in a carton.

Aclar / PVC blisters with aluminium foil backing in a pack containing 112 × 1 mg film-coated tablets in a carton.

High-density polyethylene (HDPE) blue white tablet container with polypropylene child resistant closure and an aluminium foil / polyethylene induction seal containing 56 × 1 mg film-coated tablets

Aclar / PVC blisters with aluminium foil backing in a pack containing 140 × 1 mg film-coated tablets in secondary heat sealed card packaging.

Not all pack sizes may be marketed.

6.6 Special precautions for disposal and other handling

No special requirements.

7. MARKETING AUTHORISATION HOLDER

Pfizer Limited

Ramsgate Road

Sandwich

Kent

CT13 9NJ

UK

8. MARKETING AUTHORISATION NUMBER(S)

EU/1/06/360/003

EU/1/06/360/008

EU/1/06/360/012

EU/1/06/360/006

EU/1/06/360/007

EU/1/06/360/001

EU/1/06/360/004

EU/1/06/360/005

EU/1/06/360/009

EU/1/06/360/010

EU/1/06/360/011

EU/1/06/360/002

EU/1/06/360/013

9. DATE OF FIRST AUTHORISATION/RENEWAL OF THE AUTHORISATION

26/09/2006

10. DATE OF REVISION OF THE TEXT

03/08/2009

LEGAL CATEGORY

POM

CI11_0

Chirocaine 0.625mg/ml & 1.25mg/ml solution for infusion

(Abbott Laboratories Limited)

1. NAME OF THE MEDICINAL PRODUCT

Chirocaine 0.625 mg/ml solution for infusion

Chirocaine 1.25 mg/ml solution for infusion

2. QUALITATIVE AND QUANTITATIVE COMPOSITION

Levobupivacaine hydrochloride corresponding to 0.625 mg/ml or 1.25 mg/ml Levobupivacaine.

Excipients: 3.6mg/ml of sodium per bag.

For a full list of excipients, see section 6.1.

3. PHARMACEUTICAL FORM

Solution for infusion

Clear solution

4. CLINICAL PARTICULARS

4.1 Therapeutic indications

Adults

Pain management

Continuous epidural infusion, for the management of post operative pain and labour analgesia.

4.2 Posology and method of administration

Levobupivacaine should be administered only by, or under the supervision of, a clinician having the necessary training and experience.

Chirocaine Solution for Infusion is for epidural use only. It must not be used for intravenous administration.

(see Table 1 on next page)

Careful aspiration before infusion is recommended to prevent intravascular injection. If toxic symptoms occur, the injection should be stopped immediately.

Maximum dose

The maximum dosage must be determined by evaluating the size and physical status of the patient. The maximum recommended dose during a 24 hour period is 400 mg.

For post-operative pain management, the dose should not exceed 18.75 mg/hour, however the accumulated dose for a 24 hour period should not exceed 400 mg. For labour analgesia by epidural infusion, the dose should not exceed 12.5 mg/ hour.

Children

The safety and efficacy of levobupivacaine in children for pain management has not been established.

Special Populations

Debilitated, elderly or acutely ill patients should be given reduced doses of levobupivacaine commensurate with their physical status.

In the management of post-operative pain, the dose given during surgery must be taken into account.

There are no relevant data in patients with hepatic impairment (see sections 4.4 and 5.2).

4.3 Contraindications

General contra-indications related to regional anaesthesia regardless of the local anaesthetic used, should be taken into account.

Levobupivacaine solutions are contra-indicated in patients with a known hypersensitivity to levobupivacaine, local anaesthetics of the amide type or any of the excipients (see section 4.8).

Levobupivacaine solutions are contra-indicated for intravenous regional anaesthesia (Bier's block).

Levobupivacaine solutions are contra-indicated in patients with severe hypotension such as cardiogenic or hypovolaemic shock.

Levobupivacaine solutions are contra-indicated for use in paracervical block in obstetrics (see section 4.6).

4.4 Special warnings and precautions for use

All forms of local and regional anaesthesia with levobupivacaine should be performed in well-equipped facilities and administered by staff trained and experienced in the required anaesthetic techniques and able to diagnose and treat any unwanted adverse effects that may occur.

The introduction of local anesthetics via epidural administration into the central nervous system in patients with preexisting CNS diseases may potentially exacerbate some of these disease states. Therefore, clinical judgment should be exercised when contemplating epidural anesthesia in such patients.

This medicinal product contains 3.6 mg/ml sodium in the bag or ampoule solution to be taken into consideration by patients on a controlled sodium diet.

During epidural administration of levobupivacaine, concentrated solutions (0.5-0.75%) should be administered in incremental doses of 3 to 5 ml with sufficient time between doses to detect toxic manifestations of unintentional intravascular or intrathecal injection. When a large dose is to be injected, e.g. in epidural block, a test dose of 3-5 ml lidocaine with adrenaline is recommended. An inadvertent intravascular injection may then be recognised by a temporary increase in heart rate and accidental intrathecal injection by signs of a spinal block. Syringe aspirations should also be performed before and during each supplemental injection in continuous (intermittent) catheter techniques. An intravascular injection is still possible even if aspirations for blood are negative. During the administration of epidural anesthesia, it is recommended that a test dose be administered initially and the effects monitored before the full dose is given.

Epidural anaesthesia with any local anaesthetic may cause hypotension and bradycardia. All patients must have intravenous access established. The availability of appropriate fluids, vasopressors, anaesthetics with anticonvulsant properties, myorelaxants, and atropine, resuscitation equipment and expertise must be ensured (see section 4.9).

Special populations

Debilitated, elderly or acutely ill patients: levobupivacaine should be used with caution in debilitated, elderly or acutely ill patients (see section 4.2).

Hepatic impairment: since levobupivacaine is metabolised in the liver, it should be used cautiously in patients with liver disease or with reduced liver blood flow e.g. alcoholics or cirrhotics (see section 5.2).

4.5 Interaction with other medicinal products and other forms of interaction

In vitro studies indicate that the CYP3A4 isoform and CYP1A2 isoform mediate the metabolism of levobupivacaine. Although no clinical studies have been conducted, metabolism of levobupivacaine may be affected by CYP3A4 inhibitors eg: ketoconazole, and CYP1A2 inhibitors eg: methylxanthines.

Levobupivacaine should be used with caution in patients receiving anti-arrhythmic agents with local anaesthetic activity, e.g., mexiletine, or class III anti-arrhythmic agents since their toxic effects may be additive.

No clinical studies have been completed to assess levobupivacaine in combination with adrenaline.

4.6 Pregnancy and lactation

Pregnancy

Levobupivacaine solutions are contraindicated for use in paracervical block in obstetrics. Based on experience with bupivacaine foetal bradycardia may occur following paracervical block (see section 4.3).

For levobupivacaine, there are no clinical data on first trimester-exposed pregnancies. Animal studies do not indicate teratogenic effects but have shown embryo-foetal toxicity at systemic exposure levels in the same range as those obtained in clinical use (see section 5.3). The potential risk for human is unknown. Levobupivacaine should therefore not be given during early pregnancy unless clearly necessary.

Nevertheless, to date, the clinical experience of bupivacaine for obstetrical surgery (at the term of pregnancy or for delivery) is extensive and has not shown a foetotoxic effect.

Lactation

Levobupivacaine excretion in breast milk is unknown. However, levobupivacaine is likely to be poorly transmitted in the breast milk, as for bupivacaine. Thus breast feeding is possible after local anaesthesia.

4.7 Effects on ability to drive and use machines

Levobupivacaine can have a major influence on the ability to drive or use machines. Patients should be warned not to drive or operate machinery until all the effects of the anaesthesia and the immediate effects of surgery are passed.

4.8 Undesirable effects

The adverse drug reactions for Chirocaine are consistent with those known for its respective class of medicinal products. The most commonly reported adverse drug reactions are hypotension, nausea, anaemia, vomiting, dizziness, headache, pyrexia, procedural pain, back pain and foetal distress syndrome in obstetric use (see table below).

Adverse reactions reported either spontaneously or observed in clinical trials are depicted in the following table. Within each system organ class, the adverse drug reactions are ranked under headings of frequency, using the following convention: very common (⩾1/10), common (⩾1/100, <1/10), uncommon (⩾1/1000, <1/100), not known (cannot be estimated from the available data).

System Organ Class	Frequency	Adverse Reaction
Blood and lymphatic system disorders	Very Common	Anaemia
Nervous system disorders	Common Common Not known Not known Not known	Dizziness Headache Convulsion Loss of consciousness Somnolence
Eye disorders	Not known	Vision blurred
Respiratory, thoracic and mediastinal disorders	Not known	Respiratory arrest
Gastrointestinal disorders	Very Common Common Not known	Nausea Vomiting Hypoaesthesia oral
Musculoskeletal and connective tissue disorders	Common Not known	Back pain Muscle twitching
Injury, poisoning and procedural complications	Common	Procedural pain
Vascular disorders	Very Common	Hypotension
General disorders and administration site conditions	Common	Pyrexia
Pregnancy, puerperium and perinatal conditions	Common	Foetal distress syndrome
Immune system disorders	Not known	Anaphylactic reaction

Adverse reactions with local anaesthetics of the amide type are rare, but they may occur as a result of overdosage or unintentional intravascular injection and may be serious.

Table 1

Type of Block	Concentration	Infusion Rate Per Hour	
	mg/ml	ml	mg
Continuous Infusion: Post operative pain management	0.625 1.25	20-30 10-15	12.5-18.75 12.5-18.75
Lumbar epidural (analgesia in labour)	0.625 1.25	8-20 4-10	5–12.5 5–12.5

Allergic-type reactions are rare and may occur as a result of sensitivity to the local anesthetic. These reactions are characterised by signs such as urticaria, pruritus, erythema, angioneurotic edema (including laryngeal edema), tachycardia, sneezing, nausea, vomiting, dizziness, syncope, excessive sweating, elevated temperature, and, possibly, anaphylactoid-like symptomatology (including severe hypotension). Cross-sensitivity among members of the amide-type local anesthetic group have been reported (see section 4.3).

Accidental intrathecal injection of local anaesthetics can lead to very high spinal anaesthesia possibly with apnoea, severe hypotension and loss of consciousness.

Cardiovascular effects are related to depression of the conduction system of the heart and a reduction in myocardial excitability and contractility. This results in decreased cardiac output, hypotension and ECG changes indicative of either heart block, bradycardia or ventricular tachyarrythmias that may lead to cardiac arrest. Usually these will be preceded by major CNS toxicity, i.e. convulsions, but in rare cases, cardiac arrest may occur without prodromal CNS effects.

Neurological damage is a rare but well recognised consequence of regional and particularly epidural and spinal anaesthesia. It may be due to direct injury to the spinal cord or spinal nerves, anterior spinal artery syndrome, injection of an irritant substance or an injection of a non-sterile solution. These may result in localised areas of paraesthesia or anaesthesia, motor weakness, loss of sphincter control and paraplegia. Rarely, these may be permanent.

4.9 Overdose

Accidental intravascular injection of local anaesthetics may cause immediate toxic reactions. In the event of overdose, peak plasma concentrations may not be reached until 2 hours after administration depending upon the injection site and, therefore, signs of toxicity may be delayed. The effects of the drug may be prolonged.

Systemic adverse reactions following overdose or accidental intravascular injection reported with long acting local anaesthetic agents involve both CNS and cardiovascular effects.

CNS Effects

Convulsions should be treated immediately with intravenous thiopentone or diazepam titrated as necessary. Thiopentone and diazepam also depress central nervous system, respiratory and cardiac function. Therefore, their use may result in apnoea. Neuro-muscular blockers may be used only if the clinician is confident ofmaintaining a patent airway and managing a fully paralysed patient.

If not treated promptly, convulsions with subsequent hypoxia and hypercarbia plus myocardial depression from the effects of the local anaesthetic on the heart, may result in cardiac arrhythmias, ventricular fibrillation or cardiac arrest.

Cardiovascular Effects

Hypotension may be prevented or attenuated by pre-treatment with a fluid load and/or the use of vasopressors. If hypotension occurs it should be treated with intravenous crystalloids or colloids and/or incremental doses of a vasopressor such as ephedrine 5-10 mg. Any coexisting causes of hypotension should be rapidly treated.

If severe bradycardia occurs, treatment with atropine 0.3-1.0 mg will normally restore the heart rate to an acceptable level.

Cardiac arrhythmia should be treated as required and ventricular fibrillation should be treated by cardioversion.

5. PHARMACOLOGICAL PROPERTIES

5.1 Pharmacodynamic properties

Pharmacotherapeutic group: Local anaesthetics, amide

ATC Code N01B B10

Levobupivacaine is a long acting local anaesthetic and analgesic. It blocks nerve conduction in sensory and motor nerves largely by interacting with voltage sensitive sodium channels on the cell membrane, but also potassium and calcium channels are blocked. In addition, levobupivacaine interferes with impulse transmission and conduction in other tissues where effects on the cardiovascular and central nervous systems are most important for the occurrence of clinical adverse reactions.

The dose of levobupivacaine is expressed as base, whereas, in the racemate bupivacaine the dose is expressed as hydrochloride salt. This gives rise to approximately 13% more active substance in levobupivacaine solutions compared to bupivacaine. In clinical studies at the same nominal concentrations levobupivacaine showed similar clinical effect to bupivacaine.

In a clinical pharmacology study using the ulnar nerve block model, levobupivacaine was equipotent with bupivacaine.

5.2 Pharmacokinetic properties

In human studies, the distribution kinetics of levobupivacaine following i.v. administration are essentially the same as bupivacaine. The plasma concentration of levobupivacaine following therapeutic administration depends on dose and, as absorption from the site of administration is affected by the vascularity of the tissue, on route of administration.

There are no relevant data in patients with hepatic impairment (see section 4.4).

There are no data in patients with renal impairment. Levobupivacaine is extensively metabolised and unchanged levobupivacaine is not excreted in urine.

Plasma protein binding of levobupivacaine in man was evaluated *in vitro* and was found to be > 97% at concentrations between 0.1 and 1.0 µg/ml.

In a clinical pharmacology study where 40 mg levobupivacaine was given by intravenous administration, the mean half-life was approximately 80 ± 22 minutes, C_{max} 1.4 ± 0.2 µg/ml and AUC 70 ± 27 µg•min/ml.

The mean C_{max} and AUC(0-24h) of levobupivacaine were approximately dose-proportional following epidural administration of 75 mg (0.5%) and 112.5 mg (0.75%) and following doses of 1 mg/kg (0.25%) and 2 mg/kg (0.5%) used for brachial plexus block. Following epidural administration of 112.5 mg (0.75%) the mean C_{max} and AUC values were 0.58 µg/ml and 3.56 µg•h/ml respectively.

The mean total plasma clearance and terminal half-life of levobupivacaine after intravenous infusion were 39 litres/hour and 1.3 hours, respectively. The volume of distribution after intravenous administration was 67 litres.

Levobupivacaine is extensively metabolised with no unchanged levobupivacaine detected in urine or faeces. 3-hydroxylevobupivacaine, a major metabolite of levobupivacaine, is excreted in the urine as glucuronic acid and sulphate ester conjugates. *In vitro* studies showed that CYP3A4 isoform and CYP1A2 isoform mediate the metabolism of levobupivacaine to desbutyl-levobupivacaine and 3-hydroxylevobupivacaine respectively. These studies indicate that the metabolism of levobupivacaine and bupivacaine are similar.

Following intravenous administration, recovery of levobupivacaine was quantitative with a mean total of about 95% being recovered in urine (71%) and faeces (24%) in 48 hours.

There is no evidence of *in vivo* racemisation of levobupivacaine.

5.3 Preclinical safety data

In an embryo-foetal toxicity study in rats, an increased incidence of dilated renal pelvis, dilated ureters, olfactory ventricle dilatation and extra thoraco-lumbar ribs was observed at systemic exposure levels in the same range as those obtained at clinical use. There were no treatment-related malformations.

Levobupivacaine was not genotoxic in a standard battery of assays for mutagenicity and clastogenicity. No carcinogenicity testing has been conducted.

6. PHARMACEUTICAL PARTICULARS

6.1 List of excipients

Sodium Chloride

Sodium Hydroxide

Hydrochloric acid

Water for Injections

6.2 Incompatibilities

Levobupivacaine may precipitate if diluted with alkaline solutions and should not be diluted or co-administered with sodium bicarbonate injections. This medicinal product must not be mixed with other medicinal products except those mentioned in section 6.3.

6.3 Shelf life

Shelf life as packaged for sale: 3 years

Shelf life after first opening: The product should be used immediately

Shelf life after dilution in sodium chloride solution 0.9%: Chemical and physical in-use stability has been demonstrated for both levobupivacaine 0.625 mg/ml and 1.25 mg/

ml with 8.3-8,4 µg/ml clonidine, 50 µg /ml morphine and 2 µg /ml fentanyl, respectively, stored for 30 days at either 2-8°C or 20–22°C. Chemical and physical in-use stability has been demonstrated for both levobupivacaine 0.625 mg/ml and 1.25 mg/ml with sufentanil added in the concentration of 0.4 µg /ml and stored for 30 days at 2-8°C or 7 days at 20–22°C.

From a microbiological point of view, the product should be used immediately after opening. If not used immediately, in-use storage times and conditions prior to use are the responsibility of the user and would normally not be longer than 24 hours at 2-8°C, unless the admix has been prepared in controlled and validated aseptic conditions.

6.4 Special precautions for storage

This medicinal product does not require any special storage conditions

For storage conditions of the reconstituted medicinal product, see section 6.3.

6.5 Nature and contents of container

Chirocaine is available in two presentations;

- 100 ml solution in a 100 ml flexible polyester bag with an aluminium foil overpouch.
- 200 ml solution in a 250 ml flexible polyester bag with an aluminium foil overpouch.

Each polyester bag contains one PVC admixture port and one PVC administration port.

Pack sizes: 5 bags of the 100 ml solution.

5 bags of the 200 ml solution.

24 bags of the 100 ml solution.

12 bags of the 200 ml solution.

60 bags of the 100 ml solution.

32 bags of the 200 ml solution.

Not all pack sizes may be marketed.

6.6 Special precautions for disposal and other handling

For single epidural use only. Do not use unless the solution is clear and container is undamaged. Discard any unused solution.

The solution/dilution should be inspected visually prior to use. Only clear solutions without visible particles should be used.

7. MARKETING AUTHORISATION HOLDER

Abbott Laboratories Ltd

Queenborough

Kent

ME11 5EL

United Kingdom

8. MARKETING AUTHORISATION NUMBER(S)

Chirocaine 0.625mg/ml solution for infusion PL 00037/0404

Chirocaine 1.25mg/ml solution for infusion PL 00037/0405

9. DATE OF FIRST AUTHORISATION/RENEWAL OF THE AUTHORISATION

Date of first authorisation: 20th August 2003

Date of last renewal: 18th December 2008

10. DATE OF REVISION OF THE TEXT

August 2009

Chirocaine 2.5mg/ml solution for injection/ concentrate for solution for infusion

(Abbott Laboratories Limited)

1. NAME OF THE MEDICINAL PRODUCT

Chirocaine 2.5 mg/ml solution for injection/concentrate for solution for infusion.

2. QUALITATIVE AND QUANTITATIVE COMPOSITION

One ml contains 2.5 mg levobupivacaine as levobupivacaine hydrochloride.

Each ampoule contains 25 mg in 10 ml.

Excipients: 3.6mg/ml of sodium per ampoule.

For a full list of excipients, see section 6.1.

3. PHARMACEUTICAL FORM

Solution for injection/concentrate for solution for infusion.

Clear colourless solution.

4. CLINICAL PARTICULARS

4.1 Therapeutic indications

Adults

Surgical anaesthesia

- Major, e.g. epidural (including for caesarean section), intrathecal, peripheral nerve block.

- Minor, e.g. local infiltration, peribulbar block in ophthalmic surgery.

Pain management

- Continuous epidural infusion, single or multiple bolus epidural administration for the management of pain especially post-operative pain or labour analgesia.

Children

Analgesia (ilioinguinal/iliohypogastric blocks).

4.2 Posology and method of administration

Levobupivacaine should be administered only by, or under the supervision of, a clinician having the necessary training and experience.

The table below is a guide to dosage for the more commonly used blocks. For analgesia (e.g. epidural administration for pain management), the lower concentrations and doses are recommended. Where profound or prolonged anaesthesia is required with dense motor block (e.g. epidural or peribulbar block), the higher concentrations may be used. Careful aspiration before and during injection is recommended to prevent intravascular injection.

Aspiration should be repeated before and during administration of a bolus dose, which should be injected slowly and in incremental doses, at a rate of 7.5–30 mg/min, while closely observing the patient's vital functions and maintaining verbal contact.

If toxic symptoms occur, the injection should be stopped immediately.

Maximum dose

The maximum dosage must be determined by evaluating the size and physical status of the patient, together with the concentration of the agent and the area and route of administration. Individual variation in onset and duration of block does occur. Experience from clinical studies shows onset of sensory block adequate for surgery in 10-15 minutes following epidural administration, with a time to regression in the range of 6-9 hours.

The recommended maximum single dose is 150 mg. Where sustained motor and sensory block are required for a prolonged procedure, additional doses may be required. The maximum recommended dose during a 24 hour period is 400 mg. For post-operative pain management, the dose should not exceed 18.75 mg/hour.

Obstetrics

For caesarean section, higher concentrations than the 5.0 mg/ml solution should not be used (See section 4.3). The maximum recommended dose is 150 mg.

For labour analgesia by epidural infusion, the dose should not exceed 12.5 mg/hour.

Children

In children, the maximum recommended dose for analgesia (ilioinguinal/iliohypogastric blocks) is 1.25 mg/kg/side.

The safety and efficacy of levobupivacaine in children for other indications have not been established.

Special populations

Debilitated, elderly or acutely ill patients should be given reduced doses of levobupivacaine commensurate with their physical status.

In the management of post-operative pain, the dose given during surgery must be taken into account.

There are no relevant data in patients with hepatic impairment (see sections 4.4 and 5.2).

Table of Doses

(see Table 1 below)

4.3 Contraindications

General contra-indications related to regional anaesthesia, regardless of the local anaesthetic used, should be taken into account.

Levobupivacaine solutions are contra-indicated in patients with a known hypersensitivity to levobupivacaine, local anaesthetics of the amide type or any of the excipients (see section 4.8).

Levobupivacaine solutions are contra-indicated for intravenous regional anaesthesia (Bier's block).

Levobupivacaine solutions are contra-indicated in patients with severe hypotension such as cardiogenic or hypovolaemic shock.

Levobupivacaine solutions are contra-indicated for use in paracervical block in obstetrics (see section 4.6).

4.4 Special warnings and precautions for use

All forms of local and regional anaesthesia with levobupivacaine should be performed in well-equipped facilities and administered by staff trained and experienced in the required anaesthetic techniques and able to diagnose and treat any unwanted adverse effects that may occur.

Levobupivacaine should be used with caution for regional anaesthesia in patients with impaired cardiovascular function e.g. serious cardiac arrhythmias.

The introduction of local anesthetics via either intrathecal or epidural administration into the central nervous system in patients with preexisting CNS diseases may potentially exacerbate some of these disease states. Therefore, clinical judgment should be exercised when contemplating epidural or intrathecal anesthesia in such patients.

This medicinal product contains 3.6 mg/ml sodium in the bag or ampoule solution to be taken into consideration by patients on a controlled sodium diet.

Epidural Anesthesia

During epidural administration of levobupivacaine, concentrated solutions (0.5-0.75%) should be administered in incremental doses of 3 to 5 ml with sufficient time between doses to detect toxic manifestations of unintentional intravascular or intrathecal injection. When a large dose is to be injected, e.g. in epidural block, a test dose of 3-5 ml lidocaine with adrenaline is recommended. An inadvertent intravascular injection may then be recognised by a temporary increase in heart rate and accidental intrathecal injection by signs of a spinal block.

Syringe aspirations should also be performed before and during each supplemental injection in continuous (intermittent) catheter techniques. An intravascular injection is still possible even if aspirations for blood are negative. During the administration of epidural anesthesia, it is recommended that a test dose be administered initially and the effects monitored before the full dose is given.

Epidural anaesthesia with any local anaesthetic may cause hypotension and bradycardia. All patients must have intravenous access established. The availability of appropriate fluids, vasopressors, anaesthetics with anticonvulsant properties, myorelaxants, and atropine, resuscitation equipment and expertise must be ensured (see section 4.9).

Table 1 Table of Doses

	Concentration (mg/ml)[1]	Dose	Motor Block
Surgical Anaesthesia			
Epidural (slow) bolus[2] for surgery - Adults	5.0-7.5	10-20 ml (50-150 mg)	Moderate to complete
Epidural slow injection[3] for Caesarean Section	5.0	15-30 ml (75-150 mg)	Moderate to complete
Intrathecal	5.0	3 ml (15 mg)	Moderate to complete
Peripheral Nerve	2.5-5.0	1-40 ml (2.5-150 mg max.)	Moderate to complete
Ilioinguinal/Iliohypogastric blocks in children < 12 years	2.5-5.0	0.25-0.5 ml/kg (0.625-2.5 mg/kg)	Not applicable
Ophthalmic (peribulbar block)	7.5	5–15 ml (37.5-112.5 mg)	Moderate to complete
Local Infiltration - Adults	2.5	1-60 ml (2.5-150 mg max.)	Not applicable
Pain Management[4] **Labour Analgesia (epidural bolus[5])**	2.5	6-10 ml (15-25 mg)	Minimal to moderate
Labour Analgesia (epidural infusion)	1.25[6]	4-10 ml/h (5-12.5 mg/h)	Minimal to moderate
Post-operative pain	1.25[6] 2.5	10-15ml/h (12.5-18.75mg/h) 5-7.5ml/h (12.5 –18.75mg/h)	Minimal to moderate

[1] Levobupivacaine solution for injection/concentration for solution for infusion is available in 2.5, 5.0 and 7.5 mg/ml solutions.

[2] Spread over 5 minutes (see also text).

[3] Given over 15-20 minutes.

[4] In cases where levobupivacaine is combined with other agents e.g. opioids in pain management, the levobupivacaine dose should be reduced and use of a lower concentration (e.g. 1.25 mg/ml) is preferable.

[5] The minimum recommended interval between intermittent injections is 15 minutes.

[6] For information on dilution, see section 6.6.

Major regional nerve blocks

The patient should have I.V. fluids running via an indwelling catheter to assure a functioning intravenous pathway. The lowest dosage of local anesthetic that results in effective anesthesia should be used to avoid high plasma levels and serious adverse effects. The rapid injection of a large volume of local anesthetic solution should be avoided and fractional (incremental) doses should be used when feasible.

Use in Head and Neck Area

Small doses of local anesthetics injected into the head and neck area, including retrobulbar, dental and stellate ganglion blocks, may produce adverse reactions similar to systemic toxicity seen with unintentional intravascular injections of larger doses. The injection procedures require the utmost care. Reactions may be due to intraarterial injection of the local anesthetic with retrograde flow to the cerebral circulation. They may also be due to puncture of the dural sheath of the optic nerve during retrobulbar block with diffusion of any local anesthetic along the subdural space to the midbrain. Patients receiving these blocks should have their circulation and respiration monitored and be constantly observed. Resuscitative equipment and personnel for treating adverse reactions should be immediately available.

Use in Ophthalmic Surgery

Clinicians who perform retrobulbar blocks should be aware that there have been reports of respiratory arrest following local anaesthetic injection. Prior to retrobulbar block, as with all other regional procedures, the immediate availability of equipment, drugs, and personnel to manage respiratory arrest or depression, convulsions, and cardiac stimulation or depression should be assured. As with other anesthetic procedures, patients should be constantly monitored following ophthalmic blocks for signs of these adverse reactions.

Special populations

Debilitated, elderly or acutely ill patients: levobupivacaine should be used with caution in debilitated, elderly or acutely ill patients (see section 4.2).

Hepatic impairment: since levobupivacaine is metabolised in the liver, it should be used cautiously in patients with liver disease or with reduced liver blood flow e.g. alcoholics or cirrhotics (see section 5.2).

4.5 Interaction with other medicinal products and other forms of interaction

In vitro studies indicate that the CYP3A4 isoform and CYP1A2 isoform mediate the metabolism of levobupivacaine. Although no clinical studies have been conducted, metabolism of levobupivacaine may be affected by CYP3A4 inhibitors eg: ketoconazole, and CYP1A2 inhibitors eg: methylxanthines.

Levobupivacaine should be used with caution in patients receiving anti-arrhythmic agents with local anaesthetic activity, e.g., mexiletine, or class III anti-arrhythmic agents since their toxic effects may be additive.

No clinical studies have been completed to assess levobupivacaine in combination with adrenaline.

4.6 Pregnancy and lactation

Pregnancy

Levobupivacaine solutions are contraindicated for use in paracervical block in obstetrics. Based on experience with bupivacaine foetal bradycardia may occur following paracervical block (see section 4.3).

For levobupivacaine, there are no clinical data on first trimester-exposed pregnancies. Animal studies do not indicate teratogenic effects but have shown embryo-foetal toxicity at systemic exposure levels in the same range as those obtained in clinical use (see section 5.3). The potential risk for human is unknown. Levobupivacaine should therefore not be given during early pregnancy unless clearly necessary.

Nevertheless, to date, the clinical experience of bupivacaine for obstetrical surgery (at the term of pregnancy or for delivery) is extensive and has not shown a foetotoxic effect.

Lactation

Levobupivacaine excretion in breast milk is unknown. However, levobupivacaine is likely to be poorly transmitted in the breast milk, as for bupivacaine. Thus breast feeding is possible after local anaesthesia.

4.7 Effects on ability to drive and use machines

Levobupivacaine can have a major influence on the ability to drive or use machines. Patients should be warned not to drive or operate machinery until all the effects of the anaesthesia and the immediate effects of surgery are passed.

4.8 Undesirable effects

The adverse drug reactions for Chirocaine are consistent with those known for its respective class of medicinal products. The most commonly reported adverse drug reactions are hypotension, nausea, anaemia, vomiting, dizziness, headache, pyrexia, procedural pain, back pain and foetal distress syndrome in obstetric use (see table below).

Adverse reactions reported either spontaneously or observed in clinical trials are depicted in the following table. Within each system organ class, the adverse drug reactions are ranked under headings of frequency, using the following convention: very common (≥1/10), common (≥1/100, <1/10), uncommon (≥1/1000, <1/100), not known (cannot be estimated from the available data).

System Organ Class	Frequency	Adverse Reaction
Blood and lymphatic system disorders	Very Common	Anaemia
Nervous system disorders	Common Common Not known Not known Not known	Dizziness Headache Convulsion Loss of consciousness Somnolence
Eye disorder	Not known	Vision blurred
Respiratory, thoracic and mediastinal disorders	Not known	Respiratory arrest
Gastrointestinal disorders	Very Common Common Not known	Nausea Vomiting Hypoaesthesia oral
Musculoskeletal and connective tissue	Common Not known	Back pain Muscle twitching
Injury, poisoning and procedural complications	Common	Procedural pain
Vascular disorders	Very common	Hypotension
General disorders and administration site conditions	Common	Pyrexia
Pregnancy, puerperium and perinatal conditions	Common	Foetal distress syndrome
Immune system disorders	Not known	Anaphylactic reaction

Adverse reactions with local anaesthetics of the amide type are rare, but they may occur as a result of overdosage or unintentional intravascular injection and may be serious.

Allergic-type reactions are rare and may occur as a result of sensitivity to the local anesthetic. These reactions are characterised by signs such as urticaria, pruritus, erythema, angioneurotic edema (including laryngeal edema), tachycardia, sneezing, nausea, vomiting, dizziness, syncope, excessive sweating, elevated temperature, and, possibly, anaphylactoid-like symptomatology (including severe hypotension). Cross-sensitivity among members of the amide-type local anesthetic group have been reported (see section 4.3).

Accidental intrathecal injection of local anaesthetics can lead to very high spinal anaesthesia possibly with apnoea, severe hypotension and loss of consciousness.

Cardiovascular effects are related to depression of the conduction system of the heart and a reduction in myocardial excitability and contractility. This results in decreased cardiac output, hypotension and ECG changes indicative of either heart block, bradycardia or ventricular tachyarrythmias that may lead to cardiac arrest. Usually these will be preceded by major CNS toxicity, i.e. convulsions, but in rare cases, cardiac arrest may occur without prodromal CNS effects.

Neurological damage is a rare but well recognised consequence of regional and particularly epidural and spinal anaesthesia. It may be due to direct injury to the spinal cord or spinal nerves, anterior spinal artery syndrome, injection of an irritant substance or an injection of a non-sterile solution. These may result in localised areas of paraesthesia or anaesthesia, motor weakness, loss of sphincter control and paraplegia. Rarely, these may be permanent.

4.9 Overdose

Accidental intravascular injection of local anaesthetics may cause immediate toxic reactions. In the event of overdose, peak plasma concentrations may not be reached until 2 hours after administration depending upon the injection site and, therefore, signs of toxicity may be delayed. The effects of the drug may be prolonged.

Systemic adverse reactions following overdose or accidental intravascular injection reported with long acting local anaesthetic agents involve both CNS and cardiovascular effects.

CNS Effects

Convulsions should be treated immediately with intravenous thiopentone or diazepam titrated as necessary. Thiopentone and diazepam also depress central nervous system, respiratory and cardiac function. Therefore their use may result in apnoea. Neuro-muscular blockers may be used only if the clinician is confident of maintaining a patent airway and managing a fully paralysed patient.

If not treated promptly, convulsions with subsequent hypoxia and hypercarbia plus myocardial depression from the effects of the local anaesthetic on the heart, may result in cardiac arrhythmias, ventricular fibrillation or cardiac arrest.

Cardiovascular Effects

Hypotension may be prevented or attenuated by pre-treatment with a fluid load and/or the use of vasopressors. If hypotension occurs it should be treated with intravenous crystalloids or colloids and/or incremental doses of a vasopressor such as ephedrine 5-10 mg. Any coexisting causes of hypotension should be rapidly treated.

If severe bradycardia occurs, treatment with atropine 0.3-1.0 mg will normally restore the heart rate to an acceptable level.

Cardiac arrhythmia should be treated as required and ventricular fibrillation should be treated by cardioversion.

5. PHARMACOLOGICAL PROPERTIES

5.1 Pharmacodynamic properties

Pharmacotherapeutic group: Local anaesthetics, amide

ATC Code N01B B10

Levobupivacaine is a long acting local anaesthetic and analgesic. It blocks nerve conduction in sensory and motor nerves largely by interacting with voltage sensitive sodium channels on the cell membrane, but also potassium and calcium channels are blocked. In addition, levobupivacaine interferes with impulse transmission and conduction in other tissues where effects on the cardiovascular and central nervous systems are most important for the occurrence of clinical adverse reactions.

The dose of levobupivacaine is expressed as base, whereas, in the racemate bupivacaine the dose is expressed as hydrochloride salt. This gives rise to approximately 13% more active substance in levobupivacaine solutions compared to bupivacaine. In clinical studies at the same nominal concentrations levobupivacaine showed similar clinical effect to bupivacaine.

In a clinical pharmacology study using the ulnar nerve block model, levobupivacaine was equipotent with bupivacaine.

5.2 Pharmacokinetic properties

In human studies, the distribution kinetics of levobupivacaine following i.v. administration are essentially the same as bupivacaine. The plasma concentration of levobupivacaine following therapeutic administration depends on dose and, as absorption from the site of administration is affected by the vascularity of the tissue, on route of administration.

There are no relevant data in patients with hepatic impairment (see section 4.4).

There are no data in patients with renal impairment. Levobupivacaine is extensively metabolised and unchanged levobupivacaine is not excreted in urine.

Plasma protein binding of levobupivacaine in man was evaluated *in vitro* and was found to be > 97% at concentrations between 0.1 and 1.0 μg/ml.

In a clinical pharmacology study where 40 mg levobupivacaine was given by intravenous administration, the mean half-life was approximately 80 ± 22 minutes, C_{max} 1.4 ± 0.2 μg/ml and AUC 70 ± 27 μg•min/ml.

The mean C_{max} and AUC(0-24h) of levobupivacaine were approximately dose-proportional following epidural administration of 75 mg (0.5%) and 112.5 mg (0.75%) and following doses of 1 mg/kg (0.25%) and 2 mg/kg (0.5%) used for brachial plexus block. Following epidural administration of 112.5 mg (0.75%) the mean C_{max} and AUC values were 0.58 μg/ml and 3.56 μg•h/ml respectively.

The mean total plasma clearance and terminal half-life of levobupivacaine after intravenous infusion were 39 litres/hour and 1.3 hours, respectively. The volume of distribution after intravenous administration was 67 litres.

Levobupivacaine is extensively metabolised with no unchanged levobupivacaine detected in urine or faeces. 3-hydroxylevobupivacaine, a major metabolite of levobupivacaine, is excreted in the urine as glucuronic acid and sulphate ester conjugates. *In vitro* studies showed that CYP3A4 isoform and CYP1A2 isoform mediate the metabolism of levobupivacaine to desbutyl-levobupivacaine and 3-hydroxylevobupivacaine respectively. These studies indicate that the metabolism of levobupivacaine and bupivacaine are similar.

Following intravenous administration, recovery of levobupivacaine was quantitative with a mean total of about 95% being recovered in urine (71%) and faeces (24%) in 48 hours.

There is no evidence of *in vivo* racemisation of levobupivacaine.

5.3 Preclinical safety data

In an embryo-foetal toxicity study in rats, an increased incidence of dilated renal pelvis, dilated ureters, olfactory ventricle dilatation and extra thoraco-lumbar ribs was observed at systemic exposure levels in the same range as those obtained at clinical use. There were no treatment-related malformations.

Levobupivacaine was not genotoxic in a standard battery of assays for mutagenicity and clastogenicity. No carcinogenicity testing has been conducted.

6. PHARMACEUTICAL PARTICULARS

6.1 List of excipients

Sodium Chloride

Sodium Hydroxide

Hydrochloric acid

Water for Injections

6.2 Incompatibilities

Levobupivacaine may precipitate if diluted with alkaline solutions and should not be diluted or co-administered with sodium bicarbonate injections. This medicinal product must not be mixed with other medicinal products except those mentioned in section 6.6.

6.3 Shelf life

Shelf life as packaged for sale: 3 years

Shelf life after first opening: The product should be used immediately

Shelf life after dilution in sodium chloride solution 0.9%: Chemical and physical in-use stability has been demonstrated for 7 days at 20-22°C. Chemical and physical in-use stability with clonidine, morphine or fentanyl has been demonstrated for 40 hours at 20-22°C.

From a microbiological point of view, the product should be used immediately. If not used immediately, in-use storage times and conditions prior to use are the responsibility of the user.

6.4 Special precautions for storage

Polypropylene ampoules: polypropylene ampoules do not require any special storage conditions.

For storage conditions of the reconstituted medicinal product, see section 6.3.

6.5 Nature and contents of container

Chirocaine is available in two presentations;

10 ml polypropylene ampoule in packs of 5, 10 & 20

10 ml polypropylene ampoule, in sterile blister packs of 5, 10 & 20

Not all pack sizes may be marketed.

6.6 Special precautions for disposal and other handling

For single use only. Discard any unused solution.

The solution/dilution should be inspected visually prior to use. Only clear solutions without visible particles should be used.

A sterile blister container should be chosen when a sterile ampoule surface is required. Ampoule surface is not sterile if sterile blister is pierced.

Dilutions of levobupivacaine standard solutions should be made with sodium chloride 9 mg/ml (0.9%) solution for injection using aseptic techniques.

Clonidine 8.4 μg/ml, morphine 0.05 mg/ml and fentanyl 4 μg/ml have been shown to be compatible with levobupivacaine in sodium chloride 9 mg/ml (0.9%) solution for injection.

7. MARKETING AUTHORISATION HOLDER

Abbott Laboratories Ltd

Queenborough

Kent

ME11 5EL

United Kingdom

8. MARKETING AUTHORISATION NUMBER(S)

PL 00037/0300

9. DATE OF FIRST AUTHORISATION/RENEWAL OF THE AUTHORISATION

Date of first authorisation: 06 January 2000

Date of last renewal: 18th December 2008

10. DATE OF REVISION OF THE TEXT

August 2009

Chirocaine 5mg/ml solution for injection/concentrate for solution for infusion

(Abbott Laboratories Limited)

1. NAME OF THE MEDICINAL PRODUCT

Chirocaine 5 mg/ml solution for injection/concentrate for solution for infusion

2. QUALITATIVE AND QUANTITATIVE COMPOSITION

One ml contains 5 mg levobupivacaine as levobupivacaine hydrochloride.

Each ampoule contains 50 mg in 10 ml.

Excipients: 3.6mg/ml of sodium per ampoule.

For a full list of excipients, see section 6.1.

3. PHARMACEUTICAL FORM

Solution for injection/concentrate for solution for infusion.

Clear colourless solution.

4. CLINICAL PARTICULARS

4.1 Therapeutic indications

Adults

Surgical anaesthesia

- Major, e.g. epidural (including for caesarean section), intrathecal, peripheral nerve block.

- Minor, e.g. local infiltration, peribulbar block in ophthalmic surgery.

Pain management

- Continuous epidural infusion, single or multiple bolus epidural administration for the management of pain especially post - operative pain or labour analgesia.

Children

Analgesia (ilioinguinal/iliohypogastric blocks).

4.2 Posology and method of administration

Levobupivacaine should be administered only by, or under the supervision of, a clinician having the necessary training and experience.

The table below is a guide to dosage for the more commonly used blocks. For analgesia (e.g. epidural administration for pain management), the lower concentrations and doses are recommended. Where profound or prolonged anaesthesia is required with dense motor block (e.g. epidural or peribulbar block), the higher concentrations may be used. Careful aspiration before and during injection is recommended to prevent intravascular injection.

Aspiration should be repeated before and during administration of a bolus dose, which should be injected slowly and in incremental doses, at a rate of 7.5–30 mg/min, while closely observing the patient's vital functions and maintaining verbal contact.

If toxic symptoms occur, the injection should be stopped immediately.

Maximum dose

The maximum dosage must be determined by evaluating the size and physical status of the patient, together with the concentration of the agent and the area and route of administration. Individual variation in onset and duration of block does occur. Experience from clinical studies shows onset of sensory block adequate for surgery in 10-15 minutes following epidural administration, with a time to regression in the range of 6-9 hours.

The recommended maximum single dose is 150 mg. Where sustained motor and sensory block are required for a prolonged procedure, additional doses may be required. The maximum recommended dose during a 24 hour period is 400 mg. For post-operative pain management, the dose should not exceed 18.75 mg/hour.

Obstetrics

For caesarean section, higher concentrations than the 5.0 mg/ml solution should not be used (See 4.3). The maximum recommended dose is 150 mg.

For labour analgesia by epidural infusion, the dose should not exceed 12.5 mg/hour.

Children

In children, the maximum recommended dose for analgesia (ilioinguinal/iliohypogastric blocks) is 1.25 mg/kg/side.

The safety and efficacy of levobupivacaine in children for other indications have not been established.

Special populations

Debilitated, elderly or acutely ill patients should be given reduced doses of levobupivacaine commensurate with their physical status.

In the management of post-operative pain, the dose given during surgery must be taken into account.

There are no relevant data in patients with hepatic impairment (see sections 4.4 and 5.2).

Table of Doses

(see Table 1 below)

4.3 Contraindications

General contra-indications related to regional anaesthesia, regardless of the local anaesthetic used, should be taken into account.

Levobupivacaine solutions are contra-indicated in patients with a known hypersensitivity to levobupivacaine, local anaesthetics of the amide type or any of the excipients (see section 4.8).

Levobupivacaine solutions are contra-indicated for intravenous regional anaesthesia (Bier's block).

Levobupivacaine solutions are contra-indicated in patients with severe hypotension such as cardiogenic or hypovolaemic shock.

Levobupivacaine solutions are contra-indicated for use in paracervical block in obstetrics (see section 4.6).

4.4 Special warnings and precautions for use

All forms of local and regional anaesthesia with levobupivacaine should be performed in well-equipped facilities and administered by staff trained and experienced in the required anaesthetic techniques and able to diagnose and treat any unwanted adverse effects that may occur.

Levobupivacaine should be used with caution for regional anaesthesia in patients with impaired cardiovascular function e.g. serious cardiac arrhythmias.

The introduction of local anesthetics via either intrathecal or epidural administration into the central nervous system in patients with preexisting CNS diseases may potentially exacerbate some of these disease states. Therefore, clinical judgment should be exercised when contemplating epidural or intrathecal anesthesia in such patients.

This medicinal product contains 3.6 mg/ml sodium in the bag or ampoule solution to be taken into consideration by patients on a controlled sodium diet.

Epidural Anesthesia

During epidural administration of levobupivacaine, concentrated solutions (0.5-0.75%) should be administered in incremental doses of 3 to 5 ml with sufficient time between doses to detect toxic manifestations of unintentional intravascular or intrathecal injection. When a large dose is to be injected, e.g. in epidural block, a test dose of 3-5 ml lidocaine with adrenaline is recommended. An inadvertent intravascular injection may then be recognised by a temporary increase in heart rate and accidental intrathecal injection by signs of a spinal block. Syringe aspirations should also be performed before and during each supplemental injection in continuous (intermittent) catheter techniques. An intravascular injection is still possible even if aspirations for blood are negative. During the administration of epidural anesthesia, it is recommended that a test dose be administered initially and the effects monitored before the full dose is given.

Epidural anaesthesia with any local anaesthetic may cause hypotension and bradycardia. All patients must have intravenous access established. The availability of appropriate fluids, vasopressors, anaesthetics with anticonvulsant properties, myorelaxants, and atropine, resuscitation equipment and expertise must be ensured (see section 4.9).

Major regional nerve blocks

The patient should have I.V. fluids running via an indwelling catheter to assure a functioning intravenous pathway. The

Table 1 Table of Doses

	Concentration (mg/ml)[1]	Dose	Motor Block
Surgical Anaesthesia			
Epidural (slow) bolus[2] for surgery - Adults	5.0-7.5	10-20 ml (50-150 mg)	Moderate to complete
Epidural slow injection[3] for Caesarean Section	5.0	15-30 ml (75-150 mg)	Moderate to complete
Intrathecal	5.0	3 ml (15 mg)	Moderate to complete
Peripheral Nerve	2.5-5.0	1-40 ml (2.5-150 mg max	Moderate to complete
Ilioinguinal/liohypogastric blocks in children <12 years	2.5-5.0	0.25-0.5 ml/kg (0.625-2.5 mg/kg)	Not applicable
Ophthalmic (peribulbar block)	7.5	5–15 ml (37.5-112.5 mg)	Moderate to complete
Local Infiltration - Adults	2.5	1-60 ml (2.5-150 mg max)	Not applicable
Pain Management[4] Labour Analgesia (epidural bolus[5])	2.5	6-10 ml (15-25 mg)	Minimal to moderate
Labour Analgesia (epidural infusion)	1.25[6]	4-10 ml/h (5-12.5 mg/h)	Minimal to moderate
Post-operative pain	1.25[6] 2.5	10-15ml/h (12.5-18.75mg/h) 5-7.5ml/h (12.5–18.75mg/h)	Minimal to moderate

[1] Levobupivacaine solution for injection/concentration for solution for infusion is available in 2.5, 5.0 and 7.5 mg/ml solutions.

[2] Spread over 5 minutes (see also text).

[3] Given over 15-20 minutes.

[4] In cases where levobupivacaine is combined with other agents e.g. opioids in pain management, the levobupivacaine dose should be reduced and use of a lower concentration (e.g. 1.25 mg/ml) is preferable.

[5] The minimum recommended interval between intermittent injections is 15 minutes.

[6] For information on dilution, see section 6.6.

lowest dosage of local anesthetic that results in effective anesthesia should be used to avoid high plasma levels and serious adverse effects. The rapid injection of a large volume of local anesthetic solution should be avoided and fractional (incremental) doses should be used when feasible.

Use in Head and Neck Area

Small doses of local anesthetics injected into the head and neck area, including retrobulbar, dental and stellate ganglion blocks, may produce adverse reactions similar to systemic toxicity seen with unintentional intravascular injections of larger doses. The injection procedures require the utmost care. Reactions may be due to intraarterial injection of the local anesthetic with retrograde flow to the cerebral circulation. They may also be due to puncture of the dural sheath of the optic nerve during retrobulbar block with diffusion of any local anesthetic along the subdural space to the midbrain. Patients receiving these blocks should have their circulation and respiration monitored and be constantly observed. Resuscitative equipment and personnel for treating adverse reactions should be immediately available.

Use in Ophthalmic Surgery

Clinicians who perform retrobulbar blocks should be aware that there have been reports of respiratory arrest following local anaesthetic injection. Prior to retrobulbar block, as with all other regional procedures, the immediate availability of equipment, drugs, and personnel to manage respiratory arrest or depression, convulsions, and cardiac stimulation or depression should be assured. As with other anaesthetic procedures, patients should be constantly monitored following ophthalmic blocks for signs of these adverse reactions.

Special populations

Debilitated, elderly or acutely ill patients: levobupivacaine should be used with caution in debilitated, elderly or acutely ill patients (see section 4.2).

Hepatic impairment: since levobupivacaine is metabolised in the liver, it should be used cautiously in patients with liver disease or with reduced liver blood flow e.g. alcoholics or cirrhotics (see section 5.2).

4.5 Interaction with other medicinal products and other forms of interaction

In vitro studies indicate that the CYP3A4 isoform and CYP1A2 isoform mediate the metabolism of levobupivacaine. Although no clinical studies have been conducted, metabolism of levobupivacaine may be affected by CYP3A4 inhibitors eg: ketoconazole, and CYP1A2 inhibitors eg: methylxanthines.

Levobupivacaine should be used with caution in patients receiving anti-arrhythmic agents with local anaesthetic activity, e.g., mexiletine, or class III anti-arrhythmic agents since their toxic effects may be additive.

No clinical studies have been completed to assess levobupivacaine in combination with adrenaline.

4.6 Pregnancy and lactation

Pregnancy

Levobupivacaine solutions are contraindicated for use in paracervical block in obstetrics. Based on experience with bupivacaine foetal bradycardia may occur following paracervical block (see section 4.3).

For levobupivacaine, there are no clinical data on first trimester-exposed pregnancies. Animal studies do not indicate teratogenic effects but have shown embryo-foetal toxicity at systemic exposure levels in the same range as those obtained in clinical use (see section 5.3). The potential risk for human is unknown. Levobupivacaine should therefore not be given during early pregnancy unless clearly necessary.

Nevertheless, to date, the clinical experience of bupivacaine for obstetrical surgery (at the term of pregnancy or for delivery) is extensive and has not shown a foetotoxic effect.

Lactation

Levobupivacaine excretion in breast milk is unknown. However, levobupivacaine is likely to be poorly transmitted in the breast milk, as for bupivacaine. Thus breast feeding is possible after local anaesthesia.

4.7 Effects on ability to drive and use machines

Levobupivacaine can have a major influence on the ability to drive or use machines. Patients should be warned not to drive or operate machinery until all the effects of the anaesthesia and the immediate effects of surgery are passed.

4.8 Undesirable effects

The adverse drug reactions for Chirocaine are consistent with those known for its respective class of medicinal products. The most commonly reported adverse drug reactions are hypotension, nausea, anaemia, vomiting, dizziness, headache, pyrexia, procedural pain, back pain and foetal distress syndrome in obstetric use (see table below).

Adverse reactions reported either spontaneously or observed in clinical trials are depicted in the following table Within each system organ class, the adverse drug reactions are ranked under headings of frequency, using the following convention: very common (≥1/10), common (≥1/100, <1/10), uncommon (≥1/1000, <1/100), not known (cannot be estimated from the available data).

System Organ Class	Frequency	Adverse Reaction
Blood and lymphatic system disorders	Very Common	Anaemia
Nervous system disorders	Common Common Not known Not known Not known	Dizziness Headache Convulsion Loss of consciousness Somnolence
Eye disorders	Not known	Vision blurred
Respiratory, thoracic and mediastinal disorders	Not known	Respiratory arrest
Gastrointestinal disorders	Very Common Common Not known	Nausea Vomiting Hypoasthesia oral
Musculoskeletal and connective tissue disorders	Common Not known	Back pain Muscle twitching
Injury, poisoning and procedural complications	Common	Procedural pain
Vascular disorders	Very common	Hypotension
General disorders and administration site conditions	Common	Pyrexia
Pregnancy, puerperium and perinatal conditions	Common	Foetal distress syndrome
Immune system disorders	Not known	Anaphylactic reaction

Postmarketing reports

Adverse reactions with local anaesthetics of the amide type are rare, but they may occur as a result of overdosage or unintentional intravascular injection and may be serious.

Allergic-type reactions are rare and may occur as a result of sensitivity to the local anesthetic. These reactions are characterised by signs such as urticaria, pruritus, erythema, angioneurotic edema (including laryngeal edema), tachycardia, sneezing, nausea, vomiting, dizziness, syncope, excessive sweating, elevated temperature, and, possibly, anaphylactoid-like symptomatology (including severe hypotension). Cross-sensitivity among members of the amide-type local anesthetic group have been reported (see section 4.3).

Accidental intrathecal injection of local anaesthetics can lead to very high spinal anaesthesia possibly with apnoea, severe hypotension and loss of consciousness.

Cardiovascular effects are related to depression of the conduction system of the heart and a reduction in myocardial excitability and contractility. This results in decreased cardiac output, hypotension and ECG changes indicative of either heart block, bradycardia or ventricular tachyarrythmias that may lead to cardiac arrest. Usually these will be preceded by major CNS toxicity, i.e. convulsions, but in rare cases, cardiac arrest may occur without prodromal CNS effects.

Neurological damage is a rare but well recognised consequence of regional and particularly epidural and spinal anaesthesia. It may be due to direct injury to the spinal cord or spinal nerves, anterior spinal artery syndrome, injection of an irritant substance or an injection of a non-sterile solution. These may result in localised areas of paraesthesia or anaesthesia, motor weakness, loss of sphincter control and paraplegia. Rarely, these may be permanent.

4.9 Overdose

Accidental intravascular injection of local anaesthetics may cause immediate toxic reactions. In the event of overdose, peak plasma concentrations may not be reached until 2 hours after administration depending upon the injection site and, therefore, signs of toxicity may be delayed. The effects of the drug may be prolonged.

Systemic adverse reactions following overdose or accidental intravascular injection reported with long acting local anaesthetic agents involve both CNS and cardiovascular effects.

CNS Effects

Convulsions should be treated immediately with intravenous thiopentone or diazepam titrated as necessary. Thiopentone and diazepam also depress central nervous system, respiratory and cardiac function. Therefore their use may result in apnoea. Neuro-muscular blockers may be used only if the clinician is confident of maintaining a patent airway and managing a fully paralysed patient.

If not treated promptly, convulsions with subsequent hypoxia and hypercarbia plus myocardial depression from the effects of the local anaesthetic on the heart, may result in cardiac arrhythmias, ventricular fibrillation or cardiac arrest.

Cardiovascular Effects

Hypotension may be prevented or attenuated by pre-treatment with a fluid load and/or the use of vasopressors. If hypotension occurs it should be treated with intravenous crystalloids or colloids and/or incremental doses of a vasopressor such as ephedrine 5-10 mg. Any coexisting causes of hypotension should be rapidly treated.

If severe bradycardia occurs, treatment with atropine 0.3 - 1.0 mg will normally restore the heart rate to an acceptable level.

Cardiac arrhythmia should be treated as required and ventricular fibrillation should be treated by cardioversion.

5. PHARMACOLOGICAL PROPERTIES

5.1 Pharmacodynamic properties

Pharmacotherapeutic group: Local anaesthetics, amide ATC Code N01B B10

Levobupivacaine is a long acting local anaesthetic and analgesic. It blocks nerve conduction in sensory and motor nerves largely by interacting with voltage sensitive sodium channels on the cell membrane, but also potassium and calcium channels are blocked. In addition, levobupivacaine interferes with impulse transmission and conduction in other tissues where effects on the cardiovascular and central nervous systems are most important for the occurrence of clinical adverse reactions.

The dose of levobupivacaine is expressed as base, whereas, in the racemate bupivacaine the dose is expressed as hydrochloride salt. This gives rise to approximately 13% more active substance in levobupivacaine solutions compared to bupivacaine. In clinical studies at the same nominal concentrations levobupivacaine showed similar clinical effect to bupivacaine.

In a clinical pharmacology study using the ulnar nerve block model, levobupivacaine was equipotent with bupivacaine.

5.2 Pharmacokinetic properties

In human studies, the distribution kinetics of levobupivacaine following i.v. administration are essentially the same as bupivacaine. The plasma concentration of levobupivacaine following therapeutic administration depends on dose and, as absorption from the site of administration is affected by the vascularity of the tissue, on route of administration.

There are no relevant data in patients with hepatic impairment (see section 4.4).

There are no data in patients with renal impairment. Levobupivacaine is extensively metabolised and unchanged levobupivacaine is not excreted in urine.

Plasma protein binding of levobupivacaine in man was evaluated *in vitro* and was found to be > 97% at concentrations between 0.1 and 1.0 μg/ml.

In a clinical pharmacology study where 40 mg levobupivacaine was given by intravenous administration, the mean half-life was approximately 80 ± 22 minutes, C_{max} 1.4 ± 0.2 μg/ml and AUC 70 ± 27 μg•min/ml.

The mean C_{max} and AUC(0-24h) of levobupivacaine were approximately dose-proportional following epidural administration of 75 mg (0.5%) and 112.5 mg (0.75%) and following doses of 1 mg/kg (0.25%) and 2 mg/kg (0.5%) used for brachial plexus block. Following epidural administration of 112.5 mg (0.75%) the mean C_{max} and AUC values were 0.58 μg/ml and 3.56 μg•h/ml respectively.

The mean total plasma clearance and terminal half-life of levobupivacaine after intravenous infusion were 39 litres/hour and 1.3 hours, respectively. The volume of distribution after intravenous administration was 67 litres.

Levobupivacaine is extensively metabolised with no unchanged levobupivacaine detected in urine or faeces. 3-hydroxylevobupivacaine, a major metabolite of levobupivacaine, is excreted in the urine as glucuronic acid and sulphate ester conjugates. *In vitro* studies showed that CYP3A4 isoform and CYP1A2 isoform mediate the metabolism of levobupivacaine to desbutyl-levobupivacaine and 3-hydroxylevobupivacaine respectively. These studies indicate that the metabolism of levobupivacaine and bupivacaine are similar.

Following intravenous administration, recovery of levobupivacaine was quantitative with a mean total of about 95% being recovered in urine (71%) and faeces (24%) in 48 hours.

There is no evidence of *in vivo* racemisation of levobupivacaine.

5.3 Preclinical safety data

In an embryo-foetal toxicity study in rats, an increased incidence of dilated renal pelvis, dilated ureters, olfactory ventricle dilatation and extra thoraco-lumbar ribs was observed at systemic exposure levels in the same range as those obtained at clinical use. There were no treatment-related malformations.

Levobupivacaine was not genotoxic in a standard battery of assays for mutagenicity and clastogenicity. No carcinogenicity testing has been conducted.

6. PHARMACEUTICAL PARTICULARS

6.1 List of excipients

Sodium Chloride

Sodium Hydroxide

Hydrochloric acid

Water for Injections

6.2 Incompatibilities

Levobupivacaine may precipitate if diluted with alkaline solutions and should not be diluted or co-administered with sodium bicarbonate injections. This medicinal product must not be mixed with other medicinal products except those mentioned in section 6.6.

6.3 Shelf life

Shelf life as packaged for sale: 3 years

Shelf life after first opening: The product should be used immediately

Shelf life after dilution in sodium chloride solution 0.9%: Chemical and physical in-use stability has been demonstrated for 7 days at 20-22°C. Chemical and physical in-use stability with clonidine, morphine or fentanyl has been demonstrated for 40 hours at 20-22°C.

From a microbiological point of view, the product should be used immediately. If not used immediately, in-use storage times and conditions prior to use are the responsibility of the user.

6.4 Special precautions for storage

Polypropylene ampoules: polypropylene ampoules do not require any special storage conditions.

For storage conditions of the reconstituted medicinal product, see section 6.3.

6.5 Nature and contents of container

Chirocaine is available in two presentations;

10 ml polypropylene ampoule in packs of 5, 10 & 20

10 ml polypropylene ampoule, in sterile blister packs of 5, 10 & 20

Not all pack sizes may be marketed.

6.6 Special precautions for disposal and other handling

For single use only. Discard any unused solution.

The solution/dilution should be inspected visually prior to use. Only clear solutions without visible particles should be used.

A sterile blister container should be chosen when a sterile ampoule surface is required. Ampoule surface is not sterile if sterile blister is pierced.

Dilutions of levobupivacaine standard solutions should be made with sodium chloride 9 mg/ml (0.9%) solution for injection using aseptic techniques.

Clonidine 8.4 μg/ml, morphine 0.05 mg/ml and fentanyl 4 μg/ml have been shown to be compatible with levobupivacaine in sodium chloride 9 mg/ml (0.9%) solution for injection.

7. MARKETING AUTHORISATION HOLDER

Abbott Laboratories Ltd
Queenborough
Kent
ME11 5EL
United Kingdom

8. MARKETING AUTHORISATION NUMBER(S)

PL 00037/0301

9. DATE OF FIRST AUTHORISATION/RENEWAL OF THE AUTHORISATION

Date of first authorisation: 06th January 2000

Date of last renewal: 18th December 2008

10. DATE OF REVISION OF THE TEXT

August 2009

Chirocaine 7.5mg/ml solution for injection/ concentrate for solution for infusion

(Abbott Laboratories Limited)

1. NAME OF THE MEDICINAL PRODUCT

Chirocaine 7.5 mg/ml solution for injection/concentrate for solution for infusion

2. QUALITATIVE AND QUANTITATIVE COMPOSITION

One ml contains 7.5 mg levobupivacaine as levobupivacaine hydrochloride.

Each ampoule contains 75 mg in 10 ml.

Excipients: 3.6 mg/ml of sodium per ampoule.

For a full list of excipients, see section 6.1.

3. PHARMACEUTICAL FORM

Solution for injection/concentrate for solution for infusion.

Clear colourless solution.

4. CLINICAL PARTICULARS

4.1 Therapeutic indications

Adults

Surgical anaesthesia

- Major, e.g. epidural, intrathecal, peripheral nerve block.
- Minor, e.g. local infiltration, peribulbar block in ophthalmic surgery.

Pain management

- Continuous epidural infusion, single or multiple bolus epidural administration for the management of pain especially post - operative pain or labour analgesia.

Children

Analgesia (ilioinguinal/iliohypogastric blocks).

4.2 Posology and method of administration

Levobupivacaine should be administered only by, or under the supervision of, a clinician having the necessary training and experience.

The table below is a guide to dosage for the more commonly used blocks. For analgesia (e.g. epidural administration for pain management), the lower concentrations and doses are recommended. Where profound or prolonged anaesthesia is required with dense motor block (e.g. epidural or peribulbar block), the higher concentrations may be used. Careful aspiration before and during injection is recommended to prevent intravascular injection.

Aspiration should be repeated before and during administration of a bolus dose, which should be injected slowly and in incremental doses, at a rate of 7.5–30 mg/min, while closely observing the patient's vital functions and maintaining verbal contact.

If toxic symptoms occur, the injection should be stopped immediately.

Maximum dose

The maximum dosage must be determined by evaluating the size and physical status of the patient, together with the concentration of the agent and the area and route of administration. Individual variation in onset and duration of block does occur. Experience from clinical studies shows onset of sensory block adequate for surgery in 10-15 minutes following epidural administration, with a time to regression in the range of 6-9 hours.

The recommended maximum single dose is 150 mg. Where sustained motor and sensory block are required for a prolonged procedure, additional doses may be required. The maximum recommended dose during a 24 hour period is 400mg. For post-operative pain management, the dose should not exceed 18.75 mg/hour.

Obstetrics

For caesarean section, higher concentrations than the 5.0 mg/ml solution should not be used (See section 4.3). The maximum recommended dose is 150 mg.

For labour analgesia by epidural infusion, the dose should not exceed 12.5 mg/hour.

Children

In children, the maximum recommended dose for analgesia (ilioinguinal/iliohypogastric blocks) is 1.25 mg/kg/side.

The safety and efficacy of levobupivacaine in children for other indications have not been established.

Special populations

Debilitated, elderly or acutely ill patients should be given reduced doses of levobupivacaine commensurate with their physical status.

In the management of post-operative pain, the dose given during surgery must be taken into account.

There are no relevant data in patients with hepatic impairment (see sections 4.4 and 5.2).

Table of Doses

(see Table 1 below)

4.3 Contraindications

General contra-indications related to regional anaesthesia, regardless of the local anaesthetic used, should be taken into account.

Levobupivacaine solutions are contra-indicated in patients with a known hypersensitivity to levobupivacaine, local anaesthetics of the amide type or any of the excipients (see section 4.8).

Levobupivacaine solutions are contra-indicated for intravenous regional anaesthesia (Bier's block).

Levobupivacaine solutions are contra-indicated in patients with severe hypotension such as cardiogenic or hypovolaemic shock.

The 7.5 mg/ml solution is contra-indicated for obstetric use due to an enhanced risk for cardiotoxic events based on experience with bupivacaine (see section 4.6).

Levobupivacaine solutions are contra-indicated for use in paracervical block in obstetrics (see section 4.6).

4.4 Special warnings and precautions for use

All forms of local and regional anaesthesia with levobupivacaine should be performed in well-equipped facilities and administered by staff trained and experienced in the required anaesthetic techniques and able to diagnose and treat any unwanted adverse effects that may occur.

Levobupivacaine should be used with caution for regional anaesthesia in patients with impaired cardiovascular function e.g. serious cardiac arrhythmias.

The introduction of local anesthetics via either intrathecal or epidural administration into the central nervous system in patients with preexisting CNS diseases may potentially exacerbate some of these disease states. Therefore, clinical judgment should be exercised when contemplating epidural or intrathecal anesthesia in such patients.

This medicinal product contains 3.6 mg/ml sodium in the bag or ampoule solution to be taken into consideration by patients on a controlled sodium diet.

Epidural Anesthesia

During epidural administration of levobupivacaine, concentrated solutions (0.5-0.75%) should be administered in incremental doses of 3 to 5 ml with sufficient time between doses to detect toxic manifestations of unintentional intravascular or intrathecal injection. When a large dose is to be injected, e.g. in epidural block, a test dose of 3-5 ml lidocaine with adrenaline is recommended. An inadvertent intravascular injection may then be recognised by a temporary increase in heart rate and accidental intrathecal injection by signs of a spinal block. Syringe aspirations should also be performed before and during each supplemental injection in continuous (intermittent) catheter techniques. An intravascular injection is still

Table 1 Table of Doses

	Concentration (mg/ml)[1]	Dose	Motor Block
Surgical Anaesthesia			
Epidural (slow) bolus[2] for surgery - Adults	5.0-7.5	10-20 ml (50-150 mg)	Moderate to complete
Epidural slow injection[3] for Caesarean Section	5.0	15-30 ml (75-150 mg)	Moderate to complete
Intrathecal	5.0	3 ml (15 mg)	Moderate to complete
Peripheral Nerve	2.5-5.0	1-40 ml (2.5-150 mg max	Moderate to complete
Ilioinguinal/Iliohypogastric blocks in children <12 years	2.5-5.0	0.25-0.5 ml/kg (0.625-2.5 mg/kg)	Not applicable
Ophthalmic (peribulbar block)	7.5	5–15 ml (37.5-112.5 mg)	Moderate to complete
Local Infiltration - Adults	2.5	1-60 ml (2.5-150 mg max)	Not applicable
Pain Management[4] Labour Analgesia (epidural bolus[5])	2.5	6-10ml (15-25 mg)	Minimal to moderate
Labour Analgesia (epidural infusion)	1.25[6]	4-10 ml/h (5-12.5 mg/h)	Minimal to moderate
Post-operative pain	1.25[6] 2.5	10-15ml/h (12.5-18.75mg/h) 5-7.5ml/h (12.5 –18.75mg/h)	Minimal to moderate

[1] Levobupivacaine solution for injection/concentration for solution for infusion is available in 2.5, 5.0 and 7.5 mg/ml solutions.

[2] Spread over 5 minutes (see also text).

[3] Given over 15-20 minutes.

[4] In cases where levobupivacaine is combined with other agents e.g. opioids in pain management, the levobupivacaine dose should be reduced and use of a lower concentration (e.g. 1.25 mg/ml) is preferable.

[5] The minimum recommended interval between intermittent injections is 15 minutes.

[6] For information on dilution, see section 6.6.

possible even if aspirations for blood are negative. During the administration of epidural anesthesia, it is recommended that a test dose be administered initially and the effects monitored before the full dose is given.

Epidural anaesthesia with any local anaesthetic may cause hypotension and bradycardia. All patients must have intravenous access established. The availability of appropriate fluids, vasopressors, anaesthetics with anticonvulsant properties, myorelaxants, and atropine, resuscitation equipment and expertise must be ensured (see section 4.9).

Major regional nerve blocks

The patient should have I.V. fluids running via an indwelling catheter to assure a functioning intravenous pathway. The lowest dosage of local anesthetic that results in effective anesthesia should be used to avoid high plasma levels and serious adverse effects. The rapid injection of a large volume of local anesthetic solution should be avoided and fractional (incremental) doses should be used when feasible.

Use in Head and Neck Area

Small doses of local anesthetics injected into the head and neck area, including retrobulbar, dental and stellate ganglion blocks, may produce adverse reactions similar to systemic toxicity seen with unintentional intravascular injections of larger doses. The injection procedures require the utmost care. Reactions may be due to intraarterial injection of the local anesthetic with retrograde flow to the cerebral circulation. They may also be due to puncture of the dural sheath of the optic nerve during retrobulbar block with diffusion of any local anesthetic along the subdural space to the midbrain. Patients receiving these blocks should have their circulation and respiration monitored and be constantly observed. Resuscitative equipment and personnel for treating adverse reactions should be immediately available.

Use in Ophthalmic Surgery

Clinicians who perform retrobulbar blocks should be aware that there have been reports of respiratory arrest following local anaesthetic injection. Prior to retrobulbar block, as with all other regional procedures, the immediate availability of equipment, drugs, and personnel to manage respiratory arrest or depression, convulsions, and cardiac stimulation or depression should be assured. As with other anaesthetic procedures, patients should be constantly monitored following ophthalmic blocks for signs of these adverse reactions.

Special populations

Debilitated, elderly or acutely ill patients: levobupivacaine should be used with caution in debilitated, elderly or acutely ill patients (see section 4.2).

Hepatic impairment: since levobupivacaine is metabolised in the liver, it should be used cautiously in patients with liver disease or with reduced liver blood flow e.g. alcoholics or cirrhotics (see section 5.2).

4.5 Interaction with other medicinal products and other forms of interaction

In vitro studies indicate that the CYP3A4 isoform and CYP1A2 isoform mediate the metabolism of levobupivacaine. Although no clinical studies have been conducted, metabolism of levobupivacaine may be affected by CYP3A4 inhibitors eg: ketoconazole, and CYP1A2 inhibitors eg: methylxanthines.

Levobupivacaine should be used with caution in patients receiving anti-arrhythmic agents with local anaesthetic activity, e.g., mexiletine, or class III anti-arrhythmic agents since their toxic effects may be additive.

No clinical studies have been completed to assess levobupivacaine in combination with adrenaline.

4.6 Pregnancy and lactation

Pregnancy

Levobupivacaine solutions are contraindicated for use in paracervical block in obstetrics. Based on experience with bupivacaine foetal bradycardia may occur following paracervical block (see section 4.3).

The 7.5 mg/ml solution is contra-indicated for obstetric use due to enhanced risk for cardiotoxic events based on experience with bupivacaine (see section 4.3).

For levobupivacaine, there are no clinical data on first trimester-exposed pregnancies. Animal studies do not indicate teratogenic effects but have shown embryo-foetal toxicity at systemic exposure levels in the same range as those obtained in clinical use (see section 5.3). The potential risk for human is unknown. Levobupivacaine should therefore not be given during early pregnancy unless clearly necessary.

Lactation

Levobupivacaine excretion in breast milk is unknown. However, levobupivacaine is likely to be poorly transmitted in the breast milk, as for bupivacaine. Thus breast feeding is possible after local anaesthesia.

4.7 Effects on ability to drive and use machines

Levobupivacaine can have a major influence on the ability to drive or use machines. Patients should be warned not to drive or operate machinery until all the effects of the anaesthesia and the immediate effects of surgery are passed.

4.8 Undesirable effects

The adverse drug reactions for Chirocaine are consistent with those known for its respective class of medicinal products. The most commonly reported adverse drug reactions are hypotension, nausea, anaemia, vomiting, dizziness, headache, pyrexia, procedural pain, back pain and foetal distress syndrome in obstetric use (see table below).

Adverse reactions reported either spontaneously or observed in clinical trials are depicted in the following table. Within each system organ class, the adverse drug reactions are ranked under headings of frequency, using the following convention: very common (≥1/10), common (≥1/100, <1/10), uncommon (≥1/1000, <1/100), not known (cannot be estimated from the available data).

System Organ Class	Frequency	Adverse Reaction
Blood and lymphatic system disorders	Very Common	Anaemia
Nervous system disorders	Common Common Not known Not known Not known	Dizziness Headache Convulsion Loss of consciousness Somnolence
Eye disorders	Not known	Vision blurred
Respiratory, thoracic and mediastinal disorders	Not known	Respiratory arrest
Gastrointestinal disorders	Very Common Common Not known	Nausea Vomiting Hypoaesthesia oral
Musculoskeletal and connective tissue disorders	Common Not known	Back pain Muscle twitching
Injury, poisoning and procedural complications	Common	Procedural pain
Vascular disorders	Very common	Hypotension
General disorders and administration site conditions	Common	Pyrexia
Pregnancy, puerperium and perinatal conditions	Common	Foetal distress syndrome
Immune system disorders	Not known	Anaphylactic reaction

Adverse reactions with local anaesthetics of the amide type are rare, but they may occur as a result of overdosage or unintentional intravascular injection and may be serious.

Allergic-type reactions are rare and may occur as a result of sensitivity to the local anesthetic. These reactions are characterised by signs such as urticaria, pruritus, erythema, angioneurotic edema (including laryngeal edema), tachycardia, sneezing, nausea, vomiting, dizziness, syncope, excessive sweating, elevated temperature, and, possibly, anaphylactoid-like symptomatology (including severe hypotension). Cross-sensitivity among members of the amide-type local anesthetic group have been reported (see section 4.3).

Accidental intrathecal injection of local anaesthetics can lead to very high spinal anaesthesia possibly with apnoea, severe hypotension and loss of consciousness.

Cardiovascular effects are related to depression of the conduction system of the heart and a reduction in myocardial excitability and contractility. This results in decreased cardiac output, hypotension and ECG changes indicative of either heart block, bradycardia or ventricular tachyarrythmias that may lead to cardiac arrest. Usually these will be preceded by major CNS toxicity, i.e. convulsions, but in rare cases, cardiac arrest may occur without prodromal CNS effects.

Neurological damage is a rare but well recognised consequence of regional and particularly epidural and spinal anaesthesia. It may be due to direct injury to the spinal cord or spinal nerves, anterior spinal artery syndrome, injection of an irritant substance or an injection of a non-sterile solution. These may result in localised areas of paraesthesia or anaesthesia, motor weakness, loss of sphincter control and paraplegia. Rarely, these may be permanent.

4.9 Overdose

Accidental intravascular injection of local anaesthetics may cause immediate toxic reactions. In the event of overdose, peak plasma concentrations may not be reached until 2 hours after administration depending upon the injection site and, therefore, signs of toxicity may be delayed. The effects of the drug may be prolonged.

Systemic adverse reactions following overdose or accidental intravascular injection reported with long acting local anaesthetic agents involve both CNS and cardiovascular effects.

CNS Effects

Convulsions should be treated immediately with intravenous thiopentone or diazepam titrated as necessary. Thiopentone and diazepam also depress central nervous system, respiratory and cardiac function. Therefore their use may result in apnoea. Neuro-muscular blockers may be used only if the clinician is confident of maintaining a patent airway and managing a fully paralysed patient.

If not treated promptly, convulsions with subsequent hypoxia and hypercarbia plus myocardial depression from the effects of the local anaesthetic on the heart, may result in cardiac arrhythmias, ventricular fibrillation or cardiac arrest.

Cardiovascular Effects

Hypotension may be prevented or attenuated by pre-treatment with a fluid load and/or the use of vasopressors. If hypotension occurs it should be treated with intravenous crystalloids or colloids and/or incremental doses of a vasopressor such as ephedrine 5-10 mg. Any coexisting causes of hypotension should be rapidly treated.

If severe bradycardia occurs, treatment with atropine 0.3-1.0 mg will normally restore the heart rate to an acceptable level.

Cardiac arrhythmia should be treated as required and ventricular fibrillation should be treated by cardioversion.

5. PHARMACOLOGICAL PROPERTIES

5.1 Pharmacodynamic properties

Pharmacotherapeutic group: Local anaesthetics, amide

ATC Code N01B B10

Levobupivacaine is a long acting local anaesthetic and analgesic. It blocks nerve conduction in sensory and motor nerves largely by interacting with voltage sensitive sodium channels on the cell membrane, but also potassium and calcium channels are blocked. In addition, levobupivacaine interferes with impulse transmission and conduction in other tissues where effects on the cardiovascular and central nervous systems are most important for the occurrence of clinical adverse reactions.

The dose of levobupivacaine is expressed as base, whereas, in the racemate bupivacaine the dose is expressed as hydrochloride salt. This gives rise to approximately 13% more active substance in levobupivacaine solutions compared to bupivacaine. In clinical studies at the same nominal concentrations levobupivacaine showed similar clinical effect to bupivacaine.

In a clinical pharmacology study using the ulnar nerve block model, levobupivacaine was equipotent with bupivacaine.

5.2 Pharmacokinetic properties

In human studies, the distribution kinetics of levobupivacaine following i.v. administration are essentially the same as bupivacaine. The plasma concentration of levobupivacaine following therapeutic administration depends on dose and, as absorption from the site of administration is affected by the vascularity of the tissue, on route of administration.

There are no relevant data in patients with hepatic impairment (see section 4.4).

There are no data in patients with renal impairment. Levobupivacaine is extensively metabolised and unchanged levobupivacaine is not excreted in urine.

Plasma protein binding of levobupivacaine in man was evaluated *in vitro* and was found to be > 97% at concentrations between 0.1 and 1.0 μg/ml.

In a clinical pharmacology study where 40 mg levobupivacaine was given by intravenous administration, the mean half-life was approximately 80 ± 22 minutes, C_{max} 1.4 ± 0.2 μg/ml and AUC 70 ± 27 μg•min/ml.

The mean C_{max} and AUC(0-24h) of levobupivacaine were approximately dose-proportional following epidural administration of 75 mg (0.5%) and 112.5 mg (0.75%) and following doses of 1 mg/kg (0.25%) and 2 mg/kg (0.5%) used for brachial plexus block. Following epidural administration of 112.5 mg (0.75%) the mean C_{max} and AUC values were 0.58 μg/ml and 3.56 μg•h/ml respectively.

The mean total plasma clearance and terminal half-life of levobupivacaine after intravenous infusion were 39 litres/hour and 1.3 hours, respectively. The volume of distribution after intravenous administration was 67 litres.

Levobupivacaine is extensively metabolised with no unchanged levobupivacaine detected in urine or faeces. 3-hydroxylevobupivacaine, a major metabolite of levobupivacaine, is excreted in the urine as glucuronic acid and sulphate ester conjugates. *In vitro* studies showed that CYP3A4 isoform and CYP1A2 isoform mediate the metabolism of levobupivacaine to desbutyl-levobupivacaine and 3-hydroxylevobupivacaine respectively. These studies indicate that the metabolism of levobupivacaine and bupivacaine are similar.

Following intravenous administration, recovery of levobupivacaine was quantitative with a mean total of about 95% being recovered in urine (71%) and faeces (24%) in 48 hours.

There is no evidence of *in vivo* racemisation of levobupivacaine.

5.3 Preclinical safety data

In an embryo-foetal toxicity study in rats, an increased incidence of dilated renal pelvis, dilated ureters, olfactory ventricle dilatation and extra thoraco-lumbar ribs was observed at systemic exposure levels in the same range as those obtained at clinical use. There were no treatment-related malformations.

Levobupivacaine was not genotoxic in a standard battery of assays for mutagenicity and clastogenicity. No carcinogenicity testing has been conducted.

6. PHARMACEUTICAL PARTICULARS

6.1 List of excipients

Sodium Chloride

Sodium Hydroxide

Hydrochloric acid

Water for Injections

6.2 Incompatibilities

Levobupivacaine may precipitate if diluted with alkaline solutions and should not be diluted or co-administered with sodium bicarbonate injections. This medicinal product must not be mixed with other medicinal products except those mentioned in section 6.6.

6.3 Shelf life

Shelf life as packaged for sale: 3 years

Shelf life after first opening: The product should be used immediately

Shelf life after dilution in sodium chloride solution 0,9%:

Chemical and physical in-use stability has been demonstrated for 7 days at 20-22°C. Chemical and physical in-use stability with clonidine, morphine or fentanyl has been demonstrated for 40 hours at 20-22°C.

From a microbiological point of view, the product should be used immediately. If not used immediately, in-use storage times and conditions prior to use are the responsibility of the user.

6.4 Special precautions for storage

Polypropylene ampoules: polypropylene ampoules do not require any special storage conditions.

For storage conditions of the reconstituted medicinal product, see section 6.3.

6.5 Nature and contents of container

Chirocaine is available in two presentations;

10 ml polypropylene ampoule in packs of 5, 10 & 20

10 ml polypropylene ampoule, in sterile blister packs of 5, 10 & 20

Not all pack sizes may be marketed.

6.6 Special precautions for disposal and other handling

For single use only. Discard any unused solution.

The solution/dilution should be inspected visually prior to use. Only clear solutions without visible particles should be used.

A sterile blister container should be chosen when a sterile ampoule surface is required. Ampoule surface is not sterile if sterile blister is pierced.

Dilutions of levobupivacaine standard solutions should be made with sodium chloride 9 mg/ml (0.9%) solution for injection using aseptic techniques.

Clonidine 8.4 μg/ml, morphine 0.05 mg/ml and fentanyl 4 μg/ml have been shown to be compatible with levobupivacaine in sodium chloride 9 mg/ml (0.9%) solution for injection.

7. MARKETING AUTHORISATION HOLDER

Abbott Laboratories Ltd

Queenborough

Kent

ME11 5EL

United Kingdom

8. MARKETING AUTHORISATION NUMBER(S)

PL 00037/0302

9. DATE OF FIRST AUTHORISATION/RENEWAL OF THE AUTHORISATION

Date of first authorisation: 06th January 2000

Date of last renewal: 18th December 2008

10. DATE OF REVISION OF THE TEXT

August 2009

ChloraPrep Summary of Product Characteristics

(Enturia)

1. NAME OF THE MEDICINAL PRODUCT

ChloraPrep® 2% w/v / 70% v/v cutaneous solution

2. QUALITATIVE AND QUANTITATIVE COMPOSITION

Chlorhexidine gluconate 2.0% w/v

Isopropyl alcohol 70% v/v

For excipients see 6.1

3. PHARMACEUTICAL FORM

Cutaneous Solution.

The solution appears as a clear liquid having an odour of alcohol.

4. CLINICAL PARTICULARS

4.1 Therapeutic indications

The medicinal product is to be used for disinfection of the skin prior to invasive procedures.

4.2 Posology and method of administration

For cutaneous use.

One applicator is used containing 0.67 ml, 1.5 ml, 3 ml, 10.5 ml or 26 ml of the ChloraPrep alcoholic solution.

The choice of applicator will depend on the invasive procedure being undertaken and the clinician's preference.

Applicator	Coverage Area (cm × cm)	For Procedures such as:
0.67 ml (Sepp) 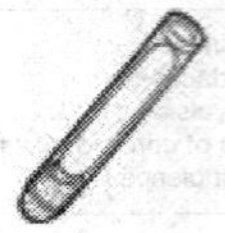	5 × 8	- Peripheral cannulation - Simple biopsy - Routine venipuncture
1.5 ml 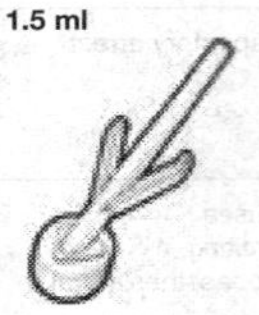 1.5 ml (Frepp) 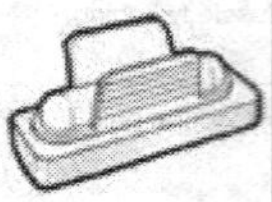	10 × 13	- Blood culture collection - Peripheral cannulation - Peripheral arterial line cannulation - Simple biopsy - Routine venipuncture - Dialysis Fistula/Graft site cleansing
3 ml 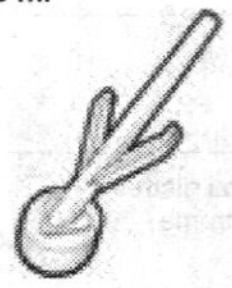	15 × 15	- Midline & Central Venous Catheter (CVC) insertion and maintenance - Peritoneal dialysis site cleansing
10.5 ml 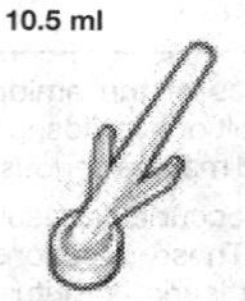 26 ml 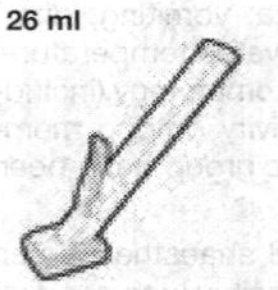	25 × 30 50 × 50	- Minor and major surgical procedures - Implantable device placement - Prosthetic device placement or removal - Midline, Peripheral Intravascular Central Catheter (PICC) & CVC insertion and maintenance - Cardiac catheterisation and Cardiac Cath Lab procedures - Interventional Radiology procedure

The applicator is removed from the wrapper and held with the sponge facing downward. The applicator is squeezed gently to break the ampoule containing the antiseptic solution, which is released onto the sponge in a controlled flow (for the 0.67 ml the barrel is squeezed; for the 26 ml applicator the lever is pressed). The broken ampoule remains safely contained within the applicator. The sponge is gently pressed against the patient's skin in order to apply the antiseptic solution. A back and forth action of the sponge should be used for 30 seconds. The 26 ml applicator includes two swabs. Clean umbilicus with enclosed swabs when applicable. (Moisten swabs by pressing against solution-soaked sponge applicator.) The area covered should be allowed to dry naturally.

4.3 Contraindications

The medicinal product is contra-indicated where patients have shown previous hypersensitivity to chlorhexidine or isopropyl alcohol.

4.4 Special warnings and precautions for use

The solution is an irritant to eyes and mucous membranes. It should therefore be kept away from these areas. If the solution comes in contact with the eyes, they should be washed promptly and thoroughly with water.

It should also not be used on open skin wounds, broken or damaged skin, for lumbar puncture or in children less than 2 months of age. In addition, contact with the brain, meninges and middle ear must be avoided.

Prolonged skin contact with alcoholic solutions should be avoided.

Rarely allergic or irritation skin reactions have been reported with chlorhexidine.

For external use only.

Do not use with electrocautery procedures until dry. Remove any soaked materials, drapes or gowns before proceeding.

4.5 Interaction with other medicinal products and other forms of interaction

Alcohol should not be brought into contact with some vaccines and skin test injections (patch tests). If in doubt, consult the vaccine manufacturers' literature.

4.6 Pregnancy and lactation

There are no studies with this product in pregnant or lactating women. However as percutaneous absorption is negligible, there is no reason why this product may not be used during pregnancy or by breast feeding mothers.

4.7 Effects on ability to drive and use machines

No effects are reported.

4.8 Undesirable effects

Rarely allergic or irritation skin reactions have been reported with chlorhexidine and isopropyl alcohol.

4.9 Overdose

There are no reports of this occurring and the nature of the product makes it unlikely.

5. PHARMACOLOGICAL PROPERTIES

5.1 Pharmacodynamic properties

ATC code D08A C52 (Chlorhexidine, combinations).

Mode of Action: Bisbiguanide antiseptics exert their lethal effect upon bacterial cells through non-specific interaction with acidic phospholipids of the cell membranes.

Since there is little percutaneous absorption of isopropyl alcohol or chlorhexidine gluconate and the medicinal product is indicated for use on pre-injection sites, pharmacodynamic studies have not been undertaken.

5.2 Pharmacokinetic properties

There is little absorption of isopropyl alcohol or of chlorhexidine gluconate through intact skin. Pharmacokinetic studies have not been conducted with the product.

5.3 Preclinical safety data

There are no preclinical data of relevance to the prescriber that are not already included elsewhere in the SPC.

6. PHARMACEUTICAL PARTICULARS

6.1 List of excipients

Purified water.

6.2 Incompatibilities

Chlorhexidine is incompatible with soap and other anionic agents

6.3 Shelf life

24 months.

6.4 Special precautions for storage

Do not store above 25°C.

Avoid freezing.

Store in the original packaging

6.5 Nature and contents of container

The alcoholic solution is contained in a borosilicate Type 1 glass ampoule which is housed in an applicator.

The applicator consists of a HDPE plastic handle/barrel containing the ampoule with the ChloraPrep solution. For the 1.5 ml (both the Frepp® and standard applicator) and 3 ml, 10.5 ml and 26 ml applicators, the handle is bonded to a Novonette film and a polyester urethane foam. For the 0.67 ml Sepp® applicator, the barrel is bonded to the polyester urethane foam which is stitch-bonded to a polyester airweave.

The applicator is wrapped in an ethyl vinyl acetate film.

The medicinal product is available as 0.67 ml, 1.5 ml, 3 ml, 10.5 ml and 26 ml fill volumes.

Pack Size:

0.67 ml (Sepp®): 200 applicators

1.5ml (Frepp®): 20 applicators

1.5 ml and 3 ml: 25 applicators

10.5 ml: 1 applicator or 25 applicators

26 ml: 1 applicator

6.6 Special precautions for disposal and other handling

The solution is flammable. Do not use while smoking, or near any naked flames or strong heat source. Avoid exposure of the container and contents to naked flames during use, storage and disposal.

This product is for single use only.

Discard after use as per clinical waste procedures.

7. MARKETING AUTHORISATION HOLDER

Insight Health Limited

1.9 Wembley Commercial Centre

East Lane

Wembley

HA9 7XX

8. MARKETING AUTHORISATION NUMBER(S)

PL 19803/0001

9. DATE OF FIRST AUTHORISATION/RENEWAL OF THE AUTHORISATION
08 /09/2005

10. DATE OF REVISION OF THE TEXT
Date of approval

Choragon 5000 U and Choragon Solvent

(Ferring Pharmaceuticals Ltd)

1. NAME OF THE MEDICINAL PRODUCT
Choragon 5000U and Choragon Solvent

2. QUALITATIVE AND QUANTITATIVE COMPOSITION
Active Ingredient

Each ampoule with dry substance contains chorionic gonadotrophin EP corresponding to 5000 units.

3. PHARMACEUTICAL FORM
Powder for injection and solvent for parenteral use.

4. CLINICAL PARTICULARS
4.1 Therapeutic indications
In the female

In the management of anovulatory infertility.

In the male

In the management of delayed puberty, undescended testes and oligospermia.

4.2 Posology and method of administration
Treatment should only commence after expert assessment.

In the female

Induction of ovulation: 10000 units mid-cycle if plasma oestrogen levels are favourable following follicular stimulation.

In the male

Delayed puberty: Dose should be titrated against plasma testosterone, starting with 500 units twice weekly. Treatment should be continued for 4 - 6 weeks.

Undescended testes: Treatment should begin before puberty, the optimum age range being 7 - 10 years. 500 units three times weekly is a suitable starting dose. This may be increased to 4000 units if necessary. Treatment should continue for 6 - 10 weeks.

In males over 17 years of age a commencing dose of 1000 units twice weekly can be given. Treatment should be continued for one or two months after testicular descent.

Oligospermia: Dose should be titrated against seminal analysis starting with 500 units two or three times weekly. Treatment should be continued for 16 weeks.

Choragon is given by intramuscular injection.

4.3 Contraindications
hCG should not be given to patients with disorders that might be exacerbated by androgen release.

4.4 Special warnings and precautions for use
hCG should be given with care to patients in whom fluid retention might be a hazard, as in asthma, epilepsy, migraine or cardiac or renal disorders.

Allergic reactions may occur and patients thought to be susceptible should be given skin tests before treatment.

hCG preparations should only be used under the supervision of a specialist having available adequate facilities for appropriate laboratory monitoring.

In the female - Use in induction of ovulation may result in ovarian enlargement or cysts, acute abdominal pain, superovulation or multiple pregnancies, particularly if endocrine monitoring is inadequate.

In the male - Treatment for undescended testes may produce precocious puberty; use should cease immediately. Gynaecomastia has been reported. A growth spurt may also be associated with use and this should be kept in mind particularly where epiphyseal growth is still potentially active.

4.5 Interaction with other medicinal products and other forms of interaction
None known.

4.6 Pregnancy and lactation
Not applicable as only recommended in females for infertility.

4.7 Effects on ability to drive and use machines
None known.

4.8 Undesirable effects
Headache, tiredness and mood changes have been described.

4.9 Overdose
See "Warnings".

5. PHARMACOLOGICAL PROPERTIES
5.1 Pharmacodynamic properties
Gonadotrophin.

5.2 Pharmacokinetic properties
hCG is not effective when taken orally and is administered by intramuscular injection.

5.3 Preclinical safety data
There are no preclinical data of relevance to the Prescriber which are additional to those already included in other sections of the SPC.

6. PHARMACEUTICAL PARTICULARS
6.1 List of excipients
Dry substance: Mannitol, sodium hydroxide for pH-adjustment.

Diluent: Isotonic sodium chloride solution (0.9% w/w), dilute hydrochloric acid for pH-adjustment.

6.2 Incompatibilities
None stated.

6.3 Shelf life
36 months as packaged for sale.

6.4 Special precautions for storage
Protect from light and store below 25°C

6.5 Nature and contents of container
Each pack contains ampoule(s) with 5000 units of hCG powder for solution for injection packaged together with ampoule(s) of 1ml Choragon solvent. Ampoules are assembled in boxes containing either 1 pair, 3 pairs or 5 pairs of ampoules and solvents.

6.6 Special precautions for disposal and other handling
The dry substance must be reconstituted with the solvent prior to use.

7. MARKETING AUTHORISATION HOLDER
Ferring Pharmaceuticals Limited
The Courtyard
Waterside Drive
Langley
Berkshire
SL3 6EZ

8. MARKETING AUTHORISATION NUMBER(S)
PL 03194/0065

9. DATE OF FIRST AUTHORISATION/RENEWAL OF THE AUTHORISATION
15/08/96

10. DATE OF REVISION OF THE TEXT
29 April 2009

Cialis 2.5mg, 5mg, 10mg & 20mg film-coated tablets

(Eli Lilly and Company Limited)

1. NAME OF THE MEDICINAL PRODUCT
CIALIS* 2.5mg, 5mg, 10mg and 20mg film-coated tablets.

2. QUALITATIVE AND QUANTITATIVE COMPOSITION
Each 2.5mg tablet contains 2.5mg tadalafil.

Excipient: Each coated tablet contains 92mg lactose monohydrate.

Each 5mg tablet contains 5mg tadalafil.

Excipient: Each coated tablet contains 127mg lactose monohydrate.

Each 10mg tablet contains 10mg tadalafil.

Excipient: Each coated tablet contains 179mg lactose monohydrate.

Each 20mg tablet contains 20mg tadalafil.

Excipient: Each coated tablet contains 245mg lactose monohydrate.

For a full list of excipients, see section 6.1.

3. PHARMACEUTICAL FORM
Film-coated tablet (tablet).

The 2.5mg tablets are light orange-yellow and almond shaped, marked 'C 2 ½' on one side.

The 5mg tablets are light yellow and almond shaped, marked 'C 5' on one side.

The 10mg tablets are light yellow and almond shaped, marked 'C 10' on one side.

The 20mg tablets are yellow and almond shaped, marked 'C 20' on one side.

4. CLINICAL PARTICULARS
4.1 Therapeutic indications
Treatment of erectile dysfunction.

In order for tadalafil to be effective, sexual stimulation is required.

CIALIS is not indicated for use by women.

4.2 Posology and method of administration
For oral use. CIALIS is available as 2.5mg, 5mg, 10mg and 20mg film-coated tablets.

Use in Adult Men

In general, the recommended dose is 10mg taken prior to anticipated sexual activity and with or without food. In those patients in whom tadalafil 10mg does not produce an adequate effect, 20mg might be tried. It may be taken at least 30 minutes prior to sexual activity.

The maximum dose frequency is once per day.

Tadalafil 10mg and 20mg is intended for use prior to anticipated sexual activity and it is not recommended for continuous daily use.

In responder patients to on-demand regimen who anticipate a frequent use of CIALIS (i.e., at least twice weekly) a once daily regimen with the lowest doses of CIALIS might be considered suitable, based on patient choice and the physician's judgement.

In these patients, the recommended dose is 5mg taken once a day at approximately the same time of day. The dose may be decreased to 2.5mg once a day based on individual tolerability.

The appropriateness of continued use of the daily regimen should be reassessed periodically.

Use in Elderly Men

Dose adjustments are not required in elderly patients.

Use in Men with Impaired Renal Function

Dose adjustments are not required in patients with mild to moderate renal impairment. For patients with severe renal impairment, 10mg is the maximum recommended dose. Once-a-day dosing of tadalafil is not recommended in patients with severe renal impairment. (See sections 4.4 and 5.2.)

Use in Men with Impaired Hepatic Function

The recommended dose of CIALIS is 10mg taken prior to anticipated sexual activity and with or without food. There is limited clinical data on the safety of CIALIS in patients with severe hepatic impairment (Child-Pugh class C); if prescribed, a careful individual benefit/risk evaluation should be undertaken by the prescribing physician. There are no available data about the administration of doses higher than 10mg of tadalafil to patients with hepatic impairment. Once-a-day dosing has not been evaluated in patients with hepatic impairment; therefore if prescribed, a careful individual benefit/risk evaluation should be undertaken by the prescribing physician. (See section 5.2.)

Use in Men with Diabetes

Dose adjustments are not required in diabetic patients.

Use in Children and Adolescents

CIALIS should not be used in individuals below 18 years of age.

4.3 Contraindications
Hypersensitivity to the active substance or to any of the excipients.

In clinical studies, tadalafil was shown to augment the hypotensive effects of nitrates. This is thought to result from the combined effects of nitrates and tadalafil on the nitric oxide/cGMP pathway. Therefore, administration of CIALIS to patients who are using any form of organic nitrate is contra-indicated. (See section 4.5.)

Agents for the treatment of erectile dysfunction, including CIALIS, must not be used in men with cardiac disease for whom sexual activity is inadvisable. Physicians should consider the potential cardiac risk of sexual activity in patients with pre-existing cardiovascular disease.

The following groups of patients with cardiovascular disease were not included in clinical trials and the use of tadalafil is therefore contra-indicated:

- Patients with myocardial infarction within the last 90 days.
- Patients with unstable angina or angina occurring during sexual intercourse.
- Patients with New York Heart Association class 2 or greater heart failure in the last 6 months.
- Patients with uncontrolled arrhythmias, hypotension (<90/50mmHg), or uncontrolled hypertension.
- Patients with a stroke within the last 6 months.

CIALIS is contra-indicated in patients who have loss of vision in one eye because of non-arteritic anterior ischaemic optic neuropathy (NAION), regardless of whether this episode was in connection or not with previous PDE5 inhibitor exposure (see section 4.4).

4.4 Special warnings and precautions for use
A medical history and physical examination should be undertaken to diagnose erectile dysfunction and determine potential underlying causes, before pharmacological treatment is considered.

Prior to initiating any treatment for erectile dysfunction, physicians should consider the cardiovascular status of their patients, since there is a degree of cardiac risk associated with sexual activity. Tadalafil has vasodilator properties, resulting in mild and transient decreases in blood pressure (see section 5.1), and as such potentiates the hypotensive effect of nitrates (see section 4.3).

Tadalafil (2.5mg and 5mg) - In patients receiving concomitant antihypertensive medicines, tadalafil may induce a blood pressure decrease. When initiating daily treatment with tadalafil, appropriate clinical considerations should be given to a possible dose adjustment of the antihypertensive therapy.

Serious cardiovascular events, including myocardial infarction, sudden cardiac death, unstable angina pectoris, ventricular arrhythmia, stroke, transient ischaemic attacks, chest pain, palpitations, and tachycardia, have been reported either post-marketing and/or in clinical trials. Most of the patients in whom these events have been reported had pre-existing cardiovascular risk factors. However, it is not possible to definitively determine whether these events are related directly to these risk factors, to CIALIS, to sexual activity, or to a combination of these or other factors.

Visual defects and cases of NAION have been reported in connection with the intake of CIALIS and other PDE5 inhibitors. The patient should be advised that in case of sudden visual defect, he should stop taking CIALIS and consult a physician immediately (see section 4.3).

Due to increased tadalafil exposure (AUC), limited clinical experience and the lack of ability to influence clearance by dialysis, once-a-day dosing of CIALIS is not recommended in patients with severe renal impairment.

There is limited clinical data on the safety of single-dose administration of CIALIS in patients with severe hepatic insufficiency (Child-Pugh class C). Once-a-day administration has not been evaluated in patients with hepatic insufficiency. If CIALIS is prescribed, a careful individual benefit/risk evaluation should be undertaken by the prescribing physician.

Patients who experience erections lasting 4 hours or more should be instructed to seek immediate medical assistance. If priapism is not treated immediately, penile tissue damage and permanent loss of potency may result.

Agents for the treatment of erectile dysfunction, including CIALIS, should be used with caution in patients with anatomical deformation of the penis (such as angulation, cavernosal fibrosis, or Peyronie's disease) or in patients who have conditions which may predispose them to priapism (such as sickle cell anaemia, multiple myeloma, or leukaemia).

The evaluation of erectile dysfunction should include a determination of potential underlying causes and the identification of appropriate treatment following an appropriate medical assessment. It is not known if CIALIS is effective in patients who have undergone pelvic surgery or radical non-nerve-sparing prostatectomy.

In patients who are taking alpha$_1$-blockers concomitant administration of CIALIS may lead to symptomatic hypotension in some patients (see section 4.5). The combination of tadalafil and doxazosin is not recommended.

Caution should be exercised when prescribing CIALIS to patients using potent CYP3A4 inhibitors (ritonavir, saquinavir, ketoconazole, itraconazole, and erythromycin), as increased tadalafil exposure (AUC) has been observed if the medicines are combined (see section 4.5).

The safety and efficacy of combinations of CIALIS and other treatments for erectile dysfunction have not been studied. Therefore, the use of such combinations is not recommended.

CIALIS contains lactose monohydrate. Patients with rare hereditary problems of galactose intolerance, the Lapp lactase deficiency or glucose-galactose malabsorption should not take this medicinal product.

4.5 Interaction with other medicinal products and other forms of interaction

Interaction studies were conducted with 10mg and/or 20mg tadalafil, as indicated below. With regard to those interaction studies where only the 10mg tadalafil dose was used, clinically relevant interactions at higher doses cannot be completely ruled out.

Effects of Other Substances on Tadalafil

Tadalafil is principally metabolised by CYP3A4. A selective inhibitor of CYP3A4, ketoconazole (200mg daily), increased tadalafil (10mg) exposure (AUC) 2-fold and C_{max} by 15%, relative to the AUC and C_{max} values for tadalafil alone. Ketoconazole (400mg daily) increased tadalafil (20mg) exposure (AUC) 4-fold and C_{max} by 22%. Ritonavir, a protease inhibitor (200mg twice daily), which is an inhibitor of CYP3A4, CYP2C9, CYP2C19, and CYP2D6, increased tadalafil (20mg) exposure (AUC) 2-fold with no change in C_{max}. Although specific interactions have not been studied, other protease inhibitors, such as saquinavir, and other CYP3A4 inhibitors, such as erythromycin, clarithromycin, itraconazole, and grapefruit juice, should be co-administered with caution, as they would be expected to increase plasma concentrations of tadalafil (see section 4.4). Consequently, the incidence of the undesirable effects listed in section 4.8 might be increased.

The role of transporters (for example, p-glycoprotein) in the disposition of tadalafil is not known. There is thus the potential of drug interactions mediated by inhibition of transporters.

A CYP3A4 inducer, rifampicin, reduced tadalafil AUC by 88%, relative to the AUC values for tadalafil alone (10mg). This reduced exposure can be anticipated to decrease the efficacy of tadalafil; the magnitude of decreased efficacy is unknown. Other inducers of CYP3A4, such as phenobarbital, phenytoin, and carbamazepine, may also decrease plasma concentrations of tadalafil.

Effects of Tadalafil on Other Medicinal Products

In clinical studies, tadalafil (5mg, 10mg and 20mg) was shown to augment the hypotensive effects of nitrates. Therefore, administration of CIALIS to patients who are using any form of organic nitrate is contra-indicated (see section 4.3). Based on the results of a clinical study in which 150 subjects received daily doses of tadalafil 20mg for 7 days and 0.4mg sublingual nitroglycerin at various times, this interaction lasted for more than 24 hours and was no longer detectable when 48 hours had elapsed after the last tadalafil dose. Thus, in a patient prescribed any dose of CIALIS (2.5mg - 20mg), where nitrate administration is deemed medically necessary in a life-threatening situation, at least 48 hours should have elapsed after the last dose of CIALIS before nitrate administration is considered. In such circumstances, nitrates should only be administered under close medical supervision with appropriate haemodynamic monitoring.

In clinical pharmacology studies, the potential for tadalafil to augment the hypotensive effects of antihypertensive agents was examined. Major classes of antihypertensive agents were studied, including calcium-channel blockers (amlodipine), angiotensin converting enzyme (ACE) inhibitors (enalapril), beta-adrenergic receptor blockers (metoprolol), thiazide diuretics (bendrofluazide), and angiotensin II receptor blockers (various types and doses, alone or in combination with thiazides, calcium-channel blockers, beta-blockers, and/or alpha-blockers). Tadalafil (10mg, except for studies with angiotensin II receptor blockers and amlodipine in which a 20mg dose was applied) had no clinically significant interaction with any of these classes. In another clinical pharmacology study, tadalafil (20mg) was studied in combination with up to 4 classes of antihypertensives. In subjects taking multiple antihypertensives, the ambulatory-blood-pressure changes appeared to relate to the degree of blood pressure control. In this regard, study subjects whose blood pressure was well controlled, the reduction was minimal and similar to that seen in healthy subjects. In study subjects whose blood pressure was not controlled, the reduction was greater, although this reduction was not associated with hypotensive symptoms in the majority of subjects. In patients receiving concomitant antihypertensive medicines, tadalafil 20mg may induce a blood pressure decrease, which (with the exception of alpha-blockers - see below) is, in general, minor and not likely to be clinically relevant. Analysis of Phase 3 clinical trial data showed no difference in adverse events in patients taking tadalafil with or without antihypertensive medicines. However, appropriate clinical advice should be given to patients regarding a possible decrease in blood pressure when they are treated with antihypertensive medicines.

The co-administration of doxazosin (4 and 8 mg daily) and tadalafil (5 mg daily dose and 20 mg as a single dose) increases the blood pressure-lowering effect of this alpha-blocker in a significant manner. This effect lasts at least twelve hours and may be symptomatic, including syncope. Therefore this combination is not recommended (see section 4.4).

In interaction studies performed in a limited number of healthy volunteers, these effects were not reported with alfuzosin or tamsulosin. However, caution should be exercised when using tadalafil in patients treated with any alpha-blockers, and notably in the elderly. Treatments should be initiated at minimal dosage and progressively adjusted.

Alcohol concentrations (mean maximum blood concentration 0.08%) were not affected by co-administration with tadalafil (10mg or 20mg). In addition, no changes in tadalafil concentrations were seen 3 hours after co-administration with alcohol. Alcohol was administered in a manner to maximise the rate of alcohol absorption (overnight fast with no food until 2 hours after alcohol). Tadalafil (20mg) did not augment the mean blood pressure decrease produced by alcohol (0.7g/kg or approximately 180ml of 40% alcohol [vodka] in an 80 kg male) but, in some subjects, postural dizziness and orthostatic hypotension were observed. When tadalafil was administered with lower doses of alcohol (0.6g/kg), hypotension was not observed and dizziness occurred with similar frequency to alcohol alone. The effect of alcohol on cognitive function was not augmented by tadalafil (10mg).

Tadalafil has been demonstrated to produce an increase in the oral bioavailability of ethinyloestradiol; a similar increase may be expected with oral administration of terbutaline, although the clinical consequence of this is uncertain.

When tadalafil 10mg was administered with theophylline (a non-selective phosphodiesterase inhibitor) in a clinical pharmacology study, there was no pharmacokinetic interaction. The only pharmacodynamic effect was a small (3.5 bpm) increase in heart rate. Although this effect is minor and was of no clinical significance in this study, it should be considered when co-administering these medicines.

Tadalafil is not expected to cause clinically significant inhibition or induction of the clearance of medicinal products metabolised by CYP450 isoforms. Studies have confirmed that tadalafil does not inhibit or induce CYP450 isoforms, including CYP3A4, CYP1A2, CYP2D6, CYP2E1, CYP2C9 and CYP2C19.

Tadalafil (10mg and 20mg) had no clinically significant effect on exposure (AUC) to S-warfarin or R-warfarin (CYP2C9 substrate), nor did tadalafil affect changes in prothrombin time induced by warfarin.

Tadalafil (10mg and 20mg) did not potentiate the increase in bleeding time caused by acetylsalicylic acid.

Specific interaction studies with antidiabetic agents were not conducted.

4.6 Pregnancy and lactation

CIALIS is not indicated for use by women.

For tadalafil, no clinical data on exposed pregnancies are available. Animal studies do not indicate direct or indirect harmful effects with respect to pregnancy, embryonal/foetal development, parturition or postnatal development (see section 5.3).

4.7 Effects on ability to drive and use machines

No studies on the effect of the ability to drive and use machines have been performed. Although the frequency of reports of dizziness in placebo and tadalafil arms in clinical trials was similar, patients should be aware of how they react to CIALIS before driving or operating machinery.

4.8 Undesirable effects

The most commonly reported adverse reactions were headache and dyspepsia. The adverse reactions reported were transient, and generally mild or moderate. Adverse reaction data are limited in patients over 75 years of age.

The table below lists the adverse reactions reported during placebo-controlled clinical trials for registration in patients treated with CIALIS on demand and daily dosing. Adverse reactions are also included that have been reported from post marketing surveillance in patients taking CIALIS on demand.

Adverse Reactions

Frequency estimate: Very common (≥1/10), Common (≥1/100 to <1/10), Uncommon (≥1/1000 to <1/100), Rare (≥1/10,000 to <1/1000), Very Rare (<1/10,000) and Not known (events not reported in registration trials cannot be estimated from post marketing spontaneous reports).

(see Table 1 on next page)

A slightly higher incidence of ECG abnormalities, primarily sinus bradycardia, has been reported in patients treated with tadalafil once a day as compared with placebo. Most of these ECG abnormalities were not associated with adverse reactions.

4.9 Overdose

Single doses of up to 500mg have been given to healthy subjects, and multiple daily doses up to 100mg have been given to patients. Adverse events were similar to those seen at lower doses.

In cases of overdose, standard supportive measures should be adopted, as required. Haemodialysis contributes negligibly to tadalafil elimination.

5. PHARMACOLOGICAL PROPERTIES

5.1 Pharmacodynamic properties

Pharmacotherapeutic group: Drugs used in erectile dysfunction. *ATC code:* G04BE.

Tadalafil is a selective, reversible inhibitor of cyclic guanosine monophosphate (cGMP)-specific phosphodiesterase type 5 (PDE5). When sexual stimulation causes the local release of nitric oxide, inhibition of PDE5 by tadalafil produces increased levels of cGMP in the corpus cavernosum. This results in smooth muscle relaxation and inflow of blood into the penile tissues, thereby producing an erection. Tadalafil has no effect in the absence of sexual stimulation.

Studies *in vitro* have shown that tadalafil is a selective inhibitor of PDE5. PDE5 is an enzyme found in corpus cavernosum smooth muscle, vascular and visceral smooth muscle, skeletal muscle, platelets, kidney, lung, and cerebellum. The effect of tadalafil is more potent on PDE5 than on other phosphodiesterases. Tadalafil is >10,000-fold more potent for PDE5 than for PDE1, PDE2, and PDE4, enzymes which are found in the heart, brain, blood vessels, liver, and other organs. Tadalafil is >10,000-fold more potent for PDE5 than for PDE3, an enzyme found in the heart and blood vessels. This selectivity for PDE5 over PDE3 is important because PDE3 is an enzyme involved in cardiac contractility. Additionally, tadalafil is approximately 700-fold more potent for PDE5 than for PDE6, an enzyme which is found in the retina and is responsible for phototransduction. Tadalafil is also >10,000-fold more potent for PDE5 than for PDE7 through PDE10.

Three clinical studies were conducted in 1,054 patients in an at-home setting to define the period of responsiveness to CIALIS. Tadalafil demonstrated statistically significant improvement in erectile function and the ability to have successful sexual intercourse up to 36 hours following dosing, as well as patients' ability to attain and maintain erections for successful intercourse compared to placebo as early as 16 minutes following dosing.

Tadalafil administered to healthy subjects produced no significant difference compared to placebo in supine systolic and diastolic blood pressure (mean maximal decrease of 1.6/0.8mmHg, respectively), in standing systolic and diastolic blood pressure (mean maximal decrease of 0.2/4.6mmHg, respectively), and no significant change in heart rate.

In a study to assess the effects of tadalafil on vision, no impairment of colour discrimination (blue/green) was detected using the Farnsworth-Munsell 100-hue test. This finding is consistent with the low affinity of tadalafil for PDE6 compared to PDE5. Across all clinical studies, reports of changes in colour vision were rare (<0.1%).

Three studies were conducted in men to assess the potential effect on spermatogenesis of CIALIS 10mg (one

Table 1

Very common (≥1/10)	**Common** (≥1/100 to <1/10)	**Uncommon** (≥1/1000 to <1/100)	**Rare** (≥1/10,000 to <1/1000)	**Not known**
System Organ Class: Immune system disorders				
		Hypersensitivity reactions		
System Organ Class: Nervous system disorders				
Headache	Dizziness		Stroke[1], Syncope, Transient ischaemic attacks[1], Migraine	Seizures, Transient amnesia
System Organ Class: Eye disorders				
		Blurred vision, Sensations described as eye pain, Swelling of eyelids, Conjunctival hyperaemia	Visual field defect	Non-arteritic anterior ischaemic optic neuropathy (NAION), Retinal vascular occlusion
System Organ Class: Ear and labyrinth disorders				
				Sudden deafness[2]
System Organ Class: Cardiac disorders[1]				
	Palpitations	Tachycardia	Myocardial infarction	Unstable angina pectoris, Ventricular arrhythmia
System Organ Class: Vascular disorders				
	Flushing	Hypotension (more commonly reported when tadalafil is given to patients who are already taking antihypertensive agents), Hypertension		
System Organ Class: Respiratory, thoracic and mediastinal disorders				
	Nasal congestion	Epistaxis		
System Organ Class: Gastro-intestinal disorders				
Dyspepsia	Abdominal pain, Gastro-oesophageal reflux			
System Organ Class: Skin and subcutaneous tissue disorders				
		Rash, Urticaria, Hyperhydrosis (sweating)		Stevens-Johnson syndrome, Exfoliative dermatitis
System Organ Class: Musculoskeletal, connective tissue and bone disorders				
	Back pain, Myalgia			
System Organ Class: Reproductive system and breast disorders				
			Prolonged erections	Priapism
System Organ Class: General disorders and administration site conditions				
		Chest pain[1]	Facial oedema	Sudden cardiac death[1]

[1] Most of the patients in whom these events have been reported had pre-existing cardiovascular risk factors (see section 4.4).

[2] Sudden decrease or loss of hearing has been reported in a small number of post marketing and clinical trial cases with the use of all PDE5 inhibitors, including tadalafil.

6-month study) and 20mg (one 6-month and one 9-month study) administered daily. In two of these studies decreases were observed in sperm count and concentration related to tadalafil treatment of unlikely clinical relevance. These effects were not associated with changes in other parameters, such as motility, morphology, and FSH.

Tadalafil at doses of 2.5mg, 5mg, and 10 mg taken once a day has been evaluated in 3 clinical studies involving 853 patients of various ages (range 21-82 years) and ethnicities, with erectile dysfunction of various severities (mild, moderate, severe) and etiologies. Most patients in all three studies were responders to previous on-demand treatment with PDE5 inhibitors. In the two primary efficacy studies of general populations, the mean per-subject proportion of successful attempts were 57 and 67% on CIALIS 5mg, 50% on CIALIS 2.5mg as compared to 31 and 37% with placebo. In the study in patients with erectile dysfunction secondary to diabetes, the mean per-subject proportion of successful attempts were 41 and 46% on CIALIS 5mg and 2.5mg, respectively, as compared to 28% with placebo.

Tadalafil at doses of 2 to 100 mg has been evaluated in 16 clinical studies involving 3250 patients, including patients with erectile dysfunction of various severities (mild, moderate, severe), etiologies, ages (range 21-86 years), and ethnicities. Most patients reported erectile dysfunction of at least 1 year in duration. In the primary efficacy studies of general populations, 81% of patients reported that CIALIS improved their erections as compared to 35% with placebo. Also, patients with erectile dysfunction in all severity categories reported improved erections whilst taking CIALIS (86%, 83%, and 72% for mild, moderate, and severe, respectively, as compared to 45%, 42%, and 19% with placebo). In the primary efficacy studies, 75% of intercourse attempts were successful in CIALIS-treated patients as compared to 32% with placebo.

In a 12-week study performed in 186 patients (142 tadalafil, 44 placebo) with erectile dysfunction secondary to spinal cord injury, tadalafil significantly improved the erectile function leading to a mean per-subject proportion of successful attempts in patients treated with tadalafil 10mg or 20 mg (flexible-dose, on demand) of 48% as compared to 17% with placebo.

5.2 Pharmacokinetic properties

Absorption

Tadalafil is readily absorbed after oral administration and the mean maximum observed plasma concentration (C_{max}) is achieved at a median time of 2 hours after dosing. Absolute bioavailability of tadalafil following oral dosing has not been determined.

The rate and extent of absorption of tadalafil are not influenced by food, thus CIALIS may be taken with or without food. The time of dosing (morning versus evening) had no clinically relevant effects on the rate and extent of absorption.

Distribution

The mean volume of distribution is approximately 63 litres, indicating that tadalafil is distributed into tissues. At therapeutic concentrations, 94% of tadalafil in plasma is bound to proteins. Protein binding is not affected by impaired renal function.

Less than 0.0005% of the administered dose appeared in the semen of healthy subjects.

Biotransformation

Tadalafil is predominantly metabolised by the cytochrome P450 (CYP) 3A4 isoform. The major circulating metabolite is the methylcatechol glucuronide. This metabolite is at least 13,000-fold less potent than tadalafil for PDE5. Consequently, it is not expected to be clinically active at observed metabolite concentrations.

Elimination

The mean oral clearance for tadalafil is 2.5 l/h and the mean half-life is 17.5 hours in healthy subjects.

Tadalafil is excreted predominantly as inactive metabolites, mainly in the faeces (approximately 61% of the dose) and to a lesser extent in the urine (approximately 36% of the dose).

Linearity/Non-Linearity

Tadalafil pharmacokinetics in healthy subjects are linear with respect to time and dose. Over a dose range of 2.5mg to 20mg, exposure (AUC) increases proportionally with dose. Steady-state plasma concentrations are attained within 5 days of once daily dosing.

Pharmacokinetics determined with a population approach in patients with erectile dysfunction are similar to pharmacokinetics in subjects without erectile dysfunction.

Special Populations

Elderly

Healthy elderly subjects (65 years or over) had a lower oral clearance of tadalafil, resulting in 25% higher exposure (AUC) relative to healthy subjects aged 19 to 45 years. This effect of age is not clinically significant and does not warrant a dose adjustment.

Renal Insufficiency

In clinical pharmacology studies using single dose tadalafil (5mg-20mg), tadalafil exposure (AUC) approximately doubled in subjects with mild (creatinine clearance 51 to 80ml/min) or moderate (creatinine clearance 31 to 50ml/min) renal impairment and in subjects with end-stage renal disease on dialysis. In haemodialysis patients, C_{max} was 41% higher than that observed in healthy subjects. Haemodialysis contributes negligibly to tadalafil elimination.

Hepatic Insufficiency

Tadalafil exposure (AUC) in subjects with mild and moderate hepatic impairment (Child-Pugh class A and B) is comparable to exposure in healthy subjects when a dose of 10mg is administered. There is limited clinical data on the safety of CIALIS in patients with severe hepatic insufficiency (Child-Pugh class C). If CIALIS is prescribed, a careful individual benefit/risk evaluation should be undertaken by the prescribing physician. There are no available data about the administration of doses higher than 10mg of tadalafil to patients with hepatic impairment. There are no available data about the administration of once-a-day dosing of tadalafil to patients with hepatic impairment. If CIALIS is prescribed once-a-day, a careful individual benefit/risk evaluation should be undertaken by the prescribing physician.

Patients with Diabetes

Tadalafil exposure (AUC) in patients with diabetes was approximately 19% lower than the AUC value for healthy subjects. This difference in exposure does not warrant a dose adjustment.

5.3 Preclinical safety data

Non-clinical data reveal no special hazard for humans based on conventional studies of safety pharmacology, repeat dose toxicity, genotoxicity, carcinogenic potential, and toxicity to reproduction.

There was no evidence of teratogenicity, embryotoxicity, or foetotoxicity in rats or mice that received up to 1000mg/kg/day tadalafil. In a rat prenatal and postnatal development study, the no observed effect dose was 30mg/kg/day. In the pregnant rat the AUC for calculated free drug at this dose was approximately 18-times the human AUC at a 20mg dose.

There was no impairment of fertility in male and female rats. In dogs given tadalafil daily for 6 to 12 months at doses of 25mg/kg/day (resulting in at least a 3-fold greater exposure [range 3.7-18.6] than seen in humans given a single 20mg dose) and above, there was regression of the seminiferous tubular epithelium that resulted in a decrease in spermatogenesis in some dogs. See also section 5.1.

6. PHARMACEUTICAL PARTICULARS

6.1 List of excipients

Tablet core:

Lactose monohydrate

Croscarmellose sodium

Hydroxypropylcellulose

Microcrystalline cellulose

Sodium laurilsulfate

Magnesium stearate

2.5mg Film-coat:

Lactose monohydrate

Hypromellose

Triacetin,

Titanium dioxide (E171)

Iron oxide yellow (E172)

Iron oxide red (E172)

Talc

5mg, 10mg and 20mg Film-coat:

Lactose monohydrate

Hypromellose

Triacetin

Titanium dioxide (E171)

Iron oxide yellow (E172)

Talc

6.2 Incompatibilities
Not applicable.

6.3 Shelf life
3 years.

6.4 Special precautions for storage
Store in the original package in order to protect from moisture. For Tadalafil 5mg - Do not store above 25°C. For Tadalafil 2.5mg, 10mg and 20mg - Do not store above 30°C.

6.5 Nature and contents of container
Aluminium/PVC/PE/ PCTFE blisters in cartons of 2, 4, 8, 12, 14 and 28 film-coated tablets.

Not all pack sizes may be marketed.

6.6 Special precautions for disposal and other handling
No special requirements.

7. MARKETING AUTHORISATION HOLDER
Eli Lilly Nederland B.V.

Grootslag 1-5, NL-3991 RA, Houten The Netherlands

8. MARKETING AUTHORISATION NUMBER(S)

EU/1/02/237/001	CIALIS 10mg × 4 film coated tablets.
EU/1/02/237/002	CIALIS 20mg × 2 film coated tablets.
EU/1/02/237/003	CIALIS 20mg × 4 film coated tablets.
EU/1/02/237/004	CIALIS 20mg × 8 film coated tablets.
EU/1/02/237/005	CIALIS 20mg × 12 film coated tablets.
EU/1/02/237/006	CIALIS 2.5mg × 28 film coated tablets.
EU/1/02/237/007	CIALIS 5mg × 14 film coated tablets.
EU/1/02/237/008	CIALIS 5mg × 28 film coated tablets.

9. DATE OF FIRST AUTHORISATION/RENEWAL OF THE AUTHORISATION
Date of first Authorisation: 12 November 2002

Date of last renewal: 12 November 2007

10. DATE OF REVISION OF THE TEXT
03 September 2008

LEGAL CATEGORY
POM

*CIALIS (tadalafil) is a trademark of Eli Lilly and Company.

CI12M

Cidomycin Adult Injectable 80mg/2ml

(sanofi-aventis)

1. NAME OF THE MEDICINAL PRODUCT
Cidomycin^{TM} Adult Injectable 80mg/2ml.

2. QUALITATIVE AND QUANTITATIVE COMPOSITION
Each ampoule or vial (2ml) contains Gentamicin Sulphate Ph Eur equivalent to 80mg Gentamicin base.

For excipients, see section 6.1

3. PHARMACEUTICAL FORM
Solution for Injection.

Clear, colourless solution.

4. CLINICAL PARTICULARS

4.1 Therapeutic indications
Gentamicin is an aminoglycoside antibiotic with broad-spectrum bactericidal activity. It is usually active against most strains of the following organisms: Escherichia coli, Klebsiella spp., Proteus spp. (indole positive and indole negative), Pseudomonas aeruginosa, Staphylococci, Enterobacter spp., Citrobacter spp and Providencia spp.

Gentamicin injection and gentamicin paediatric injection are indicated in urinary-tract infections, chest infections, bacteraemia, septicaemia, severe neonatal infections and other systemic infections due to sensitive organisms.

4.2 Posology and method of administration
ADULTS:

Serious infections: If renal function is not impaired, 5mg/kg/daily in divided doses at six or eight hourly intervals. The total daily dose may be subsequently increased or decreased as clinically indicated.

Systemic infections: If renal function is not impaired, 3-5mg/kg/day in divided doses according to severity of infection, adjusting according to clinical response and body weight.

Urinary tract infections: As "Systemic infections". Or, if renal function is not impaired, 160mg once daily may be used.

CHILDREN:

Premature infants or full term neonates up to 2 weeks or age: 3mg/kg 12 hourly.

2 weeks to 12 years: 2mg/kg 8 hourly.

THE ELDERLY:

There is some evidence that elderly patients may be more susceptible to aminoglycoside toxicity whether secondary to previous eighth nerve impairment or borderline renal dysfunction. Accordingly, therapy should be closely monitored by frequent determination of gentamicin serum levels, assessment of renal function and signs of ototoxicity.

RENAL IMPAIRMENT:

Gentamicin is excreted by simple glomerular filtration and therefore reduced dosage is necessary where renal function is impaired. Nomograms are available for the calculation of dose, which depends on the patient's age, weight and renal function. The following table may be useful when treating adults.

(see Table 1 below)

The recommended dose and precautions for intramuscular and intravenous administration are identical. Gentamicin when given intravenously should be injected directly into a vein or into the drip set tubing over no less than three minutes. If administered by infusion, this should be over no longer than 20 minutes and in no greater volume of fluid than 100ml.

4.3 Contraindications
Hypersensitivity; Myasthenia Gravis.

4.4 Special warnings and precautions for use
Ototoxicity has been recorded following the use of gentamicin. Groups at special risk include patients with impaired renal function, infants and possibly the elderly. Consequently, renal, auditory and vestibular functions should be monitored in these patients and serum levels determined so as to avoid peak concentrations above 10mg/l and troughs above 2mg/l. As there is some evidence that risk of both ototoxicity and nephrotoxicity is related to the level of total exposure, duration of therapy should be the shortest possible compatible with clinical recovery. In some patients with impaired renal function there has been a transient rise in blood-urea-nitrogen which has usually reverted to normal during or following cessation of therapy. It is important to adjust the frequency of dosage according to the degree of renal function.

Gentamicin should only be used in pregnancy if considered essential by the physician (see section 4.6 Pregnancy and Lactation.)

Gentamicin should be used with care in conditions characterised by muscular weakness.

In cases of significant obesity gentamicin serum concentrations should be closely monitored and a reduction in dose should be considered.

4.5 Interaction with other medicinal products and other forms of interaction
Concurrent administration of gentamicin and other potentially ototoxic or nephrotoxic drugs should be avoided. Potent diuretics such as etacrynic acid and furosemide are believed to enhance the risk of ototoxicity whilst amphotericin B, cisplatin and ciclosporin are potential enhancers of nephrotoxicity.

Any potential nephrotoxicity of cephalosporins, and in particular cephaloridine, may also be increased in the presence of gentamicin. Consequently, if this combination is used monitoring of kidney function is advised.

Neuromuscular blockade and respiratory paralysis have been reported from administration of aminoglycosides to patients who have received curare-type muscle relaxants during anaesthesia.

Indometacin possibly increases plasma concentrations of gentamicin in neonates.

Concurrent use with oral anticoagulants may increase the hypothrombinanaemic effect.

Concurrent use of bisphosphonates may increase the risk of hypocalcaemia.

Concurrent use of the Botulinum Toxin and gentamicin may increase the risk of toxicity due to enhanced neuromuscular block.

Antagonism of effect may occur with concomitant administration of gentamicin with either neostigmine or pyridostigmine.

4.6 Pregnancy and lactation
There are no proven cases of intrauterine damage caused by gentamicin. However, in common with most drugs known to cross the placenta, usage in pregnancy should only be considered in life threatening situations where expected benefits outweigh possible risks. In the absence of gastro-intestinal inflammation, the amount of gentamicin ingested from the milk is unlikely to result in significant blood levels in breast-fed infants.

4.7 Effects on ability to drive and use machines
Not known.

4.8 Undesirable effects
Side-effects include vestibular damage or hearing loss, particularly after exposure to ototoxic drugs or in the presence of renal dysfunction. Nephrotoxicity (usually reversible) and occasionally acute renal failure, hypersensitivity, anaemia, blood dycrasias, purpura, stomatitis, convulsions and effects on liver function occur occasionally.

Rarely hypomagnesia on prolonged therapy and antibiotic–associated colitis have been reported.

Nausea, vomiting and rash have also been reported.

Central neurotoxicity, including encephalopathy, confusion, lethargy, mental depression and hallucinations, has been reported in association with gentamicin therapy but this is extremely rare.

4.9 Overdose
Haemodialysis and peritoneal dialysis will aid the removal from blood but the former is probably more efficient. Calcium salts given intravenously have been used to counter the neuromuscular blockade caused by gentamicin.

5. PHARMACOLOGICAL PROPERTIES

5.1 Pharmacodynamic properties
Gentamicin is a mixture of antibiotic substances produced by the growth of micromonospora purpurea. It is bactericidal with greater antibacterial activity than streptomycin, neomycin or kanamycin.

Gentamicin exerts a number of effects on cells of susceptible bacteria. It affects the integrity of the plasma membrane and the metabolism of RNA, but its most important effects is inhibition of protein synthesis at the level of the 30s ribosomal subunit.

5.2 Pharmacokinetic properties
Gentamicin is not readily absorbed from the gastro-intestinal tract. Gentamicin is 70-85% bound to plasma albumin following administration and is excreted 90% unchanged in urine. The half-life for its elimination in normal patients is 2 to 3 hours.

Effective plasma concentration is 4-8 μg/ml.

The volume of distribution (vd) is 0.3 l/kg.

The elimination rate constant is:

0.02 hr^{-1} for anuric patients *

0.30 hr^{-1} normal

* Therefore in those with anuria care must be exercised following the usual initial dose, any subsequent administration being reduced in-line with plasma concentrations of gentamicin.

5.3 Preclinical safety data
Not applicable.

6. PHARMACEUTICAL PARTICULARS

6.1 List of excipients
Methyl parahydroxybenzoate (E218)

Propyl parahydroxybenzoate (E216)

Disodium Edetate

Water for Injections

2M Sodium Hydroxide

1M Sulphuric Acid

Table 1

Blood Urea (mg/100ml)	(mmol/l)	Creatinine clearance (GFR) (ml/min)	Dose & frequency of administration
< 40	6 - 7	> 70	80mg* 8 hourly
40 - 100	6 - 17	30 - 70	80mg* 12 hourly
100 - 200	17 - 34	10 - 30	80mg* daily
> 200	> 34	5 - 10	80mg* every 48 hours
Twice weekly intermittent haemodialysis		< 5	80mg* after dialysis

**60mg if body weight <60kg. Frequency of dosage in hours may also be approximated as serum creatinine (mg%) × eight or in si units, as serum creatinine (umol/l) divided by 11. If these dosage guides are used peak serum levels must be measured. Peak levels of gentamicin occur approximately one hour after intra muscular injection and intravenous injection. Trough levels are measured just prior to the next injection. Assay of peak serum levels gives confirmation of adequacy of dosage and also serves to detect levels above 10mg/l, at which the possibility of ototoxicity should be considered. One hour concentrations of gentamicin should not exceed 10mg/l (but should reach 4mg/l), while the pre dose trough concentration should be less than 2mg/l.*

6.2 Incompatibilities
In general, gentamicin injection should not be mixed. In particular the following are incompatible in mixed solution with gentamicin injection: penicillins, cephalosporins, erythromycin, heparins, sodium bicarbonate. * Dilution in the body will obviate the danger of physical and chemical incompatibility and enable gentamicin to be given concurrently with the drugs listed above either as a bolus injection into the drip tubing, with adequate flushing, or at separate sites. In the case of carbenicillin, administration should only be at a separate site.

* Carbon dioxide may be liberated on addition of the two solutions. Normally this will dissolve in the solution but under some circumstances small bubbles may form.

6.3 Shelf life
3 years

6.4 Special precautions for storage
Do not store above 25°C. Do not refrigerate or freeze.

6.5 Nature and contents of container
Cidomycin Adult Injectable is supplied in ampoules and vials.

6.6 Special precautions for disposal and other handling
Not applicable.

7. MARKETING AUTHORISATION HOLDER
Sanofi-aventis

One Onslow Street

Guildford

Surrey

UK

8. MARKETING AUTHORISATION NUMBER(S)
PL 0109/5065R

9. DATE OF FIRST AUTHORISATION/RENEWAL OF THE AUTHORISATION
24th January 1991

10. DATE OF REVISION OF THE TEXT
July 2007

Legal category:
POM

Cilest

(Janssen-Cilag Ltd)

1. NAME OF THE MEDICINAL PRODUCT
Cilest™

2. QUALITATIVE AND QUANTITATIVE COMPOSITION
Cilest are tablets for oral administration.

Each tablet contains norgestimate 0.25 mg and ethinylestradiol PhEur 0.035 mg.

3. PHARMACEUTICAL FORM
Tablets (small, round, dark blue, engraved 'C 250' on both faces).

4. CLINICAL PARTICULARS

4.1 Therapeutic indications
Contraception and the recognised indications for such oestrogen/progestogen combinations.

4.2 Posology and method of administration
For oral administration.

Adults

It is preferable that tablet intake from the first pack is started on the first day of menstruation in which case no extra contraceptive precautions are necessary.

If menstruation has already begun (that is 2, 3 or 4 days previously), tablet taking should commence on day 5 of the menstrual period. In this case additional contraceptive precautions must be taken for the first 7 days of tablet taking.

If menstruation began more than 5 days previously then the patient should be advised to wait until her next menstrual period before starting to take Cilest.

How to take Cilest:

One tablet is taken daily at the same time (preferably in the evening) without interruption for 21 days, followed by a break of 7 tablet-free days. Each subsequent pack is started after the 7 tablet-free days have elapsed. Additional contraceptive precautions are not then required.

Elderly:

Not applicable.

Children:

Not recommended.

4.3 Contraindications
Absolute contra-indications

- Pregnancy or suspected pregnancy (that cannot yet be excluded).

- Circulatory disorders (cardiovascular or cerebrovascular) such as thrombophlebitis and thrombo-embolic processes, or a history of these conditions (including history of confirmed venous thrombo-embolism (VTE), family history of idiopathic VTE and other known risk factors for VTE), moderate to severe hypertension, hyperlipoproteinaemia. In addition the presence of more than one of the risk factors for arterial disease.

- Severe liver disease, cholestatic jaundice or hepatitis (viral or non-viral) or a history of these conditions if the results of liver function tests have failed to return to normal, and for 3 months after liver function tests have been found to be normal; a history of jaundice of pregnancy or jaundice due to the use of steroids, Rotor syndrome and Dubin-Johnson syndrome, hepatic cell tumours and porphyria.

- Cholelithiasis

- Known or suspected oestrogen-dependent tumours; endometrial hyperplasia; undiagnosed vaginal bleeding.

- Systemic lupus erythematosus or a history of this condition.

- A history during pregnancy or previous use of steroids of:

- severe pruritus
- herpes gestationis
- a manifestation or deterioration of otosclerosis

Relative contra-indications:

If any relative contra-indications listed below are present, the benefits of oestrogen/progestogen-containing preparations must be weighed against the possible risk for each individual case and the patient kept under close supervision. In case of aggravation or appearance of any of these conditions whilst the patient is taking the pill, its use should be discontinued.

- Conditions implicating an increasing risk of developing venous thrombo-embolic complications, eg severe varicose veins or prolonged immobilisation or major surgery. Disorders of coagulation.

- Presence of any risk factor for arterial disease eg smoking, hyperlipidaemia or hypertension.

- Other conditions associated with an increased risk of circulatory disease such as latent or overt cardiac failure, renal dysfunction, or a history of these conditions.

- Epilepsy or a history of this condition.

- Migraine or a history of this condition.

- A history of cholelithiasis.

- Presence of any risk factor for oestrogen-dependent tumours; oestrogen-sensitive gynaecological disorders such as uterine fibromyomata and endometriosis.

- Diabetes mellitus.

- Severe depression or a history of this condition. If this is accompanied by a disturbance in tryptophan metabolism, administration of vitamin B6 might be of therapeutic value.

- Sickle cell haemoglobinopathy, since under certain circumstances, eg during infections or anoxia, oestrogen-containing preparations may induce thrombo-embolic process in patients with this condition.

- If the results of liver function tests become abnormal, use should be discontinued.

4.4 Special warnings and precautions for use
Post-partum administration

Following a vaginal delivery, oral contraceptive administration to non-breast-feeding mothers can be started 21 days post-partum provided the patient is fully ambulant and there are no puerperal complications. No additional contraceptive precautions are required. If post-partum administration begins more than 21 days after delivery, additional contraceptive precautions are required for the first 7 days of pill-taking.

If intercourse has taken place post-partum, oral contraceptive use should be delayed until the first day of the first menstrual period.

After miscarriage or abortion administration should start immediately in which case no additional contraceptive precautions are required.

Changing from a 21 day pill or another 22 day pill to Cilest:

All tablets in the old pack should be finished. The first Cilest tablet is taken the next day, ie no gap is left between taking tablets nor does the patient need to wait for her period to begin. Tablets should be taken as instructed in 'How to take Cilest' (see 4.2). Additional contraceptive precautions are not required. The patient will not have a period until the end of the first Cilest pack, but this is not harmful, nor does it matter if she experiences some bleeding on tablet-taking days.

Changing from a combined every day pill (28 day tablets) to Cilest:

Cilest should be started after taking the last active tablet from the 'Every day Pill' pack (ie after taking 21 or 22 tablets). The first Cilest tablet is taken the next day ie no gap is left between taking tablets nor does the patient need to wait for her period to begin. Tablets should be taken as instructed in 'How to take Cilest' (see 4.2). Additional contraceptive precautions are not required. Remaining tablets from the every day (ED) pack should be discarded.

The patient will not have a period until the end of the first Cilest pack, but this is not harmful, nor does it matter if she experiences some bleeding on tablet-taking days.

Changing from a progestogen-only pill (POP or mini pill) to Cilest:

The first Cilest tablet should be taken on the first day of the period, even if the patient has already taken a mini pill on that day. Tablets should be taken as instructed in 'How to take Cilest' (see 4.2). Additional contraceptive precautions are not required. All the remaining progestogen-only pills in the mini pill pack should be discarded.

If the patient is taking a mini pill, then she may not always have a period, especially when she is breast feeding. The first Cilest tablet should be taken on the day after stopping the mini pill. All remaining pills in the mini pill packet must be discarded. Additional contraceptive precautions must be taken for the first 7 days.

To skip a period

To skip a period, a new pack of Cilest should be started on the day after finishing the current pack (the patient skips the tablet-free days). Tablet-taking should be continued in the usual way.

During the use of the second pack she may experience slight spotting or break-through bleeding but contraceptive protection will not be diminished provided there are no tablet omissions.

The next pack of Cilest is started after the usual 7 tablet-free days, regardless of whether the period has completely finished or not.

Reduced reliability

When Cilest is taken according to the directions for use the occurrence of pregnancy is highly unlikely. However, the reliability of oral contraceptives may be reduced under the following circumstances:

(i) Forgotten tablets

If the patient forgets to take a tablet, she should take it as soon as she remembers and take the next one at the normal time. This may mean that two tablets are taken in one day. Provided she is less than 12 hours late in taking her tablet, Cilest will still give contraceptive protection during this cycle and the rest of the pack should be taken as usual.

If she is more than 12 hours late in taking one or more tablets then she should take the last missed pill as soon as she remembers but leave the other missed pills in the pack. She should continue to take the rest of the pack as usual but must use extra precautions (eg sheath, diaphragm, plus spermicide) and follow the '7-day rule' (see Further Information for the 7-day rule).

If there are 7 or more pills left in the pack after the missed and delayed pills then the usual 7-day break can be left before starting the next pack. If there are less than 7 pills left in the pack after the missed and delayed pills then when the pack is finished the next pack should be started the next day. If withdrawal bleeding does not occur at the end of the second pack then a pregnancy test should be performed.

(ii) Vomiting or diarrhoea

If after tablet intake vomiting or diarrhoea occurs, a tablet may not be absorbed properly by the body. If the symptoms disappear within 12 hours of tablet-taking, the patient should take an extra tablet from a spare pack and continue with the rest of the pack as usual.

However, if the symptoms continue beyond those 12 hours, additional contraceptive precautions are necessary for any sexual intercourse during the stomach or bowel upset and for the following 7 days (the patient must be advised to follow the '7-day rule').

(iii) Change in bleeding pattern

If after taking Cilest for several months there is a sudden occurrence of spotting or breakthrough bleeding (not observed in previous cycles) or the absence of withdrawal bleeding, contraceptive effectiveness may be reduced. If withdrawal bleeding fails to occur and none of the above mentioned events has taken place, pregnancy is highly unlikely and oral contraceptive use can be continued until the end of the next pack. (If withdrawal bleeding fails to occur at the end of the second cycle, tablet intake should be discontinued and pregnancy excluded before oral contraceptive use can be resumed.) However, if withdrawal bleeding is absent and any of the above mentioned events has occurred, tablet intake should be discontinued and pregnancy excluded before oral contraceptive use can be resumed.

Medical examination/consultation

Assessment of women prior to starting oral contraceptives (and at regular intervals thereafter) should include a personal and family medical history of each woman. Physical examination should be guided by this and by the contra-indications (Section 4.3) and warnings (Section 4.4) for this product. The frequency and nature of these assessments should be based upon relevant guidelines and should be adapted to the individual woman, but should include measurement of blood pressure and, if judged appropriate by the clinician, breast, abdominal and pelvic examination including cervical cytology.

Caution should be observed when prescribing oral contraceptives to young women whose cycles are not yet stabilised.

Venous thrombo-embolic disease

The use of any combined oral contraceptives (COCs) carries an increased risk for venous thrombo-embolism (VTE), including deep venous thrombosis and pulmonary embolism, compared with no use. The excess risk of VTE is highest during the first year a woman ever uses a combined oral contraceptive. This increased risk is less than the risk of VTE associated with pregnancy, which is estimated as 60 per 100,000 pregnancies. VTE is fatal in 1-2% of cases.

It is not known how Cilest influences the risk of VTE compared with other combined oral contraceptives.

However, epidemiological studies have shown that the incidence of VTE in users of oral contraceptives with low estrogen content (<50 µg ethinyl estradiol) ranges from about 20-40 cases per 100,000 women years, but this risk estimate varies according to the progestogen. This compares with 5-10 cases per 100,000 women years for non-users.

Epidemiological studies have also associated the use of combined oral contraceptives with an increased risk for arterial thrombo-embolism (eg myocardial infarction, transient ischaemic attack).

Surgery, varicose veins or immobilisation

In patients using oestrogen-containing preparations the risk of deep vein thrombosis may be temporarily increased when undergoing a major operation (eg abdominal, orthopaedic), and surgery to the legs, medical treatment for varicose veins or prolonged immobilisation. Therefore, it is advisable to discontinue oral contraceptive use at least 4 to 6 weeks prior to these procedures if performed electively and to (re)start not less than 2 weeks after full ambulation. The latter is also valid with regard to immobilisation after an accident or emergency surgery. In case of emergency surgery, thrombotic prophylaxis is usually indicated eg with subcutaneous heparin.

Chloasma

Chloasma may occasionally occur, especially in women with a history of chloasma gravidarum. Women with a tendency to chloasma should avoid exposure to the sun or ultraviolet radiation whilst taking this preparation. Chloasma is often not fully reversible.

Laboratory tests

The use of steroids may influence the results of certain laboratory tests. In the literature, at least a hundred different parameters have been reported to possibly be influenced by oral contraceptive use, predominantly by the oestrogenic component. Among these are: biochemical parameters of the liver, thyroid, adrenal and renal function, plasma levels of (carrier) proteins and lipid/lipoprotein fractions and parameters of coagulation and fibrinolysis.

Further information

Additional contraceptive precautions

When additional contraceptive precautions are required, the patient should be advised either not to have sex, or to use a cap plus spermicide or for her partner to use a condom. Rhythm methods should not be advised as the pill disrupts the usual cyclical changes associated with the natural menstrual cycle, eg changes in temperature and cervical mucus.

The 7-day rule

If any one tablet is forgotten for more than 12 hours.

If the patient has vomiting or diarrhoea for more than 12 hours.

If the patient is taking any of the drugs listed under 'Interactions':

The patient should continue to take her tablets as usual and:

– Additional contraceptive precautions must be taken for the next 7 days.

But - if these 7 days run beyond the end of the current pack, the next pack must be started as soon as the current one is finished, ie no gap should be left between packs. (This prevents an extended break in tablet taking which may increase the risk of the ovaries releasing an egg and thus reducing contraceptive protection). The patient will not have a period until the end of 2 packs but this is not harmful nor does it matter if she experiences some bleeding on tablet taking days.

4.5 Interaction with other medicinal products and other forms of interaction

Irregular cycles and reduced reliability of oral contraceptives may occur when these preparations are used concomitantly with drugs such as anticonvulsants, barbiturates, antibiotics, (eg tetracyclines, ampicillin, rifampicin, etc), griseofulvin, activated charcoal and certain laxatives. Special consideration should be given to patients being treated with antibiotics for acne. They should be advised to use a non-hormonal method of contraception, or to use an oral contraceptive containing a progestogen showing minimal androgenicity, which have been reported as helping to improve acne without using an antibiotic. Oral contraceptives may diminish glucose tolerance and increase the need for insulin or other antidiabetic drugs in diabetics.

The herbal remedy St John's Wort *(Hypericum perforatum)* should not be taken concomitantly with this medicine as this could potentially lead to a loss of contraceptive effect.

4.6 Pregnancy and lactation

Cilest is contra-indicated for use during pregnancy or suspected pregnancy, since it has been suggested that combined oral contraceptives, in common with many other substances, might be capable of affecting the normal development of the child in the early stages of pregnancy. It can be definitely concluded, however, that, if a risk of abnormality exists at all, it must be very small.

Figure 1

Estimated cumulative numbers of breast cancers per 10,000 women diagnosed in 5 years of use and up to 10 years after stopping COCs, compared with numbers of breast cancers diagnosed in 10,000 women who had never used COCs

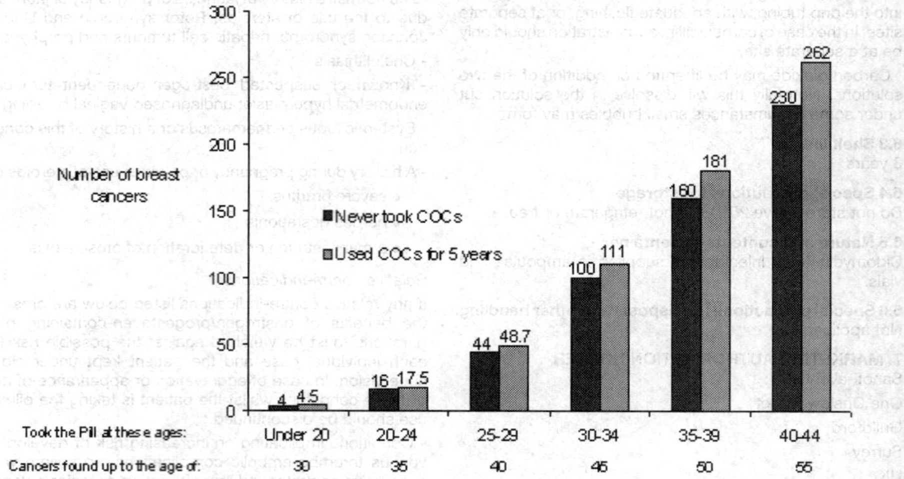

Mothers who are breast-feeding should be advised not to use the combined pill since this may reduce the amount of breast-milk, but may be advised instead to use a progestogen-only pill (POP).

4.7 Effects on ability to drive and use machines

Not applicable.

4.8 Undesirable effects

Various adverse reactions have been associated with oral contraceptive use. The first appearance of symptoms indicative of any one of these reactions necessitates immediate cessation of oral contraceptive use while appropriate diagnostic and therapeutic measures are undertaken.

Serious Adverse Reactions

There is a general opinion, based on statistical evidence, that users of combined oral contraceptives experience more often than non-users various disorders of the coagulation. How often these disorders occur in users of modern low-oestrogen oral contraceptives is unknown, but there are reasons for suggesting that they may occur less often than with the older types of pill which contain more oestrogen.

Various reports have associated oral contraceptive use with the occurrence of deep venous thrombosis, pulmonary embolism and other embolisms. Other investigations of these oral contraceptives have suggested an increased risk of oestrogen and/or progestogen dose-dependent coronary and cerebrovascular accidents, predominantly in heavy smokers. Thrombosis has very rarely been reported to occur in other veins or arteries, eg hepatic, mesenteric, renal or retinal.

It should be noted that there is no consensus about often contradictory findings obtained in early studies. The physician should bear in mind the possibility of vascular accidents occurring and that there may not be full recovery from such disorders and they may be fatal. The physician should take into account the presence of risk factors for arterial disease and deep venous thrombosis when prescribing oral contraceptives. Risk factors for arterial disease include smoking, the presence of hyperlipidaemia, hypertension or diabetes.

Signs and symptoms of a thrombotic event may include: sudden severe pain in the chest, whether or not reaching to the left arm; sudden breathlessness; and unusual severe, prolonged headache, especially if it occurs for the first time or gets progressively worse, or is associated with any of the following symptoms: sudden partial or complete loss of vision or diplopia, aphasia, vertigo, a bad fainting attack or collapse with or without focal epilepsy, weakness or very marked numbness suddenly affecting one side or one part of the body, motor disturbances; severe pain in the calf of one leg; acute abdomen.

Cigarette smoking increases the risk of serious cardiovascular adverse reactions to oral contraceptive use. The risk increases with age and with heavy smoking and is more marked in women over 35 years of age. Women who use oral contraceptives should be strongly advised not to smoke.

The use of oestrogen-containing oral contraceptives may promote growth of existing sex steroid dependent tumours. For this reason, the use of these oral contraceptives in patients with such tumours is contra-indicated. Numerous epidemiological studies have been reported on the risk of ovarian, endometrial, cervical and breast cancer in women using combined oral contraceptives. The evidence is clear that combined oral contraceptives offer substantial protection against both ovarian and endometrial cancer. An increased risk of cervical cancer in long term users of combined oral contraceptives has been reported in some studies, but there continues to be controversy about the extent to which this is attributable to the confounding effects of sexual behaviour and other factors.

A meta-analysis from 54 epidemiological studies reported that there is a slightly increased relative risk (RR = 1.24) of having breast cancer diagnosed in women who are currently using combined oral contraceptives (COCs). The observed pattern of increased risk may be due to an earlier diagnosis of breast cancer in COC users, the biological effects of COCs or a combination of both. The additional breast cancers diagnosed in current users of COCs or in women who have used COCs in the last 10 years are more likely to be localised to the breast than those in women who never used COCs.

Breast cancer is rare among women under 40 years of age whether or not they take COCs. Whilst this background risk increases with age, the excess number of breast cancer diagnoses in current and recent COC users is small in relation to the overall risk of breast cancer (see bar chart).

The most important risk factor for breast cancer in COC users is the age women discontinue the COC; the older the age at stopping, the more breast cancers are diagnosed. Duration of use is less important and the excess risk gradually disappears during the course of the 10 years after stopping COC use such that by 10 years there appears to be no excess.

The possible increase in risk of breast cancer should be discussed with the user and weighed against the benefits of COCs taking into account the evidence that they offer substantial protection against the risk of developing certain other cancers (e.g. ovarian and endometrial cancer).

(see Figure 1 above)

Malignant hepatic tumours have been reported on rare occasions in long-term users of oral contraceptives. Benign hepatic tumours have also been associated with oral contraceptive usage. A hepatic tumour should be considered in the differential diagnosis when upper abdominal pain, enlarged liver or signs of intra-abdominal haemorrhage occur.

The use of oral contraceptives may sometimes lead to the development of cholestatic jaundice or cholelithiasis.

On rare occasions the use of oral contraceptives may trigger or reactivate systemic lupus erythematosus.

A further rare complication of oral contraceptive use is the occurrence of chorea which can be reversed by discontinuing the pill. The majority of cases of oral contraceptive-induced chorea shows a pre-existing predisposition which often relates to acute rheumatism.

Other Adverse Reactions

Cardiovascular System

Rise of blood pressure. If hypertension develops, treatment should be discontinued.

Genital Tract

Intermenstrual bleeding, post-medication amenorrhoea, changes in cervical secretion, increase in size of uterine fibromyomata, aggravation of endometriosis, certain vaginal infections, eg candidiasis.

Breast

Tenderness, pain, enlargement, secretion.

Gastro-intestinal Tract

Nausea, vomiting, cholelithiasis, cholestatic jaundice.

Skin
Erythema nodosum, rash, chloasma, erythema multiforme.
Eyes
Discomfort of the cornea if contact lenses are used.
CNS
Headache, migraine, mood changes, depression.
Metabolic
Fluid retention, change in body weight, reduced glucose tolerance.
Other
Changes in libido.

4.9 Overdose
There have been no reports of serious ill-health from overdosage even when a considerable number of tablets has been taken by a small child. In general, it is therefore unnecessary to treat overdosage. However, if overdosage is discovered within two or three hours and is large, then gastric lavage can be safely used. There are no antidotes and further treatment should be symptomatic.

5. PHARMACOLOGICAL PROPERTIES
5.1 Pharmacodynamic properties
Cilest acts through the mechanism of gonadotrophin suppression by the oestrogenic and progestational actions of ethinylestradiol and norgestimate. The primary mechanism of action is inhibition of ovulation, but alterations to the cervical mucus and to the endometrium may also contribute to the efficacy of the product.

5.2 Pharmacokinetic properties
Norgestimate and ethinylestradiol are absorbed from the gastro-intestinal tract and metabolised in the liver. To obtain maximal contraceptive effectiveness the tablets should be taken as directed and at approximately the same time each day. Because the active ingredients are metabolised in the liver, reduced contraceptive efficacy has been associated with concomitant use of oral contraceptives and rifampicin. A similar association has been suggested with oral contraceptives and barbiturates, phenytoin sodium, phenylbutazone, griseofulvin and ampicillin.

5.3 Preclinical safety data
The toxicology of norgestimate and ethinylestradiol has been extensively investigated in animal studies and through long term clinical experience with widespread use in contraceptives.

6. PHARMACEUTICAL PARTICULARS
6.1 List of excipients
Lactose (anhydrous)
Magnesium Stearate
Pregelatinised Starch
F.D. & C. Blue No. 2 Lake
Methanol (does not appear in final product)

6.2 Incompatibilities
Not applicable.

6.3 Shelf life
Three years.

6.4 Special precautions for storage
Store at room temperature (below 25°C). Protect from light.

6.5 Nature and contents of container
Cartons containing 1 (Starter Pack), 3 and 6 PVC/foil blister strips of 21 tablets each.

6.6 Special precautions for disposal and other handling
Not applicable.

7. MARKETING AUTHORISATION HOLDER
Janssen-Cilag Limited
50-100 Holmers Farm Way
High Wycombe
Buckinghamshire
HP12 4EG
UK

8. MARKETING AUTHORISATION NUMBER(S)
PL 00242/0209

9. DATE OF FIRST AUTHORISATION/RENEWAL OF THE AUTHORISATION
1 July 1995 / 7 January 2009

10. DATE OF REVISION OF THE TEXT
11 February 2009
Legal category POM

Cimzia 200 mg solution for injection

(UCB Pharma Limited)

1. NAME OF THE MEDICINAL PRODUCT
▼ Cimzia 200 mg solution for injection

2. QUALITATIVE AND QUANTITATIVE COMPOSITION
Each pre-filled syringe contains 200 mg certolizumab pegol in one ml.

Certolizumab pegol is a recombinant, humanised antibody Fab' fragment against tumour necrosis factor alpha (TNFα) expressed in *Escherichia coli* and conjugated to polyethylene glycol (PEG).

For a full list of excipients, see section 6.1.

3. PHARMACEUTICAL FORM
Solution for injection in pre-filled syringe.

Clear to opalescent, colourless to yellow solution. The pH of the solution is approximately 4.7.

4. CLINICAL PARTICULARS
4.1 Therapeutic indications
Cimzia, in combination with methotrexate (MTX), is indicated for the treatment of moderate to severe, active rheumatoid arthritis (RA) in adult patients when the response to disease-modifying antirheumatic drugs (DMARDs) including methotrexate, has been inadequate.

Cimzia can be given as monotherapy in case of intolerance to methotrexate or when continued treatment with methotrexate is inappropriate.

Cimzia has been shown to reduce the rate of progression of joint damage as measured by X-ray and to improve physical function, when given in combination with methotrexate.

4.2 Posology and method of administration
Treatment should be initiated and supervised by specialist physicians experienced in the diagnosis and treatment of rheumatoid arthritis. Patients should be given the special alert card.

Posology
The recommended starting dose of Cimzia for adult patients with rheumatoid arthritis is 400 mg (as 2 injections of 200 mg each on one day) at weeks 0, 2 and 4, followed by a maintenance dose of 200 mg every 2 weeks. MTX should be continued during treatment with Cimzia where appropriate.

Available data suggest that clinical response is usually achieved within 12 weeks of treatment. Continued therapy should be carefully reconsidered in patients who show no evidence of therapeutic benefit within the first 12 weeks of treatment.

Missed dose
Patients who miss a dose should be advised to inject the next dose of Cimzia as soon as they remember and then continue injecting subsequent doses every 2 weeks as originally instructed.

Paediatric population (< 18 years old)
Cimzia is not recommended for use in children and adolescents below age 18 due to a lack of data on efficacy and safety.

Elderly (≥65 years old)
No dose adjustment is required. Population pharmacokinetic analyses showed no effect of age (see section 5.2).

Renal and hepatic impairment
Cimzia has not been studied in these patient populations. No dose recommendations can be made (see section 5.2).

Method of administration
The total content (1 ml) of the pre-filled syringe should be administered as a subcutaneous injection only. Suitable sites for injection would include the thigh or abdomen.

After proper training in injection technique, patients may self-inject if their physician determines that it is appropriate and with medical follow-up as necessary.

4.3 Contraindications
Hypersensitivity to the active substance or to any of the excipients.

Active tuberculosis or other severe infections such as sepsis or opportunistic infections (see section 4.4).

Moderate to severe heart failure (NYHA classes III/IV) (see section 4.4).

4.4 Special warnings and precautions for use
Infections
Patients must be monitored closely for signs and symptoms of infections including tuberculosis before, during and after treatment with Cimzia. Because the elimination of Cimzia may take up to 5 months, monitoring should be continued throughout this period (see section 4.3).

Treatment with Cimzia must not be initiated in patients with a clinically important active infection, including chronic or localised infections, until the infection is controlled (see section 4.3).

Patients who develop a new infection while undergoing treatment with Cimzia should be monitored closely. Administration of Cimzia should be discontinued if a patient develops a new serious infection until the infection is controlled. Physicians should exercise caution when considering the use of Cimzia in patients with a history of recurring infection or with underlying conditions which may predispose patients to infections, including the use of concomitant immunosuppressive medications.

Patients with rheumatoid arthritis may not manifest typical symptoms of infection, including fever, due to their disease and concomitant medicinal products. Therefore, early detection of any infection, particularly atypical clinical presentations of a serious infection, is critical to minimise delays in diagnosis and initiation of treatment.

Serious infections, including sepsis and tuberculosis (including miliary, disseminated and extrapulmonary disease), and opportunistic infections (e.g. histoplasmosis, nocardia, candidiasis) have been reported in patients receiving Cimzia. Some of these events have been fatal.

Tuberculosis
Before initiation of therapy with Cimzia, all patients must be evaluated for both active or inactive (latent) tuberculosis infection. This evaluation should include a detailed medical history for patients with a personal history of tuberculosis, with possible previous exposure to others with active tuberculosis, and with previous and/or current use of immunosuppressive therapy. Appropriate screening tests, e.g. tuberculin skin test and chest X -ray, should be performed in all patients (local recommendations may apply). It is recommended that the conduct of these tests should be recorded in the patient's alert card. Prescribers are reminded of the risk of false negative tuberculin skin test results, especially in patients who are severely ill or immunocompromised.

If active tuberculosis is diagnosed prior to or during treatment, Cimzia therapy must not be initiated and must be discontinued (see section 4.3).

If inactive ('latent') tuberculosis is suspected, a physician with expertise in the treatment of tuberculosis should be consulted. In all situations described below, the benefit/risk balance of Cimzia therapy should be very carefully considered.

If latent tuberculosis is diagnosed, appropriate anti-tuberculosis therapy must be started before initiating treatment with Cimzia and in accordance with local recommendations.

Use of anti-tuberculosis therapy should also be considered before the initiation of Cimzia in patients with a past history of latent or active tuberculosis in whom an adequate course of treatment cannot be confirmed, and in patients who have significant risk factors for tuberculosis despite a negative test for latent tuberculosis. Biological tests for tuberculosis screening should be considered before starting Cimzia treatment if there is any potential latent tuberculosis infection, regardless of BCG vaccination.

Patients should be instructed to seek medical advice if signs/symptoms (e.g. persistent cough, wasting/weight loss, low grade fever, listlessness) suggestive of a tuberculosis infection occur during or after therapy with Cimzia.

Hepatitis B Virus (HBV) reactivation
Reactivation of HBV has occurred in patients who are chronic carriers of this virus receiving TNF antagonists. Some cases have had a fatal outcome. As HBV infection has also been reported with Cimzia, patients at risk for HBV infection should be evaluated for prior evidence of HBV infection before initiating Cimzia therapy. Adequate data on treating patients who are carriers of HBV with TNF antagonist therapy, in conjunction with anti-viral therapy, to prevent HBV reactivation are not available. Carriers of HBV who require treatment with TNF antagonists should be closely monitored for clinical and laboratory signs of active HBV infection throughout therapy and for 5 months following termination of therapy, especially if the patient is on concomitant corticosteroid therapy.

In patients who develop HBV reactivation, Cimzia should be discontinued and effective anti-viral therapy with appropriate supportive treatment should be initiated. The safety of resuming TNF antagonist therapy after HBV reactivation is controlled is not known. Therefore, prescribers should exercise caution when considering resumption of Cimzia therapy in this situation and monitor patients closely.

Malignancies and lymphoproliferative disorders
The potential role of TNF antagonist therapy in the development of malignancies is not known. Caution should be exercised when considering TNF antagonist therapy for patients with a history of malignancy or when considering continuing treatment in patients who develop malignancy.

With the current knowledge, a possible risk for the development of lymphomas or other malignancies in patients treated with a TNF antagonist cannot be excluded.

In clinical trials with Cimzia and other TNF antagonists, more cases of lymphoma and other malignancies have been reported among patients receiving TNF antagonists than in control patients receiving placebo (see section 4.8).

Furthermore, there is an increased background lymphoma risk in rheumatoid arthritis patients with long-standing, highly active, inflammatory disease, which complicates the risk estimation. No trials have been conducted that include patients with a history of malignancy, or that continue treatment in patients who develop malignancy, while receiving Cimzia.

Chronic obstructive pulmonary disease (COPD)
In an exploratory clinical trial evaluating the use of another TNF antagonist, infliximab, in patients with moderate to severe chronic obstructive pulmonary disease (COPD), more malignancies, mostly in the lung or head and neck, were reported in infliximab-treated patients compared with control patients. All patients had a history of heavy smoking. Therefore, caution should be exercised when using any TNF antagonist in COPD patients, as well as in patients with increased risk for malignancy due to heavy smoking.

Congestive heart failure

Cimzia is contraindicated in moderate or severe heart failure (see section 4.3). In a clinical trial with another TNF antagonist, worsening congestive heart failure and increased mortality due to congestive heart failure have been observed. Cases of congestive heart failure have also been reported in rheumatoid arthritis patients receiving Cimzia. Cimzia should be used with caution in patients with mild heart failure (NYHA class I/II). Treatment with Cimzia must be discontinued in patients who develop new or worsening symptoms of congestive heart failure.

Haematological reactions

Reports of pancytopaenia, including aplastic anaemia, have been rare with TNF antagonists. Adverse reactions of the haematologic system, including medically significant cytopaenia (e.g. leukopaenia, pancytopaenia, thrombocytopaenia) have been reported with Cimzia (see section 4.8). All patients should be advised to seek immediate medical attention if they develop signs and symptoms suggestive of blood dyscrasias or infection (e.g., persistent fever, bruising, bleeding, pallor) while on Cimzia. Discontinuation of Cimzia therapy should be considered in patients with confirmed significant haematological abnormalities.

Neurological events

Use of TNF antagonists has been associated with rare cases of new onset or exacerbation of clinical symptoms and/or radiographic evidence of demyelinating disease, including multiple sclerosis. In patients with pre-existing or recent onset of demyelinating disorders, the benefits and risks of TNF antagonist treatment should be carefully considered before initiation of Cimzia therapy. Rare cases of neurological disorders, including seizure disorder, neuritis and peripheral neuropathy, have been reported in patients treated with Cimzia.

Hypersensitivity

Severe hypersensitivity reactions have been reported rarely following Cimzia administration in trials. If severe reactions occur, administration of Cimzia should be discontinued immediately and appropriate therapy instituted.

There are limited data on the use of Cimzia in patients who have experienced a severe hypersensitivity reaction towards another TNF antagonist; in these patients caution is needed.

Immunosuppression

Since tumour necrosis factor (TNF) mediates inflammation and modulates cellular immune responses, the possibility exists for TNF antagonists, including Cimzia, to cause immunosupression, affecting host defences against infections and malignancies.

Autoimmunity

Treatment with Cimzia may result in the formation of antinuclear antibodies (ANA) and, uncommonly, in the development of a lupus-like syndrome (see section 4.8). The impact of long-term treatment with Cimzia on the development of autoimmune diseases is unknown. If a patient develops symptoms suggestive of a lupus-like syndrome following treatment with Cimzia, treatment must be discontinued. Cimzia has not been studied specifically in a lupus population (see section 4.8).

Vaccinations

No data are available on the response to vaccinations or the transmission of infection by live vaccines in patients receiving Cimzia. Live vaccines or attenuated vaccines should not be administered concurrently with Cimzia.

Concomitant use with other biologics

Severe infections and neutropaenia were reported in clinical trials with concurrent use of anakinra (an interleukin-1 antagonist) or abatacept (a CD28 modulator) and another TNF antagonist, etanercept, with no added benefit compared to TNF antagonist therapy alone. Because of the nature of the adverse events seen with the combination of another TNF antagonist with either abatacept or anakinra therapy, similar toxicities may also result from the combination of anakinra or abatacept and other TNF antagonists. Therefore the use of Cimzia in combination with anakinra or abatacept is not recommended (see section 4.5).

Surgery

There is limited safety experience with surgical procedures in patients treated with Cimzia. The 14-day half-life of certolizumab pegol should be taken into consideration if a surgical procedure is planned. A patient who requires surgery while on Cimzia should be closely monitored for infections, and appropriate actions should be taken.

Activated partial thromboplastin time (aPTT) assay

Interference with certain coagulation assays has been detected in patients treated with Cimzia. Cimzia may cause erroneously elevated aPTT assay results in patients without coagulation abnormalities. This effect has been observed with the PTT-Lupus Anticoagulant (LA) test and Standard Target Activated Partial Thromboplastin time (STA-PTT) Automate tests from Diagnostica Stago, and the HemosIL APTT-SP liquid and HemosIL lyophilised silica tests from Instrumentation Laboratories. Other aPTT assays may be affected as well. There is no evidence that Cimzia therapy has an effect on coagulation *in vivo*. After patients receive Cimzia, careful attention should be given to interpretation of abnormal coagulation results. Interference with thrombin time (TT) and prothrombin time (PT) assays have not been observed.

Elderly

In the clinical trials, there was an apparently higher incidence of infections among subjects ≥65 years of age, compared to younger subjects, although experience is limited. Caution should be exercised when treating the elderly, and particular attention paid with respect to occurrence of infections.

4.5 Interaction with other medicinal products and other forms of interaction

Concomitant treatment with methotrexate, corticosteroids, nonsteroidal anti-inflammatory drugs (NSAIDs) and analgesics showed no effect on the pharmacokinetics of certolizumab pegol based on a population pharmacokinetics analysis.

The combination of Cimzia and anakinra or abatacept is not recommended (see section 4.4).

Co-administration of Cimzia with methotrexate had no significant effect on the pharmacokinetics of methotrexate. In study-to-study comparison, the pharmacokinetics of certolizumab pegol appeared similar to those observed previously in healthy subjects.

4.6 Pregnancy and lactation

Pregnancy

There are no adequate data from the use of Cimzia in pregnant women.

Animal studies using a rodent anti-rat TNFα did not reveal evidence of impaired fertility or harm to the foetus. However, these are insufficient with respect to human reproductive toxicity (see section 5.3). Due to its inhibition of TNFα, Cimzia administered during pregnancy could affect normal immune response in the newborn. Therefore, Cimzia should not be used in pregnancy.

Women of childbearing potential should use adequate contraception to prevent pregnancy and continue its use for at least 5 months after the last Cimzia administration.

Lactation

There is insufficient information on the excretion of certolizumab pegol in human or animal breast milk. Since immunoglobulins are excreted into human breast milk, a risk to the breast-feeding child cannot be excluded. A decision on whether to continue/discontinue breast-feeding or to continue/discontinue therapy with Cimzia should be made taking into account the benefit of breast-feeding to the child and the benefit of Cimzia therapy to the woman.

Fertility

Effects on sperm motility measures and a trend of reduced sperm count in male rodents have been observed with no apparent effect on fertility (see section 5.3). The clinical relevance of this finding is unknown.

4.7 Effects on ability to drive and use machines

Cimzia may have a minor influence on the ability to drive and use machines. Dizziness (including vertigo, vision disorder and fatigue) may occur following administration of Cimzia (see section 4.8)

4.8 Undesirable effects

Cimzia was studied in 2,367 patients with rheumatoid arthritis in controlled and open label trials for up to 57 months. The data in Table 1 is based on the pivotal controlled Studies involving 1,774 patients receiving Cimzia and 647 patients receiving placebo during the controlled period.

In the placebo-controlled studies, patients receiving Cimzia had an approximately 4 times greater duration of exposure compared with the placebo group. This difference in exposure is primarily due to patients on placebo being more likely to withdraw early. In addition, Studies RA-I and RA-II had a mandatory withdrawal for non-responders at Week 16, the majority of whom were on placebo.

The proportion of patients who discontinued treatment due to adverse events during the controlled trials was 5% for patients treated with Cimzia and 2.5% for patients treated with placebo.

The most common adverse reactions belonged to the system organ classes Infections and infestations, reported in 15.5% of patients on Cimzia and 7.6% of patients on placebo, and General disorders and administration site conditions, reported in 10.0% of patients on Cimzia and 9.7% of patients on placebo.

Adverse reactions reported in rheumatoid arthritis clinical trials and at least possibly related to Cimzia are listed in Table 1 below, according to frequency and system organ class. Frequency categories are defined as follows: Very common (≥ 1/10); Common (≥ 1/100 to < 1/10); Uncommon (≥ 1/1000 to < 1/100); Rare (≥ 1/10,000 to < 1/1000); Very rare (< 1/10,000), not known (cannot be estimated from the available data). Within each frequency grouping, undesirable effects are presented in order of decreasing seriousness.

Table: 1. Adverse drug reactions in clinical trials

(see Table 1 on next page)

The additional following ADRs have been observed uncommonly with Cimzia in other indications: gastrointestinal stenosis and obstructions, general physical health deterioration, grand mal convulsion, optic neuritis, abortion spontaneous and azoospermia.

Infections

The incidence of new cases of infections in placebo-controlled clinical trials in rheumatoid arthritis was 0.91 per patient-year for all Cimzia-treated patients and 0.72 per patient-year for placebo-treated patients. The infections consisted primarily of upper respiratory tract infections, herpes infections, urinary tract infections, and lower respiratory tract infections (see sections 4.3 and 4.4).

In the placebo-controlled clinical trials, there were more new cases of serious infection in the Cimzia treatment groups (0.06 per patient-year; all doses), compared with placebo (0.02 per patient-year). Serious infections included tuberculosis and invasive opportunistic infections (e.g. pneumocystosis, fungal oesophagitis, nocardiosis and herpes zoster disseminated). There is no evidence of an increased risk of infections with continued exposure over time (see section 4.4).

Malignancies and lymphoproliferative disorders

Excluding non-melanoma of the skin, 30 malignancies including 3 cases of lymphoma were observed in the Cimzia RA clinical trials in which a total of 2,367 patients were treated, representing 4,136 patient-years. Cases of lymphoma occurred at an incidence rate of 0.07 per 100 patient-years and melanoma at an incidence rate of 0.02 per 100 patient-years with Cimzia in rheumatoid arthritis clinical trials. (see section 4.4).

Autoimmunity

For subjects who were ANA negative at baseline, 16.7% of those treated with Cimzia developed positive ANA titers, compared with 12.0% of subjects in the placebo group. For subjects who were anti-dsDNA antibody negative at baseline, 2.2% of those treated with Cimzia developed positive anti-dsDNA antibody titers, compared with 1.0% of subjects in the placebo group. In both placebo-controlled and open-label follow-up clinical trials for rheumatoid arthritis, cases of lupus-like syndrome were reported uncommonly. There have been rare reports of other immune-mediated conditions; the causal relationship to Cimzia is not known. The impact of long-term treatment with Cimzia on the development of autoimmune diseases is unknown.

Injection site reactions

In the placebo-controlled rheumatoid arthritis clinical trials, 6.4% of patients treated with Cimzia developed injection site reactions (erythema, itching, haematoma, pain, swelling or bruising), compared to 6.5% of patients receiving placebo. Injection site pain was observed in 1.5% of patients treated with Cimzia with no cases leading to withdrawal.

4.9 Overdose

No dose-limiting toxicity was observed during clinical trials. Multiple doses of up to 800 mg subcutaneously and 20 mg/kg intravenously have been administered. In cases of overdose, it is recommended that patients are monitored closely for any adverse reactions or effect, and appropriate symptomatic treatment initiated immediately.

5. PHARMACOLOGICAL PROPERTIES

5.1 Pharmacodynamic properties

Pharmacotherapeutic group: Tumour necrosis factor alpha (TNFα) inhibitors, ATC code: L04AB05

Mechanism of action

Cimzia has a high affinity for human TNFα and binds with a dissociation constant (KD) of 90 pM. TNFα is a key pro-inflammatory cytokine with a central role in inflammatory processes. Cimzia selectively neutralises TNFα (IC90 of 4 ng/ml for inhibition of human TNFα in the *in vitro* L929 murine fibrosarcoma cytotoxicity assay) but does not neutralise lymphotoxin α (TNFβ).

Cimzia was shown to neutralise membrane associated and soluble human TNFα in a dose-dependant manner. Incubation of monocytes with Cimzia resulted in a dose-dependant inhibition of lipopolysaccharide (LPS)-induced TNFα and IL1β production in human monocytes.

Cimzia does not contain a fragment crystallisable (Fc) region, which is normally present in a complete antibody, and therefore does not fix complement or cause antibody-dependent cell-mediated cytotoxicity *in vitro*. It does not induce apoptosis *in vitro* in human peripheral blood-derived monocytes or lymphocytes, or neutrophil degranulation.

Clinical efficacy

The efficacy and safety of Cimzia have been assessed in 2 randomised, placebo-controlled, double-blind clinical trials in patients ≥ 18 years of age with active rheumatoid arthritis diagnosed according to American College of Rheumatology (ACR) criteria, RA-I (RAPID 1) and RA-II (RAPID 2). Patients had ≥ 9 swollen and tender joints each and had active RA for at least 6 months prior to baseline. Cimzia was administered subcutaneously in combination with oral MTX for a minimum of 6 months with stable doses of at least 10 mg weekly for 2 months in both trials. There is no experience with Cimzia in combination with DMARDs other than MTX.

Table: 2. Clinical trial description

(see Table 2 on page 396)

ACR response

The results of clinical trials RA-I and RA-II are shown in Table 3. Statistically significantly greater ACR 20 and ACR

Table 1 Adverse drug reactions in clinical trials

System Organ Class	Frequency	Adverse Drug Reactions
Infections and infestations	Common	bacterial infections (including abscess), viral infections (including herpes, papillomavirus, influenza)
	Uncommon	sepsis (including multi-organ failure, septic shock), tuberculosis, fungal infections (including candidiasis, histoplasmosis, pneumocystosis),
Neoplasms benign, malignant and unspecified (including cysts and polyps)	Uncommon	solid organ tumours, non-melanoma skin cancers, pre-cancerous lesions (including oral leukoplakia, melanocytic nevus), benign tumours and cysts (including skin papilloma)
	Rare	lymphoma, gastrointestinal tumours, melanoma
Blood and the lymphatic system disorders	Common	eosinophilic disorders, leukopaenia (including neutropaenia, lymphopaenia)
	Uncommon	anaemia, lymphadenopathy, thrombocytopaenia, thrombocytosis
	Rare	pancytopaenia, splenomegaly, erythrocytosis, white blood cell morphology abnormal
Immune system disorders	Uncommon	vasculitides, lupus erythematosus, drug hypersensitivity, allergic disorders, autoantibody positive
	Rare	angioneurotic oedema, sarcoidosis, serum sickness, panniculitis (including erythema nodosum)
Endocrine disorders	Rare	thyroid disorders
Metabolism and nutrition disorders	Uncommon	electrolyte imbalance, dyslipidaemia, appetite disorders, weight change
	Rare	haemosiderosis
Psychiatric disorders	Uncommon	anxiety (including restlessness), mood disorders
	Rare	suicide attempt, delirium, mental impairment
Nervous system disorders	Common	headaches (including migraine), sensory abnormalities
	Uncommon	peripheral neuropathies, dizziness, tremor
	Rare	acoustic neuritis, trigeminal neuralgia, impaired coordination or balance
	Not known	multiple sclerosis*
Eye disorders	Uncommon	visual disorder (including decreased vision), eye and eyelid inflammation, lacrimation disorder
Ear and labyrinth disorders	Uncommon	vertigo
	Rare	tinnitus
Cardiac disorders	Uncommon	cardiomyopathies (including heart failure), ischaemic coronary artery disorders, arrhythmias (including atrial fibrillation), palpitations
	Rare	pericarditis, atrioventricular block
Vascular disorders	Common	hypertension
	Uncommon	haemorrhage or bleeding (any site), hypercoagulation (including thrombophlebitis, pulmonary embolism), syncope, oedema (including peripheral, facial), ecchymoses (including haematoma, petechiae)
	Rare	cerebrovascular accident, arteriosclerosis, Raynaud's phenomenon, livedo reticularis, telangiectasia
Respiratory, thoracic and mediastinal disorders	Uncommon	asthma and related symptoms, pleural effusion and symptoms, respiratory tract congestion and inflammation, cough
	Rare	interstitial lung disease, pneumonitis
Gastrointestinal disorders	Uncommon	ascites, gastrointestinal ulceration and perforation, gastrointestinal tract inflammation (any site), stomatitis, dyspepsia, abdominal distension, oropharyngeal dryness
	Rare	gastrointestinal fistula, odynophagia, hypermotility
Hepatobiliary disorders	Common	hepatitis (including hepatic enzyme increased)
	Uncommon	hepatopathy (including cirrhosis), cholestasis, blood bilirubin increased
	Rare	cholelithiasis
Skin and subcutaneous tissue disorders	Common	rash
	Uncommon	alopecia, psoriasis and related conditions, dermatitis and eczema, sweat gland disorder, skin ulcer, photosensitivity, acne, skin discolouration, dry skin, nail and nail bed disorders
	Rare	skin exfoliation and desquamation, bullous conditions, hair texture disorder
Musculoskeletal, connective tissue and bone disorders	Uncommon	muscle disorders, blood creatine phosphokinase increased
Renal and urinary disorders	Uncommon	renal impairment, blood in urine, bladder and urethral symptoms
	Rare	nephropathy (including nephritis)
Reproductive system and breast disorders	Uncommon	menstrual cycle and uterine bleeding disorders (including amenorrhea), breast disorders
	Rare	sexual dysfunction
General disorders and administration site conditions	Common	pyrexia, pain (any site), asthaenia, pruritis (any site), injection site reactions
	Uncommon	chills, influenza-like illness, altered temperature perception, night sweats, flushing
Investigations	Uncommon	blood alkaline phosphatase increased, coagulation time prolonged
	Rare	blood uric acid increased
Injury, poisoning and procedural complications	Uncommon	skin injuries, impaired healing

*These events have been related to the class of TNF-antagonists, but incidence with Cimzia is not known.

Table 2 Clinical trial description

Study number	Patient numbers	Dose regimen	Study objectives
RA-I (52 weeks)	982	400 mg (0,2,4 weeks) with MTX 200 mg or 400 mg every 2 weeks with MTX	Evaluation for treatment of signs and symptoms and inhibition of structural damage. Co-primary endpoints: ACR 20 at Week 24 and change from baseline in mTSS at Week 52
RA-II (24 weeks)	619	400 mg (0,2,4 weeks) with MTX 200 mg or 400 mg every 2 weeks with MTX	Evaluation for treatment of signs and symptoms and inhibition of structural damage. Primary endpoint: ACR 20 at Week 24.

mTSS: modified Total Sharp Score

Table 3 ACR response in clinical trials RA-I and RA-II

	Study RA-I Methotrexate combination (24 and 52 weeks)		Study RA-II Methotrexate combination (24 weeks)	
Response	Placebo + MTX N=199	Cimzia 200 mg + MTX every 2 weeks N=393	Placebo + MTX N=127	Cimzia 200 mg + MTX every 2 weeks N=246
ACR 20				
Week 24	14%	59%**	9%	57%**
Week 52	13%	53%**	N/A	N/A
ACR 50				
Week 24	8%	37%**	3%	33%**
Week 52	8%	38%**	N/A	N/A
ACR 70				
Week 24	3%	21%**	1%	16%*
Week 52	4%	21%**	N/A	N/A
Major Clinical Response[a]	1%	13%**		

Cimzia vs. placebo: *$p \leqslant 0.01$, ** $p < 0.001$

[a] Major clinical response is defined as achieving ACR 70 response at every assessment over a continuous 6-month period

Wald p-values are quoted for the comparison of treatments using logistic regression with factors for treatment and region.

Percentage response based upon number of subjects contributing data (n) to that endpoint and time point which may differ from N

50 responses were achieved from Week 1 and Week 2, respectively, in both clinical trials compared to placebo. Responses were maintained through Weeks 52 (RA-I) and 24 (RA-II). Of the 783 patients initially randomised to active treatment in RA-I, 508 completed 52 weeks of placebo-controlled treatment and entered the open-label extension study. Of these, 427 completed 2 years of open-label follow-up and thus had a total exposure to Cimzia of 148 weeks overall. The observed ACR20 response rate at this timepoint was 91%. The reduction (RA-I) from Baseline in DAS28 (ESR) also was significantly greater ($p < 0.001$) at Week 52 (RA-I) and Week 24 (RA-II) compared to placebo and maintained through 2 years in the open-label extension trial to RA-I.

Table: 3. ACR response in clinical trials RA-I and RA-II

(see Table 3 above)

<ins>Radiographic response</ins>

In RA-I, structural joint damage was assessed radiographically and expressed as change in mTSS and its components, the erosion score and joint space narrowing (JSN) score, at Week 52, compared to baseline. Cimzia patients demonstrated significantly less radiographic progression than patients receiving placebo at Week 24 and Week 52 (see Table 4). In the placebo group, 52% of patients experienced no radiographic progression (mTSS $\leqslant 0.0$) at Week 52 compared to 69% in the Cimzia 200 mg treatment group.

Table: 4. Changes over 12 months in RA-I

(see Table 4 opposite)

Of the 783 patients initially randomised to active treatment in RA-I, 508 completed 52 weeks of placebo-controlled treatment and entered the open-label extension study. Sustained inhibition of progression of structural damage was demonstrated in a subset of 449 of these patients who completed at least 2 years of treatment with Cimzia (RA-I and open-label extension study) and had evaluable data at the 2-year timepoint.

<ins>Physical function response and health-related outcomes</ins>

In RA-I and RA-II, Cimzia-treated patients reported significant improvements in physical function as assessed by the Health Assessment Questionnaire – Disability Index (HAQ-DI) and in tiredness (fatigue) as reported by the Fatigue Assessment Scale (FAS) from Week 1 through to the end of the studies compared to placebo. In both clinical trials, Cimzia-treated patients reported significantly greater improvements in the SF-36 Physical and Mental Component Summaries and all domain scores. Improvements in physical function and HRQoL were maintained through 2 years in the open-label extension to RA-I. Cimzia-treated patients reported statistically significant improvements in the Work Productivity Survey compared to placebo.

<ins>Immunogenicity</ins>

The overall percentage of patients with antibodies to Cimzia detectable on at least 1 occasion was 7.7% in the Phase III RA placebo-controlled trials. Approximately one-third of antibody-positive patients (2.6% of the total population) had antibodies with neutralising activity *in vitro*. Patients treated with concomitant immunosuppressants (MTX) had a lower rate of antibody development than patients not taking immunosuppressants at baseline. Antibody formation was associated with lowered drug plasma concentration and in some patients, reduced efficacy.

A pharmacodynamic model based on the Phase III trial data predicts that around 15% of the patients develop antibodies in 6 months at the recommended dose regimen (200 mg every 2 weeks following a loading dose) without MTX co-treatment. This number decreases with increasing doses of concomitant MTX treatment. These data are reasonably in agreement with observed data.

The data reflect the percentage of patients whose test results were considered positive for antibodies to Cimzia in an ELISA, and are highly dependant on the sensitivity and specificity of the assay. Additionally, the observed incidence of antibodies in an assay may be influenced by several factors including sample handling, timing of sample collection, concomitant medicinal products, and underlying disease. For these reasons, comparison of the incidence of antibodies to Cimzia with the incidence of antibodies to other TNF antagonists is not appropriate.

Table 4 Changes over 12 months in RA-I

	Placebo + MTX N=199 Mean (SD)	Cimzia 200 mg + MTX N=393 Mean (SD)	Cimzia 200 mg + MTX – Placebo + MTX Mean Difference
mTSS			
Week 52	2.8 (7.8)	0.4 (5.7)	-2.4
Erosion Score			
Week 52	1.5 (4.3)	0.1 (2.5)	-1.4
JSN Score			
Week 52	1.4 (5.0)	0.4 (4.2)	-1.0

p-values were < 0.001 for both mTSS and erosion score and $\leqslant 0.01$ for JSN score. An ANCOVA was fitted to the ranked change from baseline for each measure with region and treatment as factors and rank baseline as a covariate.

5.2 Pharmacokinetic properties

Certolizumab pegol plasma concentrations were broadly dose-proportional. Pharmacokinetics observed in patients with rheumatoid arthritis were consistent with those seen in healthy subjects.

<ins>Absorption</ins>

Following subcutaneous administration, peak plasma concentrations of certolizumab pegol were attained between 54 and 171 hours post-injection. Certolizumab pegol has a bioavailability (F) of approximately 80% (range 76% to 88%) following subcutaneous administration compared to intravenous administration.

<ins>Distribution</ins>

The apparent volume of distribution (V/F) was estimated at 8.01 l in a population pharmacokinetic analysis of patients with rheumatoid arthritis.

<ins>Biotransformation and elimination</ins>

PEGylation, the covalent attachment of PEG polymers to peptides, delays the elimination of these entities from the circulation by a variety of mechanisms, including decreased renal clearance, decreased proteolysis, and decreased immunogenicity. Accordingly, certolizumab pegol is an antibody Fab' fragment conjugated with PEG in order to extend the terminal plasma elimination half-life of the Fab' to a value comparable with a whole antibody product. The terminal elimination phase half-life ($t_{1/2}$) was approximately 14 days for all doses tested.

Clearance following subcutaneous dosing was estimated to be 21.0 ml/h in a rheumatoid arthritis population pharmacokinetic analysis, with an inter-subject variability of 30.8% (CV) and an inter-occasion variability of 22.0%. The presence of antibodies to certolizumab pegol resulted in an approximately three-fold increase in clearance. Compared with a 70 kg person, clearance is 29% lower and 38% higher, respectively, in individual RA patients weighing 40 kg and 120 kg.

The Fab' fragment comprises protein compounds and is expected to be degraded to peptides and amino acids by proteolysis. The de-conjugated PEG component is rapidly eliminated from plasma and is to an unknown extent excreted renally.

<ins>Special populations</ins>

Renal impairment

Specific clinical trials have not been performed to assess the effect of renal impairment on the pharmacokinetics of certolizumab pegol or its PEG fraction. However, population pharmacokinetic analysis based on subjects with mild renal impairment showed no effect of creatinine clearance. There are insufficient data to provide a dosing recommendation in moderate and severe renal impairment. The pharmacokinetics of the PEG fraction of certolizumab pegol are expected to be dependent on renal function but have not been assessed in patients with renal impairment.

Hepatic impairment

Specific clinical trials have not been performed to assess the effect of hepatic impairment on the pharmacokinetics of certolizumab pegol.

Elderly (≥65 years old)

Specific clinical trials have not been performed in elderly subjects. However, no effect of age was observed in a population pharmacokinetic analysis in patients with rheumatoid arthritis in which 78 subjects (13.2% of the population) were aged 65 or greater and the oldest subject was aged 83 years.

<ins>Gender</ins>

There was no effect of gender on the pharmacokinetics of certolizumab pegol. As clearance decreases with decreasing body weight, females may generally obtain somewhat higher systemic exposure of certolizumab pegol.

<ins>Pharmacokinetic/pharmacodynamic relationship</ins>

On the basis of Phase II and Phase III clinical trial data, a population exposure-response relationship was established between average plasma concentration of certolizumab pegol during a dosing interval (C_{avg}) and efficacy (ACR 20 responder definition). The typical C_{avg} that produces half the maximum probability of ACR 20 response (EC50) was 17 μg/ml (95% CI: 10-23 μg/ml).

5.3 Preclinical safety data

The pivotal non-clinical safety studies were conducted in the cynomolgus monkey. In rats and monkeys, at doses higher than those given to humans, histopathology revealed cellular vacuolation, present mainly in macrophages, in a number of organs (lymph nodes, injection sites, spleen, adrenal, uterine, cervix, choroid plexus of the brain, and in the epithelial cells of the choroid plexus). It is likely that this finding was caused by cellular uptake of the PEG moiety. *In vitro* functional studies of human vacuolated macrophages indicated all functions tested were retained. Studies in rats indicated that >90% of the administered PEG was eliminated in 3 months following a single dose, with the urine being the main route of excretion.

Certolizumab pegol does not cross-react with rodent TNF. Therefore, reproductive toxicology studies have been performed with a homologous reagent recognising rat TNF. The value of these data to the evaluation of human risk may be limited. No adverse effects were seen on maternal well-being or female fertility, embryo-foetal and peri- and post-natal reproductive indices in rats using a rodent anti-rat TNFα PEGylated Fab' (cTN3 PF) following sustained TNFα suppression. In male rats, reduced sperm motility and a trend of reduced sperm count were observed.

Distribution studies have demonstrated that placental and milk transfer of cTN3 PF to the foetal and neonatal circulation is negligible. It is presently unknown whether the same is true for Cimzia in humans.

No mutagenic or clastogenic effects were demonstrated in preclinical studies. Carcinogenicity studies have not been performed with Cimzia.

6. PHARMACEUTICAL PARTICULARS

6.1 List of excipients

Sodium acetate

Sodium chloride

Water for injections

6.2 Incompatibilities

In the absence of compatibility studies, this medicinal product must not be mixed with other medicinal products.

6.3 Shelf life

18 months.

6.4 Special precautions for storage

Store in a refrigerator (2°C – 8°C).

Do not freeze.

Keep the pre-filled syringe in the outer carton in order to protect from light.

6.5 Nature and contents of container

One ml pre-filled syringe (type I glass) with a plunger stopper (bromobutyl rubber), containing

200 mg of certolizumab pegol.

None of the components of the syringe contain latex.

Pack size of 2 syringes and 2 alcohol wipes, and multipack containing 6 (3 packs of 2) pre-filled syringes and 6 (3 packs of 2) alcohol wipes.

Not all pack sizes may be marketed.

6.6 Special precautions for disposal and other handling

This medicinal product is for single use only.

Any unused product or waste material should be disposed of in accordance with local requirements.

Comprehensive instructions for the preparation and administration of Cimzia in a pre-filled syringe are given in the package leaflet.

7. MARKETING AUTHORISATION HOLDER

UCB Pharma SA

Allée de la Recherche 60

B-1070 Bruxelles

Belgium

8. MARKETING AUTHORISATION NUMBER(S)

EU/1/09/544/001

9. DATE OF FIRST AUTHORISATION/RENEWAL OF THE AUTHORISATION

October 2009

10. DATE OF REVISION OF THE TEXT

Detailed information on this medicinal product is available on the website of the European Medicines Agency (EMEA) http://www.emea.europa.eu.

Cipralex 5, 10 and 20 mg film-coated tablets and 10 and 20 mg/ml oral drops, solution

(Lundbeck Limited)

1. NAME OF THE MEDICINAL PRODUCT

CIPRALEX® 5 mg film-coated tablets

CIPRALEX® 10 mg film-coated tablets

CIPRALEX® 20 mg film-coated tablets

CIPRALEX® 10 mg/ml oral drops, solution

CIPRALEX® 20 mg/ml oral drops, solution

2. QUALITATIVE AND QUANTITATIVE COMPOSITION

Cipralex 5 mg: Each tablet contains 5 mg escitalopram (as oxalate)

Cipralex 10 mg: Each tablet contains 10 mg escitalopram (as oxalate)

Cipralex 20 mg: Each tablet contains 20 mg escitalopram (as oxalate)

Cipralex 10 mg/ml oral drops, solution

Each ml of solution contains:

10 mg escitalopram (as 12.78 mg escitalopram oxalate).

Each drop contains 0.5 mg escitalopram.

Cipralex 20 mg/ml oral drops, solution

Each ml of solution contains:

20 mg escitalopram (as 22.551 mg escitalopram oxalate).

Each drop contains 1 mg escitalopram.

Excipients: each drop contains 4.7 mg ethanol.

For a full list of excipients, see section 6.1.

3. PHARMACEUTICAL FORM

Film-coated tablets

Cipralex 5 mg: Round, white, film-coated tablet marked with "EK" on one side.

Cipralex 10 mg: Oval, white, scored, film-coated tablet marked with "E" and "L" on each side of the score on one side of the tablet.

Cipralex 20 mg: Oval, white, scored, film-coated tablet marked with "E" and "N" on each side of the score on one side of the tablet.

The 10 mg and 20 mg tablets can be divided into equal halves.

Oral drops, solution

10 mg/ml and 20 mg/ml oral drops, solution: Clear, nearly colourless to yellowish solution with a bitter taste.

4. CLINICAL PARTICULARS

4.1 Therapeutic indications

Treatment of major depressive episodes.

Treatment of panic disorder with or without agoraphobia.

Treatment of social anxiety disorder (social phobia).

Treatment of generalised anxiety disorder.

Treatment of obsessive-compulsive disorder.

4.2 Posology and method of administration

Safety of daily doses above 20 mg (40 drops of 10 mg/ml oral solution or 20 drops of 20 mg/ml oral solution) has not been demonstrated.

Cipralex is administered as a single daily dose and may be taken with or without food.

Cipralex oral drops, solution: A bottle with dropper applicator or an oral syringe may be used for administration. The oral syringe bears a graduation in mg referring to the escitalopram dose.

Cipralex oral drops, solution can be mixed with water, orange juice or apple juice.

Major depressive episodes

Usual dosage is 10 mg (20 drops of 10 mg/ml oral solution or 10 drops of 20 mg/ml oral solution) once daily. Depending on individual patient response, the dose may be increased to a maximum of 20 mg (40 drops of 10 mg/ml oral solution or 20 drops of 20 mg/ml oral solution) daily.

Usually 2-4 weeks are necessary to obtain antidepressant response. After the symptoms resolve, treatment for at least 6 months is required for consolidation of the response.

Panic disorder with or without agoraphobia

An initial dose of 5 mg (10 drops of 10 mg/ml oral solution or 5 drops of 20 mg/ml oral solution) is recommended for the first week before increasing the dose to 10 mg (20 drops of 10 mg/ml oral solution or 10 drops of 20 mg/ml oral solution) daily. The dose may be further increased, up to a maximum of 20 mg (40 drops of 10 mg/ml oral solution or 20 drops of 20 mg/ml oral solution) daily, dependent on individual patient response.

Maximum effectiveness is reached after about 3 months. The treatment lasts several months.

Social anxiety disorder

Usual dosage is 10 mg (20 drops of 10 mg/ml oral solution or 10 drops of 20 mg/ml oral solution) once daily. Usually 2-4 weeks are necessary to obtain symptom relief. The dose may subsequently, depending on individual patient response, be decreased to 5 mg (10 drops of 10 mg/ml oral solution or 5 drops of 20 mg/ml oral solution) or increased to a maximum of 20 mg daily (40 drops of 10 mg/ml oral solution or 20 drops of 20 mg/ml oral solution).

Social anxiety disorder is a disease with a chronic course, and treatment for 12 weeks is recommended to consolidate response. Long-term treatment of responders has been studied for 6 months and can be considered on an individual basis to prevent relapse; treatment benefits should be re-evaluated at regular intervals.

Social anxiety disorder is a well-defined diagnostic terminology of a specific disorder, which should not be confounded with excessive shyness. Pharmacotherapy is only indicated if the disorder interferes significantly with professional and social activities.

The place of this treatment compared to cognitive behavioural therapy has not been assessed. Pharmacotherapy is part of an overall therapeutic strategy.

Generalised anxiety disorder

Initial dosage is 10 mg (20 drops of 10 mg/ml oral solution or 10 drops of 20 mg/ml oral solution) once daily. Depending on the individual patient response, the dose may be increased to a maximum of 20 mg (40 drops of 10 mg/ml oral solution or 20 drops of 20 mg/ml oral solution) daily.

Long-term treatment of responders has been studied for at least 6 months in patients receiving 20 mg (40 drops of 10 mg/ml oral solution or 20 drops of 20 mg/ml oral solution) daily. Treatment benefits and dose should be re-evaluated at regular intervals (see Section 5.1).

Obsessive-compulsive disorder

Initial dosage is 10 mg (20 drops of 10 mg/ml oral solution or 10 drops of 20 mg/ml oral solution) once daily. Depending on the individual patient response, the dose may be increased to a maximum of 20 mg (40 drops of 10 mg/ml oral solution or 20 drops of 20 mg/ml oral solution) daily.

As OCD is a chronic disease, patients should be treated for a sufficient period to ensure that they are symptom free.

Treatment benefits and dose should be re-evaluated at regular intervals (see section 5.1).

Elderly patients (> 65 years of age)

Initial treatment with half the usually recommended dose and a lower maximum dose should be considered (see section 5.2).

The efficacy of Cipralex in social anxiety disorder has not been studied in elderly patients.

Children and adolescents (<18 years)

Cipralex should not be used in the treatment of children and adolescents under the age of 18 years (see section 4.4).

Reduced renal function

Dosage adjustment is not necessary in patients with mild or moderate renal impairment. Caution is advised in patients with severely reduced renal function (CL_{CR} less than 30 ml/min.) (see section 5.2).

Reduced hepatic function

An initial dose of 5 mg daily (10 drops of 10 mg/ml oral solution or 5 drops of 20 mg/ml oral solution) for the first two weeks of treatment is recommended in patients with mild or moderate hepatic impairment. Depending on individual patient response, the dose may be increased to 10 mg (20 drops of 10 mg/ml oral solution or 10 drops of 20 mg/ml oral solution) daily. Caution and extra careful dose titration is advised in patients with severely reduced hepatic function (see section 5.2).

Poor metabolisers of CYP2C19

For patients who are known to be poor metabolisers with respect to CYP2C19, an initial dose of 5 mg (10 drops of 10 mg/ml oral solution or 5 drops of 20 mg/ml oral solution) daily during the first two weeks of treatment is recommended. Depending on individual patient response, the dose may be increased to 10 mg (20 drops of 10 mg/ml oral solution or 10 drops of 20 mg/ml oral solution) daily (see section 5.2).

Discontinuation symptoms seen when stopping treatment

Abrupt discontinuation should be avoided. When stopping treatment with escitalopram the dose should be gradually reduced over a period of at least one to two weeks in order to reduce the risk of discontinuation symptoms (see section 4.4 and 4.8). If intolerable symptoms occur following a decrease in the dose or upon discontinuation of treatment, then resuming the previously prescribed dose may be considered. Subsequently, the physician may continue decreasing the dose, but at a more gradual rate.

4.3 Contraindications

Hypersensitivity to escitalopram or to any of the excipients.

Concomitant treatment with non-selective, irreversible monoamine oxidase inhibitors (MAO-inhibitors) is contraindicated due to the risk of serotonin syndrome with agitation, tremor, hyperthermia etc. (see section 4.5).

The combination of escitalopram with reversible MAO-A inhibitors (e.g. moclobemide) or the reversible non-selective MAO-inhibitor linezolid is contraindicated due to the risk of onset of a serotonin syndrome (see section 4.5).

4.4 Special warnings and precautions for use

The following special warnings and precautions apply to the therapeutic class of SSRIs (Selective Serotonin Reuptake Inhibitors).

Use in children and adolescents under 18 years of age

Cipralex should not be used in the treatment of children and adolescents under the age of 18 years. Suicide-related behaviours (suicide attempt and suicidal thoughts), and hostility (predominantly aggression, oppositional behaviour and anger) were more frequently observed in clinical trials among children and adolescents treated with antidepressants compared to those treated with placebo. If, based on clinical need, a decision to treat is nevertheless taken, the patient should be carefully monitored for the appearance of suicidal symptoms. In addition, long-term safety data in children and adolescents concerning growth, maturation and cognitive and behavioural development are lacking.

Paradoxical anxiety

Some patients with panic disorder may experience increased anxiety symptoms at the beginning of treatment with antidepressants. This paradoxical reaction usually subsides within two weeks during continued treatment. A low starting dose is advised to reduce the likelihood of an anxiogenic effect (see section 4.2).

Seizures

The medicinal product should be discontinued in any patient who develops seizures. SSRIs should be avoided in patients with unstable epilepsy and patients with controlled epilepsy should be carefully monitored. SSRIs should be discontinued if there is an increase in seizure frequency.

Mania

SSRIs should be used with caution in patients with a history of mania/hypomania. SSRIs should be discontinued in any patient entering a manic phase.

Diabetes

In patients with diabetes, treatment with an SSRI may alter glycaemic control (hypoglycaemia or hyperglycaemia). Insulin and/or oral hypoglycaemic dosage may need to be adjusted.

Suicide/suicidal thoughts or clinical worsening

Depression is associated with an increased risk of suicidal thoughts, self harm and suicide (suicide-related events). This risk persists until significant remission occurs. As improvement may not occur during the first few weeks or more of treatment, patients should be closely monitored until such improvement occurs. It is general clinical experience that the risk of suicide may increase in the early stages of recovery.

Other psychiatric conditions for which Cipralex is prescribed can also be associated with an increased risk of suicide-related events. In addition, these conditions may be co-morbid with major depressive disorder. The same precautions observed when treating patients with major depressive disorder should therefore be observed when treating patients with other psychiatric disorders.

Patients with a history of suicide-related events, or those exhibiting a significant degree of suicidal ideation prior to commencement of treatment, are known to be at greater risk of suicidal thoughts or suicide attempts, and should receive careful monitoring during treatment. A meta analysis of placebo controlled clinical trials of antidepressant drugs in adult patients with psychiatric disorders showed an increased risk of suicidal behaviour with antidepressants compared to placebo in patients less than 25 years old. Close supervision of patients and in particular those at high risk should accompany drug therapy especially in early treatment and following dose changes.

Patients (and caregivers of patients) should be alerted about the need to monitor for any clinical worsening, suicidal behaviour or thoughts and unusual changes in behaviour and to seek medical advice immediately if these symptoms present.

Akathisia/psychomotor restlessness

The use of SSRIs/SNRIs has been associated with the development of akathisia, characterised by a subjectively unpleasant or distressing restlessness and need to move often accompanied by an inability to sit or stand still. This is most likely to occur within the first few weeks of treatment. In patients who develop these symptoms, increasing the dose may be detrimental.

Hyponatraemia

Hyponatraemia, probably due to inappropriate antidiuretic hormone secretion (SIADH), has been reported rarely with the use of SSRIs and generally resolves on discontinuation of therapy. Caution should be exercised in patients at risk, such as elderly, cirrhotic patients or patients concomitantly treated with medications known to cause hyponatraemia.

Haemorrhage

There have been reports of cutaneous bleeding abnormalities, such as ecchymoses and purpura, with SSRIs. Caution is advised in patients taking SSRIs, particularly in concomitant use with oral anticoagulants, with medicinal products known to affect platelet function (e.g. atypical antipsychotics and phenothiazines, most tricyclic antidepressants, acetylsalicylic acid and non-steroidal anti-inflammatory medicinal products (NSAIDs), ticlopidine and dipyridamole) and in patients with known bleeding tendencies.

ECT (electroconvulsive therapy)

There is limited clinical experience of concurrent administration of SSRIs and ECT, therefore caution is advisable.

Serotonin syndrome

Caution is advisable if escitalopram is used concomitantly with medicinal products with serotonergic effects such as sumatriptan or other triptans, tramadol and tryptophan.

In rare cases, serotonin syndrome has been reported in patients using SSRIs concomitantly with serotonergic medicinal products. A combination of symptoms, such as agitation, tremor, myoclonus and hyperthermia may indicate the development of this condition. If this occurs treatment with the SSRI and the serotonergic medicinal product should be discontinued immediately and symptomatic treatment initiated.

St. John's Wort

Concomitant use of SSRIs and herbal remedies containing St. John's Wort (*Hypericum perforatum*) may result in an increased incidence of adverse reactions (see section 4.5).

Discontinuation symptoms seen when stopping treatment

Discontinuation symptoms when stopping treatment are common, particularly if discontinuation is abrupt (see section 4.8). In clinical trials adverse events seen on treatment discontinuation occurred in approximately 25% of patients treated with escitalopram and 15% of patients taking placebo.

The risk of discontinuation symptoms may be dependent on several factors including the duration and dose of therapy and the rate of dose reduction. Dizziness, sensory disturbances (including paraesthesia and electric shock sensations), sleep disturbances (including insomnia and intense dreams), agitation or anxiety, nausea and/or vomiting, tremor, confusion, sweating, headache, diarrhoea, palpitations, emotional instability, irritability, and visual disturbances are the most commonly reported reactions. Generally these symptoms are mild to moderate, however, in some patients they may be severe in intensity.

They usually occur within the first few days of discontinuing treatment, but there have been very rare reports of such symptoms in patients who have inadvertently missed a dose.

Generally these symptoms are self-limiting and usually resolve within 2 weeks, though in some individuals they may be prolonged (2-3 months or more). It is therefore advised that escitalopram should be gradually tapered when discontinuing treatment over a period of several weeks or months, according to the patient's needs (see "Discontinuation symptoms seen when stopping treatment", section 4.2).

Coronary heart disease

Due to limited clinical experience, caution is advised in patients with coronary heart disease (see section 5.3).

4.5 Interaction with other medicinal products and other forms of interaction

Pharmacodynamic interactions

Contra-indicated combinations:

Irreversible non-selective MAOIs

Cases of serious reactions have been reported in patients receiving an SSRI in combination with a non-selective, irreversible monoamine oxidase inhibitor (MAOI), and in patients who have recently discontinued SSRI treatment and have been started on such MAOI treatment (see section 4.3). In some cases, the patient developed serotonin syndrome (see section 4.8).

Escitalopram is contra-indicated in combination with non-selective, irreversible MAOIs. Escitalopram may be started 14 days after discontinuing treatment with an irreversible MAOI. At least 7 days should elapse after discontinuing escitalopram treatment, before starting a non-selective, irreversible MAOI.

Reversible, selective MAO-A inhibitor (moclobemide)

Due to the risk of serotonin syndrome, the combination of escitalopram with a MAO-A inhibitor such as moclobemide is contraindicated (see section 4.3). If the combination proves necessary, it should be started at the minimum recommended dosage and clinical monitoring should be reinforced.

Reversible, non-selective MAO-inhibitor (linezolid)

The antibiotic linezolid is a reversible non-selective MAO-inhibitor and should not be given to patients treated with escitalopram. If the combination proves necessary, it should be given with minimum dosages and under close clinical monitoring (see section 4.3).

Irreversible, selective MAO-B inhibitor (selegiline)

In combination with selegiline (irreversible MAO-B inhibitor), caution is required due to the risk of developing serotonin syndrome. Selegiline doses up to 10 mg/day have been safely co-administered with racemic citalopram.

Combinations requiring precautions for use:

Serotonergic medicinal products

Co-administration with serotonergic medicinal products (e.g. tramadol, sumatriptan and other triptans) may lead to serotonin syndrome.

Medicinal products lowering the seizure threshold

SSRIs can lower the seizure threshold. Caution is advised when concomitantly using other medicinal products capable of lowering the seizure threshold (e.g antidepressants (tricyclics, SSRIs), neuroleptics (phenothiazines, thioxanthenes and butyrophenones), mefloquine, bupropion and tramadol).

Lithium, tryptophan

There have been reports of enhanced effects when SSRIs have been given together with lithium or tryptophan, therefore concomitant use of SSRIs with these medicinal products should be undertaken with caution.

St. John's Wort

Concomitant use of SSRIs and herbal remedies containing St. John's Wort (*Hypericum perforatum*) may result in an increased incidence of adverse reactions (see section 4.4).

Haemorrhage

Altered anti-coagulant effects may occur when escitalopram is combined with oral anticoagulants. Patients receiving oral anticoagulant therapy should receive careful coagulation monitoring when escitalopram is started or stopped (see section 4.4).

Alcohol

No pharmacodynamic or pharmacokinetic interactions are expected between escitalopram and alcohol. However, as with other psychotropic medicinal products, the combination with alcohol is not advisable.

Pharmacokinetic interactions

Influence of other medicinal products on the pharmacokinetics of escitalopram.

The metabolism of escitalopram is mainly mediated by CYP2C19. CYP3A4 and CYP2D6 may also contribute to the metabolism although to a smaller extent. The metabolism of the major metabolite S-DCT (demethylated escitalopram) seems to be partly catalysed by CYP2D6.

Co-administration of escitalopram with omeprazole 30 mg once daily (a CYP2C19 inhibitor) resulted in moderate (approximately 50%) increase in the plasma concentrations of escitalopram.

Co-administration of escitalopram with cimetidine 400 mg twice daily (moderately potent general enzyme-inhibitor) resulted in a moderate (approximately 70%) increase in the plasma concentrations of escitalopram.

Thus, caution should be exercised when used concomitantly with CYP2C19 inhibitors (e.g. omeprazole, esomeprazole, fluvoxamine, lansoprazole, ticlopidine) or cimetidine. A reduction in the dose of escitalopram may be necessary based on monitoring of side-effects during concomitant treatment.

Effect of escitalopram on the pharmacokinetics of other medicinal products

Escitalopram is an inhibitor of the enzyme CYP2D6. Caution is recommended when escitalopram is co-administered with medicinal products that are mainly metabolised by this enzyme, and that have a narrow therapeutic index, e.g. flecainide, propafenone and metoprolol (when used in cardiac failure), or some CNS acting medicinal products that are mainly metabolised by CYP2D6, e.g. antidepressants such as desipramine, clomipramine and nortriptyline or antipsychotics like risperidone, thioridazine and haloperidol. Dosage adjustment may be warranted.

Co-administration with desipramine or metoprolol resulted in both cases in a twofold increase in the plasma levels of these two CYP2D6 substrates.

In vitro studies have demonstrated that escitalopram may also cause weak inhibition of CYP2C19. Caution is recommended with concomitant use of medicinal products that are metabolised by CYP2C19.

4.6 Pregnancy and lactation

Pregnancy

For escitalopram only limited clinical data are available regarding exposed pregnancies.

In reproductive toxicity studies performed in rats with escitalopram, embryo-fetotoxic effects, but no increased incidence of malformations, were observed (see section 5.3). Cipralex should not be used during pregnancy unless clearly necessary and only after careful consideration of the risk/benefit.

Neonates should be observed if maternal use of Cipralex continues into the later stages of pregnancy, particularly in the third trimester. Abrupt discontinuation should be avoided during pregnancy.

The following symptoms may occur in the neonate after maternal SSRI/SNRI use in later stages of pregnancy: respiratory distress, cyanosis, apnoea, seizures, temperature instability, feeding difficulty, vomiting, hypoglycaemia, hypertonia, hypotonia, hyperreflexia, tremor, jitteriness, irritability, lethargy, constant crying, somnolence and difficulty sleeping. These symptoms could be due to either serotonergic effects or discontinuation symptoms. In a majority of instances the complications begin immediately or soon (<24 hours) after delivery.

Lactation

It is expected that escitalopram will be excreted into human milk.

Consequently, breast-feeding is not recommended during treatment.

4.7 Effects on ability to drive and use machines

Although escitalopram has been shown not to affect intellectual function or psychomotor performance, any psychoactive medicinal product may impair judgement or skills. Patients should be cautioned about the potential risk of an influence on their ability to drive a car and operate machinery.

4.8 Undesirable effects

Adverse reactions are most frequent during the first or second week of treatment and usually decrease in intensity and frequency with continued treatment.

Adverse drug reactions known for SSRIs and also reported for escitalopram in either placebo-controlled clinical studies or as spontaneous post-marketing events are listed below by system organ class and frequency.

Frequencies are taken from clinical studies; they are not placebo-corrected. Frequencies are defined as: very common (≥1/10), common (≥1/100 to <1/10), uncommon (≥1/1,000 to <1/100), rare (≥1/10,000 to <1/1,000), very rare >1/10,000), or not known (cannot be estimated from the available data).

(see Table 1 below)

The following adverse drug reactions have been reported for the therapeutic class of SSRIs: psychomotor restlessness/akathisia (see section 4.4) and anorexia.

Cases of QT-prolongation have been reported during the post-marketing period, predominantly in patients with pre-existing cardiac disease. No causal relationship has been established.

Discontinuation symptoms seen when stopping treatment

Discontinuation of SSRIs/SNRIs (particularly when abrupt) commonly leads to discontinuation symptoms. Dizziness, sensory disturbances (including paraesthesia and electric shock sensations), sleep disturbances (including insomnia and intense dreams), agitation or anxiety, nausea and/or vomiting, tremor, confusion, sweating, headache, diarrhoea, palpitations, emotional instability, irritability, and visual disturbances are the most commonly reported reactions. Generally these events are mild to moderate and are self-limiting, however, in some patients they may be severe and/or prolonged. It is therefore advised that when escitalopram treatment is no longer required, gradual discontinuation by dose tapering should be carried out (see section 4.2 and 4.4).

4.9 Overdose

Toxicity

Clinical data on escitalopram overdose are limited and many cases involve concomitant overdoses of other drugs. In the majority of cases mild or no symptoms have been reported. Fatal cases of escitalopram overdose have rarely been reported with escitalopram alone; the majority of cases have involved overdose with concomitant medications. Doses between 400 and 800mg of escitalopram alone have been taken without any severe symptoms.

Symptoms

Symptoms seen in reported overdose of escitalopram include symptoms mainly related to the central nervous system (ranging from dizziness, tremor, and agitation to rare cases of serotonin syndrome, convulsion, and coma), the gastrointestinal system (nausea/vomiting), and the cardiovascular system (hypotension, tachycardia, QT prolongation, and arrhythmia) and electrolyte/fluid balance conditions (hypokalaemia, hyponatraemia).

Treatment

There is no specific antidote. Establish and maintain an airway, ensure adequate oxygenation and respiratory function. Gastric lavage and the use of activated charcoal should be considered. Gastric lavage should be carried out as soon as possible after oral ingestion. Cardiac and vital signs monitoring are recommended along with general symptomatic supportive measures.

5. PHARMACOLOGICAL PROPERTIES

5.1 Pharmacodynamic properties

Pharmacotherapeutic group: antidepressants, selective serotonin reuptake inhibitors

ATC-code: N 06 AB 10

Mechanism of action

Escitalopram is a selective inhibitor of serotonin (5-HT) reuptake with high affinity for the primary binding site. It also binds to an allosteric site on the serotonin transporter, with a 1000 fold lower affinity.

Escitalopram has no or low affinity for a number of receptors including $5\text{-}HT_{1A}$, $5\text{-}HT_2$, DA D_1 and D_2 receptors, α_1-, α_2-, β-adrenoceptors, histamine H_1, muscarine cholinergic, benzodiazepine, and opioid receptors.

The inhibition of 5-HT re-uptake is the only likely mechanism of action explaining the pharmacological and clinical effects of escitalopram.

Clinical efficacy

Major depressive episodes

Escitalopram has been found to be effective in the acute treatment of major depressive episodes in three out of four double-blind, placebo controlled short-term (8-week) studies. In a long-term relapse prevention study, 274 patients who had responded during an initial 8-week open label treatment phase with escitalopram 10 or 20 mg/day, were randomised to continuation with escitalopram at the same dose, or to placebo, for up to 36 weeks. In this study, patients receiving continued escitalopram experienced a significantly longer time to relapse over the subsequent 36 weeks compared to those receiving placebo.

Social anxiety disorder

Escitalopram was effective in both three short-term (12-week) studies and in responders in a 6 months relapse prevention study in social anxiety disorder. In a 24-week dose-finding study, efficacy of 5, 10 and 20 mg escitalopram has been demonstrated.

Generalised anxiety disorder

Escitalopram in doses of 10 and 20 mg/day was effective in four out of four placebo-controlled studies.

In pooled data from three studies with similar design comprising 421 escitalopram-treated patients and 419 placebo-treated patients there were 47.5% and 28.9% responders respectively and 37.1% and 20.8% remitters. Sustained effect was seen from week 1.

Maintenance of efficacy of escitalopram 20mg/day was demonstrated in a 24 to 76 week, randomised, maintenance of efficacy study in 373 patients who had responded during the initial 12-week open-label treatment.

Obsessive-compulsive disorder

In a randomised, double-blind, clinical study, 20 mg/day escitalopram separated from placebo on the Y-BOCS total score after 12 weeks. After 24 weeks, both 10 and 20 mg/day escitalopram were superior as compared to placebo.

Prevention of relapse was demonstrated for 10 and 20 mg/day escitalopram in patients who responded to escitalopram in a 16-week open-label period and who entered a 24-week, randomised, double-blind, placebo controlled period.

5.2 Pharmacokinetic properties

Absorption

Tablets: Absorption is almost complete and independent of food intake. (Mean time to maximum concentration (mean T_{max}) is 4 hours after multiple dosing). As with racemic citalopram, the absolute bio-availability of escitalopram is expected to be about 80%.

Oral drops, solution: Absorption is almost complete and independent of food intake. (Mean time to maximum concentration (mean T_{max}) is 4 hours after multiple dosing). The oral drops, solution is bioequivalent with Cipralex tablets, and the absolute bioavailability of escitalopram is expected to be about 80% as for citalopram.

Distribution

The apparent volume of distribution (V_d,β/F) after oral administration is about 12 to 26 L/kg. The plasma protein binding is below 80% for escitalopram and its main metabolites.

Biotransformation

Escitalopram is metabolised in the liver to the demethylated and didemethylated metabolites. Both of these are pharmacologically active. Alternatively, the nitrogen may be oxidised to form the N-oxide metabolite. Both parent substance and metabolites are partly excreted as glucuronides. After multiple dosing the mean concentrations of the demethyl and didemethyl metabolites are usually 28-31% and <5%, respectively, of the escitalopram concentration. Biotransformation of escitalopram to the demethylated metabolite is mediated primarily by CYP2C19. Some contribution by the enzymes CYP3A4 and CYP2D6 is possible.

Elimination

The elimination half-life ($t_{½}$β) after multiple dosing is about 30 hours and the oral plasma clearance (Cl_{oral}) is about 0.6 L/min. The major metabolites have a significantly longer half-life. Escitalopram and major metabolites are assumed to be eliminated by both the hepatic (metabolic) and the renal routes, with the major part of the dose excreted as metabolites in the urine.

There is linear pharmacokinetics. Steady-state plasma levels are achieved in about 1 week. Average steady-state concentrations of 50 nmol/L (range 20 to 125 nmol/L) are achieved at a daily dose of 10 mg.

Elderly patients (> 65 years)

Pappears to be eliminated more slowly in elderly patients compared to younger patients. Systemic exposure (AUC) is about 50% higher in elderly compared to young healthy volunteers (see section 4.2).

Reduced hepatic function

In patients with mild or moderate hepatic impairment (Child-Pugh Criteria A and B), the half-life of escitalopram

Table 1

	Very common	Common	Uncommon	Rare	Not known
Investigations		Weight increased	Weight decreased		Liver function test abnormal
Cardiac disorders			Tachycardia	Bradycardia	
Blood and lymphatic disorders					Thrombocytopenia
Nervous system disorders		Insomnia, somnolence, dizziness, paraesthesia, tremor	Taste disturbance, sleep disorder, syncope	Serotonin syndrome	Dyskinesia, movement disorder, convulsion
Eye disorders			Mydriasis, visual disturbance		
Ear and labyrinth disorders			Tinnitus		
Respiratory, thoracic and mediastinal disorders		Sinusitis, yawning	Epistaxis		
Gastrointestinal disorders	Nausea	Diarrhoea, constipation, vomiting, dry mouth	Gastrointestinal haemorrhages (including rectal haemorrhage)		
Renal and urinary disorders					Urinary retention
Skin and subcutaneous tissue disorders		Sweating increased	Urticaria, alopecia, rash, pruritus		Ecchymosis, angioedemas
Musculoskeletal, connective tissue and bone disorders		Arthralgia, myalgia			
Endocrine disorders					Inappropriate ADH secretion
Metabolism and nutrition disorders		Decreased appetite, increased appetite			Hyponatraemia
Vascular disorders					Orthostatic hypotension
General disorders and administration site conditions		Fatigue, pyrexia	Oedema		
Immune system disorders				Anaphylactic reaction	
Hepatobiliary disorders					Hepatitis
Reproductive system and breast disorders		Male: ejaculation disorder, impotence	Female: metrorrhagia, menorrhagia		Galactorrhoea Male: priapism,
Psychiatric disorders		Anxiety, restlessness, abnormal dreams Female and male: libido decreased Female: anorgasmia	Bruxism, agitation, nervousness, panic attack, confusional state	Aggression, depersonalisation, hallucination	Mania, suicidal ideation, suicidal behaviour[1]

[1] Cases of suicidal ideation and suicidal behaviours have been reported during escitalopram therapy or early after treatment discontinuation (see section 4.4).

was about twice as long and the exposure was about 60% higher than in subjects with normal liver function (see section 4.2).

Reduced renal function

With racemic citalopram, a longer half-life and a minor increase in exposure have been observed in patients with reduced kidney function (CL_{CR} 10-53 ml/min). Plasma concentrations of the metabolites have not been studied, but they may be elevated (see section 4.2).

Polymorphism

It has been observed that poor metabolisers with respect to CYP2C19 have twice as high a plasma concentration of escitalopram as extensive metabolisers. No significant change in exposure was observed in poor metabolisers with respect to CYP2D6 (see section 4.2).

5.3 Preclinical safety data

No complete conventional battery of preclinical studies was performed with escitalopram since the bridging toxicokinetic and toxicological studies conducted in rats with escitalopram and citalopram showed a similar profile. Therefore, all the citalopram information can be extrapolated to escitalopram.

In comparative toxicological studies in rats, escitalopram and citalopram caused cardiac toxicity, including congestive heart failure, after treatment for some weeks, when using dosages that caused general toxicity. The cardiotoxicity seemed to correlate with peak plasma concentrations rather than to systemic exposures (AUC). Peak plasma concentrations at no-effect-level were in excess (8-fold) of those achieved in clinical use, while AUC for escitalopram was only 3- to 4-fold higher than the exposure achieved in clinical use. For citalopram AUC values for the S-enantiomer were 6- to 7-fold higher than exposure achieved in clinical use. The findings are probably related to an exaggerated influence on biogenic amines i.e. secondary to the primary pharmacological effects, resulting in hemodynamic effects (reduction in coronary flow) and ischaemia. However, the exact mechanism of cardiotoxicity in rats is not clear. Clinical experience with citalopram, and the clinical trial experience with escitalopram, do not indicate that these findings have a clinical correlate.

Increased content of phospholipids has been observed in some tissues e.g. lung, epididymides and liver after treatment for longer periods with escitalopram and citalopram in rats. Findings in the epididymides and liver were seen at exposures similar to that in man. The effect is reversible after treatment cessation. Accumulation of phospholipids (phospholipidosis) in animals has been observed in connection with many cationic amphiphilic medicines. It is not known if this phenomenon has any significant relevance for man.

In the developmental toxicity study in the rat embryotoxic effects (reduced foetal weight and reversible delay of ossification) were observed at exposures in terms of AUC in excess of the exposure achieved during clinical use. No increased frequency of malformations was noted. A pre- and postnatal study showed reduced survival during the lactation period at exposures in terms of AUC in excess of the exposure achieved during clinical use.

6. PHARMACEUTICAL PARTICULARS

6.1 List of excipients

Tablet core:

Microcrystalline cellulose, colloidal anhydrous silica, talc, croscarmellose sodium, magnesium stearate.

Tablet coating:

Hypromellose, macrogol 400, titanium dioxide (E 171).

10 mg/ml oral drops, solution:

Sodium hydroxide, purified water.

20 mg/ml oral drops, solution:

Propyl gallate, citric acid (anhydrous), ethanol 96%, sodium hydroxide, purified water.

6.2 Incompatibilities

Tablets:

Not applicable.

10 mg/ml and 20 mg/ml oral drops, solution:

In the absence of compatibility studies, this medicinal product must not be mixed with other medicinal products.

6.3 Shelf life

Tablets:

3 years.

10 mg/ml oral drops, solution:

2 years.

After opening, the drops should be used within 16 weeks.

20 mg/ml oral drops, solution:

3 years.

After opening, the drops should be used within 8 weeks.

6.4 Special precautions for storage

Tablets:

No special precautions for storage.

10 mg/ml oral drops, solution:

Do not store above 25°C.

Keep the bottle in the outer container in order to protect from light.

20 mg/ml oral drops, solution:

After opening the bottle should not be stored above 25°C.

6.5 Nature and contents of container

Tablets

Blister: Transparent; PVC/PE/PVdC/Aluminium blister, pack with an outer carton; 14, 28, 56, 98 tablets - Unit dose; 49x1, 56x1, 98x1, 100x1, 500x1 tablets (5, 10 and 20 mg)

Blister: White; PVC/PE/PVdC/Aluminium blister, pack with an outer carton; 14, 20, 28, 50, 100, 200 tablets (5, 10 and 20 mg)

Polypropylene tablet container; 100 (5, 10 and 20 mg), 200 (5 and 10 mg) tablets

10 mg/ml oral drops, solution

15 ml and 28 ml in a brown glass bottle with dropper applicator (polyethylene), and child-proof screw cap (polypropylene).

15 ml and 28 ml in a brown glass bottle with adapter (polyethylene), child-proof screw cap (polypropylene) and a 1 ml syringe (polypropylene).

20 mg/ml oral drops, solution:

15 ml in a brown glass bottle with dropper applicator (polyethylene), and child-proof screw cap (polypropylene).

Not all pack sizes may be marketed.

6.6 Special precautions for disposal and other handling

No special requirements.

7. MARKETING AUTHORISATION HOLDER

H. Lundbeck A/S
Ottiliavej 7-9
DK-2500 Copenhagen-Valby
Denmark

8. MARKETING AUTHORISATION NUMBER(S)

Cipralex 5 mg PL 13761/0008

Cipralex 10 mg PL 13761/0009

Cipralex 20 mg PL 13761/0011

Cipralex 10 mg/ml oral drops, solution PL 13761/0019

Cipralex 20 mg/ml oral drops, solution PL 13761/0028

9. DATE OF FIRST AUTHORISATION/RENEWAL OF THE AUTHORISATION

Date of first authorisation

Tablets: 10 June 2002

10 mg/ml oral drops, solution: 8 December 2004

20 mg/ml oral drops, solution: 3 January 2008

Date of last renewal tablets and 10 mg/ml oral drops: 7 December 2006

10. DATE OF REVISION OF THE TEXT

16 October 2008

LEGAL CATEGORY

POM

Cipramil Drops 40 mg/ml

(Lundbeck Limited)

1. NAME OF THE MEDICINAL PRODUCT

Cipramil® Drops 40 mg/ml

2. QUALITATIVE AND QUANTITATIVE COMPOSITION

Oral drops 40 mg/ml (44.48 mg citalopram hydrochloride corresponding to 40 mg citalopram base per ml).

3. PHARMACEUTICAL FORM

Oral drops, solution.

4. CLINICAL PARTICULARS

4.1 Therapeutic indications

Treatment of depressive illness in the initial phase and as maintenance against potential relapse/recurrence.

Cipramil is also indicated in the treatment of panic disorder with or without agoraphobia.

4.2 Posology and method of administration

MAJOR DEPRESSIVE EPISODES

The recommended dose is 16 mg (8 drops) daily. In general improvement in patients starts after one week but may only become evident from the second week of therapy.

As with all antidepressant medicinal products, dosage should be reviewed and adjusted if necessary within 3 to 4 weeks of initiation of therapy and thereafter as judged clinically appropriate. Although there may be an increased potential for undesirable effects at higher doses, if after some weeks on the recommended dose insufficient response is seen some patients may benefit from having their dose increased up to a maximum of 48 mg (24 drops) a day in 16 mg (8 drops) steps according to the patient's response (see section 5.1). Dosage adjustments should be made carefully on an individual patient basis, to maintain the patient at the lowest effective dose.

Patients with depression should be treated for a sufficient period of at least 6 months to ensure that they are free from symptoms.

PANIC DISORDER

Patients should be started on 8 mg (4 drops)/day and the dose gradually increased in 8 mg (4 drops) steps according to the patient's response up to the recommended dose. The recommended dose is 16-24 mg (8 to 12 drops) daily. A low initial starting dose is recommended to minimise the potential worsening of panic symptoms, which is generally recognised to occur early in the treatment of this disorder. Although there may be an increased potential for undesirable effects at higher doses, if after some weeks on the recommended dose insufficient response is seen some patients may benefit from having their dose increased gradually up to a maximum of 48 mg (24 drops) /day (see section 5.1). Dosage adjustments should be made carefully on an individual patient basis, to maintain the patients at the lowest effective dose.

Patients with panic disorder should be treated for a sufficient period to ensure that they are free from symptoms. This period may be several months or even longer.

Elderly patients (> 65 years of age)

The recommended daily dose is 16 mg (8 drops). Dependent on individual patient response this may be increased to a maximum of 32 mg (16 drops) daily.

Children (< 18 years of age)

Citalopram should not be used in the treatment of children and adolescents under the age of 18 years (see section 4.4).

Reduced hepatic function

Dosage should be restricted to the lower end of the dose range.

Reduced renal function

Dosage adjustment is not necessary in cases of mild or moderate renal impairment. No information is available in cases of severe renal impairment (creatinine clearance <20 mL / min).

Withdrawal symptoms seen on discontinuation of citalopram

Abrupt discontinuation should be avoided. When stopping treatment with citalopram the dose should be gradually reduced over a period of at least one to two weeks in order to reduce the risk of withdrawal reactions (see section 4.4 Special Warnings and Special Precautions for Use and section 4.8 Undesirable Effects). If intolerable symptoms occur following a decrease in the dose or upon discontinuation of treatment, then resuming the previously prescribed dose may be considered. Subsequently, the physician may continue decreasing the dose, but at a more gradual rate.

For oral administration after mixing with water, orange juice or apple juice.

Cipramil Oral Drops can be taken as a single daily dose, at any time of day, without regard to food intake.

Citalopram oral drops have approximately 25% increased bioavailability compared to tablets. The tablet corresponds to the number of drops as follows:

Tablets / dose	Equivalent	Drops
10 mg	8 mg	(4 drops)
20 mg	16 mg	(8 drops)
30 mg	24 mg	(12 drops)
40 mg	32 mg	(16 drops)
60 mg	48 mg	(24 drops)

4.3 Contraindications

Hypersensitivity to citalopram.

Monoamine Oxidase Inhibitors. Cases of serious and sometimes fatal reactions have been reported in patients receiving an SSRI in combination with monoamine oxidase inhibitor (MAOI), including the selective MAOI selegiline and the reversible MAOI (RIMA), moclobemide and in patients who have recently discontinued an SSRI and have been started on a MAOI.

Some cases presented with features resembling serotonin syndrome. Symptoms of a drug interaction with a MAOI include: hyperthermia, rigidity, myoclonus, autonomic instability with possible rapid fluctuations of vital signs, mental status changes that include confusion, irritability and extreme agitation progressing to delirium and coma.

Citalopram should not be used in combination with a MAOI. Citalopram may be started 14 days after discontinuing treatment with an irreversible MAOI and at least one day after discontinuing treatment with the reversible MAOI (RIMA), moclobemide. At least 7 days should elapse after discontinuing citalopram treatment before starting a MAOI or RIMA.

Concomitant treatment with pimozide (see section 4.5).

4.4 Special warnings and precautions for use

Suicide/suicidal thoughts or clinical worsening

Depression is associated with an increased risk of suicidal thoughts, self harm and suicide (suicide-related events). This risk persists until significant remission occurs. As improvement may not occur during the first few weeks or more of treatment, patients should be closely monitored until such improvement occurs. It is general clinical experience that the risk of suicide may increase in the early stages of recovery.

Other psychiatric conditions for which Cipramil is prescribed can also be associated with an increased risk of suicide-related events. In addition, these conditions may be co-morbid with major depressive disorder. The same precautions observed when treating patients with major depressive disorder should therefore be observed when treating patients with other psychiatric disorders.

Patients with a history of suicide-related events, or those exhibiting a significant degree of suicidal ideation prior to commencement of treatment are known to be at greater risk of suicidal thoughts or suicide attempts, and should receive careful monitoring during treatment. A meta-analysis of placebo-controlled clinical trials of antidepressant drugs in adult patients with psychiatric disorders showed an increased risk of suicidal behaviour with antidepressants compared to placebo in patients less than 25 years old.

Close supervision of patients and in particular those at high risk should accompany drug therapy especially in early treatment and following dose changes. Patients (and care-givers of patients) should be alerted about the need to monitor for any clinical worsening, suicidal behaviour or thoughts and unusual changes in behaviour and to seek medical advice immediately if these symptoms present.

Use in children and adolescents under 18 years of age

Cipramil should not be used in the treatment of children and adolescents under the age of 18 years. Suicide-related behaviours (suicide attempt and suicidal thoughts) and hostility (predominantly aggression, oppositional behaviour and anger) were more frequently observed in clinical trials among children and adolescents treated with antidepressants compared to those treated with placebo. If, based on clinical need, a decision to treat is nevertheless taken; the patient should be carefully monitored for the appearance of suicidal symptoms. In addition, long-term safety data in children and adolescents concerning growth, maturation and cognitive and behavioural development are lacking.

Diabetes

In patients with diabetes, treatment with an SSRI may alter glycaemic control, possibly due to improvement of depressive symptoms. Insulin and or oral hypoglycaemic dosage may need to be adjusted.

Seizures

Seizures are a potential risk with antidepressant drugs. The drug should be discontinued in any patient who develops seizures. Citalopram should be avoided in patients with unstable epilepsy and patients with controlled epilepsy should be carefully monitored. Citalopram should be discontinued if there is an increase in seizure frequency.

ECT

There is little clinical experience of concurrent administration of citalopram and ECT, therefore caution is advisable.

Mania

Citalopram should be used with caution in patients with a history of mania/hypomania. Citalopram should be discontinued in any patient entering a manic phase.

Haemorrhage

There have been reports of cutaneous bleeding abnormalities such as ecchymoses and purpura, as well as haemorrhagic manifestations e.g. gastrointestinal haemorrhage with SSRIs. The risk of gastrointestinal haemorrhage may be increased in elderly people during treatment with SSRIs. Caution is advised in patients taking SSRIs, particularly in concomitant use with drugs known to affect platelet function (e.g. atypical antipsychotics and phenothiazines, most tricyclic antidepressants, aspirin and non-steroidal anti-inflammatory drugs (NSAIDs) as well as in patients with a history of bleeding disorders.

Experience with citalopram has not revealed any clinically relevant interactions with neuroleptics. However, as with other SSRIs, the possibility of a pharmacodynamic interaction cannot be excluded.

Consideration should be given to factors which may affect the disposition of a minor metabolite of citalopram (didemethylcitalopram) since increased levels of this metabolite could theoretically prolong the QTc interval in susceptible individuals. However, in ECG monitoring of 2500 patients in clinical trials, including 277 patients with pre-existing cardiac conditions, no clinically significant changes were noted.

As with most antidepressants, citalopram should be discontinued if the patient enters a manic phase. There is little clinical experience of concurrent use of citalopram and ECT.

Some patients with panic disorder experience an initial anxiogenic effect when starting pharmacotherapy. A low starting dose (see Posology) reduces the likelihood of this effect.

Akathisia/psychomotor restlessness

The use of citalopram has been associated with the development of akathisia, characterised by a subjectively unpleasant or distressing restlessness and need to move often accompanied by an inability to sit or stand still. This is most likely to occur within the first few weeks of treatment. In patients who develop these symptoms, increasing the dose may be detrimental.

Withdrawal symptoms seen on discontinuation of SSRI treatment

Withdrawal symptoms when treatment is discontinued are common, particularly if discontinuation is abrupt (see section 4.8 Undesirable effects). In clinical trials adverse events seen on treatment discontinuation occurred in approximately 40% of patients treated with citalopram.

The risk of withdrawal symptoms may be dependent on several factors including the duration and dose of therapy and the rate of dose reduction. Dizziness, sensory disturbances (including paraesthesia), sleep disturbances (including insomnia and intense dreams), agitation or anxiety, nausea and/or vomiting, tremor and headache are the most commonly reported reactions. Generally these symptoms are mild to moderate, however, in some patients they may be severe in intensity. They usually occur within the first few days of discontinuing treatment, but there have been very rare reports of such symptoms in patients who have inadvertently missed a dose. Generally these symptoms are self-limiting and usually resolve within 2 weeks, though in some individuals they may be prolonged (2-3 months or more). It is therefore advised that citalopram should be gradually tapered when discontinuing treatment over a period of several weeks or months, according to the patient's needs (see "Withdrawal symptoms seen on discontinuation of citalopram", Section 4.2 Posology and Method of Administration).

4.5 Interaction with other medicinal products and other forms of interaction

Monoamine Oxidase Inhibitors (MAOIs) should not be used in combination with SSRIs (see 4.3 Contraindications).

The metabolism of citalopram is only partly dependent on the hepatic cytochrome P450 isozyme CYP2D6 and, unlike some other SSRIs, citalopram is only a weak inhibitor of this important enzyme system which is involved in the metabolism of many drugs (including antiarrhythmics, neuroleptics, beta-blockers, TCAs and some SSRIs). Protein binding is relatively low (<80%). These properties give citalopram a low potential for clinically significant drug interactions.

Alcohol – The combination of citalopram and alcohol is not advisable. However clinical studies have revealed no adverse pharmacodynamic interactions between citalopram and alcohol.

Serotonergic drugs – Co-administration with serotonergic drugs (e.g. tramadol, sumatriptan) may lead to enhancement of 5-HT associated effects.

Lithium & tryptophan – There is no pharmacokinetic interaction between lithium and citalopram. However, there have been reports of enhanced serotonergic effects when SSRIs have been given with lithium or tryptophan and therefore the concomitant use of citalopram with these drugs should be undertaken with caution. Routine monitoring of lithium levels need not be adjusted.

In a pharmacokinetic study no effect was demonstrated on either citalopram or imipramine levels, although the level of desipramine, the primary metabolite of imipramine, was increased. In animal studies cimetidine had little or no influence on citalopram kinetics.

Dynamic interactions between citalopram and herbal remedy St John's Wort (*Hypericum perforatum*) can occur, resulting in an increase in undesirable effects.

A pharmacokinetic/pharmacodynamic interaction study in healthy volunteers with concomitant administration of citalopram and metoprolol (a CYP2D6 substrate) showed a twofold increase in metoprolol concentrations, but no statistically significant increase in the effect of metoprolol on blood pressure and heart rate.

No pharmacodynamic interactions have been noted in clinical studies in which citalopram has been given concomitantly with benzodiazepines, neuroleptics, analgesics, lithium, alcohol, antihistamines, antihypertensive drugs, beta-blockers and other cardiovascular drugs.

Pimozide

Co administration of a single dose of pimozide 2 mg to subjects treated with racemic citalopram 40 mg/day for 11 days caused an increase in AUC and Cmax of pimozide, although not consistently throughout the study. The co-administration of pimozide and citalopram resulted in a mean increase in the QTc interval of approximately 10 msec. Due to the interaction noted at a low dose of pimozide, concomitant administration of citalopram and pimozide is contraindicated.

4.6 Pregnancy and lactation

Pregnancy

Animal studies did not provide any evidence of teratogenicity, however the safety of citalopram during human pregnancy has not been established. As with all drugs citalopram should only be used in pregnancy if the potential benefits of treatment to the mother outweigh the possible risks to the developing foetus.

Neonates should be observed if maternal use of citalopram continues into the later stages of pregnancy, particularly in the third trimester. Abrupt discontinuation should be avoided during pregnancy.

The following symptoms may occur in the neonates after maternal SSRI/SNRI use in later stages of pregnancy: respiratory distress, cyanosis, apnoea, seizures, temperature instability, feeding difficulty, vomiting, hypoglycaemia, hypertonia, hypotonia, hyperreflexia, tremor, jitteriness, irritability, lethargy, constant crying, somnolence and difficulty sleeping. These symptoms could be due to either serotonergic effects or discontinuation symptoms. In a majority of instances the complications begin immediately or soon (<24 hours) after delivery.

Lactation

Citalopram is known to be excreted in breast milk. Its effects on the nursing infant have not been established. If treatment with citalopram is considered necessary, discontinuation of breast feeding should be considered.

4.7 Effects on ability to drive and use machines

Citalopram does not impair intellectual function and psychomotor performance. However, patients who are prescribed psychotropic medication may be expected to have some impairment of general attention and concentration either due to the illness itself, the medication or both and should be cautioned about their ability to drive a car and operate machinery.

4.8 Undesirable effects

Adverse effects observed with citalopram are in general mild and transient. They are most prominent during the first one or two weeks of treatment and usually attenuate as the depressive state improves.

The most commonly observed adverse events associated with the use of citalopram and not seen at an equal incidence among placebo-treated patients were: nausea, somnolence, dry mouth, increased sweating and tremor. The incidence of each in excess over placebo is low (<10%).

In comparative clinical trials with tricyclic antidepressants the incidence of adverse events occurring with citalopram was found to be lower in all cases.

Withdrawal reactions have been reported in association with selective serotonin reuptake inhibitors (SSRIs), including citalopram. Common symptoms include dizziness, paraesthesia, headache, anxiety and nausea. Abrupt discontinuation of treatment with Cipramil should be avoided. The majority of symptoms experienced on withdrawal of SSRIs are non-serious and self-limiting.

Treatment emergent adverse events reported in clinical trials (N=2985):

Frequent (≥5 - 20%)

Increased sweating, headache, tremor, dizziness, abnormal accommodation, somnolence, insomnia, agitation, nervousness, nausea, dry mouth, constipation, diarrhoea, palpitation, asthenia.

Less frequent (1 - <5%)

Rash, pruritus, paraesthesia, migraine, abnormal vision, taste perversion, sleep disorder, decreased libido, impaired concentration, abnormal dreaming, amnesia, anxiety, increased appetite, anorexia, apathy, impotence, suicide attempt, confusion, dyspepsia, vomiting, abdominal pain, flatulence, increased salivation, weight decrease, weight increase, postural hypotension, tachycardia, rhinitis, micturition disorder, polyuria, ejaculation failure, female anorgasmia, fatigue.

Rare (<1%)

Myalgia, movement disorders, convulsions, tinnitus, euphoria, increased libido, coughing, malaise. Psychomotor restlessness/akathisia (see section 4.4 Special Warnings and Special Precautions for Use)

Post Marketing - The following adverse reactions apply to the therapeutic class of SSRIs

Skin Disorders: Angiodema; ecchymoses. Photosensitivity reactions have been reported very rarely.

Disorders of metabolism and nutrition: Rare cases of hyponatraemia and inappropriate ADH secretion have been reported and appear to be reversible on discontinuation. The majority of the reports were associated with the older patients.

Gastrointestinal disorders: ***Gastrointestinal bleeding***.

General disorders: Anaphylactoid reactions.

Hepato-billiary disorders: Abnormal LFT's.

Musculoskeletal disorders: Arthralgia.

Neurological disorders: Serotonin syndrome.

Psychiatric disorders: Hallucinations; mania; depersonalisation; panic attacks (these symptoms may be due to the underlying disease).

Cases of suicidal ideation and suicidal behaviours have been reported during citalopram therapy or early after treatment discontinuation (see section 4.4).

Reproductive disorders: Galactorrhoea.

Withdrawal symptoms seen on discontinuation of SSRI treatment

Discontinuation of citalopram (particularly when abrupt) commonly leads to withdrawal symptoms. Dizziness, sensory disturbances (including paraesthesia), sleep disturbances (including insomnia and intense dreams), agitation or anxiety, nausea and/or vomiting, tremor and headache are the most commonly reported reactions. Generally these events are mild to moderate and are self-limiting, however, in some patients they may be severe and/or prolonged. It is therefore advised that when citalopram treatment is no longer required, gradual discontinuation by dose tapering should be carried out (see section 4.2 Posology and Method of Administration and section 4.4 Special Warnings and Special Precautions for use).

4.9 Overdose

Fatal dose is not known. Patients have survived ingestion of more than 2 g citalopram.

The effects may be potentiated by alcohol taken at the same time.

Potential interaction with TCAs, MAOIs and other SSRIs.

Symptoms

Nausea, dizziness, tachycardia, tremor, drowsiness and somnolence may occur. At higher doses convulsions may occur within a few hours after ingestion. Hyperventilation, hyperpyrexia and coma have been reported.

ECG changes including nodal rhythm, prolonged QT intervals and wide QRS complexes may occur and rarely rhabdomyolysis. Fatalities have been reported.

Prolonged bradycardia with severe hypotension and syncope has also been reported.

Rarely, features of the "serotonin syndrome" may occur in severe poisoning. This includes alteration of mental status, neuromuscular hyperactivity and autonomic instability. There may be hyperpyrexia and elevation of serum creatine kinase. Rhabdomyolysis is rare.

Treatment

There is no specific antidote.

An ECG should be taken.

Consider oral activated charcoal in adults and children who have ingested more than 5 mg/kg body weight within 1 hour. Activated charcoal given ½ hour after ingestion of citalopram has been shown to reduce absorption by 50%.

Control convulsions with intravenous diazepam if they are frequent or prolonged

Management should be symptomatic and supportive and include the maintenance of a clear airway and monitoring of cardiac and vital signs until stable.

5. PHARMACOLOGICAL PROPERTIES

5.1 Pharmacodynamic properties

ATC-code: N 06 AB 04

Biochemical and behavioural studies have shown that citalopram is a potent inhibitor of the serotonin (5-HT)-uptake. Tolerance to the inhibition of 5-HT-uptake is not induced by long-term treatment with citalopram.

Citalopram is the most Selective Serotonin Reuptake Inhibitor (SSRI) yet described, with no, or minimal, effect on noradrenaline (NA), dopamine (DA) and gamma aminobutyric acid (GABA) uptake.

In contrast to many tricyclic antidepressants and some of the newer SSRI's, citalopram has not or very low affinity for a series of receptors including 5-HT $_{1A}$, 5-HT$_2$, DA D$_1$ and D$_2$ receptors, α_1-, α_2-, β-adrenoceptors, histamine H$_1$, muscarine cholinergic, benzodiazepine, and opioid receptors. A series of functional *in vitro* tests in isolated organs as well as functional *in vivo* tests have confirmed the lack of receptor affinity. This absence of effects on receptors could explain why citalopram produces fewer of the traditional side effects such as dry mouth, bladder and gut disturbance, blurred vision, sedation, cardiotoxicity and orthostatic hypotension.

Suppression of rapid eye movement (REM) sleep is considered a predictor of antidepressant activity. Like tricyclic antidepressants, other SSRI's and MAO inhibitors, citalopram suppresses REM-sleep and increases deep slow-wave sleep.

Although citalopram does not bind to opioid receptors it potentiates the anti-nociceptive effect of commonly used opioid analgesics. There was potentiation of d-amphetamine-induced hyperactivity following administration of citalopram.

The main metabolites of citalopram are all SSRIs although their potency and selectivity ratios are lower than those of citalopram. However, the selectivity ratios of the metabolites are higher than those of many of the newer SSRIs. The metabolites do not contribute to the overall antidepressant effect.

In humans citalopram does not impair cognitive (intellectual function) and psychomotor performance and has no or minimal sedative properties, either alone or in combination with alcohol.

Citalopram did not reduce saliva flow in a single dose study in human volunteers and in none of the studies in healthy volunteers did citalopram have significant influence on cardiovascular parameters. Citalopram has no effect on the serum levels of prolactin and growth hormone.

Dose response

In the fixed dose studies there is a flat dose response curve, providing no suggestion of advantage in terms of efficacy for using higher than the recommended doses. However, it is clinical experience that up-titrating the dose might be beneficial for some patients.

5.2 Pharmacokinetic properties

Absorption

Absorption is almost complete and independent of food intake (T_{max} mean 2 hours) after ingestion of drops and T_{max} mean 3 hours after intake of tablets. Oral bioavailability is about 80% after ingestion of tablets. Relative bioavailability of drops is approximately 25% greater than the tablets.

Distribution

The apparent volume of distribution $(V_d)_\beta$ is about 12.3 L/kg. The plasma protein binding is below 80% for citalopram and its main metabolites.

Biotransformation

Citalopram is metabolized to the active demethylcitalopram, didemethylcitalopram, citalopram-N-oxide and an inactive deaminated propionic acid derivative. All the active metabolites are also SSRIs, although weaker than the parent compound. Unchanged citalopram is the predominant compound in plasma.

Elimination

The elimination half-life ($T_{½β}$) is about 1.5 days and the systemic citalopram plasma clearance (Cl_s) is about 0.33 L/min, and oral plasma clearance (Cl_{oral}) is about 0.41 L/min.

Citalopram is excreted mainly via the liver (85%) and the remainder (15%) via the kidneys. About 12% of the daily dose is excreted in urine as unchanged citalopram. Hepatic (residual) clearance is about 0.35 L/min and renal clearance about 0.068 L/min.

The kinetics are linear. Steady state plasma levels are achieved in 1-2 weeks. Average concentrations of 250 nmol/L (100-500 nmol/L) are achieved at a daily dose of 40 mg. There is no clear relationship between citalopram plasma levels and therapeutic response or side effects.

Elderly patients (⩾ 65 years)

Longer half-lives and decreased clearance values due to a reduced rate of metabolism have been demonstrated in elderly patients.

Reduced hepatic function

Citalopram is eliminated more slowly in patients with reduced hepatic function. The half-life of citalopram is about twice as long and steady state citalopram concentrations at a given dose will be about twice as high as in patients with normal liver function.

Reduced renal function

Citalopram is eliminated more slowly in patients with mild to moderate reduction of renal function, without any major impact on the pharmacokinetics of citalopram. At present no information is available for treatment of patients with severely reduced renal function (creatinine clearance <20 mL/min).

5.3 Preclinical safety data

Citalopram has low acute toxicity. In chronic toxicity studies there were no findings of concern for the therapeutic use of citalopram. Based on data from reproduction toxicity studies (segment I, II and III) there is no reason to have special concern for the use of citalopram in women of child-bearing potential. Citalopram has no mutagenic or carcinogenic potential.

6. PHARMACEUTICAL PARTICULARS

6.1 List of excipients

Methyl-parahydroxybenzoate, propyl-parahydroxybenzoate, ethyl alcohol 9% v/v, hydroxyethylcellulose, purified water.

6.2 Incompatibilities

Cipramil Drops should only be mixed with water, orange juice or apple juice.

6.3 Shelf life

24 months (there is a "use by" date on the label).

A bottle may be used for 16 weeks after first use, if stored below 25°.

6.4 Special precautions for storage

None

6.5 Nature and contents of container

Brown glass bottle containing 15 ml with screw cap and polyethylene dropper. One bottle per carton.

6.6 Special precautions for disposal and other handling

Nil.

7. MARKETING AUTHORISATION HOLDER

Lundbeck Limited

Lundbeck House

Caldecotte Lake Business Park

Caldecotte

Milton Keynes

MK7 8LF

8. MARKETING AUTHORISATION NUMBER(S)

PL 0458/0071

9. DATE OF FIRST AUTHORISATION/RENEWAL OF THE AUTHORISATION

4 August 1998

10. DATE OF REVISION OF THE TEXT

11/08/2008

Legal category: POM

Legal category

POM

Cipramil Tablets

(Lundbeck Limited)

1. NAME OF THE MEDICINAL PRODUCT

Cipramil 10 mg film-coated tablets
Citalopram 10 mg film-coated tablets

Cipramil 20 mg film-coated tablets
Citalopram 20 mg film-coated tablets

Cipramil 40 mg film-coated tablets
Citalopram 40 mg film-coated tablets

2. QUALITATIVE AND QUANTITATIVE COMPOSITION

10 mg tablet: Each tablet contains 10 mg citalopram (as 12.49 mg citalopram hydrobromide).

20 mg tablet: Each tablet contains 20mg citalopram (as 24.98 mg citalopram hydrobromide).

40 mg tablet: Each tablet contains 40mg citalopram (as 49.96 mg citalopram hydrobromide).

For a full list of excipients see section 6.1

3. PHARMACEUTICAL FORM

Film-coated tablet

10 mg tablet: White, round, film-coated tablets marked "CL" on one side.

20 mg tablet: White, oval, scored, film-coated tablets marked "C" and "N" symmetrically around the score. The tablets can be divided into equal halves.

40 mg tablet: White, oval, scored, film-coated tablets marked "C" and "R" symmetrically around the score. The tablets can be divided into equal halves.

4. CLINICAL PARTICULARS

4.1 Therapeutic indications

Treatment of depressive illness in the initial phase and as maintenance against potential relapse/recurrence.

Cipramil/citalopram is also indicated in the treatment of panic disorder with or without agoraphobia.

4.2 Posology and method of administration

Posology

MAJOR DEPRESSIVE EPISODES

The recommended dose is 20 mg daily. In general improvement in patients starts after one week but may only become evident from the second week of therapy.

As with all antidepressant medicinal products, dosage should be reviewed and adjusted if necessary within 3 to 4 weeks of initiation of therapy and thereafter as judged clinically appropriate. Although there may be an increased potential for undesirable effects at higher doses, if after some weeks on the recommended dose insufficient response is seen some patients may benefit from having their dose increased up to a maximum of 60 mg a day in 20 mg steps according to the patient's response (see section 5.1). Dosage adjustments should be made carefully on an individual patient basis, to maintain the patient at the lowest effective dose.

Patients with depression should be treated for a sufficient period of at least 6 months to ensure that they are free from symptoms.

PANIC DISORDER

Patients should be started on 10 mg/day and the dose gradually increased in 10 mg steps according to the patient's response up to the recommended dose. The recommended dose is 20-30 mg daily. A low initial starting dose is recommended to minimise the potential worsening of panic symptoms, which is generally recognised to occur early in the treatment of this disorder. Although there may be an increased potential for undesirable effects at higher doses, if after some weeks on the recommended dose insufficient response is seen some patients may benefit from having their dose increased gradually up to a maximum of 60 mg /day (see section 5.1). Dosage adjustments should be made carefully on an individual patient basis, to maintain the patients at the lowest effective dose.

Patients with panic disorder should be treated for a sufficient period to ensure that they are free from symptoms. This period may be several months or even longer.

Elderly patients (> 65 years of age)

The recommended daily dose is 20 mg. Dependent on individual patient response this may be increased to a maximum of 40 mg daily.

Children and adolescents (< 18 years of age)

Citalopram should not be used in the treatment of children and adolescents under the age of 18 years (see section 4.4).

Reduced hepatic function

Dosage should be restricted to the lower end of the dose range.

Reduced renal function

Dosage adjustment is not necessary in cases of mild or moderate renal impairment. No information is available in cases of severe renal impairment (creatinine clearance <20 mL / min).

Withdrawal symptoms seen on discontinuation of citalopram

Abrupt discontinuation should be avoided. When stopping treatment with citalopram the dose should be gradually reduced over a period of at least one to two weeks in order to reduce the risk of withdrawal reactions (see section 4.4 Special Warnings and Special Precautions for Use and section 4.8 Undesirable Effects). If intolerable symptoms occur following a decrease in the dose or upon discontinuation of treatment, then resuming the previously prescribed dose may be considered. Subsequently, the physician may continue decreasing the dose, but at a more gradual rate.

Method of administration

Citalopram tablets are administered as a single daily dose. Citalopram tablets can be taken at any time of the day without regard to food intake.

4.3 Contraindications

Hypersensitivity to citalopram.

Monoamine Oxidase Inhibitors: Cases of serious and sometimes fatal reactions have been reported in patients receiving an SSRI in combination with monoamine oxidase inhibitor (MAOI), including the selective MAOI selegiline and the reversible MAOI (RIMA), moclobemide and in patients who have recently discontinued an SSRI and have been started on a MAOI.

Some cases presented with features resembling serotonin syndrome. Symptoms of a drug interaction with a MAOI include: hyperthermia, rigidity, myoclonus, autonomic instability with possible rapid fluctuations of vital signs, mental status changes that include confusion, irritability and extreme agitation progressing to delirium and coma.

Citalopram should not be used in combination with a MAOI. Citalopram may be started 14 days after discontinuing treatment with an irreversible MAOI and at least one day after discontinuing treatment with the reversible MAOI (RIMA), moclobemide. At least 7 days should elapse after discontinuing citalopram treatment before starting a MAOI or RIMA.

Concomitant treatment with pimozide (see section 4.5).

4.4 Special warnings and precautions for use
Suicide/suicidal thoughts or clinical worsening

Depression is associated with an increased risk of suicidal thoughts, self harm and suicide (suicide-related events). This risk persists until significant remission occurs. As improvement may not occur during the first few weeks or more of treatment, patients should be closely monitored until such improvement occurs. It is general clinical experience that the risk of suicide may increase in the early stages of recovery.

Other psychiatric conditions for which Cipramil is prescribed can also be associated with an increased risk of suicide-related events. In addition, these conditions may be co-morbid with major depressive disorder. The same precautions observed when treating patients with major depressive disorder should therefore be observed when treating patients with other psychiatric disorders.

Patients with a history of suicide-related events, or those exhibiting a significant degree of suicidal ideation prior to commencement of treatment are known to be at greater risk of suicidal thoughts or suicide attempts, and should receive careful monitoring during treatment. A meta-analysis of placebo-controlled clinical trials of antidepressant drugs in adult patients with psychiatric disorders showed an increased risk of suicidal behaviour with antidepressants compared to placebo in patients less than 25 years old.

Close supervision of patients and in particular those at high risk should accompany drug therapy especially in early treatment and following dose changes. Patients (and caregivers of patients) should be alerted about the need to monitor for any clinical worsening, suicidal behaviour or thoughts and unusual changes in behaviour and to seek medical advice immediately if these symptoms present.

Use in children and adolescents under 18 years of age

Cipramil should not be used in the treatment of children and adolescents under the age of 18 years. Suicide-related behaviours (suicide attempt and suicidal thoughts) and hostility (predominantly aggression, oppositional behaviour and anger) were more frequently observed in clinical trials among children and adolescents treated with antidepressants compared to those treated with placebo. If, based on clinical need, a decision to treat is nevertheless taken; the patient should be carefully monitored for the appearance of suicidal symptoms. In addition, long-term safety data in children and adolescents concerning growth, maturation and cognitive and behavioural development are lacking.

Serotonin syndrome

If citalopram is used concomitantly with medicinal products with serotonergic effects such as sumatriptan or other triptans, tramadol and tryptophan, caution is advisable. Rarely, the occurrence of "serotonin syndrome" has been reported in patients receiving SSRIs. A combination of symptoms, possibly including agitation, confusion, tremor, myoclonus and hyperthermia, may indicate the development of this condition (see section 4.5).

Hyponatraemia

Hyponatraemia, probably due to inappropriate antidiuretic hormone secretion (SIADH), has been reported as a rare adverse reaction with the use of SSRIs. Especially elderly female patients seem to be a risk group.

Diabetes

In patients with diabetes, treatment with an SSRI may alter glycaemic control, possibly due to improvement of depressive symptoms. Insulin and or oral hypoglycaemic dosage may need to be adjusted.

Seizures

Seizures are a potential risk with antidepressant drugs. The drug should be discontinued in any patient who develops seizures. Citalopram should be avoided in patients with unstable epilepsy and patients with controlled epilepsy should be carefully monitored. Citalopram should be discontinued if there is an increase in seizure frequency.

ECT

There is little clinical experience of concurrent administration of citalopram and ECT, therefore caution is advisable.

Mania

Citalopram should be used with caution in patients with a history of mania/hypomania. Citalopram should be discontinued in any patient entering a manic phase.

Haemorrhage

There have been reports of cutaneous bleeding abnormalities such as ecchymoses and purpura, as well as haemorrhagic manifestations e.g. gastrointestinal haemorrhage with SSRIs. The risk of gastrointestinal haemorrhage may be increased in elderly people during treatment with SSRIs. Caution is advised in patients taking SSRIs, particularly in concomitant use with drugs known to affect platelet function (e.g. atypical antipsychotics and phenothiazines, most tricyclic antidepressants, aspirin and non-steroidal anti-inflammatory drugs (NSAIDs) as well as in patients with a history of bleeding disorders.

Experience with citalopram has not revealed any clinically relevant interactions with neuroleptics. However, as with other SSRIs, the possibility of a pharmacodynamic interaction cannot be excluded.

Consideration should be given to factors which may affect the disposition of a minor metabolite of citalopram (didemethylcitalopram) since increased levels of this metabolite could theoretically prolong the QTc interval in susceptible individuals. However, in ECG monitoring of 2500 patients in clinical trials, including 277 patients with pre-existing cardiac conditions, no clinically significant changes were noted.

Some patients with panic disorder experience an initial anxiogenic effect when starting pharmacotherapy. A low starting dose (see Posology) reduces the likelihood of this effect.

Glaucoma

As with other SSRIs, citalopram can cause mydriasis and should be used with caution in patients with narrow angle glaucoma or history of glaucoma.

Akathisia/psychomotor restlessness

The use of citalopram has been associated with the development of akathisia, characterised by a subjectively unpleasant or distressing restlessness and need to move often accompanied by an inability to sit or stand still. This is most likely to occur within the first few weeks of treatment. In patients who develop these symptoms, increasing the dose may be detrimental.

Withdrawal symptoms seen on discontinuation of SSRI treatment

Withdrawal symptoms when treatment is discontinued are common, particularly if discontinuation is abrupt (see section 4.8 Undesirable effects). In clinical trials adverse events seen on treatment discontinuation occurred in approximately 40% of patients treated with citalopram.

The risk of withdrawal symptoms may be dependent on several factors including the duration and dose of therapy and the rate of dose reduction. Dizziness, sensory disturbances (including paraesthesia), sleep disturbances (including insomnia and intense dreams), agitation or anxiety, nausea and/or vomiting, tremor and headache are the most commonly reported reactions. Generally these symptoms are mild to moderate, however, in some patients they may be severe in intensity. They usually occur within the first few days of discontinuing treatment, but there have been very rare reports of such symptoms in patients who have inadvertently missed a dose. Generally these symptoms are self-limiting and usually resolve within 2 weeks, though in some individuals they may be prolonged (2-3 months or more). It is therefore advised that citalopram should be gradually tapered when discontinuing treatment over a period of several weeks or months, according to the patient's needs (see "Withdrawal symptoms seen on discontinuation of citalopram", Section 4.2 Posology and Method of Administration)

Excipients

The tablets contain lactose monohydrate. Patients with rare hereditary problems of galactose intolerance, the Lapp deficiency or glucose-galactose malabsorption should not receive this medicine.

4.5 Interaction with other medicinal products and other forms of interaction

Monoamine Oxidase Inhibitors (MAOIs) should not be used in combination with SSRIs (see Contraindications).

The metabolism of citalopram is only partly dependent on the hepatic cytochrome P450 isozyme CYP2D6 and, unlike some other SSRIs, citalopram is only a weak inhibitor of this important enzyme system which is involved in the metabolism of many drugs (including antiarrhythmics, neuroleptics, beta-blockers, TCAs and some SSRIs). Protein binding is relatively low (<80%). These properties give citalopram a low potential for clinically significant drug interactions.

Alcohol – The combination of citalopram and alcohol is not advisable. However clinical studies have revealed no adverse pharmacodynamic interactions between citalopram and alcohol.

Serotonergic drugs – Co administration with serotonergic drugs (e.g. tramadol, sumatriptan) may lead to enhancement of 5-HT associated effects.

Lithium & tryptophan – There is no pharmacokinetic interaction between lithium and citalopram. However there are have been reports of enhanced effects when SSRIs have been given with lithium or tryptophan and therefore the concomitant use of citalopram with these drugs should be undertaken with caution. Routine monitoring of lithium levels need not be adjusted.

In a pharmacokinetic study no affect was demonstrated on either citalopram or imipramine levels, although the level of desipramine, the primary metabolite of imipramine, was increased. In animal studies cimetidine had little or no influence on citalopram kinetics.

Dynamic interactions between citalopram and herbal remedy St John's Wort (*Hypericum perforatum*) can occur, resulting in an increase in undesirable effects.

A pharmacokinetic/pharmacodynamic interaction study in healthy volunteers with concomitant administration of citalopram and metoprolol (a CYP2D6 substrate) showed a twofold increase in metoprolol concentrations, but no statistically significant increase in the effect of metoprolol on blood pressure and heart rate.

No pharmacodynamic interactions have been noted in clinical studies in which citalopram has been given concomitantly with benzodiazepines, neuroleptics, analgesics, lithium, alcohol, antihistamines, antihypertensive drugs, beta-blockers and other cardiovascular drugs

Pimozide

Co administration of a single dose of pimozide 2 mg to subjects treated with racemic citalopram 40 mg/day for 11 days caused an increase in AUC and Cmax of pimozide, although not consistently throughout the study. The co-administration of pimozide and citalopram resulted in a mean increase in the QTc interval of approximately 10 msec. Due to the interaction noted at a low dose of pimozide, concomitant administration of citalopram and pimozide is contraindicated.

4.6 Pregnancy and lactation

Pregnancy

Animal studies did not provide any evidence of teratogenicity, however the safety of citalopram during human pregnancy has not been established. As with all drugs citalopram should only be used in pregnancy if the potential benefits of treatment to the mother outweigh the possible risks to the developing foetus.

Neonates should be observed if maternal use of citalopram continues into the later stages of pregnancy, particularly in the third trimester. Abrupt discontinuation should be avoided during pregnancy.

The following symptoms may occur in the neonates after maternal SSRI/SNRI use in later stages of pregnancy: respiratory distress, cyanosis, apnoea, seizures, temperature instability, feeding difficulty, vomiting, hypoglycaemia, hypertonia, hypotonia, hyperreflexia, tremor, jitteriness, irritability, lethargy, constant crying, somnolence and difficulty sleeping. These symptoms could be due to either serotonergic effects or discontinuation symptoms. In a majority of instances the complications begin immediately or soon (<24 hours) after delivery.

Lactation

Citalopram is known to be excreted in breast milk. Its effects on the nursing infant have not been established. If treatment with citalopram is considered necessary, discontinuation of breast feeding should be considered.

4.7 Effects on ability to drive and use machines

Citalopram does not impair intellectual function and psychomotor performance. However, patients who are prescribed psychotropic medication may be expected to have some impairment of general attention and concentration either due to the illness itself, the medication or both and should be cautioned about their ability to drive a car and operate machinery.

4.8 Undesirable effects

Adverse effects observed with citalopram are in general mild and transient. They are most prominent during the first one or two weeks of treatment and usually attenuate as the depressive state improves.

The most commonly observed adverse events associated with the use of citalopram and not seen at an equal incidence among placebo-treated patients were: nausea, somnolence, dry mouth, increased sweating and tremor. The incidence of each in excess over placebo is low (<10%).

In comparative clinical trials with tricyclic antidepressants the incidence of adverse events occurring with citalopram was found to be lower in all cases.

Withdrawal reactions have been reported in association with selective serotonin reuptake inhibitors (SSRIs), including Cipramil. Common symptoms include dizziness, paraesthesia, headache, anxiety and nausea. Abrupt discontinuation of treatment with Cipramil should be avoided. The majority of symptoms experienced on withdrawal of SSRIs are non-serious and self-limiting.

Treatment emergent adverse events reported in clinical trials (N=2985):

Frequent ($\geqslant$5 - 20%)

Increased sweating, headache, tremor, dizziness, abnormal accommodation, somnolence, insomnia, agitation, nervousness, nausea, dry mouth, constipation, diarrhoea, palpitation, asthenia.

Less frequent (1 - <5%)

Rash, pruritus, paraesthesia, migraine, abnormal vision, taste perversion, sleep disorder, decreased libido, impaired concentration, abnormal dreaming, amnesia, anxiety, increased appetite, anorexia, apathy, impotence, suicide attempt, confusion, dyspepsia, vomiting, abdominal pain, flatulence, increased salivation, weight decrease, weight increase, postural hypotension, tachycardia, rhinitis, micturition disorder, polyuria, ejaculation failure, female anorgasmia, fatigue, eye disorders (visual disturbance, mydriasis (which may lead to acute narrow angle glaucoma), see section 4.4 Special warnings and precautions for use).

Rare (<1%)

Myalgia, movement disorders, convulsions, tinnitus, euphoria, increased libido, coughing, malaise. Psychomotor restlessness/akathisia (see section 4.4 Special Warnings and Special Precautions for Use)

Post Marketing - The following adverse reactions apply to the therapeutic class of SSRIs

Skin Disorders: Angiodema; ecchymoses. Photosensitivity reactions have been reported very rarely.

Disorders of metabolism and nutrition: Rare cases of hyponatraemia and inappropriate ADH secretion have been reported and appear to be reversible on discontinuation. The majority of the reports were associated with the older patients.

Gastrointestinal disorders: Gastrointestinal bleeding.

General disorders: Anaphylactoid reactions.

Hepato-billiary disorders: Abnormal LFT's.

Musculoskeletal disorders: Arthralgia.

Neurological disorders: Serotonin syndrome.

Psychiatric disorders: Hallucinations; mania; depersonalisation; panic attacks (these symptoms may be due to the underlying disease).

Cases of suicidal ideation and suicidal behaviours have been reported during citalopram therapy or early after treatment discontinuation (see section 4.4).

Reproductive disorders: Galactorrhoea.

Withdrawal symptoms seen on discontinuation of SSRI treatment

Discontinuation of citalopram (particularly when abrupt) commonly leads to withdrawal symptoms. Dizziness, sensory disturbances (including paraesthesia), sleep disturbances (including insomnia and intense dreams), agitation or anxiety, nausea and/or vomiting, tremor and headache are the most commonly reported reactions. Generally these events are mild to moderate and are self-limiting, however, in some patients they may be severe and/or prolonged. It is therefore advised that when citalopram treatment is no longer required, gradual discontinuation by dose tapering should be carried out (see section 4.2 Posology and Method of Administration and section 4.4 Special Warnings and Special Precautions for use).

4.9 Overdose

Fatal dose is not known. Patients have survived ingestion of more than 2 g citalopram.

The effects may be potentiated by alcohol taken at the same time.

Potential interaction with TCAs, MAOIs and other SSRIs.

Symptoms

Nausea, dizziness, tachycardia, tremor, drowsiness and somnolence may occur. At higher doses convulsions may occur within a few hours after ingestion. Hyperventilation, hyperpyrexia and coma have been reported.

ECG changes including nodal rhythm, prolonged QT intervals and wide QRS complexes may occur and rarely rhabdomyolysis. Fatalities have been reported.

Prolonged bradycardia with severe hypotension and syncope has also been reported.

Rarely, features of the "serotonin syndrome" may occur in severe poisoning. This includes alteration of mental status, neuromuscular hyperactivity and autonomic instability. There may be hyperpyrexia and elevation of serum creatine kinase. Rhabdomyolysis is rare.

Treatment

There is no specific antidote.

An ECG should be taken.

Consider oral activated charcoal in adults and children who have ingested more than 5 mg/kg body weight within 1 hour. Activated charcoal given ½ hour after ingestion of citalopram has been shown to reduce absorption by 50%.

Control convulsions with intravenous diazepam if they are frequent or prolonged

Management should be symptomatic and supportive and include the maintenance of a clear airway and monitoring of cardiac and vital signs until stable.

5. PHARMACOLOGICAL PROPERTIES

5.1 Pharmacodynamic properties

ATC-code: N 06 AB 04

Biochemical and behavioural studies have shown that citalopram is a potent inhibitor of the serotonin (5-HT)-uptake. Tolerance to the inhibition of 5-HT-uptake is not induced by long-term treatment with citalopram.

Citalopram is the most Selective Serotonin Reuptake Inhibitor (SSRI) yet described, with no, or minimal, effect on noradrenaline (NA), dopamine (DA) and gamma aminobutyric acid (GABA) uptake.

In contrast to many tricyclic antidepressants and some of the newer SSRIs, citalopram has no or very low affinity for a series of receptors including 5-HT $_{1A}$, 5-HT$_2$, DA D$_1$ and D$_2$ receptors, α_1-, α_2-, β-adrenoceptors, histamine H$_1$, muscarine cholinergic, benzodiazepine, and opioid receptors. A series of functional *in vitro* tests in isolated organs as well as functional *in vivo* tests have confirmed the lack of receptor affinity. This absence of effects on receptors could explain why citalopram produces fewer of the traditional side effects such as dry mouth, bladder and gut disturbance, blurred vision, sedation, cardiotoxicity and orthostatic hypotension.

Suppression of rapid eye movement (REM) sleep is considered a predictor of antidepressant activity. Like tricyclic antidepressants, other SSRI's and MAO inhibitors, citalopram suppresses REM-sleep and increases deep slow-wave sleep.

Although citalopram does not bind to opioid receptors it potentiates the anti-nociceptive effect of commonly used opioid analgesics. There was potentiation of d-amphetamine-induced hyperactivity following administration of citalopram.

The main metabolites of citalopram are all SSRIs although their potency and selectivity ratios are lower than those of citalopram. However, the selectivity ratios of the metabolites are higher than those of many of the newer SSRIs. The metabolites do not contribute to the overall antidepressant effect.

In humans citalopram does not impair cognitive (intellectual function) and psychomotor performance and has no or minimal sedative properties, either alone or in combination with alcohol.

Citalopram did not reduce saliva flow in a single dose study in human volunteers and in none of the studies in healthy volunteers did citalopram have significant influence on cardiovascular parameters. Citalopram has no effect on the serum levels of prolactin and growth hormone.

Dose response

In the fixed dose studies there is a flat dose response curve, providing no suggestion of advantage in terms of efficacy for using higher than the recommended doses. However, it is clinical experience that up-titrating the dose might be beneficial for some patients.

5.2 Pharmacokinetic properties

Absorption

Absorption is almost complete and independent of food intake (T_{max}average/mean 3.8 hours). Oral bioavailability is about 80%.

Distribution

The apparent volume of distribution $(V_d)_\beta$ is about 12.3 L/kg. The plasma protein binding is below 80% for citalopram and its main metabolites.

Biotransformation

Citalopram is metabolized to the active demethylcitalopram, didemethylcitalopram, citalopram-N-oxide and an inactive deaminated propionic acid derivative. All the active metabolites are also SSRIs, although weaker than the parent compound. Unchanged citalopram is the predominant compound in plasma.

Elimination

The elimination half-life ($T_{½\beta}$) is about 1.5 days and the systemic citalopram plasma clearance (Cl_s) is about 0.33 L/min, and oral plasma clearance (Cl_{oral}) is about 0.41 L/min.

Citalopram is excreted mainly via the liver (85%) and the remainder (15%) via the kidneys. About 12% of the daily dose is excreted in urine as unchanged citalopram. Hepatic (residual) clearance is about 0.35 L/min and renal clearance about 0.068 L/min.

The kinetics are linear. Steady state plasma levels are achieved in 1-2 weeks. Average concentrations of 250 nmol/L (100-500 nmol/L) are achieved at a daily dose of 40 mg. There is no clear relationship between citalopram plasma levels and therapeutic response or side effects.

Elderly patients ($\geqslant$ 65 years)

Longer half-lives and decreased clearance values due to a reduced rate of metabolism have been demonstrated in elderly patients.

Reduced hepatic function

Citalopram is eliminated more slowly in patients with reduced hepatic function. The half-life of citalopram is about twice as long and steady state citalopram concentrations at a given dose will be about twice as high as in patients with normal liver function.

Reduced renal function

Citalopram is eliminated more slowly in patients with mild to moderate reduction of renal function, without any major impact on the pharmacokinetics of citalopram. At present no information is available for treatment of patients with severely reduced renal function (creatinine clearance <20 mL/min).

5.3 Preclinical safety data

Citalopram has low acute toxicity. In chronic toxicity studies there were no findings of concern for the therapeutic use of citalopram. Based on data from reproduction toxicity studies (segment I, II and III) there is no reason to have special concern for the use of citalopram in women of child-bearing potential. Citalopram has no mutagenic or carcinogenic potential.

6. PHARMACEUTICAL PARTICULARS

6.1 List of excipients

Tablets: Maize starch, Lactose, Microcrystalline-cellulose, Copolyvidone, Glycerol, Croscarmellose Sodium Type A, Magnesium stearate, Methylhydroxypropyl-cellulose, Macrogol, Titanium dioxide.

6.2 Incompatibilities

None.

6.3 Shelf life

Each pack has an expiry date.

Citalopram tablets are valid for 5 years

6.4 Special precautions for storage

Do not store above 25°C

6.5 Nature and contents of container

Press through packs (UPVC/PVdC with aluminium closure) 28 tablets.

6.6 Special precautions for disposal and other handling

Nil.

7. MARKETING AUTHORISATION HOLDER

Lundbeck Limited

Lundbeck House

Caldecotte Lake Business Park

Caldecotte

Milton Keynes

MK7 8LF

(Manufacturer: H. Lundbeck A/S, DK-2500 Copenhagen-Valby, Denmark)

8. MARKETING AUTHORISATION NUMBER(S)

Cipramil 10 mg film-coated tablets PL 0458/0057
Citalopram 10 mg film-coated tablets

Cipramil 20 mg film-coated tablets PL 0458/0058
Citalopram 20 mg film-coated tablets

Cipramil 40mg film-coated tablets PL 0458/0059
Citalopram 40 mg film-coated tablets

9. DATE OF FIRST AUTHORISATION/RENEWAL OF THE AUTHORISATION

First authorisation: 17 March 1995

Renewal of authorisation: 24 August 2001

10. DATE OF REVISION OF THE TEXT

18/09/2009

Legal category: POM

Circadin 2mg prolonged-release tablets

(Lundbeck Limited)

1. NAME OF THE MEDICINAL PRODUCT

Circadin ▼ 2 mg prolonged-release tablets

2. QUALITATIVE AND QUANTITATIVE COMPOSITION

Each prolonged-release tablet contains 2 mg melatonin.

Excipient: each prolonged-release tablet contains 80 mg lactose monohydrate.

For a full list of excipients, see section 6.1.

3. PHARMACEUTICAL FORM

Prolonged-release tablet.

White to off-white, round, biconvex tablets

4. CLINICAL PARTICULARS

4.1 Therapeutic indications

Circadin is indicated as monotherapy for the short-term treatment of primary insomnia characterised by poor quality of sleep in patients who are aged 55 or over.

4.2 Posology and method of administration

Oral use. Tablets should be swallowed whole.

The recommended dose is 2 mg once daily, 1-2 hours before bedtime and after food. This dosage should be continued for three weeks.

Paediatric use

Circadin is not recommended for use in children and adolescents below age 18 due to insufficient data on safety and efficacy.

Renal insufficiency

The effect of any stage of renal insufficiency on melatonin pharmacokinetics has not been studied. Caution should be used when melatonin is administered to such patients.

Hepatic impairment

There is no experience of the use of Circadin in patients with liver impairment. Published data demonstrates markedly elevated endogenous melatonin levels during daytime hours due to decreased clearance in patients with hepatic impairment. Therefore, Circadin is not recommended for use in patients with hepatic impairment.

4.3 Contraindications

Hypersensitivity to the active substance or to any of the excipients.

4.4 Special warnings and precautions for use

Circadin may cause drowsiness. Therefore the product should be used with caution if the effects of drowsiness are likely to be associated with a risk to safety.

No clinical data exist concerning the use of Circadin in individuals with autoimmune diseases. Therefore Circadin is not recommended for use in patients with autoimmune diseases.

Patients with rare hereditary problems of galactose intolerance, the LAPP lactase deficiency or glucose-galactose malabsorption should not take this medicine.

4.5 Interaction with other medicinal products and other forms of interaction

Pharmacokinetic interactions

- Melatonin has been observed to induce CYP3A in vitro at supra-therapeutic concentrations. The clinical relevance of the finding is unknown. If induction occurs, this can give rise to reduced plasma concentrations of concomitantly administered drugs.
- Melatonin does not induce CYP1A enzymes in vitro at supra-therapeutic concentrations. Therefore, interactions between melatonin and other active substances as a consequence of melatonin's effect on CYP1A enzymes are not likely to be significant.
- Melatonin's metabolism is mainly mediated by CYP1A enzymes. Therefore, interactions between melatonin and other active substances as a consequence of their effect on CYP1A enzymes is possible.
- Caution should be exercised in patients on fluvoxamine, which increases melatonin levels (by 17-fold higher AUC and a 12-fold higher serum C_{max}) by inhibiting its metabolism by hepatic cytochrome P450 (CYP) isozymes CYP1A2 and CYP2C19. The combination should be avoided.
- Caution should be exercised in patients on 5- or 8-methoxypsoralen (5 and 8-MOP), which increases melatonin levels by inhibiting its metabolism.
- Caution should be exercised in patients on cimetidine a CYP2D inhibitor, which increases plasma melatonin levels, by inhibiting its metabolism.
- Cigarette smoking may decrease melantonin levels due to induction of CYP1A2.
- Caution should be exercised in patients on oestrogens (e.g. contraceptive or hormone replacement therapy), which increase melatonin levels by inhibiting its metabolism by CYP1A1 and CYP1A2.
- CYP1A2 inhibitors such as quinolones may give rise to increased melatonin exposure.
- CYP1A2 inducers such as carbamazepine and rifampicin may give rise to reduced plasma concentrations of melatonin.
- There is a large amount of data in the literature regarding the effect of adrenergic agonists/antagonists, opiate agonists/antagonists, antidepressant medicinal products, prostaglandin inhibitors, benzodiazepines, tryptophan and alcohol, on endogenous melatonin secretion. Whether or not these active substances interfere with the dynamic or kinetic effects of Circadin or vice versa has not been studied.

Pharmacodynamic interactions

- Alcohol should not be taken with Circadin, because it reduces the effectiveness of Circadin on sleep.
- Circadin may enhance the sedative properties of benzodiazepines and non-benzodiazepine hypnotics, such as zalepon, zolpidem and zopiclone. In a clinical trial, there was clear evidence for a transitory pharmacodynamic interaction between Circadin and zolpidem one hour following co-dosing. Concomitant administration resulted in increased impairment of attention, memory and co-ordination compared to zolpidem alone.
- Circadin has been co-administered in studies with thioridazine and imipramine, active substances which affect the central nervous system. No clinically significant pharmacokinetic interactions were found in each case. However, Circadin co-administration resulted in increased feelings of tranquility and difficulty in performing tasks compared to imipramine alone, and increased feelings of "muzzy-headedness" compared to thioridazine alone.

4.6 Pregnancy and lactation

For melatonin, no clinical data on exposed pregnancies are available. Animal studies do not indicate direct or indirect harmful effects with respect to pregnancy, embryonal/foetal development, parturition or postnatal development (see section 5.3). In view of the lack of clinical data, use in pregnant women and by women intended to become pregnant is not recommended.

Endogenous melatonin was measured in human breast milk thus exogenous melatonin is probably secreted into human milk. There are data in animal models including rodents, sheep, bovine and primates that indicate maternal transfer of melatonin to the foetus via the placenta or in the milk. Therefore, breast-feeding is not recommended in women under treatment with melatonin.

4.7 Effects on ability to drive and use machines

Circadin has moderate influence on the ability to drive and use machines. Circadin may cause drowsiness, therefore the product should be used with caution if the effects of drowsiness are likely to be associated with a risk to safety.

4.8 Undesirable effects

In clinical trials (in which a total of 1361 patients were taking Circadin and 1247 patients were taking placebo), 37.0% of patients receiving Circadin reported an adverse reaction compared with 31.8% taking placebo. Comparing the rate of patients with adverse reactions per 100 patient weeks, the rate was higher for placebo than Circadin (8.21 – placebo vs. 3.17 – Circadin). The most common adverse reactions were headache, pharyngitis, back pain, and asthenia, which were common, by MedDRA definition, in both the Circadin and placebo treated groups.

The following adverse reactions were reported in clinical trials and were defined as possibly, probably or definitely related to treatment. A total of 6.9% of subjects receiving Circadin reported an adverse reaction compared with 5.9% of subjects taking placebo. Only those adverse events occurring in subjects at an equivalent or greater rate than placebo have been included below.

Within each frequency grouping, undesirable effects are presented in order of decreasing seriousness.

Very common (≥ 1/10); Common (≥ 1/100 to <1/10); Uncommon (≥ 1/1,000 to <1/100); Rare (≥ 1/10,000 to <1/1,000); Very rare (<1/10,000), Not known (cannot be established from the available data).

(see Table 1 below)

4.9 Overdose

No case of overdose has been reported. Circadin has been administered at 5 mg daily doses in clinical trials over 12 months without significantly changing the nature of the adverse reactions reported.

Administration of daily doses of up to 300 mg of melatonin without causing clinically significant adverse reactions have been reported in the literature.

If overdose occurs, drowsiness is to be expected. Clearance of the active substance is expected within 12 hours after ingestion. No special treatment is required.

5. PHARMACOLOGICAL PROPERTIES

5.1 Pharmacodynamic properties

Pharmacotherapeutic group: Melatonin Receptor Agonists, ATC code: N05CH01

Melatonin is a naturally occurring hormone produced by the pineal gland and is structurally related to serotonin. Physiologically, melatonin secretion increases soon after the onset of darkness, peaks at 2-4 am and diminishes during the second half of the night. Melatonin is associated with the control of circadian rhythms and entrainment to the light-dark cycle. It is also associated with a hypnotic effect and increased propensity for sleep.

Mechanism of action

The activity of melatonin at the MT1, MT2 and MT3 receptors is believed to contribute to its sleep-promoting properties, as these receptors (mainly MT1 and MT2) are involved in the regulation of circadian rhythms and sleep regulation.

Rationale for use

Because of the role of melatonin in sleep and circadian rhythm regulation, and the age related decrease in endogenous melatonin production, melatonin may effectively improve sleep quality particularly in patients who are over 55 with primary insomnia.

Clinical efficacy

In clinical trials, where patients suffering from primary insomnia received Circadin 2 mg every evening for 3 weeks, benefits were shown in treated patients compared to placebo in sleep latency (as measured by objective and subjective means) and in subjective quality of sleep and daytime functioning (restorative sleep) with no impairment of vigilance during the day.

In a polysomnographic (PSG) study with a run-in of 2 weeks (single-blind with placebo treatment), followed by a

Table 1

System Organ Class	Very Common	Common	Uncommon	Rare
Infections and Infestations				Herpes zoster
Blood and Lymphatic System Disorders				Leukopenia, Thrombocytopenia
Metabolism and Nutrition Disorders				Hypertriglyceridaemia
Psychiatric Disorders			Irritability, Nervousness, Restlessness, Insomnia, Abnormal dreams	Mood altered, Aggression, Agitation, Crying, Early morning awakening, Libido increased
Nervous System Disorders			Migraine, Psychomotor hyperactivity, Dizziness, Somnolence	Memory impairment, Disturbance in attention, Poor quality sleep
Eye Disorders				Visual acuity reduced, Vision blurred, Lacrimation increased
Ear and Labyrinth Disorders				Vertigo positional
Vascular Disorders				Hot flush
Gastrointestinal Disorders			Abdominal pain, Constipation, Dry mouth	Gastrointestinal disorder, Gastrointestinal upset, Vomiting, Bowel sounds abnormal, Flatulence, Salivary hypersecretion, Halitosis
Hepatobiliary Disorders			Hyperbilirubinaemia	Hepatic enzyme increased, Liver function test abnormal, laboratory test abnormal
Skin and Subcutaneous Tissue Disorders			Hyperhidrosis	Eczema, Erythema, Rash pruritic, Pruritus, Dry skin, Nail disorder, Night sweats,
Musculoskeletal and Connective Tissue Disorders				Muscle cramp, Neck pain
Reproductive System and Breast Disorders				Priapism
General Disorders and Administration Site Conditions			Asthenia	Fatigue
Investigations			Weight increased	

treatment period of 3 weeks (double-blind, placebo-controlled, parallel group design) and a 3-week withdrawal period, sleep latency (SL) was shortened by 9 minutes compared to placebo. There were no modifications of sleep architecture and no effect on REM sleep duration by Circadin. Modifications in diurnal functioning did not occur with Circadin 2 mg.

In an outpatient study with 2 week run-in baseline period with placebo, a randomised, double blind, placebo controlled, parallel group treatment period of 3 weeks and 2 week withdrawal period with placebo, the rate of patients who showed a clinically significant improvement in both quality of sleep and morning alertness was 47% in the Circadin group as compared to 27% in the placebo group. In addition, quality of sleep and morning alertness significantly improved with Circadin compared to placebo. Sleep variables gradually returned to baseline with no rebound, no increase in adverse events and no increase in withdrawal symptoms.

In a second outpatient study with two week run in baseline period with placebo and a randomised, double blind, placebo controlled, parallel group treatment period of 3 weeks, the rate of patients who showed a clinically significant improvement in both quality of sleep and morning alertness was 26% in the Circadin group as compared to 15% in the placebo group. Circadin shortened patients' reported sleep latency by 24.3 minutes vs 12.9 minutes with placebo. In addition, patients' self-reported quality of sleep, number of awakenings and morning alertness significantly improved with Circadin compared to placebo. Quality of life was improved significantly with Circadin 2 mg compared to placebo.

5.2 Pharmacokinetic properties

Absorption

The absorption of orally ingested melatonin is complete in adults and may be decreased by up to 50% in the elderly. The kinetics of melatonin are linear over the range of 2-8 mg.

Bioavailability is in the order of 15%. There is a significant first pass effect with an estimated first pass metabolism of 85%. T_{max} occurs after 3 hours in a fed state. The rate of melatonin absorption and C_{max} following Circadin 2 mg oral administration is affected by food. The presence of food delayed the absorption of the melatonin resulting in a later (T_{max}=3.0 h versus T_{max}=0.75 h) and lower peak plasma concentration in the fed state (C_{max}=1020pg/ml versus C_{max}=1176 pg/ml).

Distribution

The in vitro plasma protein binding of melatonin is approximately 60%. Circadin is mainly bound to albumin, alpha$_1$-acid glycoprotein and high density lipoprotein.

Biotransformation

Experimental data suggest that isoenzymes CYP1A1, CYP1A2 and possibly CYP2C19 of the cytochrome P450 system are involved in melatonin metabolism. The principal metabolite is 6-sulphatoxy-melatonin (6-S-MT), which is inactive. The site of biotransformation is the liver. The excretion of the metabolite is completed within 12 hours after ingestion.

Elimination

Terminal half life ($t_{½}$) is 3.5-4 hours. Elimination is by renal excretion of metabolites, 89% as sulphated and glucoronide conjugates of 6-hydroxymelatonin and 2% is excreted as melatonin (unchanged drug).

Gender

A 3-4-fold increase in C_{max} is apparent for women compared to men. A five-fold variability in C_{max} between different members of the same sex has also been observed. However, no pharmacodynamic differences between males and females were found despite differences in blood levels.

Special populations

Elderly

Melatonin metabolism is known to decline with age. Across a range of doses, higher AUC and C_{max} levels have been reported in older subjects compared to younger subjects, reflecting the lower metabolism of melatonin in the elderly. C_{max} levels around 500 pg/ml in adults (18-45) versus 1200 pg/ml in elderly (55-69); AUC levels around 3,000 pg*h/mL in adults versus 5,000 pg*h/mL in the elderly.

Renal impairment

Company data indicates that there is no accumulation of melatonin after repeated dosing. This finding is compatible with the short half-life of melatonin in humans.

The levels assessed in the blood of the patients at 23:00 (2 hours after administration) following 1 and 3 weeks of daily administration were 411.4 ± 56.5 and 432.00 ± 83.2 pg/ml respectively, and are similar to those found in in healthy volunteers following a single dose of Circadin 2 mg.

Hepatic impairment

The liver is the primary site of melatonin metabolism and therefore, hepatic impairment results in higher endogenous melatonin levels.

Plasma melatonin levels in patients with cirrhosis were significantly increased during daylight hours. Patients had a significantly decreased total excretion of 6-sulfatoxymelatonin compared with controls.

5.3 Preclinical safety data

Non-clinical data revealed no special hazard for humans based on conventional studies of safety pharmacology, repeated dose toxicity and genotoxicity.

The No Observed Adverse Effect Level (NOAEL) at 15 mg/kg/day in rats, is equivalent to an AUC which is considerably higher (x 15000) than the human exposure after ingestion of Circadin 2 mg.

The carcinogenicity study in the rat did not reveal any effect which may be relevant for humans.

In reproductive toxicology, oral administration of melatonin in pregnant female mice, rats or rabbits did not result in adverse effects on their offspring, measured in terms of foetal viability, skeletal and visceral abnormalities, sex ratio, birthweight and subsequent physical, functional and sexual development. A slight effect on post-natal growth and viability was found in rats only at very high doses, equivalent to approximately 2000 mg/day in humans.

6. PHARMACEUTICAL PARTICULARS

6.1 List of excipients

Ammonio methacrylate copolymer type B

Calcium hydrogen phosphate dihydrate

Lactose monohydrate

Silica, colloidal anhydrous

Talc

Magnesium stearate

6.2 Incompatibilities

Not applicable.

6.3 Shelf life

5 years

6.4 Special precautions for storage

Do not store above 25°C. Store in the original package in order to protect from light.

6.5 Nature and contents of container

The tablets are packed in PVC/PVDC opaque blister strips with aluminium foil backing. The pack consists of one blister strip containing 20 or 21 tablets. The blisters are then packed in cardboard boxes.

Not all pack sizes may be marketed.

6.6 Special precautions for disposal and other handling

Medicines no longer required should not be disposed of via wastewater or the municipal sewage system. Return them to a pharmacy or ask your pharmacist how to dispose of them in accordance with the national regulations. These measures will help to protect the environment.

7. MARKETING AUTHORISATION HOLDER

RAD Neurim Pharmaceuticals EEC Limited

One Forbury Square

The Forbury

Reading

Berkshire RG1 3EB

United Kingdom

e-mail: neurim@neurim.com

8. MARKETING AUTHORISATION NUMBER(S)

EU/1/07/392/001

EU/1/07/392/002

9. DATE OF FIRST AUTHORISATION/RENEWAL OF THE AUTHORISATION

29/06/2007

10. DATE OF REVISION OF THE TEXT

19/03/2009

Detailed information on this product is available on the website of the European Medicines Agency (EMEA) http://www.emea.europa.eu

Cisplatin 50mg Freeze Dried Powder for Injection (Pharmacia Limited)

(Pharmacia Limited)

1. NAME OF THE MEDICINAL PRODUCT

Cisplatin 50

2. QUALITATIVE AND QUANTITATIVE COMPOSITION

Cisplatin 50.0mg

3. PHARMACEUTICAL FORM

Yellowish-white, freeze-dried cake in vials containing 50 mg cisplatin.

4. CLINICAL PARTICULARS

4.1 Therapeutic indications

Cisplatin has antitumour activity either as a single agent or in combination chemotherapy particularly in the treatment of testicular and metastatic ovarian tumours, also cervical tumours, lung carcinoma and bladder cancer.

4.2 Posology and method of administration

Route of administration: Intravenous infusion.

Cisplatin should be dissolved in water for injections such that the reconstituted solution contains 1 mg/ml of Cisplatin. This solution should then be diluted in 2 litres of 0.9% saline or a dextrose/saline solution (to which 37.5 g of mannitol may be added) and administration should be over a 6-8 hour period.

Adults and children

Single agent therapy

The usual dose regimen given as a single agent is 50 - 120 mg/m^2 by infusion once every 3 - 4 weeks or 15 - 20 mg/m^2 by infusion daily for 5 consecutive days, every 3 - 4 weeks.

Combination chemotherapy

Dosage may be adjusted if the drug is used in combination with other antitumour chemotherapy.

With multiple drug treatment schedules Cisplatin is usually given in doses 20 mg/m^2 upwards every 3 - 4 weeks.

Dosage should be reduced for patients with renal impairment or depressed bone marrow function.

Pre-treatment hydration with 1 - 2 litres of fluid infused for 8 - 12 hours prior to the Cisplatin will initiate diuresis. Adequate subsequent hydration should maintain diuresis during the 24 hours following administration.

Aluminium containing equipment should not be used for administration of Cisplatin as it may interact with metal aluminium to form a black precipitate of platinum.

4.3 Contraindications

Cisplatin is contra-indicated in patients who have previous allergic reactions to Cisplatin or other platinum compounds as anaphylactic-like reactions have been reported. Relative contra-indications are pre-existing renal impairment, hearing disorders and depressed bone marrow function which may increase toxicity.

4.4 Special warnings and precautions for use

This agent should only be administered under the direction of physicians experienced in cancer chemotherapy.

Renal function: Cisplatin produces cumulative nephrotoxicity. Renal function and serum electrolyte (magnesium, sodium, potassium and calcium) should be evaluated prior to initiating cisplatin treatment and prior to each subsequent course of therapy.

To maintain urine output and reduce renal toxicity it is recommended that Cisplatin be administered as an intravenous infusion over 6-8 hours, as indicated in section 4.2 'Posology and method of administration'. Moreover, pre-treatment intravenous hydration with 1-2 litres of fluid over 8-12 hours followed by adequate hydration for the next 24 hours is recommended.

Repeat courses of Cisplatin should not be given unless levels of serum creatinine are below 1.5 mg/100 ml (100 mcmol/l) or blood urea below 55 mg/100 ml (9 mmol/l) and circulating blood elements are at an acceptable level.

Special care has to be taken when cisplatin-treated patients are given concomitant therapies with other potentially nephrotoxic drugs (See also section 4.5 'Interaction with other medicinal products and other forms of Interaction').

In addition, adequate post-treatment hydration and urinary output should be monitored. Concomitant use of nephrotoxic drugs may seriously impair kidney function.

Bone marrow function: Peripheral blood counts should be monitored frequently in patients receiving Cisplatin. Although the haematologic toxicity is usually moderate and reversible, severe thrombocytopenia and leucopenia may occur. In patients who develop thrombocytopenia special precautions are recommended: care in performing invasive procedures; search for signs of bleeding or bruising; test of urine, stools and emesis for occult blood, avoiding aspirin and other NSAIDs. Patients who develop leucopenia should be observed carefully for signs of infection and might require antibiotic support and blood product transfusions.

Hearing function: Cisplatin may produce cumulative ototoxicity, which is more likely to occur with high-dose regimens. Audiometry should be performed prior to initiating therapy, and repeated audiograms should be performed when auditory symptoms occur or clinical hearing changes become apparent. Clinically important deterioration of auditive function may require dosage modifications or discontinuation of therapy.

CNS functions: Cisplatin is known to induce neurotoxicity; therefore, neurologic examination is warranted in patients receiving a cisplatin-containing treatment. Since neurotoxicity may result in irreversible damage, it is recommended to discontinue therapy with Cisplatin when neurologic toxic signs or symptoms become apparent.

Anaphylactic-like reactions to Cisplatin have been observed. These reactions can be controlled by administration of antihistamines, adrenaline and/or glucocorticoids.

Neurotoxicity secondary to Cisplatin administration has been reported and therefore neurological examinations are recommended. Cisplatin has been shown to be mutagenic. It may also have an anti-fertility effect. Other antineoplastic substances have been shown to be carcinogenic and this possibility should be borne in mind in long term use of Cisplatin.

Liver function should also be monitored periodically.

4.5 Interaction with other medicinal products and other forms of interaction

The nephrotoxicity, ototoxicity and myelosuppression induced by Cisplatin will be additive to existing impairment or to similar toxicity of agents such as cephaloridine, furosemide, aminoglycosides, etc administered concurrently.

4.6 Pregnancy and lactation

Cisplatin has been shown to be teratogenic and embryotoxic in animals. The use of the drug should be avoided in pregnant of nursing women if possible.

4.7 Effects on ability to drive and use machines

There are no known effects of Cisplatin on the ability to drive or operate machinery. However, the profile of undesirable effects (central nervous system and special sense) may reduce the patient's driving skills and abilities to operate machinery.

4.8 Undesirable effects

Nephrotoxicity: Acute renal toxicity, which was highly frequent in the past and represented the major dose-limiting toxicity of Cisplatin, has been greatly reduced by the use of 6 to 8-hour infusions as well as by concomitant intravenous hydration and forced diuresis. Cumulative toxicity, however, remains a problem and may be severe. Renal impairment, which is associated with tubular damage, may be first noted during the second week after a dose and is manifested by an increase in serum creatinine, blood urea nitrogen, serum uric acid and/or a decrease in creatinine clearance. Renal insufficiency is generally mild to moderate and reversible at the usual doses of the drug (recovery occurring as a rule within 2-4 weeks); however, high or repeated Cisplatin doses can increase the severity and duration of renal impairment and may produce irreversible renal insufficiency (sometimes fatal). Renal failure has been reported also following intraperitoneal instillation of the drug.

Cisplatin may also cause serious electrolyte disturbances, mainly represented by hypomagnesemia, hypocalcemia, and hypokalemia, and associated with renal tubular dysfunction. Hypomagnesemia and/or hypocalcemia may become symptomatic, with muscle irritability or cramps, clonus, tremor, carpopedal spasm, and/or tetany.

Gastrointestinal toxicity: Nausea and vomiting occur in the majority of Cisplatin-treated patients, usually starting within 1 hour of treatment and lasting up to 24 hours or longer. These side effects are only partially relieved by standard antiemetics. The severity of these systems may be reduced by dividing the total dose per cycle into smaller doses given once daily for five days.

Haematologic toxicity: Myelosuppression often occurs during Cisplatin therapy, but is mostly mild to moderate and reversible at the usual doses. Leucopenia is dose-related, possibly cumulative, and usually reversible. The onset of leucopenia occurs usually between days 6 and 26 and the time of recovery ranges from 21 to 45 days. Thrombocytopenia is also a dose-limiting effect of Cisplatin but is usually reversible. The onset of thrombocytopenia is usually from days 10 to 26 and the time of recovery ranges from about 28 to 45 days.

The incidence of Cisplatin-induced anaemia (haemoglobin drop of 2 g/100 ml) ranges from 9% to 40%, although this is a difficult toxic effect to assess because it may have a complex aetiology in cancer patients.

There have been rare reports of acute myelogenous leukemias and myelodysplastic syndromes arising in patients who have been treated with Cisplatin, mostly when given in combination with other potentially leukomogenic agents.

Ototoxicity: Unilateral or bilateral tinnitus, with or without hearing loss, occurs in about 10% of Cisplatin-treated patients and is usually reversible. The damage to the hearing system appears to be dose-related and cumulative, and it is reported more frequently in very young and very old patients.

The overall incidence of audiogram abnormalities is 24%, but large variations exist. These abnormalities usually appear within 4 days after drug administration and consist of at least a 15 decibel loss in pure tone threshold. The audiogram abnormalities are most common in the 4000-8000 Hz frequencies.

Neurotoxicity: Peripheral neuropathies occur infrequently with usual doses of the drug. These are generally sensory in nature (e.g. paresthesia of the upper and lower extremities) but can also include motor difficulties, reduced reflexes and leg weakness. Autonomic neuropathy, seizures, slurred speech, loss of taste and memory loss have also been reported. These neuropathies usually appear after prolonged therapy, but have also developed after a single drug dose. Peripheral neuropathy may be irreversible in some patients; however, it has been partially or completely reversible in others following discontinuance of Cisplatin therapy.

Hypersensitivity: Anaphylactic and anaphylactic-like reactions, such as flushing, facial oedema, wheezing, tachycardia and hypotension, have been occasionally reported. These reactions may occur within a few minutes after intravenous administration. Antihistamine, adrenaline and/or glucocorticoids control all these reactions. Rarely, urticarial or maculopapular skin rashes have also been observed.

Ocular toxicity: Optic neuritis, papilloedema, and cortical blindness have been reported rarely in patients receiving Cisplatin. These events are usually reversible after drug withdrawal.

Hepatotoxicity: Mild and transient elevations of serum AST and ALT levels may occur infrequently.

Other toxicities: Other reported toxicities are:

cardiovascular abnormalities (coronary artery disease, congestive heart failure, arrhythmias, postural hypotension, thrombotic microangiopathy, etc), hyponatremia / syndrome of inappropriate antidiuretic hormone (SIADH)), mild alopecia, myalgia, pyrexia and gingival platinum line. Pulmonary toxicity has been reported in patients treated with Cisplatin in combination with bleomycin or 5-fluorouracil.

Hyperuricaemia: Hyperuricaemia occurring with Cisplatin is more pronounced with doses greater than 50 mg/m^2. Allopurinol effectively reduces uric acid levels.

Hypomagnesemia: Asymptomatic hypomagnesemia has been documented in a certain number of patients treated with Cisplatin, symptomatic hypomagnesemia has been observed in a limited number of cases.

Convulsions: Seizures have also been reported with the use of this product.

Cardiotoxicity: Isolated cases of tachycardia and arrhythmia have been reported with Cisplatin chemotherapy.

Thromboembolism: Cancer patients are generally at an increased risk for thromboembolic events. Cerebrovascular accidents (e.g. haemorrhagic and ischaemic stroke, amaurosis fugax, sagittal sinus thrombosis) have been observed in patients receiving Cisplatin therapy.

Local effects such as phlebitis, cellulitis and skin necrosis (following extravasation of the drug) may also occur.

Cisplatin can affect male fertility. Impairment of spermatogenesis and azoospermia have been reported. Although the impairment of spermatogenesis can be reversible, males undergoing Cisplatin treatment should be warned about the possible adverse effects on male fertility.

4.9 Overdose

There are no special instructions.

5. PHARMACOLOGICAL PROPERTIES

5.1 Pharmacodynamic properties

In vitro studies indicate that DNA is the principal target molecule of cis-platinum.

The basis for the selectivity of the cis-isomer may reside in its ability to react in a specifically defined configuration with DNA.

Modification of the DNA template results in the selective inhibition of DNA synthesis.

The drug is cell cycle non-specific.

5.2 Pharmacokinetic properties

A biphasic plasma-decay pattern occurs in man after bolus administration. The initial plasma half-life in man is 25 - 49 minutes and the terminal half-life 3 - 4 days. In addition, a third excretory phase with a longer half-life may be postulated from the high plasma platinum concentration found after 21 days. During the terminal phase more than 90% of the drug is bound to plasma proteins.

The urinary elimination of the drug is incomplete: the 5-day recovery of platinum in the urine being only 27 to 45%.

Studies in man measuring free platinum species have shown a mean terminal half-life of 48 minutes after bolus injection, which probably corresponds to the initial half-life (25 - 49 minutes) seen when total platinum is monitored and reflects the distribution of the drug. Urinary excretion of filterable platinum was greater after 6 hours infusion (75%) than after a 15 minute injection (40%) of the same dose of cis-platinum.

Diuresis induced by high-volume hydration or mannitol infusion was associated with a reduction in the concentration of platinum excreted in the urine. The reduced concentration of platinum caused by the high urine volume may play a role in renal protection.

5.3 Preclinical safety data

No further preclinical safety data are available.

6. PHARMACEUTICAL PARTICULARS

6.1 List of excipients

Sodium chloride

Mannitol

6.2 Incompatibilities

None known.

6.3 Shelf life

36 months.

6.4 Special precautions for storage

The unopened vials should be stored at room temperature, protected from light.

The reconstituted solution must not be cooled or refrigerated, as cooling may result in precipitation. It should be kept at room temperature and protected from light, also during intravenous infusion. Any unused solution should be discarded.

Keep out of the reach and sight of children.

6.5 Nature and contents of container

Colourless glass vials (Type II) with bromobutyl rubber stoppers and aluminium snap-caps.

6.6 Special precautions for disposal and other handling

Cisplatin powder should be dissolved in sterile Water for Injections such that the reconstituted solution contains 1mg/ml of Cisplatin. The reconstituted solution should be diluted in 2 litres of 0.9% saline or a dextrose/saline solution (to which 37.5g of mannitol may be added).

Personnel should be trained in good technique for reconstitution and handling. Pregnant staff should be excluded from working with Cisplatin.

Care should be taken to prevent inhaling particles and exposing the skin to Cisplatin. Adequate protective clothing should be worn, such as PVC gloves, safety glasses, disposable gowns and masks.

In the event of contact with eyes, wash with water or saline. If the skin comes into contact with the drug wash thoroughly with water and in both cases seek medical advice. Seek immediate medical attention if the drug is ingested or inhaled.

All used materials, needles, syringes, vials and other items which have come into contact with cytotoxic drugs should be incinerated. Contaminated surfaces should be washed with copious amounts of water.

Administrative Data

7. MARKETING AUTHORISATION HOLDER

Pharmacia Limited

Ramsgate Road

Sandwich

CT13 9NJ

UK

8. MARKETING AUTHORISATION NUMBER(S)

PL 0032/0334

9. DATE OF FIRST AUTHORISATION/RENEWAL OF THE AUTHORISATION

25 March 2002 / 22 February 2006

10. DATE OF REVISION OF THE TEXT

July 2007

Ref CC3_1

Citanest 1%

(AstraZeneca UK Limited)

1. NAME OF THE MEDICINAL PRODUCT

Citanest 1%

2. QUALITATIVE AND QUANTITATIVE COMPOSITION

Each ml of sterile, clear, aqueous solution contains Prilocaine Hydrochloride 10mg.

For excipients, see 6.1

3. PHARMACEUTICAL FORM

Solution for injection.

4. CLINICAL PARTICULARS

4.1 Therapeutic indications

Citanest is a local anaesthetic for use in infiltration anaesthesia and nerve blocks.

4.2 Posology and method of administration

Care should be taken to prevent toxic reactions by avoiding intravascular injection. Careful aspiration before and during the injection is recommended. When a large dose is to be injected, e.g. in epidural block, a test dose of 3-5 ml of prilocaine containing adrenaline is recommended. An accidental intravascular injection may be recognised by a temporary increase in heart rate. The main dose should be injected slowly, at a rate of 100-200 mg/min, or in incremental doses, while keeping in constant verbal contact with the patient. If toxic symptoms occur, the injection should be stopped immediately.

The dose is adjusted according to the response of the patient and the site of administration.

The lowest concentration and smallest dose producing the required effect should be given.

The maximum dose of Citanest for healthy adults should not exceed 400mg.

Elderly or debilitated patients require smaller doses, commensurate with age and physical status.

In children above the age of 6 months the dosage can be calculated on a weight basis up to 5mg/kg.

Prilocaine for injection is not recommended in children under 6 months of age and for use in paracervical (PCB) block and pudendal block in the obstetric patient. There is an increased risk of methaemoglobin formation in children and in the neonate after delivery.

4.3 Contraindications

Known hypersensitivity to anaesthetics of the amide type or to any of the excipients.

Hypersensitivity to methyl and/or propyl parahydroxybenzoate (methyl-/propyl paraben), or to their metabolite para-aminobenzoic acid (PABA).

Formulations of prilocaine containing parabens should be avoided in patients allergic to ester local anaesthetics or its metabolite PABA.

Citanest should be avoided in patients with anaemia or congenital or acquired methaemoglobinaemia.

4.4 Special warnings and precautions for use

Regional anaesthetic procedures should always be performed in a properly equipped and staffed area, with the equipment and drugs necessary for monitoring an emergency resuscitation immediately available. When performing major blocks, an i.v. cannula should be inserted before the local anaesthetic is injected. Clinicians should have received adequate and appropriate training in the procedure to be performed and should be familiar with the diagnosis and treatment of side effects, systemic toxicity or other complications (see section 4.9).

Great caution must be exercised to avoid accidental intravascular injection of this compound, since it may give rise to the rapid onset of toxicity, with marked restlessness, twitching, or convulsions, followed by coma with apnoea and cardiovascular collapse.

In common with other local anaesthetics, Citanest should be used cautiously in the elderly, patients in poor health, patients with epilepsy, severe or untreated hypertension, impaired cardiac conduction, severe heart disease, impaired respiratory function, and in patients with liver or kidney damage, if the dose or site of administration is likely to result in high blood levels.

Patients treated with anti-arrhythmic drugs class III (e.g. amiodarone) should be under close surveillance and ECG monitoring considered, since cardiac effects may be additive (see section 4.5).

Citanest solution for injection is possibly porphyrinogenic and should only be prescribed to patients with acute porphyria when no safer alternative is available. Appropriate precautions should be taken in case of vulnerable patients.

Certain local anaesthetic procedures may be associated with serious adverse reactions, regardless of the local anaesthetic drug used, e.g.:

- Peribulbar injections of local anaesthetics carry a low risk of persistent ocular muscle dysfunction. The primary causes include trauma and/or local toxic effects on muscles and/or nerves. The severity of such tissue reactions is related to the degree of trauma, the concentration of the local anaesthetic and the duration of exposure of the tissue to the local anaesthetic. For this reason, as with all local anaesthetics, the lowest effective concentration and dose of local anaesthetic should be used.

- Injections in the head and neck regions may be made inadvertently into an artery, causing cerebral symptoms even at low doses.

Methaemoglobinaemia may occur at lower doses of prilocaine in patients suffering from anaemia, from congenital or acquired haemoglobinopathy (including methaemoglobinaemia), or in patients receiving concomitant therapy e.g. sulphonamides, known to cause such conditions. Infants are particularly susceptible, due to a lower activity of the enzyme which reduces methaemoglobin to haemoglobin. Hence prilocaine is not recommended for paracervical block (PCB) or pudendal block in the obstetric patient and in children under the age of 6 months.

Local anaesthetics should be avoided when there is inflammation at the site of the proposed injection.

Preservative containing solutions i.e. those supplied in multi-dose vials should not be used for intrathecal or epidural anaesthesia, intraocular or retrobulbar injections or in doses of more than 15 ml for other types of blockades.

4.5 Interaction with other medicinal products and other forms of interaction

Drugs which may predispose to methaemoglobin formation, e.g. sulfonamides (eg cotrimoxazole), antimalarials and certain nitric compounds, could potentiate this adverse effect of prilocaine.

Prilocaine should be used with caution in patients receiving other local anaesthetics or agents structurally related to amide-type anaesthetics, since the toxic effects are additive.

Specific interaction studies with prilocaine and anti-arrhythmic drugs class III (e.g. amiodarone) have not been performed, but caution is advised (see also section 4.4).

4.6 Pregnancy and lactation

Pregnancy

Although there is no evidence from animal studies of harm to the foetus, as with all drugs Citanest should not be given in early pregnancy unless the benefits are considered to outweigh the risks.

Neonatal methaemoglobinaemia has been reported after paracervical block (PCB) or pudendal block in the obstetric patient.

Foetal adverse effects due to local anaesthetics, such as foetal bradycardia, seem to be most apparent in paracervical block anaesthesia. Such effects may be due to high concentrations of anaesthetic reaching the foetus.

Lactation

Prilocaine enters the mothers milk but there is generally no risk of effects on the infant at recommended doses.

4.7 Effects on ability to drive and use machines

Besides the direct anaesthetic effect, local anaesthetics may have a very mild effect on mental function and co-ordination even in the absence of overt CNS toxicity, and may temporarily impair locomotion and alertness.

4.8 Undesirable effects

In common with other local anaesthetics, adverse reactions to Citanest are extremely rare and are usually the result of excessively high blood concentrations due to inadvertent intravascular injection, excessive dosage, rapid absorption or occasionally to hypersensitivity, idiosyncrasy or diminished tolerance on the part of the patient. In such circumstances systemic effects occur involving the central nervous system and/or the cardiovascular system.

CNS reactions are excitatory and/or depressant and may be characterised by nervousness, dizziness, blurred vision and tremors, followed by drowsiness, convulsions, unconsciousness and possibly respiratory arrest. The excitatory reactions may be very brief or may not occur at all, in which case the first manifestations of toxicity may be drowsiness, merging into unconsciousness and respiratory arrest.

Cardiovascular reactions are depressant and may be characterised by hypotension, myocardial depression, bradycardia and possibly cardiac arrest.

Allergic reactions to local anaesthetics of the amide type are extremely rare. They may be characterised by cutaneous lesions, urticaria, oedema or anaphylactoid reactions. However, other constituents of the solutions, e.g. methylparahydroxybenzoate, may cause this type of reaction. Detection of sensitivity by skin testing is of doubtful value.

Neurological complications for example nerve trauma, neuropathy, anterior spinal artery occlusion, arachnoiditis etc., have been associated with regional anaesthetic techniques, regardless of the local anaesthetic drug used.

Hypotension may occur as a physiological response to central nerve blocks.

Acute systemic toxicity

Systemic toxic reactions primarily involve the central nervous system (CNS) and the cardiovascular system (CVS). Such reactions are caused by high blood concentrations of a local anaesthetic, which may appear due to (accidental) intravascular injection, overdose or exceptionally rapid absorption from highly vascularised areas (see section 4.4). CNS reactions are similar for all amide local anaesthetics, while cardiac reactions are more dependent on the drug, both quantitatively and qualitatively.

Central nervous system toxicity is a graded response with symptoms and signs of escalating severity. The first symptoms are circumoral paraesthesia, numbness of the tongue, light-headedness, hyperacusis, tinnitus and visual disturbances. Dysarthria, muscular twitching or tremors are more serious and precede the onset of generalized convulsions. These signs must not be mistaken for neurotic behaviour. Unconsciousness and grand mal convulsions may follow which may last from a few seconds to several minutes. Hypoxia and hypercarbia occur rapidly following convulsions due to the increased muscular activity, together with the interference with respiration and possible loss of functional airways. In severe cases apnoea may occur. Acidosis, hyperkalaemia, hypocalcaemia and hypoxia increase and extend the toxic effects of local anaesthetics.

Recovery is due to redistribution of the local anaesthetic drug from the central nervous system and subsequent metabolism and excretion. Recovery may be rapid unless large amounts of the drug have been injected.

Cardiovascular system toxicity may be seen in severe cases and is generally preceded by signs of toxicity in the central nervous system. In patients under heavy sedation or receiving a general anaesthetic, prodromal CNS symptoms may be absent. Hypotension, bradycardia, arrhythmia and even cardiac arrest may occur as a result of high systemic concentrations of local anaesthetics, but in rare cases cardiac arrest has occurred without prodromal CNS effects.

In children, early signs of local anaesthetic toxicity may be difficult to detect in cases where the block is given during general anaesthesia.

Treatment of acute toxicity

If signs of acute systemic toxicity appear, injections of the local anaesthetic should be stopped immediately and CNS symptoms (convulsion, CNS depression) must promptly be treated with appropriate airway/respiratory support and the administration of anticonvulsant drugs.

If circulatory arrest should occur, immediate cardiopulmonary resuscitation should be instituted. Optimal oxygenation and ventilation and circulatory support as well as treatment of acidosis are of vital importance.

If cardiovascular depression occurs (hypotension, bradycardia), appropriate treatment with intravenous fluids, vasopressor, chronotropic and or inotropic agents should be considered. Children should be given doses commensurate with age and weight.

Methaemoglobinaemia

Methaemoglobinaemia may occur after the administration of prilocaine. The repeated administration of prilocaine, even in relatively small doses, can lead to clinically overt methaemoglobinaemia (cyanosis). Prilocaine is therefore not recommended for continuous techniques of regional anaesthesia.

Methaemoglobin has risen to clinically significant levels in patients receiving high doses of prilocaine. Cyanosis occurs when the methaemoglobin concentration in the blood reaches 1–2 g/100 ml (6–12% of the normal haemoglobin concentration). The reduction in oxygen-carrying capacity due to the administration of prilocaine in normal patients is marginal; hence the methaemoglobinaemia is usually symptomless. However, in severely anaemic patients it may cause hypoxaemia. It is important to rule out other more serious causes of cyanosis such as acute hypoxaemia and/or heart failure.

In neonates and small infants there is an increased risk of development of methaemoglobinaemia (see sections 4.2 and 4.4).

Note: Even low concentrations of methaemoglobin may interfere with pulse oximetry readings, indicating a false, low oxygen saturation.

Treatment of methaemoglobinaemia

If clinical methaemoglobinaemia occurs, it can be rapidly treated by a single intravenous injection of a 1% methylene blue solution, 1 mg/kg body weight, over a 5-minute period. Cyanosis will disappear in about 15 minutes. This dose should not be repeated as methylene blue in high concentrations acts as a haemoglobin oxidant.

4.9 Overdose

Accidental intravascular injections of local anaesthetics may cause immediate (within seconds to a few minutes) systemic toxic reactions. In the event of overdose, systemic toxicity appears later (15–60 minutes after injection) due to the slower increase in local anaesthetic blood concentration (see section 4.8 Acute systemic toxicity and Treatment of acute systemic toxicity).

5. PHARMACOLOGICAL PROPERTIES

5.1 Pharmacodynamic properties

ATC code: NO1B B04

Prilocaine is a local anaesthetic of the amide type. Local anaesthetics act by preventing transmission of impulses along nerve fibres and at nerve endings; depolarisation and ion-exchange are inhibited. The effects are reversible.

5.2 Pharmacokinetic properties

Prilocaine hydrochloride is absorbed more slowly than lidocaine (lignocaine) because of its slight vasoconstrictor action but its half-life in blood is less than that of lidocaine (lidocaine half-life approximately 10 minutes, elimination half-life approximately 2 hours).

Amidases in the liver and kidney metabolise prilocaine directly.

In the liver, prilocaine is primarily metabolised by amide hydrolysis to orthotoluidine and N-propylamine. O-Toluidine is subsequently hydroxylated to 2-amino-3-hydroxytoluene and 2-amino-5-hydroxytoluene, metabolites with long half-lives that tend to accumulate and are believed to be responsible for the occurrence of methaemoglobinaemia.

5.3 Preclinical safety data

Prilocaine hydrochloride is a well established active ingredient.

6. PHARMACEUTICAL PARTICULARS

6.1 List of excipients

Sodium chloride, sodium hydroxide/hydrochloric acid for pH adjustment, methyl parahydroxybenzoate and water for injections.

6.2 Incompatibilities

None known

6.3 Shelf life

The shelf-life is 3 years

6.4 Special precautions for storage

Do not store above 25°C.

6.5 Nature and contents of container

Multi-dose glass vials of 20ml and 50ml

6.6 Special precautions for disposal and other handling

None stated

7. MARKETING AUTHORISATION HOLDER

AstraZeneca UK Ltd
600 Capability Green,
Luton, LU1 3LU, UK.

8. MARKETING AUTHORISATION NUMBER(S)

PL 17901/0118

9. DATE OF FIRST AUTHORISATION/RENEWAL OF THE AUTHORISATION

14th May 2002

10. DATE OF REVISION OF THE TEXT

6th August 2009

CitraFleet Powder for Oral Solution

(Laboratorios Casen Fleet S.L.U)

1. NAME OF THE MEDICINAL PRODUCT

CitraFleet, Powder for oral solution in sachet

2. QUALITATIVE AND QUANTITATIVE COMPOSITION

Each sachet (16.11 g) contains the following active ingredients:

Sodium picosulfate	10.0 mg
Light magnesium oxide	3.5 g
Citric acid monohydrate	12.0 g

Each sachet also contains 5 mmol (or 195 mg) potassium (see section 4.4)

For a full list of excipients, see section 6.1.

3. PHARMACEUTICAL FORM

Powder for oral solution, in sachet.

White crystalline powder with a lemon flavour.

4. CLINICAL PARTICULARS

4.1 Therapeutic indications

For bowel cleansing prior to any diagnostic procedures requiring a clean bowel e.g. colonoscopy or x-ray examination.

4.2 Posology and method of administration

Route of administration: Oral

A low residue diet is recommended on the day prior to the hospital procedure. To avoid dehydration during treatment with CitraFleet, it is recommended to drink approximately 250 ml per hour, of water or other clear fluid while the washout effect persists.

Directions for reconstitution:

Refer to section 6.6.

Adults (including the elderly) aged 18 years and over:

One sachet reconstituted in water as directed, taken before 8 am on the day before the procedure. Second sachet 6 to 8 hours later.

4.3 Contraindications

Hypersensitivity to any of the ingredients of the product, congestive cardiac failure, severe dehydration, hypermagnesaemia, gastric retention, gastro-intestinal ulceration, toxic colitis, toxic megacolon, ileus, nausea and vomiting, ascites, acute surgical abdominal conditions such as acute appendicitis and known or suspected gastro-intestinal obstruction or perforation.

Do not use in patients with rhabdomyolysis as laxatives may induce rhabdomyolysis and may therefore exacerbate the condition.

Do not use in patients with active inflammatory bowel disease e.g. Crohn's disease, ulcerative colitis.

In patients with severely reduced renal function, accumulation of magnesium in plasma may occur. Another preparation should be used in such cases.

4.4 Special warnings and precautions for use

CitraFleet should not be used as a routine laxative.

CitraFleet could rarely lead to severe and potentially fatal cases of electrolyte disorders in fragile or debilitated elderly patients. Therefore, the benefit/risk ratio of CitraFleet needs to be carefully considered before initiating treatment in this at-risk population.

Special attention should be taken when prescribing CitraFleet to any patient with regard to known contra-indications and special attention made to the importance of adequate hydration and, in at-risk populations (as defined below), to the importance of also obtaining baseline and post-treatment electrolyte levels.

Elderly and debilitated patients, and patients at risk of hypokalaemia or hyponatraemia, may need particular attention.

CitraFleet should be used with caution in patients with known disorders of water and/or electrolyte balance or on drugs that might affect water and/or electrolyte balance e.g. diuretics, corticosteroids, lithium (see 4.5).

Care should also be taken in patients who have recently undergone gastrointestinal surgery or who have renal impairment, mild to moderate dehydration, hypotension or heart disease.

The period of bowel cleansing should not exceed 24 hours because longer preparation may increase the risk of water and electrolyte imbalance.

CitraFleet may modify the absorption of regularly prescribed oral medication and should be used with caution e.g. there have been isolated reports of seizures in patients on antiepileptics, with previously controlled epilepsy (see 4.5 and 4.8).

This medicine contains 5mmol (or 195 mg) potassium per sachet. This should be taken into consideration by patients with reduced kidney function or patients on a controlled potassium diet.

4.5 Interaction with other medicinal products and other forms of interaction

As a purgative, CitraFleet increases the gastrointestinal transit rate. Absorption of other orally administered medicines (e.g. anti-epileptics, contraceptives, anti-diabetics, antibiotics) may therefore be modified during the treatment period (see 4.4). Tetracycline and fluoroquinolone antibiotics, and pencillamine, should be taken at least 2 hours before and not less than 6 hours after administration of CitraFleet to avoid chelation with magnesium.

The efficacy of CitraFleet is lowered by bulk-forming laxatives.

Care should be taken with patients already receiving drugs which may be associated with hypokalaemia (such as diuretics or corticosteroids, or drugs where hypokalaemia is a particular risk i.e. cardiac glycosides). Caution is also advised when CitraFleet is used in patients on NSAIDs or drugs known to induce SIADH e.g. tricyclic antidepressants, selective serotonin re-uptake inhibitors, antipsychotic drugs and carbamazepine as these drugs may increase the risk of water retention and/or electrolyte imbalance.

4.6 Pregnancy and lactation

For CitraFleet neither clinical data on exposed pregnancy nor reproductive toxicity are available. As picosulfate is a stimulant laxative, for safety measure, it is preferable to avoid the use of CitraFleet during pregnancy.

There is no experience with the use of CitraFleet in nursing mothers. However, due to the pharmacokinetic properties of the active ingredients, treatment with CitraFleet may be considered for females who are breastfeeding.

4.7 Effects on ability to drive and use machines

CitraFleet may cause fatigue or dizziness, probably as a result of dehydration, and this may have a mild to moderate effect on the ability to drive or use machinery.

4.8 Undesirable effects

The most common adverse events reported in clinical trials using the combination of sodium picosulfate and magnesium citrate were related to direct effects on the bowel (abdominal pain and nausea) and the consequences of diarrhoea and dehydration (sleep disturbance, dry mouth, thirst, headache and fatigue).

Undesirable effects are presented below by MedDRA System Organ Class and Preferred Term, using the following frequency convention: very common ($\geq$ 1/10); common ($\geq$ 1/100, $<$ 1/10); uncommon ($\geq$ 1/1,000, $<$ 1/100). The frequency calculations are based on data derived from an analysis of clinical studies. Undesirable effects that were not reported in these clinical trials are described as 'Frequency not known'.

Immune system disorders

Frequency not known: Anaphylactoid reaction, hypersensitivity

Metabolism and nutrition disorders

Frequency not known: Hyponatraemia

Psychiatric disorders

Common: Sleep disorder

Nervous system disorders

Common: Headache

Uncommon: Dizziness

Frequency not known: Epilepsy, grand mal convulsion, convulsion, confusional state

Vascular disorders

Uncommon: Orthostatic hypotension

Gastrointestinal disorders

Very common: Abdominal pain

Common: Dry mouth, nausea, abdominal distension, anal discomfort, proctalgia

Uncommon: Vomiting, faecal incontinence

Frequency not known: Diarrhoea*, flatulence

* Diarrhoea is the primary clinical effect of CitraFleet

Skin and subcutaneous tissue disorders

Frequency not known: Rash (including erythematous and maculo-papular rash), urticaria, pruritus, purpura

General disorders and administrative site conditions

Common: Thirst, fatigue

Frequency not known: Pain

Hyponatraemia has been reported with or without associated convulsions (see 4.4). In epileptic patients, there have been reports of seizure/grand mal convulsion without associated hyponatraemia (see 4.4 and 4.5).

4.9 Overdose

No cases of overdose with CitraFleet, or similar combinations of sodium picosulfate and magnesium citrate, have been reported. However, because of its modes of action, an overdose of CitraFleet would be expected to cause profuse diarrhoea with dehydration and electrolyte loss. Dehydration could also lead to orthostatic hypotension and dizziness. Dehydration and electrolyte imbalances should be corrected with fluid and electrolytes as necessary.

5. PHARMACOLOGICAL PROPERTIES

5.1 Pharmacodynamic properties

A06A B58 - Sodium picosulfate, combinations.

The active components of CitraFleet are sodium picosulfate, a stimulant cathartic, active locally in the colon, and magnesium citrate which acts as an osmotic laxative by retaining moisture in the colon. The action is of a potent 'washing out' effect combined with peristaltic stimulation to clear the bowel prior to radiography, colonoscopy or surgery. The product is not intended for use as a routine laxative.

5.2 Pharmacokinetic properties

Both active components are locally active in the colon, and neither is absorbed in any detectable amounts.

In patients with severely reduced renal function, accumulation of magnesium in plasma may occur.

5.3 Preclinical safety data

Prenatal developmental studies in rats and rabbits did not reveal any teratogenic potential after oral dosing of sodium picosulfate up to 100 mg/kg/d, but embryotoxicity had been observed in both species at this dose level. In rats daily doses of 10mg/kg during late gestation (fetal development) and lactation reduced body weights and survival of the offspring. Male and female fertility was not affected by oral doses of sodium picosulfate up to 100 mg/kg.

6. PHARMACEUTICAL PARTICULARS

6.1 List of excipients

Potassium hydrogen carbonate

Saccharin sodium

Lemon Flavour (lemon flavour, maltodextrin, tocopherol E306).

6.2 Incompatibilities

Not applicable

6.3 Shelf life

Unopened sachets: 18 months

Use immediately after reconstitution.

6.4 Special precautions for storage

Do not store above 25°C.

6.5 Nature and contents of container

The powder is supplied in unit dose sachets containing 16.11 g. Sachets are packaged in cartons of 2 sachets or 50 sachets (hospital pack). The sachet is a complex formed by a polyester layer, an intermediate aluminium layer and an internal polyethylene layer.

Not all pack sizes may be marketed.

6.6 Special precautions for disposal and other handling

Directions for reconstitution:

Reconstitute the contents of one sachet in a cup of water (approximately 150 ml). The resulting solution appears turbid. Stir for 2-3 minutes and drink the solution. If it becomes hot, wait until it cools sufficiently to drink.

7. MARKETING AUTHORISATION HOLDER

E. C. De Witt & Company Limited,
Aegon House
Daresbury Park
Daresbury
Warrington
Cheshire
WA4 4HS.
United Kingdom

8. MARKETING AUTHORISATION NUMBER(S)

PL 00083/0046

9. DATE OF FIRST AUTHORISATION/RENEWAL OF THE AUTHORISATION

8th June 2005

10. DATE OF REVISION OF THE TEXT

September 2007

Clasteon 400mg Capsules

(Beacon Pharmaceuticals)

1. NAME OF THE MEDICINAL PRODUCT

CLASTEON® 400mg capsules, hard

2. QUALITATIVE AND QUANTITATIVE COMPOSITION

Each Clasteon capsule contains 400mg clodronic acid disodium salt (as the tetrahydrate). For excipients, see 6.1.

3. PHARMACEUTICAL FORM

Hard capsules for oral administration.

Clasteon Capsules are oblong, white and blue, marked "CLASTEON®".

4. CLINICAL PARTICULARS

4.1 Therapeutic indications

Clasteon is indicated for the management of osteolytic lesions, hypercalcaemia and bone pain associated with skeletal metastases in patients with carcinoma of the breast or multiple myeloma. Clasteon capsules are also indicated for the maintenance of clinically acceptable serum calcium levels in patients with hypercalcaemia of malignancy initially treated with an intravenous infusion of clodronic acid disodium salt

4.2 Posology and method of administration

Adults; The recommended dose is 4 capsules (1600mg clodronic acid disodium salt) daily. If necessary, the dosage may be increased but should not exceed a maximum of 8 capsules (3200mg clodronic acid disodium salt) daily.

The capsules may be taken as a single dose or in two equally divided doses if necessary to improve gastrointestinal tolerance. Clasteon capsules should be swallowed with a little fluid, but not milk, at least one hour before or one hour after food.

Elderly; No special dosage recommendations.

Children; Safety and efficacy in children has not been established.

Use in renal impairment; In patients with renal insufficiency with creatinine clearance between 10 and 30ml/min, the daily dose should be reduced to one half the recommended adult dose. Serum creatinine should be monitored during therapy. Clodronic acid disodium salt is contra-indicated in patients with creatinine clearance below 10ml/min.

The oral bioavailability of bisphosphonates is poor. Bioequivalence studies have shown appreciable differences in bioavailability between different oral formulations of clodronic acid disodium salt, as well as marked inter and intra patient variability. Dose adjustment may be required if the formulation is changed.

4.3 Contraindications
Hypersensitivity to clodronic acid disodium salt. Acute, severe inflammatory conditions of the gastrointestinal tract. Pregnancy and lactation. Renal failure with creatinine clearance below 10ml/min, except for short term use in the presence of purely functional renal insufficiency caused by elevated serum calcium levels. Concomitant use of other bisphosphonates.

4.4 Special warnings and precautions for use
No information is available on the potential carcinogenicity of clodronic acid disodium salt, but patients have been treated in clinical trials for up to 2 years. The duration of the treatment is therefore at the discretion of the physician, according to the status of the underlying malignancy.

Osteonecrosis of the jaw, generally associated with tooth extraction and/or local infection (including osteomyelitis) has been reported in patients with cancer receiving treatment regimens including primarily intravenously administered bisphosphonates. Many of these patients were also receiving chemotherapy and corticosteroids. Osteonecrosis of the jaw has also been reported in patients with osteoporosis receiving oral bisphosphonates.

A dental examination with appropriate preventive dentistry should be considered prior to treatment with bisphosphonates in patients with concomitant risk factors (e.g. cancer, chemotherapy, radiotherapy, corticosteroids, poor oral hygiene).

While on treatment, these patients should avoid invasive dental procedures if possible. For patients who develop osteonecrosis of the jaw while on bisphosphonate therapy, dental surgery may exacerbate the condition. For patients requiring dental procedures, there are no data available to suggest whether discontinuation of bisphosphonate treatment reduces the risk of osteonecrosis of the jaw.

Clinical judgment of the treating physician should guide the management plan of each patient based on individual benefit/risk assessment.

4.5 Interaction with other medicinal products and other forms of interaction
No other bisphosphonate drugs should be given with Clasteon capsules.

The calcium-lowering action of clodronic acid disodium salt can be potentiated by the administration of aminoglycosides either concomitantly or one to several weeks apart. Severe hypocalcaemia has been observed in some cases. Hypomagnesaemia may also occur simultaneously. Patients receiving NSAID's in addition to clodronic acid disodium salt have developed renal dysfunction. However, a synergistic action has not been established. There is no evidence from clinical experience that clodronic acid disodium salt interacts with other medication, such as steroids, diuretics, calcitonin, non NSAID analgesics, or chemotherapeutic agents. Calcium rich foods, mineral supplements and antacids may impair absorption.

4.6 Pregnancy and lactation
There are insufficient data either from animal studies or from experience in humans of the effects of clodronic acid disodium salt on the embryo and foetus. No studies have been conducted on excretion in breast milk. Consequently, clodronic acid disodium salt is contra-indicated in pregnancy and lactation.

4.7 Effects on ability to drive and use machines
No effects.

4.8 Undesirable effects
Patients may experience a mild gastrointestinal upset, usually in the form of nausea or mild diarrhoea. The symptoms may respond to the use of a twice daily dosage regime rather than a single dose. It is not normally required to withdraw therapy or to provide medication to control these effects. Asymptomatic hypocalcaemia has been noted rarely. A reversible elevation of serum parathyroid hormone may occur. In a small proportion of patients, a mild, reversible increase in serum lactate dehydrogenase and a modest transient leucopenia have been reported although these may have been associated with concurrent chemotherapy. Renal dysfunction, including renal failure has been reported. Hypersensitivity reactions have been mainly confined to the skin: pruritus, urticaria and rarely exfoliative dermatitis. However, bronchospasm has been precipitated in patients with or without a previous history of asthma.

4.9 Overdose
Symptoms and signs: There is no experience of acute overdosage in humans. The development of hypocalcaemia is possible for up to 2 or 3 days following the overdosage.

Treatment: Serum calcium should be monitored and oral or parenteral calcium supplementation may be required. Acute overdosage may be associated with gastrointestinal symptoms such as nausea and vomiting. Treatment should be symptomatic.

5. PHARMACOLOGICAL PROPERTIES
5.1 Pharmacodynamic properties
Clodronic acid disodium salt is a bisphosphonate which has a high affinity to bone. It is mainly the portion of the dose adsorbed to bone which is pharmacologically active. The pharmacological effect of clodronic acid disodium salt is to suppress osteoclast mediated bone resorption as judged by bone histology and decreases in serum calcium, urine calcium and urinary excretion of hydroxyproline, without adversely affecting mineralisation.

5.2 Pharmacokinetic properties
Oral bioavailability is in the order of 2%.

Clodronic acid disodium salt is not metabolised. The volume of distribution is approximately 0.3L/kg. Elimination from serum is rapid, 75% of the dose is recovered unchanged in urine within 24 hours.

The elimination kinetics best fit a 3 compartment model. The first two compartments have relatively short half-lives. The third compartment is probably the skeleton. Elimination half life is approximately 12 - 13 hours.

5.3 Preclinical safety data
Clodronic acid disodium salt shows relatively little toxicity either on single oral administration or after daily oral administration for a period of up to 6 months. In rats, a dose of 200mg/kg/day in the chronic toxicity test is at the limit of tolerability. In dogs, 40mg/kg/day chronically is within the tolerated range.

On daily administration of 500mg/kg for 6 weeks to rats, signs of renal failure with a clear rise in BUN, and initial liver parenchymal reaction with rises of SGOT, SGPT and AP occurred. No significant haematological changes were found in the toxicological investigations.

Investigations for mutagenic properties did not show any indication of mutagenic potency.

Reproduction toxicology investigations did not provide any indication of peri and post natal disorders, teratogenic damage or disorders of fertility.

It is not known if clodronic acid disodium salt passes into the mother's milk or through the placenta.

6. PHARMACEUTICAL PARTICULARS
6.1 List of excipients
Capsule content: Maize starch, Talc, Magnesium stearate, Sodium starch glycolate.

Capsule shell: Titanium dioxide (E171), Indigotin (E132), Gelatin.

6.2 Incompatibilities
Not applicable.

6.3 Shelf life
PVC/PVDC/aluminium blister packs:3 years.

6.4 Special precautions for storage
No special precautions for storage.

6.5 Nature and contents of container
PVC/PVDC/aluminium Blister Packs containing 30, 60 or 120 capsules.

6.6 Special precautions for disposal and other handling
No special instructions.

7. MARKETING AUTHORISATION HOLDER
Beacon Pharmaceuticals Limited

85 High Street, Tunbridge Wells, Kent TN1 1YG

8. MARKETING AUTHORISATION NUMBER(S)
PL 18157/0028

9. DATE OF FIRST AUTHORISATION/RENEWAL OF THE AUTHORISATION
15 May 2007

10. DATE OF REVISION OF THE TEXT

Clexane Forte Syringes

(sanofi-aventis)

1. NAME OF THE MEDICINAL PRODUCT
Clexane® Forte Syringes

2. QUALITATIVE AND QUANTITATIVE COMPOSITION
Pre-filled syringes:

120 mg Injection	Enoxaparin sodium 120 mg (equivalent to 12,000 IU anti-Xa activity) in 0.8 mL Water for Injections
150 mg Injection	Enoxaparin sodium 150 mg (equivalent to 15,000 IU anti-Xa activity) in 1.0 mL Water for Injections

3. PHARMACEUTICAL FORM
Solution for injection.

4. CLINICAL PARTICULARS
4.1 Therapeutic indications
The prophylaxis of thromboembolic disorders of venous origin, in particular those which may be associated with orthopaedic or general surgery.

The prophylaxis of venous thromboembolism in medical patients bedridden due to acute illness.

The treatment of venous thromboembolic disease presenting with deep vein thrombosis, pulmonary embolism or both.

The treatment of unstable angina and non-Q-wave myocardial infarction, administered concurrently with aspirin.

The prevention of thrombus formation in the extracorporeal circulation during haemodialysis.

4.2 Posology and method of administration
Adults:

Prophylaxis of venous thromboembolism:

In patients with a low to moderate risk of venous thromboembolism the recommended dosage is 20 mg (2,000 IU) once daily for 7 to 10 days, or until the risk of thromboembolism has diminished. In patients undergoing surgery, the initial dose should be given approximately 2 hours pre-operatively.

In patients with a higher risk, such as in orthopaedic surgery, the dosage should be

40 mg (4,000 IU) daily with the initial dose administered approximately 12 hours before surgery.

Prophylaxis of venous thromboembolism in medical patients:

The recommended dose of enoxaparin sodium is 40 mg (4,000 IU) once daily. Treatment with enoxaparin sodium is prescribed for a minimum of 6 days and continued until the return to full ambulation, for a maximum of 14 days.

Treatment of venous thromboembolism:

Clexane should be administered subcutaneously as a single daily injection of 1.5 mg/kg (150 IU/kg). Clexane treatment is usually prescribed for at least 5 days and until adequate oral anticoagulation is established.

Treatment of unstable angina and non-Q-wave myocardial infarction

The recommended dose is 1 mg/kg Clexane every 12 hours by subcutaneous injection, administered concurrently with oral aspirin (100 to 325 mg once daily)

Treatment with Clexane in these patients should be prescribed for a minimum of 2 days and continued until clinical stabilisation. The usual duration of treatment is 2 to 8 days.

Prevention of extracorporeal thrombus formation during haemodialysis:

A dose equivalent to 1 mg/kg (100 IU/kg) introduced into the arterial line at the beginning of a dialysis session is usually sufficient for a 4 hour session. If fibrin rings are found, such as after a longer than normal session, a further dose of 0.5 to 1 mg/kg (50 to 100 IU/kg) may be given. For patients at a high risk of haemorrhage the dose should be reduced to 0.5 mg/kg (50 IU/kg) for double vascular access or 0.75 mg/kg (75 IU/kg) for single vascular access.

Elderly: No dosage adjustments are necessary in the elderly, unless kidney function is impaired (see also section 4.2 Posology and method of administration: *Renal impairment*; section 4.4 Special warnings and precautions for use: *Haemorrhage in the elderly*; *Renal impairment and Monitoring*; section 5.2 Pharmacokinetic properties).

Children: Not recommended, as dosage not established.

Renal impairment: (See also section 4.4 Special warnings and precautions for use: *Renal impairment and Monitoring*; section 5.2 Pharmacokinetic properties).

Severe renal impairment:

A dosage adjustment is required for patients with severe renal impairment (creatinine clearance < 30 ml/min), according to the following tables, since enoxaparin sodium exposure is significantly increased in this patient population:

Dosage adjustments for therapeutic dosage ranges

Standard dosing	Severe renal impairment
1 mg/kg twice daily	1 mg/kg once daily
1.5 mg/kg once daily	1 mg/kg once daily

Dosage adjustments for prophylactic dosage ranges

Standard dosing	Severe renal impairment
40 mg once daily	20 mg once daily
20 mg once daily	20 mg once daily

The recommended dosage adjustments do not apply to the haemodialysis indication.

Moderate and mild renal impairment:

Although no dosage adjustments are recommended in patients with moderate renal impairment (creatinine clearance 30-50 ml/min) or mild renal impairment (creatinine clearance 50-80 ml/min), careful clinical monitoring is advised.

Hepatic impairment: In the absence of clinical studies, caution should be exercised.

Body weight: No dosage adjustments are recommended in obesity or low body weight (see also section 4.4 Special warnings and precautions for use: *Low body weight and Monitoring*; section 5.2 Pharmacokinetic properties).

Clexane is administered by subcutaneous injection for the prevention of venous thromboembolic disease, treatment of deep vein thrombosis or for the treatment of unstable angina and non-Q-wave myocardial infarction; and through the arterial line of a dialysis circuit for the prevention of thrombus formation in the extra-corporeal circulation during haemodialysis. It must not be administered by the intramuscular route.

Subcutaneous injection technique. The prefilled disposable syringe is ready for immediate use.

Clexane should be administered when the patient is lying down by deep subcutaneous injection. The administration should be alternated between the left and right anterolateral or posterolateral abdominal wall. The whole length of the needle should be introduced vertically into a skin fold held between the thumb and index finger. The skin fold should not be released until the injection is complete. Do not rub the injection site after administration.

4.3 Contraindications

Contraindicated in patients with acute bacterial endocarditis, active major bleeding and conditions with a high risk of uncontrolled haemorrhage, including recent haemorrhagic stroke; thrombocytopenia in patients with a positive in-vitro aggregation test in the presence of enoxaparin; active gastric or duodenal ulceration; hypersensitivity to either enoxaparin sodium, heparin or its derivatives including other Low Molecular Weight Heparins; in patients receiving heparin for treatment rather than prophylaxis, locoregional anaesthesia in elective surgical procedures is contra-indicated.

4.4 Special warnings and precautions for use

Low Molecular Weight Heparins should not be used interchangeably since they differ in their manufacturing process, molecular weights, specific anti Xa activities, units and dosage. This results in differences in pharmacokinetics and associated biological activities (e.g. anti-IIa activity, and platelet interactions). Special attention and compliance with the instructions for use specific to each proprietary medicinal product are therefore required.

Enoxaparin is to be used with extreme caution in patients with a history of heparin-induced thrombocytopenia with or without thrombosis.

As there is a risk of antibody-mediated heparin-induced thrombocytopenia also occurring with low molecular weight heparins, regular platelet count monitoring should be considered prior to and during therapy with these agents. Thrombocytopenia, should it occur, usually appears between the 5th and the 21st day following the beginning of therapy. Therefore, it is recommended that the platelet counts be measured before the initiation of therapy with enoxaparin sodium and then regularly thereafter during the treatment. In practice, if a confirmed significant decrease of the platelet count is observed (30 to 50 % of the initial value), enoxaparin sodium treatment must be immediately discontinued and the patient switched to another therapy.

Enoxaparin injection, as with any other anticoagulant therapy, should be used with caution in conditions with increased potential for bleeding, such as: impaired haemostasis, history of peptic ulcer, recent ischaemic stroke, uncontrolled severe arterial hypertension, diabetic retinopathy, recent neuro- or ophthalmologic surgery.

As with other anticoagulants, bleeding may occur at any site (see section 4.8 Undesirable effects). If bleeding occurs, the origin of the haemorrhage should be investigated and appropriate treatment instituted.

Heparin can suppress adrenal secretion of aldosterone leading to hyperkalaemia, particularly in patients such as those with diabetes mellitus, chronic renal failure, pre-existing metabolic acidosis, a raised plasma potassium or taking potassium sparing drugs. The risk of hyperkalaemia appears to increase with duration of therapy but is usually reversible. Plasma potassium should be measured in patients at risk before starting heparin therapy and monitored regularly thereafter particularly if treatment is prolonged beyond about 7 days.

As with other anti-coagulants, there have been cases of intra-spinal haematomas reported with the concurrent use of enoxaparin sodium and spinal/epidural anaesthesia or spinal puncture resulting in long term or permanent paralysis. These events are rare with enoxaparin sodium dosage regimens 40 mg od or lower. The risk is greater with higher enoxaparin sodium dosage regimens, use of post-operative indwelling catheters or the concomitant use of additional drugs affecting haemostasis such as NSAIDs (see section 4.5 Interaction with other medicinal products and other forms of interaction). The risk also appears to be increased by traumatic or repeated neuraxial puncture.

To reduce the potential risk of bleeding associated with the concurrent use of enoxaparin sodium and epidural anaesthesia/analgesia, the pharmacokinetic profile of the drug should be considered (see section 5.2 Pharmacokinetics properties). Placement and removal of the catheter is best performed when the anticoagulation effect of enoxaparin is low.

Placement or removal of a catheter should be delayed for 10 - 12 hours after administration of DVT prophylactic doses of enoxaparin sodium, whereas patients receiving higher doses of enoxaparin sodium (1.5 mg/kg once daily) will require longer delays (24 hours). The subsequent enoxaparin sodium dose should be given no sooner than 4 hours after catheter removal.

Should the physician decide to administer anticoagulation in the context of epidural/spinal anaesthesia, extreme vigilance and frequent monitoring must be exercised to detect any signs and symptoms of neurological impairment such as midline back pain, sensory and motor deficits (numbness or weakness in lower limbs) bowel and/or bladder dysfunction. Patients should be instructed to inform their nurse or physician immediately if they experience any of the above signs or symptoms. If signs or symptoms of spinal haematoma are suspected, urgent diagnosis and treatment including spinal cord decompression should be initiated.

Percutaneous coronary revascularisation procedures:

To minimise the risk of bleeding following the vascular instrumentation during the treatment of unstable angina and non-Q-wave myocardial infarction, the vascular access sheath should remain in place for 6 to 8 hours following a subcutaneous dose of enoxaparin sodium. The next scheduled dose should be given no sooner than 6 to 8 hours after sheath removal. The site of the procedure should be observed for signs of bleeding or haematoma formation.

For some patients with pulmonary embolism (e.g. those with severe haemodynamic instability) alternative treatment such as thrombolysis or surgery may be indicated.

Prosthetic Heart Valves:

There have been no adequate studies to assess the safe and effective use of enoxaparin sodium in preventing valve thrombosis in patients with prosthetic heart valves. Prophylactic doses of enoxaparin are not sufficient to prevent valve thrombosis in patients with prosthetic heart valves. Confounding factors, including underlying disease and insufficient clinical data, limit the evaluation of these cases. Therapeutic failures have been reported in pregnant women with prosthetic heart valves on full anti-coagulant doses (see section 4.6 Pregnancy and lactation). The use of enoxaparin sodium cannot be recommended for this purpose.

Haemorrhage in the elderly: No increased bleeding tendency is observed in the elderly within the prophylactic dosage ranges. Elderly patients (especially patients aged eighty years and above) may be at an increased risk for bleeding complications within the therapeutic dosage ranges. Careful clinical monitoring is advised (see also section 4.2 Posology and method of administration: Elderly; section 5.2 Pharmacokinetic properties).

Renal impairment: In patients with renal impairment, there is an increase in enoxaparin exposure which increases the risk of bleeding. Since enoxaparin exposure is significantly increased in patients with severe renal impairment (creatinine clearance < 30 ml/min) dosage adjustments are recommended in therapeutic and prophylactic dosage ranges. Although no dosage adjustments are recommended in patients with moderate (creatinine clearance 30-50 ml/min) and mild (creatinine clearance 50-80 ml/min) renal impairment, careful clinical monitoring is advised (see also section 4.2 Posology and method of administration: Renal impairment; section 5.2 Pharmacokinetic properties).

Low body weight: In low-weight women (< 45 kg) and low-weight men (< 57 kg), an increase in enoxaparin exposure has been observed within the prophylactic dosage ranges (non-weight adjusted), which may lead to a higher risk of bleeding. Therefore, careful clinical monitoring is advised in these patients (see also section 5.2 Pharmacokinetic properties).

Monitoring: Risk assessment and clinical monitoring are the best predictors of the risk of potential bleeding. Routine anti-Xa activity monitoring is usually not required. However, anti-Xa activity monitoring might be considered in those patients treated with LMWH who also have either an increased risk of bleeding (such as those with renal impairment, elderly and extremes of weight) or are actively bleeding.

Laboratory tests:

At doses used for prophylaxis of venous thromboembolism, enoxaparin sodium does not influence bleeding time and global blood coagulation tests significantly, nor does it affect platelet aggregation or binding of fibrinogen to platelets. At higher doses, increases in APTT (activated partial thromboplastin time) and ACT (activated clotting time) may occur. Increases in APTT and ACT are not linearly correlated with increasing enoxaparin sodium antithrombotic activity and therefore are unsuitable and unreliable for monitoring enoxaparin sodium activity.

4.5 Interaction with other medicinal products and other forms of interaction

It is recommended that agents which affect haemostasis should be discontinued prior to enoxaparin therapy unless their use is essential, such as: systemic salicylates, acetylsalicylic acid, NSAIDs including ketorolac, dextran, and clopidogrel, systemic glucocorticoids, thrombolytics and anticoagulants. If the combination cannot be avoided, enoxaparin should be used with careful clinical and laboratory monitoring.

4.6 Pregnancy and lactation

Pregnancy: Animal studies have not shown any evidence of foetotoxicity or teratogenicity. In the pregnant rat, the transfer of ^{35}S-enoxaparin across the maternal placenta to the foetus is minimal.

In humans, there is no evidence that enoxaparin crosses the placental barrier during the second trimester of pregnancy. There is no information available concerning the first and the third trimesters.

As there are no adequately powered and well-controlled studies in pregnant women and because animal studies are not always predictive of human response, this drug should be used during pregnancy only if the physician has established a clear need.

Pregnant women with mechanical prosthetic heart valves

The use of enoxaparin for thromboprophylaxis in pregnant women with mechanical prosthetic heart valves has not been adequately studied. In a clinical study of pregnant women with mechanical prosthetic heart valves given enoxaparin (1 mg/kg bid) to reduce the risk of thromboembolism, 2 of 8 women developed clots resulting in blockage of the valve and leading to maternal and foetal death. There have been isolated postmarketing reports of valve thrombosis in pregnant women with mechanical prosthetic heart valves while receiving enoxaparin for thromboprophylaxis. Pregnant women with mechanical prosthetic heart valves may be at higher risk for thromboembolism. Enoxaparin sodium is not recommended for use in pregnant women with prosthetic heart valves (see section 4.4 Special warnings and precautions for use: Prosthetic heart valves).

Lactation: In lactating rats, the concentration of ^{35}S-enoxaparin or its labelled metabolites in milk is very low.

It is not known whether unchanged enoxaparin is excreted in human breast milk. The oral absorption of enoxaparin is unlikely. However, as a precaution, lactating mothers receiving enoxaparin should be advised to avoid breast-feeding.

4.7 Effects on ability to drive and use machines

Enoxaparin has no effect on the ability to drive and operate machines

4.8 Undesirable effects

As with other anticoagulants bleeding may occur during enoxaparin therapy in the presence of associated risk factors such as: organic lesions liable to bleed, invasive procedures or the use of medications affecting haemostasis (see section 4.5 Interaction with other medicinal products and other forms of interaction). The origin of the bleeding should be investigated and appropriate treatment instituted.

Major haemorrhage including retroperitoneal and intracranial bleeding have been reported, in rare instances these have been fatal.

Mild, transient, asymptomatic thrombocytopenia has been reported during the first days of therapy. Rare cases of immuno-allergic thrombocytopenia with or without thrombosis have been reported. In some cases thrombosis was complicated by organ infarction or limb ischaemia (see section 4.4 Special warnings and precautions for use: Monitoring)

Pain, haematoma and mild local irritation may follow the subcutaneous injection of enoxaparin. Rarely, hard inflammatory nodules which are not cystic enclosures of enoxaparin, have been observed at the injection site. They resolve after a few days and should not cause therapy discontinuation.

Exceptional cases of skin necrosis at the injection site have been reported with heparins and low molecular weight heparins. These phenomena are usually preceded by purpura or erythematous plaques, infiltrated and painful. Treatment with enoxaparin must be discontinued.

Although rare, cutaneous (bullous eruptions) or systemic allergic reactions including anaphylactoid reactions may occur. In some cases discontinuation of therapy may be necessary.

Very rare cases of hypersensitivity cutaneous vasculitis have been reported.

Asymptomatic and reversible increases in platelet counts and liver enzyme levels have been reported.

Long term treatment with heparin has been associated with a risk of osteoporosis. Although this has not been observed with enoxaparin the risk of osteoporosis cannot be excluded.

Heparin products can cause hypoaldosteronism which may result in an increase in plasma potassium. Rarely, clinically significant hyperkalaemia may occur particularly in patients with chronic renal failure and diabetes mellitus (see section 4.4 Special warnings and precautions for use).

There have been very rare reports of intra-spinal haematomas with the concurrent use of enoxaparin and spinal/epidural anaesthesia, spinal puncture and post-operative indwelling catheters. These events have resulted in varying degrees of neurological injuries including long term or permanent paralysis. (see section 4.4 Special warnings and precautions for use)

Valve thrombosis in patients with prosthetic heart valves have been reported rarely, usually associated with inadequate dosing (see section 4.4 Special warnings and precautions for use).

4.9 Overdose

Orally administered enoxaparin is poorly absorbed and even large oral doses should not lead to any serious consequences. This may be checked by plasma assays of anti-Xa and anti-IIa activities.

Accidental overdose following parenteral administration may produce haemorrhagic complications. The anticoagulant effects can be largely neutralised by the slow intravenous injection of Protamine, but even with high doses of Protamine, the anti-Xa activity of enoxaparin sodium is never completely neutralised (maximum about 60%). The initial dose of Protamine depends on the dose of enoxaparin given and also consideration of the maximum recommended Protamine dose (50mg). Data on Protamine dosing in humans for enoxaparin overdose is extremely limited. The available data suggest that in the first 8 hours after enoxaparin administration 1mg Protamine should neutralise the effects of 1mg of enoxaparin. Where the dose of enoxaparin has exceeded 50mg, an initial dose of 50mg Protamine would be appropriate, based on the maximum recommended single protamine dose. Decisions regarding the necessity and dose of subsequent Protamine injections should be based on clinical response rather than measurement of anti Xa or anti XIIa results. The physician should also consider that the amount of enoxaparin in the body drops to 50% after 8 hours and 33% or less after 12 hours. The dose of Protamine should be adjusted depending on the length of time since enoxaparin was administered.

5. PHARMACOLOGICAL PROPERTIES

5.1 Pharmacodynamic properties

Pharmacotherapeutic group: Antithrombotic agent, heparin group. ATC code B01A B05.

Enoxaparin is a low molecular weight heparin with a mean molecular weight of approximately 4,500 daltons. The drug substance is the sodium salt. The molecular weight distribution is:

<2000 daltons ⩽ 20%

2000 to 8000 daltons ⩾ 68%

>8000 daltons ⩽ 18%

Enoxaparin sodium is obtained by alkaline depolymerization of heparin benzyl ester derived from porcine intestinal mucosa. Its structure is characterized by a 2-O-sulfo-4-enepyranosuronic acid group at the non-reducing end and a 2-N,6-O-disulfo-D-glucosamine at the reducing end of the chain. About 20% (ranging between 15% and 25%) of the enoxaparin structure contains an 1,6 anhydro derivative on the reducing end of the polysaccharide chain.

It is characterised by a higher ratio of antithrombotic activity to anticoagulant activity than unfractionated heparin. At recommended doses, it does not significantly influence platelet aggregation, binding of fibrinogen to platelets or global blood clotting tests such as APTT and prothrombin time.

5.2 Pharmacokinetic properties

Enoxaparin is rapidly and completely absorbed following subcutaneous injection. The maximum plasma anti-Xa activity occurs 1 to 4 hours after injection with peak activities in the order of 0.16 IU/mL and 0.38 IU/mL after doses of 20 mg or 40 mg respectively. The anti-Xa activity generated is localised within the vascular compartments and elimination is characterised by a half life of 4 to 5 hours. Following a 40 mg dose, anti-Xa activity may persist in the plasma for 24 hours.

A linear relationship between anti-Xa plasma clearance and creatinine clearance at steady-state has been observed, which indicates decreased clearance of enoxaparin sodium in patients with reduced renal function. In patients with severe renal impairment (creatinine clearance < 30 ml/min), the AUC at steady state is significantly increased by an average of 65% after repeated, once daily subcutaneous doses of 40mg.

Hepatic metabolism by desulphation and depolymerisation also contributes to elimination. The elimination half life may be prolonged in elderly patients although no dosage adjustment is necessary.

A study of repeated, once daily subcutaneous doses of 1.5 mg/kg in healthy volunteers suggests that no dosage adjustment is necessary in obese subjects (BMI 30-48 kg/m^2) compared to non-obese subjects.

Enoxaparin, as detected by anti-Xa activity, does not cross the placental barrier during the second trimester of pregnancy.

Low Body Weight

When non-weight adjusted dosing was administered, it was found after a single-subcutaneous 40 mg dose, that anti-Xa exposure is 52% higher in low-weight women (<45 kg) and 27% higher in low-weight men (<57 kg) when compared to normal weight control subjects (see section 4.4 Special warnings and precautions for use: Low Body Weight).

5.3 Preclinical safety data

No long-term studies in animals have been performed to evaluate the carcinogenic potential of enoxaparin.

Enoxaparin was not mutagenic in *in vitro* tests, including the Ames test, mouse lymphoma cell forward mutation test, and human lymphocyte chromosomal aberration test, and the *in vivo* rat bone marrow chromosomal aberration test.

Enoxaparin was found to have no effect on fertility or reproductive performance of male and female rats at SC doses up to 20 mg/kg/day. Teratology studies have been conducted in pregnant rats and rabbits at SC doses of enoxaparin up to 30 mg/kg/day. There was no evidence of teratogenic effects or fetotoxicity due to enoxaparin.

Besides the anticoagulant effects of enoxaparin, there was no evidence of adverse effects at 15 mg/kg/day in the 13-week subcutaneous toxicity studies both in rats and dogs and at 10 mg/kg/day in the 26-week subcutaneous and intravenous toxicity studies both in rats and monkeys.

6. PHARMACEUTICAL PARTICULARS

6.1 List of excipients

Water for Injections Ph. Eur.

6.2 Incompatibilities

Clexane should not be mixed with any other injections or infusions

6.3 Shelf life

24 months.

6.4 Special precautions for storage

Do not store above 25°C. Do not refrigerate or freeze.

Clexane prefilled syringes are single dose containers - discard any unused product.

6.5 Nature and contents of container

Solution for injection in Type I glass prefilled syringes fitted with injection needle in packs of 10.

6.6 Special precautions for disposal and other handling

See section 4.4 Posology and method of administration

7. MARKETING AUTHORISATION HOLDER

Sanofi-aventis

One Onslow Street

Guildford

Surrey, GU1 4YS

UK

8. MARKETING AUTHORISATION NUMBER(S)

PL 00012/0339

9. DATE OF FIRST AUTHORISATION/RENEWAL OF THE AUTHORISATION

04/02/2009

10. DATE OF REVISION OF THE TEXT

04/02/2009

Legal Category: POM

Clexane Syringes and Clexane Multidose Vial

(sanofi-aventis)

1. NAME OF THE MEDICINAL PRODUCT

Clexane Syringes

Clexane Multidose Vial

2. QUALITATIVE AND QUANTITATIVE COMPOSITION

Clexane pre-filled syringes:

20 mg Injection	Enoxaparin sodium 20 mg (equivalent to 2,000 IU anti-Xa activity) in 0.2 mL Water for Injections
40 mg Injection	Enoxaparin sodium 40 mg (equivalent to 4,000 IU anti-Xa activity) in 0.4 mL Water for Injections
60 mg Injection	Enoxaparin sodium 60 mg (equivalent to 6,000 IU anti-Xa activity) in 0.6 mL Water for Injections
80 mg Injection	Enoxaparin sodium 80 mg (equivalent to 8,000 IU anti-Xa activity) in 0.8 mL Water for Injections
100 mg Injection	Enoxaparin sodium 100mg (equivalent to 10,000 IU anti-Xa activity) in 1.0 mL Water for Injections

Clexane Multidose Vial

Vials containing 300 mg enoxaparin (equivalent to 30,000 IU anti-Xa activity) in 3.0 ml

3. PHARMACEUTICAL FORM

Syringes: Solution for injection.

Multidose vial: Sterile pyrogen-free solution for injection contained in a multidose vial for single patient use.

4. CLINICAL PARTICULARS

4.1 Therapeutic indications

The prophylaxis of thromboembolic disorders of venous origin, in particular those which may be associated with orthopaedic or general surgery.

The prophylaxis of venous thromboembolism in medical patients bedridden due to acute illness.

The treatment of venous thromboembolic disease presenting with deep vein thrombosis, pulmonary embolism or both.

The treatment of unstable angina and non-Q-wave myocardial infarction, administered concurrently with aspirin.

Treatment of acute ST-segment Elevation Myocardial Infarction (STEMI) including patients to be managed medically or with subsequent Percutaneous Coronary Intervention (PCI) in conjunction with thrombolytic drugs (fibrin or non-fibrin specific).

The prevention of thrombus formation in the extracorporeal circulation during haemodialysis.

4.2 Posology and method of administration

Adults:

Prophylaxis of venous thromboembolism:

In patients with a low to moderate risk of venous thromboembolism the recommended dosage is 20 mg (2,000 IU) once daily for 7 to 10 days, or until the risk of thromboembolism has diminished. In patients undergoing surgery, the initial dose should be given approximately 2 hours pre-operatively. In patients with a higher risk, such as in orthopaedic surgery, the dosage should be 40 mg (4,000 IU) daily with the initial dose administered approximately 12 hours before surgery.

Prophylaxis of venous thromboembolism in medical patients:

The recommended dose of enoxaparin sodium is 40 mg (4,000 IU) once daily. Treatment with enoxaparin sodium is prescribed for a minimum of 6 days and continued until the return to full ambulation, for a maximum of 14 days.

Treatment of venous thromboembolism:

Clexane should be administered subcutaneously as a single daily injection of 1.5 mg/kg (150 IU/kg). Clexane treatment is usually prescribed for at least 5 days and until adequate oral anticoagulation is established.

Treatment of unstable angina and non-Q-wave myocardial infarction

The recommended dose is 1 mg/kg Clexane every 12 hours by subcutaneous injection, administered concurrently with oral aspirin (100 to 325mg once daily). Treatment with Clexane in these patients should be prescribed for a minimum of 2 days and continued until clinical stabilisation. The usual duration of treatment is 2 to 8 days.

Treatment of acute ST-segment Elevation Myocardial Infarction:

The recommended dose of enoxaparin sodium is a single IV bolus of 30mg plus a 1mg/kg SC dose followed by 1mg/kg administered SC every 12 hours (max 100mg for the first two doses only, followed by 1mg/kg dosing for the remaining doses). For dosage in patients ⩾75 years of age, see section 4.2 Posology and method of administration: *Elderly*.

When administered in conjunction with a thrombolytic (fibrin specific or non-fibrin specific) enoxaparin sodium should be given between 15 minutes before and 30 minutes after the start of fibrinolytic therapy. All patients should receive acetylsalicylic acid (ASA) as soon as they are identified as having STEMI and maintained under (75 to 325mg once daily) unless contraindicated.

The recommended duration of enoxaparin sodium treatment is 8 days or until hospital discharge, whichever comes first.

For patients managed with Percutaneous Coronary Intervention (PCI): If the last enoxaparin sodium SC administration was given less than 8 hours before balloon inflation, no additional dosing is needed. If the last SC administration was given more than 8 hours before balloon inflation, an IV bolus of 0.3mg/kg of enoxaparin sodium should be administered.

Prevention of extracorporeal thrombus formation during haemodialysis:

A dose equivalent to 1 mg/kg (100 IU/kg) introduced into the arterial line at the beginning of a dialysis session is usually sufficient for a 4 hour session. If fibrin rings are found, such as after a longer than normal session, a further dose of 0.5 to 1mg/kg (50 to 100 IU/kg) may be given. For patients at a high risk of haemorrhage the dose should be reduced to 0.5 mg/kg (50 IU/kg) for double vascular access or 0.75 mg/kg (75 IU/kg) for single vascular access.

Elderly:

For treatment of acute ST-segment Elevation Myocardial Infarction in elderly patients ⩾75 years of age, do not use an initial IV bolus. Initiate dosing with 0.75mg/kg SC every 12 hours (maximum 75mg for the first two doses only, followed by 0.75mg/kg dosing for the remaining doses).

For other indications, no dosage adjustments are necessary in the elderly, unless kidney function is impaired (see also section 4.2 Posology and method of administration: *Renal impairment*; section 4.4 Special warnings and precautions for use: *Haemorrhage in the elderly*; *Renal impairment and Monitoring*; section 5.2 Pharmacokinetic properties).

Children: Not recommended, as dosage not established.

Renal impairment: (See also section 4.4 Special warnings and precautions for use: *Renal impairment and Monitoring*; section 5.2 Pharmacokinetic properties).

Severe renal impairment:

A dosage adjustment is required for patients with severe renal impairment (creatinine clearance < 30 ml/min), according to the following tables, since enoxaparin sodium exposure is significantly increased in this patient population:

Dosage adjustments for therapeutic dosage ranges

Standard dosing	Severe renal impairment
1 mg/kg SC twice daily	1 mg/kg SC once daily
1.5 mg/kg SC once daily	1 mg/kg SC once daily
30mg-single IV bolus plus a 1mg/kg SC dose followed by 1mg/kg twice daily.	30mg-single IV bolus plus a 1mg/kg SC dose followed by 1mg/kg once daily.
Elderly patients ⩾75years of age (for acute STEMI indication only)	
0.75mg/kg SC twice daily without initial bolus.	1mg/kg SC once daily without initial bolus.

Dosage adjustments for prophylactic dosage ranges

Standard dosing	Severe renal impairment
40 mg once daily	20 mg once daily
20 mg once daily	20 mg once daily

The recommended dosage adjustments do not apply to the haemodialysis indication.

Moderate and mild renal impairment:

Although no dosage adjustments are recommended in patients with moderate renal impairment (creatinine clearance 30-50 ml/min) or mild renal impairment (creatinine clearance 50-80 ml/min), careful clinical monitoring is advised.

Hepatic impairment: In the absence of clinical studies, caution should be exercised.

Body weight:

No dosage adjustments are recommended in obesity or low body weight (see also section 4.4 Special warnings and precautions for use: *Low body weight and Monitoring*; section 5.2 Pharmacokinetic properties).

Clexane is administered by subcutaneous injection for the prevention of venous thromboembolic disease, treatment of deep vein thrombosis or for the treatment of unstable angina and non-Q-wave myocardial infarction and acute ST-elevation myocardial infarction (STEMI); through the arterial line of a dialysis circuit for the prevention of thrombus formation in the extra-corporeal circulation during haemodialysis. and via intravenous (bolus) injection through an intravenous line only for the initial dose of acute STEMI indication and before PCI when needed. It must not be administered by the intramuscular route.

Subcutaneous injection technique:

The prefilled disposable syringe is ready for immediate use. When using vials of enoxaparin sodium, the volume to be injected should be measured precisely with a graduated syringe fitted with an appropriate needle for subcutaneous injection.

Clexane should be administered when the patient is lying down by deep subcutaneous injection. The administration should be alternated between the left and right anterolateral or posterolateral abdominal wall. The whole length of the needle should be introduced vertically into a skin fold held between the thumb and index finger. The skin fold should not be released until the injection is complete. Do not rub the injection site after administration.

Intravenous (Bolus) Injection Technique (for acute STEMI indication only):

For intravenous injection, the Multi dose vial should be used. Enoxaparin sodium should be administered through an intravenous line. It should not be mixed or co-administered with other medications. To avoid the possible mixture of enoxaparin sodium with all other drugs, the intravenous access chosen should be flushed with a sufficient amount of saline or dextrose solution prior to and following the intravenous bolus administration of enoxaparin sodium to clear the port of the drug. Enoxaparin sodium may be safely administered with normal saline solution (0.9%) or 5% dextrose in water.

4.3 Contraindications

Contraindicated in patients with acute bacterial endocarditis, active major bleeding and conditions with a high risk of uncontrolled haemorrhage, including recent haemorrhagic stroke, thrombocytopenia in patients with a positive in-vitro aggregation test in the presence of enoxaparin; active gastric or duodenal ulceration; hypersensitivity to either enoxaparin sodium, heparin or its derivatives including other Low Molecular Weight Heparins; hypersensitivity to benzyl alcohol; in patients receiving heparin for treatment rather than prophylaxis, locoregional anaesthesia in elective surgical procedures is contraindicated.

4.4 Special warnings and precautions for use

Low Molecular Weight Heparins should not be used interchangeably since they differ in their manufacturing process, molecular weights, specific anti Xa activities, units and dosage. This results in differences in pharmacokinetics and associated biological activities (e.g. anti-IIa activity, and platelet interactions). Special attention and compliance with the instructions for use specific to each proprietary medicinal product are therefore required.

Enoxaparin is to be used with extreme caution in patients with a history of heparin-induced thrombocytopenia with or without thrombosis.

As there is a risk of antibody-mediated heparin-induced thrombocytopenia also occurring with low molecular weight heparins, regular platelet count monitoring should be considered prior to and during therapy with these agents. Thrombocytopenia, should it occur, usually appears between the 5th and the 21st day following the beginning of therapy. Therefore, it is recommended that the platelet counts be measured before the initiation of therapy with enoxaparin sodium and then regularly thereafter during the treatment. In practice, if a confirmed significant decrease of the platelet count is observed (30 to 50 % of the initial value), enoxaparin sodium treatment must be immediately discontinued and the patient switched to another therapy.

Enoxaparin injection, as with any other anticoagulant therapy, should be used with caution in conditions with increased potential for bleeding, such as: impaired haemostasis, history of peptic ulcer, recent ischaemic stroke, uncontrolled severe arterial hypertension, diabetic retinopathy, recent neuro- or ophthalmologic surgery.

As with other anticoagulants, bleeding may occur at any site (see section 4.8 Undesirable effects). If bleeding occurs, the origin of the haemorrhage should be investigated and appropriate treatment instituted.

Heparin can suppress adrenal secretion of aldosterone leading to hyperkalaemia, particularly in patients such as those with diabetes mellitus, chronic renal failure, pre-existing metabolic acidosis, a raised plasma potassium or taking potassium sparing drugs. The risk of hyperkalaemia appears to increase with duration of therapy but is usually reversible. Plasma potassium should be measured in patients at risk before starting heparin therapy and monitored regularly thereafter particularly if treatment is prolonged beyond about 7 days.

As with other anti-coagulants, there have been cases of intra-spinal haematomas reported with the concurrent use of enoxaparin sodium and spinal/epidural anaesthesia or spinal puncture resulting in long term or permanent paralysis. These events are rare with enoxaparin sodium dosage regimens 40 mg od or lower. The risk is greater with higher enoxaparin sodium dosage regimens, use of post-operative indwelling catheters or the concomitant use of additional drugs affecting haemostasis such as NSAIDs (see section 4.5 Interaction with other medicinal products and other forms of interaction). The risk also appears to be increased by traumatic or repeated neuraxial puncture.

To reduce the potential risk of bleeding associated with the concurrent use of enoxaparin sodium and epidural anaesthesia/analgesia, the pharmacokinetic profile of the drug should be considered (see section 5.2 Pharmacokinetic properties). Placement and removal of the catheter is best performed when the anticoagulation effect of enoxaparin is low.

Placement or removal of a catheter should be delayed for 10 - 12 hours after administration of DVT prophylactic doses of enoxaparin sodium, whereas patients receiving higher doses of enoxaparin sodium (1.5 mg/kg once daily) will require longer delays (24 hours). The subsequent enoxaparin sodium dose should be given no sooner than 4 hours after catheter removal.

Should the physician decide to administer anticoagulation in the context of epidural/spinal anaesthesia, extreme vigilance and frequent monitoring must be exercised to detect any signs and symptoms of neurological impairment such as midline back pain, sensory and motor deficits (numbness or weakness in lower limbs), bowel and/or bladder dysfunction. Patients should be instructed to inform their nurse or physician immediately if they experience any of the above signs or symptoms. If signs or symptoms of spinal haematoma are suspected, urgent diagnosis and treatment including spinal cord decompression should be initiated.

The Multidose vial contains benzyl alcohol as a preservative and should not be given to premature babies or neonates. The administration of medicines containing benzyl alcohol as a preservative may cause toxic reactions and anaphylactoid reactions in children up to 3 years old.

Percutaneous coronary revascularisation procedures:

To minimise the risk of bleeding following vascular instrumentation during the treatment of unstable angina, non-Q-wave myocardial infarction and acute ST-elevation myocardial infarction, adhere precisely to the intervals recommended between enoxaparin sodium doses. It is important to achieve homeostasis at the puncture site after PCI. If a closure device is used, the sheath can be removed immediately. If a manual compression method is used, sheath should be removed 6 hours after the last IV/SC enoxaparin sodium injection. If the treatment is continued, the next scheduled dose should be given no sooner than 6 to 8 hours after sheath removal. The site of the procedure should be observed for signs of bleeding or haematoma formation.

For some patients with pulmonary embolism (e.g. those with severe haemodynamic instability) alternative treatment such as thrombolysis or surgery may be indicated.

Prosthetic Heart Valves:

There have been no adequate studies to assess the safe and effective use of enoxaparin sodium in preventing valve thrombosis in patients with prosthetic heart valves. Prophylactic doses of enoxaparin are not sufficient to prevent valve thrombosis in patients with prosthetic heart valves. Confounding factors, including underlying diseases and insufficient clinical data, limit the evaluation of these cases. Therapeutic failures have been reported in pregnant women with prosthetic heart valves on full anti-coagulant doses (see section 4.6 Pregnancy and lactation). The use of enoxaparin sodium cannot be recommended for this purpose.

Haemorrhage in the elderly: No increased bleeding tendency is observed in the elderly within the prophylactic dosage ranges. Elderly patients (especially patients aged eighty years and above) may be at an increased risk for bleeding complications within the therapeutic dosage ranges. In the treatment of acute ST-segment Elevation Myocardial Infarction (STEMI), an increase in bleeding events was observed in patients aged 65-75 years suggesting these patients might be at particular risk of bleeding. Careful clinical monitoring is advised (see also section 4.2 Posology and method of administration: Elderly; section 5.2 Pharmacokinetic properties).

Renal impairment: In patients with renal impairment, there is an increase in enoxaparin exposure which increases the risk of bleeding. Since enoxaparin exposure is significantly increased in patients with severe renal impairment (creatinine clearance < 30 ml/min) dosage adjustments are recommended in therapeutic and prophylactic dosage ranges. Although no dosage adjustments are recommended in patients with moderate (creatinine clearance 30-50 ml/min) and mild (creatinine clearance 50-80 ml/min) renal impairment, careful clinical monitoring is advised (see also section 4.2 Posology and method of administration: Renal impairment; section 5.2 Pharmacokinetic properties). In the treatment of acute ST-segment Elevation Myocardial Infarction (STEMI), the data are limited in patients with creatinine levels above 220 and 175 μmol/L for males and females respectively.

Low body weight: In low-weight women (< 45 kg) and low-weight men (< 57 kg), an increase in enoxaparin exposure has been observed within the prophylactic dosage ranges (non-weight adjusted), which may lead to a higher risk of bleeding. Therefore, careful clinical monitoring is advised in these patients (see also section 5.2 Pharmacokinetic properties).

Monitoring: Risk assessment and clinical monitoring are the best predictors of the risk of potential bleeding. Routine anti-Xa activity monitoring is usually not required. However, anti-Xa activity monitoring might be considered in those patients treated with LMWH who also have either an increased risk of bleeding (such as those with renal impairment, elderly and extremes of weight) or are actively bleeding.

Laboratory tests:

At doses used for prophylaxis of venous thromboembolism, enoxaparin sodium does not influence bleeding time and global blood coagulation tests significantly, nor does it affect platelet aggregation or binding of fibrinogen to platelets. At higher doses, increases in APTT (activated partial thromboplastin time) and ACT (activated clotting time) may occur. Increases in APTT and ACT are not linearly correlated with increasing enoxaparin sodium antithrombotic activity and therefore are unsuitable and unreliable for monitoring enoxaparin sodium activity.

4.5 Interaction with other medicinal products and other forms of interaction

It is recommended that agents which affect haemostasis should be discontinued prior to enoxaparin therapy unless their use is essential, such as: systemic salicylates, acetylsalicylic acid, NSAIDs including ketorolac, dextran, and clopidogrel, systemic glucocorticoids, thrombolytics and anticoagulants. If the combination cannot be avoided, enoxaparin should be used with careful clinical and laboratory monitoring.

4.6 Pregnancy and lactation

Pregnancy: Animal studies have not shown any evidence of foetotoxicity or teratogenicity. In the pregnant rat, the transfer of ^{35}S-enoxaparin across the maternal placenta to the foetus is minimal.

In humans, there is no evidence that enoxaparin crosses the placental barrier during the second trimester of pregnancy. There is no information available concerning the first and the third trimesters.

As there are no adequately powered and well-controlled studies in pregnant women and because animal studies are not always predictive of human response, this drug should be used during pregnancy only if the physician has established a clear need.

Pregnant women with mechanical prosthetic heart valves

The use of enoxaparin for thromboprophylaxis in pregnant women with mechanical prosthetic heart valves has not been adequately studied. In a clinical study of pregnant women with mechanical prosthetic heart valves given enoxaparin (1 mg/kg bid) to reduce the risk of thromboembolism, 2 of 8 women developed clots resulting in blockage of the valve and leading to maternal and foetal death. There have been isolated postmarketing reports of valve thrombosis in pregnant women with mechanical prosthetic heart valves while receiving enoxaparin for thromboprophylaxis. Pregnant women with mechanical prosthetic heart valves may be at higher risk for thromboembolism. Enoxaparin sodium is not recommended for use in pregnant women with prosthetic heart valves (see section 4.4 Special warnings and precautions for use: Prosthetic heart valves).

Lactation: In lactating rats, the concentration of ^{35}S-enoxaparin or its labelled metabolites in milk is very low.

It is not known whether unchanged enoxaparin is excreted in human breast milk. The oral absorption of enoxaparin is unlikely. However, as a precaution, lactating mothers receiving enoxaparin should be advised to avoid breast-feeding.

4.7 Effects on ability to drive and use machines

Enoxaparin has no effect on the ability to drive and operate machines

4.8 Undesirable effects

As with other anticoagulants bleeding may occur during enoxaparin therapy in the presence of associated risk factors such as: organic lesions liable to bleed, invasive procedures or the use of medications affecting haemostasis (see section 4.5 Interaction with other medicinal products and other forms of interaction). The origin of the bleeding should be investigated and appropriate treatment instituted.

Major haemorrhage including retroperitoneal and intracranial bleeding have been reported, in rare instances these have been fatal.

Mild, transient, asymptomatic thrombocytopenia has been reported during the first days of therapy. Rare cases of immuno-allergic thrombocytopenia with or without thrombosis have been reported. In some cases thrombosis was complicated by organ infarction or limb ischaemia (see section 4.4 Special warnings and precautions for use: Monitoring).

Pain, haematoma and mild local irritation may follow the subcutaneous injection of enoxaparin. Rarely, hard inflammatory nodules which are not cystic enclosures of enoxaparin, have been observed at the injection site. They resolve after a few days and should not cause therapy discontinuation.

Exceptional cases of skin necrosis, usually occuring at the injection site have been reported with heparins and low molecular weight heparins. These phenomena are usually preceded by purpura or erythematous plaques, infiltrated and painful. Treatment with enoxaparin must be discontinued.

Although rare, cutaneous (bullous eruptions) or systemic allergic reactions including anaphylactic/anaphylactoid reactions may occur. In some cases discontinuation of therapy may be necessary.

Very rare cases of hypersensitivity cutaneous vasculitis have been reported.

Asymptomatic and reversible increases in platelet counts and liver enzyme levels have been reported.

Long term treatment with heparin has been associated with a risk of osteoporosis. Although this has not been observed with enoxaparin the risk of osteoporosis cannot be excluded.

Heparin products can cause hypoaldosteronism which may result in an increase in plasma potassium. Rarely, clinically significant hyperkalaemia may occur particularly in patients with chronic renal failure and diabetes mellitus (see section 4.4 Special warnings and precautions for use).

There have been very rare reports of intra-spinal haematomas with the concurrent use of enoxaparin and spinal/epidural anaesthesia, spinal puncture and post-operative indwelling catheters. These events have resulted in varying degrees of neurological injuries including long term or permanent paralysis (see section 4.4 Special warnings and precautions for use).

Valve thrombosis in patients with prosthetic heart valves have been reported rarely, usually associated with inadequate dosing (see section 4.4 Special warnings and precautions for use).

4.9 Overdose

Orally administered enoxaparin is poorly absorbed and even large oral doses should not lead to any serious consequences. This may be checked by plasma assays of anti-Xa and anti-IIa activities.

Accidental overdose following parenteral administration may produce haemorrhagic complications.

The anticoagulant effects can be largely neutralised by the slow intravenous injection of Protamine, but even with high doses of Protamine, the anti-Xa activity of enoxaparin sodium is never completely neutralised (maximum about 60%). The initial dose of Protamine depends on the dose of enoxaparin given and also consideration of the maximum recommended Protamine dose (50mg). Data on Protamine dosing in humans for enoxaparin overdose is extremely limited. The available data suggest that in the first 8 hours after enoxaparin administration 1mg Protamine should neutralise the effects of 1mg of enoxaparin. Where the dose of enoxaparin has exceeded 50mg, an initial dose of 50mg Protamine would be appropriate, based on the maximum recommended single protamine dose. Decisions regarding the necessity and dose of subsequent Protamine injections should be based on clinical response rather than measurement of anti Xa or anti IIa results. The physician should also consider that the amount of enoxaparin in the body drops to 50% after 8 hours and 33% or less after 12 hours. The dose of Protamine should be adjusted depending on the length of time since enoxaparin was administered.

5. PHARMACOLOGICAL PROPERTIES

5.1 Pharmacodynamic properties

Pharmacotherapeutic group: Antithrombotic agent, heparin group. ATC code B01A B05

Enoxaparin is a low molecular weight heparin with a mean molecular weight of approximately 4,500 daltons. The drug substance is the sodium salt. The molecular weight distribution is:

$<$2000 daltons $\leqslant$ 20%

2000 to 8000 daltons $\geqslant$ 68%

$>$8000 daltons $\leqslant$ 18%

Enoxaparin sodium is obtained by alkaline depolymerization of heparin benzyl ester derived from porcine intestinal mucosa. Its structure is characterized by a 2-O-sulfo-4-enepyranosuronic acid group at the non-reducing end and a 2-N,6-O-disulfo-D-glucosamine at the reducing end of the chain. About 20% (ranging between 15% and 25%) of the enoxaparin structure contains an 1,6 anhydro derivative on the reducing end of the polysaccharide chain.

Enoxaparin sodium is characterised by a higher ratio of antithrombotic activity to anticoagulant activity than unfractionated heparin. At recommended doses, it does not significantly influence platelet aggregation, binding of fibrinogen to platelets or global blood clotting tests such as APTT and prothrombin time.

5.2 Pharmacokinetic properties

Enoxaparin is rapidly and completely absorbed following subcutaneous injection. The maximum plasma anti-Xa activity occurs 1 to 4 hours after injection with peak activities in the order of 0.16 IU/ml and 0.38 IU/ml after doses of 20 mg or 40 mg respectively. The anti-Xa activity generated is localised within the vascular compartments and elimination is characterised by a half-life of 4 to 5 hours. Following a 40 mg dose, anti-Xa activity may persist in the plasma for 24 hours.

A 30mg IV bolus immediately followed by a 1mg/kg SC every 12 hours provided initial peak anti-Factor Xa levels of 1.16IU/ml (n=16) and average exposure corresponding to 88% of steady state levels.

A linear relationship between anti-Xa plasma clearance and creatinine clearance at steady-state has been observed, which indicates decreased clearance of enoxaparin sodium in patients with reduced renal function. In patients with severe renal impairment (creatinine clearance $<$ 30 ml/min), the AUC at steady state is significantly increased by an average of 65% after repeated, once daily subcutaneous doses of 40mg.

Hepatic metabolism by desulphation and depolymerisation also contributes to elimination. The elimination half-life may be prolonged in elderly patients although no dosage adjustment is necessary.

A study of repeated, once daily subcutaneous doses of 1.5 mg/kg in healthy volunteers suggests that no dosage adjustment is necessary in obese subjects (BMI 30-48 kg/m2) compared to non-obese subjects.

Enoxaparin, as detected by anti-Xa activity, does not cross the placental barrier during the second trimester of pregnancy.

Low Body Weight

When non-weight adjusted dosing was administered, it was found after a single-subcutaneous 40 mg dose, that anti-Xa exposure is 52% higher in low-weight women ($<$45 kg) and 27% higher in low-weight men ($<$57 kg) when compared to normal weight control subjects (see section 4.4 Special warnings and precautions for use: Low Body Weight).

Pharmacokinetic interactions

No pharmacokinetic interactions were observed between enoxaparin and thrombolytics when administered concomitantly.

5.3 Preclinical safety data

No long-term studies in animals have been performed to evaluate the carcinogenic potential of enoxaparin.

Enoxaparin was not mutagenic in *in vitro* tests, including the Ames test, mouse lymphoma cell forward mutation test, and human lymphocyte chromosomal aberration test, and the *in vivo* rat bone marrow chromosomal aberration test.

Enoxaparin was found to have no effect on fertility or reproductive performance of male and female rats at SC doses up to 20 mg/kg/day. Teratology studies have been conducted in pregnant rats and rabbits at SC doses of enoxaparin up to 30 mg/kg/day. There was no evidence of teratogenic effects or fetotoxicity due to enoxaparin.

Besides the anticoagulant effects of enoxaparin, there was no evidence of adverse effects at 15 mg/kg/day in the 13-week subcutaneous toxicity studies both in rats and dogs and at 10 mg/kg/day in the 26-week subcutaneous and intravenous toxicity studies both in rats and monkeys.

6. PHARMACEUTICAL PARTICULARS

6.1 List of excipients

Clexane Syringes: Water for Injections BP

Multidose Vials: Benzyl alcohol (45mg/3ml); Water for Injections

6.2 Incompatibilities

Subcutaneous Injection:

Clexane should not be mixed with any other injections or infusions.

Intravenous (Bolus) Injection for acute STEMI indication only: Enoxaparin: sodium may be safely administered with normal saline solution (0.9%) or 5% dextrose in water.

6.3 Shelf life

Clexane syringes: 36 months

Multidose Vials: 24 months

6.4 Special precautions for storage

Clexane Syringes: Do not store above 25°C. Do not refrigerate or freeze.

Clexane pre-filled syringes are single dose containers - discard any unused product

Multidose Vials: Store below 25°C. The contents of the multidose vial should be used within 28 days of opening.

6.5 Nature and contents of container

Clexane Syringes: Solution for injection in Type I glass pre-filled syringes fitted with injection needle in packs of 10.

Multidose Vials: Boxes containing a single 3 ml multidose glass vial for single patient use.

6.6 Special precautions for disposal and other handling

See section 4.2 Posology and method of administration.

7. MARKETING AUTHORISATION HOLDER

Sanofi-aventis

One Onslow Street

Guildford

Surrey

GU1 4YS

UK

8. MARKETING AUTHORISATION NUMBER(S)

Clexane Syringes: PL 04425/0187

Clexane Multidose Vials: PL 00012/0314

9. DATE OF FIRST AUTHORISATION/RENEWAL OF THE AUTHORISATION

Clexane Syringes: 30 January 2009

Clexane Multidose Vials: August 2002

10. DATE OF REVISION OF THE TEXT

Clexane Syringes: 28 May 2009

Clexane Multidose Vials: 28 May 2009

11. LEGAL CATEGORY

POM

Clopixol Acuphase Injection

(Lundbeck Limited)

1. NAME OF THE MEDICINAL PRODUCT

Clopixol® Acuphase

2. QUALITATIVE AND QUANTITATIVE COMPOSITION

Zuclopenthixol acetate 5.0% w/v equivalent to 4.526% w/v of zuclopenthixol base.

3. PHARMACEUTICAL FORM

Oily solution for deep intramuscular injection.

4. CLINICAL PARTICULARS

4.1 Therapeutic indications

For the initial treatment of acute psychoses including mania and exacerbation of chronic psychoses, particularly where a rapid onset of action, and a duration of effect of 2-3 days is desirable.

4.2 Posology and method of administration

Dosage

Adults

Dosage should be adjusted according to the severity of the patient's illness. Clopixol Acuphase is administered by deep intramuscular injection, into the upper outer buttock or lateral thigh.

The usual dosage is 50-150 mg (1-3 ml), repeated if necessary after 2 or 3 days. Some patients may need an additional injection between 1 and 2 days after the first injection.

Clopixol Acuphase is not intended for long-term use and duration of treatment should not be more than two weeks.

The maximum accumulated dosage in a course should not exceed 400 mg and the number of injections should not exceed four.

Patients with compromised hepatic function should receive half the recommended dosages for normal patients. Where there is reduced renal function, it is not necessary to reduce the dosage but where there is renal failure dosage should be reduced to half the normal dosage.

Elderly

The dosage may need to be reduced in the elderly owing to reduced rates of metabolism and elimination. Maximum dosage per injection should be 100 mg.

Children

Not recommended for children.

Maintenance Therapy:

Clopixol Acuphase is not intended for long-term use.

A single injection of Clopixol Acuphase has an onset of sedative action shortly after injection and an antipsychotic action persisting for 2 to 3 days. In this period, maintenance treatment with tablets or a longer acting depot neuroleptic can be initiated. The possible side-effects of long-term maintenance treatment with a neuroleptic, including tardive dyskinesia, should be considered.

Maintenance treatment where required can be continued with Clopixol tablets, Clopixol injection or Clopixol conc. injection, according to the following guidelines:

1. Introduce Clopixol tablets at a dosage of 20-60 mg/day in divided doses, 2 to 3 days after the last injection of Clopixol Acuphase. If necessary increase the tablet dosage by 10-20 mg each day up to a maximum of 150 mg/day.

or

2. Concomitantly with the last injection of Clopixol Acuphase, administer 200-500 mg of Clopixol injection or Clopixol Conc. injection by deep intramuscular injection and repeat the Clopixol injection or Clopixol Conc. injection at intervals of 2 to 4 weeks. Higher dosages or a shorter interval may be necessary.

Route of Administration:

Deep intramuscular injection, into the upper outer buttock or lateral thigh.

4.3 Contraindications

Hypersensitivity to the active substance or to any of the excipients (see section 6.1).

Circulatory collapse, depressed level of consciousness due to any cause (e.g. intoxication with alcohol, barbiturates or opiates), coma.

4.4 Special warnings and precautions for use

Like other neuroleptics zuclopenthixol acetate should be used with caution in patients with convulsive disorders or advanced hepatic, renal or cardiovascular disease.

Zuclopenthixol is not suitable for patients who do not tolerate oral neuroleptic drugs or for patients suffering from Parkinson's disease.

The possibility of development of neuroleptic malignant syndrome (hyperthermia, muscle rigidity, fluctuating consciousness, instability of the autonomous nervous system) exists with any neuroleptic. The risk is possibly greater with the more potent agents. Patients with pre-existing organic brain syndrome, mental retardation and opiate and alcohol abuse are over-represented among fatal cases.

Treatment:

Discontinuation of the neuroleptic. Symptomatic treatment and use of general supportive measures. Dantrolene and bromocriptine may be helpful. Symptoms may persist for more than a week after oral neuroleptics are discontinued and somewhat longer when associated with the depot forms of the drugs.

Like other neuroleptics, zuclopenthixol should be used with caution in patients with organic brain syndrome, convulsions or advanced hepatic disease.

Blood dyscrasias have been reported rarely. Blood counts should be carried out if a patient develops signs of persistent infection.

An approximately 3-fold increased risk of cerebrovascular adverse events has been seen in randomised placebo controlled clinical trials in the dementia population with some atypical antipsychotics. The mechanism for this increased risk is not known. An increased risk cannot be excluded for other antipsychotics or other patient populations.

Zuclopenthixol should be used with caution in patients with risk factors for stroke.

As with other drugs belonging to the therapeutic class of antipsychotics, zuclopenthixol may cause QT prolongation. Persistently prolonged QT intervals may increase the risk of malignant arrhythmias. Therefore, zuclopenthixol should be used with caution in susceptible individuals (with hypokalemia, hypomagnesia or genetic predisposition) and in patients with a history of cardiovascular disorders, e.g. QT prolongation, significant bradycardia (<50 beats per minute), a recent acute myocardial infarction, uncompensated heart failure, or cardiac arrhythmia.

Concomitant treatment with other antipsychotics should be avoided (see section 4.5).

As described for other psychotropics zuclopenthixol may modify insulin and glucose responses calling for adjustment of the antidiabetic therapy in diabetic patients.

4.5 Interaction with other medicinal products and other forms of interaction

In common with other antipsychotics, zuclopenthixol enhances the response to alcohol, the effects of barbiturates and other CNS depressants.

Zuclopenthixol may potentiate the effects of general anaesthetics and anticoagulants and prolong the action of neuromuscular blocking agents.

The anticholinergic effects of atropine or other drugs with anticholinergic properties may be increased.

Concomitant use of drugs such as metoclopramide, piperazine or antiparkinson drugs may increase the risk of extrapyramidal effects such as tardive dyskinesia.

Combined use of antipsychotics and lithium or sibutramine has been associated with an increased risk of neurotoxicity.

Antipsychotics may enhance the cardiac depressant effects of quinidine; the absorption of corticosteroids and digoxin.

The hypotensive effect of vasodilator antihypertensive agents such as hydralazine and α blockers (e.g. doxazosin), or methyl-dopa may be enhanced.

Increases in the QT interval related to antipsychotic treatment may be exacerbated by the co administration of other drugs known to significantly increase the QT interval. Co-administration of such drugs should be avoided. Relevant classes include:

- class Ia and III antiarrhythmics (e.g. quinidine, amiodarone, sotalol, dofetilide)
- some antipsychotics (e.g. thioridazine)
- some macrolides (e.g. erythromycin)
- some antihistamines
- some quinolone antibiotics (e.g. moxifloxacin)

The above list is not exhaustive and other individual drugs known to significantly increase QT interval (e.g. cisapride, lithium) should be avoided. Drugs known to cause electrolyte disturbances such as thiazidediuretics (hypokalemia) and drugs known to increase the plasma concentration of zuclopenthixol should also be used with caution as they may increase the risk of QT prolongation and malignant arrhythmias (see section 4.4).

Antipsychotics may antagonise the effects of adrenaline and other sympathomimetic agents, and reverse the antihypertensive effects of guanethidine and similar adrenergic-blocking agents.

Antipsychotics may also impair the effect of levodopa, adrenergic drugs and anticonvulsants.

The metabolism of tricyclic antidepressants may be inhibited and the control of diabetes may be impaired.

Since zuclopenthixol is partly metabolised by CYP2D6 concomitant use of drugs known to inhibit this enzyme may lead to higher than expected plasma concentrations of zuclopenthixol, increasing the risk of adverse effects and cardiotoxicity.

4.6 Pregnancy and lactation

Pregnancy

Zuclopenthixol should not be administered during pregnancy unless the expected benefit to the patient outweighs the theoretical risk to the foetus.

The newborn of mothers treated with neuroleptics in late pregnancy, or labour, may show signs of intoxication such as lethargy, tremor and hyper excitability, and have a low Apgar score.

Animal-reproduction studies have not given evidence of an increased incidence of foetal damage or other deleterious effects on the reproduction process.

Lactation

As zuclopenthixol is found in breast milk in low concentrations it is not likely to affect the infant when therapeutic doses are used. The dose ingested by the infant is less than 1% of the weight related maternal dose (in mg/kg). Breast-feeding can be continued during zuclopenthixol therapy if considered of clinical importance but observation of the infant is recommended, particularly in the first 4 weeks after giving birth.

4.7 Effects on ability to drive and use machines

Zuclopenthixol is a sedative drug.

Alertness may be impaired, especially at the start of treatment, or following the consumption of alcohol; patients should be warned of this risk and advised not to drive or operate machinery until their susceptibility is known.

Patients should not drive if they have blurred vision.

4.8 Undesirable effects

Undesirable effects are for the majority dose dependent. The frequency and severity are most pronounced in the early phase of treatment and decline during continued treatment.

Extrapyramidal reactions may occur, especially in the early phase of treatment. In most cases these side effects can be satisfactorily controlled by reduction of dosage and/or use of antiparkinsonian drugs. The routine prophylactic use of antiparkinsonian drugs is not recommended. Antiparkinsonian drugs do not alleviate tardive dyskinsea and may aggravate them. Reduction in dosage or, if possible, discontinuation of zuclopenthixol therapy is recommeneded. In persistent akathisia a benzodiazepine or propranolol may be useful.

Cardiac disorders	Tachycardia, palpitations.
	Electrocardiogram QT prolonged.
Blood and lymphatic system disorders	Thrombocytopenia, neutropenia, leukopenia, agranulocytosis.
Nervous system disorders	Somnolence, akathisia, hyperkinesia, hypokinesia.
	Tremor, dystonia, hypertonia, dizziness, headache, paraesthesia, disturbance in attention, amnesia, gait abnormal.
	Tardive dyskinesia, hyperreflexia, dyskinesia, parkinsonism, syncope, ataxia, speech disorder, hypotonia, convulsion, migraine.
	Neuroleptic malignant syndrome.
Eye disorders	Accommodation disorder, vision abnormal.
	Oculogyration, mydriasis.
Ear and labyrinth disorders	Vertigo.
	Hyperacusis, tinnitus.
Respiratory, thoracic and medistianal disorders	Nasal congestion, dyspnoea.
Gastrointestinal disorders	Dry mouth.
	Salivary hypersecretion, constipation, vomiting, dyspepsia, diarrhoea.
	Abdominal pain, nausea, flatulence.
Renal and urinary disorders	Micturition disorder, urinary retention, polyuria.
Skin and subcutaneous tissue disorders	Hyperhidrosis, pruritus.
	Rash, photosensitivity reaction, pigmentation disorder, seborrhoea, dermatitis, purpura.
Musculoskeletal and connective tissue disorder	Myalgia.
	Muscle rigidity, trismus, torticollis.
Endocrine disorders	Hyperprolactinaemia.
Metabolism and nutrition disorders	Increased appetite, weight increased.
	Decreased appetite, weight decreased.
	Hyperglycaemia, glucose tolerance impaired, hyperlipidaemia.
Vascular disorders	Hypotension, hot flush.
General disorders and administration site conditions	Asthenia, fatigue, malaise, pain.
	Thirst, hypothermia, pyrexia. Injection site reaction
Immune system disorders	Hypersensitivity, anaphylactic reaction.
Hepato-biliary disorders	Liver function test abnormal.
	Cholestatic hepatitis, jaundice.
Reproductive system and breast disorders	Ejaculation failure, erectile dysfunction, female orgasmic disorder, vulvovaginal dryness.
	Gynaecomastia, galactorrhoea, amenorrhoea, priapism.
Psychiatric disorders	Insomnia, depression, anxiety, nervousness, abnormal dreams, agitation, libido decreased.
	Apathy, nightmare, libido increased, confusional state.

As with other drugs belonging to the therapeutic class of antipsychotics, rare cases of QT prolongation, ventricular arrhythmias - ventricular fibrillation, ventricular tachycardia, Torsade de Pointes and sudden unexplained death have been reported for zuclopenthixol (see section 4.4).

Abrupt discontinuation of zuclopenthixol may be accompanied by withdrawal symptoms. The most common symptoms are nausea, vomiting, anorexia, diarrhoea, rhinorrhoea, sweating, myalgias, paraesthesias, insomnia, restlessness, anxiety, and agitation. Patients may also experience vertigo, alternate feelings of warmth and coldness, and tremor. Symptoms generally begin within 1 to 4 days of withdrawal and abate within 7 to 14 days.

4.9 Overdose

Symptoms: somnolence, coma, extrapyramidal symptoms, convulsions, hypotension, shock, hyper or hypothermia. ECG changes, QT prolongation, Torsade de Pointes, cardiac arrest and ventricular arrhythmias have been reported when administered in overdose together with drugs known to affect the heart.

Treatment: treatment is symptomatic and supportive. Measures aimed at supporting the respiratory and cardiovascular systems should be instituted. Adrenaline (epinephrine) must not be used in these patients. There is no specific antidote.

5. PHARMACOLOGICAL PROPERTIES

5.1 Pharmacodynamic properties

Zuclopenthixol is a potent neuroleptic of the thioxanthene series with a piperazine side-chain. The antipsychotic effect of neuroleptics is related to their dopamine receptor blocking effect. The thioxanthenes have a high affinity for both the adenylate cyclase coupled dopamine D1 receptors and for the dopamine D2 receptors; in the phenothiazine group the affinity for D1 receptors is much lower than that for D2 receptors, whereas butyrophenones, diphenylbutylpiperidines and benzamides only have affinity for D2 receptors.

In the traditional tests for antipsychotic effect, e.g. antagonism of stereotypic behaviour induced by dopamine agonists, the chemical groups of neuroleptics mentioned reveal equal but dosage dependent activity. However, the antistereotypic effect of phenothiazines, butyrophenones, diphenylbutylpiperidines, and benzamindes is strongly counteracted by the anticholinergic drug, scopolamine, while the antisteriotypic effect of the thioxanthenes, e.g. zuclopenthixol, is not, or only very slightly, influenced by concomitant treatment with anticholinergics.

5.2 Pharmacokinetic properties

By esterification of zuclopenthixol with acetic acid, zuclopenthixol has been converted to a more lipophilic substance, zuclopenthixol acetate. When dissolved in oil and injected intramuscularly this substance diffuses slowly into the surrounding body water, where enzymatic breakdown occurs releasing the active component zuclopenthixol.

Maximum serum concentrations of zuclopenthixol are usually reached 36 hours after an injection, after which the serum levels decline slowly. The average maximum serum level corresponding to the 100 mg dose is 41 ng/ml. Three days after the injection the serum level is about one third of the maximum.

Zuclopenthixol is distributed in the body in a similar way to other neuroleptics; with the higher concentrations of drug and metabolites in liver, lungs, intestines and kidneys and lower concentrations in heart, spleen, brain and blood. The apparent volume of distribution is about 20 l/kg and the protein binding about 98%.

Zuclopenthixol crosses the placental barrier in small amounts. Zuclopenthixol is excreted in small amounts with the milk - the ratio milk concentration/serum concentration in women is on average 0.3.

The metabolism of zuclopenthixol proceeds via three main routes - sulphoxidation, side chain N-dealkylation and glucuronic acid conjugation. The metabolites are devoid of psychopharmacolical activity. The excretion proceeds mainly with the faeces but also to some degree with the urine. The systemic clearance is about 0.9 l/min.

The kinetics seem to be linear, since highly significant correlation exist between the dose and the area under the serum concentration curve.

5.3 Preclinical safety data

Zuclopenthixol has no mutagenic potential. In a rat oncogeneticity study, 30 mg/kg/day resulted in slight non statistical increases in the incidence of mammary adenocarcinomas and pancreatic islet cell adenomas and carcinomas in females and of thyroid parafollicular carcinomas. This is a common finding for D_2 antagonists which increase prolactin secretion when administered to rats. The physiological differences between rats and humans suggest that these changes are not predictive of an oncogenic risk in patients.

Local muscle damage is less pronounced with oily solutions of zuclopenthixol (including Clopixol Acuphase) then with aqueous solutions of zuclopenthixol and other neuroleptic

6. PHARMACEUTICAL PARTICULARS

6.1 List of excipients

Thin vegetable oil (derived from coconuts).

6.2 Incompatibilities

Zuclopenthixol acetate should not be mixed with other injection fluids.

6.3 Shelf life

2 years as packaged for sale.

6.4 Special precautions for storage

Store at room temperature (at or below 25°C). Protect from light.

6.5 Nature and contents of container

Clear glass ampoules containing either 1 or 2 ml of zuclopenthixol acetate 5% w/v in thin vegetable oil.

The ampoules are packed in boxes of 5.

6.6 Special precautions for disposal and other handling

Nil.

7. MARKETING AUTHORISATION HOLDER

Lundbeck Ltd

Lundbeck House

Caldecotte Lake Business Park

Caldecotte

Milton Keynes

MK7 8LF

8. MARKETING AUTHORISATION NUMBER(S)

PL 0458/0063

9. DATE OF FIRST AUTHORISATION/RENEWAL OF THE AUTHORISATION

First Authorisation: 16 March 1990

Renewal of Authorisation: 9 May 2001

10. DATE OF REVISION OF THE TEXT

24 October 2008

®Trademark Clopixol is made by H Lundbeck A/S, Denmark

Clopixol Injection and Conc Injection

(Lundbeck Limited)

1. NAME OF THE MEDICINAL PRODUCT

Clopixol® Injection

Clopixol® Conc Injection.

2. QUALITATIVE AND QUANTITATIVE COMPOSITION

Clopixol Injection

Zuclopenthixol Decanoate 20.0% w/v (equivalent to zuclopenthixol base 14.445% w/v).

Clopixol Conc Injection

Zuclopenthixol Decanoate 50.0% w/v (equivalent to zuclopenthixol base 36.1% w/v).

3. PHARMACEUTICAL FORM

Solution for Injection.

4. CLINICAL PARTICULARS

4.1 Therapeutic indications

The maintenance treatment of schizophrenia and paranoid psychoses.

4.2 Posology and method of administration

Route of administration

By deep intramuscular injection into the upper outer buttock or lateral thigh.

Note

As with all oil based injections it is important to ensure, by aspiration before injection, that inadvertent intravascular entry does not occur.

Adults

Dosage and dosage interval should be adjusted according to the patient's symptoms and response to treatment.

The usual dosage range of zuclopenthixol decanoate is 200-500 mg every one to four weeks, depending on response, but some patients may require up to 600 mg per week. In patients who have not previously received depot antipsychotics, treatment is usually started with a small dose (e.g. 100 mg) to assess tolerance. An interval, of at least one week should be allowed before the second injection is given at a dose consistent with the patient's condition.

Adequate control of severe psychotic symptoms may take up to 4 to 6 months at high enough dosage. Once stabilised lower maintenance doses may be considered, but must be sufficient to prevent relapse.

Injection volumes of greater than 2 ml should be distributed between two injection sites.

Elderly

In accordance with standard medical practice initial dosage may need to be reduced to a quarter or half the normal starting dose in the frail or elderly.

Children

Not indicated for children.

4.3 Contraindications

Hypersensitivity to the active substance or to any of the excipients (see section 6.1).

Circulatory collapse, depressed level of consciousness due to any cause (e.g. intoxication with alcohol, barbiturates or opiates), coma.

4.4 Special warnings and precautions for use

Caution should be exercised in patients having: liver disease; cardiac disease, or arrhythmias; severe respiratory disease; renal failure; epilepsy (and conditions predisposing to epilepsy, eg alcohol withdrawal or brain damage); Parkinson's disease; narrow angle glaucoma; prostatic hypertrophy; hypothyroidism; hyperthyroidism; myasthenia gravis; phaeochromocytoma and patients who have shown hypersensitivity to thioxanthenes or other antipsychotics.

The elderly require close supervision because they are especially prone to experience such adverse effects as sedation, hypotension, confusion and temperature changes.

Acute withdrawal symptoms, including nausea, vomiting, sweating and insomnia have been described after abrupt cessation of antipsychotic drugs. Recurrence of psychotic symptoms may also occur, and the emergence of involuntary movement disorders (such as akathisia, dystonia and dyskinesia) has been reported. The plasma concentrations of Clopixol Conc Injection 500mg/ml gradually decrease over several weeks which make gradual dosage tapering unnecessary.

When transferring patients from oral to depot antipsychotic treatment, the oral medication should not be discontinued immediately, but gradually withdrawn over a period of several days after administering the first injection.

The possibility of development of neuroleptic malignant syndrome (hyperthermia, muscle rigidity, fluctuating consciousness, instability of the autonomous nervous system) exists with any neuroleptic. The risk is possibly greater with the more potent agents. Patients with pre-existing organic brain syndrome, mental retardation and opiate and alcohol abuse are over-represented among fatal cases.

Treatment:

Discontinuation of the neuroleptic. Symptomatic treatment and use of general supportive measures. Dantrolene and bromocriptine may be helpful. Symptoms may persist for more than a week after oral neuroleptics are discontinued and somewhat longer when associated with the depot forms of the drugs.

Like other neuroleptics, zuclopenthixol should be used with caution in patients with organic brain syndrome, convulsions or advanced hepatic disease.

Blood dyscrasias have been reported rarely. Blood counts should be carried out if a patient develops signs of persistent infection.

An approximately 3-fold increased risk of cerebrovascular adverse events has been seen in randomised placebo controlled clinical trials in the dementia population with some atypical antipsychotics. The mechanism for this increased risk is not known. An increased risk cannot be excluded for other antipsychotics or other patient populations.

Zuclopenthixol should be used with caution in patients with risk factors for stroke.

As with other drugs belonging to the therapeutic class of antipsychotics, zuclopenthixol may cause QT prolongation. Persistently prolonged QT intervals may increase the risk of malignant arrhythmias. Therefore, zuclopenthixol should be used with caution in susceptible individuals (with hypokalemia, hypomagnesia or genetic predisposition) and in patients with a history of cardiovascular disorders, e.g. QT prolongation, significant bradycardia (<50 beats per minute), a recent acute myocardial infarction, uncompensated heart failure, or cardiac arrhythmia.

Concomitant treatment with other antipsychotics should be avoided (see section 4.5).

As described for other psychotropics zuclopenthixol may modify insulin and glucose responses calling for adjustment of the antidiabetic therapy in diabetic patients

4.5 Interaction with other medicinal products and other forms of interaction

In common with other antipsychotics, zuclopenthixol enhances the response to alcohol, the effects of barbiturates and other CNS depressants.

Zuclopenthixol may potentiate the effects of general anaesthetics and anticoagulants and prolong the action of neuromuscular blocking agents.

The anticholinergic effects of atropine or other drugs with anticholinergic properties may be increased.

Concomitant use of drugs such as metoclopramide, piperazine or antiparkinson drugs may increase the risk of extrapyramidal effects such as tardive dyskinesia.

Combined use of antipsychotics and lithium or sibutramine has been associated with an increased risk of neurotoxicity.

Antipsychotics may enhance the cardiac depressant effects of quinidine; the absorption of corticosteroids and digoxin.

The hypotensive effect of vasodilator antihypertensive agents such as hydralazine and α blockers (e.g. doxazosin), or methyl-dopa may be enhanced.

Increases in the QT interval related to antipsychotic treatment may be exacerbated by the co administration of other drugs known to significantly increase the QT interval. Co-administration of such drugs should be avoided. Relevant classes include:

- class Ia and III antiarrhythmics (e.g. quinidine, amiodarone, sotalol, dofetilide)
- some antipsychotics (e.g. thioridazine)
- some macrolides (e.g. erythromycin)

- some antihistamines
- some quinolone antibiotics (e.g. moxifloxacin)

The above list is not exhaustive and other individual drugs known to significantly increase QT interval (e.g. cisapride, lithium) should be avoided. Drugs known to cause electrolyte disturbances such as thiazidediuretics (hypokalemia) and drugs known to increase the plasma concentration of zuclopenthixol should also be used with caution as they may increase the risk of QT prolongation and malignant arrhythmias (see section 4.4).

Antipsychotics may antagonise the effects of adrenaline and other sympathomimetic agents, and reverse the antihypertensive effects of guanethidine and similar adrenergic-blocking agents.

Antipsychotics may also impair the effect of levodopa, adrenergic drugs and anticonvulsants.

The metabolism of tricyclic antidepressants may be inhibited and the control of diabetes may be impaired.

Since zuclopenthixol is partly metabolised by CYP2D6 concomitant use of drugs known to inhibit this enzyme may lead to higher than expected plasma concentrations of zuclopenthixol, increasing the risk of adverse effects and cardiotoxicity.

4.6 Pregnancy and lactation

Pregnancy

Zuclopenthixol should not be administered during pregnancy unless the expected benefit to the patient outweighs the theoretical risk to the foetus.

The newborn of mothers treated with neuroleptics in late pregnancy, or labour, may show signs of intoxication such as lethargy, tremor and hyper excitability, and have a low Apgar score.

Animal-reproduction studies have not given evidence of an increased incidence of foetal damage or other deleterious effects on the reproduction process.

Lactation

As zuclopenthixol is found in breast milk in low concentrations it is not likely to affect the infant when therapeutic doses are used. The dose ingested by the infant is less than 1% of the weight related maternal dose (in mg/kg). Breast-feeding can be continued during zuclopenthixol therapy if considered of clinical importance but observation of the infant is recommended, particularly in the first 4 weeks after giving birth.

4.7 Effects on ability to drive and use machines

Zuclopenthixol is a sedative drug.

Alertness may be impaired, especially at the start of treatment, or following the consumption of alcohol; patients should be warned of this risk and advised not to drive or operate machinery until their susceptibility is known.

Patients should not drive if they have blurred vision.

4.8 Undesirable effects

Undesirable effects are for the majority dose dependent. The frequency and severity are most pronounced in the early phase of treatment and decline during continued treatment.

Extrapyramidal reactions may occur, especially in the early phase of treatment. In most cases these side effects can be satisfactorily controlled by reduction of dosage and/or use of antiparkinsonian drugs. The routine prophylactic use of antiparkinsonian drugs is not recommended. Antiparkinsonian drugs do not alleviate tardive dyskinsea and may aggravate them. Reduction in dosage or, if possible, discontinuation of zuclopenthixol therapy is recommeneded. In persistent akathisia a benzodiazepine or propranolol may be useful.

Cardiac disorders	Tachycardia, palpitations.
	Electrocardiogram QT prolonged.
Blood and lymphatic system disorders	Thrombocytopenia, neutropenia, leukopenia, agranulocytosis.
Nervous system disorders	Somnolence, akathisia, hyperkinesia, hypokinesia.
	Tremor, dystonia, hypertonia, dizziness, headache, paraesthesia, disturbance in attention, amnesia, gait abnormal.
	Tardive dyskinesia, hyperreflexia, dyskinesia, parkinsonism, syncope, ataxia, speech disorder, hypotonia, convulsion, migraine.
	Neuroleptic malignant syndrome.
Eye disorders	Accommodation disorder, vision abnormal.
	Oculogyration, mydriasis.
Ear and labyrinth disorders	Vertigo.
	Hyperacusis, tinnitus.
Respiratory, thoracic and medistianal disorders	Nasal congestion, dyspnoea.
Gastrointestinal disorders	Dry mouth.
	Salivary hypersecretion, constipation, vomiting, dyspepsia, diarrhoea.
	Abdominal pain, nausea, flatulence.
Renal and urinary disorders	Micturition disorder, urinary retention, polyuria.
Skin and subcutaneous tissue disorders	Hyperhidrosis, pruritus.
	Rash, photosensitivity reaction, pigmentation disorder, seborrhoea, dermatitis, purpura.
Musculoskeletal and connective tissue disorder	Myalgia.
	Muscle rigidity, trismus, torticollis.
Endocrine disorders	Hyperprolactinaemia.
Metabolism and nutrition disorders	Increased appetite, weight increased.
	Decreased appetite, weight decreased.
	Hyperglycaemia, glucose tolerance impaired, hyperlipidaemia.
Vascular disorders	Hypotension, hot flush.
General disorders and administration site conditions	Asthenia, fatigue, malaise, pain.
	Thirst, hypothermia, pyrexia. Injection site reaction
Immune system disorders	Hypersensitivity, anaphylactic reaction.
Hepato-biliary disorders	Liver function test abnormal.
	Cholestatic hepatitis, jaundice.
Reproductive system and breast disorders	Ejaculation failure, erectile dysfunction, female orgasmic disorder, vulvovaginal dryness.
	Gynaecomastia, galactorrhoea, amenorrhoea, priapism.
Psychiatric disorders	Insomnia, depression, anxiety, nervousness, abnormal dreams, agitation, libido decreased.
	Apathy, nightmare, libido increased, confusional state.

As with other drugs belonging to the therapeutic class of antipsychotics, rare cases of QT prolongation, ventricular arrhythmias - ventricular fibrillation, ventricular tachycardia, Torsade de Pointes and sudden unexplained death have been reported for zuclopenthixol (see section 4.4).

Abrupt discontinuation of zuclopenthixol may be accompanied by withdrawal symptoms. The most common symptoms are nausea, vomiting, anorexia, diarrhoea, rhinorrhoea, sweating, myalgias, paraesthesias, insomnia, restlessness, anxiety, and agitation. Patients may also experience vertigo, alternate feelings of warmth and coldness, and tremor. Symptoms generally begin within 1 to 4 days of withdrawal and abate within 7 to 14 days.

4.9 Overdose

Symptoms: somnolence, coma, extrapyramidal symptoms, convulsions, hypotension, shock, hyper or hypothermia. ECG changes, QT prolongation, Torsade de Pointes, cardiac arrest and ventricular arrhythmias have been reported when administered in overdose together with drugs known to affect the heart.

Treatment: treatment is symptomatic and supportive. Measures aimed at supporting the respiratory and cardiovascular systems should be instituted. Adrenaline (epinephrine) must not be used in these patients. There is no specific antidote.

5. PHARMACOLOGICAL PROPERTIES

5.1 Pharmacodynamic properties

The action of zuclopenthixol, as with other antipsychotics is mediated through dopamine receptor blockade. Zuclopenthixol has a high affinity for D_1 and D_2 receptors and activity has been demonstrated in standard animal models used to assess antipsychotic action. Serotonergic blocking properties, a high affinity for alpha-adrenoreceptors and slight antihistamine properties have been observed.

5.2 Pharmacokinetic properties

After deep intramuscular injection of Clopixol, serum levels of zuclopenthixol increase during the first week and decline slowly thereafter. A linear relationship has been observed between Clopixol dosage and serum level. Metabolism proceeds by sulphoxidation, dealkylation and glucuronic acid conjugation. Sulphoxide metabolites are mainly excreted in the urine while unchanged drug and the dealkylated form tend to be excreted in the faeces.

5.3 Preclinical safety data

Nil of relevance

6. PHARMACEUTICAL PARTICULARS

6.1 List of excipients

Thin vegetable oil

6.2 Incompatibilities

This product may be mixed in the same syringe with other products in the Clopixol Injection range, including Clopixol Acuphase Injection (zuclopenthixol acetate 50 mg/ml).

It should not be mixed with any other injection fluids.

6.3 Shelf life

Clopixol Injection

1 ml ampoules: 36 months.

10 ml vials: 36 months (unopened), shelf life after opening vials: 1 day

Clopixol Conc Injection

48 months.

6.4 Special precautions for storage

Store at or below 25°C. Protect from light.

6.5 Nature and contents of container

Clopixol Injection

Ampoules containing 1 ml of 200 mg/ml zuclopenthixol decanoate in thin vegetable oil. Pack size: 10 ampoules per box.

10 ml clear glass vials with a rubber stopper secured with an aluminium collar having a flip-top cap. Pack size: 1 vial per box.

Clopixol Conc. Injection

Ampoules containing 1 ml of 500 mg/ml zuclopenthixol decanoate in thin vegetable oil. Pack size: 5 ampoules per box.

6.6 Special precautions for disposal and other handling

Nil.

7. MARKETING AUTHORISATION HOLDER

Lundbeck Limited
Lundbeck House
Caldecotte Lake Business Park
Caldecotte
Milton Keynes
MK7 8LF

8. MARKETING AUTHORISATION NUMBER(S)

Clopixol Injection	PL 0458/0017
Clopixol Conc Injection	PL 0458/0060

9. DATE OF FIRST AUTHORISATION/RENEWAL OF THE AUTHORISATION

	Date of first authorisation	Date of renewal
Clopixol Injection	May 1978	January 2002
Clopixol Conc Injection	November 1988	May 2004

10. DATE OF REVISION OF THE TEXT

24 October 2008

®Trademark Clopixol is made by H Lundbeck A/S, Denmark

Clopixol Tablets

(Lundbeck Limited)

1. NAME OF THE MEDICINAL PRODUCT

Clopixol® Tablets 2 mg, 10 mg and 25 mg.

2. QUALITATIVE AND QUANTITATIVE COMPOSITION

2 mg, 10 mg and 25 mg tablets (containing 2.36, 11.9 or 29.7 mg zuclopenthixol dihydrochloride equivalent to 2 mg, 10 mg or 25 mg zuclopenthixol base).

Excipients:

Lactose, hydrogenated castor oil.

For a full list of excipients see section 6.1

3. PHARMACEUTICAL FORM

Film-coated tablet

2 mg: Round, biconvex, pale red, film-coated tablet.

10 mg: Round, biconvex, light red-brown film-coated tablet.

25 mg: Round, biconvex, red-brown, film-coated tablet.

4. CLINICAL PARTICULARS

4.1 Therapeutic indications

The treatment of psychoses, especially schizophrenia.

4.2 Posology and method of administration

Route of administration: Oral.

Adults

The dosage range is 4-150 mg/day in divided doses. The usual initial dose is 20-30 mg/day (sometimes with higher dosage requirements in acute cases), increasing as necessary. The usual maintenance dose is 20-50 mg/day.

When transferring patients from oral to depot antipsychotic treatment, the oral medication should not be discontinued immediately, but gradually withdrawn over a period of several days after administering the first injection.

Elderly

In accordance with standard medical practice, initial dosage may need to be reduced to a quarter or half the normal starting dose in the frail or elderly.

Children

Not indicated for children.

4.3 Contraindications

Hypersensitivity to the active substance or to any of the excipients (see section 6.1).

Circulatory collapse, depressed level of consciousness due to any cause (e.g. intoxication with alcohol, barbiturates or opiates), coma.

4.4 Special warnings and precautions for use

Caution should be exercised in patients having: liver disease; cardiac disease or arrhythmias; severe respiratory disease; renal failure; epilepsy (and conditions predisposing to epilepsy e.g. alcohol withdrawal or brain damage); Parkinson's disease; narrow angle glaucoma; prostatic hypertrophy; hypothyroidism; hyperthyroidism; myasthenia gravis; phaeochromocytoma and patients who have shown hypersensitivity to thioxanthenes or other antipsychotics.

The elderly require close supervision because they are specially prone to experience such adverse effects as sedation, hypotension, confusion and temperature changes.

Acute withdrawal symptoms, including nausea, vomiting, sweating and insomnia have been described after abrupt cessation of antipsychotic drugs. Recurrence of psychotic symptoms may also occur, and the emergence of involuntary movement disorders (such as akathisia, dystonia and dyskinesia) has been reported. Therefore, gradual withdrawal is advisable.

The possibility of development of neuroleptic malignant syndrome (hyperthermia, muscle rigidity, fluctuating consciousness, instability of the autonomous nervous system) exists with any neuroleptic. The risk is possibly greater with the more potent agents. Patients with pre-existing organic brain syndrome, mental retardation and opiate and alcohol abuse are over-represented among fatal cases.

Treatment:

Discontinuation of the neuroleptic. Symptomatic treatment and use of general supportive measures. Dantrolene and bromocriptine may be helpful. Symptoms may persist for more than a week after oral neuroleptics are discontinued and somewhat longer when associated with the depot forms of the drugs.

Like other neuroleptics, zuclopenthixol should be used with caution in patients with organic brain syndrome, convulsions or advanced hepatic disease.

Blood dyscrasias have been reported rarely. Blood counts should be carried out if a patient develops signs of persistent infection.

An approximately 3-fold increased risk of cerebrovascular adverse events has been seen in randomised placebo controlled clinical trials in the dementia population with some atypical antipsychotics. The mechanism for this increased risk is not known. An increased risk cannot be excluded for other antipsychotics or other patient populations.

Zuclopenthixol should be used with caution in patients with risk factors for stroke.

As with other drugs belonging to the therapeutic class of antipsychotics, zuclopenthixol may cause QT prolongation. Persistently prolonged QT intervals may increase the risk of malignant arrhythmias. Therefore, zuclopenthixol should be used with caution in susceptible individuals (with hypokalemia, hypomagnesia or genetic predisposition) and in patients with a history of cardiovascular disorders, e.g. QT prolongation, significant bradycardia (<50 beats per minute), a recent acute myocardial infarction, uncompensated heart failure, or cardiac arrhythmia.

Concomitant treatment with other antipsychotics should be avoided (see section 4.5).

As described for other psychotropics zuclopenthixol may modify insulin and glucose responses calling for adjustment of the antidiabetic therapy in diabetic patients.

Excipients

The tablets contain lactose monohydrate. Patients with rare hereditary problems of galactose intolerance, the Lapp lactase deficiency or glucose-galactose malabsorption should not receive this medicine.

This medicinal product contains hydrogenated castor oil, which may cause stomach upset and diarrhoea.

4.5 Interaction with other medicinal products and other forms of interaction

In common with other antipsychotics, zuclopenthixol enhances the response to alcohol, the effects of barbiturates and other CNS depressants.

Zuclopenthixol may potentiate the effects of general anaesthetics and anticoagulants and prolong the action of neuromuscular blocking agents.

The anticholinergic effects of atropine or other drugs with anticholinergic properties may be increased.

Concomitant use of drugs such as metoclopramide, piperazine or antiparkinson drugs may increase the risk of extrapyramidal effects such as tardive dyskinesia.

Combined use of antipsychotics and lithium or sibutramine has been associated with an increased risk of neurotoxicity.

Antipsychotics may enhance the cardiac depressant effects of quinidine; the absorption of corticosteroids and digoxin.

The hypotensive effect of vasodilator antihypertensive agents such as hydralazine and α blockers (e.g. doxazosin), or methyl-dopa may be enhanced.

Increases in the QT interval related to antipsychotic treatment may be exacerbated by the co administration of other drugs known to significantly increase the QT interval. Co-administration of such drugs should be avoided. Relevant classes include:

- class Ia and III antiarrhythmics (e.g. quinidine, amiodarone, sotalol, dofetilide)
- some antipsychotics (e.g. thioridazine)
- some macrolides (e.g. erythromycin)
- some antihistamines
- some quinolone antibiotics (e.g. moxifloxacin)

The above list is not exhaustive and other individual drugs known to significantly increase QT interval (e.g. cisapride, lithium) should be avoided. Drugs known to cause electrolyte disturbances such as thiazidediuretics (hypokalemia) and drugs known to increase the plasma concentration of zuclopenthixol should also be used with caution as they may increase the risk of QT prolongation and malignant arrhythmias (see section 4.4).

Antipsychotics may antagonise the effects of adrenaline and other sympathomimetic agents, and reverse the antihypertensive effects of guanethidine and similar adrenergic-blocking agents.

Antipsychotics may also impair the effect of levodopa, adrenergic drugs and anticonvulsants.

The metabolism of tricyclic antidepressants may be inhibited and the control of diabetes may be impaired.

Since zuclopenthixol is partly metabolised by CYP2D6 concomitant use of drugs known to inhibit this enzyme may lead to higher than expected plasma concentrations of zuclopenthixol, increasing the risk of adverse effects and cardiotoxicity.

4.6 Pregnancy and lactation

Pregnancy

Zuclopenthixol should not be administered during pregnancy unless the expected benefit to the patient outweighs the theoretical risk to the foetus.

The newborn of mothers treated with neuroleptics in late pregnancy, or labour, may show signs of intoxication such as lethargy, tremor and hyper excitability, and have a low Apgar score.

Animal-reproduction studies have not given evidence of an increased incidence of foetal damage or other deleterious effects on the reproduction process.

Lactation

As zuclopenthixol is found in breast milk in low concentrations it is not likely to affect the infant when therapeutic doses are used. The dose ingested by the infant is less than 1% of the weight related maternal dose (in mg/kg). Breast-feeding can be continued during zuclopenthixol therapy if considered of clinical importance but observation of the infant is recommended, particularly in the first 4 weeks after giving birth.

4.7 Effects on ability to drive and use machines

Zuclopenthixol is a sedative drug.

Alertness may be impaired, especially at the start of treatment, or following the consumption of alcohol; patients should be warned of this risk and advised not to drive or operate machinery until their susceptibility is known.

Patients should not drive if they have blurred vision.

4.8 Undesirable effects

Undesirable effects are for the majority dose dependent. The frequency and severity are most pronounced in the early phase of treatment and decline during continued treatment.

Extrapyramidal reactions may occur, especially in the early phase of treatment. In most cases these side effects can be satisfactorily controlled by reduction of dosage and/or use of antiparkinsonian drugs. The routine prophylactic use of antiparkinsonian drugs is not recommended. Antiparkinsonian drugs do not alleviate tardive dyskinsea and may aggravate them. Reduction in dosage or, if possible, discontinuation of zuclopenthixol therapy is recommeneded. In persistent akathisia a benzodiazepine or propranolol may be useful.

Cardiac disorders	Tachycardia, palpitations.
	Electrocardiogram QT prolonged.
Blood and lymphatic system disorders	Thrombocytopenia, neutropenia, leukopenia, agranulocytosis.
Nervous system disorders	Somnolence, akathisia, hyperkinesia, hypokinesia.
	Tremor, dystonia, hypertonia, dizziness, headache, paraesthesia, disturbance in attention, amnesia, gait abnormal.
	Tardive dyskinesia, hyperreflexia, dyskinesia, parkinsonism, syncope, ataxia, speech disorder, hypotonia, convulsion, migraine.
	Neuroleptic malignant syndrome.
Eye disorders	Accommodation disorder, vision abnormal.
	Oculogyration, mydriasis.
Ear and labyrinth disorders	Vertigo.
	Hyperacusis, tinnitus.
Respiratory, thoracic and medistianal disorders	Nasal congestion, dyspnoea.
Gastrointestinal disorders	Dry mouth.
	Salivary hypersecretion, constipation, vomiting, dyspepsia, diarrhoea.
	Abdominal pain, nausea, flatulence.
Renal and urinary disorders	Micturition disorder, urinary retention, polyuria.
Skin and subcutaneous tissue disorders	Hyperhidrosis, pruritus.
	Rash, photosensitivity reaction, pigmentation disorder, seborrhoea, dermatitis, purpura.
Musculoskeletal and connective tissue disorder	Myalgia.
	Muscle rigidity, trismus, torticollis.
Endocrine disorders	Hyperprolactinaemia.
Metabolism and nutrition disorders	Increased appetite, weight increased.
	Decreased appetite, weight decreased.
	Hyperglycaemia, glucose tolerance impaired, hyperlipidaemia.
Vascular disorders	Hypotension, hot flush.
General disorders and administration site conditions	Asthenia, fatigue, malaise, pain.
	Thirst, hypothermia, pyrexia.
Immune system disorders	Hypersensitivity, anaphylactic reaction.
Hepato-biliary disorders	Liver function test abnormal.
	Cholestatic hepatitis, jaundice.
Reproductive system and breast disorders	Ejaculation failure, erectile dysfunction, female orgasmic disorder, vulvovaginal dryness.
	Gynaecomastia, galactorrhoea, amenorrhoea, priapism.
Psychiatric disorders	Insomnia, depression, anxiety, nervousness, abnormal dreams, agitation, libido decreased.
	Apathy, nightmare, libido increased, confusional state.

As with other drugs belonging to the therapeutic class of antipsychotics, rare cases of QT prolongation, ventricular arrhythmias - ventricular fibrillation, ventricular tachycardia, Torsade de Pointes and sudden unexplained death have been reported for zuclopenthixol (see section 4.4).

Abrupt discontinuation of zuclopenthixol may be accompanied by withdrawal symptoms. The most common symptoms are nausea, vomiting, anorexia, diarrhoea, rhinorrhoea, sweating, myalgias, paraesthesias, insomnia, restlessness, anxiety, and agitation. Patients may also experience vertigo, alternate feelings of warmth and coldness, and tremor. Symptoms generally begin within 1 to 4 days of withdrawal and abate within 7 to 14 days

4.9 Overdose

Overdosage may cause somnolence, or even coma, extrapyramidal symptoms, convulsions, hypotension, shock, hyper-or hypothermia. ECG changes, QT prolongation, Torsade de Pointes, cardiac arrest and ventricular arrhythmias have been reported when administered in overdose together with drugs known to affect the heart.

Treatment is symptomatic and supportive, with measures aimed at supporting the respiratory and cardiovascular systems. The following specific measures may be employed if required.

- anticholinergic antiparkinson drugs if extrapyramidal symptoms occur.

- sedation (with benzodiazepines) in the unlikely event of agitation or excitement or convulsions.

- noradrenaline in saline intravenous drip if the patient is in shock. Adrenaline must not be given.

- Gastric lavage should be considered.

5. PHARMACOLOGICAL PROPERTIES

5.1 Pharmacodynamic properties

The action of zuclopenthixol as with other antipsychotics is mediated through dopamine receptor blockage. Zuclopenthixol has a high affinity for D_1 and D_2 receptors and activity has been demonstrated in standard animal models used to assess antipsychotic action. Serotonergic blocking properties, a high affinity for alpha-adrenoreceptors and slight antihistaminergic properties have been observed.

5.2 Pharmacokinetic properties

Zuclopenthixol given orally in man is relatively quickly absorbed and maximum serum concentrations are reached in 3-6 hours. There is good correlation between the dose of zuclopenthixol and the concentrations achieved in serum. the biological half-life in man is about one day. Zuclopenthixol is distributed in the liver, lungs, intestines and kidney, with somewhat lower concentration in the brain. Small amounts of drug or metabolites cross the placenta and are excreted in milk.

Zuclopenthixol is metabolised by sulphoxidation, N-Dealkylation and glucuronic acid conjugation.

The faecal route of excretion predominates and mostly unchanged zuclopenthixol and N-dealkylated metabolite are excreted in this way.

5.3 Preclinical safety data

Nil of relevance

6. PHARMACEUTICAL PARTICULARS

6.1 List of excipients

Potato starch, Lactose, Microcrystalline cellulose, Copolyidone, Glycerol, Talc, Castor oil, hydrogenated, Magnesium Stearate, Methylhydroxypropyl Cellulose, Macrogol, Titanium Dioxide (E171) and Red Iron Oxide (E172).

6.2 Incompatibilities

None known.

6.3 Shelf life

Clopixol Tablets are stable for 2 years. Each container has an expiry date.

6.4 Special precautions for storage

Clopixol Tablets 2mg

Store in original container, protected from light and moisture, below 25°C.

Clopixol Tablets 10 mg, 25 mg

Store in the original container protected from light and moisture. Do not store above 30°C.

6.5 Nature and contents of container

Grey polypropylene container (with desiccant capsule for 2 mg strength) or glass bottle. Contents: 100 tablets.

6.6 Special precautions for disposal and other handling

Nil.

7. MARKETING AUTHORISATION HOLDER

Lundbeck Ltd

Lundbeck House

Caldecotte Lake Business Park

Caldecotte

Milton Keynes

MK7 8LF

8. MARKETING AUTHORISATION NUMBER(S)

2 mg tablets	PL 0458/0027
10 mg tablets	PL 0458/0028
25 mg tablets	PL 0458/0029

9. DATE OF FIRST AUTHORISATION/RENEWAL OF THE AUTHORISATION

First Authorisation: March 1982

Renewal of Authorisation: January 2002

10. DATE OF REVISION OF THE TEXT

01 March 2009

®Trademark Clopixol is made by H Lundbeck A/S, Denmark

Clotam Rapid

(Galen Limited)

1. NAME OF THE MEDICINAL PRODUCT

Clotam® Rapid.

2. QUALITATIVE AND QUANTITATIVE COMPOSITION

Tolfenamic acid 200 mg.

3. PHARMACEUTICAL FORM

Tablets.

4. CLINICAL PARTICULARS

4.1 Therapeutic indications

Acute migraine.

4.2 Posology and method of administration

For oral administration.

To be taken preferably with or after food.

Undesirable effects may be minimised by using the lowest effective dose for the shortest duration necessary to control symptoms (see 4.4 Special warnings and precautions for use).

ADULTS

Migraine - acute attacks:

200mg when the first symptoms of migraine appear. The treatment can be repeated once after 1-2 hours if a satisfactory response is not obtained.

CHILDREN

A paediatric dosage regimen has not yet been established.

ELDERLY

The elderly are at increased risk of the serious consequences of adverse reactions. If an NSAID is considered necessary, the lowest effective dose should be used and for the shortest possible duration. The patient should be monitored regularly for GI bleeding during NSAID therapy.

4.3 Contraindications

Hypersensitivity to tolfenamic acid or to any of the excipients.

Active, or history of recurrent peptic ulcer/haemorrhage (two or more distinct episodes of proven ulceration or bleeding).

NSAIDs are contraindicated in patients who have previously shown hypersensitivity reactions (e.g. asthma, rhinitis, angioedema or urticaria) in response to ibuprofen, aspirin, or other non-steroidal anti-inflammatory drugs.

Severe heart failure, hepatic failure and renal failure (see 4.4 Special warnings and precautions for use).

During the last trimester of pregnancy (see 4.6 Pregnancy and lactation).

History of gastrointestinal bleeding or perforation, related to previous NSAIDs therapy.

4.4 Special warnings and precautions for use

In all patients:

Undesirable effects may be minimised by using the lowest effective dose for the shortest duration necessary to control symptoms (see 4.2 Posology and administration, and GI and cardiovascular risks below).

The use of Clotam Rapid with concomitant NSAIDs including cyclooxygenase-2 selective inhibitors should be avoided (see 4.5 Interaction with other medicinal products and other forms of interaction).

Elderly:

The elderly have an increased frequency of adverse reactions to NSAIDs especially gastrointestinal bleeding and perforation which may be fatal (see 4.2 Posology and administration).

Respiratory disorders:

Caution is required if administered to patients suffering from, or with a previous history of, bronchial asthma since NSAIDs have been reported to precipitate bronchospasm in such patients.

Cardiovascular, renal and hepatic impairment:

The administration of an NSAID may cause a dose dependent reduction in prostaglandin formation and precipitate renal failure. Patients at greatest risk of this reaction are those with impaired renal function, cardiac impairment, liver dysfunction, those taking diuretics and the elderly. Renal function should be monitored in these patients (see also 4.3 Contraindications).

Cardiovascular and cerebrovascular effects:

Appropriate monitoring and advice are required for patients with a history of hypertension and/or mild to moderate congestive heart failure as fluid retention and oedema have been reported in association with NSAID therapy.

Clinical trial and epidemiological data suggest that use of some NSAIDs (particularly at high doses and in long term treatment) may be associated with a small increased risk of arterial thrombotic events (for example myocardial infarction or stroke). There are insufficient data to exclude such a risk for tolfenamic acid.

Patients with uncontrolled hypertension, congestive heart failure, established ischaemic heart disease, peripheral arterial disease, and/or cerebrovascular disease should only be treated with tolfenamic acid after careful consideration. Similar consideration should be made before initiating longer-term treatment of patients with risk factors for cardiovascular disease (e.g. hypertension, hyperlipidaemia, diabetes mellitus, smoking).

Gastrointestinal bleeding, ulceration and perforation:

GI bleeding, ulceration or perforation, which can be fatal, has been reported with all NSAIDs at any time during treatment, with or without warning symptoms or a previous history of serious GI events.

The risk of GI bleeding, ulceration or perforation is higher with increasing NSAID doses, in patients with a history of ulcer, particularly if complicated with haemorrhage or perforation (see 4.3 Contraindications), and in the elderly. These patients should commence treatment on the lowest dose available. Combination therapy with protective agents (e.g. misoprostol or proton pump inhibitors) should be considered for these patients, and also for patients requiring concomitant low dose aspirin, or other drugs likely to increase gastrointestinal risk (see below and section 4.5 Interaction with other medicinal products and other forms of interaction).

Patients with a history of GI toxicity, particularly when elderly, should report any unusual abdominal symptoms (especially GI bleeding) particularly in the initial stages of treatment.

Caution should be advised in patients receiving concomitant medications which could increase the risk of ulceration or bleeding, such as oral corticosteroids, anticoagulants such as warfarin, selective serotonin-reuptake inhibitors or anti-platelet agents such as aspirin (see 4.5 Interaction with other medicinal products and other forms of interaction).

When GI bleeding or ulceration occurs in patients receiving tolfenamic acid, the treatment should be withdrawn.

NSAIDs should be given with care to patients with a history of gastrointestinal disease (ulcerative colitis, Crohn's disease) as these conditions may be exacerbated (see 4.8 Undesirable effects).

SLE and mixed connective tissue disease:

In patients with systemic lupus erythematosus (SLE) and mixed connective tissue disorders there may be an increased risk of aseptic meningitis (see 4.8 Undesirable effects).

Dermatological:

Serious skin reactions, some of them fatal, including exfoliative dermatitis, Stevens-Johnson syndrome, and toxic epidermal necrolysis, have been reported very rarely in association with the use of NSAIDs (see 4.8 Undesirable effects). Patients appear to be at highest risk for these reactions early in the course of therapy: the onset of the reaction occurring in the majority of cases within the first month of treatment. Clotam Rapid should be discontinued at the first appearance of skin rash, mucosal lesions or any other sign of hypersensitivity.

Impaired female fertility:

The use of tolfenamic acid may impair female fertility and is not recommended in women attempting to conceive. In women who have difficulties conceiving or who are undergoing investigation of infertility, withdrawal of tolfenamic acid should be considered.

4.5 Interaction with other medicinal products and other forms of interaction

Other analgesics including cyclooxygenase-2 selective inhibitors: Avoid concomitant use of two or more NSAIDs (including aspirin) as this may increase the risk of adverse effects (see 4.4 Special warnings and precautions for use).

Anti-hypertensives:

Reduced anti-hypertensive effect.

Diuretics:

Reduced diuretic effect. Diuretics can increase the risk of nephrotoxicity of NSAIDs.

Cardiac glycosides:

NSAIDs may exacerbate cardiac failure, reduce GFR and increase plasma glycoside levels.

Lithium:

The effect of lithium may be increased due to decreased elimination of lithium.

Methotrexate:

Decreased elimination of methotrexate.

Ciclosporin:

Increased risk of nephrotoxicity.

Mifepristone:

NSAIDs should not be used for 8-12 days after mifepristone administration as NSAIDs can reduce the effect of mifepristone.

Corticosteroids:

Increased risk of gastrointestinal ulceration or bleeding (see 4.4 Special warnings and precautions for use).

Anti-coagulants:

NSAIDs may enhance the effects of anti-coagulants, such as warfarin (see 4.4 Special warnings and precautions for use). In patients treated with anti-coagulants, close monitoring of blood coagulation is recommended.

Quinolone antibiotics:

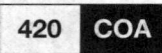

Animal data indicate that NSAIDs can increase the risk of convulsions associated with quinolone antibiotics. Patients taking NSAIDs and quinolones may have an increased risk of developing convulsions.

Anti-platelet agents and selective serotonin reuptake inhibitors (SSRIs):

Increased risk of gastrointestinal bleeding (see 4.4 Special warnings and precautions for use).

Tacrolimus:

Possible increased risk of nephrotoxicity when NSAIDs are given with tacrolimus.

Zidovudine:

Increased risk of haematological toxicity when NSAIDs are given with zidovudine. There is evidence of an increased risk of haemarthroses and haematoma in HIV(+) haemophiliacs receiving concurrent treatment with zidovudine and ibuprofen.

4.6 Pregnancy and lactation

Pregnancy:

Congenital abnormalities have been reported in association with NSAID administration in man, however, these are low in frequency and do not appear to follow any discernible pattern. In view of the known effects of NSAIDs on the foetal cardiovascular system (risk of closure of the ductus arteriosus), use in the last trimester of pregnancy is contraindicated. The onset of labour may be delayed and the duration increased with an increased bleeding tendency in both mother and child (see 4.3 Contraindications). NSAIDs should not be used during the first two trimesters of pregnancy or labour unless the potential benefit to the patient outweighs the potential risk to the foetus.

Lactation:

In limited studies so far available, NSAIDs can appear in breast milk in very low concentrations. NSAIDs should, if possible, be avoided when breastfeeding.

See 4.4 Special warnings and special precautions for use, regarding female fertility.

4.7 Effects on ability to drive and use machines

Undesirable effects such as dizziness, drowsiness, fatigue and visual disturbances are possible after taking NSAIDs. If affected, patients should not drive or operate machinery.

4.8 Undesirable effects

Tolfenamic acid is well tolerated at the recommended dosage.

The following side effects have been observed:

Gastrointestinal:

The most commonly-observed adverse events are gastrointestinal in nature. Peptic ulcers, perforation or GI bleeding, sometimes fatal, particularly in the elderly, may occur (see 4.4 Special warnings and precautions for use). Nausea, vomiting, diarrhoea, flatulence, constipation, dyspepsia, abdominal pain, melaena, haematemesis, ulcerative stomatitis, exacerbation of colitis and Crohn's disease (see 4.4 Special warnings and precautions for use) have been reported following administration. Less frequently, gastritis has been observed. Pancreatitis has been reported very rarely.

Hypersensitivity:

Hypersensitivity reactions have been reported following treatment with NSAIDs. These may consist of (a) non-specific allergic reactions and anaphylaxis (b) respiratory tract reactivity comprising asthma, aggravated asthma, bronchospasm or dyspnoea, or (c) assorted skin disorders, including rashes of various types, pruritus, urticaria, purpura, angioedema and, more rarely exfoliative and bullous dermatoses (including epidermal necrolysis and erythema multiforme).

Cardiovascular and cerebrovascular:

Oedema, hypertension and cardiac failure have been reported in association with NSAID treatment.

Clinical trial and epidemiological data suggest that use of some NSAIDs (particularly at high doses and in long term treatment) may be associated with an increased risk of arterial thrombotic events (for example myocardial infarction or stroke) (see 4.4 Special warnings and precautions for use).

Other adverse reactions reported less commonly include:

Renal:

Nephrotoxicity in various forms, including interstitial nephritis, nephrotic syndrome and renal failure. Harmless dysuria in the form of smarting during urination may occur occasionally, most commonly in males. The occurrence is correlated with the concentration of a metabolite and is most probably due to a local irritating effect of the urethra. Increased consumption of liquid or reduction of the dose diminishes the risk of smarting. The urine may, due to coloured metabolites, become a little more lemon coloured.

Hepatic:

Abnormal liver function, hepatitis and jaundice.

Neurological and special senses:

Visual disturbances, optic neuritis, headaches, paraesthesia, reports of aseptic meningitis (especially in patients with existing auto-immune disorders, such as systemic lupus erythematosus, mixed connective tissue disease), with symptoms such as stiff neck, headache, nausea, vomiting, fever or disorientation (see 4.4 Special warnings and precautions for use), depression, confusion, hallucinations, tinnitus, vertigo, tremor, euphoria, dizziness, malaise, fatigue and drowsiness.

Haematological:

Thrombocytopenia, neutropenia, agranulocytosis, aplastic anaemia and haemolytic anaemia.

Dermatological:

Bullous reactions including Stevens Johnson Syndrome and Toxic Epidermal Necrolysis (very rare). Photosensitivity.

4.9 Overdose

Symptoms

Symptoms include headache, nausea, vomiting, epigastric pain, gastrointestinal bleeding, rarely diarrhoea, disorientation, excitation, coma, drowsiness, dizziness, tinnitus, fainting, occasionally convulsions. In cases of significant poisoning acute renal failure and liver damage are possible.

Therapeutic measure

Patients should be treated symptomatically as required. Within one hour of ingestion of a potentially toxic amount, activated charcoal should be considered. Alternatively, in adults, gastric lavage should be considered within one hour of ingestion of a potentially life-threatening overdose. Good urine output should be ensured. Renal and liver function should be closely monitored. Patients should be observed for at least four hours after ingestion of potentially toxic amounts. Frequent or prolonged convulsions should be treated with intravenous diazepam. Other measures may be indicated by the patient's clinical condition.

5. PHARMACOLOGICAL PROPERTIES

5.1 Pharmacodynamic properties

NSAID with anti-inflammatory, analgesic, and antipyretic effects. Tolfenamic acid is a prostaglandin synthesis inhibitor and a leukotriene synthesis inhibitor.

5.2 Pharmacokinetic properties

Tolfenamic acid is absorbed quickly and almost completely after oral administration.

Hepatic first pass metabolism is as low as 15% (bioavailability 85%). Maximum plasma concentrations are reached after about 1-1½ hours. The half-life in plasma is about 2 hours. Tolfenamic acid is extensively bound to plasma proteins (99%). It is metabolised in the liver and tolfenamic acid as well as the metabolites is conjugated with glucuronic acid. About 90% of a given dose of tolfenamic acid is excreted in the urine as glucuronic acid conjugates, and about 10% is excreted in the faeces. Enterohepatic circulation exists.

5.3 Preclinical safety data

The therapeutic index for tolfenamic acid is high, and gastrointestinal ulceration and kidney changes have only been seen with oral doses approximately 6-10 times the maximum therapeutic dose recommended for tolfenamic acid. In human volunteers, tolfenamic acid did not affect renal function.

6. PHARMACEUTICAL PARTICULARS

6.1 List of excipients

Maize starch; Sodium starch glycollate (Type A); Macrogol 6000; Alginic acid; Cellulose, microcrystalline; Croscarmellose sodium; Silica, colloidal anhydrous;

Sodium stearyl fumarate.

6.2 Incompatibilities

None known.

6.3 Shelf life

Five years.

6.4 Special precautions for storage

Store below 25°C.

6.5 Nature and contents of container

Blister card:

Cover foil: 20 μm Al foil.

Form foil: 250 μm PVC foil

HDPE tablet container with LDPE closure.

Pack sizes: 3, 10 and 30 tablets.

6.6 Special precautions for disposal and other handling

None.

7. MARKETING AUTHORISATION HOLDER

A/S GEA Farmaceutisk Fabrik

Holger Danskes Vej 89

DK-2000 Frederiksberg

Denmark

8. MARKETING AUTHORISATION NUMBER(S)

PL 04012/0043

9. DATE OF FIRST AUTHORISATION/RENEWAL OF THE AUTHORISATION

25 April 1997

10. DATE OF REVISION OF THE TEXT

03 February 2009

CoAprovel 150/12.5 mg, 300/12.5 mg and 300/25 mg Film-Coated Tablet (sanofi-aventis)

(sanofi-aventis)

1. NAME OF THE MEDICINAL PRODUCT

CoAprovel 150/12.5 mg film-coated tablets

CoAprovel 300/12.5 mg film-coated tablets

CoAprovel 300/25 mg film-coated tablets

2. QUALITATIVE AND QUANTITATIVE COMPOSITION

CoAprovel 150/12.5 mg

Each film-coated tablet contains 150 mg of irbesartan and 12.5 mg of hydrochlorothiazide.

Excipient: 38.5 mg of lactose (as lactose monohydrate).

CoAprovel 300/12.5 mg

Each film-coated tablet contains 300 mg of irbesartan and 12.5 mg of hydrochlorothiazide.

Excipient: 89.5 mg of lactose (as lactose monohydrate).

CoAprovel 300 mg/25 mg

Each film-coated tablet contains 300 mg of irbesartan and 25 mg of hydrochlorothiazide.

Excipient: 53.3 mg of lactose (as lactose monohydrate).

For a full list of excipients, see section 6.1.

3. PHARMACEUTICAL FORM

Film-coated tablet.

CoAprovel 150/12.5 mg

Peach, biconvex, oval-shaped, with a heart debossed on one side and the number 2875 engraved on the other side.

CoAprovel 300/12.5 mg

Peach, biconvex, oval-shaped, with a heart debossed on one side and the number 2876 engraved on the other side.

CoAprovel 300 mg/25 mg

Pink, biconvex, oval-shaped, with a heart debossed on one side and the number 2788 engraved on the other side.

4. CLINICAL PARTICULARS

4.1 Therapeutic indications

Treatment of essential hypertension.

This fixed dose combination is indicated in adult patients whose blood pressure is not adequately controlled on irbesartan or hydrochlorothiazide alone (see section 5.1).

4.2 Posology and method of administration

CoAprovel can be taken once daily, with or without food.

Dose titration with the individual components (i.e. irbesartan and hydrochlorothiazide) may be recommended.

When clinically appropriate direct change from monotherapy to the fixed combinations may be considered:

- CoAprovel 150 mg/12.5 mg may be administered in patients whose blood pressure is not adequately controlled with hydrochlorothiazide or irbesartan 150 mg alone;
- CoAprovel 300 mg/12.5 mg may be administered in patients insufficiently controlled by irbesartan 300 mg or by CoAprovel 150 mg/12.5 mg.
- CoAprovel 300 mg/25 mg may be administered in patients insufficiently controlled by CoAprovel 300 mg/12.5 mg.

Doses higher than 300 mg irbesartan/25 mg hydrochlorothiazide once daily are not recommended.

When necessary, CoAprovel may be administered with another antihypertensive medicinal product (see section 4.5).

Renal impairment: due to the hydrochlorothiazide component, CoAprovel is not recommended for patients with severe renal dysfunction (creatinine clearance < 30 ml/min). Loop diuretics are preferred to thiazides in this population. No dosage adjustment is necessary in patients with renal impairment whose renal creatinine clearance is ⩾ 30 ml/min (see sections 4.3 and 4.4).

Hepatic impairment: CoAprovel is not indicated in patients with severe hepatic impairment. Thiazides should be used with caution in patients with impaired hepatic function. No dosage adjustment of CoAprovel is necessary in patients with mild to moderate hepatic impairment (see section 4.3).

Elderly patients: no dosage adjustment of CoAprovel is necessary in elderly patients.

Paediatric patients: CoAprovel is not recommended for use in children and adolescents due to a lack of data on safety and efficacy.

4.3 Contraindications

Hypersensitivity to the active substances, to any of the excipients (see section 6.1), or to other sulfonamide-derived substances (hydrochlorothiazide is a sulfonamide-derived substance)

Second and third trimesters of pregnancy (see sections 4.4 and 4.6)

Severe renal impairment (creatinine clearance < 30 ml/min)

Refractory hypokalaemia, hypercalcaemia

Severe hepatic impairment, biliary cirrhosis and cholestasis

4.4 Special warnings and precautions for use

Hypotension - Volume-depleted patients: CoAprovel has been rarely associated with symptomatic hypotension in hypertensive patients without other risk factors for hypotension. Symptomatic hypotension may be expected to occur in patients who are volume and/or sodium depleted by vigorous diuretic therapy, dietary salt restriction, diarrhoea or vomiting. Such conditions should be corrected before initiating therapy with CoAprovel.

Renal artery stenosis - Renovascular hypertension: there is an increased risk of severe hypotension and renal insufficiency when patients with bilateral renal artery stenosis or stenosis of the artery to a single functioning kidney are treated with angiotensin converting enzyme inhibitors or angiotensin-II receptor antagonists. While this is not documented with CoAprovel, a similar effect should be anticipated.

Renal impairment and kidney transplantation: when CoAprovel is used in patients with impaired renal function, a periodic monitoring of potassium, creatinine and uric acid serum levels is recommended. There is no experience regarding the administration of CoAprovel in patients with a recent kidney transplantation. CoAprovel should not be used in patients with severe renal impairment (creatinine clearance < 30 ml/min) (see section 4.3). Thiazide diuretic-associated azotemia may occur in patients with impaired renal function. No dosage adjustment is necessary in patients with renal impairment whose creatinine clearance is ⩾ 30 ml/min. However, in patients with mild to moderate renal impairment (creatinine clearance ⩾ 30 ml/min but < 60 ml/min) this fixed dose combination should be administered with caution.

Hepatic impairment: thiazides should be used with caution in patients with impaired hepatic function or progressive liver disease, since minor alterations of fluid and electrolyte balance may precipitate hepatic coma. There is no clinical experience with CoAprovel in patients with hepatic impairment.

Aortic and mitral valve stenosis, obstructive hypertrophic cardiomyopathy: as with other vasodilators, special caution is indicated in patients suffering from aortic or mitral stenosis, or obstructive hypertrophic cardiomyopathy.

Primary aldosteronism: patients with primary aldosteronism generally will not respond to anti-hypertensive medicinal products acting through inhibition of the renin-angiotensin system. Therefore, the use of CoAprovel is not recommended.

Metabolic and endocrine effects: thiazide therapy may impair glucose tolerance. In diabetic patients dosage adjustments of insulin or oral hypoglycemic agents may be required. Latent diabetes mellitus may become manifest during thiazide therapy.

Increases in cholesterol and triglyceride levels have been associated with thiazide diuretic therapy; however at the 12.5 mg dose contained in CoAprovel, minimal or no effects were reported.

Hyperuricaemia may occur or frank gout may be precipitated in certain patients receiving thiazide therapy.

Electrolyte imbalance: as for any patient receiving diuretic therapy, periodic determination of serum electrolytes should be performed at appropriate intervals.

Thiazides, including hydrochlorothiazide, can cause fluid or electrolyte imbalance (hypokalaemia, hyponatraemia, and hypochloremic alkalosis). Warning signs of fluid or electrolyte imbalance are dryness of mouth, thirst, weakness, lethargy, drowsiness, restlessness, muscle pain or cramps, muscular fatigue, hypotension, oliguria, tachycardia, and gastrointestinal disturbances such as nausea or vomiting.

Although hypokalaemia may develop with the use of thiazide diuretics, concurrent therapy with irbesartan may reduce diuretic-induced hypokalaemia. The risk of hypokalaemia is greatest in patients with cirrhosis of the liver, in patients experiencing brisk diuresis, in patients who are receiving inadequate oral intake of electrolytes and in patients receiving concomitant therapy with corticosteroids or ACTH. Conversely, due to the irbesartan component of CoAprovel hyperkalaemia might occur, especially in the presence of renal impairment and/or heart failure, and diabetes mellitus. Adequate monitoring of serum potassium in patients at risk is recommended. Potassium-sparing diuretics, potassium supplements or potassium-containing salts substitutes should be co-administered cautiously with CoAprovel (see section 4.5).

There is no evidence that irbesartan would reduce or prevent diuretic-induced hyponatraemia. Chloride deficit is generally mild and usually does not require treatment.

Thiazides may decrease urinary calcium excretion and cause an intermittent and slight elevation of serum calcium in the absence of known disorders of calcium metabolism. Marked hypercalcaemia may be evidence of hidden hyperparathyroidism. Thiazides should be discontinued before carrying out tests for parathyroid function.

Thiazides have been shown to increase the urinary excretion of magnesium, which may result in hypomagnesaemia.

Lithium: the combination of lithium and CoAprovel is not recommended (see section 4.5).

Anti-doping test: hydrochlorothiazide contained in this medicinal product could produce a positive analytic result in an anti-doping test.

General: in patients whose vascular tone and renal function depend predominantly on the activity of the renin-angiotensin-aldosterone system (e.g. patients with severe congestive heart failure or underlying renal disease, including renal artery stenosis), treatment with angiotensin converting enzyme inhibitors or angiotensin-II receptor antagonists that affect this system has been associated with acute hypotension, azotemia, oliguria, or rarely acute renal failure. As with any anti-hypertensive agent, excessive blood pressure decrease in patients with ischemic cardiopathy or ischemic cardiovascular disease could result in a myocardial infarction or stroke.

Hypersensitivity reactions to hydrochlorothiazide may occur in patients with or without a history of allergy or bronchial asthma, but are more likely in patients with such a history.

Exacerbation or activation of systemic lupus erythematosus has been reported with the use of thiazide diuretics.

Cases of photosensitivity reactions have been reported with thiazides diuretics (see section 4.8). If photosensitivity reaction occurs during treatment, it is recommended to stop the treatment. If a re-administration of the diuretic is deemed necessary, it is recommended to protect exposed areas to the sun or to artificial UVA.

Pregnancy: Angiotensin II Receptor Antagonists (AIIRAs) should not be initiated during pregnancy. Unless continued AIIRA therapy is considered essential, patients planning pregnancy should be changed to alternative anti-hypertensive treatments which have an established safety profile for use in pregnancy. When pregnancy is diagnosed, treatment with AIIRAs should be stopped immediately, and, if appropriate, alternative therapy should be started (see sections 4.3 and 4.6).

Lactose: this medicinal product contains lactose. Patients with rare hereditary problems of galactose intolerance, the Lapp lactase deficiency or glucose-galactose malabsorption should not take this medicinal product.

4.5 Interaction with other medicinal products and other forms of interaction

Other antihypertensive agents: the antihypertensive effect of CoAprovel may be increased with the concomitant use of other antihypertensive agents. Irbesartan and hydrochlorothiazide (at doses up to 300 mg irbesartan/25 mg hydrochlorothiazide) have been safely administered with other antihypertensive agents including calcium channel blockers and beta-adrenergic blockers. Prior treatment with high dose diuretics may result in volume depletion and a risk of hypotension when initiating therapy with irbesartan with or without thiazide diuretics unless the volume depletion is corrected first (see section 4.4).

Lithium: reversible increases in serum lithium concentrations and toxicity have been reported during concomitant administration of lithium with angiotensin converting enzyme inhibitors. Similar effects have been very rarely reported with irbesartan so far. Furthermore, renal clearance of lithium is reduced by thiazides so the risk of lithium toxicity could be increased with CoAprovel. Therefore, the combination of lithium and CoAprovel is not recommended (see section 4.4). If the combination proves necessary, careful monitoring of serum lithium levels is recommended.

Medicinal products affecting potassium: the potassium-depleting effect of hydrochlorothiazide is attenuated by the potassium-sparing effect of irbesartan. However, this effect of hydrochlorothiazide on serum potassium would be expected to be potentiated by other medicinal products associated with potassium loss and hypokalaemia (e.g. other kaliuretic diuretics, laxatives, amphotericin, carbenoxolone, penicillin G sodium). Conversely, based on the experience with the use of other medicinal products that blunt the renin-angiotensin system, concomitant use of potassium-sparing diuretics, potassium supplements, salt substitutes containing potassium or other medicinal products that may increase serum potassium levels (e.g. heparin sodium) may lead to increases in serum potassium. Adequate monitoring of serum potassium in patients at risk is recommended (see section 4.4).

Medicinal products affected by serum potassium disturbances: periodic monitoring of serum potassium is recommended when CoAprovel is administered with medicinal products affected by serum potassium disturbances (e.g. digitalis glycosides, antiarrhythmics).

Non-steroidal anti-inflammatory drugs: when angiotensin II antagonists are administered simultaneously with non-steroidal anti- inflammatory drugs (i.e. selective COX-2 inhibitors, acetylsalicylic acid (> 3 g/day) and non-selective NSAIDs), attenuation of the antihypertensive effect may occur.

As with ACE inhibitors, concomitant use of angiotensin II antagonists and NSAIDs may lead to an increased risk of worsening of renal function, including possible acute renal failure, and an increase in serum potassium, especially in patients with poor pre-existing renal function. The combination should be administered with caution, especially in the elderly. Patients should be adequately hydrated and consideration should be given to monitoring renal function after initiation of concomitant therapy, and periodically thereafter.

Additional information on irbesartan interactions: in clinical studies, the pharmacokinetic of irbesartan is not affected by hydrochlorothiazide. Irbesartan is mainly metabolised by CYP2C9 and to a lesser extent by glucuronidation. No significant pharmacokinetic or pharmacodynamic interactions were observed when irbesartan was coadministered with warfarin, a medicinal product metabolised by CYP2C9. The effects of CYP2C9 inducers such as rifampicin on the pharmacokinetic of irbesartan have not been evaluated. The pharmacokinetic of digoxin was not altered by co-administration of irbesartan.

Additional information on hydrochlorothiazide interactions: when administered concurrently, the following medicinal products may interact with thiazide diuretics:

Alcohol: potentiation of orthostatic hypotension may occur;

Antidiabetic medicinal products (oral agents and insulins): dosage adjustment of the antidiabetic medicinal product may be required (see section 4.4);

Colestyramine and Colestipol resins: absorption of hydrochlorothiazide is impaired in the presence of anionic exchange resins;

Corticosteroids, ACTH: electrolyte depletion, particularly hypokalaemia, may be increased;

Digitalis glycosides: thiazide induced hypokalaemia or hypomagnaesemia favour the onset of digitalis-induced cardiac arrhythmias (see section 4.4);

Non-steroidal anti-inflammatory drugs: the administration of a non-steroidal anti-inflammatory drug may reduce the diuretic, natriuretic and antihypertensive effects of thiazide diuretics in some patients;

Pressor amines (e.g. noradrenaline): the effect of pressor amines may be decreased, but not sufficiently to preclude their use;

Nondepolarizing skeletal muscle relaxants (e.g. tubocurarine): the effect of nondepolarizing skeletal muscle relaxants may be potentiated by hydrochlorothiazide;

Antigout medicinal products: dosage adjustments of antigout medicinal products may be necessary as hydrochlorothiazide may raise the level of serum uric acid. Increase in dosage of probenecid or sulfinpyrazone may be necessary. Co-administration of thiazide diuretics may increase the incidence of hypersensitivity reactions to allopurinol;

Calcium salts: thiazide diuretics may increase serum calcium levels due to decreased excretion. If calcium supplements or calcium sparing medicinal products (e.g. vitamin D therapy) must be prescribed, serum calcium levels should be monitored and calcium dosage adjusted accordingly;

Other interactions: the hyperglycaemic effect of beta-blockers and diazoxide may be enhanced by thiazides. Anticholinergic agents (e.g. atropine, beperiden) may increase the bioavailability of thiazide-type diuretics by decreasing gastrointestinal motility and stomach emptying rate. Thiazides may increase the risk of adverse effects caused by amantadine. Thiazides may reduce the renal excretion of cytotoxic medicinal products (e.g. cyclophosphamide, methotrexate) and potentiate their myelosuppressive effects.

4.6 Pregnancy and lactation

Pregnancy

The use of AIIRAs is not recommended during the first trimester of pregnancy (see section 4.4). The use of AIIRAs is contraindicated during the second and third trimester of pregnancy (see sections 4.3 and 4.4).

Epidemiological evidence regarding the risk of teratogenicity following exposure to ACE inhibitors during the first trimester of pregnancy has not been conclusive; however a small increase in risk cannot be excluded. Whilst there is no controlled epidemiological data on the risk with Angiotensin II Receptor Antagonists (AIIRAs), similar risks may exist for this class of drugs. Unless continued AIIRA therapy is considered essential, patients planning pregnancy should be changed to alternative anti-hypertensive treatments which have an established safety profile for use in pregnancy. When pregnancy is diagnosed, treatment with AIIRAs should be stopped immediately, and, if appropriate, alternative therapy should be started.

Exposure to AIIRA therapy during the second and third trimesters is known to induce human fetotoxicity (decreased renal function, oligohydramnios, skull ossification retardation) and neonatal toxicity (renal failure, hypotension, hyperkalaemia). (see section 5.3).

Should exposure to AIIRAs have occurred from the second trimester of pregnancy, ultrasound check of renal function and skull is recommended.

Infants whose mothers have taken AIIRAs should be closely observed for hypotension (see also sections 4.3 and 4.4).

Thiazides cross the placental barrier and appear in cord blood. They may cause a decrease in placental perfusion, foetal electrolyte disturbances and possibly other reactions that have occurred in the adults. Cases of neonatal thrombocytopenia, or foetal or neonatal jaundice have been reported with maternal thiazide therapy. Since CoAprovel contains hydrochlorothiazide, it is not recommended during the first trimester of pregnancy. A switch to a suitable alternative treatment should be carried out in advance of a planned pregnancy.

Lactation:

Because no information is available regarding the use of CoAprovel during breast-feeding, CoAprovel is not recommended and alternative treatments with better established safety profiles during breast-feeding are preferable, especially while nursing a newborn or preterm infant.

4.7 Effects on ability to drive and use machines

No studies on the effects on the ability to drive and use machines have been performed. Based on its pharmacodynamic properties, CoAprovel is unlikely to affect this ability. When driving vehicles or operating machines, it should be taken into account that occasionally dizziness or weariness may occur during treatment of hypertension.

4.8 Undesirable effects

Irbesartan/hydrochlorothiazide combination:

Table 1 gives the adverse reactions observed from spontaneous reporting and in placebo-controlled trials in which 898 hypertensive patients received various doses (range: 37.5 mg/6.25 mg to 300 mg/25 mg irbesartan/hydrochlorothiazide).

The frequency of adverse reactions listed below is defined using the following convention:

very common (⩾ 1/10); common (⩾ 1/100 to < 1/10); uncommon (⩾ 1/1,000 to < 1/100); rare (⩾ 1/10,000 to < 1/1,000); very rare (< 1/10,000). Within each frequency grouping, undesirable effects are presented in order of decreasing seriousness.

(see Table 1 opposite)

Table 1 Adverse Reactions in Placebo-Controlled Trials and Spontaneous Reports*

Investigations:	Common:	increases in blood urea nitrogen (BUN), creatinine and creatine kinase
	Uncommon:	decreases in serum potassium and sodium
Cardiac disorders:	Uncommon:	syncope, hypotension, tachycardia, oedema
Nervous system disorders:	Common:	dizziness
	Uncommon:	orthostatic dizziness
	Not known:	headache
Ear and labyrinth disorders:	Not known:	tinnitus
Respiratory, thoracic and mediastinal disorders:	Not known:	cough
Gastrointestinal disorders:	Common:	nausea/vomiting
	Uncommon:	diarrhoea
	Not known:	dyspepsia, dysgeusia
Renal and urinary disorders:	Common:	abnormal urination
	Not known:	impaired renal function including isolated cases of renal failure in patients at risk (see section 4.4)
Musculoskeletal and connective tissue disorders:	Uncommon:	swelling extremity
	Not known:	arthralgia, myalgia
Metabolism and nutrition disorders:	Not known:	hyperkalaemia
Vascular disorders:	Uncommon:	flushing
General disorders and administration site conditions:	Common:	fatigue
Immune system disorders:	Not known:	cases of hypersensitivity reactions such as angioedema, rash, urticaria
Hepatobiliary disorders:	Not known:	hepatitis, abnormal liver function
Reproductive system and breast disorders:	Uncommon:	sexual dysfunction, libido changes

* Frequency for adverse reactions detected by spontaneous reports is described as "not known"

Additional information on individual components: in addition to the adverse reactions listed above for the combination product, other adverse reactions previously reported with one of the individual components may be potential adverse reactions with CoAprovel. Tables 2 and 3 below detail the adverse reactions reported with the individual components of CoAprovel.

Table 2:
Adverse reactions reported with the use of **irbesartan** alone

General disorders and administration site conditions:	Uncommon:	chest pain

(see Table 3 on next page)

4.9 Overdose

No specific information is available on the treatment of overdose with CoAprovel. The patient should be closely monitored, and the treatment should be symptomatic and supportive. Management depends on the time since ingestion and the severity of the symptoms. Suggested measures include induction of emesis and/or gastric lavage. Activated charcoal may be useful in the treatment of overdose. Serum electrolytes and creatinine should be monitored frequently. If hypotension occurs, the patient should be placed in a supine position, with salt and volume replacements given quickly.

The most likely manifestations of irbesartan overdose are expected to be hypotension and tachycardia; bradycardia might also occur.

Overdose with hydrochlorothiazide is associated with electrolyte depletion (hypokalaemia, hypochloremia, hyponatraemia) and dehydration resulting from excessive diuresis. The most common signs and symptoms of overdose are nausea and somnolence. Hypokalaemia may result in muscle spasms and/or accentuate cardiac arrhythmias associated with the concomitant use of digitalis glycosides or certain anti-arrhythmic medicinal products.

Irbesartan is not removed by haemodialysis. The degree to which hydrochlorothiazide is removed by haemodialysis has not been established.

5. PHARMACOLOGICAL PROPERTIES

5.1 Pharmacodynamic properties

Pharmacotherapeutic group: angiotensin-II antagonists, combinations

ATC code: C09DA04.

CoAprovel is a combination of an angiotensin-II receptor antagonist, irbesartan, and a thiazide diuretic, hydrochlorothiazide. The combination of these ingredients has an additive antihypertensive effect, reducing blood pressure to a greater degree than either component alone.

Irbesartan is a potent, orally active, selective angiotensin-II receptor (AT_1 subtype) antagonist. It is expected to block all actions of angiotensin-II mediated by the AT_1 receptor, regardless of the source or route of synthesis of angiotensin-II. The selective antagonism of the angiotensin-II (AT_1) receptors results in increases in plasma renin levels and angiotensin-II levels, and a decrease in plasma aldosterone concentration. Serum potassium levels are not significantly affected by irbesartan alone at the recommended doses in patients without risk of electrolyte imbalance (see sections 4.4 and 4.5). Irbesartan does not inhibit ACE (kininase-II), an enzyme which generates angiotensin-II and also degrades bradykinin into inactive metabolites. Irbesartan does not require metabolic activation for its activity.

Hydrochlorothiazide is a thiazide diuretic. The mechanism of antihypertensive effect of thiazide diuretics is not fully known. Thiazides affect the renal tubular mechanisms of electrolyte reabsorption, directly increasing excretion of sodium and chloride in approximately equivalent amounts. The diuretic action of hydrochlorothiazide reduces plasma volume, increases plasma renin activity, increases aldosterone secretion, with consequent increases in urinary potassium and bicarbonate loss, and decreases in serum potassium. Presumably through blockade of the renin-angiotensin-aldosterone system, co-administration of irbesartan tends to reverse the potassium loss associated with these diuretics. With hydrochlorothiazide, onset of diuresis occurs in 2 hours, and peak effect occurs at about 4 hours, while the action persists for approximately 6-12 hours.

The combination of hydrochlorothiazide and irbesartan produces dose-related additive reductions in blood pressure across their therapeutic dose ranges. The addition of 12.5 mg hydrochlorothiazide to 300 mg irbesartan once daily in patients not adequately controlled on 300 mg irbesartan alone resulted in further placebo-corrected diastolic blood pressure reductions at trough (24 hours post-dosing) of 6.1 mm Hg. The combination of 300 mg irbesartan and 12.5 mg hydrochlorothiazide resulted in an overall placebo-subtracted systolic/diastolic reductions of up to 13.6/11.5 mm Hg.

Limited clinical data (7 out of 22 patients) suggest that patients not controlled with the 300 mg/12.5 mg combination may respond when uptitrated to 300 mg/25 mg. In these patients, an incremental blood pressure lowering effect was observed for both systolic blood pressure (SBP) and diastolic blood pressure (DBP) (13.3 and 8.3 mm Hg, respectively).

Once daily dosing with 150 mg irbesartan and 12.5 mg hydrochlorothiazide gave systolic/diastolic mean placebo-adjusted blood pressure reductions at trough (24 hours post-dosing) of 12.9/6.9 mm Hg in patients with mild-to-moderate hypertension. Peak effects occurred at 3-6 hours. When assessed by ambulatory blood pressure monitoring, the combination 150 mg irbesartan and 12.5 mg hydrochlorothiazide once daily produced consistent reduction in blood pressure over the 24 hours period with mean 24-hour placebo-subtracted systolic/diastolic reductions of 15.8/10.0 mm Hg. When measured by ambulatory blood pressure monitoring, the trough to peak effects of CoAprovel 150 mg/12.5 mg were 100%. The trough to peak effects measured by cuff during office visits were 68% and 76% for CoAprovel 150 mg/12.5 mg and CoAprovel 300 mg/12.5 mg, respectively. These 24-hour effects were observed without excessive blood pressure lowering at peak and are consistent with safe and effective blood-pressure lowering over the once-daily dosing interval.

In patients not adequately controlled on 25 mg hydrochlorothiazide alone, the addition of irbesartan gave an added placebo-subtracted systolic/diastolic mean reduction of 11.1/7.2 mm Hg.

The blood pressure lowering effect of irbesartan in combination with hydrochlorothiazide is apparent after the first dose and substantially present within 1-2 weeks, with the maximal effect occurring by 6-8 weeks. In long-term follow-up studies, the effect of irbesartan/hydrochlorothiazide was maintained for over one year. Although not specifically studied with the CoAprovel, rebound hypertension has not been seen with either irbesartan or hydrochlorothiazide.

The effect of the combination of irbesartan and hydrochlorothiazide on morbidity and mortality has not been studied. Epidemiological studies have shown that long term treatment with hydrochlorothiazide reduces the risk of cardiovascular mortality and morbidity.

There is no difference in response to CoAprovel, regardless of age or gender. As is the case with other medicinal products that affect the renin-angiotensin system, black hypertensive patients have notably less response to irbesartan monotherapy. When irbesartan is administered concomitantly with a low dose of hydrochlorothiazide (e.g. 12.5 mg daily), the antihypertensive response in black patients approaches that of non-black patients.

Efficacy and safety of CoAprovel as initial therapy for severe hypertension (defined as SeDBP ⩾ 110 mmHg) was evaluated in a multicenter, randomized, double-blind, active-controlled, 8-week, parallel-arm study. A total of 697 patients were randomized in a 2:1 ratio to either irbesartan/hydrochlorothiazide 150 mg/12.5 mg or to irbesartan 150 mg and systematically force-titrated (before assessing the response to the lower dose) after one week to irbesartan/hydrochlorothiazide 300 mg/25 mg or irbesartan 300 mg, respectively.

Table 3 Adverse reactions (regardless of relationship to medicinal product) reported with the use of hydrochlorothiazide alone

Investigations:	Not known:	electrolyte imbalance (including hypokalaemia and hyponatraemia, see section 4.4), hyperuricaemia, glycosuria, hyperglycaemia, increases in cholesterol and triglycerides
Cardiac disorders:	Not known:	cardiac arrhythmias
Blood and lymphatic system disorders:	Not known:	aplastic anaemia, bone marrow depression, neutropenia/ agranulocytosis, haemolytic anaemia, leucopenia, thrombocytopenia
Nervous system disorders:	Not known:	vertigo, paraesthesia, light-headedness, restlessness
Eye disorders:	Not known:	transient blurred vision, xanthopsia
Respiratory, thoracic and mediastinal disorders:	Not known:	respiratory distress (including pneumonitis and pulmonary oedema)
Gastrointestinal disorders:	Not known:	pancreatitis, anorexia, diarrhoea, constipation, gastric irritation, sialadenitis, loss of appetite
Renal and urinary disorders:	Not known:	interstitial nephritis, renal dysfunction
Skin and subcutaneous tissue disorders:	Not known:	anaphylactic reactions, toxic epidermal necrolysis, necrotizing angitis (vasculitis, cutaneous vasculitis), cutaneous lupus erythematosus-like reactions, reactivation of cutaneous lupus erythematosus, photosensitivity reactions, rash, urticaria
Musculoskeletal and connective tissue disorders:	Not known:	weakness, muscle spasm
Vascular disorders:	Not known:	postural hypotension
General disorders and administration site conditions:	Not known:	fever
Hepatobiliary disorders:	Not known:	jaundice (intrahepatic cholestatic jaundice)
Psychiatric disorders:	Not known:	depression, sleep disturbances

The dose dependent adverse events of hydrochlorothiazide (particularly electrolyte disturbances) may increase when titrating the hydrochlorothiazide.

The study recruited 58% males. The mean age of patients was 52.5 years, 13% were ≥ 65 years of age, and just 2% were ≥ 75 years of age. Twelve percent (12%) of patients were diabetic, 34% were hyperlipidemic and the most frequent cardiovascular condition was stable angina pectoris in 3.5% of the participants.

The primary objective of this study was to compare the proportion of patients whose SeDBP was controlled (SeDBP < 90 mmHg) at Week 5 of treatment. Forty-seven percent (47.2%) of patients on the combination achieved trough SeDBP < 90 mmHg compared to 33.2% of patients on irbesartan (p = 0.0005). The mean baseline blood pressure was approximately 172/113 mmHg in each treatment group and decreases of SeSBP/SeDBP at five weeks were 30.8/24.0 mmHg and 21.1/19.3 mmHg for irbesartan/hydrochlorothiazide and irbesartan, respectively (p < 0.0001).

The types and incidences of adverse events reported for patients treated with the combination were similar to the adverse event profile for patients on monotherapy. During the 8-week treatment period, there were no reported cases of syncope in either treatment group. There were 0.6% and 0% of patients with hypotension and 2.8% and 3.1% of patients with dizziness as adverse reactions reported in the combination and monotherapy groups, respectively.

5.2 Pharmacokinetic properties

Concomitant administration of hydrochlorothiazide and irbesartan has no effect on the pharmacokinetics of either medicinal product.

Irbesartan and hydrochlorothiazide are orally active agents and do not require biotransformation for their activity. Following oral administration of CoAprovel, the absolute oral bioavailability is 60-80% and 50-80% for irbesartan and hydrochlorothiazide, respectively. Food does not affect the bioavailability of CoAprovel. Peak plasma concentration occurs at 1.5-2 hours after oral administration for irbesartan and 1-2.5 hours for hydrochlorothiazide.

Plasma protein binding of irbesartan is approximately 96%, with negligible binding to cellular blood components. The volume of distribution for irbesartan is 53-93 litres. Hydrochlorothiazide is 68% protein-bound in the plasma, and its apparent volume of distribution is 0.83-1.14 l/kg.

Irbesartan exhibits linear and dose proportional pharmacokinetics over the dose range of 10 to 600 mg. A less than proportional increase in oral absorption at doses beyond 600 mg was observed; the mechanism for this is unknown. The total body and renal clearance are 157-176 and 3.0-3.5 ml/min, respectively. The terminal elimination half-life of irbesartan is 11-15 hours. Steady-state plasma concentrations are attained within 3 days after initiation of a once-daily dosing regimen. Limited accumulation of irbesartan (< 20%) is observed in plasma upon repeated once-daily dosing. In a study, somewhat higher plasma concentrations of irbesartan were observed in female hypertensive patients. However, there was no difference in the half-life and accumulation of irbesartan. No dosage adjustment is necessary in female patients. Irbesartan AUC and Cmax values were also somewhat greater in elderly subjects (≥ 65 years) than those of young subjects (18-40 years). However the terminal half-life was not significantly altered. No dosage adjustment is necessary in elderly patients. The mean plasma half-life of hydrochlorothiazide reportedly ranges from 5-15 hours.

Following oral or intravenous administration of ^{14}C irbesartan, 80-85% of the circulating plasma radioactivity is attributable to unchanged irbesartan. Irbesartan is metabolised by the liver via glucuronide conjugation and oxidation. The major circulating metabolite is irbesartan glucuronide (approximately 6%). *In vitro* studies indicate that irbesartan is primarily oxidised by the cytochrome P450 enzyme CYP2C9; isoenzyme CYP3A4 has negligible effect. Irbesartan and its metabolites are eliminated by both biliary and renal pathways. After either oral or intravenous administration of ^{14}C irbesartan, about 20% of the radioactivity is recovered in the urine, and the remainder in the faeces. Less than 2% of the dose is excreted in the urine as unchanged irbesartan. Hydrochlorothiazide is not metabolized but is eliminated rapidly by the kidneys. At least 61% of the oral dose is eliminated unchanged within 24 hours. Hydrochlorothiazide crosses the placental but not the blood-brain barrier, and is excreted in breast milk.

Renal impairment: in patients with renal impairment or those undergoing haemodialysis, the pharmacokinetic parameters of irbesartan are not significantly altered. Irbesartan is not removed by haemodialysis. In patients with creatinine clearance < 20 ml/min, the elimination half-life of hydrochlorothiazide was reported to increase to 21 hours.

Hepatic impairment: in patients with mild to moderate cirrhosis, the pharmacokinetic parameters of irbesartan are not significantly altered. Studies have not been performed in patients with severe hepatic impairment.

5.3 Preclinical safety data

Irbesartan/hydrochlorothiazide: the potential toxicity of the irbesartan/hydrochlorothiazide combination after oral administration was evaluated in rats and macaques in studies lasting up to 6 months. There were no toxicological findings observed of relevance to human therapeutic use.

The following changes, observed in rats and macaques receiving the irbesartan/hydrochlorothiazide combination at 10/10 and 90/90 mg/kg/day, were also seen with one of the two medicinal products alone and/or were secondary to decreases in blood pressure (no significant toxicologic interactions were observed):

- kidney changes, characterized by slight increases in serum urea and creatinine, and hyperplasia/hypertrophy of the juxtaglomerular apparatus, which are a direct consequence of the interaction of irbesartan with the renin-angiotensin system;
- slight decreases in erythrocyte parameters (erythrocytes, haemoglobin, haematocrit);
- stomach discoloration, ulcers and focal necrosis of gastric mucosa were observed in few rats in a 6 months toxicity study at irbesartan 90 mg/kg/day, hydrochlorothiazide 90 mg/kg/day, and irbesartan/hydrochlorothiazide 10/10 mg/kg/day. These lesions were not observed in macaques;
- decreases in serum potassium due to hydrochlorothiazide and partly prevented when hydrochlorothiazide was given in combination with irbesartan.

Most of the above mentioned effects appear to be due to the pharmacological activity of irbesartan (blockade of angiotensin-II-induced inhibition of renin release, with stimulation of the renin-producing cells) and occur also with angiotensin converting enzyme inhibitors. These findings appear to have no relevance to the use of therapeutic doses of irbesartan/hydrochlorothiazide in humans.

No teratogenic effects were seen in rats given irbesartan and hydrochlorothiazide in combination at doses that produced maternal toxicity. The effects of the irbesartan/hydrochlorothiazide combination on fertility have not been evaluated in animal studies, as there is no evidence of adverse effect on fertility in animals or humans with either irbesartan or hydrochlorothiazide when administered alone. However, another angiotensin-II antagonist affected fertility parameters in animal studies when given alone. These findings were also observed with lower doses of this other angiotensin-II antagonist when given in combination with hydrochlorothiazide.

There was no evidence of mutagenicity or clastogenicity with the irbesartan/hydrochlorothiazide combination. The carcinogenic potential of irbesartan and hydrochlorothiazide in combination has not been evaluated in animal studies.

Irbesartan: there was no evidence of abnormal systemic or target organ toxicity at clinically relevant doses. In non-clinical safety studies, high doses of irbesartan (≥ 250 mg/kg/day in rats and ≥ 100 mg/kg/day in macaques) caused a reduction of red blood cell parameters (erythrocytes, haemoglobin, haematocrit). At very high doses (≥ 500 mg/kg/day) degenerative changes in the kidneys (such as interstitial nephritis, tubular distention, basophilic tubules, increased plasma concentrations of urea and creatinine) were induced by irbesartan in the rat and the macaque and are considered secondary to the hypotensive effects of the medicinal product which led to decreased renal perfusion. Furthermore, irbesartan induced hyperplasia/hypertrophy of the juxtaglomerular cells (in rats at ≥ 90 mg/kg/day, in macaques at ≥ 10 mg/kg/day). All of these changes were considered to be caused by the pharmacological action of irbesartan. For therapeutic doses of irbesartan in humans, the hyperplasia/hypertrophy of the renal juxtaglomerular cells does not appear to have any relevance.

There was no evidence of mutagenicity, clastogenicity or carcinogenicity.

Animal studies with irbesartan showed transient toxic effects (increased renal pelvic cavitation, hydroureter or subcutaneous oedema) in rat foetuses, which were resolved after birth. In rabbits, abortion or early resorption was noted at doses causing significant maternal toxicity, including mortality. No teratogenic effects were observed in the rat or rabbit.

Hydrochlorothiazide: although equivocal evidence for a genotoxic or carcinogenic effect was found in some experimental models, the extensive human experience with hydrochlorothiazide has failed to show an association between its use and an increase in neoplasms.

6. PHARMACEUTICAL PARTICULARS

6.1 List of excipients

Tablet core:

Lactose monohydrate

Microcrystalline cellulose

Croscarmellose sodium

Hypromellose (CoAprovel 150/12.5mg and 300/12.5mg only)

Silicon dioxide

Magnesium stearate

(CoAprovel 300 mg/25 mg also contains pregelatinized starch and red and yellow ferric oxides)

Film-coating:

Lactose monohydrate

Hypromellose

Titanium dioxide

Macrogol 3000 (CoAprovel 300 mg/25 mg contains Macrogol 3350 instead of Macrogol 3000)

Red and yellow ferric oxides

Carnauba wax

6.2 Incompatibilities

Not applicable.

6.3 Shelf life

3 years.

6.4 Special precautions for storage

Do not store above 30°C.

Store in the original package in order to protect from moisture.

6.5 Nature and contents of container

Cartons of 28 film-coated tablets; 2 blister cards of 14 film-coated tablets in PVC/PVDC/Aluminium blisters.

6.6 Special precautions for disposal and other handling

Any unused product or waste material should be disposed of in accordance with local requirements.

7. MARKETING AUTHORISATION HOLDER

SANOFI PHARMA BRISTOL-MYERS SQUIBB SNC

174 avenue de France

F-75013 Paris - France

8. MARKETING AUTHORISATION NUMBER(S)

CoAprovel 150/12.5mg film-coated tablets: EU/1/98/086/012

CoAprovel 300/12.5mg film-coated tablets: EU/1/98/086/017

CoAprovel 300/25mg film-coated tablets: EU/1/98/086/024

9. DATE OF FIRST AUTHORISATION/RENEWAL OF THE AUTHORISATION

Date of first authorisation: 15 October 1998

Date of last renewal: 15 October 2008

10. DATE OF REVISION OF THE TEXT

31 March 2009

Detailed information on this product is available on the website of the European Medicines Agency (EMEA) http://www.emea.europa.eu/

Co-danthramer capsules and Strong Co-danthramer capsules

(Napp Pharmaceuticals Limited)

1. NAME OF THE MEDICINAL PRODUCT

Co-danthramer capsules

Strong Co-danthramer capsules

2. QUALITATIVE AND QUANTITATIVE COMPOSITION

Co-danthramer capsules contain Dantron 25 mg and Poloxamer 188 200 mg.

Strong Co-danthramer capsules contain Dantron 37.5 mg and Poloxamer 188 500 mg.

For excipients, see section 6.1.

3. PHARMACEUTICAL FORM

Capsule, hard

Co-danthramer capsules have light brown bodies, opaque orange caps and are marked CX and Napp.

Strong Co-danthramer capsules have light brown bodies, opaque green caps and are marked CXF and Napp.

4. CLINICAL PARTICULARS

4.1 Therapeutic indications

Constipation in terminally ill patients

4.2 Posology and method of administration

Adults

One or two capsules at bedtime.

Children under 12 years of age

Co-danthramer capsules: One capsule at bedtime or as recommended by the physician.

Strong Co-danthramer capsules: Not recommended.

Elderly

As recommended by the physician.

4.3 Contraindications

In common with other gastro-intestinal evacuants, Co-danthramer capsules should not be given when acute or painful conditions of the abdomen are present or when the cause of the constipation is thought to be an intestinal obstruction. Hypersensitivity to any of the constituents of the product. Peanut or soya allergies. Pregnancy and lactation.

4.4 Special warnings and precautions for use

Oral administration of dantron has been reported to cause liver or intestinal tumours in rats and mice. There is no sound evidence to conclude a no effect dose and therefore there may be a risk of such effects in humans.

Co-danthramer use should therefore be restricted to the licensed indications.

In babies, children and patients wearing nappies there may be staining of the buttocks. This may lead to superficial sloughing of the skin. Therefore, Co-danthramer should not be given to infants in nappies and should be used with caution in all incontinent patients.

4.5 Interaction with other medicinal products and other forms of interaction

None stated.

4.6 Pregnancy and lactation

Co-danthramer capsules are contraindicated in pregnant women and nursing mothers.

4.7 Effects on ability to drive and use machines

None stated.

4.8 Undesirable effects

Dantron may cause temporary harmless pink or red colouring of the urine and peri-anal skin. With prolonged high dosage the mucosa of the large intestine may become coloured.

4.9 Overdose

In case of overdosage, patients should be given plenty of fluids. An anti-cholinergic preparation such as atropine sulphate may be given to offset the excessive intestinal motility.

5. PHARMACOLOGICAL PROPERTIES

5.1 Pharmacodynamic properties

Pharmacotherapeutic group: Dantron combinations

ATC code: A06A B53

Co-danthramer owes its laxative action to the mild purgative dantron which is the subject of a monograph in the British Pharmacopeia. This is an anthraquinone derivative chemically related to emodin, the active principle of cascara and other naturally occurring products such as senna, aloes and rhubarb. It acts on the nerve endings of the myenteric plexus and stimulates the muscles of the large intestine.

Poloxamer 188 is a wetting agent which increases the penetration of water into faecal material. The surface activity of the poloxamer has a lubricant effect on the gut contents.

5.2 Pharmacokinetic properties

Like other anthraquinone compounds, dantron is partially absorbed from the small intestine. Because it does not affect the small intestine, griping and cramping do not occur. Dantron begins to act between 6-12 hours after administration.

Poloxamer 188 is not absorbed and is fully recovered in the faeces.

5.3 Preclinical safety data

There are no pre-clinical data of relevance to the prescriber which are additional to that already included in other sections of the SPC.

6. PHARMACEUTICAL PARTICULARS

6.1 List of excipients

Butylhydroxytoluene (E321)

Capsule shell

Gelatin

Erythrosine (E127)

Iron oxide (E172)

Indigo carmine (E132)

Titanium dioxide (E171)

Sodium dodecylsulphate

Printing ink

Opacode S-1-7020 HV white 005

(containing shellac, soya, lecithin, 2-ethoxyethanol, dimethicone, E171))

6.2 Incompatibilities

Not applicable.

6.3 Shelf life

Three years

6.4 Special precautions for storage

Do not store above 30°C.

6.5 Nature and contents of container

Clear or pale yellow blister packs (aluminium foil sealed to 250µm PVC with a PVdC coating of at least 40 gsm thickness), containing 60 capsules.

6.6 Special precautions for disposal and other handling

No special requirements.

7. MARKETING AUTHORISATION HOLDER

Napp Pharmaceuticals Ltd

Cambridge Science Park

Milton Road

Cambridge CB4 0GW

United Kingdom

8. MARKETING AUTHORISATION NUMBER(S)

PL 16950/0017-0018

9. DATE OF FIRST AUTHORISATION/RENEWAL OF THE AUTHORISATION

19 October 1994/9 December 2005

10. DATE OF REVISION OF THE TEXT

25 February 2009

11. Legal category

POM

® The Napp device is a Registered Trade Mark

COLESTID granules for oral suspension

(Pharmacia Limited)

1. NAME OF THE MEDICINAL PRODUCT

Colestid granules for oral suspension 5g

2. QUALITATIVE AND QUANTITATIVE COMPOSITION

Each level scoopful or sachet contains 5.0 grams of Colestipol hydrochloride BP.

For excipients see 6.1

3. PHARMACEUTICAL FORM

Granules for oral suspension.

Light yellow, tasteless and odourless granules.

4. CLINICAL PARTICULARS

4.1 Therapeutic indications

Colestid is indicated as adjunctive therapy to diet in the management of patients with elevated cholesterol levels who have not responded adequately to diet. It may be used alone or in combination with additional lipid lowering agents.

Dietary therapy specific for the type of hypercholesterolaemia should be the initial treatment of choice. Excess body weight may be an important factor and weight reduction should be attempted prior to drug therapy in the overweight. The use of drugs should be considered only when reasonable attempts have been made to obtain satisfactory results with non-drug method. When drug therapy is begun, the patient should be instructed of the importance of adhering to the correct diet.

Although Colestid is effective in all types of hypercholesterolaemia, it is medically most appropriate in patients with Fredrickson's type II hyperlipoproteinaemia.

4.2 Posology and method of administration

Route of administration: Oral, mixed with water or other fluids.

Adults:

The recommended initial daily adult dosage of colestipol hydrochloride is 5 grams either once or twice daily.

For adults colestipol hydrochloride is recommended in doses of 5 - 30 grams taken as one dose or two divided doses. Initiation of therapy is recommended at 5 grams either once or twice daily with 5 gram increments at one month intervals. Appropriate use of lipid profiles including LDL-cholesterol and triglycerides is advised so that optimal, but not excessive doses are used to obtain the desired therapeutic effect on LDL-cholesterol level. If the desired therapeutic effect is not obtained at a dose of 5 - 30 grams/day with good compliance and acceptable side-effects, combined therapy or alternate treatment should be considered.

Patients should take other drugs at least one hour before or four hours after Colestid to minimise possible interference with their absorption. However, Colestid and Gemfibrozil may be used in the same patient when administered 2 hours apart (see Interactions).

Preparation:

Colestid Granules should always be taken mixed in a liquid such as orange or tomato juice, water, skimmed milk or non-carbonated beverage. The contents of the sachet or level scoopful should be added to 100 ml or more of the preferred aqueous vehicle and mixed thoroughly until dispersed. Colestid may also be taken in soups or with cereals, pulpy fruits with a higher water content or yoghurt.

Elderly Patients:

At present there are no extensive clinical studies with colestipol in patients over the age of 65. Review of available data does not suggest that the elderly are more predisposed to side effects attributable to colestipol than the general population; however, therapy should be individualised and based on each patient's clinical characteristics and tolerance to the medication.

Children:

Dosage in children has not been established.

4.3 Contraindications

Colestipol is contra-indicated in individuals who have previously demonstrated hypersensitivity to its use.

4.4 Special warnings and precautions for use

Warnings:

Before instituting therapy with Colestid, diseases contributing to increased blood cholesterol such as hypothyroidism, diabetes mellitus, nephrotic syndrome, dysproteinaemias and obstructive liver disease should be looked for and specifically treated.

To avoid accidental inhalation or oesophageal distress, Colestid should not be taken in its dry form.

Colestid may elevate serum triglyceride levels when used as sole therapy. This elevation is generally transient but may persist in some individuals. A significant rise in triglyceride level should be considered as an indication for dose reduction, drug discontinuation, or combined or alternate therapy.

The use of Colestid in children has been limited; however, it does appear to be effective in lowering serum cholesterol in older children and young adults. Because bile acid sequestrants may interfere with the absorption of fat soluble vitamins, appropriate monitoring of growth and development is essential. Dosage and long term safety in children has not been established.

Precautions:

Because it sequesters bile acids, Colestid may interfere with normal fat absorption and thus may alter absorption of fat soluble vitamins such as A, D, E and K. A study in humans found only one patient in whom a prolonged prothombin time was noted. Most studies did not show a decrease in vitamin A, D or E levels during the administration of Colestid; however, if Colestid is to be given for a long period these vitamin levels should be monitored and supplements given if necessary.

Both clinical usage and animal studies with Colestid have provided no evidence of drug related intestinal neoplasms. Colestid is not mutagenic in the Ames test.

4.5 Interaction with other medicinal products and other forms of interaction

In man, Colestid may delay or reduce the absorption of certain concomitant oral drugs (digitalis and its glycosides, propranolol, chlorothiazide and hydrochlorothiazide, tetracycline hydrochloride, penicillin G, gemfibrozil and furosemide). Particular caution should be taken with digitalis preparations since conflicting results have been obtained for the effect of Colestid on the availability of digoxin and digitoxin. Colestid has been shown not to interfere with the absorption of clindamycin, clofibrate, asparin, tolbutamide, warfarin, methyldopa and phenytoin. The clinical response to concomitant medication should be closely monitored and appropriate adjustments made.

Repeated doses of Colestid given prior to a single dose of propranolol in human trials have been reported to decrease propranolol absorption. However, in a follow-up study in normal subjects, single dose administration of Colestid and propranolol or multiple dose administration of both agents did not affect the extent of propranolol absorption. Effects on the absorption of other beta-blockers have not been determined. Patients on propranolol should be observed when Colestid is either added or deleted from a therapeutic regimen.

4.6 Pregnancy and lactation

Safety for use in pregnant women has not been established. The use of Colestid in pregnancy or lactation or by women of childbearing age requires that the potential benefits of treatment be weighed against the possible hazards to the mother and child.

4.7 Effects on ability to drive and use machines

No adverse effect has been reported.

4.8 Undesirable effects

Side-effects

The most common adverse reactions reported with Colestid have been of a functional gastro-intestinal nature. The most frequent is constipation which is usually mild, transient and responsive to the usual adjunctive measures. At times, constipation can be severe and may be accompanied by impaction. As such, haemorrhoids can be aggravated, and infrequent blood in the stools has been reported. Less frequent gastro-intestinal complaints are abdominal discomfort, belching, flatulence, indigestion, nausea, vomiting and diarrhoea. Rarely, peptic ulceration and bleeding, cholelithiasis and cholecystitis have been reported, although these are not necessarily drug related.

Transient and modest elevation of SGOT and alkaline phosphatase have been observed. No medical significance is attached to these observed changes.

Although not necessarily drug-related, the following non gastro-intestinal medical events have been reported during clinical trials at a similar incidence to placebo.

Cardiovascular: Chest pain, angina and tachycardia have been infrequently reported.

Hypersensitivity: Rash has been infrequently reported. Urticaria and dermatitis have been rarely noted.

Musculoskeletal: Musculoskeletal pain, aches and pains in the extremities, joint pain and arthritis, and backache have been reported.

Neurological: Headache, migraine headache and sinus headache have been reported. Other infrequently reported complaints include dizziness, light-headedness, and insomnia.

Miscellaneous: Anorexia, fatigue, weakness, shortness of breath, and swelling of the hands or feet, have been infrequently reported.

4.9 Overdose

No toxic effects due to overdosage have been reported. Should overdosage occur, obstruction of the gastro-intestinal tract would be expected to occur. Treatment would be determined by the location and degree of obstruction.

5. PHARMACOLOGICAL PROPERTIES

5.1 Pharmacodynamic properties

Ion exchange resin which lowers plasma cholesterol through binding with bile acids in the intestinal lumen.

5.2 Pharmacokinetic properties

Colestid is not absorbed; its action is limited to the lumen of the gastro-intestinal tract, and it is passed in the faeces. It binds bile acids in the intestinal lumen and causes them to be excreted in the faeces together with the polymer. When the enterohepatic circulation of bile acids is interrupted, cholesterol conversion to bile acids is enhanced and plasma cholesterol levels are thereby lowered.

5.3 Preclinical safety data

Both clinical and animal studies with Colestid have provided no evidence of drug related intestinal neospasms. Colestid is not mutagenic in the Ames test.

6. PHARMACEUTICAL PARTICULARS

6.1 List of excipients

Colloidal Anhydrous Silica Ph.Eur

6.2 Incompatibilities

None

6.3 Shelf life

4 years

6.4 Special precautions for storage

None

6.5 Nature and contents of container

Paper/Aluminium foil/vinyl sachets of 5 gm in packs of 30 sachets

6.6 Special precautions for disposal and other handling

None

Administrative Data

7. MARKETING AUTHORISATION HOLDER

Pharmacia Limited

Ramsgate Road

Sandwich

Kent CT13 9NJ

United Kingdom

8. MARKETING AUTHORISATION NUMBER(S)

PL 0032/0055

9. DATE OF FIRST AUTHORISATION/RENEWAL OF THE AUTHORISATION

26 October 1992

10. DATE OF REVISION OF THE TEXT

November 2007

Company Reference: CL4_0

COLESTID Orange

(Pharmacia Limited)

1. NAME OF THE MEDICINAL PRODUCT

Colestid Orange

2. QUALITATIVE AND QUANTITATIVE COMPOSITION

Colestipol Hydrochloride USP 5.0 gram

3. PHARMACEUTICAL FORM

Granules for oral administration.

4. CLINICAL PARTICULARS

4.1 Therapeutic indications

Colestid is indicated as adjunctive therapy to diet in the management of patients with elevated cholesterol levels who have not responded adequately to diet. It may be used alone or in combination with additional lipid lowering agents.

Dietary therapy specific for the type of hypercholesterolaemia should be the initial treatment of choice. Excess body weight may be an important factor and weight reduction should be attempted prior to drug therapy in the overweight. The use of drugs should be considered only when reasonable attempts have been made to obtain satisfactory results with non-drug methods. When drug therapy is begun, the patient should be instructed of the importance of adhering to the correct diet.

Although Colestid is effective in all types of hypercholesterolaemia, it is medically most appropriate in patients with Fredrickson's type II hyperlipoproteinaemia.

4.2 Posology and method of administration

Route of administration: Oral, mixed with water or other fluids.

Adults:

The recommended initial daily adult dosage of colestipol hydrochloride is 5 grams either once or twice daily.

For adults colestipol hydrochloride is recommended in doses of 5-30 grams taken as one dose or two divided doses. Initiation of therapy is recommended at 5 grams either once or twice daily with 5 gram increments at one month intervals. Appropriate use of lipid profiles including LDL-cholesterol and triglycerides is advised so that optimal, but not excessive doses are used to obtain the desired therapeutic effect on LDL-cholesterol level. If the desired therapeutic effect is not obtained at a dose of 5-30 grams/day with good compliance and acceptable side-effects, combined therapy or alternate treatment should be considered.

Patients should take other drugs at least one hour before or four hours after Colestid to minimise possible interference with their absorption. However, Colestid and gemfibrozil may be used in the same patient when administered 2 hours apart. (See interactions).

Preparation:

Colestid should always be taken mixed in a liquid such as orange or tomato juice, water, skimmed milk or non-carbonated beverage. The contents of the sachet or level scoopful should be added to 100 ml or more of the preferred aqueous vehicle and mixed thoroughly until dispersed. Colestid may also be taken in soups or with cereals, pulpy fruits with a high water content or yoghurt.

Elderly patients:

At present there are no extensive clinical studies with colestipol in patients over the age of 65. Review of available data does not suggest that the elderly are more predisposed to side-effects attributable to colestipol than the general population; however, therapy should be individualised and based on each patient's clinical characteristics and tolerance to the medication.

Children:

Dosage in children has not been established.

4.3 Contraindications

Colestipol is contra-indicated in individuals who have previously demonstrated hypersensitivity to its use.

4.4 Special warnings and precautions for use

Warnings:

Before instituting therapy with Colestid, diseases contributing to increased blood cholesterol such as hypothyroidism, diabetes mellitus, nephrotic syndrome, dysproteinaemias and obstructive liver diseases should be looked for and specifically treated.

To avoid accidental inhalation or oesophageal distress, Colestid should not be taken in its dry form.

Colestid Orange contains 0.0325 g aspartame per sachet or level scoopful. This should be taken into consideration in patients suffering from phenylketonuria since excessive amounts of aspartame may interfere with the control of this condition.

Colestid may elevate serum triglyceride levels when used as sole therapy. This elevation is generally transient but may persist in some individuals. A significant rise in triglyceride level should be considered as an indication for dose reduction, drug discontinuation, or combined or alternate therapy.

The use of Colestid in children has been limited; however, it does appear to be effective in lowering serum cholesterol in older children and young adults. Because bile acid sequestrants may interfere with the absorption of fat-soluble vitamins, appropriate monitoring of growth and development is essential. Dosage and long term safety in children have not been established.

Precautions:

Because it sequesters bile acids, Colestid may interfere with normal fat absorption and thus may alter absorption of fat soluble vitamins such as A, D, E and K. A study in humans found only one patient in whom a prolonged prothombin time was noted. Most studies did not show a decrease in vitamin A, D or E levels during the administration of Colestid; however, if Colestid is to be given for a long period these vitamin levels should be monitored and supplements given if necessary.

4.5 Interaction with other medicinal products and other forms of interaction

In man, Colestid may delay or reduce the absorption of certain concomitant oral drugs (digitalis and its glycosides, propranolol, chlorothiazide and hydrochlorothiazide, tetracycline hydrochloride, penicillin G, gemfibrozil and furosemide). Particular caution should be taken with digitalis preparations since conflicting results have been obtained for the effect of Colestid on the availability of digoxin and digitoxin. Colestid has been shown not to interfere with the absorption of clindamycin, clofibrate, aspirin, tolbutamide, warfarin, methyldopa and phenytoin. The clinical response to concomitant medication should be closely monitored and appropriate adjustments made.

Repeated doses of Colestid given prior to a single dose of propranolol in human trials have been reported to decrease propranolol absorption. However, in a follow-up study in normal subjects, single dose administration of Colestid and propranolol or multiple dose administration of both agents did not affect the extent of propranolol absorption. Effects on the absorption of other beta-blockers have not been determined. Patients on propranolol should be observed when Colestid is either added or deleted from a therapeutic regimen.

4.6 Pregnancy and lactation

Safety for use in pregnant women has not been established. The use of Colestid in pregnancy or lactation or by women of childbearing age requires that the potential benefits of treatment be weighed against the possible hazards to the mother and child.

4.7 Effects on ability to drive and use machines

No adverse effect has been reported.

4.8 Undesirable effects

Side-effects:

The most common adverse reactions reported with Colestid have been of a functional gastro-intestinal nature. The most frequent is constipation which is usually mild, transient and responsive to the usual adjunctive measures. At times, constipation can be severe and may be accompanied by impaction. As such, haemorrhoids can be aggravated, and infrequent blood in the stools has been reported. Less frequent gastro-intestinal complaints are abdominal discomfort, belching, flatulence, indigestion, nausea, vomiting and diarrhoea. Rarely, peptic ulceration and bleeding, cholelithiasis and cholecystitis have been reported, although these are not necessarily drug related.

Transient and modest elevation of SGOT and alkaline phosphatase have been observed. No medical significance is attached to these observed changes.

Although not necessarily drug-related, the following non-gastro-intestinal medical events have been reported during clinical trials at a similar incidence to placebo.

Cardiovascular: Chest pain, angina, and tachycardia have been infrequently reported.

Hypersensitivity: Rash has been infrequently reported. Urticaria and dermatitis have been rarely noted.

Musculoskeletal: Musculoskeletal pain, aches and pains in the extremities, joint pain and arthritis, and backache have been reported.

Neurological: Headache, migraine headache and sinus headache have been reported. Other infrequently reported complaints include dizziness, light-headedness, and insomnia.

Miscellaneous: Anorexia, fatigue, weakness, shortness of breath, and swelling of the hands or feet, have been infrequently reported.

4.9 Overdose

No toxic effects due to overdosage have been reported. Should overdosage occur, obstruction of the gastro-intestinal tract would be expected to occur. Treatment should be determined by the location and degree of obstruction.

5. PHARMACOLOGICAL PROPERTIES

5.1 Pharmacodynamic properties

Ion exchange resin which lowers plasma cholesterol through binding with bile acids in the intestinal lumen.

5.2 Pharmacokinetic properties

Colestid is not absorbed; its action is limited to the lumen of the gastro-intestinal tract, and it is passed in the faeces. It binds bile acids in the intestinal lumen and causes them to be excreted in the faeces together with the polymer. When the enterohepatic circulation of bile acids is interrupted, cholesterol conversion to bile acids is enhanced and plasma cholesterol levels are thereby lowered.

5.3 Preclinical safety data

Both clinical usage and animal studies with Colestid have provided no evidence of drug related intestinal neoplasms. Colestid is not mutagenic in the ames test.

6. PHARMACEUTICAL PARTICULARS

6.1 List of excipients

Mannitol Ph. Eur.

Methylcellulose (15CPS) Ph. Eur.

Citric Acid Ph. Eur.

Orange Durarome Wonf HSE

Aspartame Powder NF

Maltol HSE

Ethyl Vanillin NF

Beta Carotene 1% HSE

Glycerol Ph. Eur.

Purified Water Ph. Eur.

6.2 Incompatibilities

None.

6.3 Shelf life

24 months.

6.4 Special precautions for storage

Store at controlled room temperature (15-30°C).

6.5 Nature and contents of container

Foil sachets in packs 30 sachets.

6.6 Special precautions for disposal and other handling

None.

7. MARKETING AUTHORISATION HOLDER

Pharmacia Limited

Ramsgate Road

Sandwich

Kent CT13 9NJ

United Kingdom

8. MARKETING AUTHORISATION NUMBER(S)

PL 0032/0172

9. DATE OF FIRST AUTHORISATION/RENEWAL OF THE AUTHORISATION

Date of Grant: 25 February 1992

Date of Renewal: 30 Oct 2002

10. DATE OF REVISION OF THE TEXT

22 June 2007

Legal Category POM

Company Reference: CL3_0

Colofac MR

(Solvay Healthcare Limited)

1. NAME OF THE MEDICINAL PRODUCT

Colofac® MR. Modified release capsule.

2. QUALITATIVE AND QUANTITATIVE COMPOSITION

Mebeverine hydrochloride 200 mg.

For excipients, see section 6.1

3. PHARMACEUTICAL FORM

Modified release capsule.

White, opaque, modified release capsule imprinted '$ 245'

4. CLINICAL PARTICULARS

4.1 Therapeutic indications

For the symptomatic relief of irritable bowel syndrome.

4.2 Posology and method of administration

Adults (including the elderly): One capsule twice a day, preferably 20 minutes before meals.

Children: Not recommended.

4.3 Contraindications

Paralytic ileus.

Hypersensitivity to any of the components of the product.

4.4 Special warnings and precautions for use

Porphyria.

4.5 Interaction with other medicinal products and other forms of interaction

None known.

4.6 Pregnancy and lactation

Pregnancy: Animal experiments have failed to show any teratogenic effects. However, the usual precautions concerning the administration of any drug during pregnancy should be observed.

Lactation: Mebeverine is excreted in milk of lactating women after therapeutic doses.

4.7 Effects on ability to drive and use machines

None.

4.8 Undesirable effects

In very rare cases allergic reactions have been reported, in particular erythematous rash, urticaria and angioedema.

4.9 Overdose

On theoretical grounds it may be predicted that CNS excitability will occur in cases of overdosage. No specific antidote is known; gastric lavage and symptomatic treatment is recommended.

5. PHARMACOLOGICAL PROPERTIES

5.1 Pharmacodynamic properties

Mebeverine is a musculotropic antispasmodic with a direct action on the smooth muscle of the gastrointestinal tract, relieving spasm without affecting normal gut motility.

5.2 Pharmacokinetic properties

Mebeverine is rapidly and completely absorbed after oral administration in the form of tablets or suspension. Mebeverine is not excreted as such, but metabolised completely. The first step in the metabolism is hydrolysis, leading to veratric acid and mebeverine alcohol. Both veratric acid and mebeverine alcohol are excreted into the urine, the latter partly as the corresponding carboxylic acid and partly as the demethylated carboxylic acid.

5.3 Preclinical safety data

None

6. PHARMACEUTICAL PARTICULARS

6.1 List of excipients

Modified release granules:

Magnesium stearate

Copolymer of ethyl acrylate and methyl methacrylate

Talc

Hypromellose

Methacrylic acid-ethyl acrylate copolymer (1:1)

Glycerol triacetate

Capsule shell:

Gelatine

Titanium dioxide (E171)

Printing inks:

Shellac (E904)

Black iron oxide (E172)

Soya lecithin (E322)

Antifoam DC

6.2 Incompatibilities

Not applicable.

6.3 Shelf life

3 years when stored in the original container.

6.4 Special precautions for storage

Do not store above 30°C.

Do not refrigerate or freeze.

Store in the original package.

6.5 Nature and contents of container

Boxes containing 10 or 60 capsules in PVC-Al press through strips.

6.6 Special precautions for disposal and other handling

None.

7. MARKETING AUTHORISATION HOLDER

Solvay Healthcare Limited

Mansbridge Road

West End

Southampton

SO18 3JD

8. MARKETING AUTHORISATION NUMBER(S)

PL 00512/0155

9. DATE OF FIRST AUTHORISATION/RENEWAL OF THE AUTHORISATION

14 August 1998/August 2003

10. DATE OF REVISION OF THE TEXT

April 2003

Legal Category

POM

Colofac Tablets 135mg

(Solvay Healthcare Limited)

1. NAME OF THE MEDICINAL PRODUCT

Colofac Tablets 135 mg

Mebeverine Tablets 135mg

Fomac Tablets 135 mg

Colofac IBS

Boots Pharmacy IBS Relief 135mg Tablets

2. QUALITATIVE AND QUANTITATIVE COMPOSITION

Mebeverine hydrochloride 135mg.

For excipients, see section 6.1

3. PHARMACEUTICAL FORM

Coated tablets.

Round white sugar coated tablets, with no superficial markings.

4. CLINICAL PARTICULARS

4.1 Therapeutic indications

Colofac Tablets/Mebeverine Tablets 135 mg/Fomac Tablets 135mg:

For the symptomatic treatment of irritable bowel syndrome and other conditions usually included in this grouping, such as: chronic irritable colon, spastic constipation, mucous colitis, spastic colitis. Colofac is effectively used to treat the symptoms of these conditions, such as: colicky abdominal pain and cramps, persistent, non-specific diarrhoea (with or without alternating constipation) and flatulence.

Colofac IBS/ Boots Pharmacy IBS Relief 135mg Tablets:

For the symptomatic relief of Irritable Bowel Syndrome.

4.2 Posology and method of administration

Colofac Tablets/Mebeverine Tablets 135 mg/Fomac Tablets 135mg:

Adults (including the elderly) and children 10 years and over:

One tablet three times a day, preferably 20 minutes before meals. After a period of several weeks, when the desired effect has been obtained, the dosage may be gradually reduced.

Children under 10 years: Not applicable.

Colofac IBS/ Boots Pharmacy IBS Relief 135mg Tablets:

Adults (including the elderly) and children 10 years and over:

One tablet three times a day, preferably 20 minutes before meals.

If symptoms persist for more than 2 weeks, consult your doctor.

Warning: Do not exceed the stated dose.

Children under 10 years: Not applicable.

4.3 Contraindications

Hypersensitivity to any component of the product.

4.4 Special warnings and precautions for use

Colofac Tablets/Mebeverine Tablets 135 mg/Fomac 135 mg:

None.

Colofac IBS / Boots Pharmacy IBS Relief 135mg Tablets:

If this is the first time you have had these symptoms, consult your doctor before using any treatment.

If any of the following apply, do not use mebeverine. It may not be the right treatment for you. See your doctor as soon as possible.

- you are aged 40 years or over
- you have passed blood form the bowel
- you are feeling sick or vomiting
- you are looking pale and feeling tired
- you are suffering from severe constipation
- you have a fever
- you have recently travelled abroad
- you are or may be pregnant

- you have abnormal vaginal bleeding or discharge
- you have difficulty or pain passing urine

Consult your doctor if you have developed new symptoms, or if your symptoms worsen, or if they do not improve after 2 weeks treatment.

4.5 Interaction with other medicinal products and other forms of interaction
None known.

4.6 Pregnancy and lactation
Animal experiments have failed to show any teratogenic effects. However, the usual precautions concerning the administration of any drug during pregnancy should be observed.

4.7 Effects on ability to drive and use machines
None.

4.8 Undesirable effects
In very rare cases allergic reactions have been reported, in particular erythematous rash, urticaria and angioedema.

4.9 Overdose
On theoretical grounds it may be predicted that CNS excitability will occur in cases of overdosage. No specific antidote is known; gastric lavage and symptomatic treatment is recommended.

5. PHARMACOLOGICAL PROPERTIES

5.1 Pharmacodynamic properties
Mebeverine is a musculotropic antispasmodic with a direct action on the smooth muscle of the gastrointestinal tract, relieving spasm without affecting normal gut motility.

5.2 Pharmacokinetic properties
Mebeverine is rapidly and completely absorbed after oral administration in the form of tablets or suspension. Mebeverine is not excreted as such, but metabolised completely. The first step in the metabolism is hydrolysis, leading to veratric acid and mebeverine alcohol. Both veratric acid and mebeverine alcohol are excreted into the urine, the latter partly as the corresponding carboxylic acid and partly as the demethylated carboxylic acid.

5.3 Preclinical safety data
Not applicable.

6. PHARMACEUTICAL PARTICULARS

6.1 List of excipients
Lactose, starch (potato or maize), povidone, talc, magnesium stearate, sucrose, gelatin, acacia, carnauba wax.

6.2 Incompatibilities
Not applicable.

6.3 Shelf life
5 years.

6.4 Special precautions for storage
Do not store above 30°C. Store in the original package.

6.5 Nature and contents of container
Boxes containing 10, 15, 84 or 100 tablets in blister strips. HDPE tamper-evident tablet container with snap on cap containing 500 tablets.

6.6 Special precautions for disposal and other handling
None.

7. MARKETING AUTHORISATION HOLDER
Solvay Healthcare Limited/Solvay Healthcare Limited trading as Mansbridge Pharmaceuticals and Boots Pharmacy
Mansbridge Road
West End
Southampton
SO18 3JD

8. MARKETING AUTHORISATION NUMBER(S)
PL 00512/0044

9. DATE OF FIRST AUTHORISATION/RENEWAL OF THE AUTHORISATION
14 March 1978/21 April 2005

10. DATE OF REVISION OF THE TEXT
May 2006

LEGAL STATUS
Colofac Tablets/ Mebeverine Tablets 135 mg/Fomac 135 mg: POM
Colofac IBS/ Boots Pharmacy IBS Relief 135mg Tablets: P

Colomycin Injection

(Forest Laboratories UK Limited)

1. NAME OF THE MEDICINAL PRODUCT
COLOMYCIN INJECTION 1 million or 2 million International Units.

Powder for solution for injection, infusion or inhalation.

2. QUALITATIVE AND QUANTITATIVE COMPOSITION
Each vial contains either 1 million or 2 million International Units Colistimethate Sodium.

For excipients, see 6.1

3. PHARMACEUTICAL FORM
Powder for solution for injection, infusion or inhalation.

1 million IU/vial: Sterile white powder in a 10ml colourless glass vial with a red 'flip-off' cap.

2 million IU/vial: Sterile white powder in a 10ml colourless glass vial with a lilac 'flip-off' cap.

4. CLINICAL PARTICULARS

4.1 Therapeutic indications
Colomycin is indicated in the treatment of the following infections where sensitivity testing suggests that they are caused by susceptible bacteria:

Treatment by inhalation of *Pseudomonas aeruginosa* lung infection in patients with cystic fibrosis (CF).

Intravenous administration for the treatment of some serious infections caused by Gram-negative bacteria, including those of the lower respiratory tract and urinary tract, when more commonly used systemic antibacterial agents may be contra-indicated or may be ineffective because of bacterial resistance.

4.2 Posology and method of administration
SYSTEMIC TREATMENT

Colomycin can be given as a 50ml intravenous infusion over a period of 30 minutes. Patients with a totally implantable venous access device (TIVAD) in place may tolerate a bolus injection of up to 2 million units in 10ml given over a minimum of 5 minutes (see section 6.6).

The dose is determined by the severity and type of infection and the age, weight and renal function of the patient. Should clinical or bacteriological response be slow the dose may be increased as indicated by the patient's condition.

Serum level estimations are recommended especially in renal impairment, neonates and cystic fibrosis patients. Levels of 10–15 mg/l (approximately 125-200 units/ml) colistimethate sodium should be adequate for most infections.

A minimum of 5 days treatment is generally recommended. For the treatment of respiratory exacerbations in cystic fibrosis patients, treatment should be continued for up to 12 days.

Children and adults (including the elderly):

Up to 60kg: 50,000 units/kg/day to a maximum of 75,000 units/kg/day. The total daily dose should be divided into three doses given at approximately 8-hour intervals.

Over 60kg: 1-2 million units three times a day. The maximum dose is 6 million units in 24 hours.

Anomalous distribution in patients with cystic fibrosis may require higher doses in order to maintain therapeutic serum levels.

Renal impairment: In moderate to severe renal impairment, excretion of colistimethate sodium is delayed. Therefore, the dose and dose interval should be adjusted in order to prevent accumulation. The table below is a guide to dose regimen modifications in patients of 60kg bodyweight or greater. It is emphasised that further adjustments may have to be made based on blood levels and evidence of toxicity.

SUGGESTED DOSAGE ADJUSTMENT IN RENAL IMPAIRMENT

Grade	Creatinine clearance (ml/min)	Over 60kg bodyweight
Mild	20-50	1-2 million units every 8hr
Moderate	10-20	1 million units every 12-18 hr
Severe	<10	1 million units every 18-24 hr

AEROSOL INHALATION

For local treatment of lower respiratory tract infections Colomycin powder is dissolved in 2-4 ml of water for injections or 0.9% sodium chloride intravenous infusion for use in a nebuliser attached to an air/oxygen supply (see section 6.6).

In small, uncontrolled clinical trials, doses of from 500,000 units twice daily up to 2 million units three times daily have been found to be safe and effective in patients with cystic fibrosis.

The following recommended doses are for guidance only and should be adjusted according to clinical response:

Children <2 years: 500,000-1 million units twice daily

Children >2 years and adults: 1-2 million units twice daily

4.3 Contraindications
Hypersensitivity to colistimethate sodium (colistin) or to polymyxin B.

Patients with myasthenia gravis.

4.4 Special warnings and precautions for use
Use with extreme caution in patients with porphyria.

Nephrotoxicity or neurotoxicity may occur if the recommended parenteral dose is exceeded.

Use with caution in renal impairment (see Section 4.2 - Posology and method of administration). It is advisable to assess baseline renal function and to monitor during treatment. Serum colistimethate sodium concentrations should be monitored.

Bronchospasm may occur on inhalation of antibiotics. This may be prevented or treated with appropriate use of beta$_2$-agonists. If troublesome, treatment should be withdrawn.

4.5 Interaction with other medicinal products and other forms of interaction
Concomitant use of colistimethate sodium with other medicinal products of neurotoxic and/or nephrotoxic potential should be avoided. These include the aminoglycoside antibiotics such as gentamicin, amikacin, netilmicin and tobramycin. There may be an increased risk of nephrotoxicity if given concomitantly with cephalosporin antibiotics.

Neuromuscular blocking drugs and ether should be used with extreme caution in patients receiving colistimethate sodium.

4.6 Pregnancy and lactation
There are no adequate data from the use of colistimethate sodium in pregnant women. Single dose studies in human pregnancy show that colistimethate sodium crosses the placental barrier and there may be a risk of foetal toxicity if repeated doses are given to pregnant patients. Animal studies are insufficient with respect to the effect of colistimethate sodium on reproduction and development (see Section 5.3 – Preclinical safety data). Colistimethate sodium should be used in pregnancy only if the benefit to the mother outweighs the potential risk to the fetus.

Colistimethate sodium is secreted in breast milk. Colistimethate sodium should be administered to breastfeeding women only when clearly needed.

4.7 Effects on ability to drive and use machines
During parenteral treatment with colistimethate sodium neurotoxicity may occur with the possibility of dizziness, confusion or visual disturbance. Patients should be warned not to drive or operate machinery if these effects occur.

4.8 Undesirable effects
Systemic treatment

The likelihood of adverse events may be related to the age, renal function and condition of the patient.

In cystic fibrosis patients neurological events have been reported in up to 27% of patients. These are generally mild and resolve during or shortly after treatment.

Neurotoxicity may be associated with overdose, failure to reduce the dose in patients with renal insufficiency and concomitant use of either neuromuscular blocking drugs or other drugs with similar neurological effects. Reducing the dose may alleviate symptoms. Effects may include apnoea, transient sensory disturbances (such as facial paraesthesia and vertigo) and, rarely, vasomotor instability, slurred speech, visual disturbances, confusion or psychosis.

Adverse effects on renal function have been reported, usually following use of higher than recommended doses in patients with normal renal function, or failure to reduce the dosage in patients with renal impairment or during concomitant use of other nephrotoxic drugs. The effects are usually reversible on discontinuation of therapy.

In cystic fibrosis patients treated within the recommended dosage limits, nephrotoxicity appears to be rare (less than 1%). In seriously ill hospitalised non-CF patients, signs of nephrotoxicity have been reported in approximately 20% of patients.

Hypersensitivity reactions including skin rash and drug fever have been reported. If these occur treatment should be withdrawn.

Local irritation at the site of injection may occur.

Inhalation treatment

Inhalation may induce coughing or bronchospasm.

Sore throat or mouth has been reported and may be due to *Candida albicans* infection or hypersensitivity. Skin rash may also indicate hypersensitivity, if this occurs treatment should be withdrawn.

4.9 Overdose
Overdose can result in neuromuscular blockade that can lead to muscular weakness, apnoea and possible respiratory arrest. Overdose can also cause acute renal failure characterised by decreased urine output and increased serum concentrations of BUN and creatinine.

There is no specific antidote, manage by supportive treatment. Measures to increase the rate of elimination of colistin e.g. mannitol diuresis, prolonged haemodialysis or peritoneal dialysis may be tried, but effectiveness is unknown.

5. PHARMACOLOGICAL PROPERTIES

5.1 Pharmacodynamic properties
Pharmacotherapeutic group: Antibacterials for systemic use.

ATC Code: JOIX B01

Mode of action

Colistimethate sodium is a cyclic polypeptide antibiotic derived from *Bacillus polymyxa var. colistinus* and belongs to the polymyxin group. The polymyxin antibiotics are cationic agents that work by damaging the cell membrane. The resulting physiological affects are lethal to the bacterium. Polymyxins are selective for Gram-negative bacteria that have a hydrophobic outer membrane.

Resistance

Resistant bacteria are characterised by modification of the phosphate groups of lipopolysaccharide that become substituted with ethanolamine or aminoarabinose. Naturally resistant Gram-negative bacteria, such as *Proteus mirabilis* and *Burkholderia cepacia*, show complete substitution of their lipid phosphate by ethanolamine or aminoarabinose.

Cross resistance

Cross resistance between colistimethate sodium and polymyxin B would be expected. Since the mechanism of action of the polymyxins is different from that of other antibiotics, resistance to colistin and polymixin by the above mechanism alone would not be expected to result in resistance to other drug classes.

Breakpoints

The suggested general MIC breakpoint to identify bacteria susceptible to colistimethate sodium is $\leq$ 4mg/l.

Bacteria for which the MIC of colistimethate sodium is $\geq$ 8mg/l should be considered resistant.

Susceptibility

The prevalence of acquired resistance may vary geographically and with time for selected species and local information on resistance is desirable, particularly when treating severe infections. As necessary, expert advice should be sought when the local prevalence of resistance is such that the utility of the agent in at least some types of infections is questionable.

Commonly susceptible species
Acinetobacter species*
Citrobacter species
Escherichia coli
Haemophilus influenzae
Pseudomonas aeruginosa
Species for which acquired resistance may be a problem
Enterobacter species
Klebsiella species
Inherently resistant organisms
Brucella species
Burkholderia cepacia and related species.
Neisseria species
Proteus species
Providencia species
Serratia species
Anaerobes
All Gram positive organisms

*In-vitro results may not correlate with clinical responses in the case of Acinetobacter spp.

5.2 Pharmacokinetic properties

Absorption

Absorption from the gastrointestinal tract does not occur to any appreciable extent in the normal individual.

When given by nebulisation, variable absorption has been reported that may depend on the aerosol particle size, nebuliser system and lung status. Studies in healthy volunteers and patients with various infections have reported serum levels from nil to potentially therapeutic concentrations of 4mg/l or more. Therefore, the possibility of systemic absorption should always be borne in mind when treating patients by inhalation.

Distribution

After the administration to patients with cystic fibrosis of 7.5 mg/kg/day in divided doses given as 30-min intravenous infusions to steady state the C max was determined to be 23$\pm$6 mg/l and C min at 8 h was 4.5$\pm$4 mg/l. In another study in similar patients given 2 million units every 8 hours for 12 days the C max was 12.9 mg/l (5.7 – 29.6 mg/l) and the C min was 2.76 mg/l (1.0 – 6.2 mg/l). In healthy volunteers given a bolus injection of 150mg (2 million units approx.) peak serum levels of 18 mg/l were observed 10 minutes after injection.

Protein binding is low. Polymyxins persist in the liver, kidney, brain, heart and muscle. One study in cystic fibrosis patients gives the steady-state volume of distribution as 0.09 L/kg.

Biotransformation

Colistimethate sodium is converted to the base *in vivo*. As 80% of the dose can be recovered unchanged in the urine, and there is no biliary excretion, it can be assumed that the remaining drug is inactivated in the tissues. The mechanism is unknown.

Elimination

The main route of elimination after parenteral administration is by renal excretion with 40% of a parenteral dose recovered in the urine within 8 hours and around 80% in 24 hours. Because colistimethate sodium is largely excreted in the urine, dose reduction is required in renal impairment to prevent accumulation. Refer to the table in Section 4.2.

After intravenous administration to healthy adults the elimination half-life is around 1.5 hrs. In a study in cystic fibrosis patients given a single 30-minute intravenous infusion the elimination half-life was 3.4 $\pm$ 1.4 hrs.

The elimination of colistimethate sodium following inhalation has not been studied. A study in cystic fibrosis patients failed to detect any colistimethate sodium in the urine after 1 million units were inhaled twice daily for 3 months.

Colistimethate sodium kinetics appear to be similar in children and adults, including the elderly, provided renal function is normal. Limited data are available on use in neonates which suggest kinetics are similar to children and adults but the possibility of higher peak serum levels and prolonged half-life in these patients should be considered and serum levels monitored.

5.3 Preclinical safety data

Data on potential genotoxicity are limited and carcinogenicity data for colistimethate sodium are lacking. Colistimethate sodium has been shown to induce chromosomal aberrations in human lymphocytes, in vitro. This effect may be related to a reduction in mitotic index, which was also observed.

Reproductive toxicity studies in rats and mice do not indicate teratogenic properties. However, colistimethate sodium given intramuscularly during organogenesis to rabbits at 4.15 and 9.3 mg/kg resulted in talipes varus in 2.6 and 2.9% of fetuses respectively. These doses are 0.5 and 1.2 times the maximum daily human dose. In addition, increased resorption occurred at 9.3 mg/kg.

There are no other preclinical safety data of relevance to the prescriber which are additional to safety data derived from patient exposure and already included in other sections of the SPC.

6. PHARMACEUTICAL PARTICULARS

6.1 List of excipients

None

6.2 Incompatibilities

Mixed infusions, injections and nebuliser solutions involving colistimethate sodium should be avoided.

6.3 Shelf life

Before opening: 3 years

Reconstituted solutions: Solutions for infusion or injection:

Chemical and physical in-use stability for 28 days at 4°C has been demonstrated.

From a microbiological point of view, solutions should be used immediately. If not used immediately in-use storage times and conditions prior to use are the responsibility of the user. They would normally be no longer than 24 hours at 2 to 8°C, unless reconstituted and diluted under controlled and validated aseptic conditions.

Solutions for nebulisation:

Solutions for nebulisation have similar in-use stability and should be treated as above. Patients self-treating with nebulised antibiotic should be advised to use solutions immediately after preparation. If this is not possible, solutions should not be stored for longer than 24hrs in a refrigerator.

6.4 Special precautions for storage

Do not store above 25°C. Keep the vials in the outer carton.

For storage of solutions following reconstitution refer to 6.3.

6.5 Nature and contents of container

1 million IU/vial: Type 1 glass vial with a red 'flip-off' cap supplied in cartons of ten vials.

2 million IU/vial: Type 1 glass vial with a lilac 'flip-off' cap supplied in cartons of ten vials.

6.6 Special precautions for disposal and other handling

Parenteral administration

The normal adult dose of 2 million units should be dissolved in 10-50ml of 0.9% sodium chloride intravenous infusion or water for injections to form a clear solution. The solution is for single use only and any remaining solution should be discarded.

Inhalation

The required amount of powder is dissolved preferably in 2-4ml 0.9% sodium chloride solution and poured into the nebuliser. Alternatively, water for injections may be used. The solution will be slightly hazy and may froth if shaken. Usually jet or ultrasonic nebulisers are preferred for antibiotic delivery. These should produce the majority of their output in the respirable particle diameter range of 0.5-5.0 microns when used with a suitable compressor. The instructions of the manufacturers should be followed for the operation and care of the nebuliser and compressor.

The output from the nebuliser may be vented to the open air or a filter may be fitted. Nebulisation should take place in a well ventilated room.

The solution is for single use only and any remaining solution should be discarded.

7. MARKETING AUTHORISATION HOLDER

Forest Laboratories UK Limited

Bourne Road

Bexley

Kent DA5 1NX

U.K.

8. MARKETING AUTHORISATION NUMBER(S)

1 million IU/vial: PL 0108/5006R

2 million IU/vial: PL 0108/0122

9. DATE OF FIRST AUTHORISATION/RENEWAL OF THE AUTHORISATION

1 million IU/vial: June 1986 / November 2006

2 million IU/vial: June 2003 / November 2006

10. DATE OF REVISION OF THE TEXT

July 2009

11. LEGAL CATEGORY

POM

Colomycin Syrup

(Forest Laboratories UK Limited)

1. NAME OF THE MEDICINAL PRODUCT

COLOMYCIN SYRUP

2. QUALITATIVE AND QUANTITATIVE COMPOSITION

Each bottle contains 4,000,000 units Colistin Sulphate, equivalent to 250,000 units/5ml when dispensed.

3. PHARMACEUTICAL FORM

Powder for syrup

4. CLINICAL PARTICULARS

4.1 Therapeutic indications

For the treatment of gastrointestinal infections caused by sensitive Gram negative organisms. Also for bowel preparation.

Colistin sulphate is not absorbed from the gastrointestinal tract except in infants under the age of 6 months, and must not be given orally for the treatment of systemic infections in any age group.

4.2 Posology and method of administration

After reconstitution, the following doses are taken orally:

Adults over 30kg (including the elderly):

1,500,000 to 3,000,000 units every 8 hours.

Colomycin Tablets may be more suitable for adults.

Children (up to 15kg):

250,000 to 500,000 units (i.e. 5-10ml syrup) every 8 hours.

Children (15-30kg):

750,000 to 1,500,000 units (i.e. 15-30ml syrup) every 8 hours.

A minimum of 5 days treatment is recommended. Dosage may be increased when clinical or bacteriological response is slow. For bowel preparation, a 24 hour course at the normal dosage above is given. Treatment should preferably finish 12 hours before surgery.

4.3 Contraindications

The preparation is contra-indicated in patients with known sensitivity to colistin and those with myasthenia gravis.

4.4 Special warnings and precautions for use

Colistin is subject to limited and unpredictable absorption from the gastrointestinal tract in infants under six months. Studies in older children and in adults have demonstrated no systemic absorption of colistin following oral administration.

Nevertheless, caution should be employed in the use of the preparation in patients with renal failure and in patients receiving curari-form muscle relaxants and patients with porphyria.

4.5 Interaction with other medicinal products and other forms of interaction

Neurotoxicity has been reported in association with the concomitant use of either curari-form agents or antibiotics with similar neurotoxic effects. Therapy need not be discontinued and reduction of dosage may alleviate symptoms.

4.6 Pregnancy and lactation

Safety in human pregnancy has not been established. Animal studies do not indicate teratogenic properties; however, parenteral single dose studies in human pregnancy show that Colomycin crosses the placental barrier and there is a risk of foetal toxicity if repeated doses are given to pregnant patients. Colomycin should only be used in pregnancy if the potential benefit justifies the potential risk.

Colomycin is secreted in breast milk and patients to whom the drug is administered should not breast-feed an infant.

4.7 Effects on ability to drive and use machines

No specific warnings

4.8 Undesirable effects

No significant systemic absorption has been found to occur in older children and adults following oral administration nor have any systemic side effects been reported.

However, since the use of colistin may be associated with unpredictable, albeit limited, absorption in infants under 6 months, the potential adverse effects of systemic administration should be noted for this patient population. These adverse effects may include transient sensory disturbances such as perioral paraesthesia and vertigo.

Neurotoxicity and adverse effects on renal function have been reported in association with systemic over-dosage, failure to reduce dosage in patients with renal insufficiency and the concomitant use of either curariform agents or antibiotics with similar neurotoxic effects.

Therapy need not be discontinued and reduction of dosage may alleviate symptoms. Permanent nerve damage such as deafness or vestibular damage has not been reported.

4.9 Overdose

No symptoms of overdosage have been reported following oral use of colistin. However, following systemic administration overdosage can result in renal insufficiency, muscle weakness and apnoea and this should be borne in mind in the oral therapy of infants under 6 months old (see 'Undesirable effects' above).

There is no specific antidote. Manage by supportive treatment and measures to increase the rate of elimination of colistin, e.g. mannitol diuresis, prolonged haemodialysis or peritoneal dialysis.

5. PHARMACOLOGICAL PROPERTIES

5.1 Pharmacodynamic properties

Colistin is a polymyxin antibiotic derived from Bacillus polymyxa var. colistinus. It has a bactericidal action on most Gram negative bacilli, including Pseudomonas aeruginosa, and use is largely free from the development or transference of resistance. It is not recommended for Proteus spp.

5.2 Pharmacokinetic properties

In adults and older children, colistin sulphate taken orally is not absorbed from the G.I. tract. However, in small infants less than 6 months old, some very limited and unpredictable absorption may occur.

Following oral administration of colistin sulphate, excretion is through faecal matter in both children and adults. Assuming minimal absorption in the intestine, only 1 to 10% of colistin is found in faeces, to that estimated from the dose administered and stool volume. Colistin faecal levels in man average 128μg/g when daily oral doses of 5-20mg/kg are administered (1mg colistin sulphate contains approx. 19,500 units).

Control studies have indicated that colistin is bound by the stool. When greater concentrations of colistin were assayed, significantly less activity, percentage-wise, was lost. This suggests that the 'binding sites' in the stool were saturated.

5.3 Preclinical safety data

There are no preclinical data of relevance to the prescriber that might add to the safety data provided in other sections of this SPC.

6. PHARMACEUTICAL PARTICULARS

6.1 List of excipients

Sucrose

Sodium Citrate

Benzoic Acid

Sodium Methylhydroxybenzoate (E219)

6.2 Incompatibilities

None stated

6.3 Shelf life

Three years

6.4 Special precautions for storage

Do not store above 25°C. Store in a dry place, protected from light.

6.5 Nature and contents of container

Colomycin Syrup powder is presented in a 4oz amber glass Winchester bottle fitted with a white polypropylene cap.

6.6 Special precautions for disposal and other handling

Colomycin Syrup powder is reconstituted by adding 58ml of water, and shaking the bottle until the powder is dissolved.

7. MARKETING AUTHORISATION HOLDER

Forest Laboratories UK Limited

Bourne Road

Bexley

Kent DA5 1NX

UK

8. MARKETING AUTHORISATION NUMBER(S)

PL 0108/5009R

9. DATE OF FIRST AUTHORISATION/RENEWAL OF THE AUTHORISATION

21 March 1991 / 07 November 2001

10. DATE OF REVISION OF THE TEXT

August 2005

11. Legal Category

POM

Colomycin Tablets

(Forest Laboratories UK Limited)

1. NAME OF THE MEDICINAL PRODUCT

COLOMYCIN TABLETS

2. QUALITATIVE AND QUANTITATIVE COMPOSITION

Colistin Sulphate BP 1.5MU per tablet.

3. PHARMACEUTICAL FORM

Tablet

4. CLINICAL PARTICULARS

4.1 Therapeutic indications

For the treatment of gastrointestinal infections caused by sensitive Gram negative organisms. Also for bowel preparation.

Colistin sulphate is not absorbed from the gastrointestinal tract and must not, therefore, be used for systemic infections.

4.2 Posology and method of administration

To be taken orally.

Adults (including the elderly) (over 30kg):

1,500,000 to 3,000,000 units every 8 hours.

Children (up to 15kg):

250,000 to 500,000 units every 8 hours.

Children (15-30kg):

750,000 to 1,500,000 units every 8 hours.

A minimum of five days treatment is recommended. Dosage may be increased when clinical or bacteriological response is slow.

For bowel preparation, a 24 hour course at the normal dosage above is given. Treatment should preferably finish 12 hours before surgery.

4.3 Contraindications

Contra-indicated in patients with known sensitivity to colistin and those with myasthenia gravis.

4.4 Special warnings and precautions for use

Colistin is subject to limited and unpredictable absorption from the GI tract in infants under six months. Studies in older children and in adults have demonstrated no systemic absorption of colistin following oral administration. Nevertheless, caution should be employed in the use of the preparation in patients with renal failure, patients receiving curari-form muscle relaxants and patients with porphyria.

4.5 Interaction with other medicinal products and other forms of interaction

Neurotoxicity has been reported in association with the concomitant use of either curariform agents or antibiotics with similar neurotoxic effects.

Therapy need not be discontinued and reduction of dosage may alleviate symptoms.

4.6 Pregnancy and lactation

Safety in human pregnancy has not been established. Animal studies do not indicate teratogenic properties; however, parenteral single dose studies in human pregnancy show that Colomycin crosses the placental barrier and there is a risk of foetal toxicity if repeated doses are given to pregnant patients. Colomycin should only be used in pregnancy if the potential benefit justifies the potential risk.

Colomycin is secreted in breast milk and patients to whom the drug is administered should not breast-feed an infant.

4.7 Effects on ability to drive and use machines

No specific warnings

4.8 Undesirable effects

No significant systemic absorption has been found to occur in older children and adults following oral administration nor have any systemic side effects been reported.

However, since the use of colistin may be associated with unpredictable, albeit limited, absorption in infants under 6 months the potential adverse effects of systemic administration should be noted for this patient population. These adverse effects may include transient sensory disturbances such as perioral parasthesia and vertigo.

Neuro-toxicity and adverse effects on renal function have been reported in association with systemic over-dosage, failure to reduce dosage in patients with renal insufficiency and the concomitant use of either curariform agents or antibiotics with similar neurotoxic effects. Therapy need not be discontinued and reduction of dosage may alleviate symptoms. Permanent nerve damage such as deafness or vestibular damage has not been reported.

4.9 Overdose

No symptoms of overdosage have been reported following oral use of colistin. However, following systemic administration overdosage can result in renal insufficiency, muscle weakness and apnoea and this should be borne in mind in the oral therapy of infants under 6 months old (see 'Undesirable Effects' above).

There is no specific antidote. Manage by supportive treatment and measures to increase the rate of elimination of colistin, e.g. mannitol diuresis, prolonged haemodialysis or peritoneal dialysis.

5. PHARMACOLOGICAL PROPERTIES

5.1 Pharmacodynamic properties

Colistin is a polypeptide antibiotic derived from Bacillus polymyxa var. colistinus.

It possesses a rapid bactericidal activity against a number of Gram-negative organisms, including Pseudomonas aeruginosa and is largely free from the development or transference of resistance.

5.2 Pharmacokinetic properties

Studies on the gastrointestinal absorption of colistin have shown no significant systemic absorption following oral administration in adults and older children.

Limited and unpredictable absorption is, however, evident in infants under 6 months.

5.3 Preclinical safety data

There are no preclinical data of relevance to the prescriber which are additional to that already included in other sections of the SPC.

6. PHARMACEUTICAL PARTICULARS

6.1 List of excipients

Microcrystalline cellulose

Starch (maize)

Colloidal silicon dioxide

Cutina HR.

6.2 Incompatibilities

None stated

6.3 Shelf life

5 years

6.4 Special precautions for storage

Do not store above 25°C. Store in the original container.

6.5 Nature and contents of container

Plastic container of 50 tablets

6.6 Special precautions for disposal and other handling

None stated

7. MARKETING AUTHORISATION HOLDER

Forest Laboratories UK Limited

Bourne Road

Bexley

Kent DA5 1NX

8. MARKETING AUTHORISATION NUMBER(S)

PL 0108/5008R

9. DATE OF FIRST AUTHORISATION/RENEWAL OF THE AUTHORISATION

30 May 1986 / 11 July 1996

10. DATE OF REVISION OF THE TEXT

July 1996

11. Legal Category

POM

Combigan

(Allergan Ltd)

1. NAME OF THE MEDICINAL PRODUCT

Combigan 2 mg/ml + 5 mg/ml eye drops, solution

2. QUALITATIVE AND QUANTITATIVE COMPOSITION

One ml solution contains:

2.0 mg brimonidine tartrate, equivalent to 1.3 mg of brimonidine

5.0 mg timolol as 6.8 mg timolol maleate

Contains benzalkonium chloride 0.05 mg/mL.

For a full list of excipients, see section 6.1

3. PHARMACEUTICAL FORM

Eye drops, solution.

Clear, greenish-yellow solution.

4. CLINICAL PARTICULARS

4.1 Therapeutic indications

Reduction of intraocular pressure (IOP) in patients with chronic open-angle glaucoma or ocular hypertension who are insufficiently responsive to topical beta-blockers.

4.2 Posology and method of administration

To avoid contamination of the eye or eye drops do not allow the dropper tip to come into contact with any surface.

Recommended dosage in adults (including the elderly)

The recommended dose is one drop of Combigan in the affected eye(s) twice daily, approximately 12 hours apart. If more than one topical ophthalmic product is to be used, the different products should be instilled at least 5 minutes apart.

As with any eye drops, to reduce possible systemic absorption, it is recommended that the lachrymal sac be compressed at the medial canthus (punctual occlusion) for one minute. This should be performed immediately following the instillation of each drop.

Use in renal and hepatic impairment

Combigan has not been studied in patients with hepatic or renal impairment. Therefore, caution should be used in treating such patients.

Use in children and adolescents

Combigan is contraindicated in neonates and infants (less than 2 years of age) (see section 4.3 Contraindications, section 4.4 Special warnings and precautions for use, section 4.8 Undesirable effects and section 4.9 Overdose).

The safety and effectiveness of Combigan in children and adolescents (2 to 17 years of age) have not been established and therefore, its use is not recommended in children or adolescents (see also section 4.4 and section 4.8).

4.3 Contraindications

• Reactive airway disease including bronchial asthma or a history of bronchial asthma, severe chronic obstructive pulmonary disease.

• Sinus bradycardia, second or third degree atrioventricular block not controlled with a pace-maker, overt cardiac failure, cardiogenic shock.

• Use in neonates and infants (less than 2 years of age) (see section 4.8)

• Patients receiving monoamine oxidase (MAO) inhibitor therapy.

• Patients on antidepressants which affect noradrenergic transmission (e.g. tricyclic antidepressants and mianserin)

• Hypersensitivity to the active substances or to any of the excipients.

4.4 Special warnings and precautions for use

Children of 2 years of age and above, especially those in the 2-7 age range and/or weighing < 20 Kg, should be treated with caution and closely monitored due to the high incidence of somnolence. The safety and effectiveness of Combigan in children and adolescents (2 to 17 years of age) have not been established (see section 4.2 and section 4.8).

Like other topically applied ophthalmic agents, Combigan may be absorbed systemically. No enhancement of the systemic absorption of the individual active substances has been observed.

Some patients have experienced ocular allergic type reactions (allergic conjunctivitis and allergic blepharitis) with Combigan in clinical trials. Allergic conjunctivitis was seen in 5.2% of patients. Onset was typically between 3 and 9 months resulting in an overall discontinuation rate of 3.1%. Allergic blepharitis was uncommonly reported (<1%). If allergic reactions are observed, treatment with Combigan should be discontinued.

Due to the beta-adrenergic component, timolol, the same types of cardiovascular and pulmonary adverse reactions as seen with systemic beta-blockers may occur.

Caution should be exercised in treating patients with severe or unstable and uncontrolled cardiovascular disease. Cardiac failure should be adequately controlled before beginning therapy. Patients with a history of severe cardiac disease should be watched for signs of cardiac failure and have their pulse rates checked. Cardiac and respiratory reactions, including death due to bronchospasm in patients with asthma, and, rarely, death in association with cardiac failures have been reported following administration of timolol maleate.

In patients with severe renal impairment on dialysis, treatment with timolol has been associated with pronounced hypotension.

Timolol may impair compensatory tachycardia and increase risk of hypotension when used in conjunction with anaesthetics. The anaesthetist must be informed if the patient is using Combigan.

Beta-blockers may also mask the signs of hyperthyroidism and cause worsening of Prinzmetal angina, severe peripheral and central circulatory disorders and hypotension. Combigan must be used with caution in patients with metabolic acidosis and untreated phaeochromocytoma.

Beta-adrenergic blocking agents should be administered with caution in patients subject to spontaneous hypoglycaemia or to uncontrolled diabetic patients (especially those with labile diabetes) as beta-blockers may mask the signs and symptoms of acute hypoglycaemia. The indicatory signs of acute hypoglycaemia may be masked, in particular tachycardia, palpitations and sweating.

Combigan should be used with caution in patients with depression, cerebral or coronary insufficiency, Raynaud's phenomenon, orthostatic hypotension, or thromboangiitis obliterans.

While taking beta-blockers, patients with a history of atopy or a history of severe anaphylactic reaction to a variety of allergens may be unresponsive to the usual dose of adrenaline used to treat anaphylactic reactions.

As with systemic beta-blockers, if discontinuation of treatment is needed in patients with coronary heart disease, therapy should be withdrawn gradually to avoid rhythm disorders, myocardial infarct or sudden death.

Choroidal detachment after filtration procedures has been reported with administration of aqueous suppressant therapy (e.g. timolol, acetazolamide).

The preservative in Combigan, benzalkonium chloride, may cause eye irritation. Remove contact lenses prior to application and wait at least 15 minutes before reinsertion. Benzalkonium chloride is known to discolour soft contact lenses. Avoid contact with soft contact lenses.

Combigan has not been studied in patients with closed-angle glaucoma.

4.5 Interaction with other medicinal products and other forms of interaction

No interaction studies have been performed. Although specific drug interactions studies have not been conducted with Combigan, the theoretical possibility of an additive or potentiating effect with CNS depressants (alcohol, barbiturates, opiates, sedatives, or anaesthetics) should be considered.

There is potential for additive effects resulting in hypotension, and/or marked bradycardia when eye drops with timolol are administered concomitantly with oral calcium channel blockers, guanethidine, or beta-blocking agents, anti-arrhythmics, digitalis glycosides or parasympathomimetics. After the application of brimonidine, very rare (<1 in 10,000) cases of hypotension have been reported. Caution is therefore advised when using Combigan with systemic antihypertensives.

Although timolol has little effect on the size of the pupil, mydriasis has occasionally been reported when timolol has been used with mydriatic agents such as adrenaline.

Beta-blockers may increase the hypoglycaemic effect of antidiabetic agents. Beta-blockers can mask the signs and symptoms of hypoglycaemia (see 4.4 Special warnings and precautions for use)

The hypertensive reaction to sudden withdrawal of clonidine can be potentiated when taking beta-blockers.

Potentiated systemic beta-blockade (e.g., decreased heart rate) has been reported during combined treatment with quinidine and timolol, possibly because quinidine inhibits the metabolism of timolol via the P450 enzyme, CYP2D6.

Concomitant use of a beta-blocker with anaesthetic drugs may attenuate compensatory tachycardia and increase the risk of hypotension (see section 4.4), and therefore the anaesthetist must be informed if the patient is using Combigan.

Caution must be exercised if Combigan is used concomitantly with iodine contrast products or intravenously administered lidocain.

Cimetidine, hydralazine and alcohol may increase the plasma concentrations of timolol.

No data on the level of circulating catecholamines after Combigan administration are available. Caution, however, is advised in patients taking medication which can affect the metabolism and uptake of circulating amines e.g. chlorpromazine, methylphenidate, reserpine.

Caution is advised when initiating (or changing the dose of) a concomitant systemic agent (irrespective of pharmaceutical form) which may interact with α-adrenergic agonists or interfere with their activity i.e. agonists or antagonists of the adrenergic receptor e.g. (isoprenaline, prazosin).

Although specific drug interactions studies have not been conducted with Combigan, the theoretical possibility of an additive IOP lowering effect with prostamides, prostaglandins, carbonic anhydrase inhibitors and pilocarpine should be considered.

Concomitant administration of MAO inhibitors is contraindicated (see section 4.3). Patients who have been receiving MAOI therapy should wait 14 days after discontinuation before commencing treatment with Combigan.

4.6 Pregnancy and lactation

Pregnancy

There are no adequate data for the use of Combigan in pregnant women.

Brimonidine tartrate

There are no adequate data from the use of brimonidine tartrate in pregnant women. Studies in animals have shown reproductive toxicity at high maternotoxic doses (see section 5.3 Preclinical safety data). The potential risk for humans is unknown.

Timolol

Studies in animals have shown reproductive toxicity at doses significantly higher than would be used in clinical practice (see 5.3). However, epidemiological studies have not revealed malformative effects but have shown a risk for intra uterine growth retardation when beta-blockers are administered by the oral route. In addition, signs and symptoms of beta-blockade (e.g. bradycardia, hypotension, respiratory distress and hypoglycaemia) have been observed in the neonate when beta-blockers have been administered until delivery. Therefore, if Combigan is administered in pregnancy up to the time of delivery, the neonate should be carefully monitored during the first days of life.

Combigan should not be used during pregnancy unless clearly necessary.

Lactation

Timolol is excreted in human milk. It is not known if brimonidine is excreted in human milk but it is excreted in the milk of the lactating rat. Combigan should not be used by women breast-feeding infants.

4.7 Effects on ability to drive and use machines

Combigan has minor influence on the ability to drive and use machines. Combigan may cause transient blurring of vision, fatigue and/or drowsiness which may impair the ability to drive or operate machines. The patient should wait until these symptoms have cleared before driving or using machinery.

4.8 Undesirable effects

Based on 12 month clinical data, the most commonly reported ADRs were conjunctival hyperaemia (approximately 15% of patients) and burning sensation in the eye (approximately 11% of patients). The majority of these cases was mild and led to discontinuation rates of only 3.4% and 0.5% respectively.

The following adverse drug reactions were reported during clinical trials with Combigan:

Eye disorders

Very Common (>1/10): conjunctival hyperaemia, burning sensation

Common (>1/100, <1/10): stinging sensation in the eye, allergic conjunctivitis, corneal erosion, superficial punctuate keratitis, eye pruritus, conjunctival folliculosis, visual disturbance, blepharitis, epiphora, eye dryness, eye discharge, eye pain, eye irritation, foreign body sensation

Uncommon (>1/1000, <1/100): visual acuity worsened, conjunctival oedema, follicular conjunctivitis, allergic blepharitis, conjunctivitis, vitreous floater, asthenopia, photophobia, papillary hypertrophy, eyelid pain, conjunctival blanching, corneal oedema, corneal infiltrates, vitreous detachment

Psychiatric disorders

Common (>1/100, <1/10): depression

Nervous system disorders

Common (>1/100, <1/10): somnolence, headache

Uncommon (>1/1000, <1/100): dizziness, syncope

Cardiac disorders

Uncommon (>1/1000, <1/100): congestive heart failure, palpitations

Vascular disorders

Common (>1/100, <1/10): hypertension

Respiratory, thoracic and mediastinal disorders

Uncommon (>1/1000, <1/100): rhinitis, nasal dryness

Gastrointestinal disorders

Common (>1/100, <1/10): oral dryness

Uncommon (>1/1000, <1/100): taste perversion

Skin and subcutaneous tissue disorders

Common (>1/100, <1/10): eyelid oedema, eyelid pruritus, eyelid erythema

Uncommon (>1/1000, <1/100): allergic contact dermatitis

General disorders and administration site conditions

Common (>1/100, <1/10): asthenic conditions

Investigations

Common (>1/100, <1/10): LFTs abnormal

The following adverse drug reactions have been reported since Combigan has been marketed:

Cardiac disorders

Not known: arrhythmia, bradycardia, tachycardia

Vascular disorders

Not known: hypotension

Additional adverse events that have been seen with one of the components and may potentially occur also with Combigan:

Brimonidine

Eye disorders: iritis, miosis

Psychiatric disorders: insomnia

Respiratory, thoracic and mediastinal disorders: upper respiratory symptoms, dyspnoea

Gastrointestinal disorders: gastrointestinal symptoms

General disorders and administration site conditions: systemic allergic reactions

In cases where brimonidine has been used as part of the medical treatment of congenital glaucoma, symptoms of brimonidine overdose such as loss of consciousness, hypotension, hypotonia, bradycardia, hypothermia, cyanosis and apnoea have been reported in neonates and infants (less than 2 years of age) receiving brimonidine (see section 4.3).

A high incidence of somnolence has been reported in children of 2 years of age and above, especially those in the 2-7 age range and/or weighing < 20 Kg (see section 4.4).

Timolol

Eye disorders: decreased corneal sensitivity, diplopia, ptosis, choroidal detachment (following filtration surgery), refractive changes (due to withdrawal of miotic therapy in some cases)

Psychiatric disorders: insomnia, nightmares, decreased libido

Nervous system disorders: memory loss, increase in signs and symptoms of myasthenia gravis, paresthaesia, cerebral ischaemia

Ear and labyrinth disorders: tinnitus

Cardiac disorders: heart block, cardiac arrest

Vascular disorders: cerebrovascular accident, claudication, Raynaud's phenomenon, cold hands and feet

Respiratory, thoracic and mediastinal disorders: bronchospasm (predominantly in patients with pre-existing bronchospastic disease), dyspnoea, cough, respiratory failure

Gastrointestinal disorders: nausea, diarrhoea, dyspepsia

Skin and subcutaneous tissue disorders: alopecia, psoriasiform rash or exacerbation of psoriasis

Musculoskeletal, connective tissue and bone disorders: systemic lupus erythematosus

Renal and urinary disorders: Peyronie's disease

General disorders and administration site conditions: oedema, chest pain

4.9 Overdose

Brimonidine

Ophthalmic overdose:

In cases where brimonidine has been used as part of the medical treatment of congenital glaucoma, symptoms of brimonidine overdose such as loss of consciousness, hypotension, hypotonia, bradycardia, hypothermia, cyanosis and apnoea have been reported in neonates and infants (less than 2 years of age) receiving brimonidine.

Systemic overdose resulting from accidental ingestion:

Several reports of serious adverse events following inadvertent ingestion of brimonidine by paediatric subjects have been published or reported to Allergan. The subjects experienced symptoms of CNS depression, typically temporary coma or low level of consciousness, hypotonia, bradycardia, hypothermia and apnoea and required admission to intensive care with intubation if indicated. All subjects were reported to have made a full recovery, usually within 6-24 hours.

Two cases of adverse effects following inadvertent ingestion of 9-10 drops of brimonidine by adult subjects have been received. The subjects experienced a hypotensive episode, followed in one instance by rebound hypertension approximately 8 hours after ingestion. Both subjects were reported to have made a full recovery within 24 hours. No adverse effects were noted in a third subject who ingested an unknown amount of brimonidine orally.

Oral overdoses of other alpha-2-agonists have been reported to cause symptoms such as hypotension, asthenia, vomiting, lethargy, sedation, bradycardia, arrhythmias, miosis, apnoea, hypotonia, hypothermia, respiratory depression and seizure.

Timolol

Symptoms of systemic timolol overdose are: bradycardia, hypotension, bronchospasm, headache, dizziness and cardiac arrest. A study of patients showed that timolol did not dialyse readily.

If overdose occurs treatment should be symptomatic and supportive.

5. PHARMACOLOGICAL PROPERTIES

5.1 Pharmacodynamic properties

Pharmacotherapeutic group: Ophthalmological – antiglaucoma preparations and miotics - beta-blocking agents – timolol, combinations

ATC code: S01ED51

Mechanism of action

Combigan consists of two active substances: brimonidine tartrate and timolol maleate. These two components decrease elevated intraocular pressure (IOP) by complementary mechanisms of action and the combined effect results in additional IOP reduction compared to either compound administered alone. Combigan has a rapid onset of action.

Brimonidine tartrate is an alpha-2 adrenergic receptor agonist that is 1000-fold more selective for the alpha-2 adrenoceptor than the alpha-1 adrenoreceptor. This selectivity results in no mydriasis and the absence of vasoconstriction in microvessels associated with human retinal xenografts.

It is thought that brimonidine tartrate lowers IOP by enhancing uveoscleral outflow and reducing aqueous humour formation.

Timolol is a $beta_1$ and $beta_2$ non-selective adrenergic receptor blocking agent that does not have significant intrinsic sympathomimetic, direct myocardial depressant, or local anaesthetic (membrane-stabilising) activity. Timolol lowers IOP by reducing aqueous humour formation. The precise mechanism of action is not clearly established, but inhibition of the increased cyclic AMP synthesis caused by endogenous beta-adrenergic stimulation is probable.

Clinical effects

In three controlled, double-masked clinical studies, Combigan (twice daily) produced a clinically meaningful additive decrease in mean diurnal IOP compared with timolol (twice daily) and brimonidine (twice daily or three times a day) when administered as monotherapy.

In a study in patients whose IOP was insufficiently controlled following a minimal 3-week run-in on any monotherapy, additional decreases in mean diurnal IOP of 4.5, 3.3 and 3.5 mmHg were observed during 3 months of treatment for Combigan (twice daily), timolol (twice daily) and brimonidine (twice daily), respectively. In this study, at trough, a significant additional decrease in IOP could only be demonstrated on comparison with brimonidine but not with timolol, however a positive trend was seen with superiority at all other timepoints. In the pooled data of the other two trials statistical superiority versus timolol was seen throughout.

In addition, the IOP-lowering effect of Combigan was consistently non-inferior to that achieved by adjunctive therapy of brimonidine and timolol (all twice daily).

The IOP-lowering effect of Combigan has been shown to be maintained in double-masked studies of up to 12 months.

5.2 Pharmacokinetic properties

Combigan

Plasma brimonidine and timolol concentrations were determined in a crossover study comparing the monotherapy treatments to Combigan treatment in healthy subjects. There were no statistically significant differences in brimonidine or timolol AUC between Combigan and the respective monotherapy treatments. Mean plasma C_{max} values for brimonidine and timolol following dosing with Combigan were 0.0327 and 0.406 ng/ml respectively.

Brimonidine

After ocular administration of 0.2% eye drops solution in humans, plasma brimonidine concentrations are low. Brimonidine is not extensively metabolised in the human eye and human plasma protein binding is approximately 29%. The mean apparent half-life in the systemic circulation was approximately 3 hours after topical dosing in man.

Following oral administration to man, brimonidine is well absorbed and rapidly eliminated. The major part of the dose (around 74% of the dose) was excreted as metabolites in urine within five days; no unchanged drug was detected in urine. In vitro studies, using animal and human liver, indicate that the metabolism is mediated largely by aldehyde oxidase and cytochrome P450. Hence, the systemic elimination seems to be primarily hepatic metabolism.

Brimonidine binds extensively and reversibly to melanin in ocular tissues without any untoward effects. Accumulation does not occur in the absence of melanin.

Brimonidine is not metabolised to a great extent in human eyes.

Timolol

After ocular administration of a 0.5% eye drops solution in humans undergoing cataract surgery, peak timolol concentration was 898 ng/ml in the aqueous humour at one hour post-dose. Part of the dose is absorbed systemically where it is extensively metabolised in the liver. The half-life of timolol in plasma is about 7 hours. Timolol is partially metabolised by the liver with timolol and its metabolites excreted by the kidney. Timolol is not extensively bound to plasma protein.

5.3 Preclinical safety data

The ocular and systemic safety profile of the individual components is well established. Non-clinical data reveal no special hazard for humans based on conventional studies of the individual components in safety pharmacology, repeated dose toxicity, genotoxicity, and carcinogenicity studies. Additional ocular repeated dose toxicity studies on Combigan also showed no special hazard for humans.

Brimonidine

Brimonidine tartrate did not cause any teratogenic effects in animals, but caused abortion in rabbits and postnatal growth reduction in rats at systemic exposures approximately 37-times and 134-times those obtained during therapy in humans, respectively.

Timolol

In animal studies, beta-blockers have been shown to produce reduced umbilical blood flow, reduced foetal growth, delayed ossification and increased foetal and postnatal death, but no teratogenicity. With timolol, embryotoxicity (resorption) in rabbit and foetotoxicity (delayed ossification) in rats have been seen at high maternal doses. Teratogenicity studies in mice, rats and rabbits, at oral doses of timolol up to 4200 times of that in the human daily dose of Combigan, showed no evidence of foetal malformation.

6. PHARMACEUTICAL PARTICULARS

6.1 List of excipients

Benzalkonium chloride

Sodium phosphate, monobasic monohydrate

Sodium phosphate, dibasic heptahydrate

Hydrochloric acid or sodium hydroxide to adjust pH

Purified water

6.2 Incompatibilities

Not applicable.

6.3 Shelf life

21 months.

After first opening: Use within 28 days.

6.4 Special precautions for storage

Keep the bottle in the outer carton in order to protect from light.

6.5 Nature and contents of container

White low density polyethylene bottles with polystyrene screw caps. Each bottle has a fill volume of 5 ml.

The following pack sizes are available: cartons containing 1 or 3 bottles of 5 ml. Not all pack sizes may be marketed.

6.6 Special precautions for disposal and other handling

No special requirements.

7. MARKETING AUTHORISATION HOLDER

Allergan Pharmaceuticals Ireland
Castlebar Road
Westport
Co. Mayo
Ireland

8. MARKETING AUTHORISATION NUMBER(S)

PL 05179/0006

9. DATE OF FIRST AUTHORISATION/RENEWAL OF THE AUTHORISATION

12th April 2005

10. DATE OF REVISION OF THE TEXT

18th November 2008

Combivent UDVs

(Boehringer Ingelheim Limited)

1. NAME OF THE MEDICINAL PRODUCT

Combivent® UDVs®

2. QUALITATIVE AND QUANTITATIVE COMPOSITION

Each 2.5 ml single dose unit contains 500 micrograms ipratropium bromide (as 520 micrograms ipratropium bromide monohydrate) and 3 mg salbutamol sulphate (corresponds to 2.5mg salbutamol base).

For excipients, see 6.1.

3. PHARMACEUTICAL FORM

Nebuliser solution.

A clear, colourless or almost colourless solution.

4. CLINICAL PARTICULARS

4.1 Therapeutic indications

The management of bronchospasm in patients suffering from chronic obstructive pulmonary disease who require regular treatment with both ipratropium and salbutamol.

4.2 Posology and method of administration

For inhalation.

COMBIVENT UDVs may be administered from a suitable nebuliser or an intermittent positive pressure ventilator. The single dose units should not be taken orally or administered parenterally.

The recommended dose is:

Adults (including elderly patients and children over 12 years):

1 single dose unit three or four times daily.

Children under 12 years:

There is no experience of the use of COMBIVENT UDVs in children under 12 years.

4.3 Contraindications

COMBIVENT UDVs are contraindicated in patients with hypertrophic obstructive cardio- myopathy or tachyarrhythmia. COMBIVENT UDVs are also contraindicated in patients with a history of hypersensitivity to ipratropium bromide, salbutamol sulphate or to atropine or its derivatives.

4.4 Special warnings and precautions for use

Immediate hypersensitivity reactions may occur after administration of COMBIVENT UDVs, as demonstrated by rare cases of urticaria, angioedema, rash, bronchospasm and oropharyngeal oedema.

There have been rare reports of ocular complications (i.e. mydriasis, blurring of vision, narrow-angle glaucoma and eye pain) when the contents of metered aerosols containing ipratropium bromide have been sprayed inadvertently into the eye.

Patients must be instructed in the correct use of COMBIVENT UDVs and warned not to allow the solution or mist to enter the eyes. This is particularly important in patients who may be pre-disposed to glaucoma. Such patients should be warned specifically to protect their eyes. Eye pain or discomfort, blurred vision, visual halos or coloured images, in association with red eyes from conjunctival congestion and corneal oedema may be signs of acute narrow-angle glaucoma. Should any combination of these symptoms develop, treatment with miotic drops should be initiated and specialist advice sought immediately.

In the following conditions COMBIVENT UDVs should only be used after careful risk/benefit assessment: insufficiently controlled diabetes mellitus, recent myocardial infarction and/or severe organic heart or vascular disorders, hyperthyroidism, pheochromocytoma, risk of narrow-angle glaucoma, prostatic hypertrophy or bladder-neck obstruction.

There is some evidence from post-marketing data and published literature of rare occurences of myocardial ischaemia associated with salbutamol. Patients with underlying severe heart disease (e.g. ischaemic heart disease, tachyarrhythmia or severe heart failure) who are receiving salbutamol for respiratory disease, should be warned to seek medical advice if they experience chest pain or other symptoms of worsening heart disease.

Potentially serious hypokalaemia may result from $beta_2$-agonist therapy. Particular caution is advised in severe airway obstruction as this effect may be potentiated by concomitant treatment with xanthine derivatives, steroids and diuretics. Additionally, hypoxia may aggravate the effects of hypokalaemia on cardiac rhythm (especially in patients receiving digoxin). It is recommended that serum potassium levels are monitored in such situations.

Patients with cystic fibrosis may be more prone to gastro-intestinal motility disturbances.

The patient should be instructed to consult a doctor immediately in the event of acute, rapidly worsening dyspnoea. In addition, the patient should be warned to seek medical advice should a reduced response become apparent.

4.5 Interaction with other medicinal products and other forms of interaction

The use of additional beta-agonists, xanthine derivatives and corticosteroids may enhance the effect of COMBIVENT UDVs. The concurrent administration of other beta-mimetics, systemically absorbed anticholinergics and xanthine derivatives may increase the severity of side effects. A potentially serious reduction in effect may occur during concurrent administration of beta-blockers.

Beta-adrenergic agonists should be administered with caution to patients being treated with monoamine oxidase inhibitors or tricyclic antidepressants, since the action of beta-adrenergic agonists may be enhanced.

Inhalation of halogenated hydrocarbon anaesthetics such as halothane, trichloroethylene and enflurane may increase the susceptibility to the cardiovascular effects of beta-agonists.

4.6 Pregnancy and lactation

Ipratropium bromide has been in general use for several years and there is no definite evidence of ill-consequence during pregnancy; animal studies have shown no hazard.

Salbutamol has been in widespread use for many years without apparent ill-consequence during pregnancy. There is inadequate published evidence of safety in the early stages of human pregnancy but in animal studies there has been evidence of some harmful effects on the foetus at very high dose levels.

As with all medicines, COMBIVENT UDVs should not be used in pregnancy, especially the first trimester, unless the expected benefit is thought to outweigh any possible risk to the foetus. Similarly, COMBIVENT UDVs should not be administered to breast-feeding mothers unless the expected benefit is thought to outweigh any possible risk to the neonate.

4.7 Effects on ability to drive and use machines

None stated.

4.8 Undesirable effects

The following side effects have been reported based on clinical trials involving 821 patients.

Frequencies

Very common	≥ 1/10
Common	≥ 1/100 < 1/10
Uncommon	≥ 1/1,000 < 1/100
Rare	≥ 1/10,000 < 1/1,000
Very Rare	< 1/10,000
Not known	cannot be estimated from the available data

Immune system disorders:	
Anaphylactic reaction	Not known
Hypersensitivity	Not known
Metabolism and nutrition disorders:	
Hypokalaemia	Not known
Psychiatric disorders:	
Nervousness	Uncommon
Mental disorder	Not known
Nervous system disorders:	
Dizziness	Uncommon
Headache	Uncommon
Tremor	Uncommon
Eye disorders:	
Angle closure glaucoma	Not known
Eye pain	Not known
Intraocular pressure increased	Not known
Mydriasis	Not known
Vision blurred	Not known

There have been isolated reports of ocular complications with symptoms mentioned above when aerosolised ipratropium bromide either alone or in combination with an adrenergic beta$_2$-agonist, has escaped into the eyes.

Cardiac disorders:	
Palpitations	Uncommon
Tachycardia	Uncommon
Arrhythmia	Very rare
Atrial fibrillation	Very rare
Myocardial ischaemia	Very rare
Blood pressure diastolic decreased	Not known
Blood pressure systolic increased	Not known
Respiratory, thoracic and mediastinal disorders:	
Cough	Uncommon
Dysphonia	Uncommon
Bronchospasm	Not known
Laryngospasm	Not known
Pharyngeal oedema	Not known
Throat irritation	Not known
Gastrointestinal disorders:	
Dry mouth	Common
Nausea	Uncommon
Oedema mouth	Not known
Gastrointestinal motility disorder	Not known
Vomiting	Not known
Skin and subcutaneous tissue disorders:	
Angioedema	Not known
Hyperhidrosis	Not known
Rash	Not known
Skin reaction	Not known
Urticaria	Not known
Musculoskeletal and connective tissue disorders	
Muscle spasms	Not known
Muscular weakness	Not known
Myalgia	Not known
Renal and urinary disorders:	
Urinary retention	Uncommon
General disorders and administration site conditions:	
Asthenia	Uncommon

4.9 Overdose

Acute effects of overdosage with ipratropium bromide are unlikely due to its poor systemic absorption after either inhalation or oral administration. Any effects of overdosage are therefore likely to be related to the salbutamol component.

Manifestations of overdosage with salbutamol may include anginal pain, hypertension, hypokalaemia and tachycardia. The preferred antidote for overdosage with salbutamol is a cardioselective beta-blocking agent but caution should be used in administering these drugs in patients with a history of bronchospasm.

5. PHARMACOLOGICAL PROPERTIES

5.1 Pharmacodynamic properties

Ipratropium bromide is an anticholinergic agent which inhibits vagally-mediated reflexes by antagonising the action of acetylcholine, the transmitter agent released from the vagus nerve. The bronchodilation following inhalation of ipratropium bromide is primarily local and site specific to the lung and not systemic in nature.

Salbutamol is a beta$_2$-adrenergic agent which acts on airway smooth muscle resulting in relaxation. Salbutamol relaxes all smooth muscle from the trachea to the terminal bronchioles and protects against bronchoconstrictor challenges.

COMBIVENT UDVs provide the simultaneous delivery of ipratropium bromide and salbutamol sulphate allowing effects on both muscarinic and beta$_2$-adrenergic receptors in the lung leading to increased bronchodilation over that provided by each agent singly.

5.2 Pharmacokinetic properties

Ipratropium bromide is not readily absorbed into the systemic circulation either from the surface of the lung or from the gastrointestinal tract as assessed by blood level and renal excretion studies. The elimination half-life of drug and metabolites is about 3 to 4 hours after inhalation or intravenous administration. Ipratropium bromide does not cross the blood-brain barrier.

Salbutamol is rapidly and completely absorbed following oral administration either by the inhaled or the gastric route. Peak plasma salbutamol concentrations are seen within three hours of administration and the drug is excreted unchanged in the urine after 24 hours. The elimination half-life is 4 hours. Salbutamol will cross the blood brain barrier reaching concentrations amounting to about five percent of the plasma concentrations.

It has been shown that co-nebulisation of ipratropium bromide and salbutamol sulphate does not potentiate the systemic absorption of either component and that therefore the additive activity of COMBIVENT UDVs is due to the combined local effect on the lung following inhalation.

5.3 Preclinical safety data

None stated.

6. PHARMACEUTICAL PARTICULARS

6.1 List of excipients

Sodium chloride

1N Hydrochloric acid

Purified water

6.2 Incompatibilities

None stated.

6.3 Shelf life

24 months.

6.4 Special precautions for storage

Store below 25°C. Do not freeze. Keep vials in the outer carton in order to protect from light.

Do not use if solution is discoloured.

6.5 Nature and contents of container

Low density polyethylene (Ph.Eur.) vials containing 2.5 ml solution, formed into strips of 10 and packed into cartons containing 10, 20, 40, 60, 80 or 100 vials.

6.6 Special precautions for disposal and other handling

i) Prepare the nebuliser by following the manufacturer's instructions and the advice of your doctor.

ii) Carefully separate a new vial from the strip. NEVER use one that has been opened already.

iii) Open the vial by simply twisting off the top, always taking care to hold it in an upright position.

iv) Unless otherwise instructed by your doctor squeeze all the contents of the plastic vial into the nebuliser chamber.

v) Assemble the nebuliser and use it as directed by your doctor.

vi) After nebulisation clean the nebuliser according to the manufacturer's instructions.

Since the single dose units contain no preservatives, it is important that the contents are used soon after opening and a fresh vial is used for each administration to avoid microbial contamination. Partly used, opened or damaged single dose units should be discarded.

It is strongly recommended not to mix COMBIVENT with other drugs in the same nebuliser.

Administrative Data

7. MARKETING AUTHORISATION HOLDER

Boehringer Ingelheim Limited

Ellesfield Avenue

Bracknell

Berkshire

RG12 8YS

United Kingdom

8. MARKETING AUTHORISATION NUMBER(S)

PL 00015/0197

9. DATE OF FIRST AUTHORISATION/RENEWAL OF THE AUTHORISATION

7 June 1995

10. DATE OF REVISION OF THE TEXT

February 2009

11. Legal Category

POM

Combivir Film Coated Tablets

(GlaxoSmithKline UK)

1. NAME OF THE MEDICINAL PRODUCT

Combivir 150 mg/300 mg film-coated tablets

2. QUALITATIVE AND QUANTITATIVE COMPOSITION

Each film-coated tablet contains 150 mg lamivudine and 300 mg zidovudine.

For a full list of excipients see section 6.1.

3. PHARMACEUTICAL FORM

Film-coated tablet

White to off-white, capsule-shaped film-coated scored tablets engraved with "GXFC3" on both sides.

4. CLINICAL PARTICULARS

4.1 Therapeutic indications

Combivir is indicated in antiretroviral combination therapy for the treatment of Human Immunodeficiency Virus (HIV) infection (see section 4.2).

4.2 Posology and method of administration

Therapy should be initiated by a physician experienced in the management of HIV infection.

Combivir may be administered with or without food.

To ensure administration of the entire dose, the tablet(s) should ideally be swallowed without crushing. For patients who are unable to swallow tablets, tablets may be crushed and added to a small amount of semi-solid food or liquid, all of which should be consumed immediately (see section 5.2).

Adults and adolescents weighing at least 30 kg: the recommended dose of Combivir is one tablet twice daily.

Children weighing between 21 kg and 30 kg: the recommended oral dose of COMBIVIR is one-half tablet taken in the morning and one whole tablet taken in the evening.

Children weighing from 14 kg to 21 kg: the recommended oral dose of COMBIVIR is one-half tablet taken twice daily.

The dosing regimen for paediatric patients weighing 14-30 kg is based primarily on pharmacokinetic modelling and supported by data from clinical studies using the individual components lamivudine and zidovudine. A pharmacokinetic overexposure of zidovudine can occur, therefore close safety monitoring is warranted in these patients. If gastrointestinal intolerance occurs in patients weighing 21-30 kg, an alternative dosing schedule with one-half tablet taken thrice daily can be applied in attempt to improve tolerability.

Combivir tablets should not be used for children weighing less than 14 kg, since doses can not be appropriately adjusted for the weight of the child. In these patients, lamivudine and zidovudine should be taken as separate formulations according to the prescribed dosing recommendations for these products. For these patients and for patients, who are unable to swallow tablets, oral solutions of lamivudine and zidovudine are available.

For situations where discontinuation of therapy with one of the active substances of Combivir, or dose reduction is necessary separate preparations of lamivudine and zidovudine are available in tablets/capsules and oral solution.

Renal impairment: Lamivudine and zidovudine concentrations are increased in patients with renal impairment due to decreased clearance. Therefore as dosage adjustment of these may be necessary it is recommended that separate preparations of lamivudine and zidovudine be administered to patients with reduced renal function (creatinine clearance $\leqslant$50 ml/min). Physicians should refer to the individual prescribing information for these medicinal products.

Hepatic impairment: Limited data in patients with cirrhosis suggest that accumulation of zidovudine may occur in patients with hepatic impairment because of decreased glucuronidation. Data obtained in patients with moderate to severe hepatic impairment show that lamivudine pharmacokinetics are not significantly affected by hepatic dysfunction. However, as dosage adjustments for zidovudine may be necessary, it is recommended that separate preparations of lamivudine and zidovudine be administered to patients with severe hepatic impairment. Physicians should refer to the individual prescribing information for these medicinal products.

Dosage adjustments in patients with haematological adverse reactions: Dosage adjustment of zidovudine may be necessary if the haemoglobin level falls below 9 g/dl or 5.59 mmol/l or the neutrophil count falls below 1.0 $\times$ 10^9/l (see sections 4.3 and 4.4). As dosage adjustment of Combivir is not possible, separate preparations of zidovudine and lamivudine should be used. Physicians should refer to the individual prescribing information for these medicinal products.

Dosage in the elderly: No specific data are available, however special care is advised in this age group due to age associated changes such as the decrease in renal function and alteration of haematological parameters.

4.3 Contraindications

Hypersensitivity to the active substances or to any of the excipients.

Zidovudine is contraindicated in patients with abnormally low neutrophil counts (<0.75 $\times$ 10^9/l), or abnormally low haemoglobin levels (<7.5 g/dl or 4.65 mmol/l). Combivir is therefore contra-indicated in these patients (see section 4.4).

4.4 Special warnings and precautions for use

The special warnings and precautions relevant to both lamivudine and zidovudine are included in this section. There are no additional precautions and warnings relevant to the combination Combivir.

It is recommended that separate preparations of lamivudine and zidovudine should be administered in cases where dosage adjustment is necessary (see section 4.2). In these cases the physician should refer to the individual prescribing information for these medicinal products.

The concomitant use of stavudine with zidovudine should be avoided (see section 4.5).

Opportunistic infections: Patients receiving Combivir or any other antiretroviral therapy may continue to develop opportunistic infections and other complications of HIV infection. Therefore patients should remain under close clinical observation by physicians experienced in the treatment of HIV infection.

Transmission of HIV: Patients should be advised that current antiretroviral therapy, including Combivir, has not been proven to prevent the risk of transmission of HIV to others through sexual contact or contamination with blood. Appropriate precautions should continue to be taken.

Haematological adverse reactions: Anaemia, neutropenia and leucopenia (usually secondary to neutropenia) can be expected to occur in patients receiving zidovudine. These occurred more frequently at higher zidovudine dosages (1200-1500 mg/day) and in patients with poor bone marrow reserve prior to treatment, particularly with advanced HIV disease. Haematological parameters should therefore be carefully monitored (see section 4.3) in patients receiving Combivir. These haematological effects are not usually observed before four to six weeks therapy. For patients with advanced symptomatic HIV disease, it is generally recommended that blood tests are performed at least every two weeks for the first three months of therapy and at least monthly thereafter.

In patients with early HIV disease haematological adverse reactions are infrequent. Depending on the overall condition of the patient, blood tests may be performed less often, for example every one to three months. Additionally dosage adjustment of zidovudine may be required if severe anaemia or myelosuppression occurs during treatment with Combivir, or in patients with pre-existing bone marrow compromise e.g. haemoglobin <9 g/dl (5.59 mmol/l) or neutrophil count <1.0 $\times$ 10^9/l (see section 4.2). As dosage adjustment of Combivir is not possible separate preparations of zidovudine and lamivudine should be used. Physicians should refer to the individual prescribing information for these medicinal products.

Pancreatitis: Cases of pancreatitis have occurred rarely in patients treated with lamivudine and zidovudine. However it is not clear whether these cases were due to the antiretroviral treatment or to the underlying HIV disease. Treatment with Combivir should be stopped immediately if clinical signs, symptoms or laboratory abnormalities suggestive of pancreatitis occur.

> *Lactic acidosis:* lactic acidosis usually associated with hepatomegaly and hepatic steatosis has been reported with the use of nucleoside analogues. Early symptoms (symptomatic hyperlactatemia) include benign digestive symptoms (nausea, vomiting and abdominal pain) non-specific malaise, loss of appetite, weight loss, respiratory symptoms (rapid and/or deep breathing) or neurological symptoms (including motor weakness).
>
> Lactic acidosis has a high mortality and may be associated with pancreatitis, liver failure, or renal failure.
>
> Lactic acidosis generally occurred after a few or several months of treatment.
>
> Treatment with nucleoside analogues should be discontinued if there is symptomatic hyperlactatemia and metabolic/lactic acidosis, progressive hepatomegaly, or rapidly elevating aminotransferase levels.
>
> Caution should be exercised when administering nucleoside analogues to any patient (particularly obese women) with hepatomegaly, hepatitis or other known risk factors for liver disease and hepatic steatosis (including certain medicinal products and alcohol). Patients co-infected with hepatitis C and treated with alpha interferon and ribavirin may constitute a special risk.
>
> Patients at increased risk should be followed closely.

Mitochondrial dysfunction: Nucleoside and nucleotide analogues have been demonstrated *in vitro* and *in vivo* to cause a variable degree of mitochondrial damage. There have been reports of mitochondrial dysfunction in HIV-negative infants exposed *in utero* and/or post-natally to nucleoside analogues. The main adverse events reported are haematological disorders (anaemia, neutropenia), metabolic disorders (hyperlactatemia, hyperlipasemia). These events are often transitory. Some late-onset neurological disorders have been reported (hypertonia, convulsion, abnormal behaviour). Whether the neurological disorders are transient or permanent is currently unknown. Any child exposed *in utero* to nucleoside and nucleotide analogues, even HIV-negative children, should have clinical and laboratory follow-up and should be fully investigated for possible mitochondrial dysfunction in case of relevant signs or symptoms. These findings do not affect current national recommendations to use antiretroviral therapy in pregnant women to prevent vertical transmission of HIV.

Lipodystrophy: Combination antiretroviral therapy has been associated with the redistribution of body fat (lipodystrophy) in HIV patients. The long-term consequences of these events are currently unknown. Knowledge about the mechanism is incomplete. A connection between visceral lipomatosis and protease inhibitors (PIs) and lipoatrophy and nucleoside reverse transcriptase inhibitors (NRTIs) has been hypothesised. A higher risk of lipodystrophy has been associated with individual factors such as older age, and with drug related factors such as longer duration of antiretroviral treatment and associated metabolic disturbances. Clinical examination should include evaluation for physical signs of fat redistribution. Consideration should be given to the measurement of fasting serum lipids and blood glucose. Lipid disorders should be managed as clinically appropriate (see section 4.8).

Immune Reactivation Syndrome: In HIV-infected patients with severe immune deficiency at the time of institution of combination antiretroviral therapy (CART), an inflammatory reaction to asymptomatic or residual opportunistic pathogens may arise and cause serious clinical conditions, or aggravation of symptoms. Typically, such reactions have been observed within the first few weeks or months of initiation of CART. Relevant examples are cytomegalovirus retinitis, generalised and/or focal mycobacterium infections, and *Pneumocystis jiroveci pneumonia* (formerly known as *Pneumocystis carinii pneumonia*). Any inflammatory symptoms should be evaluated and treatment instituted when necessary.

Liver disease: If lamivudine is being used concomitantly for the treatment of HIV and HBV, additional information relating to the use of lamivudine in the treatment of hepatitis B infection is available in the Zeffix SPC.

The safety and efficacy of zidovudine has not been established in patients with significant underlying liver disorders.

Patients with chronic hepatitis B or C and treated with combination antiretroviral therapy are at an increased risk of severe and potentially fatal hepatic adverse events. In case of concomitant antiviral therapy for hepatitis B or C, please refer also to the relevant product information for these medicinal products.

If Combivir is discontinued in patients co-infected with hepatitis B virus, periodic monitoring of both liver function tests and markers of HBV replication for 4 months is recommended, as withdrawal of lamivudine may result in an acute exacerbation of hepatitis.

Patients with pre-existing liver dysfunction, including chronic active hepatitis, have an increased frequency of liver function abnormalities during combination antiretroviral therapy, and should be monitored according to standard practice. If there is evidence of worsening liver disease in such patients, interruption or discontinuation of treatment must be considered.

Patients co-infected with hepatitis C virus: The concomitant use of ribavirin with zidovudine is not recommended due to an increased risk of anaemia (see section 4.5).

Osteonecrosis: Although the etiology is considered to be multifactorial (including corticosteroid use, alcohol consumption, severe immunosuppression, higher body mass index), cases of osteonecrosis have been reported particularly in patients with advanced HIV-disease and/or long-term exposure to combination antiretroviral therapy (CART). Patients should be advised to seek medical advice if they experience joint aches and pain, joint stiffness or difficulty in movement.

4.5 Interaction with other medicinal products and other forms of interaction

As Combivir contains lamivudine and zidovudine, any interactions that have been identified with these agents individually may occur with Combivir. The likelihood of metabolic interactions with lamivudine is low due to limited metabolism and plasma protein binding, and almost complete renal clearance. Zidovudine is primarily eliminated by hepatic conjugation to an inactive glucuronidated metabolite. Medicinal products which are primarily eliminated by hepatic metabolism especially via glucuronidation may have the potential to inhibit metabolism of zidovudine. The interactions listed below should not be considered exhaustive but are representative of the classes of medicinal products where caution should be exercised.

Lamivudine and zidovudine metabolism do not involve CYP3A, making interactions with medicinal products metabolised by this system (e.g. PIs) unlikely.

Interactions relevant to lamivudine

The possibility of interactions with other medicinal products administered concurrently with Combivir should be considered, particularly when the main route of elimination is active renal secretion, especially via the cationic transport system e.g. trimethoprim. Nucleoside analogues (e.g. zidovudine, didanosine and zalcitabine) and other medicinal products (e.g. ranitidine, cimetidine) are eliminated only in part by this mechanism and were shown not to interact with lamivudine.

Administration of trimethoprim/sulfamethoxazole 160 mg/800 mg results in a 40% increase in lamivudine exposure, because of the trimethoprim component; the sulfamethoxazole component does not interact. However, unless the patient has renal impairment, no dosage adjustment of lamivudine is necessary (see section 4.2). Lamivudine has no effect on the pharmacokinetics of trimethoprim or sulfamethoxazole. When concomitant administration with co-trimoxazole is warranted, patients should be monitored clinically. Co-administration of Combivir with high doses of co-trimoxazole for the treatment of *Pneumocystis jiroveci pneumonia* (formerly known as *Pneumocystis carinii pneumonia* [PCP]) and toxoplasmosis should be avoided.

Co-administration of lamivudine with intravenous ganciclovir or foscarnet is not recommended.

Interactions relevant to zidovudine

Limited data suggest that co-administration of zidovudine and rifampicin decreases the AUC of zidovudine by 48% ± 34%. However the clinical significance of this is unknown. Dose modifications of zidovudine in this situation have not been formally evaluated.

Limited data suggest that probenecid increases the mean half-life and area under the plasma concentration curve of zidovudine by decreasing glucuronidation. Renal excretion of the glucuronide (and possibly zidovudine itself) is reduced in the presence of probenecid. Patients receiving both medicinal products should be closely monitored for haematological toxicity.

Phenytoin blood levels have been reported to be low in some patients receiving zidovudine, while in one patient a high level was noted. These observations suggest that phenytoin concentrations should be carefully monitored in patients receiving Combivir and phenytoin.

In a pharmacokinetic study co-administration of zidovudine and atovaquone tablets showed a decrease in zidovudine clearance after oral dosing leading to a 35% ± 23% increase in plasma zidovudine AUC. The mode of interaction is unknown and as higher concentrations of atovaquone can be achieved with atovaquone suspension it is possible that greater changes in AUC values for zidovudine might be induced when atovaquone is administered as a suspension. Given the limited data available the clinical significance of this is unknown.

Valproic acid, fluconazole or methadone when co-administered with zidovudine have been shown to increase the AUC of zidovudine, with a corresponding decrease in its clearance. As only limited data are available the clinical significance is not known. If zidovudine is used concurrently with either valproic acid, fluconazole or methadone, patients should be monitored closely for potential toxicity of zidovudine.

Zidovudine and stavudine in combination are antagonistic *in vitro*, therefore the concomitant use of stavudine with Combivir should be avoided (see section 4.4).

Exacerbation of anaemia due to ribavirin has been reported when zidovudine is part of the regimen used to treat HIV although the exact mechanism remains to be elucidated. The concomitant use of ribavirin with zidovudine is not recommended due to an increased risk of anaemia (see section 4.4). Consideration should be given to replacing zidovudine in a combination ART regimen if this is already established. This would be particularly important in patients with a known history of zidovudine induced anaemia.

Concomitant treatment, especially acute therapy, with potentially nephrotoxic or myelosuppressive medicinal products (e.g. systemic pentamidine, dapsone, pyrimethamine, co-trimoxazole, amphotericin, flucytosine, ganciclovir, interferon, vincristine, vinblastine and doxorubicin) may also increase the risk of adverse reactions to zidovudine. If concomitant therapy with Combivir and any of these medicinal products is necessary then extra care should be taken in monitoring renal function and haematological parameters and, if required, the dosage of one or more agents should be reduced.

Since some patients receiving Combivir may continue to experience opportunistic infections, concomitant use of prophylactic antimicrobial therapy may have to be considered. Limited data from clinical trials do not indicate a significantly increased risk of adverse reactions to zidovudine with co-trimoxazole (see interaction information above relating to lamivudine and co-trimoxazole), aerosolised pentamidine, pyrimethamine and acyclovir at doses used in prophylaxis.

Clarithromycin tablets reduce the absorption of zidovudine. This can be avoided by separating the administration of Combivir and clarithromycin by at least two hours.

4.6 Pregnancy and lactation

Pregnancy: The safety of lamivudine in human pregnancy has not been established. No data are available for the treatment with a combination of lamivudine and zidovudine in humans or animals (see also section 5.3). The use in pregnant women of zidovudine alone, with subsequent treatment of the newborn infants, has been shown to reduce the rate of maternal-foetal transmission of HIV. However, no such data are available for lamivudine.

In humans, consistent with passive transmission of lamivudine across the placenta, lamivudine concentrations in infant serum at birth were similar to those in maternal and cord serum at delivery. Zidovudine was measured in plasma and gave similar results to those observed for lamivudine (see section 5.2).

As the active ingredients of Combivir may inhibit cellular DNA replication, any use, especially during the first trimester of pregnancy, presents a potential risk to the foetus. Consequently the administration of Combivir during pregnancy should only be considered if expected benefits outweigh any possible risks.

Pregnant women considering using Combivir during pregnancy should be made aware of the findings from animal carcinogenicity and mutagenicity studies (see section 5.3).

In men zidovudine has not been shown to affect sperm count, morphology or motility.

Lactation: Both lamivudine and zidovudine are excreted in breast milk at similar concentrations to those found in serum. It is recommended that mothers taking Combivir do not breast-feed their infants. It is recommended that HIV infected women do not breast-feed their infants under any circumstances in order to avoid transmission of HIV.

4.7 Effects on ability to drive and use machines

No studies on the effects on the ability to drive and use machines have been performed.

4.8 Undesirable effects

Adverse reactions have been reported during therapy for HIV disease with lamivudine and zidovudine separately or in combination. For many of these events, it is unclear whether they are related to lamivudine, zidovudine, the wide range of medicinal products used in the management of HIV disease, or as a result of the underlying disease process.

As Combivir contains lamivudine and zidovudine, the type and severity of adverse reactions associated with each of the compounds may be expected. There is no evidence of added toxicity following concurrent administration of the two compounds.

Cases of lactic acidosis, sometimes fatal, usually associated with severe hepatomegaly and hepatic steatosis, have been reported with the use of nucleoside analogues (see section 4.4).

Combination antiretroviral therapy has been associated with redistribution of body fat (lipodystrophy) in HIV patients including the loss of peripheral and facial subcutaneous fat, increased intra-abdominal and visceral fat, breast hypertrophy and dorsocervical fat accumulation (buffalo hump).

Combination antiretroviral therapy has been associated with metabolic abnormalities such as hypertriglyceridaemia, hypercholesterolaemia, insulin resistance, hyperglycaemia and hyperlactataemia (see section 4.4).

In HIV-infected patients with severe immune deficiency at the time of initiation of combination antiretroviral therapy (CART), an inflammatory reaction to asymptomatic or residual opportunistic infections may arise (see section 4.4).

Cases of osteonecrosis have been reported, particularly in patients with generally acknowledged risk factors, advanced HIV disease or long-term exposure to combination antiretroviral therapy (CART). The frequency of this is unknown (see section 4.4).

Lamivudine:

The adverse reactions considered at least possibly related to the treatment are listed below by body system, organ class and absolute frequency. Frequencies are defined as very common (≥1/10), common (≥1/100 to <1/10), uncommon (≥1/1000 to <1/100), rare (≥1/10,000 to <1/1000), very rare (<1/10,000). Within each frequency grouping, undesirable effects are presented in order of decreasing seriousness.

<u>Blood and lymphatic systems disorders</u>

Uncommon: Neutropenia and anaemia (both occasionally severe), thrombocytopenia

Very rare: Pure red cell aplasia

<u>Nervous system disorders</u>

Common: Headache, insomnia

Very rare: Peripheral neuropathy (or paraesthesiae)

<u>Respiratory, thoracic and mediastinal disorders</u>

Common: Cough, nasal symptoms

<u>Gastrointestinal disorders</u>

Common: Nausea, vomiting, abdominal pain or cramps, diarrhoea

Rare: Pancreatitis, rises in serum amylase

<u>Hepatobiliary disorders</u>

Uncommon: Transient rises in liver enzymes (AST, ALT)

Rare: Hepatitis

<u>Skin and subcutaneous tissue disorders</u>

Common: Rash, alopecia

<u>Musculoskeletal and connective tissue disorders</u>

Common: Arthralgia, muscle disorders

Rare: Rhabdomyolysis

<u>General disorders and administration site conditions</u>

Common: Fatigue, malaise, fever

Zidovudine:

The adverse reactions profile appears similar for adults and adolescents. The most serious adverse reactions include anaemia (which may require transfusions), neutropenia and leucopenia. These occurred more frequently at higher dosages (1200-1500 mg/day) and in patients with advanced HIV disease (especially when there is poor bone marrow reserve prior to treatment), and particularly in patients with CD4 cell counts less than 100/mm^3 (see section 4.4).

The incidence of neutropenia was also increased in those patients whose neutrophil counts, haemoglobin levels and serum vitamin B_{12} levels were low at the start of zidovudine therapy.

The adverse reactions considered at least possibly related to the treatment are listed below by body system, organ class and absolute frequency. Frequencies are defined as very common (≥1/10), common (≥1/100 to <1/10), uncommon (≥1/1000 to <1/100), rare (≥1/10,000 to <1/1000), very rare (<1/10,000). Within each frequency grouping, undesirable effects are presented in order of decreasing seriousness.

<u>Blood and lymphatic system disorders</u>

Common: Anaemia, neutropenia and leucopenia

Uncommon: Thrombocyopenia and pancytopenia (with marrow hypoplasia)

Rare: Pure red cell aplasia

Very rare: Aplastic anaemia

<u>Metabolism and nutrition disorders</u>

Rare: Lactic acidosis in the absence of hypoxaemia, anorexia

<u>Psychiatric disorders</u>

Rare: Anxiety and depression

<u>Nervous system disorders</u>

Very common: Headache

Common: Dizziness

Rare: Insomnia, paraesthesiae, somnolence, loss of mental acuity, convulsions

<u>Cardiac disorders</u>

Rare: Cardiomyopathy

<u>Respiratory, thoracic and mediastinal disorders</u>

Uncommon: Dyspnoea

Rare: Cough

<u>Gastrointestinal disorders</u>

Very common: Nausea

Common: Vomiting, abdominal pain and diarrhoea

Uncommon: Flatulence

Rare: Oral mucosa pigmentation, taste perversion and dyspepsia. Pancreatitis

<u>Hepatobiliary disorders</u>

Common: Raised blood levels of liver enzymes and bilirubin

Rare: Liver disorders such as severe hepatomegaly with steatosis

<u>Skin and subcutaneous tissue disorders</u>

Uncommon: Rash and pruritus

Rare: Nail and skin pigmentation, urticaria and sweating

<u>Musculoskeletal and connective tissue disorders</u>

Common: Myalgia

Uncommon: Myopathy

<u>Renal and urinary disorders</u>

Rare: Urinary frequency

<u>Reproductive system and breast disorders</u>

Rare: Gynaecomastia

<u>General disorders and administration site conditions</u>

Common: Malaise

Uncommon: Fever, generalised pain and asthenia

Rare: Chills, chest pain and influenza-like syndrome

The available data from both placebo-controlled and open-label studies indicate that the incidence of nausea and other frequently reported clinical adverse events consistently decreases over time during the first few weeks of therapy with zidovudine.

4.9 Overdose

There is limited experience of overdosage with Combivir. No specific symptoms or signs have been identified following acute overdose with zidovudine or lamivudine apart from those listed as undesirable effects. No fatalities occurred, and all patients recovered.

If overdosage occurs the patient should be monitored for evidence of toxicity (see section 4.8), and standard supportive treatment applied as necessary. Since lamivudine is dialysable, continuous haemodialysis could be used in the treatment of overdosage, although this has not been studied. Haemodialysis and peritoneal dialysis appear to have a limited effect on elimination of zidovudine, but enhance the elimination of the glucuronide metabolite. For more details physicians should refer to the individual prescribing information for lamivudine and zidovudine.

5. PHARMACOLOGICAL PROPERTIES

5.1 Pharmacodynamic properties

Pharmacotherapeutic group: Antivirals for treatment of HIV infections, combinations, ATC Code: J05AR01

Lamivudine and zidovudine are nucleoside analogues which have activity against HIV. Additionally, lamivudine has activity against hepatitis B virus (HBV). Both medicinal products are metabolised intracellularly to their active moieties, lamivudine 5'-triphosphate (TP) and zidovudine 5'-TP respectively. Their main modes of action are as chain terminators of viral reverse transcription. Lamivudine-TP and zidovudine-TP have selective inhibitory activity against HIV-1 and HIV-2 replication *in vitro*; lamivudine is also active against zidovudine-resistant clinical isolates of HIV. Lamivudine in combination with zidovudine exhibits synergistic anti-HIV activity against clinical isolates in cell culture.

HIV-1 resistance to lamivudine involves the development of a M184V amino acid change close to the active site of the viral reverse transcriptase (RT). This variant arises both *in vitro* and in HIV-1 infected patients treated with lamivudine-containing antiretroviral therapy. M184V mutants display greatly reduced susceptibility to lamivudine and show diminished viral replicative capacity *in vitro*. *In vitro* studies indicate that zidovudine-resistant virus isolates can become zidovudine sensitive when they simultaneously acquire resistance to lamivudine. The clinical relevance of such findings remains, however, not well defined.

In vitro data tend to suggest that the continuation of lamivudine in anti-retroviral regimen despite the development of M184V might provide residual anti-retroviral activity (likely through impaired viral fitness). The clinical relevance of these findings is not established. Indeed, the available clinical data are very limited and preclude any reliable conclusion in the field. In any case, initiation of susceptible NRTI's should always be preferred to maintenance of lamivudine therapy. Therefore, maintaining lamivudine therapy despite emergence of M184V mutation should only be considered in cases where no other active NRTIs are available

Cross-resistance conferred by the M184V RT is limited within the nucleoside inhibitor class of antiretroviral agents. Zidovudine and stavudine maintain their antiretroviral activities against lamivudine-resistant HIV-1. Abacavir maintains its antiretroviral activities against lamivudine-resistant HIV-1 harbouring only the M184V mutation. The M184V RT mutant shows a <4-fold decrease in susceptibility to didanosine and zalcitabine; the clinical significance of these findings is unknown. *In vitro* susceptibility testing has not been standardised and results may vary according to methodological factors.

Lamivudine demonstrates low cytotoxicity to peripheral blood lymphocytes, to established lymphocyte and monocyte-macrophage cell lines, and to a variety of bone marrow progenitor cells *in vitro*. Resistance to thymidine analogues (of which zidovudine is one) is well characterised and is conferred by the stepwise accumulation of up to six specific mutations in the HIV reverse transcriptase at codons 41, 67, 70, 210, 215 and 219. Viruses acquire phenotypic resistance to thymidine analogues through the combination of mutations at codons 41 and 215 or by the accumulation of at least four of the six mutations. These thymidine analogue mutations alone do not cause high-level cross-resistance to any of the other nucleosides, allowing for the subsequent use of any of the other approved reverse transcriptase inhibitors.

Two patterns of multi-drug resistance mutations, the first characterised by mutations in the HIV reverse transcriptase at codons 62, 75, 77, 116 and 151 and the second involving a T69S mutation plus a 6-base pair insert at the same position, result in phenotypic resistance to AZT as well as to the other approved NRTIs. Either of these two patterns of multinucleoside resistance mutations severely limits future therapeutic options.

Clinical Experience

In clinical trials, lamivudine in combination with zidovudine has been shown to reduce HIV-1 viral load and increase CD4 cell count. Clinical end-point data indicate that lamivudine in combination with zidovudine, results in a significant reduction in the risk of disease progression and mortality.

Lamivudine and zidovudine have been widely used as components of antiretroviral combination therapy with other antiretroviral agents of the same class (NRTIs) or different classes (PIs, non-nucleoside reverse transcriptase inhibitors).

Multiple drug antiretroviral therapy containing lamivudine has been shown to be effective in antiretrovirally-naive patients as well as in patients presenting with viruses containing the M184V mutations.

Evidence from clinical studies shows that lamivudine plus zidovudine delays the emergence of zidovudine resistant isolates in individuals with no prior antiretroviral therapy. Subjects receiving lamivudine and zidovudine with or without additional concomitant antiretroviral therapies and who already present with the M184V mutant virus also experience a delay in the onset of mutations that confer resistance to zidovudine and stavudine (Thymidine Analogue Mutations; TAMs).

The relationship between *in vitro* susceptibility of HIV to lamivudine and zidovudine and clinical response to lamivudine/zidovudine containing therapy remains under investigation.

Lamivudine at a dose of 100 mg once daily has also been shown to be effective for the treatment of adult patients with chronic HBV infection (for details of clinical studies, see the prescribing information for Zeffix). However, for the treatment of HIV infection only a 300 mg daily dose of lamivudine (in combination with other antiretroviral agents) has been shown to be efficacious.

Lamivudine has not been specifically investigated in HIV patients co-infected with HBV.

5.2 Pharmacokinetic properties

Absorption: Lamivudine and zidovudine are well absorbed from the gastrointestinal tract. The bioavailability of oral lamivudine in adults is normally between 80–85% and for zidovudine 60–70%.

A bioequivalence study compared Combivir with lamivudine 150 mg and zidovudine 300 mg tablets taken together. The effect of food on the rate and extent of absorption was also studied. Combivir was shown to be bioequivalent to lamivudine 150 mg and zidovudine 300 mg given as separate tablets, when administered to fasting subjects.

Following single dose Combivir administration in healthy volunteers, mean (CV) lamivudine and zidovudine C_{max} values were 1.6 μg/ml (32%) and 2.0 μg/ml (40%), respectively and the corresponding values for AUC were 6.1 μg h/ml (20%) and 2.4 μg h/ml (29%) respectively. The median (range) lamivudine and zidovudine t_{max} values were 0.75 (0.50-2.00) hours and 0.50 (0.25-2.00) hours respectively. The extent of lamivudine and zidovudine absorption (AUC_{∞}) and estimates of half-life following administration of Combivir with food were similar when compared to fasting subjects, although the rates of absorption (C_{max}, t_{max}) were slowed. Based on these data Combivir may be administered with or without food.

Administration of crushed tablets with a small amount of semi-solid food or liquid would not be expected to have an impact on the pharmaceutical quality, and would therefore not be expected to alter the clinical effect. This conclusion is based on the physiochemical and pharmacokinetic data assuming that the patient crushes and transfers 100% of the tablet and ingests immediately.

Distribution: Intravenous studies with lamivudine and zidovudine showed that the mean apparent volume of distribution is 1.3 and 1.6 l/kg respectively. Lamivudine exhibits linear pharmacokinetics over the therapeutic dose range and displays limited binding to the major plasma protein albumin (<36% serum albumin *in vitro*). Zidovudine plasma protein binding is 34% to 38%. Interactions involving binding site displacement are not anticipated with Combivir.

Data show that lamivudine and zidovudine penetrate the central nervous system (CNS) and reach the cerebrospinal fluid (CSF). The mean ratios of CSF/serum lamivudine and zidovudine concentrations 2-4 hours after oral administration were approximately 0.12 and 0.5 respectively. The true extent of CNS penetration of lamivudine and its relationship with any clinical efficacy is unknown.

Metabolism: Metabolism of lamivudine is a minor route of elimination. Lamivudine is predominately cleared unchanged by renal excretion. The likelihood of metabolic drug interactions with lamivudine is low due to the small extent of hepatic metabolism (5-10%) and low plasma binding.

The 5'-glucuronide of zidovudine is the major metabolite in both plasma and urine, accounting for approximately 50–80% of the administered dose eliminated by renal excretion. 3'-amino-3'-deoxythymidine (AMT) has been identified as a metabolite of zidovudine following intravenous dosing.

Elimination: The observed lamivudine half-life of elimination is 5 to 7 hours. The mean systemic clearance of lamivudine is approximately 0.32 l/h/kg, with predominantly renal clearance (>70%) via the organic cationic transport system. Studies in patients with renal impairment show lamivudine elimination is affected by renal dysfunction. Dose reduction is required for patients with creatinine clearance ⩽50 ml/min (see section 4.2).

From studies with intravenous zidovudine, the mean terminal plasma half-life was 1.1 hours and the mean systemic clearance was 1.6 l/h/kg. Renal clearance of zidovudine is estimated to be 0.34 l/h/kg, indicating glomerular filtration and active tubular secretion by the kidneys. Zidovudine concentrations are increased in patients with advanced renal failure.

Pharmacokinetics in children: In children over the age of 5-6 months, the pharmacokinetic profile of zidovudine is similar to that in adults. Zidovudine is well absorbed from the gut and at all dose levels studied in adults and children, the bioavailability was between 60-74% with a mean of 65%. Css_{max} levels were 4.45 μM (1.19 μg/ml) following a dose of 120 mg zidovudine (in solution)/m² body surface area and 7.7 μM (2.06 μg/ml) at 180 mg/m² body surface area. Dosages of 180 mg/m² four times daily in children produced similar systemic exposure (24 hour AUC 40.0 h μM or 10.7 h μg/ml) as doses of 200 mg six times daily in adults (40.7 h μM or 10.9 h μg/ml).

In six HIV-infected children from 2 to 13 years of age, zidovudine plasma pharmacokinetics were evaluated while subjects were receiving 120 mg/m² zidovudine three times daily and again after switching to 180 mg/m² twice daily. Systemic exposures (daily AUC and C_{max}) in plasma from the twice daily regimen appeared equivalent to those from the same total daily dose given in three divided doses [Bergshoeff, 2004].

In general, lamivudine pharmacokinetics in paediatric patients are similar to adults. However, absolute bioavailability (approximately 55-65%) was reduced in paediatric patients below 12 years of age. In addition, systemic clearance values were greater in younger paediatric patients and decreased with age, approaching adult values around 12 years of age. Due to these differences, the recommended dose for lamivudine in children (aged more than three months and weighing less than 30 kg) is 4 mg/kg twice a day. This dose will achieve an average AUC_{0-12} ranging from approximately 3,800 to 5,300 ng h/ml. Recent findings indicate that exposure in children <6 years of age may be reduced by about 30% compared with other age groups. Further data addressing this issue are currently awaited. At present, the available data do not suggest that lamivudine is less efficacious in this age group.

Pharmacokinetics in pregnancy: The pharmacokinetics of lamivudine and zidovudine were similar to that of non-pregnant women.

5.3 Preclinical safety data

The clinically relevant effects of lamivudine and zidovudine in combination are anaemia, neutropenia and leucopenia.

Neither lamivudine nor zidovudine are mutagenic in bacterial tests, but like many nucleoside analogues they show activity in *in vitro* mammalian tests such as the mouse lymphoma assay.

Lamivudine has not shown any genotoxic activity in *in vivo* studies at doses that gave plasma concentrations up to 40-50 times higher than clinical plasma levels. Zidovudine showed clastogenic effects in an oral repeated dose micronucleus test in mice. Peripheral blood lymphocytes from AIDS patients receiving zidovudine treatment have also been observed to contain higher numbers of chromosome breakages.

A pilot study has demonstrated that zidovudine is incorporated into leukocyte nuclear DNA of adults, including pregnant women, taking zidovudine as treatment for HIV-1 infection, or for the prevention of mother to child viral transmission. Zidovudine was also incorporated into DNA from cord blood leukocytes of infants from zidovudine-treated mothers. A transplacental genotoxicity study conducted in monkeys compared zidovudine alone with the combination of zidovudine and lamivudine at human-equivalent exposures. The study demonstrated that foetuses exposed *in utero* to the combination sustained a higher level of nucleoside analogue-DNA incorporation into multiple foetal organs, and showed evidence of more telomere shortening than in those exposed to zidovudine alone. The clinical significance of these findings is unknown.

The carcinogenic potential of a combination of lamivudine and zidovudine has not been tested.

In long-term oral carcinogenicity studies in rats and mice, lamivudine did not show any carcinogenic potential.

In oral carcinogenicity studies with zidovudine in mice and rats, late appearing vaginal epithelial tumours were observed. A subsequent intravaginal carcinogenicity study confirmed the hypothesis that the vaginal tumours were the result of long term local exposure of the rodent vaginal epithelium to high concentrations of unmetabolised zidovudine in urine. There were no other zidovudine-related tumours observed in either sex of either species.

In addition, two transplacental carcinogenicity studies have been conducted in mice. In one study, by the US National Cancer Institute, zidovudine was administered at maximum tolerated doses to pregnant mice from day 12 to 18 of gestation. One year post-natally, there was an increase in the incidence of tumours in the lung, liver and female reproductive tract of offspring exposed to the highest dose level (420 mg/kg term body weight).

In a second study, mice were administered zidovudine at doses up to 40 mg/kg for 24 months, with exposure beginning prenatally on gestation day 10. Treatment related findings were limited to late-occurring vaginal epithelial tumours, which were seen with a similar incidence and time of onset as in the standard oral carcinogenicity study. The second study thus provided no evidence that zidovudine acts as a transplacental carcinogen.

It is concluded that as the increase in incidence of tumours in the first transplacental carcinogenicity study represents a hypothetical risk, this should be balanced against the proven therapeutic benefit.

In reproductive toxicity studies lamivudine has demonstrated evidence of causing an increase in early embryonic deaths in the rabbit at relatively low systemic exposures, comparable to those achieved in man, but not in the rat even at very high systemic exposure. Zidovudine had a similar effect in both species, but only at very high systemic exposures. Lamivudine was not teratogenic in animal studies. At maternally toxic doses, zidovudine given to rats during organogenesis resulted in an increased incidence of malformations, but no evidence of foetal abnormalities was observed at lower doses.

6. PHARMACEUTICAL PARTICULARS

6.1 List of excipients

Tablet core:

Microcrystalline cellulose (E460),

sodium starch glycollate,

colloidal silicon dioxide,

magnesium stearate

Tablet film coat:

Hypromellose (E464),

titanium dioxide (E171),

macrogol 400,

polysorbate 80

6.2 Incompatibilities

Not applicable

6.3 Shelf life

2 years

6.4 Special precautions for storage

Do not store above 30°C

6.5 Nature and contents of container

Tamper-evident cartons containing opaque polyvinyl chloride/foil blister packs or white high density polyethylene (HDPE) bottle with a child-resistant closure. Each pack type contains 60 film-coated tablets.

6.6 Special precautions for disposal and other handling

No special requirements

Any unused product or waste material should be disposed of in accordance with local requirements.

7. MARKETING AUTHORISATION HOLDER

Glaxo Group Ltd

Greenford Road

Greenford

Middlesex UB6 0NN

United Kingdom

8. MARKETING AUTHORISATION NUMBER(S)

EU/1/98/058/001

EU/1/98/058/002

9. DATE OF FIRST AUTHORISATION/RENEWAL OF THE AUTHORISATION

18 March 2003

10. DATE OF REVISION OF THE TEXT
16 September 2008

Detailed information on this medicinal product is available on the website of the European Medicines Agency (EMEA) http://www.emea.europa.eu

Compound Macrogol Oral Powder Sugar Free

(Galen Limited)

1. NAME OF THE MEDICINAL PRODUCT
Compound Macrogol Oral Powder Sugar Free.

2. QUALITATIVE AND QUANTITATIVE COMPOSITION
Each sachet contains the following quantitative composition of active ingredients:

Macrogol 3350	13.125g
Sodium Chloride	350.7mg
Sodium Hydrogen Carbonate	178.5mg
Potassium Chloride	46.6mg

The content of electrolyte ions per sachet following reconstitution in 125ml of water is equivalent to:

Sodium	65mmol/l
Chloride	53mmol/l
Hydrogen Carbonate (Bicarbonate)	17mmol/l
Potassium	5.4mmol/l

For a full list of excipients, see section 6.1.

3. PHARMACEUTICAL FORM
Powder for oral solution. Single-dose sachet containing a free flowing white powder.

4. CLINICAL PARTICULARS

4.1 Therapeutic indications
For the treatment of chronic constipation. Compound Macrogol Oral Powder Sugar Free is also effective in resolving faecal impaction, defined as refractory constipation with faecal loading of the rectum and/or colon.

4.2 Posology and method of administration
Compound Macrogol Oral Powder Sugar Free is for oral use.

Chronic Constipation:

A course of treatment for chronic constipation with Compound Macrogol Oral Powder Sugar Free does not normally exceed 2 weeks, although this can be repeated if required. As for all laxatives, prolonged use is not usually recommended. Extended use may be necessary in the care of patients with severe chronic or resistant constipation, secondary to multiple sclerosis or Parkinson's Disease, or induced by regular constipating medication in particular opioids and antimuscarinics.

Adults, adolescents and the elderly: 1-3 sachets daily in divided doses, according to individual response. For extended use, the dose can be adjusted down to 1 or 2 sachets daily.

Children below 12 years old: Not recommended.

Faecal Impaction:

A course of treatment for faecal impaction with Compound Macrogol Oral Powder Sugar Free does not normally exceed 3 days.

Adults, adolescents and the elderly: 8 sachets daily, all of which should be consumed within a 6 hour period.

Children below 12 years old: Not recommended.

Patients with impaired cardiovascular function: For the treatment of faecal impaction the dose should be divided so that no more than 2 sachets are taken in any one hour.

Patients with renal insufficiency: No dosage change is necessary for the treatment of constipation or faecal impaction.

Administration:

Each sachet should be dissolved in 125 ml water. For use in faecal impaction, 8 sachets may be dissolved in 1 litre of water.

4.3 Contraindications
Compound Macrogol Oral Powder Sugar Free is contraindicated in intestinal obstruction or perforation caused by functional or structural disorder of the gut wall, ileus and in patients with severe inflammatory conditions of the intestinal tract (e.g. ulcerative colitis, Crohn's disease and toxic megacolon).

Hypersensitivity to the active substances or any of the excipients.

4.4 Special warnings and precautions for use
The faecal impaction diagnosis should be confirmed by appropriate physical or radiological examination of the rectum and abdomen.

Mild adverse drug reactions are possible as indicated in Section 4.8. If patients develop any symptoms indicating shifts of fluids/electrolytes (e.g. oedema, shortness of breath, increasing fatigue, dehydration, cardiac failure) Compound Macrogol Oral Powder Sugar Free should be stopped immediately and electrolytes measured and any abnormality should be treated appropriately.

4.5 Interaction with other medicinal products and other forms of interaction
There are no known interactions of Compound Macrogol Oral Powder Sugar Free with other medicinal products. However, macrogol 3350 raises the solubility of medicinal products that are soluble in alcohol and mainly insoluble in water. It is a theoretical possibility that absorption of these drugs could be reduced transiently. Therefore, other medicines should not be taken orally for one hour before and for one hour after taking Compound Macrogol Oral Powder Sugar Free.

4.6 Pregnancy and lactation
There is no experience with the use of Compound Macrogol Oral Powder Sugar Free during pregnancy and lactation and it should not be used during pregnancy and lactation unless clearly necessary.

4.7 Effects on ability to drive and use machines
Compound Macrogol Oral Powder Sugar Free has no influence on the ability to drive and use machines.

4.8 Undesirable effects
Immune System Disorders:

Allergic reactions are possible.

Gastro-intestinal Disorders:

Potential gastro-intestinal effects that may occur include abdominal distension and pain, borborygmi and nausea. Mild diarrhoea may also occur, but normally resolves after dose reduction.

4.9 Overdose
Severe distension or pain can be treated using nasogastric aspiration. Vomiting or diarrhoea may induce extensive fluid loss, possibly leading to electrolyte disturbances that should be treated appropriately.

5. PHARMACOLOGICAL PROPERTIES

5.1 Pharmacodynamic properties
Pharmacotherapeutic group: Osmotically acting laxatives.

ATC code: A06A D65

Macrogol 3350 induces a laxative effect through its osmotic action in the gut. This product also contains electrolytes to ensure that there is no overall gain or loss of water, potassium or sodium.

Clinical studies using the listed active substances for the treatment of chronic constipation have shown that the dose required to produce normally formed stools tends to decrease over time. For most patients, the maintenance dose will be one to two sachets per day (adjusted according to individual response).

Comparative studies in faecal impaction using active controls (e.g. enemas) have not been performed. However, results from a non-comparative study have shown that, from a population of 27 adult patients, the listed combination of active substances cleared faecal impaction in 12/27 (44%) patients after one day's treatment, increasing to 23/27 (85%) following two days' treatment and 24/27 (89%) recovered at the end of three days.

5.2 Pharmacokinetic properties
Macrogol 3350 is virtually unabsorbed from the gastro-intestinal tract and is excreted, unaltered, in faeces. Any macrogol 3350 that enters the systemic circulation is excreted in urine.

5.3 Preclinical safety data
Preclinical studies provide evidence that macrogol 3350 has no significant systemic toxicity potential, although no tests of its effects on reproduction or genotoxicity have been conducted.

There are no long-term animal toxicity or carcinogenicity studies involving macrogol 3350, although there are toxicity studies using high levels of orally administered high-molecular weight macrogols that provide evidence of safety at the recommended therapeutic dose.

6. PHARMACEUTICAL PARTICULARS

6.1 List of excipients
Acesulfame Potassium (E950)

6.2 Incompatibilities
Not applicable.

6.3 Shelf life
Sachet: Two years.

Reconstituted solution: Six hours.

6.4 Special precautions for storage
Sachet: Store below 25°C.

Reconstituted solution: Store covered in a refrigerator (2°C to 8°C).

6.5 Nature and contents of container
The sachet is composed of paper, low density polyethylene and aluminium.

Sachets are packed in cartons of 2, 8, 10, 20, 30, 50 and 100.

Not all pack sizes may be marketed.

6.6 Special precautions for disposal and other handling
No special requirements.

7. MARKETING AUTHORISATION HOLDER
Galen Limited

Seagoe Industrial Estate

Craigavon

BT63 5UA

UK

8. MARKETING AUTHORISATION NUMBER(S)
PL 21590/0088.

9. DATE OF FIRST AUTHORISATION/RENEWAL OF THE AUTHORISATION
01 May 2008

10. DATE OF REVISION OF THE TEXT
09 January 2009

Comtess 200 mg film-coated Tablets

(Orion Pharma (UK) Limited)

1. NAME OF THE MEDICINAL PRODUCT
Comtess 200 mg film-coated tablets

2. QUALITATIVE AND QUANTITATIVE COMPOSITION
Each film-coated tablet contains 200 mg entacapone.

For a full list of excipients, see section 6.1.

3. PHARMACEUTICAL FORM
Film-coated tablet

Brownish-orange, oval, biconvex film-coated tablet with "COMT" engraved on one side.

4. CLINICAL PARTICULARS

4.1 Therapeutic indications
Entacapone is indicated as an adjunct to standard preparations of levodopa/benserazide or levodopa/carbidopa for use in adult patients with Parkinson's disease and end-of-dose motor fluctuations, who cannot be stabilised on those combinations.

4.2 Posology and method of administration
Entacapone should only be used in combination with levodopa/benserazide or levodopa/carbidopa. The prescribing information for these levodopa preparations is applicable to their concomitant use with entacapone.

Posology

One 200 mg tablet is taken with each levodopa/dopa decarboxylase inhibitor dose. The maximum recommended dose is 200 mg ten times daily, i.e. 2,000 mg of entacapone.

Entacapone enhances the effects of levodopa. Hence, to reduce levodopa-related dopaminergic adverse reactions, e.g. dyskinesias, nausea, vomiting and hallucinations, it is often necessary to adjust levodopa dosage within the first days to first weeks after initiating entacapone treatment. The daily dose of levodopa should be reduced by about 10-30% by extending the dosing intervals and/or by reducing the amount of levodopa per dose, according to the clinical condition of the patient.

If entacapone treatment is discontinued, it is necessary to adjust the dosing of other antiparkinsonian treatments, especially levodopa, to achieve a sufficient level of control of the parkinsonian symptoms.

Entacapone increases the bioavailability of levodopa from standard levodopa/benserazide preparations slightly (5-10%) more than from standard levodopa/carbidopa preparations. Hence, patients who are taking standard levodopa/benserazide preparations may need a larger reduction of levodopa dose when entacapone is initiated.

Renal impairment: Renal insufficiency does not affect the pharmacokinetics of entacapone and there is no need for dose adjustment. However, for patients who are receiving dialysis therapy, a longer dosing interval may be considered (see section 5.2).

Hepatic impairment: see section 4.3.

Elderly: No dosage adjustment of entacapone is required for elderly patients.

Children: Comtess is not recommended for use in children below age 18 due to lack of data of safety and efficacy.

Method of administration

Entacapone is administered orally and simultaneously with each levodopa/carbidopa or levodopa/benserazide dose.

Entacapone can be taken with or without food (see section 5.2).

4.3 Contraindications
- Hypersensitivity to the active substance or to any of the excipients.
- Hepatic impairment.
- Phaeochromocytoma.
- Concomitant use of entacapone and non-selective monoamine oxidase (MAO-A and MAO-B) inhibitors (e.g. phenelzine, tranylcypromine).
- Concomitant use of a selective MAO-A inhibitor plus a selective MAO-B inhibitor and entacapone (see section 4.5).

- A previous history of neuroleptic malignant syndrome (NMS) and/or non-traumatic rhabdomyolysis.

4.4 Special warnings and precautions for use

Rhabdomyolysis secondary to severe dyskinesias or neuroleptic malignant syndrome (NMS) has been observed rarely in patients with Parkinson's disease.

NMS, including rhabdomyolysis and hyperthermia, is characterised by motor symptoms (rigidity, myoclonus, tremor), mental status changes (e.g. agitation, confusion, coma), hyperthermia, autonomic dysfunction (tachycardia, labile blood pressure) and elevated serum creatine phosphokinase. In individual cases, only some of these symptoms and/or findings may be evident.

Neither NMS nor rhabdomyolysis have been reported in association with entacapone treatment from controlled trials in which entacapone was discontinued abruptly. Since the introduction into the market, isolated cases of NMS have been reported, especially following abrupt reduction or discontinuation of entacapone and other concomitant dopaminergic medicinal products. When considered necessary, withdrawal of entacapone and other dopaminergic treatment should proceed slowly, and if signs and/or symptoms occur despite a slow withdrawal of entacapone, an increase in levodopa dosage may be necessary.

Because of its mechanism of action, entacapone may interfere with the metabolism of medicinal products containing a catechol group and potentiate their action. Thus, entacapone should be administered cautiously to patients being treated with medicinal products metabolised by catechol-O-methyl transferase (COMT), e.g. rimiterole, isoprenaline, adrenaline, noradrenaline, dopamine, dobutamine, alpha-methyldopa, and apomorphine (see also section 4.5).

Entacapone is always given as an adjunct to levodopa treatment. Hence, the precautions valid for levodopa treatment should also be taken into account for entacapone treatment. Entacapone increases the bioavailability of levodopa from standard levodopa/benserazide preparations 5-10% more than from standard levodopa/carbidopa preparations. Consequently, adverse dopaminergic reactions may be more frequent when entacapone is added to levodopa/benserazide treatment (see also section 4.8). To reduce levodopa-related dopaminergic adverse reactions, it is often necessary to adjust levodopa dosage within the first days to first weeks after initiating entacapone treatment, according to the clinical condition of the patient (see sections 4.2 and 4.8).

Entacapone may aggravate levodopa-induced orthostatic hypotension. Entacapone should be given cautiously to patients who are taking other medicinal products which may cause orthostatic hypotension.

In clinical studies, undesirable dopaminergic effects, e.g. dyskinesia, were more common in patients who received entacapone and dopamine agonists (such as bromocriptine), selegiline or amantadine compared to those who received placebo with this combination. The doses of other antiparkinsonian medicinal products may need to be adjusted when entacapone treatment is initiated.

Entacapone in association with levodopa has been associated with somnolence and episodes of sudden sleep onset in patients with Parkinson's disease and caution should therefore be exercised when driving or operating machines (see also section 4.7).

For patients experiencing diarrhoea, a follow-up of weight is recommended in order to avoid potential excessive weight decrease.

Pathological gambling, increased libido and hypersexuality have been reported in Parkinson's disease patients treated with dopamine agonists and other dopaminergic treatments such as entacapone in association with levodopa.

For patients who experience progressive anorexia, asthenia and weight decrease within a relatively short period of time, a general medical evaluation including liver function should be considered.

4.5 Interaction with other medicinal products and other forms of interaction

No interaction of entacapone with carbidopa has been observed with the recommended treatment schedule. Pharmacokinetic interaction with benserazide has not been studied.

In single-dose studies in healthy volunteers, no interactions were observed between entacapone and imipramine or between entacapone and moclobemide. Similarly, no interactions between entacapone and selegiline were observed in repeated-dose studies in parkinsonian patients. However, the experience of the clinical use of entacapone with several medicinal products, including MAO-A inhibitors, tricyclic antidepressants, noradrenaline reuptake inhibitors such as desipramine, maprotiline and venlafaxine, and medicinal products that are metabolised by COMT (e.g. catechol-structured compounds: rimiterole, isoprenaline, adrenaline, noradrenaline, dopamine, dobutamine, alpha-methyldopa, apomorphine, and paroxetine) is still limited. Caution should be exercised when these medicinal products are used concomitantly with entacapone (see also sections 4.3 and section 4.4).

Entacapone may be used with selegiline (a selective MAO-B inhibitor), but the daily dose of selegiline should not exceed 10 mg.

Entacapone may form chelates with iron in the gastrointestinal tract. Entacapone and iron preparations should be taken at least 2-3 hours apart (see section 4.8).

Entacapone binds to human albumin binding site II which also binds several other medicinal products, including diazepam and ibuprofen. Clinical interaction studies with diazepam and non-steroidal anti-inflammatory medicinal products have not been carried out. According to *in vitro* studies, significant displacement is not anticipated at therapeutic concentrations of the medicinal products.

Due to its affinity to cytochrome P450 2C9 *in vitro* (see section 5.2), entacapone may potentially interfere with medicinal products with metabolism dependent on this isoenzyme, such as S-warfarin.

However, in an interaction study with healthy volunteers, entacapone did not change the plasma levels of S-warfarin, while the AUC for R-warfarin increased on average by 18% [CI_{90} 11–26%]. The INR values increased on average by 13% [CI_{90} 6–19%]. Thus, control of INR is recommended when entacapone treatment is initiated for patients receiving warfarin.

4.6 Pregnancy and lactation

No overt teratogenic or primary foetotoxic effects were observed in animal studies in which the exposure levels of entacapone were markedly higher than the therapeutic exposure levels. As there is no experience in pregnant women, entacapone should not be used during pregnancy.

In animal studies entacapone was excreted in milk. The safety of entacapone in infants is unknown. Women should not breast-feed during treatment with entacapone.

4.7 Effects on ability to drive and use machines

Comtess in association with levodopa may have major influence on the ability to drive and use machines. Entacapone may, together with levodopa, cause dizziness and symptomatic orthostatism. Therefore, caution should be exercised when driving or using machines.

Patients being treated with entacapone in association with levodopa and presenting with somnolence and/or sudden sleep onset episodes must be instructed to refrain from driving or engaging in activities where impaired alertness may put themselves or others at risk of serious injury or death (e.g. operating machines) until such recurrent episodes have resolved (see also section 4.4).

4.8 Undesirable effects

The most frequent adverse reactions caused by entacapone relate to the increased dopaminergic activity and occur most commonly at the beginning of the treatment. Reduction of levodopa dosage decreases the severity and frequency of these reactions. The other major class of adverse reactions are gastrointestinal symptoms, including nausea, vomiting, abdominal pain, constipation and diarrhoea. Urine may be discoloured reddish-brown by entacapone, but this is a harmless phenomenon.

Usually the adverse reactions caused by entacapone are mild to moderate. In clinical studies the most common adverse reactions leading to discontinuation of entacapone treatment have been gastrointestinal symptoms (e.g. diarrhoea, 2.5%) and increased dopaminergic adverse reactions of levodopa (e.g. dyskinesias, 1.7%).

Dyskinesias (27%), nausea (11%), diarrhoea (8%), abdominal pain (7%) and dry mouth (4.2%) were reported significantly more often with entacapone than with placebo in pooled data from clinical studies involving 406 patients taking the medicinal product and 296 patients taking placebo.

Some of the adverse reactions, such as dyskinesia, nausea, and abdominal pain, may be more common with the higher doses (1,400 to 2,000 mg per day) than with the lower doses of entacapone.

The following adverse drug reactions, listed below in Table 1, have been accumulated both from clinical studies with entacapone and since the introduction of entacapone into the market.

Table 1. Adverse drug reactions*

Nervous system disorders Very common: Dyskinesia Common: Parkinsonism aggravated, dizziness, dystonia, hyperkinesia
Gastrointestinal disorders Very common: Nausea Common: Diarrhoea, abdominal pain, dry mouth, constipation, vomiting Very rare: Anorexia Not known: Colitis
Renal and urinary disorders Very common: Urine discoloration
Skin and subcutaneous tissue disorders Rare: Erythematous or maculopapular rash Very rare: Urticaria Not known: Skin, hair, beard and nail discolorations
General disorders and administration site conditions Common: Fatigue, sweating increased, fall Very rare: Weight decrease
Hepatobiliary disorders Rare: Hepatic function tests abnormal Not known: Hepatitis with mainly cholestatic features (see section 4.4.)
Psychiatric disorders Common: Insomnia, hallucinations, confusion, paroniria Very rare: Agitation

* Adverse reactions are ranked under headings of frequency, the most frequent first, using the following convention: Very common (≥1/10); common (≥1/100, <1/10); uncommon (≥1/1,000, <1/100); rare (≥1/10,000, <1/1,000); very rare (<1/10,000), not known (cannot be estimated from the available data, since no valid estimate can be derived from clinical trials or epidemiological studies).

Entacapone in association with levodopa has been associated with isolated cases of excessive daytime somnolence and sudden sleep onset episodes.

Parkinson's disease patients treated with dopamine agonists and other dopaminergic treatments such as entacapone in association with levodopa, especially at high doses, have been reported as exhibiting signs of pathological gambling, increased libido and hypersexuality, which were generally reversible upon reduction of the dose or treatment discontinuation.

Isolated cases of NMS have been reported following abrupt reduction or discontinuation of entacapone and other dopaminergic treatments.

Isolated cases of rhabdomyolysis have been reported.

4.9 Overdose

The post-marketing data include isolated cases of overdose in which the reported highest daily dose of entacapone has been 16,000 mg. The acute symptoms and signs in these cases of overdose included confusion, decreased activity, somnolence, hypotonia, skin discolouration and urticaria. Management of acute overdose is symptomatic.

5. PHARMACOLOGICAL PROPERTIES

5.1 Pharmacodynamic properties

Pharmacotherapeutic group: other dopaminergic agents, ATC code: NO4BX02.

Entacapone belongs to a new therapeutic class, catechol-O-methyl transferase (COMT) inhibitors. It is a reversible, specific, and mainly peripherally acting COMT inhibitor designed for concomitant administration with levodopa preparations. Entacapone decreases the metabolic loss of levodopa to 3-O-methyldopa (3-OMD) by inhibiting the COMT enzyme. This leads to a higher levodopa AUC. The amount of levodopa available to the brain is increased. Entacapone thus prolongs the clinical response to levodopa.

Entacapone inhibits the COMT enzyme mainly in peripheral tissues. COMT inhibition in red blood cells closely follows the plasma concentrations of entacapone, thus clearly indicating the reversible nature of COMT inhibition.

Clinical studies

In two phase III double-blind studies in a total of 376 patients with Parkinson's disease and end-of-dose motor fluctuations, entacapone or placebo was given with each levodopa/dopa decarboxylase inhibitor dose. The results are given in Table 2. In study I, daily ON time (hours) was measured from home diaries and in study II, the proportion of daily ON time.

Table 2. Daily ON time (Mean ± SD)

(see Table 2 on next page)

There were corresponding decreases in OFF time.

The % change from baseline in OFF time was –24% in the entacapone group and 0% in the placebo group in study I. The corresponding figures in study II were –18% and –5%.

5.2 Pharmacokinetic properties

General characteristics of the active substance

Absorption

There are large intra- and interindividual variations in the absorption of entacapone.

The peak concentration (C_{max}) in plasma is usually reached about one hour after ingestion of a 200 mg entacapone tablet. The substance is subject to extensive first-pass metabolism. The bioavailability of entacapone is about 35% after an oral dose. Food does not affect the absorption of entacapone to any significant extent.

Distribution

After absorption from the gastrointestinal tract, entacapone is rapidly distributed to the peripheral tissues with a distribution volume of 20 litres at steady state (Vd_{ss}). Approximately 92 % of the dose is eliminated during β-phase with a short elimination half-life of 30 minutes. The total clearance of entacapone is about 800 ml/min.

Entacapone is extensively bound to plasma proteins, mainly to albumin. In human plasma the unbound fraction is about 2.0% in the therapeutic concentration range. At therapeutic concentrations, entacapone does not displace other extensively bound substances (e.g. warfarin, salicylic acid, phenylbutazone, or diazepam), nor is it displaced to any significant extent by any of these substances at therapeutic or higher concentrations.

Table 2 Daily ON time (Mean ±SD)

Study I: Daily On time (h)			
	Entacapone (n=85)	Placebo (n=86)	Difference
Baseline	9.3±2.2	9.2±2.5	
Week 8-24	10.7±2.2	9.4±2.6	1 h 20 min(8.3%) $CI_{95\%}$ 45 min, 1 h 56 min
Study II: Proportion of daily On time (%)			
	Entacapone (n=103)	Placebo (n=102)	Difference
Baseline	60.0±15.2	60.8±14.0	
Week 8-24	66.8±14.5	62.8±16.80	4.5% (0 h 35 min) $CI_{95\%}$ 0.93%, 7.97%

Metabolism

A small amount of entacapone, the *(E)*-isomer, is converted to its *(Z)*-isomer. The *(E)*-isomer accounts for 95% of the AUC of entacapone. The *(Z)*-isomer and traces of other metabolites account for the remaining 5%.

Data from *in vitro* studies using human liver microsomal preparations indicate that entacapone inhibits cytochrome P450 2C9 (IC_{50}~4 µM). Entacapone showed little or no inhibition of other types of P450 isoenzymes (CYP1A2, CYP2A6, CYP2D6, CYP2E1, CYP3A and CYP2C19) (see section 4.5).

Elimination

The elimination of entacapone occurs mainly by non-renal metabolic routes. It is estimated that 80-90% of the dose is excreted in faeces, although this has not been confirmed in man. Approximately 10-20% is excreted in urine. Only traces of entacapone are found unchanged in urine. The major part (95%) of the product excreted in urine is conjugated with glucuronic acid. Of the metabolites found in urine only about 1% have been formed through oxidation.

Characteristics in patients

The pharmacokinetic properties of entacapone are similar in both young and elderly adults. The metabolism of the medicinal product is slowed in patients with mild to moderate liver insufficiency (Child-Pugh Class A and B), which leads to an increased plasma concentration of entacapone in both the absorption and elimination phases (see section 4.3). Renal impairment does not affect the pharmacokinetics of entacapone. However, a longer dosing interval may be considered for patients who are receiving dialysis therapy.

5.3 Preclinical safety data

Preclinical data revealed no special hazard for humans based on conventional studies of safety pharmacology, repeated dose toxicity, genotoxicity, and carcinogenic potential. In repeated dose toxicity studies, anaemia most likely due to iron chelating properties of entacapone was observed. Regarding reproduction toxicity, decreased foetal weight and a slightly delayed bone development were noticed in rabbits at systemic exposure levels in the therapeutic range.

6. PHARMACEUTICAL PARTICULARS

6.1 List of excipients

Tablet core:

Microcrystalline cellulose

Croscarmellose sodium

Povidone

Magnesium stearate

Film-coating:

Polyvinyl alcohol, partly hydrolysed

Talc

Macrogol

Soybean lecithin

Yellow iron oxide (E 172)

Red iron oxide (E 172)

Titanium dioxide (E 171)

6.2 Incompatibilities

Not applicable.

6.3 Shelf life

3 years.

6.4 Special precautions for storage

This medicinal product does not require any special storage conditions.

6.5 Nature and contents of container

White high-density polyethylene (HDPE) bottles with white tamper proof polypropylene (PP) closures containing 30, 60, 100 or 175 tablets.

Not all pack sizes may be marketed.

6.6 Special precautions for disposal and other handling

No special requirements.

7. MARKETING AUTHORISATION HOLDER

Orion Corporation

Orionintie 1

FI-02200 Espoo

Finland

8. MARKETING AUTHORISATION NUMBER(S)

EU/1/98/082/001-003

EU/1/98/082/005

9. DATE OF FIRST AUTHORISATION/RENEWAL OF THE AUTHORISATION

Date of first authorisation: 16.09.98

Date of last renewal: 3.9.2008

10. DATE OF REVISION OF THE TEXT

3.9.2008

Detailed information on this medicine is available on the European Medicine's Agency (EMEA) web site: http://www.emea.europa.eu

Concerta XL 18 mg - 36 mg Prolonged-Release Tablets

(Janssen-Cilag Ltd)

1. NAME OF THE MEDICINAL PRODUCT

CONCERTA XL 18 mg prolonged-release tablets.

CONCERTA XL 36 mg prolonged-release tablets.

2. QUALITATIVE AND QUANTITATIVE COMPOSITION

One tablet contains either 18 mg or 36 mg of methylphenidate hydrochloride.

Excipients: contains 6.49 mg (18 mg strength) and 14.44 mg (36 mg strength) of lactose.

For a full list of excipients, see section 6.1.

3. PHARMACEUTICAL FORM

Prolonged-release Tablet.

18 mg Tablet:

Capsule-shaped yellow tablet with "alza 18" printed on one side in black ink.

36 mg Tablet:

Capsule-shaped white tablet with "alza 36" printed on one side in black ink.

4. CLINICAL PARTICULARS

4.1 Therapeutic indications

CONCERTA® XL is indicated as part of a comprehensive treatment programme for Attention Deficit Hyperactivity Disorder (ADHD) in children (over 6 years of age) and adolescents when remedial measures alone prove insufficient. Diagnosis must be made according to DSM-IV criteria or the guidelines in ICD-10 and should be based on a complete history and evaluation of the patient. The specific aetiology of this syndrome is unknown, and there is no single diagnostic test. Adequate diagnosis requires the use of medical and special psychological, educational, and social resources. Learning may or may not be impaired. Drug treatment may not be necessary for all children with this syndrome. Therefore CONCERTA® XL treatment is not indicated in all children with ADHD and the decision to use the drug must be based on a very thorough assessment of the severity and chronicity of the child's symptoms in relation to the child's age.

Use of CONCERTA® XL should be limited to patients requiring a product with effects lasting through the day to the evening when taken in the morning. A comprehensive treatment programme for the treatment of ADHD should include other measures (psychological, educational, social) for patients with this disorder. Stimulants are not intended for use in the patient who exhibits symptoms secondary to environmental factors and/or other primary psychiatric disorders, including psychosis. Appropriate educational placement is essential, and psychosocial intervention is often helpful.

4.2 Posology and method of administration

Adults: Not applicable.

Elderly: Not applicable.

Children (under 6 years): The safety and efficacy of CONCERTA® XL in children under 6 years of age have not been established. Therefore, CONCERTA® XL should not be used in children under 6 years of age.

Children (over 6 years of age) and Adolescents: CONCERTA® XL is administered orally once daily in the morning.

CONCERTA® XL must be swallowed whole with the aid of liquids, and must not be chewed, divided, or crushed (see section 4.4 Special warnings and precautions for use).

CONCERTA® XL may be administered with or without food (see section 5.2 Pharmacokinetic properties).

Treatment must be initiated under the supervision of a specialist conversant with childhood and/or adolescence behavioural disorders.

Dosage should be individualised according to the needs and responses of the patient.

Dosage may be adjusted in 18 mg increments to a maximum of 54 mg/day taken once daily in the morning. In general, dosage adjustment may proceed at approximately weekly intervals.

Patients New to Methylphenidate: Clinical experience with CONCERTA® XL is limited in these patients (see section 5.1 Pharmacodynamic properties). CONCERTA® XL may not be indicated in all children with ADHD syndrome. Lower doses of short-acting methylphenidate formulations may be considered sufficient to treat patients new to methylphenidate. Careful dose titration by the physician in charge is required in order to avoid unnecessarily high doses of methylphenidate. The recommended starting dose of CONCERTA® XL for patients who are not currently taking methylphenidate, or for patients who are on stimulants other than methylphenidate, is 18 mg once daily.

Patients Currently Using Methylphenidate: The recommended dose of CONCERTA® XL for patients who are currently taking methylphenidate three times daily at doses of 15 to 45 mg/day is provided in Table 1. Dosing recommendations are based on current dose regimen and clinical judgement.

TABLE 1

Recommended Dose Conversion from Other Methylphenidate Regimens, where available, to CONCERTA® XL

Previous Methylphenidate Daily Dose	Recommended CONCERTA® XL Dose
5 mg Methylphenidate three times daily	18 mg once daily
10 mg Methylphenidate three times daily	36 mg once daily
15 mg Methylphenidate three times daily	54 mg once daily

Daily dosage above 54 mg is not recommended.

If improvement is not observed after appropriate dosage adjustment over a one-month period, the drug should be discontinued.

Maintenance/Extended Treatment: The long-term use of methylphenidate has not been systematically evaluated in controlled trials. The physician who elects to use CONCERTA® XL for extended periods in patients with ADHD should periodically re-evaluate the long-term usefulness of the drug for the individual patient with trial periods off medication to assess the patient's functioning without pharmacotherapy. Improvement may be sustained when the drug is either temporarily or permanently discontinued.

Dose Reduction and Discontinuation: If paradoxical aggravation of symptoms or other adverse events occur, the dosage should be reduced, or, if necessary, the drug should be discontinued. Drug treatment is usually discontinued during or after puberty.

Renal/hepatic impairment: There is no experience with the use of CONCERTA® XL in patients with renal insufficiency or hepatic insufficiency (see section 5.2 Pharmacokinetic properties).

4.3 Contraindications

CONCERTA® XL is contraindicated:

- in patients known to be hypersensitive to the active substance (methylphenidate hydrochloride) or to any of the excipients;
- in patients with marked anxiety and tension, since the drug may aggravate these symptoms;
- in patients with glaucoma;
- in patients with a family history or diagnosis of Tourette's syndrome;
- in combination with non-selective, irreversible monoamine oxidase inhibitors (MAO), and also within a minimum of 14 days following discontinuation of a non-selective, irreversible MAO inhibitor (hypertensive crises may result) (see section 4.5 Interactions with other medicinal products and other forms of interaction);

- in patients with hyperthyroidism;
- in patients with severe angina pectoris;
- in patients with cardiac arrhythmias;
- in patients with severe hypertension;
- in patients who currently exhibit severe depression, anorexia nervosa, psychotic symptoms or suicidal tendency, since the drug might worsen these conditions;
- in patients with known drug dependence or alcoholism;
- in patients during pregnancy (see sections 4.6 Pregnancy and lactation and 5.3 Preclinical safety data).

4.4 Special warnings and precautions for use

Pre-existing structural cardiac abnormalities

Sudden death has been reported in association with the use of stimulants of the central nervous system at usual doses in children with structural cardiac abnormalities. Although some structural cardiac abnormalities alone may carry an increased risk of sudden death, stimulant products are not recommended in children or adolescents with known structural cardiac abnormalities.

Hypertension and other cardiovascular conditions

Use cautiously in patients with hypertension. Blood pressure should be monitored at appropriate intervals in patients taking CONCERTA® XL, especially patients with hypertension. In the laboratory classroom clinical trials, both CONCERTA® XL and methylphenidate three times daily increased resting pulse by an average of 2 to 6 bpm and produced average increases of systolic and diastolic blood pressure of roughly 1 to 4 mm Hg during the day, relative to placebo. Therefore, caution is indicated in treating patients whose underlying medical conditions might be compromised by increases in blood pressure or heart rate.

Use in children under 6 years of age

CONCERTA® XL should not be used in children under 6 years old. The safety and efficacy of CONCERTA® XL in this age group have not been established.

Potential for gastrointestinal obstruction

Because the CONCERTA® XL tablet is nondeformable and does not appreciably change in shape in the gastrointestinal (GI) tract, it should not ordinarily be administered to patients with pre-existing severe GI narrowing (pathologic or iatrogenic) or in patients with dysphagia or significant difficulty in swallowing tablets. There have been rare reports of obstructive symptoms in patients with known strictures in association with the ingestion of drugs in nondeformable prolonged-release formulations.

Due to the prolonged-release design of the tablet, CONCERTA® XL should only be used in patients who are able to swallow the tablet whole. Patients should be informed that CONCERTA® XL must be swallowed whole with the aid of liquids. Tablets should not be chewed, divided, or crushed. The medication is contained within a nonabsorbable shell designed to release the drug at a controlled rate. The tablet shell is eliminated from the body; patients should not be concerned if they occasionally notice in their stool something that looks like a tablet.

Choice of methylphenidate formulation

The choice between treatment with either CONCERTA® XL or an immediate release formulation, containing methylphenidate, will have to be decided by the treating physician on an individual basis and depends on the intended duration of effect.

Tics

CNS stimulants, including methylphenidate, have been associated with the onset or exacerbation of motor and verbal tics. Therefore, clinical evaluation for tics in children should precede use of stimulant medication. Family history should be assessed.

Fatigue

It should not be used for the prevention or treatment of normal fatigue states.

Psychosis/Mania

Clinical experience suggests that in psychotic patients, administration of methylphenidate may exacerbate symptoms of behaviour disturbance and thought disorder.

Psychotic (e.g., hallucinations) or manic symptoms have been reported in patients without a prior history of psychotic illness or mania during treatment with CONCERTA® XL at usual doses. If such symptoms occur, consideration should be given to a possible causal role of CONCERTA® XL and discontinuation of treatment may be appropriate (see Section 4.8).

Drug dependence

CONCERTA® XL should be given cautiously to patients with a history of drug dependence or alcoholism. Chronic abusive use can lead to marked tolerance and psychological dependence with varying degrees of abnormal behaviour. Frank psychotic episodes can occur, especially with parenteral abuse. Careful supervision is required during withdrawal from abusive use since severe depression may occur. Withdrawal following chronic therapeutic use may unmask symptoms of the underlying disorder that may require follow-up.

Seizures

There is some clinical evidence that methylphenidate may lower the convulsive threshold in patients with prior history of seizures, in patients with prior EEG abnormalities in absence of seizures, and, very rarely, in absence of history of seizures and no prior EEG evidence of seizures. In the presence of seizures, the drug should be discontinued.

Aggression

Patients beginning treatment with CONCERTA® XL should be monitored for the appearance or worsening of aggressive behaviour. Aggression is frequently associated with ADHD; however, emergence or worsening of aggression has been reported during treatment with CONCERTA® XL (see Section 4.8).

Haematological monitoring

Periodic full blood count, differential, and platelet counts are advised during prolonged therapy.

Visual disturbance

Symptoms of visual disturbances have been encountered in rare cases.

Difficulties with accommodation and blurring of vision have been reported.

Long term suppression of growth

Sufficient data on the safety of long-term use of methylphenidate in children are not yet available. Although a causal relationship has not been established, suppression of growth (ie, weight gain, and/or height) has been reported with the long-term use of stimulants in children. Therefore, patients requiring long-term therapy should be carefully monitored. Patients who are not growing or gaining weight as expected should have their treatment interrupted temporarily.

Use in sports persons

Sport: This product contains methylphenidate which results in a positive result during drug testing.

Use of contraception

Females of child-bearing potential (females post-menarche) should use effective contraception (see section 4.6 Pregnancy and lactation).

Galactose intolerance

This medicinal product contains lactose: patients with rare hereditary problems of galactose intolerance, the Lapp lactase deficiency or glucose-galactose malabsorption should not take this medicine.

4.5 Interaction with other medicinal products and other forms of interaction

CONCERTA® XL should not be used in patients being treated (currently or within the preceding 2 weeks) with non-selective, irreversible MAO inhibitors (see section 4.3 Contraindications).

Because of possible increases in blood pressure, CONCERTA® XL should be used cautiously with vasopressor agents (see section 4.4 Special warnings and precautions for use).

Formal drug-drug interaction studies have not been performed with CONCERTA® XL. Hence, the interaction potential is not fully elucidated. It is not known how methylphenidate may affect plasma concentrations of concomitantly administered drugs. Caution is recommended at combination of methylphenidate with other drugs, especially those with a narrow therapeutic window. Case reports have indicated that methylphenidate may inhibit the metabolism of coumarin anticoagulants, anticonvulsants (eg, phenobarbital, phenytoin, primidone), and some antidepressants (tricyclics and selective serotonin reuptake inhibitors). Downward dose adjustment of these drugs may be required when given concomitantly with methylphenidate. It may be necessary to adjust the dosage and monitor plasma drug concentrations (or, in the case of coumarin, coagulation times), when initiating or discontinuing concomitant methylphenidate.

Halogenated anaesthetics: There is a risk of sudden blood pressure increase during surgery. If surgery is planned, methylphenidate treatment should not be used on the day of surgery.

Alcohol may exacerbate the adverse CNS effect of psychoactive drugs, including CONCERTA®XL. It is therefore advisable for patients to abstain from alcohol during treatment.

4.6 Pregnancy and lactation

Women of childbearing potential/Contraception

Females of child-bearing potential (females post-menarche) should use effective contraception.

Pregnancy

CONCERTA® XL is contraindicated during pregnancy (see section 4.3 Contraindications).

There are no adequate data from the use of methylphenidate in pregnant women.

Studies in animals have shown reproductive toxicity (teratogenic effects) of methylphenidate (see section 5.3 Preclinical safety data). The potential risk for humans is unknown.

From observations in humans there are indications that amfetamines could be harmful to the foetus.

Lactation

It is not known whether methylphenidate or its metabolites pass into breast milk, but for safety reasons breast-feeding mothers should not use CONCERTA®XL.

4.7 Effects on ability to drive and use machines

No studies have been performed on the effects of CONCERTA® XL on the ability to drive and use machines. However, CONCERTA® XL may cause dizziness. It is therefore advisable to exercise caution when driving, operating machinery, or engaging in other potentially hazardous activities.

4.8 Undesirable effects

The most commonly reported adverse drug reaction is headache occurring in approximately 13% of patients.

Frequency estimate: very common ($\geq$ 1/10); common ($\geq$ 1/100 to $<$ 1/10); uncommon ($\geq$ 1/1000 to $<$ 1/100); rare ($\geq$ 1/10,000 to $<$1/1000); very rare ($<$1/10,000), not known (cannot be estimated from the available data).

(see Table 2 on next page)

Undesirable effects noted with other methylphenidate formulations:

In addition to the above reactions observed with CONCERTA® XL, the following adverse reactions have been noted with the use of other methylphenidate products:

Nervous system disorders: Choreoathetoid movements, Tourette's syndrome, poorly documented neuroleptic malignant syndrome (NMS).

Hepatobiliary disorders: Hepatic coma.

Vascular disorders: Cerebral arteritis, and/or occlusion.

Miscellaneous: Growth retardation during prolonged use in children.

4.9 Overdose

The prolonged release of methylphenidate from CONCERTA® XL should be considered when treating patients with overdose.

Signs and Symptoms: Signs and symptoms of acute methylphenidate overdosage, resulting principally from overstimulation of the CNS and from excessive sympathomimetic effects, may include the following: vomiting, agitation, tremors, hyperreflexia, muscle twitching, convulsions (may be followed by coma), euphoria, confusion, hallucinations, delirium, sweating, flushing, headache, hyperpyrexia, tachycardia, palpitations, cardiac arrhythmias, hypertension, mydriasis, and dryness of mucous membranes.

Recommended Treatment: Treatment consists of appropriate supportive measures. The patient must be protected against self-injury and against external stimuli that would aggravate overstimulation already present. Gastric contents may be evacuated by gastric lavage as indicated. Before performing gastric lavage, control agitation and seizures if present and protect the airway. Other measures to detoxify the gut include administration of activated charcoal and a cathartic. Intensive care must be provided to maintain adequate circulation and respiratory exchange; external cooling procedures may be required for hyperpyrexia.

Efficacy of peritoneal dialysis or extracorporeal haemodialysis for CONCERTA® XL overdosage has not been established.

5. PHARMACOLOGICAL PROPERTIES

5.1 Pharmacodynamic properties

Pharmacotherapeutic group: psychoanaleptics, psychostimulants and nootropics, centrally acting sympathomimetics: ATC code: N06BA04

Methylphenidate HCl is a mild central nervous system (CNS) stimulant. The mode of therapeutic action in Attention Deficit Hyperactivity Disorder (ADHD) is not known. Methylphenidate is thought to block the reuptake of noradrenaline and dopamine into the presynaptic neurone and increase the release of these monoamines into the extraneuronal space. Methylphenidate is a racemic mixture comprised of the d- and l-isomers. The d-isomer is more pharmacologically active than the l-isomer.

In the pivotal clinical studies, CONCERTA® XL was assessed in 321 patients already stabilised with immediate release preparations (IR) of methylphenidate and in 95 patients not previously treated with IR preparations of methylphenidate.

Clinical studies showed that the effects of CONCERTA® XL were maintained until 12 hours after dosing when the product was taken once daily in the morning.

5.2 Pharmacokinetic properties

Absorption: Methylphenidate is readily absorbed. Following oral administration of CONCERTA® XL to adults the drug overcoat dissolves, providing an initial maximum drug concentration at about 1 to 2 hours. The methylphenidate contained in the two internal drug layers is gradually released over the next several hours. Peak plasma concentrations are achieved at about 6 to 8 hours, after which plasma levels of methylphenidate gradually decrease. CONCERTA® XL taken once daily minimises the fluctuations between peak and trough concentrations associated with immediate-release methylphenidate three times daily. The extent of absorption of CONCERTA® XL once daily is generally comparable to conventional immediate release preparations.

Following the administration of CONCERTA® XL 18 mg once daily in 36 adults, the mean pharmacokinetic parameters were: C_{max} 3.7 ± 1.0 (ng/mL), T_{max} 6.8 ± 1.8 (h), AUC_{inf} 41.8 ± 13.9 (ng.h/mL), and $t_{½}$ 3.5 ± 0.4 (h).

Table 2

System Organ Class	Adverse Drug Reaction				
	Frequency				
	Very common	Common	Uncommon	Rare	Not known
Infections and infestations		Nasopharyngitis			
Blood and lymphatic system disorders					Leucopenia, Pancytopenia, Thrombocytopenia, Thrombocytopenic purpura
Metabolism and nutrition disorders			Anorexia, Decreased appetite		
Psychiatric disorders		Insomnia, Tic, Aggression, Anxiety, Affect lability	Depression, Sleep disorder, Mood altered, Mood swings, Anger, Agitation, Hypervigilance, Tearfulness, Drug-induced psychosis (e.g. hallucinations), Restlessness, Nervousness, Suicidal ideation[1]	Disorientation, Mania	Confusional state, Suicide attempt[1]
Nervous system disorders	Headache	Dizziness	Somnolence, Psychomotor hyperactivity, Tremor, Sedation		Convulsions, Grand mal convulsions
Eye disorders			Vision blurred, Diplopia	Mydriasis, Visual disturbance	
Cardiac disorders			Tachycardia, Palpitation		Angina pectoris, Bradycardia, Extrasystoles, Supraventricular tachycardia, Ventricular extrasystoles
Vascular disorders			Hypertension		Raynaud's phenomenon
Respiratory, thoracic and mediastinal disorders		Cough, Pharyngolaryngeal pain	Dyspnoea		
Gastrointestinal disorders		Abdominal pain, Vomiting, Nausea, Diarrhoea, Stomach discomfort	Constipation		
Skin and subcutaneous tissue disorders			Alopecia, Rash	Erythema, Hyperhidrosis, Rash macular	
Musculoskeletal, connective tissue and bone disorders			Myalgia, Arthralgia, Muscle twitching		
Immune System Disorders			Hypersensitivity reactions such as Angioedema, Anaphylactic reactions, Auricular swelling, Bullous conditions, Exfoliative conditions, Urticarias, Pruritus, Rashes, and Eruptions		
General disorders and administration site conditions		Irritability, Pyrexia	Fatigue, Chest pain		Chest discomfort, Hyperpyrexia
Investigations		Weight decreased	Blood pressure increased, Cardiac murmur, Hepatic enzyme increased		Blood alkaline phosphatase increased, Blood bilirubin increased, Platelet count decreased, White blood cell count abnormal

[1]Reports of suicidal ideation and/or suicide attempt have been received in patients treated with CONCERTA® XL. The role of CONCERTA® XL in these cases is uncertain.

No differences in the pharmacokinetics of CONCERTA® XL were noted following single and repeated once daily dosing, indicating no significant drug accumulation. The AUC and $t_{1/2}$ following repeated once daily dosing are similar to those following the first dose of CONCERTA® XL 18 mg.

Following administration of CONCERTA® XL in single doses of 18, 36, and 54 mg/day to adults, C_{max} and $AUC_{(0-inf)}$ of methylphenidate were proportional to dose.

Distribution: Plasma methylphenidate concentrations in adults decline biexponentially following oral administration. The half-life of methylphenidate in adults following oral administration of CONCERTA® XL was approximately 3.5 h. The rate of protein binding of methylphenidate and of its metabolites is approximately 15%. The apparent volume of distribution of methylphenidate is approximately 13 litres/kg.

Metabolism: In humans, methylphenidate is metabolised primarily by de-esterification to alpha-phenyl-piperidine acetic acid (PPA, approximately 50 fold the level of the unchanged substance) which has little or no pharmacologic activity. In adults the metabolism of CONCERTA® XL once daily as evaluated by metabolism to PPA is similar to that of methylphenidate three times daily. The metabolism of single and repeated once daily doses of CONCERTA® XL is similar.

Excretion: The elimination half-life of methylphenidate in adults following administration of CONCERTA® XL was approximately 3.5 hours. After oral administration, about 90% of the dose is excreted in urine and 1 to 3% in faeces, as metabolites within 48 to 96 hours. Small quantities of unchanged methylphenidate are recovered in urine (less than 1%). The main urinary metabolite is alpha-phenyl-piperidine acetic acid (60-90%).

After oral dosing of radiolabelled methylphenidate in humans, about 90% of the radioactivity was recovered in urine. The main urinary metabolite was PPA, accounting for approximately 80% of the dose.

Food Effects: In patients, there were no differences in either the pharmacokinetics or the pharmacodynamic performance of CONCERTA® XL when administered after a high fat breakfast on an empty stomach.

Special Populations

Gender: In healthy adults, the mean dose-adjusted $AUC_{(0-inf)}$ values for CONCERTA® XL were 36.7 ng.h/mL in men and 37.1 ng.h/mL in women, with no differences noted between the two groups.

Race: In healthy adults receiving CONCERTA® XL, dose-adjusted $AUC_{(0-inf)}$ was consistent across ethnic groups; however, the sample size may have been insufficient to detect ethnic variations in pharmacokinetics.

Age: The pharmacokinetics of CONCERTA® XL has not been studied in children younger than 6 years of age. In children 7-12 years of age, the pharmacokinetics of CONCERTA® XL after 18, 36 and 54 mg were (mean±SD): C_{max} 6.0±1.3, 11.3±2.6, and 15.0±3.8 ng/mL, respectively, T_{max} 9.4±0.02, 8.1±1.1, 9.1±2.5 h, respectively, and $AUC_{0-11.5}$ 50.4±7.8, 87.7±18.2, 121.5±37.3 ng.h/mL, respectively.

Renal Insufficiency: There is no experience with the use of CONCERTA® XL in patients with renal insufficiency. After oral administration of radiolabelled methylphenidate in humans, methylphenidate was extensively metabolised and approximately 80% of the radioactivity was excreted in the urine in the form of PPA. Since renal clearance is not an important route of methylphenidate clearance, renal insufficiency is expected to have little effect on the pharmacokinetics of CONCERTA® XL.

Hepatic Insufficiency: There is no experience with the use of CONCERTA® XL in patients with hepatic insufficiency.

5.3 Preclinical safety data

There is evidence that methylphenidate may be a teratogen in two species. Spina bifida and limb malformations have been reported in rabbits whilst in the rat, equivocal evidence of induction of abnormalities of the vertebrae was found.

Methylphenidate did not affect reproductive performance or fertility at low multiples (2-5 times) of the therapeutic human dose.

There was no evidence of carcinogenicity in the rat. In mice, methylphenidate caused an increase in hepatocellular adenomas, in animals of both sexes and, in males only, hepatoblastomas. In the absence of exposure data, the significance of these findings to humans is not known.

The weight of evidence from the genotoxicity studies reveals no special hazard for humans.

6. PHARMACEUTICAL PARTICULARS

6.1 List of excipients

Butylhydroxytoluene (E321)

Cellulose acetate 398-10

Hypromellose 3cp

Phosphoric acid concentrated

Poloxamer 188

Polyethylene oxides 200K and 7000K

Povidone K29-32

Sodium chloride

Stearic acid

Succinic acid

Black iron oxide (E172)

Ferric oxide yellow (E172)

Film Coat:

Ferric oxide yellow (E172) (18 mg tablet only)

Hypromellose 15cp

Lactose monohydrate

Stearic acid (18 mg tablet only)

Titanium dioxide (E171)

Triacetin

Clear Coat:

Carnauba wax

Hypromellose 6cp

Macrogol 400

Printing Ink:

Black iron oxide (E172)

Hypromellose 6cp

Isopropyl alcohol

Propylene glycol

Purified water

6.2 Incompatibilities

Not applicable.

6.3 Shelf life

3 years

6.4 Special precautions for storage

Keep the bottle tightly closed. Do not store above 30°C.

6.5 Nature and contents of container

High-density polyethylene (HDPE) bottle with a child-resistant polypropylene closure with one or two desiccants enclosed.

28 or 30 tablets.

Not all pack sizes may be marketed.

6.6 Special precautions for disposal and other handling

No special requirements.

7. MARKETING AUTHORISATION HOLDER

Janssen-Cilag Limited

50-100 Holmers Farm Way

High Wycombe

Buckinghamshire

HP12 4EG

UK

8. MARKETING AUTHORISATION NUMBER(S)

18 mg Tablets: PL 00242/0372

36 mg Tablets: PL 00242/0373

9. DATE OF FIRST AUTHORISATION/RENEWAL OF THE AUTHORISATION

Date of first authorisation: 19 February 2002

Date of last renewal: 6 June 2007

10. DATE OF REVISION OF THE TEXT

29th July 2008

Concerta XL 27 mg Prolonged-Release Tablets

(Janssen-Cilag Ltd)

1. NAME OF THE MEDICINAL PRODUCT

CONCERTA® XL 27 mg prolonged-release tablets.

2. QUALITATIVE AND QUANTITATIVE COMPOSITION

One prolonged release tablet contains 27 mg of methylphenidate hydrochloride.

Excipients: contains 4.94mg lactose.

For a full list of excipients, see section 6.1.

3. PHARMACEUTICAL FORM

Prolonged-release Tablet.

Capsule-shaped grey tablet with "alza 27" printed on one side in black ink.

4. CLINICAL PARTICULARS

4.1 Therapeutic indications

CONCERTA® XL is indicated as part of a comprehensive treatment programme for Attention Deficit Hyperactivity Disorder (ADHD) in children (over 6 years of age) and adolescents when remedial measures alone prove insufficient. Diagnosis must be made according to DSM-IV criteria or the guidelines in ICD-10 and should be based on a complete history and evaluation of the patient. The specific aetiology of this syndrome is unknown, and there is no single diagnostic test. Adequate diagnosis requires the use of medical and special psychological, educational, and social resources. Learning may or may not be impaired. Medicinal product treatment may not be necessary for all children with this syndrome. Therefore CONCERTA® XL treatment is not indicated in all children with ADHD and the decision to use the medicinal product must be based on a very thorough assessment of the severity and chronicity of the child's symptoms in relation to the child's age.

Use of CONCERTA® XL should be limited to patients requiring a product with effects lasting through the day to the evening when taken in the morning. A comprehensive treatment programme for the treatment of ADHD should include other measures (psychological, educational, social) for patients with this disorder. Stimulants are not intended for use in the patient who exhibits symptoms secondary to environmental factors and/or other primary psychiatric disorders, including psychosis. Appropriate educational placement is essential, and psychosocial intervention is often helpful.

4.2 Posology and method of administration

Adults: Not applicable.

Elderly: Not applicable.

Children (under 6 years): The safety and efficacy of CONCERTA XL in children under 6 years of age have not been established. Therefore, CONCERTA XL should not be used in children under 6 years of age.

Children (over 6 years of age) and Adolescents: CONCERTA® XL is administered orally once daily in the morning.

CONCERTA® XL must be swallowed whole with the aid of liquids, and must not be chewed, divided, or crushed (see section 4.4.).

CONCERTA® XL may be administered with or without food (see section 5.2.).

Treatment must be initiated under the supervision of a specialist conversant with childhood and/or adolescence behavioural disorders.

Dosage should be individualised according to the needs and responses of the patient.

Dosage may be adjusted in 18 mg increments to a maximum of 54 mg/day taken once daily in the morning. A 27 mg dosage strength is available for those who wish to prescribe between the 18 mg and 36 mg dosages. In general, dosage adjustment may proceed at approximately weekly intervals.

Patients New to Methylphenidate: Clinical experience with CONCERTA® XL is limited in these patients (see section 5.1). CONCERTA® XL may not be indicated in all children with ADHD syndrome. Lower doses of short-acting methylphenidate formulations may be considered sufficient to treat patients new to methylphenidate. Careful dose titration by the physician in charge is required in order to avoid unnecessarily high doses of methylphenidate. The recommended starting dose of CONCERTA® XL for patients who are not currently taking methylphenidate, or for patients who are on stimulants other than methylphenidate, is 18 mg once daily.

Patients Currently Using Methylphenidate: The recommended dose of CONCERTA® XL for patients who are currently taking methylphenidate three times daily at doses of 15 to 45 mg/day is provided in Table 1. Dosing recommendations are based on current dose regimen and clinical judgement.

TABLE 1
Recommended Dose Conversion from Other Methylphenidate hydrochloride Regimens, where available, to CONCERTA® XL

Previous Methylphenidate Daily Dose	Recommended CONCERTA® XL Dose
5 mg methylphenidate three times daily	18 mg once daily
10 mg methylphenidate three times daily	36 mg once daily
15 mg methylphenidate three times daily	54 mg once daily

Daily dosage above 54 mg is not recommended.

If improvement is not observed after appropriate dosage adjustment over a one-month period, the medicinal product should be discontinued.

Maintenance/Extended Treatment: The long-term use of methylphenidate has not been systematically evaluated in controlled trials. The physician who elects to use CONCERTA® XL for extended periods in patients with ADHD should periodically re-evaluate the long-term usefulness of the medicinal product for the individual patient with trial periods off medication to assess the patient's functioning without pharmacotherapy. Improvement may be sustained when the medicinal product is either temporarily or permanently discontinued.

Dose Reduction and Discontinuation: If paradoxical aggravation of symptoms or other adverse events occur, the dosage should be reduced, or, if necessary, the medicinal product should be discontinued. Medicinal product treatment is usually discontinued during or after puberty.

Renal or hepatic impairment: There is no experience with the use of CONCERTA XL in patients with renal insufficiency or hepatic insufficiency (see section 5.2).

4.3 Contraindications

CONCERTA® XL is contraindicated:

- in patients with hypersensitivity to the active substance or to any other excipients;
- in patients with marked anxiety and tension, since the active ingredient may aggravate these symptoms;
- in patients with glaucoma;
- in patients with a family history or diagnosis of Tourette's syndrome;
- in combination with non-selective, irreversible monoamine oxidase inhibitors (MAO), and also within a minimum of 14 days following discontinuation of a non-selective, irreversible MAO inhibitor (hypertensive crises may result) (see section 4.5.)
- in patients with hyperthyroidism;
- in patients with severe angina pectoris;
- in patients with cardiac arrhythmias;
- in patients with severe hypertension;
- in patients who currently exhibit severe depression, anorexia nervosa, psychotic symptoms or suicidal tendency, since the active ingredient might worsen these conditions;
- in patients with known drug dependence or alcoholism;
- in patients during pregnancy (see sections 4.6. and 5.3.).

4.4 Special warnings and precautions for use

Pre-existing structural cardiac abnormalities

Sudden death has been reported in association with the use of stimulants of the central nervous system at usual doses in children with structural cardiac abnormalities. Although some structural cardiac abnormalities alone may carry an increased risk of sudden death, stimulant products are not recommended in children or adolescents with known structural cardiac abnormalities.

Hypertension and other cardiovascular conditions

Use cautiously in patients with hypertension. Blood pressure should be monitored at appropriate intervals in patients taking CONCERTA® XL, especially patients with hypertension. In the laboratory classroom clinical trials, both CONCERTA® XL and methylphenidate three times daily increased resting pulse by an average of 2 to 6 bpm and produced average increases of systolic and diastolic blood pressure of roughly 1 to 4 mm Hg during the day, relative to placebo. Therefore, caution is indicated in treating patients whose underlying medical conditions might be compromised by increases in blood pressure or heart rate.

Use in children under 6 years of age

CONCERTA® XL should not be used in children under 6 years old. The safety and efficacy of CONCERTA® XL in this age group have not been established.

Potential for gastrointestinal obstruction

Because the CONCERTA® XL tablet is nondeformable and does not appreciably change in shape in the gastrointestinal (GI) tract, it should not ordinarily be administered to patients with pre-existing severe GI narrowing (pathologic or iatrogenic) or in patients with dysphagia or significant difficulty in swallowing tablets. There have been rare reports of obstructive symptoms in patients with known strictures in association with the ingestion of medicinal products in nondeformable prolonged-release formulations.

Due to the prolonged-release design of the tablet, CONCERTA® XL should only be used in patients who are able to swallow the tablet whole. Patients should be informed that CONCERTA® XL must be swallowed whole with the aid of liquids. Tablets should not be chewed, divided, or crushed. The medication is contained within a nonabsorbable shell designed to release the active ingredient at a controlled rate. The tablet shell is eliminated from the body; patients should not be concerned if they occasionally notice in their stool something that looks like a tablet.

Choice of methylphenidate formulation

The choice between treatment with either CONCERTA® XL or an immediate release formulation, containing methylphenidate, will have to be decided by the treating physician on an individual basis and depends on the intended duration of effect.

Tics

CNS stimulants, including methylphenidate, have been associated with the onset or exacerbation of motor and verbal tics. Therefore, clinical evaluation for tics in children should precede use of stimulant medication. Family history should be assessed.

Fatigue

It should not be used for the prevention or treatment of normal fatigue states.

Psychosis/Mania

Clinical experience suggests that in psychotic patients, administration of methylphenidate may exacerbate symptoms of behaviour disturbance and thought disorder.

Psychotic (e.g., hallucinations) or manic symptoms have been reported in patients without a prior history of psychotic illness or mania during treatment with CONCERTA® XL at usual doses. If such symptoms occur, consideration should be given to a possible causal role of CONCERTA® XL and discontinuation of treatment may be appropriate (see Section 4.8).

Drug dependence

CONCERTA® XL should be given cautiously to patients with a history of drug dependence or alcoholism. Chronic abusive use can lead to marked tolerance and psychological dependence with varying degrees of abnormal behaviour. Frank psychotic episodes can occur, especially with parenteral abuse. Careful supervision is required during withdrawal from abusive use since severe depression may occur. Withdrawal following chronic therapeutic use may unmask symptoms of the underlying disorder that may require follow-up.

Seizures

There is some clinical evidence that methylphenidate may lower the convulsive threshold in patients with prior history of seizures, in patients with prior EEG abnormalities in absence of seizures, and, very rarely, in absence of history of seizures and no prior EEG evidence of seizures. In the presence of seizures, the medicinal product should be discontinued.

Aggression

Patients beginning treatment with CONCERTA® XL should be monitored for the appearance or worsening of aggressive behaviour. Aggression is frequently associated with ADHD; however, emergence or worsening of aggression has been reported during treatment with CONCERTA® XL (see Section 4.8).

Haematological monitoring

Periodic full blood count, differential, and platelet counts are advised during prolonged therapy.

Visual disturbance

Symptoms of visual disturbances have been encountered in rare cases.

Difficulties with accommodation and blurring of vision have been reported.

Long term suppression of growth

Sufficient data on the safety of long-term use of methylphenidate in children are not yet available. Although a causal relationship has not been established, suppression of growth (ie, weight gain, and/or height) has been reported with the long-term use of stimulants in children. Therefore, patients requiring long-term therapy should be carefully monitored. Patients who are not growing or gaining weight as expected should have their treatment interrupted temporarily.

Use in sports persons

Sport: This product contains methylphenidate which results in a positive result during drug testing.

Use of contraception

Females of child-bearing potential (females post-menarche) should use effective contraception.

Galactose intolerance

This medicinal product contains lactose: patients with rare hereditary problems of galactose intolerance, the Lapp lactase deficiency or glucose-galactose malabsorption should not take this medicine.

4.5 Interaction with other medicinal products and other forms of interaction

CONCERTA® XL must not be used in patients being treated (currently or within the preceding 2 weeks) with non-selective, irreversible MAO inhibitors (see section 4.3).

Because of possible increases in blood pressure, CONCERTA® XL should be used cautiously with vasopressor agents (see section 4.4).

Formal drug-drug interaction studies have not been performed with CONCERTA® XL. Hence, the interaction potential is not fully elucidated. It is not known how methylphenidate may affect plasma concentrations of concomitantly administered medicinal products. Caution is recommended at combination of methylphenidate with other medicinal products, especially those with a narrow therapeutic window. Case reports have indicated that methylphenidate may inhibit the metabolism of coumarin anticovaulants, anticonvulsants (eg, phenobarbital, phenytoin, primidone), and some antidepressants (tricyclics and selective serotonin reuptake inhibitors). Downward dose adjustment of these medicinal products may be required when given concomitantly with methylphenidate. It may be necessary to adjust the dosage and monitor plasma active ingredient concentrations (or, in the case of coumarin, coagulation times), when initiating or discontinuing concomitant methylphenidate.

Halogenated anaesthetics: There is a risk of sudden blood pressure increase during surgery. If surgery is planned, methylphenidate treatment should not be used on the day of surgery.

Alcohol may exacerbate the adverse CNS effect of psychoactive medicinal products, including CONCERTA® XL. It is therefore advisable for patients to abstain from alcohol during treatment.

4.6 Pregnancy and lactation

Pregnancy

There are no adequate data from the use of methylphenidate in pregnant women.

Studies in animals have shown reproductive toxicity (teratogenic effects) of methylphenidate (see section 5.3.). The potential risk for humans is unknown.

From observations in humans there are indications that amfetamines could be harmful to the foetus.

CONCERTA® XL is contraindicated during pregnancy (see section 4.3).

Females of child-bearing potential (females post-menarche) should use effective contraception.

Lactation

It is not known whether methylphenidate or its metabolites pass into breast milk, but for safety reasons breast-feeding mothers should not use CONCERTA® XL.

4.7 Effects on ability to drive and use machines

No studies on the effects of CONCERTA® XL on the ability to drive and use machines have been performed. However, CONCERTA® XL may cause dizziness. It is therefore advisable to exercise caution when driving, operating machinery, or engaging in other potentially hazardous activities.

4.8 Undesirable effects

The most commonly reported adverse drug reaction is headache occurring in approximately 13% of patients.

Frequency estimate: very common (⩾ 1/10); common (⩾ 1/100 to < 1/10); uncommon (⩾ 1/1000 to < 1/100); rare (⩾ 1/10,000 to < 1/1000); very rare (< 1/10,000), not known (cannot be estimated from the available data).

Within each frequency grouping, undesirable effects are presented in order of decreasing seriousness.

(see Table 2 opposite)

Undesirable effects noted with other methylphenidate formulations:

In addition to the above reactions observed with CONCERTA® XL, the following adverse reactions have been noted with the use of other methylphenidate products:

Nervous system disorders: Choreoathetoid movements, Tourette's syndrome, poorly documented neuroleptic malignant syndrome (NMS).

Hepatobiliary disorders: Hepatic coma.

Vascular disorders: Cerebral arteritis, and/or occlusion.

Table 2

System Organ Class	Adverse Drug Reaction				
	Frequency				
	Very common	Common	Uncommon	Rare	Not known
Infections and infestations		Nasopharyngitis			
Blood and lymphatic system disorders					Pancytopenia Thrombocytopenic purpura Thrombocytopenia Leucopenia,
Metabolism and nutrition disorders			Anorexia, Decreased appetite		
Psychiatric disorders		Aggression, Anxiety, Affect lability Tic Insomnia	Drug-induced psychosis (e.g. hallucinations), Suicidal ideation[1], Depression, Hypervigilance, Agitation, Anger, Mood swings, Mood altered, Restlessness, Nervousness, Sleep disorder, Tearfulness,	Mania, Disorientation,	Suicide attempt[1], Confusional state,
Nervous system disorders	Headache	Dizziness	Somnolence, Sedation, Tremor, Psychomotor hyperactivity,		Grand mal convulsions, Convulsions,
Eye disorders			Diplopia, Vision blurred,	Visual disturbance, Mydriasis,	
Cardiac disorders			Tachycardia, Palpitation		Angina pectoris, Ventricular extrasystoles Supraventricular tachycardia, Bradycardia, Extrasystoles,
Vascular disorders			Hypertension		Raynaud's phenomenon
Respiratory, thoracic and mediastinal disorders		Cough, Pharyngolaryngeal pain	Dyspnoea		
Gastrointestinal disorders		Abdominal pain, Stomach discomfort, Diarrhoea, Vomiting, Nausea,	Constipation		
Skin and subcutaneous tissue disorders			Alopecia, Rash	Erythema, Hyperhidrosis, Rash macular	
Musculoskeletal and connective tissue disorders			Arthralgia, Myalgia, Muscle twitching		
Immune System Disorders			Hypersensitivity reactions such as Anaphylactic reactions, Exfoliative conditions, Angioedema, Bullous conditions, Auricular swelling, Eruptions, Rashes, Pruritus Urticarias,		
General disorders and administration site conditions		Irritability, Pyrexia	Chest pain, Fatigue		Chest discomfort, Hyperpyrexia
Investigations		Weight decreased	Blood pressure increased, Cardiac murmur, Hepatic enzyme increased		Blood bilirubin increased, Platelet count decreased, White blood cell count abnormal, Blood alkaline phosphatase increased

[1]Reports of suicidal ideation and/or suicide attempt have been received in patients treated with CONCERTA® XL. The role of CONCERTA® XL in these cases is uncertain.

Miscellaneous: Growth retardation during prolonged use in children.

4.9 Overdose

The prolonged release of methylphenidate from CONCERTA® XL should be considered when treating patients with overdose.

Signs and Symptoms: Signs and symptoms of acute methylphenidate overdose, resulting principally from overstimulation of the CNS and from excessive sympathomimetic effects, may include the following: vomiting, agitation, tremors, hyperreflexia, muscle twitching, convulsions (may be followed by coma), euphoria, confusion, hallucinations, delirium, sweating, flushing, headache, hyperpyrexia, tachycardia, palpitations, cardiac arrhythmias, hypertension, mydriasis, and dryness of mucous membranes.

Recommended Treatment: Treatment consists of appropriate supportive measures. The patient must be protected against self-injury and against external stimuli that would aggravate overstimulation already present. Gastric contents may be evacuated by gastric lavage as indicated. Before performing gastric lavage, control agitation and seizures if present and protect the airway. Other measures to detoxify the gut include administration of activated charcoal and a cathartic. Intensive care must be provided to maintain adequate circulation and respiratory exchange; external cooling procedures may be required for hyperpyrexia.

Efficacy of peritoneal dialysis or extracorporeal haemodialysis for CONCERTA® XL overdose has not been established.

5. PHARMACOLOGICAL PROPERTIES

5.1 Pharmacodynamic properties

Pharmacotherapeutic group: centrally acting sympathomimetics: ATC code: N06BA04

Methylphenidate HCl is a mild central nervous system (CNS) stimulant. The mode of therapeutic action in Attention Deficit Hyperactivity Disorder (ADHD) is not known. Methylphenidate is thought to block the reuptake of noradrenaline and dopamine into the presynaptic neurone and increase the release of these monoamines into the extraneuronal space. Methylphenidate is a racemic mixture comprised of the d- and l-isomers. The d-isomer is more pharmacologically active than the l-isomer.

In the pivotal clinical studies, CONCERTA® XL was assessed in 321 patients already stabilised with immediate release preparations (IR) of methylphenidate and in 95 patients not previously treated with IR preparations of methylphenidate.

Clinical studies showed that the effects of CONCERTA® XL were maintained until 12 hours after dosing when the product was taken once daily in the morning.

5.2 Pharmacokinetic properties

Absorption: Methylphenidate is readily absorbed. Following oral administration of CONCERTA® XL to adults the drug overcoat dissolves, providing an initial maximum active ingredient concentration at about 1 to 2 hours. The methylphenidate contained in the two internal drug layers is gradually released over the next several hours. Peak plasma concentrations are achieved at about 6 to 8 hours, after which plasma levels of methylphenidate gradually decrease. CONCERTA® XL taken once daily minimises the fluctuations between peak and trough concentrations associated with immediate-release methylphenidate three times daily. The extent of absorption of CONCERTA® XL once daily is generally comparable to conventional immediate release preparations.

Following the administration of CONCERTA® XL 18 mg once daily in 36 adults, the mean pharmacokinetic parameters were: C_{max} 3.7 ± 1.0 (ng/mL), T_{max} 6.8 ± 1.8 (h), AUCinf 41.8 ± 13.9 (ng.h/mL), and $t_{½}$ 3.5 ± 0.4 (h).

No differences in the pharmacokinetics of CONCERTA® XL were noted following single and repeated once daily dosing, indicating no significant active ingredient accumulation. The AUC and $t_{1/2}$ following repeated once daily dosing are similar to those following the first dose of CONCERTA® XL 18 mg.

Following administration of CONCERTA® XL in single doses of 18, 36, and 54 mg/day to adults, C_{max} and $AUC_{(0-inf)}$ of methylphenidate were proportional to dose.

Distribution: Plasma methylphenidate concentrations in adults decline biexponentially following oral administration. The half-life of methylphenidate in adults following oral administration of CONCERTA® XL was approximately 3.5 h. The rate of protein binding of methylphenidate and of its metabolites is approximately 15%. The apparent volume of distribution of methylphenidate is approximately 13 litres/kg.

Metabolism: In humans, methylphenidate is metabolised primarily by de-esterification to alpha-phenyl-piperidine acetic acid (PPA, approximately 50 fold the level of the unchanged substance) which has little or no pharmacologic activity. In adults the metabolism of CONCERTA® XL once daily as evaluated by metabolism to PPA is similar to that of methylphenidate three times daily. The metabolism of single and repeated once daily doses of CONCERTA® XL is similar.

Excretion: The elimination half-life of methylphenidate in adults following administration of CONCERTA® XL was approximately 3.5 hours. After oral administration, about 90% of the dose is excreted in urine and 1 to 3% in faeces, as metabolites within 48 to 96 hours. Small quantities of unchanged methylphenidate are recovered in urine (less than 1%). The main urinary metabolite is alpha-phenyl-piperidine acetic acid (60-90%).

After oral dosing of radiolabelled methylphenidate in humans, about 90% of the radioactivity was recovered in urine. The main urinary metabolite was PPA, accounting for approximately 80% of the dose.

Food Effects: In patients, there were no differences in either the pharmacokinetics or the pharmacodynamic performance of CONCERTA® XL when administered after a high fat breakfast on an empty stomach.

Special Populations

Gender: In healthy adults, the mean dose-adjusted $AUC_{(0-inf)}$ values for CONCERTA® XL were 36.7 ng.h/mL in men and 37.1 ng.h/mL in women, with no differences noted between the two groups.

Race: In healthy adults receiving CONCERTA® XL, dose-adjusted $AUC_{(0-inf)}$ was consistent across ethnic groups; however, the sample size may have been insufficient to detect ethnic variations in pharmacokinetics.

Age: The pharmacokinetics of CONCERTA® XL has not been studied in children younger than 6 years of age. In children 7-12 years of age, the pharmacokinetics of CONCERTA® XL after 18, 36 and 54 mg were (mean±SD): C_{max} 6.0±1.3, 11.3±2.6, and 15.0±3.8 ng/mL, respectively, T_{max} 9.4±0.02, 8.1±1.1, 9.1±2.5 h, respectively, and $AUC_{0-11.5}$ 50.4±7.8, 87.7±18.2, 121.5±37.3 ng.h/mL, respectively.

Renal Insufficiency: There is no experience with the use of CONCERTA® XL in patients with renal insufficiency. After oral administration of radiolabelled methylphenidate in humans, methylphenidate was extensively metabolised and approximately 80% of the radioactivity was excreted in the urine in the form of PPA. Since renal clearance is not an important route of methylphenidate clearance, renal insufficiency is expected to have little effect on the pharmacokinetics of CONCERTA® XL.

Hepatic Insufficiency: There is no experience with the use of CONCERTA® XL in patients with hepatic insufficiency.

5.3 Preclinical safety data

There is evidence that methylphenidate may be a teratogen in two species. Spina bifida and limb malformations have been reported in rabbits whilst in the rat, equivocal evidence of induction of abnormalities of the vertebrae was found.

Methylphenidate did not affect reproductive performance or fertility at low multiples (2-5 times) of the therapeutic human dose.

There was no evidence of carcinogenicity in the rat. In mice, methylphenidate caused an increase in hepatocellular adenomas, in animals of both sexes and, in males only, hepatoblastomas. In the absence of exposure data, the significance of these findings to humans is not known.

The weight of evidence from the genotoxicity studies reveals no special hazard for humans.

6. PHARMACEUTICAL PARTICULARS

6.1 List of excipients

Butylhydroxytoluene (E321)

Cellulose acetate

Hypromellose (E646)

Phosphoric acid concentrated

Poloxamer 188

Polyethylene oxides 200K and 7000K

Povidone K29-32

Sodium chloride

Stearic acid

Succinic acid

Iron oxide black (E172)

Iron oxide red(E172)

Iron oxide yellow (E172).

Film Coat:

Iron oxide black(E172)

Hypromellose (E464)

Lactose monohydrate

Titanium dioxide (E171)

Triacetin.

Clear Coat:

Carnauba wax

Hypromellose (E464)

Macrogol 400

Printing Ink:

Iron oxide black (E172)

Hypromellose (E646)

Propylene glycol.

6.2 Incompatibilities

Not applicable.

6.3 Shelf life

2 years

6.4 Special precautions for storage

Keep the bottle tightly closed in order to protect from moisture.

6.5 Nature and contents of container

High-density polyethylene (HDPE) bottle with a child-resistant polypropylene closure with one or two silica gel desiccant pouches enclosed.

28 or 30 prolonged-release tablets.

Not all pack sizes may be marketed.

6.6 Special precautions for disposal and other handling

No special requirements.

7. MARKETING AUTHORISATION HOLDER

Janssen-Cilag Limited

50-100 Holmers Farm Way

High Wycombe

Buckinghamshire

HP12 4EG

UK

8. MARKETING AUTHORISATION NUMBER(S)

PL 00242/0400

9. DATE OF FIRST AUTHORISATION/RENEWAL OF THE AUTHORISATION

09/03/2007

10. DATE OF REVISION OF THE TEXT

4th September 2008

Conotrane Cream

(Astellas Pharma Ltd)

1. NAME OF THE MEDICINAL PRODUCT

Conotrane Cream.

2. QUALITATIVE AND QUANTITATIVE COMPOSITION

A smooth white cream containing benzalkonium chloride 0.1% w/w and Dimeticone 22.0% w/w.

3. PHARMACEUTICAL FORM

Cream for topical administration.

4. CLINICAL PARTICULARS

4.1 Therapeutic indications

Conotrane is used for protection of the skin from moisture, irritants, chafing and contamination with bacteria or yeasts.

It may be used in situations such as in the prevention/treatment of napkin rash, the prevention of pressure sores and in the management of incontinence.

4.2 Posology and method of administration

The cream should be applied to the affected area several times a day, as necessary or after every napkin change.

4.3 Contraindications

Known hypersensitivity to benzalkonium chloride.

4.4 Special warnings and precautions for use

Cetostearyl alcohol may cause local skin reactions (e.g. contact dermatitis).

4.5 Interaction with other medicinal products and other forms of interaction

None stated.

4.6 Pregnancy and lactation

Not applicable.

4.7 Effects on ability to drive and use machines

None stated.

4.8 Undesirable effects

Local hypersensitivity to benzalkonium chloride is rare.

4.9 Overdose

Not applicable.

5. PHARMACOLOGICAL PROPERTIES

5.1 Pharmacodynamic properties

This is a remedy suitable for both prescription and for self medication. It is a cream for topical application containing dimeticone and benzalkonium chloride. The dimeticone is water repellent allowing transpiration of water vapour from the skin. The benzalkonium chloride is a quaternary ammonium compound, active against bacteria and yeasts.

5.2 Pharmacokinetic properties

Not applicable.

5.3 Preclinical safety data

None stated.

6. PHARMACEUTICAL PARTICULARS

6.1 List of excipients

Cetostearyl alcohol

Macrogol cetostearyl ether

White soft paraffin

Light liquid paraffin

Deionised water

Macrogol 300

Potassium dihydrogen orthophosphate

Geranium SC45

6.2 Incompatibilities

None stated.

6.3 Shelf life

3 years.

6.4 Special precautions for storage

Do not store above 25°C.

6.5 Nature and contents of container

(i) 7 g, 15 g, 50 g and 100 g in white LDPE tubes.

(ii) 500 g white polypropylene pot with screw lid.

6.6 Special precautions for disposal and other handling

None stated.

Administrative Data

7. MARKETING AUTHORISATION HOLDER

Astellas Pharma Limited

Lovett House

Lovett Road

Staines

TW18 3AZ

United Kingdom

8. MARKETING AUTHORISATION NUMBER(S)
PL 0166/0178.

9. DATE OF FIRST AUTHORISATION/RENEWAL OF THE AUTHORISATION
1 July 1998 / 16th July 2003

10. DATE OF REVISION OF THE TEXT
18 January 2008

11. Legal category
GSL

Copegus 200mg Film-coated Tablets

(Roche Products Limited)

1. NAME OF THE MEDICINAL PRODUCT
Copegus 200 mg film-coated tablet

2. QUALITATIVE AND QUANTITATIVE COMPOSITION
Each film-coated tablet contains 200 milligrams of ribavirin.

For a full list of excipients, see section 6.1.

3. PHARMACEUTICAL FORM
Film-coated tablet

Light pink, flat oval-shaped film-coated tablet (marked with RIB 200 on one side and ROCHE on the opposite side).

4. CLINICAL PARTICULARS

4.1 Therapeutic indications
Copegus is indicated for the treatment of chronic hepatitis C and must only be used as part of a combination regimen with peginterferon alfa-2a or with interferon alfa-2a. Copegus monotherapy must not be used.

The combination of Copegus with peginterferon alfa-2a or interferon alfa-2a is indicated in adult patients who are positive for serum HCV-RNA, including patients with compensated cirrhosis. (See section 4.4) The combination with peginterferon alfa-2a is also indicated in patients co-infected with clinically stable HIV, including patients with compensated cirrhosis (See section 4.3). The combination regimens are indicated in previously untreated patients as well as in patients who have previously responded to interferon alpha therapy and subsequently relapsed after treatment was stopped.

Please refer to the Summary of Product Characteristics (SPC) of peginterferon alfa-2a or interferon alfa-2a for prescribing information particular to either of these products.

4.2 Posology and method of administration
Treatment should be initiated, and monitored, by a physician experienced in the management of chronic hepatitis C.

Method of Administration
Copegus film-coated tablets are administered orally in two divided doses with food (morning and evening). Due to the teratogenic potential of ribavirin, the tablets should not be broken or crushed.

Posology
Copegus is used in combination with peginterferon alfa-2a or interferon alfa-2a. The exact dose and duration of treatment depend on the interferon product used.

Please refer to the SPC of peginterferon alfa-2a or interferon alfa-2a for further information on dosage and duration of treatment when Copegus is to be used in combination with either of these products.

Posology in combination with peginterferon alfa-2a:

Dose to be administered

The recommended dose of Copegus in combination with peginterferon alfa-2a solution for injection depends on viral genotype and the patient's body weight (see Table 1).

Duration of treatment

The duration of combination therapy with peginterferon alfa-2a depends on viral genotype. Patients infected with HCV genotype 1 who have detectable HCV RNA at week 4 regardless of pre-treatment viral load should receive 48 weeks of therapy.

Treatment for 24 weeks may be considered in patients infected with

- genotype 1 with low viral load (LVL) (≤ 800,000 IU/mL) at baseline or

- genotype 4 who become HCV RNA negative at week 4 and remain HCV RNA negative at week 24. However, an overall 24 weeks treatment duration may be associated with a higher risk of relapse than a 48 weeks treatment duration (see 5.1). In these patients, tolerability to combination therapy and additional prognostic factors such as degree of fibrosis should be taken into account when deciding on treatment duration. Shortening the treatment duration in patients with genotype 1 and high viral load (HVL) (> 800, 000 IU/ml) at baseline who become HCV RNA negative at week 4 and remain HCV RNA negative at week 24 should be considered with even more caution since the limited data available suggest that this may significantly negatively impact the sustained virologic response.

Patients infected with HCV genotype 2 or 3 who have detectable HCV RNA at week 4, regardless of pre-treatment viral load should receive 24 weeks of therapy. Treatment for only 16 weeks may be considered in selected patients infected with genotype 2 or 3 with LVL (≤ 800,000 IU/mL) at baseline who become HCV negative by week 4 of treatment and remain HCV negative by week 16. Overall 16 weeks of treatment may be associated with a lower chance of response and is associated with a higher risk of relapse than a 24 week treatment duration (see section 5.1). In these patients, tolerability to combination therapy and the presence of additional clinical or prognostic factors such as degree of fibrosis should be taken into account when considering deviations from standard 24 weeks treatment duration. Shortening the treatment duration in patients infected with genotype 2 or 3 with HVL (> 800,000 IU/mL) at baseline who become HCV negative by week 4 should be considered with more caution as this may significantly negatively impact the sustained virological response (see Table 1).

Available data for patients infected with genotype 5 or 6 are limited; therefore combination treatment with 1000/1200 mg of ribavirin for 48 weeks is recommended.

(see Table 1 above)

The ultimate clinical impact of a shortened initial treatment of 16 weeks instead of 24 weeks is unknown, taking into account the need for retreating non-responding and relapsing patients.

HIV-HCV Co-infection

The recommended dosage for Copegus in combination with 180 micrograms once weekly of peginterferon alfa-2a is 800 milligrams, daily for 48 weeks, regardless of genotype. The safety and efficacy of combination therapy with ribavirin doses greater than 800 milligrams daily or a duration of therapy less than 48 weeks has not been studied.

Predictability of response and non-response

Early virological response by week 12, defined as a 2 log viral load decrease or undetectable levels of HCV RNA has been shown to be predictive for sustained response (see Table 2).

(see Table 2 above)

A similar negative predictive value has been observed in HIV-HCV co-infected patients treated with peginterferon alfa-2a monotherapy or in combination with ribavirin (100% (130/130) or 98% (83/85), respectively). Positive predictive values of 45% (50/110) and 70% (59/84) were observed for genotype 1 and genotype 2/3 HIV-HCV co-infected patients receiving combination therapy.

Posology in combination with interferon alfa-2a:

Dose to be administered

The recommended dose of Copegus in combination with interferon alfa-2a solution for injection depends on the patient's body weight (see Table 3).

Table 1 Copegus Dosing Recommendations in Combination with Peginterferon alfa-2a for HCV patients

Genotype	Daily Copegus Dose	Duration of treatment	Number of 200/400 mg tablets
Genotype 1 LVL with RVR*	< 75 kg = 1,000 mg ≥ 75 kg = 1,200 mg	24 weeks or 48 weeks	5 × 200 mg (2 morning, 3 evening) 6 × 200 mg (3 morning, 3 evening)
Genotype 1 HVL with RVR*	<75 kg = 1000 mg ≥75 kg = 1200 mg	48 weeks	5 × 200 mg (2 morning, 3 evening) 6 × 200 mg (3 morning, 3 evening)
Genotype 4 with RVR*	<75 kg = 1000 mg ≥75 kg = 1200 mg	24 weeks or 48 weeks	5 × 200 mg (2 morning, 3 evening) 6 × 200 mg (3 morning, 3 evening)
Genotype 1 or 4 without RVR*	<75 kg = 1000 mg ≥75 kg = 1200 mg	48 weeks	5 × 200 mg (2 morning, 3 evening) 6 × 200 mg (3 morning, 3 evening)
Genotype 2 or 3 LVL with RVR**	800 mg	16 weeks or 24 weeks	4 × 200 mg (2 morning, 2 evening) or 2 × 400 mg (1 morning, 1 evening)
Genotype 2 or 3 HVL with RVR**	800 mg	24 weeks	4 × 200 mg (2 morning, 2 evening) or 2 × 400 mg (1 morning, 1 evening)
Genotype 2 or 3 without RVR**	800 mg	24 weeks	4 × 200 mg (2 morning, 2 evening) or 2 × 400 mg (1 morning, 1 evening)

*RVR = rapid viral response (HCV RNA undetectable) at week 4 and HCV RNA undetectable at week 24;
**RVR = rapid viral response (HCV RNA negative) by week 4
LVL= ≤ 800,000 IU/mL; HVL= > 800,000 IU/mL

Table 2 Predictive Value of Week 12 Virological Response at the Recommended Dosing Regimen while receiving Copegus and peginterferon Combination Therapy

Genotype	Negative			Positive		
	No response by week 12	No sustained response	Predictive Value	Response by week 12	Sustained response	Predictive Value
Genotype 1 (N= 569)	102	97	**95%** (97/102)	467	271	**58%** (271/467)
Genotype 2 and 3 (N=96)	3	3	**100%** (3/3)	93	81	**87%** (81/93)

Table 3 Copegus Dosing Recommendations in Combination with Interferon alfa-2a

Patient weight (kg)	Daily Copegus dose	Duration of treatment	Number of 200 mg tablets
<75	1,000 mg	24 or 48 weeks	5 (2 morning, 3 evening)
≥75	1,200 mg	24 or 48 weeks	6 (3 morning, 3 evening)

Duration of treatment:

Patients should be treated with combination therapy with interferon alfa-2a for at least six months. Patients with HCV genotype 1 infections should receive 48 weeks of combination therapy. In patients infected with HCV of other genotypes, the decision to extend therapy to 48 weeks should be based on other prognostic factors (such as high viral load at baseline, male gender, age > 40 years and evidence of bridging fibrosis).

(see Table 3 above)

Dosage modification for adverse reactions

Please refer to the SPC of peginterferon alfa-2a or interferon alfa-2a for further information on dose adjustment and discontinuation of treatment for either of these products.

If severe adverse reactions or laboratory abnormalities develop during therapy with Copegus and peginterferon alfa-2a or interferon alfa-2a, modify the dosages of each product, until the adverse reactions abate. Guidelines were developed in clinical trials for dose modification (see **Dosage Modification Guidelines for Management of Treatment-Emergent Anaemia**, Table 4).

If intolerance persists after dose adjustment, discontinuation of Copegus or both Copegus and peginterferon alfa-2a or interferon alfa-2a may be needed.

Table 4 Dosage Modification Guidelines for Management of Treatment-Emergent Anaemia

Laboratory Values	Reduce only Copegus dose to 600 mg/day* if:	Discontinue Copegus if:**
Haemoglobin in Patients with No Cardiac Disease	<10 g/dl	<8.5 g/dl
Haemoglobin: Patients with History of Stable Cardiac Disease	≥2 g/dl decrease in haemoglobin during any 4 week period during treatment (permanent dose reduction)	<12 g/dl despite 4 weeks at reduced dose

*Patients whose dose of Copegus is reduced to 600 mg daily receive one 200 mg tablet in the morning and two 200 mg tablets or one 400 mg tablet in the evening.

**If the abnormality is reversed, Copegus may be restarted at 600 mg daily, and further increased to 800 mg daily at the discretion of the treating physician. However, a return to higher doses is not recommended.

Special populations

Use in renal impairment: The recommended dose regimens (adjusted by the body weight cut off of 75 kg) of ribavirin give rise to substantial increases in plasma concentrations of ribavirin in patients with renal impairment.

There are insufficient data on the safety and efficacy of ribavirin in patients with serum creatinine > 2 mg/dl or creatinine clearance < 50 ml/min, whether or not on haemodialysis, to support recommendations for dose adjustments. Therefore, ribavirin should be used in such patients only when this is considered to be essential. Therapy should be initiated (or continued if renal impairment develops while on therapy) with extreme caution and intensive monitoring of haemoglobin concentrations, with corrective action as may be necessary, should be employed throughout the treatment period. (see section 4.4 and section 5.2).

Use in hepatic impairment: Hepatic function does not affect the pharmacokinetics of ribavirin (see section 5.2). Therefore, no dose adjustment of Copegus is required in patients with hepatic impairment. The use of peginterferon alfa-2a and interferon alfa-2a is contraindicated in patients with decompensated cirrhosis and other forms of severe hepatic impairment.

Use in elderly patients over the age of 65: There does not appear to be a significant age-related effect on the pharmacokinetics of ribavirin. However, as in younger patients, renal function must be determined prior to administration of Copegus.

Use in patients under the age of 18 years: Treatment with Copegus is not recommended for use in children and adolescents (<18 years) due to insufficient data on safety and efficacy in combination with peginterferon alfa-2a and interferon alfa-2a.

4.3 Contraindications

See peginterferon alfa-2a or interferon alfa-2a prescribing information for contraindications related to either of these products.

- hypersensitivity to ribavirin or to any of the excipients.
- pregnant women (see section 4.4). Copegus must not be initiated until a report of a negative pregnancy test has been obtained immediately prior to initiation of therapy.
- women who are breast-feeding (see section 4.6).
- a history of severe pre-existing cardiac disease, including unstable or uncontrolled cardiac disease, in the previous six months.
- severe hepatic dysfunction or decompensated cirrhosis of the liver.
- haemoglobinopathies (e.g. thalassaemia, sickle-cell anaemia).
- Initiation of peginterferon alfa-2a is contraindicated in HIV-HCV patients with cirrhosis and a Child-Pugh score ⩾ 6 (Please refer to the SPC of peginterferon alfa-2a for Child-Pugh assessment).

4.4 Special warnings and precautions for use

Psychiatric and Central Nervous System (CNS): Severe CNS effects, particularly depression, suicidal ideation and attempted suicide have been observed in some patients during Copegus combination therapy with peginterferon alfa-2a or interferon alfa-2a, and even after treatment discontinuation mainly during the 6-month follow-up period. Other CNS effects including aggressive behaviour (sometimes directed against others), confusion and alterations of mental status have been observed with alpha interferons. Patients should be closely monitored for any signs or symptoms of psychiatric disorders. If such symptoms appear, the potential seriousness of these undesirable effects must be borne in mind by the prescribing physician and the need for adequate therapeutic management should be considered. If psychiatric symptoms persist or worsen, or suicidal ideation is identified, it is recommended that treatment with Copegus and peginterferon alfa-2a or interferon alfa-2a be discontinued, and the patient followed, with psychiatric intervention as appropriate.

Patients with existence of, or history of severe psychiatric conditions: If treatment with Copegus in combination with peginterferon alfa-2a or interferon alfa-2a is judged necessary in patients with existence or history of severe psychiatric conditions, this should only be initiated after having ensured appropriate individualised diagnostic and therapeutic management of the psychiatric condition.

Please refer to the SPC of peginterferon alfa-2a or interferon alfa-2a for further information on special warnings and precautions for use related to either of these products.

All patients in the chronic hepatitis C studies had a liver biopsy before inclusion, but in certain cases (ie, patients with genotype 2 or 3), treatment may be possible without histological confirmation. Current treatment guidelines should be consulted as to whether a liver biopsy is needed prior to commencing treatment.

In patients with normal ALT, progression of fibrosis occurs on average at a slower rate than in patients with elevated ALT. This should be considered in conjunction with other factors, such as HCV genotype, age, extrahepatic manifestations, risk of transmission, etc. which influence the decision to treat or not.

Teratogenic risk: See **4.6 Pregnancy and lactation.**

Prior to initiation of treatment with ribavirin the physician must comprehensively inform the patient of the teratogenic risk of ribavirin, the necessity of effective and continuous contraception, the possibility that contraceptive methods may fail and the possible consequences of pregnancy should it occur during treatment with ribavirin. For laboratory monitoring of pregnancy please refer to Laboratory tests.

Carcinogenicity: Ribavirin is mutagenic in some *in vivo* and *in vitro* genotoxicity assays. A potential carcinogenic effect of ribavirin cannot be excluded (see section 5.3).

Haemolysis and Cardiovascular system: A decrease in haemoglobin levels to <10 g/dl was observed in up to 15% of patients treated for 48 weeks with Copegus 1000/1200 milligrams in combination with peginterferon alfa-2a and up to 19% of patients in combination with interferon alfa-2a. When Copegus 800 milligram was combined with peginterferon alfa-2a for 24 weeks, 3% of patients had a decrease in haemoglobin levels to <10 g/dl. The risk of developing anaemia is higher in the female population. Although ribavirin has no direct cardiovascular effects, anaemia associated with Copegus may result in deterioration of cardiac function, or exacerbation of the symptoms of coronary disease, or both. Thus, Copegus must be administered with caution to patients with pre-existing cardiac disease. Cardiac status must be assessed before start of therapy and monitored clinically during therapy; if any deterioration occurs, stop therapy (see section 4.2). Patients with a history of congestive heart failure, myocardial infarction, and/or previous or current arrhythmic disorders must be closely monitored. It is recommended that those patients who have pre-existing cardiac abnormalities have electrocardiograms taken prior to and during the course of treatment. Cardiac arrhythmias (primarily supraventricular) usually respond to conventional therapy but may require discontinuation of therapy.

Acute hypersensitivity: If an acute hypersensitivity reaction (e.g. urticaria, angioedema, bronchoconstriction, anaphylaxis) develops, Copegus must be discontinued immediately and appropriate medical therapy instituted. Transient rashes do not necessitate interruption of treatment.

Liver function: In patients who develop evidence of hepatic decompensation during treatment, Copegus in combination with peginterferon alfa-2a or interferon alfa-2a should be discontinued. When the increase in ALT levels is progressive and clinically significant, despite dose reduction, or is accompanied by increased direct bilirubin, therapy should be discontinued.

Renal impairment: The pharmacokinetics of ribavirin are altered in patients with renal dysfunction due to reduction of apparent clearance in these patients (see section 5.2). Therefore, it is recommended that renal function be evaluated in all patients prior to initiation of Copegus, preferably by estimating the patient's creatinine clearance. Substantial increases in ribavirin plasma concentrations are seen at the recommended dosing regimen in patients with serum creatinine >2 mg/dl or with creatinine clearance <50 ml/minute. There are insufficient data on the safety and efficacy of Copegus in such patients to support recommendations for dose adjustments. Copegus therapy should not be initiated (or continued if renal impairment occurs while on treatment) in such patients, whether or not on haemodialysis, unless it is considered to be essential. Extreme caution is required. Haemoglobin concentrations should be monitored intensively during treatment and corrective action taken as necessary (see section 4.2. and section 5.2).

Ocular changes: Copegus is used in combination therapy with alpha interferons. Retinopathy including retinal haemorrhages, cotton wool spots, papilloedema, optic neuropathy and retinal artery or vein obstruction which may result in loss of vision have been reported in rare instances with combination therapy with alpha interferons. All patients should have a baseline eye examination. Any patient complaining of decrease or loss of vision must have a prompt and complete eye examination. Patients with preexisting ophthalmologic disorders (eg, diabetic or hypertensive retinopathy) should receive periodic ophthalmologic exams during combination therapy with alpha interferons. Combination therapy with alpha interferons should be discontinued in patients who develop new or worsening ophthalmologic disorders.

HIV/HCV Co-infection: Please refer to the respective Summary of Product Characteristics of the antiretroviral medicinal products that are to be taken concurrently with HCV therapy for awareness and management of toxicities specific for each product and the potential for overlapping toxicities with peginterferon alfa-2a with or without ribavirin. In study NR15961, patients concurrently treated with stavudine and interferon therapy with or without ribavirin, the incidence of pancreatitis and/or lactic acidosis was 3% (12/398).

Chronic hepatitis C patients co-infected with HIV and receiving Highly Active Anti-Retroviral Therapy (HAART) may be at increased risk of serious adverse effects (e.g. lactic acidosis; peripheral neuropathy; pancreatitis).

Co-infected patients with advanced cirrhosis receiving HAART may also be at increased risk of hepatic decompensation and possibly death if treated with Copegus in combination with interferons. Baseline variables in co-infected cirrhotic patients that may be associated with hepatic decompensation include: increased serum bilirubin, decreased haemoglobin, increased alkaline phosphatase or decreased platelet count, and treatment with didanosine (ddI). Caution should therefore be exercised when adding peginterferon alfa-2a and Copegus to HAART (see section 4.5).

Co-infected patients should be closely monitored, assessing their Child-Pugh score during treatment, and should be immediately discontinued if they progress to a Child-Pugh score of 7 or greater.

Co-administration of Copegus and didanosine is not recommended due to the risk of mitochondrial toxicity (see Section 4.5). Moreover, co-adminstration of Copegus and stavudine should be avoided to limit the risk of overlapping mitochondrial toxicity.

Patients treated with Copegus and alpha interferon (standard and pegylated) combination therapy and zidovudine could be at increased risk of developing anaemia.

Laboratory tests: Standard haematologic tests and blood chemistries (complete blood count [CBC] and differential, platelet count, electrolytes, serum creatinine, liver function tests, uric acid) must be conducted in all patients prior to initiating therapy. Acceptable baseline values that may be considered as a guideline prior to initiation of Copegus in combination with peginterferon alfa-2a or interferon alfa-2a:

Haemoglobin ⩾12 g/dl (females); ⩾13 g/dl (males)

Platelets ⩾ 90,000/mm^3

Neutrophil Count ⩾1,500/mm^3

In patients co-infected with HIV-HCV, limited efficacy and safety data (N = 51) are available in subjects with CD4 counts less than 200 cells/μL. Caution is therefore warranted in the treatment of patients with low CD4 counts.

Laboratory evaluations are to be conducted at weeks 2 and 4 of therapy, and periodically thereafter as clinically appropriate.

For women of childbearing potential: Female patients must have a routine pregnancy test performed monthly during treatment and for 4 months thereafter. Female partners of male patients must have a routine pregnancy test performed monthly during treatment and for 7 months thereafter.

Uric acid may increase with Copegus due to haemolysis and therefore predisposed patients should be carefully monitored for development of gout.

Dental and periodontal disorders: Dental and periodontal disorders, which may lead to loss of teeth, have been reported in patients receiving Copegus and peginterferon alfa-2a combination therapy. In addition, dry mouth could have a damaging effect on teeth and mucous membranes of the mouth during long-term treatment with the combination of Copegus and peginterferon alfa-2a. Patients should brush their teeth thoroughly twice daily and have regular dental examinations. In addition some patients may experience vomiting. If this reaction occurs, they should be advised to rinse out their mouth thoroughly afterwards.

4.5 Interaction with other medicinal products and other forms of interaction

Interaction studies have been conducted with ribavirin in combination with peginterferon alfa-2a, interferon alfa-2b and antacids. Ribavirin concentrations are similar when given alone or concomitantly with interferon alfa-2b or peginterferon alfa-2a.

Any potential for interactions may persist for up to 2 months (5 half lives for ribavirin) after cessation of Copegus therapy due to the long half-life.

Results of *in vitro* studies using both human and rat liver microsome preparations indicated no cytochrome P450 enzyme mediated metabolism of ribavirin. Ribavirin does not inhibit cytochrome P450 enzymes. There is no evidence from toxicity studies that ribavirin induces liver enzymes. Therefore, there is a minimal potential for P450 enzyme-based interactions.

Antacid: The bioavailability of ribavirin 600 milligrams was decreased by co-administration with an antacid containing magnesium, aluminium and methicone; AUC_{tf} decreased 14%. It is possible that the decreased bioavailability in this study was due to delayed transit of ribavirin or modified pH. This interaction is not considered to be clinically relevant.

Nucleoside analogues: Ribavirin was shown *in vitro* to inhibit phosphorylation of zidovudine and stavudine. The clinical significance of these findings is unknown. However, these *in vitro* findings raise the possibility that concurrent use of Copegus with either zidovudine or stavudine might lead to increased HIV plasma viraemia. Therefore, it is recommended that plasma HIV RNA levels be closely monitored in patients treated with Copegus concurrently with either of these two agents. If HIV RNA levels increase, the use of Copegus concomitantly with reverse transcriptase inhibitors must be reviewed.

Didanosine (ddI): Co-administration of ribavirin and didanosine is not recommended. Exposure to didanosine or its active metabolite (dideoxyadenosine 5'-triphosphate) is increased *in vitro* when didanosine is co-administered with ribavirin. Reports of fatal hepatic failure as well as peripheral neuropathy, pancreatitis, and symptomatic hyperlactataemia/lactic acidosis have been reported with use of ribavirin.

HIV-HCV co-infected patients

No apparent evidence of drug interaction was observed in 47 HIV-HCV co-infected patients who completed a 12

Table 5 Undesirable Effects Reported with Copegus in combination with Peginterferon alfa-2a for HCV Patients

Body system	Very Common ⩾1 /10	Common ⩾1 /100 to < 1 /10	Uncommon ⩾1 /1000 to < 1 /100	Rare ⩾1 /10,000 to < 1 /1000	Very rare <1/10,000
Infections and infestations		Upper respiratory infection, bronchitis, oral candidiasis, herpes simplex	Lower respiratory tract infection, urinary tract infection, skin infection	Endocarditis, Otitis externa	
Neoplasms benign and malignant			Malignant hepatic neoplasm		
Blood and lymphatic system disorders	Anaemia	Thrombocytopenia, lymphadenopathy		Pancytopenia	Aplastic anaemia
Immune system disorders			Sarcoidosis, thyroiditis	Anaphylaxis, systemic lupus erythematosus, rheumatoid arthritis	idiopathic or thrombotic thrombocytopenic purpura
Endocrine disorders		Hypothyroidism, hyperthyroidism	Diabetes		
Metabolism and Nutrition Disorders	Anorexia		Dehydration		
Psychiatric disorders	Depression, insomnia	Mood alteration, emotional disorders, anxiety, aggression, nervousness, libido decreased	Suicidal ideation, hallucinations, anger	Suicide, psychotic disorder	
Nervous system disorders	Headache, dizziness, concentration impaired	Memory impairment, syncope, weakness, migraine, hypoaesthesia, hyperaesthesia, paraesthesia, tremor, taste disturbance, nightmares, somnolence	Hearing loss, peripheral neuropathy	Coma, convulsions, facial palsy	
Eye disorders		Vision blurred, eye pain, eye inflammation, xerophthalmia	Retinal haemorrhage,	Optic neuropathy, papilloedema, retinal vascular disorder, retinopathy, corneal ulcer	Vision loss
Ear and labyrinth disorders		Vertigo, earache			
Cardiac disorders		Tachycardia, palpitations, oedema peripheral		Myocardial infarction, congestive heart failure, angina, Supraventricular tachycardia arrhythmia, atrial fibrillation, pericarditis	
Vascular disorders		Flushing	Hypertension	Cerebral haemorrhage	
Respiratory, thoracic and mediastinal disorders	Dyspnoea, cough	Dyspnoea exertional, epistaxis, nasopharyngitis, sinus congestion, nasal congestion, rhinitis, sore throat	Wheezing	Interstitial pneumonitis with fatal outcome, pulmonary embolism	
Gastrointestinal disorders	Diarrhoea, nausea, abdominal pain	Vomiting, dyspepsia, dysphagia, mouth ulceration, gingival bleeding, glossitis, stomatitis, flatulence, constipation, dry mouth	Gastrointestinal bleeding, cheilitis, gingivitis	Peptic ulcer, pancreatitis	
Hepato-biliary disorders			Hepatic dysfunction	Hepatic failure, cholangitis, fatty liver	
Skin and subcutaneous tissue disorders	Alopecia, dermatitis, pruritus, dry skin	Rash, sweating increased, psoriasis, urticaria, eczema, skin disorder, photosensitivity reaction, night sweats			Toxic epidermal necrolysis, Stevens-Johnson syndrome, angioedema, erythema multiforme
Musculoskeletal connective tissue and bone disorders	Myalgia, arthralgia	Back pain, arthritis, muscle weakness, bone pain, neck pain, musculoskeletal pain, muscle cramps		Myositis	
Reproductive system and breast disorders		Impotence			
General disorders and administration site conditions	Pyrexia, rigors, pain, asthenia, fatigue, injection site reaction, irritability	Chest pain, influenza like illness, malaise, lethargy, hot flushes, thirst			
Investigations		Weight decreased			
Injury and poisoning				Substance overdose	

week pharmacokinetic substudy to examine the effect of ribavirin on the intracellular phosphorylation of some nucleoside reverse transcriptase inhibitors (lamivudine and zidovudine or stavudine). However, due to high variability, the confidence intervals were quite wide. Plasma exposure of ribavirin did not appear to be affected by concomitant administration of nucleoside reverse transcriptase inhibitors (NRTIs).

4.6 Pregnancy and lactation

Preclinical data: Significant teratogenic and/or embryocidal potential have been demonstrated for ribavirin in all animal species in which adequate studies have been conducted, occurring at doses well below the recommended human dose. Malformations of the skull, palate, eye, jaw, limbs, skeleton and gastrointestinal tract were noted. The incidence and severity of teratogenic effects increased with escalation of the ribavirin dose. Survival of foetuses and offspring was reduced.

Female patients: Copegus must not be used by women who are pregnant (see section 4.3 and section 4.4). Extreme care must be taken to avoid pregnancy in female patients. Copegus therapy must not be initiated until a report of a negative pregnancy test has been obtained immediately prior to initiation of therapy. Any birth control method can fail. Therefore, it is critically important that women of childbearing potential and their partners must use 2 forms of effective contraception simultaneously, during treatment and for 4 months after treatment has been concluded; routine monthly pregnancy tests must be performed during this time. If pregnancy does occur during treatment or within 4 months from stopping treatment the patient must be advised of the significant teratogenic risk of ribavirin to the foetus.

Male patients and their female partners: Extreme care must be taken to avoid pregnancy in partners of male patients taking Copegus. Ribavirin accumulates intracellularly and is cleared from the body very slowly. In animal studies, ribavirin produced changes in sperm at doses below the clinical dose. It is unknown whether the ribavirin that is contained in sperm will exert its known teratogenic effects upon fertilisation of the ova. Male patients and their female partners of childbearing age must, therefore, be counselled to use 2 forms of effective contraception simultaneously during treatment with Copegus and for 7 months after treatment has been concluded. A pregnancy test must be performed before therapy is started. Men whose partners are pregnant must be instructed to use a condom to minimise delivery of ribavirin to the partner.

Lactation: It is not known whether ribavirin is excreted in human milk. Because of the potential for adverse reactions in nursing infants, nursing must be discontinued prior to initiation of treatment.

4.7 Effects on ability to drive and use machines

Copegus has no or negligible influence on the ability to drive and use machines. However, peginterferon alfa-2a or interferon alfa-2a used in combination with Copegus may have an effect. Please refer to the SPC of peginterferon alfa-2a or interferon alfa-2a for further information.

4.8 Undesirable effects

See peginterferon alfa-2a or interferon alfa-2a prescribing information for additional undesirable effects for either of these products.

Adverse events reported in patients receiving Copegus in combination with interferon alfa-2a are essentially the same as for those reported for Copegus in combination with peginterferon alfa-2a.

Within each frequency grouping, undesirable effects are presented in order of decreasing seriousness.

Chronic Hepatitis C

The most frequently reported adverse events with Copegus in combination with peginterferon alfa-2a 180 micrograms were mostly mild to moderate in severity and were manageable without the need for modification of doses or discontinuation of therapy.

Chronic Hepatitis C and Human Immunodeficiency Virus Co-infection

In HIV-HCV co-infected patients, the clinical adverse event profiles reported for peginterferon alfa-2a, alone or in combination with ribavirin, were similar to those observed in HCV mono-infected patients. For HIV-HCV patients receiving Copegus and peginterferon alfa-2a combination therapy other undesirable effects have been reported in ⩾ 1% to ⩽ 2% of patients: hyperlactacidaemia/lactic acidosis, influenza, pneumonia, affect lability, apathy, tinnitus, pharyngolaryngeal pain, cheilitis, acquired lipodystrophy and chromaturia. Peginterferon alfa-2a treatment was associated with decreases in absolute CD4+ cell counts within the first 4 weeks without a reduction in CD4+ cell percentage. The decrease in CD4+ cell counts was reversible upon dose reduction or cessation of therapy. The use of peginterferon alfa-2a had no observable negative impact on the control of HIV viraemia during therapy or follow-up. Limited safety data (N= 51) are available in co-infected patients with CD4+ cell counts < 200/µl (see peginterferon alfa-2a SPC).

Table 5 shows the undesirable effects reported in patients who have received Copegus and peginterferon alfa-2a or interferon alfa-2a therapy.

(see Table 5 on previous page)

Laboratory values: In clinical trials of Copegus in combination with peginterferon alfa-2a or interferon alfa-2a, the majority of cases of abnormal laboratory values were managed with dose modifications (see section 4.2). With peginterferon alfa-2a and Copegus combination treatment, up to 2% of patients experienced increased ALT levels that led to dose modification or discontinuation of treatment.

Haemolysis is the dose limiting toxicity of ribavirin therapy. A decrease in haemoglobin levels to <10 g/dl was observed in up to 15% of patients treated for 48 weeks with Copegus 1000/1200 milligrams in combination with peginterferon alfa-2a and up to 19% of patients in combination with interferon alfa-2a. When Copegus 800 milligram was combined with peginterferon alfa-2a for 24 weeks, 3% of patients had a decrease in haemoglobin levels to <10 g/dl. It is not expected that patients will need to discontinue therapy because of decrease in haemoglobin levels alone. In most cases the decrease in haemoglobin occurred early in the treatment period and stabilised concurrently with a compensatory increase in reticulocytes.

Most cases of anaemia, leucopenia and thrombocytopenia were mild (WHO grade 1). WHO grade 2 laboratory changes were reported for haemoglobin (4% of patients), leucocytes (24% of patients) and thrombocytes (2% of patients). Moderate (absolute neutrophil count (ANC): 0.749-0.5x109/L) and severe (ANC: <0.5x109/L) neutropenia was observed in 24% (216/887) and 5% (41/887) of patients receiving 48 weeks of Copegus 1000/1200 milligrams in combination with peginterferon alfa-2a.

An increase in uric acid and indirect bilirubin values associated with haemolysis were observed in some patients treated with Copegus used in combination with peginterferon alfa-2a or interferon alfa-2a and values returned to baseline levels within 4 weeks after the end of therapy. In rare cases (2/755) this was associated with clinical manifestation (acute gout).

Laboratory values for HIV-HCV co-infected patients

Although haematological toxicities of neutropenia, thrombocytopenia and anaemia occurred more frequently in HIV-HCV patients, the majority could be managed by dose modification and the use of growth factors and infrequently required premature discontinuation of treatment. Decrease in ANC levels below 500 cells/mm^3 was observed in 13% and 11% of patients receiving peginterferon alfa-2a monotherapy and combination therapy, respectively. Decrease in platelets below 50,000/mm^3 was observed in 10% and 8% of patients receiving peginterferon alfa-2a monotherapy and combination therapy, respectively. Anaemia (haemoglobin < 10g/dL) was reported in 7% and 14% of patients treated with peginterferon alfa-2a monotherapy or in combination therapy, respectively.

4.9 Overdose

No cases of overdose of Copegus have been reported in clinical trials. Hypocalcaemia and hypomagnesaemia have been observed in persons administered dosages greater than four times the maximal recommended dosages. In many of these instances ribavirin was administered intravenously. Ribavirin is not effectively removed by haemodialysis.

5. PHARMACOLOGICAL PROPERTIES

5.1 Pharmacodynamic properties

Pharmacotherapeutic group: Nucleosides and nucleotides (excl. reverse transcriptase inhibitors), ATC code: J05A B04.

Table 6 Virological Response in the overall population (including non-cirrhotic and cirrhotic patients)

	Study NV15942	Study NV15801	
	Copegus 1,000/1,200 mg & Peginterferon alfa-2a 180 micrograms	Copegus 1,000/1,200 mg & Peginterferon alfa-2a 180 micrograms	Ribavirin 1,000/1,200 mg & Interferon alfa-2b 3 MIU
	(N=436) 48 weeks	(N=453) 48 weeks	(N=444) 48 weeks
Response at End of Treatment	68%	69%	52%
Overall Sustained Response	63%	54%*	45%*

*95% CI for difference: 3% to 16% p-value (stratified Cochran-Mantel-Haenszel test) = 0.003

Mechanism of Action: Ribavirin is a synthetic nucleoside analog that shows *in vitro* activity against some RNA and DNA viruses. The mechanism by which ribavirin in combination with peginterferon alfa-2a or interferon alfa-2a exerts its effects against HCV is unknown.

HCV RNA levels decline in a biphasic manner in responding patients with hepatitis C who have received treatment with 180 micrograms peginterferon alfa-2a. The first phase of decline occurs 24 to 36 hours after the first dose of peginterferon alfa-2a and is followed by the second phase of decline which continues over the next 4 to 16 weeks in patients who achieve a sustained response. Copegus had no significant effect on the initial viral kinetics over the first 4 to 6 weeks in patients treated with the combination of Copegus and pegylated interferon alfa-2a or interferon alfa.

Oral formulations of ribavirin monotherapy have been investigated as therapy for chronic hepatitis C in several clinical trials. Results of these investigations showed that ribavirin monotherapy had no effect on eliminating hepatitis virus (HCV-RNA) or improving hepatic histology after 6 to 12 months of therapy and 6 months of follow-up.

Clinical Trial Results

Copegus in combination with peginterferon alfa-2a

Predictability of response

Please refer to section 4.2, Table 2.

Study results

Efficacy and safety of the combination of Copegus and peginterferon alfa-2a were established in two pivotal studies (NV15801 + NV15942), including a total of 2405 patients. The study population comprised interferon-naïve patients with CHC confirmed by detectable levels of serum HCV RNA, elevated levels of ALT, and a liver biopsy consistent with chronic hepatitis C infection. Only HIV-HCV co-infected patients were included in the study NR15961 (see Table 12). These patients had stable HIV disease and mean CD4 T-cell count was about 500 cells/µl.

Study NV15801 (1121 patients treated) compared the efficacy of 48 weeks of treatment with peginterferon alfa-2a (180 mcg once weekly) and Copegus (1000/1200 mg daily) with either peginterferon alfa-2a monotherapy or combination therapy with interferon-alfa-2b and ribavirin. The combination of peginterferon alfa-2a and Copegus was significantly more efficacious than either the combination of interferon alfa-2b and ribavirin or peginterferon alfa-2a monotherapy.

Study NV15942 (1284 patients treated) compared the efficacy of two durations of treatment (24 weeks with 48

Table 7 Sustained Virological Response based on Genotype and Pre-treatment Viral Load after Copegus Combination Therapy with peginterferon alfa-2a

	Study NV15942				Study NV15801	
	Copegus 800 mg & **PEG-IFN alfa-2a** 180 mcg 24 weeks	**Copegus** 1000/1200 mg & **PEG-IFN alfa-2a** 180 mcg 24 weeks	**Copegus** 800 mg & **PEG-IFN alfa-2a** 180 mcg 48 weeks	**Copegus** 1000/1200 mg & **PEG-IFN alfa-2a** 180 mcg 48 weeks	**Copegus** 1000/1200 mg & **PEG-IFN alfa-2a** 180 mcg 48 weeks	**Ribavirin** 1000/1200 mg & **Interferon alfa-2b** 3 MIU 48 weeks
Genotype 1	29 % (29/101)	42 % (49/118)†	41 % (102/250)*	**52 %** (142/271)*†	45 % (134/298)	36 % (103/285)
Low viral load	41 % (21/51)	52 % (37/71)	55 % (33/60)	**65 %** (55/85)	53 % (61/115)	44 % (41/94)
High viral load	16 % (8/50)	26 % (12/47)	36 % (69/190)	**47 %** (87/186)	40 % (73/182)	33 % (62/189)
Genotype 2/3	**84 %** (81/96)	81 % (117/144)	79 % (78/99)	80 % (123/153)	71 % (100/140)	61 % (88/145)
Low viral load	**85 %** (29/34)	83 % (39/47)	88 % (29/33)	77 % (37/48)	76 % (28/37)	65 % (34/52)
High viral load	**84 %** (52/62)	80 % (78/97)	74 % (49/66)	82 % (86/105)	70 % (72/103)	58 % (54/93)
Genotype 4	0 % (0/5)	67 % (8/12)	63 % (5/8)	82 % (9/11)	77 % (10/13)	45 % (5/11)

Low viral load= ⩽ 800,000 IU/mL; High viral load= > 800,000 IU/mL

*Copegus 1000/1200 mg + peginterferon alfa-2a 180 mcg, 48 w vs. Copegus 800 mg + peginterferon alfa-2a 180 mcg, 48 w: Odds Ratio (95% CI) = 1.52 (1.07 to 2.17) P-value (stratified Cochran-Mantel-Haenszel test) = 0.020

†Copegus 1000/1200 mg + peginterferon alfa-2a 180 mcg, 48 w vs. Copegus 1000/1200 mg + peginterferon alfa-2a 180 mcg, 24 w: Odds Ratio (95% CI) = 2.12 (1.30 to 3.46) P-value (stratified Cochran-Mantel-Haenszel test) = 0.002

weeks) and two dosages of Copegus (800 mg with 1000/1200 mg).

For HCV monoinfected patients and HIV-HCV co-infected patients, for treatment regimens, duration of therapy and study outcome see tables 6, 7, 8 and 12, respectively. Virological response was defined as undetectable HCV RNA as measured by the COBAS AMPLICOR® HCV Test, version 2.0 (limit of detection 100 copies/ml equivalent to 50 International Units/ml) and sustained response as one negative sample approximately 6 months after the end of therapy.

(see Table 6 on previous page)

The virological responses of HCV monoinfected patients treated with Copegus and peginterferon alfa-2a combination therapy in relation to genotype and pre-treatment viral load and in relation to genotype, pre-treatment viral load and rapid virological response at week 4 are summarised in Table 7 and Table 8 respectively. The results of study NV15942 provide the rationale for recommending treatment regimens based on genotype, baseline viral load and virological response at week 4 (see Tables 1, 7 and 8).

The difference between treatment regimens was in general not influenced by presence/absence of cirrhosis; therefore treatment recommendations for genotype 1, 2 or 3 are independent of this baseline characteristic.

(see Table 7 on previous page)

The possibility to consider shortening treatment duration to 24 weeks in genotype 1 and 4 patients was examined based on a sustained rapid virological response observed in patients with rapid virological response at week 4 in studies NV15942 and ML17131 (see Table 8).

(see Table 8 above)

Although limited, data indicated that shortening treatment to 24 weeks might be associated with a higher risk of relapse (see Table 9).

(see Table 9 opposite)

The possibility of shortening treatment duration to 16 weeks in genotype 2 or 3 patients was examined based on the sustained rapid virological response observed in patients with rapid virological response by week 4 in study NV17317 (see Table 10).

In study NV17317 in patients infected with viral genotype 2 or 3, all patients received peginterferon alfa-2a 180 µg sc qw and a Copegus dose of 800 mg and were randomised to treatment for either 16 or 24 weeks. Overall treatment for 16 weeks resulted in lower sustained viral response (65%) than treatment for 24 weeks (76%) ($p < 0.0001$).

The sustained viral response achieved with 16 weeks of treatment and with 24 weeks of treatment was also examined in a retrospective subgroup analysis of patients who were HCV RNA negative by week 4 and had a LVL at baseline (see Table 10).

(see Table 10 opposite)

The data indicated that shortening treatment to 16 weeks is associated with a higher risk of relapse (see Table 11)

(see Table 11 on next page)

HCV patients with normal ALT

In study NR16071, HCV patients with normal ALT values were randomised to receive peginterferon alfa-2a 180 micrograms/week with a Copegus dose of 800 milligrams/day for either 24 or 48 weeks followed by a 24 week treatment free follow-up period or an untreated control group for 72 weeks. The SVRs reported in the treatment arms of this study were similar to the corresponding treatment arms from study NV15942.

HIV-HCV co-infected patients

The virological responses of patients treated with Copegus and peginterferon alfa-2a combination therapy in relation to genotype and pre-treatment viral load for HIV-HCV co-infected patients are summarised below in Table 12.

(see Table 12 on next page)

Ribavirin in combination with interferon alfa-2a

The therapeutic efficacy of interferon alfa-2a alone and in combination with oral ribavirin was compared in clinical trials in naïve (previously untreated) and relapsed patients who had virologically, biochemically and histologically documented chronic hepatitis C. Six months after end of treatment sustained biochemical and virological response as well as histological improvement were assessed.

A statistically significant 10-fold increase (from 4% to 43%; $p < 0.01$) in sustained virological and biochemical response was observed in relapsed patients (M23136; N=99). The favourable profile of the combination therapy was also reflected in the response rates relative to HCV genotype or baseline viral load. In the combination and interferon monotherapy arms, respectively, the sustained response rates in patients with HCV genotype-1 were 28% versus 0% and with genotype non-1 were 58% versus 8%. In addition the histological improvement favoured the combination therapy. Supportive favourable results (monotherapy vs combination; 6% vs 48%, $p < 0.04$) from a small published study in naïve patients (N=40) were reported using interferon alfa-2a (3 MIU 3 times per week) with ribavirin.

5.2 Pharmacokinetic properties

Ribavirin is absorbed rapidly following oral administration of a single dose of Copegus (median T_{max} = 1-2 hours). The

Table 8 Sustained Virological Response Based on Rapid Viral Response at week 4 for Genotype 1 and 4 after Copegus Combination Therapy with Peginterferon alfa-2a in HCV Patients

Study NV15942			Study ML17131
	Copegus 1000/1200 mg & Peginterferon alfa-2a 180 mcg 24 weeks	Copegus 1000/1200 mg & Peginterferon alfa-2a 180 mcg 48 weeks	Copegus 1000/1200 mg & Peginterferon alfa-2a 180 mcg 24 weeks
Genotype 1 RVR	90% (28/31)	92% (47/51)	77% (59/77)
Low viral load	93% (25/27)	96% (26/27)	80% (52/65)
High viral load	75% (3/4)	88% (21/24)	58% (7/12)
Genotype 1 non RVR	24% (21/87)	43% (95/220)	-
Low viral load	27% (12/44)	50% (31/62)	-
High viral load	21% (9/43)	41% (64/158)	-
Genotype 4 RVR	(5/6)	(5/5)	92% (22/24)
Genotype 4 non RVR	(3/6)	(4/6)	-

Low viral load= ≤ 800,000 IU/mL; High viral load= > 800,000 IU/mL

RVR = rapid viral response (HCV RNA undetectable) at week 4 and HCV RNA undetectable at week 24

Table 9 Relapse of Virological Response at the End of Treatment for Rapid Virological Response Population

Study NV15942			Study NV15801
	Copegus 1000/1200 mg & Peginterferon alfa-2a 180 mcg 24 weeks	Copegus 1000/1200 mg & Peginterferon alfa-2a 180 mcg 48 weeks	Copegus 1000/1200 mg & Peginterferon alfa-2a 180 mcg 48 weeks
Genotype 1 RVR	6.7% (2/30)	4.3% (2/47)	0% (0/24)
Low viral load	3.8% (1/26)	0% (0/25)	0% (0/17)
High viral load	25% (1/4)	9.1% (2/22)	0% (0/7)
Genotype 4 RVR	(0/5)	(0/5)	0% (0/4)

Table 10 Sustained Virological Response Overall and Based on Rapid Viral Response by Week 4 for Genotype 2 or 3 after Copegus Combination Therapy with Peginterferon alfa-2a in HCV Patients

Study NV17317	Copegus 800 mg & Peginterferon alfa-2a 180 mcg 16 weeks	Copegus 800 mg & Peginterferon alfa-2a 180 mcg 24 weeks	Treatment difference 95% CI	p value
Genotype 2 or 3	65% (443/679)	76% (478/630)	-10.6% [-15.5%; -0.06%]	P<0.0001
Genotype 2 or 3 RVR	82% (378/461)	90% (370/410)	-8.2% [-12.8%; -3.7%]	P=0.0006
Low viral load	89% (147/166)	94% (141/150)	-5.4% [-12%; 0.9%]	P=0.11
High viral load	78% (231/295)	88% (229/260)	-9.7% [-15.9%; -3.6%]	P=0.002

Low viral load= ≤ 800,000 IU/mL at baseline; High viral load= > 800,000 IU/mL at baseline

RVR = rapid viral response (HCV RNA negative) by week 4

mean terminal phase half-life of ribavirin following single doses of Copegus range from 140 to 160 hours. Ribavirin data from the literature demonstrates absorption is extensive with approximately 10% of a radiolabelled dose excreted in the faeces. However, absolute bioavailability is approximately 45%-65%, which appears to be due to first pass metabolism. There is an approximately linear relationship between dose and AUC_{tf} following single doses of 200-1,200 milligrams ribavirin. Mean apparent oral clearance of ribavirin following single 600 milligram doses of Copegus ranges from 22 to 29 litres/hour. Volume of distribution is approximately 4,500 litres following administration of Copegus. Ribavirin does not bind to plasma proteins.

Ribavirin has been shown to produce high inter- and intra-subject pharmacokinetic variability following single oral doses of Copegus(intra-subject variability of ≤25% for both AUC and C_{max}), which may be due to extensive first pass metabolism and transfer within and beyond the blood compartment.

Ribavirin transport in non-plasma compartments has been most extensively studied in red cells, and has been identified to be primarily via an e_s-type equilibrative nucleoside transporter. This type of transporter is present on virtually all cell types and may account for the high volume of distribution of ribavirin. The ratio of whole blood: plasma ribavirin concentrations is approximately 60:1; the excess of ribavirin in whole blood exists as ribavirin nucleotides sequestered in erythrocytes.

Ribavirin has two pathways of metabolism: 1) a reversible phosphorylation pathway, 2) a degradative pathway involving deribosylation and amide hydrolysis to yield a triazole carboxyacid metabolite. Ribavirin and both its triazole carboxamide and triazole carboxylic acid metabolites are excreted renally.

Upon multiple dosing, ribavirin accumulates extensively in plasma with a six-fold ratio of multiple-dose to single-dose AUC_{12hr} based on literature data. Following oral dosing with 600 milligrams BID, steady-state was reached by approximately 4 weeks, with mean steady state plasma concentrations of approximately 2,200 ng/ml. Upon discontinuation of dosing the half-life was approximately 300 hours, which probably reflects slow elimination from non-plasma compartments.

Food effect: The bioavailability of a single oral 600 mg dose Copegus was increased by coadministration of a high

Table 11 Relapse of Virological Response after the End of Treatment in Genotype 2 or 3 Patients with a Rapid Viral Response

Study NV17317				
	Copegus 800 mg & **Peginterferon alfa-2a** 180 mcg 16 weeks	**Copegus** 800 mg & **Peginterferon alfa-2a** 180 mcg 24 weeks	**Treatment difference** $_{95\%}$ **CI**	**p value**
Genotype 2 or 3 RVR	15% (67/439)	6% (23/386)	9.3% [5.2%; 13.6%]	P<0.0001
Low viral load	6% (10/155)	1% (2/141)	5% [0.6%; 10.3%]	P=0.04
High viral load	20% (57/284)	9% (21/245)	11.5% [5.6%; 17.4%]	P=0.0002

Table 12 Sustained Virological Response based on Genotype and Pre-treatment Viral Load after Copegus Combination Therapy with peginterferon alfa-2a in HIV-HCV co-infected patients

Study NR15961			
	Interferon alfa-2a 3 MIU & **Copegus 800 mg** 48 weeks	**Peginterferon alfa-2a** 180 mcg & **Placebo** 48 weeks	**Peginterferon alfa-2a** 180 mcg & **Copegus 800 mg** 48 weeks
All patients	12% (33/285)*	20% (58/286)*	40% (116/289)*
Genotype 1	7% (12/171)	14% (24/175)	29% (51/176)
Low viral load	19% (8/42)	38% (17/45)	61% (28/46)
High viral load	3% (4/129)	5% (7/130)	18% (23/130)
Genotype 2-3	20% (18/89)	36% (32/90)	62% (59/95)
Low viral load	27% (8/30)	38% (9/24)	61% (17/28)
High viral load	17% (10/59)	35% (23/66)	63% (42/67)

Low viral load= ⩽ 800,000 IU/mL; High viral load= > 800,000 IU/mL

* peginterferon alfa-2a 180 mcg Copegus 800mg vs. Interferon alfa-2a 3MIU ribavirin 800mg: Odds Ratio (95% CI) = 5.40 (3.42 to 8.54), ...P-value (stratified Cochran-Mantel-Haenszel test) = < 0.0001

* peginterferon alfa-2a 180 mcg Copegus 800mg vs. peginterferon alfa-2a 180μg: Odds Ratio (95% CI) = 2.89 (1.93 to 4.32),. . ..P-value (stratified Cochran-Mantel-Haenszel test) = < 0.0001

* Interferon alfa-2a 3MIU Copegus 800mg vs. peginterferon alfa-2a 180mcg: Odds Ratio (95% CI) = 0.53 (0.33 to 0.85), . . .P-value (stratified Cochran-Mantel-Haenszel test) = < 0.0084.

fat meal. The ribavirin exposure parameters of $AUC_{(0-192h)}$ and C_{max} increased by 42% and 66%, respectively, when Copegus was taken with a high fat breakfast compared to being taken in the fasted state. The clinical relevance of results from this single dose study is unknown. Ribavirin exposure after multiple dosing when taken with food was comparable in patients receiving peginterferon alfa-2a and Copegus and interferon alfa-2b and ribavirin. In order to achieve optimal ribavirin plasma concentrations, it is recommended to take ribavirin with food.

Renal function: Single-dose ribavirin pharmacokinetics were altered (increased AUC_{tf} and C_{max}) in patients with renal dysfunction compared with control subjects whose creatinine clearance was greater than 90 ml/minute. The clearance of ribavirin is substantially reduced in patients with serum creatinine > 2 mg/dl or creatinine clearance < 50 ml/min. There are insufficient data on the safety and efficacy of ribavirin in such patients to support recommendations for dose adjustments. Plasma concentrations of ribavirin are essentially unchanged by haemodialysis.

Hepatic function: Single-dose pharmacokinetics of ribavirin in patients with mild, moderate or severe hepatic dysfunction (Child-Pugh Classification A, B or C) are similar to those of normal controls.

Use in elderly patients over the age of 65: Specific pharmacokinetic evaluations for elderly subjects have not been performed. However, in a published population pharmacokinetic study, age was not a key factor in the kinetics of ribavirin; renal function is the determining factor.

Patients under the age of 18 years: The pharmacokinetic properties of ribavirin have not been fully evaluated in patients under the age of 18 years. Copegus in combination with peginterferon alfa-2 or interferon alfa-2a is indicated for the treatment of chronic hepatitis C only in patients 18 years of age or older.

Population Pharmacokinetics: A population pharmacokinetic analysis was performed using plasma concentration values from five clinical trials. While body weight and race were statistically significant covariates in the clearance model, only the effect of body weight was clinically significant. Clearance increased as a function of body weight and was predicted to vary from 17.7 to 24.8 L/h over a weight range of 44 to 155 kg. Creatinine clearance (as low as 34 ml/min) did not affect ribavirin clearance.

5.3 Preclinical safety data

Ribavirin is embryotoxic and/or teratogenic at doses well below the recommended human dose in all animal species in which adequate studies have been conducted. Malformations of the skull, palate, eye, jaw, limbs, skeleton and gastrointestinal tract were noted. The incidence and severity of teratogenic effects increased with escalation of the dose. Survival of foetuses and offspring is reduced.

Erythrocytes are a primary target of toxicity for ribavirin in animal studies, including studies in dogs and monkeys. Anaemia occurs shortly after initiation of dosing, but is rapidly reversible upon cessation of treatment. Hypoplastic anaemia was observed only in rats at the high dose of 160 milligrams/kg/day in the subchronic study.

Reduced leucocyte and/or lymphocyte counts were consistently noted in the repeat-dose rodent and dog toxicity studies with ribavirin and transiently in monkeys administered ribavirin in the subchronic study. Repeat-dose rat toxicity studies showed thymic lymphoid depletion and/or depletion of thymus-dependent areas of the spleen (periarteriolar lymphoid sheaths, white pulp) and mesenteric lymph node. Following repeat-dosing of dogs with ribavirin, increased dilatation/necrosis of the intestinal crypts of the duodenum was noted, as well as chronic inflammation of the small intestine and erosion of the ileum.

In repeat dose studies in mice to investigate ribavirin-induced testicular and sperm effects, abnormalities in sperm occurred at doses in animals well below therapeutic doses. Upon cessation of treatment, essentially total recovery from ribavirin-induced testicular toxicity occurred within one or two spermatogenic cycles.

Genotoxicity studies have demonstrated that ribavirin does exert some genotoxic activity. Ribavirin was active in an *in vitro* Transformation Assay. Genotoxic activity was observed in *in vivo* mouse micronucleus assays. A dominant lethal assay in rats was negative, indicating that if mutations occurred in rats they were not transmitted through male gametes. Ribavirin is a possible human carcinogen.

Administration of ribavirin and peginterferon alfa-2a in combination did not produce any unexpected toxicity in monkeys. The major treatment-related change was reversible mild to moderate anaemia, the severity of which was greater than that produced by either active substance alone.

6. PHARMACEUTICAL PARTICULARS

6.1 List of excipients

Tablet core:

Pregelatinised maize starch

Sodium starch glycolate (type A)

Microcrystalline cellulose

Maize starch

Magnesium stearate

Film-coating:

Hypromellose

Talc

Titanium dioxide (E171)

Yellow iron oxide (E172)

Red iron oxide (E172)

Ethylcellulose aqueous dispersion

Triacetin

6.2 Incompatibilities

Not applicable

6.3 Shelf life

4 years

6.4 Special precautions for storage

This medicinal product does not require any special storage conditions

6.5 Nature and contents of container

Copegus is supplied in high density polyethylene (HDPE) bottles with a child-resistant polypropylene screw cap containing 28, 42, 112 or 168 tablets. Not all pack sizes may be marketed.

6.6 Special precautions for disposal and other handling

No special requirements

7. MARKETING AUTHORISATION HOLDER

Roche Products Limited
6 Falcon Way
Shire Park
Welwyn Garden City
AL7 1TW
United Kingdom

8. MARKETING AUTHORISATION NUMBER(S)

PL 00031/0604
PA 50/153/1

9. DATE OF FIRST AUTHORISATION/RENEWAL OF THE AUTHORISATION

UK: 13 November 2002 / 9 April 2007

Ireland: 4 April 2003 / 9 April 2007

10. DATE OF REVISION OF THE TEXT

UK: 15 July 2009
Ireland: 15 July 2009

LEGAL STATUS

POM

Copegus 400mg Film-coated Tablets

(Roche Products Limited)

1. NAME OF THE MEDICINAL PRODUCT

Copegus 400 mg film-coated tablet

2. QUALITATIVE AND QUANTITATIVE COMPOSITION

Each film-coated tablet contains 400 milligrams of ribavirin.

For a full list of excipients, see section 6.1.

3. PHARMACEUTICAL FORM

Film-coated tablet

Reddish brown, flat oval-shaped film-coated tablet (marked with RIB 400 on one side and ROCHE on the opposite side).

4. CLINICAL PARTICULARS

4.1 Therapeutic indications

Copegus is indicated for the treatment of chronic hepatitis C and must only be used as part of a combination regimen with peginterferon alfa-2a or with interferon alfa-2a. Copegus monotherapy must not be used.

The combination of Copegus with peginterferon alfa-2a or interferon alfa-2a is indicated in adult patients who are positive for serum HCV-RNA, including patients with compensated cirrhosis. (See section 4.4) The combination with peginterferon alfa-2a is also indicated in patients co-infected with clinically stable HIV, including patients with compensated cirrhosis (See section 4.3). The combination regimens are indicated in previously untreated patients as well as in patients who have previously responded to interferon alpha therapy and subsequently relapsed after treatment was stopped.

Please refer to the Summary of Product Characteristics (SPC) of peginterferon alfa-2a or interferon alfa-2a for prescribing information particular to either of these products.

4.2 Posology and method of administration

Treatment should be initiated, and monitored, by a physician experienced in the management of chronic hepatitis C.

Method of Administration

Copegus film-coated tablets are administered orally in two divided doses with food (morning and evening). Due to the teratogenic potential of ribavirin, the tablets should not be broken or crushed. As Copegus is available in a 200 mg tablet, there is no need for dividing or cutting the 400 mg tablet in half.

Posology

Copegus is used in combination with peginterferon alfa-2a or interferon alfa-2a. The exact dose and duration of treatment depend on the interferon product used.

Please refer to the SPC of peginterferon alfa-2a or interferon alfa-2a for further information on dosage and duration of treatment when Copegus is to be used in combination with either of these products.

Posology in combination with peginterferon alfa-2a:

Dose to be administered

The recommended dose of Copegus in combination with peginterferon alfa-2a solution for injection depends on viral genotype and the patient's body weight (see Table 1).

Duration of treatment

The duration of combination therapy with peginterferon alfa-2a depends on viral genotype. Patients infected with HCV genotype 1 who have detectable HCV RNA at week 4 regardless of pre-treatment viral load should receive 48 weeks of therapy.

Treatment for 24 weeks may be considered in patients infected with

- genotype 1 with low viral load (LVL) (≤ 800,000 IU/mL) at baseline or

- genotype 4 who become HCV RNA negative at week 4 and remain HCV RNA negative at week 24. However, an overall 24 weeks treatment duration may be associated with a higher risk of relapse than a 48 weeks treatment duration (see 5.1). In these patients, tolerability to combination therapy and additional prognostic factors such as degree of fibrosis should be taken into account when deciding on treatment duration. Shortening the treatment duration in patients with genotype 1 and high viral load (HVL) (>800, 000 IU/ml) at baseline who become HCV RNA negative at week 4 and remain HCV RNA negative at week 24 should be considered with even more caution since the limited data available suggest that this may significantly negatively impact the sustained virologic response.

Patients infected with HCV genotype 2 or 3 who have detectable HCV RNA at week 4, regardless of pre-treatment viral load should receive 24 weeks of therapy. Treatment for only 16 weeks may be considered in selected patients infected with genotype 2 or 3 with LVL (≤ 800,000 IU/mL) at baseline who become HCV negative by week 4 of treatment and remain HCV negative by week 16. Overall 16 weeks of treatment may be associated with a lower chance of response and is associated with a higher risk of relapse than a 24 week treatment duration (see section 5.1). In these patients, tolerability to combination therapy and the presence of additional clinical or prognostic factors such as degree of fibrosis should be taken into account when considering deviations from standard 24 weeks treatment duration. Shortening the treatment duration in patients infected with genotype 2 or 3 with HVL (> 800,000 IU/mL) at baseline who become HCV negative by week 4 should be considered with more caution as this may significantly negatively impact the sustained virological response (see Table 1).

Available data for patients infected with genotype 5 or 6 are limited; therefore combination treatment with 1000/1200 mg of ribavirin for 48 weeks is recommended.

(see Table 1 above)

The ultimate clinical impact of a shortened initial treatment of 16 weeks instead of 24 weeks is unknown, taking into account the need for retreating non-responding and relapsing patients.

HIV-HCV Co-infection

The recommended dosage for Copegus in combination with 180 micrograms once weekly of peginterferon alfa-2a is 800 milligrams, daily for 48 weeks, regardless of genotype. The safety and efficacy of combination therapy with ribavirin doses greater than 800 milligrams daily or a duration of therapy less than 48 weeks has not been studied.

Predictability of response and non-response

Early virological response by week 12, defined as a 2 log viral load decrease or undetectable levels of HCV RNA has been shown to be predictive for sustained response (see Table 2).

(see Table 2 above)

A similar negative predictive value has been observed in HIV-HCV co-infected patients treated with peginterferon alfa-2a monotherapy or in combination with ribavirin (100 %(130/130) or 98%(83/85), respectively). Positive predictive values of 45 %(50/110) and 70%(59/84) were observed for genotype 1 and genotype 2/3 HIV-HCV co-infected patients receiving combination therapy.

Table 1 Copegus Dosing Recommendations in Combination with Peginterferon alfa-2a for HCV patients

Genotype	Daily Copegus Dose	Duration of treatment	Number of 200/400 mg tablets
Genotype 1 LVL with RVR*	<75 kg = 1000 mg ≥75 kg = 1200 mg	24 weeks or 48 weeks	5 × 200 mg (2 morning, 3 evening) 6 × 200 mg (3 morning, 3 evening)
Genotype 1 HVL with RVR*	<75 kg = 1000 mg ≥75 kg = 1200 mg	48 weeks	5 × 200 mg (2 morning, 3 evening) 6 × 200 mg (3 morning, 3 evening)
Genotype 4 with RVR*	<75 kg = 1000 mg ≥75 kg = 1200 mg	24 weeks or 48 weeks	5 × 200 mg (2 morning, 3 evening) 6 × 200 mg (3 morning, 3 evening)
Genotype 1 or 4 without RVR*	< 75 kg = 1,000 mg ≥ 75 kg = 1,200 mg	48 weeks	5 × 200 mg (2 morning, 3 evening) 6 × 200 mg (3 morning, 3 evening)
Genotype 2 or 3 LVL with RVR**	800 mg	16 weeks or 24 weeks	4 × 200 mg (2 morning, 2 evening) or 2 × 400 mg (1 morning, 1 evening)
Genotype 2 or 3 HVL with RVR**	800 mg	24 weeks	4 × 200 mg (2 morning, 2 evening) or 2 × 400 mg (1 morning, 1 evening)
Genotype 2 or 3 without RVR**	800 mg	24 weeks	4 × 200 mg (2 morning, 2 evening) or 2 × 400 mg (1 morning, 1 evening)

*RVR = rapid viral response (HCV RNA undetectable) at week 4 and HCV RNA undetectable at week 24;
**RVR = rapid viral response (HCV RNA negative) by week 4
LVL= ≤ 800,000 IU/mL; HVL= > 800,000 IU/mL

Table 2 Predictive Value of Week 12 Virological Response at the Recommended Dosing Regimen while receiving Copegus and peginterferon Combination Therapy

Genotype	Negative			Positive		
	No response by week 12	No sustained response	Predictive Value	Response by week 12	Sustained response	Predictive Value
Genotype 1 (N= 569)	102	97	**95 %** (97/102)	467	271	**58 %** (271/467)
Genotype 2 and 3 (N=96)	3	3	**100 %** (3/3)	93	81	**87 %** (81/93)

Table 3 Copegus Dosing Recommendations in Combination with Interferon alfa-2a

Patient weight (kg)	Daily Copegus dose	Duration of treatment	Number of 200 mg tablets
< 75	1,000 mg	24 or 48 weeks	5 (2 morning, 3 evening)
≥ 75	1,200 mg	24 or 48 weeks	6 (3 morning, 3 evening)

Posology in combination with interferon alfa-2a:

Dose to be administered

The recommended dose of Copegus in combination with interferon alfa-2a solution for injection depends on the patient's body weight (see Table 3).

Duration of treatment:

Patients should be treated with combination therapy with interferon alfa-2a for at least six months. Patients with HCV genotype 1 infections should receive 48 weeks of combination therapy. In patients infected with HCV of other genotypes, the decision to extend therapy to 48 weeks should be based on other prognostic factors (such as high viral load at baseline, male gender, age > 40 years and evidence of bridging fibrosis).

(see Table 3 above)

Dosage modification for adverse reactions

Please refer to the SPC of peginterferon alfa-2a or interferon alfa-2a for further information on dose adjustment and discontinuation of treatment for either of these products.

If severe adverse reactions or laboratory abnormalities develop during therapy with Copegus and peginterferon alfa-2a or interferon alfa-2a, modify the dosages of each product, until the adverse reactions abate. Guidelines were developed in clinical trials for dose modification (see **Dosage Modification Guidelines for Management of Treatment-Emergent Anaemia**, Table 4).

If intolerance persists after dose adjustment, discontinuation of Copegus or both Copegus and peginterferon alfa-2a or interferon alfa-2a may be needed.

Table 4 Dosage Modification Guidelines for Management of Treatment-Emergent Anaemia

Laboratory Values	Reduce only Copegus dose to 600 mg/day* if:	Discontinue Copegus if:**
Haemoglobin in Patients with No Cardiac Disease	< 10 g/dl	< 8.5 g/dl
Haemoglobin: Patients with History of Stable Cardiac Disease	≥ 2 g/dl decrease in haemoglobin during any 4 week period during treatment (permanent dose reduction)	< 12 g/dl despite 4 weeks at reduced dose

*Patients whose dose of Copegus is reduced to 600 mg daily receive one 200 mg tablet in the morning and either two 200 mg tablets or one 400 mg tablet in the evening.

**If the abnormality is reversed, Copegus may be restarted at 600 mg daily, and further increased to 800 mg daily at the discretion of the treating physician. However, a return to higher doses is not recommended.

Special populations

Use in renal impairment: The recommended dose regimens (adjusted by the body weight cut off of 75 kg) of ribavirin give rise to substantial increases in plasma concentrations of ribavirin in patients with renal impairment. There are insufficient data on the safety and efficacy of ribavirin in patients with serum creatinine > 2 mg/dl or creatinine clearance < 50 ml/min, whether or not on haemodialysis, to support recommendations for dose adjustments. Therefore, ribavirin should be used in such patients only when this is considered to be essential. Therapy should be initiated (or continued if renal impairment develops while on therapy) with extreme caution and intensive monitoring of haemoglobin concentrations, with corrective action as may be necessary, should be employed throughout the treatment period. (see section 4.4 and section 5.2).

Use in hepatic impairment: Hepatic function does not affect the pharmacokinetics of ribavirin (see section 5.2). Therefore, no dose adjustment of Copegus is required in patients with hepatic impairment. The use of peginterferon alfa-2a and interferon alfa-2a is contraindicated in patients with decompensated cirrhosis and other forms of severe hepatic impairment.

Use in elderly patients over the age of 65: There does not appear to be a significant age-related effect on the pharmacokinetics of ribavirin. However, as in younger patients, renal function must be determined prior to administration of Copegus.

Use in patients under the age of 18 years: Treatment with Copegus is not recommended for use in children and adolescents (<18 years) due to insufficient data on safety and efficacy in combination with peginterferon alfa-2a and interferon alfa-2a.

4.3 Contraindications

See peginterferon alfa-2a or interferon alfa-2a prescribing information for contraindications related to either of these products.

- hypersensitivity to ribavirin or to any of the excipients.
- pregnant women (see section 4.4). Copegus must not be initiated until a report of a negative pregnancy test has been obtained immediately prior to initiation of therapy.
- women who are breast-feeding (see section 4.6).

- a history of severe pre-existing cardiac disease, including unstable or uncontrolled cardiac disease, in the previous six months.

- severe hepatic dysfunction or decompensated cirrhosis of the liver.

- haemoglobinopathies (e.g. thalassaemia, sickle-cell anaemia).

- Initiation of peginterferon alfa-2a is contraindicated in HIV-HCV patients with cirrhosis and a Child-Pugh score ⩾ 6 (Please refer to the SPC of peginterferon alfa-2a for Child-Pugh assessment).

4.4 Special warnings and precautions for use

Psychiatric and Central Nervous System (CNS): Severe CNS effects, particularly depression, suicidal ideation and attempted suicide have been observed in some patients during Copegus combination therapy with peginterferon alfa-2a or interferon alfa-2a, and even after treatment discontinuation mainly during the 6-month follow-up period. Other CNS effects including aggressive behaviour (sometimes directed against others), confusion and alterations of mental status have been observed with alpha interferons. Patients should be closely monitored for any signs or symptoms of psychiatric disorders. If such symptoms appear, the potential seriousness of these undesirable effects must be borne in mind by the prescribing physician and the need for adequate therapeutic management should be considered. If psychiatric symptoms persist or worsen, or suicidal ideation is identified, it is recommended that treatment with Copegus and peginterferon alfa-2a or interferon alfa-2a be discontinued, and the patient followed, with psychiatric intervention as appropriate.

Patients with existence of, or history of severe psychiatric conditions: If treatment with Copegus in combination with peginterferon alfa-2a or interferon alfa-2a is judged necessary in patients with existence or history of severe psychiatric conditions, this should only be initiated after having ensured appropriate individualised diagnostic and therapeutic management of the psychiatric condition.

Please refer to the SPC of peginterferon alfa-2a or interferon alfa-2a for further information on special warnings and precautions for use related to either of these products.

All patients in the chronic hepatitis C studies had a liver biopsy before inclusion, but in certain cases (ie, patients with genotype 2 or 3), treatment may be possible without histological confirmation. Current treatment guidelines should be consulted as to whether a liver biopsy is needed prior to commencing treatment.

In patients with normal ALT, progression of fibrosis occurs on average at a slower rate than in patients with elevated ALT. This should be considered in conjunction with other factors, such as HCV genotype, age, extrahepatic manifestations, risk of transmission, etc. which influence the decision to treat or not.

Teratogenic risk: See **4.6 Pregnancy and lactation**.

Prior to initiation of treatment with ribavirin the physician must comprehensively inform the patient of the teratogenic risk of ribavirin, the necessity of effective and continuous contraception, the possibility that contraceptive methods may fail and the possible consequences of pregnancy should it occur during treatment with ribavirin. For laboratory monitoring of pregnancy please refer to Laboratory tests.

Carcinogenicity: Ribavirin is mutagenic in some *in vivo* and *in vitro* genotoxicity assays. A potential carcinogenic effect of ribavirin cannot be excluded (see section 5.3).

Haemolysis and Cardiovascular system: A decrease in haemoglobin levels to < 10 g/dl was observed in up to 15 %of patients treated for 48 weeks with Copegus 1000/1200 milligrams in combination with peginterferon alfa-2a and up to 19 %of patients in combination with interferon alfa-2a. When Copegus 800 milligram was combined with peginterferon alfa-2a for 24 weeks, 3 % of patients had a decrease in haemoglobin levels to < 10 g/dl. The risk of developing anaemia is higher in the female population. Although ribavirin has no direct cardiovascular effects, anaemia associated with Copegus may result in deterioration of cardiac function, or exacerbation of the symptoms of coronary disease, or both. Thus, Copegus must be administered with caution to patients with pre-existing cardiac disease. Cardiac status must be assessed before start of therapy and monitored clinically during therapy; if any deterioration occurs, stop therapy (see section 4.2). Patients with a history of congestive heart failure, myocardial infarction, and/or previous or current arrhythmic disorders must be closely monitored. It is recommended that those patients who have pre-existing cardiac abnormalities have electrocardiograms taken prior to and during the course of treatment. Cardiac arrhythmias (primarily supraventricular) usually respond to conventional therapy but may require discontinuation of therapy.

Acute hypersensitivity: If an acute hypersensitivity reaction (e.g. urticaria, angioedema, bronchoconstriction, anaphylaxis) develops, Copegus must be discontinued immediately and appropriate medical therapy instituted. Transient rashes do not necessitate interruption of treatment.

Liver function: In patients who develop evidence of hepatic decompensation during treatment, Copegus in combination with peginterferon alfa-2a or interferon alfa-2a should be discontinued. When the increase in ALT levels is progressive and clinically significant, despite dose reduction, or is accompanied by increased direct bilirubin, therapy should be discontinued.

Renal impairment: The pharmacokinetics of ribavirin are altered in patients with renal dysfunction due to reduction of apparent clearance in these patients (see section 5.2). Therefore, it is recommended that renal function be evaluated in all patients prior to initiation of Copegus, preferably by estimating the patient's creatinine clearance. Substantial increases in ribavirin plasma concentrations are seen at the recommended dosing regimen in patients with serum creatinine > 2 mg/dl or with creatinine clearance < 50 ml/minute. There are insufficient data on the safety and efficacy of Copegus in such patients to support recommendations for dose adjustments. Copegus therapy should not be initiated (or continued if renal impairment occurs while on treatment) in such patients, whether or not on haemodialysis, unless it is considered to be essential. Extreme caution is required. Haemoglobin concentrations should be monitored intensively during treatment and corrective action taken as necessary (see section 4.2. and section 5.2).

Ocular changes: Copegus is used in combination therapy with alpha interferons. Retinopathy including retinal haemorrhages, cotton wool spots, papilloedema, optic neuropathy and retinal artery or vein obstruction which may result in loss of vision have been reported in rare instances with combination therapy with alpha interferons. All patients should have a baseline eye examination. Any patient complaining of decrease or loss of vision must have a prompt and complete eye examination. Patients with preexisting ophthalmologic disorders (eg, diabetic or hypertensive retinopathy) should receive periodic ophthalmologic exams during combination therapy with alpha interferons. Combination therapy with alpha interferons should be discontinued in patients who develop new or worsening ophthalmologic disorders.

HIV/HCV Co-infection: Please refer to the respective Summary of Product Characteristics of the antiretroviral medicinal products that are to be taken concurrently with HCV therapy for awareness and management of toxicities specific for each product and the potential for overlapping toxicities with peginterferon alfa-2a with or without ribavirin. In study NR15961, patients concurrently treated with stavudine and interferon therapy with or without ribavirin, the incidence of pancreatitis and/or lactic acidosis was 3 % (12/398).

Chronic hepatitis C patients co-infected with HIV and receiving Highly Active Anti-Retroviral Therapy (HAART) may be at increased risk of serious adverse effects (e.g. lactic acidosis; peripheral neuropathy; pancreatitis).

Co-infected patients with advanced cirrhosis receiving HAART may also be at increased risk of hepatic decompensation and possibly death if treated with Copegus in combination with interferons. Baseline variables in co-infected cirrhotic patients that may be associated with hepatic decompensation include: increased serum bilirubin, decreased haemoglobin, increased alkaline phosphatase or decreased platelet count, and treatment with didanosine (ddI). Caution should therefore be exercised when adding peginterferon alfa-2a and Copegus to HAART (see section 4.5).

Co-infected patients should be closely monitored, assessing their Child-Pugh score during treatment, and should be immediately discontinued if they progress to a Child-Pugh score of 7 or greater.

Co-administration of Copegus and didanosine is not recommended due to the risk of mitochondrial toxicity (see Section 4.5). Moreover, co-adminstration of Copegus and stavudine should be avoided to limit the risk of overlapping mitochondrial toxicity.

Patients treated with Copegus and alpha interferon (standard and pegylated) combination therapy and zidovudine could be at increased risk of developing anaemia.

Laboratory tests: Standard haematologic tests and blood chemistries (complete blood count [CBC] and differential, platelet count, electrolytes, serum creatinine, liver function tests, uric acid) must be conducted in all patients prior to initiating therapy. Acceptable baseline values that may be considered as a guideline prior to initiation of Copegus in combination with peginterferon alfa-2a or interferon alfa-2a:

Haemoglobin ⩾ 12 g/dl (females); ⩾ 13 g/dl (males)

Platelets ⩾ 90,000/mm^3

Neutrophil Count ⩾ 1,500/mm^3

In patients co-infected with HIV-HCV, limited efficacy and safety data (N = 51) are available in subjects with CD4 counts less than 200 cells/μL. Caution is therefore warranted in the treatment of patients with low CD4 counts.

Laboratory evaluations are to be conducted at weeks 2 and 4 of therapy, and periodically thereafter as clinically appropriate.

For women of childbearing potential: Female patients must have a routine pregnancy test performed monthly during treatment and for 4 months thereafter. Female partners of male patients must have a routine pregnancy test performed monthly during treatment and for 7 months thereafter.

Uric acid may increase with Copegus due to haemolysis and therefore predisposed patients should be carefully monitored for development of gout.

Dental and periodontal disorders: Dental and periodontal disorders, which may lead to loss of teeth, have been reported in patients receiving Copegus and peginterferon alfa-2a combination therapy. In addition, dry mouth could have a damaging effect on teeth and mucous membranes of the mouth during long-term treatment with the combination of Copegus and peginterferon alfa-2a. Patients should brush their teeth thoroughly twice daily and have regular dental examinations. In addition some patients may experience vomiting. If this reaction occurs, they should be advised to rinse out their mouth thoroughly afterwards.

4.5 Interaction with other medicinal products and other forms of interaction

Interaction studies have been conducted with ribavirin in combination with peginterferon alfa-2a, interferon alfa-2b and antacids. Ribavirin concentrations are similar when given alone or concomitantly with interferon alfa-2b or peginterferon alfa-2a.

Any potential for interactions may persist for up to 2 months (5 half lives for ribavirin) after cessation of Copegus therapy due to the long half-life.

Results of *in vitro* studies using both human and rat liver microsome preparations indicated no cytochrome P450 enzyme mediated metabolism of ribavirin. Ribavirin does not inhibit cytochrome P450 enzymes. There is no evidence from toxicity studies that ribavirin induces liver enzymes. Therefore, there is a minimal potential for P450 enzyme-based interactions.

Antacid: The bioavailability of ribavirin 600 milligrams was decreased by co-administration with an antacid containing magnesium, aluminium and methicone; AUC_{tf} decreased 14 %. It is possible that the decreased bioavailability in this study was due to delayed transit of ribavirin or modified pH. This interaction is not considered to be clinically relevant.

Nucleoside analogues: Ribavirin was shown *in vitro* to inhibit phosphorylation of zidovudine and stavudine. The clinical significance of these findings is unknown. However, these *in vitro* findings raise the possibility that concurrent use of Copegus with either zidovudine or stavudine might lead to increased HIV plasma viraemia. Therefore, it is recommended that plasma HIV RNA levels be closely monitored in patients treated with Copegus concurrently with either of these two agents. If HIV RNA levels increase, the use of Copegus concomitantly with reverse transcriptase inhibitors must be reviewed.

Didanosine (ddI): Co-administration of ribavirin and didanosine is not recommended. Exposure to didanosine or its active metabolite (dideoxyadenosine 5'-triphosphate) is increased in vitro when didanosine is co-administered with ribavirin. Reports of fatal hepatic failure as well as peripheral neuropathy, pancreatitis, and symptomatic hyperlactataemia/lactic acidosis have been reported with use of ribavirin.

HIV-HCV co-infected patients

No apparent evidence of drug interaction was observed in 47 HIV-HCV co-infected patients who completed a 12 week pharmacokinetic substudy to examine the effect of ribavirin on the intracellular phosphorylation of some nucleoside reverse transcriptase inhibitors (lamivudine and zidovudine or stavudine). However, due to high variability, the confidence intervals were quite wide. Plasma exposure of ribavirin did not appear to be affected by concomitant administration of nucleoside reverse transcriptase inhibitors (NRTIs).

4.6 Pregnancy and lactation

Preclinical data: Significant teratogenic and/or embryocidal potential have been demonstrated for ribavirin in all animal species in which adequate studies have been conducted, occurring at doses well below the recommended human dose. Malformations of the skull, palate, eye, jaw, limbs, skeleton and gastrointestinal tract were noted. The incidence and severity of teratogenic effects increased with escalation of the ribavirin dose. Survival of foetuses and offspring was reduced.

Female patients: Copegus must not be used by women who are pregnant (see section 4.3 and section 4.4). Extreme care must be taken to avoid pregnancy in female patients. Copegus therapy must not be initiated until a report of a negative pregnancy test has been obtained immediately prior to initiation of therapy. Any birth control method can fail. Therefore, it is critically important that women of childbearing potential and their partners must use 2 forms of effective contraception simultaneously, during treatment and for 4 months after treatment has been concluded; routine monthly pregnancy tests must be performed during this time. If pregnancy does occur during treatment or within 4months from stopping treatment the patient must be advised of the significant teratogenic risk of ribavirin to the foetus.

Male patients and their female partners: Extreme care must be taken to avoid pregnancy in partners of male patients taking Copegus. Ribavirin accumulates intracellularly and is cleared from the body very slowly. In animal studies, ribavirin produced changes in sperm at doses below the clinical dose. It is unknown whether the ribavirin that is

Table 5 Undesirable Effects Reported with Copegus in combination with Peginterferon alfa-2a for HCV Patients

Body system	Very Common ≥1 /10	Common ≥1 /100 to < 1 /10	Uncommon ≥1 /1000 to < 1 /100	Rare ≥1 /10,000 to < 1 /1000	Very rare <1/10,000
Infections and infestations		Upper respiratory infection, bronchitis, oral candidiasis, herpes simplex	Lower respiratory tract infection, urinary tract infection, skin infection	Endocarditis, Otitis externa	
Neoplasms benign and malignant			Malignant hepatic neoplasm		
Blood and lymphatic system disorders	Anaemia	Thrombocytopenia, lymphadenopathy		Pancytopenia	Aplastic anaemia
Immune system disorders			Sarcoidosis, thyroiditis	Anaphylaxis, systemic lupus erythematosus, rheumatoid arthritis	idiopathic or thrombotic thrombocytopenic purpura
Endocrine disorders		Hypothyroidism, hyperthyroidism	Diabetes		
Metabolism and Nutrition Disorders	Anorexia		Dehydration		
Psychiatric disorders	Depression, insomnia	Mood alteration, emotional disorders, anxiety, aggression, nervousness, libido decreased	Suicidal ideation, hallucinations, anger	Suicide, psychotic disorder	
Nervous system disorders	Headache, dizziness, concentration impaired	Memory impairment, syncope, weakness, migraine, hypoaesthesia, hyperaesthesia, paraesthesia, tremor, taste disturbance, nightmares, somnolence	Hearing loss, peripheral neuropathy	Coma, convulsions, facial palsy	
Eye disorders		Vision blurred, eye pain, eye inflammation, xerophthalmia	Retinal haemorrhage	Optic neuropathy, papilloedema, retinal vascular disorder, retinopathy, corneal ulcer	Vision loss
Ear and labyrinth disorders		Vertigo, earache			
Cardiac disorders		Tachycardia, palpitations, oedema peripheral		Myocardial infarction, congestive heart failure, angina, Supraventricular tachycardia arrhythmia, atrial fibrillation, pericarditis	
Vascular disorders		Flushing	Hypertension	Cerebral haemorrhage	
Respiratory, thoracic and mediastinal disorders	Dyspnoea, cough	Dyspnoea exertional, epistaxis, nasopharyngitis, sinus congestion, nasal congestion, rhinitis, sore throat	Wheezing	Interstitial pneumonitis with fatal outcome, pulmonary embolism	
Gastrointestinal disorders	Diarrhoea, nausea, abdominal pain	Vomiting, dyspepsia, dysphagia, mouth ulceration, gingival bleeding, glossitis, stomatitis, flatulence, constipation, dry mouth	Gastrointestinal bleeding, cheilitis, gingivitis	Peptic ulcer, pancreatitis	
Hepato-biliary disorders			Hepatic dysfunction	Hepatic failure, cholangitis, fatty liver	
Skin and subcutaneous tissue disorders	Alopecia, dermatitis, pruritus, dry skin	Rash, sweating increased, psoriasis, urticaria, eczema, skin disorder, photosensitivity reaction, night sweats			Toxic epidermal necrolysis, Stevens-Johnson syndrome, angioedema, erythema multiforme
Musculoskeletal connective tissue and bone disorders	Myalgia, arthralgia	Back pain, arthritis, muscle weakness, bone pain, neck pain, musculoskeletal pain, muscle cramps		Myositis	
Reproductive system and breast disorders		Impotence			
General disorders and administration site conditions	Pyrexia, rigors, pain, asthenia, fatigue, injection site reaction, irritability	Chest pain, influenza like illness, malaise, lethargy, hot flushes, thirst			
Investigations		Weight decreased			
Injury and poisoning				Substance overdose	

contained in sperm will exert its known teratogenic effects upon fertilisation of the ova. Male patients and their female partners of childbearing age must, therefore, be counselled to use 2 forms of effective contraception simultaneously during treatment with Copegus and for 7 months after treatment has been concluded. A pregnancy test must be performed before therapy is started. Men whose partners are pregnant must be instructed to use a condom to minimise delivery of ribavirin to the partner.

Lactation: It is not known whether ribavirin is excreted in human milk. Because of the potential for adverse reactions in nursing infants, nursing must be discontinued prior to initiation of treatment.

4.7 Effects on ability to drive and use machines

Copegus has no or negligible influence on the ability to drive and use machines. However, peginterferon alfa-2a or interferon alfa-2a used in combination with Copegus may have an effect. Please refer to the SPC of peginterferon alfa-2a or interferon alfa-2a for further information.

4.8 Undesirable effects

See peginterferon alfa-2a or interferon alfa-2a prescribing information for additional undesirable effects for either of these products.

Adverse events reported in patients receiving Copegus in combination with interferon alfa-2a are essentially the same as for those reported for Copegus in combination with peginterferon alfa-2a.

Within each frequency grouping, undesirable effects are presented in order of decreasing seriousness.

Chronic Hepatitis C

The most frequently reported adverse events with Copegus in combination with peginterferon alfa-2a 180 micrograms were mostly mild to moderate in severity and were manageable without the need for modification of doses or discontinuation of therapy.

Chronic Hepatitis C and Human Immunodeficiency Virus Co-infection

In HIV-HCV co-infected patients, the clinical adverse event profiles reported for peginterferon alfa-2a, alone or in combination with ribavirin, were similar to those observed in HCV mono-infected patients. For HIV-HCV patients receiving Copegus and peginterferon alfa-2a combination therapy other undesirable effects have been reported in ≥ 1% to ⩽ 2% of patients: hyperlactacidaemia/lactic acidosis, influenza, pneumonia, affect lability, apathy, tinnitus, pharyngolaryngeal pain, cheilitis, acquired lipodystrophy and chromaturia. Peginterferon alfa-2a treatment was associated with decreases in absolute CD4+ cell counts within the first 4 weeks without a reduction in CD4+ cell percentage. The decrease in CD4+ cell counts was reversible upon dose reduction or cessation of therapy. The use of peginterferon alfa-2a had no observable negative impact on the control of HIV viraemia during therapy or follow-up. Limited safety data (N= 51) are available in co-infected patients with CD4+ cell counts < 200/µl (see peginterferon alfa-2a SPC).

Table 5 shows the undesirable effects reported in patients who have received Copegus and peginterferon alfa-2a or interferon alfa-2a therapy.

(see Table 5 on previous page)

Laboratory values: In clinical trials of Copegus in combination with peginterferon alfa-2a or interferon alfa-2a, the majority of cases of abnormal laboratory values were managed with dose modifications (see section 4.2). With peginterferon alfa-2a and Copegus combination treatment, up to 2 % of patients experienced increased ALT levels that led to dose modification or discontinuation of treatment.

Haemolysis is the dose limiting toxicity of ribavirin therapy. A decrease in haemoglobin levels to < 10 g/dl was observed in up to 15 % of patients treated for 48 weeks with Copegus 1000/1200 milligrams in combination with peginterferon alfa-2a and up to 19 % of patients in combination with interferon alfa-2a. When Copegus 800 milligram was combined with peginterferon alfa-2a for 24 weeks, 3 % of patients had a decrease in haemoglobin levels to < 10 g/dl. It is not expected that patients will need to discontinue therapy because of decrease in haemoglobin levels alone. In most cases the decrease in haemoglobin occurred early in the treatment period and stabilised concurrently with a compensatory increase in reticulocytes.

Most cases of anaemia, leucopenia and thrombocytopenia were mild (WHO grade 1). WHO grade 2 laboratory changes were reported for haemoglobin (4 % of patients), leucocytes (24 % of patients) and thrombocytes (2 % of patients). Moderate (absolute neutrophil count (ANC): 0.749-0.5x109/L) and severe (ANC: <0.5x109/L) neutropenia was observed in 24 % (216/887) and 5 % (41/887) of patients receiving 48 weeks of Copegus 1000/1200 milligrams in combination with peginterferon alfa-2a.

An increase in uric acid and indirect bilirubin values associated with haemolysis were observed in some patients treated with Copegus used in combination with peginterferon alfa-2a or interferon alfa-2a and values returned to baseline levels within 4 weeks after the end of therapy. In rare cases (2/755) this was associated with clinical manifestation (acute gout).

Laboratory values for HIV-HCV co-infected patients

Although haematological toxicities of neutropenia, thrombocytopenia and anaemia occurred more frequently in HIV-HCV patients, the majority could be managed by dose modification and the use of growth factors and infrequently required premature discontinuation of treatment. Decrease in ANC levels below 500 cells/mm^3 was observed in 13 % and 11 % of patients receiving peginterferon alfa-2a monotherapy and combination therapy, respectively. Decrease in platelets below 50,000/mm^3 was observed in 10 % and 8 % of patients receiving peginterferon alfa-2a monotherapy and combination therapy, respectively. Anaemia (haemoglobin < 10g/dL) was reported in 7 % and 14 % of patients treated with peginterferon alfa-2a monotherapy or in combination therapy, respectively.

4.9 Overdose

No cases of overdose of Copegus have been reported in clinical trials. Hypocalcaemia and hypomagnesaemia have been observed in persons administered dosages greater than four times the maximal recommended dosages. In many of these instances ribavirin was administered intravenously. Ribavirin is not effectively removed by haemodialysis.

Table 6 Virological Response in the overall population (including non-cirrhotic and cirrhotic patients)

	Study NV15942	Study NV15801	
	Copegus 1,000/1,200 mg & Peginterferon alfa-2a 180 micrograms	Copegus 1,000/1,200 mg & Peginterferon alfa-2a 180 micrograms	Ribavirin 1,000/1,200 mg & Interferon alfa-2b 3 MIU
	(N=436) 48 weeks	(N=453) 48 weeks	(N=444) 48 weeks
Response at End of Treatment	68%	69%	52%
Overall Sustained Response	63%	54%*	45%*

*95% CI for difference: 3% to 16% p-value (stratified Cochran-Mantel-Haenszel test) = 0.003

5. PHARMACOLOGICAL PROPERTIES

5.1 Pharmacodynamic properties

Pharmacotherapeutic group: Nucleosides and nucleotides (excl. reverse transcriptase inhibitors), ATC code: J05A B04.

Mechanism of Action: Ribavirin is a synthetic nucleoside analog that shows *in vitro* activity against some RNA and DNA viruses. The mechanism by which ribavirin in combination with peginterferon alfa-2a or interferon alfa-2a exerts its effects against HCV is unknown.

HCV RNA levels decline in a biphasic manner in responding patients with hepatitis C who have received treatment with 180 micrograms peginterferon alfa-2a. The first phase of decline occurs 24 to 36 hours after the first dose of peginterferon alfa-2a and is followed by the second phase of decline which continues over the next 4 to 16 weeks in patients who achieve a sustained response. Copegus had no significant effect on the initial viral kinetics over the first 4 to 6 weeks in patients treated with the combination of Copegus and pegylated interferon alfa-2a or interferon alfa.

Oral formulations of ribavirin monotherapy have been investigated as therapy for chronic hepatitis C in several clinical trials. Results of these investigations showed that ribavirin monotherapy had no effect on eliminating hepatitis virus (HCV-RNA) or improving hepatic histology after 6 to 12 months of therapy and 6 months of follow-up.

Clinical Trial Results

Copegus in combination with peginterferon alfa-2a

Predictability of response

Please refer to section 4.2, Table 2.

Study results

Efficacy and safety of the combination of Copegus and peginterferon alfa-2a were established in two pivotal studies (NV15801 + NV15942), including a total of 2405 patients. The study population comprised interferon-naïve patients with CHC confirmed by detectable levels of serum HCV RNA, elevated levels of ALT, and a liver biopsy consistent with chronic hepatitis C infection. Only HIV-HCV co-infected patients were included in the study NR15961 (see Table 12). These patients had stable HIV disease and mean CD4 T-cell count was about 500 cells/µl.

Study NV15801 (1121 patients treated) compared the efficacy of 48 weeks of treatment with peginterferon alfa-2a (180 mcg once weekly) and Copegus (1000/1200 mg daily) with either peginterferon alfa-2a monotherapy or combination therapy with interferon-alfa-2b and ribavirin. The combination of peginterferon alfa-2a and Copegus was significantly more efficacious than either the combination of interferon alfa-2b and ribavirin or peginterferon alfa-2a monotherapy.

Study NV15942 (1284 patients treated) compared the efficacy of two durations of treatment (24 weeks with 48 weeks) and two dosages of Copegus (800 mg with 1000/1200 mg).

For HCV monoinfected patients and HIV-HCV co-infected patients, for treatment regimens, duration of therapy and study outcome see tables 6, 7, 8 and 12, respectively. Virological response was defined as undetectable HCV RNA as measured by the COBAS AMPLICOR™ HCV Test, version 2.0 (limit of detection 100 copies/ml equivalent to 50 International Units/ml) and sustained response as one negative sample approximately 6 months after the end of therapy.

(see Table 6 above)

The virological responses of HCV monoinfected patients treated with Copegus and peginterferon alfa-2a combination therapy in relation to genotype and pre-treatment viral load and in relation to genotype, pre-treatment viral load and rapid virological response at week 4 are summarised in Table 7 and Table 8 respectively. The results of study NV15942 provide the rationale for recommending treatment regimens based on genotype, baseline viral load and virological response at week 4 (see Tables 1, 7 and 8).

The difference between treatment regimens was in general not influenced by presence/absence of cirrhosis; therefore treatment recommendations for genotype 1, 2 or 3 are independent of this baseline characteristic.

(see Table 7 below)

The possibility to consider shortening treatment duration to 24 weeks in genotype 1 and 4 patients was examined based on a sustained rapid virological response observed in patients with rapid virological response at week 4 in studies NV15942 and ML17131 (see Table 8).

(see Table 8 on next page)

Although limited, data indicated that shortening treatment to 24 weeks might be associated with a higher risk of relapse (see Table 9).

(see Table 9 on next page)

The possibility of shortening treatment duration to 16 weeks in genotype 2 or 3 patients was examined based on the sustained rapid virological response observed in

Table 7 Sustained Virological Response based on Genotype and Pre-treatment Viral Load after Copegus Combination Therapy with peginterferon alfa-2a

	Study NV15942				Study NV15801	
	Copegus 800 mg & **PEG-IFN alfa-2a** 180 mcg 24 weeks	**Copegus** 1000/1200 mg & **PEG-IFN alfa-2a** 180 mcg 24 weeks	**Copegus** 800 mg & **PEG-IFN alfa-2a** 180 mcg 48 weeks	**Copegus** 1000/1200 mg & **PEG-IFN alfa-2a** 180 mcg 48 weeks	**Copegus** 1000/1200 mg & **PEG-IFN alfa-2a** 180 mcg 48 weeks	**Ribavirin** 1000/1200 mg & **Interferon alfa-2b** 3 MIU 48 weeks
Genotype 1	29 % (29/101)	42 % (49/118)†	41 % (102/250)*	**52 %** (142/271)*†	45 % (134/298)	36 % (103/285)
Low viral load	41 % (21/51)	52 % (37/71)	55 % (33/60)	**65 %** (55/85)	53 % (61/115)	44 % (41/94)
High viral load	16 % (8/50)	26 % (12/47)	36 % (69/190)	**47 %** (87/186)	40 % (73/182)	33 % (62/189)
Genotype 2/3	**84 %** (81/96)	81 % (117/144)	79 % (78/99)	80 % (123/153)	71 % (100/140)	61 % (88/145)
Low viral load	**85 %** (29/34)	83 % (39/47)	88 % (29/33)	77 % (37/48)	76 % (28/37)	65 % (34/52)
High viral load	**84 %** (52/62)	80 % (78/97)	74 % (49/66)	82 % (86/105)	70 % (72/103)	58 % (54/93)
Genotype 4	0 % (0/5)	67 % (8/12)	63 % (5/8)	82 % (9/11)	77 % (10/13)	45 % (5/11)

Low viral load= ⩽ 800,000 IU/mL; High viral load= > 800,000 IU/mL

*Copegus 1000/1200 mg + peginterferon alfa-2a 180 mcg, 48 w vs. Copegus 800 mg + peginterferon alfa-2a 180 mcg, 48 w: Odds Ratio (95% CI) = 1.52 (1.07 to 2.17) P-value (stratified Cochran-Mantel-Haenszel test) = 0.020

†Copegus 1000/1200 mg + peginterferon alfa-2a 180 mcg, 48 w vs. Copegus 1000/1200 mg + peginterferon alfa-2a 180 mcg, 24 w: Odds Ratio (95% CI) = 2.12 (1.30 to 3.46) P-value (stratified Cochran-Mantel-Haenszel test) = 0.002

Table 8 Sustained Virological Response Based on Rapid Viral Response at week 4 for Genotype 1 and 4 after Copegus Combination Therapy with Peginterferon alfa-2a in HCV Patients

Study NV15942			Study ML17131
	Copegus 1000/1200 mg & Peginterferon alfa-2a 180 mcg 24 weeks	Copegus 1000/1200 mg & Peginterferon alfa-2a 180 mcg 48 weeks	Copegus 1000/1200 mg & Peginterferon alfa-2a 180 mcg 24 weeks
Genotype 1 RVR Low viral load	90% (28/31) 93% (25/27)	92% (47/51) 96% (26/27)	77% (59/77) 80% (52/65)
High viral load	75% (3/4)	88% (21/24)	58% (7/12)
Genotype 1 non RVR	24% (21/87)	43% (95/220)	-
Low viral load	27% (12/44)	50% (31/62)	-
High viral load	21% (9/43)	41% (64/158)	-
Genotype 4 RVR	(5/6)	(5/5)	92% (22/24)
Genotype 4 non RVR	(3/6)	(4/6)	-

Low viral load= ⩽ 800,000 IU/mL; High viral load= > 800,000 IU/mL
RVR = rapid viral response (HCV RNA undetectable) at week 4 and HCV RNA undetectable at week 24

Table 9 Relapse of Virological Response at the End of Treatment for Rapid Virological Response Population

	Study NV15942		Study NV15801
	Copegus 1000/1200 mg & Peginterferon alfa-2a 180 mcg 24 weeks	Copegus 1000/1200 mg & Peginterferon alfa-2a 180 mcg 48 weeks	Copegus 1000/1200 mg & Peginterferon alfa-2a 180 mcg 48 weeks
Genotype 1 RVR	6.7% (2/30)	4.3% (2/47)	0% (0/24)
Low viral load	3.8% (1/26)	0% (0/25)	0% (0/17)
High viral load	25% (1/4)	9.1% (2/22)	0% (0/7)
Genotype 4 RVR	(0/5)	(0/5)	0% (0/4)

Table 10 Sustained Virological Response Overall and Based on Rapid Viral Response by Week 4 for Genotype 2 or 3 after Copegus Combination Therapy with Peginterferon alfa-2a in HCV Patients

Study NV17317				
	Copegus 800 mg & Peginterferon alfa-2a 180 mcg 16 weeks	Copegus 800 mg & Peginterferon alfa-2a 180 mcg 24 weeks	Treatment difference 95% CI	p value
Genotype 2 or 3	65% (443/679)	76% (478/630)	-10.6% [-15.5%; -0.06%]	P<0.0001
Genotype 2 or 3 RVR	82% (378/461)	90% (370/410)	-8.2% [-12.8%; -3.7%]	P=0.0006
Low viral load	89% (147/166)	94% (141/150)	-5.4% [-12%; 0.9%]	P=0.11
High viral load	78% (231/295)	88% (229/260)	-9.7% [-15.9%; -3.6%]	P=0.002

Low viral load= ⩽ 800,000 IU/mL at baseline; High viral load= > 800,000 IU/mL at baseline
RVR = rapid viral response (HCV RNA negative) by week 4

patients with rapid virological response by week 4 in study NV17317 (see Table 10).

In study NV17317 in patients infected with viral genotype 2 or 3, all patients received peginterferon alfa-2a 180 μg sc qw and a Copegus dose of 800 mg and were randomised to treatment for either 16 or 24 weeks. Overall treatment for 16 weeks resulted in lower sustained viral response (65%) than treatment for 24 weeks (76%) ($p < 0.0001$).

The sustained viral response achieved with 16 weeks of treatment and with 24 weeks of treatment was also examined in a retrospective subgroup analysis of patients who were HCV RNA negative by week 4 and had a LVL at baseline (see Table 10).

(see Table 10 above)

The data indicated that shortening treatment to 16 weeks is associated with a higher risk of relapse (see Table 11)

(see Table 11 opposite)

HCV patients with normal ALT

In study NR16071, HCV patients with normal ALT values were randomised to receive peginterferon alfa-2a 180 micrograms/week with a Copegus dose of 800 milligrams/day for either 24 or 48 weeks followed by a 24 week treatment free follow-up period or an untreated control group for 72 weeks. The SVRs reported in the treatment arms of this study were similar to the corresponding treatment arms from study NV15942.

Table 11 Relapse of Virological Response after the End of Treatment in Genotype 2 or 3 Patients with a Rapid Viral Response

Study NV17317				
	Copegus 800 mg & Peginterferon alfa-2a 180 mcg 16 weeks	Copegus 800 mg & Peginterferon alfa-2a 180 mcg 24 weeks	Treatment difference 95% CI	p value
Genotype 2 or 3 RVR	15% (67/439)	6% (23/386)	9.3% [5.2%; 13.6%]	P<0.0001
Low viral load	6% (10/155)	1% (2/141)	5% [0.6%; 10.3%]	P=0.04
High viral load	20% (57/284)	9% (21/245)	11.5% [5.6%; 17.4%]	P=0.0002

HIV-HCV co-infected patients

The virological responses of patients treated with Copegus and peginterferon alfa-2a combination therapy in relation to genotype and pre-treatment viral load for HIV-HCV co-infected patients are summarised below in Table 12.

(see Table 12 on next page)

Ribavirin in combination with interferon alfa-2a

The therapeutic efficacy of interferon alfa-2a alone and in combination with oral ribavirin was compared in clinical trials in naïve (previously untreated) and relapsed patients who had virologically, biochemically and histologically documented chronic hepatitis C. Six months after end of treatment sustained biochemical and virological response as well as histological improvement were assessed.

A statistically significant 10-fold increase (from 4 % to 43 %; $p < 0.01$) in sustained virological and biochemical response was observed in relapsed patients (M23136; N=99). The favourable profile of the combination therapy was also reflected in the response rates relative to HCV genotype or baseline viral load. In the combination and interferon monotherapy arms, respectively, the sustained response rates in patients with HCV genotype-1 were 28 % versus 0 % and with genotype non-1 were 58 % versus 8 %. In addition the histological improvement favoured the combination therapy. Supportive favourable results (monotherapy vs combination; 6 % vs 48 %, $p < 0.04$) from a small published study in naïve patients (N=40) were reported using interferon alfa-2a (3 MIU 3 times per week) with ribavirin.

5.2 Pharmacokinetic properties

Ribavirin is absorbed rapidly following oral administration of a single dose of Copegus (median T_{max} = 1-2 hours). The mean terminal phase half-life of ribavirin following single doses of Copegus range from 140 to 160 hours. Ribavirin data from the literature demonstrates absorption is extensive with approximately 10 % of a radiolabelled dose excreted in the faeces. However, absolute bioavailability is approximately 45 % -65 %, which appears to be due to first pass metabolism. There is an aproximately linear relationship between dose and AUC_{tf} following single doses of 200-1,200 milligrams ribavirin. Mean apparent oral clearance of ribavirin following single 600 milligram doses of Copegus ranges from 22 to 29 litres/hour. Volume of distribution is approximately 4,500 1itres following administration of Copegus. Ribavirin does not bind to plasma proteins.

Ribavirin has been shown to produce high inter- and intra-subject pharmacokinetic variability following single oral doses of Copegus(intra-subject variability of ⩽ 25 % for both AUC and C_{max}), which may be due to extensive first pass metabolism and transfer within and beyond the blood compartment.

Ribavirin transport in non-plasma compartments has been most extensively studied in red cells, and has been identified to be primarily via an e_s-type equilibrative nucleoside transporter. This type of transporter is present on virtually all cell types and may account for the high volume of distribution of ribavirin. The ratio of whole blood: plasma ribavirin concentrations is approximately 60:1; the excess of ribavirin in whole blood exists as ribavirin nucleotides sequestered in erythrocytes.

Ribavirin has two pathways of metabolism: 1) a reversible phosphorylation pathway, 2) a degradative pathway involving deribosylation and amide hydrolysis to yield a triazole carboxyacid metabolite. Ribavirin and both its triazole carboxamide and triazole carboxylic acid metabolites are excreted renally.

Upon multiple dosing, ribavirin accumulates extensively in plasma with a six-fold ratio of multiple-dose to single-dose AUC_{12hr} based on literature data. Following oral dosing with 600 milligrams BID, steady-state was reached by approximately 4 weeks, with mean steady state plasma concentrations of approximately 2,200 ng/ml. Upon discontinuation of dosing the half-life was approximately 300 hours, which probably reflects slow elimination from non-plasma compartments.

Food effect: The bioavailability of a single oral 600 mg dose Copegus was increased by coadministration of a high fat meal. The ribavirin exposure parameters of $AUC_{(0-192h)}$

Table 12 Sustained Virological Response based on Genotype and Pre-treatment Viral Load after Copegus Combination Therapy with peginterferon alfa-2a in HIV-HCV co-infected patients

Study NR15961			
	Interferon alfa-2a 3 MIU & **Copegus 800 mg** 48 weeks	**Peginterferon alfa-2a** 180 mcg & **Placebo** 48 weeks	**Peginterferon alfa-2a** 180 mcg & **Copegus 800 mg** 48 weeks
All patients	12% (33/285)*	20% (58/286)*	40% (116/289)*
Genotype 1	7% (12/171)	14% (24/175)	29% (51/176)
Low viral load	19% (8/42)	38% (17/45)	61% (28/46)
High viral load	3% (4/129)	5% (7/130)	18% (23/130)
Genotype 2-3	20% (18/89)	36% (32/90)	62% (59/95)
Low viral load	27% (8/30)	38% (9/24)	61% (17/28)
High viral load	17% (10/59)	35% (23/66)	63% (42/67)

Low viral load= ⩽ 800,000 IU/mL; High viral load= > 800,000 IU/mL

* peginterferon alfa-2a 180 mcg Copegus 800mg vs. Interferon alfa-2a 3MIU ribavirin 800 mg: Odds Ratio (95 % CI) = 5.40 (3.42 to 8.54), P-value (stratified Cochran-Mantel-Haenszel test) = < 0.0001

* peginterferon alfa-2a 180 mcg Copegus 800mg vs. peginterferon alfa-2a 180 μg: Odds Ratio (95 % CI) = 2.89 (1.93 to 4.32), P-value (stratified Cochran-Mantel-Haenszel test) = < 0.0001

* Interferon alfa-2a 3MIU Copegus 800mg vs. peginterferon alfa-2a 180mcg: Odds Ratio (95 % CI) = 0.53 (0.33 to 0.85), P-value (stratified Cochran-Mantel-Haenszel test) = < 0.0084.

and C_{max} increased by 42 % and 66 %, respectively, when Copegus was taken with a high fat breakfast compared to being taken in the fasted state. The clinical relevance of results from this single dose study is unknown. Ribavirin exposure after multiple dosing when taken with food was comparable in patients receiving peginterferon alfa-2a and Copegus and interferon alfa-2b and ribavirin. In order to achieve optimal ribavirin plasma concentrations, it is recommended to take ribavirin with food.

Renal function: Single-dose ribavirin pharmacokinetics were altered (increased AUC_{tf} and C_{max}) in patients with renal dysfunction compared with control subjects whose creatinine clearance was greater than 90 ml/minute. The clearance of ribavirin is substantially reduced in patients with serum creatinine > 2 mg/dl or creatinine clearance < 50 ml/min. There are insufficient data on the safety and efficacy of ribavirin in such patients to support recommendations for dose adjustments. Plasma concentrations of ribavirin are essentially unchanged by haemodialysis.

Hepatic function: Single-dose pharmacokinetics of ribavirin in patients with mild, moderate or severe hepatic dysfunction (Child-Pugh Classification A, B or C) are similar to those of normal controls.

Use in elderly patients over the age of 65: Specific pharmacokinetic evaluations for elderly subjects have not been performed. However, in a published population pharmacokinetic study, age was not a key factor in the kinetics of ribavirin; renal function is the determining factor.

Patients under the age of 18 years: The pharmacokinetic properties of ribavirin have not been fully evaluated in patients under the age of 18 years. Copegus in combination with peginterferon alfa-2 or interferon alfa-2a is indicated for the treatment of chronic hepatitis C only in patients 18 years of age or older.

Population Pharmacokinetics: A population pharmacokinetic analysis was performed using plasma concentration values from five clinical trials. While body weight and race were statistically significant covariates in the clearance model, only the effect of body weight was clinically significant. Clearance increased as a function of body weight and was predicted to vary from 17.7 to 24.8 L/h over a weight range of 44 to 155 kg. Creatinine clearance (as low as 34 ml/min) did not affect ribavirin clearance.

5.3 Preclinical safety data

Ribavirin is embryotoxic and/or teratogenic at doses well below the recommended human dose in all animal species in which adequate studies have been conducted. Malformations of the skull, palate, eye, jaw, limbs, skeleton and gastrointestinal tract were noted. The incidence and severity of teratogenic effects increased with escalation of the dose. Survival of foetuses and offspring is reduced.

Erythrocytes are a primary target of toxicity for ribavirin in animal studies, including studies in dogs and monkeys. Anaemia occurs shortly after initiation of dosing, but is rapidly reversible upon cessation of treatment. Hypoplastic anaemia was observed only in rats at the high dose of 160 milligrams/kg/day in the subchronic study.

Reduced leucocyte and/or lymphocyte counts were consistently noted in the repeat-dose rodent and dog toxicity studies with ribavirin and transiently in monkeys administered ribavirin in the subchronic study. Repeat-dose rat toxicity studies showed thymic lymphoid depletion and/or depletion of thymus-dependent areas of the spleen (periarteriolar lymphoid sheaths, white pulp) and mesenteric lymph node. Following repeat-dosing of dogs with ribavirin, increased dilatation/necrosis of the intestinal crypts of the duodenum was noted, as well as chronic inflammation of the small intestine and erosion of the ileum.

In repeat dose studies in mice to investigate ribavirin-induced testicular and sperm effects, abnormalities in sperm occurred at doses in animals well below therapeutic doses. Upon cessation of treatment, essentially total recovery from ribavirin-induced testicular toxicity occurred within one or two spermatogenic cycles.

Genotoxicity studies have demonstrated that ribavirin does exert some genotoxic activity. Ribavirin was active in an *in vitro* Transformation Assay. Genotoxic activity was observed in *in vivo* mouse micronucleus assays. A dominant lethal assay in rats was negative, indicating that if mutations occurred in rats they were not transmitted through male gametes. Ribavirin is a possible human carcinogen.

Administration of ribavirin and peginterferon alfa-2a in combination did not produce any unexpected toxicity in monkeys. The major treatment-related change was reversible mild to moderate anaemia, the severity of which was greater than that produced by either active substance alone.

6. PHARMACEUTICAL PARTICULARS

6.1 List of excipients

Tablet core:

Pregelatinised maize starch

Sodium starch glycolate (type A)

Microcrystalline cellulose

Maize starch

Magnesium stearate

Film-coating:

Hypromellose

Talc

Titanium dioxide (E171)

Yellow iron oxide (E172)

Red iron oxide (E172)

Triacetin

6.2 Incompatibilities

Not applicable

6.3 Shelf life

4 years

6.4 Special precautions for storage

This medicinal product does not require any special storage conditions

6.5 Nature and contents of container

Copegus is supplied in high density polyethylene (HDPE) bottles with a child-resistant polypropylene screw cap containing 14 or 56 tablets. Not all pack sizes may be marketed.

6.6 Special precautions for disposal and other handling

No special requirements

7. MARKETING AUTHORISATION HOLDER

Roche Products Limited
6 Falcon Way
Shire Park
Welwyn Garden City
AL7 1TW
United Kingdom

8. MARKETING AUTHORISATION NUMBER(S)

PL 00031/0827

PA 50/153/2

9. DATE OF FIRST AUTHORISATION/RENEWAL OF THE AUTHORISATION

UK: October 2006 / 9 April 2007

Ireland: 8 December 2006 / 9 April 2007

10. DATE OF REVISION OF THE TEXT

UK: 15 July 2009
Ireland: 15 July 2009

LEGAL STATUS

POM

Coracten SR Capsules 10mg or 20mg

(UCB Pharma Limited)

1. NAME OF THE MEDICINAL PRODUCT

Coracten SR Capsules 10mg

BIDNIF 10

Coracten SR Capsules 20mg

BIDNIF 20

2. QUALITATIVE AND QUANTITATIVE COMPOSITION

Each capsule contains 10mg Nifedipine USP in sustained release form.

Each capsule contains 20mg Nifedipine USP in sustained release form.

For excipients, see 6.1

3. PHARMACEUTICAL FORM

Modified-release capsule, hard

10 mg - Sustained release capsules with opaque grey body and opaque brownish-pink cap, overprinted in white with 'Coracten' on the body and '10mg' on the cap, and filled with yellow pellets.

20 mg - Sustained release capsules with opaque brownish-pink body and opaque reddish-brown cap, overprinted in white with 'Coracten' on the body and '20mg' on the cap, and filled with yellow pellets.

4. CLINICAL PARTICULARS

4.1 Therapeutic indications

Coracten SR Capsules are indicated for the prophylaxis of chronic stable angina pectoris and the treatment of hypertension.

They are also indicated for the treatment of Prinzmetal (variant) angina when diagnosed by a cardiologist.

4.2 Posology and method of administration

Adults only: The recommended starting dose of Coracten SR Capsules is 10mg every 12 hours swallowed with water with subsequent titration of dosage according to response. The dose may be adjusted to 40mg every 12 hours.

Children: Coracten SR Capsules are not recommended for use in children.

Elderly: The pharmacokinetics of nifedipine are altered in the elderly so that lower maintenance doses of nifedipine may be required compared to younger patients.

Hepatic impairment: Caution should be exercised in treating patients with hepatic impairment. In these patients the use of one 10mg Coracten SR Capsule every 12 hours, together with careful monitoring, is suggested when commencing therapy.

Renal impairment: Dosage adjustments are not usually required in patients with renal impairment.

4.3 Contraindications

Coracten SR Capsules are contra-indicated in patients with known hypersensitivity to nifedipine or other dihydropyridines because of the theoretical risk of cross reactivity. They should not be used in women who are or who may become pregnant (see section 4.6. Pregnancy and Lactation).

Coracten SR Capsules should not be used in clinically significant aortic stenosis, unstable angina, or during or within one month of a myocardial infarction. They should not be used in patients in cardiogenic shock.

Coracten SR Capsules should not be used for the treatment of acute attacks of angina, or in patients who have had ischaemic pain following its administration previously.

The safety of Coracten SR Capsules in malignant hypertension has not been established.

Coracten SR Capsules should not be used for secondary prevention of myocardial infarction.

Coracten SR Capsules are contra-indicated in patients with acute porphyria.

Coracten SR Capsules should not be administered concomitantly with rifampicin since effective plasma levels of nifedipine may not be achieved owing to enzyme induction.

4.4 Special warnings and precautions for use

The dose of nifedipine should be reduced in patients with hepatic impairment (***see section 4.2. Posology and Method of Administration***). Nifedipine should be used with caution in patients who are hypotensive; in patients with poor cardiac reserve; in patients with heart failure or significantly impaired left ventricular function as their condition may deteriorate; in diabetic patients as they may require adjustment of their diabetic therapy; and in dialysis patients with malignant hypertension and irreversible renal failure with hypovolaemia, since a significant drop in blood pressure may occur due to the vasodilator effects of nifedipine.

Excessive falls in blood pressure may result in transient blindness. If affected the patient should not attempt to drive or use machinery (see section 4.8. Undesirable Effects).

Since nifedipine has no beta-blocking activity, it gives no protection against the dangers of abrupt withdrawal of beta-blocking drugs. Withdrawal of any previously prescribed beta-blockers should be gradual, preferably over 8 to 10 days.

The dose of nifedipine should be reduced in patients with hepatic impairment (see section 4.2. Posology and Method of Administration).

Nifedipine may be used in combination with beta-blockers and other antihypertensive agents, but the possibility of an additive effect resulting in postural hypotension and/or cardiac failure must be borne in mind.

4.5 Interaction with other medicinal products and other forms of interaction

As with other dihydropyridines, nifedipine should not be taken with grapefruit juice because bioavailability is increased.

The simultaneous administration of nifedipine and digoxin may lead to reduced digoxin clearance and hence an increase in the plasma digoxin. Digoxin levels should be monitored and, if necessary, the digoxin dose reduced.

Nifedipine may increase the spectrophotometric values of urinary vanillylmandelic acid falsely. However, HPLC measurements are unaffected.

Coracten SR Capsules should not be administered concomitantly with rifampicin since effective plasma levels of nifedipine may not be achieved owing to enzyme induction (see section 4.3. Contra-indications).

Increased plasma levels of nifedipine have been reported during concomitant use of H_2-receptor antagonists (specifically cimetidine), other calcium channel blockers (specifically diltiazem), alcohol, cyclosporin, macrolide antibiotics, gingko biloba and ginseng. Azole antifungals may increase serum concentrations of nifedipine.

Plasma levels of nifedipine are possibly decreased by the concomitant use of antiepileptics and St John's Wort.

When used in combination with nifedipine, plasma concentrations of quinidine have been shown to be suppressed regardless of quinidine dosage. The plasma concentrations of phenytoin, theophylline and non-depolarising muscle relaxants (e.g. tubocurarine) are increased when used in combination with nifedipine. Tacrolimus concentrations may be increased by nifedipine.

Enhanced hypotensive effect of nifedipine may occur with: aldesleukin, alprostadil, anaesthetics, antipsychotics, diuretics, phenothiazides, prazosin and intravenous ionic X-ray contrast medium. Profound hypotension has been reported with nifedipine and intravenous magnesium sulphate in the treatment of pre-eclampsia.

Ritonavir and quinupristin/dalfopristin may result in increased plasma concentrations of nifedipine.

Effective plasma levels of nifedipine may not be achieved due to enzyme induction with concurrent administration of erythromycin carbamazepine and phenobarbitone.

There is an increased risk of excessive hypotension, bradycardia and heart failure with β-blockers.

An increased rate of absorption of nifedipine from sustained release preparation may occur if given concurrently with cisapride.

Nifedipine may result in increased levels of mizolastine due to inhibition of cytochrome CYP3A4.

Nifedipine may increase the neuromuscular blocking effects of vecuronium.

4.6 Pregnancy and lactation

Pregnancy

Because animal studies show embryotoxicity and teratogenicity, Coracten SR Capsules are contra-indicated during pregnancy (see also section 4.3. Contra-indications). Embryotoxicity was noted at 6 to 20 times the maximum recommended dose for Coracten SR Capsules given to rats, mice and rabbits, and teratogenicity was noted in rabbits given 20 times the maximum recommended dose for Coracten SR Capsules.

Lactation

Nifedipine is excreted in breast milk, therefore Coracten SR Capsules are not recommended during lactation.

4.7 Effects on ability to drive and use machines

Dizziness and lethargy are potential undesirable effects. If affected do not attempt to drive or use machinery (see also section 4.8. Undesirable Effects).

Excessive falls in blood pressure may result in transient blindness. If affected do not attempt to drive or use machinery (see also section 4.8. Undesirable Effects).

4.8 Undesirable effects

Most side-effects are consequences of the vasodilatory effects of nifedipine.

Side-effects are generally transient and mild, and usually occur at the start of treatment only. They include headache, flushing and, usually at higher dosages, nausea, dyspepsia, heartburn, constipation, diarrhoea, dizziness, lethargy, skin reactions (such as rash, pruritus and urticaria), paraesthesia, hypotension, palpitation, tachycardia, dependent oedema, increased frequency of micturition, eye pain, depression, fever, gingival hyperplasia, telangiectasia and erythema multiforme

Other less frequently reported side effects include myalgia, tremor, pemphigoid reaction and visual disturbances. Impotence may occur rarely. Mood changes may occur rarely.

Excessive falls in blood pressure may result in cerebral or myocardial ischaemia or transient blindness.

As with other sustained release dihydropyridines, exacerbation of angina pectoris may occur rarely at the start of treatment with sustained release formulations of nifedipine. The occurrence of myocardial infarction has been described although it is not possible to distinguish such an event from the natural course of ischaemic heart disease.

Ischaemic pain has been reported in a small proportion of patients following the introduction of nifedipine therapy. Although a 'steal' effect has not been demonstrated, patients experiencing this effect should discontinue nifedipine therapy.

There are reports in older men on long-term therapy of gynaecomastia, which usually regresses upon withdrawal of therapy.

Side-effects which may occur in isolated cases are photosensitivity, exfoliative dermatitis, systemic allergic reactions, purpura and a worsening of myasthenia gravis. Usually, these regress after discontinuation of the drug.

Rare cases of hypersensitivity-type jaundice have been reported. In addition, disturbances of liver function such as intra-hepatic cholestasis may occur. These regress after discontinuation of therapy.

4.9 Overdose

Human experience:

Reports of nifedipine overdosage are limited and symptoms are not necessarily dose-related. Severe hypotension due to vasodilation, and tachycardia or bradycardia are the most likely manifestations of overdose.

Metabolic disturbances include hyperglycaemia, metabolic acidosis and hypo- or hyperkalaemia.

Cardiac effects may include heart block, AV dissociation and asystole, and cardiogenic shock with pulmonary oedema.

Other toxic effects include nausea, vomiting, drowsiness, dizziness, confusion, lethargy, flushing, hypoxia, unconsciousness and coma.

Management of overdose in man:

As far as treatment is concerned, elimination of nifedipine and the restoration of stable cardiovascular conditions have priority.

After oral ingestion, gastric lavage is indicated, if necessary in combination with irrigation of the small intestine. Ipecacuanha should be given to children.

Elimination must be as complete as possible, including the small intestine, to prevent the otherwise inevitable subsequent absorption of the active substance.

Activated charcoal should be given in 4-hourly doses of 25g for adults, 10g for children.

Blood pressure, ECG, central arterial pressure, pulmonary wedge pressure, urea and electrolytes should be monitored.

Hypotension as a result of cardiogenic shock and arterial vasodilation should be treated with elevation of the feet and plasma expanders. If these measures are ineffective, hypotension may be treated with 10% calcium gluconate 10-20 ml intravenously over 5-10 minutes. If the effects are inadequate, the treatment can be continued, with ECG monitoring. In addition, beta-sympathomimetics may be given, e.g. isoprenaline 0.2 mg slowly i.v. or as a continuous infusion of 5μg/min. If an insufficient increase in blood pressure is achieved with calcium and isoprenaline, vasoconstricting sympathomimetics such as dopamine or noradrenaline should be administered. The dosage of these drugs should be determined by the patient's response.

Bradycardia may be treated with atropine, beta-sympathomimetics or a temporary cardiac pacemaker, as required. Additional fluids should be administered with caution to avoid cardiac overload.

5. PHARMACOLOGICAL PROPERTIES

5.1 Pharmacodynamic properties

ATC Code: C08C A05

Nifedipine is a potent calcium-channel blocker which, by dilating peripheral arterial smooth muscle, decreases cardiac work and myocardial oxygen requirement. It also dilates coronary arteries, thereby improving myocardial perfusion and reducing coronary artery spasm. In hypertension, it reduces blood pressure but has little or no effect in normotensive subjects. It has no therapeutic antiarrhythmic effect.

5.2 Pharmacokinetic properties

Coracten SR Capsules are a sustained release formulation of nifedipine designed to provide less fluctuation and more prolonged nifedipine blood concentrations than standard immediate release preparations.

Nifedipine is highly protein bound. It undergoes hepatic oxidation to inactive metabolites which are excreted in the urine (80%) and faeces (20%).

5.3 Preclinical safety data

There are no pre-clinical data of relevance to the prescriber which are additional to that already included in other sections of the Summary of Product Characteristics.

6. PHARMACEUTICAL PARTICULARS

6.1 List of excipients

Capsule contents:

Sucrose Ph.Eur., Maize Starch Ph.Eur., Lactose Ph.Eur., Povidone K30 Ph.Eur., Methacrylic acid copolymer type A (Eudragit L100) NF, Talc Ph.Eur., Purified Water Ph.Eur.

Capsule shells 10 mg:

Gelatin, Red iron oxide (E172), Yellow iron oxide (E172), Black iron oxide (E172), Titanium dioxide (E171).

Capsule shells 20 mg:

Gelatin, Red iron oxide (E172), Yellow iron oxide (E172), Titanium dioxide (E171).

6.2 Incompatibilities

None known.

6.3 Shelf life

36 months.

6.4 Special precautions for storage

Store in original pack at a temperature not exceeding 30°C and protect from light.

6.5 Nature and contents of container

Coracten SR Capsules are presented in blister strips packed in cartons containing 60 capsules. The blister strips are formed from PVC with a coating of PVdC backed with aluminium foil.

(Cartons of 10, 15, 30, 56, 100, 150, 250, 500 and 600 capsules are licenced but not marketed.)

6.6 Special precautions for disposal and other handling

None.

7. MARKETING AUTHORISATION HOLDER

UCB Pharma Limited

208 Bath Road

Slough

Berkshire

SL1 3WE

UK

8. MARKETING AUTHORISATION NUMBER(S)

10 mg - PL 00039/0365

20 mg - PL 00039/0367

9. DATE OF FIRST AUTHORISATION/RENEWAL OF THE AUTHORISATION

31 July 1991

10. DATE OF REVISION OF THE TEXT

April 2009

POM

Coracten XL Joint SPC 30mg, 60mg

(UCB Pharma Limited)

1. NAME OF THE MEDICINAL PRODUCT

Coracten XL 30mg.

Coracten XL 60mg.

2. QUALITATIVE AND QUANTITATIVE COMPOSITION

Each capsule contains 30mg Nifedipine Ph.Eur in sustained release form.

Each capsule contains 60mg Nifedipine Ph.Eur in sustained release form.

For excipients, see 6.1

3. PHARMACEUTICAL FORM

Prolonged release capsule, hard

4. CLINICAL PARTICULARS

4.1 Therapeutic indications

Coracten XL capsules are indicated for the treatment of hypertension and the prophylaxis of chronic stable angina pectoris.

4.2 Posology and method of administration

The capsules are for oral administration and should be swallowed whole with a little fluid.

Dosage - Angina Pectoris and Hypertension

Adults only: Normally treatment is initiated with one 30mg Coracten XL capsule every 24 hours. Dosage may be titrated to a higher level as clinically warranted. The dose may be adjusted to 90mg every 24 hours.

Children: Coracten XL capsules are not recommended for use in children.

Elderly: The pharmacokinetics of nifedipine are altered in the elderly so that lower maintenance doses of nifedipine may be required compared to younger patients.

Hepatic impairment: As Coracten XL is a long acting formulation, it should not be administered to patients with hepatic impairment.

Renal impairment: Dosage adjustments are not usually required in patients with renal impairment.

4.3 Contraindications

Coracten XL capsules are contra-indicated in patients with known hypersensitivity to nifedipine or other dihydropyridines because of the theoretical risk of cross reactivity. They should not be used in nursing mothers and women who are or who may become pregnant (see section 4.6. Pregnancy and Lactation).

Coracten XL capsules should not be used in clinically significant aortic stenosis, unstable angina, or during or within one month of a myocardial infarction. They should not be used in patients in cardiogenic shock.

Coracten XL capsules should not be used for the treatment of acute attacks of angina, or in patients who have had ischaemic pain following its administration previously.

The safety of Coracten XL capsules in malignant hypertension has not been established.

Coracten XL capsules should not be used for secondary prevention of myocardial infarction.

Coracten XL capsules are contra-indicated in patients with acute porphyria.

Coracten XL capsules should not be administered concomitantly with rifampicin since effective plasma levels of nifedipine may not be achieved owing to enzyme induction.

As Coracten XL is a long acting formulation, it should not be administered to patients with hepatic impairment.

4.4 Special warnings and precautions for use

The dose of nifedipine should be reduced in patients with hepatic impairment (***see section 4.2. Posology and Method of Administration***). Nifedipine should be used with caution in patients who are hypotensive; in patients with poor cardiac reserve; in patients with heart failure or significantly impaired left ventricular function as their condition may deteriorate; in diabetic patients as they may require adjustment of their diabetic therapy; and in dialysis patients with malignant hypertension and irreversible renal failure with hypovolaemia, since a significant drop in blood pressure may occur due to the vasodilator effects of nifedipine.

Excessive falls in blood pressure may result in transient blindness. If affected do not attempt to drive or use machinery (see also section 4.8. Undesirable Effects).

Since nifedipine has no beta-blocking activity, it gives no protection against the dangers of abrupt withdrawal of beta-blocking drugs. Withdrawal of any previously prescribed beta-blockers should be gradual, preferably over 8 to 10 days.

The dose of nifedipine should be reduced in patients with hepatic impairment (see section 4.2. Posology and Method of Administration).

Nifedipine may be used in combination with beta-blocking drugs and other antihypertensive agents, but the possibility of an additive effect resulting in postural hypotension should be borne in mind. Nifedipine will not prevent possible rebound effects after cessation of other anti-hypertensive therapy.

4.5 Interaction with other medicinal products and other forms of interaction

As with other dihydropyridines, nifedipine should not be taken with grapefruit juice because bioavailability is increased.

The simultaneous administration of nifedipine and digoxin may lead to reduced digoxin clearance and hence an increase in the plasma digoxin. Digoxin levels should be monitored and, if necessary, the digoxin dose reduced.

Nifedipine may increase the spectrophotometric values of urinary vanillylmandelic acid falsely. However, HPLC measurements are unaffected.

Coracten XL capsules should not be administered concomitantly with rifampicin since effective plasma levels of nifedipine may not be achieved owing to enzyme induction (see section 4.3. Contra-indications).

Increased plasma levels of nifedipine have been reported during concomitant use of H_2-receptor antagonists (specifically cimetidine), other calcium channel blockers (specifically diltiazem), alcohol, cyclosporin, macrolide antibiotics, gingko biloba and ginseng. Azole antifungals may increase serum concentrations of nifedipine.

Decreased plasma levels of nifedipine have been reported during concomitant use of antibacterials (specifically rifampicin), and probably also antiepileptics and St John's Wort.

When used in combination with nifedipine, plasma concentrations of quinidine have been shown to be suppressed regardless of quinidine dosage. The plasma concentrations of phenytoin, theophylline, non-depolarising muscle relaxants (e.g. tubocurarine) and possibly digoxin are increased when used in combination with nifedipine. Tacrolimus concentrations may be increased by nifedipine.

Enhanced hypotensive effect of nifedipine may occur with: aldesleukin, alprostadil, anaesthetics, antipsychotics, diuretics, phenothiazides, prazosin and intravenous ionic X-ray contrast medium. Profound hypotension has been reported with nifedipine and intravenous magnesium sulphate in the treatment of pre-eclampsia.

Ritonavir and quinupristin/dalfopristin may result in increased plasma concentrations of nifedipine.

Effective plasma levels of nifedipine may not be achieved due to enzyme induction with concurrent administration of erythromycin, carbamazepine and phenobarbitone.

There is an increased risk of excessive hypotension, bradycardia and heart failure with β-blockers.

An increased rate of absorption of nifedipine from sustained release preparation may occur if given concurrently with cisapride.

Nifedipine may result in increased levels of mizolastine due to inhibition of cytochrome CYP3A4.

Nifedipine may increase the neuromuscular blocking effects of vecuronium.

4.6 Pregnancy and lactation

Pregnancy

Because animal studies show embryotoxicity and teratogenicity, nifedipine is contraindicated during pregnancy (see also section 4.3. Contra-indications). Embryotoxicity was noted at 6 to 20 times the maximum recommended dose for nifedipine given to rats, mice and rabbits, and teratogenicity was noted in rabbits given 20 times the maximum recommended dose for nifedipine.

Lactation

Nifedipine is secreted in breast milk, therefore, Coracten XL capsules are not recommended during lactation.

4.7 Effects on ability to drive and use machines

Dizziness and lethargy are potential undesirable effects. If affected do not attempt to drive or use machinery (see also section 4.8. Undesirable Effects).

Excessive falls in blood pressure may result in transient blindness. If affected do not attempt to drive or use machinery (see also section 4.8. Undesirable Effects).

4.8 Undesirable effects

Most side-effects are consequences of the vasodilatory effects of nifedipine.

Side-effects are generally transient and mild, and usually occur at the start of treatment only. They include headache, flushing and, usually at higher dosages, nausea, dyspepsia, heartburn, constipation, diarrhoea, dizziness, lethargy, skin reactions (rash, urticaria and pruritus), paraesthesia, hypotension, palpitation, tachycardia, dependent oedema, increased frequency of micturition, eye pain, depression, fever, gingival hyperplasia, telangiectasia and erythema multiforme.

Other less frequently reported side-effects include myalgia, tremor, pemphigoid reaction and visual disturbances. Impotence may occur rarely. Mood changes may occur rarely.

Excessive falls in blood pressure may result in cerebral or myocardial ischaemia or transient blindness.

As with other sustained release dihydropyridines, exacerbation of angina pectoris may occur rarely at the start of treatment with sustained release formulations of nifedipine. The occurrence of myocardial infarction has been described although it is not possible to distinguish such an event from the natural course of ischaemic heart disease. Ischaemic pain has been reported in a small proportion of patients following the introduction of nifedipine therapy. Although a 'steal' effect has not been demonstrated, patients experiencing this effect should discontinue nifedipine therapy.

There are reports in older men on long-term therapy of gynaecomastia which usually regresses upon withdrawal of therapy.

Side-effects which may occur in isolated cases are photosensitivity, exfoliative dermatitis, systemic allergic reactions, purpura and a worsening of myasthenia gravis. Usually, these regress after discontinuation of the drug.

Rare cases of hypersensitivity-type jaundice have been reported. In addition, disturbances of liver function such as intra-hepatic cholestasis may occur. These regress after discontinuation of therapy.

4.9 Overdose

Clinical effects

Reports of nifedipine overdosage are limited and symptoms are not necessarily dose-related. Severe hypotension due to vasodilation, and tachycardia and bradycardia are the most likely manifestations of overdose.

Metabolic disturbances include hyperglycaemia, metabolic acidosis and hypo- or hyperkalaemia.

Cardiac effects may include heart block, AV dissociation and asystole, and cardiogenic shock with pulmonary oedema.

Other toxic effects include nausea, vomiting, drowsiness, dizziness, confusion, lethargy, flushing, hypoxia and unconsciousness to the point of coma.

Treatment

As far as treatment is concerned, elimination of nifedipine and the restoration of stable cardiovascular conditions have priority.

After oral ingestion, gastric lavage is indicated, if necessary in combination with irrigation of the small intestine. Ipecacuanha should be given to children.

Elimination must be as complete as possible, including the small intestine, to prevent the otherwise inevitable subsequent absorption of the active substance.

Activated charcoal should be given in 4-hourly doses of 25g for adults, 10g for children.

Blood pressure, ECG, central arterial pressure, pulmonary wedge pressure, urea and electrolytes should be monitored.

Hypotension as a result of cardiogenic shock and arterial vasodilation should be treated with elevation of the feet and plasma expanders. If these measures are ineffective, hypotension may be treated with 10% calcium gluconate 10-20 ml intravenously over 5-10 minutes. If the effects are inadequate, the treatment can be continued, with ECG monitoring. In addition, beta-sympathomimetics may be given, e.g. isoprenaline 0.2 mg slowly i.v. or as a continuous infusion of 5μg/min. If an insufficient increase in blood pressure is achieved with calcium and isoprenaline, vasoconstricting sympathomimetics such as dopamine or noradrenaline should be administered. The dosage of these drugs should be determined by the patient's response.

Bradycardia may be treated with atropine, beta-sympathomimetics or a temporary cardiac pacemaker, as required.

Additional fluids should be administered with caution to avoid cardiac overload.

5. PHARMACOLOGICAL PROPERTIES

5.1 Pharmacodynamic properties

ATC Code: C08C A05

Nifedipine is a potent calcium-channel blocker which, by dilating peripheral arterial smooth muscle, decreases cardiac work and myocardial oxygen requirement. It also dilates coronary arteries, thereby improving myocardial perfusion and reducing coronary artery spasm. In hypertension, it reduces blood pressure but has little or no effect in normotensive subjects. It has no therapeutic antiarrhythmic effect.

5.2 Pharmacokinetic properties

Coracten XL capsules are a sustained release formulation of nifedipine designed to provide less fluctuation and more prolonged nifedipine blood concentrations than standard immediate release preparations.

Nifedipine is highly protein bound. It undergoes hepatic oxidation to inactive metabolites which are excreted in the urine (80%) and faeces (20%).

5.3 Preclinical safety data

There are no pre-clinical data of relevance to the prescriber which are additional to that already included in other sections of the Summary of Product Characteristics.

6. PHARMACEUTICAL PARTICULARS

6.1 List of excipients

Capsule contents:

Lactose monohydrate

Microcrystalline Cellulose

Hydroxylpropyl methylcellulose K100

Povidone K30

Magnesium Stearate

Hydroxypropylcellulose

Ammonio methacrylate copolymer type B

Polyethylene Glycol 6000

Dibutylphthalate

Titanium dioxide E171

Talc

30 mg - Capsule shells (size 3):

Yellow iron oxide E172

Red iron oxide E172

Titanium dioxide E171

Gelatin

60 mg - Capsule shells (size 1)

Red iron oxide E172

Titanium dioxide E171

Gelatin

The printing ink is made of shellac, purified water, black iron oxide (E172) with 2-ethoxyethanol, soya lecithin, antifoam and IMS or with ethyl alcohol, isopropyl alcohol, n-butyl alcohol, propylene glycol, ammonium hydroxide and potassium hydroxide.

6.2 Incompatibilities

None known.

6.3 Shelf life

36 months.

6.4 Special precautions for storage

Do not store above 25°C. Store in the original package.

6.5 Nature and contents of container

Coracten XL capsules are available in blister strips packed in cartons containing 28, 30, 56 and 60 capsules. The blister strips are formed from PVC with a coating of PVdC backed with aluminium foil.

6.6 Special precautions for disposal and other handling
None.

7. MARKETING AUTHORISATION HOLDER
UCB Pharma Limited
208 Bath Road
Slough
Berkshire
SL1 3WE
UK

8. MARKETING AUTHORISATION NUMBER(S)
30 mg - PL 00039/0506
60 mg - PL 00039/0507

9. DATE OF FIRST AUTHORISATION/RENEWAL OF THE AUTHORISATION
7 October 1998

10. DATE OF REVISION OF THE TEXT
April 2009
POM

Cordarone X 100, Cordarone X 200

(sanofi-aventis)

1. NAME OF THE MEDICINAL PRODUCT
Cordarone X 100.
Cordarone X 200.

2. QUALITATIVE AND QUANTITATIVE COMPOSITION
Cordarone X 100 contain 100mg of amiodarone hydrochloride.

Cordarone X 200 contain 200mg of amiodarone hydrochloride.

For excipients, see 6.1

3. PHARMACEUTICAL FORM
Tablet.

Round, white tablet with a breakline on one side, imprinted with 100 or 200 on the other.

4. CLINICAL PARTICULARS

4.1 Therapeutic indications
Treatment should be initiated and normally monitored only under hospital or specialist supervision. Oral Cordarone X is indicated only for the treatment of severe rhythm disorders not responding to other therapies or when other treatments cannot be used.

Tachyarrhythmias associated with Wolff-Parkinson-White Syndrome.

Atrial flutter and fibrillation when other drugs cannot be used.

All types of tachyarrhythmias of paroxysmal nature including: supraventricular, nodal and ventricular tachycardias, ventricular fibrillation: when other drugs cannot be used.

4.2 Posology and method of administration

Adults

It is particularly important that the minimum effective dose be used. In all cases the patient's management must be judged on the individual response and well being. The following dosage regimen is generally effective.

Initial Stabilisation

Treatment should be started with 200mg, three times a day and may be continued for 1 week. The dosage should then be reduced to 200mg, twice daily for a further week.

Maintenance

After the initial period the dosage should be reduced to 200mg daily, or less if appropriate. Rarely, the patient may require a higher maintenance dose. The scored 100mg tablet should be used to titrate the minimum dosage required to maintain control of the arrhythmia. The maintenance dose should be regularly reviewed, especially where this exceeds 200mg daily.

General Considerations

Initial dosing

A high dose is needed in order to achieve adequate tissue levels rapidly.

Maintenance

Too high a dose during maintenance therapy can cause side effects which are believed to be related to high tissue levels of amiodarone and its metabolites.

Amiodarone is strongly protein bound and has an average plasma half life of 50 days (reported range 20-100 days). It follows that sufficient time must be allowed for a new distribution equilibrium to be achieved between adjustments of dosage. In patients with potentially lethal arrhythmias the long half life is a valuable safeguard, as omission of occasional doses does not significantly influence the overall therapeutic effect. It is particularly important that the minimum effective dosage is used and the patient is monitored regularly to detect the clinical features of excess amiodarone dosage. Therapy may then be adjusted accordingly.

Dosage reduction/withdrawal

Side effects slowly disappear as tissue levels fall. Following drug withdrawal, residual tissue bound amiodarone may protect the patient for up to a month. However, the likelihood of recurrence of arrhythmia during this period should be considered.

Paediatric population

No controlled paediatric studies have been undertaken. In published uncontrolled studies effective doses for children were:

- Loading dose: 10 to 20mg/kg/day for 7 to 10 days (or 500mg/m^2/day if expressed per square metre)
- Maintenance dose: the minimum effective dosage should be used; according to individual response, it may range between 5 to 10 mg/kg/day (or 250mg/m^2/day if expressed per square metre).

Elderly

As with all patients it is important that the minimum effective dose is used. Whilst there is no evidence that dosage requirements are different for this group of patients they may be more susceptible to bradycardia and conduction defects if too high a dose is employed. Particular attention should be paid to monitoring thyroid function. *(see sections 4.3, 4.4 and 4.8).*

Cordarone X 100 and 200 are for oral administration.

4.3 Contraindications
Sinus bradycardia and sino-atrial heart block. In patients with severe conduction disturbances (high grade AV block, bifascicular or trifascicular block) or sinus node disease, Cordarone X should be used only in conjunction with a pacemaker.

Evidence or history of thyroid dysfunction. Thyroid function tests should be performed in all patients prior to therapy.

Known hypersensitivity to iodine or to amiodarone, or to any of the excipients. (One 100mg tablet contains approximately 37.5mg iodine).

The combination of Cordarone X with drugs which may induce torsades de pointes is contra-indicated *(see section 4.5).*

Pregnancy - except in exceptional circumstances *(see section 4.6)*

Lactation *(see section 4.6).*

4.4 Special warnings and precautions for use
Patients with rare hereditary problems of galactose intolerance, the Lapp lactase deficiency or glucose-galactose malabsorption should not take this medicine.

Amiodarone can cause serious adverse reactions affecting the eyes, heart, lung, liver, thyroid gland, skin and peripheral nervous system *(see section 4.8.).* Because these reactions may be delayed, patients on long-term treatment should be carefully supervised. As undesirable effects are usually dose-related, the minimum effective maintenance dose should be given.

Before surgery, the anaesthetist should be informed that the patient is taking amiodarone *(see sections 4.5 and 4.8).*

Cardiac disorders *(see section 4.8):*

Too high a dosage may lead to severe bradycardia and to conduction disturbances with the appearance of an idioventricular rhythm, particularly in elderly patients or during digitalis therapy. In these circumstances, Cordarone X treatment should be withdrawn. If necessary beta-adrenostimulants or glucagon may be given. Because of the long half-life of amiodarone, if bradycardia is severe and symptomatic the insertion of a pacemaker should be considered.

Oral Cordarone X is not contra-indicated in patients with latent or manifest heart failure but caution should be exercised as, occasionally, existing heart failure may be worsened. In such cases, Cordarone X may be used with other appropriate therapies.

The pharmacological action of amiodarone induces ECG changes: QT prolongation (related to prolonged repolarisation) with the possible development of U-waves and deformed T-waves; these changes do not reflect toxicity.

In the elderly, heart rate may decrease markedly.

Treatment should be discontinued in case of onset of 2nd or 3rd degree A-V block, sino-atrial block, or bifascicular block.

Amiodarone has a low pro-arrhythmic effect. Onsets of new arrhythmias or worsening of treated arrhythmias, sometimes fatal, have been reported. It is important, but difficult, to differentiate a lack of efficacy of the drug from a proarrhythmic effect, whether or not this is associated with a worsening of the cardiac condition. Proarrhythmic effects generally occur in the context of drug interactions and/or electrolytic disorders *(see sections 4.5. and 4.8).*

Before starting amiodarone, it is recommended to perform an ECG and serum potassium measurement. Monitoring of ECG is recommended during treatment.

Amiodarone may increase the defibrillation threshold and/or pacing threshold in patients with an implantable cardioverter defibrillator or a pacemaker, which may adversely affect the efficacy of the device. Regular tests are recommended to ensure the proper function of the device after initiation of treatment or change in posology.

Endocrine disorders *(see section 4.8)*

Amiodarone may induce hypothyroidism or hyperthyroidism, particularly in patients with a personal history of thyroid disorders. Clinical and biological [including ultrasensitive TSH (usTSH)] monitoring should be performed prior to therapy in all patients. Monitoring should be carried out during treatment, at six-monthly intervals, and for several months following its discontinuation. This is particularly important in the elderly. In patients whose history indicates an increased risk of thyroid dysfunction, regular assessment is recommended. Serum usTSH level should be measured when thyroid dysfunction is suspected.

Amiodarone contains iodine and thus may interfere with radio-iodine uptake. However, thyroid function tests (free-T_3, free-T_4, usTSH) remain interpretable. Amiodarone inhibits peripheral conversion of levothyroxine (T_4) to triiodothyronine (T_3) and may cause isolated biochemical changes (increase in serum free-T_4, free-T_3 being slightly decreased or even normal) in clinically euthyroid patients. There is no reason in such cases to discontinue amiodarone treatment if there is no clinical or further biological (usTSH) evidence of thyroid disease.

Hypothyroidism

Hypothyroidism should be suspected if the following clinical signs occur: weight gain, cold intolerance, reduced activity, excessive bradycardia. The diagnosis is supported by an increase in serum usTSH and an exaggerated TSH response to TRH. T_3 and T_4 levels may be low. Euthyroidism is usually obtained within 3 months following the discontinuation of treatment. In life-threatening situations, amiodarone therapy can be continued, in combination with levothyroxine. The dose of levothyroxine is adjusted according to TSH levels.

Hyperthyroidism

Hyperthyroidism may occur during amiodarone treatment, or, up to several months after discontinuation. Clinical features, such as weight loss, asthenia, restlessness, increase in heart rate, onset of arrhythmia, angina, congestive heart failure should alert the physician. The diagnosis is supported by a decrease in serum usTSH level, an elevated T_3 and a reduced TSH response to thyrotropin releasing hormone. Elevation of reverse T_3 (rT_3) may also be found.

In the case of hyperthyroidism, therapy should be withdrawn. Clinical recovery usually occurs within a few months, although severe cases, sometimes resulting in fatalities, have been reported. Clinical recovery precedes the normalisation of thyroid function tests.

Courses of anti-thyroid drugs have been used for the treatment of severe thyroid hyperactivity; large doses may be required initially. These may not always be effective and concomitant high dose corticosteroid therapy (e.g. 1mg/kg prednisolone) may be required for several weeks.

Eye disorders *(see section 4.8)*

If blurred or decreased vision occurs, complete ophthalmologic examination including fundoscopy should be promptly performed. Appearance of optic neuropathy and/or optic neuritis requires amiodarone withdrawal due to the potential progression to blindness. Unless blurred or decreased vision occurs, opthamological examination is recommended annually.

Hepato-biliary disorders *(see section 4.8):*

Amiodarone may be associated with a variety of hepatic effects, including cirrhosis, hepatitis, jaundice and hepatic failure. Some fatalities have been reported, mainly following long-term therapy, although rarely they have occurred soon after starting treatment particularly after Cordarone X intravenous. It is advisable to monitor liver function particularly transaminases before treatment and six monthly thereafter.

At the beginning of therapy, elevation of serum transaminases which can be in isolation (1.5 to 3 times normal) may occur. These may return to normal with dose reduction, or sometimes spontaneously.

Isolated cases of acute liver disorders with elevated serum transaminases and/or jaundice may occur; in such cases treatment should be discontinued.

There have been reports of chronic liver disease. Alteration of laboratory tests which may be minimal (transaminases elevated 1.5 to 5 times normal) or clinical signs (possible hepatomegaly) during treatment for longer than 6 months should suggest this diagnosis. Routine monitoring of liver function tests is therefore advised. Abnormal clinical and laboratory test results usually regress upon cessation of treatment, but fatal cases have been reported. Histological findings may resemble pseudo-alcoholic hepatitis, but they can be variable and include cirrhosis.

Although there have been no literature reports on the potentiation of hepatic adverse effects of alcohol, patients should be advised to moderate their alcohol intake while taking Cordarone X.

Nervous system disorders *(see section 4.8):*

Amiodarone may induce peripheral sensorimotor neuropathy and/or myopathy. Both these conditions may be severe, although recovery usually occurs within several months after amiodarone withdrawal, but may sometimes be incomplete.

Respiratory, thoracic and mediastinal disorders (*see section 4.8*):

Onset of dyspnoea or non-productive cough may be related to pulmonary toxicity (hypersensitivity pneumonitis, alveolar/interstitial pneumonitis or fibrosis, pleuritis, bronchiolitis obliterans organising pneumonitis. Presenting features can include dyspnoea (which may be severe and unexplained by the current cardiac status), non-productive cough and deterioration in general health (fatigue, weight loss and fever). The onset is usually slow but may be rapidly progressive. Whilst the majority of cases have been reported with long term therapy, a few have occurred soon after starting treatment.

Patients should be carefully evaluated clinically and consideration given to chest X-rays before starting therapy. During treatment, if pulmonary toxicity is suspected, this should be repeated and associated with lung function testing including, where possible, measurement of transfer factor. Initial radiological changes may be difficult to distinguish from pulmonary venous congestion. Pulmonary toxicity has usually been reversible following early withdrawal of amiodarone therapy, with or without corticosteroid therapy. Clinical symptoms often resolve within a few weeks followed by slower radiological and lung function improvement. Some patients can deteriorate despite discontinuing Cordarone X.

Skin and subcutaneous tissue disorders (*see section 4.8*)

Patients should be instructed to avoid exposure to sun and to use protective measures during therapy as patients taking Cordarone X can become unduly sensitive to sunlight, which may persist after several months of discontinuation of Cordarone X. In most cases symptoms are limited to tingling, burning and erythema of sun-exposed skin but severe phototoxic reactions with blistering may be seen.

Drug interactions (*see section 4.5*)

Concomitant use of amiodarone is not recommended with the following drugs: beta-blockers, heart rate lowering calcium channel inhibitors (verapamil, diltiazem), stimulant laxative agents which may cause hypokalaemia.

Increased plasma levels of flecainide have been reported with co-administration of amiodarone. The flecainide dose should be reduced accordingly and the patient closely monitored.

4.5 Interaction with other medicinal products and other forms of interaction

Some of the more important drugs that interact with amiodarone include warfarin, digoxin, phenytoin and any drug which prolongs the QT interval.

Amiodarone raises the plasma concentrations of oral anticoagulants (warfarin) and phenytoin by inhibition of CYP 2C9. The dose of warfarin should be reduced accordingly. More frequent monitoring of prothrombin time both during and after amiodarone treatment is recommended. Phenytoin dosage should be reduced if signs of overdosage appear, and plasma levels may be measured.

Administration of Cordarone X to a patient already receiving digoxin will bring about an increase in the plasma digoxin concentration and thus precipitate symptoms and signs associated with high digoxin levels. Clinical, ECG and biological monitoring is recommended and digoxin dosage should be halved. A synergistic effect on heart rate and atrioventricular conduction is also possible.

Combined therapy with the following drugs which prolong the QT interval is contra-indicated (*see section 4.3*) due to the increased risk of torsades de pointes; for example:

- Class Ia anti-arrhythmic drugs e.g. quinidine, procainamide, disopyramide
- Class III anti-arrhythmic drugs e.g. sotalol, bretylium
- intravenous erythromycin, co-trimoxazole or pentamidine injection
- some anti-psychotics e.g. chlorpromazine, thioridazine, fluphenazine, pimozide, haloperidol, amisulpiride and sertindole
- lithium and tricyclic anti-depressants e.g. doxepin, maprotiline, amitriptyline
- certain antihistamines e.g. terfenadine, astemizole, mizolastine
- anti-malarials e.g. quinine, mefloquine, chloroquine, halofantrine.
- Moxifloxacin

Fluoroquinolones

There have been rare reports of QTc interval prolongation, with or without torsades de pointes, in patients taking amiodrone with fluoroquinolones. Concomitant use of amiodarone with fluoroquinolones should be avoided (concomitant use with moxifloxacin is contra-indicated, see above).

Combined therapy with the following drugs is not recommended:

eta blockers and certain calcium channel inhibitors azem, verapamil); potentiation of negative chronotropic properties and conduction slowing effects may occur.

ulant laxatives, which may cause hypokalaemia thus sing the risk of torsades de pointes; other types of es should be used.

Caution should be exercised over combined therapy with the following drugs which may also cause hypokalaemia and/or hypomagnesaemia, e.g. diuretics, systemic corticosteroids, tetracosactide, intravenous amphotericin.

In cases of hypokalaemia, corrective action should be taken and QT interval monitored. In case of torsades de pointes antiarrhythmic agents should not be given; pacing may be instituted and IV magnesium may be used.

Caution is advised in patients undergoing general anaesthesia, or receiving high dose oxygen therapy.

Potentially severe complications have been reported in patients taking amiodarone undergoing general anaesthesia: bradycardia unresponsive to atropine, hypotension, disturbances of conduction, decreased cardiac output.

A few cases of adult respiratory distress syndrome, most often in the period immediately after surgery, have been observed. A possible interaction with a high oxygen concentration may be implicated.

Grapefruit juice inhibits cytochrome P450 3A4 and may increase the plasma concentration of amiodarone. Grapefruit juice should be avoided during treatment with oral amiodarone.

Drugs metabolised by cytochrome P450 3A4

When drugs are co-administered with amiodarone, an inhibitor of CYP 3A4, this may result in a higher level of their plasma concentrations, which may lead to a possible increase in their toxicity:

- Ciclosporin: plasma levels of ciclosporin may increase as much as 2-fold when used in combination. A reduction in the dose of ciclosporin may be necessary to maintain the plasma concentration within the therapeutic range.
- Statins: the risk of muscular toxicity is increased by concomitant administration of amiodarone with statins metabolised by CYP 3A4 such as simvastatin, atorvastatin and lovastatin. It is recommended to use a statin not metabolised by CYP 3A4 when given with amiodarone.
- Other drugs metabolised by cytochrome P450 3A4: examples of such drugs are lidocaine, tacrolimus, sildenafil, fentanyl, midazolam, triazolam, dihydroergotamine and ergotamine.

Flecainide

Given that flecainide is mainly metabolised by CYP 2D6, by inhibiting this isoenzyme, amiodarone may increase flecainide plasma levels; it is advised to reduce the flecainide dose by 50% and to monitor the patient closely for adverse effects. Monitoring of flecainide plasma levels is strongly recommended in such circumstances.

Interaction with substrates of other CYP 450 isoenzymes

In vitro studies show that amiodarone also has the potential to inhibit CYP 1A2, CYP 2C19 and CYP 2D6 through its main metabolite. When co-administered, amiodarone would be expected to increase the plasma concentration of drugs whose metabolism is dependent upon CYP 1A2, CYP 2C19 and CYP 2D6.

4.6 Pregnancy and lactation

Pregnancy

There are insufficient data on the use of amiodarone during pregnancy in humans to judge any possible toxicity. However, in view of its effect on the foetal thyroid gland, amiodarone is contraindicated during pregnancy, except in exceptional circumstances.

If, because of the long half life of amiodarone, discontinuation of the drug is considered prior to planned conception, the real risk of reoccurrence of life threatening arrhythmias should be weighed against the possible hazard for the foetus.

Lactation

Amiodarone is excreted into the breast milk in significant quantities and breast-feeding is contra-indicated.

4.7 Effects on ability to drive and use machines

The ability to drive or to operate machinery may be impaired in patients with clinical symptoms of amiodarone-induced eye disorders.

4.8 Undesirable effects

The following adverse reactions are classified by system organ class and ranked under heading of frequency using the following convention: very common (>= 10%), common (>= 1% and < 10%); uncommon (>= 0.1% and < 1%); rare (>= 0.01% and < 0.1%), very rare (< 0.01%), not known (cannot be estimated from the available data).

Blood and lymphatic system disorders:

- Very rare:

- haemolytic anemia

- aplastic anaemia

- thrombocytopenia.

In patients taking amiodarone there have been incidental findings of bone marrow granulomas. The clinical significance of this is unknown.

Cardiac disorders:

- Common: bradycardia, generally moderate and dose-related.
- Uncommon:

- onset or worsening of arrhythmia, sometimes followed by cardiac arrest (*see sections 4.4 and 4.5.*)

- conduction disturbances (sinoatrial block, AV block of various degrees) (*see section 4.4*)

- Very rare: marked bradycardia or sinus arrest in patients with sinus node dysfunction and/or in elderly patients.

Endocrine disorders (*see section 4.4*):

- Common:

- hypothyroidism

- hyperthyroidism, sometimes fatal

- Very rare

- syndrome of inappropriate antidiuretic hormone secretion (SIADH)

Eye disorders:

- Very common: corneal microdeposits usually limited to the area under the pupil, which are usually only discernable by slit-lamp examinations. They may be associated with colored halos in dazzling light or blurred vision. Corneal micro-deposits consist of complex lipid deposits and are reversible following discontinuation of treatment. The deposits are considered essentially benign and do not require discontinuation of amiodarone.
- Very rare: optic neuropathy/neuritis that may progress to blindness (*see section 4.4*).

Gastrointestinal disorders:

- Very common: benign gastrointestinal disorders (nausea, vomiting, dysgeusia) usually occurring with loading dosage and resolving with dose reduction.

Hepato-biliary disorders: (*see section 4.4*).

- Very common: isolated increase in serum transaminases, which is usually moderate (1.5 to 3 times normal range), occurring at the beginning of therapy. It may return to normal with dose reduction or even spontaneously.
- Common: acute liver disorders with high serum transaminases and/or jaundice, including hepatic failure, which are sometimes fatal
- Very rare: chronic liver disease (pseudo alcoholic hepatitis, cirrhosis), sometimes fatal.

Immune system disorders:

Angioedema (there have been some reports of angioedema, although exact frequencies are not known)

Investigations:

- Very rare: increase in blood creatinine.

Nervous system disorders:

- Common:

- extrapyramidal tremor, for which regression usually occurs after reduction of dose or withdrawal

- nightmares

- sleep disorders.

- Uncommon: peripheral sensorimotor neuropathy and/or myopathy, usually reversible on withdrawal of the drug (*see section 4.4*).
- Very rare:

- cerebellar ataxia, for which regression usually occurs after reduction of dose or withdrawal

- benign intracranial hypertension (pseudo- tumor cerebri)

- headache

- vertigo.

Reproductive system and breast disorders:

- Very rare:

- epididymo-orchitis

- impotence.

Respiratory, thoracic and mediastinal disorders:

- Common: pulmonary toxicity [hypersensitivity pneumonitis, alveolar/interstitial pneumonitis or fibrosis, pleuritis, bronchiolitis obliterans organising pneumonia (BOOP)], sometimes fatal (*see section 4.4*).
- Very rare:

- bronchospasm in patients with severe respiratory failure and especially in asthmatic patients

- surgery (possible interaction with a high oxygen concentration) (*see sections 4.4 and 4.5*).

Pulmonary haemorrhage (there have been some reports of pulmonary haemorrhage, although exact frequencies are not known)

Skin and subcutaneous tissue disorders:

- Very common: photosensitivity (*see section 4.4*).
- Common: slate grey or bluish pigmentations of light-exposed skin, particularly the face, in case of prolonged treatment with high daily dosages; such pigmentations slowly disappear following treatment discontinuation.
- Very rare:

- erythema during the course of radiotherapy

- skin rashes, usually non- specific

- exfoliative dermatitis

- alopecia.

- Not known: urticaria

Vascular disorders:

- Very rare: vasculitis.

4.9 Overdose
Little information is available regarding acute overdosage with oral amiodarone. Few cases of sinus bradycardia, heart block, attacks of ventricular tachycardia, torsades de pointes, circulatory failure and hepatic injury have been reported.

In the event of overdose treatment should be symptomatic, gastric lavage may be employed to reduce absorption in addition to general supportive measures. The patient should be monitored and if bradycardia occurs beta-adrenostimulants or glucagon may be given. Spontaneously resolving attacks of ventricular tachycardia may also occur. Due to the pharmacokinetics of amiodarone, adequate and prolonged surveillance of the patient, particularly cardiac status, is recommended. Neither amiodarone nor its metabolites are dialysable.

5. PHARMACOLOGICAL PROPERTIES
5.1 Pharmacodynamic properties
Amiodarone hydrochloride is an antiarrhythmic.

5.2 Pharmacokinetic properties
Amiodarone is strongly protein bound and the plasma half life is usually of the order of 50 days. However there may be considerable inter-patient variation; in individual patients a half life of less than 20 days and a half life of more than 100 days has been reported. High doses of Cordarone X, for example 600mg/day, should be given initially to achieve effective tissue levels as rapidly as possible. Owing to the long half life of the drug, a maintenance dose of only 200mg/day, or less is usually necessary. Sufficient time must be allowed for a new distribution equilibrium to be achieved between adjustments of dose.

The long half life is a valuable safeguard for patients with potentially lethal arrhythmias as omission of occasional doses does not significantly influence the protection afforded by Cordarone X.

5.3 Preclinical safety data
There are no pre-clinical data of relevance to the prescriber which are additional to that already included in other sections of the SPC.

6. PHARMACEUTICAL PARTICULARS
6.1 List of excipients
Lactose monohydrate, Maize starch, Povidone, Colloidal anhydrous silica, Magnesium stearate.

6.2 Incompatibilities
Not applicable.

6.3 Shelf life
60 months.

6.4 Special precautions for storage
The tablets should be protected from light.

6.5 Nature and contents of container
Cordarone X tablets are supplied in blister packs of 28 tablets packed in cardboard cartons.

6.6 Special precautions for disposal and other handling
Not applicable

7. MARKETING AUTHORISATION HOLDER
Sanofi-aventis

One Onslow Street

Guildford

Surrey

GU1 4YS

UK

8. MARKETING AUTHORISATION NUMBER(S)
Cordarone X 100: PL 11723/0012.

Cordarone X 200: PL 11723/0013.

9. DATE OF FIRST AUTHORISATION/RENEWAL OF THE AUTHORISATION
Cordarone 100: 15 January 2001.

Cordarone 200: 18 June 2003

10. DATE OF REVISION OF THE TEXT
30 March 2009

Legal category: POM

Cordarone X Intravenous

(sanofi-aventis)

1. NAME OF THE MEDICINAL PRODUCT
Cordarone X Intravenous.

2. QUALITATIVE AND QUANTITATIVE COMPOSITION
Each 3ml ampoule contains 150mg amiodarone hydrochloride.

For excipients, see 6.1

3. PHARMACEUTICAL FORM
Solution for injection.

4. CLINICAL PARTICULARS
4.1 Therapeutic indications
Treatment should be initiated and normally monitored only under hospital or specialist supervision. Cordarone X Intravenous is indicated only for the treatment of severe rhythm disorders not responding to other therapies or when other treatments cannot be used.

Tachyarrhythmias associated with Wolff-Parkinson-White syndrome.

All types of tachyarrhythmias including supraventricular, nodal and ventricular tachycardias; atrial flutter and fibrillation; ventricular fibrillation; when other drugs cannot be used.

Cordarone X Intravenous can be used where a rapid response is required or where oral administration is not possible.

4.2 Posology and method of administration
Cordarone X Intravenous should only be used when facilities exist for cardiac monitoring, defibrillation, and cardiac pacing.

Cordarone X Intravenous may be used prior to DC cardioversion.

The standard recommended dose is 5mg/kg bodyweight given by intravenous infusion over a period of 20 minutes to 2 hours. This should be administered as a dilute solution in 250ml 5% dextrose. This may be followed by repeat infusion up to 1200mg (approximately 15mg/kg bodyweight) in up to 500ml 5% dextrose per 24 hours, the rate of infusion being adjusted on the basis of clinical response. (see section 4.4).

In extreme clinical emergency the drug may, at the discretion of the clinician, be given as a slow injection of 150-300mg in 10-20ml 5% dextrose over a minimum of 3 minutes. This should not be repeated for at least 15 minutes. Patients treated in this way with Cordarone X Intravenous must be closely monitored, e.g. in an intensive care unit.(see section 4.4).

Changeover from Intravenous to Oral therapy

As soon as an adequate response has been obtained, oral therapy should be initiated concomitantly at the usual loading dose (i.e. 200mg three times a day). Cordarone X Intravenous should then be phased out gradually.

Paediatric population

Due to the presence of benzyl alcohol, intravenous amiodarone is usually contraindicated in neonates and premature babies (see section 4.3).

No controlled paediatric studies have been undertaken. In published uncontrolled studies effective doses for children were (see section 4.4):

- Loading dose: 5mg/kg body weight over 20 minutes to 2 hours
- Maintenance dose: 10 to 15mg/kg/day from a few hours to several days.

If needed, oral therapy may be initiated concomitantly.

Elderly

As with all patients it is important that the minimum effective dose is used. Whilst there is no evidence that dosage requirements are different for this group of patients they may be more susceptible to bradycardia and conduction defects if too high a dose is employed. Particular attention should be paid to monitoring thyroid function (see sections 4.3, 4.4 and 4.8).

Cardiopulmonary resuscitation

The recommended dose for ventricular fibrillations/pulseless ventricular tachycardia resistant to defibrillation is 300 mg (or 5 mg/kg body-weight) diluted in 20 ml 5% dextrose and rapidly injected. An additional 150 mg (or 2.5 mg/kg body-weight) IV dose may be considered if ventricular fibrillation persists.

See section 6.2 for information on incompatibilities

4.3 Contraindications

- Sinus bradycardia and sino-atrial heart block. In patients with severe conduction disturbances (high grade AV block, bifascicular or trifascicular block) or sinus node disease, Cordarone X should be used only in conjunction with a pacemaker.
- Evidence or history of thyroid dysfunction. Thyroid function tests should be performed where appropriate prior to therapy in all patients.
- Severe respiratory failure, circulatory collapse, or severe arterial hypotension; hypotension, heart failure and cardiomyopathy are also contra-indications when using Cordarone X Intravenous as a bolus injection.
- Known hypersensitivity to iodine or to amiodarone, or to any of the excipients. (One ampoule contains approximately 56mg iodine).
- The combination of Cordarone X with drugs which may induce torsades de pointes is contra-indicated (*see section 4.5*).
- Cordarone X Intravenous ampoules contain benzyl alcohol. There have been reports of fatal 'gasping syndrome' in neonates (hypotension, bradycardia and cardiovascular collapse) following the administration of intravenous solution containing this preservative. Cordarone X Intravenous should not be given to neonates or premature babies unless the rhythm disturbance is life threatening and either resistant to other medication or alternative therapy is deemed inappropriate.
- Pregnancy - except in exceptional circumstances *(see section 4.6)*
- Lactation *(see section 4.6)*

All these above contra-indications do not apply to the use of amiodarone for cardiopulmonary resuscitation of shock resistant ventricular fibrillation.

4.4 Special warnings and precautions for use
Benzyl alcohol may cause toxic reactions and allergic reactions in infants and children up to 3 years old.

Cordarone X Intravenous should only be used in a special care unit under continuous monitoring (ECG and blood pressure).

IV infusion is preferred to bolus due to the haemodynamic effects sometimes associated with rapid injection (*see section 4.8*). Circulatory collapse may be precipitated by too rapid administration or overdosage (atropine has been used successfully in such patients presenting with bradycardia).

Repeated or continuous infusion via peripheral veins may lead to injection site reactions *(see section 4.8).* When repeated or continuous infusion is anticipated, administration by a central venous catheter is recommended.

When given by infusion Cordarone X may reduce drop size and, if appropriate, adjustments should be made to the rate of infusion.

Anaesthesia (*see section 4.5*): Before surgery, the anaesthetist should be informed that the patient is taking amiodarone.

Cardiac disorders:

Caution should be exercised in patients with hypotension and decompensated cardiomyopathy and severe heart failure *(also see section 4.3).*

Amiodarone has a low pro-arrhythmic effect. Onsets of new arrhythmias or worsening of treated arrhythmias, sometimes fatal, have been reported. It is important, but difficult to differentiate a lack of efficacy of the drug from a proarrhythmic effect, whether or not this is associated with a worsening of the cardiac condition. Proarrhythmic effects generally occur in the context of drug interactions and/or electrolytic disorders (*see sections 4.5 and 4.8*).

Too high a dosage may lead to severe bradycardia and to conduction disturbances with the appearance of an idioventricular rhythm, particularly in elderly patients or during digitalis therapy. In these circumstances, Cordarone X treatment should be withdrawn. If necessary beta-adrenostimulants or glucagon may be given. Because of the long half-life of amiodarone, if bradycardia is severe and symptomatic the insertion of a pacemaker should be considered.

The pharmacological action of amiodarone induces ECG changes: QT prolongation (related to prolonged repolarisation) with the possible development of U-waves and deformed T-waves; these changes do not reflect toxicity.

Respiratory, thoracic and mediastinal disorders *(see section 4.8)*:

Very rare cases of interstitial pneumonitis have been reported with intravenous amiodarone. When the diagnosis is suspected, a chest X-ray should be performed. Amiodarone therapy should be re-evaluated since interstitial pneumonitis is generally reversible following early withdrawal of amiodarone, and corticosteroid therapy should be considered *(see section 4.8).* Clinical symptoms often resolve within a few weeks followed by slower radiological and lung function improvement. Some patients can deteriorate despite discontinuing Cordarone X. Fatal cases of pulmonary toxicity have been reported.

Very rare cases of severe respiratory complications, sometimes fatal, have been observed usually in the period immediately following surgery (adult acute respiratory distress syndrome); a possible interaction with a high oxygen concentration may be implicated *(see sections 4.5 and 4.8).*

Hepato-biliary disorders *(see section 4.8)*

Severe hepatocellular insufficiency may occur within the first 24 hours of IV amiodarone, and may sometimes be fatal. Close monitoring of transaminases is therefore recommended as soon as amiodarone is started.

Drug interactions *(see section 4.5)*

Concomitant use of amiodarone with the following drugs is not recommended; beta-blockers, heart rate lowering calcium channel inhibitors (verapamil, diltiazem), stimulant laxative agents which may cause hypokalaemia.

Increased plasma levels of flecainide have been reporte[d] with co-administration of amiodarone. The flecainide dos[e] should be reduced accordingly and the patient clos[ely] monitored.

4.5 Interaction with other medicinal products and [other] forms of interaction
Some of the more important drugs that interact wit[h amio]darone include warfarin, digoxin, phenytoin and a[ny drug] which prolongs the QT interval.

Amiodarone raises the plasma concentrations of [oral antic]oagulants (warfarin) and phenytoin by inhibiti[ng CYP] 2C9. The dose of warfarin should be reduced [...] More frequent monitoring of prothrombin time [...] and after amiodarone treatment is recomme[nded ...] toin dosage should be reduced if signs [...] appear, and plasma levels may be measu[red ...]

Administration of Cordarone X to a patie[nt ...] ing digoxin will bring about an increa[se ...]

digoxin concentration and thus precipitate symptoms and signs associated with high digoxin levels. Clinical, ECG and biological monitoring is recommended and digoxin dosage should be halved. A synergistic effect on heart rate and atrioventricular conduction is also possible.

Combined therapy with the following drugs which prolong the QT interval is contra-indicated (*see section 4.3*) due to the increased risk of torsades de pointes; for example:

• Class Ia anti-arrhythmic drugs e.g. quinidine, procainamide, disopyramide

• Class III anti-arrhythmic drugs e.g. sotalol, bretylium

• intravenous erythromycin, co-trimoxazole or pentamidine injection

• some anti-psychotics e.g. chlorpromazine, thioridazine, fluphenazine, pimozide, haloperidol, amisulpiride and sertindole

• lithium and tricyclic anti-depressants e.g. doxepin, maprotiline, amitriptyline

• certain antihistamines e.g. terfenadine, astemizole, mizolastine

• anti-malarials e.g. quinine, mefloquine, chloroquine, halofantrine.

• Moxifloxacin

Fluoroquinolones

There have been rare reports of QTc interval prolongation, with or without torsades de pointes, in patients taking amiodrone with fluoroquinolones. Concomitant use of amidarone with fluoroquinolones should be avoided (concomitant use with moxifloxacin is contra-indicated, see above).

Combined therapy with the following drugs is not recommended:

• Beta blockers and certain calcium channel inhibitors (diltiazem, verapamil); potentiation of negative chronotropic properties and conduction slowing effects may occur.

• Stimulant laxatives, which may cause hypokalaemia thus increasing the risk of torsades de pointes; other types of laxatives should be used.

Caution should be exercised over combined therapy with the following drugs which may also cause hypokalaemia and/or hypomagnesaemia, e.g. diuretics, systemic corticosteroids, tetracosactide, intravenous amphotericin.

In cases of hypokalaemia, corrective action should be taken and QT interval monitored. In case of torsades de pointes antiarrhythmic agents should not be given; pacing may be instituted and IV magnesium may be used.

Caution is advised in patients undergoing general anaesthesia, or receiving high dose oxygen therapy.

Potentially severe complications have been reported in patients taking amiodarone undergoing general anaesthesia: bradycardia unresponsive to atropine, hypotension, disturbances of conduction, decreased cardiac output.

A few cases of adult respiratory distress syndrome, most often in the period immediately after surgery, have been observed. A possible interaction with a high oxygen concentration may be implicated.

Grapefruit juice inhibits cytochrome P450 3A4 and may increase the plasma concentration of amiodarone. Grapefruit juice should be avoided during treatment with oral amiodarone.

Drugs metabolised by cytochrome P450 3A4

When drugs are co-administered with amiodarone, an inhibitor of CYP 3A4, this may result in a higher level of their plasma concentrations, which may lead to a possible increase in their toxicity:

• Ciclosporin: plasma levels of ciclosporin may increase as much as 2-fold when used in combination. A reduction in the dose of ciclosporin may be necessary to maintain the plasma concentration within the therapeutic range.

• Statins: the risk of muscular toxicity is increased by concomitant administration of amiodarone with statins metabolised by CYP 3A4 such as simvastatin, atorvastatin and lovastatin. It is recommended to use a statin not metabolised by CYP 3A4 when given with amiodarone.

• Other drugs metabolised by cytochrome P450 3A4: examples of such drugs are lidocaine, tacrolimus, sildenafil, fentanyl, midazolam, triazolam, dihydroergotamine and ergotamine.

Flecainide

Given that flecainide is mainly metabolised by CYP 2D6, by inhibiting this isoenzyme, amiodarone may increase flecainide plasma levels; it is advised to reduce the flecainide dose by 50% and to monitor the patient closely for adverse effects. Monitoring of flecainide plasma levels is strongly recommended in such circumstances.

Interaction with substrates of other CYP 450 isoenzymes

In vitro studies show that amiodarone also has the potential to inhibit CYP 1A2, CYP 2C19 and CYP 2D6 through its main metabolite. When co-administered, amiodarone would be expected to increase the plasma concentration of drugs whose metabolism is dependent upon CYP 1A2, CYP 2C19 and CYP 2D6.

4.6 Pregnancy and lactation

Pregnancy

There are insufficient data on the use of amiodarone during pregnancy in humans to judge any possible toxicity. However, in view of its effect on the foetal thyroid gland, amiodarone is contraindicated during pregnancy, except in exceptional circumstances.

Lactation

Amiodarone is excreted into the breast milk in significant quantities and breast-feeding is contra-indicated.

4.7 Effects on ability to drive and use machines

Not relevant

4.8 Undesirable effects

The following adverse reactions are classified by system organ class and ranked under heading of frequency using the following convention: very common (> = 10%), common (> = 1% and < 10%); uncommon (> = 0.1% and < 1%); rare (> = 0.01% and < 0.1%), very rare (< 0.01%), not known (cannot be estimated from the available data).

Blood and lymphatic system disorders:

• In patients taking amiodarone there have been incidental findings of bone marrow granulomas. The clinical significance of this is unknown

Cardiac disorders:

• Common: bradycardia, generally moderate.

• Very rare:

- marked bradycardia, sinus arrest requiring discontinuation of amiodarone, especially in patients with sinus node dysfunction and/or in elderly patients

- onset of worsening of arrythmia, sometimes followed by cardiac arrest *(see sections 4.4 and 4.5)*.

Gastrointestinal disorders:

• Very rare: nausea.

General disorders and administration site conditions:

• Common: injection site reactions such as pain, erythema, oedema, necrosis, extravasation, infiltration, inflammation, induration, thrombophlebitis, phlebitis, cellulitis, infection, pigmentation changes.

Hepato-biliary disorders:

• Very rare:

- isolated increase in serum transaminases, which is usually moderate (1.5 to 3 times normal range) at the beginning of therapy. They may return to normal with dose reduction or even spontaneously.

- acute liver disorders with high serum transaminases and/or jaundice, including hepatic failure, sometimes fatal *(see section 4.4)*.

Immune system disorders:

• Very rare: anaphylactic shock.

Angioedema (there have been some reports of angioedema, although exact frequencies are not known)

Nervous system disorders:

• Very rare: benign intra-cranial hypertension (pseudo tumor cerebri), headache.

Respiratory, thoracic and mediastinal disorders:

• Very rare:

- interstitial pneumonitis *(see section 4.4)*

- severe respiratory complications (adult acute respiratory distress syndrome), sometimes fatal *(see sections 4.4 and 4.5)*

- bronchospasm and/or apnoea in case of severe respiratory failure, and especially in asthmatic patients.

Skin and subcutaneous tissue disorders:

• Very rare: sweating.

• Not known: urticaria

Vascular disorders:

• Common: decrease in blood pressure, usually moderate and transient. Cases of hypotension or collapse have been reported following overdosage or a too rapid injection.

• Very rare: hot flushes.

4.9 Overdose

There is no information regarding overdosage with intravenous amiodarone.

Little information is available regarding acute overdosage with oral amiodarone. Few cases of sinus bradycardia, heart block, attacks of ventricular tachycardia, torsades de pointes, circulatory failure and hepatic injury have been reported.

In the event of overdose, treatment should be symptomatic, in addition to general supportive measures. The patient should be monitored and if bradycardia occurs beta-adrenostimulants or glucagon may be given.

Spontaneously resolving attacks of ventricular tachycardia may also occur. Due to the pharmacokinetics of amiodarone, adequate and prolonged surveillance of the patient, particularly cardiac status, is recommended.

Neither amiodarone nor its metabolites are dialysable.

5. PHARMACOLOGICAL PROPERTIES

5.1 Pharmacodynamic properties

Cordarone is a product for the treatment of tachyarrhythmias and has complex pharmacological actions. Its effects are anti-adrenergic (partial alpha and beta blocker). It has haemodynamic effects (increased blood flow and systemic/coronary vasodilation). The drug reduces myocardial oxygen consumption and has been shown to have a sparing effect of rat myocardial ATP utilisation, with decreased oxidative processes. Amiodarone inhibits the metabolic and biochemical effects of catecholamines on the heart and inhibits Na^+ and K^+ activated ATP-ase.

5.2 Pharmacokinetic properties

Pharmacokinetics of amiodarone are unusual and complex, and have not been completely elucidated. Absorption following oral administration is variable and may be prolonged, with enterohepatic cycling. The major metabolite is desethylamiodarone. Amiodarone is highly protein bound (> 95%). Renal excretion is minimal and faecal excretion is the major route. A study in both healthy volunteers and patients after intravenous administration of amiodarone reported that the calculated volumes of distribution and total blood clearance using a two-compartment open model were similar for both groups. Elimination of amiodarone after intravenous injection appeared to be biexponential with a distribution phase lasting about 4 hours. The very high volume of distribution combined with a relatively low apparent volume for the central compartment suggests extensive tissue distribution. A bolus IV injection of 400mg gave a terminal T½ of approximately 11 hours.

5.3 Preclinical safety data

There are no pre-clinical data of relevance to the prescriber which are additional to that already included in other sections of the SPC.

6. PHARMACEUTICAL PARTICULARS

6.1 List of excipients

Benzyl alcohol,

Polysorbate and

Water for Injections.

6.2 Incompatibilities

Cordarone X Intravenous is incompatible with saline and should be administered solely in 5% dextrose solution. Cordarone X Intravenous, diluted with 5% dextrose solution to a concentration of less than 0.6mg/ml, is unstable. Solutions containing less than 2 ampoules Cordarone X Intravenous in 500ml dextrose 5% are unstable and should not be used.

The use of administration equipment or devices containing plasticizers such as DEHP (di-2-ethylhexylphthalate) in the presence of amiodarone may result in leaching out of DEHP. In order to minimise patient exposure to DEHP, the final amiodarone dilution for infusion should preferably be administered through non DEHP-containing sets.

6.3 Shelf life

24 months.

6.4 Special precautions for storage

Do not store above 25°C. Store in the original container.

6.5 Nature and contents of container

Each carton contains ten glass ampoules.

6.6 Special precautions for disposal and other handling

Refer to 4.2 above.

7. MARKETING AUTHORISATION HOLDER

Sanofi-aventis

One Onslow Street

Guildford

Surrey

GU1 4YS

UK.

8. MARKETING AUTHORISATION NUMBER(S)

PL 11723/0014

9. DATE OF FIRST AUTHORISATION/RENEWAL OF THE AUTHORISATION

2 September 2002

10. DATE OF REVISION OF THE TEXT

30 March 2009

Legal category: POM

Corgard Tablets 80mg

(sanofi-aventis)

1. NAME OF THE MEDICINAL PRODUCT

Corgard Tablets 80mg

2. QUALITATIVE AND QUANTITATIVE COMPOSITION

The tablets contain Nadolol 80.0mg.

3. PHARMACEUTICAL FORM

Tablet.

White, capsule-shaped, biconvex tablet engraved "80" on one side and with a break line on the other side.

4. CLINICAL PARTICULARS

4.1 Therapeutic indications

Corgard is indicated in the management of:

Angina Pectoris:

For the long-term management of patients with angina pectoris by continuous medication.

Hypertension:

For the long-term management of essential hypertension, either alone or in combination with other antihypertensive agents, especially thiazide-type diuretics.

Arrhythmias:

For the treatment of cardiac tachyarrhythmias.

Migraine:

For the prophylactic management of migraine headache. The efficacy of Corgard in the treatment of a migraine attack that has already started has not been established, and Corgard is not indicated for such use.

Thyrotoxicosis:

For the relief of the symptoms of hyperthyroidism and the pre- operative preparation of patients for surgery. Nadolol may be used in conjunction with conventional antithyroid therapy.

4.2 Posology and method of administration

Adults:

Dosage should be titrated gradually with at least a week between increments to assess response; individuals show considerable variation in their response to beta-adrenergic blockade.

Corgard may be given in a once daily dosage without regard to meals. The dosage interval should be increased when creatinine clearance is below 50ml/min/1.73m^2.

If Corgard is to be discontinued, reduce dosage over a period of at least two weeks (see warnings).

Angina pectoris:	Initially 40mg once daily. This may be increased at weekly intervals until an adequate response is obtained or excessive bradycardia occurs. Most patients respond to 160mg or less daily. The value and safety of daily doses exceeding 240mg have not been established.
Hypertension:	Initially 80mg once daily. This may be increased by a weekly increment of 80mg or less until an optimum response is obtained. Many patients respond to 80mg daily, and most patients respond to 240mg or less, daily, but higher doses have been required for a few patients. In some patients it is necessary to administer a diuretic, peripheral vasolidator and/or other antihypertensive agents in conjunction with nadolol in order to achieve satisfactory response.
	Treatment of hypertension associated with phaeochromocytoma may require the addition of an alpha-blocking agent.
Cardiac-tachyarrhythmias:	Initially 40mg once daily. This may be increased if necessary to 160mg once daily. If bradycardia occurs dosage should be reduced to 40mg once daily.
Migraine:	The initial dose of nadolol is 40mg once daily. Dosage may be gradually increased in 40mg increments until optimum migraine prophylaxis is achieved. The usual maintenance dose is 80 to 160mg administered once daily. After 4 to 6 weeks at the maximum dose if a satisfactory response is not obtained, therapy with nadolol should be withdrawn gradually.
Thyrotoxicosis:	The dosage range is 80-160mg once daily. It has been found that most patients require a dose of 160mg once daily. Nadolol may be used together with conventional anti-thyroid treatment. For the preparation of patients for partial thyroidectomy, nadolol should be administered in conjunction with potassium iodide for a period of 10 days prior to operation. Nadolol should be administered on the morning of operation. Post-operatively, nadolol dosage should be slowly reduced and then withdrawn following clinical stability.

Children:

Safety and effectiveness in children have not been established.

Elderly:

In elderly patients a low initial dose should be used so that sensitivity to side-effects may be assessed.

Renal or hepatic impairment

As with all drugs patients with impaired renal or hepatic function should be monitored.

4.3 Contraindications

- Bronchial asthma or a history of asthma
- Sinus bradycardia
- Greater than first degree atrioventricular conduction block
- Cardiogenic shock
- Right ventricular failure secondary to pulmonary hypertension
- Overt cardiac failure (see 4.4 – Special warnings and special precautions for use)
- Previously demonstrated hypersensitivity to nadolol

4.4 Special warnings and precautions for use

Warnings

Exacerbation of Ischaemic Heart Disease Following Abrupt Withdrawal

Hypersensitivity to catecholamines has been observed in patients withdrawn from beta-blocker therapy; exacerbation of angina, hypertension, and, in some cases, myocardial infarction have occurred after *abrupt* discontinuation of such therapy. When discontinuing chronically administered nadolol, particularly in patients with ischaemic heart disease, the dosage should be gradually reduced over a period of one to two weeks, and the patient should be carefully monitored. If angina markedly worsens or acute coronary insufficiency develops, nadolol administration should be re-instituted promptly (at least temporarily), and other measures appropriate for the management of unstable angina should be taken. Patients should be warned against interruption or discontinuation of therapy without the physician's advice. Because coronary artery disease is common and may be unrecognised, it may be prudent not to discontinue nadolol therapy abruptly, even in patients under treatment for hypertension alone.

Patients with a History of Cardiac Failure - Sympathetic stimulation may be a vital component supporting circulatory function in patients with congestive heart failure, and beta-blockade may worsen failure.

Although beta-blockers including nadolol should be avoided in overt congestive heart failure, they can be cautiously used, if necessary, in patients with a history of heart failure who are well compensated (usually with digitalis and diuretics). Beta-adrenergic blocking agents do not abolish the inotropic action of digitalis on heart muscle.

Patients Without a History of Heart Failure - Continued depression of the myocardium with beta blockade over a period of time can, in some cases, lead to cardiac failure. At the first sign or symptom of impending heart failure, the patient should be fully digitalised and/or treated with diuretics, and the response observed closely.

If cardiac failure continues despite adequate digitalisation and diuresis, Corgard should be withdrawn (gradually, if possible).

Major Surgery - Beta-blockade impairs the ability of the heart to respond to reflex stimuli and may increase the risks of general anaesthesia and surgical procedures, resulting in protracted hypotension or low cardiac output. It has generally been suggested that beta blocker therapy should be withdrawn several days prior to surgery. Recognition of the increased sensitivity to catecholamines of patients recently withdrawn from beta-blocker therapy, however, has made this recommendation controversial. If possible, beta-blockers including nadolol should be withdrawn well before surgery takes place.

In no circumstances should beta-blockers be discontinued prior to surgery in patients with phaeochromocytoma or thyrotoxicosis.

In the event of emergency surgery, the anaesthesiologist should be informed that the patient is on beta-blocker therapy. The effects of nadolol can be reversed by administration of beta-receptor agonists such as isoprenaline or dobutamine. However, such patients may be subject to protracted severe hypotension. Difficulty in restarting and maintaining the heart beat has also been reported with beta-adrenergic receptor blocking agents.

(An exception to the above paragraph is thyroid surgery—see under 'Thyrotoxicosis' in section 4.1 Indications and section 4.2 Posology and method of administration).

Nonallergic Bronchospasm (e.g. chronic bronchitis, emphysema) - Patients with bronchospastic diseases should not, in general, receive beta-blockers since they may block bronchodilation produced by endogenous or exogenous catecholamine stimulation of beta receptors.

(NOTE: Corgard is contra-indicated in asthmatic patients.)

Diabetes and Hypoglycaemia - Beta-adrenergic blockade may prevent the appearance of warning signs and symptoms (e.g. tachycardia and blood pressure changes) of acute hypoglycaemia. This is especially important with labile diabetics. Beta-blockade also reduces the release of insulin in response to hyperglycaemia; therefore, it may be necessary to adjust the dose of anti-diabetic drugs.

Occasionally causes hypoglycaemia, even in non-diabetic patients, e.g., neonates, infants, children, elderly patients, patients on haemodialysis or patients suffering from chronic liver disease and patients suffering from overdose. Severe hypoglycaemia associated with nadolol has rarely presented with seizures and/or coma in isolated patients.

Skin Rashes - There have been reports of skin rashes (including a psoriasiform type) and/or ocular changes (conjunctivitis and 'dry eye') associated with the use of beta-adrenergic blocking drugs. The reported incidence is small and in most cases the symptoms have cleared when the treatment was withdrawn. Discontinuation of the drug should be considered if any such reaction is not otherwise explicable. Cessation of the therapy with a beta-adrenergic blocker should be gradual.

Treatment for Anaphylactic Reaction - While taking beta-blockers, patients with a history of severe anaphylactic reaction may be more reactive to repeated challenge, either accidental, diagnostic, or therapeutic. Such patients may be unresponsive to the usual doses of epinephrine used to treat allergic reaction.

(NOTE: Epinephrine combined with non cardio-selective beta blockers such as nadolol can cause a hypertensive episode followed by bradycardia.)

Thyrotoxicosis - Beta-adrenergic blockade may mask certain clinical signs of hyperthyroidism (e.g. tachycardia). Abrupt withdrawal of nadolol in thyroid patients can precipitate thyroid storm.

Precautions

Occasionally, beta-blockade with drugs such as nadolol may produce hypotension and/or marked bradycardia, resulting in vertigo, syncope or orthostatic hypotension.

Impaired Renal or Hepatic Function - Nadolol should be used with caution in patients with impaired renal or hepatic function (see section 4.2 Posology and method of administration).

Carcinogenesis, Mutagenesis, Impairment of Fertility - In chronic oral toxicologic studies lasting one to two years, nadolol did not produce any significant toxic effects in mice, rats, or dogs. In two-year oral carcinogenic studies in rats and mice, nadolol did not produce any neoplastic, pre-neoplastic, or non-neoplastic pathologic lesions. In fertility and general reproductive performance studies in rats, nadolol caused no adverse effects.

4.5 Interaction with other medicinal products and other forms of interaction

General anaesthetics - Those which cause myocardial depression such as chloroform, cyclopropane, trichlorethylene and ether should be avoided as the patient may be subject to protracted severe hypotension. (see Major Surgery in section 4.4 Special warnings and special precautions for use).

Myocardial depressants such as lidocaine and procainamide may subject the patient to protracted severe hypotension.

Adrenoceptor Stimulants - Beta-adrenoceptor stimulants such as isoprenaline and verapamil, or alpha-adrenoceptor stimulants such as noradrenaline and adrenaline, will reverse the hypotensive effects and increase vasoconstrictor activity.

Catecholamine Depleting Drugs - Additive effects may occur with nadolol; monitor closely for evidence of hypotension and/or excessive bradycardia (e.g. vertigo, syncope, postural hypotension).

Antihypertensives (*e.g. neurone-blocking drugs, vasodilators, diuretics*) Additive hypotensive effect.

Clonidine - If Corgard and clonidine are given concurrently, clonidine should not be discontinued until several days after Corgard withdrawal.

Antidiabetic drugs *(oral agents and insulin)* - Hypoglycaemia or hyperglycaemia; adjust dosage of anti-diabetic drug accordingly (see Diabetes and Hypoglycaemia in section 4.4 Special warnings and special precautions for use).

Monoamine oxidase inhibitors (MAOIs) - Isolated cases of bradycardia have occurred during concurrent use of beta blockers and MAOIs.

Antimuscarinic agents - May counteract the bradycardia caused by beta blockers.

Calcium-channel blockers - Calcium channel blockers generally potentiate the pharmacologic effects of beta-blockers. Patients taking both agents should be carefully monitored for adverse cardiovascular events.

Other antiarrhythmic agents - Additive or antagonistic effects may occur with nadolol.

Lidocaine, IV - Significant reduction of lidocaine clearance can occur when a beta blocker is administered concurrently.

Non-steroidal anti-inflammatory agents (NSAIDs) - The antihypertensive effects of beta blockers may be reduced during concurrent administration of indometacin and possibly other NSAIDs.

Phenothiazines and other antipsychotic agents - Additive antihypertensive effects have occurred with other beta blockers when they were given concurrently with phenothiazines or haloperidol.

Vasoconstrictor Agents - Effects with nadolol can be additive (e.g. with ergot alkaloids).

4.6 Pregnancy and lactation

Pregnancy

There are no adequate and well-controlled studies in pregnant women. In animal reproduction studies with nadolol, evidence of embryo- and foetotoxicity was found in rabbits, but not in rats or hamsters, at doses 5 to 10 times greater (on a mg/kg basis) than the maximum indicated human dose. No teratogenic potential was observed in any of these species.

Nadolol should be used during pregnancy only if the potential benefit justifies the potential risk to the foetus.

Neonates whose mothers are receiving nadolol at parturition have exhibited bradycardia, hypoglycaemia, and associated symptoms.

Lactation

Nadolol is excreted in human milk. Because of the potential for adverse effects in nursing infants, a decision should be made whether to discontinue nursing or to discontinue therapy, taking into account the importance of nadolol to the mother.

4.7 Effects on ability to drive and use machines

There are no studies on the effect of this medicine on the ability to drive. When driving vehicles or operating machines it should be taken into account that occasionally dizziness or fatigue may occur.

4.8 Undesirable effects

Most adverse effects have been mild and transient and have rarely required withdrawal of therapy. The percentages given below were based on a population of 1440 patients taking nadolol in clinical trials.

Cardiovascular:

Bradycardia (heart rate <60 BPM) occurs commonly in nadolol-treated patients; heart rate <40 BPM and/or symptomatic bradycardia occurred in approximately 2% of patients; Symptoms of peripheral vascular insufficiency, usually of the Raynaud type (approximately 2%);

Cardiac failure, hypotension, and rhythm/conduction disturbances (about 1%). Single instances of first-degree and third-degree heart block have been reported; intensification of AV block is a known effect of beta-blockers (see also section 4.3 Contra-indications, and section 4.4 Special warnings and special precautions for use).

Central Nervous System:

Dizziness or fatigue has been reported in approximately 2% of patients; paraesthesias, sedation, and change in behaviour have each been reported in approximately 0.6% of patients. Light-headedness, insomnia and cold extremities have also been reported.

Gastrointestinal:

Nausea, diarrhoea, abdominal discomfort, constipation, vomiting, indigestion, anorexia, bloating and flatulence have been reported in 0.1% to 0.5% of patients.

Respiratory:

Bronchospasm has been reported in approximately 0.1% of patients (see section 4.3 Contraindications and section 4.4 Special warnings and precautions for use).

Endocrine:

Hypoglycaemia in neonates, infants, children, elderly patients, patients on haemodialysis, patients on concomitant anti-diabetic therapy, patients with prolonged fasting and patients with chronic liver disease has been reported (see section 4.4).

Miscellaneous:

Each of the following has been reported in 0.1% to 0.5% of patients: rash; pruritus; headache; dry mouth, eyes or skin; impotence or decreased libido; facial swelling; weight gain; slurred speech; cough; nasal stuffiness; sweating; tinnitus; blurred vision. Reversible alopaecia has been reported infrequently.

The events listed below have also occurred with nadolol and/or other beta-adrenergic blocking agents; however, no causal relationship to nadolol was established:

Central Nervous System - Reversible depression progressing to catatonia; visual disturbances; hallucinations; an acute reversible syndrome characterised by disorientation for time and place, short-term memory loss, emotional lability, slightly clouded sensorium, and decreased performance on neuropsychologic tests.

Gastrointestinal - Mesenteric arterial thrombosis; ischaemic colitis; elevated liver enzymes.

Haematologic - Agranulocytosis; thrombocytopaenic or non-thrombocytopaenic purpura.

Allergic - Fever combined with aching, and sore throat; laryngospasm; respiratory distress.

Miscellaneous - Pemphigoid rash; hypertensive reaction in patients with pheochromocytoma; sleep disturbances; Peyronie's disease.

4.9 Overdose

In the event of overdosage, nadolol may cause excessive bradycardia, cardiac failure, hypotension, or bronchospasm.

Transitory increase in BUN has been reported, and serum electrolyte changes may occur, especially in patients with impaired renal function.

Treatment

Nadolol can be removed from the general circulation by haemodialysis. In determining the duration of corrective therapy, note must be taken of the long duration of the effect of nadolol.

In addition to gastric lavage, the following measures should be employed, as appropriate:

Excessive Bradycardia - Administer atropine (0.25 to 1.0 mg). If there is no response to vagal blockade, administer isoprenaline cautiously.

Cardiac Failure - Administer a digitalis glycoside and diuretic. It has been reported that glucagon may also be useful in this situation.

Hypotension - If fluid administration is ineffective, administer vasopressors such as dopamine, dobutamine or adrenaline.

Bronchospasm - **Administer** a beta-2-agonist agent and/or a theophylline derivative.

Stupor or coma - Supportive therapy as warranted.

Gastrointestinal Effects - Symptomatic treatment as needed.

BUN and/or Serum Electrolyte Abnormalities - Institute supportive measures as required to maintain hydration, electrolyte balance, respiration, and cardiovascular and renal function.

5. PHARMACOLOGICAL PROPERTIES

5.1 Pharmacodynamic properties

Nadolol is a beta-adrenergic receptor blocking agent with a prolonged activity, permitting once-daily dosage in angina, hypertension, cardiac arrhythmias, the prophylaxis of migraine, and the relief of hyperthyroid symptoms.

Nadolol is not metabolised. It has no membrane stabilising or intrinsic sympathomimetic activity, and its only effect on the autonomic nervous system is one of beta-adrenergic blockade. Nadolol is nonselective.

Receptor blockade by nadolol results in protection from excessive inappropriate sympathetic activity. Nadolol reduces the number and severity of attacks of angina pectoris by blocking response to catecholamine stimulation and thus lowers the oxygen requirement of the heart at any given level of effort.

Nadolol reduces both supine and erect blood pressure. Like other beta-blockers nadolol exerts an antiarrhythmic action. Nadolol has been shown to reduce the rapid ventricular response which accompanies atrial fibrillation/flutter by slowing conduction through the A-V node. Beta-blockade is of particular value in arrhythmias caused by increased levels of, or sensitivity of the heart to, circulating catecholamines, e.g. arrhythmias associated with phaeochromocytoma, thyrotoxicosis, or exercise. Nadolol is effective in reducing ventricular premature beats in selected patients.

Nadolol exerts an effect in the prophylaxis of migraine by a mechanism which may involve prevention of vasoconstriction in the area served by the internal carotid artery and prevention of excessive adrenergic vasodilation in the external carotid artery.

Nadolol alleviates the symptoms of thyrotoxicosis and provides symptomatic control before and during thyroid surgery.

Beta-blocking agents have been shown in large scale studies to reduce mortality by preventing reinfarction and sudden death in patients surviving their first myocardial infarction.

5.2 Pharmacokinetic properties

About 30 percent of an oral dose of Corgard is absorbed. Peak serum concentrations usually occur in 3 to 4 hours after drug administration. The presence of food in the gastrointestinal tract does not affect the rate or extent of Corgard absorption. Approximately 30 percent of the Corgard present in serum is reversibly bound to plasma protein. Unlike most available beta-blocking agents, Corgard is not metabolised, and is excreted unchanged principally by the kidneys. The serum half-life of therapeutic doses of Corgard is relatively long, ranging from 20 to 24 hours (permitting once daily dosage). A significant correlation between minimum steady-state serum concentrations of Corgard and total oral daily dose has been demonstrated in hypertensive patients; however, the observed dose-response range is wide and proper dosage requires individual titration.

5.3 Preclinical safety data

None stated.

6. PHARMACEUTICAL PARTICULARS

6.1 List of excipients

The tablets also contain microcrystalline cellulose and magnesium stearate.

6.2 Incompatibilities

Not applicable.

6.3 Shelf life

36 months.

6.4 Special precautions for storage

Do not store above 25°C.

6.5 Nature and contents of container

PVC/aluminium foil blister packs in cartons containing 28 tablets.

6.6 Special precautions for disposal and other handling

None stated.

7. MARKETING AUTHORISATION HOLDER

Sanofi-aventis
One Onslow Street
Guildford
Surrey
GU1 4YS
UK

8. MARKETING AUTHORISATION NUMBER(S)

PL 11723/0100.

9. DATE OF FIRST AUTHORISATION/RENEWAL OF THE AUTHORISATION

24 November 1995/23 September 2004

10. DATE OF REVISION OF THE TEXT

January 2009

Legal Category: POM

Corlan Pellets

(UCB Pharma Limited)

1. NAME OF THE MEDICINAL PRODUCT

Corlan Pellets

2. QUALITATIVE AND QUANTITATIVE COMPOSITION

Each pellet contains 2.5mg Hydrocortisone in the form of the ester hydrocortisone sodium succinate

For excipients, see 6.1

3. PHARMACEUTICAL FORM

Muco-adhesive buccal tablet

Small white pellet engraved 'Corlan Evans' on one side

4. CLINICAL PARTICULARS

4.1 Therapeutic indications

Local use in previously diagnosed aphthous ulceration of the mouth, whether simple or occurring as a complication in diseases such as sprue, idiopathic steatorrhoea or ulcerative colitis.

4.2 Posology and method of administration

Adults and elderly:

Corlan Pellets should not be sucked, but kept in the mouth and allowed to dissolve slowly in close proximity to the ulcers. One pellet should be used in this way four times a day. If the ulcers have not healed after 5 days of treatment (completion of one pack), or if they recur quickly after healing, a doctor should be consulted.

Children under 12 years of age:

Children under 12 years old must see a doctor before starting each course of Corlan Pellets.

4.3 Contraindications

Corlan Pellets should not be used in the presence of oral infection unless effective appropriate anti-infective therapy is also employed. Hypersensitivity to any component of the product.

4.4 Special warnings and precautions for use

If aphthous ulceration is severe or recurring, serious underlying disease should be excluded.

4.5 Interaction with other medicinal products and other forms of interaction

None known.

4.6 Pregnancy and lactation

There is inadequate evidence of safety in human pregnancy. Topical administration of corticosteroids to pregnant animals can cause abnormalities of foetal development including cleft palate and intra-uterine growth retardation. There may, therefore, be a very small risk of such effects in the human foetus.

4.7 Effects on ability to drive and use machines

None known.

4.8 Undesirable effects

Corticosteroids may worsen diabetes.

Occasionally, topical therapy may result in an exacerbation of local infection.

Hypersensitivity reactions have occurred with corticosteroids, mainly when administered topically.

Most topically applied corticosteroids may, under certain circumstances, be absorbed in sufficient amounts to produce systemic effects.

4.9 Overdose

Treatment is unlikely to be needed in cases of acute overdosage.

5. PHARMACOLOGICAL PROPERTIES

5.1 Pharmacodynamic properties

ATC Code: A01A C03

None stated.

5.2 Pharmacokinetic properties

None stated.

5.3 Preclinical safety data

None stated.

6. PHARMACEUTICAL PARTICULARS

6.1 List of excipients

Lactose

Acacia

Magnesium Stearate

6.2 Incompatibilities

None known.

6.3 Shelf life

3 years.

6.4 Special precautions for storage

Store below 25°C. Replace cap firmly after use.

6.5 Nature and contents of container
Tamper evident polypropylene container with polythene lid containing 20 pellets.

Tubular glass vials with snap-plug closure containing 20 pellets.

6.6 Special precautions for disposal and other handling
None.

7. MARKETING AUTHORISATION HOLDER
UCB Pharma Limited

208 Bath Road

Slough

Berkshire

SL1 3WE

UK

8. MARKETING AUTHORISATION NUMBER(S)
PL 00039/0397

9. DATE OF FIRST AUTHORISATION/RENEWAL OF THE AUTHORISATION
20 January 1993

10. DATE OF REVISION OF THE TEXT
June 2005

Cortisone acetate 25mg (sanofi-aventis)

(sanofi-aventis)

1. NAME OF THE MEDICINAL PRODUCT
Cortisone Acetate 25mg Tablets

2. QUALITATIVE AND QUANTITATIVE COMPOSITION
Each tablet contains 25mg of Cortisone Acetate BP

3. PHARMACEUTICAL FORM
Tablet

4. CLINICAL PARTICULARS

4.1 Therapeutic indications
Replacement therapy as in Addison's disease or when the adrenals have been removed surgically or damaged as result of haemorrhage or shock.

4.2 Posology and method of administration
Adults

Acute episodes: doses up to 300mg daily for several days may be required.

Maintenance dosage: 12.5 to 37.5mg daily with, if necessary 0.1mg daily of fludrocortisone to supplement the salt retaining properties of cortisone acetate.

Children

The use of cortisone acetate in children would be limited, as in adults to replacement therapy. Dosage should be limited to a single dose on alternate days to lessen retardation of growth and to minimise suppression of the hypothalamo-pituitary axis.

Elderly

Treatment of elderly patients, particularly if long term, should be planned bearing in mind the more serious consequences of the common side effects of corticosteroids in old age, especially osteoporosis, diabetes, hypertension, susceptibility to infection and thinning of the skin.

4.3 Contraindications
This product is intended for use solely as replacement therapy. Corticosteroids are contraindicated in systemic fungal and viral infections, acute bacterial infections unless specific anti-infective therapy is given.

4.4 Special warnings and precautions for use
Corticosteroids should be given with care to patients with a history of tuberculosis or the characteristic appearance of tuberculous disease on X-ray. The emergence of tuberculosis can however be prevented by the prophylactic use of anti-tuberculosis therapy.

Administration of corticosteroids may impair the ability to resist and counteract infections: in addition, the clinical signs of and symptoms of infection may be suppressed.

Prolonged corticosteroid treatment is likely to reduce the response of the Pituitary-Adrenal Axis to stress, and relative insufficiency may persist for a year after withdrawal of therapy.

Cortisone acetate should be used with care in diabetes, osteoporosis (post-menopausal women are especially at risk), hypertension, patients with a history of severe affective disorders (especially a history of steroid psychosis), glaucoma or a family history of glaucoma, previous steroid myopathy and epilepsy.

Patients/and or carers should be warned that potentially sever psychiatric adverse reactions may occur with systemic steroids (see section 4.8). Symptoms typically emerge within a few days or weeks of starting the treatment. Risks may be higher with high doses/systemic exposure (see also section 4.5 pharmacokinetic interactions that can increase the risk of side effects), although dose levels do not allow prediction of the onset, type, severity or duration of reactions. Most reactions recover after either dose reduction or withdrawal, although specific treatment may be necessary. Patients/carers should be encouraged to seek medical advice if worrying psychological symptoms develop, especially if depressed mood or suicidal ideation is suspected. Patients/carers should also be alert to possible psychiatric disturbances that may occur either during or immediately after dose tapering/withdrawal of systemic steroids, although such reactions have been reported infrequently.

Particular care is required when considering the use of systemic corticosteroids in patient with existing or previous history of severe affective disorders in themselves or in their first degree relatives. These would include depressive or manic-depressive illness and previous steroid psychosis.

In patients who have received more than physiological doses of systemic corticosteroids (approximately 40mg cortisone or equivalent) for greater than 3 weeks, withdrawal should not be abrupt. How dose reduction should be carried out depends largely on whether the disease is likely to relapse as the dose of systemic corticosteroids is reduced. Clinical assessment of disease activity may be needed during withdrawal. If the disease is unlikely to relapse on withdrawal of systemic corticosteroids but there is uncertainty about HPA suppression, the dose of systemic corticosteroid may be reduced rapidly to physiological doses. Once a daily dose equivalent to 40mg of cortisone is reached, dose reduction should be slower to allow the HPA-axis to recover.

Abrupt withdrawal of systemic corticosteroid treatment, which has continued up to 3 weeks is appropriate if it is considered that the disease is unlikely to relapse. Abrupt withdrawal of doses of up to 200mg daily cortisone, or equivalent for 3 weeks is unlikely to lead to clinically relevant HPA-axis suppression, in the majority of patients. In the following patient groups, gradual withdrawal of systemic corticosteroid therapy should be considered even after courses lasting 3 weeks or less:

* patients who have had repeated courses of systemic corticosteroids, particularly if taken for greater than 3 weeks.

* when a short course has been prescribed within one year of cessation of long term therapy.

* patients who may have reasons for adrenocortical insufficiency other than exogenous corticosteroid therapy.

* patients receiving doses of systemic corticosteroid greater than 40mg daily of prednisolone or equivalent.

* patients repeatedly taking doses in the evening.

4.5 Interaction with other medicinal products and other forms of interaction
The effectiveness of anti-coagulants may be increased or decreased with concurrent corticosteroid therapy.

Serum levels of salicylates may increase considerably if corticosteroid therapy is withdrawn, possibly causing intoxication. Since both salicylates and corticosteroids are ulcerogenic, it is possible that there will be an increased rate of gastro-intestinal ulceration.

The action of hypoglycaemic drugs are antagonised by the hypoglycaemic action of corticosteroids.

Since both amphotericin and corticosteroids have potassium depleting effects, signs of hypokalaemia should be looked for during their concurrent use.

There is a small amount of evidence that the use of corticosteroids and methotrexate simultaneously, may cause increased methotrexate toxicity and possible death, although the combination of drugs has been used successfully.

Barbiturates, phenytoin and rifampicin are known to reduce the effects of corticosteroids.

Live virus vaccines should not be administered to patients on immunosuppressant doses of corticosteroids. If inactivated vaccines are administered to such individuals the expected serum antibody response may not be obtained.

In patients treated with systemic corticosteroids, use of non-depolarizing muscle relaxants can result in prolonged relaxation and acute myopathy. Risk factors for this include prolonged and high dose corticosteroids treatment and prolonged duration of muscle paralysis. This interaction is more likely to occur following prolonged ventililation (such as in an ITU setting).

Corticosteroid requirements may be reduced in patients taking estrogens (eg contraceptive products)

4.6 Pregnancy and lactation
Pregnancy

The ability of corticosteroids to cross the placenta varies between individual drugs, however cortisone readily crosses the placenta. Administration of corticosteroids to pregnant animals can cause abnormalities of foetal development including cleft palate, intra-uterine growth retardation and affects on brain growth and development. There is no evidence that corticosteroids cause an increased incidence of congenital abnormalities, such as cleft palate/lip in man. However, when administered for prolonged periods or repeatedly during pregnancy, corticosteroids may increase the risk of intrauterine growth retardation. Hypoadrenalism may occur in the neonate following prenatal exposure to corticosteroids but usually resolves spontaneously following birth and is rarely clinically important. As with all drugs, corticosteroids should only be prescribed when the benefits to the mother and child outweigh the risks. When corticosteroids are essential, however, patients with abnormal pregnancies may be treated as though they were in the non-gravid state.

Lactation

Corticosteroids are excreted in breast milk. However, doses of up to 200mg daily of cortisone are unlikely to cause systemic effects in the infant. Infants of mothers taking higher doses than this may have a degree of adrenal suppression but the benefits of breast feeding are likely to out-weigh any theoretical risk.

4.7 Effects on ability to drive and use machines
Not applicable.

4.8 Undesirable effects
The following side-effects may be associated with the long-term systemic use of corticosteroids:-

Gastro-intestinal: perforations and haemorrhage from peptic ulcer may be presenting features. Fatalities have been reported: perforation of the small and large bowel, particularly in patients with inflammatory bowel disease; other gastro-intestinal side effects include dyspepsia, abdominal distension, oesophageal ulceration candidiasis and acute pancreatitis.

Musculo-skeletal: muscle weakness, wasting and loss of muscle mass, osteoporosis, vertebral compression fractures, avascular necrosis of bone, pathological fractures of the long bones and tendon rupture. Acute myopathy may be precipitated in patients administered non-depolarising muscle relaxants (See section 4.5).

Endocrine and metabolic: suppression of growth in childhood and adolescence, menstrual irregularities, amenorrhoea, cushingoid face, hirsuitism and weight gain, decreased carbohydrate tolerance with development of classical symptoms of diabetes mellitus, increased need for insulin or oral hypoglycaemic agents in diabetics, negative nitrogen balance due to protein catabolism.

Fluid and electrolyte disturbance: sodium and water retention leading to congestive heart failure in susceptible subjects, hypertension, potassium loss and hypokalaemic alkalosis.

Dermatological: impaired wound healing, skin atrophy, patechial haemorrhage and ecchymoses, erythema, telangiectasia, skin striae and acne.

Neuropsychiatric:

Potentially severe Psychiatric reactions:

A wide range of psychiatric reactions including affective disorders (such as irritable, euphoric, depressed and labile mood, and suicidal thoughts), psychotic reactions (including mania, delusions, hallucinations, and aggravation of schizophrenia) behavioural disturbances, irritability, anxiety, sleep disturbances, and cognitive dysfunction including confusion and amnesia have been reported. Reactions are common and may occur in both adults and children. In adults, the frequency of severe reactions has been estimated to be 5-6%. Psychological effects have been reported on withdrawal of corticosteroids; the frequency is unknown.

Other psychiatric reactions:

There is an increased risk of increased intracranial pressure and papilloedema in children. Psychological dependence may be marked.

Ophthalmic: increased intra-ocular pressure with the development of glaucoma, papilloedema, posterior subcapsular cataracts, corneal and scleral thinning or perforation after prolonged use. Viral ophthalmic disease may be re-ignited or spread.

Miscellaneous: opportunistic infections occur more frequently in corticosteroids recipients; hypersensitivity; thromboembolism and increased appetite have also been reported. Clinical reactivation of previously dormant tuberculosis, leukocytosis (sometimes an almost leukaemoid-like reaction) may occur and there may be a suppression of the hypothalamic-pituitary axis on stopping treatment. Withdrawal after prolonged therapy may result in the characteristic withdrawal symptoms including fever, myalgia, arthralgia and malaise. These may occur even without evidence of adrenal insufficiency. The latter arises from too rapid withdrawal of long-term corticosteroids and may be minimised by gradual reduction of dosage.

4.9 Overdose
Treatment is symptomatic but is unlikely to be required. Blood electrolytes should be observed.

5. PHARMACOLOGICAL PROPERTIES

5.1 Pharmacodynamic properties
Cortisone is a glucocorticoid. It has appreciable mineralocorticoid properties and is used mainly for replacement therapy in Addison's disease or chronic adrenocortical insufficiency secondary to hypopituitarism.

5.2 Pharmacokinetic properties
Cortisone acetate is readily absorbed from the gastro-intestinal tract and the cortisone is rapidly converted in the liver to its active metabolite hydrocortisone. The biological half-life of cortisone itself is about 30 minutes.

It is metabolised mainly in the liver, but also in the kidney. It is excreted in the urine.

5.3 Preclinical safety data
Not applicable.

6. PHARMACEUTICAL PARTICULARS

6.1 List of excipients

Lactose

Maize Starch

Povidone

Soluble Starch (Amisol)

Colloidal Silicon Dioxide (Aerosil)

Magnesium Stearate

Purified Talc.

6.2 Incompatibilities

None.

6.3 Shelf life

Blister packs: 3 years

6.4 Special precautions for storage

Protect from light.

Additionally, for blister packs, store below 25°C in a dry place.

6.5 Nature and contents of container

Opaque PVC blister sealed with an aluminium foil: packs of 56 tablets.

6.6 Special precautions for disposal and other handling

Not applicable.

7. MARKETING AUTHORISATION HOLDER

Sanofi-aventis

One Onslow Street

Guildford

Surrey, GU1 4YS, UK

8. MARKETING AUTHORISATION NUMBER(S)

PL 04425/0332

08/03/02

9. DATE OF FIRST AUTHORISATION/RENEWAL OF THE AUTHORISATION

08/03/02

10. DATE OF REVISION OF THE TEXT

May 2008

11. LEGAL CATEGORY

POM

Cosopt Ophthalmic Solution

(Merck Sharp & Dohme Limited)

1. NAME OF THE MEDICINAL PRODUCT

COSOPT® 20 mg/ml + 5 mg/ml, eye drops, solution

2. QUALITATIVE AND QUANTITATIVE COMPOSITION

Each ml contains 22.26 mg of dorzolamide hydrochloride corresponding to 20 mg dorzolamide and 6.83 mg of timolol maleate corresponding to 5 mg timolol.

Excipients: Benzalkonium chloride 0.075 mg/ml

For a full list of excipients, see section 6.1.

3. PHARMACEUTICAL FORM

Eye drops, solution.

Clear, colourless to nearly colourless, slightly viscous solution.

4. CLINICAL PARTICULARS

4.1 Therapeutic indications

Indicated in the treatment of elevated intraocular pressure (IOP) in patients with open-angle glaucoma or pseudoexfoliative glaucoma when topical beta-blocker monotherapy is not sufficient.

4.2 Posology and method of administration

The dose is one drop of COSOPT in the (conjunctival sac of the) affected eye(s) two times daily.

If another topical ophthalmic agent is being used, COSOPT and the other agent should be administered at least ten minutes apart.

Patients should be instructed to wash their hands before use and avoid allowing the tip of the container to come into contact with the eye or surrounding structures.

Patients should also be instructed that ocular solutions, if handled improperly, can become contaminated by common bacteria known to cause ocular infections. Serious damage to the eye and subsequent loss of vision may result from using contaminated solutions.

Patients should be informed of the correct handling of the OCUMETER PLUS bottles.

Usage Instructions

1 Before using the medication for the first time, be sure the Safety Strip on the front of the bottle is unbroken. A gap between the bottle and the cap is normal for an unopened bottle.

2 Tear off the Safety Strip to break the seal.

3 To open the bottle, unscrew the cap by turning as indicated by the arrows on the top of the cap. Do not pull the cap directly up and away from the bottle. Pulling the cap directly up will prevent your dispenser from operating properly.

4 Tilt your head back and pull your lower eyelid down slightly to form a pocket between your eyelid and eye.

5. Invert the bottle, and press lightly with the thumb or index finger over the "Finger Push Area" until a single drop is dispensed into the eye as directed by your doctor. DO NOT TOUCH YOUR EYE OR EYELID WITH THE DROPPER TIP.

6. If drop dispensing is difficult after opening for the first time, replace the cap on the bottle and tighten (do not overtighten) and then remove by turning the cap in the opposite directions as indicated by the arrows on the top of the cap.

7. Repeat steps 4 & 5 with the other eye if instructed to do so by your doctor.

8. Replace the cap by turning until it is firmly touching the bottle. The arrow on the left side of the cap must be aligned with the arrow on the left side of the bottle label for proper closure. Do not overtighten or you may damage the bottle and cap.

9. The dispenser tip is designed to provide a single drop; therefore, do NOT enlarge the hole of the dispenser tip.

10. After you have used all doses, there will be some COSOPT left in the bottle. You should not be concerned since an extra amount of COSOPT has been added and you will get the full amount of COSOPT that your doctor prescribed. Do not attempt to remove the excess medicine from the bottle.

Paediatric Use

Efficacy in paediatric patients has not been established.

Safety in paediatric patients below the age of two years has not been established. (For information regarding safety in paediatric patients $\geq$ 2 and $<$ 6 years of age, see section 5.1).

4.3 Contraindications

COSOPT is contraindicated in patients with:

- reactive airway disease, including bronchial asthma or a history of bronchial asthma, or severe chronic obstructive pulmonary disease
- sinus bradycardia, second- or third-degree atrioventricular block, overt cardiac failure, cardiogenic shock
- severe renal impairment (CrCl $<$ 30 ml/min) or hyperchloraemic acidosis
- hypersensitivity to one or both active substances or to any of the excipients.

The above are based on the components and are not unique to the combination.

4.4 Special warnings and precautions for use

Cardiovascular/Respiratory Reactions

As with other topically-applied ophthalmic agents, this medicinal product may be absorbed systemically. The timolol component is a beta-blocker. Therefore, the same types of adverse reactions found with systemic administration of beta-blockers may occur with topical administration, including worsening of Prinzmetal's angina, worsening of severe peripheral and central circulatory disorders, and hypotension.

Because of the timolol maleate component, cardiac failure should be adequately controlled before beginning therapy with COSOPT. In patients with a history of severe cardiac disease, signs of cardiac failure should be watched for and pulse rates should be checked.

Respiratory reactions and cardiac reactions, including death due to bronchospasm in patients with asthma and rarely death in association with cardiac failure, have been reported following administration of timolol maleate.

Hepatic Impairment

COSOPT has not been studied in patients with hepatic impairment and should therefore be used with caution in such patients.

Immunology and Hypersensitivity

As with other topically-applied ophthalmic agents, this medicinal product may be absorbed systemically. Dorzolamide contains a sulfonamido group, which also occurs in sulphonamides. Therefore, the same types of adverse reactions found with systemic administration of sulphonamides may occur with topical administration. If signs of serious reactions or hypersensitivity occur, discontinue use of this preparation.

Local ocular adverse effects, similar to those observed with dorzolamide hydrochloride eye drops, have been seen with COSOPT. If such reactions occur, discontinuation of COSOPT should be considered.

While taking beta-blockers, patients with a history of atopy or a history of severe anaphylactic reaction to a variety of allergens may be more reactive to accidental, diagnostic, or therapeutic repeated challenge with such allergens. Such patients may be unresponsive to the usual doses of epinephrine used to treat anaphylactic reactions.

Concomitant Therapy

The following concomitant medication is not recommended:

– dorzolamide and oral carbonic anhydrase inhibitors

– topical beta-adrenergic blocking agents.

Withdrawal of Therapy

As with systemic beta-blockers, if discontinuation of ophthalmic timolol is needed in patients with coronary heart disease, therapy should be withdrawn gradually.

Additional Effects of Beta-Blockade

Therapy with beta-blockers may mask certain symptoms of hypoglycaemia in patients with diabetes mellitus or hypoglycaemia.

Therapy with beta-blockers may mask certain symptoms of hyperthyroidism. Abrupt withdrawal of beta-blocker therapy may precipitate a worsening of symptoms.

Therapy with beta-blockers may aggravate symptoms of myasthenia gravis.

Additional Effects of Carbonic Anhydrase Inhibition

Therapy with oral carbonic anhydrase inhibitors has been associated with urolithiasis as a result of acid-base disturbances, especially in patients with a prior history of renal calculi. Although no acid-base disturbances have been observed with COSOPT, urolithiasis has been reported infrequently. Because COSOPT contains a topical carbonic anhydrase inhibitor that is absorbed systemically, patients with a prior history of renal calculi may be at increased risk of urolithiasis while using COSOPT.

Other

The management of patients with acute angle-closure glaucoma requires therapeutic interventions in addition to ocular hypotensive agents. COSOPT has not been studied in patients with acute angle-closure glaucoma.

Corneal oedema and irreversible corneal decompensation have been reported in patients with pre-existing chronic corneal defects and/or a history of intraocular surgery while using dorzolamide. Topical dorzolamide should be used with caution in such patients.

Choroidal detachment concomitant with ocular hypotony have been reported after filtration procedures with administration of aqueous suppressant therapies.

As with the use of other antiglaucoma drugs, diminished responsiveness to ophthalmic timolol maleate after prolonged therapy has been reported in some patients. However, in clinical studies in which 164 patients have been followed for at least three years, no significant difference in mean intraocular pressure has been observed after initial stabilisation.

Contact Lens Use

COSOPT contains the preservative benzalkonium chloride, which may cause eye irritation. Remove contact lenses prior to application and wait at least 15 minutes before reinsertion. Benzalkonium chloride is known to discolour soft contact lenses.

Paediatric use

See section 5.1.

4.5 Interaction with other medicinal products and other forms of interaction

Specific drug interaction studies have not been performed with COSOPT.

In clinical studies, COSOPT was used concomitantly with the following systemic medications without evidence of adverse interactions: ACE-inhibitors, calcium channel blockers, diuretics, non-steroidal anti-inflammatory drugs including aspirin, and hormones (e.g. oestrogen, insulin, thyroxine).

However, the potential exists for additive effects and production of hypotension and/or marked bradycardia when timolol maleate ophthalmic solution is administered together with oral calcium channel blockers, catecholamine-depleting drugs or beta-adrenergic blocking agents, antiarrhythmics (including amiodarone), digitalis glycosides, parasympathomimetics, narcotics, and monoamine oxidase (MAO) inhibitors.

Potentiated systemic beta-blockade (e.g., decreased heart rate, depression) has been reported during combined treatment with CYP2D6 inhibitors (e.g. quinidine, SSRIs) and timolol.

Although COSOPT alone has little or no effect on pupil size, mydriasis resulting from concomitant use of ophthalmic timolol maleate and epinephrine (adrenaline) has been reported occasionally.

Beta-blockers may increase the hypoglycaemic effect of antidiabetic agents.

Oral beta-adrenergic blocking agents may exacerbate the rebound hypertension which can follow the withdrawal of clonidine.

4.6 Pregnancy and lactation

Use During Pregnancy

COSOPT should not be used during pregnancy.

Dorzolamide

No adequate clinical data in exposed pregnancies are available. In rabbits, dorzolamide produced teratogenic effect at maternotoxic doses (see Section 5.3).

Timolol

Well controlled epidemiological studies with systemic beta-blockers showed no evidence of teratogenic effects, but some pharmacological effects such as bradycardia were observed in foetuses or neonates. If COSOPT is administered until delivery, the neonate should be carefully monitored during the first days of life.

Use During Lactation

It is not known whether dorzolamide is excreted in human milk. In lactating rats receiving dorzolamide, decreases in the body weight gain of offspring were observed. Timolol does appear in human milk. If treatment with COSOPT is required, then lactation is not recommended.

4.7 Effects on ability to drive and use machines

No studies on the effects on the ability to drive and use machines have been performed. Possible side effects such as blurred vision may affect some patients' ability to drive and/or operate machinery.

4.8 Undesirable effects

In clinical studies no adverse experiences specific to COSOPT have been observed; adverse reactions have been limited to those that were reported previously with dorzolamide hydrochloride and/or timolol maleate.

During clinical studies, 1035 patients were treated with COSOPT. Approximately 2.4% of all patients discontinued therapy with COSOPT because of local ocular adverse reactions, approximately 1.2% of all patients discontinued because of local adverse reactions suggestive of allergy or hypersensitivity (such as lid inflammation and conjunctivitis).

The following adverse reactions have been reported with COSOPT or one of its components either during clinical trials or during post-marketing experience:

[Very Common: (≥ 1/10), Common: (≥ 1/100 to < 1/10), Uncommon: ≥ 1/1000 to < 1/100), and Rare: (≥ 1/10,000 to < 1/1000)]

Musculoskeletal and connective tissue disorders:

Timolol maleate eye drops, solution:

Rare: systemic lupus erythematosus

Nervous system disorders:

Dorzolamide hydrochloride eye drops, solution:

Common: headache*

Rare: dizziness*, paraesthesia*

Timolol maleate eye drops, solution:

Common: headache*

Uncommon: dizziness*, depression*

Rare: insomnia*, nightmares*, memory loss, paraesthesia*, increase in signs and symptoms of myasthenia gravis, decreased libido*, cerebrovascular accident*

Eye disorders:

COSOPT:

Very Common: burning and stinging

Common: conjunctival injection, blurred vision, corneal erosion, ocular itching, tearing

Dorzolamide hydrochloride eye drops, solution:

Common: eyelid inflammation*, eyelid irritation*

Uncommon: iridocyclitis*

Rare: irritation including redness*, pain*, eyelid crusting*, transient myopia (which resolved upon discontinuation of therapy), corneal oedema*, ocular hypotony*, choroidal detachment (following filtration surgery)*

Timolol maleate eye drops, solution:

Common: signs and symptoms of ocular irritation including blepharitis*, keratitis*, decreased corneal sensitivity, and dry eyes*

Uncommon: visual disturbances including refractive changes (due to withdrawal of miotic therapy in some cases)*

Rare: ptosis, diplopia, choroidal detachment (following filtration surgery)*

Ear and labyrinth disorders:

Timolol maleate eye drops, solution:

Rare: tinnitus*

Cardiac and vascular disorders:

Timolol maleate eye drops, solution:

Uncommon: bradycardia*, syncope*

Rare: hypotension*, chest pain*, palpitation*, oedema*, arrhythmia*, congestive heart failure*, heart block*, cardiac arrest*, cerebral ischaemia, claudication, Raynaud's phenomenon*, cold hands and feet*

Respiratory, thoracic, and mediastinal disorders:

COSOPT:

Common: sinusitis

Rare: shortness of breath, respiratory failure, rhinitis

Dorzolamide hydrochloride eye drops, solution:

Rare: epistaxis*

Timolol maleate eye drops, solution:

Uncommon: dyspnoea*

Rare: bronchospasm (predominantly in patients with pre-existing bronchospastic disease)*, cough*

Gastro-intestinal disorders:

COSOPT:

Very Common: taste perversion

Dorzolamide hydrochloride eye drops, solution:

Common: nausea*

Rare: throat irritation, dry mouth*

Timolol maleate eye drops, solution:

Uncommon: nausea*, dyspepsia*

Rare: diarrhoea, dry mouth*

Skin and subcutaneous tissue disorders:

COSOPT:

Rare: contact dermatitis

Dorzolamide hydrochloride eye drops, solution:

Rare: rash*

Timolol maleate eye drops, solution:

Rare: alopecia*, psoriasiform rash or exacerbation of psoriasis*

Renal and urinary disorders:

COSOPT:

Uncommon: urolithiasis

Reproductive system and breast disorders:

Timolol maleate eye drops, solution:

Rare: Peyronie's disease*

General disorders and administration site conditions:

COSOPT:

Rare: signs and symptoms of systemic allergic reactions, including angioedema, urticaria, pruritus, rash, anaphylaxis, rarely bronchospasm

Dorzolamide hydrochloride eye drops, solution:

Common: asthenia/fatigue*

Timolol maleate eye drops, solution:

Uncommon: asthenia/fatigue*

*These adverse reactions were also observed with COSOPT during post-marketing experience.

Laboratory findings

COSOPT was not associated with clinically meaningful electrolyte disturbances in clinical studies.

4.9 Overdose

No data are available in humans in regard to overdose by accidental or deliberate ingestion of COSOPT.

Symptoms

There have been reports of inadvertent overdoses with timolol maleate ophthalmic solution resulting in systemic effects similar to those seen with systemic beta-adrenergic blocking agents such as dizziness, headache, shortness of breath, bradycardia, bronchospasm, and cardiac arrest. The most common signs and symptoms to be expected with overdoses of dorzolamide are electrolyte imbalance, development of an acidotic state, and possibly central nervous system effects.

Only limited information is available with regard to human overdose by accidental or deliberate ingestion of dorzolamide hydrochloride. With oral ingestion, somnolence has been reported. With topical application the following have been reported: nausea, dizziness, headache, fatigue, abnormal dreams, and dysphagia.

Treatment

Treatment should be symptomatic and supportive. Serum electrolyte levels (particularly potassium) and blood pH levels should be monitored. Studies have shown that timolol does not dialyse readily.

5. PHARMACOLOGICAL PROPERTIES

5.1 Pharmacodynamic properties

Pharmacotherapeutic group: Antiglaucoma preparations and miotics, Beta blocking agents, Timolol, combinations, ATC code: S01ED51

Mechanism of Action

COSOPT is comprised of two components: dorzolamide hydrochloride and timolol maleate. Each of these two components decreases elevated intraocular pressure by reducing aqueous humor secretion, but does so by a different mechanism of action.

Dorzolamide hydrochloride is a potent inhibitor of human carbonic anhydrase II. Inhibition of carbonic anhydrase in the ciliary processes of the eye decreases aqueous humor secretion, presumably by slowing the formation of bicarbonate ions with subsequent reduction in sodium and fluid transport. Timolol maleate is a non-selective beta-adrenergic receptor blocking agent. The precise mechanism of action of timolol maleate in lowering intraocular pressure is not clearly established at this time, although a fluorescein study and tonography studies indicate that the predominant action may be related to reduced aqueous formation. However, in some studies a slight increase in outflow facility was also observed. The combined effect of these two agents results in additional intraocular pressure (IOP) reduction compared to either component administered alone.

Following topical administration, COSOPT reduces elevated intraocular pressure, whether or not associated with glaucoma. Elevated intraocular pressure is a major risk factor in the pathogenesis of optic nerve damage and glaucomatous visual field loss. COSOPT reduces intraocular pressure without the common side effects of miotics such as night blindness, accommodative spasm and pupillary constriction.

Pharmacodynamic effects

Clinical effects:

Clinical studies of up to 15 months duration were conducted to compare the IOP-lowering effect of COSOPT b.i.d. (dosed morning and bedtime) to individually- and concomitantly-administered 0.5% timolol and 2.0% dorzolamide in patients with glaucoma or ocular hypertension for whom concomitant therapy was considered appropriate in the trials. This included both untreated patients and patients inadequately controlled with timolol monotherapy. The majority of patients were treated with topical beta-blocker monotherapy prior to study enrollment. In an analysis of the combined studies, the IOP-lowering effect of COSOPT b.i.d. was greater than that of monotherapy with either 2% dorzolamide t.i.d. or 0.5% timolol b.i.d. The IOP-lowering effect of COSOPT b.i.d. was equivalent to that of concomitant therapy with dorzolamide b.i.d. and timolol b.i.d. The IOP-lowering effect of COSOPT b.i.d. was demonstrated when measured at various time points throughout the day and this effect was maintained during long-term administration.

Paediatric use

A 3 month controlled study, with the primary objective of documenting the safety of 2% dorzolamide hydrochloride ophthalmic solution in children under the age of 6 years has been conducted. In this study, 30 patients under 6 and greater than or equal to 2 years of age whose IOP was not adequately controlled with monotherapy by dorzolamide or timolol received COSOPT in an open label phase. Efficacy in those patients has not been established. In this small group of patients, twice daily administration of COSOPT was generally well tolerated with 19 patients completing the treatment period and 11 patients discontinuing for surgery, a change in medication, or other reasons.

5.2 Pharmacokinetic properties

Dorzolamide hydrochloride:

Unlike oral carbonic anhydrase inhibitors, topical administration of dorzolamide hydrochloride allows for the active substance to exert its effects directly in the eye at substantially lower doses and therefore with less systemic exposure. In clinical trials, this resulted in a reduction in IOP without the acid-base disturbances or alterations in electrolytes characteristic of oral carbonic anhydrase inhibitors.

When topically applied, dorzolamide reaches the systemic circulation. To assess the potential for systemic carbonic anhydrase inhibition following topical administration, active substance and metabolite concentrations in red blood cells (RBCs) and plasma and carbonic anhydrase inhibition in RBCs were measured. Dorzolamide accumulates in RBCs during chronic dosing as a result of selective binding to CA-II while extremely low concentrations of free active substance in plasma are maintained. The parent active substance forms a single N-desethyl metabolite that inhibits CA-II less potently than the parent active substance but also inhibits a less active isoenzyme (CA-I). The metabolite also accumulates in RBCs where it binds primarily to CA-I. Dorzolamide binds moderately to plasma proteins (approximately 33%). Dorzolamide is primarily excreted unchanged in the urine; the metabolite is also excreted in urine. After dosing ends, dorzolamide washes out of RBCs non-linearly, resulting in a rapid decline of active substance concentration initially, followed by a slower elimination phase with a half-life of about four months.

When dorzolamide was given orally to simulate the maximum systemic exposure after long term topical ocular administration, steady state was reached within 13 weeks. At steady state, there was virtually no free active substance or metabolite in plasma; CA inhibition in RBCs was less than that anticipated to be necessary for a pharmacological effect on renal function or respiration. Similar pharmacokinetic results were observed after chronic, topical administration of dorzolamide hydrochloride. However, some elderly patients with renal impairment (estimated CrCl 30-60 ml/min) had higher metabolite concentrations in RBCs, but no meaningful differences in carbonic anhydrase inhibition and no clinically significant systemic side effects were directly attributable to this finding.

Timolol maleate:

In a study of plasma active substance concentration in six subjects, the systemic exposure to timolol was determined following twice daily topical administration of timolol maleate ophthalmic solution 0.5%. The mean peak plasma concentration following morning dosing was 0.46 ng/ml and following afternoon dosing was 0.35 ng/ml.

5.3 Preclinical safety data

The ocular and systemic safety profile of the individual components is well established.

Dorzolamide

In rabbits given maternotoxic doses of dorzolamide associated with metabolic acidosis, malformations of the vertebral bodies were observed

Timolol

Animal studies have not shown teratogenic effect.

Furthermore, no adverse ocular effects were seen in animals treated topically with dorzolamide hydrochloride and timolol maleate ophthalmic solution or with concomitantly-administered dorzolamide hydrochloride and timolol maleate. *In vitro* and *in vivo* studies with each of the components did not reveal a mutagenic potential. Therefore, no significant risk for human safety is expected with therapeutic doses of COSOPT.

6. PHARMACEUTICAL PARTICULARS

6.1 List of excipients

Benzalkonium chloride

Hydroxyethyl cellulose

Mannitol (E421)

Sodium citrate (E331)

Sodium hydroxide (E524) for pH adjustment

Water for injections

6.2 Incompatibilities

Not applicable.

6.3 Shelf life

2 years.

COSOPT should be used no longer than 28 days after first opening the container.

6.4 Special precautions for storage

Keep the bottle in the outer carton, in order to protect from light.

6.5 Nature and contents of container

The OCUMETER Plus Ophthalmic Dispenser consists of a translucent, high-density polyethylene container with a sealed dropper tip, a flexible fluted side area which is depressed to dispense the drops, and a 2-piece cap assembly. The 2-piece cap mechanism punctures the sealed dropper tip upon initial use, then locks together to provide a single cap during the usage period. Tamper evidence is provided by a safety strip on the container label. The OCUMETER Plus ophthalmic dispenser contains 5 ml of solution.

COSOPT is available in the following packaging configurations:

1 × 5 ml (single 5-ml container)

3 × 5 ml (three 5-ml containers)

6 × 5 ml (six 5-ml containers)

Not all pack sizes may be marketed.

6.6 Special precautions for disposal and other handling

No special requirements.

7. MARKETING AUTHORISATION HOLDER

Merck Sharp & Dohme Limited

Hertford Road, Hoddesdon, Hertfordshire EN11 9BU, UK.

8. MARKETING AUTHORISATION NUMBER(S)

PL 0025/0373

9. DATE OF FIRST AUTHORISATION/RENEWAL OF THE AUTHORISATION

04 August 1998 / 10 December 2008.

10. DATE OF REVISION OF THE TEXT

June 2009

LEGAL CATEGORY

POM

® denotes registered trademark of Merck & Co., Inc., Whitehouse Station, NJ, USA.

MSD

Merck Sharp & Dohme Limited

Hertford Road, Hoddesdon, Hertfordshire EN11 9BU, UK

SPC.CST.07.UK.2464 (II-033; II-034; II-036; R2)

Cosopt Preservative-Free, Single Dose Eye Drops

(Merck Sharp & Dohme Limited)

1. NAME OF THE MEDICINAL PRODUCT

COSOPT® Preservative-Free 20 mg/ml + 5 mg/ml, eye drops, solution, single-dose container

2. QUALITATIVE AND QUANTITATIVE COMPOSITION

Each ml contains 22.26 mg of dorzolamide hydrochloride corresponding to 20 mg dorzolamide and 6.83 mg of timolol maleate corresponding to 5 mg timolol.

For a full list of excipients, see section 6.1.

3. PHARMACEUTICAL FORM

Eye drops, solution, single dose container

Clear, colourless to nearly colourless, slightly viscous solution.

4. CLINICAL PARTICULARS

4.1 Therapeutic indications

Indicated in the treatment of elevated intraocular pressure (IOP) in patients with open-angle glaucoma or pseudoexfoliative glaucoma when topical beta-blocker monotherapy is not sufficient.

4.2 Posology and method of administration

The dose is one drop of COSOPT Preservative-Free in the (conjunctival sac of the) affected eye(s) two times daily.

If another topical ophthalmic agent is being used, COSOPT Preservative-Free and the other agent should be administered at least ten minutes apart.

COSOPT Preservative-Free is a sterile solution that does not contain a preservative. The solution from one individual single dose container is to be used immediately after opening for administration to the affected eye(s). Since sterility cannot be maintained after the individual single dose container is opened, any remaining contents must be discarded immediately after administration.

Patients should be instructed to avoid allowing the tip of the container to come into contact with the eye or surrounding structures.

Patients should also be instructed that ocular solutions, if handled improperly, can become contaminated by common bacteria known to cause ocular infections. Serious damage to the eye and subsequent loss of vision may result from using contaminated solutions.

Usage Instructions

1. Open the sachet which contains 15 individual single dose containers. There are three strips of 5 single dose containers each in the sachet.

2. First wash your hands then break off one single dose container from the strip and twist open the top.

3. Tilt your head back and pull your lower eyelid down slightly to form a pocket between your eyelid and eye.

4. Instill one drop in the affected eye(s) as directed by your physician. Each single dose container contains enough solution for both eyes.

5. After instillation, discard the used single dose container even if there is solution remaining.

6. Store the remaining single dose containers in the sachet; the remaining single dose containers must be used within 15 days after opening of the sachet.

Paediatric Use

Efficacy in paediatric patients has not been established.

Safety in paediatric patients below the age of 2 years has not been established. (For information regarding safety in paediatric patients ≥ 2 and < 6 years of age, see section 5.1)

4.3 Contraindications

COSOPT Preservative-Free is contraindicated in patients with:

- reactive airway disease, including bronchial asthma or a history of bronchial asthma, or severe chronic obstructive pulmonary disease
- sinus bradycardia, second- or third-degree atrioventricular block, overt cardiac failure, cardiogenic shock
- severe renal impairment (CrCl < 30 ml/min) or hyperchloraemic acidosis
- hypersensitivity to one or both active substances or to any of the excipients.

The above are based on the components and are not unique to the combination.

4.4 Special warnings and precautions for use

Cardiovascular/Respiratory Reactions

As with other topically-applied ophthalmic agents, this medicinal product may be absorbed systemically. The timolol component is a beta-blocker. Therefore, the same types of adverse reactions found with systemic administration of beta-blockers may occur with topical administration, including worsening of Prinzmetal angina, worsening of severe peripheral and central circulatory disorders, and hypotension.

Because of the timolol maleate component, cardiac failure should be adequately controlled before beginning therapy with COSOPT Preservative-Free. In patients with a history of severe cardiac disease, signs of cardiac failure should be watched for and pulse rates should be checked.

Respiratory reactions and cardiac reactions, including death due to bronchospasm in patients with asthma and rarely death in association with cardiac failure, have been reported following administration of timolol maleate.

Hepatic Impairment

COSOPT Preservative-Free has not been studied in patients with hepatic impairment and should therefore be used with caution in such patients.

Immunology and Hypersensitivity

As with other topically-applied ophthalmic agents, COSOPT Preservative-Free may be absorbed systemically. Dorzolamide contains a sulfonamido group, which also occurs in sulfonamides. Therefore, the same types of adverse reactions found with systemic administration of sulfonamides may occur with topical administration. If signs of serious reactions or hypersensitivity occur, discontinue use of this preparation.

Local ocular adverse effects, similar to those observed with dorzolamide hydrochloride eye drops, have been seen with COSOPT Preservative-Free. If such reactions occur, discontinuation of COSOPT Preservative-Free should be considered.

While taking beta-blockers, patients with a history of atopy or a history of severe anaphylactic reaction to a variety of allergens may be more reactive to accidental, diagnostic, or therapeutic repeated challenge with such allergens. Such patients may be unresponsive to the usual doses of epinephrine used to treat anaphylactic reactions.

Concomitant Therapy

The following concomitant medication is not recommended:

- dorzolamide and oral carbonic anhydrase inhibitors
- topical beta-adrenergic blocking agents

Withdrawal of Therapy

As with systemic beta-blockers, if discontinuation of ophthalmic timolol is needed in patients with coronary heart disease, therapy should be withdrawn gradually.

Additional Effects of Beta-Blockade

Therapy with beta-blockers may mask certain symptoms of hypoglycaemia in patients with diabetes mellitus or hypoglycaemia.

Therapy with beta-blockers may mask certain symptoms of hyperthyroidism. Abrupt withdrawal of beta-blocker therapy may precipitate a worsening of symptoms.

Therapy with beta-blockers may aggravate symptoms of myasthenia gravis.

Additional Effects of Carbonic Anhydrase Inhibition

Therapy with oral carbonic anhydrase inhibitors has been associated with urolithiasis as a result of acid-base disturbances, especially in patients with a prior history of renal calculi. Although no acid-base disturbances have been observed with COSOPT (preserved formulation), urolithiasis has been reported infrequently. Because COSOPT Preservative-Free contains a topical carbonic anhydrase inhibitor that is absorbed systemically, patients with a prior history of renal calculi may be at increased risk of urolithiasis while using COSOPT Preservative-Free.

Other

The management of patients with acute angle-closure glaucoma requires therapeutic interventions in addition to ocular hypotensive agents. COSOPT Preservative-Free has not been studied in patients with acute angle-closure glaucoma.

Corneal oedema and irreversible corneal decompensation have been reported in patients with pre-existing chronic corneal defects and/or a history of intraocular surgery while using dorzolamide. Topical dorzolamide should be used with caution in such patients.

Choroidal detachment concomitant with ocular hypotony have been reported after filtration procedures with administration of aqueous suppressant therapies.

As with the use of other antiglaucoma drugs, diminished responsiveness to ophthalmic timolol maleate after prolonged therapy has been reported in some patients. However, in clinical studies in which 164 patients have been followed for at least three years, no significant difference in mean intraocular pressure has been observed after initial stabilisation.

Contact Lens Use

COSOPT Preservative-Free has not been studied in patients wearing contact lenses.

Paediatric Use

See section 5.1

4.5 Interaction with other medicinal products and other forms of interaction

Specific drug interaction studies have not been performed with COSOPT Preservative-Free.

In a clinical study, COSOPT Preservative-Free was used concomitantly with the following systemic medications without evidence of adverse interactions: ACE-inhibitors, calcium channel blockers, diuretics, non-steroidal anti-inflammatory drugs including aspirin, and hormones (e.g., oestrogen, insulin, thyroxine).

However, the potential exists for additive effects and production of hypotension and/or marked bradycardia when timolol maleate ophthalmic solution is administered together with oral calcium channel blockers, catecholamine-depleting drugs or beta-adrenergic blocking agents, antiarrhythmics(including amiodarone), digitalis glycosides, parasympathomimetics, narcotics, and monoamine oxidase (MAO) inhibitors.

Potentiated systemic beta-blockade (e.g., decreased heart rate, depression) has been reported during combined treatment with CYP2D6 inhibitors (e.g. quinidine, SSRIs) and timolol.

Although COSOPT (preserved formulation) alone has little or no effect on pupil size, mydriasis resulting from concomitant use of ophthalmic timolol maleate and epinephrine (adrenaline) has been reported occasionally.

Beta-blockers may increase the hypoglycaemic effect of antidiabetic agents.

Oral beta-adrenergic blocking agents may exacerbate the rebound hypertension which can follow the withdrawal of clonidine.

4.6 Pregnancy and lactation

Use During Pregnancy

COSOPT Preservative-Free should not be used during pregnancy.

Dorzolamide

No adequate clinical data in exposed pregnancies are available. In rabbits, dorzolamide produced teratogenic effect at maternotoxic doses (see Section 5.3).

Timolol

Well controlled epidemiological studies with systemic beta-blockers showed no evidence of teratogenic effects, but some pharmacological effects such as bradycardia were observed in foetuses or neonates. If COSOPT Preservative-Free is administered until delivery, the neonate should be carefully monitored during the first days of life.

Use During Lactation

It is not known whether dorzolamide is excreted in human milk. In lactating rats receiving dorzolamide, decreases in the body weight gain of offspring were observed. Timolol does appear in human milk. If treatment with COSOPT Preservative-Free is required, then lactation is not recommended.

4.7 Effects on ability to drive and use machines

No studies on the effects on the ability to drive and use machines have been performed. Possible side effects such as blurred vision may affect some patients' ability to drive and/or operate machinery.

4.8 Undesirable effects

In a clinical study no adverse experiences specificto COSOPT Preservative-Free have been observed; adverse reactions have been limited to those that were reported previously with COSOPT (preserved formulation), dorzolamide hydrochloride and/or timolol maleate.

During clinical studies, 1035 patients were treated with COSOPT (preserved formulation). Approximately 2.4% of all patients discontinued therapy with COSOPT (preserved formulation) because of local ocular adverse reactions; approximately 1.2% of all patients discontinued because of local adverse reactions suggestive of allergy or hypersensitivity (such as lid inflammation and conjunctivitis).

COSOPT Preservative-Free has been shown to have a similar safety profile to COSOPT (preservative containing formulation) in a repeat dose double-masked, comparative study.

The following adverse reactions have been reported with COSOPT or one of its components either during clinical trials or during post-marketing experience:

[Very Common: (≥ 1/10), Common: (≥ 1/100, <1/10), Uncommon: (≥ 1/1000, <1/100), and Rare: (≥ 1/10,000, <1/1000)]

Musculoskeletal and connective tissue disorders:

Timolol maleate eye drops, solution:

Rare: systemic lupus erythematosus

Nervous system disorders:

Dorzolamide hydrochloride eye drops, solution:

Common: headache*

Rare: dizziness*, paraesthesia*

Timolol maleate eye drops, solution:

Common: headache*

Uncommon: dizziness*, depression*

Rare: insomnia*, nightmares*, memory loss, paraesthesia*, increase in signs and symptoms of myasthenia gravis, decreased libido*, cerebrovascular accident*

Eye disorders:

COSOPT:

Very Common: burning and stinging

Common: conjunctival injection, blurred vision, corneal erosion, ocular itching, tearing

Dorzolamide hydrochloride eye drops, solution:

Common: eyelid inflammation*, eyelid irritation*

Uncommon: iridocyclitis*

Rare: irritation including redness*, pain*, eyelid crusting*, transient myopia (which resolved upon discontinuation of therapy), corneal oedema*, ocular hypotony*, choroidal detachment (following filtration surgery)*

Timolol maleate eye drops, solution:

Common: signs and symptoms of ocular irritation including blepharitis*, keratitis*, decreased corneal sensitivity, and dry eyes*

Uncommon: visual disturbances including refractive changes (due to withdrawal of miotic therapy in some cases)*

Rare: ptosis, diplopia, choroidal detachment (following filtration surgery)*

Ear and labyrinth disorders:

Timolol maleate eye drops, solution:

Rare: tinnitus*

Cardiac and vascular disorders:

Timolol maleate eye drops, solution:

Uncommon: bradycardia*, syncope*

Rare: hypotension*, chest pain*, palpitation*, oedema*, arrhythmia*, congestive heart failure*, heart block*, cardiac arrest*, cerebral ischaemia, claudication, Raynaud's phenomenon*, cold hands and feet*

Respiratory, thoracic, and mediastinal disorders:

COSOPT:

Common: sinusitis

Rare: shortness of breath, respiratory failure, rhinitis

Dorzolamide hydrochloride eye drops, solution:

Rare: epistaxis*

Timolol maleate eye drops, solution:

Uncommon: dyspnoea*

Rare: bronchospasm (predominantly in patients with pre-existing bronchospastic disease)*, cough*

Gastro-intestinal disorders:

COSOPT:

Very Common: taste perversion

Dorzolamide hydrochloride eye drops, solution:

Common: nausea*

Rare: throat irritation, dry mouth*

Timolol maleate eye drops, solution:

Uncommon: nausea*, dyspepsia*

Rare: diarrhoea, dry mouth*

Skin and subcutaneous tissue disorders:

COSOPT:

Rare: contact dermatitis

Dorzolamide hydrochloride eye drops, solution:

Rare: rash*

Timolol maleate eye drops, solution:

Rare: alopecia*, psoriasiform rash or exacerbation of psoriasis*

Renal and urinary disorders:

COSOPT:

Uncommon: urolithiasis

Reproductive system and breast disorders:

Timolol maleate eye drops, solution:

Rare: Peyronie's disease*

General disorders and administration site disorders:

COSOPT:

Rare: signs and symptoms of systemic allergic reactions, including angioedema, urticaria, pruritus, rash, anaphylaxis, rarely bronchospasm

Dorzolamide hydrochloride eye drops, solution:

Common: asthenia/fatigue*

Timolol maleate eye drops, solution:

Uncommon: asthenia/fatigue*

*These adverse reactions were also observed with COSOPT (preserved formulation) during post-marketing experience.

Laboratory Findings

COSOPT (preserved formulation) was not associated with clinically meaningful electrolyte disturbances in clinical studies.

4.9 Overdose

No data are available in humans in regard to overdose by accidental or deliberate ingestion of COSOPT (preserved formulation) or COSOPT Preservative-Free.

Symptoms

There have been reports of inadvertent overdoses with timolol maleate ophthalmic solution resulting in systemic effects similar to those seen with systemic beta-adrenergic blocking agents such as dizziness, headache, shortness of breath, bradycardia, bronchospasm, and cardiac arrest. The most common signs and symptoms to be expected with overdoses of dorzolamide are electrolyte imbalance, development of an acidotic state, and possibly central nervous system effects.

Only limited information is available with regard to human overdose by accidental or deliberate ingestion of dorzolamide hydrochloride. With oral ingestion, somnolence has been reported. With topical application the following have been reported: nausea, dizziness, headache, fatigue, abnormal dreams, and dysphagia.

Treatment

Treatment should be symptomatic and supportive. Serum electrolyte levels (particularly potassium) and blood pH levels should be monitored. Studies have shown that timolol does not dialyse readily.

5. PHARMACOLOGICAL PROPERTIES

5.1 Pharmacodynamic properties

Pharmacotherapeutic group: Antiglaucoma preparations and miotics, Beta blocking agents, Timolol, combinations, ATC code: S01E D51.

Mechanism of Action

COSOPT Preservative-Free is comprised of two components: dorzolamide hydrochloride and timolol maleate. Each of these two components decreases elevated intraocular pressure by reducing aqueous humor secretion, but does so by a different mechanism of action.

Dorzolamide hydrochloride is a potent inhibitor of human carbonic anhydrase II. Inhibition of carbonic anhydrase in the ciliary processes of the eye decreases aqueous humor secretion, presumably by slowing the formation of bicarbonate ions with subsequent reduction in sodium and fluid transport. Timolol maleate is a non-selective beta-adrenergic receptor blocking agent. The precise mechanism of action of timolol maleate in lowering intraocular pressure is not clearly established at this time, although a fluorescein study and tonography studies indicate that the predominant action may be related to reduced aqueous formation. However, in some studies a slight increase in outflow facility was also observed. The combined effect of these two agents results in additional intraocular pressure reduction (IOP) compared to either component administered alone.

Following topical administration, COSOPT Preservative-Free reduces elevated intraocular pressure, whether or not associated with glaucoma. Elevated intraocular pressure is a major risk factor in the pathogenesis of optic nerve damage and glaucomatous visual field loss. COSOPT Preservative-Free reduces intraocular pressure without the common side effects of miotics such as night blindness, accommodative spasm and pupillary constriction.

Pharmacodynamic effects

Clinical Effects

Clinical studies of up to 15 months duration were conducted to compare the IOP-lowering effect of COSOPT (preserved formulation) b.i.d. (dosed morning and bedtime) to individually- and concomitantly-administered 0.5% timolol and 2.0% dorzolamide in patients with glaucoma or ocular hypertension for whom concomitant therapy was considered appropriate in the trials. This included both untreated patients and patients inadequately controlled with timolol monotherapy. The majority of patients were treated with topical beta-blocker monotherapy prior to study enrolment. In an analysis of the combined studies, the IOP-lowering effect of COSOPT (preserved formulation) b.i.d. was greater than that of monotherapy with either 2% dorzolamide t.i.d. or 0.5% timolol b.i.d. The IOP-lowering effect of COSOPT (preserved formulation) b.i.d. was equivalent to that of concomitant therapy with dorzolamide b.i.d. and timolol b.i.d. The IOP-lowering effect of COSOPT (preserved formulation) b.i.d. was demonstrated when measured at various time points throughout the day and this effect was maintained during long-term administration.

In an active-treatment-controlled, parallel, double-masked study in 261 patients with elevated intraocular pressure ≥ 22 mmHg in one or both eyes, COSOPT Preservative-Free had an IOP-lowering effect equivalent to that of COSOPT (preserved formulation). The safety profile of COSOPT Preservative-Free was similar to COSOPT (preserved formulation).

Paediatric use

A 3 month controlled study, with the primary objective of documenting the safety of 2% dorzolamide hydrochloride ophthalmic solution in children under the age of 6 years has been conducted. In this study, 30 patients under 6 and greater than or equal to 2 years of age whose IOP was not adequately controlled with monotherapy by dorzolamide or timolol received COSOPT (preserved formulation) in an open label phase. Efficacy in those patients has not been established. In this small group of patients, twice daily administration of COSOPT (preserved formulation) was generally well tolerated with 19 patients completing the treatment period and 11 patients discontinuing for surgery, a change in medication, or other reasons.

5.2 Pharmacokinetic properties

Dorzolamide Hydrochloride

Unlike oral carbonic anhydrase inhibitors, topical administration of dorzolamide hydrochloride allows for the active substance to exert its effects directly in the eye at substantially lower doses and therefore with less systemic exposure. In clinical trials, this resulted in a reduction in IOP without the acid-base disturbances or alterations in electrolytes characteristic of oral carbonic anhydrase inhibitors.

When topically applied, dorzolamide reaches the systemic circulation. To assess the potential for systemic carbonic anhydrase inhibition following topical administration, active substance and metabolite concentrations in red blood cells (RBCs) and plasma and carbonic anhydrase inhibition in RBCs were measured. Dorzolamide accumulates in RBCs during chronic dosing as a result of selective binding to CA-II while extremely low concentrations of free active substance in plasma are maintained. The parent active substance forms a single N-desethyl metabolite that inhibits CA-II less potently than the parent active substance but also inhibits a less active isoenzyme (CA-I). The metabolite also accumulates in RBCs where it binds primarily to CA-I. Dorzolamide binds moderately to plasma proteins (approximately 33%). Dorzolamide is primarily excreted unchanged in the urine; the metabolite is also excreted in urine. After dosing ends, dorzolamide washes out of RBCs non-linearly, resulting in a rapid decline of active substance concentration initially, followed by a slower elimination phase with a half-life of about four months.

When dorzolamide was given orally to simulate the maximum systemic exposure after long term topical ocular administration, steady state was reached within 13 weeks. At steady state, there was virtually no free active substance or metabolite in plasma; CA inhibition in RBCs was less than that anticipated to be necessary for a pharmacological effect on renal function or respiration. Similar pharmacokinetic results were observed after chronic, topical administration of dorzolamide hydrochloride. However, some elderly patients with renal impairment (estimated CrCl 30-60 ml/min) had higher metabolite concentrations in RBCs, but no meaningful differences in carbonic anhydrase inhibition and no clinically significant systemic side effects were directly attributable to this finding.

Timolol Maleate

In a study of plasma active substance concentration in six subjects, the systemic exposure to timolol was determined following twice daily topical administration of timolol maleate ophthalmic solution 0.5%. The mean peak plasma concentration following morning dosing was 0.46 ng/ml and following afternoon dosing was 0.35 ng/ml.

5.3 Preclinical safety data

The ocular and systemic safety profile of the individual components is well established.

Dorzolamide

In rabbits given maternotoxic doses of dorzolamide associated with metabolic acidosis, malformations of the vertebral body were observed.

Timolol

Animal studies have not shown teratogenic effect.

Furthermore, no adverse ocular effects were seen in animals treated topically with dorzolamide hydrochloride and timolol maleate ophthalmic solution or with concomitantly-administered dorzolamide hydrochloride and timolol maleate. *In vitro* and *in vivo* studies with each of the components did not reveal a mutagenic potential. Therefore, no significant risk for human safety is expected with therapeutic doses of COSOPT Preservative-Free.

6. PHARMACEUTICAL PARTICULARS

6.1 List of excipients

Hydroxyethyl cellulose

Mannitol (E421)

Sodium citrate (E331)

Sodium hydroxide (E524) for pH adjustment

Water for injections.

6.2 Incompatibilities

Not applicable.

6.3 Shelf life

2 years.

After first opening of the sachet: 15 days. Discard any unused single dose containers after that time.

Discard the opened single dose container immediately after first use.

6.4 Special precautions for storage

Do not store above 30°C.

Do not freeze.

Store in the original package in order to protect from light.

6.5 Nature and contents of container

COSOPT Preservative-Free is available in 0.2 ml low density polyethylene single dose containers in an aluminium sachet containing 15 single-dose containers.

Pack sizes:

30 × 0.2 ml (2 sachets with 15 single dose containers)

60 × 0.2 ml (4 sachets with 15 single dose containers)

120 × 0.2 ml (8 sachets with 15 single dose containers)

Not all pack sizes may be marketed.

6.6 Special precautions for disposal and other handling

No special requirements.

7. MARKETING AUTHORISATION HOLDER

Merck Sharp & Dohme Limited

Hertford Road, Hoddesdon, Hertfordshire EN11 9BU, UK.

8. MARKETING AUTHORISATION NUMBER(S)

PL 0025/0698

9. DATE OF FIRST AUTHORISATION/RENEWAL OF THE AUTHORISATION

9 August 2006 / 10 December 2008

10. DATE OF REVISION OF THE TEXT

February 2009

LEGAL CATEGORY

POM

® denotes registered trademark of Merck & Co., Inc., Whitehouse Station, NJ, USA.

MSD (logo)

Merck Sharp & Dohme Limited

Hertford Road, Hoddesdon, Hertfordshire EN11 9BU, UK

SPC.CST-PF.07.UK.2465 (II-036 + R2) F.T. 04.03.09

Coversyl Arginine

(Servier Laboratories Limited)

1. NAME OF THE MEDICINAL PRODUCT

COVERSYL ARGININE 2.5 mg tablets

COVERSYL ARGININE 5 mg tablets

COVERSYL ARGININE 10 mg tablets

2. QUALITATIVE AND QUANTITATIVE COMPOSITION

Perindopril arginine.

2.5mg One film-coated tablet contains 1.6975 mg perindopril corresponding to 2.5 mg perindopril arginine.

5mg One film-coated tablet contains 3.395 mg perindopril corresponding to 5 mg perindopril arginine.

10mg One film-coated tablet contains 6.790 mg perindopril corresponding to 10 mg perindopril arginine.

Excipient: lactose.

For a full list of excipients, see section 6.1.

3. PHARMACEUTICAL FORM

Film-coated tablet.

2.5 mg White, round, convex, film-coated tablet.

5mg Light-green, rod-shaped film-coated tablet engraved with on one face and scored on both edges. The tablet can be divided into equal halves.

10mg Green, round, biconvex, film-coated tablet engraved with on one face and on the other face.

4. CLINICAL PARTICULARS

4.1 Therapeutic indications

Hypertension:

Treatment of hypertension.

Heart failure:

Treatment of symptomatic heart failure.

Stable coronary artery disease:

Reduction of risk of cardiac events in patients with a history of myocardial infarction and/or revascularisation.

4.2 Posology and method of administration

It is recommended that COVERSYL ARGININE is taken once daily in the morning before a meal.

The dose should be individualised according to the patient profile (see section 4.4) and blood pressure response.

Hypertension:

COVERSYL ARGININE may be used in monotherapy or in combination with other classes of anti-hypertensive therapy.

The recommended starting dose is 5 mg given once daily in the morning.

Patients with a strongly activated renin-angiotensin-aldosterone system (in particular, renovascular hypertension, salt and/or volume depletion, cardiac decompensation or severe hypertension) may experience an excessive drop in blood pressure following the initial dose. A starting dose of 2.5 mg is recommended in such patients and the initiation of treatment should take place under medical supervision.

The dose may be increased to 10 mg once daily after one month of treatment.

Symptomatic hypotension may occur following initiation of therapy with COVERSYL ARGININE; this is more likely in patients who are being treated concurrently with diuretics. Caution is therefore recommended since these patients may be volume and/or salt depleted.

If possible, the diuretic should be discontinued 2 to 3 days before beginning therapy with COVERSYL ARGININE (see section 4.4).

In hypertensive patients in whom the diuretic cannot be discontinued, therapy with COVERSYL ARGININE should be initiated with a 2.5 mg dose. Renal function and serum potassium should be monitored. The subsequent dosage of COVERSYL ARGININE should be adjusted according to blood pressure response. If required, diuretic therapy may be resumed.

In elderly patients treatment should be initiated at a dose of 2.5 mg which may be progressively increased to 5 mg after one month then to 10 mg if necessary depending on renal function (see table below).

Symptomatic heart failure:

It is recommended that COVERSYL ARGININE, generally associated with a non-potassium-sparing diuretic and/or digoxin and/or a beta-blocker, be introduced under close medical supervision with a recommended starting dose of 2.5 mg taken in the morning. This dose may be increased after 2 weeks to 5 mg once daily if tolerated. The dose adjustment should be based on the clinical response of the individual patient.

In severe heart failure and in other patients considered to be at high risk (patients with impaired renal function and a tendency to have electrolyte disturbances, patients receiving simultaneous treatment with diuretics and/or treatment with vasodilating agents), treatment should be initiated under careful supervision (see section 4.4).

Patients at high risk of symptomatic hypotension e.g. patients with salt depletion with or without hyponatraemia, patients with hypovolaemia or patients who have been receiving vigorous diuretic therapy should have these conditions corrected, if possible, prior to therapy with COVERSYL ARGININE. Blood pressure, renal function and serum potassium should be monitored closely, both before and during treatment with COVERSYL ARGININE (see section 4.4).

Stable coronary artery disease:

COVERSYL ARGININE should be introduced at a dose of 5 mg once daily for two weeks, then increased to 10 mg once daily, depending on renal function and provided that the 5 mg dose is well tolerated.

Elderly patients should receive 2.5 mg once daily for one week, then 5 mg once daily the next week, before increasing the dose up to 10 mg once daily depending on renal function (see Table 1 "Dosage adjustment in renal impairment"). The dose should be increased only if the previous lower dose is well tolerated.

Dosage adjustment in renal impairment:

Dosage in patients with renal impairment should be based on creatinine clearance as outlined in table 1 below:

Table 1: dosage adjustment in renal impairment

Creatinine clearance (ml/min)	Recommended dose
$Cl_{CR} \geq 60$	5 mg per day
$30 < Cl_{CR} < 60$	2.5 mg per day
$15 < Cl_{CR} < 30$	2.5 mg every other day
Haemodialysed patients *	
$Cl_{CR} < 15$	2.5 mg on the day of dialysis

* Dialysis clearance of perindoprilat is 70 ml/min.

For patients on haemodialysis, the dose should be taken after dialysis.

Dosage adjustment in hepatic impairment:

No dosage adjustment is necessary in patients with hepatic impairment (see sections 4.4 and 5.2).

Children and adolescents (less than 18 years of age):

Efficacy and safety of use in children and adolescents have not been established. Therefore, use in children and adolescents is not recommended.

4.3 Contraindications

- Hypersensitivity to perindopril, to any of the excipients or to any other ACE inhibitor;
- History of angioedema associated with previous ACE inhibitor therapy;
- Hereditary or idiopathic angioedema;
- Second and third trimesters of pregnancy (see sections 4.4 and 4.6).

4.4 Special warnings and precautions for use

Stable coronary artery disease:

If an episode of unstable angina pectoris (major or not) occurs during the first month of perindopril treatment, a careful appraisal of the benefit/risk should be performed before treatment continuation.

Hypotension:

ACE inhibitors may cause a fall in blood pressure. Symptomatic hypotension is seen rarely in uncomplicated hypertensive patients and is more likely to occur in patients who have been volume-depleted e.g. by diuretic therapy, dietary salt restriction, dialysis, diarrhoea or vomiting, or who have severe renin-dependent hypertension (see sections 4.5 and 4.8). In patients with symptomatic heart failure, with or without associated renal insufficiency, symptomatic hypotension has been observed. This is most likely to occur in those patients with more severe degrees of heart failure, as reflected by the use of high doses of loop diuretics, hyponatraemia or functional renal impairment. In patients at increased risk of symptomatic hypotension, initiation of therapy and dose adjustment should be closely monitored (see sections 4.2 and 4.8). Similar considerations apply to patients with ischaemic heart or cerebrovascular disease in whom an excessive fall in blood pressure could result in a myocardial infarction or cerebrovascular accident.

If hypotension occurs, the patient should be placed in the supine position and, if necessary, should receive an intravenous infusion of sodium chloride 9 mg/ml (0.9%) solution. A transient hypotensive response is not a contraindication to further doses, which can be given usually without difficulty once the blood pressure has increased after volume expansion. In some patients with congestive heart failure who have normal or low blood pressure, additional lowering of systemic blood pressure may occur with COVERSYL ARGININE. This effect is anticipated and is usually not a reason to discontinue treatment. If hypotension becomes symptomatic, a reduction of dose or discontinuation of COVERSYL ARGININE may be necessary.

Aortic and mitral valve stenosis / hypertrophic cardiomyopathy:

As with other ACE inhibitors, COVERSYL ARGININE should be given with caution to patients with mitral valve stenosis and obstruction in the outflow of the left ventricle such as aortic stenosis or hypertrophic cardiomyopathy.

Renal impairment:

In cases of renal impairment (creatinine clearance < 60 ml/min) the initial perindopril dosage should be adjusted according to the patient's creatinine clearance (see section

4.2) and then as a function of the patient's response to treatment. Routine monitoring of potassium and creatinine are part of normal medical practice for these patients (see section 4.8).

In patients with symptomatic heart failure, hypotension following the initiation of therapy with ACE inhibitors may lead to some further impairment in renal function. Acute renal failure, usually reversible, has been reported in this situation.

In some patients with bilateral renal artery stenosis or stenosis of the artery to a solitary kidney, who have been treated with ACE inhibitors, increases in blood urea and serum creatinine, usually reversible upon discontinuation of therapy, have been seen. This is especially likely in patients with renal insufficiency. If renovascular hypertension is also present there is an increased risk of severe hypotension and renal insufficiency. In these patients, treatment should be started under close medical supervision with low doses and careful dose titration. Since treatment with diuretics may be a contributory factor to the above, they should be discontinued and renal function should be monitored during the first weeks of COVERSYL ARGININE therapy.

Some hypertensive patients with no apparent pre-existing renal vascular disease have developed increases in blood urea and serum creatinine, usually minor and transient, especially when COVERSYL ARGININE has been given concomitantly with a diuretic. This is more likely to occur in patients with pre-existing renal impairment. Dosage reduction and/or discontinuation of the diuretic and/or COVERSYL ARGININE may be required.

Haemodialysis patients:

Anaphylactoid reactions have been reported in patients dialysed with high flux membranes, and treated concomitantly with an ACE inhibitor. In these patients consideration should be given to using a different type of dialysis membrane or different class of anti-hypertensive agent.

Kidney transplantation:

There is no experience regarding the administration of COVERSYL ARGININE in patients with a recent kidney transplantation.

Hypersensitivity/Angioedema:

Angioedema of the face, extremities, lips, mucous membranes, tongue, glottis and/or larynx has been reported rarely in patients treated with ACE inhibitors, including COVERSYL ARGININE (see section 4.8). This may occur at any time during therapy. In such cases, COVERSYL ARGININE should promptly be discontinued and appropriate monitoring should be initiated and continued until complete resolution of symptoms has occurred. In those instances where swelling was confined to the face and lips the condition generally resolved without treatment, although antihistamines have been useful in relieving symptoms.

Angioedema associated with laryngeal oedema may be fatal. Where there is involvement of the tongue, glottis or larynx, likely to cause airway obstruction, emergency therapy should be administered promptly. This may include the administration of adrenaline and/or the maintenance of a patent airway. The patient should be under close medical supervision until complete and sustained resolution of symptoms has occurred.

Patients with a history of angioedema unrelated to ACE inhibitor therapy may be at increased risk of angioedema while receiving an ACE inhibitor (see section 4.3).

Intestinal angioedema has been reported rarely in patients treated with ACE inhibitors. These patients presented with abdominal pain (with or without nausea or vomiting); in some cases there was no prior facial angioedema and C-1 esterase levels were normal. The angioedema was diagnosed by procedures including abdominal CT scan, or ultrasound or at surgery and symptoms resolved after stopping the ACE inhibitor. Intestinal angioedema should be included in the differential diagnosis of patients on ACE inhibitors presenting with abdominal pain.

Anaphylactoid reactions during low-density lipoproteins (LDL) apheresis:

Rarely, patients receiving ACE inhibitors during low-density lipoprotein (LDL) apheresis with dextran sulphate have experienced life-threatening anaphylactoid reactions. These reactions were avoided by temporarily withholding ACE inhibitor therapy prior to each apheresis.

Anaphylactic reactions during desensitisation:

Patients receiving ACE inhibitors during desensitisation treatment (e.g. hymenoptera venom) have experienced anaphylactoid reactions. In the same patients, these reactions have been avoided when the ACE inhibitors were temporarily withheld, but they reappeared upon inadvertent rechallenge.

Hepatic failure:

Rarely, ACE inhibitors have been associated with a syndrome that starts with cholestatic jaundice and progresses to fulminant hepatic necrosis and (sometimes) death. The mechanism of this syndrome is not understood. Patients receiving ACE inhibitors who develop jaundice or marked elevations of hepatic enzymes should discontinue the ACE inhibitor and receive appropriate medical follow-up (see section 4.8).

Neutropenia/Agranulocytosis/Thrombocytopenia/Anaemia:

Neutropenia/agranulocytosis, thrombocytopenia and anaemia have been reported in patients receiving ACE inhibitors. In patients with normal renal function and no other complicating factors, neutropenia occurs rarely. Perindopril should be used with extreme caution in patients with collagen vascular disease, immunosuppressant therapy, treatment with allopurinol or procainamide, or a combination of these complicating factors, especially if there is pre-existing impaired renal function. Some of these patients developed serious infections, which in a few instances did not respond to intensive antibiotic therapy. If perindopril is used in such patients, periodic monitoring of white blood cell counts is advised and patients should be instructed to report any sign of infection (e.g. sore throat, fever).

Race:

ACE inhibitors cause a higher rate of angioedema in black patients than in non-black patients.

As with other ACE inhibitors, perindopril may be less effective in lowering blood pressure in black people than in non-blacks, possibly because of a higher prevalence of low-renin states in the black hypertensive population.

Cough:

Cough has been reported with the use of ACE inhibitors. Characteristically, the cough is non-productive, persistent and resolves after discontinuation of therapy. ACE inhibitor-induced cough should be considered as part of the differential diagnosis of cough.

Surgery/Anaesthesia:

In patients undergoing major surgery or during anaesthesia with agents that produce hypotension, COVERSYL ARGININE may block angiotensin II formation secondary to compensatory renin release. The treatment should be discontinued one day prior to the surgery. If hypotension occurs and is considered to be due to this mechanism, it can be corrected by volume expansion.

Hyperkalaemia:

Elevations in serum potassium have been observed in some patients treated with ACE inhibitors, including perindopril. Risk factors for the development of hyperkalaemia include those with renal insufficiency, worsening of renal function, age (> 70 years), diabetes mellitus, inter-current events, in particular dehydration, acute cardiac decompensation, metabolic acidosis and concomitant use of potassium-sparing diuretics (e.g. spironolactone, eplerenone, triamterene, or amiloride), potassium supplements or potassium-containing salt substitutes; or those patients taking other drugs associated with increases in serum potassium (e.g. heparin). The use of potassium supplements, potassium-sparing diuretics, or potassium-containing salt substitutes particularly in patients with impaired renal function may lead to a significant increase in serum potassium. Hyperkalaemia can cause serious, sometimes fatal arrhythmias. If concomitant use of the above-mentioned agents is deemed appropriate, they should be used with caution and with frequent monitoring of serum potassium (see section 4.5).

Diabetic patients:

In diabetic patients treated with oral antidiabetic agents or insulin, glycaemic control should be closely monitored during the first month of treatment with an ACE inhibitor (see section 4.5).

Lithium:

The combination of lithium and perindopril is generally not recommended (see section 4.5).

Potassium sparing diuretics, potassium supplements or potassium-containing salt substitutes

The combination of perindopril and potassium sparing diuretics, potassium supplements or potassium-containing salt substitutes is generally not recommended (see section 4.5).

Pregnancy:

ACE inhibitors should not be initiated during pregnancy. Unless continued ACE inhibitor therapy is considered essential, patients planning pregnancy should be changed to alternative anti-hypertensive treatments which have an established safety profile for use in pregnancy. When pregnancy is diagnosed, treatment with ACE inhibitors should be stopped immediately, and, if appropriate, alternative therapy should be started (see sections 4.3 and 4.6).

Excipients:

Due to the presence of lactose, patients with rare hereditary problems of galactose intolerance, glucose-galactose malabsorption, or the Lapp lactase deficiency should not take this medicinal product.

4.5 Interaction with other medicinal products and other forms of interaction

Diuretics:

Patients on diuretics, and especially those who are volume and/or salt depleted, may experience excessive reduction in blood pressure after initiation of therapy with an ACE inhibitor. The possibility of hypotensive effects can be reduced by discontinuation of the diuretic, by increasing volume or salt intake prior to initiating therapy with low and progressive doses of perindopril.

Potassium sparing diuretics, potassium supplements or potassium-containing salt substitutes:

Although serum potassium usually remains within normal limits, hyperkalaemia may occur in some patients treated with perindopril. Potassium sparing diuretics (e.g. spironolactone, triamterene, or amiloride), potassium supplements, or potassium-containing salt substitutes may lead to significant increases in serum potassium. Therefore the combination of perindopril with the above-mentioned drugs is not recommended (see section 4.4). If concomitant use is indicated because of demonstrated hypokalaemia they should be used with caution and with frequent monitoring of serum potassium.

Lithium:

Reversible increases in serum lithium concentrations and toxicity have been reported during concomitant administration of lithium with ACE inhibitors. Concomitant use of thiazide diuretics may increase the risk of lithium toxicity and enhance the already increased risk of lithium toxicity with ACE inhibitors. Use of perindopril with lithium is not recommended, but if the combination proves necessary, careful monitoring of serum lithium levels should be performed (see section 4.4).

Non-steroidal anti-inflammatory medicinal products (NSAIDs) including aspirin ⩾ 3 g/day:

When ACE-inhibitors are administered simultaneously with non-steroidal anti-inflammatory drugs (i.e. acetylsalicylic acid at anti-inflammatory dosage regimens, COX-2 inhibitors and non-selective NSAIDs), attenuation of the anti-hypertensive effect may occur. Concomitant use of ACE-inhibitors and NSAIDs may lead to an increased risk of worsening of renal function, including possible acute renal failure, and an increase in serum potassium, especially in patients with poor pre-existing renal function. The combination should be administered with caution, especially in the elderly. Patients should be adequately hydrated and consideration should be given to monitoring renal function after initiation of concomitant therapy, and periodically thereafter.

Anti-hypertensive agents and vasodilators:

Concomitant use of these agents may increase the hypotensive effects of perindopril. Concomitant use with nitroglycerin and other nitrates, or other vasodilators, may further reduce blood pressure.

Antidiabetic agents:

Epidemiological studies have suggested that concomitant administration of ACE inhibitors and antidiabetic medicines (insulins, oral hypoglycaemic agents) may cause an increased blood-glucose lowering effect with risk of hypoglycaemia. This phenomenon appeared to be more likely to occur during the first weeks of combined treatment and in patients with renal impairment.

Tricyclic antidepressants/Antipsychotics/Anaesthetics:

Concomitant use of certain anaesthetic medicinal products, tricyclic antidepressants and antipsychotics with ACE inhibitors may result in further reduction of blood pressure (see section 4.4).

Sympathomimetics:

Sympathomimetics may reduce the anti-hypertensive effects of ACE inhibitors.

Acetylsalicylic acid, thrombolytics, beta-blockers, nitrates:

Perindopril may be used concomitantly with acetylsalicylic acid (when used as a thrombolytic), thrombolytics, beta-blockers and/or nitrates.

Gold:

Nitritoid reactions (symptoms include facial flushing, nausea, vomiting and hypotension) have been reported rarely in patients on therapy with injectable gold (sodium aurothiomalate) and concomitant ACE inhibitor therapy including perindopril.

4.6 Pregnancy and lactation

Pregnancy:

The use of ACE inhibitors is not recommended during the first trimester of pregnancy (see section 4.4). The use of ACE inhibitors is contra-indicated during the 2nd and 3rd trimesters of pregnancy (see sections 4.3 and 4.4).

Epidemiological evidence regarding the risk of teratogenicity following exposure to ACE inhibitors during the first trimester of pregnancy has not been conclusive; however a small increase in risk cannot be excluded. Unless continued ACE inhibitor therapy is considered essential, patients planning pregnancy should be changed to alternative anti-hypertensive treatments which have an established safety profile for use in pregnancy. When pregnancy is diagnosed, treatment with ACE inhibitors should be stopped immediately, and, if appropriate, alternative therapy should be started.

Exposure to ACE inhibitor therapy during the second and third trimesters is known to induce human foeto-toxicity (decreased renal function, oligohydramnios, skull ossification retardation) and neonatal toxicity (renal failure, hypotension, hyperkalaemia) (see section 5.3). Should exposure to ACE inhibitor have occurred from the second trimester of pregnancy, ultrasound check of renal function and skull is recommended. Infants whose mothers have taken ACE inhibitors should be closely observed for hypotension (see also sections 4.3 and 4.4).

Lactation:

Because no information is available regarding the use of COVERSYL ARGININE during breast-feeding, COVERSYL ARGININE is not recommended and alternative treatments with better established safety profiles during breast-feeding are preferable, especially while nursing a newborn or preterm infant.

4.7 Effects on ability to drive and use machines

COVERSYL ARGININE has no direct influence on the ability to drive and use machines but individual reactions related to low blood pressure may occur in some patients, particularly at the start of treatment or in combination with another anti-hypertensive medication.

As a result the ability to drive or operate machinery may be impaired.

4.8 Undesirable effects

The following undesirable effects have been observed during treatment with perindopril and ranked under the following frequency:

Very common ($\geqslant$1/10); common ($\geqslant$1/100, $<$1/10); uncommon ($\geqslant$1/1000, $<$1/100); rare ($\geqslant$1/10000, $<$1/1000); very rare ($<$1/10000); not known (cannot be estimated from the available data).

Blood and lymphatic system disorders:

Decreases in haemoglobin and haematocrit, thrombocytopenia, leucopenia/neutropenia, and cases of agranulocytosis or pancytopenia, have been reported very rarely. In patients with a congenital deficiency of G-6PDH, very rare cases of haemolytic anaemia have been reported (see section 4.4).

Metabolism and nutrition disorders:

Not known: hypoglycaemia (see sections 4.4 and 4.5).

Psychiatric disorders:

Uncommon: mood or sleep disturbances.

Nervous system disorders:

Common: headache, dizziness, vertigo, paresthaesia.

Very rare: confusion.

Eye disorders:

Common: vision disturbance.

Ear and labyrinth disorders:

Common: tinnitus.

Cardiac disorders:

Very rare: arrhythmia, angina pectoris and myocardial infarction, possibly secondary to excessive hypotension in high-risk patients (see section 4.4).

Vascular disorders:

Common: hypotension and effects related to hypotension.

Very rare: stroke, possibly secondary to excessive hypotension in high-risk patients (see section 4.4).

Not known: vasculitis.

Respiratory, thoracic and mediastinal disorders:

Common: cough, dyspnoea.

Uncommon: bronchospasm.

Very rare: eosinophilic pneumonia, rhinitis.

Gastro-intestinal disorders:

Common: nausea, vomiting, abdominal pain, dysgeusia, dyspepsia, diarrhoea, constipation.

Uncommon: dry mouth.

Very rare: pancreatitis.

Hepato-biliary disorders:

Very rare: hepatitis either cytolytic or cholestatic (see section 4.4).

Skin and subcutaneous tissue disorders:

Common: rash, pruritus.

Uncommon: angioedema of face, extremities, lips, mucous membranes, tongue, glottis and/or larynx, urticaria (see section 4.4).

Very rare: erythema multiforme.

Musculoskeletal and connective tissue disorders:

Common: muscle cramps.

Renal and urinary disorders:

Uncommon: renal insufficiency.

Very rare: acute renal failure.

Reproductive system and breast disorders:

Uncommon: impotence.

General disorders and administration site conditions:

Common: asthenia.

Uncommon: sweating.

Investigations:

Increases in blood urea and plasma creatinine, hyperkalaemia reversible on discontinuation may occur, especially in the presence of renal insufficiency, severe heart failure and renovascular hypertension. Elevation of liver enzymes and serum bilirubin have been reported rarely.

Clinical trials:

During the randomised period of the EUROPA study, only serious adverse events were collected. Few patients experienced serious adverse events: 16 (0.3%) of the 6122 perindopril patients and 12 (0.2%) of the 6107 placebo patients. In perindopril-treated patients, hypotension was observed in 6 patients, angioedema in 3 patients and sudden cardiac arrest in 1 patient. More patients withdrew for cough, hypotension or other intolerance on perindopril than on placebo, 6.0% (n=366) versus 2.1% (n=129) respectively.

4.9 Overdose

Limited data are available for overdosage in humans. Symptoms associated with overdosage of ACE inhibitors may include hypotension, circulatory shock, electrolyte disturbances, renal failure, hyperventilation, tachycardia, palpitations, bradycardia, dizziness, anxiety, and cough.

The recommended treatment of overdosage is intravenous infusion of sodium chloride 9 mg/ml (0.9%) solution. If hypotension occurs, the patient should be placed in the shock position. If available, treatment with angiotensin II infusion and/or intravenous catecholamines may also be considered. Perindopril may be removed from the general circulation by haemodialysis (see section 4.4). Pacemaker therapy is indicated for therapy-resistant bradycardia. Vital signs, serum electrolytes and creatinine concentrations should be monitored continuously.

5. PHARMACOLOGICAL PROPERTIES

5.1 Pharmacodynamic properties

Pharmacotherapeutic group: ACE inhibitor, plain, ATC code: C09A A04

Perindopril is an inhibitor of the enzyme that converts angiotensin I into angiotensin II (Angiotensin Converting Enzyme ACE). The converting enzyme, or kinase, is an exopeptidase that allows conversion of angiotensin I into the vasoconstrictor angiotensin II as well as causing the degradation of the vasodilator bradykinin into an inactive heptapeptide. Inhibition of ACE results in a reduction of angiotensin II in the plasma, which leads to increased plasma renin activity (by inhibition of the negative feedback of renin release) and reduced secretion of aldosterone. Since ACE inactivates bradykinin, inhibition of ACE also results in an increased activity of circulating and local kallikrein-kinin systems (and thus also activation of the prostaglandin system). It is possible that this mechanism contributes to the blood pressure-lowering action of ACE inhibitors and is partially responsible for certain of their side effects (e.g. cough).

Perindopril acts through its active metabolite, perindoprilat. The other metabolites show no inhibition of ACE activity *in vitro*.

Hypertension:

Perindopril is active in all grades of hypertension: mild, moderate, severe; a reduction in systolic and diastolic blood pressures in both supine and standing positions is observed.

Perindopril reduces peripheral vascular resistance, leading to blood pressure reduction. As a consequence, peripheral blood flow increases, with no effect on heart rate.

Renal blood flow increases as a rule, while the glomerular filtration rate (GFR) is usually unchanged.

The anti-hypertensive activity is maximal between 4 and 6 hours after a single dose and is sustained for at least 24 hours: trough effects are about 87-100 % of peak effects.

The decrease in blood pressure occurs rapidly. In responding patients, normalisation is achieved within a month and persists without the occurrence of tachyphylaxis.

Discontinuation of treatment does not lead to a rebound effect.

Perindopril reduces left ventricular hypertrophy.

In man, perindopril has been confirmed to demonstrate vasodilatory properties. It improves large artery elasticity and decreases the media: lumen ratio of small arteries.

An adjunctive therapy with a thiazide diuretic produces an additive-type of synergy. The combination of an ACE inhibitor and a thiazide also decreases the risk of hypokalaemia induced by the diuretic treatment.

Heart failure:

Perindopril reduces cardiac work by a decrease in pre-load and after-load.

Studies in patients with heart failure have demonstrated:

- decreased left and right ventricular filling pressures,
- reduced total peripheral vascular resistance,
- increased cardiac output and improved cardiac index.

In comparative studies, the first administration of 2.5 mg of perindopril arginine to patients with mild to moderate heart failure was not associated with any significant reduction of blood pressure as compared to placebo.

Patients with stable coronary artery disease:

The EUROPA study was a multicentre, international, randomised, double-blind, placebo-controlled clinical trial lasting 4 years.

Twelve thousand two hundred and eighteen (12218) patients aged over 18 were randomised to 8 mg perindopril tert-butylamine (equivalent to 10 mg perindopril arginine) (n=6110) or placebo (n=6108).

The trial population had evidence of coronary artery disease with no evidence of clinical signs of heart failure. Overall, 90% of the patients had a previous myocardial infarction and/or a previous coronary revascularisation. Most of the patients received the study medication on top of conventional therapy including platelet inhibitors, lipid lowering agents and beta-blockers.

The main efficacy criterion was the composite of cardiovascular mortality, non-fatal myocardial infarction and/or cardiac arrest with successful resuscitation. The treatment with 8 mg perindopril tert-butylamine (equivalent to 10 mg perindopril arginine) once daily resulted in a significant absolute reduction in the primary endpoint of 1.9% (relative risk reduction of 20%, 95%CI [9.4; 28.6] – $p<0.001$).

In patients with a history of myocardial infarction and/or revascularisation, an absolute reduction of 2.2% corresponding to a RRR of 22.4% (95%CI [12.0; 31.6] – $p<0.001$) in the primary endpoint was observed by comparison to placebo.

5.2 Pharmacokinetic properties

After oral administration, the absorption of perindopril is rapid and the peak concentration is achieved within 1 hour. The plasma half-life of perindopril is equal to 1 hour.

Perindopril is a pro-drug. Twenty seven percent of the administered perindopril dose reaches the bloodstream as the active metabolite perindoprilat. In addition to active perindoprilat, perindopril yields five metabolites, all inactive. The peak plasma concentration of perindoprilat is achieved within 3 to 4 hours.

As ingestion of food decreases conversion to perindoprilat, hence bioavailability, perindopril arginine should be administered orally in a single daily dose in the morning before a meal.

It has been demonstrated a linear relationship between the dose of perindopril and its plasma exposure.

The volume of distribution is approximately 0.2 l/kg for unbound perindoprilat. Protein binding of perindoprilat to plasma proteins is 20%, principally to angiotensin converting enzyme, but is concentration-dependent.

Perindoprilat is eliminated in the urine and the terminal half-life of the unbound fraction is approximately 17 hours, resulting in steady-state within 4 days.

Elimination of perindoprilat is decreased in the elderly, and also in patients with heart or renal failure. Dosage adjustment in renal insufficiency is desirable depending on the degree of impairment (creatinine clearance).

Dialysis clearance of perindoprilat is equal to 70 ml/min.

Perindopril kinetics are modified in patients with cirrhosis: hepatic clearance of the parent molecule is reduced by half. However, the quantity of perindoprilat formed is not reduced and therefore no dosage adjustment is required (see sections 4.2 and 4.4).

5.3 Preclinical safety data

In the chronic oral toxicity studies (rats and monkeys), the target organ is the kidney, with reversible damage.

No mutagenicity has been observed in *in vitro* or *in vivo* studies.

Reproduction toxicology studies (rats, mice, rabbits and monkeys) showed no sign of embryotoxicity or teratogenicity. However, angiotensin converting enzyme inhibitors, as a class, have been shown to induce adverse effects on late foetal development, resulting in foetal death and congenital effects in rodents and rabbits: renal lesions and an increase in peri- and postnatal mortality have been observed.

No carcinogenicity has been observed in long-term studies in rats and mice.

6. PHARMACEUTICAL PARTICULARS

6.1 List of excipients

Core:

Lactose monohydrate

Magnesium stearate

Maltodextrin

Hydrophobic colloidal silica

Sodium starch glycolate (type A)

Film-coating:

Glycerol

Hypromellose

Copper chlorophyllin (not 2.5 mg)

Macrogol

Magnesium stearate

Titanium dioxide.

6.2 Incompatibilities

Not applicable.

6.3 Shelf life

3 years.

6.4 Special precautions for storage

Keep the container tightly closed in order to protect from moisture.

6.5 Nature and contents of container

5, 10, 14, 20, 30 or 50 tablets in a white polypropylene tablet container equipped with a polyethylene flow reducer and a white opaque stopper containing a desiccant gel.

Box of 1 container of 5, 10, 14, 20, 30 or 50 tablets.

Box of 2 containers of 30 or 50 tablets.

Box of 3 containers of 30 tablets.

Box of 4 containers of 30 tablets.

Box of 10 containers of 50 tablets.

Not all pack sizes may be marketed.

6.6 Special precautions for disposal and other handling

Medicines no longer required should not be disposed of via the wastewater or the municipal sewage system. Return them to a pharmacy or ask your pharmacist how to dispose of them in accordance with the national regulations. These measures will help to protect the environment.

7. MARKETING AUTHORISATION HOLDER

Les Laboratoires Servier
22, rue Garnier
92200 Neuilly-sur-Seine
France

8. MARKETING AUTHORISATION NUMBER(S)

2.5mg	PL 05815/0035
5mg	PL 05815/0036
10mg	PL 05815/0037

9. DATE OF FIRST AUTHORISATION/RENEWAL OF THE AUTHORISATION

28/02/2007

10. DATE OF REVISION OF THE TEXT

May 2009

Coversyl Arginine Plus

(Servier Laboratories Limited)

1. NAME OF THE MEDICINAL PRODUCT

COVERSYL ARGININE PLUS 5mg/1.25mg Tablets.

2. QUALITATIVE AND QUANTITATIVE COMPOSITION

One tablet contains 3.395 mg perindopril corresponding to 5 mg perindopril arginine and 1.25 mg indapamide.

Excipient: 71.33 mg lactose monohydrate

For a full list of excipients, see section 6.1.

3. PHARMACEUTICAL FORM

Film-coated tablet.

White, rod-shaped film-coated tablet.

4. CLINICAL PARTICULARS

4.1 Therapeutic indications

Treatment of essential hypertension, COVERSYL ARGININE PLUS 5mg/1.25mg tablet is indicated in patients whose blood pressure is not adequately controlled on perindopril alone.

4.2 Posology and method of administration

Oral route

One COVERSYL ARGININE PLUS 5mg/1.25mg tablet per day as a single dose, preferably to be taken in the morning, and before a meal.

When possible individual dose titration with the components is recommended. COVERSYL ARGININE PLUS 5mg/1.25mg tablet should be used when blood pressure is not adequately controlled on COVERSYL ARGININE PLUS 2.5mg/0.625mg tablet (where available). When clinically appropriate, direct change from monotherapy to COVERSYL ARGININE PLUS 5mg/1.25mg tablet may be considered.

Elderly (see section 4.4)

Treatment should be initiated after considering blood pressure response and renal function.

Patients with renal impairment (see section 4.4)

In severe renal impairment (creatinine clearance below 30 ml/min), treatment is contraindicated.

In patients with moderate renal impairment (creatinine clearance 30-60 ml/min), it is recommended to start treatment with the adequate dosage of the free combination.

In patients with creatinine clearance greater than or equal to 60 ml/min, no dose modification is required. Usual medical follow-up will include frequent monitoring of creatinine and potassium.

Patients with hepatic impairment (see sections 4.3, 4.4 and 5.2)

In severe hepatic impairment, treatment is contraindicated.

In patients with moderate hepatic impairment, no dose modification is required.

Children and adolescents

COVERSYL ARGININE PLUS 5mg/1.25mg should not be used in children and adolescents as the efficacy and tolerability of perindopril in children and adolescents, alone or in combination, have not been established.

4.3 Contraindications

Linked to perindopril:

- Hypersensitivity to perindopril or any other ACE inhibitor
- History of angioedema (Quincke's oedema) associated with previous ACE inhibitor therapy
- Hereditary/idiopathic angioedema
- Second and third trimesters of pregnancy (see section 4.6)

Linked to indapamide:

- Hypersensitivity to indapamide or to any other sulphonamides
- Severe renal impairment (creatinine clearance below 30 ml/min)
- Hepatic encephalopathy
- Severe hepatic impairment
- Hypokalaemia
- As a general rule, this medicine is inadvisable in combination with non antiarrhythmic agents causing torsades de pointes (see section 4.5)
- Lactation (see section 4.6).

Linked to COVERSYL ARGININE PLUS 5mg/1.25mg:

- Hypersensitivity to any of the excipients

Due to the lack of sufficient therapeutic experience, COVERSYL ARGININE PLUS 5mg/1.25mg should not be used in:

- Dialysis patients
- Patients with untreated decompensated heart failure.

4.4 Special warnings and precautions for use

Special warnings

Common to perindopril and indapamide:

Lithium:

The combination of lithium and the combination of perindopril and indapamide is usually not recommended (see section 4.5).

Linked to perindopril:

Risk of neutropenia/agranulocytosis in immuno-suppressed patients: The risk of neutropenia appears to be dose- and type-related and is dependent on patient's clinical status. It is rarely seen in uncomplicated patients but may occur in patients with some degree of renal impairment especially when it is associated with collagen vascular disease e.g. systemic lupus erythematosus, scleroderma and therapy with immunosuppressive agents. It is reversible after discontinuation of the ACE inhibitor.

Strict compliance with the predetermined dose seems to be the best way to prevent the onset of these events. However, if an angiotensin converting enzyme inhibitor is to be administered to this type of patient, the risk/benefit ratio should be evaluated carefully.

Angioedema (Quincke's oedema):

Angioedema of the face, extremities, lips, tongue, glottis and/or larynx has been reported rarely in patients receiving treatment with angiotensin converting enzyme inhibitors, including perindopril. In such cases, treatment with perindopril should be stopped immediately and the patient should be monitored until the oedema has disappeared.

When the oedema only affects the face and the lips, the effect generally recedes without treatment, even though anti-histamines may be used to relieve symptoms.

Angioedema combined with laryngeal oedema may be fatal. Involvement of tongue, glottis or larynx may lead to an obstruction of the airways. A subcutaneous injection of adrenaline at 1:1000 (0.3 ml to 0.5 ml) should be administered quickly and other appropriate measures taken.

The prescription of an angiotensin converting enzyme inhibitor should not subsequently be considered in these patients (see section 4.3).

Patients with a previous history of Quincke's oedema which was not linked to taking an angiotensin converting enzyme inhibitor have an increased risk of Quincke's oedema with an angiotensin converting enzyme inhibitor.

Anaphylactoid reactions during desensitisation:

There have been isolated reports of patients experiencing sustained, life-threatening anaphylactoid reactions while receiving ACE inhibitors during desensitisation treatment with hymenoptera (bees, wasps) venom. ACE inhibitors should be used with caution in allergic patients treated with desensitisation, and avoided in those undergoing venom immunotherapy. However these reactions could be prevented by temporary withdrawal of ACE inhibitor for at least 24 hours before treatment in patients who require both ACE inhibitors and desensitisation.

Anaphylactoid reactions during membrane exposure:

There have been reports of patients experiencing sustained, life-threatening anaphylactoid reactions while receiving ACE inhibitors during dialysis with high-flux membranes or low-density lipoprotein apheresis with dextran sulphate adsorption. ACE inhibitors should be avoided in such patients. However these reactions could be prevented by temporary withdrawal of ACE inhibitor for at least 24 hours before treatment in patients who require both ACE inhibitors and LDL apheresis.

Potassium-sparing diuretics, potassium salts:

The combination of perindopril and potassium-sparing diuretics, potassium salts is usually not recommended (see section 4.5).

Linked to indapamide:

When liver function is impaired, thiazide diuretics and thiazide-related diuretics may cause hepatic encephalopathy. Administration of the diuretic should be stopped immediately if this occurs.

Sultopride:

The combination of indapamide and sultopride is usually not recommended (see section 4.5).

Precautions for use

Common to perindopril and indapamide:

Renal impairment:

In cases of severe renal impairment (creatinine clearance < 30 ml/min), treatment is contraindicated.

In certain hypertensive patients without pre-existing apparent renal lesions and for whom renal blood tests show functional renal insufficiency, treatment should be stopped and possibly restarted either at a low dose or with one constituent only. In these patients usual medical follow-up will include frequent monitoring of potassium and creatinine, after two weeks of treatment and then every two months during therapeutic stability period. Renal failure has been reported mainly in patients with severe heart failure or underlying renal failure including renal artery stenosis.

The drug is usually not recommended in case of bilateral renal artery stenosis or a single functioning kidney.

Hypotension and water and electrolyte depletion:

There is a risk of sudden hypotension in the presence of pre-existing sodium depletion (in particular in individuals with renal artery stenosis). Therefore systematic testing should be carried out for clinical signs of water and electrolyte depletion, which may occur with an intercurrent episode of diarrhoea or vomiting. Regular monitoring of plasma electrolytes should be carried out in such patients.

Marked hypotension may require the implementation of an intravenous infusion of isotonic saline.

Transient hypotension is not a contraindication to continuation of treatment. After re-establishment of a satisfactory blood volume and blood pressure, treatment can be started again either at a reduced dose or with only one of the constituents.

Potassium levels:

The combination of perindopril and indapamide does not prevent the onset of hypokalaemia particularly in diabetic patients or in patients with renal failure. As with any antihypertensive agent in combination with a diuretic, regular monitoring of plasma potassium levels should be carried out.

Excipients:

COVERSYL ARGININE PLUS 5mg/1.25mg should not be administered to patients with rare hereditary problems of galactose intolerance, the Lapp lactase deficiency or glucose-galactose malabsorption.

Linked to perindopril:

Cough:

A dry cough has been reported with the use of angiotensin converting enzyme inhibitors. It is characterised by its persistence and by its disappearance when treatment is withdrawn. An iatrogenic aetiology should be considered in the event of this symptom. If the prescription of an angiotensin converting enzyme inhibitor is still preferred, continuation of treatment may be considered.

Children and adolescents:

The efficacy and tolerability of perindopril in children and adolescents, alone or in combination, have not been established.

Risk of arterial hypotension and/or renal insufficiency (in cases of cardiac insufficiency, water and electrolyte depletion, etc.):

Marked stimulation of the renin-angiotensin-aldosterone system has been observed particularly during marked water and electrolyte depletions (strict sodium restricted diet or prolonged diuretic treatment), in patients whose blood pressure was initially low, in cases of renal artery stenosis, congestive heart failure or cirrhosis with oedema and ascites.

The blocking of this system with an angiotensin converting enzyme inhibitor may therefore cause, particularly at the time of the first administration and during the first two weeks of treatment, a sudden drop in blood pressure and/or an increase in plasma levels of creatinine, showing a functional renal insufficiency. Occasionally this can be acute in onset, although rare, and with a variable time to onset.

In such cases, the treatment should then be initiated at a lower dose and increased progressively.

Elderly:

Renal function and potassium levels should be tested before the start of treatment. The initial dose is subsequently adjusted according to blood pressure response, especially in cases of water and electrolyte depletion, in order to avoid sudden onset of hypotension.

Patients with known atherosclerosis:

The risk of hypotension exists in all patients but particular care should be taken in patients with ischaemic heart disease or cerebral circulatory insufficiency, with treatment being started at a low dose.

Renovascular hypertension:

The treatment for renovascular hypertension is revascularisation. Nonetheless, angiotensin converting enzyme inhibitors can be beneficial in patients presenting with renovascular hypertension who are awaiting corrective surgery or when such a surgery is not possible.

If COVERSYL ARGININE PLUS 5mg/1.25mg is prescribed to patients with known or suspected renal artery stenosis, treatment should be started in a hospital setting at a low dose and renal function and potassium levels should be monitored, since some patients have developed a functional renal insufficiency which was reversed when treatment was stopped.

Other populations at risk:

In patients with severe cardiac insufficiency (grade IV) or in patients with insulin dependent diabetes mellitus (spontaneous tendency to increased levels of potassium), treatment should be started under medical supervision with a reduced initial dose. Treatment with beta-blockers in hypertensive patients with coronary insufficiency should not be stopped: the ACE inhibitor should be added to the beta-blocker.

Anaemia:

Anaemia has been observed in patients who have had a kidney transplant or have been undergoing dialysis. The reduction in haemoglobin levels is more apparent as initial values were high. This effect does not seem to be dose-dependent but may be linked to the mechanism of action of angiotensin converting enzyme inhibitors.

This reduction in haemoglobin is slight, occurs within 1 to 6 months, and then remains stable. It is reversible when treatment is stopped. Treatment can be continued with regular haematological testing.

Surgery:

Angiotensin converting enzyme inhibitors can cause hypotension in cases of anaesthesia, especially when the anaesthetic administered is an agent with hypotensive potential.

It is therefore recommended that treatment with long-acting angiotensin converting enzyme inhibitors such as perindopril should be discontinued where possible one day before surgery.

Aortic stenosis / hypertrophic cardiomyopathy:

ACE inhibitors should be used with caution in patient with an obstruction in the outflow tract of the left ventricle.

Hepatic failure:

Rarely, ACE inhibitors have been associated with a syndrome that starts with cholestatic jaundice and progresses to fulminant hepatic necrosis and (sometimes) death. The mechanism of this syndrome is not understood. Patients receiving ACE inhibitors who develop jaundice or marked elevations of hepatic enzymes should discontinue the ACE inhibitor and receive appropriate medical follow-up (see section 4.8).

Hyperkalaemia:

Elevations in serum potassium have been observed in some patients treated with ACE inhibitors, including perindopril. Patients at risk for the development of hyperkalaemia include those with renal insufficiency, uncontrolled diabetes mellitus, or those using concomitant potassium-sparing diuretics, potassium supplements or potassium-containing salt substitutes; or those patients taking other drugs associated with increases in serum potassium (e.g. heparin). If concomitant use of the above mentioned agents is deemed appropriate, regular monitoring of serum potassium is recommended. The drug is usually not recommended in case of raised plasma levels of potassium.

Linked to indapamide:

Water and electrolyte balance:

Sodium levels:

These should be tested before treatment is started, then at regular intervals. All diuretic treatment can cause a reduction in sodium levels, which may have serious consequences. Reduction in sodium levels can be initially asymptomatic and regular testing is therefore essential. Testing should be more frequent in elderly and cirrhotic patients (see sections 4.8 and 4.9).

Potassium levels:

Potassium depletion with hypokalaemia is a major risk with thiazide diuretics and thiazide-related diuretics. The risk of onset of lowered potassium levels (< 3.4 mmol/l) should be prevented in some high risk populations such as elderly and/or malnourished subjects, whether or not they are taking multiple medications, cirrhotic patients with oedema and ascites, coronary patients and patients with heart failure.

In such cases hypokalaemia increases the cardiac toxicity of cardiac glycosides and the risk of rhythm disorders.

Subjects presenting with a long QT interval are also at risk, whether the origin is congenital or iatrogenic. Hypokalaemia, as with bradycardia, acts as a factor which favours the onset of severe rhythm disorders, in particular torsades de pointes, which may be fatal.

In all cases more frequent testing of potassium levels is necessary. The first measurement of plasma potassium levels should be carried out during the first week following the start of treatment.

If low potassium levels are detected, correction is required.

Calcium levels:

Thiazide diuretics and thiazide-related diuretics may reduce urinary excretion of calcium and cause a mild and transient increase in plasma calcium levels. Markedly raised levels of calcium may be related to undiagnosed hyperparathyroidism. In such cases the treatment should be stopped before investigating the parathyroid function.

Blood glucose:

Monitoring of blood glucose is important in diabetic patients, particularly when potassium levels are low.

Uric acid:

Tendency to gout attacks may be increased in hyperuricaemic patients.

Renal function and diuretics:

Thiazide diuretics and thiazide-related diuretics are only fully effective when renal function is normal or only slightly impaired (creatinine levels lower than approximately 25 mg/l, i.e. 220 μmol/l for an adult).

In the elderly the value of plasma creatinine levels should be adjusted to take account of the age, weight and sex of the patient, according to the Cockroft formula:

clcr = (140 - age) × body weight / 0.814 × plasma creatinine level

with: age expressed in years

body weight in kg

plasma creatinine level in micromol/l

This formula is suitable for an elderly male and should be adapted for women by multiplying the result by 0.85.

Hypovolaemia, resulting from the loss of water and sodium caused by the diuretic at the start of treatment, causes a reduction in glomerular filtration. It may result in an increase in blood urea and creatinine levels. This transitory functional renal insufficiency is of no adverse consequence in patients with normal renal function but may however worsen a pre-existing renal impairment.

Athletes:

Athletes should note that this product contains an active substance which may cause a positive reaction in doping tests.

4.5 Interaction with other medicinal products and other forms of interaction

Common to perindopril and indapamide:

Concomitant use not recommended:

Lithium: reversible increases in serum lithium concentrations and toxicity have been reported during concomitant administration of lithium with ACE inhibitors. Concomitant use of thiazide diuretics may further increase lithium levels and enhance the risk of lithium toxicity with ACE inhibitors. Use of perindopril combined with indapamide with lithium is not recommended, but if the combination proves necessary, careful monitoring of serum lithium levels should be performed (see section 4.4).

Concomitant use which requires special care:

- Baclofen: Potentiation of antihypertensive effect. Monitoring of blood pressure and renal function, and dose adaptation of the antihypertensive if necessary.

- Non-steroidal anti-inflammatory medicinal products (included acetylsalicylic acid at high doses): the administration of a non-steroidal anti-inflammatory medicinal product may reduce the diuretic, natriuretic and antihypertensive effects in some patients. In elderly patients and patients who may be dehydrated there is a risk of acute renal failure, therefore monitoring of renal function at the initiation of treatment is recommended. Patients should be well hydrated.

Concomitant use which requires some care:

- Imipramine-like antidepressants (tricyclics), neuroleptics: Increased antihypertensive effect and increased risk of orthostatic hypotension (additive effect).

- Corticosteroids, tetracosactide: Reduction in antihypertensive effect (salt and water retention due to corticosteroids).

- other antihypertensive agents: use of other antihypertensive medicinal products with perindopril/indapamide could result in additional blood pressure lowering effect.

Linked to perindopril:

Concomitant use not recommended:

- Potassium-sparing diuretics (spironolactone, triamterene, alone or in combination), potassium (salts): ACE inhibitors attenuate diuretic induced potassium loss. Potassium-sparing diuretics e.g. spironolactone, triamterene, or amiloride, potassium supplements, or potassium-containing salt substitutes may lead to significant increases in serum potassium (potentially lethal). If concomitant use is indicated because of documented hypokalaemia they should be used with caution and with frequent monitoring of serum potassium and by ECG.

Concomitant use which requires special care:

- Antidiabetic agents (insulin, hypoglycaemic sulphonamides): Reported with captopril and enalapril.

The use of angiotensin converting enzyme inhibitors may increase the hypoglycaemic effect in diabetics receiving treatment with insulin or with hypoglycaemic sulphonamides. The onset of hypoglycaemic episodes is very rare (improvement in glucose tolerance with a resulting reduction in insulin requirements).

Concomitant use which requires some care:

- Allopurinol, cytostatic or immunosuppressive agents, systemic corticosteroids or procainamide: Concomitant administration with ACE inhibitors may lead to an increased risk for leucopenia.

- Anaesthetic drugs: ACE inhibitors may enhance the hypotensive effects of certain anaesthetic drugs.

- Diuretics (thiazide or loop diuretics): Prior treatment with high dose diuretics may result in volume depletion and in a risk of hypotension when initiating therapy with perindopril.

Linked to indapamide:

Concomitant use not recommended:

- Sultopride: Increased risk of ventricular arrhythmia, especially torsades de pointes (hypokalaemia favours the occurrence of this adverse event) (see section 4.4).

Concomitant use which requires special care:

- Torsades de pointes inducing drugs: Due to the risk of hypokalaemia, indapamide should be administered with caution when associated with medicinal products that induced torsades de pointes such as class IA antiarrhythmic agents (quinidine, hydroquinidine, disopyramide); class III antiarrhythmic agents (amiodarone, dofetilide, ibutilide, bretylium, sotalol); some neuroleptics (chlorpromazine, cyamemazine, levomepromazine, thioridazine, trifluoperazine), benzamides (amisulpride, sulpiride, tiapride), butyrophenones (droperidol, haloperidol), other neuroleptics (pimozide); other substances such as bepridil, cisapride, diphemanil, IV erythromycin, halofantrine, mizolastine, moxifloxacin, pentamidine, sparfloxacin, IV vincamine, methadone, astemizole, terfenadine. Prevention of low potassium levels and correction if necessary: monitoring of the QT interval.

- Potassium-lowering drugs: amphotericin B (IV route), glucocorticoids and mineralocorticoids (systemic route), tetracosactide, stimulant laxatives: Increased risk of low potassium levels (additive effect). Monitoring of potassium levels, and correction if necessary; particular consideration required in cases of treatment with cardiac glycosides. Non stimulant laxatives should be used.

- Cardiac glycosides: Low potassium levels favour the toxic effects of cardiac glycosides. Potassium levels and ECG should be monitored and treatment reconsidered if necessary.

Concomitant use which requires some care:

- Metformin: Lactic acidosis due to metformin caused by possible functional renal insufficiency linked to diuretics and in particular to loop diuretics. Do not use metformin when plasma creatinine levels exceed 15 mg/l (135 micromol/l) in men and 12 mg/l (110 micromol/l) in women.

- Iodinated contrast media: In cases of dehydration caused by diuretics, there is an increased risk of acute renal insufficiency, particularly when high doses of iodinated contrast media are used. Rehydration should be carried out before the iodinated compound is administered.

- Calcium (salts): Risk of increased levels of calcium due to reduced elimination of calcium in the urine.

- Ciclosporin: Risk of increased creatinine levels with no change in circulating levels of ciclosporin, even when there is no salt and water depletion.

4.6 Pregnancy and lactation

Pregnancy:

COVERSYL ARGININE PLUS 5mg/1.25mg should not be used during the first trimester of pregnancy. When a pregnancy is planned or confirmed the switch to an alternative treatment should be initiated as soon as possible. Controlled studies with ACE inhibitors have not been done in humans, but in a limited number of cases with first trimester exposure there do not appear to have been any malformations consistent with human fetotoxicity as described below.

COVERSYL ARGININE PLUS 5mg/1.25mg is contraindicated during the second and third trimesters of pregnancy (see section 4.3).

Prolonged ACE inhibitors exposure during the second and third trimesters is known to induce human fetotoxicity (decreased renal function, oligohydramnios, retardation of skull ossification) and neonatal toxicity (renal failure, hypotension, hyperkalaemia) (see section 5.3).

Prolonged exposure to thiazide during the third trimester of pregnancy can reduce maternal plasma volume as well as uteroplacental blood flow, which may cause a feto-placental ischaemia and growth retardation. Moreover, rare cases of hypoglycemia and thrombocytopenia in neonates have been reported following exposure near term.

Should exposure to COVERSYL ARGININE PLUS 5mg/1.25mg have occurred from the second trimester of pregnancy, an ultrasound check of renal function and the skull is recommended.

Lactation:

COVERSYL ARGININE PLUS 5mg/1.25mg is contraindicated during lactation.

The excretion of perindopril into breast milk is unknown.

Indapamide is excreted in human milk. Indapamide is closely related to thiazide diuretics which have been associated, during breast-feeding, with decrease or even suppression of milk lactation. Hypersensitivity to sulfonamide-derived drugs, hypokalaemia and nuclear icterus might occur.

As, with both drugs, serious adverse reactions might occur in nursing infants, a decision should be made whether to discontinue nursing or to discontinue therapy taking account the importance of this therapy for the mother.

4.7 Effects on ability to drive and use machines

Linked to perindopril, indapamide and COVERSYL ARGININE PLUS 5mg/1.25mg:

Neither the two active substances nor COVERSYL ARGININE PLUS 5mg/1.25mg affect alertness but individual reactions related to low blood pressure may occur in some patients, particularly at the start of treatment or in combination with another antihypertensive medication.

As a result the ability to drive or operate machinery may be impaired.

4.8 Undesirable effects

The administration of perindopril inhibits the renin-angiotensin-aldosterone axis and tends to reduce the potassium loss caused by indapamide. Four percent of the patients on treatment with COVERSYL ARGININE PLUS 5mg/1.25mg experience hypokalaemia (potassium level < 3.4 mmol/l).

Blood and the lymphatic system disorders:

Very rare (< 1/10,000):

- Thrombocytopenia, leucopenia, agranulocytosis, aplastic anaemia, haemolytic anaemia.

- Anaemia (see section 4.4) has been reported with angiotensin converting enzyme inhibitors in specific circumstances (patients who have had kidney transplants, patients undergoing haemodialysis).

Nervous system disorders:

Uncommon (> 1/1,000, < 1/100):

- Paresthesia, headache, asthenia, feelings of dizziness, mood disturbances and/or sleep disturbances.

Vascular disorders:

Uncommon (> 1/1,000, < 1/100):

- Hypotension whether orthostatic or not (see section 4.4).

Respiratory, thoracic and mediastinal disorders:

Common (> 1/100, < 1/10):

- A dry cough has been reported with the use of angiotensin converting enzyme inhibitors. It is characterised by its persistence and by its disappearance when treatment is withdrawn. An iatrogenic aetiology should be considered in the presence of this symptom.

Gastrointestinal disorders:

Common (> 1/100, < 1/10):

- constipation, dry mouth, nausea, epigastric pain, anorexia, abdominal pains, taste disturbance

Very rare (< 1/10,000):

- pancreatitis

In case of hepatic insufficiency, there is a possibility of onset of hepatic encephalopathy (see sections 4.3 and 4.4)

Skin and subcutaneous tissue disorders:

Uncommon (> 1/1,000, < 1/100):

- Hypersensitivity reactions, mainly dermatological, in subjects with a predisposition to allergic and asthmatic reactions

- Maculopapular eruptions, purpura, possible aggravation of pre-existing acute disseminated lupus erythematosus

- Skin rash

Very rare (< 1/10,000):

- Angioedema (Quincke's oedema) (see section 4.4)

Musculoskeletal, connective tissue and bone disorders:

Uncommon (> 1/1,000, < 1/100):

- Cramps.

Investigations:

- Potassium depletion with particularly serious reduction in levels of potassium in some at risk populations (see section 4.4).

- Reduced sodium levels with hypovolaemia causing dehydration and orthostatic hypotension.

- Increase in uric acid levels and in blood glucose levels during treatment.

- Slight increase in urea and in plasma creatinine levels, reversible when treatment is stopped. This increase is more frequent in cases of renal artery stenosis, arterial hypertension treated with diuretics, renal insufficiency.

- Increased levels of potassium, usually transitory.

Rare (> 1/10,000, < 1/1,000):

- raised plasma calcium levels.

4.9 Overdose

The most likely adverse reaction in cases of overdose is hypotension, sometimes associated with nausea, vomiting, cramps, dizziness, sleepiness, mental confusion, oliguria which may progress to anuria (due to hypovolaemia). Salt and water disturbances (low sodium levels, low potassium levels) may occur.

The first measures to be taken consist of rapidly eliminating the product(s) ingested by gastric lavage and/or administration of activated charcoal, then restoring fluid and electrolyte balance in a specialised centre until they return to normal.

If marked hypotension occurs, this can be treated by placing the patient in a supine position with the head lowered. If necessary an intravenous infusion of isotonic saline may be given, or any other method of volaemic expansion may be used.

Perindoprilat, the active form of perindopril, can be dialysed (see section 5.2).

5. PHARMACOLOGICAL PROPERTIES

5.1 Pharmacodynamic properties

Pharmacotherapeutic group: perindopril and diuretics, ATC code: C09BA04

COVERSYL ARGININE PLUS 5mg/1.25mg is a combination of perindopril arginine salt, an angiotensin converting enzyme inhibitor, and indapamide, a chlorosulphamoyl diuretic. Its pharmacological properties are derived from those of each of the components taken separately, in addition to those due to the additive synergic action of the two products when combined.

Pharmacological mechanism of action

Linked to COVERSYL ARGININE PLUS 5mg/1.25mg:

COVERSYL ARGININE PLUS 5mg/1.25mg produces an additive synergy of the antihypertensive effects of the two components.

Linked to perindopril:

Perindopril is an inhibitor of the angiotensin converting enzyme (ACE inhibitor) which converts angiotensin I to angiotensin II, a vasoconstricting substance; in addition the enzyme stimulates the secretion of aldosterone by the adrenal cortex and stimulates the degradation of bradykinin, a vasodilatory substance, into inactive heptapeptides.

This results in:

- a reduction in aldosterone secretion,

- an increase in plasma renin activity, since aldosterone no longer exercises negative feedback,

- a reduction in total peripheral resistance with a preferential action on the vascular bed in muscle and the kidney, with no accompanying salt and water retention or reflex tachycardia, with chronic treatment.

The antihypertensive action of perindopril also occurs in patients with low or normal renin concentrations.

Perindopril acts through its active metabolite, perindoprilat. The other metabolites are inactive.

Perindopril reduces the work of the heart:

- by a vasodilatory effect on veins, probably caused by changes in the metabolism of prostaglandins: reduction in pre-load,

- by reduction of the total peripheral resistance: reduction in afterload.

Studies carried out on patients with cardiac insufficiency have shown:

- a reduction in left and right ventricular filling pressures,

- a reduction in total peripheral vascular resistance,

- an increase in cardiac output and an improvement in the cardiac index,

- an increase in regional blood flow in muscle.

Exercise test results also showed improvement.

Linked to indapamide:

Indapamide is a sulphonamide derivative with an indole ring, pharmacologically related to the thiazide group of diuretics. Indapamide inhibits the reabsorption of sodium in the cortical dilution segment. It increases the urinary excretion of sodium and chlorides and, to a lesser extent, the excretion of potassium and magnesium, thereby increasing urine output and having an antihypertensive action.

Characteristics of antihypertensive action

Linked to COVERSYL ARGININE PLUS *5mg/1.25mg:*

In hypertensive patients regardless of age, COVERSYL ARGININE PLUS 5mg/1.25mg exerts a dose-dependent antihypertensive effect on diastolic and systolic arterial pressure whilst supine or standing. This antihypertensive effect lasts for 24 hours. The reduction in blood pressure is obtained in less than one month without tachyphylaxis; stopping treatment has no rebound effect. During clinical trials, the concomitant administration of perindopril and indapamide produced antihypertensive effects of a synergic nature in relation to each of the products administered alone.

Linked to perindopril:

Perindopril is active in all grades of hypertension: mild to moderate or severe. A reduction in systolic and diastolic arterial pressure is observed in the lying and standing position.

The antihypertensive activity after a single dose is maximal at between 4 and 6 hours and is maintained over 24 hours.

There is a high degree of residual blocking of angiotensin converting enzyme at 24 hours, approximately 80%.

In patients who respond, normalised blood pressure is reached after one month and is maintained without tachyphylaxis.

Withdrawal of treatment has no rebound effect on hypertension.

Perindopril has vasodilatory properties and restores elasticity of the main arterial trunks, corrects histomorphometric changes in resistance arteries and produces a reduction in left ventricular hypertrophy.

If necessary, the addition of a thiazide diuretic leads to an additive synergy. The combination of an angiotensin converting enzyme inhibitor with a thiazide diuretic decreases the hypokalaemia risk associated with the diuretic alone.

Linked to indapamide:

Indapamide, as monotherapy, has an antihypertensive effect which lasts for 24 hours. This effect occurs at doses at which the diuretic properties are minimal. Its antihypertensive action is proportional to an improvement in arterial compliance and a reduction in total and arteriolar peripheral vascular resistance. Indapamide reduces left ventricular hypertrophy.

When a dose of thiazide diuretic and thiazide-related diuretics is exceeded, the antihypertensive effect reaches a plateau, whereas the adverse effects continue to increase. If the treatment is ineffective, the dose should not be increased.

Furthermore, it has been shown that in the short-term, mid-term and long-term in hypertensive patients, indapamide:

- has no effect on lipid metabolism: triglycerides, LDL-cholesterol and HDL-cholesterol,

- has no effect on carbohydrate metabolism, even in diabetic hypertensive patients.

5.2 Pharmacokinetic properties

Linked to COVERSYL ARGININE PLUS 5mg/1.25mg:

The co-administration of perindopril and indapamide does not change their pharmacokinetic properties by comparison to separate administration.

Linked to perindopril:

After oral administration, the absorption of perindopril is rapid and the peak concentration is achieved within 1 hour. The plasma half-life of perindopril is equal to 1 hour.

Perindopril is a prodrug. Twenty seven percent of the administered perindopril dose reaches the bloodstream as the active metabolite perindoprilat. In addition to active perindoprilat, perindopril yields five metabolites, all inactive. The peak plasma concentration of perindoprilat is achieved within 3 to 4 hours.

As ingestion of food decreases conversion to perindoprilat, hence bioavailability, perindopril arginine should be administered orally in a single daily dose in the morning before a meal.

It has been demonstrated a linear relationship between the dose of perindopril and its plasma exposure.

The volume of distribution is approximately 0.2 l/kg for unbound perindoprilat. Protein binding of perindoprilat to plasma proteins is 20%, principally to angiotensin converting enzyme, but is concentration-dependent. Perindoprilat is eliminated in the urine and the terminal half-life of the unbound fraction is approximately 17 hours, resulting in steady-state within 4 days. Elimination of perindoprilat is decreased in the elderly, and also in patients with heart or renal failure. Dosage adjustment in renal insufficiency is desirable depending on the degree of impairment (creatinine clearance).

Dialysis clearance of perindoprilat is equal to 70 ml/min. Perindopril kinetics are modified in patients with cirrhosis: hepatic clearance of the parent molecule is reduced by half. However, the quantity of perindoprilat formed is not reduced and therefore no dosage adjustment is required (see sections4.2 and 4.4).

Linked to indapamide:

Indapamide is rapidly and completely absorbed from the digestive tract. The peak plasma level is reached in humans approximately one hour after oral administration of the product. Plasma protein binding is 79 %.

The elimination half-life is between 14 and 24 hours (average 18 hours). Repeated administration does not produce accumulation. Elimination is mainly in the urine (70 % of the dose) and faeces (22 %) in the form of inactive metabolites. The pharmacokinetics are unchanged in patients with renal insufficiency.

5.3 Preclinical safety data

COVERSYL ARGININE PLUS 5mg/1.25mg has slightly increased toxicity than that of its components. Renal manifestations do not seem to be potentiated in the rat. However, the combination produces gastro-intestinal toxicity in the dog and the toxic effects on the mother seem to be increased in the rat (compared to perindopril).

Nonetheless, these adverse effects are shown at dose levels corresponding to a very marked safety margin by comparison to the therapeutic doses used. Preclinical studies performed separately with perindopril and indapamide did not show genotoxic, carcinogenic or teratogenic potential.

6. PHARMACEUTICAL PARTICULARS

6.1 List of excipients

Core:

Lactose monohydrate

Magnesium stearate (E470B)

Maltodextrin

Silica colloidal anhydrous (E551)

Sodium starch glycolate (type A)

Film-coating:
Glycerol (E422)
Hypromellose (E464)
Macrogol 6000
Magnesium stearate (E470B)
Titanium dioxide (E171)

6.2 Incompatibilities
Not applicable.

6.3 Shelf life
3 years.

6.4 Special precautions for storage
Keep the container tightly closed in order to protect from moisture.

6.5 Nature and contents of container
14, 20, 28, 30 or 50 tablets in polypropylene white container equipped with a low density polyethylene flow reducer and a low density polyethylene blue opaque stopper containing a white desiccant gel.

Box of 1 container of 14, 20, 28, 30 or 50 tablets.

Box of 2 containers of 28, 30 or 50 tablets.

Box of 3 containers of 30 tablets.

Box of 10 containers of 50 tablets.

Not all pack sizes may be marketed.

6.6 Special precautions for disposal and other handling
No special requirements.

7. MARKETING AUTHORISATION HOLDER
Les Laboratoires Servier
22, rue Garnier
92200 Neuilly-sur-Seine
France

8. MARKETING AUTHORISATION NUMBER(S)
PL 05815/0052

9. DATE OF FIRST AUTHORISATION/RENEWAL OF THE AUTHORISATION
13/09/2007

10. DATE OF REVISION OF THE TEXT
01/10/2007

Cozaar - Comp 50/12.5mg, 100/12.5mg and 100/25mg Film-Coated Tablets

(Merck Sharp & Dohme Limited)

1. NAME OF THE MEDICINAL PRODUCT
Cozaar Comp 50 mg/12.5 mg film-coated tablets
Cozaar Comp 100 mg/12.5 mg film-coated tablets
Cozaar Comp 100 mg/25 mg film-coated tablets

2. QUALITATIVE AND QUANTITATIVE COMPOSITION
Cozaar Comp 50 mg/12.5 mg
Each tablet contains 50 mg of losartan potassium and 12.5 mg of hydrochlorothiazide (HCTZ) as the active ingredients.

Cozaar Comp 100 mg/12.5 mg
Each tablet contains 100 mg of losartan potassium and 12.5 mg of hydrochlorothiazide (HCTZ) as the active ingredients.

Cozaar Comp 100 mg/25 mg
Each tablet contains 100 mg of losartan potassium and 25 mg of hydrochlorothiazide (HCTZ) as the active ingredients.

Excipients
Cozaar Comp 50 mg/12.5 mg: Each tablet contains 63.13 mg lactose monohydrate.
Cozaar Comp 100 mg/12.5 mg: Each tablet contains 88.40 mg lactose monohydrate.
Cozaar Comp 100 mg/25 mg: Each tablet contains 126.26 mg lactose monohydrate.
For a full list of excipients, see section 6.1.

3. PHARMACEUTICAL FORM
Film coated tablets
Cozaar Comp 50 mg/12.5 mg
Yellow, oval film-coated tablets marked 717 on one side and plain or scored on the other.

The scoreline is only to facilitate breaking for ease of swallowing and not to divide into equal doses.

Cozaar Comp 100 mg/12.5 mg
White, oval film-coated tablets marked 745 on one side and plain on the other.

Cozaar Comp 100 mg/25 mg
Light yellow, oval film-coated tablets marked 747 on one side and plain on the other.

4. CLINICAL PARTICULARS
4.1 Therapeutic indications
Cozaar Comp is indicated for the treatment of essential hypertension in patients whose blood pressure is not adequately controlled on losartan or hydrochlorothiazide alone.

4.2 Posology and method of administration
Cozaar Comp may be administered with other antihypertensive agents.

Cozaar Comp tablets should be swallowed with a glass of water.

Cozaar Comp may be administered with or without food.

Hypertension

Losartan and hydrochlorothiazide is not for use as initial therapy, but in patients whose blood pressure is not adequately controlled by losartan potassium or hydrochlorothiazide alone.

Dose titration with the individual components (losartan and hydrochlorothiazide) is recommended.

When clinically appropriate, direct change from monotherapy to the fixed combination may be considered in patients whose blood pressure is not adequately controlled.

The usual maintenance dose of Cozaar Comp is one tablet of Cozaar Comp 50 mg/12.5 mg (losartan 50 mg/HCTZ 12.5 mg) once daily. For patients who do not respond adequately to Cozaar Comp 50 mg/12.5 mg, the dosage may be increased to one tablet of Cozaar Comp 100 mg/ 25 mg (losartan 100 mg/ HCTZ 25 mg) once daily. The maximum dose is one tablet of Cozaar Comp 100 mg/ 25 mg once daily. In general, the antihypertensive effect is attained within three to four weeks after initiation of therapy. Cozaar Comp 100/12.5 (losartan 100 mg/ HCTZ 12.5 mg) is available for those patients titrated to 100 mg of Cozaar Comp who require additional blood pressure control.

Use in patients with renal impairment and haemodialysis patients

No initial dosage adjustment is necessary in patients with moderate renal impairment (i.e. creatinine clearance 30-50 ml/min). Losartan and hydrochlorothiazide tablets are not recommended for haemodialysis patients. Losartan/ HCTZ tablets must not be used in patients with severe renal impairment (i.e. creatinine clearance <30 ml/min) (see section 4.3).

Use in patients with intravascular volume depletion

Volume and /or sodium depletion should be corrected prior to administration of Losartan/HCTZ tablets.

Use in patients with hepatic impairment

Losartan/HCTZ is contraindicated in patients with severe hepatic impairment (see section 4.3.).

Use in the elderly

Dosage adjustment is not usually necessary for the elderly.

Use in children and adolescents (< 18 years)

There is no experience in children and adolescents. Therefore, losartan/hydrochlorothiazide should not be administered to children and adolescents.

4.3 Contraindications

- Hypersensitivity to losartan, sulphonamide-derived substances (as hydrochlorothiazide) or to any of the excipients
- Therapy resistant hypokalaemia or hypercalcaemia
- Severe hepatic impairment; Cholestasis and biliary obstructive disorders
- Refractory hyponatraemia
- Symtomatic hyperuricaemia/gout
- 2nd and 3rd trimester of pregnancy (see section 4.4 and 4.6)
- Lactation (see section 4.6)
- Severe renal impairment (i.e. creatinine clearance <30 ml/min)
- Anuria.

4.4 Special warnings and precautions for use
Losartan

Angiooedema

Patients with a history of angiooedema (swelling of the face, lips, throat, and/or tongue) should be closely monitored (see section 4.8).

Hypotension and Intravascular volume depletion

Symptomatic hypotension, especially after the first dose, may occur in patients who are volume- and/or sodium-depleted by vigorous diuretic therapy, dietary salt restriction, diarrhoea or vomiting. Such conditions should be corrected before the administration of Cozaar Comp tablets (see sections 4.2. and 4.3).

Electrolyte imbalances

Electrolyte imbalances are common in patients with renal impairment, with or without diabetes, and should be addressed. Therefore, the plasma concentrations of potassium and creatinine clearance values should be closely monitored; especially patients with heart failure and a creatinine clearance between 30-50 ml/ min should be closely monitored.

The concomitant use of potassium sparing diuretics, potassium supplements and potassium containing salt substitutes with losartan/ hydrochlorothiazide is not recommended (see section 4.5).

Liver function impairment

Based on pharmacokinetic data which demonstrate significantly increased plasma concentrations of losartan in cirrhotic patients, Cozaar Comp should be used with caution in patients with a history of mild to moderate hepatic impairment. There is no therapeutic experience with losartan in patients with severe hepatic impairment. Therefore Cozaar Comp is contraindicated in patients with severe hepatic impairment (see sections 4.2, 4.3 and 5.2).

Renal function impairment

As a consequence of inhibiting the renin-angiotensin-aldosterone system, changes in renal function, including renal failure, have been reported (in particular, in patients whose renal function is dependent on the renin-angiotensin-aldosterone system, such as those with severe cardiac insufficiency or pre-existing renal dysfunction).

As with other drugs that affect the renin-angiotensin-aldosterone system, increases in blood urea and serum creatinine have also been reported in patients with bilateral renal artery stenosis or stenosis of the artery to a solitary kidney; these changes in renal function may be reversible upon discontinuation of therapy. Losartan should be used with caution in patients with bilateral renal artery stenosis or stenosis of the artery to a solitary kidney.

Renal transplantation

There is no experience in patients with recent kidney transplantation.

Primary hyperaldosteronism

Patients with primary aldosteronism generally will not respond to antihypertensive drugs acting through inhibition of the renin-angiotensin system. Therefore, the use of Cozaar Comp tablets is not recommended.

Coronary heart disease and cerebrovascular disease:

As with any antihypertensive agents, excessive blood pressure decrease in patients with ischaemic cardiovascular and cerebrovascular disease could result in a myocardial infarction or stroke.

Heart failure:

In patients with heart failure, with or without renal impairment, there is - as with other drugs acting on the renin-angiotensin system - a risk of severe arterial hypotension, and (often acute) renal impairment.

Aortic and mitral valve stenosis, obstructive hypertrophic cardiomyopathy

As with other vasodilators, special caution is indicated in patients suffering from aortic or mitral stenosis, or obstructive hypertrophic cardiomyopathy.

Ethnic differences

As observed for angiotensin converting enzyme inhibitors, losartan and the other angiotensin antagonists are apparently less effective in lowering blood pressure in black people than in non-blacks, possibly because of higher prevalence of low-renin states in the black hypertensive population.

Pregnancy

Cozaar Comp should not be initiated during pregnancy. Unless continued Losartan/HTCZ therapy is considered essential, patients planning pregnancy should be changed to alternative anti-hypertensive treatments which have an established safety profile for use in pregnancy. When pregnancy is diagnosed, treatment with Cozaar Comp should be stopped immediately, and, if appropriate, alternative therapy should be started (see sections 4.3 and 4.6).

Hydrochlorothiazide

Hypotension and electrolyte/fluid imbalance

As with all antihypertensive therapy, symptomatic hypotension may occur in some patients. Patients should be observed for clinical signs of fluid or electrolyte imbalance, e.g., volume depletion, hyponatremia, hypochloremic alkalosis, hypomagnesemia or hypokalemia which may occur during intercurrent diarrhea or vomiting. Periodic determination of serum electrolytes should be performed at appropriate intervals in such patients. Dilutional hyponatraemia may occur in oedematous patients in hot weather.

Metabolic and endocrine effects

Thiazide therapy may impair glucose tolerance. Dosage adjustment of antidiabetic agents, including insulin, may be required (see section 4.5). Latent diabetes mellitus may become manifest during thiazide therapy.

Thiazides may decrease urinary calcium excretion and may cause intermittent and slight elevation of serum calcium. Marked hypercalcemia may be evidence of hidden hyperparathyroidism. Thiazides should be discontinued before carrying out tests for parathyroid function.

Increases in cholesterol and triglyceride levels may be associated with thiazide diuretic therapy.

Thiazide therapy may precipitate hyperuricemia and/or gout in certain patients. Because losartan decreases uric acid, losartan in combination with hydrochlorothiazide attenuates the diuretic-induced hyperuricemia.

Hepatic impairment

Thiazides should be used with caution in patients with impaired hepatic function or progressive liver disease, as it may cause intrahepatic cholestasis, and since minor alterations of fluid and electrolyte balance may precipitate hepatic coma.

Cozaar Comp is contraindicated for patients with severe hepatic impairment (see section 4.3 and 5.2).

Other

In patients receiving thiazides, hypersensitivity reactions may occur with or without a history of allergy or bronchial asthma. Exacerbation or activation of systemic lupus erythematosus has been reported with the use of thiazides.

Excipient

Patients with rare hereditary problems of galactose intolerance, the Lapp lactase deficiency or glucose-galactose malabsorption should not take this medicine (see section 6.1).

4.5 Interaction with other medicinal products and other forms of interaction

Losartan

Rifampicin and fluconazole have been reported to reduce levels of active metabolite. The clinical consequences of these interactions have not been evaluated.

As with other drugs that block angiotensin II or its effects, concomitant use of potassium-sparing diuretics (e.g., spironolactone, triamterene, amiloride), potassium supplements, or salt substitutes containing potassium may lead to increases in serum potassium. Co-medication is not advisable.

As with other medicines which affect the excretion of sodium, lithium excretion may be reduced. Therefore, serum lithium levels should be monitored carefully if lithium salts are to be co-administered with angiotensin II receptor antagonists.

When angiotensin II antagonists are administered simultaneously with NSAIDs (i.e. selective COX-2 inhibitors, acetylsalicylic acid at anti-inflammatory doses) and non-selective NSAIDs, attenuation of the antihypertensive effect may occur. Concomitant use of angiotensin II antagonists or diuretics and NSAIDs may lead to an increased risk of worsening of renal function, including possible acute renal failure, and an increase in serum potassium, especially in patients with poor pre-existing renal function. The combination should be administered with caution, especially in the elderly. Patients should be adequately hydrated and consideration should be given to monitoring renal function after initiation of concomitant therapy, and periodically thereafter.

In some patients with compromised renal function who are being treated with non-steroidal anti-inflammatory drugs, including selective cyclooxygenase-2 inhibitors, the co-administration of angiotensin II receptor antagonists may result in a further deterioration of renal function. These effects are usually reversible.

Other substances inducing hypotension like tricyclic antidepressants, antipsychotics, baclofene, amifostine: Concomitant use with these drugs that lower blood pressure, as main or side-effect, may increase the risk of hypotension.

Hydrochlorothiazide

When given concurrently, the following drugs may interact with thiazide diuretics:

Alcohol, barbiturates, narcotics or antidepressants:

Potentiation of orthostatic hypotension may occur.

Antidiabetic drugs (oral agents and insulin):

The treatment with a thiazide may influence the glucose tolerance. Dosage adjustment of the antidiabetic drug may be required. Metformin should be used with caution because of the risk of lactic acidosis induced by possible functional renal failure linked to hydrochlorothiazide.

Other antihypertensive drugs

Additive effect.

Cholestyramine and colestipol resins:

Absorption of hydrochlorothiazide is impaired in the presence of anionic exchange resins. Single doses of either cholestyramine or colestipol resins bind the hydrochlorothiazide and reduce its absorption from the gastrointestinal tract by up to 85 and 43 percent, respectively.

Corticosteroids, ACTH

Intensified electrolyte depletion, particularly hypokalemia.

Pressor amines (e.g., adrenaline)

Possible decreased response to pressor amines but not sufficient to preclude their use.

Skeletal muscle relaxants, nondepolarizing (e.g., tubocurarine)

Possible increased responsiveness to the muscle relaxant.

Lithium

Diuretic agents reduce the renal clearance of lithium and add a high risk of lithium toxicity; concomitant use is not recommended.

Medicinal products used in the treatment of gout (probenecid, sulfinpyrazone and allopurinol)

Dosage adjustment of uricosuric medicinal products may be necessary since hydrochlorothiazide may raise the level of serum uric acid. Increase in dosage of probenecid or sulfinpyrazone may be necessary. Coadministration of a thiazide may increase the incidence of hypersensitivity reactions to allopurinol.

Anticholinergic agents (e.g. atropine, biperiden)

Increase of the bioavailability to thiazide-type diuretics by decreasing gastrointestinal motility and stomach emptying rate.

Cytotoxic agents (eg cyclophosphamide, methotrexate)

Thiazides may reduce the renal excretion of cytotoxic medicinal products and potentiate their myelosuppressive effects.

Salicylates

In case of high dosages of salicylates hydrochlorothiazide may enhance the toxic effect of the salicylates on the central nervous system.

Methyldopa

There have been isolated reports of haemolytic anaemia occurring with concomitant use of hydrochlorothiazide and methyldopa.

Ciclosporin

Concomitant treatment with ciclosporin may increase the risk of hyperuricaemia and gout-type complications.

Digitalis glycosides

Thiazide-induced hypokalaemia or hypomagnesaemia may favour the onset of digitalis-induced cardiac arrhythmias.

Medicinal products affected by serum potassium disturbances

Periodic monitoring of serum potassium and ECG is recommended when Losartan/hydrochlorothiazide is administered with medicinal products affected by serum potassium disturbances (e.g. digitalis glycosides and antiarrhythmics) and with the following torsades de pointes (ventricular tachycardia)-inducing medicinal products (including some antiarrhythmics), hypokalaemia being a predisposing factor to torsades de pointes (ventricular tachycardia):

- Class Ia antiarrythmics (eg quinidine, hydroquinidine, disopyramide).
- Class III antiarrythmics (eg amiodarone, sotalol, dofetilide, ibutilide).
- Some antipsychotics (eg thioridazine, chlorpromazine, levomepromazine, trifluoperazine, cyamemazine, sulpiride, sultopride, amisulpride, tiapride, pimozide, haloperidol, droperidol).
- Others (eg bepridil, cisapride, diphemanil, erythromycin IV, halofantrin, mizolastin, pentamidine, terfenadine, vincamine IV).

Calcium salts

Thiazide diuretics may increase serum calcium levels due to decreased excretion. If calcium supplements must be prescribed, serum calcium levels should be monitored and calcium dosage should be adjusted accordingly.

Laboratory Test Interactions

Because of their effects on calcium metabolism, thiazides may interfere with tests for parathyroid function (see section 4.4).

Carbamazepine

Risk of symptomatic hyponatremia. Clinical and biological monitoring is required.

Iodine Contrast Media

In case of diuretic-induced dehydration, there is an increased risk of acute renal failure, especially with high doses of the iodine product.

Patients should be rehydrated before the administration.

Amphotericin B (parenteral), corticosteroids, ACTH or stimulant laxatives

Hydrochlorothiazide may intensify electrolyte imbalance, particularly hypokalaemia.

4.6 Pregnancy and lactation

Pregnancy

The use of Cozaar Comp is not recommended during the first trimester of pregnancy (see section 4.4). The use of Cozaar Comp is contra-indicated during the 2nd and 3rd trimester of pregnancy (see section 4.3 and 4.4).

Epidemiological evidence regarding the risk of teratogenicity following exposure to ACE inhibitors during the first trimester of pregnancy has not been conclusive; however a small increase in risk cannot be excluded. Whilst there is no controlled epidemiological data on the risk with Angiotensin II Receptor Inhibitors (AIIRAs), similar risks may exist for this class of drugs. Unless continued AIIRA therapy is considered essential, patients planning pregnancy should be changed to alternative anti-hypertensive treatments which have an established safety profile for use in pregnancy. When pregnancy is diagnosed, treatment with Cozaar Comp should be stopped immediately and, if appropriate, alternative therapy should be started.

Cozaar Comp therapy exposure during the second and third trimesters is known to induce human fetotoxicity (decreased renal function, oligohydramnios, skull ossification retardation) and neonatal toxicity (renal failure, hypotension, hyperkalaemia) (see also 5.3 'Preclinical safety data'). Should exposure to Cozaar Comp have occurred from the second trimester of pregnancy, ultrasound check of renal function and skull is recommended.

Infants whose mothers have taken Cozaar Comp should be closely observed for hypotension (see also section 4.3 and 4.4).

Hydrochlorothiazide may reduce both plasma volume and uteroplacental blood flow. Thiazides pass the placental barrier and are found in cord blood. They may cause fetal electrolyte disturbances and possibly other reactions that have been observed in adults. Cases of thrombocytopenia in neonates and fetal or neonatal jaundice were reported after treating the mothers with thiazides.

Lactation

It is not known whether losartan is excreted in human milk. However, losartan is excreted in the milk of lactating rats. Thiazides pass into human milk and may inhibit lactation. Because of the potential for adverse effects on the nursing infant, Cozaar Comp is contraindicated during breast-feeding (see section 4.3).

4.7 Effects on ability to drive and use machines

No studies on the effects on the ability to drive and use machines have been performed.

However, when driving vehicles or operating machinery it must be borne in mind that dizziness or drowsiness may occasionally occur when taking antihypertensive therapy, in particular during initiation of treatment or when the dose is increased.

4.8 Undesirable effects

The adverse events below are classified where appropriate by system organ class and frequency according to the following convention:

Very common: ⩾ 1/10

Common: ⩾ 1/100, < 1/10

Uncommon: ⩾ 1/1,000, ⩽ 1/100

Rare: ⩾ 1/10,000, ⩽ 1/1,000

Very rare: ⩽ 1/10,000

Not known: ⩽ 1/10,000

(cannot be estimated from the available data)

In clinical trials with losartan potassium salt and hydrochlorothiazide, no adverse events peculiar to this combination of substances were observed. The adverse events were restricted to those which were formerly observed with losartan potassium salt and/or hydrochlorothiazide.

In controlled clinical trials for essential hypertension, dizziness was the only adverse experience reported as substance-related that occurred with an incidence greater than placebo in 1% or more of patients treated with losartan and hydrochlorothiazide.

Next to these effects, there are further adverse reactions reported after the introduction of the product to the market as follows:

Hepato-biliary disorders

Rare: Hepatitis

Investigations

Rare: Hyperkalaemia, elevation of ALT

Additional adverse events that have been seen with one of the individual components and may be potential adverse events with losartan potassium/ hydrochlorothiazide are the following:

Losartan

Blood and lymphatic system disorders

Uncommon: Anaemia, Henoch-Schönlein purpura, ecchymosis, haemolysis

Immune system disorders

Rare: Anaphylactic reactions, angioedema, urticaria

Metabolism and nutrition disorders

Uncommon: Anorexia, gout

Psychiatric disorders

Common: Insomnia

Uncommon: Anxiety, anxiety disorder, panic disorder, confusion, depression, abnormal dreams, sleep disorder, somnolence, memory impairment

Nervous system disorders

Common: Headache, dizziness

Uncommon: Nervousness, paraesthesia, peripheral neuropathy, tremor, migraine, syncope

Eye disorders

Uncommon: Blurred vision, burning/stinging in the eye, conjunctivitis, decrease in visual acuity

Ear and labyrinth disorders

Uncommon: Vertigo, tinnitus

Cardiac disorders

Uncommon: Hypotension, orthostatic hypotension, sternalgia, angina pectoris, grade II-AV block, cerebrovascular event, myocardial infarction, palpitation, arrhythmias (atrial fibrillations, sinus bradycardia, tachycardia, ventricular tachycardia, ventricular fibrillation)

Vascular disorders

Uncommon: Vasculitis

Respiratory, thoracic and mediastinal disorders

Common: Cough, upper respiratory infection, nasal congestion, sinusitis, sinus disorder

Uncommon: Pharyngeal discomfort, pharyngitis, laryngitis, dyspnoea, bronchitis, epistaxis, rhinitis, respiratory congestion

Gastrointestinal disorders

Common: Abdominal pain, nausea, diarrhoea, dyspepsia

Uncommon: Constipation, dental pain, dry mouth, flatulence, gastritis, vomiting

Hepato-biliary disorders

Not known: Liver function abnormalities

Skin and subcutaneous tissue disorders

Uncommon: Alopecia, dermatitis, dry skin, erythema, flushing, photosensitivity, pruritus, rash, urticaria, sweating

Musculoskeletal and connective tissue disorders

Common: Muscle cramp, back pain, leg pain, myalgia

Uncommon: Arm pain, joint swelling, knee pain, musculoskeletal pain, shoulder pain, stiffness, arthralgia, arthritis, coxalgia, fibromyalgia, muscle weakness

Renal and urinary disorders

Uncommon: Nocturia, urinary frequency, urinary tract infection

Reproductive system and breast disorders

Uncommon: Decreased libido, impotence

General disorders and administration site conditions

Common: Asthenia, fatigue, chest pain

Uncommon: Facial oedema, fever

Investigations

Common: Hyperkalaemia, mild reduction of haematocrit and haemoglobin

Uncommon: Mild increase in urea and creatinine serum levels

Very rare: Increase in hepatic enzymes and bilirubin.

Hydrochlorothiazide

Blood and lymphatic system disorders

Uncommon: Agranulocytosis, aplastic anaemia, haemolytic anaemia, leukopenia, purpura, thrombocytopenia

Immune system disorders

Rare: Anaphylactic reaction

Metabolism and nutrition disorders

Uncommon: Anorexia, hyperglycaemia, hyperuricaemia, hypokalaemia, hyponatraemia

Psychiatric disorders

Uncommon: Insomnia

Nervous system disorders

Common: Cephalalgia

Eye disorders

Uncommon: Transient blurred vision, xanthopsia

Vascular disorders

Uncommon: Necrotising angiitis (vasculitis, cutaneous vasculitis)

Respiratory, thoracic and mediastinal disorders

Uncommon: Respiratory distress including pneumonitis and pulmonary oedema

Gastrointestinal disorders

Uncommon: Sialoadenitis, spasms, stomach irritation, nausea, vomiting, diarrhoea, constipation

Hepato-biliary disorders

Uncommon: Icterus (intrahepatic cholestatis), pancreatitis

Skin and subcutaneous tissue disorders

Uncommon: Photosensitivity, urticaria, toxic epidermal necrolysis

Musculoskeletal and connective tissue disorders

Uncommon: Muscle cramps

Renal and urinary disorders

Uncommon: Glycosuria, interstitial nephritis, renal dysfunction, renal failure

General disorders and administration site conditions

Uncommon: Fever, dizziness

4.9 Overdose

No specific information is available on the treatment of overdosage with Cozaar Comp. Treatment is symptomatic and supportive. Therapy with Cozaar Comp should be discontinued and the patient observed closely. Suggested measures include induction of emesis if ingestion is recent, and correction of dehydration, electrolyte imbalance, hepatic coma and hypotension by established procedures.

Losartan

Limited data are available in regard to overdosage in humans. The most likely manifestation of overdosage would be hypotension and tachycardia; bradycardia could occur from parasympathetic (vagal) stimulation. If symptomatic hypotension should occur, supportive treatment should be instituted.

Neither losartan nor the active metabolite can be removed by hemodialysis.

Hydrochlorothiazide

The most common signs and symptoms observed are those caused by electrolyte depletion (hypokalemia, hypochloremia, hyponatremia) and dehydration resulting from excessive diuresis. If digitalis has also been administered, hypokalemia may accentuate cardiac arrhythmias.

The degree to which hydrochlorothiazide is removed by hemodialysis has not been established.

5. PHARMACOLOGICAL PROPERTIES

5.1 Pharmacodynamic properties

Pharmacotherapeutic group: Combination containing an angiotensin II-receptor(type AT1)-antagonist and a thiazide diuretic, Antihypertensive, ATC code: C09DA01

Losartan-Hydrochlorothiazide

The components of Cozaar Comp have been shown to have an additive effect on blood pressure reduction, reducing blood pressure to a greater degree than either component alone. This effect is thought to be a result of the complimentary actions of both components. Further, as a result of its diuretic effect, hydrochlorothiazide increases plasma renin activity, increases aldosterone secretion, decreases serum potassium, and increases the levels of angiotensin II. Administration of losartan blocks all the physiologically relevant actions of angiotensin II and through inhibition of aldosterone could tend to attenuate the potassium loss associated with the diuretic.

Losartan has been shown to have a mild and transient uricosuric effect. Hydrochlorothiazide has been shown to cause modest increases in uric acid; the combination of losartan and hydrochlorothiazide tends to attenuate the diuretic-induced hyperuricemia.

The antihypertensive effect of Cozaar Comp is sustained for a 24-hour period. In clinical studies of at least one year's duration, the antihypertensive effect was maintained with continued therapy. Despite the significant decrease in blood pressure, administration of Cozaar Comp had no clinically significant effect on heart rate. In clinical trials, after 12 weeks of therapy with losartan 50 mg /hydrochlorothiazide 12.5 mg, trough sitting diastolic blood pressure was reduced by an average of up to 13.2 mmHg.

Cozaar Comp is effective in reducing blood pressure in males and females, blacks and non-blacks and in younger (<65 years) and older (⩾65 years) patients and is effective in all degrees of hypertension.

Losartan

Losartan is a synthetically produced oral angiotensin-II receptor (type AT_1) antagonist. Angiotensin II, a potent vasoconstrictor, is the primary active hormon of the renin-angiotensin system and an important determinant of the pathophysiology of hypertension. Angiotensin II binds to the AT_1 receptor found in many tissues (e.g. vascular smooth muscle, adrenal gland, kidneys and the heart) and elicits several important biological actions, including vasoconstriction and the release of aldosterone. Angiotensin II also stimulates smooth-muscle cell proliferation.

Losartan selectively blocks the AT_1 receptor. *In vitro* and *in vivo* losartan and its pharmacologically active carboxylic acid metabolite E-3174 block all physiologically relevant actions of angiotensin II, regardless of the source or route of its synthesis.

Losartan does not have an agonist effect nor does it block other hormone receptors or ion channels important in cardiovascular regulation. Furthermore, losartan does not inhibit ACE (kininase II), the enzyme that degrades bradykinin. Consequently, there is thus no increase in bradykinin-mediated undesirable effects.

During the administration of losartan the removal of the angiotensin II negative feedback on renin secretion leads to increased plasma-renin activity (PRA). Increase in the PRA leads to an increase in angiotensin II in plasma. Despite these increases, antihypertensive activity and suppression of the plasma aldosterone concentration are maintained, indicating effective angiotensin II receptor blockade. After the discontinuation of losartan, PRA and angiotensin II values fell within 3 days to the baseline values.

Both losartan and its principal active metabolite have a far greater affinity for the AT_1 receptor than for the AT_2 receptor. The active metabolite is 10- to 40-times more active than losartan on a weight for weight basis.

In a study specifically designed to assess the incidence of cough in patients treated with losartan as compared to patients treated with ACE inhibitors, the incidence of cough reported by patients receiving losartan or hydrochlorothiazide was similar and was significantly less than in patients treated with an ACE inhibitor. In addition, in an overall analysis of 16 double-blind clinical trials in 4131 patients, the incidence of spontaneously reported cough in patients treated with losartan was similar (3.1%) to that of patients treated with placebo (2.6%) or hydrochlorothiazide (4.1%), whereas the incidence with ACE inhibitors was 8.8%.

In nondiabetic hypertensive patients with proteinuria, the administration of losartan potassium significantly reduces proteinuria, fractional excretion of albumin and IgG. Losartan maintains glomerular filtration rate and reduces filtration fraction. Generally losartan causes a decrease in serum uric acid (usually <0.4 mg/dL) which was persistent in chronic therapy.

Losartan has no effect on autonomic reflexes and no sustained effect on plasma norepinephrine.

In patients with left ventricular failure, 25 mg and 50 mg doses of losartan produced positive hemodynamic and neurohormonal effects characterized by an increase in cardiac index and decreases in pulmonary capillary wedge pressure, systemic vascular resistance, mean systemic arterial pressure and heart rate and a reduction in circulating levels of aldosterone and norepinephrine, respectively. The occurrence of hypotension was dose related in these heart failure patients.

Hypertension Studies

In controlled clinical studies, once-daily administration of Losartan to patients with mild to moderate essential hypertension produced statistically significant reductions in systolic and diastolic blood pressure. Measurements of blood pressure 24 hours post-dose relative to 5 – 6 hours post-dose demonstrated blood pressure reduction over 24 hours; the natural diurnal rhythm was retained. Blood pressure reduction at the end of the dosing interval was 70 – 80 % of the effect seen 5-6 hours post-dose.

Discontinuation of Losartan in hypertensive patients did not result in an abrupt rise in blood pressure (rebound). Despite the marked decrease in blood pressure, Losartan had no clinically significant effects on heart rate.

Losartan is equally effective in males and females, and in younger (below the age of 65 years) and older hypertensive patients.

LIFE Study

The Losartan Intervention For Endpoint reduction in hypertension (LIFE) study was a randomised, triple-blind, active-controlled study in 9193 hypertensive patients aged 55 to 80 years with ECG-documented left ventricular hypertrophy. Patients were randomised to once daily losartan 50 mg or once daily atenolol 50 mg. If goal blood pressure (<140/90 mmHg) was not reached, hydrochlorothiazide (12.5 mg) was added first and, if needed, the dose of losartan or atenolol was then increased to 100 mg once daily. Other antihypertensives, with the exception of ACE inhibitors, angiotensin II antagonists or beta-blockers were added if necessary to reach the goal blood pressure.

The mean length of follow up was 4.8 years.

The primary endpoint was the composite of cardiovascular morbidity and mortality as measured by a reduction in the combined incidence of cardiovascular death, stroke and myocardial infarction. Blood pressure was significantly lowered to similar levels in the two groups. Treatment with losartan resulted in a 13.0% risk reduction (p=0.021, 95 % confidence interval 0.77-0.98) compared with atenolol for patients reaching the primary composite endpoint. This was mainly attributable to a reduction of the incidence of stroke. Treatment with losartan reduced the risk of stroke by 25% relative to atenolol (p=0.001 95% confidence interval 0.63-0.89). The rates of cardiovascular death and myocardial infarction were not significantly different between the treatment groups.

Hydrochlorothiazide

Hydrochlorothiazide is a thiazide diuretic. The mechanism of the antihypertensive effect of thiazide diuretics is not fully known. Thiazides affect the renal tubular mechanisms of electrolyte reabsorption, directly increasing excretion of sodium and chloride in approximately equivalent amounts. The diuretic action of hydrochlorothiazide reduces plasma volume, increases plasma renin activity and increases aldosterone secretion, with consequent increases in urinary potassium and bicarbonate loss, and decreases in serum potassium. The renin-aldosterone link is mediated by angiotensin II and therefore coadministration of an angiotensin II receptor antagonist tends to reverse the potassium loss associated with thiazide diuretics.

After oral use, diuresis begins within 2 hours, peaks in about 4 hours and lasts about 6 to 12 hours the antihypertensive effect persists for up to 24 hours.

5.2 Pharmacokinetic properties

Absorption

Losartan

Following oral administration, losartan is well absorbed and undergoes first-pass metabolism, forming an active carboxylic acid metabolite and other inactive metabolites. The systemic bioavailability of losartan tablets is approximately 33%. Mean peak concentrations of losartan and its active metabolite are reached in 1 hour and in 3-4 hours, respectively. There was no clinically significant effect on the plasma concentration profile of losartan when the drug was administered with a standardized meal.

Distribution

Losartan

Both losartan and its active metabolite are ⩾99% bound to plasma proteins, primarily albumin. The volume of distribution of losartan is 34 liters. Studies in rats indicate that losartan crosses the blood-brain barrier poorly, if at all.

Hydrochlorothiazide

Hydrochlorothiazide crosses the placental but not the blood-brain barrier and is excreted in breast milk.

Biotransformation

Losartan

About 14% of an intravenously- or orally-administered dose of losartan is converted to its active metabolite. Following oral and intravenous administration of ^{14}C-labelled losartan potassium, circulating plasma radioactivity primarily is attributed to losartan and its active metabolite. Minimal conversion of losartan to its active metabolite was seen in about one percent of individuals studied.

In addition to the active metabolite, inactive metabolites are formed, including two major metabolites formed by hydroxylation of the butyl side chain and a minor metabolite, an N-2 tetrazole glucuronide.

Elimination

Losartan

Plasma clearance of losartan and its active metabolite is about 600 mL/min and 50 mL/min, respectively. Renal clearance of losartan and its active metabolite is about 74 mL/min and 26 mL/min, respectively. When losartan is administered orally, about 4% of the dose is excreted unchanged in the urine, and about 6% of the dose is excreted in the urine as active metabolite. The pharmacokinetics of losartan and its active metabolite are linear with oral losartan potassium doses up to 200 mg.

Following oral administration, plasma concentrations of losartan and its active metabolite decline polyexponentially with a terminal half-life of about 2 hours and 6-9 hours, respectively. During once-daily dosing with 100 mg, neither losartan nor its active metabolite accumulates significantly in plasma.

Both biliary and urinary excretion contribute to the elimination of losartan and its metabolites. Following an oral dose of ^{14}C-labelled losartan in man, about 35% of radioactivity is recovered in the urine and 58% in the faeces.

Hydrochlorothiazide

Hydrochlorothiazide is not metabolized but is eliminated rapidly by the kidney. When plasma levels have been followed for at least 24 hours, the plasma half-life has been observed to vary between 5.6 and 14.8 hours. At least 61 percent of the oral dose is eliminated unchanged within 24 hours.

Characteristics in Patients

Losartan-Hydrochlorothiazide

The plasma concentrations of losartan and its active metabolite and the absorption of hydrochlorothiazide in elderly hypertensives are not significantly different from those in young hypertensives.

Losartan

Following oral administration in patients with mild to moderate alcoholic cirrhosis of the liver, plasma concentrations of losartan and its active metabolite were, respectively, 5-fold and 1.7-fold greater than those seen in young male volunteers.

Neither losartan nor the active metabolite can be removed by hemodialysis.

5.3 Preclinical safety data

Preclinical data reveal no special hazard for humans based on conventional studies of general pharmacology, genotoxicity and carcinogenic potential. The toxic potential of the combination of losartan/hydrochlorothiazide was evaluated in chronic toxicity studies for up to six months duration in rats and dogs after oral administration, and the changes observed in these studies with the combination were mainly produced by the losartan component. The administration of the losartan/hydrochlorothiazide combination induced a decrease in the red blood cell parameters (erythrocytes, haemoglobin, haematocrit), a rise in urea-N in the serum, a decrease in heart weight (without a histological correlate) and gastrointestinal changes (mucous membrane lesions, ulcers, erosions, haemorrhages). There was no evidence of teratogenicity in rats or rabbits treated with the losartan/hydrochlorothiazide combination. Foetal toxicity in rats, as evidenced by a slight increase in supernumerary ribs in the F_1 generation, was observed when females were treated prior to and throughout gestation. As observed in studies with losartan alone, adverse foetal and neonatal effects, including renal toxicity and foetal death, occurred when pregnant rate were treated with the losartan/hydrochlorothiazide combination during late gestation and/or lactation.

6. PHARMACEUTICAL PARTICULARS

6.1 List of excipients

Cozaar Comp 50 mg/12.5 mg, Cozaar Comp 100 mg/12.5 mg and Cozaar Comp 100 mg/25 mg:

Each tablet contains the following inactive ingredients:

microcrystalline cellulose(E460),

lactose monohydrate,

pregelatinized maize starch,

magnesium stearate (E572),

hydroxypropyl cellulose (E463),

hypromellose(E464).

Cozaar Comp 50 mg/12.5 mg contains 4.24 mg (0.108 mEq) of potassium.

Cozaar Comp 100 mg/12.5 mg mg contains 8.48 mg (0.216 mEq) of potassium.

and Cozaar Comp 100 mg/25 mg contains 8.48 mg (0.216 mEq) of potassium.

Cozaar Comp 50 mg/12.5 mg and Cozaar Comp 100 mg/25 mg also contain, Titanium dioxide (E171), Quinoline yellow aluminum lake (E104), and Carnauba wax (E903)

Cozaar Comp 100 mg/12.5 mg also contain: white color concentrate (or the individual ingredients of the concentrate: hydroxypropyl cellulose, hypromellose and titanium dioxide) and carnauba wax. Carnauba wax (E903), Titanium dioxide (E171)

Cozaar Comp 100 mg/25 mg also contain:, Titanium dioxide (E171), Quinoline yellow aluminum lake (E104), and Carnauba wax (E903)

6.2 Incompatibilities

Not applicable.

6.3 Shelf life

3 years

6.4 Special precautions for storage

Blisters; Do not store above 30°C. Store in the original package.

HDPE bottle: Do not store above 25 °C. Store in the original container. Keep the bottle tightly closed.

6.5 Nature and contents of container

Cozaar Comp 50 mg/12.5 mg - PVC/PE/PVDC blister packages with aluminum foil lidding in packs of 4, 7, 10, 14, 20, 28, 30, 50, 56, 84, 98, or 280 tablets. HDPE bottles of 100 tablets.

Cozaar Comp 100 mg/12.5 mg - PVC/PE/PVDC blister packages with aluminum foil lidding in packs of 14, 15, 28, 30, 50, 56, 84, 90, 98, 280 tablets. HDPE bottles of 100 tablets.

Cozaar Comp 100 mg/25 mg > - PVC/PE/PVDC blister packages with aluminum foil lidding in packs of 7, 14, 28, 30, 50, 56, 84, 90, 98, or 280 tablets. HDPE bottles of 100 tablets.

Not all pack sizes may be marketed.

6.6 Special precautions for disposal and other handling

No special requirements.

7. MARKETING AUTHORISATION HOLDER

Merck Sharp & Dohme Limited

Hertford Road

Hoddesdon

Hertfordshire

EN11 9BU

8. MARKETING AUTHORISATION NUMBER(S)

Cozaar Comp 50 mg/12.5 mg film-coated tablets: PL 0025/0338

Cozaar Comp 100 mg/12.5 mg film-coated tablets: PL 0025/0473

Cozaar Comp 100 mg/25 mg film-coated tablets PL 0025/0374

9. DATE OF FIRST AUTHORISATION/RENEWAL OF THE AUTHORISATION

Cozaar Comp 50 mg/12.5 mg film-coated tablets: 12 April 1996

Cozaar Comp 100 mg/12.5 mg film-coated tablets: 17 October 2007

Cozaar Comp 100 mg/25 mg film-coated tablets 21 December 2004

10. DATE OF REVISION OF THE TEXT

January 2009

® denotes registered trademark of E. I. du Pont de Nemours and Company, Wilmington, Delaware, USA.

SPC.HYZ.08.UK.2917 Art 30

COZAAR 12.5 mg, 25 mg, 50 mg and 100 mg Film-Coated Tablets

(Merck Sharp & Dohme Limited)

1. NAME OF THE MEDICINAL PRODUCT

Cozaar®▼* 12.5 mg film-coated tablets

Cozaar®▼* 25 mg film-coated tablets

Cozaar®▼* 50 mg film-coated tablets

Cozaar®▼* 100 mg film-coated tablets

** Intensive monitoring is requested only when used for the recently-licensed indication in chronic heart failure*

2. QUALITATIVE AND QUANTITATIVE COMPOSITION

Each COZAAR 12.5 mg Tablet contains 12.5 mg of losartan potassium.

Each COZAAR 25 mg Tablet contains 25 mg of losartan potassium.

Each COZAAR 50 mg Tablet contains 50 mg of losartan potassium.

Each COZAAR 100 mg Tablet contains 100 mg of losartan potassium.

Each COZAAR 12.5 mg tablet contains 25.25 mg lactose monohydrate.

Each COZAAR 25 mg tablet contains 12.75 mg lactose monohydrate.

Each COZAAR 50 mg tablet contains 25.5 mg lactose monohydrate.

Each COZAAR 100 mg tablet contains 51.0 mg lactose monohydrate.

For a full list of excipients, see section 6.1.

3. PHARMACEUTICAL FORM

Film-coated tablets

COZAAR 12.5 mg tablet

Blue, oval film-coated tablets marked 11 on one side and plain on the other.

COZAAR 25 mg tablet

White, oval unscored film-coated tablets marked 951 on one side and plain on the other.

COZAAR 50 mg tablet

White, oval film-coated tablets marked 952 on one side and scored on the other.

The tablet can be divided into equal halves.

COZAAR 100 mg tablet

White, teardrop-shaped film-coated tablets marked 960 on one side and plain on the other.

4. CLINICAL PARTICULARS

4.1 Therapeutic indications

- Treatment of essential hypertension in adults and in children and adolescents 6-18 years of age.
- Treatment of renal disease in adult patients with hypertension and type 2 diabetes mellitus with proteinuria ⩾ 0.5 g/day as part of an antihypertensive treatment.
- Treatment of chronic heart failure (in patients ⩾ 60 years), when treatment with Angiotensin converting enzyme (ACE) inhibitors is not considered suitable due to incompatibility, *especially cough,* or contraindication. Patients with heart failure who have been stabilised with an ACE inhibitor should not be switched to losartan. The patients should have a left ventricular ejection fraction ⩽ 40% and should be clinically stable and on an established treatment regimen for chronic heart failure.
- Reduction in the risk of stroke in adult hypertensive patients with left ventricular hypertrophy documented by ECG (see section 5.1 LIFE study, Race).

4.2 Posology and method of administration

Losartan tablets should be swallowed with a glass of water. COZAAR may be administered with or without food.

Hypertension

The usual starting and maintenance dose is 50 mg once daily for most patients. The maximal antihypertensive effect is attained 3-6 weeks after initiation of therapy. Some patients may receive an additional benefit by increasing the dose to 100 mg once daily (in the morning).

Losartan may be administered with other antihypertensive agents, especially with diuretics (e.g. hydrochlorothiazide).

Hypertensive type II diabetic patients with proteinuria ⩾ 0.5 g/day

The usual starting dose is 50 mg once daily. The dose may be increased to 100 mg once daily based on blood pressure response from one month onwards after initiation of therapy. Losartan may be administered with other antihypertensive agents (e.g. diuretics, calcium channel blockers, alpha- or beta-blockers, and centrally acting agents) as well as with insulin and other commonly used hypoglycemic agents (e.g.sulfonylureas, glitazones and glucosidase inhibitors).

Heart failure

The usual initial dose of losartan in patients with heart failure is 12.5 mg once daily. The dose should generally be titrated at weekly intervals (i.e. 12.5 mg daily, 25 mg daily, 50 mg daily) to the usual maintenance dose of 50 mg once daily, as tolerated by the patient.

Reduction in the risk of stroke in hypertensive patients with left ventricular hypertrophy documented by ECG

The usual starting dose is 50 mg of losartan once daily. A low dose of hydrochlorothiazide should be added and/ or the dose of losartan should be increased to 100 mg once daily based on blood pressure response.

Special populations

Use in patients with intravascular volume depletion:

For patients with intravascular volume-depletion (e.g. those treated with high-dose diuretics), a starting dose of 25 mg once daily should be considered (see section 4.4).

Use in patients with renal impairment and haemodialysis patients:

No initial dosage adjustment is necessary in patients with renal impairment and in haemodialysis patients.

Use in patients with hepatic impairment:

A lower dose should be considered for patients with a history of hepatic impairment. There is no therapeutic experience in patients with severe hepatic impairment. Therefore, losartan is contraindicated in patients with severe hepatic impairment (see sections 4.3 and 4.4).

Use in paediatric patients

There are limited data on the efficacy and safety of losartan in children and adolescents aged 6-18 years old for the treatment of hypertension (see section 5.1). Limited pharmacokinetic data are available in hypertensive children above one month of age (see section 5.2).

For patients who can swallow tablets, the recommended dose is 25 mg once daily in patients >20 to <50 kg. (In exceptional cases the dose can be increased to a maximum of 50 mg once daily). Dosage should be adjusted according to blood pressure response.

In patients >50 kg, the usual dose is 50 mg once daily. In exceptional cases the dose can be adjusted to a maximum of 100 mg once daily. Doses above 1.4 mg/ kg (or in excess of 100 mg) daily have not been studied in paediatric patients.

Losartan is not recommended for use in children under 6 years old, as limited data are available in these patient groups.

It is not recommended in children with glomerular filtration rate < 30 ml/ min / 1.73 m^2, as no data are available (see also section 4.4).

Losartan is also not recommended in children with hepatic impairment (see also section 4.4).

Use in Elderly

Although consideration should be given to initiating therapy with 25 mg in patients over 75 years of age, dosage adjustment is not usually necessary for the elderly.

4.3 Contraindications

Hypersensitivity to the active substance or to any of the excipients (see section 4.4 and 6.1).

2nd and 3rd trimester of pregnancy (see section 4.4 and 4.6).

Severe hepatic impairment.

4.4 Special warnings and precautions for use

Hypersensitivity

Angio-oedema. Patients with a history of angio-oedema (swelling of the face, lips, throat, and/ or tongue) should be closely monitored (see section 4.8).

Hypotension and electrolyte/fluid imbalance

Symptomatic hypotension, especially after the first dose and after increasing of the dose, may occur in patients who are volume- and/or sodium-depleted by vigorous diuretic therapy, dietary salt restriction, diarrhoea or vomiting. These conditions should be corrected prior to administration of losartan, or a lower starting dose should be used (see section 4.2). This also applies to children 6 to 18 years of age.

Electrolyte imbalances

Electrolyte imbalances are common in patients with renal impairment, with or without diabetes, and should be addressed. In a clinical study conducted in type 2 diabetic patients with nephropathy, the incidence of hyperkalemia was higher in the group treated with losartan as compared to the placebo group (see section 4.8). Therefore, the plasma concentrations of potassium as well as creatinine clearance values should be closely monitored, especially patients with heart failure and a creatinine clearance between 30-50 ml/ min should be closely monitored.

The concomitant use of potassium-sparing diuretics, potassium supplements and potassium-containing salt substitutes with losartan is not recommended (see section 4.5).

Hepatic impairment

Based on pharmacokinetic data which demonstrate significantly increased plasma concentrations of losartan in cirrhotic patients, a lower dose should be considered for patients with a history of hepatic impairment. There is no therapeutic experience with losartan in patients with severe hepatic impairment. Therefore losartan must not be administered in patients with severe hepatic impairment (see sections 4.2, 4.3 and 5.2).

Losartan is not recommended in children with hepatic impairment (see section 4.2).

Renal impairment

As a consequence of inhibiting the renin-angiotensin system, changes in renal function including renal failure have been reported (in particular, in patients whose renal function is dependent on the renin- angiotensin-aldosterone system such as those with severe cardiac insufficiency or pre-existing renal dysfunction). As with other medicinal products that affect the renin-angiotensin-aldosterone system, increases in blood urea and serum creatinine have also been reported in patients with bilateral renal artery stenosis or stenosis of the artery to a solitary kidney; these changes in renal function may be reversible upon discontinuation of therapy. Losartan should be used with caution in patients with bilateral renal artery stenosis or stenosis of the artery to a solitary kidney.

Use in paediatric patients with renal impairment

Losartan is not recommended in children with glomerular filtration rate < 30 ml/ min/ 1.73 m^2 as no data are available (see section 4.2).

Renal function should be regularly monitored during treatment with losartan as it may deteriorate. This applies particularly when losartan is given in the presence of other conditions (fever, dehydration) likely to impair renal function.

Concomitant use of losartan and ACE-inhibitors has shown to impair renal function. Therefore, concomitant use is not recommended (see section 4.5).

Renal transplantation

There is no experience in patients with recent kidney transplantation.

Primary hyperaldosteronism

Patients with primary aldosteronism generally will not respond to antihypertensive medicinal products acting through inhibition of the renin-angiotensin system. Therefore, the use of losartan is not recommended.

Coronary heart disease and cerebrovascular disease

As with any antihypertensive agents, excessive blood pressure decrease in patients with ischaemic cardiovascular and cerebrovascular disease could result in a myocardial infarction or stroke.

Heart failure

In patients with heart failure, with or without renal impairment, there is - as with other medicinal products acting on the renin-angiotensin system - a risk of severe arterial hypotension, and (often acute) renal impairment.

There is no sufficient therapeutic experience with losartan in patients with heart failure and concomitant severe renal impairment, in patients with severe heart failure (NYHA class IV) as well as in patients with heart failure and symptomatic life threatening cardiac arrhythmias. Therefore, losartan should be used with caution in these patient groups. The combination of losartan with a beta-blocker should be used with caution (see section 5.1).

Aortic and mitral valve stenosis, obstructive hypertrophic cardiomyopathy

As with other vasodilators, special caution is indicated in patients suffering from aortic or mitral stenosis, or obstructive hypertrophic cardiomyopathy.

Excipients

This medicinal product contains lactose. Patients with rare hereditary problems of galactose intolerance, the Lapp lactase deficiency or glucose-galactose malabsorption should not take this medicine.

Pregnancy

Losartan should not be initiated during pregnancy. Unless continued losartan therapy is considered essential, patients planning pregnancy should be changed to alternative anti-hypertensive treatments which have an established safety profile for use in pregnancy. When pregnancy is diagnosed, treatment with losartan should be stopped immediately, and, if appropriate, alternative therapy should be started (see sections 4.3 and 4.6).

Other warnings and precautions

As observed for angiotensin converting enzyme inhibitors, losartan and the other angiotensin antagonists are apparently less effective in lowering blood pressure in black people than in non-blacks, possibly because of higher prevalence of low-renin states in the black hypertensive population.

4.5 Interaction with other medicinal products and other forms of interaction

Other antihypertensive agents may increase the hypotensive action of losartan. Concomitant use with other substances which may induce hypotension as an adverse reaction (like tricyclic antidepressants, antipsychotics, baclofen and amifostine) may increase the risk of hypotension.

Losartan is predominantly metabolised by cytochrome P450 (CYP) 2C9 to the active carboxy-acid metabolite. In a clinical trial it was found that fluconazole (inhibitor of CYP2C9) decreases the exposure to the active metabolite by approximately 50%. It was found that concomitant treatment of losartan with rifampicin (inducer of metabolism enzymes) gave a 40% reduction in plasma concentration of the active metabolite. The clinical relevance of this effect is unknown. No difference in exposure was found with concomitant treatment with fluvastatin (weak inhibitor of CYP2C9).

As with other medicinal products that block angiotensin II or its effects, concomitant use of other medicinal products which retain potassium (e.g. potassium-sparing diuretics: amiloride, triamterene, spironolactone) or may increase potassium levels (e.g. heparin), potassium supplements or salt substitutes containing potassium may lead to increases in serum potassium. Co-medication is not advisable.

Reversible increases in serum lithium concentrations and toxicity have been reported during concomitant administration of lithium with ACE inhibitors. Very rare cases have also been reported with angiotensin II receptor antagonists. Co-administration of lithium and losartan should be undertaken with caution. If this combination proves essential, serum lithium level monitoring is recommended during concomitant use.

When angiotensin II antagonists are administered simultaneously with NSAIDs (i.e. selective COX-2 inhibitors, acetylsalicylic acid at anti-inflammatory doses and non-selective NSAIDs), attenuation of the antihypertensive effect may occur. Concomitant use of angiotensin II antagonists or diuretics and NSAIDs may lead to an increased risk of worsening of renal function, including possible acute renal failure, and an increase in serum potassium, especially in patients with poor pre-existing renal function. The combination should be administered with caution, especially in the elderly. Patients should be adequately hydrated and consideration should be given to monitoring renal function after initiation of concomitant therapy, and periodically thereafter.

4.6 Pregnancy and lactation

Pregnancy

The use of losartan is not recommended during the first trimester of pregnancy (see section 4.4). The use of losartan is contra-indicated during the 2nd and 3rd trimester of pregnancy (see section 4.3 and 4.4).

Epidemiological evidence regarding the risk of teratogenicity following exposure to ACE inhibitors during the first trimester of pregnancy has not been conclusive; however a small increase in risk cannot be excluded. Whilst there is no controlled epidemiological data on the risk with Angiotensin II Receptor Inhibitors (AIIRAs), similar risks may exist for this class of medicinal products. Unless continued AIIRA therapy is considered essential, patients planning pregnancy should be changed to alternative anti-hypertensive treatments which have an established safety profile for use in pregnancy. When pregnancy is diagnosed, treatment with losartan should be stopped immediately and, if appropriate, alternative therapy should be started.

Exposure to AIIA therapy during the second and third trimesters is known to induce human fetotoxicity (decreased renal function, oligohydramnios, skull ossification retardation) and neonatal toxicity (renal failure, hypotension, hyperkalaemia) (see also 5.3). Should exposure to losartan have occurred from the second trimester of pregnancy, ultrasound check of renal function and skull is recommended.

Infants whose mothers have taken losartan should be closely observed for hypotension (see also section 4.3 and 4.4).

Lactation

Because no information is available regarding the use of losartan during breastfeeding, losartan is not recommended and alternative treatments with better established safety profiles during breastfeeding are preferable, especially while nursing a newborn or preterm infant.

4.7 Effects on ability to drive and use machines

No studies on the effects on the ability to drive and use machines have been performed. However, when driving vehicles or operating machinery it must be borne in mind that dizziness or drowsiness may occasionally occur when taking antihypertensive therapy, in particular during initiation of treatment or when the dose is increased.

4.8 Undesirable effects

Losartan has been evaluated in clinical studies as follows:

- in controlled clinical trials in approximately 3300 adult patients 18 years of age and older for essential hypertension,
- in a controlled clinical trial in 9193 hypertensive patients 55 to 80 years of age with left ventricular hypertrophy
- in a controlled clinical trial in approximately 3900 patients 20 years of age and older with chronic heart failure
- in a controlled clinical trial in 1513 type 2 diabetic patients 31 years of age and older with proteinuria
- in a controlled clinical trial in 177 hypertensive paediatric patients 6 to 16 years of age

In these clinical trials, the most common adverse reaction was dizziness.

The frequency of adverse reactions listed below is defined using the following convention:

very common (⩾ 1/10); common (⩾ 1/100, to < 1/10); uncommon (⩾ 1/1,000, to < 1/100); rare (⩾ 1/10,000, to < 1/1,000); very rare (< 1/10,000), not known (cannot be estimated from the available data).

Hypertension

In controlled clinical trials of approximately 3300 adult patients 18 years of age and older, for essential hypertension with losartan, the following adverse reactions were reported

Nervous system disorders:

common: dizziness, vertigo

uncommon: somnolence, headache, sleep disorders

Cardiac disorder:

uncommon: palpitations, angina pectoris

Vascular disorders:

uncommon: symptomatic hypotension (especially in patients with intravascular volume depletion, e.g. patients with severe heart failure or under treatment with high dose diuretics), dose-related orthostatic effects, rash.

Gastro-intestinal disorders:

uncommon: abdominal pain, obstipation

General disorders and administration site conditions:

uncommon: asthenia, fatigue, oedema

Investigations:

In controlled clinical trials, clinically important changes in standard laboratory parameters were rarely associated with administration of losartan tablets. Elevations of ALT occurred rarely and usually resolved upon discontinuation of therapy. Hyperkalaemia (serum potassium >5.5 mmol/l) occurred in 1.5% of patients in hypertension clinical trials.

Hypertensive patients with left ventricular hypertrophy

In a controlled clinical trial in 9193 hypertensive patients 55 to 80 years of age, with left ventricular hypertrophy, the following adverse reactions were reported:

Nervous system disorders:

common: dizziness

Ear and labyrinth disorders:

common: vertigo

General disorders and administration site conditions:

common: asthenia/fatigue

Chronic heart failure

In a controlled clinical trial in approximately 3900 patients 20 years of age and older, with cardiac insufficiency, the following adverse reactions were reported:

Nervous system disorders:

uncommon: dizziness, headache

rare: paraesthesia

Cardiac disorders:

rare: syncope, atrial fibrillation, cerebrovascular accident

Vascular disorders:

uncommon: hypotension, including orthostatic hypotension

Respiratory, thoracic and mediastinal disorders:

uncommon: dyspnoea

Gastro-intestinal disorders:

uncommon: diarrhoea, nausea, vomiting

Skin and subcutaneous tissue disorders:

uncommon: urticaria, pruritus, rash

General disorders and administration site conditions:

uncommon: asthenia/fatigue

Investigations:

uncommon: increase in blood urea, serum creatinine and serum potassium has been reported.

Hypertension and type 2 diabetes with renal disease

In a controlled clinical trial in 1513 type 2 diabetic patients 31 years of age and older, with proteinuria (RENAAL study, see section 5.1), the most common drug-related adverse events which were reported for losartan are as follows:

Nervous system disorders:

common: dizziness

Vascular disorders:

common: hypotension

General disorders and administration site conditions:

common: asthenia/fatigue

Investigations:

common: hypoglycaemia, hyperkalaemia

The following adverse reactions occurred more often in patients receiving losartan than placebo:

Blood and lymphatic system disorders:

not known: anaemia

Cardiac disorders:

not known: syncope, palpitations

Vascular disorders:

not known: orthostatic hypotension

Gastro-intestinal disorders:

not known: diarrhoea

Musculoskeletal and connective tissue disorders:

not known: back pain

Renal and urinary disorders:

not known: urinary tract infections

General disorders and administration site conditions:

not known: flu-like symptoms

Investigations:

In a clinical study conducted in type 2 diabetic patients with nephropathy, 9.9% of patients treated with losartan tablets developed hyperkalaemia >5.5 mEq/l and 3.4% of patients treated with placebo.

Post-marketing experience

The following adverse reactions have been reported in post-marketing experience:

Blood and lymphatic system disorders:

not known: anaemia, thrombocytopenia

Ear and labyrinth disorders:

not known: tinnitus

Immune system disorders:

rare: hypersensitivity: anaphylactic reactions, angio-oedema including swelling of the larynx and glottis causing airway obstruction and/or swelling of the face, lips, pharynx, and/or tongue; in some of these patients angio-oedema had been reported in the past in connection with the administration of other medicines, including ACE inhibitors; vasculitis, including Henoch-Schonlein purpura.

Nervous system disorders:

not known: migraine

Respiratory, thoracic and mediastinal disorders:

not known: cough

Gastro-intestinal disorders:

not known: diarrhoea, pancreatitis

General disorders and administration site conditions:

not known: malaise

Hepatobiliary disorders:

rare: hepatitis

not known: liver function abnormalities

Skin and subcutaneous tissue disorders:

not known: urticaria, pruritus, rash, photosensitivity

Musculoskeletal and connective tissue disorders:

not known: myalgia, arthralgia, rhabdomyolysis

Reproductive system and breast disorders:

not known: erectile dysfunction/impotence

Renal and urinary disorders:

As a consequence of inhibiting the renin-angiotensin-aldosterone system, changes in renal function including renal failure have been reported in patients at risk; these changes in renal function may be reversible upon discontinuation of therapy (see section 4.4)

Psychiatric disorders:

not known: depression

Investigations:

not known: hyponatraemia

Paediatric population

The adverse reaction profile for paediatric patients appears to be similar to that seen in adult patients. Data in the paediatric population are limited.

4.9 Overdose

Symptoms of intoxication

No case of overdose has been reported. The most likely symptoms, depending on the extent of overdose, are hypotension, tachycardia, possibly bradycardia.

Treatment of intoxication

Measures are depending on the time of medicinal product intake and kind and severity of symptoms. Stabilisation of the cardiovascular system should be given priority. After oral intake, the administration of a sufficient dose of activated charcoal is indicated. Afterwards, close monitoring of the vital parameters should be performed. Vital parameters should be corrected if necessary.

Neither losartan nor the active metabolite can be removed by haemodialysis.

5. PHARMACOLOGICAL PROPERTIES

Pharmacotherapeutic group: Angiotensin II antagonists, plain ATC code: C09CA01

5.1 Pharmacodynamic properties

Losartan is a synthetic oral angiotensin-II receptor (type AT_1) antagonist. Angiotensin II, a potent vasoconstrictor, is the primary active hormone of the renin/angiotensin system and an important determinant of the pathophysiology of hypertension. Angiotensin II binds to the AT_1 receptor found in many tissues (e.g. vascular smooth muscle, adrenal gland, kidneys and the heart) and elicits several important biological actions, including vasoconstriction and the release of aldosterone. Angiotensin II also stimulates smooth muscle cell proliferation.

Losartan selectively blocks the AT_1 receptor. *In vitro* and *in vivo* losartan and its pharmacologically active carboxylic acid metabolite E-3174 block all physiologically relevant actions of angiotensin II, regardless of the source or route of its synthesis.

Losartan does not have an agonist effect nor does it block other hormone receptors or ion channels important in cardiovascular regulation. Furthermore losartan does not inhibit ACE (kininase II), the enzyme that degrades bradykinin. Consequently, there is no potentiation of undesirable bradykinin-mediated effects.

During administration of losartan, removal of the angiotensin II negative feedback on renin secretion leads to increased plasma renin activity (PRA). Increase in the PRA leads to an increase in angiotensin II in plasma. Despite these increases, antihypertensive activity and suppression of plasma aldosterone concentration are maintained, indicating effective angiotensin II receptor blockade. After discontinuation of losartan, PRA and angiotensin II values fell within three days to the baseline values.

Both losartan and its principal active metabolite have a far greater affinity for the AT_1-receptor than for the AT_2-receptor. The active metabolite is 10- to 40- times more active than losartan on a weight for weight basis.

Hypertension studies

In controlled clinical studies, once-daily administration of losartan to patients with mild to moderate essential hypertension produced statistically significant reductions in systolic and diastolic blood pressure. Measurements of blood pressure 24 hours post-dose relative to 5 – 6 hours post-dose demonstrated blood pressure reduction over 24 hours; the natural diurnal rhythm was retained. Blood pressure reduction at the end of the dosing interval was 70 – 80 % of the effect seen 5-6 hours post-dose.

Discontinuation of losartan in hypertensive patients did not result in an abrupt rise in blood pressure (rebound). Despite the marked decrease in blood pressure, losartan had no clinically significant effects on heart rate.

Losartan is equally effective in males and females, and in younger (below the age of 65 years) and older hypertensive patients.

LIFE-study

The Losartan Intervention For Endpoint Reduction in Hypertension [LIFE] study was a randomised, triple-blind, active-controlled study in 9193 hypertensive patients aged 55 to 80 years with ECG-documented left-ventricular hypertrophy. Patients were randomised to once daily losartan 50 mg or once daily atenolol 50 mg. If goal blood pressure (< 140/90 mmHg) was not reached, hydrochlorothiazide (12.5 mg) was added first and, if needed, the dose of losartan or atenolol was then increased to 100 mg once daily. Other antihypertensives, with the exception of ACE-inhibitors, angiotensin II antagonists or beta-blockers were added if necessary to reach the goal blood pressure.

The mean length of follow up was 4.8 years.

The primary endpoint was the composite of cardiovascular morbidity and mortality as measured by a reduction in the combined incidence of cardiovascular death, stroke and myocardial infarction. Blood pressure was significantly lowered to similar levels in the two groups. Treatment with losartan resulted in a 13.0% risk reduction (p=0.021, 95 % confidence interval 0.77-0.98) compared with atenolol for patients reaching the primary composite endpoint. This was mainly attributable to a reduction of the incidence of stroke. Treatment with losartan reduced the risk of stroke by 25% relative to atenolol (p=0.001 95% confidence interval 0.63-0.89). The rates of cardiovascular death and myocardial infarction were not significantly different between the treatment groups.

Race

In the LIFE-Study black patients treated with losartan had a higher risk of suffering the primary combined endpoint, i.e. a cardiovascular event (e.g. cardiac infarction, cardiovascular death) and especially stroke, than the black patients treated with atenolol. Therefore the results observed with losartan in comparison with atenolol in the LIFE study with regard to cardiovascular morbidity/mortality do not apply for black patients with hypertension and left ventricular hypertrophy.

RENAAL-study

The Reduction of Endpoints in NIDDM with the Angiotensin II Receptor Antagonist losartan RENAAL study was a controlled clinical study conducted worldwide in 1513 Type 2 diabetic patients with proteinuria, with or without hypertension. 751 patients were treated with losartan. The objective of the study was to demonstrate a nephroprotective effect of losartan potassium over and above the benefit of lowering blood pressure.

Patients with proteinuria and a serum creatinine of 1.3 – 3.0 mg/dl were randomised to receive losartan 50 mg once a day, titrated if necessary, to achieve blood pressure response, or to placebo, on a background of conventional antihypertensive therapy excluding ACE-inhibitors and angiotensin II antagonists.

Investigators were instructed to titrate the study medication to 100 mg daily as appropriate; 72 % of patients were taking the100 mg daily dose for the majority of the time. Other antihypertensive agents (diuretics, calcium antagonists, alpha- and beta-receptor blockers and also centrally acting antihypertensives) were permitted as supplementary treatment depending on the requirement in both groups. Patients were followed up for up to 4.6 years (3.4 years on average).

The primary endpoint of the study was a composite endpoint of doubling of the serum creatinine end-stage renal failure (need for dialysis or transplantation) or death.

The results showed that the treatment with losartan (327 events) as compared with placebo (359 events) resulted in a16.1 % risk reduction (p = 0.022) in the number of patients reaching the primary composite endpoint. For the following individual and combined components of the primary endpoint, the results showed a significant risk reduction in the group treated with losartan: 25.3 % risk reduction for doubling of the serum creatinine (p = 0.006); 28.6 % risk reduction for end-stage renal failure (p = 0.002); 19.9 % risk reduction for end-stage renal failure or death (p = 0.009); 21.0 % risk reduction for doubling of serum creatinine or end-stage renal failure (p = 0.01).

All-cause mortality rate was not significantly different between the two treatment groups. In this study losartan was generally well tolerated, as shown by a therapy discontinuation rate on account of adverse reactions that was comparable to the placebo group.

ELITE I and ELITE II studies

In the ELITE Study carried out over 48 weeks in722 patients with heart failure (NYHA Class II-IV), no difference was observed between the patients treated with losartan and those treated with captopril with regard to the primary endpoint of a long-term change in renal function. The observation of the ELITE I Study, that, compared with captopril, losartan reduced the mortality risk, was not confirmed in the subsequent ELITE II Study.

In the ELITE II Study losartan 50 mg once daily (starting dose 12.5 mg, increased to 25 mg, then 50 mg once daily) was compared with captopril 50 mg three times daily (starting dose 12.5 mg, increased to 25 mg and then to 50 mg three times daily). The primary endpoint of this prospective study was the all-cause mortality.

In this study, 3152 patients with heart failure (NYHA Class II-IV) were followed for almost two years (median: 1.5 years) in order to determine whether losartan is superior to captopril in reducing all cause mortality. The primary endpoint did not show any statistically significant difference between losartan and captopril in reducing all-cause mortality.

In both comparator-controlled (not placebo-controlled) clinical studies on patients with heart failure the tolerability of losartan was superior to that of captopril, measured on the basis of a significantly lower rate of discontinuations of therapy on account of adverse reactions and a significantly lower frequency of cough.

An increased mortality was observed in ELITE II in the small subgroup (22% of all HF patients) taking beta-blockers at baseline.

Paediatric Population

Paediatric hypertension

The antihypertensive effect of losartan was established in a clinical study involving 177 hypertensive paediatric patients 6 to 16 years of age with a body weight > 20 kg and a glomerular filtration rate > 30 ml/ min/ 1.73 m^2. Patients who weighed > 20kg to < 50 kg received either 2.5, 25 or 50 mg of losartan daily and patients who weighed > 50 kg received either 5, 50 or 100 mg of losartan daily. At the end of three weeks, losartan administration once daily lowered trough blood pressure in a dose-dependent manner.

Overall, there was a dose-response. The dose-response relationship became very obvious in the low dose group compared to the middle dose group (period I: -6.2 mmHg vs. -11.65 mmHg), but was attenuated when comparing the middle dose group with the high dose group (period I: -11.65 mmHg vs. -12.21 mmHg). The lowest doses studied, 2.5 mg and 5 mg, corresponding to an average daily dose of 0.07 mg/ kg, did not appear to offer consistent antihypertensive efficacy.

These results were confirmed during period II of the study where patients were randomised to continue losartan or placebo, after three weeks of treatment. The difference in blood pressure increase as compared to placebo was largest in the middle dose group (6.70 mmHg middle dose vs. 5.38 mmHg high dose). The rise in trough diastolic blood pressure was the same in patients receiving placebo and in those continuing losartan at the lowest dose in each group, again suggesting that the lowest dose in each group did not have significant antihypertensive effect.

Long-term effects of losartan on growth, puberty and general development have not been studied. The long-term efficacy of antihypertensive therapy with losartan in childhood to reduce cardiovascular morbidity and mortality has also not been established.

In hypertensive (N=60) and normotensive (N=246) children with proteinuria, the effect of losartan on proteinuria was evaluated in a 12-week placebo- and active-controlled (amlodipine) clinical study. Proteinuria was defined as urinary protein/creatinine ratio of ⩾0.3. The hypertensive patients (ages 6 through 18 years) were randomised to receive either losartan (n=30) or amlodipine (n=30). The normotensive patients (ages 1 through 18 years) were randomised to receive either losartan (n=122) or placebo (n=124). Losartan was given at doses of 0.7 mg/kg to 1.4 mg/kg (up to maximum dose of 100 mg per day). Amlodipine was given at doses of 0.05 mg/kg to 0.2 mg/kg (up to a maximum dose of 5 mg per day).

Overall, after 12 weeks of treatment, patients receiving losartan experienced a statistically significant reduction from baseline in proteinuria of 36% versus 1% increase in placebo/amlodipine group (p⩽0.001). Hypertensive patients receiving losartan experienced a reduction from baseline proteinuria of -41.5% (95% CI -29.9;-51.1) versus +2.4% (95% CI -22.2;14.1) in the amlodipine group. The decline in both systolic blood pressure and diastolic blood pressure was greater in the losartan group (-5.5/-3.8 mmHg) versus the amlodipine group (-0.1/+0.8 mm Hg). In normotensive children a small decrease in blood pressure was observed in the losartan group (-3.7/-3.4 mm Hg) compared to placebo. No significant correlation between the decline in proteinuria and blood pressure was noted, however it is possible that the decline in blood pressure was responsible, in part, for the decline in proteinuria in the losartan treated group. Long-term effects of reduction of proteinuria in children have not been studied.

5.2 Pharmacokinetic properties

Absorption

Following oral administration, losartan is well absorbed and undergoes first-pass metabolism, forming an active carboxylic acid metabolite and other inactive metabolites. The systemic bioavailability of losartan tablets is approximately 33%. Mean peak concentrations of losartan and its active metabolite are reached in 1 hour and in 3-4 hours, respectively.

Distribution

Both losartan and its active metabolite are ⩾99% bound to plasma proteins, primarily albumin. The volume of distribution of losartan is 34 litres.

Biotransformation

About 14% of an intravenously- or orally-administered dose of losartan is converted to its active metabolite. Following oral and intravenous administration of ^{14}C-labelled losartan potassium, circulating plasma radioactivity primarily is attributed to losartan and its active metabolite. Minimal conversion of losartan to its active metabolite was seen in about 1% of individuals studied.

In addition to the active metabolite, inactive metabolites are formed.

Elimination

Plasma clearance of losartan and its active metabolite is about 600 ml/min and 50 ml/min, respectively. Renal clearance of losartan and its active metabolite is about 74 ml/min and 26 ml/min, respectively. When losartan is administered orally, about 4% of the dose is excreted unchanged in the urine, and about 6% of the dose is excreted in the urine as active metabolite. The pharmacokinetics of losartan and its active metabolite are linear with oral losartan potassium doses up to 200 mg.

Following oral administration, plasma concentrations of losartan and its active metabolite decline polyexponentially, with a terminal half-life of about 2 hours and 6-9 hours, respectively. During once-daily dosing with 100 mg, neither losartan nor its active metabolite accumulates significantly in plasma.

Both biliary and urinary excretions contribute to the elimination of losartan and its metabolites. Following an oral dose/intravenous administration of ^{14}C-labelled losartan in man, about 35% / 43% of radioactivity is recovered in the urine and 58%/ 50% in the faeces.

Characteristics in patients

In elderly hypertensive patients the plasma concentrations of losartan and its active metabolite do not differ essentially from those found in young hypertensive patients.

In female hypertensive patients the plasma levels of losartan were up to twice as high as in male hypertensive patients, while the plasma levels of the active metabolite did not differ between men and women.

In patients with mild to moderate alcohol-induced hepatic cirrhosis, the plasma levels of losartan and its active metabolite after oral administration were respectively 5 and 1.7 times higher than in young male volunteers (see section 4.2 and 4.4).

Plasma concentrations of losartan are not altered in patients with a creatinine clearance above 10 ml/minute. Compared to patients with normal renal function, the AUC for losartan is about 2-times higher in haemodialysis dialysis patients.

The plasma concentrations of the active metabolite are not altered in patients with renal impairment or in haemodialysis patients.

Neither losartan nor the active metabolite can be removed by haemodialysis.

Pharmacokinetics in paediatric patients

The pharmacokinetics of losartan have been investigated in 50 hypertensive paediatric patients > 1 month to < 16 years of age following once daily oral administration of approximately 0.54 to 0.77 mg/ kg of losartan (mean doses).

The results showed that the active metabolite is formed from losartan in all age groups. The results showed roughly similar pharmacokinetic parameters of losartan following oral administration in infants and toddlers, preschool children, school age children and adolescents. The pharmacokinetic parameters for the metabolite differed to a greater extent between the age groups. When comparing preschool children with adolescents these differences became statistically significant. Exposure in infants/ toddlers was comparatively high.

5.3 Preclinical safety data

Preclinical data reveal no special hazard for humans based on conventional studies of general pharmacology, genotoxicity and carcinogenic potential. In repeated dose toxicity studies, the administration of losartan induced a decrease in the red blood cell parameters (erythrocytes, haemoglobin, haematocrit), a rise in urea-N in the serum and occasional rises in serum creatinine, a decrease in heart weight (without a histological correlate) and gastrointestinal changes (mucous membrane lesions, ulcers, erosions, haemorrhages). Like other substances that directly affect the renin-angiotensin system, losartan has been shown to induce adverse effects on the late foetal development, resulting in foetal death and malformations.

6. PHARMACEUTICAL PARTICULARS

6.1 List of excipients

microcrystalline cellulose (E460)

lactose monohydrate

pregelatinized maize starch

magnesium stearate (E572)

hydroxypropyl cellulose (E463)

hypromellose (E464)

COZAAR 12.5 mg, 25 mg, 50 mg and 100 mg contain potassium in the following amounts: 1.06 mg (0.027 mEq), 2.12 mg (0.054 mEq), 4.24 mg (0.108 mEq) and 8.48 mg (0.216 mEq) respectively.

COZAAR 12.5 mg tablets also contain carnauba wax (E903), titanium dioxide (E171), indigo carmine (E132) aluminum lake.

COZAAR 25 mg tablets also contain carnauba wax (E903), titanium dioxide (E171).

COZAAR 50 mg tablets also contain carnauba wax (E903), titanium dioxide (E171).

COZAAR 100 mg tablets also contain carnauba wax (E903), titanium dioxide (E171).

6.2 Incompatibilities

Not applicable.

6.3 Shelf life

3 years

6.4 Special precautions for storage

Blisters: Store in the original package in order to protect from light and moisture. HDPE Bottle: do not store above 25°C. Store in original container. Keep the bottle tightly closed in order to protect from light and moisture.

6.5 Nature and contents of container

COZAAR 12.5 mg - PVC/PE/PVDC blister packages with aluminum foil lidding in cartons containing 7, 14, 21, 28, 50, 98, 210 or 500 tablets. HDPE bottles of 100 tablets.

COZAAR 25 mg - PVC/PE/PVDC blister packages with aluminum foil lidding in cartons containing 7 or 28 tablets.

COZAAR 50 mg - PVC/PE/PVDC blister packages with aluminum foil lidding in cartons containing 7, 10, 14, 20, 28, 30, 50, 56, 84, 90, 98, 280 or 500 tablets. HDPE bottles of 100 or 300 tablets.

COZAAR 100 mg - PVC/PE/PVDC blister packages with aluminum foil lidding in cartons containing 7, 10, 14, 15, 20, 28, 30, 50, 56, 84, 90, 98 or 280 tablets. HDPE bottles of 100 tablets.

Not all pack sizes may be marketed.

6.6 Special precautions for disposal and other handling

No special requirements.

7. MARKETING AUTHORISATION HOLDER

Merck Sharp & Dohme Limited

Hertford Road

Hoddesdon

Herts

EN11 9BU

8. MARKETING AUTHORISATION NUMBER(S)

12.5 mg: PL 0025/0515

25 mg: PL 0025/0336

50 mg: PL 0025/0324

100 mg: PL 0025/0416

9. DATE OF FIRST AUTHORISATION/RENEWAL OF THE AUTHORISATION

12.5 mg: 6 January 2009

25 mg/50 mg: 15 December 1994

100 mg: 28 November 2001

10. DATE OF REVISION OF THE TEXT

August 2009

® denotes registered trademark of E. I. du Pont de Nemours and Company, Wilmington, Delaware, USA.

SPC.CZR.08.UK.3005-II-003

COZAAR 2.5 mg/ml powder and solvent for oral suspension

(Merck Sharp & Dohme Limited)

1. NAME OF THE MEDICINAL PRODUCT

COZAAR®▼ 2.5 mg/ml powder and solvent for oral suspension

2. QUALITATIVE AND QUANTITATIVE COMPOSITION

Each sachet of powder for oral suspension delivers 500 mg of losartan potassium. After reconstitution, each ml suspension contains 2.5 mg of losartan potassium.

One bottle of reconstituted suspension (200 ml) contains 500 mg of losartan potassium.

Excipient:

Each ml suspension contains 0.296 mg methylhydroxybenzoate, 0.041 mg propylhydroxybenzoate, 50.6 mg sorbitol, and 1.275 mg lactose.

For a full list of excipients, see section 6.1.

3. PHARMACEUTICAL FORM

Powder and solvent for oral suspension.

White to off-white powder.

The solvent is a cloudy, colorless liquid.

4. CLINICAL PARTICULARS

4.1 Therapeutic indications

• Treatment of essential hypertension in adults and in children and adolescents 6 – 16 years of age.

• Treatment of renal disease in adult patients with hypertension and type 2 diabetes mellitus with proteinuria ⩾ 0.5 g/day as part of an antihypertensive treatment.

• Treatment of chronic heart failure (in patients ⩾ 60 years), when treatment with Angiotensin-converting enzyme (ACE) inhibitors is not considered suitable due to incompatibility, *especially cough,* or contraindication. Patients with heart failure who have been stabilised with an ACE inhibitor should not be switched to losartan. The patients should have a left ventricular ejection fraction ⩽ 40 % and should be stabilised under the treatment of the chronic heart failure.

• Reduction in the risk of stroke in adult hypertensive patients with left-ventricular hypertrophy documented by ECG (see section 5.1 LIFE study, Race).

4.2 Posology and method of administration

Hypertension

The usual starting and maintenance dose is 50 mg once daily for most patients. The maximal antihypertensive effect is attained 3-6 weeks after initiation of therapy. Some patients may receive an additional benefit by increasing the dose to 100 mg once daily (in the morning).

Losartan may be administered with other antihypertensive agents, especially with diuretics (e.g. hydrochlorothiazide).

Paediatric hypertension

Use in children and adolescents (6 to 16 years):

There are limited data on the efficacy and safety of losartan in children and adolescents aged 6-16 years old for the treatment of hypertension (see section 5.1). Limited pharmacokinetic data are available in hypertensive children above one month of age (see section 5.2).

The recommended starting dose in patients >20 to <50 kg is 0.7 mg/kg once daily (up to 25 mg total, in exceptional cases where target doses above 25 mg are required, the maximal dose is 50 mg). Dosage should be adjusted according to blood pressure response.

In patients >50 kg, the usual dose is 50 mg once daily. In exceptional cases the dose can be adjusted to a maximum of 100 mg once daily. Doses above 1.4 mg/kg (or in excess of 100 mg) daily have not been studied in paediatric patients.

For patients who can swallow tablets, this dosage form is also available.

Paediatric patients

Losartan is not recommended for use in children below 6 years old due to insufficient data on safety and/or efficacy in these patient groups.

It is not recommended in children with glomerular filtration rate < 30 ml/ min / 1.73 m^2, as no data are available (see also section 4.4).

Losartan is also not recommended in children with hepatic impairment (see also section 4.4).

Hypertensive type II diabetic patients with proteinuria ≥ 0.5 g/day

The usual starting dose is 50 mg once daily. The dose may be increased to 100 mg once daily based on blood pressure response from one month onwards after initiation of therapy. Losartan may be administered with other antihypertensive agents (e.g. diuretics, calcium channel blockers, alpha- or beta-blockers, and centrally acting agents) as well as with insulin and other commonly used hypoglycemic agents (e.g.sulfonylureas, glitazones and glucosidase inhibitors).

Heart failure

The usual initial dose of losartan in patients with heart failure is 12.5 mg once daily. The dose should generally be titrated at weekly intervals (i.e. 12.5 mg daily, 25 mg daily, 50 mg daily) to the usual maintenance dose of 50 mg once daily, as tolerated by the patient.

Reduction in the risk of stroke in hypertensive patients with left-ventricular hypertrophy documented by ECG

The usual starting dose is 50 mg of losartan once daily. A low dose of hydrochlorothiazide should be added and/ or the dose of losartan should be increased to 100 mg once daily based on blood pressure response.

Special populations

Use in patients with intravascular volume depletion:

For patients with intravascular volume-depletion (e.g. those treated with high-dose diuretics), a starting dose of 25 mg once daily should be considered (see section 4.4).

Use in patients with renal impairment and haemodialysis patients:

No initial dosage adjustment is necessary in patients with renal impairment and in haemodialysis patients.

Use in patients with hepatic impairment:

A lower dose should be considered for patients with a history of hepatic impairment. There is no therapeutic experience in patients with severe hepatic impairment. Therefore, losartan is contraindicated in patients with severe hepatic impairment (see sections 4.3 and 4.4).

Use in elderly

Although consideration should be given to initiating therapy with 25 mg in patients over 75 years of age, dosage adjustment is not usually necessary for the elderly.

Administration of the oral suspension

Shake the closed bottle of losartan oral suspension well before use. Push the plunger of the dispenser completely down toward the tip of the dispenser. Insert the dispenser into the adapter on the medication bottle until a tight seal is made between the bottle and the adapter. With the dispenser, adapter, and bottle attached, turn the entire assembly upside down. Pull out the plunger to withdraw the medication medicinal product into the dispenser. Return the entire assembly to the upright position. Remove the dispenser and administer the medication. Replace the original cap onto the bottle.

For reconstitution see section 6.6.

Losartan may be administered with or without food.

4.3 Contraindications

• Hypersensitivity to the active substance or to any of the excipients (see section 4.4 and 6.1).

• 2nd and 3rd trimester of pregnancy (see section 4.6).

• Severe hepatic impairment.

4.4 Special warnings and precautions for use

Hypersensitivity

Angio-edema. Patients with a history of angio-oedema (swelling of the face, lips, throat, and/ or tongue) should be closely monitored (see section 4.8).

Hypotension and electrolyte/fluid imbalance

Symptomatic hypotension, especially after the first dose and after increasing of the dose, may occur in patients who are volume- and/or sodium-depleted by vigorous diuretic therapy, dietary salt restriction, diarrhoea or vomiting. These conditions should be corrected prior to administration of losartan, or a lower starting dose should be used (see section 4.2). This also applies to children 6 to 16 years of age.

Electrolyte imbalances

Electrolyte imbalances are common in patients with renal impairment, with or without diabetes, and should be addressed. In a clinical study conducted in type 2 diabetic patients with nephropathy, the incidence of hyperkalemia was higher in the group treated with losartan as compared to the placebo group (see section 4.8). Therefore, the plasma concentrations of potassium as well as creatinine clearance values should be closely monitored especially patients with heart failure and a creatinine clearance between 30-50 ml/min should be closely monitored.

The concomitant use of potassium sparing diuretics, potassium supplements and potassium containing salt substitutes with losartan is not recommended (see section 4.5).

Hepatic impairment

Based on pharmacokinetic data which demonstrate significantly increased plasma concentrations of losartan in cirrhotic patients, a lower dose should be considered for patients with a history of hepatic impairment. There is no therapeutic experience with losartan in patients with severe hepatic impairment. Therefore losartan must not be administered in patients with severe hepatic impairment (see sections 4.2, 4.3 and 5.2).

Losartan is not recommended in children with hepatic impairment (see section 4.2).

Renal impairment

As a consequence of inhibiting the renin-angiotensin system, changes in renal function including renal failure have been reported (in particular, in patients whose renal function is dependent on the renin angiotensin aldosterone system such as those with severe cardiac insufficiency or pre-existing renal dysfunction). As with other medicinal products that affect the renin-angiotensin-aldosterone system, increases in blood urea and serum creatinine have also been reported in patients with bilateral renal artery stenosis or stenosis of the artery to a solitary kidney; these changes in renal function may be reversible upon discontinuation of therapy. Losartan should be used with caution in patients with bilateral renal artery stenosis or stenosis of the artery to a solitary kidney.

Use in paediatric patients with renal impairment

Losartan is not recommended in children with glomerular filtration rate < 30 ml/ min/1.73 m^2 as no data are available (see section 4.2).

Renal function should be regularly monitored during treatment with losartan as it may deteriorate. This applies particularly when losartan is given in the presence of other conditions (fever, dehydration) likely to impair renal function.

Concomitant use of losartan and ACE-inhibitors has been shown to impair renal function. Therefore, concomitant use is not recommended (see section 4.5).

Renal transplantation

There is no experience in patients with recent kidney transplantation.

Primary hyperaldosteronism

Patients with primary aldosteronism generally will not respond to antihypertensive medicinal products acting through inhibition of the renin-angiotensin system. Therefore, the use of losartan is not recommended.

Coronary heart disease and cerebrovascular disease

As with any antihypertensive agents, excessive blood pressure decrease in patients with ischaemic cardiovascular and cerebrovascular disease could result in a myocardial infarction or stroke.

Heart failure

In patients with heart failure, with or without renal impairment, there is, as with other medicinal products acting on the renin-angiotensin system, a risk of severe arterial hypotension, and (often acute) renal impairment.

There is no sufficient therapeutic experience with losartan in patients with heart failure and concomitant severe renal impairment, in patients with severe heart failure (NYHA class IV) as well as in patients with heart failure and symptomatic life-threatening cardiac arrhythmias. Therefore, losartan should be used with caution in these patient groups. The combination of losartan with a beta-blocker should be used with caution (see section 5.1).

Aortic and mitral valve stenosis, obstructive hypertrophic cardiomyopathy

As with other vasodilators, special caution is indicated in patients suffering from aortic or mitral stenosis, or obstructive hypertrophic cardiomyopathy.

Pregnancy

Losartan should not be initiated during pregnancy. Unless continued losartan therapy is considered essential, patients planning pregnancy should be changed to alternative anti-hypertensive treatments which have an established safety profile for use in pregnancy. When pregnancy is diagnosed, treatment with losartan should be stopped immediately, and, if appropriate, alternative therapy should be started (see sections 4.3 and 4.6).

Other warnings and precautions:

As observed for angiotensin converting enzyme inhibitors, losartan and the other angiotensin antagonists are apparently less effective in lowering blood pressure in black people than in non-blacks, possibly because of higher prevalence of low-renin states in the black hypertensive population.

Galactose intolerance, Lapp lactase deficiency, glucose-galactose malabsorption

Patients with rare hereditary problems of galactose intolerance, the Lapp lactase deficiency or glucose-galactose malabsorption should not take this medicine.

Sorbitol/Fructose intolerance

The solvent contains sorbitol. Patients with rare hereditary problems of fructose intolerance should not take this medicine.

Methylhydroxybenzoate and propylhydroxybenzoate

May cause allergic reactions (possibly delayed).

4.5 Interaction with other medicinal products and other forms of interaction

Other antihypertensive agents may increase the hypotensive action of losartan. Concomitant use with other substances which may induce hypotension as an adverse reaction (like tricyclic antidepressants, antipsychotics, baclofen, and amifostine) may increase the risk of hypotension.

Losartan is predominantly metabolised by cytochrome P450 (CYP) 2C9 to the active carboxy-acid metabolite. In a clinical trial it was found that fluconazole (inhibitor of CYP2C9) decreases the exposure to the active metabolite by approximately 50 %. It was found that concomitant treatment of losartan with rifampicin (inducer of metabolism enzymes) gave a 40 % reduction in plasma concentration of the active metabolite. The clinical relevance of this effect is unknown. No difference in exposure was found with concomitant treatment with fluvastatin (weak inhibitor of CYP2C9).

As with other medicinal products that block angiotensin II or its effects, concomitant use of other medicinal products which retain potassium (e.g. potassium-sparing diuretics: amiloride, triamterene, spironolactone), or may increase potassium levels (e.g. heparin, potassium supplements or salt substitutes containing potassium), may lead to increases in serum potassium. Co-medication is not advisable.

Reversible increases in serum lithium concentrations and toxicity have been reported during concomitant administration of lithium with ACE inhibitors. Very rare cases have also been reported with angiotensin II receptor antagonists. Co-administration of lithium and losartan should be undertaken with caution. If this combination proves essential, serum lithium level monitoring is recommended during concomitant use.

When angiotensin II antagonists are administered simultaneously with NSAIDs (i.e. selective COX-2 inhibitors, acetylsalicylic acid at anti-inflammatory doses and non-selective NSAIDs), attenuation of the antihypertensive effect may occur. Concomitant use of angiotensin II antagonists or diuretics and NSAIDs may lead to an increased risk of worsening of renal function, including possible acute renal failure, and an increase in serum potassium, especially in patients with poor pre-existing renal function. The combination should be administered with caution, especially in the elderly. Patients should be adequately hydrated and consideration should be given to monitoring renal function after initiation of concomitant therapy, and periodically thereafter.

4.6 Pregnancy and lactation

Pregnancy

The use of losartan is not recommended during the first trimester of pregnancy (see section 4.4). The use of losartan is contraindicated during the 2nd and 3rd trimester of pregnancy (see section 4.3 and 4.4).

Epidemiological evidence regarding the risk of teratogenicity following exposure to ACE inhibitors during the first trimester of pregnancy has not been conclusive; however a small increase in risk cannot be excluded. Whilst there is no controlled epidemiological data on the risk with Angiotensin II Receptor Inhibitors (AIIRAs), similar risks may exist for this class of medicinal products. Unless continued AIIRA therapy is considered essential, patients planning pregnancy should be changed to alternative anti-hypertensive treatments which have an established safety profile for use in pregnancy. When pregnancy is diagnosed, treatment with losartan should be stopped immediately and, if appropriate, alternative therapy should be started.

Exposure to AIIRA therapy during the second and third trimesters is known to induce human fetotoxicity (decreased renal function, oligohydramnios, skull ossification retardation) and neonatal toxicity (renal failure, hypotension, hyperkalaemia) (see also section 5.3). Should exposure to losartan have occurred from the second trimester of pregnancy, ultrasound check of renal function and skull is recommended.

Infants whose mothers have taken losartan should be closely observed for hypotension.

Lactation

Because no information is available regarding the use of losartan during breast-feeding, losartan is not recommended and alternative treatments with better established safety profiles during breast feeding are preferable, especially while nursing a newborn or preterm infant.

4.7 Effects on ability to drive and use machines

No studies on the effects on the ability to drive and use machines have been performed. However, when driving vehicles or operating machines it must be borne in mind that dizziness or drowsiness may occasionally occur when taking antihypertensive therapy, in particular during initiation of treatment or when the dose is increased.

4.8 Undesirable effects

Losartan has been evaluated in clinical studies as follows:

- In controlled clinical trials in approximately 3300 adult patients 18 years of age and older for essential hypertension
- In a controlled clinical trial in 9193 hypertensive patients 55 to 80 years of age with left ventricular hypertrophy
- In a controlled clinical trial in approximately 3900 patients 20 years of age and older with chronic heart failure
- In a controlled clinical trial in 1513 type 2 diabetic patients 31 years of age and older with proteinuria
- In a controlled clinical trial in 177 hypertensive paediatric patients 6 to 16 years of age

In these clinical trials, the most common adverse event was dizziness.

The frequency of adverse events listed below is defined using the following convention:

very common (⩾ 1/10); common (⩾ 1/100, to < 1/10); uncommon (⩾ 1/1,000, to < 1/100); rare (⩾ /10,000, to < 1/1,000); very rare (< 1/10,000), not known (cannot be estimated from the available data).

Hypertension

In controlled clinical trials of approximately 3300 adult patients 18 years of age and older for essential hypertension with losartan the following adverse events were reported:

Nervous system disorders:

Common: dizziness, vertigo

Uncommon: somnolence, headache, sleep disorders

Cardiac disorder:

Uncommon: palpitations, angina pectoris

Vascular disorders:

Uncommon: symptomatic hypotension (especially in patients with intravascular volume depletion, e.g. patients with severe heart failure or under treatment with high-dose diuretics), dose-related orthostatic effects, rash.

Gastro-intestinal disorders:

Uncommon: abdominal pain, obstipation

General disorders and administration site conditions:

Uncommon: asthenia, fatigue, oedema

Investigations:

In controlled clinical trials, clinically important changes in standard laboratory parameters were rarely associated with administration of losartan tablets. Elevations of ALT occurred rarely and usually resolved upon discontinuation of therapy. Hyperkalaemia (serum potassium >5.5 mmol/l) occurred in 1.5 % of patients in hypertension clinical trials.

Hypertensive patients with left-ventricular hypertrophy

In a controlled clinical trial in 9193 hypertensive patients 55 to 80 years of age with left-ventricular hypertrophy the following adverse events were reported:

Nervous system disorders:

common: dizziness

Ear and labyrinth disorders:

common: vertigo

General disorders and administration site conditions:

common: asthenia/fatigue

Chronic heart failure

In a controlled clinical trial in approximately 3900 patients 20 years of age and older with cardiac insufficiency the following adverse events were reported:

Nervous system disorders:

uncommon: dizziness, headache

rare: paraesthesia

Cardiac disorders:

rare: syncope, atrial fibrillation, cerebrovascular accident

Vascular disorders:

uncommon: hypotension, including orthostatic hypotension

Respiratory, thoracic and mediastinal disorders:

uncommon: dyspnoea

Gastrointestinal disorders:

uncommon: diarrhoea, nausea, vomiting

Skin and subcutaneous tissue disorders:

uncommon: urticaria, pruritus, rash

General disorders and administration site conditions:

uncommon: asthenia/fatigue

Investigations:

uncommon: increase in blood urea, serum creatinine and serum potassium has been reported.

Hypertension and type 2 diabetes with renal disease

In a controlled clinical trial in 1513 type 2 diabetic patients 31 years of age and older with proteinuria (RENAAL study, see section 5.1) the most common drug-related adverse reactions which were reported for losartan are as follows:

Nervous system disorders:

common: dizziness

Vascular disorders:

common: hypotension

General disorders and administration site conditions:

common: asthenia/fatigue

Investigations:

common: hypoglycaemia, hyperkalaemia

The following adverse events occurred more often in patients receiving losartan than placebo:

Blood and lymphatic system disorders:

not known: anaemia

Cardiac disorders:

not known: syncope, palpitations

Vascular disorders:

not known: orthostatic hypotension

Gastrointestinal disorders:

not known: diarrhoea

Muscoskeletal and connective tissue disorders:

not known: back pain

Renal and urinary disorders:

not known: urinary tract infections

General disorders and administration site conditions:

not known: flu-like symptoms

Investigations:

In a clinical study conducted in type 2 diabetic patients with nephropathy, 9.9 % of patients treated with losartan tablets developed hyperkalaemia >5.5 mEq/l and 3.4 % of patients treated with placebo

Post-marketing experience

The following adverse events have been reported in post-marketing experience:

Blood and lymphatic system disorders:

not known: anaemia, thrombocytopenia

Immune system disorders:

rare: hypersensitivity: anaphylactic reactions, angiooedema including swelling of the larynx and glottis causing airway obstruction and/or swelling of the face, lips, pharynx, and/or tongue; in some of these patients angiooedema had been reported in the past in connection with the administration of other medicines, including ACE inhibitors; vasculitis, including Henoch-Schönlein purpura.

Nervous system disorders:

not known: migraine

Respiratory, thoracic and mediastinal disorders:

not known: cough

Gastrointestinal disorders:

not known: diarrhoea

Hepatobiliary disorders:

rare: hepatitis

not known: liver function abnormalities

Skin and subcutaneous tissue disorders:

not known: urticaria, pruritus, rash

Musculoskeletal and connective tissue disorders:

not known: myalgia, arthralgia

Renal and urinary disorders:

As a consequence of inhibiting the renin-angiotensin-aldosterone system, changes in renal function including renal failure have been reported in patients at risk; these changes in renal function may be reversible upon discontinuation of therapy (see section 4.4)

Paediatric population

The adverse experience profile for paediatric patients appears to be similar to that seen in adult patients. Data in the paediatric population are limited.

4.9 Overdose

Symptoms of intoxication

No case of overdose has been reported. The most likely symptoms, depending on the extent of overdose, are hypotension, tachycardia, possibly bradycardia.

Treatment of intoxication

Measures are depending on the time of medicinal product intake and kind and severity of symptoms. Stabilisation of the cardiovascular system should be given priority. After oral intake the administration of a sufficient dose of activated charcoal is indicated. Afterwards, close monitoring of the vital parameters should be performed. Vital parameters should be corrected if necessary.

Neither losartan nor the active metabolite can be removed by haemodialysis.

5. PHARMACOLOGICAL PROPERTIES

Pharmacotherapeutic group: Angiotensin II antagonists, plain, ATC code: C09CA01

5.1 Pharmacodynamic properties

Losartan is a synthetic oral angiotensin-II receptor (type AT_1) antagonist. Angiotensin II, a potent vasoconstrictor, is the primary active hormone of the renin/angiotensin system and an important determinant of the pathophysiology of hypertension. Angiotensin II binds to the AT_1 receptor found in many tissues (e.g. vascular smooth muscle, adrenal gland, kidneys and the heart) and elicits several important biological actions, including vasoconstriction and the release of aldosterone. Angiotensin II also stimulates smooth muscle cell proliferation.

Losartan selectively blocks the AT_1 receptor. *In vitro* and *in vivo* losartan and its pharmacologically active carboxylic acid metabolite E-3174 block all physiologically relevant actions of angiotensin II, regardless of the source or route of its synthesis.

Losartan does not have an agonist effect nor does it block other hormone receptors or ion channels important in cardiovascular regulation. Furthermore losartan does not inhibit ACE (kininase II), the enzyme that degrades bradykinin. Consequently, there is no potentiation of undesirable bradykinin-mediated effects.

During administration of losartan, removal of the angiotensin II negative feedback on renin secretion leads to increased plasma renin activity (PRA). Increase in the PRA leads to an increase in angiotensin II in plasma. Despite these increases, antihypertensive activity and suppression of plasma aldosterone concentration are maintained, indicating effective angiotensin II receptor blockade. After discontinuation of losartan, PRA and angiotensin II values fell within three days to the baseline values.

Both losartan and its principal active metabolite have a far greater affinity for the AT_1-receptor than for the AT_2-receptor. The active metabolite is 10- to 40- times more active than losartan on a weight for weight basis.

Hypertension studies

In controlled clinical studies, once-daily administration of losartan to patients with mild to moderate essential hypertension produced statistically significant reductions in systolic and diastolic blood pressure. Measurements of blood pressure 24 hours post-dose relative to 5 – 6 hours post-dose demonstrated blood pressure reduction over 24 hours; the natural diurnal rhythm was retained. Blood pressure reduction at the end of the dosing interval was 70 – 80 % of the effect seen 5-6 hours post-dose.

Discontinuation of losartan in hypertensive patients did not result in an abrupt rise in blood pressure (rebound). Despite the marked decrease in blood pressure, losartan had no clinically significant effects on heart rate.

Losartan is equally effective in males and females, and in younger (below the age of 65 years) and older hypertensive patients.

LIFE-Study

The losartan Intervention For Endpoint Reduction in Hypertension [LIFE] study was a randomised, triple-blind, active-controlled study in 9193 hypertensive patients aged 55 to 80 years with ECG-documented left-ventricular hypertrophy. Patients were randomised to once daily losartan 50 mg or once daily atenolol 50 mg. If goal blood pressure (< 140/90 mmHg) was not reached, hydrochlorothiazide (12.5 mg) was added first and, if needed, the dose of losartan or atenolol was then increased to 100 mg once daily. Other antihypertensives, with the exception of ACE-inhibitors, angiotensin II antagonists or beta-blockers were added if necessary to reach the goal blood pressure.

The mean length of follow-up was 4.8 years.

The primary endpoint was the composite of cardiovascular morbidity and mortality as measured by a reduction in the combined incidence of cardiovascular death, stroke and myocardial infarction. Blood pressure was significantly lowered to similar levels in the two groups. Treatment with losartan resulted in a 13.0 % risk reduction (p=0.021, 95 % confidence interval 0.77-0.98) compared with atenolol for patients reaching the primary composite endpoint. This was mainly attributable to a reduction of the incidence of stroke. Treatment with losartan reduced the risk of stroke by 25 % relative to atenolol (p=0.001 95 % confidence interval 0.63-0.89). The rates of cardiovascular death and myocardial infarction were not significantly different between the treatment groups.

Race

In the LIFE-Study black patients treated with losartan had a higher risk of suffering the primary combined endpoint, i.e. a cardiovascular event (e.g. cardiac infarction, cardiovascular death) and especially stroke, than the black patients treated with atenolol. Therefore the results observed with losartan in comparison with atenolol in the LIFE study with regard to cardiovascular morbidity/mortality do not apply for black patients with hypertension and left-ventricular hypertrophy.

RENAAL-Study

The Reduction of Endpoints in NIDDM with the Angiotensin II Receptor Antagonist losartan RENAAL study was a controlled clinical study conducted worldwide in 1513 Type 2 diabetic patients with proteinuria, with or without hypertension. 751 patients were treated with losartan.

The objective of the study was to demonstrate a nephroprotective effect of losartan potassium over and above the benefit of lowering blood pressure. Patients with proteinuria and a serum creatinine of 1.3 – 3.0 mg/dl were randomised to receive losartan 50 mg once a day, titrated if necessary, to achieve blood pressure response, or to placebo, on a background of conventional antihypertensive therapy excluding ACE-inhibitors and angiotensin II antagonists.

Investigators were instructed to titrate the study medication to 100 mg daily as appropriate; 72 % of patients were taking the100 mg daily dose for the majority of the time. Other antihypertensive agents (diuretics, calcium antagonists, alpha- and beta-receptor blockers and also centrally acting antihypertensives) were permitted as supplementary treatment depending on the requirement in both groups. Patients were followed up for up to 4.6 years (3.4 years on average).

The primary endpoint of the study was a composite endpoint of doubling of the serum creatinine end-stage renal failure (need for dialysis or transplantation) or death.

The results showed that the treatment with losartan (327 events) as compared with placebo (359 events) resulted in a16.1 % risk reduction (p = 0.022) in the number of patients reaching the primary composite endpoint. For the following individual and combined components of the primary endpoint, the results showed a significant risk reduction in the group treated with losartan: 25.3 % risk reduction for doubling of the serum creatinine (p = 0.006); 28.6 % risk reduction for end-stage renal failure (p = 0.002); 19.9 % risk reduction for end-stage renal failure or death (p = 0.009); 21.0 % risk reduction for doubling of serum creatinine or end-stage renal failure (p = 0.01).

All-cause mortality rate was not significantly different between the two treatment groups. In this study losartan was generally well tolerated, as shown by a therapy discontinuation rate on account of adverse events that was comparable to the placebo group.

ELITE I and ELITE II Study

In the ELITE Study carried out over 48 weeks in722 patients with heart failure (NYHA Class II-IV), no difference was observed between the patients treated with losartan and those treated with captopril with regard to the primary endpoint of a long-term change in renal function. The observation of the ELITE Study, that, compared with captopril, losartan reduced the mortality risk, was not confirmed in the subsequent ELITE II Study.

In the ELITE II Study losartan 50 mg once daily (starting dose 12.5 mg, increased to 25 mg, then 50 mg once daily) was compared with captopril 50 mg three times daily (starting dose 12.5 m, increased to 25 mg and then to 50 mg three times daily). The primary endpoint of this prospective study was the all-cause mortality.

In this study 3152 patients with heart failure (NYHA Class II-IV) were followed for almost two years (median: 1.5 years) in order to determine whether losartan is superior to captopril in reducing all cause mortality. The primary endpoint did not show any statistically significant difference between Losartan and captopril in reducing all-cause mortality.

In both comparator-controlled (not placebo-controlled) clinical studies on patients with heart failure the tolerability of losartan was superior to that of captopril, measured on the basis of a significantly lower rate of discontinuations of therapy on account of adverse events and a significantly lower frequency of cough.

An increased mortality was observed in ELITE II in the small subgroup (22 % of all HF patients) taking beta-blockers at baseline.

Paediatric Hypertension

The antihypertensive effect of losartan was established in a clinical study involving 177 hypertensive paediatric patients 6 to 16 years of age with a body weight > 20 kg and a glomerular filtration rate > 30 ml/ min/ 1.73 m^2. Patients who weighed >20 kg to < 50 kg received either 2.5, 25 or 50 mg of losartan daily and patients who weighed > 50 kg received either 5, 50 or 100 mg of losartan daily. At the end of three weeks, losartan administration once daily lowered trough blood pressure in a dose-dependent manner.

Overall, there was a dose-response. The dose-response relationship became very obvious in the low dose group compared to the middle dose group (period I: -6.2 mmHg vs. -11.65 mmHg), but was attenuated when comparing the middle dose group with the high dose group (period I: -11.65 mmHg vs. -12.21 mmHg). The lowest doses studied, 2.5 mg and 5 mg, corresponding to an average daily dose of 0.07 mg/ kg, did not appear to offer consistent antihypertensive efficacy.

These results were confirmed during period II of the study where patients were randomized to continue losartan or placebo, after three weeks of treatment. The difference in blood pressure increase as compared to placebo was largest in the middle dose group (6.70 mmHg middle dose vs. 5.38 mmHg high dose). The rise in trough diastolic blood pressure was the same in patients receiving placebo and in those continuing losartan at the lowest dose in each group, again suggesting that the lowest dose in each group did not have significant antihypertensive effect.

Long-term effects of losartan on growth, puberty and general development have not been studied. The long-term efficacy of antihypertensive therapy with losartan in childhood to reduce cardiovascular morbidity and mortality has also not been established.

The European Medicines Agency has deferred the obligation to submit the results of studies with Cozaar in one or more subsets of the paediatric population in Hypertension and Proteinuria. See 4.2 for information on paediatric use.

5.2 Pharmacokinetic properties

Absorption

Following oral administration, losartan is well absorbed and undergoes first-pass metabolism, forming an active carboxylic acid metabolite and other inactive metabolites. The systemic bioavailability of losartan tablets is approximately 33 %. Mean peak concentrations of losartan and its active metabolite are reached in 1 hour and in 3-4 hours, respectively.

Distribution

Both losartan and its active metabolite are ⩾99 % bound to plasma proteins, primarily albumin. The volume of distribution of losartan is 34 litres.

Biotransformation

About 14 % of an intravenously- or orally-administered dose of losartan is converted to its active metabolite. Following oral and intravenous administration of ^{14}C-labelled losartan potassium, circulating plasma radioactivity primarily is attributed to losartan and its active metabolite. Minimal conversion of losartan to its active metabolite was seen in about one percent of individuals studied.

In addition to the active metabolite, inactive metabolites are formed.

Elimination

Plasma clearance of losartan and its active metabolite is about 600 ml/min and 50 ml/min, respectively. Renal clearance of losartan and its active metabolite is about 74 ml/min and 26 ml/min, respectively. When losartan is administered orally, about 4 % of the dose is excreted unchanged in the urine, and about 6 % of the dose is excreted in the urine as active metabolite. The pharmacokinetics of losartan and its active metabolite are linear with oral losartan potassium doses up to 200 mg.

Following oral administration, plasma concentrations of losartan and its active metabolite decline polyexponentially with a terminal half-life of about 2 hours and 6-9 hours, respectively. During once-daily dosing with 100 mg, neither losartan nor its active metabolite accumulates significantly in plasma.

Both biliary and urinary excretions contribute to the elimination of losartan and its metabolites. Following an oral dose/intravenous administration of ^{14}C-labelled losartan in man, about 35 % / 43 % of radioactivity is recovered in the urine and 58 %/ 50 % in the faeces.

Characteristics in patients

In elderly hypertensive patients the plasma concentrations of losartan and its active metabolite do not differ essentially from those found in young hypertensive patients.

In female hypertensive patients the plasma levels of losartan were up to twice as high as in male hypertensive patients, while the plasma levels of the active metabolite did not differ between men and women.

In patients with mild to moderate alcohol-induced hepatic cirrhosis, the plasma levels of losartan and its active metabolite after oral administration were respectively 5 and 1.7 times higher than in young male volunteers (see section 4.2 and 4.4).

Plasma concentrations of losartan are not altered in patients with a creatinine clearance above 10 ml/minute. Compared to patients with normal renal function, the AUC for losartan is about 2-times higher in haemodialysis dialysis patients.

The plasma concentrations of the active metabolite are not altered in patients with renal impairment or in haemodialysis patients.

Neither losartan nor the active metabolite can be removed by haemodialysis.

Pharmacokinetics in paediatric patients

The pharmacokinetics of losartan have been investigated in 50 hypertensive paediatric patients > 1 month to < 16 years of age following once daily oral administration of approximately 0.54 to 0.77 mg/ kg of losartan (mean doses). The results showed that the active metabolite is formed from losartan in all age groups. The results showed roughly similar pharmacokinetic parameters of losartan following oral administration in infants and toddlers, preschool children, school-age children and adolescents. The pharmacokinetic parameters for the metabolite differed to a greater extent between the age groups. When comparing preschool children with adolescents these differences became statistically significant. Exposure in infants/ toddlers was comparatively high.

5.3 Preclinical safety data

Preclinical data reveal no special hazard for humans based on conventional studies of general pharmacology, genotoxicity and carcinogenic potential. In repeated dose toxicity studies, the administration of losartan induced a decrease in the red blood cell parameters (erythrocytes, haemoglobin, haematocrit), a rise in urea-N in the serum and occasional rises in serum creatinine, a decrease in heart weight (without a histological correlate) and gastrointestinal changes (mucous membrane lesions, ulcers, erosions, haemorrhages). Like other substances that directly affect the renin-angiotensin system, losartan has been shown to induce adverse effects on the late foetal development, resulting in foetal death and malformations.

6. PHARMACEUTICAL PARTICULARS

6.1 List of excipients

Powder

microcrystalline cellulose (E460)

lactose monohydrate

pregelatinized maize starch

magnesium stearate (E572)

hydroxypropyl cellulose (E463)

hypromellose (E464)

titanium dioxide (E171)

Solvent

microcrystalline cellulose

carboxymethylcellulose sodium

citric acid anhydrous

purified water

xantham gum (E415)

methylhydroxybenzoate (E218)

sodium phosphate monobasic monohydrate

potassium sorbate (E202)

carrageenan calcium sulfate, trisodium phosphate

flavor berry citrus sweet

glycerin

propylhydroxybenzoate (E216)

sodium citrate anhydrous

saccharin sodium

sorbitol (E420)antifoam AF emulsion (contains water, polydimethylsiloxane, C-14-18, mono- and di-glycerides, polyethylene glucol stearate, and polyethylene glycol.)

6.2 Incompatibilities

Not applicable.

6.3 Shelf life

2 years

After reconstitution: 4 weeks.

6.4 Special precautions for storage

Kit: Do not store above 25°C. Store in the original package.

Store the prepared suspension in a refrigerator at 2-8°C.

6.5 Nature and contents of container

The following components are packed in a kit:

• A single aluminum foil sachet filled with powder containing 500 mg losartan potassium The sachet material consists of the following materials, from outside to inside and product contact layer: PET/Ink/ Adhesive/ Foil/ Adhesive/ PE

• a 473 ml white, high-density polyethylene (HDPE) bottle of solvent,

• a 240 ml amber polyethylene terephthalate (PET) bottle with polypropylene child resistant closure for mixing the suspension,

• a 10 ml oral dosing polypropylene syringe packed individually with a low density polyethylene push-in bottle neck adapter (PIBA) in a poly bag.

6.6 Special precautions for disposal and other handling

Losartan suspension is a white to off-white liquid when reconstituted with the supplied solution.

Reconstitution of COZAAR oral suspension [for 200 ml of a 2.5 mg/ml suspension]:

Add 200 ml of solvent to the 240 ml amber polyethylene terephthalate (PET) bottle provided. Before opening the sachet gently tap on the side of the sachet to facilitate transfer of the material. Carefully add the complete contents of the sachet into the PET container bottle containing the solvent, tapping the side of the sachet and inverting as necessary. It is normal to have a small amount of residual powder adhering to the interior surfaces of the sachet. The sachet should NOT be rinsed. Place the screw cap on the bottle and shake the contents well to disperse. After reconstitution, losartan suspension is an off-white liquid. Remove the screw cap, place the push-in bottle neck adaptor on the bottle, and re-cap the bottle. The suspension should be stored in a refrigerator at 2-8°C for up to 4 weeks. Shake the suspension prior to each use and return promptly to the refrigerator.

Discard the excess solvent not used in the preparation of the suspension.

7. MARKETING AUTHORISATION HOLDER

Merck Sharp and Dohme Limited
Hertford Road
Hoddesdon
Hertfordshire
EN11 9BU
UK

8. MARKETING AUTHORISATION NUMBER(S)

PL 00025/0530

9. DATE OF FIRST AUTHORISATION/RENEWAL OF THE AUTHORISATION

10 March 2009

10. DATE OF REVISION OF THE TEXT

10 March 2009

® denotes registered trademark of E. I. du Pont de Nemours and Company, Wilmington, Delaware, USA.

SPC.CZR-OS.09.UK.3016

Creon 10000 Capsules

(Solvay Healthcare Limited)

1. NAME OF THE MEDICINAL PRODUCT

Creon® 10000 Capsules

2. QUALITATIVE AND QUANTITATIVE COMPOSITION

Each capsule contains:

Lipase	10,000	PhEur units
Amylase	8,000	PhEur units
Protease	600	PhEur units

3. PHARMACEUTICAL FORM

Brown/clear capsules containing gastro-resistant granules.

4. CLINICAL PARTICULARS

4.1 Therapeutic indications

For the treatment of pancreatic exocrine insufficiency.

4.2 Posology and method of administration

Adults (including the elderly) and children:

Initially one to two capsules with each meal. Dose increases, if required, should be added slowly, with careful monitoring of response and symptomatology.

It is important to ensure adequate hydration of patients at all times whilst dosing Creon.

The capsules can be swallowed whole, or for ease of administration they may be opened and the granules taken with fluid or soft food, but without chewing. If the granules are mixed with food it is important that they are taken immediately, otherwise dissolution of the enteric coating may result.

Colonic damage has been reported in patients with cystic fibrosis taking in excess of 10,000 units of lipase/kg/day (see Undesirable effects).

4.3 Contraindications

Patients with known hypersensitivity to porcine proteins.

4.4 Special warnings and precautions for use

The product is of porcine origin.

Oral medications should not be administered during the early stages of acute pancreatitis.

4.5 Interaction with other medicinal products and other forms of interaction

None known.

4.6 Pregnancy and lactation

Pregnancy

For pancreatic enzymes no clinical data on exposed pregnancies are available.

Animal studies show no evidence for any absorption of porcine pancreatic enzymes. Therefore, no reproductive or developmental toxicity is to be expected.

Caution should be exercised when prescribing to pregnant women.

Lactation

No effects on the suckling child are anticipated since animal studies suggest no systemic exposure of the breastfeeding woman to pancreatic enzymes. Pancreatic enzymes can be used during breastfeeding.

If required during pregnancy or lactation Creon should be used in doses sufficient to provide adequate nutritional status.

4.7 Effects on ability to drive and use machines

None known.

4.8 Undesirable effects

Diarrhoea, constipation, gastric discomfort, nausea and skin reactions have been reported occasionally in patients receiving enzyme replacement therapy.

Rarely cases of hyper-uricosuria and hyper-uricaemia have been reported with very high doses of pancreatin.

Stricture of the ileo-caecum and large bowel and colitis has been reported in children with cystic fibrosis taking high doses of pancreatic enzyme supplements. To date, Creon has not been implicated in the development of colonic damage. However, unusual abdominal symptoms or changes in abdominal symptoms should be reviewed to exclude the possibility of colonic damage - especially if the patient is taking in excess of 10,000 units of lipase/kg/day.

4.9 Overdose

Most cases respond to supportive measures including stopping enzyme therapy, ensuring adequate rehydration.

5. PHARMACOLOGICAL PROPERTIES

5.1 Pharmacodynamic properties

Replacement therapy in pancreatic enzyme deficiency states. The enzymes have hydrolytic activity on fat, carbohydrates and proteins.

5.2 Pharmacokinetic properties

Pharmacokinetic data are not available as the enzymes act locally in the gastro-intestinal tract. After exerting their action, the enzymes are digested themselves in the intestine.

5.3 Preclinical safety data

None stated.

6. PHARMACEUTICAL PARTICULARS

6.1 List of excipients

Granules:

Macrogol 4000
Hypromellose phthalate
Dimeticone
Cetyl alcohol
Triethyl citrate

Capsule shell:

Gelatin,
Anhydrous iron (III) oxide, E172
Hydrated iron (III) oxide, E172
Iron (II, III) oxide (E172)
Titanium dioxide (E171)
Sodium lauryl sulphate

6.2 Incompatibilities

Not applicable.

6.3 Shelf life

2 years.

6.4 Special precautions for storage

Do not store above 30°C.

6.5 Nature and contents of container

HDPE container with tamper-evident PP cap. Containers hold 100, 250 or 300 capsules.

6.6 Special precautions for disposal and other handling

No special instructions.

Administrative Data

7. MARKETING AUTHORISATION HOLDER

Solvay Healthcare Limited
Mansbridge Road
West End
Southampton
SO18 3JD
United Kingdom

8. MARKETING AUTHORISATION NUMBER(S)

PL 00512/0149

9. DATE OF FIRST AUTHORISATION/RENEWAL OF THE AUTHORISATION

01 January 2001

10. DATE OF REVISION OF THE TEXT

May 2009

Creon 25000 Capsules

(Solvay Healthcare Limited)

1. NAME OF THE MEDICINAL PRODUCT

Creon® 25000 Capsules

2. QUALITATIVE AND QUANTITATIVE COMPOSITION

Each capsule contains pancreatin PhEur 300 mg equivalent to:

Lipase	25,000	PhEur units
Amylase	18,000	PhEur units
Protease	1,000	PhEur units

3. PHARMACEUTICAL FORM

Orange/colourless capsules filled with brownish minimicrospheres.

4. CLINICAL PARTICULARS

4.1 Therapeutic indications

For the treatment of pancreatic exocrine insufficiency.

4.2 Posology and method of administration

Adults (including the elderly) and children:

Initially one capsule with meals. Dose increases, if required, should be added slowly, with careful monitoring of response and symptomatology.

It is important to ensure adequate hydration of patients at all times whilst dosing Creon 25000.

The capsules can be swallowed whole, or for ease of administration they may be opened and the granules taken with fluid or soft food. If the granules are mixed with food, it is important that they are taken immediately, otherwise dissolution of the enteric coating may result. In order to protect the enteric coating, it is important that the granules are not crushed or chewed.

Colonic damage has been reported in patients with cystic fibrosis taking in excess of 10,000 units of lipase/kg/day (see Undesirable Effects).

4.3 Contraindications

Patients with known hypersensitivity to porcine proteins.

4.4 Special warnings and precautions for use

The product is of porcine origin.

Oral medications should not be administered during the early stages of acute pancreatitis.

4.5 Interaction with other medicinal products and other forms of interaction

None known.

4.6 Pregnancy and lactation

Pregnancy

For pancreatic enzymes no clinical data on exposed pregnancies are available.

Animal studies show no evidence for any absorption of porcine pancreatic enzymes. Therefore, no reproductive or developmental toxicity is to be expected.

Caution should be exercised when prescribing to pregnant women.

Lactation

No effects on the suckling child are anticipated since animal studies suggest no systemic exposure of the breastfeeding woman to pancreatic enzymes. Pancreatic enzymes can be used during breastfeeding.

If required during pregnancy or lactation Creon should be used in doses sufficient to provide adequate nutritional status.

4.7 Effects on ability to drive and use machines

None known.

4.8 Undesirable effects

Diarrhoea, constipation, gastric discomfort, nausea and skin reactions have been reported occasionally in patients receiving enzyme replacement therapy.

Rarely cases of hyper-uricosuria and hyper-uricaemia have been reported with very high doses of Pancreatin

Stricture of the ileo-caecum and large bowel and colitis has been reported in children with cystic fibrosis taking high doses of pancreatic enzyme supplements. To date, Creon 25000 has not been implicated in the development of colonic damage. However, unusual abdominal symptoms or changes in abdominal symptoms should be reviewed to exclude the possibility of colonic damage - especially if the patient is taking in excess of 10,000 units of lipase/kg/day.

4.9 Overdose

Most cases respond to supportive measures including stopping enzyme therapy, ensuring adequate rehydration.

5. PHARMACOLOGICAL PROPERTIES

5.1 Pharmacodynamic properties

Replacement therapy in pancreatic enzyme deficiency states. The enzymes have hydrolytic activity on fat, carbohydrates and proteins.

5.2 Pharmacokinetic properties

Pharmacokinetic data are not available as the enzymes act locally in the gastro-intestinal tract. After exerting their action, the enzymes are digested themselves in the intestine.

5.3 Preclinical safety data

Not applicable.

6. PHARMACEUTICAL PARTICULARS

6.1 List of excipients

Granules:

Macrogol 4000
Hypromellose phthalate
Dimeticone
Cetyl alcohol
Triethyl citrate

Capsules:

Gelatin,
Anhydrous iron (III) oxide, E172
Hydrated iron (III) oxide, E172
Titanium dioxide, E171
Sodium lauryl sulphate

6.2 Incompatibilities
None known.

6.3 Shelf life
3 years

6.4 Special precautions for storage
Store below 30°C.

6.5 Nature and contents of container
HDPE container with tamper-evident PP cap. Each container contains 100 capsules.

6.6 Special precautions for disposal and other handling
No special instructions.

Administrative Data

7. MARKETING AUTHORISATION HOLDER
Solvay Healthcare Limited
Mansbridge Road
West End
Southampton
SO18 3JD
United Kingdom

8. MARKETING AUTHORISATION NUMBER(S)
PL 00512/0150

9. DATE OF FIRST AUTHORISATION/RENEWAL OF THE AUTHORISATION
01 January 2001

10. DATE OF REVISION OF THE TEXT
May 2009

Legal category
POM

Creon 40000 Capsules

(Solvay Healthcare Limited)

1. NAME OF THE MEDICINAL PRODUCT
Creon® 40000 Capsules

2. QUALITATIVE AND QUANTITATIVE COMPOSITION
Each capsule contains pancreatin PhEur 400 mg equivalent to:
Lipase 40,000 PhEur units
Amylase 25,000 PhEur units
Protease 1,600 PhEur units

3. PHARMACEUTICAL FORM
Capsules.

Brown/clear size 00 capsules containing light brown, gastro-resistant granules.

4. CLINICAL PARTICULARS

4.1 Therapeutic indications
For the treatment of pancreatic exocrine insufficiency.

4.2 Posology and method of administration
Adults (including the elderly) and children:
Creon 40000 should only be used if the patient requires equal to or more than 40,000 lipase units per meal or snack. Creon 40000 should only be used in patients in whom the minimum effective dose has already been determined using lower strength pancreatic enzyme products.

Initially one or two capsules with meals. The capsules should be swallowed whole. Dose increases, if required, should be added slowly, with careful monitoring of response and symptomatology.

It is important to ensure adequate hydration of patients at all times whilst dosing Creon 40000.

Colonic damage has been reported in patients with cystic fibrosis taking in excess of 10,000 units of lipase/kg/day (see Undesirable Effects).

4.3 Contraindications
Patients with known hypersensitivity to porcine proteins.

4.4 Special warnings and precautions for use
The product is of porcine origin.

Oral medications should not be administered during the early stages of acute pancreatitis.

4.5 Interaction with other medicinal products and other forms of interaction
None known.

4.6 Pregnancy and lactation
Pregnancy

For pancreatic enzymes no clinical data on exposed pregnancies are available.

Animal studies show no evidence for any absorption of porcine pancreatic enzymes. Therefore, no reproductive or developmental toxicity is to be expected.

Caution should be exercised when prescribing to pregnant women.

Lactation

No effects on the suckling child are anticipated since animal studies suggest no systemic exposure of the breastfeeding woman to pancreatic enzymes. Pancreatic enzymes can be used during breastfeeding.

If required during pregnancy or lactation Creon should be used in doses sufficient to provide adequate nutritional status.

4.7 Effects on ability to drive and use machines
Creon 40000 has no influence on the ability to drive or use machines.

4.8 Undesirable effects
Diarrhoea, constipation, gastric discomfort, nausea and skin reactions have been reported occasionally in patients receiving enzyme replacement therapy.

Rarely cases of hyper-uricosuria and hyperuricaemia have been reported with very high doses of pancreatin.

Stricture of the ileocaecum and large bowel and colitis has been reported in children with cystic fibrosis taking high doses of pancreatic enzyme supplements. To date, Creon 10000 and 25000 have not been implicated in the development of colonic damage. Experience with Creon 40000 in clinical use is limited. Unusual abdominal symptoms or changes in abdominal symptoms should be reviewed to exclude the possibility of colonic damage - especially if the patient is taking in excess of 10,000 units of lipase/kg/day.

4.9 Overdose
Most cases respond to supportive measures including stopping enzyme therapy, ensuring adequate rehydration.

5. PHARMACOLOGICAL PROPERTIES

5.1 Pharmacodynamic properties
The ATC code is A09A A (Enzyme preparations).

Replacement therapy in pancreatic enzyme deficiency states. The enzymes have hydrolytic activity on fat, carbohydrates and proteins.

5.2 Pharmacokinetic properties
Pharmacokinetic data are not available as the enzymes act locally in the gastro-intestinal tract. After exerting their action, the enzymes are digested themselves in the intestine.

5.3 Preclinical safety data
None stated.

6. PHARMACEUTICAL PARTICULARS

6.1 List of excipients
Granules:
Macrogol 4000
Hypromellose phthalate
Dimeticone
Cetyl alcohol
Triethyl citrate
Capsules:
Gelatin
Anhydrous iron (III) oxide (E172)
Hydrated iron (III) oxide (E172)
Iron (II, III) oxide (E172)
Titanium dioxide E171
Sodium lauryl sulphate

6.2 Incompatibilities
None known.

6.3 Shelf life
3 years.

6.4 Special precautions for storage
Do not store above 25°C. Keep container tightly closed.

6.5 Nature and contents of container
HDPE container with tamper-evident PP cap. Each container contains 100 capsules.

6.6 Special precautions for disposal and other handling
No special instructions.

7. MARKETING AUTHORISATION HOLDER
Solvay Healthcare Limited
Mansbridge Road
West End
Southampton
SO18 3JD
United Kingdom

8. MARKETING AUTHORISATION NUMBER(S)
PL 00512/0177

9. DATE OF FIRST AUTHORISATION/RENEWAL OF THE AUTHORISATION
25/02/2009

10. DATE OF REVISION OF THE TEXT
May 2009

Legal Category
POM

Creon Micro

(Solvay Healthcare Limited)

1. NAME OF THE MEDICINAL PRODUCT
Creon® Micro Pancreatin 60.12 mg Gastro-resistant Granules

2. QUALITATIVE AND QUANTITATIVE COMPOSITION
Each 100 mg of gastro-resistant granules (equivalent to one measuring spoonful) contains 60.12mg of pancreatin, containing the following pancreatic enzymes:

Lipase	5,000 PhEur units
Amylase	3,600 PhEur units
Protease	200 PhEur units

For excipients, see 6.1.

3. PHARMACEUTICAL FORM
Gastro-resistant granules.

Round, light brown gastro-resistant granules.

4. CLINICAL PARTICULARS

4.1 Therapeutic indications
For the treatment of pancreatic exocrine insufficiency.

4.2 Posology and method of administration
Initially 100 mg (5000 lipase units) of gastro-resistant granules (one measure) should be taken with each feed or meal. Dose increases, if required, should be added slowly, with careful monitoring of response and symptomatology. The maximum daily dosage should not exceed 10,000 units lipase/kg/day. The required quantity of gastro-resistant granules should be dispensed using the measuring scoop contained in the pack which holds 100 mg.

In young infants, Creon Micro granules should be mixed with a small amount of apple juice and given from a spoon directly before the feed. In weaned infants, granules should be taken with acidic liquids or soft foods (e.g. mixed with apple juice or apple puree), but without chewing, directly before the meal. When giving Creon Micro to young or weaned infants the apple juice should not be diluted.

It is important to ensure adequate hydration of patients at all times whilst dosing with Creon.

Colonic damage has been reported in patients with cystic fibrosis taking in excess of 10000 units of lipase/kg/day (see Undesirable effects).

4.3 Contraindications
Patients with known hypersensitivity to porcine proteins or to any of the excipients.

4.4 Special warnings and precautions for use
The product is of porcine origin.

Oral medications should not be administered during the early stages of acute pancreatitis.

4.5 Interaction with other medicinal products and other forms of interaction
None known.

4.6 Pregnancy and lactation
Pregnancy

For pancreatic enzymes no clinical data on exposed pregnancies are available.

Animal studies show no evidence for any absorption of porcine pancreatic enzymes. Therefore, no reproductive or developmental toxicity is to be expected.

Caution should be exercised when prescribing to pregnant women.

Lactation

No effects on the suckling child are anticipated since animal studies suggest no systemic exposure of the breastfeeding woman to pancreatic enzymes. Pancreatic enzymes can be used during breastfeeding.

If required during pregnancy or lactation Creon should be used in doses sufficient to provide adequate nutritional status

4.7 Effects on ability to drive and use machines
Creon has no influence on the ability to drive or use machines.

4.8 Undesirable effects
In pooled data from clinical trials, the overall incidence of adverse drug events reported with Creon was the same as with placebo. The incidence tended to reflect the general symptomatology of the underlying disease.

Very common (*Frequency* $>10\%$):

Gastrointestinal disorders: abdominal pain

Common (*Frequency 1-10%*):

Gastrointestinal disorders: diarrhoea, constipation, abnormal stool, nausea and vomiting.

Skin and subcutaneous tissue: allergic or hypersensitivity reactions.

Stricture of the ileo-caecum and large bowel an colitis has been reported in children with cystic fibrosis taking high doses of pancreatic enzyme supplements. To date, Creon 10000 and 25000 have not been implicated in the development of colonic damage. Experience with Creon 40000 and Creon Micro in clinical use is limited. Unusual abdominal symptoms or changes in abdominal symptoms should be reviewed to exclude the possibility of colonic damage especially if the patient is taking in excess of 10,000 units lipase/kg/day.

4.9 Overdose
Most cases respond to supportive measures including stopping enzyme therapy, ensuring adequate rehydration. Rarely cases of hyperuricosuria and hyperuricaemia have been reported with very high doses of pancreatin.

5. PHARMACOLOGICAL PROPERTIES

5.1 Pharmacodynamic properties

The ATC code is A09A A (Enzyme preparations).

Replacement therapy in pancreatic enzyme deficiency states. The enzymes have hydrolytic activity on fat, carbohydrates and proteins.

5.2 Pharmacokinetic properties

Pharmacokinetic data are not available as the enzymes act locally in the gastro-intestinal tract. After exerting their action, the enzymes are digested themselves in the intestine.

5.3 Preclinical safety data

None stated.

6. PHARMACEUTICAL PARTICULARS

6.1 List of excipients

Hypromellose phthalate

Macrogol 4000

Dimeticone

Cetyl alcohol

Triethyl citrate

6.2 Incompatibilities

Not applicable.

6.3 Shelf life

2 years. 12 weeks after first opening.

6.4 Special precautions for storage

Do not store above 30°C.

Keep the container tightly closed in order to protect from moisture.

6.5 Nature and contents of container

Glass bottle with LDPE stopper. Containers hold 20 g of gastro-resistant granules.

6.6 Special precautions for disposal and other handling

No special requirements.

7. MARKETING AUTHORISATION HOLDER

Solvay Healthcare Limited
Mansbridge Road
West End
Southampton
SO18 3JD
United Kingdom

8. MARKETING AUTHORISATION NUMBER(S)

PL 00512/0179

9. DATE OF FIRST AUTHORISATION/RENEWAL OF THE AUTHORISATION

August 2004

10. DATE OF REVISION OF THE TEXT

May 2009

Legal category

P

Crestor 5mg, 10mg, 20mg and 40mg film-coated tablets

(AstraZeneca UK Limited)

1. NAME OF THE MEDICINAL PRODUCT

Crestor 5 mg, 10 mg, 20 mg and 40 mg film-coated tablets.

2. QUALITATIVE AND QUANTITATIVE COMPOSITION

Each tablet contains either 5 mg, 10 mg, 20 mg or 40 mg rosuvastatin (as rosuvastatin calcium).

Each 5 mg tablet contains 94.88 mg lactose monohydrate.

Each 10 mg tablet contains 91.3 mg lactose monohydrate.

Each 20 mg tablet contains 182.6 mg lactose monohydrate.

Each 40 mg tablet contains 168.32 mg lactose monohydrate.

For a full list of excipients, see Section 6.1.

3. PHARMACEUTICAL FORM

Film-coated tablet.

5 mg tablet:

Round, yellow coloured tablets, intagliated with 'ZD4522' and '5' on one side and plain on the reverse.

10 mg tablet:

Round, pink coloured tablets, intagliated with 'ZD4522' and '10' on one side and plain on the reverse.

20 mg tablet:

Round, pink coloured tablets, intagliated with 'ZD4522' and '20' on one side and plain on the reverse.

40 mg tablet:

Oval, pink coloured tablets, intagliated with 'ZD4522' on one side and '40' on the reverse.

4. CLINICAL PARTICULARS

4.1 Therapeutic indications

Primary hypercholesterolaemia (type IIa including heterozygous familial hypercholesterolaemia) or mixed dyslipidaemia (type IIb) as an adjunct to diet when response to diet and other non-pharmacological treatments (e.g. exercise, weight reduction) is inadequate.

Homozygous familial hypercholesterolaemia as an adjunct to diet and other lipid lowering treatments (e.g. LDL apheresis) or if such treatments are not appropriate.

4.2 Posology and method of administration

Before treatment initiation the patient should be placed on a standard cholesterol-lowering diet that should continue during treatment. The dose should be individualised according to the goal of therapy and patient response, using current consensus guidelines.

The recommended start dose is 5 mg or 10 mg orally once daily in both statin naïve or patients switched from another HMG CoA reductase inhibitor. The choice of start dose should take into account the individual patient's cholesterol level and future cardiovascular risk as well as the potential risk for adverse reactions (see below). A dose adjustment to the next dose level can be made after 4 weeks, if necessary (see Section 5.1). In light of the increased reporting rate of adverse reactions with the 40 mg dose compared to lower doses (see Section 4.8), a final titration to the maximum dose of 40 mg should only be considered in patients with severe hypercholesterolaemia at high cardiovascular risk (in particular those with familial hypercholesterolaemia), who do not achieve their treatment goal on 20 mg, and in whom routine follow-up will be performed (see Section 4.4). Specialist supervision is recommended when the 40 mg dose is initiated.

Crestor may be given at any time of day, with or without food.

Paediatric use

Safety and efficacy have not been established in children. Paediatric experience is limited to a small number of children (aged 8 years or above) with homozygous familial hypercholesterolaemia. Therefore, Crestor is not recommended for paediatric use at this time.

Use in the elderly

A start dose of 5 mg is recommended in patients >70 years (see Section 4.4). No other dose adjustment is necessary in relation to age.

Dosage in patients with renal insufficiency

No dose adjustment is necessary in patients with mild to moderate renal impairment. The recommended start dose is 5 mg in patients with moderate renal impairment (creatinine clearance of <60 ml/min). The 40 mg dose is contraindicated in patients with moderate renal impairment. The use of Crestor in patients with severe renal impairment is contraindicated for all doses (See Section 4.3 and Section 5.2).

Dosage in patients with hepatic impairment

There was no increase in systemic exposure to rosuvastatin in subjects with Child-Pugh scores of 7 or below. However, increased systemic exposure has been observed in subjects with Child-Pugh scores of 8 and 9 (see Section 5.2). In these patients an assessment of renal function should be considered (see Section 4.4). There is no experience in subjects with Child-Pugh scores above 9. Crestor is contraindicated in patients with active liver disease (see Section 4.3).

Race

Increased systemic exposure has been seen in Asian subjects (see Section 4.4 and Section 5.2). The recommended start dose is 5 mg for patients of Asian ancestry. The 40 mg dose is contraindicated in these patients.

Dosage in patients with pre-disposing factors to myopathy

The recommended start dose is 5 mg in patients with predisposing factors to myopathy (see Section 4.4).

The 40 mg dose is contraindicated in some of these patients (see Section 4.3).

4.3 Contraindications

Crestor is contraindicated:

- in patients with hypersensitivity to rosuvastatin or to any of the excipients.

- in patients with active liver disease including unexplained, persistent elevations of serum transaminases and any serum transaminase elevation exceeding 3 × the upper limit of normal (ULN).

- in patients with severe renal impairment (creatinine clearance <30 ml/min).

- in patients with myopathy.

- in patients receiving concomitant ciclosporin.

- during pregnancy and lactation and in women of childbearing potential not using appropriate contraceptive measures.

The 40 mg dose is contraindicated in patients with predisposing factors for myopathy/rhabdomyolysis. Such factors include:

– moderate renal impairment (creatinine clearance < 60 ml/min)

– hypothyroidism

– personal or family history of hereditary muscular disorders

– previous history of muscular toxicity with another HMG-CoA reductase inhibitor or fibrate

– alcohol abuse

– situations where an increase in plasma levels may occur

– Asian patients

– concomitant use of fibrates.

(see Sections 4.4, 4.5 and 5.2)

4.4 Special warnings and precautions for use

Renal Effects

Proteinuria, detected by dipstick testing and mostly tubular in origin, has been observed in patients treated with higher doses of Crestor, in particular 40 mg, where it was transient or intermittent in most cases. Proteinuria has not been shown to be predictive of acute or progressive renal disease (see Section 4.8). The reporting rate for serious renal events in post-marketing use is higher at the 40 mg dose. An assessment of renal function should be considered during routine follow-up of patients treated with a dose of 40 mg.

Skeletal Muscle Effects

Effects on skeletal muscle e.g. myalgia, myopathy and, rarely, rhabdomyolysis have been reported in Crestor-treated patients with all doses and in particular with doses > 20 mg. Very rare cases of rhabdomyolysis have been reported with the use of ezetimibe in combination with HMG-CoA reductase inhibitors. A pharmacodynamic interaction cannot be excluded (see Section 4.5) and caution should be exercised with their combined use.

As with other HMG-CoA reductase inhibitors, the reporting rate for rhabdomyolysis associated with Crestor in post-marketing use is higher at the 40 mg dose.

Creatine Kinase Measurement

Creatine Kinase (CK) should not be measured following strenuous exercise or in the presence of a plausible alternative cause of CK increase which may confound interpretation of the result. If CK levels are significantly elevated at baseline (>5xULN) a confirmatory test should be carried out within 5 – 7 days. If the repeat test confirms a baseline CK>5xULN, treatment should not be started.

Before Treatment

Crestor, as with other HMG-CoA reductase inhibitors, should be prescribed with caution in patients with predisposing factors for myopathy/rhabdomyolysis. Such factors include:

- renal impairment
- hypothyroidism
- personal or family history of hereditary muscular disorders
- previous history of muscular toxicity with another HMG-CoA reductase inhibitor or fibrate
- alcohol abuse
- age >70 years
- situations where an increase in plasma levels may occur (see Section 5.2)
- concomitant use of fibrates.

In such patients the risk of treatment should be considered in relation to possible benefit and clinical monitoring is recommended. If CK levels are significantly elevated at baseline (>5xULN) treatment should not be started.

Whilst on Treatment

Patients should be asked to report inexplicable muscle pain, weakness or cramps immediately, particularly if associated with malaise or fever. CK levels should be measured in these patients. Therapy should be discontinued if CK levels are markedly elevated (>5xULN) or if muscular symptoms are severe and cause daily discomfort (even if CK levels are ⩽ 5x ULN). If symptoms resolve and CK levels return to normal, then consideration should be given to re-introducing Crestor or an alternative HMG-CoA reductase inhibitor at the lowest dose with close monitoring. Routine monitoring of CK levels in asymptomatic patients is not warranted.

In clinical trials there was no evidence of increased skeletal muscle effects in the small number of patients dosed with Crestor and concomitant therapy. However, an increase in the incidence of myositis and myopathy has been seen in patients receiving other HMG-CoA reductase inhibitors together with fibric acid derivatives including gemfibrozil, ciclosporin, nicotinic acid, azole antifungals, protease inhibitors and macrolide antibiotics. Gemfibrozil increases the risk of myopathy when given concomitantly with some HMG-CoA reductase inhibitors. Therefore, the combination of Crestor and gemfibrozil is not recommended. The benefit of further alterations in lipid levels by the combined use of Crestor with fibrates or niacin should be carefully weighed against the potential risks of such combinations. The 40 mg dose is contraindicated with concomitant use of a fibrate.

(See Section 4.5 and Section 4.8)

Crestor should not be used in any patient with an acute, serious condition suggestive of myopathy or predisposing to the development of renal failure secondary to rhabdomyolysis (e.g. sepsis, hypotension, major surgery, trauma, severe metabolic, endocrine and electrolyte disorders; or uncontrolled seizures).

Liver Effects

As with other HMG-CoA reductase inhibitors, Crestor should be used with caution in patients who consume excessive quantities of alcohol and/or have a history of liver disease.

It is recommended that liver function tests be carried out prior to, and 3 months following, the initiation of treatment. Crestor should be discontinued or the dose reduced if the level of serum transaminases is greater than 3 times the upper limit of normal. The reporting rate for serious hepatic events (consisting mainly of increased hepatic transaminases) in post-marketing use is higher at the 40 mg dose.

In patients with secondary hypercholesterolaemia caused by hypothyroidism or nephrotic syndrome, the underlying disease should be treated prior to initiating therapy with Crestor.

Race

Pharmacokinetic studies show an increase in exposure in Asian subjects compared with Caucasians (see Section 4.2 and Section 5.2)

Protease inhibitors

The concomitant use with protease inhibitors is not recommended (see Section 4.5).

Lactose intolerance

Patients with rare hereditary problems of galactose intolerance, the Lapp lactase deficiency or glucose-galactose malabsorption should not take this medicine.

4.5 Interaction with other medicinal products and other forms of interaction

Ciclosporin: During concomitant treatment with Crestor and ciclosporin, rosuvastatin AUC values were on average 7 times higher than those observed in healthy volunteers (see Section 4.3).

Concomitant administration did not affect plasma concentrations of ciclosporin.

Vitamin K antagonists: As with other HMG-CoA reductase inhibitors, the initiation of treatment or dosage up-titration of Crestor in patients treated concomitantly with vitamin K antagonists (e.g. warfarin or another coumarin anticoagulant) may result in an increase in International Normalised Ratio (INR). Discontinuation or down-titration of Crestor may result in a decrease in INR. In such situations, appropriate monitoring of INR is desirable.

Ezetimibe: Concomitant use of Crestor and ezetimibe resulted in no change to AUC or Cmax for either drug. However, a pharmacodynamic interaction, in terms of adverse effects, between Crestor and ezetimibe cannot be ruled out (see Section 4.4).

Gemfibrozil and other lipid-lowering products: Concomitant use of Crestor and gemfibrozil resulted in a 2-fold increase in rosuvastatin C_{max} and AUC (see Section 4.4).

Based on data from specific interaction studies no pharmacokinetic relevant interaction with fenofibrate is expected, however a pharmacodynamic interaction may occur. Gemfibrozil, fenofibrate, other fibrates and lipid lowering doses (> or equal to 1g/day) of niacin (nicotinic acid) increase the risk of myopathy when given concomitantly with HMG-CoA reductase inhibitors, probably because they can produce myopathy when given alone. The 40 mg dose is contraindicated with concomitant use of a fibrate (see Section 4.3 and Section 4.4). These patients should also start with the 5 mg dose.

Protease inhibitors: Although the exact mechanism of interaction is unknown, concomitant protease inhibitor use may strongly increase rosuvastatin exposure. In a pharmacokinetic study, co-administration of 20 mg rosuvastatin and a combination product of two protease inhibitors (400 mg lopinavir / 100 mg ritonavir) in healthy volunteers was associated with an approximately two-fold and five-fold increase in rosuvastatin steady-state $AUC_{(0-24)}$ and Cmax respectively. Therefore, concomitant use of rosuvastatin in HIV patients receiving protease inhibitors is not recommended (see also Section 4.4).

Antacid: The simultaneous dosing of Crestor with an antacid suspension containing aluminium and magnesium hydroxide resulted in a decrease in rosuvastatin plasma concentration of approximately 50%. This effect was mitigated when the antacid was dosed 2 hours after Crestor. The clinical relevance of this interaction has not been studied.

Erythromycin: Concomitant use of Crestor and erythromycin resulted in a 20% decrease in AUC (0-t) and a 30% decrease in C_{max} of rosuvastatin. This interaction may be caused by the increase in gut motility caused by erythromycin.

Oral contraceptive/hormone replacement therapy (HRT): Concomitant use of Crestor and an oral contraceptive resulted in an increase in ethinyl estradiol and norgestrel AUC of 26% and 34%, respectively. These increased plasma levels should be considered when selecting oral contraceptive doses. There are no pharmacokinetic data available in subjects taking concomitant Crestor and HRT and therefore a similar effect cannot be excluded. However, the combination has been extensively used in women in clinical trials and was well tolerated.

Other medicinal products: Based on data from specific interaction studies no clinically relevant interaction with digoxin is expected.

Cytochrome P450 enzymes: Results from *in vitro* and *in vivo* studies show that rosuvastatin is neither an inhibitor nor an inducer of cytochrome P450 isoenzymes. In addition, rosuvastatin is a poor substrate for these isoenzymes. No clinically relevant interactions have been observed between rosuvastatin and either fluconazole (an inhibitor of CYP2C9 and CYP3A4) or ketoconazole (an inhibitor of CYP2A6 and CYP3A4). Concomitant administration of itraconazole (an inhibitor of CYP3A4) and rosuvastatin resulted in a 28% increase in AUC of rosuvastatin. This small increase is not considered clinically significant. Therefore, drug interactions resulting from cytochrome P450-mediated metabolism are not expected.

4.6 Pregnancy and lactation

Crestor is contraindicated in pregnancy and lactation.

Women of child bearing potential should use appropriate contraceptive measures.

Since cholesterol and other products of cholesterol biosynthesis are essential for the development of the foetus, the potential risk from inhibition of HMG-CoA reductase outweighs the advantage of treatment during pregnancy. Animal studies provide limited evidence of reproductive toxicity (see Section 5.3). If a patient becomes pregnant during use of this product, treatment should be discontinued immediately.

Rosuvastatin is excreted in the milk of rats. There are no data with respect to excretion in milk in humans. (see Section 4.3).

4.7 Effects on ability to drive and use machines

Studies to determine the effect of Crestor on the ability to drive and use machines have not been conducted. However, based on its pharmacodynamic properties, Crestor is unlikely to affect this ability. When driving vehicles or operating machines, it should be taken into account that dizziness may occur during treatment.

4.8 Undesirable effects

The adverse events seen with Crestor are generally mild and transient. In controlled clinical trials, less than 4% of Crestor-treated patients were withdrawn due to adverse events.

The frequencies of adverse events are ranked according to the following: Common (>1/100, <1/10); Uncommon (>1/1,000, <1/100); Rare (>1/10,000, <1/1000); Very rare (<1/10,000); Not known (cannot be estimated from the available data).

Immune system disorders

Rare: hypersensitivity reactions including angioedema

Nervous system disorders

Common: headache, dizziness

Gastrointestinal disorders

Common: constipation, nausea, abdominal pain

Rare: pancreatitis

Skin and subcutaneous tissue disorders

Uncommon: pruritus, rash and urticaria

Musculoskeletal, connective tissue and bone disorders

Common: myalgia

Rare: myopathy (including myositis) and rhabdomyolysis

General disorders

Common: asthenia

As with other HMG-CoA reductase inhibitors, the incidence of adverse drug reactions tends to be dose dependent.

Renal Effects: Proteinuria, detected by dipstick testing and mostly tubular in origin, has been observed in patients treated with Crestor. Shifts in urine protein from none or trace to ++ or more were seen in <1% of patients at some time during treatment with 10 and 20 mg, and in approximately 3% of patients treated with 40 mg. A minor increase in shift from none or trace to + was observed with the 20 mg dose. In most cases, proteinuria decreases or disappears spontaneously on continued therapy. Review of data from clinical trials and post-marketing experience to date has not identified a causal association between proteinuria and acute or progressive renal disease.

Haematuria has been observed in patients treated with Crestor and clinical trial data show that the occurrence is low.

Skeletal muscle effects: Effects on skeletal muscle e.g. myalgia, myopathy (including myositis) and, rarely, rhabdomyolysis with and without acute renal failure have been reported in Crestor-treated patients with all doses and in particular with doses > 20 mg.

A dose-related increase in CK levels has been observed in patients taking rosuvastatin; the majority of cases were mild, asymptomatic and transient. If CK levels are elevated (>5xULN), treatment should be discontinued (see Section 4.4).

Liver Effects: As with other HMG-CoA reductase inhibitors, a dose-related increase in transaminases has been observed in a small number of patients taking rosuvastatin; the majority of cases were mild, asymptomatic and transient.

Post Marketing Experience:

In addition to the above, the following adverse events have been reported during post marketing experience for CRESTOR:

Gastrointestinal disorders: Not known: diarrhoea.

Hepatobiliary disorders: Very rare: jaundice, hepatitis; *rare:* increased transaminases.

Musculoskeletal disorders: Very rare: arthralgia.

Nervous system disorders: Very rare: polyneuropathy, memory loss.

Renal disorders: Very rare: haematuria.

Skin and subcutaneous tissue disorders: Not known: Stevens-Johnson syndrome.

The reporting rates for rhabdomyolysis, serious renal events and serious hepatic events (consisting mainly of increased hepatic transaminases) is higher at the 40 mg dose.

4.9 Overdose

There is no specific treatment in the event of overdose. In the event of overdose, the patient should be treated symptomatically and supportive measures instituted as required. Liver function and CK levels should be monitored. Haemodialysis is unlikely to be of benefit.

5. PHARMACOLOGICAL PROPERTIES

5.1 Pharmacodynamic properties

Pharmacotherapeutic group: HMG-CoA reductase inhibitors

ATC code: C10A A07

Mechanism of action

Rosuvastatin is a selective and competitive inhibitor of HMG-CoA reductase, the rate-limiting enzyme that converts 3-hydroxy-3-methylglutaryl coenzyme A to mevalonate, a precursor for cholesterol. The primary site of action of rosuvastatin is the liver, the target organ for cholesterol lowering.

Rosuvastatin increases the number of hepatic LDL receptors on the cell-surface, enhancing uptake and catabolism of LDL and it inhibits the hepatic synthesis of VLDL, thereby reducing the total number of VLDL and LDL particles.

Pharmacodynamic effects

Crestor reduces elevated LDL-cholesterol, total cholesterol and triglycerides and increases HDL-cholesterol. It also lowers ApoB, nonHDL-C, VLDL-C, VLDL-TG and increases ApoA-I (see Table 1). Crestor also lowers the LDL-C/HDL-C, total C/HDL-C and nonHDL-C/HDL-C and the ApoB/ApoA-I ratios.

Table 1 Dose response in patients with primary hypercholesterolaemia (type IIa and IIb) (adjusted mean percent change from baseline)

(see Table 1 below)

A therapeutic effect is obtained within 1 week following treatment initiation and 90% of maximum response is achieved in 2 weeks. The maximum response is usually achieved by 4 weeks and is maintained after that.

Clinical efficacy

Crestor is effective in adults with hypercholesterolaemia, with and without hypertriglyceridaemia, regardless of race, sex, or age and in special populations such as diabetics, or patients with familial hypercholesterolaemia.

From pooled phase III data, Crestor has been shown to be effective at treating the majority of patients with type IIa and IIb hypercholesterolaemia (mean baseline LDL-C about 4.8 mmol/l) to recognised European Atherosclerosis Society (EAS; 1998) guideline targets; about 80% of patients treated with 10 mg reached the EAS targets for LDL-C levels (<3 mmol/l).

In a large study, 435 patients with heterozygous familial hypercholesterolaemia were given Crestor from 20 mg to 80 mg in a force-titration design. All doses showed a beneficial effect on lipid parameters and treatment to target goals. Following titration to a daily dose of 40 mg (12 weeks of treatment), LDL-C was reduced by 53%. 33% of

Table 1 Dose response in patients with primary hypercholesterolaemia (type IIa and IIb) (adjusted mean percent change from baseline)

Dose	N	LDL-C	Total-C	HDL-C	TG	nonHDL-C	ApoB	ApoA-I
Placebo	13	-7	-5	3	-3	-7	-3	0
5	17	-45	-33	13	-35	-44	-38	4
10	17	-52	-36	14	-10	-48	-42	4
20	17	-55	-40	8	-23	-51	-46	5
40	18	-63	-46	10	-28	-60	-54	0

patients reached EAS guidelines for LDL-C levels (<3 mmol/l).

In a force-titration, open label trial, 42 patients with homozygous familial hypercholesterolaemia were evaluated for their response to Crestor 20 - 40 mg. In the overall population, the mean LDL-C reduction was 22%.

In clinical studies with a limited number of patients, Crestor has been shown to have additive efficacy in lowering triglycerides when used in combination with fenofibrate and in increasing HDL-C levels when used in combination with niacin (see Section 4.4).

Rosuvastatin has not been proven to prevent the associated complications of lipid abnormalities, such as coronary heart disease as mortality and morbidity studies with Crestor have not yet been completed.

In a multi-centre, double-blind, placebo-controlled clinical study (METEOR), 984 patients between 45 and 70 years of age and at low risk for coronary heart disease (defined as Framingham risk <10% over 10 years), with a mean LDL-C of 4.0 mmol/l (154.5 mg/dL), but with subclinical atherosclerosis (detected by Carotid Intima Media Thickness) were randomised to 40 mg rosuvastatin once daily or placebo for 2 years. Rosuvastatin significantly slowed the rate of progression of the maximum CIMT for the 12 carotid artery sites compared to placebo by -0.0145 mm/year [95% confidence interval -0.0196, -0.0093; p<0.0001]. The change from baseline was -0.0014 mm/year (-0.12%/year (non-significant)) for rosuvastatin compared to a progression of +0.0131 mm/year (1.12%/year (p<0.0001)) for placebo. No direct correlation between CIMT decrease and reduction of the risk of cardiovascular events has yet been demonstrated. The population studied in METEOR is low risk for coronary heart disease and does not represent the target population of Crestor 40mg. The 40mg dose should only be prescribed in patients with severe hypercholesterolaemia at high cardiovascular risk (see Section 4.2).

5.2 Pharmacokinetic properties

Absorption: Maximum rosuvastatin plasma concentrations are achieved approximately 5 hours after oral administration. The absolute bioavailability is approximately 20%.

Distribution: Rosuvastatin is taken up extensively by the liver which is the primary site of cholesterol synthesis and LDL-C clearance. The volume of distribution of rosuvastatin is approximately 134 L. Approximately 90% of rosuvastatin is bound to plasma proteins, mainly to albumin.

Metabolism: Rosuvastatin undergoes limited metabolism (approximately 10%). *In vitro* metabolism studies using human hepatocytes indicate that rosuvastatin is a poor substrate for cytochrome P450-based metabolism. CYP2C9 was the principal isoenzyme involved, with 2C19, 3A4 and 2D6 involved to a lesser extent. The main metabolites identified are the N-desmethyl and lactone metabolites. The N-desmethyl metabolite is approximately 50% less active than rosuvastatin whereas the lactone form is considered clinically inactive. Rosuvastatin accounts for greater than 90% of the circulating HMG-CoA reductase inhibitor activity.

Excretion: Approximately 90% of the rosuvastatin dose is excreted unchanged in the faeces (consisting of absorbed and non-absorbed active substance) and the remaining part is excreted in urine. Approximately 5% is excreted unchanged in urine. The plasma elimination half-life is approximately 19 hours. The elimination half-life does not increase at higher doses. The geometric mean plasma clearance is approximately 50 litres/hour (coefficient of variation 21.7%). As with other HMG-CoA reductase inhibitors, the hepatic uptake of rosuvastatin involves the membrane transporter OATP-C. This transporter is important in the hepatic elimination of rosuvastatin.

Linearity: Systemic exposure of rosuvastatin increases in proportion to dose. There are no changes in pharmacokinetic parameters following multiple daily doses.

Special populations:

Age and sex: There was no clinically relevant effect of age or sex on the pharmacokinetics of rosuvastatin.

Race: Pharmacokinetic studies show an approximate 2-fold elevation in median AUC and C_{max} in Asian subjects (Japanese, Chinese, Filipino, Vietnamese and Koreans) compared with Caucasians; Asian-Indians show an approximate 1.3-fold elevation in median AUC and Cmax. A population pharmacokinetic analysis revealed no clinically relevant differences in pharmacokinetics between Caucasian and Black groups.

Renal insufficiency: In a study in subjects with varying degrees of renal impairment, mild to moderate renal disease had no influence on plasma concentration of rosuvastatin or the N-desmethyl metabolite. Subjects with severe impairment (CrCl <30 ml/min) had a 3-fold increase in plasma concentration and a 9-fold increase in the N-desmethyl metabolite concentration compared to healthy volunteers. Steady-state plasma concentrations of rosuvastatin in subjects undergoing haemodialysis were approximately 50% greater compared to healthy volunteers.

Hepatic insufficiency: In a study with subjects with varying degrees of hepatic impairment there was no evidence of increased exposure to rosuvastatin in subjects with Child-Pugh scores of 7 or below. However, two subjects with Child-Pugh scores of 8 and 9 showed an increase in systemic exposure of at least 2-fold compared to subjects with lower Child-Pugh scores. There is no experience in subjects with Child-Pugh scores above 9.

5.3 Preclinical safety data

Preclinical data reveal no special hazard for humans based on conventional studies of safety pharmacology, genotoxicity and carcinogenicity potential. Specific tests for effects on hERG have not been evaluated. Adverse reactions not observed in clinical studies, but seen in animals at exposure levels similar to clinical exposure levels were as follows: In repeated-dose toxicity studies histopathologic liver changes likely due to the pharmacologic action of rosuvastatin were observed in mouse, rat, and to a lesser extent with effects in the gall bladder in dogs, but not in monkeys. In addition, testicular toxicity was observed in monkeys and dogs at higher dosages. Reproductive toxicity was evident in rats, with reduced litter sizes, litter weight and pup survival observed at maternally toxic doses, where systemic exposures were several times above the therapeutic exposure level.

6. PHARMACEUTICAL PARTICULARS

6.1 List of excipients

Tablet core

Lactose monohydrate

Microcrystalline cellulose

Calcium phosphate

Crospovidone

Magnesium stearate

Tablet coat

Lactose monohydrate

Hypromellose

Triacetin

Titanium dioxide (E171)

Ferric oxide, yellow (E172) (5 mg tablet)

Ferric oxide, red (E172) (10 mg, 20 mg and 40 mg tablets)

6.2 Incompatibilities

Not applicable.

6.3 Shelf life

3 years.

6.4 Special precautions for storage

Blisters: Store below 30°C. Store in the original package.

HDPE containers: Store below 30°C. Keep container tightly closed.

6.5 Nature and contents of container

Blisters of aluminium laminate/aluminium foil of 7, 14, 15, 20, 28, 30, 42, 50, 56, 60, 84, 90, 98 and 100 tablets and HDPE containers of 30 and 100 tablets.

Not all pack sizes may be marketed.

6.6 Special precautions for disposal and other handling

No special requirements.

7. MARKETING AUTHORISATION HOLDER

AstraZeneca UK Ltd

600 Capability Green

Luton

LU1 3LU

United Kingdom

8. MARKETING AUTHORISATION NUMBER(S)

5 mg: PL 17901/0243

10 mg: PL 17901/0201

20 mg: PL 17901/0202

40 mg: PL 17901/0203

9. DATE OF FIRST AUTHORISATION/RENEWAL OF THE AUTHORISATION

21st March 2003/6th November 2007

10. DATE OF REVISION OF THE TEXT

28th April 2009

Crinone 8% Progesterone Vaginal Gel

(Merck Serono)

1. NAME OF THE MEDICINAL PRODUCT

CRINONE® 8% Progesterone Vaginal Gel.

2. QUALITATIVE AND QUANTITATIVE COMPOSITION

Active Ingredient

	mg/dose	% w/w
Progesterone	90	8.0

3. PHARMACEUTICAL FORM

Vaginal gel.

4. CLINICAL PARTICULARS

4.1 Therapeutic indications

Treatment of infertility due to inadequate luteal phase.

For use during in-vitro fertilisation, where infertility is mainly due to tubal, idiopathic or endometriosis linked sterility associated with normal ovulatory cycles.

4.2 Posology and method of administration

Intravaginal application.

Treatment of infertility due to inadequate luteal phase: one application (1.125g 8% gel) every day, starting after documented ovulation or arbitrarily on the 18th-21st day of the cycle.

When used during in-vitro fertilisation, daily application of Crinone 8% gel should be continued for 30 days if there is laboratory evidence of pregnancy.

Children: Not applicable.

The Elderly: Not applicable.

4.3 Contraindications

Known allergy to any of the excipients.

Undiagnosed uterine bleeding.

Porphyria

4.4 Special warnings and precautions for use

Cautious use in severe hepatic insufficiency.

The product should not be used concurrently with other local intravaginal therapy.

4.5 Interaction with other medicinal products and other forms of interaction

No interaction reported.

4.6 Pregnancy and lactation

In case of corpus luteum deficiency, CRINONE can be used during the first month of pregnancy.

Do not use during lactation.

4.7 Effects on ability to drive and use machines

Drivers and users of machines are warned that risk of somnolence may occur.

4.8 Undesirable effects

Rare cases of somnolence.

Occasional spotting.

4.9 Overdose

Not applicable.

5. PHARMACOLOGICAL PROPERTIES

5.1 Pharmacodynamic properties

The pharmacological particulars of the product are those of the naturally occurring progesterone with induction of a full secretory endometrium.

5.2 Pharmacokinetic properties

The progesterone vaginal gel is based on a polycarbophil delivery system which attaches to the vaginal mucosa and provides a prolonged release of progesterone for at least three days.

5.3 Preclinical safety data

In rabbits, Crinone was an eye irritant categorised class IV (minimal effects clearing in less than 24 hours), but not a dermal irritant.

A moderate vaginal irritation was found in rabbits after application of 2.0ml/day of 8% gel for 5 days.

6. PHARMACEUTICAL PARTICULARS

6.1 List of excipients

Glycerin, Light Liquid Paraffin, Hydrogenated Palm Oil Glyceride, Carbopol 974P, Sorbic acid, Polycarbophil, Sodium hydroxide, Purified water.

6.2 Incompatibilities

No incompatibilities were found with the usual contraceptive devices.

6.3 Shelf life

36 months.

6.4 Special precautions for storage

Store below 25°C.

6.5 Nature and contents of container

A single use, one piece, white polyethylene applicator with a twist-off top, designed for intravaginal application.

Each applicator contains 1.45 g of gel and delivers 1.125g of gel. Each one is wrapped up and sealed in a paper/aluminium/polyethylene foil overwrap.

The applicators are packed in cardboard boxes containing 6 or 15 units of Crinone 8% progesterone vaginal gel.

6.6 Special precautions for disposal and other handling

Crinone is applied directly from the specially designed sealed applicator into the vagina. Remove the applicator from the sealed wrapper. DO NOT remove the twist-off cap at this time.

1. Grip the applicator firmly by the thick end. Shake down like a thermometer to ensure that the contents are at the thin end.

2. Twist off the tab and discard.

3. The applicator may be inserted while you are in a sitting position or when lying on your back with the knees bent. Gently insert the thin end of applicator well into the vagina.

4. Press the thick end of the applicator firmly to deposit gel. Remove the applicator and discard in a waste container.

5. CRINONE coats the vaginal mucosa to provide long-lasting release of progesterone.

7. MARKETING AUTHORISATION HOLDER
Serono Ltd

Bedfont Cross

Stanwell Road

Feltham

Middlesex TW14 8NX

United Kingdom

Tel: 020 8818 7200

8. MARKETING AUTHORISATION NUMBER(S)
PL 03400/0081

9. DATE OF FIRST AUTHORISATION/RENEWAL OF THE AUTHORISATION
Granted: 26th January 2000

Renewed: 26th June 2004

10. DATE OF REVISION OF THE TEXT
June 2004

CRIXIVAN 200 mg and 400 mg hard capsules

(Merck Sharp & Dohme Limited)

1. NAME OF THE MEDICINAL PRODUCT
CRIXIVAN 200 mg hard capsules

CRIXIVAN 400 mg hard capsules

2. QUALITATIVE AND QUANTITATIVE COMPOSITION
CRIXIVAN 200 mg:

Each hard capsule contains indinavir sulphate corresponding to 200 mg of indinavir.

Excipient: Each 200 mg capsule contains 74.8 mg lactose

CRIXIVAN 400 mg:

Each hard capsule contains indinavir sulphate corresponding to 400 mg of indinavir.

Excipient: Each 400 mg capsule contains 149.6 mg lactose

For full list of excipients, see section 6.1

3. PHARMACEUTICAL FORM
Hard capsule.

CRIXIVAN 200 mg: The capsules are semi–translucent white and coded CRIXIVAN™ 200 mg in blue.

CRIXIVAN 400 mg: The capsules are semi–translucent white and coded CRIXIVAN™ 400 mg in green.

4. CLINICAL PARTICULARS

4.1 Therapeutic indications
CRIXIVAN is indicated in combination with antiretroviral nucleoside analogues for the treatment of HIV–1 infected adults, adolescents, and children 4 years of age and older. In adolescents and children, the benefit of indinavir therapy versus the increased risk of nephrolithiasis should particularly be considered (see section 4.4).

4.2 Posology and method of administration
CRIXIVAN should be administered by physicians who are experienced in the treatment of HIV infection. On the basis of current pharmacodynamic data, indinavir must be used in combination with other antiretroviral agents. When indinavir is administered as monotherapy resistant viruses rapidly emerge (see section 5.1).

Adults

The recommended dosage of CRIXIVAN is 800 mg orally every 8 hours.

Data from published studies suggest that CRIXIVAN 400 mg in combination with ritonavir 100 mg, both administered orally twice daily, may be an alternative dosing regimen. The suggestion is based on limited published data (see section 5.2).

If co-administered with ritonavir, CRIXIVAN may be administered with or without food.

Children and adolescents (4 to 17 years of age)

The recommended dosage of CRIXIVAN for patients 4 to 17 years of age is 500 mg/m^2 (dose adjusted from calculated body surface area [BSA] based on height and weight) orally every 8 hours (see table below). This dose should not exceed the equivalent of the adult dose of 800 mg every 8 hours. CRIXIVAN hard capsules should only be given to children who are able to swallow hard capsules. CRIXIVAN has not been studied in children under the age of 4 years (see section 5.1 and 5.2).

Paediatric dose (500 mg/m^2) to be administered every 8 hours

Body Surface Area (m^2)	CRIXIVAN dose Every 8 hours (mg)
0.50	300
0.75	400
1.00	500
1.25	600
1.50	800

General administration recommendations

The hard capsules should be swallowed whole.

Since CRIXIVAN must be taken at intervals of 8 hours, a schedule convenient for the patient should be developed. For optimal absorption, CRIXIVAN should be administered without food but with water 1 hour before or 2 hours after a meal. Alternatively, CRIXIVAN may be administered with a low–fat, light meal.

To ensure adequate hydration, it is recommended that adults drink at least 1.5 litres of liquids during the course of 24 hours. It is also recommended that children who weigh less than 20 kg drink at least 75 ml/kg/day and that children who weigh 20 to 40 kg drink at least 50 ml/kg/day.

Medical management in patients with one or more episodes of nephrolithiasis must include adequate hydration and may include temporary interruption of therapy (e.g., 1 to 3 days) during the acute episode of nephrolithiasis or discontinuation of therapy (see section 4.4).

Special dosing considerations in adults

A dosage reduction of CRIXIVAN to 600 mg every 8 hours should be considered when administering itraconazole or ketoconazole concurrently (see section 4.5).

In patients with mild–to–moderate hepatic impairment due to cirrhosis, the dosage of CRIXIVAN should be reduced to 600 mg every 8 hours. The recommendation is based on limited pharmacokinetic data (see section 5.2). Patients with severe hepatic impairment have not been studied; therefore, no dosing recommendations can be made (see section 4.4).

Safety in patients with impaired renal function has not been studied; however, less than 20 % of indinavir is excreted in the urine as unchanged drug or metabolites (see section 4.4).

4.3 Contraindications
Hypersensitivity to the active substance or to any of the excipients.

Indinavir with or without ritonavir should not be administered concurrently with medicinal products with narrow therapeutic windows and which are substrates of CYP3A4. Inhibition of CYP3A4 by both CRIXIVAN and ritonavir could result in elevated plasma concentrations of these medicines, potentially causing serious or life–threatening reactions.

CRIXIVAN with or without ritonavir should not be administered concurrently with amiodarone, terfenadine, cisapride, astemizole, alprazolam, triazolam, midazolam administered orally (for caution on parenterally administered midazolam, see section 4.5), pimozide, ergot derivatives, simvastatin or lovastatin (see section 4.4).

Combination of rifampicin with CRIXIVAN with or without concomitant low-dose ritonavir is contraindicated (see section 4.5). Concurrent use of indinavir with herbal preparations containing St John's wort (hypericum perforatum) is contraindicated (see section 4.5).

In addition, indinavir with ritonavir should not be administered with alfuzosin, meperidine, piroxicam, propoxyphene, bepridil, encainide, flecanide, propafenone, quinidine, fusidic acid, clozapine, clorazepate, diazepam, estazolam and flurazepam.

Ritonavir should not be given with indinavir to patients with decompensated liver disease as ritonavir is principally metabolised and eliminated by the liver (see section 4.4).

When CRIXIVAN is used with ritonavir, consult the Summary of Product Characteristics of ritonavir for additional contraindications.

4.4 Special warnings and precautions for use
Nephrolithiasis and tubulointerstitial nephritis

Nephrolithiasis has occurred with indinavir therapy in adult and paediatric patients. The frequency of nephrolithiasis is higher in paediatric patients than in adult patients. In some cases, nephrolithiasis has been associated with renal insufficiency or acute renal failure; in the majority of these cases renal insufficiency and acute renal failure were reversible. If signs and symptoms of nephrolithiasis, including flank pain with or without haematuria (including microscopic haematuria) occur, temporary interruption of therapy (e.g. for 1–3 days) during the acute episode of nephrolithiasis or discontinuation of therapy may be considered. Paediatric patients who experience flank pain should be evaluated for the possibility of nephrolithiasis. Evaluation may consist of urinalysis, serum BUN and creatinine, and ultrasound of the bladder and kidneys. The long–term effects of nephrolithiasis in paediatric patients are unknown. Adequate hydration is recommended in all patients on indinavir (see section 4.2 and 4.8).

Cases of interstitial nephritis with medullary calcification and cortical atrophy have been observed in patients with asymptomatic severe leucocyturia (> 100 cells/high power field). In patients at increased risk such as children, urinary screening should be considered. If persistent severe leucocyturia is found, further investigation might be warranted.

Medicinal product interactions

Indinavir should be used cautiously with other medicinal products that are potent inducers of CYP3A4. Co–administration may result in decreased plasma concentrations of indinavir and as a consequence an increased risk for suboptimal treatment and facilitation of development of resistance (see section 4.5).

If indinavir is given with ritonavir, the potential drug interaction may be increased. The Interactions section of the SPC for ritonavir should also be consulted for information about potential interactions.

Concomitant use of indinavir with lovastatin or simvastatin is not recommended due to an increased risk of myopathy including rhabdomyolysis. Based on an interaction study with lopinavir/ritonavir, combination of rosuvastatin and protease inhibitors is not recommended. Caution must also be exercised if indinavir is used concurrently with atorvastatin. The interaction of indinavir or indinavir/ritonavir with pravastatin or fluvastatin is not known (see section 4.5).

Co–administration of CRIXIVAN with sildenafil, tadalafil and vardenafil (PDE5 inhibitors) are expected to substantially increase the plasma concentrations of these compounds and may result in an increase in PDE5 inhibitor-associated adverse events, including hypotension, visual changes, and priapism (see section 4.5).

Acute haemolytic anaemia

Acute haemolytic anaemia has been reported which in some cases was severe and progressed rapidly. Once a diagnosis is apparent, appropriate measures for the treatment of haemolytic anaemia should be instituted which may include discontinuation of indinavir.

Hyperglycaemia

New onset diabetes mellitus, hyperglycaemia or exacerbation of existing diabetes mellitus has been reported in patients receiving protease inhibitors (PIs). In some of these the hyperglycaemia was severe and in some cases also associated with ketoacidosis. Many patients had confounding medical conditions, some of which required therapy with agents that have been associated with the development of diabetes mellitus or hyperglycaemia.

Fat redistribution

Combination antiretroviral therapy has been associated with the redistribution of body fat (lipodystrophy) in HIV patients. The long term-consequences of these events are currently unknown. Knowledge about the mechanism is incomplete. A connection between visceral lipomatosis and PIs and lipoatrophy and nucleoside reverse transcriptase inhibitors (NRTIs) has been hypothesised. A higher risk of lipodystrophy has been associated with individual factors such as older age, and with drug related factors such as longer duration of antiretroviral treatment and associated metabolic disturbances. Clinical examination should include evaluation for physical signs of fat redistribution. Consideration should be given to the measurement of fasting serum lipids and blood glucose. Lipid disorders should be managed as clinically appropriate (see section 4.8).

Liver disease

The safety and efficacy of indinavir has not been established in patients with significant underlying liver disorders. Patients with chronic hepatitis B or C and treated with combination antiretroviral therapy are at an increased risk for severe and potentially fatal hepatic adverse events. In case of concomitant antiviral therapy for hepatitis B or C, please refer also to the relevant product information for these medicinal products.

The safety and efficacy of indinavir/ritonavir has not been established in patients with significant underlying liver disorders and should not be used in this patient population.

Patients with pre-existing liver dysfunction including chronic active hepatitis have an increased frequency of liver function abnormalities during combination antiretroviral therapy and should be monitored according to standard practice. If there is evidence of worsening liver disease in such patients, interruption or discontinuation of treatment must be considered.

An increased incidence of nephrolithiasis has been observed in patients with underlying liver disorders when treated with indinavir.

Immune Reactivation Syndrome

In HIV-infected patients with severe immune deficiency at the time of institution of combination antiretroviral therapy (CART), an inflammatory reaction to asymptomatic or residual opportunistic pathogens may arise and cause serious clinical conditions, or aggravation of symptoms. Typically, such reactions have been observed within the first few weeks or months of initiation of CART. Relevant examples are cytomegalovirus retinitis, generalised and/or focal myobacterial infections, and *Pneumocystis carinii* pneumonia. Any inflammatory symptoms should be evaluated and treatment instituted when necessary.

Patients with coexisting conditions

There have been reports of increased bleeding, including spontaneous skin haematomas and haemarthroses, in haemophiliac patients type A and B treated with PIs. In some patients additional factor VIII was given. In more than a half of the reported cases, treatment with PIs was continued or re-introduced if treatment had been discontinued. A causal relationship has been evoked, although the mechanism of action has not been elucidated. Haemophiliac patients should therefore be made aware of the possibility of increased bleeding.

Patients with mild–to–moderate hepatic insufficiency due to cirrhosis will require a dosage reduction of indinavir due to decreased metabolism of indinavir (see section 4.2). Patients with severe hepatic impairment have not been studied. In the absence of such studies, caution should be exercised as increased levels of indinavir may occur.

Safety in patients with impaired renal function has not been studied; however, less than 20 % of indinavir is excreted in the urine as unchanged drug or metabolites (see section 4.2).

Osteonecrosis:

Although the etiology is considered to be multifactorial (including corticosteroid use, alcohol consumption, severe immunosuppression, higher body mass index), cases of osteonecrosis have been reported particularly in patients with advanced HIV-disease and/or long-term exposure to combination antiretroviral therapy (CART). Patients should be advised to seek medical advice if they experience joint aches and pain, joint stiffness or difficulty in movement.

Lactose

This medicinal product contains 299.2 mg of lactose in each 800-mg dose (maximum single dose). This quantity is not likely to induce symptoms of lactose intolerance (milk intolerance).

Patients with rare hereditary problems of galactose intolerance, the Lapp lactose deficiency or glucose-galactose malabsorption should not take this medicine.

4.5 Interaction with other medicinal products and other forms of interaction

Interaction studies have only been performed in adults. The relevance of the results from these studies in paediatric patients is unknown.

The metabolism of indinavir is mediated by the cytochrome P450 enzyme CYP3A4. Therefore, other substances that either share this metabolic pathway or modify CYP3A4 activity may influence the pharmacokinetics of indinavir. Similarly, indinavir might also modify the pharmacokinetics of other substances that share this metabolic pathway. Boosted indinavir (indinavir with ritonavir) may have additive pharmacokinetic effects on substances that share the CYP3A4 pathway as both ritonavir and indinavir inhibit the cytochrome P450 enzyme CYP3A4.

Indinavir with or without ritonavir should not be administered concurrently with medicinal products with narrow therapeutic windows and which are substrates of CYP3A4. Inhibition of CYP3A4 by both CRIXIVAN and ritonavir could result in elevated plasma concentrations of these medicines, potentially causing serious or life-threatening reactions. CRIXIVAN with or without ritonavir should not be administered concurrently with amiodarone, terfenadine, cisapride, astemizole, alprazolam, triazolam, midazolam administered orally (for caution on parenterally administered midazolam, see Table 1 and 2 below), pimozide, ergot derivatives, simvastatin or lovastatin. In addition, indinavir with ritonavir should not be administered with alfuzosin, meperidine, piroxicam, propoxyphene, bepridil, encainide, flecanide, propafenone, quinidine, fusidic acid, clozapine, clorazepate, diazepam, estazolam and flurazepam.

Concurrent use of indinavir with rifampicin or herbal preparations containing St John's wort (hypericum perforatum) is contraindicated.

Drugs listed above are not repeated in Table 1 and 2 unless specific interaction data is available.

Refer also to sections 4.2 and 4.3.

Table 1. Interactions and dose recommendations with other medical products – UNBOOSTED INDINAVIR

Interactions between indinavir and other medicinal products are listed in the tables below (increase is indicated as "↑", decrease as "↓", no change (≤±/- 20%) as "↔", single dose as "SD", once daily as "QD", twice daily as "BID", three times daily as "TID", and four times as "QID").

(see Table 1 below)

Table 2. Interactions and dose recommendations with other medical products – INDINAVIR BOOSTED WITH RITONAVIR. *No specific interaction studies have been performed with the boosted dose 400 mg indinavir with 100 mg ritonavir.*

Interactions between indinavir/ritonavir and other medicinal products are listed in the tables below (increase is indicated as "↑", decrease as "↓", no change (≤±/- 20%) as "↔", single dose as "SD", once daily as "QD", twice daily as "BID", three times daily as "TID", and four times as "QID").

(see Table 2 on page 494)

For information regarding diet or the effect of food on indinavir absorption (see section 4.2 and 5.2).

4.6 Pregnancy and lactation

Use during pregnancy

There are no adequate and well-controlled studies in pregnant patients. Indinavir should be used during pregnancy only if the potential benefit justifies the potential risk to the foetus. Given that substantially lower antepartum exposures have been observed in a small study of HIV-infected pregnant patients and the limited data in this patient population, indinavir use is not recommended in HIV-infected pregnant patients (see section 5.2).

Hyperbilirubinaemia, reported predominantly as elevated indirect bilirubin, has occurred in 14 % of patients during treatment with indinavir. Because it is unknown whether indinavir will exacerbate physiologic hyperbilirubinaemia in neonates, careful consideration must be given to the use of indinavir in pregnant women at the time of delivery (see section 4.8).

In Rhesus monkeys, administration of indinavir to neonates caused a mild exacerbation of the transient physiologic hyperbilirubinaemia seen in this species after birth. Administration of indinavir to pregnant Rhesus monkeys during the third trimester did not cause a similar exacerbation in neonates; however, only limited placental transfer of indinavir occurred.

Use during lactation

It is recommended that HIV–infected women do not breast–feed their infants under any circumstances in order to avoid transmission of HIV. It is not known whether indinavir is excreted in human milk. Mothers should be instructed to discontinue breast–feeding during treatment.

4.7 Effects on ability to drive and use machines

No studies on the effects on the ability to drive and use machines have been performed. There are no data to suggest that indinavir affects the ability to drive and use machines. However, patients should be informed that dizziness and blurred vision have been reported during treatment with indinavir.

Table 1 Interactions and dose recommendations with other medical products – UNBOOSTED INDINAVIR

Medicinal products by therapeutic areas	Interaction	Recommendations concerning co-administration
ANTI-INFECTIVES		
Antiretrovirals		
NRTIs		
Didanosine Formulation with buffer	No formal interaction study has been performed. A normal (acidic) gastric pH may be necessary for optimum absorption of indinavir whereas acid rapidly degrades didanosine which is formulated with buffering agents to increase pH. Antiretroviral activity was unaltered when didanosine was administered 3 hours after treatment with indinavir.	Indinavir and didanosine formulations containing buffer should be administered at least one hour apart on an empty stomach.
Didanosine enteric-coated 400 mg SD (Indinavir 800 mg SD)	Indinavir: ↔ (Relative to Indinavir 800 mg SD alone) Didanosine: ↔	Can be administered without any restrictions with respect to time of administration or food.
Stavudine 40 mg BID (Indinavir 800 mg TID)	Indinavir AUC: ↔ Indinavir C_{min}: ↔ (Relative to Indinavir 800 mg TID alone) Stavudine AUC: ↑ 21% Staudine C_{min}: not evaluated	Indinavir and NRTIs can be co-administered without dose adjustment
Zidovudine 200 mg TID (Indinavir 1000 mg TID)	Indinavir AUC: ↔ Indinavir C_{min}: ↔ (Relative to Indinavir 1000 mg TID alone) Zidovudine AUC: ↔ Zidovudine C_{min}: ↑ 51%	
Zidovudine/Lamivudine 200/150 mg TID (Indinavir 800 mg TID)	Indinavir AUC: ↔ Indinavir C_{min}: ↔ (Relative to Indinavir 800 mg TID alone) Zidovudine AUC: ↑ 39% Zidovudine C_{min}: ↔ Lamivudine AUC: ↔ Lamivudine C_{min}: ↔	
NNRTIs		
Delavirdine 400 mg TID (Indinavir 600 mg TID) Delavirdine 400 mg TID Indinavir 400 mg TID	Indinavir AUC: ↑ 53% Indinavir C_{min} ↑ 298% (Relative to Indinavir 800 mg TID alone) Indinavir AUC: ↔ Indinavir C_{min}: ↑ 118% (Relative to Indinavir 800 mg TID alone) Delavirdine: ↔	Dose reduction of CRIXIVAN to 400-600 mg every 8 hours should be considered.
Efavirenz 600 mg QD (Indinavir 1000 mg TID) Efavirenz 200 mg QD(Indinavir 800 mg TID)	Indinavir AUC: ↓ 46% Indinavir C_{min}: ↓ 57% (Relative to Indinavir 800 mg TID alone) An increased dose (1000mg TID) of indinavir does not compensate for the inducing effect of efavirenz. Indinavir AUC: ↓ 31% Indinavir C_{min}: ↓ 40% Efavirenz AUC: ↔	No specific dose recommendation can be given.
Nevirapine 200 mg BID (Indinavir 800 mg TID)	Indinavir AUC: ↓ 28 % Nevirapine: ↔ (CYP3A induction)	A dose increase of indinavir to 1000 mg every 8 hours should be considered if given with nevirapine.
PIs		
Amprenavir 1200 mg BID (Indinavir 1200 mg BID)	Amprenavir AUC: ↑ 90% Indinavir: ↔	The appropriate doses for this combination, with respect to efficacy and safety, have not been established.

Medicinal products by therapeutic areas	Interaction	Recommendations concerning co-administration
Ritonavir 100 mg BID (Indinavir 800 mg BID)	**Indinavir AUC_{24hr}: ↑ 178% Indinavir C_{min}: ↑ 11-fold; (Relative to Indinavir 800 mg TID alone*) Ritonavir AUC: ↑ 72% Ritonavir C_{min}: ↑ 62%**	**The appropriate doses for this combination, with respect to efficacy and safety, have not been established. Preliminary clinical data suggest that CRIXIVAN 400 mg in combination with ritonavir 100 mg, both administered orally twice daily, may be an alternative dosing regimen (see section 5.2). A boosted dose of 800 mg indinavir/100 mg ritonavir twice daily results in increased risk of adverse events.**
Ritonavir 200 mg BID (Indinavir 800 mg BID)	**Indinavir AUC_{24hr}: ↑ 266% Indinavir C_{min}: ↑ 24-fold; (Relative to Indinavir 800 mg TID alone*) Ritonavir AUC: ↑ 96% Ritonavir C_{min}: ↑ 371%**	
Ritonavir 400 mg BID (Indinavir 800 mg BID)	**Indinavir AUC_{24hr}: ↑ 220% Indinavir C_{min}: ↑ 24-fold (Relative to Indinavir 800 mg TID alone*) Ritonavir AUC_{24hr}: ↔**	
Ritonavir 400 mg BID (Indinavir 400 mg BID)	**Indinavir AUC_{24hr}: ↑ 68% Indinavir C_{min}: ↑ 10-fold (Relative to Indinavir 800 mg TID alone*) Ritonavir AUC_{24hr}: ↔**	
Ritonavir 100 mg BID (Indinavir 400 mg BID)	**Indinavir AUC and C_{min}: ↔ (Relative to Indinavir 800 mg TID alone*) (*historical controls**	
Saquinavir 600 mg SD (hard gel capsule formulation) (Indinavir 800 mg TID)	**Saquinavir AUC: ↑ 500% Saquinavir C_{min}: ↑ 190% (Relative to saquinavir 600 mg SD (hard gel formulation) alone)**	**The appropriate doses for this combination, with respect to efficacy and safety, have not been established.**
Saquinavir 800 mg SD (soft gel capsule formulation) (Indinavir 800 mg TID)	**Saquinavir AUC: ↑ 620% Saquinavir C_{min}: ↑ 450% (Relative to saquinavir 800 mg SD (soft gel formulation) alone)**	
Saquinavir 1200 mg SD (soft gel capsule formulation) (Indinavir 800 mg TID)	**Saquinavir AUC: ↑ 360% Saquinavir C_{min}: ↑ 450% (Relative to saquinavir 1200 mg (soft gel formulation) alone) The design of the study does not allow for definitive evaluation of the effect of saquinavir on indinavir, but suggests there is less than a two-fold increase in indinavir AUC_{8h} during co-administration with saquinavir.**	
Antibiotics		
Sulphamethoxazole/ Trimethoprim 800 mg/160 mg BID (Indinavir 400 mg QID)	**Indinavir AUC and C_{min}: ↔ (Relative to Indinavir 400 mg QID alone) Sulphamethoxazole AUC and C_{min}: ↔**	**Indinavir and sulphamethoxazole/ trimethoprim can be co-administered without dose adjustment.**
Antifungals		
Fluconazole 400 mg QD (Indinavir 1000 mg TID)	**Indinavir AUC: ↓ 24% Indinavir C_{min}: ↔ (Relative to Indinavir 1000 mg TID alone)**	**Indinavir and fluconazole can be co-administered without dose adjustment**
Itraconazole 200 mg BID (Indinavir 600 mg TID)	**Indinavir AUC: ↔ Indinavir C_{min}: ↑ 49% (Relative to Indinavir 800 mg TID alone)**	**Dose reduction of CRIXIVAN to 600 mg every 8 hours is recommended with administering itraconazole concurrently.**
Ketoconazole 400 mg QD (Indinavir 600 mg TID) Ketoconazole 400 mg QD(Indinavir 400 mg TID)	**Indinavir AUC: ↓ 20% Indinavir C_{min}: ↑ 29% (Relative to Indinavir 800 mg TID alone) Indinavir AUC ↓ 56% Indinavir C_{min}↓ 27% (Relative to Indinavir 800 mg TID alone)**	**Dose reduction of CRIXIVAN to 600 mg every 8 hours should be considered.**
Anti-Mycobacterial		
Isoniazid 300 mg QD (Indinavir 800 mg TID)	**Indinavir AUC and C_{min}: ↔ (Relative to Indinavir 800 mg TID alone) Isoniazid AUC and C_{min}: ↔**	**Indinavir and isoniazid can be co-administered without dose adjustment.**
Rifabutin 300 mg QD (Indinavir 800 mg TID)	**Indinavir AUC ↓ 34% Indinavir C_{min} : ↓ 39% (Relative to Indinavir 800 mg TID alone) Rifabutin AUC: ↑ 173% Rifabutin C_{min}: ↑ 244% (Relative to rifabutin 300 mg QD alone)**	**Dose reduction of rifabutin and dose increase of CRIXIVAN has not been confirmed in clinical studies. Therefore co-administration is not recommended. If rifabutin treatment is required, alternative agents for treating HIV infection should be sought.**
Rifabutin 150 mg QD (Indinavir 800 mg TID)	**Indinavir AUC: ↓ 32% Indinavir C_{min}: ↓ 40% (Relative to Indinavir 800 mg TID alone) Rifabutin AUC*: ↑ 54% Rifabutin C_{min}: ↑ 99% (*Relative to rifabutin 300 mg QD alone. No data has been obtained comparing rifabutin 150 mg QD in combination with indinavir 800 mg TID with a reference dose of 150 mg rifabutin alone)**	
Rifampicin 600 mg QD (Indinavir 800 mg TID)	**Indinavir AUC: ↓ 92% (Relative to Indinavir 800 mg TID alone) This effect is due to an induction of CYP3A4 by rifampicin.**	**The use of rifampicin with indinavir is contraindicated.**
ANALGESICS		
Methadone 20-60 mg QD (Indinavir 800 mg TID)	**Indinavir AUC: ↔ (Relative to Indinavir 800 mg TID historical controls) Methadone AUC and C_{min}: ↔**	**Indinavir and methadone can be co-administered without dose adjustment.**
ANTIARRHYTHMICS		
Quinidine 200 mg SD (Indinavir 400 mg SD)	**Indinavir AUC and C_{min}: ↔ (Relative to Indinavir 400 mg SD) ↑ Quinidine concentration expected (CYP3A4 inhibition by indinavir)**	**Caution is warranted and therapeutic concentration monitoring is recommended for quinidine when coadministered with CRIXIVAN. The use of indinavir/ritonavir with quinidine is contraindicated.**
ANTIASTHMATIC		
Theophylline 250 mg SD (Indinavir 800 mg TID)	**Theophylline AUC and C_{min}: ↔**	**Indinavir and theophylline can be co-administered without dose adjustment.**
ANTICOAGULANT		
Warfarin	**Not studied, combined administration may result in increased warfarin levels.**	**Dose adjustment of warfarin may be required.**
ANTICONVULSANTS		
Carbamazepine, phenobarbital phenytoin	**Indinavir inhibits CYP3A4 and as a result is expected to increase the plasma concentrations of these anticonvulsants. Concomitant use of medicinal products that are inducers of CYP3A4, such as carbamazepine, phenobarbital and phenytoin may reduce indinavir plasma concentrations.**	**Careful monitoring of therapeutic and adverse effects is recommended when these medicines are concomitantly administered with indinavir.**

Medicinal products by therapeutic areas	Interaction	Recommendations concerning co-administration
ANTIDEPRESSANTS		
Venlafaxine 50 mg TID (Indinavir 800 mg SD)	**Indinavir AUC: $\downarrow$ 28% (Relative to Indinavir 800 mg SD alone) Venlafaxine and active metabolite O-desmethyl-venlafaxine: $\leftrightarrow$**	**The clinical significance of this finding is unknown**
CALCIUM CHANNEL BLOCKERS		
Dihydropyridine: e.g., felodipine, nifedipine, nicardipine	**$\uparrow$ dihydropyridine calcium channel blocker concentration. Calcium channel blockers are metabolised by CYP3A4 which is inhibited by indinavir**	**Caution is warranted and clinical monitoring of patients is recommended.**
HERBAL MEDICATIONS		
St. John's wort (Hypericum perforatum) 300 mg TID (Indinavir 800 mg TID)	**Indinavir AUC: $\downarrow$ 54% Indinavir C_{min}: $\downarrow$ 81% (Relative to Indinavir 800 mg TID alone) Reduction in indinavir concentrations due to induction of drug metabolising and/or transport proteins by St. John's wort.**	**Herbal preparations containing St. John's wort are contraindicated with Crixivan. If a patient is already taking St. John's wort, stop St. John's wort, check viral levels and if possible indinavir levels. Indinavir levels may increase on stopping St. John's wort, and the dose of CRIXIVAN may need adjusting. The inducing effect may persist up to 2 weeks after cessation of treatment with St. John's wort.**
HISTAMINE H_2 Antagonist		
Cimetidine 600 mg BID (Indinavir 400 mg SD)	**Indinavir AUC and C_{min}: $\leftrightarrow$ (Relative to Indinavir 400 mg SD alone)**	**Indinavir and cimetidine can be co-administered without dose adjustment**
HMG-CoA REDUCTASE INHIBITIORS		
Lovastatin, simvastatin	**Indinavir inhibits CYP3A4 and as a result is expected to markedly increase the plasma concentrations of these HMG-CoA reductase inhibitors, which are highly dependent on CYP3A4 metabolism.**	**Combination contraindicated due to an increased risk of myopathy including rhabdomyolysis.**
Rosuvastatin	**Interaction not studied. Interaction study with Lopinavir/ritonavir + rosuvastatin: Rosuvastatin AUC $\uparrow$ 2.08 -fold Rosuvastatin Cmax $\uparrow$ 4.66 -fold (Mechanism unknown)**	**Combination not recommended.**
Atorvastatin	**$\uparrow$ atorvastatin concentration Atorvastatin is less dependent on CYP3A4 for metabolism than lovastatin or simvastatin.**	**Use the lowest possible dose of atorvastatin with careful monitoring. Caution is advised.**
Pravastatin, fluvastatin	**Interaction not studied. Metabolism of pravastatin and fluvastatin is not dependent on CYP3A4. Interaction via effects on transport proteins cannot be excluded.**	**Interaction unknown. If no alternative treatment is available, use with careful monitoring.**
IMMUNOSUPPRESSIVES		
Ciclosporin A	**Ciclospori A (CsA) levels markedly increase in patients on PIs, including indinavir.**	**CsA levels require progressive dose adjustment using therapeutic drug monitoring.**
ORAL CONTRACEPTIVES		
Norethindrone/ethinyl estradiol 1/35 1 mcg QD (Indinavir 800 mg TID)	**Norethindrone AUC: $\uparrow$ 26% Norethindrone AUC $\uparrow$ 26%**	**Indinavir and norethindrone/ethinyl estradiol 1/35 can be co-administered without dose adjustment.**
PDE5 INHIBITOR		
Sildenafil 25 mg SD (Indinavir 800 mg TID)	**Indinavir AUC: $\uparrow$ 11% Sildenafil AUC $\uparrow$ 340% Coadministration of CRIXIVAN with sildenafil is likely to result in an increase of sildenafil by competitive inhibition of metabolism.**	**Sildenafil dose should not exceed a maximum of 25 mg in a 48-hour period in patients receiving concomitant indinavir therapy.**
Vardenafil 10 mg SD (Indinavir 800 mg TID)	**Vardenafil AUC: $\uparrow$ 16-fold Coadministration of CRIXIVAN with vardenafil is likely to result in an increase of vardenafil by competitive inhibition of metabolism.**	**Vardenafil dose should not exceed a maximum of 2.5 mg in a 24-hour period in patients receiving concomitant indinavir therapy.**
Tadalafil	**Interaction not studied. Coadministration of CRIXIVAN with tadalafil is likely to result in an increase of tadalafil by competitive inhibition of metabolism.**	**Tadalafil dose should not exceed a maximum of 10 mg in a 72 hour period in patients receiving concomitant indinavir therapy.**
SEDATIVES/HYPNOTICS		
Midazolam (parenteral)	**Not studied, combined administrations are expected to significantly increase concentrations of midazolam, particularly when midazolam is given orally. Midazolam is extensively metabolised by CYP3A4.**	**CRIXIVAN and oral midazolam should not be coadministered (see section 4.3). Caution should be used with coadministration of CRIXIVAN and parenteral midazolam. If CRIXIVAN is coadministered with parenteral midazolam, it should be done in an intensive care unit with close clinical monitoring in case of respiratory depression and/or prolonged sedation. Dosage adjustment for midazolam should be considered, especially if more than a single dose of midazolam is administered.**
STEROIDS		
Dexamethasone	**Interaction not studied. $\uparrow$ dexamethasone exposure expected (CYP3A inhibition). $\downarrow$ indinavir plasma concentrations may be expected (CYP3A induction).**	**Careful monitoring of therapeutic and adverse effects is recommended when dexamethasone is concomitantly administered with indinavir.**

4.8 Undesirable effects

In controlled clinical trials conducted world–wide, indinavir was administered alone or in combination with other antiretroviral agents (zidovudine, didanosine, stavudine, and/or lamivudine) to approximately 2,000 patients, the majority of whom were adult Caucasian males (15 % females).

Indinavir did not alter the type, frequency, or severity of known major adverse effects associated with the use of zidovudine, didanosine, or lamivudine.

Clinical adverse reactions reported by the investigators as possibly, probably, or definitely related to CRIXIVAN in ⩾ 5 % of patients treated with CRIXIVAN alone or in combination (n = 309) for 24 weeks are listed below. Many of these adverse reactions were also identified as common pre–existing or frequently occurring medical conditions in this population. These adverse reactions were: nausea (35.3 %), headache (25.2 %), diarrhoea (24.6 %), asthenia/fatigue (24.3 %), rash (19.1 %), taste perversion (19.1 %), dry skin (16.2 %), abdominal pain (14.6 %), vomiting (11.0 %), dizziness (10.7 %). With the exception of dry skin, rash, and taste perversion, the incidence of clinical adverse reactions was similar or higher among patients treated with antiretroviral nucleoside analogue controls than among patients treated with CRIXIVAN alone or in combination. This overall safety profile remained similar for 107 patients treated with CRIXIVAN alone or in combination for up to 48 weeks. Adverse reactions, including nephrolithiasis, may lead to treatment interruption.

Adverse reactions have also been reported during post-marketing experience* as they are derived from spontaneous reports, incidences cannot be determined.

The following adverse reactions have been reported during clinical studies and/or post–marketing use for CRIXIVAN.

Very Common (⩾ 1/10); Common (⩾ 100, < 1/10); Uncommon (⩾ 1/1,000, < 1/100); Rare (⩾ 1/10,000, < 1/1,000); Very rare (< 1/10,000); not known (cannot be estimated from the available data).

Blood and the lymphatic system disorders:

*Not known**: increased spontaneous bleeding in patients with haemophilia; anaemia including acute haemolytic anaemia; thrombocytopenia (see section 4.4).

Immune system disorders:

*Not known**: anaphylactoid reactions.

Metabolism and nutrition disorders:

*Not known**: new onset diabetes mellitus or hyperglycaemia, or exacerbation of pre-existing diabetes mellitus (see section 4.4).

Nervous system disorders:

Very Common: headache, dizziness

Common: insomnia; hypoaesthesia; paraesthesia.

*Not known**: oral paraesthesia.

Gastrointestinal disorders:

Very Common: nausea; vomiting; diarrhoea; dyspepsia.

Common: flatulence; dry mouth; acid regurgitation.

*Not known**: hepatitis, including reports of hepatic failure; pancreatitis

Skin and subcutaneous tissue disorders:

Very Common: rash, dry skin

Common: pruritus.

*Not known**: rash including erythema multiforme and Stevens Johnson syndrome; hypersensitivity vasculitis; alopecia, hyperpigmentation; urticaria; ingrown toenails and/or paronychia

Musculoskeletal, connective tissue and bone disorders:

Common: myalgia.

*Not known**: myositis; rhabdomyolysis.

Renal and urinary disorders:

Very Common: nephrolithiasis in paediatric patients 3 years of age and older.

Common: nephrolithiasis in adults; dysuria.

Nephrolithiasis, including flank pain with or without haematuria (including microscopic haematuria), has been

Table 2 Interactions and dose recommendations with other medical products – INDINAVIR BOOSTED WITH RITONAVIR

Medicinal products by therapeutic areas	Interaction	Recommendations concerning co-administration
ANTI-INFECTIVES		
Antiretrovirals		
Amprenavir	Amprenavir 1200 mg BID AUC ↑ 90% with 800 mg TID indinavir alone (see Table 1). Amprenavir 600 mg BID AUC ↓ 64% with 100 mg BID ritonavir alone (relative to amprenavir 1200 mg BID alone). Ritonavir increases the serum levels of amprenavir as a result of CYP3A4 inhibition. There are no interaction data available on the coadministration of indinavir/ritonavir and amprenavir.	The appropriate doses for this combination, with respect to efficacy and safety, have not been established. Ritonavir oral solution should not be co-administered with amprenavir oral solution to children due to the risk of toxicity from excipients in the two formulations.
Efavirenz 600mg QD (Indinavir/ritonavir 800/100 BID)	Indinavir AUC: ↓ 25% Indinavir C_{min} ↓ 50% (Relative to Indinavir/ritonavir 800/100 BID alone) Ritonavir AUC ↓ 36% Ritonavir C_{min}: ↓ 39% Efavirenz AUC and C_{min}: ↔	Dose increases of indinavir/ritonavir when given in combination with efavirenz have not been studied.
Anti-Mycobacterial		
Rifabutin	Interaction with indinavir/ritonavir not studied. Decreased indinavir concentrations and increased rifabutin concentrations are expected.	No dose recommendations for indinavir/ritonavir with rifabutin could be given, therefore the combination is not recommended. If rifabutin treatment is required, alternative agents for treating HIV infection should be sought.
Rifampicin	Rifampicin is a strong CYP3A4 inducer and has been shown to cause a 92% decrease in indinavir AUC which can result in virological failure and resistance development. During attempts to overcome the decreased exposure by increasing the dose of other protease inhibitors with ritonavir, a high frequency of liver reactions was seen.	The combination of rifampicin and CRIXIVAN with concomitant low-dose ritonavir is contraindicated (see section 4.3).
Other Anti-infectives		
Atovaquone	Interaction with indinavir/ritonavir not studied. Ritonavir induces glucuronidation and as a result is expected to decrease the plasma concentrations of atovaquone.	Careful monitoring of therapeutic and adverse effects is recommended when atovaquone is concomitantly administered with indinavir/ritonavir.
Erythromycin, Itraconazole	Interaction with indinavir/ritonavir not studied Indinavir and ritonavir inhibit CYP3A4 and as a result are expected to increase the plasma concentrations of erythromycin and itraconazole.	Careful monitoring of therapeutic and adverse effects is recommended when erythromycin or itraconazole are concomitantly administered with indinavir/ritonavir.
Ketoconazole	Interaction with indinavir/ritonavir not studied. Indinavir and ritonavir inhibit CYP3A4 and as a result are expected to increase the plasma concentrations of ketoconazole. Co-administration of ritonavir and ketoconazole caused an increased incidence of gastrointestinal and hepatic adverse events.	Careful monitoring of therapeutic and adverse effects is recommended when ketoconazole is concomitantly administered with indinavir/ritonavir. A dose reduction of ketoconazole should be considered when co-administered with indinavir/ritonavir.
ANALGESICS		
Fentanyl	Interaction with indinavir/ritonavir not studied. Indinavir and ritonavir inhibit CYP3A4 and as a result are expected to increase the plasma concentrations of fentanyl.	Careful monitoring of therapeutic and adverse effects is recommended when fentanyl is concomitantly administered with indinavir/ritonavir.
Methadone	Interaction with indinavir/ritonavir not studied. There is no significant effect of unboosted indinavir on methadone AUC (see Table 1 above). Decreases in methadone AUC has been observed with other ritonavir-boosted protease inhibitors. Ritonavir may induce glucuronidation of methadone.	Increased methadone dose may be necessary when concomitantly administered with indinavir/ritonavir. Dose adjustment should be considered based on the patient's clinical response to methadone therapy.
Morphine	Interaction with indinavir/ritonavir not studied. Morphine levels may be decreased due to induction of glucuronidation by coadministered ritonavir.	Careful monitoring of therapeutic and adverse effects is recommended when morphine is concomitantly administered with indinavir/ritonavir.
ANTIARRTHYMICS		
Digoxin 0.4 mg SD Ritonavir 200 mg BID	Interaction with indinavir/ritonavir not studied. Digoxin AUC: ↑ 22%	Ritonavir may increase digoxin levels due to modification of P-glycoprotein mediated digoxin efflux. Careful monitoring of digoxin levels is recommended when digoxin is concomitantly administered with indinavir/ritonavir.
ANTICOAGULANT		
Warfarin Ritonavir 400 mg BID	Interaction with indinavir/ritonavir not studied. R-warfarin levels may be decreased leading to reduced anticoagulation due to induction of CYP1A2 and CYP2C9 by ritonavir.	Anticoagulation parameters should be monitored when warfarin is co-administered with indinavir/ritonavir.
ANTICONVULSANTS		
Carbamazepine	Interaction with indinavir/ritonavir not studied. Indinavir and ritonavir inhibit CYP3A4 and as a result are expected to increase the plasma concentrations of carbamazepine.	Careful monitoring of therapeutic and adverse effects is recommended when carbamazepine is concomitantly administered with indinavir/ritonavir.
Divalproex, lamotrigine, phenytoin	Interaction with indinavir/ritonavir not studied. Ritonavir induces oxidation by CYP2C9 and glucuronidation and as a result is expected to decrease the plasma concentrations of anticonvulsants.	Careful monitoring of serum levels or therapeutic effects is recommended when these medicines are concomitantly administered with indinavir/ritonavir. Phenytoin may decrease serum levels of ritonavir.
ANTIDEPRESSANTS		
Trazodone 50 mg SD Ritonavir 200 mg BID	Interaction with indinavir/ritonavir not studied. Trazodone AUC: ↑ 2.4-fold An increase in the incidence in trazodone-related adverse events was noted when coadministered with ritonavir.	The combination of trazodone with indinavir/ritonavir should be used with caution, initiating trazodone at the lowest dosage and monitoring for clinical response and tolerability.
ANTIHISTAMINES		
Fexofenadine	Interaction with indinavir/ritonavir not studied. Ritonavir may modify P-glycoprotein mediated fexofenadine efflux when coadministered resulting in increased concentrations of fexofenadine.	Careful monitoring of therapeutic and adverse effects is recommended when fexofenadine is concomitantly administered with indinavir/ritonavir.
Loratidine	Interaction with indinavir/ritonavir not studied. Indinavir and ritonavir inhibit CYP3A4 and as a result are expected to increase the plasma concentrations of loratidine.	Careful monitoring of therapeutic and adverse effects is recommended when loratidine is concomitantly administered with indinavir/ritonavir.
CALCIUM CHANNEL BLOCKERS		
Dilitazem 120 mg QD (Indinavir/ritonavir 800/100 BID)	Dilitazem $AUC_{0\text{-}24hr}$: ↑ 43% Indinavir/ritonavir AUCs: ↔	Dose modification of calcium channel blockers should be considered when co-administered with indinavir/ritonavir as it may result in an increased response.
Amlodipine 5 mg QD (Indinavir/ritonavir 800/100 BID)	Amlodipine $AUC_{0\text{-}24hr}$: ↑ 80% Indinavir/ritonavir AUCs: ↔	
HMG-CoA REDUCTASE INHIBITORS		Same recommendations as for indinavir without ritonavir boosting (see Table 1).
IMMUNOSUPPRESSIVES		
Ciclosporin A (Indinavir/ritonavir 800/100 BID)	Following initiation of indinavir/ritonavir 800/100 BID or lopinavir/ritonavir 400/100 BID, dose reduction of ciclosporin A to 5-20% of prior dose was needed to maintain ciclosporin A levels within therapeutic range in one study.	Ciclosporin A dose adjustments should be made according to measured ciclosporin A trough blood levels.

Medicinal products by therapeutic areas	Interaction	Recommendations concerning co-administration
Tacrolimus	Interaction with indinavir/ritonavir not studied. Indinavir and ritonavir inhibit CYP3A4 and as a result are expected to increase the plasma concentrations of tacrolimus.	Careful monitoring of therapeutic and adverse effects is recommended when tacrolimus is concomitantly administered with indinavir/ritonavir.
PDE5 INHIBITOR		
Sildenafil, tadalafil	Interaction not studied.	For sildenafil and tadalafil, same recommendations as for indinavir without ritonavir boosting (see Table 1).
Vardenafil	Interaction not studied.	Vardenafil dose should not exceed a maximum of 2.5 mg in a 72-hour period when given with a boosted protease inhibitor.
SEDATIVES/HYPNOTICS		
Buspirone	Interaction with indinavir/ritonavir not studied. Indinavir and ritonavir inhibit CYP3A4 and as a result are expected to increase the plasma concentrations of buspirone.	Careful monitoring of therapeutic and adverse effects is recommended when buspirone is concomitantly administered with indinavir/ritonavir.
Midazolam (parenteral)	Interaction with indinavir/ritonavirnot studied, Combined administrations are expected to significantly increase concentrations of midazolam, particularly when midazolam is given orally (CYP3A4 inhibition).	CRIXIVAN with ritonavir and oral midazolam should not be co-administered (see section 4.3). Caution should be used with co-administration of CRIXIVAN with ritonavir and parenteral midazolam. If CRIXIVAN with ritonavir is co-administered with parenteral midazolam, it should be done in an intensive care unit with close clinical monitoring in case of respiratory depression and/or prolonged sedation. Dosage adjustment for midazolam should be considered, especially if more than a single dose of midazolam is administered.
STEROIDS		
Dexamethasone	Interaction with indinavir/ritonavir not studied. ↑ dexamethasone exposure expected (CYP3A inhibition). ↓ indinavir plasma concentrations may be expected (CYP3A induction).	Careful monitoring of therapeutic and adverse effects is recommended when dexamethasone is concomitantly administered with indinavir/ritonavir.

reported in approximately 10 % (252/2,577) of patients receiving CRIXIVAN in clinical trials at the recommended dose compared to 2.2 % in the control arms. In general, these events were not associated with renal dysfunction and resolved with hydration and temporary interruption of therapy (e.g., 1–3 days).

In clinical trials in paediatric patients 3 years of age and older, the adverse experience profile was similar to that for adult patients except for a higher frequency of nephrolithiasis of 29 % (20/70) in paediatric patients who were treated with CRIXIVAN at the recommended dose of 500 mg/m^2 every 8 hours.

*Not known**: nephrolithiasis, in some cases with renal insufficiency or acute renal failure; pyelonephritis; interstitial nephritis, sometimes associated with indinavir crystal deposits. In some patients, resolution of the interstitial nephritis did not occur following discontinuation of indinavir therapy; renal insufficiency; renal failure; leucocyturia (see section 4.4).

General disorders and administration site conditions:

Very Common: asthenia/fatigue; taste perversion; abdominal pain.

*Not known**: Combination antiretroviral therapy has been associated with redistribution of body fat (lipodystrophy) in HIV patients, including the loss of peripheral and facial subcutaneous fat, increased intra-abdominal fat and visceral fat, breast hypertrophy and dorsocervical fat accumulation (buffalo hump).

Combination antiretroviral therapy has been associated with metabolic abnormalities such as hypertriglyceridaemia, hypercholesterolaemia, insulin resistance, hyperglycaemia and hyperlactataemia (see section 4.4).

Cases of osteonecrosis have been reported, particularly in patients with generally acknowledged risk factors, advanced HIV disease or long-term exposure to combination antiretroviral therapy (CART). The frequency of this is unknown (see section 4.4).

In HIV-infected patients with severe immune deficiency at the time of initiation of combination antiretroviral therapy (CART), an inflammatory reaction to asymptomatic or residual opportunistic infections may arise (see section 4.4).

Laboratory test findings

The laboratory abnormalities reported by the investigators as possibly, probably, or definitely related to CRIXIVAN in ⩾ 10 % of patients treated with CRIXIVAN alone or in combination were:

Very Common (> 10 %)

Blood and lymphatic system disorders: increases in MCV, decreases in neutrophils.

Renal and urinary disorders: haematuria, proteinuria, crystalluria; pyuria in paediatric patients 3 years of age and older.

Hepato-biliary disorders: isolated asymptomatic hyperbilirubinaemia (total bilirubin ⩾ 2.5 mg/dl, 43 mcmol/l), reported predominantly as elevated indirect bilirubin and rarely associated with elevations in ALT, AST, or alkaline phosphatase, has occurred in approximately 14 % of patients treated with CRIXIVAN alone or in combination with other antiretroviral agents. Most patients continued treatment with CRIXIVAN without dosage reduction and bilirubin values gradually declined toward baseline. Hyperbilirubinaemia occurred more frequently at doses exceeding 2.4 g/day compared to doses less than 2.4 g/day. Increased ALT and AST.

In clinical trials with CRIXIVAN in paediatric patients 3 years of age and older, asymptomatic pyuria of unknown etiology was noted in 10.9 % (6/55) of patients who received CRIXIVAN at the recommended dose of 500 mg/m^2 every 8 hours. Some of these events were associated with mild elevation of serum creatinine.

The following additional laboratory abnormalities have been reported during post-marketing experience; they are derived from spontaneous reports for which precise incidences cannot be determined:

Metabolic and nutritional disorders: increased serum triglycerides, increased serum cholesterol.

Hepato-biliary disorders: liver function abnormalities.

Musculoskeletal and connective tissue and bone disorders: increased CPK.

4.9 Overdose

There have been reports of human overdose with CRIXIVAN. The most commonly reported symptoms were gastro-intestinal (e.g., nausea, vomiting, diarrhoea) and renal (e.g., nephrolithiasis, flank pain, haematuria).

It is not known whether indinavir is dialysable by peritoneal or haemodialysis.

5. PHARMACOLOGICAL PROPERTIES

5.1 Pharmacodynamic properties

Pharmacotherapeutic group: Protease inhibitor, ATC code JO5AE02

Mechanism of action

Indinavir inhibits recombinant HIV–1 and HIV–2 protease with an approximate tenfold selectivity for HIV–1 over HIV–2 proteinase. Indinavir binds reversibly to the protease active site and inhibits competitively the enzyme, thereby preventing cleavage of the viral precursor polyproteins that occurs during maturation of the newly formed viral particle. The resulting immature particles are non–infectious and are incapable of establishing new cycles of infection. Indinavir did not significantly inhibit the eukaryotic proteases human renin, human cathepsin D, human elastase, and human factor Xa.

Microbiology

Indinavir at concentrations of 50 to 100 nM mediated 95 % inhibition (IC_{95}) of viral spread (relative to an untreated virus–infected control) in human T–lymphoid cell cultures and primary human monocytes/macrophages infected with HIV−1 variants LAI, MN, RF, and a macrophage–tropic variant SF–162, respectively. Indinavir at concentrations of 25 to 100 nM mediated 95 % inhibition of viral spread in cultures of mitogen–activated human peripheral blood mononuclear cells infected with diverse, primary clinical isolates of HIV−1, including isolates resistant to zidovudine and non–nucleoside reverse transcriptase inhibitors (NNRTIs). Synergistic antiretroviral activity was observed when human T–lymphoid cells infected with the LAI variant of HIV–1 were incubated with indinavir and either zidovudine, didanosine, or NNRTIs.

Drug resistance

Loss of suppression of viral RNA levels occurred in some patients; however, CD4 cell counts were often sustained above pre–treatment levels. When loss of viral RNA suppression occurred, it was typically associated with replacement of circulating susceptible virus with resistant viral variants. Resistance was correlated with the accumulation of mutations in the viral genome that resulted in the expression of amino acid substitutions in the viral protease.

At least eleven amino acid sites in the protease have been associated with indinavir resistance: L10, K20, L24, M46, I54, L63, I64, A71, V82, I84, and L90. The basis for their contributions to resistance, however, is complex. None of these substitutions was either necessary or sufficient for resistance. For example, no single substitution or pair of substitutions was capable of engendering measurable (⩾ four–fold) resistance to indinavir, and the level of resistance was dependent on the ways in which multiple substitutions were combined. In general, however, higher levels of resistance resulted from the co–expression of greater numbers of substitutions at the eleven identified positions. Among patients experiencing viral RNA rebound during indinavir monotherapy at 800 mg q8h, substitutions at only three of these sites were observed in the majority of patients: V82 (to A or F), M46 (to I or L), and L10 (to I or R). Other substitutions were observed less frequently. The observed amino acid substitutions appeared to accumulate sequentially and in no consistent order, probably as a result of ongoing viral replication.

It should be noted that the decrease in suppression of viral RNA levels was seen more frequently when therapy with indinavir was initiated at doses lower than the recommended oral dose of 2.4 g/day. **Therefore, therapy with indinavir should be initiated at the recommended dose to increase suppression of viral replication and therefore inhibit the emergence of resistant virus.**

The concomitant use of indinavir with nucleoside analogues (to which the patient is naive) may lessen the risk of the development of resistance to both indinavir and the nucleoside analogues. In one comparative trial, combination therapy with nucleoside analogues (triple therapy with zidovudine plus didanosine) conferred protection against the selection of virus expressing at least one resistance–associated amino acid substitution to both indinavir (from 13/24 to 2/20 at therapy week 24) and to the nucleoside analogues (from 10/16 to 0/20 at therapy week 24).

Cross resistance

HIV−1 patient isolates with reduced susceptibility to indinavir expressed varying patterns and degrees of cross–resistance to a series of diverse HIV PIs, including ritonavir and saquinavir. Complete cross−resistance was noted between indinavir and ritonavir; however, cross−resistance to saquinavir varied among isolates. Many of the protease amino acid substitutions reported to be associated with resistance to ritonavir and saquinavir were also associated with resistance to indinavir.

Pharmacodynamic effects

Adults

Treatment with indinavir alone or in combination with other antiretroviral agents (i.e., nucleoside analogues) has so far been documented to reduce viral load and increase CD4 lymphocytes in patients with CD4 cell counts below 500 cells/mm^3.

In one published study, 20 HIV-infected patients with undetectable plasma viral load (<200 copies /ml) receiving indinavir 800 mg every 8 hours were switched in an open, cross-over design to indinavir/ritonavir 400/100 mg every 12 hours. Eighteen patients completed the study to week 48. Viral load remained <200 copies/mL for 48 weeks in all patients.

Another published study evaluated the efficacy and safety of indinavir/ritonavir 400/100 mg every 12 hours in 40 antiretroviral-naïve patients. Thirty subjects completed 48 weeks of treatment. At week 4, the indinavir Cmin was 500 ng/mL with substantial trough variability (range 5 to 8100 ng/mL). By intent to treat analysis 65% of patients had HIV RNA <400 copies/mL and 50% had viral load < 50 copies/mL; by on-treatment analysis 96% of patients had HIV RNA <400 copies/mL and 74% had viral load <50 copies/mL.

Eighty antiretroviral naïve patients were entered into a third published study. In this open label non-randomised single arm study, patients were treated with stavudine and lamivudine plus indinavir/ritonavir 400/100 mg every 12 hours. Sixty-two patients completed the study to week 96. In the intent to treat and on treatment analyses the proportion of patients with HIV RNA of <50 copies/mL was 68.8% and 88.7%, respectively, at week 96.

Indinavir alone or in combination with nucleoside analogues (zidovudine/stavudine and lamivudine) has been shown to delay clinical progression rate compared with nucleoside analogues and to provide a sustained effect on viral load and CD4 count.

In zidovudine experienced patients, indinavir, zidovudine and lamivudine in combination compared with lamivudine added to zidovudine reduced the probability of AIDS defining illness or death (ADID) at 48 weeks from 13 % to 7 %. Similarly, in antiretroviral naive patients, indinavir with and without zidovudine compared with zidovudine alone reduced the probability of ADID at 48 weeks from 15 % with zidovudine alone to approximately 6 % with indinavir alone or in combination with zidovudine.

Effects on viral load were consistently more pronounced in patients treated with indinavir in combination with nucleoside analogues, but the proportion of patients with serum viral RNA below the limit of quantification (500 copies/ml) varied between studies, at week 24 from 40 % to more than 80 %. This proportion tends to remain stable over prolonged periods of follow-up. Similarly, effects on CD4 cell count tend to be more pronounced in patients treated with indinavir in combination with nucleoside analogues compared with indinavir alone. Within studies, this effect is sustained also after prolonged periods of follow-up.

Paediatric patients

Two ongoing clinical trials in 41 paediatric patients (4 to 15 years of age) were designed to characterise the safety, antiretroviral activity, and pharmacokinetics of indinavir in combination with stavudine and lamivudine. In one study, at week 24, the proportion of patients with plasma viral RNA below 400 copies/ml was 60 %; the mean increase in CD4 cell counts was 242 cells/mm^3; and the mean increase in percent CD4 cell counts was 4.2 %. At week 60, the proportion of patients with plasma viral RNA below 400 copies/ml was 59 %. In another study, at week 16, the proportion of patients with plasma viral RNA below 400 copies/ml was 59 %; the mean increase in CD4 cell counts was 73 cells/mm^3; and the mean increase in percent CD4 cell counts was 1.2 %. At week 24, the proportion of patients with plasma viral RNA below 400 copies/ml was 60 %.

5.2 Pharmacokinetic properties

Absorption

Indinavir is rapidly absorbed in the fasted state with a time to peak plasma concentration of 0.8 hours ± 0.3 hours (mean ± S.D.). A greater than dose-proportional increase in indinavir plasma concentrations was observed over the 200 – 800 mg dose range. Between 800-mg and 1,000-mg dose levels, the deviation from dose-proportionality is less pronounced. As a result of the short half-life, 1.8 ± 0.4 hours, only a minimal increase in plasma concentrations occurred after multiple dosing. The bioavailability of a single 800-mg dose of indinavir was approximately 65 % (90 % CI, 58 – 72 %).

Data from a steady state study in healthy volunteers indicate that there is a diurnal variation in the pharmacokinetics of indinavir. Following a dosage regimen of 800 mg every 8 hours, measured peak plasma concentrations (C_{max}) after morning, afternoon and evening doses were 15,550 nM, 8,720 nM and 8,880 nM, respectively. Corresponding plasma concentrations at 8 hours post dose were 220 nM, 210 nM and 370 nM, respectively. The relevance of these findings for ritonavir boosted indinavir is unknown. At steady state following a dosage regimen of 800 mg every 8 hours, HIV-seropositive adult patients in one study achieved geometric means of: $AUC_{0\text{-}8h}$ of 27,813 nM*h (90% confidence interval = 22,185, 34,869), peak plasma concentrations 11,144 nM (90% confidence interval = 9,192, 13,512) and plasma concentrations at 8 hours post dose 211 nM (90% confidence interval = 163, 274).

Food effect

At steady state following a dosage regimen of 800 mg/100 mg of indinavir/ritonavir every 12 hours with a low-fat meal, healthy volunteers in one study achieved geometric means: $AUC_{0\text{-}12h}$ 116,067 nM*h (90% confidence interval = 101,680, 132,490), peak plasma concentrations 19,001 nM (90% confidence interval = 17,538, 20,588), and plasma concentrations at 12 hours post dose 2,274 nM (90% confidence interval = 1,701, 3,042). No significant difference in exposure was seen when the regimen was given with a high-fat meal.

Indinavir boosted regimen. Limited data are available on the pharmacokinetics of indinavir in association with low dose ritonavir. The pharmacokinetics of indinavir (400 mg) with ritonavir (100 mg) dosed twice daily was examined in two studies. Pharmacokinetic analysis in one study was performed on 19 of the patients, with a median (range) indinavir AUC 0-12hr, Cmax, and Cmin of 25421 nM*h (21489-36236 nM*h), 5758 nM (5056-6742 nM) and 239 (169-421 nM), respectively. The pharmacokinetic parameters in the second study were comparable.

In HIV–infected paediatric patients, a dosage regimen of indinavir hard capsules, 500 mg/m^2 every 8 hours, produced $AUC_{0\text{-}8hr}$ values of 27,412 nM *h, peak plasma concentrations of 12,182 nM, and plasma concentrations at 8 hours post dose of 122 nM. The AUC and peak plasma concentrations were generally similar to those previously observed in HIV-infected adults receiving the recommended dose of 800 mg every 8 hours; it should be observed that the plasma concentrations 8 hours post dose were lower.

During pregnancy, it has been demonstrated that the systemic exposure of indinavir is relevantly decreased (PACTG 358. Crixivan, 800 mg every 8 hours + zidovudine 200 mg every 8 hours and lamivudine 150 mg twice a day). The mean indinavir plasma $AUC_{0\text{-}8hr}$ at week 30-32 of gestation (n=11) was 9,231 nM*hr, which is 74% (95% CI: 50%, 86%) lower than that observed 6 weeks postpartum. Six of these 11 (55%) patients had mean indinavir plasma concentrations 8 hours post-dose (C_{min}) below assay threshold of reliable quantification. The pharmacokinetics of indinavir in these 11 patients at 6 weeks postpartum were generally similar to those observed in non-pregnant patients in another study (see section 4.6).

Administration of indinavir with a meal high in calories, fat, and protein resulted in a blunted and reduced absorption with an approximate 80 % reduction in AUC and an 86 % reduction in C_{max}. Administration with light meals (e.g., dry toast with jam or fruit conserve, apple juice, and coffee with skimmed or fat-free milk and sugar or corn flakes, skimmed or fat-free milk and sugar) resulted in plasma concentrations comparable to the corresponding fasted values.

The pharmacokinetics of indinavir taken as indinavir sulphate salt (from opened hard capsules) mixed in apple sauce were generally comparable to the pharmacokinetics of indinavir taken as hard capsules, under fasting conditions. In HIV-infected paediatric patients, the pharmacokinetic parameters of indinavir in apple sauce were: $AUC_{0\text{-}8hr}$ of 26,980 nM *h peak plasma concentration of 13,711 nM; and plasma concentration at 8 hours post dose of 146 nM.

Distribution

Indinavir was not highly bound to human plasma proteins (39 % unbound).

There are no data concerning the penetration of indinavir into the central nervous system in humans.

Biotransformation

Seven major metabolites were identified and the metabolic pathways were identified as glucuronidation at the pyridine nitrogen, pyridine-N-oxidation with and without 3'-hydroxylation on the indane ring, 3'-hydroxylation of indane, p-hydroxylation of phenylmethyl moiety, and N-depyridomethylation with and without the 3'-hydroxylation. *In vitro* studies with human liver microsomes indicated that CYP3A4 is the only P450 isozyme that plays a major role in the oxidative metabolism of indinavir. Analysis of plasma and urine samples from subjects who received indinavir indicated that indinavir metabolites had little proteinase inhibitory activity.

Elimination

Over the 200–1,000-mg dose range administered in both volunteers and HIV infected patients, there was a slightly greater than dose-proportional increase in urinary recovery of indinavir. Renal clearance (116 ml/min) of indinavir is concentration-independent over the clinical dose range. Less than 20 % of indinavir is excreted renally. Mean urinary excretion of unchanged drug following single dose administration in the fasted state was 10.4 % following a 700-mg dose, and 12.0 % following a 1,000-mg dose. Indinavir was rapidly eliminated with a half-life of 1.8 hours.

Characteristics in patients

Pharmacokinetics of indinavir do not appear to be affected by race.

There are no clinically significant differences in the pharmacokinetics of indinavir in HIV seropositive women compared to HIV seropositive men.

Patients with mild-to-moderate hepatic insufficiency and clinical evidence of cirrhosis had evidence of decreased metabolism of indinavir resulting in approximately 60 % higher mean AUC following a 400-mg dose. The mean half-life of indinavir increased to approximately 2.8 hours.

5.3 Preclinical safety data

Crystals have been seen in the urine of rats, one monkey, and one dog. The crystals have not been associated with drug-induced renal injury. An increase in thyroidal weight and thyroidal follicular cell hyperplasia, due to an increase in thyroxine clearance, was seen in rats treated with indinavir at doses ⩾ 160 mg/kg/day. An increase in hepatic weight occurred in rats treated with indinavir at doses ⩾ 40 mg/kg/day and was accompanied by hepatocellular hypertrophy at doses ⩾ 320 mg/kg/day.

The maximum non-lethal oral dose of indinavir was at least 5,000 mg/kg in rats and mice, the highest dose tested in acute toxicity studies.

Studies in rats indicated that uptake into brain tissue was limited, distribution into and out of the lymphatic system was rapid, and excretion into the milk of lactating rats was extensive. Distribution of indinavir across the placental barrier was significant in rats, but limited in rabbits.

Mutagenicity

Indinavir did not have any mutagenic or genotoxic activity in studies with or without metabolic activation.

Carcinogenicity

No carcinogenicity was noted in mice at the maximum tolerated dose, which corresponded to a systemic exposure approximately 2 to 3 times higher than the clinical exposure. In rats, at similar exposure levels, an increased incidence of thyroid adenomas was seen, probably related to an increase in release of thyroid stimulating hormone secondary to an increase in thyroxine clearance. The relevance of the findings to humans is likely limited.

Developmental Toxicity

Developmental toxicity studies were performed in rats, rabbits and dogs (at doses which produced systemic exposures comparable to or slightly greater than human exposure) and revealed no evidence of teratogenicity. No external or visceral changes were observed in rats, however, increases in the incidence of supernumerary ribs and of cervical ribs were seen. No external, visceral, or skeletal changes were observed in rabbits or dogs. In rats and rabbits, no effects on embryonic/foetal survival or foetal weights were observed. In dogs, a slight increase in resorptions was seen; however, all foetuses in medication-treated animals were viable, and the incidence of live foetuses in medication-treated animals was comparable to that in controls.

6. PHARMACEUTICAL PARTICULARS

6.1 List of excipients

Capsule content

- anhydrous lactose
- magnesium stearate

Capsule shell:

- gelatin
- titanium dioxide (E171)
- silicon dioxide
- sodium lauryl sulphate

CRIXIVAN 200 mg: printing ink: indigo carmine (E 132).

CRIXIVAN 400 mg: printing ink: titanium dioxide (E 171), indigo carmine (E 132) and iron oxide (E172).

6.2 Incompatibilities

Not applicable.

6.3 Shelf life

CRIXIVAN 200 mg	3 years
CRIXIVAN 400 mg	2 years for HDPE bottles containing 18 hard capsules
	3 years for HDPE bottles containing 90 and 180 hard capsules

6.4 Special precautions for storage

Store in the original bottle. Keep the bottle tightly closed in order to protect from moisture.

6.5 Nature and contents of container

CRIXIVAN 200 mg: HDPE bottles with a polypropylene cap and a foil induction cap containing 180, 270 or 360 capsules.

CRIXIVAN 400 mg: HDPE bottles with a polypropylene cap and a foil induction cap containing 18, 90 or 180 capsules.

Not all pack sizes may be marketed.

6.6 Special precautions for disposal and other handling

The bottles contain desiccant canisters that should remain in the container.

Any unused product or waste material should be disposed of in accordance with local requirements.

7. MARKETING AUTHORISATION HOLDER

Merck Sharp and Dohme Limited

Hertford Road, Hoddesdon

Hertfordshire EN11 9BU

United Kingdom

8. MARKETING AUTHORISATION NUMBER(S)

CRIXIVAN 200 mg

EU/1/96/024/001

EU/1/96/024/002

EU/1/96/024/003

CRIXIVAN 400 mg

EU/1/96/024/004

EU/1/96/024/005

EU/1/96/024/008

9. DATE OF FIRST AUTHORISATION/RENEWAL OF THE AUTHORISATION

Date of first authorisation: 04/10/1996

Date of latest renewal: 07/10/2006

10. DATE OF REVISION OF THE TEXT

29 October 2008.

SPC.CRX.08.UK.2938 (II/78)

Crystapen Injection

(Genus Pharmaceuticals)

1. NAME OF THE MEDICINAL PRODUCT

Crystapen Injection

2. QUALITATIVE AND QUANTITATIVE COMPOSITION

Benzylpenicillin sodium BP available as 600 mg and 1200 mg vials.

3. PHARMACEUTICAL FORM

White crystalline, water-soluble sterile powder for injection.

4. CLINICAL PARTICULARS

4.1 Therapeutic indications

Crystapen is indicated for most wound infections, pyogenic infections of the skin, soft tissue infections and infections of the nose, throat, nasal sinuses, respiratory tract and middle ear, etc.

It is also indicated for the following infections caused by penicillin-sensitive microorganisms: Generalised infections, septicaemia and pyaemia from susceptible bacteria. Acute and chronic osteomyelitis, sub-acute bacterial endocarditis and meningitis caused by susceptible organisms. Suspected meningococcal disease. Gas gangrene, tetanus, actinomycosis, anthrax, leptospirosis, rat-bite fever, listeriosis, severe Lyme disease, and prevention of neonatal group B streptococcal infections. Complications secondary to gonorrhoea and syphilis (e.g. gonococcal arthritis or endocarditis, congenital syphilis and neurosyphilis). Diphtheria, brain abscesses and pasteurellosis.

Consideration should be given to official local guidance (e.g. national recommendations) on the appropriate use of antibacterial agents.

Susceptibility of the causative organism to the treatment should be tested (if possible), although therapy may be initiated before the results are available.

4.2 Posology and method of administration

Route of administration:

Intramuscular, intravenous.

Preparation of solutions:

Pharmaceutical preparation

Only freshly prepared solutions should be used. Reconstituted solutions of benzylpenicillin sodium BP are intended for immediate administration.

600 mg vial

Intramuscular injection: 600 mg (1 mega unit) is usually dissolved in 1.6 to 2.0 ml of Water for Injections BP.

600 mg and 1200 mg vials

Intravenous Injection: A suitable concentration is 600 mg (1 mega unit) dissolved in 4 to 10 ml of Water for Injections BP or Sodium Chloride Injection BP and 1200 mg (2 mega units) dissolved in at least 8 ml of Sodium Chloride Injection BP or Water for Injections BP.

Intravenous Infusion: It is recommended that 600 mg (1 mega unit) should be dissolved in at least 10 ml of Sodium Chloride Injection BP or Water for Injections BP and 1200 mg (2 mega units) should be dissolved in at least 20 ml of Sodium Chloride Injection BP or Water for Injections BP.

Sodium overload and/or heart failure may occur if benzylpenicillin sodium BP is administered in sodium-containing solvents to patients who suffer from renal failure and/or heart failure. Therefore, for such patients, benzylpenicillin sodium BP should not be reconstituted in sodium-containing liquids such as Sodium Chloride Injection BP or Ringer's solution.

Dosage and administration:

The following dosages apply to both intramuscular and intravenous injection.

Alternate sites should be used for repeated injections.

Adults

600 to 3,600 mg (1 to 6 mega units) daily, divided into 4 to 6 doses, depending on the indication. Higher doses (up to 14.4 g/day (24 mega units) in divided doses) may be given in serious infections such as adult meningitis by the intravenous route.

In bacterial endocarditis, 7.2 to 12 g (12 to 20 mega units) or more may be given daily in divided doses by the intravenous route, often by infusion.

Doses up to 43.2 g (72 mega units) per day may be necessary for patients with rapidly spreading gas gangrene.

High doses should be administered by intravenous injection or infusion, with intravenous doses in excess of 1.2g (2 mega units) being given slowly, taking at least one minute for each 300 mg (0.5 mega unit) to avoid high levels causing irritation of the central nervous system and/or electrolyte imbalance.

High dosage of benzylpenicillin sodium BP may result in hypernatraemia and hypokalaemia unless the sodium content is taken into account.

For the prevention of Group B Streptococcal disease of the newborn, a 3 g (5 mega units) loading dose should be given to the mother initially, followed by 1.5 g (2.5 mega units) every 4 hours until delivery.

Children aged 1 month to 12 years

100 mg/kg/day in 4 divided doses; not exceeding 4 g/day.

Infants 1-4 weeks

75 mg/kg/day in 3 divided doses.

Newborn Infants

50 mg/kg/day in 2 divided doses.

Meningococcal disease

Children 1 month to 12 years:	180-300 mg/kg/day in 4-6 divided doses, not exceeding 12 g/day.
Infants 1-4 weeks:	150 mg/kg/day in 3 divided doses.
Newborn infants:	100 mg/kg/day in 2 divided doses.
Adults and children over 12 years:	2.4 g every 4 hours

Suspected meningococcal disease

If meningococcal disease is suspected general practitioners should give a single dose of benzylpenicillin sodium BP, before transferring the patient to hospital, as follows:

Adults and children over 10 years:	1,200 mg IV (or IM)
Children 1-9 years:	600 mg IV (or IM)
Children under 1 year:	300 mg IV (or IM)

Premature babies and neonates

Dosing should not be more frequent than every 8 or 12 hours in this age group, since renal clearance is reduced at this age and the mean half-life of benzylpenicillin may be as long as 3 hours.

Since infants have been found to develop severe local reactions to intramuscular injections, intravenous treatment should preferably be used.

Patients with renal insufficiency

For doses of 0.6-1.2 g (1-2 mega units) the dosing interval should be no more frequent than every 8-10 hours.

For high doses e.g. 14.4 g (24 mega units) required for the treatment of serious infections such as meningitis, the dosage and dose interval of benzylpenicillin sodium BP should be adjusted in accordance with the following schedule:

(see Table 1 below)

The dose in the above table should be further reduced to 300 mg (0.5 mega units) 8 hourly if advanced liver disease is associated with severe renal failure.

If haemodialysis is required, an additional dose of 300 mg (0.5 mega units) should be given 6 hourly during the procedure.

Elderly Patients

Elimination may be delayed in elderly patients and dose reduction may be necessary.

4.3 Contraindications

Allergy to penicillins. Hypersensitivity to any ingredient of the preparation.

Cross allergy to other beta-lactams such as cephalosporins should be taken into account.

4.4 Special warnings and precautions for use

600 mg benzylpenicillin contains 1.68 mmol of sodium. Massive doses of Benzylpenicillin Sodium BP can cause hypokalaemia and sometimes hypernatraemia. Use of a potassium-sparing diuretic may be helpful. In patients undergoing high-dose treatment for more than 5 days, electrolyte balance, blood counts and renal functions should be monitored.

In the presence of impaired renal function, large doses of penicillin can cause cerebral irritation, convulsions and coma.

Skin sensitisation may occur in persons handling the antibiotic and care should be taken to avoid contact with the substance.

It should be recognised that any patient with a history of allergy, especially to drugs, is more likely to develop a hypersensitivity reaction to penicillin. Patients should be observed for 30 minutes after administration and if an allergic reaction occurs the drug should be withdrawn and appropriate treatment given.

Delayed absorption from the intramuscular depot may occur in diabetics.

Prolonged use of benzylpenicillin may occasionally result in an overgrowth of non-susceptible organisms or yeast and patients should be observed carefully for superinfections.

Pseudomembranous colitis should be considered in patients who develop severe and persistent diarrhoea during or after receiving benzylpenicillin. In this situation, even if Clostridium difficile is only suspected, administration of benzylpenicillin should be discontinued and appropriate treatment given.

4.5 Interaction with other medicinal products and other forms of interaction

The efficacy of oral contraceptives may be impaired under concomitant administration of benzylpenicillin sodium BP, which may result in unwanted pregnancy. Women taking oral contraceptives should be aware of this and should be informed about alternative methods of contraception.

There is reduced excretion of methotrexate (and therefore increased risk of methotrexate toxicity) when used with benzylpenicillin sodium BP.

Probenecid inhibits tubular secretion of benzylpenicillin sodium BP and so may be given to increase the plasma concentrations.

Penicillins may interfere with:

- Urinary glucose tests
- Coomb's tests
- Tests for urinary or serum proteins
- Tests which use bacteria e.g. Guthrie test

4.6 Pregnancy and lactation

Benzylpenicillin sodium BP has been taken by a large number of pregnant women and women of childbearing age without an increase in malformations or other direct or indirect harmful effects on the foetus having been observed.

Although it is not known if benzylpenicillin sodium BP may be excreted into the breast milk of nursing mothers, it is actively transported from the blood to milk in animals and trace amounts of other penicillins in human milk have been detected.

4.7 Effects on ability to drive and use machines

None

4.8 Undesirable effects

Blood and Lymphatic System Disorders

Rare (0.01% - 0.1%)

Haemolytic anaemia and granulocytopenia (neutropenia), agranulocytosis, leucopenia and thrombocytopenia, have been reported in patients receiving prolonged high doses of benzylpenicillin sodium BP (eg. Subacute bacterial endocarditis).

Immune System Disorders

Very Common (>10%)

Patients undergoing treatment for syphilis or neurosyphilis with benzylpenicillin may develop a Jarisch-Herxheimer reaction.

Common (1-10%)

Hypersensitivity to penicillin in the form of rashes (all types), fever, and serum sickness may occur (1-10% treated patients). These may be treated with antihistamine drugs.

Rare (0.01%-0.1%)

More rarely, anaphylactic reactions have been reported (<0.05% treated patients).

Nervous System Disorders

Rare (0.01%-0.1%)

Central nervous system toxicity, including convulsions, has been reported with massive doses over 60 g per day and in patients with severe renal impairment.

Renal and Urinary Disorders

Rare (0.01%-0.1%)

Interstitial nephritis has been reported after intravenous benzylpenicillin sodium BP at doses of more than 12 g per day.

4.9 Overdose

Excessive blood levels of benzylpenicillin sodium BP can be corrected by haemodialysis.

5. PHARMACOLOGICAL PROPERTIES

5.1 Pharmacodynamic properties

Pharmacotherapeutic group: Beta-lactamase sensitive penicillins.

ATC code: J01 CE01.

General Properties:

Benzylpenicillin sodium BP is a beta-lactam antibiotic. It is bactericidal by inhibiting bacterial cell wall biosynthesis.

Table 1

Creatinine clearance (ml per minute)	Dose (g)	Dose (mega units)	Dosing interval (hours)
125	1.2 or 1.8	2 or 3	2 3
60	1.2	2	4
40	0.9	1.5	4
20	0.6	1.0	4
10	0.6	1.0	6
Nil	0.3 or 0.6	0.5 or 1.0	6 8

Table 2

Organism	S ≤ (mg/L)	I (mg/L)	R ≥ (mg/L)
Streptococcus pneumoniae Neisseria gonorrhoeae	0.06	0.12-1.0	2.0
Neisseria meningitides	0.06		0.12
Haemolytic streptococci Staphylococci Moraxella catarrhalis Haemophilus influenzae	0.12		0.25
Rapidly growing anaerobes	1.0		2.0

S = Susceptible, I = Intermediate susceptibility, R = Resistant

Table 3

Type of Micro-organism	Micro-organism	Range of acquired resistance
Susceptible and intermediately susceptible micro-organisms		
Aerobic Gram-positive micro-organisms	• Bacillus anthracis	0%**
	• Corynebacterium diphtheriae	0%*
	• Haemolytic streptococci (including Streptococcus pyogenes)	0%*-3%**
	• Listeria monocytogenes	0%**
	• Streptococcus pneumoniae	4%*-40%**
	• Streptococcus viridans	3-32%*
Aerobic Gram-negative micro-organisms	• Neisseria gonorrhoeae	9-10%*
	• Neisseria meningitidis	18%*
	• Pasteurella multocida	0%***
Anaerobic micro-organisms	• Actinomyces israelii	8%**
	• Fusobacterium nucleatum and Fusobacterium necrophorum	Usually sensitive
	• Gram-positive sporing bacilli (including Clostridium tetani and Clostridium perfringens (welchii))	14%**
	• Gram-positive cocci (including peptostreptococcus)	7%*
Other micro-organisms	• Borrelia bugdorferi	Usually sensitive
	• Capnocytophaga canimorosus	Usually sensitive
	• Leptospirae	Usually sensitive
	• Streptobacillus moniliformis and spirillum minus	Usually sensitive
	• Treponema pallidum	0%***
Insusceptible micro-organisms		
Aerobic Gram-positive microorganisms	• Coagulase negative Staphylococcus	71-81%*
	• Enterococcus Spp	Resistant
	• Staphylococcus aureus	79-87%*
Aerobic Gram-negative microorganisms	• Acinetobacter	Resistant
	• Bordetella pertussis	Generally resistant
	• Brucella spp.	Resistant
	• Enterobacteriaceae (including Escherichia coli, Salmonella, Shigella, Enterobacter, Klebsiella, Proteus, Citrobacter).	Generally resistant
	• Haemophilus influenzae	Resistant
	• Pseudomonas	Resistant
Anaerobic microorganisms	• Bacteroides fragilis	100%***

* UK data; ** European data, *** Global data

Breakpoints:

The tentative breakpoints (British Society for Antimicrobial Chemotherapy, BSAC) for benzylpenicillin sodium BP are as follows:

(see Table 2 above)

Susceptibility:

The prevalence of resistance may vary geographically and with time for selected species and local information on resistance is desirable, particularly when treating severe infections. The following table gives only approximate guidance on probabilities whether microorganisms will be susceptible to benzylpenicillin sodium BP or not.

(see Table 3 above)

Other Information:

Known Resistance Mechanisms and Cross-resistance

Penicillin resistance can be mediated by alteration of penicillin binding proteins or development of beta-lactamases.

Resistance to penicillin may be associated with cross-resistance to a variety of other beta lactam antibiotics either due to a shared target site that is altered, or due to a beta-lactamase with a broad range of substrate molecules. In addition to this, cross resistance to unrelated antibiotics can develop due to more than one resistance gene being present on a mobile section of DNA (e.g. plasmid, transposon etc) resulting in two or more resistance mechanisms being transferred to a new organism at the same time.

5.2 Pharmacokinetic properties

Benzylpenicillin sodium BP rapidly appears in the blood following intramuscular injection of water-soluble salts and maximum concentrations are usually reached in 15-30 minutes. Peak plasma concentrations of about 12 mcg/ml have been reported after doses of 600 mg with therapeutic plasma concentrations for most susceptible organisms detectable for about 5 hours. Approximately 60% of the dose injected is reversibly bound to plasma protein.

In adults with normal renal function the plasma half-life is about 30 minutes. Most of the dose (60-90%) undergoes renal elimination, 10% by glomerular filtration and 90% by tubular secretion. Tubular secretion is inhibited by probenecid, which is sometimes given to increase plasma penicillin concentrations. Biliary elimination of benzylpenicillin sodium BP accounts for only a minor fraction of the dose.

5.3 Preclinical safety data

There are no pre-clinical data of relevance to the prescriber which are additional to that already included in other sections of the SmPC.

6. PHARMACEUTICAL PARTICULARS

6.1 List of excipients

None

6.2 Incompatibilities

Benzylpenicillin sodium BP and solutions that contain metal ions should be administered separately.

Benzylpenicillin sodium should not be administered in the same syringe / giving set as amphotericin B, cimetidine, cytarabine, flucloxacillin, hydroxyzine, methylprednisolone, or promethazine since it is incompatible with these drugs.

6.3 Shelf life

Unopened 36 months.

Reconstituted product should be used immediately.

6.4 Special precautions for storage

Store below 25°C.

6.5 Nature and contents of container

Tubular type III glass vials sealed with bromobutyl rubber plugs with aluminium overseals or plastic 'flip-top' caps. This product is supplied in vials containing 600 mg and 1.2 g of powder in boxes containing 10, 25, 50, and 100 vials, and "GP pack" containing 2 vials of 600 mg.

6.6 Special precautions for disposal and other handling

After contact with skin, wash immediately with water. In case of contact with eyes, rinse immediately with plenty of water and seek medical advice if discomfort persists.

7. MARKETING AUTHORISATION HOLDER

Genus Pharmaceuticals

Park View House

65 London Road

Newbury

Berkshire RG14 1JN

United Kingdom

8. MARKETING AUTHORISATION NUMBER(S)

PL 06831/0213

9. DATE OF FIRST AUTHORISATION/RENEWAL OF THE AUTHORISATION

3 July 2008

10. DATE OF REVISION OF THE TEXT

3 July 2008

Cuprofen for Children

(SSL International plc)

1. NAME OF THE MEDICINAL PRODUCT

Cuprofen For Children

2. QUALITATIVE AND QUANTITATIVE COMPOSITION

Ibuprofen 100mg / 5ml

For excipients see 6.1

3. PHARMACEUTICAL FORM

Oral Suspension

A white, opaque smooth suspension

4. CLINICAL PARTICULARS

4.1 Therapeutic indications

For reduction in fever (including post immunization fever) and relief of mild to moderate pain such as headache, sore throat, earache, teething pain and toothache, cold and flu symptoms, minor aches and sprains.

4.2 Posology and method of administration

For oral administration and short term use only, as required:

Children 8 to 12 years: 10ml three to four times daily.

Children 3 to 7 years: 5ml three to four times daily.

Children 1 to 2 years: 2.5ml three to four times daily.

Infants 6 months to 1 year: 2.5ml three times daily.

Leave at least four hours between doses.

Not recommended for children under 6 months of age.

For post immunization fever: 2.5ml followed by one further 2.5ml 6 hours later, if necessary. No more than 2 doses in 24 hours. If fever is not reduced, consult your doctor.

If the child's symptoms persist for more than 3 days consult your doctor.

4.3 Contraindications

Hypersensitivity to ibuprofen or any of the constituents in the product.

Patients who have previously shown hypersensitivity reactions (e.g. asthma, rhinitis, or urticaria) in response to aspirin or other non-steroidal anti-inflammatory drugs.

Table 2

Kidney	Very rare	Acute renal failure, papillary necrosis, especially in long-term use, associated with increased serum urea and oedema
Liver	Very rare	Liver disorders
Blood	Very rare	Haematopoietic disorders (anaemia, leucopenia, thrombocytopenia, pancytopenia, agranulocytosis). First signs are: fever, sore throat, superficial mouth ulcers, flu-like symptoms, severe exhaustion, unexplained bleeding and bruising.
Skin	Uncommon	Various skin rashes.
	Very rare	Severe forms of skin reactions such as erythema multiforme and epidermal necrolysis can occur.
Immune System	Very rare	In patients with existing auto-immune disorders (such as systemic lupus erythematosus, mixed connective tissue disease) during treatment with ibuprofen, single cases of symptoms of aseptic meningitis, such as stiff neck, headache, nausea, vomiting, fever or disorientation have been observed (see section 4.4 special warnings and precautions for use).
Hypersensitivity reactions	Uncommon	Hypersensitivity reactions with urticaria and pruritus.
	Very rare	Severe hypersensitivity reactions. Symptoms could be: facial, tongue and laryngeal swelling, dyspnoea, tachycardia, hypotension (anaphylaxis, angioedema or severe shock). Exacerbation of asthma and bronchospasm.

Active or previous peptic ulcer.

History of upper gastrointestinal bleeding or perforation, related to previous NSAIDs therapy.

Use with concomitant NSAIDs including cyclo-oxygenase-2 specific inhibitors (see section 4.5 Interactions)

Severe hepatic failure, renal failure or heart failure (see section 4.4 Special warnings and precautions for use)

Last trimester of pregnancy (see section 4.6 Pregnancy and lactation).

Severe heart failure.

4.4 Special warnings and precautions for use

Bronchospasm may be precipitated in patients suffering from or with a previous history of bronchial asthma or allergic disease.

Undesirable effects may be minimized by using the minimum effective dose for the shortest possible duration.

The elderly are at increased risk of the serious consequences of adverse reactions.

Systemic lupus erythematosus and mixed connective tissue disease – increased risk of aseptic meningitis (see section 4.8 Undesirable effects).

Chronic inflammatory intestinal disease (ulcerative colitis, Crohn's disease) – as these conditions may be exacerbated (see section 4.8 Undesirable effects).

Hypertension and/or cardiac impairment as renal function may deteriorate and/or fluid retention occur.

Renal impairment as renal function may further deteriorate (see section 4.3 Contraindications and section 4.8 Undesirable effects).

Hepatic dysfunction (see section 4.3 Contraindications and section 4.8 Undesirable effects).

There is limited evidence that drugs which inhibit cyclo-oxygenase/prostaglandin synthesis may cause impairment of female fertility by an effect on ovulation. This is reversible on withdrawal of treatment.

GI bleeding, ulceration or perforation, which can be fatal, has been reported with all NSAIDs at anytime during treatment, with or without warning symptoms or a previous history of serious GI events.

Patients with a history of GI toxicity, particularly when elderly, should report any unusual abdominal symptoms (especially GI bleeding) particularly in the initial stages of treatment.

Caution should be advised in patients receiving concomitant medications which could increase the risk of gastrotoxicity or bleeding, such as corticosteroid, or anticoagulants such as warfarin or anti-platelet agents such as aspirin (see section 4.5 Interactions).

Where GI bleeding or ulceration occurs in patients receiving ibuprofen, the treatment should be withdrawn.

Contains Liquid Maltitol (E965). Patients with rare hereditary problems of fructose intolerance should not take this medicine.

Caution (discussion with doctor or pharmacist) is required prior to starting treatment in patients with a history of hypertension and/or heart failure as fluid retention, hypertension and oedema have been reported in association with NSAID therapy.

Undesirable effects may be minimised by using the lowest effective dose for the shortest duration necessary to control symptoms (see GI and cardiovascular risks below).

Cardiovascular and cerebrovascular effects

Clinical trial and epidemiological data suggest that use of ibuprofen, particularly at high doses (2400mg daily) and in long-term treatment may be associated with a small increased risk of arterial thrombotic events (for example myocardial infarction or stroke). Overall, epidemiological studies do not suggest that low dose ibuprofen (e.g. $\leqslant$ 1200mg daily) is associated with an increased risk of myocardial infarction.

The label will include:

Read the enclosed leaflet before taking this product.

Do not use if your child

• has or has ever had a stomach ulcer, perforation or bleeding

• is allergic to ibuprofen or any other ingredient of the product, aspirin or other related painkillers

• is taking other NSAID painkillers, or aspirin with a daily dose above 75mg

• is in the last three months of pregnancy

Talk to a pharmacist or your doctor before using this product if your child

• has asthma, liver, heart, kidney problems

• has stomach or bowel disorders

• is in the first 6 months of pregnancy

Do not exceed the stated dose. Keep all medicines out of the reach and sight of children.

If symptoms persist for more than 3 days, consult a doctor.

4.5 Interaction with other medicinal products and other forms of interaction

Ibuprofen should not be used in combination with:

Aspirin: Unless low-dose aspirin (not above 75mg daily) has been advised by a doctor, as this may increase the risk of adverse reactions (see section 4.3 contraindications).

Other NSAIDs: As these may increase the risk of adverse effects (see section 4.3 contraindications).

Ibuprofen should be used with caution in combination with:

Anticoagulants: NSAIDs may enhance the effects of anti-coagulants, such as warfarin (see section 4.4 special warnings and precautions for use).

Antihypertensives and diuretics: NSAIDs may diminish the effect of these drugs.

Corticosteroids: May increase the risk of adverse reactions in the gastrointestinal tract (see section 4.4 special warnings and precautions for use).

Lithium: There is evidence for potential increases in plasma levels of lithium.

Methotrexate: There is a potential for an increase in plasma methotrexate.

Zidovudine: There is evidence of an increased risk of haemarthroses and haematoma in HIV (+) haemophiliacs receiving concurrent treatment with zidovudine and ibuprofen.

4.6 Pregnancy and lactation

Children under 9 years are unlikely to become pregnant or breast feed. However, whilst no teratogenic effects have been demonstrated in animal experiments, the use of the suspension should, if possible, be avoided during the first 6 months of pregnancy.

During the 3rd trimester, there is a risk of premature closure of the foetal ductus arteriosus with possible persistent pulmonary hypertension. The onset of labour may be delayed and the duration increased with an increased bleeding tendency in both mother and child (see section 4.3 Contraindications).

In limited studies, ibuprofen appears in the breast milk in very low concentration and is unlikely to affect the breast-fed infant adversely.

See section 4.4 regarding female fertility.

4.7 Effects on ability to drive and use machines

None expected at recommended doses and duration of therapy.

4.8 Undesirable effects

Hypersensitivity reactions have been reported and these may consist of:

a) Non-specific allergic reactions and anaphylaxis,

b) Respiratory tract reactivity e.g. asthma, aggravated asthma, bronchospasm, dyspnoea

c) Various skin reactions e.g. pruritis, urticaria, angioedema and more rarely exfoliative and bullous dermatoses (including epidermal necrolysis and erythema multiforme).

The following list of adverse effects relates to those experienced with ibuprofen at OTC doses, for short-term use. In the treatment of chronic conditions, under long-term treatment, additional adverse effects may occur.

Gastrointestinal Disorders	Uncommon	Abdominal pain, nausea and dyspepsia
	Rare	Diarrhoea, flatulence, constipation and vomiting
	Very rare	Peptic ulcer, perforation or gastrointestinal haemorrhage, sometimes fatal, particularly in the elderly. Exacerbation of ulcerative colitis and Crohn's disease (see section 4.4 special warnings and precautions for use)
Nervous System	Uncommon	Headache

(see Table 2 opposite)

Oedema, hypertension, and cardiac failure, have been reported in association with NSAID treatment.

Clinical trial and epidemiological data suggest that use of ibuprofen (particularly at high doses 2400mg daily) and in long-term treatment may be associated with a small increased risk of arterial thrombotic events (for example myocardial infarction or stroke) (see section 4.4).

4.9 Overdose

In children ingestion of more than 400 mg/kg may cause symptoms. In adults the dose response effect is less clear cut. The half-life in overdose is 1.5-3 hours.

Symptoms

Most patients who have ingested clinically important amounts of NSAIDs will develop no more than nausea, vomiting, epigastric pain, or more rarely diarrhoea. Tinnitus, headache and gastrointestinal bleeding are also possible. In more serious poisoning, toxicity is seen in the central nervous system, manifesting as drowsiness, occasionally excitation and disorientation or coma. Occasionally patients develop convulsions. In serious poisoning metabolic acidosis may occur and the prothrombin time / INR may be prolonged, probably due to interference with the actions of circulating clotting factors. Acute renal failure and liver damage may occur. Exacerbation of asthma is possible in asthmatics.

Management

Management should be symptomatic and supportive and include the maintenance of a clear airway and monitoring of cardiac and vital signs until stable. Consider oral administration of activated charcoal if the patient presents within 1 hour of ingestion of a potentially toxic amount. If frequent or prolonged, convulsions should be treated with intravenous diazepam or lorazepam. Give bronchodilators for asthma.

5. PHARMACOLOGICAL PROPERTIES

5.1 Pharmacodynamic properties

Pharmacotherapeutic group: Antiinflammatory and anti-rheumatic products, non-steroids, propionic acid derivatives.

ATC code: M01A E01

Ibuprofen is a propionic acid derivative NSAID that has demonstrated its efficacy by inhibition of prostaglandin synthesis. Ibuprofen has analgesic, antipyretic and anti-inflammatory properties.

5.2 Pharmacokinetic properties

Ibuprofen is rapidly absorbed following administration and is rapidly distributed throughout the whole body. The excretion is rapid and complete via the kidneys.

Maximum plasma concentrations are reached 45 minutes after ingestion if taken on an empty stomach. When taken with food, high peak levels are observed after 1 to 2 hours. These times may vary with different dosage forms.

The half life of ibuprofen is about 2 hours.

In limited studies, ibuprofen appears in the breast milk in very low concentrations.

5.3 Preclinical safety data

No relevant information additional to that contained elsewhere in the SPC.

6. PHARMACEUTICAL PARTICULARS

6.1 List of excipients

Sodium Methyl Parahydroxybenzoate (E219)

Sodium Propyl Parahydroxybenzoate (E217)

Citric Acid Anhydrous

Saccharin Sodium

Sodium Benzoate (E211)

Dispersible Cellulose

Orange Juicy Flavour

Polysorbate 80

Liquid Maltitol (E965)

Xanthan Gum

Purified Water.

6.2 Incompatibilities

None.

6.3 Shelf life
Amber glass or PET bottles with PP closures: 2 years.

6.4 Special precautions for storage
Do not store above 25°C. Store in the original container.

6.5 Nature and contents of container
Amber glass or PET bottles with polypropylene child resistant screw closures, containing 100 or 150ml enclosed in an outer carton. A measuring spoon is provided.

6.6 Special precautions for disposal and other handling
Not applicable.

7. MARKETING AUTHORISATION HOLDER
Galpharm Healthcare Ltd
Hugh House
Upper Cliffe Road
Dodworth Business Park
Dodworth
South Yorkshire
S75 3SP

8. MARKETING AUTHORISATION NUMBER(S)
PL 16028/0075

9. DATE OF FIRST AUTHORISATION/RENEWAL OF THE AUTHORISATION
10/02/2006

10. DATE OF REVISION OF THE TEXT
03/04/2007

Cuprofen Maximum Strength Tablets

(SSL International plc)

1. NAME OF THE MEDICINAL PRODUCT
Cuprofen Maximum Strength Tablets

2. QUALITATIVE AND QUANTITATIVE COMPOSITION
Ibuprofen 400mg/tablet

3. PHARMACEUTICAL FORM
Coated tablets

4. CLINICAL PARTICULARS

4.1 Therapeutic indications
For the relief of rheumatic, muscular, dental and period pains and pain in backache, neuralgia, migraine and headache, and for the symptomatic relief of colds, flu and feverishness.

4.2 Posology and method of administration
Route of administration: Oral.

Adults and children over 12 years of age:

Initial dose: one tablet to be taken with water. The initial dose may be followed by further doses of one tablet not more frequently than every four hours.

Maximum daily dose: three tablets in 24 hours.

Not suitable for children under 12 years of age.

To be taken preferably after food.

4.3 Contraindications
Hypersensitivity to any of the constituents

Hypersensitivity to aspirin or other NSAIDS including asthma, rhinitis or urticaria

Current or previous peptic ulceration

Severe heart failure

4.4 Special warnings and precautions for use
Caution should be exercised in administering ibuprofen to patients with asthma and especially patients who have developed bronchospasm with other non-steroidal agents. Special care should be taken when using ibuprofen in elderly patients, in whom increased tissue levels may result with an attendant increase in the risk of adverse reactions.

Undesirable effects may be minimised by using the minimum effective dose for the shortest possible duration. In patients with renal, cardiac or hepatic impairment caution is required, since the use of non-steroidal anti-inflammatory drugs may result in deterioration of renal function. The dose should be kept as low as possible and renal function should be monitored. Do not take Cuprofen with any lithium-containing medication.

Caution (discussion with doctor or pharmacist) is required prior to starting treatment in patients with a history of hypertension and/or heart failure as fluid retention, hypertension and oedema have been reported in association with NSAID therapy.

Undesirable effects may be minimised by using the lowest effective dose for the shortest duration necessary to control symptoms (see GI and cardiovascular risks below).

Cardiovascular and cerebrovascular effects
Clinical trial and epidemiological data suggest that use of ibuprofen, particularly at high doses (2400mg daily) and in long-term treatment may be associated with a small increased risk of arterial thrombotic events (for example myocardial infarction or stroke). Overall, epidemiological studies do not suggest that low dose ibuprofen (e.g. ⩽ 1200mg daily) is associated with an increased risk of myocardial infarction.

The label will state:

1. Do not exceed the stated dose.
2. Consult your doctor if you are asthmatic, sensitive to aspirin or other NSAIDs or are pregnant.
3. If symptoms persist consult your doctor.
4. Do not take if you have a stomach ulcer or other stomach disorders.
5. Keep out of the reach of children.
6. Not suitable for children under 12 years of age.

4.5 Interaction with other medicinal products and other forms of interaction
NSAIDS may enhance the effects of anticoagulants and diminish the effects of antihypertensives or thiazide diuretics.

Concurrent aspirin or other NSAIDS may result in an increased incidence of adverse reaction. Lithium excretion reduced by ibuprofen, risk of toxicity, avoid concomitant use.

4.6 Pregnancy and lactation
Whilst no teratogenic effects have been demonstrated in animal studies, ibuprofen should be avoided during pregnancy. The onset of labour may be delayed and duration of labour increased. Ibuprofen appears in breast milk in very low concentrations and is unlikely to affect the breast-fed infant adversely.

4.7 Effects on ability to drive and use machines
None known.

4.8 Undesirable effects
Adverse effects reported include dyspepsia, gastrointestinal intolerance and bleeding, and skin rashes. Less frequently, thrombocytopenia has occurred. Very rarely toxic amblyopia has occurred; on cessation of treatment recovery has occurred. Non-steroidal anti-inflammatory drugs have been reported to cause nephrotoxicity in various forms and their use can lead to interstitial nephritis, nephrotic syndrome and renal failure.

Skin rashes, pruritis, urticaria, rarely exfoliative dermatitis and epidermal necrolysis, headache, dizziness, and hearing disturbance.

Oedema, hypertension, and cardiac failure, have been reported in association with NSAID treatment

Clinical trial and epidemiological data suggest that use of ibuprofen (particularly at high doses 2400mg daily) and in long-term treatment may be associated with a small increased risk of arterial thrombotic events (for example myocardial infarction or stroke) (see section 4.4).

4.9 Overdose
Symptoms include headache, vomiting, drowsiness and hypotension. Gastric lavage and correction of severe electrolyte abnormalities should be considered.

5. PHARMACOLOGICAL PROPERTIES

5.1 Pharmacodynamic properties
Ibuprofen is a non-steroidal anti-inflammatory agent which exhibits analgesic and antipyretic properties.

It is an effective inhibitor of cyclo-oxygenase responsible for the biosynthesis of prostaglandins which forms part of the inflammatory process. It also inhibits the same enzymes in the gastric mucosa.

Clinical trials have shown that, with ibuprofen, onset of pain relief is rapid and may be felt by 30 minutes after dosing.

5.2 Pharmacokinetic properties
Ibuprofen is rapidly absorbed following oral administration:

t max = approximately 2 hours

t ½ = 2 ± 0.5 hours

Clearance = 0.75 ± 0.20 ml / min / kg

Vd = 0.15 L/ kg

The excretion of ibuprofen is rapid and complete. Greater than 90% of an ingested dose is excreted and no ibuprofen per se is found in the urine.

The major metabolites are a hydroxylated and a carboxylated compound.

5.3 Preclinical safety data
Not applicable.

6. PHARMACEUTICAL PARTICULARS

6.1 List of excipients
Lactose

Ac-di-sol

Methyl cellulose (methocel A4C)

Magnesium stearate

Water

IMS

Polyethylene glycol

Methyl cellulose (methocel E15)

Sepisperse rose AP 5002 or

Mastercote pink FA 0430

Purified water

6.2 Incompatibilities
None known.

6.3 Shelf life
Three years.

6.4 Special precautions for storage
Store at or below 25°C.

6.5 Nature and contents of container
a. Polypropylene containers with a low density polythene tamper evident lid (21, 100, 250, 500, 1000 tablets).

b. Polythene bags free from additives, inside a cardboard outer (5,000, 10,000 tablets).

c. Blister packs comprised of 250μ plain white rigid UPVC and 20μ hard temper aluminium foil (12, 24, 36, 48, 96 tablets).

6.6 Special precautions for disposal and other handling
Not applicable

7. MARKETING AUTHORISATION HOLDER
Cupal Limited
Venus
1 Old Park Lane
Trafford Park
Manchester
M41 7HA

8. MARKETING AUTHORISATION NUMBER(S)
PL 00338/0085

9. DATE OF FIRST AUTHORISATION/RENEWAL OF THE AUTHORISATION
04/07/94 / 12/01/01

10. DATE OF REVISION OF THE TEXT
March 2007

Cuprofen Plus

(SSL International plc)

1. NAME OF THE MEDICINAL PRODUCT
Cuprofen PLUS

2. QUALITATIVE AND QUANTITATIVE COMPOSITION
Ibuprofen Ph Eur 200 mg

Codeine Phosphate Hemihydrate Ph Eur 12.8 mg

3. PHARMACEUTICAL FORM
White film-coated capsule-shaped tablets.

4. CLINICAL PARTICULARS

4.1 Therapeutic indications
Symptomatic relief of mild to moderate pain in such conditions as soft tissue injuries, including sprains, strains and musculo-tendonitis, backache, non-serious arthritic and rheumatic conditions. Also for the relief of mild to moderate pain in neuralgia, migraine, headache, dental pain and dysmenorrhoea.

4.2 Posology and method of administration
Dosage:

Do not take for more than 3 days continuously without medical review.

Adults:

The minimum effective dose should be used for the shortest time necessary to relieve symptoms.

One or two tablets every four to six hours.

Not more than 6 tablets should be taken in 24 hours.

Children under 12 years:

Not recommended

Elderly:

No specific dosage recommendations are required unless renal or hepatic function is impaired, in which case dosage should be assessed individually.

Route of Administration:

For oral administration and short-term use only.

4.3 Contraindications
Cuprofen PLUS are contraindicated in individuals with hypersensitivity to the active ingredients or any of the constituents in the product.

Patients who have previously shown hypersensitivity reactions (e.g. asthma, rhinitis, angioedema or urticaria) in response to aspirin or other non-steroidal anti-inflammatory drugs.

Active or previous peptic ulcer.

History of upper gastrointestinal bleeding or perforation, related to previous NSAIDs therapy.

Use with concomitant NSAIDs including cyclo-oxygenase-2 specific inhibitors (see section 4.5 Interactions).

Severe hepatic failure, renal failure or severe heart failure (see section 4.4, Special warnings and precautions for use).

Last trimester of pregnancy (See section 4.6 Pregnancy and lactation).

4.4 Special warnings and precautions for use
Cuprofen PLUS should be used with caution in patients with gastro-intestinal disease. In patients receiving anti-coagulant therapy, prothrombin time should be monitored daily for the first few days of combined treatment.

Bronchospasm may be precipitated in patients suffering from, or with a history of, bronchial asthma or allergic disease. The possibility of cross-sensitivity with aspirin and other non-steroidal anti-inflammatory agents should be considered.

The elderly are at increased risk of the serious consequences of adverse reactions.

Patients should be advised to consult their doctor if their headaches become persistent.

Systemic lupus erythematosus and mixed connective tissue disease – increased risk of aseptic meningitis (see section 4.8 Undesirable effects)

Chronic inflammatory intestinal disease (ulcerative colitis, Crohn's disease) – as these conditions may be exacerbated (See section 4.8 Undesirable effects)

Caution (discussion with a doctor or pharmacist) is required prior to starting treatment in patients with a history of hypertension and/or heart failure as fluid retention, hypertension and oedema have been reported in association with NSAID therapy.

Renal impairment as renal function may further deteriorate (See section 4.3 Contraindications and Section 4.8 Undesirable effects)

Hepatic dysfunction (See section 4.3 Contraindications and section 4.8 Undesirable effects)

There is limited evidence that drugs which inhibit cyclo-oxygenase / prostaglandin synthesis may cause impairment of female fertility by an effect on ovulation. This is reversible upon withdrawal of the treatment.

GI bleeding, ulceration or perforation, which can be fatal, has been reported with all NSAIDs at anytime during treatment, with or without warning symptoms or a previous history of serious GI events.

Patients with a history of GI toxicity, particularly when elderly, should report any unusual abdominal symptoms (especially GI bleeding) particularly in the initial stages of treatment.

Caution should be advised in patients receiving concomitant medications which could increase the risk of gastrotoxicity or bleeding, such as corticosteroids, or anticoagulants such as warfarin or anti-platelet agents such as aspirin (see section 4.5 Interactions).

When GI bleeding or ulceration occurs in patients receiving ibuprofen, the treatment should be withdrawn.

Cardiovascular and cerebrovascular effects

Clinical trial and epidemiological data suggest that use of ibuprofen, particularly at high doses (2400 mg daily) and in long-term treatment may be associated with a small increased risk of arterial thrombotic events (for example myocardial infarction or stroke). Overall, epidemiological studies do not suggest that low dose ibuprofen (e.g. ⩽ 1200 mg daily) is associated with an increased risk of myocardial infarction.

Undesirable effects may be minimised by using the lowest effective dose for the shortest duration necessary to control symptoms (see GI and cardiovascular risks below).

The leaflet will state in a prominent position in the 'before taking' section:

- If you need to use this medicine for more than three days at a time, see your doctor, pharmacist or health care professional.
- Taking codeine regularly for a long time can lead to addiction, which might cause you to feel restless and irritable when you stop the tablets.
- Taking a painkiller for headaches too often or for too long can make them worse.

The label will state (To be displayed prominently on outer pack -not boxed):

- If you need to use this medicine for more than three days at a time, see your doctor or pharmacist. Taking codeine regularly for a long time can lead to addiction.
- Taking a painkiller for headaches too often or for too long can make them worse.

Read the enclosed leaflet before taking this product.

Do not take if you

- have or have ever had a stomach ulcer, perforation or bleeding
- are allergic to ibuprofen or any other ingredient of the product, aspirin or other related painkillers
- are taking other NSAID painkillers, or aspirin with a daily dose above 75mg
- are in the last 3 months of pregnancy

Speak to a pharmacist or your doctor before you take this product if you

- have asthma, liver, heart, kidney or bowel problems
- are in the first 6 months of pregnancy

If symptoms persist or worsen, consult your doctor

4.5 Interaction with other medicinal products and other forms of interaction

Caution should be exercised in patients taking monoamine oxidase inhibitors.

Ibuprofen should not be used in combination with:

Aspirin: Unless low-dose aspirin (not above 75mg daily) has been advised by a doctor, as this may increase the risk of adverse reactions (See 4.3 Contraindications).

Other NSAIDS: As these may increase the risk of adverse effects (See section 4.3 Contraindications).

Ibuprofen should be used with caution in combination with:

Anticoagulants: NSAIDS may enhance the effects of anti-coagulants, such as warfarin (See section 4.4).

Antihypertensives and diuretics: NSAIDS may diminish the effects of these drugs.

Corticosteroids: May increase the risk of adverse reactions in the gastrointestinal tract (See section 4.4 Special warnings).

Lithium: There is evidence for potential increases in plasma levels of lithium.

Methotrexate: There is a potential for an increase in plasma methotrexate.

Zidovudine: There is evidence of an increased risk of haemarthroses and haematoma in HIV (+) haemophiliacs receiving concurrent treatment with zidovudine and ibuprofen.

4.6 Pregnancy and lactation

Based on animal studies and clinical experience there is no evidence to suggest that foetal abnormalities are associated with the use of ibuprofen or codeine. As with all drugs, use should be avoided in pregnancy and lactation unless essential.

During the 3rd trimester, ibuprofen is contraindicated as there is a risk of premature closure of the foetal ductus arteriosus with possible persistent pulmonary hypertension. The onset of labour may be delayed and its duration increased with an increased bleeding tendency in both mother and child. (See section 4.3 Contraindications).

See section 4.4 regarding female fertility.

4.7 Effects on ability to drive and use machines

Patients should be advised not to drive or operate machinery if affected by dizziness or sedation.

4.8 Undesirable effects

Codeine may cause constipation, nausea, dizziness and drowsiness according to dosage and individual susceptibility.

Regular prolonged use of codeine is known to lead to addiction and symptoms of restlessness and irritability may result when treatment is then stopped.

Prolonged use of a painkiller for headaches can make them worse.

Hypersensitivity reactions have been reported and these may consist of:

a) Non-specific allergic reactions and anaphylaxis

b) Respiratory tract reactivity, e.g. asthma, aggravated asthma, bronchospasm, dyspnoea

c) Various skin reactions, e.g. pruritus, urticaria, angioedema and more rarely exfoliative and bullous dermatoses (including epidermal necrolysis and erythema multiforme)

The following list of adverse effects relates to those experienced with ibuprofen at OTC doses, for short term use. In treatment of chronic conditions, under long-term treatment, additional adverse effects may occur.

Hypersensitivity reactions:

Uncommon: Hypersensitivity reactions with urticaria and pruritus.

Very rare: severe hypersensitivity reactions. Symptoms could be: facial, tongue and laryngeal swelling, dyspnoea, tachycardia, hypotension (anaphylaxis, angioedema or severe shock).

Exacerbation of asthma and bronchospasm.

Gastrointestinal:

Uncommon: abdominal pain, nausea and dyspepsia.

Rare: diarrhoea, flatulence, constipation and vomiting.

Very rare: peptic ulcer, perforation or gastrointestinal haemorrhage, sometimes fatal, particularly in the elderly. Exacerbation of ulcerative colitis and Crohn's disease (See section 4.4).

Nervous system:

Uncommon: Headache

Renal:

Very Rare: Acute renal failure, papillary necrosis, especially in long-term use, associated with increased serum urea and oedema.

Hepatic:

Very rare: liver disorders.

Haematological:

Very rare: Haematopoietic disorders (anaemia, leucopenia, thrombocytopenia, pancytopenia, agranulocytosis). First signs are: fever, sore throat, superficial mouth ulcers, flu-like symptoms, severe exhaustion, unexplained bleeding and bruising.

Skin:

Uncommon: Various skin rashes

Very rare: Severe forms of skin reactions such as erythema multiforme and epidermal necrolysis can occur.

Immune system:

In patients with existing auto-immune disorders (such as systemic lupus erythematosus, mixed connective tissue disease) during treatment with ibuprofen, single cases of symptoms of aseptic meningitis, such as stiff neck, headache, nausea, vomiting, fever or disorientation have been observed (See section 4.4)

Others:

Hearing disturbance.

Oedema, hypertension, and cardiac failure, have been reported in association with NSAID treatment.

Clinical trial and epidemiological data suggest that use of ibuprofen (particularly at high doses 2400 mg daily) and in long-term treatment may be associated with a small increased risk of arterial thrombotic events (for example myocardial infarction or stroke) (see section 4.4).

4.9 Overdose

Overuse of this product, defined as consumption of quantities in excess of the recommended dose, or consumption for a prolonged period of time may lead to physical or psychological dependency. Symptoms of restlessness and irritability may result when treatment is stopped.

Codeine

The effects in overdosage will be potentiated by simultaneous ingestion of alcohol and psychotropic drugs.

Symptoms

Central nervous system depression, including respiratory depression, may develop but is unlikely to be severe unless other sedative agents have been co-ingested, including alcohol, or the overdose is very large. The pupils may be pin-point in size; nausea and vomiting are common. Hypotension and tachycardia are possible but unlikely.

Management

This should include general symptomatic and supportive measures including a clear airway and monitoring of vital signs until stable. Consider activated charcoal if an adult presents within one hour of ingestion of more than 350 mg or a child more than 5 mg/kg.

Give naloxone if coma or respiratory depression is present. Naloxone is a competitive antagonist and has a short half-life, so large and repeated doses may be required in a seriously poisoned patient. Observe for at least four hours after ingestion, or eight hours if a sustained release preparation has been taken.

Ibuprofen

In children ingestion of more than 400 mg/kg may cause symptoms. In adults the dose response effect is less clear cut. The half-life in overdose is 1.5-3 hours.

Symptoms:

Most patients who have ingested clinically important amounts of NSAIDs will develop no more than nausea, vomiting, epigastric pain, or more rarely diarrhoea. Tinnitus, headache and gastrointestinal bleeding are also possible. In more serious poisoning, toxicity is seen in the central nervous system, manifesting as drowsiness, occasionally excitation and disorientation or coma. Occasionally patients develop convulsions. In serious poisoning metabolic acidosis may occur and the prothrombin time/INR may be prolonged, probably due to interference with the actions of circulating clotting factors. Acute renal failure and liver damage may occur. Exacerbation of asthma is possible in asthmatics.

Management:

Management should be symptomatic and supportive and include the maintenance of a clear airway and monitoring of cardiac and vital signs until stable. Consider oral administration of activated charcoal if the patient presents within 1 hour of ingestion of a potentially toxic amount. If frequent or prolonged, convulsions should be treated with intravenous diazepam or lorazepam. Give bronchodilators for asthma.

5. PHARMACOLOGICAL PROPERTIES

5.1 Pharmacodynamic properties

Ibuprofen is a propionic acid derivative NSAID that has demonstrated its efficacy by inhibition of prostaglandin synthesis. In humans ibuprofen reduces inflammatory pain, swellings and fever. Furthermore, ibuprofen reversibly inhibits platelet aggregation.

Codeine is a centrally-acting opioid analgesic.

5.2 Pharmacokinetic properties

Ibuprofen is rapidly absorbed following administration and is distributed throughout the whole body. The excretion is rapid and complete via kidneys.

Maximum plasma concentrations are reached 45 minutes after ingestion if taken on an empty stomach. When taken with food, peak levels are observed after 1-2 hours. These times may vary with different dosage forms.

The half-life of ibuprofen is about 2 hours.

In limited studies, ibuprofen appears in the breast milk in very low concentrations.

Codeine phosphate is absorbed from the gastrointestinal tract, with a relative bioavailability (versus parenteral administration) of about 75%. The half-life in plasma is about 2.5 - 3 hours, whilst its analgesic effect occurs from 15 minutes up to 4 - 6 hours after oral administration. Peak plasma concentrations occur about one hour post-dose. Codeine and its metabolites are excreted almost entirely via the kidneys.

5.3 Preclinical safety data

Both ibuprofen and codeine are well established analgesics with well-documented preclinical safety profiles.

6. PHARMACEUTICAL PARTICULARS

6.1 List of excipients

Microcrystalline cellulose

Hydrogenated vegetable oil

Sodium starch glycollate

Colloidal silicon dioxide

Cellactose 80

Hydroxypropyl methyl cellulose

Polyethylene glycol 400

6.2 Incompatibilities

Not applicable.

6.3 Shelf life

Three years.

6.4 Special precautions for storage

None.

6.5 Nature and contents of container

White opaque polyvinyl chloride (250μm)/aluminium foil (20μm) blister packs containing 4, 6, 12, 24, 48 or 96 tablets.

6.6 Special precautions for disposal and other handling

Not applicable.

7. MARKETING AUTHORISATION HOLDER

SmithKline Beecham (SWG) Limited

980 Great West Road

Brentford

Middlesex

TW8 9GS

United Kingdom

Trading as: GlaxoSmithKline Consumer Healthcare, Brentford, TW8 9GS, U.K.

8. MARKETING AUTHORISATION NUMBER(S)

PL 00071/0431

9. DATE OF FIRST AUTHORISATION/RENEWAL OF THE AUTHORISATION

8 February 1996

10. DATE OF REVISION OF THE TEXT

10 April 2007

Cuprofen Tablets

(SSL International plc)

1. NAME OF THE MEDICINAL PRODUCT

Cuprofen Tablets

2. QUALITATIVE AND QUANTITATIVE COMPOSITION

Ibuprofen 200mg/tablet

3. PHARMACEUTICAL FORM

Film coated tablets

4. CLINICAL PARTICULARS

4.1 Therapeutic indications

For the relief of rheumatic, muscular, dental and period pains and pain in backache, neuralgia, migraine and headache, and for the symptomatic relief of colds, flu and feverishness.

4.2 Posology and method of administration

For oral use. Tablets to be taken preferably after food.

Adults and children over 12 years:

Initial dose: 2 tablets to be taken with water.

The initial dose may be followed by further doses of 1 or 2 tablets every four hours.

Maximum daily dose - 6 tablets in 24 hours.

Not suitable for children under 12 years of age.

4.3 Contraindications

Patients with a history of peptic ulceration or bleeding disorders. Bronchospasm may be precipitated in patients suffering from a previous history of bronchial asthma. Cuprofen should not be given to patients in whom aspirin or other NSAID induce the symptoms; rhinitis or urticaria.

Severe heart failure

4.4 Special warnings and precautions for use

Bronchospasm may be precipitated in patients suffering from or with a previous history of bronchial asthma or allergic disease. Undesirable effects may be minimised by using the minimum effective dose for the shortest possible duration. The elderly are at an increased risk of the serious consequences of adverse reactions.

Caution is required in patients with renal, cardiac or hepatic impairment since renal function may deteriorate.

Do not take Cuprofen with any lithium-containing medication.

Caution (discussion with doctor or pharmacist) is required prior to starting treatment in patients with a history of hypertension and/or heart failure as fluid retention, hypertension and oedema have been reported in association with NSAID therapy.

Undesirable effects may be minimised by using the lowest effective dose for the shortest duration necessary to control symptoms (see GI and cardiovascular risks below).

Cardiovascular and cerebrovascular effects

Clinical trial and epidemiology data suggest that use of ibuprofen, particularly at high doses (2400mg daily) and in long-term treatment may be associated with a small increased risk of arterial thrombotic event (for example myocardial infarction or stroke). Overall, epidemiological studies do not suggest that low dose ibuprofen (e.g. ⩽ 1200mg daily) is associated with an increased risk of myocardial infarction.

The label will state:

1. Do not exceed the stated dose.
2. Consult a doctor if you are asthmatic, sensitive to aspirin or other NSAIDs or are pregnant.
3. If symptoms persist, consult your doctor.
4. Do not take if you have a stomach ulcer or other stomach disorders.
5. Keep out of the reach of children.
6. Not suitable for children under 12 years of age.

4.5 Interaction with other medicinal products and other forms of interaction

NSAIDS may enhance the effects of anticoagulants and diminish the effects of anti-hypertensives or thiazide diuretics.

Concurrent aspirin or other NSAIDS may result in an increased incidence of an adverse reaction. Lithium excretion reduced by ibuprofen, risk of toxicity, avoid concomitant use.

4.6 Pregnancy and lactation

Whilst no teratogenic effects have been demonstrated in animal studies, ibuprofen should be avoided during pregnancy. The onset of labour may be delayed and duration of labour increased. Ibuprofen appears in breast milk in very low concentrations and is unlikely to affect the breast-fed infant adversely.

4.7 Effects on ability to drive and use machines

None stated.

4.8 Undesirable effects

The most frequent adverse effects which may occur are gastrointestinal disturbances, including dyspepsia, abdominal discomfort or pain, nausea, vomiting, gastro-intestinal bleeding or activation of peptic ulcers.

Skin: rashes, pruritis, urticaria, rarely exfoliative dermatitis and epidermal necrolysis.

CNS related side effects which may occur include dizziness, headache, drowsiness, depression, nervousness, insomnia and tinnitus.

More rarely, hypersensitivity reactions may occur, including fever and rashes. Hepatotoxicity and aseptic meningitis rarely may occur may also be hypersensitivity reactions.

Renal: papillary necrosis which can lead to renal failure.

Other adverse effects include anaemias, thrombocytopenia, neutropenia, eosinophilia, agranulocytosis, abnormalities in liver function tests, blurred vision, changes in visual colour perception, toxic amblyopia, cystitis and haematuria.

Non-steroidal anti-inflammatory drugs have been reported to cause nephrotoxicity in various forms and their use can lead to interstitial nephritis, nephrotic syndrome and renal failure.

Oedema, hypertension, and cardiac failure, have been reported in association with NSAID treatment.

Clinical trial and epidemiological data suggest that use of ibuprofen (particularly at high doses 2400mg daily) and in long-term treatment may be associated with a small increased risk of arterial thrombotic events (for example myocardial infarction or stroke) (see section 4.4).

4.9 Overdose

In case of overdose, supportive measures should be taken, such as gastric lavage and correction of serum electrolytes if necessary.

5. PHARMACOLOGICAL PROPERTIES

5.1 Pharmacodynamic properties

Ibuprofen has analgesic, anti-inflammatory and antipyretic properties, it is an inhibitor prostaglandin synthetase.

Clinical trials have shown that, with ibuprofen, onset of pain relief is rapid and may be felt by 30 minutes after dosing.

5.2 Pharmacokinetic properties

Following oral administration, ibuprofen is rapidly and almost completely absorbed. Peak serum levels are achieved between 1 and 2 hours after dosing. The relationship between the administered dose and the area of the total ibuprofen concentration-time curve appears to be non-linear, though a linear relationship does exist between free ibuprofen plasma concentration and dose. This plasma protein binding of the drug may be non-linear. Total urinary excretion of ibuprofen and its metabolites is a linear function of dosage. The absorption and elimination of ibuprofen are not affected by the dosage regimen. Peak serum levels are lower and later when the drug is taken after food. Ibuprofen is rapidly eliminated from the plasma with a half-life of about 2 hours.

Except at very high concentrations, about 99% of ibuprofen is bound to a single site on plasma albumin although a second primary site can be occupied. The high plasma protein binding of ibuprofen results in relatively low volume of distribution, about 0.1L kg^{-1}. Only very small amounts of ibuprofen are excreted in breast milk, not sufficient to have any effect on the infant. It is not known if the drug crosses the placenta.

Ibuprofen is extensively metabolised in the liver, with more than 90% of the dose excreted in the urine and the remainder presumably in the faeces. Less than 10% of the dose is excreted unchanged. Excretion is essentially complete within 24 hours.

Renal impairment has no effect on the kinetics of the drug, rapid elimination still occurring as a consequence of metabolism.

There is no accumulation of ibuprofen or its metabolites in normal subjects on repeated administration of the drug. Old age has no significant effect on the elimination of ibuprofen.

Summary: Oral absorption: >95%.

Plasma half life: 2h

Volume of distribution: 0.1L kg^{-1}.

Plasma protein binding: 99%.

5.3 Preclinical safety data

None stated.

6. PHARMACEUTICAL PARTICULARS

6.1 List of excipients

Core:

Lactose

Ac-di-Sol

Methyl Cellulose (Methocel A4C)

Magnesium Stearate

Industrial Methylated Spirits

Purified Water

Coating:

Methyl Cellulose (Methocel E15)

Polyethylene Glycol 400

Sepisperse Rose AP 5002 or

Mastercoat Pink FA0430

Purified Water

6.2 Incompatibilities

None stated.

6.3 Shelf life

36 months unopened

6.4 Special precautions for storage

In glass bottle – normal storage conditions

In blister pack - store below 25°C in a dry place.

6.5 Nature and contents of container

15ml Amber Glass Universal Tablet containing 18 tablets

30ml Amber Glass Universal Tablet containing 36 tablets

60ml Amber Glass Universal Tablet containing 50/96 tablets

All above fitted with child resistant cap

Thermoformed blister pack of 6 tablets constructed of:-

a) Plain 250μ white rigid UPVC

b) 20μ hard temper aluminium foil containing 12, 24, 36, 48 or 96 tablets

6.6 Special precautions for disposal and other handling

Not applicable.

7. MARKETING AUTHORISATION HOLDER

SSL International PLC

Venus

1 Old Park Lane

Trafford Park

Manchester

M41 7HA

8. MARKETING AUTHORISATION NUMBER(S)

PL 00338/0055.

9. DATE OF FIRST AUTHORISATION/RENEWAL OF THE AUTHORISATION

24/10/85 / 12/01/01

10. DATE OF REVISION OF THE TEXT

March 2007

Curanail 5% Nail Lacquer

(Galderma (U.K) Ltd)

1. NAME OF THE MEDICINAL PRODUCT

Curanail 5% Nail Lacquer

2. QUALITATIVE AND QUANTITATIVE COMPOSITION

Curanail 5% nail lacquer contains 5% w/v amorolfine in the form of hydrochloride. Amorolfine is chemically described as *cis*-4-[(RS)-3[4-(1,1-Dimethylpropyl)phenyl]-2-methylpropyl]-2,6-dimethylmorpholine.

Amorolfine hydrochloride HSE 6.40 %w/w

3. PHARMACEUTICAL FORM

Medicated Nail Lacquer.

4. CLINICAL PARTICULARS

4.1 Therapeutic indications

Treatment of mild cases of distal and lateral subungual onychomycoses caused by dermatophytes, yeasts and moulds limited up to 2 nails.

4.2 Posology and method of administration

Adults and Elderly

The nail lacquer should be applied to the affected finger or toe nails once weekly.

The patient should apply the nail lacquer as follows:

1. Before the first application of Curanail 5% nail lacquer, it is essential that the affected areas of nail (particularly the nail surfaces) should be filed down as thoroughly as possible using a nail file. The surface of the nail should then be cleansed and degreased using an alcohol cleaning pad. Before repeat application of Curanail 5% nail lacquer, the affected nails should be filed down again as required, following cleansing with a cleaning pad to remove any remaining lacquer.

Caution: Nail files used for affected nails must not be used for healthy nails.

2. With one of the reusable applicators supplied, apply the nail lacquer to the entire surface of the affected nails and allow it to dry. After use, clean the applicator with the same cleaning pad used before for nail cleaning. Keep the bottle tightly closed.

For each nail to be treated, dip the applicator into the nail lacquer without wiping off any of the lacquer on the bottle neck.

Caution: When working with organic solvents (thinners, white spirit, etc.) wear impermeable gloves in order to protect the Curanail 5% nail lacquer on the nails.

Treatment should be continued without interruption until the nail is regenerated and the affected areas are finally cured. The required frequency and duration of treatment depends essentially on intensity and localisation of the infection. In general, it is six months (finger nails) and nine to twelve months (toe nails). A review of the treatment is recommended at intervals of approximately three months.

Co-existent tinea pedis should be treated with an appropriate antimycotic cream.

Children

Due to the lack of clinical experience available, Curanail 5% nail lacquer is not recommended for patients below the age of 18 years.

4.3 Contraindications

Curanail 5% nail lacquer must not be reused by patients who have shown hypersensitivity to the treatment.

No experience exists of use during pregnancy and nursing, therefore, the use of Curanail 5% nail lacquer should be avoided during pregnancy and lactation.

4.4 Special warnings and precautions for use

Avoid contact of the lacquer with eyes, ears and mucous membranes.

Patients with underlying conditions predisposing to fungal nail infections should be referred to a doctor. Such conditions include peripheral circulatory disorders, diabetes mellitus, and immunosuppression.

Patients with nail dystrophy and destroyed nail plate should be referred to their doctor.

4.5 Interaction with other medicinal products and other forms of interaction

There are no specific studies involving concomitant treatment with other topical medicines.

Use of nail varnish or artificial nails should be avoided during treatment.

4.6 Pregnancy and lactation

Reproductive toxicology studies showed no evidence of teratogenicity in laboratory animals but embryotoxicity was observed at high oral doses. The systemic absorption of amorolfine during and after topical administration is very low and therefore the risk to the human foetus appears to be negligible. However, because there is no relevant experience, Curanail 5% nail lacquer should be avoided during pregnancy and breast feeding.

4.7 Effects on ability to drive and use machines

None.

4.8 Undesirable effects

Adverse drug reactions are rare. Nail disorders (e.g. nail discoloration, broken nails, brittle nails) may occur. These reactions can also be linked to the onychomycosis itself.

System Organ Class	Frequency	Adverse drug reaction
Skin and subcutaneous tissue disorders	Rare (⩾ 1/10000, ⩽ 1/1000)	Nail disorder, nail discoloration, onychoclasia
	Very rare (⩽ 1/10000)	Skin burning sensation, contact dermatitis

4.9 Overdose

Accidental oral ingestion

Curanail 5% nail lacquer is for topical use. In the event of accidental oral ingestion, an appropriate method of gastric emptying may be used.

5. PHARMACOLOGICAL PROPERTIES

5.1 Pharmacodynamic properties

Curanail 5% nail lacquer is a topical antimycotic. Amorolfine belongs to a new chemical class, and its fungicidal action is based on an alteration of the fungal cell membrane targeted primarily on sterol biosynthesis. The ergosterol content is reduced, and at the same time unusual sterically nonplanar sterols accumulate.

Amorolfine is a broad spectrum antimycotic. It is highly active (MIC < 2mcg/ml) *in vitro* against

yeasts:Candida, Cryptococcus, Malassezia

dermatophytes: Trichophyton, Microsporum, Epidermophyton

moulds: Hendersonula, Alternaria, Scopulariopsis

dematiacea: Cladosporium, Fonsecaea, Wangiella

dimorphic fungi: Coccidioides, Histoplasma, Sporothrix

With the exception of *Actinomyces*, bacteria are not sensitive to amorolfine. *Propionibacterium acnes* is only slightly sensitive.

5.2 Pharmacokinetic properties

Amorolfine from nail lacquer penetrates into and diffuses through the nail plate and is thus able to eradicate poorly accessible fungi in the nail bed. Systemic absorption of the active ingredient is very low with this type of application.

Following prolonged use of Curanail 5% Nail Lacquer, there is no indication of drug accumulation in the body.

5.3 Preclinical safety data

None stated.

6. PHARMACEUTICAL PARTICULARS

6.1 List of excipients

Ammonio methacrylate copolymer A, triacetin, butyl acetate, ethyl acetate, ethanol absolute.

6.2 Incompatibilities

None.

6.3 Shelf life

3 years.

6.4 Special precautions for storage

Curanail 5% nail lacquer should be stored below 30°C. Protect from heat. Keep bottle tightly closed after use.

6.5 Nature and contents of container

Amber glass bottle with screw thread and plastic screw closure.

Pack Size: 3ml

All packs contain spatulas.

6.6 Special precautions for disposal and other handling

No special instructions.

Administrative Data

7. MARKETING AUTHORISATION HOLDER

Galderma (UK) Limited

Meridien House

69-71 Clarendon Road

Watford

Herts

WD17 1DS

UK

8. MARKETING AUTHORISATION NUMBER(S)

PL 10590/0049

9. DATE OF FIRST AUTHORISATION/RENEWAL OF THE AUTHORISATION

07/04/2006

10. DATE OF REVISION OF THE TEXT

November 2008

Cutivate Cream 0.05%

(GlaxoSmithKline UK)

1. NAME OF THE MEDICINAL PRODUCT

Cutivate Cream 0.05%.

2. QUALITATIVE AND QUANTITATIVE COMPOSITION

Fluticasone Propionate (micronised) HSE 0.05% w/w.

3. PHARMACEUTICAL FORM

Cream

4. CLINICAL PARTICULARS

4.1 Therapeutic indications

Adults:

For the relief of the inflammatory and pruritic manifestations of corticosteroid-responsive dermatoses such as: eczema including atopic and discoid eczemas; prurigo nodularis; psoriasis (excluding widespread plaque psoriasis); neurodermatoses including lichen simplex; lichen planus; seborrhoeic dermatitis; contact sensitivity reactions; discoid lupus erythematosus; an adjunct to systemic steroid therapy in generalised erythroderma; insect bite reactions; or prickly heat.

Children:

For children and infants aged three months and over who are unresponsive to lower potency corticosteroids Cutivate Cream is indicated for the relief of the inflammatory and pruritic manifestations of atopic dermatitis under the supervision of a specialist. Expert opinion should be sought prior to the use of Cutivate Cream in other corticosteroid responsive dermatoses in children.

4.2 Posology and method of administration

Eczema/Dermatitis

For adults, children and infants aged three months and over, apply a thin film of Cutivate Cream to the affected skin areas once daily.

Other indications

Apply a thin film of Cutivate Cream to the affected skin areas twice daily

Duration of use:

Daily treatment should be continued until adequate control of the condition is achieved. Frequency of application should thereafter be reduced to the lowest effective dose.

When Cutivate is used in the treatment of children, if there is no improvement within 7 – 14 days, treatment should be withdrawn and the child re-evaluated. Once the condition has been controlled (usually within 7-14 days), frequency of application should be reduced to the lowest effective dose for the shortest possible time. Continuous daily treatment for longer than 4 weeks is not recommended

For topical administration.

4.3 Contraindications

Rosacea, acne vulgaris, perioral dermatitis, primary cutaneous viral infections (e.g. herpes simplex, chickenpox). Hypersensitivity to any of the ingredients. Perianal and genital pruritus. The use of fluticasone propionate skin preparations is not indicated in the treatment of primarily infected skin lesions caused by infection with fungi or bacteria. Dermatoses in infants under three months of age, including dermatitis and napkin eruptions.

4.4 Special warnings and precautions for use

Fluticasone propionate has a very low propensity for systemic absorption, nevertheless, prolonged application of high doses to large areas of body surface, especially in infants and small children, might lead to adrenal suppression. Children and infants have a greater surface area to body weight ratio compared with adults. Therefore, in comparison with adults, children and infants may absorb proportionally larger amounts of topical corticosteroids and thus be more susceptible to systemic toxicity. Care should be taken when using Cutivate Cream to ensure the amount applied is the minimum that provides therapeutic benefit.

Long-term continuous use should be avoided in children and infants. The safety and efficacy of fluticasone propionate when used continuously for longer than 4 weeks has not been established.

The face, more than other areas of the body may exhibit atrophic changes after prolonged treatment with potent topical corticosteroids. This must be borne in mind when treating such conditions as psoriasis, discoid lupus erythematosus and severe eczema.

If applied to the eyelids, care is needed to ensure that the preparation does not enter the eye so as to avoid the risk of local irritation or glaucoma.

Topical steroids may be hazardous in psoriasis for a number of reasons, including rebound relapses, development of tolerance, risk of generalised pustular psoriasis and development of local or systemic toxicity due to impaired barrier function of the skin. If used in psoriasis careful patient supervision is important and referral to a dermatologist is required before using Cutivate Cream to treat psoriasis in children and infants.

Appropriate antimicrobial therapy should be used whenever treating inflammatory lesions, which have become infected. Any infection requires withdrawal of topical corticosteroid therapy and systemic administration of antimicrobial agents. Bacterial infection is encouraged by the warm, moist conditions induced by occlusive dressing, and so the skin should be cleansed before a fresh dressing is applied.

Cutivate Cream contains the excipient, imidurea, which releases traces of formaldehyde as a breakdown product. Formaldehyde may cause allergic sensitization or irritation upon contact with the skin.

4.5 Interaction with other medicinal products and other forms of interaction

None known.

4.6 Pregnancy and lactation

Pregnancy: Topical administration of corticosteroids to pregnant animals can cause abnormalities of foetal development, but in humans there is no convincing evidence that systemic corticosteroids cause an increased incidence of congenital abnormalities. However, administration of fluticasone propionate during pregnancy should only be considered if the expected benefit to the mother is greater than any possible risk to the foetus.

Lactation: The excretion of fluticasone propionate into human breast milk has not been investigated. When measurable, plasma levels were obtained in lactating laboratory rats following subcutaneous administration, there was evidence of fluticasone propionate in the breast milk. However plasma levels in patients following dermal application of fluticasone propionate at recommended doses are likely to be low.

When fluticasone propionate is used in breast feeding mothers, the therapeutic benefits must be weighed against the potential hazards to mother and baby.

4.7 Effects on ability to drive and use machines

None known.

4.8 Undesirable effects

Adverse events are listed below by system organ class and frequency. Frequencies are defined as: very common (≥1/10), common (≥1/100 and <1/10), uncommon (≥1/1000 and <1/100), rare (≥1/10,000 and <1/1000) and very rare (<1/10,000) including isolated reports. Very common, common and uncommon events were generally determined from clinical trial data. The background rates in placebo and comparator groups were not taken into account when assigning frequency categories to adverse events derived from clinical trial data, since these rates were generally comparable to those in the active treatment group. Rare and very rare events were generally derived from spontaneous data.

Infections and infestations

Very rare: Secondary infection.

Secondary infections, particularly when occlusive dressings are used or when skin folds are involved have been reported with corticosteroid use.

Immune system disorders

Very rare: Hypersensitivity.

If signs of hypersensitivity appear, application should stop immediately.

Endocrine disorders

Very rare: Features of hypercortisolism.

Prolonged use of large amounts of corticosteroids, or treatment of extensive areas, can result in sufficient systemic absorption to produce the features of hypercortisolism. This effect is more likely to occur in infants and children, and if occlusive dressings are used. In infants, the napkin may act as an occlusive dressing (See 4.4 Special Warnings and Special Precautions for Use).

Vascular disorders

Very rare: Dilation of superficial blood vessels.

Prolonged and intensive treatment with potent corticosteroid preparations may cause dilation of the superficial blood vessels.

Skin and subcutaneous tissue disorders

Common: Pruritus.

Uncommon: Local burning.

Very rare: Allergic contact dermatitis, exacerbation of signs and symptoms of dermatoses, pustular psoriasis. Prolonged and intensive treatment wih potent corticosteroid preparations may cause thinning, striae, hypertrichosis and hypopigmentation.

Treatment of psoriasis with a corticosteroid (or its withdrawal) may provoke the pustular form of the disease.

4.9 Overdose

Acute overdosage is very unlikely to occur, however, in the case of chronic overdosage or misuse, the features of hypercortisolism may appear and in this situation, topical steroids should be discontinued gradually. However, because of the risk of acute adrenal suppression this should be done under medical supervision.

5. PHARMACOLOGICAL PROPERTIES

5.1 Pharmacodynamic properties

Fluticasone propionate is a glucocorticoid with high topical anti-inflammatory potency but low HPA-axis suppressive activity after dermal administration. It therefore has a therapeutic index which is greater than most of the commonly available steroids.

It shows high systemic glucocorticoid potency after subcutaneous administration but very weak oral activity, probably due to metabolic inactivation. *In vitro* studies show a strong affinity for, and agonist activity at, human glucocorticoid receptors.

Fluticasone propionate has no unexpected hormonal effects, and no overt, marked effects upon the central and peripheral nervous systems, the gastrointestinal system, or the cardiovascular or respiratory systems.

5.2 Pharmacokinetic properties

Pharmacokinetic data for the rat and dog indicate rapid elimination and extensive metabolic clearance. Bioavailability is very low after topical or oral administration, due to limited absorption through the skin or from the gastrointestinal tract, and because of extensive first-pass metabolism. Distribution studies have shown that only minute traces of orally administered compound reach the systemic circulation, and that any systemically-available radiolabel is rapidly eliminated in the bile and excreted in the faeces.

Fluticasone propionate does not persist in any tissue, and does not bind to melanin. The major route of metabolism is hydrolysis of the S-fluoromethyl carbothioate group, to yield a carboxylic acid (GR36264), which has very weak glucocorticoid or anti-inflammatory activity. In all test animal species, the route of excretion of radioactivity is independent of the route of administration of radiolabelled fluticasone propionate. Excretion is predominantly faecal and is essentially complete within 48 hours.

In man too, metabolic clearance is extensive, and elimination is consequently rapid. Thus drug entering the systemic circulation via the skin, will be rapidly inactivated. Oral bioavailability approaches zero, due to poor absorption and extensive first-pass metabolism. Therefore systemic exposure to any ingestion of the topical formulation will be low.

5.3 Preclinical safety data

Reproductive studies suggest that administration of corticosteroids to pregnant animals can result in abnormalities of foetal development including cleft palate/lip. However, in humans, there is no convincing evidence of congenital abnormalities, such as cleft palate or lip.

Studies of safety pharmacology, repeated dose toxicity, genotoxicity, carcinogenic potential, fertility and general reproductive performance revealed no special hazard for humans, other than that anticipated for a potent steroid.

6. PHARMACEUTICAL PARTICULARS

6.1 List of excipients

Liquid Paraffin

Cetostearyl Alcohol

Isopropyl Myristate

Cetomacrogol 1000

Propylene Glycol

Imidurea

Sodium Phosphate

Citric Acid Monohydrate

Purified Water

6.2 Incompatibilities

None reported.

6.3 Shelf life

24 months.

6.4 Special precautions for storage

Store below 30°C.

6.5 Nature and contents of container

15g, 30g, 50g and 100g collapsible internally-laquered, blind-end aluminium tubes, with latex bands and closed with polypropylene caps.

Not all pack sizes may be marketed

6.6 Special precautions for disposal and other handling

No special instructions.

Administrative Data

7. MARKETING AUTHORISATION HOLDER

Glaxo Wellcome UK Ltd T/A Glaxo Laboratories

and / or GlaxoSmithKline UK

Stockley Park West

Uxbridge

Middlesex, UB11 1BT.

8. MARKETING AUTHORISATION NUMBER(S)

PL 10949/0013.

9. DATE OF FIRST AUTHORISATION/RENEWAL OF THE AUTHORISATION

30 May 2008

10. DATE OF REVISION OF THE TEXT

30 May 2008

11. Legal Status

POM.

Cutivate Ointment 0.005%

(GlaxoSmithKline UK)

1. NAME OF THE MEDICINAL PRODUCT

Cutivate Ointment 0.005%.

2. QUALITATIVE AND QUANTITATIVE COMPOSITION

Fluticasone Propionate (micronised) HSE 0.005% w/w.

3. PHARMACEUTICAL FORM

Ointment.

4. CLINICAL PARTICULARS

4.1 Therapeutic indications

Adults:

For the relief of the inflammatory and pruritic manifestations of corticosteroid-responsive dermatoses such as: eczema including atopic and discoid eczemas; prurigo nodularis; psoriasis (excluding widespread plaque psoriasis); neurodermatoses including lichen simplex; lichen planus; seborrhoeic dermatitis; contact sensitivity reactions; discoid lupus erythematosus; an adjunct to systemic steroid therapy in generalised erythroderma; insect bite reactions; or prickly heat.

Children:

For children and infants aged three months and over who are unresponsive to lower potency corticosteroids Cutivate Ointment is indicated for the relief of the inflammatory and pruritic manifestations of atopic dermatitis under the supervision of a specialist. Expert opinion should be sought prior to the use of Cutivate Ointment in other corticosteroid responsive dermatoses in children.

4.2 Posology and method of administration

For adults, children and infants aged three months and over, apply a thin film of Cutivate Ointment to the affected skin areas twice daily.

Duration of use:

Daily treatment should be continued until adequate control of the condition is achieved. Frequency of application should thereafter be reduced to the lowest effective dose.

When Cutivate is used in the treatment of children, if there is no improvement within 7 - 14 days, treatment should be withdrawn and the child re-evaluated. Once the condition has been controlled (usually within 7 -14 days), frequency of application should be reduced to the lowest effective dose for the shortest possible time. Continuous daily treatment for longer than 4 weeks is not recommended.

For topical administration.

4.3 Contraindications

Rosacea, acne vulgaris, perioral dermatitis, primary cutaneous viral infections (e.g. herpes simplex, chickenpox).

Hypersensitivity to any of the ingredients.

Perianal and genital pruritus.

The use of fluticasone propionate skin preparations is not indicated in the treatment of

- primarily infected skin lesions caused by infection with fungi or bacteria
- dermatoses in infants under three months of age, including dermatitis and napkin eruptions.

4.4 Special warnings and precautions for use

Prolonged applications of high doses to large areas of body surface, especially in infants and small children, might lead to adrenal suppression. Children and infants have a greater surface area to body weight ratio compared with adults. Therefore, in comparison with adults, children may absorb proportionally larger amounts of topical corticosteroids and thus be more susceptible to systemic toxicity. Care should be taken when using Cutivate Ointment to ensure the amount applied is the minimum that provides therapeutic benefit.

Long-term continuous use should be avoided in children and infants. The safety and efficacy of fluticasone propionate when used continuously for longer than 4 weeks has not been established.

The face, more than other areas of the body may exhibit atrophic changes after prolonged treatment with potent topical corticosteroids. This must be borne in mind when treating such conditions as psoriasis, discoid lupus erythematosus and severe eczema.

If applied to the eyelids, care is needed to ensure that the preparation does not enter the eye so as to avoid the risk of local irritation or glaucoma.

Topical steroids may be hazardous in psoriasis for a number of reasons, including rebound relapses, development of tolerance, risk of generalised pustular psoriasis and development of local or systemic toxicity due to impaired barrier function of the skin. If used in psoriasis careful patient supervision is important and referral to a dermatologist is required before using Cutivate Ointment to treat psoriasis in children and infants.

Appropriate antimicrobial therapy should be used whenever treating inflammatory lesions, which have become infected. Any infection requires withdrawal of topical corticosteroid therapy and systemic administration of antimicrobial agents. Bacterial infection is encouraged by the warm, moist conditions induced by occlusive dressing, and so the skin should be cleansed before a fresh dressing is applied.

4.5 Interaction with other medicinal products and other forms of interaction

None known.

4.6 Pregnancy and lactation

Pregnancy: Topical administration of corticosteroids to pregnant animals can cause abnormalities of foetal development, but in humans there is no convincing evidence that systemic corticosteroids cause an increased incidence of congenital abnormalities. However, administration of fluticasone propionate during pregnancy should only be considered if the expected benefit to the mother is greater than any possible risk to the foetus.

Lactation: The excretion of fluticasone propionate into human breast milk has not been investigated. When measurable, plasma levels were obtained in lactating laboratory rats following subcutaneous administration, there was evidence of fluticasone propionate in the breast milk. However plasma levels in patients following dermal application of fluticasone propionate at recommended doses are likely to be low.

When fluticasone propionate is used in breast feeding mothers, the therapeutic benefits must be weighed against the potential hazards to mother and baby.

4.7 Effects on ability to drive and use machines
None known.

4.8 Undesirable effects
Adverse events are listed below by system organ class and frequency. Frequencies are defined as: very common (≥1/10), common (≥1/100 and <1/10), uncommon (≥1/1000 and <1/100), rare (≥1/10,000 and <1/1000) and very rare (<1/10,000) including isolated reports. Very common, common and uncommon events were generally determined from clinical trial data. The background rates in placebo and comparator groups were not taken into account when assigning frequency categories to adverse events derived from clinical trial data, since these rates were generally comparable to those in the active treatment group. Rare and very rare events were generally derived from spontaneous data.

Infections and infestations

Very rare: Secondary infection.

Secondary infections, particularly when occlusive dressings are used or when skin folds are involved have been reported with corticosteroid use.

Immune system disorders

Very rare: Hypersensitivity.

If signs of hypersensitivity appear, application should stop immediately.

Endocrine disorders

Very rare: Hypothalamic-pituitary-adrenal (HPA) axis suppression

Features of hypercortisolism.

Prolonged use of large amounts of corticosteroids, or treatment of extensive areas, can result in sufficient systemic absorption to produce the features of hypercortisolism. This effect is more likely to occur in infants and children, and if occlusive dressings are used. In infants, the napkin may act as an occlusive dressing (See 4.4 Special Warnings and Special Precautions for Use).

Vascular disorders

Very rare: Dilation of superficial blood vessels.

Prolonged and intensive treatment with potent corticosteroid preparations may cause dilation of the superficial blood vessels.

Skin and subcutaneous tissue disorders

Common: Pruritus.

Uncommon: Local burning.

Very rare: Allergic contact dermatitis, exacerbation of signs and symptoms of dermatoses, pustular psoriasis. Prolonged and intensive treatment wih potent corticosteroid preparations may cause thinning, striae, hypertrichosis and hypopigmentation.

Treatment of psoriasis with a corticosteroid (or its withdrawal) may provoked the pustular form of the disease.

4.9 Overdose
Acute overdosage is very unlikely to occur, however, in the case of chronic overdosage or misuse, the features of hypercortisolism may appear and in this situation, topical steroids should be discontinued gradually. However, because of the risk of acute adrenal suppression this should be done under medical supervision.

5. PHARMACOLOGICAL PROPERTIES

5.1 Pharmacodynamic properties
Fluticasone propionate is a glucocorticoid with high topical anti-inflammatory potency but low HPA-axis suppressive activity after dermal administration. It therefore has a therapeutic index which is greater than most of the commonly available steroids.

It shows high systemic glucocorticoid potency after subcutaneous administration but very weak oral activity, probably due to metabolic inactivation. *In vitro* studies show a strong affinity for and agonist activity at, human glucocorticoid receptors.

Fluticasone propionate has no unexpected hormonal effects, and no overt, marked effects upon the central and peripheral nervous systems, the gastrointestinal system, or the cardiovascular or respiratory systems.

5.2 Pharmacokinetic properties
Pharmacokinetic data for the rat and dog indicate rapid elimination and extensive metabolic clearance. Bioavailability is very low after topical or oral administration, due to limited absorption through the skin or from the gastrointestinal tract, and because of extensive first-pass metabolism. Distribution studies have shown that only minute traces of orally administered compound reach the systemic circulation, and that any systemically-available radiolabel is rapidly eliminated in the bile and excreted in the faeces.

Fluticasone propionate does not persist in any tissue, and does not bind to melanin. The major route of metabolism is hydrolysis of the S-fluoromethyl carbothioate group, to yield a carboxylic acid (GR36264), which has very weak glucocorticoid or anti-inflammatory activity. In all test animal species, the route of excretion of radioactivity is independent of the route of administration of radiolabelled fluticasone propionate. Excretion is predominantly faecal and is essentially complete within 48 hours.

In man too, metabolic clearance is extensive, and elimination is consequently rapid. Thus drug entering the systemic circulation via the skin, will be rapidly inactivated. Oral bioavailability approaches zero, due to poor absorption and extensive first-pass metabolism. Therefore systemic exposure to any ingestion of the topical formulation will be low.

5.3 Preclinical safety data
Reproductive studies suggest that administration of corticosteroids to pregnant animals can result in abnormalities of foetal development including cleft palate/lip. However, in humans, there is no convincing evidence of congenital abnormalities, such as cleft palate or lip.

Studies of safety pharmacology, repeated dose toxicity, genotoxicity, carcinogenic potential, fertility and general reproductive performance revealed no special hazard for humans, other than that anticipated for a potent steroid.

6. PHARMACEUTICAL PARTICULARS

6.1 List of excipients
Propylene Glycol
Sorbitan Sesquioleate
Microcrystalline Wax
Liquid Paraffin

6.2 Incompatibilities
None reported.

6.3 Shelf life
24 months.

6.4 Special precautions for storage
Store below 30°C.

6.5 Nature and contents of container
15g, 30g, 50g and 100g collapsible blind-end aluminium tubes, with latex bands and closed with polypropylene caps.

Not all pack sizes may be marketed

6.6 Special precautions for disposal and other handling
None.

Administrative Data

7. MARKETING AUTHORISATION HOLDER
Glaxo Wellcome UK Ltd T/A Glaxo Laboratories
and / or GlaxoSmithKline UK
Stockley Park West
Uxbridge
Middlesex, UB11 1BT.

8. MARKETING AUTHORISATION NUMBER(S)
PL 10949/0012

9. DATE OF FIRST AUTHORISATION/RENEWAL OF THE AUTHORISATION
30 May 2008.

10. DATE OF REVISION OF THE TEXT
30 May 2008

11. Legal Status
POM

Cyclogest 200mg

(Actavis UK Ltd)

1. NAME OF THE MEDICINAL PRODUCT
CYCLOGEST 200mg

2. QUALITATIVE AND QUANTITATIVE COMPOSITION
Each pessary contains 200mg Progesterone PhEur.

3. PHARMACEUTICAL FORM
Off-white pessaries.

4. CLINICAL PARTICULARS

4.1 Therapeutic indications
1) Treatment of premenstrual syndrome, including premenstrual tension and depression.

2) Treatment of puerperal depression.

4.2 Posology and method of administration
Posology

200mg daily to 400mg twice a day, by vaginal or rectal insertion. For premenstrual syndrome commence treatment on day 14 of menstrual cycle and continue treatment until onset of menstruation. If symptoms are present at ovulation commence treatment on day 12.

Children: Not applicable.

Elderly: Not applicable.

Method of Administration
For rectal or vaginal insertion.

4.3 Contraindications
Undiagnosed vaginal bleeding.

4.4 Special warnings and precautions for use
Use rectally if barrier methods of contraception are used.

Use vaginally if patients suffer from colitis or faecal incontinence. Use rectally if patients suffer from vaginal infection (especially moniliasis) or recurrent cystitis. Use rectally in patients who have recently given birth.

Progesterone is metabolised in the liver and should be used with caution in patients with hepatic dysfunction.

Cyclogest contains the hormone progesterone which is present in significant concentrations in women during the second half of the menstrual cycle and during pregnancy. This should be borne in mind when treating patients with conditions that may be hormone-sensitive.

4.5 Interaction with other medicinal products and other forms of interaction
None known.

4.6 Pregnancy and lactation
Due to the indications of the product, it is anticipated that it will not be administered to pregnant women. As progesterone is a natural hormone, it is not expected to have adverse effects, however, no evidence is available to this effect.

4.7 Effects on ability to drive and use machines
None known.

4.8 Undesirable effects
Menstruation may occur earlier than expected, or, more rarely, menstruation may be delayed.

Soreness, diarrhoea and flatulence may occur with rectal administration.

As with other vaginal and rectal preparations, some leakage of the pessary base may occur.

4.9 Overdose
There is a wide margin of safety with Cyclogest pessaries, but overdosage may produce euphoria or dysmenorrhoea.

5. PHARMACOLOGICAL PROPERTIES

5.1 Pharmacodynamic properties
ATC code: G03D A

Progesterone is a progestational steroid.

5.2 Pharmacokinetic properties
Not applicable.

5.3 Preclinical safety data
Not applicable.

6. PHARMACEUTICAL PARTICULARS

6.1 List of excipients
Also contains: vegetable fat.

6.2 Incompatibilities
None known.

6.3 Shelf life
Shelf-life

Three years from the date of manufacture.

Shelf-life after dilution/reconstitution

Not applicable.

Shelf-life after first opening

Not applicable.

6.4 Special precautions for storage
Store below 25°C in a dry place.

6.5 Nature and contents of container
The product may be supplied in strip packs contained in cartons:

Carton: White backed folding box board printed on white.

Strip pack: Aluminium foil lacquer-laminated to 20μm polypropylene foil and coated on the reverse with polythene (20mg/m^2). The alternative is thermoplastic film and laminated PVC to 95μm and polyethylene to 27-30μm.

Pack sizes: 5s, 12s, 15s

6.6 Special precautions for disposal and other handling
Not applicable.

Administrative Data

7. MARKETING AUTHORISATION HOLDER
Actavis UK Limited
(Trading style: Actavis)
Whiddon Valley
Barnstaple
North Devon
EX32 8NS
United Kingdom

8. MARKETING AUTHORISATION NUMBER(S)
PL 00142/0507

9. DATE OF FIRST AUTHORISATION/RENEWAL OF THE AUTHORISATION
23 August 2000

10. DATE OF REVISION OF THE TEXT
February 2007

Cyclogest 400mg

(Actavis UK Ltd)

1. NAME OF THE MEDICINAL PRODUCT
CYCLOGEST 400mg

2. QUALITATIVE AND QUANTITATIVE COMPOSITION
Each pessary contains 400mg Progesterone PhEur.

3. PHARMACEUTICAL FORM
Off-white pessaries.

4. CLINICAL PARTICULARS

4.1 Therapeutic indications

1) Treatment of premenstrual syndrome, including premenstrual tension and depression.

2) Treatment of puerperal depression.

4.2 Posology and method of administration

Posology

200mg daily to 400mg twice a day, by vaginal or rectal insertion. For premenstrual syndrome commence treatment on day 14 of menstrual cycle and continue treatment until onset of menstruation. If symptoms are present at ovulation commence treatment on day 12.

Children: Not applicable.

Elderly: Not applicable.

Method of Administration

For rectal or vaginal insertion.

4.3 Contraindications

Undiagnosed vaginal bleeding.

4.4 Special warnings and precautions for use

Use rectally if barrier methods of contraception are used.

Use vaginally if patients suffer from colitis or faecal incontinence. Use rectally if patients suffer from vaginal infection (especially moniliasis) or recurrent cystitis. Use rectally in patients who have recently given birth.

Progesterone is metabolised in the liver and should be used with caution in patients with hepatic dysfunction.

Cyclogest contains the hormone progesterone which is present in significant concentrations in women during the second half of the menstrual cycle and during pregnancy. This should be borne in mind when treating patients with conditions that may be hormone-sensitive.

4.5 Interaction with other medicinal products and other forms of interaction

None known.

4.6 Pregnancy and lactation

Due to the indications of the product, it is anticipated that it will not be administered to pregnant women. As progesterone is a natural hormone, it is not expected to have adverse effects, however, no evidence is available to this effect.

4.7 Effects on ability to drive and use machines

None known.

4.8 Undesirable effects

Menstruation may occur earlier than expected, or, more rarely, menstruation may be delayed.

Soreness, diarrhoea and flatulence may occur with rectal administration.

As with other vaginal and rectal preparations, some leakage of the pessary base may occur.

4.9 Overdose

There is a wide margin of safety with Cyclogest pessaries, but overdosage may produce euphoria or dysmenorrhoea.

5. PHARMACOLOGICAL PROPERTIES

5.1 Pharmacodynamic properties

ATC code: G03D A

Progesterone is a progestational steroid.

5.2 Pharmacokinetic properties

Not applicable.

5.3 Preclinical safety data

Not applicable.

6. PHARMACEUTICAL PARTICULARS

6.1 List of excipients

Also contains: vegetable fat.

6.2 Incompatibilities

None known.

6.3 Shelf life

Shelf-life

Three years from the date of manufacture.

Shelf-life after dilution/reconstitution

Not applicable.

Shelf-life after first opening

Not applicable.

6.4 Special precautions for storage

Store below 25°C in a dry place.

6.5 Nature and contents of container

The product may be supplied in strip packs contained in cartons:

Carton: White backed folding box board printed on white.

Strip pack: Aluminium foil lacquer-laminated to 20μm polypropylene foil and coated on the reverse with polythene (20mg/m^2). The alternative is thermoplastic film and laminated PVC to 95μm and polyethylene to 27-30μm.

Pack sizes: 5s, 12s, 15s

6.6 Special precautions for disposal and other handling

Not applicable.

Administrative Data

7. MARKETING AUTHORISATION HOLDER

Actavis UK Limited

(Trading style: Actavis)

Whiddon Valley

Barnstaple

North Devon

EX32 8NS

United Kingdom

8. MARKETING AUTHORISATION NUMBER(S)

PL 00142/0508

9. DATE OF FIRST AUTHORISATION/RENEWAL OF THE AUTHORISATION

23 August 2000

10. DATE OF REVISION OF THE TEXT

February 2007

Cyclophosphamide 50 Tablets (Pharmacia Limited)

(Pharmacia Limited)

1. NAME OF THE MEDICINAL PRODUCT

Cyclophosphamide Tablets.

2. QUALITATIVE AND QUANTITATIVE COMPOSITION

Cyclophosphamide monohydrate BP 53.50 mg equivalent to 50 mg anhydrous cyclophosphamide.

3. PHARMACEUTICAL FORM

Sugar-coated tablets

4. CLINICAL PARTICULARS

4.1 Therapeutic indications

Alkylating, antineoplastic agent. Cyclophosphamide has been used successfully to induce and maintain regressions in a wide range of neoplastic conditions, including leukaemias, lymphomas, soft tissue and osteogenic sarcomas, paediatric malignancies and adult solid tumours; in particular, breast and lung carcinomas.

Cyclophosphamide is frequently used in combination chemotherapy regimens involving other cytotoxic drugs.

4.2 Posology and method of administration

Route of administration: Oral.

Adults and children:

The recommended dose for cyclophosphamide tablets is 50-250 mg/m^2 daily (doses towards the upper end of this range should be used only for short courses).

The dose may be amended at the discretion of the physician.

It is recommended that the calculated dose of cyclophosphamide be reduced when it is given in combination with other antineoplastic agents or radiotherapy, and in patients with bone marrow depression.

Cyclophosphamide tablets should be swallowed whole, preferably on an empty stomach, but if gastric irritation is severe, they may be taken with meals.

A minimum output of 100 ml/hour should be maintained during therapy with conventional doses to avoid cystitis. If the larger doses are used, an output of at least this level should be maintained for 24 hours following administration, if necessary by forced diuresis. Alkalisation of the urine is not recommended.

Cyclophosphamide should be given early in the day and the bladder voided frequently. The patient should be well hydrated and maintained in fluid balance.

Mesna (Uromitexan) can be used concurrently with cyclophosphamide to reduce urotoxic effects (for dosage see Uromitexan data sheet). If Mesna (Uromitexan) is used to reduce uroethelial toxicity, frequent emptying of the bladder should be avoided.

If the leucocyte count is below 4,000/mm^3 or the platelet count is below 100,000/mm^3, treatment with cyclophosphamide should be temporarily withheld until the blood count returns to normal levels.

4.3 Contraindications

Hypersensitivity and haemorrhagic cystitis.

4.4 Special warnings and precautions for use

Cyclophosphamide should be withheld in the presence of severe bone marrow depression and reduced doses should be used in the presence of lesser degrees of bone marrow depression. Regular blood counts should be performed in patients receiving cyclophosphamide.

It should not normally be given to patients with severe infections and should be withdrawn if such infections become life threatening.

Cyclophosphamide should be used with caution in debilitated patients and those with renal and/or hepatic failure. Cyclophosphamide is not recommended in patients with a plasma creatinine greater than 120 μmol/l (1.5 mg/100 ml) bilirubin greater than 17 μmol/l (1 mg/100 ml); or serum transaminases or alkaline phosphatase more than 2-3 times the upper limit of normal. In all such cases, dosage should be reduced.

Cyclophosphamide should be used only under the directions of physicians experienced in cytotoxic or immunosuppressant therapy.

<u>*Further Information:*</u>

The dosage regimen for mesna (Uromitexan) varies according to the dose of cyclophosphamide administered. In general i.v. Uromitexan is given as 60% w/w of the dose of i.v. Cyclophosphamide in three equal doses of 20% at 0, 4 and 8 hours. With the higher doses of cyclophosphamide, the dose and frequency of administration may need to be increased. Uromitexan Tablets are also available; full prescribing information for both presentation is available on the appropriate data sheet.

4.5 Interaction with other medicinal products and other forms of interaction

Oral hypoglycaemic agents may be potentiated by cyclophosphamide.

4.6 Pregnancy and lactation

This product should not normally be administered to patients who are pregnant or to mothers who are breast feeding. Alkylating agents, including cyclophosphamide, have been shown to possess mutagenic, teratogenic and carcinogenic potential. Pregnancy should therefore be avoided during cyclophosphamide therapy and for three months thereafter.

4.7 Effects on ability to drive and use machines

None known.

4.8 Undesirable effects

Single doses will produce a leucopenia which may be severe but usually returns to normal within 21 days.

Depression of the reticuloendothelial system with granulopoiesis and lymphopoiesis being more affected than thrombopoiesis and erythropoiesis. This depression, however, is reversible.

Amenorrhoea and azoospermia often occur during treatment with cyclophosphamide but in most cases are reversible.

Haematuria may occur during or after therapy with Cyclophosphamide. Cyclophosphamide is excreted mainly in the urine, largely in the form of active metabolites which may give rise to a chemical cystitis which may be haemorrhagic. Acute sterile haemorrhagic cystitis may occur in up to 10% of patients not given mesna (Uromitexan) in conjunction with Cyclophosphamide. Late sequelae of this cystitis are bladder contracture and fibrosis.

Because of this, a high fluid intake should be maintained with frequent emptying of the bladder. Cyclophosphamide therapy may lead to inappropriate secretion of anti-diuretic hormone, fluid retention and hyponatremia, with subsequent water intoxication. Should this arise, a diuretic may be given. Cyclophosphamide may cause myocardial toxicity, especially at high dosage.

Cyclophosphamide may induce permanent sterility in children.

In addition to those noted above, the following may accompany cyclophosphamide therapy: hair loss, which may be total, although generally reversible; mucosal ulcertation; anorexia, nausea and vomiting; pigmentation, typically affecting the palms and nails of the hands and the soles of the feet, and interstitial pulmonary fibrosis.

Hepatic toxicity has rarely been reported.

Cyclophosphamide has been shown to be mutagenic, teratogenic, and carcinogenic in certain laboratory tests and as with other cytotoxic agents, there have been reports of possible drug-induced neoplasia. There is an excessive risk of acute leukaemia and bladder cancer following cyclophosphamide therapy.

An alteration in carbohydrate metabolism may be seen in patients on cyclophosphamide. Other side effects, such as pancreatitis, macrocytosis, and induction of hyperglycaemia or hypoglycaemia have been reported.

There are certain complications such as veno-occlusive disease, thromboembolism, disseminated intravascular coagulation or haemolytic uraemic syndrome, that may also be induced by the underlying disease, but which might occur with an increased frequency during chemotherapy that includes cyclophosphamide.

Side effects have occasionally occurred after cessation of therapy.

4.9 Overdose

Myelosuppression (particularly granulocytopenia) and haemorrhagic cystitis are the most serious consequences of overdosage. Recovery from myelosuppression will occur by the 21st day after the overdosage in the great majority of patients (at doses up to 200 mg/kg i.v.) while granulocytopenia is usually seen by day 6 and lasts for a mean period of 12 days (up to 18 days). A broad spectrum antibiotic may be administered until recovery occurs. Transfusion of whole-blood, platelets or white cells and reverse barrier nursing may be necessary.

If the drug has been taken in the form of tablets, early gastric lavage may reduce the amount of drug absorbed.

During the first 24 hours and possibly up to 48 hours after overdosage, i.v. mensa may be beneficial in ameliorating damage to the urinary system. Normal supportive measures such as analgesics and maintenance of fluid balance should be instituted. If the cystitis does not resolve more intensive treatment may be necessary.

No further courses should be given until the patient has fully recovered.

5. PHARMACOLOGICAL PROPERTIES

5.1 Pharmacodynamic properties

Cyclophosphamide is an antineoplastic agent which is converted in the body to an active alkylating metabolite. It also possesses marked immunosuppressant properties. The principal site of cyclophosphamide activation is the liver. The chemotherapeutic and immunosuppressant activity of cyclophosphamide is thought to be mediated by the cytotoxic intermediates produced by activation by mixed function oxidases in hepatic microsomes. Non-enzymatic cleavage, possibly taking place in the tumour cells, results in the formulation of highly cytotoxic forms of the drug.

5.2 Pharmacokinetic properties

Cyclophosphamide may be incompletely absorbed from the gastro-intestinal tract. It rapidly disappears from the plasma and peak concentrations occur about 1 hour after an oral dose.

The metabolites of cyclophosphamide are excreted in the urine and these have an irritant effect on the bladder mucosa. Unchanged drug is also excreted in the urine and accounts for only 5-25% of the administered dose.

Metabolites have been found to be more protein bound than the parent compound.

5.3 Preclinical safety data

No further preclinical data are available.

6. PHARMACEUTICAL PARTICULARS

6.1 List of excipients

Maize starch

Pregelatinised starch

Lactose monohydrate

Gelatin

Microcrystalline cellulose

Sodium stearyl fumarate

Magnesium stearate

Coating

Polyethylene glycol

Sucrose

Maize starch

Calcium carbonate

Povidone

Opalux AS-9486 consisting of

- titanium dioxide
- red iron oxide
- yellow iron oxide
- sucrose
- purified water
- polyvinylpyrrolidone
- sodium benzoate

Carnauba wax

6.2 Incompatibilities

None stated.

6.3 Shelf life

60 months.

6.4 Special precautions for storage

Do not store above 25°C. Store in the original container in order to protect from moisture.

6.5 Nature and contents of container

White polyethylene containers with polyethylene snap-caps, containing a white capsule of desiccant.

6.6 Special precautions for disposal and other handling

None stated.

Administrative Data

7. MARKETING AUTHORISATION HOLDER

Pharmacia Limited

Ramsgate Road

Sandwich

Kent CT13 9NJ

UK

8. MARKETING AUTHORISATION NUMBER(S)

PL 00032/0335

9. DATE OF FIRST AUTHORISATION/RENEWAL OF THE AUTHORISATION

16 August 2002

10. DATE OF REVISION OF THE TEXT

20 August 2007

Ref: CP4_0 SPC

CYCLOSERINE

(King Pharmaceuticals Ltd)

1. NAME OF THE MEDICINAL PRODUCT

CYCLOSERINE

2. QUALITATIVE AND QUANTITATIVE COMPOSITION

Each capsule contains as active ingredient 250mg of cycloserine.

3. PHARMACEUTICAL FORM

Capsule

4. CLINICAL PARTICULARS

4.1 Therapeutic indications

Actions: Cycloserine inhibits cell wall synthesis in susceptible strains of Gram-positive and Gram-negative bacteria and in *Mycobacterium tuberculosis*.

Indications: Cycloserine is indicated in the treatment of active pulmonary and extra-pulmonary tuberculosis (including renal disease) when the organisms are susceptible to this drug and after failure of adequate treatment with the primary medications (streptomycin, isoniazid, rifampicin and ethambutol). Like all anti-tuberculous drugs, cycloserine should be administered in conjunction with other effective chemotherapy and not as the sole therapeutic agent.

Cycloserine may be effective in the treatment of acute urinary tract infections caused by susceptible strains of Gram-positive and Gram-negative bacteria, especially *Klebsiella/Enterobacter* species and *Escherichia coli*. It is generally no more and may be less effective than other antimicrobial agents in the treatment of urinary tract infections caused by bacteria other than mycobacteria. Use of cycloserine in these infections should be considered only when the more conventional therapy has failed and when the organism has been demonstrated to be sensitive to the drug.

4.2 Posology and method of administration

Adults: the usual dosage is 500mg to 1g daily in divided doses, monitored by blood level determinations. The initial adult dosage most frequently given is 250mg twice daily at 12-hour intervals for the first two weeks. A daily dosage of 1g should not be exceeded.

Children: the usual starting dose is 10mg/ kg/ day, then adjusted according to blood levels obtained and therapeutic response.

The elderly: as for adults but reduce dosage if renal function is impaired.

4.3 Contraindications

Cycloserine is contra-indicated in the presence of any of the following: hypersensitivity to cycloserine; epilepsy; depression, severe anxiety or psychosis; severe renal insufficiency; alcohol abuse.

4.4 Special warnings and precautions for use

Administration of cycloserine should be discontinued or the dosage reduced if the patient develops allergic dermatitis or symptoms of central nervous system toxicity such as convulsions, psychosis, somnolence, depression, confusion, hyper-reflexia, headache, tremor, vertigo, paresis or dysarthria.

Toxicity is usually associated with blood levels of greater than 30mg/l, which may be the result of high dosage or inadequate renal clearance. The therapeutic index for this drug is low. The risk of convulsions is increased in chronic alcoholics (see 'Precautions' section).

Patients should be monitored by haematological, renal excretion, blood level and liver function studies.

Before treatment with cycloserine is begun, cultures should be taken and the susceptibility of the organism to the drug should be established. In tuberculous infections, sensitivity to the other anti-tuberculous agents in the regimen should also be demonstrated.

Blood levels should be determined at least weekly for patients having reduced renal function, for individuals receiving a daily dosage of more than 500mg, and for those showing signs and symptoms suggestive of toxicity. The dosage should be adjusted to keep the blood level below 30mg/l.

Anticonvulsant drugs or sedatives may be effective in controlling symptoms of central nervous system toxicity, such as convulsions, anxiety or tremor. Patients receiving more than 500mg of cycloserine daily should be closely observed for such symptoms. The value of pyridoxine in preventing CNS toxicity from cycloserine has not been proven.

Administration of cycloserine and other anti-tuberculous drugs has been associated in a few instances with vitamin B_{12} and/or folic acid deficiency, megaloblastic anaemia and sideroblastic anaemia. If evidence of anaemia develops during treatment, appropriate investigations and treatment should be carried out.

Cycloserine has been associated with clinical exacerbations of porphyria and is not recommended in porphyric patients.

4.5 Interaction with other medicinal products and other forms of interaction

Drug interactions: Concurrent administration of ethionamide has been reported to potentiate neurotoxic side-effects. Alcohol and cycloserine are incompatible, especially during a regimen calling for large doses of the latter. Alcohol increases the possibility and risk of epileptic episodes. Patients receiving cycloserine and isoniazid should be monitored for signs of CNS toxicity, such as dizziness and drowsiness, as these drugs have a combined toxic action on the CNS. Dosage adjustments may be necessary.

4.6 Pregnancy and lactation

Usage in pregnancy: Concentrations in fetal blood approach those found in the serum. A study in 2 generations of rats given doses up to 100mg/ kg/ day demonstrated nc teratogenic effect in offspring. It is not known whether cycloserine can cause fetal harm when administered to a pregnant woman or can affect reproductive capability. Cycloserine should be given to a pregnant woman only if clearly needed.

Usage in nursing mothers: Concentrations in the mother's milk approach those found in the serum. A decision should be made whether to discontinue nursing or to discontinue the drug, taking into account the importance of the drug to the mother.

4.7 Effects on ability to drive and use machines

None known

4.8 Undesirable effects

Most side-effects occurring during treatment with cycloserine involve the nervous system or are manifestations of drug hypersensitivity. The following side-effects have been observed: nervous system manifestations, which appear to be related to higher dosages of drug, i.e. more than 500mg daily, can be convulsions, drowsiness, somnolence, headache, tremor, dysarthria, vertigo, confusion and disorientation with loss of memory, psychosis, possibly with suicidal tendencies, character changes, hyper-irritability, aggression, paresis, hyper-reflexia, paraesthesiae, major and minor localised clonic seizures and coma.

Other reported side-effects include allergy, rash, megaloblastic anaemia and elevated serum aminotransferases, especially in patients with pre-existing liver disease.

Sudden development of congestive heart failure, in patients receiving 1 to 1.5g of cycloserine daily, has been reported.

4.9 Overdose

Signs and symptoms: Acute toxicity can occur if more than 1g is ingested by an adult. Chronic toxicity is dose related and can occur if more than 500mg is administered daily. For patients with renal impairment see 'Contra-indications' and 'Warnings'. Toxicity commonly affects the central nervous system. Effects may include headache, vertigo, confusion, drowsiness, hyper-irritability, paraesthesias, dysarthria and psychosis. Following larger ingestions, paresis, convulsions and coma often occur. Ethanol may increase the risk of seizures.

Treatment: Symptomatic and supportive therapy is recommended. Activated charcoal may be more effective in reducing absorption than emesis or lavage. In adults, many neurotoxic effects can be both treated and prevented with 200-300mg of pyridoxine daily. Haemodialysis removes cycloserine from the bloodstream but should be reserved for life-threatening toxicity.

5. PHARMACOLOGICAL PROPERTIES

5.1 Pharmacodynamic properties

Actions: Cycloserine inhibits cell wall synthesis (by competing with D-alanine for incorporation into the cell wall) in susceptible strains of Gram-positive and Gram-negative bacteria and in *Mycobacterium tuberculosis*.

Indications: Cycloserine is indicated in the treatment of active pulmonary and extra-pulmonary tuberculosis (including renal disease) when the organisms are susceptible to this drug and after failure of adequate treatment with the primary medications (streptomycin, isoniazid, rifampicin and ethambutol). Like all anti-tuberculous drugs, cycloserine should be administered in conjunction with other effective chemotherapy and not as the sole therapeutic agent.

Cycloserine may be effective in the treatment of acute urinary tract infections caused by susceptible strains of Gram-positive and Gram-negative bacteria, especially *Klebsiella/Enterobacter* species and *Escherichia coli*. It is generally no more and may be less effective than other antimicrobial agents in the treatment of urinary tract infections caused by bacteria other than mycobacteria. Use of cycloserine in these infections should be considered only when the more conventional therapy has failed and when the organism has been demonstrated to be sensitive to the drug.

5.2 Pharmacokinetic properties

Cycloserine is rapidly and almost completely absorbed from the GI tract after oral administration. Following the administration of a 250mg dose plasma levels are detectable within an hour and peak plasma concentrations of approximately 10mg/l are achieved 3-4 hours after dosage administration. It is widely distributed throughout body fluids and tissues.

There is no appreciable blood-brain barrier, and CSF levels are approximately the same as plasma levels. It is found in the sputum of tuberculous patients and has been detected in pleural and ascitic fluids, bile, amniotic fluid and fetal blood, breast milk, lung and lymph tissues.

Cycloserine is excreted into the urine, levels appearing within half an hour of oral ingestion. Approximately 66 per cent of a dose appears unchanged in the urine in 24 hours. A further 10 per cent is excreted over the next 48 hours. It is not significantly excreted in the faeces.

Approximately 35 per cent is metabolised, but the metabolites have not yet been identified.

The half-life of cycloserine is in the range 8-12 hours.

5.3 Preclinical safety data
A study in two generations of rats given doses up to 100mg/ kg/ day demonstrated no teratogenic effect in offspring.

6. PHARMACEUTICAL PARTICULARS

6.1 List of excipients
Talc
Ponceau 4R
Yellow Iron Oxide
Titanium Dioxide
Black Iron Oxide
Edible Printing Ink (trace)
Gelatin

6.2 Incompatibilities
None known

6.3 Shelf life
2 years when stored appropriately.

6.4 Special precautions for storage
Keep tightly closed. Protect from moisture. Store below 25°C.

6.5 Nature and contents of container
HDPE bottles of 100 capsules and HDPE bottles with an extruded polyethylene (PE) / PET / Al foil Liner for Induction Heat Seal also containing 100 capsules.

6.6 Special precautions for disposal and other handling
For oral administration

Administrative Data

7. MARKETING AUTHORISATION HOLDER
King Pharmaceuticals Ltd
Donegal Street
Ballybofey
County Donegal
Ireland

8. MARKETING AUTHORISATION NUMBER(S)
PL 14385/0005

9. DATE OF FIRST AUTHORISATION/RENEWAL OF THE AUTHORISATION
October 1996

10. DATE OF REVISION OF THE TEXT
March 2007

Legal Category
POM

Cyklokapron Injection
(Pharmacia Limited)

1. NAME OF THE MEDICINAL PRODUCT
Cyklokapron Injection

2. QUALITATIVE AND QUANTITATIVE COMPOSITION
Active ingredient: Tranexamic Acid Ph.Eur 500 mg

3. PHARMACEUTICAL FORM
Ampoules containing 5ml colourless solution

4. CLINICAL PARTICULARS

4.1 Therapeutic indications
Local fibrinolysis
For short term use in prophylaxis and treatment in patients at high risk of per - and post-operative haemorrhage following:
a) prostatectomy
b) conisation of the cervix
c) surgical procedures and dental extractions in haemophiliacs

General fibrinolysis
a) haemorrhagic complications in association with thrombolytic therapy.
b) Haemorrhage associated with disseminated intravascular coagulation with predominant activation of the fibrinolytic system.

4.2 Posology and method of administration
Route of administration: by slow intravenous injection.

Local fibrinolysis: the recommended standard dose is 5-10ml (500-1000mg) by slow intravenous injection (1 ml/min), three times daily. If treatment continues for more than three days, consideration should be given to the use of Cyklokapron tablets or syrup. Alternatively, following an initial intravenous injection, subsequent treatment may proceed by intravenous infusion. Following addition to a suitable diluent (see Section 4.5), Cyklokapron may be administered at a rate of 25-50 mg/kg body wt/day.

Children: According to body weight (10mg/kg body wt/ 2-3 times daily)

Elderly patients: No reduction in dosage is necessary unless there is evidence of renal failure.

General fibrinolysis
1 In disseminated intravascular coagulation with predominant activation of the fibrinolytic system, usually a single dose of 10ml (1g) is sufficient to control bleeding.
2 Neutralisation of thrombolytic therapy; 10mg/kg body wt by slow intravenous injection.

4.3 Contraindications
Cyklokapron is contra-indicated in patients with a history of thromboembolic disease.

4.4 Special warnings and precautions for use
In patients with renal insufficiency, because of the risk of accumulation. The dose should be reduced according to the following table:

Serum Creatinine	Dose iv	Dose Frequency
120-250 mcmol/l	10 mg/kg	Twice daily
250-500 mcmol/l	10 mg/kg	Every 24th hour
> 500 mcmol/l	5 mg/kg	Every 24th hour

In massive haematuria from the upper urinary tract (especially in haemophilia) since, in a few cases, ureteric obstruction has been reported.

In patients with disseminated intravascular coagulation (DIC) treatment must be restricted to those in whom there is predominant activation of the fibrinolytic system with acute severe bleeding. Characteristically, the haematological profile approximates to the following: reduced euglobulin clot lysis time; prolonged prothrombin time; reduced plasma levels of fibrinogen, factors V and VIII, plasminogen and alpha-2 macroglobulin; normal plasma levels of P and P complex; i.e. factors II (prothrombin), VIII and X; increased plasma levels of fibrinogen degradation products; a normal platelet count. The foregoing presumes that the underlying disease state does not of itself modify the various elements in this profile. In such acute cases a single dose of 1g tranexamic acid is frequently sufficient to control bleeding. The fibrinolytic activity in the blood will be reduced for about 4 hours if renal function is normal. Anticoagulation with heparin should be instigated in order to prevent further fibrin deposition. Administration of Cyklokapron in DIC should be considered only when appropriate haematological laboratory facilities and expertise are available. Cyklokapron must not be administered in DIC with predominant activation of the coagulation system.

4.5 Interaction with other medicinal products and other forms of interaction
The solution for injection may be mixed with the following solutions: isotonic sodium chloride; isotonic glucose; 20% fructose; 10% invertose; dextran 40; dextran 70; ringer's solution.

Cyklokapron solution for injection may be mixed with Heparin.

4.6 Pregnancy and lactation
Although there is no evidence from animal studies of a teratogenic effect, the usual caution with the use of drugs in pregnancy should be observed.

Tranexamic acid passes into breast milk to a concentration of approximately one hundredth of the concentration in the maternal blood. An antifibrinolytic effect in the infant is unlikely.

4.7 Effects on ability to drive and use machines
None known.

4.8 Undesirable effects
Gastro-intestinal disorders (nausea, vomiting, diarrhoea) may occur but disappear when the dosage is reduced. Rapid intravenous injection may cause dizziness and/or hypotension. Rare cases of thromboembolic events have been reported.

4.9 Overdose
No cases of overdosage have been reported. Symptoms may be nausea, vomiting, orthostatic symptoms and/or hypotension. Maintain a high fluid intake to promote renal excretion.

5. PHARMACOLOGICAL PROPERTIES

5.1 Pharmacodynamic properties
Tranexamic acid is an antifibrinolytic agent, which competitively inhibits the activation of plasminogen to plasmin.

5.2 Pharmacokinetic properties
Approximately 90% of an intravenously administered tranexamic acid dose is excreted, largely unchanged, in the urine within 24 hours. The plasma half-life is approximately 2 hours.

5.3 Preclinical safety data
There are no preclinical data of relevance to the prescriber which are additional to that already included in other sections of the Summary of Product Characteristics.

6. PHARMACEUTICAL PARTICULARS

6.1 List of excipients
Water for injections

6.2 Incompatibilities
Cyklokapron solution for injection should not be added to blood for transfusion, or to injections containing penicillin.

6.3 Shelf life
3 years.

6.4 Special precautions for storage
None.

6.5 Nature and contents of container
Type I glass 5ml ampoules packed in outer cardboard carton.

6.6 Special precautions for disposal and other handling
See Section 4.2

Administrative Data

7. MARKETING AUTHORISATION HOLDER
Pharmacia Limited
Ramsgate Road
Sandwich
CT13 9NJ
UK

8. MARKETING AUTHORISATION NUMBER(S)
PL 00032/0314

9. DATE OF FIRST AUTHORISATION/RENEWAL OF THE AUTHORISATION
9th February 1987

10. DATE OF REVISION OF THE TEXT
July 2007

Company Ref: CK1_0

Cymalon
(Actavis UK Ltd)

1. NAME OF THE MEDICINAL PRODUCT
Cymalon

2. QUALITATIVE AND QUANTITATIVE COMPOSITION
Each sachet of 6.76g of granules contain the following actives:

Citric Acid (anhydrous) EP	1063.00mg
Sodium Citrate dihydrate EP	2819.00mg
Sodium Carbonate EP	130.00mg
Sodium Bicarbonate EP	1200.00mg

3. PHARMACEUTICAL FORM
Granules for solution.

4. CLINICAL PARTICULARS

4.1 Therapeutic indications
Cymalon is indicated for the relief of symptoms due to cystitis in adult females only.

4.2 Posology and method of administration
Route of administration: Oral
Adults One sachet to be taken in water, three times a day over 48 hours.
Children Cymalon is not recommended for children.

4.3 Contraindications
Cymalon should not be taken in cases of pregnancy, heart disease, high blood pressure, any form of kidney disease or whenever a restricted salt intake is indicated.

4.4 Special warnings and precautions for use
Patients should be advised against repeated use. If symptoms persist 48 hours after treatment is completed you are advised to consult your doctor. Do not exceed the stated dose. Keep out of the reach of children.

4.5 Interaction with other medicinal products and other forms of interaction
Sodium containing preparations should be avoided by patients on lithium because sodium is preferentially absorbed by the kidney resulting in increased lithium excretion and reduced plasma levels.

Urinary alkalinisers should not be used with hexamine because it is only effective in acid urine.

The effects of a number of drugs may be reduced or increased by the alkalinisination of the urine and reduction in gastric pH brought about by the active ingredients in the product.

4.6 Pregnancy and lactation
Do not use during pregnancy and lactation.

4.7 Effects on ability to drive and use machines
None stated.

4.8 Undesirable effects
Sodium bicarbonate may cause flatulence.

Mild diuresis may occur.

4.9 Overdose
Excessive administration of sodium citrate may cause gastrointestinal discomfort and diarrhoea. Excessive doses of sodium salts may lead to sodium overloading and hyperosmolality. Excessive administration of bicarbonate may lead to hypokalaemia and metabolic alkalosis, especially in patients with impaired renal function. Treatment is symptomatic and consists of appropriate correction of fluid and electrolyte balance.

5. PHARMACOLOGICAL PROPERTIES

5.1 Pharmacodynamic properties

Sodium Bicarbonate increases the alkali reserve of the plasma and increases excretion of urine, which is rendered less acidic. Sodium Citrate is used to make the urine alkaline in the treatment of urinary tract infections. Citric acid increases the secretion of urine and renders it less acidic. It is also used in the preparation of effervescent granules to aid effervescence.

5.2 Pharmacokinetic properties

Cymalon is administered in the form of a solution.

5.3 Preclinical safety data

Not applicable.

6. PHARMACEUTICAL PARTICULARS

6.1 List of excipients

Castor Sugar EP

Saccharin Sodium BP

Flavour Lemon Natural (F309)

6.2 Incompatibilities

There are no known records of incompatibilities.

6.3 Shelf life

36 months

6.4 Special precautions for storage

Protect from moisture.

6.5 Nature and contents of container

Cymalon granules are packed into low density polythene, aluminium foil and paper (PPFP) laminate sachets, each containing 6.76g granules. These are further packed into cardboard cartons each containing 6 sachets.

6.6 Special precautions for disposal and other handling

Not applicable.

7. MARKETING AUTHORISATION HOLDER

Actavis Group PTC ehf

Reykjavíkurvegi 76-78

220 Hafnarfjordur

Iceland.

8. MARKETING AUTHORISATION NUMBER(S)

PL 30306/0066

9. DATE OF FIRST AUTHORISATION/RENEWAL OF THE AUTHORISATION

22 July 2002

10. DATE OF REVISION OF THE TEXT

Cymalon Cranberry Liquid

(Actavis UK Ltd)

1. NAME OF THE MEDICINAL PRODUCT

Cymalon Cranberry Liquid

2. QUALITATIVE AND QUANTITATIVE COMPOSITION

Potassium Citrate 1.5g/5ml

3. PHARMACEUTICAL FORM

Solution

A pale yellow/brown opaque viscous liquid.

4. CLINICAL PARTICULARS

4.1 Therapeutic indications

For the symptomatic relief of dysuria associated with mild urinary tract infections, especially cystitis.

Indications stated on label: For the relief of the symptoms of cystitis and other mild urinary tract infections.

4.2 Posology and method of administration

Oral:

Recommended Doses

Unless directed otherwise by a doctor:

Adults including the elderly, and children over 6 years: 10ml.

Not recommended for use in children under 6 years.

It should be taken well diluted with water, after meals.

Shake the bottle before use.

Dosage Schedule

The dose may be taken three times a day.

4.3 Contraindications

Contraindicated in hyperkalaemia, renal dysfunction, ventricular arrhythmics and Addison's Disease.

Contraindicated in known hypersensitivity to potassium citrate or any other ingredient.

4.4 Special warnings and precautions for use

Cymalon Cranberry Liquid provides symptomatic relief only and is not anti-bacterial. Effective anti-bacterial therapy should be co-prescribed. It should be used with caution when renal or cardiac dysfunction is present.

Citrate mobilises calcium from bones and increases its urinary excretion. This together with raised urinary pH may predispose to formation of stones in the urinary tract.

This medicinal product contains small amounts of ethanol (alcohol), less than 100mg per 10ml dose. This product contains 2.2g of sucrose per10ml dose. This should be taken into account in patients with diabetes mellitus.

Patients with rare hereditary problems of fructose intolerance, glucose-galactose malabsorption or sucrase-isomaltase insufficiency should not take this medicine.

Labels to state: If symptoms persist after 2 days, consult your doctor. Discard any unused mixture 2 months after opening.

4.5 Interaction with other medicinal products and other forms of interaction

Concurrent administration of potassium-containing or sparing medications may lead to hyperkalaemia. May interact with cardiac glycosides.

Citrates alkalinize the urine and thus may alter the urinary excretion of a number of drugs. Particularly noteworthy is the diminished anti-bacterial activity of nitrofurantoin.

4.6 Pregnancy and lactation

There are no adequate data from the use of Cymalon Cranberry Liquid in pregnant women. Animal studies are insufficient with respect to effects on pregnancy. The potential risk to humans is unknown. Cymalon Cranberry Liquid should not be used during pregnancy unless clearly necessary and on the advice of a physician.

(Treatment with Cymalon Cranberry Liquid is adjunctive and secondary to anti-bacterial treatment of urinary tract infection).

4.7 Effects on ability to drive and use machines

No effect on mental alertness.

4.8 Undesirable effects

Mild nausea and occasionally vomiting may occur due to gastric irritation. Other side effects are those due to hyperkalaemia (if this occurs).

4.9 Overdose

Overdosage is accompanied by nausea, vomiting, abdominal pain and symptoms due to hyperkalaemia and metabolic acidosis. Fluid and electrolyte balance together with ECG should be closely monitored.

Treatment is symptomatic and supportive. Moderate to severe hyperkalaemia is a medical emergency requiring prompt correction.

5. PHARMACOLOGICAL PROPERTIES

5.1 Pharmacodynamic properties

Citrate and Citric acid solutions are systematic and urinary alkalinizers thereby providing symptomatic relief of dysuria.

5.2 Pharmacokinetic properties

Potassium Citrate is absorbed and the citrate is metabolised to bicarbonate. Citric acid is metabolised to carbon dioxide and water. Oxidation is virtually complete with less than 5% of citrate being excreted unchanged in the urine.

5.3 Preclinical safety data

There are no preclinical data of relevance to the prescriber which are additional to that already included in other sections of the Summary of Product Characteristics.

6. PHARMACEUTICAL PARTICULARS

6.1 List of excipients

Citric acid monohydrate, quillaia tincture, cranberry flavour FV 4249, cranberry flavour FV 6247, ethanol (96%), chloroform, purified water, syrup.

6.2 Incompatibilities

Incompatible with calcium and strontium salts.

6.3 Shelf life

60ml: 3 years unopened. 2 months after first opening.

6.4 Special precautions for storage

Store below 25°C.

6.5 Nature and contents of container

60ml: Amber type III glass bottle with a 28mm R3 polypropylene white cap with EPE/aluminium/melinex liner and a double ended 2.5ml/5ml polypropylene spoon, inside a cardboard carton.

Or

60ml: Amber type III glass sirop bottle with a 28mm tamper evident polypropylene white cap with EPE/Aluminium/Melinex liner and a 15ml dosing cup, inside a cardboard container.

6.6 Special precautions for disposal and other handling

None

7. MARKETING AUTHORISATION HOLDER

Actavis Group PTC ehf

Reykjavíkurvegi 76-78

220 Hafnarfjordur

Iceland.

8. MARKETING AUTHORISATION NUMBER(S)

PL 30306/0065

9. DATE OF FIRST AUTHORISATION/RENEWAL OF THE AUTHORISATION

1st March 2004

10. DATE OF REVISION OF THE TEXT

Cymbalta 30mg hard gastro-resistant capsules, Cymbalta 60mg hard gastro-resistant capsules

(Eli Lilly and Company Limited)

1. NAME OF THE MEDICINAL PRODUCT

CYMBALTA*▼ 30 mg hard gastro-resistant capsules.

CYMBALTA ▼ 60 mg hard gastro-resistant capsules.

2. QUALITATIVE AND QUANTITATIVE COMPOSITION

Each capsule contains 30 mg of duloxetine (as hydrochloride).

Excipients 30 mg: each capsule contains 8.6 mg sucrose.

Each capsule contains 60 mg of duloxetine (as hydrochloride).

Excipients 60 mg: each capsule contains 17.2 mg sucrose.

For a full list of excipients, see section 6.1.

3. PHARMACEUTICAL FORM

Hard gastro-resistant capsule.

30 mg:

Opaque white body, imprinted with '30 mg' and an opaque blue cap, imprinted with '9543'.

60 mg:

Opaque green body, imprinted with '60 mg' and an opaque blue cap, imprinted with '9542'.

4. CLINICAL PARTICULARS

4.1 Therapeutic indications

Treatment of major depressive episodes.

Treatment of diabetic peripheral neuropathic pain in adults.

Treatment of generalised anxiety disorder.

4.2 Posology and method of administration

Adults

Major Depressive Episodes: The starting and recommended maintenance dose is 60 mg once daily with or without food. Dosages above 60 mg once daily, up to a maximum dose of 120 mg per day have been evaluated from a safety perspective in clinical trials. However, there is no clinical evidence suggesting that patients not responding to the initial recommended dose may benefit from dose up-titrations.

Therapeutic response is usually seen after 2-4 weeks of treatment.

After consolidation of the antidepressive response, it is recommended to continue treatment for several months, in order to avoid relapse.

Generalised Anxiety Disorder: The recommended starting dose in patients with generalised anxiety disorder is 30 mg once daily with or without food. In patients with insufficient response, the dose should be increased to 60 mg, which is the usual maintenance dose in most patients.

In patients with co-morbid major depressive episodes, the starting and maintenance dose is 60 mg once daily (please see also dosing recommendation above).

Doses up to 120 mg per day have been shown to be efficacious and have been evaluated from a safety perspective in clinical trials. In patients with insufficient response to 60 mg, escalation up to 90 mg or 120 mg may therefore be considered. Dose escalation should be based upon clinical response and tolerability.

After consolidation of the response, it is recommended to continue treatment for several months, in order to avoid relapse.

Diabetic Peripheral Neuropathic Pain: The starting and recommended maintenance dose is 60 mg daily with or without food. Dosages above 60 mg once daily, up to a maximum dose of 120 mg per day administered in evenly divided doses, have been evaluated from a safety perspective in clinical trials. The plasma concentration of duloxetine displays large inter-individual variability (see section 5.2). Hence, some patients that respond insufficiently to 60 mg may benefit from a higher dose.

Response to treatment should be evaluated after 2 months. In patients with inadequate initial response, additional response after this time is unlikely.

The therapeutic benefit should be reassessed regularly (at least every three months) (see section 5.1).

Method of Administration

For oral use.

Elderly

No dosage adjustment is recommended for elderly patients solely on the basis of age. However, as with any medicine, caution should be exercised when treating the elderly, especially with CYMBALTA 120 mg per day for major depressive episodes, for which data are limited (see sections 4.4 and 5.2).

Children and Adolescents

Duloxetine is not recommended for use in children and adolescents due to insufficient data on safety and efficacy (see section 4.4).

Hepatic Impairment

CYMBALTA must not be used in patients with liver disease resulting in hepatic impairment (see sections 4.3 and 5.2).

Renal Impairment

No dosage adjustment is necessary for patients with mild or moderate renal dysfunction (creatinine clearance 30 to 80 ml/min). CYMBALTA must not be used in patients with severe renal impairment (creatinine clearance <30 ml/min; see section 4.3).

Discontinuation of Treatment

Abrupt discontinuation should be avoided. When stopping treatment with CYMBALTA the dose should be gradually reduced over a period of at least one to two weeks in order to reduce the risk of withdrawal reactions (see sections 4.4 and 4.8). If intolerable symptoms occur following a decrease in the dose or upon discontinuation of treatment, then resuming the previously prescribed dose may be considered. Subsequently, the physician may continue decreasing the dose, but at a more gradual rate.

4.3 Contraindications

Hypersensitivity to the active substance or to any of the excipients.

Concomitant use of CYMBALTA with non-selective, irreversible monoamine oxidase inhibitors (MAOIs) is contraindicated (see section 4.5).

Liver disease resulting in hepatic impairment (see section 5.2).

CYMBALTA should not be used in combination with fluvoxamine, ciprofloxacin or enoxacine (i.e., potent CYP1A2 inhibitors), since the combination results in elevated plasma concentrations of duloxetine (see section 4.5).

Severe renal impairment (creatinine clearance <30 ml/min) (see section 4.4).

The initiation of treatment with CYMBALTA is contraindicated in patients with uncontrolled hypertension that could expose patients to a potential risk of hypertensive crisis (see sections 4.4 and 4.8).

4.4 Special warnings and precautions for use

Mania and Seizures

CYMBALTA should be used with caution in patients with a history of mania or a diagnosis of bipolar disorder, and/or seizures.

Mydriasis

Mydriasis has been reported in association with duloxetine, therefore, caution should be used when prescribing CYMBALTA to patients with increased intra-ocular pressure or those at risk of acute narrow-angle glaucoma.

Blood Pressure and Heart Rate

Duloxetine has been associated with an increase in blood pressure, and clinically significant hypertension in some patients. This may be due to the noradrenergic effect of duloxetine. Cases of hypertensive crisis have been reported with duloxetine, especially in patients with pre-existing hypertension. Therefore, in patients with known hypertension and/or other cardiac disease, blood pressure monitoring is recommended, especially during the first month of treatment. Duloxetine should be used with caution in patients whose conditions could be compromised by an increased heart rate or by an increase in blood pressure. Caution should also be exercised when duloxetine is used with medicinal products that may impair its metabolism (see section 4.5). For patients who experience a sustained increase in blood pressure while receiving duloxetine, either dose reduction or gradual discontinuation should be considered (see section 4.8). In patients with uncontrolled hypertension, duloxetine should not be initiated (see section 4.3).

Renal Impairment

Increased plasma concentrations of duloxetine occur in patients with severe renal impairment on haemodialysis (creatinine clearance <30 ml/min). For patients with severe renal impairment, see section 4.3. See section 4.2 for information on patients with mild or moderate renal dysfunction.

Use With Antidepressants

Caution should be exercised when using CYMBALTA in combination with antidepressants. In particular the combination with selective reversible MAOIs is not recommended.

St John's Wort

Adverse reactions may be more common during concomitant use of CYMBALTA and herbal preparations containing St John's Wort (*Hypericum perforatum*).

Suicide

Major Depressive Episodes and Generalised Anxiety Disorder: Depression is associated with an increased risk of suicidal thoughts, self-harm, and suicide (suicide-related events). This risk persists until significant remission occurs. As improvement may not occur during the first few weeks or more of treatment, patients should be closely monitored until such improvement occurs. It is general clinical experience that the risk of suicide may increase in the early stages of recovery.

Other psychiatric conditions for which CYMBALTA is prescribed can also be associated with an increased risk of suicide-related events. In addition, these conditions may be co-morbid with major depressive disorder. The same precautions observed when treating patients with major depressive disorder should therefore be observed when treating patients with other psychiatric disorders.

Patients with a history of suicide-related events or those exhibiting a significant degree of suicidal thoughts prior to commencement of treatment, are known to be at greater risk of suicidal thoughts or suicidal behaviour, and should receive careful monitoring during treatment. A meta-analysis of placebo-controlled clinical trials of antidepressant medicinal products in psychiatric disorders showed an increased risk of suicidal behaviour with antidepressants compared to placebo in patients less than 25 years old.

Cases of suicidal thoughts and suicidal behaviours have been reported during duloxetine therapy or early after treatment discontinuation (see section 4.8).

Close supervision of patients, and in particular those at high risk, should accompany drug therapy especially in early treatment and following dose changes. Patients (and caregivers of patients) should be alerted about the need to monitor for any clinical worsening, suicidal behaviour or thoughts, and unusual changes in behaviour, and to seek medical advice immediately if these symptoms present.

Diabetic Peripheral Neuropathic Pain

As with other medicinal products with similar pharmacological action (antidepressants), isolated cases of suicidal ideation and suicidal behaviours have been reported during duloxetine therapy or early after treatment discontinuation. Concerning risk factors for suicidality in depression, see above. Physicians should encourage patients to report any distressing thoughts or feelings at any time.

Use in Children and Adolescents Under 18 Years of Age

No clinical trials have been conducted with duloxetine in paediatric populations. CYMBALTA should not be used in the treatment of children and adolescents under the age of 18 years. Suicide-related behaviours (suicide attempts and suicidal thoughts) and hostility (predominantly aggression, oppositional behaviour, and anger) were more frequently observed in clinical trials among children and adolescents treated with antidepressants compared to those treated with placebo. If, based on clinical need, a decision to treat is nevertheless taken, the patient should be carefully monitored for the appearance of suicidal symptoms. In addition, long-term safety data in children and adolescents concerning growth, maturation, and cognitive and behavioural development are lacking.

Haemorrhage

There have been reports of bleeding abnormalities, such as ecchymoses, purpura, and gastrointestinal haemorrhage, with selective serotonin reuptake inhibitors (SSRIs) and serotonin/noradrenaline reuptake inhibitors (SNRIs). Caution is advised in patients taking anticoagulants and/or medicinal products known to affect platelet function, and in patients with known bleeding tendencies.

Hyponatraemia

Hyponatraemia has been reported rarely, predominantly in the elderly, when administering CYMBALTA. Caution is required in patients at increased risk for hyponatraemia, such as elderly, cirrhotic, or dehydrated patients, or patients treated with diuretics. Hyponatraemia may be due to a syndrome of inappropriate anti-diuretic hormone secretion (SIADH).

Discontinuation of Treatment

Withdrawal symptoms when treatment is discontinued are common, particularly if discontinuation is abrupt (see section 4.8). In clinical trials, adverse events seen on abrupt treatment discontinuation occurred in approximately 45% of patients treated with CYMBALTA and 23% of patients taking placebo.

The risk of withdrawal symptoms seen with SSRIs and SNRIs may be dependent on several factors, including the duration and dose of therapy and the rate of dose reduction. The most commonly reported reactions are listed in section 4.8. Generally, these symptoms are mild to moderate; however, in some patients they may be severe in intensity. They usually occur within the first few days of discontinuing treatment, but there have been very rare reports of such symptoms in patients who have inadvertently missed a dose. Generally, these symptoms are self-limiting and usually resolve within 2 weeks, though in some individuals they may be prolonged (2-3 months or more). It is therefore advised that duloxetine should be gradually tapered when discontinuing treatment over a period of no less than 2 weeks, according to the patient's needs (see section 4.2).

Elderly

Data on the use of CYMBALTA 120 mg in elderly patients with major depressive disorders are limited. Therefore, caution should be exercised when treating the elderly with the maximum dosage (see sections 4.2 and 5.2). Data on the use of CYMBALTA in elderly patients with generalised anxiety disorder are limited.

Akathisia/Psychomotor Restlessness

The use of duloxetine has been associated with the development of akathisia, characterised by a subjectively unpleasant or distressing restlessness and need to move, often accompanied by an inability to sit or stand still. This is most likely to occur within the first few weeks of treatment. In patients who develop these symptoms, increasing the dose may be detrimental.

Medicinal Products Containing Duloxetine

Duloxetine is used under different trademarks in several indications (treatment of diabetic neuropathic pain, major depressive episodes, generalised anxiety disorder, as well as stress urinary incontinence). The use of more than one of these products concomitantly should be avoided.

Hepatitis/Increased Liver Enzymes

Cases of liver injury, including severe elevations of liver enzymes (>10-times upper limit of normal), hepatitis, and jaundice have been reported with duloxetine (see section 4.8). Most of them occurred during the first months of treatment. The pattern of liver damage was predominantly hepatocellular. Duloxetine should be used with caution in patients treated with other medicinal products associated with hepatic injury.

Sucrose

CYMBALTA hard gastro-resistant capsules contain sucrose. Patients with rare hereditary problems of fructose intolerance, glucose-galactose malabsorption or sucrose-isomaltase insufficiency should not take this medicine.

4.5 Interaction with other medicinal products and other forms of interaction

CNS Medicinal Products

The risk of using duloxetine in combination with other CNS-active medicinal products has not been systematically evaluated, except in the cases described in this section. Consequently, caution is advised when CYMBALTA is taken in combination with other centrally-acting medicinal products and substances, including alcohol and sedative medicinal products (e.g., benzodiazepines, morphinomimetics, antipsychotics, phenobarbital, sedative antihistamines).

Monoamine Oxidase Inhibitors (MAOIs)

Due to the risk of serotonin syndrome, duloxetine should not be used in combination with non-selective, irreversible monoamine oxidase inhibitors (MAOIs) or within at least 14 days of discontinuing treatment with an MAOI. Based on the half-life of duloxetine, at least 5 days should be allowed after stopping CYMBALTA before starting an MAOI (see section 4.3).

For selective, reversible MAOIs, like moclobemide, the risk of serotonin syndrome is lower. However, the concomitant use of CYMBALTA with selective, reversible MAOIs is not recommended (see section 4.4).

Serotonin Syndrome

In rare cases, serotonin syndrome has been reported in patients using SSRIs (e.g., paroxetine, fluoxetine) concomitantly with serotonergic medicinal products. Caution is advisable if CYMBALTA is used concomitantly with serotonergic antidepressants like SSRIs, tricyclics like clomipramine or amitriptyline, St John's Wort (*Hypericum perforatum*), venlafaxine, or triptans, tramadol, pethidine, and tryptophan.

Effect of Duloxetine on Other Medicinal Products

Medicinal products metabolised by CYP1A2: The pharmacokinetics of theophylline, a CYP1A2 substrate, were not significantly affected by co-administration with duloxetine (60 mg twice daily).

Medicinal products metabolised by CYP2D6: Duloxetine is a moderate inhibitor of CYP2D6. When duloxetine was administered at a dose of 60 mg twice daily with a single dose of desipramine, a CYP2D6 substrate, the AUC of desipramine increased 3-fold. The co-administration of duloxetine (40 mg twice daily) increases steady-state AUC of tolterodine (2 mg twice daily) by 71%, but does not affect the pharmacokinetics of its active 5-hydroxyl metabolite and no dosage adjustment is recommended. Caution is advised if CYMBALTA is co-administered with medicinal products that are predominantly metabolised by CYP2D6 (risperidone, tricyclic antidepressants [TCAs], such as nortriptyline, amitriptyline, and imipramine), particularly if they have a narrow therapeutic index (such as flecainide, propafenone, and metoprolol).

Oral contraceptives and other steroidal agents: Results of *in vitro* studies demonstrate that duloxetine does not induce the catalytic activity of CYP3A. Specific *in vivo* drug interaction studies have not been performed.

Anticoagulants and antiplatelet agents: Caution should be exercised when duloxetine is combined with oral anticoagulants or antiplatelet agents due to a potential increased risk of bleeding attributable to a pharmacodynamic interaction. Furthermore, increases in INR values have been reported when duloxetine was co-administered to patients treated with warfarin. However, concomitant administration of duloxetine with warfarin under steady state conditions, in healthy volunteers, as part of a clinical pharmacology study, did not result in a clinically significant change in INR from baseline or in the pharmacokinetics of R- or S-warfarin.

Effects of Other Medicinal Products on Duloxetine

Antacids and H_2 antagonists: Co-administration of duloxetine with aluminium- and magnesium-containing antacids, or duloxetine with famotidine, had no significant effect on the rate or extent of duloxetine absorption after administration of a 40 mg oral dose.

Inhibitors of CYP1A2: Because CYP1A2 is involved in duloxetine metabolism, concomitant use of duloxetine with potent inhibitors of CYP1A2 is likely to result in higher concentrations of duloxetine. Fluvoxamine (100 mg once daily), a potent inhibitor of CYP1A2, decreased the apparent plasma clearance of duloxetine by about 77% and increased AUC_{o-t} 6-fold. Therefore, CYMBALTA should

For additional & updated information visit www.emc.medicines.org.uk

Table 1 Adverse reactions

Very common	Common	Uncommon	Rare	Very Rare	Frequency not known
Infections and Infestations					
		Laryngitis			
Immune System Disorders					
			Anaphylactic reaction Hyper-sensitivity disorder		
Endocrine Disorders					
			Hypo-thyroidism		
Metabolism and Nutrition Disorders					
	Decreased appetite	Hyperglycaemia (reported especially in diabetic patients)	Dehydration Hyponatraemia		SIADH
Psychiatric Disorders					
	Insomnia Agitation Libido decreased Anxiety Orgasm abnormal Abnormal dreams	Sleep disorder Bruxism Disorientation Apathy	Mania Hallucinations Aggression and anger[4]		Suicidal ideation [5] Suicidal[5] behaviour
Nervous System Disorders					
Headache (14.3%) Somnolence (10.7%) Dizziness (10.2%)	Tremor Paraesthesia	Myoclonus Nervousness Disturbance in attention Lethargy Dysgeusia Dyskinesia Restless legs syndrome Poor quality sleep	Convulsions[1]		Serotonin syndrome Extra-pyramidal symptoms Akathisia Psychomotor restlessness
Eye Disorders					
	Blurred vision	Mydriasis Visual disturbance	Glaucoma		
Ear and Labyrinth Disorders					
	Tinnitus[1]	Vertigo Ear pain			
Cardiac Disorders					
	Palpitations	Tachycardia Supra-ventricular arrhythmia, mainly atrial fibrillation			
Vascular Disorders					
	Flushing	Blood pressure increase Peripheral coldness Orthostatic hypotension[2] Syncope[2]			Hypertension Hypertensive crisis
Respiratory, Thoracic and Mediastinal Disorders					
	Yawning	Throat tightness Epistaxis			
Gastrointestinal Disorders					
Nausea (24.3%) Dry mouth (12.8%)	Constipation Diarrhoea Vomiting Dyspepsia Flatulence	Gastroenteritis Eructation Gastritis	Stomatitis Breath odour Haematochezia		Gastrointestinal haemorrhage
Hepato-biliary Disorders					
		Elevated liver enzymes (ALT, AST, alkaline phosphatase) Hepatitis[3] Acute liver injury			Jaundice Hepatic failure
Skin and Subcutaneous Tissue Disorders					
	Sweating increased Rash	Night sweats Urticaria Dermatitis contact Cold sweat Photo-sensitivity reactions Increased tendency to bruise			Angio-neurotic oedema Stevens-Johnson Syndrome
Musculoskeletal and Connective Tissue Disorders					
	Musculo-skeletal pain Muscle tightness Muscle spasm	Muscle twitching	Trismus		
Renals and Urinary Disorders					
		Urinary retention Dysuria Urinary hesitation Nocturia Polyuria Urine flow decreased	Urine odour abnormal		
Reproductive System and Breast Disorders					
	Erectile dysfunction	Ejaculation disorder Ejaculation delayed Sexual dysfunction Gynaecological haemorrhage	Menopausal symptoms		
General Disorders and Administration Site Conditions					
	Fatigue Abdominal pain	Feeling abnormal Feeling cold Thirst Chills Malaise Feeling hot Gait disturbance			Chest pain
Investigations					
	Weight decrease	Weight increase Creatine phosphokinase increased	Blood cholesterol increased		

[1] Cases of convulsion and cases of tinnitus have also been reported after treatment discontinuation.
[2] Cases of orthostatic hypotension and syncope have been reported especially at the initiation of treatment.
[3] See section 4.4.
[4] Cases of aggression and anger have been reported particularly early in treatment or after treatment discontinuation.
[5] Cases of suicidal ideation and suicidal behaviours have been reported during duloxetine therapy or early after treatment discontinuation (see section 4.4).

not be administered in combination with potent inhibitors of CYP1A2 like fluvoxamine (see section 4.3).

Inducers of CYP1A2: Population pharmacokinetic analyses have shown that smokers have almost 50% lower plasma concentrations of duloxetine compared with non-smokers.

4.6 Pregnancy and lactation

Pregnancy

There are no adequate data on the use of duloxetine in pregnant women. Studies in animals have shown reproductive toxicity at systemic exposure levels (AUC) of duloxetine lower than the maximum clinical exposure (see section 5.3).

The potential risk for humans is unknown. As with other serotonergic medicinal products, discontinuation symptoms may occur in the neonate after maternal duloxetine use near term. CYMBALTA should be used in pregnancy only if the potential benefit justifies the potential risk to the foetus. Women should be advised to notify their physician if they become pregnant, or intend to become pregnant, during therapy.

Breast-Feeding

Duloxetine is very weakly excreted into human milk, based on a study of 6 lactating patients who did not breast-feed their children. The estimated daily infant dose on a mg/kg basis is approximately 0.14% of the maternal dose (see section 5.2). As the safety of duloxetine in infants is not known, the use of CYMBALTA while breast-feeding is not recommended.

4.7 Effects on ability to drive and use machines

No studies on the effects on the ability to drive and use machines have been performed. CYMBALTA may be associated with sedation and dizziness. Patients should be instructed that if they experience sedation or dizziness they should avoid potentially hazardous tasks such as driving or operating machinery.

4.8 Undesirable effects

Table 1 gives the adverse reactions observed from spontaneous reporting and in placebo-controlled clinical trials (comprising a total of 6828 patients, 4199 on duloxetine and 2629 on placebo) in depression, generalised anxiety disorder and diabetic neuropathic pain.

The most commonly reported adverse reactions in patients treated with CYMBALTA were nausea, headache, dry mouth, somnolence and dizziness. However, the majority of common adverse reactions were mild to moderate; they usually started early in therapy, and most tended to subside even as therapy was continued.

Table 1: Adverse reactions

Frequency estimate: Very common (≥1/10), common (≥1/100 to <1/10), uncommon (≥1/1,000 to <1/100), rare (≥1/10,000 to <1/1,000), very rare (<1/10,000), not known (cannot be estimated from the available data).

Within each frequency grouping, undesirable effects are presented in order of decreasing seriousness.

(see Table 1 on previous page)

Discontinuation of duloxetine (particularly when abrupt) commonly leads to withdrawal symptoms. Dizziness, sensory disturbances (including paraesthesia), sleep disturbances (including insomnia and intense dreams), fatigue, agitation or anxiety, nausea and/or vomiting, tremor, headache, irritability, diarrhoea, hyperhydrosis and vertigo are the most commonly reported reactions.

Generally, for SSRIs and SNRIs, these events are mild to moderate and self-limiting; however, in some patients they may be severe and/or prolonged. It is therefore advised that when duloxetine treatment is no longer required, gradual discontinuation by dose tapering should be carried out (see sections 4.2 and 4.4).

In the 12-week acute phase of three clinical trials of duloxetine in patients with diabetic neuropathic pain, small but statistically significant increases in fasting blood glucose were observed in duloxetine-treated patients. HbA_{1c} was stable in both duloxetine-treated and placebo-treated patients. In the extension phase of these studies, which lasted up to 52 weeks, there was an increase in HbA_{1c} in both the duloxetine and routine care groups, but the mean increase was 0.3% greater in the duloxetine-treated group. There was also a small increase in fasting blood glucose and in total cholesterol in duloxetine-treated patients, while those laboratory tests showed a slight decrease in the routine care group.

The heart rate-corrected QT interval in duloxetine-treated patients did not differ from that seen in placebo-treated patients. No clinically significant differences were observed for QT, PR, QRS, or QTcB measurements between duloxetine-treated and placebo-treated patients.

4.9 Overdose

Cases of overdoses, alone or in combination with other medicinal products, with duloxetine doses of 5400 mg were reported. Some fatalities have occurred, primarily with mixed overdoses, but also with duloxetine alone at a dose of approximately 1000 mg. Signs and symptoms of overdose (duloxetine alone or in combination with other medicinal products) included somnolence, coma, serotonin syndrome, seizures, vomiting and tachycardia.

No specific antidote is known for duloxetine, but if serotonin syndrome ensues, specific treatment (such as with cyproheptadine and/or temperature control) may be considered. A free airway should be established. Monitoring of cardiac and vital signs is recommended, along with appropriate symptomatic and supportive measures. Gastric lavage may be indicated if performed soon after ingestion or in symptomatic patients. Activated charcoal may be useful in limiting absorption. Duloxetine has a large volume of distribution and forced diuresis, haemoperfusion, and exchange perfusion are unlikely to be beneficial.

5. PHARMACOLOGICAL PROPERTIES

5.1 Pharmacodynamic properties

Pharmacotherapeutic group: Other antidepressants. *ATC code:* N06AX21.

Duloxetine is a combined serotonin (5-HT) and noradrenaline (NA) reuptake inhibitor. It weakly inhibits dopamine reuptake, with no significant affinity for histaminergic, dopaminergic, cholinergic, and adrenergic receptors. Duloxetine dose-dependently increases extracellular levels of serotonin and noradrenaline in various brain areas of animals.

Duloxetine normalised pain thresholds in several preclinical models of neuropathic and inflammatory pain and attenuated pain behaviour in a model of persistent pain. The pain inhibitory action of duloxetine is believed to be a result of potentiation of descending inhibitory pain pathways within the central nervous system.

Major Depressive Episodes

CYMBALTA was studied in a clinical programme involving 3,158 patients (1,285 patient-years of exposure) meeting DSM-IV criteria for major depression. The efficacy of CYMBALTA at the recommended dose of 60 mg once a day was demonstrated in three out of three randomised, double-blind, placebo-controlled, fixed-dose acute studies in adult outpatients with major depressive disorder. Overall, CYMBALTA's efficacy has been demonstrated at daily doses between 60 and 120 mg in a total of five out of seven randomised, double-blind, placebo-controlled, fixed-dose acute studies in adult outpatients with major depressive disorder.

CYMBALTA demonstrated statistical superiority over placebo as measured by improvement in the 17-item Hamilton Depression Rating Scale (HAM-D) total score (including both the emotional and somatic symptoms of depression). Response and remission rates were also statistically significantly higher with CYMBALTA compared with placebo. Only a small proportion of patients included in pivotal clinical trials had severe depression (baseline HAM-D >25).

In a relapse prevention study, patients responding to 12 weeks of acute treatment with open-label CYMBALTA 60 mg once daily were randomised to either CYMBALTA 60 mg once daily or placebo for a further 6 months. CYMBALTA 60 mg once daily demonstrated a statistically significant superiority compared to placebo ($p = 0.004$) on the primary outcome measure, the prevention of depressive relapse, as measured by time to relapse. The incidence of relapse during the 6-months double-blind, follow-up period was 17% and 29% for duloxetine and placebo, respectively.

The effect of CYMBALTA 60 mg once a day in elderly depressed patients (≥65 years) was specifically examined in a study that showed a statistically significative difference in the reduction of the HAM-D17 score for duloxetine-treated patients compared to placebo. Tolerability of CYMBALTA 60 mg once daily in elderly patients was comparable to that seen in the younger adults. However, data on elderly patients exposed to the maximum dose (120 mg per day) are limited and thus, caution is recommended when treating this population.

Generalised Anxiety Disorder

CYMBALTA demonstrated statistically significant superiority over placebo in five out of five studies including four randomised, double-blind, placebo-controlled acute studies and a relapse prevention study in adult patients with generalised anxiety disorder.

CYMBALTA demonstrated statistically significant superiority over placebo as measured by improvement in the Hamilton Anxiety Scale (HAM-A) total score and by the Sheehan Disability Scale (SDS) global functional impairment score. Response and remission rates were also higher with CYMBALTA compared to placebo. CYMBALTA showed comparable efficacy results to venlafaxine in terms of improvements on the HAM-A total score.

In a relapse prevention study, patients responding to 6 months of acute treatment with open-label CYMBALTA were randomised to either CYMBALTA or placebo for a further 6 months. CYMBALTA 60 mg to 120 mg once daily demonstrated statistically significant superiority compared to placebo ($p < 0.001$) on the prevention of relapse, as measured by time to relapse. The incidence of relapse during the 6-months double-blind, follow-up period was 14% for CYMBALTA and 42% for placebo.

Diabetic Peripheral Neuropathic Pain

The efficacy of CYMBALTA as a treatment for diabetic neuropathic pain was established in 2 randomised, 12-week, double-blind, placebo-controlled, fixed-dose studies in adults (22 to 88 years) having diabetic neuropathic pain for at least 6 months. Patients meeting diagnostic criteria for major depressive disorder were excluded from these trials. The primary outcome measure was the weekly mean of 24-hour average pain, which was collected in a daily diary by patients on an 11-point Likert scale.

In both studies, CYMBALTA 60 mg once daily and 60 mg twice daily significantly reduced pain compared with placebo. The effect in some patients was apparent in the first week of treatment. The difference in mean improvement between the two active treatment arms was not significant. At least 30% reported pain reduction was recorded in approximately 65% of duloxetine-treated patients versus 40% for placebo. The corresponding figures for at least 50% pain reduction were 50% and 26%, respectively. Clinical response rates (50% or greater improvement in pain) were analysed according to whether or not the patient experienced somnolence during treatment. For patients not experiencing somnolence, clinical response was observed in 47% of patients receiving duloxetine and 27% of patients on placebo. Clinical response rates in patients experiencing somnolence were 60% on duloxetine and 30% on placebo. Patients not demonstrating a pain reduction of 30% within 60 days of treatment were unlikely to reach this level during further treatment.

In an open-label, long-term uncontrolled study, the pain reduction in patients responding to 8 weeks of acute treatment of CYMBALTA 60 mg once daily was maintained for a further 6 months as measured by change on the Brief Pain Inventory (BPI) 24-hour average pain item.

5.2 Pharmacokinetic properties

Duloxetine is administered as a single enantiomer. Duloxetine is extensively metabolised by oxidative enzymes (CYP1A2 and the polymorphic CYP2D6), followed by conjugation. The pharmacokinetics of duloxetine demonstrate large intersubject variability (generally 50-60%), partly due to gender, age, smoking status, and CYP2D6 metaboliser status.

Absorption: Duloxetine is well absorbed after oral administration, with a C_{max} occurring 6 hours post-dose. The absolute oral bioavailability of duloxetine ranged from 32% to 80% (mean of 50%). Food delays the time to reach the peak concentration from 6 to 10 hours and it marginally decreases the extent of absorption (approximately 11%). These changes do not have any clinical significance.

Distribution: Duloxetine is approximately 96% bound to human plasma proteins. Duloxetine binds to both albumin and $alpha_1$-acid glycoprotein. Protein binding is not affected by renal or hepatic impairment.

Biotransformation: Duloxetine is extensively metabolised and the metabolites are excreted principally in urine. Both cytochromes P450-2D6 and 1A2 catalyse the formation of the two major metabolites, glucuronide conjugate of 4-hydroxy duloxetine and sulphate conjugate of 5-hydroxy, 6-methoxy duloxetine. Based upon *in vitro* studies, the circulating metabolites of duloxetine are considered pharmacologically inactive. The pharmacokinetics of duloxetine in patients who are poor metabolisers with respect to CYP2D6 has not been specifically investigated. Limited data suggest that the plasma levels of duloxetine are higher in these patients.

Elimination: The elimination half-life of duloxetine ranges from 8 to 17 hours (mean of 12 hours). After an intravenous dose the plasma clearance of duloxetine ranges from 22 l/hr to 46 l/hr (mean of 36 l/hr). After an oral dose the apparent plasma clearance of duloxetine ranges from 33 to 261 l/hr (mean 101 l/hr).

Special Populations

Gender: Pharmacokinetic differences have been identified between males and females (apparent plasma clearance is approximately 50% lower in females). Based upon the overlap in the range of clearance, gender-based pharmacokinetic differences do not justify the recommendation for using a lower dose for female patients.

Age: Pharmacokinetic differences have been identified between younger and elderly females (≥65 years) (AUC increases by about 25% and half-life is about 25% longer in the elderly), although the magnitude of these changes is not sufficient to justify adjustments to the dose. As a general recommendation, caution should be exercised when treating the elderly (see sections 4.2 and 4.4).

Renal impairment: End stage renal disease (ESRD) patients receiving dialysis had 2-fold higher duloxetine C_{max} and AUC values compared with healthy subjects. Pharmacokinetic data on duloxetine is limited in patients with mild or moderate renal impairment.

Hepatic impairment: Moderate liver disease (Child-Pugh Class B) affected the pharmacokinetics of duloxetine. Compared with healthy subjects, the apparent plasma clearance of duloxetine was 79% lower, the apparent terminal half-life was 2.3-times longer, and the AUC was 3.7-times higher in patients with moderate liver disease. The pharmacokinetics of duloxetine and its metabolites have not been studied in patients with mild or severe hepatic insufficiency.

Breast-feeding mothers: The disposition of duloxetine was studied in 6 lactating women who were at least 12-weeks postpartum. Duloxetine is detected in breast milk, and steady-state concentrations in breast milk are about one-fourth those in plasma. The amount of duloxetine in breast milk is approximately 7µg/day while on 40 mg twice-daily dosing. Lactation did not influence duloxetine pharmacokinetics.

5.3 Preclinical safety data

Duloxetine was not genotoxic in a standard battery of tests and was not carcinogenic in rats.

Multinucleated cells were seen in the liver in the absence of other histopathological changes in the rat carcinogenicity study. The underlying mechanism and the clinical relevance are unknown. Female mice receiving duloxetine for 2 years had an increased incidence of hepatocellular adenomas and carcinomas at the high dose only (144 mg/kg/day), but these were considered to be secondary to hepatic microsomal enzyme induction. The relevance of this mouse data to humans is unknown. Female rats receiving duloxetine (45 mg/kg/day) before and during mating and early pregnancy had a decrease in maternal food consumption and body weight, oestrous cycle disruption, decreased live birth indices and progeny survival, and progeny growth retardation at systemic exposure levels estimated to be at the most at maximum clinical exposure (AUC). In an embryotoxicity study in the rabbit, a higher incidence of cardiovascular and skeletal malformations was observed at systemic exposure levels below the maximum clinical exposure (AUC). No malformations were observed in another study testing a higher dose of a different salt of duloxetine. In prenatal/postnatal toxicity studies in the rat, duloxetine induced adverse behavioural effects in the offspring at exposures below maximum clinical exposure (AUC).

6. PHARMACEUTICAL PARTICULARS

6.1 List of excipients

Capsule Content

Hypromellose

Hypromellose acetate succinate

Sucrose

Sugar spheres

Talc

Titanium dioxide (E171)

Triethyl citrate

Capsule Shell

30 mg:

Gelatin, sodium lauryl sulphate, titanium dioxide (E171), indigo carmine (E132), edible green ink. Edible green ink contains: black iron oxide - synthetic (E172), yellow iron oxide - synthetic (E172), propylene glycol, shellac.

60 mg:

Gelatin, sodium lauryl sulphate, titanium dioxide (E171), indigo carmine (E132), yellow iron oxide (E172), edible white ink. Edible white ink contains: titanium dioxide (E171), propylene glycol, shellac, povidone.

6.2 Incompatibilities

Not applicable.

6.3 Shelf life

3 years.

6.4 Special precautions for storage

Store in the original package in order to protect from moisture. Do not store above 30°C.

6.5 Nature and contents of container

Polyvinylchloride (PVC), polyethylene (PE), and polychlorotrifluoroethylene (PCTFE) blister sealed with an aluminium foil.

CYMBALTA 30 mg is available in packs of 7, 28 and 98 capsules.

CYMBALTA 60 mg is available in packs of 28, 56, 84, 98, 100 (Each pack contains 5 cartons of 20 capsules) and 500 capsules (Each pack contains 25 cartons of 20 capsules).

Not all pack sizes may be marketed.

6.6 Special precautions for disposal and other handling

No special requirements.

7. MARKETING AUTHORISATION HOLDER

Eli Lilly Nederland BV, Grootslag 1-5, NL-3991 RA Houten, The Netherlands.

8. MARKETING AUTHORISATION NUMBER(S)

30 mg, 7 capsules: EU/1/04/296/006

30 mg, 28 capsules: EU/1/04/296/001

30 mg, 98 capsules: EU/1/04/296/009

60 mg, 28 capsules: EU/1/04/296/002

60 mg, 56 capsules: EU/1/04/296/005

60 mg, 84 capsules: EU/1/04/296/003

60 mg, 98 capsules: EU/1/04/296/004

60 mg, 100 capsules: EU/1/04/296/008

60 mg, 500 capsules: EU/1/04/296/007

9. DATE OF FIRST AUTHORISATION/RENEWAL OF THE AUTHORISATION

Date of first authorisation: 17 December 2004

Date of latest renewal: 24 June 2009

10. DATE OF REVISION OF THE TEXT

06 July 2009

Detailed information on this medicine is available on the European Medicines Agency (EMEA) web site: http://www.emea.europa.eu

LEGAL CATEGORY

POM

*CYMBALTA (duloxetine) is a trademark of Eli Lilly and Company. CYM12M

Cymevene IV

(Roche Products Limited)

1. NAME OF THE MEDICINAL PRODUCT

Cymevene® powder for infusion.

2. QUALITATIVE AND QUANTITATIVE COMPOSITION

Ganciclovir 500mg (as ganciclovir sodium 546mg).

3. PHARMACEUTICAL FORM

Sterile, freeze-dried powder for reconstitution with Water for Injection.

4. CLINICAL PARTICULARS

4.1 Therapeutic indications

Cymevene is indicated for the treatment of life-threatening or sight-threatening cytomegalovirus (CMV) infections in immunocompromised individuals. These states include acquired immunodeficiency syndrome (AIDS), iatrogenic immunosuppression associated with organ transplantation, or chemotherapy for neoplasia.

Cymevene may also be used for the prevention of CMV disease, specifically in those patients receiving immunosuppressive therapy secondary to organ transplantation.

4.2 Posology and method of administration

For intravenous infusion following reconstitution with 10ml Water for Injection BP. Based on patient weight and therapeutic indication the appropriate calculated dose volume should be removed from the vial (ganciclovir concentration 50mg/ml) and added to an acceptable infusion fluid (typically 100ml) for delivery over the course of 1 hour. Infusion concentrations greater than 10mg/ml are not recommended. (See section 6.6 *Instructions for use/handling*).

Adults

Treatment of CMV infection

Initial (induction) treatment: 5mg/kg infused at a constant rate over 1 hour every 12 hours (10mg/kg/day) for 14 to 21 days.

Long-term (maintenance) treatment: For immunocompromised patients at risk of relapse of CMV retinitis a course of maintenance therapy may be given. Intravenous infusion of 6mg/kg once daily 5 days per week, or 5mg/kg once daily 7 days per week is recommended.

Treatment of disease progression: Indefinite treatment may be required in patients with AIDS, but even with continued maintenance treatment, patients may have progression of retinitis. Any patient in whom the retinitis progresses, either while on maintenance treatment or because treatment with Cymevene has been withdrawn, may be re-treated using the induction treatment regimen.

Prevention of CMV disease

Induction regimen: 5mg/kg infused every 12 hours (10mg/kg/day) for 7 to 14 days.

Maintenance regimen: Intravenous infusion of 6mg/kg once daily 5 days per week, or 5mg/kg once daily 7 days per week is recommended.

Special dosage instructions

Patients with renal impairment:

Serum creatinine levels or creatinine clearance should be monitored carefully. Dosage adjustment is required according to creatinine clearance as shown in the table below (see section *4.4 Special warnings and precautions for use and section 5.2 Pharmacokinetic properties*).

An estimated creatinine clearance (ml/min) can be related to serum creatinine by the following formulae:

$$\text{For males} = \frac{(140 - \text{age[years]}) \times (\text{body weight [kg]})}{(72 \times (0.011 \times \text{serum creatinine [micromol/L]})}$$

For females = 0.85 x male value

CrCl	Induction dose of ganciclovir
≥ 70ml/min	5.0mg/kg every 12 hours
50 - 69ml/min	2.5mg/kg every 12 hours
25 - 49ml/min	2.5mg/kg/day
10 - 24ml/min	1.25mg/kg/day
< 10ml/min	1.25mg/kg/day after haemodialysis

Elderly patients

No studies on the efficacy or safety of Cymevene in elderly patients have been conducted. Since elderly individuals often have reduced renal function, Cymevene should be administered to elderly patients with special consideration for their renal status (see above).

Paediatric patients

There has been limited clinical experience in treating patients under the age of 12 years (see section *4.4 Special warnings and precautions for use* and *5.2 Pharmacokinetic properties*). Reported adverse events were similar to those seen in adults. However, the use of Cymevene in children warrants extreme caution due to the potential for long-term carcinogenicity and reproductive toxicity. The benefits of treatment should outweigh the risks. Cymevene is not indicated for the treatment of congenital or neonatal CMV infections.

Dosage reductions

For less severe neutropenia or other cytopenias a reduction in the total daily dose should be considered. Cell counts usually normalise within 3 to 7 days after discontinuing the drug or decreasing the dose. As evidence of marrow recovery becomes apparent gradual increases in dose, with careful monitoring of white blood cell counts, may be appropriate.

Patients with severe leucopenia, neutropenia, anaemia, thrombocytopenia and pancytopenia

See section *4.4 Special warnings and precautions for use* before initiation of therapy.

If there is a significant deterioration of blood cell counts during therapy with Cymevene, treatment with haematopoetic growth factors and/or dose interruption should be considered (see section *4.4 Special warnings and precautions for use* and section *4.8 Undesirable effects*).

Method of administration

Cymevene is a powder for solution for intravenous infusion. For directions on the preparation of the infusion solution, see section *6.6 Instructions for use and handling, and disposal*.

Cymevene must only be given by intravenous infusion, preferably via a plastic cannula, into a vein with adequate blood flow.

Caution - do not administer by rapid or bolus i.v. injection! The toxicity of Cymevene may be increased as a result of excessive plasma levels.

Caution - i.m. or s.c. injection may result in severe tissue irritation due to the high pH (~11) of ganciclovir solutions.

The recommended dosage, frequency, or infusion rates should not be exceeded.

Caution should be exercised in the handling of Cymevene, see section *6.6 Instructions for use and handling, and disposal*.

4.3 Contraindications

Cymevene is contra-indicated in patients with hypersensitivity to ganciclovir or valganciclovir or to any of the excipients.

Due to the similarity of the chemical structure of Cymevene and that of aciclovir and valaciclovir, a cross-hypersensitivity reaction between these drugs is possible. Therefore, Cymevene is contra-indicated in patients with hypersensitivity to aciclovir and valaciclovir.

Cymevene is contra-indicated during pregnancy and lactation (see section *4.6 Pregnancy and lactation*).

4.4 Special warnings and precautions for use

Prior to initiation of ganciclovir treatment, patients should be advised of the potential risks to the foetus. In animal studies ganciclovir was found to be mutagenic, teratogenic, aspermatogenic and carcinogenic and a suppressor of female fertility. Cymevene should therefore be considered a potential teratogen and carcinogen in humans with the potential to cause birth defects and cancers (see section *5.3 Preclinical safety data*). It is also considered likely that Cymevene causes temporary or permanent inhibition of spermatogenesis. Women of child bearing potential must be advised to use effective contraception during treatment. Men must be advised to practise barrier contraception during treatment, and for at least 90 days thereafter, unless it is certain that the female partner is not at risk of pregnancy (see section *4.6 Pregnancy and lactation*, section *4.8 Undesirable effects* and section *5.3 Preclinical safety data*).

The use of Cymevene in children and adolescents warrants extreme caution due to the potential for long-term carcinogenicity and reproductive toxicity. The benefits of treatment should outweigh the risks.

Severe leucopenia, neutropenia, anaemia, thrombocytopenia, pancytopenia, bone marrow depression and aplastic anaemia have been observed in patients treated with Cymevene. Therapy should not be initiated if the absolute neutrophil count is less than 500 cells/μL, or the platelet count is less than 25000/μL, or the haemoglobin level is less than 8g/dL (see section 4.2 Posology and method of administration, Special dosage instructions and section 4.8 Undesirable effects).

Cymevene should be used with caution in patients with pre-existing haematological cytopenia or a history of drug-related haematological cytopenia and in patients receiving radiotherapy.

It is recommended that complete blood counts and platelet counts be monitored during therapy. Increased haematological monitoring may be warranted in patients with renal impairment. In patients developing severe leucopenia, neutropenia, anaemia and/or thrombocytopenia, it is recommended that treatment with haematopoietic growth factors and/or dose interruption be considered (see section *4.2 Posology and method of administration*, Special dosage instructions and section *4.8 Undesirable effects*).

In patients with impaired renal function, dosage adjustments based on creatinine clearance are required (see section *4.2 Posology and method of administration*, Special dosage instructions and section *5.2 Pharmacokinetic properties, Pharmacokinetics in special populations*).

Convulsions have been reported in patients taking imipenem-cilastatin and ganciclovir. Cymevene should not be used concomitantly with imipenem-cilastatin unless the potential benefits outweigh the potential risks (see section *4.5 Interaction with other medicinal products and other forms of interaction*).

Patients treated with Cymevene and (a) didanosine, (b) drugs that are known to be myelosuppressive (e.g. zidovudine), or (c) substances affecting renal function, should be closely monitored for signs of added toxicity (see section *4.5 Interaction with other medicinal products and other forms of interaction*).

4.5 Interaction with other medicinal products and other forms of interaction

Imipenem-cilastatin

Convulsions have been reported in patients taking ganciclovir and imipenem-cilastatin concomitantly. These drugs should not be used concomitantly unless the potential benefits outweigh the potential risks (see section *4.4 Special warnings and precautions for use*).

Probenecid

Probenecid given with oral ganciclovir resulted in statistically significantly decreased renal clearance of ganciclovir (20%) leading to statistically significantly increased exposure (40%). These changes were consistent with a mechanism of interaction involving competition for renal tubular secretion. Therefore, patients taking probenecid and Cymevene should be closely monitored for ganciclovir toxicity.

Zidovudine

When zidovudine was given in the presence of oral ganciclovir there was a small (17%), but statistically significant increase in the AUC of zidovudine. There was also a trend towards lower ganciclovir concentrations when administered with zidovudine, although this was not statistically significant. However, since both zidovudine and ganciclovir have the potential to cause neutropenia and anaemia, some patients may not tolerate concomitant therapy at full dosage (see section *4.4 Special warnings and precautions for use*).

Didanosine

Didanosine plasma concentrations were found to be consistently raised when given with ganciclovir (both intravenous and oral). At ganciclovir oral doses of 3 and 6g/day, an increase in the AUC of didanosine ranging from 84 to 124% has been observed, and likewise at intravenous doses of 5 and 10 mg/kg/day, an increase in the AUC of didanosine ranging from 38 to 67% has been observed. There was no clinically significant effect on ganciclovir concentrations. Patients should be closely monitored for didanosine toxicity (see section *4.4 Special warnings and precautions for use*).

Mycophenolate Mofetil

Based on the results of a single dose administration study of recommended doses of oral mycophenolate mofetil (MMF) and intravenous ganciclovir and the known effects of renal impairment on the pharmacokinetics of MMF and ganciclovir, it is anticipated that co-administration of these agents (which have the potential to compete for renal tubular secretion) will result in increases in phenolic glucuronide of mycophenolic acid (MPAG) and ganciclovir concentration. No substantial alteration of mycophenolic acid (MPA) pharmacokinetics is anticipated and MMF dose adjustment is not required. In patients with renal impairment to whom MMF and ganciclovir are co-administered, the dose recommendation of ganciclovir should be observed and the patients monitored carefully.

Zalcitabine

No clinically significant pharmacokinetic changes were observed after concomitant administration of ganciclovir and zalcitabine. Both valganciclovir and zalcitabine have the potential to cause peripheral neuropathy and patients should be monitored for such events.

Stavudine

No clinically significant interactions were observed when stavudine and oral ganciclovir were given in combination.

Trimethoprim

No clinically significant pharmacokinetic interaction was observed when trimethoprim and oral ganciclovir were given in combination. However, there is a potential for toxicity to be enhanced since both drugs are known to be myelosuppressive and therefore both drugs should be used concomitantly only if the potential benefits outweigh the risks.

Other antiretrovirals

At clinically relevant concentrations, there is unlikely to be either a synergistic or antagonistic effect on the inhibition of either HIV in the presence of ganciclovir or CMV in the presence of a variety of antiretroviral drugs. Metabolic interactions with, for example, protease inhibitors and non-nucleoside reverse transcriptase inhibitors (NNRTIs) are unlikely due to the lack of P450 involvement in the metabolism of ganciclovir.

Other potential drug interactions

Toxicity may be enhanced when ganciclovir is co-administered with, or is given immediately before or after, other drugs that inhibit replication of rapidly dividing cell populations such as occur in the bone marrow, testes and germinal layers of the skin and gastrointestinal mucosa. Examples of these types of drugs are dapsone, pentamidine, flucytosine, vincristine, vinblastine, adriamycin, amphotericin B, trimethoprim/sulpha combinations, nucleoside analogues and hydroxyurea.

Since ganciclovir is excreted through the kidney (section *5.2*), toxicity may also be enhanced during co-administration of ganciclovir with drugs that might reduce the renal clearance of ganciclovir and hence increase its exposure. The renal clearance of ganciclovir might be inhibited by two mechanisms: (a) nephrotoxicity, caused by drugs such as cidofovir and foscarnet, and (b) competitive inhibition of active tubular secretion in the kidney by, for example, other nucleoside analogues.

Therefore, all of these drugs should be considered for concomitant use with ganciclovir only if the potential benefits outweigh the potential risks (see section *4.4 Special warnings and precautions for use*).

4.6 Pregnancy and lactation

The safety of Cymevene for use in human pregnancy has not been established. Ganciclovir readily diffuses across the human placenta. Based on its pharmacological mechanism of action and reproductive toxicity observed in animal studies with ganciclovir (see section *5.3 Preclinical safety data*), there is a theoretical risk of teratogenicity in humans. Therefore, Cymevene should not be given to pregnant women as there is a high likelihood of damage to the developing foetus.

Women of childbearing potential must be advised to use effective contraception during treatment. Male patients should be advised to practise barrier contraception during, and for at least 90 days following treatment unless it is certain that the female partner is not at risk of pregnancy (see section *5.3 Preclinical safety data*).

It is unknown if ganciclovir is excreted in breast milk, but the possibility of ganciclovir being excreted in the breast milk and causing serious adverse reactions in the nursing infant cannot be discounted. Therefore, breastfeeding must be discontinued.

4.7 Effects on ability to drive and use machines

No studies on the effects on the ability to drive and use machines have been performed.

Convulsion, sedation, dizziness, ataxia and/or confusion have been reported with the use of Cymevene. If they occur, such effects may affect tasks requiring alertness including the patient's ability to drive and operate machinery.

4.8 Undesirable effects

In patients who were being treated with ganciclovir the most common haematological side effects were neutropenia, anaemia and thrombocytopenia.

Adverse reactions reported with i.v. ganciclovir, oral ganciclovir and valganciclovir are presented in the table below. Valganciclovir is a pro-drug of ganciclovir, and adverse reactions associated with valganciclovir can be expected to occur with ganciclovir. The frequency groupings of these adverse events are based upon the frequency recorded in clinical trials with CMV retinitis patients with AIDS and in clinical trials with solid organ transplant patients.

(see Table 1 on next page)

4.9 Overdose

Overdose experience with intravenous ganciclovir

Reports of overdoses with intravenous ganciclovir have been received from clinical trials and during post-marketing experience. In some of these cases no adverse events were reported. The majority of patients experienced one or more of the following adverse events:

– *Haematological toxicity* - pancytopenia, bone marrow depression, medullary aplasia, leucopenia, neutropenia, granulocytopenia.

– *Hepatotoxicity* - hepatitis, liver function disorder.

– *Renal toxicity* - worsening of haematuria in a patient with pre-existing renal impairment, acute renal failure, elevated creatinine.

– *Gastrointestinal toxicity* - abdominal pain, diarrhoea, vomiting.

– *Neurotoxicity* - generalised tremor, convulsion.

In addition, one adult received an excessive volume of i.v. ganciclovir solution by intravitreal injection, and experienced temporary loss of vision and central retinal artery occlusion secondary to increased intraocular pressure related to the injected fluid volume.

Haemodialysis and hydration may be of benefit in reducing blood plasma levels in patients who receive an overdose of ganciclovir (see section 5.2 Pharmacokinetic properties, Patients undergoing haemodialysis).

Overdose experience with valganciclovir

One adult developed fatal bone marrow depression (medullary aplasia) after several days of dosing that was at least 10-fold greater than recommended for the patient's degree of renal impairment (decreased creatinine clearance).

5. PHARMACOLOGICAL PROPERTIES

5.1 Pharmacodynamic properties

Pharmacotherapeutic group: ATC code: J 05 A B 06 (anti-infectives for systemic use, antivirals for systemic use, direct acting antivirals, nucleosides and nucleotides excluding reverse transcriptase inhibitors).

Ganciclovir is a synthetic analogue of 2'-deoxyguanosine which inhibits replication of herpes viruses *in vitro* and *in vivo*. Sensitive human viruses include human cytomegalovirus (HCMV), herpes simplex virus-1 and -2 (HSV-1 and HSV-2), human herpes virus-6, 7 and 8 (HHV-6, HHV-7, HHV-8), Epstein-Barr virus (EBV) and varicella zoster virus (VZV) and hepatitis B virus. Clinical studies have been limited to assessment of efficacy in patients with CMV infection.

In CMV infected cells ganciclovir is initially phosphorylated to ganciclovir monophosphate by the viral protein kinase, UL97. Further phosphorylation occurs by several cellular kinases to produce ganciclovir triphosphate, which is then slowly metabolised intracellularly. This has been shown to occur in HSV- and HCMV-infected cells with half-lives of 18 and between 6 and 24 hours respectively after removal of extracellular ganciclovir. As the phosphorylation is largely dependent on the viral kinase, phosphorylation of ganciclovir occurs preferentially in virus-infected cells.

The virustatic activity of ganciclovir is due to the inhibition of viral DNA synthesis by: (1) competitive inhibition of incorporation of deoxyguanosine triphosphate into DNA by DNA polymerase and (2) incorporation of ganciclovir triphosphate into viral DNA causing termination of, or very limited, viral DNA elongation. The *in vitro* anti-viral activity, measured as IC_{50} of ganciclovir against CMV, is in the range of 0.08μM (0.02μg/ml) to 14 μM (3.5μg/ml).

Viral resistance

The possibility of viral resistance should be considered for patients who repeatedly show poor clinical response or experience persistent viral excretion during therapy. CMV resistant to ganciclovir can arise after prolonged treatment or prophylaxis with ganciclovir by selection of mutations in either the viral protein kinase gene (UL97) responsible for ganciclovir monophosphorylation and/or, but less frequently, in the viral polymerase gene (UL54). Virus with mutations in the UL97 gene are resistant to ganciclovir alone, whereas virus with mutations in the UL54 gene may show cross-resistance to other antivirals with a similar mechanism of action and vice versa.

The working definition of CMV resistance to ganciclovir based on *in vitro* antiviral assays is an IC_{50} value $\geqslant$ 12.0μM with values $>$ 6.0μM $<$ 12.0μM being considered as indicating intermediate resistance. By these definitions up to 4% of untreated patients have CMV isolates with IC_{50} values that meet the criteria for either resistance or intermediate resistance.

In a prospective study of 76 previously untreated severely immunocompromised AIDS patients with CMV retinitis starting therapy with ganciclovir (i.v. induction / i.v. maintenance or i.v. induction / oral maintenance), the number of patients carrying resistant virus (IC_{50} $>$ 6.0μM) increased with time of treatment; 3.7%, 5.4%, 11.4% and 27.5% of those still on treatment at baseline, 3, 6 and 12 months respectively. Similarly in another study of AIDS patients with CMV retinitis treated for $\geqslant$ 3 months with i.v. ganciclovir 7.8% of patients carried virus with IC_{50} $\geqslant$ 12.0μM. Combined data from 4 clinical studies of the treatment of CMV retinitis indicated an incidence of resistance (IC_{50} $>$ 6.0μM) of 3.2% (median exposure 75 days) for i.v. ganciclovir and 6.5% (median exposure 165 days) for oral ganciclovir.

5.2 Pharmacokinetic properties

Systemic exposure

The systemic exposure (AUC_{0-24}) reported following dosing with a single 1-hour i.v. infusion of 5mg/kg ganciclovir in HIV+/CMV+ patients ranged from 21.4 ± 3.1 (N=16) to 26.0 ± 6.06 (N=16) μg.h/ml. In this patient population peak plasma concentration (C_{max}) ranged from 8.27 ± 1.02 (N=16) to 9.03 ± 1.42 (N=16)μg/ml.

Distribution

For i.v. ganciclovir, the volume of distribution is correlated with body weight with values for the steady state volume of distribution ranging from 0.536 ± 0.078 (N=15) to 0.870 ± 0.116 (N=16) L/kg. Cerebrospinal fluid concentrations obtained 0.25 - 5.67 hours post-dose in 2 patients who received 2.5mg/kg ganciclovir i.v. every 8 hours or every 12 hours ranged from 0.50 to 0.68μg/ml representing 24 - 67% of the respective plasma concentrations. Binding to plasma proteins was 1 - 2% over ganciclovir concentrations of 0.5 and 51μg/ml.

Intra-ocular concentrations of ganciclovir range from 40 to 200% of those measured simultaneously in plasma following administration of i.v. ganciclovir. Average intravitreal concentrations following induction and maintenance dosing with i.v. ganciclovir were 1.15 and 1.0 μg/ml respectively. Half-life of ganciclovir within the eye is much longer

Table 1

Infections and infestations:	
Common (≥ 1/100, < 1/10):	Sepsis (bacteraemia, viraemia), cellulitis, urinary tract infection, oral candidiasis.
Blood and lymphatic disorders:	
Very common (≥ 1/10):	neutropenia, anaemia.
Common (≥ 1/100, < 1/10):	thrombocytopenia, leucopenia, pancytopenia.
Uncommon (≥ 1/1000, < 1/100):	bone marrow depression.
Immune system disorders:	
Uncommon (≥ 1/1000, < 1/100):	anaphylactic reaction.
Metabolic and nutrition disorders:	
Common (≥ 1/100, < 1/10):	appetite decreased, anorexia.
Psychiatric disorders:	
Common (≥ 1/100, < 1/10):	depression, anxiety, confusion, abnormal thinking.
Uncommon (≥ 1/1000, < 1/100):	agitation, psychotic disorder
Nervous system disorders:	
Common (≥ 1/100, < 1/10):	headache, insomnia, dysgeusia (taste disturbance), hypoaesthesia, paraesthesia, peripheral neuropathy, convulsions, dizziness (excluding vertigo).
Uncommon (≥ 1/1000, < 1/100):	tremor.
Eye disorders:	
Common (≥ 1/100, < 1/10):	macular oedema, retinal detachment, vitreous floaters, eye pain.
Uncommon (≥ 1/1000, < 1/100):	vision abnormal, conjunctivitis.
Ear and labyrinth disorders:	
Common (≥ 1/100, < 1/10):	ear pain
Uncommon (≥ 1/1000, < 1/100):	deafness.
Cardiac disorders:	
Uncommon (≥ 1/1000, < 1/100):	arrhythmias.
Vascular disorders:	
Uncommon (≥ 1/1000, < 1/100):	hypotension.
Respiratory, thoracic and mediastinal disorders:	
Very common (≥ 1/10):	dyspnoea.
Common (≥ 1/100, < 1/10):	cough.
Gastrointestinal disorders:	
Very common (≥ 1/10):	diarrhoea.
Common (≥ 1/100, < 1/10):	nausea, vomiting, abdominal pain, abdominal pain upper, constipation, flatulence, dysphagia, dyspepsia.
Uncommon (≥1/1000, <1/100):	abdominal distention, mouth ulcerations, pancreatitis.
Hepato-biliary disorders:	
Common (≥ 1/100, < 1/10):	hepatic function abnormal, blood alkaline phosphatase increased, aspartate aminotransferase increased.
Uncommon (≥ 1/1000, < 1/100):	alanine aminotransferase increased.
Skin and subcutaneous tissues disorders:	
Common (≥ 1/100, < 1/10):	dermatitis, night sweats, pruritus.
Uncommon (≥ 1/1000, < 1/100):	alopecia, urticaria, dry skin.
Musculo-skeletal and connective tissue disorders:	
Common (≥ 1/100, < 1/10):	back pain, myalgia, arthralgia, muscle cramps.
Renal and urinary disorders:	
Common (≥ 1/100, < 1/10):	creatinine clearance renal decreased, renal impairment.
Uncommon (≥ 1/1000, < 1/100):	haematuria, renal failure.
Reproductive system and breast disorders:	
Uncommon (≥ 1/1000, < 1/100):	male infertility.
General disorders and administration site conditions:	
Common (≥ 1/100, < 1/10):	fatigue, pyrexia, rigors, pain, chest pain, malaise, asthenia, injection site reaction (intravenous ganciclovir only).
Investigations:	
Common (≥ 1/100, < 1/10):	weight decreased, blood creatinine increased.

than that in plasma with estimates ranging from 13.3 to 18.8 hours.

Metabolism and elimination

When administered i.v., ganciclovir exhibits linear pharmacokinetics over the range of 1.6 - 5.0mg/kg. Renal excretion of unchanged drug by glomerular filtration and active tubular secretion is the major route of elimination of ganciclovir. In patients with normal renal function, 89.6 ± 5.0% (N=4) of i.v. administered ganciclovir was recovered unmetabolised in the urine. In subjects with normal renal function, systemic clearance ranged from 2.64 ± 0.38ml/min/kg (N=15) to 4.52 ± 2.79ml/min/kg (N=6) and renal clearance ranged from 2.57 ± 0.69ml/min/kg (N=15) to 3.48 ± 0.68ml/min/kg (N=16), corresponding to 90% - 101% of administered ganciclovir. Half-lives in subjects without renal impairment ranged from 2.73 ± 1.29 (N=6) to 3.98 ± 1.78 hours (N=8).

Pharmacokinetics in special populations

Renal impairment

Renal impairment leads to altered kinetics of ganciclovir as indicated below.

Serum creatinine (micromol/l)	Ganciclovir Systemic plasma clearance (ml/min/kg)	Plasma half-life (hours)
< 124 (n = 22)	3.64	2.9
125 - 225 (n = 9)	2.00	5.3
226 - 398 (n = 3)	1.11	9.7
> 398 (n = 5)	0.33	28.5

Patients undergoing haemodialysis

Haemodialysis reduces plasma concentrations of ganciclovir by about 50% after both i.v. and oral administration (see section *4.9 Overdosage*).

During intermittent haemodialysis, estimates for the clearance of ganciclovir ranged from 42 to 92 ml/min, resulting in intra-dialytic half-lives of 3.3 to 4.5 hours. Estimates of ganciclovir clearance for continuous dialysis were lower (4.0 to 29.6 ml/min) but resulted in greater removal of ganciclovir over a dose interval. For intermittent haemodialysis, the fraction of ganciclovir removed in a single dialysis session varied from 50% to 63%.

Paediatric patients

Ganciclovir pharmacokinetics were also studied in 10 children, aged 9 months to 12 years. The pharmacokinetic characteristics of ganciclovir are similar after single and multiple (every 12 hours) i.v. doses (5mg/kg). After the administration of a 5mg/kg single dose, exposure as measured by mean AUC∞ was 19.4 ± 7.1 μg.h/ml, the steady-state volume of distribution reported was 0.68 ± 0.20 l/kg, C_{max} was 7.59 ± 3.21μg/ml, systemic clearance was 4.66 ± 1.72ml/min/kg, and $t_{1/2}$ was 2.49 ± 0.57 hours. The pharmacokinetics of i.v. ganciclovir in children are similar to those observed in adults.

Elderly patients

No studies have been conducted in adults older than 65 years of age.

5.3 Preclinical safety data

Ganciclovir was mutagenic in mouse lymphoma cells and clastogenic in mammalian cells. Such results are consistent with the positive mouse carcinogenicity study with ganciclovir. Ganciclovir is a potential carcinogen.

Ganciclovir causes impaired fertility and teratogenicity in animals (see section 4.4 *Special warnings and precautions for use*).

Based upon animal studies where aspermatogenesis was induced at ganciclovir systemic exposures below therapeutic levels, it is considered likely that ganciclovir could cause inhibition of human spermatogenesis.

Data obtained using an *ex vivo* human placental model show that ganciclovir crosses the placenta and that simple diffusion is the most likely mechanism of transfer. The transfer was not saturable over a concentration range of 1 to 10 mg/ml and occurred by passive diffusion.

6. PHARMACEUTICAL PARTICULARS

6.1 List of excipients

None.

6.2 Incompatibilities

The dry powder should not be reconstituted with bacteriostatic water containing parabens, since these are incompatible with ganciclovir sterile powder and may cause precipitation.

6.3 Shelf life

36 months.

6.4 Special precautions for storage

Undiluted vials: Do not store above 30°C.

From a microbiological point of view, the product should be used immediately after reconstitution and dilution. If the product is not used immediately, the in-use storage times and conditions prior to use are the responsibility of the user. Following reconstitution and dilution, the following in-use storage times should be followed unless reconstitution and dilution has taken place in controlled and validated aseptic conditions.

In-use storage time for the reconstituted vial should not be longer than 12 hours. Do not refrigerate.

In-use storage time for the infusion solution should not be longer than 24 hours when stored in a refrigerator at 2 - 8°C. Freezing is not recommended.

6.5 Nature and contents of container

10ml multidose vials (type I, clear glass) with a grey butyl siliconised stopper in quantities of 5 or 25 vials.

6.6 Special precautions for disposal and other handling

Caution should be exercised in the handling of Cymevene

Since Cymevene is considered a potential teratogen and carcinogen in humans, caution should be exercised in its handling (see section *4.4 Special warnings and precautions for use*). Avoid inhalation or direct contact of the powder contained in the vials or direct contact of the reconstituted solution with the skin or mucous membranes. Cymevene solutions are alkaline (pH approximately 11). If such contact occurs, wash thoroughly with soap and water, rinse eyes thoroughly with sterile water, or plain water if sterile water is unavailable.

Method of preparation of Cymevene solution

1. Lyophilised Cymevene should be reconstituted by injecting 10ml of sterile Water for Injections into the vial. **Do not use bacteriostatic water for injection containing parabens (para-hydroxybenzoates), since these are incompatible with Cymevene sterile powder and may cause precipitation.**

2. The vial should be shaken to dissolve the drug.

3. Reconstituted solution should be inspected for particulate matter prior to proceeding with the admixture preparation.

4. Reconstituted solution in the vial is stable at room temperature for 12 hours. It should not be refrigerated.

Preparation and administration of infusion solution

Based on patient weight the appropriate calculated dose volume should be removed from the Cymevene vial (concentration 50 mg/ml) and added to an acceptable infusion fluid. Normal saline, dextrose 5% in water, Ringer's or lactated Ringer's solution are determined chemically or physically compatible with Cymevene. Infusion concentrations greater than 10mg/ml are not recommended.

Cymevene should not be mixed with other i.v. products.

Because Cymevene is reconstituted with nonbacteriostatic sterile water, the infusion solution should be used as soon as possible and within 24 hours of dilution in order to reduce the risk of bacterial contamination.

The infusion solution should be refrigerated. Freezing is not recommended.

Any unused product or waste material should be disposed of in accordance with local requirements.

7. MARKETING AUTHORISATION HOLDER

Roche Products Limited, 6 Falcon Way, Shire Park, Welwyn Garden City, AL7 1TW, United Kingdom

8. MARKETING AUTHORISATION NUMBER(S)

PL 0031/0465

9. DATE OF FIRST AUTHORISATION/RENEWAL OF THE AUTHORISATION

June 1998/1st February 2006

10. DATE OF REVISION OF THE TEXT

February 2006

LEGAL STATUS

POM

Cymevene is a registered trade mark

Cymex Cream

(Actavis UK Ltd)

1. NAME OF THE MEDICINAL PRODUCT

Cymex Cream

Own Label Supplier:

Superdrug Lip & Cold Sore Cream

Boots Lip & Cold Sore Cream

2. QUALITATIVE AND QUANTITATIVE COMPOSITION

Urea BP	1.0% w/w
Cetrimide BP	0.5% w/w
Dimeticone 350 BPC	9.0% w/w
Chlorocresol BP	0.1% w/w

For excipients, see 6.1.

3. PHARMACEUTICAL FORM

Emollient White Cream

4. CLINICAL PARTICULARS

4.1 Therapeutic indications

For the application to cold sores and cracked lips.

Topical Application Only.

4.2 Posology and method of administration

Apply sparingly every hour for the relief of cold sores and cracked lips.

4.3 Contraindications

None known.

4.4 Special warnings and precautions for use

Keep out of the reach of children.

For External use only.

If symptoms persist consult a Doctor.

4.5 Interaction with other medicinal products and other forms of interaction

None known.

4.6 Pregnancy and lactation

Can be used during pregnancy and lactation.

4.7 Effects on ability to drive and use machines

Not applicable.

4.8 Undesirable effects

None.

4.9 Overdose

Not known.

5. PHARMACOLOGICAL PROPERTIES

5.1 Pharmacodynamic properties

Urea has keratolytic properties, Cetrimide is a quaternary ammonium disinfectant, Chlorocresol is a mild disinfectant while Dimeticone 350 acts as a water repellent.

5.2 Pharmacokinetic properties

Not applicable.

5.3 Preclinical safety data

No particular remarks.

6. PHARMACEUTICAL PARTICULARS

6.1 List of excipients

Deionised Water

Liquid paraffin BP

Cetosteryl Alcohol BP

6.2 Incompatibilities

Not applicable.

6.3 Shelf life

36 months

6.4 Special precautions for storage

Store below 25°C.

6.5 Nature and contents of container

5 g White Aluminium tubes with Elongated nozzles and caps. Internally lacquered.

6.6 Special precautions for disposal and other handling

See 4.2 Posology and Method of Administration.

7. MARKETING AUTHORISATION HOLDER

Actavis Group PTC ehf

Reykjavíkurvegi 76-78

220 Hafnarfjordur

Iceland.

Own label supplier:

Superdrug Stores plc

Admail 838

Croydon

Surrey

CR9 4WZ

England

Own label supplier:

Boots the Chemist plc

1 Thane Road

Nottingham

NG2 3AA

England

8. MARKETING AUTHORISATION NUMBER(S)

PL 30306/0028

9. DATE OF FIRST AUTHORISATION/RENEWAL OF THE AUTHORISATION

13th December 2007

10. DATE OF REVISION OF THE TEXT

Cystrin 3mg Tablets, Cystrin 5mg Tablets

(sanofi-aventis)

1. NAME OF THE MEDICINAL PRODUCT

Cystrin 3mg Tablets

Cystrin 5mg Tablets

2. QUALITATIVE AND QUANTITATIVE COMPOSITION

Oxybutynin hydrochloride 3.00mg

Oxybutynin hydrochloride 5.00mg

3. PHARMACEUTICAL FORM

Tablet

4. CLINICAL PARTICULARS

4.1 Therapeutic indications

Cystrin is indicated for urinary incontinence, urgency and frequency in unstable bladder conditions due either to idiopathic detrusor instability or neurogenic bladder disorders (detrusor hyperreflexia) in conditions such as spina bifida and multiple sclerosis.

In addition, for children over 5 years of age, oxybutynin may be used in nocturnal enuresis in conjunction with non-drug therapy where this alone, or in conjunction with other drug treatment, has failed.

4.2 Posology and method of administration

Children under 5 years of age: Not recommended

Children over 5 years of age:

Neurogenic bladder disorders: The usual dose is 5mg twice a day. This may be increased to a maximum of 5mg three times a day to obtain a clinical response provided that the side effects are tolerated.

Nocturnal enuresis: The usual dose is 5mg two or three times a day. The last dose should be given before bedtime.

In children the maintenance dose may be achieved by upward titration from an initial dose of 3mg twice daily.

Adults: The usual dose is 5mg two or three times a day. This may be increased to a maximum dosage of 5mg four times a day (20mg) to obtain a satisfactory clinical response provided that the side effects are tolerated.

Elderly: The elimination half-life may be increased in some elderly patients, therefore, dosage should be individually titrated commencing at 3mg twice a day. The final dosage will depend on response and tolerance to side-effects. As with other anticholinergic drugs caution should be observed in frail and elderly patients.

4.3 Contraindications

Hypersensitivity to oxybutynin or any component.

Myasthenia gravis.

Narrow-angle glaucoma or shallow anterior chamber.

Gastrointestinal obstruction including paralytic ileus, intestinal atony.

Patients with toxic megacolon, severe ulcerative colitis.

Patients with bladder outflow obstruction where urinary retention may be precipitated.

4.4 Special warnings and precautions for use

Oxybutynin should be used with caution in the frail elderly and children who may be more sensitive to the effects of the product and in patients with autonomic neuropathy, hepatic or renal impairment and severe gastro-intestinal motility disorders (also see section 4.3).

Oxybutynin may aggravate the symptoms of hyperthyroidism, congestive heart failure, coronary heart disease, cardiac arrhythmia, tachycardia, hypertension and prostatic hypertrophy.

Oxybutynin can cause decreased sweating; in high environmental temperatures this can lead to heat prostration.

The use of oxybutynin in children under 5 years of age is not recommended; it has not been established whether oxybutynin can be safely used in this age group.

Special care should be taken in patients with hiatus hernia associated with reflux oesophagitis, as anticholinergic drugs can aggravate this condition.

4.5 Interaction with other medicinal products and other forms of interaction

Care should be taken if other anticholinergic agents are administered together with Cystrin, as potentiation of anticholinergic effects could occur.

Occasional cases of interaction between anticholinergics and phenothiazines, amantidine, butyrophenones, L-dopa, digitalis and tricyclic antidepressants have been reported and care should be taken if Cystrin is administered concurrently with such drugs.

By reducing gastric motility, oxybutynin may affect absorption of other drugs.

4.6 Pregnancy and lactation

Pregnancy

There is no experience of the use of oxybutynin during pregnancy in humans, however, in foetal toxicity and fertility studies in animals, effects were seen on reproductive processes at dosages associated with maternal toxicity. Cystrin should, therefore, only be prescribed during pregnancy if considered essential.

Lactation

Small amounts of oxybutynin have been found in mother's milk of lactating animals. Breast feeding while using oxybutynin is therefore not recommended.

4.7 Effects on ability to drive and use machines

As Cystrin may produce drowsiness or blurred vision, the patient should be cautioned regarding activities requiring mental alertness such as driving, operating machinery or performing hazardous work while taking this drug.

4.8 Undesirable effects

Gastro-intestinal disorders

Nausea, diarrhoea, constipation, dry mouth, abdominal discomfort, anorexia, vomiting, gastroesophageal reflux.

CNS and psychiatric disorders

Agitation, headache, dizziness, drowsiness, disorientation, hallucinations, nightmares, convulsions.

Cardiovascular disorders

Tachycardia, cardiac arrythmia.

Vision disorders

Blurred vision, mydriasis, intraocular hypertension, onset of narrow-angle glaucoma, dry eyes.

Renal and urinary disorders

Urinary retention, difficulty in micturition.

Skin and appendages

Facial flushing which may be more marked in children, dry skin, allergic reactions such as rash, urticaria, angioedema, photosensitivity.

4.9 Overdose

The symptoms of overdosage with oxybutynin progress from an intensification of the usual side-effects of CNS disturbances (from restlessness and excitement to psychotic behaviour), circulatory changes (flushing, fall in blood pressure, circulatory failure etc), respiratory failure, paralysis and coma.

Measures to be taken are:

(1) immediate gastric lavage and

(2) physostigmine by slow intravenous injection

Adults: 0.5 to 2.0 mg of physostigmine by slow intravenous administration. Repeat after 5 minutes, if necessary up to a maximum total dose of 5mg

Children: 30 micrograms/kg of physostigmine by slow intravenous administration. Repeat after 5 minutes, if necessary up to a maximum total dose of 2mg.

Fever should be treated symptomatically with tepid sponging or ice packs.

In pronounced restlessness or excitation, diazepam 10mg may be given by intravenous injection. Tachycardia may be treated with intravenous propanolol and urinary retention managed by bladder catheterization.

In the event of progression of the curare-like effect to paralysis of the respiratory muscles, mechanical ventilation will be required.

5. PHARMACOLOGICAL PROPERTIES

5.1 Pharmacodynamic properties

Oxybutynin hydrochloride is an anticholinergic agent which also exerts a direct antispasmodic effect on smooth muscle. It inhibits bladder contraction and relieves spasm induced by various stimuli; it increases bladder volume, diminishes the frequency of contractions and delays the desire to void in the disturbance of neurogenic bladder. The relaxation of smooth muscle results from the papaverin like effect of the antagonism of the processes distal to the neuromuscular junction in addition to the anticholinergic blocking action of the muscarinic type receptors. In addition oxybutynin hydrochloride has local anaesthetic properties.

5.2 Pharmacokinetic properties

Pharmacodynamic reports show oxybutynin to be rapidly absorbed from the gastrointestinal tract following oral administration with maximum plasma concentrations reached in less than 1 hour subsequently falling bioexponentially with a half-life of between 2 and 3 hours. Maximum effect can be seen within 3-4 hours with some effect still evident after 10 hours.

Repeated oral administration achieved steady state after eight days. Oxybutynin does not appear to accumulate in elderly patients and the pharmacokinetics are similar to those in other adults. Some excretion via the biliary system has been observed in the rabbit and partial first-pass metabolism occurs, the metabolites also appearing to have antimuscarinic properties. The main elimination route is via the kidneys with only 0.3-0.4% of unchanged drug appearing in the urine of the rat after 24 hours and 1% appearing in the urine of the dog after 48 hours. In rats and dogs therefore, oxybutynin appears to be almost completely absorbed.

5.3 Preclinical safety data

No additional data available.

6. PHARMACEUTICAL PARTICULARS

6.1 List of excipients

Lactose anhydrous, microcrystalline cellulose, calcium stearate, indigo carmine aluminium lake (E132).

6.2 Incompatibilities

None known

6.3 Shelf life

3 years

6.4 Special precautions for storage

Do not store above 30°C.

6.5 Nature and contents of container

Cystrin 3mg: 56 tablets in aluminium/PVC blister strips which are contained within a printed Cardboard carton.

Cystrin 5mg: 84 tablets in aluminium/PVC blister strips which are contained within a printed cardboard carton.

6.6 Special precautions for disposal and other handling

No relevance.

7. MARKETING AUTHORISATION HOLDER

Sanofi-aventis

One Onslow Street

Guildford

Surrey

GU1 4YS

UK

8. MARKETING AUTHORISATION NUMBER(S)

Cystrin 3mg: PL 04425/0192

Cystrin 5mg: PL 04425/0193

9. DATE OF FIRST AUTHORISATION/RENEWAL OF THE AUTHORISATION

25th March 2009

10. DATE OF REVISION OF THE TEXT

25 March 2009

Legal Category: POM

Cytamen Injection 1000mcg

(UCB Pharma Limited)

1. NAME OF THE MEDICINAL PRODUCT

Cytamen Injection 1000mcg

2. QUALITATIVE AND QUANTITATIVE COMPOSITION

Cyanocobalamin 1.0mg

3. PHARMACEUTICAL FORM

Solution for injection.

4. CLINICAL PARTICULARS

4.1 Therapeutic indications

Addisonian pernicious anaemia. Prophylaxis and treatment of other macrocytic anaemias associated with vitamin B_{12} deficiency. Schilling test.

Not indicated for treatment of toxic amblyopias - use Neo-Cytamen.

4.2 Posology and method of administration

Route of administration: intramuscular.

Adults and Children

Addisonian pernicious anaemia and other macrocytic anaemias without neurological involvement:

Initially: 250 to 1000mcg intramuscularly on alternate days for one to two weeks, then 250mcg weekly until the blood count is normal.

Maintenance: 1000mcg monthly.

Addisonian pernicious anaemia and other macrocytic anaemias with neurological complications:

Initially: 1000mcg intramuscularly on alternate days as long as improvement is occurring.

Maintenance: 1000mcg monthly.

Prophylaxis of macrocytic anaemia associated with vitamin B_{12} deficiency resulting from gastrectomy, some malabsorption syndromes and strict vegetarianism:

250mcg - 1000mcg monthly.

Schilling Test:

An intramuscular injection of 1000mcg cyanocobalamin is an essential part of this test.

4.3 Contraindications

Hypersensitivity to cyanocobalamin or any other constitutents.

Cytomen should not be used for the treatment of megaloblastic anaemia of pregnancy unless vitamin B12 deficiency has been demonstrated.

Not indicated for treatment of toxic amblyopias - use Neo-Cytamen.

4.4 Special warnings and precautions for use

Precautions:

The dosage schemes given above are usually satisfactory, but regular examination of the blood is advisable. If megaloblastic anaemia fails to respond to Cytamen, folate metabolism should be investigated. Doses in excess of 10mcg daily may produce an incomplete haematological response in patients with folate deficiency. Indiscriminate administration may mask the true diagnosis. The haematological and neurological state should be monitored regularly to ensure adequacy of therapy. Cardiac arrhythmias secondary to hypokalaemia during initial therapy have been reported. Plasma potassium should therefore be monitored during this period. Platelet count should be monitored during the first weeks of use in megaloblastic anaemia due to the possible occurrence of reactive thrombocytosis.

4.5 Interaction with other medicinal products and other forms of interaction

Chloramphenicol-treated patients may respond poorly to Cytamen. Serum concentrations of cyanocobalamin may be lowered by oral contraceptives but this interaction is unlikely to have clinical significance.

Antimetabolites and most antibiotics invalidate vitamin B_{12} assays by microbiological techniques.

4.6 Pregnancy and lactation

Cytamen should not be used for the treatment of megaloblastic anaemia of pregnancy unless vitamin B_{12} deficiency has been demonstrated. Cytamen is secreted into breast milk but this is unlikely to harm the infant, and may be beneficial if the mother and infant are vitamin B_{12} deficient.

4.7 Effects on ability to drive and use machines

None stated.

4.8 Undesirable effects

Hypersensitivity reactions have been reported including skin reactions (e.g. rash, itching) and exceptionally anaphylaxis. Other symptoms reported include fever, chills, hot flushing, dizziness, malaise, nausea, acneiform and bullous eruptions, tremor and injection site reactions including injection site pain, injection site induration and injection site necrosis. Reactive thrombocytosis can occur during the first weeks of use in megaloblastic anaemia

4.9 Overdose

Treatment is unlikely to be needed in cases of overdosage.

5. PHARMACOLOGICAL PROPERTIES

5.1 Pharmacodynamic properties

Cyanocobalamin is a form of vitamin B_{12}.

5.2 Pharmacokinetic properties

Cobalamins are absorbed from the gastro-intestinal tract, but may be irregularly absorbed when given in large therapeutic doses. Absorption is impaired in patients with an absence of intrinsic factor, with a malabsorption syndrome or with a disease or abnormality of the gut, or after gastrectomy.

After injection of cyanocobalamin a large proportion is excreted in the urine within 24 hours; the body retains only 55% of a 100-microgram dose and 15% of a 1000-microgram dose. Vitamin B12 is extensively bound to specific plasma proteins called transcobalamins; transcobalamin II appears to be involved in the rapid transport of the cobalamins to tissues. Vitamin B12 is stored in the liver, excreted in the bile, and undergoes extensive enterohepatic recycling; part of an administered dose is excreted in the urine, most of it in the first 8 hours; urinary excretion, however, accounts for only a small fraction in the reduction of total body stores acquired by dietary means. Vitamin B12 diffuses across the placenta and also appears in breast milk.

5.3 Preclinical safety data

None stated.

6. PHARMACEUTICAL PARTICULARS

6.1 List of excipients

Sodium chloride

Acetic acid

Water for injections

6.2 Incompatibilities

None.

6.3 Shelf life

36 months.

6.4 Special precautions for storage

Protect from light. Do not store above 25°C

6.5 Nature and contents of container

1ml glass ampoules in packs of 5.

6.6 Special precautions for disposal and other handling

Not applicable.

7. MARKETING AUTHORISATION HOLDER

UCB Pharma Limited

208 Bath Road

Slough

Berkshire

SL1 3WE

UK

8. MARKETING AUTHORISATION NUMBER(S)

PL 00039/0403

9. DATE OF FIRST AUTHORISATION/RENEWAL OF THE AUTHORISATION

17 December 1992 / 17 December 1997

10. DATE OF REVISION OF THE TEXT

September 2008

Cytarabine Injection Solution 20mg/ml and 100mg/ml (Pharmacia Limited)

(Pharmacia Limited)

1. NAME OF THE MEDICINAL PRODUCT

Cytarabine 20mg/ml

Cytarabine 100mg/ml

2. QUALITATIVE AND QUANTITATIVE COMPOSITION

1 ml of solution containing 20mg of cytarabine

1 ml of solution contains 100mg of cytarabine.

For a full list of excipients see section 6.1

3. PHARMACEUTICAL FORM

Solution for infusion or injection.

4. CLINICAL PARTICULARS

4.1 Therapeutic indications

Cytotoxic. For induction of remission in acute myeloid leukaemia in adults and for other acute leukaemias of adults and children.

4.2 Posology and method of administration

By intravenous infusion or injection, or subcutaneous injection.

Dosage recommendations may be converted from those in terms of bodyweight to those related to surface area by means of nomograms, as presented in Documenta Geigy.

1) Remission induction:

a) Continuous treatment:

i) Rapid injection - 2 mg/kg/day is a judicious starting dose. Administer for 10 days. Obtain daily blood counts. If no antileukaemic effect is noted and there is no apparent toxicity, increase to 4 mg/kg/day and maintain until therapeutic response or toxicity is evident. Almost all patients can be carried to toxicity with these doses.

ii) 0.5 - 1.0 mg/kg/day may be given in an infusion of up to 24 hours duration. Results from one-hour infusions have been satisfactory in the majority of patients. After 10 days this initial daily dose may be increased to 2 mg/kg/day subject to toxicity. Continue to toxicity or until remission occurs.

b) Intermittent treatment:

3 - 5 mg/kg/day are administered intravenously on each of five consecutive days. After a two to nine-day rest period, a further course is given. Continue until response or toxicity occurs.

The first evidence of marrow improvement has been reported to occur 7 - 64 days (mean 28 days) after the beginning of therapy.

In general, if a patient shows neither toxicity nor remission after a fair trial, the cautious administration of higher doses is warranted. As a rule, patients have been seen to tolerate higher doses when given by rapid intravenous injection as compared with slow infusion. This difference is due to the rapid metabolism of Cytarabine and the consequent short duration of action of the high dose.

2) Maintenance therapy: Remissions which have been induced by Cytarabine, or by other drugs, may be maintained by intravenous or subcutaneous injection of 1 mg/kg once or twice weekly.

Children: Children appear to tolerate higher doses than adults and, where dose ranges are quoted, the children should receive the higher dose and the adults the lower.

Elderly Patients: There is no information to suggest that a change in dosage is warranted in the elderly. Nevertheless, the elderly patient does not tolerate drug toxicity as well as the younger patient, and particular attention should thus be given to drug induced leucopenia, thrombocytopenia, and anaemia, with appropriate initiation of supportive therapy when indicated.

4.3 Contraindications

Therapy with Cytarabine should not be considered in patients with pre-existing drug-induced bone marrow suppression, unless the clinician feels that such management offers the most hopeful alternative for the patient. Cytarabine should not be used in the management of non-malignant disease, except for immunosuppression.

4.4 Special warnings and precautions for use

Warnings: Cytarabine is a potent bone marrow suppressant. Therapy should be started cautiously in patients with pre-existing drug-induced bone marrow suppression. Patients receiving this drug must be under close medical supervision and, during induction therapy, should have leucocyte and platelet counts performed daily. Bone marrow examinations should be performed frequently after blasts have disappeared from the peripheral blood.

Facilities should be available for management of complications, possibly fatal, of bone marrow suppression (infection resulting from granulocytopenia and other impaired body defences, and haemorrhage secondary to thrombocytopenia). Anaphylactic reactions have occurred with cytarabine treatment. Anaphylaxis that resulted in acute cardiopulmonary arrest and required resuscitation has been reported. This occurred immediately after the intravenous administration of Cytarabine.

Severe and at times fatal CNS, GI and pulmonary toxicity (different from that seen with conventional therapy regimens of Cytarabine) has been reported following some experimental Cytarabine dose schedules. These reactions include reversible corneal toxicity; cerebral and cerebellar dysfunction, usually reversible; somnolence; convulsion; severe gastro-intestinal ulceration, including pneumatosis cystoides intestinalis, leading to peritonitis; sepsis and liver abscess; and pulmonary oedema.

Cytarabine has been shown to be carcinogenic in animals. The possibility of a similar effect should be borne in mind when designing the long-term management of the patient.

Precautions: Patients receiving Cytarabine must be monitored closely. Frequent platelet and leucocyte counts are mandatory. Suspend or modify therapy when drug-induced marrow depression has resulted in a platelet count under 50,000 or a polymorphonuclear count under 1,000 per cubic mm. Counts of formed elements in the peripheral blood may continue to fall after the drug is stopped, and reach lowest values after drug-free intervals of five to seven days. If indicated, restart therapy when definite signs of marrow recovery appear (on successive bone marrow studies). Patients whose drug is withheld until 'normal' peripheral blood values are attained may escape from control.

Peripheral motor and sensory neuropathies after consolidation with high doses of cytarabine, daunorubicin, and asparaginase have occurred in adult patients with acute non lymphocytic leukemia. Patients treated with high doses of cytarabine should be observed for neuropathy since dose schedule alterations may be needed to avoid irreversible neurologic disorders.

Severe and sometimes fatal pulmonary toxicity, adult respiratory distress syndrome and pulmonary oedema have occurred following high dose schedules with cytarabine therapy.

When intravenous doses are given quickly, patients are frequently nauseated and may vomit for several hours afterwards. This problem tends to be less severe when the drug is infused.

Abdominal tenderness (peritonitis) and guaiac positive colitis, with concurrent neutropenia and thrombocytopenia, have been reported in patients treated with conventional doses of cytarabine in combination with other drugs. Patients have responded to nonoperative medical management. Delayed progressive ascending paralysis resulting in death has been reported in children with AML following intrathecal and intravenous cytarabine at conventional doses in combination with other drugs.

The human liver apparently detoxifies a substantial fraction of an administered dose of cytarabine. Use the drug with caution and at reduced doses in patients whose liver function is poor.

Periodic checks of bone marrow, liver and kidney functions should be performed in patients receiving Cytarabine.

The safety of this drug for use in infants is not established.

Like other cytotoxic drugs, Cytarabine may induce hyperuricaemia secondary to rapid lysis of neoplastic cells. The clinician should monitor the patient's blood uric acid level and be prepared to use such supportive and pharmacological measures as may be necessary to control this problem.

Immunosuppressant Effects/Increased Susceptibility to Infections. Administration of live or live-attenuated vaccines in patients immunocompromised by chemotherapeutic agents including cytarabine, may result in serious or fatal infections. Vaccination with a live vaccine should be avoided in patients receiving cytarabine. Killed or inactivated vaccines may be administered; however, the response to such vaccines may be diminished.

4.5 Interaction with other medicinal products and other forms of interaction

5-Fluorocytosine should not be administered with Cytarabine as the therapeutic efficacy of 5-Fluorocytosine has been shown to be abolished during such therapy.

Reversible decreases in steady-state plasma digoxin concentrations and renal glycoside excretion were observed in patients receiving beta-acetyldigoxin and chemotherapy regimens containing cyclophosphamide, vincristine and prednisone with or without Cytarabine or procarbazine. Steady-state plasma digitoxin concentrations did not appear to change. Therefore, monitoring of plasma digoxin levels may be indicated in patients receiving similar combination chemotherapy regimens. The utilisation of digitoxin for such patients may be considered as an alternative.

An *in-vitro* interaction study between gentamicin and Cytarabine showed a Cytarabine related antagonism for the susceptibility of *K. pneumoniae* strains. In patients on Cytarabine being treated with gentamicin for a *K.pneumoniae* infection, a lack of a prompt therapeutic response may indicate the need for re-evaluation of antibacterial therapy.

4.6 Pregnancy and lactation

Cytarabine is known to be teratogenic in some animal species. The use of Cytarabine in women who are, or who may become, pregnant should be undertaken only after due consideration of the potential benefits and hazards.

This product should not normally be administered to patients who are pregnant or to mothers who are breast-feeding.

4.7 Effects on ability to drive and use machines

Cytarabine has no effect on intellectual function or psychomotor performance. Nevertheless, patients receiving chemotherapy may have an impaired ability to drive or operate machinery and should be warned of the possibility and advised to avoid such tasks if so affected.

4.8 Undesirable effects

Because Cytarabine is a bone marrow suppressant, anaemia, leucopenia, thrombocytopenia, megaloblastosis and reduced reticulocytes can be expected as a result of its administration. The severity of these reactions are dose and schedule dependent. Cellular changes in the morphology of bone marrow and peripheral smears can be expected.

Most frequent adverse reactions include nausea, vomiting, diarrhoea, fever, rash, anorexia, oral and anal inflammation or ulceration, and hepatic dysfunction.

Infections and infestations: Pneumonia, sepsis, cellulitis at injection site, liver abscess

Immune system disorders: Anaphylaxis, allergic oedema

Metabolism and nutrition disorders: Anorexia

Nervous system disorders: Neural toxicity, neuritis, dizziness, headache

Eye disorders: Conjunctivitis (may occur with rash)

Cardiac disorders: Pericarditis

Vascular disorders: Thrombophlebitis

Respiratory, thoracic and mediastinal disorders: Shortness of breath, sore throat

Gastrointestinal disorders: Pancreatitis, esophageal ulceration, abdominal pain, diarrhea, esophagitis, nausea/vomiting, oral and anal inflammation or ulceration

Hepatobiliary disorders: Hepatic dysfunction, jaundice

Skin and subcutaneous tissue disorders: Skin ulceration, alopecia, freckling, rash, pruritus, urticaria

Renal and urinary disorders: Renal dysfunction, urinary retention

General disorders and administration site conditions: Chest pain, fever

<u>**High Dose Therapy (see section 4.4)**</u>

Infections and infestations: Sepsis, liver abscess

Nervous system disorders: cerebral and cerebellar dysfunction including personality changes, somnolence, and convulsion; peripheral motor and sensory neuropathies.

Eye disorders: Corneal toxicity

Cardiac disorders: Cardiomyopathy with subsequent death

Respiratory, thoracic and mediastinal disorders: Adult respiratory distress syndrome, pulmonary oedema

Skin and subcutaneous tissue disorders: Skin rash leading to desquamation, alopecia

Viral, bacterial, fungal, parasitic, or saprophytic infections, in any location in the body, may be associated with the use of Cytarabine alone or in combination with other immunosuppressive agents following immunosuppressant doses that affect cellular or humoral immunity. These infections may be mild, but can be severe.

A Cytarabine syndrome has been described. It is characterised by fever, myalgia, bone pain, occasionally chest pain, maculopapular rash, conjunctivitis and malaise. It usually occurs 6 - 12 hours following drug administration. Corticosteroids have been shown to be beneficial in treating or preventing this syndrome. If the symptoms of the syndrome are serious enough to warrant treatment, corticosteroids should be contemplated as well as continuation of therapy with Cytarabine.

Cases of pancreatitis have been observed with the induction of Cytarabine.

Cytarabine is not recommended for intrathecal use; however, the following side-effects have been reported with such use. Expected systemic reactions: bone marrow depression, nausea, vomiting. Occasionally, severe spinal cord toxicity even leading to quadriplegia and paralysis, necrotising encephalopathy, blindness and other isolated neurotoxicities have been reported.

4.9 Overdose

Cessation of therapy, followed by management of ensuing bone marrow depression including whole blood or platelet transfusion and antibiotics as required.

5. PHARMACOLOGICAL PROPERTIES

5.1 Pharmacodynamic properties

ATC Code: L01BC01

Cytarabine, a pyrimidine nucleoside analogue, is an antineoplastic agent which inhibits the synthesis of deoxyribonucleic acid. It also has antiviral and immunosuppressant properties. Detailed studies on the mechanism of cytotoxicity in vitro suggests that the primary action of Cytarabine is inhibition of deoxycytidine synthesis, although inhibition of cytidylic kinases and incorporation of the compound into nucleic acids may also play a role in its cytostatic and cytocidal actions.

5.2 Pharmacokinetic properties

Cytarabine is deaminated to arabinofuranosyl uracil in the liver and kidneys. After intravenous administration to humans, only 5.8% of the administered doses is excreted unaltered in urine within 12-24 hours, 90% of the dose is excreted as the deaminated product. Cytarabine appears to be metabolised rapidly, primarily by the liver and perhaps by the kidney. After single high intravenous doses, blood levels fall to unmeasurable levels within 15 minutes in most patients. Some patients have indemonstrable circulating drug as early as 5 minutes after injection.

5.3 Preclinical safety data

There are no preclinical data of relevance to the prescriber which are additional to that already included in other sections of the Summary of Product Characteristics.

6. PHARMACEUTICAL PARTICULARS

6.1 List of excipients

Hydrochloric Acid

Sodium Hydroxide

Nitrogen

Water for injections

Sodium Chloride

6.2 Incompatibilities

In the absence of compatibility studies, this medicinal product must not be mixed with other medicinal products except those mentioned in section 6.6.

6.3 Shelf life

12 months

6.4 Special precautions for storage

Store at 15°C - 25°C. Keep container in outer carton.

Cytarabine should not be stored at refrigerated temperatures (2-8°C).

6.5 Nature and contents of container

Polypropylene vials, closed with either a West S63/1704 Grey EPDM rubber stopper or a West 4110/40 Grey FlurroTec® Plus-faced rubber stopper, and sealed with an aluminium crimp with a plastic flip-off top.

Cytarabine is supplied as vials containing 20mg/ml cytarabine in 5 ml (100mg) in packs of 5, or 25ml (500mg) as single vials.

Cytarabine is supplied as single vials containing 100mg/ml cytarabine in 10ml (1g) or 20ml (2g).

6.6 Special precautions for disposal and other handling

Cytarabine 100mg/ml only:

Prior to use, vials of Cytarabine 100mg/ml must be warmed to 55°C, for 30 minutes, with adequate shaking, and allowed to cool to room temperature.

Cytarabine 20mg/ml & 100mg/ml:

Once opened, the contents of each vial must be used immediately and not stored. Discard any unused portion.

Water for injections, 0.9% saline or 5% dextrose are commonly used infusion fluids for Cytarabine. Compatibility must be assured before mixing with any other substance.

Infusion fluids containing Cytarabine should be used immediately.

Disposal and Spills: To destroy, place in a high risk (for cytotoxics) waste disposal bag and incinerate at 1100°C. If spills occur, restrict access to the affected area and adequate protection including gloves and safety spectacles should be worn. Limit the spread and clean the area with absorbent paper/material. Spills may also be treated with 5% sodium hypochlorite. The spill area should be cleaned with copious amounts of water. Place the contaminated material in a leak proof disposal bag for cytotoxics and incinerate at 1100°C.

7. MARKETING AUTHORISATION HOLDER

Pharmacia Limited

Ramsgate Road

Sandwich, Kent

CT13 9NJ

UK

8. MARKETING AUTHORISATION NUMBER(S)

Cytarabine 20mg/ml PL 0032/0197

Cytarabine 100mg/ml PL 0032/0198

9. DATE OF FIRST AUTHORISATION/RENEWAL OF THE AUTHORISATION

03 June 1999

10. DATE OF REVISION OF THE TEXT

15th December 2008

LEGAL CATEGORY

POM

CCAB 6_0

Cytotec Tablets

(Pharmacia Limited)

1. NAME OF THE MEDICINAL PRODUCT

Cytotec 200mcg tablets.

2. QUALITATIVE AND QUANTITATIVE COMPOSITION

Each tablet contains 200 micrograms misoprostol.

For excipients, see 6.1.

3. PHARMACEUTICAL FORM

White to off-white hexagonal tablets scored both sides, engraved SEARLE 1461 on one side for oral administration.

4. CLINICAL PARTICULARS

4.1 Therapeutic indications

Cytotec is indicated for the healing of duodenal ulcer and gastric ulcer including those induced by nonsteroidal anti-inflammatory drugs (NSAID) in arthritic patients at risk, whilst continuing their NSAID therapy. In addition, Cytotec can be used for the prophylaxis of NSAID-induced ulcers.

4.2 Posology and method of administration

Adults

Healing of duodenal ulcer, gastric ulcer and NSAID-induced peptic ulcer: 800 micrograms daily in two or four divided doses taken with breakfast and / or each main meal and at bedtime.

Treatment should be given initially for at least 4 weeks even if symptomatic relief has been achieved sooner. In most patients ulcers will be healed in 4 weeks but treatment may be continued for up to 8 weeks if required. If the ulcer relapses further treatment courses may be given.

Prophylaxis of NSAID-induced peptic ulcer: 200 micrograms twice daily, three times daily or four times daily. Treatment can be continued as required. Dosage should be individualised according to the clinical condition of each patient.

Elderly

The usual dosage may be used.

Renal impairment: Available evidence indicates that no adjustment of dosage is necessary in patients with renal impairment.

Hepatic impairment: Cytotec is metabolised by fatty acid oxidising systems present in organs throughout the body. Its metabolism and plasma levels are therefore unlikely to be affected markedly in patients with hepatic impairment.

Children

Use of Cytotec in children has not yet been evaluated in the treatment of peptic ulceration or NSAID-induced peptic ulcer disease.

4.3 Contraindications

Use in pregnancy and lactation:

Cytotec is contraindicated in pregnant women and in women planning a pregnancy as it increases uterine tone and contractions in pregnancy which may cause partial or complete expulsion of the products of conception. Use in pregnancy has been associated with birth defects.

It is also contraindicated in patients with a known allergy to prostaglandins.

4.4 Special warnings and precautions for use

Warnings

Use in pre-menopausal women (see also Contraindications): Cytotec should not be used in pre-menopausal women unless the patient requires nonsteroidal anti-inflammatory (NSAID) therapy and is at high risk of complications from NSAID-induced ulceration.

In such patients it is advised that Cytotec should only be used if the patient:

- takes effective contraceptive measures
- has been advised of the risks of taking Cytotec if pregnant (see Contraindications)

If pregnancy is suspected the product should be discontinued.

Precautions

The results of clinical studies indicate that Cytotec does not produce hypotension at dosages effective in promoting the healing of gastric and duodenal ulcers. Nevertheless, Cytotec should be used with caution in the presence of disease states where hypotension might precipitate severe complications, e.g., cerebrovascular disease, coronary artery disease or severe peripheral vascular disease including hypertension.

There is no evidence that Cytotec has adverse effects on glucose metabolism in human volunteers or patients with diabetes mellitus.

4.5 Interaction with other medicinal products and other forms of interaction

Cytotec is predominantly metabolised via fatty acid oxidising systems and has shown no adverse effect on the hepatic microsomal mixed function oxidase (P450) enzyme system. In specific studies no clinically significant pharmacokinetic interaction has been demonstrated with antipyrine, diazepam and propranolol. In extensive clinical studies no drug interactions have been attributed to Cytotec. Additional evidence shows no clinically important pharmacokinetic or pharmacodynamic interaction with nonsteroidal anti-inflammatory drugs including aspirin, diclofenac and ibuprofen.

4.6 Pregnancy and lactation

Pregnancy

See Contraindications.

Lactation

It is not known if the active metabolite of Cytotec is excreted in breast milk; therefore Cytotec should not be administered during breast feeding.

4.7 Effects on ability to drive and use machines

Not applicable.

4.8 Undesirable effects

Gastrointestinal system: Diarrhoea has been reported and is occasionally severe and prolonged and may require withdrawal of the drug. It can be minimised by using single doses not exceeding 200 micrograms with food and by avoiding the use of predominantly magnesium containing antacids when an antacid is required.

Abdominal pain with or without associated dyspepsia or diarrhoea can follow misoprostol therapy.

Other gastrointestinal adverse effects reported include dyspepsia, flatulence, nausea and vomiting.

Female reproductive system: Menorrhagia, vaginal bleeding and intermenstrual bleeding have been reported in pre-and post-menopausal women.

Other adverse events: Skin rashes have been reported. Dizziness has been infrequently reported.

The pattern of adverse events associated with Cytotec is similar when an NSAID is given concomitantly.

A number of side effects have been reported in clinical studies or in the literature following use of misoprostol for non-approved indications. These include abnormal uterine contractions, uterine haemorrhage, retained placenta, amniotic fluid embolism, incomplete abortion and premature birth.

4.9 Overdose

Intensification of pharmacological effects may occur with overdose. In the event of overdosage symptomatic and supportive therapy should be given as appropriate. In clinical trials patients have tolerated 1200 micrograms daily for three months without significant adverse effects.

5. PHARMACOLOGICAL PROPERTIES

5.1 Pharmacodynamic properties

Cytotec is an analogue of naturally occurring prostaglandin E_1 which promotes peptic ulcer healing and symptomatic relief.

Cytotec protects the gastroduodenal mucosa by inhibiting basal, stimulated and nocturnal acid secretion and by reducing the volume of gastric secretions, the proteolytic activity of the gastric fluid, and increasing bicarbonate and mucus secretion.

5.2 Pharmacokinetic properties

Cytotec is rapidly absorbed following oral administration, with peak plasma levels of the active metabolite (misoprostol acid) occurring after about 30 minutes. The plasma elimination half-life of misoprostol acid is 20-40 minutes. No accumulation of misoprostol acid in plasma occurs after repeated dosing of 400 micrograms twice daily.

5.3 Preclinical safety data

In single and repeat-dose studies in dogs, rats and mice at multiples of the human dose, toxicological findings were consistent with the known pharmacological effects of the E-type prostaglandins, the main symptoms being diarrhoea, vomiting, mydriasis, tremors and hyperpyrexia. Gastric mucosal hyperplasia was also observed in the mouse, rat and the dog. In the rat and the dog the hyperplasia was reversible on discontinuation of misoprostol following one year of dosing. Histological examination of gastric biopsies in humans has shown no adverse tissue response after up to one year's treatment. In studies of fertility, teratogenicity and peri/post-natal toxicity in rats and rabbits there were no major findings. A decrease in implantations and some pup growth retardation was observed at doses greater than 100 times the human dose. It was concluded that misoprostol does not significantly affect fertility, is not teratogenic or embryotoxic and does not affect rat pups in the peri/post-natal period.

Misoprostol was negative in a battery of 6 in vitro assays and one in vivo test to assess mutagenic potential. In carcinogenicity studies in the rat and mouse it was concluded that there was no risk of carcinogenic hazard.

6. PHARMACEUTICAL PARTICULARS

6.1 List of excipients

Microcrystalline cellulose,

Sodium starch glycolate (Type A),

Hydrogenated castor oil,

Hypromellose.

6.2 Incompatibilities

Not applicable.

6.3 Shelf life

3 years.

6.4 Special precautions for storage

Do not store above 30°C. Store in the original package.

6.5 Nature and contents of container

Cold-formed aluminium blister packs of 56, 60, 112, 120 or 140 tablets.

Not all pack sizes may be marketed.

6.6 Special precautions for disposal and other handling

No Special Requirements.

7. MARKETING AUTHORISATION HOLDER

Pharmacia Limited

Ramsgate Road

Sandwich, Kent

CT13 9NJ

United Kingdom

8. MARKETING AUTHORISATION NUMBER(S)

PL 00032/0404

9. DATE OF FIRST AUTHORISATION/RENEWAL OF THE AUTHORISATION

First authorised: 10 May 2002

10. DATE OF REVISION OF THE TEXT

June 2007.

Dacarbazine 100mg, 200mg, 500mg, 1000mg (medac UK)

(medac GmbH)

1. NAME OF THE MEDICINAL PRODUCT
Dacarbazine medac 100 mg, Powder for solution for injection or infusion

Dacarbazine medac 200 mg, Powder for solution for injection or infusion

Dacarbazine medac 500 mg, Powder for solution for infusion

Dacarbazine medac 1000 mg, Powder for solution for infusion

2. QUALITATIVE AND QUANTITATIVE COMPOSITION
Each single-dose vial of Dacarbazine medac 100 mg (-200 mg, -500 mg, -1000 mg) contains 100 mg (200 mg, 500 mg, 1000 mg) dacarbazine (as dacarbazine citrate, formed in situ).

After reconstitution, Dacarbazine medac 100 mg (-200 mg) contains 10 mg/ml dacarbazine (see 6.6 a).

After reconstitution and final dilution, Dacarbazine medac 500 mg (-1000 mg) contains

1.4 – 2.0 mg/ml (2.8 – 4.0 mg/ml) dacarbazine (see 6.6 b).

For excipients, see section 6.1.

3. PHARMACEUTICAL FORM
Dacarbazine medac 100 mg (-200 mg-): Powder for solution for injection or infusion.

Dacarbazine medac 500 mg (-1000 mg-): Powder for solution for infusion.

Dacarbazine medac is a white or pale yellow powder.

4. CLINICAL PARTICULARS

4.1 Therapeutic indications
Dacarbazine is indicated for the treatment of patients with metastasized malignant melanoma.

Further indications for dacarbazine as part of a combination chemotherapy are:

- advanced Hodgkin's disease,
- advanced adult soft tissue sarcomas (except mesothelioma, Kaposi sarcoma).

4.2 Posology and method of administration
The use of dacarbazine should be confined to physicians experienced in oncology or haematology respectively.

Dacarbazine is sensitive to light exposure. All reconstituted solutions should be suitably protected from light also during administration (light-resistant infusion set).

Care should be taken of administration of the injection to avoid extravasation into tissues since this will cause local pain and tissue damage. If extravasation occurs, the injection should be discontinued immediately and any remaining portion of the dose should be introduced into another vein.

The following regimes can be used. For further details cf. current scientific literature.

Malignant Melanoma

Dacarbazine can be administered as single agent in doses of 200 to 250 mg/m^2 body surface area/day as an i.v. injection for 5 days every 3 weeks.

As an alternative to an intravenous bolus injection dacarbazine can be administered as a short-term infusion (over 15 - 30 minutes).

It is also possible to give 850 mg/m^2 body surface area on day 1 and then once every 3 weeks as intravenous infusion.

Hodgkin's disease

Dacarbazine is administered in a daily dose of 375 mg/m^2 body surface area i.v. every 15 days in combination with doxorubicin, bleomycin and vinblastine (ABVD regimen).

Adult soft tissue sarcoma

For adult soft tissue sarcomas dacarbazine is given in daily doses of 250 mg/m^2 body surface area i.v. (days 1 - 5) in combination with doxorubicin every 3 weeks (ADIC regimen).

During dacarbazine treatment frequent monitoring of blood counts should be conducted as well as monitoring of hepatic and renal function. Since severe gastrointestinal reactions frequently occur, antiemetic and supportive measures are advisable.

Because severe gastrointestinal and haematological disturbances can occur, an extremely careful benefit-risk analysis has to be made before every course of therapy with dacarbazine.

Duration of therapy

The treating physician should individually decide about the duration of therapy taking into account the type and stage of the underlying disease, the combination therapy administered and the response to and adverse effects of dacarbazine. In advanced Hodgkin's disease, a usual recommendation is to administer 6 cycles of ABVD combination therapy. In metastasized malignant melanoma and in advanced tissue sarcoma, the duration of treatment depends on the efficacy and tolerability in the individual patient.

Rate of administration

Doses up to 200 mg/m^2 may be given as a slow intravenous injection. Larger doses (ranging from 200 to 850 mg/m^2) should be administered as an i.v. infusion over 15 - 30 minutes.

It is recommended to test the patency of the vein first with a 5- to 10-ml flush of sodium chloride infusion solution or glucose 5 %. The same solutions should be used after infusion to flush any remaining drug from the tubing.

After reconstitution with water for injection without further dilution with sodium chloride infusion solution or glucose 5 %, dacarbazine 100 mg and 200 mg preparations are hypo-osmolar (ca. 100 mOsmol/kg) and should therefore be given by slow intravenous injection e.g. over 1 minute rather than rapid intravenous bolus over a few seconds.

Special populations

Patients with kidney/liver insufficiency:

If there is mild to moderate renal or hepatic insufficiency alone, a dose reduction is not usually required. In patients with combined renal and hepatic impairment elimination of dacarbazine is prolonged. However, no validated recommendations on dose reductions can be given currently.

Elderly patients:

As limited experience in elderly patients is available no special instructions for the use in elderly patients can be given.

Children:

No special recommendations for the use of dacarbazine in the paediatric age group can be given until further data become available.

4.3 Contraindications
Dacarbazine is contraindicated in patients

- who have a history of hypersensitivity reactions to dacarbazine or to any of the excipients,
- in pregnant or breastfeeding women,
- in patients with leucopenia and/or thrombocytopenia,
- in patients with severe liver or kidney diseases.

4.4 Special warnings and precautions for use
It is recommended that dacarbazine should only be administered under the supervision of a physician specialised in oncology, having the facilities for regular monitoring of clinical, biochemical and haematological effects, during and after therapy.

If symptoms of a liver or kidney functional disorder or symptoms of a hypersensitivity reaction are observed, immediate cessation of therapy is required. If veno-occlusive disease of the liver occurs, further therapy with dacarbazine is contra-indicated.

Note: The responsible physician should be aware of a rarely observed severe complication during therapy resulting from liver necrosis due to occlusion of intrahepatic veins. Therefore, frequent monitoring of liver size, function and blood counts (especially eosinophils) is required. In single cases of suspected veno-occlusive disease early therapy with high-dose corticosteroids (for example hydrocortisone 300mg/day) with or without fibrinolytic agents like heparin or tissue plasminogen activator was successful (see 4.8).

Long-term therapy can cause cumulative bone marrow toxicity.

The possible bone marrow depression requires careful monitoring of white blood cells, red blood cells and platelet levels. Hemopoetic toxicity may warrant temporary suspension or cessation of therapy.

Extravasation of the drug during i.v. administration may result in tissue damage and severe pain.

Furthermore dacarbazine is a moderate immunosuppressive agent.

Hepatotoxic drugs and alcohol should be avoided during chemotherapy.

Contraceptive measures:

Men are advised to take contraceptive measures during and for 6 months after cessation of therapy.

Administration of dacarbazine in the paediatric age group:

Dacarbazine is not recommended for use in the paediatric age group until further data become available.

Handling of dacarbazine:

Dacarbazine should be handled according to standard procedures for cytostatics that have mutagenic, carcinogenic and teratogenic effects.

4.5 Interaction with other medicinal products and other forms of interaction
In case of previous or concomitant treatment having adverse effects on the bone marrow (particularly cytostatic agents, irradiation) myelotoxic interactions are possible.

Studies to investigate the presence of phenotypic metabolism have not been undertaken but hydroxylation of the parent compound to metabolites with anti-tumour activity has been identified.

Dacarbazine is metabolised by cytochrome P450 (CYP1A1, CYP1A2, and CYP2E1). This has to be taken into account if other drugs are co-administered which are metabolised by the same hepatic enzymes.

Dacarbazine can enhance the effects of methoxypsoralen because of photosensitization.

4.6 Pregnancy and lactation
Pregnancy/Lactation:

Dacarbazine has been shown to be mutagenic, teratogenic and carcinogenic in animals. It must be assumed that an increased risk for teratogenic effects exists in humans. Therefore dacarbazine must not be used during pregnancy and during breastfeeding (see: 4.3 und 4.4).

Women of child bearing potential:

Women of child bearing age must avoid pregnancy during dacarbazine treatment.

4.7 Effects on ability to drive and use machines
Dacarbazine may influence the ability to drive or operate machines because of its central nervous side effects or because of nausea and vomiting.

4.8 Undesirable effects
Frequencies

Very common (>1/10)

Common (>1/100, <1/10)

Uncommon (>1/1,000, <1/100)

Rare (>1/10,000, <1/1,000)

Very rare (<1/10,000), including isolated reports

The most commonly reported ADRs are gastrointestinal disorders (anorexia, nausea and vomiting) and blood and lymphatic system disorders as anemia, leukopenia and thrombocytopenia. The latter are dose-dependant and delayed, with the nadirs often only occurring after 3 to 4 weeks.

Blood and lymphatic system disorders	Common (>1/100, <1/10) Anemia, leukopenia, thrombocytopenia Rare (>1/10,000, <1/1,000) Pancytopenia, agranulocytosis
Immune system disorders	Rare (>1/10,000, <1/1,000) Anaphylactic reactions
Nervous system disorders	Rare (>1/10,000, <1/1,000) Headaches, impaired vision, confusion, lethargy, convulsions, facial paraesthesia
Vascular disorders	Rare (>1/10,000, <1/1,000) Facial flushing
Gastrointestinal disorders	Common (>1/100, <1/10) Anorexia, nausea, vomiting Rare (>1/10,000, <1/1,000) Diarrhoea
Hepatobiliary disorders	Rare (>1/10,000, <1/1,000) Hepatic necrosis due to veno-occlusive disease (VOD) of the liver
Renal and urinary disorders	Rare (>1/10,000, <1/1,000) Impaired renal function
Skin and subcutaneous tissue disorders	Uncommon (>1/1,000, <1/100) Alopecia, hyperpigmentation, photosensitivity Rare (>1/10,000, <1/1,000) Erythema, maculopapular exanthema, urticaria
General disorders and administration site conditions	Uncommon (>1/1,000, <1/100) Flu-like symptoms Rare (>1/10,000, <1/1,000) Application site irritation
Investigations	Rare (>1/10,000, <1/1,000) Elevation of liver enzymes

Disturbances of the digestive tract such as anorexia, nausea and vomiting are common and severe. In rare cases diarrhoea has been observed.

Changes in blood counts often observed (anemia, leukopenia, thrombocytopenia) are dose-dependent and delayed, with the nadirs often only occurring after 3 to 4 weeks. In rare cases pancytopenia and agranulocytosis have been described.

Flu-like symptoms with exhaustion, chills, fever and muscular pain are occasionally observed during or often only days after dacarbazine administration. These disturbances may recur with the next infusion.

Elevation of liver enzymes (e.g. alkaline phosphatase) is observed in rare cases.

Rarely liver necrosis due to occlusion of intrahepatic veins (veno-occlusive disease of the liver) has been observed after administration of dacarbazine in monotherapy or in combined treatment modalities. In general the syndrome occurred during the second cycle of therapy. Symptoms included fever, eosinophilia, abdominal pain, enlarged liver, jaundice and shock which worsened rapidly over a few hours or days. As fatal outcome has been described special care has to be taken of frequently monitoring of liver size, function and blood counts (especially eosinophils). In single cases of suspected veno-occlusive disease early therapy with high-dose corticosteroids (for example hydrocortisone 300mg/day) with or without fibrinolytic agents like heparin or tissue plasminogen activator was successful (see 4.2 and 4.4).

Application site irritations and some of the systemic adverse reactions are thought to result from formation of photo-degradation products.

Impaired renal function with increased blood levels of substances obligatory excreted by urine is rare.

Central nervous side effects such as headaches, impaired vision, confusion, lethargy and convulsions rarely may occur. Facial paraesthesia and flushing may occur shortly after injection.

Allergic reactions of the skin in the form of erythema, maculopapular exanthema or urticaria are observed rarely. Infrequently alopecia, hyperpigmentation and photosensitivity of the skin may occur. In rare cases anaphylactic reactions have been described.

Inadvertent paravenous injection is expected to cause local pain and necrosis.

4.9 Overdose

The primary anticipated complications of overdose are severe bone marrow suppression, eventually bone marrow aplasia which may be delayed by up to two weeks.

Time to occurrence of nadirs of leucocytes and thrombocytes can be 4 weeks. Even if overdosage is only suspected, long-term careful hematologic monitoring is essential. There is no known antidote for dacarbazine overdose. Therefore, special care has to be taken to avoid overdose of this drug.

5. PHARMACOLOGICAL PROPERTIES

5.1 Pharmacodynamic properties

Pharmacotherapeutic group: Alkylating agents, ATC code: L01AX04.

Dacarbazine is a cytostatic agent. The antineoplastic effect is due to an inhibition of cell growth which is independent of the cell cycle and due to an inhibition of DNA synthesis. An alkylating effect has also been shown and other cytostatic mechanisms may also be influenced by dacarbazine.

Dacarbazine is considered not to show an antineoplastic effect by itself. However by microsomal N-demethylation it is quickly converted to 5-amino-imidazole-4-carboxamide and a methyl cation, which is responsible for the alkylating effect of the drug.

5.2 Pharmacokinetic properties

After intravenous administration dacarbazine is quickly distributed into tissue. Plasma protein binding is 5%. Kinetics in plasma are biphasic; the initial (distribution) half-life is only 20 minutes, terminal half-life is 0.5 - 3.5 hours.

Dacarbazine is inactive until metabolised in the liver by cytochromes P450 to form the reactive N-demethylated species HMMTIC and MTIC. This is catalysed by CYP1A1, CYP1A2, and CYP2E1. MTIC is further metabolised to 5-aminoimidazole-4-carboxamide (AIC).

Dacarbazine is metabolised mainly in the liver by both hydroxylation and demethylation, approx. 20-50% of the drug is excreted unmodified by the kidney via renal tubular secretion.

5.3 Preclinical safety data

Because of its pharmacodynamic properties dacarbazine shows mutagenic, carcinogenic and teratogenic effects which are detectable in experimental test systems.

6. PHARMACEUTICAL PARTICULARS

6.1 List of excipients

Citric acid, anhydrous, and mannitol.

6.2 Incompatibilities

Dacarbazine-solution is chemically incompatible with heparin, hydrocortisone, L-cysteine and sodium hydrogen carbonate.

6.3 Shelf life

The shelf-life is 3 years.

Shelf life of the reconstituted solution of Dacarbazine medac 100 mg (-200 mg):

A chemical and physical in-use stability has been demonstrated for 24 hours at 20°C protected from light.

From a microbiological point of view, the product should be used immediately. If not used immediately, in-use storage times and conditions prior to use are the responsibility of the user and would normally be no longer than 24 hours at 2 to 8°C, unless reconstitution has taken place in controlled and validated aseptic conditions.

Shelf life of the reconstituted and further diluted solution of Dacarbazine medac 100 mg (-200 mg):

The reconstituted and further diluted solution must be used immediately.

Shelf life of the reconstituted and further diluted solution of Dacarbazine medac 500 mg (-1000 mg):

The reconstituted and further diluted solution must be used immediately.

6.4 Special precautions for storage

Do not store above 25°C, keep the vial in outer carton in order to protect from light. Reconstituted solutions should also be protected from light.

For storage of the reconstituted product, see 6.3.

6.5 Nature and contents of container

Dacarbazine medac 100 mg (-200 mg) is supplied as a sterile powder for solution for injection or infusion in single-dose vials made of amber glass (Type I, Ph.Eur.) and closed with butyl rubber stoppers. Each carton of Dacarbazine medac 100 mg (-200 mg) contains 10 vials.

Dacarbazine medac 500 mg (-1000 mg) is supplied as a sterile powder for solution for infusion in single-dose vials made of amber glass (Type I, Ph.Eur.) and closed with butyl rubber stoppers. Each carton of Dacarbazine medac 500 mg (-1000 mg) contains one vial.

6.6 Special precautions for disposal and other handling

Recommendations for the safe handling:

Dacarbazine is an antineoplastic agent. Before commencing, local cytotoxic guidelines should be referred to.

Dacarbazine should only be opened by trained staff and as with all cytotoxic agents, precautions should be taken to avoid exposing staff. Handling of cytotoxic drugs should be generally avoided during pregnancy. Preparation of solution for administration should be carried out in a designated handling area and working over a washable tray or disposable plastic-backed absorbent paper.

Suitable eye protection, disposable gloves, face mask and disposable apron should be worn. Syringes and infusion sets should be assembled carefully to avoid leakage (use of Luer lock fittings is recommended).

On completion, any exposed surface should be thoroughly cleaned and hands and face washed.

In the event of spillage, operators should put on gloves, face masks, eye-protection and disposable apron and mop up the spilled material with an absorbent material tapped in the area for that purpose. The area should then be cleaned and all contaminated material transferred to a cytotoxic spillage bag or bin or sealed for incineration.

Preparation for the intravenous administration:

Dacarbazine solutions are prepared immediately before use.

Dacarbazine is sensitive to light exposure. During administration, the infusion container and administration set should be protected from exposure to daylight, e.g. by using light-resistant PVC-infusion sets. Normal infusion sets should be wrapped up in e.g. UV-resistant foils.

a) Preparation of Dacarbazine medac 100 mg (-200 mg):

Aseptically transfer the required amount of water for injection (Dacarbazine medac 100 mg: 10 ml; Dacarbazine medac 200 mg: 20 ml) into the vial and shake until a solution is obtained. This freshly prepared solution (dacarbazine: 10 mg/ml*) is administered as a slow injection.

For preparation of Dacarbazine medac 100 mg (-200 mg) for i.v. infusion the freshly prepared solution is further diluted with 200-300 ml sodium chloride infusion solution or glucose 5%. This solution is given as a short term infusion over a period between 15-30 minutes.

b) Preparation of Dacarbazine medac 500 mg (-1000 mg):

Aseptically transfer the required amount of 50 ml water for injection into the Dacarbazine medac 500 mg (-1000 mg) vial and shake until a solution is obtained⁺. The resulting solution has to be further diluted with 200-300 ml sodium chloride infusion solution or glucose 5%. The obtained infusion solution is ready for i.v. administration (Dacarbazine medac 500 mg: 1.4 - 2.0 mg/ml; Dacarbazine medac 1000 mg: 2.8 - 4.0 mg/ml) and should be given within 20-30 minutes.

Dacarbazine medac 100 mg (-200 mg, -500 mg, -1000 mg) is for single use only.

The diluted solution for infusion should be visually inspected and only clear solutions practically free from particles should be used. Do not use the solution if particles are present.

Any portion of the contents remaining after use should be discarded, as well as solutions where the visual appearance of the product has changed.

Disposal: All materials that have been utilized for dilution and administration should be disposed of according to standard procedures (incineration).

* Density of the solution:
ρ = 1.007 mg/ml

⁺ Density of the solution:
ρ = 1.007 mg/ml (Dacarbazine medac 500 mg)
ρ = 1.015 mg/ml (Dacarbazine medac 1000 mg)

Administrative Data

7. MARKETING AUTHORISATION HOLDER

medac

Gesellschaft für klinische Spezialpräparate mbH

Fehlandtstraße 3

D-20354 Hamburg

8. MARKETING AUTHORISATION NUMBER(S)

Dacarbazine medac 100 mg: PL 11587/0008

Dacarbazine medac 200 mg: PL 11587/0009

Dacarbazine medac 500 mg: PL 11587/0010

Dacarbazine medac 1000 mg: PL 11587/0011

9. DATE OF FIRST AUTHORISATION/RENEWAL OF THE AUTHORISATION

Date of first authorisation: November 28, 1997

Date of last renewal: April 24, 2005

10. DATE OF REVISION OF THE TEXT

November 20, 2006

Full information is available on request from medac UK

Scion House

Stirling University Innovation Park

Stirling FK9 4NF

Tel: 01786 458 086

Daktacort Cream & Ointment

(Janssen-Cilag Ltd)

1. NAME OF THE MEDICINAL PRODUCT

Daktacort™ Cream

Daktacort™ Ointment

2. QUALITATIVE AND QUANTITATIVE COMPOSITION

Miconazole nitrate 2% w/w and hydrocortisone 1% w/w.

3. PHARMACEUTICAL FORM

Cream: White, homogenous cream.

Ointment: White, odourless, fatty ointment.

4. CLINICAL PARTICULARS

4.1 Therapeutic indications

For the topical treatment of inflamed dermatoses where infection by susceptible organisms and inflammation coexist, eg intertrigo and infected eczema.

Moist or dry eczema or dermatitis including atopic eczema, primary irritant or contact allergic eczema or seborrhoeic eczema including that associated with acne.

Intertriginous eczema including inframammary intertrigo, perianal and genital dermatitis.

Organisms which are susceptible to miconazole are dermatophytes and pathogenic yeasts (eg *Candida* spp.). Also many Gram-positive bacteria including most strains of *Streptococcus* and *Staphylococcus*.

The properties of Daktacort indicate it particularly for the initial stages of treatment. Once the inflammatory symptoms have disappeared (after about 7 days), treatment can be continued where necessary with Daktarin™ Cream or Daktarin™ Powder.

4.2 Posology and method of administration

For topical administration.

Cream:

Apply the cream two or three times a day to the affected area, rubbing in gently until the cream has been absorbed by the skin.

Ointment:

Daktacort Ointment should be applied topically two or three times daily.

The same dosage applies to both adults and children.

Use in elderly:

Natural thinning of the skin occurs in the elderly, hence corticosteroids should be used sparingly and for short periods of time.

In infants, long term continuous topical corticosteroid therapy should be avoided.

If after about 7 days' application, no improvement has occurred, cultural isolation of the offending organism should be followed by appropriate local or systemic antimicrobial therapy.

4.3 Contraindications

True hypersensitivity to any of the ingredients. Tubercular or viral infections of the skin or those caused by Gram-negative bacteria.

4.4 Special warnings and precautions for use

When Daktacort is used by patients taking oral anticoagulants, the anticoagulant effect should be carefully monitored.

As with any topical corticosteroid, care is advised with infants and children when Daktacort is to be applied to extensive surface areas or under occlusive dressings including baby napkins; similarly, application to the face should be avoided.

In infants, long term continuous topical corticosteroid therapy should be avoided. Adrenal suppression can occur even without occlusion.

4.5 Interaction with other medicinal products and other forms of interaction

Miconazole administered systemically is known to inhibit CYP3A4/2C9. Due to the limited systemic availability after topical application (see Section 5.2 Pharmacokinetic properties), clinically relevant interactions are rare. However, in patients on oral anticoagulants, such as warfarin, caution should be exercised and anticoagulant effect should be monitored.

Miconazole is a CYP3A4 inhibitor that can decrease the rate of metabolism of hydrocortisone. Serum concentrations of hydrocortisone may be higher with the use of Daktacort compared with topical preparations containing hydrocortisone alone.

4.6 Pregnancy and lactation

In animals, miconazole nitrate has shown no teratogenic effects but is foetotoxic at high oral doses and administration of corticosteroids to pregnant animals can cause abnormalities of foetal development. The relevance of these findings to humans has not been established. However, combinations of topical steroids with imidazoles should be used in pregnant women only if the practitioner considers it to be necessary.

4.7 Effects on ability to drive and use machines

None known.

4.8 Undesirable effects

Rarely, local sensitivity may occur requiring discontinuation of treatment.

Additional adverse drug reactions reported in postmarketing reports with DAKTACORT CREAM but not with DAKTACORT OINTMENT are included in Table 1. The frequencies are based on spontaneous reporting rates, according to the following convention:

Very common ⩾1/10

Common ⩾1/100 and < 1/10

Uncommon ⩾1/1,000 and <1/100

Rare ⩾1/10,000, <1/1,000

Very rare <1/10,000, including isolated reports

Table 1. Adverse Drug Reactions Identified During Postmarketing Experience with Daktacort Cream by Frequency Category Estimated from Spontaneous Reporting Rates

Immune system disorders	
Very rare	Anaphylactic reaction
Skin and Subcutaneous Tissue Disorders	
Very rare Contact	dermatitis, Erythema, Rash

Review of adverse events reported with Daktacort Ointment did not find sufficient evidence to assess any of the events as adverse drug reactions associated with the use of Daktacort Ointment.

4.9 Overdose

Topically applied corticosteroids can be absorbed in sufficient amounts to produce systemic effects. If accidental ingestion of large quantities of the product occurs, an appropriate method of gastric emptying may be used if considered necessary.

5. PHARMACOLOGICAL PROPERTIES

5.1 Pharmacodynamic properties

Miconazole nitrate is a potent broad-spectrum antifungal and antibacterial agent with marked activity against dermatophytes, pathogenic yeasts (eg *Candida* spp) and many Gram-positive bacteria including most strains of *Streptococcus* and *Staphylococcus*.

Hydrocortisone is a widely used topical anti-inflammatory of value in the treatment of inflammatory skin conditions including atrophic and infantile eczema, contact sensitivity reactions and intertrigo.

5.2 Pharmacokinetic properties

Absorption

Miconazole remains in the skin after topical application for up to 4 days. Systemic absorption of miconazole is limited, with a bioavailability of less than 1% following topical application of miconazole. Plasma concentrations of miconazole and/or its metabolites were measurable 24 and 48 hours after application. Approximately 3% of the dose of hydrocortisone is absorbed after application on the skin.

Distribution

Absorbed miconazole is bound to plasma proteins (88.2%) and red blood cells (10.6%). More than 90% of hydrocortisone is bound to plasma proteins.

Metabolism and elimination

The small amount of miconazole that is absorbed is eliminated predominantly in faeces as both unchanged drug and metabolites over a four-day post-administration period. Smaller amounts of unchanged drug and metabolites also appear in urine.

The half-life of hydrocortisone is about 100 minutes. Metabolism takes place in the liver and tissues and the metabolites are excreted with the urine, mostly as glucuronides, together with a very small fraction of unchanged hydrocortisone.

5.3 Preclinical safety data

Not applicable.

6. PHARMACEUTICAL PARTICULARS

6.1 List of excipients

Cream:

PEG-6, PEG-32 and glycol stearate

Oleoyl macroglycerides

Mineral oil

Benzoic acid

Disodium edetate

Butylated hydroxyanisole

Purified water

Ointment:

Polyethylene 5.5%

liquid paraffin gel

6.2 Incompatibilities

None known.

6.3 Shelf life

36 months.

6.4 Special precautions for storage

Cream: Store in a refrigerator (2-8°C).

Ointment: Store at or below 25°C.

6.5 Nature and contents of container

Aluminium tube with polypropylene cap.

Cream: Each tube contains 30 g cream.

Ointment: Each tube contains 30 g ointment.

6.6 Special precautions for disposal and other handling

None.

7. MARKETING AUTHORISATION HOLDER

Janssen-Cilag Ltd

50-100 Holmers Farm Way

High Wycombe

Buckinghamshire

HP12 4EG

UK

8. MARKETING AUTHORISATION NUMBER(S)

Cream: PL 00242/0042

Ointment: PL 00242/0130

9. DATE OF FIRST AUTHORISATION/RENEWAL OF THE AUTHORISATION

Date of First Authorisation:

Cream: 04/02/77

Ointment: 05/03/87

Renewal of Authorisation:

Cream: 24/02/09

Ointment: 28/03/03

10. DATE OF REVISION OF THE TEXT

Cream: 26th March 2009

Ointment: 26th March 2009

Legal category: POM.

Daktarin Cream

(Janssen-Cilag Ltd)

1. NAME OF THE MEDICINAL PRODUCT

Daktarin Cream.

2. QUALITATIVE AND QUANTITATIVE COMPOSITION

Miconazole nitrate 2% w/w.

(Each gram of cream contains 20mg of miconazole nitrate)

For excipients, see Section 6.1

3. PHARMACEUTICAL FORM

Cream

White homogeneous cream.

4. CLINICAL PARTICULARS

4.1 Therapeutic indications

For the treatment of mycotic infections of the skin and nails and superinfections due to Gram-positive bacteria.

4.2 Posology and method of administration

Route of administration:

Cutaneous use.

Recommended dosage:

For all ages:

Skin infections: Apply the cream twice daily to the lesions. Treatment should be prolonged for 10 days after all lesions have disappeared to prevent relapse.

Nail infections: Apply the cream once or twice daily to the lesions. Treatment should be prolonged for 10 days after all lesions have disappeared to prevent relapse.

4.3 Contraindications

Daktarin Cream is contraindicated in individuals with a known hypersensitivity to miconazole or another ingredient in this product.

4.4 Special warnings and precautions for use

Daktarin Cream must not come into contact with the eyes.

If a reaction suggesting sensitivity or irritation should occur, the treatment should be discontinued.

4.5 Interaction with other medicinal products and other forms of interaction

Miconazole administered systemically is known to inhibit CYP3A4/2C9. Due to the limited systemic availability after topical application, clinically relevant interactions are rare. However, in patients on oral anticoagulants, such as warfarin, caution should be exercised and anticoagulant effect should be monitored.

4.6 Pregnancy and lactation

Pregnancy

In animals miconazole nitrate has shown no teratogenic effects but is foetotoxic at high oral doses. Only small amounts of miconazole nitrate are absorbed following topical administration. However, as with other imidazoles, miconazole nitrate should be used with caution during pregnancy.

Lactation

Topically applied miconazole is minimally absorbed into the systemic circulation, and it is not known whether miconazole is excreted in human breast milk. Caution should be exercised when using topically applied miconazole products during lactation.

4.7 Effects on ability to drive and use machines

Not applicable.

4.8 Undesirable effects

Adverse drug reactions from spontaneous reports during the worldwide postmarketing experience with Daktarin that meet threshold criteria are included. The adverse drug reactions are ranked by frequency, using the following convention:

Very common ⩾ 1/10

Common ⩾1/100 and < 1/10

Uncommon ⩾1/1,000 and <1/100

Rare ⩾1/10,000, <1/1,000

Very rare <1/10,000, including isolated reports

The frequencies provided below reflect reporting rates for adverse drug reactions from spontaneous reports, and do not represent more precise estimates of incidence that might be obtained in clinical or epidemiological studies.

Immune system disorders

Very rare: anaphylactic reaction, hypersensitivity, angioneurotic edema

Skin and subcutaneous tissue disorders

Very rare: urticaria, contact dermatitis, rash, erythema, pruritus, skin burning sensation

General disorders and administration site conditions

Rare: application site reactions, including application site irritation

4.9 Overdose

Symptoms

Cutaneous use: Excessive use can result in skin irritation, which usually disappears after discontinuation of therapy.

Treatment

Daktarin Cream is intended for cutaneous use, not for oral use. If accidental ingestion of large quantities of the product occurs, an appropriate method of gastric emptying may be used if considered necessary.

5. PHARMACOLOGICAL PROPERTIES

5.1 Pharmacodynamic properties

Pharmacotherapeutic classification: (Antifungals for dermatological/topical use; imidazole derivative) *ATC code:* D01A C02.

Miconazole nitrate is an imidazole antifungal agent and may act by interfering with the permeability of the fungal cell membrane. It possesses a wide antifungal spectrum and has some antibacterial activity.

5.2 Pharmacokinetic properties

Absorption: There is little absorption through skin or mucous membranes when miconazole nitrate is applied topically.

Distribution: Absorbed miconazole is bound to plasma proteins (88.2%) and red blood cells (10.6%).

Metabolism and Excretion: The small amount of miconazole that is absorbed is eliminated predominantly in faeces as both unchanged drug and metabolites.

5.3 Preclinical safety data

Preclinical data reveal no special hazard for humans based on conventional studies of local irritation, single and repeated dose toxicity, genotoxicity, and toxicity to reproduction.

6. PHARMACEUTICAL PARTICULARS

6.1 List of excipients

PEG-6, PEG-32 and glycol stearate

Oleoyl macroglycerides

Liquid paraffin

Benzoic acid (E210)

Butylated hydroxyanisole (E320)

Purified water

6.2 Incompatibilities

None known.

6.3 Shelf life

24 months.

6.4 Special precautions for storage

Do not store above 25°C.

6.5 Nature and contents of container

Aluminium tube inner lined with heat polymerised epoxy-phenol resin with a white polypropylene cap containing 15 g, 30 g or 70 g* of cream, or aluminium tube inner lined with heat polymerised epoxy-phenol resin with a high density polyethylene cap containing 5 g of cream.

*Not all pack sizes may be marketed

6.6 Special precautions for disposal and other handling

Not applicable.

7. MARKETING AUTHORISATION HOLDER

Janssen-Cilag Ltd,

50-100 Holmers Farm Way

High Wycombe

Buckinghamshire

HP12 4EG

UK

8. MARKETING AUTHORISATION NUMBER(S)

PL 00242/0016

9. DATE OF FIRST AUTHORISATION/RENEWAL OF THE AUTHORISATION

13 May 1974 / 08 December 2008

10. DATE OF REVISION OF THE TEXT

08 December 2008

Daktarin Oral Gel

(Janssen-Cilag Ltd)

1. NAME OF THE MEDICINAL PRODUCT

DAKTARIN® Oral Gel

2. QUALITATIVE AND QUANTITATIVE COMPOSITION

Each gram of Daktarin Oral Gel contains 20 mg of miconazole.

For excipients, see 6.1.

3. PHARMACEUTICAL FORM

Oral gel.

White gel with orange taste.

4. CLINICAL PARTICULARS

4.1 Therapeutic indications

POM

Oral treatment and prevention of fungal infections of the oropharynx and gastrointestinal tract, and of super infections due to Gram-positive bacteria.

P

Oral treatment and prevention of fungal infections of the oropharynx and of superinfections due to Gram-positive bacteria.

4.2 Posology and method of administration

POM only

For oral administration.

Dosage is based on 15 mg/kg/day (0.625 ml/kg/day).

Adults:

1-2 spoonfuls (5-10 ml) of gel four times per day.

Elderly:

As for adults.

Children aged 6 years and over:

One spoonful (5 ml) of gel four times per day.

Children aged 2-6 years:

One spoonful (5 ml) of gel twice per day.

Infants 4 months- 2 years:

Half a spoonful (2.5 ml) of gel twice per day. Each dose should be divided into smaller portions (see section 4.4)

The lower age limit should be increased by 1-2 months for infants who are pre-term, or infants exhibiting slow neuromuscular development.

POM and P

For localised lesions of the mouth, a small amount of gel may be applied directly to the affected area with a clean finger.

For topical treatment of the oropharynx, the gel should be kept in the mouth for as long as possible.

Treatment should be continued for up to 2 days after the symptoms have cleared.

For oral candidosis, dental prostheses should be removed at night and brushed with the gel.

4.3 Contraindications

Known hypersensitivity to miconazole or to any of the excipients.

In infants less than 4 months of age or in those whose swallowing reflex is not yet sufficiently developed.

In patients with liver dysfunction.

Coadministration of the following drugs that are subject to metabolism by CYP3A4: (See Section 4.5 Interactions with Other Medicinal Products and Other Forms of Interaction)

- Substrates known to prolong the QT-interval e.g., astemizole, cisapride, dofetilide, mizolastine, pimozide, quinidine, sertindole and terfenadine
- Ergot alkaloids
- HMG-CoA reductase inhibitors such as simvastatin and lovastatin
- Triazolam and oral midazolam.

4.4 Special warnings and precautions for use

If the concomitant use of Daktarin and anticoagulants is envisaged, the anti-coagulant effect should be carefully monitored and titrated. (see section 4.5)

It is advisable to monitor miconazole and phenytoin levels, if these two drugs are used concomitantly.

In patients using certain oral hypoglycaemics such as sulphonylureas, an enhanced therapeutic effect leading to hypoglycaemia may occur during concomitant treatment with miconazole and appropriate measures should be considered (See Section 4.5 Interactions with Other Medicinal Products and Other Forms of Interaction).

Particularly in infants and young children, caution is required to ensure that the gel does not obstruct the throat. Hence, the gel should not be applied to the back of the throat and each dose should be divided into smaller portions. Observe the patient for possible choking.

The lower age limit should be increased by 1-2 months for infants who are pre-term, or infants exhibiting slow neuromuscular development.

4.5 Interaction with other medicinal products and other forms of interaction

When using any concomitant medication the corresponding label should be consulted for information on the route of metabolism. Miconazole can inhibit the metabolism of drugs metabolised by the CYP3A4 and CYP2C9 enzyme systems. This can result in an increase and/or prolongation of their effects, including adverse effects.:

Oral miconazole is contraindicated with the coadministration of the following drugs that are subject to metabolism by CYP3A4 (See Section 4.3 Contraindications);

- Substrates known to prolong the QT-interval e.g., astemizole, cisapride, dofetilide, mizolastine, pimozide, quinidine, sertindole and terfenadine
- Ergot alkaloids
- HMG-CoA reductase inhibitors such as simvastatin and lovastatin
- Triazolam and oral midazolam

When coadministered with oral miconazole the following drugs should be used with caution because of a possible increase or prolongation of the therapeutic outcome and/or adverse events. If necessary, their dosage should be reduced and, where appropriate, plasma levels monitored:

Drugs subject to metabolism by CYP2C9 (see Section 4.4 Special Warnings and Precautions for Use);

- Oral anticoagulants such as warfarin
- Oral hypoglycaemics such as sulphonylureas
- Phenytoin

Other drugs subject to metabolism by CYP3A4;

- HIV Protease Inhibitors such as saquinavir;
- Certain antineoplastic agents such as vinca alkaloids, busulfan and docetaxel;
- Certain calcium channel blockers such as dihydropyridines and verapamil;
- Certain immunosuppressive agents: cyclosporin, tacrolimus, sirolimus (= rapamycin)
- Others:, carbamazepine, cilostazol, disopyramide, buspirone, alfentanil, sildenafil, alprazolam, brotizolam, midazolam IV, rifabutin, methylprednisolone, trimetrexate, ebastine and reboxetine.

4.6 Pregnancy and lactation

In animals, miconazole has shown no teratogenic effects but is foetotoxic at high oral doses. The significance of this to man is unknown. However, as with other imidazoles, Daktarin Oral Gel should be avoided in pregnant women if possible. The potential hazards should be balanced against the possible benefits.

It is not known whether miconazole is excreted in human milk. Caution should be exercised when prescribing Daktarin Oral Gel to nursing mothers.

4.7 Effects on ability to drive and use machines

Daktarin should not affect alertness or driving ability.

4.8 Undesirable effects

Adverse drug reactions from spontaneous reports during the worldwide postmarketing experience with Daktarin that meet threshold criteria are included in Table 2below. The adverse drug reactions are ranked by frequency, using the following convention:

Very common ⩾1/10

Common ⩾1/100 and <1/10

Uncommon ⩾1/1,000 and <1/100

Rare ⩾1/10,000 and <1/1,000

Very rare <1/10,000, including isolated reports

The frequencies provided below reflect reporting rates for adverse drug reactions from spontaneous reports, and do not represent more precise estimates of incidence that might be obtained in clinical or epidemiological studies.

Immune system disorders

Very rare Allergic conditions, including angioneurotic edema and anaphylactic reactions; Lyell syndrome (Toxic Epidermal Necrolysis), Stevens Johnson syndrome, urticaria, rash

Gastrointestinal system disorders

Very rare Choking (see Section 4.3 Contraindications), nausea*, vomiting* and diarrhoea

Hepatobiliary disorders

Very rare Hepatitis

*Nausea and vomiting were observed commonly during clinical trials.

4.9 Overdose

Symptoms:

In the event of accidental overdose, vomiting and diarrhoea may occur.

Treatment:

Treatment is symptomatic and supportive. A specific antidote is not available.

In the event of accidental ingestion of large quantities of Daktarin an appropriate method of gastic emptying may be used, if considered necessary (See Section 4.5 Interactions with Other Medicinal Products and Other Forms of Interaction.)

5. PHARMACOLOGICAL PROPERTIES

5.1 Pharmacodynamic properties

ATC Code: A01A B09 and A07A C01

Miconazole possesses an antifungal activity against the common dermatophytes and yeasts as well as an antibacterial activity against certain gram-positive bacilli and cocci.

Its activity is based on the inhibition of the ergosterol biosynthesis in fungi and the change in the composition of the lipid components in the membrane, resulting in fungal cell necrosis.

5.2 Pharmacokinetic properties

Absorption:

Miconazole is systemically absorbed after administration as the oral gel. Administration of a 60 mg dose of miconazole as the oral gel results in peak plasma concentrations of 31 to 49 ng/mL, occurring approximately two hours post-dose.

Distribution:

Absorbed miconazole is bound to plasma proteins (88.2%), primarily to serum albumin and red blood cells (10.6%).

Metabolism and Elimination:

The absorbed portion of miconazole is largely metabolized; less than 1% of an administered dose is excreted unchanged in the urine. The terminal half-life of plasma miconazole is 20 to 25 hours in most patients. The elimination half-life of miconazole is similar in renally impaired patients. Plasma concentrations of miconazole are moderately reduced (approximately 50%) during hemodialysis. About 50% of an oral dose may be excreted in the faeces partly metabolized and partly unchanged.

5.3 Preclinical safety data

Preclinical data reveal no special hazard for humans based on conventional studies of local irritation, single and repeated dose toxicity, genotoxicity, and toxicity to reproduction.

6. PHARMACEUTICAL PARTICULARS

6.1 List of excipients

Purified water

Pregelatinised potato starch

Alcohol

Polysorbate 20

Sodium saccharin

Cocoa flavour

Orange flavour

Glycerol

6.2 Incompatibilities

None known.

6.3 Shelf life

3 years.

6.4 Special precautions for storage

Do not Store above 30°C.

6.5 Nature and contents of container
Aluminium tubes containing 5 g*, 15 g*, 40 *g or 80 g gel.

A 5 ml plastic spoon, marked with a 2.5 ml graduation is provided.

* *not marketed*

6.6 Special precautions for disposal and other handling
Not applicable.

Administrative Data

7. MARKETING AUTHORISATION HOLDER
Janssen-Cilag Limited

50-100 Holmers Farm Way

High Wycombe

Buckinghamshire

HP12 4EG

UK

8. MARKETING AUTHORISATION NUMBER(S)
PL 0242/0048

9. DATE OF FIRST AUTHORISATION/RENEWAL OF THE AUTHORISATION
Date of First Authorisation: 19 July 1977

Date of Renewal of Authorisation: 22 September 2002

10. DATE OF REVISION OF THE TEXT
24th September 2008

Legal category POM/P.

External use: Pharmacy Medicine Only.

Other: Prescription Only Medicine.

Dalacin C Capsules 75mg and 150mg

(Pharmacia Limited)

1. NAME OF THE MEDICINAL PRODUCT
Dalacin C Capsules 75 & 150 mg or Clindamycin Hydrochloride Capsules 75 & 150 mg

2. QUALITATIVE AND QUANTITATIVE COMPOSITION
Each capsule contains clindamycin hydrochloride equivalent to 75 &150 mg Clindamycin.

For excipients, see section 6.1

3. PHARMACEUTICAL FORM
Capsule

Hard capsule (Green/White) with markings of 'CLIN 75 & Pfizer'on cap and body.

Hard capsule (white/white) with markings 'CLIN 150 and Pfizer'. On cap and body

4. CLINICAL PARTICULARS

4.1 Therapeutic indications
Antibacterial. Serious infections caused by susceptible Gram-positive organisms, staphylococci (both penicillinase- and non-penicillinase-producing), streptococci (except *Streptococcus faecalis*) and pneumococci. It is also indicated in serious infections caused by susceptible anaerobic pathogens.

Clindamycin does not penetrate the blood/brain barrier in therapeutically effective quantities.

4.2 Posology and method of administration
Oral. Dalacin C Capsules should always be taken with a full glass of water. Absorption of Dalacin C is not appreciably modified by the presence of food.

Adults: Moderately severe infection, 150 - 300 mg every six hours; severe infection, 300 - 450 mg every six hours.

Elderly patients: The half-life, volume of distribution and clearance, and extent of absorption after administration of clindamycin hydrochloride are not altered by increased age. Analysis of data from clinical studies has not revealed any age-related increase in toxicity. Dosage requirements in elderly patients, therefore, should not be influenced by age alone.

Children: 3 - 6 mg/kg every six hours depending on the severity of the infection.

Dosage in Renal /Hepatic Impairment: Clindamycin dosage modification is not necessary in patients with renal or hepatic insufficiency.

Note: In cases of beta-haemolytic streptococcal infection, treatment with Dalacin C should continue for at least 10 days to diminish the likelihood of subsequent rheumatic fever or glomerulonephritis.

4.3 Contraindications
Dalacin C is contra-indicated in patients previously found to be sensitive to clindamycin, lincomycin or to any component of the formulation.

4.4 Special warnings and precautions for use
Warnings: Dalacin C should only be used in the treatment of serious infections. In considering the use of the product, the practitioner should bear in mind the type of infection and the potential hazard of the diarrhoea which may develop, since cases of colitis have been reported during, or even two or three weeks following, the administration of clindamycin.

Studies indicate a toxin(s) produced by clostridia (especially *Clostridium difficile*) is the principal direct cause of antibiotic-associated colitis. These studies also indicate that this toxigenic clostridium is usually sensitive *in vitro* to vancomycin. When 125 mg to 500 mg of vancomycin are administered orally four times a day for 7 - 10 days, there is a rapid observed disappearance of the toxin from faecal samples and a coincident clinical recovery from the diarrhoea. (Where the patient is receiving cholestyramine in addition to vancomycin, consideration should be given to separating the times of administration).

Colitis is a disease which has a clinical spectrum from mild, watery diarrhoea to severe, persistent diarrhoea, leucocytosis, fever, severe abdominal cramps, which may be associated with the passage of blood and mucus. If allowed to progress, it may produce peritonitis, shock and toxic megacolon. This may be fatal.

The appearance of marked diarrhoea should be regarded as an indication that the product should be discontinued immediately. The disease is likely to follow a more severe course in older patients or patients who are debilitated. Diagnosis is usually made by the recognition of the clinical symptoms, but can be substantiated by endoscopic demonstration of pseudomembranous colitis. The presence of the disease may be further confirmed by culture of the stool for *Clostridium difficile* on selective media and assay of the stool specimen for the toxin(s) of *C. difficile*.

Precautions: Caution should be used when prescribing Dalacin C to individuals with a history of gastro-intestinal disease, especially colitis.

Periodic liver and kidney function tests should be carried out during prolonged therapy. Such monitoring is also recommended in neonates and infants.

Prolonged administration of Dalacin C, as with any anti-infective, may result in super-infection due to organisms resistant to clindamycin.

Care should be observed in the use of Dalacin C in atopic individuals.

4.5 Interaction with other medicinal products and other forms of interaction
Clindamycin has been shown to have neuromuscular blocking properties that may enhance the action of other neuromuscular blocking agents. It should be used with caution, therefore, in patients receiving such agents.

Antagonism has been demonstrated between clindamycin and erythromycin *in vitro*. Because of possible clinical significance the two drugs should not be administered concurrently.

4.6 Pregnancy and lactation
Safety for use in pregnancy has not yet been established.

Clindamycin is excreted in human milk. Caution should be exercised when Dalacin C is administered to a nursing mother. It is unlikely that a nursing infant can absorb a significant amount of clindamycin from its gastro-intestinal tract.

4.7 Effects on ability to drive and use machines
The effect of clindamycin on the ability to drive or operate machinery has not been systemically evaluated.

4.8 Undesirable effects
Blood and the Lymphatic System Disorders: Transient neutropenia (leucopenia), eosinophilia, agranulocytosis and thrombocytopenia have been reported. No direct aetiologic relationship to concurrent clindamycin therapy could be made in any of the foregoing.

Immune System Disorders: A few cases of anaphylactoid reactions have been reported.

Gastro-intestinal Disorders: Oesophageal ulcers have been reported as serious adverse events; oesophagitis with oral preparations, nausea, vomiting, abdominal pain and diarrhoea (see Section 4.4 *Special Warnings and Special Precautions for Use, Warnings*).

Hepatobiliary Disorders: Jaundice and abnormalities in liver function tests have been observed during clindamycin therapy.

Skin and Subcutaneous Tissue Disorders: Maculopapular rash and urticaria have been observed during drug therapy. Generalised mild to moderate morbilliform-like skin rashes are the most frequently reported reactions. Rare instances of erythema multiforme, some resembling Stevens-Johnson syndrome, have been associated with clindamycin. Pruritus, vaginitis and rare instances of exfoliative and vesiculobullous dermatitis have been reported. Serious cutaneous adverse reaction (SCAR) and rare cases of toxic epidermal necrolysis have been reported during post-marketing surveillance.

Nervous System Disorders: Frequent cases of Dysgeusia have been observed upon systemic administration of clindamycin using injectables (IM or IV), capsules, or oral granulate solutions, which include a few (non-frequent) serious adverse **events**.

4.9 Overdose
In cases of overdosage no specific treatment is indicated.

The serum biological half-life of clindamycin is 2.4 hours. Clindamycin cannot readily be removed from the blood by dialysis or peritoneal dialysis.

If an allergic adverse reaction occurs, therapy should be with the usual emergency treatments, including corticosteroids, adrenaline and antihistamines.

5. PHARMACOLOGICAL PROPERTIES

5.1 Pharmacodynamic properties
Clindamycin is a lincosamide antibiotic with a primarily bacteriostatic action against Gram-positive aerobes and a wide range of anaerobic bacteria. Most Gram-negative aerobic bacteria, including the Enterobacteriaceae, are resistant to clindamycin. Lincosamides such as clindamycin bind to the 50S subunit of the bacterial ribosome similarly to macrolides such as erythromycin and inhibit the early stages of protein synthesis. The action of clindamycin is predominantly bacteriostatic although high concentrations may be slowly bactericidal against sensitive strains.

5.2 Pharmacokinetic properties
General characteristics of active substance

About 90% of a dose of clindamycin hydrochloride is absorbed from the gastro-intestinal tract; concentrations of 2 to 3 micrograms per ml occur within one hour after a 150 mg dose of clindamycin, with average concentrations of about 0.7 micrograms per ml after 6 hours. After doses of 300 and 600 mg peak plasma concentrations of 4 and 8 micrograms per ml, respectively, have been reported. Absorption is not significantly diminished by food in the stomach but the rate of absorption may be reduced.

Clindamycin is widely distributed in body fluids and tissues, including bone, but it does not reach the csf in significant concentrations. It diffuses across the placenta into the foetal circulation and has been reported to appear in breast milk. High concentrations occur in bile. It accumulates in leucocytes and macrophages. Over 90% of clindamycin in the circulation is bound to plasma proteins. The half-life is 2 to 3 hours, although this may be prolonged in pre-term neonates and patients with severe renal impairment.

Clindamycin undergoes metabolism, presumably in the liver, to the active *N*-demethyl and sulphoxide metabolites, and also some inactive metabolites. About 10% of a dose is excreted in the urine as active drug or metabolites and about 4% in the faeces; the remainder is excreted as inactive metabolites. Excretion is slow, and takes place over several days. It is not effectively removed from the blood by dialysis.

Characteristics in patients

No special characteristics. See section 4.4 "Special warnings and special precautions for use" for further information.

6. PHARMACEUTICAL PARTICULARS

6.1 List of excipients
Lactose

Maize starch

Talc

Magnesium stearate

Capsule shell:

Gelatin

Indigo carmine (E132)

Quinoline yellow (E104)

Capsule cap and body:

Titanium dioxide (E 171)

Printing ink:

Shellac

Soya lecithin

Dimeticone (Antifoam DC 1510)

Black Iron Oxide (E 172)

6.2 Incompatibilities
Not applicable.

6.3 Shelf life
Bottle: 60 months

Blister: 60 months

6.4 Special precautions for storage
Do not store above 25°C.

6.5 Nature and contents of container
Dalacin C Capsules 75 & 150 mg are available in blister packs (aluminium foil/PVC) of 24 capsules and bottle packs (high density polyethylene or amber glass) of 24, 100 or 500 capsules.

Not all pack sizes may be marketed.

6.6 Special precautions for disposal and other handling
None stated.

Administrative Data

7. MARKETING AUTHORISATION HOLDER
Pharmacia Limited

Ramsgate Road

Sandwich, Kent

CT13 9NJ

UK

8. MARKETING AUTHORISATION NUMBER(S)
PL 00032/5006R

PL 00032/5007R

9. DATE OF FIRST AUTHORISATION/RENEWAL OF THE AUTHORISATION
20 February 1989/22nd May 2001/7th August 2009

10. DATE OF REVISION OF THE TEXT
September 2009

Legal category: POM

DA3R_0

Dalacin C Phosphate

(Pharmacia Limited)

1. NAME OF THE MEDICINAL PRODUCT
Dalacin C Phosphate Sterile Solution

2. QUALITATIVE AND QUANTITATIVE COMPOSITION
Each ml of solution contains clindamycin phosphate equivalent to 150 mg clindamycin.

For excipients, see section 6.1.

3. PHARMACEUTICAL FORM
Solution for Injection

Clear, colourless, sterile solution.

4. CLINICAL PARTICULARS
4.1 Therapeutic indications
Antibacterial. Serious infections caused by susceptible Gram-positive organisms, staphylococci (both penicillinase- and non-penicillinase-producing), streptococci (except *Streptococcus faecalis*) and pneumococci. It is also indicated in serious infections caused by susceptible anaerobic pathogens such as *Bacteroides* spp, *Fusobacterium* spp, *Propionibacterium* spp, *Peptostreptococcus* spp. and microaerophilic streptococci.

Clindamycin does not penetrate the blood/brain barrier in therapeutically effective quantities.

4.2 Posology and method of administration
Parenteral (IM or IV administration). Dalacin C Phosphate **must** be diluted prior to IV administration and should be infused over at least 10-60 minutes.

Adults: Serious infections: 600 mg - 1.2 g/day in two, three or four equal doses.

More severe infections: 1.2-2.7 g/day in two, three or four equal doses.

Single IM injections of greater than 600 mg are not recommended nor is administration of more than 1.2 g in a single one-hour infusion.

For more serious infections, these doses may have to be increased. In life-threatening situations, doses as high as 4.8 g daily have been given intravenously to adults.

Alternatively, the drug may be administered in the form of a single rapid infusion of the first dose followed by continuous IV infusion.

Children (over 1 month of age): Serious infections: 15-25 mg/kg/day in three or four equal doses.

More severe infections: 25-40 mg/kg/day in three or four equal doses. In severe infections it is recommended that children be given no less than 300 mg/day regardless of body weight.

Elderly patients: The half-life, volume of distribution and clearance, and extent of absorption after administration of clindamycin phosphate are not altered by increased age. Analysis of data from clinical studies has not revealed any age-related increase in toxicity. Dosage requirements in elderly patients should not be influenced, therefore, by age alone.

Dosage in Renal/Hepatic Impairment: clindamycin dosage modification is not necessary in patients with renal or hepatic insufficiency.

Treatment for infections caused by beta-haemolytic streptococci should be continued for at least 10 days to guard against subsequent rheumatic fever or glomerulonephritis.

The concentration of clindamycin in diluent for infusion should not exceed 18 mg per mL and INFUSION RATES SHOULD NOT EXCEED 30 MG PER MINUTE. The usual infusion rates are as follows:

Dose	Diluent	Time
300 mg	50 mL	10 min
600 mg	50 mL	20 min
900 mg	50-100 mL	30 min
1200 mg	100 mL	40 min

4.3 Contraindications
Dalacin C Phosphate is contra-indicated in patients previously found to be sensitive to clindamycin, lincomycin or to any component of the formulation.

4.4 Special warnings and precautions for use
Warnings

This product contains benzyl alcohol. Benzyl alcohol has been reported to be associated with a fatal "Gasping syndrome" in premature infants.

Dalacin C Phosphate should only be used in the treatment of serious infections. In considering the use of the product, the practitioner should bear in mind the type of infection and the potential hazard of the diarrhoea which may develop, since cases of colitis have been reported during, or even two or three weeks following, the administration of clindamycin.

Studies indicate a toxin(s) produced by clostridia (especially *Clostridium difficile*) is the principal direct cause of antibiotic-associated colitis. These studies also indicate that this toxigenic clostridium is usually sensitive *in vitro* to vancomycin. When 125 mg to 500 mg of vancomycin are administered orally four times a day for 7 - 10 days, there is a rapid observed disappearance of the toxin from faecal samples and a coincident clinical recovery from the diarrhoea. (Where the patient is receiving colestyramine in addition to vancomycin, consideration should be given to separating the times of administration).

Colitis is a disease, which has a clinical spectrum from mild, watery diarrhoea to severe, persistent diarrhoea, leucocytosis, fever, severe abdominal cramps, which may be associated with the passage of blood and mucus. If allowed to progress, it may produce peritonitis, shock and toxic megacolon. This may be fatal. The appearance of marked diarrhoea should be regarded as an indication that the product should be discontinued immediately. The disease is likely to follow a more severe course in older patients or patients who are debilitated. Diagnosis is usually made by the recognition of the clinical symptoms, but can be substantiated by endoscopic demonstration of pseudomembranous colitis. The presence of the disease may be further confirmed by culture of the stool for *C. difficile* on selective media and assay of the stool specimen for the toxin(s) of *C. difficile*.

Precautions

Caution should be used when prescribing Dalacin C Phosphate to individuals with a history of gastro-intestinal disease, especially colitis.

Periodic liver and kidney function tests should be carried out during prolonged therapy. Such monitoring is also recommended in neonates and infants. Safety and appropriate dosage in infants less than one month old have not been established.

Prolonged administration of Dalacin C Phosphate, as with any anti-infective, may result in super-infection due to organisms resistant to clindamycin.

Care should be observed in the use of Dalacin C Phosphate in atopic individuals.

4.5 Interaction with other medicinal products and other forms of interaction
Clindamycin has been shown to have neuromuscular blocking properties that may enhance the action of other neuromuscular blocking agents. It should be used with caution, therefore, in patients receiving such agents.

Antagonism has been demonstrated between clindamycin and erythromycin *in vitro*. Because of possible clinical significance, the two drugs should not be administered concurrently.

4.6 Pregnancy and lactation
Safety for use in pregnancy has not been established.

Clindamycin is excreted in human milk. Caution should be exercised when Dalacin C Phosphate is administered to a nursing mother. It is unlikely that a nursing infant can absorb a significant amount of clindamycin from its gastro-intestinal tract.

4.7 Effects on ability to drive and use machines
The effect of clindamycin on the ability to drive or operate machinery has not been systematically evaluated.

4.8 Undesirable effects
Gastro-intestinal Disorders: Oesophageal ulcers have been reported as serious adverse events during postmarketing surveillance and oesophagitis with oral preparations, nausea, vomiting, abdominal pain and diarrhoea (See Section 4.4 Special Warnings and Special Precautions for Use: *Warnings*).

Blood and Lymphatic System Disorders: Transient neutropenia (leucopenia), eosinophilia, agranulocytosis and thrombocytopenia have been reported. No direct aetiologic relationship to concurrent clindamycin therapy could be made in any of the foregoing.

Immune System Disorders: A few cases of anaphylactoid reactions have been reported.

Skin and Subcutaneous Tissue Disorders: Maculopapular rash and urticaria have been observed during drug therapy. Generalised mild to moderate morbilliform-like skin rashes are the most frequently reported reactions. Rare instances of erythema multiforme, some resembling Stevens-Johnson syndrome, have been associated with clindamycin. Pruritus, vaginitis and rare instances of exfoliative and vesiculobullous dermatitis have been reported. Serious cutaneous adverse reaction (SCAR) and rare cases of toxic epidermal necrolysis have been reported during postmarketing surveillance.

Hepatobiliary disorders: Jaundice and abnormalities in liver function tests have been observed during clindamycin therapy.

Cardiac Disorders: Rare instances of cardiopulmonary arrest and hypotension have been reported following too rapid intravenous administration. (See Section 4.2 Posology and Method of Administration)

Nervous System Disorders: Frequent cases of Dysgeusia have been observed upon systemic administration of clindamycin using injectables (IM or IV), capsules, or oral granulate solutions, which include a few (non-frequent) serious adverse events.

General Disorders and Administration Site Conditions: Local irritation, pain, abscess formation have been observed in conjunction with IM injection. These reactions can be minimized by deep IM injection and avoiding the use of an indwelling catheter.

Thrombophlebitis has been reported with IV injection.

4.9 Overdose
In cases of overdosage no specific treatment is indicated.

The serum biological half-life of lincomycin is 2.4 hours. Clindamycin cannot readily be removed from the blood by dialysis or peritoneal dialysis.

If an allergic adverse reaction occurs, therapy should be with the usual emergency treatments, including corticosteroids, adrenaline and antihistamines.

5. PHARMACOLOGICAL PROPERTIES
5.1 Pharmacodynamic properties
Clindamycin is a lincosamide antibiotic with a primarily bacteriostatic action against Gram-positive aerobes and a wide range of anaerobic bacteria. Lincosamides such as clindamycin bind to the 50S subunit of the bacterial ribosome similarly to macrolides such as erythromycin and inhibit the early stages of protein synthesis. The action of clindamycin is predominantly bacteriostatic although high concentrations may be slowly bactericidal against sensitive strains.

Most Gram-negative aerobic bacteria, including the Enterobacteriaceae, are resistant to clindamycin. Clindamycin demonstrates cross-resistance with lincomycin. When tested by *in vitro* methods, some staphylococcal strains originally resistant to erythromycin rapidly developed resistance to clindamycin. The mechanisms for resistance are the same as for erythromycin, namely methylation of the ribosomal binding site, chromosomal mutation of the ribosomal protein and in a few staphylococcal isolates enzymatic inactivation by a plasmid-mediated adenyltransferase.

5.2 Pharmacokinetic properties
General characteristics of active substance

Following parenteral administration, the biologically inactive clindamycin phosphate is hydrolysed to clindamycin. When the equivalent of 300 mg of clindamycin is injected intramuscularly, a mean peak plasma concentration of 6 microgram/ml is achieved within three hours; 600 mg gives a peak concentration of 9 microgram/ml. In children, peak concentration may be reached within one hour. When the same doses are infused intravenously, peak concentrations of 7 and 10 micrograms per ml respectively are achieved by the end of infusion.

Clindamycin is widely distributed in body fluids and tissues, including bone, but it does not reach the cerebrospinal fluid in significant concentrations. It diffuses across the placenta into the foetal circulation and appears in breast milk. High concentrations occur in bile. It accumulates in leucocytes and macrophages. Over 90% of clindamycin in the circulation is bound to plasma proteins. The half-life is 2 to 3 hours, although this may be prolonged in pre-term neonates and patients with severe renal impairment.

Clindamycin undergoes metabolism, to the active *N*-demethyl and sulphoxide metabolites and also some inactive metabolites. About 10% of the drug is excreted in the urine as active drug or metabolites and about 4% in the faeces; the remainder is excreted as inactive metabolites. Excretion is slow and takes place over several days. It is not effectively removed from the blood by dialysis.

Characteristics in patients

No special characteristics. See section 4.4 "**Special warnings and special precautions for use**" for further information.

6. PHARMACEUTICAL PARTICULARS
6.1 List of excipients
Benzyl alcohol

Disodium edetate

Sterilised water for injections

6.2 Incompatibilities
Solutions of clindamycin salts have a low pH and incompatibilities may reasonably be expected with alkaline preparations or drugs unstable at low pH. Incompatibility has been reported with: ampicillin sodium, aminophylline, barbiturates, calcium gluconate, ceftriaxone sodium, ciprofloxacin, diphenylhydantoin, idarubicin hydrochloride, magnesium sulphate, phenytoin sodium and ranitidine hydrochloride.

6.3 Shelf life
24 months

6.4 Special precautions for storage
Do not store above 25°C. Do not refrigerate or freeze.

6.5 Nature and contents of container
Type 1 flint glass ampoule containing 2 ml or 4 ml sterile, aqueous solution, packed in cardboard carton, together with a leaflet.

6.6 Special precautions for disposal and other handling
Dalacin C Phosphate has been shown to be physically and chemically compatible for at least 24 hours in dextrose 5% water and sodium chloride injection solutions containing the following antibiotics in usually administered concentrations: Amikacin sulphate, aztreonam, cefamandole nafate,

cephazolin sodium, cefotaxime sodium, cefoxitin sodium, ceftazidime sodium, ceftizoxime sodium, gentamicin sulphate, netilmicin sulphate, piperacillin and tobramycin.

The compatibility and duration of stability of drug admixtures will vary depending upon concentration and other conditions.

7. MARKETING AUTHORISATION HOLDER
Pharmacia Limited
Ramsgate Road
Sandwich, Kent
CT13 9NJ
UK

8. MARKETING AUTHORISATION NUMBER(S)
PL 00032/0042R

9. DATE OF FIRST AUTHORISATION/RENEWAL OF THE AUTHORISATION
27th December 1997 / 22nd May 2002/7th August 2009

10. DATE OF REVISION OF THE TEXT
September 2009

Legal category: POM

DA3R_0

Dalacin Cream 2%

(Pharmacia Limited)

1. NAME OF THE MEDICINAL PRODUCT
Dalacin Cream 2%.

2. QUALITATIVE AND QUANTITATIVE COMPOSITION
Each gram of cream contains clindamycin phosphate equivalent to 20 mg or 2.0% w/w clindamycin.

For Excipients, see section 6.1

3. PHARMACEUTICAL FORM
Cream
White, semi-solid.

4. CLINICAL PARTICULARS

4.1 Therapeutic indications
Antibiotic for the treatment of bacterial vaginosis.

4.2 Posology and method of administration
One applicator full (approximately 5 grams) intravaginally at bedtime for 7 consecutive days.

In patients in whom a shorter treatment course is desirable, a 3 day regimen has been shown to be effective.

Children and the elderly: No clinical studies have been conducted in populations younger than 15 or older than 60. Dalacin Cream is not recommended in children under 12 years of age.

4.3 Contraindications
Dalacin Cream is contra-indicated in patients previously found to be hypersensitive to preparations containing clindamycin or any of the components of the cream base (see "Presentation"). Although cross-sensitisation to lincomycin has not been demonstrated, it is recommended that Dalacin Cream should not be used in patients who have demonstrated lincomycin sensitivity. Dalacin Cream 2% is also contraindicated individuals with a history of inflammatory bowel disease or a history of antibiotic-associated colitis.

4.4 Special warnings and precautions for use
As there are no data available on the use of Dalacin Cream in patients younger than 12 years of age, it should not be used in this population. The use of clindamycin may result in the overgrowth of non-susceptible organisms, particularly yeasts.

Virtually all antibiotics have been associated with diarrhoea and in some cases pseudomembranous colitis. Therefore, even though only a minimal amount of drug is absorbed, if significant diarrhoea occurs, the drug should be discontinued and appropriate diagnostic procedures and treatment provided as necessary.

Dalacin Cream contains oil-based components. Some of these have been shown to weaken the rubber of condoms and diaphragms and make them less effective as a barrier method of contraception or as protection from sexually transmitted disease, including AIDS. Do not rely on condoms and diaphragms when using Dalacin Cream.

4.5 Interaction with other medicinal products and other forms of interaction
Cross resistance has been demonstrated between clindamycin and lincomycin, and erythromycin and clindamycin. Antagonism has been demonstrated between clindamycin and erythromycin *in vitro*.

Clindamycin has been shown to have neuromuscular blocking properties that may enhance the action of other neuromuscular blocking agents. Therefore, it should be used with caution in patients receiving such agents.

No information is available on concomitant use with other intravaginal products, which is not recommended.

4.6 Pregnancy and lactation
Pregnancy
Reproduction studies have been performed in rats and mice using subcutaneous and oral doses of clindamycin ranging from 20 to 600 mg/kg/day and have revealed no evidence of impaired fertility or harm to the foetus due to clindamycin. In one mouse strain, cleft palates were observed in treated foetuses; this response was not produced in other mouse strains or in other species, and is therefore considered to be a strain specific effect.

There are no adequate and well-controlled studies in pregnant women during their first trimester, and because animal reproduction studies are not always predictive of human response, this drug should be used during the first trimester of pregnancy only if clearly needed. In a clinical trial in pregnant women during the second trimester, Dalacin Cream was effective in treating bacterial vaginosis, and no drug-related medical events were reported in the neonates. However, as with any drug used during pregnancy, a careful risk-benefit assessment should take place beforehand.

Lactation
It is not known if clindamycin is excreted in breast milk following the use of vaginally administered clindamycin phosphate. However, orally and parenterally administered clindamycin has been reported to appear in breast milk. Therefore, a full assessment of benefit-risk should be made when consideration is given to using vaginal clindamycin phosphate in a nursing mother.

4.7 Effects on ability to drive and use machines
Not applicable.

4.8 Undesirable effects
In clinical trials medical events judged to be related, probably related, or possibly related to vaginally administered clindamycin phosphate cream were reported for (24%) of patients as indicated below:

Genital tract:	cervicitis/vaginitis (14%); vulvo-vaginal irritation (6%).
Central nervous system:	dizziness, headache, vertigo.
Gastro-intestinal:	heartburn, nausea, vomiting, diarrhoea, constipation, abdominal pain.
Dermatological:	rash, exanthema.
Hypersensitivity:	urticaria.

(Events without percentages were reported by less than 1% of the patients.)

4.9 Overdose
Vaginally applied clindamycin phosphate vaginal cream 2% can be absorbed in sufficient amounts to produce systemic effects.

5. PHARMACOLOGICAL PROPERTIES

5.1 Pharmacodynamic properties
Clindamycin is an antimicrobial agent which has been shown to be effective in the treatment of infection caused by susceptible anaerobic bacteria or susceptible strains of Gram positive aerobic bacteria. It has been shown to have *in-vitro* activity against the following organisms which are associated with bacterial vaginosis:

Gardnerella vaginalis;
Mobiluncus spp;
Bacteroides spp;
Mycoplasma hominis;
Peptostreptococcus spp.

5.2 Pharmacokinetic properties
Following once a day dosing of 100 mg of vaginally administered clindamycin phosphate, at a concentration equivalent to 20 mg of clindamycin per gram of cream, peak serum clindamycin levels average 20 nanograms/ml (range 3-93 nanograms/ml in normal volunteers. Approximately 3% (range 0.1-7%) of the administered dose is absorbed systematically.

In women with bacterial vaginosis, the amount of clindamycin absorbed following vaginal administration of 100 mg of Dalacin Cream (20 mg/g) is 4% (range 0.8-8%), which is approximately the same as in normal women.

Characteristics in patients
No special characteristics. See section 4.4 **"Special warnings and special precautions for use"** for further information.

6. PHARMACEUTICAL PARTICULARS

6.1 List of excipients
Sorbitan stearate
polysorbate 60
propylene glycol
stearic acid
cetostearyl alcohol
cetyl palmitate
liquid paraffin
benzyl alcohol
water.

6.2 Incompatibilities
Not applicable.

6.3 Shelf life
2 years

6.4 Special precautions for storage
Do not store above 25°C. Do not freeze.

6.5 Nature and contents of container
Laminate tube (consisting of LMDPE and aluminium foil) with polypropylene cap containing 7.8 g, 20 g or 40 g cream, packed in cardboard carton, together with a leaflet.

Not all pack sizes may be marketed.

6.6 Special precautions for disposal and other handling
None

Administrative Data

7. MARKETING AUTHORISATION HOLDER
Pharmacia Limited
Ramsgate Road
Sandwich Kent
CT13 9NJ
United Kingdom

8. MARKETING AUTHORISATION NUMBER(S)
PL 0032/0176

9. DATE OF FIRST AUTHORISATION/RENEWAL OF THE AUTHORISATION
Date of first authorisation: 27 April 1993 / Renewal 21st May 2001/ 7th August 2009

10. DATE OF REVISION OF THE TEXT
September 2009

Legal category
POM

DA4_0

Dalacin T Topical Lotion or Clindamycin Phosphate Topical Lotion

(Pharmacia Limited)

1. NAME OF THE MEDICINAL PRODUCT
Dalacin T Topical Lotion
Clindamycin Phosphate Topical Lotion

2. QUALITATIVE AND QUANTITATIVE COMPOSITION
One ml of Dalacin T Topical Lotion contains the equivalent of 10mg clindamycin.

For excipients see Section 6.1 ('List of excipients').

3. PHARMACEUTICAL FORM
Topical Emulsion.

White to off-white aqueous emulsion.

4. CLINICAL PARTICULARS

4.1 Therapeutic indications
Dalacin T Topical is indicated for the treatment of acne vulgaris.

4.2 Posology and method of administration
Apply a thin film of Dalacin T Topical Lotion twice daily to the affected area.

4.3 Contraindications
Topical clindamycin is contraindicated in individuals with a history of hypersensitivity to clindamycin or lincomycin. Clindamycin topical is contraindicated in individuals with a history of inflammatory bowel disease or a history of antibiotic-associated colitis.

4.4 Special warnings and precautions for use
Oral and parenteral clindamycin, as well as most other antibiotics, have been associated with severe pseudomembranous colitis. However, post-marketing studies have indicated a very low incidence of colitis with Dalacin T Solution. The physician should, nonetheless, be alert to the development of antibiotic-associated diarrhoea or colitis. If diarrhoea occurs, the product should be discontinued immediately.

Diarrhea, colitis, and pseudomembranous colitis have been observed to begin up to several weeks following cessation of oral and parenteral therapy with clindamycin.

Studies indicate a toxin(s) produced by *Clostridium difficile* is the major cause of antibiotic-associated colitis. Colitis is usually characterized by persistent, severe diarrhoea and abdominal cramps. Endoscopic examination may reveal pseudomembranous colitis. Stool culture for *C. difficile* and/or assay for *C. difficile* toxin may be helpful to diagnosis.

Vancomycin is effective in the treatment of antibiotic-associated colitis produced by *C. difficile*. The usual dose is 125 - 500 mg orally every 6 hours for 7 - 10 days. Additional supportive medical care may be necessary.

Mild cases of colitis may respond to discontinuance of clindamycin alone. Colestyramine and colestipol resins have been shown to bind *C. difficile* toxin *in vitro*, and cholestyramine has been effective in the treatment of some mild cases of antibiotic-associated colitis. Colestyramine resins have been shown to bind vancomycin; therefore, when both colestyramine and vancomycin are used concurrently, their administration should be separated by at least two hours.

The lotion has an unpleasant taste and caution should be exercised when applying medication around the mouth.

Topical clindamycin should be prescribed with caution to atopic individuals.

4.5 Interaction with other medicinal products and other forms of interaction

Clindamycin has been shown to have neuromuscular blocking properties that may enhance the action of other neuromuscular blocking agents. Therefore, it should be used with caution in patients receiving such agents.

4.6 Pregnancy and lactation

Reproduction studies have been performed in rats and mice using subcutaneous and oral doses of clindamycin ranging from 100 to 600 mg/kg/day and have revealed no evidence of impaired fertility or harm to the foetus due to clindamycin. There are, however, no adequate and well-controlled studies in pregnant women. Because animal reproduction studies are not always predictive of human response, this drug should be used during pregnancy only if clearly needed.

It is not known whether clindamycin is excreted in human milk following use of Dalacin T Topical Lotion. However, orally and parenterally administered clindamycin has been reported to appear in breast milk. As a general rule, breast-feeding should not be undertaken while a patient is on a drug since many drugs are excreted in human milk.

4.7 Effects on ability to drive and use machines

None.

4.8 Undesirable effects

Skin dryness is the most common adverse reaction seen with the solution. In addition, the following adverse effects have been reported with the use of topical clindamycin.

Eye disorders: stinging of the eye

Gastrointestinal disorders: abdominal pain, gastrointestinal disturbances

Infections and infestations: gram-negative folliculitis

Skin and subcutaneous skin disorders: skin irritation, contact dermatitis, skin oiliness, urticaria

4.9 Overdose

Topically applied clindamycin can be absorbed in sufficient amounts to produce systemic effects.

5. PHARMACOLOGICAL PROPERTIES

Anti-infectives for treatment of acne. D10A F

5.1 Pharmacodynamic properties

The active constituent, clindamycin, is a known antibiotic. When applied topically it is found in comedone samples at sufficient levels to be active against most strains of *P. acnes*.

5.2 Pharmacokinetic properties

When applied topically in an alcoholic solution, clindamycin has been shown to be absorbed from the skin in small amounts. Very low levels, more than 1,000 times lower than those from normal systemic doses of clindamycin, have been found in the plasma. Using a sensitive RIA method, clindamycin has been detected in the urine at levels of < 1 to 53 ng/ml, 0.15-0.25% of the cumulative dose being recovered from the urine. No clindamycin has been detected in the serum following topical application.

5.3 Preclinical safety data

None stated.

6. PHARMACEUTICAL PARTICULARS

6.1 List of excipients

Glycerol,

sodium lauroyl sarcosinate,

stearic acid,

tegin,

cetostearyl alcohol,

isostearyl alcohol,

methylparaben,

purified water.

6.2 Incompatibilities

None.

6.3 Shelf life

36 months.

6.4 Special precautions for storage

Do not store above 25°C.

6.5 Nature and contents of container

HDPE/LDPE bottles and polypropylene cap containing, 15 ml, 30 ml and 60 ml of Dalacin T Topical lotion and HDPE bottle, polypropylene roller-ball and cap containing 15 ml, 30 ml and 50 ml of Dalacin Topical Lotion.

Only the 30 ml and 50 ml packs are marketed in the UK.

6.6 Special precautions for disposal and other handling

None.

7. MARKETING AUTHORISATION HOLDER

Pharmacia Limited

Ramsgate Road

Sandwich Kent

CT13 9NJ

United Kingdom

8. MARKETING AUTHORISATION NUMBER(S)

PL 00032/0156

9. DATE OF FIRST AUTHORISATION/RENEWAL OF THE AUTHORISATION

18th September 1990/21st May 2001/ 7th August 2009

10. DATE OF REVISION OF THE TEXT

September 2009

11. LEGAL CATEGORY

POM

DA4_0

Dalacin T Topical Solution

(Pharmacia Limited)

1. NAME OF THE MEDICINAL PRODUCT

Dalacin® T Topical Solution

Clindamycin Phosphate Topical Solution.

2. QUALITATIVE AND QUANTITATIVE COMPOSITION

One ml of Dalacin T Topical Solution contains the equivalent of 10 mg Clindamycin.

For excipients see Section 6.1 ('List of excipients').

3. PHARMACEUTICAL FORM

Topical solution.

Clear colourless aqueous solution.

4. CLINICAL PARTICULARS

4.1 Therapeutic indications

Dalacin T Topical Solution is indicated in the treatment of acne vulgaris

4.2 Posology and method of administration

Apply a thin film of Dalacin T Topical Solution twice daily to the affected area.

4.3 Contraindications

Topical clindamycin is contraindicated in individuals with a history of hypersensitivity to clindamycin or lincomycin. Clindamycin topical is contraindicated in individuals with a history of inflammatory bowel disease or a history of antibiotic-associated colitis.

4.4 Special warnings and precautions for use

Products containing benzoyl peroxide should not be used concurrently with Dalacin T Topical Solution.

Oral and parenteral clindamycin, as well as most other antibiotics, have been associated with severe pseudo-membranous colitis. Post-marketing studies, however, have indicated a very low incidence of colitis with Dalacin T Topical Solution. The physician should, nonetheless, be alert to the development of antibiotic associated diarrhoea or colitis. If significant or prolonged diarrhoea occurs, the product should be discontinued immediately.

Diarrhoea, colitis, and pseudomembranous colitis have been observed to begin up to several weeks following cessation of oral and parenteral therapy with clindamycin.

Studies indicate a toxin(s) produced by *Clostridium difficile* is the major cause of antibiotic associated colitis. Colitis is usually characterised by persistent, severe diarrhoea and abdominal cramps. Endoscopic examination may reveal pseudomembranous colitis. Stool culture for *C. difficile* and/or assay for *C. difficile* toxin may be helpful to diagnosis.

Vancomycin is effective in the treatment of antibiotic-associated colitis produced by *C. difficile*. The usual dose is 125-500 mg orally every 6 hours for 7-10 days. Additional supportive medical care may be necessary.

Mild cases of colitis may respond to discontinuance of clindamycin alone. Colestyramine and colestipol resins have been shown to bind *C. difficile* toxin *in vitro*, and colestyramine has been effective in the treatment of some mild cases of antibiotic-associated colitis. Colestyramine resins have been shown to bind vancomycin; therefore, when both colestyramine and vancomycin are used concurrently, their administration should be separated by at least two hours.

Dalacin T Topical Solution contains an alcohol base which can cause burning and irritation of the eye. In the event of accidental contact with sensitive surfaces (eye, abraded skin, mucous membranes), bathe with copious amounts of cool tap water. The solution has an unpleasant taste and caution should be exercised when applying medication around the mouth.

Topical clindamycin should be prescribed with caution to atopic individuals.

4.5 Interaction with other medicinal products and other forms of interaction

Clindamycin has been shown to have neuromuscular blocking properties that may enhance the action of other neuromuscular blocking agents. Therefore, it should be used with caution in patients receiving such agents.

4.6 Pregnancy and lactation

Reproduction studies have been performed in rats and mice using subcutaneous and oral doses of clindamycin ranging from 100 to 600 mg/kg/day and have revealed no evidence of impaired fertility or harm to the foetus due to clindamycin. There are, however, no adequate and well-controlled studies in pregnant women. Because animal reproduction studies are not always predictive of human response, this drug should be used during pregnancy only if clearly needed.

It is not known whether clindamycin is excreted in human milk following use of Dalacin T Topical Solution. However, orally and parenterally administered clindamycin has been reported to appear in breast milk. As a general rule, breast-feeding should not be undertaken while a patient is on a drug since many drugs are excreted in human milk.

4.7 Effects on ability to drive and use machines

Not applicable.

4.8 Undesirable effects

Skin dryness is the most common adverse reaction seen with the solution. In addition, the following adverse effects have been reported with the use of topical clindamycin.

Eye disorders: stinging of the eye

Gastrointestinal disorders: abdominal pain, gastrointestinal disturbances

Infections and infestations: gram-negative folliculitis

Skin and subcutaneous skin disorders: skin irritation, contact dermatitis, skin oiliness, urticaria

4.9 Overdose

Topically applied clindamycin can be absorbed in sufficient amounts to produce systemic effects.

5. PHARMACOLOGICAL PROPERTIES

Anti-infectives for treatment of acne. D10A F

5.1 Pharmacodynamic properties

The active constituent, clindamycin, is a known antibiotic. When applied topically it is found in comedone samples at sufficient levels to be active against most strains of *Propionibacterium acnes*.

5.2 Pharmacokinetic properties

When applied topically, clindamycin has been shown to be absorbed from the skin in small amounts.

Very low levels, more than 1000 times lower than those from normal systemic doses of clindamycin, have been found in the plasma. Using a sensitive RIA method clindamycin has been detected in the urine at levels of < 1 to 53 nanograms/ml, 0.15 - 0.25% of the cumulative dose being recovered from the urine. No clindamycin has been detected in the serum following topical applications.

5.3 Preclinical safety data

No further pre-clinical safety data are available.

6. PHARMACEUTICAL PARTICULARS

6.1 List of excipients

Isopropyl alcohol

Propylene glycol

Purified water

Hydrochloric acid (10%)

Sodium hydroxide (10%)

6.2 Incompatibilities

Not applicable.

6.3 Shelf life

24 months.

6.4 Special precautions for storage

Store below 25°C

6.5 Nature and contents of container

Bottle - White high density polyethylene bottle containing 30 ml, 50 ml or 60 ml

Cap– Prolypropylene, linerless screw caps

Or

Prolypropylene, screw cap with polyvinylidene chloride film liner

Applicator– Low-density polyethylene applicator made by Dab-O-Matic

6.6 Special precautions for disposal and other handling

None

7. MARKETING AUTHORISATION HOLDER

Pharmacia Limited

Ramsgate Road

Sandwich Kent

CT13 9NJ

United Kingdom

8. MARKETING AUTHORISATION NUMBER(S)

PL 0032/0135

9. DATE OF FIRST AUTHORISATION/RENEWAL OF THE AUTHORISATION

Date of first authorisation: 18 January 1988

Date of renewal of authorisation: 22nd May 2001

Date of renewal of authorisation: 7th August 2009

10. DATE OF REVISION OF THE TEXT

September 2009

LEGAL CATEGORY

POM

DA5_0

Danol 100mg Capsules, Danol 200mg Capsules

(sanofi-aventis)

1. NAME OF THE MEDICINAL PRODUCT

Danol 100mg Capsules

Danol 200mg Capsules

2. QUALITATIVE AND QUANTITATIVE COMPOSITION

Danazol 100mg

Danazol 200mg

For excipients see 6.1

3. PHARMACEUTICAL FORM

Capsule

4. CLINICAL PARTICULARS

4.1 Therapeutic indications

Danol capsules are recommended for the treatment of:

Endometriosis: treatment of endometriosis-associated symptoms or/and to reduce the extent of endometriosis foci. Danazol may be used either in conjunction with surgery or, as sole hormonal therapy, in patients not responding to other treatments.

Benign fibrocystic breast disease: symptomatic relief of severe pain and tenderness. Danazol should be used only in patients not responsive to other therapeutic measures or for whom such measures are inadvisable.

4.2 Posology and method of administration

Adults:

Danol capsules should be given as a continuous course, dosage being adjusted according to the severity of the condition and the patient's response. A reduction in dosage once a satisfactory response has been achieved may prove possible. In fertile females, Danol capsules should be started during menstruation, preferably on the first day, to avoid exposing a pregnancy to its possible effects. Where doubt exists, appropriate checks should be made to exclude pregnancy before starting medication. Females of child-bearing age should employ non-hormonal contraception throughout the course of treatment.

In endometriosis the recommended dosage is 200mg to 800mg daily in a course of treatment lasting normally three to six months. Dosage should be increased if normal cyclical bleeding still persists after two months therapy, a higher dosage (not exceeding 800mg per day) may also be needed for severe disease.

In benign fibrocystic breast disease, treatment should commence at a dose of 300mg daily, a course of treatment normally lasting 3 to 6 months.

Elderly: Danol is not recommended.

Children: Danol is not recommended.

The capsules are for oral administration.

4.3 Contraindications

1. Pregnancy
2. Breast feeding
3. Markedly impaired hepatic, renal or cardiac function
4. Porphyria
5. Active thrombosis or thromboembolic disease and a history of such events
6. Androgen dependent tumour
7. Undiagnosed abnormal genital bleeding.

4.4 Special warnings and precautions for use

4.4.1 Special warnings

In the event of virilisation, Danol should be withdrawn. Androgenic reactions generally prove reversible, but continued use of Danol after evidence of androgenic virilisation increases the risk of irreversible androgenic effects.

Danol should be stopped if any clinically significant adverse event arises, and particularly if there is evidence of papilloedema, headache, visual disturbances or other signs or symptoms of raised intracranial pressure, jaundice or other indication of significant hepatic disturbance, thrombosis or thromboembolism.

Whilst a course of therapy may need to be repeated, care should be observed as no safety data are available in relation to repeated courses of treatment over time. The long-term risk of 17-alkylated steroids (including benign hepatic adenomata, peliosis hepatis and hepatic carcinoma), should be considered when danazol, which is chemically related to those compounds, is used.

Data, from two case-control epidemiological studies, were pooled to examine the relationship between endometriosis, endometriosis treatments and ovarian cancer. These preliminary results suggest that the use of danazol might increase the baseline risk of ovarian cancer in - patients treated for endometriosis.

Patients with rare hereditary problems of galactose intolerance, the Lapp lactase deficiency or glucose-galactose malabsorption should not take this medicine.

4.4.2 Precautions

In view of its pharmacology, known interactions and side effects, particular care should be observed when using Danol in patients with hepatic or renal disease, hypertension or other cardiovascular disease and in any state which may be exacerbated by fluid retention as well as in diabetes mellitus, polycythaemia, epilepsy, lipoprotein disorder, and in those who have shown marked or persistent androgenic reaction to previous gonadal steroid therapy.

Caution is advised in patients with migraine.

Until more is known, caution is advised in the use of Danol in the presence of known or suspected malignant disease (see also contra-indications). Before treatment initiation, the presence of hormone-dependent carcinoma should be excluded at least by careful clinical examination, as well as if breast nodules persist or enlarge during danazol treatment.

In addition to clinical monitoring in all patients, appropriate laboratory monitoring should be considered which may include periodic measurement of hepatic function and haematological state. For long-term treatment (> 6 months) or repeated courses of treatment, biannual hepatic ultrasonography is recommended.

Danazol should be initiated during menstruation. An effective, non-hormonal method of contraception should be employed (see Section 4.2 and 4.6 Pregnancy and Lactation).

The lowest effective dose of Danol should always be sought.

4.5 Interaction with other medicinal products and other forms of interaction

Anti-convulsant therapy: Danol may affect the plasma level of carbamazepine and possibly the patient's response to this agent and to phenytoin. With phenobarbital it is likely that similar interaction would occur.

Anti-diabetic therapy: Danol can cause insulin resistance.

Oral anti-coagulant therapy: Danol can potentiate the action of warfarin.

Anti-hypertensive therapy: Possibly through promotion of fluid retention, Danol can oppose the action of anti-hypertensive agents.

Ciclosporin and tacrolimus: Danol can increase the plasma level of ciclosporin and tacrolimus, leading to an increase of the renal toxicity of these drugs.

Concomitant steroids: Although specific instances have not been described, it is likely that interactions will occur between Danol and gonadal steroid therapy.

Migraine therapy: Danol may itself provoke migraine and possibly reduce the effectiveness of medication to prevent that condition.

Ethyl alcohol: Subjective intolerance in the form of nausea and shortness of breath has been reported.

Alpha calcidol: Danol may increase the calcaemic response in primary hypoparathyroidism necessitating a reduction in dosage of this agent.

Interactions with laboratory function tests: Danazol treatment may interfere with laboratory determination of testosterone or plasma proteins (See also section 4.8 Undesirable effects)

4.6 Pregnancy and lactation

There is epidemiological and toxicological evidence of hazard in human pregnancy. Danazol is known to be associated with the risk of virilisation to the female foetus if administered during human pregnancy. Danazol should not be used during pregnancy. Women of childbearing age should be advised to use an effective, non-hormonal, method of contraception. If the patient conceives during therapy, danazol should be stopped. Danazol has the theoretical potential for androgenic effects in breast-fed infants and therefore either danazol therapy or breast-feeding should be discontinued.

4.7 Effects on ability to drive and use machines

No special warning is felt necessary.

4.8 Undesirable effects

Androgenic effects include weight gain, increased appetite, acne and seborrhoea. Hirsutism, hair loss, voice change, which may take the form of hoarseness, sore throat or of instability or deepening of pitch may occur. Hypertrophy of the clitoris as well as fluid retention are rare.

Other possible endocrine effects include menstrual disturbances in the form of spotting, alteration of the timing of the cycle and amenorrhoea. Although cyclical bleeding and ovulation usually return within 60-90 days after Danol, persistent amenorrhoea has occasionally been reported. Flushing, vaginal dryness, changes in libido, irritation and reduction in breast size may reflect a lowering of oestrogen. In the male a modest reduction in spermatogenesis may be evident during treatment.

Insulin resistance may be increased in diabetes mellitus but symptomatic hypoglycaemia in non-diabetic patients has also been reported as has an increase in plasma glucagon level. Coupled with elevated plasma insulin levels, danazol can also cause a mild impairment of glucose tolerance.

Danol may aggravate epilepsy and expose the condition in those so predisposed.

Cutaneous reactions include rashes, which may be maculopapular, petechial or purpuric or may take an urticarial form and may be accompanied by facial oedema. Associated fever has also been reported. Rarely, sun-sensitive rash has been noted. Inflammatory erythematous nodules, changes in skin pigmentation, exfoliative dermatitis and erythema multiforme have also been reported.

Musculo-skeletal reactions include backache and muscle cramps which can be severe, creatine phosphokinase levels may also rise. Muscle tremors, fasciculation, limb pain, joint pain and joint swelling have also been reported.

Cardiovascular reactions may include hypertension, palpitations and tachycardia.

Thrombotic events have also been observed. Sagittal sinus and cerebrovascular thrombosis as well as arterial thrombosis have been observed. Cases of myocardial infarction have been reported.

Benign intracranial hypertension, visual disturbances such as blurring of vision, difficulty in focusing, difficulty in wearing contact lenses and refraction disorders requiring correction have been noted.

Haematological responses include an increase in red cell and platelet count. Reversible polycythaemia may be provoked. Eosinophilia, leucopenia thrombocytopenia and splenic peliosis have also been noted.

Hepatic–pancreatic reactions include isolated increases in serum transaminase levels and rarely cholestatic jaundice and benign hepatic adenomata and pancreatitis. Very rarely peliosis hepatitis as well as malignant hepatic tumour have been observed with long term use.

Fluid retention may explain the occasional reports of carpal tunnel syndrome. Danol capsules may also provoke migraine.

Possible psychical reactions include emotional lability, anxiety, depressed mood and nervousness. Dizziness, vertigo, nausea, headache, fatigue and epigastric and pleuritic pain have also been noted.

A temporary alteration of lipoproteins in the form of an increase in LDL cholesterol, a decrease in HDL cholesterol, affecting all subfractions, and a decrease in apolipoproteins AI and AII have been reported with Danol in the female.

Other metabolic events have been reported, including induction of aminolevulinic acid (ALA) synthetase, and reduction in thyroid binding globulin, T4, with increased uptake of T3 but without disturbance of thyroid stimulating hormone or free levothyroxine index, is also likely during therapy.

Haematuria has rarely been reported with prolonged use in patients with hereditary angioedema. Cases of interstitial pneumonitis have been reported

4.9 Overdose

Available evidence suggests that acute overdosage would be unlikely to give rise to immediate serious reaction.

In the case of acute overdose consideration should be given to reducing the absorption of the drug with activated charcoal and the patient should be kept under observation in case of any delayed reactions.

5. PHARMACOLOGICAL PROPERTIES

5.1 Pharmacodynamic properties

Danazol, 17a-pregna-2,4-dien-20-yno(2,3-d)-isoxazol-17-ol, is a synthetic steroid derived from ethisterone. Its pharmacological properties include:

1. Relatively marked affinity for androgen receptors, less marked affinity for progesterone receptors and least affinity for oestrogen receptors. Danazol is a weak androgen but in addition antiandrogenic, progestogenic, antiprogestogenic, oestrogenic and antioestrogenic actions have been observed.

2. Interference with the synthesis of gonadal steroids, possibly by inhibition of the enzymes of steroidogenesis, including 3β hydroxysteroid dehydrogenase, 17β hydroxysteroid dehydrogenase, 17 hydroxylase, 17, 20 lyase, 11β hydroxylase, 21 hydroxylase and cholesterol side chain cleavage enzymes, or alternatively by inhibition of the cyclic AMP accumulation usually induced by gonadotrophic hormones in granulosa and luteal cells.

3. Inhibition of the mid-cycle surge of FSH and LH as well as alterations in the pulsatility of LH. Danazol can also reduce the mean plasma levels of these gonadotrophins after the menopause.

4. A wide range of actions on plasma proteins, including increasing prothrombin, plasminogen, antithrombin III, alpha-2 macroglobulin, C1 esterase inhibitor, and erythropoietin and reducing fibrinogen, thyroid binding and sex hormone binding globulins. Danazol increases the proportion and concentration of testosterone carried unbound in plasma.

5 The suppressive effects of danazol on the hypothalmic-pituitary-gonadal axis are reversible, cyclical activity reappearing normally within 60-90 days after therapy.

5.2 Pharmacokinetic properties

Danazol is absorbed from the gastrointestinal tract, peak plasma concentrations of 50-80ng/ml being reached approximately 2-3 hours after dosing. Compared to the fasting state, the bioavailability has been shown to increase 3 fold when the drug is taken with a meal with a high fat content. It is thought that food stimulates bile flow which facilitates the dissolution and absorption of danazol, a highly lipophilic compound.

The apparent plasma elimination half life of danazol in a single dose is approximately 3-6 hours. With multiple doses this may increase to approximately 26 hours.

None of the metabolites of danazol, which have been isolated, exhibits pituitary inhibiting activity comparable to that of danazol.

Few data on excretion routes and rates exist. In the monkey 36% of a radioactive dose was recoverable in the urine and 48% in the faeces within 96 hours.

5.3 Preclinical safety data

There are no pre-clinical data of relevance to the prescriber which are additional to that already included in other sections of the SPC.

6. PHARMACEUTICAL PARTICULARS

6.1 List of excipients

Capsule

Maize Starch

Lactose monohydrate

Purified talc

Magnesium stearate

Cap -100mg

Titanium dioxide

Gelatin

Black iron oxide

Cap – 200mg

Gelatin

Titanium dioxide

Red iron oxide

Yellow iron oxide

Ink

Shellac

Shellac glaze

Propylene glycol

Black iron oxide

6.2 Incompatibilities

None.

6.3 Shelf life

60 months.

6.4 Special precautions for storage

None.

6.5 Nature and contents of container

PVC blister pack compound of polyvinyl chloride (thickness 250μm) sealed to aluminium foil (thickness 20μm). The blisters are then packed in a cardboard carton.

Pack sizes: 60 capsules.

6.6 Special precautions for disposal and other handling

Not applicable.

7. MARKETING AUTHORISATION HOLDER

Sanofi-aventis

One Onslow Street

Guildford, Surrey

GU1 4YS

8. MARKETING AUTHORISATION NUMBER(S)

Danol 100mg: PL 11723/0015

Danol 200mg: PL 11723/0016

9. DATE OF FIRST AUTHORISATION/RENEWAL OF THE AUTHORISATION

28th October 1993

10. DATE OF REVISION OF THE TEXT

July 2007

Legal category: POM

Dantrium 100mg Capsules

(SpePharm UK Ltd)

1. NAME OF THE MEDICINAL PRODUCT

Dantrium Capsules 100mg

2. QUALITATIVE AND QUANTITATIVE COMPOSITION

Each capsule contains 100mg Dantrolene Sodium.

3. PHARMACEUTICAL FORM

Capsule

4. CLINICAL PARTICULARS

4.1 Therapeutic indications

Dantrium is indicated for the treatment of chronic, spasticity of skeletal muscle in adults.

4.2 Posology and method of administration

Dosage for use in spasticity for Adults

For the individual patient the lowest dose compatible with optimal response recommended. A recommended dosage increment scale is shown below:

1st week	One 25mg capsule daily.
2nd week	One 25mg capsule twice daily.
3rd week	Two 25mg capsules twice daily.
4th week	Two 25mg capsules three daily.
5th week	Three 25mg capsules three times daily.
6th week	Three 25mg capsules four times daily.
7th week	One 100mg capsule four times daily.

Each dosage level should be maintained for seven days in order to determine the patient's response. Therapy with a dose four times may offer maximum benefit to some patients. Maximum daily should not exceed 400mg. In view of the potential for hepatotoxicity in long term use, if no observable benefit is derived from the administration of Dantrium after a total of 45 days, therapy should be discontinued.

A similar dosage titration schedule should be used with the elderly.

Dantrium is not recommended for use in children.

4.3 Contraindications

Dantrium is contraindicated where spasticity is utilised to sustain upright posture and balance in locomotion or whenever spasticity is utilised to obtain or maintain increased function.

Dantrium is contraindicated in patients with evidence of hepatic dysfunction. Dantrium is not indicated for the treatment of acute skeletal muscle spasms. Dantrium should not be administered to children.

4.4 Special warnings and precautions for use

Fatal and non-fatal liver disorders of an idiosyncratic or hypersensitivity type may occur with Dantrium therapy.

Patients should be instructed to contact their physician should signs or symptoms of hepatotoxicity (e.g., discolored feces, generalized pruritus, jaundice, anorexia, nausea, vomiting) occur during therapy.

Factors that may increase the risk of developing hepatotoxicity include:

- Higher daily doses (doses exceeding 400 mg daily)
- Duration of therapy (most frequently reported between 2 and 12 months of treatment)
- Female gender
- Age greater than 30 years
- Prior history of liver disease/dysfunction
- Receiving other hepatotoxic therapies concomitantly.

Spontaneous reports also suggest a higher proportion of hepatic events with fatal outcome in elderly patients.

At the start of Dantrium therapy, it is desirable to do liver function studies (SGOT/ALT, SGPT/AST, alkaline phosphatase, total bilirubin) for a baseline or to establish whether there is pre-existing liver disease. If baseline liver abnormalities exist and are confirmed, there is a clear possibility that the potential for Dantrium hepatotoxicity could be enhanced, although such a possibility has not yet been established.

Liver functions studies (e.g. serum, SGOT/AST, SGPT/ALT) should be performed at appropriate intervals during Dantrium therapy. If such studies reveal abnormal values, therapy should generally be discontinued. Only where benefits of the drug have been of major importance to the patient, should re-introduction or continuation of therapy be considered. Some patients have revealed a return to normal laboratory values in the face of continued therapy while others have not.

If symptoms compatible with hepatitis, accompanied by abnormalities in liver function tests or jaundice appear, Dantrium should be discontinued. If caused by Dantrium and detected early, the abnormalities in liver function have reverted to normal when the drug was discontinued.

Dantrium has been re-introduced in a few patients who have developed clinical signs, or elevated serum enzymes, of hepatocellular injury.

Re-introduction of Dantrium therapy should only be contemplated in patients who clearly need the drug, and only after complete reversal of the signs of hepatotoxicity and liver function tests. Patients being re-challenged with Dantrium should be hospital in-patients, and small, gradually increasing doses should be used. Laboratory test monitoring should be frequent, and the drug should be withdrawn immediately if there is any indication of recurrent liver abnormality. Some patients have reacted with unmistakable signs of liver abnormality upon administration of a challenge dose, whilst others have not.

The use of Dantrium with other potentially hepatotoxic drugs should be avoided.

There are isolated cases of possibly significant effects of Dantrium on the cardiovascular and respiratory systems. These cases also have other features suggesting a predisposition to cardiovascular disease, and impaired respiratory function, particularly obstructive pulmonary disease. Dantrium should be used with caution in such patients.

Dantrolene sodium showed some evidence of tumourgenicity at high dose levels in Sprague-Dawley female rats. However, these effects were not seen in other studies in Fischer 344 rats or HaM/ICR mice. There is no clinical evidence of carcinogenicity in humans, however, this possibility cannot be absolutely excluded.

Caution should be exercised in the simultaneous administration of tranquillising agents and alcohol.

This medicine contains lactose. Patients with rare hereditary problems of galactose intolerance, the Lapp lactase deficiency or glucose-galactose malabsorption should not take this medicine.

The colouring agent E110 can cause allergic-type reactions including asthma. Allergy is more common in those people who are allergic to aspirin.

4.5 Interaction with other medicinal products and other forms of interaction

Hyperkalemia and myocardial depression have been observed in malignant hyperthermia-susceptible patients receiving intravenous dantrolene and concomitant calcium channel blockers

The effects of non-depolarizing muscle relaxants may be potentiated in patients administered Dantrium.

4.6 Pregnancy and lactation

Dantrolene crosses the placenta, and has been detected in human milk. Although teratological studies in animals have proved satisfactory, the use of Dantrium is not advised in pregnant or nursing mothers.

4.7 Effects on ability to drive and use machines

Patients should be advised not to drive a motor vehicle or to undertake potentially dangerous work until Dantrium therapy has been stabilised, because some patients drowsiness and dizziness.

4.8 Undesirable effects

The most frequently reported unwanted effects associated with the use of Dantrium have been drowsiness, dizziness, weakness, general malaise, fatigue and diarrhoea. These effects are generally transient, occur early in treatment, and can often be obviated by careful determination and regulation of the dosage. Diarrhoea may be severe, and may necessitate temporary withdrawal of Dantrium. If diarrhoea recurs upon re-introduction of Dantrium, then Dantrium therapy should probably be withdrawn permanently.

Other undesirable effects reported by > 1% or < 1% in post-marketing adverse drug reaction reports are:

Metabolism and nutrition disorders:

> 1%: Anorexia

Psychiatric disorders:

< 1%: Mental depression, mental confusion, nervousness, insomnia

Nervous system disorders:

> 1%: Seizure, visual disturbances, speech disturbance, headache

Cardiac disorders:

> 1%: Pericarditis

< 1%: Exacerbation of cardiac insufficiency, tachycardia

Vascular disorders:

< 1%: Labile blood pressure

Respiratory, thoracic and mediastinal disorders:

> 1%: Pleural effusion with associated eosinophilia, respiratory depression

< 1%: Dyspnoea

Gastrointestinal disorders:

> 1%: Nausea and/or vomiting, abdominal pain

<1%: Dysphagia, constipation (rarely progressing to signs of intestinal obstruction)

Hepato-biliary disorders:

> 1%: Hepatotoxicity (see section 4.4), liver function test disturbances

Skin and subcutaneous tissue disorders:

> 1%: Acne-like rash, skin rash

< 1%: Sweating

Renal and urinary disorders:

<1%: Incontinence, increased urinary frequency, urinary retention, haematuria, crystalluria

General disorders and administration site conditions:

> 1%: Chills and /or fever

Dantrium has a potential for hepatotoxicity. Symptomatic hepatitis (fatal and non-fatal) has been reported at various dose levels although the incidence is greater in patients taking more than 400 mg/day. Liver dysfunction as evidenced by blood chemical abnormalities alone (liver enzyme elevation) has been observed in patients exposed to Dantrium for varying periods of time.

Overt hepatitis has occurred at varying intervals after initiation of therapy, but has most frequently been observed between the second and twelfth month of treatment. The risk of hepatic injury appears to be greater in females, in patients over 30 years old and in patients taking concomitant medication. There is some evidence that hepatic injury is more likely in patients using concomitant oral oestrogen.

4.9 Overdose

There is no known constellation of symptoms with acute overdose. Symptoms that may occur include, but are not limited to, muscular weakness, alterations in the state of consciousness (e.g. lethargy, coma), vomiting, and diarrhoea. For acute overdosage, general supportive measures and gastric lavage should be employed as well as measures to reduce the absorption of Dantrium. The theoretical possibility of crystalluria in overdose has not been reported for Dantrium, but would be treated according to general principles, including administration of fluids. The value of dialysis in dantrolene overdose is not known.

5. PHARMACOLOGICAL PROPERTIES

5.1 Pharmacodynamic properties

Molecular Pharmacology

The receptor molecule for dantrolene has not been identified. Radiolabelled dantrolene sodium binds to specific components of the striated muscle cell, namely the t-tubules and the sarcoplastic reticulum; however the kinetics of binding varies between these two organelles. The binding of ryanodine is thought to compete with the binding of calcium in these organelles; further evidence for the specificity of binding is that dantrolene inhibits the binding of the insecticide ryanodine to heavy sarcoplastic reticulum vesicles from rabbit skeletal muscle. Under some conditions, dantrolene will lower intra-sarcoplasmic calcium concentrations in the resting state. This may be more important in diseased muscle (e.g. in malignant hyperthermia in humans and swine stress syndrome) than in muscle with normal function.

Dantrolene does not bind to the same sites as calcium channel blocking drugs such as nitrendipine or calmodulin. There is no electrophysiological evidence that dantrolene interferes with the influx of calcium from outside the cell. This may be one reason why paralysis by dantrolene has never been reported in animals or man; the muscle cell has alternative sources of calcium which are not influenced by dantrolene.

Biochemical Pharmacology

Whatever the molecular mechanism, the cardinal property of dantrolene sodium is that it lowers intracellular calcium concentration in skeletal muscle. Calcium concentrations may be lower in both the quiescent state, and as a result of a reduction in the release of calcium form the sarcoplasmic reticulum in response to a standard stimulus. This effect has been observed in striated muscle fibres from several species, and is not seen in myocardium. Fast fibres may be more sensitive than slow fibres to the action of dantrolene sodium.

Diverse other properties of dantrolene sodium have been observed *in-vitro*, and in animal studies. Dantrolene sodium may inhibit the release of calcium from the smooth endoplasmic reticulum of smooth muscle, but the significance of this observation is questionable; for example, dantrolene sodium has no effect on isolated human urinary bladder smooth muscle. Calcium dependent, pre-synaptic neurotransmitter release may also be inhibited by dantrolene sodium. Again, the clinical significance of this has not been demonstrated.

Studies on Isolated, Functional Muscle

Elevation of intracellular, free calcium ion concentration is an obligatory step in excitation-contraction coupling of skeletal muscle. Dantrolene sodium, therefore, acts as a muscle relaxant by a peripheral mechanism which is quite different, and easily distinguishable from neuromuscular junction blocking drugs. In contrast with compounds that relax skeletal muscle by acting principally on the central nervous system, dantrolene sodium acts directly on skeletal muscle cells. In rabbit atria, dantrolene sodium has no effect alone, but it may antagonise inotropic agents which act by increasing intramyocardial cell calcium e.g. the experimental drug anthopleurin-A.

5.2 Pharmacokinetic properties

Absorption

Dantrium is easily and almost completely absorbed from the gastrointestinal tract. After dosing on an empty stomach, plasma dantrolene levels peak within three hours in most subjects.

Distribution

Dantrolene sodium is a highly lipophobic drug. In addition it lacks hydrophilicity. Dantrolene sodium binds to human serum albumin (HSA) with a molar ratio of 0.95 to 1.68 *in-vitro*. The association constant *in-vitro* is higher (2.3 to 5.4×10^{-5} per mol). *In-vitro* dantrolene sodium can be displaced from HSA by warfarin, clofibrate and tolbutamide but these interactions have not been confirmed in humans (re. manufacturer's database). Single intravenous dose studies suggest that the primary volume of distribution is about 15 litres. Single oral doses achieve peak plasma concentration of about a quarter of that for a similarly sized intravenous dose.

Metabolism and Excretion

The biological half life in plasma in most human subjects is between 5 and 9 hours, although half-lives as long as 12.1 ± 1.9 hours have been reported after a single intravenous dose. Inactivation is by hepatic metabolism in the first instance. There are two alternative pathways. Most of the drug is hydroxylated to 5-hydroxy-dantrolene. The minor pathway involves nitro-reduction to amino-dantrolene which is then acetylated (compound F-490). The 5-hydroxy metabolite is a muscle relaxant with nearly the same potency as the parent molecule, and may have a longer half life than the parent compound. Compound F-490 is much less potent and is probably inactive at the concentrations achieved in clinical samples. Metabolites are subsequently excreted in the urine in the ratio of 79 5-hydroxy-dantrolene:17 compound F-490: 4 unaltered dantrolene (salt or free acid). The proportion of drug excreted in the faeces depends upon dose size.

5.3 Preclinical safety data

Sprague-Dawley female rats fed dantrolene sodium for 18 months at dosage levels of 15, 30 and 60 mg/kg/day showed an increased incidence of benign and malignant mammary tumors compared with concurrent controls. At the highest dose level, there was an increase in the incidence of benign hepatic lymphatic neoplasms. In a 30-month study at the same dose levels also in Sprague-Dawley rats, dantrolene sodium produced a decrease in the time of onset of mammary neoplasms. Female rats at the highest dose level showed an increased incidence of hepatic lymphangiomas and hepatic angiosarcomas.

The only drug-related effect seen in a 30-month study in Fischer-344 rats was a dose-related reduction in the time of onset of mammary and testicular tumors. A 24-month study in HaM/ICR mice revealed no evidence of carcinogenic activity.

The significance of carcinogenicity data relative to use of dantrolene sodium in humans is unknown.

Dantrolene sodium has produced positive results in the Ames S. Typhimurium bacterial mutagenesis assay in the presence and absence of a liver activating system.

Dantrolene sodium administered to male and female rats at dose levels up to 45 mg/kg/day showed no adverse effects on fertility or general reproductive performance.

6. PHARMACEUTICAL PARTICULARS

6.1 List of excipients

Gelatin, starch, talc, magnesium stearate, lactose, E110, E171 and E172.

6.2 Incompatibilities

None.

6.3 Shelf life

Three years.

6.4 Special precautions for storage

Store below 30°C.

6.5 Nature and contents of container

Dantrium 100mg capsules are supplied in high density polyethylene (HDPE) bottles with tinplate caps containing 100 capsules each and polypropylene securitainers with polyethylene caps containing 100 capsules each.

Not all packaging versions may be marketed.

6.6 Special precautions for disposal and other handling

A patient leaflet is provided for details of use and handling of the product.

7. MARKETING AUTHORISATION HOLDER

Procter & Gamble Pharmaceuticals UK Limited
Rusham Park
Whitehall Lane
Egham
Surrey TW20 9NW
UK

8. MARKETING AUTHORISATION NUMBER(S)

PL 0364/0016R

9. DATE OF FIRST AUTHORISATION/RENEWAL OF THE AUTHORISATION

25 October 1989

10. DATE OF REVISION OF THE TEXT

30/09/2008

Dantrium 25mg Capsules

(SpePharm UK Ltd)

1. NAME OF THE MEDICINAL PRODUCT

Dantrium Capsules 25mg

2. QUALITATIVE AND QUANTITATIVE COMPOSITION

Each capsule contains 25mg Dantrolene Sodium.

3. PHARMACEUTICAL FORM

Caspsule

4. CLINICAL PARTICULARS

4.1 Therapeutic indications

Dantrium is indicated for the treatment of chronic, severe spasticity of skeletal muscle in adults.

4.2 Posology and method of administration

Dosage for Use in Spasticity for Adults

For the individual patient the lowest dose compatible with response is recommended. A recommended dosage increment scale is shown below:

1st week	One 25mg capsule daily
2nd week	One 25mg capsule twice daily
3rd week	Two 25mg capsules twice daily
4th week	Two 25mg capsules three times daily
5th week	Three 25mg capsules three times daily
6th week	Three 25mg capsules four times daily
7th week	One 100mg capsule four times daily.

Each dosage level should be maintained for seven days in order to determine the patient's response. Therapy with a dose four times daily may offer maximum benefit to some patients. Maximum daily dose should not exceed 400mg. In view of the potential for hepatotoxicity in long term use, if no observable benefit is derived from the administration of dantrium after a total of 45 days, therapy should be discontinued.

A similar dosage titration schedule should be used with the elderly.

Dantrium is not recommended for use in children.

4.3 Contraindications

Dantrium is contraindicated where spasticity is utilised to sustain upright posture and balance in locomotion or whenever spasticity is utilised to obtain or maintain increased function. Dantrium is contraindicated in patients with evidence of hepatic dysfunction. Dantrium is not indicated for the treatment of acute skeletal muscle spasms. Dantrium should not be administered to children.

4.4 Special warnings and precautions for use

Fatal and non-fatal liver disorders of an idiosyncratic or hypersensitivity type may occur with Dantrium therapy.

Patients should be instructed to contact their physician should signs or symptoms of hepatotoxicity (e.g., discolored feces, generalized pruritus, jaundice, anorexia, nausea, vomiting) occur during therapy.

Factors that may increase the risk of developing hepatotoxicity include:

- Higher daily doses (doses exceeding 400 mg daily)
- Duration of therapy (most frequently reported between 2 and 12 months of treatment)
- Female gender
- Age greater than 30 years
- Prior history of liver disease/dysfunction
- Receiving other hepatotoxic therapies concomitantly.

Spontaneous reports also suggest a higher proportion of hepatic events with fatal outcome in elderly patients.

At the start of Dantrium therapy, it is desirable to do liver function studies (SGOT/ALT, SGPT/AST, alkaline phosphatase, total bilirubin) for a baseline or to establish whether there is pre-existing liver disease. If baseline liver abnormalities exist and are confirmed, there is a clear possibility that the potential for Dantrium hepatotoxicity could be enhanced, although such a possibility has not yet been established.

Liver functions studies (e.g. serum, SGOT/AST, SGPT/ALT) should be performed at appropriate intervals during Dantrium therapy. If such studies reveal abnormal values, therapy should generally be discontinued. Only where benefits of the drug have been of major importance to the patient, should re-introduction or continuation of therapy be considered. Some patients have revealed a return to normal laboratory values in the face of continued therapy while others have not.

If symptoms compatible with hepatitis, accompanied by abnormalities in liver function tests or jaundice appear, Dantrium should be discontinued. If caused by Dantrium and detected early, the abnormalities in liver function have reverted to normal when the drug was discontinued.

Dantrium has been re-introduced in a few patients who have developed clinical signs, or elevated serum enzymes, of hepatocellular injury.

Re-introduction of Dantrium therapy should only be contemplated in patients who clearly need the drug, and only after complete reversal of the signs of hepatotoxicity and liver function tests. Patients being re-challenged with Dantrium should be hospital in-patients, and small, gradually increasing doses should be used. Laboratory test monitoring should be frequent, and the drug should be withdrawn immediately if there is any indication of recurrent liver abnormality. Some patients have reacted with unmistakable signs of liver abnormality upon administration of a challenge dose, whilst others have not.

The use of Dantrium with other potentially hepatotoxic drugs should be avoided.

There are isolated cases of possibly significant effects of Dantrium on the cardiovascular and respiratory systems. These cases also have other features suggesting a pre-disposition to cardiovascular disease, and impaired respiratory function, particularly obstructive pulmonary disease. Dantrium should be used with caution in such patients.

Dantrolene sodium showed some evidence of tumourgenicity at high dose levels in Sprague-Dawley female rats. However, these effects were not seen in other studies in Fischer 344 rats or HaM/ICR mice. There is no clinical evidence of carcinogenicity in humans, however, this possibility cannot be absolutely excluded.

Caution should be exercised in the simultaneous administration of tranquillising agents and alcohol.

This medicine contains lactose. Patients with rare hereditary problems of galactose intolerance, the Lapp lactase deficiency or glucose-galactose malabsorption should not take this medicine.

The colouring agent E110 can cause allergic-type reactions including asthma. Allergy is more common in those people who are allergic to aspirin.

4.5 Interaction with other medicinal products and other forms of interaction

Hyperkalemia and myocardial depression have been observed in malignant hyperthermia-susceptible patients receiving intravenous dantrolene and concomitant calcium channel blockers

The effects of non-depolarizing muscle relaxants may be potentiated in patients administered Dantrium.

4.6 Pregnancy and lactation

Dantrolene crosses the placenta, and has been detected in human milk. Although teratological studies in animals have proved satisfactory, the use of Dantrium is not advised in pregnant or nursing mothers.

4.7 Effects on ability to drive and use machines

Patients should be advised not to drive a motor vehicle or undertake potentially dangerous work until dantrium therapy has been stabilised, because some patients experience drowsiness and dizziness.

4.8 Undesirable effects

The most frequently reported unwanted effects associated with the use of Dantrium have been drowsiness, dizziness, weakness, general malaise, fatigue and diarrhoea. These effects are generally transient, occur early in treatment, and can often be obviated by careful determination and regulation of the dosage. Diarrhoea may be severe, and may necessitate temporary withdrawal of Dantrium. If diarrhoea recurs upon re-introduction of Dantrium, then Dantrium therapy should probably be withdrawn permanently.

Other undesirable effects reported by > 1% or < 1% in post-marketing adverse drug reaction reports are:

Metabolism and nutrition disorders:

> 1%: Anorexia

Psychiatric disorders:

< 1%: Mental depression, mental confusion, nervousness, insomnia

Nervous system disorders:

> 1%: Seizure, visual disturbances, speech disturbance, headache

Cardiac disorders:

> 1%: Pericarditis

< 1%: Exacerbation of cardiac insufficiency, tachycardia

Vascular disorders:

< 1%: Labile blood pressure

Respiratory, thoracic and mediastinal disorders:

> 1%: Pleural effusion with associated eosinophilia, respiratory depression

< 1%: Dyspnoea

Gastrointestinal disorders:

> 1%: Nausea and/or vomiting, abdominal pain

< 1%: Dysphagia, constipation (rarely progressing to signs of intestinal obstruction)

Hepato-biliary disorders:

> 1%: Hepatotoxicity (see section 4.4), liver function test disturbances

Skin and subcutaneous tissue disorders:

> 1%: Acne-like rash, skin rash

< 1%: Sweating

Renal and urinary disorders:

<1%: Incontinence, increased urinary frequency, urinary retention, haematuria, crystalluria

General disorders and administration site conditions:

> 1%: Chills and /or fever

Dantrium has a potential for hepatotoxicity. Symptomatic hepatitis (fatal and non-fatal) has been reported at various dose levels although the incidence is greater in patients taking more than 400 mg/day. Liver dysfunction as evidenced by blood chemical abnormalities alone (liver enzyme elevation) has been observed in patients exposed to Dantrium for varying periods of time.

Overt hepatitis has occurred at varying intervals after initiation of therapy, but has most frequently been observed between the second and twelfth month of treatment. The risk of hepatic injury appears to be greater in females, in patients over 30 years old and in patients taking concomitant medication. There is some evidence that hepatic injury is more likely in patients using concomitant oral oestrogen.

4.9 Overdose

There is no known constellation of symptoms with acute overdose. Symptoms that may occur include, but are not limited to, muscular weakness, alterations in the state of consciousness (e.g. lethargy, coma), vomiting, and diarrhoea. For acute overdosage, general supportive measures and gastric lavage should be employed as well as measures to reduce the absorption of Dantrium. The theoretical possibility of crystalluria in overdose has not been reported for Dantrium, but would be treated according to general principles, including administration of fluids. The value of dialysis in dantrolene overdose is not known.

5. PHARMACOLOGICAL PROPERTIES

5.1 Pharmacodynamic properties

Molecular Pharmacology

The receptor molecule for dantrolene has not been identified. Radiolabelled dantrolene sodium binds to specific components of the striated muscle cell, namely the t-tubules and the sarcoplastic reticulum; however the kinetics of binding varies between these two organelles. The binding of ryanodine is thought to compete with the binding of calcium in these organelles; further evidence for the specificity of binding is that dantrolene inhibits the binding of the insecticide ryanodine to heavy sarcoplastic reticulum vesicles from rabbit skeletal muscle. Under some conditions, dantrolene will lower intra-sarcoplasmic calcium concentrations in the resting state. This may be more important in diseased muscle (e.g. in malignant hyperthermia in humans and swine stress syndrome) than in muscle with normal function.

Dantrolene does not bind to the same sites as calcium channel blocking drugs such as nitrendipine or calmodulin. There is no electrophysiological evidence that dantrolene interferes with the influx of calcium from outside the cell. This may be one reason why paralysis by dantrolene has never been reported in animals or man; the muscle cell has alternative sources of calcium which are not influenced by dantrolene.

Biochemical Pharmacology

Whatever the molecular mechanism, the cardinal property of dantrolene sodium is that it lowers intracellular calcium concentration in skeletal muscle. Calcium concentrations may be lower in both the quiescent state, and as a result of a reduction in the release of calcium form the sarcoplasmic reticulum in response to a standard stimulus. This effect has been observed in striated muscle fibres from several species, and is not seen in myocardium. Fast fibres may be more sensitive than slow fibres to the action of dantrolene sodium.

Diverse other properties of dantrolene sodium have been observed in-vitro, and in animal studies. Dantrolene sodium may inhibit the release of calcium from the smooth endoplasmic reticulum of smooth muscle, but the significance of this observation is questionable; for example, dantrolene sodium has no effect on isolated human urinary bladder smooth muscle. Calcium dependent, pre-synaptic neurotransmitter release may also be inhibited by dantrolene sodium. Again, the clinical significance of this has not been demonstrated.

Studies on Isolated, Functional Muscle

Elevation of intracellular, free calcium ion concentration is an obligatory step in excitation-contraction coupling of skeletal muscle. Dantrolene sodium, therefore, acts as a muscle relaxant by a peripheral mechanism which is quite different, and easily distinguishable from neuromuscular junction blocking drugs. In contrast with compounds that relax skeletal muscle by acting principally on the central nervous system, dantrolene sodium acts directly on skeletal muscle cells. In rabbit atria, dantrolene sodium has no effect alone, but it may antagonise inotropic agents which act by increasing intramyocardial cell calcium e.g. the experimental drug anthopleurin-A.

5.2 Pharmacokinetic properties

Absorption

Dantrium is easily and almost completely absorbed from the gastrointestinal tract. After dosing on an empty stomach, plasma dantrolene levels peak within three hours in most subjects.

Distribution

Dantrolene sodium is a highly lipophobic drug. In addition it lacks hydrophilicity. Dantrolene sodium binds to human serum albumin (HSA) with a molar ratio of 0.95 to 1.68 *in-vitro*. The association constant *in-vitro* is higher (2.3 to 5.4×10^{-5} per mol). *In-vitro* dantrolene sodium can be displaced from HSA by warfarin, clofibrate and tolbutamide but these interactions have not been confirmed in humans (re. manufacturer's database). Single intravenous dose studies suggest that the primary volume of distribution is about 15 litres. Single oral doses achieve peak plasma concentration of about a quarter of that for a similarly sized intravenous dose.

Metabolism and Excretion

The biological half life in plasma in most human subjects is between 5 and 9 hours, although half-lives as long as 12.1 ± 1.9 hours have been reported after a single intravenous dose. Inactivation is by hepatic metabolism in the first instance. There are two alternative pathways. Most of the drug is hydroxylated to 5-hydroxy-dantrolene. The minor pathway involves nitro-reduction to amino-dantrolene which is then acetylated (compound F-490). The 5-hydroxy metabolite is a muscle relaxant with nearly the same potency as the parent molecule, and may have a longer half life than the parent compound. Compound F-490 is much less potent and is probably inactive at the concentrations achieved in clinical samples. Metabolites are subsequently excreted in the urine in the ratio of 79 5-hydroxy-dantrolene:17 compound F-490: 4 unaltered dantrolene (salt or free acid). The proportion of drug excreted in the faeces depends upon dose size.

5.3 Preclinical safety data

Sprague-Dawley female rats fed dantrolene sodium for 18 months at dosage levels of 15, 30 and 60 mg/kg/day showed an increased incidence of benign and malignant mammary tumors compared with concurrent controls. At the highest dose level, there was an increase in the incidence of benign hepatic lymphatic neoplasms. In a 30-month study at the same dose levels also in Sprague-Dawley rats, dantrolene sodium produced a decrease in the time of onset of mammary neoplasms. Female rats at the highest dose level showed an increased incidence of hepatic lymphangiomas and hepatic angiosarcomas.

The only drug-related effect seen in a 30-month study in Fischer-344 rats was a dose-related reduction in the time of onset of mammary and testicular tumors. A 24-month study in HaM/ICR mice revealed no evidence of carcinogenic activity.

The significance of carcinogenicity data relative to use of dantrolene sodium in humans is unknown.

Dantrolene sodium has produced positive results in the Ames S. Typhimurium bacterial mutagenesis assay in the presence and absence of a liver activating system.

Dantrolene sodium administered to male and female rats at dose levels up to 45 mg/kg/day showed no adverse effects on fertility or general reproductive performance.

6. PHARMACEUTICAL PARTICULARS

6.1 List of excipients

Gelatin, starch, talc, magnesium stearate, lactose, E110, E171 and E172.

6.2 Incompatibilities

None.

6.3 Shelf life

Three years.

6.4 Special precautions for storage

Store below 30°C.

6.5 Nature and contents of container

Dantrium 25mg capsules are supplied in high density polyethylene (HDPE) bottles with tinplate caps containing 100 capsules each and polypropylene securitainers with polyethylene caps containing 100 capsules each.

Not all packaging versions may be marketed.

6.6 Special precautions for disposal and other handling

A patient leaflet is provided for details of use and handling of the product.

7. MARKETING AUTHORISATION HOLDER

Procter & Gamble Pharmaceuticals UK Limited

Rusham Park

Whitehall Lane

Egham

Surrey TW20 9NW

UK

8. MARKETING AUTHORISATION NUMBER(S)

PL 0364/0015R

9. DATE OF FIRST AUTHORISATION/RENEWAL OF THE AUTHORISATION

25 October 1989

10. DATE OF REVISION OF THE TEXT

30/09/2008

Dantrium Intravenous

(SpePharm UK Ltd)

1. NAME OF THE MEDICINAL PRODUCT

Dantrium Intravenous

2. QUALITATIVE AND QUANTITATIVE COMPOSITION

Each vial contains 20 mg dantrolene sodium. For excipients, see 6.1

3. PHARMACEUTICAL FORM

Powder for solution for injection.

4. CLINICAL PARTICULARS

4.1 Therapeutic indications

For the treatment of malignant hyperthermia.

4.2 Posology and method of administration

As soon as the malignant hyperthermia syndrome is recognised all anaesthetic agents should be discontinued. An initial Dantrium intravenous dose of 1 mg/kg should be given rapidly into the vein. If the physiological and metabolic abnormalities persist or reappear, this dose may be repeated up to a cumulative dose of 10 mg/kg. Clinical experience to date has shown that the average dose of Dantrium intravenous required to reverse the manifestations of malignant hyperthermia has been 2.5 mg/kg. If a relapse or recurrence occurs, Dantrium intravenous should be readministered at the last effect dose.

4.3 Contraindications

None stated.

4.4 Special warnings and precautions for use

In some subjects as much as 10 mg/kg of Dantrium intravenous has been needed to reverse the crisis. In a 70 kg man this dose would require approximately 36 vials. Such a volume has been administered in approximately one and a half hours.

When mannitol is used for prevention or treatment of renal complication of malignant hyperthermia, the 3 grams of mannitol present as an excipient in each 20 mg vial of intravenous dantrolene sodium should be taken into consideration when calculating total mannitol dose to be administered.

Because of the high pH of the intravenous formulation of Dantrium and potential for tissue necrosis, care must be taken to prevent extravasation of the intravenous solution into the surrounding tissues.

The use of Dantrium intravenous in the management of malignant hyperthermia is not a substitute for previously known supportive measures. It will be necessary to discontinue the suspect triggering agents, attend to increased oxygen requirements and manage the metabolic acidosis.

When necessary institute cooling, attend to urinary output and monitor for electrolyte imbalance.

Hepatic dysfunction, including hepatitis and fatal hepatic failure, has been reported with dantrolene sodium therapy. Whilst the licensed indications of intravenous dantrolene do not generally necessitate prolonged therapy, the risk of hepatic dysfunction may increase with dose and duration of treatment, based on experience with oral therapy. However in some patients it is of an idiosyncratic or hypersensitivity type, and could occur after a single dose.

4.5 Interaction with other medicinal products and other forms of interaction

The combination of therapeutic doses of intravenous dantrolene sodium and verapamil in halothane/alpha-chloralose anaesthetised swine has resulted in ventricular fibrillation and cardiovascular collapse in association with marked hyperkalaemia. Hyperkalaemia and myocardial depression have also been reported rarely in malignant hyperthermia-susceptible patients receiving intravenous dantrolene and concomitant calcium channel blockers. It is recommended that the combination of intravenous dantrolene sodium and calcium channel blockers, such as verapamil, is not used during the reversal of a malignant hyperthermia crisis until the relevance of these findings to humans is established.

Administration of dantrolene may potentiate vecuronium-induced neuromuscular block.

4.6 Pregnancy and lactation

The safety of Dantrium intravenous in pregnant women has not been established. Dantrolene crosses the placenta, and should be given only when the potential benefits have been weighed against the possible risk to mother and child.

Dantrolene has been detected in human milk at low concentrations (less than 2 micrograms per milliliter) during repeat intravenous administration over 3 days. Dantrium Intravenous should be used by nursing mothers only if the potential benefit justifies the potential risk to the infant.

4.7 Effects on ability to drive and use machines

A decrease in grip strength and weakness of leg muscles, especially walking down stairs, can be expected post-operatively. In addition, symptoms such as "lightheadedness" may be noted. Since some of these symptoms may persist for up to 48 hours, patients must not operate an automobile or engage in other hazardous activity during this time.

4.8 Undesirable effects

There have been occasional reports of death following malignant hyperthermia crisis even when treated with intravenous dantrolene sodium; incidence figures are not available (the pre-dantrolene mortality of malignant hyperthermia crisis was approximately 50%). Most of these deaths can be accounted for by late recognition, delayed treatment, inadequate dosage, lack of supportive therapy, intercurrent disease and/or the development of delayed complications such as renal failure or disseminated intravascular coagulopathy. In some cases there are insufficient data to completely rule out therapeutic failure of dantrolene sodium.

The administration of intravenous dantrolene sodium to human volunteers is associated with loss of grip strength and weakness in the legs, as well as subjective central nervous system complaints.

There are rare reports of pulmonary oedema developing during the treatment of malignant hyperthermia crisis in which the diluent volume and mannitol needed to deliver i.v. dantrolene sodium possibly contributed.

Injection site reactions including erythema, rash, swelling, localised pain and thrombophlebitis may occur following administration of intravenous dantrolene sodium. Extravasation may lead to tissue necrosis (see section 4.4).

Hepatic dysfunction may occur, including fatal hepatic failure (see section 4.4).

4.9 Overdose

None stated.

5. PHARMACOLOGICAL PROPERTIES

5.1 Pharmacodynamic properties

Molecular Pharmacology

The receptor molecule for dantrolene has not been identified. Radiolabelled dantrolene sodium binds to specific components of the striated muscle cell, namely the t-tubules and the sarcoplasmic reticulum. However, the kinetics of binding vary between these two organelles. The binding of ryanodine is thought to compete with the binding of calcium in these organelles; further evidence for the specificity of binding is that dantrolene inhibits the binding of ryanodine to heavy sarcoplasmic reticulum vesicles from rabbit skeletal muscle. Under some conditions, dantrolene will lower intra-sarcoplasmic calcium concentrations in the resting state. This may be more important in diseased muscle [e.g. in malignant hyperthermia in humans and swine stress syndrome] than in muscle with normal function.

Dantrolene does not bind to the same sites as calcium channel blocking drugs such as nitrendipine or calmodulin. There is no electrophysiological evidence that dantrolene interferes with the influx of calcium from outside the cell. This may be one reason why paralysis by dantrolene has never been reported in animals or man; the muscle cell has alternative sources of calcium which are not influenced by dantrolene.

Biochemical Pharmacology

Whatever the molecular mechanism, the cardinal property of dantrolene sodium is that it lowers intracellular calcium concentration in skeletal muscle. Calcium concentrations may be lower in both the quiescent state, and as a result of a reduction in the release of calcium from the sarcoplasmic reticulum in response to a standard stimulus. This effect has been observed in striated muscle fibres from several species, and is not seen in myocardium. Fast fibres may be more sensitive than slow fibres to the action of dantrolene sodium.

Diverse other properties of dantrolene sodium have been observed *in vitro*, and in animal studies. Dantrolene sodium may inhibit the release of calcium from the smooth endoplasmic reticulum of smooth muscle, but the significance of this observation is questionable; for example, dantrolene sodium has no effect on isolated human urinary bladder smooth muscle. Calcium dependent, pre-synaptic neurotransmitter release may also be inhibited by dantrolene sodium. Again, the clinical significance of this has not been demonstrated.

Studies on Isolated, Functional Muscle

Elevation of intracellular, free calcium ion concentration is an obligatory step in excitation-contraction coupling of skeletal muscle. Dantrolene sodium, therefore, acts as a muscle relaxant by a peripheral mechanism which is quite different, and easily distinguishable from neuromuscular junction blocking drugs. In contrast with compounds that relax skeletal muscle by acting principally on the central nervous system, dantrolene sodium acts directly on skeletal muscle cells. In rabbit atria, dantrolene sodium has no effect alone, but it may antagonise inotropic agents which act by increasing intramyocardial cell calcium e.g. anthopleurin-a.

5.2 Pharmacokinetic properties

Distribution

Dantrolene sodium is a highly lipophobic drug. In addition, it lacks hydrophilicity. Dantrolene sodium binds to human serum albumin (HSA) with a molar ratio of 0.95 to 1.68 *in vitro*. The association constant *in vitro* is 2.3 to 5.4 $\times$ 10^{-5} per mol. *In vitro* dantrolene sodium can be displaced from HSA by warfarin, clofibrate and tolbutamide but these interactions have not been confirmed in humans (re. manufacturer's database). Single intravenous dose studies suggest that the primary volume of distribution is about 15 litres.

Metabolism and Excretion

The biological half life in plasma in most human subjects is between 5 and 9 hours, although half-lives as long as 12.1 $\pm$ 1.9 hours have been reported after a single intravenous dose. Inactivation is by hepatic metabolism in the first instance. There are two alternative pathways. Most of the drug is hydroxylated to 5-hydroxy-dantrolene. The minor pathway involves nitro-reduction to amino-dantrolene which is then acetylated (compound F-490). The 5-hydroxy metabolite is a muscle relaxant with nearly the same potency as the parent molecule, and may have a longer half life than the parent compound. Compound F-490 is much less potent and is probably inactive at the concentrations achieved in clinical samples. Metabolites are subsequently excreted in the urine in the ratio of 79 5-hydroxy dantrolene: 17 compound F-490: 4 unaltered dantrolene (salt or free acid). The proportion of drug excreted in the faeces depends upon dose size.

5.3 Preclinical safety data

Whilst there is no clinical evidence of carcinogenicity in humans, this possibility cannot be absolutely excluded. Dantrolene sodium has shown some evidence of tumourgenicity at high dose levels in Sprague-Dawley female rats, but these effects have not been seen in other studies in Fischer 344 rats or HaM/ICR mice.

6. PHARMACEUTICAL PARTICULARS

6.1 List of excipients

Mannitol and sodium hydroxide.

6.2 Incompatibilities

Dantrium intravenous should not be mixed with other intravenous infusions.

6.3 Shelf life

Three years. The reconstituted solution should be used within six hours.

6.4 Special precautions for storage

Unopened product: Do not store above 30°C. Reconstituted solution: Do not store above 30°C. Do not refrigerate or freeze. Protect from direct light.

Because of the nature of the freeze-drying process used in the manufacture of Dantrium intravenous, the freeze-dried cake of Dantrium intravenous may have a mottled orange/white appearance or be in the form of loose aggregates. This is an entirely normal artefact and in no way compromises the stability of the product.

6.5 Nature and contents of container

Type I glass vial with butyl rubber stopper and aluminium seal. Twelve vials per carton.

6.6 Special precautions for disposal and other handling

Each vial of Dantrium IV should be reconstituted by adding 60ml of water for injection PhEur, and shaken until the solution is clear. Any unused portion of the reconstituted solution should be discarded. There are no special requirements relating to the disposal of the container or contents.

7. MARKETING AUTHORISATION HOLDER

Procter & Gamble Pharmaceuticals UK Limited
Rusham Park
Whitehall Lane
Egham
Surrey
TW20 9NW, UK

8. MARKETING AUTHORISATION NUMBER(S)

PL 0364/0030

9. DATE OF FIRST AUTHORISATION/RENEWAL OF THE AUTHORISATION

14 February 1980

10. DATE OF REVISION OF THE TEXT

July 2008

Daraprim Tablets

(GlaxoSmithKline UK)

1. NAME OF THE MEDICINAL PRODUCT

Daraprim 25mg Tablets

2. QUALITATIVE AND QUANTITATIVE COMPOSITION

Pyrimethamine 25.0 mg

For excipients see 6.1.

3. PHARMACEUTICAL FORM

Tablet

Each tablet is white and round with the markingGS A3A.

4. CLINICAL PARTICULARS

4.1 Therapeutic indications

Malaria prophylaxis

Daraprim is indicated for chemoprophylaxis of malaria due to susceptible strains of Plasmodia. However, since resistance to pyrimethamine is increasing worldwide, Daraprim can only be considered suitable for use in individuals who are resident in areas where pyrimethamine is acknowledged to be effective. It is not suitable as a prophylactic for travellers.

Toxoplasmosis

Treatment is not normally required for asymtomatic or mild toxoplasma infection. Daraprim, in conjunction with a sulphonamide, is effective in the treatment of the following conditions associated with toxoplasma infections:

Toxoplasmic encephalitis and other manifestations in immune deficient individuals including those with AIDS.

Ocular infections where there is considered to be a risk of visual damage.

Proven foetal infection following maternal infection during pregnancy.

For the treatment of toxoplasmosis, Daraprim should not be used as monotherapy. It must be combined with a synergistic agent, normally an orally administered sulphonamide as recommended in section 4.2, Posology and Method of Administration.

4.2 Posology and method of administration

Malaria Prophylaxis:

Adults: 1 tablet regularly each week.

Children: Over 10 years: 1 tablet regularly each week.

5 to 10 years: ½ tablet regularly each week.

Under 5 years: Formulation not applicable.

Daraprim is rapidly absorbed and therefore prophylactic cover can be expected shortly after the first dose. Prophylaxis should commence before arrival in an endemic area and be continued once weekly. On returning to a non-malarious area dosage should be maintained for a further four weeks.

Toxoplasmosis treatment:

Daraprim should be given concurrently with sulphadiazine or another appropriate sulphonamide. Data on the extent to which other combinations might be better than pyrimethamine alone are limited. For patients who are intolerant of sulphonamides however, consideration should be given to substituting the sulphonamide for another agent such as clindamycin.

In the treatment of toxoplasmosis, all patients receiving Daraprim should be given a folate supplement to reduce the risk of bone marrow depression. Whenever possible calcium folinate should be administered. Folic acid is likely to be less effective than calcium folinate.

Daraprim treatment should generally be given for 3 to 6 weeks and not less than three weeks in immunosuppressed patients. If further therapy is indicated, a period of two weeks should elapse between treatments.

There have been no dose response studies of pyrimethamine in the treatment of toxoplasmosis. The following recommendations are therefore for guidance only.

Dosage for Toxoplasmic encephalitis and other manifestations in immune-deficient patients (adults and children over 5 years)

Daraprim

A loading dose of 100 mg – 200 mg daily should be given for the first 2 - 3 days of treatment.

The optimal dose subsequently for the treatment of toxoplasmic encephalitis in AIDS patients is not fully established but is generally in the range 25mg-75mg/day. Doses up to 100mg/day have been used successfully. The duration of treatment of the acute infection will depend on the clinical response and tolerability, but should normally be not less than three to six weeks.

Maintenance treatment is required indefinitely in immunocompromised patients if relapses are to be avoided. There is insufficient evidence to establish the optimal dose regimen, but doses of 25-100mg daily have been employed successfully.

Sulphadiazine 2 - 6 g per day in divided doses.

Dosage for treatment of ocular infections (adults and children over 5 years)

Daraprim

A loading dose of 100mg for 1-2 days followed by maintenance doses of 25-50mg daily. The optimal maintenance dose has not been clearly established.

Sulphadiazine 2-4g daily in divided doses.

• Dosage for treatment of foetal toxoplasmosis during pregnancy

See Section 4.4 Special Warnings and Precautions for Use and Section 4.6 Pregnancy and Lactation

Daraprim:	***25 - 50 mg daily***
Sulphadiazine	***2 - 4 g daily in divided doses***

Children under 5 years

There is insufficient data to provide specific dose recommendations in children. This formulation is not suitable for children under 5 years.

Use in the elderly

There is no definitive information on the effect of Daraprim on elderly individuals. It is theoretically possible that elderly patients might be more susceptible to folate depression associated with the daily administration of Daraprim in the treatment of toxoplasmosis, and folate supplements are therefore essential (See Special Warnings and Precautions for Use).

4.3 Contraindications

Daraprim should not be given to patients with a history of pyrimethamine sensitivity.

Daraprim should not be used during the first trimester of pregnancy. (See Section 4.6 Pregnancy and Lactation).

Breast-feeding should be avoided during toxoplasmosis treatment. (See Section 4.6 Pregnancy and Lactation).

4.4 Special warnings and precautions for use

During pregnancy and in other conditions predisposing to folate deficiency, a folate supplement should be given. The co-administration of a folate supplement is necessary for treatment of toxoplasmosis (see Dosage & Method of Administration). Full blood counts should be carried out weekly during therapy and for a further two weeks after treatment is stopped. In immunosuppressed patients, full blood counts should be carried out twice weekly. Should signs of folate deficiency develop, treatment must be discontinued and high doses of calcium folinate administered. Calcium folinate should be used because folic acid does not correct folate deficiency due to dihydrofolate reductase inhibitors.

Daraprim may exacerbate folate deficiency in subjects predisposed to this condition through disease or malnutrition. Accordingly, a calcium folinate supplement should be given to such individuals. In patients with megaloblastic anaemia due to folate deficiency the risks versus benefits of administering Daraprim require careful consideration.

Caution should be exercised in administering Daraprim to patients with a history of seizures; large loading doses should be avoided in such patients (see Undesirable Effects).

When a sulphonamide is given an adequate fluid intake should be ensured to minimise the risk of crystalluria.

Since pyrimethamine is administered with a sulphonamide for the conditions indicated the general precautions applicable to sulphonamides should be observed.

Occasional reports suggest that individuals taking pyrimethamine as malarial prophylaxis at doses in excess of 25 mg weekly may develop megaloblastic anaemia if co-trimoxazole is prescribed concurrently.

Use in renal impairment

The kidney is not the major route of excretion of pyrimethamine and excretion is not significantly altered in patients with renal failure. There are, however, no substantial data on the use of Daraprim in renally impaired subjects. Due to lack of data on the theoretical possibility of active metabolites with prolonged treatment, caution should be exercised in renally impaired patients. It is not known if Daraprim is dialyzable. Since Daraprim is co-administered with a sulphonamide, care should be taken to avoid accumulation of the sulphonamide in renally impaired patients.

Use in hepatic impairment

The liver is the main route for metabolism of pyrimethamine. Data on the use of pyrimethamine in patients with liver disease are limited. Daraprim in combination with sulphonamides has been used effectively to treat toxoplasmosis in a patient with mild hepatic disease. There are no general recommendations for dosage reductions for liver-impaired states but consideration should be given to dose adjustment for individual cases.

4.5 Interaction with other medicinal products and other forms of interaction

Daraprim, by its mode of action, may further depress folate metabolism in patients receiving treatment with other folate inhibitors, or agents associated with myelosuppression, including co-trimoxazole, trimethoprim, proguanil, zidovudine, or cytostatic agents (eg. methotrexate). Cases of fatal bone marrow aplasia have been associated with the administration of daunorubicin, cytosine arabinoside and pyrimethamine to individuals suffering from acute myeloid leukaemia. Megaloblastic anaemia has been reported occasionally in individuals who took pyrimethamine in excess of 25 mg weekly concurrently with a trimethoprim/sulphonamide combination.

Convulsions have occurred after concurrent administration of methotrexate and pyrimethamine to children with central nervous system leukaemia. Also, seizures have occasionally been reported when pyrimethamine was used in combination with other antimalarial drugs.

The concurrent administration of lorazepam and Daraprim may induce hepatotoxicity.

In vitro data suggest that antacid salts and the anti-diarrhoeal agent kaolin reduce the absorption of pyrimethamine.

The high protein binding exhibited by pyrimethamine may prevent protein binding by other compounds (eg. quinine or warfarin). This could affect the efficacy or toxicity of the concomitant drug depending on the levels of unbound drug.

4.6 Pregnancy and lactation

Pregnancy

Pyrimethamine in combination with sulphonamide has been used for many years in the treatment of toxoplasmosis during pregnancy. This infection carries a high risk to the foetus. Pyrimethamine crosses the placenta and, although there is a theoretical risk of foetal abnormalities from all folate inhibitors given during pregnancy, there have been no reports that have shown with any certainty that pyrimethamine is associated with human teratogenicity. Nevertheless, caution should be exercised in the administration of pyrimethamine. A folate supplement should be given to pregnant women receiving Daraprim.

Consideration should be given to the treatment of all suspected cases of acquired toxoplasmosis in pregnancy. The risks associated with the administration of Daraprim must be balanced against the dangers of abortion or foetal malformation due to the infection.

Treatment with pyrimethamine and sulfadiazine during pregnancy is indicated in the presence of confirmed placental or foetal infection or when the mother is at risk of serious sequelae. However, in view of the theoretical risk of foetal abnormality arising from the use of Daraprim in early pregnancy, its use in combination therapy should be restricted to the second and third trimesters. Alternative therapy is therefore advised in the first trimester of pregnancy and until diagnosis has been confirmed.

Lactation

Pyrimethamine enters human breast milk. It has been estimated that over a 9-day period an average weight infant would receive about 45% of the dose ingested by the mother. In view of the high doses of pyrimethamine and concurrent sulphonamides needed in toxoplasmosis treatment, breast feeding should be avoided for the duration of treatment.

4.7 Effects on ability to drive and use machines

Not known.

4.8 Undesirable effects

At the recommended dose for malaria prophylaxis, side-effects are rare. Occasionally, rashes have been observed. At the doses required for treatment of toxoplasmosis, pyrimethamine may produce myelosuppression with anaemia, leucopenia and thrombocytopenia.

Precipitation of a grand mal attack in one patient predisposed to epilepsy has been reported but the clinical significance has not been defined.

Since a concurrent sulphonamide is to be taken with pyrimethamine for the indications listed the relevant sulphonamide data sheet/SPC or published literature should be consulted for sulphonamide associated adverse events.

4.9 Overdose

Symptoms and signs:-

Vomiting and convulsions occur in cases of severe, acute overdoses. Ataxia, tremor and respiratory depression can also occur. There have been isolated cases with fatal outcomes following acute overdose of pyrimethamine.

Chronic excess doses can result in bone marrow depression (eg. megaloblastic anaemia, leucopenia, thrombocytopenia) resulting from folic acid deficiency.

Management:-

Routine supportive treatment, including maintenance of a clear airway and control of convulsions.

Adequate fluids should be given to ensure optimal diuresis.

Gastric lavage may be of value only if instituted within two hours of ingestion in view of the rapid absorption of Daraprim.

To counteract possible folate deficiency, calcium folinate should be given until signs of toxicity have subsided. There may a delay of 7 to 10 days before the full leucopenic side effects become evident, therefore calcium folinate therapy should be continued for the period at risk.

5. PHARMACOLOGICAL PROPERTIES

5.1 Pharmacodynamic properties

Pyrimethamine is an antiparasitic agent.

Group: diaminopyrimidines

ATC code:- P01B D01

Mode of Action:-

The antiparasitic action of pyrimethamine is due to its specific activity on folic acid metabolism in the Plasmodium and Toxoplasma parasites. In this respect it competitively inhibits the dihydrofolate reductase enzyme with an affinity far greater for the protozoal than for the human enzyme.

5.2 Pharmacokinetic properties

Absorption:-

Pyrimethamine is rapidly absorbed from the gastrointestinal tract after administration. Time to peak plasma concentration is 2 to 4 hours in healthy volunteers. Peak plasma concentrations vary widely between individuals and can range from 260 to 1411ng/ml after daily doses of 25mg. A similar degree of inter-patient variability in serum levels has been noted in patients with AIDS.

Distribution:-

The volume of distribution for pyrimethamine is approximately 2L/kg. In patients with HIV infection, population pharmacokinetic analysis has indicated that the mean volume of distribution (corrected for bioavailability) is 246+/-64L.

About 87% of the drug is bound to plasma proteins. Pyrimethamine has been shown to reach the cerebrospinal fluid of patients with AIDS given daily doses, achieving concentrations approximately one fifth of those in serum.

Metabolism and elimination:-

Pyrimethamine is predominantly eliminated by metabolism, with up to 30% recovered in the urine as parent compound over a period of several weeks. The mean elimination half-life is 85 hours (ranging from 35 to 175 hours). In AIDS patients, the total clearance is 1.28+/-0.41L/h resulting in an elimination half life of 139+/-34h. Data are lacking on the nature of the metabolites of pyrimethamine, their route/rate of formation and elimination in man and any pharmacological activity, particularly after prolonged daily dosing.

Multiple dose studies indicate that steady state is achieved in 12 to 20 days with daily dosing. It is theoretically possible that metabolic pathways might be saturable, leading to excessive accumulation of the drug in some patients. However, it has been demonstrated that plasma levels are approximately proportional to dose at steady state so this appears unlikely. Genetic variation in the exposure to pyrimethamine has been reported but these data are unsubstantiated.

Some studies in patients with AIDS have indicated shorter half lives than those noted above: these are very likely to be a consequence of inappropriate sampling and analytical techniques. However, if there are patients in whom the half-life is particularly short, steady state therapeutic levels might be inadequate.

5.3 Preclinical safety data

Mutagenicity:-

In microbial tests, pyrimethamine was found to be non-mutagenic in the Ames Salmonella assay whereas DNA damage was seen in the Escherichia coli repair assay.

Further in vitro data indicate that pyrimethamine induces mutagenic activity in mouse lymphoma cells in the absence, but not in the presence of metabolic activation.

Pyrimethamine also showed clastogenic activity in mammalian lymphocytes in the absence of metabolic activation. Following intraperitoneal administration, pyrimethamine has been shown to induce chromosomal damage in male rodent germ cells although studies in somatic cells (micronucleus tests) are either negative or inconclusive. Studies following oral administration of pyrimethamine in rodents showed negative results in female germ cells and in male and female bone marrow/peripheral blood cells.

Carcinogenicity

A study in mice (dosed with either 500 or 1000 ppm pyrimethamine in the diet for 5 days per week, for 78 weeks) showed no evidence of carcinogenicity in females. Survival in the male mice did not allow for an assessment of carcinogenicity in this sex.

A similar study in rats dosed at 200 or 400 ppm pyrimethamine showed no evidence of carcinogenicity.

Teratogenicity

No changes in early development were seen in embryos from 15 mice given a single intra-gastric dose of pyrimethamine (50mg/kg bodyweight) on the first day of gestation. However development of mouse and rat embryos in culture was severely hindered by pyrimethamine in a dose-dependent manner.

Pyrimethamine was teratogenic in rodents and in the Gottingen minipig in a dose-dependent manner.

Other studies in rats dosed at either 1mg/kg or 10mg/kg bodyweight showed some inhibition of developmental processes but no teratological effects.

Pyrimethamine was not teratogenic in rabbits at dose levels up to 100mg/kg bodyweight/day administered on days 6 to 18 of pregnancy. Pyrimethamine markedly reduced early stage cell division in rabbit embryos but implantation and foetal development were normal.

Fertility

A study in rats dosed with 5mg/kg bodyweight/day for 6 weeks resulted in reduced sperm concentrations and testis weights, but there were no effects on fertility. Reversible arrest of spermatogenesis was shown in a study on mice dosed with 200mg/kg/day for 50 days. However, this dose is far in excess of human therapeutic doses.

6. PHARMACEUTICAL PARTICULARS

6.1 List of excipients

Lactose Monohydrate

Maize Starch

Hydrolysed Starch

Docusate sodium

Magnesium stearate

6.2 Incompatibilities

Not applicable

6.3 Shelf life

5 years

6.4 Special precautions for storage

Do not store above 30°C.

Store in the original container.

6.5 Nature and contents of container

Vinyl - lacquered aluminium foil strip-packs.

Pack size: 30 tablets

6.6 Special precautions for disposal and other handling

Not applicable

Administrative Data

7. MARKETING AUTHORISATION HOLDER

The Wellcome Foundation Ltd t/a GlaxoSmithKline UK
Glaxo Wellcome House
Berkeley Avenue
Greenford
Middlesex
UB6 ONN

Stockley Park West, Uxbridge
Middlesex, UB11 1BT

8. MARKETING AUTHORISATION NUMBER(S)

PL 00003/5026R

9. DATE OF FIRST AUTHORISATION/RENEWAL OF THE AUTHORISATION

21 December 2005

10. DATE OF REVISION OF THE TEXT

21 December 2005

DDAVP Melt 60mcg, 120mcg and 240mcg oral lyophilisate

(Ferring Pharmaceuticals Ltd)

1. NAME OF THE MEDICINAL PRODUCT

DDAVP Melt ▼60 micrograms oral lyophilisate

DDAVP Melt ▼120 micrograms oral lyophilisate

DDAVP Melt ▼240 micrograms oral lyophilisate

2. QUALITATIVE AND QUANTITATIVE COMPOSITION

Each unit contains 60, 120 or 240 micrograms desmopressin (as acetate).

For excipients, see 6.1

3. PHARMACEUTICAL FORM

Oral lyophilisate

DDAVP Melt 60 micrograms oral lyophilisate

White, round, oral lyophilisate marked with a drop shaped figure on one side.

DDAVP Melt 120 micrograms oral lyophilisate

White, round, oral lyophilisate marked with two drop shaped figures on one side.

DDAVP Melt 240 micrograms oral lyophilisate

White, round, oral lyophilisate marked with three drop shaped figure on one side.

4. CLINICAL PARTICULARS

4.1 Therapeutic indications

DDAVP Melt is indicated for the treatment of vasopressin-sensitive cranial diabetes insipidus or in the treatment of post-hypophysectomy polyuria/polydipsia.

4.2 Posology and method of administration

DDAVP Melt is for sublingual use.

Treatment of diabetes insipidus:

Dosage is individual in diabetes insipidus but the total daily sublingual dose normally lies in the range of 120 micrograms to 720 micrograms. A suitable starting dose in adults and children is 60 micrograms three times daily, administered sublingually. This dosage regimen should then be adjusted in accordance with the patient's response. For the majority of patients, the maintenance dose is 60 micrograms to 120 micrograms sublingually three times daily.

Post-hypophysectomy polyuria/polydipsia:

The dose of DDAVP Melt should be controlled by measurement of urine osmolality.

4.3 Contraindications

DDAVP Melt is contraindicated in cases of cardiac insufficiency and other conditions requiring treatment with diuretic agents.

Before prescribing DDAVP Melt, the diagnoses of psychogenic polydipsia and alcohol abuse should be excluded.

4.4 Special warnings and precautions for use

Care should be taken with patients who have reduced renal function and/or cardiovascular disease. In chronic renal disease the antidiuretic effect of DDAVP Melt would be less than normal.

Precautions to prevent fluid overload must be taken in:

- conditions characterised by fluid and/or electrolyte imbalance

- patients at risk for increased intracranial pressure.

4.5 Interaction with other medicinal products and other forms of interaction

Substances which are known to induce SIADH e.g. tricyclic antidepressants, selective serotonin re-uptake inhibitors, chlorpromazine and carbamazepine, may cause an additive antidiuretic effect leading to an increased risk of water retention and/or hyponatraemia.

NSAIDs may induce water retention and/or hyponatraemia.

Concomitant treatment with loperamide may result in a 3-fold increase of desmopressin plasma concentrations, which may lead to an increased risk of water retention and/or hyponatraemia. Although not investigated, other drugs slowing intestinal transport might have the same effect.

A standardised 27% fat meal significantly decreased the absorption (rate and extent) of a 0.4mg dose of oral desmopressin tablets. Although it did not significantly affect the pharmacodynamic effect (urine production and osmolality), there is the potential for this to occur at lower doses. If a diminution of effect is noted, then the effect of food should be considered before increasing the dose.

4.6 Pregnancy and lactation

Pregnancy:

Data on a limited number (n=53) of exposed pregnancies in women with diabetes insipidus indicate rare cases of malformations in children treated during pregnancy. To date, no other relevant epidemiological data are available. Animal studies do not indicate direct or indirect harmful effects with respect to pregnancy, embryonal/fetal development, parturition or postnatal development.

Caution should be exercised when prescribing to pregnant women. Blood pressure monitoring is recommended due to the increased risk of pre-eclampsia.

Lactation:

Results from analyses of milk from nursing mothers receiving high dose desmopressin (300 micrograms intranasally) indicate that the amounts of desmopressin that may be transferred to the child are considerably less than the amounts required to influence diuresis.

4.7 Effects on ability to drive and use machines

None

4.8 Undesirable effects

Side-effects include headache, stomach pain and nausea. Isolated cases of allergic skin reactions and more severe general allergic reactions have been reported. Very rare cases of emotional disorders including aggression in children have been reported. Treatment with desmopressin without concomitant reduction of fluid intake may lead to water retention/hyponatraemia with accompanying symptoms of headache, nausea, vomiting, weight gain, decreased serum sodium and in serious cases, convulsions.

4.9 Overdose

An overdose of DDAVP Melt leads to a prolonged duration of action with an increased risk of water retention and/or hyponatraemia.

Treatment:

Although the treatment of hyponatraemia should be individualised, the following general recommendations can be given. Hyponatraemia is treated by discontinuing the desmopressin treatment, fluid restriction and symptomatic treatment if needed

5. PHARMACOLOGICAL PROPERTIES

5.1 Pharmacodynamic properties

Pharmacotherapeutic group: vasopressin and analogues

ATC code: H01B A02

In its main biological effects, DDAVP does not differ qualitatively from vasopressin. However, DDAVP is characterised by a high antidiuretic activity whereas the uterotonic and vasopressor actions are extremely low.

5.2 Pharmacokinetic properties

The overall mean systemic bioavailability of desmopressin administered sublingually as Melts at doses of 200, 400 and 800 micrograms is 0.25% with a 95% confidence interval of 0.21% - 0.31%. The C_{max} was 14, 30 and 65pg/ml after administration of 200, 400 and 800 micrograms respectively. t_{max} was observed at 0.5 – 2.0 hours after dosing. The geometric mean terminal half-life is 2.8 (CV = 24%) hours.

Correlation table between desmopressin in Tablet and Melt forms:

(see Table 1 below)

The distribution volume of desmopressin after intravenous administration is 33 L (0.41 L/kg). Desmopressin does not cross the blood-brain barrier. Desmopressin exhibits a moderate to high variability in bioavailability, both within and between subjects. Concomitant use of food decreases the rate and extent of absorption by 40%.

In vitro, in human liver microsome preparations, it has been shown that no significant amount of desmopressin is metabolised in the liver and thus human liver metabolism *in vivo* is not likely to occur.

It is unlikely that desmopressin will interact with drugs affecting hepatic metabolism, since desmopressin has been shown not to undergo significant liver metabolism in *in vitro* studies with human microsomes. However, formal *in vivo* interaction studies have not been performed.

5.3 Preclinical safety data

There are no pre-clinical data of relevance to the prescriber which are additional to that already included in other sections of the SPC.

6. PHARMACEUTICAL PARTICULARS

6.1 List of excipients

Gelatin

Mannitol

Citric acid, anhydrous

6.2 Incompatibilities

Not applicable

6.3 Shelf life

24 months

6.4 Special precautions for storage

Store in the original package.

6.5 Nature and contents of container

PVC/Polyamide/Aluminium/Polyamide/PVC blisters. Top foil consists of Paper/Polyester teraphthalate/Aluminium/heat seal lacquer. Strips of 10 oral lyophilisates in packs of 100 oral lyophilisates.

6.6 Special precautions for disposal and other handling

None.

7. MARKETING AUTHORISATION HOLDER

Ferring Pharmaceuticals Ltd.

The Courtyard

Waterside Drive

Langley

Berkshire SL3 6EZ

United Kingdom.

Table 1 Correlation table between desmopressin in Tablet and Melt forms

Tablet	Tablet	Melt	Melt
Desmopressin acetate	Desmopressin free base	Desmopressin free base	Desmopressin acetate
0.1mg	89 micrograms	60 micrograms	Approx. 67 micrograms +
0.2mg	178 micrograms	120 micrograms	Approx. 135 micrograms +
0.4mg	356 micrograms	240 micrograms	Approx. 270 micrograms +

+ calculated for comparative purposes

8. MARKETING AUTHORISATION NUMBER(S)
DDAVP Melt 60 micrograms oral lyophilisate PL 03194/0091
DDAVP Melt 120 micrograms oral lyophilisate PL 03194/0092
DDAVP Melt 240 micrograms oral lyophilisate PL 03194/0093

9. DATE OF FIRST AUTHORISATION/RENEWAL OF THE AUTHORISATION
19th January 2006

10. DATE OF REVISION OF THE TEXT
May 2008

11. LEGAL CATEGORY
POM

* DDAVP is a trademark of Ferring BV.

DDAVP Tablets 0.1mg

(Ferring Pharmaceuticals Ltd)

1. NAME OF THE MEDICINAL PRODUCT
DDAVP® Tablets 0.1mg.

2. QUALITATIVE AND QUANTITATIVE COMPOSITION
Each tablet contains 0.1mg Desmopressin acetate
For excipients, see 6.1

3. PHARMACEUTICAL FORM
Tablet
Uncoated, white, oval, convex tablets scored on one side and engraved '0.1' on the other side.

4. CLINICAL PARTICULARS

4.1 Therapeutic indications
DDAVP Tablets are indicated for the treatment of vasopressin-sensitive cranial diabetes insipidus or in the treatment of post-hypophysectomy polyuria/polydipsia.

4.2 Posology and method of administration
Treatment of Diabetes Insipidus:
Dosage is individual in diabetes insipidus but clinical experience has shown that the total daily dose normally lies in the range of 0.2 to 1.2mg. A suitable starting dose in adults and children is 0.1mg three times daily. This dosage regimen should then be adjusted in accordance with the patient's response. For the majority of patients, the maintenance dose is 0.1mg to 0.2mg three times daily.

Post-hypophysectomy polyuria/polydipsia:
The dose of DDAVP Tablets should be controlled by measurement of urine osmolality.

4.3 Contraindications
DDAVP Tablets are contraindicated in cases of cardiac insufficiency and other conditions requiring treatment with diuretic agents.
Before prescribing DDAVP Tablets the diagnoses of psychogenic polydipsia and alcohol abuse should be excluded.

4.4 Special warnings and precautions for use
Care should be taken with patients who have reduced renal function and/or cardiovascular disease. In chronic renal disease the antidiuretic effect of DDAVP Tablets would be less than normal.
Precautions to prevent fluid overload must be taken in:
- conditions characterised by fluid and/or electrolyte imbalance
- patients at risk for increased intracranial pressure

4.5 Interaction with other medicinal products and other forms of interaction
Substances which are known to induce SIADH e.g. tricyclic antidepressants, selective serotonin re-uptake inhibitors, chlorpromazine and carbamazepine, may cause an additive antidiuretic effect leading to an increased risk of water retention and/or hyponatraemia.
NSAIDs may induce water retention and/or hyponatraemia.
Concomitant treatment with loperamide may result in a 3-fold increase of desmopressin plasma concentrations, which may lead to an increased risk of water retention and/or hyponatraemia. Although not investigated, other drugs slowing transport might have the same effect.
A standardised 27% fat meal significantly decreased the absorption (rate and extent) of a 0.4mg dose of oral desmopressin. Although it did not significantly affect the pharmacodynamic effect (urine production and osmolality), there is the potential for this to occur at lower doses. If a diminution of effect is noted, then the effect of food should be considered before increasing the dose.

4.6 Pregnancy and lactation
Pregnancy:
Data on a limited number (n=53) of exposed pregnancies in women with diabetes insipidus indicate rare cases of malformations in children treated during pregnancy. To date, no other relevant epidemiological data are available. Animal studies do not indicate direct or indirect harmful effects with respect to pregnancy, embryonal/fetal development, parturition or postnatal development.
Caution should be exercised when prescribing to pregnant women. Blood pressure monitoring is recommended due to the increased risk of pre-eclampsia.
Lactation:
Results from analyses of milk from nursing mothers receiving high dose desmopressin (300 micrograms intranasally) indicate that the amounts of desmopressin that may be transferred to the child are considerably less than the amounts required to influence diuresis.

4.7 Effects on ability to drive and use machines
None

4.8 Undesirable effects
Side-effects include headache, stomach pain and nausea. Isolated cases of allergic skin reactions and more severe general allergic reactions have been reported. Very rare cases of emotional disorders including aggression in children have been reported. Treatment with desmopressin without concomitant reduction of fluid intake may lead to water retention/hyponatraemia with accompanying symptoms of headache, nausea, vomiting, weight gain, decreased serum sodium and in serious cases, convulsions.

4.9 Overdose
An overdose of DDAVP Tablets leads to a prolonged duration of action with an increased risk of water retention and/or hyponatraemia.
Treatment:
Although the treatment of hyponatraemia should be individualised, the following general recommendations can be given. Hyponatraemia is treated by discontinuing the desmopressin treatment, fluid restriction and symptomatic treatment if needed.

5. PHARMACOLOGICAL PROPERTIES

5.1 Pharmacodynamic properties
In its main biological effects, DDAVP does not differ qualitatively from vasopressin. However, DDAVP is characterised by a high antidiuretic activity whereas the uterotonic and vasopressor actions are extremely low.
In a modelling study in which intravenous desmopressin was infused over two hours in healthy adult male subjects, the EC_{50} value was calculated as 1.7pg/ml based on urinary osmolality and 2.4pg/ml based on urinary volume.

5.2 Pharmacokinetic properties
The absolute bioavailability of orally administered desmopressin varies between 0.08% and 0.16%. Mean maximum plasma concentration is reached within 2 hours. The distribution volume is 0.2 – 0.32 l/kg. Desmopressin does not cross the blood-brain barrier. The oral terminal half-life varies between 2.0 and 3.11 hours.
After oral administration of a single dose of 2 × 200 micrograms desmopressin tablets to healthy subjects, 25% of the subjects had plasma concentrations of desmopressin above 1pg/ml up to at least 14 hours post dosing.
In *in vitro* studies in human liver microsome preparations, it has been shown that no significant amount of desmopressin is metabolised, and thus human liver metabolism *in vivo* is not likely to occur. Consequently it is also unlikely that desmopressin will interact with drugs affecting hepatic metabolism. However, formal *in vivo* interaction studies have not been performed.
About 65% of the amount of desmopressin absorbed after oral administration could be recovered in the urine within 24 hours.

5.3 Preclinical safety data
There are no pre-clinical data of relevance to the prescriber which are additional to that already included in other sections of the SPC.

6. PHARMACEUTICAL PARTICULARS

6.1 List of excipients
Lactose monohydrate
Potato starch
Povidone
Magnesium stearate

6.2 Incompatibilities
Not applicable

6.3 Shelf life
36 months

6.4 Special precautions for storage
Do not store above 25°C. Keep the container tightly closed.

6.5 Nature and contents of container
30ml High Density Polyethylene (HDPE) bottle with a tamper-proof, twist-off polypropylene (PP) closure with a silica gel desiccant insert. Each bottle contains either 30 or 90 tablets.
Not all pack sizes may be marketed.

6.6 Special precautions for disposal and other handling
None

7. MARKETING AUTHORISATION HOLDER
Ferring Pharmaceuticals Ltd.
The Courtyard
Waterside Drive
Langley
Berkshire SL3 6EZ.

8. MARKETING AUTHORISATION NUMBER(S)
PL 03194/0040

9. DATE OF FIRST AUTHORISATION/RENEWAL OF THE AUTHORISATION
12th January 2003

10. DATE OF REVISION OF THE TEXT
May 2008

DDAVP Tablets 0.2mg

(Ferring Pharmaceuticals Ltd)

1. NAME OF THE MEDICINAL PRODUCT
DDAVP® Tablets 0.2mg.

2. QUALITATIVE AND QUANTITATIVE COMPOSITION
Each tablet contains 0.2mg Desmopressin acetate
For excipients, see 6.1

3. PHARMACEUTICAL FORM
Tablet
Uncoated, white, round, convex tablets scored on one side and engraved '0.2' on the other side.

4. CLINICAL PARTICULARS

4.1 Therapeutic indications
DDAVP Tablets are indicated for the treatment of vasopressin-sensitive cranial diabetes insipidus or in the treatment of post-hypophysectomy polyuria/polydipsia.

4.2 Posology and method of administration
Treatment of Diabetes Insipidus:
Dosage is individual in diabetes insipidus but clinical experience has shown that the total daily dose normally lies in the range of 0.2 to 1.2mg. A suitable starting dose in adults and children is 0.1mg three times daily. This dosage regimen should then be adjusted in accordance with the patient's response. For the majority of patients, the maintenance dose is 0.1mg to 0.2mg three times daily.

Post-hypophysectomy polyuria/polydipsia:
The dose of DDAVP Tablets should be controlled by measurement of urine osmolality.

4.3 Contraindications
DDAVP Tablets are contraindicated in cases of cardiac insufficiency and other conditions requiring treatment with diuretic agents.
Before prescribing DDAVP Tablets the diagnoses of psychogenic polydipsia and alcohol abuse should be excluded.

4.4 Special warnings and precautions for use
Care should be taken with patients who have reduced renal function and/or cardiovascular disease. In chronic renal disease the antidiuretic effect of DDAVP Tablets would be less than normal.
Precautions to prevent fluid overload must be taken in:
- conditions characterised by fluid and/or electrolyte imbalance
- patients at risk for increased intracranial pressure

4.5 Interaction with other medicinal products and other forms of interaction
Substances which are known to induce SIADH e.g. tricyclic antidepressants, selective serotonin re-uptake inhibitors, chlorpromazine and carbamazepine, may cause an additive antidiuretic effect leading to an increased risk of water retention and/or hyponatraemia.
NSAIDs may induce water retention and/or hyponatraemia.
Concomitant treatment with loperamide may result in a 3-fold increase of desmopressin plasma concentrations, which may lead to an increased risk of water retention and/or hyponatraemia. Although not investigated, other drugs slowing transport might have the same effect.
A standardised 27% fat meal significantly decreased the absorption (rate and extent) of a 0.4mg dose of oral desmopressin. Although it did not significantly affect the pharmacodynamic effect (urine production and osmolality), there is the potential for this to occur at lower doses. If a diminution of effect is noted, then the effect of food should be considered before increasing the dose.

4.6 Pregnancy and lactation
Pregnancy:
Data on a limited number (n=53) of exposed pregnancies in women with diabetes insipidus indicate rare cases of malformations in children treated during pregnancy. To date, no other relevant epidemiological data are available. Animal studies do not indicate direct or indirect harmful effects with respect to pregnancy, embryonal/fetal development, parturition or postnatal development.
Caution should be exercised when prescribing to pregnant women. Blood pressure monitoring is recommended due to the increased risk of pre-eclampsia.
Lactation:
Results from analyses of milk from nursing mothers receiving high dose desmopressin (300 micrograms intranasally) indicate that the amounts of desmopressin that may be

transferred to the child are considerably less than the amounts required to influence diuresis.

4.7 Effects on ability to drive and use machines
None

4.8 Undesirable effects
Side-effects include headache, stomach pain and nausea. Isolated cases of allergic skin reactions and more severe general allergic reactions have been reported. Very rare cases of emotional disorders including aggression in children have been reported. Treatment with desmopressin without concomitant reduction of fluid intake may lead to water retention/hyponatraemia with accompanying symptoms of headache, nausea, vomiting, weight gain, decreased serum sodium and in serious cases, convulsions.

4.9 Overdose
An overdose of DDAVP Tablets leads to a prolonged duration of action with an increased risk of water retention and/or hyponatraemia.

Treatment:

Although the treatment of hyponatraemia should be individualised, the following general recommendations can be given. Hyponatraemia is treated by discontinuing the desmopressin treatment, fluid restriction and symptomatic treatment if needed.

5. PHARMACOLOGICAL PROPERTIES

5.1 Pharmacodynamic properties
In its main biological effects, DDAVP does not differ qualitatively from vasopressin. However, DDAVP is characterised by a high antidiuretic activity whereas the uterotonic and vasopressor actions are extremely low.

In a modelling study in which intravenous desmopressin was infused over two hours in healthy adult male subjects, the EC_{50} value was calculated as 1.7pg/ml based on urinary osmolality and 2.4pg/ml based on urinary flow.

5.2 Pharmacokinetic properties
The absolute bioavailability of orally administered desmopressin varies between 0.08% and 0.16%. Mean maximum plasma concentration is reached within 2 hours. The distribution volume is 0.2 – 0.32 l/kg. Desmopressin does not cross the blood-brain barrier. The oral terminal half-life varies between 2.0 and 3.11 hours.

After oral administration of a single dose of 2 × 200 micrograms desmopressin tablets to healthy subjects, 25% of the subjects had plasma concentrations of desmopressin above 1pg/ml up to at least 14 hours post dosing.

In *in vitro* studies in human liver microsome preparations, it has been shown that no significant amount of desmopressin is metabolised, and thus human liver metabolism *in vivo* is not likely to occur. Consequently it is also unlikely that desmopressin will interact with drugs affecting hepatic metabolism. However, formal *in vivo* interaction studies have not been performed.

About 65% of the amount of desmopressin absorbed after oral administration could be recovered in the urine within 24 hours.

5.3 Preclinical safety data
There are no pre-clinical data of relevance to the prescriber which are additional to that already included in other sections of the SPC.

6. PHARMACEUTICAL PARTICULARS

6.1 List of excipients
Lactose monohydrate

Potato starch

Povidone

Magnesium stearate

6.2 Incompatibilities
Not applicable

6.3 Shelf life
36 months.

6.4 Special precautions for storage
Do not store above 25°C. Keep the container tightly closed.

6.5 Nature and contents of container
30ml High Density Polyethylene (HDPE) bottle with a tamper-proof, twist-off polypropylene (PP) closure with a silica gel desiccant insert. Each bottle contains either 30 or 90 tablets.

Not all pack sizes may be marketed.

6.6 Special precautions for disposal and other handling
None

7. MARKETING AUTHORISATION HOLDER
Ferring Pharmaceuticals Ltd.

The Courtyard

Waterside Drive

Langley

Berkshire SL3 6EZ.

8. MARKETING AUTHORISATION NUMBER(S)
PL 03194/0041

9. DATE OF FIRST AUTHORISATION/RENEWAL OF THE AUTHORISATION
12th January 2003.

10. DATE OF REVISION OF THE TEXT
May 2008

DDAVP/Desmopressin Injection

(Ferring Pharmaceuticals Ltd)

1. NAME OF THE MEDICINAL PRODUCT
DDAVP®/Desmopressin Injection.

2. QUALITATIVE AND QUANTITATIVE COMPOSITION
Each 1ml ampoule contains Desmopressin acetate 4 micrograms per ml.

3. PHARMACEUTICAL FORM
Solution for injection.

4. CLINICAL PARTICULARS

4.1 Therapeutic indications
DDAVP®/Desmopressin Injection is indicated as follows:

1) Diagnosis and treatment of cranial diabetes insipidus.

2) To increase Factor VIII:C and Factor VIII:Ag in patients with mild to moderate haemophilia or von Willebrand's disease undergoing surgery or following trauma.

3) To establish renal concentration capacity.

4) To treat headache resulting from a lumbar puncture.

5) To test for fibrinolytic response.

4.2 Posology and method of administration
Treatment of Cranial Diabetes Insipidus:

By subcutaneous, intramuscular or intravenous injection.

Adults:

The usual dose is 1 to 4 micrograms given once daily.

Children and infants:

Doses from 0.4 micrograms (0.1ml) may be used.

Diagnosis of Cranial Diabetes Insipidus:

The diagnostic dose in adults and children is 2 micrograms given by subcutaneous or intramuscular injection. Failure to elaborate a concentrated urine after water deprivation, followed by the ability to do so after the administration of Desmopressin confirms a diagnosis of cranial diabetes insipidus. Failure to concentrate after the administration suggests nephrogenic diabetes insipidus.

Mild to moderate haemophilia and von Willebrand's disease:

By intravenous administration.

The dose for adults, children and infants is 0.4 micrograms per kilogram body weight administered by intravenous infusion. Further doses may be administered at 12 hourly intervals so long as cover is required. As some patients have shown a diminishing response to successive doses, it is recommended that monitoring of Factor VIII levels should continue. The dose should be diluted in 50ml of 0.9% sodium chloride for injection and given over 20 minutes. This dose should be given immediately prior to surgery or following trauma. During administration of intravenous Desmopressin, vasodilation may occur resulting in decreased blood pressure and tachycardia with facial flushing in some patients.

Increase of Factor VIII levels are dependent on basal levels and are normally between 2 and 5 times the pre-treatment levels. If results from a previous administration of Desmopressin are not available then blood should be taken predose and 20 minutes post-dose for assay of Factor VIII levels in order to monitor response.

Unless contraindicated, when surgery is undertaken, tranexamic acid may be given orally at the recommended dose from 24 hours beforehand until healing is complete.

Renal Function Testing:

By subcutaneous or intramuscular injection.

Adults and children can be expected to achieve urine concentrations above 700mOsm/kg in the period of 5 to 9 hours following a dose of 2 micrograms DDAVP®/Desmopressin Injection. It is recommended that the bladder should be emptied at the time of administration.

In normal infants, a urine concentration of 600mOsm/kg should be achieved in the five hour period following a dose of 0.4 micrograms DDAVP®/Desmopressin Injection. The fluid intake at the two meals following the administration should be restricted to 50% of the ordinary intake to avoid water overload.

Post Lumbar Puncture Headache:

By subcutaneous or intramuscular injection.

Where a headache is thought to be due to a lumbar puncture, an adult patient can be given a dose of 4 micrograms DDAVP®/Desmopressin Injection which may be repeated 24 hours later if necessary. Alternatively, a prophylactic dose of 4 micrograms can be given immediately prior to the lumbar puncture and repeated 24 hours later.

Fibrinolytic Response Testing:

By intravenous administration.

The dose for adults and children is 0.4 micrograms per kilogram body weight administered by intravenous infusion. The dose should be diluted in 50ml of 0.9% sodium chloride for injection and given over 20 minutes.

A sample of venous blood should be taken 20 minutes after the infusion. In patients with a normal response the sample should show fibrinolytic activity of euglobulin clot precipitate on fibrin plates of at least $240mm^2$.

4.3 Contraindications
DDAVP®/Desmopressin Injection is contraindicated in cases of:

GENERAL:

- habitual and psychogenic polydipsia

RENAL FUNCTION TESTING, TREATMENT OF LUMBAR PUNCTURE HEADACHE OR FIBRINOLYTIC RESPONSE TESTING:

- should not be carried out in patients with hypertension, heart disease, cardiac insufficiency and other conditions requiring treatment with diuretic agents

FOR HAEMOSTATIC USE

- unstable angina pectoris

- decompensated cardiac insufficiency

- von Willebrand's Disease Type IIB where the administration of Desmopressin may result in pseudothrombocytopenia due to the release of clotting factors which cause platelet aggregation.

4.4 Special warnings and precautions for use
GENERAL

Precautions to prevent fluid overload must be taken in:

- conditions characterised by fluid and/or electrolyte imbalance

- patients at risk for increased intracranial pressure

Care should be taken with patients who have reduced renal function and/or cardiovascular disease.

When DDAVP®/Desmopressin Injection is used for diagnostic purposes, fluid intake must be limited and not exceed 0.5 litres from 1 hour before until 8 hours after administration.

Renal concentration capacity testing in children below the age of 1 year should only be performed under carefully supervised conditions in hospital.

FOR HAEMOSTATIC USE

When repeated doses are used to control bleeding in haemophilia or von Willebrand's disease, care should be taken to prevent fluid overload. Fluid should not be forced, orally or parenterally, and patients should only take as much fluid as they require to satisfy thirst. Intravenous infusions should not be left up as a routine after surgery. Fluid accumulation can be readily monitored by weighing the patient or by determining plasma sodium or osmolality.

Measures to prevent fluid overload must be taken in patients with conditions requiring treatment with diuretic agents.

Special attention must be paid to the risk of water retention. The fluid intake should be restricted to the least possible and the body weight should be checked regularly.

If there is a gradual increase of the body weight, decrease of serum sodium to below 130mmol/l or plasma osmolality to below 270mOsm/kg, the fluid intake must be reduced drastically and the administration of DDAVP®/Desmopressin Injection interrupted.

During infusion of DDAVP®/Desmopressin Injection for haemostatic use, it is recommended that the patient's blood pressure is monitored continuously.

DDAVP®/Desmopressin Injection does not reduce prolonged bleeding time in thrombocytopenia.

4.5 Interaction with other medicinal products and other forms of interaction
Substances which are known to induce SIADH e.g. tricyclic antidepressants, selective serotonin re-uptake inhibitors, chlorpromazine and carbamazepine, may cause an additive antidiuretic effect leading to an increased risk of water retention and/or hyponatraemia.

NSAIDs may induce water retention and/or hyponatraemia.

4.6 Pregnancy and lactation
Pregnancy:

Data on a limited number (n=53) of exposed pregnancies in women with diabetes insipidus indicate rare cases of malformations in children treated during pregnancy. To date, no other relevant epidemiological data are available. Animal studies do not indicate direct or indirect harmful effects with respect to pregnancy, embryonal/fetal development, parturition or postnatal development.

Caution should be exercised when prescribing to pregnant women. Blood pressure monitoring is recommended due to the increased risk of pre-eclampsia.

Lactation:

Results from analyses of milk from nursing mothers receiving high dose Desmopressin (300 micrograms intranasally) indicate that the amounts of Desmopressin that may be transferred to the child are considerably less than the amounts required to influence diuresis or haemostasis.

4.7 Effects on ability to drive and use machines
None

4.8 Undesirable effects
Side-effects include headache, stomach pain and nausea. Isolated cases of allergic skin reactions and more severe general allergic reactions have been reported. Very rare cases of emotional disorders including aggression in children have been reported. Treatment with Desmopressin without concomitant reduction of fluid intake may lead

to water retention/hyponatraemia with accompanying symptoms of headache, nausea, vomiting, weight gain, decreased serum sodium and in serious cases, convulsions.

4.9 Overdose
An overdose of DDAVP®/Desmopressin injection leads to a prolonged duration of action with an increased risk of water retention and/or hyponatraemia.

Treatment:

Although the treatment of hyponatraemia should be individualised, the following general recommendations can be given. Hyponatraemia is treated by discontinuing the desmopressin treatment, fluid restriction and symptomatic treatment if needed.

5. PHARMACOLOGICAL PROPERTIES

5.1 Pharmacodynamic properties
Desmopressin is a structural analogue of vasopressin in which the antidiuretic activity has been enhanced by the order of 10, while the vasopressor effect has been reduced by the order of 1500. The clinical advantage of this highly changed ratio of antidiuretic to vasopressor effect is that clinically active antidiuretic doses are far below the threshold for a vasopressor effect.

Like vasopressin, Desmopressin also increases concentrations of Factor VIII:C, Factor VIII:Ag and Plasminogen Activator.

5.2 Pharmacokinetic properties
Following intravenous injection, plasma concentrations of Desmopressin follow a biexponential curve. The initial fast phase of a few minutes duration and with a half life of less than 10 minutes is thought mainly to represent the diffusion of Desmopressin from plasma to its volume of distribution. The second phase with a half life of 51-158 minutes represents the elimination rate of Desmopressin from the body.

As a comparison, the half life of vasopressin is less than 10 minutes.

In vitro, in human liver microsome preparations, it has been shown that no significant amount of desmopressin is metabolised in the liver and thus human liver metabolism *in vivo* is not likely to occur.

It is unlikely that desmopressin will interact with drugs affecting hepatic metabolism, since desmopressin has been shown not to undergo significant liver metabolism in *in vitro* studies with human microsomes. However, formal *in vivo* interaction studies have not been performed.

5.3 Preclinical safety data
There are no pre-clinical data of relevance to the prescriber which are additional to those already included in other sections of the SPC.

6. PHARMACEUTICAL PARTICULARS

6.1 List of excipients
Sodium Chloride EP

Hydrochloric Acid EP

Water for Injection EP

6.2 Incompatibilities
None known

6.3 Shelf life
Shelf life of unopened ampoule: 24 months.

6.4 Special precautions for storage
To be stored in a refrigerator at 2°C to 8°C.

6.5 Nature and contents of container
Carton containing 10 × 1ml clear Type I glass ampoules. Each ampoule contains 1ml of a sterile, clear, colourless solution for injection.

6.6 Special precautions for disposal and other handling
As indicated under the posology and method of administration section.

7. MARKETING AUTHORISATION HOLDER
Ferring Pharmaceuticals Limited

The Courtyard

Waterside Drive

Langley

Berkshire SL3 6EZ.

8. MARKETING AUTHORISATION NUMBER(S)
PL 03194/0002

9. DATE OF FIRST AUTHORISATION/RENEWAL OF THE AUTHORISATION
10th September 1998

10. DATE OF REVISION OF THE TEXT
March 2009

DDAVP/Desmopressin Intranasal Solution

(Ferring Pharmaceuticals Ltd)

1. NAME OF THE MEDICINAL PRODUCT
DDAVP®/Desmopressin Intranasal Solution

2. QUALITATIVE AND QUANTITATIVE COMPOSITION
Desmopressin acetate 0.01% w/v

3. PHARMACEUTICAL FORM
Aqueous solution for intranasal administration

4. CLINICAL PARTICULARS

4.1 Therapeutic indications
DDAVP®/Desmopressin Intranasal Solution is indicated for:

1) The diagnosis and treatment of vasopressin-sensitive cranial diabetes insipidus.

2) The treatment of nocturia associated with multiple sclerosis where other treatments have failed.

3) Establishing renal concentration capacity.

4.2 Posology and method of administration

Treatment of Diabetes Insipidus:

Dosage is individual but clinical experience has shown that the average maintenance doses are as follows:

Adults: 10 to 20 micrograms once or twice daily.

Elderly: 10 to 20 micrograms once or twice daily.

Children: 5 to 20 micrograms daily, (a lower dose may be required for infants).

Diagnosis of Diabetes Insipidus:

The diagnostic dose in adults and children is 20 micrograms. Failure to elaborate a concentrated urine after water deprivation, followed by the ability to do so after the administration of Desmopressin confirms the diagnosis of cranial diabetes insipidus. Failure to concentrate after the administration suggests nephrogenic diabetes insipidus.

Treatment of nocturia:

For multiple sclerosis patients up to 65 years of age with normal renal function suffering from nocturia the dose is 10 to 20 micrograms at bed time. Not more than one dose should be used in any 24 hour period.

Renal Function Testing:

To establish renal concentration capacity, the following single doses are recommended:

Adults: 40 micrograms

Elderly: 40 micrograms

Children (1 - 15 years): 20 micrograms

Infants (to 1 year): 10 micrograms

Adults and children with normal renal function can be expected to achieve concentrations above 700mOsm/kg in the period of 5-9 hours following administration of DDAVP®/Desmopressin Intranasal Solution. It is recommended that the bladder should be emptied at the time of administration.

In normal infants a urine concentration of 600mOsm/kg should be achieved in the 5 hour period following the administration of DDAVP®/Desmopressin Intranasal Solution. The fluid intake at the two meals following the administration should be restricted to 50% of the ordinary intake in order to avoid water overload.

4.3 Contraindications
DDAVP®/Desmopressin Intranasal Solution is contraindicated in cases of:

- cardiac insufficiency and other conditions requiring treatment with diuretic agents.

- hypersensitivity to the preservative.

Before prescribing DDAVP®/Desmopressin Intranasal the diagnoses of psychogenic polydipsia and alcohol abuse should be excluded.

When used to control nocturia in patients with multiple sclerosis, Desmopressin should not be used in patients with hypertension or cardiovascular disease.

Desmopressin should not be prescribed to patients over the age of 65 for the treatment of nocturia associated with multiple sclerosis.

4.4 Special warnings and precautions for use
Care should be taken with patients who have reduced renal function and/or cardiovascular disease or cystic fibrosis.

When DDAVP®/Desmopressin Intranasal Solution is used for the treatment of nocturia associated with multiple sclerosis, fluid intake must be limited from 1 hour before until 8 hours after administration. Periodic assessments should be made of blood pressure and weight to monitor the possibility of fluid overload.

When used for diagnostic purposes, fluid intake must be limited and not exceed 0.5 litres from 1 hour before until 8 hours after administration.

Following diagnostic testing for diabetes insipidus or renal concentration, care should be taken to prevent fluid overload. Fluid should not be forced, orally or parenterally, and patients should only take as much fluid as they require to satisfy thirst.

Precautions to prevent fluid overload must be taken in:

- conditions characterised by fluid and/or electrolyte imbalance.

- patients at risk for increased intracranial pressure.

Renal concentration capacity testing in children below the age of 1 year should only be performed under carefully supervised conditions in hospital.

4.5 Interaction with other medicinal products and other forms of interaction
Substances which are known to induce SIADH e.g. tricyclic antidepressants, selective serotonin re-uptake inhibitors, chlorpromazine and carbamazepine, may cause an additive antidiuretic effect leading to an increased risk of water retention and/or hyponatraemia.

NSAIDs may induce water retention and/or hyponatraemia.

4.6 Pregnancy and lactation
Pregnancy:

Data on a limited number (n=53) of exposed pregnancies in women with diabetes insipidus indicate rare cases of malformations in children treated during pregnancy. To date, no other relevant epidemiological data are available. Animal studies do not indicate direct or indirect harmful effects with respect to pregnancy, embryonal/fetal development, parturition or postnatal development.

Caution should be exercised when prescribing to pregnant women. Blood pressure monitoring is recommended due to the increased risk of pre-eclampsia.

Lactation:

Results from analyses of milk from nursing mothers receiving high dose Desmopressin (300 micrograms intranasally) indicate that the amounts of Desmopressin that may be transferred to the child are considerably less than the amounts required to influence diuresis.

4.7 Effects on ability to drive and use machines
None

4.8 Undesirable effects
Side-effects include headache, stomach pain, nausea, nasal congestion, rhinitis and epistaxis. Isolated cases of allergic skin reactions and more severe general allergic reactions have been reported. Very rare cases of emotional disorders including aggression in children have been reported. Treatment with Desmopressin without concomitant reduction of fluid intake may lead to water retention/hyponatraemia with accompanying symptoms of headache, nausea, vomiting, weight gain, decreased serum sodium and in serious cases, convulsions.

4.9 Overdose
An overdose of DDAVP®/Desmopressin Intranasal Solution leads to a prolonged duration of action with an increased risk of water retention and/or hyponatraemia.

Treatment:

Although the treatment of hyponatraemia should be individualised, the following general recommendations can be given. Hyponatraemia is treated by discontinuing the desmopressin treatment, fluid restriction and symptomatic treatment if needed.

5. PHARMACOLOGICAL PROPERTIES

5.1 Pharmacodynamic properties
Desmopressin is a structural analogue of vasopressin, with two chemical changes namely desamination of the N-terminal and replacement of the 8-L-Arginine by 8-D-Arginine. These changes have increased the antidiuretic activity and prolonged the duration of action. The pressor activity is reduced to less than 0.01% of the natural peptide as a result of which side-effects are rarely seen.

5.2 Pharmacokinetic properties
Following intranasal administration, the bioavailability of Desmopressin is of the order of 10%.

Pharmacokinetic parameters following intravenous administration were reported as follows:

Total clearance: 2.6ml/min/kg body weight.

$T_{½}$: 55 mins

Plasma kinetics of DDAVP in man

H.Vilhardt, S. Lundin, J. Falch.

Acta Pharmacol. ET. Toxicol. 1986, 58, 379-381

In vitro, in human liver microsome preparations, it has been shown that no significant amount of desmopressin is metabolised in the liver and thus human liver metabolism *in vivo* is not likely to occur.

It is unlikely that desmopressin will interact with drugs affecting hepatic metabolism, since desmopressin has been shown not to undergo significant liver metabolism in *in vitro* studies with human microsomes. However, formal *in vivo* interaction studies have not been performed.

5.3 Preclinical safety data
There are no pre-clinical data of relevance to the prescriber which are additional to those already included in other sections of the SPC.

6. PHARMACEUTICAL PARTICULARS

6.1 List of excipients
Sodium Chloride BP

Chlorobutanol EP

Hydrochloric Acid EP

Purified Water EP

6.2 Incompatibilities
None.

6.3 Shelf life
36 months.

6.4 Special precautions for storage
Store in a refrigerator at a temperature of 2° to 8°C. Protect from light.

6.5 Nature and contents of container
Brown glass vial, 1st hydrolytic glass. Fitted with a dropper set composed of poly-propylene and a cap of polyethylene.

6.6 Special precautions for disposal and other handling
None.

7. MARKETING AUTHORISATION HOLDER
Ferring Pharmaceuticals Limited
The Courtyard,
Waterside Drive,
Langley,
Berkshire SL3 6EZ

8. MARKETING AUTHORISATION NUMBER(S)
PL 03194/0001R

9. DATE OF FIRST AUTHORISATION/RENEWAL OF THE AUTHORISATION
28th April 1997

10. DATE OF REVISION OF THE TEXT
May 2008

Decapeptyl SR 11.25mg

(Ipsen Ltd)

1. NAME OF THE MEDICINAL PRODUCT
DECAPEPTYL SR 11.25 mg, powder for suspension for injection.

2. QUALITATIVE AND QUANTITATIVE COMPOSITION
Triptorelin (I.N.N.) 15 mg, as triptorelin acetate.

The vial contains an overage to ensure that a dose of 11.25 mg is administered to the patient.

For excipients, see 6.1.

3. PHARMACEUTICAL FORM
Powder for suspension for injection, sustained release formulation.

4. CLINICAL PARTICULARS
4.1 Therapeutic indications
Treatment of patients with locally advanced, non-metastatic prostate cancer, as an alternative to surgical castration (see section 5.1).

Treatment of metastatic prostate cancer

Treatment of endometriosis.

Treatment of precocious puberty (onset before 8 years in girls and 9 years in boys).

4.2 Posology and method of administration
Prostate cancer

One intramuscular injection should be administered every 3 months.

No dosage adjustment is necessary in the elderly.

Endometriosis

One intramuscular injection should be administered every 3 months. The treatment must be initiated in the first five days of the menstrual cycle. Treatment duration depends on the initial severity of the endometriosis and the changes observed in the clinical features (functional and anatomical) during treatment. The maximum duration of treatment should be 6 months (two injections).

A second course of treatment with DECAPEPTYL SR 11.25 mg or with other GnRH analogues should not be undertaken due to concerns about bone density losses.

Precocious puberty

One intramuscular injection of Decapeptyl *SR* 11.25mg repeated every 3 months.

Treatment should be stopped around the physiological age of puberty in boys and girls and should not be continued in girls with a bone maturation of more than 12 years. There are limited data available in boys relating to the optimum time to stop treatment based on bone age, however it is advised that treatment is stopped in boys with a bone maturation age of 13-14 years.

4.3 Contraindications
Hypersensitivity of GnRH analogues or to any of the excipients.

In prostate cancer, DECAPEPTYL SR 11.25 mg is contraindicated in patients presenting with spinal cord compression or evidence of spinal metastases.

In endometriosis, confirm that the patient is not pregnant before beginning treatment.

4.4 Special warnings and precautions for use
In adults the prolonged use of GnRH analogues may lead to bone loss which enhances the risk of osteoporosis.

Prostate cancer

Initially, DECAPEPTYL SR 11.25 mg like other GnRH analogues causes a transient increase in serum testosterone and consequent worsening of symptoms including increase in bone pain (and serum acid phosphatase levels).

Continued treatment with DECAPEPTYL SR 11.25 mg leads to suppression of testosterone (and dihydrotestosterone) and consequent improvement in the disease.

During the first month of treatment, patients presenting with, or at particular risk of developing, urinary tract obstruction should be carefully monitored, as should those at risk of developing spinal cord compression. Consideration should be given to the use of an anti-androgen for three days prior to DECAPEPTYL SR 11.25 mg treatment, to counteract this initial rise in serum testosterone levels.

Endometriosis

At the recommended dose, DECAPEPTYL SR 11.25 mg causes a persistent hypogonadotrophic amenorrhoea. A supervening metrorrhagia in the course of treatment, other than in the first month, should lead to measurement of plasma oestradiol levels. Should this level be less than 50 pg/mL, possible associated organic lesions should be sought. After withdrawal of treatment, ovarian function resumes, with ovulation expected to occur approximately 5 months after the last injection.

A non-hormonal method of contraception should be used throughout treatment including for 3 months after the last injection.

Due to concerns about bone density losses, DECAPEPTYL SR 11.25 mg should be used with caution in women with known metabolic bone disease.

Precocious puberty (in girls)

Initial ovarian stimulation at treatment initiation, followed by the treatment-induced oestrogen withdrawal, may lead, in the first month, to vaginal bleeding of mild or moderate intensity.

4.5 Interaction with other medicinal products and other forms of interaction
Drugs which raise prolactin levels should not be prescribed concomitantly as they reduce the level of LHRH receptors in the pituitary.

4.6 Pregnancy and lactation
Animal studies have not revealed any teratogenic effects. During post-marketing surveillance and in a limited number of pregnant women who were exposed inadvertently to triptorelin, there were no reports of malformation or foetotoxicity attributable to the product. However, as the number of patients is too small to draw conclusions regarding the risk of foetal malformations or foetotoxicity, if a patient becomes pregnant while receiving triptorelin, therapy should be discontinued.

Triptorelin is not recommended for use during lactation.

4.7 Effects on ability to drive and use machines
No effects on ability to drive and use machines have been observed.

4.8 Undesirable effects
Prostate cancer

The most frequently occurring side-effects of treatment with triptorelin are hot flushes, decreased libido and impotence, each reported by > 10 % of patients in clinical trials using DECAPEPTYL SR 11.25 mg.

At the beginning of treatment increased bone pain, worsening of genito-urinary obstruction symptoms (haematuria, urinary disorders) and/or worsening of neurological signs of vertebral metastases (back pain, weakness or paresthesia of the lower limbs) are commonly observed, resulting from the initial and transient increase in plasma testosterone. These symptoms disappear in one or two weeks.

The following uncommon adverse reactions have been observed during clinical trials with other triptorelin formulations: hypertension, gynaecomastia, insomnia, mood disorders, emergence of psychiatric disorders, vertigo, dizziness.

Additional rare adverse reactions reported among patients treated with other marketed triptorelin formulations are: allergic reactions (rash, pruritus, urticaria, and very occasionally Quincke's oedema), phlebitis, dry mouth or excessive salivation, headaches, recurrence of asthma, fever, sweating, weight increase, pain/erythema/induration at injection site, gastralgia, gastric disturbance, nausea, vomiting, slight hair loss, visual disturbances.

Endometriosis

At the beginning of treatment the symptoms of endometriosis (pelvic pain, dysmenorrhoea) may be exacerbated during the initial and transient increase in plasma oestradiol levels. These symptoms should disappear in one or two weeks. Genital haemorrhage including menorrhagia, metrorrhagia or spotting may occur in the month following the first injection.

During clinical trials the adverse reactions showed a general pattern of hypo-oestrogenic events related to pituitary-ovarian blockade such as hot flushes, sweating, sleep disturbances, headache, mood changes, vaginal dryness, dyspareunia, and decreased libido.

Transient pain, redness or local inflammation at the injection site may occur.

The following adverse reactions have been observed during clinical trials with other triptorelin formulations: breast pain, muscle cramps, joint pain, weight gain, nausea, abdominal pain or discomfort, asthenia, increased blood pressure, episodes of blurred or abnormal vision, cutaneous rash, oedema, hair loss.

As with any GnRH analogue, a small loss in bone density, specifically trabecular bone density, occurs during six months of DECAPEPTYL SR 11.25 mg treatment. Clinical data suggests that this loss is reversible.

Precocious puberty

Mild or moderate withdrawal bleeding (common) may occur in girls in the first month of treatment. Additional common adverse reactions may be observed such as injection site reactions and arthralgia.

According to the cumulative safety experience with triptorelin in children treated for precocious puberty, in addition the following rare reactions have been reported from post-marketing surveillance: allergic reactions, headache, weight gain, increased blood pressure, episodes of blurred or abnormal vision, gastrointestinal tract discomfort with abdominal pain and vomiting, epistaxis, malaise, myalgia, emotional lability, nervousness.

4.9 Overdose
No case of overdose has been reported. Animal data do not predict any effects other than those on sex hormone concentration and consequent effect on the reproductive tract. If overdose occurs, symptomatic management is indicated.

5. PHARMACOLOGICAL PROPERTIES
5.1 Pharmacodynamic properties
Pharmacotherapeutic group:

Gonadotrophin-Releasing Hormone analogue

L 02 A E 04: Antineoplastic and immunomodulator

Triptorelin is a synthetic decapeptide analogue of natural GnRH.

Prostate cancer

The first administration of DECAPEPTYL SR 11.25 mg stimulates the release of pituitary gonadotrophins with a transient increase in testosterone levels ("flare-up") in men and in oestradiol levels in women. Prolonged administration leads to a suppression of gonadotrophins and a fall in plasma testosterone or oestradiol to castrate levels after approximately 20 days, which is maintained for as long as the product is administered.

The efficacy and safety of triptorelin has been determined in clinical studies involving 645 patients with locally advanced or metastatic prostate cancer.

Of these, three long term controlled studies compared the efficacy and safety of triptorelin to bilateral orchidectomy as an initial therapy in patients with locally advanced or metastatic prostate cancer (stage C or D). In one of these three long term studies, 7 patients in the triptorelin group and 7 patients in the orchidectomy group had also undergone prostatectomy. Triptorelin induced biochemical castration at least as rapidly as surgical pulpectomy and was as effective as surgical castration in the long term palliative treatment of locally advanced or metastatic prostate cancer. Both the triptorelin and orchidectomy groups showed improvements in dysuria and pain, and reduction in volume of prostate. Analysis after six and eight years in two of the studies showed that there was no significant difference in the median survival rates in the triptorelin group versus the orchidectomy group.

A study assessing the pharmacodynamic equivalence between triptorelin 3-month and 28-day prolonged release formulations in patients with locally advanced or metastatic prostate cancer, found that equivalent testosterone suppression was achieved, whether 3 doses of Decapeptyl SR 3mg (n=68) or a single dose of Decapeptyl SR 11.25mg (n=63) was given. The percentage of patients who achieved a testosterone castrate level ⩽ 0.5 ng/mL at D84 was similar in the two treatment groups (98% and 96% in the 3-month and 28-day formulation groups, respectively). The time to achieve chemical castration was not significantly different between the two groups.

Endometriosis

The first administration of DECAPEPTYL SR 11.25 mg stimulates the release of pituitary gonadotrophins with a transient increase in testosterone levels ("flare-up") in men and in oestradiol levels in women. Prolonged administration leads to a suppression of gonadotrophins and a fall in plasma testosterone or oestradiol to castrate levels after approximately 20 days, which is maintained for as long as the product is administered.

Continued administration of DECAPEPTYL SR 11.25 mg induces suppression of oestrogen secretion and thus enables resting of ectopic endometrial tissue.

Precocious puberty

Inhibition of the increased hypophyseal gonadotropic activity in children with precocious puberty leads to suppression of oestradiol and testosterone secretion in girls and boys, respectively, and to lowering of the LH peak due to the LHRH stimulation test. The consequence is a regression or stabilisation of secondary sex characteristics and an improvement in median predicted adult height of 2.3cm after one year's treatment.

5.2 Pharmacokinetic properties
Following intramuscular injection of DECAPEPTYL SR 11.25 mg in patients (men and women), a peak of plasma triptorelin is observed in the first 3 hours after injection.

After a phase of decrease, the circulating triptorelin levels remain stable at around 0.04-0.05ng/ml in endometriosis patients and around 0.1ng/ml in prostate cancer patients until day 90.

5.3 Preclinical safety data

The compound did not demonstrate any specific toxicity in animal toxicological studies. The effects observed are related to the pharmacological properties of triptorelin on the endocrine system.

6. PHARMACEUTICAL PARTICULARS

6.1 List of excipients

D,L lactide-glycolide copolymer

Mannitol

Carmellose sodium

Polysorbate 80.

6.2 Incompatibilities

This medicinal product must not be mixed with other medicinal products except the one mentioned in 6.6.

6.3 Shelf life

2 years.

The product should be used immediately after reconstitution.

6.4 Special precautions for storage

Do not store above 25°C. Keep container in the outer carton.

6.5 Nature and contents of container

A type I, 4 ml capacity glass vial with an elastomer stopper and an aluminium cap containing the powder.

A type I, 3 ml capacity glass ampoule containing 2 ml of the suspension vehicle.

One syringe and 2 needles.

Box containing 1 vial and 1 ampoule with 1 syringe and 2 needles. The injection needle is equipped with a safety shield.

6.6 Special precautions for disposal and other handling

The suspension for injection must be reconstituted following the aseptic technique and using exclusively the provided ampoule of mannitol solution 0.8% for injection, suspension vehicle for DECAPEPTYL SR 11.25 mg.

The suspension vehicle should be drawn into the syringe provided using the pink needle and transferred to the vial containing the powder for injection. The vial should be gently shaken and the mixture then drawn back into the syringe without inverting the vial. The needle should then be changed and the green needle used to administer the injection immediately. The vial is intended for single use only and any remaining product should be discarded.

7. MARKETING AUTHORISATION HOLDER

Ipsen Limited

190 Bath Road

Slough

Berkshire

SL1 3XE

United Kingdom

8. MARKETING AUTHORISATION NUMBER(S)

06958/0016

9. DATE OF FIRST AUTHORISATION/RENEWAL OF THE AUTHORISATION

16/03/2009

10. DATE OF REVISION OF THE TEXT

16/03/2009

Decapeptyl SR 3mg

(Ipsen Ltd)

1. NAME OF THE MEDICINAL PRODUCT

DECAPEPTYL SR 3mg, powder for suspension for injection.

2. QUALITATIVE AND QUANTITATIVE COMPOSITION

Triptorelin (I.N.N.) 4.2 mg, as triptorelin acetate.

The vial contains an overage to ensure that a dose of 3mg is administered to the patient.

For excipients, see 6.1.

3. PHARMACEUTICAL FORM

Powder for suspension for injection, sustained release formulation.

4. CLINICAL PARTICULARS

4.1 Therapeutic indications

Treatment of patients with locally advanced, non-metastatic prostate cancer, as an alternative to surgical castration (see section 5.1).

Treatment of metastatic prostate cancer.

Treatment of endometriosis.

Treatment of uterine fibroids prior to surgery or when surgery is not appropriate

4.2 Posology and method of administration

Prostate cancer

One intramuscular injection should be administered every 4 weeks (28 days). No dosage adjustment is necessary in the elderly.

Endometriosis and uterine fibroids

One intramuscular injection every 28 days. For the treatment of endometriosis and uterine fibroids the treatment must be initiated in the first five days of the cycle. The maximum duration of treatment should be 6 months. For patients with uterine fibroids DECAPEPTYL SR 3mg should be administered for a minimum of 3 months.

A second course of treatment by DECAPEPTYL SR 3mg or by other GnRH analogues should not be undertaken due to concerns about bone density losses.

4.3 Contraindications

Hypersensitivity of GnRH analogues or to any of the excipients.

In prostate cancer, DECAPEPTYL SR 3mg should not be prescribed in patients presenting with spinal cord compression or evidence of spinal metastases.

In endometriosis and uterine fibroid treatment, confirm that the patient is not pregnant before beginning treatment.

4.4 Special warnings and precautions for use

Prostate cancer

Initially, DECAPEPTYL 3mg causes a transient increase in serum testosterone and consequent worsening of symptoms including increase in bone pain (and acid phosphatase levels). Consideration should be given to the use of an anti-androgen for three days prior to DECAPEPTYL SR 3mg treatment, to counteract this initial rise in serum testosterone levels. During the first month of treatment, patients presenting with, or at particular risk of developing, ureteric obstruction should be carefully monitored, as should those at risk of developing spinal cord compression. Continued treatment with DECAPEPTYL SR 3mg leads to suppression of testosterone (and dihydrotestosterone) and consequent improvement in the disease.

Endometriosis and uterine fibroids-

Regular administration, every 28 days of one vial of DECAPEPTYL SR 3mg causes a persistent hypogonadotrophic amenorrhoea. During the first month of treatment, a non-hormonal contraception should be given. A supervening metrorrhagia in the course of treatment, other than in the first month, should lead to measurement of plasma oestradiol levels. Should this level be less than 50 pg/ml, possible associated organic lesions should be sought. After withdrawal of treatment, ovarian function resumes and ovulation occurs on average 58 days after the last injection, with first menses occurring on average 70 days after the last injection. Contraception may therefore be required. Due to concerns about bone density losses, DECAPEPTYL SR 3mg should be used with caution in women with known metabolic bone disease.

With uterine fibroid patients it is important to monitor the early response to GnRH analogues and if there is no change or even an increase in uterine volume then the possibility of uterine leiomyosarcoma should be considered.

4.5 Interaction with other medicinal products and other forms of interaction

Drugs which raise prolactin levels should not be prescribed concomitantly as they reduce the level of LHRH receptors in the pituitary.

4.6 Pregnancy and lactation

Reproductive studies in primates have shown no maternal toxicity or embryotoxicity, and there was no effect on parturition. Inadvertent administration of triptorelin during human pregnancy has not demonstrated a teratogenic or other foetal risk. However, it is recommended that DECAPEPTYL SR 3mg should not be used during pregnancy or lactation.

4.7 Effects on ability to drive and use machines

There is no evidence that DECAPEPTYL SR 3mg has any effect on the ability to drive or operate machinery.

4.8 Undesirable effects

Prostate cancer

In prostate cancer patients, the most frequent side-effects of hot flushes, decreased libido, and impotence are a result of the decrease in testosterone levels. Bone pain, as a result of "disease flare", occurs occasionally. Pain and erythema at injection site, phlebitis and moderate and transient hypertension have been reported. On rare occasions the following have been reported: gynaecomastia, gastralgia, dry mouth, headaches, recurrence of asthma, increased dysuria, fever, pruritus, sweating, paresthesias, dizziness, insomnia, excessive salivation, gastric disturbance, nausea, vertigo, slight hair loss, induration at injection site.

Endometriosis and uterine fibroid patients

In endometriosis and uterine fibroid patients, adverse effects such as hot flushes, menorrhagia and vaginal dryness, reflect the efficacy of pituitary-ovarian blockade. Cutaneous rash, hair loss, asthenia, headache, weight gain, oedema, arthralgia, myalgia, transient sight disturbances and temporary hypertension may occur. As with any GnRH analogue, a small loss in bone density, specifically trabecular bone density, occurs during six months of DECAPEPTYL SR 3mg treatment. Clinical data suggests that this loss is reversible.

In the studies of uterine fibroids, surgical intervention as a result of an increase in vaginal haemorrhage was a rare complication of GnRH therapy.

4.9 Overdose

There is no human experience of overdosage. Animal data do not predict any effects other than those on sex hormone concentration and consequent effect on the reproductive tract. If overdosage occurs, symptomatic management is indicated.

5. PHARMACOLOGICAL PROPERTIES

5.1 Pharmacodynamic properties

Pharmacotherapeutic group: Gonadotrophin-Releaseing Hormone analogue

L 02 A E 04: Antineoplastic and immunomodulator

Triptorelin is a decapeptide analogue of GnRH which initially stimulates release of pituitary gonadotrophins.

Prostate cancer patients

This results in an increase in peripheral circulating levels of testosterone and dihydrotestosterone. Continued administration (over 7 days) however, leads to suppression of gonadotrophins and a consequent fall in plasma testosterone. In prostate cancer patients, plasma testosterone levels fall to castrate levels after 2-3 weeks of treatment, frequently resulting in an improvement of function and objective symptoms.

The efficacy and safety of triptorelin has been determined in clinical studies involving 645 patients with locally advanced or metastatic prostate cancer.

Of these, three long term controlled studies compared the efficacy and safety of triptorelin to bilateral orchidectomy as an initial therapy in patients with locally advanced or metastatic prostate cancer (stage C or D). In one of these three long term studies, 7 patients in the triptorelin group and 7 patients in the orchidectomy group had also undergone prostatectomy. Triptorelin induced biochemical castration at least as rapidly as surgical pulpectomy and was as effective as surgical castration in the long term palliative treatment of locally advanced or metastatic prostate cancer. Both the triptorelin and orchidectomy groups showed improvements in dysuria and pain, and reduction in volume of prostate. Analysis after six and eight years in two of the studies showed that there was no significant difference in the median survival rates in the triptorelin group versus the orchidectomy group.

A study assessing the pharmacodynamic equivalence between triptorelin 3-month and 28-day prolonged release formulations in patients with locally advanced or metastatic prostate cancer, found that equivalent testosterone suppression was achieved, whether 3 doses of Decapeptyl SR 3mg (n=68) or a single dose of Decapeptyl SR 11.25mg (n=63) was given. The percentage of patients who achieved a testosterone castrate level $\leqslant$ 0.5 ng/ml at D84 was similar in the two treatment groups (98% and 96% in the 3-month and 28-day formulation groups, respectively). The time to achieve chemical castration was not significantly different between the two groups.

Endometriosis and Uterine fibroid patients

Continued administration of DECAPEPTYL SR 3mg induces suppression of oestrogen secretion and thus enables resting of ectopic endometrial tissue. In pre-operative therapy for uterine fibroids there appears to be a beneficial effect on the blood loss at surgery. Studies have demonstrated a consistent and marked reduction in uterine and/or fibroid volume becoming maximal in a three to six month treatment period. Clinical studies have shown that 90-100% of fibroid patients become amenorrhoeic within two months of treatment and triptorelin provides relief from the symptoms of abdominal pain, dysmenorrhoea and menorrhagia associated with uterine fibroids

5.2 Pharmacokinetic properties

SUBCUTANEOUS FORM

In healthy volunteers:

Subcutaneously administered triptorelin (100 μg) is rapidly absorbed (Tmax = 0.63 ± 0.26 hr for peak plasma concentration = 1.85 ± 0.23 ng/ml). Elimination is effected with a biological half-life of 7.6 ± 1.6 hr, after a 3 to 4 hr distribution phase. Total plasma clearance is: 161 ± 28 ml/min. Distribution volume is 104.1 ± 11.7 litres.

In prostate cancer patients:

With subcutaneous administration (100 μg), triptorelin blood levels oscillate between maximum values of 1.28 ± 0.24 ng/ml (Cmax) obtained in general one hour after injection (Tmax) and minimum values of 0.28 ± 0.15 ng/ml (Cmin) obtained 24 hrs after injection.

The biological half-life is on average 11.7 ± 3.4 hr but varies according to patients. Plasma clearance (118 ± 32 ml/min) reflects slower elimination in patients, whilst distribution volumes are close to those of healthy volunteers (113.4 ± 21.6 litres).

SUSTAINED RELEASE FORM

Prostate cancer patients

Following intramuscular injection of the sustained release form, an initial phase of release of the active principle present on the surface of the microspheres is observed, followed by further fairly regular release (Cmax = 0.32 ± 0.12 ng/ml), with a mean rate of release of triptorelin of 46.6 ± 7.1 μg/day. The bioavailability of the microparticles is approximately 53% at one month.

Endometriosis and uterine fibroid patients

After intramuscular injection of DECAPEPTYL SR 3mg in endometriosis and uterine fibroid patients the maximum blood level of triptorelin is obtained between 2 to 6 hours after injection, the peak value reached is 11 ng/ml. There was no evidence of accumulation of the product following monthly injections over six months. The minimum blood level oscillates between 0.1 and 0.2 ng/ml. The bioavailability of the sustained release product is approximately 50%.

5.3 Preclinical safety data

Preclinical findings were only those related to the expected pharmacological activity of triptorelin, namely down-regulation of the hypothalamic-pituitary-gonadal axis. These included atrophy of the testes and genital tract, with resultant suppression of spermatogenesis, together with decreased weight of the prostate gland. These findings were largely reversible within the recovery period. In a small number of rats, in a 24 months oncogenicity study, a low incidence of benign histological changes were seen in the non-glandular part of the fore stomach. Erosions, ulcers, necrosis and inflammation were seen at varying degrees of severity. The clinical relevance of these findings is unknown. The increased incidence of adenomatous tumours in the rat pituitary observed with DECAPEPTYL following long-term repeated dosing is thought to be a class specific action of GnRH analogues due to an hormonally-mediated mechanism and has not been found in the mouse nor has it been described in man.

Standard mutagenicity testing revealed no mutagenic activity of triptorelin

6. PHARMACEUTICAL PARTICULARS

6.1 List of excipients

D,L-lactide/glycolide copolymer

Mannitol

Carmellose sodium

Polysorbate 80

6.2 Incompatibilities

This medicinal product must not be mixed with other medicinal products except those mentioned in 6.6.

6.3 Shelf life

18 months.

The product should be used immediately after reconstitution

6.4 Special precautions for storage

Do not store above 25°C. Keep the container in the outer carton.

6.5 Nature and contents of container

A type I, 5ml capacity glass vial with an elastomer stopper and an aluminium cap containing the powder.

Type I, 3ml capacity glass ampoule containing 2ml of the suspension vehicle.

Box containing 1 vial and 1 ampoule with 1 syringe and 2 needles. The injection needle is equipped with a safety shield.

6.6 Special precautions for disposal and other handling

The suspension for injection must be reconstituted following the aseptic technique and using exclusively the provided ampoule of mannitol solution 0.8% for injection, suspension vehicle for DECAPEPTYL SR 3 mg.

The suspension for injection must be reconstituted following the aseptic technique and using exclusively the provided ampoule of mannitol solution 0.8% for injection, suspension vehicle for DECAPEPTYL SR 3mg.

The vehicle should be drawn into the syringe provided using the pink needle and transferred to the vial containing the powder for injection. The vial should be gently shaken and the mixture then drawn back into the syringe without inverting the vial. The needle should then be changed and the green needle used to administer the injection immediately.

7. MARKETING AUTHORISATION HOLDER

Ipsen Limited

190 Bath Road

Slough

Berkshire

SL1 3XE

United Kingdom

8. MARKETING AUTHORISATION NUMBER(S)

PL 06958/0017

9. DATE OF FIRST AUTHORISATION/RENEWAL OF THE AUTHORISATION

10 January 2002

10. DATE OF REVISION OF THE TEXT

October 2007

Deltacortril Gastro-resistant Tablets

(Alliance Pharmaceuticals)

1. NAME OF THE MEDICINAL PRODUCT

Deltacortril® 2.5mg Gastro-resistant Tablets

Deltacortril® 5mg Gastro-resistant Tablets

Prednisolone 2.5mg Gastro-resistant Tablets

Prednisolone 5mg Gastro-resistant Tablets.

2. QUALITATIVE AND QUANTITATIVE COMPOSITION

Prednisolone 2.5mg

Prednisolone 5mg

Excipients: also includes lactose.

For full list of excipients see section 6.1.

3. PHARMACEUTICAL FORM

Gastro-resistant Tablets 2.5 mg, uniformly brown in colour.

Gastro-resistant Tablets 5mg, uniformly maroon in colour.

4. CLINICAL PARTICULARS

4.1 Therapeutic indications

Allergy and anaphylaxis: bronchial asthma, drug hypersensitivity reactions, serum sickness, angioneurotic oedema, anaphylaxis.

Arteritis/collagenosis: giant cell arteritis/polymyalgia rheumatica, mixed connective tissue disease, polyarteritis nodosa, polymyositis.

Blood disorders: haemolytic anaemia (auto-immune), leukaemia (acute and chronic lymphocytic), lymphoma, multiple myeloma, idiopathic thrombocytopenic purpura.

Cardiovascular disorders: post-myocardial infarction syndrome, rheumatic fever with severe carditis.

Endocrine disorders: primary and secondary adrenal insufficiency, congenital adrenal hyperplasia.

Gastro-intestinal disorders: Crohn's disease, ulcerative colitis, persistent coeliac syndrome (coeliac disease unresponsive to gluten withdrawal), auto-immune chronic active hepatitis, multisystem disease affecting liver, biliary peritonitis.

Hypercalcaemia: sarcoidosis, vitamin D excess.

Infections (with appropriate chemotherapy): helminthic infestations, Herxheimer reaction, infectious mononucleosis, miliary tuberculosis, mumps orchitis (adult), tuberculous meningitis, rickettsial disease.

Muscular disorders: polymyositis, dermatomyositis.

Neurological disorders: infantile spasms, Shy-Drager syndrome, sub-acute demyelinating polyneuropathy.

Ocular disease: scleritis, posterior uveitis, retinal vasculitis, pseudo-tumours of the orbit, giant cell arteritis, malignant ophthalmic Graves disease.

Renal disorders: lupus nephritis, acute interstitial nephritis, minimal change glomerulonephritis.

Respiratory disease: allergic pneumonitis, asthma, occupational asthma, pulmonary aspergillosis, pulmonary fibrosis, pulmonary alveolitis, aspiration of foreign body, aspiration of stomach contents, pulmonary sarcoid, drug induced lung disease, adult respiratory distress syndrome, spasmodic croup.

Rheumatic disorders: rheumatoid arthritis, polymyalgia rheumatica, juvenile chronic arthritis, systemic lupus erythematosus, dermatomyositis, mixed connective tissue disease.

Skin disorders: pemphigus vulgaris, bullous pemphigoid, systemic lupus erythematosus, pyoderma gangrenosum.

Miscellaneous: sarcoidosis, hyperpyrexia, Behçets disease, immunosuppression in organ transplantation.

4.2 Posology and method of administration

The initial dosage of Deltacortril Gastro-resistant Tablets may vary from 5mg to 60mg daily depending on the disorder being treated. Divided daily dosage is usually used.

The following therapeutic guidelines should be kept in mind for all therapy with corticosteroids:

Corticosteroids are palliative symptomatic treatment by virtue of their anti-inflammatory effects; they are never curative.

The appropriate individual dose must be determined by trial and error and must be re-evaluated regularly according to activity of the disease.

As corticosteroid therapy becomes prolonged and as the dose is increased, the incidence of disabling side-effects increases.

In general, initial dosage shall be maintained or adjusted until the anticipated response is observed. The dose should be gradually reduced until the lowest dose which will maintain an adequate clinical response is reached. Use of the lowest effective dose may also minimise side-effects (see 'Special warnings and special precautions for use').

In patients who have received more than physiological dose for systemic corticosteroids (approximately 7.5mg prednisolone or equivalent) for greater than 3 weeks, withdrawal should not be abrupt. How dose reduction should be carried out depends largely on whether the disease is likely to relapse as the dose of systemic corticosteroids is reduced. Clinical assessment of disease activity may be needed during withdrawal. If the disease is unlikely to relapse on withdrawal of systemic corticosteroids but there is uncertainty about hypothalamic-pituitary-adrenal (HPA) suppression, the dose of corticosteroid may be reduced rapidly to physiological doses. Once a daily dose equivalent to 7.5mg of prednisolone is reached, dose reduction should be slower to allow the HPA-axis to recover.

Abrupt withdrawal of systemic corticosteroid treatment, which has continued up to 3 weeks is appropriate if it is considered that the disease is unlikely to relapse. Abrupt withdrawal of doses of up to 40mg daily of prednisolone, or equivalent for 3 weeks is unlikely to lead to clinically relevant HPA-axis suppression, in the majority of patients. In the following patient groups, gradual withdrawal of systemic corticosteroid therapy should be considered even after courses lasting 3 weeks or less:

- patients who have had repeated courses of systemic corticosteroids, particularly if taken for greater than 3 weeks.
- when a short course has been prescribed within one year of cessation of long-term therapy (months or years).
- patients who may have reasons for adrenocortical insufficiency other than exogenous corticosteroid therapy.
- patients receiving doses of systemic corticosteroid greater than 40mg daily of prednisolone (or equivalent).
- patients repeatedly taking doses in the evening.

(See 'Special warnings and special precautions for use' and 'Undesirable effects')

During prolonged therapy, dosage may need to be temporarily increased during periods of stress or during exacerbations of the disease (see 'Special warnings and special precautions for use')

If there is lack of a satisfactory clinical response to Gastro-resistant Tablets, the drug should be gradually discontinued and the patient transferred to alternative therapy.

Intermittent dosage regimen A single dose of Gastro-resistant Tablets in the morning on alternate days or at longer intervals is acceptable therapy for some patients. When this regimen is practical, the degree of pituitary-adrenal suppression can be minimised.

Specific dosage guidelines The following recommendations for some corticosteroid-responsive disorders are for guidance only. Acute or severe disease may require initial high dose therapy with reduction to the lowest effective maintenance dose as soon as possible. Dosage reductions should not exceed 5-7.5mg daily during chronic treatment.

Allergic and skin disorders Initial doses of 5-15mg daily are commonly adequate.

Collagenosis Initial doses of 20-30mg daily are frequently effective. Those with more severe symptoms may require higher doses.

Rheumatoid arthritis The usual initial dose is 10-15mg daily. The lowest daily maintenance dose compatible with tolerable symptomatic relief is recommended.

Blood disorders and lymphoma An initial daily dose of 15-60mg is often necessary with reduction after an adequate clinical or haematological response. Higher doses may be necessary to induce remission in acute leukaemia.

Use in children Although appropriate fractions of the actual dose may be used, dosage will usually be determined by clinical response as in adults (see also 'Special warnings and special precautions for use'). Alternate day dosage is preferable where possible.

Use in elderly Treatment of elderly patients, particularly if long-term, should be planned bearing in mind the more serious consequences of the common side-effects of corticosteroids in old age (see also 'Special warnings and special precautions for use').

4.3 Contraindications

Systemic infections unless specific anti-infective therapy is employed. Hypersensitivity to any ingredient. Ocular herpes simplex because of possible perforation.

4.4 Special warnings and precautions for use

Patients/ and or carers should be warned that potentially severe psychiatric adverse reactions may occur with systemic steroids (see section 4.8). Symptoms typically emerge within a few days or weeks of starting the treatment. Risks may be higher with high doses/ systemic exposure (see also section 4.5 pharmacokinetic interactions that can increase the risk of side effects), although dose levels do not allow prediction of the onset, type, severity or duration of reactions. Most reactions recover after either dose reduction or withdrawal, although specific treatment may be necessary. Patients/carers should be encouraged to seek medical advice if worrying psychological symptoms develop, especially if depressed mood or suicidal ideation is suspected. Patients/carers should also be alert to possible psychiatric disturbances that may occur either during or immediately after dose tapering/ withdrawal of systemic steroids, although such reactions have been reported infrequently.

Particular care is required when considering the use of systemic corticosteroids in patients with existing or previous history of severe affective disorders in themselves or in their first degree relatives. These would include depressive or manic-depressive illness and previous steroid psychosis.

Caution is necessary when oral corticosteroids, including Deltacortril Gastro-resistant Tablets, are prescribed in patients with the following conditions, and frequent patient monitoring is necessary.

- Tuberculosis: Those with a previous history of, or X-ray changes characteristic of, tuberculosis. The emergence of active tuberculosis can, however, be prevented by the prophylactic use of anti-tuberculosis therapy.

- Hypertension.
- Congestive heart failure.
- Liver failure.
- Renal insufficiency.
- Diabetes mellitus or in those with a family history of diabetes.
- Osteoporosis: This is of special importance in post-menopausal females who are at particular risk.
- Patients with a history of severe affective disorders and particularly those with a previous history of steroid-induced psychoses.
- Also, existing emotional instability or psychotic tendencies may be aggravated by corticosteroids including prednisolone.
- Epilepsy, and/or seizure disorders
- Peptic ulceration.
- Previous steroid myopathy.
- Glucocorticoids should be used cautiously in patients with myasthenia gravis receiving anticholinesterase therapy.
- Because cortisone has been reported rarely to increase blood coagulability and to precipitate intravascular thrombosis, thromboembolism, and thrombophlebitis, corticosteroids should be used with caution in patients with thromboembolic disorders.
- Duchenne's muscular dystrophy: transient rhabdomyolysis and myoglobinuria may occur following strenuous physical activity. It is not known whether this is due to prednisolone itself or the increased physical activity.

Undesirable effects may be minimised by using the lowest effective dose for the minimum period and by administering the daily requirement as a single morning dose on alternate days. Frequent patient review is required to titrate the dose appropriately against disease activity (see 'Posology and method of administration').

Adrenocortical Insufficiency Pharmacologic doses of corticosteroids administered for prolonged periods may result in hypothalamic-pituitary-adrenal (HPA) suppression (secondary adrenocortical insufficiency). The degree and duration of adrenocortical insufficiency produced is variable among patients and depends on the dose, frequency, time of administration, and duration of glucocorticoid therapy.

In addition, acute adrenal insufficiency leading to a fatal outcome may occur if glucocorticoids are withdrawn abruptly. Drug-induced secondary adrenocortical insufficiency may therefore be minimized by gradual reduction of dosage. This type of relative insufficiency may persist for months after discontinuation of therapy; therefore, in any situation of stress occurring during that period, hormone therapy should be reinstituted. Since mineralocorticoid secretion may be impaired, salt and/or a mineralocorticoid should be administered concurrently. During prolonged therapy any intercurrent illness, trauma, or surgical procedure will require a temporary increase in dosage; if corticosteroids have been stopped following prolonged therapy they may need to be temporarily re-introduced.

Patients should carry "Steroid treatment" cards which give clear guidance on the precautions to be taken to minimise risk and which provide details of prescriber, drug, dosage and the duration of treatment.

Anti-inflammatory/Immunosuppressive effects and Infection Suppression of the inflammatory response and immune function increases the susceptibility to infections and their severity. The clinical presentation may often be atypical and serious infection such as septicaemia and tuberculosis may be masked and may reach an advanced stage before being recognised when corticosteroids including prednisolone are used. The immunosuppressive effects of glucocorticoids may result in activation of latent infection or exacerbation of intercurrent infections.

Chickenpox Chickenpox is of particular concern since this normally minor illness may be fatal in immunosuppressed patients. Patients (or parents of children) without a definite history of chickenpox should be advised to avoid close personal contact with chickenpox or herpes zoster and if exposed they should seek urgent medical attention. Passive immunisation with varicella-zoster immunoglobulin (VZIG) is needed by exposed non-immune patients who are receiving systemic corticosteroids or who have used them within the previous 3 months; this should be given within 10 days of exposure to chickenpox. If a diagnosis of chickenpox is confirmed, the illness warrants specialist care and urgent treatment. Corticosteroids should not be stopped and the dose may need to be increased. The effect of corticosteroids may be enhanced in patients with hypothyroidism and in those with chronic liver disease with impaired hepatic function.

Measles Patients should be advised to take particular care to avoid exposure to measles, and to seek immediate medical advice if exposure occurs. Prophylaxis with intramuscular normal immunoglobulin may be needed.

Administration of Live Vaccines Live vaccines should not be given to individuals on high doses of corticosteroids, due to impaired immune response. Live vaccines should be postponed until at least 3 months after stopping corticosteroid therapy. (See also section 4.5 Interactions).

Ocular Effects Prolonged use of corticosteroids may produce posterior subcapsular cataracts and nuclear cataracts (particularly in children), exophthalmos, or increased intraocular pressure, which may result in glaucoma with possible damage to the optic nerves. Establishment of secondary fungal and viral infections of the eye may also be enhanced in patients receiving glucocorticoids.

Corticosteroids should be used cautiously in patients with ocular herpes simplex because of possible perforation.

Cushing's disease Because glucocorticoids can produce or aggravate *Cushing's syndrome*, glucocorticoids should be avoided in patients with Cushing's disease

There is an enhanced effect of corticosteroids in patients with hypothyroidism and in those with cirrhosis.

Psychic derangements may appear when corticosteroids, including prednisolone, are used, ranging from euphoria, insomnia, mood swings, personality changes, and severe depression, to frank psychotic manifestations.

Use in children Corticosteroids cause growth retardation in infancy, childhood and adolescence, which may be irreversible, and therefore long-term administration of pharmacological doses should be avoided. If prolonged therapy is necessary, treatment should be limited to the minimum suppression of the hypothalamo-pituitary adrenal axis and growth retardation. The growth and development of infants and children should be closely monitored. Treatment should be administered where possible as a single dose on alternate days

Use in the elderly Treatment of elderly patients, particularly if long term, should be planned bearing in mind the more serious consequences of the common side-effects of corticosteroids in old age, especially osteoporosis, diabetes, hypertension, hypokalaemia, susceptibility to infection and thinning of the skin. Close clinical supervision is required to avoid life threatening reactions.

Patients with rare hereditary problems of galactose intolerance, the Lapp lactase deficiency or glucose-galactose malabsorption should not take this medicine.

4.5 Interaction with other medicinal products and other forms of interaction

Hepatic microsomal enzyme inducers Drugs that induce hepatic enzyme cytochrome P-450 (CYP) isoenzyme 3A4 such as phenobarbital, phenytoin, rifampicin, rifabutin, carbamazepine, primidone and aminoglutethimide may reduce the therapeutic efficacy of corticosteroids by increasing the rate of metabolism. Lack of expected response may be observed and dosage of Deltacortril Gastro-resistant Tablets may need to be increased.

Hepatic microsomal enzyme inhibitors Drugs that inhibit hepatic enzyme cytochrome P-450 (CYP) isoenzyme 3A4 (e.g. ketoconazole, troleandomycin) may decrease glucocorticoid clearance. Dosages of glucocorticoids given in combination with such drugs may need to be decreased to avoid potential adverse effects.

Antidiabetic agents Glucocorticoids may increase blood glucose levels. Patients with diabetes mellitus receiving concurrent insulin and/or oral hypoglycemic agents may require dosage adjustments of such therapy.

Non-steroidal anti-inflammatory drugs Concomitant administration of ulcerogenic drugs such as indomethacin during corticosteroid therapy may increase the risk of GI ulceration. Aspirin should be used cautiously in conjunction with glucocorticoids in patients with hypoprothrombinaemia. Although concomitant therapy with salicylate and corticosteroids does not appear to increase the incidence or severity of GI ulceration, the possibility of this effect should be considered.

Serum salicylate concentrations may decrease when corticosteroids are administered concomitantly. The renal clearance of salicylates is increased by corticosteroids and steroid withdrawal may result in salicylate intoxication. Salicylates and corticosteroids should be used concurrently with caution. Patients receiving both drugs should be observed closely for adverse effects of either drug.

Antibacterials Rifamycins accelerate metabolism of corticosteroids and thus may reduce their effect. Erythromycin inhibits metabolism of methylprednisolone and possibly other corticosteroids.

Anticoagulants Response to anticoagulants may be reduced or, less often, enhanced by corticosteroids. Close monitoring of the INR or prothrombin time is required to avoid spontaneous bleeding.

Antiepileptics Carbamazepine, phenobarbital, phenytoin, and primidone accelerate metabolism of corticosteroids and may reduce their effect.

Antifungals Risk of hypokalaemia may be increased with amphotericin, therefore concomitant use with corticosteroids should be avoided unless corticosteroids are required to control reactions; ketoconazole inhibits metabolism of methylprednisolone and possibly other corticosteroids.

Antivirals Ritonavir possibly increases plasma concentrations of prednisolone and other corticosteroids.

Cardiac Glycosides Increased toxicity if hypokalaemia occurs with corticosteroids.

Ciclosporin Concomitant administration of prednisolone and ciclosporin may result in decreased plasma clearance of prednisolone (i.e. increased plasma concentration of prednisolone). The need for appropriate dosage adjustment should be considered when these drugs are administered concomitantly.

Cytotoxics Increased risk of haematological toxicity with methotrexate.

Mifepristone Effect of corticosteroids may be reduced for 3-4 days after mifepristone.

Vaccines Live vaccines should not be given to individuals with impaired immune responsiveness. The antibody response to other vaccines may be diminished.

Oestrogens Oestrogens may potentiate the effects of glucocorticoids and dosage adjustments may be required if oestrogens are added to or withdrawn from a stable dosage regimen.

Somatropin Growth promoting effect may be inhibited.

Sympathomimetics Increased risk of hypokalaemia if high doses of corticosteroids given with high doses of bambuterol, fenoteral, formoterol, ritodrine, salbutamol, salmeterol and terbutaline.

Other The desired effects of hypoglycaemic agents (including insulin), antihypertensives and diuretics are antagonised by corticosteroids; and the hypokalaemic effect of acetazolamide, loop diuretics, thiazide diuretics, carbenoxolone and theophylline are enhanced.

4.6 Pregnancy and lactation

Use in pregnancy The ability of corticosteroids to cross the placenta varies between individual drugs, however, 88% of prednisolone is inactivated as it crosses the placenta. Administration of corticosteroids to pregnant animals can cause abnormalities of foetal development including cleft palate, intra-uterine growth retardation and effects on brain growth and development. There is no evidence that corticosteroids result in an increased incidence of congenital abnormalities, such as cleft palate/lip in man. However, when administered for prolonged periods or repeatedly during pregnancy, corticosteroids may increase the risk of intra-uterine growth retardation. Hypoadrenalism may, in theory, occur in the neonate following prenatal exposure to corticosteroids but usually resolves spontaneously following birth and is rarely clinically important. Cataracts have been observed in infants born to mothers treated with long-term prednisolone during pregnancy. As with all drugs, corticosteroids should only be prescribed when the benefits to the mother and child outweigh the risks. When corticosteroids are essential however, patients with normal pregnancies may be treated as though they were in the non-gravid state.

Patients with pre-eclampsia or fluid retention require close monitoring.

Use in lactation Corticosteroids are excreted in small amounts in breast milk. Corticosteroids distributed into breast milk may suppress growth and interfere with endogenous glucocorticoid production in nursing infants. Since adequate reproductive studies have not been performed in humans with glucocorticoids, these drugs should be administered to nursing mothers only if the benefits of therapy are judged to outweigh the potential risks to the infant.

4.7 Effects on ability to drive and use machines

The effect of Deltacortril Gastro-resistant Tablets on the ability to drive or use machinery has not been evaluated. There is no evidence to suggest that prednisolone may affect these abilities.

4.8 Undesirable effects

A wide range of psychiatric reactions including affective disorders (such as irritable, euphoric, depressed and labile mood, and suicidal thoughts), psychotic reactions (including mania, delusions, hallucinations, and aggravation of schizophrenia), behavioural disturbances, irritability, anxiety, sleep disturbances, and cognitive dysfunction including confusion and amnesia have been reported. Reactions are common and may occur in both adults and children. In adults, the frequency of severe reactions has been estimated to be 5-6%. Psychological effects have been reported on withdrawal of corticosteroids; the frequency is unknown.

The incidence of predictable undesirable effects, including hypothalamic-pituitary adrenal suppression correlates with the relative potency of the drug, dosage, timing of administration and the duration of treatment (see 'Special warnings and special precautions for use').

Body as a Whole Leucocytosis, hypersensitivity including anaphylaxis, thromboembolism, fatigue, malaise.

Cardiovascular congestive heart failure in susceptible patients, hypertension

Gastro-intestinal Dyspepsia, nausea, peptic ulceration with perforation and haemorrhage, abdominal distension, abdominal pain, increased appetite which may result in weight gain, diarrhoea, oesophageal ulceration, oesophageal candidiasis, acute pancreatitis.

Musculo-skeletal Proximal myopathy, osteoporosis, vertebral and long bone fractures, avascular osteonecrosis, tendon rupture, myalgia.

Metabolic/Nutritional Sodium and water retention, hypokalaemic alkalosis, potassium loss, negative nitrogen and calcium balance.

Skin/Appendages Impaired healing, hirsutism, skin atrophy, bruising, striae, telangiectasia, acne, increased sweating, may suppress reactions to skin tests, pruritis, rash, urticaria.

Endocrine Suppression of the hypothalamo-pituitary adrenal axis particularly in times of stress, as in trauma, surgery or illness, growth suppression in infancy, childhood and adolescence, menstrual irregularity and amenorrhoea. Cushingoid facies, weight gain, impaired carbohydrate tolerance with increased requirement for antidiabetic therapy, manifestation of latent diabetes mellitus, Increased appetite.

Central and Peripheral Nervous System Euphoria, psychological dependence, depression, insomnia, dizziness, headache, vertigo. Raised intracranial pressure with papilloedema (pseudotumor cerebri) in children, usually after treatment withdrawal. Aggravation of schizophrenia. Aggravation of epilepsy.

Vision Increased intra-ocular pressure, glaucoma, papilloedema, posterior subcapsular cataracts, exophthalmos, corneal or scleral thinning, exacerbation of ophthalmic viral or fungal disease.

Anti-inflammatory and immunosuppressive effects Increases susceptibility to, and severity of infections with suppression of clinical symptoms and signs, opportunistic infections, recurrence of dormant tuberculosis (see 'Special warnings and special precautions for use').

Withdrawal symptoms Too rapid a reduction of corticosteroid dosage following prolonged treatment can lead to acute adrenal insufficiency, hypotension and death (see 'Special warnings and special precautions for use' and 'Posology and method of administration'). A steroid "withdrawal syndrome" seemingly unrelated to adrenocortical insufficiency may also occur following abrupt discontinuance of glucocorticoids. This syndrome includes symptoms such as: anorexia, nausea, vomiting, lethargy, headache, fever, joint pain, desquamation, myalgia, arthralgia, rhinitis, conjunctivitis, painful itchy skin nodules weight loss, and/or hypotension. These effects are thought to be due to the sudden change in glucocorticoid concentration rather than to low corticosteroid levels.

4.9 Overdose
Reports of acute toxicity and/or death following overdosage of glucocorticoids are rare. No specific antidote is available; treatment is supportive and symptomatic. Serum electrolytes should be monitored.

5. PHARMACOLOGICAL PROPERTIES

5.1 Pharmacodynamic properties
Naturally occurring glucocorticoids (hydrocortisone and cortisone), which also have salt- retaining properties, are used as replacement therapy in adrenocortical deficiency states. Their synthetic analogs are primarily used for their potent anti-inflammatory effects in disorders of many organ systems.

Glucocorticoids cause profound and varied metabolic effects. In addition, they modify the body's immune responses to diverse stimuli.

5.2 Pharmacokinetic properties
Prednisolone is rapidly and apparently almost completely absorbed after oral administration; it reaches peak plasma concentrations after 1-3 hours. There is however wide inter-subject variation suggesting impaired absorption in some individuals. Plasma half-life is about 3 hours in adults and somewhat less in children. Its initial absorption, but not its overall bioavailability, is affected by food. Prednisolone has a biological half-life lasting several hours, making it suitable for alternate-day administration regimens.

Although peak plasma prednisolone levels are somewhat lower after administration of Deltacortril Gastro-resistant Tablets and absorption is delayed, total absorption and bioavailability are the same as after plain prednisolone. Prednisolone shows dose dependent pharmacokinetics, with an increase in dose leading to an increase in volume of distribution and plasma clearance. The degree of plasma protein binding determines the distribution and clearance of free, pharmacologically active drug. Reduced doses are necessary in patients with hypoalbuminaemia.

Prednisolone is metabolised primarily in the liver to a biologically inactive compound. Liver disease prolongs the half-life of prednisolone and, if the patient has hypoalbuminaemia, also increases the proportion of unbound drug and may thereby increase adverse effects.

Prednisolone is excreted in the urine as free and conjugated metabolites, together with small amounts of unchanged prednisolone.

6. PHARMACEUTICAL PARTICULARS

6.1 List of excipients
Core: calcium carbonate, lactose, magnesium stearate, maize starch

2.5 mg Coating:
polyvinyl alcohol, titanium dioxide (E171), purified talc, lecithin, xanthan gum (E415), polyvinyl acetate phthalate, polyethylene glycol, sodium hydrogen carbonate, triethyl citrate, purified stearic acid, sodium alginate (E401), colloidal silicon dioxide, lactose, methylcellulose (E461), sodium carboxymethyl cellulose, iron oxide (E172), beeswax (E901), carnauba wax (E903), polysorbate 20 (E432) and sorbic acid (E200).

5 mg Coating:
polyvinyl alcohol, titanium dioxide (E171), purified talc, lecithin, xanthan gum (E415), polyvinyl acetate phthalate, polyethylene glycol, sodium hydrogen carbonate, triethyl citrate, purified stearic acid, sodium alginate (E401), colloidal silicon dioxide, lactose monohydrate, methylcellulose (E461), sodium carboxymethyl cellulose, carmine (E120), indigo carmine aluminium lake (E132), beeswax (E901), carnauba wax (E903), polysorbate 20 (E432) and sorbic acid (E200).

6.2 Incompatibilities
None.

6.3 Shelf life
24 months.

6.4 Special precautions for storage
Store below 25°C.

6.5 Nature and contents of container
2.5mg

100 tablets in white HDPE bottles with a white polypropylene child resistant, tamper evident screw cap.

28, 30, 56, 60,100 or 500 tablets in HDPE containers with HDPE/polypropylene child resistant cap with PVDC faced pulp board wad.

30 tablets in aluminium /PVC blister strips with an aluminium foil (2 blisters per carton).

Not all pack sizes may be marketed.

5mg

28, 30, 56, 60 or 100 tablets in HDPE containers with HDPE/polypropylene child resistant cap with PVDC faced pulp board wad.

30 tablets in aluminium/PVC blister strips with an aluminium foil (2 blisters per carton).

500 tablets in polypropylene containers

Not all pack sizes may be marketed.

6.6 Special precautions for disposal and other handling
None.

7. MARKETING AUTHORISATION HOLDER
Alliance Pharmaceuticals Limited

Avonbridge House,

Bath Road

Chippenham

Wiltshire

SN15 2BB

United Kingdom

For Prednisolone 2.5mg and 5mg Gastro-resistant Tablets trading as: Alliance Generics, Avonbridge House, Bath Road, Chippenham, Wiltshire, SN15 2BB, United Kingdom.

8. MARKETING AUTHORISATION NUMBER(S)
Deltacortril 2.5 mg Gastro-resistant Tablets, Prednisolone 2.5mg Gastro-resistant Tablets - PL16853/0092

Deltacortril 5mg Gastro-resistant Tablets, Prednisolone 5mg Gastro-resistant Tablets - PL16853/0093

9. DATE OF FIRST AUTHORISATION/RENEWAL OF THE AUTHORISATION
20 December 2006

10. DATE OF REVISION OF THE TEXT
16th July 2009

De-Noltab

(Astellas Pharma Ltd)

1. NAME OF THE MEDICINAL PRODUCT
DE-NOLTAB

2. QUALITATIVE AND QUANTITATIVE COMPOSITION
Tri-potassium di-citrato bismuthate equivalent to 120mg Bi_2O_3

3. PHARMACEUTICAL FORM
Film-coated tablet

4. CLINICAL PARTICULARS

4.1 Therapeutic indications
For the treatment of gastric and duodenal ulcers.

4.2 Posology and method of administration
For Adults, and the Elderly:

One tablet to be taken four times a day, half an hour before each of the three main meals and two hours after the last meal of the day, or

Two tablets to be taken twice daily, half an hour before breakfast and half an hour before the evening meal, or

As directed by the physician

The maximum duration for one course of treatment is two months; De-Noltab should not be used for maintenance therapy.

For children:

Not recommended.

4.3 Contraindications
In cases of severe renal insufficiency.

Harmful to people on a low potassium diet.

Hypersensitivity to the active substance(s) or to any of the excipients.

4.4 Special warnings and precautions for use
Prolonged use of high doses of bismuth compounds is not recommended because this has occasionally led to reversible encephalopathy. It is, not advisable to take other bismuth-containing drugs concomitantly.

Contains approximately 2 mmol (approximately 40 mg) potassium per tablet. To be taken into consideration by patients with reduced kidney function or patients on a controlled potassium diet.

4.5 Interaction with other medicinal products and other forms of interaction
No other medicines, food or drink, in particular antacids, milk, fruit or fruit juices, should be consumed within half an hour before or after a dose of De-Nol as they may influence its effect. The efficacy of oral tetracyclines may be inhibited.

4.6 Pregnancy and lactation
On theoretical grounds De-Noltab is contraindicated in pregnancy. No information is available on excretion in breast milk.

4.7 Effects on ability to drive and use machines
None reported.

4.8 Undesirable effects
(see Table 1 on next page)

4.9 Overdose
Extremely few cases of overdosage have been reported; contact the company for further information.

5. PHARMACOLOGICAL PROPERTIES

5.1 Pharmacodynamic properties
The active constituent exerts a local healing effect at the ulcer site, and by eradication or reduction of *Helicobacter pylori* defers relapse.

5.2 Pharmacokinetic properties
The action is local in the gastro-intestinal tract.

5.3 Preclinical safety data
No relevant pre-clinical safety data has been generated.

6. PHARMACEUTICAL PARTICULARS

6.1 List of excipients
Povidone K 30

Polacrillin potassium

Macrogol 6000

Magnesium stearate

Maize starch

Hypromellose

6.2 Incompatibilities
None

6.3 Shelf life
Four years

6.4 Special precautions for storage
Do not store above 25°C

6.5 Nature and contents of container
Amber glass bottles and/or aluminium foil strips, containing 112 tablets

6.6 Special precautions for disposal and other handling
None

7. MARKETING AUTHORISATION HOLDER
Astellas Pharma Ltd

Lovett House

Lovett Road

Staines

TW18 3AZ

United Kingdom

8. MARKETING AUTHORISATION NUMBER(S)
PL0166/0124

9. DATE OF FIRST AUTHORISATION/RENEWAL OF THE AUTHORISATION
1 December 1986;11th January 2007.

10. DATE OF REVISION OF THE TEXT
18 July 2008

11. LEGAL CATEGORY
P

DENTINOX CRADLE CAP TREATMENT SHAMPOO

(DDD Limited)

1. NAME OF THE MEDICINAL PRODUCT
DENTINOX CRADLE CAP TREATMENT SHAMPOO

2. QUALITATIVE AND QUANTITATIVE COMPOSITION
Sodium lauryl ether sulpho-succinate 6.00 % w/w

Sodium lauryl ether sulphate 2.70 % w/w

For full list of excipients see section 6.1

Table 1 Undesirable effects

System Organ Class	Common >1/100, <1/10	Uncommon >1/1000, <1/100	Very rare <1/10,000, Not known (cannot be estimated from the available data)
Immune system disorders			anaphylactic reaction
Gastrointestinal disorders	blackening of the stool	nausea, vomiting, constipation, diarrhoea	
Skin and subcutaneous tissue disorders		rash, pruritus	

3. PHARMACEUTICAL FORM

Shampoo

Colourless viscous liquid

4. CLINICAL PARTICULARS

4.1 Therapeutic indications

For the treatment of infant cradle cap, and general care of infant scalp, and hair.

4.2 Posology and method of administration

Two shampoo applications of between 2 - 3ml. Repeat at each bath-time until the scalp is clear. Then use as necessary.

Wet the baby's head with warm water. Squeeze a little Dentinox Cradle Cap Treatment Shampoo onto your palm, and massage gently but firmly over the entire scalp. Do not be afraid of touching the soft area of the scalp(fontanelle). Rinse off and repeat application. Rinse well and dry.

4.3 Contraindications

Hypersensitivity to the active substances or to any of the excipients

Avoid contact with the eyes.

4.4 Special warnings and precautions for use

For external application only.

Keep all medicines out of the reach of children.

4.5 Interaction with other medicinal products and other forms of interaction

Not applicable.

4.6 Pregnancy and lactation

Not applicable.

4.7 Effects on ability to drive and use machines

Not applicable.

4.8 Undesirable effects

There have been very rare reports of erythema and skin irritation

4.9 Overdose

Overdosage by external application will not be a problem. Shampoo is non-toxic if ingested.

5. PHARMACOLOGICAL PROPERTIES

5.1 Pharmacodynamic properties

Pharmacotherapeutic Group: Other Dermatological preparations

ATC Code: D11 AX.

Dentinox Cradle Cap Treatment Shampoo contains two principal cleansing surfactants.

a) sodium lauryl ether sulphate - an anionic surfactant widely used in cosmetics and toiletries,

and

b) sodium lauryl ether sulpho-succinate - a secondary anionic surfactant employed on account of its exceptionally mild character.

A clinical trial carried out by Huntingdon Research Centre found that the product was effective in 25 out of 26 patients treated. A 1% cetavlon placebo was used as a control, which was effective in only 6 patients out of 19 treated.

The product is non-toxic, and has similar eye irritation potential to typical family shampoo's though less than anti-dandruff shampoos.

5.2 Pharmacokinetic properties

Not applicable.

Dentinox Cradle Cap Treatment Shampoo has a cleansing action. The product is massaged into the scalp with a little water, then rinsed off.

5.3 Preclinical safety data

N/A

6. PHARMACEUTICAL PARTICULARS

6.1 List of excipients

Sodium Salt of Coconut Imidazoline, Oleic Acid Diethanolamide, Sodium Chloride,

Rose Perfume, Purified Water.

6.2 Incompatibilities

None known.

6.3 Shelf life

3 years

6.4 Special precautions for storage

Do not store above 25°C

6.5 Nature and contents of container

White high density polythene bottle with snap fit closure in white polypropylene.

Pack size 125ml

2.7g sachet of 40gsm Craft Paper, 10gsm Polyethylene, 8 micrometer Aluminum Foil and 30gsm Surlyn. Pack size 2.7g

Not all pack sizes may be marketed

6.6 Special precautions for disposal and other handling

Special precautions for disposal

7. MARKETING AUTHORISATION HOLDER

DDD LIMITED,

94, Rickmansworth Road, Watford, Hertfordshire, United Kingdom, WDI 7JJ

8. MARKETING AUTHORISATION NUMBER(S)

PL 0133/0030

9. DATE OF FIRST AUTHORISATION/RENEWAL OF THE AUTHORISATION

Date of last renewal 20 July 2006

10. DATE OF REVISION OF THE TEXT

20 July 2006

Dentinox Infant Colic Drops

(DDD Limited)

1. NAME OF THE MEDICINAL PRODUCT

Dentinox Infant Colic Drops

2. QUALITATIVE AND QUANTITATIVE COMPOSITION

Activated Dimeticone 42.00 mg/5ml

For excipients, see 6.1

3. PHARMACEUTICAL FORM

Oral suspension

Translucent white liquid

4. CLINICAL PARTICULARS

4.1 Therapeutic indications

For the gentle relief of wind and griping pains in infants, caused by the accumulation of ingested air. Facilitates eructation. Can be used from birth onwards.

4.2 Posology and method of administration

2½ ml (one measured dose of the syringe) with or after each feed. May be added to the infant's bottle or given orally directly from the syringe. Maximum 6 doses per day. For infants can be used from birth onwards.

4.3 Contraindications

Hypersensitivity to the active substances or to any of the excipients

Contains sucrose. Patients with rare hereditary problems of fructose intolerance, glucose-galactose malabsorption or sucrase-isomaltase insufficiency should not take this medicine.

4.4 Special warnings and precautions for use

Keep all medicines out of the reach of children.

If symptoms persist obtain medical advice.

4.5 Interaction with other medicinal products and other forms of interaction

None known.

4.6 Pregnancy and lactation

Not applicable.

4.7 Effects on ability to drive and use machines

Not applicable.

4.8 Undesirable effects

None known.

4.9 Overdose

From the literature it would appear that all the silicone will be excreted unchanged and that there was no increase of urinary silicate output or of absorption of the silicone.

It was concluded that the Activated Dimeticone carried no significant carcinogenic hazard, and that no other significant toxic effect attributable to Activated Dimeticone has been observed.

Overdosage may prove a problem with diabetics because of the sugar content.

5. PHARMACOLOGICAL PROPERTIES

5.1 Pharmacodynamic properties

Excessive swallowing of air results in collection of gas in the intestine. This can be the result of too rapid eating, excessive use of a pacifier (dummy), finger sucking or yelling. When the swallowed air is in the intestine, bubbles are formed, which makes it more difficult for the gas to pass through the intestine canal, resulting in abdominal distension and pain. Activated Dimeticone is a surface active substance which changes the surface tension of the intestinal mucus. Thus, the air bubbles burst and the gas is released. The elimination of the gas, air or foam from the gastro-intestinal tract, relieves abdominal distension and dyspepsia.

5.2 Pharmacokinetic properties

Activated Dimeticone is chemically inert and is not absorbed. Its effect is local on the intestinal contents.

No side effects from the substance are reported from the literature.

From the toxicity trials undertaken by Dow Corning, it has been demonstrated in the rat that all the Dimeticone was recovered in the faeces and that there was no increase in urinary salicate output.

In four human subjects given 376.5mg of Activated Dimeticone, twice daily for 10 days, it was found that there was no increase in their urinary silicate output and no evidence of absorption of the silicone.

5.3 Preclinical safety data

There are no pre-clinical data of relevance to the prescriber which are additional to that already included in other sections of the SPC

6. PHARMACEUTICAL PARTICULARS

6.1 List of excipients

Purified Water, Sucrose, Carbomer, Dill Oil, Sodium Hydroxide, Nipasept [Methylhydroxybenzoate, Ethylhydroxybenzoate, Propylhydroxybenzoate].

6.2 Incompatibilities

None known.

6.3 Shelf life

2 years

6.4 Special precautions for storage

Do not store above 25 °C.

6.5 Nature and contents of container

Pack size 100ml

100ml - HDPE round bottle with a jay cap tamper evident closure, with 2.5ml oral dosing syringe.

Pack size 2.5ml

Sample sachets:

40gsm craft paper, 10 gsm polyethylene, 8gsm aluminium foil and 30gsm surlyn.

6.6 Special precautions for disposal and other handling

After use, rinse the syringe with warm water and dry.

ADMINISTRATION DETAILS

7. MARKETING AUTHORISATION HOLDER

DDD Limited,

94, Rickmansworth Road

Watford

Hertfordshire, WD18 7JJ.

8. MARKETING AUTHORISATION NUMBER(S)

PL 0133/0022

9. DATE OF FIRST AUTHORISATION/RENEWAL OF THE AUTHORISATION

Date of first authorisation: 29th November 1976

Date of last renewal: 9th September 2008

10. DATE OF REVISION OF THE TEXT

July 2009

Dentinox Teething Gel

(DDD Limited)

1. NAME OF THE MEDICINAL PRODUCT

Dentinox Teething Gel

2. QUALITATIVE AND QUANTITATIVE COMPOSITION

Lidocaine Hydrochloride BP 0.33 % w/w

Cetylpyridinium Chloride BP 0.10 % w/w

For full list of excipients, see section 6.1.

3. PHARMACEUTICAL FORM

Dental gel

Greenish yellow brown gel.

4. CLINICAL PARTICULARS

4.1 Therapeutic indications

Dentinox Gel relieves the pain of baby's teething and soothes the gums.

4.2 Posology and method of administration

Place a small quantity of Dentinox Teething Gel on a pad of cotton wool or a clean finger and rub gently on baby's gum. Repeat after 20 minutes if necessary. Use when necessary during the teething period.

4.3 Contraindications
Hypersensitivity to the active substances or to any of the excipients.

Contains sorbitol. Patients with rare hereditary problems of fructose intolerance should not take this medicine.

4.4 Special warnings and precautions for use
Keep all medicines out of the sight and reach of children.

Do not use if seal on nozzle is broken.

4.5 Interaction with other medicinal products and other forms of interaction
None known.

4.6 Pregnancy and lactation
Not applicable.

4.7 Effects on ability to drive and use machines
Not applicable.

4.8 Undesirable effects
None known.

4.9 Overdose
We are not aware of any problems caused by overdosage.

5. PHARMACOLOGICAL PROPERTIES

5.1 Pharmacodynamic properties
Pharmacotherapeutic group: Stomatological Preparation, ATC code: A01AD

Cetylpyridium Chloride is a cationic disinfectant which is used for minor wounds, treating superficial infections of the mouth and preserving the product.

Lidocaine Hydrochloride is a local anaesthetic. It works by blocking nerve conduction when applied topically to nerve tissue. It acts on any part of the nervous system and on every type of nerve fibre. For example, when it is applied to the motor cortex, impulse transmission from that area stops, and when it is injected into the skin it prevents the initiation and the transmission of the sensory impulses. A local anaesthetic in contact with a nerve trunk can cause both sensory and motor paralysis in the area innervated. Many kinds of compounds interfere with conduction, but they often permanently damage the nerve cells. The great practical advantage of the local anaesthetics is that their use is reversible, their use is followed by complete recovery in nerve function with no evidence of structural damage to nerve fibres or cells.

5.2 Pharmacokinetic properties
Lidocaine produces more prompt, more intense, longer-lasting and more intense anaesthesia than does an equal concentration of procaine. Unlike procaine it is an aminoethylamide. It is an agent of choice, therefore, in individuals sensitive to ester-type local anaesthetics. Lidocaine is relatively quickly absorbed. Lidocaine is metabolised in the liver by mixed-function oxidases by dealkylation to monoethyl glycine and xylidide. The latter compound retains significant local anaesthetic and toxic activity. In man about 75% of xylidide is excreted in the urine as the further metabolite 4-hydroxy-2,6-dimethylaniline. The typical dose of Dentinox gel is about 150mg containing about 0.5mg of lidocaine hydrochloride (which approximates to about 0.1 mg/kg of bodyweight). Martindale recommends that the total dose of lidocaine hydrochloride should not exceed 200mg (3mg per kg of bodyweight). Thus the dosage of Dentinox Gel is well within this level.

5.3 Preclinical safety data
Not applicable.

6. PHARMACEUTICAL PARTICULARS

6.1 List of excipients

Purified Water BP	43.31 % w/w
Sorbitol Solution 70 % (non-crystallising) BP	21.00 % w/w
Xylitol HSE	14.00 % w/w
Ethanol 96% BP	9.36 % w/w
Glycerol BP	7.00 % w/w
Hydroxethylcellulose BP	2.50 % w/w
Polyoxyl 40 hydrogenated castor oils	1.00 % w/w
Pharmaceutical Liquid Flavour	0.48 % w/w
Hydroxypolyethoxy Dodecane	0.33 % w/w
Macrogol 300	0.33 % w/w
Sodium Saccharin	0.10 % w/w
Caramel E150	0.10 % w/w
Levomenthol	0.06 % w/w

6.2 Incompatibilities
Not applicable

6.3 Shelf life
3 years

6.4 Special precautions for storage
Do not store above 25°C

6.5 Nature and contents of container
Internally lacquered aluminium tube, the nozzle of which contains a membrane.

Sachet- 40gsm craft paper, 10 gsm polyethylene, 8 gsm aluminium foil and 30 gsm surlyn.

Pack size 15g (tube), 10g (tube), 1 g sachet

Not all pack sizes may be marketed.

6.6 Special precautions for disposal and other handling
No special requirements.

7. MARKETING AUTHORISATION HOLDER
DDD Limited,

94, Rickmansworth Road,

Watford,

Hertfordshire,

United Kingdom,

WD1 7JJ.

8. MARKETING AUTHORISATION NUMBER(S)
PL 00133/5010R

9. DATE OF FIRST AUTHORISATION/RENEWAL OF THE AUTHORISATION
26 November 1996

10. DATE OF REVISION OF THE TEXT
December 2007

Depakote tablets

(sanofi-aventis)

1. NAME OF THE MEDICINAL PRODUCT
Depakote 250mg Tablets.

Depakote 500mg Tablets.

2. QUALITATIVE AND QUANTITATIVE COMPOSITION
Containing 269.10mg of valproate semisodium* per tablet (equivalent to 250mg of valproic acid).

Containing 538.20mg of valproate semisodium* per tablet (equivalent to 500mg of valproic acid).

*Valproate semisodium is a stable coordination compound comprised of sodium valproate and valproic acid in a 1:1 molar relationship. It is also known as divalproex sodium (USAN).

3. PHARMACEUTICAL FORM
Gastro-resistant tablets.

4. CLINICAL PARTICULARS

4.1 Therapeutic indications
Depakote is indicated for the acute treatment of a manic episode associated with bipolar disorder.

4.2 Posology and method of administration
For oral administration. The tablets should be swallowed whole with a drink of water, and not crushed or chewed.

The daily dosage should be established according to age and body weight. The wide variation in individual sensitivity to Depakote should also be considered.

There is no clear correlation between daily dose, plasma concentration and therapeutic effect. Optimum dosage should be determined mainly by clinical response. Measurement of valproate plasma levels may be considered in addition to clinical monitoring when adequate therapeutic effect is not achieved or adverse effects are suspected.

In mania it is generally agreed that plasma levels around 45 to 50μg/ml are needed to allow efficacy; most patients receiving Depakote during controlled clinical trials achieved a maximum plasma concentration of greater than 75μg/ml.

Dosage

Adults

The recommended initial dose is 750mg daily in 2 to 3 divided doses. From day 2 the dose should be increased as rapidly as possible to achieve the lowest therapeutic dose which produces the desired clinical effect. Daily doses usually range between 1000 and 2000mg (i.e. 20 – 30 mg/kg/day body weight). Where adequate control is not achieved within this range the dose may be increased.

Patients receiving daily doses higher than 45mg/kg/day body weight should be carefully monitored.

Elderly

Although the pharmacokinetics of Depakote are modified in the elderly, they have limited clinical significance and dosage should be determined on the basis of clinical response.

Children and adolescents

The safety and effectiveness of Depakote for the treatment of manic episodes have not been studied in individuals below the age of 18 years.

In patients with renal insufficiency

It may be necessary to decrease dosage. Dosage should be adjusted according to clinical monitoring since monitoring of plasma concentrations may be misleading (see section 5.2 Pharmacokinetic Properties).

In patients with hepatic insufficiency

Salicylates should not be used concomitantly with Depakote since they employ the same metabolic pathway (see also sections 4.4 Special Warnings and Precautions for Use and 4.8 Undesirable Effects).

Liver dysfunction, including hepatic failure resulting in fatalities, has occurred in patients whose treatment included valproic acid (see sections 4.3 Contraindications and 4.4 Special Warnings and Precautions for Use).

Salicylates should not be used in children under 16 years (see aspirin/salicylate product information on Reye's syndrome). In addition in conjunction with Depakote, concomitant use in children under 3 years can increase the risk of liver toxicity (see section 4.4.1 Special warnings).

Combined Therapy

When starting Depakote in patients, already on anticonvulsants, these should be tapered slowly; if clinically possible; initiation of Depakote therapy should then be gradual, with target dose being reached after about 2 weeks. Faster titration may be permissible if plasma level monitoring is available. In certain cases it may be necessary to raise the dose by 5 to 10mg/kg/day when used in combination with anticonvulsants which induce liver enzyme activity, e.g. phenytoin, phenobarbital and carbamazepine. Once known enzyme inducers have been withdrawn it may be possible to maintain control on a reduced dose of Depakote. When barbiturates are being administered concomitantly and particularly if sedation is observed the dosage of barbiturate should be reduced.

When using Depakote with other psycotropics, a reduced dose may be required, (see 4.5.1 Effects of Depakote on other drugs)

Optimum dosage is mainly determined by control. However, a method for measurement of plasma levels is available and may be helpful where there is poor control or side effects are suspected (see section 5.2 Pharmacokinetic Properties).

4.3 Contraindications
Active liver disease

Personal or family history of severe hepatic dysfunction, drug related

Hypersensitivity to valproate semisodium or any other ingredient of the preparation.

Porphyria

4.4 Special warnings and precautions for use
To ensure the correct medication is prescribed for the patient's condition, care must be taken not to confuse Depakote with Epilim or sodium valproate. Patients with bipolar disorder and epilepsy are distinct populations. These differences are reflected in the patient information leaflets which clearly indicate specific indications for these differing medications.

Although there is no specific evidence of sudden recurrence of underlying symptoms following withdrawal of valproate, discontinuation should normally only be done under the supervision of a specialist in a gradual manner. This is due to the possibility of sudden alterations in plasma concentrations giving rise to a recurrence of symptoms. NICE has advised that generic switching of valproate preparations is not normally recommended due to the clinical implications of possible variations in plasma concentrations.

4.4.1 Special Warnings

Liver dysfunction:

Conditions of occurrence:

Severe liver damage, including hepatic failure sometimes resulting in fatalities, has been very rarely reported. Experience in epilepsy has indicated that patients most at risk are infants and in particular young children under the age of 3 and those with severe seizure disorders, organic brain disease, and (or) congenital metabolic or degenerative disease associated with mental retardation.

After the age of 3, the incidence of occurrence is significantly reduced and progressively decreases with age.

The concomitant use of salicylates should be avoided in children under 3 due to the risk of liver toxicity. Additionally, salicylates should not be used in children under 16 years (see aspirin/salicylate product information on Reye's syndrome).

In most cases, such liver damage occurred during the first 6 months of therapy, the period of maximum risk being 2-12 weeks.

Suggestive signs:

Clinical symptoms are essential for early diagnosis. In particular, the following conditions which may precede jaundice should be taken into consideration, especially in patients at risk (see above: 'Conditions of occurrence'):

- non specific symptoms, usually of sudden onset, such as asthenia, malaise, anorexia, lethargy, oedema and drowsiness, which are sometimes associated with repeated vomiting and abdominal pain.

- in patients with epilepsy, recurrence of seizures,

These are an indication for immediate withdrawal of the drug. Patients (or their family for children) should be instructed to report immediately any such signs to a physician should they occur. Investigations including clinical examination and biological assessment of liver function should be undertaken immediately.

Detection:

Liver function should be measured before and then periodically monitored during the first 6 months of therapy, especially in those who seem most at risk, and those with a prior history of liver disease. Amongst usual investigations, tests which reflect protein synthesis, particularly prothrombin rate, are most relevant. Confirmation of an abnormally low prothrombin rate, particularly in association with other biological abnormalities (significant decrease in fibrinogen and coagulation factors; increased bilirubin level and raised transaminases) requires cessation of treatment. As a matter of precaution and in case they are taken concomitantly salicylates should also be discontinued since they employ the same metabolic pathway.

Increased liver enzymes are common, particularly at the beginning of therapy; they are also transient.

More extensive biological investigations (including prothrombin rate) are recommended in these patients; a reduction in dosage may be considered when appropriate and tests should be repeated as necessary.

Pancreatitis: Pancreatitis, which may be severe and result in fatalities, has been very rarely reported. Patients experiencing nausea, vomiting or acute abdominal pain should have a prompt medical evaluation (including measurement of serum amylase). Young children are at particular risk; this risk decreases with increasing age. Hepatic failure with pancreatitis increases the risk of fatal outcome. In case of pancreatitis, Depakote should be discontinued.

Suicidal ideation and behaviour:

Suicidal ideation and behaviour have been reported in patients treated with anti-epileptic agents in several indications. A meta-analysis of randomised placebo controlled trials of anti-epileptic drugs has also shown a small increased risk of suicidal ideation and behaviour. The mechanism of this risk is not known and the available data do not exclude the possibility of an increased risk for valproate semisodium.

Therefore patients should be monitored for signs of suicidal ideation and behaviours and appropriate treatment should be considered. Patients (and caregivers of patients) should be advised to seek medical advice should signs of suicidal ideation or behaviour emerge.

4.4.2 Precautions

Haematological: Blood tests (blood cell count, including platelet count, bleeding time and coagulation tests) are recommended prior to initiation of therapy or before surgery, and in case of spontaneous bruising or bleeding (see section 4.8. Undesirable Effects).

Renal insufficiency: In patients with renal insufficiency, it may be necessary to decrease dosage. As monitoring of plasma concentrations may be misleading, dosage should be adjusted according to clinical monitoring (see sections 4.2 Posology and Method of Administration and 5.2. Pharmacokinetic Properties).

Systemic lupus erythematosus: Although immune disorders have only rarely been noted during the use of Depakote, the potential benefit of Depakote should be weighed against its potential risk in patients with systemic lupus erythematosus (see also section 4.8 Undesirable Effects).

Hyperammonaemia: When a urea cycle enzymatic deficiency is suspected, metabolic investigations should be performed prior to treatment because of the risk of hyperammonaemia with Depakote.

Weight gain: Depakote very commonly causes weight gain, which may be marked and progressive. Patients should be warned of the risk of weight gain at the initiation of therapy and appropriate strategies should be adopted to minimise it (see section 4.8 Undesirable Effects).

Pregnancy: Women of child-bearing potential should not be started on Depakote without specialist psychiatric advice. Adequate counselling should be made available to all women with bipolar disorder of childbearing potential regarding the risks associated with pregnancy because of the potential teratogenic risk to the foetus (see also section 4.6 Pregnancy and Lactation).

Diabetic patients: Depakote is eliminated mainly through the kidneys, partly in the form of ketone bodies; this may give false positives in the urine testing of possible diabetics.

4.5 Interaction with other medicinal products and other forms of interaction

4.5.1 Effects of Depakote on other drugs

- Clozapine, haloperidol, lithium

No significant interaction was observed when clozapine and haloperidol were administered concurrently with Depakote. Co-administration of Depakote and lithium does not appear to affect the steady state kinetics of lithium.

- Antipsychotics, MAO inhibitors, antidepressants and benzodiazepines

Depakote may potentiate the effect of other psychotropics such as antipsychotics, MAO inhibitors, antidepressants and benzodiazepines; therefore, clinical monitoring is advised and the dosage of the other psychotropics should be adjusted when appropriate.

In particular, a clinical study has suggested that adding olanzapine to valproate or lithium therapy may significantly increase the risk of certain adverse events associated with olanzapine e.g. neutropenia, tremor, dry mouth, increased appetite and weight gain, speech disorder and somnolence.

- Phenobarbital

Depakote increases phenobarbital plasma concentrations (due to inhibition of hepatic catabolism) and sedation may occur. Therefore, clinical monitoring is recommended throughout the first 15 days of combined treatment with immediate reduction of phenobarbital doses if sedation occurs and determination of phenobarbital plasma levels when appropriate.

- Primidone

Depakote increases primidone plasma levels with exacerbation of its adverse effects (such as sedation); these signs cease with long term treatment. Clinical monitoring is recommended especially at the beginning of combined therapy with dosage adjustment when appropriate.

- Phenytoin

Depakote decreases phenytoin total plasma concentration. Moreover Depakote increases phenytoin free form with possible overdosage symptoms (valproic acid displaces phenytoin from its plasma protein binding sites and reduces its hepatic catabolism). Therefore clinical monitoring is recommended; when phenytoin plasma levels are determined, the free form should be evaluated.

- Carbamazepine

Clinical toxicity has been reported when Depakote was administered with carbamazepine as Depakote may potentiate toxic effects of carbamazepine. Clinical monitoring is recommended especially at the beginning of combined therapy with dosage adjustment when appropriate.

- Lamotrigine

Depakote may reduce the metabolism of lamotrigine and increase the mean half-life. Dose should be adjusted (lamotrigine dosage decreased) when appropriate. Co-administration of lamotrigine and Depakote might increase the risk of rash.

- Zidovudine

Depakote may raise zidovudine plasma concentration leading to increased zidovudine toxicity.

- Vitamin K-dependent anticoagulants

The anticoagulant effect of warfarin and other coumarin anticoagulants may be increased following displacement from plasma protein binding sites by valproic acid. The prothrombin time should be closely monitored.

- Temozolomide

Co-administration of temozolomide and Depakote may cause a small decrease in the clearance of temozolomide that is not thought to be clinically relevant.

4.5.2 Effects of other drugs on Depakote

Antiepileptics with enzyme inducing effects (including ***phenytoin, phenobarbital, carbamazepine***) decrease valproic acid plasma concentrations. Dosages should be adjusted according to blood levels in case of combined therapy. On the other hand, combination of ***felbamate*** and Depakote may increase valproic acid plasma concentration. Depakote dosage should be monitored.

Mefloquine and ***Chloroquine*** increase valproic acid metabolism. Accordingly, the dosage of Depakote may need adjustment.

In case of concomitant use of Depakote and ***highly protein bound agents (e.g. aspirin),*** free valproic acid plasma levels may be increased.

Valproic acid plasma levels may be increased (as a result of reduced hepatic metabolism) in case of concomitant use with ***cimetidine or erythromycin.***

Carbapenem antibiotics such as ***panipenem***, *imipenem* and *meropenem*: Decrease in valproic acid blood level, sometimes associated with convulsions, has been observed when panipenem, imipenem or meropenem were combined. If these antibiotics have to be administered, close monitoring of valproic acid blood level is recommended.

Colestyramine may decrease the absorption of Depakote.

4.5.3 Other interactions

Depakote usually has no enzyme inducing effect; as a consequence, Depakote does not reduce efficacy of oestroprogestative agents in women receiving hormonal contraception, including the oral contraceptive pill.

4.6 Pregnancy and lactation

Women of child-bearing potential should not be started on Depakote without specialist psychiatric advice.

Adequate counselling should be made available to all women with bipolar disorder of childbearing potential regarding the risks associated with pregnancy because of the potential teratogenic risk to the foetus (see also section 4.6.1).

Women who are taking Depakote and who may become pregnant should receive specialist psychiatric advice and the benefits of its use should be weighed against the risks.

If pregnancy is planned, consideration should be given to cessation of Depakote treatment, if appropriate.

When Depakote treatment is deemed necessary, precautions to minimize the potential teratogenic risk should be followed. (See also section 4.6.1 paragraph entitled "In view of the above")

In offspring born to mothers with epilepsy receiving any antiepileptic treatment, the overall rate of malformations has been demonstrated to be 2 to 3 times higher than the rate (approximately 3 %) reported in the general population. An increased number of children with malformations have been reported in cases of multiple drug therapy. Malformations most frequently encountered are cleft lip and cardio-vascular malformations.

Epidemiological studies have suggested an association between in-utero exposure to Depakote and a risk of developmental delay. Developmental delay has been reported in children born to mothers with epilepsy. It is not possible to differentiate what may be due to genetic, social, environmental factors, maternal epilepsy or antiepileptic treatment.

Notwithstanding those potential risks, no sudden discontinuation in the bipolar therapy should be undertaken as this may lead to an immediate relapse of the underlying symptoms.

4.6.1 Pregnancy

From experience in treating mothers with epilepsy, the risk associated with the use of Depakote during pregnancy has been described as follows:

- Risk associated with valproate

In animals: teratogenic effects have been demonstrated in the mouse, rat and rabbit.

There is animal experimental evidence that high plasma peak levels and the size of an individual dose are associated with neural tube defects.

In humans: Valproate use is associated with neural tube defects such as myelomeningocele and spina bifida. The frequency of this effect is estimated to be 1 to 2%. An increased incidence of minor or major malformations including neural tube defects, craniofacial defects, malformation of the limbs, cardiovascular malformations, hypospadias and multiple anomalies involving various body systems has been reported in offspring born to mothers treated with valproate.

Some data from studies, of women with epilepsy, have suggested an association between in-utero exposure to valproate and the risk of developmental delay (frequently associated with craniofacial abnormalities), particularly of verbal IQ.

- In view of the above data

When a woman is planning pregnancy, this provides an opportunity to review the need for treatment. Women of childbearing age should be informed of the risks and benefits of continuing treatment throughout pregnancy.

Folate supplementation, **prior** to pregnancy, has been demonstrated to reduce the incidence of neural tube defects in the offspring of women at high risk. Although no direct evidence exists of such effects in women receiving Depakote, women should be advised to start taking folic acid supplementation (5mg) as soon as contraception is discontinued.

Dosage should be reviewed before conception and the lowest effective dose used, in divided doses, as abnormal pregnancy outcome tends to be associated with higher total daily dosage and with the size of an individual dose. The incidence of neural tube defects rises with increasing dosage, particularly above 1000mg daily. The administration in several divided doses over the day is preferable in order to avoid high peak plasma levels.

Nevertheless, specialised prenatal monitoring should be instituted in order to detect the possible occurrence of a neural tube defect or any other malformation. Pregnancies should be carefully screened by ultrasound, and other techniques if appropriate (see Section 4.4 Special Warnings and Precautions for Use).

- Risk in the neonate

Very rare cases of haemorrhagic syndrome have been reported in neonates whose mothers have taken valproate during pregnancy. This haemorrhagic syndrome is related to hypofibrinogenemia; afibrinogenemia has also been reported and may be fatal. These are possibly associated with a decrease of coagulation factors. However, this syndrome has to be distinguished from the decrease of the vitamin-K factors induced by phenobarbital and other enzyme inducing drugs.

Therefore, platelet count, fibrinogen plasma level, coagulation tests and coagulation factors should be investigated in neonates.

4.6.2 Lactation

Excretion of Depakote in breast milk is low, with a concentration between 1 % to 10 % of total maternal serum levels; up to now children breast fed that have been monitored during the neonatal period have not experienced clinical effects. There appears to be no contra-indication to breast feeding by patients on Depakote.

4.7 Effects on ability to drive and use machines

Patients should be warned of the risk of transient drowsiness, especially in cases of polytherapy or association with benzodiazepines (see section 4.5 Interactions with Other Medicaments and Other Forms of Interaction).

4.8 Undesirable effects

The following adverse events have been described from experience of sodium valproate in epilepsy; no other adverse event that could be specifically associated with the use of Depakote in the treatment of manic episodes have been identified.

Congenital and familial/genetic disorders: (see section 4.6. Pregnancy and Lactation)

Hepato-biliary disorders: rare cases of liver dysfunction (see section 4.4.1 Special Warnings)

Severe liver damage, including hepatic failure sometimes resulting in death, has been reported (see also sections 4.2, 4.3 and 4.4.1). Increased liver enzymes are common, particularly early in treatment, and may be transient (see section 4.4.1 Special Warnings).

Gastrointestinal disorders: (nausea, gastralgia, diarrhoea) frequently occur at the start of treatment, but they usually disappear after a few days without discontinuing treatment. These problems can usually be overcome by taking Depakote Tablets with or after food.

Very rare cases of pancreatitis, sometimes lethal, have been reported (see section 4.4 Special Warnings and Precautions for Use).

Nervous system disorders: Sedation has been reported occasionally. In monotherapy it occurred early in treatment on rare occasions and is usually transient. Rare cases of lethargy and confusion occasionally progressing to stupor, sometimes with associated hallucinations or convulsions have been reported. Encephalopathy and coma have very rarely been observed. These cases have often been associated with too high a starting dose or too rapid a dose escalation or concomitant use of anticonvulsants, notably phenobarbital. They have usually been reversible on withdrawal of treatment or reduction of dosage.

Very rare cases of reversible extrapyramidal symptoms including parkinsonism, or reversible dementia associated with reversible cerebral atrophy have been reported. Dose-related ataxia and fine postural tremor have occasionally been reported.

An increase in alertness may occur; this is generally beneficial but occasionally aggression, hyperactivity and behavioural deterioration have been reported.

Metabolic disorders:Cases of isolated and moderate hyperammonaemia without change in liver function tests may occur frequently, but they are usually transient and should not cause treatment discontinuation. However, they may present clinically as vomiting, ataxia, and increasing clouding of consciousness. Should these symptoms occur Depakote should be discontinued. Very rare cases of hyponatraemia have been reported.

Hyperammonaemia associated with neurological symptoms has also been reported (see section 4.4.2. Precautions). In such cases further investigations should be considered.

Blood and lymphatic system disorders: frequent occurrence of thrombocytopenia, rare cases of anaemia, leucopenia or pancytopenia. The blood picture returned to normal when the drug was discontinued.

Isolated reduction of fibrinogen or reversible increase in bleeding time have been reported, usually without associated clinical signs and particularly with high doses (Depakote has an inhibitory effect on the second phase of platelet aggregation). Spontaneous bruising or bleeding is an indication for withdrawal of medication pending investigations (see also section 4.6 Pregnancy and Lactation).

Skin and subcutaneous tissue disorders: cutaneous reactions such as exanthematous rash rarely occur with Depakote. In very rare cases, toxic epidermal necrolysis, Stevens-Johnson syndrome and erythema multiforme have been reported.

Transient hair loss, which may sometimes be dose-related, has often been reported. Regrowth normally begins within six months, although the hair may become more curly than previously. Hirsutism and acne have been very rarely reported.

Reproductive system and breast disorders: Amenorrhea and irregular periods have been reported. Very rarely gynaecomastia has occurred.

Vascular disorders: the occurrence of vasculitis has occasionally been reported.

Ear disorders: hearing loss, either reversible or irreversible, has been reported rarely; however a cause and effect relationship has not been established.

Renal and urinary disorders: there have been isolated reports of a reversible Fanconi's syndrome (a defect in proximal renal tubular function giving rise to glycosuria, amino aciduria, phosphaturia, and uricosuria) associated with Depakote therapy, but the mode of action is as yet unclear. Very rare cases of enuresis have been reported.

Immune system disorders: allergic reactions (ranging from rash to hypersensitivity reactions) have been reported

General disorders: very rare cases of non severe peripheral oedema have been reported.

Increase in weight may also occur. Weight gain being a risk factor for polycystic ovary syndrome, it should be carefully monitored (see section 4.4 Special Warnings and Precautions for Use).

4.9 Overdose

Signs of acute massive overdose, i.e. plasma concentration 10 to 20 times maximum therapeutic levels, usually include CNS depression, or coma with muscular hypotonia, hyporeflexia, miosis, impaired respiratory functions and metabolic acidosis.

Symptoms may however be variable and seizures have been reported in the presence of very high plasma levels in epileptic patients. Cases of intracranial hypertension related to cerebral oedema have been reported.

Hospital management of overdose should be symptomatic, including cardio-respiratogastric monitoring. Gastric lavage may be useful up to 10 to 12 hours following ingestion.

Haemodialysis and haemoperfusion have been used successfully.

Naloxone has been successfully used in a few isolated cases, sometimes in association with activated charcoal given orally.

Deaths have occurred following massive overdose; nevertheless, a favourable outcome is usual.

5. PHARMACOLOGICAL PROPERTIES

5.1 Pharmacodynamic properties

Depakote exerts its effects mainly on the central nervous system.

The most likely mode of action for Depakote is potentiation of the inhibitory action of gamma amino butyric acid (GABA) through an action on the further synthesis or further metabolism of GABA.

The effectiveness of Depakote in acute mania was demonstrated in two, 3-week, double-blind, placebo-controlled trials conducted in bipolar patients. Depakote was initiated at a dose of 250mg tid and subsequently titrated up to a maximum daily dose not exceeding 2500mg; the concomitant use of a benzodiazepine was allowed during the first 10 days of treatment to manage associated symptoms such as severe agitation.

Pharmacological studies have demonstrated activity in experimental models of animal behaviour in mania.

5.2 Pharmacokinetic properties

Following oral administration of Depakote the absolute bioavailability of valproic acid approaches 100%. Mean terminal half life is about 14 hours, steady state conditions usually being achieved within 3 to 4 days. Peak plasma concentrations are achieved within 3 to 5 hours. Administration with food increases T_{max} by about 4 hours but does not modify the extent of absorption.

Depakote is extensively metabolised in the liver with less than 3% of an administered dose excreted unchanged in the urine. Principal metabolites found in urine are those originating from β-oxidation (up to 45% of the dose) and glucuronidation (up to 60% of the dose). Plasma clearance ranges from 0.4 to 0.6L/h and is independent of hepatic blood flow.

Plasma protein binding of Depakote ranges from 85 to 94% over plasma drug concentrations of 40 to 100 mcg/ml. It is concentration-dependent and the free fraction increases non-linearly with plasma drug concentration.

In elderly patients and those with liver cirrhosis (including alcoholic), acute hepatitis or renal failure the elimination of valproic acid is reduced. Reduction in intrinsic clearance and protein binding are reported. Thus, monitoring of total concentrations may be misleading and dosage adjustment may need to be considered according to clinical response.

Haemodialysis reduces serum valproic acid concentrations by about 20%.

5.3 Preclinical safety data

There are no pre-clinical data of relevance to the prescriber which are additional to that already included in other sections of the SPC.

6. PHARMACEUTICAL PARTICULARS

6.1 List of excipients

Depakote 250 mg: Colloidal silica, hydrated; starch pregelatinised; povidone; titanium dioxide (E171); talc; hypromellose phthalate; diacetylated monoglycerides; sunset yellow aluminium lake (E110); vanillin.

Depakote 500 mg: Colloidal silica, hydrated; starch pregelatinised; povidone; titanium dioxide (E171); talc; hypromellose phthalate; diacetylated monoglycerides; ponceau 4R aluminium lake (E124); indigo carmine aluminium lake (E132); vanillin.

6.2 Incompatibilities

Not relevant.

6.3 Shelf life

3 years.

6.4 Special precautions for storage

None.

6.5 Nature and contents of container

Aluminium/aluminium blister packs containing 90 tablets.

6.6 Special precautions for disposal and other handling

None.

7. MARKETING AUTHORISATION HOLDER

Sanofi-aventis

One Onslow Street

Guildford

Surrey

GU1 4YS

8. MARKETING AUTHORISATION NUMBER(S)

Depakote 250 mg: 11723/0251

Depakote 500 mg: 11723/0252

9. DATE OF FIRST AUTHORISATION/RENEWAL OF THE AUTHORISATION

Depakote 250mg: 1 June 2009

Depakote 500mg: 24 March 2009

10. DATE OF REVISION OF THE TEXT

1st June 2009

11 Legal classification

POM

Depixol Injection and Conc Injection

(Lundbeck Limited)

1. NAME OF THE MEDICINAL PRODUCT

Depixol® Injection and Depixol® Conc. Injection

2. QUALITATIVE AND QUANTITATIVE COMPOSITION

Depixol Injection

20 mg/mL (2% w/v) cis(Z)-flupentixol decanoate in thin vegetable oil. Ampoules 1mL and 2 mL, Syringes 1 mL and 2 mL and Vial 10 mL.

Depixol Conc. Injection

100 mg/mL (10%w/v) cis (Z)-flupentixol decanoate in thin vegetable oil. Ampoules 0.5 mL and 1 mL and Vial 5 mL.

3. PHARMACEUTICAL FORM

Oily solution for deep intramuscular injection.

4. CLINICAL PARTICULARS

4.1 Therapeutic indications

The treatment of schizophrenia and other psychoses.

4.2 Posology and method of administration

Route of administration

Deep intramuscular injection into the upper outer buttock or lateral thigh. Dosage and dosage interval should be adjusted according to the patients' symptoms and response to treatment.

Note: As with all oil based injections it is important to ensure, by aspiration before injection, that inadvertent intravascular entry does not occur.

Adults

The usual dosage of flupentixol decanoate lies between 50 mg every 4 weeks and 300 mg every 2 weeks, but some patients may require up to 400 mg weekly. Other patients may be adequately maintained on dosages of 20-40 mg flupentixol decanoate every 2-4 weeks. In patients who have not previously received depot antipsychotic, treatment is usually started with a small dose (e.g. 20 mg) to assess tolerability. An interval of at least one week should be allowed before the second injection is given at a dose consistent with the patients' condition.

Adequate control of severe psychotic symptoms may take up to 4 to 6 months at high enough dosage. Once stabilised lower maintenance doses may be considered, but must be sufficient to prevent relapse.

The appropriate presentation of Depixol should be selected to achieve an injection volume which does not exceed 2 mL. Volumes greater than 2 mL should be distributed between two injection sites.

Elderly

In accordance with standard medical practice, initial dosage may need to be reduced to a quarter or half the normal starting dose in the frail or elderly.

Children

Depixol Injection and Depixol Conc. Injection are not indicated for children.

4.3 Contraindications

Hypersensitivity to the active substance or to any of the excipients (see section 6.1).

Circulatory collapse, depressed level of consciousness due to any cause (e.g. intoxication with alcohol, barbiturates or opiates), coma

Not recommended for excitable or agitated patients.

4.4 Special warnings and precautions for use

Caution should be exercised in patients having: liver disease; cardiac disease or arrhythmias; severe respiratory disease; renal failure; epilepsy (and conditions predisposing to epilepsy e.g. alcohol withdrawal or brain damage); Parkinson's disease; narrow angle glaucoma; prostatic hypertrophy; hypothyroidism; hyperthyroidism; myasthenia gravis; phaeochromocytoma and patients who have shown hypersensitivity to thioxanthenes or other antipsychotics.

The elderly require close supervision because they are specially prone to experience such adverse effects as sedation, hypotension, confusion and temperature changes.

The possibility of development of neuroleptic malignant syndrome (hyperthermia, muscle rigidity, fluctuating consciousness, instability of the autonomous nervous system) exists with any neuroleptic. The risk is possibly greater with the more potent agents. Patients with pre-existing organic brain syndrome, mental retardation, and opiate and alcohol abuse are over-represented among fatal cases.

Treatment: Discontinuation of the neuroleptic. Symptomatic treatment and use of general supportive measures. Dantrolene and bromocriptine may be helpful.

Symptoms may persist for more than a week after oral neuroleptics are discontinued and somewhat longer when associated with the depot forms of the drugs.

Blood dyscrasias, including thrombocytopenia, have been reported rarely. Blood counts should be carried out if a patient develops signs of persistent infection.

As described for other psychotropics flupentixol may modify insulin and glucose responses calling for adjustment of the antidiabetic therapy in diabetic patients.

When transferring patients from oral to depot antipsychotic treatment, the oral medication should not be discontinued immediately, but gradually withdrawn over a period of several days after administering the first injection.

An approximately 3-fold increased risk of cerebrovascular adverse events have been seen in randomised placebo controlled clinical trials in the dementia population with some atypical antipsychotics. The mechanism for this increased risk is not known. An increased risk cannot be excluded for other antipsychotics or other patient populations.

Flupentixol should be used with caution in patients with risk factors for stroke.

As with other drugs belonging to the therapeutic class of antipsychotics, flupentixol may cause QT prolongation. Persistently prolonged QT intervals may increase the risk of malignant arrhythmias. Therefore, flupentixol should be used with caution in susceptible individuals (with hypokalaemia, hypomagnesia or genetic predisposition) and in patients with a history of cardiovascular disorders, e.g. QT prolongation, significant bradycardia (<50 beats per minute), a recent acute myocardial infarction, uncompensated heart failure, or cardiac arrhythmia.

Concomitant treatment with other antipsychotics should be avoided (see section 4.5).

Suicide/suicidal thoughts or clinical worsening

Depression is associated with an increased risk of suicidal thoughts, self harm and suicide (suicide-related events). This risk persists until significant remission occurs. As improvement may not occur during the first few weeks or more of treatment, patients should be closely monitored until such improvement occurs. It is general clinical experience that the risk of suicide may increase in the early stages of recovery.

Other psychiatric conditions for which Flupentixol is prescribed can also be associated with an increased risk of suicide-related events. In addition, these conditions may be co-morbid with major depressive disorder. The same precautions observed when treating patients with major depressive disorder should therefore be observed when treating patients with other psychiatric disorders.

Patients with a history of suicide-related events, or those exhibiting a significant degree of suicidal ideation prior to commencement of treatment are known to be at greater risk of suicidal thoughts or suicide attempts, and should receive careful monitoring during treatment. A meta-analysis of placebo-controlled clinical trials of antidepressant drugs in adult patients with psychiatric disorders showed an increased risk of suicidal behaviour with antidepressants compared to placebo in patients less than 25 years old.

Close supervision of patients and in particular those at high risk should accompany drug therapy especially in early treatment and following dose changes. Patients (and caregivers of patients) should be alerted about the need to monitor for any clinical worsening, suicidal behaviour or thoughts and unusual changes in behaviour and to seek medical advice immediately if these symptoms present.

4.5 Interaction with other medicinal products and other forms of interaction

In common with other antipsychotics, flupentixol enhances the response to alcohol, the effects of barbiturates and other CNS depressants. Flupentixol may potentiate the effects of general anaesthetics and anticoagulants and prolong the action of neuromuscular blocking agents.

The anticholinergic effects of atropine or other drugs with anticholinergic properties may be increased. Concomitant use of drugs such as metoclopramide, piperazine or antiparkinson drugs may increase the risk of extrapyramidal effects such as tardive dyskinesia. Combined use of antipsychotics and lithium or sibutramine has been associated with an increased risk of neurotoxicity.

Antipsychotics may enhance the cardiac depressant effects of quinidine; the absorption of corticosteroids and digoxin. The hypotensive effect of vasodilator antihypertensive agents such as hydralazine and α-blockers (e.g. doxazosin), or methyl-dopa may be enhanced.

Increases in the QT interval related to antipsychotic treatment may be exacerbated by the co-administration of other drugs known to significantly increase the QT interval. Co-administration of such drugs should be avoided. Relevant classes include:

- class Ia and III antiarrhythmics (e.g. quinidine, amiodarone, sotalol, dofetilide)
- some antipsychotics (e.g. thioridazine)
- some macrolides (e.g. erythromycin)
- some antihistamines
- some quinolone antibiotics (e.g. moxifloxacin)

The above list is not exhaustive and other individual drugs known to significantly increase QT interval (e.g. cisapride, lithium) should be avoided.

Drugs known to cause electrolyte disturbances such as thiazide diuretics (hypokalaemia) and drugs known to increase the plasma concentration of flupentixol should also be used with caution as they may increase the risk of QT prolongation and malignant arrythmias (see section 4.4).

Antipsychotics may antagonise the effects of adrenaline and other sympathomimetic agents, and reverse the antihypertensive effects of guanethidine and similar adrenergic-blocking agents. Antipsychotics may also impair the effect of levodopa, adrenergic drugs and anticonvulsants.

The metabolism of tricyclic antidepressants may be inhibited and the control of diabetes may be impaired.

4.6 Pregnancy and lactation

As the safety of this drug during pregnancy has not been established, use during pregnancy, especially the first and last trimesters, should be avoided, unless the expected benefit to the patient outweighs the potential risk to the foetus.

Flupentixol is excreted into the breast milk. If the use of Depixol is considered essential, nursing mothers should be advised to stop breast feeding.

The newborn of mothers treated with antipsychotics in late pregnancy, or labour, may show signs of intoxication such as lethargy, tremor and hyperexcitability, and have a low apgar score.

4.7 Effects on ability to drive and use machines

Alertness may be impaired, especially at the start of treatment, or following the consumption of alcohol; patients should be warned of this risk and advised not to drive or operate machinery until their susceptibility is known. Patients should not drive if they have blurred vision.

4.8 Undesirable effects

Cases of suicidal ideation and suicidal behaviours have been reported during Flupentixol therapy or early after treatment discontinuation (see section 4.4).

Undesirable effects are for the majority dose dependent. The frequency and severity are most pronounced in the early phase of treatment and decline during continued treatment.

Extrapyramidal reactions may occur, especially in the early phase of treatment. In most cases these side effects can be satisfactorily controlled by reduction of dosage and/or use of antiparkinsonian drugs. The routine prophylactic use of antiparkinsonian drugs is not recommended. Antiparkinsonian drugs do not alleviate tardive dyskinesia and may aggravate them. Reduction in dosage or, if possible, discontinuation of zuclopenthixol therapy is recommended. In persistent akathisia a benzodiazepine or propranolol may be useful.

Cardiac disorders	Tachycardia, palpitations. Electrocardiogram QT prolonged.
Blood and lymphatic system disorders	Thrombocytopenia, neutropenia, leukopenia, agranulocytosis
Nervous system disorders	Somnolence, akathisia, hyperkinesia, hypokinesia. Tremor, dystonia, dizziness, headache, disturbance in attention. Tardive dyskinesia, dyskinesia, parkinsonism, speech disorder, convulsion. Neuroleptic malignant syndrome.
Eye disorders	Accommodation disorder, vision abnormal. Oculogyration.
Respiratory, thoracic and mediastinal disorders	Dyspnoea.
Gastrointestinal disorders	Dry mouth. Salivary hypersecretion, constipation, vomiting, dyspepsia, diarrhoea. Abdominal pain, nausea, flatulence.
Renal and urinary disorders	Micturition disorder, urinary retention.
Skin and subcutaneous tissue disorders	Hyperhidrosis, pruritus. Rash, photosensitivity reaction, dermatitis.
Musculoskeletal and connective tissue disorder	Myalgia. Muscle rigidity.
Endocrine disorder	Hyperprolactinaemia.
Metabolism and nutrition disorders	Increased appetite, weight increased. Decreased appetite. Hyperglycaemia, glucose tolerance abnormal.
Vascular disorders	Hypotension, hot flush.
General disorders and administration site conditions	Asthenia, fatigue. Injection site reactions
Immune system disorders	Hypersensitivity, anaphylactic reaction.
Hepatobiliary disorders	Liver function test abnormal. Jaundice.
Reproductive system and breast disorders	Ejaculation failure, erectile dysfunction. Gynaecomastia, galactorrhoea, amenorrhoea.
Psychiatric disorders	Insomnia, depression, nervousness, agitation, libido decreased. Confusional state.

As with other drugs belonging to the therapeutic class of antipsychotics, rare cases of QT prolongation, ventricular arrhythmias - ventricular fibrillation, ventricular tachycardia, Torsade de Pointes and sudden unexplained death have been reported for flupentixol (see section 4.4).

Abrupt discontinuation of flupentixol may be accompanied by withdrawal symptoms. The most common symptoms are nausea, vomiting, anorexia, diarrhoea, rhinorrhoea, sweating, myalgias, paraesthesias, insomnia, restlessness, anxiety, and agitation. Patients may also experience vertigo, alternate feelings of warmth and coldness, and tremor. Symptoms generally begin within 1 to 4 days of withdrawal and abate within 7 to 14 days.

4.9 Overdose

Overdosage may cause somnolence, or even coma, extrapyramidal symptoms, convulsions, hypotension, shock, hyper-or hypothermia. ECG changes, QT prolongation, Torsade de Pointes, cardiac arrest and ventricular arrhythmias have been reported when administered in overdose together with drugs known to affect the heart.

Treatment is symptomatic and supportive, with measures aimed at supporting the respiratory and cardiovascular systems. The following specific measures may be employed if required.

- anticholinergic antiparkinson drugs if extrapyramidal symptoms occur.
- sedation (with benzodiazepines) in the unlikely event of agitation or excitement or convulsions.
- noradrenaline in saline intravenous drip if the patient is in shock. Adrenaline must not be given.

5. PHARMACOLOGICAL PROPERTIES

5.1 Pharmacodynamic properties

Flupentixol is a non-sedating antipsychotics drug of the thioxanthene group. Its primary pharmacological action is dopamine blockade. Flupentixol has a high affinity for D_1 and D_2 receptors.

5.2 Pharmacokinetic properties

After intramuscular injection, the ester is slowly released from the oil depot and is rapidly hydrolysed to release flupentixol. Flupentixol is widely distributed in the body and extensively metabolised in the liver. Peak circulating levels occur around 7 days after administration.

5.3 Preclinical safety data

Nil of relevance

6. PHARMACEUTICAL PARTICULARS

6.1 List of excipients

Thin vegetable oil "Viscoleo" (fractionated coconut oil).

6.2 Incompatibilities

This product may be mixed in the same syringe with other products in the Depixol Injection range. It should not be mixed with any other injection fluids.

6.3 Shelf life

Depixol Injection:	
Ampoules 1 mL and 2 mL	4 years
Syringes 1 mL and 2 mL	2 years
Vial 10 mL	3 years (shelf-life after opening: 1 day)
Depixol Conc. Injection:	
Ampoule 0.5 mL	2 years
Ampoule 1 mL	4 years
Vial 5 mL	3 years

6.4 Special precautions for storage
Store at or below 25°C. Protect from light.

6.5 Nature and contents of container
Depixol Injection:

Ampoules containing 1 mL and 2 mL of 20 mg/mL (2% w/v) cis (Z)-flupentixol decanoate in thin vegetable oil. Pack size = 10 ampoules per box.

Syringes containing 1 mL and 2 mL of 20 mg/mL (2%w/v) cis (Z)-flupentixol decanoate in thin vegetable oil. Pack size = 5 syringes per box.

Vial containing 10 mL of 20 mg/mL (2%w/v) cis (Z)-flupentixol decanoate in thin vegetable oil. Pack size = 1 vial per box.

Depixol Conc. Injection:

Ampoules containing 0.5 mL and 1 mL of 100 mg/ml (10% w/v) cis (Z)-flupentixol decanoate in thin vegetable oil. Pack size = 10 ampoules per box.

Vial containing 5 mL of 100 mg/ml (10%) cis(Z)- flupentixol decanoate in thin vegetable oil. Pack size = 1 vial per box.

6.6 Special precautions for disposal and other handling
Nil

7. MARKETING AUTHORISATION HOLDER
Lundbeck Limited

Lundbeck House

Caldecotte Lake Business Park

Caldecotte

Milton Keynes

MK7 8LF

8. MARKETING AUTHORISATION NUMBER(S)
Depixol Injection: PL 0458/0007R

Depixol Conc. Injection: PL 0458/0015R

9. DATE OF FIRST AUTHORISATION/RENEWAL OF THE AUTHORISATION
First Authorised 28 January 1987

Renewed 17 March 2002

10. DATE OF REVISION OF THE TEXT
28 January 2009

Legal category: POM

® Trademark

Depixol Injection and Depixol Conc Injection are made by H Lundbeck A/S, Denmark

Depixol Low Volume Injection

(Lundbeck Limited)

1. NAME OF THE MEDICINAL PRODUCT
Depixol® Low Volume Injection

2. QUALITATIVE AND QUANTITATIVE COMPOSITION
200 mg/ml (20% w/v) cis-(Z)-flupentixol decanoate in thin vegetable oil. Ampoules 1 ml and 2 ml and Glass Vial 5 ml.

3. PHARMACEUTICAL FORM
Oily solution for deep intramuscular injection.

4. CLINICAL PARTICULARS

4.1 Therapeutic indications
The treatment of schizophrenia and other psychoses.

4.2 Posology and method of administration
Route of administration

Deep intramuscular injection into the upper outer buttock or lateral thigh. Dosage and dosage interval should be adjusted according to the patients' symptoms and response to treatment.

Note: As with all oil based injections it is important to ensure, by aspiration before injection, that inadvertent intravascular entry does not occur.

Adults

The usual dosage of flupentixol decanoate lies between 50 mg every 4 weeks and 300 mg every 2 weeks, but some patients may require up to 400 mg weekly. Other patients may be adequately maintained on dosages of 20-40 mg flupentixol decanoate every 2-4 weeks. In patients who have not previously received depot antipsychotic, treatment is usually started with a small dose (e.g. 20 mg) to assess tolerability. An interval of at least one week should be allowed before the second injection is given at a dose consistent with the patients' condition.

Adequate control of severe psychotic symptoms may take up to 4 to 6 months at high enough dosage. Once stabilised lower maintenance doses may be considered, but must be sufficient to prevent relapse.

The appropriate presentation of Depixol should be selected to achieve an injection volume which does not exceed 2 ml. Volumes greater than 2 ml should be distributed between two injection sites.

Elderly

In accordance with standard medical practice, initial dosage may need to be reduced to a quarter or half the normal starting dose in the frail or elderly.

Children

Depixol Low Volume Injection is not indicated for children.

4.3 Contraindications
Hypersensitivity to the active substance or to any of the excipients (see section 6.1).

Circulatory collapse, depressed level of consciousness due to any cause (e.g. intoxication with alcohol, barbiturates or opiates), coma

Not recommended for excitable or agitated patients.

4.4 Special warnings and precautions for use
Caution should be exercised in patients having: liver disease; cardiac disease or arrhythmias; severe respiratory disease; renal failure; epilepsy (and conditions predisposing to epilepsy e.g. alcohol withdrawal or brain damage); Parkinson's disease; narrow angle glaucoma; prostatic hypertrophy; hypothyroidism; hyperthyroidism; myasthenia gravis; phaeochromocytoma and patients who have shown hypersensitivity to thioxanthenes or other antipsychotics.

The elderly require close supervision because they are specially prone to experience such adverse effects as sedation, hypotension, confusion and temperature changes.

The possibility of development of neuroleptic malignant syndrome (hyperthermia, muscle rigidity, fluctuating consciousness, instability of the autonomous nervous system) exists with any neuroleptic. The risk is possibly greater with the more potent agents. Patients with pre-existing organic brain syndrome, mental retardation, and opiate and alcohol abuse are over-represented among fatal cases.

Treatment: Discontinuation of the neuroleptic. Symptomatic treatment and use of general supportive measures. Dantrolene and bromocriptine may be helpful.

Symptoms may persist for more than a week after oral neuroleptics are discontinued and somewhat longer when associated with the depot forms of the drugs.

Blood dyscrasias, including thrombocytopenia, have been reported rarely. Blood counts should be carried out if a patient develops signs of persistent infection.

As described for other psychotropics flupentixol may modify insulin and glucose responses calling for adjustment of the antidiabetic therapy in diabetic patients.

When transferring patients from oral to depot antipsychotic treatment, the oral medication should not be discontinued immediately, but gradually withdrawn over a period of several days after administering the first injection.

An approximately 3-fold increased risk of cerebrovascular adverse events have been seen in randomised placebo controlled clinical trials in the dementia population with some atypical antipsychotics. The mechanism for this increased risk is not known. An increased risk cannot be excluded for other antipsychotics or other patient populations.

Flupentixol should be used with caution in patients with risk factors for stroke.

As with other drugs belonging to the therapeutic class of antipsychotics, flupentixol may cause QT prolongation. Persistently prolonged QT intervals may increase the risk of malignant arrhythmias. Therefore, flupentixol should be used with caution in susceptible individuals (with hypokalaemia, hypomagnesia or genetic predisposition) and in patients with a history of cardiovascular disorders, e.g. QT prolongation, significant bradycardia (<50 beats per minute), a recent acute myocardial infarction, uncompensated heart failure, or cardiac arrhythmia.

Concomitant treatment with other antipsychotics should be avoided (see section 4.5).

Suicide/suicidal thoughts or clinical worsening

Depression is associated with an increased risk of suicidal thoughts, self harm and suicide (suicide-related events). This risk persists until significant remission occurs. As improvement may not occur during the first few weeks or more of treatment, patients should be closely monitored until such improvement occurs. It is general clinical experience that the risk of suicide may increase in the early stages of recovery.

Other psychiatric conditions for which Flupentixol is prescribed can also be associated with an increased risk of suicide-related events. In addition, these conditions may be co-morbid with major depressive disorder. The same precautions observed when treating patients with major depressive disorder should therefore be observed when treating patients with other psychiatric disorders.

Patients with a history of suicide-related events, or those exhibiting a significant degree of suicidal ideation prior to commencement of treatment are known to be at greater risk of suicidal thoughts or suicide attempts, and should receive careful monitoring during treatment. A meta-analysis of placebo-controlled clinical trials of antidepressant drugs in adult patients with psychiatric disorders showed an increased risk of suicidal behaviour with antidepressants compared to placebo in patients less than 25 years old.

Close supervision of patients and in particular those at high risk should accompany drug therapy especially in early treatment and following dose changes. Patients (and care-givers of patients) should be alerted about the need to monitor for any clinical worsening, suicidal behaviour or thoughts and unusual changes in behaviour and to seek medical advice immediately if these symptoms present.

4.5 Interaction with other medicinal products and other forms of interaction
In common with other antipsychotics, flupentixol enhances the response to alcohol, the effects of barbiturates and other CNS depressants. Flupentixol may potentiate the effects of general anaesthetics and anticoagulants and prolong the action of neuromuscular blocking agents.

The anticholinergic effects of atropine or other drugs with anticholinergic properties may be increased. Concomitant use of drugs such as metoclopramide, piperazine or antiparkinson drugs may increase the risk of extrapyramidal effects such as tardive dyskinesia. Combined use of antipsychotics and lithium or sibutramine has been associated with an increased risk of neurotoxicity.

Antipsychotics may enhance the cardiac depressant effects of quinidine; the absorption of corticosteroids and digoxin. The hypotensive effect of vasodilator antihypertensive agents such as hydralazine and α-blockers (e.g. doxazosin), or methyl-dopa may be enhanced.

Increases in the QT interval related to antipsychotic treatment may be exacerbated by the co-administration of other drugs known to significantly increase the QT interval. Co-administration of such drugs should be avoided. Relevant classes include:

- class Ia and III antiarrhythmics (e.g. quinidine, amiodarone, sotalol, dofetilide)
- some antipsychotics (e.g. thioridazine)
- some macrolides (e.g. erythromycin)
- some antihistamines
- some quinolone antibiotics (e.g.moxifloxacin)

The above list is not exhaustive and other individual drugs known to significantly increase QT interval (e.g. cisapride, lithium) should be avoided.

Drugs known to cause electrolyte disturbances such as thiazide diuretics (hypokalaemia) and drugs known to increase the plasma concentration of flupentixol should also be used with caution as they may increase the risk of QT prolongation and malignant arrythmias (see section 4.4).

Antipsychotics may antagonise the effects of adrenaline and other sympathomimetic agents, and reverse the antihypertensive effects of guanethidine and similar adrenergic-blocking agents. Antipsychotics may also impair the effect of levodopa, adrenergic drugs and anticonvulsants.

The metabolism of tricyclic antidepressants may be inhibited and the control of diabetes may be impaired.

4.6 Pregnancy and lactation
As the safety of this drug during pregnancy has not been established, use during pregnancy, especially the first and last trimesters, should be avoided, unless the expected benefit to the patient outweighs the potential risk to the foetus.

Flupentixol is excreted into the breast milk. If the use of Depixol is considered essential, nursing mothers should be advised to stop breast feeding.

The newborn of mothers treated with antipsychotics in late pregnancy, or labour, may show signs of intoxication such as lethargy, tremor and hyperexcitability, and have a low apgar score.

4.7 Effects on ability to drive and use machines
Alertness may be impaired, especially at the start of treatment, or following the consumption of alcohol; patients should be warned of this risk and advised not to drive or operate machinery until their susceptibility is known. Patients should not drive if they have blurred vision.

4.8 Undesirable effects
Cases of suicidal ideation and suicidal behaviours have been reported during Flupentixol therapy or early after treatment discontinuation (see section 4.4).

Undesirable effects are for the majority dose dependent. The frequency and severity are most pronounced in the early phase of treatment and decline during continued treatment.

Extrapyramidal reactions may occur, especially in the early phase of treatment. In most cases these side effects can be satisfactorily controlled by reduction of dosage and/or use of antiparkinsonian drugs. The routine prophylactic use of antiparkinsonian drugs is not recommended. Antiparkinsonian drugs do not alleviate tardive dyskinesia and may aggravate them. Reduction in dosage or, if possible, discontinuation of zuclopenthixol therapy is recommended. In persistent akathisia a benzodiazepine or propranolol may be useful.

Cardiac disorders	Tachycardia, palpitations. Electrocardiogram QT prolonged.
Blood and lymphatic system disorders	Thrombocytopenia, neutropenia, leukopenia, agranulocytosis

Nervous system disorders	Somnolence, akathisia, hyperkinesia, hypokinesia. Tremor, dystonia, dizziness, headache, disturbance in attention. Tardive dyskinesia, dyskinesia, parkinsonism, speech disorder, convulsion. Neuroleptic malignant syndrome.
Eye disorders	Accommodation disorder, vision abnormal. Oculogyration.
Respiratory, thoracic and mediastinal disorders	Dyspnoea.
Gastrointestinal disorders	Dry mouth. Salivary hypersecretion, constipation, vomiting, dyspepsia, diarrhoea. Abdominal pain, nausea, flatulence.
Renal and urinary disorders	Micturition disorder, urinary retention.
Skin and subcutaneous tissue disorders	Hyperhidrosis, pruritus. Rash, photosensitivity reaction, dermatitis.
Musculoskeletal and connective tissue disorder	Myalgia. Muscle rigidity.
Endocrine disorder	Hyperprolactinaemia.
Metabolism and nutrition disorders	Increased appetite, weight increased. Decreased appetite. Hyperglycaemia, glucose tolerance abnormal.
Vascular disorders	Hypotension, hot flush.
General disorders and administration site conditions	Asthenia, fatigue. Injection site reactions
Immune system disorders	Hypersensitivity, anaphylactic reaction.
Hepatobiliary disorders	Liver function test abnormal. Jaundice.
Reproductive system and breast disorders	Ejaculation failure, erectile dysfunction. Gynaecomastia, galactorrhoea, amenorrhoea.
Psychiatric disorders	Insomnia, depression, nervousness, agitation, libido decreased. Confusional state

As with other drugs belonging to the therapeutic class of antipsychotics, rare cases of QT prolongation, ventricular arrhythmias - ventricular fibrillation, ventricular tachycardia, Torsade de Pointes and sudden unexplained death have been reported for flupentixol (see section 4.4).

Abrupt discontinuation of flupentixol may be accompanied by withdrawal symptoms. The most common symptoms are nausea, vomiting, anorexia, diarrhoea, rhinorrhoea, sweating, myalgias, paraesthesias, insomnia, restlessness, anxiety, and agitation. Patients may also experience vertigo, alternate feelings of warmth and coldness, and tremor. Symptoms generally begin within 1 to 4 days of withdrawal and abate within 7 to 14 days.

4.9 Overdose

Overdosage may cause somnolence, or even coma, extrapyramidal symptoms, convulsions, hypotension, shock, hyper-or hypothermia. ECG changes, QT prolongation, Torsade de Pointes, cardiac arrest and ventricular arrhythmias have been reported when administered in overdose together with drugs known to affect the heart.

Treatment is symptomatic and supportive, with measures aimed at supporting the respiratory and cardiovascular systems. The following specific measures may be employed if required.

- anticholinergic antiparkinson drugs if extrapyramidal symptoms occur.

- sedation (with benzodiazepines) in the unlikely event of agitation or excitement or convulsions.

- noradrenaline in saline intravenous drip if the patient is in shock. Adrenaline must not be given.

5. PHARMACOLOGICAL PROPERTIES

5.1 Pharmacodynamic properties

Cis-(Z)-flupentixol is an antipsychotic of the thioxanthene series.

The antipsychotic effect of antipsychotics is related to their dopamine receptor blocking effect. The thioxanthenes have high affinity for both the adenylate cyclase coupled dopamine D_1 receptors and for the dopamine D_2 receptors; in the phenothiazine group the affinity for D_1 receptors is much lower than that for D_2 receptors, whereas butyrophenones, diphenylbutylpiperidines and benzamides only have affinity for D_2 receptors.

In the traditional tests for antipsychotic effect, eg. antagonism of stereotypic behaviour induced by dopamine agonists, the chemical groups of antipsychotics mentioned reveal equal but dosage-dependent activity. However, the antistereotypic effects of phenothiazines, butyrophenones, diphenylbutylpiperidines, and benzamides is strongly counteracted by the anticholinergic drug scopolamine, while the antistereotypic effect of thioxanthenes, eg cis-(Z)-flupentixol is not, or only very slightly, influenced by concomitant treatment with anticholinergics.

5.2 Pharmacokinetic properties

By esterification of cis-(Z)-flupentixol with decanoic acid cis-(Z)-flupentixol has been converted to a highly lipophilic substance, cis-(Z)-flupentixol decanoate. When dissolved in oil and injected intramuscularly this substance diffuses slowly into the surrounding body water, where enzymatic breakdown occurs releasing the active component cis(Z)-flupentixol. The duration of action is 2-4 weeks with maximum serum levels being reached by the end of the first week after injection.

Cis-(Z)-flupentixol is distributed in the body in a similar way to other antipsychotics; with the highest concentrations of drug and metabolites in liver, lungs, intestines and kidneys and lower concentrations in heart, spleen, brain and blood. The apparent volume of distribution is about 14 l/kg and the protein binding >95%.

Cis-(Z)-flupentixol crosses the placental barrier in small amounts; it is also excreted in breast milk in very small amounts.

The metabolism of cis-(Z)-flupentixol proceeds via three main routes - sulphoxidation, side chain N-dealkylation and glucuronic acid conjugation. The metabolites are devoid of psychopharmacological activity. The excretion proceeds mainly with the faeces but also to some degree with the urine. Systemic clearance is about 0.4-0.5 l/min.

5.3 Preclinical safety data

Nil of relevance

6. PHARMACEUTICAL PARTICULARS

6.1 List of excipients

Thin vegetable oil "Viscoleo" (fractionated coconut oil).

6.2 Incompatibilities

This product may be mixed in the same syringe with other products in the Depixol Injection range. It should not be mixed with any other injection fluids.

6.3 Shelf life

Ampoule 1 ml and 2 ml: 2 years

Vial 5 ml: 2 years

6.4 Special precautions for storage

Store below 25°C. Protect from light.

6.5 Nature and contents of container

Ampoules containing 1 ml and 2 ml of 200 mg/ml (20% w/v) cis-(Z)-flupentixol in thin vegetable oil. Pack size = 5 ampoules per box.

Vial containing 5 ml of 200 mg/ml (20%) cis-(Z)-flupentixol decanoate in thin vegetable oil. Pack size = 1 vial per box.

6.6 Special precautions for disposal and other handling

Nil

7. MARKETING AUTHORISATION HOLDER

Lundbeck Limited

Lundbeck House

Caldecotte Lake Business Park

Caldecotte

Milton Keynes

MK7 8LF

8. MARKETING AUTHORISATION NUMBER(S)

PL 0458/0065

9. DATE OF FIRST AUTHORISATION/RENEWAL OF THE AUTHORISATION

First Authorised: 23 October 1991

Renewed: 22 January 2002

10. DATE OF REVISION OF THE TEXT

28 January 2009

Legal category: POM

® Trademark

Depixol Injection is made by H Lundbeck A/S, Denmark

Depixol Tablets 3mg

(Lundbeck Limited)

1. NAME OF THE MEDICINAL PRODUCT

Depixol® Tablets 3 mg

2. QUALITATIVE AND QUANTITATIVE COMPOSITION

3.504 mg flupentixol dihydrochloride corresponding to 3 mg flupentixol base.

3. PHARMACEUTICAL FORM

Round, biconvex, yellow, sugar-coated tablets.

4. CLINICAL PARTICULARS

4.1 Therapeutic indications

The treatment of schizophrenia and other psychoses.

4.2 Posology and method of administration

Route of administration

Oral.

Adults

1 - 3 tablets twice daily to a maximum of 18 mg (6 tablets) per day. It is recommended that commencement of treatment and increase in dosage should be carried out under close supervision. As with all antipsychotic drugs, the dose of Depixol should be titrated to the needs of each patient.

When transferring patients from oral to depot antipsychotic treatment, the oral medication should not be discontinued immediately, but gradually withdrawn over a period of several days after administering the first injection.

Elderly

In accordance with standard medical practice, initial dosage may need to be reduced to a quarter or half the normal starting dose in the frail or elderly.

Children

Not indicated for children.

4.3 Contraindications

Hypersensitivity to the active substance or to any of the excipients (see section 6.1).

Circulatory collapse, depressed level of consciousness due to any cause (e.g. intoxication with alcohol, barbiturates or opiates), coma

Not recommended for excitable or agitated patients.

4.4 Special warnings and precautions for use

Caution should be exercised in patients having: liver disease; cardiac disease or arrhythmias; severe respiratory disease; renal failure; epilepsy (and conditions predisposing to epilepsy e.g. alcohol withdrawal or brain damage); Parkinson's disease; narrow angle glaucoma; prostatic hypertropy; hypothyroidism; hyperthyroidism; myasthenia gravis; phaeochromocytoma and patients who have shown hypersensitivity to thioxanthenes or other antipsychotics.

The elderly require close supervision because they are specially prone to experience such adverse effects as sedation, hypotension, confusion and temperature changes.

The possibility of development of neuroleptic malignant syndrome (hyperthermia, muscle rigidity, fluctuating consciousness, instability of the autonomous nervous system) exists with any neuroleptic. The risk is possibly greater with the more potent agents. Patients with pre-existing organic brain syndrome, mental retardation, and opiate and alcohol abuse are over-represented among fatal cases.

Treatment: Discontinuation of the neuroleptic. Symptomatic treatment and use of general supportive measures. Dantrolene and bromocriptine may be helpful.

Symptoms may persist for more than a week after oral neuroleptics are discontinued and somewhat longer when associated with the depot forms of the drugs.

Blood dyscrasias, including thrombocytopenia, have been reported rarely. Blood counts should be carried out if a patient develops signs of persistent infection.

As described for other psychotropics flupentixol may modify insulin and glucose responses calling for adjustment of the antidiabetic therapy in diabetic patients.

Acute withdrawal symptoms, including nausea, vomiting, sweating and insomnia have been described after abrupt cessation of antipsychotic drugs. Recurrence of psychotic symptoms may also occur, and the emergence of involuntary movement disorders (such as akathisia, dystonia and dyskinesia) has been reported. Therefore, gradual withdrawal is advisable.

When transferring patients from oral to depot antipsychotic treatment, the oral medication should not be discontinued immediately, but gradually withdrawn over a period of several days after administering the first injection.

An approximately 3-fold increased risk of cerebrovascular adverse events have been seen in randomised placebo controlled clinical trials in the dementia population with some atypical antipsychotics. The mechanism for this increased risk is not known. An increased risk cannot be excluded for other antipsychotics or other patient populations.

Flupentixol should be used with caution in patients with risk factors for stroke.

As with other drugs belonging to the therapeutic class of antipsychotics, flupentixol may cause QT prolongation. Persistently prolonged QT intervals may increase the risk of malignant arrhythmias. Therefore, flupentixol should be used with caution in susceptible individuals (with hypokalaemia, hypomagnesia or genetic predisposition) and in patients with a history of cardiovascular disorders, e.g. QT prolongation, significant bradycardia (<50 beats per minute), a recent acute myocardial infarction, uncompensated heart failure, or cardiac arrhythmia.

Concomitant treatment with other antipsychotics should be avoided (see section 4.5).

Suicide/suicidal thoughts or clinical worsening

Depression is associated with an increased risk of suicidal thoughts, self harm and suicide (suicide-related events). This risk persists until significant remission occurs. As improvement may not occur during the first few weeks or more of treatment, patients should be closely monitored until such improvement occurs. It is general clinical experience that the risk of suicide may increase in the early stages of recovery.

Other psychiatric conditions for which Flupentixol is prescribed can also be associated with an increased risk of suicide-related events. In addition, these conditions may be co-morbid with major depressive disorder. The same precautions observed when treating patients with major depressive disorder should therefore be observed when treating patients with other psychiatric disorders.

Patients with a history of suicide-related events, or those exhibiting a significant degree of suicidal ideation prior to commencement of treatment are known to be at greater risk of suicidal thoughts or suicide attempts, and should receive careful monitoring during treatment. A meta-analysis of placebo-controlled clinical trials of antidepressant drugs in adult patients with psychiatric disorders showed an increased risk of suicidal behaviour with antidepressants compared to placebo in patients less than 25 years old.

Close supervision of patients and in particular those at high risk should accompany drug therapy especially in early treatment and following dose changes. Patients (and caregivers of patients) should be alerted about the need to monitor for any clinical worsening, suicidal behaviour or thoughts and unusual changes in behaviour and to seek medical advice immediately if these symptoms present.

4.5 Interaction with other medicinal products and other forms of interaction

In common with other antipsychotics, flupentixol enhances the response to alcohol, the effects of barbiturates and other CNS depressants. Flupentixol may potentiate the effects of general anaesthetics and anticoagulants and prolong the action of neuromuscular blocking agents.

The anticholinergic effects of atropine or other drugs with anticholinergic properties may be increased. Concomitant use of drugs such as metoclopramide, piperazine or antiparkinson drugs may increase the risk of extrapyramidal effects such as tardive dyskinesia. Combined use of antipsychotics and lithium or sibutramine has been associated with an increased risk of neurotoxicity.

Antipsychotics may enhance the cardiac depressant effects of quinidine; the absorption of corticosteroids and digoxin. The hypotensive effect of vasodilator antihypertensive agents such as hydralazine and α-blockers (e.g. doxazosin), or methyl-dopa may be enhanced.

Increases in the QT interval related to antipsychotic treatment may be exacerbated by the co-administration of other drugs known to significantly increase the QT interval. Co-administration of such drugs should be avoided. Relevant classes include:

- class Ia and III antiarrhythmics (e.g. quinidine, amiodarone, sotalol, dofetilide)
- some antipsychotics (e.g. thioridazine)
- some macrolides (e.g. erythromycin)
- some antihistamines (e.g. terfenadine, astemizole)
- some quinolone antibiotics (e.g. gatifloxacin, moxifloxacin)

The above list is not exhaustive and other individual drugs known to significantly increase QT interval (e.g. cisapride, lithium) should be avoided.

Drugs known to cause electrolyte disturbances such as thiazide diuretics (hypokalaemia) and drugs known to increase the plasma concentration of flupentixol should also be used with caution as they may increase the risk of QT prolongation and malignant arrythmias (see section 4.4).

Antipsychotics may antagonise the effects of adrenaline and other sympathomimetic agents, and reverse the antihypertensive effects of guanethidine and similar adrenergic-blocking agents. Antipsychotics may also impair the effect of levodopa, adrenergic drugs and anticonvulsants.

The metabolism of tricyclic antidepressants may be inhibited and the control of diabetes may be impaired.

4.6 Pregnancy and lactation

As the safety of this drug during pregnancy has not been established, use during pregnancy, especially the first and last trimesters, should be avoided, unless the expected benefit to the patient outweighs the potential risk to the foetus.

Flupentixol is excreted into the breast milk. If the use of Depixol is considered essential, nursing mothers should be advised to stop breast feeding.

The newborn of mothers treated with antipsychotics in late pregnancy, or labour, may show signs of intoxication such as lethargy, tremor and hyperexcitability, and have a low apgar score.

4.7 Effects on ability to drive and use machines

Alertness may be impaired, especially at the start of treatment, or following the consumption of alcohol; patients should be warned of this risk and advised not to drive or operate machinery until their susceptibility is known. Patients should not drive if they have blurred vision.

4.8 Undesirable effects

Cases of suicidal ideation and suicidal behaviours have been reported during Flupentixol therapy or early after treatment discontinuation (see section 4.4).

Undesirable effects are for the majority dose dependent. The frequency and severity are most pronounced in the early phase of treatment and decline during continued treatment.

Extrapyramidal reactions may occur, especially in the early phase of treatment. In most cases these side effects can be satisfactorily controlled by reduction of dosage and/or use of antiparkinson drugs. The routine prophylactic use of antiparkinson drugs is not recommended. Antiparkinson drugs do not alleviate tardive dyskinesia and may aggravate them. Reduction in dosage or, if possible, discontinuation of zuclopenthixol therapy is recommended. In persistent akathisia a benzodiazepine or propranolol may be useful.

Cardiac disorders	Tachycardia, palpitations. Electrocardiogram QT prolonged.
Blood and lymphatic system disorders	Thrombocytopenia, neutropenia, leukopenia, agranulocytosis
Nervous system disorders	Somnolence, akathisia, hyperkinesia, hypokinesia. Tremor, dystonia, dizziness, headache, disturbance in attention. Tardive dyskinesia, dyskinesia, parkinsonism, speech disorder, convulsion. Neuroleptic malignant syndrome.
Eye disorders	Accommodation disorder, vision abnormal. Oculogyration.
Respiratory, thoracic and mediastinal disorders	Dyspnoea.
Gastrointestinal disorders	Dry mouth. Salivary hypersecretion, constipation, vomiting, dyspepsia, diarrhoea. Abdominal pain, nausea, flatulence.
Renal and urinary disorders	Micturition disorder, urinary retention.
Skin and subcutaneous tissue disorders	Hyperhidrosis, pruritus. Rash, photosensitivity reaction, dermatitis.
Musculoskeletal and connective tissue disorder	Myalgia. Muscle rigidity.
Endocrine disorder	Hyperprolactinaemia.
Metabolism and nutrition disorders	Increased appetite, weight increased. Decreased appetite. Hyperglycaemia, glucose tolerance abnormal.
Vascular disorders	Hypotension, hot flush.
General disorders and administration site conditions	Asthenia, fatigue.
Immune system disorders	Hypersensitivity, anaphylactic reaction.
Hepatobiliary disorders	Liver function test abnormal. Jaundice.
Reproductive system and breast disorders	Ejaculation failure, erectile dysfunction. Gynaecomastia, galactorrhoea, amenorrhoea.
Psychiatric disorders	Insomnia, depression, nervousness, agitation, libido decreased. Confusional state.

As with other drugs belonging to the therapeutic class of antipsychotics, rare cases of QT prolongation, ventricular arrhythmias - ventricular fibrillation, ventricular tachycardia, Torsade de Pointes and sudden unexplained death have been reported for flupentixol (see section 4.4).

Abrupt discontinuation of flupentixol may be accompanied by withdrawal symptoms. The most common symptoms are nausea, vomiting, anorexia, diarrhoea, rhinorrhoea, sweating, myalgias, paraesthesias, insomnia, restlessness, anxiety, and agitation. Patients may also experience vertigo, alternate feelings of warmth and coldness, and tremor. Symptoms generally begin within 1 to 4 days of withdrawal and abate within 7 to 14 days.

4.9 Overdose

Overdosage may cause somnolence, or even coma, extrapyramidal symptoms, convulsions, hypotension, shock, hyper-or hypothermia. ECG changes, QT prolongation, Torsade de Pointes, cardiac arrest and ventricular arrhythmias have been reported when administered in overdose together with drugs known to affect the heart.

Treatment is symptomatic and supportive, with measures aimed at supporting the respiratory and cardiovascular systems. The following specific measures may be employed if required.

- anticholinergic antiparkinson drugs if extrapyramidal symptoms occur.

- sedation (with benzodiazepines) in the unlikely event of agitation or excitement or convulsions.

- noradrenaline in saline intravenous drip if the patient is in shock. Adrenaline must not be given.

- ingestion of activated charcoal and gastric lavage should be considered.

5. PHARMACOLOGICAL PROPERTIES

5.1 Pharmacodynamic properties

Flupentixol is an antipsychotic of the thioxanthene series.

The antipsychotic effect of antipsychotics is believed to be related to their dopamine receptor blocking effect. The thioxanthenes have high affinity for D_1 and D_2 receptors.

5.2 Pharmacokinetic properties

Oral administration to volunteers (8 mg single dose and 1.5 mg/day) and patients (5-60 mg/d) resulted in serum drug concentration curves with a maximum around four hours after administration. Mean biological half-life was about 35 hours in patients. No difference was seen in patients between half-lives estimated after single-dose administration and those estimated after repeated administration. Mean oral bioavailability of flupentixol varied between 40% and 55%.

5.3 Preclinical safety data

Nil of relevance

6. PHARMACEUTICAL PARTICULARS

6.1 List of excipients

Potato starch, lactose, gelatin, talc, magnesium stearate, sucrose and yellow iron oxide (E172).

6.2 Incompatibilities

Not applicable.

6.3 Shelf life

Depixol tablets are stable for 2 years. Each container has an expiry date.

6.4 Special precautions for storage

Store in original container, protected from light and moisture. Do not store above 25°C.

6.5 Nature and contents of container

Grey polypropylene container with screw cap or glass bottles with white plastic stoppers. Contents 100 tablets.

6.6 Special precautions for disposal and other handling

Nil

7. MARKETING AUTHORISATION HOLDER

Lundbeck Limited
Lundbeck House
Caldecotte Lake Business Park
Caldecotte
Milton Keynes
MK7 8LF

8. MARKETING AUTHORISATION NUMBER(S)

PL 0458/0013R

9. DATE OF FIRST AUTHORISATION/RENEWAL OF THE AUTHORISATION

First Authorised 29 January 1987

Renewed 17 March 2002

10. DATE OF REVISION OF THE TEXT

20 November 2008

Legal Category: POM

® Trademark

Depixol is made by H Lundbeck A/S, Denmark

DepoCyte 50 mg suspension for injection

(Napp Pharmaceuticals Limited)

1. NAME OF THE MEDICINAL PRODUCT

DepoCyte® 50 mg suspension for injection

2. QUALITATIVE AND QUANTITATIVE COMPOSITION

Each 5ml vial contains 50 mg cytarabine (10mg/ml).

For a full list of excipients, see section 6.1.

Table 1: Adverse events possibly reflecting meningeal irritation in Phase II, III, and IV patients (n [%] of cycles* of therapy)

MedDRA preferred term	**DepoCyte** (n = 929 cycles)	Methotrexate (n = 258 cycles)	Cytarabine (n = 99 cycles)
Headache NOS	24%	16%	14%
Nausea	18%	12%	15%
Vomiting NOS	17%	11%	11%
Arachnoiditis	16%	7%	13%
Pyrexia	12%	7%	16%
Back Pain	7%	7%	6%
Convulsions NOS	6%	5%	2%
Neck pain	4%	3%	3%
Neck stiffness	3%	<1%	4%
Hydrocephalus acquired	2%	1%	0%
CSF Pleocytosis	1%	0%	0%
Meningism	<1%	1%	1%

* Cycle length was 2 weeks during which the patient received either 1 dose of **DepoCyte** or 4 doses of cytarabine or methotrexate. Cytarabine and methotrexate patients not completing all 4 doses are counted as a fraction of a cycle.

3. PHARMACEUTICAL FORM

A white to off-white suspension for injection.

4. CLINICAL PARTICULARS

4.1 Therapeutic indications

Intrathecal treatment of lymphomatous meningitis. In the majority of patients such treatment will be part of symptomatic palliation of the disease.

4.2 Posology and method of administration

DepoCyte should be administered only under the supervision of a physician experienced in the use of cancer chemotherapeutic agents

Adults and the elderly

For the treatment of lymphomatous meningitis, the dose for adults is 50 mg (one vial) administered intrathecally (lumbar puncture or intraventricularly via an Ommaya reservoir). The following regimen of induction, consolidation and maintenance therapy is recommended:

Induction therapy: 50 mg administered every 14 days for 2 doses (weeks 1 and 3).

Consolidation therapy: 50 mg administered every 14 days for 3 doses (weeks 5, 7 and 9) followed by an additional dose of 50 mg at week 13.

Maintenance therapy: 50 mg administered every 28 days for 4 doses (weeks 17, 21, 25 and 29).

Method of administration: ***DepoCyte*** is to be administered by slow injection over a period of 1-5 minutes directly into the cerebrospinal fluid (CSF) via either an intraventricular reservoir or by direct injection into the lumbar sac. Following administration by lumbar puncture, it is recommended that the patient should be instructed to lie flat for one hour. Patients should be started on dexamethasone 4 mg twice daily orally or intravenously for 5 days beginning on the day of injection of ***DepoCyte***.

DepoCyte must not be administered by any other route of administration.

DepoCyte must be used as supplied; do not dilute (see also Section 6.2).

Patients should be observed by the physician for immediate toxic reactions.

If neurotoxicity develops the dose should be reduced to 25 mg. If it persists, treatment with ***DepoCyte*** should be discontinued.

Children and adolescents

Safety and efficacy in children have not been adequately demonstrated (see section 5.1). ***Depocyte*** is not recommended for use in children and adolescents until further data become available.

4.3 Contraindications

Hypersensitivity to the active substance or any of the excipients.

Patients with active meningeal infection.

4.4 Special warnings and precautions for use

Patients receiving ***DepoCyte*** should be concurrently treated with corticosteroids (e.g. dexamethasone) to mitigate the symptoms of arachnoiditis (see section 4.8) which is a common adverse event.

Arachnoiditis is a syndrome manifested primarily by nausea, vomiting, headache and fever. If left untreated, chemical arachnoiditis may be fatal.

Patients should be informed about the expected adverse reactions of headache, nausea, vomiting and fever, and about the early signs and symptoms of neurotoxicity. The importance of concurrent dexamethasone administration should be emphasised at the initiation of each cycle of ***DepoCyte*** treatment. Patients should be instructed to seek medical attention if signs or symptoms of neurotoxicity develop, or if oral dexamethasone is not well tolerated.

Cytarabine, when administered intrathecally, has been associated with nausea, vomiting and serious central nervous system toxicity which can lead to a permanent deficit, this includes blindness, myelopathy and other neurological toxicity.

Administration of ***DepoCyte*** in combination with other neurotoxic chemotherapeutic agents or with cranial/spinal irradiation may increase the risk of neurotoxicity.

Infectious meningitis may be associated with intrathecal administration. Hydrocephalus has also been reported, possibly precipitated by arachnoiditis.

Blockage of CSF flow may result in increased free cytarabine concentrations in the CSF with increased risk of neurotoxicity.

Although significant systemic exposure to free cytarabine is not expected following intrathecal treatment, some effects on bone marrow function cannot be excluded. Systemic toxicity due to intravenous administration of cytarabine consists primarily of bone marrow suppression with leucopenia, thrombocytopenia and anaemia. Therefore monitoring of the haemopoietic system is advised.

Anaphylactic reactions following intravenous administration of free cytarabine have been rarely reported.

Since ***DepoCyte's*** particles are similar in size and appearance to white blood cells, care must be taken in interpreting CSF examination following ***DepoCyte*** administration.

4.5 Interaction with other medicinal products and other forms of interaction

No definite interactions between ***DepoCyte*** delivered intrathecally and other drugs have been established.

Concomitant administration of ***DepoCyte*** with other antineoplastic agents administered by the intrathecal route has not been studied.

Intrathecal co-administration of cytarabine with other cytotoxic agents may increase the risk of neurotoxicity.

4.6 Pregnancy and lactation

Teratology studies in animals have not been conducted with ***DepoCyte*** and there are no adequate and well controlled studies in pregnant women; however cytarabine can cause foetal harm when administered during pregnancy. Therefore, women of childbearing potential should not receive the treatment until pregnancy is excluded and should be advised to use a reliable contraceptive method.

Given that cytarabine has a mutagenic potential which could induce chromosomal damage in the human spermatozoa, males undergoing ***DepoCyte*** treatment and their partner should be advised to use a reliable contraceptive method.

It is not known whether cytarabine is excreted in human milk following intrathecal administration. The systemic exposure to free cytarabine following intrathecal treatment with ***DepoCyte*** was negligible. Because of possible excretion in human milk and because of the potential for serious adverse reactions in nursing infants, the use of ***DepoCyte*** is not recommended in breast-feeding women.

4.7 Effects on ability to drive and use machines

There have been no reports explicitly relating to effects of ***DepoCyte*** treatment on the ability to drive or use machines. However, on the basis of reported adverse reactions, patients should be advised against driving or using machines during treatment.

4.8 Undesirable effects

DepoCyte has the potential of producing serious toxicity. All patients receiving ***DepoCyte*** should be treated concurrently with corticosteroids (e.g., dexamethasone) to mitigate the symptoms of arachnoiditis. Toxic effects may be related to a single dose or to cumulative doses. Because toxic effects can occur at any time during therapy (although they are most likely within 5 days of administration), patients receiving ***DepoCyte*** therapy should be monitored continuously for the development of neurotoxicity. If patients develop neurotoxicity, subsequent doses of ***DepoCyte*** should be reduced, and ***DepoCyte*** should be discontinued if toxicity persists.

Arachnoiditis, a syndrome manifested primarily by headache, nausea, vomiting, fever, neck rigidity, neck or back pain, meningism, convulsions, hydrocephalus, CSF pleocytosis, with or without altered state of consciousness, is a common adverse event. Arachnoiditis can be fatal if left untreated.

The incidence of adverse reactions possibly reflecting meningeal irritation determined from all the patients treated with 50 mg **DepoCyte** in the Phase II-IV clinical trials is given in Table 1 below:

(see Table 1 opposite)

The incidence of all adverse reactions occurring in > 10 % of cycles in either treatment group in Phase 1-4 studies in patients with lymphomatous meningitis receiving **DepoCyte** or cytarabine is given in Table 2 below:

Table 2: Adverse reactions occurring in > 10% of cycles in either treatment group in Phase 1 – 4 study patients with lymphomatous meningitis receiving DepoCyte 50mg or cytarabine (% of cycles* of therapy)

	Number of cycles	
System Organ Class MedDRA Preferred Term	DepoCyte (n=151 cycles)	Cytarabine (n=99 cycles)
Nervous System Disorders		
Headache NOS	23%	14%
Arachnoiditis	16%	13%
Confusion	11%	3%
Gastrointestinal Disorders		
Nausea	13%	15%
Vomiting NOS	12%	11%
Diarrhoea NOS	11%	10%
General Disorders and Administrative Site Conditions		
Weakness	13%	17%
Pyrexia	14%	16%
Fatigue	6%	14%
Blood and Lymphatic System Disorders		
Thrombocytopenia	10%	13%

* Induction and Maintenance cycle lengths were 2 and 4 weeks, respectively, during which the patient received either 1 dose of **DepoCyte** or 4 doses of cytarabine. Cytarabine patients not completing all 4 doses within a cycle are counted as a complete cycle.

Intrathecal administration of cytarabine may cause myelopathy and other neurologic toxicity sometimes leading to a permanent neurological deficit. Following intrathecal administration of **DepoCyte**, serious central nervous system toxicity, including persistent extreme somnolence, confusion, hemiplegia, visual disturbances including blindness, deafness and cranial nerve palsies have been reported. Symptoms and signs of peripheral neuropathy, such as pain, numbness, paresthesia, hypoaesthesia, weakness, and impaired bowel and bladder control (incontinence) have also been observed.

Adverse reactions more commonly associated with **DepoCyte** are headache, arachnoiditis and confusion. In addition, in Phase 1 – 4 studies, the patient incidence of convulsions was higher in the **DepoCyte** group (7/33, 21%) than in the cytarabine group (1/28, 4%).

Transient elevations in CSF protein and white blood cells have also been observed in patients following ***DepoCyte*** administration and also been noted after intrathecal treatment with methotrexate or cytarabine.

4.9 Overdose

No overdosages with ***DepoCyte*** have been reported. An overdose with ***DepoCyte*** may be associated with severe arachnoiditis including encephalopathy.

In an early uncontrolled study without dexamethasone prophylaxis, single doses up to 125 mg were administered. One patient at the 125 mg dose level died of encephalopathy 36 hours after receiving ***DepoCyte*** intraventricularly. This patient, however, was also receiving concomitant whole brain irradiation and had previously received intraventricular methotrexate.

There is no antidote for intrathecal ***DepoCyte*** or unencapsulated cytarabine released from ***DepoCyte***. Exchange of cerebrospinal fluid with isotonic saline has been carried out in a case of intrathecal overdose of free cytarabine and such a procedure may be considered in the case of ***DepoCyte*** overdose. Management of overdose should be directed at maintaining vital functions.

5. PHARMACOLOGICAL PROPERTIES

5.1 Pharmacodynamic properties

Pharmacotherapeutic group: Antimetabolite (pyrimidine analogue). ATC code L01B C01

DepoCyte is a sustained-release formulation of cytarabine, designed for direct administration into the cerebrospinal fluid (CSF).

Cytarabine is a cell-cycle phase specific antineoplastic agent, affecting cells only during the S-phase of cell division. Intracellularly, cytarabine is converted into cytarabine-5'-triphosphate (ara-CTP), which is the active metabolite. The mechanism of action is not completely understood, but it appears that ara-CTP acts primarily through inhibition of DNA synthesis. Incorporation into DNA and RNA may also contribute to cytarabine cytotoxicity. Cytarabine is cytotoxic to a wide variety of proliferating mammalian cells in culture.

For cell-cycle phase specific antimetabolites the duration of exposure of neoplastic cells to cytotoxic concentrations is an important determination of drug efficacy.

In vitro studies, examining more than 60 cell lines, demonstrated that the median cytarabine concentration resulting in 50% growth inhibition (IC_{50}) was approximately 10 μM (2.4 μg/ml) for two days of exposure and 0.1 μM (0.024 μg/ml) for 6 days of exposure. The studies also demonstrated susceptibility of many solid tumour cell lines to cytarabine, particularly after longer periods of exposure to cytarabine.

In an open-label, active-controlled, multicentre clinical study, 35 patients with lymphomatous meningitis (with malignant cells found on CSF cytology) were randomised to intrathecal therapy with either ***DepoCyte*** (n=18) or unencapsulated cytarabine (n=17). During the 1 month Induction phase of treatment, ***DepoCyte*** was administered intrathecally as 50 mg every 2 weeks, and unencapsulated cytarabine as 50 mg twice a week. Patients who did not respond discontinued protocol treatment after 4 weeks. Patients who achieved a response (defined as clearing of the CSF of malignant cells in the absence of progression of neurological symptoms) went on to receive Consolidation and Maintenance therapy for up to 29 weeks.

Responses were observed in 13/18 (72%, 95% confidence intervals: 47, 90) of ***DepoCyte*** patients versus 3/17 (18% patients, 95% confidence intervals: 4, 43) in the unencapsulated cytarabine arm. A statistically significant association between treatment and response was observed (Fisher's exact test p-value = 0.002). The majority of ***DepoCyte*** patients went on beyond Induction to receive additional therapy. ***DepoCyte*** patients received a median of 5 cycles (doses) per patient (range 1 to 10 doses) with a median time on therapy of 90 days (range 1 to 207 days).

No statistically significant differences were noted in secondary endpoints such as duration of response, progression-free survival, neurological signs and symptoms, Karnofsky performance status, quality of life and overall survival. Median progression-free survival (defined as time to neurological progression or death) for all treated patients was 77 versus 48 days for ***DepoCyte*** versus unencapsulated cytarabine, respectively. The proportion of patients alive at 12 months was 24% for ***DepoCyte*** versus 19% for unencapsulated cytarabine.

In an open-label non-comparative dose escalation study in 18 paediatric patients (4 to 19 years) with leukaemic meningitis or neoplastic meningitis due to primary brain tumour, an intrathecal dose of 35 mg was identified as the maximum tolerated dose.

5.2 Pharmacokinetic properties

Analysis of the available pharmacokinetic data shows that following intrathecal ***DepoCyte*** administration in patients, either via the lumbar sac or by intraventricular reservoir, peaks of free cytarabine were observed within 5 hours in both the ventricle and lumbar sac. These peaks were followed by a biphasic elimination profile consisting of an initial sharp decline and subsequent slow decline with a terminal phase half-life of 100 to 263 hours over a dose-range of 12.5 mg to 75 mg. In contrast, intrathecal administration of 30 mg free cytarabine has shown a biphasic CSF concentration profile with a terminal phase half-life of about 3.4 hours.

Pharmacokinetic parameters of ***DepoCyte*** (75 mg) in neoplastic meningitis patients in whom the drug was administered either intraventricularly or by lumbar puncture suggest that exposure to the drug in the ventricular or lumbar spaces is similar regardless of the route of administration. In addition, compared with free cytarabine, the formulation increases the biological half-life by a factor of 27 to 71 depending upon the route of administration and the compartment sampled. Encapsulated cytarabine concentrations and the counts of the lipid particles in which the cytarabine is encapsulated in ***DepoCyte*** followed a similar distribution pattern. AUCs of free and encapsulated cytarabine after ventricular injection of ***DepoCyte*** appeared to increase linearly with increasing dose, indicating that the release of cytarabine from ***DepoCyte*** and the pharmacokinetics of cytarabine are linear in human CSF.

The transfer rate of cytarabine from CSF to plasma is slow and the conversion to uracil arabinoside (ara-U), the inactive metabolite, in the plasma is fast. Systemic exposure to cytarabine was determined to be negligible following intrathecal administration of 50 mg and 75 mg of ***DepoCyte***.

Metabolism and Elimination

The primary route of elimination of cytarabine is metabolism to the inactive compound ara-U, (1-β-D-arabinofuranosyluracil or uracil arabinoside) followed by urinary excretion of ara-U. In contrast with systemically administered cytarabine which is rapidly metabolised to ara-U, conversion to ara-U in the CSF is negligible after intrathecal administration because of the significantly lower cytidine deaminase activity in the CNS tissues and CSF. The CSF clearance rate of cytarabine is similar to the CSF bulk flow rate of 0.24 ml/min.

The distribution and clearance of cytarabine and of the predominant phospholipid component of the lipid particle (DOPC) following intrathecal administration of ***DepoCyte*** was evaluated in rodents. Radiolabels for cytarabine and DOPC were distributed rapidly throughout the neuraxis. More than 90% of cytarabine was excreted by day 4 and an additional 2.7% by 21 days. The results suggest that the lipid components undergo hydrolysis and are largely incorporated in the tissues following breakdown in the intrathecal space.

5.3 Preclinical safety data

A review of the toxicological data available for the constituent lipids (DOPC and DPPG) or similar phospholipids to those in ***DepoCyte*** indicates that such lipids are well tolerated in various animal species even when administered for prolonged periods at doses in the g/kg range.

The results of acute and subacute toxicity studies performed in monkeys suggested that intrathecal ***DepoCyte*** was tolerated up to a dose of 10 mg (comparable to a human dose of 100 mg). Slight to moderate inflammation of the meninges in the spinal cord and brain and/or astrocytic activation were observed in animals receiving intrathecal ***DepoCyte***. These changes were believed to be consistent with the toxic effects of other intrathecal agents such as unencapsulated cytarabine. Similar changes (generally described as minimal to slight) were also observed in some animals receiving DepoFoam alone (***DepoCyte*** vesicles without cytarabine) but not in saline control animals. Mouse, rat and dog studies have shown that free cytarabine is highly toxic for the haemopoietic system.

No carcinogenicity, mutagenicity or impairment of fertility studies have been conducted with ***DepoCyte***. The active ingredient of ***DepoCyte***, cytarabine, was mutagenic in *in vitro* tests and was clastogenic *in vitro* (chromosome aberrations and sister chromatid exchange in human leukocytes) and *in vivo* (chromosome aberrations and sister chromatid exchange assay in rodent bone marrow, mouse micronucleus assay). Cytarabine caused the transformation of hamster embryo cells and rat H43 cells *in vitro*. Cytarabine was clastogenic to meiotic cells; a dose-dependent increase in sperm-head abnormalities and chromosomal aberrations occurred in mice given i.p. cytarabine. No studies assessing the impact of cytarabine on fertility are available in the literature. Because the systemic exposure to free cytarabine following intrathecal treatment with ***DepoCyte*** was negligible, the risk of impaired fertility is likely to be low.

6. PHARMACEUTICAL PARTICULARS

6.1 List of excipients

Cholesterol

Triolein,

Dioleylphosphatidylcholine (DOPC),

Dipalmitoylphosphatidylglycerol (DPPG),

Sodium chloride,

Water for injections.

6.2 Incompatibilities

No formal assessments of pharmacokinetic drug-drug interactions between ***DepoCyte*** and other agents have been conducted. ***DepoCyte*** should not be diluted or mixed with any other medicinal products, as any change in concentration or pH may affect the stability of the microparticles.

6.3 Shelf life

18 months

6.4 Special precautions for storage

Store at 2°C - 8°C (in a refrigerator).

Do not freeze.

6.5 Nature and contents of container

DepoCyte is supplied in individual cartons each containing one single-dose Type I glass vial containing 50 mg (in 5ml), closed with a fluororesin faced butyl rubber stopper and sealed with an aluminium flip-off seal.

6.6 Special precautions for disposal and other handling

Preparation of ***DepoCyte***

Given its toxic nature, special precautions should be taken in handling ***DepoCyte***. See 'Precautions for the handling and disposal of ***DepoCyte***' below.

Vials of ***DepoCyte*** should be allowed to warm to room temperature (18°C -22°C) for a minimum of 30 minutes and be gently inverted to resuspend the particles immediately prior to withdrawal from the vial. Avoid vigorous shaking. No further reconstitution or dilution is required.

DepoCyte administration

DepoCyte must only be administered by the intrathecal route

DepoCyte should be withdrawn from the vial immediately before administration. Since it is a single use vial and does not contain any preservative, the drug should be used within 4 hours of withdrawal from the vial. Unused drug must be discarded and not used subsequently. Do not mix ***DepoCyte*** with any other medicinal products (see Section 6.2). Do not dilute the suspension.

In-line filters must not be used when administering ***DepoCyte***. ***DepoCyte*** is administered directly into the CSF via an intraventricular reservoir or by direct injection into the lumbar sac. ***DepoCyte*** should be injected slowly over a period of 1-5 minutes. Following drug administration by lumbar puncture, the patient should be instructed to lie flat for one hour. Patients should be observed by the physician for immediate toxic reactions.

Patients should be started on corticosteroids (e.g. dexamethasone 4 mg twice daily either orally or intravenously) for 5 days beginning on the day of ***DepoCyte*** injection.

Precautions for the handling and disposal of ***DepoCyte***

The following protective recommendations are given due to the toxic nature of this substance:

- personnel should be trained in good technique for handling anticancer agents
- male and female staff who are trying to conceive and female staff who are pregnant should be excluded from working with the substance
- personnel must wear protective clothing: goggles, gowns, disposable gloves and masks
- a designated area should be defined for preparation (preferably under a laminar flow system). The work surface should be protected by disposable, plastic backed, absorbent paper
- all items used during administration or cleaning, should be placed in high risk, waste-disposal bags for high temperature incineration
- in the event of accidental contact with the skin, exposed areas should be washed immediately with soap and water
- in the event of accidental contact with the mucous membranes, exposed areas should be treated immediately by copious lavage with water; medical attention should be sought.

7. MARKETING AUTHORISATION HOLDER

Pacira Ltd

West Forest Gate

Wellington Road

Wokingham

Berkshire

RG40 2AQ

United Kingdom

8. MARKETING AUTHORISATION NUMBER(S)

EU/1/01/187/001

9. DATE OF FIRST AUTHORISATION/RENEWAL OF THE AUTHORISATION

Date of first authorisation: 11 July 2001

Date of last renewal: 11 July 2006

10. DATE OF REVISION OF THE TEXT

28 May 2009

11. LEGAL CATEGORY

POM

® The Napp device and ***DepoCyte*** are Registered Trade Marks.

Depo-Medrone 40mg/ml

(Pharmacia Limited)

1. NAME OF THE MEDICINAL PRODUCT

Depo-Medrone 40 mg/ml.

2. QUALITATIVE AND QUANTITATIVE COMPOSITION
Methylprednisolone Acetate BP 40 mg/ml.

3. PHARMACEUTICAL FORM
Sterile, aqueous suspension.

4. CLINICAL PARTICULARS

4.1 Therapeutic indications
Depo-Medrone may be used locally or systemically, particularly where oral therapy is not feasible.

Depo-Medrone may be used by any of the following routes: intramuscular, intra-articular, periarticular, intrabursal, intralesional or into the tendon sheath. It must not be used by the intrathecal or intravenous routes (see Contra-indications and Undesirable effects).

Intramuscular administration:

1. Rheumatic disorders

Rheumatoid arthritis

2. Collagen diseases/arteritis

Systemic lupus erythematosus

3. Dermatological diseases

Severe erythema multiforme (Stevens-Johnson syndrome)

4. Allergic states

Bronchial asthma

Severe seasonal and perennial allergic rhinitis

Drug hypersensitivity reactions

Angioneurotic oedema

5. Gastro-intestinal diseases

Ulcerative colitis

Crohn's disease

6. Respiratory diseases

Fulminating or disseminated tuberculosis (with appropriate antituberculous chemotherapy)

Aspiration of gastric contents

7. Miscellaneous

TB meningitis (with appropriate antituberculous chemotherapy)

Intra-articular administration:

Rheumatoid arthritis

Osteo-arthritis with an inflammatory component

Soft tissue administration (intrabursal, periarticular, into tendon sheath):

Synovitis not associated with infection

Epicondylitis

Tenosynovitis

Plantar fasciitis

Bursitis

Intralesional:

Keloids

Localized lichen planus

Localized lichen simplex

Granuloma annulare

Discoid lupus erythematosus

Alopecia areata

4.2 Posology and method of administration
Depo-Medrone should not be mixed with any other suspending agent or solution. Parenteral drug products should be inspected visually for particulate matter and discoloration prior to administration, whenever suspension and container permit. Depo-Medrone may be used by any of the following routes: intramuscular, intra-articular, periarticular, intrabursal, intralesional and into the tendon sheath. It must not be used by the intrathecal or intravenous routes (see Contra-indications and Undesirable effects).

Undesirable effects may be minimised by using the lowest effective dose for the minimum period (see Special warnings and special precautions for use).

Depo-Medrone vials are intended for single dose use only.

Intramuscular - for sustained systemic effect: Allergic conditions (severe seasonal and perennial allergic rhinitis, asthma, drug reactions), 80 - 120 mg (2 - 3 ml).

Dermatological conditions, 40 - 120 mg (1 - 3 ml).

Rheumatic disorders and collagen diseases (rheumatoid arthritis, SLE), 40 - 120 mg (1 - 3 ml) per week.

Dosage must be individualized and depends on the condition being treated and its severity.

Note: Depo-Medrone is not intended for the prophylaxis of severe seasonal and perennial allergic rhinitis or other seasonal allergies and should be administered only when symptoms are present.

The frequency of intramuscular injections should be determined by the duration of clinical response.

In the case of seasonal allergic rhinitis a single injection is frequently sufficient. If necessary, however, a second injection may be given after two to three weeks.

On average the effect of a single 2 ml (80 mg) injection may be expected to last approximately two weeks.

Intra-articular: Rheumatoid arthritis, osteo-arthritis. The dose of Depo-Medrone depends upon the size of the joint and the severity of the condition. Repeated injections, if needed, may be given at intervals of one to five or more weeks depending upon the degree of relief obtained from the initial injection. A suggested dosage guide is: large joint (knee, ankle, shoulder), 20 - 80 mg (0.5 - 2 ml); medium joint (elbow, wrist), 10 - 40 mg (0.25 - 1 ml); small joint (metacarpophalangeal, interphalangeal, sternoclavicular, acromioclavicular), 4 - 10 mg (0.1 - 0.25 ml).

Intrabursal: Subdeltoid bursitis, prepatellar bursitis, olecranon bursitis. For administration directly into bursae, 4 - 30 mg (0.1 - 0.75 ml). In most cases, repeat injections are not needed.

Intralesional: Keloids, localised lichen planus, localized lichen simplex, granuloma annulare, alopecia areata, and discoid lupus erythematosus. For administration directly into the lesion for local effect in dermatological conditions, 20 - 60 mg (0.5 - 1.5 ml). For large lesions, the dose may be distributed by repeated local injections of 20 - 40 mg (0.5 - 1 ml). One to four injections are usually employed. Care should be taken to avoid injection of sufficient material to cause blanching, since this may be followed by a small slough.

Peri-articular: Epicondylitis. Infiltrate 4 - 30 mg (0.1 - 0.75 ml) into the affected area.

Into the tendon sheath: Tenosynovitis, epicondylitis. For administration directly into the tendon sheath, 4 - 30 mg (0.1 - 0.75 ml). In recurrent or chronic conditions, repeat injections may be necessary.

Special precautions should be observed when administering Depo-Medrone. Intramuscular injections should be made deeply into the gluteal muscles. The usual technique of aspirating prior to injection should be employed to avoid intravascular administration. Doses recommended for intramuscular injection must not be administered superficially or subcutaneously.

Intra-articular injections should be made using precise, anatomical localisation into the synovial space of the joint involved. The injection site for each joint is determined by that location where the synovial cavity is most superficial and most free of large vessels and nerves. Suitable sites for intra-articular injection are the knee, ankle, wrist, elbow, shoulder, phalangeal and hip joints. The spinal joints, unstable joints and those devoid of synovial space are not suitable. Treatment failures are most frequently the result of failure to enter the joint space. Intra-articular injections should be made with care as follows: ensure correct positioning of the needle into the synovial space and aspirate a few drops of joint fluid. The aspirating syringe should then be replaced by another containing Depo-Medrone. To ensure position of the needle, synovial fluid should be aspirated and the injection made. After injection the joint is moved slightly to aid mixing of the synovial fluid and the suspension. Subsequent to therapy care should be taken for the patient not to overuse the joint in which benefit has been obtained. Negligence in this matter may permit an increase in joint deterioration that will more than offset the beneficial effects of the steroid.

Intrabursal injections should be made as follows: the area around the injection site is prepared in a sterile way and a wheal at the site made with 1 per cent procaine hydrochloride solution. A 20 to 24 gauge needle attached to a dry syringe is inserted into the bursa and the fluid aspirated. The needle is left in place and the aspirating syringe changed for a small syringe containing the desired dose. After injection, the needle is withdrawn and a small dressing applied. In the treatment of tenosynovitis care should be taken to inject Depo-Medrone into the tendon sheath rather than into the substance of the tendon. Due to the absence of a true tendon sheath, the Achilles tendon should not be injected with Depo-Medrone.

Children: Dosage may be reduced for infants and children but should be governed more by the severity of the condition and response of the patient, than by age or size.

Elderly patients: When used according to instructions, there is no information to suggest that a change in dosage is warranted in the elderly. However, treatment of elderly patients, particularly if long-term, should be planned bearing in mind the more serious consequences of the common side-effects of corticosteroids in old age and close clinical supervision is required (see Special warnings and special precautions for use).

4.3 Contraindications
Depo-medrone is contra-indicated where there is known hypersensitivity to components and in systemic infection unless specific anti-infective therapy is employed.

Due to its potential for neurotoxicity, Depo-Medrone must not be given by the intrathecal route. In addition, as the product is a suspension it must not be given by the intravenous route (see Undesirable effects).

4.4 Special warnings and precautions for use
Warnings and Precautions:

1. A Patient Information Leaflet is provided in the pack by the manufacturer.

2. Undesirable effects may be minimised by using the lowest effective dose for the minimum period. Frequent patient review is required to appropriately titrate the dose against disease activity (see Posology and method of administration).

3. Patients should carry 'Steroid Treatment' cards which give clear guidance on the precautions to be taken to minimise risk and which provide details of prescriber, drug, dosage and the duration of treatment.

4. Depo-Medrone vials are intended for single dose use only. Any multidose use of the product may lead to contamination.

5. Depo-Medrone is not recommended for epidural, intranasal, intra-ocular, or any other unapproved route of administration. See Undesirable effects section for details of side-effects reported from some non-recommended routes of administration.

6. Due to the absence of a true tendon sheath, the Achilles tendon should not be injected with Depo-Medrone.

7. While crystals of adrenal steroids in the dermis suppress inflammatory reactions, their presence may cause disintegration of the cellular elements and physiochemical changes in the ground substance of the connective tissue. The resultant infrequently occurring dermal and/or subdermal changes may form depressions in the skin at the injection site. The degree to which this reaction occurs will vary with the amount of adrenal steroid injected. Regeneration is usually complete within a few months or after all crystals of the adrenal steroid have been absorbed. In order to minimize the incidence of dermal and subdermal atrophy, care must be exercised not to exceed recommended doses in injections. Multiple small injections into the area of the lesion should be made whenever possible. The technique of intra-articular and intramuscular injection should include precautions against injection or leakage into the dermis. Injection into the deltoid muscle should be avoided because of a high incidence of subcutaneous atrophy.

8. Intralesional doses should not be placed too superficially, particularly in easily visible sites in patients with deeply pigmented skins, since there have been rare reports of subcutaneous atrophy and depigmentation.

9. Systemic absorption of methylprednisolone occurs following intra-articular injection of Depo-Medrone. Systemic as well as local effects can therefore be expected.

10. Intra-articular corticosteroids are associated with a substantially increased risk of inflammatory response in the joint, particularly bacterial infection introduced with the injection. Charcot-like arthropathies have been reported particularly after repeated injections. Appropriate examination of any joint fluid present is necessary to exclude any bacterial infection, prior to injection.

11. Following a single dose of Depo-Medrone, plasma cortisol levels are reduced and there is evidence of hypothalamic-pituitary-adrenal (HPA) axis suppression. This suppression lasts for a variable period of up to 4 weeks. The usual dynamic tests of HPA axis function can be used to diagnose evidence of impaired activity (e.g. Synacthen test).

12. Adrenal cortical atrophy develops during prolonged therapy and may persist for months after stopping treatment. In patients who have received more than physiological doses of systemic corticosteroids (approximately 6 mg methylprednisolone) for greater than 3 weeks, withdrawal should not be abrupt. How dose reduction should be carried out depends largely on whether the disease is likely to relapse as the dose of systemic corticosteroids is reduced. Clinical assessment of disease activity may be needed during withdrawal. If the disease is unlikely to relapse on withdrawal of systemic corticosteroids, but there is uncertainty about HPA suppression, the dose of systemic corticosteroid may be reduced rapidly to physiological doses. Once a daily dose of 6 mg methylprednisolone is reached, dose reduction should be slower to allow the HPA-axis to recover.

Abrupt withdrawal of systemic corticosteroid treatment, which has continued up to 3 weeks is appropriate if it considered that the disease is unlikely to relapse. Abrupt withdrawal of doses up to 32 mg daily of methylprednisolone for 3 weeks is unlikely to lead to clinically relevant HPA-axis suppression, in the majority of patients. In the following patient groups, gradual withdrawal of systemic corticosteroid therapy should be *considered* even after courses lasting 3 weeks or less:

- Patients who have had repeated courses of systemic corticosteroids, particularly if taken for greater than 3 weeks.
- When a short course has been prescribed within one year of cessation of long-term therapy (months or years).
- Patients who may have reasons for adrenocortical insufficiency other than exogenous corticosteroid therapy.
- Patients receiving doses of systemic corticosteroid greater than 32 mg daily of methylprednisolone.
- Patients repeatedly taking doses in the evening.

13. Since mineralocorticoid secretion may be impaired, salt and/or a mineralocorticoid should be administered concurrently.

14. Because rare instances of anaphylactic reactions have occurred in patients receiving parenteral corticosteroid therapy, appropriate precautionary measures should be taken prior to administration, especially when the patient has a history of drug allergy.

15. Corticosteroids may mask some signs of infection, and new infections may appear during their use. Suppression of the inflammatory response and immune function increases the susceptibility to fungal, viral and bacterial

infections and their severity. The clinical presentation may often be atypical and may reach an advanced stage before being recognised.

16. Chickenpox is of serious concern since this normally minor illness may be fatal in immunosuppressed patients. Patients (or parents of children) without a definite history of chickenpox should be advised to avoid close personal contact with chickenpox or herpes zoster and if exposed they should seek urgent medical attention. Passive immunization with varicella/zoster immunoglobin (VZIG) is needed by exposed non-immune patients who are receiving systemic corticosteroids or who have used them within the previous 3 months; this should be given within 10 days of exposure to chickenpox. If a diagnosis of chickenpox is confirmed, the illness warrants specialist care and urgent treatment. Corticosteroids should not be stopped and the dose may need to be increased.

17. Live vaccines should not be given to individuals with impaired immune responsiveness. The antibody response to other vaccines may be diminished.

18. The use of Depo-Medrone in active tuberculosis should be restricted to those cases of fulminating or disseminated tuberculosis in which the corticosteroid is used for the management of the disease in conjunction with an appropriate antituberculous regimen. If corticosteroids are indicated in patients with latent tuberculosis or tuberculin reactivity, close observation is necessary as reactivation of the disease may occur. During prolonged corticosteroid therapy, these patients should receive chemoprophylaxis.

19. Care should be taken for patients receiving cardioactive drugs such as digoxin because of steroid induced electrolyte disturbance/potassium loss (see Undesirable effects).

20. *The following precautions apply for parenteral corticosteroids:* Following intra-articular injection, the occurrence of a marked increase in pain accompanied by local swelling, further restriction of joint motion, fever, and malaise are suggestive of septic arthritis. If this complication occurs and the diagnosis of sepsis is confirmed, appropriate antimicrobial therapy should be instituted.

Local injection of a steroid into a previously infected joint is to be avoided.

Corticosteroids should not be injected into unstable joints.

Sterile technique is necessary to prevent infections or contamination.

The slower rate of absorption by intramuscular administration should be recognised.

Special precautions:

Particular care is required when considering the use of systemic corticosteroids in patients with the following conditions and frequent patient monitoring is necessary.

1. Osteoporosis (post-menopausal females are particularly at risk).
2. Hypertension or congestive heart failure.
3. Existing or previous history of severe affective disorders (especially previous steroid psychosis).
4. Diabetes mellitus (or a family history of diabetes).
5. History of tuberculosis.
6. Glaucoma (or a family history of glaucoma).
7. Previous corticosteroid-induced myopathy.
8. Liver failure or cirrhosis.
9. Renal insufficiency.
10. Epilepsy.
11. Peptic ulceration.
12. Fresh intestinal anastomoses.
13. Predisposition to thrombophlebitis.
14. Abscess or other pyogenic infections.
15. Ulcerative colitis.
16. Diverticulitis.
17. Myasthenia gravis.
18. Ocular herpes simplex, for fear of corneal perforation.
19. Hypothyroidism.
20. Patients and/or carers should be warned that potentially severe psychiatric adverse reactions may occur with systemic steroids (see section 4.8). Symptoms typically emerge within a few days or weeks of starting treatment. Risks may be higher with high doses/systemic exposure (see also section 4.5 Interaction with Other Medicaments and Other Forms of Interaction that can increase the risk of side effects), although dose levels do not allow prediction of the onset, type, severity or duration of reactions. Most reactions recover after either dose reduction or withdrawal, although specific treatment may be necessary. Patients/carers should be encouraged to seek medical advice if worrying psychological symptoms develop, especially if depressed mood or suicidal ideation is suspected. Patients/carers should be alert to possible psychiatric disturbances that may occur either during or immediately after dose tapering/withdrawal of systemic steroids, although such reactions have been reported infrequently.

Particular care is required when considering the use of systemic corticosteroids in patients with existing or previous history of severe affective disorders in themselves or in their first degree relatives. These would include depressive or manic-depressive illness and previous steroid psychosis.

Use in Children: Corticosteroids cause growth retardation in infancy, childhood and adolescence which may be irreversible. Treatment should be limited to the minimum dosage for the shortest possible time.

Use in the elderly: The common adverse effects of systemic corticosteroids may be associated with more serious consequences in old age, especially osteoporosis, hypertension, hypokalaemia, diabetes, susceptibility to infection and thinning of the skin. Close clinical supervision is required to avoid life-threatening reactions.

4.5 Interaction with other medicinal products and other forms of interaction

1. Convulsions have been reported with concurrent use of methylprednisolone and cyclosporin. Since concurrent administration of these agents results in a mutual inhibition of metabolism, it is possible that convulsions and other adverse effects associated with the individual use of either drug may be more apt to occur.

2. Drugs that induce hepatic enzymes, such as rifampicin, rifabutin, carbamazepine, phenobarbitone, phenytoin, primidone, and aminoglutethimide enhance the metabolism of corticosteroids and its therapeutic effects may be reduced.

3. Drugs such as erythromycin and ketoconazole may inhibit the metabolism of corticosteroids and thus decrease their clearance.

4. Steroids may reduce the effects of anticholinesterases in myasthenia gravis. The desired effects of hypoglycaemic agents (including insulin), anti-hypertensives and diuretics are antagonised by corticosteroids, and the hypokalaemic effects of acetazolamide, loop diuretics, thiazide diuretics and carbenoxolone are enhanced.

5. The efficacy of coumarin anticoagulants may be enhanced by concurrent corticosteroid therapy and close monitoring of the INR or prothrombin time is required to avoid spontaneous bleeding.

6. The renal clearance of salicylates is increased by corticosteroids and steroid withdrawal may result in salicylate intoxication. Salicylates and non-steroidal anti-inflammatory agents should be used cautiously in conjunction with corticosteroids in hypothrombinaemia.

7. Steroids have been reported to interact with neuromuscular blocking agents such as pancuronium with partial reversal of the neuromuscular block.

4.6 Pregnancy and lactation

Pregnancy

The ability of corticosteroids to cross the placenta varies between individual drugs, however, methylprednisolone does cross the placenta.

Administration of corticosteroids to pregnant animals can cause abnormalities of foetal development including cleft palate, intra-uterine growth retardation and affects on brain growth and development. There is no evidence that corticosteroids result in an increased incidence of congenital abnormalities, such as cleft palate in man, however, when administered for long periods or repeatedly during pregnancy, corticosteroids may increase the risk of intra-uterine growth retardation. Hypoadrenalism may, in theory, occur in the neonate following prenatal exposure to corticosteroids but usually resolves spontaneously following birth and is rarely clinically important. As with all drugs, corticosteroids should only be prescribed when the benefits to the mother and child outweigh the risks. When corticosteroids are essential, however, patients with normal pregnancies may be treated as though they were in the non-gravid state.

Lactation

Corticosteroids are excreted in small amounts in breast milk, however, doses of up to 40 mg daily of methylprednisolone are unlikely to cause systemic effects in the infant. Infants of mothers taking higher doses than this may have a degree of adrenal suppression, but the benefits of breastfeeding are likely to outweigh any theoretical risk.

4.7 Effects on ability to drive and use machines

None stated.

4.8 Undesirable effects

The incidence of predictable undesirable side-effects associated with the use of corticosteroids, including hypothalamic-pituitary-adrenal suppression correlates with the relative potency of the drug, dosage, timing of administration and duration of treatment (see Special warnings and special precautions for use).

PARENTERAL CORTICOSTEROID THERAPY - Anaphylactic reaction or allergic reactions, hypopigmentation or hyperpigmentation, subcutaneous and cutaneous atrophy, sterile abscess, post injection flare (following intra-articular use), Charcot-like arthropathy, rare instances of blindness associated with intralesional therapy around the face and head.

GASTRO-INTESTINAL - Dyspepsia, peptic ulceration with perforation and haemorrhage, abdominal distension, oesophageal ulceration, oesophageal candidiasis, acute pancreatitis, perforation of bowel.

Increases in alanine transaminase (ALT, SGPT) aspartate transaminase (AST, SGOT) and alkaline phosphatase have been observed following corticosteroid treatment. These changes are usually small, not associated with any clinical syndrome and are reversible upon discontinuation.

ANTI-INFLAMMATORY AND IMMUNOSUPPRESSIVE EFFECTS - Increased susceptibility and severity of infections with suppression of clinical symptoms and signs, opportunistic infections, may suppress reactions to skin tests, recurrence of dormant tuberculosis (see Special warnings and special precautions for use).

MUSCULOSKELETAL - Proximal myopathy, osteoporosis, vertebral and long bone fractures, avascular osteonecrosis, tendon rupture, aseptic necrosis, muscle weakness.

FLUID AND ELECTROLYTE DISTURBANCE - Sodium and water retention, potassium loss, hypertension, hypokalaemic alkalosis, congestive heart failure in susceptible patients.

DERMATOLOGICAL - Impaired healing, petechiae and ecchymosis, thin fragile skin, skin atrophy, bruising, striae, telangiectasia, acne.

ENDOCRINE/METABOLIC - Suppression of the hypothalamo-pituitary-adrenal axis, growth suppression in infancy, childhood and adolescence, menstrual irregularity and amenorrhoea. Cushingoid facies, hirsutism, weight gain, impaired carbohydrate tolerance with increased requirement for antidiabetic therapy, negative nitrogen and calcium balance. Increased appetite.

NEUROPSYCHIATRIC - A wide range of psychiatric reactions including affective disorders (such as irritable, euphoric, depressed and labile mood psychological dependence and suicidal thoughts), psychotic reactions (including mania, delusions, hallucinations and aggravation of schizophrenia), behavioural disturbances, irritability, anxiety, sleep disturbances, and cognitive dysfunction including confusion and amnesia have been reported for all corticosteroids. Reactions are common and may occur in both adults and children. In adults, the frequency of severe reactions was estimated to be 5-6% for corticosteroids in 1983, primarily based upon data from prednisone administration. Psychological effects have been reported on withdrawal of corticosteroids; the frequency is unknown. Increased intra-cranial pressure with papilloedema in children (pseudotumour cerebri) has been reported, usually after treatment withdrawal of methylprednisolone.

OPHTHALMIC - Increased intra-ocular pressure, glaucoma, papilloedema, cataracts with possible damage to the optic nerve, corneal or scleral thinning, exacerbation of ophthalmic viral or fungal disease, exophthalmos.

GENERAL - Leucocytosis, hypersensitivity including anaphylaxis, thrombo-embolism, nausea, vertigo.

WITHDRAWAL SYMPTOMS - Too rapid a reduction of corticosteroid dosage following prolonged treatment can lead to acute adrenal insufficiency, hypotension and death. However, this is more applicable to corticosteroids with an indication where continuous therapy is given (see Special warnings and special precautions for use).

A 'withdrawal syndrome' may also occur including, fever, myalgia, arthralgia, rhinitis, conjunctivitis, painful itchy skin nodules and loss of weight.

CERTAIN SIDE-EFFECTS REPORTED WITH SOME NON-RECOMMENDED ROUTES OF ADMINISTRATION.

Intrathecal: Usual systemic corticoid adverse reactions, headache, meningismus, meningitis, paraplegia, spinal fluid abnormalities, nausea, vomiting, sweating, arachnoiditis, convulsions.

Extradural: Wound dehiscence, loss of sphincter control.

Intranasal: Permanent/temporary blindness, rhinitis.

Ophthalmic: (Subconjunctival) - Redness and itching, abscess, slough at injection site, residue at injection site, increased intra-ocular pressure, decreased vision - blindness, infection.

Miscellaneous injection sites - Scalp, tonsillar fauces, sphenopalatine ganglion: blindness.

4.9 Overdose

There is no clinical syndrome of acute overdosage with Depo-Medrone. Following overdosage the possibility of adrenal suppression should be guarded against by gradual diminution of dose levels over a period of time. In such event the patient may require to be supported during any further traumatic episode.

5. PHARMACOLOGICAL PROPERTIES

5.1 Pharmacodynamic properties

Methylprednisolone acetate is a synthetic glucocorticoid. An aqueous suspension may be injected directly into joints and soft tissues in the treatment of rheumatoid arthritis, osteoarthritis, bursitis and similar inflammatory conditions. For prolonged systemic effect it may be administered intramuscularly.

5.2 Pharmacokinetic properties

Methylprednisolone acetate is absorbed from joints in a few days, with peak serum levels being reached 2-12 hours after injection.

It is more slowly absorbed following deep intramuscular injection with plasma levels detected up to 17 days afterwards.

Methylprednisolone acetate is less soluble than methylprednisolone.

6. PHARMACEUTICAL PARTICULARS

6.1 List of excipients

Polyethylene glycol, sodium chloride, myristyl-gamma-picolinium chloride and sterile water for injections.

6.2 Incompatibilities

None stated.

6.3 Shelf life

Shelf-life of the medicinal product as packaged for sale: 60 months.

Depo-Medrone should not be mixed with any other fluid. Discard any remaining suspension after use.

6.4 Special precautions for storage

Depo-Medrone should be protected from freezing.

6.5 Nature and contents of container

Type I flint glass vial with a butyl rubber plug and metal seal. Each vial contains 1 ml, 2ml, or 3 ml of Depo-Medrone 40 mg/ml.

6.6 Special precautions for disposal and other handling

No special requirements.

7. MARKETING AUTHORISATION HOLDER

Pharmacia Ltd
Ramsgate Road
Sanwich
Kent CT13 9NJ
UK

8. MARKETING AUTHORISATION NUMBER(S)

PL 0032/5038

9. DATE OF FIRST AUTHORISATION/RENEWAL OF THE AUTHORISATION

Date of first authorisation: 7 March 1989.

Last renewal date: 5 September 1996

10. DATE OF REVISION OF THE TEXT

March 2008

Ref: DM4_0 UK

Depo-Medrone with Lidocaine

(Pharmacia Limited)

1. NAME OF THE MEDICINAL PRODUCT

Depo-Medrone with Lidocaine

2. QUALITATIVE AND QUANTITATIVE COMPOSITION

Methyprednisolone BP 4%, Lidocaine Hydrochloride BP 1%

3. PHARMACEUTICAL FORM

White, sterile aqueous suspension for injection

4. CLINICAL PARTICULARS

4.1 Therapeutic indications

Corticosteroid (glucocorticoid). Depo-Medrone with Lidocaine is indicated in conditions requiring a glucocorticoid effect: e.g. anti-inflammatory or anti-rheumatic. It is recommended for local use where the added anaesthetic effect would be considered advantageous.

Depo-Medrone with Lidocaine may be used as follows:

<u>Intra-articular administration</u>

Rheumatoid arthritis

Osteo-arthritis with an inflammatory component

<u>Periarticular administration</u>

Epicondylitis

<u>Intrabursal administration</u>

Subacromial bursitis

Prepatellar bursitis

Olecranon bursitis

<u>Tendon sheath administration</u>

Tendinitis

Tenosynovitis

Epicondylitis

Therapy with Depo-Medrone with Lidocaine does not obviate the need for the conventional measures usually employed. Although this method of treatment will ameliorate symptoms, it is in no sense a cure and the hormone has no effect on the cause of the inflammation.

4.2 Posology and method of administration

Depo-Medrone with Lidocaine should not be mixed with any other preparation as flocculation of the product may occur. Parenteral drug products should be inspected visually for particulate matter and discoloration prior to administration whenever suspension and container permit. Depo-Medrone with Lidocaine may be used by any of the following routes: intra-articular, periarticular, intrabursal, and into the tendon sheath. It <u>must not</u> be used by the intrathecal or intravenous routes (see Contra-indications and Side-effects)

Adults

Intra-articular: Rheumatoid arthritis, osteo-arthritis. The dose of Depo-Medrone with Lidocaine depends on the size of the joint and the severity of the condition. Repeated injections, if needed, may be given at intervals of one to five or more weeks depending upon the degree of relief obtained from the initial injection. A suggested dosage guide is: large joint (knee, ankle, shoulder), 0.5 - 2 ml (20 - 80 mg of steroid); medium joint (elbow, wrist), 0.25 - 1 ml (10 - 40 mg of steroid); small joint (metacarpophalangeal, interphalangeal, sternoclavicular, acromioclavicular), 0.1 - 0.25 ml (4 - 10 mg of steroid).

Periarticular: Epicondylitis. Infiltrate 0.1 - 0.75 ml (4 - 30 mg of steroid) into the affected area.

Intrabursal: Subdeltoid bursitis, prepatellar bursitis, olecranon bursitis. For administration directly into bursae, 0.1 - 0.75 ml (4 - 30 mg of steroid). In most acute cases, repeat injections are not needed.

Into the tendon sheath: Tendinitis, tenosynovitis, epicondylitis. For administration directly into the tendon sheath, 0.1 - 0.75 ml (4 - 30 mg of steroid). In recurrent or chronic conditions, repeat injections may be necessary.

Children:

For infants and children, the recommended dosage should be reduced, but dosage should be governed by the severity of the condition rather than by strict adherence to the ratio indicated by age or body weight.

Elderly:

When used according to instructions, there is no information to suggest that a change in dosage is warranted in the elderly. However, treatment of elderly patients, particularly if long-term, should be planned bearing in mind the more serious consequences of the common side-effects of corticosteroids in old age and close clinical supervision is required (see Other special warnings and precautions).

Special precautions should be observed when administering Depo-Medrone with Lidocaine:

Intra-articular injections should be made using precise, anatomical localisation into the synovial space of the joint involved. The injection site for each joint is determined by that location where the synovial cavity is most superficial and most free of large vessels and nerves. Suitable sites for intra-articular injection are the knee, ankle, wrist, elbow, shoulder, phalangeal and hip joints. The spinal joints, unstable joints and those devoid of synovial space are not suitable. Treatment failures are most frequently the result of failure to enter the joint space. Intra-articular injections should be made with care as follows: ensure correct positioning of the needle into the synovial space and aspirate a few drops of joint fluid. The aspirating syringe should then be replaced by another containing Depo-Medrone with Lidocaine. To ensure position of the needle synovial fluid should be aspirated and the injection made.

After injection the joint is moved slightly to aid mixing of the synovial fluid and the suspension. Subsequent to therapy care should be taken for the patient not to overuse the joint in which benefit has been obtained. Negligence in this matter may permit an increase in joint deterioration that will more than offset the beneficial effects of the steroid.

Intrabursal injections should be made as follows: the area around the injection site is prepared in a sterile way and a wheal at the site made with 1 percent procaine hydrochloride solution. A 20 to 24 gauge needle attached to a dry syringe is inserted into the bursa and the fluid aspirated. The needle is left in place and the aspirating syringe changed for a small syringe containing the desired dose. After injection, the needle is withdrawn and a small dressing applied. In the treatment of tenosynovitis and tendinitis, care should be taken to inject Depo-Medrone with Lidocaine into the tendon sheath rather than into the substance of the tendon. Due to the absence of a true tendon sheath, the Achilles tendon should not be injected with Depo-Medrone with Lidocaine.

4.3 Contraindications

Depo-Medrone with Lidocaine is contra-indicated where there is known hypersensitivity to components or to any local anaesthetics of the amide type and in systemic infection unless anti-infective therapy is employed.

Due to its potential for neurotoxicity, Depo-Medrone with Lidocaine <u>must not</u> be given by the intrathecal route. In addition, as the product is a suspension it <u>must not</u> be given by the intravenous route (see Side-effects).

4.4 Special warnings and precautions for use

1. Undesirable effects may be minimised by using the lowest effective dose for the minimum period. Frequent patient review is required to appropriately titrate the dose against disease activity (see Dosage and administration).

2. Patients should carry 'Steroid Treatment' cards which give clear guidance on the precautions to be taken to minimise risk and which provide details of prescriber, drug, dosage and the duration of treatment.

3. Depo-Medrone with Lidocaine vials are intended for single dose use only. Any multidose use of the product may lead to contamination.

4. Depo-Medrone with Lidocaine is not recommended for epidural, intranasal, intra-ocular, or any other unapproved route of administration. See Side-effects section for details of side-effects reported from some non-recommended routes of administration.

5. Due to the absence of a true tendon sheath, the Achilles tendon should not be injected with Depo-Medrone with Lidocaine.

6. While crystals of adrenal steroids in the dermis suppress inflammatory reactions, their presence may cause disintegration of the cellular elements and physiochemical changes in the ground substance of the connective tissue. The resultant infrequently occurring dermal and/or subdermal changes may form depressions in the skin at the injection site and the possibility of depigmentation. The degree to which this reaction occurs will vary with the amount of adrenal steroid injected. Regeneration is usually complete within a few months or after all crystals of the adrenal steroid have been absorbed. In order to minimize the incidence of dermal and subdermal atrophy, care must be exercised not to exceed recommended doses in injections. Multiple small injections into the area of the lesion should be made whenever possible. The technique of intra-articular injection should include precautions against injection or leakage into the dermis.

7. Systemic absorption of methylprednisolone occurs following intra-articular injection of Depo-Medrone with Lidocaine. Systemic as well as local effects can therefore be expected.

8. Intra-articular corticosteroids are associated with a substantially increased risk of inflammatory response in the joint, particularly bacterial infection introduced with the injection. Charcot-like arthropathies have been reported particularly after repeated injections. Appropriate examination of any joint fluid present is necessary to exclude any bacterial infection, prior to injection.

9 Following a single dose of Depo-Medrone with Lidocaine, plasma cortisol levels are reduced and there is evidence of hypothalamic-pituitary-adrenal axis (HPA) suppression. This suppression lasts for a variable period of up to 4 weeks. The usual dynamic tests of HPA axis function can be used to diagnose evidence of impaired activity (e.g. Synacthen test).

10. Adrenal cortical atrophy develops during prolonged therapy and may persist for months after stopping treatment. In patients who have received more than physiological doses of systemic corticosteroids (approximately 6 mg methylprednisolone) for greater than 3 weeks, withdrawal should not be abrupt. How dose reduction should be carried out depends largely on whether the disease is likely to relapse as the dose of systemic corticosteroids is reduced. Clinical assessment of disease activity may be needed during withdrawal. If the disease is unlikely to relapse on withdrawal of systemic corticosteroids, but there is uncertainty about HPA suppression, the dose of systemic corticosteroid <u>may</u> be reduced rapidly to physiological doses. Once a daily dose of 6 mg methylprednisolone is reached, dose reduction should be slower to allow the HPA-axis to recover.

Abrupt withdrawal of systemic corticosteroid treatment, which has continued up to 3 weeks is appropriate if it considered that the disease is unlikely to relapse. Abrupt withdrawal of doses up to 32 mg daily of methylprednisolone for 3 weeks is unlikely to lead to clinically relevant HPA-axis suppression, in the majority of patients. In the following patient groups, gradual withdrawal of systemic corticosteroid therapy should be *considered* even after courses lasting 3 weeks or less:

- Patients who have had repeated courses of systemic corticosteroids, particularly if taken for greater than 3 weeks.
- When a short course has been prescribed within one year of cessation of long-term therapy (months or years).
- Patients who may have reasons for adrenocortical insufficiency other than exogenous corticosteroid therapy.
- Patients receiving doses of systemic corticosteroid greater than 32 mg daily of methylprednisolone.
- Patients repeatedly taking doses in the evening.

11. Since mineralocorticoid secretion may be impaired, salt and/or a mineralocorticoid should be administered concurrently.

12. Because rare instances of anaphylactic reactions have occurred in patients receiving parenteral corticosteroid therapy, appropriate precautionary measures should be taken prior to administration, especially when the patient has a history of drug allergy.

13. Corticosteroids may mask some signs of infection, and new infections may appear during their use. Suppression of the inflammatory response and immune function increases the susceptibility to fungal, viral and bacterial infections and their severity. The clinical presentation may often be atypical and may reach an advanced stage before being recognised.

14. Chickenpox is of serious concern since this normally minor illness may be fatal in immunosuppressed patients. Patients (or parents of children) without a definite history of chickenpox should be advised to avoid close personal contact with chickenpox or herpes zoster and if exposed they should seek urgent medical attention. Passive immunization with varicella/zoster immunoglobin (VZIG) is needed by exposed non-immune patients who are receiving systemic corticosteroids or who have used them within the previous 3 months; this should be given within 10 days of exposure to chickenpox. If a diagnosis of chickenpox is confirmed, the illness warrants specialist care and urgent treatment. Corticosteroids should not be stopped and the dose may need to be increased.

15. Live vaccines should not be given to individuals with impaired immune responsiveness. The antibody response to other vaccines may be diminished.

16. If corticosteroids are indicated in patients with latent tuberculosis or tuberculin reactivity, close observation is necessary as reactivation of the disease may occur. During prolonged corticosteroid therapy, these patients should receive chemoprophylaxis.

17. This product contains benzyl alcohol. Benzyl alcohol has been reported to be associated with a fatal "Gasping Syndrome" in premature infants.

18. Care should be taken for patients receiving cardioactive drugs such as digoxin because of steroid induced electrolyte disturbance/potassium loss (see Side-effects).

19. *The following precautions apply for parenteral corticosteroids:* Following intra-articular injection, a marked increase in pain accompanied by local swelling, further restriction of joint motion, fever, and malaise are suggestive of septic arthritis. If this complication occurs and the diagnosis of sepsis is confirmed, appropriate antimicrobial therapy should be instituted.

No additional benefit derives from the intramuscular administration of Depo-Medrone with Lidocaine. Where parenteral corticosteroid therapy for sustained systemic effect is desired, plain Depo-Medrone should be used.

Local injection of a steroid into a previously infected joint is to be avoided.

Corticosteroids should not be injected into unstable joints.

Sterile technique is necessary to prevent infections or contamination.

Special precautions:

Particular care is required when considering the use of systemic corticosteroids in patients with the following conditions and frequent patient monitoring is necessary.

1. Osteoporosis (post-menopausal females are particularly at risk).
2. Hypertension or congestive heart failure.
3. Existing or previous history of severe affective disorders (especially previous steroid psychosis).
4. Diabetes mellitus (or a family history of diabetes).
5. History of tuberculosis.
6. Glaucoma (or a family history of glaucoma).
7. Previous corticosteroid-induced myopathy.
8. Liver failure or cirrhosis.
9. Renal insufficiency.
10. Epilepsy.
11. Peptic ulceration.
12. Fresh intestinal anastomoses.
13. Predisposition to thrombophlebitis.
14. Abscess or other pyogenic infections.
15. Ulcerative colitis.
16. Diverticulitis.
17. Myasthenia gravis.
18. Ocular herpes simplex, for fear of corneal perforation.
19. Hypothyroidism.
20. Patients and/or carers should be warned that potentially severe psychiatric adverse reactions may occur with systemic steroids (see section 4.8). Symptoms typically emerge within a few days or weeks of starting treatment. Risks may be higher with high doses/systemic exposure (see also section 4.5 Interaction with Other Medicaments and Other Forms of Interaction that can increase the risk of side effects), although dose levels do not allow prediction of the onset, type, severity or duration of reactions. Most reactions recover after either dose reduction or withdrawal, although specific treatment may be necessary. Patients/carers should be encouraged to seek medical advice if worrying psychological symptoms develop, especially if depressed mood or suicidal ideation is suspected. Patients/carers should be alert to possible psychiatric disturbances that may occur either during or immediately after dose tapering/withdrawal of systemic steroids, although such reactions have been reported infrequently.

Particular care is required when considering the use of systemic corticosteroids in patients with existing or previous history of severe affective disorders in themselves or in their first degree relatives. These would include depressive or manic-depressive illness and previous steroid psychosis.

Use in children: Corticosteroids cause growth retardation in infancy, childhood and adolescence which may be irreversible. Treatment should be limited to the minimum dosage for the shortest possible time.

Use in the elderly: The common adverse effects of systemic corticosteroids may be associated with more serious consequences in old age, especially osteoporosis, hypertension, hypokalaemia, diabetes, susceptibility to infection and thinning of the skin. Close clinical supervision is required to avoid life-threatening reactions.

4.5 Interaction with other medicinal products and other forms of interaction

1. Convulsions have been reported with concurrent use of methylprednisolone and cyclosporin. Since concurrent administration of these agents results in a mutual inhibition of metabolism, it is possible that convulsions and other adverse effects associated with the individual use of either drug may be more apt to occur.

2. Drugs that induce hepatic enzymes, such as rifampicin, rifabutin, carbamazepine, phenobarbitone, phenytoin, primidone, and aminoglutethimide enhance the metabolism of corticosteroids and its therapeutic effects may be reduced.

3. Drugs such as erythromycin and ketoconazole may inhibit the metabolism of corticosteroids and thus decrease their clearance.

4. Steroids may reduce the effects of anticholinesterases in myasthenia gravis. The desired effects of hypoglycaemic agents (including insulin), anti-hypertensives and diuretics are antagonised by corticosteroids, and the hypokalaemic effects of acetazolamide, loop diuretics, thiazide diuretics and carbenoxolone are enhanced.

5. The efficacy of coumarin anticoagulants may be enhanced by concurrent corticosteroid therapy and close monitoring of the INR or prothrombin time is required to avoid spontaneous bleeding.

6. The renal clearance of salicylates is increased by corticosteroids and steroid withdrawal may result in salicylate intoxication. Salicylates and non-steroidal anti-inflammatory agents should be used cautiously in conjunction with corticosteroids in hypothrombinaemia.

7. Steroids have been reported to interact with neuromuscular blocking agents such as pancuronium with partial reversal of the neuromuscular block.

4.6 Pregnancy and lactation

Pregnancy

The ability of corticosteroids to cross the placenta varies between individual drugs, however, methylprednisolone does cross the placenta.

Administration of corticosteroids to pregnant animals can cause abnormalities of foetal development including cleft palate, intra-uterine growth retardation and affects on brain growth and development. There is no evidence that corticosteroids result in an increased incidence of congenital abnormalities, such as cleft palate in man, however, when administered for long periods or repeatedly during pregnancy, corticosteroids may increase the risk of intra-uterine growth retardation. Hypoadrenalism may, in theory, occur in the neonate following prenatal exposure to corticosteroids but usually resolves spontaneously following birth and is rarely clinically important. As with all drugs, corticosteroids should only be prescribed when the benefits to the mother and child outweigh the risks. When corticosteroids are essential, however, patients with normal pregnancies may be treated as though they were in the non-gravid state.

The use of local anaesthetics such as lidocaine during labour and delivery may be associated with adverse effects on mother and foetus. Lidocaine readily crosses the placenta.

Lactation

Corticosteroids are excreted in small amounts in breast milk, however, doses of up to 40 mg daily of methylprednisolone are unlikely to cause systemic effects in the infant. Infants of mothers taking higher doses than this may have a degree of adrenal suppression, but the benefits of breast-feeding are likely to outweigh any theoretical risk.

It is not known whether lidocaine is excreted in human breast milk.

4.7 Effects on ability to drive and use machines

None stated.

4.8 Undesirable effects

The incidence of predictable undesirable side-effects associated with the use of corticosteroids, including hypothalamic-pituitary-adrenal suppression correlates with the relative potency of the drug, dosage, timing of administration and duration of treatment (See other special warnings and precautions).

Side-effects for the Depo-Medrone component may be observed including:

PARENTERAL CORTICOSTEROID THERAPY - Anaphylactic reaction or allergic reactions, hypopigmentation or hyperpigmentation, subcutaneous and cutaneous atrophy, sterile abscess, post injection flare (following intra-articular use), charcot-like arthropathy.

GASTRO-INTESTINAL - Dyspepsia, peptic ulceration with perforation and haemorrhage, abdominal distension, oesophageal ulceration, oesophageal candidiasis, acute pancreatitis, perforation of bowel.

Increases in alanine transaminase (ALT, SGPT) aspartate transaminase (AST, SGOT) and alkaline phosphatase have been observed following corticosteroid treatment. These changes are usually small, not associated with any clinical syndrome and are reversible upon discontinuation.

ANTI-INFLAMMATORY AND IMMUNOSUPPRESSIVE EFFECTS - Increased susceptibility and severity of infections with suppression of clinical symptoms and signs, opportunistic infections, may suppress reactions to skin tests, recurrence of dormant tuberculosis (see Other special warnings and precautions).

MUSCULOSKELETAL - Proximal myopathy, osteoporosis, vertebral and long bone fractures, avascular osteonecrosis, tendon rupture, aseptic necrosis, muscle weakness.

FLUID AND ELECTROLYTE DISTURBANCE - Sodium and water retention, potassium loss, hypertension, hypokalaemic alkalosis, congestive heart failure in susceptible patients.

DERMATOLOGICAL - Impaired healing, petechiae and ecchymosis, thin fragile skin, skin atrophy, bruising, striae, telangiectasia, acne.

ENDOCRINE/METABOLIC - Suppression of the hypothalamo-pituitary-adrenal axis; growth suppression in infancy, childhood and adolescence; menstrual irregularity and amenorrhoea. Cushingoid facies, hirsutism, weight gain, impaired carbohydrate tolerance with increased requirement for antidiabetic therapy, negative nitrogen and calcium balance. Increased appetite.

NEUROPSYCHIATRIC - A wide range of psychiatric reactions including affective disorders (such as irritable, euphoric, depressed and labile mood psychological dependence and suicidal thoughts), psychotic reactions (including mania, delusions, hallucinations and aggravation of schizophrenia), behavioural disturbances, irritability, anxiety, sleep disturbances, and cognitive dysfunction including confusion and amnesia have been reported for all corticosteroids. Reactions are common and may occur in both adults and children. In adults, the frequency of severe reactions was estimated to be 5-6% for corticosteroids in 1983, primarily based upon data from prednisone administration. Psychological effects have been reported on withdrawal of corticosteroids; the frequency is unknown. Increased intra-cranial pressure with papilloedema in children (pseudotumour cerebri) has been reported, usually after treatment withdrawal of methylprednisolone.

OPHTHALMIC - Increased intra-ocular pressure, glaucoma, papilloedema, cataracts with possible damage to the optic nerve, corneal or scleral thinning, exacerbation of ophthalmic viral or fungal disease, exophthalmos.

GENERAL - Leucocytosis, hypersensitivity including anaphylaxis, thrombo-embolism, nausea, vertigo.

WITHDRAWAL SYMPTOMS - Too rapid a reduction of corticosteroid dosage following prolonged treatment can lead to acute adrenal insufficiency, hypotension and death. However, this is more applicable to corticosteroids with an indication where continuous therapy is given (see Other special warnings and precautions).

A 'withdrawal syndrome' may also occur including, fever, myalgia, arthralgia, rhinitis, conjunctivitis, painful itchy skin nodules and loss of weight.

Side-effects for the Lidocaine component include:

CENTRAL NERVOUS SYSTEM - Lightheadedness, nervousness, apprehension, euphoria, confusion, dizziness, drowsiness, tinnitus, blurred or double vision, vomiting, sensation of heat, cold, numbness, twitching, tremors, convulsions, loss of consciousness, respiratory depression, respiratory arrest.

CARDIOVASCULAR SYSTEM - Bradycardia, hypotension, cardiovascular collapse, cardiac arrest.

ALLERGIC REACTIONS - Cutaneous lesions, urticaria, oedema, anaphylactic reactions.

CERTAIN SIDE-EFFECTS REPORTED WITH SOME NON RECOMMENDED ROUTES OF ADMINISTRATION:

Intrathecal: Usual systemic corticoid adverse reactions, headache, meningismus, meningitis, paraplegia, spinal fluid abnormalities, nausea, vomiting, sweating, arachnoiditis, convulsions.

Extradural: Wound dehiscence, loss of sphincter control.

Intranasal: Permanent/temporary blindness, allergic reactions, rhinitis.

Ophthalmic (Subconjunctival): Redness and itching, abscess, slough at injection site, residue at injection site, increased intra-ocular pressure, decreased vision - blindness, infection.

Miscellaneous: Scalp, tonsillar fauces, sphenopalatine ganglion: blindness.

4.9 Overdose

There is no clinical syndrome of acute overdosage with Depo-Medrone with Lidocaine. Following overdosage the possibility of adrenal suppression should be guarded against by gradual diminution of dose levels over a period of time. In such event the patient may require to be supported during any further traumatic episode.

5. PHARMACOLOGICAL PROPERTIES

5.1 Pharmacodynamic properties

Methylprednisolone acetate is a synthetic glucocorticoid with the actions and use of natural corticosteroids. However the slower metabolism of the synthetic corticosteroid with their lower protein-binding affinity may account for their increased potency compared with the natural corticosteroids.

Lidocaine has the actions of a local anaesthetic.

5.2 Pharmacokinetic properties

Administration of methylprednisolone acetate 40 mg intramuscularly produced measurable plasma concentrations of methylprednisolone for 11-17 days. The average peak plasma concentration was 14.8 ng per ml and occurred after 6-8 hours.

Plasma concentrations of lidocaine decline rapidly after an intravenous dose with an initial half life of less than 30 minutes; the elimination half life is 1-2 hours.

5.3 Preclinical safety data
Due to the age and well established safety nature of this product, preclinical data has not been included.

6. PHARMACEUTICAL PARTICULARS
6.1 List of excipients
Sodium chloride, myristyl-gamma-picolinium chloride, benzyl alcohol, ***macrogol***, sodium hydroxide, hydrochloric acid and water for injection.

6.2 Incompatibilities
None

6.3 Shelf life
24 months

6.4 Special precautions for storage
Store at room temperature. Protect from freezing.

6.5 Nature and contents of container
Glass vials with rubber cap containing 1 or 2 ml of suspension.

6.6 Special precautions for disposal and other handling
None

Administrative Data
7. MARKETING AUTHORISATION HOLDER
Pharmacia Limited,
Ramsgate Road,
Sandwich,
Kent CT13 9NJ
U.K.

8. MARKETING AUTHORISATION NUMBER(S)
PL 0032/0076

9. DATE OF FIRST AUTHORISATION/RENEWAL OF THE AUTHORISATION
MA granted: 03 March 1981
MA renewed: 25 November 1991

10. DATE OF REVISION OF THE TEXT
March 2008

11. Legal category
POM

Ref: DML4_0 UK

Deponit 10

(UCB Pharma Limited)

1. NAME OF THE MEDICINAL PRODUCT
Deponit 10

2. QUALITATIVE AND QUANTITATIVE COMPOSITION
One patch contains glyceryl trinitrate 37.4 mg

The average amount of glyceryl trinitrate absorbed from each patch in 24 hours is 10 mg.

3. PHARMACEUTICAL FORM
Transdermal patch
White, translucent square patch with convex round corners with "Deponit 10" marked on the outer face.

4. CLINICAL PARTICULARS
4.1 Therapeutic indications
Prophylaxis of angina pectoris alone or in combination with other anti-anginal therapy.

4.2 Posology and method of administration
Dermal
Adults: Treatment should be initiated with one patch daily. If necessary the dosage may be increased to two patches.

It is recommended that the patch is applied to healthy, undamaged, relatively crease free and hairless skin. The best places to apply Deponit patches are the easily reached, fairly static areas at the front or side of the chest. However, Deponit patches may also be applied to the upper arm, thigh, abdomen or shoulder. Skin care products should not be used before applying the patch. The replacement patch should be applied to a new area of skin. Allow several days to elapse before applying a fresh patch to the same area of skin.

Tolerance may occur during chronic nitrate therapy. Tolerance is likely to be avoided by allowing a patch-free period of 8-12 hours each day, usually at night. Additional anti-anginal therapy with drugs not containing nitro compounds should be considered for the nitrate-free interval if required.

As with any nitrate therapy, treatment with these patches should not be stopped abruptly. If the patient is being changed to another type of treatment, the two should overlap.

Elderly: No specific information on use in the elderly is available, however there is no evidence to suggest that an alteration in dose is required.

Children: The safety and efficacy of this patch in children has yet to be established

4.3 Contraindications
- Known hypersensitivity to nitrates or to the adhesives used in the patch
- Raised intracranial pressure including that caused by head trauma or cerebral haemorrhage
- Marked anaemia
- Closed angle glaucoma
- Hypotensive conditions and hypovolaemia
- Hypertrophic obstructive cardiomyopathy
- Aortic stenosis and mitral stenosis
- Constrictive pericarditis
- Cardiac tamponade
- Concomitant use of phosphodiesterase type-5 inhibitors. Phosphodiesterase type-5 inhibitors (e.g. sildenafil, tadalafil, vardenafil) have been shown to potentiate the hypotensive effects of nitrates, and their co-administration with nitrates or nitric oxide donors is therefore contra-indicated.

4.4 Special warnings and precautions for use
This patch should be used with caution in patients with
- Severe hepatic or renal impairment
- Hypothyroidism
- Hypothermia
- Malnutrition
- A recent history of myocardial infarction
- Hypoxaemia or a ventilation/perfusion imbalance due to lung disease or ischaemic heart failure.

The patch is not indicated for use in acute angina attacks. In the event of an acute angina attack, sublingual treatment such as a spray or tablet should be used. As with all nitrate preparations withdrawal of long-term treatment should be gradual by replacement with decreasing doses of long acting oral nitrates.

If the patches are not used as indicated (see Section 4.2) tolerance to the medication could develop.

4.5 Interaction with other medicinal products and other forms of interaction
Concomitant treatment with other vasodilators, calcium antagonists, ACE inhibitors, beta-blockers, diuretics, antihypertensives, tricyclic antidepressants and major tranquillisers, as well as the consumption of alcohol, may potentiate the hypotensive effect of the preparation.

The blood pressure lowering effect of these patches will be increased if used together with phosphodiesterase inhibitors (e.g. sildenafil) which are used for erectile dysfunction (see Section 4.3). This might lead to life threatening cardiovascular complications. Patients who are on nitrate therapy must not use phosphodiesterase inhibitors (e.g. sildenafil).

If administered concurrently, these patches may increase the blood level of dihydroergotamine and lead to coronary vasoconstriction.

The possibility that ingestion of acetylsalicylic acid and non-steroidal anti-inflammatory drugs might diminish the therapeutic response to the patch cannot be excluded.

4.6 Pregnancy and lactation
These patches should not be used during pregnancy or lactation unless considered absolutely essential by the physician.

It is not known whether the active substance passes into the breast milk. Benefits to the mother must be weighed against risk to the child.

4.7 Effects on ability to drive and use machines
Glyceryl trinitrate can cause postural hypotension and dizziness. Patients should not drive or operate machinery if they feel affected.

4.8 Undesirable effects
A very common (> 10% of patients) adverse reaction to the patch is headache. The incidence of headache diminishes gradually with time and continued use.

At start of therapy or when the dosage is increased, hypotension and/or light-headedness on standing are observed commonly (i.e. in 1-10% of patients). These symptoms may be associated with dizziness, drowsiness, reflex tachycardia, and a feeling of weakness.

Infrequently (i.e. in less than 1% of patients), nausea, vomiting, flushing and allergic skin reaction (e.g. rash), which may be severe can occur. Exfoliative dermatitis has been reported

Severe hypotensive responses have been reported for organic nitrates and include nausea, vomiting, restlessness, pallor and excessive perspiration. Uncommonly collapse may occur (sometimes accompanied by bradyarrhythmia and syncope). Uncommonly severe hypotension may lead to enhanced angina symptoms.

A few reports of heartburn, most likely due to a nitrate-induced sphincter relaxation, have been recorded.

Allergic skin reactions to glyceryl trinitrate and ingredients can occur, but they are uncommon (i.e. > 0.1% but < 1%). Patients may commonly experience slight itching or burning at the site of application. Slight reddening usually disappears without therapeutic measures after the patch has been removed. Allergic contact dermatitis is uncommon.

During the treatment with these patches, a temporary hypoxaemia may occur due to a relative redistribution of the blood flow in hypoventilated alveolar areas. Particularly in patients with coronary artery disease this may lead to a myocardial hypoxia.

4.9 Overdose
In view of the transdermal mode of delivery, an overdose of glyceryl trinitrate is unlikely to occur. However, in the unlikely event of an overdose, the symptoms could include the following:
- Fall in blood pressure ≤ 90 mmHg
- Paleness
- Sweating
- Weak pulse
- Tachycardia
- Flushing
- Light-headedness on standing
- Headache
- Weakness
- Dizziness
- Nausea
- Vomiting
- Methaemoglobinaemia has been reported in patients receiving other organic nitrates. During glyceryl trinitrate biotransformation nitrite ions are released, which may induce methaemoglobinaemia and cyanosis with subsequent tachypnoea, anxiety, loss of consciousness and cardiac arrest. It can not be excluded that an overdose of glyceryl trinitrate may cause this adverse reaction
- In very high doses the intracranial pressure may be increased. This might lead to cerebral symptoms

General procedure:
- Stop delivery of the drug. Since these patches are applied to the skin, removing the patch immediately stops delivery of the drug.
- General procedures in the event of nitrate-related hypotension

- Patient should be kept horizontal with the head lowered and legs raised
- Supply oxygen
- Expand plasma volume
- For specific shock treatment admit patient to intensive care unit

Special procedure:
- Raising the blood pressure if the blood pressure is very low
- Treatment of methaemoglobinaemia

Treatment with intravenous methylene blue
- Initially 1 to 2 mg/kg, not exceeding 4 mg/kg of a 1% solution over 5 minutes.
- Repeat dose in 60 minutes if there is no response.
- Administer oxygen (if necessary)
- Initiate artificial ventilation

Treatment with methylene blue is contraindicated in patients with glucose-6-phosphate dehydrogenase (G-6-PD) deficiency or methaemaglobin reductase deficiency.

Where treatment with methylene blue is contraindicated or is not effective, exchange transfusion and / or transfusion of packed red blood cells is recommended.

Resuscitation measures:

In case of signs of respiratory and circulatory arrest, initiate resuscitation measures immediately.

5. PHARMACOLOGICAL PROPERTIES
5.1 Pharmacodynamic properties
ATC Code: C01DA02, Vasodilators used in Cardiac Diseases, organic nitrates.

The main pharmacological activity of organic nitrates is the relaxation of smooth vascular muscles. The systemic vasodilation induces an increase of venous capacitance. Venous return is reduced. Ventricular volume, filling pressures and diastolic wall tension are diminished (preload reduction).

A diminished ventricular radius and reduced wall tension, lower myocardial energy and oxygen consumption, respectively.

The dilation of the large arteries near the heart leads to a decrease in both the systemic (reduction of afterload) and the pulmonary vascular resistance. In addition, this relieves the myocardium and lowers oxygen demands.

By dilating the large epicardial coronary arteries, glyceryl trinitrate enhances blood supply to the myocardium, improving its pump function and increasing the oxygen supply.

At molecular level, nitrates form nitric oxide (NO), which corresponds to the physical EDRF (endothelium derived relaxing factor). EDRF mediated production of cyclic guanosine monophosphate (CGMP) leads to relaxation of smooth muscle cells.

5.2 Pharmacokinetic properties
(a) *General characteristics of the active substance*
The transdermal absorption of glyceryl trinitrate circumvents the extensive hepatic first pass metabolism so the bioavailability is about 70% of that achieved after i.v. administration.

The steady-state concentration in the plasma depends on the patch dosage and the corresponding rate of absorption. At a rate of absorption of 0.4 mg/h, the steady-state concentration is about 0.2 μg/l on average. Plasma protein binding is about 60%. Glyceryl trinitrate is metabolized to 1,2- and 1,3-dinitroglycerols. The dinitrates exert less vasodilatory activity than glyceryl trinitrate. The contribution to the overall effect is not known. The dinitrates are further metabolized to inactive mononitrates, glyceryl and carbon dioxide.

The elimination half-life of glyceryl trinitrate is 2-4 min. The metabolism of glyceryl trinitrate, which is effected in the liver, but also in many other cells, e.g. the red blood cells, includes the separation of one or more nitrate groups. In addition to the metabolism of glyceryl trinitrate, there is a renal excretion of the catabolites.

(b) *Characteristics in patients*

There is no evidence that a dosage adjustment is required in the elderly or in diseases such as renal failure or hepatic insufficiency.

5.3 Preclinical safety data

Glyceryl trinitrate is a well-known active substance, established for more than a hundred years. Thus new preclinical studies have not been carried out with Deponit 10.

6. PHARMACEUTICAL PARTICULARS

6.1 List of excipients

Acrylate/vinyl acetate copolymer (adhesive matrix)

Polypropylene (backing foil)

Polyethylene (siliconised release liner)

6.2 Incompatibilities

No incompatibilities have so far been demonstrated.

6.3 Shelf life

Shelf life of the product as packaged for sale: 36 months.

6.4 Special precautions for storage

Do not store above 25°C

6.5 Nature and contents of container

Multilaminate film/foil pouch with heat-sealed edges.

28 patches per carton.

6.6 Special precautions for disposal and other handling

The patch should be removed from the package just before application. After removal of the protective foil, the patch should be applied to unbroken, clean and dry skin that is smooth and with few hairs. The same area of skin should not be used again for some days.

7. MARKETING AUTHORISATION HOLDER

UCB Pharma Limited

208 Bath Road

Slough

Berkshire

SL1 3WE

United Kingdom

8. MARKETING AUTHORISATION NUMBER(S)

PL 00039/0736

9. DATE OF FIRST AUTHORISATION/RENEWAL OF THE AUTHORISATION

28 February 2008

10. DATE OF REVISION OF THE TEXT

Deponit 5

(UCB Pharma Limited)

1. NAME OF THE MEDICINAL PRODUCT

Deponit 5

2. QUALITATIVE AND QUANTITATIVE COMPOSITION

One patch contains glyceryl trinitrate 18.7 mg

The average amount of glyceryl trinitrate absorbed from each patch in 24 hours is 5 mg.

3. PHARMACEUTICAL FORM

Transdermal patch

White, translucent square patch with convex round corners with "Deponit 5" marked on the outer face.

4. CLINICAL PARTICULARS

4.1 Therapeutic indications

Prophylaxis of angina pectoris alone or in combination with other anti-anginal therapy.

4.2 Posology and method of administration

Dermal

Adults: Treatment should be initiated with one patch daily. If necessary the dosage may be increased to two patches.

It is recommended that the patch is applied to healthy, undamaged, relatively crease free and hairless skin. The best places to apply Deponit patches are the easily reached, fairly static areas at the front or side of the chest. However, Deponit patches may also be applied to the upper arm, thigh, abdomen or shoulder. Skin care products should not be used before applying the patch. The replacement patch should be applied to a new area of skin. Allow several days to elapse before applying a fresh patch to the same area of skin.

Tolerance may occur during chronic nitrate therapy. Tolerance is likely to be avoided by allowing a patch-free period of 8-12 hours each day, usually at night.

Additional anti-anginal therapy with drugs not containing nitro compounds should be considered for the nitrate-free interval if required.

As with any nitrate therapy, treatment with these patches should not be stopped abruptly. If the patient is being changed to another type of treatment, the two should overlap.

Elderly: No specific information on use in the elderly is available, however there is no evidence to suggest that an alteration in dose is required.

Children: The safety and efficacy of this patch in children has yet to be established.

4.3 Contraindications

- Known hypersensitivity to nitrates or to the adhesives used in the patch
- Raised intracranial pressure including that caused by head trauma or cerebral haemorrhage
- Marked anaemia
- Closed angle glaucoma
- Hypotensive conditions and hypovolaemia
- Hypertrophic obstructive cardiomyopathy
- Aortic stenosis and mitral stenosis
- Constrictive pericarditis
- Cardiac tamponade
- Concomitant use of phosphodiesterase type-5 inhibitors. Phosphodiesterase type-5 inhibitors (e.g. sildenafil, tadalafil, vardenafil) have been shown to potentiate the hypotensive effects of nitrates, and their co-administration with nitrates or nitric oxide donors is therefore contra-indicated.

4.4 Special warnings and precautions for use

This patch should be used with caution in patients with

- Severe hepatic or renal impairment
- Hypothyroidism
- Hypothermia
- Malnutrition
- A recent history of myocardial infarction
- Hypoxaemia or a ventilation/perfusion imbalance due to lung disease or ischaemic heart failure.

The patch is not indicated for use in acute angina attacks. In the event of an acute angina attack, sublingual treatment such as a spray or tablet should be used. As with all nitrate preparations withdrawal of long-term treatment should be gradual by replacement with decreasing doses of long acting oral nitrates.

If the patches are not used as indicated (see Section 4.2) tolerance to the medication could develop.

4.5 Interaction with other medicinal products and other forms of interaction

Concomitant treatment with other vasodilators, calcium antagonists, ACE inhibitors, beta-blockers, diuretics, antihypertensives, tricyclic antidepressants and major tranquillisers, as well as the consumption of alcohol, may potentiate the hypotensive effect of the preparation.

The blood pressure lowering effect of these patches will be increased if used together with phosphodiesterase inhibitors (e.g. sildenafil) which are used for erectile dysfunction (see Section 4.3). This might lead to life threatening cardiovascular complications. Patients who are on nitrate therapy must not use phosphodiesterase inhibitors (e.g. sildenafil).

If administered concurrently, these patches may increase the blood level of dihydroergotamine and lead to coronary vasoconstriction.

The possibility that ingestion of acetylsalicylic acid and non-steroidal anti-inflammatory drugs might diminish the therapeutic response to the patch cannot be excluded.

4.6 Pregnancy and lactation

These patches should not be used during pregnancy or lactation unless considered absolutely essential by the physician.

It is not known whether the active substance passes into the breast milk. Benefits to the mother must be weighed against risk to the child.

4.7 Effects on ability to drive and use machines

Glyceryl trinitrate can cause postural hypotension and dizziness. Patients should not drive or operate machinery if they feel affected.

4.8 Undesirable effects

A very common (> 10% of patients) adverse reaction to the patch is headache. The incidence of headache diminishes gradually with time and continued use.

At start of therapy or when the dosage is increased, hypotension and/or light-headedness on standing are observed commonly (i.e. in 1-10% of patients). These symptoms may be associated with dizziness, drowsiness, reflex tachycardia, and a feeling of weakness.

Infrequently (i.e. in less than 1% of patients), nausea, vomiting, flushing and allergic skin reaction (e.g. rash), which may be severe can occur. Exfoliative dermatitis has been reported.

Severe hypotensive responses have been reported for organic nitrates and include nausea, vomiting, restlessness, pallor and excessive perspiration. Uncommonly collapse may occur (sometimes accompanied by bradyarrhythmia and syncope). Uncommonly severe hypotension may lead to enhanced angina symptoms.

A few reports of heartburn, most likely due to a nitrate-induced sphincter relaxation, have been recorded.

Allergic skin reactions to glyceryl trinitrate and ingredients can occur, but they are uncommon (i.e. > 0.1% but < 1%). Patients may commonly experience slight itching or burning at the site of application. Slight reddening usually disappears without therapeutic measures after the patch has been removed. Allergic contact dermatitis is uncommon.

During the treatment with these patches, a temporary hypoxaemia may occur due to a relative redistribution of the blood flow in hypoventilated alveolar areas. Particularly in patients with coronary artery disease this may lead to a myocardial hypoxia.

4.9 Overdose

In view of the transdermal mode of delivery, an overdose of glyceryl trinitrate is unlikely to occur. However, in the unlikely event of an overdose, the symptoms could include the following:

- Fall in blood pressure ⩽ 90 mmHg
- Paleness
- Sweating
- Weak pulse
- Tachycardia
- Flushing
- Light-headedness on standing
- Headache
- Weakness
- Dizziness
- Nausea
- Vomiting
- Methaemoglobinaemia has been reported in patients receiving other organic nitrates. During glyceryl trinitrate biotransformation nitrite ions are released, which may induce methaemoglobinaemia and cyanosis with subsequent tachypnoea, anxiety, loss of consciousness and cardiac arrest. It can not be excluded that an overdose of glyceryl trinitrate may cause this adverse reaction
- In very high doses the intracranial pressure may be increased. This might lead to cerebral symptoms

General procedure:

- Stop delivery of the drug. Since these patches are applied to the skin, removing the patch immediately stops delivery of the drug.
- General procedures in the event of nitrate-related hypotension

- Patient should be kept horizontal with the head lowered and legs raised

- Supply oxygen

- Expand plasma volume

- For specific shock treatment admit patient to intensive care unit

Special procedure:

- Raising the blood pressure if the blood pressure is very low
- Treatment of methaemoglobinaemia

Treatment with intravenous methylene blue

- Initially 1 to 2 mg/kg, not exceeding 4 mg/kg of a 1% solution over 5 minutes.

- Repeat dose in 60 minutes if there is no response.

- Administer oxygen (if necessary)

- Initiate artificial ventilation

Treatment with methylene blue is contraindicated in patients with glucose-6-phosphate dehydrogenase (G-6-PD) deficiency or methaemaglobin reductase deficiency.

Where treatment with methylene blue is contraindicated or is not effective, exchange transfusion and / or transfusion of packed red blood cells is recommended.

Resuscitation measures:

In case of signs of respiratory and circulatory arrest, initiate resuscitation measures immediately.

5. PHARMACOLOGICAL PROPERTIES

5.1 Pharmacodynamic properties

ATC Code: C01DA02, Vasodilators used in Cardiac Diseases, organic nitrates.

The main pharmacological activity of organic nitrates is the relaxation of smooth vascular muscles. The systemic vasodilation induces an increase of venous capacitance. Venous return is reduced. Ventricular volume, filling pressures and diastolic wall tension are diminished (preload reduction).

A diminished ventricular radius and reduced wall tension, lower myocardial energy and oxygen consumption, respectively.

The dilation of the large arteries near the heart leads to a decrease in both the systemic (reduction of afterload) and the pulmonary vascular resistance. In addition, this relieves the myocardium and lowers oxygen demands.

By dilating the large epicardial coronary arteries, glyceryl trinitrate enhances blood supply to the myocardium, improving its pump function and increasing the oxygen supply.

At molecular level, nitrates form nitric oxide (NO), which corresponds to the physical EDRF (endothelium derived relaxing factor). EDRF mediated production of cyclic guanosine monophosphate (CGMP) leads to relaxation of smooth muscle cells.

5.2 Pharmacokinetic properties

(a) *General characteristics of the active substance*

The transdermal absorption of glyceryl trinitrate circumvents the extensive hepatic first pass metabolism so the bioavailability is about 70% of that achieved after i.v. administration.

The steady-state concentration in the plasma depends on the patch dosage and the corresponding rate of absorption. At a rate of absorption of 0.4 mg/h, the steady-state concentration is about 0.2 µg/l on average. Plasma protein binding is about 60%. Glyceryl trinitrate is metabolized to 1,2- and 1,3-dinitroglycerols. The dinitrates exert less vasodilatory activity than glyceryl trinitrate. The contribution to the overall effect is not known. The dinitrates are further metabolized to inactive mononitrates, glyceryl and carbon dioxide.

The elimination half-life of glyceryl trinitrate is 2-4 min. The metabolism of glyceryl trinitrate, which is effected in the liver, but also in many other cells, e.g. the red blood cells, includes the separation of one or more nitrate groups. In addition to the metabolism of glyceryl trinitrate, there is a renal excretion of the catabolites.

(b) *Characteristics in patients*

There is no evidence that a dosage adjustment is required in the elderly or in diseases such as renal failure or hepatic insufficiency.

5.3 Preclinical safety data

Glyceryl trinitrate is a well-known active substance, established for more than a hundred years. Thus new preclinical studies have not been carried out with Deponit 5.

6. PHARMACEUTICAL PARTICULARS

6.1 List of excipients

Acrylate/vinyl acetate copolymer (adhesive matrix)

Polypropylene (backing foil)

Polyethylene (siliconised release liner)

6.2 Incompatibilities

No incompatibilities have so far been demonstrated.

6.3 Shelf life

Shelf life of the product as packaged for sale: 36 months.

6.4 Special precautions for storage

Do not store above 25°C.

6.5 Nature and contents of container

Multi-laminate film/foil pouch with heat-sealed edges.

28 patches per carton.

6.6 Special precautions for disposal and other handling

Each patch should be removed from the package just before application. After removal of the protective foil, the patch should be applied to unbroken, clean and dry skin that is smooth and with few hairs. The same area of skin should not be used again for some days.

7. MARKETING AUTHORISATION HOLDER

UCB Pharma Limited

208 Bath Road

Slough

Berkshire

SL1 3WE

United Kingdom

8. MARKETING AUTHORISATION NUMBER(S)

PL 00039/0735

9. DATE OF FIRST AUTHORISATION/RENEWAL OF THE AUTHORISATION

28 February 2008

10. DATE OF REVISION OF THE TEXT

Depo-Provera 150mg/ml Injection

(Pharmacia Limited)

1. NAME OF THE MEDICINAL PRODUCT

Depo-Provera 150 mg/ml

2. QUALITATIVE AND QUANTITATIVE COMPOSITION

Each ml of suspension contains 150 mg medroxyprogesterone acetate Ph. Eur.

For excipients, see section 6.1

3. PHARMACEUTICAL FORM

Sterile suspension for injection.

4. CLINICAL PARTICULARS

4.1 Therapeutic indications

Progestogen: for contraception.

Depo-Provera is a long-term contraceptive agent suitable for use in women who have been appropriately counselled concerning the likelihood of menstrual disturbance and the potential for a delay in return to full fertility.

Depo-Provera may also be used for short-term contraception in the following circumstances:

(i) For partners of men undergoing vasectomy, for protection until the vasectomy becomes effective.

(ii) In women who are being immunised against rubella, to prevent pregnancy during the period of activity of the virus.

(iii) In women awaiting sterilisation.

Since loss of bone mineral density (BMD) may occur in females of all ages who use Depo-Provera injection long-term (see section 4.4 Special Warnings and Special Precautions for Use), a risk/benefit assessment, which also takes into consideration the decrease in BMD that occurs during pregnancy and/or lactation, should be considered.

Use in adolescents (12-18 years)

In adolescents, Depo-Provera may be used, but only after other methods of contraception have been discussed with the patient and considered unsuitable or unacceptable.

It is of the greatest importance that adequate explanations of the long-term nature of the product, of its possible side-effects and of the impossibility of immediately reversing the effects of each injection are given to potential users and that every effort is made to ensure that each patient receives such counselling as to enable her to fully understand these explanations. Patient information leaflets are supplied by the manufacturer. It is recommended that the doctor uses these leaflets to aid counselling of the patient.

Consistent with good clinical practice a general medical as well as gynaecological examination should be undertaken before administration of Depo-Provera and at appropriate intervals thereafter.

4.2 Posology and method of administration

The sterile aqueous suspension of Depo-Provera should be vigorously shaken just before use to ensure that the dose being given represents a uniform suspension of Depo-Provera.

Doses should be given by deep intramuscular injection. Care should be taken to ensure that the depot injection is given into the muscle tissue, preferably the gluteus maximus, but other muscle issue such as the deltoid may be used.

The site of injection should be cleansed using standard methods prior to administration of the injection.

Adults:

First injection: To provide contraceptive cover in the first cycle of use, an injection of 150 mg i.m. should be given during the first five days of a normal menstrual cycle. If the injection is carried out according to these instructions, no additional contraceptive cover is required.

Post Partum: To increase assurance that the patient is not pregnant at the time of first administration, this injection should be given within 5 days post partum if not breast-feeding.

There is evidence that women prescribed Depo-Provera in the immediate puerperium can experience prolonged and heavy bleeding. Because of this, the drug should be used with caution in the puerperium. Women who are considering use of the product immediately following delivery or termination should be advised that the risk of heavy or prolonged bleeding may be increased. Doctors are reminded that in the non breast-feeding, post partum patient, ovulation may occur as early as week 4.

If the puerperal woman will be breast-feeding, the initial injection should be given no sooner than six weeks post partum, when the infant's enzyme system is more fully developed. Further injections should be given at 12 week intervals.

Further doses: These should be given at 12 week intervals, however, as long as the injection is given no later than five days after this time, no additional contraceptive measures (e.g. barrier) are required. (N.B. For partners of men undergoing vasectomy a second injection of 150 mg i.m. 12 weeks after the first may be necessary in a small proportion of patients where the partner's sperm count has not fallen to zero.) If the interval from the preceding injection is greater than 89 days (12 weeks and five days) for any reason, then pregnancy should be excluded before the next injection is given and the patient should use additional contraceptive measures (e.g. barrier) for fourteen days after this subsequent injection.

Elderly: Not appropriate.

Children: Depo-Provera is not indicated before menarche (see section 4.1 Therapeutic Indications)

Data in adolescent females (12-18 years) is available (see section 4.4 Special Warnings and Special Precautions for Use). Other than concerns about loss of BMD, the safety and effectiveness of Depo-Provera is expected to be the same for adolescents after menarche and adult females

4.3 Contraindications

Depo-Provera is contra-indicated in patients with a known sensitivity to medroxyprogesterone acetate or any ingredient of the vehicle.

Depo-Provera should not be used during pregnancy, either for diagnosis or therapy.

Depo-Provera is contra-indicated as a contraceptive at the above dosage in known or suspected hormone-dependent malignancy of breast or genital organs.

Whether administered alone or in combination with oestrogen, Depo-Provera should not be employed in patients with abnormal uterine bleeding until a definite diagnosis has been established and the possibility of genital tract malignancy eliminated.

4.4 Special warnings and precautions for use

Warnings:

Loss of Bone Mineral Density: Use of Depo-Provera injection reduces serum oestrogen levels and is associated with significant loss of BMD due to the known effect of oestrogen deficiency on the bone remodelling system. Bone loss is greater with increasing duration of use and appears to be at least partially reversible after Depo-Provera injection is discontinued and ovarian oestrogen production increases.

This loss of BMD is of particular concern during adolescence and early adulthood, a critical period of bone accretion (see section 4.1 Therapeutic Indications) It is unknown if use of Depo-Provera injection by younger women will reduce peak bone mass and increase the risk for osteoporotic fracture in later life.

A study to assess the reversibility of loss of BMD in adolescent females is ongoing. In adolescents, Depo-Provera may be used, but only after other methods of contraception have been discussed with the patients and considered to be unsuitable or unacceptable. In women of all ages, careful re-evaluation of the risks and benefits of treatment should be carried out in those who wish to continue use for more than 2 years. In women with significant lifestyle and/or medical risk factors for osteoporosis, other methods of contraception should be considered prior to Depo-Provera.

Menstrual Irregularity: The administration of Depo-Provera usually causes disruption of the normal menstrual cycle. Bleeding patterns include amenorrhoea (present in up to 30% of women during the first 3 months and increasing to 55% by month 12 and 68% by month 24); irregular bleeding and spotting; prolonged (>10 days) episodes of bleeding (up to 33% of women in the first 3 months of use decreasing to 12% by month 12). Rarely, heavy prolonged bleeding may occur. Evidence suggests that prolonged or heavy bleeding requiring treatment may occur in 0.5-4 occasions per 100 women years of use. If abnormal bleeding persists or is severe, appropriate investigation should take place to rule out the possibility of organic pathology and appropriate treatment should be instituted when necessary. Excessive or prolonged bleeding can be controlled by the co-administration of oestrogen. This may be delivered either in the form of a low dose (30 micrograms oestrogen) combined oral contraceptive pill or in the form of oestrogen replacement therapy such as conjugated equine oestrogen (0.625-1.25 mg daily). Oestrogen therapy may need to be repeated for 1-2 cycles. Long-term co-administration of oestrogen is not recommended.

Return to Fertility: There is no evidence that Depo-Provera causes permanent infertility. Pregnancies have occurred as early as 14 weeks after a preceding injection, however, in clinical trials, the mean time to return of ovulation was 5.3 months following the preceding injection. Women should be counselled that there is a potential for delay in return to full fertility following use of the method, regardless of the duration of use, however, 83% of women may be expected to conceive within 12 months of the first "missed" injection (i.e. 15 months after the last injection administered). The median time to conception was 10 months (range 4-31) after the last injection.

Cancer Risks: Long-term case-controlled surveillance of Depo-Provera users found no overall increased risk of ovarian, liver, or cervical cancer and a prolonged, protective effect of reducing the risk of endometrial cancer in the population of users. A meta-analysis in 1996 from 54 epidemiological studies[1] reported that there is a slight increased relative risk of having breast cancer diagnosed in women who are currently using hormonal contraceptives. The observed pattern of increased risk may be due to an earlier diagnosis of breast cancer in hormonal contraceptive users, biological effects or a combination of both. The additional breast cancers diagnosed in current users of hormonal contraceptives or in women who have used them in the last ten years are more likely to be localised to the breast than those in women who never used hormonal contraceptives.

Breast cancer is rare among women under 40 years of age whether or not they use hormonal contraceptives. In the meta-analysis the results for injectable progestogens (1.5% of the data) and progestogen only pills (0.8% of the data) did not reach significance although there was no evidence that they differed from other hormonal contraceptives. Whilst the background risk of breast cancer increases with age, the excess number of breast cancer diagnoses in current and recent injectable progestogen (IP) users is small in relation to the overall risk of breast cancer, possibly of similar magnitude to that associated with combined oral contraceptives. However, for IPs, the evidence is based on much smaller populations of users (less than 1.5% of the data) and is less conclusive than for combined oral contraceptives. It is not possible to infer from these data whether it is due to an earlier diagnosis of breast cancer in ever-users, the biological effects of hormonal contraceptives, or a combination of reasons.

The most important risk factor for breast cancer in IP users is the age women discontinue the IP; the older the age at stopping, the more breast cancers are diagnosed. Duration of use is less important and the excess risk gradually disappears during the course of the 10 years after stopping IP use, such that by 10 years there appears to be no excess.

The evidence suggests that compared with never-users, among 10,000 women who use IPs for up to 5 years but stop by age 20, there would be much less than 1 extra case of breast cancer diagnosed up to 10 years afterwards. For those stopping by age 30 after 5 years use of the IP, there would be an estimated 2-3 extra cases (additional to the 44 cases of breast cancer per 10,000 women in this age group never exposed to oral contraceptives). For those stopping by age 40 after 5 years use, there would be an estimated 10 extra cases diagnosed up to 10 years afterwards (additional to the 160 cases of breast cancer per 10,000 never-exposed women in this age group).

It is important to inform patients that users of all hormonal contraceptives appear to have a small increase in the risk of being diagnosed with breast cancer, compared with non-users of hormonal contraceptives, but that this has to be weighed against the known benefits.

Weight Gain: There is a tendency for women to gain weight while on Depo-Provera therapy. Studies indicate that over the first 1-2 years of use, average weight gain was 5-8 lbs. Women completing 4-6 years of therapy gained an average of 14-16.5 lbs. There is evidence that weight is gained as a result of increased fat and is not secondary to an anabolic effect or fluid retention.

Anaphylaxis: Very few reports of anaphylactoid reactions have been received.

Thrombo-embolic Disorders: Should the patient experience pulmonary embolism, cerebrovascular disease or retinal thrombosis while receiving Depo-Provera, the drug should not be readministered.

Psychiatric Disorders: Patients with a history of endogenous depression should be carefully monitored. Some patients may complain of premenstrual-type depression while on Depo-Provera therapy.

Abscess formation: As with any intramuscular injection, especially if not administered correctly, there is a risk of abscess formation at the site of injection, which may require medical and/or surgical intervention.

Precautions:

History or emergence of the following conditions require careful consideration and appropriate investigation: migraine or unusually severe headaches, acute visual disturbances of any kind, pathological changes in liver function and hormone levels. Patients with thromboembolic or coronary vascular disease should be carefully evaluated before using Depo-Provera.

A decrease in glucose tolerance has been observed in some patients treated with progestogens. The mechanism for this decrease is obscure. For this reason, diabetic patients should be carefully monitored while receiving progestogen therapy.

Rare cases of thrombo-embolism have been reported with use of Depo-Provera, but causality has not been established.

The effects of medroxyprogesterone acetate on lipid metabolism have been studied with no clear impact demonstrated. Both increases and decreases in total cholesterol, triglycerides and low-density lipoprotein (LDL) cholesterol have been observed in studies. The use of Depo-Provera appears to be associated with a 15-20% reduction in serum high density lipoprotein (HDL) cholesterol levels which may protect women from cardiovascular disease. The clinical consequences of this observation are unknown. The potential for an increased risk of coronary disease should be considered prior to use.

Doctors should carefully consider the use of Depo-Provera in patients with recent trophoblastic disease before levels of human chorionic gonadotrophin have returned to normal.

Physicians should be aware that pathologists should be informed of the patient's use of Depo-Provera if endometrial or endocervical tissue is submitted for examination.

The results of certain laboratory tests may be affected by the use of Depo-Provera. These include gonadotrophin levels (decreased), plasma progesterone levels (decreased), urinary pregnanediol levels (decreased), plasma oestrogen levels (decreased), plasma cortisol levels (decreased), glucose tolerance test, metyrapone test, liver function tests (may increase), thyroid function tests (protein bound iodine levels may increase and T3 uptake levels may decrease). Coagulation test values for prothrombin (Factor II), and Factors VII, VIII, IX and X may increase.

4.5 Interaction with other medicinal products and other forms of interaction

Aminoglutethimide administered concurrently with Depo-Provera may significantly depress the bioavailability of Depo-Provera.

Interactions with other medicinal treatments (including oral anticoagulants) have rarely been reported, but causality has not been determined. The possibility of interaction should be borne in mind in patients receiving concurrent treatment with other drugs.

The clearance of medroxyprogesterone acetate is approximately equal to the rate of hepatic blood flow. Because of this fact, it is unlikely that drugs which induce hepatic enzymes will significantly affect the kinetics of medroxyprogesterone acetate. Therefore, no dose adjustment is recommended in patients receiving drugs known to affect hepatic metabolising enzymes.

4.6 Pregnancy and lactation

Doctors should check that patients are not pregnant before initial injection of Depo-Provera, and also if administration of any subsequent injection is delayed beyond 89 days (12 weeks and five days).

Infants from accidental pregnancies that occur 1-2 months after injection of Depo-Provera may be at an increased risk of low birth weight, which in turn is associated with an increased risk of neonatal death. The attributable risk is low because such pregnancies are uncommon.

Children exposed to medroxyprogesterone acetate *in utero* and followed to adolescence, showed no evidence of any adverse effects on their health including their physical, intellectual, sexual or social development.

Medroxyprogesterone acetate and/or its metabolites are secreted in breast milk, but there is no evidence to suggest that this presents any hazard to the child. Infants exposed to medroxyprogesterone via breast milk have been studied for developmental and behavioural effects to puberty. No adverse effects have been noted.

4.7 Effects on ability to drive and use machines

None

4.8 Undesirable effects

In a large clinical trial of over 3900 women, who were treated with Depo-Provera for up to 7 years, the following adverse events were reported.

The following adverse events were commonly (by more than 5% of subjects) reported: menstrual irregularities (bleeding and/or amenorrhoea), weight changes, headache, nervousness, abdominal pain or discomfort, dizziness, asthenia (weakness or fatigue).

Adverse events reported by 1% to 5% of subjects using Depo-Provera were: decreased libido or anorgasmia, backache, leg cramps, depression, nausea, insomnia, leucorrhoea, acne, vaginitis, pelvic pain, breast pain, no hair growth or alopecia, bloating, rash, oedema, hot flushes.

Other events were reported infrequently (by fewer than 1 % of subjects), and included: galactorrhoea, melasma, chloasma, convulsions, changes in appetite, gastrointestinal disturbances, jaundice, genitourinary infections, vaginal cysts, dyspareunia, paraesthesia, chest pain, pulmonary embolus, allergic reactions, anaemia, syncope, dyspnoea, thirst, hoarseness, somnolence, decreased glucose tolerance, hirsutism, pruritus, arthralgia, pyrexia, pain at injection site, injection site abscess, blood dyscrasia, rectal bleeding, changes in breast size, breast lumps or nipple bleeding, axillary swelling, prevention of lactation, sensation of pregnancy, lack of return to fertility, paralysis, facial palsy, scleroderma, osteoporosis, uterine hyperplasia, varicose veins, dysmenorrhoea, thrombophlebitis, deep vein thrombosis.

In postmarketing experience, there have been rare cases of osteoporosis including osteoporotic fractures reported in patients taking Depo-Provera.

4.9 Overdose

No positive action is required other than cessation of therapy.

5. PHARMACOLOGICAL PROPERTIES

5.1 Pharmacodynamic properties

Medroxyprogesterone acetate exerts anti-oestrogenic, anti-androgenic and antigonadotrophic effects.

BMD Changes in Adult Women

In a controlled, clinical study adult women using Depo-Provera injection (150 mg IM) for up to 5 years showed spine and hip mean BMD decreases of 5-6%, compared to no significant change in BMD in the control group. The decline in BMD was more pronounced during the first two years of use, with smaller declines in subsequent years. Mean changes in lumbar spine BMD of –2.86%, -4.11%, -4.89%, -4.93% and –5.38% after 1, 2, 3, 4 and 5 years, respectively, were observed. Mean decreases in BMD of the total hip and femoral neck were similar.

After stopping use of Depo-Provera injection (150 mg IM), there was partial recovery of BMD toward baseline values during the 2-year post-therapy period. A longer duration of treatment was associated with a slower rate of BMD recovery.

Table 1. Mean Percent Change from Baseline in BMD in Adults by Skeletal Site and Cohort after 5 Years of Therapy with Depo-Provera 150mg IM and After 2 Years Post-Therapy or 7 Years of Observation (Control)

(see Table 1 below)

BMD Changes in Adolescent Females (12-18 years)

Preliminary results from an ongoing, open-label clinical study of Depo-Provera injectable (150 mg IM every 12 weeks for up to 5 years) in adolescent females (12-18 years) also showed that Depo-Provera IM use was associated with a significant decline in BMD from baseline. The mean decrease in lumbar spine BMD was 4.2% after 5 years; mean decreases for the total hip and femoral neck were 6.9% and 6.1%, respectively. In contrast, most adolescent girls will significantly increase bone density during this period of growth following menarche. Preliminary data from a small number of adolescents have shown partial recovery of BMD during the 2-year follow-up period.

5.2 Pharmacokinetic properties

Parenteral medroxyprogesterone acetate (MPA) is a long acting progestational steroid. The long duration of action results from its slow absorption from the injection site. Immediately after injection of 150 mg/ml MPA, plasma levels were 1.7 ± 0.3 nmol/l. Two weeks later, levels were 6.8 ± 0.8 nmol/l. Concentrations fell to the initial levels by the end of 12 weeks. At lower doses, plasma levels of MPA appear directly related to the dose administered. Serum accumulation over time was not demonstrated. MPA is eliminated via faecal and urinary excretion. Plasma half-life is about six weeks after a single intramuscular injection. At least 11 metabolites have been reported. All are excreted in the urine, some, but not all, conjugated.

6. PHARMACEUTICAL PARTICULARS

6.1 List of excipients

Excipients are methylparaben, macrogol 3350, polysorbate 80, propylparaben, sodium chloride, hydrochloric acid, sodium hydroxide and water for injections.

6.2 Incompatibilities

None known.

6.3 Shelf life

Syringe: 36 months.

Vial: 18 months

6.4 Special precautions for storage

Do not store above 25°C.

Do not freeze.

6.5 Nature and contents of container

1 ml disposable syringe with plunger stopper and tip cap.

1 ml vial with stopper and tip cap.

6.6 Special precautions for disposal and other handling

No special instructions are applicable.

Administrative Data

7. MARKETING AUTHORISATION HOLDER

Pharmacia Limited

Ramsgate Road

Sandwich

CT13 9NJ

UK

8. MARKETING AUTHORISATION NUMBER(S)

PL 0032/0082

9. DATE OF FIRST AUTHORISATION/RENEWAL OF THE AUTHORISATION

Date of Grant: 27 August 1991

Date of Renewal: 6 February 1997

Table 1 Mean Percent Change from Baseline in BMD in Adults by Skeletal Site and Cohort after 5 Years of Therapy with Depo-Provera 150mg IM and After 2 Years Post-Therapy or 7 Years of Observation (Control)

Time In Study	Spine		Total Hip		Femoral Neck	
	Depo-Provera	Control	Depo-Provera	Control	Depo-Provera	Control
5 Years*	n=33 -5.38%	n=105 0.43%	n=21 -5.16%	n=65 0.19%	n=34 -6.12%	n=106 -0.27%
7 Years**	n=12 -3.13%	n=60 0.53%	n=7 -1.34%	n=39 0.94%	n=13 -5.38%	n=63 -0.11%

*The treatment group consisted of women who received Depo-Provera Contraceptive injection for 5 years and the control group consisted of women who did not use hormonal contraception for this time period.

**The treatment group consisted of women who received Depo-Provera Contraceptive injection for 5 years and then were followed up for 2 years post-use control group consisted of women who did not use hormonal contraception for 7 years.

10. DATE OF REVISION OF THE TEXT
July 2007

Company Reference: DP2_0

Derbac M Liquid

(SSL International plc)

1. NAME OF THE MEDICINAL PRODUCT
Derbac M Liquid

2. QUALITATIVE AND QUANTITATIVE COMPOSITION
Malathion 0.5% w/w

For excipients, see 6.1.

3. PHARMACEUTICAL FORM
Liquid emulsion.

4. CLINICAL PARTICULARS

4.1 Therapeutic indications
For the eradication of head lice, pubic lice and their eggs. Treatment of scabies.

4.2 Posology and method of administration
For topical external use only.

Adults, the elderly and children aged 6 months and over:

As this product does not contain alcohol, it may be more suitable for those with asthma or eczema.

1. Treatment of head lice:

Rub the liquid into the scalp until all the hair and scalp is thoroughly moistened. Leave the hair to dry naturally in a warm but well ventilated room. After 12 hours, or the next day if preferred, shampoo the hair in the normal way.

Rinse the hair and comb whilst wet to remove the dead lice and eggs (nits) using the Derbac Nit Comb.

Treatment should be repeated after 7 days.

2. Treatment of crab (pubic) lice:

Apply Derbac M Liquid to the entire skin surface. Pay particular attention to all hairy areas including beards and moustaches.

Avoid any other areas above the neck. Leave on for at least one hour before washing but preferably Derbac M Liquid should be left on overnight. Wash off in the usual manner.

Treatment should be repeated after 7 days.

3. Treatment of scabies:

Apply Derbac M Liquid to the entire skin surface. In adults it may not be necessary to apply above the neck but children under the age of two years should have a thin film of Derbac M Liquid applied to the scalp, face and ears, avoiding the eyes and mouth.

Do not wash off or bathe for 24 hours. If hands or any other parts must be washed during this period, the treatment must be reapplied to those areas immediately.

Treatment should be repeated after 7 days.

No special sterilisation of clothing is necessary: ordinary laundering or dry cleaning with hot iron pressing are sufficient.

The infestation is cleared by the treatment. However, the itching and rash may persist for up to 7 days. An anti-irritant cream can be applied if necessary.

Family members and close contacts should also be treated simultaneously.

Children aged 6 months and under:

Under medical supervision only.

4.3 Contraindications
Known sensitivity to malathion. Not to be used on infants less than 6 months except on medical advice.

4.4 Special warnings and precautions for use
Avoid contact with the eyes. For external use only. Keep out of the reach of children. If inadvertently swallowed, a doctor or casualty department should be contacted at once.

When Derbac M Liquid is used by a school nurse or other health officer in the mass treatment of large numbers of children, it is advisable that protective plastic or rubber gloves be worn.

Continued prolonged treatment with this product should be avoided. It should be used not more than once a week and for not more than 3 consecutive weeks.

4.5 Interaction with other medicinal products and other forms of interaction
None stated.

4.6 Pregnancy and lactation
No known effects in pregnancy and lactation. However, as with all medicines, use with caution.

4.7 Effects on ability to drive and use machines
None stated.

4.8 Undesirable effects
Skin irritation and hypersensitivity reactions such as anaphylaxis, angioedema, and swollen eyes have been reported with malathion products. Chemical burns have also been reported.

4.9 Overdose
It is most unlikely that a toxic dose of malathion will be ingested. Treatment consists of gastric lavage, assisted respiration and, if necessary in the event of massive ingestion, administration of atropine together with pralidoxime.

5. PHARMACOLOGICAL PROPERTIES

5.1 Pharmacodynamic properties
Pharmacotherapeutic group: Malathion, ATC code: P03AX03

Derbac M Liquid contains malathion, a widely used organophosphorus insecticide which is active by cholinesterase inhibition. It is effective against a wide range of insects, but is one of the least toxic organophosphorus insecticides since it is rapidly detoxified by plasma carboxylesterases.

5.2 Pharmacokinetic properties
None stated. Derbac M Liquid is applied topically to the affected area.

5.3 Preclinical safety data
None stated.

6. PHARMACEUTICAL PARTICULARS

6.1 List of excipients
Methyl hydroxybenzoate

Propyl hydroxybenzoate

Lanette Wax SX

Potassium citrate

Citric acid

Perfume HT 52

Water

6.2 Incompatibilities
None stated

6.3 Shelf life
Two and a half years unopened

6.4 Special precautions for storage
Store at or below 25°C. Protect from light.

6.5 Nature and contents of container
Cartoned, clear or amber glass bottles with polyethylene caps and polypropylene faced wads containing either 50, 2 × 50, 55, 100, 200 or 210 ml of product.

Not all pack sizes may be marketed.

6.6 Special precautions for disposal and other handling
None stated.

7. MARKETING AUTHORISATION HOLDER
Seton Products Limited, Tubiton House, Oldham, OL1 3HS.

8. MARKETING AUTHORISATION NUMBER(S)
PL 11314/0046.

9. DATE OF FIRST AUTHORISATION/RENEWAL OF THE AUTHORISATION
13/10/95 / 11/09/00

10. DATE OF REVISION OF THE TEXT
February 2008

Dermalo Bath Emollient

(Dermal Laboratories Limited)

1. NAME OF THE MEDICINAL PRODUCT
DERMALO® BATH EMOLLIENT

2. QUALITATIVE AND QUANTITATIVE COMPOSITION
Liquid Paraffin 65.0% w/w; Acetylated Wool Alcohols 5.0% w/w.

3. PHARMACEUTICAL FORM
Bath additive. Dye- and fragrance-free colourless to straw coloured clear oily liquid.

4. CLINICAL PARTICULARS

4.1 Therapeutic indications
For the symptomatic relief of contact dermatitis, atopic dermatitis, senile pruritus, ichthyosis and related dry skin disorders.

4.2 Posology and method of administration
Adults, including the elderly: Add 15 to 20 ml (1½ to 2 capfuls) to a standard bath of water (8 inch depth). Immerse and cover the affected areas with the bath water and soak for 10 to 20 minutes. Pat dry with a towel. Alternatively, use a similar amount smoothed onto wet skin following a shower. Rinse off thoroughly and pat dry with a towel.

Infants and children: Add 5 to 10 ml (½ to 1 capful) to a small bath or wash basin of water. Immerse and cover the affected areas with the bath water and soak for 10 to 20 minutes. Alternatively, repeatedly gently sponge over the affected areas. Pat dry with a towel.

There is no differentiation between the dosage quantities for the symptomatic relief of the conditions listed.

4.3 Contraindications
Sensitivity to any of the ingredients.

4.4 Special warnings and precautions for use
Take care not to slip in the bath or shower. Surfaces that have been in contact with the product should be cleaned with a proprietary detergent. Keep out of the reach of children. For external use only.

4.5 Interaction with other medicinal products and other forms of interaction
None known.

4.6 Pregnancy and lactation
The constituents are not percutaneously absorbed or toxic if ingested. There is no evidence of safety of the drug used in pregnancy or lactation, but the active constituents have been in widespread use and in similar preparations for many years without apparent ill consequence.

4.7 Effects on ability to drive and use machines
None known.

4.8 Undesirable effects
Contact sensitivity reactions or mild irritant reactions may occur occasionally. In either case, treatment should be discontinued.

4.9 Overdose
Accidental ingestion may result in a purgative action due to the liquid paraffin and the oily nature of the product. Treat symptomatically. Fluid and electrolyte replacement may be necessary.

5. PHARMACOLOGICAL PROPERTIES

5.1 Pharmacodynamic properties
For dry skin conditions it is important to use an emollient while bathing. Dermalo Bath Emollient contains 65% Liquid Paraffin and 5% Acetylated Wool Alcohols for their moisturising and skin softening properties, and is specially formulated to facilitate dispersion in bath water or for ease of application after a shower.

5.2 Pharmacokinetic properties
The active constituents are not absorbed percutaneously. Pharmacokinetic particulars are thus not relevant.

5.3 Preclinical safety data
No relevant information additional to that contained elsewhere in the SPC.

6. PHARMACEUTICAL PARTICULARS

6.1 List of excipients
Isopropyl Myristate; Macrogol 3 Lauryl Ether.

6.2 Incompatibilities
None known.

6.3 Shelf life
36 months.

6.4 Special precautions for storage
Do not store above 25°C.

6.5 Nature and contents of container
500 ml white plastic bottle fitted with a dispensing plug and screw cap. Supplied in original packs (OP).

6.6 Special precautions for disposal and other handling
Not applicable.

7. MARKETING AUTHORISATION HOLDER
Dermal Laboratories

Tatmore Place, Gosmore

Hitchin, Herts SG4 7QR, UK.

8. MARKETING AUTHORISATION NUMBER(S)
00173/0182.

9. DATE OF FIRST AUTHORISATION/RENEWAL OF THE AUTHORISATION
29 August 2008.

10. DATE OF REVISION OF THE TEXT
August 2008.

Dermamist

(Alliance Pharmaceuticals)

1. NAME OF THE MEDICINAL PRODUCT
Dermamist

2. QUALITATIVE AND QUANTITATIVE COMPOSITION
White Soft Paraffin BP 10.0% w/w.

3. PHARMACEUTICAL FORM
Pressurised aerosol

4. CLINICAL PARTICULARS

4.1 Therapeutic indications
Treatment of dry skin conditions including eczema, ichthyosis and pruritus of the elderly.

4.2 Posology and method of administration
Adults, children and the elderly: Shake before use. Bathe or shower for not more than ten minutes. Pat dry and apply spray without delay. Do not spray on face. Spray from a distance of approximately 8 inches. Spray away from the face and move the can while spraying to achieve a very light coverage of the body. Spray sparingly; over application may cause the skin to feel oily.

4.3 Contraindications
Hypersensitivity to any of the ingredients.

4.4 Special warnings and precautions for use
For external use only. Keep out of reach of children. Do not spray on face. Use in a ventilated area. Avoid inhalation. Guard against slipping. Discontinue use if the condition is made worse. Do not apply to broken skin.

Patients being dispensed or treated with large quantities (> 100g) of any paraffin based product should be advised to regularly change clothing or bedding impregnated with the product and keep away from naked flames as there is a fire hazard.

4.5 Interaction with other medicinal products and other forms of interaction
None.

4.6 Pregnancy and lactation
Can be used.

4.7 Effects on ability to drive and use machines
Not relevant.

4.8 Undesirable effects
Not relevant

4.9 Overdose
None

5. PHARMACOLOGICAL PROPERTIES

5.1 Pharmacodynamic properties
Emollients are fats or oils used for their local action on the skin and, occasionally, the mucous membranes. These oleaginous substances, also known as occlusive agents and humectants, are employed as protectives and as agents for softening the skin and rendering it more pliable. White soft paraffin forms an effective occlusive lipid film. The mechanism of action is by occluding water loss from the outer layer of skin.

5.2 Pharmacokinetic properties
White soft paraffin exerts its physiological effects by forming an occlusive layer on the surface of the skin. It is effective because it is not subject to absorption or subsequent distribution in the body, excretion or metabolism. Pharmacokinetic particulars are not appropriate in these circumstances.

5.3 Preclinical safety data
No relevant pre-clinical data has been generated.

6. PHARMACEUTICAL PARTICULARS

6.1 List of excipients
Liquid paraffin BP

Fractionated coconut oil BP

Butane 40 (butane: isobutane: propane) HSE

6.2 Incompatibilities
None

6.3 Shelf life
60 months.

6.4 Special precautions for storage
Store below 25°C. Pressurised container. Highly flammable, Protect from sunlight and do not puncture, burn or expose to temperatures over 50°C even when empty. Do not spray on a naked flame or any incandescent material.

6.5 Nature and contents of container
Pressurised aerosol. Pack sizes 50 ml, 250 ml, 75 ml, 150 ml, 200 ml, 300 ml, 400 ml, and 500 ml. (75 ml, 150 ml, 200 ml, 300 ml, 400 ml, and 500 ml are currently not marketed.)

6.6 Special precautions for disposal and other handling
No special instructions for use or handling.

7. MARKETING AUTHORISATION HOLDER
Alliance Pharmaceuticals Limited

Avonbridge House

Bath Road

Chippenham

Wiltshire

England

SN15 2BB

8. MARKETING AUTHORISATION NUMBER(S)
PL 16853/0098

9. DATE OF FIRST AUTHORISATION/RENEWAL OF THE AUTHORISATION
15/03/94

10. DATE OF REVISION OF THE TEXT
23rd June 2009

Dermax Therapeutic Shampoo

(Dermal Laboratories Limited)

1. NAME OF THE MEDICINAL PRODUCT
DERMAX® THERAPEUTIC SHAMPOO

2. QUALITATIVE AND QUANTITATIVE COMPOSITION
Benzalkonium Chloride 0.5% w/w

3. PHARMACEUTICAL FORM
Clear, pale yellow to straw coloured viscous shampoo

4. CLINICAL PARTICULARS

4.1 Therapeutic indications
For the topical treatment of pityriasis capitis and other seborrhoeic scalp conditions, where there is scaling and dandruff.

4.2 Posology and method of administration
For adults, children and the elderly.

Wet the hair. Apply a liberal quantity of the shampoo to the scalp and, with the tips of the fingers, rub in thoroughly. Rinse. Repeat the application and massage to produce a rich lather. Remove as much lather as possible with the hands, before rinsing thoroughly under running water.

4.3 Contraindications
Not to be used in cases of sensitivity to any of the ingredients.

4.4 Special warnings and precautions for use
Keep away from the eyes.

4.5 Interaction with other medicinal products and other forms of interaction
None known.

4.6 Pregnancy and lactation
No special precautions.

4.7 Effects on ability to drive and use machines
None known.

4.8 Undesirable effects
None known.

4.9 Overdose
There are no known toxic effects resulting from excessive use of Dermax Therapeutic Shampoo.

5. PHARMACOLOGICAL PROPERTIES

5.1 Pharmacodynamic properties
The surface active cationic germicide, benzalkonium chloride, is adsorbed on to dry skin scales, which are a feature of pityriasis capitis and other seborrhoeic scalp conditions. The scales are thereby loosened and attain a net positive charge. In the presence of the anionic foaming agent, sodium lauryl ether sulphate, the dandruff scales are then levitated into the negatively charged surface of the foam, and are thus washed from the hair.

The benzalkonium chloride also acts as a mild antiseptic which improves clinical performance where the condition is exacerbated by the presence of microbes. The major site of action against micro-organisms appears to be the cell membrane, where permeability is altered.

5.2 Pharmacokinetic properties
The effect of Dermax Therapeutic Shampoo is entirely superficial since it acts on the outer surface of the stratum corneum, treating the external manifestations of the recommended clinical indications. For this reason, no pharmacokinetic studies have been undertaken.

5.3 Preclinical safety data
No relevant information additional to that included elsewhere in the SPC.

6. PHARMACEUTICAL PARTICULARS

6.1 List of excipients
Sodium Lauryl Ether Sulphate; Coconut Diethanolamide; Dilute Hydrochloric Acid; Phenoxyethanol; Sodium Chloride, Lauryldimonium Hydroxypropyl Hydrolyzed Collagen; Coconut Oil; Purified Water.

6.2 Incompatibilities
None known.

6.3 Shelf life
36 months.

6.4 Special precautions for storage
Do not store above 25°C. Keep bottle in outer carton.

6.5 Nature and contents of container
250 ml white high density polyethylene bottle with a polypropylene dispensing screw cap. This is supplied as an original pack (OP).

6.6 Special precautions for disposal and other handling
Not applicable.

7. MARKETING AUTHORISATION HOLDER
Dermal Laboratories

Tatmore Place, Gosmore

Hitchin, Herts, SG4 7QR, UK.

8. MARKETING AUTHORISATION NUMBER(S)
00173/0198

9. DATE OF FIRST AUTHORISATION/RENEWAL OF THE AUTHORISATION
18 May 2005

10. DATE OF REVISION OF THE TEXT
December 2005

Dermidex Dermatological Cream (Actavis UK Ltd)

(Actavis UK Ltd)

1. NAME OF THE MEDICINAL PRODUCT
Dermidex Dermatological Cream.

2. QUALITATIVE AND QUANTITATIVE COMPOSITION
Dermidex Dermatological Cream contains:

Lidocaine 1.20% w/w

Aluminium Chlorhydroxyallantoinate 0.25% w/w

Chorobutanol 1.00% w/w

Cetrimide 0.50% w/w

For excipients, see 6.1

3. PHARMACEUTICAL FORM
Cream. A smooth white cream, free from lumps, non greasy with an even distribution of emulsion droplets.

4. CLINICAL PARTICULARS

4.1 Therapeutic indications
Antiseptic, anaesthetic, anti-irritant, and emollient agent. For the treatment of mild pain caused by minor skin cuts, scratches and grazes (chapping) and soreness caused by detergents, soaps, deodorants and jewellery and bites and stings.

4.2 Posology and method of administration
Adults, Children (age 4 and above) and the Elderly:

Apply to the affected area every 3 hours

Not suitable for children aged less than 4 years.

Route of administration: Cream for cutaneous use.

4.3 Contraindications
Dermidex Cream is contraindicated where there is hypersensitivity to cetrimide, chlorobutanol, lidocaine or other local anaesthetics of the amide type, or any of the other ingredients.

4.4 Special warnings and precautions for use
For external use only. Keep out of reach and sight of children.

The product should not be used for longer than 7 days without seeking medical advice.

Avoid contact with the eyes.

4.5 Interaction with other medicinal products and other forms of interaction
None known.

4.6 Pregnancy and lactation
Lidocaine crosses the placenta and is distributed into breast milk. As with all medicines use with care.

4.7 Effects on ability to drive and use machines
No or negligible influence.

4.8 Undesirable effects
Occasionally there have been reports of skin reaction with all such preparations.

4.9 Overdose
Overdose is unlikely.

Accidental ingestion may result in anaesthesia of the upper respiratory tract, nausea, vomiting and abdominal discomfort. Ingestion of very large quantities could result in CNS and cardiovascular toxicity. Treatment should be symptomatic and supportive.

5. PHARMACOLOGICAL PROPERTIES

5.1 Pharmacodynamic properties
Other dermatologicals D11A

Not applicable.

5.2 Pharmacokinetic properties
Not applicable

5.3 Preclinical safety data
There are no pre-clinical data of relevance to the prescriber which are additional to that already included in other sections of the SPC.

6. PHARMACEUTICAL PARTICULARS

6.1 List of excipients
Cetyl Alcohol

Glyceryl Monostearate

Isopropyl Myristate

Light Liquid Paraffin

Purified Water

Phenoxyethanol

Sorbitol Solution

Stearyl Alcohol 1895

Perfume Sport 14412C

6.2 Incompatibilities
None known

6.3 Shelf life
36 months unopened

6.4 Special precautions for storage
None

6.5 Nature and contents of container
Lacquered covex tube with a low or medium density Polyethylene cap in a carton. Aluminium tubes with a Polyamide internal lacquer, a membrane nozzle fitted with a full skirted, spiked white Polyethylene cap in a carton.

Pack sizes: 3g, 4g, 5g, 7.5g, 10g, 30g & 50g.

6.6 Special precautions for disposal and other handling
For external use only.

7. MARKETING AUTHORISATION HOLDER
Actavis Group PTC ehf

Reykjavikurvegi 76-78

220 Hafnarfjordur

Iceland.

8. MARKETING AUTHORISATION NUMBER(S)
PL 30306/0068

9. DATE OF FIRST AUTHORISATION/RENEWAL OF THE AUTHORISATION
2 December 2002

10. DATE OF REVISION OF THE TEXT

11 DOSIMETRY (IF APPLICABLE)
Not Applicable

12 INSTRUCTIONS FOR PREPARATION OF RADIOPHARMACEUTICALS (IF APPLICABLE)
Not Applicable

Dermol 200 Shower Emollient

(Dermal Laboratories Limited)

1. NAME OF THE MEDICINAL PRODUCT
DERMOL® 200 SHOWER EMOLLIENT

2. QUALITATIVE AND QUANTITATIVE COMPOSITION
Liquid Paraffin 2.5% w/w; Isopropyl Myristate 2.5% w/w; Benzalkonium Chloride 0.1% w/w; Chlorhexidine Dihydrochloride 0.1% w/w.

3. PHARMACEUTICAL FORM
White, non-greasy cutaneous emulsion.

4. CLINICAL PARTICULARS

4.1 Therapeutic indications
An antimicrobial shower emollient for the management of dry and pruritic skin conditions, especially eczema and dermatitis. Dermol 200 Shower Emollient is for direct application onto the skin and is suitable for use as a soap substitute.

4.2 Posology and method of administration
For adults, children and the elderly: For application to the skin (eg after showering): Apply to the affected areas as required. Massage into the skin, until absorbed. For use as a soap substitute in the shower: As required, use the shower emollient instead of an ordinary shower gel or soap. Pat dry.

4.3 Contraindications
Do not use in cases of known sensitivity to any of the ingredients.

4.4 Special warnings and precautions for use
Avoid contact with the eyes, especially when used on the face. Take care to avoid slipping in the shower or bath. The excipient cetostearyl alcohol may on rare occasions give rise to local skin reactions (e.g. contact dermatitis) in sensitive people.

4.5 Interaction with other medicinal products and other forms of interaction
None known.

4.6 Pregnancy and lactation
No special precautions.

4.7 Effects on ability to drive and use machines
None known.

4.8 Undesirable effects
Although the shower emollient has been specially formulated for use on dry or problem skin, in the unlikely event of a reaction, discontinue treatment. These reactions are very rare (<1/10,000, based on spontaneous reporting) and may be irritant or allergic in nature. Reactions have been observed occasionally when used excessively as a leave-on application in areas of folded skin such as the anogenital area.

4.9 Overdose
Not applicable.

5. PHARMACOLOGICAL PROPERTIES

5.1 Pharmacodynamic properties
Bacteria (especially *Staphylococcus aureus*) are implicated in the pathogenesis of inflammatory dry skin conditions such as atopic eczema and dermatitis.

Dermol 200 Shower Emollient contains 5% of emollient oils in a non-greasy aqueous system which also contains the well-known and effective antiseptics benzalkonium chloride and chlorhexidine dihydrochloride. Its antimicrobial properties assist in overcoming infection, whether from *Staph aureus*, the pathogen which often complicates eczema and associated pruritus, or secondary infection caused by scratching.

The emollients, liquid paraffin and isopropyl myristate, permit rehydration of dry skin by forming an occlusive barrier within the skin surface, thus reducing drying from evaporation of water that diffuses from the underlying layers.

Patients with dry skin conditions have a deficiency of the natural oils which assist in the retention of moisture.

A non-ionic emollient soap substitute such as Dermol 200 Shower Emollient, will cleanse the skin, helping to remove surface debris without removing the skin's natural oils.

5.2 Pharmacokinetic properties
The active ingredients are presented in an aqueous emulsion system and so are readily absorbed into the stratum corneum when the product is gently massaged over the areas of dry skin. The antiseptic ingredients are in intimate contact with the skin, and as they are in solution, their availability is optimal.

5.3 Preclinical safety data
No special information.

6. PHARMACEUTICAL PARTICULARS

6.1 List of excipients
Cetostearyl Alcohol; Cetomacrogol 1000; Phenoxyethanol; Purified Water.

6.2 Incompatibilities
None known.

6.3 Shelf life
30 months.

6.4 Special precautions for storage
Do not store above 25°C.

6.5 Nature and contents of container
Plastic 200 ml bottle with a hooked overcap. This is supplied as an original pack (OP).

6.6 Special precautions for disposal and other handling
Not applicable.

7. MARKETING AUTHORISATION HOLDER
Dermal Laboratories

Tatmore Place, Gosmore

Hitchin, Herts SG4 7QR, UK.

8. MARKETING AUTHORISATION NUMBER(S)
00173/0156.

9. DATE OF FIRST AUTHORISATION/RENEWAL OF THE AUTHORISATION
20 February 2009.

10. DATE OF REVISION OF THE TEXT
February 2009.

Dermol 500 Lotion

(Dermal Laboratories Limited)

1. NAME OF THE MEDICINAL PRODUCT
DERMOL® 500 LOTION

2. QUALITATIVE AND QUANTITATIVE COMPOSITION
Benzalkonium Chloride 0.1% w/w; Chlorhexidine Dihydrochloride 0.1% w/w; Liquid Paraffin 2.5% w/w; Isopropyl Myristate 2.5% w/w.

3. PHARMACEUTICAL FORM
White, non-greasy cutaneous emulsion.

4. CLINICAL PARTICULARS

4.1 Therapeutic indications
An antimicrobial emollient for the management of dry and pruritic skin conditions, especially eczema and dermatitis. The lotion is suitable for direct application, and for use as a soap substitute.

4.2 Posology and method of administration
For adults, children and the elderly: For application to the skin: apply the lotion to the affected areas as required. Massage into the skin, until absorbed. For use as a soap substitute: use as a cleanser in the bath or shower, or for other toiletry purposes, instead of ordinary soap or shower gel.

4.3 Contraindications
Do not use in cases of known sensitivity to any of the ingredients.

4.4 Special warnings and precautions for use
Avoid contact with the eyes. The excipient cetostearyl alcohol may on rare occasions give rise to local skin reactions (e.g. contact dermatitis) in sensitive people.

4.5 Interaction with other medicinal products and other forms of interaction
None known.

4.6 Pregnancy and lactation
No special precautions.

4.7 Effects on ability to drive and use machines
None known.

4.8 Undesirable effects
Although the lotion has been specially formulated for use on dry or problem skin, in the unlikely event of a reaction discontinue treatment. These reactions are very rare (<1/10,000, based on spontaneous reporting) and may be irritant or allergic in nature. Reactions have been observed occasionally when used excessively as a leave-on application in areas of folded skin such as the anogenital area.

4.9 Overdose
Not applicable.

5. PHARMACOLOGICAL PROPERTIES

5.1 Pharmacodynamic properties
Bacteria (especially *Staphylococcus aureus*) are implicated in the pathogenesis of inflammatory dry skin conditions such as atopic eczema or dermatitis. Dermol 500 Lotion contains 5% of emollient oils in a non-greasy aqueous lotion which also contains the well-known and effective antiseptics benzalkonium chloride and chlorhexidine dihydrochloride. Its antimicrobial properties assist in overcoming infection, whether from *Staph. aureus*, the pathogen which often complicates eczema and associated pruritus, or secondary infection caused by scratching.

Massaged into the skin, the emollients, liquid paraffin and isopropyl myristate, permit rehydration of dry skin by forming an occlusive barrier within the skin surface, thus reducing drying from evaporation of water that diffuses from the underlying layers.

5.2 Pharmacokinetic properties
The active ingredients are presented in an aqueous lotion and so are readily absorbed into the stratum corneum when the product is gently massaged over the areas of dry skin. The antiseptic ingredients are in intimate contact with the skin, and as they are in solution, their availability is optimal.

5.3 Preclinical safety data
No special information.

6. PHARMACEUTICAL PARTICULARS

6.1 List of excipients
Cetostearyl Alcohol; Cetomacrogol 1000; Phenoxyethanol; Purified Water.

6.2 Incompatibilities
None known.

6.3 Shelf life
30 months.

6.4 Special precautions for storage
Do not store above 25°C. Replace cap after use.

6.5 Nature and contents of container
Plastic 500 ml bottle with a white pump dispenser. Supplied as an original pack (OP).

6.6 Special precautions for disposal and other handling
Not applicable.

7. MARKETING AUTHORISATION HOLDER
Dermal Laboratories

Tatmore Place, Gosmore

Hitchin, Herts SG4 7QR, UK.

8. MARKETING AUTHORISATION NUMBER(S)
00173/0051.

9. DATE OF FIRST AUTHORISATION/RENEWAL OF THE AUTHORISATION
1 October 2007.

10. DATE OF REVISION OF THE TEXT
February 2009.

Dermol 600 Bath Emollient

(Dermal Laboratories Limited)

1. NAME OF THE MEDICINAL PRODUCT
DERMOL® 600 BATH EMOLLIENT

2. QUALITATIVE AND QUANTITATIVE COMPOSITION
Liquid Paraffin 25.0% w/w; Isopropyl Myristate 25.0% w/w; Benzalkonium Chloride 0.5% w/w.

3. PHARMACEUTICAL FORM
White bath additive.

4. CLINICAL PARTICULARS

4.1 Therapeutic indications
An antimicrobial bath emollient for use as an aid in the treatment of dry and pruritic skin conditions, especially eczema, dermatitis, ichthyosis or xeroderma. It permits the rehydration of the keratin by replacing lost lipids, and its antiseptic properties assist in overcoming secondary infection.

4.2 Posology and method of administration
For use in the bath: For adults, children and the elderly: Add up to 30 ml to a bath of warm water (more or less according to the size of the bath and individual patient requirements). For infants: Add up to 15ml to a bath of warm water (more or less according to the size of the bath and individual patient requirements). Soak for 5 to 10 minutes. Pat dry.

4.3 Contraindications
Sensitivity to any of the ingredients.

4.4 Special warnings and precautions for use
Keep away from the eyes. For external use only. Keep out of the reach and sight of children. Take care to avoid slipping in the bath.

4.5 Interaction with other medicinal products and other forms of interaction
None known.

4.6 Pregnancy and lactation
No special precautions.

4.7 Effects on ability to drive and use machines
None known.

4.8 Undesirable effects
Although the bath emollient has been specially formulated for use on dry or problem skin, in the unlikely event of a reaction discontinue treatment.

These reactions are very rare (<1/10,000, based on spontaneous reporting) and may be irritant or allergic in nature.

4.9 Overdose
Not applicable.

5. PHARMACOLOGICAL PROPERTIES

5.1 Pharmacodynamic properties
For dry skin conditions it is important to add an emollient to the bath water. Dermol 600 Bath Emollient contains 50% of oils emulsified in water as well as the well-known antiseptic, benzalkonium chloride which assists in overcoming secondary infection.

5.2 Pharmacokinetic properties
Dermol 600 Bath Emollient contains 0.5% of the quaternary ammonium antiseptic, benzalkonium chloride. The large positively charged cation is readily adsorbed from the formulation onto negatively charged bacterial cell surfaces, thereby conferring substantial antimicrobial activity. Even at extended dilution, it is particularly effective against *Staphylococcus aureus*, a bacterium which is known to colonise the skin in large numbers in patients with eczema, especially atopic eczema. Apart from its emollient properties, Dermol 600 Bath Emollient therefore also helps to prevent and overcome secondary infection which may exacerbate the eczematous condition.

5.3 Preclinical safety data
The safety and efficacy of the emollients (liquid paraffin and isopropyl myristate) and the antiseptic (benzalkonium chloride) in topical dosage forms have been well established over many years of widespread clinical usage.

6. PHARMACEUTICAL PARTICULARS

6.1 List of excipients
Sorbitan Stearate; Polysorbate 60; Industrial Methylated Spirit 95%; Purified Water.

6.2 Incompatibilities
None known.

6.3 Shelf life
36 months.

6.4 Special precautions for storage
Do not store above 25°C. Always replace the cap after use.

6.5 Nature and contents of container
600 ml plastic bottle with a measuring cap.

6.6 Special precautions for disposal and other handling
Not applicable.

7. MARKETING AUTHORISATION HOLDER
Dermal Laboratories

Tatmore Place, Gosmore

Hitchin, Herts SG4 7QR, UK.

8. MARKETING AUTHORISATION NUMBER(S)
00173/0155.

9. DATE OF FIRST AUTHORISATION/RENEWAL OF THE AUTHORISATION
13 July 2009.

10. DATE OF REVISION OF THE TEXT
July 2009.

Dermol Cream
(Dermal Laboratories Limited)

1. NAME OF THE MEDICINAL PRODUCT
DERMOL® CREAM

2. QUALITATIVE AND QUANTITATIVE COMPOSITION
Liquid Paraffin 10.0% w/w; Isopropyl Myristate 10.0% w/w; Benzalkonium Chloride 0.1% w/w; Chlorhexidine Dihydrochloride 0.1% w/w.

3. PHARMACEUTICAL FORM
Cream.

White non-greasy topical emulsion.

4. CLINICAL PARTICULARS

4.1 Therapeutic indications
An antimicrobial emollient cream for the management of dry and pruritic skin conditions, especially eczema and dermatitis. The cream is suitable for direct application, and for use as a soap substitute.

4.2 Posology and method of administration
For external use only.

Before using the 500g pump bottle, turn the top of the pump dispenser anti-clockwise to unlock it.

For adults, the elderly, infants and children.

For application to the skin

Apply Dermol Cream to the affected areas as often as necessary.

For use as a soap substitute

Dermol Cream may also be used as a cleanser in the bath or shower, or for other toiletry purposes, instead of ordinary soap or shower gel.

4.3 Contraindications
Do not use in cases of known sensitivity to any of the ingredients.

4.4 Special warnings and precautions for use
Avoid contact with the eyes. The excipient cetostearyl alcohol may on rare occasions give rise to local skin reactions (e.g. contact dermatitis) in sensitive people.

4.5 Interaction with other medicinal products and other forms of interaction
None known.

4.6 Pregnancy and lactation
No special precautions.

4.7 Effects on ability to drive and use machines
None known.

4.8 Undesirable effects
Although the cream has been specially formulated for use on dry or problem skin, in the unlikely event of a reaction discontinue treatment. These reactions are very rare (<1/10,000, based on spontaneous reporting) and may be irritant or allergic in nature. Reactions have been observed occasionally when used excessively as a leave-on application in areas of folded skin such as the anogenital area.

4.9 Overdose
Excessive topical use is very unlikely to cause any untoward effects other than making the skin feel greasy.

In the event of a significant quantity being accidentally swallowed, nausea and vomiting may occur but serious effects are unlikely. Unless there are signs that give cause for concern, treatment should be conservative.

5. PHARMACOLOGICAL PROPERTIES

5.1 Pharmacodynamic properties
ATC Code: D02AX - Dermatologicals, other emollients and protectives.

Bacteria (especially *Staphylococcus aureus*) are implicated in the pathogenesis of inflammatory dry skin conditions such as atopic eczema or dermatitis.

Dermol Cream contains 20% of emollient oils in a non-greasy aqueous cream which also contains the well-known and effective antiseptics benzalkonium chloride and chlorhexidine dihydrochloride. Its antimicrobial properties assist in overcoming infection, whether from *Staph aureus*, the pathogen which often complicates eczema and associated pruritus, or secondary infection caused by scratching.

Massaged into the skin, the emollients, liquid paraffin and isopropyl myristate, permit rehydration of dry skin by forming an occlusive barrier within the skin surface, thus reducing drying from evaporation of water that diffuses from the underlying layers.

5.2 Pharmacokinetic properties
The active ingredients are presented in an aqueous cream and so are readily absorbed into the stratum corneum when the product is gently massaged over the areas of dry skin. The antiseptic ingredients are in intimate contact with the skin, and as they are in solution, their availability is optimal.

5.3 Preclinical safety data
No special information.

6. PHARMACEUTICAL PARTICULARS

6.1 List of excipients
Cetostearyl Alcohol; Glycerol; Cetomacrogol 1000; Phenoxyethanol; Disodium Phosphate Dodecahydrate; Sodium Dihydrogen Phosphate Dihydrate; Purified Water.

6.2 Incompatibilities
None known.

6.3 Shelf life
36 months – for 500g pack.

24 months - for 100g pack.

6.4 Special precautions for storage
Do not store above 30°C. Replace cap after use.

6.5 Nature and contents of container
High density polyethylene bottle (500g) with a polypropylene metering pump.

High density polyethylene tube (100g) with a polypropylene screw cap.

6.6 Special precautions for disposal and other handling
Not applicable.

7. MARKETING AUTHORISATION HOLDER
Dermal Laboratories

Tatmore Place, Gosmore

Hitchin, Herts SG4 7QR, UK.

8. MARKETING AUTHORISATION NUMBER(S)
00173/0171.

9. DATE OF FIRST AUTHORISATION/RENEWAL OF THE AUTHORISATION
16 February 2009.

10. DATE OF REVISION OF THE TEXT
February 2009.

Dermovate Cream
(GlaxoSmithKline UK)

1. NAME OF THE MEDICINAL PRODUCT
Dermovate Cream

2. QUALITATIVE AND QUANTITATIVE COMPOSITION
Clobetasol propionate 0.0525% w/w

3. PHARMACEUTICAL FORM
Cream

4. CLINICAL PARTICULARS

4.1 Therapeutic indications
Clobetasol propionate is a very active topical corticosteroid which is of particular value when used in short courses for the treatment of more resistant dermatoses such as psoriasis (excluding widespread plaque psoriasis), recalcitrant eczemas, lichen planus, discoid lupus erythematosus, and other skin conditions which do not respond satisfactorily to less active steroids.

4.2 Posology and method of administration
Apply sparingly to the affected area once or twice daily until improvement occurs. As with other highly active topical steroid preparations, therapy should be discontinued when control is achieved. In the more responsive conditions this may be within a few days.

If no improvement is seen within two to four weeks, reassessment of the diagnosis, or referral, may be necessary.

Repeated short courses of Dermovate may be used to control exacerbations. If continuous steroid treatment is necessary, a less potent preparation should be used.

In very resistant lesions, especially where there is hyperkeratosis, the anti-inflammatory effect of Dermovate can be enhanced, if necessary, by occluding the treatment area with polythene film. Overnight occlusion only is usually adequate to bring about a satisfactory response. Thereafter improvement can usually be maintained by application without occlusion.

For topical administration.

4.3 Contraindications
Rosacea.

Acne vulgaris.

Perioral dermatitis.

Perianal and genital pruritus.

Primary cutaneous viral infections (e.g. herpes simplex, chickenpox).

Hypersensitivity to the preparation.

The use of Dermovate skin preparations is not indicated in the treatment of primary infected skin lesions caused by infection with fungi (e.g. candidiasis, tinea) or bacteria (e.g. impetigo); or dermatoses in children under one year of age, including dermatitis and napkin eruptions.

4.4 Special warnings and precautions for use
Long-term continuous therapy should be avoided where possible, particularly in infants and children, as adrenal suppression can occur even without occlusion. If Dermovate is required for use in children, it is recommended that the treatment should be reviewed weekly. It should be noted that the infant's napkin may act as an occlusive dressing.

If used in childhood or on the face, courses should be limited if possible to five days and occlusion should not be used.

The face, more than other areas of the body, may exhibit atrophic changes after prolonged treatment with potent topical corticosteroids. This must be borne in mind when treating such conditions as psoriasis, discoid lupus erythematosus and severe eczema.

If applied to the eyelids, care is needed to ensure that the preparation does not enter the eye, as glaucoma might result. If Dermovate Cream does enter the eye, the affected eye should be bathed in copious amounts of water.

Topical steroids may be hazardous in psoriasis for a number of reasons including rebound relapses, development of tolerance, risk of generalised pustular psoriasis and development of local or systemic toxicity due to impaired barrier function of the skin. If used in psoriasis careful patient supervision is important.

Appropriate antimicrobial therapy should be used whenever treating inflammatory lesions which have become infected. Any spread of infection requires withdrawal of topical corticosteroid therapy and systemic administration of antimicrobial agents. Bacterial infection is encouraged by the warm, moist conditions induced by occlusive dressings, and so the skin should be cleansed before a fresh dressing is applied.

4.5 Interaction with other medicinal products and other forms of interaction
None reported.

4.6 Pregnancy and lactation
There is inadequate evidence of safety in human pregnancy. Topical administration of corticosteroids to pregnant animals can cause abnormalities of foetal development including cleft palate and intrauterine growth retardation. The relevance of this finding to humans has not been established, therefore, topical steroids should not be used extensively in pregnancy, i.e. in large amounts or for prolonged periods.

The safe use of clobetasol propionate during lactation has not been established.

4.7 Effects on ability to drive and use machines
Clobetasol propionate is not expected to have any effects.

4.8 Undesirable effects
The following adverse reactions have been identified during post-approval use of clobetasol propionate. Because these reactions are reported voluntarily from a population of uncertain size, it is not always possible to reliably estimate their frequency or establish a causal relationship to drug exposure. The frequency of these adverse events has therefore been classified as "unknown".

Immune system disorders

Hypersensitivity

Local hypersensitivity reactions such as erythema, rash, pruritus, urticaria and allergic contact dermatitis may occur at the site of application and may resemble symptoms of the condition under treatment.

If signs of hypersensitivity appear, application should be stopped immediately.

Endocrine disorders

Features of Cushing's syndrome

As with other topical corticosteroids, prolonged use of large amounts, or treatment of extensive areas can result in sufficient systemic absorption to produce the features of Cushing's syndrome. This effect is more likely to occur in infants and children, and if occlusive dressings are used. In infants, the nappy may act as an occlusive dressing.

Provided the weekly dosage is less than 50g in adults, any suppression of the HPA axis is likely to be transient with a rapid return to normal values once the short course of steroid therapy has ceased. The same applies to children given proportionate dosage.

Vascular disorders

Dilatation of the superficial blood vessels

Prolonged and intensive treatment with highly-active corticosteroid preparations may cause dilatation of the superficial blood vessels, particularly when occlusive dressings are used, or when skin folds are involved.

Skin and subcutaneous tissue disorders

Local skin burning, local atrophy, striae, thinning, pigmentation changes, hypertrichosis, exacerbation of underlying symptoms, pustular psoriasis.

Prolonged and intensive treatment with highly-active corticosteroid preparations may cause local atrophic changes, such as thinning and striae.

Treatment of psoriasis with corticosteroids (or its withdrawal) is thought to have provoked the pustular form of the disease.

4.9 Overdose
Acute overdosage is very unlikely to occur, however, in the case of chronic overdosage or misuse, the features of hypercortisolism may appear and in this situation topical steroids should be reduced or discontinued gradually, under medical supervision.

5. PHARMACOLOGICAL PROPERTIES

5.1 Pharmacodynamic properties
Clobetasol propionate is a highly active corticosteroid with topical anti-inflammatory activity. The major effect of clobetasol propionate on skin is a non-specific anti-inflammatory response, partially due to vasoconstriction and decrease in collagen synthesis.

5.2 Pharmacokinetic properties
Percutaneous penetration of clobetasol propionate varies among individuals and can be increased by the use of occlusive dressings, or when the skin is inflamed or diseased.

Mean peak plasma clobetasol propionate concentrations of 0.63 ng/ml occurred in one study eight hours after the second application (13 hours after an initial application) of 30 g clobetasol propionate 0.05% ointment to normal individuals with healthy skin. Following the application of a second dose of 30 g clobetasol propionate cream 0.05% mean peak plasma concentrations were slightly higher than the ointment and occurred 10 hours after application.

In a separate study, mean peak plasma concentrations of approximately 2.3 ng/ml and 4.6 ng/ml occurred respectively in patients with psoriasis and eczema three hours after a single application of 25 g clobetasol propionate 0.05% ointment.

Following percutaneous absorption of clobetasol propionate, the drug probably follows the metabolic pathway of systemically administered corticosteroids, i.e. metabolised primarily by the liver and then excreted by the kidneys. However, systemic metabolism of clobetasol has never been fully characterised or quantified.

5.3 Preclinical safety data
There are no preclinical data of relevance to the prescriber which are additional to that in other sections of the SmPC.

6. PHARMACEUTICAL PARTICULARS

6.1 List of excipients
Cetostearyl alcohol

Glyceryl monostearate

Arlacel 165

Beeswax substitute 6621

Propylene glycol

Chlorocresol

Sodium citrate

Citric acid monohydrate

Purified water

6.2 Incompatibilities
None reported.

6.3 Shelf life
24 months.

6.4 Special precautions for storage
Store below 25°C.

6.5 Nature and contents of container
Collapsible latex banded aluminium tube internally coated with epoxy resin based lacquer, with polypropylene cap.
Pack sizes: 25 g, 30 g or 100 g.

Not all pack sizes may be marketed.

6.6 Special precautions for disposal and other handling
Patients should be advised to wash their hands after applying Dermovate unless it is the hands that are being treated.

Administrative Data

7. MARKETING AUTHORISATION HOLDER
Glaxo Wellcome UK Ltd

trading as

Glaxo Laboratories and/or GlaxoSmithKline UK

Stockley Park West

Uxbridge

Middlesex

UB11 1BT

8. MARKETING AUTHORISATION NUMBER(S)
PL 10949/0025

9. DATE OF FIRST AUTHORISATION/RENEWAL OF THE AUTHORISATION
6 August 2004

10. DATE OF REVISION OF THE TEXT
27 November 2007

Dermovate Ointment

(GlaxoSmithKline UK)

1. NAME OF THE MEDICINAL PRODUCT
Dermovate Ointment

2. QUALITATIVE AND QUANTITATIVE COMPOSITION
Clobetasol 17-propionate 0.05375% w/w

3. PHARMACEUTICAL FORM
Ointment

4. CLINICAL PARTICULARS

4.1 Therapeutic indications
Clobetasol propionate is a very active topical corticosteroid which is of particular value when used in short courses for the treatment of more resistant dermatoses such as psoriasis (excluding widespread plaque psoriasis), recalcitrant eczemas, lichen planus, discoid lupus erythematosus, and other conditions which do not respond satisfactorily to less active steroids.

4.2 Posology and method of administration
Apply sparingly to the affected area once or twice daily until improvement occurs. As with other highly active topical steroid preparations, therapy should be discontinued when control is achieved. In the more responsive conditions this may be within a few days.

If no improvement is seen within two to four weeks, reassessment of the diagnosis, or referral, may be necessary.

Repeated short courses of Dermovate may be used to control exacerbations. If continuous steroid treatment is necessary, a less potent preparation should be used.

In very resistant lesions, especially where there is hyperkeratosis, the anti-inflammatory effect of Dermovate can be enhanced, if necessary, by occluding the treatment area with polythene film. Overnight occlusion only is usually adequate to bring about a satisfactory response. Thereafter improvement can usually be maintained by application without occlusion.

For topical administration.

4.3 Contraindications
Rosacea.

Acne vulgaris.

Perioral dermatitis.

Perianal and genital pruritus.

Primary cutaneous viral infections (e.g. herpes simplex, chickenpox).

Hypersensitivity to the preparation.

The use of Dermovate skin preparations is not indicated in the treatment of primary infected skin lesions caused by infection with fungi (e.g. candidiasis, tinea), or bacteria (e.g. impetigo); or dermatoses in children under one year of age, including dermatitis and napkin eruptions.

4.4 Special warnings and precautions for use
Long term continuous topical therapy should be avoided where possible, particularly in infants and children, as adrenal suppression can occur readily even without occlusion. If Dermovate is required for use in children, it is recommended that the treatment should be reviewed weekly. It should be noted that the infant's napkin may act as an occlusive dressing.

If used in childhood or on the face, courses should be limited if possible to five days and occlusion should not be used.

The face, more than other areas of the body, may exhibit atrophic changes after prolonged treatment with potent topical corticosteroids. This must be borne in mind when treating such conditions as psoriasis, discoid lupus erythematosus and severe eczema.

If applied to the eyelids, care is needed to ensure that the preparation does not enter the eye, as glaucoma might result. If Dermovate Ointment does enter the eye, the affected eye should be bathed in copious amounts of water.

Topical corticosteroids may be hazardous in psoriasis for a number of reasons including rebound relapses, development of tolerance, risk of generalised pustular psoriasis and development of local or systemic toxicity due to impaired barrier function of the skin. If used in psoriasis careful patient supervision is important.

Appropriate antimicrobial therapy should be used whenever treating inflammatory lesions which have become infected. Any spread of infection requires withdrawal of topical corticosteroid therapy and systemic administration of antimicrobial agents. Bacterial infection is encouraged by the warm, moist conditions induced by occlusive dressings, and so the skin should be cleansed before a fresh dressing is applied.

4.5 Interaction with other medicinal products and other forms of interaction
None reported.

4.6 Pregnancy and lactation
There is inadequate evidence of safety in human pregnancy. Topical administration of corticosteroids to pregnant animals can cause abnormalities of fetal development including cleft palate and intrauterine growth retardation. The relevance of this finding to humans has not been established, therefore, topical steroids should not be used extensively in pregnancy, i.e. in large amounts or for prolonged periods.

The safe use of clobetasol propionate during lactation has not been established.

4.7 Effects on ability to drive and use machines
Clobetasol propionate is not expected to have any effects.

4.8 Undesirable effects
The following adverse reactions have been identified during post-approval use of clobetasol propionate. Because these reactions are reported voluntarily from a population of uncertain size, it is not always possible to reliably estimate their frequency or establish a causal relationship to drug exposure. The frequency of these adverse events has therefore been classified as "unknown".

Immune system disorders

Hypersensitivity

Local hypersensitivity reactions such as erythema, rash, pruritus, urticaria and allergic contact dermatitis may occur at the site of application and may resemble symptoms of the condition under treatment.

If signs of hypersensitivity appear, application should be stopped immediately.

Endocrine disorders

Features of Cushing's syndrome

As with other topical corticosteroids, prolonged use of large amounts, or treatment of extensive areas can result in sufficient systemic absorption to produce the features of Cushing's syndrome. This effect is more likely to occur in infants and children, and if occlusive dressings are used. In infants, the nappy may act as an occlusive dressing.

Provided the weekly dosage is less than 50g in adults, any suppression of the HPA axis is likely to be transient with a rapid return to normal values once the short course of steroid therapy has ceased. The same applies to children given proportionate dosage.

Vascular disorders

Dilatation of the superficial blood vessels

Prolonged and intensive treatment with highly-active corticosteroid preparations may cause dilatation of the superficial blood vessels, particularly when occlusive dressings are used, or when skin folds are involved.

Skin and subcutaneous tissue disorders

Local skin burning, local atrophy, striae, thinning, pigmentation changes, hypertrichosis, exacerbation of underlying symptoms, pustular psoriasis.

Prolonged and intensive treatment with highly-active corticosteroid preparations may cause local atrophic changes, such as thinning and striae.

Treatment of psoriasis with corticosteroids (or its withdrawal) is thought to have provoked the pustular form of the disease.

4.9 Overdose

Acute overdosage is very unlikely to occur, however, in the case of chronic overdosage or misuse, the features of hypercortisolism may appear and in this situation topical steroids should be reduced or discontinued gradually, under medical supervision.

5. PHARMACOLOGICAL PROPERTIES

5.1 Pharmacodynamic properties

Clobetasol propionate is a highly active corticosteroid with topical anti-inflammatory activity. The major effect of clobetasol propionate on skin is a non-specific anti-inflammatory response, partially due to vasoconstriction and decrease in collagen synthesis.

5.2 Pharmacokinetic properties

Percutaneous penetration of clobetasol propionate varies among individuals and can be increased by the use of occlusive dressings, or when the skin is inflamed or diseased.

Mean peak plasma clobetasol propionate concentrations of 0.63 ng/ml occurred in one study eight hours after the second application (13 hours after an initial application) of 30 g clobetasol propionate 0.05% ointment to normal individuals with healthy skin. Following the application of a second dose of 30 g clobetasol propionate cream 0.05% mean peak plasma concentrations were slightly higher than the ointment and occurred 10 hours after application.

In a separate study, mean peak plasma concentrations of approximately 2.3 ng/ml and 4.6 ng/ml occurred respectively in patients with psoriasis and eczema three hours after a single application of 25 g clobetasol propionate 0.05% ointment.

Following percutaneous absorption of clobetasol propionate, the drug probably follows the metabolic pathway of systemically administered corticosteroids, i.e. metabolised primarily by the liver and then excreted by the kidneys. However, systemic metabolism of clobetasol has never been fully characterised or quantified.

5.3 Preclinical safety data

There are no preclinical data of relevance to the prescriber which are additional to that in other sections of the SmPC.

6. PHARMACEUTICAL PARTICULARS

6.1 List of excipients

Propylene glycol

Sorbitan sesquioleate

White soft paraffin

6.2 Incompatibilities

None known.

6.3 Shelf life

24 months.

6.4 Special precautions for storage

Store below 30°C.

6.5 Nature and contents of container

Collapsible tubes either internally coated with epoxy resin based lacquer or uncoated with wadless polypropylene caps.

Pack sizes: 25 g, 30 g or 100 g.

<u>Not all pack sizes may be marketed</u>

6.6 Special precautions for disposal and other handling

Patients should be advised to wash their hands after applying Dermovate Ointment unless it is the hands that are being treated.

Administrative Data

7. MARKETING AUTHORISATION HOLDER

Glaxo Wellcome UK Ltd

trading as

Glaxo Laboratories and/or GlaxoSmithKline UK

Stockley Park West

Uxbridge

Middlesex

UB11 1BT

8. MARKETING AUTHORISATION NUMBER(S)

PL 10949/0028

9. DATE OF FIRST AUTHORISATION/RENEWAL OF THE AUTHORISATION

6 August 2004

10. DATE OF REVISION OF THE TEXT

27 November 2007

Dermovate Scalp Application

(GlaxoSmithKline UK)

1. NAME OF THE MEDICINAL PRODUCT

Dermovate Scalp Application

2. QUALITATIVE AND QUANTITATIVE COMPOSITION

Clobetasol propionate 0.05 % $^w/w$

3. PHARMACEUTICAL FORM

Scalp application

4. CLINICAL PARTICULARS

4.1 Therapeutic indications

Psoriasis and recalcitrant eczemas of the scalp.

Clobetasol propionate is a highly active topical corticosteroid which is indicated for use in short courses for conditions which do not respond satisfactorily to less active steroids.

4.2 Posology and method of administration

Route of administration: Topical, on the scalp.

Apply sparingly to the scalp night and morning until improvement occurs. As with other highly active topical steroid preparations, therapy should be discontinued when control is achieved. Repeated short courses of Dermovate Scalp Application may be used to control exacerbations. If continuous steroid treatment is necessary, a less potent preparation should be used.

These recommendations apply to both children and adults, including the elderly.

4.3 Contraindications

Infections of the scalp.

Hypersensitivity to the preparation.

Dermatoses in children under one year of age, including dermatitis.

4.4 Special warnings and precautions for use

Care must be taken to keep the preparation away from the eyes. Do not use near a naked flame.

Long-term continuous topical therapy should be avoided, particularly in infants and children, as adrenal suppression can occur readily even without occlusion.

Development of secondary infection requires withdrawal of topical corticosteroid therapy and commencement of appropriate systemic antimicrobial therapy.

Topical corticosteroids may be hazardous in psoriasis for a number of reasons, including rebound relapses, development of tolerance, risk of generalised pustular psoriasis and development of local or systemic toxicity due to impaired barrier function of the skin. If used in psoriasis careful patient supervision is important.

The least potent corticosteroid which will control the disease should be selected. The viscosity of the scalp application has been adjusted so that the preparation spreads easily without being too fluid. The specially designed bottle and nozzle allow easy application direct to the scalp through the hair.

4.5 Interaction with other medicinal products and other forms of interaction

None known.

4.6 Pregnancy and lactation

There is inadequate evidence of safety in human pregnancy. Topical administration of corticosteroids to pregnant animals can cause abnormalities of foetal development, including cleft palate and intrauterine growth retardation. The relevance of this finding to human beings has not been established; therefore, topical steroids should not be used extensively in pregnancy, i.e. in large amounts or for prolonged periods.

The safe use of clobetasol propionate during lactation has not been established.

4.7 Effects on ability to drive and use machines

None known.

4.8 Undesirable effects

The following adverse reactions have been identified during post-approval use of clobetasol propionate. Because these reactions are reported voluntarily from a population of uncertain size, it is not always possible to reliably estimate their frequency or establish a causal relationship to drug exposure. The frequency of these adverse events has therefore been classified as "unknown".

Immune system disorders

Hypersensitivity

Local hypersensitivity reactions such as erythema, rash, pruritus, urticaria and allergic contact dermatitis may occur at the site of application and may resemble symptoms of the condition under treatment.

If signs of hypersensitivity appear, application should be stopped immediately.

Endocrine disorders

Features of Cushing's syndrome

As with other topical corticosteroids, prolonged use of large amounts, or treatment of extensive areas can result in sufficient systemic absorption to produce the features of Cushing's syndrome. This effect is more likely to occur in infants and children, and if occlusive dressings are used.

Skin and subcutaneous tissue disorders

Local skin burning, local atrophy, pustular psoriasis.

Local atrophy may occur after prolonged treatment.

Treatment of psoriasis with corticosteroids (or its withdrawal) is thought to have provoked the pustular form of the disease.

4.9 Overdose

Acute overdosage is very unlikely to occur, however, in the case of chronic overdosage or misuse, the features of hypercortisolism may appear and in this situation topical steroids should be reduced or discontinued gradually, under medical supervision.

5. PHARMACOLOGICAL PROPERTIES

5.1 Pharmacodynamic properties

Clobetasol propionate is a highly active corticosteroid with topical anti-inflammatory activity. The major effect of clobetasol propionate on skin is a non-specific anti-inflammatory response partially due to vasoconstriction and decrease in collagen synthesis.

5.2 Pharmacokinetic properties

Percutaneous penetration of clobetasol propionate varies among individuals and can be increased by the use of occlusive dressings, or when the skin is inflamed or diseased.

Following percutaneous absorption of clobetasol propionate the drug follows the metabolic pathway of systemically administered corticosteroids, i.e. metabolised primarily by the liver and then excreted by the kidneys. However, systemic metabolism of clobetasol has never been fully characterised or quantified.

5.3 Preclinical safety data

There are no preclinical data of relevance to the prescriber which are additional to that in other sections of the SmPC.

6. PHARMACEUTICAL PARTICULARS

6.1 List of excipients

Carbomer

Isopropyl Alcohol

Sodium Hydroxide

Purified Water

6.2 Incompatibilities

None known.

6.3 Shelf life

24 months

6.4 Special precautions for storage

None.

6.5 Nature and contents of container

White opaque low density polyethylene squeeze bottle with a polyethylene nozzle and either a polystyrene or high density polyethylene cap

or

White High Density Polyethylene (HDPE) Hostalen GF4750 and Remafin white CEG 020 container with a polyethylene nozzle and either a polystyrene or polyethylene cap.

Pack size: 25ml, 30ml, 100ml.

6.6 Special precautions for disposal and other handling

Patients should be advised to wash their hands after applying Dermovate Scalp Application.

For detailed instructions for use refer to the Patient Information Leaflet in every pack.

Do not use near a naked flame.

Administrative Data

7. MARKETING AUTHORISATION HOLDER

Glaxo Wellcome UK Ltd

trading as

Glaxo Laboratories and/or GlaxoSmithKline UK

Stockley Park West

Uxbridge

Middlesex

UB11 1BT

8. MARKETING AUTHORISATION NUMBER(S)
PL 10949/0046

9. DATE OF FIRST AUTHORISATION/RENEWAL OF THE AUTHORISATION
10 November 1999

10. DATE OF REVISION OF THE TEXT
27 November 2007

Deseril Tablets 1mg

(Alliance Pharmaceuticals)

1. NAME OF THE MEDICINAL PRODUCT
Deseril® tablets 1mg

2. QUALITATIVE AND QUANTITATIVE COMPOSITION
Methysergide maleate BP 1.33 mg.

3. PHARMACEUTICAL FORM
White, biconvex, sugar-coated tablet, branded DSL on one side.

4. CLINICAL PARTICULARS

4.1 Therapeutic indications
Prophylactic treatment of migraine with or without aura, and cluster headache and other vascular headaches in patients who, despite attempts at control, experience headaches of such severity or regularity that social or economic life is seriously disrupted. (Note: Deseril is not recommended for treatment of the acute attack).

Diarrhoea caused by carcinoid disease.

4.2 Posology and method of administration
Prophylactic treatment of headache: 1 or 2 tablets three times a day with meals. Treatment should start with one tablet at bedtime and dosage should then be increased gradually over about two weeks until effective levels are reached. The minimum effective dose should be used, often that which will prevent 75% of attacks rather than all headaches.

From the outset, patients should understand that regular clinical supervision and periodic withdrawal of treatment are essential so that adverse effects can be recognised and minimised (see Section 4.4 Special warnings and precautions for use).

Carcinoid Syndrome: High doses are usually necessary. In most reported cases, dosage ranged between 12 and 20 tablets daily.

Children: Not recommended.

Elderly: No evidence exists that elderly patients require different dosage from younger patients.

4.3 Contraindications
Hypersensitivity to methysergide or any of the excipients of Deseril, pregnancy, lactation, peripheral vascular disorders, progressive arteriosclerosis, inadequately controlled hypertension, coronary heart disease, valvular heart disease, phlebitis or cellulitis of the lower extremities, impaired kidney or liver function, temporal arteritis, hemiplegic or basilar migraine, history of drug – induced fibrotic disorders (e.g. retroperitoneal fibrosis), pulmonary fibrosis, collagen diseases, obstructive diseases of the urinary tract, cachectic or septic conditions.

Concomitant treatment with macrolide antibiotics, HIV-protease or reverse-transcriptase inhibitors, azole antifungals (see section 4.5 Interaction with other medicinal products and other forms of interaction).

Concomitant treatment with vasoconstrictive agents (including ergot alkaloids), sumatriptan and other 5HT$_1$-receptor agonists (see section 4.5 Interaction with other medicinal products and other forms of interaction).

4.4 Special warnings and precautions for use
Continuous Deseril administration should not exceed six months without a drug-free interval of at least one month for re-assessment; dosage should be reduced gradually over two to three weeks to avoid rebound headaches. In patients undergoing treatment with Deseril the dose of ergotamine required to control acute attacks may have to be reduced.

Regular clinical supervision of patients treated with Deseril is essential. Particular attention should be paid to complaints of urinary dysfunction, pain in the loin, flank or chest, and pain, coldness or numbness in the limbs. Patients should be regularly examined for the presence of cardiac murmurs, vascular bruits, pleural or pericardial friction rubs and abdominal or flank masses or tenderness. Caution is also advised during drug administration to patients with a past history of peptic ulceration.

At the first signs of impaired peripheral circulation, prompt withdrawal of the drug is recommended.

In carcinoid syndrome the risk of adverse reactions due to the higher dosage must be weighed against the therapeutic benefit.

4.5 Interaction with other medicinal products and other forms of interaction
Concomitant use of Deseril and vasoconstrictors or vasopressors, including ergot alkaloids, sumatriptan and other 5-HT$_1$-receptor agonists, and nicotine (e.g. heavy smoking) must be avoided since this may result in enhanced vasoconstriction (see section 4.3 Contra-indications). Methysergide should not be administered within six hours of therapy with 5-HT$_1$ receptor agonists. In addition, use of 5-HT$_1$ receptor agonists should be avoided for at least 24 hours after the last methysergide dose.

The concomitant use of cytochrome P450 3A (CYP3A) inhibitors such as macrolide antibiotics (e.g. troleandomycin, erythromycin, clarithromycin), HIV protease or reverse transcriptase inhibitors (e.g. ritonavir, indinavir, nelfinavir, delavirdine), azole antifungals (e.g. ketoconazole, itraconazole, voriconazole) or cimetidine and Deseril must be avoided (see 4.3 Contra-indications), since this can result in an elevated exposure to methysergide and ergot toxicity (vasospasm and ischemia of the extremities and other tissues). Ergot alkaloids have also been shown to be inhibitors of CYP3A. No pharmacokinetic interactions involving other cytochrome P450 isoenzymes are known.

4.6 Pregnancy and lactation
Deseril is contra-indicated during pregnancy. It is likely that methysergide is excreted in breast milk. Deseril is therefore contra-indicated for nursing mothers.

4.7 Effects on ability to drive and use machines
Patients should be warned of the potential hazards of driving or operating machinery if they experience side effects such as dizziness, drowsiness or disturbances in vision.

4.8 Undesirable effects
General: The most commonly reported side-effects are nausea, heartburn, abdominal discomfort, vomiting, dizziness, lassitude and drowsiness. These side-effects can often be minimised by taking Deseril with food. Tissue oedema, insomnia, vertigo, leg cramps and weight gain have occurred, and skin eruptions or loss of scalp hair have occasionally been reported. Mental and behavioural disturbances have occurred in isolated instances.

Fibrosis: Continuous long-term Deseril administration has been associated with the development of fibrosis particularly of the pleura and retroperitoneum but, in rare cases also of the pericardium and the cardiac valves.

Retroperitoneal fibrosis: May present with symptoms of urinary tract obstruction such as general malaise, backache, persistent loin or flank pain, oliguria, dysuria, increased blood nitrogen and vascular insufficiency of the lower limbs. Deseril must be withdrawn if retroperitoneal fibrosis develops; drug withdrawal is often associated with clinical improvement over a few days to several weeks.

Fibrosis in other areas: Fibrotic processes involving lungs, pleura, heart valves and major vessels have been reported. Fibrosis of the pericardium and cardiac valves is very rare when the drug was given for less than 6 months. Pleuropulmonary fibrosis may present with chest pain, dyspnoea or pleural friction rub and pleural effusion. Cardiac valve fibrosis may be noticed by cardiac murmurs, which may lead to impaired cardiac function. Appearance of these symptoms demands immediate withdrawal of Deseril. These fibrotic manifestations are often reversible although less readily so than retroperitoneal fibrosis.

Vascular: Vascular reactions, (affecting both large and small arteries) including arterial spasm, have been seen in some patients. The following have all been described; arterial spasm in a limb causing coldness, numbness, pain or intermittent claudication with or without paraesthesia and diminished or absent pulse; renal artery spasm giving rise to transitory hypertension; mesenteric artery spasm causing abdominal pain; retinal artery spasm causing reversible loss of vision; coronary artery spasm causing angina. Arterial spasm is rapidly reversible following drug withdrawal. There have been isolated reports of myocardial infarction particularly in patients not adhering to the contraindications of coronary heart disease or the use of other vasoconstrictive drugs.

4.9 Overdose
Experience with cases of overdoses with Deseril is limited. Symptoms: headache, agitation, hyperactivity, nausea, vomiting, abdominal pain, mydriasis, tachycardia, cyanosis, peripheral vasospasm with diminished pulses and coldness of extremities.

Treatment: Treatment is essentially symptomatic and supportive. Administration of activated charcoal is recommended; in case of very recent intake, gastric lavage may be considered. For controlling hyperactivity, conventional sedative measures may be used. In the event of severe vasospastic reactions, i.v. administration of a peripheral vasodilator such as nitroprusside, phentolamine, local administration of warmth to the affected area and nursing care to prevent tissue damage are recommended. In the case of coronary constriction, appropriate treatment should be initiated.

5. PHARMACOLOGICAL PROPERTIES

5.1 Pharmacodynamic properties
Deseril is effective in the prevention of migraine chiefly on account of its marked 5–HT receptor antagonism, probably by inhibition of 5-HT$_{2B}$ receptors (inhibition of pain-facilitating and permeability-increasing actions of 5-HT).

5.2 Pharmacokinetic properties
Methysergide is rapidly and well absorbed. The parent drug is metabolised in the liver mainly to methylergometrine. Unchanged parent drug and metabolites are excreted predominantly via the kidney; the elimination is biphasic, with a half-life of 2.7 hours for the α-phase and 10 hours for the β-phase. Protein binding is moderate (66%).

5.3 Preclinical safety data
There are no findings of relevance to the prescriber which are additional to those already included in other sections of the SmPC.

6. PHARMACEUTICAL PARTICULARS

6.1 List of excipients
Maleic acid, gelatin, stearic acid, talc, maize starch, lactose. The coating constituents are gum acacia, sugar, talc, titanium dioxide, silica, carnauba wax and printing ink (consisting of Shellac, black iron oxide, ethanol and isopropanol).

6.2 Incompatibilities
None.

6.3 Shelf life
5 years.

6.4 Special precautions for storage
None.

6.5 Nature and contents of container
Aluminium/PVdC blister strips of 60 tablets.

6.6 Special precautions for disposal and other handling
None.

Administrative Data

7. MARKETING AUTHORISATION HOLDER
Alliance Pharmaceuticals Ltd

Avonbridge House

Bath Road

Chippenham

Wiltshire

SN15 2BB

8. MARKETING AUTHORISATION NUMBER(S)
PL16853/0006

9. DATE OF FIRST AUTHORISATION/RENEWAL OF THE AUTHORISATION
25 June 1998

10. DATE OF REVISION OF THE TEXT
December 2006

11. Legal status
POM

Alliance, Alliance Pharmaceuticals and associated devices are registered Trademarks of Alliance Pharmaceuticals Ltd.

DesmoMelt 120mcg and 240mcg oral lyophilisate

(Ferring Pharmaceuticals Ltd)

1. NAME OF THE MEDICINAL PRODUCT
DesmoMelt* ▼ 120 micrograms oral lyophilisate

DesmoMelt* ▼ 240 micrograms oral lyophilisate

2. QUALITATIVE AND QUANTITATIVE COMPOSITION
Each unit contains 120 or 240 micrograms desmopressin (as acetate).

For excipients, see 6.1

3. PHARMACEUTICAL FORM
Oral lyophilisate

DesmoMelt 120 micrograms oral lyophilisate

White, round, oral lyophilisate marked with two drop shaped figures on one side.

DesmoMelt* 240 micrograms oral lyophilisate

White, round, oral lyophilisate marked with three drop shaped figures on one side.

4. CLINICAL PARTICULARS

4.1 Therapeutic indications
DesmoMelt is indicated for the treatment of primary nocturnal enuresis.

4.2 Posology and method of administration
DesmoMelt is for sublingual use.

Children (from 5 years of age) and adults (up to 65 years of age) with normal urine concentrating ability who have primary nocturnal enuresis should take 120 micrograms at bedtime administered sublingually and only if needed should the dose be increased to 240 micrograms sublingually.

The need for continued treatment should be reassessed after 3 months by means of a period of at least 1 week without DesmoMelt.

4.3 Contraindications
DesmoMelt is contraindicated in cases of cardiac insufficiency and other conditions requiring treatment with diuretic agents. DesmoMelt should only be used in patients with normal blood pressure.

Before prescribing DesmoMelt, the diagnoses of psychogenic polydipsia and alcohol abuse should be excluded.

Desmopressin should not be prescribed to patients over the age of 65 for the treatment of primary nocturnal enuresis.

4.4 Special warnings and precautions for use

Care should be taken with patients who have reduced renal function and/or cardiovascular disease or cystic fibrosis. In chronic renal disease the antidiuretic effect of DesmoMelt would be less than normal.

When DesmoMelt is used for the treatment of enuresis, fluid intake must be limited from 1 hour before until 8 hours after administration.

Patients being treated for primary nocturnal enuresis should be warned to avoid ingesting water while swimming and to discontinue DesmoMelt during an episode of vomiting and/or diarrhoea until their fluid balance is once again normal.

Precautions to prevent fluid overload must be taken in:

- conditions characterised by fluid and/or electrolyte imbalance
- patients at risk for increased intracranial pressure

4.5 Interaction with other medicinal products and other forms of interaction

Substances which are known to induce SIADH e.g. tricyclic antidepressants, selective serotonin re-uptake inhibitors, chlorpromazine and carbamazepine, may cause an additive antidiuretic effect leading to an increased risk of water retention and/or hyponatraemia.

NSAIDs may induce water retention and/or hyponatraemia.

Concomitant treatment with loperamide may result in a 3-fold increase of desmopressin plasma concentrations, which may lead to an increased risk of water retention and/or hyponatraemia. Although not investigated, other drugs slowing intestinal transport might have the same effect.

A standardised 27% fat meal significantly decreased the absorption (rate and extent) of a 0.4mg dose of oral desmopressin tablets. Although it did not significantly affect the pharmacodynamic effect (urine production and osmolality) there is the potential for this to occur at lower doses. If a diminution of effect is noted, then the effect of food should be considered before increasing the dose.

4.6 Pregnancy and lactation

Pregnancy:

Data on a limited number (n=53) of exposed pregnancies in women with diabetes insipidus indicate rare cases of malformations in children treated during pregnancy. To date, no other relevant epidemiological data are available. Animal studies do not indicate direct or indirect harmful effects with respect to pregnancy, embryonal/fetal development, parturition or postnatal development.

Caution should be exercised when prescribing to pregnant women. Blood pressure monitoring is recommended due to the increased risk of pre-eclampsia.

Lactation:

Results from analyses of milk from nursing mothers receiving high dose desmopressin (300 micrograms intranasally) indicate that the amounts of desmopressin that may be transferred to the child are considerably less than the amounts required to influence diuresis.

4.7 Effects on ability to drive and use machines

None

4.8 Undesirable effects

Side-effects include headache, stomach pain and nausea. Isolated cases of allergic skin reactions and more severe general allergic reactions have been reported. Very rare cases of emotional disorders including aggression in children have been reported. Treatment with desmopressin without concomitant reduction of fluid intake may lead to water retention/hyponatraemia with accompanying symptoms of headache, nausea, vomiting, weight gain, decreased serum sodium and in serious cases, convulsions.

4.9 Overdose

An overdose of DesmoMelt leads to a prolonged duration of action with an increased risk of water retention and/or hyponatraemia.

Treatment:

Although the treatment of hyponatraemia should be individualised, the following general recommendations can be given. Hyponatraemia is treated by discontinuing the desmopressin treatment, fluid restriction and symptomatic treatment if needed.

5. PHARMACOLOGICAL PROPERTIES

5.1 Pharmacodynamic properties

Pharmacotherapeutic group: vasopressin and analogues

ATC code: H01B A02

In its main biological effects, desmopressin does not differ qualitatively from vasopressin. However, desmopressin is characterised by a high antidiuretic activity whereas the uterotonic and vasopressor actions are extremely low.

5.2 Pharmacokinetic properties

The overall mean systemic bioavailability of desmopressin administered sublingually as Melts at doses of 200, 400 and 800 micrograms is 0.25% with a 95% confidence interval of 0.21% - 0.31%. The C_{max} was 14, 30 and 65pg/ml after administration of 200, 400 and 800 micrograms respectively. t_{max} was observed at 0.5 – 2.0 hours after dosing. The geometric mean terminal half-life is 2.8 (CV= 24%) hours.

Correlation table between desmopressin in Tablet and Melt forms:

(see Table 1 below)

The distribution volume of desmopressin after intravenous administration is 33 L (0.41 L/kg). Desmopressin does not cross the blood-brain barrier. Desmopressin exhibits a moderate to high variability in bioavailability, both within and between subjects. Concomitant use of food decreases the rate and extent of absorption by 40%.

In vitro, in human liver microsome preparations, it has been shown that no significant amount of desmopressin is metabolised in the liver and thus human liver metabolism *in vivo* is not likely to occur.

It is unlikely that desmopressin will interact with drugs affecting hepatic metabolism, since desmopressin has been shown not to undergo significant liver metabolism in *in vitro* studies with human microsomes. However, formal *in vivo* interaction studies have not been performed.

5.3 Preclinical safety data

There are no pre-clinical data of relevance to the prescriber which are additional to that already included in other sections of the SPC.

6. PHARMACEUTICAL PARTICULARS

6.1 List of excipients

Gelatin

Mannitol

Citric acid, anhydrous

6.2 Incompatibilities

Not applicable

6.3 Shelf life

24 months

6.4 Special precautions for storage

Store in the original package.

6.5 Nature and contents of container

PVC/Polyamide/Aluminium/Polyamide/PVC blisters. Top foil consists of Paper/Polyester teraphthalate/Aluminium/heat seal lacquer. Strips of 10 oral lyophilisates in packs of 30 oral lyophilisates.

6.6 Special precautions for disposal and other handling

None.

Administrative Data

7. MARKETING AUTHORISATION HOLDER

Ferring Pharmaceuticals Ltd.

The Courtyard

Waterside Drive

Langley

Berkshire SL3 6EZ

United Kingdom

8. MARKETING AUTHORISATION NUMBER(S)

DesmoMelt 120 micrograms oral lyophilisate PL 03194/0094

DesmoMelt 240 micrograms oral lyophilisate PL 03194/0095

9. DATE OF FIRST AUTHORISATION/RENEWAL OF THE AUTHORISATION

19th January 2006

Table 1 Correlation table between desmopressin in Tablet and Melt forms

Tablet	Tablet	Melt	Melt
Desmopressin acetate	Desmopressin free base	Desmopressin free base	Desmopressin acetate
0.1mg	89 micrograms	60 micrograms	Approx. 67 micrograms *
0.2mg	178 micrograms	120 micrograms	Approx. 135 micrograms *
0.4mg	356 micrograms	240 micrograms	Approx. 270 micrograms *

*calculated for comparative purposes

10. DATE OF REVISION OF THE TEXT

MAY 2008

* DesmoMelt is a trademark of Ferring BV.

Desmospray, Desmopressin Nasal Spray

(Ferring Pharmaceuticals Ltd)

1. NAME OF THE MEDICINAL PRODUCT

DESMOSPRAY®, Desmopressin Nasal Spray.

2. QUALITATIVE AND QUANTITATIVE COMPOSITION

DESMOSPRAY contains 10 micrograms of Demopressin acetate per actuation.

3. PHARMACEUTICAL FORM

Nasal spray.

4. CLINICAL PARTICULARS

4.1 Therapeutic indications

DESMOSPRAY is indicated for:

i) The treatment of nocturia associated with multiple sclerosis where other treatments have failed.

ii) The diagnosis and treatment of vasopressin-sensitive cranial diabetes insipidus.

iii) Establishing renal concentration capacity.

4.2 Posology and method of administration

Treatment of Nocturia:

When DESMOSPRAY is used for the treatment of nocturia associated with multiple sclerosis, fluid intake must be limited to a minimum from 1 hour before using the spray at bedtime until the next morning and in any case for a minimum of 8 hours after administration.

For multiple sclerosis patients up to 65 years of age with normal renal function suffering from nocturia the dose is one or two sprays intranasally (10 to 20 micrograms) at bedtime. Not more than one dose should be used in any 24 hour period. If a dose of two sprays is required, this should be as one spray into each nostril.

Treatment of Diabetes Insipidus:

Dosage is individual but clinical experience has shown that the average maintenance dose in adults and children is one or two sprays (10 to 20 micrograms) once or twice daily. If a dose of two sprays is required, this should be as one spray into each nostril.

Diagnosis of Diabetes Insipidus:

The diagnostic dose in adults and children is two sprays (20 micrograms). Failure to elaborate a concentrated urine after water deprivation, followed by the ability to do so after the administration of DESMOSPRAY confirms the diagnosis of cranial diabetes insipidus. Failure to concentrate after the administration suggests nephrogenic diabetes insipidus.

Renal Function Testing:

Recommended doses for the renal concentration capacity test:

Adults: Two sprays into each nostril (a total of 40 micrograms)

Children: (1-15 years): One spray into each nostril (a total of 20 micrograms).

Infants (to 1 year): One spray (10 micrograms).

Adults and children with normal renal function can be expected to achieve concentrations above 700mOsm/kg in the period of 5-9 hours following administration of DESMOSPRAY. It is recommended that the bladder should be emptied at the time of administration.

In normal infants a urine concentration of 600mOsm/kg should be achieved in the 5 hour period following the administration of DESMOSPRAY. The fluid intake at the two meals following the administration should be restricted to 50% of the ordinary intake in order to avoid water overload.

4.3 Contraindications

DESMOSPRAY is contraindicated in cases of:

- syndrome of inappropriate ADH secretion (SIADH)
- known hyponatraemia
- a history of known or suspected cardiac insufficiency and other conditions requiring treatment with diuretics
- moderate and severe renal insufficiency (creatinine clearance below 50ml/min)
- hypersensitivity to desmopressin or to any of the excipients of DESMOSPRAY.

Before prescribing DESMOSPRAY, the diagnoses of habitual or psychogenic polydipsia (resulting in a urine production exceeding 40mg/kg/24 hours) and alcohol abuse should be excluded.

When used to control nocturia in patients with multiple sclerosis, desmopressin should not be used in patients with hypertension or cardiovascular disease.

Desmopressin should not be prescribed to patients over the age of 65 for the treatment of nocturia associated with multiple sclerosis.

4.4 Special warnings and precautions for use

DESMOSPRAY should only be used in patients where orally administered formulations are not suitable.

When DESMOSPRAY is prescribed, it is recommended:

- to start at the lowest dose
- to ensure compliance with fluid restriction instructions
- to increase dosage progressively, with caution
- to ensure that in children, administration is under adult supervision in order to control the dose intake.

Care should be taken with patients who have reduced renal function and/or cardiovascular disease or cystic fibrosis.

Severe bladder dysfunction and outlet obstruction should be considered before starting treatment.

When DESMOSPRAY is used for the treatment of nocturia associated with multiple sclerosis, periodic assessments should be made of blood pressure and weight to monitor the possibility of fluid overload. Treatment with desmopressin should be interrupted during acute intercurrent illness characterised by fluid and/or electrolyte imbalance (such as vomiting, diarrhoea, systemic infections, fever, gastroenteritis).

In the event of signs or symptoms of water retention and/or hyponatraemia (headache, nausea/vomiting, weight gain and in severe cases, convulsions) treatment should be interrupted until the patient has fully recovered. When restarting treatment, strict fluid restriction should be enforced.

Elderly patients and patients with low serum sodium levels may have an increased risk of hyponatraemia.

Precautions to avoid hyponatraemia, including careful attention to fluid restriction and more frequent monitoring of serum sodium, must be taken in case of concomitant treatment with drugs which are known to induce SIADH e.g. tricyclic antidepressants, selective serotonin reuptake inhibitors, chlorpromazine, carbamazepine and NSAIDs.

When used for diagnostic purposes, fluid intake must be limited and not exceed 0.5 litres from 1 hour before until 8 hours after administration.

Following diagnostic testing for diabetes insipidus or renal concentration capacity, care should be taken to prevent fluid overload. Fluid should not be forced, orally or parenterally, and patients should only take as much fluid as they require to satisfy thirst.

There is some evidence from post-marketing data for the occurrence of severe hyponatraemia in association with the nasal spray formulation of desmopressin, when it is used in the treatment of cranial diabetes insipidus.

Precautions to prevent fluid overload must be taken in:

- conditions characterised by fluid and/or electrolyte imbalance
- patients at risk for increased intracranial pressure

Renal concentration capacity testing in children below the age of 1 year should only be performed under carefully supervised conditions in hospital.

4.5 Interaction with other medicinal products and other forms of interaction

Substances which are known to induce SIADH e.g. tricyclic antidepressants, selective serotonin re-uptake inhibitors, chlorpromazine and carbamazepine, may cause an additive antidiuretic effect leading to an increased risk of water retention and/or hyponatraemia (see 4.4).

NSAIDs may induce water retention and/or hyponatraemia (see 4.4).

4.6 Pregnancy and lactation

Pregnancy:

Data on a limited number (n=53) of exposed pregnancies in women with diabetes insipidus indicate rare cases of malformations in children treated during pregnancy. To date, no other relevant epidemiological data are available. Animal studies do not indicate direct or indirect harmful effects with respect to pregnancy, embryonal/fetal development, parturition or postnatal development.

Caution should be exercised when prescribing to pregnant women. Blood pressure monitoring is recommended due to the increased risk of pre-eclampsia.

Lactation:

Results from analyses of milk from nursing mothers receiving high dose desmopressin (300 micrograms intranasally) indicate that the amounts of desmopressin that may be transferred to the child are considerably less than the amounts required to influence diuresis.

4.7 Effects on ability to drive and use machines

None

4.8 Undesirable effects

Side-effects include headache, stomach pain, nausea, nasal congestion, rhinitis and epistaxis. Isolated cases of allergic skin reactions and more severe general allergic reactions have been reported. Very rare cases of emotional disorders including aggression in children have been reported. Treatment without concomitant reduction of fluid intake may lead to water retention/hyponatraemia with or without accompanying warning signs and symptoms (headache, nausea/vomiting, weight gain, decreased serum sodium and in severe cases, convulsions).

4.9 Overdose

An overdose of DESMOSPRAY leads to a prolonged duration of action with an increased risk of water retention and/ or hyponatraemia.

Treatment:

Although the treatment of hyponatraemia should be individualised, the following general recommendations can be given. Hyponatraemia is treated by discontinuing the desmopressin treatment, fluid restriction and symptomatic treatment if needed.

5. PHARMACOLOGICAL PROPERTIES

5.1 Pharmacodynamic properties

Desmopressin is a structural analogue of vasopressin, with two chemical changes, namely desamination of the N-terminal and replacement of the 8-L-Arginine by D-8-Arginine. These changes have increased the antidiuretic activity and prolonged the duration of action. The pressor activity is reduced to less than 0.01% of the natural peptide as a result of which side-effects are rarely seen.

5.2 Pharmacokinetic properties

Following intranasal administration, the bioavailability of desmopressin is of the order of 10%.

Pharmacokinetic parameters following intravenous administration have been reported as follows:

Total clearance: 2.6ml/ min/kg body wt.

$T_{½}$: 55mins

Plasma kinetics of DDAVP in man

H. Vilhardt, S. Lundin, J. Falch

Acta Pharmacol et Toxicol, 1986, 58, 379-381

In vitro, in human liver microsome preparations, it has been shown that no significant amount of desmopressin is metabolised in the liver and thus human liver metabolism *in vivo* is not likely to occur.

It is unlikely that desmopressin will interact with drugs affecting hepatic metabolism, since desmopressin has been shown not to undergo significant liver metabolism in *in vitro* studies with human microsomes. However, formal *in vivo* interaction studies have not been performed.

5.3 Preclinical safety data

There are no pre-clinical data of relevance to the prescriber which are additional to that already included in other sections of the SPC.

6. PHARMACEUTICAL PARTICULARS

6.1 List of excipients

Sodium Chloride EP

Citric Acid Monohydrate EP

Disodium Phosphate Dihydrate EP

Benzalkonium Chloride Solution 50% EP

Purified Water EP.

6.2 Incompatibilities

None known.

6.3 Shelf life

3 years.

6.4 Special precautions for storage

Store at room temperature (up to 25°C). Protect from light.

6.5 Nature and contents of container

The spray pack comprises of a 10ml amber glass injection vial fitted with a snap-on tamper-proof pre-compression pump spray device, to which a 20mm nasal adaptor is attached. It contains a clear, colourless solution of desmopressin acetate 0.1mg/ml. The fill volume is 7.1ml including overage to allow delivery of 60 doses of 0.1ml.

6.6 Special precautions for disposal and other handling

None.

7. MARKETING AUTHORISATION HOLDER

Ferring Pharmaceuticals Ltd.,

The Courtyard

Waterside Drive

Langley

Berkshire

SL3 6EZ

8. MARKETING AUTHORISATION NUMBER(S)

PL 03194/0024

9. DATE OF FIRST AUTHORISATION/RENEWAL OF THE AUTHORISATION

First authorisation: 1 April 1987

Renewal: 30th April 2002

10. DATE OF REVISION OF THE TEXT

May 2008

Desmotabs 0.2mg

(Ferring Pharmaceuticals Ltd)

1. NAME OF THE MEDICINAL PRODUCT

DESMOTABS® 0.2mg

2. QUALITATIVE AND QUANTITATIVE COMPOSITION

Each tablet contains 0.2mg desmopressin acetate

For excipients, see 6.1

3. PHARMACEUTICAL FORM

Tablet

Uncoated, white, round, convex tablets scored on one side and engraved '0.2' on the other side.

4. CLINICAL PARTICULARS

4.1 Therapeutic indications

Desmopressin tablets are indicated for the treatment of primary nocturnal enuresis.

4.2 Posology and method of administration

Children (from 5 years of age) and adults (up to 65 years of age) with normal urine concentrating ability who have primary nocturnal enuresis should take 0.2mg at bedtime and only if needed should the dose be increased to 0.4mg.

The need for continued treatment should be reassessed after 3 months by means of a period of at least 1 week without desmopressin tablets.

4.3 Contraindications

Desmopressin tablets are contraindicated in cases of cardiac insufficiency and other conditions requiring treatment with diuretic agents. Desmopressin tablets should only be used in patients with normal blood pressure.

Before prescribing desmopressin tablets the diagnoses of psychogenic polydipsia and alcohol abuse should be excluded.

Desmopressin should not be prescribed to patients over the age of 65 for the treatment of primary nocturnal enuresis.

4.4 Special warnings and precautions for use

Care should be taken with patients who have reduced renal function and/or cardiovascular disease or cystic fibrosis. In chronic renal disease the antidiuretic effect of desmopressin tablets would be less than normal.

When desmopressin tablets are used for the treatment of enuresis, fluid intake must be limited from 1 hour before taking the tablets at bedtime until the next morning and in any case for a minimum of 8 hours after administration.

Patients being treated for primary nocturnal enuresis should be warned to avoid ingesting water while swimming and to discontinue desmopressin tablets during an episode of vomiting and/or diarrhoea until their fluid balance is once again normal.

Precautions to prevent fluid overload must be taken in:

- conditions characterised by fluid and/or electrolyte imbalance
- patients at risk for increased intracranial pressure

4.5 Interaction with other medicinal products and other forms of interaction

Substances which are known to induce SIADH e.g. tricyclic antidepressants, selective serotonin re-uptake inhibitors, chlorpromazine and carbamazepine, may cause an additive antidiuretic effect leading to an increased risk of water retention and/or hyponatraemia.

NSAIDs may induce water retention and/or hyponatraemia.

Concomitant treatment with loperamide may result in a 3-fold increase of desmopressin plasma concentrations, which may lead to an increased risk of water retention and/or hyponatraemia. Although not investigated, other drugs slowing transport might have the same effect.

A standardised 27% fat meal significantly decreased the absorption (rate and extent) of a 0.4mg dose of oral desmopressin. Although it did not significantly affect the pharmacodynamic effect (urine production and osmolality), there is the potential for this to occur at lower doses. If a diminution of effect is noted, then the effect of food should be considered before increasing the dose.

4.6 Pregnancy and lactation

Pregnancy:

Data on a limited number (n=53) of exposed pregnancies in women with diabetes insipidus indicate rare cases of malformations in children treated during pregnancy. To date, no other relevant epidemiological data are available. Animal studies do not indicate direct or indirect harmful effects with respect to pregnancy, embryonal/fetal development, parturition or postnatal development.

Caution should be exercised when prescribing to pregnant women. Blood pressure monitoring is recommended due to the increased risk of pre-eclampsia.

Lactation:

Results from analyses of milk from nursing mothers receiving high dose desmopressin (300 micrograms intranasally) indicate that the amounts of desmopressin that may be transferred to the child are considerably less than the amounts required to influence diuresis.

4.7 Effects on ability to drive and use machines

None

4.8 Undesirable effects

Side-effects include headache, stomach pain and nausea. Isolated cases of allergic skin reactions and more severe general allergic reactions have been reported. Very rare cases of emotional disorders including aggression in children have been reported. Treatment with desmopressin without concomitant reduction of fluid intake may lead to water retention/hyponatraemia with accompanying symptoms of headache, nausea, vomiting, weight gain, decreased serum sodium and in serious cases, convulsions.

4.9 Overdose

An overdose of desmopressin tablets leads to a prolonged duration of action with an increased risk of water retention and/or hyponatraemia.

Treatment:

Although the treatment of hyponatraemia should be individualised, the following general recommendations can be given. Hyponatraemia is treated by discontinuing the desmopressin treatment, fluid restriction and symptomatic treatment if needed.

5. PHARMACOLOGICAL PROPERTIES

5.1 Pharmacodynamic properties

In its main biological effects, desmopressin does not differ qualitatively from vasopressin. However, desmopressin is characterised by a high antidiuretic activity whereas the uterotonic and vasopressor actions are extremely low.

In a modelling study in which intravenous desmopressin was infused over two hours in healthy adult male subjects, the EC_{50} value was calculated as 1.7pg/ml based on urinary osmolality and 2.4pg/ml based on urinary volume.

5.2 Pharmacokinetic properties

The absolute bioavailability of orally administered desmopressin varies between 0.08% and 0.16%. Mean maximum plasma concentration is reached within 2 hours. The distribution volume is 0.2 – 0.32 l/kg. Desmopressin does not cross the blood-brain barrier. The oral terminal half-life varies between 2.0 and 3.11 hours.

After oral administration of a single dose of 2 × 200 micrograms desmopressin tablets to healthy subjects, 25% of the subjects had plasma concentrations of desmopressin above 1pg/ml up to at least 14 hours post dosing.

In *in vitro* studies in human liver microsome preparations, it has been shown that no significant amount of desmopressin is metabolised, and thus human liver metabolism *in vivo* is not likely to occur. Consequently it is also unlikely that desmopressin will interact with drugs affecting hepatic metabolism. However, formal *in vivo* interaction studies have not been performed.

About 65% of the amount of desmopressin absorbed after oral administration could be recovered in the urine within 24 hours.

5.3 Preclinical safety data

There are no pre-clinical data of relevance to the prescriber which are additional to that already included in other sections of the SPC.

6. PHARMACEUTICAL PARTICULARS

6.1 List of excipients

Lactose monohydrate

Potato starch

Povidone

Magnesium stearate

6.2 Incompatibilities

Not applicable

6.3 Shelf life

36 months.

6.4 Special precautions for storage

Do not store above 25°C. Keep the container tightly closed.

6.5 Nature and contents of container

30ml High Density Polyethylene (HDPE) bottle with a tamper-proof, twist-off polypropylene (PP) closure with a silica gel desiccant insert. Each bottle contains 7, 30 or 90 tablets.

Not all pack sizes may be marketed.

6.6 Special precautions for disposal and other handling

None.

7. MARKETING AUTHORISATION HOLDER

Ferring Pharmaceuticals Ltd.,

The Courtyard

Waterside Drive

Langley

Berkshire SL3 6EZ.

8. MARKETING AUTHORISATION NUMBER(S)

PL 03194/0046

9. DATE OF FIRST AUTHORISATION/RENEWAL OF THE AUTHORISATION

19th April 1999.

10. DATE OF REVISION OF THE TEXT

May 2008

DESTOLIT 150 mg tablets

(Norgine Limited)

1. NAME OF THE MEDICINAL PRODUCT

Destolit 150 mg tablets

2. QUALITATIVE AND QUANTITATIVE COMPOSITION

Each tablet contains 150 mg ursodeoxycholic acid (UDCA)

3. PHARMACEUTICAL FORM

Tablet

4. CLINICAL PARTICULARS

4.1 Therapeutic indications

The dissolution of radiolucent (i.e. non-radio opaque) cholesterol gallstones in patients with a functioning gallbladder

4.2 Posology and method of administration

Adults and the elderly

Dissolution of gallstones:

A daily dose of 8 to 12mg/kg UDCA will produce cholesterol desaturation in the majority of cases. The measurement of the lithogenic index on bile-rich duodenal drainage fluid after 4-6 weeks of therapy may be useful for determining the minimum effective dose. The lowest effective dose has been found to be 4 mg/kg. The daily dose for most patients is 3 or 4 tablets, according to body weight. The dose should be divided into two administrations after meals, with one administration always after the evening meal.

The duration of treatment needed to achieve dissolution will not usually exceed 2 years, and should be monitored with regular cholecystograms. Treatment should be continued for 3-4 months after the radiological disappearance of gallstones.

Any temporary discontinuation of treatment, if prolonged for 3-4 weeks, will allow the bile to return to a state of supersaturation, and will extend the total time taken for litholysis. In some cases stones may recur after successful treatment.

Children and adolescents

Not recommended.

For oral administration.

4.3 Contraindications

Active gastric or duodenal ulcers, a non-functioning gall bladder, radio-opaque gall stones and inflammatory bowel disease are contraindicated, as are hepatic and intestinal conditions interfering with the enterohepatic circulation of bile acids (ileal resection and stoma, regional ileitis, extra and intra-hepatic cholestasis, severe, acute, and chronic liver diseases).

4.4 Special warnings and precautions for use

Excessive dietary intake of calories and cholesterol should be avoided; a low cholesterol diet will probably improve the effectiveness of Destolit tablets.

4.5 Interaction with other medicinal products and other forms of interaction

Drugs such as cholestyramine and some antacids bind bile acids in vitro, and may inhibit the absorption of UDCA.

There is a possibility of increased serum ciclosporin levels in some patients taking ursodeoxycholic acid and ciclosporin simultaneously.

It is recommended that drugs known to increase cholesterol elimination in bile, such as oestrogenic hormones, oral contraceptive agents and certain blood cholesterol lowering agents, such as clofibrate, should also not be prescribed concomitantly.

4.6 Pregnancy and lactation

It is advised that women of child bearing age should use adequate nonhormonal or low oestrogen oral contraceptive measures during treatment with UDCA, and that the drug should not be given during the first trimester of pregnancy unless, in the opinion of the physician, the benefit outweighs the risk.

There are no clinical data available on the safety of UDCA in women who are breast-feeding. Therefore, Destolit is not recommended in this patient group.

4.7 Effects on ability to drive and use machines

None known

4.8 Undesirable effects

Destolit is normally well tolerated. Diarrhoea has been found to occur only occasionally. No significant alterations have so far been observed in liver function. Nausea, vomiting, pruritus and gallstone calcification may occur.

4.9 Overdose

It is unlikely that overdosage will cause serious adverse effects. Diarrhoea may occur and it is recommended that liver function tests be monitored. Ion-exchange resins may be useful to bind bile acids in the intestine.

5. PHARMACOLOGICAL PROPERTIES

5.1 Pharmacodynamic properties

Ursodeoxycholic acid is a gallstone dissolving agent which acts by reducing the content of cholesterol in bile. This may be due either to a reduction in hepatic cholesterol synthesis or reduced absorption of cholesterol or both.

5.2 Pharmacokinetic properties

Intestinal absorption after an oral dose of UDCA is high, with a first-pass clearance of about 50 to 60%. Studies show that passive diffusion occurs, whereupon the drug enters the enterohepatic circulation and is subject to an efficient hepatic extraction mechanism. The 'spillover' into the systemic blood supply is therefore minimal. Plasma levels are not clinically important but may be useful in estimating patient compliance; they reach maximum concentrations at about 60 minutes after ingestion with another peak recorded at 3 hours.

Ursodeoxycholic acid is rapidly conjugated with glycine and taurine in the liver. Microbial biotransformation of the drug and its metabolites occurs when they leave the enterohepatic circulation and is responsible for high levels of faecal lithocholic and 7-ketolithocholic acids during ursodeoxycholic acid therapy. Intestinal flora also hydrolyse conjugated drug back to the parent compound and interconvert ursodeoxycholic and chenodeoxycholic acids.

5.3 Preclinical safety data

UDCA has not shown teratogenic potential in rats and rabbits; embryotoxicity seen in the rat at high doses appears to occur early in gestation.

UDCA was not genotoxic in bacterial mutation tests. It has shown genotoxic potential in vitro in a mammalian chromosome aberration study and in a gene mutation study using yeast, however, the relevance of this is questionable since UDCA was not carcinogenic in long term studies in mice and rats.

Bile acids act as tumour promoters in colon carcinogenesis, but there is no evidence that they are direct carcinogens. In two year carcinogenicity studies UDCA was not tumourigenic in mice. In rats an increase in adrenal phaeochromocytomas was observed which is not considered to be clinically significant

6. PHARMACEUTICAL PARTICULARS

6.1 List of excipients

Lactose, pregelatinised maize starch, acacia gum, talc, magnesium stearate, purified water.

6.2 Incompatibilities

None known

6.3 Shelf life

3 years

6.4 Special precautions for storage

None

6.5 Nature and contents of container

Blister pack of 60 tablets

6.6 Special precautions for disposal and other handling

None

7. MARKETING AUTHORISATION HOLDER

Norgine Ltd

Chaplin House

Widewater Place

Moorhall Road

Harefield

Uxbridge

Middlesex

UB9 5NS

8. MARKETING AUTHORISATION NUMBER(S)

PL 00322/0076

9. DATE OF FIRST AUTHORISATION/RENEWAL OF THE AUTHORISATION

22 August 2002

10. DATE OF REVISION OF THE TEXT

January 2009

Legal category POM

Detrusitol 1mg & 2mg film-coated tablets

(Pharmacia Limited)

1. NAME OF THE MEDICINAL PRODUCT

Detrusitol 1 mg filmcoated tablets

Detrusitol 2 mg filmcoated tablets

2. QUALITATIVE AND QUANTITATIVE COMPOSITION

Each filmcoated tablet contains tolterodine tartrate 1 mg or 2 mg corresponding to 0.68 mg and 1.37 mg tolterodine, respectively

For a full list of excipients, see section 6.1

3. PHARMACEUTICAL FORM

Filmcoated tablets

The filmcoated tablets are white, round and biconvex. The 1 mg tablet is engraved with arcs above and below the letters TO and the 2 mg tablet is engraved with arcs above and below the letters DT.

4. CLINICAL PARTICULARS

4.1 Therapeutic indications

Symptomatic treatment of urge incontinence and/or increased urinary frequency and urgency as may occur in patients with overactive bladder syndrome.

4.2 Posology and method of administration

Adults (including elderly):

The recommended dose is 2 mg twice daily except in patients with impaired liver function or severely impaired renal function (GFR$\leq$30 ml/min) for whom the recommended dose is 1 mg twice daily (see section 4.4). In case of troublesome side effects the dose may be reduced from 2 mg to 1 mg twice daily.

The effect of treatment should be re-evaluated after 2-3 months (see section 5.1).

Paediatric patients:

Efficacy of Detrusitol has not been demonstrated in children (See section 5.1). Therefore, Detrusitol is not recommended for children.

4.3 Contraindications

Tolterodine is contraindicated in patients with

- Urinary retention
- Uncontrolled narrow angle glaucoma
- Myasthenia gravis
- Known hypersensitivity to tolterodine or excipients
- Severe ulcerative colitis
- Toxic megacolon

4.4 Special warnings and precautions for use

Tolterodine shall be used with caution in patients with

- Significant bladder outlet obstruction at risk of urinary retention
- Gastrointestinal obstructive disorders, e.g. pyloric stenosis
- Renal impairement (see section 4.2)
- Hepatic disease. (see section 4.2 and 5.2)
- Autonomic neuropathy
- Hiatus hernia
- Risk for decreased gastrointestinal motility

Multiple oral total daily doses of immediate release 4 mg (therapeutic) and 8 mg (supratherapeutic) tolterodine have been shown to prolong the QTc interval (see section 5.1). The clinical relevance of these findings is unclear and will depend on individual patient risk factors and susceptibilities present.

Tolterodine should be used with caution in patients with risk factors for QT-prolongation including:

- Congenital or documented acquired QT prolongation
- Electrolyte disturbances such as hypokalaemia, hypomagnesaemia and hypocalcaemia
- Bradycardia
- Relevant pre-existing cardiac diseases (i.e. cardiomyopathy, myocardial ischaemia, arrhythmia, congestive heart failure)
- Concomitant administration of drugs known to prolong QT-interval including Class IA (e. g. quinidine, procainamide) and Class III (e. g. amiodarone, sotalol) anti-arrhythmics

This especially holds true when taking potent CYP3A4 inhibitors (see section 5.1).

Concomitant treatment with potent CYP3A4 inhibitors should be avoided (see section 4.5, Interactions).

As with all treatments for symptoms of urgency and urge incontinence, organic reasons for urge and frequency should be considered before treatment.

4.5 Interaction with other medicinal products and other forms of interaction

Concomitant systemic medication with potent CYP3A4 inhibitors such as macrolide antibiotics (e.g. erythromycin and clarithromycin), antifungal agents (e.g. ketoconazole and itraconazole) and antiproteases is not recommended due to increased serum concentrations of tolterodine in poor CYP2D6 metabolisers with (subsequent) risk of overdosage (see section 4.4).

Concomitant medication with other drugs that possess antimuscarinic properties may result in more pronounced therapeutic effect and side-effects. Conversely, the therapeutic effect of tolterodine may be reduced by concomitant administration of muscarinic cholinergic receptor agonists.

The effect of prokinetics like metoclopramide and cisapride may be decreased by tolterodine.

Concomitant treatment with fluoxetine (a potent CYP2D6 inhibitor) does not result in a clinically significant interaction since tolterodine and its CYP2D6-dependent metabolite, 5-hydroxymethyl tolterodine are equipotent.

Drug interaction studies have shown no interactions with warfarin or combined oral contraceptives (ethinyl estradiol/levonorgestrel).

A clinical study has indicated that tolterodine is not a metabolic inhibitor of CYP2D6, 2C19, 2C9, 3A4 or 1A2. Therefore an increase of plasma levels of drugs metabolised by these isoenzymes is not expected when dosed in combination with tolterodine.

4.6 Pregnancy and lactation

Pregnancy

There are no adequate data from the use of tolterodine in pregnant women.

Studies in animals have shown reproductive toxicity (see section 5.3). The potential risk for humans is unknown.

Consequently, Detrusitol is not recommended during pregnancy.

Lactation

No data concerning the excretion of tolterodine into human milk are available. Tolterodine should be avoided during lactation.

4.7 Effects on ability to drive and use machines

Since this drug may cause accommodation disturbances and influence reaction time, the ability to drive and use machines may be negatively affected.

4.8 Undesirable effects

Due to the pharmacological effect of tolterodine it may cause mild to moderate antimuscarinic effects, like dryness of the mouth, dyspepsia and dry eyes.

The table below reflects the data obtained with Detrusitol in clinical trials and from postmarketing experience. The most commonly reported adverse reaction was dry mouth, which occurred in 35% of patients treated with Detrusitol tablets and in 10% of placebo treated patients. Headaches were also reported very commonly and occurred in 10.1% of patients treated with Detrusitol tablets and in 7.4% of placebo treated patients.

(see Table 1 below)

Cases of aggravation of symptoms of dementia (e.g. confusion, disorientation, delusion) have been reported after tolterodine therapy was initiated in patients taking cholinesterase inhibitors for the treatment of dementia.

Paediatric patients

In two paediatric phase III randomised, placebo-controlled, double-blind studies conducted over 12 weeks where a total of 710 paediatric patients were recruited, the proportion of patients with urinary tract infections, diarrhoea and abnormal behaviour was higher in patients treated with tolterodine than placebo (urinary tract infection: tolterodine 6.8 %, placebo 3.6 %; diarrhoea: tolterodine 3.3 %, placebo 0.9 %; abnormal behaviour: tolterodine 1.6 %, placebo 0.4 %). (See section 5.1)

4.9 Overdose

The highest dose given to human volunteers of tolterodine L-tartrate is 12.8 mg as single dose. The most severe adverse events observed were accommodation disturbances and micturition difficulties.

In the event of tolterodine overdose, treat with gastric lavage and give activated charcoal. Treat symptoms as follows:

- Severe central anticholinergic effects (e.g. hallucinations, severe excitation): treat with physostigmine
- Convulsions or pronounced excitation: treat with benzodiazepines
- Respiratory insufficiency: treat with artificial respiration
- Tachycardia: treat with beta-blockers
- Urinary retention: treat with catheterization
- Mydriasis: treat with pilocarpine eye drops and/or place patient in dark room

An increase in QT interval was observed at a total daily dose of 8 mg immediate release tolterodine (twice the recommended daily dose of the immediate release formulation and equivalent to three times the peak exposure of the prolonged release capsule formulation) administered over four days. In the event of tolterodine overdose, standard supportive measures for managing QT prolongation should be adopted.

5. PHARMACOLOGICAL PROPERTIES

5.1 Pharmacodynamic properties

Pharmacotherapeutic group: Urinary antispasmodics

ATC code: G04B D07

Tolterodine is a competitive, specific muscarinic receptor antagonist with a selectivity for the urinary bladder over salivary glands in vivo. One of the tolterodine metabolites (5-hydroxymethyl derivative) exhibits a pharmacological profile similar to that of the parent compound. In extensive metabolisers this metabolite contributes significantly to the therapeutic effect (see 5.2).

Effect of the treatment can be expected within 4 weeks.

Effect of treatment with Detrusitol 2 mg twice daily after 4 and 12 weeks, respectively, compared with placebo (pooled data). Absolute change and percentage change relative to baseline.

(see Table 2 on next page)

The effect of tolterodine was evaluated in patients, examined with urodynamic assessment at baseline and, depending on the urodynamic result, they were allocated to a urodynamic positive (motor urgency) or a urodynamic negative (sensory urgency) group. Within each group, the patients were randomised to receive either tolterodine or placebo. The study could not provide convincing evidence that tolterodine had effects over placebo in patients with sensory urgency.

The clinical effects of tolterodine on QT interval were studied in ECGs obtained from over 600 treated patients, including the elderly and patients with pre-existing cardiovascular disease. The changes in QT intervals did not significantly differ between placebo and treatment groups.

The effect of tolterodine on QT-prolongation was investigated further in 48 healthy male and female volunteers aged 18 – 55 years. Subjects were administered 2 mg BID and 4 mg BID tolterodine as the immediate release formulations. The results (Fridericia corrected) at peak tolterodine concentration (1 hour) showed mean QTc interval increases of 5.0 and 11.8 msec for tolterodine doses of 2 mg BID 4 mg BID respectively and 19.3 msec for moxifloxacin (400mg) which was used as an active internal control. A pharmacokinetic/pharmacodynamic model estimated that QTc interval increases in poor metabolisers

Table 1

	Very Common (⩾ 1/10)	Common (⩾ 1/100 and < 1/10)	Uncommon (⩾ 1/1000 and < 1/100)	Not known (cannot be estimated from the available data)
Infections and infestations		Bronchitis		
Immune system disorders			Hypersensitivity not otherwise specified	Anaphylactoid reactions
Psychiatric disorders			Nervousness	Confusion, hallucinations, disorientation
Nervous system disorders	Headaches	Dizziness, somnolence, paresthesia	Memory impairment	
Eye disorders		Dry eyes, abnormal vision including abnormal accommodation		
Ear and labyrinth disorders		Vertigo		
Cardiac disorders		Palpitations	Tachycardia, cardiac failure, arrhythmia	
Vascular disorders				Flushing
Gastrointestinal disorders	Dry mouth	Dyspepsia, constipation, abdominal pain, flatulence, vomiting, diarrhoea	Gastroesophageal reflux	
Skin and subcutaneous tissue disorders		Dry skin		Angioedema
Renal and urinary disorders		Dysuria, urinary retention		
General disorders		Fatigue, chest pain, peripheral oedema		
Investigations		Increased weight		

Table 2

Variable	4-week studies			12-week studies		
	Detrusitol 2 mg b.i.d.	Placebo	Statistical significance vs. placebo	Detrusitol 2 mg b.i.d.	Placebo	Statistical significance vs. placebo
Number of micturitions per 24 hours	-1.6 (-14%) n=392	-0.9 (-8%) n=189	*	-2.3 (-20%) n=354	-1.4 (-12%) n=176	**
Number of incontinence episodes per 24 hours	-1.3 (-38%) n=288	-1.0 (-26%) n=151	n.s.	-1.6 (-47%) n=299	-1.1 (-32%) n=145	*
Mean volume voided per micturition (ml)	+25 (+17%) n=385	+12 (+8%) n=185	***	+35 (+22%) n=354	+10 (+6%) n=176	***
Number of patients with no or minimal bladder problems after treatment (%)	16% n=394	7% n=190	**	19% n=356	15% n=177	n.s.

n.s.=not significant; *=$p \leq 0.05$; **= $p \leq 0.01$; ***= $p \leq 0.001$

(devoid of CYP2D6) treated with tolterodine 2mg BID are comparable to those observed in extensive metabolisers receiving 4mg BID. At both doses of tolterodine, no subject, irrespective of their metabolic profile, exceeded 500 msec for absolute QTcF or 60 msec for change from baseline that are considered thresholds of particular concern. The 4mg BID dose corresponds to a peak exposure (C_{max}) of three times that obtained with the highest therapeutic dose of Detrusitol XL capsules.

Paediatric patients

Efficacy in the paediatric population has not been demonstrated. Two paediatric phase 3 randomised, placebo-controlled, double-blind 12 week studies were conducted using tolterodine extended release capsules. A total of 710 paediatric patients (486 on tolterodine and 224 on placebo) aged 5-10 years with urinary frequency and urge urinary incontinence were studied. No significant difference between the two groups was observed in either study with regard to change from baseline in total number of incontinence episodes/week. (See section 4.8)

5.2 Pharmacokinetic properties

Pharmacokinetic characteristics specific for this formulation: Tolterodine is rapidly absorbed. Both tolterodine and the 5-hydroxymethyl metabolite reach maximal serum concentrations 1-3 hours after dose. The half-life for tolterodine given as the tablet is 2-3 hours in extensive and about 10 hours in poor metabolisers (devoid of CYP2D6). Steady state concentrations are reached within 2 days after administration of the tablets.

Food does not influence the exposure to the unbound tolterodine and the active 5-hydroxymethyl metabolite in extensive metabolisers, although the tolterodine levels increase when taken with food. Clinically relevant changes are likewise not expected in poor metabolisers.

Absorption: After oral administration tolterodine is subject to CYP2D6 catalysed first-pass metabolism in the liver, resulting in the formation of the 5-hydroxymethyl derivative, a major pharmacologically equipotent metabolite.

The absolute bioavailability of tolterodine is 17 % in extensive metabolisers, the majority of the patients, and 65% in poor metabolisers (devoid of CYP2D6).

Distribution: Tolterodine and the 5-hydroxymethyl metabolite bind primarily to orosomucoid. The unbound fractions are 3.7% and 36%, respectively. The volume of distribution of tolterodine is 113 l.

Elimination: Tolterodine is extensively metabolised by the liver following oral dosing. The primary metabolic route is mediated by the polymorphic enzyme CYP2D6 and leads to the formation of the 5-hydroxymethyl metabolite. Further metabolism leads to formation of the 5-carboxylic acid and N-dealkylated 5-carboxylic acid metabolites, which account for 51 % and 29 % of the metabolites recovered in the urine, respectively. A subset (about 7%) of the population is devoid of CYP2D6 activity. The identified pathway of metabolism for these individuals (poor metabolisers) is dealkylation via CYP3A4 to N-dealkylated tolterodine, which does not contribute to the clinical effect. The remainder of the population is referred to as extensive metabolisers. The systemic clearance of tolterodine in extensive metabolisers is about 30 L/h. In poor metabolisers the reduced clearance leads to significantly higher serum concentrations of tolterodine (about 7-fold) and negligible concentrations of the 5-hydroxymethyl metabolite are observed.

The 5-hydroxymethyl metabolite is pharmacologically active and equipotent with tolterodine. Because of the differences in the protein-binding characteristics of tolterodine and the 5-hydroxymethyl metabolite, the exposure (AUC) of unbound tolterodine in poor metabolisers is similar to the combined exposure of unbound tolterodine and the 5-hydroxymethyl metabolite in patients with CYP2D6 activity given the same dosage regimen. The safety, tolerability and clinical response are similar irrespective of phenotype.

The excretion of radioactivity after administration of [^{14}C]-tolterodine is about 77% in urine and 17% in faeces. Less than 1% of the dose is recovered as unchanged drug, and about 4% as the 5-hydroxymethyl metabolite. The carboxylated metabolite and the corresponding dealkylated metabolite account for about 51% and 29% of the urinary recovery, respectively.

The pharmacokinetics is linear in the therapeutic dosage range.

Specific patient groups:

Impaired liver function: About 2-fold higher exposure of unbound tolterodine and the 5-hydroxymethyl metabolite is found in subjects with liver cirrhosis (see section 4.2 and 4.4).

Impaired renal function: The mean exposure of unbound tolterodine and its 5-hydroxymethyl metabolite is doubled in patients with severe renal impairment (inulin clearance GFR ≤ 30 ml/min). The plasma levels of other metabolites were markedly (up to 12-fold) increased in these patients. The clinical relevance of the increased exposure of these metabolites is unknown. There is no data in mild to moderate renal impairment (see section 4.2 and 4.4).

Paediatric patients

The exposure of the active moiety per mg dose is similar in adults and adolescents. The mean exposure of the active moiety per mg dose is approximately two-fold higher in children between 5-10 years than in adults (See sections 4.2 and 5.1).

5.3 Preclinical safety data

In toxicity, genotoxicity, carcinogenicity and safety pharmacology studies no clinically relevant effects have been observed, except those related to the pharmacological effect of the drug.

Reproduction studies have been performed in mice and rabbits.

In mice, there was no effect of tolterodine on fertility or reproductive function. Tolterodine produced embryo death and malformations at plasma exposures (C_{max} or AUC) 20 or 7 times higher than those seen in treated humans.

In rabbits, no malformative effect was seen, but the studies were conducted at 20 or 3 times higher plasma exposure (C_{max} or AUC) than those expected in treated humans.

Tolterodine, as well as its active human metabolites prolong action potential duration (90% repolarisation) in canine purkinje fibres (14 - 75 times therapeutic levels) and block the K+-current in cloned human ether-a-go-go-related gene (hERG) channels (0.5 – 26.1 times therapeutic levels). In dogs prolongation of the QT interval has been observed after application of tolterodine and its human metabolites (3.1 – 61.0 times therapeutic levels). The clinical relevance of these findings is unknown.

6. PHARMACEUTICAL PARTICULARS

6.1 List of excipients

Core:

Cellulose, microcrystalline

Calcium hydrogen phosphate dihydrate

Sodium starch glycollate (Type B)

Magnesium stearate

Colloidal anhydrous silica

Film coating:

Coating granules containing

Hypromellose

Cellulose, microcrystalline

Stearic acid

Titanium dioxide E171

6.2 Incompatibilities

Not applicable.

6.3 Shelf life

3 years.

6.4 Special precautions for storage

No special precautions for storage

6.5 Nature and contents of container

Tablets are packed in either blister package made of PVC/PVDC and aluminium foil with a heat seal coating of PVDC or HDPE bottles with LDPE closures.

Pack sizes:

Detrusitol tablets are available in blisters of 2x10, 3x10, 5x10 and 10x10 tablets, 1x14, 2x14 and 4x14 tablets, 280 and 560 tablets and in bottles of 60 and 500 tablets.

Not all pack sizes may be marketed.

6.6 Special precautions for disposal and other handling

Any unused product or waste material should be disposed of in accordance with local requirements.

7. MARKETING AUTHORISATION HOLDER

Pharmacia Ltd

Ramsgate Road

Sandwich

Kent

CT 13 9NJ

UK

8. MARKETING AUTHORISATION NUMBER(S)

PL 00032/0222

PL 00032/0223

9. DATE OF FIRST AUTHORISATION/RENEWAL OF THE AUTHORISATION

3rd February 1998/ 23rd March 2006

10. DATE OF REVISION OF THE TEXT

February 2009

11 Legal category

POM

Ref: DT A 7_0

Detrusitol XL 4mg

(Pharmacia Limited)

1. NAME OF THE MEDICINAL PRODUCT

Detrusitol XL 4 mg, prolonged-release capsules, hard

2. QUALITATIVE AND QUANTITATIVE COMPOSITION

Each prolonged-release capsule contains tolterodine tartrate 4 mg corresponding to 2.74 mg tolterodine.

Each 4 mg prolonged-release capsule contains a maximum of 123.07 mg of sucrose.

For a full list of excipients see section 6.1

3. PHARMACEUTICAL FORM

Prolonged-release capsule, hard

The 4 mg prolonged-release capsule is blue with white printing (symbol and 4).

4. CLINICAL PARTICULARS

4.1 Therapeutic indications

Symptomatic treatment of urge incontinence and/or increased urinary frequency and urgency as may occur in patients with overactive bladder syndrome.

4.2 Posology and method of administration

Adults (including the elderly):

The recommended dose is 4 mg once daily except in patients with impaired liver function or severely impaired renal function (GFR ≤ 30 ml/min) for whom the recommended dose is 2 mg once daily (see sections 4.4 and 5.2). In case of troublesome side-effects the dose may be reduced from 4 mg to 2 mg once daily.

The prolonged-release capsules can be taken with or without food and must be swallowed whole.

The effect of treatment should be re-evaluated after 2-3 months (see section 5.1).

Paediatric patients:

Efficacy of Detrusitol XL has not been demonstrated in children (See section 5.1). Therefore, Detrusitol XL is not recommended for children.

4.3 Contraindications

Tolterodine is contraindicated in patients with

- Urinary retention
- Uncontrolled narrow angle glaucoma
- Myasthenia gravis
- Known hypersensitivity to tolterodine or excipients
- Severe ulcerative colitis
- Toxic megacolon

4.4 Special warnings and precautions for use

Tolterodine shall be used with caution in patients with

- Significant bladder outlet obstruction at risk ofurinary retention
- Gastrointestinal obstructive disorders, e.g. pyloric stenosis
- Renal impairment (see sections 4.2 and 5.2)
- Hepatic disease (see sections 4.2 and 5.2)
- Autonomic neuropathy
- Hiatus hernia

- Risk of decreased gastrointestinal motility

Multiple oral total daily doses of immediate release 4 mg (therapeutic) and 8 mg (supratherapeutic) tolterodine have been shown to prolong the QTc interval (see section 5.1). The clinical relevance of these findings is unclear and will depend on individual patient risk factors and susceptibilities present.

Tolterodine should be used with caution in patients with risk factors for QT prolongation including:

- Congenital or documented acquired QT prolongation
- Electrolyte disturbances such as hypokalaemia, hypomagnesaemia and hypocalcaemia
- Bradycardia
- Relevant pre-existing cardiac diseases (i.e. cardiomyopathy, myocardial ischaemia, arrhythmia, congestive heart failure)
- Concomitant administration of drugs known to prolong QT-interval including Class IA (e.g. quinidine, procainamide) and Class III (e.g. amiodarone, sotalol) anti-arrhythmics.

This especially holds true when taking potent CYP3A4 inhibitors (see section 5.1).

Concomitant treatment with potent CYP3A4 inhibitors should be avoided (see section 4.5, Interactions).

As with all treatments for symptoms of urgency and urge incontinence, organic reasons for urge and frequency should be considered before treatment.

Patients with rare hereditary problems of fructose intolerance, glucose-galactose malabsorption or sucrase-isomaltase insufficiency should not take this medicine.

4.5 Interaction with other medicinal products and other forms of interaction

Concomitant systemic medication with potent CYP3A4 inhibitors such as macrolide antibiotics (erythromycin and clarithromycin), antifungal agents (e.g. ketoconazole and itraconazole) and antiproteases is not recommended due to increased serum concentrations of tolterodine in poor CYP2D6 metabolisers with (subsequent) risk of overdosage (see section 4.4).

Concomitant medication with other drugs that possess antimuscarinic properties may result in more pronounced therapeutic effect and side-effects. Conversely, the therapeutic effect of tolterodine may be reduced by concomitant administration of muscarinic cholinergic receptor agonists.

The effect of prokinetics like metoclopramide and cisapride may be decreased by tolterodine.

Concomitant treatment with fluoxetine (a potent CYP2D6 inhibitor) does not result in a clinically significant interaction since tolterodine and its CYP2D6-dependent metabolite, 5-hydroxymethyl tolterodine are equipotent.

Drug interaction studies have shown no interactions with warfarin or combined oral contraceptives (ethinyl estradiol/levonorgestrel).

A clinical study has indicated that tolterodine is not a metabolic inhibitor of CYP2D6, 2C19, 2C9, 3A4 or 1A2. Therefore an increase of plasma levels of drugs metabolised by these isoenzymes is not expected when dosed in combination with tolterodine.

4.6 Pregnancy and lactation

Pregnancy

There are no adequate data from the use of tolterodine in pregnant women.

Studies in animals have shown reproductive toxicity (see section 5.3). The potential risk for humans is unknown.

Consequently, Detrusitol XL is not recommended during pregnancy.

Lactation

No data concerning the excretion of tolterodine into human milk are available. Tolterodine should be avoided during lactation.

4.7 Effects on ability to drive and use machines

Since this drug may cause accommodation disturbances and influence reaction time, the ability to drive and use machines may be negatively affected.

4.8 Undesirable effects

Due to the pharmacological effect of tolterodine it may cause mild to moderate antimuscarinic effects, like dryness of the mouth, dyspepsia and dry eyes.

The table below reflects the data obtained with Detrusitol in clinical trials and from post marketing experience. The most commonly reported adverse reaction was dry mouth, which occurred in 23.4 % of patients treated with Detrusitol XL and in 7.7 % of placebo-treated patients.

(see Table 1 opposite)

Cases of aggravation of symptoms of dementia (e.g. confusion, disorientation, delusion) have been reported after tolterodine therapy was initiated in patients taking cholinesterase inhibitors for the treatment of dementia.

Paediatric patients

In two paediatric phase III randomised, placebo-controlled, double-blind studies conducted over 12 weeks where a total of 710 paediatric patients were recruited, the proportion of patients with urinary tract infections, diarrhoea and abnormal behaviour was higher in patients treated with tolterodine than placebo (urinary tract infection: tolterodine 6.8 %, placebo 3.6 %; diarrhoea: tolterodine 3.3 %, placebo 0.9 %; abnormal behaviour: tolterodine 1.6 %, placebo 0.4 %). (See section 5.1)

4.9 Overdose

The highest dose given to human volunteers of tolterodine tartrate is 12.8 mg as a single dose of the immediate release formulation. The most severe adverse events observed were accommodation disturbances and micturition difficulties.

In the event of tolterodine overdose, treat with gastric lavage and give activated charcoal. Treat symptoms as follows:

- Severe central anticholinergic effects (e.g. hallucinations, severe excitation): treat with physostigmine
- Convulsions or pronounced excitation: treat with benzodiazepines
- Respiratory insufficiency: treat with artificial respiration
- Tachycardia: treat with beta-blockers
- Urinary retention: treat with catheterisation
- Mydriasis: treat with pilocarpine eye drops and/or place patient in dark room

An increase in QT interval was observed at a total daily dose of 8 mg immediate release tolterodine (twice the recommended daily dose of the immediate release formulation and equivalent to three times the peak exposure of the prolonged release capsule formulation) administered over four days. In the event of tolterodine overdose, standard supportive measures for managing QT prolongation should be adopted

5. PHARMACOLOGICAL PROPERTIES

5.1 Pharmacodynamic properties

Pharmacotherapeutic group: Urinary antispasmodics

ATC code: G04B D07

Tolterodine is a competitive, specific muscarinic receptor antagonist with a selectivity for the urinary bladder over salivary glands in vivo. One of the tolterodine metabolites (5-hydroxymethyl derivative) exhibits a pharmacological profile similar to that of the parent compound. In extensive metabolisers this metabolite contributes significantly to the therapeutic effect (see 5.2).

Effect of the treatment can be expected within 4 weeks.

In the Phase III program, the primary endpoint was reduction of incontinence episodes per week and the secondary endpoints were reduction of micturitions per 24 hours and increase of mean volume voided per micturition. These parameters are presented in the following table.

Effect of treatment with Detrusitol XL 4 mg once daily after 12 weeks, compared with placebo. Absolute change and percentage change relative to baseline. Treatment difference Detrusitol vs. placebo: Least Squares estimated mean change and 95% confidence interval.

(see Table 2 on next page)

After 12 weeks of treatment 23.8% (121/507) in the Detrusitol XL group and 15.7% (80/508) in the placebo group reported that they subjectively had no or minimal bladder problems.

The effect of tolterodine was evaluated in patients, examined with urodynamic assessment at baseline and, depending on the urodynamic result, they were allocated to a urodynamic positive (motor urgency) or a urodynamic negative (sensory urgency) group. Within each group, the patients were randomised to receive either tolterodine or placebo. The study could not provide convincing evidence that tolterodine had effects over placebo in patients with sensory urgency.

The clinical effects of tolterodine on QT interval were studied in ECGs obtained from over 600 treated patients, including the elderly and patients with pre-existing cardiovascular disease. The changes in QT intervals did not significantly differ between placebo and treatment groups.

The effect of tolterodine on QT-prolongation was investigated further in 48 healthy male and female volunteers aged 18 – 55 years. Subjects were administered 2 mg BID and 4 mg BID tolterodine as the immediate release formulations. The results (Fridericia corrected) at peak tolterodine concentration (1 hour) showed mean QTc interval increases of 5.0 and11.8 msec for tolterodine doses of 2 mg BID and 4 mg BID respectively and 19.3 msec for moxifloxacin (400mg) which was used as an active internal control. A pharmacokinetic/pharmacodynamic model estimated that QTc interval increases in poor metabolisers (devoid of CYP2D6) treated with tolterodine 2mg BID are comparable to those observed in extensive metabolisers receiving 4mg BID. At both doses of tolterodine, no subject, irrespective of their metabolic profile, exceeded 500 msec for absolute QTcF or 60 msec for change from baseline that are considered thresholds of particular concern. The 4mg BID dose corresponds to a peak exposure (C_{max}) of three times that obtained with the highest therapeutic dose of Detrusitol XL capsules.

Paediatric patients

Efficacy in the paediatric population has not been demonstrated. Two paediatric phase 3 randomised, placebo-controlled, double-blind 12 week studies were conducted using tolterodine extended release capsules. A total of 710 paediatric patients (486 on tolterodine and 224 on placebo) aged 5-10 years with urinary frequency and urge urinary incontinence were studied. No significant difference between the two groups was observed in either study with regard to change from baseline in total number of incontinence episodes/week. (See section 4.8)

Table 1

	Very Common ($\geq$1/10)	Common ($\geq$1/100 and <1/10)	Uncommon ($\geq$1/1000 and <1/100)	**Not known** (cannot be estimated from the available data)
Infections and infestations		Sinusitis		
Immune system disorders			Hypersensitivity not otherwise specified	Anaphylactoid reactions
Psychiatric disorders			Nervousness	Confusion, hallucinations, disorientation
Nervous system disorders		Dizziness, somnolence, headache	Paresthesia, memory impairment	
Eye disorders		Dry eyes, abnormal vision (including abnormal accomodation)		
Ear and labyrinth disorders			Vertigo	
Cardiac disorders			Palpitations, cardiac failure, arrhythmia	Tachycardia
Vascular disorders				Flushing
Gastrointestinal disorders	Dry mouth	Dyspepsia, constipation, abdominal pain, flatulence, diarrhoea		Gastroesophageal reflux, vomiting
Skin and subcutaneous tissue disorders				Angioedema, dry skin
Renal and urinary disorders		Dysuria	Urinary retention	
General disorders		Fatigue, peripheral oedema	Chest pain	

Table 2

	Detrusitol XL 4 mg once daily (n=507)	Placebo (n=508)	Treatment difference vs. placebo: Mean change and 95% CI	Statistical significance vs. placebo (p-value)
Number of incontinence episodes per week	-11.8 (-54%)	-6.9 (-28%)	-4.8 (-7.2; -2.5)*	<0.001
Number of micturitions per 24 hours	-1.8 (-13%)	-1.2 (-8%)	-0.6 (-1.0; -0.2)	0.005
Mean volume voided per micturition (ml)	+34 (+27%)	+14 (+12%)	+20 (14; 26)	<0.001

*) 97.5% confidence interval according to Bonferroni

5.2 Pharmacokinetic properties

Pharmacokinetic characteristics specific for this formulation: Tolterodine prolonged-release capsules give a slower absorption of tolterodine than the immediate-release tablets do. As a result, the maximum serum concentrations are observed 4 (2-6) hours after administration of the capsules. The apparent half-life for tolterodine given as the capsule is about 6 hours in extensive and about 10 hours in poor metabolisers (devoid of CYP2D6). Steady state concentrations are reached within 4 days after administration of the capsules.

There is no effect of food on the bioavailability of the capsules.

Absorption: After oral administration tolterodine is subject to CYP2D6 catalysed first-pass metabolism in the liver, resulting in the formation of the 5-hydroxymethyl derivative, a major pharmacologically equipotent metabolite.

The absolute bioavailability of tolterodine is 17 % in extensive metabolisers, the majority of the patients, and 65% in poor metabolisers (devoid of CYP2D6).

Distribution: Tolterodine and the 5-hydroxymethyl metabolite bind primarily to orosomucoid. The unbound fractions are 3.7% and 36%, respectively. The volume of distribution of tolterodine is 113 l.

Elimination: Tolterodine is extensively metabolised by the liver following oral dosing. The primary metabolic route is mediated by the polymorphic enzyme CYP2D6 and leads to the formation of the 5-hydroxymethyl metabolite. Further metabolism leads to formation of the 5-carboxylic acid and N-dealkylated 5-carboxylic acid metabolites, which account for 51 % and 29 % of the metabolites recovered in the urine, respectively. A subset (about 7%) of the population is devoid of CYP2D6 activity. The identified pathway of metabolism for these individuals (poor metabolisers) is dealkylation via CYP3A4 to N-dealkylated tolterodine, which does not contribute to the clinical effect. The remainder of the population is referred to as extensive metabolisers. The systemic clearance of tolterodine in extensive metabolisers is about 30 L/h. In poor metabolisers the reduced clearance leads to significantly higher serum concentrations of tolterodine (about 7-fold) and negligible concentrations of the 5-hydroxymethyl metabolite are observed.

The 5-hydroxymethyl metabolite is pharmacologically active and equipotent with tolterodine. Because of the differences in the protein-binding characteristics of tolterodine and the 5-hydroxymethyl metabolite, the exposure (AUC) of unbound tolterodine in poor metabolisers is similar to the combined exposure of unbound tolterodine and the 5-hydroxymethyl metabolite in patients with CYP2D6 activity given the same dosage regimen. The safety, tolerability and clinical response are similar irrespective of phenotype.

The excretion of radioactivity after administration of [^{14}C]-tolterodine is about 77% in urine and 17% in faeces. Less than 1% of the dose is recovered as unchanged drug, and about 4% as the 5-hydroxymethyl metabolite. The carboxylated metabolite and the corresponding dealkylated metabolite account for about 51% and 29% of the urinary recovery, respectively.

The pharmacokinetics is linear in the therapeutic dosage range.

Specific patient groups:

Impaired liver function: About 2-fold higher exposure of unbound tolterodine and the 5-hydroxymethyl metabolite is found in subjects with liver cirrhosis (see section 4.2 and 4.4).

Impaired renal function: The mean exposure of unbound tolterodine and its 5-hydroxymethyl metabolite is doubled in patients with severe renal impairment (inulin clearance GFR ⩽ 30 ml/min). The plasma levels of other metabolites were markedly (up to 12-fold) increased in these patients. The clinical relevance of the increased exposure of these metabolites is unknown. There is no data in mild to moderate renal impairment (see section 4.2 and 4.4).

Paediatric patients

The exposure of the active moiety per mg dose is similar in adults and adolescents. The mean exposure of the active moiety per mg dose is approximately two-fold higher in children between 5-10 years than in adults (See sections 4.2 and 5.1).

5.3 Preclinical safety data

In toxicity, genotoxicity, carcinogenicity and safety pharmacology studies no clinically relevant effects have been observed except those related to the pharmacological effect of the drug.

Reproduction studies have been performed in mice and rabbits.

In mice, there was no effect of tolterodine on fertility or reproductive function. Tolterodine produced embryo death and malformations at plasma exposures (C_{max} or AUC) 20 or 7 times higher than those seen in treated humans.

In rabbits, no malformative effect was seen, but the studies were conducted at 20 or 3 times higher plasma exposure (C_{max} or AUC) than those expected in treated humans.

Tolterodine, as well as its active human metabolites prolong action potential duration (90% repolarisation) in canine purkinje fibres (14 - 75 times therapeutic levels) and block the K+-current in cloned human ether-a-go-go-related gene (hERG) channels (0.5 – 26.1 times therapeutic levels). In dogs prolongation of the QT interval has been observed after application of tolterodine and its human metabolites (3.1 – 61.0 times therapeutic levels). The clinical relevance of these findings is unknown.

6. PHARMACEUTICAL PARTICULARS

6.1 List of excipients

Prolonged release capsule contents:

Sugar spheres (containing sucrose and maize starch)

Hypromellose

Surelease E-7-9010 clear:

Ethylcellulose

Medium Chain Triglycerides

Oleic acid

Prolonged release capsule shell contents:

Gelatin

Printing ink:

Shellac glaze

Titanium dioxide, E 171

Propylene glycol

Simeticone

Colorants in the blue 4 mg prolonged release capsule:

Indigo carmine, E132

Titanium dioxide, E 171

6.2 Incompatibilities

Not applicable.

6.3 Shelf life

2 years

6.4 Special precautions for storage

Do not store above 30°C

Bottles: Store in the original container.

Blisters: Keep container in the outer carton.

6.5 Nature and contents of container

Detrusitol XL prolonged-release capsules are packed in either blisters made of PVC/PVDC and aluminium foil with a heat seal coating of PVDC or HDPE bottles with LDPE closures.

Pack sizes:

Detrusitol XL prolonged release capsules of 4 mg are available in blisters of 1 × 7, 2 × 7, 4 × 7, 7 × 7, 12 × 7, 14 × 7, 40 × 7 capsules and in bottles of 30, 100 and 200. Hospital packs are available in blisters of 10 × 2 × 4, 20 × 2 × 4 and 40 × 2 × 4 capsules.

Not all pack sizes may be marketed.

6.6 Special precautions for disposal and other handling

Any unused product or waste material should be disposed of in accordance with local requirements.

7. MARKETING AUTHORISATION HOLDER

Pharmacia Limited

Ramsgate Road

Sandwich

Kent

CT13 9NJ

UK

8. MARKETING AUTHORISATION NUMBER(S)

PL 00032/ 0287

9. DATE OF FIRST AUTHORISATION/RENEWAL OF THE AUTHORISATION

14th August 2001

10. DATE OF REVISION OF THE TEXT

February 2009

11 LEGAL CATEGORY

POM

DTB 7_0

Dexedrine Tablets 5mg

(UCB Pharma Limited)

1. NAME OF THE MEDICINAL PRODUCT

Dexedrine Tablets 5mg

2. QUALITATIVE AND QUANTITATIVE COMPOSITION

Dexamfetamine Sulphate 5mg

For excipients see 6.1

3. PHARMACEUTICAL FORM

Tablets for oral administration

4. CLINICAL PARTICULARS

4.1 Therapeutic indications

Dexedrine is a symphathomimetic amine with central stimulant and anorectic activity. It is indicated in narcolepsy. It is also indicated for children with refractory hyperkinetic states under the supervision of a physician specialising in child psychiatry.

4.2 Posology and method of administration

Adults: In narcolepsy, the usual starting dose is 10mg Dexedrine a day, given in divided doses. Dosage may be increased if necessary by 10mg a day at weekly intervals to a suggested maximum of 60mg a day.

Elderly: Start with 5mg a day, and increase by increments of 5mg at weekly intervals.

Children: In hyperkinetic states, the usual starting dosage for children aged 3-5 years is 2.5mg a day, increased if necessary by 2.5mg a day at weekly intervals; for children aged 6 years and over, the usual starting dose is 5-10mg a day increasing if necessary by 5mg at weekly intervals.

The usual upper limit is 20mg a day though some older children have needed 40mg or more for optimal response.

4.3 Contraindications

- Hypersensitivity to dexamfetamine or other amfetamine derivatives or any of the excipients.
- Patients with symptomatic cardiovascular disease, structural cardiac abnormalities and/or moderate or severe hypertensive disease.
- Patients with advanced arteriosclerosis.
- During or for 14 days after treatment with an MAO inhibitor.
- Patients with a history of drug abuse or alcohol abuse.
- Patients with hyperthyroidism, glaucoma, porphyria or hyperexcitability.
- Patients with Gilles de la Tourette syndrome or similar dystonias.
- Dexedrine tablets include lactose. Patients with rare hereditary problems of galactose intolerance, the Lapp lactase deficiency or glucose-galactose malabsorption should not take this medicine.
- Dexedrine tablets include sucrose. Patients with rare hereditary problems of fructose intolerance, glucose-galactose malabsorption or sucrase-isomaltase insufficiency should not take this medicine.
- Pregnancy and lactation.

4.4 Special warnings and precautions for use

Use with caution in patients on guanethidine and patients with mild hypertension or a family history of dystonias. If tics develop, discontinue treatment with dexedrine. Dexamfetamine is likely to reduce the convulsant threshold therefore caution is advised in patients with epilepsy. Height and weight should be carefully monitored in children as growth retardation may occur. Children who are not gaining weight as expected should have their treatment interrupted temporarily.

Caution should be used when administering dexamfetamine to patients with impaired kidney function or unstable personality.

Drug dependence, with consumption of increasing doses to levels many times those recommended, may occur as tolerance develops. At such levels, a psychosis which may be clinically indistinguishable from schizophrenia can occur.

Treatment should be stopped gradually since abrupt cessation may produce extreme fatigue and mental depression.

Cardiomyopathy has been reported with chronic amfetamine use.

Due to the potential decreased appetite associated with dexamfetamine use, caution is advised in the presence of anorexia nervosa.

Pre-existing structural cardiac abnormalities: Sudden death has been reported in association with the use of stimulants of the central nervous system at usual doses in children with structural cardiac abnormalities. Although some structural cardiac abnormalities alone may carry an increased risk of sudden death, stimulant products are not recommended in children, adolescents, or adults with known structural cardiac abnormalities (*see 4.3, Contraindications*).

Blood pressure should be monitored at appropriate intervals in all patients taking dexamfetamine, especially those with hypertension.

Psychiatric adverse events:

• Administration of stimulants may exacerbate symptoms of behaviour disturbance and thought disorders in patients with a pre-existing psychotic disorder.

• Particular care should be taken in using stimulants to treat ADHD in patients with comorbid bipolar disorder because of concern for possible induction of a mixed/manic episode in such patients. Prior to initiating treatment with a stimulant, patients with comorbid depressive symptoms should be adequately screened to determine if they are at risk for bipolar disorder; such screening should include a detailed psychiatric history, including a family history of suicide, bipolar disorder and depression.

• Treatment emergent psychotic or manic symptoms, e.g. hallucinations, delusional thinking or mania in children or adolescents without a prior history of psychotic illness or mania can be caused by stimulants at usual doses. If such symptoms occur, consideration should be given to a possible causal role of the stimulant and discontinuation of treatment may be appropriate.

• Patients beginning treatment with stimulants for ADHD should be monitored for the appearance, or worsening of, aggressive behaviour or hostility.

4.5 Interaction with other medicinal products and other forms of interaction

Adrenoreceptor blocking agents (e.g. propanolol), lithium and α methyltyrosine may antagonise the effects of dexamfetamine. Disulfiram may inhibit metabolism and excretion.

The concurrent use of tricyclic antidepressants may increase the risk of cardiovascular side effects.

Concurrent use of MAOI's or use within the preceding 14 days may precipitate a hypertensive crisis.

Concurrent use of beta-blockers may result in severe hypertension and dexamfetamine may result in diminished effect of other anti-hypertensives such as guanethidine.

Phenothiazines may inhibit the actions of dexamfetamine.

Amfetamines may delay the absorption of ethosuximide, phenobarbital and phenytoin.

Acute dystonia has been noted with concurrent administration of haloperidol.

Haloperidol blocks dopamine and norepinephrine reuptake, thus inhibiting the central stimulant effects of amfetamines.

The analgesic effect of morphine may be increased and its respiratory depressant effects decreased with concurrent use of morphine and dexamfetamine.

Amfetamines potentiate the analgesic effects of meperidine.

Concomitant administration of clonidine and dexamfetamine may result in an increased duration of action of dexamfetamine.

Gastrointestinal acidifying agents (guanethidine, reserpine, glutamic acid HCl, ascorbic acid, fruit juices, etc.) lower absorption of dexamfetamine. Urinary acidifying agents (ammonium chloride, sodium acid phosphate, etc.) increase urinary excretion of dexamfetamine. Both groups of agents lower blood levels and efficacy of dexamfetamine.

Gastrointestinal alkalizing agents (sodium bicarbonate, etc) increase the absorption of amfetamines. Urinary alkalizing agents (acetazolamide, some thiazides) increase the concentration of the non-ionized species of the amfetamine molecule, thereby decreasing urinary excretion. Both groups of agents increase blood levels and efficacy of amfetamines.

Alcohol may exacerbate the CNS adverse reactions of psychoactive drugs, including dexamfetamine. It is therefore advisable for patients to abstain from alcohol during treatment.

Chlorpromazine blocks dopamine and norepinephrine reuptake, thus inhibiting the central stimulant effects of amfetamines, and can be used to treat amfetamine poisoning.

4.6 Pregnancy and lactation

Dexamfetamine has been thought to produce embryotoxic effects in rodents and retrospective evidence of certain significance in man has suggested a similar possibility.

Dexedrine is contraindicated during pregnancy.

Dexedrine passes into breast milk.

Because of the potential for adverse reactions in nursing infants from dexamfetamine, a decision should be made whether to discontinued nursing or discontinue the drug, taking into account the importance of the drug to the mother.

4.7 Effects on ability to drive and use machines

Dexedrine may affect ability to drive or operate machinery.

4.8 Undesirable effects

Cardiac disorders: cardiomyopathy, myocardial infarction, palpitations, tachycardia

Eye disorders: mydriasis, visual disturbance

Gastrointestinal disorders: abdominal cramps, colitis ischaemic, diarrhea, dry mouth, nausea

General disorders and administration site conditions: chest pain, death due to cardiovascular collapse, growth retardation, hyperpyrexia, hypersensitivity including angioedema and anaphylaxis, sudden death (*see 4.4, Special Warnings and Special Precautions for Use).*

Investigations: blood pressure decreased, blood pressure increased

Metabolism and nutrition disorders: acidosis, anorexia, weight loss.

Musculoskeletal and connective tissue disorders: rhabdomyolysis

Nervous system disorders: ataxia, choreoathetoid movements, concentration difficulties, convulsion, dizziness, dyskinesia, dysgeusia, fatigue, headache, hyperactivity, hyperreflexia, intracranial haemorrhage, neuroleptic malignant syndrome, stroke, tremor, Tourette's syndrome

Psychiatric disorders: aggressive behaviour, anxiety, confusion, delirium, depression, drug dependence, dysphoria, emotional lability, euphoria, hallucination, impaired cognitive test performance, insomnia, irritability, libido altered, nervousness, night terrors, obsessive-compulsive behavior, panic states, paranoia, psychosis/ psychotic reactions, restlessness, tics

Renal and urinary disorders: renal damage

Reproductive system and breast disorders: impotence

Skin and subcutaneous tissue disorders: alopecia, rash, sweating, urticaria

Vascular disorders: cardiovascular collapse, cerebral vasculitis

A toxic hypermetabolic state, characterised by transient hyperactivity, hyperpyrexia, acidosis and death due to cardiovascular collapse have been reported.

Cessation of, or reduction in, amfetamine use that has been heavy and prolonged can result in withdrawal symptoms. Symptoms include dysphoric mood, fatigue, vivid and unpleasant dreams, insomnia or hypersomnia, increased appetite, psychomotor retardation or agitation, anhedonia and drug craving.

4.9 Overdose

In acute overdosage, the adverse effects are accentuated and may be accompanied by hyperpyrexia, mydriasis, hyperreflexia, chest pain, tachycardia, cardiac arrhythmias, confusion, panic states, aggressive behaviour, hallucinations, delirium, convulsions, respiratory depression, coma, circulatory collapse, and death.

Individual patient response may vary widely and toxic manifestations may occur with quite small overdoses.

Treatment consists of the induction of vomiting and/or gastric lavage together with supportive and symptomatic measures. Excessive stimulation or convulsions may be treated with diazepam. Excretion of dexamfetamine may be increased by forced acid diuresis. Chlorpromazine antagonises the central stimulant effects of amfetamines and can be used to treat amfetamine intoxication.

5. PHARMACOLOGICAL PROPERTIES

5.1 Pharmacodynamic properties

Dexedrine is a sympathomimetic amine with a central stimulant and anorectic activity.

5.2 Pharmacokinetic properties

Dexamfetamine is readily absorbed from the gastrointestinal tract. It is resistant to metabolism by monoamine oxidase. It is excreted in the urine as unchanged parent drug together with some hydroxylated metabolites. Elimination is increased in acidic urine. After high doses, elimination in the urine may take several days.

5.3 Preclinical safety data

Dexamfetamine has been thought to produce embryotoxic effects in rodents, and retrospective evidence of uncertain significance in man has suggested a similar possibility. Dexedrine passes into breast milk.

6. PHARMACEUTICAL PARTICULARS

6.1 List of excipients

Stearic acid

Acacia powder

Lactose

Paraffin, Light Liquid

Maize starch

Sucrose

Purified talc

Purified water

6.2 Incompatibilities

None stated.

6.3 Shelf life

5 years

6.4 Special precautions for storage

No special storage precautions are necessary.

6.5 Nature and contents of container

Polypropylene securitainers, amber glass bottles or polythene vials containing 1000 and 100 tablets. Blister packs containing 100 and 28 tablets

6.6 Special precautions for disposal and other handling

None

7. MARKETING AUTHORISATION HOLDER

UCB Pharma Ltd., 208 Bath Road, Slough, Berkshire, SL1 3WE, UK.

8. MARKETING AUTHORISATION NUMBER(S)

PL 0039/0385

9. DATE OF FIRST AUTHORISATION/RENEWAL OF THE AUTHORISATION

13 October 1992

10. DATE OF REVISION OF THE TEXT

Approved: September 2008

Dexsol 2mg/5ml Oral Solution

(Rosemont Pharmaceuticals Limited)

1. NAME OF THE MEDICINAL PRODUCT

Dexsol 2mg/5ml Oral Solution

2. QUALITATIVE AND QUANTITATIVE COMPOSITION

Dexamethasone 2mg/5ml (as dexamethasone sodium phosphate)

For excipients, see section 6.1

3. PHARMACEUTICAL FORM

Oral Solution

A colourless to faint yellow solution with odour of mint.

4. CLINICAL PARTICULARS

4.1 Therapeutic indications

Dexamethasone is a corticosteroid. It is designed for use in certain endocrine and non-endocrine disorders, in certain cases of cerebral oedema and for diagnostic testing of adrenocortical hyperfunction.

Endocrine disorders:

Endocrine exophthalmos.

Non-endocrine disorders:

Dexamethasone may be used in the treatment of non-endocrine corticosteroid responsive conditions including:

Allergy and anaphylaxis: Anaphylaxis.

Arteritis collagenosis: Polymyalgia rheumatica, polyarteritis nodosa.

Haematological disorders: Haemolytic anaemia (also auto immune), leukaemia, myeloma, idiopathic thrombocytopenic purpura in adults, reticulolymphoproliferative disorders (see also under oncological disorders).

Gastroenterological disorders: For treatment during the critical stage in: ulcerative colitis (rectal only); regional enteritis (Crohn's disease), certain forms of hepatitis.

Muscular disorders: Polymyositis.

Neurological disorders: Raised intra-cranial pressure secondary to cerebral tumours, acute exacerbations of multiple sclerosis.

Ocular disorders: Anterior and posterior uveitis, optic neuritis, chorioretinitis, iridocyclitis, temporal arteritis, orbital pseudotumour.

Renal disorders: Nephrotic syndrome

Pulmonary disorders: Chronic bronchial asthma, aspiration pneumonitis, chronic obstructive pulmonary disease (COPD), sarcoidosis, allergic pulmonary disease such as farmer's and pigeon breeder's lung, Löffler's syndrome, cryptogenic fibrosing alveolitis.

Rheumatic disorders: some cases or specific forms (Felty's syndrome, Sjörgen's syndrome) of rheumatoid arthritis, including juvenile rheumatoid arthritis, acute rheumatism, lupus erythematosus disseminatus, temporal arteritis (polymyalgia rheumatica).

Skin disorders: Pemphigus vulgaris, bullous pemphigoid, erythrodermas, serious forms of erythema multiforme (Stevens-Johnson syndrome), mycosis fungoides, bullous dermatitis herpetiformis.

Oncological Disorders: lymphatic leukaemia, especially acute forms, malignant lymphoma (Hodgkin's disease, non-Hodgkin's lymphoma), metastasized breast cancer, hypercalcaemia as a result of bone metastasis or Kahler's disease, Kahler's disease.

Various: intense allergic reactions; as immunosuppressant in organ transplantation; as an adjuvant in the prevention of nausea and vomiting and in the treatment of cancer with oncolytics that have a serious emetic effect.

4.2 Posology and method of administration

Adults

General considerations:

The dosage should be titrated to the individual response and the nature of the disease. In order to minimise side effects, the lowest effective possible dosage should be used (see 'Side effects').

The initial dosage varies from 0.5 – 9mg a day depending on the disease being treated. In more severe diseases, doses higher than 9mg may be required. The initial dosage should be maintained or adjusted until the patient's response is satisfactory. Both the dose in the evening, which is useful in alleviating morning stiffness, and the divided dosage regimen are associated with greater suppression of the hypothalamo-pituitary-adrenal axis. If satisfactory clinical response does not occur after a reasonable period of time, discontinue treatment with dexamethasone and transfer the patient to another therapy.

If the initial response is favourable, the maintenance dosage should be determined by lowering the dose gradually to the lowest dose required to maintain an adequate clinical response. Chronic dosage should preferably not exceed 1.5mg dexamethasone daily.

Patients should be monitored for signs that may require dosage adjustment. These may be changes in clinical status resulting from remissions or exacerbations of the disease, individual drug responsiveness and the effect of stress (e.g. surgery, infection, trauma). During stress it may be necessary to increase dosage temporarily.

If the drug is to be stopped after more than a few days of treatment, it should be withdrawn gradually.

The following equivalents facilitate changing to dexamethasone from other glucocorticoids:

Milligram for milligram, dexamethasone is approximately equivalent to betamethasone, 4 to 6 times more potent than methylprednisolone and triamcinolone, 6 to 8 times more potent than prednisone and prednisolone, 25 to 30 times more potent than hydrocortisone, and about 35 times more potent than cortisone.

Acute, self-limiting allergic disorders or acute exacerbations of chronic allergic disorders.

The following dosage schedule combining parenteral and oral therapy is suggested:

First day:	Dexamethasone sodium phosphate injection 4mg or 8mg (1ml or 2ml) intramuscularly.
Second day:	1mg (2.5ml) Dexamethasone Oral Solution twice a day.
Third day:	1mg (2.5ml) Dexamethasone Oral Solution twice a day.
Fourth day:	500micrograms (1.25ml) Dexamethasone Oral Solution twice a day.
Fifth day:	500micrograms (1.25ml) Dexamethasone Oral Solution twice a day.
Sixth day:	500micrograms (1.25ml) Dexamethasone Oral Solution.
Seventh day:	500micrograms (1.25ml) Dexamethasone Oral Solution.
Eighth day:	Re-assessment.

If a dose of less than 5ml is required, an oral dosing device should be employed.

This schedule is designed to ensure adequate therapy during acute episodes whilst minimising the risk of overdosage in chronic cases.

Raised intracranial pressure: Initial therapy is usually by injection. When maintenance therapy is required, this should be changed to dexamethasone oral solution as soon as possible. For the palliative management of patients with recurrent or inoperable brain tumours, maintenance dosage should be calculated individually. A dosage of 2mg two or three times a day may be effective. The smallest dosage necessary to control symptoms should always be used.

Dexamethasone suppression tests:

1. Tests for Cushing's syndrome:

2mg (5ml) Dexamethasone Oral Solution should be administered at 11pm. Blood samples are then taken at 8am the next morning for plasma cortisol determination.

If greater accuracy is required, 500 micrograms (1.25ml) Dexamethasone Oral Solution should be administered every 6 hours for 48 hours. Blood should be drawn at 8am for plasma cortisol determination on the third morning.

24-hour urine collection should be employed for 17-hydroxycorticosteroid excretion determination.

2. Test to distinguish Cushing's syndrome caused by pituitary ACTH excess from the syndrome induced by other causes:

2mg (5ml) Dexamethasone Oral Solution should be administered every 6 hours for 48 hours. Blood should be drawn at 8am for plasma cortisol determination on the third morning.

24-hour urine collection should be employed for 17-hydroxycorticosteroid excretion determination.

Children:

Dosage should be limited to a single dose on alternate days to lessen retardation of growth and minimize suppression of hypothalamo-pituitary-adrenal axis.

Elderly:

Treatment of elderly patients, particularly if long term, should be planned bearing in mind the more serious consequences of the common side effects of corticosteroids in old age.

4.3 Contraindications

- Hypersensitivity to dexamethasone or any of the excipients listed.
- Systemic infection unless specific anti-infective therapy is employed.
- Systemic fungal infections.
- Stomach ulcer or duodenal ulcer
- Infection with tropical worms

4.4 Special warnings and precautions for use

Patients should carry 'steroid treatment' cards, which give clear guidance on the precautions to be taken to minimise risk, and which provides details of prescriber, drug, dosage and the duration of treatment.

Undesirable effects may be minimised by using the lowest effective dose for the minimum period. Dexamethasone Oral Solution may be given in divided doses as appropriate. Frequent patient review is required to appropriately titrate the dose against disease activity. When reduction in dosage is possible, the reduction should be gradual (Refer to 'Posology and Administration').

Anti-inflammatory/Immunosuppressive effects/Infection

Corticosteroids may exacerbate systemic fungal infections and should not be used unless they are needed to control drug reactions due to amphotericin. There have also been reports in which concomitant use of amphotericin and hydrocortisone was followed by cardiac enlargement and heart failure.

Administration of live virus vaccines is contra-indicated in individuals receiving immunosuppressive doses of corticosteroids. If inactivated viral or bacterial vaccines are administered to individuals receiving immunosuppressive doses of corticosteroids, the expected serum antibody response may not be obtained.

Suppression of the inflammatory response and immune function increases the susceptibility to infections and their severity. The clinical presentation may be atypical, and serious infections such as septicaemia and tuberculosis may be masked and may reach an advanced stage before being recognised.

Appropriate anti-microbial therapy should accompany glucocorticoid therapy when necessary e.g. in tuberculosis and viral and fungal infections of the eye.

There may be decreased resistance and inability to localise infection in patients on corticosteroids.

Chickenpox is of particular concern, since this normally minor illness may be fatal in immunosuppressed patients. Patients (or parents of children) without a definite history of chickenpox should be advised to avoid close personal contact with chickenpox or herpes zoster, and if exposed they should seek urgent medical attention. Passive immunisation with varicella/zoster immunoglobulin (VZIG) is needed by exposed non-immune patients who are receiving systemic corticosteroids or who have used them within the previous three months; this should be given within ten days of exposure to chickenpox. *If a diagnosis of chickenpox is confirmed, the illness warrants specialist care and urgent treatment. Corticosteroids should not be stopped and the dose may need to be increased.*

Measles can have a more serious or even fatal course in immunosuppressed patients. In such children or adults particular care should be taken to avoid exposure to measles. If exposed, prophylaxis with intramuscular pooled immunoglobulin (IG) may be indicated. Exposed patients should be advised to seek medical advice without delay.

Corticosteroids may activate latent amoebiasis or strongyloidiasis or exacerbate active disease. Latent disease may be activated or there may be an exacerbation of intercurrent infections due to pathogens, including those caused by Amoeba, Candida, Cryptococcus, Mycobacterium, Nocardia, Pneumocystis or Toxoplasma. It is recommended that these are ruled out before initiating corticosteroid therapy particularly in those patients who have spent time in the tropics or those with unexplained diarrhoea.

Prolonged use of corticosteroids may produce subcapsular cataracts, glaucoma with possible damage to the optic nerves, and may enhance the establishment of secondary ocular infections due to fungi or viruses.

General

A report shows that the use of corticosteroids in cerebral malaria is associated with a prolonged coma and an increased incidence of pneumonia and gastro-intestinal bleeding and therefore corticosteroids should not be used in cerebral malaria.

Average and large doses of hydrocortisone or cortisone can cause elevation of blood pressure, retention of salt and water, and increased excretion of potassium, but these effects are less likely to occur with synthetic derivatives, except when used in large doses. Dietary salt restriction and potassium supplementation may be necessary with corticosteroid therapy. All corticosteroids increase calcium excretion.

Adrenal Suppression:

Adrenal cortical atrophy develops during prolonged therapy and may persist for years after stopping treatment. Withdrawal of corticosteroids after prolonged therapy must therefore always be gradual to avoid acute adrenal insufficiency, being tapered off over weeks or months according to the dose and duration of treatment.

During prolonged therapy, any intercurrent illness, trauma, stressor surgical procedure will require a temporary increase in dosage; if corticosteroids have been stopped following prolonged therapy they may need to be temporarily re-introduced.

Patients under stress may require increased doses of corticosteroids prior, during and after the period of stressful situation.

Stopping corticosteroids after prolonged therapy may cause withdrawal symptoms including fever, myalgia, arthralgia and malaise. This may occur in patients even without evidence of adrenal insufficiency.

There is an enhanced effect of corticosteroids in patients with hypothyroidism and in those with cirrhosis.

Particular care is required when considering the use of systemic corticosteroids in patients with the following conditions and frequent patient monitoring is necessary:

- renal insufficiency
- hypertension or congestive heart failure
- diabetes mellitus (or a family history of diabetes)
- osteoporosis (especially post-menopausal females)
- previous corticosteroid-induced myopathy
- glaucoma (or family history of glaucoma)
- myasthenia gravis
- non-specific ulcerative colitis, diverticulitis or fresh intestinal anastomosis
- peptic ulceration
- existing or previous history of severe affective disorders (especially previous steroid psychosis)
- liver failure
- epilepsy
- migraine
- history of allergy to corticosteroids
- ocular herpes simplex, because of possible corneal perforation
- tuberculosis
- herpes simplex
- psychiatric disorders

Fat embolism has been reported as a possible complication of hypercortisonism.

Large doses of corticosteroids may mask the symptoms of gastro-intestinal perforation.

Reports in the literature suggest an apparent association between use of corticosteroids and left-ventricular free-wall rupture after a recent myocardial infarction; therefore, corticosteroids should be used with great caution in these patients.

Rare cases of anaphylactoid or hypersensitivity reactions have been reported especially with parenteral administration of corticosteroids. Prophylactic measures should be taken especially if the patient has a history of allergic reactions to medicines.

In rare cases, decrease or withdrawal of orally administered corticosteroids could reveal underlying disease that are accompanied by eosinophilia (e.g. Churg Strauss Syndrome) in patients with asthma.

Patients and/or carers should be warned that potentially severe psychiatric adverse reactions may occur with systemic steroids (see section 4.8). Symptoms typically emerge within a few days or weeks of starting the treatment. Risks may be higher with high doses/systemic exposure (see also section 4.5 pharmacokinetic interactions that can increase the risk of side effects), although dose levels do not allow prediction of the onset, type, severity or duration of reactions. Most reactions recover after either dose reduction or withdrawal, although specific treatment may be necessary. Patients/carers should be encouraged to seek medical advice if worrying psychological symptoms develop, especially if depressed mood or suicidal ideation is suspected. Patients/carers should also be alert to possible psychiatric disturbances that may occur either during or immediately after dose tapering/withdrawal of systemic steroids, although such reactions have been reported infrequently.

Particular care is required when considering the use of systemic corticosteroids in patients with existing or previous history of severe affective disorders in themselves or in their first degree relatives. These would include depressive or manic-depressive illness and previous steroid psychosis.

Use in Children

Corticosteroids cause growth retardation. Treatment should be limited to the minimum dose for the shortest period.

Children on prolonged therapy should be carefully monitored.

Excipient Warnings

The medicine contains benzoic acid which is a mild irritant to the skin, eyes and mucous membrane. It may also increase the risk of jaundice in newborn babies.

It also contains 0.7g sorbitol in each 5ml. When given according to the recommended dosage instructions, each dose will provide up to 3.1g of sorbitol. It is unsuitable in hereditary fructose intolerance and can cause stomach upset and diarrhoea.

It also contains liquid maltitol which may cause diarrhoea.

4.5 Interaction with other medicinal products and other forms of interaction

Effects of other medicinal products on dexamethasone:

Dexamethasone is metabolized via cytochrome P450 3A4 (CYP3A4). Concomitant administration of dexamethasone with inducers of CYP3A4, such as phenytoin, barbiturates, ephedrine, rifabutin, carbamazepine and rifampicin may lead to decreased plasma concentrations of dexamethasone and the dose may need to be increased. Concomitant administration of inhibitors of CYP3A4 such as ketoconazole, ritonavir and erythromycin may lead to increased plasma concentrations of dexamethasone.

These interactions may also interfere with dexamethasone suppression tests, which therefore should be interpreted with caution during administration of substances that affect the metabolism of dexamethasone.

Ketoconazole may increase plasma concentrations of dexamethasone by inhibition of CYP3A4, but may also suppress corticosteroid synthesis in the adrenal and thereby cause adrenal insufficiency at withdrawal of corticosteroid treatment.

Ephedrine may increase the metabolic clearance of corticosteroids, resulting in decreased plasma levels. An increase of the corticosteroid dose might be necessary.

False-negative results in the dexamethasone suppression test inpatients being treated with indometacin have been reported.

Antibiotics: Macrolide antibiotics have been reported to cause a significant decrease in corticosteroid clearance

Anticholinesterases: Concomitant use of anticholinesterase agents and corticosteroids may produce severe weakness in patients with myasthenia gravis. If possible, anticholinesterase agents should be withdrawn at least 24 hours before initiating corticosteroid therapy.

Colestyramine: Colestyramine may decrease the absorption of dexamethasone.

Estrogens, including oral contraceptives: Estrogens may decrease the hepatic metabolism of certain corticosteroids, thereby increasing their effect

Aminoglutethimide: Decrease of dexamethasone efficacy, due to its metabolism increase. An adjustment of dexamethasone dosage may be required.

Gastrointestinal topicals, antacids, charcoal: A decrease in digestive absorption of glucocorticoids have been reported with prednisolone and dexamethasone. Therefore, glucocorticoids should be taken separately from gastrointestinal topicals, antacids or charcoal, with an interval between treatment of at least two hours.

Effects of dexamethasone on other medicinal products

Dexamethasone is a moderate inducer of CYP3A4. Concomitant administration of dexamethasone with substances that are metabolised via CYP3A4 could lead to increased clearance and decreased plasma concentrations of these substances.

The renal clearance of salicylates is increased by corticosteroids and therefore, salicylate dosage should be reduced along with steroidal withdrawal.

The desired effects of hypoglycaemic agents (including insulin), anti-hypertensives and diuretics are antagonised by corticosteroids.

The hypokalaemic effects of acetazolamide, loop diuretics, thiazide diuretics, amphotericin B injection, potassium depleting agents, corticosteroids (gluco-mineralo), tetracosactide and carbenoxolone are enhanced. Hypokalaemia predisposes to cardiac arrhythmia especially "torsade de pointes" and increase the toxicity of cardiac glycosides. Hypokalemia should be corrected before corticosteroid treatment initiation. In addition, there have been cases reported in which concomitant use of amphotericin B and hydrocortisone was followed by cardiac enlargement and congestive heart failure.

Sultopride has been linked to ventricular arrhythmias, especially torsade de pointes. This combination is not recommended.

Patients taking NSAID's should be monitored since the incidence and/or severity of gastro-ulceration may increase. Aspirin should also be used cautiously in conjunction with corticosteroids in hypoprothrombinaemia.

Antitubercular drugs: Serum concentrations of isoniazid may be decreased.

Ciclosporin: Increased activity of both ciclosporin and corticosteroids may occur when the two are used concurrently. Convulsions have been reported with this concurrent use.

Thalidomide: Co-administration with thalidomide should be employed cautiously, as toxic epidermal necrolysis has been reported with concomitant use.

Corticosteroids may affect the nitrobuletetrazolium test for bacterial infection and produce false-negative results.

Vaccines attenuated live

Risk of fatal systemic disease

Praziquantel:

Decrease in praziquantel plasmatic concentrations, with a risk of treatment failure, due to its hepatic metabolism increased by dexamethasone.

Oral anticoagulants:

Possible impact of corticosteroid therapy on the metabolism of oral anticoagulants and on clotting factors. At high doses or with treatment for more than 10 days, there is a risk of bleeding specific to corticosteroid therapy (gastro-intestinal mucosa, vascular fragility). Patients taking corticosteroids associated with oral anticoagulants should be closely monitored (biological investigations on 8th day, then every 2 weeks during treatment and after treatment discontinuation)

Insulin, sulfonylureas, metformin:

Increase in blood glucose, with sometimes diabetic ketosis, since corticosteroids impair carbohydrate tolerance. Therefore, blood and urine self-monitoring should be reinforced by the patient, in particular at the start of treatment

Isoniazid:

A decrease in plasma isoniazid levels have been reported with prednisolone. The suggested mechanism is an increase in hepatic metabolism of isoniazid and a decrease in the hepatic metabolism of isoniazid and a decrease in the hepatic metabolism of glucocorticoids. Patients taking isoniazid should be closely monitored.

4.6 Pregnancy and lactation

Since adequate human reproduction studies have not been performed with corticosteroids, dexamethasone should not be used during pregnancy for maternal indications, unless it is clearly necessary. The lowest effective dose needed to maintain adequate disease control should be used.

Infants born of mothers who have received substantial doses of corticosteroids during pregnancy should be carefully observed for signs of hypoadrenalism.

Patients with pre-eclampsia or fluid retention require close monitoring.

Placental transfer in considerable: foetal serum concentrations are similar to maternal concentrations.

Corticosteroids are excreted in small amounts in breast milk and may suppress growth, interfere with endogenous corticosteroid production or cause other unwanted effects. A decision on whether to continue/discontinue breast feeding or to continue/discontinue therapy with dexamethasone should be made taking into account the benefit of breast feeding to the child and the benefit of dexamethasone therapy to the woman.

There is evidence of harmful effects on pregnancy in animals (see section 5.3)

4.7 Effects on ability to drive and use machines

There are some side effects associated with this product that may affect some patients' ability to drive or operate machinery (see 4.8 Undesirable effects).

4.8 Undesirable effects

The incidence of predictable undesirable effects, including hypothalamic-pituitary-adrenal suppression correlates with the relative potency of the drug, dosage, timing of administration and the duration of treatment (refer to Special Warnings and Precautions).

Reports in the literature suggest an apparent association between use of corticosteroids and left ventricular free wall rupture after a recent myocardial infarction; therefore corticosteroids should be used with great caution in these patients.

Fluid and electrolyte disturbances

Sodium retention, fluid retention, congestive heart failure in susceptible patients, potassium loss, hypokalaemic alkalosis, hypertension, increased calcium excretion.

Musculoskeletal

Osteoporosis, vertebral and long bone fractures, avascular necrosis, tendon rupture. Proximal myopathy. Muscle weakness, aseptic necrosis of femoral and humeral heads, loss of muscle mass.

Gastro-intestinal

Dyspepsia, peptic ulceration with perforation and haemorrhage, acute pancreatitis, candidiasis. Abdominal distension and vomiting. Ulcerative oesophagitis. Perforation of the small and large bowel particularly in patients with inflammatory bowel disease.

Dermatological

Impaired wound healing, thin fragile skin, petechiae and ecchymoses, erythema, striae, telangiectasia, acne, increased sweating, suppressed reaction to skin tests, other cutaneous reactions such as allergic dermatitis, urticaria, angioneurotic oedema, thinning scalp hair.

Ophthalmic

Posterior subcapsular cataracts, increased intra-ocular pressure, glaucoma, papilloedema, corneal or scleral thinning, exacerbation of ophthalmic viral or fungal diseases, exopthalmos.

Anti-inflammatory and immunosuppressive effects

Increased susceptibility and severity of infections with suppression of clinical symptoms and signs, opportunistic infections, recurrence of dormant tuberculosis. Decreased resistance to infection

Endocrine/metabolic

Menstrual irregularities and amenorrhoea, suppression of the hypothalamic-pituitary-adrenal axis, growth suppression in children and adolescents, premature epiphyseal closure, development of Cushingoid state, hirsutism, weight gain, impaired carbohydrate tolerance with increased requirement for anti-diabetic therapy. Negative protein and calcium balance. Secondary adrenocortical and pituitary unresponsiveness (particularly in times of stress, as in trauma, surgery or illness).

Neurological

Convulsions and aggravation of epilepsy, vertigo, headache, increased intra-cranial pressure with papilloedema in children (Pseudotumour cerebri), usually after treatment withdrawal, psychological dependence, depression, insomnia, aggravation of schizophrenia and psychic disturbances ranging from euphoria to frank psychotic manifestations.

A wide range of psychiatric reactions including affective disorders (such as irritable, euphoric, depressed and labile mood and suicidal thoughts), psychotic reactions (including mania, delusions, hallucinations and aggravation of schizophrenia), behavioural disturbances, irritability, anxiety, sleep disturbances and cognitive dysfunction including confusion and amnesia have been reported. Reactions are common and may occur in both adults and children. In adults, the frequency of severe reactions has been estimated to be 5-6%. Psychological effects have been reported on withdrawal of corticosteroids; the frequency is unknown.

General

Hypersensitivity including anaphylaxis has been reported. Leucocytosis, thromboembolism, increased appetite, nausea, malaise, hiccups, abnormal fat deposits, increased or decreased motility and number of spermatozoa.

Withdrawal symptoms and signs

Too rapid a reduction of corticosteroid dosage following prolonged treatment can lead to acute adrenal insufficiency, hypotension and death (See 'Special Warnings and Precautions').

A 'withdrawal syndrome' may also occur including fever, myalgia, arthralgia, rhinitis, conjunctivitis, painful itchy skin nodules and loss of weight.

4.9 Overdose

Reports of acute toxicity and/or deaths following overdosage with glucocorticoids are rare. No antidote is available. Treatment is probably not indicated for reactions due to chronic poisoning unless the patient has a condition that would render him unusually susceptible to ill effects from corticosteroids. In this case, the stomach should be emptied and symptomatic treatment should be instituted as necessary. Anaphylactic and hypersensitivity reactions may be treated with epinephrine (adrenaline), positive-pressure artificial respiration and aminophylline. The patient should be kept warm and quiet. The biological half life of dexamethasone in plasma is about 190 minutes.

5. PHARMACOLOGICAL PROPERTIES

5.1 Pharmacodynamic properties

ATC Code: H02A B02

Pharmacotherapeutic Group: Corticosteroid

Dexamethasone is a highly potent and long-acting glucocorticoid with negligible sodium retaining properties and is therefore, particularly suitable for the use in patients with cardiac failure and hypertension. It's anti-inflammatory potency is 7 times greater than prednisolone and like other glucocorticoids, dexamethasone also has anti-allergic, antipyretic and immunosuppressive properties.

Dexamethasone has a biological half life of 36 - 54 hours and therefore is suitable in conditions where continuous glucocorticoid action is required.

5.2 Pharmacokinetic properties

Dexamethasone is well absorbed when given by mouth; peak plasma levels are reached between 1 and 2 hours after ingestion and show wide interindividual variations. The mean plasma half life is 3.6 ± 0.9h. Dexamethasone is bound (to about 77%) to plasma proteins, mainly albumins. Percentage protein binding of dexamethasone, unlike that of cortisol, remains practically unchanged with increasing steroid concentrations. Corticosteroids are rapidly distributed to all body tissues. Dexamethasone is metabolised mainly in the liver but also in the kidney. Dexamethasone and its metabolites are excreted in the urine.

5.3 Preclinical safety data

Toxicity: Cleft palate is observed in rats, mice, hamsters, rabbits, dogs and primates. It is not observed in horses and sheep. Sometime abnormalities were accompanied by defects from the central nervous system and the heart. In primates, brain damage was observed at antenatal exposure (Schardein). Additionally, intrauterine growth was inhibited (Reprotox). These effects were observed after use of high doses of dexamethasone.

There are no further preclinical data considered relevant to clinical safety beyond data included in other section of the SPC.

6. PHARMACEUTICAL PARTICULARS

6.1 List of excipients

Benzoic acid, propylene glycol, citric acid monohydrate, liquid maltitol, garden mint flavour (containing isopropanol and propylene glycol), liquid sorbitol non-crystallising, sodium citrate and purified water.

6.2 Incompatibilities

Not applicable

6.3 Shelf life

Shelf Life: 2 years

Shelf life after first opening the container:3 months

6.4 Special precautions for storage

Do not store above 25°C. Do not refrigerate.

The storage at temperatures higher than 25°C could allow precipitation inside the solution. Do not use the product if solid particles are observed inside the solution.

6.5 Nature and contents of container

Bottles: 150ml in Amber Type III) glass.

Closures: HDPE, EPE wadded, tamper evident, child resistant closure.

6.6 Special precautions for disposal and other handling

No special requirements

7. MARKETING AUTHORISATION HOLDER

Rosemont Pharmaceuticals Ltd., Rosemont House, Yorkdale Industrial Park, Braithwaite Street, Leeds, LS11 9XE, UK

8. MARKETING AUTHORISATION NUMBER(S)

PL 00427/0137

9. DATE OF FIRST AUTHORISATION/RENEWAL OF THE AUTHORISATION

Date of first authorisation: 08th March 2005

10. DATE OF REVISION OF THE TEXT

05th March 2008

DHC Continus prolonged release tablets 60mg, 90mg and 120 mg

(Napp Pharmaceuticals Limited)

1. NAME OF THE MEDICINAL PRODUCT

DHC® Continus® prolonged release tablets 60 mg, 90 mg, 120 mg.

2. QUALITATIVE AND QUANTITATIVE COMPOSITION

Dihydrocodeine tartrate 60 mg, 90 mg, 120 mg.

3. PHARMACEUTICAL FORM

Prolonged release tablet.

White capsule shaped tablets, 60 mg are marked DHC 60, 90 mg are marked DHC 90 and 120 mg are marked DHC 120.

4. CLINICAL PARTICULARS

4.1 Therapeutic indications

For the relief of severe pain in cancer and other chronic conditions.

4.2 Posology and method of administration

Adults and children over 12 years: 60 mg - 120 mg every 12 hours.

Elderly: Dosage should be reduced.

Children 12 years or under: Not recommended.

Method of administration

Oral.

4.3 Contraindications

Hypersensitivity to dihydrocodeine or any of the tablet constituents; respiratory depression; obstructive airways disease; paralytic ileus; head injury; raised intracranial pressure; acute alcoholism. As dihydrocodeine may cause the release of histamine, it should not be given during an asthma attack and should be given with caution to asthmatics.

Patients with rare hereditary problems of galactose intolerance, the Lapp lactase deficiency or glucose-galactose malabsorption should not take this medicine.

4.4 Special warnings and precautions for use

Dosage should be reduced in the elderly, in hypothyroidism, chronic hepatic disease and renal insufficiency.

Dihydrocodeine should be administered with caution to patients with a history of opioid abuse, biliary tract disorders, prostatic hypertrophy, pancreatitis, constipation, obstructive bowel disorder and severe cor pulmonale.

Dihydrocodeine has a recognised abuse and addiction profile similar to other opioids. Tolerance to analgesic effects may develop upon repeated administration.

The risk-benefit of continued use should be assessed regularly by the prescriber, and in particular the prescriber should take care to avoid any unnecessary increase in dosage especially where there is evidence of a previous history of drug dependence or abuse.

DHC Continus tablets must be swallowed whole, and not broken, chewed or crushed. The administration of broken, chewed or crushed tablets may lead to a rapid release and absorption of a potential overdose of dihydrocodeine (see Section 4.9).

4.5 Interaction with other medicinal products and other forms of interaction

Other central nervous system depressants, including sedatives or hypnotics, phenothiazines, other tranquillisers and alcohol, may result in respiratory depression or sedation. Dihydrocodeine should be used with caution in patients taking monoamine oxidase inhibitors or within two weeks of such therapy.

4.6 Pregnancy and lactation

There is little published evidence on safety in human pregnancy but dihydrocodeine has been used for many years without apparent ill effects. Dihydrocodeine has not been reported to be excreted in breast milk. However, it is advisable that dihydrocodeine only be administered to breast-feeding mothers if considered essential.

4.7 Effects on ability to drive and use machines

Dihydrocodeine may cause drowsiness and, if affected, patients should not drive or operate machinery.

4.8 Undesirable effects

Common adverse drug reactions seen during therapy are constipation, nausea, vomiting, headache, somnolence, pruritus and rash.

Uncommon adverse reactions are urinary retention, ureteric or biliary spasm, dry mouth, mood changes, blurred vision, sweating, decreased libido, flushing, abdominal pain, hypotension, paraesthesia, confusion, dizziness, hallucinations, urticaria, paralytic ileus and respiratory depression.

Dependence may occur. Regular prolonged use of dihydrocodeine is known to lead to addiction and tolerance. Symptoms of restlessness and irritability may result when treatment is stopped.

Prolonged use of a painkiller for headaches can make them worse.

4.9 Overdose

Acute overdosage with dihydrocodeine can be manifested by somnolence progressing to stupor or coma, miotic pupils, rhabdomyolysis, non-cardiac pulmonary oedema, bradycardia, hypotension and respiratory depression or apnoea.

Primary attention should be given to the establishment of a patent airway and institution of assisted or controlled ventilation.

In the case of massive overdosage, administer naloxone intravenously (0.4 to 2 mg for an adult and 0.01 mg/kg body weight for children) if the patient is in a coma or respiratory depression is present. Repeat the dose at 2 minute intervals if there is no response, or by an infusion. An infusion of 60% of the initial dose per hour is a useful starting point. A solution of 10 mg made up in 50 ml dextrose will produce 200 micrograms/ml for infusion using an IV pump (dose adjusted to the clinical response). Infusions are not a substitute for frequent review of the patient's clinical state. Intramuscular naloxone is an alternative in the event that IV access is not possible.

As the duration of action of naloxone is relatively short, the patient must be carefully monitored until spontaneous respiration is reliably re-established. Naloxone is a competitive antagonist and large doses (4 mg) may be required in seriously poisoned patients. For less severe overdosage, administer naloxone 0.2 mg intravenously followed by increments of 0.1 mg every 2 minutes if required.

Naloxone should not be administered in the absence of clinically significant respiratory or circulatory depression secondary to dihydrocodeine overdosage. Naloxone should be administered cautiously to persons who are known, or suspected, to be physically dependent on dihydrocodeine. In such cases, an abrupt or complete reversal of opioid effects may precipitate pain and an acute withdrawal syndrome.

Additional/other considerations:

- Consider activated charcoal (50 g for adults, 10-15 g for children), if a substantial amount has been ingested within 1 hour, provided the airway can be protected. It may be reasonable to assume that late administration of activated charcoal may be beneficial for prolonged release preparations but there is no evidence to support this.
- *DHC Continus* tablets will continue to release and add to the dihydrocodeine load for up to 12 hours after administration and the management of overdosage should be modified accordingly. Gastric contents may therefore need to be emptied, as this can be useful in removing unabsorbed drug, particularly when a prolonged release formulation has been taken.

5. PHARMACOLOGICAL PROPERTIES

5.1 Pharmacodynamic properties

Dihydrocodeine is a semisynthetic narcotic analgesic with a potency between morphine and codeine. It acts on opioid receptors in the brain to reduce the patient's perception of pain and improve the psychological reaction to pain by reducing the associated anxiety.

5.2 Pharmacokinetic properties

Dihydrocodeine is well absorbed from the gastrointestinal tract following administration of *DHC Continus* tablets and plasma levels are maintained throughout the twelve hour dosing interval.

Like other phenanthrene derivatives, dihydrocodeine is mainly metabolised in the liver with the resultant metabolites being excreted mainly in the urine. Metabolism of dihydrocodeine includes o-demethylation, n-demethylation and 6-keto reduction.

5.3 Preclinical safety data

There are no pre-clinical data of relevance to the prescriber which are additional to that already included in other sections of the SPC.

6. PHARMACEUTICAL PARTICULARS

6.1 List of excipients

Lactose (anhydrous)

Hydroxyethylcellulose

Cetostearyl alcohol

Magnesium stearate

Purified talc

Purified water

6.2 Incompatibilities

None known.

6.3 Shelf life

Three years.

6.4 Special precautions for storage

Do not store above 25°C.

6.5 Nature and contents of container

Polypropylene containers with polyethylene lids (56 tablets)

6.6 Special precautions for disposal and other handling

None stated.

7. MARKETING AUTHORISATION HOLDER

Napp Pharmaceuticals Limited

Cambridge Science Park

Milton Road

Cambridge

CB4 0GW

8. MARKETING AUTHORISATION NUMBER(S)

PL 16950/0019 - 0021

9. DATE OF FIRST AUTHORISATION/RENEWAL OF THE AUTHORISATION

60 mg 5 November 1986 / 5 March 2001

90 mg and 120 mg 12 July 1990 / 5 March 2001

10. DATE OF REVISION OF THE TEXT

February 2007

Legal Category

POM

® The Napp device, DHC and DHC CONTINUS are Registered Trade Marks

Diamicron

(Servier Laboratories Limited)

1. NAME OF THE MEDICINAL PRODUCT

DIAMICRON®

2. QUALITATIVE AND QUANTITATIVE COMPOSITION

Gliclazide 80 mg

3. PHARMACEUTICAL FORM

Tablets.

4. CLINICAL PARTICULARS

4.1 Therapeutic indications

Non insulin dependent diabetes mellitus.

4.2 Posology and method of administration

Oral administration.

Adults: The total daily dose may vary from 40 to 320 mg taken orally. The dose should be adjusted according to the individual patient's response, commencing with 40-80 mg daily (1/2 - 1 tablet) and increasing until adequate control is achieved. A single dose should not exceed 160 mg (2 tablets). When higher doses are required, DIAMICRON® should be taken twice daily and according to the main meals of the day.

In obese patients or those not showing adequate response to DIAMICRON® alone, additional therapy may be required.

Elderly: Plasma clearance of gliclazide is not altered in the elderly and steady state plasma levels can therefore be expected to be similar to those in adults under 65 years. Clinical experience in the elderly to date shows that DIAMICRON® is effective and well tolerated. Care should be exercised, however, when prescribing sulphonylureas in the elderly due to a possible age-related increased risk of hypoglycaemia.

Children: DIAMICRON® as with other sulphonylureas, is not indicated for the treatment of juvenile onset diabetes mellitus.

4.3 Contraindications

DIAMICRON® should not be used in:

- Juvenile onset diabetes.
- Diabetes complicated by ketosis and acidosis.
- Pregnancy.
- Diabetics undergoing surgery, after severe trauma or during infections.
- Patients known to have hypersensitivity to other sulphonylureas and related drugs.
- Diabetic pre-coma and coma.
- Severe renal or hepatic insufficiency.

4.4 Special warnings and precautions for use

Hypoglycaemia: all sulphonylurea drugs are capable of producing moderate or severe hypoglycaemia, particularly in the following conditions:

- in patients controlled by diet alone,
- in cases of accidental overdose,
- when calorie or glucose intake is deficient,
- in patients with hepatic and/or renal impairment; however, in long-term clinical trials, patients with renal insufficiency have been treated satisfactorily, using DIAMICRON® at reduced doses.

In order to reduce the risk of hypoglycaemia it is therefore recommended:

- to initiate treatment for non-insulin dependent diabetics by diet alone, if this is possible,
- to take into account the age of the patient: blood sugar levels not strictly controlled by diet alone might be acceptable in the elderly,
- to adjust the dose of DIAMICRON® according to the blood glucose response and to the 24 hour urinary glucose during the first days of treatment.

Dosage adjustments may be necessary:

- on the occurrence of mild symptoms of hypoglycaemia (sweating, pallor, hunger pangs, tachycardia, sensation of malaise). Such findings should be treated with oral glucose and adjustments made in drug dosage and/or meal patterns,
- on the occurrence of severe hypoglycaemic reactions (coma or neurological impairment, see overdose),
- loss of control of blood glucose (hyperglycaemia). When a patient stabilised on any diabetic regimen is exposed to stress such as fever, trauma, infection or surgery, a loss of control may occur. At such times, it may be necessary to increase progressively the dosage of DIAMICRON® and if this is insufficient, to discontinue the treatment with DIAMICRON® and to administer insulin. As with other sulphonylureas, hypoglycaemia will occur if the patients' dietary intake is reduced or if they are receiving a larger dose of DIAMICRON® than required.

Care should be exercised in patients with hepatic and/or renal impairment and a small starting dose should be used with careful patient monitoring.

4.5 Interaction with other medicinal products and other forms of interaction

Care should be taken when giving DIAMICRON® with drugs which are known to alter the diabetic state or potentiate the drug's action.

The hypoglycaemic effect of DIAMICRON® may be potentiated by phenylbutazone, salicylates, sulphonamides, coumarin derivatives, MAOIs, beta adrenergic blocking agents, tetracycline compounds, chloramphenicol, clofibrate, disopyramide, miconazole (oral forms) and cimetidine.

It may be diminished by corticosteroids, oral contraceptives, thiazide diuretics, phenothiazine derivatives, thyroid hormones and abuse of laxatives.

4.6 Pregnancy and lactation

Pregnancy: See "Contra-indications".

Lactation: It has not been established whether gliclazide is transferred to human milk. However, other sulphonylureas have been found in milk and there is no evidence to suggest that gliclazide differs from the group in this respect.

4.7 Effects on ability to drive and use machines

Patients should be informed that their concentration may be affected if their diabetes is not satisfactorily controlled, especially at the beginning of treatment (see special warnings and precautions).

4.8 Undesirable effects

- Hypoglycaemia (see special warnings and precautions).
- Abnormalities of hepatic function are not uncommon during DIAMICRON® therapy. There are rare reports of hepatic failure, hepatitis and jaundice following treatment with DIAMICRON®.
- Mild gastro-intestinal disturbances including nausea, dyspepsia, diarrhoea, constipation have been reported but this type of adverse reaction can be avoided if DIAMICRON® is taken during a meal.
- Skin reactions including rash, pruritus, erythema, bullous eruption; blood dyscrasia including anaemia, leukopenia, thrombocytopenia and granulocytopenia have been observed during treatment with DIAMICRON® but are not known to be directly attributable to the drug.

4.9 Overdose

The symptom to be expected of overdose would be hypoglycaemia. The treatment is gastric lavage and correction of the hypoglycaemia by appropriate means with continual monitoring of the patient's blood sugar until the effect of the drug has ceased.

5. PHARMACOLOGICAL PROPERTIES

5.1 Pharmacodynamic properties

Gliclazide is a hypoglycaemic sulphonylurea differing from other related compounds by the addition of an azabicyclo-octane ring.

In man, apart from having similar hypoglycaemic effect to the other sulphonylureas, gliclazide has been shown to reduce platelet adhesiveness and aggregation and increase fibrinolytic activity. These factors are thought to be implicated in the pathogenesis of long-term complications of diabetes mellitus.

Gliclazide primarily enhances the first phase of insulin secretion, but also to a lesser degree its second phase. Both phases are diminished in non-insulin dependent diabetes mellitus.

5.2 Pharmacokinetic properties

The drug is well absorbed and its half-life in man is approximately 10-12 hours. Gliclazide is metabolised in the liver; less than 5% of the dose is excreted unchanged in the urine.

5.3 Preclinical safety data

No findings in the preclinical testing which could be of relevance for the prescriber.

6. PHARMACEUTICAL PARTICULARS

6.1 List of excipients

Lactose monohydrate, maize starch, pregelatinised maize starch, talc, magnesium stearate.

6.2 Incompatibilities

None

6.3 Shelf life

5 years

6.4 Special precautions for storage

None

6.5 Nature and contents of container

Blister strip (PVC/Aluminium) of 20 tablets. 3 strips per carton.

Blister strip (PVC/Aluminium) of 28 tablets. 1 strip per carton.

Blister strip (PVC/Aluminium) of 28 tablets. 2 strips per carton.

Blister strip (PVC/Aluminium) of 28 tablets. 4 strips per carton.

6.6 Special precautions for disposal and other handling

Not applicable.

7. MARKETING AUTHORISATION HOLDER

Servier Laboratories Limited

Gallions, Wexham Springs,

Framewood Road, Wexham

Slough

SL3 6RJ

8. MARKETING AUTHORISATION NUMBER(S)

PL 0093/0024

9. DATE OF FIRST AUTHORISATION/RENEWAL OF THE AUTHORISATION

21 December 1979

10. DATE OF REVISION OF THE TEXT

5 July 2005

Diamicron 30 mg MR

(Servier Laboratories Limited)

1. NAME OF THE MEDICINAL PRODUCT

DIAMICRON 30 mg MR Tablets

2. QUALITATIVE AND QUANTITATIVE COMPOSITION

One tablet contains gliclazide 30 mg

For excipients, see section 6.1.

3. PHARMACEUTICAL FORM

Modified release tablet.

White, oblong tablet engraved on both faces, 'DIA 30' on one face and on the other.

4. CLINICAL PARTICULARS

4.1 Therapeutic indications

Non insulin-dependent diabetes (type 2) in adults when dietary measures, physical exercise and weight loss alone are not sufficient to control blood glucose.

4.2 Posology and method of administration

Oral use.

For adult use only.

The daily dose may vary from 1 to 4 tablets per day, *i.e.* from 30 to 120 mg taken orally in a single intake at breakfast time.

It is recommended that the tablet(s) be swallowed whole.

If a dose is forgotten, there must be no increase in the dose taken the next day.

As with any hypoglycaemic agent, the dose should be adjusted according to the individual patient's metabolic response (blood glucose, HbAlc)

• Initial dose

The recommended starting dose is 30 mg daily.

If blood glucose is effectively controlled, this dose may be used for maintenance treatment.

If blood glucose is not adequately controlled, the dose may be increased to 60, 90 or 120 mg daily, in successive steps. The interval between each dose increment should be at least 1 month except in patients whose blood glucose has not reduced after two weeks of treatment. In such cases, the dose may be increased at the end of the second week of treatment.

The maximum recommended daily dose is 120 mg.

• Switching from Diamicron 80 mg tablets to Diamicron 30 mg modified release tablets:

1 tablet of Diamicron 80 mg is comparable to 1 tablet of Diamicron 30 mg MR. Consequently the switch can be performed provided a careful blood monitoring.

• Switching from another oral antidiabetic agent to Diamicron 30 mg MR Tablets:

Diamicron 30 mg MR Tablets can be used to replace other oral antidiabetic agents.

The dosage and the half-life of the previous antidiabetic agent should be taken into account when switching to Diamicron 30 mg MR Tablets.

A transitional period is not generally necessary. A starting dose of 30 mg should be used and this should be adjusted to suit the patient's blood glucose response, as described above.

When switching from a hypoglycaemic sulphonylurea with a prolonged half-life, a treatment free period of a few days may be necessary to avoid an additive effect of the two products, which might cause hypoglycaemia. The procedure described for initiating treatment should also be used when switching to treatment with Diamicron 30 mg MR Tablets, *i.e.* a starting dose of 30 mg/day, followed by a stepwise increase in dose, depending on the metabolic response.

• Combination treatment with other antidiabetic agents:

Diamicron 30 mg MR Tablets can be given in combination with biguanides, alpha glucosidase inhibitors or insulin.

In patients not adequately controlled with Diamicron 30 mg MR Tablets, concomitant insulin therapy can be initiated under close medical supervision.

• In the elderly (over 65), Diamicron 30 mg MR Tablets should be prescribed using the same dosing regimen recommended for patients under 65 years of age. In patients with mild to moderate renal insufficiency the same dosing regimen can be used as in patients with normal renal function with careful patient monitoring. These data have been confirmed in clinical trials.

• In patients at risk of hypoglycaemia:

- undernourished or malnourished,
- severe or poorly compensated endocrine disorders (hypopituitarism, hypothyroidism, adrenocorticotrophic insufficiency),
- withdrawal of prolonged and/or high dose corticosteroid therapy,
- severe vascular disease (severe coronary heart disease, severe carotid impairment, diffuse vascular disease);

It is recommended that the minimum daily starting dose of 30 mg is used.

There are no data and clinical studies available in children.

4.3 Contraindications

• known hypersensitivity to gliclazide or to any of the excipients, other sulphonylureas, sulphonamides,

• type 1 diabetes,

• diabetic pre-coma and coma, diabetic keto-acidosis,

• severe renal or hepatic insufficiency: in these cases the use of insulin is recommended,

• treatment with miconazole (see Section "Interactions with other medicinal products and other forms of interaction"),

• lactation (see Section "Pregnancy and Lactation").

4.4 Special warnings and precautions for use

HYPOGLYCAEMIA:

This treatment should be prescribed only if the patient is likely to have a regular food intake (including breakfast). It is important to have a regular carbohydrate intake due to the increased risk of hypoglycaemia if a meal is taken late, if an inadequate amount of food is consumed or if the food is low in carbohydrate. Hypoglycaemia is more likely to occur during low-calorie diets, following prolonged or strenuous exercise, alcohol intake or if a combination of hypoglycaemic agents is being used.

Hypoglycaemia may occur following administration of sulphonylureas (see 4.8. Undesirable effects). Some cases may be severe and prolonged. Hospitalisation may be necessary and glucose administration may need to be continued for several days.

Careful selection of patients, of the dose used, and clear patient directions are necessary to reduce the risk of hypoglycaemic episodes.

Factors which increase the risk of hypoglycaemia:

- patient refuses or (particularly in elderly subjects) is unable to co-operate,
- malnutrition, irregular mealtimes, skipping meals, periods of fasting or dietary changes,
- imbalance between physical exercise and carbohydrate intake,
- renal insufficiency,
- severe hepatic insufficiency,
- overdose of Diamicron 30 mg MR Tablets,
- certain endocrine disorders: thyroid disorders, hypopituitarism and adrenal insufficiency,
- concomitant administration of certain other medicines (see Interactions).

Renal and hepatic insufficiency: the pharmacokinetics and/or pharmacodynamics of gliclazide may be altered in patients with hepatic insufficiency or severe renal failure. A hypoglycaemic episode occurring in these patients may be prolonged, so appropriate management should be initiated.

Patient information:

The risks of hypoglycaemia, together with its symptoms, treatment, and conditions that predispose to its development, should be explained to the patient and to family members.

The patient should be informed of the importance of following dietary advice, of taking regular exercise, and of regular monitoring of blood glucose levels.

Poor blood glucose control: blood glucose control in a patient receiving antidiabetic treatment may be affected by any of the following: fever, trauma, infection or surgical intervention. In some cases, it may be necessary to administer insulin.

The hypoglycaemic efficacy of any oral antidiabetic agent, including gliclazide, is attenuated over time in many patients: this may be due to progression in the severity of the diabetes, or to a reduced response to treatment. This phenomenon is known as secondary failure which is distinct from primary failure, when an active substance is ineffective as first-line treatment. Adequate dose adjustment and dietary compliance should be considered before classifying the patient as secondary failure.

Laboratory tests: Measurement of glycated haemoglobin levels (or fasting venous plasma glucose) is recommended in assessing blood glucose control. Blood glucose self-monitoring may also be useful.

Treatment of patients with G6PD-deficiency with sulphonylurea agents can lead to haemolytic anaemia. Since gliclazide belongs to the chemical class of sulphonylurea drugs, caution should be used in patients with G6PD-deficiency and a non- sulphonylurea alternative should be considered.

4.5 Interaction with other medicinal products and other forms of interaction

1) The following products are likely to increase the risk of hypoglycaemia

Contra-indicated combination

- **Miconazole** (systemic route, oromucosal gel): increases the hypoglycaemic effect with possible onset of hypoglycaemic symptoms, or even coma.

Combinations which are not recommended

- Phenylbutazone (systemic route): increases the hypoglycaemic effect of sulphonylureas (displaces their binding to plasma proteins and/or reduces their elimination).
- It is preferable to use a different anti-inflammatory agent, or else to warn the patient and emphasise the importance of self-monitoring. Where necessary, adjust the dose during and after treatment with the anti-inflammatory agent.
- **Alcohol:** increases the hypoglycaemic reaction (by inhibiting compensatory reactions) that can lead to the onset of hypoglycaemic coma.

Avoid alcohol or medicines containing alcohol.

Combinations requiring precautions for use

Potentiation of the blood glucose lowering effect and thus, in some instances, hypoglycaemia may occur when one of the following drugs is taken, for example:

Other antidiabetic agents (insulins, acarbose, biguanides), beta-blockers, fluconazole, angiotensin converting enzyme inhibitors (captopril, enalapril), H2-receptor antagonists, MAOIs, sulfonamides, and nonsteroidal anti-inflammatory agents.

2) The following products may cause an increase in blood glucose levels

Combination which is not recommended

- **Danazol**: diabetogenic effect of danazol.

If the use of this active substance cannot be avoided, warn the patient and emphasise the importance of urine and blood glucose monitoring. It may be necessary to adjust the dose of the antidiabetic agent during and after treatment with danazol.

Combinations requiring precautions during use

- **Chlorpromazine** (neuroleptic agent): high doses (>100 mg per day of chlorpromazine) increase blood glucose levels (reduced insulin release).

Warn the patient and emphasise the importance of blood glucose monitoring. It may be necessary to adjust the dose of the antidiabetic active substance during and after treatment with the neuroleptic agent.

- **Glucocorticoids** (systemic and local route: intra-articular, cutaneous and rectal preparations) and tetracosactrin: increase in blood glucose levels with possible ketosis (reduced tolerance to carbohydrates due to glucocorticoids).

Warn the patient and emphasise the importance of blood glucose monitoring, particularly at the start of treatment. It may be necessary to adjust the dose of the antidiabetic active substance during and after treatment with glucocorticoids.

- **Ritodrine, salbutamol, terbutaline: (I.V.)**

Increased blood glucose levels due to beta-2 agonist effects.

Emphasise the importance of monitoring blood glucose levels. If necessary, switch to insulin.

3) Combination which must be taken into account

- **Anticoagulant therapy** (Warfarin.):

Sulphonylureas may lead to potentiation of anticoagulation during concurrent treatment.

Adjustment of the anticoagulant may be necessary.

4.6 Pregnancy and lactation

Pregnancy

There is no experience with the use of gliclazide during pregnancy in humans, even though there are few data with other sulphonylureas.

In animal studies, gliclazide is not teratogenic.

Control of diabetes should be obtained before the time of conception to reduce the risk of congenital abnormalities linked to uncontrolled diabetes.

Oral hypoglycaemic agents are not suitable, insulin is the drug of first choice for treatment of diabetes during pregnancy. It is recommended that oral hypoglycaemic therapy is changed to insulin before a pregnancy is attempted, or as soon as pregnancy is discovered.

Lactation

It is not known whether gliclazide or its metabolites are excreted in breast milk. Given the risk of neonatal hypoglycaemia, the product is contra-indicated in breast-feeding mothers.

4.7 Effects on ability to drive and use machines

Patients should be made aware of the symptoms of hypoglycaemia and should be careful if driving or operating machinery, especially at the beginning of treatment.

4.8 Undesirable effects

Based on the experience with gliclazide and with other sulphonylureas, the following undesirable effects have to be mentioned.

Hypoglycaemia

As for other sulphonylureas, treatment with Diamicron 30 mg MR Tablets can cause hypoglycaemia, if mealtimes are irregular and, in particular, if meals are skipped. Possible symptoms of hypoglycaemia are: headache, intense hunger, nausea, vomiting, lassitude, sleep disorders, agitation, aggression, poor concentration, reduced awareness and slowed reactions, depression, confusion, visual and speech disorders, aphasia, tremor, paresis, sensory disorders, dizziness, feeling of powerlessness, loss of self-control, delirium, convulsions, shallow respiration, bradycardia, drowsiness and loss of consciousness, possibly resulting in coma and lethal outcome.

In addition, signs of adrenergic counter-regulation may be observed: sweating, clammy skin, anxiety, tachycardia, hypertension, palpitations, angina pectoris and cardiac arrhythmia.

Usually, symptoms disappear after intake of carbohydrates (sugar). However, artificial sweeteners have no effect. Experience with other sulphonylureas shows that hypoglycaemia can recur even when measures prove effective initially.

If a hypoglycaemic episode is severe or prolonged, and even if it is temporarily controlled by intake of sugar, immediate medical treatment or even hospitalisation are required.

Gastrointestinal disturbances, including abdominal pain, nausea, vomiting dyspepsia, diarrhoea, and constipation have been reported: if these should occur they can be avoided or minimised if gliclazide is taken with breakfast.

The following undesirable effects have been more rarely reported:

- Skin and subcutaneous tissue disorders: rash, pruritus, urticaria, erythema, maculopapular rashes, bullous reactions.
- Blood and lymphatic system disorders: Changes in haematology are rare. They may include anaemia, leucopenia, thrombocytopenia, granulocytopenia. These are in general reversible upon discontinuation of medication.
- Hepato-biliary disorders: raised hepatic enzyme levels (AST, ALT, alkaline phosphatase), hepatitis (isolated reports). Discontinue treatment if cholestatic jaundice appears.

These symptoms usually disappear after discontinuation of treatment.

- Eye disorders

Transient visual disturbances may occur especially on initiation of treatment, due to changes in blood glucose levels.

- Class attribution effects:

Cases of erythrocytopenia, agranulocytosis, haemolytic anaemia, pancytopenia and allergic vasculitis, have been described for other sulphonylureas.

With other sulphonylureas cases were also observed of elevated liver enzyme levels and even impairment of liver function (e.g. with cholestasis and jaundice) and hepatitis which regressed after withdrawal of the sulphonylurea or led to life-threatening liver failure in isolated cases.

4.9 Overdose

An overdose of sulphonylureas may cause hypoglycaemia.

Moderate symptoms of hypoglycaemia, without any loss of consciousness or neurological signs, must be corrected by carbohydrate intake, dose adjustment and/or change of diet. Strict monitoring should be continued until the doctor is sure that the patient is out of danger.

Severe hypoglycaemic reactions, with coma, convulsions or other neurological disorders are possible and must be treated as a medical emergency, requiring immediate hospitalisation.

If hypoglycaemic coma is diagnosed or suspected, the patient should be given a rapid I.V. injection of 50 mL of concentrated glucose solution (20 to 30 %). This should be followed by continuous infusion of a more dilute glucose solution (10 %) at a rate that will maintain blood glucose levels above 1 g/L. Patients should be monitored closely and, depending on the patient's condition after this time, the doctor will decide if further monitoring is necessary.

Dialysis is of no benefit to patients due to the strong binding of gliclazide to proteins.

5. PHARMACOLOGICAL PROPERTIES

5.1 Pharmacodynamic properties

SULFONAMIDES, UREA DERIVATIVES

ATC code: A10BB09

Gliclazide is a hypoglycaemic sulphonylurea oral antidiabetic active substance differing from other related compounds by an N-containing heterocyclic ring with an endocyclic bond.

Gliclazide reduces blood glucose levels by stimulating insulin secretion from the β-cells of the islets of Langerhans. Increase in postprandial insulin and C-peptide secretion persists after two years of treatment.

In addition to these metabolic properties, gliclazide has haemovascular properties.

Effects on insulin release

In type 2 diabetics, gliclazide restores the first peak of insulin secretion in response to glucose and increases the second phase of insulin secretion. A significant increase in insulin response is seen in response to stimulation induced by a meal or glucose.

Haemovascular properties:

Gliclazide decreases microthrombosis by two mechanisms which may be involved in complications of diabetes:

- a partial inhibition of platelet aggregation and adhesion, with a decrease in the markers of platelet activation (beta thromboglobulin, thromboxane B_2).
- an action on the vascular endothelium fibrinolytic activity with an increase in tPA activity.

5.2 Pharmacokinetic properties

Plasma levels increase progressively during the first 6 hours, reaching a plateau which is maintained from the sixth to the twelfth hour after administration.

Intra-individual variability is low.

Gliclazide is completely absorbed. Food intake does not affect the rate or degree of absorption.

The relationship between the dose administered ranging up to 120 mg and the area under the concentration time curve is linear.

Plasma protein binding is approximately 95%.

Gliclazide is mainly metabolised in the liver and excreted in the urine: less than 1% of the unchanged form is found in the urine. No active metabolites have been detected in plasma.

The elimination half-life of gliclazide varies between 12 and 20 hours.

The volume of distribution is around 30 litres.

No clinically significant changes in pharmacokinetic parameters have been observed in elderly patients.

A single daily dose of Diamicron 30 mg MR Tablets maintains effective gliclazide plasma concentrations over 24 hours.

5.3 Preclinical safety data
Preclinical data reveal no special hazards for humans based on conventional studies of repeated dose toxicity and genotoxicity. Long term carcinogenicity studies have not been done. No teratogenic changes have been shown in animal studies, but lower fœtal body weight was observed in animals receiving doses 25 fold higher than the maximum recommended dose in humans.

6. PHARMACEUTICAL PARTICULARS
6.1 List of excipients
Calcium hydrogen phosphate dihydrate,

Maltodextrin,

Hypromellose,

Magnesium stearate,

Anhydrous colloidal silica.

6.2 Incompatibilities
Not applicable.

6.3 Shelf life
3 years.

6.4 Special precautions for storage
Store in the original package.

6.5 Nature and contents of container
Aluminium/Poly(vinylchloride) blister, packed in cardboard boxes.

Pack sizes
7, 10, 14, 20, 28, 30, 56, 60, 84, 90, 100, 112, 120, 180 and 500 tablets.

Not all pack sizes may be marketed.

6.6 Special precautions for disposal and other handling
No special requirements.

7. MARKETING AUTHORISATION HOLDER
Les Laboratoires Servier

22, rue Garnier

92200 Neuilly Sur Seine

France

8. MARKETING AUTHORISATION NUMBER(S)
PL 05815/0019

9. DATE OF FIRST AUTHORISATION/RENEWAL OF THE AUTHORISATION
7th December 2000 / 29th March 2005

10. DATE OF REVISION OF THE TEXT
May 2008

Diazemuls

(Actavis UK Ltd)

1. NAME OF THE MEDICINAL PRODUCT
Diazemuls

2. QUALITATIVE AND QUANTITATIVE COMPOSITION
Each emulsion contains Diazepam 0.5w/v

3. PHARMACEUTICAL FORM
Sterile, milky white emulsion

4. CLINICAL PARTICULARS
4.1 Therapeutic indications
1. Sedation prior to procedures such as endoscopy, dentistry, cardiac catheterisation and cardioversion.

2. Premedication prior to general anaesthesia.

3. Control of acute muscle spasm due to tetanus or poisoning.

4. Control of convulsions; status epilepticus.

5. Management of severe acute anxiety or agitation including delirium tremens.

4.2 Posology and method of administration
Diazemuls may be administered by slow intravenous injection (1ml per min), or by continuous infusion. Diazemuls should be drawn into the syringe immediately prior to administration.

Sedation: 0.1-0.2mg diazepam/kg body weight by iv injection. The normal adult dose is 10-20 mg, but dosage should be titrated to the patient's response.

Premedication: 0.1-0.2mg diazepam/kg body weight by iv injection. Dosage should be titrated to the patient's response. In this indication, prior treatment with diazepam leads to a reduction in fasciculations and postoperative myalgia associated with the use of suxamethonium.

Tetanus: 0.1-0.3mg diazepam/kg body weight by iv injection repeated every 1-4 hours as required. Alternatively, continuous infusion of 3-10mg/kg body weight over 24 hours may be infused.

Status epilepticus: An initial dose 0.15-0.25mg/kg body weight by iv injection repeated in 30 to 60 minutes if required, and followed if necessary by infusion (see below) of up to 3mg/kg body weight over 24 hours.

Anxiety and tension, acute muscle spasm, acute states of excitation, delirium tremens: The usual dose is 10mg repeated at intervals of 4 hours, or as required.

Elderly or debilitated patients: Elderly and debilitated patients are particularly sensitive to benzodiazepines. Dosage should initially be reduced to one half of the normal recommendations.

If a continuous infusion is required, Diazemuls can be added to dextrose solution 5% or 10% to achieve a final diazepam concentration within the range 0.1-0.4mg/ml (i.e. 2-8ml Diazemuls per 100ml dextrose solution). A dextrose solution containing Diazemuls should be used within 6 hours of the admixture. Diazemuls can be mixed in all proportions with intralipid 10% or 20% but not with saline solutions. It can be injected into the infusion tube during an ongoing infusion of isotonic saline or dextrose solution 5% or 10%. As with other diazepam injections, adsorption may occur to plastic infusion equipment. This adsorption may occur to a lesser degree with Diazemuls than with aqueous diazepam injection preparations when mixed with dextrose solutions.

4.3 Contraindications
1. Should not be used in phobic or obsessional states since there is inadequate evidence of efficacy and safety.

2. Should not be used in the treatment of chronic psychosis.

3. Hypersensitivity to diazepam or any of the excipients. Hypersensitivity to egg or soybean as egg phospholipid and soybean oil are included in the preparation.

4. Acute porphyria.

4.4 Special warnings and precautions for use
Use with caution in patients with impairment of renal or hepatic function and in patients with pulmonary insufficiency or myasthenia gravis.

Should not be used alone to treat depression or anxiety associated with depression.

Amnesia may occur. In cases of loss or bereavement psychological adjustment may be inhibited by benzodiazepines.

Disinhibiting effects may be manifested in various ways. Suicide may be precipitated in patients who are depressed and aggressive behaviour toward self and others may be precipitated. Extreme caution should therefore be used in prescribing benzodiazepines in patients with personality disorders.

Physiological and psychological symptoms of withdrawal including depression may be associated with discontinuation of benzodiazepines even after normal therapeutic doses for short periods of time.

4.5 Interaction with other medicinal products and other forms of interaction
Not recommended: Concomitant intake with alcohol.

The sedative effects may be enhanced when the product is used in combination with alcohol. This affects the ability to drive or use machines. Concomitant use of neuroleptics (antipsychotics), hypnotics, sedative antihistamines, and central nervous system depressants, e.g. general anaesthetics, narcotic analgesics, or antidepressants, including MAOI's will result in accentuation of their sedative effects. When Diazemuls is combined with centrally depressant drugs administered parenterally, severe respiratory and cardiovascular depression may occur. It is recommended that Diazemuls is administered following the analgesic, and that the dose should be carefully titrated to the patient's response. Diazepam clearance is increased by concomitant administration of phenobarbitone, and is decreased by administration of cimetidine. Omeprazole and Isoniazid inhibit diazepam metabolism. Concurrent use of zidovudine with benzodiazepines may decrease zidovudine clearance.

4.6 Pregnancy and lactation
If Diazemuls is prescribed to a woman of childbearing potential, she should be warned to contact her physician regarding discontinuance of Diazemuls if she intends to become, or suspects that she is pregnant.

If, for compelling medical reasons, Diazemuls is administered during the late phase of pregnancy, or during labour at high doses, effects on neonate, such as hypothermia, hypotonia and moderate respiratory depression; can be expected, due to the pharmacological action of Diazemuls.

Moreover, infants borne to mothers who took benzodiazepines chronically during the latter stages of pregnancy may have developed physical dependence and may be at some risk for developing withdrawal symptoms in the postnatal period.

Since benzodiazepines are found in the breast milk, benzodiazepines should not be given to breast feeding mothers.

4.7 Effects on ability to drive and use machines
Sedation, amnesia, impaired concentration, and impaired muscular function may adversely affect the ability to drive or use machines. If insufficient sleep duration occurs, the likelihood of impaired alertness may be increased (see also Interactions).

4.8 Undesirable effects
This formulation may rarely cause local pain of thrombophlebitis in the vein used for administration.

Rare instances have been reported of a local painless erythematous rash round the site of injection, which has resolved in 1-2 days. Urticaria and, rarely anaphylaxis have been reported following the injection of Diazemuls.

Dose related adverse effects which occur commonly with diazepam and which may persist into the following day, even after a single dose include sedation, drowsiness, unsteadiness and ataxia.

The elderly are particularly sensitive to the effects of centrally-depressant drugs and may experience confusion, especially if organic brain changes are present.

Less commonly, headache, vertigo, hypotension, gastrointestinal disturbances, visual disturbances, changes in libido and urinary retention have been reported. Isolated cases of blood dyscrasias and jaundice have been reported.

Abnormal psychological reactions have been reported and are more likely to occur in children and the elderly.

4.9 Overdose
Symptoms of diazepam overdosage are mainly an intensification of its therapeutic effects - sedation, muscle weakness, profound sleep or paradoxical excitation. In more severe cases, symptoms may include ataxia, hypotonia, hypotension, respiratory depression, and rarely, coma and death. When combined with other CNS depressants, including alcohol, the effects of overdosage are likely to be severe and may prove fatal.

Treatment is symptomatic.

Respiratory and cardiovascular functions should be carefully monitored in intensive care. If excitation occurs, barbiturates should not be used. Flumazenil, a specific competitive inhibitor of the central effects of benzodiazepines, may be useful as an antidote. Benzodiazepines are not significantly removed from the body by dialysis.

5. PHARMACOLOGICAL PROPERTIES
5.1 Pharmacodynamic properties
Diazepam is a potent anxiolytic, anticonvulsant and central muscle relaxant mediating its effects mainly via the limbic system as well as the postsynaptic spinal reflexes. Diazemuls contains diazepam dissolved in the oil phase of an oil-in-water emulsion. Release of the diazepam from the lipid particles of the emulsion has been demonstrated by clinical studies showing comparable efficacy with injectable diazepam preparations.

5.2 Pharmacokinetic properties
Diazepam is metabolised to two active metabolites, one of which, desmethyldiazepam, has an extended half-life. Diazepam is therefore a long acting benzodiazepine and repeated doses may lead to accumulation.

Diazepam is metabolised in the liver and excreted via the kidney. Impaired hepatic or renal function may prolong the duration of action of diazepam. It is recommended that elderly and debilitated patients receive initially one half the normal recommended dose.

During prolonged administration, for example in the treatment of tetanus, the dosage should generally be reduced after 6-7 days, to reduce the likelihood of accumulation and prolonged CNS depression.

5.3 Preclinical safety data
Not applicable.

6. PHARMACEUTICAL PARTICULARS
6.1 List of excipients
Fractionated soy bean oil, diacetylated monoglycerides, fractionated egg phospholipids, glycerol (anhydrous), sodium hydroxide (to pH8), water for injections (to 2ml).

6.2 Incompatibilities
Diazemuls should only be mixed in the same container or syringe with dextrose solution 5% or 10% or intralipid 10% or 20%. The contents of the ampoule should not be mixed with any drugs other than the infusion solutions mentioned above. Store at room temperature. Do not freeze.

6.3 Shelf life
24 months.

6.4 Special precautions for storage
Store below 25°C. Do not freeze.

6.5 Nature and contents of container
2ml glass type 1 ampoules in cartons of 10.

6.6 Special precautions for disposal and other handling
Not applicable.

Administrative Data
7. MARKETING AUTHORISATION HOLDER
Actavis Group PTC ehf.

Reykjavikurvegi 76-78

220 Hafnarfjordur

Iceland

8. MARKETING AUTHORISATION NUMBER(S)
PL 30306/0038

9. DATE OF FIRST AUTHORISATION/RENEWAL OF THE AUTHORISATION
15.3.89

Renewed: 10.2.97; 10.2.02

10. DATE OF REVISION OF THE TEXT
31 July 2007

Diclomax Retard

(Galen Limited)

1. NAME OF THE MEDICINAL PRODUCT
Diclomax Retard.

2. QUALITATIVE AND QUANTITATIVE COMPOSITION
Each Diclomax Retard capsule contains diclofenac sodium 100mg.

For excipients, see 6.1.

3. PHARMACEUTICAL FORM
Modified release capsules for oral use.

4. CLINICAL PARTICULARS

4.1 Therapeutic indications
For rheumatoid arthritis; osteoarthritis; low back pain; acute musculo-skeletal disorders and trauma such as periarthritis (especially frozen shoulder), tendinitis, tenosynovitis, bursitis, sprains, strains and dislocations; relief of pain in fractures; ankylosing spondylitis; acute gout; control of pain and inflammation in orthopaedic, dental and other minor surgery.

4.2 Posology and method of administration
For oral use.

Undesirable effects may be minimised by using the lowest effective dose for the shortest duration necessary to control symptoms (see section 4.4).

Adults
One 100mg capsule taken whole daily, preferably with food or after food.

Children

Not recommended.

Elderly
The elderly are at an increased risk of serious consequences of adverse reactions. Studies indicate the pharmacokinetics of diclofenac sodium are not impaired to any clinical extent in the elderly, however, as with all non-steroidal anti-inflammatory drugs, Diclomax should be used with caution in elderly patients and the lowest effective dose used for the shortest possible duration. These patients should be monitored regularly for GI bleeding during NSAID therapy.

4.3 Contraindications
Diclomax is contraindicated in patients with a known hypersensitivity to diclofenac sodium or to any the excipients, patients with a history of/or active peptic ulcer, history of/or upper gastro-intestinal bleeding or perforation related to previous NSAID therapy. NSAIDs are contraindicated in patients who have previously shown hypersensitivity reactions (e.g. asthma, rhinitis, angioedema or urticaria) in response to ibuprofen, aspirin, or other non-steroidal anti-inflammatory drugs.

Diclomax should not be used in patients with severe hepatic, renal or cardiac failure (see section 4.4) or during the last trimester of pregnancy (see section 4.6).

As Diclomax contains lactose and sucrose, patients with rare hereditary problems of fructose/galactose intolerance, Lapp lactase deficiency, glucose-galactose malabsorption or sucrase-isomaltase insufficiency should not take this medicine.

4.4 Special warnings and precautions for use
As with all non-steroidal anti-inflammatory drugs (NSAIDs) Diclomax should only be given to the elderly after other forms of treatment have been carefully considered, as the elderly have an increased frequency of adverse reactions to NSAIDs especially gastro-intestinal bleeding and perforation which may be fatal (see section 4.2).

Undesirable effects may be minimised by using the lowest effective dose for the shortest duration necessary to control symptoms (see section 4.2, and GI and cardiovascular risks below).

<u>Renal and Hepatic impairment:</u>
The administration of an NSAID may cause a dose dependent reduction in prostaglandin formation and precipitate renal failure. Patients at greatest risk of this reaction are those with impaired renal function, cardiac impairment, liver dysfunction, those taking diuretics and the elderly. Renal function should be monitored in these patients (see section 4.3).

All patients who are receiving long-term treatment with NSAIDs should be monitored as a precautionary measure, e.g. renal, hepatic function (elevation of liver enzymes may occur) and blood counts.

If abnormal liver function tests persist or worsen, clinical signs or symptoms consistent with liver disease develop or if other manifestations occur (eosinophilia, rash), Diclomax should be discontinued.

<u>Cardiovascular and cerebrovascular effects:</u>
Appropriate monitoring and advice are required for patients with a history of hypertension and/or mild to moderate congestive heart failure as fluid retention and oedema have been reported in association with NSAID therapy.

Clinical trial and epidemiological data suggest that use of diclofenac, particularly at high dose (150mg daily) and in long term treatment may be associated with a small increased risk of arterial thrombotic events (for example myocardial infarction or stroke).

Patients with uncontrolled hypertension, congestive heart failure, established ischaemic heart disease, peripheral arterial disease, and/or cerebrovascular disease should only be treated with diclofenac after careful consideration. Similar consideration should be made before initiating longer-term treatment of patients with risk factors for cardiovascular events (e.g. hypertension, hyperlipidaemia, diabetes mellitus, smoking).

<u>Respiratory disorders:</u>
Caution is required if administered to patients suffering from, or with a previous history of, bronchial asthma since NSAIDs have been reported to cause bronchospasm in such patients.

<u>Gastro-intestinal bleeding, ulceration and perforation:</u>
Diclomax should be used with caution in patients with gastro-intestinal disorders or haematological abnormalities, as GI bleeding, ulceration or perforation, which can be fatal, has been reported with NSAID therapy at any time during treatment, with or without warning symptoms or a previous history of serious GI events.

Patients with a history of GI toxicity, particularly the elderly, should report any unusual abdominal symptoms (especially GI bleeding) particularly in the initial stages of treatment. Caution is advised in patients receiving concomitant medications which could increase the risk of gastrotoxicity or bleeding, such as corticosteroids, or anticoagulants such as warfarin or anti-platelet agents such as aspirin (see section 4.5).

When GI bleeding or ulceration occurs in patients receiving Diclomax, the treatment should be withdrawn.

NSAIDs should be given with care to patients with a history of gastro-intestinal disease (ulcerative colitis, Crohn's disease) as these conditions may be exacerbated (see section 4.8).

<u>Haematological:</u>
Diclomax, in common with other NSAIDs, can reversibly inhibit platelet aggregation.

<u>SLE and mixed connective tissue disease:</u>
In patients with systemic lupus erythematosus (SLE) and mixed connective tissue disorders there may be an increased risk of aseptic meningitis (see section 4.8).

<u>Female fertility:</u>
The use of Diclomax may impair female fertility and is not recommended in women attempting to conceive. In women who have difficulties conceiving or who are undergoing investigation of infertility, withdrawal of Diclomax should be considered.

4.5 Interaction with other medicinal products and other forms of interaction
Lithium: Diclomax may increase plasma concentrations and decrease elimination of lithium.

Cardiac glycosides: NSAIDs may exacerbate cardiac failure, reduce GFR and increase plasma glycoside levels.

Anticoagulants: NSAIDS may enhance the effects of anticoagulants, such as warfarin (see section 4.4)

Antidiabetic agents: Clinical studies have shown that Diclomax can be given together with oral hypoglycaemic agents without influencing their clinical effect. However, there have been isolated reports of hyperglycaemic and hypoglycaemic effects, which have required adjustments to the dosage of hypoglycaemic agents.

Ciclosporin: Ciclosporin nephrotoxicity may be increased by the effect of NSAIDs on renal prostaglandins.

Mifepristone: NSAIDs should not be used for 8-12 days after mifepristone administration as NSAIDs can reduce the effect of mifepristone.

Methotrexate: Caution should be exercised if NSAIDs and methotrexate are administered within 24 hours of each other, since NSAIDs may increase methotrexate plasma levels with decreased elimination, resulting in increased toxicity.

Quinolone antibiotics: Animal data indicate that the NSAIDs can increase the risk of convulsions associated with quinolone antibiotics. Patients taking NSAIDs and quinolones may have an increased risk of developing convulsions.

Anti-platelet agents and selective serotonin reuptake inhibitors (SSRIs): Increased risk of GI bleeding (see section 4.4).

Other analgesics including cyclooxygenase-2 selective inhibitors: Avoid concomitant use of two or more NSAIDs (including aspirin) as this may increase the risk of adverse events (see section 4.4).

Corticosteroids: Corticosteroids can increase the risk of GI ulceration or bleeding (see section 4.4).

Diuretics: Various NSAIDs are liable to inhibit the activity of diuretics. Diuretics can increase the risk of nephrotoxicity of NSAIDs. Concomitant treatment with potassium-sparing diuretics may be associated with increased serum potassium levels, hence serum potassium should be monitored.

Anti-hypertensives: Reduced anti-hypertensive effect.

Tacrolimus: Possible increased risk of nephrotoxicity when NSAIDs are given with tacrolimus.

Zidovudine: Increased risk of haematological toxicity when NSAIDs are given with zidovudine. There is evidence of an increased risk of haemarthroses and haematoma in HIV (+) haemophiliacs receiving concurrent treatment with zidovudine and ibuprofen.

4.6 Pregnancy and lactation
Congenital abnormalities have been reported in association with NSAID administration in man; however, these are low in frequency and do not appear to follow any discernible pattern. In view of the known effects of NSAIDs on the foetal cardiovascular system (risk of closure of the ductus arteriosus), use in the last trimester of pregnancy is contraindicated. The onset of labour may be delayed and the duration increased with increased bleeding tendency in both mother and child (see section 4.3). NSAIDs should not be used during the first two trimesters of pregnancy or labour unless the potential benefit to the patient outweighs the potential risk to the foetus.

In limited studies so far available, NSAIDs can appear in breast milk in very low concentrations with traces of diclofenac sodium found in breast milk following oral doses of 50mg every 8 hours. NSAIDs should, if possible, be avoided when breastfeeding (see section 4.4 regarding female fertility).

4.7 Effects on ability to drive and use machines
Undesirable effects such as dizziness, drowsiness, fatigue and visual disturbances are possible after taking NSAIDs. If affected, patients should not drive or operate machinery.

4.8 Undesirable effects
The following adverse events have been reported with NSAIDs:

<u>Gastro-intestinal:</u>
The most commonly observed adverse events are gastro-intestinal in nature. Peptic ulcers, perforation or GI bleeding, sometimes fatal, particularly in the elderly, may occur (see section 4.4). Nausea, vomiting, diarrhoea, flatulence, constipation, dyspepsia, abdominal pain, melaena, haematemesis, ulcerative stomatitis, exacerbation of colitis and Crohn's disease (see section 4.4) have been reported following administration. Less frequently, gastritis has been observed. Pancreatitis has been reported very rarely.

<u>Hypersensitivity:</u>
Hypersensitivity reactions have been reported following treatment with NSAIDs. These may consist of a) non-specific allergic reactions and anaphylaxis b) respiratory tract reactivity comprising asthma, aggravated asthma, bronchospasm or dyspnoea, or c) assorted skin disorders, including rashes of various types, pruritus, urticaria, purpura, angioedema and, more rarely exfoliative and bullous dermatoses (including epidermal necrolysis and erythema multiforme).

<u>Cardiovascular and cerebrovascular:</u>
Oedema, hypertension and cardiac failure have been reported in association with NSAID treatment.

Clinical trial and epidemiological data suggest that use of diclofenac, particularly at high doses (150mg daily) and in long term treatment may be associated with a small increased risk of arterial thrombotic events (for example myocardial infarction or stroke) (see section 4.4).

Other adverse events reported less commonly include:

<u>Renal:</u>
Nephrotoxicity in various forms, including interstitial nephritis, nephrotic syndrome and renal failure.

<u>Hepatic:</u>
Abnormal liver function, hepatitis and jaundice.

<u>Neurological and special senses:</u>
Visual disturbances, optic neuritis, headaches, paraesthesia, reports of aseptic meningitis (especially in patients with existing auto-immune disorders, such as systemic lupus erythematosus, mixed connective tissue disease), with symptoms such as stiff neck, headache, nausea, vomiting, fever or disorientation (see section 4.4), depression, confusion, hallucinations, tinnitus, vertigo, dizziness, malaise, fatigue and drowsiness.

<u>Haematological:</u>
Thrombocytopenia, neutropenia, agranulocytosis, aplastic anaemia and haemolytic anaemia.

<u>Dermatological:</u>
Photosensitivity.

4.9 Overdose
(a) <u>Symptoms</u>

Symptoms include headache, nausea, vomiting, epigastric pain, gastro-intestinal bleeding, rarely diarrhoea, disorientation, excitation, coma, drowsiness, dizziness, tinnitus, fainting, occasionally convulsions. In cases of significant poisoning acute renal failure and liver damage are possible.

(b) <u>Therapeutic Measures</u>

Patients should be treated symptomatically as required.

Within one hour of ingestion of a potentially toxic amount, activated charcoal should be considered. Alternatively, in adults, gastric lavage should be considered within one hour of ingestion of a potentially life-threatening overdose.

Good urine output should be ensured.

Renal and liver function should be closely monitored.

Patients should be observed for at least four hours after ingestion of potentially toxic amounts.

Frequent or prolonged convulsions should be treated with intravenous diazepam.

Other measures may be indicated by the patient's clinical condition.

5. PHARMACOLOGICAL PROPERTIES

5.1 Pharmacodynamic properties

Diclofenac Sodium is a non-steroidal agent with marked analgesic/anti-inflammatory and anti-pyretic properties. It is an inhibitor of prostaglandin synthetase (cyclo-oxygenase).

5.2 Pharmacokinetic properties

Diclofenac Sodium is rapidly absorbed from the gut and is subject to first-pass metabolism. Capsules give peak plasma concentrations after approximately 2.5 hours. The active substance is 99.7% protein bound and plasma half-life for the terminal elimination phase is 1-2 hours. Approximately 60% of the administered dose is excreted via the kidneys in the form of metabolites and less than 1% in unchanged form. About 30% of the dose is excreted via the bile in metabolised form.

The Diclomax slow release preparation:

- Increases the duration of action of the drug
- Maintains relatively constant rate of absorption in the gastro-intestinal tract over a longer period of time
- Increases the fraction of the ingested dose absorbed in the GI tract
- Regulates the rate at which the drug is made available for absorption, thereby reducing the possibility of malabsorption and occurrence of side-effects.

5.3 Preclinical safety data

The results of the preclinical tests do not add anything of further significance to the prescriber.

6. PHARMACEUTICAL PARTICULARS

6.1 List of excipients

Sucrose

Maize starch

Polyethylene glycol 6000

Ammonio methacrylate copolymer type A

Talc

Lactose

Polysorbate 80

Purified water

Ethanol 96%

Acetone

Capsule Shell Constituents:

Gelatin

Titanium dioxide (E171)

Overprint Ink Constituents:

Shellac glaze

Propylene glycol

Black iron oxide (E172)

6.2 Incompatibilities

None known.

6.3 Shelf life

24 months – PVC/PE/PVDC blister packs.

18 months – PVC blister packs.

60 months – Polyamide/Al/PVC-Al blister packs.

6.4 Special precautions for storage

PVC/PE/PVDC and PVC blister packs: Store between 10°C and 25°C. Protect from moisture. Do not refrigerate.

Polyamide/Al/PVC-Al blister packs: This medicinal product does not require any special storage conditions.

6.5 Nature and contents of container

White opaque PVC/Al blister strips or white opaque PVC/PE/PVDC/Al blister strips or Polyamide/Al/PVC-Al blister strips.

Packs of 4 or 28 capsules.

6.6 Special precautions for disposal and other handling

None.

7. MARKETING AUTHORISATION HOLDER

Galen Limited

Seagoe Industrial Estate

Craigavon

BT63 5UA

UK.

8. MARKETING AUTHORISATION NUMBER(S)

PL 27827/0005.

9. DATE OF FIRST AUTHORISATION/RENEWAL OF THE AUTHORISATION

09 March 1993.

10. DATE OF REVISION OF THE TEXT

17 July 2009.

Diclomax SR

(Galen Limited)

1. NAME OF THE MEDICINAL PRODUCT

Diclomax SR.

2. QUALITATIVE AND QUANTITATIVE COMPOSITION

Each Diclomax SR capsule contains diclofenac sodium 75mg.

For excipients, see 6.1.

3. PHARMACEUTICAL FORM

Modified release capsules for oral use.

4. CLINICAL PARTICULARS

4.1 Therapeutic indications

For rheumatoid arthritis; osteoarthritis; low back pain; acute musculo-skeletal disorders and trauma such as periarthritis (especially frozen shoulder), tendinitis, tenosynovitis, bursitis, sprains, strains and dislocations; relief of pain in fractures; ankylosing spondylitis; acute gout; control of pain and inflammation in orthopaedic, dental and other minor surgery.

4.2 Posology and method of administration

For oral use.

Undesirable effects may be minimised by using the lowest effective dose for the shortest duration necessary to control symptoms (see section 4.4).

Adults

One or two 75mg capsules daily taken whole in single or divided doses preferably with food or after food.

Children

Not recommended.

Elderly

The elderly are at an increased risk of serious consequences of adverse reactions. Studies indicate the pharmacokinetics of diclofenac sodium are not impaired to any clinical extent in the elderly, however, as with all non-steroidal anti-inflammatory drugs, Diclomax should be used with caution in elderly patients and the lowest effective dose used for the shortest possible duration. These patients should be monitored regularly for GI bleeding during NSAID therapy.

4.3 Contraindications

Diclomax is contraindicated in patients with a known hypersensitivity to diclofenac sodium or to any the excipients, patients with a history of/or active peptic ulcer, history of/or upper gastro-intestinal bleeding or perforation related to previous NSAID therapy. NSAIDs are contraindicated in patients who have previously shown hypersensitivity reactions (e.g. asthma, rhinitis, angioedema or urticaria) in response to ibuprofen, aspirin, or other non-steroidal anti-inflammatory drugs.

Diclomax should not be used in patients with severe hepatic, renal or cardiac failure (see section 4.4) or during the last trimester of pregnancy (see section 4.6).

As Diclomax contains lactose and sucrose, patients with rare hereditary problems of fructose/galactose intolerance, Lapp lactase deficiency, glucose-galactose malabsorption or sucrase-isomaltase insufficiency should not take this medicine.

4.4 Special warnings and precautions for use

As with all non-steroidal anti-inflammatory drugs (NSAIDs) Diclomax should only be given to the elderly after other forms of treatment have been carefully considered, as the elderly have an increased frequency of adverse reactions to NSAIDs especially gastro-intestinal bleeding and perforation which may be fatal (see section 4.2).

Undesirable effects may be minimised by using the lowest effective dose for the shortest duration necessary to control symptoms (see section 4.2, and GI and cardiovascular risks below).

<u>Renal and Hepatic impairment:</u>

The administration of an NSAID may cause a dose dependent reduction in prostaglandin formation and precipitate renal failure. Patients at greatest risk of this reaction are those with impaired renal function, cardiac impairment, liver dysfunction, those taking diuretics and the elderly. Renal function should be monitored in these patients (see section 4.3).

All patients who are receiving long-term treatment with NSAIDs should be monitored as a precautionary measure, e.g. renal, hepatic function (elevation of liver enzymes may occur) and blood counts.

If abnormal liver function tests persist or worsen, clinical signs or symptoms consistent with liver disease develop or if other manifestations occur (eosinophilia, rash), Diclomax should be discontinued.

<u>*Cardiovascular and cerebrovascular effects:*</u>

Appropriate monitoring and advice are required for patients with a history of hypertension and/or mild to moderate congestive heart failure as fluid retention and oedema have been reported in association with NSAID therapy.

Clinical trial and epidemiological data suggest that use of diclofenac, particularly at high dose (150mg daily) and in long term treatment may be associated with a small increased risk of arterial thrombotic events (for example myocardial infarction or stroke).

Patients with uncontrolled hypertension, congestive heart failure, established ischaemic heart disease, peripheral arterial disease, and/or cerebrovascular disease should only be treated with diclofenac after careful consideration. Similar consideration should be made before initiating longer-term treatment of patients with risk factors for cardiovascular events (e.g. hypertension, hyperlipidaemia, diabetes mellitus, smoking).

<u>*Respiratory disorders:*</u>

Cautions is required if administered to patients suffering from, or with a previous history of, bronchial asthma since NSAIDs have been reported to cause bronchospasm in such patients.

<u>*Gastro-intestinal bleeding, ulceration and perforation:*</u>

Diclomax should be used with caution in patients with gastro-intestinal disorders or haematological abnormalities, as GI bleeding, ulceration or perforation, which can be fatal, has been reported with NSAID therapy at any time during treatment, with or without warning symptoms or a previous history of serious GI events.

Patients with a history of GI toxicity, particularly the elderly, should report any unusual abdominal symptoms (especially GI bleeding) particularly in the initial stages of treatment. Caution is advised in patients receiving concomitant medications which could increase the risk of gastrotoxicity or bleeding, such as corticosteroids, or anticoagulants such as warfarin or anti-platelet agents such as aspirin (see section 4.5).

When GI bleeding or ulceration occurs in patients receiving Diclomax, the treatment should be withdrawn.

NSAIDs should be given with care to patients with a history of gastro-intestinal disease (ulcerative colitis, Crohn's disease) as these conditions may be exacerbated (see section 4.8).

<u>*Haematological:*</u>

Diclomax, in common with other NSAIDs, can reversibly inhibit platelet aggregation.

<u>*SLE and mixed connective tissue disease:*</u>

In patients with systemic lupus erythematosus (SLE) and mixed connective tissue disorders there may be an increased risk of aseptic meningitis (see section 4.8).

<u>*Female fertility:*</u>

The use of Diclomax may impair female fertility and is not recommended in women attempting to conceive. In women who have difficulties conceiving or who are undergoing investigation of infertility, withdrawal of Diclomax should be considered.

4.5 Interaction with other medicinal products and other forms of interaction

Lithium: Diclomax may increase plasma concentrations and decrease elimination of lithium.

Cardiac glycosides: NSAIDs may exacerbate cardiac failure, reduce GFR and increase plasma glycoside levels.

Anticoagulants: NSAIDS may enhance the effects of anti-coagulants, such as warfarin (see section 4.4)

Antidiabetic agents: Clinical studies have shown that Diclomax can be given together with oral hypoglycaemic agents without influencing their clinical effect. However, there have been isolated reports of hyperglycaemic and hypoglycaemic effects, which have required adjustments to the dosage of hypoglycaemic agents.

Ciclosporin: Ciclosporin nephrotoxicity may be increased by the effect of NSAIDs on renal prostaglandins.

Mifepristone: NSAIDs should not be used for 8-12 days after mifepristone administration as NSAIDs can reduce the effect of mifepristone.

Methotrexate: Caution should be exercised if NSAIDs and methotrexate are administered within 24 hours of each other, since NSAIDs may increase methotrexate plasma levels with decreased elimination, resulting in increased toxicity.

Quinolone antibiotics: Animal data indicate that the NSAIDs can increase the risk of convulsions associated with quinolone antibiotics. Patients taking NSAIDs and quinolones may have an increased risk of developing convulsions.

Anti-platelet agents and selective serotonin reuptake inhibitors (SSRIs): Increased risk of GI bleeding (see section 4.4).

Other analgesics including cyclooxygenase-2 selective inhibitors: Avoid concomitant use of two or more NSAIDs (including aspirin) as this may increase the risk of adverse events (see section 4.4).

Corticosteroids: Corticosteroids can increase the risk of GI ulceration or bleeding (see section 4.4).

Diuretics: Various NSAIDs are liable to inhibit the activity of diuretics. Diuretics can increase the risk of nephrotoxicity of NSAIDs. Concomitant treatment with potassium-sparing diuretics may be associated with increased serum potassium levels, hence serum potassium should be monitored.

Anti-hypertensives: Reduced anti-hypertensive effect.

Tacrolimus: Possible increased risk of nephrotoxicity when NSAIDs are given with tacrolimus.

Zidovudine: Increased risk of haematological toxicity when NSAIDs are given with zidovudine. There is evidence of an increased risk of haemarthroses and haematoma in HIV (+) haemophiliacs receiving concurrent treatment with zidovudine and ibuprofen.

4.6 Pregnancy and lactation

Congenital abnormalities have been reported in association with NSAID administration in man; however, these are low in frequency and do not appear to follow any discernible pattern. In view of the known effects of NSAIDs on the foetal cardiovascular system (risk of closure of the ductus arteriosus), use in the last trimester of pregnancy is contraindicated. The onset of labour may be delayed and the duration increased with increased bleeding tendency in both mother and child (see Section 4.3). NSAIDs should not be used during the first two trimesters of pregnancy or labour unless the potential benefit to the patient outweighs the potential risk to the foetus.

In limited studies so far available, NSAIDs can appear in breast milk in very low concentrations with traces of diclofenac sodium found in breast milk following oral doses of 50mg every 8 hours. NSAIDs should, if possible, be avoided when breastfeeding (see section 4.4 regarding female fertility).

4.7 Effects on ability to drive and use machines

Undesirable effects such as dizziness, drowsiness, fatigue and visual disturbances are possible after taking NSAIDs. If affected, patients should not drive or operate machinery.

4.8 Undesirable effects

The following adverse events have been reported with NSAIDs:

Gastro-intestinal:

The most commonly observed adverse events are gastrointestinal in nature. Peptic ulcers, perforation or GI bleeding, sometimes fatal, particularly in the elderly, may occur (see section 4.4). Nausea, vomiting, diarrhoea, flatulence, constipation, dyspepsia, abdominal pain, melaena, haematemesis, ulcerative stomatitis, exacerbation of colitis and Crohn's disease (see section 4.4) have been reported following administration. Less frequently, gastritis has been observed. Pancreatitis has been reported very rarely.

Hypersensitivity:

Hypersensitivity reactions have been reported following treatment with NSAIDs. These may consist of a) non-specific allergic reactions and anaphylaxis b) respiratory tract reactivity comprising asthma, aggravated asthma, bronchospasm or dyspnoea, or c) assorted skin disorders, including rashes of various types, pruritus, urticaria, purpura, angioedema and, more rarely exfoliative and bullous dermatoses (including epidermal necrolysis and erythema multiforme).

Cardiovascular and cerebrovascular:

Oedema, hypertension and cardiac failure have been reported in association with NSAID treatment.

Clinical trial and epidemiological data suggest that use of diclofenac, particularly at high doses (150mg daily) and in long term treatment may be associated with a small increased risk of arterial thrombotic events (for example myocardial infarction or stroke) (see section 4.4).

Other adverse events reported less commonly include:

Renal:

Nephrotoxicity in various forms, including interstitial nephritis, nephrotic syndrome and renal failure.

Hepatic:

Abnormal liver function, hepatitis and jaundice.

Neurological and special senses:

Visual disturbances, optic neuritis, headaches, paraesthesia, reports of aseptic meningitis (especially in patients with existing auto-immune disorders, such as systemic lupus erythematosus, mixed connective tissue disease), with symptoms such as stiff neck, headache, nausea, vomiting, fever or disorientation (see section 4.4), depression, confusion, hallucinations, tinnitus, vertigo, dizziness, malaise, fatigue and drowsiness.

Haematological:

Thrombocytopenia, neutropenia, agranulocytosis, aplastic anaemia and haemolytic anaemia.

Dermatological:

Photosensitivity.

4.9 Overdose

(a) Symptoms

Symptoms include headache, nausea, vomiting, epigastric pain, gastro-intestinal bleeding, rarely diarrhoea, disorientation, excitation, coma, drowsiness, dizziness, tinnitus, fainting, occasionally convulsions. In cases of significant poisoning acute renal failure and liver damage are possible.

(b) Therapeutic Measures

Patients should be treated symptomatically as required.

Within one hour of ingestion of a potentially toxic amount, activated charcoal should be considered. Alternatively, in adults, gastric lavage should be considered within one hour of ingestion of a potentially life-threatening overdose.

Good urine output should be ensured.

Renal and liver function should be closely monitored.

Patients should be observed for at least four hours after ingestion of potentially toxic amounts.

Frequent or prolonged convulsions should be treated with intravenous diazepam.

Other measures may be indicated by the patient's clinical condition.

5. PHARMACOLOGICAL PROPERTIES

5.1 Pharmacodynamic properties

Diclofenac Sodium is a non-steroidal agent with marked analgesic/anti-inflammatory and anti-pyretic properties. It is an inhibitor of prostaglandin synthetase (cyclo-oxygenase).

5.2 Pharmacokinetic properties

Diclofenac Sodium is rapidly absorbed from the gut and is subject to first-pass metabolism. Capsules give peak plasma concentrations after approximately 2.5 hours. The active substance is 99.7% protein bound and plasma half-life for the terminal elimination phase is 1-2 hours. Approximately 60% of the administered dose is excreted via the kidneys in the form of metabolites and less than 1% in unchanged form. About 30% of the dose is excreted via the bile in metabolised form.

The Diclomax slow release preparation:

- Increases the duration of action of the drug
- Maintains relatively constant rate of absorption in the gastro-intestinal tract over a longer period of time
- Increases the fraction of the ingested dose absorbed in the GI tract
- Regulates the rate at which the drug is made available for absorption, thereby reducing the possibility of malabsorption and occurrence of side-effects.

5.3 Preclinical safety data

The results of the preclinical tests do not add anything of further significance to the prescriber.

6. PHARMACEUTICAL PARTICULARS

6.1 List of excipients

Sucrose

Maize starch

Polyethylene glycol 6000

Ammonio methacrylate copolymer type A

Talc

Lactose

Polysorbate 80

Purified water

Ethanol 96%

Acetone

Capsule Shell Constituents:

Gelatin

Yellow iron oxide (E172)

Titanium dioxide (E171)

Overprint Ink Constituents:

Shellac glaze

Propylene glycol

Black iron oxide (E172)

6.2 Incompatibilities

None known.

6.3 Shelf life

24 months – PVC/PE/PVDC blister packs.

18 months – PVC blister packs.

60 months – Polyamide/Al/PVC-Al blister packs.

6.4 Special precautions for storage

PVC/PE/PVDC and PVC blister packs: Store between 10°C and 25°C. Protect from moisture. Do not refrigerate.

Polyamide/Al/PVC-Al blister packs: This medicinal product does not require any special storage conditions.

6.5 Nature and contents of container

White opaque PVC blister pack with hard tempered foil or white opaque PVC/PE/PVDC/hard tempered foil blister strips or Polyamide/Al/PVC-Al blister strips.

Packs of 4 and 56 capsules.

6.6 Special precautions for disposal and other handling

No special instructions needed.

7. MARKETING AUTHORISATION HOLDER

Galen Limited

Seagoe Industrial Estate

Craigavon

BT63 5UA

UK.

8. MARKETING AUTHORISATION NUMBER(S)

PL 27827/0004.

9. DATE OF FIRST AUTHORISATION/RENEWAL OF THE AUTHORISATION

12 January 1995.

10. DATE OF REVISION OF THE TEXT

17 July 2009.

Dicobalt Edetate Injection 300mg

(Cambridge Laboratories)

1. NAME OF THE MEDICINAL PRODUCT

Dicobalt Edetate Injection 300mg

2. QUALITATIVE AND QUANTITATIVE COMPOSITION

Each ampoule contains 300mg Dicobalt Edetate INN (15mg/ml)

3. PHARMACEUTICAL FORM

Solution for Injection

4. CLINICAL PARTICULARS

4.1 Therapeutic indications

Dicobalt Edetate Injection is a specific antidote for acute cyanide poisoning. In view of the difficulty of certain diagnosis in emergency situations, it is recommended that Dicobalt Edetate Injection only be given when the patient is tending to lose or has lost consciousness. The product should not be used as a precautionary measure.

4.2 Posology and method of administration

Cyanide poisoning must be treated as quickly as possible and intensive supportive measures must be instituted: clear airways and adequate ventilation are essential. 100% oxygen should be administered concurrently with Dicobalt Edetate.

Expert advice on the treatment of poisoning is available at the local poisons centre.

Adults

One 300mg ampoule intravenously over approximately one minute. If the patient shows inadequate response, a second ampoule may be given. If there is no response after a further five minutes, a third ampoule maybe administered.

Each ampoule of Dicobalt Edetate Injection may be followed immediately by 50ml Glucose Intravenous Infusion BP 500g/l.

When the patient's condition is less severe but in the physician's judgement still warrants the use of Dicobalt Edetate Injection, the period over which the injection is given should be extended to 5 minutes.

Children

There is no clinical experience of the use of Dicobalt Edetate Injection in children. As with adults the dose required will be related to the quantity of cyanide ingested.

The elderly

There is no clinical evidence of the use of Dicobalt Edetate Injection in the elderly, but there is no reason to believe that the dosage schedule should be different from that for adults.

4.3 Contraindications

None.

4.4 Special warnings and precautions for use

There is a reciprocal antidote action between cyanide and cobalt. Thus in the absence of cyanide, Dicobalt Edetate Injection itself is toxic. It is therefore essential that the product only be used in cases of cyanide poisoning. When the patient is fully conscious, it is unlikely that the extent of poisoning warrants the use of Dicobalt Edetate Injection.

4.5 Interaction with other medicinal products and other forms of interaction

No information is available.

4.6 Pregnancy and lactation

No information is available.

4.7 Effects on ability to drive and use machines

Not applicable.

4.8 Undesirable effects

The initial effects of Dicobalt Edetate Injection are vomiting, a fall in blood pressure and compensatory tachycardia. After this the patient should recover.

4.9 Overdose

Signs and symptoms – these may be due to cobalt toxicity or to an anaphylactic type reaction, which may be dramatic. Oedema (particularly of the face and neck), vomiting, chest pain, sweating, hypotension, cardiac irregularities and rashes may occur.

Treatment – intensive supportive therapy is required.

5. PHARMACOLOGICAL PROPERTIES

5.1 Pharmacodynamic properties

Cyanide blocks intracellular respiration by binding to cytochrome oxidase. Dicobalt Edetate Injection forms a stable complex with the cyanide thereby acting as an antidote.

5.2 Pharmacokinetic properties

Only very limited data are available. Intravenous infusion of Dicobalt Edetate Injection is likely to result in rapid distribution in the extracellular fluid compartment. Excretion is entirely via the kidneys within 24 hours and it is not metabolised.

5.3 Preclinical safety data

There are no pre-clinical data of relevance to the prescriber which are additional to that already included in other sections of the SPC.

6. PHARMACEUTICAL PARTICULARS

6.1 List of excipients

Dextrose Monohydrate

Water for Injections

6.2 Incompatibilities

Not applicable.

6.3 Shelf life

Three years.

6.4 Special precautions for storage

Store below 25°C away from light.

6.5 Nature and contents of container

Packs of six Ph.Eur Type 1 glass ampoules each containing 20ml of rose-violet coloured sterile pyrogen free solution.

6.6 Special precautions for disposal and other handling

None.

Administrative Data

7. MARKETING AUTHORISATION HOLDER

Medicis Limited

The Cricketers

Turgis Green

Nr Basingstoke

RG27 0AH

8. MARKETING AUTHORISATION NUMBER(S)

PL: 14945/0001

9. DATE OF FIRST AUTHORISATION/RENEWAL OF THE AUTHORISATION

18 March 2003

10. DATE OF REVISION OF THE TEXT

November 2003

Dicynene 500 Tablets

(sanofi-aventis)

1. NAME OF THE MEDICINAL PRODUCT

Dicynene 500 Tablets

2. QUALITATIVE AND QUANTITATIVE COMPOSITION

Each tablet contains 500mg etamsylate as the active ingredient.

For a full list of excipients, see section 6.1.

3. PHARMACEUTICAL FORM

Tablet.

White capsule-shaped tablet imprinted "D500" on one face, with a break-mark on the other.

4. CLINICAL PARTICULARS

4.1 Therapeutic indications

Dicynene is used clinically for the short term treatment of blood loss in primary and IUCD-induced menorrhagia.

4.2 Posology and method of administration

Adults only

The usual dosage is 500mg four times daily from the start of bleeding until menstruation ceases.

Route of administration: oral

4.3 Contraindications

Treatment should only be undertaken following exclusion of other pelvic pathology, in particular the presence of fibroids. Use in patients with a known hypersensitivity to etamsylate or to any of the excipients. Use in patients with porphyria.

4.4 Special warnings and precautions for use

The drug contains:

• Sulfites which may cause anaphylactic reactions (see 4.8 Undesirable effects).

• Wheat starch which may contain gluten but only in trace amounts and is therefore considered safe for patients with coeliac disease. Patients with wheat allergy (different from coeliac disease) should not take this medicine.

If the patient develops a fever then treatment should be discontinued.

In patients receiving Dicynene for menorrhagia the use of the product before onset of bleeding is not recommended.

4.5 Interaction with other medicinal products and other forms of interaction

None stated.

4.6 Pregnancy and lactation

Clinical use in pregnancy is not relevant for this indication. Studies in animals have revealed no teratogenic effect of etamsylate however there is inadequate evidence of safety in human pregnancy.

Etamsylate is secreted in breast milk and administration to nursing mothers is not recommended.

4.7 Effects on ability to drive and use machines

None stated.

4.8 Undesirable effects

Fever may occur.

Occasional headaches or skin rashes may also occur but usually disappear on reduced dosage. A few patients may experience gastrointestinal disturbances such as nausea, vomiting or diarrhoea; however this may be overcome by administering the dose after food.

Due to the presence of sulfites, allergic reactions may occur including anaphylactic symptoms ranging from rash to anaphylactic shock (see 4.4 Special warnings and precautions for use).

4.9 Overdose

There is no experience of overdosage with Dicynene 500 tablets.

5. PHARMACOLOGICAL PROPERTIES

5.1 Pharmacodynamic properties

Pharmacotherapeutic group: Vitamin K and Other Hemostatics, Other systemic hemostatics. ATC code B02BX01.

Dicynene is a non-hormonal agent which reduces capillary exudation and blood loss. Dicynene does not affect the normal coagulation mechanism since administration is without effect on prothrombin times, fibrinolysis, platelet count or function.

Dicynene is thought to act by increasing capillary vascular wall resistance and platelet adhesiveness; in the presence of a vascular lesion, it inhibits the biosynthesis and action of those prostaglandins which cause platelet disaggregation, vasodilation and increased capillary permeability. Dicynene does not have a vasoconstricting action.

5.2 Pharmacokinetic properties

Dicynene is fully absorbed when given orally and is excreted unchanged, largely by the urinary route.

5.3 Preclinical safety data

No further information is available.

6. PHARMACEUTICAL PARTICULARS

6.1 List of excipients

Sodium sulphite anhydrous

Sodium dihydrogen citrate

Microcrystalline cellulose

Povidone

Wheat starch

Stearic acid

6.2 Incompatibilities

Not applicable.

6.3 Shelf life

3 years.

6.4 Special precautions for storage

Do not store above 25°C. Securitainer - Keep the bottle in the outer carton.

6.5 Nature and contents of container

Securitainer with lid and foam wad or moulded pack insert (jayfilla) containing 100 tablets.

6.6 Special precautions for disposal and other handling

No special requirements.

7. MARKETING AUTHORISATION HOLDER

Sanofi-aventis

One Onslow Street

Guildford

Surrey

GU1 4YS, UK

8. MARKETING AUTHORISATION NUMBER(S)

PL 04425/0206

9. DATE OF FIRST AUTHORISATION/RENEWAL OF THE AUTHORISATION

20 February 2009

10. DATE OF REVISION OF THE TEXT

February 2009

Legal category: POM

Didronel 200mg Tablets

(Procter & Gamble Pharmaceuticals UK Limited)

1. NAME OF THE MEDICINAL PRODUCT

Didronel 200mg Tablets.

2. QUALITATIVE AND QUANTITATIVE COMPOSITION

Each tablet contains 200mg of Etidronate Disodium, USP.

3. PHARMACEUTICAL FORM

White rectangular tablets marked with 'P&G' on one face and '402' on the other.

4. CLINICAL PARTICULARS

4.1 Therapeutic indications

Paget's disease of bone:

Effectiveness has been demonstrated primarily in patients with polyostotic Paget's disease with symptoms of pain and with clinically significant elevations of urinary hydroxyproline and serum alkaline phosphatase. In other circumstances in which there is extensive involvement of the skull or the spine with the prospect of irreversible neurological damage, or when a weight-bearing bone may be involved, the use of Didronel may also be considered.

4.2 Posology and method of administration

5mg/kg/day to 20mg/kg/day as detailed below.

Didronel should be given on an empty stomach. It is recommended that patients take the therapy with water, at the mid point of a four hour fast (ie. two hours before and two after food).

Adults and Elderly:

The recommended initial dose of Didronel for most patients is 5mg/kg body weight/day, for a period not exceeding six months. Doses above 10mg/kg should be reserved for use when there is an overriding requirement for suppression of increased bone turnover associated with Paget's disease or when the patient requires more prompt reduction of elevated cardiac output. Treatment with doses above 10mg/kg/day should be approached cautiously and should not exceed three months duration. Doses in excess of 20mg/kg/day are not recommended.

Re-treatment should be undertaken only after a drug-free period of at least three months and after it is evident that reactivation of the disease has occurred and biochemical indices of the disease have become substantially re-elevated or approach pretreatment values (approximately twice the upper limit of normal or 75% of pre-treatment value). In no case should duration of treatment exceed the maximum duration of the initial treatment. Premature re-treatment should be avoided. In clinical trials the biochemical improvements obtained during drug therapy have generally persisted for a period of three months to 2 years after drug withdrawal.

Daily Dosage Guide

Body Weight		Required Daily Regimen of 200mg Tablets		
Kilogrames	Stones	5mg/kg*	10mg/kg*	20mg/kg+
50	8	1	3	5
60	9.5	2	3	6
70	11	2	4	7
80	12.5	2	4	8
90	14	2	5	9

* Course of therapy - 6 months

+ Course of therapy - 3 months

Children:

Disorders of bone in children, referred to as juvenile Paget's disease, have been reported rarely. The relationship to adult Paget's disease has not been established. Didronel has not been studied in children for Paget's disease.

4.3 Contraindications

Known hypersensitivity to the drug. Clinically overt osteomalacia.

4.4 Special warnings and precautions for use

In Pagetic patients the physician should adhere to the recommended dose regimen in order to avoid over- treatment with Didronel. The response to therapy may be of slow onset and may continue even for months after treatment with the drug has been discontinued. Dosage should not be increased prematurely nor should treatment be resumed before there is clear evidence of reactivation of the disease process. Re-treatment should not be initiated until the patient has had at least a three-month drug-free interval.

Didronel is not metabolised but excreted unchanged via the kidney; therefore, a reduced dose should be used in patients with mild renal impairment and treatment of patients with moderate to severe renal impairment should be avoided. Caution should be taken in patients with a history of renal stone formation. In patients with impaired renal function or a history of renal stone formation, serum and urinary calcium should be monitored regularly.

It is recommended that serum phosphate, serum alkaline phosphatase and if possible urinary hydroxyproline be measured before commencing medication and at three month intervals during treatment. If after three months of medication the pre-treatment levels have not been reduced by at least 25%, the patient may be relatively resistant to therapy. If the serum phosphate level is unchanged in the "resistant" patient, consideration should be given to increasing the dose since the absorption of pharmacologically active amounts of Didronel is typically accompanied by a rise in serum phosphate. This rise usually correlates with reductions in the biochemical indices of disease activity. If after three or more months of medication elevations of serum phosphate above the upper limit of normal are not accompanied by clinical or biochemical evidence of reduced activity, resistance of the disease to the action of Didronel is probable and termination of Didronel medication should be considered. Etidronate disodium suppresses bone turnover and may retard mineralisation of osteoid laid down during the bone accretion process. These effects are dose and time dependent. Osteoid, which may accumulate noticeably at doses of 10-20 mg/kg/day, mineralises normally post-therapy. Patients in whom serum phosphate elevations are high and reductions of disease activity are low may be particularly prone to retarded mineralisation of new osteoid. In those cases where 200mg per day (a single tablet) may be excessive, doses may be administered less frequently.

Patients with Paget's disease of bone should maintain an adequate intake of calcium and vitamin D. Patients with low vitamin D and calcium intake may be particularly sensitive to drugs that affect calcium homeostasis and should be closely monitored during Didronel therapy.

Etidronate disodium does not adversely affect serum levels of parathyroid hormone or calcium.

Hyperphosphataemia has been observed in patients receiving etidronate disodium, usually in association with doses of 10-20mg/kg/day. No adverse effects have been traced to this, and it does not constitute grounds for discontinuing therapy. It is apparently due to a drug-related increase in renal tubular reabsorption of phosphate. Serum phosphate levels generally return to normal 2-4 weeks post therapy.

Patients with significant chronic diarrhoeal disease may experience increased frequency of bowel movements and diarrhoea, particularly at higher doses.

Increased or recurrent bone pain at existing Pagetic sites and/or the appearance of pain at sites previously asymptomatic have been reported at a dose of 5mg/kg/day.

Fractures are recognised as a common feature in patients with Paget's disease. There has been no evidence of increased risk of fractures at the recommended dose of 5mg/kg/day for six months. At doses of 20mg/kg/day in excess of three months' duration, mineralisation of newly formed osteoid may be impaired and the risk of fracture may be increased. The risk of fracture may also be greater in patients with extensive and severe disease, a history of multiple fractures, and/or rapidly advancing osteolytic lesions. It is therefore recommended that the drug is discontinued when fractures occur and therapy not reinstated until the fracture healing is complete.

Patients with predominantly lytic lesions should be monitored radiographically and biochemically to permit termination of etidronate disodium in those patients unresponsive to treatment. The incidence of osteogenic sarcoma is known to be increased in Paget's disease. Pagetic lesions, with or without therapy, may appear by X-ray to progress markedly, possibly with some loss of definition of periosteal margins. Such lesions should be evaluated carefully to differentiate these from osteogenic sarcoma.

Osteonecrosis of the jaw, generally associated with tooth extraction and/or local infection (including osteomyelitis) has been reported in patients with cancer receiving treatment regimens including primarily intravenously administered bisphosphonates. Many of these patients were also receiving chemotherapy and corticosteroids. Osteonecrosis of the jaw has also been reported in patients with osteoporosis receiving bisphosphonates.

A dental examination with appropriate preventive dentistry should be considered prior to treatment with bisphosphonates in patient with concominant risk factors (e.g. cancer, chemotherapy, radiotherapy, corticosteroids, poor oral hygiene).

While on treatment, these patients should avod invasive dental procedures if possible. For patients who develop osteonecrosis of the jaw while on bisphosphonate therapy, dental surgery may exacerbate the condition. For patients requiring dental procedures, there are no data available to suggest whether discontinuation of bisphosphonate treatment reduces risk of osteonecrosis of the jaw.

Clinical judgement of the treating physician should guide the management plan of each patient based on individual benefit/risk assessment.

4.5 Interaction with other medicinal products and other forms of interaction

Food in the stomach or upper portions of the small intestine, particularly materials with a high calcium content such as milk, may reduce absorption of etidronate disodium. Vitamins with mineral supplements such as iron, calcium supplements, laxatives containing magnesium, or antacids containing calcium or aluminium should not be taken within two hours of dosing etidronate disodium.

There have been isolated reports of patients experiencing changes in their prothrombin times when etidronate was added to warfarin therapy. The majority of these reports concerned variable elevations in prothrombin times without clinically significant sequelae. Although the relevance of these reports and any mechanism of coagulation alterations is unclear, patients on warfarin should have their prothrombin time monitored.

4.6 Pregnancy and lactation

The safety of this medicinal product for use in human pregnancy has not been established. Reproductive studies have shown skeletal abnormalities in rats. It is therefore recommended that Didronel should not be used in women of childbearing potential unless adequate contraceptive measures are taken.

It is not known whether this drug is excreted in human milk, and therefore caution should be exercised when Didronel is administered to a nursing woman.

4.7 Effects on ability to drive and use machines

Etidronate disodium does not interfere with the ability to drive or use machines.

4.8 Undesirable effects

Gastro-intestinal

The most common effects reported are diarrhoea and nausea. Reports of exacerbation of peptic ulcer with complications in a few patients.

Dermatological/hypersensitivity

Hypersensitivity reactions, including angio-oedema/urticaria, rash and/or pruritus, have been reported rarely.

Nervous System

Paresthesia, confusion, have been reported rarely.

Haematological

In patients receiving etidronate disodium, there have been rare reports of leucopenia, agranulocytosis and pancytopenia.

Other

Less common effects believed to be related to therapy include arthropathies (arthralgia and arthritis), and rarely burning of the tongue, alopecia, erythema multiforme and exacerbation of asthma.

4.9 Overdose

Overdose would manifest as the signs and symptoms of hypocalcaemia. Treatment should involve cessation of therapy and correction of hypocalcaemia with administration of Ca^{2+} intravenously.

5. PHARMACOLOGICAL PROPERTIES

5.1 Pharmacodynamic properties

Etidronate acts primarily on bone. It can inhibit the formation, growth and dissolution of hydroxyapatite crystals and amorphous precursors by chemisorption to calcium phosphate surfaces. Inhibition of crystal resorption occurs at lower doses than are required for the inhibition of crystal growth. Both effects increase as dose increases.

5.2 Pharmacokinetic properties

Etidronate is not metabolised. Absorption averages about 1% of an oral dose of 5mg/kg body weight/day. This increases to about 1.5% at 10mg/kg/day and 6% at 20mg/kg/day. Most of the drug is cleared from the blood within 6 hours. Within 24 hours about half of the absorbed dose is excreted in the urine. The remainder is chemically absorbed to bone, especially to areas of elevated osteogenesis, and is slowly eliminated. Unabsorbed drug is excreted in the faeces.

5.3 Preclinical safety data

In long term studies in mice and rats, there was no evidence of carcinogenicity with etidronate disodium. All *in vitro* and *in vivo* assays conducted to assess the mutagenic potential of etidronate disodium have been negative.

6. PHARMACEUTICAL PARTICULARS

6.1 List of excipients

Starch, magnesium stearate and microcrystalline cellulose.

6.2 Incompatibilities

See section 4.5 Interactions with other medicaments and other forms of interaction.

6.3 Shelf life

Four years.

6.4 Special precautions for storage

None.

6.5 Nature and contents of container

Supplied in high density polypropylene bottles or blister packs of 60 tablets.

6.6 Special precautions for disposal and other handling

None.

7. MARKETING AUTHORISATION HOLDER

Procter & Gamble Pharmaceuticals UK Limited

Rusham Park

Whitehall Lane

Egham

Surrey

TW20 9NW

UK

8. MARKETING AUTHORISATION NUMBER(S)

PL 0364/0039

9. DATE OF FIRST AUTHORISATION/RENEWAL OF THE AUTHORISATION

26th November 1987

10. DATE OF REVISION OF THE TEXT

October 2006

Didronel PMO

(Procter & Gamble Pharmaceuticals UK Limited)

1. NAME OF THE MEDICINAL PRODUCT

Didronel PMO.

2. QUALITATIVE AND QUANTITATIVE COMPOSITION

A two component therapy consisting of 14 Didronel 400mg tablets and 76 Cacit 500mg effervescent tablets (equivalent to 500mg elemental calcium). Each Didronel tablet contains 400mg of etidronate disodium, USP. Each Cacit 500mg effervescent tablet contains 1250mg of calcium carbonate, Ph.Eur, which when dispersed in water provides 500mg of elemental calcium as calcium citrate.

3. PHARMACEUTICAL FORM

Each Didronel 400mg tablet is white, capsule-shaped and marked with "NE" on one face and "406" on the other. The Cacit 500mg effervescent tablet is round, flat, white with pink speckles and has a distinctive orange flavour.

4. CLINICAL PARTICULARS

4.1 Therapeutic indications

Treatment of osteoporosis, and prevention of bone loss in postmenopausal women considered at risk of developing osteoporosis. Didronel PMO is particularly indicated in patients who are unable or unwilling to take oestrogen replacement therapy. Didronel PMO is also indicated for the prevention and treatment of corticosteroid - induced osteoporosis.

4.2 Posology and method of administration

Didronel PMO therapy is a long-term cyclical regimen administered in 90-day cycles. Each cycle consists of Didronel 400mg tablets for the first 14 days, followed by Cacit 500mg tablets for the remaining 76 days.

The majority of patients have been treated for 3 years, with a small number of patients treated for up to 7 years, with no clinical safety concerns. The optimum duration of treatment has not been established.

***Didronel 400mg component:**

One tablet should be taken each day for 14 consecutive days on an empty stomach. It is recommended that patients take the tablet with water at the midpoint of a four hour fast (ie. two hours before and two hours after food).

***Cacit 500mg component:**

Following 14 days treatment with Didronel 400mg tablets, one Cacit tablet should be taken on a daily basis. The Cacit tablet should be dissolved in water and drunk immediately after complete dissolution.

Adults and Elderly

The patient should adhere to the prescribed regimen above. Modification of the dosage for the elderly is not required.

Children

No data exists in the use of this therapy in juvenile osteoporosis.

4.3 Contraindications

Known hypersensitivity to any of the ingredients. Treatment of patients with severe renal impairment. Patients with hypercalcaemia or hypercalciuria. Clinically overt osteomalacia. Use in pregnancy and lactation.

4.4 Special warnings and precautions for use

Clinicians should advise patients to adhere to the recommended treatment regimen, and compliance pack.

In long-term trials no clinical osteomalacia was observed in patients receiving cyclical etidronate. Following long-term therapy in excess of 4 years, analysis of bone biopsies showed an increased prevalence of peritrabecular fibrosis and histologically defined atypical and focal osteomalacia (not to be confused with the syndrome associated with "clinical osteomalacia" due to vitamin D deficiency). In addition, these laboratory findings were not associated with any clinical consequences. Osteoid, which may accumulate at high doses of continuous etidronate therapy (10-20mg/kg/day) mineralises normally after discontinuation of therapy. Continuous administration of etidronate should be avoided.

Patients with significant chronic diarrhoeal disease may experience increased frequency of bowel movements and diarrhoea. Therapy should be withheld from patients with enterocolitis because of increased frequency of bowel movements.

Caution should be taken in patients with impaired renal function, or a history of renal stone formation. In these patients, serum and urinary calcium should be monitored regularly.

Etidronate disodium does not adversely effect serum levels of parathyroid hormone or calcium.

Hyperphosphataemia has been observed in patients receiving etidronate disodium, usually in association with doses of 10-20mg/kg/day. No adverse effects have been traced to this, and it does not constitute grounds for discontinuing therapy. It is apparently due to a drug-related increase in renal tubular re absorption of phosphate. Serum phosphate levels generally return to normal 2-4 weeks post therapy.

Osteonecrosis of the jaw, generally associated with tooth extraction and/or local infection (including osteomyelitis) has been reported in patients with cancer receiving treatment regimens including primarily intravenously administered bisphosphonates. Many of these patients were also receiving chemotherapy and corticosteroids. Osteonecrosis of the jaw has also been reported in patients with osteoporosis receiving bisphosphonates.

A dental examination with appropriate preventive dentistry should be considered prior to treatment with bisphosphonates in patient with concominant risk factors (e.g. cancer, chemotherapy, radiotherapy, corticosteroids, poor oral hygiene).

While on treatment, these patients should avoid invasive dental procedures if possible. For patients who develop osteonecrosis of the jaw while on bisphosphonate therapy, dental surgery may exacerbate the condition. For patients requiring dental procedures, there are no data available to suggest whether discontinuation of bisphosphonate treatment reduces risk of osteonecrosis of the jaw.

Clinical judgement of the treating physician should guide the management plan of each patient based on individual benefit/risk assessment.

Patients with rare hereditary problems of fructose intolerance should not take this medicine.

4.5 Interaction with other medicinal products and other forms of interaction

Food in the stomach or upper gastrointestinal tract, particularly materials with a high calcium content such as milk, may reduce absorption of etidronate disodium. Vitamins with mineral supplements such as iron, calcium supplements, laxatives containing magnesium, or antacids containing calcium or aluminium should not be taken within two hours of dosing etidronate disodium.

A small number of patients in clinical trials (involving more than 600 patients) received either thiazide diuretics or intravaginal oestrogen while on this treatment. The concomitant use of either of these agents did not interfere with the positive effects of the therapy on vertebral bone mass or fracture rates.

Calcium salts may reduce the absorption of some drugs, eg. tetracyclines. It is therefore suggested that administration of Cacit tablets be separated from these products by at least three hours.

Vitamin D causes an increase in calcium absorption and plasma calcium levels may continue to rise after stopping vitamin D therapy. Concomitant administration of Cacit tablets and vitamin D should therefore be carried out with caution.

The effects of digoxin and other cardiac glycosides may be accentuated by calcium and toxicity may be produced, especially in combination with vitamin D therapy.

There have been isolated reports of patients experiencing changes in their prothrombin times when etidronate was added to warfarin therapy. The majority of these reports concerned variable elevations in prothrombin times without clinically significant sequelae. Although the relevance of these reports and any mechanism of coagulation alterations is unclear, patients on warfarin should have their prothrombin time monitored.

4.6 Pregnancy and lactation

Contra-indicated.

4.7 Effects on ability to drive and use machines

Etidronate disodium does not interfere with the ability to drive or use machines.

4.8 Undesirable effects

Gastro-intestinal

In clinical studies of 2-3 years duration, the incidence of these events were comparable to placebo. The most common effects reported in order of incidence were diarrhoea, nausea, flatulence, dyspepsia, abdominal pain, gastritis, constipation and vomiting. Reports of exacerbation of peptic ulcer with complications in a few patients.

Dermatological/hypersensitivity

Hypersensitivity reactions including angio-oedema, urticaria, rash and/or pruritus have been reported rarely. The colouring agent E110 can cause allergic-type reactions including asthma. Allergy is more common in those people who are allergic to aspirin.

Nervous System

Headache, and rarely paresthesia, peripheral neuropathy and confusion.

Haematological

There have been rare reports of leucopenia, agranulocytosis and pancytopenia

Other

Less common effects believed to be related to therapy include arthropathies (arthralgia and arthritis), and rarely burning of the tongue, alopecia, erythema multiforme and exacerbation of asthma.

Occasional mild leg cramps have been reported in less than 5% of patients on the Didronel PMO regimen. These cramps were transient, often nocturnal and generally associated with other underlying conditions.

4.9 Overdose

Clinical experience of acute overdosage with etidronate is limited and unlikely with this compliance kit. Theoretically it would be manifested as the signs and symptoms of hypocalcaemia and possibly paresthesia of the fingers. Treatment would consist of gastric lavage to remove unabsorbed drug along with correction of hypocalcaemia with administration of Ca^{2+} intravenously.

Prolonged continuous treatment (chronic overdose) has been reported to cause nephrotic syndrome and fractures.

5. PHARMACOLOGICAL PROPERTIES

5.1 Pharmacodynamic properties

Etidronate in an intermittent cyclical regimen, works indirectly to increase bone mass. By timing delivery and withdrawal, the etidronate disodium component acts to modulate osteoclasts and reduce the mean resorption depth of the affected basic multicellular units (BMU). Calcium is an essential element which has been shown to help prevent bone loss.

Epidemiological studies have suggested that there are a number of risk factors associated with postmenopausal osteoporosis, such as early menopause, a family history of osteoporosis, prolonged exposure to corticosteroid therapy, small and thin skeletal frame and excessive cigarette smoking.

5.2 Pharmacokinetic properties

Within 24 hours, about one half of the absorbed dose of etidronate is excreted in the urine. The remainder is chemically absorbed on bone and is slowly eliminated. Unabsorbed drug is excreted in the faeces. Etidronate disodium is not metabolised. After oral doses of up to 1600mg of the disodium salt, the amount of drug absorbed is approximately 3-4%. In normal subjects, plasma half life (t½) of etidronate, based on non-compartmental pharmacokinetics is 1-6 hours.

Calcium carbonate is converted into soluble calcium salts in the stomach under the influence of hydrochloric acid. 30-80% of orally ingested calcium is absorbed both by active transport (primarily in the upper small intestine) and by passive diffusion. The distribution of calcium in the body is subject to the mechanism of physiological regulation controlled by parathyroid hormone, calcitonin, calciferol and other hormones.

When calcium effervescent tablets are added to water, insoluble calcium carbonate is converted into calcium citrate.

5.3 Preclinical safety data

In long-term studies in mice and rats, there was no evidence of carcinogenicity with etidronate disodium. All *in vitro* and *in vivo* assays conducted to assess the mutagenic potential of etidronate disodium have been negative.

6. PHARMACEUTICAL PARTICULARS

6.1 List of excipients

Etidronate disodium tablets contain microcrystalline cellulose, pregelatinised starch and magnesium stearate. Cacit tablets contain citric acid, sodium saccharin, sodium cyclamate, sunset yellow (E110) and orange flavouring.

6.2 Incompatibilities

None.

6.3 Shelf life

The expiry date for the compliance pack should not exceed 3 years from the date of its manufacture.

6.4 Special precautions for storage

Store in a dry place below 30°C. Since Cacit 500mg tablets are hygroscopic, the stopper should be carefully replaced after use.

6.5 Nature and contents of container

14 Didronel 400mg tablets in a blister plus four polypropylene tubes, each containing 19 Cacit 500mg tablets, all packaged in a compliance kit.

6.6 Special precautions for disposal and other handling

None.

7. MARKETING AUTHORISATION HOLDER

Procter & Gamble Pharmaceuticals UK Limited

Rusham Park

Whitehall Lane

Egham

Surrey TW20 9NW

UK

8. MARKETING AUTHORISATION NUMBER(S)

PL 0364/0051

9. DATE OF FIRST AUTHORISATION/RENEWAL OF THE AUTHORISATION

1 November 1991

10. DATE OF REVISION OF THE TEXT

June 2006

Differin Cream

(Galderma (U.K) Ltd)

1. NAME OF THE MEDICINAL PRODUCT

Differin Cream 0.1% w/w

2. QUALITATIVE AND QUANTITATIVE COMPOSITION

Adapalene 0.1% w/w.

For excipients, see 6.1

3. PHARMACEUTICAL FORM

Cream

White shiny cream

4. CLINICAL PARTICULARS

4.1 Therapeutic indications

Differin Cream is proposed for the cutaneous treatment of mild to moderate acne vulgaris where comedones, papules and pustules predominate. Differin Cream is best suited for use on dry and fair skin. Acne of the face, chest or back is appropriate for treatment.

4.2 Posology and method of administration

Differin Cream should be applied to the acne affected areas once a day before retiring and after washing. A thin film of cream should be applied, with the fingertips, avoiding the eyes and lips (see 4.4 *Special warnings and special precautions for use*, below). Ensure that the affected areas are dry before application.

Since it is customary to alternate therapies in the treatment of acne, it is recommended that the physician assess the continued improvement of the patient after three months of treatment with Differin Cream.

With patients for whom it is necessary to reduce the frequency of application or to temporarily discontinue treatment, frequency of application may be restored or therapy resumed once it is judged that the patient can again tolerate the treatment.

If patients use cosmetics, these should be non-comedogenic and non-astringent.

The safety and effectiveness of Differin Cream have not been studied in neonates and young children.

4.3 Contraindications

Hypersensitivity to any ingredient of the product.

4.4 Special warnings and precautions for use

If a reaction suggesting sensitivity or severe irritation occurs, use of the medication should be discontinued. If the degree of local irritation warrants, patients should be directed to use the medication less frequently, to discontinue use temporarily, or to discontinue use altogether. Differin Cream should not come into contact with the eyes, mouth, angles of the nose or mucous membranes.

If product enters the eye, wash immediately with warm water. The product should not be applied to either broken (cuts and abrasions), sunburnt or eczematous skin, nor should it be used in patients with severe acne, or acne involving large areas of the body, especially in women of child bearing age who are not on effective contraception.

Exposure to sunlight and artificial UV irradiation, including sunlamps, should be minimised during use of adapalene. Patients who normally experience high levels of sun exposure and those with inherent sensitivity to sun, should be warned to exercise caution. Use of sunscreen products and protective clothing over treated areas is recommended when exposure cannot be avoided.

Methyl parahydroxybenzoate (E218) and propyl parahydroxybenzoate (E216) may cause allergic reactions which can possibly be delayed.

4.5 Interaction with other medicinal products and other forms of interaction

There are no known interactions with other medications which might be used cutaneously and concurrently with Differin Cream; however, other retinoids or drugs with a similar mode of action should not be used concurrently with adapalene.

Adapalene is essentially stable to oxygen and light and is chemically non-reactive. Whilst extensive studies in animals and man have shown neither phototoxic nor photoallergic potential for adapalene, the safety of using adapalene during repeated exposure to sunlight or UV irradiation has not been established in either animals or man. Exposure to excessive sunlight or UV irradiation should be avoided.

Absorption of adapalene through human skin is low (see Pharmacokinetic Properties) and therefore interaction with systemic medications is unlikely. There is no evidence that the efficacy of oral drugs such as contraceptives and antibiotics is influenced by the cutaneous use of Differin Cream.

Differin Cream has a potential for mild local irritation, and therefore it is possible that concomitant use of peeling agents, astringents or irritant products may produce additive irritant effects. However, cutaneous antiacne treatment e.g. erythromycin (up to 4%) or clindamycin phosphate (1% as the base) solutions or benzoyl peroxide water based gels up to 10% may be used in the morning when Differin Cream is used at night as there is no mutual degradation or cumulative irritation.

4.6 Pregnancy and lactation

No information on the effects of Adapalene in pregnant women is available and therefore this product should not be used during pregnancy, unless considered essential by the physician. Because of the risk of teratogenicity shown in animal studies and since there is no information on the use of adapalene in pregnant women, it should not be used in women of child bearing age unless they are using an effective means of contraception.

Adapalene produces teratogenic effects by the oral route in rats and rabbits. At cutaneous doses up to 200-fold the therapeutic dose, producing circulating plasma levels of adapalene at least 35 to 120 times higher than plasma levels demonstrated in therapeutic use, adapalene increased the incidence of additional ribs in rats and rabbits, without increasing the incidence of major malformations.

It is not known whether adapalene is secreted in animal or human milk. In animal studies, infant rats suckled by mother with circulating levels of adapalene at least 300 times those demonstrated in clinical use developed normally.

Its use in women breast feeding infants should be avoided but when it is used in breast feeding women, to avoid contact exposure of the infant, application of adapalene to the chest should be avoided.

4.7 Effects on ability to drive and use machines
Based upon the pharmacodynamic profile and clinical experience, performance related to driving and using machines should not be affected.

4.8 Undesirable effects
Side effects include skin irritation (erythema, dryness, scaling, burning) and stinging at the site of application which is reversible when treatment is reduced in frequency or discontinued. Eyelid oedema as well as eye irritation when the product comes into contact with the eyes have been reported rarely.

4.9 Overdose
Differin Cream is not to be taken orally and is for cutaneous use only. If the medication is applied excessively, no more rapid or better results will be obtained and marked redness, peeling or discomfort may occur.

The acute oral dose of Differin Cream required to produce toxic effects in mice is greater than 10 g/kg. Nevertheless, unless the amount accidentally ingested is small, an appropriate method of gastric emptying should be considered.

5. PHARMACOLOGICAL PROPERTIES

5.1 Pharmacodynamic properties
Adapalene is a retinoid-like compound which in, in vivo and in vitro models of inflammation, has been demonstrated to possess anti-inflammatory properties. Adapalene is essentially stable to oxygen and light and is chemically non-reactive. Mechanically, adapalene binds like tretinoin to specific retinoic acid nuclear receptors but, unlike tretinoin not to cytosolic receptor binding proteins.

Adapalene applied cutaneously is comedolytic in the rhino mouse model and also has effects on the abnormal processes of epidermal keratinisation and differentiation, both of which are present in the pathogenesis of acne vulgaris. The mode of action of adapalene is suggested to be a normalisation of differentiation of follicular epithelial cells resulting in decreased microcomedone formation.

Adapalene is superior to reference retinoids in standard anti-inflammatory assays, both in vivo and in vitro. Mechanistically, it inhibits chemotactic and chemokinetic responses of human polymorphonuclear leucocytes and also the metabolism by lipoxidation of arachidonic acid to pro-inflammatory mediators. This profile suggests that the cell mediated inflammatory component of acne may be modified by adapalene. Studies in human patients provide clinical evidence that cutaneous adapalene is effective in reducing the inflammatory components of acne (papules and pustules).

5.2 Pharmacokinetic properties
Absorption of adapalene through human skin is low, in clinical trials measurable plasma adapalene levels were not found following chronic cutaneous application to large areas of acneic skin with an analytical sensitivity of 0.15 ng/ml.

After administration of [^{14}C]-adapalene in rats (IV, IP, oral and cutaneous), rabbits (IV, oral and cutaneous) and dogs (IV and oral), radioactivity was distributed in several tissues, the highest levels being found in liver, spleen, adrenals and ovaries. Metabolism in animals has been tentatively identified as being mainly by O-demethylation, hydroxylation and conjugation, and excretion is primarily by the biliary route.

5.3 Preclinical safety data
In animal studies, adapalene was well tolerated on cutaneous application for periods of up to six months in rabbits and for up to two years in mice. The major symptoms of toxicity found in all animal species by the oral route were related to an hypervitaminosis A syndrome, and included bone dissolution, elevated alkaline phosphatase and a slight anaemia. Large oral doses of adapalene produced no adverse neurological, cardiovascular or respiratory effects in animals. Adapalene is not mutagenic. Lifetime studies with adapalene have been completed in mice at cutaneous doses of 0.6, 2 and 6 mg/kg/day and in rats at oral doses of 0.15, 0.5 and 1.5 mg/kg/day. The only significant finding was a statistically significant increase of benign phaeochromocytomas of the adrenal medulla among male rats receiving adapalene at 1.5 mg/kg/day. These changes are unlikely to be of relevance to the cutaneous use of adapalene.

6. PHARMACEUTICAL PARTICULARS

6.1 List of excipients
Carbomer 934P
Macrogol-20 methyl glucose sesquistearate
Glycerol (E422)
Natural squalane
Methyl parahydroxybenzoate (E218)
Propyl parahydroxybenzoate (E216)
Disodium edetate
Methyl glucose sesquistearate
Phenoxyethanol
Cyclomethicone
Sodium hydroxide
Purified water

6.2 Incompatibilities
None known.

6.3 Shelf life
The shelf life expiry date for this product shall not exceed three years from the date of its manufacture.

6.4 Special precautions for storage
Do not store above 25°C.

Do not freeze.

Keep out of the reach and sight of children.

6.5 Nature and contents of container
Collapsible Aluminium tube coated internally with an epoxy-phenolic resin and fitted with a white Polypropylene screw cap. Pack sizes 5g (Sample Pack), 30g, 45g and 50g.

6.6 Special precautions for disposal and other handling
A thin film of the cream should be applied, avoiding eyes, lips and mucous membranes.

7. MARKETING AUTHORISATION HOLDER
Galderma (UK) Limited
Meridien House
69-71 Clarendon Road
Watford
Herts.
WD17 1DS
UK

8. MARKETING AUTHORISATION NUMBER(S)
PL 10590/0029

9. DATE OF FIRST AUTHORISATION/RENEWAL OF THE AUTHORISATION
9 January 1998

10. DATE OF REVISION OF THE TEXT
February 2006

11. Legal Category
POM

Differin Gel

(Galderma (U.K) Ltd)

1. NAME OF THE MEDICINAL PRODUCT
Differin Gel 0.1% w/w

2. QUALITATIVE AND QUANTITATIVE COMPOSITION
Adapalene 0.1% w/w

For excipients, see 6.1

3. PHARMACEUTICAL FORM
Topical Gel

A smooth white gel

4. CLINICAL PARTICULARS

4.1 Therapeutic indications
Differin Gel is proposed for the cutaneous treatment of mild to moderate acne where comedones, papules and pustules predominate. Acne of the face, chest or back is appropriate for treatment.

4.2 Posology and method of administration
Differin Gel should be applied to the acne affected areas once a day before retiring and after washing. A thin film of gel should be applied, with the fingertips, avoiding the eyes and lips (see 4.4 Special Warnings and Special Precautions for Use, below). Ensure that the affected areas are dry before application.

Since it is customary to alternate therapies in the treatment of acne, it is recommended that the physician assess the continued improvement of the patient after three months of treatment with Differin Gel.

With patients for whom it is necessary to reduce the frequency of application or to temporarily discontinue treatment, frequency of application may be restored or therapy resumed once it is judged that the patient can again tolerate the treatment.

If patients use cosmetics, these should be non-comedogenic and non-astringent.

The safety and effectiveness of Differin Gel have not been studied in neonates and young children. Differin gel should not be used in patients with severe acne.

4.3 Contraindications
Hypersensitivity to any ingredient of the product.

4.4 Special warnings and precautions for use
If a reaction suggesting sensitivity or severe irritation occurs, use of the medication should be discontinued. If the degree of local irritation warrants, patients should be directed to use the medication less frequently, to discontinue use temporarily, or to discontinue use altogether. Differin Gel should not come into contact with the eyes, mouth, nostrils or mucous membranes.

If product enters the eye, wash immediately with warm water. The product should not be applied to either broken (cut and abrasions) or eczematous skin, nor should it be used in patients with severe acne involving large areas of the body, especially in women of child bearing age who are not on effective contraception.

The excipient propylene glycol (E1520) may cause skin irritation and methyl parahydroxybenzoate (E218) may cause allergic reactions which can possibly be delayed.

4.5 Interaction with other medicinal products and other forms of interaction
There are no known interactions with other medications which might be used cutaneously and concurrently with Differin Gel, however, other retinoids or drugs with a similar mode of action should not be used concurrently with adapalene.

Adapalene is essentially stable to oxygen and light and is chemically non-reactive. Whilst extensive studies in animals and man have shown neither phototoxic nor photoallergic potential for adapalene, the safety of using adapalene during repeated exposure to sunlight or UV irradiation has not been established in either animals or man. Exposure to excessive sunlight or UV irradiation should be avoided.

Absorption of adapalene through human skin is low (see 5.2 Pharmacokinetic Properties) and therefore interaction with systemic medications is unlikely. There is no evidence that the efficacy of oral drugs such as contraceptives and antibiotics is influenced by the cutaneous use of Differin Gel.

Differin Gel has a potential for mild local irritation, and therefore it is possible that concomitant use of peeling agents, abrasive cleansers, strong drying agents, astringents or irritant products (aromatic and alcoholic agents) may produce additive irritant effects. However, cutaneous antiacne treatment (eg erythromycin up to 4%) or clindamycin phosphate (1% as the base) solutions or benzoyl peroxide water based gels up to 10% may be used in the morning when Differin Gel is used at night as there is no mutual degradation or cumulative irritation.

4.6 Pregnancy and lactation
No information on the effects of Adapalene in pregnant women is available and therefore this product should not be used during pregnancy, unless considered essential by the physician. Because of the risk of teratogenicity shown in animal studies and since there is no information on the use of adapalene in pregnant women, it should not be used in women of child bearing age unless they are using an effective means of contraception.

Adapalene produces teratogenic effects by the oral route in rats and rabbits. At cutaneous doses up to 200-fold the therapeutic dose, producing circulating plasma levels of adapalene at least 35 to 120 times higher than plasma levels demonstrated in therapeutic use, adapalene increased the incidence of additional ribs in rats and rabbits, without increasing the incidence of major malformations.

It is not known whether adapalene is secreted in animal or human milk. In animal studies, infant rats suckled by mother with circulating levels of adapalene at least 300 times those demonstrated in clinical use developed normally.

Its use in women breast feeding infants should be avoided but when it is used in breast feeding women, to avoid contact exposure of the infant, application of adapalene to the chest should be avoided.

4.7 Effects on ability to drive and use machines
Based upon the pharmodynamic profile and clinical experience, performance related to driving and using machines should not be affected.

4.8 Undesirable effects
Local reactions include burning, erythema, stinging, pruritus, dry or peeling skin. Eye irritation and oedema, and blistering or crusting of skin have been reported rarely.

The major undesirable effect which may occur is irritation of the skin which is reversible when treatment is reduced in frequency or discontinued.

4.9 Overdose
Differin Gel is not to be taken orally and is for cutaneous use only. If the medication is applied excessively, no more rapid or better results will be obtained and marked redness, peeling or discomfort may occur.

The acute oral dose of Differin Gel required to produce toxic effects in mice is greater that 10 mg/kg. Nevertheless, unless the amount accidentally ingested is small, an appropriate method of gastric emptying should be considered.

5. PHARMACOLOGICAL PROPERTIES

5.1 Pharmacodynamic properties
Adapalene is a retinoid-like compound which in, in vivo and in vitro models of inflammation, has been demonstrated to possess anti-inflammatory properties. Adapalene is essentially stable to oxygen and light and is chemically non-reactive. Mechanically, adapalene binds like tretinoin to specific retinoic acid nuclear receptors but, unlike tretinoin not to cytosolic receptor binding proteins.

Adapalene applied cutaneously is comedolytic in the rhino mouse model and also has effects on the abnormal processes of epidermal keratinization and differentiation, both of which are present in the pathogenesis of acne vulgaris. The mode of action of adapalene is suggested to be a normalisation of differentiation of follicular epithelial cells resulting in decreased microcomedone formation.

Adapalene is superior to reference retinoids in standard anti-inflammatory assays, both in vivo and in vitro. Mechanistically, it inhibits chemotactic and chemokinetic responses of human polymorphonuclear leucocytes and also the metabolism by lipoxidation of arachidonic acid to pro-inflammatory mediators. This profile suggests that the cell mediated inflammatory component of acne may be modified by adapalene.

5.2 Pharmacokinetic properties

Absorption of adapalene through human skin is low, in clinical trial measurable plasma adapalene levels where not found following chronic cutaneous application to large areas of acneic skin with an analytical sensitivity of 0.15 ng/ml.

After administration of [^{14}C] adapalene in rats (IV, IP, oral and cutaneous), rabbits (IV, oral and cutaneous) and dogs (IV and oral), radioactivity was distributed in several tissues, the highest levels being found in liver, spleen, adrenals and ovaries. Metabolism in animals has been tentatively identified as being mainly by O-demethylation, hydroxylation and conjugation, and excretion is primarily by the biliary route.

5.3 Preclinical safety data

In animal studies, adapalene was well tolerated on cutaneous application for periods of up to six months in rabbits and for up to two years in mice. The major symptom of toxicity found in all animal species by the oral route were related to a hypervitaminosis A syndrome, and included bone dissolution, elevated alkaline phosphatase and a slight anaemia. Large oral doses of adapalene produced no adverse neurological, caridovascular or respiratory effects in animals. Adapalene is not mutagenic. Lifetime studies with adapalene have been completed in mice at cutaneous doses of 0.6,2 and 6 mg/kg/day and in rats at oral doses of 0.15, 0.5 and 1.5 mg/kg/day. The only significant finding was a statistically significant increase of benign phaeochromocytomas of the adrenal medulla among male rats receiving adapalene at 1.5 mg/kg/day. These changes are unlikely to be of relevance to the cutaneous use of adapalene.

6. PHARMACEUTICAL PARTICULARS

6.1 List of excipients

Carbomer 940

Propylene Glycol (E1520)

Poloxamer 182

Disodium Edetate

Methyl Parahydroxybenzoate (E218)

Phenoxyethanol

Sodium Hydroxide

Purified Water

6.2 Incompatibilities

None Known

6.3 Shelf life

The shelf life expiry date for this product shall not exceed three years from the date of its manufacture.

6.4 Special precautions for storage

Do not store above 25°C.

Do not freeze.

Keep out of the reach and sight of children

6.5 Nature and contents of container

White LDPE tube with white PP screw cap. Pack size 30g, 45g & 50g

6.6 Special precautions for disposal and other handling

A thin film of the gel should be applied, avoiding eyes, lips and mucous membranes

7. MARKETING AUTHORISATION HOLDER

Galderma (UK) Limited

Meridien House

69-71 Clarendon Road

Watford

Herts.

WD17 1DS

UK

8. MARKETING AUTHORISATION NUMBER(S)

PL 10590/0015

9. DATE OF FIRST AUTHORISATION/RENEWAL OF THE AUTHORISATION

10. DATE OF REVISION OF THE TEXT

February 2006

Diflucan 150 Capsules

(Pfizer Limited)

1. NAME OF THE MEDICINAL PRODUCT

DIFLUCAN™ 150 CAPSULE.

2. QUALITATIVE AND QUANTITATIVE COMPOSITION

Diflucan 150 capsule contains as its active ingredient fluconazole 150mg.

3. PHARMACEUTICAL FORM

Diflucan 150 capsules are light turquoise blue, coded 'FLU 150' and 'PFIZER'.

4. CLINICAL PARTICULARS

4.1 Therapeutic indications

Diflucan 150 is indicated for the treatment of the following conditions:

Genital candidiasis. Vaginal candidiasis, acute or recurrent. Candidal balanitis. The treatment of partners who present with symptomatic genital candidiasis should be considered.

4.2 Posology and method of administration

In adults Vaginal candidiasis or candidal balanitis - 150mg single oral dose.

In children Despite extensive data supporting the use of Diflucan in children there are limited data available on the use of Diflucan for genital candidiasis in children below 16 years. Use at present is not recommended unless antifungal treatment is imperative and no suitable alternative agent exists.

Use in elderly The normal adult dose should be used.

Use in renal impairment Fluconazole is excreted predominantly in the urine as unchanged drug. No adjustments in single dose therapy are required.

4.3 Contraindications

Diflucan 150 should not be used in patients with known hypersensitivity to fluconazole or to related azole compounds or any other ingredient in the formulation.

Fluconazole should not be co-adminstered with cisapride or terfenadine which are known to both prolong the QT – interval and are metabolised by CYP3A4 (See "Interactions with other medicinal products and other forms of interaction".)

4.4 Special warnings and precautions for use

In some patients, particularly those with serious underlying diseases such as AIDS and cancer, abnormalities in haematological, hepatic, renal and other biochemical function test results have been observed during treatment with Diflucan but the clinical significance and relationship to treatment is uncertain.

Very rarely, patients who died with severe underlying disease and who had received multiple doses of Diflucan had post-mortem findings which included hepatic necrosis. These patients were receiving multiple concomitant medications, some known to be potentially hepatotoxic, and/or had underlying diseases which could have caused the hepatic necrosis.

In cases of hepatotoxicity, no obvious relationship to total daily dose of Diflucan, duration of therapy, sex or age of the patient has been observed; the abnormalities have usually been reversible on discontinuation of Diflucan therapy.

As a causal relationship with Diflucan cannot be excluded, patients who develop abnormal liver function tests during Diflucan therapy should be monitored for the development of more serious hepatic injury. Diflucan should be discontinued if clinical signs or symptoms consistent with liver disease develop during treatment with Diflucan.

Patients have rarely developed exfoliative cutaneous reactions, such as Stevens-Johnson Syndrome and toxic epidermal necrolysis, during treatment with fluconazole. AIDS patients are more prone to the development of severe cutaneous reactions to many drugs.

If a rash develops in a patient which is considered attributable to Diflucan 150, further therapy with this agent is not recommended.

In rare cases, as with other azoles, anaphylaxis has been reported.

Some azoles, including fluconazole, have been associated with prolongation of the QT interval on the electrocardiogram. During post-marketing surveillance, there have been very rare cases of QT prolongation and torsade de pointes in patients taking fluconazole. Although the association of fluconazole and QT-prolongation has not been fully established, fluconazole should be used with caution in patients with potentially proarrythmic conditions such as:

- Congenital or documented acquired QT prolongation
- Cardiomyopathy, in particular when heart failure is present
- Sinus bradycardia
- Existing symptomatic arrythmias
- Concomitant medication not metabolized by CY34A but known to prolong QT interval
- Electrolyte disturbances such as hypokalaemia, hypomagnesaemia and hypocalaemia

(See Section 4.5 Interactions with other medicinal products and other forms of interaction)

4.5 Interaction with other medicinal products and other forms of interaction

The following drug interactions relate to the use of multiple-dose fluconazole, and the relevance to single-dose Diflucan 150 has not yet been established:

Rifampicin Concomitant administration of Diflucan and rifampicin resulted in a 25% decrease in the AUC and 20% shorter half-life of fluconazole. In patients receiving concomitant rifampicin, an increase in the Diflucan dose should be considered.

Hydrochlorothiazide In a kinetic interaction study, co-administration of multiple-dose hydrochlorothiazide to healthy volunteers receiving Diflucan increased plasma concentrations of fluconazole by 40%. An effect of this magnitude should not necessitate a change in the Diflucan dose regimen in subjects receiving concomitant diuretics, although the prescriber should bear it in mind.

Anticoagulants In an interaction study, fluconazole increased the prothrombin time (12%) after warfarin administration in healthy males. In post-marketing experience, as with other azole antifungals, bleeding events (bruising, epistaxis, gastrointestinal bleeding, hematuria and melena) have been reported in association with increases in prothrombin time in patients receiving fluconazole concurrently with warfarin. Prothrombin time in patients receiving coumarin-type anticoagulants should be carefully monitored.

Benzodiazepines (Short Acting) Following oral administration of midazolam, fluconazole resulted in substantial increases in midazolam concentrations and psychomotor effects. This effect on midazolam appears to be more pronounced following oral administration of fluconazole than with fluconazole administered intravenously. If concomitant benzodiazepine therapy is necessary in patients being treated with fluconazole, consideration should be given to decreasing the benzodiazepine dosage and the patients should be appropriately monitored.

Sulphonylureas Fluconazole has been shown to prolong the serum half-life of concomitantly administered oral sulphonylureas (chlorpropamide, glibenclamide, glipizide and tolbutamide) in healthy volunteers. Fluconazole and oral sulphonylureas may be co-administered to diabetic patients, but the possibility of a hypoglycaemic episode should be borne in mind.

Phenytoin Concomitant administration of fluconazole and phenytoin may increase the levels of phenytoin to a clinically significant degree. If it is necessary to administer both drugs concomitantly, phenytoin levels should be monitored and the phenytoin dose adjusted to maintain therapeutic levels.

Oral contraceptives Two kinetic studies with combined oral contraceptives have been performed using multiple doses of fluconazole. There were no relevant effects on either hormone level in the 50mg fluconazole study, while at 200mg daily the AUCs of ethinyloestradiol and levonorgestrel were increased 40% and 24% respectively. Thus multiple dose use of fluconazole at these doses is unlikely to have an effect on the efficacy of the combined oral contraceptive.

In a 300 mg once weekly fluconazole study, the AUCs of ethinyl estradiol and norethindrone were increased by 24% and 13%, respectively.

Endogenous steroid Fluconazole 50mg daily does not affect endogenous steroid levels in females: 200-400mg daily has no clinically significant effect on endogenous steroid levels or on ACTH stimulated response in healthy male volunteers.

Cyclosporin A kinetic study in renal transplant patients found fluconazole 200mg daily to slowly increase cyclosporin concentrations. However, in another multiple dose study with 100mg daily, fluconazole did not affect cyclosporin levels in patients with bone marrow transplants. Cyclosporin plasma concentration monitoring in patients receiving fluconazole is recommended.

Theophylline In a placebo controlled interaction study, the administration of fluconazole 200mg for 14 days resulted in an 18% decrease in the mean plasma clearance of theophylline. Patients who are receiving high doses of theophylline or who are otherwise at increased risk for theophylline toxicity should be observed for signs of theophylline toxicity while receiving fluconazole, and the therapy modified appropriately if signs of toxicity develop.

Terfenadine Because of the occurrence of serious dysrhythmias secondary to prolongation of the QTc interval in patients receiving other azole antifungals in conjunction with terfenadine, interactions studies have been performed. One study at a 200mg daily dose of fluconazole failed to demonstrate a prolongation in QTc interval. Another study at a 400mg and 800mg daily dose of fluconazole demonstrated that fluconazole taken in multiple doses of 400mg per day or greater significantly increased plasma levels of terfenadine when taken concomitantly. There have been spontaneously reported cases of palpitations, tachycardia, dizziness, and chest pain in patients taking concomitant fluconazole and terfenadine where the relationship of the reported adverse events to drug therapy or underlying medical conditions was not clear. Because of the potential seriousness of such an interaction, it is recommended that terfenadine not be taken in combination with fluconazole. (See "Contra-indications".)

Cisapride There have been reports of cardiac events including torsades de pointes in patients to whom fluconazole and cisapride were co-administered. A controlled study found that concomitant fluconazole 200 mg once daily and cisapride 20 mg four times a day yielded a significant increase in cisapride plasma levels and prolongation of QTc interval. In most of these cases, the patients appear to have been predisposed to arrhythmias or had serious underlying illnesses, and the relationship of the reported events to a possible fluconazole-cisapride drug interaction is unclear. Because of the potential seriousness of such an interaction, co-administration of cisapride is contra-indicated in patients receiving fluconazole. (See "Contra-indications".)

Zidovudine Two kinetic studies resulted in increased levels of zidovudine most likely caused by the decreased conversion of zidovudine to its major metabolite. One study determined zidovudine levels in AIDS or ARC patients before and following fluconazole 200mg daily for 15 days. There was a significant increase in zidovudine AUC (20%). A second randomised, two-period, two-treatment cross-over study examined zidovudine levels in HIV infected patients. On two occasions, 21 days apart, patients received zidovudine 200mg every eight hours either with or without fluconazole 400mg daily for seven days. The AUC of zidovudine significantly increased (74%) during co-administration with fluconazole. Patients receiving this combination should be monitored for the development of zidovudine-related adverse reactions.

Rifabutin There have been reports that an interaction exists when fluconazole is administered concomitantly with rifabutin, leading to increased serum levels of rifabutin. There have been reports of uveitis in patients to whom fluconazole and rifabutin were co-administered. Patients receiving rifabutin and fluconazole concomitantly should be carefully monitored.

Tacrolimus There have been reports that an interaction exists when fluconazole is administered concomitantly with tacrolimus, leading to increased serum levels of tacrolimus. There have been reports of nephrotoxicity in patients to whom fluconazole and tacrolimus were co-administered. Patients receiving tacrolimus and fluconazole concomitantly should be carefully monitored.

The use of fluconazole in patients concurrently taking astemizole or other drugs metabolised by the cytochrome P450 system may be associated with elevations in serum levels of these drugs. In the absence of definitive information, caution should be used when co-administering fluconazole. This is particularly important for drugs known to prolong QT interval. Patients should be carefully monitored.

Interaction studies have shown that when oral fluconazole is co-administered with food, cimetidine, antacids or following total body irradiation for bone marrow transplantation, no clinically significant impairment of fluconazole absorption occurs.

Physicians should be aware that drug-drug interaction studies with other medications have not been conducted, but that such interactions may occur.

4.6 Pregnancy and lactation

Use during pregnancy There are no adequate and well controlled studies in pregnant women. There have been reports of multiple congenital abnormalities in infants whose mothers were being treated for 3 or more months with high dose (400-800 mg/day) fluconazole therapy for coccidioidomycosis. The relationship between fluconazole and these events is unclear. Accordingly, Diflucan 150 should not be used in pregnancy, or in women of child-bearing potential unless adequate contraception is employed.

Use during lactation Fluconazole is found in human breast milk at concentrations similar to plasma, hence its use in nursing mothers is not recommended.

4.7 Effects on ability to drive and use machines

Experience with Diflucan indicates that therapy is unlikely to impair a patient's ability to drive or use machinery.

4.8 Undesirable effects

Fluconazole is generally well tolerated. The most common undesirable effects observed during clinical trials and associated with fluconazole are:

Nervous System Disorders: Headache.

Skin and Subcutaneous Tissue Disorders: Rash.

Gastrointestinal Disorders: Abdominal pain, diarrhoea, flatulence, nausea.

In some patients, particularly those with serious underlying diseases such as AIDS and cancer, changes in renal and haematological function test results and hepatic abnormalities have been observed during treatment with fluconazole and comparative agents, but the clinical significance and relationship to treatment is uncertain (see Section 4.4 "Special warnings and special precautions for use").

Hepatobiliary Disorders: Hepatic toxicity including rare cases of fatalities, elevated alkaline phosphatase, elevated bilirubin, elevated SGOT, elevated SGPT.

In addition, the following undesirable effects have occurred during post-marketing:

Nervous System Disorders: Dizziness, seizures, taste perversion.

Skin and Subcutaneous Tissue Disorders: Alopecia, exfoliative skin disorders including Stevens-Johnson syndrome and toxic epidermal necrosis.

Gastrointestinal Disorders: Dyspepsia, vomiting.

Blood and Lymphatic System Disorders: Leukopenia including neutropenia and agranulocytosis, thrombocytopenia.

Immune System Disorders:

Allergic reaction: Anaphylaxis (including angioedema, face oedema, pruritus), urticaria.

Hepatobiliary Disorders: Hepatic failure, hepatitis, hepatocellular necrosis, jaundice.

Metabolism and Nutrition Disorders: Hypercholesterolaemia, hypertriglyceridaemia, hypokalaemia.

Cardiac Disorders: QT prolongation, torsade de pointes (see section 4.4 **Special Warnings and Special Precautions for Use**).

4.9 Overdose

There have been reports of overdosage with fluconazole and in one case, a 42 year-old patient infected with human immunodeficiency virus developed hallucinations and exhibited paranoid behaviour after reportedly ingesting 8200mg of fluconazole, unverified by his physician. The patient was admitted to the hospital and his condition resolved within 48 hours.

In the event of overdosage, supportive measures and symptomatic treatment, with gastric lavage if necessary, may be adequate.

As fluconazole is largely excreted in the urine, forced volume diuresis would probably increase the elimination rate. A three hour haemodialysis session decreases plasma levels by approximately 50%.

5. PHARMACOLOGICAL PROPERTIES

5.1 Pharmacodynamic properties

Pharmacotherapeutic group: Triazole derivatives, ATC code J02AC.

Fluconazole, a member of the triazole class of antifungal agents, is a potent and selective inhibitor of fungal enzymes necessary for the synthesis of ergosterol.

Fluconazole shows little pharmacological activity in a wide range of animal studies. Some prolongation of pentobarbitone sleeping times in mice (p.o.), increased mean arterial and left ventricular blood pressure and increased heart rate in anaesthetised cats (i.v.) occurred. Inhibition of rat ovarian aromatase was observed at high concentrations.

Both orally and intravenously administered fluconazole was active in a variety of animal fungal infection models. Activity has been demonstrated against opportunistic mycoses, such as infections with *Candida* spp. Including systemic candidiasis in immunocompromised animals; with *Cryptococcus neoformans,* including intracranial infections; with *Microsporum* spp. and with *Trichophyton* spp. Fluconazole has also been shown to be active in animal models of endemic mycoses, including infections with *Blastomyces dermatitides;* with *Coccidoides immitis,* including intracranial infection and with *Histoplasma capsulatum* in normal and immunosuppressed animals.

There have been reports of cases of superinfection with *Candida* species other than *C. albicans*, which are often inherently not susceptible to fluconazole (e.g. *Candida krusei).* Such cases may require alternative antifungal therapy.

Fluconazole is highly specific for fungal cytochrome P-450 dependent enzymes. Fluconazole 50mg daily given up to 28 days has been shown not to affect testosterone plasma concentrations in males or steroid concentrations in females of child-bearing age. Fluconazole 200-400mg daily has no clinically significant effect on endogenous steroid levels or on ACTH stimulated response in healthy male volunteers. Interaction studies with antipyrine indicate that single or multiple doses of fluconazole 50mg do not affect its metabolism.

5.2 Pharmacokinetic properties

The pharmacokinetic properties of fluconazole are similar following administration by the intravenous or oral route. After oral administration fluconazole is well absorbed and plasma levels (and systemic bioavailability) are over 90% of the levels achieved after intravenous administration. Oral absorption is not affected by concomitant food intake. Peak plasma concentrations in the fasting state occur between 0.5 and 1.5 hours post-dose with a plasma elimination half-life of approximately 30 hours. Plasma concentrations are proportional to dose. Ninety percent steady-state levels are reached by day 4 -5 with multiple once daily dosing.

Administration of loading dose (on day 1) of twice the usual daily dose enables plasma levels to approximate to 90% steady-state levels by day 2. The apparent volume of distribution approximates to total body water. Plasma protein binding is low (11-12%).

Fluconazole achieves good penetration in all body fluids studied. The levels of fluconazole in saliva and sputum are similar to plasma levels. In patients with fungal meningitis, fluconazole levels in the CSF are approximately 80% of the corresponding plasma levels.

High skin concentrations of fluconazole, above serum concentrations, are achieved in the stratum corneum, epidermis-dermis and eccrine sweat. Fluconazole accumulates in the stratum corneum. At a dose of 50mg once daily, the concentration of fluconazole after 12 days was 73 microgram/g and 7 days after cessation of treatment the concentration was still 5.8 microgram/g.

The major route of excretion is renal, with approximately 80% of the administered dose appearing in the urine as unchanged drug. Fluconazole clearance is proportional to creatinine clearance. There is no evidence of circulating metabolites.

The long plasma elimination half-life provides the basis for single dose therapy for genital candidiasis.

A study compared the saliva and plasma concentrations of a single fluconazole 100mg dose administration in a capsule or in an oral suspension by rinsing and retaining in mouth for 2 minutes and swallowing. The maximum concentration of fluconazole in saliva after the suspension was observed 5 minutes after ingestion, and was 182 times higher than the maximum saliva concentration after the capsule which occurred 4 hours after ingestion. After about 4 hours, the saliva concentrations of fluconazole were similar. The mean AUC (0-96) in saliva was significantly greater after the suspension compared to the capsule. There was no significant difference in the elimination rate from saliva or the plasma pharmacokinetic parameters for the two formulations.

Pharmacokinetics in Children

In children, the following pharmacokinetics data have been reported:

(see Table 1 below)

In premature new-borns (gestational age around 28 weeks), intravenous administration of fluconazole of 6mg/kg was given every third day for a maximum of five doses while the premature new-borns remained in the intensive care unit. The mean half-life (hours) was 74 (range 44-185) on day 1 which decreased with time to a mean of 53 (range 30-131) on day 7 and 47 (range 27-68) on day 13.

The area under the curve (microgram.h/ml) was 271 (range 173-385) on day 1 and increased with a mean of 490 (range 292-734) on day 7 and decreased with a mean of 360 (range 167-566) on day 13.

The volume of distribution (ml/kg) was 1183 (range 1070-1470) on day 1 and which increased with time to a mean of 1184 (range 510-2130) on day 7 and 1328 (range 1040-1680) on day 13.

5.3 Preclinical safety data

Reproductive toxicity Increases in fetal anatomical variants (supernumerary ribs, renal pelvis dilation) and delays in ossification were observed at 25 and 50mg/kg and

Table 1

Age Studied	Dose (mg/kg)	Half-life (hours)	AUC (microgram.h/ml)
11 days- 11 months	Single-IV 3mg/kg	23	110.1
9 months- 13 years	Single-Oral 2mg/kg	25.0	94.7
9 months- 13 years	Single-Oral 8mg/kg	19.5	362.5
5 years- 15 years	Multiple-IV 2mg/kg	17.4*	67.4
5 years- 15 years	Multiple-IV 4mg/kg	15.2*	139.1
5 years- 15 years	Multiple-IV 8mg/kg	17.6*	196.7
Mean age 7 years	Multiple-Oral 3mg/kg	15.5	41.6

*Denotes final day

higher doses. At doses ranging from 80mg/kg (approximately 20-60x the recommended human dose) to 320mg/kg embryolethality in rats was increased and fetal abnormalities included wavy ribs, cleft palate and abnormal craniofacial ossification.

These effects are consistent with the inhibition of oestrogen synthesis in rats and may be a result of known effects of lowered oestrogen on pregnancy, organogenesis and parturition.

Carcinogenesis Fluconazole showed no evidence of carcinogenic potential in mice and rats treated orally for 24 months at doses of 2.5, 5 or 10mg/kg/day. Male rats treated with 5 and 10mg/ kg/day had an increased incidence of hepatocellular adenomas.

Mutagenesis Fluconazole, with or without metabolic activation, was negative in tests for mutagenicity in 4 strains of S.typhimurium and in the mouse lymphoma L5178Y system. Cytogenetic studies in vivo (murine bone marrow cells, following oral administration of fluconazole) and in vitro (human lymphocytes exposed to fluconazole at 1000µg/ml) showed no evidence of chromosomal mutations.

Impairment of fertility Fluconazole did not affect the fertility of male or female rats treated orally with daily doses of 5, 10 or 20mg/kg or with parenteral doses of 5, 25 or 75mg/kg, although the onset of parturition was slightly delayed at 20mg/kg p.o. In an intravenous perinatal study in rats at 5, 20 and 40mg/kg, dystocia and prolongation of parturition were observed in a few dams at 20mg/kg and 40mg/kg, but not at 5mg/kg. The disturbances in parturition were reflected by a slight increase in the number of still-born pups and decrease of neonatal survival at these dose levels. The effects on parturition in rats are consistent with the species specific oestrogen-lowering property produced by high doses of fluconazole. Such a hormone change has not been observed in women treated with Diflucan.

6. PHARMACEUTICAL PARTICULARS

6.1 List of excipients

Diflucan 150 capsules contain lactose, maize starch, colloidal silicon dioxide, magnesium stearate and sodium lauryl sulphate as excipients.

In addition, capsule shells contain: patent blue V (E131), titanium dioxide (E171) and gelatin.

6.2 Incompatibilities

No specific incompatibilities have been noted.

6.3 Shelf life

Current stability data support a shelf life of 5 years.

6.4 Special precautions for storage

Store below 30°C.

6.5 Nature and contents of container

Diflucan 150 capsules will be supplied as a pack containing one capsule in clear or opaque PVC blister packs with aluminium foil backing.

6.6 Special precautions for disposal and other handling

Diflucan 150 capsules should be swallowed whole.

7. MARKETING AUTHORISATION HOLDER

Pfizer Limited
Sandwich
Kent CT13 9NJ
United Kingdom

8. MARKETING AUTHORISATION NUMBER(S)

PL 00057/0290

9. DATE OF FIRST AUTHORISATION/RENEWAL OF THE AUTHORISATION

11 January 2000

10. DATE OF REVISION OF THE TEXT

November 2004

Legal Category

POM

Company Reference: DF11_0

Diflucan Capsules 50mg and 200mg, Powder for Oral Suspension 50mg/5ml and 200mg/5ml, Intravenous Infusion 2mg/ml

(Pfizer Limited)

1. NAME OF THE MEDICINAL PRODUCT

DIFLUCAN™ CAPSULES 50MG

DIFLUCAN™ CAPSULES 200MG

DIFLUCAN™ POWDER FOR ORAL SUSPENSION 50MG/5ML

DIFLUCAN™ POWDER FOR ORAL SUSPENSION 200MG/5ML

DIFLUCAN™ INTRAVENOUS INFUSION 2MG/ML

2. QUALITATIVE AND QUANTITATIVE COMPOSITION

Diflucan contains as its active ingredient fluconazole 50mg and 200mg as capsules, 50mg or 200mg per 5ml as powder for oral suspension on reconstitution with water, and as 2mg/ml in a saline solution for intravenous infusion.

3. PHARMACEUTICAL FORM

Diflucan Capsules 50mg are light turquoise blue and white, coded 'FLU 50' and 'PFIZER'.

Diflucan Capsules 200mg are purple and white, coded 'FLU 200' and 'PFIZER'.

Diflucan Powder for Oral Suspension is a dry white to off-white powder which yields, on reconstitution with water (24ml), an orange flavoured suspension containing the equivalent of 50mg or 200mg fluconazole per 5ml.

Diflucan Intravenous Infusion 2mg/ml is available in a 0.9% aqueous sodium chloride solution, presented in glass infusion vials (25 or 100ml).

4. CLINICAL PARTICULARS

4.1 Therapeutic indications

Therapy may be instituted before the results of the cultures and other laboratory studies are known; however, once these results become available, anti-infective therapy should be adjusted accordingly.

Diflucan is indicated for the treatment of the following conditions:

1. Genital candidiasis. Vaginal candidiasis, acute or recurrent. Candidal balanitis. The treatment of partners who present with symptomatic genital candidiasis should be considered.

2. Mucosal candidiasis. These include oropharyngeal, oesophageal, non-invasive bronchopulmonary infections, candiduria, mucocutaneous and chronic oral atrophic candidiasis (denture sore mouth). Normal hosts and patients with compromised immune function may be treated.

3. Tinea pedis, tinea corporis, tinea cruris, tinea versicolor and dermal *Candida* infections. Diflucan is not indicated for nail infections and tinea capitis.

4. Systemic candidiasis including candidaemia, disseminated candidiasis and other forms of invasive candidal infection. These include infections of the peritoneum, endocardium and pulmonary and urinary tracts. Candidal infections in patients with malignancy, in intensive care units or those receiving cytotoxic or immunosuppressive therapy may be treated.

5. Cryptococcosis, including cryptococcal meningitis and infections of other sites (e.g. pulmonary, cutaneous). Normal hosts, and patients with AIDS, organ transplants or other causes of immunosuppression may be treated. Diflucan can be used as maintenance therapy to prevent relapse of cryptococcal disease in patients with AIDS.

6. For the prevention of fungal infections in immunocompromised patients considered at risk as a consequence of neutropenia following cytotoxic chemotherapy or radiotherapy, including bone marrow transplant patients.

4.2 Posology and method of administration

Diflucan may be administered either orally or by intravenous infusion at a rate of approximately 5-10ml/min, the route being dependent on the clinical state of the patient. On transferring from the intravenous route to the oral route or vice versa, there is no need to change the daily dose. Diflucan intravenous infusion is formulated in 0.9% sodium chloride solution, each 200mg (100ml bottle) containing 15mmol each of Na^+ and Cl^-.

The daily dose of Diflucan should be based on the nature and severity of the fungal infection. Most cases of vaginal candidiasis respond to single dose therapy. Therapy for those types of infections requiring multiple dose treatment should be continued until clinical parameters or laboratory tests indicate that active fungal infection has subsided. An inadequate period of treatment may lead to recurrence of active infection. Patients with AIDS and cryptococcal meningitis usually require maintenance therapy to prevent relapse.

Use in adults

1. Candidal vaginitis or balanitis - 150mg single oral dose.

2. Mucosal Candidiasis

Oropharyngeal candidiasis - the usual dose is 50mg once daily for 7 - 14 days. Treatment should not normally exceed 14 days except in severely immunocompromised patients.

For atrophic oral candidiasis associated with dentures - the usual dose is 50mg once daily for 14 days administered concurrently with local antiseptic measures to the denture.

For other candidal infections of mucosa except genital candidiasis (see above), e.g. oesophagitis, non-invasive bronchopulmonary infections, candiduria, mucocutaneous candidiasis etc., the usual effective dose is 50mg daily, given for 14 - 30 days.

In unusually difficult cases of mucosal candidal infections the dose may be increased to 100mg daily.

3. For tinea pedis, corporis, cruris, versicolor and dermal *Candida* infections the recommended dosage is 50mg once daily. Duration of treatment is normally 2 to 4 weeks but tinea pedis may require treatment for up to 6 weeks. Duration of treatment should not exceed 6 weeks.

4. For candidaemia, disseminated candidiasis and other invasive candidal infections the usual dose is 400mg on the first day followed by 200mg daily. Depending on the clinical response the dose may be increased to 400mg daily. Duration of treatment is based upon the clinical response.

5a. For cryptococcal meningitis and cryptococcal infections at other sites, the usual dose is 400mg on the first day followed by 200mg - 400mg once daily. Duration of treatment for cryptococcal infections will depend on the clinical and mycological response, but is usually at least 6-8 weeks for cryptococcal meningitis.

5b. For the prevention of relapse of cryptococcal meningitis in patients with AIDS, after the patient receives a full course of primary therapy, Diflucan may be administered indefinitely at a daily dose of 100 - 200mg.

6. For the prevention of fungal infections in immunocompromised patients considered at risk as a consequence of neutropenia following cytotoxic chemotherapy or radiotherapy, the dose should be 50 to 400mg once daily, based on the patient's risk for developing fungal infection. For patients at high risk of systemic infection, e.g. patients who are anticipated to have profound or prolonged neutropenia such as during bone marrow transplantation, the recommended dose is 400mg once daily. Diflucan administration should start several days before the anticipated onset of neutropenia, and continue for 7 days after the neutrophil count rises above 1000 cells per mm^3.

Use in children

As with similar infections in adults, the duration of treatment is based on the clinical and mycological response. Diflucan is administered as a single daily dose each day.

For children with impaired renal function, see dosing in "Use in patients with impaired renal function".

Children over four weeks of age The recommended dose of Diflucan for mucosal candidiasis is 3mg/kg daily. A loading dose of 6mg/kg may be used on the first day to achieve steady state levels more rapidly.

For the treatment of systemic candidiasis and cryptococcal infections, the recommended dosage is 6-12mg/kg daily, depending on the severity of the disease.

For the prevention of fungal infections in immunocompromised patients considered at risk as a consequence of neutropenia following cytotoxic chemotherapy or radiotherapy, the dose should be 3-12mg/kg daily, depending on the extent and duration of the induced neutropenia (see adult dosing).

A maximum dosage of 400mg daily should not be exceeded in children.

Despite extensive data supporting the use of Diflucan in children there are limited data available on the use of Diflucan for genital candidiasis in children below 16 years. Use at present is not recommended unless antifungal treatment is imperative and no suitable alternative agent exists.

Children four weeks of age and younger Neonates excrete fluconazole slowly. In the first two weeks of life, the same mg/kg dosing as in older children should be used but administered every 72 hours. During weeks 3 and 4 of life, the same dose should be given every 48 hours.

A maximum dosage of 12mg/kg every 72 hours should not be exceeded in children in the first two weeks of life. For children between 3 and 4 weeks of life, 12mg/kg every 48 hours should not be exceeded.

To facilitate accurate measurement of doses less than 10mg, Diflucan should only be administered to children in hospital using the 50mg/5ml suspension orally or the intravenous infusion, depending on the clinical condition of the child. A suitable measuring device should be used for administration of the suspension. Once reconstituted the suspension should not be further diluted.

Use in the elderly The normal dose should be used if there is no evidence of renal impairment. In patients with renal impairment (creatinine clearance less than 50ml/min) the dosage schedule should be adjusted as described below.

Use in patients with impaired renal function Fluconazole is excreted predominantly in the urine as unchanged drug. No adjustments in single dose therapy are required. In patients (including children) with impaired renal function who will receive multiple doses of Diflucan, the normal recommended dose (according to indication) should be given on day 1, followed by a daily dose based on the following table:

Creatinine clearance (ml/min)	***Percent of recommended dose***
>50	100%
≤50 (no dialysis)	50%
Regular dialysis	100% after each dialysis

Compatibility of intravenous infusion

Although further dilution is unnecessary Diflucan Intravenous Infusion is compatible with the following administration fluids:

a) Dextrose 20%

b) Ringer's solution

c) Hartmann's solution

d) Potassium chloride in dextrose

e) Sodium bicarbonate 4.2%

f) Normal saline (0.9%)

Diflucan may be infused through an existing line with one of the above listed fluids. No specific incompatibilities have been noted, although mixing with any other drug prior to infusion is not recommended.

4.3 Contraindications
Diflucan should not be used in patients with known hypersensitivity to fluconazole or to related azole compounds or any other ingredient in the formulation.

Fluconazole should not be co-adminstered with cisapride or terfenadine which are known to both prolong the QT – interval and are metabolised by CYP3A4 (See "Interactions with other medicinal products and other forms of interaction").

4.4 Special warnings and precautions for use
In some patients, particularly those with serious underlying diseases such as AIDS and cancer, abnormalities in haematological, hepatic, renal and other biochemical function test results have been observed during treatment with Diflucan but the clinical significance and relationship to treatment is uncertain.

Very rarely, patients who died with severe underlying disease and who had received multiple doses of Diflucan had post-mortem findings which included hepatic necrosis. These patients were receiving multiple concomitant medications, some known to be potentially hepatotoxic, and/or had underlying diseases which could have caused the hepatic necrosis.

In cases of hepatotoxicity, no obvious relationship to total daily dose of Diflucan, duration of therapy, sex or age of the patient has been observed; the abnormalities have usually been reversible on discontinuation of Diflucan therapy.

As a causal relationship with Diflucan cannot be excluded, patients who develop abnormal liver function tests during Diflucan therapy should be monitored for the development of more serious hepatic injury. Diflucan should be discontinued if clinical signs or symptoms consistent with liver disease develop during treatment with Diflucan.

Patients have rarely developed exfoliative cutaneous reactions, such as Stevens-Johnson Syndrome and toxic epidermal necrolysis, during treatment with fluconazole. AIDS patients are more prone to the development of severe cutaneous reactions to many drugs. If a rash develops in a patient treated for a superficial fungal infection which is considered attributable to Diflucan, further therapy with this agent should be discontinued. If patients with invasive/systemic fungal infections develop rashes, they should be monitored closely and Diflucan discontinued if bullous lesions or erythema multiforme develop.

In rare cases, as with other azoles, anaphylaxis has been reported.

Some azoles, including fluconazole, have been associated with prolongation of the QT interval on the electrocardiogram. During post-marketing surveillance, there have been very rare cases of QT prolongation and torsade de pointes in patients taking fluconazole. Although the association of fluconazole and QT-prolongation has not been fully established, fluconazole should be used with caution in patients with potentially proarrythmic conditions such as:

- Congenital or documented acquired QT prolongation
- Cardiomyopathy, in particular when heart failure is present
- Sinus bradycardia
- Existing symptomatic arrythmias
- Concomitant medication not metabolized by CY34A but known to prolong QT interval
- Electrolyte disturbances such as hypokalaemia, hypomagnesaemia and hypocalaemia

(See Section 4.5 Interactions with other medical products and other forms of interaction)

4.5 Interaction with other medicinal products and other forms of interaction
The following drug interactions relate to the use of multiple-dose fluconazole, and the relevance to single-dose 150mg fluconazole has not yet been established.

Rifampicin Concomitant administration of fluconazole and rifampicin resulted in a 25% decrease in the AUC and 20% shorter half-life of fluconazole. In patients receiving concomitant rifampicin, an increase in the fluconazole dose should be considered.

Hydrochlorothiazide In a kinetic interaction study, co-administration of multiple-dose hydrochlorothiazide to healthy volunteers receiving fluconazole increased plasma concentrations of fluconazole by 40%. An effect of this magnitude should not necessitate a change in the fluconazole dose regimen in subjects receiving concomitant diuretics, although the prescriber should bear it in mind.

Anticoagulants In an interaction study, fluconazole increased the prothrombin time (12%) after warfarin administration in healthy males. In post-marketing experience, as with other azole antifungals, bleeding events (bruising, epistaxis, gastrointestinal bleeding, hematuria and melaena) have been reported in association with increases in prothrombin time in patients receiving fluconazole concurrently with warfarin. Prothrombin time in patients receiving coumarin-type anticoagulants should be carefully monitored.

Benzodiazepines (Short Acting) Following oral administration of midazolam, fluconazole resulted in substantial increases in midazolam concentrations and psychomotor effects. This effect on midazolam appears to be more pronounced following oral administration of fluconazole than with fluconazole administered intravenously. If concomitant benzodiazepine therapy is necessary in patients being treated with fluconazole, consideration should be given to decreasing the benzodiazepine dosage and the patients should be appropriately monitored.

Sulphonylureas Fluconazole has been shown to prolong the serum half-life of concomitantly administered oral sulphonylureas (chlorpropamide, glibenclamide, glipizide and tolbutamide) in healthy volunteers. Fluconazole and oral sulphonylureas may be co-administered to diabetic patients, but the possibility of a hypoglycaemic episode should be borne in mind.

Phenytoin Concomitant administration of fluconazole and phenytoin may increase the levels of phenytoin to a clinically significant degree. If it is necessary to administer both drugs concomitantly, phenytoin levels should be monitored and the phenytoin dose adjusted to maintain therapeutic levels.

Oral contraceptives Two kinetic studies with combined oral contraceptives have been performed using multiple doses of fluconazole. There were no relevant effects on either hormone level in the 50mg fluconazole study, while at 200mg daily the AUCs of ethinyloestradiol and levonorgestrel were increased 40% and 24% respectively. Thus multiple dose use of fluconazole at these doses is unlikely to have an effect on the efficacy of the combined oral contraceptive.

In a 300 mg once weekly fluconazole study, the AUCs of ethinyl estradiol and norethindrone were increased by 24% and 13%, respectively.

Endogenous steroid Fluconazole 50mg daily does not affect endogenous steroid levels in females: 200-400mg daily has no clinically significant effect on endogenous steroid levels or on ACTH stimulated response in healthy male volunteers.

Ciclosporin A kinetic study in renal transplant patients found fluconazole 200mg daily to slowly increase ciclosporin concentrations. However, in another multiple dose study with 100mg daily, fluconazole did not affect ciclosporin levels in patients with bone marrow transplants. Ciclosporin plasma concentration monitoring in patients receiving fluconazole is recommended.

Theophylline In a placebo controlled interaction study, the administration of fluconazole 200mg for 14 days resulted in an 18% decrease in the mean plasma clearance of theophylline. Patients who are receiving high doses of theophylline or who are otherwise at increased risk for theophylline toxicity should be observed for signs of theophylline toxicity while receiving fluconazole, and the therapy modified appropriately if signs of toxicity develop.

Terfenadine Because of the occurrence of serious dysrhythmias secondary to prolongation of the QTc interval in patients receiving other azole antifungals in conjunction with terfenadine, interactions studies have been performed. One study at a 200mg daily dose of fluconazole failed to demonstrate a prolongation in QTc interval. Another study at a 400mg and 800mg daily dose of fluconazole demonstrated that fluconazole taken in multiple doses of 400mg per day or greater significantly increased plasma levels of terfenadine when taken concomitantly. There have been spontaneously reported cases of palpitations, tachycardia, dizziness, and chest pain in patients taking concomitant fluconazole and terfenadine where the relationship of the reported adverse events to drug therapy or underlying medical conditions was not clear. Because of the potential seriousness of such an interaction, it is recommended that terfenadine not be taken in combination with fluconazole. (See "Contra-indications".)

Cisapride There have been reports of cardiac events including torsades de pointes in patients to whom fluconazole and cisapride were co-administered. A controlled study found that concomitant fluconazole 200 mg once daily and cisapride 20 mg four times a day yielded a significant increase in cisapride plasma levels and prolongation of QTc interval. In most of these cases, the patients appear to have been predisposed to arrhythmias or had serious underlying illnesses, and the relationship of the reported events to a possible fluconazole-cisapride drug interaction is unclear. Because of the potential seriousness of such an interaction, co-administration of cisapride is contra-indicated in patients receiving fluconazole. (See "Contra-indications".)

Zidovudine Two kinetic studies resulted in increased levels of zidovudine most likely caused by the decreased conversion of zidovudine to its major metabolite. One study determined zidovudine levels in AIDS or ARC patients before and following fluconazole 200mg daily for 15 days. There was a significant increase in zidovudine AUC (20%). A second randomised, two-period, two-treatment cross-over study examined zidovudine levels in HIV infected patients. On two occasions, 21 days apart, patients received zidovudine 200mg every eight hours either with or without fluconazole 400mg daily for seven days. The AUC of zidovudine significantly increased (74%) during co-administration with fluconazole. Patients receiving this combination should be monitored for the development of zidovudine-related adverse reactions.

Rifabutin There have been reports that an interaction exists when fluconazole is administered concomitantly with rifabutin, leading to increased serum levels of rifabutin. There have been reports of uveitis in patients to whom fluconazole and rifabutin were co-administered. Patients receiving rifabutin and fluconazole concomitantly should be carefully monitored.

Tacrolimus There have been reports that an interaction exists when fluconazole is administered concomitantly with tacrolimus, leading to increased serum levels of tacrolimus. There have been reports of nephrotoxicity in patients to whom fluconazole and tacrolimus were co-administered. Patients receiving tacrolimus and fluconazole concomitantly should be carefully monitored.

The use of fluconazole in patients concurrently taking astemizole or other drugs metabolised by the cytochrome P450 system may be associated with elevations in serum levels of these drugs. In the absence of definitive information, caution should be used when co-administering fluconazole. This is particularly important for drugs known to prolong QT interval. Patients should be carefully monitored.

Interaction studies have shown that when oral fluconazole is co-administered with food, cimetidine, antacids or following total body irradiation for bone marrow transplantation, no clinically significant impairment of fluconazole absorption occurs.

Physicians should be aware that drug-drug interaction studies with other medications have not been conducted, but that such interactions may occur.

4.6 Pregnancy and lactation
Use during pregnancy There are no adequate and well controlled studies in pregnant women. There have been reports of multiple congenital abnormalities in infants whose mothers were being treated for 3 or more months with high dose (400-800 mg/day) fluconazole therapy for coccidioidomycosis. The relationship between fluconazole and these events is unclear.

Accordingly, Diflucan should not be used in pregnancy, or in women of childbearing potential unless adequate contraception is employed.

Use during lactation Fluconazole is found in human breast milk at concentrations similar to plasma, hence its use in nursing mothers is not recommended.

4.7 Effects on ability to drive and use machines
Experience with Diflucan indicates that therapy is unlikely to impair a patient's ability to drive or use machinery.

4.8 Undesirable effects
Fluconazole is generally well tolerated. The most common undesirable effects observed during clinical trials and associated with fluconazole are:

Nervous System Disorders: Headache.

Skin and Subcutaneous Tissue Disorders: Rash.

Gastrointestinal Disorders: Abdominal pain, diarrhoea, flatulence, nausea.

In some patients, particularly those with serious underlying diseases such as AIDS and cancer, changes in renal and haematological function test results and hepatic abnormalities have been observed during treatment with fluconazole and comparative agents, but the clinical significance and relationship to treatment is uncertain (see Section 4.4 "Special warnings and special precautions for use").

Hepatobiliary Disorders: Hepatic toxicity including rare cases of fatalities, elevated alkaline phosphatase, elevated bilirubin, elevated SGOT, elevated SGPT.

In addition, the following undesirable effects have occurred during post-marketing:

Nervous System Disorders: Dizziness, seizures, taste perversion.

Skin and Subcutaneous Tissue Disorders: Alopecia, exfoliative skin disorders including Stevens-Johnson syndrome and toxic epidermal necrolysis.

Gastrointestinal Disorders: Dyspepsia, vomiting.

Blood and Lymphatic System Disorders: Leukopenia including neutropenia and agranulocytosis, thrombocytopenia.

Immune System Disorders:

Allegic reaction: Anaphylaxis(including angioedema, face oedema, pruritus), urticaria.

Hepatobiliary Disorders: Hepatic failure, hepatitis, hepatocellular necrosis, jaundice.

Metabolism and Nutrition Disorders: Hypercholesterolaemia, hypertriglyceridaemia, hypokalaemia.

Cardiac Disorders: QT prolongation, torsade de pointes (see section 4.4 Special Warnings and Special Precautions for Use).

4.9 Overdose
There have been reports of overdosage with fluconazole and in one case, a 42 year-old patient infected with human immunodeficiency virus developed hallucinations and exhibited paranoid behaviour after reportedly ingesting 8200mg of fluconazole, unverified by his physician. The patient was admitted to the hospital and his condition resolved within 48 hours.

In the event of overdosage, supportive measures and symptomatic treatment, with gastric lavage if necessary, may be adequate.

As fluconazole is largely excreted in the urine, forced volume diuresis would probably increase the elimination rate. A three hour haemodialysis session decreases plasma levels by approximately 50%.

5. PHARMACOLOGICAL PROPERTIES

5.1 Pharmacodynamic properties

Pharmacotherapeutic group: Triazole derivatives, ATC code J02AC.

Fluconazole, a member of the triazole class of antifungal agents, is a potent and selective inhibitor of fungal enzymes necessary for the synthesis of ergosterol.

Fluconazole shows little pharmacological activity in a wide range of animal studies. Some prolongation of pentobarbital sleeping times in mice (p.o.), increased mean arterial and left ventricular blood pressure and increased heart rate in anaesthetised cats (i.v.) occurred. Inhibition of rat ovarian aromatase was observed at high concentrations.

Both orally and intravenously administered fluconazole was active in a variety of animal fungal infection models. Activity has been demonstrated against opportunistic mycoses, such as infections with *Candida* spp. including systemic candidiasis in immunocompromised animals; with *Cryptococcus neoformans*, including intracranial infections; with *Microsporum* spp. and with *Trichophyton* spp. Fluconazole has also been shown to be active in animal models of endemic mycoses, including infections with *Blastomyces dermatitides;* with *Coccidioides immitis,* including intracranial infection and with *Histoplasma capsulatum* in normal and immunosuppressed animals.

There have been reports of cases of superinfection with *Candida* species other than *C. albicans*, which are often inherently not susceptible to fluconazole (e.g. *Candida krusei*). Such cases may require alternative antifungal therapy.

Fluconazole is highly specific for fungal cytochrome P-450 dependent enzymes. Fluconazole 50mg daily given up to 28 days has been shown not to affect testosterone plasma concentrations in males or steroid concentrations in females of child-bearing age. Fluconazole 200-400mg daily has no clinically significant effect on endogenous steroid levels or on ACTH stimulated response in healthy male volunteers. Interaction studies with antipyrine indicate that single or multiple doses of fluconazole 50mg do not affect its metabolism.

The efficacy of fluconazole in tinea capitis has been studied in 2 randomised controlled trials in a total of 878 patients comparing fluconazole with griseofulvin. Fluconazole at 6 mg/kg/day for 6 weeks was not superior to griseofulvin administered at 11 mg/kg/day for 6 weeks. The overall success rate at week 6 was low (fluconazole 6 weeks: 18.3%; fluconazole 3 weeks: 14.7%; griseofulvin: 17.7%) across all treatment groups. These findings are not inconsistent with the natural history of tinea capitis without therapy.

5.2 Pharmacokinetic properties

The pharmacokinetic properties of fluconazole are similar following administration by the intravenous or oral route. After oral administration fluconazole is well absorbed and plasma levels (and systemic bioavailability) are over 90% of the levels achieved after intravenous administration. Oral absorption is not affected by concomitant food intake. Peak plasma concentrations in the fasting state occur between 0.5 and 1.5 hours post-dose with a plasma elimination half-life of approximately 30 hours. Plasma concentrations are proportional to dose. Ninety percent steady-state levels are reached by day 4 -5 with multiple once daily dosing.

Administration of a loading dose (on day 1) of twice the usual daily dose enables plasma levels to approximate to 90% steady-state levels by day 2. The apparent volume of distribution approximates to total body water. Plasma protein binding is low (11-12%).

Fluconazole achieves good penetration in all body fluids studied. The levels of fluconazole in saliva and sputum are similar to plasma levels. In patients with fungal meningitis, fluconazole levels in the CSF are approximately 80% of the corresponding plasma levels.

High skin concentrations of fluconazole, above serum concentrations, are achieved in the stratum corneum, epidermis-dermis and eccrine sweat. Fluconazole accumulates in the stratum corneum. At a dose of 50mg once daily, the concentration of fluconazole after 12 days was 73 microgram/g and 7 days after cessation of treatment the concentration was still 5.8 microgram/g.

The major route of excretion is renal, with approximately 80% of the administered dose appearing in the urine as unchanged drug. Fluconazole clearance is proportional to creatinine clearance. There is no evidence of circulating metabolites.

The long plasma elimination half-life provides the basis for single dose therapy for genital candidiasis and once daily dosing for other indications.

A study compared the saliva and plasma concentrations of a single fluconazole 100mg dose administration in a capsule or in an oral suspension by rinsing and retaining in mouth for 2 minutes and swallowing. The maximum concentration of fluconazole in saliva after the suspension was observed 5 minutes after ingestion, and was 182 times higher than the maximum saliva concentration after the capsule which occurred 4 hours after ingestion. After about 4 hours, the saliva concentrations of fluconazole were similar. The mean AUC (0-96) in saliva was significantly greater after the suspension compared to the capsule. There was no significant difference in the elimination rate from saliva or the plasma pharmacokinetic parameters for the two formulations.

Pharmacokinetics in Children

In children, the following pharmacokinetic data have been reported:

(see Table 1 below)

In premature new-borns (gestational age around 28 weeks), intravenous administration of fluconazole of 6mg/kg was given every third day for a maximum of five doses while the premature new-borns remained in the intensive care unit. The mean half-life (hours) was 74 (range 44-185) on day 1 which decreased with time to a mean of 53 (range 30-131) on day 7 and 47 (range 27-68) on day 13.

The area under the curve (microgram.h/ml) was 271 (range 173-385) on day 1 and increased with a mean of 490 (range 292-734) on day 7 and decreased with a mean of 360 (range 167-566) on day 13.

The volume of distribution (ml/kg) was 1183 (range 1070-1470) on day 1 and increased with time to a mean of 1184 (range 510-2130) on day 7 and 1328 (range 1040-1680) on day 13.

5.3 Preclinical safety data

Reproductive Toxicity Increases in fetal anatomical variants (supernumerary ribs, renal pelvis dilation) and delays in ossification were observed at 25 and 50mg/kg and higher doses. At doses ranging from 80mg/kg (approximately 20-60x the recommended human dose) to 320mg/kg embryolethality in rats was increased and fetal abnormalities included wavy ribs, cleft palate and abnormal craniofacial ossification. These effects are consistent with the inhibition of oestrogen synthesis in rats and may be a result of known effects of lowered oestrogen on pregnancy, organogenesis and parturition.

Carcinogenesis Fluconazole showed no evidence of carcinogenic potential in mice and rats treated orally for 24 months at doses of 2.5, 5 or 10mg/kg/day. Male rats treated with 5 and 10mg/kg/day had an increased incidence of hepatocellular adenomas.

Mutagenesis Fluconazole, with or without metabolic activation, was negative in tests for mutagenicity in 4 strains of S.typhimurium and in the mouse lymphoma L5178Y system. Cytogenetic studies in vivo (murine bone marrow cells, following oral administration of fluconazole) and in vitro (human lymphocytes exposed to fluconazole at 1000μg/ml) showed no evidence of chromosomal mutations.

Impairment of fertility Fluconazole did not affect the fertility of male or female rats treated orally with daily doses of 5, 10 or 20mg/kg or with parenteral doses of 5, 25 or 75mg/kg, although the onset of parturition was slightly delayed at 20mg/kg p.o. In an intravenous perinatal study in rats at 5, 20 and 40mg/kg, dystocia and prolongation of parturition were observed in a few dams at 20mg/kg and 40mg/kg, but not at 5mg/kg. The disturbances in parturition were reflected by a slight increase in the number of still-born pups and decrease of neonatal survival at these dose levels. The effects on parturition in rats are consistent with the species specific oestrogen-lowering property produced by high doses of fluconazole. Such a hormone change has not been observed in women treated with fluconazole.

6. PHARMACEUTICAL PARTICULARS

6.1 List of excipients

Diflucan Capsules (all strengths) contain lactose, maize starch, colloidal silicon dioxide, magnesium stearate and sodium lauryl sulphate as excipients.

In addition, capsule shells contain:

50mg - patent blue V (E131), titanium dioxide (E171) and gelatin.

200mg - titanium dioxide (E171), erythrosine (E127), indigotine (E132) and gelatin.

Diflucan Intravenous Infusion is a sterile aqueous solution which is made iso-osmotic with sodium chloride.

Diflucan Powder for Oral Suspension contains sucrose (2.88g per 50mg dose; 2.73g per 200mg dose), colloidal silicon dioxide, titanium dioxide, xanthan gum, sodium citrate dihydrate, citric acid anhydrous, sodium benzoate and natural orange flavour.

6.2 Incompatibilities

No specific incompatibilities have been noted.

6.3 Shelf life

Current stability data support a shelf life of 5 years for the capsules, 5 years for the intravenous infusion and 2 years for the dry powder for oral suspension. There is a use period of 14 days for the reconstituted suspension.

6.4 Special precautions for storage

Store below 30°C.

Reconstituted suspension should be stored at 5°C - 30°C.

Do not freeze reconstituted suspension or intravenous infusion.

6.5 Nature and contents of container

Diflucan Capsules will be supplied in clear or opaque PVC blister packs with aluminium foil backing, as follows:

7 × 50mg or 200mg Diflucan capsules for multiple dose therapy.

Diflucan Intravenous Infusion will be supplied in clear Type I glass infusion vials (25 or 100ml) sealed with rubber bungs on crimping with aluminium over-caps.

Diflucan Powder for Oral Suspension will be supplied in high density polyethylene bottles with child resistant closures, containing 35ml of suspension (50mg/5ml or 200mg/5ml) on reconstitution with 24ml of water.

6.6 Special precautions for disposal and other handling

Diflucan Capsules should be swallowed whole.

Diflucan Intravenous Infusion Do not freeze. The infusion does not contain any preservative. It is for single use only. Discard any remaining solution.

To reconstitute the ***Diflucan Powder for Oral Suspension***: Tap the bottle to loosen powder. Add 24ml of water. Shake well. Shake immediately prior to use. Where doses of less than 5ml are required, a suitable measuring device should be used. Dilution is not appropriate.

7. MARKETING AUTHORISATION HOLDER

Pfizer Limited

Sandwich

Kent CT13 9NJ

United Kingdom

8. MARKETING AUTHORISATION NUMBER(S)

Diflucan Capsules 50mg PL 00057/0289

Diflucan Capsules 200mg PL 00057/0317

Diflucan Intravenous Infusion 2mg/ml PL 00057/0315

Diflucan Powder for Oral Suspension 50mg/5ml PL 00057/0343

Diflucan Powder for Oral Suspension 200mg/5ml PL 00057/0344

9. DATE OF FIRST AUTHORISATION/RENEWAL OF THE AUTHORISATION

Diflucan Capsules 50mg	11 January 2000
Diflucan Capsules 200mg	30 May 1996
Diflucan IV Infusion	24 November 1994
Diflucan POS	18 December 1996

10. DATE OF REVISION OF THE TEXT

April 2007

Table 1

Age Studied	Dose (mg/kg)	Half-life (hours)	AUC (microgram.h/ml)
11 days- 11 months	Single-IV 3mg/kg	23	110.1
9 months- 13 years	Single-Oral 2mg/kg	25.0	94.7
9 months- 13 years	Single-Oral 8mg/kg	19.5	362.5
5 years- 15 years	Multiple IV 2mg/kg	17.4*	67.4
5 years- 15 years	Multiple IV 4mg/kg	15.2*	139.1
5 years- 15 years	Multiple IV 8mg/kg	17.6*	196.7
Mean Age 7 Years	Multiple Oral 3mg/kg	15.5	41.6

* Denotes final day

Legal Category
POM

Company Reference: DF12_0

DIGIBIND*

(GlaxoSmithKline UK)

DATA SHEET

DIGIBIND*

DIGOXIN-SPECIFIC ANTIBODY FRAGMENTS (FAB)

Presentation Each vial of Digibind contains a sterile, lyophilised, crystalline off-white powder, comprising 38 mg of antigen-binding fragments (Fab) derived from specific anti-digoxin antibodies raised in sheep, approximately 75 mg Sorbitol BP and approximately 28 mg Sodium Chloride BP.

Uses Digibind is indicated for the treatment of known or strongly suspected digoxin or digitoxin toxicity, where measures beyond the withdrawal of the digitalis glycoside and correction of any serum electrolyte abnormality are felt to be necessary.

Dosage and administration

Dosage: The dosage of Digibind varies according to the amount of digoxin (or digitoxin) to be neutralised. The average dose used during clinical testing was 10 vials. When determining the dose for Digibind, the following guidelines should be considered:

• Dosage estimates are based on a steady-state volume of distribution of 5 l/kg for digoxin (0.5 l/kg for digitoxin) to convert serum digitalis concentration to the amount of digitalis in the body. These volumes are population averages and vary widely among individuals. Many patients may require higher doses for complete neutralisation. Doses should ordinarily be rounded up to the next whole vial.

• Erroneous calculations may result from inaccurate estimates of the amount of digitalis ingested or absorbed or from non steady-state serum digitalis concentrations. Inaccurate serum digitalis concentration measurements are a possible source of error; this is especially so for very high values, since most digoxin assay kits are not designed to measure values above 5 nanogram/ml.

• If after several hours toxicity has not adequately reversed or appears to recur, re-administration of Digibind at a dose guided by clinical judgement may be required.

Acute ingestion of unknown amount of glycoside: Adults and children over 20 kg: If a patient presents with potentially life-threatening digitalis toxicity after acute ingestion of an unknown amount of digoxin or digitoxin, and neither a serum digoxin concentration nor an estimate of the ingested amount of glycoside is available, 20 vials of Digibind can be administered. This amount will be adequate to treat most life-threatening ingestions in adults and large children.

As an alternative, the physician may consider administering 10 vials of Digibind, observing the patient's response, and following with an additional 10 vials if clinically indicated.

Infants and children ⩽ 20 kg: In infants and small children (⩽ 20 kg) with potentially life- threatening digitalis toxicity after acute ingestion of an unknown amount of digoxin or digitoxin, when neither a serum concentration nor an estimate of the ingested amount is available, clinical judgement must be exercised to estimate an appropriate number of vials of Digibind to administer.

This estimate should be based on the maximum likely total body load of glycoside and the neutralising capacity of Digibind (one vial of Digibind per 0.5 mg of digoxin or digitoxin). It is important to monitor for volume overload during administration of Digibind.

Acute ingestion of known amount of glycoside: Each vial of Digibind contains 38 mg of purified digoxin-specific Fab fragments which will bind approximately 0.5 mg of digoxin or digitoxin. Thus one can calculate the total number of vials required by dividing the total digitalis body load in mg by 0.5 (see formula 1).

Table 3: Infants and Small Children Dose Estimates of Digibind (in mg) from Steady-State Serum Digoxin Concentration

Patient Weight (kg)	Serum Digoxin Concentration (ng/ml)						
	1	2	4	8	12	16	20
1	0.4mg*	1mg*	1.5mg*	3mg	5mg	6mg	8mg
3	1mg*	2mg*	5mg	9mg	14mg	18mg	23mg
5	2mg*	4mg	8mg	15mg	23mg	30mg	38mg
10	4mg	8mg	15mg	30mg	46mg	61mg	76mg
20	8mg	15mg	30mg	61mg	91mg	122mg	152mg

* Dilution of reconstituted vial to 1 mg/ml may be desirable.

Formula 1

$$\text{Dose (in number of vials)} = \frac{\text{Total body load (mg)}}{0.5}$$

For toxicity from an acute ingestion, total body load in milligrams will be approximately equal to the amount ingested in milligrams for digitoxin, or the amount ingested in milligrams multiplied by 0.80 (to account for incomplete absorption) for digoxin. Table 1 gives Digibind doses based on an estimate of the number of digoxin tablets (0.25 mg) ingested as a single dose and is applicable to children or adults.

TABLE 1: Approximate Digibind Dose for Reversal of a Single Large Digoxin Overdose

Number of Digoxin Tablets*	Digibind dose number of vials
25	10
50	20
75	30
100	40
150	60
200	80

* 0.25 mg tablets with 80% bioavailability.

Toxicity during chronic therapy: Adults and children over 20 kg: In adults and children over 20 kg with digitalis toxicity resulting from chronic digoxin or digitoxin therapy and for whom a steady-state serum concentration is not available, a dose of 6 vials of Digibind will usually be adequate to reverse toxicity.

Table 2 gives dosage estimates in number of vials for adult patients for whom a steady-state serum digoxin concentration is known. The Digibind dose (in number of vials) represented in Table 2 can be approximated using the following formula:

Formula 2

$$\text{Dose (in number of vials)} = \frac{\text{(serum digoxin concentration in ng/ml x weight in kg)}}{100}$$

TABLE 2: Adult Dose Estimate of Digibind (in number of vials) from Steady-State Serum Digoxin Concentration

(see Table 2 below)

In patients for whom a steady-state serum digitoxin concentration is known the Digibind dose (in number of vials) can be approximated using the following formula:

Formula 3

$$\text{Dose (in number of vials)} = \frac{\text{(serum digitoxin concentration in ng/ml x weight in kg)}}{1000}$$

Infants and children ⩽ 20kg: In infants and small children with toxicity resulting from chronic digoxin or digitoxin therapy and for whom a steady-state serum concentration is not available, a dose of one vial of Digibind will usually suffice.

Clinical experience in children has indicated that the calculation of dose of Digibind from steady-state serum digoxin concentration may be carried out as for adults.

Table 3 (see next page) gives dosage estimates in milligrams for infants and small children based on the steady-state serum digoxin concentration. The Digibind dose represented in Table 3 can be estimated by multiplying the dose (in number of vials) calculated from Formula 2, by the amount of Digibind contained in a vial (38 mg/vial).

Formula 4

$$\text{Dose (in mg)} = 38 \times \text{dose (in number of vials)}$$

TABLE 3: Infants and Small Children Dose Estimates of Digibind (in mg) from Steady-State Serum Digoxin Concentration

(see Table 3 above)

For very small doses, it may be necessary to dilute the reconstituted vial with sterile isotonic saline to achieve a concentration of 1 mg/ml, and to administer the dose with a tuberculin syringe.

Use in the elderly: Clinical experience has indicated that Digibind is effective and that calculation of dose may be carried out as for adults.

Use in renal impairment: See Precautions.

Administration: The contents of each vial to be used should be dissolved in 4 ml of sterile Water for Injections BP, by gentle mixing, thus producing an approximately isosmotic solution with a protein concentration of between 8.5 and 10.5mg/ml. This may be diluted further to any convenient volume with sterile saline suitable for infusion.

The final solution of Digibind should be infused intravenously over a 30 minute period. Infusion through a 0.22 micron membrane filter is recommended to remove any incompletely dissolved aggregates of Digibind. If cardiac arrest seems imminent, Digibind can be given as a bolus intravenous injection.

Pharmacology: The affinity constant (K_D) of Fab for digoxin is high ($10^{11}M^{-1}$) and greater than that of digoxin for its receptor (Na-K ATPase). The affinity constant of Fab for digitoxin is also high (fifteen fold lower than for digoxin). Digoxin and digitoxin are therefore attracted away from the receptor on heart tissue (and presumably other tissues as well, though this has not been studied) and their rate of elimination is changed from that governed by the kinetics of receptor binding to that governed by the kinetics of access and elimination of Fab.

In dogs, anti-digoxin Fab reverses arrhythmic manifestations of digoxin toxicity much more quickly than does IgG. There is a suggestion that reversal of inotropy with Fab lags behind reversal of cardiac electrophysiological effects.

The plasma elimination (β) half-life of ovine digoxin-specific Fab in the baboon is 9 to l3h and that of the parent IgG antibody is 61h. The total volume of distribution of Digibind in the baboon appears to be about 9 times greater than that of IgG and more ready diffusion of the smaller moiety sufficiently accounts for this.

About 93% of radioactively labelled Fab, injected into baboons, was recovered in the urine within 24h and the corresponding amount of recoverable digoxin-specific IgG was less than 1%. Much of the urinary Fab was not intact; after glomerular filtration, low molecular weight proteins are taken into proximal renal tubular cells and catabolised.

Corresponding information on human patients is sparse, but the close relationship of therapeutic performance to predictions suggest that the animal data will be helpful. The human plasma elimination half-life after intravenous administration of Digibind is about l6 to 20h with good renal function.

Ordinarily, following administration of Digibind, improvements in signs and symptoms of digitalis intoxication begins within 30 minutes.

Contra-indications, warnings, etc

Contra-indications: None known.

Precautions: Failure to respond to Digibind raises the possibility that the clinical problem is not caused by digitalis intoxication. If there is no response to an adequate dose of Digibind, the diagnosis of digitalis toxicity should be questioned.

Although allergic reactions have been reported rarely, the possibility of anaphylactic, hypersensitive or febrile reactions should be borne in mind. The likelihood of an allergic

Table 2: Adult Dose Estimate of Digibind (in number of vials) from Steady-State Serum Digoxin Concentration

Patient Weight (kg)	Serum Digoxin Concentration (ng/ml)						
	1	2	4	8	12	16	20
40	0.5v	1v	2v	3v	5v	7v	8v
60	0.5v	1v	3v	5v	7v	10v	12v
70	1v	2v	3v	6v	9v	11v	14v
80	1v	2v	3v	7v	10v	13v	16v
100	1v	2v	4v	8v	12v	16v	20v

v = vials

reaction is distinctly greater where there is a history of allergy to antibiotics or asthma. Since papain is used to cleave the whole antibody into Fab and Fc fragments, and traces of papain or inactivated papain residues may be present in Digibind, patients with known allergies to papain, chymopapain or other papaya extracts would be at particular risk, as would those allergic to ovine proteins. However, as the Fab fragment of the antibody lacks the antigenic determinants of the Fc fragment it should present less of an immunogenic threat to patients than does an intact immunoglobulin molecule.

Many patients with mild or moderate renal dysfunction and some with severe renal dysfunction have been treated successfully with Digibind. There has been no evidence that administration of Digibind to patients with renal dysfunction will exacerbate that dysfunction; the dominant pattern of serial serum creatinine measurements has been one of stable or improved renal function after Digibind administration. The time course and general pattern of therapeutic effect have not been different in patients with severe renal dysfunction, although excretion of the Fab-digoxin complexes from the body is slowed in this situation. A theoretical possibility exists that digoxin could be released after some days from Fab-digoxin complexes which remained in the circulation because their excretion was prevented by renal failure. However, this phenomenon has proved to be rare.

Patients previously dependent on the inotropism of digoxin may develop signs of heart failure when treated with Digibind. After successful management of poisoning, digoxin has had to be reinstituted in some cases. If deemed absolutely necessary, additional inotropic support can be obtained from a non-glycoside inotropic drug such as dopamine or dobutamine, but caution is required as catecholamines and catecholamine analogues can aggravate arrhythmias caused by cardiac glycosides.

Parenteral drug products should be inspected visually for particulate matter and discoloration prior to administration, whenever solution and container permit.

Monitoring and laboratory tests: Patients should have continuous electrocardiographic monitoring during and for at least 24 hours after administration of Digibind.

Presence of the exogenous antibody fragments will interfere with radioimmunoassay measurements of digoxin.

The total serum digoxin concentration may rise precipitously following administration of Digibind, but this will be almost entirely bound to the Fab fragment and therefore not able to react with receptors in the body.

Serum potassium concentrations should be followed carefully, since severe digitalis intoxication can cause life-threatening elevation in serum potassium concentration by shifting it from within the cells. When the effect of digitalis is reversed by Digibind, potassium returns to the cell causing the serum potassium concentrations to fall. It is possible for there to be a total body deficit of potassium in the presence of digitalis toxicity-induced hyperkalaemia and Digibind treatment could result in a significant hypokalaemia.

Side- and adverse effects: Allergic responses of possible or probable attribution to Digibind have been reported rarely. The development of a pruritic rash (either with or without facial flushing and swelling) or shaking or chills without fever, have occurred on the day of treatment. Urticaria and thrombocytopenia have occurred up to 16 days post treatment. There are no reports of any allergic reactions to re-administration of Digibind in the same patient, but there are few instances on which information is available.

Use in pregnancy and lactation: To date there is no evidence that Digibind administered during human pregnancy causes foetal abnormalities; however, the use of Digibind should be considered only if the expected clinical benefit of treatment to the mother outweighs any possible risk to the developing foetus.

Carcinogenesis, mutagenesis, impairment of fertility: There have been no long-term studies performed in animals to evaluate carcinogenic or mutagenic potential or effects on fertility.

Drug interactions: No drug interactions have been identified.

Toxicity and treatment of overdosage: Not relevant.

Pharmaceutical precautions Store between 2 & 8°C. Protect from light. After reconstitution store between 2 and 8°C for up to 4 hours.

Reconstituted product should be used promptly. If it is not used immediately, it may be stored under refrigeration between 2 and 8°C for up to 4 hours. The reconstituted product may be diluted with sterile isotonic saline to a convenient volume.

Legal category POM.

Package quantities Single vial of lyophilised powder containing 38 mg of antigen-binding fragments (Fab).

Further information Digoxin-specific antibody Fab fragments have been used successfully to treat a case of lanatoside C intoxication. Reversal of ß-methyl digoxin and ß-acetyl digoxin-induced arrhythmias by Digibind has been verified in guinea-pigs.

Product licence number 00003/0207

Product licence holder

The Wellcome Foundation Limited
Glaxo Wellcome House
Berkeley Avenue
Greenford
Middlesex
UB6 0NN

Trading as GlaxoSmithKline UK, Stockley Park West, Uxbridge, Middlesex UB11 1BT

Date of Revision of Text: 2 April 2003

Digitoxin Tablets BP 100mcg (UCB Pharma Limited)

(UCB Pharma Limited)

1. NAME OF THE MEDICINAL PRODUCT
Digitoxin Tablets BP 100 micrograms.

2. QUALITATIVE AND QUANTITATIVE COMPOSITION
Digitoxin BP 0.10 mg.

3. PHARMACEUTICAL FORM
White, biconvex uncoated tablets, engraved EVANS 128 on one side and plain on the obverse.

4. CLINICAL PARTICULARS
4.1 Therapeutic indications
Digitoxin tablets are indicated in the treatment of heart failure and supraventricular arrhythmias particularly atrial fibrillation.

Digitoxin is metabolised in the liver and is therefore preferable to digoxin in patients with impaired renal function.

4.2 Posology and method of administration
Adults and the elderly

Initial dose:

a) Rapid digitalisation (titrated to individual patients needs)

1 to 1.5 mg in divided doses over 24 hours.

b) Slow digitalisation

200 micrograms twice daily for 4 days.

Maintenance dose: 100 to 200 micrograms once a day (usually 10% of loading dose).

The elderly and those of low body weight may be particularly susceptible to digitoxin toxicity. Close monitoring of serum digitoxin levels is advised.

Renal Disease

These patients may be maintained at lower serum digitoxin concentrations than other patients.

Children

There is no dosage recommendation in children.

Route of administration:

Oral

4.3 Contraindications
Supraventricular arrhythmias caused by Wolff-Parkinson-White syndrome.

Ventricular fibrillation; ventricular tachycardia, unless congestive failure supervenes after a protracted episode not due to digitalis; presence of digitalis toxicity; Beri Beri, heart disease and some instances of hypersensitive carotid sinus syndrome. There may be cross-sensitivity between different formulations of cardiac glycosides.

4.4 Special warnings and precautions for use
Digitoxin should be used with caution in patients with abnormalities of thyroid function or impaired hepatic function. Digitoxin should also be used with caution in heart block; complete heart block may be induced if cardiac glycosides are used in partial heart block. Almost any deterioration in the conditions of the heart or circulation may increase the sensitivity to digitoxin.

4.5 Interaction with other medicinal products and other forms of interaction
Concomitant administration of some drugs may increase serum levels of digitoxin or the risk of toxicity:

There is a risk of increased toxicity with digitoxin if hypokalaemia occurs. This is likely with loop diuretics, thiazides, acetazolamide, carbenoxolone, antifungals and corticosteroids.

NSAIDs may exacerbate heart failure, reduce GFR and increase cardiac glycoside concentrations.

Macrolide antibiotics (such as azithromycin, erythromycin and clarithromycin) may cause digitoxin toxicity.

Quinidine, amiodarone and propafenone appear to increase digitoxin serum levels by reducing its non-renal clearance.

Calcium channel blockers (eg verapamil or diltiazem) may lead to increased digitoxin serum levels.

Beta blockers can cause increased AV block and bradycardia.

Edrophonium and other anticholinesterase drugs (eg neostigmine and pyridostigmine) may cause excessive bradycardia and AV-block in patients on digitalis glycosides.

The use of suxamethonium or pancuronium in digitalised patients may cause arrhythmias.

Intravenous calcium should be avoided in patients on cardiac glycosides as arrhythmias may be precipitated.

Anti-malarial drugs such as quinine, hydroxychloroquine and possibly chloroquine can increase the plasma concentration of digoxin. Mefloquine may increase the risk of bradycardia.

Other drugs may reduce serum levels of digitoxin:

The absorption of digitoxin may be reduced by concomitant administration of cholestyramine and colestipol.

Rifampicin, phenytoin, barbiturates and aminoglutethimide accelerate the metabolism of digitoxin, thus lowering its serum level.

In healthy volunteers the AUC of digoxin has been shown to be decreased by 18% with concurrent administration of St John's Wort.

4.6 Pregnancy and lactation
Safety for use in pregnancy and lactation has not been established hence digitoxin should not be given to pregnant or lactating women.

4.7 Effects on ability to drive and use machines
Digitoxin can cause fatigue, dizziness and drowsiness and patients should be advised not to drive or to use machines.

4.8 Undesirable effects
Cardiac glycosides commonly produce side effects because the margin between the therapeutic and toxic doses is small.

The most serious adverse effects are those on the heart. Toxic doses may cause or aggravate heart failure. Atrial or ventricular arrhythmias and defects of conduction are common and may be an early indication of excessive dosage.

In general, the incidence and severity of arrhythmias is related to the severity of the underlying heart disease. Almost any arrhythmia may ensue, but particular note should be made of supraventricular tachycardia, especially atrioventricular (AV) junctional tachycardia and atrial tachycardia and block.

Nausea, vomiting, anorexia, abdominal pain, diarrhoea, headache, fatigue, weakness, dizziness, drowsiness, disorientation, mental confusion, chorea, hypersensitivity reactions (skin desquamation, urticaria, angioneurotic oedema, eosiniphilia and fever), facial pain and rarely delirium. Acute psychoses, bad dreams and hallucinations may also occur.

Disturbances of vision have been reported, as have occasional reports of convulsions, gynaecomastia or thrombocytopenia.

4.9 Overdose
The main effects of overdose are cardiac and consist of arrhythmias (usually ventricular) in combination with heart block. Hyperkalaemia may develop because of Na^+K^+-ATPase inhibition.

Perform gastric lavage or induce emesis immediately following ingestion of a single toxic dose. Oral administration of activated charcoal or an insoluble stero-binding resin such as colestipol or cholestyramine has also been advocated. Monitor ECG continuously and potassium regularly. Specific antidigitoxin antibody fragments may be appropriate.

5. PHARMACOLOGICAL PROPERTIES
5.1 Pharmacodynamic properties
Digitoxin is a cardiac glycoside. Cardiac glycosides have a positive inotropic effect on myocardial cells, increasing the force and velocity of myocardial systolic contraction. In patients with congestive cardiac failure this results in increased cardiac output, more complete systolic emptying and a decreased diastolic heart size. Cardiac glycosides reduce the conductivity of the heart, particularly by reducing conduction through the atrioventricular node. At the cellular level, cardiac glycosides inhibit the activity of the enzyme Na^+K^+-ATPase, thus increasing plasma K^+.

5.2 Pharmacokinetic properties
Digitoxin is well absorbed orally with a bioavailability of more than 90%. Peak plasma concentrations occur 1.5 - 2.5 hours after an oral dose.

Digitoxin is more than 90% bound to plasma protein. Digitoxin is not removed by haemodialysis.

Digitoxin is widely distributed to all body tissues except fat. High concentrations are found in the kidney, liver, skeletal muscle and ventricular myocardium. It is not known if digitoxin is distributed into milk.

Steady-state plasma concentrations of digitoxin range from 10 to 35 nanograms per mL.

Digitoxin is extensively metabolised in the liver and undergoes some enterohepatic recirculation. The intermediate metabolites of digitoxin have pharmacological activity. At steady-state about 25% of a dose is excreted unchanged. The clearance of digitoxin is prolonged in hypothyroid patients and decreased in hyperthyroid patients. The excretion of digitoxin appears unaltered by renal impairment. The plasma half-life of digitoxin averages about 7.5 days.

5.3 Preclinical safety data
Not applicable since Digitoxin Tablets have been used in clinical practice for many years and its effects in man are well known.

6. PHARMACEUTICAL PARTICULARS

6.1 List of excipients

Maize Starch BP

Lactose BP

Magnesium Stearate BP

Purified Water BP

6.2 Incompatibilities

None.

6.3 Shelf life

36 months.

6.4 Special precautions for storage

Store below 25°C.

6.5 Nature and contents of container

Pigmented polypropylene containers fitted with a tamper evident closure of low density polyethylene containing 28 or 250 tablets.

6.6 Special precautions for disposal and other handling

No special precautions are required.

7. MARKETING AUTHORISATION HOLDER

UCB Pharma Ltd

208 Bath Road

Slough

Berkshire

Sl1 3WE

United Kingdom

8. MARKETING AUTHORISATION NUMBER(S)

PL 00039/0544

9. DATE OF FIRST AUTHORISATION/RENEWAL OF THE AUTHORISATION

5 September 2005

10. DATE OF REVISION OF THE TEXT

28 November 2006.

Dilzem SR 60, 90 and 120mg Hard Capsules

(Cephalon Limited)

1. NAME OF THE MEDICINAL PRODUCT

Dilzem SR 60mg Prolonged-release Hard Capsules

Dilzem SR 90mg Prolonged release Hard Capsules

Dilzem SR 120mg Prolonged-release Hard Capsules

2. QUALITATIVE AND QUANTITATIVE COMPOSITION

Each Dilzem SR 60mg capsule contains diltiazem hydrochloride 60mg.

Each Dilzem SR 90mg capsule contains diltiazem hydrochloride 90mg.

Each Dilzem SR 120mg capsule contains diltiazem hydrochloride 120mg.

Excipients: Sucrose 12.6mg in each SR 60mg capsule.

Sucrose 18.9mg in each SR 90mg capsule.

Sucrose 25.2mg in each SR 120mg capsule.

For *full list of* excipients, see *Section* 6.1.

3. PHARMACEUTICAL FORM

Prolonged-release capsule, hard.

Buff coloured, hard gelatin capsules, printed with 60mg and containing roughly spherical white to off-white beads.

Buff coloured, hard gelatin capsules, printed with 90mg and containing roughly spherical white to off-white beads.

Buff coloured, hard gelatin capsules, printed with 120mg and containing roughly spherical white to off-white beads.

4. CLINICAL PARTICULARS

4.1 Therapeutic indications

Treatment of angina pectoris including Prinzmetal's angina.

Treatment of mild to moderate hypertension.

4.2 Posology and method of administration

Oral use only.

Adults:

Hypertension: The usual initial dose is 90 mg twice daily (corresponding to 180 mg of diltiazem hydrochloride). Depending upon clinical response the patient's dosage may be increased to 180 mg twice daily if required.

Angina Pectoris: The usual initial dose is 90 mg twice daily (corresponding to 180 mg of diltiazem hydrochloride). Depending upon clinical response the patient's dosage may be increased to 180 mg twice daily if required.

Elderly patients and those with renal or hepatic impairment:

Dosage should commence at the lower level of 60 mg twice daily and be increased slowly. Do not increase the dose if the heart rate falls below 50 beats per minute.

Children:

This product is not recommended for use in children.

4.3 Contraindications

- Use in women of child-bearing potential

- Concomitant administration of dantrolene infusion due to the risk of ventricular fibrillation

- Shock

- Acute cardiac infarct with complications (bradycardia, severe hypotension, left heart insufficiency)

- Bradycardia (pulse rate, at rest, of less than 50 bpm), hypotension (less than 90 mm Hg systole), second or third degree heart block or sick sinus syndrome, except in the presence of a functioning ventricular pacemaker

- Atrial fibrillation/flutter and simultaneous presence of a WPW (Wolff-Parkinson-White) syndrome (increased risk of triggering a ventricular tachycardia)

- Manifest myocardial insufficiency

- Left ventricular failure with stasis

- Hypersensitivity to diltiazem or any of the excipients

4.4 Special warnings and precautions for use

- Capsules should not be sucked or chewed.

- The use of diltiazem hydrochloride in diabetic patients may require adjustment of their control.

- The product should be used with caution in patients with hepatic dysfunction. Abnormalities of liver function may occur during therapy. Very occasional reports of abnormal liver function have been received, these reactions have been reversible upon discontinuation of therapy.

- First degree AV block or prolonged PR interval. Diltelan prolongs AV node refractory periods without significantly prolonging sinus node recovery time, except in patients with sick sinus syndrome. This effect may rarely result in abnormally slow heart rates (particularly in patients with sick sinus syndrome) or second or third degree AV block (see interactions section for information concerning beta-blockers and digitalis).

- Mild bradycardia.

- Patients with reduced left ventricular function.

- Renally impaired patients.

- Owing to the presence of sucrose, patients with rare hereditary problems of fructose intolerance, glucose-galactose malabsorption or sucrase-isomaltase insufficiency should not take this medicine.

As with any drug given over prolonged periods, laboratory parameters should be monitored at regular intervals.

4.5 Interaction with other medicinal products and other forms of interaction

Diltiazem undergoes biotransformation by the hepatic cytochrome P-450 mixed function oxidase system. The principal isoenzyme involved is CYP3A4. Hence, co-administration with other agents that are also substrates for CYP3A4 may result in competitive inhibition of the metabolism of the concomitant agent.

Simultaneous administration with enzyme inducers such as rifampicin and phenobarbital may lead to reduced activity of diltiazem.

Diltiazem hydrochloride should only be administered with great care to patients receiving concurrent treatment with antihypertensives or other hypotensive agents including halogenated anaesthetics or drugs with moderate protein binding.

Diltiazem hydrochloride will not protect against effects of withdrawal of β-adrenoceptor blocking agents, nor the rebound effects seen with various antihypertensives. Combination with β-adrenoceptor blockers having a significant "first pass" loss, e.g. propranolol may require a decrease in their dose and may lead to bradycardia. There may be an additive effect when used with drugs which may induce bradycardia or with other antihypertensives. Concomitant H_2 antagonist therapy may increase diltiazem blood levels.

Diltiazem may affect the blood levels of concomitant carbamazepine, theophylline, ciclosporin and digoxin. Careful attention should therefore be given to signs of overdosage. The levels should be determined and the dose of carbamazepine, theophylline, ciclosporin, or digoxin reduced if necessary. Patients receiving β-blockers, diuretics, ACE inhibitors or other antihypertensive agents should be regularly monitored. Use with alpha blockers should be strictly monitored.

The simultaneous administration of diltiazem with drugs such as β-blockers, antiarrhythmics or heart glycosides may cause a greater degree of AV blocking, reduce the heart rate or induce a hypotensive effect. Intravenous administration of β-blockers should be discontinued during therapy with diltiazem.

Anaesthetists should be warned that a patient is on a calcium antagonist. The depression of cardiac contractility, conductivity, and automaticity as well as the vascular dilation associated with anaesthetics may be potentiated by calcium channel blockers. When used concomitantly, anaesthetics and calcium channel blockers should be titrated carefully.

There have been reports in the literature of diltiazem interactions with warfarin and lithium.

Cautious use with simvastatin and atorvastatin at the lowest effective dose, with patient monitoring for signs and symptoms of rhabdomyolysis, is recommended when co-administration with diltiazem is considered.

There is an increased risk of bradycardia, AV block and myocardial depression when diltiazem and amiodarone are given together.

4.6 Pregnancy and lactation

Diltiazem must not be taken during pregnancy as experimental studies have shown indications of teratogenicity. There is no experience of its effects in humans. As diltiazem is known to enter the breast milk and there is no experience of possible effects in infants, infants should be weaned if treatment of the mother with diltiazem is necessary.

4.7 Effects on ability to drive and use machines

Not applicable.

4.8 Undesirable effects

In studies carried out to date, serious adverse reactions with diltiazem have been rare; however, it should be recognised that patients with impaired ventricular function and cardiac conduction abnormalities have usually been excluded from these studies.

In 900 patients with hypertension, the most common adverse events were oedema (9%), headache (8%), dizziness (6%), asthenia (5%), sinus bradycardia (3%), flushing (3%), and first degree AV block (3%). Only oedema and perhaps bradycardia were dose related. The most common adverse events (>1%) observed in clinical studies of over 2100 angina and hypertensive patients receiving diltiazem were: oedema (5.4%), headache (4.5%), dizziness (3.4%), asthenia (2.8%), first-degree AV block (1.8%), flushing (1.7%), nausea (1.6%), bradycardia (1.5%) and rash (1.5%).

Less common adverse events have included the following:

Cardiovascular: angina, arrhythmia, AV block (second or third degree), congestive heart failure, hypotension, palpitations, syncope.

Nervous system: amnesia, depression, gait abnormality, hallucinations, insomnia, nervousness, paraesthesia, personality change, somnolence, tinnitus, tremor.

Gastrointestinal: anorexia, constipation, diarrhoea, dyspepsia, mild elevations of alkaline phosphatase, SGOT, SGPT and LDH (see Special Warnings and Precautions), vomiting, weight increase, gingivitis and gingival hypertrophy.

Dermatologic: petechiae, pruritus, photosensitivity, urticaria, Stevens-Johnson syndrome. Allergic skin reactions including erythema multiforme, vasculitis, lymphadenopathy and eosinophilia have been observed in isolated cases. Dermatological events may be transient and may disappear despite continued use of diltiazem. Should a dermatologic reaction persist, the drug should be discontinued.

Other: amblyopia, CK elevation, dyspnoea, epistaxis, eye irritation, hyperglycaemia, nasal congestion, nocturia, osteoarticular pain, muscle pain, polyuria, sexual difficulties, thrombocytopenia, gynaecomastia.

4.9 Overdose

Experience of overdosage in man is limited but cases of spontaneous recovery have been reported. However, it is recommended that patients with suspected overdose should be placed under observation in a coronary care unit with facilities available for treatment of any possible hypotension and conduction disturbances that may occur. Most patients suffering from overdosage of diltiazem become hypotensive within 8 hours of ingestion. With bradycardia and first to third degree atrioventricular block also developing cardiac arrest may ensue. Hyperglycaemia is also a recognised complication. The elimination half-life of diltiazem after overdosage is estimated to be about 5.5 - 10.2 hours. If a patient presents early after overdose, gastric lavage should be performed and activated charcoal administered to reduce diltiazem absorption.

Hypotension should be corrected with plasma expanders, intravenous calcium gluconate and inotropic agents (dopamine, dobutamine or isoprenaline). Symptomatic bradycardia and high grade AV block may respond to atropine, isoprenaline or occasionally cardiac pacing which may be useful if cardiac standstill occurs.

5. PHARMACOLOGICAL PROPERTIES

5.1 Pharmacodynamic properties

Diltiazem has pharmacologic actions similar to those of other calcium channel blocking agents such as nifedipine or verapamil. The principal physiologic action of diltiazem is to inhibit the transmembrane influx of extracellular calcium ions across the membranes of myocardial cells and vascular smooth muscle cells.

Calcium plays important roles in the excitation-contraction coupling processes of the heart and vascular smooth muscle cells and in the electrical discharge of the specialised conduction cells of the heart. The membranes of these cells contain numerous channels that carry a slow inward current and that are selective for calcium.

By inhibiting calcium influx, diltiazem inhibits the contractile processes of cardiac and vascular smooth muscle, thereby dilating the main coronary and systemic arteries. Dilation of systemic arteries by diltiazem results in a decrease in total peripheral resistance, a decrease in systemic blood pressure and a decrease in the afterload of the heart. The reduction in afterload, seen at rest and with exercise, and its resultant decrease in myocardial oxygen consumption are thought to be responsible for the beneficial effects of diltiazem in patients with chronic stable angina pectoris. In patients with prinzmetal variant angina, inhibition of spontaneous and ergonovine-induced coronary artery spasm by diltiazem results in increased myocardial oxygen delivery.

5.2 Pharmacokinetic properties

a) General Characteristics

Absorption: Capsules seem to have a similar bioavailability to tablets (30-40%), with peak concentrations for the prolonged release product after 8-11 hours compared with 1-2 hours after the conventional release product. The relatively low bioavailability is due to first pass metabolism in the liver to an active metabolite.

Distribution: Diltiazem hydrochloride is lipophilic and has a high volume of distribution. Typical study results are in the range of 3-8 litres/kg. Protein binding is about 80% and is not concentration-dependent at levels likely to be found clinically. Protein binding does not appear to be influenced by phenylbutazone, warfarin, propranolol, salicylic acid or digoxin.

Metabolism: Diltiazem hydrochloride is extensively metabolised in the liver. N-monodesmethyl diltiazem is the predominant metabolite followed quantitatively by the desacetyl metabolite, which has some pharmacological activity. The efficacy of the metabolites, desacetyl diltiazem and N-monodesmethyl diltiazem is 25-50% and about 20% respectively of that of diltiazem. In liver function disorders delayed metabolism in the liver is likely. These metabolites are converted to conjugates, generally the glucuronide or the sulphate.

Elimination: Diltiazem is excreted in the form of its metabolites (about 35%) and in the non-metabolised form (about 2-4%) via the kidneys while about 60% is excreted via the faeces. The average elimination half life period for diltiazem is 6-8 hours but may vary between 2 and 11 hours. Although the elimination half life is not changed after repeated oral administration, diltiazem and also the desacetyl metabolite show a slight accumulation in the plasma.

b) Characteristics in Patients

Decreased first-pass metabolism in the elderly tends to result in increased plasma concentrations of calcium antagonists but no major changes have been found with diltiazem. Renal impairment did not cause significant changes in diltiazem pharmacokinetics. Plasma concentrations of diltiazem also tend to be higher in hepatic cirrhosis due to impaired oxidative metabolism.

5.3 Preclinical safety data

Chronic toxicity studies in rats revealed no remarkable changes at oral doses up to 125 mg/kg/day although there was a 60% mortality at this dose. In dogs chronically treated with oral doses of 20 mg/kg/day, transient rises in SGPT were observed. Embryotoxicity has been reported in mice, rats and rabbits following i.p. administration of diltiazem. Main types of malformations included limb and tail defects with a small number of vertebral and rib deformities also noted.

6. PHARMACEUTICAL PARTICULARS

6.1 List of excipients

Fumaric acid

Talc

Povidone

Sugar spheres (containing sucrose and maize starch)

Ammonio methacrylate copolymer Type B

Ammonio methacrylate copolymer Type A

The capsule shell contains:

Yellow iron oxide (E172)

Erythrosine (E127)

Titanium dioxide (E171)

Gelatin

The printing ink contains:

Shellac

Black iron oxide (E172)

Propylene glycol (E1520)

6.2 Incompatibilities

Not applicable.

6.3 Shelf life

Three years from date of manufacture for all presentations.

6.4 Special precautions for storage

Do not store above 25°C. Store in the original package.

6.5 Nature and contents of container

Securitainer containing 30 or 100 capsules.

Clear PVC blister pack containing 4 or 60 or 100 capsules.

Opaque PVC/PVDC blister pack containing 56, 60 or 100 capsules.

6.6 Special precautions for disposal and other handling

Not applicable.

7. MARKETING AUTHORISATION HOLDER

Cephalon Limited

1 Albany Place

Hyde Way

Welwyn Garden City

Hertfordshire

AL7 3BT

8. MARKETING AUTHORISATION NUMBER(S)

Dilzem SR 60 mg – PL 21799/0006

Dilzem SR 90 mg – PL 21799/0007

Dilzem SR 120 mg – PL 21799/0008

9. DATE OF FIRST AUTHORISATION/RENEWAL OF THE AUTHORISATION

30 January 2006

10. DATE OF REVISION OF THE TEXT

August 2009

11. LEGAL CATEGORY

POM

Dilzem XL 120, 180 and 240mg hard-capsules

(Cephalon Limited)

1. NAME OF THE MEDICINAL PRODUCT

Dilzem XL 120mg Prolonged-release Hard Capsules

Dilzem XL 180mg Prolonged-release Hard Capsules

Dilzem XL 240mg Prolonged-release Hard Capsules

2. QUALITATIVE AND QUANTITATIVE COMPOSITION

Each Dilzem XL 120mg capsule contains diltiazem hydrochloride 120mg.

Each Dilzem XL 180mg capsule contains diltiazem hydrochloride 180mg.

Each Dilzem XL 240mg capsule contains diltiazem hydrochloride 240mg.

Excipients: Sucrose 25.2mg in each XL 120mg capsule.

Sucrose 37.8mg in each XL 180mg capsule.

Sucrose 50.4mg in each XL 240mg capsule.

For full list of excipients, see Section 6.1.

3. PHARMACEUTICAL FORM

Prolonged-release capsule, hard.

White, hard gelatin capsules, printed with e120 and containing roughly spherical white to off-white beads.

White, hard gelatin capsules, printed with e180 and containing roughly spherical white to off-white beads.

White, hard gelatin capsules, printed with e240 and containing roughly spherical white to off-white beads.

4. CLINICAL PARTICULARS

4.1 Therapeutic indications

Prophylaxis and treatment of angina pectoris.

Treatment of mild to moderate hypertension.

4.2 Posology and method of administration

Oral use only.

Adults:

Hypertension: The usual initial dose is one 180mg capsule per day (corresponding to 180mg of diltiazem hydrochloride once daily). Depending upon the clinical response the dosage may be increased stepwise to 360mg/day if required.

Angina Pectoris: The usual initial dose is one 180mg capsule per day (corresponding to 180mg of diltiazem hydrochloride once daily). Depending upon the clinical response the dosage may be increased stepwise to 360mg/day if required.

Elderly patients and those with renal or hepatic impairment:

Dosage should commence at the lower level of 120mg once daily and be increased slowly. Do not increase the dose if the heart rate falls below 50 beats per minute.

Children:

This product is not recommended for use in children.

4.3 Contraindications

- Use in women of child-bearing potential
- Concomitant administration of dantrolene infusion due to the risk of ventricular fibrillation
- Shock
- Acute cardiac infarct with complications (bradycardia, severe hypotension, left heart insufficiency)
- Bradycardia (pulse rate, at rest, of less than 50 bpm), hypotension (less than 90 mm Hg systole), second or third degree heart block or sick sinus syndrome, except in the presence of a functioning ventricular pacemaker
- Atrial fibrillation/flutter and simultaneous presence of a WPW (Wolff-Parkinson-White) syndrome (increased risk of triggering a ventricular tachycardia)
- Manifest myocardial insufficiency
- Left ventricular failure with stasis
- Hypersensitivity to diltiazem or any of the excipients

4.4 Special warnings and precautions for use

- Capsules should not be sucked or chewed.
- The use of diltiazem hydrochloride in diabetic patients may require adjustment of their control.
- The product should be used with caution in patients with hepatic dysfunction. Abnormalities of liver function may occur during therapy. Very occasional reports of abnormal liver function have been received, these reactions have been reversible upon discontinuation of therapy.
- First degree AV block or prolonged PR interval. Diltelan prolongs AV node refractory periods without significantly prolonging sinus node recovery time, except in patients with sick sinus syndrome. This effect may rarely result in abnormally slow heart rates (particularly in patients with sick sinus syndrome) or second or third degree AV block (see interactions section for information concerning beta-blockers and digitalis).
- Mild bradycardia.
- Patients with reduced left ventricular function.
- Renally impaired patients.
- Owing to the presence of sucrose, patients with rare hereditary problems of fructose intolerance, glucose-galactose malabsorption or sucrose-isomaltase insufficiency should not take this medicine.

As with any drug given over prolonged periods, laboratory parameters should be monitored at regular intervals.

4.5 Interaction with other medicinal products and other forms of interaction

Diltiazem undergoes biotransformation by the hepatic cytochrome P-450 mixed function oxidase system. The principal isoenzyme involved is CYP3A4. Hence, co-administration with other agents that are also substrates for CYP3A4 may result in competitive inhibition of the metabolism of the concomitant agent.

Simultaneous administration with enzyme inducers such as rifampicin and phenobarbital may lead to reduced activity of diltiazem.

Diltiazem hydrochloride should only be administered with great care to patients receiving concurrent treatment with antihypertensives or other hypotensive agents including halogenated anaesthetics or drugs with moderate protein binding.

Diltiazem hydrochloride will not protect against effects of withdrawal of β-adrenoceptor blocking agents, nor the rebound effects seen with various antihypertensives. Combination with β-adrenoceptor blockers having a significant "first pass" loss, e.g. propranolol may require a decrease in their dose and may lead to bradycardia. There may be an additive effect when used with drugs which may induce bradycardia or with other antihypertensives. Concomitant H_2 antagonist therapy may increase diltiazem blood levels.

Diltiazem may affect the blood levels of concomitant carbamazepine, theophylline, ciclosporin and digoxin. Careful attention should therefore be given to signs of overdosage. The levels should be determined and the dose of carbamazepine, theophylline, ciclosporin, or digoxin reduced if necessary. Patients receiving β-blockers, diuretics, ACE inhibitors or other antihypertensive agents should be regularly monitored. Use with alpha blockers should be strictly monitored.

The simultaneous administration of diltiazem with drugs such as β-blockers, antiarrhythmics or heart glycosides may cause a greater degree of AV blocking, reduce the heart rate or induce a hypotensive effect. Intravenous administration of β-blockers should be discontinued during therapy with diltiazem.

Anaesthetists should be warned that a patient is on a calcium antagonist. The depression of cardiac contractility, conductivity, and automaticity as well as the vascular dilation associated with anaesthetics may be potentiated by calcium channel blockers. When used concomitantly, anaesthetics and calcium channel blockers should be titrated carefully.

There have been reports in the literature of diltiazem interactions with warfarin and lithium.

Cautious use with simvastatin and atorvastatin at the lowest effective dose, with patient monitoring for signs and symptoms of rhabdomyolysis, is recommended when co-administration with diltiazem is considered.

There is an increased risk of bradycardia, AV block and myocardial depression when diltiazem and amiodarone are given together.

4.6 Pregnancy and lactation

Diltiazem must not be taken during pregnancy as experimental studies have shown indications of teratogenicity. There is no experience of its effects in humans. As diltiazem is known to enter the breast milk and there is no experience of possible effects in infants, infants should be weaned if treatment of the mother with diltiazem is necessary.

4.7 Effects on ability to drive and use machines

Not applicable.

4.8 Undesirable effects

In studies carried out to date, serious adverse reactions with diltiazem have been rare; however, it should be recognised that patients with impaired ventricular function and cardiac conduction abnormalities have usually been excluded from these studies.

In 900 patients with hypertension, the most common adverse events were oedema (9%), headache (8%), dizziness (6%), asthenia (5%), sinus bradycardia (3%), flushing (3%), and first degree AV block (3%). Only oedema and perhaps bradycardia were dose related. The most common adverse events (>1%) observed in clinical studies of over 2100 angina and hypertensive patients receiving diltiazem were: oedema (5.4%), headache (4.5%), dizziness (3.4%), asthenia (2.8%), first-degree AV block (1.8%), flushing (1.7%), nausea (1.6%), bradycardia (1.5%) and rash (1.5%).

Less common adverse events have included the following:

Cardiovascular: angina, arrhythmia, AV block (second or third degree), congestive heart failure, hypotension, palpitations, syncope.

Nervous system: amnesia, depression, gait abnormality, hallucinations, insomnia, nervousness, paraesthesia, personality change, somnolence, tinnitus, tremor.

Gastrointestinal: anorexia, constipation, diarrhoea, dyspepsia, mild elevations of alkaline phosphatase, SGOT, SGPT and LDH (see Special Warnings and Precautions), vomiting, weight increase, gingivitis and gingival hypertrophy.

Dermatologic: petechiae, pruritus, photosensitivity, urticaria, Stevens-Johnson syndrome. Allergic skin reactions including erythema multiforme, vasculitis, lymphadenopathy and eosinophilia have been observed in isolated cases. Dermatological events may be transient and may disappear despite continued use of diltiazem. Should a dermatologic reaction persist, the drug should be discontinued.

Other: amblyopia, CK elevation, dyspnoea, epistaxis, eye irritation, hyperglycaemia, nasal congestion, nocturia, osteoarticular pain, muscle pain, polyuria, sexual difficulties, thrombocytopenia, gynaecomastia.

4.9 Overdose

Experience of overdosage in man is limited but cases of spontaneous recovery have been reported. However, it is recommended that patients with suspected overdose should be placed under observation in a coronary care unit with facilities available for treatment of any possible hypotension and conduction disturbances that may occur. Most patients suffering from overdosage of diltiazem become hypotensive within 8 hours of ingestion. With bradycardia and first to third degree atrioventricular block also developing cardiac arrest may ensue. Hyperglycaemia is also a recognised complication. The elimination half-life of diltiazem after overdosage is estimated to be about 5.5 - 10.2 hours. If a patient presents early after overdose, gastric lavage should be performed and activated charcoal administered to reduce diltiazem absorption.

Hypotension should be corrected with plasma expanders, intravenous calcium gluconate and inotropic agents (dopamine, dobutamine or isoprenaline). Symptomatic bradycardia and high grade AV block may respond to atropine, isoprenaline or occasionally cardiac pacing which may be useful if cardiac standstill occurs.

5. PHARMACOLOGICAL PROPERTIES

5.1 Pharmacodynamic properties

Diltiazem has pharmacologic actions similar to those of other calcium channel blocking agents such as nifedipine or verapamil. The principal physiologic action of diltiazem is to inhibit the transmembrane influx of extracellular calcium ions across the membranes of myocardial cells and vascular smooth muscle cells.

Calcium plays important roles in the excitation-contraction coupling processes of the heart and vascular smooth muscle cells and in the electrical discharge of the specialised conduction cells of the heart. The membranes of these cells contain numerous channels that carry a slow inward current and that are selective for calcium.

By inhibiting calcium influx, diltiazem inhibits the contractile processes of cardiac and vascular smooth muscle, thereby dilating the main coronary and systemic arteries. Dilation of systemic arteries by diltiazem results in a decrease in total peripheral resistance, a decrease in systemic blood pressure and a decrease in the afterload of the heart. The reduction in afterload, seen at rest and with exercise, and its resultant decrease in myocardial oxygen consumption are thought to be responsible for the beneficial effects of diltiazem in patients with chronic stable angina pectoris. In patients with prinzmetal variant angina, inhibition of spontaneous and ergonovine-induced coronary artery spasm by diltiazem results in increased myocardial oxygen delivery.

5.2 Pharmacokinetic properties

a) General Characteristics

Absorption: Capsules seem to have a similar bioavailability to tablets (30-40%), with peak concentrations for the prolonged release product after 8-11 hours compared with 1-2 hours after the conventional release product. The relatively low bioavailability is due to first pass metabolism in the liver to an active metabolite.

Distribution: Diltiazem hydrochloride is lipophilic and has a high volume of distribution. Typical study results are in the range of 3-8 litres/kg. Protein binding is about 80% and is not concentration-dependent at levels likely to be found clinically. Protein binding does not appear to be influenced by phenylbutazone, warfarin, propranolol, salicylic acid or digoxin.

Metabolism: Diltiazem hydrochloride is extensively metabolised in the liver. N-monodesmethyl diltiazem is the predominant metabolite followed quantitatively by the desacetyl metabolite, which has some pharmacological activity. The efficacy of the metabolites, desacetyl diltiazem and N-monodesmethyl diltiazem is 25-50% and about 20% respectively of that of diltiazem. In liver function disorders delayed metabolism in the liver is likely. These metabolites are converted to conjugates, generally the glucuronide or the sulphate.

Elimination: Diltiazem is excreted in the form of its metabolites (about 35%) and in the non-metabolised form (about 2-4%) via the kidneys while about 60% is excreted via the faeces. The average elimination half life period for diltiazem is 6-8 hours but may vary between 2 and 11 hours. Although the elimination half life is not changed after repeated oral administration, diltiazem and also the desacetyl metabolite show a slight accumulation in the plasma.

b) Characteristics in Patients

Decreased first-pass metabolism in the elderly tends to result in increased plasma concentrations of calcium antagonists but no major changes have been found with diltiazem. Renal impairment did not cause significant changes in diltiazem pharmacokinetics. Plasma concentrations of diltiazem also tend to be higher in hepatic cirrhosis due to impaired oxidative metabolism.

5.3 Preclinical safety data

Chronic toxicity studies in rats revealed no remarkable changes at oral doses up to 125 mg/kg/day although there was a 60% mortality at this dose. In dogs chronically treated with oral doses of 20 mg/kg/day, transient rises in SGPT were observed. Embryotoxicity has been reported in mice, rats and rabbits following i.p. administration of diltiazem. Main types of malformations included limb and tail defects with a small number of vertebral and rib deformities also noted.

6. PHARMACEUTICAL PARTICULARS

6.1 List of excipients

Fumaric acid

Talc

Povidone

Sugar spheres (containing sucrose and maize starch)

Ammonio methacrylate copolymer Type B

Ammonio methacrylate copolymer Type A

The capsule shell contains:

Gelatin

Titanium dioxide (E171)

The printing ink contains:

Shellac

Black iron oxide (E172)

Propylene glycol (E1520)

6.2 Incompatibilities

Not applicable.

6.3 Shelf life

Two years from the date of manufacture.

6.4 Special precautions for storage

Do not store above 25°C. Store in the original package.

6.5 Nature and contents of container

Jaysquare container, containing 7, 20, 30, 50, 60 or 100 capsules.

PVC/PVDC blister pack, containing 4, 28 or 30 capsules.

6.6 Special precautions for disposal and other handling

Not applicable.

7. MARKETING AUTHORISATION HOLDER

Cephalon Limited

1 Albany Place

Hyde Way

Welwyn Garden City

Hertfordshire

AL7 3BT

8. MARKETING AUTHORISATION NUMBER(S)

Dilzem XL 120 mg – PL 21799/0003

Dilzem XL 180 mg – PL 21799/0004

Dilzem XL 240 mg – PL 21799/0005

9. DATE OF FIRST AUTHORISATION/RENEWAL OF THE AUTHORISATION

30 January 2006

10. DATE OF REVISION OF THE TEXT

August 2009

11. LEGAL CATEGORY

POM

Dioctyl Capsules

(UCB Pharma Limited)

1. NAME OF THE MEDICINAL PRODUCT

Dioctyl 100 mg Capsules.

DulcoEase, 100 mg capsules

2. QUALITATIVE AND QUANTITATIVE COMPOSITION

Docusate sodium 100 mg.

For excipients, see Section 6.1.

3. PHARMACEUTICAL FORM

Capsules

A two colour (opaque white and opaque yellow) soft, oval, gelatin capsule with a clear, colourless liquid fill.

4. CLINICAL PARTICULARS

4.1 Therapeutic indications

a) To prevent and treat chronic constipation.

(i) to soften hard, dry stools in order to ease defaecation and reduce straining at stool; and

(ii) in the presence of haemorrhoids and anal fissure, to prevent hard, dry stools and reduce straining.

b) As an adjunct in abdominal radiological procedures.

4.2 Posology and method of administration

Route of administration: Oral

Adults and elderly:

Up to 500 mg should be taken daily in divided doses. Treatment should be commenced with large doses, which should be decreased as the condition of the patient improves.

For use with barium meals:

400 mg to be taken with the meal.

Children under 12 years:

Not recommended.

4.3 Contraindications

These capsules should not be administered when abdominal pain, nausea, vomiting or intestinal obstruction is present.

This product should not be given to patients with a known hypersensitivity to Dioctyl capsules or any of the components.

Patients with rare hereditary problems of fructose intolerance should not take this medicine.

4.4 Special warnings and precautions for use

Organic disorders should be excluded prior to the administration of any laxative.

The treatment of constipation with any medicinal product is only adjuvant to a healthy lifestyle and diet, for example:

- Increased intake of fluids and dietary fibre.
- Advice on appropriate physical activity

If laxatives are needed every day, or if there is persistent abdominal pain, consult your doctor.

Contains sorbitol: do not use this medicine if you are intolerant to small quantities of sugar (sorbitol, fructose).

Contains colouring E110 which may cause allergic reactions.

4.5 Interaction with other medicinal products and other forms of interaction

These capsules should not be taken concurrently with mineral oil.

4.6 Pregnancy and lactation

There are no adequate data from the use of the drug in pregnant women. Animal studies are insufficient with respect to effects on pregnancy and embryonic foetal development. The potential risk for humans is unknown. During wide use, no adverse consequences have been reported.

Use in pregnancy only if the benefits outweigh the risks.

Docusate sodium is excreted in breast milk and should therefore, be used with caution in lactating mothers.

4.7 Effects on ability to drive and use machines

None known.

4.8 Undesirable effects

Rarely, these capsules can cause diarrhoea, nausea, abdominal cramps or skin rash.

4.9 Overdose

In rare cases of overdose, excessive loss of water and electrolytes should be treated by encouraging the patient to drink plenty of fluid. Electrolyte loss should be replenished where appropriate.

5. PHARMACOLOGICAL PROPERTIES

5.1 Pharmacodynamic properties

ATC code: A06A02 Laxatives, softeners, emollients

Docusate sodium is an anionic wetting agent, which acts as a faecal softener by lowering the surface tension and allowing penetration of accumulated hard dry faeces by water and salts.

Docusate Sodium also possesses stimulant activity.

5.2 Pharmacokinetic properties

Docusate sodium exerts its clinical effect in the gastrointestinal tract. There is some evidence that docusate sodium is absorbed and is excreted in the bile. There is also evidence that docusate sodium is capable of enhancing absorption of certain compounds administered concomitantly.

5.3 Preclinical safety data

None Stated

6. PHARMACEUTICAL PARTICULARS

6.1 List of excipients

Macrogol 400

Propylene glycol

Gelatin 195 bloom

Purified water

Sorbitol special

Glycerol

Titanium dioxide E171

Quinoline yellow E104

Sunset yellow E110

6.2 Incompatibilities

None.

6.3 Shelf life

3 years.

6.4 Special precautions for storage

Do not store above 25°C. Store in the original package in order to protect from moisture.

6.5 Nature and contents of container

PVC/PVdC blister packs with aluminium foil containing 10, 20, 30, 40 or 50 capsules.

Polyethylene / polypropylene containers, e.g.: securitainers / tampertainers containing 30, 100 and 250 capsules.

Not all pack sizes may be marketed.

6.6 Special precautions for disposal and other handling

None

7. MARKETING AUTHORISATION HOLDER

UCB Pharma Limited

208 Bath Road

Slough

Berkshire

SL1 3WE

United Kingdom

8. MARKETING AUTHORISATION NUMBER(S)

PL 00039/0737

9. DATE OF FIRST AUTHORISATION/RENEWAL OF THE AUTHORISATION

28 February 2008

10. DATE OF REVISION OF THE TEXT

Dioderm 0.1% w/w Cream

(Dermal Laboratories Limited)

1. NAME OF THE MEDICINAL PRODUCT

DIODERM™ 0.1% w/w CREAM

2. QUALITATIVE AND QUANTITATIVE COMPOSITION

Hydrocortisone 0.1% w/w.

3. PHARMACEUTICAL FORM

Smooth white aqueous cream.

4. CLINICAL PARTICULARS

4.1 Therapeutic indications

For the topical treatment of eczema and dermatitis.

4.2 Posology and method of administration

For adults, children and the elderly: Apply to the affected areas twice daily. For infants, the treatment period should not normally exceed 7 days.

4.3 Contraindications

As with all topical steroids, Dioderm is not to be used where there is bacterial, viral or fungal infection.

Not to be used on open wounds, ulcers or broken skin.

Not to be used in cases of sensitivity to any of the ingredients.

4.4 Special warnings and precautions for use

Although generally regarded as safe, even for long-term administration in adults, there is a potential for overdosage in infancy. Extreme caution is required in dermatoses in infancy, including napkin eruption. In such patients, courses of treatment should not normally exceed 7 days.

Prolonged or extensive uninterrupted application should be avoided, particularly if used on the face or with occlusive dressings.

The excipient propylene glycol may on rare occasions cause skin irritation in sensitive people.

Keep out of the reach and sight of children. Keep away from the eyes. For external use only.

4.5 Interaction with other medicinal products and other forms of interaction

None known.

4.6 Pregnancy and lactation

There is inadequate evidence of safety in human pregnancy. Topical administration of corticosteroids to pregnant animals can cause abnormalities of foetal development including cleft palate and intra-uterine growth retardation. There may therefore be a very small risk of such effects in the human foetus.

4.7 Effects on ability to drive and use machines

None known.

4.8 Undesirable effects

Reported side effects of corticosteroids include skin thinning and striae. Although rare, these could occur even with hydrocortisone, especially when used under occlusion or in the folds of the skin.

Dioderm is usually well tolerated but in the event of a hypersensitivity reaction (allergic contact dermatitis) treatment should be discontinued.

4.9 Overdose

Under exceptional circumstances, if Dioderm is used excessively, particularly in young children, it is theoretically possible that adrenal suppression and skin thinning may occur. The symptoms are normally reversible on cessation of treatment.

5. PHARMACOLOGICAL PROPERTIES

5.1 Pharmacodynamic properties

Corticosteroids are used in pharmacological doses for their anti-inflammatory and immunosuppressive glucocorticoid properties which suppress the clinical manifestations of a wide range of diseases. Although many synthetic derivatives have been developed, hydrocortisone is still used widely in topical formulations for inflammatory dermatoses. It has the advantage over its synthetic derivatives that it is metabolised in the skin and therefore cannot accumulate to form a depot which may result in local side effects.

5.2 Pharmacokinetic properties

The cream formulation of Dioderm was developed in order to optimise the release and partition of its active ingredient, hydrocortisone, into the skin. The hydrocortisone is presented as a saturated or near saturated solution in aqueous propylene glycol, which represents the continuous phase of the emulsion system. It has been shown, by the vasoconstrictor assay on normal skin, that, in this environment, a 0.1% concentration of the hydrocortisone is equivalent to the 1.0% concentration of the official cream formulations appearing in the British Pharmacopoeia where the drug substance is in suspension. Clinical studies have confirmed that 0.1% Dioderm is equivalent to 1.0% Hydrocortisone Cream BP whilst the reduced strength of Dioderm increases the margin of safety.

5.3 Preclinical safety data

No special information.

6. PHARMACEUTICAL PARTICULARS

6.1 List of excipients

Citric Acid; Emulsifying Ointment; Propylene Glycol; Purified Water.

6.2 Incompatibilities

None known.

6.3 Shelf life

24 months.

6.4 Special precautions for storage

Do not store above 25°C. Replace cap tightly after use.

6.5 Nature and contents of container

30 g collapsible tube. This is supplied as an original pack (OP).

6.6 Special precautions for disposal and other handling

Not applicable.

7. MARKETING AUTHORISATION HOLDER

Dermal Laboratories

Tatmore Place, Gosmore

Hitchin, Herts SG4 7QR, UK.

8. MARKETING AUTHORISATION NUMBER(S)

00173/0047.

9. DATE OF FIRST AUTHORISATION/RENEWAL OF THE AUTHORISATION

9 May 2008.

10. DATE OF REVISION OF THE TEXT

September 2008.

Dioralyte Relief Apricot

(sanofi-aventis)

1. NAME OF THE MEDICINAL PRODUCT

Dioralyte Relief Apricot.

2. QUALITATIVE AND QUANTITATIVE COMPOSITION

Active ingredients per sachet:

Pre-cooked Rice Powder	6g
Sodium Citrate PhEur	580mg
Sodium Chloride PhEur	350mg
Potassium Chloride PhEur	300mg

For excipients, see 6.1.

3. PHARMACEUTICAL FORM

Sachet containing powder for mixing with water prior to administration.

4. CLINICAL PARTICULARS

4.1 Therapeutic indications

Oral correction of fluid and electrolyte loss in infants aged 3 months upwards, children and adults.

Treatment of watery diarrhoea of various aetiologies including gastroenteritis in all age groups from 3 months upwards.

Dioralyte Relief is particularly recommended in the case of too loose or frequent stools where it enables over-loose stools to revert to normal.

4.2 Posology and method of administration

Method of Use

Pour the contents of one sachet into a large glass of drinking water (200ml). Mix well and drink the whole glassful. For infants and where drinking water is not available, the water should be freshly boiled and cooled. The solution should be made up immediately before use.

Adults and children:

5 sachets per day for 3 to 4 days following a loose motion.

Infants from 3 months to one year under medical advice:

In the event of diarrhoea and depending on the extent of dehydration (loss of weight assessed at less than 10%) 150 to 200 ml/kg/24 hours of preparation may be given.

- half the volume is to be given during the first 8 hours, and the other half during the next 16 hours.
- in the event of vomiting accompanying the diarrhoea, the amount administered can be divided up (5 to 10 ml every 5 minutes) and this may be gradually increased until the infant can drink normally.

4.3 Contraindications

Dioralyte Relief should not be used in patients with phenylketonuria.

However, there may be a number of conditions where treatment with Dioralyte Relief may be inappropriate, e.g. intestinal obstruction requiring surgical intervention, cases of severe renal or hepatic impairment.

4.4 Special warnings and precautions for use

For oral administration only. Dioralyte Relief should not be reconstituted in diluents other than water.

Each sachet should always be dissolved in 200ml water.

Dioralyte Relief should not be administered to infants under 3 months and for those aged 3 months to 1 year under medical advice.

If diarrhoea persists unremittingly for longer than 36 hours the patient should be reassessed by the physician.

No specific precautions are necessary in the elderly. However, care should be taken when administering Dioralyte Relief solution in cases of severe renal or hepatic impairment or other conditions where normal electrolyte balance may be disturbed.

4.5 Interaction with other medicinal products and other forms of interaction

None known.

4.6 Pregnancy and lactation

Dioralyte Relief is not contraindicated in pregnancy or lactation but should be used on medical advice.

4.7 Effects on ability to drive and use machines

Dioralyte Relief could not be expected to affect the ability to drive or use machines.

4.8 Undesirable effects

None known.

4.9 Overdose

In the event of significant overdose, serum electrolytes should be evaluated as soon as possible, appropriate steps taken to correct any abnormalities and levels monitored until return to normal levels is established. This is particularly important in the very young.

5. PHARMACOLOGICAL PROPERTIES

5.1 Pharmacodynamic properties

ATC code: Electrolytes with carbohydrates A07C.

Dioralyte Relief contains a balanced amount of electrolytes, starch and proteins in water. Oral rehydration therapy with Dioralyte Relief enables a dehydrated subject to be rehydrated rapidly. The presence of pre-cooked rice in the formulation enables watery stools to return to normal more rapidly.

The advantages of Dioralyte Relief are bound with its composition.

•*Water:* the appropriate amount is essential to correct dehydration.

•*Starch:* low osmotic capacity (unlike pure glucose) thus preventing any additional loss of fluid through the stools. Rice starch contains 20% amylose and 80% amylopectin.

•*Proteins:* specific nutritional properties.

•*Electrolytes:* essential for restoring the ionic equilibrium. The role of citrate is to correct the acidosis that occurs as a result of diarrhoea. Citrate also enhances the absorption of Na^+ and is more stable than bicarbonate.

5.2 Pharmacokinetic properties

Content of electrolytes in the reconstituted preparation:

Na^+	60 mmol/l
Cl^-	50 mmol/l
K^+	20 mmol/l
Citrate	10 mmol/l (or 30 meq/l)
Osmolarity	140 mosm/l

5.3 Preclinical safety data

Not applicable.

6. PHARMACEUTICAL PARTICULARS

6.1 List of excipients

Apricot Flavour

Hypromellose

Aspartame

Ethanol 96%

Purified Water

6.2 Incompatibilities

None known.

6.3 Shelf life

A shelf life of 36 months is given for unopened sachets of the product when stored under the conditions given in section 6.4. Once reconstituted, any solution should be used within one hour, or within 24 hours if stored in a refrigerator.

6.4 Special precautions for storage

Store in a dry place under 25°C.

6.5 Nature and contents of container

Carton containing paper/PVDC sachets of Dioralyte Relief Apricot powder. Dioralyte Relief Apricot is available in packs of 20 sachets.

6.6 Special precautions for disposal and other handling

See section 4.2 for instructions on reconstitution.

7. MARKETING AUTHORISATION HOLDER

Sanofi-aventis

One Onslow Street

Guildford

Surrey

GU1 4YS

UK

8. MARKETING AUTHORISATION NUMBER(S)

PL 004425/0272

9. DATE OF FIRST AUTHORISATION/RENEWAL OF THE AUTHORISATION

3 March 2009

10. DATE OF REVISION OF THE TEXT

March 2009

11 LEGAL CLASSIFICATION

P

Dioralyte Sachets Plain, Blackcurrant & Citrus P

(sanofi-aventis)

1. NAME OF THE MEDICINAL PRODUCT

Dioralyte Sachets Natural, Blackcurrant and Citrus.

2. QUALITATIVE AND QUANTITATIVE COMPOSITION

Glucose	3.56g
Sodium chloride	0.47g
Potassium chloride	0.30g
Disodium hydrogen citrate	0.53g

3. PHARMACEUTICAL FORM

Powder for reconstitution with 200ml water.

4. CLINICAL PARTICULARS

4.1 Therapeutic indications

Oral correction of fluid and electrolyte loss in infants, children and adults. Treatment of watery diarrhoea of various aetiologies including gastro-enteritis in all age groups.

4.2 Posology and method of administration

Route of administration: Oral

RECONSTITUTION

The contents of each sachet should be dissolved in 200ml (approx. 7 fl oz ounces) of drinking water. Use fresh drinking water for adults and children. For infants, and where drinking water is unavailable, the water should be freshly boiled and cooled. The solution should be made up immediately before use and may be stored for up to 24 hours in a refrigerator, otherwise any solution remaining an hour after reconstitution should be discarded. The solution must not be boiled.

A basic principle of treatment of diarrhoea is to replace lost fluid and electrolytes and then to maintain sufficient fluid intake to replace fluid loss from stools. The amount of reconstituted Dioralyte administered should be adapted to the age and weight of the patient and the stage and severity of the condition.

Severe dehydration may need to be corrected by parenteral fluids initially, followed by oral maintenance if indicated. If the loss of fluid in the diarrhoea is excessive, medical advice should be sought.

Daily intake may be based on a volume of 150ml/kg body weight for infants up to the age of 2 and 20-40ml/kg body weight for adults and children. A reasonable approximation is:

Infants up to the age of 2: One to one and a half times the usual 24 hour feed volume.

Children: One sachet dissolved in 200ml of water after every loose motion

Adults (including elderly): One or two sachets after every loose motion. Each sachet should be dissolved in 200ml of water.

More may be required initially to ensure early and full volume repletion.

In the initial stages of treatment of diarrhoea all foods, including cow's or artificial milk should be stopped. However, breast milk need not be withheld. In breast fed infants it is suggested that the infant is given the same volume of Dioralyte as the bottle fed baby and then put to the breast until satisfied. Expression of residual milk from the breasts may be necessary during this period. After 24-48 hours, when symptoms have subsided, the normal diet should be resumed but this should be gradual to avoid exacerbation of the condition.

When vomiting is present with the diarrhoea it is advisable that small amounts of Dioralyte be taken frequently. However, it is important that the whole of the required volume of Dioralyte be taken. Where the kidneys are functioning normally, it is difficult to over-hydrate by mouth and where there is doubt about the dosage, more rather than less should be taken. If no improvement is seen within 24-48 hours it is recommended that the patient be seen by a physician.

4.3 Contraindications

There are no known contraindications to Dioralyte. However, there may be a number of conditions where treatment with Dioralyte will be inappropriate, e.g. intestinal obstruction requiring surgical intervention.

4.4 Special warnings and precautions for use

For oral administration only.

Dioralyte should not be reconstituted in diluents other than water.

Each sachet should always be dissolved in 200ml of water. A weaker solution than recommended will not contain the optimal glucose and electrolyte concentration and a stronger solution than recommended may give rise to electrolyte imbalance. If diarrhoea persists unremittingly for longer than 24-48 hours the patient should be seen by a physician. Dioralyte should not be used for the self treatment of chronic or persistent diarrhoea except under medical supervision. Infants under the age of 2 years with diarrhoea should be seen by a physician as soon as possible. No specific precautions are necessary in the elderly.

Dioralyte should not be used for self treatment by patients with liver or kidney disease, patients on low potassium or sodium diets or patients with diabetes. The use of Dioralyte in patients with these conditions should be supervised by a physician.

4.5 Interaction with other medicinal products and other forms of interaction

None stated.

4.6 Pregnancy and lactation

Dioralyte is not contraindicated in pregnancy or lactation.

4.7 Effects on ability to drive and use machines

Dioralyte could not be expected to affect the ability to drive or use machines.

4.8 Undesirable effects

None stated.

4.9 Overdose

In the event of significant overdose, serum electrolytes should be evaluated as soon as possible, appropriate steps taken to correct any abnormalities and levels monitored until return to normal levels is established. This is particularly important in the very young and in cases of severe hepatic or renal failure.

5. PHARMACOLOGICAL PROPERTIES

5.1 Pharmacodynamic properties

Dioralyte is an oral rehydration therapy. The combination of electrolytes stimulates water and electrolyte absorption from the GI tract and therefore prevents or reverses dehydration in diarrhoea.

5.2 Pharmacokinetic properties

Sodium and glucose are actively transported via the membrane into the enterocytes. Sodium is then extruded into the intercellular spaces and the resulting osmotic gradient causes water and electrolytes to be drawn from the gut and then into the circulation.

5.3 Preclinical safety data

No relevant data.

6. PHARMACEUTICAL PARTICULARS

6.1 List of excipients

Natural: Silicon dioxide and saccharin sodium.

Blackcurrant: Silicon dioxide, Saccharin sodium and Blackcurrant flavour.

Citrus: Silicon dioxide, Saccharin sodium and Lemon and Lime flavour.

6.2 Incompatibilities

None stated.

6.3 Shelf life

Foil/laminate sachets: 24 months

6.4 Special precautions for storage

Store in a cool dry place.

6.5 Nature and contents of container

Foil/laminate sachets containing powder for reconstitution with 200ml of water.

6.6 Special precautions for disposal and other handling

The contents of each sachet should be dissolved in 200ml (approximately 7 fluid ounces) of drinking water.

7. MARKETING AUTHORISATION HOLDER

Sanofi-aventis

One Onslow Street

Guildford

Surrey GU1 4YS

8. MARKETING AUTHORISATION NUMBER(S)

Dioralyte Natural: PL 04425/0270

Dioralyte Blackcurrant: PL 04425/0211

Dioralyte Citrus: PL 04425/0260

9. DATE OF FIRST AUTHORISATION/RENEWAL OF THE AUTHORISATION

7 February 2009

10. DATE OF REVISION OF THE TEXT

February 2009

Legal Classification:

Packs of 20 sachets - P

Dipentum Capsules 250 mg, Dipentum Tablets 500 mg

(UCB Pharma Limited)

1. NAME OF THE MEDICINAL PRODUCT

Dipentum Capsules 250 mg

Dipentum Tablets 500 mg

2. QUALITATIVE AND QUANTITATIVE COMPOSITION

Each capsule or tablet contains 250mg or 500mg olsalazine sodium.

For excipients, see 6.1.

3. PHARMACEUTICAL FORM

Capsule, hard

Tablet

4. CLINICAL PARTICULARS

4.1 Therapeutic indications

Oral treatment of mild active ulcerative colitis and maintenance of remission.

4.2 Posology and method of administration

Oral.

General

Olsalazine taken on an empty stomach may sometimes lead to loose stools or diarrhoea. By taking the drug at the end of a meal, this may be avoided.

Acute Mild Disease

Adults including the elderly: Commence on 1 g daily in divided doses taken at the end of meals. Depending on the patient's response, the dose may be titrated upwards over a period of one week to a maximum of 3g daily.

A single dose should not exceed 1 g.

Remission

Adults including the elderly: A dose of 0.5g should be taken twice daily, at the end of meals.

Olsalazine has been used concomitantly with gluco-corticosteroids.

4.3 Contraindications

Hypersensitivity to olsalazine or other salicylates or any other of the excipients.

There is no experience of the use of olsalazine in patients with significant renal impairment. Olsalazine is contra-indicated in patients with significant renal impairment.

4.4 Special warnings and precautions for use

It is recommended to monitor patients with impaired kidney or liver function.

Patients suffering from severe allergy or asthma should be observed for signs of worsening of these conditions.

Serious blood dyscrasias have been reported very rarely with olsalazine. Haematological investigations should be performed if the patient develops unexplained bleeding, bruising, purpura, anaemia, fever or sore throat. Treatment should be stopped if there is a suspicion or evidence of a blood dyscrasia.

4.5 Interaction with other medicinal products and other forms of interaction

The coadministration of salicylates and low molecular weight heparins or heparinoids may result in an increased risk of bleeding, more specifically hematomas following neuraxial anesthesia. Salicylates should be discontinued prior to the initiation of a low molecular weight heparin or heparinoid. If this is not possible, it is recommended to monitor patients closely for bleeding.

Increased prothrombin time in patients taking concomitant warfarin has been reported.

The coadministration of olsalazine and 6-mercaptopurine or thioguanine may result in an increased risk of myelo-suppression. If coadministered with 6-mercaptopurine, it is recommended to use the lowest possible doses of each drug and to monitor the patient, especially for leukopenia. In case of coadministration with thioguanine, careful monitoring of blood counts is recommended.

It is recommended not to give salicylates for six weeks after the varicella vaccine to avoid a possible increased risk of developing Reye's syndrome.

4.6 Pregnancy and lactation

Pregnancy:

Olsalazine has been shown to produce fetal developmental toxicity as indicated by reduced fetal weights, retarded ossifications and immaturity of the fetal visceral organs when given during organogenesis to pregnant rats in doses 5 to 20 times the human dose (100 to 400 mg/kg).

There are no adequate and well-controlled studies in pregnant women. Olsalazine should be used during pregnancy only if the potential benefit justifies the potential risk to the foetus.

There is a reported risk of stillborn or pre-term birth but with no substantial risk of malformation.

Lactation:

Small amounts of the active metabolite of olsalazine (5-ASA) may pass into breast milk. Harmful infant effects (diarrhea) have been reported when 5-ASA was used during breastfeeding. Unless the benefit of the treatment outweighs the risks, olsalazine should not be taken by breast-feeding women, or patients should be advised to discontinue breastfeeding if using olsalazine.

4.7 Effects on ability to drive and use machines

On the basis of the pharmacodynamic profile and reported adverse events, olsalazine has minor or moderate influence on the ability to drive and use machines in patients that experience dizziness and /or blurred vision when taking olsalazine. Caution is recommended in patients that experience these symptoms.

4.8 Undesirable effects

The most common side effect is diarrhoea which is usually transient. Where it does not, taking the drug at the end of a more substantial meal, dose titration or dose reduction are usually effective. Withdrawal in clinical studies when the drug was taken at the end of meals was around 3%. Where diarrhoea persists, the drug should be stopped.

In addition, the following undesirable effects have been reported:

General disorders and administration site conditions: headache, pyrexia

Blood and lymphatic system disorders: aplastic anaemia, eosinophilia, haemolytic anemia, leukopenia, neutropenia, pancytopenia, thrombocytopenia

Gastrointestinal disorders: abdominal pain upper, diarrhoea, dyspepsia, nausea, pancreatitis, vomiting

Hepatobiliary disorders: hepatic enzyme increased, hepatitis, increased bilirubin

Skin and subcutaneous tissue disorders: alopecia, angioneurotic oedema, photosensitivity reaction, pruritus, rash, urticaria,

Cardiac disorders: myocarditis, palpitations, pericarditis, tachycardia

Renal and urinary disorders: interstitial nephritis

Respiratory, thoracic and mediastinal disorders: dyspnoea

Musculoskeletal and connective tissue disorders: arthralgia, myalgia

Nervous system disorders: dizziness, paraesthesia

Eye disorders: vision blurred

4.9 Overdose

The knowledge of overdosage is limited. Possible overdose symptoms include nausea, vomiting and diarrhoea. It is recommended to check hematology, acid-base, electrolyte, liver and kidney status, and to provide supportive treatment. There is no specific antidote to Dipentum.

As a salicylate, interference in biochemical and other tests characteristic of salicylates may occur.

5. PHARMACOLOGICAL PROPERTIES

5.1 Pharmacodynamic properties

ATC Code: A07E C 03, Aminosalicylic acid and similar agents.

Olsalazine is itself a relatively inert compound. Absorption in the small intestine is slight. On entering the colon it is split by bacteria into two molecules of 5-amino salicylate (5-ASA, mesalazine). 5-ASA is believed to be principal active fragment of sulphasalazine, which has been in use for 40 years in the treatment of ulcerative colitis. 5-ASA is believed to be the active form of Dipentum as olsalazine has little effect in in-vitro tests or on experimental animals. The clinical benefits of sulphasalazine, 5-ASA and olsalazine are evident in ulcerative colitis, but the pharmacological mechanism is not established.

5.2 Pharmacokinetic properties

Studies in man and animals indicate a low uptake of olsalazine and its metabolites, which is in keeping with the desired aim to deliver a high local concentration of 5-ASA to the colon.

In man an oral dose of olsalazine is negligibly absorbed in the gut. Bacteria split olsalazine in the colon into two molecules of 5-ASA. Local concentrations of 5-ASA in the colon can be 1000 times the plasma levels. Uptake by colonic mucosal cells leads to acetyl 5-ASA generation (the principle metabolite), traces of 5-ASA and olsalazine-O-SO_4 also being found in plasma. 500 mg b.d. in 6 volunteers gave a steady state level of amino salicylate of 0.8-2.9 mcg/ml after 6-9 days. In ileostomised patients almost all the olsalazine could be recovered in ileal fluid. Intravenous administration of olsalazine showed bilary excretion and traces of Ac-5-ASA in the urine and a half life of 56 minutes. Olsalazine given with or without food was taken up to the extent of 1.3 or 1.6% respectively. After a 1 g dose p.o. a maximum plasma level of 12.2 mcg/ml was noted at 1 hour of olsalazine. 22-33% of an oral dose appears in the urine almost all as Ac-5-ASA. The metabolite olsalazine-O-SO_4 is 99% plasma bound and has a half life of 6-10 days. Olsalazine does not penetrate red cells nor displace warfarin, naproxen, diazepam or digitoxin from plasma binding.

Autoradiography in rats showed no activity in the brain, testes, placenta or foetus, some activity in the bile duct and kidney and high activity in the gut.

5.3 Preclinical safety data

None stated

6. PHARMACEUTICAL PARTICULARS

6.1 List of excipients

Dipentum Capsules 250mg:

Magnesium stearate

Gelatin

Dipentum Tablets 500mg:

Magnesium stearate

Colloidal silicon dioxide

Polyvidone 30

Crospovidone

Ethanol 99.5%

6.2 Incompatibilities

As a salicylate, interference in biochemical and other tests characteristics of salicylates may occur.

6.3 Shelf life

Capsules – 60 months, unopened

Tablets - 48 months, unopened.

6.4 Special precautions for storage

Capsules – Store at room temperature in a dry place

Tablets - Store in a dry place.

6.5 Nature and contents of container

Capsules:

White, square, polyethylene bottles with knurled tamper evident cap containing 112 capsules, with a label incorporating a pull-out leaflet.

Tablets:

HD polyethylene securitainers with cap,

or

HD polyethylene square section pots with child and tamper resistant cap.

Packs of 60 tablets

Packs of 100 tablets (not marketed)

6.6 Special precautions for disposal and other handling

None stated.

7. MARKETING AUTHORISATION HOLDER

UCB Pharma Limited

208 Bath Road

Slough

Berkshire

SL1 3WE

United Kingdom

8. MARKETING AUTHORISATION NUMBER(S)

Dipentum Capsules 250mg: PL 00039/0526

Dipentum Tablets 500mg: PL 00039/0527

9. DATE OF FIRST AUTHORISATION/RENEWAL OF THE AUTHORISATION

31st October 2002

10. DATE OF REVISION OF THE TEXT

Approved: September 2008

Diprivan 1%

(AstraZeneca UK Limited)

1. NAME OF THE MEDICINAL PRODUCT

Diprivan 10 mg/ml (1%) emulsion for injection or infusion

2. QUALITATIVE AND QUANTITATIVE COMPOSITION

Propofol 10 mg/ml

3. PHARMACEUTICAL FORM

Emulsion for injection or infusion.

White aqueous isotonic oil-in-water emulsion.

4. CLINICAL PARTICULARS

4.1 Therapeutic indications

'Diprivan' 1% is a short-acting intravenous anaesthetic agent suitable for induction and maintenance of general anaesthesia.

Diprivan' 1% may also be used for sedation of ventilated patients receiving intensive care.

'Diprivan' 1% may also be used for sedation for surgical and diagnostic procedures.

4.2 Posology and method of administration

For specific guidance relating to the administration of 'Diprivan' 1% with a target controlled infusion (TCI) device, which incorporates 'Diprifusor' TCI Software, see Section 4.2.5. Such use is restricted to induction and maintenance of anaesthesia in adults. The 'Diprifusor' TCI system is not recommended for use in ICU sedation or sedation for surgical and diagnostic procedures, or in children.

4.2.1 Induction of General Anaesthesia

Adults

In unpremedicated and premedicated patients, it is recommended that 'Diprivan' 1% should be titrated (approximately 4 ml [40 mg] every 10 seconds in an average healthy adult by bolus injection or infusion) against the response of the patient until the clinical signs show the onset of anaesthesia. Most adult patients aged less than 55 years are likely to require 1.5 to 2.5 mg/kg of 'Diprivan' 1%. The total dose required can be reduced by lower rates of administration (2 to 5 ml/min [20 to 50 mg/min]). Over this age, the requirement will generally be less. In patients of ASA Grades 3 and 4, lower rates of administration should be used (approximately 2 ml [20 mg] every 10 seconds).

Elderly Patients

In elderly patients the dose requirement for induction of anaesthesia with 'Diprivan' 1% is reduced. The reduction should take into account of the physical status and age of the patient. The reduced dose should be given at a slower rate and titrated against the response.

Children

'Diprivan' 1% is not recommended for induction of anaesthesia in children aged less than 1 month.

When used to induce anaesthesia in children, it is recommended that 'Diprivan' 1% be given slowly until the clinical signs show the onset of anaesthesia. The dose should be adjusted for age and/or weight. Most patients over 8 years of age are likely to require approximately 2.5 mg/kg of 'Diprivan' 1% for induction of anaesthesia. Under this age the requirement may be more. Lower dosage is recommended for children of ASA grades 3 and 4.

Administration of 'Diprivan' 1% by a 'Diprifusor' TCI system is not recommended for induction of general anaesthesia in children.

4.2.2 Maintenance Of General Anaesthesia

Adults

Anaesthesia can be maintained by administering 'Diprivan' 1% either by continuous infusion or by repeat bolus injections to prevent the clinical signs of light anaesthesia. Recovery from anaesthesia is typically rapid and it is therefore important to maintain 'Diprivan' 1% administration until the end of the procedure.

Continuous Infusion

The required rate of administration varies considerably between patients, but rates in the region of 4 to 12 mg/kg/h usually maintain satisfactory anaesthesia.

Repeat Bolus Injections

If a technique involving repeat bolus injections is used, increments of 25 mg (2.5 ml) to 50 mg (5.0 ml) may be given according to clinical need.

Elderly Patients

When 'Diprivan' 1% is used for maintenance of anaesthesia the rate of infusion or 'target concentration' should also be reduced. Patients of ASA grades 3 and 4 will require further reductions in dose and dose rate. Rapid bolus administration (single or repeated) should not be used in the elderly as this may lead to cardiorespiratory depression.

Children

'Diprivan' 1% is not recommended for maintenance of anaesthesia in children less than 1 month old.

Anaesthesia can be maintained by administering 'Diprivan' 1% by infusion or repeat bolus injection to prevent the clinical signs of light anaesthesia. The required rate of administration varies considerably between patients, but rates in the region of 9 to 15 mg/kg/h usually achieve satisfactory anaesthesia. Younger children, less than 3 years, may have higher dosage requirements within the range of recommended dosages, as compared with older paediatric patients. Dosage should be adjusted individually and particular attention paid to the need for adequate analgesia. A maximum duration of use of approximately 60 minutes should not be exceeded except where there is a specific indication for longer use e.g. malignant hyperthermia where volatile agents must be avoided.

Administration of 'Diprivan' 1% by a 'Diprifusor' TCI system is not recommended for maintenance of general anaesthesia in children.

4.2.3 Sedation During Intensive Care

Adults

For sedation during intensive care it is advised that Diprivan 1% should be administered by continuous infusion. The infusion rate should be determined by the desired depth of sedation. In most patients sufficient sedation can be obtained with a dosage of 0.3 - 4 mg/kg/h of Diprivan 1% (See 4.4 Special warnings and precautions for use). Diprivan 1% is not indicated for sedation in intensive care of patients of 16 years of age or younger (see 4.3 Contraindications). Administration of Diprivan 1% by Diprifusor TCI system is not advised for sedation in the intensive care unit.

Diprivan' 1% may be diluted with 5% Dextrose (see "Dilution and Co-administration" table below).

It is recommended that blood lipid levels be monitored should 'Diprivan' 1% be administered to patients thought to be at particular risk of fat overload. Administration of 'Diprivan' 1% should be adjusted appropriately if the monitoring indicates that fat is being inadequately cleared from the body. If the patient is receiving other intravenous lipid concurrently, a reduction in quantity should be made in order to take account of the amount of lipid infused as part of the 'Diprivan' 1% formulation; 1.0 ml of 'Diprivan' 1% contains approximately 0.1g of fat.

If the duration of sedation is in excess of 3 days, lipids should be monitored in all patients.

Elderly Patients

When 'Diprivan' 1% is used for sedation the rate of infusion should also be reduced. Patients of ASA grades 3 and 4 will require further reductions in dose and dose rate. Rapid bolus administration (single or repeated) should not be used in the elderly as this may lead to cardiorespiratory depression.

Children

'Diprivan' 1% is contraindicated for the sedation of ventilated children aged 16 years or younger receiving intensive care.

4.2.4 Sedation For Surgical And Diagnostic Procedures

Adults

To provide sedation for surgical and diagnostic procedures, rates of administration should be individualised and titrated to clinical response.

Most patients will require 0.5 to 1 mg/kg over 1 to 5 minutes for onset of sedation.

Maintenance of sedation may be accomplished by titrating 'Diprivan' 1% infusion to the desired level of sedation - most patients will require 1.5 to 4.5 mg/kg/h. In addition to the infusion, bolus administration of 10 to 20 mg may be used if a rapid increase in the depth of sedation is required. In patients of ASA Grades 3 and 4 the rate of administration and dosage may need to be reduced.

Administration of 'Diprivan' 1% by a 'Diprifusor' TCI system is not recommended for sedation for surgical and diagnostic procedures.

Elderly Patients

When 'Diprivan' 1% is used for sedation the rate of infusion or 'target concentration' should also be reduced. Patients of ASA grades 3 and 4 will require further reductions in dose and dose rate. Rapid bolus administration (single or repeated) should not be used in the elderly as this may lead to cardiorespiratory depression.

Children

'Diprivan' 1% is not recommended for sedation in children as safety and efficacy have not been demonstrated.

4.2.5 Administration

'Diprivan' 1% has no analgesic properties and therefore supplementary analgesic agents are generally required in addition to 'Diprivan' 1%.

'Diprivan' 1% can be used for infusion undiluted from glass containers, plastic syringes or 'Diprivan' 1% pre-filled syringes or diluted with 5% Dextrose (Intravenous Infusion BP) only, in PVC infusion bags or glass infusion bottles. Dilutions, which must not exceed 1 in 5 (2 mg propofol per ml) should be prepared aseptically immediately before administration and must be used within 6 hours of preparation.

It is recommended that, when using diluted 'Diprivan' 1%, the volume of 5% Dextrose removed from the infusion bag during the dilution process is totally replaced in volume by 'Diprivan' 1% emulsion. (see "Dilution and Co-administration" table below).

The dilution may be used with a variety of infusion control techniques, but a giving set used alone will not avoid the risk of accidental uncontrolled infusion of large volumes of diluted 'Diprivan' 1%. A burette, drop counter or volumetric pump must be included in the infusion line. The risk of uncontrolled infusion must be taken into account when deciding the maximum amount of 'Diprivan' 1% in the burette.

When 'Diprivan' 1% is used undiluted to maintain anaesthesia, it is recommended that equipment such as syringe pumps or volumetric infusion pumps should always be used to control infusion rates.

'Diprivan' 1% may be administered via a Y-piece close to the injection site into infusions of the following:

- Dextrose 5% Intravenous Infusion B.P.
- Sodium Chloride 0.9% Intravenous Infusion B.P.
- Dextrose 4% with Sodium Chloride 0.18% Intravenous Infusion B.P.

The glass pre-filled syringe (PFS) has a lower frictional resistance than plastic disposable syringes and operates more easily. Therefore, if 'Diprivan' 1% is administered using a hand held pre-filled syringe, the line between the syringe and the patient must not be left open if unattended.

When the pre-filled syringe presentation is used in a syringe pump appropriate compatibility should be ensured. In particular, the pump should be designed to prevent syphoning and should have an occlusion alarm set no greater than 1000 mm Hg. If using a programmable or equivalent pump that offers options for use of different syringes then choose only the 'B-D' 50/60 ml 'PLASTIPAK' setting when using the 'Diprivan' 1% pre-filled syringe.

'Diprivan' 1% may be premixed with alfentanil injection containing 500 micrograms/ml alfentanil in the ratio of 20:1 to 50:1 v/v. Mixtures should be prepared using sterile technique and used within 6 hours of preparation.

In order to reduce pain on initial injection, 'Diprivan' 1% may be mixed with preservative-free Lidocaine Injection 0.5% or 1%; (see "Dilution and Co-administration" table below).

Target Controlled Infusion - Administration of 'Diprivan' 1% by a 'Diprifusor' TCI System in Adults

Administration of 'Diprivan' 1% by a 'Diprifusor' TCI system is restricted to induction and maintenance of general anaesthesia in adults. It is not recommended for use in ICU sedation or sedation for surgical and diagnostic procedures, or in children.

'Diprivan' 1% may be administered by TCI only with a 'Diprifusor' TCI system incorporating 'Diprifusor' TCI software. Such systems will operate only on recognition of electronically tagged pre-filled syringes containing 'Diprivan' 1% or 2% Injection. The 'Diprifusor' TCI system will automatically adjust the infusion rate for the concentration of 'Diprivan' recognised. Users must be familiar with the infusion pump users' manual, and with the administration of 'Diprivan' 1% by TCI and with the correct use of the syringe identification system.

The system allows the anaesthetist or intensivist to achieve and control a desired speed of induction and depth of anaesthesia by setting and adjusting target (predicted) blood concentrations of propofol.

The 'Diprifusor' TCI system assumes that the initial blood propofol concentration in the patient is zero. Therefore, in patients who have received prior propofol, there may be a need to select a lower initial target concentration when commencing 'Diprifusor' TCI. Similarly, the immediate recommencement of 'Diprifusor' TCI is not recommended if the pump has been switched off.

Guidance on propofol target concentrations is given below. In view of interpatient variability in propofol pharmacokinetics and pharmacodynamics, in both premedicated and unpremedicated patients the target propofol concentration should be titrated against the response of the patient in order to achieve the depth of anaesthesia required.

Induction and Maintenance of General Anaesthesia

In adult patients under 55 years of age anaesthesia can usually be induced with target propofol concentrations in the region of 4 to 8 microgram/ml. An initial target of 4 microgram/ml is recommended in premedicated patients and in unpremedicated patients an initial target of 6 microgram/ml is advised. Induction time with these targets is generally within the range of 60 to 120 seconds. Higher targets will allow more rapid induction of anaesthesia but may be associated with more pronounced haemodynamic and respiratory depression.

A lower initial target concentration should be used in patients over the age of about 55 years and in patients of ASA grades 3 and 4. The target concentration can then be increased in steps of 0.5 to 1.0 microgram/ml at intervals of 1 minute to achieve a gradual induction of anaesthesia.

Supplementary analgesia will generally be required and the extent to which target concentrations for maintenance of anaesthesia can be reduced will be influenced by the amount of concomitant analgesia administered. Target propofol concentrations in the region of 3 to 6 microgram/ml usually maintain satisfactory anaesthesia.

The predicted propofol concentration on waking is generally in the region of 1.0 to 2.0 microgram/ml and will be influenced by the amount of analgesia given during maintenance.

Sedation during intensive care

Target blood propofol concentration settings in the range of 0.2 to 2.0 μg/ml will generally be required. Administration should begin at low target setting which should be titrated against the response of the patient to achieve the depth of sedation desired.

Dilution and CoAdministration of 'Diprivan' 1% with Other Drugs or Infusion Fluids (see also 'Additional Precautions' Section)

(see Table 1 below)

4.3 Contraindications

Diprivan is contraindicated in patients with a known hypersensitivity to propofol or any of the excipients.

Diprivan 1% is contraindicated for sedation in intensive care of patients of 16 years of age or younger (See 4.4 Special warnings and precautions for use).

Diprivan 1% contains soya oil and should not be used in patients who are hypersensitive to peanut or soya.

4.4 Special warnings and precautions for use

'Diprivan' 1% should be given by those trained in anaesthesia or, where appropriate, doctors trained in the care of

Table 1

Co-administration Technique	Additive or Diluent	Preparation	Precautions
Pre-mixing.	Dextrose 5% Intravenous Infusion	Mix 1 part of 'Diprivan' 1% with up to 4 parts of Dextrose 5% Intravenous Infusion B.P in either PVC infusion bags or glass infusion bottles. When diluted in PVC bags it is recommended that the bag should be full and that the dilution be prepared by withdrawing a volume of infusion fluid and replacing it with an equal volume of 'Diprivan' 1%.	Prepare aseptically immediately before administration. The mixture is stable for up to 6 hours.
	Lidocaine hydrochloride injection (0.5% or 1% without preservatives).	Mix 20 parts of 'Diprivan' 1% with up to 1 part of either 0.5% or 1% lidocaine hydrochloride injection.	Prepare mixture aseptically immediately prior to administration. Use for Induction only.
	Alfentanil injection (500 microgram/ml).	Mix 'Diprivan' 1% with alfentanil injection in a ratio of 20:1 to 50:1 v/v.	Prepare mixture aseptically; use within 6 hours of preparation.
Co-administration via a Y-piece connector.	Dextrose 5% intravenous infusion	Co-administer via a Y-piece connector.	Place the Y-piece connector close to the injection site.
	Sodium chloride 0.9% intravenous infusion	As above	As above
	Dextrose 4% with sodium chloride 0.18% intravenous infusion	As above	As above

patients in Intensive Care. Patients should be constantly monitored and facilities for maintenance of a patient airway, artificial ventilation, oxygen enrichment and other resuscitative facilities should be readily available at all times. 'Diprivan' 1% should not be administered by the person conducting the diagnostic or surgical procedure.

When 'Diprivan' 1% is administered for sedation for surgical and diagnostic procedures patients should be continually monitored for early signs of hypotension, airway obstruction and oxygen desaturation.

As with other sedative agents, when Diprivan is used for sedation during operative procedures, involuntary patient movements may occur. During procedures requiring immobility these movements may be hazardous to the operative site.

As with other intravenous anaesthetic and sedative agents, patients should be instructed to avoid alcohol before and for at least 8 hours after administration of 'Diprivan' 1%.

'Diprivan' 1% should be used with caution when used to sedate patients undergoing some procedures where spontaneous movements are particularly undesirable, such as ophthalmic surgery.

As with other intravenous sedative agents, when 'Diprivan' 1% is given along with central nervous system depressants, such as potent analgesics, the sedative effect may be intensified and the possibility of severe respiratory or cardiovascular depression should be considered.

During bolus administration for operative procedures, extreme caution should be exercised in patients with acute pulmonary insufficiency or respiratory depression.

Concomitant use of central nervous system depressants e.g., alcohol, general anaesthetics, narcotic analgesics will result in accentuation of their sedative effects. When 'Diprivan' 1% is combined with centrally depressant drugs administered parenterally, severe respiratory and cardiovascular depression may occur. It is recommended that 'Diprivan' 1% is administered following the analgesic and the dose should be carefully titrated to the patient's response (see Section 4.5).

During induction of anaesthesia, hypotension and transient apnoea may occur depending on the dose and use of premedicants and other agents.

Occasionally, hypotension may require use of intravenous fluids and reduction of the rate of administration of 'Diprivan' 1% during the period of anaesthetic maintenance.

An adequate period is needed prior to discharge of the patient to ensure full recovery after general anaesthesia. Very rarely the use of 'Diprivan' may be associated with the development of a period of post-operative unconsciousness, which may be accompanied by an increase in muscle tone. This may or may not be preceded by a period of wakefulness. Although recovery is spontaneous, appropriate care of an unconscious patient should be administered.

When 'Diprivan' 1% is administered to an epileptic patient, there may be a risk of convulsion.

As with other intravenous anaesthetic agents, caution should be applied in patients with cardiac, respiratory, renal or hepatic impairment or in hypovolaemic, elderly or debilitated patients.

The risk of relative vagal overactivity may be increased because 'Diprivan' 1% lacks vagolytic activity; it has been associated with reports of bradycardia (occasionally profound) and also asystole. The intravenous administration of an anticholinergic agent before induction, or during maintenance of anaesthesia should be considered, especially in situations where vagal tone is likely to predominate, or when 'Diprivan' 1% is used in conjunction with other agents likely to cause a bradycardia.

Appropriate care should be applied in patients with disorders of fat metabolism and in other conditions where lipid emulsions must be used cautiously.

Use is not recommended with electroconvulsive treatment.

As with other anaesthetics, sexual disinhibition may occur during recovery.

Diprivan 1% is not advised for general anaesthesia in children younger than 1 month of age. The safety and efficacy of Diprivan 1% for (background) sedation in children younger than 16 years of age have not been demonstrated. Although no causal relationship has been established, serious undesirable effects with (background) sedation in patients younger than 16 years of age (including cases with fatal outcome) have been reported during unlicensed use. In particular these effects concerned occurrence of metabolic acidosis, hyperlipidemia, rhabdomyolysis and/or cardiac failure. These effects were most frequently seen in children with respiratory tract infections who received dosages in excess of those advised in adults for sedation in the intensive care unit.

Diprivan is not recommended for use in neonates for induction and maintenance of anaesthesia. Data from 'off-label' use have indicated that if the paediatric (1 month to 16 years of age) dose regimen is applied in neonates, a relative overdose could occur which may result in cardio-respiratory depression.

Similarly very rare reports have been received of occurrence of metabolic acidosis, rhabdomyolysis, hyperkalaemia and/or rapidly progressive cardiac failure (in some cases with fatal outcome) in adults who were treated for more than 58 hours with dosages in excess of 5 mg/kg/h. This exceeds the maximum dosage of 4 mg/kg/h currently advised for sedation in the intensive care unit. The patients affected were mainly (but not only) seriously head-injured patients with raised ICP. The cardiac failure in such cases was usually unresponsive to inotropic supportive treatment. Treating physicians are reminded if possible not to exceed the dosage of 4 mg/kg/h. Prescribers should be alert to these possible undesirable effects and consider decreasing the Diprivan 1% dosage or switching to an alternative sedative at the first sign of occurrence of symptoms. Patients with raised ICP should be given appropriate treatment to support the cerebral perfusion pressure during these treatment modifications.

Diprivan 1% contains 0.0018 mmol sodium per ml.

EDTA is a chelator of metal ions, including zinc. The need for supplemental zinc should be considered during prolonged administration of Diprivan, particularly in patients who are predisposed to zinc deficiency, such as those with burns, diarrhoea and/or major sepsis.

Additional Precautions

'Diprivan' 1% contains no antimicrobial preservatives and supports growth of micro-organisms. When 'Diprivan' 1% is to be aspirated, it must be drawn aseptically into a sterile syringe or giving set immediately after opening the ampoule or breaking the vial seal. Administration must commence without delay. Asepsis must be maintained for both 'Diprivan' 1% and infusion equipment throughout the infusion period. Any drugs or fluids added to the 'Diprivan' 1% line must be administered close to the cannula site. 'Diprivan' 1% must not be administered via a microbiological filter.

'Diprivan' 1% and any syringe containing 'Diprivan' 1% are for single use in an individual patient. For use in long term maintenance of anaesthesia or sedation in intensive care it is recommended that the infusion line and reservoir of 'Diprivan' 1% be discarded and replaced at regular intervals.

4.5 Interaction with other medicinal products and other forms of interaction

'Diprivan' 1% has been used in association with spinal and epidural anaesthesia and with commonly used premedicants, neuromuscular blocking drugs, inhalational agents and analgesic agents; no pharmacological incompatibility has been encountered. Lower doses of 'Diprivan' 1% may be required where general anaesthesia is used as an adjunct to regional anaesthetic techniques.

The concurrent administration of other CNS depressants such as pre-medication drugs, inhalation agents, analgesic agents may add to the sedative, anaesthetic and cardiorespiratory depressant effects of propofol (see Section 4.4).

4.6 Pregnancy and lactation

Pregnancy

The safety of Diprivan during pregnancy has not been established. Therefore Diprivan should not be used in pregnancy unless clearly necessary. Diprivan has been used, however, during termination of pregnancy in the first trimester.

Obstetrics

'Diprivan' 1% crosses the placenta and may be associated with neonatal depression. It should not be used for obstetric anaesthesia unless clearly necessary.

Lactation

Safety to the neonate has not been established following the use of 'Diprivan' 1% in mothers who are breast feeding.

4.7 Effects on ability to drive and use machines

Patients should be advised that performance at skilled tasks, such as driving and operating machinery, may be impaired for some time after general anaesthesia.

4.8 Undesirable effects

General

Induction of anaesthesia is generally smooth with minimal evidence of excitation. The most commonly reported ADRs are pharmacologically predictable side effects of an anaesthetic agent, such as hypotension. Given the nature of anaesthesia and those patients receiving intensive care, events reported in association with anaesthesia and intensive care may also be related to the procedures being undertaken or the recipient's condition.

Very common (>1/10)	*General disorders and administration site conditions:*	Local pain on induction [1]
Common (>1/100, <1/10)	*Vascular disorder:*	Hypotension [2]
	Cardiac disorders:	Bradycardia [3]
	Respiratory, thoracic and mediastinal disorders:	Transient apnoea during induction
	Gastrointestinal disorders:	Nausea and vomiting during recovery phase
	Nervous system disorders:	Headache during recovery phase
	General disorders and administration site conditions:	Withdrawal symptoms in children [4]
	Vascular disorders:	Flushing in children [4]
Uncommon (>1/1000, <1/100)	*Vascular disorders:*	Thrombosis and phlebitis
Rare (>1/10 000, <1/1000)	*Nervous system disorders:*	Epileptiform movements, including convulsions and opisthotonus during induction, maintenance and recovery
Very rare (<1/10 000)	*Musculoskeletal and connective tissue disorders:*	Rhabdomyolysis [5]
	Gastrointestinal disorders:	Pancreatitis
	Injury, poisoning and procedural complications:	Post-operative fever
	Renal and urinary disorders:	Discolouration of urine following prolonged administration
	Immune system disorders:	Anaphylaxis – may include angioedema, bronchospasm, erythema and hypotension
	Reproductive system and breast disorders:	Sexual disinhibition
	Cardiac disorders:	Pulmonary oedema
	Nervous system disorders:	Postoperative unconsciousness

(1) May be minimised by using the larger veins of the forearm and antecubital fossa. With Diprivan 1% local pain can also be minimised by the co-administration of lidocaine.

(2) Occasionally, hypotension may require use of intravenous fluids and reduction of the administration rate of Diprivan.

(3) Serious bradycardias are rare. There have been isolated reports of progression to asystole.

(4) Following abrupt discontinuation of Diprivan during intensive care.

(5) Very rare reports of rhadbomyolysis have been received where Diprivan has been given at doses greater than 4 mg/kg/hr for ICU sedation.

Pulmonary oedema, hypotension, asystole, bradycardia, and convulsions, have been reported. In very rare cases rhabdomyolysis, metabolic acidosis, hyperkalaemia or cardiac failure, sometimes with fatal outcome, have been observed when propofol was administered at dosages in excess of 4 mg/kg/h for sedation in the intensive care unit (see 4.4 Special warnings and precautions for use). Dystonia/dyskinesia have been reported.

Reports from off-label use of Diprivan for induction of anaesthesia in neonates indicates that cardio-respiratory depression may occur if the paediatric dose regimen is applied.

Local

The local pain which may occur during the induction phase of 'Diprivan' 1% anaesthesia can be minimised by the co-administration of lidocaine (see "Dosage and Administration") and by the use of the larger veins of the forearm and antecubital fossa. Thrombosis and phlebitis are rare. Accidental clinical extravasation and animal studies showed minimal tissue reaction. Intra-arterial injection in animals did not induce local tissue effects.

4.9 Overdose

Accidental overdosage is likely to cause cardiorespiratory depression. Respiratory depression should be treated by artificial ventilation with oxygen. Cardiovascular depression would require lowering of the patient's head and, if severe, use of plasma expanders and pressor agents.

5. PHARMACOLOGICAL PROPERTIES

5.1 Pharmacodynamic properties

Propofol (2, 6-diisopropylphenol) is a short-acting general anaesthetic agent with a rapid onset of action of approximately 30 seconds. Recovery from anaesthesia is usually rapid. The mechanism of action, like all general anaesthetics, is poorly understood. However, propofol is thought to produce its sedative/anaesthetic effects by the positive modulation of the inhibitory function of the neurotransmitter GABA through the ligand-gated $GABA_A$ receptors.

In general, falls in mean arterial blood pressure and slight changes in heart rate are observed when 'Diprivan' 1% is administered for induction and maintenance of anaesthesia. However, the haemodynamic parameters normally remain relatively stable during maintenance and the incidence of untoward haemodynamic changes is low.

Although ventilatory depression can occur following administration of 'Diprivan' 1%, any effects are qualitatively similar to those of other intravenous anaesthetic agents and are readily manageable in clinical practice.

'Diprivan' 1% reduces cerebral blood flow, intracranial pressure and cerebral metabolism. The reduction in intracranial pressure is greater in patients with an elevated baseline intracranial pressure.

Recovery from anaesthesia is usually rapid and clear headed with a low incidence of headache and post-operative nausea and vomiting.

In general, there is less post-operative nausea and vomiting following anaesthesia with 'Diprivan' 1% than following anaesthesia with inhalational agents. There is evidence that this may be related to a reduced emetic potential of propofol.

'Diprivan' 1%, at the concentrations likely to occur clinically, does not inhibit the synthesis of adrenocortical hormones.

5.2 Pharmacokinetic properties

The decline in propofol concentrations following a bolus dose or following the termination of an infusion can be described by a three compartment open model with very rapid distribution (half-life 2 to 4 minutes), rapid elimination (half-life 30 to 60 minutes), and a slower final phase, representative of redistribution of propofol from poorly perfused tissue.

Propofol is extensively distributed and rapidly cleared from the body (total body clearance 1.5 to 2 litres/minute). Clearance occurs by metabolic processes, mainly in the liver, to form inactive conjugates of propofol and its corresponding quinol, which are excreted in urine.

When 'Diprivan' 1% is used to maintain anaesthesia, blood concentrations asymptotically approach the steady-state value for the given administration rate. The pharmacokinetics are linear over the recommended range of infusion rates of 'Diprivan' 1%.

5.3 Preclinical safety data

Propofol is a drug on which extensive clinical experience has been obtained. All relevant information for the prescriber is provided elsewhere in the Summary of Product Characteristics.

6. PHARMACEUTICAL PARTICULARS

6.1 List of excipients

Glycerol Ph Eur

Purified Egg Phosphatide

Sodium Hydroxide Ph Eur

Soya-bean Oil, Refined Ph Eur

Water for Injections Ph Eur

Nitrogen Ph Eur

Disodium Edetate Ph Eur

6.2 Incompatibilities

The neuromuscular blocking agents, atracurium and mivacurium should not be given through the same intravenous line as 'Diprivan' 1% without prior flushing.

6.3 Shelf life

6.3.1 Shelf life of the product as packaged for sale

Ampoules - 3 years

Vials - 3 years

Pre-filled syringe - 2 years.

6.3.2 Shelf life after dilution

Use of diluted Diprivan must begin immediately following dilution.

6.4 Special precautions for storage

Store between 2°C and 25°C.

Do not freeze.

6.5 Nature and contents of container

a) Clear neutral glass ampoules of 20 ml in boxes of 5

b) Clear neutral glass vials of 50 ml and 100 ml

c) Type 1 glass pre-filled syringe of 50 ml

6.6 Special precautions for disposal and other handling In-use precautions

Containers should be shaken before use.

Any portion of the contents remaining after use should be discarded.

'Diprivan' 1% should not be mixed prior to administration with injections or infusion fluids other than 5% Dextrose or Lidocaine Injection (see Section 4.2.5).

7. MARKETING AUTHORISATION HOLDER

AstraZeneca UK Limited,

600 Capability Green,

Luton, LU1 3LU, UK.

8. MARKETING AUTHORISATION NUMBER(S)

PL 17901/0007

9. DATE OF FIRST AUTHORISATION/RENEWAL OF THE AUTHORISATION

8th July 2000 / 24th September 2004

10. DATE OF REVISION OF THE TEXT

28th July 2009

Diprivan 2%

(AstraZeneca UK Limited)

1. NAME OF THE MEDICINAL PRODUCT

Diprivan 20 mg/ml (2%) emulsion for injection or infusion

2. QUALITATIVE AND QUANTITATIVE COMPOSITION

Propofol 20 mg/ml

3. PHARMACEUTICAL FORM

Emulsion for injection or infusion

White aqueous isotonic oil-in-water emulsion

4. CLINICAL PARTICULARS

4.1 Therapeutic indications

Diprivan 2% is a short-acting intravenous anaesthetic agent suitable for induction and maintenance of general anaesthesia.

Diprivan 2% may also be used for sedation of ventilated patients receiving intensive care.

4.2 Posology and method of administration

For specific guidance relating to the administration of Diprivan 2% with a target controlled infusion (TCI) device, which incorporates 'Diprifusor' TCI Software, see Section 4.2.4. Such use is restricted to induction and maintenance of anaesthesia in adults. The 'Diprifusor' TCI system is not recommended for use in ICU sedation or in children.

4.2.1 Induction of General Anaesthesia

Adults

Diprivan 2% may be used to induce anaesthesia by infusion.

Administration of Diprivan 2% by bolus injection is not recommended.

Diprivan 2% may be used to induce anaesthesia by infusion but only in those patients who will receive Diprivan 2% for maintenance of anaesthesia.

In unpremedicated and premedicated patients, it is recommended that Diprivan 2% should be titrated (approximately 2 ml [40 mg] every 10 seconds in an average healthy adult by infusion) against the response of the patient until the clinical signs show the onset of anaesthesia. Most adult patients aged less than

55 years are likely to require 1.5 to 2.5 mg/kg of Diprivan 2%. The total dose required can be reduced by lower rates of administration (1 to 2.5 ml/min [20 to 50 mg/min]). Over this age, the requirement will generally be less. In patients of ASA Grades 3 and 4, lower rates of administration should be used (approximately 1 ml [20 mg] every 10 seconds).

Elderly Patients

In elderly patients the dose requirement for induction of anaesthesia with Diprivan 2% is reduced. The reduction should take into account of the physical status and age of the patient. The reduced dose should be given at a slower rate and titrated against the response.

Children

Diprivan 2% is not recommended for induction of anaesthesia in children less than 3 years of age.

When used to induce anaesthesia in children, it is recommended that Diprivan 2% be given by slow infusion until the clinical signs show the onset of anaesthesia. The dose should be adjusted for age and/or weight. Most patients over 8 years of age are likely to require approximately 2.5 mg/kg of Diprivan 2% for induction of anaesthesia. Under this age the requirement may be more. Lower dosage is recommended for children of ASA grades 3 and 4.

Administration of Diprivan 2% by a 'Diprifusor' TCI system is not recommended for induction of general anaesthesia in children.

4.2.2 Maintenance Of General Anaesthesia

Anaesthesia can be maintained by administering Diprivan 2% by continuous infusion to prevent the clinical signs of light anaesthesia. Administration of Diprivan 2% by bolus injection is not recommended. Recovery from anaesthesia is typically rapid and it is therefore important to maintain Diprivan 2% administration until the end of the procedure.

Adults

The required rate of administration varies considerably between patients, but rates in the region of 4 to 12 mg/kg/h usually maintain satisfactory anaesthesia.

Elderly Patients

When Diprivan 2% is used for maintenance of anaesthesia the rate of infusion or 'target concentration' should also be reduced. Patients of ASA grades 3 and 4 will require further reductions in dose and dose rate. Rapid bolus administration (single or repeated) should not be used in the elderly as this may lead to cardiorespiratory depression.

Children

Diprivan 2% is not recommended for maintenance of anaesthesia in children less than 3 years of age.

The required rate of administration varies considerably between patients but rates in the region of 9 to 15 mg/kg/h usually achieve satisfactory anaesthesia.

Administration of Diprivan 2% by a 'Diprifusor' TCI System is not recommended for maintenance of general anaesthesia in children.

4.2.3 Sedation During Intensive Care

Adults

For sedation during intensive care it is advised that Diprivan 2% should be administered by continuous infusion. The infusion rate should be determined by the desired depth of sedation. In most patients sufficient sedation can be obtained with a dosage of 0.3 - 4 mg/kg/h of Diprivan 2% (See 4.4 Special warnings and precautions for use). Diprivan 2% is not indicated for sedation in intensive care of patients of 16 years of age or younger (see 4.3 Contraindications). Administration of Diprivan 2% by Diprifusor TCI system is not advised for sedation in the intensive care unit.

It is recommended that blood lipid levels be monitored should Diprivan 2% be administered to patients thought to be at particular risk of fat overload.

Administration of Diprivan 2% should be adjusted appropriately if the monitoring indicates that fat is being inadequately cleared from the body. If the patient is receiving other intravenous lipid concurrently, a reduction in quantity should be made in order to take account of the amount of lipid infused as part of the Diprivan 2% formulation: 1.0 ml of Diprivan 2% contains approximately 0.1 g of fat.

If the duration of sedation is in excess of 3 days, lipids should be monitored in all patients.

Elderly Patients

When Diprivan 2% is used for sedation of anaesthesia the rate of infusion should also be reduced. Patients of ASA grades 3 and 4 will require further reductions in dose and dose rate. Rapid bolus administration (single or repeated) should not be used in the elderly as this may lead to cardiorespiratory depression.

Children

Diprivan 2% is contra-indicated for the sedation of ventilated children aged 16 years or younger receiving intensive care.

4.2.4 Administration

Diprivan 2% has no analgesic properties and therefore supplementary analgesic agents are generally required in addition to Diprivan 2%.

Diprivan has been used in association with spinal and epidural anaesthesia and with commonly used premedicants, neuromuscular blocking drugs, inhalational agents and analgesic agents; no pharmacological incompatibility has been encountered. Lower doses of Diprivan 2% may be required where general anaesthesia is used as an adjunct to regional anaesthetic techniques.

Diprivan 2% should not be diluted. Diprivan 2% can be used for infusion undiluted from glass containers, plastic syringes or Diprivan 2% pre-filled syringes.

When Diprivan 2% is used to maintain anaesthesia, it is recommended that equipment such as syringe pumps or volumetric infusion pumps should always be used to control infusion rates.

Diprivan 2% should not be mixed prior to administration with injections or infusion fluids. However, Diprivan 2% may be co-administered via a Y-piece connector close to the injection site into infusions of the following:

- Dextrose 5% Intravenous Infusion B.P.
- Sodium Chloride 0.9% Intravenous Infusion B.P.
- Dextrose 4% with Sodium Chloride 0.18% Intravenous Infusion B.P.

The glass pre-filled syringe (PFS) has a lower frictional resistance than plastic disposable syringes and operates more easily. Therefore, if 'Diprivan' 2% is administered using a hand held pre-filled syringe, the line between the syringe and the patient must not be left open if unattended.

When the pre-filled syringe presentation is used in a syringe pump appropriate compatibility should be ensured. In particular, the pump should be designed to prevent siphoning and should have an occlusion alarm set no greater than 1000 mm Hg. If using a programmable or equivalent pump that offers options for use of different syringes then choose only the 'B-D' 50/60 ml 'PLASTIPAK' setting when using the Diprivan 2% pre-filled syringe.

Target Controlled Infusion - Administration of Diprivan 2% by a 'Diprifusor' TCI System in Adults

Administration of Diprivan 2% by a 'Diprifusor' TCI system is restricted to induction and maintenance of general anaesthesia in adults. It is not recommended for use in ICU sedation or in children.

Diprivan may be administered by TCI only with a Diprifusor TCI system incorporating Diprifusor TCI software

Such systems will operate only on recognition of electronically tagged prefilled syringes containing Diprivan 1% or 2% Injection. The 'Diprifusor' TCI system will automatically adjust the infusion rate for the concentration of Diprivan recognised. Users must be familiar with the infusion pump users manual, and with the administration of Diprivan 2% by TCI and with the correct use of the syringe identification system.

The system allow the anaesthetist or intensivist to achieve and control a desired speed of induction and depth of anaesthesia by setting and adjusting target (predicted) blood concentrations of propofol.

The 'Diprifusor' TCI system assumes that the initial blood propofol concentration in the patient is zero. Therefore, in patients who have received prior propofol, there may be a need to select a lower initial target concentration when commencing 'Diprifusor' TCI. Similarly, the immediate recommencement of 'Diprifusor' TCI is not recommended if the pump has been switched off.

Guidance on propofol target concentrations is given below. In view of interpatient variability in propofol pharmacokinetics and pharmacodynamics, in both premedicated and unpremedicated patients the target propofol concentration should be titrated against the response of the patient in order to achieve the depth of anaesthesia required.

In adult patients under 55 years of age anaesthesia can usually be induced with target propofol concentrations in the region of 4 to 8 microgram/ml. An initial target of 4 microgram/ml is recommended in premedicated patients and in unpremedicated patients an initial target of 6 microgram/ml is advised. Induction time with these targets is generally within the range of 60 to 120 seconds. Higher targets will allow more rapid induction of anaesthesia but may be associated with more pronounced haemodynamic and respiratory depression.

A lower initial target concentration should be used in patients over the age of about 55 years and in patients of ASA Grades 3 and 4. The target concentration can then be increased in steps of 0.5 to 1.0 microgram/ml at intervals of 1 minute to achieve a gradual induction of anaesthesia.

Supplementary analgesia will generally be required and the extent to which target concentrations for maintenance of anaesthesia can be reduced will be influenced by the amount of concomitant analgesia administered. Target propofol concentrations in the region of 3 to 6 microgram/ml usually maintain satisfactory anaesthesia.

The predicted propofol concentration on waking is generally in the region of 1.0 to 2.0 microgram/ml and will be influenced by the amount of analgesia given during maintenance.

Sedation during intensive care

Target blood propofol concentration settings in the range of 0.2 to 2.0 μg/ml will generally be required. Administration should begin at a low target setting which should be titrated against the response of the patient to achieve the depth of sedation desired.

4.3 Contraindications

Diprivan is contraindicated in patients with a known hypersensitivity to propofol or any of the excipients.

Diprivan 2% is contra-indicated for sedation in intensive care of patients of 16 years of age or younger (See 4.4 Special warnings and precautions for use).

Diprivan 2% contains soya oil and should not be used in patients who are hypersensitive to peanut or soya.

4.4 Special warnings and precautions for use

Diprivan 2% should be given by those trained in anaesthesia, or where appropriate, doctors trained in the care of patients in Intensive Care. Facilities for maintenance of a patent airway, artificial ventilation and oxygen enrichment should be available.

During induction of anaesthesia, hypotension and transient apnoea may occur depending on the dose and use of premedicants and other agents.

Occasionally, hypotension may require use of intravenous fluids and reduction of the rate of administration of Diprivan 2% during the period of anaesthetic maintenance.

As with other sedative agents, when Diprivan is used for sedation during operative procedures, involuntary patient movements may occur. During procedures requiring immobility these movements may be hazardous to the operative site.

An adequate period is needed prior to discharge of the patient to ensure full recovery after general anaesthesia. Very rarely the use of Diprivan may be associated with the development of a period of post-operative unconsciousness, which may be accompanied by an increase in muscle tone. This may or may not be preceded by a period of wakefulness. Although recovery is spontaneous, appropriate care of an unconscious patient should be administered.

When Diprivan 2% is administered to an epileptic patient, there may be a risk of convulsion.

As with other intravenous anaesthetic agents, caution should be applied in patients, with cardiac, respiratory, renal or hepatic impairment or in hypovolaemic or debilitated patients.

The risk of relative vagal overactivity may be increased because Diprivan 2% lacks vagolytic activity. Diprivan has been associated with reports of bradycardia (occasionally profound) and also asystole. The intravenous administration of an anticholinergic agent before induction, or during maintenance of anaesthesia should be considered, especially in situations where vagal tone is likely to predominate or when Diprivan 2% is used in conjunction with other agents likely to cause a bradycardia.

Appropriate care should be applied in patients with disorders of fat metabolism and in other conditions where lipid emulsions must be used cautiously.

Use is not recommended with electroconvulsive treatment.

As with other anaesthetics sexual disinhibition may occur during recovery.

Diprivan 2% is not advised for general anaesthesia in children younger than 1 month of age. The safety and efficacy of Diprivan 2% for (background) sedation in children younger than 16 years of age have not been demonstrated. Although no causal relationship has been established, serious undesirable effects with (background) sedation in patients younger than 16 years of age (including cases with fatal outcome) have been reported during unlicensed use. In particular these effects concerned occurrence of metabolic acidosis, hyperlipidemia, rhabdomyolysis and/or cardiac failure. These effects were most frequently seen in children with respiratory tract infections who received dosages in excess of those advised in adults for sedation in the intensive care unit.

Similarly very rare reports have been received of occurrence of metabolic acidosis, rhabdomyolysis, hyperkalaemia and/or rapidly progressive cardiac failure (in some cases with fatal outcome) in adults who were treated for more than 58 hours with dosages in excess of 5 mg/kg/h. This exceeds the maximum dosage of 4 mg/kg/h currently advised for sedation in the intensive care unit. The patients affected were mainly (but not only) seriously head-injured patients with raised ICP. The cardiac failure in such cases was usually unresponsive to inotropic supportive treatment. Treating physicians are reminded if possible not to exceed the dosage of 4 mg/kg/h. Prescribers should be alert to these possible undesirable effects and consider decreasing the Diprivan 2% dosage or switching to an alternative sedative at the first sign of occurrence of symptoms. Patients with raised ICP should be given appropriate treatment to support the cerebral perfusion pressure during these treatment modifications.

Diprivan 2% contains 0.0018 mmol sodium per ml.

EDTA is a chelator of metal ions, including zinc. The need for supplemental zinc should be considered during prolonged administration of Diprivan, particularly in patients who are predisposed to zinc deficiency, such as those with burns, diarrhoea and/or major sepsis.

Additional Precautions

Diprivan 2% contains no antimicrobial preservatives and supports growth of micro-organisms. Asepsis must be maintained for both Diprivan 2% and infusion equipment throughout the infusion period. Any drugs or fluids added to the Diprivan 2% infusion line must be administered close to the cannula site. Diprivan 2% must not be administered via a microbiological filter.

Diprivan 2% and any syringe containing Diprivan 2% are for single use in an individual patient. For use in long-term maintenance of anaesthesia or sedation in intensive care it is recommended that the infusion line and reservoir of Diprivan 2% be discarded and replaced at regular intervals.

4.5 Interaction with other medicinal products and other forms of interaction

See Section 4.2.4 Administration.

4.6 Pregnancy and lactation

Pregnancy Teratology studies in rats and rabbits showed no teratogenic effects. Diprivan has been used during termination of pregnancy in the first trimester. Diprivan 2% should not be used in pregnancy.

Obstetrics Diprivan crosses the placenta and may be associated with neonatal depression. It should not be used for obstetric anaesthesia.

Lactation Safety to the neonate has not been established following the use of Diprivan 2% in mothers who are breast feeding. Diprivan 2% should be avoided, or mothers should stop breast feeding.

4.7 Effects on ability to drive and use machines

Patients should be advised that performance at skilled tasks, such as driving and operating machinery, may be impaired for some time after general anaesthesia.

4.8 Undesirable effects

General

Induction of anaesthesia is generally smooth with minimal evidence of excitation. The most commonly reported ADRs are pharmacologically predictable side effects of an anaesthetic agent, such as hypotension. Given the nature of anaesthesia and those patients receiving intensive care, events reported in association with anaesthesia and intensive care may also be related to the procedures being undertaken or the recipient's condition.

Very common (>1/10)	*General disorders and administration site conditions:*	Local pain on induction [1]
Common (>1/100, <1/10)	*Vascular disorder:*	Hypotension [2]
	Cardiac disorders:	Bradycardia [3]
	Respiratory, thoracic and mediastinal disorders:	Transient apnoea during induction
	Gastrointestinal disorders:	Nausea and vomiting during recovery phase
	Nervous system disorders:	Headache during recovery phase
	General disorders and administration site conditions:	Withdrawal symptoms in children [4]
	Vascular disorders:	Flushing in children [4]
Uncommon (>1/1000, <1/100)	*Vascular disorders:*	Thrombosis and phlebitis
Rare (>1/10 000, <1/1000)	*Nervous system disorders:*	Epileptiform movements, including convulsions and opisthotonus during induction, maintenance and recovery
Very rare (<1/10 000)	*Musculoskeletal and connective tissue disorders:*	Rhabdomyolysis [5]
	Gastrointestinal disorders:	Pancreatitis
	Injury, poisoning and procedural complications:	Post-operative fever
	Renal and urinary disorders:	Discolouration of urine Following prolonged administration
	Immune system disorders:	Anaphylaxis – may include angioedema, bronchospasm, erythema and hypotension
	Reproductive system and breast disorders:	Sexual disinhibition
	Cardiac disorders:	Pulmonary oedema
	Nervous system disorders:	Postoperative unconsciousness

(1) May be minimised by using the larger veins of the forearm and antecubital fossa. With Diprivan 1% local pain can also be minimised by the co-administration of lidocaine.

(2) Occasionally, hypotension may require use of intravenous fluids and reduction of the administration rate of Diprivan.

(3) Serious bradycardias are rare. There have been isolated reports of progression to asystole.

(4) Following abrupt discontinuation of Diprivan during intensive care.

(5) Very rare reports of rhadbomyolysis have been received where Diprivan has been given at doses greater than 4 mg/kg/hr for ICU sedation.

Pulmonary edema, hypotension, asystole, bradycardia, and convulsions, have been reported. In very rare cases rhabdomyolysis, metabolic acidosis, hyperkalaemia or cardiac failure, sometimes with fatal outcome, have been observed when propofol was administered at dosages in excess of 4 mg/kg/h for sedation in the intensive care unit (see 4.4 Special warnings and precautions for use). Dystonia/dyskinesia have been reported.

Reports from off-label use of Diprivan for induction of anaesthesia in neonates indicates that cardio-respiratory depression may occur if the paediatric dose regimen is applied.

Local

The local pain which may occur during the induction phase can be minimised by the use of the larger veins of the forearm and antecubital fossa. Thrombosis and phlebitis are rare. Accidental clinical extravasation and animal studies showed minimal tissue reaction. Intra-arterial injection in animals did not induce local tissue effects.

4.9 Overdose

Accidental overdosage is likely to cause cardiorespiratory depression. Respiratory depression should be treated by artificial ventilation with oxygen. Cardiovascular depression would require lowering of the patient's head and, if severe, use of plasma expanders and pressor agents.

5. PHARMACOLOGICAL PROPERTIES

5.1 Pharmacodynamic properties

Propofol (2, 6-diisopropylphenol) is a short-acting general anaesthetic agent with a rapid onset of action of approximately 30 seconds. Recovery from anaesthesia is usually rapid. The mechanism of action, like all general anaesthetics, is poorly understood. However, propofol is thought to produce its sedative/anaesthetic effects by the positive modulation of the inhibitory function of the neurotransmitter GABA through the ligand-gated $GABA_A$ receptors.

In general, falls in mean arterial blood pressure and slight changes in heart rate are observed when Diprivan 2% is administered for induction and maintenance of anaesthesia. However, the haemodynamic parameters normally remain relatively stable during maintenance and the incidence of untoward haemodynamic changes is low.

Although ventilatory depression can occur following administration of Diprivan 2%, any effects are qualitatively similar to those of other intravenous anaesthetic agents and are readily manageable in clinical practice.

Diprivan 2% reduces cerebral blood flow, intracranial pressure and cerebral metabolism. The reduction in intracranial pressure is greater in patients with an elevated baseline intracranial pressure.

Recovery from anaesthesia is usually rapid and clear headed with a low incidence of headache and post-operative nausea and vomiting.

In general, there is less post-operative nausea and vomiting following anaesthesia with Diprivan 2% than following anaesthesia with inhalational agents. There is evidence that this may be related to a reduced emetic potential of propofol.

Diprivan 2%, at the concentrations likely to occur clinically, does not inhibit the synthesis of adrenocortical hormones.

5.2 Pharmacokinetic properties

The decline in propofol concentrations following a bolus dose or following the termination of an infusion can be described by a three compartment open model with very rapid distribution (half-life 2 to 4 minutes), rapid elimination (half-life 30 to 60 minutes), and a slower final phase, representative of redistribution of propofol from poorly perfused tissue.

Propofol is extensively distributed and rapidly cleared from the body (total body clearance 1.5 to 2 litres/minute). Clearance occurs by metabolic processes, mainly in the liver, to form inactive conjugates of propofol and its corresponding quinol, which are excreted in urine.

When Diprivan 2% is used to maintain anaesthesia, blood concentrations asymptotically approach the steady-state value for the given administration rate. The pharmacokinetics are linear over the recommended range of infusion rates of Diprivan 2%.

5.3 Preclinical safety data

Propofol is a drug on which extensive clinical experience has been obtained. All relevant information for the prescriber is provided elsewhere in this document.

6. PHARMACEUTICAL PARTICULARS

6.1 List of excipients

Glycerol Ph Eur

Purified Egg Phosphatide

Sodium Hydroxide Ph Eur

Soya-Bean Oil, Refined Ph Eur

Water for Injections Ph Eur

Nitrogen Ph Eur

Disodium Edetate Ph Eur

6.2 Incompatibilities

Diprivan 2% should not be mixed prior to administration with injections or infusion fluids. However, Diprivan 2% may be co-administered via a Y-piece connector close to the injection site into infusions of the following:

- Dextrose 5% Intravenous Infusion B.P.
- Sodium Chloride 0.9% B.P.
- Dextrose 4% with Sodium Chloride 0.18% Intravenous Infusion B.P.

The neuromuscular blocking agents, atracurium and mivacurium should not be given through the same intravenous line as Diprivan 2% without prior flushing.

6.3 Shelf life

6.3.1 Shelf life of the product as packaged for sale

2 years.

6.3.2 Shelf life after dilution:

Diprivan 2% should not be diluted.

6.4 Special precautions for storage

Store between 2°C and 25°C. Do not freeze.

6.5 Nature and contents of container

Emulsion for injection:

a) 10 ml pre-filled syringe containing propofol 20 mg/ml

b) 50 ml pre-filled syringe containing propofol 20 mg/ml.

6.6 Special precautions for disposal and other handling In use precautions:

Containers should be shaken before use. Any portion of the contents remaining after use should be discarded.

Diprivan 2% should not be mixed prior to administration with injections or infusion fluids. However, Diprivan 2% may be co-administered via a Y-piece connector close to the injection site into infusions of the following:

- Dextrose 5% Intravenous Infusion B.P.
- Sodium Chloride 0.9% Intravenous Infusion B.P.
- Dextrose 4% with Sodium Chloride 0.18% Intravenous Infusion B.P.

When the pre-filled syringe presentation is used in a syringe pump, appropriate compatibility should be ensured. In particular, the pump should be designed to prevent siphoning and should have an occlusion arm set no greater than 1000 mm Hg. If using a programmable or equivalent pump that offers options for use of different syringes then choose only the "B – D" 50/60 ml "PLASTIPAK" setting when using the Diprivan pre-filled syringe.

Additional precautions:

Diprivan 2% contains no antimicrobial preservatives and supports growth of micro-organisms. Asepsis must be maintained for both Diprivan 2% and infusion equipment throughout the infusion period. Any drugs or fluids added to the Diprivan 2% infusion line must be administered close to the cannula site. Diprivan 2% must not be administered via a microbiological filter.

Diprivan 2% and any syringe containing Diprivan 2% are for single use in an individual patient. For use in long-term maintenance of anaesthesia or sedation in intensive care it is recommended that the infusion line and reservoir of Diprivan 2% be discarded and replaced at regular intervals.

7. MARKETING AUTHORISATION HOLDER

AstraZeneca UK Limited,

600 Capability Green,

Luton, LU1 3LU, UK.

8. MARKETING AUTHORISATION NUMBER(S)

PL 17901/0008

9. DATE OF FIRST AUTHORISATION/RENEWAL OF THE AUTHORISATION

8th July 2000 / 26th February 2002

10. DATE OF REVISION OF THE TEXT

28th July 2009

Diprivan 2% (vials)

(AstraZeneca UK Limited)

1. NAME OF THE MEDICINAL PRODUCT

Diprivan 20 mg/ml (2%) emulsion for injection or infusion

2. QUALITATIVE AND QUANTITATIVE COMPOSITION

Propofol 20 mg/ml

3. PHARMACEUTICAL FORM

Emulsion for injection or infusion.

White aqueous isotonic oil-in-water emulsion.

4. CLINICAL PARTICULARS

4.1 Therapeutic indications

Diprivan 2% is a short-acting intravenous anaesthetic agent suitable for induction and maintenance of general anaesthesia.

Diprivan 2% may also be used for sedation of ventilated patients receiving intensive care.

4.2 Posology and method of administration

4.2.1 Induction of General Anaesthesia

Adults

Diprivan 2% may be used to induce anaesthesia by infusion.

Administration of Diprivan 2% by bolus injection is not recommended.

Diprivan 2% may be used to induce anaesthesia by infusion but only in those patients who will receive Diprivan 2% for maintenance of anaesthesia.

In unpremedicated and premedicated patients, it is recommended that Diprivan 2% should be titrated (approximately 2 ml [40 mg] every 10 seconds in an average healthy adult by infusion) against the response of the patient until the clinical signs show the onset of anaesthesia. Most adult patients aged less than 55 years are likely to require 1.5 to 2.5 mg/kg of Diprivan 2%. The total dose required can be reduced by lower rates of administration (1 to 2.5 ml/min [20 to 50 mg/min]). Over this age, the requirement will generally be less. In patients of ASA Grades 3 and 4, lower rates of administration should be used (approximately 1 ml [20 mg] every 10 seconds).

Elderly Patients

In elderly patients the dose requirement for induction of anaesthesia with Diprivan 2% is reduced. The reduction should take into account of the physical status and age of the patient. The reduced dose should be given at a slower rate and titrated against the response.

Children

Diprivan 2% is not recommended for induction of anaesthesia in children less than 3 years of age.

When used to induce anaesthesia in children, it is recommended that Diprivan 2% be given by slow infusion until the clinical signs show the onset of anaesthesia. The dose should be adjusted for age and/or weight. Most patients over 8 years of age are likely to require approximately 2.5 mg/kg of Diprivan 2% for induction of anaesthesia. Under this age the requirement may be more. Lower dosage is recommended for children of ASA grades 3 and 4.

4.2.2 Maintenance of General Anaesthesia

Anaesthesia can be maintained by administering Diprivan 2% by continuous infusion to prevent the clinical signs of light anaesthesia. Administration of Diprivan 2% by bolus injection is not recommended. Recovery from anaesthesia is typically rapid and it is therefore important to maintain Diprivan 2% administration until the end of the procedure.

Adults

The required rate of administration varies considerably between patients, but rates in the region of 4 to 12 mg/kg/h usually maintain satisfactory anaesthesia.

Elderly Patients

When Diprivan 2% is used for maintenance of anaesthesia the rate of infusion should also be reduced. Patients of ASA grades 3 and 4 will require further reductions in dose and dose rate. Rapid bolus administration (single or repeated) should not be used in the elderly as this may lead to cardiorespiratory depression.

Children

Diprivan 2% is not recommended for maintenance of anaesthesia in children less than 3 years of age.

The required rate of administration varies considerably between patients but rates in the region of 9 to 15 mg/kg/h usually achieve satisfactory anaesthesia.

4.2.3 Sedation During Intensive Care

Adults

For sedation during intensive care it is advised that Diprivan 2% should be administered by continuous infusion. The infusion rate should be determined by the desired depth of sedation. In most patients sufficient sedation can be obtained with a dosage of 0.3 - 4 mg/kg/h of Diprivan 2% (See 4.4 Special warnings and precautions for use). Diprivan 2% is not indicated for sedation in intensive care of patients of 16 years of age or younger (see 4.3 Contraindications).

It is recommended that blood lipid levels be monitored should Diprivan 2% be administered to patients thought to be at particular risk of fat overload.

Administration of Diprivan 2% should be adjusted appropriately if the monitoring indicates that fat is being inadequately cleared from the body. If the patient is receiving other intravenous lipid concurrently, a reduction in quantity should be made in order to take account of the amount of lipid infused as part of the Diprivan 2% formulation: 1.0 ml of Diprivan 2% contains approximately 0.1 g of fat.

If the duration of sedation is in excess of 3 days, lipids should be monitored in all patients.

Elderly Patients

When Diprivan 2% is used for sedation of anaesthesia the rate of infusion should also be reduced. Patients of ASA grades 3 and 4 will require further reductions in dose and dose rate. Rapid bolus administration (single or repeated) should not be used in the elderly as this may lead to cardiorespiratory depression.

Children

Diprivan 2% is contra-indicated for the sedation of ventilated children aged 16 years or younger receiving intensive care.

4.2.4 Administration

Diprivan 2% has no analgesic properties and therefore supplementary analgesic agents are generally required in addition to Diprivan 2%.

Diprivan has been used in association with spinal and epidural anaesthesia and with commonly used premedicants, neuromuscular blocking drugs, inhalational agents and analgesic agents; no pharmacological incompatibility has been encountered. Lower doses of Diprivan 2% may be required where general anaesthesia is used as an adjunct to regional anaesthetic techniques.

Diprivan 2% should not be diluted.

When Diprivan 2% is used to maintain anaesthesia, it is recommended that equipment such as syringe pumps or volumetric infusion pumps should always be used to control infusion rates.

Diprivan 2% should not be mixed prior to administration with injections or infusion fluids. However, Diprivan 2% may be co-administered via a Y-piece connector close to the injection site with the following:

- Dextrose 5% Intravenous Infusion B.P.
- Sodium Chloride 0.9% Intravenous Infusion B.P.
- Dextrose 4% with Sodium Chloride 0.18% Intravenous Infusion B.P.

4.3 Contraindications

Diprivan is contraindicated in patients with a known hypersensitivity to propofol or any of the excipients.

Diprivan 2% is contra-indicated for sedation in intensive care of patients of 16 years of age or younger (See 4.4 Special warnings and precautions for use).

Diprivan 2% contains soya oil and should not be used in patients who are hypersensitive to peanut or soya.

4.4 Special warnings and precautions for use

Diprivan 2% should be given by those trained in anaesthesia, or where appropriate, doctors trained in the care of patients in Intensive Care. Facilities for maintenance of a patent airway, artificial ventilation and oxygen enrichment should be available.

During induction of anaesthesia, hypotension and transient apnoea may occur depending on the dose and use of premedicants and other agents.

Occasionally, hypotension may require use of intravenous fluids and reduction of the rate of administration of Diprivan 2% during the period of anaesthetic maintenance.

An adequate period is needed prior to discharge of the patient to ensure full recovery after general anaesthesia. Very rarely, the use of Diprivan may be associated with the development of a period of post-operative unconsciousness, which may be accompanied by an increase in muscle tone. This may or may not be preceded by a period of wakefulness. Although recovery is spontaneous, appropriate care of an unconscious patient should be administered.

When Diprivan 2% is administered to an epileptic patient, there may be a risk of convulsion.

As with other sedative agents, when Diprivan is used for sedation during operative procedures, involuntary patient movements may occur. During procedures requiring immobility these movements may be hazardous to the operative site.

As with other intravenous anaesthetic agents, caution should be applied in patients with cardiac, respiratory, renal or hepatic impairment or in hypovolaemic or debilitated patients.

The risk of relative vagal overactivity may be increased because Diprivan 2% lacks vagolytic activity. Diprivan has been associated with reports of bradycardia (occasionally profound) and also asystole. The intravenous administration of an anticholinergic agent before induction, or during maintenance of anaesthesia should be considered, especially in situations where vagal tone is likely to predominate or when Diprivan 2% is used in conjunction with other agents likely to cause a bradycardia.

Appropriate care should be applied in patients with disorders of fat metabolism and in other conditions where lipid emulsions must be used cautiously.

Use is not recommended with electroconvulsive treatment.

As with other anaesthetics sexual disinhibition may occur during recovery.

Diprivan 2% is not advised for general anaesthesia in children younger than 1 month of age. The safety and efficacy of Diprivan 2% for (background) sedation in children younger than 16 years of age have not been demonstrated. Although no causal relationship has been established, serious undesirable effects with (background) sedation in patients younger than 16 years of age (including cases with fatal outcome) have been reported during unlicensed use. In particular these effects concerned occurrence of metabolic acidosis, hyperlipidemia, rhabdomyolysis and/or cardiac failure. These effects were most frequently seen in children with respiratory tract infections who received dosages in excess of those advised in adults for sedation in the intensive care unit.

Similarly very rare reports have been received of occurrence of metabolic acidosis, rhabdomyolysis, hyperkalaemia and/or rapidly progressive cardiac failure (in some cases with fatal outcome) in adults who were treated for more than 58 hours with dosages in excess of 5 mg/kg/h. This exceeds the maximum dosage of 4 mg/kg/h currently advised for sedation in the intensive care unit. The patients affected were mainly (but not only) seriously head-injured patients with raised ICP. The cardiac failure in such cases was usually unresponsive to inotropic supportive treatment. Treating physicians are reminded if possible not to exceed the dosage of 4 mg/kg/h. Prescribers should be alert to these possible undesirable effects and consider decreasing the Diprivan 2% dosage or switching to an alternative sedative at the first sign of occurrence of symptoms. Patients with raised ICP should be given appropriate treatment to support the cerebral perfusion pressure during these treatment modifications.

Diprivan 2% contains 0.0018 mmol sodium per ml.

EDTA is a chelator of metal ions, including zinc. The need for supplemental zinc should be considered during prolonged administration of Diprivan, particularly in patients who are predisposed to zinc deficiency, such as those with burns, diarrhoea and/or major sepsis.

Additional Precautions

Diprivan 2% contains no antimicrobial preservatives and supports growth of micro-organisms. Asepsis must be maintained for both Diprivan 2% and infusion equipment throughout the infusion period. Any drugs or fluids added to the Diprivan 2% infusion line must be administered close to the cannula site. Diprivan 2% must not be administered via a microbiological filter.

Diprivan 2% and any syringe containing Diprivan 2% are for single use in an individual patient. For use in long-term maintenance of anaesthesia or sedation in intensive care it is recommended that the infusion line and reservoir of Diprivan 2% be discarded and replaced at regular intervals.

4.5 Interaction with other medicinal products and other forms of interaction

See Section 4.2.4 Administration.

4.6 Pregnancy and lactation

Pregnancy Teratology studies in rats and rabbits showed no teratogenic effects. Diprivan has been used during termination of pregnancy in the first trimester. Diprivan 2% should not be used in pregnancy.

Obstetrics Diprivan crosses the placenta and may be associated with neonatal depression. It should not be used for obstetric anaesthesia.

Lactation Safety to the neonate has not been established following the use of Diprivan 2% in mothers who are breast feeding. Diprivan 2% should be avoided, or mothers should stop breast feeding.

4.7 Effects on ability to drive and use machines

Patients should be advised that performance at skilled tasks, such as driving and operating machinery, may be impaired for some time after general anaesthesia.

4.8 Undesirable effects

General

Induction of anaesthesia is generally smooth with minimal evidence of excitation.

Side effects during induction, maintenance and recovery occur uncommonly.

The most commonly reported ADRs are pharmacologically predictable side effects of an anaesthetic agent, such as hypotension. Given the nature of anaesthesia and those patients receiving intensive care, events reported in association with anaesthesia and intensive care may also be related to the procedures being undertaken or the recipient's condition.

Very common (>1/10)	*General disorders and administration site conditions:*	Local pain on induction [(1)]
Common (>1/100, <1/10)	*Vascular disorder:*	Hypotension [(2)]
	Cardiac disorders:	Bradycardia [(3)]
	Respiratory, thoracic and mediastinal disorders:	Transient apnoea during induction
	Gastrointestinal disorders:	Nausea and vomiting during recovery phase
	Nervous system disorders:	Headache during recovery phase
	General disorders and administration site conditions:	Withdrawal symptoms in children [(4)]
	Vascular disorders:	Flushing in children [(4)]
Uncommon (>1/1000, <1/100)	*Vascular disorders:*	Thrombosis and phlebitis
Rare (>1/10 000, <1/1000)	*Nervous system disorders:*	Epileptiform movements, including convulsions and opisthotonus during induction, maintanence and recovery
Very rare (<1/10 000)	*Musculoskeletal and connective tissue disorders:*	Rhabdomyolysis [(5)]
	Gastrointestinal disorders:	Pancreatitis
	Injury, poisoning and procedural complications:	Post-operative fever
	Renal and urinary disorders:	Discolouration of urine Following prolonged administration
	Immune system disorders:	Anaphylaxis – may include angioedema, bronchospasm, erythema and hypotension
	Reproductive system and breast disorders:	Sexual disinhibition
	Cardiac disorders:	Pulmonary oedema
	Nervous system disorders:	Postoperative unconsciousness

(1) May be minimised by using the larger veins of the forearm and antecubital fossa. With Diprivan 1% local pain can also be minimised by the co-administration of lidocaine.

(2) Occasionally, hypotension may require use of intravenous fluids and reduction of the administration rate of Diprivan.

(3) Serious bradycardias are rare. There have been isolated reports of progression to asystole.

(4) Following abrupt discontinuation of Diprivan during intensive care.

(5) Very rare reports of rhadbomyolysis have been received where Diprivan has been given at doses greater than 4 mg/kg/hr for ICU sedation.

Pulmonary edema, hypotension, asystole, bradycardia, and convulsions, have been reported. In very rare cases rhabdomyolysis, metabolic acidosis, hyperkalaemia or cardiac failure, sometimes with fatal outcome, have been observed when propofol was administered at dosages in excess of 4 mg/kg/h for sedation in the intensive care unit (see 4.4 Special warnings and precautions for use). Dystonia/dyskinesia have been reported.

Reports from off-label use of Diprivan for induction of anaesthesia in neonates indicates that cardio-respiratory depression may occur if the paediatric dose regimen is applied.

Local

The local pain which may occur during the induction phase can be minimised by the use of the larger veins of the forearm and antecubital fossa. Thrombosis and phlebitis are rare. Accidental clinical extravasation and animal studies showed minimal tissue reaction. Intra-arterial injection in animals did not induce local tissue effects.

4.9 Overdose

Accidental overdosage is likely to cause cardiorespiratory depression. Respiratory depression should be treated by artificial ventilation with oxygen. Cardiovascular depression would require lowering of the patient's head and, if severe, use of plasma expanders and pressor agents.

5. PHARMACOLOGICAL PROPERTIES

5.1 Pharmacodynamic properties

Propofol (2, 6-diisopropylphenol) is a short-acting general anaesthetic agent with a rapid onset of action of approximately 30 seconds. Recovery from anaesthesia is usually rapid. The mechanism of action, like all general anaesthetics, is poorly understood.

In general, falls in mean arterial blood pressure and slight changes in heart rate are observed when Diprivan 2% is administered for induction and maintenance of anaesthesia. However, the haemodynamic parameters normally remain relatively stable during maintenance and the incidence of untoward haemodynamic changes is low.

Although ventilatory depression can occur following administration of Diprivan 2%, any effects are qualitatively similar to those of other intravenous anaesthetic agents and are readily manageable in clinical practice.

Diprivan 2% reduces cerebral blood flow, intracranial pressure and cerebral metabolism. The reduction in intracranial pressure is greater in patients with an elevated baseline intracranial pressure.

Recovery from anaesthesia is usually rapid and clear headed with a low incidence of headache and post-operative nausea and vomiting.

In general, there is less post-operative nausea and vomiting following anaesthesia with Diprivan 2% than following anaesthesia with inhalational agents. There is evidence that this may be related to a reduced emetic potential of propofol.

Diprivan 2%, at the concentrations likely to occur clinically, does not inhibit the synthesis of adrenocortical hormones.

5.2 Pharmacokinetic properties

The decline in propofol concentrations following a bolus dose or following the termination of an infusion can be described by a three compartment open model with very rapid distribution (half-life 2 to 4 minutes), rapid elimination (half-life 30 to 60 minutes), and a slower final phase, representative of redistribution of propofol from poorly perfused tissue.

Propofol is extensively distributed and rapidly cleared from the body (total body clearance 1.5 to 2 litres/minute). Clearance occurs by metabolic processes, mainly in the liver, to form inactive conjugates of propofol and its corresponding quinol, which are excreted in urine.

When Diprivan 2% is used to maintain anaesthesia, blood concentrations asymptotically approach the steady-state value for the given administration rate. The pharmacokinetics are linear over the recommended range of infusion rates of Diprivan 2%.

5.3 Preclinical safety data

Propofol is a drug on which extensive clinical experience has been obtained. All relevant information for the prescriber is provided elsewhere in the Summary of Product Characteristics.

6. PHARMACEUTICAL PARTICULARS

6.1 List of excipients

Glycerol Ph Eur

Nitrogen Ph Eur

Purified Egg Phosphatide

Sodium Hydroxide Ph Eur

Soya-Bean Oil, Refined Ph Eur

Water for Injections Ph Eur

Disodium Edetate Ph Eur

6.2 Incompatibilities

Diprivan' 2% should not be mixed prior to administration with injections or infusion fluids. However, Diprivan 2% may be co-administered via a Y-piece connector close to the injection site into infusions of the following:

- Dextrose 5% Intravenous Infusion B.P.
- Sodium Chloride 0.9% Intravenous Infusion B.P.
- Dextrose 4% with Sodium Chloride 0.18% Intravenous Infusion B.P.

The neuromuscular blocking agents, atracurium and mivacurium should not be given through the same intravenous line as Diprivan 2% without prior flushing.

6.3 Shelf life

6.3.1 Shelf life of the product as packaged for sale

2 years.

6.3.2 Shelf life after dilution

Diprivan 2% should not be diluted.

6.4 Special precautions for storage
Store between 2°C and 25°C. Do not freeze.

6.5 Nature and contents of container
Emulsion for injection:

50 ml vial containing propofol 20 mg/ml.

6.6 Special precautions for disposal and other handling
In-use precautions:

Containers should be shaken before use. Any portion of the contents remaining after use should be discarded.

Diprivan 2% should not be mixed prior to administration with injections or infusion fluids. However, Diprivan 2% may be co-administered via a Y-piece connector close to the injection site into infusions of the following:

- Dextrose 5% Intravenous Infusion B.P.
- Sodium Chloride 0.9% Intravenous Infusion B.P.
- Dextrose 4% with Sodium Chloride 0.18% Intravenous Infusion B.P.

7. MARKETING AUTHORISATION HOLDER
AstraZeneca UK Limited,

600 Capability Green,

Luton, LU1 3LU, UK.

8. MARKETING AUTHORISATION NUMBER(S)
PL 17901/0009

9. DATE OF FIRST AUTHORISATION/RENEWAL OF THE AUTHORISATION
8th July 2000 / 26th February 2002

10. DATE OF REVISION OF THE TEXT
21st August 2008

Dipyridamole 50mg/5ml Oral Suspension (Rosemont Pharmaceuticals Ltd)

(Rosemont Pharmaceuticals Limited)

1. NAME OF THE MEDICINAL PRODUCT
Dypridisol

Dipyridamole 50mg/5ml Oral Suspension

2. QUALITATIVE AND QUANTITATIVE COMPOSITION
Dipyridamole 50mg/5ml

For excipients see section 6.1

3. PHARMACEUTICAL FORM
Oral Suspension

Bright yellow suspension with odour of almond.

4. CLINICAL PARTICULARS
4.1 Therapeutic indications
An adjunct to oral anticoagulation for prophylaxis of thromboembolism associated with prosthetic heart valves.

4.2 Posology and method of administration
Administration:

For oral use only.

Dipyridamole suspension should usually be taken before meals.

Adults: 300mg to a maximum of 600mg daily in three or four doses.

Children: Dipyridamole is not recommend for children.

4.3 Contraindications
Hypersensitivity to any of the ingredients in the product.

4.4 Special warnings and precautions for use
Among other properties, dipyridamole acts as a vasodilator. It should be used with caution in patients with severe coronary artery disease, including unstable angina and/or recent myocardial infarction, left ventricular outflow obstruction or haemodynamic instability (e.g. decompensated heart failure).

Dipyridamole should be used with caution in patients with coagulation disorders.

In patients with myasthenia gravis, readjustment of therapy may be necessary after changes in dipyridamole dosage (see Drug Interactions).

Patients treated with regular oral doses of dipyridamole should not receive additional intravenous dipyridamole. If pharmacological stress testing with intravenous dipyridamole for coronary artery disease is considered necessary, then oral dipyridamole should be discontinued 24 hours prior to testing.

Excipients in the formulation
Dipyridamole suspension contains liquid maltitol. Patients with a rare hereditary problem of fructose intolerance should not take this medicine.

The medicine also contains parahydroxybenzoates which are known to cause urticaria, generally delayed type reactions such as contact dermatitis and rarely, immediate reaction with urticaria and bronchospasm.

4.5 Interaction with other medicinal products and other forms of interaction
Adenosine:

Dipyridamole increases plasma levels and cardiovascular effects of adenosine. Adjustment of adenosine dosage should be considered if use with dipyridamole is unavoidable.

Aspirin:

There is evidence that the effects of aspirin and dipyridamole on platelet behaviour are additive.

Antacids:

The administration of antacids may reduce the efficacy of dipyridamole.

Anticoagulants:

It is possible that dipyridamole may enhance the effects of oral anticoagulants. When dipyridamole is used in combination with anticoagulants and acetylsalicylic acid, the statements on intolerance and risks for these preparations must be observed. Addition of dipyridamole to acetylsalicylic acid does not increase the incidence of bleeding events. When dipyridamole was administered concomitantly with warfarin, bleeding was no greater in frequency or severity than that observed when warfarin was administered alone.

Anti-Hypertensives:

Dipyridamole may increase the hypotensive effect of drugs which reduce blood pressure.

Anti-cholinesterases:

Dipyridamole may counteract the anticholinesterase effect of cholinesterase inhibitors thereby potentially aggravating myasthenia gravis.

4.6 Pregnancy and lactation
There is inadequate evidence of safety in human pregnancy but dipyridamole has been used for many years without apparent ill consequence. Animal studies have shown no hazard. Medicines should not be used in pregnancy, especially in the first trimester, unless the expected benefit is thought to outweigh the possible risk to the foetus.

Dipyridamole is excreted in breast milk at levels approximately 6% of the plasma concentration. Therefore, dipyridamole should only be used during lactation if considered essential by the physician.

4.7 Effects on ability to drive and use machines
None stated.

4.8 Undesirable effects
If side effects do occur, it is usually during the early part of treatment.

Blood and the lymphatic system disorders

Isolated cases of thrombocytopenia have been reported in conjunction with treatment of dipyridamole.

Cardiac Disorders

In rare cases, worsening of symptoms of coronary heart disease has been observed.

Vascular Disorders

The vasodilating properties may occasionally produce a vascular headache which normally disappears with long-term use.

As a result of its vasodilator properties, dipyridamole may cause hypotension, hot flushes and tachycardia.

Hepato-biliary disorders

Dipyridamole has been shown to be incorporated into gallstones.

General Disorders

Vomiting, diarrhoea and symptoms such as dizziness, faintness, nausea, dyspepsia, and myalgia have been observed.

Hypersensitivity reactions such as rash, urticaria, severe bronchospasm and angio-oedema have been reported.

Surgical and medical procedures

In very rare cases, increased bleeding during or after surgery has been observed.

4.9 Overdose
Due to the low number of observations, experience with dipyridamole overdose is limited. Symptoms such as a warm feeling, flushes, sweating, restlessness, feeling of weakness, dizziness and anginal complaints can be expected. A drop in blood pressure and tachycardia might be observed.

Symptomatic therapy is recommended. Administration of xanthine derivatives (e.g. aminophylline) may reverse the haemodynamic effects of dipyridamole overdose. Due to its wide distribution to tissues and its predominantly hepatic elimination, dipyridamole is not likely to be accessible to enhanced removal procedures.

5. PHARMACOLOGICAL PROPERTIES
5.1 Pharmacodynamic properties
Dipyridamole has an antithrombotic action based on its ability to modify various aspects of platelet function, such as platelet aggregation, adhesion and survival, which have been shown to be factors associated with the initiation of thrombus formation. Dipyridamole also has coronary vasodilator properties.

5.2 Pharmacokinetic properties
Oral administration of dipyridamole gives a peak plasma level 0.5 - 2 hours after dosing. The drug has an apparent bioavailability of 37-66%. These figures were obtained with other oral immediate release forms of dipyridamole.

The volume of distribution is 2.43 ± 1.1l/kg. When given orally the elimination half life is 9 –12 hours. The major route of excretion of dipyridamole is in the bile.

5.3 Preclinical safety data
There are no preclinical data of relevance to the prescriber additional to those already included in other sections of the SPC.

6. PHARMACEUTICAL PARTICULARS
6.1 List of excipients
Methyl hydroxybenzoate (E218), propyl hydroxybenzoate (E216), propylene glycol (E1520), xanthan gum (E415), ammonium glycyrrhizinate, almond flavour (including propylene glycol and ethanol), levomenthol, liquid maltitol (E965), polysorbate 80 (E433), simethicone emulsion, aluminium magnesium silicate, disodium hydrogen phosphate (E339), citric acid monohydrate (E330) and purified water.

6.2 Incompatibilities
Not applicable.

6.3 Shelf life
24 months

1 month - once open

6.4 Special precautions for storage
Do not store above 25°C.

6.5 Nature and contents of container
Bottle: Amber (Type III) glass

Closure:

HDPE, EPE wadded, tamper evident screw cap

HDPE, EPE wadded, tamper evident child resistant closure.

Capacity: 150ml or 500ml

Not all pack sizes may be marketed

6.6 Special precautions for disposal and other handling
This product may settle during storage. Please shake the bottle thoroughly before use.

Administrative Data
7. MARKETING AUTHORISATION HOLDER
Rosemont Pharmaceuticals Ltd, Rosemont House, Yorkdale Industrial Park, Braithwaite Street, Leeds, LS11 9XE, UK

8. MARKETING AUTHORISATION NUMBER(S)
PL 00427/0133

9. DATE OF FIRST AUTHORISATION/RENEWAL OF THE AUTHORISATION
8/8/02

10. DATE OF REVISION OF THE TEXT
September 2007

Disipal Tablets

(Astellas Pharma Ltd)

1. NAME OF THE MEDICINAL PRODUCT
DISIPAL TABLETS

2. QUALITATIVE AND QUANTITATIVE COMPOSITION
Orphenadrine hydrochloride BP 50 mg

3. PHARMACEUTICAL FORM
Tablet

4. CLINICAL PARTICULARS
4.1 Therapeutic indications
Anti-cholinergic, for the treatment of all forms of Parkinsonism, including drug-induced extrapyramidal symptoms (neuroleptic syndrome).

4.2 Posology and method of administration
For Adults, and the Elderly:

Initially 150 mg daily in divided doses, increasing by 50 mg every two or three days until maximum benefit is obtained. Optimal dosage is usually 250 - 300 mg daily in divided doses in idiopathic and post-encephalitic Parkinsonism, 100 - 300 mg daily in divided doses in the neuroleptic syndrome. Maximal dosage, 400 mg daily in divided doses. The elderly may be more susceptible to side-effects at doses which are clinically optimal.

For children:

A dosage for children has not been established.

4.3 Contraindications
Contraindicated in patients with tardive dyskinesia, glaucoma, or prostatic hypertrophy, untreated urinary retention, gastro-intestinal obstruction, porphyria.

Hypersensitivity to the active substance or to any of the excipients.

4.4 Special warnings and precautions for use
Use with caution in patients with micturition difficulties, in pregnancy and breast feeding, and in the presence of cardiovascular disease and hepatic or renal impairment. Use in caution in the elderly (see 4.2). Avoid abrupt discontinuation of treatment. For some patients, orphenadrine may be a drug of abuse.

Patients with rare hereditary problems of fructose and galactose intolerance, the Lapp lactase deficiency or glucose-galactose malabsorption or sucrase-isomaltase insufficiency should not take this medicine.

The colours sunset yellow (E110), tartrazine (E102) and amaranth (E123) may cause allergic reactions.

4.5 Interaction with other medicinal products and other forms of interaction
Concomitant use of other antimuscarinic drugs can lead to an increase in side effects such as dry mouth and urine retention.

4.6 Pregnancy and lactation
No recommendations; if considered necessary, it should be used with caution, see 4.4.

4.7 Effects on ability to drive and use machines
Patients must be advised to exercise caution while driving or operating machinery or whilst carrying out other skilled tasks.

4.8 Undesirable effects
(see Table 1 below)

4.9 Overdose
Toxic effects are anti-cholinergic in nature and the treatment is gastric lavage, cholinergics such as carbachol, anticholinesterases such as physostigmine, and general non-specific treatment.

5. PHARMACOLOGICAL PROPERTIES
5.1 Pharmacodynamic properties
Orphenadrine, which is a congener of diphenhydramine without sharing its soporific effect, is an antimuscarinic agent. It also has weak antihistaminic and local anaesthetic properties.

Orphenadrine is used as the hydrochloride in the symptomatic treatment of Parkinsonism. It is also used to alleviate the extrapyramidal syndrome induced by drugs such as the phenothiazine derivatives, but is of no value in tardive dyskinesia, which may be exacerbated.

5.2 Pharmacokinetic properties
Orphenadrine is readily absorbed from the gastro-intestinal tract, and very readily absorbed following intramuscular injection. It is rapidly distributed in tissues and most of a dose is metabolised and excreted in the urine along with a small proportion of unchanged drug. A half life of 14 hours has been reported.

5.3 Preclinical safety data
No relevant pre-clinical safety data has been generated

6. PHARMACEUTICAL PARTICULARS
6.1 List of excipients
Lactose
Sucrose
Acacia
Maize starch
Tribasic calcium phosphate
Stearic acid
Magnesium stearate
Opaseal P-17-0200 (containing IMS, polyvinylacetate phthalate and stearic acid)
Calcium carbonate
Talc
Kaolin
Titanium dioxide
Gelatin
Opalux yellow AS 3026 (containing sucrose, titanium dioxide, tartrazine E102, sunset yellow E110, povidone, amaranth E123 and sodium benzoate E211)
Opaglos 6000 (containing ethanol, shellac, beeswax and yellow carnuba wax)
Black printing ink Opacode black S-1-27794 (containing shellac, IMS, black iron oxide E172, N-butyl alcohol, propylene glycol E1520, isopropyl alcohol)

6.2 Incompatibilities
None

6.3 Shelf life
Three years

6.4 Special precautions for storage
Store at room temperature (15°C - 25°C)

6.5 Nature and contents of container
Amber glass click-lock bottles and/or securitainers and/or plastic lid-seal containers, containing 100, 250, 1,000, or 10,000 tablets.

6.6 Special precautions for disposal and other handling
None

Administrative Data
7. MARKETING AUTHORISATION HOLDER
Astellas Pharma Ltd
Lovett House
Lovett Road
Staines
TW18 3AZ
United Kingdom

8. MARKETING AUTHORISATION NUMBER(S)
PL 0166/5001R

9. DATE OF FIRST AUTHORISATION/RENEWAL OF THE AUTHORISATION
6 May 1987; renewed March 2003.

10. DATE OF REVISION OF THE TEXT
12th June 2009

11. Legal Category
POM

Table 1 Undesirable effects

System Organ Class	Common >1/100 <1/10	Uncommon >1/1000 <1/100	Rare >1/10,000 <1/1000
Immune system disorder		Hypersensitivity	
Nervous system disorder	Dizziness	Sedation, confusion, nervousness, hallucinations, convulsions, insomnia, euphoria	Memory disturbances
Eye disorders	Accommodation disorders		
Cardiac disorders		Tachycardia	
Gastrointestinal disorders	Dry mouth, gastrointestinal disturbances		
Renal and urinary disorders		Urinary retention	

Distamine 125mg Film-coated tablets

(Alliance Pharmaceuticals)

1. NAME OF THE MEDICINAL PRODUCT
Distamine 125mg Film-coated tablets.

Penicillamine 125mg Film-coated tablets

2. QUALITATIVE AND QUANTITATIVE COMPOSITION
Each tablet contains 125mg D-penicillamine.

For excipients see section 6.1

3. PHARMACEUTICAL FORM
Film-coated Tablet.

White, film-coated tablet with a diameter of 8mm, marked "DS" on one face and "125" on the other.

4. CLINICAL PARTICULARS
4.1 Therapeutic indications
a) Severe active rheumatoid arthritis, including juvenile forms
b) Wilson's disease (hepatolenticular degeneration)
c) Cystinuria – dissolution and prevention of cystine stones
d) Lead poisoning
e) Chronic active hepatitis

4.2 Posology and method of administration
For oral administration.

Distamine should be taken on an empty stomach at least half an hour before meals, or on retiring.

a) Rheumatoid arthritis

Adults: 125 to 250mg daily for the first month. Increase by the same amount every four to 12 weeks until remission occurs. The minimum maintenance dose to achieve suppression of symptoms should be used and treatment should be discontinued if no benefit is obtained within 12 months. Improvement may not occur for some months.

The usual maintenance dose is 500 to 750mg daily. Up to 1500mg daily may be required.

If remission is established and has been sustained for six months, gradual reduction by 125 to 250mg amounts every 12 weeks may be attempted.

The elderly: Initial dose should not exceed 125mg daily for the first month, increasing by similar increments every four to 12 weeks until the minimum maintenance dose to suppress symptoms is reached. Daily dosage should not exceed 1000mg (see Section 4.4, "Special Warnings and Precautions for Use").

Children: The usual maintenance dose is 15 to 20mg/kg/day. The initial dose should be lower (2.5 to 5mg/kg/day) and increased every four weeks over a period of three to six months. Please note that as the smallest available tablet is 125mg, this may not be suitable for children under eight years (or less than 26kg in weight).

Renal insufficiency: Distamine therapy should be initiated at a low dose with intervals between dose increase of at least twelve weeks. Fortnightly monitoring for toxicity is mandatory throughout treatment for rheumatoid arthritis.

b) Wilson's disease

Patients must be maintained in negative copper balance and the minimum dose of Distamine required to achieve this should be given.

Adults: 1500 to 2000mg daily in divided doses. Dose may be reduced to 750 to 1000mg daily when control of the disease is achieved. It is advisable that a dose of 2000mg/day should not be continued for more than a year.

The elderly: 20mg/kg/day in divided doses adjusting the dose to minimal level necessary to control disease.

Children: Up to 20mg/kg/day in divided doses. Minimum dose 500mg/day.

Renal insufficiency: Extra precautions should be taken to monitor for adverse effects in patients with Wilson's disease and renal insufficiency.

c) Cystinuria

Ideally, establish the lowest effective dose by quantitative amino acid chromatography of urine.

(i) Dissolution of cystine stones:

Adults: 1000 to 3000mg daily in divided doses.

Urine cystine levels of not more than 200mg/l should be maintained.

(ii) Prevention of cystine stones:

Adults: 500 to 1000mg on retiring. Fluid intake should be not less than 3 litres/day. Urine cystine levels of not more than 300mg/l should be maintained.

The elderly: Use the minimum dose to maintain urinary cystine levels below 200mg/l.

Children: No dose range established, but urinary cystine levels must be kept below 200mg/l. The minimum dose of Distamine required to achieve this should be given.

Renal insufficiency: If renal insufficiency is present at the onset of therapy, the starting dose should be lower, but it will be necessary to give sufficient Distamine to achieve urine cystine levels of not more than 300mg/l. The maintenance dose should be reviewed at intervals of not more than four weeks.

d) Lead poisoning

Adults: 1000 to 1500mg daily in divided doses until urinary lead is stabilised at less than 0.5mg/day.

The elderly: 20mg/kg/day in divided doses until urinary lead is stabilised at less than 0.5mg/day.

Children: 20mg/kg/day.

e) Chronic active hepatitis

Adults: For maintenance treatment after the disease process has been brought under control with corticosteroids. The initial dose of 500mg daily, in divided doses, should be increased gradually over three months to a maintenance dose of 1250mg daily. During this period, the dose of corticosteroids should be phased out. Throughout therapy, liver function tests should be carried out periodically to assess the disease status.

The elderly: Not recommended.

4.3 Contraindications
Hypersensitivity to penicillamine or any of the ingredients.

Agranulocytosis or severe thrombocytopenia due to penicillamine.

Lupus erythematosus.

Moderate or severe renal impairment.

4.4 Special warnings and precautions for use
Full blood and platelet counts should be performed and renal function should be assessed prior to treatment with penicillamine.

During the first eight weeks of therapy full blood counts should be carried out weekly or fortnightly and also in the week after any increase in dose, otherwise monthly thereafter. In cystinuria or Wilson's disease, longer intervals may be adequate.

Withdrawal of treatment should be considered if platelets fall below 120,000/mm^3 or white blood cells below 2,500/mm^3, or if three successive falls are noted within the normal range. Treatment may be restarted at a reduced dose when counts return to normal, but should be permanently withdrawn on recurrence of leucopenia or thrombocytopenia.

In patients with normal renal function, urinalysis for detection of haematuria and proteinuria should be carried out weekly at first, and following each increase in dose, then monthly, although longer intervals may be adequate for cystinuria and Wilson's disease. Increasing or persistent proteinuria may necessitate withdrawal of therapy.

Care should be exercised in patients with renal insufficiency; modification of dosage may be necessary (see Section 4.2, "Posology and Method of Administration").

Especially careful monitoring is necessary in the elderly since increased toxicity has been observed in this patient population regardless of renal function.

Concomitant use of NSAIDs and other nephrotoxic drugs may increase the risk of renal damage.

Penicillamine should be used with caution in patients who have had adverse reactions to gold.

Concomitant or previous treatment with gold may increase the risk of side effects with penicillamine treatment. Therefore penicillamine should be used with caution in patients who have previously had adverse reactions to gold and concomitant treatment with gold should be avoided.

If concomitant oral iron therapy is indicated, this should not be given within two hours of taking penicillamine.

Antihistamines, steroid cover, or temporary reduction of dose will control urticarial reactions.

Reversible loss of taste may occur. Mineral supplements to overcome this are not recommended.

Haematuria is rare, but if it occurs in the absence of renal stones or other known cause, treatment should be stopped immediately.

A late rash, described as acquired epidermolysis bullosa and penicillamine dermopathy, may occur after several months or years of therapy. This may necessitate a reduction in dosage.

Breast enlargement has been reported as a rare complication of penicillamine therapy in both women and men. Danazol has been used successfully to treat breast enlargement which does not regress on drug discontinuation.

4.5 Interaction with other medicinal products and other forms of interaction

Concomitant iron and penicillamine treatment: oral absorption of penicillamine may be reduced by concomitant administration of iron (see Section 4.4 "Special Warnings and Precautions for Use").

Concomitant use of NSAIDs and other nephrotoxic drugs may increase the risk of renal damage (see Section 4.4 "Special Warnings and Precautions for Use").

Concomitant gold and penicillamine treatment: concomitant use not recommended (see Section 4.4 "Special Warnings and Precautions for Use").

4.6 Pregnancy and lactation

Usage in pregnancy: The safety of penicillamine for use during pregnancy has not been established (see Section 5.3, "Preclinical Safety Data").

Wilson's disease: There have been several cases of reversible cutis laxa in infants born to mothers taking penicillamine throughout pregnancy. Although there have been no controlled studies on the use of penicillamine during pregnancy, two retrospective studies have reported the successful delivery of 43 normal infants to 28 women receiving between 500 and 2000mg of penicillamine daily. There are also anecdotal reports both of congenital abnormalities and of successful outcomes in patients who have remained on penicillamine during pregnancy. If treatment with penicillamine is to be continued following a risk-benefit analysis, consideration should be given to reducing the dose of penicillamine to the lowest effective dose.

Cystinuria: Whilst normal infants have been delivered, there is one report of a severe connective tissue abnormality in the infant of a mother who received 2000mg penicillamine daily throughout pregnancy. Whenever possible, penicillamine should be withheld during pregnancy, but if stones continue to form, the benefit of resuming treatment must be weighed against the possible risk to the foetus.

Rheumatoid arthritis or chronic active hepatitis: Penicillamine should not be administered to patients who are pregnant, and therapy should be stopped when pregnancy is diagnosed or suspected, unless considered to be absolutely essential by the physician.

Usage in lactation: Due to the lack of data on use in breast feeding patients and the possibility that penicillamine may be transmitted to newborns through breast milk, Distamine should only be used in breast feeding patients when it is considered absolutely essential by the physician.

4.7 Effects on ability to drive and use machines

None known.

4.8 Undesirable effects

NB: The incidence and severity of some of the adverse reactions, noted below, varies according to the dosage and nature of the disease under treatment.

Nausea, anorexia, fever and rash may occur early in therapy, especially when full doses are given from the start.

Urticarial reactions have been reported (see Section 4.4, "Special Warnings and Precautions for Use").

Reversible loss of taste may occur (see Section 4.4, "Special Warnings and Precautions for Use").

Rarely, mouth ulceration/stomatitis has occurred.

Thrombocytopenia occurs commonly and leucopenia less often. These reactions may occur at any time during treatment and are usually reversible (see Section 4.4, "Special Warnings and Precautions for Use").

Deaths from agranulocytosis and aplastic anaemia have occurred.

Deterioration of the neurological symptoms of Wilson's disease (dystonia, rigidity, tremor, dysarthria) have been reported following introduction of penicillamine in patients treated for this condition. This may be a consequence of mobilisation and redistribution of copper from the liver to the brain.

Proteinuria occurs in up to 30% of patients and is partially dose-related (see Section 4.4, "Special Warnings and Precautions for Use").

Haematuria may occur rarely (see Section 4.4, "Special Warnings and Precautions for Use").

Other rare adverse reactions are as follows: alopecia and inflammatory conditions of the respiratory system, such as bronchiolitis and pneumonitis.

Other complications have included haemolytic anaemia, nephrotic syndrome, glomerulonephritis, pulmonary haemorrhage, Goodpasture's syndrome, pancreatitis, cholestatic jaundice (including raised liver function tests), drug induced lupus erythematosus, and conditions closely resembling myasthenia gravis, polymyositis (with rare cardiac involvement), dermatomyositis, pemphigus, Stevens-Johnson syndrome and rheumatoid arthritis.

A late rash, described as acquired epidermolysis bullosa and penicillamine dermopathy, may occur after several months or years of therapy (see Section 4.4, "Special Warnings and Precautions for Use").

Pseudoxanthoma elasticum, elastosis perforans and skin laxity have been reported rarely. Breast enlargement has been reported as a rare complication of penicillamine therapy in both women and men. In some patients breast enlargement was considerable and/or prolonged with poor resolution and others required surgery (see Section 4.4, "Special Warnings and Precautions for Use").

The use of DMARDs, including penicillamine, has been linked to the development of septic arthritis in patients with rheumatoid arthritis, although rheumatoid arthritis is a stronger predictor for the development of septic arthritis than the use of a DMARD.

4.9 Overdose

No instances of adverse reactions to an overdose of penicillamine have been recorded and no specific measures are indicated.

5. PHARMACOLOGICAL PROPERTIES

5.1 Pharmacodynamic properties

Pharmacotherapeutic group: M01C C

1. Penicillamine is used to treat severe active rheumatoid arthritis not adequately controlled by NSAID therapy.

2. Penicillamine is a chelating agent which aids the elimination from the body of certain heavy metal ions, including copper, lead and mercury, by forming stable soluble complexes with them that are readily excreted by the kidney.

3. It is used in the treatment of Wilson's disease (hepatolenticular degeneration), in conjunction with a low copper diet, to promote the excretion of copper.

4. It may be used to treat asymptomatic lead intoxication.

5. Penicillamine is used as an adjunct to diet and urinary alkalinisation in the management of cystinuria. By reducing urinary concentrations of cystine, penicillamine prevents the formation of calculi and promotes the gradual dissolution of existing calculi.

6. Desensitisation. Should the physician deem it necessary to attempt to desensitise a patient to penicillamine, it should be noted that this formulation is not suitable for this purpose.

5.2 Pharmacokinetic properties

Penicillamine is a thiol-group containing chelating agent, variably absorbed from the gastrointestinal tract. The drug undergoes a rapid distribution phase, followed by a slower elimination phase.

Penicillamine is strongly plasma-protein bound. Most penicillamine is bound to albumin but some is bound to α-globulins or ceruloplasmin.

Penicillamine is not extensively metabolised in man.

About 80% of the absorbed dose is excreted rapidly in the urine, mostly as mixed disulphides. Some of the dose is excreted as a penicillamine copper complex and some as the S-methyl derivative.

5.3 Preclinical safety data

Penicillamine has been shown to be teratogenic in rats when given in doses several times higher than those recommended for human use.

There is no known LD50 value for penicillamine. In studies some rats died after oral administration of 10,000mg/kg, but intra-peritoneal injections of a dose of 660mg/kg caused no deaths.

6. PHARMACEUTICAL PARTICULARS

6.1 List of excipients

Tablet Core

Microcrystalline cellulose

Sodium starch glycolate (Type A)

Povidone

Magnesium stearate

Tablet Coating

Glycerol

Titanium dioxide (E171)

Hypromellose

6.2 Incompatibilities

Not applicable.

6.3 Shelf life

3 years

6.4 Special precautions for storage

Do not store above 25°C. Keep the bottle tightly closed.

6.5 Nature and contents of container

HDPE bottle with screw cap, containing 100 tablets.

6.6 Special precautions for disposal and other handling

No special requirements.

7. MARKETING AUTHORISATION HOLDER

Alliance Pharmaceuticals Ltd
Avonbridge House
Bath Road
Chippenham
Wiltshire
SN15 2BB
United Kingdom

8. MARKETING AUTHORISATION NUMBER(S)

PL 16853/0057

9. DATE OF FIRST AUTHORISATION/RENEWAL OF THE AUTHORISATION

12th October 2005

10. DATE OF REVISION OF THE TEXT

27th March 2009

Distamine 250mg Film-coated tablets

(Alliance Pharmaceuticals)

1. NAME OF THE MEDICINAL PRODUCT

Distamine 250mg Film-coated tablets.

Penicillamine 250mg Film-coated tablets

2. QUALITATIVE AND QUANTITATIVE COMPOSITION

Each tablet contains 250mg D-penicillamine.

For excipients see section 6.1

3. PHARMACEUTICAL FORM

Film-coated Tablet.

White, film-coated tablet with a diameter of 10mm, marked "DM" on one face and "250" on the other.

4. CLINICAL PARTICULARS

4.1 Therapeutic indications

a) Severe active rheumatoid arthritis, including juvenile forms

b) Wilson's disease (hepatolenticular degeneration)

c) Cystinuria – dissolution and prevention of cystine stones

d) Lead poisoning

e) Chronic active hepatitis

4.2 Posology and method of administration

For oral administration.

Distamine should be taken on an empty stomach at least half an hour before meals, or on retiring.

a) Rheumatoid arthritis

Adults: 125 to 250mg daily for the first month. Increase by the same amount every four to 12 weeks until remission occurs. The minimum maintenance dose to achieve suppression of symptoms should be used and treatment should be discontinued if no benefit is obtained within 12 months. Improvement may not occur for some months.

The usual maintenance dose is 500 to 750mg daily. Up to 1500mg daily may be required.

If remission is established and has been sustained for six months, gradual reduction by 125 to 250mg amounts every 12 weeks may be attempted.

The elderly: Initial dose should not exceed 125mg daily for the first month, increasing by similar increments every four to 12 weeks until the minimum maintenance dose to suppress symptoms is reached. Daily dosage should not exceed 1000mg (see Section 4.4, "Special Warnings and Precautions for Use").

Children: The usual maintenance dose is 15 to 20mg/kg/day. The initial dose should be lower (2.5 to 5mg/kg/day) and increased every four weeks over a period of three to six months. Please note that as the smallest available tablet is

125mg, this may not be suitable for children under eight years (or less than 26kg in weight).

Renal insufficiency: Distamine therapy should be initiated at a low dose with intervals between dose increase of at least twelve weeks. Fortnightly monitoring for toxicity is mandatory throughout treatment for rheumatoid arthritis.

b) Wilson's disease

Patients must be maintained in negative copper balance and the minimum dose of Distamine required to achieve this should be given.

Adults: 1500 to 2000mg daily in divided doses. Dose may be reduced to 750 to 1000mg daily when control of the disease is achieved. It is advisable that a dose of 2000mg/day should not be continued for more than a year.

The elderly: 20mg/kg/day in divided doses adjusting the dose to minimal level necessary to control disease.

Children: Up to 20mg/kg/day in divided doses. Minimum dose 500mg/day.

Renal insufficiency: Extra precautions should be taken to monitor for adverse effects in patients with Wilson's disease and renal insufficiency.

c) Cystinuria

Ideally, establish the lowest effective dose by quantitative amino acid chromatography of urine.

(i) Dissolution of cystine stones:

Adults: 1000 to 3000mg daily in divided doses.

Urine cystine levels of not more than 200mg/l should be maintained.

(ii) Prevention of cystine stones:

Adults: 500 to 1000mg on retiring. Fluid intake should be not less than 3 litres/day. Urine cystine levels of not more than 300mg/l should be maintained.

The elderly: Use the minimum dose to maintain urinary cystine levels below 200mg/l.

Children: No dose range established, but urinary cystine levels must be kept below 200mg/l. The minimum dose of Distamine required to achieve this should be given.

Renal insufficiency: If renal insufficiency is present at the onset of therapy, the starting dose should be lower, but it will be necessary to give sufficient Distamine to achieve urine cystine levels of not more than 300mg/l. The maintenance dose should be reviewed at intervals of not more than four weeks.

d) Lead poisoning

Adults: 1000 to 1500mg daily in divided doses until urinary lead is stabilised at less than 0.5mg/day.

The elderly: 20mg/kg/day in divided doses until urinary lead is stabilised at less than 0.5mg/day.

Children: 20mg/kg/day.

e) Chronic active hepatitis

Adults: For maintenance treatment after the disease process has been brought under control with corticosteroids. The initial dose of 500mg daily, in divided doses, should be increased gradually over three months to a maintenance dose of 1250mg daily. During this period, the dose of corticosteroids should be phased out. Throughout therapy, liver function tests should be carried out periodically to assess the disease status.

The elderly: Not recommended.

4.3 Contraindications

Hypersensitivity to penicillamine or any of the ingredients.

Agranulocytosis or severe thrombocytopenia due to penicillamine.

Lupus erythematosus.

Moderate or severe renal impairment.

4.4 Special warnings and precautions for use

Full blood and platelet counts should be performed and renal function should be assessed prior to treatment with penicillamine.

During the first eight weeks of therapy full blood counts should be carried out weekly or fortnightly and also in the week after any increase in dose, otherwise monthly thereafter. In cystinuria or Wilson's disease, longer intervals may be adequate.

Withdrawal of treatment should be considered if platelets fall below 120,000/mm^3 or white blood cells below 2,500/mm^3, or if three successive falls are noted within the normal range. Treatment may be restarted at a reduced dose when counts return to normal, but should be permanently withdrawn on recurrence of leucopenia or thrombocytopenia.

In patients with normal renal function, urinalysis for detection of haematuria and proteinuria should be carried out weekly at first, and following each increase in dose, then monthly, although longer intervals may be adequate for cystinuria and Wilson's disease. Increasing or persistent proteinuria may necessitate withdrawal of therapy.

Care should be exercised in patients with renal insufficiency; modification of dosage may be necessary (see Section 4.2, "Posology and Method of Administration").

Especially careful monitoring is necessary in the elderly since increased toxicity has been observed in this patient population regardless of renal function.

Concomitant use of NSAIDs and other nephrotoxic drugs may increase the risk of renal damage.

Penicillamine should be used with caution in patients who have had adverse reactions to gold.

Concomitant or previous treatment with gold may increase the risk of side effects with penicillamine treatment. Therefore penicillamine should be used with caution in patients who have previously had adverse reactions to gold and concomitant treatment with gold should be avoided.

If concomitant oral iron therapy is indicated, this should not be given within two hours of taking penicillamine.

Antihistamines, steroid cover, or temporary reduction of dose will control urticarial reactions.

Reversible loss of taste may occur. Mineral supplements to overcome this are not recommended.

Haematuria is rare, but if it occurs in the absence of renal stones or other known cause, treatment should be stopped immediately.

A late rash, described as acquired epidermolysis bullosa and penicillamine dermopathy, may occur after several months or years of therapy. This may necessitate a reduction in dosage.

Breast enlargement has been reported as a rare complication of penicillamine therapy in both women and men. Danazol has been used successfully to treat breast enlargement which does not regress on drug discontinuation.

4.5 Interaction with other medicinal products and other forms of interaction

Concomitant iron and penicillamine treatment: oral absorption of penicillamine may be reduced by concomitant administration of iron (see Section 4.4 "Special Warnings and Precautions for Use").

Concomitant use of NSAIDs and other nephrotoxic drugs may increase the risk of renal damage (see Section 4.4 "Special Warnings and Precautions for Use").

Concomitant gold and penicillamine treatment: concomitant use not recommended (see Section 4.4 "Special Warnings and Precautions for Use").

4.6 Pregnancy and lactation

Usage in pregnancy: The safety of penicillamine for use during pregnancy has not been established (see Section 5.3, "Preclinical Safety Data").

Wilson's disease: There have been several cases of reversible cutis laxa in infants born to mothers taking penicillamine throughout pregnancy. Although there have been no controlled studies on the use of penicillamine during pregnancy, two retrospective studies have reported the successful delivery of 43 normal infants to 28 women receiving between 500 and 2000mg of penicillamine daily. There are also anecdotal reports both of congenital abnormalities and of successful outcomes in patients who have remained on penicillamine during pregnancy. If treatment with penicillamine is to be continued following a risk-benefit analysis, consideration should be given to reducing the dose of penicillamine to the lowest effective dose.

Cystinuria: Whilst normal infants have been delivered, there is one report of a severe connective tissue abnormality in the infant of a mother who received 2000mg penicillamine daily throughout pregnancy. Whenever possible, penicillamine should be withheld during pregnancy, but if stones continue to form, the benefit of resuming treatment must be weighed against the possible risk to the foetus.

Rheumatoid arthritis or chronic active hepatitis: Penicillamine should not be administered to patients who are pregnant, and therapy should be stopped when pregnancy is diagnosed or suspected, unless considered to be absolutely essential by the physician.

Usage in lactation: Due to the lack of data on use in breast feeding patients and the possibility that penicillamine may be transmitted to newborns through breast milk, Distamine should only be used in breast feeding patients when it is considered absolutely essential by the physician.

4.7 Effects on ability to drive and use machines

None known.

4.8 Undesirable effects

NB: The incidence and severity of some of the adverse reactions, noted below, varies according to the dosage and nature of the disease under treatment.

Nausea, anorexia, fever and rash may occur early in therapy, especially when full doses are given from the start.

Urticarial reactions have been reported (see Section 4.4, "Special Warnings and Precautions for Use").

Reversible loss of taste may occur (see Section 4.4, "Special Warnings and Precautions for Use").

Rarely, mouth ulceration/stomatitis has occurred.

Thrombocytopenia occurs commonly and leucopenia less often. These reactions may occur at any time during treatment and are usually reversible (see Section 4.4, "Special Warnings and Precautions for Use").

Deaths from agranulocytosis and aplastic anaemia have occurred.

Deterioration of the neurological symptoms of Wilson's disease (dystonia, rigidity, tremor, dysarthria) have been reported following introduction of penicillamine in patients treated for this condition. This may be a consequence of mobilisation and redistribution of copper from the liver to the brain.

Proteinuria occurs in up to 30% of patients and is partially dose-related (see Section 4.4, "Special Warnings and Precautions for Use").

Haematuria may occur rarely (see Section 4.4, "Special Warnings and Precautions for Use").

Other rare adverse reactions are as follows: alopecia and inflammatory conditions of the respiratory system, such as bronchiolitis and pneumonitis.

Other complications have included haemolytic anaemia, nephrotic syndrome, glomerulonephritis, pulmonary haemorrhage, Goodpasture's syndrome, pancreatitis, cholestatic jaundice (including raised liver function tests), drug induced lupus erythematosus, and conditions closely resembling myasthenia gravis, polymyositis (with rare cardiac involvement), dermatomyositis, pemphigus, Stevens-Johnson syndrome and rheumatoid arthritis.

A late rash, described as acquired epidermolysis bullosa and penicillamine dermopathy, may occur after several months or years of therapy (see Section 4.4, "Special Warnings and Precautions for Use").

Pseudoxanthoma elasticum, elastosis perforans and skin laxity have been reported rarely. Breast enlargement has been reported as a rare complication of penicillamine therapy in both women and men. In some patients breast enlargement was considerable and/or prolonged with poor resolution and others required surgery (see Section 4.4, "Special Warnings and Precautions for Use").

The use of DMARDs, including penicillamine, has been linked to the development of septic arthritis in patients with rheumatoid arthritis, although rheumatoid arthritis is a stronger predictor for the development of septic arthritis than the use of a DMARD.

4.9 Overdose

No instances of adverse reactions to an overdose of penicillamine have been recorded and no specific measures are indicated.

5. PHARMACOLOGICAL PROPERTIES

5.1 Pharmacodynamic properties

Pharmacotherapeutic group: M01C C

1. Penicillamine is used to treat severe active rheumatoid arthritis not adequately controlled by NSAID therapy.

2. Penicillamine is a chelating agent which aids the elimination from the body of certain heavy metal ions, including copper, lead and mercury, by forming stable soluble complexes with them that are readily excreted by the kidney.

3. It is used in the treatment of Wilson's disease (hepatolenticular degeneration), in conjunction with a low copper diet, to promote the excretion of copper.

4. It may be used to treat asymptomatic lead intoxication.

5. Penicillamine is used as an adjunct to diet and urinary alkalinisation in the management of cystinuria. By reducing urinary concentrations of cystine, penicillamine prevents the formation of calculi and promotes the gradual dissolution of existing calculi.

6. Desensitisation. Should the physician deem it necessary to attempt to desensitise a patient to penicillamine, it should be noted that this formulation is not suitable for this purpose.

5.2 Pharmacokinetic properties

Penicillamine is a thiol-group containing chelating agent, variably absorbed from the gastrointestinal tract. The drug undergoes a rapid distribution phase, followed by a slower elimination phase.

Penicillamine is strongly plasma-protein bound. Most penicillamine is bound to albumin but some is bound to α-globulins or ceruloplasmin.

Penicillamine is not extensively metabolised in man.

About 80% of the absorbed dose is excreted rapidly in the urine, mostly as mixed disulphides. Some of the dose is excreted as a penicillamine copper complex and some as the S-methyl derivative.

5.3 Preclinical safety data

Penicillamine has been shown to be teratogenic in rats when given in doses several times higher than those recommended for human use.

There is no known LD50 value for penicillamine. In studies some rats died after oral administration of 10,000mg/kg, but intra-peritoneal injections of a dose of 660mg/kg caused no deaths.

6. PHARMACEUTICAL PARTICULARS

6.1 List of excipients

Tablet Core

Microcrystalline cellulose

Sodium starch glycolate (Type A)

Povidone

Magnesium stearate

Tablet Coating

Glycerol

Titanium dioxide (E171)

Hypromellose

6.2 Incompatibilities

Not applicable.

6.3 Shelf life

3 years

6.4 Special precautions for storage

Do not store above 25°C. Keep the bottle tightly closed.

6.5 Nature and contents of container

HDPE bottle with screw cap, containing 100 tablets.

6.6 Special precautions for disposal and other handling

No special requirements.

7. MARKETING AUTHORISATION HOLDER

Alliance Pharmaceuticals Ltd

Avonbridge House

Bath Road

Chippenham

Wiltshire

SN15 2BB

United Kingdom

8. MARKETING AUTHORISATION NUMBER(S)

PL 16853/0058

9. DATE OF FIRST AUTHORISATION/RENEWAL OF THE AUTHORISATION

12th October 2005

10. DATE OF REVISION OF THE TEXT

27th March 2009

Dithrocream

(Dermal Laboratories Limited)

1. NAME OF THE MEDICINAL PRODUCT

DITHROCREAM™

2. QUALITATIVE AND QUANTITATIVE COMPOSITION

Dithranol 0.1%, 0.25%, 0.5%, 1.0% or 2.0% w/w.

3. PHARMACEUTICAL FORM

Yellow aqueous cream.

4. CLINICAL PARTICULARS

4.1 Therapeutic indications

For the topical treatment of subacute and chronic psoriasis including psoriasis of the scalp.

4.2 Posology and method of administration

Dithranol therapy customarily involves titrating the concentration applied to skin to suit individual patient's circumstances. Dithrocream is, therefore, available in five strengths. The different packs are colour coded as follows:

0.1%	pale blue
0.25%	red
0.5%	purple
1.0%	brown
2.0%	yellow

For adults and the elderly: It is important to determine each patient's optimal treatment strength, as too high a strength may induce a burning sensation. Where the response to Dithrocream has not previously been established, always commence with Dithrocream 0.1%, continuing for at least one week and then, if necessary, increase to the 0.25% followed by the 0.5%, the 1.0% and finally the 2.0% strength. The aim should be to build up gradually over approximately 4 weeks to the highest tolerated strength to produce the optimum therapeutic effect. This optimum concentration will depend upon such factors as the thickness and location of the psoriatic plaques, as well as the variation between individual patients in their reaction to dithranol.

Dithrocream should be applied sparingly, and only to the affected areas, once every 24 hours, at any convenient time of the day or evening. Rub the cream gently and carefully into the skin until completely absorbed. For use on the scalp, first comb the hair to remove scalar debris and, after suitably parting, rub the cream well into the affected areas. Remove by washing off the skin or scalp, usually no more than one hour after application (Short Contact Therapy). Alternatively, it may be applied at night before retiring and washed off in the morning.

Treatment should be continued until the skin is entirely clear, i.e. when there is nothing to feel with the fingers and the texture is normal. By gradually increasing the strength of cream applied, it should be possible to clear psoriasis patches within 4 to 6 weeks.

For children No additional special precautions necessary. However, use cautiously as described above for adults and the elderly, with regular supervision.

4.3 Contraindications

Not to be used on the face, or for acute or pustular psoriasis.

Not to be used in cases of sensitivity to any of the ingredients.

4.4 Special warnings and precautions for use

Dithrocream 0.5%, Dithrocream 1.0% and Dithrocream 2.0% should only be used for those patients who have failed to respond to lower strengths of dithranol. Dithrocream 1.0% and 2.0% should normally only be applied for 'short contact' periods.

Dithrocream 0.5%, Dithrocream 1.0% and Dithrocream 2.0% should always be used under medical supervision.

It is most important to avoid applying an excessive amount of the cream, which may cause unnecessary soiling and staining of the clothing and/or bed linen. After each period of treatment, a bath/shower should be taken to remove any residual cream. To prevent the possibility of discolouration, particularly where Dithrocream 1.0% or 2.0% has been used, always rinse the bath/shower with hot water immediately after washing/showering and then use a suitable cleanser to remove any deposit on the surface of the bath/shower.

After use on the scalp, a shampoo may be used to remove the Dithrocream residue. Great care must be taken when washing out the shampoo (which may contain some Dithrocream residue), to ensure that it does not get into the eyes or on the face. This is particularly important when the higher strengths of Dithrocream have been used.

Although a feeling of warmth at the application site is normal, if this amounts to a burning sensation, or if the lesions spread, treatment should be stopped at once, and the dosage re-evaluated by a doctor.

Dithrocream is not normally recommended for use on areas of folded skin such as the groin and beneath the breasts. Do not use high strengths on these sites.

Keep away from the eyes and mucous membranes.

Always wash the hands after use.

As long term use of topical corticosteroids is known to destabilise psoriasis, and withdrawal may give rise to a rebound phenomenon, an interval of at least one week should be allowed between the discontinuance of such steroids and the commencement of Dithrocream therapy. A suitably bland emollient may usefully be applied in the intervening period.

The excipients, chlorocresol and cetostearyl alcohol may on rare occasions give rise to allergic or local skin reactions (eg. contact dermatitis) in sensitive people.

Contact with fabrics, plastics and other materials may cause permanent staining and should be avoided.

4.5 Interaction with other medicinal products and other forms of interaction

None known.

4.6 Pregnancy and lactation

Although there is no experimental evidence to support the safety of the drug in pregnancy or during lactation, no adverse effects have been reported.

4.7 Effects on ability to drive and use machines

None known.

4.8 Undesirable effects

Some skin irritation and/or a feeling of warmth at the site of application is normally associated with dithranol therapy. Dithrocream applied at too high a strength or left in contact with the skin for too long may induce a burning sensation.

Dithrocream may cause temporary staining of the skin and/or hair.

4.9 Overdose

Dithranol is a cathartic (laxative) and if accidentally swallowed, it should be removed by gastric lavage.

5. PHARMACOLOGICAL PROPERTIES

5.1 Pharmacodynamic properties

Dithranol has been used in the treatment of sub-acute and chronic psoriasis for over 70 years and, during that time, it has become established as a safe and effective form of therapy. Its precise mode of action is still to be confirmed, although it has been shown to inhibit DNA replication, cellular respiration and key cellular enzymes eg glucose-6-phosphate dehydrogenase.

Because dithranol causes staining and irritation, it is now widely used in short contact therapy where the preparation is washed off the skin after periods of one hour or less. For this purpose, Dithrocream is particularly suitable, as it is convenient to apply and washes off easily in a bath or shower.

5.2 Pharmacokinetic properties

The traditional formulations of dithranol are based on soft paraffin from which it is effectively released into the skin. In Dithrocream, during manufacture, the oily paraffin phase of the cream is heated until the dithranol entirely dissolves so that, on cooling, it is retained solely within the paraffin phase and does not spread into the aqueous phase. After application of Dithrocream to the skin, the water is lost through absorption and evaporation, leaving the oily phase which then acts in the same way as a dithranol ointment. However, since the cream may be rubbed into the skin more effectively than the ointment, it is convenient to apply and, owing to the presence of the emulsifying components, is easier to wash off.

The availability of the dithranol has now been confirmed in numerous publications detailing the results of clinical trials.

5.3 Preclinical safety data

No special information.

6. PHARMACEUTICAL PARTICULARS

6.1 List of excipients

White Soft Paraffin; Cetostearyl Alcohol; Salicylic Acid; Ascorbic Acid; Sodium Laurilsulfate; Chlorocresol; Purified Water.

Dithrocream 2.0% also contains Liquid Paraffin.

6.2 Incompatibilities

None known.

6.3 Shelf life

48 months.

6.4 Special precautions for storage

Do not store above 25°C. Replace cap tightly after use.

6.5 Nature and contents of container

All strengths of Dithrocream are supplied in collapsible tubes containing 50 g. These are supplied as original packs (OP).

6.6 Special precautions for disposal and other handling

Not applicable.

7. MARKETING AUTHORISATION HOLDER

Dermal Laboratories

Tatmore Place, Gosmore

Hitchin, Herts SG4 7QR, UK.

8. MARKETING AUTHORISATION NUMBER(S)

Dithrocream 0.1%	00173/0029
Dithrocream 0.25%	00173/0028
Dithrocream 0.5%	00173/0027
Dithrocream 1.0%	00173/0039
Dithrocream 2.0%	00173/0045

9. DATE OF FIRST AUTHORISATION/RENEWAL OF THE AUTHORISATION

31 July 2008.

10. DATE OF REVISION OF THE TEXT

October 2006.

Ditropan Elixir 2.5mg/5ml

(sanofi-aventis)

1. NAME OF THE MEDICINAL PRODUCT

Ditropan elixir 2.5mg/5ml

2. QUALITATIVE AND QUANTITATIVE COMPOSITION

Ditropan elixir contains 2.5mg oxybutynin hydrochloride per 5ml.

3. PHARMACEUTICAL FORM

Ditropan elixir is a clear and colourless elixir.

4. CLINICAL PARTICULARS

4.1 Therapeutic indications

For use in urinary incontinence, urgency and frequency in the unstable bladder; whether due to neurogenic bladder disorders (detrusor hyperreflexia) in conditions such as multiple sclerosis and spina bifida or to idiopathic detrusor instability (motor urge incontinence).

Children over 5 years of age: In addition to neurogenic bladder disorders, Ditropan may also be used in nocturnal enuresis in conjunction with non-drug therapy where this alone, or in conjunction with other drug treatment, has failed.

4.2 Posology and method of administration

Dosage and administration:

Adults: The usual dose is 5mg (10ml) two or three times a day. This may be increased to a maximum of 5 mg four times a day to obtain a clinical response provided that the side effects are tolerated.

Elderly: The elimination half-life is increased in the elderly, therefore, a dose of 2.5mg (5ml) twice a day, particularly if the patient is frail, is likely to be adequate. This dose may be titrated upwards to 5mg two times a day to obtain a clinical response provided the side effects are tolerated.

Children (under 5 years of age): Not recommended.

Children (over 5 years of age): Neurogenic bladder: the usual dose is 2.5mg (5ml) twice a day. This dose may be titrated upwards to 5mg (10ml) two or three times a day to obtain a clinical response provided that the side effects are tolerated. Nocturnal enuresis: the usual dose is 2.5mg (5ml) twice a day. This dose may be titrated upwards to 5mg (10ml) two or three times a day to obtain a clinical response provided that the side effects are tolerated. The last dose should be given before bedtime.

4.3 Contraindications

Hypersensitivity to oxybutynin or any component.

Myasthenia gravis.

Narrow-angle glaucoma or shallow anterior chamber.

Gastrointestinal obstruction including paralytic ileus, intestinal atony.

Patients with toxic megacolon, severe ulcerative colitis.

Patients with bladder outflow obstruction where urinary retention may be precipitated.

4.4 Special warnings and precautions for use

Oxybutynin should be used with caution in the frail elderly and children who may be more sensitive to the effects of the product and in patients with autonomic neuropathy, hepatic or renal impairment and severe gastro-intestinal motility disorders (also see section 4.3).

Oxybutynin may aggravate the symptoms of hyperthyroidism, congestive heart failure, coronary heart disease, cardiac arrhythmias, tachycardia, hypertension and prostatic hypertrophy.

Oxybutynin can cause decreased sweating; in high environmental temperatures this can lead to heat prostration.

The use of oxybutynin in children under 5 years of age is not recommended; it has not been established whether oxybutynin can be safely used in this age group.

Special care should be taken in patients with hiatus hernia associated with reflux oesophagitis, as anticholinergic drugs can aggravate this condition.

4.5 Interaction with other medicinal products and other forms of interaction

Care should be taken if other anticholinergic agents are administered together with Ditropan as potentiation of anticholinergic effects could occur.

Occasional cases of interaction between anticholinergics and phenothiazines, amantidine, butyrophenones, L-dopa, digitalis and tricyclic antidepressants have been reported and care should be taken if Ditropan is administered concurrently with such drugs.

By reducing gastric motility, oxybutynin may affect the absorption of other drugs.

4.6 Pregnancy and lactation

Pregnancy

There is no evidence as to the safety of Ditropan in human pregnancy nor is there evidence from animal work that it is totally free from hazard. Avoid in pregnancy unless there is no safer alternative.

Lactation

Small amounts of oxybutynin have been found in mother's milk of lactating animals. Breast feeding while using oxybutynin is therefore not recommended.

4.7 Effects on ability to drive and use machines

As Ditropan may produce drowsiness or blurred vision, the patient should be cautioned regarding activities requiring mental alertness such as driving, operating machinery or performing hazardous work while taking this drug.

4.8 Undesirable effects

Gastro-intestinal disorders

Nausea, diarrhoea, constipation, dry mouth, abdominal discomfort, anorexia, vomiting, gastroesophageal reflux.

CNS and psychiatric disorders

Agitation, headache, dizziness, drowsiness, disorientation, hallucinations, nightmares, convulsions.

Cardiovascular disorders

Tachycardia, cardiac arrythmia.

Vision disorders

Blurred vision, mydriasis, intraocular hypertension, onset of narrow-angle glaucoma, dry eyes.

Renal and urinary disorders

Urinary retention, difficulty in micturition.

Skin and appendages

Facial flushing which may be more marked in children, dry skin, allergic reactions such as rash, urticaria, angioedema, photosensitivity.

4.9 Overdose

The symptoms of overdosage with oxybutynin progress from an intensification of the usual side effects of CNS disturbances (from restlessness and excitement to psychotic behaviour), circulatory changes (flushing, fall in blood pressure, circulatory failure etc), respiratory failure, paralysis and coma.

Measures to be taken are:

1) immediate gastric lavage

2) physostigmine by slow intravenous injection

Adults: 0.5 to 2.0 mg of physostigmine by slow intravenous administration. Repeat after 5 minutes, if necessary up to a maximum total dose of 5mg.

Children: 30 micrograms/kg of physostigmine by slow intravenous administration. Repeat after 5 minutes, if necessary up to a maximum total dose of 2mg.

Fever should be treated symptomatically with tepid sponging or ice packs.

In pronounced restlessness or excitation, diazepam 10mg may be given by intravenous injection, tachycardia may be treated by intravenous injection of propranolol and urinary retention can be managed by catheterisation.

In the event of progression of the curare like effect to the paralysis of the respiratory muscles, mechanical ventilation will be required.

5. PHARMACOLOGICAL PROPERTIES

5.1 Pharmacodynamic properties

Oxybutynin hydrochloride has both direct antispasmodic action on the smooth muscle of the bladder detrusor muscle as well as an anticholinergic action in blocking the muscarinic effects of acetylcholine on smooth muscle. These properties cause relaxation of the detrusor muscle of the bladder in patients with an unstable bladder. Ditropan increases bladder capacity and reduces the incidence of spontaneous contractions of the detrusor muscle.

5.2 Pharmacokinetic properties

Oxybutynin is poorly absorbed from the gastrointestinal tract. It is highly bound to plasma proteins, the peak plasma level is reached between 0.5 to 1 hour after administration. The half life is biexponential, the first phase being about 40 minutes and the second about 2-3 hours. The elimination half life may be increased in the elderly, particularly if they are frail.

Oxybutynin and its metabolites are excreted in the faeces and urine. There is no evidence of accumulation.

5.3 Preclinical safety data

No data of therapeutic relevance.

6. PHARMACEUTICAL PARTICULARS

6.1 List of excipients

Ditropan elixir contains citric acid, sodium citrate, sucrose (1.3g per 5ml dose), sorbitol, glycerol, sodium methyl-*p*-hydroxybenzoate (E219), purified water.

6.2 Incompatibilities

None known.

6.3 Shelf life

Ditropan Elixir 2.5mg/5ml has a 30 month shelf life.

6.4 Special precautions for storage

Ditropan Elixir 2.5mg/5ml: Store below 25°C. Protect from light

Discard any medicine remaining 28 days after opening the bottle

6.5 Nature and contents of container

Ditropan Elixir 2.5mg/5ml: 30ml (sample size) and 150ml amber glass bottle with a child resistant screw cap.

6.6 Special precautions for disposal and other handling

No special requirements.

7. MARKETING AUTHORISATION HOLDER

sanofi-aventis

One Onslow Street

Guildford

Surrey GU1 4YS

8. MARKETING AUTHORISATION NUMBER(S)

PL 04425/0286

9. DATE OF FIRST AUTHORISATION/RENEWAL OF THE AUTHORISATION

6 February 2009

10. DATE OF REVISION OF THE TEXT

February 2009

Legal Category: POM

Ditropan Tablets 2.5mg, Ditropan Tablets 5mg

(sanofi-aventis)

1. NAME OF THE MEDICINAL PRODUCT

Ditropan tablets 2.5mg

Ditropan tablets 5mg

2. QUALITATIVE AND QUANTITATIVE COMPOSITION

Each tablet contains 2.5mg or 5mg oxybutynin hydrochloride as the active ingredient.

3. PHARMACEUTICAL FORM

Ditropan tablets 2.5mg are pale blue oval bi-convex tablets 8 mm × 5.5 mm, marked OXB2.5 on one side.

Ditropan tablets 5mg are pale blue circular tablets with a 8.0mm nominal diameter, with a centre breakline on one side, and marked OXB5 on the reverse.

4. CLINICAL PARTICULARS

4.1 Therapeutic indications

Urinary incontinence, urgency and frequency in the unstable bladder, whether due to neurogenic bladder disorders (detrusor hyperreflexia) in conditions such as multiple sclerosis and spina bifida, or to idiopathic detrusor instability (motor urge incontinence).

Children over 5 years of age: In addition to neurogenic bladder disorders, Ditropan may also be used in nocturnal enuresis in conjunction with non-drug therapy where this alone, or in conjunction with other drug treatment, has failed.

4.2 Posology and method of administration

Dosage and administration:

Adults: The usual dose is 5mg two or three times a day. This may be increased to a maximum of 5 mg four times a day to obtain a clinical response provided that the side effects are tolerated.

Elderly (including frail elderly): The elimination half-life is increased in the elderly. Therefore, a dose of 2.5mg twice a day, particularly if the patient is frail, is likely to be adequate. This dose may be titrated upwards to 5mg two times a day to obtain a clinical response provided the side effects are well tolerated.

Children (under 5 years of age): Not recommended

Children (over 5 years of age): Neurogenic bladder instability: the usual dose is 2.5mg twice a day. This dose may be titrated upwards to 5mg two or three times a day to obtain a clinical response provided the side effects are well tolerated. Nocturnal enuresis: the usual dose is 2.5mg twice a day. This dose may be titrated upwards to 5mg two or three times a day to obtain a clinical response provided the side effects are tolerated. The last dose should be given before bedtime.

4.3 Contraindications

Hypersensitivity to oxybutynin or any component.

Myasthenia gravis.

Narrow-angle glaucoma or shallow anterior chamber.

Gastrointestinal obstruction including paralytic ileus, intestinal atony.

Patients with toxic megacolon, severe ulcerative colitis.

Patients with bladder outflow obstruction where urinary retention may be precipitated.

4.4 Special warnings and precautions for use

Oxybutynin should be used with caution in the frail elderly and children who may be more sensitive to the effects of the product and in patients with autonomic neuropathy, hepatic or renal impairment and severe gastro-intestinal motility disorders (also see section 4.3).

Oxybutynin may aggravate the symptoms of hyperthyroidism, congestive heart failure, coronary heart disease, cardiac arrhythmias, tachycardia, hypertension and prostatic hypertrophy.

Oxybutynin can cause decreased sweating; in high environmental temperatures this can lead to heat prostration.

The use of oxybutynin in children under 5 years of age is not recommended; it has not been established whether oxybutynin can be safely used in this age group.

Special care should be taken in patients with hiatus hernia associated with reflux oesophagitis, as anticholinergic drugs can aggravate this condition.

4.5 Interaction with other medicinal products and other forms of interaction

Care should be taken if other anticholinergic agents are administered together with Ditropan, as potentiation of anticholinergic effects could occur.

Occasional cases of interaction between anticholinergics and phenothiazines, amantidine, butyrophenones, L-dopa, digitalis and tricyclic antidepressants have been reported and care should be taken if Ditropan is administered concurrently with such drugs.

By reducing gastric motility, oxybutynin may affect the absorption of other drugs.

4.6 Pregnancy and lactation

Pregnancy

There is no evidence as to the safety of Ditropan in human pregnancy nor is there evidence from animal work that it is totally free from hazard. Avoid in pregnancy unless there is no safer alternative.

Lactation

Small amounts of oxybutynin have been found in mother's milk of lactating animals. Breast feeding while using oxybutynin is therefore not recommended.

4.7 Effects on ability to drive and use machines

As Ditropan may produce drowsiness or blurred vision, the patient should be cautioned regarding activities requiring mental alertness such as driving, operating machinery or performing hazardous work while taking this drug.

4.8 Undesirable effects

Gastro-intestinal disorders

Nausea, diarrhoea, constipation, dry mouth, abdominal discomfort, anorexia, vomiting, gastroesophageal reflux.

CNS and psychiatric disorders

Agitation, headache, dizziness, drowsiness, disorientation, hallucinations, nightmares, convulsions.

Cardiovascular disorders

Tachycardia, cardiac arrythmia.

Vision disorders

Blurred vision, mydriasis, intraocular hypertension, onset of narrow-angle glaucoma, dry eyes.

Renal and urinary disorders

Urinary retention, difficulty in micturition.

Skin and appendages

Facial flushing which may be more marked in children, dry skin, allergic reactions such as rash, urticaria, angioedema, photosensitivity.

4.9 Overdose

The symptoms of overdose with oxybutynin progress from an intensification of the usual side effects of CNS disturbances (from restlessness and excitement to psychotic behaviour), circulation changes (flushing, fall in blood pressure, circulatory failure etc), respiratory failure, paralysis and coma.

Measures to be taken are:

1) Immediate gastric lavage

2) physostigmine by slow intravenous injection

Adults: 0.5 to 2.0 mg of physostigmine by slow intravenous administration. Repeat after 5 minutes, if necessary up to a maximum total dose of 5mg.

Children: 30 micrograms/kg of physostigmine by slow intravenous administration. Repeat after 5 minutes, if necessary up to a maximum total dose of 2mg.

Fever should be treated symptomatically with tepid sponging or ice packs.

In pronounced restlessness or excitation, diazepam 10mg may be given by intravenous injection, tachycardia may be treated by intravenous injection of propranolol and urinary retention can be managed by catheterisation.

In the event of progression of the curare- like effect to the paralysis of the respiratory muscles, mechanical ventilation will be required.

5. PHARMACOLOGICAL PROPERTIES

5.1 Pharmacodynamic properties

Oxybutynin has both direct antispasmodic action on the smooth muscle of the bladder detrusor muscle as well as an anticholinergic action in blocking the muscarinic effects of acetylcholine on smooth muscle. These properties cause relaxation of the detrusor muscle of the bladder in patients with an unstable bladder. Ditropan increases bladder capacity and reduces the incidence of spontaneous contractions of the detrusor muscle.

5.2 Pharmacokinetic properties

Oxybutynin is poorly absorbed from the gastrointestinal tract. It is highly bound to plasma proteins, the peak plasma level is reached between 0.5 to 1 hour after administration. The half life is biexponential, the first phase being about 40 minutes and the second about 2-3 hours. The elimination half life may be increased in the elderly, particularly if they are frail.

Oxybutynin and its metabolites are excreted in the faeces and urine. There is no evidence of accumulation.

5.3 Preclinical safety data

No data of therapeutic relevance.

6. PHARMACEUTICAL PARTICULARS

6.1 List of excipients

Ditropan tablets contain lactose, cellulose, calcium stearate and indigo carmine (E132).

6.2 Incompatibilities

None known.

6.3 Shelf life

4 years

6.4 Special precautions for storage

Store at or below 30°C.

6.5 Nature and contents of container

Cartons containing 84 tablets in blister strips.

6.6 Special precautions for disposal and other handling

No special requirements.

7. MARKETING AUTHORISATION HOLDER

sanofi-aventis

One Onslow Street

Guildford

Surrey

GU1 4YS

UK

8. MARKETING AUTHORISATION NUMBER(S)

Ditropan 2.5mg tablets PL 04425/0289

Ditropan 5mg tablets PL 04425/0290

9. DATE OF FIRST AUTHORISATION/RENEWAL OF THE AUTHORISATION

26 March 2009

10. DATE OF REVISION OF THE TEXT

26 March 2009

Legal Category: POM

Dolmatil Tablets 200mg, Dolmatil 400mg Tablets

(sanofi-aventis)

1. NAME OF THE MEDICINAL PRODUCT

Dolmatil Tablets 200mg

Dolmatil Tablets 400mg

2. QUALITATIVE AND QUANTITATIVE COMPOSITION

Dolmatil Tablets 200mg: active ingredient is sulpiride 200mg.

Dolmatil Tablets 400mg: active ingredient is sulpiride 400mg

Sulpiride is a benzamide derivative.

3. PHARMACEUTICAL FORM

Dolmatil Tablets 200mg: Plain white round tablet with a transverse breakline on one side and D200 on the other.

Dolmatil Tablets 400mg: White film coated stick shaped tablets with break bar engraved SLP 400 on one side.

4. CLINICAL PARTICULARS

4.1 Therapeutic indications

Acute and chronic schizophrenia.

4.2 Posology and method of administration

Adults

A starting dose of 400mg to 800mg daily, given as one or two tablets twice daily (morning and early evening) is recommended.

Predominantly positive symptoms (formal thought disorder, hallucinations, delusions, incongruity of affect) respond to higher doses, and a starting dose of at least 400mg twice daily is recommended, increasing if necessary up to a suggested maximum of 1200mg twice daily. Increasing the dose beyond this level has not been shown to produce further improvement.

Predominantly negative symptoms (flattening of affect, poverty of speech, anergia, apathy, as well as depression) respond to doses below 800mg daily; therefore, a starting dose of 400mg twice daily is recommended. Reducing this dose towards 200mg twice daily will normally increase the alerting effect of Dolmatil.

Patients with mixed positive and negative symptoms, with neither predominating, will normally respond to dosage of 400-600mg twice daily.

Children

Clinical experience in children under 14 years of age is insufficient to permit specific recommendations.

Elderly

The same dose ranges are applicable in the elderly, but the dose should be reduced if there is evidence of renal impairment.

4.3 Contraindications

Phaeochromocytoma and acute porphyria.

Hypersensitivity to the active ingredient or to other ingredients of the medicinal product.

Concomitant prolactin-dependent tumours e.g. pituitary gland prolactinomas and breast cancer (See 4.8 Undesirable effects).

Association with levodopa (See 4.5 Interactions with other medicinal products and other forms of interaction).

4.4 Special warnings and precautions for use

Warnings:

Increased motor agitation has been reported at high dosage in a small number of patients: in aggressive, agitated or excited phases of the disease process, low doses of Dolmatil may aggravate symptoms. Care should be exercised where hypomania is present.

Extrapyramidal reactions, principally akathisia have been reported in a small number of cases. If warranted, reduction in dosage or anti-parkinsonian medication may be necessary.

As with other neuroleptics, neuroleptic malignant syndrome, a potentially fatal complication, which is characterised by hyperthermia, muscle rigidity, autonomic instability, altered consciousness and elevated CPK levels, has been reported. In such an event, all antipsychotic drugs, including Dolmatil, should be discontinued.

Elderly patients are more susceptible to postural hypotension, sedation and extrapyramidal effects.

In patients with aggressive behaviour or agitation with impulsiveness, sulpiride could be given with a sedative.

Acute withdrawal symptoms, including nausea, vomiting, sweating and insomnia have been described after abrupt cessation of antipsychotic drugs. Recurrence of psychotic symptoms may also occur, and the emergence of involuntary movement disorders (such as akathisia, dystonia and dyskinesia) have been reported. Therefore, gradual withdrawal is advisable.

Precautions:

In elderly patients, as with other neuroleptics, sulpiride should be used with particular caution (see 4.2 Posology and method of administration).

In children, efficacy and safety of sulpiride have not been thoroughly investigated. Therefore, caution should be exercised when prescribing to children (see 4.2 Posology and method of administration).

When neuroleptic treatment is absolutely necessary in a patient with Parkinson's disease, sulpiride can be used, although caution is in order.

Neuroleptics may lower the epileptogenic threshold. Cases of convulsions, sometimes in patients with no previous history, have been reported with sulpiride. Caution is advised in prescribing it for patients with unstable epilepsy, and patients with a history of epilepsy should be closely monitored during therapy with sulpiride.

In patients requiring Dolmatil who are receiving anti-convulsant therapy, the dose of the anti-convulsant should not be changed.

Cases of convulsions, sometimes in patients with no previous history, have been reported.

Dolmatil has no significant anticholinergic effect. As with all drugs for which the kidney is the major elimination pathway, the dose should be reduced and titrated in small steps in cases of renal insufficiency.

Prolongation of the QT interval:

Sulpiride induces a prolongation of the QT interval (see section 4.8). This effect is known to potentiate the risk of serious ventricular arrhythmias such as torsade de pointes.

Before any administration, and if possible according to the patient's clinical status, it is recommended to monitor factors which could favour the occurrence of this rhythm disorder, for example:

- Bradycardia less than 55 bpm
- Electrolyte imbalance in particular hypokalaemia
- Congenital prolongation of the QT interval
- On-going treatment with a medication likely to produce pronounced bradycardia (< 55 bpm), hypokalaemia, decreased intracardiac conduction, or prolongation of the QTc interval (see section 4.5)

Sulpiride should be prescribed with caution in patients presenting with these factors and patients with cardiovascular disorders which may predispose to prolongation of the QT interval.

Avoid concomitant treatment with other neuroleptics (see section 4.5).

Stroke:

In randomised clinical trials versus placebo performed in a population of elderly patients with dementia and treated with certain atypical antipsychotic drugs, a 3-fold increase of the risk of cerebrovascular events has been observed. The mechanism of such risk increase is not known. An increase in the risk with other antipsychotic drugs or other populations of patients cannot be excluded. Sulpiride should be used with caution in patients with stroke risk factors.

4.5 Interaction with other medicinal products and other forms of interaction

4.5.1 Associations contra-indicated

Levodopa: reciprocal antagonism of effects between levodopa and neuroleptics.

4.5.2 Associations not recommended.

Alcohol: alcohol enhances the sedative effects of neuroleptics.

Avoid the consumption of alcoholic beverages and drugs containing alcohol.

Combination with the following medications which could induce torsades de pointes or prolong the QT interval (see section 4.4):

– Bradycardia-inducing medications such as beta-blockers, bradycardia-inducing calcium channel blockers such as diltiazem and verapamil, clonidine; digitalis.

– Medications which induce electrolyte imbalance, in particular those causing hypokalaemia: hypokalaemic diuretics, stimulant laxatives, IV amphotericin B, glucocorticoids, tetracosactides.

Electrolyte balance should be corrected

– Class Ia antiarrhythmic agents such as quinidine, disopyramide.

– Class III antiarrhythmic agents such as amiodarone, sotalol.

– Other medications such as pimozide, haloperidol; methadone, imipramine antidepressants; lithium, cisapride, thioridazine, IV erythromycin, halofantrine, pentamidine.

4.5.3 Associations to be taken into account.

Antihypertensive agents: antihypertensive effect and possibility of enhanced postural hypotension (additive effect).

CNS depressants including narcotics, analgesics, sedative H1 antihistamines, barbiturates, benzodiazepines and other anxiolytics, clonidine and derivatives.

Antacids or sucralfate: The absorption of sulpiride is decreased after co-administration. Therefore, sulpiride should be administered two hours before these drugs

Lithium increases the risk of extrapyramidal side effects.

Sulpiride may reduce the effectiveness of ropinorole.

4.6 Pregnancy and lactation

Pregnancy:

A decrease in fertility linked to the pharmacological effects of the drug (prolactin mediated effect) was observed in treated animals. Animal studies do not indicate direct or indirect harmful effects with respect to pregnancy, embyonal/fetal development and/or postnatal development. In humans, very limited clinical data on exposed pregnancies are available In almost all cases of foetal or neonatal disorders reported in the context of sulpiride use during pregnancy, alternative explanations can be suggested and seem more likely. Therefore the use of sulpiride is not recommended during pregnancy because of the limited experience. If sulpiride is used during pregnancy, appropriate monitoring of the neonate should be considered in view of sulpiride safety profile.

Lactation:

Sulpiride has been found in the breast milk of treated women. Therefore breast-feeding is not recommended during treatment.

4.7 Effects on ability to drive and use machines

Even used as recommended, sulpiride may cause sedation so that the ability to drive vehicles or operate machinery can be impaired. (see section 4.8)

4.8 Undesirable effects

Cardiovascular disorders:

- Postural hypotension

- QT interval prolongation and ventricular arrhythmias such as torsade de pointes and ventricular tachycardia, which may result in ventricular fibrillation or cardiac arrest, sudden death. (see section 4.4)

Endocrine disorders:

- Hyperprolactinaemia

General disorders and administration site conditions:

- As with all neuroleptics, malignant syndrome (see section 4.4) which is a potentially fatal complication

- Weight gainHepatobiliary disorders:

- Increase in hepatic enzymes

Nervous system disorders:

- Sedation or drowsiness. Insomnia has been reported.

- Extrapyramidal symptoms and related disorders:

- parkinsonism and related symptoms: tremor, hypertonia, hypokinesia, hypersalivation

- acute dyskinesia and dystonia (spasm torticollis, oculogyric crisis, trismus)

- akathisia

These symptoms are generally reversible upon administration of antiparkinsonian medication.

- Tardive dyskinesia (characterised by rhythmic, involuntary movements primarily of the tongue and/or the face) have been reported, as with all neuroleptics, after a neuroleptic administration of more than 3 months. Antiparkinsonian medication is ineffective or may induce aggravation of the symptoms.

- Convulsions have been reported, in particular in patients with epilepsy. (see section 4.4)

Reproductive system and breast disorders: Disorders related to hyperprolactinaemia:

- Galactorrhoea
- Amenorrhoea
- Gynaecomastia
- Breast enlargement and breast pain
- Orgasmic dysfunction and erectile dysfunction.

Skin and subcutaneous tissue disorders:

- Maculo-papular rash

4.9 Overdose

Experience with sulpiride in overdosage is limited

The range of single toxic doses is 1 to 16g but no death has occurred even at the 16g dose.

The clinical manifestations of poisoning vary depending upon the size of the dose taken. After single doses of 1 to 3g restlessness and clouding of consciousness have been reported and (rarely) extrapyramidal symptoms. Doses of 3 to 7g may produce a degree of agitation, confusion and extrapyramidal symptoms (see section 4.8 Undesirable Effects); more than 7g can cause, in addition, coma and low blood pressure.

The duration of intoxication is generally short, the symptoms disappearing within a few hours. Comas which have occurred after large doses have lasted up to four days.

No haematological or hepatic toxicity has been reported.

Sulpiride is partly removed by haemodialysis.

There is no specific antidote to sulpiride. Treatment is only symptomatic. Appropriate supportive measures should therefore be instituted, close supervision of vital functions and cardiac monitoring (risk of QT interval prolongation and subsequent ventricular arrythmias) is recommended until the patient recovers.

If severe extrapyramidal symptoms occur anticholinergics should be administrated.

Overdose may be treated with alkaline osmotic diuresis and, if necessary, anti-parkinsonian drugs. Coma needs appropriate nursing, and cardiac monitoring is recommended until the patient recovers. Emetic drugs are unlikely to be effective in Dolmatil overdosage.

5. PHARMACOLOGICAL PROPERTIES

5.1 Pharmacodynamic properties

Dolmatil is a member of the group of substituted benzamides, which are structurally distinct from the phenothiazines, butyrophenones and thioxanthenes. Current evidence suggests that the actions of Dolmatil hint at an important distinction between different types of dopamine receptors or receptor mechanisms in the brain.

Behaviourally and biochemically, Dolmatil shares with these classical neuroleptics a number of properties indicative of cerebral dopamine receptor antagonism. Essential and intriguing differences include lack of catalepsy at doses active in other behavioural tests, lack of effect in the dopamine sensitive adenylate cyclase systems, lack of effect upon noradrenaline or 5HT turnover, negligible anticholinesterase activity, no effect on muscarinic or GABA receptor binding, and a radical difference in the binding of tritiated sulpiride to striatal preparations in-vitro, compared to ^{3}H-spiperone or ^{3}H-haloperidol. These findings indicate a major differentiation between Dolmatil and classical neuroleptics which lack such specificity.

One of the characteristics of Dolmatil is its bimodal activity, as it has both antidepressant and neuroleptic properties. Schizophrenia characterised by a lack of social contact can benefit strikingly. Mood elevation is observed after a few days treatment, followed by disappearance of the florid schizophrenic symptoms. The sedation and lack of affect characteristically associated with classical neuroleptics of the phenothiazine or butyrophenone type are not features of Dolmatil therapy.

5.2 Pharmacokinetic properties

Peak sulpiride serum levels are reached 3 - 6 hours after an oral dose. The plasma half-life in man is approximately 8 hours. Approximately 40% sulpiride is bound to plasma proteins. 95% of the compound is excreted in the urine and faeces as unchanged sulpiride.

5.3 Preclinical safety data

In long-term animal studies with neuroleptic drugs, including sulpiride, an increased incidence of various endocrine tumours (some of which have occasionally been malignant) has been seen in some but not all strains of rats and mice studied. The significance of these findings to man is not known; there is no current evidence of an association between neuroleptic use and tumour risk in man.

6. PHARMACEUTICAL PARTICULARS

6.1 List of excipients

Dolmatil Tablets 200mg: Starch, lactose, methylcellulose, magnesium stearate, talc, silica.

Dolmatil Tablets 400mg: Lactose, sodium starch glycollate, microcrystalline cellulose, hydroxypropymethyl-cellulose and magnesium stearate

6.2 Incompatibilities

None known.

6.3 Shelf life

5 years.

6.4 Special precautions for storage

Store at or below 25°C.

6.5 Nature and contents of container

Dolmatil Tablets 200mg: Cartons containing 100 tablets in blister strips

Dolmatil Tablets 400mg: strip-wrapped in a moulded bubble blister pack in 200µg PVC, heat sealed with 0.02mm printed laminated aluminium foil. Contains 100 tablets.

6.6 Special precautions for disposal and other handling

Not applicable.

7. MARKETING AUTHORISATION HOLDER

sanofi-aventis

One Onslow Street

Guildford

Surrey

GU1 4YS

8. MARKETING AUTHORISATION NUMBER(S)

Dolmatil Tablets 200mg: PL 04425/0291

Dolmatil Tablets 400mg: PL 04425/0292

9. DATE OF FIRST AUTHORISATION/RENEWAL OF THE AUTHORISATION

Dolmatil Tablets 200mg:22 December 2008

Dolmatil Tablets 400mg: 22 December 2008

10. DATE OF REVISION OF THE TEXT

Legal Category: POM

Dopacard

(Cephalon Limited)

1. NAME OF THE MEDICINAL PRODUCT

Dopacard 50mg/5ml Concentrate for Solution for Infusion

2. QUALITATIVE AND QUANTITATIVE COMPOSITION

Dopexamine hydrochloride as a 1% solution (w/v). Each 5 ml ampoule contains 50 mg of dopexamine hydrochloride.

3. PHARMACEUTICAL FORM

Concentrate for solution for infusion.

4. CLINICAL PARTICULARS

4.1 Therapeutic indications

Dopacard is indicated for short-term intravenous administration to patients in whom afterload reduction, (through peripheral vasodilatation, and/or renal and mesenteric vasodilatation), combined with a mild positive inotropic effect is required for the treatment of exacerbations of chronic heart failure, or heart failure associated with cardiac surgery.

4.2 Posology and method of administration

For intravenous use only.

Dopacard must be diluted before use.

Dosage

Adults and the elderly:

Infusion should begin at a dose of 0.5 microgram/kg/min and may be increased to 1 microgram/kg/min and then in increments (0.5-1 microgram/kg/min) up to 6 micrograms/kg/min at not less than 15 minute intervals according to the patient's haemodynamic and clinical response. Smaller increments (0.5 microgram/kg/min) may be justified in certain patients according to haemodynamic and clinical response.

Children:

The safety and efficacy of Dopacard for use in children have not been established.

Administration

Dopacard should only be administered intravenously by infusion through a cannula or catheter in a central or large peripheral vein. Contact with metal parts in infusion apparatus should be minimised. A device which provides accurate control of the rate of flow is essential.

Central administration: Dopacard can be administered via a cannula or catheter sited in a central vein. The concentration of the infusion solution for administration via this route must not exceed 4mg/ml.

Peripheral administration: Dopacard can be administered via a cannula in a large peripheral vein. The concentration of the infusion solution for administration via this route must not exceed 1mg/ml. Thrombophlebitis has been reported with peripheral administration using concentrations of Dopacard exceeding 1mg/ml.

During the administration of Dopacard, as with any parenteral catecholamine, the rate of administration and duration of therapy should be adjusted according to the patient's response as determined by heart rate and rhythm (ECG), blood pressure, urine flow and, whenever possible, measurement of cardiac output.

It is recommended that the infusion of Dopacard is reduced gradually rather than withdrawn abruptly.

The duration of therapy is dependent upon the patient's overall response to treatment. Extended therapy beyond 48 hours has not been fully evaluated.

4.3 Contraindications

Known hypersensitivity to dopexamine hydrochloride or excipients (disodium edetate).

Patients who are receiving monoamine oxidase inhibitors (MAOIs).

Phaeochromocytoma.

Thrombocytopenia.

Patients with left ventricular outlet obstruction such as hypertrophic obstructive cardiomyopathy or aortic stenosis. In such patients, positive inotropic activity may increase left ventricular outflow obstruction and sudden vasodilatation may cause hypotension.

4.4 Special warnings and precautions for use

Correction of hypovolaemia must be achieved prior to administration of Dopacard. Hypovolaemia should also be corrected during therapy as vasodilatation occurs due to treatment.

Care should be exercised so as to restrict the sodium and fluid load during administration of Dopacard.

Dopacard should not be administered to patients with severe hypotension or a markedly reduced systemic vascular resistance until specific resuscitative measures have been taken to restore blood pressure to a clinically acceptable level.

In patients with a marked reduction in systemic vascular resistance, Dopacard should not be used as a direct substitute for pressor agents or other inotropes.

As with other catecholamines, Dopacard should be administered with caution to patients with a clinical history of ischaemic heart disease especially following acute myocardial infarction or recent episodes of angina pectoris as a tachycardia may increase myocardial oxygen demand and further exacerbate myocardial ischaemia.

As has been observed with other β_2-adrenergic agonists, a small reversible fall in circulating platelet numbers has been observed in some patients. No adverse effects attributable to alterations in platelet count have been seen in clinical studies.

Care must be exercised when administering Dopacard in the presence of hypokalaemia or hyperglycaemia. In common with other β_2-agonists, Dopacard depresses plasma potassium and raises plasma glucose. These effects are minor and reversible.

Monitoring of potassium and glucose is advisable in patients likely to be at risk from such changes, e.g. diabetics, patients with myocardial infarction or patients being treated with diuretics or cardiac glycosides.

Benign arrhythmias such as ventricular premature beats and, more rarely, serious arrhythmias have been reported in some patients. If excessive tachycardia occurs during Dopacard administration, then a reduction or temporary discontinuation of the infusion should be considered.

As with other parenteral catecholamines, there have been occasional reports of partial tolerance, with some attenuation of the haemodynamic response developing during long-term infusions of Dopacard.

The risk of thrombophlebitis and local necrosis may be increased if the concentration of Dopacard administered via a peripheral vein exceeds 1 mg/ml. Thrombophlebitis is rare when the concentration of drug used for peripheral administration is less than 1 mg/ml.

4.5 Interaction with other medicinal products and other forms of interaction

As Dopacard inhibits the Uptake-1 mechanism, it may potentiate the effects of exogenous catecholamines such as noradrenaline. Caution is recommended when these agents are administered concomitantly with Dopacard or soon after its discontinuation.

There is no evidence of an interaction with dopamine, other than possible attenuation of the indirect sympathomimetic inotropic effects of higher doses of dopamine due to Uptake-1 blockade by Dopacard.

Concomitant use with β_2-adrenergic and dopamine receptor antagonists requires caution since possible attenuation of the pharmacological effects of Dopacard may occur.

4.6 Pregnancy and lactation
There is no experience of the use of Dopacard in pregnant or lactating women and therefore its safety in these situations has not been established. There is insufficient evidence from animal studies to indicate it is free from hazard. Dopacard is not therefore currently recommended for use in pregnant or lactating women.

4.7 Effects on ability to drive and use machines
Not applicable.

4.8 Undesirable effects
The most common undesirable effect reported with Dopacard administration in studies of use in heart failure is tachycardia (11.8% in studies of exacerbations of chronic heart failure; 19.4% in studies of use in cardiac surgery). The increases in heart rate are dose-related and, in most cases, not clinically significant.

Hypertension and transient hypotension have been reported after cardiac surgery (at an incidence of 8.8% and 7.0% respectively). These events, however, are not uncommon as compensatory mechanisms following cardiac surgery. Transient hypotension was reported in studies of exacerbations of chronic heart failure at an incidence of 6.3%.

Other undesirable effects reported in clinical trials in both exacerbations of chronic heart failure and cardiac surgery at an incidence of 1% or more include:

Cardiovascular: A number of tachyarrhythmias such as premature ventricular contractions (PVCs) and atrial fibrillation, bradycardia, both sinus and nodal, worsening heart failure leading to asystole and cardiac arrest, angina, myocardial infarction, cardiac enzyme changes and non-specific ECG changes have occurred.

Non-cardiovascular: Nausea and vomiting, tremor, headache, diaphoresis and dyspnoea.

Careful titration of the dose may minimise the incidence of adverse events.

More rarely a number of serious adverse events have been reported in patients undergoing cardiac surgery: renal failure, respiratory failure, acute respiratory distress syndrome (ARDS), pulmonary oedema, pulmonary hypertension, bleeding and septicaemia. However, such events may also be due to the condition of the patients in such populations.

4.9 Overdose
The half-life of Dopacard in blood is short. Consequently, the effects of overdosage are likely to be short-lived provided that administration is discontinued. However, in some cases, it may be necessary to initiate prompt supportive measures.

Effects of overdosage are likely to be related to the pharmacological actions and include tachycardia, tremulousness and tremor, nausea and vomiting, and anginal pain. Treatment should be supportive and directed to these symptoms.

5. PHARMACOLOGICAL PROPERTIES

5.1 Pharmacodynamic properties
The primary actions of Dopacard (dopexamine hydrochloride) are the stimulation of adrenergic $\beta 2$-receptors and peripheral dopamine receptors of DA_1 and DA_2 subtypes. In addition, Dopacard is an inhibitor of neuronal re-uptake of noradrenaline (Uptake-1). These pharmacological actions result in an increase in cardiac output mediated by afterload reduction (β_2, DA_1) and mild positive inotropism (β_2, Uptake-1 inhibition) together with an increase in blood flow to vascular beds (DA_1) such as the renal and mesenteric beds. Dopacard therefore provides an increase in systemic and regional oxygen delivery. Dopacard is not an α-adrenergic agonist and does not cause vasoconstriction and is not a pressor agent.

5.2 Pharmacokinetic properties
Dopacard is rapidly eliminated from blood with a half-life of approximately 6-7 minutes in healthy volunteers and around 11 minutes in patients with cardiac failure. Subsequent elimination of the metabolites is by urinary and biliary excretion. The response to Dopacard is rapid in onset and effects subside rapidly on discontinuation of the infusion.

5.3 Preclinical safety data
There is no information relevant to the prescriber, which has not been included in other sections of this Summary of Product Characteristics.

6. PHARMACEUTICAL PARTICULARS

6.1 List of excipients
Disodium edetate, Hydrochloric acid, Water for Injections.

6.2 Incompatibilities
Dopacard should only be diluted with 0.9% Sodium Chloride Injection, 5% Dextrose Injection, Hartmann's Solution (Compound Sodium Lactate Intravenous Infusion) or Dextrose 4%/Saline 0.18% Injection, and should not be added to sodium bicarbonate or any other strongly alkaline solutions as inactivation will occur.

Dopacard should not be mixed with any other drugs before administration.

Contact with metal parts, in infusion apparatus for example, should be minimised.

6.3 Shelf life
The shelf life of unopened ampoules is 3 years.

Prepared intravenous solutions in 0.9% Sodium Chloride Injection or 5% Dextrose Injection are stable for 24 hours at room temperature.

6.4 Special precautions for storage
Do not store above 25°C, protect from light.

6.5 Nature and contents of container
Box of 10 clear glass ampoules each containing 5ml of 1% (w/v) solution of dopexamine hydrochloride (50mg per ampoule).

6.6 Special precautions for disposal and other handling
The contents of four ampoules (20ml) should be injected aseptically into one of the following:

0.9%	Sodium Chloride Injection	500 or 250 ml
5%	Dextrose Injection	500 or 250 ml

These dilutions give a concentration for administration as follows:-

4 ampoules of Dopacard diluted to 500ml = 400 micrograms/ml

4 ampoules of Dopacard diluted to 250ml = 800 micrograms/ml

Dopacard, in common with other catecholamines, may turn slightly pink in prepared solutions. There is no significant loss of potency associated with this change.

Administrative Data

7. MARKETING AUTHORISATION HOLDER
Cephalon Limited
1 Albany Place
Hyde Way
Welwyn Garden City
Hertfordshire
AL7 3BT

8. MARKETING AUTHORISATION NUMBER(S)
PL 21799/0009

9. DATE OF FIRST AUTHORISATION/RENEWAL OF THE AUTHORISATION
1 October 2005

10. DATE OF REVISION OF THE TEXT
October 2007

11. LEGAL CATEGORY
POM

Doribax 500mg powder for solution for infusion

(Janssen-Cilag Ltd)

1. NAME OF THE MEDICINAL PRODUCT
Doribax ▼ 500mg powder for solution for infusion

2. QUALITATIVE AND QUANTITATIVE COMPOSITION
Each vial contains doripenem monohydrate equivalent to 500mg doripenem.

The medicinal product does not contain any excipients.

3. PHARMACEUTICAL FORM
Powder for solution for infusion (Powder for infusion)

A white to slightly yellowish off-white crystalline powder

4. CLINICAL PARTICULARS

4.1 Therapeutic indications
Doribax is indicated for the treatment of the following infections in adults (see sections 4.4 and 5.1):

- Nosocomial pneumonia (including ventilator–associated pneumonia)
- Complicated intra-abdominal infections
- Complicated urinary tract infections

Consideration should be given to official guidance on the appropriate use of antibacterial agents.

4.2 Posology and method of administration
The recommended dosage and administration by infection is shown in the following table:

(see Table 1 below)

The usual treatment duration of doripenem therapy is 5-14 days and should be guided by the severity, site of the infection and the patient's clinical response. Doripenem was given for up to 14 days in clinical studies and the safety of longer durations of therapy has not been established. After commencing treatment with intravenous doripenem, a switch to appropriate oral therapy to complete the treatment course is possible once clinical improvement has been established.

Dosage in paediatric patients

Doribax is not recommended for use in children below 18 years of age due to a lack of safety and efficacy data.

Dosage in patients with impaired renal function

In patients with mild renal impairment (i.e. creatinine clearance (CrCl) is 51-79 ml/min), no dosage adjustment is necessary. In patients with moderate renal impairment (CrCl 30 to < 50 ml/min), the dosage of Doribax should be 250mg every 8 hours. In patients with severe renal impairment (CrCl < 30ml/min), the dosage of Doribax should be 250mg every 12 hours. Due to limited clinical data and an expected increased exposure of doripenem and its metabolite, Doribax should be used with caution in patients with severe renal impairment (see section 5.2).

Dosage in patients on dialysis

Doribax is haemodialysable; however, there is insufficient information to make dose adjustment recommendations in patients on dialysis. Therefore, Doribax is not recommended for patients on any type of dialysis (see section 5.2).

Dosage in elderly patients (⩾ 65 years of age)

No dosage adjustment is necessary in elderly patients, except in cases of moderate to severe renal insufficiency (see *Dosage in patients with impaired renal function* above and section 5.2).

Dosage in patients with impaired hepatic function

No dosage adjustment is necessary.

Method for administration

Doribax is to be reconstituted and then further diluted (see section 6.6) prior to administration by intravenous infusion over a period of one or four hours.

4.3 Contraindications

- Hypersensitivity to the active substance
- Hypersensitivity to any other carbapenem antibacterial agent
- Severe hypersensitivity (e.g. anaphylactic reaction, severe skin reaction) to any other type of beta-lactam antibacterial agent (e.g. penicillins or cephalosporins).

4.4 Special warnings and precautions for use
Serious and occasionally fatal hypersensitivity (anaphylactic) reactions have occurred in patients receiving beta-lactam antibiotics. Before therapy with Doribax is started, careful inquiry should be made concerning a previous history of hypersensitivity reactions to other active substances in this class or to beta-lactam antibiotics. Doribax should be used with caution in patients with such a history. Should a hypersensitivity reaction to Doribax occur, it should be discontinued immediately and appropriate measures taken. Serious acute hypersensitivity (anaphylactic) reactions require immediate emergency treatment.

Seizures have infrequently been reported during treatment with other carbapenems.

Pseudomembranous colitis due to *Clostridium difficile* has been reported with Doribax as with nearly all anti-bacterial agents and may range in severity from mild to life-threatening. Therefore, it is important to consider this diagnosis in patients who present with diarrhoea during or subsequent to the administration of Doribax (see section 4.8).

Administration of doripenem, like other antibiotics, has been associated with emergence and selection of strains with reduced susceptibility. Patients should be carefully monitored during therapy. If superinfection occurs, appropriate measures should be taken. Prolonged use of Doribax should be avoided.

The concomitant use of doripenem and valproic acid/sodium valproate is not recommended (see section 4.5).

Table 1

Infection	Dosage	Frequency	Infusion Time
Nosocomial pneumonia including ventilator–associated pneumonia	500mg	every 8 hours	1 or 4 hours*
Complicated intra-abdominal infection	500mg	every 8 hours	1 hour
Complicated UTI, including pyelonephritis	500mg	every 8 hours	1 hour

*Based mainly on PK/PD considerations, a 4-hour infusion time may be more suitable for infection with less susceptible pathogens (see section 5.1). This dosing regimen should also be considered in particularly severe infections.

For infusion solution shelf life see section 6.3.

When Doribax was used investigationally *via* inhalation, pneumonitis occurred. Therefore, Doribax should not be administered by this route.

Description of the patient population treated in clinical studies

In two clinical trials of patients with nosocomial pneumonia (N=979), 60% of the clinically-evaluable Doribax-treated patients had ventilator-associated pneumonia (VAP). Of these, 50% had late-onset VAP (defined as that occurring after five days of mechanical ventilation), 54% had an APACHE (Acute Physiology And Chronic Health Evaluation) II score >15 and 32% received concomitant aminoglycosides (76% for more than 3 days).

In two clinical trials of patients with complicated intra-abdominal infections (N=962) the most common anatomical site of infection in microbiologically-evaluable Doribax-treated patients was the appendix (62%). Of these, 51% had generalised peritonitis at baseline. Other sources of infection included colon perforation (20%), complicated cholecystitis (5%) and infections at other sites (14%). Eleven percent had an APACHE II score of >10, 9.5% had post-operative infections, 27% had single or multiple intra-abdominal abscesses and 4% had concurrent bacteraemia at baseline.

In two clinical trials of patients with complicated urinary tract infections (N=1179), 52% of microbiologically-evaluable Doribax-treated patients had complicated lower urinary tract infections and 48% had pyelonephritis, of which 16% were complicated. Overall, 54% of patients had a persistent complication, 9% had concurrent bacteraemia and 23% were infected with a levofloxacin resistant uropathogen at baseline.

The experience in patients who are severely immunocompromised, receiving immunosuppressive therapy, and patients with severe neutropenia is limited since this population was excluded from phase 3 trials.

4.5 Interaction with other medicinal products and other forms of interaction

Doripenem undergoes little to no Cytochrome P450 (CYP450) mediated metabolism. Based on *in vitro* studies it is not expected that doripenem will inhibit or induce the activities of CYP450. Therefore, no CYP450-related drug interactions are to be expected (see section 5.2).

It has been shown that co-administration of doripenem and valproic acid significantly reduces serum valproic acid levels below the therapeutic range. The lowered valproic acid levels can lead to inadequate seizure control. In an interaction study, the serum concentrations of valproic acid were markedly reduced (AUC was reduced by 63%) following co-administration of doripenem and valproic acid. The interaction had a fast onset. Since patients were administered only four doses of doripenem, a further decrease of valproic acid levels with longer concomitant administration cannot be excluded.

Decreases in valproic acid levels have also been reported when co-administered with other carbapenem agents, achieving a 60 -100 % decrease in valproic acid levels in about two days. Therefore alternative antibacterial or supplemental anticonvulsant therapies should be considered.

Probenecid competes with doripenem for renal tubular secretion and reduces the renal clearance of doripenem. In an interaction study, the mean doripenem AUC increased by 75% following co-administration with probenecid. Therefore, co-administration of probenecid with Doribax is not recommended. An interaction with other drugs eliminated by renal tubular secretion cannot be excluded.

4.6 Pregnancy and lactation

For doripenem, limited clinical data on exposed pregnancies are available. Animal studies are insufficient with respect to pregnancy, embryonal/foetal development, parturition or postnatal development (see section 5.3). The potential risk for humans is unknown. Doribax should not be used during pregnancy unless clearly necessary.

It is unknown whether doripenem is excreted in human breast milk. A study in rats has shown that doripenem and its metabolite are transferred to milk. A decision on whether to continue/discontinue breast-feeding or to continue/discontinue therapy with Doribax should be made taking into account the benefit of breast-feeding to the child and the benefit of Doribax therapy to the woman.

4.7 Effects on ability to drive and use machines

No studies on the effects of Doribax on the ability to drive and use machines have been performed. Based on reported adverse drug reactions, it is not anticipated that Doribax will affect the ability to drive and use machines.

4.8 Undesirable effects

In 3,142 adult patients (1817 of which received Doribax) evaluated for safety in phase 2 and phase 3 clinical trials, adverse reactions due to Doribax 500 mg every 8 hours occurred at a rate of 32%. Doribax was discontinued because of adverse drug reactions in 0.1% of patients overall. Adverse drug reactions that led to Doribax discontinuation were nausea (0.1%), diarrhoea (0.1%), pruritus (0.1%), vulvomycotic infection (0.1%), hepatic enzyme increased (0.2 %) and rash (0.2%). The most common adverse reactions were headache (10%), diarrhoea (9%) and nausea (8%).

Adverse drug reactions due to Doribax 500mg are listed below by frequency category. Frequency categories are defined as follows: Very common (≥ 1/10); Common (≥1/100 to <1/10); Uncommon (≥1/1,000 to <1/100).

Within each frequency grouping, undesirable effects are presented in order of decreasing seriousness.

Adverse Drug Reactions Identified During Clinical Trials with Doribax	
Infections and infestation	Common: oral candidiasis, vulvomycotic infection
Immune system disorders	Uncommon: hypersensitivity reactions (see section 4.4)
Nervous system disorders	Very common: headache
Vascular disorders	Common: phlebitis
Gastrointestinal disorders	Common: nausea, diarrhoea Uncommon: *C. difficile* colitis (see section 4.4)
Hepato-biliary disorders	Common: hepatic enzyme increased
Skin and subcutaneous tissue disorders	Common: pruritus, rash
Adverse Drug Reactions Identified During Post-marketing Experience with Doribax	
Blood and the lymphatic system disorders	Frequency not known: neutropenia
Immune system disorders	Frequency not known: anaphylaxis (see section 4.4)

4.9 Overdose

No case of overdose has been reported. In the event of overdose, Doribax should be discontinued and general supportive treatment given until renal elimination takes place. Doribax can be removed by haemodialysis (see section 5.2); however, no information is available on the use of haemodialysis to treat overdose.

5. PHARMACOLOGICAL PROPERTIES

5.1 Pharmacodynamic properties

Pharmacotherapeutic group: Carbapenems, ATC code: J01DH04.

Mode of action

Doripenem is a synthetic carbapenem antibacterial agent.

Doripenem exerts its bactericidal activity by inhibiting bacterial cell wall biosynthesis. Doripenem inactivates multiple essential penicillin-binding proteins (PBPs) resulting in inhibition of cell wall synthesis with subsequent cell death.

In vitro doripenem showed little potential to antagonise or be antagonised by other antibacterial agents. Additive activity or weak synergy with amikacin and levofloxacin has been seen for *Pseudomonas aeruginosa* and for gram-positive bacteria with daptomycin, linezolid, levofloxacin, and vancomycin.

Pharmacokinetic/pharmacodynamic relationship

Similar to other beta-lactam antimicrobial agents, the time that the plasma concentration of doripenem exceeds the minimum inhibitory concentration (%T>MIC) of the infecting organism has been shown to best correlate with efficacy in pre-clinical pharmacokinetic/pharmacodynamic (PK/PD) studies. Monte Carlo simulations using pathogen susceptibility results from completed phase 3 trials and population PK data indicated that the %T>MIC target of 35% was achieved in greater than 90% of patients with nosocomial pneumonia, complicated urinary tract infections and complicated intra-abdominal infections, for all degrees of renal function.

Extending the infusion time of Doribax to 4 hours maximises the %T>MIC for a given dose and is the basis for the option to administer 4-hour infusions in patients with nosocomial pneumonia including ventilator-associated pneumonia. In seriously ill patients or those with an impaired immune response, a 4-hour infusion time may be more suitable when the MIC of doripenem for the known or suspected pathogen(s) has been shown or is expected to be >0.5mg/l, in order to reach a target attainment of 50% T>MIC in at least 95% of the patients (see section 4.2). Monte Carlo simulations supported the use of 500mg 4-hour infusions every 8 hours in subjects with normal renal function for target pathogens with doripenem MICs ≤4mg/l.

Mechanisms of resistance

Bacterial resistance mechanisms that effect doripenem include active substance inactivation by carbapenem-hydrolysing enzymes, mutant or acquired PBP's, decreased outer membrane permeability and active efflux. Doripenem is stable to hydrolysis by most beta-lactamases, including penicillinases and cephalosporinases produced by gram-positive and gram-negative bacteria, with the exception of relatively rare carbapenem hydrolysing beta-lactamases. Species resistant to other carbapenems do generally express co-resistance to doripenem. Methicillin-resistant staphylococci should always be considered as resistant to doripenem. As with other antimicrobial agents, including carbapenems, doripenem has been shown to select for resistant bacterial strains.

Breakpoints

Minimum inhibitory concentration (MIC) breakpoints established by the European Committee on Antimicrobial Susceptibility Testing (EUCAST) are as follows:

Non species related	S ≤1mg/l and R>4mg/l
Staphylococci	inferred from the methicillin breakpoint
Enterobacteriaceae	S ≤1mg/l and R>4mg/l
Acinetobacter spp.	S ≤1mg/l and R>4mg/l
Pseudomonas spp.	S ≤1mg/l and R>4mg/l
Streptococcus spp. other than *S. pneumoniae*	S ≤1mg/l and R>1mg/l
S. pneumoniae	S ≤ 1mg/l and R>1mg/l
Enterococci	"inappropriate target"
Haemophilus spp.	S ≤ 1mg/l and R>1mg/l
N. gonorrhoeae	IE (insufficient evidence)
Anaerobes	S ≤1mg/l and R>1mg/l

Susceptibility

The prevalence of acquired resistance may vary geographically and with time for selected species and local information on resistance is desirable, particularly when treating severe infections. As necessary, expert advice should be sought when the local prevalence of resistance is such that the utility of the agent in at least some types of infections is questionable.

Localised clusters of infections due to carbapenem-resistant organisms have been reported in the European Union. The information below gives only approximate guidance on the probability as to whether the micro-organism will be susceptible to doripenem or not.

Commonly Susceptible Species:

Gram Positive Aerobes

*Enterococcus faecalis**$

Staphylococcus aureus (methicillin susceptible strains only)*^

Staphylococcus spp. (methicillin susceptible strains only)^

*Streptococcus pneumoniae**

Streptococcus spp.

Gram Negative Aerobes

Citrobacter diversus

Citrobacter freundii

Enterobacter aerogenes

*Enterobacter cloacae**

*Haemophilus influenzae**

*Escherichia coli**

*Klebsiella pneumoniae**

Klebsiella oxytoca

Morganella morganii

*Proteus mirabilis**

Proteus vulgaris

Providencia rettgeri

Providencia stuartii

Salmonella species

Serratia marcescens

Shigella species

Anaerobes

*Bacteroides fragilis**

*Bacteroides caccae**

Bacteroides ovatus

*Bacteroides uniformis**

*Bacteroides thetaiotaomicron**

*Bacteroides vulgatus**

Bilophila wadsworthia

Peptostreptococcus magnus

*Peptostreptococcus micros**

Porphyromonas spp.

Prevotella spp.

Sutterella wadsworthenis

Species for which acquired resistance may be a problem:

*Acinetobacter baumannii**

Acinetobacter spp.

Burkholderia cepacia$+

*Pseudomonas aeruginosa**

Inherently resistant organisms:

Gram Positive Aerobes

Enterococcus faecium

Gram Negative Aerobes

Stenotrophomonas maltophilia

Legionella spp.

*species against which activity has been demonstrated in clinical studies

$species that show natural intermediate susceptibility

+species with >50% acquired resistance in one or more Member State

^all methicillin-resistant staphylococci should be regarded as resistant to doripenem

5.2 Pharmacokinetic properties

The mean C_{max} and $AUC_{0-\infty}$ of doripenem in healthy subjects across studies following administration of 500mg over 1 hour are approximately 23 μg/ml and 36 μg.h/ml, respectively. The mean C_{max} and $AUC_{-\infty}$ of doripenem in healthy subjects across studies following administration of 500mg and 1g over 4 hours are approximately 8 μg/ml and 17 μg/ml, and 34 μg.h/ml and 68 μg.h/ml, respectively. There is no accumulation of doripenem following multiple intravenous infusions of either 500mg or 1g administered every 8 hours for 7 to 10 days in patients with normal renal function.

Distribution

The average binding of doripenem to plasma proteins was approximately 8.1% and is independent of plasma concentrations. The volume of distribution at steady state is approximately 16.8L, similar to extracellular fluid volume in man. Doripenem penetrates well into several body fluids and tissues, such as uterine tissue, retroperitoneal fluid, prostatic tissue, gallbladder tissue and urine.

Metabolism

Metabolism of doripenem to a microbiologically inactive ring-opened metabolite occurs primarily via dehydropeptidase-I. Doripenem undergoes little to no Cytochrome P450 (CYP450) mediated metabolism. *In vitro* studies have determined that doripenem does not inhibit or induce the activities of CYP isoforms 1A2, 2A6, 2C9, 2C19, 2D6, 2E1 or 3A4.

Elimination

Doripenem is primarily eliminated unchanged by the kidneys. Mean plasma terminal elimination half-life of doripenem in healthy young adults is approximately 1-hour and plasma clearance is approximately 15.9 l/hour. Mean renal clearance is 10.3 l/hour. The magnitude of this value, coupled with the significant decrease in the elimination of doripenem seen with concomitant probenecid administration, suggests that doripenem undergoes glomerular filtration, tubular secretion and re-absorption. In healthy young adults given a single 500mg dose of Doribax, 71% and 15% of the dose was recovered in urine as unchanged active substance and ring-opened metabolite, respectively. Following the administration of a single 500mg dose of radiolabeled doripenem to healthy young adults, less than 1% of the total radioactivity was recovered in faeces. The pharmacokinetics of doripenem are linear over a dose range of 500mg to 1g when intravenously infused over either 1 or 4 hours.

Renal insufficiency

Following a single 500mg dose of Doribax, doripenem AUC increased 1.6-fold, 2.8-fold, and 5.1-fold in subjects with mild (CrCl 51-79 ml/min), moderate (CrCl 31-50 ml/min), and severe renal impairment (CrCl ≤ 30 ml/min), respectively, compared to age-matched healthy subjects with normal renal function (CrCl> 80 ml/min). AUC of the microbiologically inactive ring-opened metabolite is expected to be considerably increased in patients with severe renal impairment compared with healthy subjects. Dosage adjustment is necessary in patients with moderate and severe renal impairment (see section 4.2).

AUCs of doripenem and of the microbiologically inactive ring-opened metabolite are substantially increased in patients who require haemodialysis compared with healthy subjects. In a study where six subjects with end stage renal disease on haemodialysis received a single dose of 500mg doripenem by i.v. infusion, the amount of doripenem removed during the four-hour haemodialysis session was 231mg (46% of the dose).

Hepatic impairment

The pharmacokinetics of doripenem in patients with hepatic impairment have not been established. As doripenem does not appear to undergo hepatic metabolism, the pharmacokinetics of Doribax are not expected to be affected by hepatic impairment.

Elderly

The impact of age on the pharmacokinetics of doripenem was evaluated in healthy elderly male and female subjects (66-84 years of age). Doripenem AUC increased 49% in elderly adults relative to young adults. These changes were mainly attributed to age-related changes in renal function. No dosage adjustment is necessary in elderly patients, except in cases of moderate to severe renal insufficiency (see section 4.2).

Gender

The effect of gender on the pharmacokinetics of doripenem was evaluated in healthy male and female subjects. Doripenem AUC was 15% higher in females compared to males. No dose adjustment is recommended based on gender.

Race

The effect of race on doripenem pharmacokinetics was examined through a population pharmacokinetic analysis. No significant difference in mean doripenem clearance was observed across race groups and therefore, no dosage adjustment is recommended for race.

5.3 Preclinical safety data

Non-clinical data reveal no special hazard for humans based on conventional studies of safety pharmacology and genotoxicity. However, because of the design of the repeat dose toxicity studies and differences in pharmacokinetics in animals and humans, continuous exposure of animals was not assured in these studies.

No reproductive toxicity was observed in studies performed in rats and rabbits. However, these studies are of limited relevance because studies were performed with single daily dosing resulting in less than one tenth of daily doripenem exposure duration in animals.

6. PHARMACEUTICAL PARTICULARS

6.1 List of excipients

None

6.2 Incompatibilities

This medicinal product must not be mixed with other medicinal products except those mentioned in section 6.3.

6.3 Shelf life

3 years.

Storage of reconstituted solutions: Upon reconstitution with sterile water for injections or sodium chloride 9 mg/ml (0.9%) solution for injection, Doribax suspension in the vial may be held for up to 1 hour below 30°C prior to transfer and dilution in the infusion bag.

Following dilution in the infusion bag with sodium chloride 9 mg/ml (0.9%) solution for injection or dextrose 50 mg/ml (5%) solution for injection, Doribax infusions stored at controlled room temperature or under refrigeration should be completed according to the times in the following table:

Time by which reconstitution, dilution and infusion must complete for Doribax infusion solutions

Infusion solution	Solution stored at room temperature	Solution stored in a refrigerator (2°C-8°C)
sodium chloride 9 mg/ml (0.9%) solution for injection	12 hours	72 hours*
+dextrose 50 mg/ml (5%) solution for injection	4 hours	24 hours*

* Once removed from the refrigerator, infusions should be completed within the room temperature stability time, provided the total refrigeration time, time to reach room temperature and infusion time does not exceed refrigeration stability time.

+ Dextrose 50 mg/ml (5%) solution for injection should not be used for infusion durations greater than 1 hour.

Chemical and physical in-use stability has been demonstrated for the times and solutions shown in the above table.

From a microbiological point of view, the product should be used immediately. If not used immediately, in-use storage times and conditions prior to use are the responsibility of the user and would normally not be longer than 24 hours at 2°C-8°C, unless reconstitution/dilution has taken place in controlled and validated aseptic conditions.

6.4 Special precautions for storage

This medicinal product does not require any special storage conditions.

For storage conditions of the reconstituted medicinal product, and infusion solutions see section 6.3.

6.5 Nature and contents of container

Clear 20 ml Type I glass vial.

The medicinal product is supplied in cartons containing 10 vials.

6.6 Special precautions for disposal and other handling

Each vial is for single use only.

Doribax is reconstituted and then further diluted prior to infusion.

Preparation of 500 mg dose of solution for infusion

1. Add 10 ml of sterile water for injections or sodium chloride 9 mg/ml (0.9%) solution for injection to the vial and shake it to form a suspension.

2. Inspect the suspension visually for foreign matter. Note: the suspension is not for direct infusion.

3. Withdraw the suspension using a syringe and needle and add it to an infusion bag containing 100 ml of either sodium chloride 9 mg/ml (0.9%) solution for injection or dextrose 50 mg/ml (5%) solution for injection and mix to complete dissolution. Infuse all of this solution to administer a 500 mg dose of doripenem.

Preparation of 250 mg dose of solution for infusion for patients with moderate or severe renal impairment

1. Add 10ml of sterile water for injections or sodium chloride 9 mg/ml (0.9%) solution for injection to the vial and shake it to form a suspension.

2. Inspect the suspension visually for foreign matter. Note: the suspension is not for direct infusion.

3. Withdraw the suspension using a syringe and needle and add it to an infusion bag containing 100ml either sodium chloride 9 mg/ml (0.9%) solution for injection or dextrose 50 mg/ml (5%) solution for injection and mix to complete dissolution. Remove 55ml of this solution from the infusion bag and discard. Infuse all of the remaining solution to administer a 250 mg dose of doripenem.

Doribax solutions for infusion range from clear, colourless solutions to solutions that are clear and slightly yellow. Variations in colour within this range do not affect the potency of the product.

Any unused product or waste material should be disposed of in accordance with local requirements.

7. MARKETING AUTHORISATION HOLDER

Janssen-Cilag International NV

Turnhoutseweg, 30

B-2340 Beerse

Belgium

8. MARKETING AUTHORISATION NUMBER(S)

EU/1/08/467/001

9. DATE OF FIRST AUTHORISATION/RENEWAL OF THE AUTHORISATION

Date of first authorisation: 25th July 2008

10. DATE OF REVISION OF THE TEXT

08/2009

Detailed information on this medicinal product is available on the website of the European Medicines Agency (EMEA) http://www.emea.europa.eu /.

Dostinex Tablets

(Pharmacia Limited)

1. NAME OF THE MEDICINAL PRODUCT

DOSTINEX

2. QUALITATIVE AND QUANTITATIVE COMPOSITION

One DOSTINEX tablet contains 0.5 mg cabergoline.

For excipients see Section 6.1 ('List of Excipients').

3. PHARMACEUTICAL FORM

Tablet.

Flat, capsule-shaped, 4 × 8 mm, scored, white tablets.

4. CLINICAL PARTICULARS

4.1 Therapeutic indications

Inhibition/suppression of physiological lactation

DOSTINEX is indicated for the inhibition of physiological lactation soon after delivery and for suppression of already established lactation:

1. After parturition, when the mother elects not to breast feed the infant or when breast feeding is contraindicated due to medical reasons related to the mother or the newborn.

2. After stillbirth or abortion.

DOSTINEX prevents/suppresses physiological lactation by inhibiting prolactin secretion.

In controlled clinical trials, DOSTINEX given as a single 1 mg administration during the first day post-partum, was effective in inhibiting milk secretion, as well as breast engorgement and pain in 70 - 90% of the women. Less than 5% of women experienced rebound breast symptomatology during the third post-partum week (which was usually mild in severity).

Suppression of milk secretion and relief of breast engorgement and pain are obtained in approximately 85% of nursing women treated with a total dose of 1 mg DOSTINEX given in four divided doses over two days. Rebound breast symptomatology after day 10 is uncommon (approximately 2% of cases).

Treatment of hyperprolactinaemic disorders

DOSTINEX is indicated for the treatment of dysfunctions associated with hyperprolactinaemia, including amenorrhoea, oligomenorrhoea, anovulation and galactorrhoea. DOSTINEX is indicated in patients with prolactin-secreting pituitary adenomas (micro- and macroprolactinomas), idiopathic hyperprolactinaemia, or empty sella syndrome with associated hyperprolactinaemia, which represent the basic underlying pathologies contributing to the above clinical manifestations.

On chronic therapy, DOSTINEX at doses ranging between 1 and 2 mg per week, was effective in normalising serum prolactin levels in approximately 84% of hyperprolactinaemic patients. Regular cycles were resumed in 83% of previously amenorrhoeic women. Restoration of ovulation was documented in 89% of women with progesterone levels monitored during the luteal phase. Galactorrhoea disappeared in 90% of cases showing this symptom before therapy. Reduction in tumour size was obtained in 50 - 90% of female and male patients with micro- or macroprolactinoma.

4.2 Posology and method of administration

DOSTINEX is to be administered by the oral route. Since in clinical studies DOSTINEX has been mainly administered with food and since the tolerability of this class of compounds is improved with food, it is recommended that DOSTINEX be preferably taken with meals for all the therapeutic indications.

Inhibition/suppression of physiological lactation

For inhibition of lactation DOSTINEX should be administered during the first day post-partum. The recommended therapeutic dose is 1 mg (two 0.5 mg tablets) given as a single dose.

For suppression of established lactation the recommended therapeutic dosage regimen is 0.25 mg (one-half 0.5 mg tablet) every 12 hours for two days (1 mg total dose). This dosage regimen has been demonstrated to be better tolerated than the single dose regimen in women electing to suppress lactation having a lower incidence of adverse events, in particular of hypotensive symptoms.

Treatment of hyperprolactinaemic disorders

The recommended initial dosage of DOSTINEX is 0.5 mg per week given in one or two (one-half of one 0.5 mg tablet) doses (e.g. on Monday and Thursday) per week. The weekly dose should be increased gradually, preferably by adding 0.5 mg per week at monthly intervals until an optimal therapeutic response is achieved. The therapeutic dosage is usually 1 mg per week and ranges from 0.25 mg to 2 mg per week. Doses of DOSTINEX up to 4.5 mg per week have been used in hyperprolactinaemic patients.

The maximum dose should not exceed 3mg per day.

The weekly dose may be given as a single administration or divided into two or more doses per week according to patient tolerability. Division of the weekly dose into multiple administrations is advised when doses higher than 1 mg per week are to be given since the tolerability of doses greater than 1 mg taken as a single weekly dose has been evaluated only in a few patients.

Patients should be evaluated during dose escalation to determine the lowest dosage that produces the therapeutic response. Monitoring of serum prolactin levels at monthly intervals is advised since, once the effective therapeutic dosage regimen has been reached, serum prolactin normalisation is usually observed within two to four weeks.

After DOSTINEX withdrawal, recurrence of hyperprolactinaemia is usually observed. However, persistent suppression of prolactin levels has been observed for several months in some patients. Of the group of women followed up, 23/29 had ovulatory cycles which continued for greater than 6 months after DOSTINEX discontinuation.

Use in children

The safety and efficacy of DOSTINEX has not been established in subjects less than 16 years of age.

Use in the elderly

As a consequence of the indications for which DOSTINEX is presently proposed, the experience in elderly is very limited. Available data do not indicate a special risk.

4.3 Contraindications

Hypersensitivity to any ergot alkaloid.

DOSTINEX is contraindicated in patients with hepatic insufficiency and with toxaemia of pregnancy. DOSTINEX should not be co-administered with anti-psychotic medications or administered to women with a history of puerperal psychosis.

For long-term treatment: Evidence of cardiac valvulopathy as determined by pre-treatment echocardiography.

4.4 Special warnings and precautions for use

General

The safety and efficacy of DOSTINEX have not yet been established in patients with renal and hepatic disease. DOSTINEX should be given with caution to subjects with cardiovascular disease, Raynaud's syndrome, renal insufficiency, peptic ulcer, gastrointestinal bleeding, or a history of serious, particularly psychotic, mental disease. Particular care should be taken when patients are taking concomitant psychoactive medication.

Symptomatic hypotension can occur with DOSTINEX administration for any indication. Care should be exercised when administering DOSTINEX concomitantly with other drugs known to lower blood pressure.

The effects of alcohol on overall tolerability of DOSTINEX are currently unknown.

Before DOSTINEX administration, pregnancy should be excluded and after treatment pregnancy should be prevented for at least one month.

Cabergoline has been associated with somnolence and episodes of sudden sleep onset, particularly in patients with Parkinson's disease. Sudden onset of sleep during daily activities, in some cases without awareness or warning signs, has been reported uncommonly. Patients must be informed of this and advised to exercise caution while driving or operating machines during treatment with cabergoline. Patients who have experienced somnolence and/or an episode of sudden sleep onset must refrain from driving or operating machines. Furthermore a reduction of dosage or termination of therapy may be considered.

Pathological gambling, increased libido and hypersexuality have been reported in patients treated with dopamine agonists for Parkinson's disease, including cabergoline.

Inhibition/suppression of physiological lactation

By analogy with other ergot alkaloids, DOSTINEX should not be used in women with pre-eclampsia and should be used with caution in patients with post-partum hypertension.

In post-partum studies with DOSTINEX, blood pressure decreases were mostly asymptomatic and were frequently observed on a single occasion 2 to 4 days after treatment. Since decreases in blood pressure are frequently noted during the puerperium, independently of drug therapy, it is likely that many of the observed decreases in blood pressure after DOSTINEX administration were not drug-induced. However, periodic monitoring of blood pressure, particularly during the first few days after DOSTINEX administration, is advised.

DOSTINEX should not be administered as a single dose greater than 0.25 mg in nursing women treated for suppression of established lactation since a clinical study exploring the efficacy and tolerability of 0.5 mg of DOSTINEX given as a single dose for suppression of lactation has shown that the risk of side effects is approximately doubled in this indication if the drug is administered as a single dose of 0.5 mg.

In rats DOSTINEX and/or its metabolites are excreted in milk. Therefore, while no information on the excretion of DOSTINEX in maternal milk in humans is available, puerperal women should be advised not to breast-feed in case of failed lactation inhibition/suppression by DOSTINEX.

Treatment of hyperprolactinaemic disorders

Since hyperprolactinaemia with amenorrhoea/galactorrhoea and infertility may be associated with pituitary tumours, a complete evaluation of the pituitary is indicated before treatment with DOSTINEX is initiated.

DOSTINEX restores ovulation and fertility in women with hyperprolactinaemic hypogonadism: since pregnancy might occur prior to reinitiation of menses, a pregnancy test is recommended at least every four weeks during the amenorrhoeic period and, once menses are reinitiated, every time a menstrual period is delayed by more than three days. Women not seeking pregnancy should be advised to use mechanical contraception during treatment and after DOSTINEX withdrawal until recurrence of anovulation. Before administration of Dostinex, pregnancy should be excluded. Because clinical experience is still limited and the product has a long half-life, as a precautionary measure it is recommended that once regular ovulatory cycles have been achieved women seeking pregnancy discontinue Dostinex one month before intended conception. Should pregnancy occur during treatment, DOSTINEX is to be discontinued. As a precautionary measure, women who become pregnant should be monitored to detect signs of pituitary enlargement since expansion of pre-existing pituitary tumours may occur during gestation.

Regular gynaecological assessment, including cervical and endometrial cytology, is recommended for patients taking DOSTINEX for extensive periods.

Fibrosis/Valvulopathy

Fibrosis and cardiac valvulopathy and possibly related clinical phenomena:

Fibrotic and serosal inflammatory disorders such as pleuritis, pleural effusion, pleural fibrosis, pulmonary fibrosis, pericarditis, pericardial effusion, cardiac valvulopathy involving one or more valves (aortic, mitral and tricuspid) or retroperitoneal fibrosis have occurred after prolonged usage of ergot derivatives with agonist activity at the serotonin $5HT_{2B}$ receptor, such as cabergoline. In some cases, symptoms or manifestations of cardiac valvulopathy improved after discontinuation of cabergoline.

Erythrocyte sedimentation rate (ESR) has been found to be abnormally increased in association with pleural effusion/fibrosis. Chest x-ray examination is recommended in cases of unexplained ESR increases to abnormal values.

Valvulopathy has been associated with cumulative doses, therefore, patients should be treated with the lowest effective dose. At each visit, the risk benefit profile of cabergoline treatment for the patient should be reassessed to determine the suitability of continued treatment with cabergoline.

Before initiating long-term treatment:

All patients must undergo a cardiovascular evaluation, including echocardiogram, to assess the potential presence of asymptomatic valvular disease. It is also appropriate to perform baseline investigations of erythrocyte sedimentation rate or other inflammatory markers, lung function/chest X-ray and renal function prior to initiation of therapy.

In patients with valvular regurgitation, it is not known whether cabergoline treatment might worsen the underlying disease. If fibrotic valvular disease is detected, the patient should not be treated with cabergoline (see section 4.3).

During long-term treatment:

Fibrotic disorders can have an insidious onset and patients should be regularly monitored for possible manifestations of progressive fibrosis.

Therefore, during treatment, attention should be paid to the signs and symptoms of:

- Pleuro-pulmonary disease such as dyspnoea, shortness of breath, persistent cough or chest pain.
- Renal insufficiency or ureteral/abdominal vascular obstruction that may occur with pain in the loin/flank and lower limb oedema as well as any possible abdominal masses or tenderness that may indicate retroperitoneal fibrosis.
- Cardiac failure; cases of valvular and pericardial fibrosis have often manifested as cardiac failure. Therefore, valvular fibrosis (and constrictive pericarditis) should be excluded if such symptoms occur.

Clinical diagnostic monitoring for development of fibrotic disorders, as appropriate, is essential. Following treatment initiation, the first echocardiogram must occur within 3-6 months, thereafter, the frequency of echocardiographic monitoring should be determined by appropriate individual clinical assessment with particular emphasis on the above-mentioned signs and symptoms, but must occur at least every 6 to 12 months.

Cabergoline should be discontinued if an echocardiogram reveals new or worsened valvular regurgitation, valvular restriction or valve leaflet thickening (see section 4.3).

The need for other clinical monitoring (e.g. physical examination including, cardiac auscultation, X-ray, CT scan) should be determined on an individual basis.

Additional appropriate investigations such as erythrocyte sedimentation rate, and serum creatinine measurements should be performed if necessary to support a diagnosis of a fibrotic disorder.

4.5 Interaction with other medicinal products and other forms of interaction

The concomitant use of other drugs during early puerperium, particularly of ergot alkaloids, was not associated with detectable interactions modifying the efficacy and safety of DOSTINEX.

Although there is no conclusive evidence of an interaction between DOSTINEX and other ergot alkaloids the concomitant use of these medications during long term treatment with DOSTINEX is not recommended.

Since DOSTINEX exerts its therapeutic effect by direct stimulation of dopamine receptors, it should not be concurrently administered with drugs which have dopamine antagonist activity (such as phenothiazines, butyrophenones, thioxanthenes, metoclopramide) since these might reduce the prolactin-lowering effect of DOSTINEX.

By analogy with other ergot derivatives, DOSTINEX should not be used in association with macrolide antibiotics (e.g. erythromycin) since the systemic bioavailability and also adverse effects could increase.

4.6 Pregnancy and lactation

Pregnancy

DOSTINEX crossed the placenta in rats: it is unknown whether this occurs in humans. Studies in animal models have not demonstrated any teratogenic effect or effects on overall reproductive performance. However, there are no adequate and well-controlled studies in pregnant women. DOSTINEX should be used during pregnancy only if clearly needed.

In clinical studies there have been over 100 pregnancies in women treated for hyperprolactinaemic disorders. DOSTINEX was generally taken during the first 8 weeks after conception. Among the pregnancies evaluable so far, there were approximately 85% live births and about 10% spontaneous abortions. Three cases of congenital abnormalities (Down's Syndrome, hydrocephalus, malformation of lower limbs) which led to therapeutic abortion and three cases of minor abnormalities in live births were observed. These incidence rates are comparable with those quoted for normal populations and for women exposed to other ovulation-inducing drugs. Based on the above data, the use of DOSTINEX does not appear to be associated with an increased risk of abortion, premature delivery, multiple pregnancy, or congenital abnormalities.

Because clinical experience is still limited and the drug has a long half-life, as a precautionary measure it is recommended that once regular ovulatory cycles have been achieved women seeking pregnancy discontinue DOSTINEX one month before intended conception.

This will prevent possible foetal exposure to the drug and will not interfere with the possibility of conception since ovulatory cycles persist in some cases for six months after drug withdrawal. If conception occurs during therapy, treatment is to be discontinued as soon as pregnancy is confirmed to limit foetal exposure to the drug.

Before DOSTINEX administration, pregnancy should be excluded and after treatment pregnancy should be prevented for at least one month.

Lactation

DOSTINEX should not be administered to mothers who elect to breast-feed their infants since it prevents lactation and no information is available on excretion of the drug in maternal milk.

4.7 Effects on ability to drive and use machines

During the first days of DOSTINEX administration, patients should be cautioned about re-engaging in activities requiring rapid and precise responses such as driving an automobile or operating machinery.

Patients being treated with cabergoline and presenting with somnolence and/or sudden sleep episodes must be informed to refrain from driving or engaging in activities where impaired alertness may put themselves and others at risk of serious injury or death (e.g. operating machines) until such recurrent episodes and somnolence have resolved see also section 4.4 ('Special Warnings and Special Precautions for Use').

4.8 Undesirable effects

Adverse events are generally dose-related. In patients known to be intolerant to dopaminergic drugs, the likelihood of adverse events may be lessened by starting therapy with DOSTINEX at reduced doses, e.g. 0.25mg once a week, with subsequent gradual increase until the therapeutic dosage is reached. If persistent or severe adverse events occur, temporary reduction of dosage followed by a more gradual increase, e.g. increments of 0.25mg/week every two weeks, may increase tolerability.

Inhibition/Suppression of lactation:

Approximately 14% of women treated with a single 1 mg dose of DOSTINEX for inhibition of physiological lactation complained of at least one side effect. All side effects were mild to moderate in severity and of a transient nature.

Hyperprolactinaemic disorders:

Data obtained in a controlled clinical trial of 6 months therapy with doses ranging between 1 and 2 mg per week given in two weekly administrations, indicate a 68% incidence of adverse events during DOSTINEX therapy; this was significantly lower than the incidence observed for the reference standard compound. Moreover, the symptoms were generally mild to moderate in degree, mainly appearing during the first two weeks of therapy, and mostly disappearing despite continued therapy. Severe adverse events were reported at least once during therapy by 14% of patients, but therapy was discontinued because of adverse events in only approximately 3% of patients. DOSTINEX withdrawal results in reversal of side effects, usually within a few days after discontinuation.

Patients treated with dopamine agonists for treatment of Parkinson's disease including cabergoline, especially at high doses, have been reported as exhibiting signs of pathological gambling, increased libido and hypersexuality, generally reversible upon reduction of the dose or treatment discontinuation.

The following undesirable effects have been observed and reported during treatment with Dostinex with the following frequencies: Very common ($\geq$1/10); common ($\geq$1/100 to $<$1/10); uncommon ($\geq$1/1,000 to $<$1/100); rare ($\geq$1/10,000 to $<$1/1,000); very rare ($\leq$1/10,000), not known (cannot be estimated from the available data).

Cardiovascular system disorders:

Very common (>10%): cardiac valvulopathy (including regurgitation) and related disorders (pericarditis and pericardial effusion).

Uncommon: decrease in haemoglobin in amenorrhoeic women after menses resumption. Asymptomatic decreases in blood pressure may occur usually once during the first 3-4 days post-partum.

Rare: cardiovascular regulation (hypotension) in chronic treatment, palpitations, epistaxis.

Central and peripheral nervous system disorders:

Common: headache, dizziness/vertigo, syncope, breast pain.

rare: paraesthesia, digital vasospasm, leg cramps.

Psychiatric disorders:

Very common: somnolence.

uncommon: excessive daytime somnolence and episodes of sudden sleep onset.

Common: depression.

rare: hot flushes.

Vision disorders:

rare: transient hemianopia.

Gastrointestinal disorders:

Very common: nausea.

Common: abdominal pain/dyspepsia/gastritis, constipation.

rare: vomiting.

Skin and appendages disorders:

uncommon: dermal reactions, e.g. alopecia, pruritus, rash.

Musculo-Skeletal system disorders:

rare: muscle weakness/fatigue.

Body as a whole:

rare: allergic skin reactions.

Post-Marketing Surveillance

The following events have been reported in association with cabergoline: alopecia, blood creatinine phosphokinase increased, delusions, dyspnea, oedema, hepatic function abnormal, hypersensitivity reaction, liver function tests abnormal, rash, respiratory disorder and respiratory failure.

Cardiovascular system disorders: Valvulopathy

Respiratory, Thoracic and Mediastinal system disorders: Pleural effusion, pulmonary fibrosis

4.9 Overdose

There is no experience in humans of overdosage with DOSTINEX in the proposed indications: it is likely to lead to symptoms due to overstimulation of dopamine receptors. These might include nausea, vomiting, gastric complaints, hypotension, confusion/psychosis or hallucinations.

General supportive measures should be undertaken to remove any unabsorbed drug and maintain blood pressure if necessary. In addition, the administration of dopamine antagonist drugs may be advisable.

5. PHARMACOLOGICAL PROPERTIES

5.1 Pharmacodynamic properties

DOSTINEX is a dopaminergic ergoline derivative endowed with a potent and long-lasting PRL-lowering activity. It acts by direct stimulation of the D_2-dopamine receptors on pituitary lactotrophs, thus inhibiting PRL secretion. In rats the compound decreases PRL secretion at oral doses of 3-25 mcg/kg, and *in-vitro* at a concentration of 45 pg/ml. In addition, DOSTINEX exerts a central dopaminergic effect via D_2 receptor stimulation at oral doses higher than those effective in lowering serum PRL levels. The long lasting PRL-lowering effect of DOSTINEX is probably due to its long persistence in the target organ as suggested by the slow elimination of total radioactivity from the pituitary after single oral dose in rats ($t_{½}$ of approximately 60 hours).

The pharmacodynamic effects of DOSTINEX have been studied in healthy volunteers, puerperal women and hyperprolactinaemic patients. After a single oral administration of DOSTINEX (0.3 - 1.5 mg), a significant decrease in serum PRL levels was observed in each of the populations studied. The effect is prompt (within 3 hours from administration) and persistent (up to 7 - 28 days in healthy volunteers and hyperprolactinaemic patients, and up to 14 - 21 days in puerperal women). The PRL-lowering effect is dose-related both in terms of degree of effect and duration of action.

With regard to the endocrine effects of DOSTINEX not related to the antiprolactinaemic effect, available data from humans confirm the experimental findings in animals indicating that the test compound is endowed with a very selective action with no effect on basal secretion of other pituitary hormones or cortisol. The pharmacodynamic actions of DOSTINEX not correlated with the therapeutic effect only relate to blood pressure decrease. The maximal hypotensive effect of DOSTINEX as single dose usually occurs during the first 6 hours after drug intake and is dose-dependent both in terms of maximal decrease and frequency.

5.2 Pharmacokinetic properties

The pharmacokinetic and metabolic profiles of DOSTINEX have been studied in healthy volunteers of both sexes and in female hyperprolactinaemic patients.

After oral administration of the labelled compound, radioactivity was rapidly absorbed from the gastrointestinal tract as the peak of radioactivity in plasma was between 0.5 and 4 hours.

Ten days after administration about 18% and 72% of the radioactive dose was recovered in urine and faeces, respectively. Unchanged drug in urine accounted for 2-3% of the dose.

In urine, the main metabolite identified was 6-allyl-8β-carboxy-ergoline, which accounted for 4-6% of the dose. Three additional metabolites were identified in urine, which accounted overall for less than 3% of the dose. The metabolites have been found to be much less potent than DOSTINEX in inhibiting prolactin secretion *in vitro*. DOSTINEX biotransformation was also studied in plasma of healthy male volunteers treated with [^{14}C]-cabergoline: a rapid and extensive biotransformation of cabergoline was shown.

The low urinary excretion of unchanged DOSTINEX has been confirmed also in studies with non-radioactive product. The elimination half-life of DOSTINEX, estimated from urinary excretion rates, is long (63-68 hours in healthy volunteers (using a radio-immuno assay), 79-115 hours in hyperprolactinaemic patients (using a HPLC method).

On the basis of the elimination half-life, steady state conditions should be achieved after 4 weeks, as confirmed by the mean peak plasma levels of DOSTINEX obtained after a single dose (37 ± 8 pg/ml) and after a 4 week multiple regimen (101 ± 43 pg/ml).

In vitro experiments showed that the drug at concentrations of 0.1-10 ng/ml is 41-42% bound to plasma proteins. Food does not appear to affect absorption and disposition of DOSTINEX.

5.3 Preclinical safety data

Almost all the findings noted throughout the series of preclinical safety studies are a consequence of the central dopaminergic effects or the long-lasting inhibition of PRL in species (rodents) with a specific hormonal physiology different to man. Preclinical safety studies of DOSTINEX indicate a large safety margin for this compound in rodents and in monkeys, as well as a lack of teratogenic, mutagenic or carcinogenic potential.

6. PHARMACEUTICAL PARTICULARS

6.1 List of excipients

Lactose

Leucine

6.2 Incompatibilities

Not applicable.

6.3 Shelf life

24 months.

6.4 Special precautions for storage

Do not store above 25°C.

6.5 Nature and contents of container

The tablets are contained in type I amber glass bottles with tamper resistant screw caps and containing silica gel desiccant.

Each bottle contains 2, 4 or 8 tablets and is enclosed in an outer cardboard carton.

6.6 Special precautions for disposal and other handling

Bottles of DOSTINEX are supplied with desiccant in caps. This desiccant must not be removed.

7. MARKETING AUTHORISATION HOLDER

Pharmacia Limited

Ramsgate Road

Sandwich

Kent

CT13 9JN

8. MARKETING AUTHORISATION NUMBER(S)

PL 00032/0372

9. DATE OF FIRST AUTHORISATION/RENEWAL OF THE AUTHORISATION

24 June 2002

10. DATE OF REVISION OF THE TEXT

April 2009

Ref Code: DX7_4 UK

Doublebase Emollient Bath Additive

(Dermal Laboratories Limited)

1. NAME OF THE MEDICINAL PRODUCT

DOUBLEBASE™ EMOLLIENT BATH ADDITIVE

2. QUALITATIVE AND QUANTITATIVE COMPOSITION

Liquid Paraffin 65.0% w/w.

For excipients see Section 6.1.

3. PHARMACEUTICAL FORM

Bath additive. Dye- and fragrance-free white to off-white mobile liquid.

4. CLINICAL PARTICULARS

4.1 Therapeutic indications

For the symptomatic relief of contact dermatitis, atopic dermatitis, senile pruritus, ichthyosis and related dry skin disorders.

4.2 Posology and method of administration

Adults, including the elderly:

Shake the bottle to mix contents and add 15 to 20 ml (1 ½ to 2 inner capfuls) to a standard bath of water (20 cm/8 inch depth). Immerse and cover the affected areas with the bath water and soak for 10 to 20 minutes. Pat dry with a towel.

Infants and children:

Shake the bottle to mix contents and add 5 to 10 ml (½ to 1 inner capful) to a small bath or wash basin of water. Immerse and cover the affected areas with the bath water and soak for 10 to 20 minutes. Alternatively, repeatedly gently sponge over the affected areas. Pat dry with a towel.

There is no differentiation between the dosage quantities for the symptomatic relief of the conditions listed.

4.3 Contraindications

Sensitivity to any of the ingredients.

4.4 Special warnings and precautions for use

Take care not to slip in the bath. Surfaces that have been in contact with the product should be cleaned with a proprietary detergent. Keep out of the reach of children. For external use only.

4.5 Interaction with other medicinal products and other forms of interaction

None known.

4.6 Pregnancy and lactation

The constituents are not percutaneously absorbed or toxic if ingested. There is no evidence of safety of the drug used in pregnancy or lactation, but the active constituent has been in widespread use and in similar preparations for many years without apparent ill consequence.

4.7 Effects on ability to drive and use machines
None known.

4.8 Undesirable effects
Contact sensitivity reactions or mild irritant reactions may occur occasionally. In either case, treatment should be discontinued.

4.9 Overdose
Accidental ingestion may result in a purgative action due to the liquid paraffin and the oily nature of the product. Treat symptomatically. Fluid and electrolyte replacement may be necessary.

5. PHARMACOLOGICAL PROPERTIES

5.1 Pharmacodynamic properties
ATC Code: D02AX - Other emollients

For dry skin conditions it is important to use an emollient while bathing. Doublebase Emollient Bath Additive contains 65% Liquid Paraffin for its moisturising and skin softening properties, and is specially formulated to disperse in bath water.

5.2 Pharmacokinetic properties
The active constituent is not absorbed percutaneously. Pharmacokinetic particulars are thus not relevant.

5.3 Preclinical safety data
No relevant information additional to that contained elsewhere in the SPC.

6. PHARMACEUTICAL PARTICULARS

6.1 List of excipients
Isopropyl Myristate; Glycerol; Cetomacrogol 1000; Cetostearyl Alcohol; Phenoxyethanol; Purified Water.

6.2 Incompatibilities
None known.

6.3 Shelf life
30 months.

6.4 Special precautions for storage
This medicinal product does not require any special storage conditions.

6.5 Nature and contents of container
500 ml white high density polyethylene BOTTLE fitted with a polypropylene SCREW CAP. This is supplied as an original pack (OP).

6.6 Special precautions for disposal and other handling
Not applicable.

7. MARKETING AUTHORISATION HOLDER
Dermal Laboratories
Tatmore Place, Gosmore
Hitchin, Herts SG4 7QR, UK.

8. MARKETING AUTHORISATION NUMBER(S)
00173/0200.

9. DATE OF FIRST AUTHORISATION/RENEWAL OF THE AUTHORISATION
28 March 2006.

10. DATE OF REVISION OF THE TEXT
September 2007.

Doublebase Emollient Shower Gel
(Dermal Laboratories Limited)

1. NAME OF THE MEDICINAL PRODUCT
DOUBLEBASE™ EMOLLIENT SHOWER GEL

2. QUALITATIVE AND QUANTITATIVE COMPOSITION
Isopropyl Myristate 15% w/w; Liquid Paraffin 15% w/w.

For excipients, see section List of excipients.

3. PHARMACEUTICAL FORM
White opaque GEL.

4. CLINICAL PARTICULARS

4.1 Therapeutic indications
A highly emollient and protective hydrating base for regular first-line treatment and prophylaxis of dry or chapped skin conditions which may also be pruritic (itchy) or inflamed. Doublebase Emollient Shower Gel may also be used as an adjunct to other topical treatments.

4.2 Posology and method of administration
For adults, the elderly and children, who normally shower. For external use only. Use regularly and as often as necessary.

Doublebase Emollient Shower Gel may be applied before, during or after showering, with or without a normal cleanser (according to personal preference), to help prevent the drying and irritant effects of normal showering.

Doublebase Emollient Shower Gel can be used in one or more of the following ways:

• Before showering, apply the gel to dry skin areas using a few gentle strokes.

• During showering, apply the gel using a gentle washing action, rinse off any excess and pat the skin dry using a soft towel (avoid rubbing as this can irritate the skin). If a cleanser is to be used, apply the emollient gel afterwards.

• After showering, apply the gel to dry skin areas, using a few gentle strokes across the skin in the same direction as hair growth. If necessary, allow time for any excess to soak in. Do not rub vigorously.

4.3 Contraindications
Do not use in cases of known sensitivity to any of the ingredients.

4.4 Special warnings and precautions for use
Take care not to slip in the bath or shower. Surfaces that have been in contact with the product should be cleaned with a proprietary detergent.

4.5 Interaction with other medicinal products and other forms of interaction
None known.

4.6 Pregnancy and lactation
No special precautions.

4.7 Effects on ability to drive and use machines
No special precautions.

4.8 Undesirable effects
Although Doublebase Emollient Shower Gel has been specially formulated for use on dry, problem or sensitive skin, local skin reactions can occur in rare cases. In this event, treatment should be discontinued.

4.9 Overdose
Not applicable.

5. PHARMACOLOGICAL PROPERTIES

5.1 Pharmacodynamic properties
The oily ingredients, isopropyl myristate and liquid paraffin, encourage rehydration and softening of dry skin by forming an occlusive barrier within the skin surface, thus reducing drying from evaporation of water that diffuses from the underlying layers.

5.2 Pharmacokinetic properties
Because Doublebase Emollient Shower Gel is designed to deliver the emollient ingredients into the stratum corneum when gently applied to areas of dry skin, it is relatively non-greasy despite its high oil content.

5.3 Preclinical safety data
No relevant information additional to that contained elsewhere in this SPC.

6. PHARMACEUTICAL PARTICULARS

6.1 List of excipients
Glycerol; Carbomer; Sorbitan Laurate; Triethanolamine; Phenoxyethanol; Cetomacrogol 1000; Purified Water.

6.2 Incompatibilities
None known.

6.3 Shelf life
24 months.

6.4 Special precautions for storage
Do not store above 25°C. Do not freeze.

6.5 Nature and contents of container
Plastic bottle (200g) with polypropylene/silicone valve cap and plastic hooked overcap.

6.6 Special precautions for disposal and other handling
Not applicable.

7. MARKETING AUTHORISATION HOLDER
Dermal Laboratories
Tatmore Place, Gosmore
Hitchin, Herts SG4 7QR, UK.

8. MARKETING AUTHORISATION NUMBER(S)
00173/0196.

9. DATE OF FIRST AUTHORISATION/RENEWAL OF THE AUTHORISATION
6 December 2004.

10. DATE OF REVISION OF THE TEXT
February 2008.

Doublebase Emollient Wash Gel
(Dermal Laboratories Limited)

1. NAME OF THE MEDICINAL PRODUCT
DOUBLEBASE™ EMOLLIENT WASH GEL

2. QUALITATIVE AND QUANTITATIVE COMPOSITION
Isopropyl Myristate 15% w/w; Liquid Paraffin 15% w/w.

3. PHARMACEUTICAL FORM
White opaque gel.

4. CLINICAL PARTICULARS

4.1 Therapeutic indications
A highly emollient and protective hydrating base for regular first-line treatment and prophylaxis of dry or chapped skin conditions which may also be pruritic (itchy) or inflamed. The product may also be used as an adjunct to other topical treatments.

4.2 Posology and method of administration
For adults, the elderly and children. For cutaneous use only. Use regularly and as often as necessary.

• Use the product to gently wash the skin.

• Rinse off and pat the skin dry using a soft towel. (Avoid rubbing as this can irritate the skin).

4.3 Contraindications
Do not use in cases of known sensitivity to any of the ingredients.

4.4 Special warnings and precautions for use
Take care not to slip if using the product in the bath or shower. Surfaces that have been in contact with the product should be cleaned with a proprietary detergent.

4.5 Interaction with other medicinal products and other forms of interaction
None known.

4.6 Pregnancy and lactation
No special precautions.

4.7 Effects on ability to drive and use machines
No special precautions.

4.8 Undesirable effects
Although the product has been specially formulated for use on dry, problem or sensitive skin, local skin reactions can occur in rare cases. In this event, treatment should be discontinued.

4.9 Overdose
Not applicable.

5. PHARMACOLOGICAL PROPERTIES

5.1 Pharmacodynamic properties
ATC code: D02A, emollients and protectives.

The oily ingredients, isopropyl myristate and liquid paraffin, encourage rehydration and softening of dry skin by forming an occlusive barrier within the skin surface, thus reducing drying from evaporation of water that diffuses from the underlying layers. The product is also suitable for use as a soap substitute owing to the presence of a non-ionic emulsifier (cetomacrogol).

5.2 Pharmacokinetic properties
Because the product is designed to deliver the emollient ingredients into the stratum corneum when gently applied to areas of dry skin, it is relatively non-greasy despite its high oil content.

5.3 Preclinical safety data
There are no preclinical data of relevance to the prescriber, which are additional to those already included in other sections of the SmPC.

6. PHARMACEUTICAL PARTICULARS

6.1 List of excipients
Glycerol; Carbomer; Sorbitan Laurate; Triethanolamine; Phenoxyethanol; Cetomacrogol 1000; Purified Water.

6.2 Incompatibilities
None known.

6.3 Shelf life
24 months.

6.4 Special precautions for storage
Do not store above 25°C. Do not freeze.

6.5 Nature and contents of container
200g plastic bottle with pump dispenser.

6.6 Special precautions for disposal and other handling
Not applicable.

7. MARKETING AUTHORISATION HOLDER
Dermal Laboratories
Tatmore Place, Gosmore
Hitchin, Herts SG4 7QR, UK.

8. MARKETING AUTHORISATION NUMBER(S)
00173/0402.

9. DATE OF FIRST AUTHORISATION/RENEWAL OF THE AUTHORISATION
8 September 2008.

10. DATE OF REVISION OF THE TEXT
March 2009.

Doublebase Gel
(Dermal Laboratories Limited)

1. NAME OF THE MEDICINAL PRODUCT
DOUBLEBASE™ GEL

2. QUALITATIVE AND QUANTITATIVE COMPOSITION
Isopropyl Myristate 15% w/w; Liquid Paraffin 15% w/w.

For excipients see List of Excipients.

3. PHARMACEUTICAL FORM
White opaque gel.

4. CLINICAL PARTICULARS

4.1 Therapeutic indications
A highly emollient and protective hydrating base for regular first-line treatment and prophylaxis of dry or chapped skin

conditions which may also be pruritic (itchy) or inflamed. Doublebase may also be used as an adjunct to other topical treatments.

4.2 Posology and method of administration
For external use only. Before using the 500 g bottle, turn the top of the pump dispenser anti-clockwise to unlock it.

For adults, the elderly, infants and children:

• Apply Doublebase to the affected areas as often as necessary. For best results use a few gentle strokes to smooth Doublebase across the skin in the same direction as hair growth. If necessary, allow time for any excess to soak in. Do not rub vigorously.

• Doublebase may also be applied before washing, showering or having a bath to prevent further drying of the skin.

If additional topical treatments are being used on the same skin areas, Doublebase should be applied between these applications.

4.3 Contraindications
Do not use in cases of known sensitivity to any of the ingredients.

4.4 Special warnings and precautions for use
None.

4.5 Interaction with other medicinal products and other forms of interaction
None known.

4.6 Pregnancy and lactation
No special precautions.

4.7 Effects on ability to drive and use machines
No special precautions.

4.8 Undesirable effects
Although Doublebase has been specially formulated for use on dry, problem or sensitive skin, local skin reactions can occur in rare cases. In this event, treatment should be discontinued.

4.9 Overdose
Not applicable.

5. PHARMACOLOGICAL PROPERTIES

5.1 Pharmacodynamic properties
The oily ingredients, isopropyl myristate and liquid paraffin, encourage rehydration and softening of dry skin by forming an occlusive barrier within the skin surface, thus reducing drying from evaporation of water that diffuses from the underlying layers.

5.2 Pharmacokinetic properties
Because Doublebase is designed to deliver the emollient ingredients into the stratum corneum when gently applied to areas of dry skin, it is relatively non-greasy despite its high oil content.

5.3 Preclinical safety data
No relevant information additional to that contained elsewhere in this SPC.

6. PHARMACEUTICAL PARTICULARS

6.1 List of excipients
Glycerol; Carbomer; Sorbitan Laurate; Triethanolamine; Phenoxyethanol; Purified Water.

6.2 Incompatibilities
None known.

6.3 Shelf life
36 months.

6.4 Special precautions for storage
Do not store above 25°C. Do not freeze.

6.5 Nature and contents of container
500 g plastic bottle with pump dispenser or 100 g plastic laminate tube with screw cap.

6.6 Special precautions for disposal and other handling
Not applicable.

7. MARKETING AUTHORISATION HOLDER
Dermal Laboratories
Tatmore Place, Gosmore
Hitchin, Herts SG4 7QR, UK.

8. MARKETING AUTHORISATION NUMBER(S)
00173/0183.

9. DATE OF FIRST AUTHORISATION/RENEWAL OF THE AUTHORISATION
21 March 2006.

10. DATE OF REVISION OF THE TEXT
July 2006.

Dovobet Ointment

(Leo Laboratories Limited)

1. NAME OF THE MEDICINAL PRODUCT
Dovobet® 50 microgram/g + 0.5 mg/g ointment

2. QUALITATIVE AND QUANTITATIVE COMPOSITION
Calcipotriol 50 microgram/g (as hydrate), betamethasone 0.5 mg/g (as dipropionate).

For excipients, see section 6.1.

3. PHARMACEUTICAL FORM
Ointment.

Off-white to yellow.

4. CLINICAL PARTICULARS

4.1 Therapeutic indications
Topical treatment of stable plaque psoriasis vulgaris amenable to topical therapy.

4.2 Posology and method of administration
Dovobet® should be applied to the affected area once daily. The recommended treatment period is 4 weeks. After this period repeated treatment with Dovobet® can be initiated under medical supervision.

The maximum daily dose should not exceed 15 g, the maximum weekly dose should not exceed 100 g, and the treated area should not be more than 30% of the body surface.

Dovobet® is not recommended for the use in children and adolescents below the age of 18 years.

4.3 Contraindications
Known hypersensitivity to the active substances or to any of the excipients.

Due to the content of calcipotriol Dovobet® is contraindicated in patients with known disorders of calcium metabolism.

Due to the content of corticosteroid Dovobet® is contraindicated in the following conditions: Viral (e.g. herpes or varicella) lesions of the skin, fungal or bacterial skin infections, parasitic infections, skin manifestations in relation to tuberculosis or syphilis, rosacea, perioral dermatitis, acne vulgaris, atrophic skin, striae atrophicae, fragility of skin veins, ichthyosis, acne rosacea, ulcers, wounds, perianal and genital pruritus.

Dovobet® is contraindicated in guttate, erythrodermic, exfoliative and pustular psoriasis.

Dovobet® is contraindicated in patients with severe renal insufficiency or severe hepatic disorders.

4.4 Special warnings and precautions for use
The patient must be instructed in correct use of the product to avoid application and accidental transfer to the scalp, face, mouth and eyes. Hands must be washed after each application.

Treatment of more than 30% of the body surface should be avoided.

The risk of hypercalcaemia is minimal when the recommendations relevant to calcipotriol are fulfilled. Due to the content of calcipotriol hypercalcaemia may occur if the maximum weekly dose (100 g) is exceeded. Serum calcium is quickly normalised, however, when treatment is discontinued.

Dovobet® contains a strong potent group III-steroid and concurrent treatment with other steroids must be avoided. Adverse effects found in connection with systemic corticosteroid treatment such as adrenocortical suppression or impact on the metabolic control of diabetes mellitus may occur also during topical corticosteroid treatment due to systemic absorption.

Application on large areas of damaged skin and under occlusive dressings or on mucous membranes or in skin folds should be avoided since it increases the systemic absorption of corticosteroids. Skin of the face and genitals are very sensitive to corticosteroids. Long-term treatment of these parts of the body should be avoided. These areas should only be treated with the weaker corticosteroids. When lesions become secondarily infected, they should be treated with antimicrobiological therapy. However, when infection worsens, treatment with corticosteroids should be stopped.

When treating psoriasis with topical corticosteroids there may be a risk of generalised pustular psoriasis or of rebound effects when discontinuing treatment. Medical supervision should therefore continue in the post-treatment period.

With long-term use there is an increased risk of local and systemic corticosteroid undesirable effects. The treatment should be discontinued in case of undesirable effects related to long-term use of corticosteroid, see section 4.8.

There may be a risk of rebound when discontinuing a long-term treatment with corticosteroids.

There is no experience for the use of this product on the scalp. There is no experience with concurrent use of other anti-psoriatic products administered locally or systemically or with phototherapy.

During Dovobet®treatment physicians are recommended to advise patients to limit or avoid excessive exposure to either natural or artificial sunlight. Topical calcipotriol should be used with UV radiation only if the physician and patient consider that the potential benefits outweigh the potential risks (see section 5.3).

4.5 Interaction with other medicinal products and other forms of interaction
None known.

4.6 Pregnancy and lactation
Pregnancy

There are no adequate data from the use of Dovobet® in pregnant women. Studies in animals with glucocorticoids have shown reproductive toxicity (see section 5.3), but a number of epidemiological studies have not revealed congenital anomalies among infants born to women treated with corticosteroids during pregnancy. The potential risk for humans is uncertain. Therefore, during pregnancy, Dovobet® should only be used when the potential benefit justifies the potential risk.

Lactation

Betamethasone passes into breast milk but risk of an adverse effect on the infant seems unlikely with therapeutic doses. There are no data on the excretion of calcipotriol in breast milk. Caution should be exercised when prescribing Dovobet® to women who breast feed. The patient should be instructed not to use Dovobet® on the breast when breast feeding.

4.7 Effects on ability to drive and use machines
Dovobet® has no or negligible influence on the ability to drive and to use machines.

4.8 Undesirable effects
Very common >1/10

Common >1/100 and <1/10

Uncommon >1/1,000 and <1/100

Rare >1/10,000 and <1/1000

Very rare <1/10,000

The trial programme for Dovobet® ointment has so far included more than 2,500 patients and has shown that approximately 10% of patients can be expected to experience a non-serious undesirable effect.

Based on data from clinical trials and postmarket use the common undesirable effects are pruritus, rash and burning sensation of skin. Uncommon undesirable effects are skin pain or irritation, dermatitis, erythema, exacerbation of psoriasis, folliculitis and application site pigmentation changes. Pustular psoriasis is a rare undesirable effect.

The undesirable effects are listed by MedDRA SOC and the individual undesirable effects are listed starting with the most frequently reported.

• Skin and subcutaneous tissue disorders

Common: Pruritus

Common: Rash

Common: Burning sensation of skin

Uncommon: Skin pain or irritation

Uncommon: Dermatitis

Uncommon: Erythema

Uncommon: Exacerbation of psoriasis

Uncommon: Folliculitis

Uncommon: Application site pigmentation changes

Rare: Pustular psoriasis

Undesirable effects observed for calcipotriol and betamethasone, respectively:

Calcipotriol

Undesirable effects include application site reactions, pruritus, skin irritation, burning and stinging sensation, dry skin, erythema, rash, dermatitis, eczema, psoriasis aggravated, photosensitivity and hypersensitivity reactions including very rare cases of angioedema and facial oedema.

Systemic effects after topical use may appear very rarely causing hypercalcaemia or hypercalciuria, cf. section 4.4.

Betamethasone (as dipropionate)

This product contains a potent corticosteroid.

Local reactions can occur after topical use, especially during prolonged application, including skin atrophy, telangiectasia, striae, folliculitis, hypertrichosis, perioral dermatitis, allergic contact dermatitis, depigmentation and colloid milia. When treating psoriasis there may be a risk of generalised pustular psoriasis.

Systemic effects due to topical use of corticosteroids are rare in adults, however they can be severe. Adrenocortical suppression, cataract, infections and increase of intraocular pressure can occur, especially after long term treatment. Systemic effects occur more frequently when applied under occlusion (plastic, skin folds), when applied on large areas and during long term treatment, cf. section 4.4.

4.9 Overdose
Use above the recommended dose may cause elevated serum calcium which should rapidly subside when treatment is discontinued.

Excessive prolonged use of topical corticosteroids may suppress the pituitary-adrenal functions resulting in secondary adrenal insufficiency which is usually reversible. In such cases symptomatic treatment is indicated.

In case of chronic toxicity the corticosteroid treatment must be discontinued gradually.

It has been reported that due to misuse one patient with extensive erythrodermic psoriasis treated with 240g of Dovobet® ointment weekly (maximum dose 100 g weekly, cf. section 4.2 and 4.4) for 5 months developed Cushing's syndrome and pustular psoriasis after abruptly stopping treatment.

5. PHARMACOLOGICAL PROPERTIES

5.1 Pharmacodynamic properties

DO5AX52 Calcipotriol, combinations.

Calcipotriol is a vitamin D analogue. In vitro data suggests that calcipotriol induces differentiation and suppresses proliferation of keratinocytes. This is the proposed basis for its effect in psoriasis.

Like other topical corticosteroids, betamethasone dipropionate has anti-inflammatory, antipruritic, vasoconstrictive and immunosuppresive properties, however, without curing the underlying condition. Through occlusion the effect can be enhanced due to increased penetration of the stratum corneum (approximately by a factor of 10). The incidence of adverse events will increase because of this. The mechanism of the anti-inflammatory activity of the topical steroids, in general, is unclear.

A safety study in 634 psoriasis patients has investigated repeated courses of Dovobet® used once daily as required, either alone or alternating with Dovonex®, for up to 52 weeks, compared with Dovonex® used alone for 48 weeks after an initial course of Dovobet®. Adverse drug reactions were reported by 21.7% of the patients in the Dovobet® group, 29.6% in the Dovobet®/Dovonex® alternating group and 37.9% in the Dovonex® group. The adverse drug reactions that were reported by more than 2% of the patients in the Dovobet® group were pruritus (5.8%) and psoriasis (5.3%). Adverse events of concern possibly related to long-term corticosteroid use were reported by 4.8% of the patients in the Dovobet® group, 2.8% in the Dovobet®/Dovonex® alternating group and 2.9% in the Dovonex® group.

5.2 Pharmacokinetic properties

Clinical studies with radiolabelled ointment indicate that the systemic absorption of calcipotriol and betamethasone from Dovobet® is less than 1% of the dose (2.5 g) when applied to normal skin (625 cm^2) for 12 hours. Application to psoriasis plaques and under occlusive dressings may increase the absorption of topical corticosteroids.

Absorption through damaged skin is approx 24%. Protein binding is approx 64%. Plasma elimination half-life after intravenous application is 5-6 hours. Due to the formation of a depot in the skin elimination after dermal application is in order of days. Betamethasone is metabolised especially in the liver, but also in the kidneys to glucuronide and sulphate esters. Excretion takes place by urine and faeces.

5.3 Preclinical safety data

Studies of corticosteroids in animals have shown reproductive toxicity (cleft palate, skeletal malformations). In reproduction toxicity studies with long-term oral administration of corticosteroids to rats prolonged gestation and prolonged and difficult labour was detected. Moreover reduction in offspring survival, in body weight and body weight gain was observed. There was no impairment of fertility. The relevance for humans is unknown.

A dermal carcinogenicity study in mice revealed no special hazard to humans.

In a study where albino hairless mice were repeatedly exposed to both ultraviolet (UV) radiation and dermally administered calcipotriol for 40 weeks at dose levels corresponding to 9, 30 and 90 μg/m^2/day (equivalent to 0.25, 0.84, 2.5 times the maximum recommended daily dose for a 60 kg adult, respectively), a reduction in the time required for UV radiation to induce the formation of skin tumours was observed (statistically significant in males only), suggesting that calcipotriol may enhance the effect of UV radiation to induce skin tumours. The clinical relevance of this finding is unknown.

No carcinogenicity or photocarcinogenicity studies have been performed with betamethasone dipropionate.

6. PHARMACEUTICAL PARTICULARS

6.1 List of excipients

Liquid paraffin

Polyoxypropylene-15-stearyl ether

α-tocopherol

White soft paraffin

6.2 Incompatibilities

Not to be mixed with other medicinal products.

6.3 Shelf life

Unopened container: 2 years.

After first opening of container: 12 months.

6.4 Special precautions for storage

Do not store above 25°C.

6.5 Nature and contents of container

Aluminium/epoxyphenol tubes with polyethylene screw cap.

Tube sizes: 3 (sample), 15, 30, 60, 100 and 120 g.

Not all pack sizes may be marketed.

6.6 Special precautions for disposal and other handling

No special requirements.

7. MARKETING AUTHORISATION HOLDER

LEO Pharmaceutical Products
Industriparken 55
DK-2750 Ballerup
Denmark

8. MARKETING AUTHORISATION NUMBER(S)

PL 05293/0003

9. DATE OF FIRST AUTHORISATION/RENEWAL OF THE AUTHORISATION

15 March 2006

10. DATE OF REVISION OF THE TEXT

4 January 2007

Dovonex Cream

(Leo Laboratories Limited)

1. NAME OF THE MEDICINAL PRODUCT

Dovonex® Cream

2. QUALITATIVE AND QUANTITATIVE COMPOSITION

Calcipotriol 50 micrograms per g (as the hydrate)

For full list of excipients, see section 6.1

3. PHARMACEUTICAL FORM

Cream

Soft white cream

4. CLINICAL PARTICULARS

4.1 Therapeutic indications

Dovonex® Cream is indicated for the topical treatment of plaque psoriasis (psoriasis vulgaris) amenable to topical therapy.

4.2 Posology and method of administration

Adults:	Dovonex® Cream should be applied to the affected area once or twice daily. For maximum benefit use the cream twice daily. Maximum weekly dose should not exceed 100g.
Children over 12 years:	Dovonex® Cream should be applied to the affected area twice daily. Maximum weekly dose should not exceed 75g.
Children aged 6 to 12 years:	Dovonex® Cream should be applied to the affected area twice daily. Maximum weekly dose should not exceed 50g.
Children under 6 years:	There is limited experience of the use of Dovonex® in this age group. A maximum safe dose has not been established.

These dose recommendations are based on extensive experience in adults. In respect of children, clinical experience in children has shown Dovonex® to be safe and effective over eight weeks at a mean dose of 15g per week but with wide variability in dose among patients. Individual dose requirement depends on the extent of psoriasis but should not exceed the above recommendations. There is no experience of use of Dovonex® in combination with other therapies in children.

4.3 Contraindications

Dovonex® Cream is contra-indicated in patients with known disorders of calcium metabolism. As with other topical preparations, Dovonex® Cream is contra-indicated in patients with hypersensitivity to any of the ingedients.

4.4 Special warnings and precautions for use

Dovonex® Cream should not be used on the face. Patients should be advised to wash their hands after applying the cream and to avoid inadvertent transfer to other body areas, especially the face. Care should be exercised in patients with other types of psoriasis, since hypercalcaemia, which rapidly reversed on cessation of treatment, has been reported in patients with generalized pustular or erythrodermic exfoliative psoriasis.

During treatment with Dovonex® Cream physicians are recommended to advise patients to limit or avoid excessive exposure to either natural or artificial sunlight. Topical calcipotriol should be used with UV radiation only if the physician and patient consider that the potential benefits outweigh the potential risks (see section 5.3).

4.5 Interaction with other medicinal products and other forms of interaction

There is no experience of concomitant therapy with other antipsoriatic products applied to the same skin area at the same time.

4.6 Pregnancy and lactation

Safety for use during human pregnancy has not yet been established, although studies in experimental animals have not shown teratogenic effects. Avoid use in pregnancy unless there is no safer alternative. It is not known whether calcipotriol is excreted in breast milk.

4.7 Effects on ability to drive and use machines

Not applicable.

4.8 Undesirable effects

Very common	>1/10
Common	>1/100 and <1/10
Uncommon	>1/1,000 and <1/100
Rare	>1/10,000 and <1/1,000
Very rare	<1/10,000

Approximately 25% of the patients treated with Dovonex®-Cream could experience an adverse reaction. These reactions are usually mild.

Immune system disorders

Very rare:	allergic reactions (including angioedema)

Metabolism and nutrition disorders

Very rare:	hypercalcaemia, hypercalciuria, especially if the total recommended dose is exceeded (see section 4.2).

Skin and subcutaneous tissue disorders

Very common:	skin irritation
Common:	rash*, burning sensation, stinging sensation, dry skin, pruritus, erythema, contact dermatitis including facial and perioral.
Uncommon:	psoriasis aggravated, eczema
Unknown frequency:	transient changes in skin pigmentation, transient photosensitivity, urticaria, angioedema, periorbital or face oedema.

*Various types of rash reactions such as scaly, erythematous, maculo-papular, pustular, bullous have been reported.

4.9 Overdose

Hypercalcaemia should not occur at the recommended dose of Dovonex® Cream.

Excessive use may cause elevated serum calcium which rapidly subsides when the treatment is discontinued.

5. PHARMACOLOGICAL PROPERTIES

5.1 Pharmacodynamic properties

ATC Code: D05A X02

Pharmacotherapeutic group: Antipsoriatics for topical use

Calcipotriol is a vitamin D derivative. *In vitro* data suggest that calcipotriol induces differentiation and suppresses proliferation of keratinocytes. This is the proposed basis for its effect in psoriasis.

5.2 Pharmacokinetic properties

Calcipotriol is only slightly absorbed from the skin.

5.3 Preclinical safety data

The effect on calcium metabolism is approximately 100 times less than that of the hormonally active form of vitamin D_3.

A dermal carcinogenicity study in mice revealed no special hazard to humans.

In a study where albino hairless mice were repeatedly exposed to both ultraviolet (UV) radiation and dermally administered calcipotriol for 40 weeks at dose levels corresponding to 9, 30 and 90μg/m^2/day (equivalent to 0.25, 0.84, 2.5 times the maximum recommended daily dose for a 60 kg adult, respectively), a reduction in the time required for UV radiation to induce the formation of skin tumours was observed (statistically significant in males only), suggesting that calcipotriol may enhance the effect of UV radiation to induce skin tumours. The clinical relevance of these findings is unknown.

6. PHARMACEUTICAL PARTICULARS

6.1 List of excipients

Macrogol cetostearyl ether, cetostearyl alcohol, chloroallylhexaminium chloride, disodium edetate, disodium phosphate dihydrate, glycerol 85%, liquid paraffin, purified water, white soft paraffin.

6.2 Incompatibilities

Should not be mixed with other medicinal products.

6.3 Shelf life

2 years.

6.4 Special precautions for storage

Store below 25°C

6.5 Nature and contents of container

Aluminium tubes of 30g (OP), 60g (OP), 100g(OP) and 120g (OP).

Physician Sample Packs: Aluminium tubes of 15g

Polyethylene - aluminium laminate tubes with screw cap of 240g (OP).

Not all pack sizes may be marketed.

6.6 Special precautions for disposal and other handling

No special requirements.

7. MARKETING AUTHORISATION HOLDER

LEO Laboratories Limited

Longwick Road

Princes Risborough

Bucks

HP27 9RR

8. MARKETING AUTHORISATION NUMBER(S)

PL 0043/0188

9. DATE OF FIRST AUTHORISATION/RENEWAL OF THE AUTHORISATION

10 August 1993

10. DATE OF REVISION OF THE TEXT

October 2008

Dovonex Scalp Solution

(Leo Laboratories Limited)

1. NAME OF THE MEDICINAL PRODUCT

Dovonex® Scalp Solution

2. QUALITATIVE AND QUANTITATIVE COMPOSITION

Calcipotriol 50 micrograms per ml (as the hydrate)

For full list of excipients, see section 6.1.

3. PHARMACEUTICAL FORM

Solution

Colourless, slightly viscous solution.

4. CLINICAL PARTICULARS

4.1 Therapeutic indications

Dovonex® Scalp Solution is indicated for the topical treatment of scalp psoriasis.

4.2 Posology and method of administration

Adults: Dovonex® Scalp Solution should be applied twice daily (morning and evening) to the affected areas. Maximum weekly dose should not exceed 60 ml.

When used together with Dovonex® Cream or Ointment, the total dose of calcipotriol should not exceed 5mg in any week, e.g. 60 ml of Scalp Solution plus 30g of Cream or Ointment, or 30ml of Scalp Solution plus 60g of Cream or Ointment.

Children: Not recommended as there is no experience of the use of Dovonex® Scalp Solution in children.

4.3 Contraindications

Dovonex® Scalp Solution is contraindicated in patients with known disorders of calcium metabolism. As with other topical preparations, Dovonex® Scalp Solution is contraindicated in patients with hypersensitivity to any of its constituents.

4.4 Special warnings and precautions for use

Application of Dovonex® to the face may cause local irritation. Dovonex® Scalp Solution should not therefore be applied directly to the face. Patients should be advised to wash their hands after applying the scalp solution and to avoid inadvertent transfer to the face. Patients should be advised to use no more than the maximum weekly dose since hypercalcaemia, which rapidly reverses on cessation of treatment, may occur.

During treatment with Dovonex® Scalp Solution physicians are recommended to advise patients to limit or avoid excessive exposure to either natural or artificial sunlight. Topical calcipotriol should be used with UV radiation only if the physician and patient consider that the potential benefits outweigh the potential risks (see section 5.3).

4.5 Interaction with other medicinal products and other forms of interaction

There is no experience of concomitant therapy with other antipsoriatic products applied to the same skin area at the same time.

4.6 Pregnancy and lactation

Safety for use during human pregnancy has not yet been established, although studies in experimental animals have not shown teratogenic effects. Avoid use in pregnancy unless there is no safer alternative. It is not known whether calcipotriol is excreted in breast milk.

4.7 Effects on ability to drive and use machines

Not applicable

4.8 Undesirable effects

Very common	>1/10
Common	>1/100 and <1/10
Uncommon	>1/1,000 and <1/100
Rare	>1/10,000 and <1/1,000
Very rare	<1/10,000

Approximately 25% of the patients treated with Dovonex®Scalp Solution could experience an adverse reaction. These reactions are usually mild.

Immune system disorders

Very rare:	allergic reactions (including angioedema).

Metabolism and nutrition disorders

Very rare:	hypercalcaemia, hypercalciuria, especially if the total recommended dose is exceeded (see section 4.2).

Skin and subcutaneous tissue disorders

Very common:	skin irritation
Common:	rash*, burning sensation, stinging sensation, dry skin, pruritus, erythema, contact dermatitis including facial and perioral.
Uncommon:	psoriasis aggravated, eczema
Unknown frequency:	transient changes in skin pigmentation, transient photosensitivity, urticaria, angioedema, periorbital or face oedema.

*Various types of rash reactions such as scaly, erythematous, maculo-papular, pustular, bullous have been reported.

4.9 Overdose

Hypercalcaemia may occur in patients with plaque psoriasis who use more than 100g of Dovonex® Ointment weekly and has been reported at lower doses in patients with generalised pustular or erythrodermic exfoliative psoriasis.

5. PHARMACOLOGICAL PROPERTIES

5.1 Pharmacodynamic properties

ATC Code: D05A X02.

Pharmacotherapeutic group: Antipsoriatics for topical use.

Calcipotriol is a vitamin D derivative. *In vitro* data suggest that calcipotriol induces differentiation and suppresses proliferation of keratinocytes. This effect is the proposed basis for its effect in psoriasis.

5.2 Pharmacokinetic properties

Calcipotriol is only slightly absorbed from the skin.

5.3 Preclinical safety data

The effect on the calcium metabolism is approximately 100 times less than that of the hormonally active form of vitamin D_3.

A dermal carcinogenicity study in mice revealed no special hazard to humans.

In a study where albino hairless mice were repeatedly exposed to both ultraviolet (UV) radiation and dermally administered calcipotriol for 40 weeks at dose levels corresponding to 9, 30 and 90μg/m²/day (equivalent to 0.25, 0.84, 2.5 times the maximum recommended daily dose for a 60 kg adult, respectively), a reduction in the time required for UV radiation to induce the formation of skin tumours was observed (statistically significant in males only), suggesting that calcipotriol may enhance the effect of UV radiation to induce skin tumours. The clinical relevance of these findings is unknown.

6. PHARMACEUTICAL PARTICULARS

6.1 List of excipients

Hydroxypropyl cellulose, isopropyl alcohol, levomenthol, sodium citrate, propylene glycol, purified water.

6.2 Incompatibilities

Should not be mixed with other medicinal products.

6.3 Shelf life

2 years.

6.4 Special precautions for storage

Store below 25°C.

The alcohol base is flammable.

6.5 Nature and contents of container

30ml, 60ml, 100ml and 120ml polyethylene bottles with nozzle.

Not all pack sizes may be marketed.

6.6 Special precautions for disposal and other handling

No special requirements.

7. MARKETING AUTHORISATION HOLDER

LEO Laboratories Limited,

Longwick Road,

Princes Risborough,

Buckinghamshire

HP27 9RR

United Kingdom.

8. MARKETING AUTHORISATION NUMBER(S)

PL 0043/0190

9. DATE OF FIRST AUTHORISATION/RENEWAL OF THE AUTHORISATION

8th June 1994

10. DATE OF REVISION OF THE TEXT

October 2008

Doxorubicin Rapid Dissolution

(Pharmacia Limited)

1. NAME OF THE MEDICINAL PRODUCT

Doxorubicin Rapid Dissolution 10 mg, 20 mg, 50 mg and 150 mg.

2. QUALITATIVE AND QUANTITATIVE COMPOSITION

Doxorubicin Hydrochloride HSE 10.0 mg

Doxorubicin Hydrochloride HSE 20.0 mg

Doxorubicin Hydrochloride HSE 50.0 mg

Doxorubicin Hydrochloride HSE 150.0 mg

3. PHARMACEUTICAL FORM

Freeze-dried powder for injection.

4. CLINICAL PARTICULARS

4.1 Therapeutic indications

The treatment of a wide range of neoplastic diseases including acute leukaemia, lymphoma, paediatric malignancies and adult solid tumours, in particular, breast and lung carcinomas.

4.2 Posology and method of administration

Route of administration: The proposed routes of administration are intravenous and intra-arterial injection and intravesical instillation. Doxorubicin cannot be used as an antibacterial agent.

Intravesical doxorubicin is an option for use in the treatment of superficial bladder cancer, comprising transitional cell carcinoma, papillary bladder tumours, and carcinoma-in-situ, or as adjuvant treatment of low-grade Ta bladder cancers following trans-urethral resection.

<u>Adults and Children</u>:

Intravenous Administration:

The reconstituted solution is given via the tubing of a freely-running intravenous infusion, taking not less than 3 minutes and not more than 10 minutes over the injection. Commonly used acceptable solutions are sodium chloride injection, dextrose injection 5% or sodium chloride and dextrose injection. A direct push injection is not recommended due to the risk of extravasation, which may occur even in the presence of adequate blood return upon needle aspiration (see section 4.4 Special Warnings and Precautions for use).

The total doxorubicin dose per cycle may differ according to its use within a specific treatment regimen (e.g. given as a single agent or in combination with other cytotoxic drugs) and according to the indication.

Dosage is usually calculated on the basis of body surface area. As a single agent, the recommended standard starting dose of doxorubicin per cycle in adults is 60-90 mg/m² of body surface area. The total starting dose per cycle may be given as a single dose or divided over 3 successive days or in divided doses given on days 1 and 8. Under conditions of normal recovery from drug-induced toxicity (particularly bone marrow depression and stomatitis), each treatment cycle could be repeated every 3 to 4 weeks. If it is used in combination with other antitumour agents having overlapping toxicity, the dosage for doxorubicin may need to be reduced to 30-40 mg/m² every three weeks.

If dosage is to be calculated on the basis of body weight, 1.2-2.4 mg/kg should be given as a single dose every three weeks.

It has been shown that giving doxorubicin as a single dose every three weeks greatly reduces the distressing toxic effect, mucositis; however there are still some who believe that dividing the dose over three successive days (0.4-0.8 mg/kg or 20-25 mg/m² on each day) gives greater effectiveness even though at the cost of high toxicity.

Administration of doxorubicin in a weekly regimen has been shown to be as effective as the 3-weekly regimen. The recommended dosage is 20 mg/m² weekly although objective responses have been seen at 6-12 mg/m². Weekly administration leads to a reduction in cardiotoxicity.

Dosage may need to be reduced for patients who have had prior treatment with other cytotoxic agents. Dosage may also need to be reduced in children, obese patients and the elderly.

Lower starting doses or longer intervals between cycles may need to be considered for heavily pre-treated patients, or patients with neoplastic bone marrow infiltration (see section 4.4 Special Warnings and Precautions for Use).

Hepatic dysfunction

If hepatic function is impaired, doxorubicin should be reduced according to the following table:

Serum bilirubin levels	Recommended dose
1.2-3.0 mg/100 ml	50% normal dose
> 3.0 mg/100 ml	25% normal dose

Doxorubicin should not be administered to patients with severe hepatic impairment (see section 4.3 Contra-indications).

Intra-arterial Administration:

Intra-arterial injection has been used in attempts to produce intense local activity while keeping the total dose low and therefore reducing general toxicity. It should be emphasised that this technique is potentially extremely hazardous and can lead to widespread necrosis of the perfuse tissue unless due precautions are taken. Drug doses administered and dosing intervals utilized for intra-arterial perfusion vary.

Intra-arterial injection should only be attempted by those fully conversant with this technique.

Intravesical Administration:

Doxorubicin is being increasingly used by intravesical administration for the treatment of transitional cell carcinoma, papillary bladder tumours and carcinoma-in-situ. It should not be employed in this way for the treatment of invasive tumours which have penetrated the bladder wall. It has also been found useful to instil doxorubicin into the bladder at intervals after transurethral resection of a tumour in order to reduce the probability of recurrence. Instillations of 30-50 mg in 25-50 mL of saline solution are recommended. In the case of local toxicity (chemical cystitis), the dose should be instilled in 50-100 mL of saline solution. Patients may continue to receive instillations in weekly to monthly intervals.

While at present many regimens are in use, making interpretation difficult, the following may be helpful guides:

- The concentration of doxorubicin in the bladder should be 50 mg per 50 ml.
- To avoid undue dilution with urine, the patient should be instructed not to drink any fluid in the 12 hours prior to instillation.
- This should limit urine production to approximately 50 ml per hour. The patient should be rotated a quarter turn every 15 minutes while the drug is in situ.

Exposure to the drug solution for one hour is generally adequate and the patient should be instructed to void at the end of this time.

4.3 Contraindications

Hypersensitivity to doxorubicin or any other component of the product, other anthracyclines or anthracenediones.

Intravenous (IV) use:

- persistent myelosuppression
- severe hepatic impairment
- severe myocardial insufficiency
- recent myocardial infarction
- severe arrhythmias
- previous treatment with maximum cumulative doses of doxorubicin, daunorubicin, epirubicin, idarubicin and/or other anthracyclines and anthracenediones (see section 4.4 Special Warnings and Precautions for use)

Intravesical use:

- urinary infections
- inflammation of the bladder

4.4 Special warnings and precautions for use

Doxorubicin should be administered only under the supervision of physicians experienced in the use of cytotoxic therapy.

Patients should recover from acute toxicities of prior cytotoxic treatment (such as stomatitis, neutropenia, thrombocytopenia, and generalised infections) before beginning treatment with doxorubicin.

The systemic clearance of doxorubicin is reduced in obese patients (i.e. > 130% ideal body weight) (see section 4.2 Posology and Method of Administration).

Cardiac Function

Cardiotoxicity is a risk of anthracycline treatment that may be manifested by early (i.e. acute) or late (i.e. delayed) events.

Early (i.e. Acute) Events: Early cardiotoxicity of doxorubicin consists mainly of sinus tachycardia and/or ECG abnormalities such as non-specific ST-T wave changes. Tachyarrhythmias, including premature ventricular contractions and ventricular tachycardia, bradycardia, as well as atrioventricular and bundle-branch block have also been reported. These effects do not usually predict subsequent development of delayed cardiotoxicity and are generally not a consideration for discontinuation of doxorubicin treatment.

Late (i.e. Delayed) Events: Delayed cardiotoxicity usually develops late in the course of therapy with doxorubicin or within 2 to 3 months after treatment termination, but later events, several months to years after completion of treatment, have also been reported. Delayed cardiomyopathy is manifested by reduced left ventricular ejection fraction (LVEF) and/or signs and symptoms of congestive heart failure (CHF) such as dyspnoea, pulmonary oedema, dependent oedema, cardiomegaly and hepatomegaly, oliguria, ascites, pleural effusion and gallop rhythm. Subacute effects such as pericarditis/myocarditis have also been reported. Life-threatening CHF is the most severe form of anthracycline-induced cardiomyopathy and represents the cumulative dose-limiting toxicity of the drug.

Cardiac function should be assessed before patients undergo treatment with doxorubicin and must be monitored throughout therapy to minimize the risk of incurring severe cardiac impairment. The risk may be decreased through regular monitoring of LVEF during the course of treatment with prompt discontinuation of doxorubicin at the first sign of impaired function. The appropriate quantitative method for repeated assessment of cardiac function (evaluation of LVEF) includes multi-gated radionuclide angiography (MUGA) or echocardiography (ECHO). A baseline cardiac evaluation with an ECG and either a MUGA scan or an ECHO is recommended, especially in patients with risk factors for increased cardiotoxicity. Repeated MUGA or ECHO determinations of LVEF should be performed, particularly with higher, cumulative anthracycline doses. The technique used for assessment should be consistent throughout follow-up.

The probability of developing CHF, estimated around 1% to 2% at a cumulative dose of 300 mg/m^2, slowly increases up to the total cumulative dose of 450-550 mg/m^2. Thereafter, the risk of developing CHF increases steeply and it is recommended not to exceed a maximum cumulative dose of 550 mg/m^2.

Risk factors for cardiac toxicity include active or dormant cardiovascular disease, prior or concomitant radiotherapy to the mediastinal/pericardial area, previous therapy with other anthracyclines or anthracenediones and concomitant use of drugs with the ability to suppress cardiac contractility or cardiotoxic drugs (e.g., trastuzumab). Anthracyclines including doxorubicin should not be administered in combination with other cardiotoxic agents unless the patient's cardiac function is closely monitored. Patients receiving anthracyclines after stopping treatment with other cardiotoxic agents, especially those with long half-lives such as trastuzumab, may also be at an increased risk of developing cardiotoxicity. The half-life of trastuzumab is approximately 28.5 days and may persist in the circulation for up to 24 weeks. Therefore, physicians should avoid anthracycline-based therapy for up to 24 weeks after stopping trastuzumab when possible. If anthracyclines are used before this time, careful monitoring of cardiac function is recommended.

Cardiac function must be carefully monitored in patients receiving high cumulative doses and in those with risk factors. However, cardiotoxicity with doxorubicin may occur at lower cumulative doses whether or not cardiac risk factors are present.

Children and adolescents are at an increased risk for developing delayed cardiotoxicity following doxorubicin administration. Females may be at greater risk than males. Follow-up cardiac evaluations are recommended periodically to monitor for this effect.

It is probable that the toxicity of doxorubicin and other anthracyclines or anthracenediones is additive.

Haematologic Toxicity

Doxorubicin may produce myelosuppression. Haematologic profiles should be assessed before and during each cycle of therapy with doxorubicin, including differential white blood cell (WBC) counts. A dose-dependent, reversible leucopenia and/or granulocytopenia (neutropenia) is the predominant manifestation of doxorubicin haematologic toxicity and is the most common acute dose-limiting toxicity of this drug. Leucopenia and neutropenia generally reach the nadir between days 10 and 14 after drug administration; the WBC/neutrophil counts return to normal values in most cases by day 21. Thrombocytopenia and anaemia may also occur. Clinical consequences of severe myelosuppression include fever, infections, sepsis/septicaemia, septic shock, haemorrhage, tissue hypoxia or death.

Secondary Leukaemia

Secondary leukaemia, with or without a preleukaemic phase, has been reported in patients treated with anthracyclines. Secondary leukaemia is more common when such drugs are given in combination with DNA-damaging antineoplastic agents, when patients have been heavily pretreated with cytotoxic drugs or when doses of the anthracyclines have been escalated. These leukaemias can have a 1 to 3 year latency period.

Carcinogenesis, Mutagenesis and Impairment of Fertility

Doxorubicin was genotoxic and mutagenic in *in vitro* or *in vivo* tests.

In women, doxorubicin may cause infertility during the time of drug administration. Doxorubicin may cause amenorrhoea. Ovulation and menstruation appear to return after termination of therapy, although premature menopause can occur.

Doxorubicin is mutagenic and can induce chromosomal damage in human spermatozoa. Oligospermia or azoospermia may be permanent; however, sperm counts have been reported to return to normospermic levels in some instances. This may occur several years after the end of therapy. Men undergoing doxorubicin treatment should use effective contraceptive methods.

Liver function

The major route of elimination of doxorubicin is the hepatobiliary system. Serum total bilirubin should be evaluated before and during treatment with doxorubicin. Patients with elevated bilirubin may experience slower clearance of the drug with an increase in overall toxicity. Lower doses are recommended in these patients (see section 4.2 Posology and Method of Administration). Patients with severe hepatic impairment should not receive doxorubicin (see section 4.3 Contraindications).

Other

Doxorubicin may potentiate the toxicity of other anticancer therapies. Exacerbation of cyclophosphamide-induced haemorrhagic cystitis and enhanced hepatotoxicity of 6-mercaptopurine have been reported. Radiation-induced toxicities (myocardium, mucosae, skin and liver) have also been reported.

As with other cytotoxic agents, thrombophlebitis and thromboembolic phenomena including pulmonary embolism (in some cases fatal) have been coincidentally reported with the use of doxorubicin.

Tumor-Lysis Syndrome

Doxorubicin may induce hyperuricaemia as a consequence of the extensive purine catabolism that accompanies drug-induced rapid lysis of neoplastic cells (tumour-lysis syndrome). Blood uric acid levels, potassium, calcium phosphate and creatinine should be evaluated after initial treatment. Hydration, urine alkalinization, and prophylaxis with allopurinol to prevent hyperuricaemia may minimize potential complications of tumour lysis syndrome.

Vaccinations

Administration of live or live-attenuated vaccines in patients immunocompromised by chemotherapeutic agents, including doxorubicin, may result in serious or fatal infections. Vaccination with a live vaccine should be avoided in patients receiving doxorubicin. Killed or inactivated vaccines may be administered; however, the response to such vaccines may be diminished

Administration of doxorubicin by the intravesical route may produce symptoms of chemical cystitis (such as dysuria, polyuria, nocturia, stranguria, hematuria, bladder discomfort, necrosis of the bladder wall) and bladder constrictions. Special attention is required for catherisation problems (e.g. urethral obstruction due to massive intravesical tumours).

Intra-arterial administration of doxorubicin (transcatheter arterial embolisation) may be employed for the localized or regional therapy of primary hepatocellularcarcinoma or liver metastases. Intra-arterial administration may produce (in addition to systemic toxicity qualitatively similar to that observed following intravenous administration of doxorubicin) gastro-duodenal ulcers (probably due to reflux of the drugs into the gastric artery) and narrowing of bile ducts due to drug-induced sclerosing cholangitis. This route of administration can lead to widespread necrosis of the perfused tissue.

4.5 Interaction with other medicinal products and other forms of interaction

High dose cyclosporin increases the serum levels and myelotoxicity of doxorubicin.

Doxorubicin is mainly used in combination with other cytotoxic drugs. Additive toxicity may occur especially with regard to bone marrow/haematologic and gastrointestinal effects (see section 4.4 Special Warnings and Precautions for Use). The use of doxorubicin in combination chemotherapy with other potentially cardiotoxic drugs, as well as the concomitant use of other cardioactive compounds (e.g. calcium channel blockers), require monitoring of cardiac function throughout treatment. Changes in hepatic function induced by concomitant therapies may affect doxorubicin metabolism, pharmacokinetics, therapeutic efficacy and/or toxicity.

Paclitaxel can cause increased plasma-concentrations of doxorubicin and/or its metabolites when given prior to doxorubicin. Certain data indicate a smaller increase is observed when doxorubicin is administered prior to paclitaxel.

4.6 Pregnancy and lactation

Doxorubicin has harmful pharmacological effects on pregnancy and/or the foetus/newborn child.

Due to the embryotoxic potential of doxorubicin, this drug should not be used during pregnancy unless clearly necessary. If a woman receives doxorubicin during pregnancy or becomes pregnant whilst taking the drug, she should be warned of the potential hazard to the foetus. Women of childbearing potential have to use effective contraception during treatment (see section 4.4 Special Warnings and Precautions for Use).

Doxorubicin is secreted into breast milk. Women should not breastfeed while undergoing treatment with doxorubicin.

4.7 Effects on ability to drive and use machines

None stated.

4.8 Undesirable effects

The following adverse events (not listed in order of frequency) have been reported in association with doxorubicin therapy:

Neoplasms Benign and Malignant (including cysts and polyps):

The occurrence of secondary acute myeloid leukaemia with or without a pre-leukaemic phase has been reported rarely in patients concurrently treated with doxorubicin in association with DNA-damaging antineoplastic agents. Such cases could have a short (1-3 year) latency period. Acute lymphocytic leukaemia and acute myelogenous leukaemia.

Blood and Lymphatic System Disorders:

Haematological monitoring should be undertaken regularly in both haematological and non haematological conditions, because of the possibility of bone-marrow depression which may become evident around ten days from the time of administration. Clinical consequences of doxorubicin bone marrow/haematological toxicity may be fever, infections, sepsis/septicaemia, septic shock, haemorrhages, tissue hypoxia or death. Leucopenia, neutropenia, anaemia and thrombocytopenia.

Immune System Disorders:

Anaphylaxis.

Metabolism and Nutrition Disorders:

Anorexia, dehydration and hyperuricaemia.

Eye Disorders:

Conjunctivitis / keratitis and lacrimation.

Cardiac Disorders:

Cardiotoxicity may be manifested in tachycardia including supraventricular tachycardia and ECG changes. Routine ECG monitoring is recommended and caution should be exercised in patients with impaired cardiac function. Severe cardiac failure may occur suddenly without premonitory ECG changes. Tachyarrhythmias, atrio-ventricular and bundle branch block, asymptomatic reduction in left ventricular ejection fraction and congestive heart failure.

Vascular Disorders:

Phlebitis, thrombophlebitis, thromboembolism, hot flushes and shock.

Gastrointestinal Disorders:

Nausea, vomiting and mucositis/stomatitis, hyperpigmentation of oral mucosa, oesophagitis, abdominal pain, gastric erosions, gastrointestinal tract bleeding, diarrhoea and colitis.

Hepatobiliary Disorders:

Changes in transaminase levels.

Skin and Subcutaneous Tissue Disorders:

Alopecia occurs frequently, including the interruption of beard growth, but all hair growth normally resumes after treatment is stopped. Skin rashes/itch, local toxicity, skin changes, skin and nail hyperpigmentation, photosensitivity, hypersensitivity to irradiated skin ('radiation recall reaction'), urticaria, acral erythema and plantar-palmar dysaesthesia.

Renal and Urological Disorders:

Doxorubicin may impart a red colour to urine particularly to the first specimen passed after the injection and patients should be advised that this is no cause for alarm. Following intravesical administration, side-effects include symptoms of bladder irritation, haematuria, haemorrhagic cystitis and necrosis of the bladder wall.

Reproductive System and Breast Disorders:

Amenorrhoea, oligospermia and azoospermia.

General Disorders and Administration Site Conditions:

The risk of thrombophlebitis at the injection site may be minimised by following the procedure for administration recommended above. A stinging or burning sensation at the site of administration signifies a small degree of extravasation and the infusion should be stopped and re-started in another vein. Fever, malaise, asthenia and chills.

Investigations:

ECG abnormalities.

4.9 Overdose

Single doses of 250 mg and 500 mg of doxorubicin have proved fatal. Such doses may cause acute myocardial degeneration within 24 hours and severe myelosuppression (mainly leucopoenia and thrombocytopenia), the effects of which are greatest between 10 and 15 days after administration. Treatment should aim to support the patient during this period and should utilise such measures as blood transfusions and reverse barrier nursing.

Acute overdose with doxorubicin will result in gastrointestinal toxic effects (mainly mucositis). This generally appears early after drug administration, but most patients recover from this within three weeks.

Delayed cardiac failure may occur up to six months after the overdose. Patients should be observed carefully and should signs of cardiac failure arise, be treated along conventional lines.

5. PHARMACOLOGICAL PROPERTIES

5.1 Pharmacodynamic properties

ATC code: L01DB01

Doxorubicin is an antitumour agent. Tumour cells are probably killed through drug-induced alterations of nucleic acid synthesis although the exact mechanism of action has not yet been clearly elucidated.

Proposed mechanism of action include:

DNA intercalation (leading to an inhibition of synthesis of DNA, RNA and proteins), formation of highly reactive free-radicals and superoxides, chelation of divalent cations, the inhibition of Na-K ATPase and the binding of doxorubicin to certain constituents of cell membranes (particularly to the membrane lipids, spectrin and cardiolipin). Highest drug concentrations are attained in the lung, liver, spleen, kidney, heart, small intestine and bone-marrow. Doxorubicin does not cross the blood-brain barrier.

5.2 Pharmacokinetic properties

After i.v. administration, the plasma disappearance curve of doxorubicin is triphasic with half-lives of 12 minutes, 3.3 hours and 30 hours. The relatively long terminal elimination half-life reflects doxorubicin's distribution into a deep tissue compartment. Only about 33 to 50% of fluorescent or tritiated drug (or degradation products), respectively, can be accounted for in urine, bile and faeces for up to 5 days after i.v. administration. The remainder of the doxorubicin and degradation products appear to be retained for long periods of time in body tissues.

In cancer patients, doxorubicin is reduced to adriamycinol, which is an active cytotoxic agent. This reduction appears to be catalysed by cytoplasmic nadph-dependent aldo-keto reductases that are found in all tissues and play an important role in determining the overall pharmacokinetics of doxorubicin.

Microsomal glycosidases present in most tissues split doxorubicin and adriamycinol into inactive aglycones. The aglycones may then undergo O-demethylation, followed by conjugation to sulphate or glucuronide esters, and excretion in the bile.

5.3 Preclinical safety data

No further preclinical safety data available.

6. PHARMACEUTICAL PARTICULARS

6.1 List of excipients

Lactose Ph. Eur.

Methyl hydroxybenzoate Ph. Eur.

Water for Injections Ph. Eur.

6.2 Incompatibilities

Doxorubicin Rapid Dissolution should not be mixed with heparin as a precipitate may form and it is not recommended that Doxorubicin Rapid Dissolution be mixed with other drugs. Prolonged contact with any solution of an alkaline pH should be avoided as it will result in hydrolysis of the drug.

6.3 Shelf life

The shelf-life for Doxorubicin Rapid Dissolution is 48 months. Once reconstituted, the solution should be used straight away. If not it may be stored for up to 24 hours.

6.4 Special precautions for storage

None

6.5 Nature and contents of container

Glass vial, type III, with white or grey rubber stopper, aluminium seal and snap cap (10, 20, 50 and 150 mg vials).

6.6 Special precautions for disposal and other handling

The vial contents are under a negative pressure to minimise aerosol formation during reconstitution, particular care should be taken when the needle is inserted. Inhalation of any aerosol produced during reconstitution must be avoided.

The following protective recommendations are given due to the toxic nature of this substance:

- Personnel should be trained in good technique for reconstitution and handling.
- Pregnant staff should be excluded from working with this drug.
- Personnel handling doxorubicin should wear protective clothing: goggles, gowns and disposable gloves and masks.
- A designated area should be defined for reconstitution (preferably under a laminar flow system). The work surface should be protected by disposable plastic-backed absorbent paper.
- All items used for reconstitution, administration or cleaning, including gloves, should be placed in high-risk waste-disposal bags for high temperature incineration.
- Always wash hands after removing gloves.
- In case of skin contact, thoroughly wash the affected area with soap and water or sodium bicarbonate solution. However, do not graze the skin by using a scrubbing brush.
- In case of contact with the eye(s), hold back the eyelid(s) and flush the affected eye(s) with copious amounts of water for at least 15 minutes. Then seek medical evaluation by a physician.
- Spillage or leakage should be treated with dilute sodium hypochlorite (1% available chlorine) solution, preferably soaking overnight and then water. All cleaning materials should be disposed of as indicated previously.

Intravenous administration:

The vial contents must be reconstituted before use with water for injections or normal saline. For reconstitution the contents of the 10mg vial may be dissolved in 5mL Water for injections or Sodium Chloride Injection and those of the 20mg vial in 10mL of the same solvents; 50mg vial in 25mL of the same solvents and 150mg vial in 75mL of the same solvents.

After adding the diluent, the vial contents will dissolve with gentle shaking, without inversion, within 30 seconds. The approximate displacement value of the contents of a 50mg vial, after 25mL of solvent has been added is 0.15mL.

The reconstituted solution contains 0.02% methylhydroxybenzoate. This is not a preservative solution. Discard any unused solution.

Intravesical administration:

Doxorubicin should be instilled using a catheter and retained intravesically for 1-2 hours. During instillation, the patient should be rotated to ensure that the vesical mucosa of the pelvis receives the most extensive contact with the solution. To avoid undue solution with urine, the patients should be instructed not to drink any fluid in the 12 hours prior to instillation. The patient should be instructed to void at the end of the instillation.

Administrative Data

7. MARKETING AUTHORISATION HOLDER

Farmitalia Carlo Erba Limited

Ramsgate Road

Sandwich

Kent

CT13 9NJ

8. MARKETING AUTHORISATION NUMBER(S)

PL 3433/0110

9. DATE OF FIRST AUTHORISATION/RENEWAL OF THE AUTHORISATION

25 June 1987/29 April 1998

10. DATE OF REVISION OF THE TEXT

July 2009

11. Legal Category

POM

Ref: DOB6.0

Doxorubicin Solution for Injection

(Pharmacia Limited)

1. NAME OF THE MEDICINAL PRODUCT

Doxorubicin Solution for Injection

2. QUALITATIVE AND QUANTITATIVE COMPOSITION

Doxorubicin Hydrochloride 2mg/ml

3. PHARMACEUTICAL FORM

Solution for intravenous use

4. CLINICAL PARTICULARS

4.1 Therapeutic indications

Antimitotic and cytotoxic. Doxorubicin has been used successfully to produce regression in a wide range of neoplastic conditions including acute leukaemia, lymphomas, soft-tissue and osteogenic sarcomas, paediatric malignancies and adult solid tumours; in particular breast and lung carcinomas.

Doxorubicin is frequently used in combination chemotherapy regimens with other cytotoxic drugs. Doxorubicin cannot be used as an antibacterial agent.

4.2 Posology and method of administration

The total doxorubicin dose per cycle may differ according to its use within a specific treatment regimen (e.g. given as a single agent or in combination with other cytotoxic drugs) and according to the indication.

The solution is given via the tubing of a freely running intravenous infusion, taking not less than 3 minutes and not more than 10 minutes over the injection. This technique minimises the risk of thrombosis or perivenous extravasation which can lead to severe cellulitis, vesication and necrosis. A direct push injection is not recommended due to the risk of extravasation, which may occur even in the presence of adequate blood return upon needle aspiration (see section 4.4 Special Warnings and Precaution for Use).

Dosage is usually calculated on the basis of body surface area. As a single agent, the recommended standard starting dose of doxorubicin per cycle in adults is 60-90mg/m^2 of body surface area. The total starting dose per cycle may be given as a single dose or divided over 3 successive days or in divided doses given on days 1 and 8. Under conditions of normal recovery from drug-induced toxicity (particularly bone marrow depression and stomatitis), each treatment cycle can be repeated every 3 to 4 weeks. If it is used in combination with other antitumour agents having overlapping toxicity, the dosage of doxorubicin may need to be reduced to 30-60mg/m^2 every three weeks.

If dosage is calculated on the basis of body weight, it has been shown that giving doxorubicin as a single dose every three weeks greatly reduces the distressing toxic effect, mucositis. However, there are still some who believe that dividing the dose over three successive days (0.4-0.8mg/kg or 20-25mg/m^2 on each day) gives greater effectiveness though at the cost of higher toxicity. If dosage is to be calculated on the basis of body weight, 1.2-2.4 mg/kg should be given as a single dose every three weeks.

Administration of doxorubicin in a weekly regimen has been shown to be as effective as the 3-weekly regimen. The recommended dosage is 20mg/m^2 weekly, although, objective responses have been seen at 16mg/m^2. Weekly administration leads to a reduction in cardiotoxicity.

Dosage may also need to be reduced in children, obese patients and the elderly.

Lower starting doses or longer intervals between cycles may need to be considered for heavily pre-treated patients, or patients with neoplastic bone marrow infiltration (see section 4.4 Special Warnings and Precautions for Use).

Hepatic dysfunction

If hepatic function is impaired, doxorubicin dosage should be reduced according to the following table:

Serum Bilirubin Levels	Recommended Dose
1.2 – 3.0 mg/100mL	50% Normal dose
> 3.0 mg/100ml	25% Normal Dose

Doxorubicin should not be administered to patients with severe hepatic impairment (see section 4.3 Contra-indications).

4.3 Contraindications

Hypersensitivity to doxorubicin or any other component of the product, other anthracyclines or anthracenediones.

Intravenous (IV) use:

- persistent myelosuppression
- severe hepatic impairment
- severe myocardial insufficiency
- recent myocardial infarction
- severe arrhythmias
- previous treatment with maximum cumulative doses of doxorubicin, daunorubicin, epirubicin, idarubicin, and/or other anthracyclines and anthracenediones (see section 4.4 Special Warnings and Precautions for Use)

4.4 Special warnings and precautions for use

Doxorubicin should be administered only under the supervision of physicians experienced in the use of cytotoxic therapy.

Patients should recover from the acute toxicities of prior cytotoxic treatment (such as stomatitis, neutropenia, thrombocytopenia, and generalized infections) before beginning treatment with doxorubicin.

The systemic clearance of doxorubicin is reduced in obese patients (i.e. > 130% ideal body weight) (see section 4.2 Posology and Method of Administration).

Cardiac Function

Cardiotoxicity is a risk of anthracycline treatment that may be manifested by early (i.e. acute) or late (i.e. delayed) events.

Early (i.e. Acute) Events: Early cardiotoxicity of doxorubicin consists mainly of sinus tachycardia and/or ECG abnormalities such as non-specific ST-T wave changes. Tachyarrhythmias, including premature ventricular contractions and ventricular tachycardia, bradycardia, as well as atrioventricular and bundle-branch block have also been reported. These effects do not usually predict subsequent development of delayed cardiotoxicity, and are generally not a consideration for discontinuation of doxorubicin treatment.

Late (i.e. Delayed) Events: Delayed cardiotoxicity usually develops late in the course of therapy with doxorubicin or within 2 to 3 months after treatment termination, but later events, several months to years after completion of treatment, have also been reported. Delayed cardiomyopathy is manifested by reduced left ventricular ejection fraction (LVEF) and/or signs and symptoms of congestive heart failure (CHF) such as dyspnoea, pulmonary oedema, dependent oedema, cardiomegaly and hepatomegaly, oliguria, ascites, pleural effusion and gallop rhythm. Subacute effects such as pericarditis/myocarditis have also been reported. Life-threatening CHF is the most severe form of anthracycline-induced cardiomyopathy and represents the cumulative dose-limiting toxicity of the drug.

Cardiac function should be assessed before patients undergo treatment with doxorubicin and must be monitored throughout therapy to minimize the risk of incurring severe cardiac impairment. The risk may be decreased through regular monitoring of LVEF during the course of treatment with prompt discontinuation of doxorubicin at the first sign of impaired function. The appropriate quantitative method for repeated assessment of cardiac function (evaluation of LVEF) includes multi-gated radionuclide angiography (MUGA) or echocardiography (ECHO). A baseline cardiac evaluation with an ECG and either a MUGA scan or an ECHO is recommended, especially in patients with risk factors for increased cardiotoxicity. Repeated MUGA or ECHO determinations of LVEF should be performed, particularly with higher, cumulative anthracycline doses. The technique used for assessment should be consistent throughout follow-up.

The probability of developing CHF, estimated around 1% to 2% at a cumulative dose of 300 mg/m^2 slowly increases up to the total cumulative dose of 450-550 mg/m^2. Thereafter, the risk of developing CHF increases steeply and it is recommended not to exceed a maximum cumulative dose of 550 mg/m^2.

Risk factors for cardiac toxicity include active or dormant cardiovascular disease, prior or concomitant radiotherapy to the mediastinal/pericardial area, previous therapy with other anthracyclines or anthracenediones and concomitant use of drugs with the ability to suppress cardiac contractility or cardiotoxic drugs (e.g., trastuzumab). Anthracyclines including doxorubicin should not be administered in combination with other cardiotoxic agents unless the patient's cardiac function is closely monitored. Patients receiving anthracyclines after stopping treatment with other cardiotoxic agents, especially those with long half-lives such as trastuzumab, may also be at an increased risk of developing cardiotoxicity. The half-life of trastuzumab is approximately 28.5 days and may persist in the circulation for up to 24 weeks. Therefore, physicians should avoid anthracycline-based therapy for up to 24 weeks after stopping trastuzumab when possible. If anthracyclines are used before this time, careful monitoring of cardiac function is recommended.

Cardiac function must be carefully monitored in patients receiving high cumulative doses and in those with risk factors. However, cardiotoxicity with doxorubicin may occur at lower cumulative doses whether or not cardiac risk factors are present.

Children and adolescents are at an increased risk for developing delayed cardiotoxicity following doxorubicin administration. Females may be at greater risk than males. Follow-up cardiac evaluations are recommended periodically to monitor for this effect.

It is probable that the toxicity of doxorubicin and other anthracyclines or anthracenediones is additive.

Haematologic Toxicity

Doxorubicin may produce myelosuppression. Haematologic profiles should be assessed before and during each cycle of therapy with doxorubicin, including differential white blood cell (WBC) counts. A dose-dependent, reversible leucopenia and/or granulocytopenia (neutropenia) is the predominant manifestation of doxorubicin haematologic toxicity and is the most common acute dose-limiting toxicity of this drug. Leucopenia and neutropenia generally reach the nadir between days 10 and 14 after drug administration; the WBC/neutrophil counts return to normal values in most cases by day 21. Thrombocytopenia and anaemia may also occur. Clinical consequences of severe myelosuppression include fever, infections, sepsis/septicaemia, septic shock, haemorrhage, tissue hypoxia or death.

Secondary Leukaemia

Secondary leukaemia, with or without a preleukaemic phase, has been reported in patients treated with anthracyclines. Secondary leukaemia is more common when such drugs are given in combination with DNA-damaging antineoplastic agents, when patients have been heavily pretreated with cytotoxic drugs or when doses of the anthracyclines have been escalated. These leukaemias can have a 1 to 3 year latency period.

Carcinogenesis, Mutagenesis and Impairment of Fertility

Doxorubicin was genotoxic and mutagenic *in vitro* and *in vivo* tests.

In women, doxorubicin may cause infertility during the time of drug administration. Doxorubicin may cause amenorrhoea. Ovulation and menstruation appear to return after termination of therapy, although premature menopause can occur.

Doxorubicin is mutagenic and can induce chromosomal damage in human spermatozoa. Oligospermia or azoospermia may be permanent; however, sperm counts have been reported to return to normospermic levels in some instances. This may occur several years after the end of therapy. Men undergoing doxorubicin treatment should use effective contraceptive methods.

Liver function

The major route of elimination of doxorubicin is the hepatobiliary system. Serum total bilirubin should be evaluated before and during treatment with doxorubicin. Patients with elevated bilirubin may experience slower clearance of the drug with an increase in overall toxicity. Lower doses are recommended in these patients (see section 4.2 Posology and Method of Administration). Patients with severe hepatic impairment should not receive doxorubicin (see section 4.3 Contraindications).

Other

Doxorubicin may potentiate the toxicity of other anticancer therapies. Exacerbation of cyclophosphamide-induced haemorrhagic cystitis and enhanced hepatotoxicity of 6-mercaptopurine have been reported. Radiation-induced toxicities (myocardium, mucosae, skin and liver) have also been reported.

As with other cytotoxic agents, thrombophlebitis and thromboembolic phenomena including pulmonary embolism (in some cases fatal) have been coincidentally reported with the use of doxorubicin.

Tumor-Lysis Syndrome

Doxorubicin may induce hyperuricaemia as a consequence of the extensive purine catabolism that accompanies drug-induced rapid lysis of neoplastic cells (tumour-lysis syndrome). Blood uric acid levels, potassium, calcium phosphate and creatinine should be evaluated after initial treatment. Hydration, urine alkalinisation, and prophylaxis with allopurinol to prevent hyperuricaemia may minimize potential complications of tumour lysis syndrome.

Vaccinations

Administration of live or live-attenuated vaccines in patients immunocompromised by chemotherapeutic agents, including doxorubicin, may result in serious or fatal infections. Vaccination with a live vaccine should be avoided in patients receiving doxorubicin. Killed or inactivated vaccines may be administered; however, the response to such vaccines may be diminished

4.5 Interaction with other medicinal products and other forms of interaction

High dose cyclosporin increases the serum levels and myelotoxicity of doxorubicin.

Doxorubicin is mainly used in combination with other cytotoxic drugs. Additive toxicity may occur especially with regard to bone marrow/haematologic and gastrointestinal effects (see section 4.4 Special Warnings and Precautions for Use). The use of doxorubicin in combination chemotherapy with other potentially cardiotoxic drugs, as well as the concomitant use of other cardioactive compounds (e.g. calcium channel blockers), require monitoring of cardiac function throughout treatment. Changes in hepatic function induced by concomitant therapies may affect doxorubicin metabolism, pharmacokinetics, therapeutic efficacy and/or toxicity.

Paclitaxel can cause increased plasma-concentrations of doxorubicin and/or its metabolites when given prior to doxorubicin. Certain data indicate that a smaller increase is observed when doxorubicin is administered prior to paclitaxel.

4.6 Pregnancy and lactation

Doxorubicin has harmful pharmacological effects on pregnancy and/or the foetus/newborn child.

Due to the embryotoxic potential of doxorubicin, this drug should not be used during pregnancy unless clearly necessary. If a woman receives doxorubicin during pregnancy or becomes pregnant whilst taking the drug, she should be warned of the potential hazard to the foetus. Women of childbearing potential have to use effective contraception during treatment (see section 4.4 Special Warnings and Precautions for Use).

Doxorubicin is secreted into breast milk. Women should not breastfeed while undergoing treatment with doxorubicin.

4.7 Effects on ability to drive and use machines

None stated

4.8 Undesirable effects

The following adverse events (not listed in order of frequency) have been reported in association with doxorubicin therapy:

Neoplasms Benign and Malignant (including cysts and polyps):

The occurrence of secondary acute myeloid leukaemia with or without a pre-leukaemic phase has been reported rarely in patients concurrently treated with doxorubicin in association with DNA-damaging antineoplastic agents. Such cases could have a short (1-3 year) latency period. Acute lymphocytic leukaemia and acute myelogenous leukaemia.

Blood and Lymphatic System Disorders:

Haematological monitoring should be undertaken regularly in both haematological and non haematological conditions, because of the possibility of bone-marrow depression which may become evident around ten days from the time of administration. Clinical consequences of doxorubicin bone marrow/haematological toxicity may be fever, infections, sepsis/septicaemia, septic shock, haemorrhages, tissue hypoxia or death. Leucopenia, neutropenia, anaemia and thrombocytopenia.

Immune System Disorders:

Anaphylaxis.

Metabolism and Nutrition Disorders:

Anorexia, dehydration and hyperuricaemia.

Eye Disorders:

Conjunctivitis / keratitis and lacrimation.

Cardiac Disorders:

Cardiotoxicity may be manifested in tachycardia including supraventricular tachycardia and ECG changes. Routine ECG monitoring is recommended and caution should be exercised in patients with impaired cardiac function. Severe cardiac failure may occur suddenly without premonitory ECG changes. Tachyarrhythmias, atrio-ventricular and bundle branch block, asymptomatic reduction in left ventricular ejection fraction and congestive heart failure.

Vascular Disorders:

Phlebitis, thrombophlebitis, thromboembolism, hot flushes and shock.

Gastrointestinal Disorders:

Nausea, vomiting and mucositis/stomatitis, hyperpigmentation of oral mucosa, oesophagitis, abdominal pain, gastric erosions, gastrointestinal tract bleeding, diarrhoea and colitis.

Hepatobiliary Disorders:

Changes in transaminase levels.

Skin and Subcutaneous Tissue Disorders:

Alopecia occurs frequently, including the interruption of beard growth, but all hair growth normally resumes after treatment is stopped. Skin rashes/itch, local toxicity, skin changes, skin and nail hyperpigmentation, photosensitivity, hypersensitivity to irradiated skin ('radiation recall reaction'), urticaria, acral erythema and plantar-palmar dysaesthesia.

Renal and Urological Disorders:

Doxorubicin may impart a red colour to urine particularly to the first specimen passed after the injection and patients should be advised that this is no cause for alarm.

Reproductive System and Breast Disorders:

Amenorrhoea, oligospermia and azoospermia.

General Disorders and Administration Site Conditions:

The risk of thrombophlebitis at the injection site may be minimised by following the procedure for administration recommended above. A stinging or burning sensation at the site of administration signifies a small degree of extravasation and the infusion should be stopped and re-started in another vein. Fever, malaise, asthenia and chills.

Investigations:

ECG abnormalities.

4.9 Overdose

Single doses of 250mg and 500mg of doxorubicin have proved fatal. Such doses may cause acute myocardial degeneration within 24 hours and severe myelosupression (mainly leucopenia and thrombocytopenia), the effects of which are greatest between 10 and 15 days after administration. Treatment should aim to support the patient during this period and should utilise such measures as blood transfusions and reverse barrier nursing.

Acute overdose with doxorubicin will result in gastrointestinal toxic effects (mainly mucositis). This generally appears early after drug administration, but most patients recover from this within three weeks.

Delayed cardiac failure may occur up to six months after the overdosage. Patients should be observed carefully and should signs of cardiac failure arise, be treated along conventional lines.

5. PHARMACOLOGICAL PROPERTIES

5.1 Pharmacodynamic properties

ATC code: L01DB01

Doxorubicin is an antitumour agent. Tumour cells are probably killed through drug-induced alterations of nucleic acid synthesis although the exact mechanism of action has not yet been clearly elucidated.

Proposed mechanism of action include:

DNA intercalation (leading to an inhibition of synthesis of DNA, RNA and proteins), formation of highly reactive free-radicals and superoxides, chelation of divalent cations, the inhibition of Na-K ATPase and the binding of doxorubicin to certain constituents of cell membranes (particularly to the membrane lipids, spectrin and cardiolipin). Highest drug concentrations are attained in the lung, liver, spleen, kidney, heart, small intestine and bone-marrow. Doxorubicin does not cross the blood-brain barrier.

5.2 Pharmacokinetic properties

After i.v. administration, the plasma disappearance curve of doxorubicin is triphasic with half-lives of 12 minutes, 3.3 hours and 30 hours. The relatively long terminal elimination half-life reflects doxorubicin's distribution into a deep tissue compartment. Only about 33 to 50% of fluorescent or tritiated drug (or degradation products), respectively, can be accounted for in urine, bile and faeces for up to 5 days after i.v. administration. The remainder of the doxorubicin and degradation products appear to be retained for long periods of time in body tissues.

In cancer patients, doxorubicin is reduced to adriamycinol, which is an active cytotoxic agent. This reduction appears to be catalysed by cytoplasmic nadph-dependent aldo-keto reductases that are found in all tissues and play an important role in determining the overall pharmacokinetics of doxorubicin.

Microsomal glycosidases present in most tissues split doxorubicin and adriamycinol into inactive aglycones. The aglycones may then undergo 0-demethylation, followed by conjugation to sulphate or glucuronide esters, and excretion in the bile.

5.3 Preclinical safety data

No information in addition to that presented elsewhere in this Summary of Product Characteristics is available.

6. PHARMACEUTICAL PARTICULARS

6.1 List of excipients

Water for Injections Ph Eur

Sodium chloride Ph Eur

Hydrochloric acid Ph Eur

6.2 Incompatibilities

Doxorubicin should not be mixed with heparin as a precipitate may form and it is not recommended that doxorubicin be mixed with other drugs. Prolonged contact with any solution of an alkaline pH should be avoided as it will result in hydrolysis of the drug.

6.3 Shelf life

2 years

6.4 Special precautions for storage

Store refrigerated between 2- 8°C

6.5 Nature and contents of container

Single glass vials of 5ml (10mg), 10ml (20mg), 25ml (50mg) and 100ml (200mg)

Single Cytosafe® polypropylene vials of 5ml (10mg), 10ml (20mg), 25ml (50mg) and 100ml (200mg)

6.6 Special precautions for disposal and other handling

The following protective recommendations are given due to the toxic nature of this substance:

- Personnel should be trained in good technique for reconstitution and handling.
- Pregnant staff should be excluded from working with this drug.
- Personnel handling doxorubicin should wear protective clothing: goggles, gowns, disposable gloves and masks.
- A designated area should be defined for reconstitution (preferably under a laminar flow system). The work surface should be protected by disposable, plastic-backed and absorbent paper.
- All items for reconstitution, administration or cleaning, including gloves, should be placed in high-risk waste-disposal bags for high temperature incineration.
- Spillage or leakage should be treated with dilute sodium hypochlorite (1% available chlorine) solution, preferably soaking and then water.
- All cleaning materials should be disposed of as indicated previously.
- In case of skin contact, thoroughly wash the affected area with soap and water or sodium bicarbonate solution. However, do not graze the skin by using a scrubbing brush.
- In case of contact with eye(s), hold back the eyelid(s) and flush the affected eyes with copious amounts of water for at least 15 minutes. Then seek medical evaluation by a physician.
- Always wash hands after removing gloves.

Administrative Data

7. MARKETING AUTHORISATION HOLDER

Farmitalia Carlo Erba Limited

Ramsgate Road

Sandwich

Kent

CT13 9NJ

United Kingdom

8. MARKETING AUTHORISATION NUMBER(S)

PL 03433/0127

9. DATE OF FIRST AUTHORISATION/RENEWAL OF THE AUTHORISATION

Renewed 25 January 1995

10. DATE OF REVISION OF THE TEXT

July 2009

Legal Category

POM

Ref: DOA 6.0

Doxorubin 0.2%

(medac GmbH)

1. NAME OF THE MEDICINAL PRODUCT

Doxorubin 0.2%

2. QUALITATIVE AND QUANTITATIVE COMPOSITION

Doxorubin 0.2% injection contains doxorubicin hydrochloride 2 mg/ml.

3. PHARMACEUTICAL FORM

Solution for Injection.

4. CLINICAL PARTICULARS

4.1 Therapeutic indications

In combination with other antineoplastic drugs, doxorubicin is intended for the treatment of acute lymphocytic leukaemia, except acute lymphatic leukaemia of low risk in children, acute myeloid leukaemia (Hodgkin- and non-Hodgkin lymphomas) osteosarcoma, Ewing sarcoma, adult soft tissue sarcoma, metastatic breastcarcinoma, gastric carcinoma, small-cell lung cancer, neuroblastoma, Wilms tumour and bladder carcinoma.

Doxorubicin may be used intravesically as single agent for treatment and prophylaxis of superficial bladder carcinoma.

4.2 Posology and method of administration

Dosage depends on tumour type, hepatic function, and concurrent chemo-therapy.

The commonly recommended dosage schedule as a single agent is 60-75 mg/m^2 by intravenous injection, once every 3 weeks. An alternative dose schedule is 20 mg/m^2 intravenously, on 3 consecutive days, once every 3 weeks.

In combination with other cytotoxic agents doses of 50-75 mg/m^2 are administered. Myelosuppression may be more pronounced because of the additive effects of the drugs.

The risk of development of cardiomyopathy gradually increases with the dosage. A cumulative dose of 550 mg/m^2 should not be exceeded. The administration of doxorubicin should be monitored by electrocardiography, echocardiography and carotid pulse curve: when the voltage of the QRS wave decreases by 30% or at a fractional shortening of 5% it is recommended that treatment is stopped.

If a patient received mediastinal irradiation, has concomitant heart disease, or is also treated with other cardiotoxic, non-anthracyclinecytotoxic agents, a maximal cumulative dose of 400 mg/m^2 is recommended. Doxorubicin dosage should be reduced if the bilirubin is elevated as follows: serum bilirubin 12 to 30 mg/l - give $^1/_2$ of the normal dose, biliru-bin > 30 mg/l - give $^1/_4$ of the normal dose.

In general, impaired renal function does not require dose reduction.

Doxorubicin may be given by intravenous bolus injection, or as continuous infusion. Bolus injection causes higher peak plasma concentrations and therefore is probably more cardiotoxic.

Doxorubicin should not be administered intramuscularly or subcutaneously.

Intravenous administration occurs preferably through a running intravenous infusion, over 3 to 5 minutes.

Patients at increased risk for cardiotoxicity should be considered for treatment with a 24 hours continuous infusion, rather than bolus injection. In this way, cardiotoxicity may be less frequent, without a reduction in therapeutic efficacy. In these patients, the ejection fraction should be measured before each course.

Dosage in children:

Dosage in children may be lowered, since they have an increased risk for late cardiotoxicity. Myelotoxicity should be anticipated, with nadirs at 10 to 12 days after start of treatment, but is usually followed by a rapid recovery due to the large bone marrow reserve of children as compared to adults.

Superficial bladder carcinoma and bladder carcinoma in situ:

The recommended dosage is 50 mg in 50 ml normal saline, administered via a sterile catheter. Initially, this dose is given weekly, later on, monthly. The optimal duration of treatment has not yet been determined; it ranges from 6 to 12 months.

Restrictions regarding the maximal cumulative dose, as with intravenous administration, do not apply to intravesical administration, because systemic absorption of doxorubicin is negligible.

4.3 Contraindications

Myelosuppression, pre-existing heart disease, previous treatment with complete cumulative doses of doxorubicin or other anthracyclines.

Doxorubicin should not be used intravesically for the treatment of bladder carcinoma in patients with urethral stenosis who can not be catheterised.

4.4 Special warnings and precautions for use

Nausea, vomiting and mucositis are often severe and should be treated appropriately.

Doxorubicin should not be administered intramuscularly or subcutaneously.

Extravasation results in a severe and progressive tissue necrosis. If extravasation occurs, the injection should be terminated immediately and restarted in another vein. Flooding with normal saline, local infiltration with corticosteroids, or sodium hydrogen carbonate solution (8.4%), and application of dimethylsulphoxide have been reported with varying success. The advice of the plastic surgery consultant should be asked for, and wide excision of the involved area should be considered.

Exceeding the maximum cumulative dose of 550 mg/m^2 increases the risk of severe, irreversible and therapy-resistant cardiomyopathy and resulting congestive heart failure. Age over 70 or below 15 years should be considered a risk factor, as well as concomitant heart disease. In addition, ECG changes may occur including a reduction in the voltage of the QRS wave, and a prolongation of the systolic time interval, and the ejection fraction may be reduced.

In patients previously treated with other anthracyclines or cyclophos-phamide, mitomycin C or dacarbazine and patients who received radiotherapy to the mediastinal area, cardiotoxicity may occur at doses lower than the recommended cumulative limit.

Acute severe arrhythmias have been reported to occur during or within a few hours after doxorubicin administration.

Heart function should be assessed before, during and after doxorubicin therapy, e.g., by ECG, echocardiography or determination of the ejection fraction.

The high incidence of bone marrow depression requires careful haematologic monitoring. Doxorubicin therapy should not be started or continued when polynuclear granulocyte counts are below 2000/mm^3, except in the treatment of acute leukaemia, where lower limits may be applied.

Careful haematologic monitoring is also required because of the risk of secondary leukaemias after treatment with cytotoxic agents (see section 4.8 "Undesirable effects"). These leukaemias can be cured when detected at an early stage.

Hepatic function should be evaluated before and during therapy.

Doxorubicin may induce hyperuricemia. The blood uric acid level should be monitored; sufficient fluid intake should be ascertained (with a daily minimum of 3 l/m^2). If necessary, a xanthine-oxidase inhibitor (allopurinol) may be administered.

Men as well as woment should take effective contraceptive measures during and for at least 3 months after doxorubicin therapy.

Doxorubicin may impart a red coloration to the urine.

4.5 Interaction with other medicinal products and other forms of interaction

Doxorubicin cardiotoxicity is enhanced by previous or concurrent use of other anthracyclines, mitomycin C, dacarbazine, dactinomycin and, possibly, cyclophosphamide.

Doxorubicin may cause exacerbations of haemorragic cystitis caused by previous cyclophosphamide therapy.

The effects of radiation may be enhanced, and recall of these reactions may occur with doxorubicin therapy, even some time after termination of radiotherapy.

Inducers of the enzyme cytochrome P-450 (e.g. rifampicin and barbiturates) may stimulate the metabolism of doxorubicin, with a possible decrease in efficacy.

Inhibitors of cytochrome P-450 (e.g. cimetidine) may decrease the metabolism of doxorubicin, with a possible increase in toxic effects.

4.6 Pregnancy and lactation

Clinical evidence suggests a possible adverse effect on the foetus. In animals doxorubicin has embryotoxic and teratogenic effects.

Doxorubicin is excreted in breast milk. Usage during pregnancy and lactation is therefore not recommended.

4.7 Effects on ability to drive and use machines

Due to the frequent occurrence of nausea and vomiting, driving and operation of machinery should be discouraged.

4.8 Undesirable effects

Dose limiting toxicities of therapy are myelosuppression and cardio-toxicity. Myelosuppression includes a transient leukopenia, anemia and thrombocytopenia, reaching its nadir at 10 to 14 days after treatment.

Cardiotoxicity may occur as arrhythmia directly following drug administration; ECG changes, including T-wave flattening and S-T depression, may last up to 2 weeks after administration.

The risk of cardiomyopathy increases at cumulative doses higher than 550 mg/m^2. Age over 70 or below 15 years should be regarded as a risk factor. Also, concomitant or previous treatment with mitomycin C, cyclophosphamide or dacarbazine has been reported to potentiate doxorubicin induced cardiomyopathy.

Cardiotoxicity may be encountered several weeks or months after discontinuation of doxorubicin therapy.

Other adverse reactions reported are: a generally reversible alopecia; gastrointestinal disturbances, including nausea, vomiting and diarrhea. Mucositis (stomatitis or esophagitis) may occur 5 to 10 days after administration.

Hypersensitivity reactions, such as fever, urticaria and anaphylaxis have been occasionally reported. Doxorubicin influences and potentiates normal tissue reactions to radiation. Also, late ("recall") reactions may occur when doxorubicin is administered some time after irradiation.

Facial flushing may occur if the injection is given too rapidly.

Thrombophlebitis and conjunctivitis have been reported.

Slight transient increases of liver enzymes have been reported. Concomitant irradiation of the liver may cause severe hepatotoxicity, sometimes progressing to cirrhosis

As with other cytotoxic agents, myelodysplastic syndrome and acute myeloid leukaemia have been observed after treatment with combination therapy including doxorubicin. With topoisomerase II inhibitors, secondary leukaemias have been reported more frequently than expected in the form of acute myeloid leukaemia classification 2, 3, and 4. These forms of leukaemia can have a short period of latency (1 to 3 years). They can be cured when detected at an early stage and with an appropriate curative treatment (see section 4.4 "Special warnings and special precautions for use").

Intravesical administration may cause the following adverse reactions: haematuria, vesical and urethral irritation, stranguria and pollakisuria. These reactions are usually of moderate severity and of short duration.

Intravesical administration of doxorubicin may cause a sometimes hemorrhagic cystitis; this may cause a decrease in bladder capacity.

Doxorubicin may impart a red colouration to the urine.

4.9 Overdose

Acute overdosage of doxorubicin enhances the toxic effects of mucositis, leukopenia and thrombocytopenia. Overdosage at intravesical administration may cause severe cystitis. Treatment of acute overdosage consists of treatment of the severely myelosuppressed patient with hospitalization, antibiotics and transfusions after consultation with an oncologist.

Chronic overdosage with cumulative doses exceeding 550 mg/m^2 increases the risk of cardiomyopathy and resultant congestive heart failure. Treatment consists of vigorous management of congestive heart failure with digitalis preparations and diuretics.

Administration of a very high single dose may cause myocardial degeneration within 24 hours.

5. PHARMACOLOGICAL PROPERTIES

5.1 Pharmacodynamic properties

Doxorubicin is a cytotoxic anthracycline antibiotic isolated from cultures of *Streptomyces peucetius var. caesius*. Animal studies have shown a cytotoxic action in several solid and haematologic tumours. The mechanism of action is not completely elucidated. A major mechanism is probably inhibition of topoisomerase II, resulting in DNA breakage. Intercalation and free-radical formation is probably of minor importance. Drug resistance, due to increased expression of the MDR-1 gene encoding for a multidrug efflux pump, has been reported regularly.

5.2 Pharmacokinetic properties

The intravenous administration of doxorubicin is followed by a rapid plasma clearance (t½ approx. 10 min.) and significant tissue binding. The terminal half-life is approximately 30 hours.

Doxorubicin is partly metabolised, mainly to doxorubicinol and to a lesser extent, to the aglycon, and is conjugated to the glucuronide and sulfate. Biliary and fecal excretion represents the major excretion route. About 5% of the dose is eliminated by renal excretion. Plasma protein binding of doxorubicin ranges from 50-85%. The volume of distribution is 800-3500 l/m^2.

Doxorubicin is not absorbed after oral administration; it does not cross the blood-brain barrier.

Impairment of liver function may decrease the clearance of doxorubicin and its metabolites.

5.3 Preclinical safety data

Non stated.

6. PHARMACEUTICAL PARTICULARS

6.1 List of excipients

Sodium chloride, hydrochloric acid/sodium hydroxide, water for injections.

6.2 Incompatibilities

Doxorubicin should not be mixed with 5-fluorouracil or heparin. Contact with aluminium should be avoided.

6.3 Shelf life

Following the special precautions for storage (see section 6.4) the shelf-life of the 5 ml, 10 ml, and 25 ml vials is 36 months and the shelf life of the 100 ml vial is 24 months as printed on the label.

The injection may be diluted with 0.9% sodium chloride solution or 5% glucose solution.

Chemical and physical in-use stability has been demonstrated for 7 days at room temperature (15-25°C) and protected from light.

From a microbiological point of view, the product should be used immediately. If not used immediately, in-use storage times and conditions prior to use are the responsibility of the user and would normally not be longer than 24 hours at 2 to 8°C, unless dilution has taken place in controlled and validated aseptic conditions.

6.4 Special precautions for storage

Doxorubin 0.2%, injection should be stored at 2-8°C, protected from light.

6.5 Nature and contents of container

Doxorubin 0.2%, injection is supplied as a red-orange, sterile solution in injection vials containing 5 ml (10 mg), 10 ml (20 mg), 25 ml (50 mg), or 100 ml (200 mg), respectively, of doxorubicin hydrochloride 2 mg/ml.

6.6 Special precautions for disposal and other handling

Any contact with the solution should be avoided. During preparation and reconstitution a strictly aseptic working technique should be used; protective measures should include the use of gloves, mask, safety goggles and protective clothing. Use of a vertical laminair airflow (LAF) hood is recommended.

Gloves should be worn during administration. Waste-disposal procedures should take into account the cytotoxic nature of this substance.

If doxorubicin solution contacts skin, mucosae, or eyes, immediately wash thoroughly with water. Soap may be used for skin cleansing.

7. MARKETING AUTHORISATION HOLDER

Pharmachemie B.V.

Postbus 552

2003 RN Haarlem

The Netherlands.

8. MARKETING AUTHORISATION NUMBER(S)

PL 4946/0016.

9. DATE OF FIRST AUTHORISATION/RENEWAL OF THE AUTHORISATION

4 January 1996

10. DATE OF REVISION OF THE TEXT

January 2001

Doxorubin 10 mg, 50 mg

(medac GmbH)

1. NAME OF THE MEDICINAL PRODUCT

Doxorubin 10 mg.

Doxorubin 50 mg.

2. QUALITATIVE AND QUANTITATIVE COMPOSITION

Doxorubin 10 mg:

Doxorubin, powder for solution for injection contains 10 mg of doxorubicin hydrochloride E.P.

Doxorubin 50 mg:

Doxorubin, powder for solution for injection contains 50 mg of doxorubicin hydrochloride E.P.

3. PHARMACEUTICAL FORM

Powder for solution for injection.

4. CLINICAL PARTICULARS

4.1 Therapeutic indications

In combination with other antineoplastic drugs, doxorubicin is intended for the treatment of acute lymphocytic leukaemia, (except acute lymphatic leukaemia of low risk in children), acute myeloid leukaemia, Hodgkin- and non-Hodgkin lymphomas, osteosarcoma, Ewing sarcoma, adult soft tissue sarcoma, metastatic breast carcinoma, gastric carcinoma, small-cell lung cancer, neuroblastoma, Wilms tumour and bladder carcinoma.

Doxorubicin may be used intravesically as single agent for treatment and prophylaxis of superficial bladder carcinoma.

4.2 Posology and method of administration

The route of administration is by intravenous injection.

The vial contents must be reconstituted before use with water for injection or normal saline (see Section 6.6 Instructions for Use/Handling).

Doxorubicin should **not** be administered intramuscularly or subcutaneously.

INTRAVENOUS ADMINISTRATION

Doxorubicin may be given by intravenous bolus injection, or as continuous infusion. Bolus injection causes higher peak plasma concentration and therefore is probably more cardiotoxic. Intravenous administration occurs preferably through a running, recently applied intravenous infusion, of sodium chloride injection, dextrose injection 5% or sodium chloride and dextrose injection over 3 to 5 minutes.

Patients with an increased risk for cardiotoxicity (see section 4.4 Special warnings and precautions for use) should be considered for treatment with a 24 hours continuous infusion, rather than bolus injection. In this way, cardiotoxicity may be less frequent, without a reduction in therapeutic efficacy. In these patients, the ejection fraction should be measured before each course.

ADULTS

Dosage depends on tumour type, hepatic function, and concurrent chemotherapy.

The commonly recommended dosage schedule as single agent is 60-75 mg/m^2 by intravenous injection, once every 3 weeks. An alternative dose schedule is 20 mg/m^2 intravenously, during 3 consecutive days, once every 3 weeks.

Lower doses may be required in patients with inadequate marrow reserves and in patients who have had prior treatment with other cytotoxic agents. When used in combination with other chemotherapeutic agents the dosage of 30-60 mg/m^2 are administered. Myelosuppression may be more pronounced because of the additive effect of the drugs.

The risk of development of cardiomyopathy gradually increases with the dosage. The maximum cumulative dose of 450 mg/m^2 should not be exceeded. The administration of doxorubicin should be monitored by electrocardiography, echocardiography and carotid pulse curve: When the voltage of the QRS wave decreases by 30% or at a fractional shortening of 5% it is recommended to stop treatment.

If a patient receives mediastinal irradiation, has concomitant heart disease, or is also treated with other cardiotoxic, non-anthracycline oncolytics, a maximal cumulative dose of 400 mg/m^2 is recommended.

Doxorubicin dosage should be reduced if the bilirubin is elevated. When bilirubin is 12 to 30 mg/l - half the dosage should be given; when bilirubin concentrations $>$ 30 mg/l, one quarter of the dosage should be given.

In general, impaired renal function does not require dose reduction.

CHILDREN

Dosage for children may be lowered, since they have an increased risk for late cardiotoxicity. Myelotoxicity should be anticipated, with nadirs at 10 to 14 days after start of treatment, but is usually followed by a rapid recovery due to the large bone marrow reserve of children as compared to adults.

SUPERFICIAL BLADDER CARCINOMA AND BLADDER CARCINOMA IN SITU:

The recommended dosage is 50 mg in 50 ml normal saline, administered via a sterile catheter. Initially, this dose is given weekly, later on monthly. The optimal duration of treatment has not yet been determined; it ranges from 6 to 12 months.

Restrictions regarding the maximal cumulative dose, as with intravenous administration, do not apply to intravesical administration, because systemic absorption of doxorubicin is negligible.

4.3 Contraindications

Doxorubicin therapy should not be started in the following cases:

1. Marked myelosuppression induced by previous chemotherapy or by radiotherapy.
2. Pre-existing heart disease.
3. Previous treatment with complete cumulative doses of doxorubicin or other anthracyclines.
4. Doxorubicin should not be used intravesically for the treatment of bladder carcinoma in patients with urethral stenosis who can not be catheterised.

4.4 Special warnings and precautions for use

General precautions

Doxorubicin should only be used under supervision of a physician who is experienced in cytotoxic therapy. Nausea, vomiting and mucositis are often severe and should be treated appropriately.

Doxorubicin should **not** be administered intramuscularly or subcutaneously.

The total dose of doxorubicin administered to the individual patient should take into account any previous or concomitant therapy with related compounds such as daunorubicin.

Extravasation

Extravasation results in a severe and progressive tissue necrosis. If extravasation occurs, the injection should be terminated immediately and restarted in another vein. Flooding with normal saline, local infiltration with corticosteroids with or without sodium hydrogen carbonate solution (8.4%), and application of dimethylsulfoxide have been reported with varying success. The advice of a plastic surgeon should be sought, and wide excision of the involved area should be considered.

Cardiotoxicity

Congestive heart failure and/or cardiomyopathy may be encountered several weeks after discontinuation of doxorubicin therapy. Severe cardiac failure may occur precipitously without antecedent ECG change.

The risk of severe, irreversible and therapy-resistant cardiomyopathy and resulting congestive heart failure gradually increases with increasing dosages. A cumulative dose of 450 mg/m^2 should not be exceeded.

Age over 70 or below 15 years and female gender in children should be considered a risk factor, as well as concomitant heart disease. In addition, ECG changes may occur including a reduction in the voltage of the QRS wave, and a prolongation of the systolic time interval, and the ejection fraction may be reduced.

In patients previously treated with other anthracyclines or cyclophosphamide, mitomycin C or dacarbazine, and patients who received radiotherapy to the mediastinal area, cardiotoxicity may occur at doses lower than the recommended cumulative limit. The concurrent use of trastuzumab and anthracyclines (like doxorubicin) is not recommended (see section 4.5).

Acute severe arrhythmias have been reported to occur during or within a few hours after doxorubicin administration.

Heart function should be assessed before, during and after doxorubicin therapy, e.g., by ECG, echocardiography or determination of the ejection fraction. If test results indicate change in cardiac function associated with doxorubicin the benefit of continued therapy must be carefully evaluated against the risk of producing irreversible cardiac damage.

Myelosuppression

The high incidence of bone marrow depression requires careful haematologic monitoring. The nadir is reached between 10-14 days after administration. Blood values usually return to normal within 21 days after administration. Doxorubicin therapy should not be started or continued when polynuclear granulocyte counts are below 2000/mm^3, except in the treatment of acute leukaemia, where lower limits may be applied, depending on the circumstances.

Careful haematologic monitoring is also required because of the risk of secondary leukaemias after treatment with cytotoxic agents (see section 4.8 Undesirable effects). A remission of acute leukaemia can be achieved when detected at an early stage.

Hepatic impairment

Hepatic function (SGOT, SGPT, alkaline phosphatase and bilirubin) should be evaluated before and during therapy.

Hyperuricaemia

Doxorubicin may induce hyperuricemia. The blood uric acid level should be monitored. Sufficient fluid intake should be ascertained (with a daily minimum of 3 l/m^2). If necessary, a xanthine-oxidase inhibitor (allopurinol) may be administered.

Discoloration of urine

Doxorubicin may impart a red coloration to the urine.

4.5 Interaction with other medicinal products and other forms of interaction

Doxorubicin cardiotoxicity is enhanced by previous or concurrent use of other anthracyclines, mitomycin C, dacarbazine, dactinomycin and, possibly, cyclophosphamide. Also the risk of cardiotoxicity is increased if trastuzumab is given with or after doxorubicin. Trastuzumab and anthracyclines should not be used concurrently in combination except in a well-controlled clinical trial setting with cardiac monitoring. Furthermore, paclitaxel decreases the elimination of doxorubicin. Care should be taken in case of co- administration of both drugs, because of an increased risk of cardiotoxic effects of doxorubicin. The severity of neutropenia or stomatitis may also be increased.

Doxorubicin may cause exacerbations of haemorrhagic cystitis caused by previous cyclophosphamide therapy.

Doxorubicin may enhance the hepatotoxicity of 6-mercaptopurine.

The effects of radiation may be enhanced, and recall of these reactions may occur with doxorubicin therapy, even some time after termination of radiotherapy.

Inducers of the enzyme cytochrome P-450 (e.g. rifampicin and barbiturates) may stimulate the metabolism of doxorubicin, with a possible decrease in efficacy.

Inhibitors of cytochrome P-450 (e.g. cimetidine) may decrease the metabolism of doxorubicin, with a possible increase in toxic effects.

4.6 Pregnancy and lactation

Clinical evidence suggests a possible adverse effect on the foetus. In animals doxorubicin has embryotoxic and teratogenic effects.

Doxorubicin is excreted into breast milk. Usage during pregnancy and lactation is therefore not recommended.

Men as well as women should take effective contraceptive measures during and for at least three months after doxorubicin therapy.

4.7 Effects on ability to drive and use machines

Due to the frequent occurrence of nausea and vomiting, driving cars and operation of machinery should be discouraged.

4.8 Undesirable effects

Dose limiting toxicities of therapy are myelosuppression and cardiotoxicity.

Blood and Lymphatic System Disorder

Myelosuppression includes a transient leucopenia very commonly. Anaemia and thrombocytopenia are less common. Myelosuppression reaches its nadir at 10 to 14 days after treatment. Blood levels usually return to normal within 21 days after administration.

Myelodysplastic syndrome and acute myeloid leukaemia have been observed after treatment with combination therapy including doxorubicin. With topoisomerase II inhibitors, secondary leukaemias have been reported more frequently than expected in the form of acute myeloid leukaemia classification 2, 3, and 4. These forms of leukaemia can have a short period of latency (1 to 3 years) but much longer periods have been reported. They can be cured when detected at an early stage and with an appropriate curative treatment (see section 4.4 Special warnings and special precautions for use).

Immune Disorder

Hypersensitivity reactions, such as fever, urticaria and anaphylaxis occur rarely. Doxorubicin influences and potentiates normal tissue reactions to radiation. Also, late (recall) reactions may occur when doxorubicin is administered some time after irradiation. Facial flushing may occur if the injection is given too rapidly.

Cardiac Disorder

Cardiotoxicity may occur as arrhythmia directly following drug administration; ECG changes, including T-wave flattening and S-T depression, may last up to 2 weeks after administration.

The risk of cardiomyopathy increases with an increasing dosage. Severe cardiotoxicity is more likely after high cumulative doses of doxorubicin (see section 4.4 Special Warnings and Precautions for Use) and may occur months or years after administration.

Gastrointestinal Disorder

Nausea and vomiting are very common and diarrhoea occurs occasionally.

Mucositis (stomatitis or oesophagitis) may occur 5 to 10 days after administration.

Hepato-biliary Disorder

Slight transient increases of liver enzymes have been reported. Concomitant irradiation of the liver may cause severe hepatotoxicity, sometimes progressing to cirrhosis.

Other adverse reactions:

A generally reversible alopecia is very common.

A red colouration of the urine, imparted by doxorubicin, is very common.

Thrombophlebitis and conjunctivitis have been reported.

Doxorubicin may induce hyperuricemia.

Intravesical Administration

Intravesical administration may cause the following adverse reactions: haematuria, vesical and urethral irritation, dysuria, stranguria and pollakisuria. These reactions are usually of moderate severity and of short duration. Intravesical administration of doxorubicin may sometimes cause a haemorrhagic cystitis; this may cause a decrease in bladder capacity.

4.9 Overdose

Acute overdose of doxorubicin enhances the toxic effects, particularly-mucositis, leucopenia and thrombocytopenia. Overdose of intravesical administration may result in more severe cystitis. Treatment of acute overdose consists of treatment of the severely myelosuppressed patient with hospitalisation, antibiotics and transfusions after consultation of an oncologist.

Chronic overdosage with cumulative doses exceeding 450 mg/m^2 increases the risk of cardiomyopathy and resultant congestive heart failure. Treatment consists of vigorous management of congestive heart failure with digitalis preparations and diuretics. Single doses of 250 mg and 500 mg of doxorubicin have proved fatal. Such doses may cause acute myocardial degeneration within 24 hours and severe myelosuppression, the effects of which are greatest between 10 and 15 days after administration. Treatment should be symptomatic and supportive. Delayed cardiac failure may occur up to six months after the overdose.

5. PHARMACOLOGICAL PROPERTIES

5.1 Pharmacodynamic properties

Doxorubicin is an oncolytic drug of the anthracycline group. It is isolated from cultures of Streptomyces peucetius var. caesius. Animal studies have shown an oncolytic action in several solid and haematologic tumours. The mechanism of action is not completely elucidated. A major mechanism is probably inhibition of topoisomerase II, resulting in DNA breakage. Intercalation and free-radical formation is probably of minor importance. Drug resistance, due to increased expression of the MDR-1 gene encoding for a multidrug efflux pump, has been reported regularly.

5.2 Pharmacokinetic properties

The intravenous administration of doxorubicin is followed by a rapid plasma clearance (t1/2 ~ 10 min.) and significant tissue binding. The terminal half-life is approximately 30 hours.

Doxorubicin is partly metabolised, mainly to doxorubicinol and to a lesser extent, to the aglycone, and is conjugated to the glucuronide and sulphate. Biliary and faecal excretion represents the major excretion route. About 10% of the dose is eliminated by renal excretion. Plasma protein binding of doxorubicin ranges from 50-85%. The volume of distribution is 800-3500 1/m^2.

Doxorubicin is not absorbed after oral administration; it does not cross the blood-brain barrier.

Impairment of liver function may decrease the clearance of doxorubicin and its metabolites.

5.3 Preclinical safety data

There are no preclinical safety data of relevance to the prescriber which are additional to those already stated in other sections of the SPC.

6. PHARMACEUTICAL PARTICULARS

6.1 List of excipients

Lactose

6.2 Incompatibilities

Doxorubicin should not be mixed with other drugs. Alkaline solutions may hydrolyse doxorubicin. Doxorubicin should not be mixed with heparin or 5-fluorouracil. Contact with aluminium should be avoided.

6.3 Shelf life

Following the special precautions for storage (see below) the shelf life for the powder for solution for injection is 5 years. The expiration date is printed on the label.

Chemical and physical in-use stability of the reconstituted solution in 0.9% sodium chloride solution has been demonstrated for 7 days at 15-25 C and for 14 days under refrigeration (2-8 C).

Chemical and physical in-use stability of a 0.5 mg/ml solution in water for injections has been demonstrated for 24 hours at temperatures below 25 C.

Chemical and physical in-use stability of solutions in the range 0.05 mg/ml to 5 mg/ml in 0.9% sodium chloride solution has been demonstrated for 7 days at room temperature (15-25 C).

From a microbiological point of view, the product should be used immediately. If not used immediately, in-use storage times and conditions prior to use are the responsibility of the user and would normally not be longer than 24 hours at 2 to 8 C, unless reconstitution has taken place in controlled and validated aseptic conditions.

6.4 Special precautions for storage

Doxorubin, powder for solution for injection, 10 mg (50 mg) should be stored at 15-25 C, protected from light.

6.5 Nature and contents of container

Doxorubin, powder for solution for injection, 10 mg (50 mg) is supplied as a red-orange, sterile, lyophilized powder, in glass injection vials with aluminium seal. The package size is 1 or 10 vials.

6.6 Special precautions for disposal and other handling

Instructions for reconstitution:

For intravenous injection, Doxorubicin powder for solution for injection should be reconstituted to a concentration of 2 mg/ml in water for injections immediately before use. Alternatively, sodium chloride for injections may be used as a solvent, however, the product may take longer to dissolve.

In order to reconstitute the product, ensure the powder, solutions and equipment are at room temperature, add 5 (25) ml to the 10 (50) mg vial and shake for at least 60 seconds and leave to stand at room temperature for at least 5 minutes before administration to get a clear red mobile liquid. If gelatinous fragments are seen, leave the solution to stand for 5 minutes and shake again. Should the fragments still be visible, discard the solution.

When water for injections is used, immediate dilution to a concentration of less than 0.4mg/ml doxorubicin with 0.9% sodium chloride solution or 5% glucose solution is needed in order to obtain an isotonic solution.

Due to the toxic nature of doxorubicin it is recommended that the following protective measures be taken:

- *General instructions for safe use of cytotoxics:*
- Training in good techniques for reconstitution and handling should be given to relevant personnel.
- Pregnant staff should be excluded from working with this drug
- Protective clothing should be worn while administering, handling or reconstituting doxorubicin
- Contact with skin or eyes should be avoided. If it occurs, the affected area should be washed immediately with water, soap and water or sodium bicarbonate solution.
- Any spillages should be cleaned with dilute sodium hypochlorite solution.
- All equipment used for the handling, preparation and administration of doxorubicin should be incinerated.

Unused products should be disposed of in a suitable labelled container, marked as hazardous waste.

7. MARKETING AUTHORISATION HOLDER

Pharmachemie B.V.

Swensweg 5

PO Box 552

2003 RN Haarlem

The Netherlands.

8. MARKETING AUTHORISATION NUMBER(S)

Doxorubin 10 mg: PL 4946/0001

Doxorubin 50 mg: PL 4946/0002

9. DATE OF FIRST AUTHORISATION/RENEWAL OF THE AUTHORISATION

12-July-1993

10. DATE OF REVISION OF THE TEXT

April 2005

Driclor

(Stiefel Laboratories (UK) Limited)

1. NAME OF THE MEDICINAL PRODUCT

Driclor

2. QUALITATIVE AND QUANTITATIVE COMPOSITION

Aluminium Chloride Hexahydrate 20% w/w

For a full list of excipients, see section 6.1

3. PHARMACEUTICAL FORM

Solution for topical application

4. CLINICAL PARTICULARS

4.1 Therapeutic indications

Driclor is indicated for the treatment of hyperhidrosis.

4.2 Posology and method of administration

Apply Driclor last thing at night after drying the affected areas carefully. Wash off in the morning. Do not re-apply the product during the day.

Initially the product may be applied each night until sweating stops during the day. The frequency of application may then be reduced to twice a week or less.

4.3 Contraindications

Hypersensitivity to the active substance or to any of the excipients.

4.4 Special warnings and precautions for use

Ensure that the affected areas to be treated are completely dry before application.

Do not apply Driclor to broken, irritated or recently shaven skin. Avoid contact with eyes.

Avoid direct contact with clothing and polished metal surfaces.

4.5 Interaction with other medicinal products and other forms of interaction

None known

4.6 Pregnancy and lactation

There are no restrictions on the use of Driclor during pregnancy or lactation.

4.7 Effects on ability to drive and use machines

None

4.8 Undesirable effects

Driclor may cause irritation which may be alleviated by use of a weak corticosteroid cream.

4.9 Overdose

Not applicable.

5. PHARMACOLOGICAL PROPERTIES

5.1 Pharmacodynamic properties

Aluminium chloride hexahydrate acts locally, in the stratum corneum and in the terminal duct, to relieve hyperhidrosis.

5.2 Pharmacokinetic properties

Not applicable.

5.3 Preclinical safety data

Not applicable.

6. PHARMACEUTICAL PARTICULARS

6.1 List of excipients

	% w/w
Ethanol	75.45
Purified water	4.55

6.2 Incompatibilities

None

6.3 Shelf life

a) For the product as packaged for sale

3 years

b) After first opening the container

Comply with expiry date.

6.4 Special precautions for storage

Store in a cool place below 25 °C. Keep away from naked flame. Store upright.

6.5 Nature and contents of container

High density polyethylene bottle with roll-on applicator.

Pack size: 30ml, 40ml, 45ml, 50ml and 60ml

High density polyethylene bottle with polypropylene cap.

LDPE housing containing polypropylene roller-ball with over-cap for self-assembly.

Pack Size: 75ml

Not all pack sizes may be marketed.

6.6 Special precautions for disposal and other handling

The 75ml pack should be assembled according to the instructions in the package leaflet.

7. MARKETING AUTHORISATION HOLDER

Stiefel Laboratories (UK) Ltd

Eurasia Headquarters

Concorde Road

Maidenhead

SL6 4BY

UK

8. MARKETING AUTHORISATION NUMBER(S)

PL 0174/0044

9. DATE OF FIRST AUTHORISATION/RENEWAL OF THE AUTHORISATION

31st August 1981/ 7th January 2005

10. DATE OF REVISION OF THE TEXT

August 2009

Duac Once Daily 10mg/g + 50mg/g Gel

(Stiefel Laboratories (UK) Limited)

1. NAME OF THE MEDICINAL PRODUCT

Duac Once Daily 10mg/g + 50mg/g Gel

2. QUALITATIVE AND QUANTITATIVE COMPOSITION

1g of gel contains:

10mg clindamycin as clindamycin phosphate

50mg anhydrous benzoyl peroxide as hydrous benzoyl peroxide

For a full list of excipients, see section 6.1.

3. PHARMACEUTICAL FORM

Gel

White to slightly yellow homogeneous gel

4. CLINICAL PARTICULARS

4.1 Therapeutic indications

Mild to moderate acne vulgaris, particularly inflammatory lesions.

See section 5.1

4.2 Posology and method of administration

For application to the skin. For external use only.

Adults and adolescents

Duac Once Daily Gel should be applied once daily in the evening, to affected areas after the skin has been thoroughly washed, rinsed with warm water and gently patted dry.

Use in Children

The safety and efficacy of Duac Once Daily Gel has not been established in prepubescent children (under 12 years of age), since acne vulgaris rarely presents in this age group.

Use in the Elderly

No specific recommendations.

Treatment with Duac Once Daily Gel should not exceed more than 12 weeks of continuous use.

4.3 Contraindications

Duac Once Daily Gel must not be administered to patients with known hypersensitivity to:

- clindamycin
- lincomycin
- benzoyl peroxide
- any of the excipients in the formulation.

4.4 Special warnings and precautions for use

Contact with the mouth, eyes and mucous membranes and with abraded or eczematous skin should be avoided. Application to sensitive areas of skin should be made with caution. In the event of accidental contact with the eyes, bathe with copious amounts of water.

Duac Once Daily Gel should be used with caution in patients with a history of regional enteritis or ulcerative colitis, or a history of antibiotic-associated colitis. It should also be used with caution in atopic patients, in whom further skin drying may occur.

The frequency of application should be reduced if excessive irritation or dryness develops.

If prolonged or significant diarrhoea occurs or the patient suffers from abdominal cramps, treatment with Duac Once Daily Gel should be discontinued immediately, as the symptoms may indicate antibiotic-associated colitis. Suitable diagnostic methods, such as the determination of *Clostridium difficile* and toxin and, if necessary, colonoscopy should be employed and treatment options for colitis considered.

The product may bleach hair or coloured fabrics.

It is recommended that exposure to sun or sunlamps should be minimised.

Patients should be advised that, in some cases, 4-6 weeks of treatment may be required before the full therapeutic effect is observed.

Cross-resistance may occur with other antibiotics such as lincomycin and erythromycin when using antibiotic monotherapy.

Local recommendations about antibiotic use and prevalence of acquired resistance should be taken into consideration.

4.5 Interaction with other medicinal products and other forms of interaction

Concomitant topical antibiotics, medicated or abrasive soaps and cleansers, soaps and cosmetics that have a strong drying effect, and products with high concentrations of alcohol and/or astringents, should be used with caution as a cumulative irritant effect may occur.

Simultaneous application of Duac Once Daily Gel and topical acne preparations containing vitamin A derivatives should be avoided.

Potential synergism exists between clindamycin and gentamycin.

4.6 Pregnancy and lactation

There are no adequate data from the use of Duac Once Daily Gel in pregnant women. Animal reproductive/developmental studies have not been conducted with Duac Once Daily Gel or benzoyl peroxide. Data from a limited number of pregnancies exposed in the first trimester to clindamycin indicate no adverse effects of clindamycin on pregnancy or on the health of the foetus/new-born child. Reproduction studies in rats and mice, using subcutaneous and oral doses of clindamycin, revealed no evidence of impaired fertility or harm to the foetus due to clindamycin.

The safety of Duac Once Daily Gel in human pregnancy is not established. Therefore, Duac Once Daily Gel should only be prescribed to pregnant women after careful risk/benefit assessment by the physician in charge.

Women of child-bearing potential

There are no contraindications in women of child-bearing potential who are practising adequate contraception. However, due to the lack of clinical studies in pregnant women, Duac Once Daily Gel should be used with caution when adequate contraception is not being practised.

Use during lactation

There is no restriction on the use of benzoyl peroxide during lactation.

It is not known whether clindamycin is excreted in human milk following the use of Duac Once Daily Gel, but oral and parenteral administration of clindamycin has been reported to result in the appearance of clindamycin in breast milk. For this reason, treatment of nursing mothers with Duac Once Daily is not recommended.

4.7 Effects on ability to drive and use machines

Not relevant

4.8 Undesirable effects

Duac Once Daily Gel may cause:

Skin and Subcutaneous Tissue Disorders; erythema, peeling, dryness, and pruritus at the site of application.

Very rarely:

Nervous System Disorders; paraesthesia,

Skin and Subcutaneous Tissue Disorders; worsening of acne and contact dermatitis can occur.

These localised effects are typically mild to moderate. Reported frequencies in clinical trials are:

Very common (>1/10)

Skin and Subcutaneous Tissue Disorders; Erythema, Peeling, Dryness

Common (>1/100, <1/10)

Skin and Subcutaneous Tissue Disorders; Burning, Pruritus

Uncommon (>1/1000, <1/100)

Nervous System Disorder; Paraesthesia

Skin and Subcutaneous Tissue Disorders; Worsening of acne

Post marketing data have shown a much lower incidence of these localised effects.

In a few susceptible individuals there have been isolated reports of pseudomembraneous colitis or diarrhoea due to other topical treatments containing clindamycin. This is unlikely to occur with Duac Once Daily Gel, as plasma levels have been determined and the percutaneous absorption of clindamycin is clinically negligible.

With long term use of Duac Once Daily Gel resistance may occur.

Immune System Disorders

In the post-marketing environment there have been isolated instances of allergic reactions which can be sudden and severe.

4.9 Overdose

No case of overdose has been reported.

5. PHARMACOLOGICAL PROPERTIES

5.1 Pharmacodynamic properties

Pharmacotherapeutic group: Clindamycin, combinations

ATC Code: D10AF51

Clindamycin is a lincosamide antibiotic with bacteriostatic action against Gram-positive aerobes and a wide range of anaerobic bacteria. Lincosamides such as clindamycin bind to the 23S subunit of the bacterial ribosome and inhibit the early stages of protein synthesis. The action of clindamycin is predominantly bacteriostatic although high concentrations may be slowly bactericidal against sensitive strains.

Although clindamycin phosphate is inactive *in-vitro*, rapid *in-vivo* hydrolysis converts this compound to the antibacterial active clindamycin. Clindamycin activity has been demonstrated clinically in comedones from acne patients at sufficient levels to be active against most strains of *Propionibacterium acnes*. Clindamycin *in-vitro* inhibits all *Propionibacterium acnes* cultures tested (MIC 0.4mcg/ml). Free fatty acids on the skin surface have been decreased from approximately 14% to 2% following application of clindamycin.

Benzoyl peroxide is mildly keratolytic acting against comedones at all stages of their development. It is an oxidising agent with bactericidal activity against *Propionibacterium acnes*, the organism implicated in acne vulgaris. Furthermore it is sebostatic, counteracting the excessive sebum production associated with acne.

Duac Once Daily Gel has a combination of mild keratolytic and antibacterial properties providing activity particularly against inflamed lesions of mild to moderate acne vulgaris.

The prevalence of acquired resistance may vary geographically and with time for selected species. Local information of resistance is desirable, particularly when treating severe infections.

The inclusion of benzoyl peroxide reduces the potential for the emergence of organisms resistant to Clindamycin.

The presentation of both active ingredients in one product is more convenient and ensures patient compliance.

In five randomised double-blind clinical studies of 1318 patients with facial acne vulgaris with both inflammatory and non-inflammatory lesions, 396 used Duac, 396 used benzoyl peroxide, 349 used clindamycin and 177 used vehicle. Treatment was applied once daily for 11 weeks and patients were evaluated and lesions counted at 2, 5, 8 and 11 weeks.

The mean percentage reduction in the number of lesions after 11 weeks is shown in the table.

Mean percent reduction in number of lesions from baseline after 11 weeks

(see Table 1 below)

Statistically significant differences highlighted in **bold.**

The reduction in total lesions was significantly greater with Duac Once Daily Gel than clindamycin or vehicle in all five studies. The improvement was consistently greater with Duac Once Daily Gel than benzoyl peroxide, but the difference did not achieve statistical significance in individual studies.

Against inflammatory lesions, Duac Once Daily Gel was significantly superior to clindamycin alone in four of five studies and to benzoyl peroxide alone in three of five studies. Against non-inflammatory lesions, Duac Once Daily Gel was significantly better than clindamycin in four of five studies, and tended to be better than benzoyl peroxide alone.

Overall improvement in acne was assessed by the physician and was significantly better with Duac Once Daily Gel than with either benzoyl peroxide or clindamycin alone in three of five studies.

5.2 Pharmacokinetic properties

In a maximised percutaneous absorption study the mean plasma clindamycin levels during a four-week dosing period for Duac Once Daily Gel were negligible (0.043% of applied dose).

The presence of benzoyl peroxide in the formulation did not have an effect on the percutaneous absorption of clindamycin.

Radio-label studies have shown that absorption of benzoyl peroxide through the skin can only occur following its conversion to benzoic acid. Benzoic acid is mostly conjugated to form hippuric acid, which is excreted via the kidneys.

5.3 Preclinical safety data

Duac Once Daily Gel

Repeat-dose dermal toxicity studies conducted on Duac Once Daily Gel, in two species, for up to 90 days, revealed no toxic effects, apart from minor local irritation.

An ocular irritation study found Duac Once Daily Gel to be only very slightly irritant. No other preclinical studies have been performed with Duac Once Daily Gel, but only for the single substances benzoyl peroxide and clindamycin.

Benzoyl peroxide

In animal toxicity studies, benzoyl peroxide was well tolerated when applied topically.

Although high doses of benzoyl peroxide have been shown to induce DNA strand breaks, the available data from other mutagenicity studies, carcinogenicity studies and a photo co-carcinogenicity study indicate that benzoyl peroxide is not a carcinogen or a photocarcinogen.

No reproductive toxicity data are available.

Clindamycin

In-vitro and in-vivo studies did not reveal any mutagenic potential of clindamycin. No long-term animal studies investigating the tumorigenic potential of clindamycin have been conducted. Otherwise, preclinical data reveal no special hazard for humans based on conventional studies of single and repeat-dose toxicity and toxicity to reproduction.

Table 1 Mean percent reduction in number of lesions from baseline after 11 weeks

	Study 150 (n = 120)	Study 151 (n = 273)	Study 152 (n = 280)	Study 156 (n = 287)	Study 158* (n = 358)
Inflammatory lesions					
Duac Once Daily Gel	65	56	42	57	52
Benzoyl peroxide	**36**	**37**	32	57	**41**
Clindamycin	**34**	**30**	38	**49**	**33**
Vehicle	**19**	**-0.4**	29	29	**29**
Non-inflammatory lesions					
Duac Once Daily Gel	27	37	24	39	25
Benzoyl peroxide	12	30	16	**29**	23
Clindamycin	**-4**	**13**	**11**	**18**	17
Vehicle	**-9**	**-5**	17	-	-7
Total lesions (inflammatory plus non-inflammatory lesions)					
Duac Once Daily Gel	41	45	31	50	41
Benzoyl peroxide	20	35	23	43	34
Clindamycin	**11**	**22**	**22**	**33**	**26**
Vehicle	**1**	**-1**	**22**	-	**16**

*** pivotal study**

6. PHARMACEUTICAL PARTICULARS

6.1 List of excipients

Carbomer (50000mPa.s)

Dimeticone (100mm^2.s^{-1})

Disodium Lauryl Sulfosuccinate

Edetate Disodium

Glycerol

Silica, Colloidal Hydrated

Poloxamer 182

Purified Water

Sodium Hydroxide

6.2 Incompatibilities

Not applicable

6.3 Shelf life

Shelf life of medicinal product as packaged for sale

18 months

Shelf life of medicinal product after dispensing

2 months

6.4 Special precautions for storage

Store in a refrigerator (2°C-8°C). Do not freeze.

Storage conditions after dispensing

Do not store above 25°C.

6.5 Nature and contents of container

Internally lacquered membrane-sealed aluminium tubes fitted with a polyethylene screw-cap, packed into a carton.

Pack sizes: 6, 15, 25, 30, 50, 55, 60 and 70 grams.

Not all pack sizes may be marketed.

6.6 Special precautions for disposal and other handling

No special requirements.

7. MARKETING AUTHORISATION HOLDER

Stiefel Laboratories (UK) Ltd

Eurasia Headquarters

Concorde Road,

Maidenhead

SL6 4BY

8. MARKETING AUTHORISATION NUMBER(S)

PL0174/0217

9. DATE OF FIRST AUTHORISATION/RENEWAL OF THE AUTHORISATION

17 September 2003 / 16 September 2008

10. DATE OF REVISION OF THE TEXT

November 2008/June 2009

Duodopa intestinal gel

(Solvay Healthcare Limited)

1. NAME OF THE MEDICINAL PRODUCT

Duodopa, 20 mg/ml + 5 mg/ml, intestinal gel▼

2. QUALITATIVE AND QUANTITATIVE COMPOSITION

1 ml contains 20 mg levodopa and 5 mg carbidopa monohydrate.

100 ml contain 2000 mg levodopa and 500 mg carbidopa monohydrate.

For a full list of excipients, see section 6.1.

3. PHARMACEUTICAL FORM

Intestinal gel.

White to slightly yellow gel.

4. CLINICAL PARTICULARS

4.1 Therapeutic indications

Treatment of advanced levodopa-responsive Parkinson's disease with severe motor fluctuations and hyper-/dyskinesia when available combinations of Parkinson medicinal products have not given satisfactory results.

A positive test of the clinical response to Duodopa administered via a temporary nasoduodenal tube is required before a permanent tube is inserted.

4.2 Posology and method of administration

Duodopa is a gel for continuous intestinal administration. For long-term administration, the gel should be administered with a portable pump directly into the duodenum or upper jejunum by a permanent tube *via* percutaneous endoscopic gastrostomy with an outer transabdominal tube and an inner intestinal tube. Alternatively, a radiological gastrojejunostomy may be considered if percutaneous endoscopic gastrostomy is not suitable for any reason. Establishment of the transabdominal port and dose adjustments should be carried out in association with a neurological clinic.

A temporary nasoduodenal tube is recommended to find out if the patient responds favourably to this method of treatment and to adjust the dose before treatment with a permanent tube is started.

The dose should be adjusted to an optimal clinical response for the individual patient, which means maximizing the functional ON-time during the day by minimizing the number of OFF episodes and the time OFF (bradykinesia) and minimizing ON-time with disabling dyskinesia.

See recommendations under *Dosage.*

Duodopa should be given initially as monotherapy. If required other medicinal products for Parkinson's disease can be taken concurrently. For administration of Duodopa only the CADD-legacy Duodopa pump (CE 0473) should be used. *A manual with instructions for using the portable pump is delivered together with the pump.*

Treatment with Duodopa using a permanent tube can be discontinued at any time by withdrawing the tube and letting the wound heal. Treatment should then continue with oral medicinal products including levodopa/carbidopa.

Dosage:

The total dose/day of Duodopa is composed of three individually adjusted doses: the morning bolus dose, the continuous maintenance dose and extra bolus doses.

Morning dose: The morning bolus dose is administered by the pump to rapidly achieve the therapeutic dose level (within 10-30 minutes). The dose should be based on the patient's previous morning intake of levodopa + the volume to fill the tubing. The total morning dose is usually 5-10 ml, corresponding to 100-200 mg levodopa. The total morning dose should not exceed 15 ml (300 mg levodopa).

Continuous maintenance dose: The maintenance dose is adjustable in steps of 2 mg/hour (0.1 ml/hour). The dose should be calculated according to the patient's previous daily intake of levodopa. When supplementary medicines are discontinued the Duodopa dose should be adjusted. The continuous maintenance dose is adjusted individually. It should be kept within a range of 1-10 ml/hour (20-200 mg levodopa/hour) and is usually 2-6 ml/hour (40-120 mg levodopa/hour). In exceptional cases a higher dose may be needed.

Example:

Daily intake of levodopa as Duodopa: 1640 mg/day

Morning bolus dose: 140 mg = 7 ml (including the volume to fill the intestinal tube)

Continuous maintenance dose: 1500 mg/day

1500 mg/day: 20 mg/ml = 75 ml Duodopa per day

The intake is calculated over 16 hours: 75 ml/16 hours = 4.7 ml/hour.

Extra bolus doses: To be given as required if the patient becomes hypokinetic during the day. The extra dose should be adjusted individually, normally 0.5-2.0 ml. In rare cases a higher dose may be needed. If the need for extra bolus doses exceeds 5 per day the maintenance dose should be increased.

After the initial dose setting, fine adjustments of the morning bolus dose, the maintenance dose and extra bolus doses should be carried out over a few weeks.

If medically justified Duodopa may be administered during the night.

Monitoring of treatment: A sudden deterioration in treatment response with recurring motor fluctuations should lead to the suspicion that the distal part of the tube has become displaced from the duodenum into the stomach. The location of the tube should be determined by X-ray and the end of the tube repositioned to the duodenum under radiological control.

Paediatric population

There is no relevant indication for use of Duodopa in children and adolescents.

Geriatric Population

There is a considerable experience in the use of levodopa/carbidopa in elderly patients. The dosage recommendations set out above reflect the clinical data derived from this experience.

Renal/hepatic impairment

No dose adjustment is necessary.

Interruption of therapy

Patients should be carefully observed in case a sudden reduction of the dose is required or if it becomes necessary to discontinue treatment with Duodopa, particularly if the patient is receiving antipsychotics, see section 4.4.

In the case of *suspected or diagnosed* dementia with a decreased confusion threshold, the pump of the patient should be handled only by the nursing staff or a close relative capable of doing so.

When a cassette is about to be used, it should be attached to the portable pump and the system connected to the nasoduodenal tube or the transabdominal port/duodenal tube for administration, according to the instructions given. The drug cassettes are for single use only and should not be used for longer than one day (up to 16 hours) even if some medicinal product remains. Do not reuse an opened cassette.

By the end of the storage time the gel might become slightly yellow. This does not influence the concentration of the drug or the treatment.

4.3 Contraindications

Duodopa is contraindicated in patients with:

- hypersensitivity to levodopa, carbidopa or any of the excipients
- narrow-angle glaucoma
- severe liver and renal insufficiency
- severe heart failure
- severe cardiac arrhythmia
- acute stroke
- Non-selective MAO inhibitors and selective MAO type A inhibitors must not be given concomitantly, and should be withdrawn at least two weeks before initiation of Duodopa, see section 4.5.
- Conditions in which adrenergics are contraindicated, e.g. pheochromocytoma, hyperthyroidism and Cushing's syndrome.

4.4 Special warnings and precautions for use

Several warnings and precautions below are generic for levodopa and, therefore, also for Duodopa.

- Duodopa is not recommended for the treatment of drug-induced extrapyramidal reactions.
- Duodopa therapy should be administered with caution to patients with severe cardiovascular or pulmonary disease, bronchial asthma, renal, hepatic or endocrine disease, or history of peptic ulcer disease or of convulsions.
- In patients with a history of myocardial infarction who have residual atrial nodal or ventricular arrhythmias, cardiac function should be monitored with particular care during the period of initial dosage adjustments.
- All patients treated with Duodopa should be monitored carefully for the development of mental changes, depression with suicidal tendencies, and other serious mental changes. Patients with past or current psychosis should be treated with caution.
- Concomitant administration of antipsychotics with dopamine receptor blocking properties, particularly D_2 receptor antagonists should be carried out with caution, and the patient carefully observed for loss of antiparkinsonian effect or worsening of parkinsonian symptoms, see section 4.5.
- Patients with chronic wide-angle glaucoma may be treated with Duodopa with caution, provided the intra-ocular pressure is well controlled and the patient is monitored carefully for changes in intra-ocular pressure.
- Duodopa may induce orthostatic hypotension. Therefore Duodopa should be given cautiously to patients who are taking other medicinal products which may cause orthostatic hypotension, see section 4.5.
- Levodopa has been associated with somnolence and episodes of sudden sleep onset in patients with Parkinson's disease and caution should therefore be exercised when driving and operating machines.
- A symptom complex resembling Neuroleptic Malignant Syndrome (NMS), including muscular rigidity, increased body temperature, mental changes (e.g. agitation, confusion, coma) and increased serum creatine phosphokinase, has been reported when anti-Parkinsonian medicinal products were withdrawn abruptly. Rhabdomyolysis secondary to Neuroleptic Malignant Syndrome or severe dyskinesias have been observed rarely in patients with Parkinson's disease. Therefore, patients should be carefully observed when the dose of levodopa/carbidopa combinations are abruptly reduced or discontinued, especially if the patient is receiving anti-psychotics. Neither NMS nor rhabdomyolysis has been reported in association with Duodopa.
- Pathologic gambling, increased libido and hypersexuality have been reported in patients treated with dopamine agonists for Parkinson's disease, including levodopa/carbidopa.
- If general anaesthesia is required, treatment with Duodopa may be continued for as long as the patient is permitted to take fluids and medicinal products by mouth. If therapy has to be stopped temporarily, Duodopa at the same dose as before may be restarted as soon as oral intake of fluid is allowed.
- The dose of Duodopa may need to be adjusted downwards in order to avoid levodopa induced dyskinesias.
- Periodic evaluation of hepatic, haematopoietic, cardiovascular and renal function is recommended during extended therapy with Duodopa.
- Previous surgery in the upper part of the abdomen may lead to difficulty in performing gastrostomy or jejunostomy
- Reduced ability to handle the system (pump, tube connections) can lead to complications. In such patients a caregiver (e.g. nurse, assistant nurse, or close relative) should assist the patient.
- A sudden or gradual worsening of bradykinesia may indicate an obstruction in the device for whatever reason and needs to be explored.

4.5 Interaction with other medicinal products and other forms of interaction

No interaction studies have been performed with Duodopa. The following interactions are known from the generic combination of levodopa/carbidopa.

Caution is needed in concomitant administration of Duodopa with the following medicinal products:

Antihypertensives

Symptomatic postural hypotension has occurred when combinations of levodopa and a decarboxylase inhibitor are added to the treatment of patients already receiving anti-hypertensives. Dosage adjustment of the antihypertensive agent may be required.

Antidepressants

There have been rare reports of adverse reactions, including hypertension and dyskinesia, resulting from the concomitant administration of tricyclic antidepressants and carbidopa/levodopa preparations, see section 4.3.

Anticholinergics

Anticholinergics may act synergistically with levodopa to decrease tremor. However, combined use may exacerbate abnormal involuntary movements. Anticholinergics may decrease the effects of levodopa by delaying its absorption. An adjustment of the dose of Duodopa may be needed.

COMT inhibitors (tolcapone, entacapone)

Concomitant use of COMT (Catechol-O-Methyl Transferase) inhibitors and Duodopa can increase the bioavailability of levodopa. The dose of Duodopa may need adjustment.

Other medicinal products

Dopamine receptor antagonists (some antipsychotics, e.g. phenothiazines, butyrophenons and risperidone and antiemetics, e.g. metoclopramide), benzodiazepines, isoniazide, phenytoin and papaverine can reduce the therapeutic effect of levodopa. Patients taking these medicinal products together with Duodopa should be observed carefully for loss of therapeutic response.

Duodopa can be taken concomitantly with the recommended dose of an MAO inhibitor, which is selective for MAO type B (for instance selegiline-HCl).

Concomitant use of selegiline and levodopa-carbidopa has been associated with serious orthostatic hypotension.

Amantadine has synergic effect with levodopa and may increase levodopa related adverse events. An adjustment of the dose of Duodopa may be needed.

Sympathicomimetics may increase cardiovascular adverse events related to levodopa.

Levodopa forms a chelate with iron in the gastrointestinal tract leading to reduced absorption of levodopa.

As levodopa is competitive with certain amino acids, the absorption of levodopa can be disturbed in patients who are on a protein rich diet.

The effect of administration of antacids and Duodopa on the bioavailability of levodopa has not been studied.

4.6 Pregnancy and lactation

Pregnancy

There are no adequate data from the use of levodopa/carbidopa in pregnant women. Data from animal studies have shown reproduction toxicity, see section 5.3. The potential risk for humans is unknown. Duodopa should not be used during pregnancy unless the benefits for the mother outweigh the possible risks to the foetus.

Lactation

Levodopa is excreted in the breast milk. There is evidence that lactation is suppressed during treatment with levodopa. It is unknown whether carbidopa is excreted in human breast milk. Animal studies have shown excretion of carbidopa in breast milk. The safety of levodopa and carbidopa in the infant is not known. Duodopa should not be used during breast-feeding.

4.7 Effects on ability to drive and use machines

Levodopa and carbidopa may cause dizziness and orthostatic hypotension. Therefore, caution should be exercised when driving or using machines. Patients being treated with Duodopa and presenting with somnolence and/or sudden sleep episodes must be advised to refrain from driving or engaging in activities where impaired alertness may put them, or others, at risk of serious injury or death (e.g. operating machines) until such recurrent episodes and somnolence have resolved, see also section 4.4.

4.8 Undesirable effects

Undesirable effects that occur frequently with levodopa/carbidopa are those due to central neuropharmacological activity of dopamine. These reactions can usually be diminished by levodopa dosage reduction.

(see Table 1 below)

Laboratory values: The following laboratory abnormalities have been reported with levodopa/carbidopa treatment and should, therefore, be acknowledged when treating patients with Duodopa: elevated urea nitrogen, alkaline phosphatases, S-AST, S-ALT, LDH, bilirubin, blood sugar, creatinine, uric acid and positive Coomb's test, and lowered values of haemoglobin and haematocrit. Leucocytes, bacteria and blood in the urine have been reported. Levodopa/carbidopa, and thus Duodopa, may cause a false positive result when a dipstick is used to test for urinary ketone; this reaction is not altered by boiling the urine sample. The use of glucose oxidase methods may give false negative results for glucosuria.

Patients treated with dopamine agonists for treatment of Parkinson's disease, including levodopa/carbidopa, especially at high doses, have been reported as showing pathological gambling, increased libido and hypersexuality, generally reversible upon reduction of the dose or treatment discontinuation.

The device: Complications with the device are very common (>1/10), e.g. connector leakage, dislocation of the intestinal tube. Dislocation of the intestinal tube backwards into the stomach leads to reappearance of motor fluctuations (due to erratic gastric emptying of Duodopa into the small intestines). In general, relocation of the tube can be done using a guide-wire to steer the tube into the duodenum under fluoroscopy. Occlusion, kinks, or knots of the intestinal tube lead to high pressure signals from the pump. Occlusions are usually remedied by flushing the tube with tap water; kinking, knotting, or a tube displacement may need readjustment of the tubing. Should complete failure of the intestinal tube or pump occur the patient must be treated with oral levodopa/carbidopa until the problem is solved. The stoma usually heals without complications. However, abdominal pain, infection and leakage of gastric fluid may occur shortly after surgery; it is rarely a problem long-term. Reported complications include perforation of adjacent anatomical structures especially during PEG placement and bleeding, wound infection (the most common complication) and peritonitis. Local infections around the stoma are treated conservatively with a disinfectant. Treatment with antibiotics is rarely needed.

Table 1

MedDRA system organ class	Common >1/100, <1/10	Uncommon >1/1,000, <1/100	Rare >1/10,000, <1/1,000	Very rare <1/10,000 incl. isolated reports
Blood and lymphatic system disorders			Leucopenia, haemolytic and non-haemolytic anaemia, thrombocytopenia	Agranulocytosis
Metabolism and nutrition disorders	Anorexia	Loss of weight, increased weight		
Psychiatric disorders	Hallucinations, confusion, nightmares, sleepiness, fatigue, sleeplessness, depression with very rare suicide attempts, euphoria, dementia, psychotic episodes, feeling of stimulation		Agitation, fear, reduced thinking capacity, disorientation, increased libido, numbness	
Nervous system disorders	Dyskinesias, choreatic movements and dystonia, "ON-OFF" episodes, dizziness, bradykinesia ("ON-OFF" episodes)[1], somnolence[2]	Ataxia, increased tremor of the hands	Neuroleptic malignant syndrome, paraesthesias, falling, walking defects, trismus, headache, convulsions	
Eye disorders			Blurred vision, blepharospasm (see section 4.9), activation of a latent Horner's syndrome, double vision, dilated pupils, oculogyric crises	
Cardiac disorders	Palpitations, irregular heartbeat			
Vascular disorders	Orthostatic hypotension, inclination to faint, syncope	Hypertension	Phlebitis	
Respiratory, thoracic and medastinal disorders		Hoarseness, chest pain	Dyspnoea, abnormal breathing pattern	
Gastrointestinal disorders	Nausea, vomiting, dry mouth, bitter taste	Constipation, diarrhea, sialorrhoea. Dysphagia, flatulence	Dyspepsia, gastrointestinal pain, dark saliva, bruxism, hiccups, gastrointestinal bleeding, burning sensation of the tongue, duodenal ulceration	
Skin and subcutaneous tissue disorders		Oedema	Angioedema, urticaria, pruritus, facial redness, hair loss, exanthema, increased perspiration, dark perspiration fluid, malignant melanoma, Schönlein-Henoch purpura	
Musculoskeletal, connective tissue and bone disorders		Muscle spasms		
Renal and urinary disorders		Dark urine	Urinary retention, urinary incontinence, priapism	
General disorders and administration site reactions		Weakness, malaise,		

[1] Bradykinesia ("ON-OFF" episodes) may appear some months to years after the beginning of treatment with levodopa and is probably related to the progression of the disease. The adaption of dose schedule and dose intervals may be required.

[2] Levodopa/carbidopa is associated with somnolence and has been associated very rarely with excessive daytime somnolence and sudden sleep onset episodes.

4.9 Overdose

Most prominent clinical symptoms of an overdose with levodopa/carbidopa are dystonia and dyskinesia. Blepharospasms can be an early sign of overdose.

The treatment of an acute overdose of Duodopa is in general the same as that of an acute overdose of levodopa: However, pyridoxine has no effect on the reversal of the action of Duodopa. Electrocardiographic monitoring should be used and the patient observed carefully for the development of cardiac arrhythmias; if necessary an appropriate antiarrhythmic therapy should be given. The possibility that the patient took other medicinal products together with Duodopa should be taken into consideration. To date experiences with dialysis have not been reported, therefore its value in the treatment of overdose is unknown.

5. PHARMACOLOGICAL PROPERTIES

5.1 Pharmacodynamic properties

Pharmacotherapeutic group: Anti-Parkinson drugs, levodopa and decarboxylase inhibitor

ATC code: N04BA02.

Duodopa is a combination of levodopa and carbidopa (ratio 4:1) in a gel for continuous intestinal infusion in advanced Parkinson's disease with severe motor fluctuations and hyper-/dyskinesia. Levodopa relieves symptoms of Parkinson's disease following decarboxylation to dopamine in the brain. Carbidopa, which does not cross the blood-brain barrier, inhibits the extracerebral decarboxylation of levodopa, which means that a larger amount of levodopa becomes available for transportation to the brain and transformation into dopamine. Without the simultaneous administration of carbidopa much larger amounts of levodopa would be required to achieve the desired effect.

Intestinal therapy with Duodopa reduces the motor fluctuations and increases the "ON"-time for patients with advanced Parkinson's disease who have received tablet treatment with levodopa/decarboxylase inhibitor for many years. The motor fluctuations and hyper-/dyskinesias are reduced due to the fact that the plasma concentrations of levodopa are being kept at a steady level within the individual therapeutic window. Therapeutic effects on motor fluctuations and hyper-/dyskinesias are often achieved during the first treatment day.

5.2 Pharmacokinetic properties

Absorption

Duodopa is administered *via* an inserted tube directly into the duodenum. Levodopa is absorbed quickly and effectively from the intestine through a high capacity transport system for amino acids. Levodopa given as Duodopa has the same bioavailability as levodopa given as tablets (81-98 %). The variation in plasma concentration within an individual is considerably smaller for Duodopa due to the fact that it is given by continuous intestinal administration in which the gastric emptying rate has no influence on the absorption rate. With an initial high morning dose of Duodopa the therapeutic plasma level of levodopa is reached within 10-30 minutes.

Distribution

Levodopa is co-administered with carbidopa, a decarboxylase inhibitor, which increases the bioavailability and decreases clearance for levodopa. Clearance and volume of distribution for levodopa is 0.3 l/hour/kg and 0.9-1.6 l/kg, respectively, when given together with a decarboxylase inhibitor. The protein binding of levodopa in plasma is negligible.

Metabolism and elimination

The elimination half-life for levodopa is approximately 1-2 hours. Levodopa is eliminated completely through metabolism and the metabolites formed are excreted mainly in the urine. Four metabolic pathways are known, decarboxylation being predominant for levodopa administered without any enzyme inhibitor. When levodopa is co-administered with carbidopa the decarboxylase enzyme is inhibited so that metabolism via catechol-O-methyl-transferase (COMT) becomes the dominant metabolic pathway.

Pharmacokinetic-pharmacodynamic relationship

The reduced fluctuations in the plasma concentration of levodopa reduce fluctuations in the treatment response. The levodopa dose needed varies considerably in advanced Parkinson's disease and it is important that the dose is individually adjusted based on the clinical response. Development of tolerance over time has not been observed with Duodopa. On the contrary, many patients, after a period of satisfactory treatment with Duodopa, may find that a lower dose of levodopa will provide a satisfactory clinical response.

5.3 Preclinical safety data

Non-clinical data reveal no special hazard for humans based on conventional studies of safety, pharmacology, repeated dose toxicity, genotoxicity, carcinogenic potential, toxicity to reproduction. In reproductive toxicity studies both levodopa and the combination of carbidopa/

levodopa have caused visceral and skeletal malformations in rabbits.

6. PHARMACEUTICAL PARTICULARS

6.1 List of excipients

Carmellose sodium

Purified water

6.2 Incompatibilities

Not applicable.

6.3 Shelf life

Unopened: 15 weeks.

Once opened: Use immediately. Discard any unused portion.

Chemical and physical in-use stability has been demonstrated for 16 hours at 40°C.

6.4 Special precautions for storage

Store in a refrigerator (2°C-8°C).

Keep the cassette in the outer carton in order to protect from light.

6.5 Nature and contents of container

Total amount of 100 ml in PVC bag inside a hard plastic cassette for protection, carton with 7 cassettes.

6.6 Special precautions for disposal and other handling

Cassettes are for single use only.

Do not re-use an opened cassette.

Any unused product or waste material should be disposed of in accordance with local requirements.

Empty/used cassettes should be returned to the pharmacy for destruction.

7. MARKETING AUTHORISATION HOLDER

Solvay Pharmaceuticals GmbH

Hans-Boeckler-Allee 20

D-30173 Hannover

Germany

8. MARKETING AUTHORISATION NUMBER(S)

PL 05727/0016

9. DATE OF FIRST AUTHORISATION/RENEWAL OF THE AUTHORISATION

21 January 2004

10. DATE OF REVISION OF THE TEXT

22 May 2009

Duofilm

(Stiefel Laboratories (UK) Limited)

1. NAME OF THE MEDICINAL PRODUCT

Duofilm

2. QUALITATIVE AND QUANTITATIVE COMPOSITION

Salicylic acid BP 16.7% w/w

Lactic acid BP 16.7% w/w

3. PHARMACEUTICAL FORM

Solution for topical administration.

4. CLINICAL PARTICULARS

4.1 Therapeutic indications

Duofilm is indicated for the treatment of warts

4.2 Posology and method of administration

Adults and the elderly:

Apply daily to the affected areas only.

Children:

Children under the age of 12 years should be treated under supervision. Treatment of infants under the age of 2 years is not recommended.

4.3 Contraindications

Duofilm should not be used on the face or anogenital regions. Avoid applying to normal skin.

4.4 Special warnings and precautions for use

None.

4.5 Interaction with other medicinal products and other forms of interaction

None known

4.6 Pregnancy and lactation

There are no restrictions on the use of Duofilm during pregnancy or lactation.

4.7 Effects on ability to drive and use machines

None.

4.8 Undesirable effects

None

4.9 Overdose

Not Applicable.

5. PHARMACOLOGICAL PROPERTIES

5.1 Pharmacodynamic properties

Lactic acid affects the keratinisation process, reducing the hyperkeratosis which is characteristic of warts. It is caustic, leading to the destruction of the keratotic tissue of the wart and of the causative virus.

Salicylic acid is keratolytic, producing desquamation by solubilising the intercellular cement in the stratum corneum.

5.2 Pharmacokinetic properties

Not applicable.

5.3 Preclinical safety data

Not applicable.

6. PHARMACEUTICAL PARTICULARS

6.1 List of excipients

Flexible Collodion

6.2 Incompatibilities

None

6.3 Shelf life

a) For the product as packaged for sale

3 years

b) After first opening the container

Comply with expiry date

6.4 Special precautions for storage

Do not store above 25°C. Keep away from naked flame.

6.5 Nature and contents of container

Amber screw capped applicator bottle containing 15ml.

6.6 Special precautions for disposal and other handling

There are no special instructions for use or handling of Duofilm.

7. MARKETING AUTHORISATION HOLDER

Stiefel Laboratories (UK) Ltd

Eurasia Headquarters

Concorde Road

Maidenhead

SL6 4BY

UK

8. MARKETING AUTHORISATION NUMBER(S)

PL 0174/0025R

9. DATE OF FIRST AUTHORISATION/RENEWAL OF THE AUTHORISATION

14th February 1990

10. DATE OF REVISION OF THE TEXT

August 2009

Duovent UDVs

(Boehringer Ingelheim Limited)

1. NAME OF THE MEDICINAL PRODUCT

Duovent UDVs

2. QUALITATIVE AND QUANTITATIVE COMPOSITION

Each single dose unit contains Fenoterol Hydrobromide 1.25 mg and Ipratropium Bromide 0.5 mg.

For excipients, see Section 6.1.

3. PHARMACEUTICAL FORM

Nebuliser solution.

A clear, colourless or almost colourless solution.

4. CLINICAL PARTICULARS

4.1 Therapeutic indications

The management of acute severe asthma or acute exacerbation of chronic asthma presenting as an emergency requiring treatment by nebuliser.

4.2 Posology and method of administration

DUOVENT UDVs may be administered from an intermittent positive pressure ventilator or from a properly maintained and functioning nebuliser.

The recommended dose for adults and children over 14 years is one vial (4 ml) to be nebulised immediately upon presentation. Each dose should be inhaled to dryness from the nebuliser. Repeat dosing may be given at the discretion of the treating physician, up to a maximum of 4 vials in 24 hours.

In acute severe asthma additional doses may be necessary depending on clinical response. Nebuliser treatment of acute severe asthma should be replaced by standard inhaler devices 24 - 48 hours before discharge unless the patient requires a nebuliser at home.

Clinical trials have included patients over 65 years. No adverse reactions specific to this age group have been reported.

Administration

DUOVENT UDVs should only be used in a nebuliser approved by your doctor.

1. The nebuliser or ventilator unit should be prepared by following the manufacturer's instructions and /or the advice of the physician.

2. A new single dose unit should be carefully separated from the strip. NEVER use one which has been previously opened.

3. Open the single dose unit by simply twisting off the top, always taking care to hold it in an upright position.

4. Unless otherwise instructed, all the contents of the single dose unit should be squeezed into the nebuliser chamber. If dilution of the single dose unit contents is necessary this should be done using ONLY sterile sodium chloride 0.9% solution as directed by the physician.

5. Use your nebuliser as directed by your doctor.

6. After nebulisation has finished, throw away any remaining solution from the single dose unit or nebuliser chamber.

7. Follow the manufacturer's instructions for cleaning the nebuliser. It is important that the nebuliser is kept clean.

4.3 Contraindications

Hypertrophic obstructive cardiomyopathy, tachyarrhythmia. Hypersensitivity to fenoterol hydrobromide or atropine-like substances or to any of the excipients of the product.

4.4 Special warnings and precautions for use

Patients must be instructed in the correct use of a nebuliser and warned not to exceed the prescribed dose. The patient must be instructed to seek medical advice in the event of DUOVENT failing to provide relief of bronchospasm. In the case of acute, rapidly worsening dyspnoea (difficulty in breathing) a doctor should be consulted immediately.

For prolonged use, on demand (symptom-oriented) treatment may be preferable to regular use. Patients should be evaluated for the addition or the increase of anti-inflammatory therapy (e.g. inhaled corticosteroids) to control airway inflammation and to prevent deterioration of disease control.

The use of increasing amounts of beta$_2$-agonist containing products such as DUOVENT on a regular basis to control symptoms of bronchial obstruction may suggest declining disease control. If bronchial obstruction deteriorates it is inappropriate and possibly hazardous to simply increase the use of beta$_2$-agonist containing products such as DUOVENT, beyond the recommended dose over extended periods of time. In this situation, the patient's therapy plan, and in particular the adequacy of anti-inflammatory therapy with inhaled corticosteroids should be reviewed to prevent potentially life threatening deterioration of disease control.

Other sympathomimetic bronchodilators should only be used with DUOVENT under medical supervision.

In the following conditions DUOVENT should only be used after careful risk/benefit assessment, especially when doses higher than recommended are used:

Insufficiently controlled diabetes mellitus, myocardial insufficiency, angina, cardiac dysrhythmias, hypertension, recent myocardial infarction, hypertrophic subvalvular aortic stenosis, severe organic heart or vascular disorders, hyperthyroidism, pheochromocytoma.

Cardiovascular effects may be seen with sympathicomimetic drugs, including **DUOVENT**. There is some evidence from post-marketing data and published literature of rare occurrences of myocardial ischaemia associated with beta-agonists. Patients with underlying severe heart disease (e.g.ischaemic heart disease, arrhythmia or severe heart failure) who are receiving **DUOVENT**, should be warned to seek medical advice if they experience chest pain or other symptoms of worsening heart disease. Attention should be paid to assessment of symptoms such as dyspnoea and chest pain, as they may be of either respiratory or cardiac origin.

The administration of nebuliser solutions has occasionally been associated with cases of paradoxical bronchoconstriction.

Potentially serious hypokalemia may result from beta$_2$-agonist therapy. Caution is advocated in the use of anticholinergic agents in patients predisposed to or with narrow-angle glaucoma or with bladder neck obstruction or with prostatic hyperplasia.

Patients must be instructed in the correct administration of DUOVENT UDVs. Care should be taken to prevent the solution or mist from entering the eyes. It is recommended that the nebulised solution be administered via a mouth piece. If this is not available and a nebuliser mask is used, it must fit properly. Patients who may be predisposed to glaucoma should be warned specifically to protect their eyes.

There have been isolated reports of ocular complications (i.e. mydriasis, increased intra-ocular pressure, narrow-angle glaucoma, eye pain) when aerosolised ipratropium bromide either alone or in combination with an adrenergic beta$_2$-agonist was sprayed into the eyes.

Inhaled doses of ipratropium bromide nebuliser solution up to 1 mg have not been associated with elevation of intra-ocular pressure.

Eye pain or discomfort, blurred vision, visual halos or coloured images in association with red eyes from conjunctival congestion and corneal oedema may be signs of acute narrow-angle glaucoma.

Should any combination of these symptoms develop, treatment with miotic eye drops should be initiated and specialist advice sought immediately.

As patients with cystic fibrosis may be more prone to gastro-intestinal motility disturbances, DUOVENT as with other anticholinergics should be used with caution in these patients.

Immediate hypersensitivity reactions may occur after administration of DUOVENT, as demonstrated by rare cases of urticaria, angio-oedema, rash, bronchospasm, oropharyngeal oedema and anaphylaxis.

4.5 Interaction with other medicinal products and other forms of interaction

In view of a possible interaction between sympathomimetic amines and monoamine oxidase inhibitors or tricyclic antidepressants, care should be exercised if it is proposed to administer these compounds concurrently with DUOVENT UDVs.

DUOVENT UDVs should be used with caution in patients already receiving other sympathomimetic agents as cardiovascular effects may be additive.

Other beta-adrenergics and anticholinergics and xanthine derivatives (such as theophylline) may enhance the bronchodilatory effect. The concurrent administration of other beta-mimetics, systemically available anticholinergics and xanthine derivatives (e.g. theophylline) may increase the adverse reactions.

Beta-adrenergic blocking agents may antagonise fenoterol hydrobromide and potentially seriously reduce its bronchodilator effect if administered concurrently.

Beta-agonist induced hypokalemia may be increased by concomitant treatment with xanthine derivatives, corticosteroids and diuretics. This should be taken into account particularly in patients with severe airway obstruction.

Hypokalemia may result in an increased susceptibility to arrhythmias in patients receiving digoxin. Additionally, hypoxia may aggravate the effect of hypokalemia on cardiac rhythm. It is recommended that serum potassium levels are monitored in such situations.

Inhalation of halogenated hydrocarbon anaesthetics such as halothane, trichloroethylene and enflurane may increase the susceptibility to the cardiovascular effects of beta-agonists.

4.6 Pregnancy and lactation

Although both fenoterol hydrobromide and ipratropium bromide have been in general use for several years, there is no definite evidence of ill-consequence during human pregnancy; animal studies have shown no hazard. Medicines should, however, not be used in pregnancy, especially during the first trimester, unless the expected benefit is thought to outweigh any possible risk to the foetus.

Beta-adrenergic agents have been shown to prolong pregnancy and inhibit labour. The inhibitory effect of fenoterol hydrobromide on uterine contraction should be taken into account when considering the risk:benefit balance.

Preclinical studies have shown that fenoterol hydrobromide is excreted in breast milk. It is unknown whether ipratropium is excreted into breast milk. A decision on whether to continue/discontinue breast-feeding or to continue/discontinue therapy with DUOVENT should be made taking into account the benefit of breast-feeding to the child and the benefit of DUOVENT therapy to the mother.

4.7 Effects on ability to drive and use machines

None stated.

4.8 Undesirable effects

The following side effects have been reported. The frequencies given below are based on clinical trials involving 2009 patients who have been treated with fenoterol and ipratropium combinations.

Frequencies	
Very common	≥ 1/10
Common	≥ 1/100 < 1/10
Uncommon	≥ 1/1,000 < 1/100
Rare	≥ 1/10,000 < 1/1,000
Very rare	< 1/10,000
Not known	Cannot be estimated from the available data

Immune system disorders	
Anaphylactic reaction [1]	Rare [1]
Allergic type reactions	Rare
Skin rash	Rare
Urticaria	Rare
Angio-oedema of tongue, lips and face	Not known
Metabolism and nutrition disorders	
Hypokalaemia	Not known
Psychiatric disorders	
Psychological alterations	Rare
Nervousness	Rare
Nervous system disorders	
Headache	Rare
Dizziness	Rare
Fine Tremor	Rare
Hyperactivity in children	Not known
Eye disorders	
Narrow Angle Glaucoma[2]	Rare
Ocular accommodation disturbances	Not known
Increased Intraocular pressure[2]	Not known
Eye pain[2]	Not known
Mydriasis[2]	Not known
Cardiac Disorders	
Tachycardia, increased heart rate	Uncommon
Arrhythmias	Uncommon
Atrial fibrillation	Rare
Palpitations	Rare
Supraventricular tachycardia	Rare
Decrease in diastolic blood pressure	Not known
Increase in systolic blood pressure	Not known
Myocardial ischaemia	Not known
Respiratory, Thoracic and Mediastinal Disorders	
Cough	Common[3]
Local irritation	
- Pharyngitis	Common[3]
- Throat irritation	Rare[3]
Laryngospasm[1]	Rare[1]
Inhalation induced bronchospasm	Not known
Gastro-intestinal Disorders	
Dryness of mouth	Uncommon
Nausea (with or without vomiting)	Uncommon
Gastro-intestinal motility disturbances[4]	Uncommon
Skin and Subcutaneous Disorders	
Skin reactions	Uncommon
Sweating	Not known
Musculosceletal and Connective Tissue Disorders	
Myalgia	Rare
Muscle cramps	Rare
Weakness (muscle)	Not known
Renal and Urinary Disorders	
Urinary retention	Rare

[1] observed in trials with the mono-compound ipratropium bromide

[2] See section 4.4.

[3] verum frequency only for local side effects

[4] e.g. constipation, diarrhoea

4.9 Overdose

Symptoms

The effects of overdosage are expected to be primarily related to fenoterol. The expected symptoms of overdosage are those of excessive beta-adrenergic-stimulation, the most prominent being tachycardia, palpitation, hypertension, hypotension, widening of the pulse pressure, anginal pain, arrhythmias, flushing, nausea, restlessness, dizziness, headache and tremor.

Hypokalaemia may occur following overdose with fenoterol. Serum potassium levels should be monitored.

Inhaled doses of 5 mg ipratropium produce an increase in heart rate and palpitation but single doses of 2 mg have been given to adults and 1 mg to children without causing side-effects. Single doses of ipratropium bromide 30 mg by mouth cause anticholinergic side-effects but these are not severe and do not require specific reversal.

Therapy

It is suggested that the patient should be treated symptomatically. Beta$_1$-selective beta-adrenergic blocking agents should be chosen and blood pressure should be monitored. Should the administration of a beta-adrenergic blocking agent be considered necessary to counteract the effects of overdosage, its use in a patient liable to bronchospasm should be carefully monitored because of the risk of precipitating severe bronchospasm, which may be fatal.

5. PHARMACOLOGICAL PROPERTIES

5.1 Pharmacodynamic properties

Fenoterol hydrobromide is a direct acting sympathomimetic agent where the catechol nucleus of isoprenaline has been replaced by a resorcinol nucleus, and the substituent moiety on the amino group is larger. This substitution has the effect of depressing the affinity of the molecule to the beta-$_1$ (cardiac and lipolytic) adrenergic receptors and enhancing the affinity towards the beta-$_2$ (bronchial, vascular and intestinal) adrenergic receptors.

Ipratropium bromide affects airway function primarily through its neural effect on the parasympathetic nervous system. Ipratropium bromide blocks the acetylcholine receptors on smooth muscle in the lung. Stimulation of these receptors normally produces contraction and, depending on the degree of actuation, bronchoconstriction. Thus, even in normal subjects, ipratropium bromide will cause bronchodilatation.

5.2 Pharmacokinetic properties

Fenoterol hydrobromide: In man fenoterol is very rapidly distributed through the tissues following intravenous administration. The kidneys excrete up to 65% mainly in the form of acidic conjugates. Following oral administration, the plasma levels reach their maximum 2 hours after ingestion and then drop exponentially. Renal excretion is 39% following peroral administration and over 98% of the renal excretory products consist of acidic conjugates. The half life for total excretion is 7.2 hours and absorption was calculated to be 60%.

The duration of action following use of a metered dose aerosol is considerably larger and can be explained by the dose independent absorption in the upper bronchial tree. The concentration-independent absorption at this site, from the depot produced by the metered dose aerosol is maintained for several hours.

Ipratropium bromide: It is a quaternary ammonium compound which is poorly absorbed from the gastro-intestinal tract and is slow to cross mucous membranes and the blood brain barrier. Following inhalation, uptake into the plasma is minimal, a peak blood concentration is attained 1 ½ to 3 hours after inhalation (and similarly for oral administration). Excretion is chiefly via the kidneys.

5.3 Preclinical safety data

None stated.

6. PHARMACEUTICAL PARTICULARS

6.1 List of excipients

Sodium chloride

Hydrochloric acid

Purified water

6.2 Incompatibilities

Not applicable.

6.3 Shelf life

3 years.

As the product contains no preservative, a fresh vial should be used for each dose and the vial should be opened immediately before administration. Any solution left in the vial should be discarded.

6.4 Special precautions for storage

Do not store above 25°C. Protect from heat. Keep vials in the outer carton.

6.5 Nature and contents of container

Low density polyethylene (LDPE) vials formed in strips of 10 packed into cartons containing 10, 20, 30, 50, 60, 80, 100, 120, 150, 200, 500 and 1000 vials. Each vial contains 4 ml of solution.

Not all pack sizes may be marketed.

6.6 Special precautions for disposal and other handling

No special requirements

7. MARKETING AUTHORISATION HOLDER

Boehringer Ingelheim Limited,
Ellesfield Avenue,
Bracknell,
Berkshire,
RG12 8YS,
United Kingdom.

8. MARKETING AUTHORISATION NUMBER(S)

PL 00015/0164

9. DATE OF FIRST AUTHORISATION/RENEWAL OF THE AUTHORISATION

09/06/93

10. DATE OF REVISION OF THE TEXT

January 2009

11. Legal Category

POM

Duphalac

(Solvay Healthcare Limited)

1. NAME OF THE MEDICINAL PRODUCT

Lactulose Solution BP /Duphalac®.

2. QUALITATIVE AND QUANTITATIVE COMPOSITION

Lactulose 3.35 g/5 ml.

For excipients, see 6.1

3. PHARMACEUTICAL FORM

A colourless to brownish yellow, clear or not more than slightly opalescent liquid.

4. CLINICAL PARTICULARS

4.1 Therapeutic indications

1. For the treatment of constipation.

2. For the treatment of hepatic encephalopathy (portal systemic encephalopathy); hepatic coma.

4.2 Posology and method of administration

Constipation:

Adults (including the elderly): initially 15 ml twice daily

Children 5 to 10 years: 10 ml twice daily

Children under 5 years:5 ml twice daily

Babies under 1 year: 2.5 ml twice daily

All dosages should subsequently be adjusted to the needs of the individual. Each dose may if necessary be taken with water or fruit juices, etc.

Hepatic encephalopathy:

Adults (including the elderly): Initially 30 - 50 ml (6-10 × 5 ml spoonfuls) three times a day. Subsequently adjust the dose to produce two or three soft stools each day.

Children: no dosage recommendations for this indication.

4.3 Contraindications

Contraindicated in patients with galactosaemia and in cases of gastro-intestinal obstruction.

4.4 Special warnings and precautions for use

The lactose content should be taken into account when treating patients with lactose intolerance.

4.5 Interaction with other medicinal products and other forms of interaction

None known.

4.6 Pregnancy and lactation

Pregnancy: Wide clinical experience, together with data from animal reproduction studies has not revealed any increase in embryotoxic hazard to the foetus, if used in the recommended dosage during pregnancy. If drug therapy is needed during pregnancy, the use of this drug is acceptable.

Lactation: This product can be used by nursing mothers feeding their offspring.

4.7 Effects on ability to drive and use machines

Not known.

4.8 Undesirable effects

Flatulence may occur during the first few days of treatment. As a rule it disappears after a couple of days. When dosages higher than instructed are used, abdominal pain and diarrhoea may occur. In such a case the dosage should be decreased. See also overdose section 4.9.

If high doses (normally only associated with portosystemic encephalopathy, PSE) are used for an extended period of time, the patient may experience an electrolyte imbalance due to diarrhoea. Dosage should then be adjusted to obtain two or three formed stools per day.

Gastrointestinal disorders

Flatulence, abdominal pain, nausea and vomiting. If dosed too high, diarrhoea.

Investigations

Electrolyte imbalance due to diarrhoea.

4.9 Overdose

If the dose is too high, the following may occur:

Symptom: diarrhoea and abdominal pain.

Treatment: cessation of treatment or dose reduction. Extensive fluid loss by diarrhoea or vomiting may require correction of electrolyte disturbances.

No specific antidote. Symptomatic treatment should be given.

5. PHARMACOLOGICAL PROPERTIES

5.1 Pharmacodynamic properties

The active ingredient, lactulose, is metabolised in the colon by the sacchrolytic bacteria, producing low molecular weight organic acids, mainly lactic acid, which lower the pH of the colon contents, promote the retention of water by an osmotic effect, thus increasing peristaltic activity.

5.2 Pharmacokinetic properties

Lactulose is minimally absorbed; therefore, the kinetics of the absorbed material are not relevant to the principal therapeutic action.

5.3 Preclinical safety data

The results of acute, sub-chronic and chronic toxicity studies in various species indicate that the compound has very low toxicity. The effects observed appear to be more related to the effect of bulk in gastrointestinal tract than to a more specific toxic activity.

6. PHARMACEUTICAL PARTICULARS

6.1 List of excipients

None.

6.2 Incompatibilities

None known.

6.3 Shelf life

HDPE: 2 years. Other containers: 3 years.

6.4 Special precautions for storage

Do not store above 25°C. Do not refrigerate or freeze.

6.5 Nature and contents of container

Brown glass and white HDPE bottles containing 200, 300, 500 and 1000 ml; polyethylene bottles containing 5 litres; 15 ml foil sachets.

6.6 Special precautions for disposal and other handling

None.

7. MARKETING AUTHORISATION HOLDER

Solvay Healthcare Limited/Solvay Healthcare Ltd trading as Mansbridge Pharmaceuticals

Mansbridge Road

West End

Southampton

SO18 3JD

8. MARKETING AUTHORISATION NUMBER(S)

PL 00512/5001R

9. DATE OF FIRST AUTHORISATION/RENEWAL OF THE AUTHORISATION

14.03.88 / 23.07.99

10. DATE OF REVISION OF THE TEXT

May 2009

Durogesic DTrans 12/25/50/75/100 mcg/hr Transdermal Patch

(Janssen-Cilag Ltd)

1. NAME OF THE MEDICINAL PRODUCT

Durogesic® DTrans® 12/25/50/75/100 mcg/hr Transdermal Patch

2. QUALITATIVE AND QUANTITATIVE COMPOSITION

Each Durogesic DTrans 12/25/50/75/100 patch contains fentanyl 2.1/4.2/8.4/12.6/16.8 mg.

Release rate approximately 12/25/50/75/100 μg/h; active surface area 5.25/10.5/21.0/31.5/42.0 cm^2.

For excipients, see 6.1

3. PHARMACEUTICAL FORM

Transdermal patch.

4. CLINICAL PARTICULARS

4.1 Therapeutic indications

Durogesic DTrans is indicated

- in the management of chronic intractable pain due to cancer

- in the management of chronic intractable pain

4.2 Posology and method of administration

For transdermal use.

Durogesic DTrans should be applied to non-irritated and non-irradiated skin on a flat surface of the torso or upper arm. In young children, the upper back is the preferred location to apply the patch, to minimise the potential of the child removing the patch. A non-hairy area should be selected. If this is not possible, hair at the application site should be clipped (not shaved) prior to application. If the site of Durogesic DTrans application requires to be cleansed prior to application of the patch, this should be done with water. Soaps, oils, lotions or any other agent that might irritate the skin or alter its characteristics should not be used. The skin should be completely dry before the patch is applied. Patches should be inspected prior to use. Patches that are cut, divided, or damaged in any way should not be used.

The Durogesic DTrans patch should be removed from the protective pouch by first folding the notch (located close to the tip of the arrow on the pouch label) and then carefully tearing the pouch material. If scissors are used to open the pouch, this should be done close to the sealed edge so as not to damage the patch inside.

Durogesic DTrans should be applied immediately after removal from the sealed pouch. Avoid touching the adhesive side of the patch. Following removal of both parts of the protective liner, the transdermal patch should be pressed firmly in place with the palm of the hand for approximately 30 seconds, making sure the contact is complete, especially around the edges. Then wash hands with clean water.

Durogesic DTrans should be worn continuously for 72 hours. A new patch should then be applied to a different skin site after removal of the previous transdermal patch. Several days should elapse before a new patch is applied to the same area of skin.

The need for continued treatment should be assessed at regular intervals.

Adults:

Initial dose selection

It is recommended that Durogesic DTrans be used in patients who have previously tolerated opioids. The initial Durogesic DTrans dose should be based on the patient's opioid history, including the degree of opioid tolerance, if any, as well as on the current general condition and medical status of the patient.

In strong opioid-naive patients, Durogesic DTrans dose 25 μg/h should be used as the initial dose.

Clinical experience with Durogesic DTrans is limited in opioid-naïve patients. If therapy with Durogesic DTrans is considered appropriate in opioid-naïve patients, it is recommended that these patients be titrated with low doses of short-acting opioids initially. Patients can then be converted to Durogesic DTrans 25 mcg/hr. The dose may subsequently be titrated upwards or downwards, if required, in increments of 12 or 25 mcg/hr to achieve the lowest appropriate dose of Durogesic DTrans depending on the response and supplementary analgesic requirements (see also section 4.4).

In opioid-tolerant patients, the initial dose of Durogesic DTrans should be based on the previous 24 hour opioid analgesic requirement. A recommended conversion scheme from oral morphine to Durogesic DTrans is given below in Table 1:

Table 1: Recommended Durogesic DTrans dose based upon daily oral morphine dose

Oral 24-Hour Morphine (mg/day)	Durogesic DTrans (μg/h)
<90	25
90 – 134	37
135 – 189	50
190 – 224	62
225 – 314	75
315 – 404	100
405 – 494	125
495 – 584	150
585 – 674	175
675 – 764	200
765 – 854	225
855 – 944	250
945 – 1034	275
1035 – 1124	300

Previous analgesic therapy should be phased out gradually from the time of the first patch application until analgesic efficacy with Durogesic DTrans is attained. For both strong opioid-naïve and opioid tolerant patients, the initial evaluation of the analgesic effect of Durogesic DTrans should not be made until the patch has been worn for 24 hours due to the gradual increase in serum fentanyl concentrations up to this time.

Dose titration and maintenance therapy

The Durogesic DTrans patch should be replaced every 72 hours. The dose should be titrated individually until analgesic efficacy is attained. If analgesia is insufficient at the end of the initial application period, the dose may be increased. Dose adjustment, when necessary, should normally be performed in the following titration steps from 25 μg/h up to 75 μg/h: 25 μg/h, 37 μg/h, 50 μg/h, 62 μg/h and 75 μg/h; thereafter dose adjustments should normally be performed in 25 μg/h increments, although the supplementary analgesic requirements (oral morphine 90 mg/day ≈ Durogesic DTrans 25 μg/h) and pain status of the patient should be taken into account. More than one Durogesic DTrans patch may be used to achieve the desired dose. Patients may require periodic supplemental doses of a short-acting analgesic for 'breakthrough' pain. Additional or alternative methods of analgesia should be considered when the Durogesic DTrans dose exceeds 300 μg/h.

Discontinuation of Durogesic DTrans

If discontinuation of Durogesic DTrans is necessary, any replacement with other opioids should be gradual, starting at a low dose and increasing slowly. This is because fentanyl levels fall gradually after Durogesic DTrans is removed. After system removal, serum fentanyl concentrations decline gradually with mean terminal half-life ranging from 22-25 hours. As a general rule, the discontinuation of opioid analgesia should be gradual, in order to prevent withdrawal symptoms.

Opioid withdrawal symptoms (See section 4.8) are possible in some patients after conversion or dose adjustment.

Use in elderly patients

Data from intravenous studies with fentanyl suggest that elderly patients may have reduced clearance, a prolonged half-life and they may be more sensitive to the drug than younger patients. Studies of Durogesic DTrans in elderly patients demonstrated fentanyl pharmacokinetics which did not differ significantly from young patients although serum concentrations tended to be higher. Elderly, cachectic, or debilitated patients should be observed carefully for signs of fentanyl toxicity and the dose reduced if necessary.

Paediatric Patients:

Durogesic DTrans should be administered only to **opioid-tolerant paediatric patients (ages 2 to 16 years)** who are already receiving at least 30 mg oral morphine equivalents per day. To convert paediatric patients from oral opioids to Durogesic DTrans refer to Table 2, Recommended Durogesic DTrans dose based upon daily oral morphine dose.

Table 2: Recommended Durogesic DTrans dose based upon daily oral morphine dose[1]

Oral 24-Hour Morphine (mg/day)	Durogesic DTrans (μg/h)
For paediatric patients[2]	
30 - 44	12
45 - 134	25

[1] In clinical trials these ranges of daily oral morphine doses were used as a basis for conversion to Durogesic DTrans

[2] Conversion to Durogesic DTrans doses greater than 25 μg/h is the same for adult and paediatric patients

For children who receive more than 90 mg oral morphine a day, only limited information is currently available from clinical trials. In the paediatric studies, the required fentanyl transdermal patch dose was calculated conservatively: 30 mg to 44 mg oral morphine per day or its equivalent opioid dose was replaced by one Durogesic DTrans 12 patch. It should be noted that this conversion schedule for children only applies to the switch from oral morphine (or its equivalent) to Durogesic DTrans patches. The conversion schedule should not be used to convert from Durogesic DTrans into other opioids, as overdosing could then occur.

The analgesic effect of the first dose of Durogesic DTrans patches will not be optimal within the first 24 hours. Therefore, during the first 12 hours after switching to Durogesic DTrans, the patient should be given the previous regular dose of analgesics. In the next 12 hours, these analgesics should be provided based on clinical need.

Since peak fentanyl levels occur after 12 to 24 hours of treatment, monitoring of the patient for adverse events, which may include hypoventilation, is recommended for at least 48 hours after initiation of Durogesic DTrans therapy or up-titration of the dose (see also section 4.4).

Dose titration and maintenance

If the analgesic effect of Durogesic DTrans is insufficient, supplementary morphine or another short-duration opioid should be administered. Depending on the additional analgesic needs and the pain status of the child, it may be decided to increase the dose. Dose adjustments should be done in 12 μg/hour steps.

4.3 Contraindications

Durogesic DTrans is contraindicated in patients with known hypersensitivity to fentanyl or to the adhesive in the patch.

Durogesic DTrans is a sustained-release preparation indicated for the treatment of chronic intractable pain and is contraindicated in acute pain because of the lack of opportunity for dosage titration during short term use and the possibility of significant or life-threatening respiratory depression.

4.4 Special warnings and precautions for use

It is not possible to ensure the interchangeability of different makes of fentanyl transdermal patches in individual patients. Therefore, it should be emphasised that patients should not be changed from one make of fentanyl transdermal patches to another without specific counselling on the change from their healthcare professionals.

Patients who have experienced serious adverse events should be monitored for up to 24 hours after Durogesic DTrans removal since serum fentanyl concentrations decline gradually with mean terminal half-life ranging from 22-25 hours.

Durogesic DTrans should be kept out of reach and sight of children at all times before and after use.

Durogesic DTrans patches should not be cut. No data are available on cut or divided patches.

Use of Durogesic DTrans in opioid-naïve patients has been associated with very rare cases of significant respiratory depression and/or fatality when used as initial opioid therapy. The potential for serious or life-threatening hypoventilation exists even if the lowest dose of Durogesic DTrans is used in initiating therapy in opioid-naïve patients. It is recommended that Durogesic DTrans be used in patients who have demonstrated opioid tolerance (See Section 4.2).

When Durogesic DTrans is administered for chronic intractable pain that will require prolonged treatment, it is strongly recommended that the physician defines treatment outcomes with regards to pain relief and functional improvement in accordance with locally defined pain management guidelines. Physician and patient should agree to discontinue treatment if these objectives are not met.

Respiratory depression

As with all potent opioids, some patients may experience significant respiratory depression with Durogesic DTrans; patients must be observed for these effects. Respiratory depression may persist beyond the removal of the Durogesic DTrans patch. The incidence of respiratory depression increases as the Durogesic DTrans dose is increased (see Section 4.9). CNS active drugs may increase the respiratory depression (see section 4.5).

Interactions with CYP3A4 Inhibitors

The concomitant use of Durogesic DTrans with cytochrome P450 3A4 inhibitors (e.g. ritonavir, ketoconazole, itraconazole, clarithromycin, erythromycin, nelfinavir, verapamil, diltiazem and amiodarone) may result in an increase in fentanyl plasma concentrations, which could increase or prolong both the therapeutic and adverse effects, and may cause serious respiratory depression. In this situation special patient care and observation are appropriate. Therefore the concomitant use of transdermal fentanyl and cytochrome P450 3A4 inhibitors is not recommended unless the patient is closely monitored. Patients, especially those who are receiving Durogesic DTrans and CYP3A4 inhibitors, should be monitored for signs of respiratory depression and dosage adjustments should be made if warranted.

Chronic pulmonary disease

Fentanyl, like other opioids, may have more severe adverse effects in patients with chronic obstructive or other pulmonary disease. In such patients, they may decrease respiratory drive and increase airway resistance.

Drug dependence and potential for abuse

Tolerance, physical dependence and psychological dependence may develop upon repeated administration of opioids such as fentanyl. Iatrogenic addiction following opioid administration is rare.

Fentanyl can be abused in a manner similar to other opioid agonists. Abuse or intentional misuse of Durogesic DTrans may result in overdose and/or death. Patients at increased risk of opioid abuse may still be appropriately treated with modified-release opioid formulations; however, these patients will require monitoring for signs of misuse, abuse, or addiction.

Increased intracranial pressure

Durogesic DTrans should be used with caution in patients who may be particularly susceptible to the intracranial effects of CO_2 retention such as those with evidence of increased intracranial pressure, impaired consciousness or coma. Durogesic DTrans should be used with caution in patients with brain tumours.

Cardiac disease

Fentanyl may produce bradycardia and Durogesic DTrans should therefore be administered with caution to patients with bradyarrhythmias.

Hepatic disease

Because fentanyl is metabolised to inactive metabolites in the liver, hepatic disease might delay its elimination. In patients with hepatic cirrhosis, the pharmacokinetics of a single application of Durogesic DTrans were not altered although serum concentrations tended to be higher in these patients. Patients with hepatic impairment should be observed carefully for signs of fentanyl toxicity and the dose of Durogesic DTrans reduced if necessary.

Renal disease

Less than 10% of fentanyl is excreted unchanged by the kidney and, unlike morphine, there are no known active metabolites eliminated by the kidney. Data obtained with intravenous fentanyl in patients with renal failure suggest that the volume of distribution of fentanyl may be changed by dialysis. This may affect serum concentrations. If patients with renal impairment receive Durogesic DTrans, they should be observed carefully for signs of fentanyl toxicity and the dose reduced if necessary.

Patients with fever/external heat

Patients who develop fever should be monitored for opioid side effects since significant increases in body temperature can potentially increase fentanyl delivery rate.

Patients should also be advised to avoid exposing the Durogesic DTrans application site to direct external heat sources such as heating pads, hot water bottles, electric blankets, heated water beds, heat or tanning lamps, intensive sun bathing, prolonged hot baths, saunas or hot whirlpool spa baths while wearing the patch, since there is potential for temperature dependent increases in release of fentanyl from the patch.

Use in paediatric patients

Durogesic DTrans should not be administered to opioid-naïve paediatric patients (see section 4.2). The potential for serious or life-threatening hypoventilation exists regardless of the dose of Durogesic DTrans administered (see Table 2 in section 4.2).

Durogesic DTrans has not been studied in children under 2 years of age and so should not be used in these children. Durogesic DTrans should be administered only to opioid-tolerant children age 2 years or older (see section 4.2).

To guard against accidental ingestion by children, use caution when choosing the application site for Durogesic DTrans (see section 4.2) and monitor adhesion of the patch closely.

Patch disposal

Used patches may contain significant residues of active substance. After removal, therefore, used patches should be folded firmly in half, adhesive side inwards, so that the adhesive is not exposed, and then discarded safely and out of the reach of children according to the instructions in the pack.

4.5 Interaction with other medicinal products and other forms of interaction

The concomitant use of other CNS depressants, including opioids, anxiolytics, hypnotics, general anaesthetics, antipsychotics, skeletal muscle relaxants, sedating antihistamines and alcoholic beverages may produce additive depressant effects; hypoventilation, hypotension and profound sedation, coma or death may occur. Therefore, the use of any of the above mentioned concomitant drugs requires special care and observation.

Fentanyl, a high clearance drug, is rapidly and extensively metabolised mainly by CYP3A4.

The concomitant use of CYP3A4 inhibitors with transdermal fentanyl may result in an increase in fentanyl plasma concentrations, which could increase or prolong both the therapeutic and adverse effects, and may cause serious respiratory depression. In this situation, special patient care and observation are appropriate. The concomitant use of CYP3A4 inhibitors and transdermal fentanyl is not recommended, unless the patient is closely monitored (see Section 4.4).

Monoamine Oxidase Inhibitors (MAOI)

Durogesic DTrans is not recommended for use in patients who require the concomitant administration of an MAOI. Severe and unpredictable interactions with MAOIs, involving the potentiation of opiate effects or the potentiation of serotoninergic effects, have been reported.

4.6 Pregnancy and lactation

The safety of fentanyl in pregnancy has not been established. Studies in animals have shown some reproductive toxicity. The potential risk for humans is unknown. Neonatal withdrawal syndrome has been reported in newborn infants with chronic maternal use of Durogesic DTrans during pregnancy. Durogesic DTrans should not be used during pregnancy unless clearly necessary.

Use of Durogesic DTrans during childbirth is not recommended because fentanyl passes through the placenta and may cause respiratory depression in the newborn child.

Fentanyl is excreted into breast milk and may cause sedation/respiratory depression in the newborn/infant, hence Durogesic DTrans should not be used by women who are breast feeding.

4.7 Effects on ability to drive and use machines

Durogesic DTrans may impair the mental or physical ability required to perform potentially hazardous tasks such as driving or operating machinery.

4.8 Undesirable effects

Undesirable effects listed below in Table 3 have been reported in a clinical trial and/or from spontaneous reports from post-marketing experience.

A multicentre, double-blind, randomised, placebo-controlled clinical study (FEN-EMA-1) of Durogesic DTrans examined patients (> 40 years of age) with severe pain induced by osteoarthritis of the hip or knee and who were in need of and waiting for joint replacement. Patients were treated for 6 weeks with Durogesic DTrans by titrating to adequate pain control starting from 25 μg/hr to a maximum dose of 100 μg/hr in 25 μg/hr increments. This treatment was preceded by a 1-week washout period and followed by a tapering-off period of no more than 12 days. The adverse events, regardless of causality, reported by 1% or more of the patients treated with Durogesic DTrans during the trial and reported at a frequency greater than with placebo are presented in Table 3.

The adverse events are ranked by frequency, using the following convention:

Very common ≥1/10

Common ≥1/100 and <1/10

Uncommon ≥1/1,000 and <1/100

Rare ≥1/10,000 and <1/1,000

Very Rare <1/10,000

Unknown

Adverse drug reactions from spontaneous reports during worldwide postmarketing experience involving all indications with Durogesic DTrans that met threshold criteria are also included in Table 3. Unlike for clinical trials, precise frequencies cannot be provided for spontaneous reports. The frequency for these reports is therefore classified as 'not known'.

Table 3

Adverse Events, Regardless of Causality, Reported by ≥1% of Patients and Reported More Frequently with Durogesic DTrans than with Placebo during Double-Blind Treatment and Adverse Drug Reactions from Postmarketing Spontaneous Reports

Body System/ Organ Class *Frequency Category*	Clinical trials	Spontaneous Reports[a]
Immune system disorders		
Not known		Anaphylactic shock, anaphylactic reaction, anaphylactoid reaction
Metabolism and nutrition disorders		
Common	Anorexia	

Psychiatric Disorders		
Very common	Somnolence, insomnia	
Common	Anxiety, depression	
Not known		Confusional state, hallucination, euphoric mood, agitation
Nervous system disorders		
Very common	Dizziness	
Common	Muscle contractions involuntary, hypoaesthesia	
Not known		Convulsions (including clonic convulsions and grand mal convulsion), amnesia, headache, tremor, paraesthesia
Eye disorders		
Common	Conjunctivitis	
Cardiac disorders		
Common	Palpitations	
Not known		Tachycardia, bradycardia
Vascular Disorders		
Not known		Hypotension, hypertension
Respiratory, thoracic, and mediastinal disorders		
Common	Yawning, rhinitis	
Not known		Respiratory depression (including respiratory distress, apnoea, and bradypnoea; (see Section 4.9), hypoventilation, dyspnoea
Gastrointestinal disorders		
Very common	Nausea, vomiting, constipation	
Common	Abdominal pain, dyspepsia, dry mouth	
Not known		Diarrhoea
Skin and subcutaneous tissue disorders		
Common	Pruritis, skin disorder, hyperhidrosis	
Not known		Rash, erythema
Renal and urinary disorders		
Common	Urinary tract infection	
Not known		Urinary retention
Reproductive system and breast disorders		
Not known		Sexual dysfunction
General disorders and administration site conditions		
Common	Feeling of body temperature change, fatigue, malaise, influenza like illness, oedema peripheral, asthenia, drug withdrawal syndrome	Application site reaction

a: Listed are only those adverse drug reactions that were not identified during FEN-EMA-1.

As with other opioid analgesics, tolerance, physical dependence, and psychological dependence can develop on repeated use of Durogesic DTrans (see Section 4.4).

Opioid withdrawal symptoms (such as nausea, vomiting, diarrhoea, anxiety, and shivering) are possible in some patients after conversion from their previous opioid analgesic to Durogesic DTrans or if therapy is stopped suddenly (see Section 4.2).

There have been reports of newborn infants experiencing neonatal withdrawal syndrome when mothers chronically used Durogesic DTrans during pregnancy (see Section 4.6).

The adverse event profile in children and adolescents treated with Durogesic DTrans was similar to that observed in adults. No risk was identified in the paediatric population beyond that expected with the use of opioids for the relief of pain associated with serious illness. There does not appear to be any paediatric-specific risk associated with Durogesic DTrans use in children as young as 2 years old when used as directed. Very common adverse events reported in paediatric clinical trials were fever, vomiting, and nausea.

4.9 Overdose

Symptoms

The symptoms of fentanyl overdosage are an extension of its pharmacological actions, the most serious effect being respiratory depression.

Treatment

For management of respiratory depression, immediate countermeasures include removing Durogesic DTrans and physically or verbally stimulating the patient. These actions can be followed by administration of a specific opioid antagonist such as naloxone. The interval between IV antagonist doses should be carefully chosen and repeated administration or a continuous infusion of naloxone may be necessary because of continued absorption of fentanyl from the skin after patch removal, which may result in prolonged respiratory depression. Reversal of the narcotic effect may result in acute onset of pain and release of catecholamines.

A patent airway should be established and maintained. An oropharyngeal airway or endotracheal tube and oxygen should be administered and respiration assisted or controlled, as appropriate. Adequate body temperature and fluid intake should be maintained.

If severe or persistent hypotension occurs, hypovolaemia should be considered, and the condition should be managed with appropriate parenteral fluid therapy.

5. PHARMACOLOGICAL PROPERTIES

5.1 Pharmacodynamic properties

Pharmacotherapeutic group: opioid analgesic

ATC code: N02AB03

Fentanyl is an opioid analgesic with a high affinity for the μ-opioid receptor.

Paediatric Patients

The safety of Durogesic DTrans was evaluated in three open-label trials in 293 paediatric patients with chronic pain, 2 years of age through to 18 years of age, of which 66 children were aged to 2 to 6 years. In these studies, 30 mg to 44 mg oral morphine per day was replaced by one Durogesic 12 μg/h patch. Starting doses of 25 μg/h and higher were used by 181 patients who had been on prior daily opioid doses of at least 45 mg per dose of oral morphine.

5.2 Pharmacokinetic properties

Adults

Durogesic DTrans provides continuous systemic delivery of fentanyl over the 72 hour administration period. After the first Durogesic DTrans application, serum fentanyl concentrations increase gradually, generally levelling off between 12 and 24 hours, and remaining relatively constant for the remainder of the 72-hour application period. The serum fentanyl concentrations attained are proportional to the Durogesic DTrans patch size. For all practical purposes, by the second 72-hour application, a steady state serum concentration is reached and is maintained during subsequent applications of a patch of the same size.

After Durogesic DTrans is removed, serum fentanyl concentrations decline gradually, with mean terminal half-life ranging from 22-25 hours. Continued absorption of fentanyl from the skin accounts for a slower disappearance of the drug from the serum than is seen after an IV infusion. Fentanyl is metabolised primarily in the liver. Around 75% of fentanyl is excreted into the urine, mostly as metabolites, with less than 10% as unchanged drug. About 9% of the dose is recovered in the faeces, primarily as metabolites. The major metabolite, norfentanyl, is inactive. Mean values for unbound fractions of fentanyl in plasma are estimated to be between 13 and 21%.

Paediatric Patients

Adjusting for body weight, clearance (L/hr/Kg) in paediatric patients appears to be 82% higher in children 2 to 5 years old and 25% higher in children 6 to 10 years old when compared to children 11 to 16 years old, who are likely to have the same clearance as adults. These findings have been taken into consideration in determining the dosing recommendations for paediatric patients.

5.3 Preclinical safety data

No relevant information other than that contained elsewhere in the Summary of Product Characteristics.

6. PHARMACEUTICAL PARTICULARS

6.1 List of excipients

Polyacrylate adhesive

Polyethylene terephthalate/ethyl vinyl acetate film

Orange/Red/Green/Blue/Grey printing ink

Siliconised polyester film

6.2 Incompatibilities

To prevent interference with the adhesive properties of Durogesic DTrans, no creams, oils, lotions or powder should be applied to the skin area when the Durogesic DTrans transdermal patch is applied.

6.3 Shelf life

2 years.

6.4 Special precautions for storage

This medicinal product does not require any special storage precautions.

6.5 Nature and contents of container

Each patch is packed in a heat-sealed pouch made acrylonitrate film, polyethylene terephthalate (PET), low density polyethylene/aluminium foil and adhesive (Adcote 548). Five pouches are assembled in cardboard cartons.

6.6 Special precautions for disposal and other handling

Please refer to section 4.2 for instructions on how to apply the patch. There are no safety and pharmacokinetic data available for other application sites.

After removal, the used patch should be folded in half, adhesive side inwards so that the adhesive is not exposed, placed in the original sachet and then discarded safely out of reach of children.

Wash hands after applying or removing the patch.

7. MARKETING AUTHORISATION HOLDER

Janssen-Cilag Limited

50-100 Holmers Farm Way

High Wycombe

Buckinghamshire

HP12 4EG

UK

8. MARKETING AUTHORISATION NUMBER(S)

PL 00242/0409; PL 00242/0192-5

9. DATE OF FIRST AUTHORISATION/RENEWAL OF THE AUTHORISATION

Durogesic DTrans 12: 28 October 2005

Durogesic DTrans 25, 50, 75, 100: 4 March 1994/3 March 2009

10. DATE OF REVISION OF THE TEXT

Durogesic DTrans 12: 17 August 2009

Durogesic DTrans 25, 50, 75, 100: 17 August 2009

Legal category POM/CD2

Dynastat 20mg & 40mg Powder for Solution for Injection, Dynastat 20mg & 40mg Powder & Solvent for Solution for Injection

(Pfizer Limited)

1. NAME OF THE MEDICINAL PRODUCT

Dynastat ▼ 20 mg powder for solution for injection

Dynastat ▼ 20 mg powder and solvent for solution for injection

Dynastat ▼ 40 mg powder for solution for injection

Dynastat ▼ 40 mg powder and solvent for solution for injection

2. QUALITATIVE AND QUANTITATIVE COMPOSITION

20 mg vial: Each vial contains 20 mg parecoxib (present as 21.18 mg parecoxib sodium) for reconstitution. After reconstitution, the final concentration of parecoxib is 20 mg/ml.

When reconstituted in sodium chloride 9 mg/ml (0.9%) solution, Dynastat contains approximately 0.22 mEq of sodium per vial.

40 mg vial: Each vial contains 40 mg parecoxib (present as 42.36 mg parecoxib sodium) for reconstitution. After reconstitution, the final concentration of parecoxib is 20 mg/ml.

When reconstituted in sodium chloride 9 mg/ml (0.9%) solution, Dynastat contains approximately 0.44 mEq of sodium per vial.

For a full list of excipients, see section 6.1.

3. PHARMACEUTICAL FORM

Powder for solution for injection

Powder and solvent for solution for injection

White to off-white powder

Solvent: clear and colourless solution

4. CLINICAL PARTICULARS

4.1 Therapeutic indications

For the short-term treatment of postoperative pain.

The decision to prescribe a selective COX-2 inhibitor should be based on an assessment of the individual patient's overall risks (see sections 4.3 and 4.4).

4.2 Posology and method of administration

The recommended dose is 40 mg administered intravenously (IV) or intramuscularly (IM), followed every 6 to 12 hours by 20 mg or 40 mg as required, not to exceed 80 mg/day. The IV bolus injection may be given rapidly and directly into a vein or into an existing IV line. The IM injection should be given slowly and deeply into the muscle (see section 6.6 for instructions for reconstitution).

Concomitant Use with Opioid Analgesics: Opioid analgesics can be used concurrently with parecoxib, dosing as described in the paragraph above. In all clinical assessments parecoxib was administered at a fixed time interval whereas the opioids were administered on as needed basis (PRN).

As the cardiovascular risk of cyclooxygenase-2 (COX-2) specific inhibitors may increase with dose and duration of exposure, the shortest duration possible and the lowest effective daily dose should be used.

Precipitation may occur when Dynastat is combined in solution with other medicinal products and therefore Dynastat must not be mixed with any other drug, either during reconstitution or injection. In those patients where the same IV line is to be used to inject another medicinal product, the line must be adequately flushed prior to and after Dynastat injection with a solution of known compatibility.

IV line solution compatibility

After reconstitution with acceptable solvents, Dynastat may only be injected IV or IM, or into IV lines delivering:

sodium chloride 9 mg/ml (0.9%) solution

glucose 50 g/l (5%) solution for infusion

sodium chloride 4.5 mg/ml (0.45%) and glucose 50 g/l (5%) solution for injection

Ringer-Lactate solution for injection

Injection into an IV line delivering glucose 50 g/l (5%) in Ringer-Lactate solution for injection, or other IV fluids not listed above, is **not** recommended as this may cause precipitation from solution.

Elderly: No dosage adjustment is generally necessary in elderly patients (⩾ 65 years). However, for elderly patients weighing less than 50 kg, initiate treatment with half the usual recommended dose of Dynastat and reduce the maximum daily dose to 40 mg (see section 5.2).

Hepatic Impairment: No dosage adjustment is generally necessary in patients with mild hepatic impairment (Child-Pugh score 5-6). Introduce Dynastat with caution and at half the usual recommended dose in patients with moderate hepatic impairment (Child-Pugh score 7-9) and reduce the maximum daily dose to 40 mg. There is no clinical experience in patients with severe hepatic impairment (Child-Pugh score ⩾10), therefore its use is contraindicated in these patients (see sections 4.3 and 5.2).

Renal Impairment: On the basis of pharmacokinetics, no dosage adjustment is necessary in patients with mild to moderate renal impairment (creatinine clearance of 30-80 ml/min.). In patients with severe renal impairment (creatinine clearance < 30 ml/min.) or patients who may be predisposed to fluid retention parecoxib should be initiated at the lowest recommended dose and the patient's kidney function closely monitored (see sections 4.4 and 5.2).

Children and adolescents: There is no experience in children and adolescents. Therefore, its use is not recommended in these patients.

4.3 Contraindications

Hypersensitivity to the active substance or to any of the excipients (see section 6.1).

History of previous serious allergic drug reaction of any type, especially cutaneous reactions such as Stevens-Johnson syndrome, toxic epidermal necrolysis, erythema multiforme or patients with known hypersensitivity to sulphonamides (see sections 4.4 and 4.8).

Active peptic ulceration or gastrointestinal (GI) bleeding.

Patients who have experienced bronchospasm, acute rhinitis, nasal polyps, angioneurotic oedema, urticaria or other allergic-type reactions after taking acetylsalicylic acid or NSAIDs including COX-2 (cyclooxygenase-2) inhibitors.

The third trimester of pregnancy and breast-feeding (see sections 4.6 and 5.3).

Severe hepatic dysfunction (serum albumin <25 g/l or Child-Pugh score ⩾ 10).

Inflammatory bowel disease.

Congestive heart failure (NYHA II-IV).

Treatment of post-operative pain following coronary artery bypass graft (CABG) surgery (see sections 4.8 and 5.1).

Established ischaemic heart disease, peripheral arterial disease and/or cerebrovascular disease

4.4 Special warnings and precautions for use

There is limited clinical experience with Dynastat treatment beyond three days.

Because of the possibility for increased adverse reactions at higher doses of parecoxib, other COX-2 inhibitors and NSAIDs, patients treated with parecoxib should be reviewed following dose increase and, in the absence of an increase in efficacy, other therapeutic options should be considered (see section 4.2).

COX-2 inhibitors have been associated with increased risk of cardiovascular and thrombotic adverse events when taken long term. The exact magnitude of the risk associated with a single dose has not been determined, nor has the exact duration of therapy associated with increased risk.

Patients with significant risk factors for cardiovascular events (e.g. hypertension, hyperlipidaemia, diabetes mellitus, smoking) should only be treated with parecoxib sodium after careful consideration (see section 5.1).

Appropriate measures should be taken and discontinuation of parecoxib therapy should be considered if there is clinical evidence of deterioration in the condition of specific clinical symptoms in these patients (see section 5.1). Dynastat has not been studied in cardiovascular revascularization procedures other than coronary artery bypass graft procedures. Studies in other surgeries than CABG procedures included patients with ASA (American Society of Anaesthesiology) Physical Status Class I-III only.

COX-2 inhibitors are not a substitute for acetylsalicylic acid for prophylaxis of cardiovascular thrombo-embolic diseases because of their lack of antiplatelet effects. Therefore, antiplatelet therapies should not be discontinued (see section 5.1).

Upper gastrointestinal complications [perforations, ulcers or bleedings (PUBs)], some of them resulting in fatal outcome, have occurred in patients treated with parecoxib. Caution is advised in the treatment of patients most at risk of developing a gastrointestinal complication with NSAIDs; the elderly, patients using any other NSAID or acetylsalicylic acid concomitantly or patients with a prior history of gastrointestinal disease, such as ulceration and GI bleeding. There is further increase in the risk of gastrointestinal adverse effects (gastrointestinal ulceration or other gastrointestinal complications), when parecoxib sodium is taken concomitantly with acetylsalicylic acid (even at low doses).

Dynastat has been studied in dental, orthopaedic, gynaecologic (principally hysterectomy) and coronary artery bypass graft surgery. There is little experience in other types of surgery, for example gastrointestinal or urological surgery.

Serious skin reactions, including erythema multiforme, exfoliative dermatitis and Stevens-Johnson syndrome some of them fatal) have been reported through post marketing surveillance in patients receiving parecoxib. Additionally, fatal reports of toxic epidermal necrolysis, have been reported through postmarketing surveillance in patients receiving valdecoxib (the active metabolite of parecoxib) and cannot be ruled out for parecoxib (see section 4.8). Patients appear to be at highest risk for these reactions early in the course of therapy; the onset of the reaction occurring in the majority of cases within the first month of treatment.

Appropriate measures should be taken by physicians to monitor for any serious skin reactions with therapy, e.g. additional patient consultations. Patients should be advised to immediately report any emergent skin condition to their physician.

Parecoxib should be discontinued at the first appearance of skin rash, mucosal lesions, or any other sign of hypersensitivity. Serious skin reactions are known to occur with NSAIDs including COX-2 selective inhibitors as well as other medications. However, the reported rate of serious skin events appears to be greater for valdecoxib (the active metabolite of parecoxib) as compared to other COX-2 selective inhibitors. Patients with a history of sulphonamide allergy may be at greater risk of skin reactions (see section 4.3). Patients without a history of sulphonamide allergy may also be at risk for serious skin reactions.

Hypersensitivity reactions (anaphylaxis and angioedema) have been reported in post-marketing experience with valdecoxib and parecoxib (see section 4.8). Some of these reactions have occurred in patients with a history of allergic-type reactions to sulphonamides (see section 4.3). Parecoxib should be discontinued at the first sign of hypersensitivity.

Acute renal failure has been reported through post-marketing surveillance in patients receiving parecoxib (see section 4.8). Since prostaglandin synthesis inhibition may result in deterioration of renal function and fluid retention, caution should be observed when administering Dynastat in patients with impaired renal function (see section 4.2) or hypertension, or in patients with compromised cardiac or hepatic function or other conditions predisposing to fluid retention.

Caution should be used when initiating treatment with Dynastat in patients with dehydration. In this case, it is advisable to rehydrate patients first and then start therapy with Dynastat.

Dynastat should be used with caution in patients with moderate hepatic dysfunction (Child-Pugh score 7-9) (see section 4.2).

If during treatment, patients deteriorate in any of the organ system functions described above, appropriate measures should be taken and discontinuation of parecoxib sodium therapy should be considered.

Dynastat may mask fever and other signs of inflammation (see section 5.1). In isolated cases, an aggravation of soft tissue infections has been described in connection with the use of NSAIDs and in nonclinical studies with Dynastat (see section 5.3). Caution should be exercised with respect to monitoring the incision for signs of infection in surgical patients receiving Dynastat.

Caution should be exercised when co-administering Dynastat with warfarin and other oral anticoagulants (see section 4.5).

The use of Dynastat, as with any medicinal product known to inhibit cyclooxygenase/prostaglandin synthesis, is not recommended in women attempting to conceive (see sections 4.6 and 5.1).

4.5 Interaction with other medicinal products and other forms of interaction

Interaction studies have only been performed in adults.

Pharmacodynamic interactions

Anticoagulant therapy should be monitored, particularly during the first few days after initiating Dynastat therapy in patients receiving warfarin or other anticoagulants, since these patients have an increased risk of bleeding complications. Therefore, patients receiving oral anticoagulants should be closely monitored for their prothrombin time INR, particularly in the first few days when therapy with parecoxib is initiated or the dose of parecoxib is changed (see section 4.4).

Dynastat had no effect on acetylsalicylic acid-mediated inhibition of platelet aggregation or bleeding times. Clinical trials indicate that Dynastat can be given with low dose acetylsalicylic acid (⩽ 325 mg). In the submitted studies, as with other NSAIDs, an increased risk of gastrointestinal ulceration or other gastrointestinal complications compared to use of parecoxib alone was shown for concomitant administration of low-dose acetylsalicylic acid (see section 5.1).

Co-administration of parecoxib sodium and heparin did not affect the pharmacodynamics of heparin (activated partial thromboplastin time) compared to heparin alone.

NSAIDs may reduce the effect of diuretics and antihypertensive medicinal products. As for NSAIDs, the risk of acute renal insufficiency may be increased when ACE inhibitors or diuretics are co-administered with parecoxib sodium.

Co-administration of NSAIDs and cyclosporin or tacrolimus has been suggested to increase the nephrotoxic effect of cyclosporin and tacrolimus. Renal function should be monitored when parecoxib sodium and any of these medicinal products are co-administered.

Dynastat may be co-administered with opioid analgesics. In clinical trials, the daily requirement for PRN opioids was significantly reduced when coadministered with parecoxib.

Effects of other medicinal products on the pharmacokinetics of parecoxib (or its active metabolite valdecoxib)

Parecoxib is rapidly hydrolysed to the active metabolite valdecoxib. In humans, studies demonstrated that valdecoxib metabolism is predominantly mediated via CYP3A4 and 2C9 isozymes.

Plasma exposure (AUC and C_{max}) to valdecoxib was increased (62% and 19%, respectively) when co-administered with fluconazole (predominantly a CYP2C9 inhibitor), indicating that the dose of parecoxib sodium should be reduced in those patients who are receiving fluconazole therapy.

Plasma exposure (AUC and C_{max}) to valdecoxib was increased (38% and 24%, respectively) when co-administered with ketoconazole (CYP3A4 inhibitor); however, a dosage adjustment should not generally be necessary for patients receiving ketoconazole.

The effect of enzyme induction has not been studied. The metabolism of valdecoxib may increase when co-administered with enzyme inducers such as rifampicin, phenytoin, carbamazepine or dexamethasone.

Effect of parecoxib (or its active metabolite valdecoxib) on the pharmacokinetics of other medicinal products

Treatment with valdecoxib (40 mg twice daily for 7 days) produced a 3-fold increase in plasma concentrations of dextromethorphan (CYP2D6 substrate). Therefore, caution should be observed when co-administering Dynastat and medicinal products that are predominantly metabolised by CYP2D6 and which have narrow therapeutic margins (e.g. flecainide, propafenone, metoprolol).

Plasma exposure of omeprazole (CYP 2C19 substrate) 40 mg once daily was increased by 46% following administration of valdecoxib 40 mg twice daily for 7 days, while the plasma exposure to valdecoxib was unaffected. These results indicate that although valdecoxib is not metabolised by CYP2C19, it may be an inhibitor of this isoenzyme. Therefore, caution should be observed when administering Dynastat with medicinal products known to be substrates of CYP2C19 (e.g. phenytoin, diazepam, or imipramine).

In interaction studies in rheumatoid arthritis patients receiving weekly methotrexate intramuscularly, orally administered valdecoxib (40 mg twice daily) did not have a clinically significant effect on the plasma concentrations of methotrexate. However, adequate monitoring of methotrexate-related toxicity should be considered when co-administering these two medicinal products.

Co-administration of valdecoxib and lithium produced significant decreases in lithium serum clearance (25%) and renal clearance (30%) with a 34% higher serum exposure compared to lithium alone. Lithium serum concentration should be monitored closely when initiating or changing parecoxib sodium therapy in patients receiving lithium.

Co-administration of valdecoxib with glibenclamide (CYP3A4 substrate) did not affect either the pharmacokinetics (exposure) or the pharmacodynamics (blood glucose and insulin levels) of glibenclamide.

Injectable anaesthetics: Coadministration of IV parecoxib sodium 40 mg with propofol (CYP2C9 substrate) or midazolam (CYP3A4 substrate) did not affect either the pharmacokinetics (metabolism and exposure) or the pharmacodynamics (EEG effects, psychomotor tests and waking from sedation) of IV propofol or IV midazolam. Additionally, coadministration of valdecoxib had no clinically significant effect on the hepatic or intestinal CYP 3A4-mediated metabolism of orally administered midazolam. Administration of IV parecoxib sodium 40 mg had no significant effect on the pharmacokinetics of either IV fentanyl or IV alfentanil (CYP3A4 substrates).

Inhalation anaesthetics: No formal interaction studies have been done. In surgery studies in which parecoxib sodium was administered pre-operatively, no evidence of pharmacodynamic interaction was observed in patients receiving parecoxib sodium and the inhalation anaesthetic agents nitrous oxide and isoflurane (see section 5.1).

4.6 Pregnancy and lactation

Pregnancy:

Parecoxib sodium is suspected to cause serious birth defects when administered during the last trimester of pregnancy because as with other medicinal products known to inhibit prostaglandin synthesis, it may cause premature closure of the ductus arteriosus or uterine inertia (see sections 4.3, 5.1 and 5.3).

Dynastat is contraindicated (see section 4.3) in the last trimester of pregnancy.

Like other medicinal products that inhibit COX-2, Dynastat is not recommended in women attempting to conceive (see sections 4.4, 5.1 and 5.3).

There are no adequate data from the use of parecoxib sodium in pregnant women or during labour. Studies in animals have shown reproductive toxicity (see sections 5.1 and 5.3). The potential risk for humans is unknown. Dynastat should not be used during the first two trimesters of pregnancy unless clearly necessary (i.e. the potential benefit to the patient outweighs the potential risk to the foetus).

Lactation:

Parecoxib, valdecoxib (its active metabolite) and a valdecoxib active metabolite are excreted in the milk of rats. It is not known whether valdecoxib is excreted in human milk. Dynastat should not be administered to women who breast-feed (see sections 4.3 and 5.3).

4.7 Effects on ability to drive and use machines

No studies on the effect of Dynastat on the ability to drive or use machines have been performed. However, patients who experience dizziness, vertigo or somnolence after receiving Dynastat should refrain from driving or operating machines.

4.8 Undesirable effects

Within each frequency grouping, undesirable effects are presented in order of decreasing seriousness.

Of the Dynastat treated patients in controlled trials, 1962 were patients with post-surgical pain.

The following undesirable effects had a rate greater than placebo and have been reported among 1543 patients administered Dynastat 20 or 40 mg as a single or multiple dose (up to 80 mg/day) in 12 placebo controlled studies, including dental, gynaecologic, orthopaedic surgery or coronary artery bypass graft surgery as well as pre-operative administration in dental and orthopaedic surgeries. The discontinuation rate due to adverse events in these studies was 5.0 % for patients receiving Dynastat and 4.3% for patients receiving placebo.

[Very Common (≥1/10), Common (≥1/100, <1/10) Uncommon (≥1/1000, <1/100) Rare (≥1/10,000, <1/1000) Very rare (<1/10,000), not known (cannot be estimated from the available data *including isolated cases)]*

Infections and infestations

Uncommon: abnormal sternal serous wound drainage, wound infection.

Blood and lymphatic system disorders

Common: post-operative anaemia

Uncommon: thrombocytopenia

Metabolism and nutrition disorders

Common: hypokalaemia

Pyschiatric disorders:

Common: agitation, insomnia

Nervous system disorders

Common: hypoaesthesia

Uncommon: cerebrovascular disorder

Cardiac disorders

Uncommon: bradycardia

Vascular disorders

Common: hypertension, hypotension

Uncommon: aggravated hypertension

Respiratory, thoracic and mediastinal disorders

Common: respiratory insufficiency, pharyngitis

Gastrointestinal disorders

Common: alveolar osteitis (dry socket), dyspepsia, flatulence

Uncommon: gastroduodenal ulceration

Skin and subcutaneous tissue disorders

Common: pruritus

Uncommon: ecchymosis

Musculoskeletal and connective tissue disorders

Common: back pain

Renal and urinary disorders

Common: oliguria

General disorders and administration site conditions

Common: peripheral oedema

Investigations

Common: blood creatinine increased

Uncommon: SGOT increased, SGPT increased, blood urea nitrogen increased

The following rare, serious adverse events have been reported in association with the use of NSAIDs and cannot be ruled out for Dynastat: bronchospasm and hepatitis.

Following coronary artery bypass graft surgery, patients administered Dynastat have a higher risk of adverse events, such as cardiovascular/ thromboembolic events, deep surgical infections and sternal wound healing complications. Cardiovascular/thromboembolic events include myocardial infarction, stroke/TIA, pulmonary embolus and deep vein thrombosis (see section 4.3 and 5.1).

In post-marketing experience, the following reactions have been reported in association with the use of parecoxib:

Rare: acute renal failure, renal failure, myocardial infarction, congestive heart failure, abdominal pain, nausea, vomiting, dyspnoea and tachycardia and Stevens-Johnson syndrome.

Very rare: erythema multiforme, exfoliative dermatitis and hypersensitivity reactions including anaphylaxis and angioedema (see section 4.4).

In post marketing experience, the following reactions have been reported in association with the use of valdecoxib, and cannot be ruled out for parecoxib: toxic epidermal necrolysis (see section 4.4).

4.9 Overdose

No case of parecoxib overdose has been reported.

In case of overdose, patients should be managed by symptomatic and supportive care. Valdecoxib is not removed by haemodialysis. Diuresis or alkalisation of urine may not be useful due to high protein binding of valdecoxib.

5. PHARMACOLOGICAL PROPERTIES

5.1 Pharmacodynamic properties

Pharmacotherapeutic group: Coxib, ATC code: M01AH04

Parecoxib is a prodrug of valdecoxib. Valdecoxib is a selective cyclooxygenase-2 (COX-2) inhibitor within the clinical dose range. Cyclooxygenase is responsible for generation of prostaglandins. Two isoforms, COX-1 and COX-2, have been identified. COX-2 is the isoform of the enzyme that has been shown to be induced by pro-inflammatory stimuli and has been postulated to be primarily responsible for the synthesis of prostanoid mediators of pain, inflammation, and fever. COX-2 is also involved in ovulation, implantation and closure of the ductus arteriosus, regulation of renal function, and central nervous system functions (fever induction, pain perception and cognitive function). It may also play a role in ulcer healing. COX-2 has been identified in tissue around gastric ulcers in man but its relevance to ulcer healing has not been established.

The difference in antiplatelet activity between some COX-1 inhibiting NSAIDs and COX-2 selective inhibitors may be of clinical significance in patients at risk of thrombo-embolic reactions. COX-2 selective inhibitors reduce the formation of systemic (and therefore possibly endothelial) prostacyclin without affecting platelet thromboxane. The clinical relevance of these observations has not been established.

The efficacy of Dynastat was established in studies of dental, gynaecologic (hysterectomy), orthopaedic (knee and hip replacement), and coronary artery bypass graft surgical pain. The first perceptible analgesic effect occurred in 7 -13 minutes, with clinically meaningful analgesia demonstrated in 23-39 minutes and a peak effect within 2 hours following administration of single doses of 40 mg IV or IM Dynastat. The magnitude of analgesic effect of the 40 mg dose was comparable with that of ketorolac 60 mg IM or ketorolac 30 mg IV. After a single dose, the duration of analgesia was dose and clinical pain model dependent, and ranged from 6 to greater than 12 hours.

Opioid-sparing Effects: In a placebo-controlled, orthopedic and general surgery study (n =1050), patients received Dynastat at an initial parenteral dose of 40 mg IV followed by 20 mg twice daily for a minimum of 72 hours in addition to receiving standard care including supplemental patient controlled opioids. The reduction in opioid use with Dynastat treatment on Days 2 and 3 was 7.2 mg and 2.8 mg (37% and 28% respectively). This reduction in opioid use was accompanied by significant reductions in patient-reported opioid symptom distress. Added pain relief compared to opioids alone was shown. Additional studies in other surgical settings provided similar observations. There are no data indicating less overall adverse events associated with the use of parecoxib compared to placebo when used in conjunction with opioids.

Gastrointestinal studies: In short-term studies (7 days), the incidence of endoscopically observed gastroduodenal ulcers or erosions in healthy young and elderly (≥ 65 years) subjects administered Dynastat (5-21%), although higher than placebo (5-12%), was statistically significantly lower than the incidence observed with NSAIDs (66-90%).

CABG post-operative Safety Studies: In addition to routine adverse event reporting, pre-specified event categories, adjudicated by an independent expert committee, were examined in two placebo-controlled safety studies in which patients received parecoxib sodium for at least 3 days and then were transitioned to oral valdecoxib for a total duration of 10-14 days. All patients received standard of care analgesia during treatment.

Patients received low-dose acetylsalicylic acid prior to randomization and throughout the two CABG surgery studies.

The first CABG surgery study evaluated patients treated with IV parecoxib sodium 40 mg bid for a minimum of 3 days, followed by treatment with valdecoxib 40 mg bid (parecoxib sodium/valdecoxib group) (n=311) or placebo/placebo (n=151) in a 14-day, double-blind placebo-controlled study. Nine pre-specified adverse event categories were evaluated (cardiovascular thromboembolic events, pericarditis, new onset or exacerbation of congestive heart failure, renal failure/dysfunction, upper GI ulcer complications, major non-GI bleeds, infections, non-infectious pulmonary complications, and death). There was a significantly ($p<0.05$) greater incidence of cardiovascular/thromboembolic events (myocardial infarction, ischemia, cerebrovascular accident, deep vein thrombosis and pulmonary embolism) detected in the parecoxib/valdecoxib treatment group compared to the placebo/placebo treatment group for the IV dosing period (2.2% and 0.0% respectively) and over the entire study period (4.8% and 1.3% respectively). Surgical wound complications (most involving the sternal wound) were observed at an increased rate with parecoxib/valdecoxib treatment.

In the second CABG surgery study, four pre-specified event categories were evaluated (cardiovascular/thromboembolic; renal dysfunction/renal failure; upper GI ulcer/bleeding; surgical wound complication). Patients were randomized within 24-hours post-CABG surgery to: parecoxib initial dose of 40 mg IV, then 20 mg IV Q12H for a minimum of 3 days followed by valdecoxib PO (20 mg Q12H) (n=544) for the remainder of a 10 day treatment period; placebo IV followed by valdecoxib PO (n=544); or placebo IV followed by placebo PO (n=548). A significantly ($p=0.033$) greater incidence of events in the cardiovascular/thromboembolic category was detected in the parecoxib /valdecoxib treatment group (2.0%) compared to the placebo/placebo treatment group (0.5%). Placebo/valdecoxib treatment was also associated with a higher incidence of CV thromboembolic events versus placebo treatment, but this difference did not reach statistical significance. Three of the six cardiovascular thromboembolic events in the placebo/valdecoxib treatment group occurred during the placebo treatment period; these patients did not receive valdecoxib. Pre-specified events that occurred with the highest incidence in all three treatment groups involved the category of surgical wound complications, including deep surgical infections and sternal wound healing events.

There were no significant differences between active treatments and placebo for any of the other pre-specified event categories (renal dysfunction/failure, upper GI ulcer complications or surgical wound complications).

General Surgery: In a large (N=1050) major orthopedic/general surgery trial, patients received an initial dose of parecoxib 40 mg IV, then 20 mg IV Q12H for a minimum of 3 days followed by valdecoxib PO (20 mg Q12H) (n=525) for the remainder of a 10 day treatment period, or placebo IV followed by placebo PO (n=525). There were no significant differences in the overall safety profile, including the four pre-specified event categories described above for the second CABG surgery study, for parecoxib sodium/valdecoxib compared to placebo treatment in these post-surgical patients.

Platelet studies: In a series of small, multiple dose studies in healthy young and elderly subjects, Dynastat 20 mg or 40 mg twice daily had no effect on platelet aggregation or bleeding compared to placebo. In young subjects, Dynastat 40 mg twice daily had no clinically significant effect on acetylsalicylic acid -mediated inhibition of platelet function. (See section 4.5)

5.2 Pharmacokinetic properties

Following IV or IM injection, parecoxib is rapidly converted to valdecoxib, the pharmacologically active substance, by enzymatic hydrolysis in the liver.

Absorption

Exposure of valdecoxib following single doses of Dynastat, as measured by both the area under the plasma concentration vs. time curve (AUC) and peak concentration (C_{max}), is approximately linear in the range of clinical doses. AUC and C_{max} following twice daily administration is linear up to 50 mg IV and 20 mg IM. Steady state plasma concentrations of valdecoxib were reached within 4 days with twice daily dosing.

Following single IV and IM doses of parecoxib sodium 20 mg, C_{max} of valdecoxib is achieved in approximately 30 minutes and approximately 1 hour, respectively. Exposure to valdecoxib was similar in terms of AUC and C_{max} following IV and IM administration. Exposure to parecoxib was similar after IV or IM administration in terms of AUC. Average C_{max} of parecoxib after IM dosing was lower compared to bolus IV dosing, which is attributed to slower extravascular absorption after IM administration. These decreases were not considered clinically important since C_{max} of valdecoxib is comparable after IM and IV parecoxib sodium administration.

Distribution

The volume of distribution of valdecoxib after its IV administration is approximately 55 litres. Plasma protein binding is approximately 98% over the concentration range achieved with the highest recommended dose, 80 mg/day. Valdecoxib, but not parecoxib, is extensively partitioned into erythrocytes.

Metabolism

Parecoxib is rapidly and almost completely converted to valdecoxib and propionic acid in vivo with a plasma half-life of approximately 22 minutes. Elimination of valdecoxib is by extensive hepatic metabolism involving multiple pathways, including cytochrome P 450 (CYP) 3A4 and CYP2C9 isoenzymes and glucuronidation (about 20%) of the sulphonamide moiety. A hydroxylated metabolite of valdecoxib (via the CYP pathway) has been identified in human plasma that is active as a COX-2 inhibitor. It represents approximately 10% of the concentration of valdecoxib; because of this metabolite's low concentration, it is not expected to contribute a significant clinical effect after administration of therapeutic doses of parecoxib sodium.

Elimination

Valdecoxib is eliminated via hepatic metabolism with less than 5% unchanged valdecoxib recovered in the urine. No unchanged parecoxib is detected in urine and only trace amounts in the faeces. About 70% of the dose is excreted in the urine as inactive metabolites. Plasma clearance (CL_p) for valdecoxib is about 6 l/hr. After IV or IM dosing of parecoxib sodium, the elimination half-life ($t_{1/2}$) of valdecoxib is about 8 hours.

Elderly Subjects: Dynastat has been administered to 335 elderly patients (65-96 years of age) in pharmacokinetic and therapeutic trials. In healthy elderly subjects, the apparent oral clearance of valdecoxib was reduced, resulting in an approximately 40% higher plasma exposure of valdecoxib compared to healthy young subjects. When adjusted for body weight, steady state plasma exposure of valdecoxib was 16% higher in elderly females compared to elderly males (see section 4.2).

Renal Impairment: In patients with varying degrees of renal impairment administered 20 mg IV Dynastat, parecoxib was rapidly cleared from plasma. Because renal elimination of valdecoxib is not important to its disposition, no changes in valdecoxib clearance were found even in patients with severe renal impairment or in patients undergoing dialysis (see section 4.2).

Hepatic Impairment: Moderate hepatic impairment did not result in a reduced rate or extent of parecoxib conversion to valdecoxib. In patients with moderate hepatic impairment (Child-Pugh score 7-9), treatment should be initiated with half the usual recommended dose of Dynastat and the maximum daily dose should be reduced to 40 mg since valdecoxib exposures were more than doubled (130%) in these patients. Patients with severe hepatic impairment have not been studied and therefore the use of Dynastat in patients with severe hepatic impairment is not recommended (see sections 4.2 and 4.3).

5.3 Preclinical safety data

Non-clinical data reveal no special hazard for humans based on conventional studies of safety pharmacology or repeated dose toxicity at 2-fold the maximum human exposure to parecoxib. However, in the repeated dose toxicity studies in dogs and rats, the systemic exposures to valdecoxib (the active metabolite of parecoxib) were approximately 0.8-fold the systemic exposure in elderly human subjects at the maximum recommended therapeutic dose of 80 mg daily. Higher doses were associated with aggravation and delayed healing of skin infections, an effect probably associated with COX-2 inhibition.

In reproduction toxicity tests, the incidence of post-implantation losses, resorptions and foetal body weight retardation occurred at doses not producing maternal toxicity in the rabbit studies. No effects of parecoxib on male or female fertilities were found in rats.

The effects of parecoxib have not been evaluated in late pregnancy or in the pre- and postnatal period. Parecoxib sodium administered intravenously to lactating rats as a single dose showed concentrations of parecoxib, valdecoxib and a valdecoxib active metabolite in milk similar to that of maternal plasma.

The carcinogenic potential of parecoxib sodium has not been evaluated.

6. PHARMACEUTICAL PARTICULARS

6.1 List of excipients

Powder

Disodium hydrogen phosphate

Phosphoric acid and/or sodium hydroxide (for pH adjustment).

Solvent

Sodium chloride

Hydrochloric acid or sodium hydroxide (for pH adjustment)

Water for injections.

6.2 Incompatibilities

This medicinal product must **not** be mixed with other medicinal products except for those mentioned in section 6.6.

Dynastat and opioids should not be administered together in the same syringe.

Use of Ringer-Lactate solution for injection or glucose 50 g/l (5%) in Ringer Lactate solution for injection for reconstitution will cause the parecoxib to precipitate from solution and therefore is **not** recommended.

Use of Sterile Water for Injection is **not** recommended, as the resulting solution is not isotonic.

Do not inject Dynastat into an IV line delivering any other drug. The IV line must be adequately flushed prior to and after Dynastat injection with a solution of known compatibility (see section 6.6).

Injection into an IV line delivering glucose 50 g/l (5%) in Ringer-Lactate solution for injection, or other IV fluids not listed in 6.6, is **not** recommended as this may cause precipitation from solution.

6.3 Shelf life

3 years.

Chemical and physical in-use stability of the reconstituted solution has been demonstrated for 24 hours at 25°C. From a microbiological point of view, the aseptically prepared product should be used immediately. If not used immediately, in-use storage times and conditions prior to use are the responsibility of the user and would not normally be longer than 12 hours at 25°C, unless reconstitution has taken place in controlled and validated aseptic conditions.

6.4 Special precautions for storage

This medicinal product does not require special storing conditions prior to reconstitution.

Do not refrigerate or freeze reconstituted solutions.

For storage conditions of the reconstituted medicinal product see section 6.3.

6.5 Nature and contents of container

20 mg powder for solution for injection:

Parecoxib sodium vials

20 mg vials: Type I colourless glass vials (2 ml) with a laminated stopper, sealed with a yellow flip-off cap on the aluminium overseal.

Dynastat is available in packs containing 10 vials.

20 mg powder and solvent for solution for injection:

Parecoxib sodium vials

20 mg vials: Type I colourless glass vials (2 ml) with a laminated stopper, sealed with a yellow flip-off cap on the aluminium overseal.

Solvent ampoules

2 ml ampoule: colourless neutral glass, Type I.

Dynastat is supplied as a sterile, single unit-of-use vial that is packaged with a 2 ml ampoule with a fill volume of 1 ml sodium chloride 9mg/ml (0.9%) solution (see below for various pack sizes and configurations).

Pack sizes

1 × 1 pack: contains 1 vial with parecoxib 20 mg and 1 ampoule with 1 ml sodium chloride 9 mg/ml (0.9%) solution.

3 × 3 pack: contains 3 vials of parecoxib 20 mg and 3 ampoule with 1 ml sodium chloride 9 mg/ml (0.9%) solution.

5 × 5 pack: contains 5 vials of parecoxib 20 mg and 5 ampoule with 1 ml sodium chloride 9 mg/ml (0.9%) solution.

Not all pack sizes may be marketed.

40 mg powder for solution for injection:

Parecoxib sodium vials

40 mg vials: Type I colourless glass vials (5 ml) with a laminated stopper, sealed with a purple flip-off cap on the aluminium overseal.

Dynastat is available in packs containing 10 vials.

40 mg powder and solvent for solution for injection:

Parecoxib sodium vials

40 mg vials: Type I colourless glass vials (5 ml) with a laminated stopper, sealed with a purple flip-off cap on the aluminium overseal.

Solvent ampoules

2 ml ampoule: colourless neutral glass, Type I.

Dynastat is supplied as a sterile, single unit-of-use vial that is packaged with a 2 ml ampoule with a fill volume of 2 ml sodium chloride 9 mg/ml (0.9%) solution (see below for various pack sizes and configurations).

Pack Sizes

1 × 1 pack: contains 1 vial with parecoxib 40 mg and 1 ampoule with 2 ml sodium chloride 9 mg/ml (0.9%) solution.

3 × 3 pack: contains 3 vials with parecoxib 40 mg and 3 ampoule with 2 ml sodium chloride 9 mg/ml (0.9%) solution.

5 × 5 pack: contains 5 vials with parecoxib 40 mg and 5 ampoule with 2 ml sodium chloride 9 mg/ml (0.9%) solution.

Not all pack sizes may be marketed.

6.6 Special precautions for disposal and other handling

Dynastat must be reconstituted before use. Dynastat is preservative free. Aseptic technique is required for its preparation.

Reconstitution solvents

Reconstitute Dynastat 20 mg with 1 ml sodium chloride 9 mg/ml (0.9%) solution. The **only** other acceptable solvents for reconstitution are:

glucose 50 g/l (5%) solution for infusion

sodium chloride 4.5 mg/ml (0.45%) and glucose 50 g/l (5%) solution for injection

Reconstitute Dynastat 40 mg with 2 ml sodium chloride 9 mg/ml (0.9%) solution. The **only** other acceptable solvents for reconstitution are:

glucose 50 g/l (5%) solution for infusion

sodium chloride 4.5 mg/ml (0.45%) and glucose 50 g/l (5%) solution for injection

Reconstitution process

Use aseptic technique to reconstitute lyophilised parecoxib (as parecoxib sodium).

20 mg vial

Remove the purple flip-off cap to expose the central portion of the rubber stopper of the 20 mg parecoxib vial. Withdraw, with a sterile needle and syringe, 1 ml of an acceptable solvent and insert the needle through the central portion of the rubber stopper transferring the solvent into the 20 mg vial.

40 mg vial

Remove the purple flip-off cap to expose the central portion of the rubber stopper of the 40 mg parecoxib vial. Withdraw, with a sterile needle and syringe, 2 ml of an acceptable solvent and insert the needle through the central portion of the rubber stopper transferring the solvent into the 40 mg vial.

Dissolve the powder completely using a gentle swirling motion and inspect the reconstituted product before use. The entire contents of the vial should be withdrawn for a single administration.

After reconstitution, Dynastat should be inspected visually for particulate matter and discoloration prior to administration. The solution should not be used if discolored or cloudy, or if particulate matter is observed. Dynastat should be administered within 24 hours of reconstitution (see Section 6.3), or discarded.

The reconstituted product is isotonic.

IV line solution compatibility

After reconstitution with acceptable solvents, Dynastat may **only** be injected IV or IM, or into IV lines delivering:

sodium chloride 9 mg/ml (0.9%) solution

glucose 50 g/l (5%) solution for infusion

sodium chloride 4.5 mg/ml (0.45%) and glucose 50 g/l (5%) solution for injection

Ringer-Lactate solution for injection

For single use only. Any unused product or waste material should be disposed of in accordance with local requirements.

7. MARKETING AUTHORISATION HOLDER

Pfizer Limited
Sandwich
Kent CT13 9NJ
United Kingdom

8. MARKETING AUTHORISATION NUMBER(S)

EU/1/02/209/001 – Dynastat 20 mg powder for solution for injection

EU/1/02/209/002 – Dynastat 20 mg powder and solvent for solution for injection, 1 × 1 pack

EU/1/02/209/003 – Dynastat 20 mg powder and solvent for solution for injection, 3 × 3 pack

EU/1/02/209/004 – Dynastat 20 mg powder and solvent for solution for injection, 5 × 5 pack

EU/1/02/209/005 – Dynastat 40 mg powder for solution for injection

EU/1/02/209/006 – Dynastat 40 mg powder and solvent for solution for injection, 1 × 1 pack

EU/1/02/209/007 – Dynastat 40 mg powder and solvent for solution for injection, 3 × 3 pack

EU/1/02/209/008 – Dynastat 40 mg powder and solvent for solution for injection, 5 × 5 pack

9. DATE OF FIRST AUTHORISATION/RENEWAL OF THE AUTHORISATION

22nd March 2002/22nd March 2007

10. DATE OF REVISION OF THE TEXT

23rd July 2009

Detailed information on this product is available on the website of the European Medicines Agency (EMEA) http://www.emea.europa.eu

Company Ref: DY 10_0

Dysport

(Ipsen Ltd)

1. NAME OF THE MEDICINAL PRODUCT

Dysport.

2. QUALITATIVE AND QUANTITATIVE COMPOSITION

	Per Vial
Active Constituent	
Clostridium botulinum type A toxin-haemagglutinin complex	500U *
Other Constituents	
Albumin solution	125 mcg
Lactose	2.5 mg

* One unit (U) is defined as the median lethal intraperitoneal dose in mice.

3. PHARMACEUTICAL FORM

Injection.

4. CLINICAL PARTICULARS

4.1 Therapeutic indications

Dysport is indicated for focal spasticity, including the treatment of:

- arm symptoms associated with focal spasticity in conjunction with physiotherapy;

and

- dynamic equinus foot deformity due to spasticity in ambulant paediatric cerebral palsy patients, two years of age or older, only in hospital specialist centres with appropriately trained personnel.

Dysport is also indicated for the following treatments:

- Spasmodic torticollis in adults
- Blepharospasm in adults
- Hemifacial spasm in adults.

4.2 Posology and method of administration

The units of Dysport are specific to the preparation and are not interchangeable with other preparations of botulinum toxin.

Training: Dysport should only be administered by appropriately trained physicians.

Ipsen can facilitate training in administration of Dysport injections.

The exposed central portion of the rubber stopper should be cleaned with alcohol immediately prior to piercing the septum. A sterile 23 or 25 gauge needle should be used.

Arm spasticity

Posology

Adults: The recommended dose is 1000 units in total, distributed amongst the following five muscles:

(see Table 1 below)

The sites of injection should be guided by standard locations used for electromyography, although actual location of the injection site will be determined by palpation. All muscles except the biceps brachii (BB) should be injected at one site, whilst the biceps should be injected at two sites.

The dose should be lowered if there is evidence to suggest that this dose may result in excessive weakness of the target muscles, such as for patients whose target muscles are small, where the BB muscle is not to be injected or patients who are to be administered multi-level injections. Clinical improvement may be expected within two weeks after injection. Data on repeated and long term treatment are limited.

Children: The safety and effectiveness of Dysport in the treatment of arm spasticity in children have not been demonstrated.

Method of administration

When treating arm spasticity, Dysport is reconstituted with 1.0 mL of sodium chloride injection B.P. (0.9%) to yield a solution containing 500 units per mL of botulinum toxin type A.

Dysport is administered by intramuscular injection into the five muscles detailed above when treating arm spasticity.

Paediatric cerebral palsy spasticity

Posology

The initial recommended dose is 20 units/kg body weight given as a divided dose between both calf muscles. If only one calf is affected, a dose of 10 units/kg bodyweight should be used. Consideration should be given to lowering this starting dose if there is evidence to suggest that this dose may result in excessive weakness of the target muscles, such as for patients whose target muscles are small or patients who require concomitant injections to other muscle groups. Following evaluation of response to the starting dose, subsequent treatment may be titrated within the range 10 units/kg and 30 units/kg divided between both legs. The maximum dose administered must not exceed 1000 units/patient.

Administration should primarily be targeted to the gastrocnemius, although injections of the soleus and injection of the tibialis posterior should also be considered.

The use of electromyography (EMG) is not routine clinical practice but may assist in identifying the most active muscles.

Clinical improvement may be expected within two weeks after injection. Injections may be repeated approximately every 16 weeks or as required to maintain response, but not more frequently than every 12 weeks.

Method of administration

When treating paediatric cerebral palsy spasticity, Dysport is reconstituted with 1.0 mL of sodium chloride injection B.P. (0.9%) to yield a solution containing 500 units per mL of botulinum toxin type A.

Dysport is administered by intramuscular injection into the calf muscles when treating spasticity.

Spasmodic torticollis

Posology

Adults and elderly: The doses recommended for torticollis are applicable to adults of all ages providing the adults are of normal weight with no evidence of low neck muscle mass. A reduced dose may be appropriate if the patient is markedly underweight or in the elderly, where reduced muscle mass may exist.

The initial recommended dose for the treatment of spasmodic torticollis is 500 units per patient given as a divided dose and administered to the two or three most active neck muscles.

• For rotational torticollis distribute the 500 units by administering 350 units into the splenius capitis muscle, ipsilateral to the direction of the chin/head rotation and 150 units into the sternomastoid muscle, contralateral to the rotation.

• For laterocollis, distribute the 500 units by administering 350 units into the ipsilateral splenius capitis muscle and 150 units into the ipsilateral sternomastoid muscle. In cases associated with shoulder elevation the ipsilateral trapezoid or levator scapulae muscles may also require treatment, according to visible hypertrophy of the muscle or electromyographic (EMG) findings. Where injections of three muscles are required, distribute the 500 units as follows, 300 units splenius capitis, 100 units sternomastoid and 100 units to the third muscle.

• For retrocollis distribute the 500 units by administering 250 units into each of the splenius capitis muscles. This may be followed by bilateral trapezius injections (up to 250 units per muscle) after 6 weeks, if there is insufficient response. Bilateral splenii injections may increase the risk of neck muscle weakness.

• All other forms of torticollis are highly dependent on specialist knowledge and EMG to identify and treat the most active muscles. EMG should be used diagnostically for all complex forms of torticollis, for reassessment after unsuccessful injections in non complex cases, and for guiding injections into deep muscles or in overweight patients with poorly palpable neck muscles.

On subsequent administration, the doses may be adjusted according to the clinical response and side effects observed. Doses within the range of 250-1000 units are recommended, although the higher doses may be accompanied by an increase in side effects, particularly dysphagia. Doses above 1000 units are not recommended.

The relief of symptoms of torticollis may be expected within a week after the injection. Injections should be repeated approximately every 12 weeks or as required to prevent recurrence of symptoms.

Children: The safety and effectiveness of Dysport in the treatment of spasmodic torticollis in children have not been demonstrated.

Method of administration

When treating spasmodic torticollis Dysport is reconstituted with 1.0 mL of sodium chloride injection B.P. (0.9%) to yield a solution containing 500 units per mL of botulinum toxin type A.

Dysport is administered by intramuscular injection as above when treating spasmodic torticollis.

Blepharospasm and hemifacial spasm

Posology

Adults and elderly: In the treatment of bilateral blepharospasm the recommended initial dose is 120 units per eye.

Injection of 0.1 mL (20 units) should be made medially and of 0.2.mL (40 units) should be made laterally into the junction between the preseptal and orbital parts of both the upper and lower orbicularis oculi muscles of each eye.

For injections into the upper lid the needle should be directed away from its centre to avoid the levator muscle. A diagram to aid placement of these injections is provided. The relief of symptoms may be expected to begin within two to four days with maximal effect within two weeks.

Injections should be repeated approximately every 12 weeks or as required to prevent recurrence of symptoms. On such subsequent administrations the dose may need to be reduced to 80 units per eye - viz -: 0.1 mL (20 units) medially and 0.1 mL (20 units) laterally above and below each eye in the manner previously described. The dose may be further reduced to 60 units per eye by omitting the medial lower lid injection.

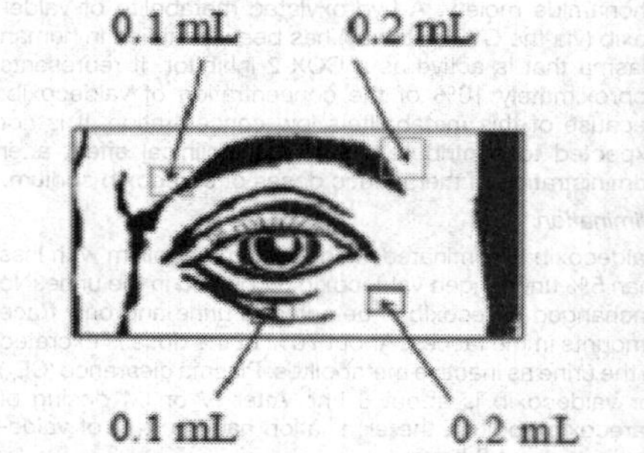

In cases of unilateral blepharospasm the injections should be confined to the affected eye. Patients with hemifacial spasm should be treated as for unilateral blepharospasm. The doses recommended are applicable to adults of all ages including the elderly.

Children: The safety and effectiveness of Dysport in the treatment of blepharospasm and hemifacial spasm in children have not been demonstrated.

Method of administration

When treating blepharospasm and hemifacial spasm, Dysport is reconstituted with 2.5 mL of sodium chloride injection BP (0.9%) to yield a solution containing 200 units per mL of botulinum toxin type A.

Dysport is administered by subcutaneous injection medially and laterally into the junction between the preseptal and orbital parts of both the upper and lower orbicularis oculi muscles of the eyes.

4.3 Contraindications

Dysport is contraindicated in individuals with known hypersensitivity to any components of Dysport.

4.4 Special warnings and precautions for use

Dysport should only be used with caution and under close supervision in patients with subclinical or clinical evidence of marked defective neuromuscular transmission (e.g. myasthenia gravis). Such patients may have an increased sensitivity to agents such as Dysport which may result in excessive muscle weakness with therapeutic doses. Patients with underlying neurological disorders are at increased risk of this side effect.

Patients with a history of dysphagia and aspiration should be treated with extreme caution. Swallowing or breathing disorders can worsen due to the spread of toxin distant from the site of administration. Aspiration has occurred in rare cases and is a risk when treating patients who have a chronic respiratory disorder. Dysport should be used under specialist supervision in all such patients and should only be used if the benefit of treatment is considered to outweigh the risk.

Side effects related to spread of toxin distant from the site of administration have been reported (see section 4.8), which in some cases was associated with dysphagia, pneumonia and /or significant debility resulting in death very rarely. Patients and their care-givers must be warned

Table 1

Biceps brachii (BB)	Flexor digitorum profundus (FDP)	Flexor digitorum superficialis (FDS)	Flexor carpi ulnaris (FCU)	Flexor carpi radialis FCR)	Total Dose
300-400 units (0.6-0.8 mL)	150 units (0.3 mL)	150-250 units (0.3-0.5 mL)	150 units (0.3 mL)	150 units (0.3 mL)	1000 units (2.0 mL)

of the necessity of immediate medical treatment in case of problems with swallowing, speech or respiratory disorders.

Careful consideration should be given before the injection of patients who have experienced a previous allergic reaction to a product containing botulinum toxin type A. The risk of a further allergic reaction must be considered in relation to the benefit of treatment.

Antibody formation to botulinum toxin has been noted rarely in patients receiving Dysport. Clinically, neutralising antibodies have been detected by a substantial deterioration in response to therapy and /or a need for consistently increasing doses.

For the treatment of cerebral palsy in children, Dysport should only be used in children over 2 years of age.

The recommended posology and frequency of administration for Dysport must not be exceeded (see section 4.2).

Dysport should only be used to treat a single patient, during a single session. Specific precautions must be taken for the preparation and administration of the product (see section 4.2) and for the inactivation and disposal of any unused reconstituted solution (see section 6.6).

As with any intramuscular injection, Dysport should be used only where strictly necessary in patients with prolonged bleeding times, infection or inflammation at the proposed injection site.

This product contains a small amount of human albumin. The risk of transmission of viral infection cannot be excluded with absolute certainty following the use of human blood or blood products.

4.5 Interaction with other medicinal products and other forms of interaction

The effects of botulinum toxin may be enhanced by drugs interfering directly or indirectly with the neuromuscular function (e.g. aminoglycosides, curare-like non-depolarising blockers) and such drugs should be used with caution in patients treated with botulinum toxin.

4.6 Pregnancy and lactation

Teratological and other reproductive studies have not been performed with Dysport. The safety of its use in pregnant or lactating women has not been demonstrated.

Dysport should not be used in pregnant or lactating women, unless clearly necessary.

4.7 Effects on ability to drive and use machines

Dysport may impair the ability to drive or operate machinery in case of adverse reactions such as muscle weakness and eye disorders (diplopia, blurred vision, eyelid ptosis).

4.8 Undesirable effects

Very common $>1/10$: Common $>1/100$, $<1/10$: Uncommon $>1/1000$, $<1/100$:

Rare $>1/10\,000$, $<1/1000$: Very rare $<1/10\,000$.

Side effects related to spread of toxin distant from the site of administration have been reported (exaggerated muscle weakness, dysphagia, aspiration/aspiration pneumonia, with fatal outcome in some very rare cases) (see section 4.4).

General

In the clinical trial programme, approximately 28% of the patients treated with Dysport experienced an adverse event.

The following adverse reactions were seen in patients treated across a variety of indications including blepharospasm, hemifacial spasm, torticollis and spasticity associated with either cerebral palsy or stroke:

Nervous system disorders

Rare: Neuralgic amyotrophy

Skin and subcutaneous tissue disorders

Uncommon: Itching

Rare: Skin rashes

General disorders and administration site conditions

Common: Generalised weakness, fatigue, flu-like syndrome, pain / bruising at injection site.

In addition, the following adverse reactions specific to individual indications were reported:

Arm spasticity

Gastrointestinal disorders

Common: Dysphagia

Musculoskeletal and connective tissue disorders

Common: Arm muscle weakness

Injury, poisoning and procedural complications

Common: Accidental injury/falls

Paediatric cerebral palsy spasticity

Gastrointestinal disorders

Common: Diarrhoea, vomiting

Musculoskeletal and connective tissue disorders

Common: Leg muscle weakness

Renal and urinary disorders

Common: Urinary incontinence

General disorders and administration site conditions

Common: Abnormal gait

Injury, poisoning and procedural complications

Common: Accidental injury due to falling

Accidental injury due to falling and abnormal gait may have been due to the over-weakening of the target muscle and / or the local spread of Dysport to other muscles involved in ambulation and balance.

Spasmodic torticollis

Nervous system disorders

Common: Dysphonia

Uncommon: Headache

Eye disorders

Uncommon: Diplopia, blurred vision

Respiratory, thoracic and mediastinal disorders

Rare: Respiratory disorders

Gastrointestinal disorders

Very common: Dysphagia

Uncommon: Dry mouth

Musculoskeletal and connective tissue disorders

Common: Neck muscle weakness

Dysphagia appeared to be dose related and occurred most frequently following injection into the sternomastoid muscle. A soft diet may be required until symptoms resolve.

These side effects may be expected to resolve within two to four weeks.

Blepharospasm and hemifacial spasm

Nervous system disorders

Common: Facial muscle weakness

Uncommon: Facial nerve paresis

Eye disorders

Very common: Ptosis

Common: Diplopia, dry eyes, tearing

Rare: Ophthalmoplegia

Skin and subcutaneous tissue disorders

Common: Eyelid oedema

Rare: Entropion

Side effects may occur due to deep or misplaced injections of Dysport temporarily paralysing other nearby muscle groups.

Post-marketing experience

The profile of adverse reactions reported to the company during post-marketing use reflects the pharmacology of the product and those seen during clinical trials. In addition, hypersensitivity reactions have been reported.

4.9 Overdose

Excessive doses may produce distant and profound neuromuscular paralysis. Respiratory support may be required where excessive doses cause paralysis of respiratory muscles. There is no specific antidote; antitoxin should not be expected to be beneficial and general supportive care is advised. Overdose could lead to an increased risk of the neurotoxin entering the bloodstream and may cause complications associated with the effects of oral botulinum poisoning (e.g. deglutition and dysphonia).

Symptomatic treatment should be instituted if necessary. In the event of an overdose the patient should be medically monitored for several weeks for symptoms of systemic weakness or muscle paralysis.

5. PHARMACOLOGICAL PROPERTIES

5.1 Pharmacodynamic properties

Clostridium botulinum type A toxin-haemagglutinin complex blocks peripheral cholinergic transmission at the neuromuscular junction by a presynaptic action at a site proximal to the release of acetylcholine. The toxin acts within the nerve ending to antagonise those events that are triggered by Ca^{2+} which culminate in transmitter release. It does not affect postganglionic cholinergic transmission or postganglionic sympathetic transmission.

The action of toxin involves an initial binding step whereby the toxin attaches rapidly and avidly to the presynaptic nerve membrane. Secondly, there is an internalisation step in which toxin crosses the presynaptic membrane, without causing onset of paralysis. Finally the toxin inhibits the release of acetylcholine by disrupting the Ca^{2+} mediated acetylcholine release mechanism, thereby diminishing the endplate potential and causing paralysis.

Recovery of impulse transmission occurs gradually as new nerve terminals sprout and contact is made with the post synaptic motor endplate, a process which takes 6 - 8 weeks in the experimental animal.

5.2 Pharmacokinetic properties

Pharmacokinetic studies with botulinum toxin pose problems in animals because of the high potency, the minute doses involved, the large molecular weight of the compound and the difficulty of labelling toxin to produce sufficiently high specific activity. Studies using I125 labelled toxin have shown that the receptor binding is specific and saturable, and the high density of toxin receptors is a contributory factor to the high potency. Dose and time responses in monkeys showed that at low doses there was a delay of 2 - 3 days with peak effect seen 5 - 6 days after injection. The duration of action, measured by changes of ocular alignment and muscle paralysis varied between 2 weeks and 8 months. This pattern is also seen in man, and is attributed to the process of binding, internalisation and changes at the neuromuscular junction.

5.3 Preclinical safety data

There is no further pre-clinical information relevant to the prescribing physician that has not been included in other sections of the Summary of Product Characteristics.

6. PHARMACEUTICAL PARTICULARS

6.1 List of excipients

Albumin and Lactose.

6.2 Incompatibilities

None known.

6.3 Shelf life

The shelf life of the packaged product is 24 months at 2-8°C.

The product may be stored for up to 8 hours at 2-8°C following reconstitution.

Since the product does not contain an antimicrobial agent, from a microbiological point of view, it is recommended that the product should be used immediately following reconstitution.

6.4 Special precautions for storage

Unopened vials must be maintained at temperatures between 2°C and 8°C. Dysport must be stored in a refrigerator at the hospital where the injections are to be carried out and should not be given to the patient to store.

Reconstituted Dysport may be stored in a refrigerator (2-8°C) for up to 8 hours prior to use. Dysport should not be frozen.

6.5 Nature and contents of container

Nature of container/closure:

Type 1 glass vials 3 mL capacity. 13 mm chlorbutyl freeze-drying closures oversealed by 13 mm aluminium overseals with centre hole, crimped over.

Contents of container:

A white lyophilised powder for reconstitution.

6.6 Special precautions for disposal and other handling

Immediately after treatment of the patient, any residual Dysport which may be present in either vial or syringe should be inactivated with dilute hypochlorite solution (1% available chlorine). Thereafter, all items should be disposed of in accordance with standard hospital practice.

Spillage of Dysport should be wiped up with an absorbent cloth soaked in dilute hypochlorite solution.

7. MARKETING AUTHORISATION HOLDER

Ipsen Limited

190 Bath Road

Slough

Berkshire

SL1 3XE

United Kingdom

8. MARKETING AUTHORISATION NUMBER(S)

PL 06958/0005

9. DATE OF FIRST AUTHORISATION/RENEWAL OF THE AUTHORISATION

9th December 1990

10. DATE OF REVISION OF THE TEXT

28th April 2009

of the benefit of intramuscular product treatment in case of problems with swallowing, speech or respiratory disorders.

Careful consideration should be given before the injection of patients who have experienced a previous allergic reaction to a product containing botulinum toxin type A. The risk of a further allergic reaction must be considered in relation to the benefit of treatment.

Antibody formation to botulinum toxin has been noted rarely in patients receiving Dysport. Clinically, neutralising antibodies have been detected by a substantial deterioration in response to therapy and / or a need for consistently increasing doses.

For the treatment of cerebral palsy in children, Dysport should only be used in children over 2 years of age.

The recommended posology and frequency of administration for Dysport must not be exceeded (see section 4.2).

Dysport should only be used to treat a single patient, during a single session. Specific precautions must be taken for the preparation and administration of the product (see section 4.2) and for the inactivation and disposal of any unused reconstituted solution (see section 6.6).

As with any intramuscular injection, Dysport should be used only where strictly necessary in patients with prolonged bleeding times, infection or inflammation at the proposed injection site.

This product contains a small amount of human albumin. The risk of transmission of viral infection cannot be excluded with absolute certainty following the use of human blood or blood products.

4.5 Interaction with other medicinal products and other forms of interaction

The effects of botulinum toxin may be enhanced by drugs interfering either directly or indirectly with neuromuscular function (e.g. aminoglycosides, curare-like non-depolarising blockers) and such drugs should be used with caution in patients treated with botulinum toxin.

4.6 Pregnancy and lactation

There are clinical data from the use of Dysport. Animal studies have not been performed with Dysport. The safety of its use in pregnant or lactating women has not been demonstrated.

Dysport should not be used in pregnant or lactating women unless clearly necessary.

4.7 Effects on ability to drive and use machines

Dysport may impair the ability to drive or operate machinery in the case of adverse reactions such as muscle weakness and vision disorders (diplopia, blurred vision, eyelid ptosis).

4.8 Undesirable effects

Very common ≥ 1/10; Common ≥ 1/100 < 1/10; Uncommon ≥ 1/1000 < 1/100;

Rare ≥ 1/10,000 < 1/1000; Very rare < 1/10 000

Side effects related to spread of toxin distant from the site of administration have been reported (exaggerated muscle weakness, dysphagia, aspiration pneumonia, pneumonia with fatal outcome in some very rare cases) (see section 4.4).

General

In the clinical trial programme, approximately 21% of the patients treated with Dysport experienced an adverse event.

The following adverse reactions were seen in patients treated across a variety of indications including blepharospasm, hemifacial spasm, torticollis and spasticity associated with either cerebral palsy or stroke:

Nervous system disorders

Rare: Neuralgic amyotrophy

Skin and subcutaneous tissue disorders

Uncommon: Itching

Rare: Skin rashes

General disorders and administration site conditions

Common: Generalised weakness, fatigue, flu-like syndrome, pain / bruising at injection site

In addition, the following adverse reactions specific to individual indications were reported:

Arm spasticity

Gastrointestinal disorders

Common: Dysphagia

Musculoskeletal and connective tissue disorders

Common: Arm muscle weakness

Injury, poisoning and procedural complications

Common: Accidental injury/falls

Paediatric cerebral palsy spasticity

Gastrointestinal disorders

Common: Diarrhoea, vomiting

Musculoskeletal and connective tissue disorders

Common: Leg muscle weakness

Renal and urinary disorders

Common: Urinary incontinence

General disorders and administration site conditions

Common: Abnormal gait

Injury, poisoning and procedural complications

Common: Accidental injury due to falling

Accidental injury due to falling and abnormal gait may have been due to the over-weakening of the target muscle and / or the local spread of Dysport to other muscles involved in ambulation and balance.

Spasmodic torticollis

Nervous system disorders

Common: Dysphonia

Uncommon: Headache

Dysfunction

Uncommon: Diplopia, blurred vision

Respiratory, thoracic and mediastinal disorders

Rare: Respiratory disorders

Gastrointestinal disorders

Very common: Dysphagia

Uncommon: Dry mouth

Musculoskeletal and connective tissue disorders

Common: Neck muscle weakness

Dysphagia appeared to be dose related and occurred most frequently following injection into the sternomastoid muscle. A soft diet may be required until symptoms resolve.

These side effects may be expected to resolve within two to four weeks.

Blepharospasm and hemifacial spasm

Nervous system disorders

Common: Facial muscle weakness

Uncommon: Facial nerve paresis

Eye disorders

Very common: Ptosis

Common: Diplopia, dry eyes, tearing

Rare: Ophthalmoplegia

Skin and subcutaneous tissue disorders

Common: Eyelid oedema

Rare: Entropion

Side effects may occur due to deep or misplaced injections of Dysport temporarily paralysing other nearby muscle groups.

Post-marketing experience

The profile of adverse reactions reported to the company during post-marketing use reflects the pharmacology of the product and those seen during clinical trials. In addition, hypersensitivity reactions have been reported.

4.9 Overdose

Excessive doses may produce distant and profound neuromuscular paralysis. Respiratory support may be required where excessive doses cause paralysis of respiratory muscles. There is no specific antidote; antitoxin should not be expected to be beneficial and general supportive care is advised. Overdose could lead to an increased risk of the neurotoxin entering the bloodstream and may cause complications associated with the effects of oral botulinum poisoning (e.g. deglutition and dysphonia).

Symptomatic treatment should be instituted if necessary. In the event of an overdose the patient should be medically monitored for several weeks for symptoms of systemic weakness or muscle paralysis.

5. PHARMACOLOGICAL PROPERTIES

5.1 Pharmacodynamic properties

Clostridium botulinum type A toxin-haemagglutinin complex blocks peripheral cholinergic transmission at the neuromuscular junction by a presynaptic action at a site proximal to the release of acetylcholine. The toxin acts within the nerve ending to antagonise those events that are triggered by Ca^{2+} which culminate in transmitter release. It does not affect postganglionic cholinergic transmission or postganglionic sympathetic transmission.

The action of toxin involves an initial binding step whereby the toxin attaches rapidly and avidly to the presynaptic nerve membrane. Secondly, there is an internalisation step in which toxin crosses the presynaptic membrane, without causing onset of paralysis. Finally, the toxin inhibits the release of acetylcholine by disrupting the Ca^{2+} mediated acetylcholine release mechanism, thereby diminishing the endplate potential and causing paralysis.

Recovery of impulse transmission occurs gradually as new nerve terminals sprout and contact is made with the post synaptic motor endplate, a process which takes 6 - 8 weeks in the experimental animal.

5.2 Pharmacokinetic properties

Pharmacokinetic studies with botulinum toxin pose problems in animals because of the high potency, the minute doses involved, the large molecular weight of the compound and the difficulty of labelling toxin to produce sufficiently high specific activity. Studies using I^{125} labelled toxin have shown that the receptor binding is specific and saturable, and the high density of toxin receptors is a contributory factor to the high potency. Dose and time responses in monkeys showed that at low doses there was a delay of 2-3 days with peak effect seen 5-6 days after injection. The duration of action, measured by changes of ocular alignment and muscle paralysis, varied between 2 weeks and 8 months. This pattern is also seen in man, and is attributed to the process of binding, internalisation and changes at the neuromuscular junction.

5.3 Preclinical safety data

There are no further pre-clinical information relevant to the prescribing physician that has not been included in other sections of the Summary of Product Characteristics.

6. PHARMACEUTICAL PARTICULARS

6.1 List of excipients

Albumin and Lactose

6.2 Incompatibilities

None known.

6.3 Shelf life

The shelf-life of the packaged product is 24 months at 2-8°C.

The product may be stored for up to 8 hours at 2-8°C following reconstitution.

Since the product does not contain an antimicrobial agent, from a microbiological point of view, it is recommended that the product should be used immediately following reconstitution.

6.4 Special precautions for storage

Unopened vials must be maintained at temperatures between 2°C and 8°C. Dysport must be stored in the refrigerator at the hospital where the injections are to be carried out and should not be given to the patient to store.

Reconstituted Dysport may be stored in a refrigerator (2-8°C) for up to 8 hours prior to use. Dysport should not be frozen.

6.5 Nature and contents of container

Nature of container and closure:

Type I glass vials of nominal capacity 3 ml and chlorobutyl freeze-drying closure, overseal by 13 mm aluminium overseals with central hole, crimped over.

Contents of container:

A white lyophilised powder for reconstitution.

6.6 Special precautions for disposal and other handling

Immediately after treatment of the patient, any residual Dysport which may be present in either vial or syringe should be inactivated with dilute hypochlorite solution (1% available chlorine). Thereafter, all items should be disposed of in accordance with standard hospital practice.

Spillage of Dysport should be wiped up with an absorbent cloth soaked in dilute hypochlorite solution.

7. MARKETING AUTHORISATION HOLDER

Ipsen Limited

190 Bath Road

Slough

Berkshire

SL1 3XE

United Kingdom

8. MARKETING AUTHORISATION NUMBER(S)

PL 06958/0005

9. DATE OF FIRST AUTHORISATION/RENEWAL OF THE AUTHORISATION

5th December 1990

10. DATE OF REVISION OF THE TEXT

13th April 2009

Easyhaler Beclometasone 200 micrograms/dose inhalation powder

(Orion Pharma (UK) Limited)

1. NAME OF THE MEDICINAL PRODUCT

Easyhaler® Beclometasone 200 micrograms/dose inhalation powder

2. QUALITATIVE AND QUANTITATIVE COMPOSITION

Name of ingredient	Amount in metered dose	Amount in delivered dose
Beclomethasone dipropionate	200 micrograms	180 micrograms

For excipients, see section 6.1

3. PHARMACEUTICAL FORM

Inhalation powder administered from multidose powder inhaler.

4. CLINICAL PARTICULARS

4.1 Therapeutic indications

Beclomethasone dipropionate given by inhalation offers preventative treatment for asthma. It provides effective anti-inflammatory action in the lungs without the problems of systemic corticosteroid treatment.

Easyhaler® Beclometasone 200 micrograms/dose is indicated in the prophylactic management of mild, moderate, or severe asthma in adults.

Mild asthma: Patients requiring symptomatic bronchodilator asthma medication on a regular basis.

Moderate asthma: Patients with unstable or worsening asthma despite prophylactic therapy or bronchodilator alone.

Severe asthma: Patients with severe chronic asthma and those who are dependent on systemic corticosteroids for adequate control of symptoms. Many patients who are dependent on systemic corticosteroids for adequate control of symptoms may be able to reduce significantly, or eliminate, their requirement for oral corticosteroids when they are transferred to high dose inhaled beclomethasone dipropionate.

4.2 Posology and method of administration

Easyhaler® Beclometasone 200 micrograms/dose is for oral inhalation use only. Patients should be given a starting dose of inhaled beclomethasone dipropionate appropriate to the severity of their disease. The dose may then be adjusted until control is achieved, or reduced to the minimum effective dose according to individual response.

Adults (including the elderly): The usual starting dose is 200 micrograms twice a day. In more severe cases the starting dose may need to increase to 600 to 800 micrograms per day which may then be reduced when the patient's asthma has stabilised. The total daily dose may be administered as two, three, or four divided doses.

Easyhaler® Beclometasone 200 micrograms/dose is not recommended for children.

4.3 Contraindications

Hypersensitivity to any of the components.

Special care is necessary in patients with active or quiescent pulmonary tuberculosis.

4.4 Special warnings and precautions for use

Patients should be instructed in the proper use of the inhaler, and their technique checked, to ensure that the drug reaches the target areas within the lungs. They should also be made aware that Easyhaler® Beclometasone 200 micrograms/dose has to be used regularly, every day, even when they are asymptomatic, for optimum benefit.

Easyhaler® Beclometasone 200 micrograms/dose is not designed to relieve acute asthma symptoms for which an inhaled short-acting bronchodilator is required. Patients should be advised to have such relief medication available.

Severe asthma requires regular medical assessment, including lung-function testing, as patients are at risk of severe attacks and even death. Patients must be instructed to seek medical attention if short-acting relief bronchodilator treatment becomes less effective, or more inhalations than usual are required as this may indicate deterioration of asthma control. In this situation, patients should be assessed and the need for increased anti-inflammatory therapy (e.g. higher doses of inhaled corticosteroid or a course of oral corticosteroid) considered.

Severe exacerbations of asthma must be treated in the normal way, e.g. by increasing the dose of inhaled beclomethasone dipropionate and, if necessary by giving a systemic steroid, and/or an antibiotic if there is an infection, and by use of β-agonist therapy.

Treatment with Easyhaler®Beclometasone 200 micrograms/dose should not be stopped abruptly.

Significant adrenal suppression rarely occurs before doses of 1,500 micrograms per day of inhaled beclomethasone dipropionate are exceeded. Reduction of plasma cortisol levels has been reported in some patients taking 2,000 micrograms per day. In such patients, the risks of developing adrenal suppression should be balanced against the therapeutic advantages, and precautions taken to provide systemic steroid cover in situations of prolonged stress. Prolonged suppression of the hypothalamic-pituitary-adrenal (HPA) axis may eventually lead to systemic effects, including growth retardation in children and adolescents.

The transfer to Easyhaler® Beclometasone 200 micrograms/dose of patients who have been treated with systemic steroids for long periods of time, or at a high dose, needs special care, since recovery from any adrenocortical suppression sustained may take a considerable time. Approximately one week after initiating treatment with Easyhaler® Beclometasone 200 micrograms/dose, reduction of the dose of systemic steroid can be commenced. The size of the reduction should correspond to the maintenance dose of systemic steroid. Reductions in dose of not more than 1mg are suitable for patients receiving maintenance doses of 10mg daily or less of prednisolone or its equivalent. Larger reductions in dose may be appropriate for higher maintenance doses. The reductions in dose should be introduced at not less than weekly intervals. Adrenocortical function should be monitored regularly as the dose of systemic steroid is gradually reduced.

Some patients feel unwell in a non-specific way during the withdrawal phase despite maintenance or even improvement of the respiratory function. They should be encouraged to persevere with inhaled beclomethasone dipropionate and to continue withdrawal of systemic steroid, unless there are objective signs of adrenal insufficiency.

Patients weaned off oral steroids whose adrenocortical function is impaired should carry a steroid warning card indicating that they may need supplementary systemic steroid during periods of stress, e.g. worsening asthma attacks, chest infections, major intercurrent illness, surgery, trauma, etc.

Replacement of systemic steroid treatment with inhaled therapy sometimes unmasks allergies such as allergic rhinitis or eczema previously controlled by the systemic drug. These allergies should be symptomatically treated with antihistamine and/or topical preparations, including topical steroids.

As with all inhaled corticosteroids, special care is necessary in patients with active or quiescent pulmonary tuberculosis.

4.5 Interaction with other medicinal products and other forms of interaction

None reported.

4.6 Pregnancy and lactation

There is inadequate evidence of safety in human pregnancy. Administration of corticosteroids to pregnant animals can cause abnormalities of fetal development including cleft palate and intra-uterine growth retardation. There may therefore be a very small risk of such effects in the human fetus. It should be noted, however, that the fetal changes in animals occur after relatively high systemic exposure. Easyhaler® Beclometasone 200 micrograms/dose delivers the drug directly to the lungs by the inhaled route and so avoids the high level of exposure that occurs when corticosteroids are given by systemic routes.

The use of beclomethasone dipropionate in pregnancy requires that the possible benefits of the drug be weighed against the possible hazards.

No specific studies examining the transference of beclomethasone dipropionate into the milk of lactating animals have been performed. It is reasonable to assume that beclomethasone dipropionate is secreted in milk, but at the dosages used for direct inhalation there is low potential for significant levels in breast milk.

The use of beclomethasone dipropionate in mothers breast feeding their babies requires that the therapeutic benefits of the drug be weighed against the potential hazards to the mother and baby.

4.7 Effects on ability to drive and use machines

None reported.

4.8 Undesirable effects

As with other inhalation therapy, paradoxical bronchospasm may occur with an immediate increase in wheezing after dosing. This should be treated immediately with a fast-acting inhaled bronchodilator. Easyhaler® Beclometasone 200 micrograms/dose should be discontinued immediately, the patient assessed and, if necessary, alternative therapy instituted.

Hypersensitivity reactions including anaphylactic shock, urticaria, rashes, angioedema, pruritus and erythema, and oedema of the eyes, face, lips and throat, have been reported.

Candidiasis of the mouth and throat (thrush) occurs in some patients, the incidence increasing with doses greater that 400 micrograms of beclomethasone dipropionate per day. Patients with high blood levels of *Candida precipitins*, indicating a previous infection, are most likely to develop this complication. Patients may find it helpful to rinse their mouth thoroughly with water after using the inhaler. Symptomatic candidiasis can be treated with topical anti-fungal therapy whilst still continuing with Easyhaler® Beclometasone 200 micrograms/dose.

In some patients inhaled beclomethasone dipropionate may cause hoarseness, cough, throat irritation and sore throat. It may be helpful to rinse the mouth out with water immediately after inhalation.

Miscellaneous undesirable effects - eosinophilic pneumonia, disturbance of growth in children, behavioural changes in children, subcapsular cataracts, easy bruising, skin thinning, decrease of bone metabolism.

With higher than the recommended doses or during long-term therapy in rare cases systemic undesirable effects like increase of intraocular pressure, glaucoma, and osteoporosis can occur.

4.9 Overdose

Acute: Inhalation of the drug in doses in excess of those recommended may lead to temporary suppression of adrenal function. This does not require emergency action. In these patients treatment should be continued at a dose sufficient to control asthma; adrenal function recovers in a few days and can be verified by measuring plasma cortisol.

Chronic: Use of inhaled beclomethasone dipropionate in daily doses in excess of 1,500 micrograms over prolonged periods may lead to some degree of adrenal suppression. Monitoring of adrenal reserve may be indicated. Treatment should be continued at a dose sufficient to control asthma.

In case of an overdose, the contra-indications, side effects and warnings with regard to systemically applied corticosteroids should be taken into account.

5. PHARMACOLOGICAL PROPERTIES

5.1 Pharmacodynamic properties

Beclomethasone dipropionate is a synthetic steroid derivative. It has a potent local anti-inflammatory effect on the respiratory mucosa when administered topically. Long-term studies have shown that after the initiation of inhaled Beclomethasone in patients with bronchial asthma, the dose of systemic corticosteroids may be gradually reduced. There is no evidence that the drug damages tracheobronchial mucosa or increases the incidence of respiratory infections.

The exact mechanisms responsible for the anti-inflammatory effect of Beclomethasone dipropionate are unknown.

5.2 Pharmacokinetic properties

Approximately 10-25 % of the inhaled drug dose reaches the lungs and the biggest fraction of the dose is retained in the upper airways and mouth and is swallowed. The drug absorbed from the lungs is ultimately metabolized in the liver. Beclomethasone dipropionate is metabolized to active 17-Beclomethasone mono-propionate, and free Beclomethasone and metabolites are mainly excreted to faeces. Less than 10 % of the drug and its metabolites is excreted in urine.

5.3 Preclinical safety data

Preclinical data were confined to those associated with over-stimulation of the recognised pharmacological action, which is the only safety concern for human use derived from animal studies. Reproduction toxicity studies in animals have, as with other glucocorticoids, revealed teratological and embryocidal effects and evidence of impaired fertility. No data concerning mutagenicity are available. No evidence of carcinogenicity was observed in a 95-week study in rats. Beclomethasone dipropionate is non-genotoxic.

6. PHARMACEUTICAL PARTICULARS

6.1 List of excipients

Lactose monohydrate

6.2 Incompatibilities

None

6.3 Shelf life

2 years in aluminium foil and 6 months after opening of the foil.

6.4 Special precautions for storage

Do not store above 25°C.

6.5 Nature and contents of container

The Easyhaler inhaler, which consists of seven plastic parts and a stainless steel spring, is wrapped in aluminium foil. The inhaler with aluminium foil and the protective cover are packed in a cardboard box.

Packages:

Easyhaler® Beclometasone 200 micrograms/dose inhalation powder:

200 doses protective cover

200 doses

2 × 200 doses

6.6 Special precautions for disposal and other handling
Patients have to be instructed to perform a rapid and forced inhalation through the Easyhaler device. Patients have to be instructed not to exhale into the device. Illustrated user's instructions for use accompany each package.

7. MARKETING AUTHORISATION HOLDER
Orion Corporation
PO Box 65
02101 Espoo
Finland

8. MARKETING AUTHORISATION NUMBER(S)
PL 27925/0001

9. DATE OF FIRST AUTHORISATION/RENEWAL OF THE AUTHORISATION
21 December 1999/August 2004

10. DATE OF REVISION OF THE TEXT
27 February 2007

Easyhaler Budesonide 100mcg

(Orion Pharma (UK) Limited)

1. NAME OF THE MEDICINAL PRODUCT
Easyhaler Budesonide 100 micrograms/dose inhalation powder.

2. QUALITATIVE AND QUANTITATIVE COMPOSITION
One metered dose contains 100 micrograms of budesonide.

With the Easyhaler device the delivered dose (ex-actuator) contains the same quantity of active substance as the metered dose (ex-reservoir).

Excipient: Lactose monohydrate.

For a full list of excipients, see section 6.1.

3. PHARMACEUTICAL FORM
Inhalation powder.

White or almost white powder.

4. CLINICAL PARTICULARS
4.1 Therapeutic indications
Treatment of mild, moderate, and severe persistent asthma.

(Note: Easyhaler Budesonide is not suitable for the treatment of acute asthma attacks.)

4.2 Posology and method of administration
Method of administration: For inhalation use. For optimum response, Easyhaler Budesonide inhalation powder should be used regularly.

The therapeutic effect begins after a few days treatment and reaches its maximum after some weeks of treatment.

When transferring a patient to Easyhaler Budesonide from other inhalation devices, the treatment should be individualised. The previous active substance, dose regimen, and method of delivery should be considered.

The patients should be prescribed a starting dose of inhaled budesonide which is appropriate for the severity or level of control of their disease. The dose should be adjusted until control is achieved and then titrated to the lowest dose at which effective control of asthma is maintained.

The starting dose for adults (including the elderly and children/adolescents over 12 years of age) with mild asthma (Step 2) and for children 6 to 12 years of age is 200-400 micrograms/day. If needed, the dose can be increased up to 800 micrograms/day. For adult patients with moderate (Step 3) and severe (Step 4) asthma the starting dose can be up to 1600 micrograms/day. The maintenance dose should be adjusted to meet the requirements of an individual patient taking into account the severity of the disease and the clinical response of the patient. **Twice daily dosing**

Adults with mild, moderate or severe asthma (including the elderly and children/adolescents over 12 years of age): The usual maintenance dose is 100-400 micrograms twice daily. During periods of severe asthma, the daily dose may be increased up to 1600 micrograms administered in divided (two) doses and subsequently reduced when asthma has stabilised.

Children 6 to 12 years: The usual maintenance dose is 100-200 micrograms twice daily. If needed, the daily dose may be increased up to 800 micrograms administered in divided (two) doses and subsequently reduced when asthma has stabilised.

Once daily dosing

Adults with mild to moderate asthma (including the elderly and children/adolescents over 12 years of age): In patients who have not previously received inhaled corticosteroids the usual maintenance dose is 200-400 micrograms once daily. In patients already controlled on inhaled corticosteroids (eg budesonide or beclometasone dipropionate) administered twice daily, once daily dosing up to 800 micrograms may be used.

Children 6 to 12 with mild to moderate asthma: In steroid naive patients or patients controlled on inhaled corticosteroids (eg budesonide or beclometasone dipropionate) administered twice daily the usual maintenance dose is 200-400 micrograms once daily.

The patient should be transferred to once daily dosing at the same equivalent total daily dose (with consideration of the drug and the method of delivery). The dose should be subsequently reduced to the minimum needed to maintain good asthma control. Patients should be instructed to take the once daily dose in the evening. It is important that the dose is taken consistently and at the same time each evening.

There are insufficient data to make recommendations for the transfer of patients from newer inhaled corticosteroids to once daily Easyhaler Budesonide.

Patients, in particular those receiving once daily treatment, should be advised that if their asthma deteriorates (e.g. increased frequency of bronchodilator use or persistent respiratory symptoms) they should double their corticosteroid dose by administering twice daily. They should be advised to contact their doctor as soon as possible.

A rapid-acting inhaled bronchodilator should be available for the relief of acute symptoms of asthma at all times.

Instructions for use and handling

It should be ensured that the patient is instructed in the use of the inhaler by a doctor or pharmacist.

Easyhaler is an inspiratory flow-driven device. This means that when the patient inhales through the mouthpiece, the substance will follow the inspired air into the airways.

Note: It is important to instruct the patient

- To carefully read the instructions for use in the patient information leaflet which is packed together with each inhaler.

- That it is recommended to keep the device in the protective cover after opening the laminate pouch to enhance the stability of the product during use and makes the inhaler more tamper proof.

- To shake and actuate the device prior to each inhalation.

- In the sitting or standing position, to breathe in forcefully and deeply through the mouthpiece to ensure that an optimal dose is delivered to the lungs.

- Never to breathe out through the mouthpiece as this will result in a reduction in the delivered dose. Should this happen the patient is instructed to tap the mouthpiece onto a table top or the palm of a hand to empty the powder, and then to repeat the dosing procedure.

- Never to actuate the device more than once without inhalation of the powder. Should this happen the patient is instructed to tap the mouthpiece onto a table top or the palm of a hand to empty the powder, and then to repeat the dosing procedure.

- To always replace the dust cap and close the protective cover after use to prevent accidental actuation of the device (which could result in either overdosing or under dosing the patient when subsequently used).

- To rinse the mouth out with water or brush the teeth after inhaling the prescribed dose to minimise the risk of oropharyngeal candidiasis and hoarseness.

- To clean the mouthpiece with a dry cloth at regular intervals. Water should never be used for cleaning because the powder is sensitive to moisture.

- To replace Easyhaler Budesonide when the counter reaches zero even though powder can still be observed within the device.

4.3 Contraindications
Hypersensitivity to budesonide or milk proteins (the excipient lactose contains milk proteins).

4.4 Special warnings and precautions for use
Easyhaler Budesonide is not indicated for the treatment of acute dyspnoea or status asthmaticus. These conditions should be treated in the normal way.

Patients should be aware that Easyhaler Budesonide inhalation powder is prophylactic therapy and therefore has to be used regularly even when asymptomatic for optimum benefit and should not be stopped abruptly.

The transfer of patients treated with oral corticosteroids to the inhaled corticosteroid and their subsequent management requires special care. The patients should be in a reasonably stable state before initiating a high dose of inhaled corticosteroid through twice daily dosing in addition to their usual maintenance dose of systemic corticosteroid. After about 10 days, withdrawal of the systemic corticosteroid is started by reducing the daily dose gradually (by for example 2.5 milligrams prednisolone or the equivalent each month) to the lowest possible level. It may be possible to completely replace the oral corticosteroid with inhaled corticosteroid. Transferred patients whose adrenocortical function is impaired may need supplementary systemic corticosteroid during periods of stress e.g. surgery, infection or worsening asthma attacks. This applies also to patients who have received prolonged treatment with high doses of inhaled corticosteroids. They may also have impaired adrenocortical function which may result in clinically significant adrenal suppression and may need systemic corticosteroid cover during periods of stress.

During transfer from oral therapy to inhaled budesonide symptoms may appear that had previously been suppressed by systemic treatment with glucocorticosteroids, for example symptoms of allergic rhinitis, eczema, muscle and joint pain. Specific treatment should be co-administered to treat these conditions.

Some patients may feel unwell in a non-specific way during the withdrawal of systemic corticosteroids despite maintenance or even improvement in respiratory function. Such patients should be encouraged to continue treatment with inhaled budesonide and withdrawal of oral corticosteroid unless there are clinical signs to indicate the contrary, for example signs which might indicate adrenal insufficiency.

As with other inhalation therapies paradoxical bronchospasm may occur, manifest by an immediate increase in wheezing and shortness of breath after dosing. Paradoxical bronchospasm responds to a rapid-acting inhaled bronchodilator and should be treated straightaway. Budesonide should be discontinued immediately, the patient should be assessed and, if necessary, alternative treatment instituted.

When despite a well monitored treatment, an acute episode of dyspnoea occurs, a rapid-acting inhaled bronchodilator should be used and medical reassessment should be considered. If despite maximum doses of inhaled corticosteroids asthma symptoms are not adequately controlled, patients may require short-term treatment with systemic corticosteroids. In such a case, it is necessary to maintain the inhaled corticosteroid therapy in association with treatment by the systemic route.

Systemic effects of inhaled corticosteroids may occur, particularly at high doses prescribed for prolonged periods. These effects are much less likely to occur than with oral corticosteroids. Possible systemic effects include adrenal suppression, growth retardation in children and adolescents, decrease in bone mineral density, cataract and glaucoma. It is important, therefore, that the dose of inhaled corticosteroid is titrated to the lowest dose at which effective control of asthma is maintained.

It is recommended that the height of children receiving prolonged treatment with inhaled corticosteroids is regularly monitored. If growth is slowed, therapy should be reviewed with the aim of reducing the dose of inhaled corticosteroid, if possible, to the lowest dose at which effective control of asthma is maintained. In addition, consideration should be given to referring the patient to a paediatric respiratory specialist.

Patients who have previously been dependent on oral corticosteroids may, as a result of prolonged systemic corticosteroid therapy, experience effects of impaired adrenal function. Recovery may take a considerable amount of time after cessation of oral corticosteroid therapy and hence oral steroid-dependent patients transferred to budesonide may remain at risk from impaired adrenocortical function for some considerable time. In such circumstances hypothalamic pituitary adrenocortical (HPA) axis function should be monitored regularly.

To reduce the risk of oral candidiasis and hoarseness patients should be advised to rinse out the mouth properly or brush the teeth after each administration of inhaled corticosteroid. Oral candidiasis can be rapidly controlled by local antimycotic treatment, without the need to discontinue the treatment with inhaled budesonide.

Exacerbation of clinical symptoms of asthma may be due to acute respiratory tract bacterial infections and treatment with appropriate antibiotics may be required. Such patients may need to increase the dose of inhaled budesonide and a short course of oral corticosteroids may be required. A rapid-acting inhaled bronchodilator should be used as "rescue" medication to relieve acute asthma symptoms.

Special care and adequate specific therapeutic control of patients with active and quiescent pulmonary tuberculosis is necessary before commencing treatment with Easyhaler Budesonide. Similarly patients with fungal, viral or other infections of the airways require close observation and special care and should use Easyhaler Budesonide only if they are also receiving adequate treatment for such infections.

In patients with excessive mucous secretion in the respiratory tract, short-term therapy with oral corticosteroids may be necessary.

In patients with severe hepatic dysfunction, treatment with inhaled budesonide can result in a reduced elimination rate and hence enhanced systemic availability. Possible systemic effects may then result and therefore HPA axis function in these patients should be monitored at regular intervals.

Concomitant treatment with ketoconazole or other potent CYP3A4 inhibitors should be avoided (see Section 4.5 Interaction with other medicinal products and other forms of interaction). If this is not possible the time interval between administration of the interacting drugs should be as long as possible.

Patients with rare hereditary problems of galactose intolerance, the Lapp lactase deficiency or glucose-galactose malabsorption should not take this medicine.

4.5 Interaction with other medicinal products and other forms of interaction

The metabolic conversion of budesonide is impeded by substances metabolised by CYP3A4 (e.g. itraconazole, ketoconazole, ritonavir, nelfinavir, ciclosporin, ethinylestradiol and troleandomycin). The concomitant administration of these inhibitors of CYP3A4 may increase plasma levels of budesonide. This is of little clinical significance for a short term treatment (1–2 weeks), but should be taken into account for long term treatment.

4.6 Pregnancy and lactation

Data on approximately 2000 exposed pregnancies indicate no increased teratogenic risk associated with the use of inhaled budesonide. In animal studies glucocorticosteroids have been shown to induce malformations (see Section 5.3 Preclinical safety data). This is not likely to be relevant for humans given recommended doses.

Animal studies have also identified an involvement of excess prenatal glucocorticoids in increased risks for intrauterine growth retardation, adult cardiovascular disease and permanent changes in glucocorticoid receptor density, neurotransmitter turnover and behaviour at exposures below the teratogenic dose range.

During pregnancy, inhaled budesonide should only be used when the benefits outweigh the potential risks. The lowest effective dose of budesonide needed to maintain adequate asthma control should be used.

It is not known whether budesonide passes into human breast milk. Administration of inhaled budesonide to women who are breast-feeding should only be considered if the expected benefit to the mother is greater than any possible risk to the child.

4.7 Effects on ability to drive and use machines

No effects on ability to drive and use machines have been observed.

4.8 Undesirable effects

The possible adverse reactions are presented in system organ class order sorted by frequency.

(see Table 1 below)

Treatment with inhaled budesonide may result in candida infection in the oropharynx. Experience has shown that candida infection occurs less often when inhalation is performed before meals and/or when the mouth is rinsed after inhalation. In most cases this condition responds to topical anti-fungal therapy without discontinuing treatment with inhaled budesonide.

Systemic effects of inhaled corticosteroids may occur, particularly at high doses prescribed for prolonged periods. These may include adrenal suppression, growth retardation in children and adolescents, decrease in bone mineral density, cataract and glaucoma, and susceptibility to infections. The ability to adapt to stress may be impaired. The systemic effects described, however, are much less likely to occur with inhaled budesonide than with oral corticosteroids.

Lactose, the excipient in the product, contains small amounts of milk proteins and can therefore cause allergic reactions.

4.9 Overdose

Symptoms of overdose

The acute toxicity of budesonide is low. Chronic use in excessive doses can result in systemic glucocorticosteroid effects, such as increased susceptibility to infection, hypercorticism and adrenal suppression. Atrophy of the adrenal cortex can occur and the ability to adapt to stress can be impaired.

Therapeutic management of overdose

For acute overdosage, no special emergency action needs to be taken. The treatment with inhaled budesonide should be continued at the recommended dose to control asthma. HPA axis function recovers in a few days.

In stress situations, it may be necessary to administer corticosteroids as a precaution (eg high doses of hydrocortisone). Patients with adrenocortical atrophy are regarded as being steroid-dependent and must be adjusted to the adequate maintenance therapy of a systemic corticosteroid until the condition has stabilised.

5. PHARMACOLOGICAL PROPERTIES

5.1 Pharmacodynamic properties

Pharmacotherapeutic group: Glucocorticoids. ATC code: R03BA02.

Budesonide is a glucocorticosteroid which possesses a high local anti-inflammatory action.

Topical anti-inflammatory effect

The exact mechanism of action of glucocorticosteroids in the treatment of asthma is not fully understood. Anti-inflammatory actions, such as inhibition of inflammatory mediator release and inhibition of cytokine-mediated immune response are probably important.

Onset of effect

After a single dose of orally inhaled budesonide, delivered via dry powder inhaler, improvement of the lung function is achieved within a few hours. After therapeutic use of orally inhaled budesonide delivered via dry powder inhaler, improvement in lung function has been shown to occur within 2 days of initiation of treatment, although maximum benefit may not be achieved for up to 4 weeks.

Airway reactivity

Budesonide has also been shown to decrease airway reactivity to histamine and methacholine in hyper-reactive patients.

Exercise-induced asthma

Therapy with inhaled budesonide has effectively been used for prevention of exercise-induced asthma.

Growth

Limited data from long term studies suggest that most children and adolescents treated with inhaled budesonide ultimately achieve their adult target height. However, an initial small but transient reduction in growth (approximately 1 cm) has been observed. This generally occurs within the first year of treatment (see section 4.4).

HPA axis function

A study in healthy volunteers with Easyhaler Budesonide has shown dose-related effects on plasma and urinary cortisol. At recommended doses, budesonide causes less effect on the adrenal function than prednisolone 10mg, as shown by ACTH tests.

5.2 Pharmacokinetic properties

The activity of Easyhaler Budesonide is due to the parent active substance, budesonide, which is provided as a mixture of two epimers (22R and 22S). In glucocorticoid receptor affinity studies, the 22R form is twice as active as the 22S epimer. These two forms of budesonide do not interconvert. The terminal half-life is the same for both epimers (2-3 hours). In asthmatic patients, approximately 15-25% of the inhaled budesonide dose from Easyhaler reaches the lungs. The largest fraction of the inhaled dose is retained in the oropharynx and swallowed if the mouth is not rinsed out.

Absorption:

After oral administration of budesonide, peak plasma concentration is achieved in about 1-2 hours and the absolute systemic availability is 6-13%. In plasma, 85-95% of budesonide is bound to proteins. In contrast, peak plasma concentration is reached approximately 30 minutes after inhalation. Most of budesonide delivered to the lungs is systemically absorbed.

Metabolism:

Budesonide is mainly eliminated by metabolism. Budesonide is rapidly and extensively metabolised in liver via cytochrome P4503A4 to two major metabolites. The *in vitro* glucocorticoid activity of these metabolites is less than 1% of that of the parent compound. Negligible metabolic inactivation has been observed in human lung and serum preparations.

Excretion:

Budesonide is excreted in urine and faeces in the form of conjugated and non-conjugated metabolites.

Special patient populations

The exposure to budesonide may be increased in patients with liver disease. In children the elimination half-life from plasma is markedly lower than in adults.

5.3 Preclinical safety data

Preclinical data with budesonide reveal no special hazard for humans based on conventional studies of safety pharmacology, repeated dose toxicity, genotoxicity, or carcinogenic potential.

In animal studies on reproductive toxicity, glucocorticosteroids such as budesonide have been shown to induce malformations (cleft palate, skeletal malformations). However, these animal results do not seem to be relevant for humans given recommended doses.

6. PHARMACEUTICAL PARTICULARS

6.1 List of excipients

Lactose monohydrate (which contains small amounts of milk proteins).

6.2 Incompatibilities

Not applicable.

6.3 Shelf life

Shelf life of the medicinal product as packaged for sale: 3 years.

Shelf life after first opening the laminate pouch: 6 months.

6.4 Special precautions for storage

As packaged for sale

Store in the original package.

In use

Do not store above 30°C and store protected from moisture.

6.5 Nature and contents of container

The multidose powder inhaler consists of seven plastic parts and a stainless steel spring. The plastic materials of the inhaler are: overcap - polyester; bulk chamber cover -LDPE; bulk chamber -polycarbonate; metering cylinder and counter wheel -acetal; mouthpiece - styrene butadiene; dust cap-polypropylene. The plastic materials of the protective cover are polypropylene and thermoplastic elastomer. The inhaler is sealed in a laminate pouch (PET, Al and PE) and packed with or without a protective cover in a cardboard box.

Packages:

Easyhaler Budesonide 100 micrograms/dose inhalation powder:

- 200 doses + protective cover
- 200 doses
- 2 × 200 doses

6.6 Special precautions for disposal and other handling

No special requirements.

7. MARKETING AUTHORISATION HOLDER

Orion Corporation

Orionintie 1

FI-02200 Espoo

Finland

Table 1

	Very common (≥1/10)	Common (≥1/100 to <1/10)	Un-common (≥1/1000 to <1/100)	Rare (≥1/10 000 to <1/1000)	Very rare (<1/10 000), not known (cannot be estimated from the available data)
Infections and infestations		oropharyngeal candidiasis			
Immune system disorders				hypersensitivity reactions, anaphylactic shock	
Endocrine disorders				hypocorticism, hypercorticism	adrenal suppression
Psychiatric disorders				depression, aggressive reactions, irritability, anxiety, psychosis, behavioural changes in children, restlessness, increased motorial activity	nervousness
Eye disorders					cataract, glaucoma
Respiratory, thoracic and mediastinal disorders		hoarseness, cough, throat irritation		bronchospasm (see Section 4.4 Special warnings and precautions for use)	
Gastrointestinal disorders		difficulty in swallowing			
Skin and subcutaneous tissue disorders				rash, urticaria, pruritus, dermatitis, erythema, angioedema	
Musculoskeletal and connective tissue disorders				growth retardation	decreased bone density

8. MARKETING AUTHORISATION NUMBER(S)
PL27925/0008

9. DATE OF FIRST AUTHORISATION/RENEWAL OF THE AUTHORISATION
29/11/2007

10. DATE OF REVISION OF THE TEXT
04/2009

Easyhaler Budesonide 200mcg

(Orion Pharma (UK) Limited)

1. NAME OF THE MEDICINAL PRODUCT
Easyhaler Budesonide 200 micrograms/dose inhalation powder.

2. QUALITATIVE AND QUANTITATIVE COMPOSITION
One metered dose contains 200 micrograms of budesonide.

With the Easyhaler device the delivered dose (ex-actuator) contains the same quantity of active substance as the metered dose (ex-reservoir).

Excipient: Lactose monohydrate.

For a full list of excipients, see section 6.1.

3. PHARMACEUTICAL FORM
Inhalation powder.

White or almost white powder.

4. CLINICAL PARTICULARS
4.1 Therapeutic indications
Treatment of mild, moderate, and severe persistent asthma.

(Note: Easyhaler Budesonide is not suitable for the treatment of acute asthma attacks.)

4.2 Posology and method of administration
Method of administration: For inhalation use. For optimum response, Easyhaler Budesonide inhalation powder should be used regularly.

The therapeutic effect begins after a few days treatment and reaches its maximum after some weeks of treatment.

When transferring a patient to Easyhaler Budesonide from other inhalation devices, the treatment should be individualised. The previous active substance, dose regimen, and method of delivery should be considered.

The patients should be prescribed a starting dose of inhaled budesonide which is appropriate for the severity or level of control of their disease. The dose should be adjusted until control is achieved and then titrated to the lowest dose at which effective control of asthma is maintained.

Lower strengths of Easyhaler Budesonide are available for appropriate dose adjustment, if necessary.

The starting dose for adults (including the elderly and children/adolescents over 12 years of age) with mild asthma (Step 2) and for children 6 to 12 years of age is 200-400 micrograms/day. If needed, the dose can be increased up to 800 micrograms/day. For adult patients with moderate (Step 3) and severe (Step 4) asthma the starting dose can be up to 1600 micrograms/day. The maintenance dose should be adjusted to meet the requirements of an individual patient taking into account the severity of the disease and the clinical response of the patient.

Twice daily dosing

Adults with mild, moderate or severe asthma (including the elderly and children/adolescents over 12 years of age): The usual maintenance dose is 100-400 micrograms twice daily. During periods of severe asthma, the daily dose may be increased up to 1600 micrograms administered in divided (two) doses and subsequently reduced when asthma has stabilised.

Children 6 to 12 years: The usual maintenance dose is 100-200 micrograms twice daily. If needed, the daily dose may be increased up to 800 micrograms administered in divided (two) doses and subsequently reduced when asthma has stabilised.

Once daily dosing

Adults with mild to moderate asthma (including the elderly and children/adolescents over 12 years of age): In patients who have not previously received inhaled corticosteroids the usual maintenance dose is 200-400 micrograms once daily. In patients already controlled on inhaled corticosteroids (eg budesonide or beclometasone dipropionate) administered twice daily, once daily dosing up to 800 micrograms may be used.

Children 6 to 12 with mild to moderate asthma: In steroid naive patients or patients controlled on inhaled corticosteroids (eg budesonide or beclometasone dipropionate) administered twice daily the usual maintenance dose is 200-400 micrograms once daily.

The patient should be transferred to once daily dosing at the same equivalent total daily dose (with consideration of the drug and the method of delivery). The dose should be subsequently reduced to the minimum needed to maintain good asthma control. Patients should be instructed to take the once daily dose in the evening. It is important that the dose is taken consistently and at the same time each evening.

There are insufficient data to make recommendations for the transfer of patients from newer inhaled corticosteroids to once daily Easyhaler Budesonide.

Patients, in particular those receiving once daily treatment, should be advised that if their asthma deteriorates (e.g. increased frequency of bronchodilator use or persistent respiratory symptoms) they should double their corticosteroid dose by administering twice daily. They should be advised to contact their doctor as soon as possible.

A rapid-acting inhaled bronchodilator should be available for the relief of acute symptoms of asthma at all times.

Instructions for use and handling

It should be ensured that the patient is instructed in the use of the inhaler by a doctor or pharmacist.

Easyhaler is an inspiratory flow-driven device. This means that when the patient inhales through the mouthpiece, the substance will follow the inspired air into the airways.

Note: It is important to instruct the patient

- To carefully read the instructions for use in the patient information leaflet which is packed together with each inhaler.
- That it is recommended to keep the device in the protective cover after opening the laminate pouch to enhance the stability of the product during use and makes the inhaler more tamper proof.
- To shake and actuate the device prior to each inhalation.
- In the sitting or standing position, to breathe in forcefully and deeply through the mouthpiece to ensure that an optimal dose is delivered to the lungs.
- Never to breathe out through the mouthpiece as this will result in a reduction in the delivered dose. Should this happen the patient is instructed to tap the mouthpiece onto a table top or the palm of a hand to empty the powder, and then to repeat the dosing procedure.
- Never to actuate the device more than once without inhalation of the powder. Should this happen the patient is instructed to tap the mouthpiece onto a table top or the palm of a hand to empty the powder, and then to repeat the dosing procedure.
- To always replace the dust cap and close the protective cover after use to prevent accidental actuation of the device (which could result in either overdosing or under dosing the patient when subsequently used).
- To rinse the mouth out with water or brush the teeth after inhaling the prescribed dose to minimise the risk of oropharyngeal candidiasis and hoarseness.
- To clean the mouthpiece with a dry cloth at regular intervals. Water should never be used for cleaning because the powder is sensitive to moisture.
- To replace Easyhaler Budesonide when the counter reaches zero even though powder can still be observed within the device.

4.3 Contraindications
Hypersensitivity to budesonide or milk proteins (the excipient lactose contains milk proteins).

4.4 Special warnings and precautions for use
Easyhaler Budesonide is not indicated for the treatment of acute dyspnoea or status asthmaticus. These conditions should be treated in the normal way.

Patients should be aware that Easyhaler Budesonide inhalation powder is prophylactic therapy and therefore has to be used regularly even when asymptomatic for optimum benefit and should not be stopped abruptly.

The transfer of patients treated with oral corticosteroids to the inhaled corticosteroid and their subsequent management requires special care. The patients should be in a reasonably stable state before initiating a high dose of inhaled corticosteroid through twice daily dosing in addition to their usual maintenance dose of systemic corticosteroid. After about 10 days, withdrawal of the systemic corticosteroid is started by reducing the daily dose gradually (by for example 2.5 milligrams prednisolone or the equivalent each month) to the lowest possible level. It may be possible to completely replace the oral corticosteroid with inhaled corticosteroid. Transferred patients whose adrenocortical function is impaired may need supplementary systemic corticosteroid during periods of stress e.g. surgery, infection or worsening asthma attacks. This applies also to patients who have received prolonged treatment with high doses of inhaled corticosteroids. They may also have impaired adrenocortical function which may result in clinically significant adrenal suppression and may need systemic corticosteroid cover during periods of stress.

During transfer from oral therapy to inhaled budesonide symptoms may appear that had previously been suppressed by systemic treatment with glucocorticosteroids, for example symptoms of allergic rhinitis, eczema, muscle and joint pain. Specific treatment should be co-administered to treat these conditions.

Some patients may feel unwell in a non-specific way during the withdrawal of systemic corticosteroids despite maintenance or even improvement in respiratory function. Such patients should be encouraged to continue treatment with inhaled budesonide and withdrawal of oral corticosteroid unless there are clinical signs to indicate the contrary, for example signs which might indicate adrenal insufficiency.

As with other inhalation therapies paradoxical bronchospasm may occur, manifest by an immediate increase in wheezing and shortness of breath after dosing. Paradoxical bronchospasm responds to a rapid-acting inhaled bronchodilator and should be treated straightaway. Budesonide should be discontinued immediately, the patient should be assessed and, if necessary, alternative treatment instituted.

When despite a well monitored treatment, an acute episode of dyspnoea occurs, a rapid-acting inhaled bronchodilator should be used and medical reassessment should be considered. If despite maximum doses of inhaled corticosteroids asthma symptoms are not adequately controlled, patients may require short-term treatment with systemic corticosteroids. In such a case, it is necessary to maintain the inhaled corticosteroid therapy in association with treatment by the systemic route.

Systemic effects of inhaled corticosteroids may occur, particularly at high doses prescribed for prolonged periods. These effects are much less likely to occur than with oral corticosteroids. Possible systemic effects include adrenal suppression, growth retardation in children and adolescents, decrease in bone mineral density, cataract and glaucoma. It is important, therefore, that the dose of inhaled corticosteroid is titrated to the lowest dose at which effective control of asthma is maintained.

It is recommended that the height of children receiving prolonged treatment with inhaled corticosteroids is regularly monitored. If growth is slowed, therapy should be reviewed with the aim of reducing the dose of inhaled corticosteroid, if possible, to the lowest dose at which effective control of asthma is maintained. In addition, consideration should be given to referring the patient to a paediatric respiratory specialist.

Patients who have previously been dependent on oral corticosteroids may, as a result of prolonged systemic corticosteroid therapy, experience effects of impaired adrenal function. Recovery may take a considerable amount of time after cessation of oral corticosteroid therapy and hence oral steroid-dependent patients transferred to budesonide may remain at risk from impaired adrenocortical function for some considerable time. In such circumstances hypothalamic pituitary adrenocortical (HPA) axis function should be monitored regularly.

To reduce the risk of oral candidiasis and hoarseness patients should be advised to rinse out the mouth properly or brush the teeth after each administration of inhaled corticosteroid. Oral candidiasis can be rapidly controlled by local antimycotic treatment, without the need to discontinue the treatment with inhaled budesonide.

Exacerbation of clinical symptoms of asthma may be due to acute respiratory tract bacterial infections and treatment with appropriate antibiotics may be required. Such patients may need to increase the dose of inhaled budesonide and a short course of oral corticosteroids may be required. A rapid-acting inhaled bronchodilator should be used as "rescue" medication to relieve acute asthma symptoms.

Special care and adequate specific therapeutic control of patients with active and quiescent pulmonary tuberculosis is necessary before commencing treatment with Easyhaler Budesonide. Similarly patients with fungal, viral or other infections of the airways require close observation and special care and should use Easyhaler Budesonide only if they are also receiving adequate treatment for such infections.

In patients with excessive mucous secretion in the respiratory tract, short-term therapy with oral corticosteroids may be necessary.

In patients with severe hepatic dysfunction, treatment with inhaled budesonide can result in a reduced elimination rate and hence enhanced systemic availability. Possible systemic effects may then result and therefore HPA axis function in these patients should be monitored at regular intervals.

Concomitant treatment with ketoconazole or other potent CYP3A4 inhibitors should be avoided (see Section 4.5 Interaction with other medicinal products and other forms of interaction). If this is not possible the time interval between administration of the interacting drugs should be as long as possible.

Patients with rare hereditary problems of galactose intolerance, the Lapp lactase deficiency or glucose-galactose malabsorption should not take this medicine.

4.5 Interaction with other medicinal products and other forms of interaction
The metabolic conversion of budesonide is impeded by substances metabolised by CYP3A4 (e.g. itraconazole, ketoconazole, ritonavir, nelfinavir, ciclosporin, ethinylestradiol and troleandomycin). The concomitant administration of these inhibitors of CYP3A4 may increase plasma levels of budesonide. This is of little clinical significance for a short term treatment (1−2 weeks), but should be taken into account for long term treatment.

4.6 Pregnancy and lactation
Data on approximately 2000 exposed pregnancies indicate no increased teratogenic risk associated with the use of

inhaled budesonide. In animal studies glucocorticosteroids have been shown to induce malformations (see Section 5.3 Preclinical safety data). This is not likely to be relevant for humans given recommended doses.

Animal studies have also identified an involvement of excess prenatal glucocorticoids in increased risks for intrauterine growth retardation, adult cardiovascular disease and permanent changes in glucocorticoid receptor density, neurotransmitter turnover and behaviour at exposures below the teratogenic dose range.

During pregnancy, inhaled budesonide should only be used when the benefits outweigh the potential risks. The lowest effective dose of budesonide needed to maintain adequate asthma control should be used.

It is not known whether budesonide passes into human breast milk. Administration of inhaled budesonide to women who are breast-feeding should only be considered if the expected benefit to the mother is greater than any possible risk to the child.

4.7 Effects on ability to drive and use machines

No effects on ability to drive and use machines have been observed.

4.8 Undesirable effects

The possible adverse reactions are presented in system organ class order sorted by frequency.

(see Table 1 below)

Treatment with inhaled budesonide may result in candida infection in the oropharynx. Experience has shown that candida infection occurs less often when inhalation is performed before meals and/or when the mouth is rinsed after inhalation. In most cases this condition responds to topical anti-fungal therapy without discontinuing treatment with inhaled budesonide.

Systemic effects of inhaled corticosteroids may occur, particularly at high doses prescribed for prolonged periods. These may include adrenal suppression, growth retardation in children and adolescents, decrease in bone mineral density, cataract and glaucoma, and susceptibility to infections. The ability to adapt to stress may be impaired. The systemic effects described, however, are much less likely to occur with inhaled budesonide than with oral corticosteroids.

Lactose, the excipient in the product, contains small amounts of milk proteins and can therefore cause allergic reactions.

4.9 Overdose

Symptoms of overdose

The acute toxicity of budesonide is low. Chronic use in excessive doses can result in systemic glucocorticosteroid effects, such as increased susceptibility to infection, hypercorticism and adrenal suppression. Atrophy of the adrenal cortex can occur and the ability to adapt to stress can be impaired.

Therapeutic management of overdose

For acute overdosage, no special emergency action needs to be taken. The treatment with inhaled budesonide should be continued at the recommended dose to control asthma. HPA axis function recovers in a few days.

In stress situations, it may be necessary to administer corticosteroids as a precaution (eg high doses of hydrocortisone). Patients with adrenocortical atrophy are regarded as being steroid-dependent and must be adjusted to the adequate maintenance therapy of a systemic corticosteroid until the condition has stabilised.

5. PHARMACOLOGICAL PROPERTIES

5.1 Pharmacodynamic properties

Pharmacotherapeutic group: Glucocorticoids. ATC code: R03BA02.

Budesonide is a glucocorticosteroid which possesses a high local anti-inflammatory action.

Topical anti-inflammatory effect

The exact mechanism of action of glucocorticosteroids in the treatment of asthma is not fully understood. Anti-inflammatory actions, such as inhibition of inflammatory mediator release and inhibition of cytokine-mediated immune response are probably important.

Onset of effect

After a single dose of orally inhaled budesonide, delivered via dry powder inhaler, improvement of the lung function is achieved within a few hours. After therapeutic use of orally inhaled budesonide delivered via dry powder inhaler, improvement in lung function has been shown to occur within 2 days of initiation of treatment, although maximum benefit may not be achieved for up to 4 weeks.

Airway reactivity

Budesonide has also been shown to decrease airway reactivity to histamine and methacholine in hyper-reactive patients.

Exercise-induced asthma

Therapy with inhaled budesonide has effectively been used for prevention of exercise-induced asthma.

Growth

Limited data from long term studies suggest that most children and adolescents treated with inhaled budesonide ultimately achieve their adult target height. However, an initial small but transient reduction in growth (approximately 1 cm) has been observed. This generally occurs within the first year of treatment (see section 4.4).

HPA axis function

A study in healthy volunteers with Easyhaler Budesonide has shown dose-related effects on plasma and urinary cortisol. At recommended doses, budesonide causes less effect on the adrenal function than prednisolone 10mg, as shown by ACTH tests.

5.2 Pharmacokinetic properties

The activity of Easyhaler Budesoonide is due to the parent active substance, budesonide, which is provided as a mixture of two epimers (22R and 22S). In glucocorticoid receptor affinity studies, the 22R form is twice as active as the 22S epimer. These two forms of budesonide do not interconvert. The terminal half-life is the same for both epimers (2-3 hours). In asthmatic patients, approximately 15-25% of the inhaled budesonide dose from Easyhaler reaches the lungs. The largest fraction of the inhaled dose is retained in the oropharynx and swallowed if the mouth is not rinsed out.

Absorption:

After oral administration of budesonide, peak plasma concentration is achieved in about 1-2 hours and the absolute systemic availability is 6-13%. In plasma, 85-95% of budesonide is bound to proteins. In contrast, peak plasma concentration is reached approximately 30 minutes after inhalation. Most of budesonide delivered to the lungs is systemically absorbed.

Metabolism:

Budesonide is mainly eliminated by metabolism. Budesonide is rapidly and extensively metabolised in liver via cytochrome P4503A4 to two major metabolites. The *in vitro* glucocorticoid activity of these metabolites is less than 1% of that of the parent compound. Negligible metabolic inactivation has been observed in human lung and serum preparations.

Excretion:

Budesonide is excreted in urine and faeces in the form of conjugated and non-conjugated metabolites.

Special patient populations

The exposure to budesonide may be increased in patients with liver disease. In children the elimination half-life from plasma is markedly lower than in adults.

5.3 Preclinical safety data

Preclinical data with budesonide reveal no special hazard for humans based on conventional studies of safety pharmacology, repeated dose toxicity, genotoxicity, or carcinogenic potential.

In animal studies on reproductive toxicity, glucocorticosteroids such as budesonide have been shown to induce malformations (cleft palate, skeletal malformations). However, these animal results do not seem to be relevant for humans given recommended doses.

6. PHARMACEUTICAL PARTICULARS

6.1 List of excipients

Lactose monohydrate (which contains small amounts of milk proteins).

6.2 Incompatibilities

Not applicable.

6.3 Shelf life

Shelf life of the medicinal product as packaged for sale: 3 years.

Shelf life after first opening the laminate pouch: 6 months.

6.4 Special precautions for storage

As packaged for sale

Store in the original package.

In use

Do not store above 30°C and store protected from moisture.

6.5 Nature and contents of container

The multidose powder inhaler consists of seven plastic parts and a stainless steel spring. The plastic materials of the inhaler are: overcap - polyester; bulk chamber cover -LDPE; bulk chamber -polycarbonate; metering cylinder and counter wheel -acetal; mouthpiece - styrene butadiene; dust cap-polypropylene. The plastic materials of the protective cover are polypropylene and thermoplastic elastomer. The inhaler is sealed in a laminate pouch (PET, Al and PE) and packed with or without a protective cover in a cardboard box.

Packages:

Easyhaler Budesonide 200 micrograms/dose inhalation powder:

- 200 doses + protective cover
- 200 doses
- 2 × 200 doses

6.6 Special precautions for disposal and other handling

No special requirements.

7. MARKETING AUTHORISATION HOLDER

Orion Corporation

Orionintie 1

FI-02200 Espoo

Finland

8. MARKETING AUTHORISATION NUMBER(S)

PL27925/0009

9. DATE OF FIRST AUTHORISATION/RENEWAL OF THE AUTHORISATION

29/11/2007

10. DATE OF REVISION OF THE TEXT

04/2009

Table 1

	Very common (≥1/10)	Common (≥1/100 to <1/10)	Un-common (≥1/1000 to <1/100)	Rare (≥1/10 000 to <1/1000)	Very rare (<1/10 000), not known (cannot be estimated from the available data)
Infections and infestations		oropharyngeal candidiasis			
Immune system disorders				hypersensitivity reactions, anaphylactic shock	
Endocrine disorders				hypocorticism, hypercorticism	adrenal suppression
Psychiatric disorders				depression, aggressive reactions, irritability, anxiety, psychosis, behavioural changes in children, restlessness, increased motorial activity	nervousness
Eye disorders					cataract, glaucoma
Respiratory, thoracic and mediastinal disorders		hoarseness, cough, throat irritation		bronchospasm (see Section 4.4 Special warnings and precautions for use)	
Gastrointestinal disorders		difficulty in swallowing			
Skin and subcutaneous tissue disorders				rash, urticaria, pruritus, dermatitis, erythema, angioedema	
Musculoskeletal and connective tissue disorders				growth retardation	decreased bone density

Easyhaler Budesonide 400mcg

(Orion Pharma (UK) Limited)

1. NAME OF THE MEDICINAL PRODUCT
Easyhaler Budesonide 400 micrograms/dose inhalation powder.

2. QUALITATIVE AND QUANTITATIVE COMPOSITION
One metered dose contains 400 micrograms of budesonide.

With the Easyhaler device the delivered dose (ex-actuator) contains the same quantity of active substance as the metered dose (ex-reservoir).

Excipient: Lactose monohydrate.

For a full list of excipients, see section 6.1.

3. PHARMACEUTICAL FORM
Inhalation powder.

White or almost white powder.

4. CLINICAL PARTICULARS

4.1 Therapeutic indications
Treatment of mild, moderate, and severe persistent asthma.

(Note: Easyhaler Budesonide is not suitable for the treatment of acute asthma attacks.)

4.2 Posology and method of administration
Method of administration: For inhalation use. For optimum response, Easyhaler Budesonide inhalation powder should be used regularly.

The therapeutic effect begins after a few days treatment and reaches its maximum after some weeks of treatment.

When transferring a patient to Easyhaler Budesonide from other inhalation devices, the treatment should be individualised. The previous active substance, dose regimen, and method of delivery should be considered.

The patients should be prescribed a starting dose of inhaled budesonide which is appropriate for the severity or level of control of their disease. The dose should be adjusted until control is achieved and then titrated to the lowest dose at which effective control of asthma is maintained.

Lower strengths of Easyhaler Budesonide are available for appropriate dose adjustment, if necessary.

The starting dose for adults (including the elderly and children/adolescents over 12 years of age) with mild asthma (Step 2) and for children 6 to 12 years of age is 200-400 micrograms/day. If needed, the dose can be increased up to 800 micrograms/day. For adult patients with moderate (Step 3) and severe (Step 4) asthma the starting dose can be up to 1600 micrograms/day. The maintenance dose should be adjusted to meet the requirements of an individual patient taking into account the severity of the disease and the clinical response of the patient.

Twice daily dosing

Adults with mild, moderate or severe asthma (including the elderly and children/adolescents over 12 years of age): The usual maintenance dose is 100-400 micrograms twice daily. During periods of severe asthma, the daily dose may be increased up to 1600 micrograms administered in divided (two) doses and subsequently reduced when asthma has stabilised.

Children 6 to 12 years: The usual maintenance dose is 100-200 micrograms twice daily. If needed, the daily dose may be increased up to 800 micrograms administered in divided (two) doses and subsequently reduced when asthma has stabilised.

Once daily dosing

Adults with mild to moderate asthma (including the elderly and children/adolescents over 12 years of age): In patients who have not previously received inhaled corticosteroids the usual maintenance dose is 200-400 micrograms once daily. In patients already controlled on inhaled corticosteroids (eg budesonide or beclometasone dipropionate) administered twice daily, once daily dosing up to 800 micrograms may be used.

Children 6 to 12 with mild to moderate asthma: In steroid naive patients or patients controlled on inhaled corticosteroids (eg budesonide or beclometasone dipropionate) administered twice daily the usual maintenance dose is 200-400 micrograms once daily.

The patient should be transferred to once daily dosing at the same equivalent total daily dose (with consideration of the drug and the method of delivery). The dose should be subsequently reduced to the minimum needed to maintain good asthma control. Patients should be instructed to take the once daily dose in the evening. It is important that the dose is taken consistently and at the same time each evening.

There are insufficient data to make recommendations for the transfer of patients from newer inhaled corticosteroids to once daily Easyhaler Budesonide.

Patients, in particular those receiving once daily treatment, should be advised that if their asthma deteriorates (e.g. increased frequency of bronchodilator use or persistent respiratory symptoms) they should double their corticosteroid dose by administering twice daily. They should be advised to contact their doctor as soon as possible.

A rapid-acting inhaled bronchodilator should be available for the relief of acute symptoms of asthma at all times.

Instructions for use and handling

It should be ensured that the patient is instructed in the use of the inhaler by a doctor or pharmacist.

Easyhaler is an inspiratory flow-driven device. This means that when the patient inhales through the mouthpiece, the substance will follow the inspired air into the airways.

Note: It is important to instruct the patient

- To carefully read the instructions for use in the patient information leaflet which is packed together with each inhaler.

- That it is recommended to keep the device in the protective cover after opening the laminate pouch to enhance the stability of the product during use and makes the inhaler more tamper proof.

- To shake and actuate the device prior to each inhalation.

- In the sitting or standing position, to breathe in forcefully and deeply through the mouthpiece to ensure that an optimal dose is delivered to the lungs.

- Never to breathe out through the mouthpiece as this will result in a reduction in the delivered dose. Should this happen the patient is instructed to tap the mouthpiece onto a table top or the palm of a hand to empty the powder, and then to repeat the dosing procedure.

- Never to actuate the device more than once without inhalation of the powder. Should this happen the patient is instructed to tap the mouthpiece onto a table top or the palm of a hand to empty the powder, and then to repeat the dosing procedure.

- To always replace the dust cap and close the protective cover after use to prevent accidental actuation of the device (which could result in either overdosing or under dosing the patient when subsequently used).

- To rinse the mouth out with water or brush the teeth after inhaling the prescribed dose to minimise the risk of oropharyngeal candidiasis and hoarseness.

- To clean the mouthpiece with a dry cloth at regular intervals. Water should never be used for cleaning because the powder is sensitive to moisture.

- To replace Easyhaler Budesonide when the counter reaches zero even though powder can still be observed within the device.

4.3 Contraindications
Hypersensitivity to budesonide or milk proteins (the excipient lactose contains milk proteins).

4.4 Special warnings and precautions for use
Easyhaler Budesonide is not indicated for the treatment of acute dyspnoea or status asthmaticus. These conditions should be treated in the normal way.

Patients should be aware that Easyhaler Budesonide inhalation powder is prophylactic therapy and therefore has to be used regularly even when asymptomatic for optimum benefit and should not be stopped abruptly.

The transfer of patients treated with oral corticosteroids to the inhaled corticosteroid and their subsequent management requires special care. The patients should be in a reasonably stable state before initiating a high dose of inhaled corticosteroid through twice daily dosing in addition to their usual maintenance dose of systemic corticosteroid. After about 10 days, withdrawal of the systemic corticosteroid is started by reducing the daily dose gradually (by for example 2.5 milligrams prednisolone or the equivalent each month) to the lowest possible level. It may be possible to completely replace the oral corticosteroid with inhaled corticosteroid. Transferred patients whose adrenocortical function is impaired may need supplementary systemic corticosteroid during periods of stress e.g. surgery, infection or worsening asthma attacks. This applies also to patients who have received prolonged treatment with high doses of inhaled corticosteroids. They may also have impaired adrenocortical function which may result in clinically significant adrenal suppression and may need systemic corticosteroid cover during periods of stress.

During transfer from oral therapy to inhaled budesonide symptoms may appear that had previously been suppressed by systemic treatment with glucocorticosteroids, for example symptoms of allergic rhinitis, eczema, muscle and joint pain. Specific treatment should be co-administered to treat these conditions.

Some patients may feel unwell in a non-specific way during the withdrawal of systemic corticosteroids despite maintenance or even improvement in respiratory function. Such patients should be encouraged to continue treatment with inhaled budesonide and withdrawal of oral corticosteroid unless there are clinical signs to indicate the contrary, for example signs which might indicate adrenal insufficiency.

As with other inhalation therapies paradoxical bronchospasm may occur, manifest by an immediate increase in wheezing and shortness of breath after dosing. Paradoxical bronchospasm responds to a rapid-acting inhaled bronchodilator and should be treated straightaway. Budesonide should be discontinued immediately, the patient should be assessed and, if necessary, alternative treatment instituted.

When despite a well monitored treatment, an acute episode of dyspnoea occurs, a rapid-acting inhaled bronchodilator should be used and medical reassessment should be considered. If despite maximum doses of inhaled corticosteroids asthma symptoms are not adequately controlled, patients may require short-term treatment with systemic corticosteroids. In such a case, it is necessary to maintain the inhaled corticosteroid therapy in association with treatment by the systemic route.

Systemic effects of inhaled corticosteroids may occur, particularly at high doses prescribed for prolonged periods. These effects are much less likely to occur than with oral corticosteroids. Possible systemic effects include adrenal suppression, growth retardation in children and adolescents, decrease in bone mineral density, cataract and glaucoma. It is important, therefore, that the dose of inhaled corticosteroid is titrated to the lowest dose at which effective control of asthma is maintained.

It is recommended that the height of children receiving prolonged treatment with inhaled corticosteroids is regularly monitored. If growth is slowed, therapy should be reviewed with the aim of reducing the dose of inhaled corticosteroid, if possible, to the lowest dose at which effective control of asthma is maintained. In addition, consideration should be given to referring the patient to a paediatric respiratory specialist.

Patients who have previously been dependent on oral corticosteroids may, as a result of prolonged systemic corticosteroid therapy, experience effects of impaired adrenal function. Recovery may take a considerable amount of time after cessation of oral corticosteroid therapy and hence oral steroid-dependent patients transferred to budesonide may remain at risk from impaired adrenocortical function for some considerable time. In such circumstances hypothalamic pituitary adrenocortical (HPA) axis function should be monitored regularly.

To reduce the risk of oral candidiasis and hoarseness patients should be advised to rinse out the mouth properly or brush the teeth after each administration of inhaled corticosteroid. Oral candidiasis can be rapidly controlled by local antimycotic treatment, without the need to discontinue the treatment with inhaled budesonide.

Exacerbation of clinical symptoms of asthma may be due to acute respiratory tract bacterial infections and treatment with appropriate antibiotics may be required. Such patients may need to increase the dose of inhaled budesonide and a short course of oral corticosteroids may be required. A rapid-acting inhaled bronchodilator should be used as "rescue" medication to relieve acute asthma symptoms.

Special care and adequate specific therapeutic control of patients with active and quiescent pulmonary tuberculosis is necessary before commencing treatment with Easyhaler Budesonide. Similarly patients with fungal, viral or other infections of the airways require close observation and special care and should use Easyhaler Budesonide only if they are also receiving adequate treatment for such infections.

In patients with excessive mucous secretion in the respiratory tract, short-term therapy with oral corticosteroids may be necessary.

In patients with severe hepatic dysfunction, treatment with inhaled budesonide can result in a reduced elimination rate and hence enhanced systemic availability. Possible systemic effects may then result and therefore HPA axis function in these patients should be monitored at regular intervals.

Concomitant treatment with ketoconazole or other potent CYP3A4 inhibitors should be avoided (see Section 4.5 Interaction with other medicinal products and other forms of interaction). If this is not possible the time interval between administration of the interacting drugs should be as long as possible.

Patients with rare hereditary problems of galactose intolerance, the Lapp lactase deficiency or glucose-galactose malabsorption should not take this medicine.

4.5 Interaction with other medicinal products and other forms of interaction
The metabolic conversion of budesonide is impeded by substances metabolised by CYP3A4 (e.g. itraconazole, ketoconazole, ritonavir, nelfinavir, ciclosporin, ethinylestradiol and troleandomycin). The concomitant administration of these inhibitors of CYP3A4 may increase plasma levels of budesonide. This is of little clinical significance for a short term treatment (1 – 2 weeks), but should be taken into account for long term treatment.

4.6 Pregnancy and lactation
Data on approximately 2000 exposed pregnancies indicate no increased teratogenic risk associated with the use of inhaled budesonide. In animal studies glucocorticosteroids have been shown to induce malformations (see Section 5.3 Preclinical safety data). This is not likely to be relevant for humans given recommended doses.

Animal studies have also identified an involvement of excess prenatal glucocorticoids in increased risks for intrauterine growth retardation, adult cardiovascular disease and permanent changes in glucocorticoid receptor

Table 1

	Very common (≥1/10)	Common (≥1/100 to <1/10)	Un-common (≥1/1000 to <1/100)	Rare (≥1/10 000 to <1/1000)	Very rare (<1/10 000), not known (cannot be estimated from the available data)
Infections and infestations		oropharyngeal candidiasis			
Immune system disorders				hypersensitivity reactions, anaphylactic shock	
Endocrine disorders				hypocorticism, hypercorticism	adrenal suppression
Psychiatric disorders				depression, aggressive reactions, irritability, anxiety, psychosis, behavioural changes in children, restlessness, increased motorial activity	nervousness
Eye disorders					cataract, glaucoma
Respiratory, thoracic and mediastinal disorders		hoarseness, cough, throat irritation		bronchospasm (see Section 4.4 Special warnings and precautions for use)	
Gastrointestinal disorders		difficulty in swallowing			
Skin and subcutaneous tissue disorders				rash, urticaria, pruritus, dermatitis, erythema, angioedema	
Musculoskeletal and connective tissue disorders				growth retardation	decreased bone density

density, neurotransmitter turnover and behaviour at exposures below the teratogenic dose range.

During pregnancy, inhaled budesonide should only be used when the benefits outweigh the potential risks. The lowest effective dose of budesonide needed to maintain adequate asthma control should be used.

It is not known whether budesonide passes into human breast milk. Administration of inhaled budesonide to women who are breast-feeding should only be considered if the expected benefit to the mother is greater than any possible risk to the child.

4.7 Effects on ability to drive and use machines

No effects on ability to drive and use machines have been observed.

4.8 Undesirable effects

The possible adverse reactions are presented in system organ class order sorted by frequency.

(see Table 1 above)

Treatment with inhaled budesonide may result in candida infection in the oropharynx. Experience has shown that candida infection occurs less often when inhalation is performed before meals and/or when the mouth is rinsed after inhalation. In most cases this condition responds to topical anti-fungal therapy without discontinuing treatment with inhaled budesonide.

Systemic effects of inhaled corticosteroids may occur, particularly at high doses prescribed for prolonged periods. These may include adrenal suppression, growth retardation in children and adolescents, decrease in bone mineral density, cataract and glaucoma, and susceptibility to infections. The ability to adapt to stress may be impaired. The systemic effects described, however, are much less likely to occur with inhaled budesonide than with oral corticosteroids.

Lactose, the excipient in the product, contains small amounts of milk proteins and can therefore cause allergic reactions.

4.9 Overdose

Symptoms of overdose

The acute toxicity of budesonide is low. Chronic use in excessive doses can result in systemic glucocorticosteroid effects, such as increased susceptibility to infection, hypercorticism and adrenal suppression. Atrophy of the adrenal cortex can occur and the ability to adapt to stress can be impaired.

Therapeutic management of overdose

For acute overdosage, no special emergency action needs to be taken. The treatment with inhaled budesonide should be continued at the recommended dose to control asthma. HPA axis function recovers in a few days.

In stress situations, it may be necessary to administer corticosteroids as a precaution (eg high doses of hydrocortisone). Patients with adrenocortical atrophy are regarded as being steroid-dependent and must be adjusted to the adequate maintenance therapy of a systemic corticosteroid until the condition has stabilised.

5. PHARMACOLOGICAL PROPERTIES

5.1 Pharmacodynamic properties

Pharmacotherapeutic group: Glucocorticoids. ATC code: R03BA02.

Budesonide is a glucocorticosteroid which possesses a high local anti-inflammatory action.

Topical anti-inflammatory effect

The exact mechanism of action of glucocorticosteroids in the treatment of asthma is not fully understood. Anti-inflammatory actions, such as inhibition of inflammatory mediator release and inhibition of cytokine-mediated immune response are probably important.

Onset of effect

After a single dose of orally inhaled budesonide, delivered via dry powder inhaler, improvement of the lung function is achieved within a few hours. After therapeutic use of orally inhaled budesonide delivered via dry powder inhaler, improvement in lung function has been shown to occur within 2 days of initiation of treatment, although maximum benefit may not be achieved for up to 4 weeks.

Airway reactivity

Budesonide has also been shown to decrease airway reactivity to histamine and methacholine in hyper-reactive patients.

Exercise-induced asthma

Therapy with inhaled budesonide has effectively been used for prevention of exercise-induced asthma.

Growth

Limited data from long term studies suggest that most children and adolescents treated with inhaled budesonide ultimately achieve their adult target height. However, an initial small but transient reduction in growth (approximately 1 cm) has been observed. This generally occurs within the first year of treatment (see section 4.4).

HPA axis function

A study in healthy volunteers with Easyhaler Budesonide has shown dose-related effects on plasma and urinary cortisol. At recommended doses, budesonide causes less effect on the adrenal function than prednisolone 10mg, as shown by ACTH tests.

5.2 Pharmacokinetic properties

The activity of Easyhaler Budesonide is due to the parent active substance, budesonide, which is provided as a mixture of two epimers (22R and 22S). In glucocorticoid receptor affinity studies, the 22R form is twice as active as the 22S epimer. These two forms of budesonide do not interconvert. The terminal half-life is the same for both epimers (2-3 hours). In asthmatic patients, approximately 15-25% of the inhaled budesonide dose from Easyhaler reaches the lungs. The largest fraction of the inhaled dose is retained in the oropharynx and swallowed if the mouth is not rinsed out.

Absorption:

After oral administration of budesonide, peak plasma concentration is achieved in about 1-2 hours and the absolute systemic availability is 6-13%. In plasma, 85-95% of budesonide is bound to proteins. In contrast, peak plasma concentration is reached approximately 30 minutes after inhalation. Most of budesonide delivered to the lungs is systemically absorbed.

Metabolism:

Budesonide is mainly eliminated by metabolism. Budesonide is rapidly and extensively metabolised in liver via cytochrome P4503A4 to two major metabolites. The *in vitro* glucocorticoid activity of these metabolites is less than 1% of that of the parent compound. Negligible metabolic inactivation has been observed in human lung and serum preparations.

Excretion:

Budesonide is excreted in urine and faeces in the form of conjugated and non-conjugated metabolites.

Special patient populations

The exposure to budesonide may be increased in patients with liver disease. In children the elimination half-life from plasma is markedly lower than in adults.

5.3 Preclinical safety data

Preclinical data with budesonide reveal no special hazard for humans based on conventional studies of safety pharmacology, repeated dose toxicity, genotoxicity, or carcinogenic potential.

In animal studies on reproductive toxicity, glucocorticosteroids such as budesonide have been shown to induce malformations (cleft palate, skeletal malformations). However, these animal results do not seem to be relevant for humans given recommended doses.

6. PHARMACEUTICAL PARTICULARS

6.1 List of excipients

Lactose monohydrate (which contains small amounts of milk proteins).

6.2 Incompatibilities

Not applicable.

6.3 Shelf life

Shelf life of the medicinal product as packaged for sale: 3 years.

Shelf life after first opening the laminate pouch: 6 months.

6.4 Special precautions for storage

As packaged for sale

Store in the original package.

In use

Do not store above 30°C and store protected from moisture.

6.5 Nature and contents of container

The multidose powder inhaler consists of seven plastic parts and a stainless steel spring. The plastic materials of the inhaler are: overcap - polyester; bulk chamber cover -LDPE; bulk chamber -polycarbonate; metering cylinder and counter wheel -acetal; mouthpiece - styrene butadiene; dust cap-polypropylene. The plastic materials of the protective cover are polypropylene and thermoplastic elastomer. The inhaler is sealed in a laminate pouch (PET, Al and PE) and packed with or without a protective cover in a cardboard box.

Packages:

Easyhaler Budesonide 400 micrograms/dose inhalation powder:

- 100 doses + protective cover
- 100 doses
- 2 × 100 doses

6.6 Special precautions for disposal and other handling

No special requirements.

7. MARKETING AUTHORISATION HOLDER

Orion Corporation

Orionintie 1

FI-02200 Espoo

Finland

8. MARKETING AUTHORISATION NUMBER(S)

PL27925/0010

9. DATE OF FIRST AUTHORISATION/RENEWAL OF THE AUTHORISATION

29/11/2007

10. DATE OF REVISION OF THE TEXT

04/2009

Easyhaler Salbutamol 100mcg

(Orion Pharma (UK) Limited)

1. NAME OF THE MEDICINAL PRODUCT

Easyhaler Salbutamol Sulphate 100 micrograms per actuation inhalation powder

2. QUALITATIVE AND QUANTITATIVE COMPOSITION

Metered dose delivery 100 mcg of Salbutamol per actuation as Salbutamol Sulphate Ph.Eur.

3. PHARMACEUTICAL FORM

White or almost white odourless powder intended for respiratory use by oral inhalation.

4. CLINICAL PARTICULARS

4.1 Therapeutic indications

Symptomatic treatment of acute asthma attack. Prevention of exercise-induced bronchospasm. Symptomatic treatment of broncho-asthma and other conditions associated with reversible airways obstruction.

Salbutamol provides a short-acting bronchodilation with fast onset of action in reversible airways obstruction due to asthma.

Easyhaler Salbutamol Sulphate should be used to relieve symptoms when they occur and to prevent them in those circumstances recognised by the patient to precipitate an attack (e.g. before exercise or unavoidable allergen exposure).

Salbutamol is valuable as a rescue medication in mild, moderate or severe asthma, provided that reliance on it does not delay the introduction and use of regular inhaled corticosteroid therapy.

4.2 Posology and method of administration

The preparation is intended for oral inhalation only.

This preparation is particularly useful for patients unable to use metered dose inhalers properly and for patients to whom the use of an inhalation aerosol causes irritation of airways. The lowest effective doses of inhaled Salbutamol are recommended to be used in the treatment of asthma. In long term treatment, it is recommended instead of continual use, to use inhaled Salbutamol when needed.

Adults and Elderly:

For the relief of acute bronchospasm and for managing intermittent episodes of asthma, one inhalation (100 micrograms) may be administered as a single starting dose, this may be increased to two inhalations (200 micrograms) if necessary.

To prevent exercise-induced bronchospasm or allergen bronchospasm two inhalations (200 micrograms) should be taken before challenge, this dose (200 micrograms) may be repeated if necessary.

Children:

One to two inhalations (100 - 200 micrograms) is the recommended starting dose for relief of acute bronchospasm, or before exercise or allergen exposure.

On demand use of Easyhaler Salbutamol Sulphate should not exceed eight inhalations (800 micrograms) in any 24 hour period.

For optimum results in most patients Easyhaler Salbutamol Sulphate inhaler should be used regularly during asthmatic attacks. The bronchodilator effect of each administration of inhaled salbutamol lasts for four hours, except in patients whose asthma is becoming worse. Such patients should be warned not to increase their usage of salbutamol, but should seek medical advice in case treatment with an inhaled and/or systemic glucocorticosteroid is indicated.

4.3 Contraindications

A history of hypersensitivity to any components of the product. Intravenous or oral salbutamol is used for the management of premature labour uncomplicated by conditions such as placenta praevia, ante-partum haemorrhage or toxaemia of pregnancy, however inhaled salbutamol is not appropriate for management of premature labour.

Salbutamol preparations should not be used for threatened abortion.

4.4 Special warnings and precautions for use

Bronchodilators should not be the only or main treatment in patients with severe or unstable asthma. Severe asthma requires regular medical assessment including lung function testing as the patients are at risk of severe attacks and even death. Physicians should consider using oral corticosteroid therapy or the maximum use of inhaled corticosteroids. Increasing use of bronchodilators, particularly short-acting inhaled β2-agonists to relieve symptoms indicates deteriorating asthma control. If patients find that short-acting relief bronchodilator treatment becomes less effective or they need more inhalations than usual, medical attention must be sought. In this situation patients should be reassessed and consideration given to an increase in their anti-inflammatory therapy, (e.g. higher doses of inhaled corticosteroids or a course of oral corticosteroids). Severe episodes of asthma must be treated in the normal way.

In the event of a previous effective dose of inhaled salbutamol failing to give relief for at least three hours, the patient should be advised to seek medical advice in order that any necessary additional steps may be taken; need for increased anti-inflammatory therapy. As there may be adverse effects associated with excessive dosing, the dosage and frequency of administration should only be increased on medical advice.

Salbutamol should be administered with caution in patients with thyrotoxicosis.

Potentially serious hypokalaemia may result from β2 agonist therapy, mainly from parenteral and nebulised therapy. Particular caution is advised in acute severe asthma, as this effect may be potentiated by concomitant treatment with xanthine derivatives, steroids, diuretics and by hypoxia. It is recommended that serum potassium levels are monitored in such situations.

4.5 Interaction with other medicinal products and other forms of interaction

Concomitant administration of salbutamol and non-selective β-blocking drugs such as Propranolol is not recommended.

Patients treated with monoamine oxidase inhibitors or tricyclic antidepressants should be followed clinically in the beginning of salbutamol treatment, because the action of salbutamol on the vascular system may be potentiated.

4.6 Pregnancy and lactation

Administration of drugs during pregnancy should only be considered if the expected benefit to the mother is greater than any possible risk to the foetus. Salbutamol has been in widespread use for many years in human beings without apparent ill consequences; this includes its well established use in the management of premature labour. However, as with the majority of drugs, there is little published evidence of its safety in the early stages of human pregnancy, but in animal studies there is evidence of some harmful effects on the foetus at very high doses.

As salbutamol is probably excreted in breast milk, its use in nursing mothers requires careful consideration. It is not known whether salbutamol has a harmful effect on the neonate, and so its use should be restricted to situations where it is felt that the expected benefit to the mother outweighs any potential risk to the neonate.

4.7 Effects on ability to drive and use machines

None Known.

4.8 Undesirable effects

Inhaled Salbutamol is well tolerated. The side-effects caused by normally used inhaled doses of Salbutamol are mild. Typical for sympathomimetic agents, and they usually disappear with continued treatment.

Frequent (>1%)

Cardiovascular - palpitation; Muscular - tremor.

Less frequent (1-0.1%)

General - headache, hypersensitivity reactions (angioedema, urticaria, hypotension and collapse).

Rare (<0.1%)

Respiratory tract - bronchospasm, irritation of mouth and throat.

Metabolic - hypokalaemia.

Muscular - muscle cramps

CNS - restlessness, dizziness.

4.9 Overdose

The preferred antidote for overdosage with salbutamol is a cardioselective beta-blocking agent, but beta-blocking drugs should be used with caution in patients with a history of bronchospasm. Hypokalaemia may occur following overdose with salbutamol. Serum potassium levels should be monitored.

5. PHARMACOLOGICAL PROPERTIES

5.1 Pharmacodynamic properties

Salbutamol is a selective β2-adrenergic receptor agonist. The pharmacological effects of salbutamol are at least in part attributable to stimulation through beta-adrenergic receptors of intracellular adenyl cyclase, the enzyme that catalyses the conversion of adenosine triphosphate (ATP) to cyclic-3',5',-adenosine monophosphate (cyclic AMP). Increased cyclic AMP levels are associated with relaxation of bronchial smooth muscle and inhibition of release of mediators of immediate hypersensitivity from cells, especially from mast cells. Salbutamol also stimulates mucous secretion and mucociliary transport in the respiratory tract. Bronchial effects of inhaled salbutamol can be detected after a few minutes and duration of action is normally 4-6 hours.

Like other β2-adrenoceptor agonists salbutamol also has cardiovascular effects in some patients as measured by changes in pulse rate, blood pressure, symptoms and ECG changes. These effects can especially be detected after oral and intravenous administration of salbutamol. Furthermore oral and intravenous salbutamol causes reduction in uterine tonicity which has been associated with pain relief in pregnancy. In addition, salbutamol has some metabolic effects. Especially intravenous and nebulised salbutamol decreases serum potassium concentrations although the effect is generally mild and transient. Salbutamol has also lipolytic effects and it has been shown to cause increases in blood glucose and insulin probably by stimulating glycogenolysis and having a stimulatory effect on β2-receptors in pancreas cells.

5.2 Pharmacokinetic properties

Orally administered salbutamol is well absorbed with peak plasma concentrations occurring 1 to 4 hours after administration. The major proportion of inhaled Salbutamol is swallowed. The fraction that is distributed to the lung (approx. 10-25%) is rapidly seen in the circulation as free unmetabolised drug. The plasma concentrations of inhaled Salbutamol are, however, lower than those produced by usual oral doses.

Salbutamol and its metabolites are rapidly excreted in the urine and faeces with about 80% of the dose being recovered in urine within 24 hours. The elimination half-life of Salbutamol is 2.7 - 5.5 hours after oral and inhaled administration.

5.3 Preclinical safety data

The short term toxicity has been tested in different animal species - the mouse, the rat and the dog - at doses extending to several thousand fold higher than the intended human therapeutic dose - maximally in the region of 15 µg/kg daily. The lethal doses via the intravenous route in the rodents range from 50mg/kg, via the peroral route to around 2000 mg/kg and even higher. Thus the agent exhibits low acute systemic toxicity.

Local toxicity on the airway has not been exclusively studied, but the historical evidence based on long clinical use suggests good airway tolerance.

The subacute toxic effects on the cardiac muscle are seen at doses ranging from 0.2 to 3mg/kg. This is a manifestation of the pharmacodynamics of salbutamol at grossly elevated doses.

The doses administered in subchronic toxicity studies have been in the milligram ranges per kilogram - 0.15 to 50 - via the oral route or by inhalation. The species have been the rat (p.o. administration), and the dog (p.o. and inhalation). The toxic signs and symptoms exhibited were, as noted in the paragraph above, related to the mode of action on the adrenergic receptor.

The chronic toxicity, again, is manifested as exaggerated pharmacodynamic effects in animals.

Animal data on reproductive toxicity is quite limited. Sympathomimetics, including salbutamol, are widely used in clinical medicine in patients of fertile age. In spite of this fact, no adverse reproductive effects attributable to salbutamol are reported in the literature.

Embryotoxicity in animal studies seems to be related only to the mouse. In this species the union of the flat bones of the lower part of the skull seem to be involved. The specific mechanism of this has not been fully elucidated.

Foetal toxicity at high single or elevated chronic doses are related to energy metabolism from glycogen. Catecholamines liberate energy in the form of glucose from glycogen stored in liver and muscle. This action is mediated by glycogen synthase and phosphorylase of these tissues. Elevated foetal insulin and glucose levels suggest a higher sensitivity of the foetal pancreas to this stimulation of β-adrenergic receptors.

The classic airways of mutagenic potential by which this agent has been tested have exhibited no increase in the incidence of mutations.

The potential of increase in the number of neoplasms shows a species and even a strain specificity, as did the effect on the delay in union flat jaw bones. Ovarian leiomyomas, benign tumours of smooth muscle, occur with a significantly higher frequency in the rat, particularly of the Spraque-Dawley strain. The other rodent species do not appear to be affected, suggesting a difference in the susceptibility of the uterine muscle of Spraque-Dawley to β-adrenergic stimulation.

6. PHARMACEUTICAL PARTICULARS

6.1 List of excipients

Lactose Ph.Eur.

6.2 Incompatibilities

None

6.3 Shelf life

Unopened: 3 Years

After first opening of foil pouch: 6 months.

6.4 Special precautions for storage

Store in a dry place at a temperature not exceeding 25°C. Use if the protective cover of the Easyhaler inhaler is recommended once the laminate foil has been opened.

6.5 Nature and contents of container

The multidose powder inhaler (Easyhaler) consists of seven plastic parts and a stainless steel spring.

The plastic materials of the inhaler are polyester, LDPE, polycarbonate, acetal, styrene butadiene, polypropylene.

The inhaler is wrapped in laminate foil and packed in a cardboard box.

The starting package contains an inhaler and a protective cover. The maintenance pack contains the dry powder inhaler only.

Pack size: 200 actuations.

6.6 Special precautions for disposal and other handling

Patients are instructed to perform a rapid and forced inhalation through the Easyhaler device. Patients are instructed not to exhale into the device. Illustrated instructions for use accompany each package.

7. MARKETING AUTHORISATION HOLDER

Orion Corporation,

Orionintie 1,

FIN-02200 Espoo,

Finland.

8. MARKETING AUTHORISATION NUMBER(S)
PL 27925/0002

9. DATE OF FIRST AUTHORISATION/RENEWAL OF THE AUTHORISATION
2 June 1998/ 1 June 2003

10. DATE OF REVISION OF THE TEXT
November 2006

Easyhaler Salbutamol 200mcg

(Orion Pharma (UK) Limited)

1. NAME OF THE MEDICINAL PRODUCT
Easyhaler Salbutamol Sulphate 200 micrograms per actuation inhalation powder

2. QUALITATIVE AND QUANTITATIVE COMPOSITION
Metered dose delivery 200 mcg of Salbutamol per actuation as Salbutamol Sulphate Ph.Eur.

3. PHARMACEUTICAL FORM
White or almost white odourless powder intended for respiratory use by oral inhalation.

4. CLINICAL PARTICULARS

4.1 Therapeutic indications
Symptomatic treatment of acute asthma attack. Prevention of exercise-induced bronchospasm. Symptomatic treatment of broncho-asthma and other conditions associated with reversible airways obstruction.

Salbutamol provides a short-acting bronchodilation with fast onset of action in reversible airways obstruction due to asthma.

Easyhaler Salbutamol Sulphate should be used to relieve symptoms when they occur and to prevent them in those circumstances recognised by the patient to precipitate an attack (e.g. before exercise or unavoidable allergen exposure).

Salbutamol is valuable as a rescue medication in mild, moderate or severe asthma, provided that reliance on it does not delay the introduction and use of regular inhaled corticosteroid therapy.

4.2 Posology and method of administration
The preparation is intended for oral inhalation only.

This preparation is particularly useful for patients unable to use metered dose inhalers properly and for patients to whom the use of an inhalation aerosol causes irritation of airways. The lowest effective doses of inhaled Salbutamol are recommended to be used in the treatment of asthma. In long term treatment, it is recommended instead of continual use, to use inhaled Salbutamol only when needed.

Adults and Elderly:

For the relief of acute bronchospasm and for managing intermittent episodes of asthma one inhalation (200 micrograms) may be administered as a single starting dose, this may be increased to two inhalations (400 micrograms).

To prevent exercise-induced bronchospasm or allergen bronchospasm one inhalations (200 micrograms) should be taken before challenge, this dose (200 micrograms) may be repeated if necessary.

Children:

One inhalation (200 micrograms) is the recommended starting dose for the relief of acute bronchospasm, or before exercise or allergen exposure.

On demand use of Easyhaler Salbutamol Sulphate should not exceed four inhalations (800 micrograms) in any 24 hour period.

For optimum results in most patients Easyhaler Salbutamol Sulphate inhaler should be used regularly during asthmatic attacks. The bronchodilator effect of each administration of inhaled salbutamol lasts for four hours, except in patients whose asthma is becoming worse. Such patients should be warned not to increase their usage of salbutamol, but should seek medical advice in case treatment with an inhaled and/or systemic glucocorticosteroid is indicated.

4.3 Contraindications
A history of hypersensitivity to any components of the product. Intravenous or oral salbutamol is used for the management of premature labour uncomplicated by conditions such as placenta praevia, ante-partum haemorrhage or toxaemia of pregnancy; however inhaled salbutamol is not appropriate for management of premature labour. Salbutamol preparations should not be used for threatened abortion.

4.4 Special warnings and precautions for use
Bronchodilators should not be the only or main treatment in patients with severe or unstable asthma. Severe asthma requires regular medical assessment including lung function testing as the patients are at risk of severe attacks and even death. Physicians should consider using oral corticosteroid therapy or the maximum use of inhaled corticosteroids. Increasing use of bronchodilators, particularly short-acting inhaled β2-agonists to relieve symptoms indicates deteriorating asthma control. If patients find that short-acting relief bronchodilator treatment becomes less effective or they need more inhalations than usual, medical attention must be sought. In this situation patients should be reassessed and consideration given to an increase in their anti-inflammatory therapy, (e.g. higher doses of inhaled corticosteroids or a course of oral corticosteroids). Severe episodes of asthma must be treated in the normal way.

In the event of a previous effective dose of inhaled salbutamol failing to give relief for at least three hours, the patient should be advised to seek medical advice in order that any necessary additional steps may be taken; need for increased anti-inflammatory therapy. As there may be adverse effects associated with excessive dosing, the dosage and frequency of administration should only be increased on medical advice.

Salbutamol should be administered with caution in patients with thyrotoxicosis.

Potentially serious hypokalaemia may result from β2-agonist therapy, mainly from parenteral and nebulised therapy. Particular caution is advised in acute severe asthma, as this effect may be potentiated by concomitant treatment with xanthine derivatives, steroids, diuretics and by hypoxia. It is recommended that serum potassium levels are monitored in such situations.

4.5 Interaction with other medicinal products and other forms of interaction
Concomitant administration of salbutamol and non-selective β -blocking drugs such as Propranolol is not recommended.

Patients treated with monoamine oxidase inhibitors or tricyclic antidepressants should be followed clinically in the beginning of salbutamol treatment, because the action of salbutamol on the vascular system may be potentiated.

4.6 Pregnancy and lactation
Administration of drugs during pregnancy should only be considered if the expected benefit to the mother is greater than any possible risk to the foetus. Salbutamol has been in widespread use for many years in human beings without apparent ill consequences; this includes its well established use in the management of premature labour. However, as with the majority of drugs, there is little published evidence of its safety in the early stages of human pregnancy, but in animal studies there is evidence of some harmful effects on the foetus at very high doses.

As salbutamol is probably excreted in breast milk, its use in nursing mothers requires careful consideration. It is not known whether salbutamol has a harmful effect on the neonate, and so its use should be restricted to situations where it is felt that the expected benefit to the mother outweighs any potential risk to the neonate.

4.7 Effects on ability to drive and use machines
None Known.

4.8 Undesirable effects
Inhaled Salbutamol is well tolerated. The side-effects caused by normally used inhaled doses of Salbutamol are mild. Typical for sympathomimetic agents, and they usually disappear with continued treatment.

Frequent (>1%)

Cardiovascular - palpitation; Muscular - tremor.

Less frequent (1-0.1%)

General - headache, hypersensitivity reactions (angioedema, urticaria, hypotension and collapse).

Rare (<0.1%)

Respiratory tract - bronchospasm, irritation of mouth and throat.

Metabolic - hypokalaemia.

Muscular - muscle cramps

CNS - restlessness, dizziness.

4.9 Overdose
The preferred antidote for overdosage with salbutamol is a cardio-selective beta-blocking agent, but beta-blocking drugs should be used with caution in patients with a history of bronchospasm. Hypokalaemia may occur following overdose with salbutamol. Serum potassium levels should be monitored.

5. PHARMACOLOGICAL PROPERTIES

5.1 Pharmacodynamic properties
Salbutamol is a selective β 2-adrenergic receptor agonist. The pharmacological effects of salbutamol are at least in part attributable to stimulation through beta-adrenergic receptors of intracellular adenyl cyclase, the enzyme that catalyses the conversion of adenosine triphosphate (ATP) to cyclic-3',5',-adenosine monophosphate (cyclic AMP). Increased cyclic AMP levels are associated with relaxation of bronchial smooth muscle and inhibition of release of mediators of immediate hypersensitivity from cells, especially from mast cells. Salbutamol also stimulates mucous secretion and mucociliary transport in the respiratory tract. Bronchial effects of inhaled salbutamol can be detected after a few minutes and duration of action is normally 4-6 hours.

Like other β 2-adrenoceptor agonists salbutamol also has cardiovascular effects in some patients as measured by changes in pulse rate, blood pressure, symptoms and ECG changes. These effects can especially be detected after oral and intravenous administration of salbutamol. Furthermore oral and intravenous salbutamol causes reduction in uterine tonicity which has been associated with pain relief in pregnancy. In addition, salbutamol has some metabolic effects. Especially intravenous and nebulised salbutamol decreases serum potassium concentrations although the effect is generally mild and transient. Salbutamol has also lipolytic effects and it has been shown to cause increases in blood glucose and insulin probably by stimulating glycogenolysis and having a stimulatory effect on β 2-receptors in pancreas cells.

5.2 Pharmacokinetic properties
Orally administered salbutamol is well absorbed with peak plasma concentrations occurring 1 to 4 hours after administration. The major proportion of inhaled Salbutamol is swallowed. The fraction that is distributed to the lung (approx. 10-25%) is rapidly seen in the circulation as free unmetabolised drug. The plasma concentrations of inhaled Salbutamol are, however, lower than those produced by usual oral doses.

Salbutamol and its metabolites are rapidly excreted in the urine and faeces with about 80% of the dose being recovered in urine within 24 hours. The elimination half-life of Salbutamol is 2.7 - 5.5 hours after oral and inhaled administration.

5.3 Preclinical safety data
The short term toxicity has been tested in different animal species - the mouse, the rat and the dog - at doses extending to several thousand fold higher than the intended human therapeutic dose - maximally in the region of 15 µg/kg daily. The lethal doses via the intravenous route in the rodents range from 50mg/kg, via the per oral route to around 2000 mg/kg and even higher. Thus the agent exhibits low acute systemic toxicity.

Local toxicity on the airway has not been exclusively studied, but the historical evidence based on long clinical use suggests good airway tolerance.

The sub-acute toxic effects on the cardiac muscle are seen at doses ranging from 0.2 to 3mg/kg. This is a manifestation of the pharmacodynamics of salbutamol at grossly elevated doses.

The doses administered in sub-chronic toxicity studies have been in the milligram ranges per kilogram - 0.15 to 50 - via the oral route or by inhalation. The species have been the rat (p.o. administration), and the dog (p.o. and inhalation). The toxic signs and symptoms exhibited were, as noted in the paragraph above, related to the mode of action on the adrenergic receptor.

The chronic toxicity, again, is manifested as exaggerated pharmacodynamic effects in animals.

Animal data on reproductive toxicity is quite limited. Sympathomimetics, including salbutamol, are widely used in clinical medicine in patients of fertile age. In spite of this fact, no adverse reproductive effects attributable to salbutamol are reported in the literature.

Embryotoxicity in animal studies seems to be related only to the mouse. In this species the union of the flat bones of the lower part of the skull seem to be involved. The specific mechanism of this has not been fully elucidated.

Foetal toxicity at high single or elevated chronic doses are related to energy metabolism from glycogen. Catecholamines liberate energy in the form of glucose from glycogen stored in liver and muscle. This action is mediated by glycogen synthase and phosphorylase of these tissues. Elevated foetal insulin and glucose levels suggest a higher sensitivity of the foetal pancreas to this stimulation of β - adrenergic receptors.

The classic airways of mutagenic potential by which this agent has been tested have exhibited no increase in the incidence of mutations.

The potential of increase in the number of neoplasms shows a species and even a strain specificity, as did the effect on the delay in union flat jaw bones. Ovarian leiomyomas, benign tumours of smooth muscle, occur with a significantly higher frequency in the rat, particularly of the Spraque-Dawley strain. The other rodent species do not appear to be affected, suggesting a difference in the susceptibility of the uterine muscle of Spraque-Dawley to β - adrenergic stimulation.

6. PHARMACEUTICAL PARTICULARS

6.1 List of excipients
Lactose Ph.Eur.

6.2 Incompatibilities
None

6.3 Shelf life
Unopened: 3 Years

After first opening of foil pouch: 6 months.

6.4 Special precautions for storage
Store in a dry place at a temperature not exceeding 25°C

6.5 Nature and contents of container
The multidose powder inhaler (Easyhaler) consists of seven plastic parts and a stainless steel spring.

The plastic materials of the inhaler are polyester, LDPE, polycarbonate, acetal, styrene butadiene, polypropylene.

The inhaler is wrapped in laminate foil and packed in a cardboard box.

The starting package contains an inhaler and a protective cover. The maintenance pack contains the dry powder inhaler only.

Pack size: 200 actuations.

6.6 Special precautions for disposal and other handling

Patients are instructed to perform a rapid and forced inhalation through the Easyhaler device. Patients are instructed not to exhale into the device. Illustrated instructions for use accompany each package.

7. MARKETING AUTHORISATION HOLDER

Orion Corporation,

Orionintie 1,

FIN-02200 Espoo,

Finland.

8. MARKETING AUTHORISATION NUMBER(S)

PL 27925/0003

9. DATE OF FIRST AUTHORISATION/RENEWAL OF THE AUTHORISATION

2 June 1998/ 1 June 2003

10. DATE OF REVISION OF THE TEXT

March 2007

Ebixa 10 mg/g oral drops, 20mg and 10 mg Tablets and Treatment Initiation Pack

(Lundbeck Limited)

1. NAME OF THE MEDICINAL PRODUCT

Ebixa 10 mg/g oral drops, solution

Ebixa 5 mg film-coated tablets

Ebixa 10 mg film-coated tablets

Ebixa 15 mg film-coated tablets

Ebixa 20 mg film-coated tablets

2. QUALITATIVE AND QUANTITATIVE COMPOSITION

Oral drops, solution

1 g of solution contains 10 mg memantine hydrochloride (equivalent to 8.31 mg memantine). One drop of solution is equivalent to 0.5 mg memantine hydrochloride.

Excipients: 1 g of solution contains 100 mg of sorbitol E420 and 0.5 mg of potassium, see section 4.4.

Film-coated tablets

Each 5 mg film-coated tablet contains 5 mg of memantine hydrochloride equivalent to 4.15 mg memantine.

Each 10 mg film-coated tablet contains 10 mg of memantine hydrochloride equivalent to 8.31 mg memantine.

Each 15 mg film-coated tablet contains 15 mg of memantine hydrochloride equivalent to 12.46 mg memantine.

Each 20 mg film-coated tablet contains 20 mg of memantine hydrochloride equivalent to 16.62 mg memantine.

Excipient: The 10 mg film-coated tablet contains 166 mg lactose, see section 4.4.

For a full list of excipients, see section 6.1.

3. PHARMACEUTICAL FORM

Oral drops, solution.

The solution is clear and colourless to light yellowish.

Film-coated tablets.

The 5 mg film-coated tablets are white to off-white, oval-oblong film-coated tablets with imprint '5' on one side and imprint 'MEM' on the other side.

The 10 mg film-coated tablets are white to off-white film-coated tablets, centrally tapered oblong, biconvex, with a single breakline on both sides. The tablet can be divided into equal halves.

The 15 mg film-coated tablets are orange to grey-orange, oval-oblong film-coated tablets with imprint '15' on one side and imprint 'MEM' on the other side.

The 20 mg film-coated tablets are pale red to grey-red, oval-oblong film-coated tablets with imprint '20' on one side and imprint 'MEM' on the other side.

4. CLINICAL PARTICULARS

4.1 Therapeutic indications

Treatment of patients with moderate to severe Alzheimer's disease.

4.2 Posology and method of administration

Treatment should be initiated and supervised by a physician experienced in the diagnosis and treatment of Alzheimer's dementia. Therapy should only be started if a caregiver is available who will regularly monitor the intake of the medicinal product by the patient. Diagnosis should be made according to current guidelines.

Ebixa should be administered once a day and should be taken at the same time every day. The drops and film-coated tablets can be taken with or without food.

Adults:

Dose titration

Treatment Initiation Pack:

The recommended starting dose is 5 mg per day, which is stepwise increased over the first 4 weeks of treatment reaching the recommended maintenance dose as follows:

Week 1 (day 1-7):

The patient should take one 5 mg film-coated tablet per day (white to off-white, oval-oblong) for 7 days.

Week 2 (day 8-14):

The patient should take one 10 mg film-coated tablet per day (white to off-white, centrally tapered oblong, biconvex, with a single breakline on both sides) for 7 days.

Week 3 (day 15-21):

The patient should take one 15 mg film-coated tablet per day (grey-orange, oval-oblong film) for 7 days.

Week 4 (day 22-28):

The patient should take one 20 mg film-coated tablet per day (grey-red, oval-oblong film) for 7 days.

The maximum daily dose is 20 mg per day.

Tablet packs of 10 mg and 20 mg and Dropper pack of 10mg/g:

The maximum daily dose is 20 mg daily. In order to reduce the risk of undesirable effects the maintenance dose is achieved by upward titration of 5 mg per week over the first 3 weeks as follows:

Week 1 (day 1-7):

The patient should take one 5 mg tablet/half a 10 mg tablet/10 drops (5 mg) per day for 7 days.

Week 2 (day 8-14):

The patient should take one 10 mg tablet/20 drops (10 mg) per day for 7 days.

Week 3 (day 15-21):

The patient should take one 15 mg tablet/one and a half 10 mg tablets/30 drops (15 mg) per day for 7 days.

From Week 4 on:

The patient should take one 20 mg tablet/two 10 mg tablets/40 drops (20 mg) once a day.

Maintenance dose

The recommended maintenance dose is 20 mg per day.

Elderly: On the basis of the clinical studies, the recommended dose for patients over the age of 65 years is 20 mg per day (one 20 mg tablet/two 10 mg tablets/40 drops) as described above.

Children and adolescents under the age of 18 years: Ebixa is not recommended for use in children below 18 years due to a lack of data on safety and efficacy.

Renal impairment: In patients with mildly impaired renal function (creatinine clearance 50 – 80 ml/min) no dosage adjustment is required. In patients with moderate renal impairment (creatinine clearance 30 - 49 ml/min) daily dose should be 10 mg per day. If tolerated well after at least 7 days of treatment, the dose could be increased up to 20 mg/day according to standard titration scheme. In patients with severe renal impairment (creatinine clearance 5 – 29 ml/min) daily dose should be 10 mg per day.

Hepatic impairment: In patients with mild or moderate hepatic impaired function (Child-Pugh A and Child-Pugh B) no dosage adjustment is needed. No data on the use of memantine in patients with severe hepatic impairment are available. Administration of Ebixa is not recommended in patients with severe hepatic impairment.

4.3 Contraindications

Hypersensitivity to the active substance or to any of the excipients.

4.4 Special warnings and precautions for use

Caution is recommended in patients with epilepsy, former history of convulsions or patients with predisposing factors for epilepsy.

Concomitant use of N-methyl-D-aspartate (NMDA)-antagonists such as amantadine, ketamine or dextromethorphan should be avoided. These compounds act at the same receptor system as memantine, and therefore adverse drug reactions (mainly CNS-related) may be more frequent or more pronounced (see also section 4.5).

Some factors that may raise urine pH (see section 5.2 "Elimination") may necessitate careful monitoring of the patient. These factors include drastic changes in diet, e.g. from a carnivore to a vegetarian diet, or a massive ingestion of alkalising gastric buffers. Also, urine pH may be elevated by states of renal tubulary acidosis (RTA) or severe infections of the urinary tract with *Proteus* bacteria.

In most clinical trials, patients with recent myocardial infarction, uncompensated congestive heart failure (NYHA III-IV), or uncontrolled hypertension were excluded. As a consequence, only limited data are available and patients with these conditions should be closely supervised.

Excipients– oral drops: The oral solution contains sorbitol. Patients with rare hereditary problems of fructose intolerance should not take this medicine.

Excipients– tablets: The 10 mg tablets contain lactose monohydrate. Patients with rare hereditary problems of galactose intolerance, the Lapp lactase deficiency or glucose-galactose malabsorption should not take this medicine.

4.5 Interaction with other medicinal products and other forms of interaction

Due to the pharmacological effects and the mechanism of action of memantine the following interactions may occur:

• The mode of action suggests that the effects of L-dopa, dopaminergic agonists, and anticholinergics may be enhanced by concomitant treatment with NMDA-antagonists such as memantine. The effects of barbiturates and neuroleptics may be reduced. Concomitant administration of memantine with the antispasmodic agents, dantrolene or baclofen, can modify their effects and a dosage adjustment may be necessary.

• Concomitant use of memantine and amantadine should be avoided, owing to the risk of pharmacotoxic psychosis. Both compounds are chemically related NMDA-antagonists. The same may be true for ketamine and dextromethorphan (see also section 4.4). There is one published case report on a possible risk also for the combination of memantine and phenytoin.

• Other active substances such as such as cimetidine, ranitidine, procainamide, quinidine, quinine and nicotine that use the same renal cationic transport system as amantadine may also possibly interact with memantine leading to a potential risk of increased plasma levels.

• There may be a possibility of reduced serum level of hydrochlorothiazide (HCT) when memantine is co-administered with HCT or any combination with HCT.

• In post-marketing experience isolated cases with INR increases have been reported in patients concomitantly treated with warfarin. Although no causal relationship has been established, close monitoring of prothrombin time or INR is advisable for patients concomitantly treated with oral anticoagulants.

In single dose PK studies in young healthy subjects no relevant drug-drug interaction of memantine with glyburide/metformin or donepezil was observed.

In a clinical study in young healthy volunteers no relevant effect of memantine on the pharmacokinetics of galantamine was observed.

Memantine did not inhibit CYP 1A2, 2A6, 2C9, 2D6, 2E1, 3A, flavin-containing monooxygenase, epoxide hydrolase or sulphation *in vitro*.

4.6 Pregnancy and lactation

Pregnancy: For memantine, no clinical data on exposed pregnancies are available. Animal studies indicate a potential for reducing intrauterine growth at exposure levels that are identical or slightly higher than at human exposure (see section 5.3). The potential risk for humans is unknown. Memantine should not be used during pregnancy unless clearly necessary.

Lactation: It is not known whether memantine is excreted in human breast milk but, taking into consideration the lipophilicity of the substance, this probably occurs. Women taking memantine should not breast-feed.

4.7 Effects on ability to drive and use machines

Moderate to severe Alzheimer's disease usually causes impairment of driving performance and compromises the ability to use machinery. Furthermore, Ebixa has minor or moderate influence on the ability to drive and use machines, such that outpatients should take special care.

4.8 Undesirable effects

In clinical trials in mild to severe dementia, involving 1,784 patients treated with Ebixa and 1,595 patients treated with placebo, the overall incidence rate of adverse events with Ebixa did not differ from those with placebo; the adverse events were usually mild to moderate in severity. The most frequently occurring adverse events with a higher incidence in the Ebixa group than in the placebo group were dizziness (6.3% vs 5.6%, respectively), headache (5.2% vs 3.9%), constipation (4.6% vs 2.6%), somnolence (3.4% vs 2.2%) and hypertension (4.1% vs 2.8%).

The following Adverse Drug Reactions listed in the Table below have been accumulated in clinical studies with Ebixa and since its introduction in the market. Within each frequency grouping, undesirable effects are presented in order of decreasing seriousness.

Adverse reactions are ranked according to system organ class, using the following convention: very common (≥1/10), common (≥1/100 to < 1/10), uncommon (≥ 1/1,000 to < 1/100), rare (≥1/10,000 to < 1/1,000), very rare (< 1/10,000), not known (cannot be estimated from the available data).

Infections and infestations	Uncommon	Fungal infections
Psychiatric disorders	Common	Somnolence
	Uncommon	Confusion
	Uncommon	Hallucinations[1]
	Not known	Psychotic reactions[2]
Nervous system disorders	Common	Dizziness
	Uncommon	Gait abnormal
	Very rare	Seizures
Cardiac disorders	Uncommon	Cardiac failure
Vascular disorders	Common	Hypertension
	Uncommon	Venous thrombosis/ thromboembolism

Respiratory, thoracic and mediastinal disorders	Common	Dyspnoea
Gastrointestinal disorders	Common	Constipation
	Uncommon	Vomiting
	Not known	Pancreatitis[2]
General disorders and administration site conditions	Common	Headache
	Uncommon	Fatigue

[1] Hallucinations have mainly been observed in patients with severe Alzheimer's disease.

[2] Isolated cases reported in post-marketing experience.

Alzheimer's disease has been associated with depression, suicidal ideation and suicide. In post-marketing experience these events have been reported in patients treated with Ebixa.

4.9 Overdose

Only limited experience with overdose is available from clinical studies and post-marketing experience.

Symptoms: Relatively large overdoses (200 mg and 105 mg/day for 3 days, respectively) have been associated with either only symptoms of tiredness, weakness and/or diarrhoea or no symptoms. In the overdose cases below 140 mg or unknown dose the patients revealed symptoms from central nervous system (confusion, drowsiness, somnolence, vertigo, agitation, aggression, hallucination, and gait disturbance) and/or of gastrointestinal origin (vomiting and diarrhoea).

In the most extreme case of overdosage, the patient survived the oral intake of a total of 2000 mg memantine with effects on the central nervous system (coma for 10 days, and later diplopia and agitation). The patient received symptomatic treatment and plasmapheresis. The patient recovered without permanent sequelae.

In another case of a large overdose, the patient also survived and recovered. The patient had received 400 mg memantine orally. The patient experienced central nervous system symptoms such as restlessness, psychosis, visual hallucinations, proconvulsiveness, somnolence, stupor, and unconsciousness.

Treatment: In the event of overdosage, treatment should be symptomatic. No specific antidote for intoxication or overdose is available. Standard clinical procedures to remove active substance material, e.g. gastric lavage, carbo medicinalis (interruption of potential entero-hepatic recirculation), acidification of urine, forced diuresis should be used as appropriate.

In case of signs and symptoms of general CNS overstimulation, careful symptomatic clinical treatment should be considered.

5. PHARMACOLOGICAL PROPERTIES

5.1 Pharmacodynamic properties

Pharmacotherapeutic group: Anti-dementia drugs, ATC code: N06DX01.

There is increasing evidence that malfunctioning of glutamatergic neurotransmission, in particular at NMDA-receptors, contributes to both expression of symptoms and disease progression in neurodegenerative dementia.

Memantine is a voltage-dependent, moderate-affinity uncompetitive NMDA-receptor antagonist. It modulates the effects of pathologically elevated tonic levels of glutamate that may lead to neuronal dysfunction.

Clinical studies: A pivotal monotherapy study in a population of patients suffering from moderate to severe Alzheimer's disease (mini mental state examination (MMSE) total scores at baseline of 3 - 14) included a total of 252 outpatients. The study showed beneficial effects of memantine treatment in comparison to placebo at 6 months (observed cases analysis for the clinician's interview based impression of change (CIBIC-plus): p=0.025; Alzheimer's disease cooperative study – activities of daily living (ADCS-ADLsev): p=0.003; severe impairment battery (SIB): p=0.002).

A pivotal monotherapy study of memantine in the treatment of mild to moderate Alzheimer's disease (MMSE total scores at baseline of 10 to 22) included 403 patients. Memantine-treated patients showed a statistically significantly better effect than placebo-treated patients on the primary endpoints: Alzheimer's disease assessment scale (ADAS-cog) (p=0.003) and CIBIC-plus (p=0.004) at week 24 (last observation carried forward (LOCF)). In another monotherapy study in mild to moderate Alzheimer's disease a total of 470 patients (MMSE total scores at baseline of 11-23) were randomised. In the prospectively defined primary analysis statistical significance was not reached at the primary efficacy endpoint at week 24.

A meta-analysis of patients with moderate to severe Alzheimer's disease (MMSE total scores < 20) from the six phase III, placebo-controlled, 6-month studies (including monotherapy studies and studies with patients on a stable dose of acetylcholinesterase inhibitors) showed that there was a statistically significant effect in favour of memantine treatment for the cognitive, global, and functional domains. When patients were identified with concurrent worsening in all three domains, results showed a statistically significant effect of memantine in preventing worsening, as twice as many placebo-treated patients as memantine-treated patients showed worsening in all three domains (21% vs. 11%, $p<0.0001$).

5.2 Pharmacokinetic properties

Absorption: Memantine has an absolute bioavailability of approximately 100%. t_{max} is between 3 and 8 hours. There is no indication that food influences the absorption of memantine.

Distribution: Daily doses of 20 mg lead to steady-state plasma concentrations of memantine ranging from 70 to 150 ng/ml (0.5 - 1 μmol) with large interindividual variations. When daily doses of 5 to 30 mg were administered, a mean cerebrospinal fluid (CSF)/serum ratio of 0.52 was calculated. The volume of distribution is around 10 l/kg. About 45% of memantine is bound to plasma-proteins.

Biotransformation: In man, about 80% of the circulating memantine-related material is present as the parent compound. Main human metabolites are N-3,5-dimethyl-gludantan, the isomeric mixture of 4- and 6-hydroxy-memantine, and 1-nitroso-3,5-dimethyl-adamantane. None of these metabolites exhibit NMDA-antagonistic activity. No cytochrome P 450 catalysed metabolism has been detected *in vitro.*

In a study using orally administered ^{14}C-memantine, a mean of 84% of the dose was recovered within 20 days, more than 99% being excreted renally.

Elimination: Memantine is eliminated in a monoexponential manner with a terminal $t_{½}$ of 60 to 100 hours. In volunteers with normal kidney function, total clearance (Cl_{tot}) amounts to 170 ml/min/1.73 m^2 and part of total renal clearance is achieved by tubular secretion.

Renal handling also involves tubular reabsorption, probably mediated by cation transport proteins. The renal elimination rate of memantine under alkaline urine conditions may be reduced by a factor of 7 to 9 (see section 4.4). Alkalisation of urine may result from drastic changes in diet, e.g. from a carnivore to a vegetarian diet, or from the massive ingestion of alkalising gastric buffers.

Linearity: Studies in volunteers have demonstrated linear pharmacokinetics in the dose range of 10 to 40 mg.

Pharmacokinetic/pharmacodynamic relationship: At a dose of memantine of 20 mg per day the cerebrospinal fluid (CSF) levels match the k_i-value (k_i = inhibition constant) of memantine, which is 0.5 μmol in human frontal cortex.

5.3 Preclinical safety data

In short term studies in rats memantine like other NMDA-antagonists have induced neuronal vacuolisation and necrosis (Olney lesions) only after doses leading to very high peak serum concentrations. Ataxia and other preclinical signs have preceded the vacuolisation and necrosis. As the effects have neither been observed in long term studies in rodents nor in non-rodents, the clinical relevance of these findings is unknown.

Ocular changes were inconsistently observed in repeat dose toxicity studies in rodents and dogs, but not in monkeys. Specific ophthalmoscopic examinations in clinical studies with memantine did not disclose any ocular changes.

Phospholipidosis in pulmonary macrophages due to accumulation of memantine in lysosomes was observed in rodents. This effect is known from other drugs with cationic amphiphilic properties. There is a possible relationship between this accumulation and the vacuolisation observed in lungs. This effect was only observed at high doses in rodents. The clinical relevance of these findings is unknown.

No genotoxicity has been observed following testing of memantine in standard assays. There was no evidence of any carcinogenicity in life long studies in mice and rats. Memantine was not teratogenic in rats and rabbits, even at maternally toxic doses, and no adverse effects of memantine were noted on fertility. In rats, foetal growth reduction was noted at exposure levels that are identical or slightly higher than at human exposure.

6. PHARMACEUTICAL PARTICULARS

6.1 List of excipients

Oral drops, solution:

Potassium sorbate

Sorbitol E420

Purified water

Tablets:

Tablet cores for 5/15/20 mg film-coated tablets:

Microcrystalline cellulose

Croscarmellose sodium

Colloidal anhydrous silica

Magnesium stearate

Tablet coat for 5/15/20 mg film-coated tablets:

Hypromellose

Macrogol 400

Titanium dioxide (E 171)

Additional for 15 mg and 20 mg film-coated tablets:

Iron oxide yellow and red (E 172)

Tablet core for 10 mg film-coated tablet:

Lactose monohydrate

Microcrystalline cellulose

Colloidal anhydrous silica

Talc

Magnesium stearate

Tablet coat for 10 mg film-coated tablet:

Methacrylic acid - ethyl acrylate copolymer (1:1)

Sodium lauryl sulphate

Polysorbate 80

Talc

Triacetin

Simethicone emulsion

6.2 Incompatibilities

Not applicable.

6.3 Shelf life

Oral drops, solution: 4 years.

Once opened, the contents of the bottle should be used within 3 months.

Film-coated tablets: 4 years.

6.4 Special precautions for storage

Oral drops, solution: Do not store above 30°C. The bottle with the mounted pump may only be kept and transported in a vertical position.

Film-coated tablets: This medicinal product does not require any special storage conditions.

6.5 Nature and contents of container

Oral drops, solution: Brown glass bottles (Hydrolytic Class III) containing either 50, 100 g or 10 × 50 g solution.

Treatment Initiation Pack: Each pack contains 28 film-coated tablets in 4 PVDC/PE/PVC/Al-blister or PP/Al-blisters with 7 film-coated tablets of 5 mg, 7 film-coated tablets of 10 mg, 7 film-coated tablets of 15 mg and 7 film-coated tablets of 20 mg.

10 mg Tablet packs: Blister packs containing either 7, 10, 14 or 20 tablets per blister strip. Pack sizes of 14, 28, 30, 42, 49 × 1, 50, 56, 56 × 1, 70, 84, 98, 98 × 1, 100, 100 × 1, 112, 980 (10 × 98) or 1000 (20 × 50) tablets are presented. The pack sizes 49 × 1, 56 x1, 98 × 1 and 100 × 1 film-coated tablets are presented in unit dose blister.

20 mg Tablet packs: Blister packs containing 14 film-coated tablets per PVDC/PE/PVC/Al-blister or PP/Al-blister strip. Pack sizes of 14, 28, 42, 49 × 1, 56, 56 × 1, 70, 84, 98, 98 × 1, 100 × 1, 112 or 840 (20 × 42) film-coated tablets are presented. The pack sizes 49 × 1, 56 x1, 98 × 1 and 100 × 1 film-coated tablets are presented in unit dose blister.

Not all pack sizes may be marketed.

6.6 Special precautions for disposal and other handling

No special requirements.

7. MARKETING AUTHORISATION HOLDER

H. Lundbeck A/S

Ottiliavej 9,

DK-2500 Valby

Denmark

8. MARKETING AUTHORISATION NUMBER(S)

Oral Drops, solution: EU/1/02/219/004-6, EU/1/02/219/013

Treatment Initiation Pack: EU/1/02/218/022, EU/1/02/218/036

10 mg Tablets: EU/1/02/219/001-3, EU/1/02/219/007-012, EU/1/02/219/014-021

20 mg Tablets: EU/1/02/219/023-035, EU/1/02/219/037-049

9. DATE OF FIRST AUTHORISATION/RENEWAL OF THE AUTHORISATION

10 mg tablets and 10 mg/g oral drops:

Date of authorisation: 15/05/2002

Date of last renewal: 15/05/2007

Treatment Initiation Pack and 20 mg tablets:

Date of authorisation: 08/05/2008

10. DATE OF REVISION OF THE TEXT

30/07/2009

Detailed information on this product is available on the website of the European Medicines Agency (EMEA) http://www.emea.europa.eu

ECALTA 100mg powder and solvent for concentrate for solution for infusion

(Pfizer Limited)

1. NAME OF THE MEDICINAL PRODUCT

ECALTA ®▼ 100 mg powder and solvent for concentrate for solution for infusion.

2. QUALITATIVE AND QUANTITATIVE COMPOSITION

Each vial contains 100 mg anidulafungin.

The reconstituted solution contains 3.33 mg/ml anidulafungin and the diluted solution contains 0.36 mg/ml anidulafungin.

Excipients: Fructose 102.5 mg per vial
Ethanol 6 g per vial

For a full list of excipients, see section 6.1.

3. PHARMACEUTICAL FORM

Powder and solvent for concentrate for solution for infusion.

Powder: White to off-white lyophilised solid.

Solvent: Clear colourless solution.

The reconstituted solution has a pH of 4.0 to 6.0.

4. CLINICAL PARTICULARS

4.1 Therapeutic indications

Treatment of invasive candidiasis in adult non-neutropenic patients.

ECALTA has been studied primarily in patients with candidaemia and only in a limited number of patients with deep tissue *Candida* infections or with abscess-forming disease (see section 4.4 and section 5.1).

4.2 Posology and method of administration

Treatment with ECALTA should be initiated by a physician experienced in the management of invasive fungal infections. Specimens for fungal culture should be obtained prior to therapy. Therapy may be initiated before culture results are known and can be adjusted accordingly once they are available.

A single 200 mg loading dose should be administered on Day 1, followed by 100 mg daily thereafter. Duration of treatment should be based on the patient's clinical response. In general, antifungal therapy should continue for at least 14 days after the last positive culture.

ECALTA should be reconstituted with the solvent to a concentration of 3.33 mg/ml and subsequently diluted to a concentration of 0.36 mg/ml before use according to the instructions given in section 6.6.

It is recommended that ECALTA be administered at a rate of infusion that does not exceed 1.1 mg/minute (equivalent to 3.0 ml/minute). Infusion associated reactions are infrequent when the rate of anidulafungin infusion does not exceed 1.1 mg/minute.

ECALTA should not be administered as a bolus injection.

Renal and hepatic impairment

No dosing adjustments are required for patients with mild, moderate, or severe hepatic impairment. No dosing adjustments are required for patients with any degree of renal insufficiency, including those on dialysis. ECALTA can be given without regard to the timing of haemodialysis (see section 5.2).

Duration of treatment

There are insufficient data to support the 100 mg dose for longer than 35 days of treatment.

Other special populations

No dosing adjustments are required for adult patients based on gender, weight, ethnicity, HIV positivity, or geriatric status (see section 5.2).

Children and adolescents

ECALTA is not recommended for use in children below 18 due to insufficient data on safety and efficacy (see section 5.2).

4.3 Contraindications

Hypersensitivity to the active substance, or to any of the excipients.

Hypersensitivity to other medicinal products of the echinocandin class.

4.4 Special warnings and precautions for use

The efficacy of ECALTA in neutropenic patients with candidaemia and in patients with deep tissue *Candida* infections or intra-abdominal abscess and peritonitis has not been established.

Clinical efficacy has been evaluated primarily in non-neutropenic patients with *C. albicans* infections and in a smaller number of patients infected with non-albicans, mainly *C. glabrata*, *C. parapsilosis* and *C. tropicalis.* Patients with candida endocarditis, osteomyelitis or meningitis and known *C.krusei* infection have not been studied.

Hepatic effects

Increased levels of hepatic enzymes have been seen in healthy subjects and patients treated with anidulafungin. In some patients with serious underlying medical conditions who were receiving multiple concomitant medicines along with anidulafungin, clinically significant hepatic abnormalities have occurred. Isolated cases of significant hepatic dysfunction, hepatitis, or worsening hepatic failure have been reported. Patients with increased hepatic enzymes during anidulafungin therapy should be monitored for evidence of worsening hepatic function and evaluated for risk/benefit of continuing anidulafungin therapy.

Infusion-related reactions

Exacerbation of infusion-related reactions by coadministration of anaesthetics has been seen in a non-clinical (rat) study (see section 5.3). The clinical relevance of this is unknown. Nevertheless, care should be taken when co-administering anidulafungin and anaesthetic agents.

Alcohol content

This medicinal product contains 24 vol% ethanol (alcohol); this is equivalent to 6 g ethanol in the 100 mg maintenance dose (administered over a 1.5-hour period), and 12 g ethanol in the 200 mg loading dose (administered over a 3-hour period). Ethanol could be harmful for those suffering from alcoholism. This should be taken into account in pregnant or breast-feeding women, children, and in high-risk groups such as those with liver disease or epilepsy.

The amount of alcohol in this medicinal product may alter the effects of other medicines.

The amount of alcohol in this medicinal product may impair the ability to drive or use machines.

Fructose content

Patients with rare hereditary problems of fructose intolerance should not take this medicine.

4.5 Interaction with other medicinal products and other forms of interaction

Anidulafungin is not a clinically relevant substrate, inducer, or inhibitor of cytochrome P450 isoenzymes (1A2, 2B6, 2C8, 2C9, 2C19, 2D6, 3A). Of note, *in vitro* studies do not fully exclude possible *in vivo* interactions.

Drug interaction studies were performed with anidulafungin and other medicinal products likely to be co-administered. No dosage adjustment of either medicinal product is recommended when anidulafungin is co-administered with ciclosporin, voriconazole or tacrolimus, and no dosage adjustment for anidulafungin is recommended when co-administered with amphotericin B or rifampicin.

4.6 Pregnancy and lactation

There are no data regarding the use of anidulafungin in pregnant women. Slight developmental effects have been observed in rabbits administered anidulafungin during pregnancy, in the presence of maternal toxicity (see section 5.3). The potential risk for humans is unknown. Therefore anidulafungin is not recommended in pregnancy.

Animal studies have shown excretion of anidulafungin in breast milk. It is not known whether anidulafungin is excreted in human breast milk. A decision on whether to continue/discontinue breast-feeding or therapy with anidulafungin should be made taking into account the benefit of breast-feeding to the child and the benefit of anidulafungin to the mother.

4.7 Effects on ability to drive and use machines

No studies on the effects on the ability to drive and use machines have been performed.

The amount of alcohol in this medicinal product may impair the ability to drive or use machines.

4.8 Undesirable effects

Nine hundred and twenty-nine (929) subjects received single or multiple doses of intravenous anidulafungin in clinical trials: 672 in Phase 2/3 trials (287 patients with candidaemia/invasive candidiasis, 355 patients with oral/oesophageal candidiasis, 30 patients with invasive aspergillosis), and 257 in Phase I studies.

Three studies (one comparative vs fluconazole, two non-comparative) assessed the efficacy of anidulafungin in patients with candidaemia and a limited number of patients with deep tissue *Candida* infections. A total of 204 patients received the recommended daily dose of 100 mg; the mean duration of intravenous treatment in these patients was 13.5 days (range, 1 to 38 days). One hundred and nineteen patients received ⩾ 14 days of anidulafungin. Adverse reactions were typically mild to moderate and seldom led to discontinuation.

Infusion-related adverse reactions have been reported with anidulafungin; in the pivotal ICC study, these included flushing/hot flush (2.3%), pruritus (2.3%), rash (1.5%), and urticaria (0.8%). Other treatment-related adverse reactions that occurred in ⩾ 1% of patients in the pivotal study included hypokalemia (3.1%), diarrhoea (3.1%), ALT increased (2.3%), hepatic enzyme increased (1.5%), blood alkaline phosphatase increased (1.5%), and blood bilirubin increased (1.5%).

In the 100 mg ICC database (N = 204), the drug-related adverse reactions (MedDRA) listed below were reported with frequencies corresponding to Common (⩾1/100 to <1/10) or Uncommon (⩾1/1,000 to <1/100). Within each frequency grouping, undesirable effects are presented in order of decreasing seriousness.

Blood and lymphatic system disorders

Common: Coagulopathy

Nervous system disorders

Common: Convulsion, headache

Gastrointestinal disorders

Common: Diarrhoea, vomiting, nausea
Uncommon: Abdominal pain upper

Renal and urinary disorders

Common: Blood creatinine increased

Skin and subcutaneous tissue disorders

Common: Rash, pruritus
Uncommon: Urticaria

Metabolism and nutrition disorders

Common: Hypokalaemia
Uncommon: Hyperglycaemia

Vascular disorders

Common: Flushing
Uncommon: Hypertension, hot flush

General disorders and administration site conditions

Uncommon: Infusion site pain

Hepatobiliary disorders

Common: Alanine aminotransferase increased, blood alkaline phosphatase increased, aspartate aminotransferase increased, blood bilirubin increased, gamma-glutamyltransferase increased
Uncommon: Cholestasis

4.9 Overdose

As with any overdose, general supportive measures should be utilised as necessary. In case of overdose, adverse reactions may occur as mentioned in section 4.8.

During clinical trials, a single 400 mg dose of anidulafungin was inadvertently administered as a loading dose. No clinical adverse reactions were reported. No dose limiting toxicity was observed in a study of 10 healthy subjects administered a loading dose of 260 mg followed by 130 mg daily; 3 of the 10 subjects experienced transient, asymptomatic transaminase elevations (⩽3 × Upper Limit of Normal (ULN)).

ECALTA is not dialysable.

5. PHARMACOLOGICAL PROPERTIES

5.1 Pharmacodynamic properties

General properties

Pharmacotherapeutic group: Other antimycotics for systemic use, ATC code: JO2AX06

Anidulafungin is a semi-synthetic echinocandin, a lipopeptide synthesised from a fermentation product of *Aspergillus nidulans*.

Anidulafungin selectively inhibits 1,3-β-D glucan synthase, an enzyme present in fungal, but not mammalian cells. This results in inhibition of the formation of 1,3-β-D-glucan, an essential component of the fungal cell wall. Anidulafungin has shown fungicidal activity against *Candida* species and activity against regions of active cell growth of the hyphae of *Aspergillus fumigatus*.

Activity *in vitro*

Anidulafungin exhibited *in-vitro* activity against *C. albicans, C. glabrata, C. parapsilosis,* and *C. tropicalis.* Susceptibility breakpoints for 1,3- β-D-glucan synthesis inhibitors have not been established. For the clinical relevance of these findings see below under clinical studies.

Minimum inhibitory concentration (MIC) determinations were performed according to the Clinical and Laboratory Standards Institute methods M27 and M38. *Candida* isolates with reduced susceptibility to anidulafungin have not been isolated from treated patients. Among a number of isolates with elevated echinocandin MICs isolated from patients treated with other echinocandins, only two *Candida* isolates were reported to also have elevated anidulafungin MICs, suggesting the lack of complete cross resistance among echinocandins.

Activity *in vivo*

Parenterally administered anidulafungin was effective against *Candida* spp. in immunocompetent and immunocompromised mouse and rabbit models. Anidulafungin treatment prolonged survival and also reduced the organ burden of *Candida* spp., when determined at intervals from 24 to 96 hours after the last treatment.

Experimental infections included disseminated *C. albicans* infection in neutropenic rabbits, oesophageal/oropharyngeal infection of neutropenic rabbits with fluconazole-resistant *C. albicans* and disseminated infection of neutropenic mice with fluconazole-resistant *C. glabrata.*

Information from clinical studies

Candidaemia and other forms of Invasive Candidiasis

The safety and efficacy of anidulafungin were evaluated in a pivotal Phase 3, randomised, double-blind, multicentre, multinational study of primarily non-neutropenic patients with candidaemia and a limited number of patients with deep tissue Candida infections or with abscess-forming disease. [Patients with *Candida* endocarditis, osteomyelitis or meningitis, or those with infection due to *C. krusei*, were specifically excluded from the study]. Patients were randomised to receive either anidulafungin (200 mg intravenous loading dose followed by 100 mg intravenous daily) or fluconazole (800 mg intravenous loading dose followed by 400 mg intravenous daily), and were stratified by APACHE II score (⩽20 and >20) and the presence or absence of neutropenia. Treatment was administered for at least 14 and not more than 42 days. Patients in both study arms were permitted to switch to oral fluconazole after at least

Table 1. Global success in the MITT population: primary and secondary endpoints

	Anidulafungin	Fluconazole	Between group difference [a] (95% CI)
End of IV Therapy (1° endpoint)	**96/127 (75.6%)**	**71/118 (60.2%)**	**15.42 (3.9, 27.0)**
Candidaemia only	88/116 (75.9%)	63/103 (61.2%)	14.7 (2.5, 26.9)
Other sterile sites[b]	8/11 (72.7%)	8/15 (53.3%)	-
Peritoneal fluid/IA[c] abscess	6/8	5/8	
Other	2/3	3/7	
C. albicans[d]	60/74 (81.1%)	38/61 (62.3%)	-
Non-*albicans* species[d]	32/45 (71.1%)	27/45 (60.0%)	-
Apache II score $\leqslant$ 20	82/101 (81.2%)	60/98 (61.2%)	-
Apache II score > 20	14/26 (53.8%)	11/20 (55.0%)	-
Non-neutropenic **(ANC, cells/mm^3 > 500)**	94/124 (75.8%)	69/114 (60.5%)	-
Neutropenic **(ANC, cells/mm^3 $\leqslant$ 500)**	2/3	2/4	-
At Other Endpoints			
End of All Therapy	94/127 (74.0%)	67/118 (56.8%)	17.24 (2.9, 31.6)[e]
2 Week Follow-up	82/127 (64.6%)	58/118 (49.2%)	15.41 (0.4, 30.4)[e]
6 Week Follow-up	71/127 (55.9%)	52/118 (44.1%)	11.84 (-3.4, 27.0)[e]

[a] Calculated as anidulafungin minus fluconazole
[b] With or without concurrent candidaemia
[c] Intra-abdominal
[d] Data presented for patients with a single baseline pathogen.
[e] 98.3% confidence intervals, adjusted post hoc for multiple comparisons of secondary time points.

10 days of intravenous therapy, provided that they were able to tolerate oral medication and were afebrile for at least 24 hours, and that the most recent blood cultures were negative for *Candida* species.

Patients who received at least one dose of study medication and who had a positive culture for *Candida* species from a normally sterile site before study entry were included in the modified intent-to-treat (MITT) population. In the primary efficacy analysis, global response in the MITT populations at the end of intravenous therapy, anidulafungin was compared to fluconazole in a pre-specified two-step statistical comparison (non-inferiority followed by superiority). A successful global response required clinical improvement and microbiological eradication. Patients were followed for six weeks beyond the end of all therapy.

Two hundred and fifty-six patients, ranging from 16 to 91 years in age, were randomised to treatment and received at least one dose of study medication. The most frequent species isolated at baseline were *C. albicans* (63.8% anidulafungin, 59.3% fluconazole), followed by *C. glabrata* (15.7%, 25.4%), *C. parapsilosis* (10.2%, 13.6%) and *C. tropicalis* (11.8%, 9.3%) - with 20, 13 and 15 isolates of the last 3 species, respectively, in the anidulafungin group. The majority of patients had Apache II scores $\leqslant$ 20 and very few were neutropenic.

Efficacy data, both overall and by various subgroups, are presented below in Table 1.

(see Table 1 above)

Mortality rates in both the anidulafungin and fluconazole arms are presented below in Table 2:

Table 2. Mortality

	Anidulafungin	Fluconazole
Overall study mortality	**29/127 (22.8%)**	**37/118 (31.4%)**
Mortality during study therapy	10/127 (7.9%)	17/118 (14.4%)
Mortality attributed to *Candida* infection	2/127 (1.6%)	5/118 (4.2%)

5.2 Pharmacokinetic properties

General pharmacokinetic characteristics

The pharmacokinetics of anidulafungin have been characterised in healthy subjects, special populations and patients. A low intersubject variability in systemic exposure (coefficient of variation ~25%) was observed. The steady state was achieved on the first day after a loading dose (twice the daily maintenance dose).

Distribution

The pharmacokinetics of anidulafungin are characterised by a rapid distribution half-life (0.5-1 hour) and a volume of distribution, 30-50 l, which is similar to total body fluid volume. Anidulafungin is extensively bound (>99%) to human plasma proteins. No specific tissue distribution studies of anidulafungin have been done in humans. Therefore, no information is available about the penetration of anidulafungin into the cerebrospinal fluid (CSF) and/or across the blood-brain barrier.

Biotransformation

Hepatic metabolism of anidulafungin has not been observed. Anidulafungin is not a clinically relevant substrate, inducer, or inhibitor of cytochrome P450 isoenzymes. It is unlikely that anidulafungin will have clinically relevant effects on the metabolism of drugs metabolised by cytochrome P450 isoenzymes.

Anidulafungin undergoes slow chemical degradation at physiologic temperature and pH to a ring-opened peptide that lacks antifungal activity. The *in vitro* degradation half-life of anidulafungin under physiologic conditions is approximately 24 hours. *In vivo*, the ring-opened product is subsequently converted to peptidic degradants and eliminated mainly through biliary excretion.

Elimination

The clearance of anidulafungin is about 1 l/h. Anidulafungin has a predominant elimination half-life of approximately 24 hours that characterizes the majority of the plasma concentration-time profile, and a terminal half-life of 40-50 hours that characterises the terminal elimination phase of the profile.

In a single-dose clinical study, radiolabeled (^{14}C) anidulafungin (~88 mg) was administered to healthy subjects. Approximately 30% of the administered radioactive dose was eliminated in the faeces over 9 days, of which less than 10% was intact drug. Less than 1% of the administered radioactive dose was excreted in the urine, indicating negligible renal clearance. Anidulafungin concentrations fell below the lower limits of quantitation 6 days post-dose. Negligible amounts of drug-derived radioactivity were recovered in blood, urine, and faeces 8 weeks post-dose.

Linearity

Anidulafungin displays linear pharmacokinetics across a wide range of once daily doses (15-130 mg).

Special populations

Patients with fungal infections

The pharmacokinetics of anidulafungin in patients with fungal infections are similar to those observed in healthy subjects based on population pharmacokinetic analyses. With the 200/100 mg daily dose regimen at an infusion rate of 1.1 mg/min, the steady state C_{max} and trough concentrations (C_{min}) could reach approximately 7 and 3 mg/l, respectively, with an average steady state AUC of approximately 110 mg•h/l.

Weight

Although weight was identified as a source of variability in clearance in the population pharmacokinetic analysis, weight has little clinical relevance on the pharmacokinetics of anidulafungin.

Gender

Plasma concentrations of anidulafungin in healthy men and women were similar. In multiple-dose patient studies, drug clearance was slightly faster (approximately 22%) in men.

Elderly

The population pharmacokinetic analysis showed that median clearance differed slightly between the elderly group (patients $\geqslant$ 65, median CL = 1.07 l/h) and the non-elderly group (patients < 65, median CL = 1.22 l/h), however the range of clearance was similar.

Ethnicity

Anidulafungin pharmacokinetics were similar among Caucasians, Blacks, Asians, and Hispanics.

HIV positivity

Dosage adjustments are not required based on HIV positivity, irrespective of concomitant anti-retroviral therapy.

Hepatic insufficiency

Anidulafungin is not hepatically metabolised. Anidulafungin pharmacokinetics were examined in subjects with Child-Pugh class A, B or C hepatic insufficiency. Anidulafungin concentrations were not increased in subjects with any degree of hepatic insufficiency. Although a slight decrease in AUC was observed in patients with Child-Pugh C hepatic insufficiency, the decrease was within the range of population estimates noted for healthy subjects.

Renal insufficiency

Anidulafungin has negligible renal clearance (<1%). In a clinical study of subjects with mild, moderate, severe or end stage (dialysis-dependent) renal insufficiency, anidulafungin pharmacokinetics were similar to those observed in subjects with normal renal function. Anidulafungin is not dialysable and may be administered without regard to the timing of hemodialysis.

Paediatric

The pharmacokinetics of anidulafungin after at least 5 daily doses were investigated in 24 immunocompromised paediatric (2 to 11 years old) and adolescent (12 to 17 years old) patients with neutropenia. Steady state was achieved on the first day after a loading dose (twice the maintenance dose), and steady state C_{max} and AUC_{ss} increase in a dose-proportional manner. Systemic exposure following daily maintenance dose of 0.75 and 1.5 mg/kg/day in this population were comparable to those observed in adults following 50 and 100 mg/day, respectively. Both regimens were well-tolerated by these patients.

5.3 Preclinical safety data

In 3 month studies, evidence of liver toxicity, including elevated enzymes and morphologic alterations, was observed in both rats and monkeys at doses 4- to 6-fold higher than the anticipated clinical therapeutic exposure. *In vitro* and *in vivo* genotoxicity studies with anidulafungin provided no evidence of genotoxic potential. Long-term studies in animals have not been conducted to evaluate the carcinogenic potential of anidulafungin.

Administration of anidulafungin to rats did not indicate any effects on reproduction, including male and female fertility.

Anidulafungin crossed the placental barrier in rats and was detected in foetal plasma.

Embryo-foetal development studies were conducted with doses between 0.2- and 2-fold (rats) and between 1- and 4-fold (rabbits) the proposed therapeutic maintenance dose of 100 mg/day. Anidulafungin did not produce any drug-related developmental toxicity in rats at the highest dose tested. Developmental effects observed in rabbits (slightly reduced foetal weights) occurred only at the highest dose tested, a dose that also produced maternal toxicity.

Crossing of the blood-brain barrier by anidulafungin was limited in healthy rats; however, in rabbits with disseminated candidiasis, anidulafungin has been shown to cross the blood-brain barrier and reduce fungal burden in the brain.

Rats were dosed with anidulafungin at three dose levels and anesthetised within one hour using a combination of ketamine and xylazine. Rats in the high dose group experienced infusion-related reactions that were exacerbated by anaesthesia. Some rats in the mid dose group experienced similar reactions but only after administration of anaesthesia. There were no adverse reactions in the low-dose animals in the presence or absence of anaesthesia, and no infusion-related reactions in the mid-dose group in the absence of anaesthesia.

6. PHARMACEUTICAL PARTICULARS

6.1 List of excipients

Powder:

Fructose

Mannitol

Polysorbate 80

Tartaric acid

Sodium hydroxide (for pH-adjustment)

Hydrochloric acid (for pH-adjustment)

Solvent:

Ethanol anhydrous

Water for injections

6.2 Incompatibilities

This medicinal product must not be mixed with other medicinal products or electrolytes except those mentioned in section 6.6.

6.3 Shelf life

Powder and solvent: 3 years

Table 3 Dilution requirements for ECALTA administration

Dose	Number of boxes	Total reconstituted volume	Infusion volume A	Total infusion volume	Infusion solution concentration	Rate of infusion
100 mg	1	30 ml (1 box)	250 ml	280 ml	0.36 mg/ml	3.0 ml/min
200 mg	2	60 ml (2 boxes)	500 ml	560 ml	0.36 mg/ml	3.0 ml/min

A Either 9 mg/ml (0.9%) sodium chloride for infusion or 50 mg/ml (5%) glucose for infusion.

Reconstituted solution:

The reconstituted solution should be further diluted within an hour. Chemical and physical in-use stability of the reconstituted solution has been demonstrated for 3 hours at 25°C and for 2 hours at 5°C.

Infusion solution:

Chemical and physical in-use stability of the infusion solution has been demonstrated for 24 hours at 25°C.

From a microbiological point of view, the product should be used immediately. If not used immediately, in-use storage times and conditions are the responsibility of the user.

6.4 Special precautions for storage

Powder and solvent:

Do not store above 25°C.

For storage conditions of the reconstituted medicinal product, see section 6.3.

6.5 Nature and contents of container

Powder:

30 ml Type 1 glass vial with an elastomeric stopper and aluminium seal with flip-off cap.

Solvent:

30 ml of 20 % (w/w) ethanol anhydrous in water for injections in a Type 1 glass vial with an elastomeric stopper and aluminium seal with flip-off cap.

ECALTA will be available as a box containing 1 vial of 100 mg powder and 1 vial of 30 ml solvent.

6.6 Special precautions for disposal and other handling

ECALTA must be reconstituted with the solvent (20% (w/w) ethanol anhydrous in water for injections) and subsequently diluted with ONLY 9 mg/ml (0.9%) sodium chloride for infusion or 50 mg/ml (5%) glucose for infusion. The compatibility of reconstituted ECALTA with intravenous substances, additives, or medicines other than 9 mg/ml (0.9%) sodium chloride for infusion or 50 mg/ml (5%) glucose for infusion has not been established.

Reconstitution

Aseptically reconstitute each vial with the solvent (20% (w/w) ethanol anhydrous in water for injections) to provide a concentration of 3.33 mg/ml. The reconstitution time can be up to 5 minutes. The reconstituted solution should be clear and free from visible particulates. After subsequent dilution, the solution is to be discarded if particulate matter or discoloration is identified.

The reconstituted solution must be further diluted within an hour and administered within 24 hours.

Dilution and infusion

Aseptically transfer the contents of the reconstituted vial(s) into an intravenous bag (or bottle) containing either 9 mg/ml (0.9%) sodium chloride for infusion or 50 mg/ml (5%) glucose for infusion obtaining an anidulafungin concentration of 0.36 mg/ml. The table below provides the volumes required for each dose.

Dilution requirements for ECALTA administration

(see Table 3 above)

Parenteral medicinal products should be inspected visually for particulate matter and discoloration prior to administration, whenever solution and container permit. If either particulate matter or discolouration are identified, discard the solution.

For single use only. Waste materials should be disposed of in accordance with local requirements.

7. MARKETING AUTHORISATION HOLDER

Pfizer Limited, Ramsgate Road, Sandwich, Kent, CT13 9NJ, United Kingdom.

8. MARKETING AUTHORISATION NUMBER(S)

EU/1/07/416/001

9. DATE OF FIRST AUTHORISATION/RENEWAL OF THE AUTHORISATION

20th September 2007

10. DATE OF REVISION OF THE TEXT

24 February 2009

Detailed information on this medicinal product is available on the website of the European Medicines Agency (EMEA) http://www.emea.europa.eu/.

Edronax 4mg Tablets

(Pharmacia Limited)

1. NAME OF THE MEDICINAL PRODUCT

EDRONAX 4 mg Tablets

2. QUALITATIVE AND QUANTITATIVE COMPOSITION

One tablet contains 4mg of reboxetine

For full list of excipients, see section 6.1.

3. PHARMACEUTICAL FORM

Tablet

White, round, convex tablet with a breakline on one side. A 'P' is marked on the left side of the breakline. A 'U' is marked on the right side of the breakline. The side opposite the breakline is marked '7671'. The tablet can be divided into equal halves.

4. CLINICAL PARTICULARS

4.1 Therapeutic indications

Reboxetine is indicated for the acute treatment of depressive illness/major depression and for maintaining the clinical improvement in patients initially responding to treatment.

4.2 Posology and method of administration

Edronax is for oral use.

Use in adults

The recommended therapeutic dose is 4 mg twice a day (b.i.d.) i.e.8 mg/day administered orally. The full therapeutic dose can be given upon starting treatment. After 3-4 weeks, this dose can be increased to 10 mg/day in case of incomplete clinical response. The maximum daily dose should not exceed 12 mg. The minimum effective dose has not yet been established.

Use in the elderly

Elderly patients have been studied in clinical trials at doses of 2 mg b.i.d. However, safety and efficacy have not been evaluated in placebo-controlled conditions. Therefore, as for other antidepressants that have not been studied in placebo-controlled conditions, reboxetine cannot be recommended.

Use in children and adolescents under the age of 18 years

Edronax should not be used in the treatment of children and adolescents under the age of 18 years (see section 4.4).

Use in patients with renal or hepatic insufficiency

The starting dose in patients with renal or hepatic insufficiency should be 2 mg b.i.d which can be increased based on patient tolerance.

4.3 Contraindications

Known hypersensitivity to reboxetine or any of the components of the product.

4.4 Special warnings and precautions for use

Use in children and adolescents under 18 years of age

Reboxetine should not be used in the treatment of children and adolescents under the age of 18 years. Suicide-related behaviours (suicide attempt and suicidal thoughts), and hostility (predominantly aggression, oppositional behaviour and anger) were more frequently observed in clinical trials among children and adolescents treated with antidepressants compared to those treated with placebo. If, based on clinical need, a decision to treat is nevertheless taken, the patient should be carefully monitored for the appearance of suicidal symptoms. In addition, long-term safety data in children and adolescents concerning growth, maturation and cognitive and behavioural development are lacking.

As reboxetine has not been tested in patients with convulsive disorders in clinical studies and since rare cases of seizures have been reported in clinical studies, it should be given under close supervision to subjects with a history of convulsive disorders and it must be discontinued if the patient develops seizures.

Concomitant use of MAO-inhibitors and reboxetine should be avoided in view of the potential risk (tyramine-like effect) based on their mechanisms of action.

Concomitant use of reboxetine with other antidepressants (tricyclics, MAO inhibitors, SSRIs and lithium) has not been evaluated during clinical trials.

As with all antidepressants, switches to mania/hypomania have occurred during the clinical studies. Close supervision of bipolar patients is, therefore, recommended.

Suicide/suicidal thoughts or clinical worsening:

Depression is associated with an increased risk of suicidal thoughts, self harm and suicide (suicide-related events). This risk persists until significant remission occurs. As improvement may not occur during the first few weeks or more of treatment, patients should be closely monitored until such improvement occurs. It is general clinical experience that the risk of suicide may increase in the early stages of recovery.

Patients with a history of suicide-related events, or those exhibiting a significant degree of suicidal ideation prior to commencement of treatment are known to be at greater risk of suicidal thoughts or suicide attempts, and should receive careful monitoring during treatment. A meta-analysis of placebo-controlled clinical trials of antidepressant drugs in adult patients with psychiatric disorders showed an increased risk of suicidal behaviour with antidepressants compared to placebo in patients less than 25 years old.

Close supervision of patients and in particular those at high risk should accompany drug therapy especially in early treatment and following dose changes. Patients (and caregivers of patients) should be alerted about the need to monitor for any clinical worsening, suicidal behaviour or thoughts and unusual changes in behaviour and to seek medical advice immediately if these symptoms present.

Clinical experience with reboxetine in patients affected by serious concomitant systemic illnesses is limited. Close supervision should be applied in patients with current evidence of urinary retention, prostatic hypertrophy, glaucoma and history of cardiac disease.

At doses higher than the maximum recommended, orthostatic hypotension has been observed with greater frequency than that observed at recommended doses. Particular attention should be paid when administering reboxetine with other drugs known to lower blood pressure.

Clinical experience with reboxetine in the long-term treatment of elderly patients is, at present, limited. In this population, lowering of mean potassium levels was found starting from week 14; the magnitude of this reduction did not exceed 0.8 mmol/litre and potassium levels never dropped below normal limits.

4.5 Interaction with other medicinal products and other forms of interaction

In vitro metabolism studies indicate that reboxetine is primarily metabolised by the CYP3A4 isozyme of cytochrome P450; reboxetine is not metabolized by CYP2D6. Therefore potent inhibitors of CYP3A4 (ketoconazole, nefazodone, erythromycin and fluvoxamine), would be expected to increase plasma concentrations of reboxetine. In a study in healthy volunteers, ketoconazole, a potent inhibitor of CYP3A4, was found to increase plasma concentrations of the reboxetine enantiomers by approximately 50%. Because of reboxetine's narrow therapeutic margin, inhibition of elimination is a major concern. Reboxetine, therefore should not be given together with drugs known to inhibit CYP3A4 such as azole antifungal agents, macrolide antibiotics such as erythromycin, or fluvoxamine

In vitro studies have shown that reboxetine does not inhibit the activity of the following P450 isoenzymes: CYP1A2, CYP2C9, CYP2C19 and CYP2E1. Pharmacokinetic interactions would not be expected with compounds metabolised by these enzymes. At concentrations which exceed those in clinical use, reboxetine inhibits CYP2D6 and CYP3A4, however, the results of *in vivo* studies suggest that interactions with other drugs metabolised by these enzymes are unlikely.

No significant reciprocal pharmacokinetic interaction has been found between reboxetine and lorazepam. During their co-administration in healthy volunteers, mild to moderate drowsiness and short lasting orthostatic acceleration of heart rate have been observed.

Reboxetine does not appear to potentiate the effect of alcohol on cognitive functions in healthy volunteers.

Concomitant use of MAO-inhibitors and reboxetine should be avoided in view of the potential risk (tyramine-like effect) based on their mechanisms of action.

Concomitant use of reboxetine with other antidepressants (tricyclics, MAO inhibitors, SSRIs and lithium) has not been evaluated during clinical trials.

Concomitant use of ergot derivatives and reboxetine might result in increased blood pressure.

Food intake delayed the absorption of reboxetine, but did not significantly influence the extent of absorption.

Although data are not available from clinical studies, the possibility of hypokalaemia with concomitant use of potassium losing diuretics should be considered.

4.6 Pregnancy and lactation

PREGNANCY

No clinical trial data on exposure to reboxetine during pregnancy are available. However, postmarketing safety data on a very limited number of exposed pregnancies indicate no adverse effects of reboxetine on pregnancy or on the health of the foetus/newborn child.

Animal studies in general do not indicate direct or indirect harmful effects with respect to pregnancy, embryonal/foetal development or parturition. Some impairment of growth and development has been noted in rat neonates (see section 5.3).

Reboxetine should only be used in pregnancy if the potential benefits of treatment to the mother outweigh the possible risks to the developing foetus.

LACTATION

Reboxetine is known to be excreted in breast milk. The level of active substance transferred in breast milk is anticipated to be very low, however there is insufficient information to exclude a risk to the nursing infant. The use of reboxetine during breastfeeding can be considered if the potential benefits outweigh the risk for the child.

4.7 Effects on ability to drive and use machines

Although reboxetine has been shown to have negligible effect on psychomotor performance in healthy volunteers, any psychoactive drug can impair judgement or skills. Patients should be cautioned about driving or operating hazardous machinery until reasonably certain that their performance has not been affected.

4.8 Undesirable effects

Over 2100 patients received reboxetine in clinical studies, approximately 250 of which received reboxetine for at least 1 year.

Common adverse events causing withdrawal at least twice as often on reboxetine than placebo include insomnia, dizziness, dry mouth, nausea, sweating, sensation of incomplete bladder emptying (males only), urinary hesitancy (males only) and headache.

The information below refers to short-term controlled studies. Very common or common adverse events that are at least two times higher on reboxetine than placebo are listed below.

[Very common (⩾ 1/10, Common (⩾ 1/100, < 1/10)]

Nervous system disorders:

Very common: insomnia, Common: vertigo

Cardiac disorders:

Common: tachycardia, palpitation, vasodilation, postural hypotension

Eye disorders:

Common: abnormality of accommodation

Gastrointestinal disorders:

Very common: dry mouth, constipation

Common: lack or loss of appetite

Skin and subcutaneous disorders:

Very common: sweating

Renal and urinary disorders:

Common: urinary hesitancy, sensation of incomplete bladder emptying, urinary tract infection

Reproductive system and breast disorders:

Common: erectile dysfunction (males only), ejaculatory pain (males only), ejaculatory delay (males only), testicular disorder-primarily pain (males only)

General disorders and administrative site conditions:

Common: chills

In addition there have been spontaneous reports of agitation, anxiety, irritability, aggressive behaviour, hallucination, cold extremities, nausea, vomiting, allergic dermatitis/rash, paraesthesia and hypertension.

Cases of suicidal ideation and suicidal behaviours have been reported during reboxetine therapy or early after treatment discontinuation (see section 4.4).

As for long-term tolerability, 143 reboxetine-treated and 140 placebo-treated adult patients participated in a long term placebo controlled study. Adverse events newly emerged on long term treatment in 28% of the reboxetine treated patients and 23% of the placebo-treated patients and caused discontinuation in 4% and 1% of the cases respectively. There was a similar risk of the development of individual events with reboxetine and placebo. In the long term studies, no individual events were seen which have not been seen on short term treatment.

In short-term controlled studies of patients with depression, no clinically significant between-gender differences were noted in the frequency of treatment emergent symptoms, with the exception of urologic events (such as the sensation of incomplete bladder emptying, urinary hesitancy and urinary frequency), which were reported in a higher percentage of reboxetine-treated male patients (31.4% [143/456]) than reboxetine-treated female patients (7.0% [59/847]). In contrast, the frequency of urologic-related events was similar among male (5.0% [15/302]) and female (8.4% [37/440]) placebo-treated patients.

In the elderly population, frequency of total adverse events, as well as of individual events, was no higher than that reported above.

In pre-marketing clinical studies, signs and symptoms newly reported on abrupt discontinuation were infrequent and less frequent in patients treated with reboxetine (4%) than in those treated with placebo (6%). In post-marketing experience, there have been a few spontaneous reports of withdrawal symptoms including headache, dizziness, nervousness and nausea; however, no consistent pattern of events on cessation of treatment with reboxetine was evident in these reports.

In those short-term studies in depression where heart rate was assessed with ECG, reboxetine was associated with mean increases in heart rate, compared to placebo, of 6 to 12 beats per minute.

In all short-term controlled studies in depression, the mean change in pulse (in beats per minute) for reboxetine-treated patients was 3.0, 6.4 and 2.9 in the standing, sitting and supine positions respectively, compared with 0, 0, and −0.5 for placebo-treated patients in the corresponding positions. In these same studies, 0.8% of reboxetine-treated patients discontinued the drug because of tachycardia compared with 0.1% of placebo-treated patients.

4.9 Overdose

The acute toxicity studies carried out in animals indicate a very low toxicity, with a wide safety margin with respect to the pharmacologically active doses. Clinical signs and cause of death were related to CNS stimulation (mainly convulsive symptoms).

In a few cases doses higher than those recommended were administered to patients (12 mg to 20 mg/day) for a period ranging from a few days to some weeks during clinical studies: newly reported complaints include postural hypotension, anxiety and hypertension. Elderly might be particularly vulnerable to overdose.

In premarketing clinical studies, there were 5 reports of reboxetine overdose alone or in combination with other pharmacologic agents. The amount of reboxetine ingested was 52 mg as the sole agent by 1 patient and 20 mg in combination with other agents by another patient. The remaining 3 patients ingested unknown quantities of reboxetine. All 5 patients recovered fully. There were no reports of ECG abnormalities, coma, or convulsions following overdose with reboxetine alone.

In postmarketing experience, there have been few reports of overdose in patients taking reboxetine alone; none of these have proved fatal. Non-fatal overdoses in patients have been reported for patients taking up to 240 mg of reboxetine. One fatal overdose was reported in a patient who ingested reboxetine in combination with amitriptyline (doses unknown).

In case of overdose, monitoring of cardiac function and vital signs is recommended. General symptomatic supportive and/or emetic measures might be required.

5. PHARMACOLOGICAL PROPERTIES

5.1 Pharmacodynamic properties

Pharmacotherapeutic group: Other Antidepressants

ATC code: NO6A X18

Reboxetine is a highly selective and potent inhibitor of noradrenaline reuptake. It has only a weak effect on the 5-HT reuptake and does not affect the uptake of dopamine.

Noradrenaline reuptake inhibition and the consequent increase of noradrenaline availability in the synaptic cleft and modification of noradrenergic transmission, reportedly is among the most relevant mechanisms of action of known antidepressant drugs.

In vitro, studies have shown that reboxetine has no significant affinity for adrenergic (α_1, α_2, β) and muscarinic receptors; antagonism of such receptors has been described to be associated with cardiovascular, anticholinergic and sedative side effects of other antidepressant drugs. Reboxetine is devoid of *in vitro* binding affinity for either α_1 or α_2 adrenoceptors, however, a functional interference with α-adrenoceptors at high doses *in vivo* cannot be excluded.

5.2 Pharmacokinetic properties

After oral administration of a single 4 mg reboxetine dose to healthy volunteers, peak levels of about 130 ng/ml are achieved within 2 h post-dosing. Data indicate that absolute bioavailability is at least 60%.

Reboxetine plasma levels decreased monoexponentially with a half-life of about 13 h. Steady-state conditions are observed within 5 days. Linearity of the pharmacokinetics was shown in the range of single oral doses in the clinically recommended dose-ranges.

The drug appears to be distributed into total body water. Reboxetine is 97 % bound to human plasma proteins in young and 92% in elderly(with affinity markedly higher for α_1 acid glycoprotein than albumin), with no significant dependence of the concentration of drug.

Reboxetine is predominantly metabolised *in vitro* via cytochrome P4503A (CYP3A4). *In vitro* studies have shown that reboxetine does not inhibit the activity of the following isozymes of cytochrome P450: CYP1A2, CYP2C9, CYP2C19, and CYP2E1. Reboxetine inhibits both CYP2D6 and CYP3A4 with low binding affinities, but has shown no effect on the *in vivo* clearance of drugs metabolized by these enzymes. Reboxetine should be co-prescribed with caution with potent inhibitors of CYP3A4.

The amount of radioactivity excreted in urine accounts for 78 % of the dose. Even though unchanged drug is predominant in the systemic circulation (70% of total radioactivity, in terms of AUC), only 10% of the dose is excreted as unchanged drug in urine. These findings suggest that biotransformation rules the overall elimination of reboxetine and that metabolites excretion is limited by their formation. The main metabolic pathways identified are 2-O-dealkylation, hydroxylation of the ethoxyphenoxy ring and oxidation of the morpholine ring, followed by partial or complete glucuro- or sulpho-conjugation.

The drug is available as a racemic mixture (with both enantiomers being active in the experimental models): no chiral inversion, nor reciprocal pharmacokinetic interferences between enantiomers have been observed. Plasma levels of the more potent SS enantiomer are about two times lower and urinary excretion two times higher than those of the enantiomeric counterpart. No significant differences were observed in the terminal half-lives of the two enantiomers.

Increases in systemic exposure and half-life of approximately two-fold are observed in patients with renal insufficiency and hepatic insufficiency. Similar or somewhat greater (3-fold) increases in systemic exposure also occur in elderly patients relative to young healthy volunteers.

5.3 Preclinical safety data

Reboxetine did not induce gene mutations in bacterial or mammalian cells *in vitro* but induced chromosomal aberrations in human lymphocytes *in vitro*. Reboxetine did not cause DNA damage in yeast cells or rat hepatocytes *in vitro*. Reboxetine did not cause chromosomal damage in an *in vivo* mouse micronucleus test, and did not increase tumor incidence in carcinogenecity studies in mice and rats.

Haemosiderosis was reported in toxicity studies in rats only.

Studies in animals have not demonstrated any teratogenic effect or any effect of the compound on global reproductive performance. Dosages that produced plasma concentrations within the therapeutic range for humans induced an impairment of growth and development and long term behavioural changes in offspring of rats.

In rats reboxetine is excreted in milk.

6. PHARMACEUTICAL PARTICULARS

6.1 List of excipients

Cellulose microcrystalline

Calcium hydrogen phosphate dihydrate

Crospovidone

Silica, colloidal hydrated

Magnesium stearate

6.2 Incompatibilities

Not applicable

6.3 Shelf life

3 years

6.4 Special precautions for storage

Do not store above 25° C.

6.5 Nature and contents of container

The tablets are contained either in amber glass, type III, bottle, closed with an aluminium pilfer-proof screw cap equipped with a polyethylene undercap or in aluminium-PVDC / PVC-PVDC opaque blisters.

Each pack contains: 10, 20, 50, 60, 100, 120, and 180 tablets in blisters;
and 60 tablets in glass bottles.

Multipacks of 3x60, 5x60 and 10x60 tablets in blisters; and 3x60, 5x60 and 10x60 tablets in glass bottles.

Not all pack sizes may be marketed.

6.6 Special precautions for disposal and other handling

No special requirements.

7. MARKETING AUTHORISATION HOLDER

Pharmacia Limited

Ramsgate Road

Sandwich

Kent

CT13 9NJ

United Kingdom

8. MARKETING AUTHORISATION NUMBER(S)

PL 00032/0216

9. DATE OF FIRST AUTHORISATION/RENEWAL OF THE AUTHORISATION

Date of first authorisation: 10 April 1997

Date of last renewal: 10 April 2007

10. DATE OF REVISION OF THE TEXT

July 2008

Legal category

POM

Company Ref: ED 8_0

Edrophonium Injection BP 10mg/1ml (Cambridge Laboratories)

(Cambridge Laboratories)

1. NAME OF THE MEDICINAL PRODUCT

Edrophonium Injection BP 10mg/1ml.

2. QUALITATIVE AND QUANTITATIVE COMPOSITION

Each ampoule contains 10mg Edrophonium Chloride BP in 1ml of solution.

3. PHARMACEUTICAL FORM

Ampoules

4. CLINICAL PARTICULARS

4.1 Therapeutic indications

Myasthenia gravis, as a diagnostic test; to distinguish between overdosage and underdosage of cholinergic drugs in myasthenic patients; diagnosis of suspected 'dual block'; antagonist to non-depolarising neuromuscular blockade.

4.2 Posology and method of administration

Edrophonium Injection BP is for intramuscular or intravenous injection. In view of the possibility of provoking a cholinergic crisis it is recommended that facilities for resuscitation should be available whenever Edrophonium Injection BP is administered.

Adults - Test for myasthenia gravis:

A syringe is filled with the contents of 1 ampoule (10mg) and 2mg is given intravenously, the needle and syringe being left in situ. If no response occurs within 30 seconds, the remaining 8mg is injected. In adults with unsuitable veins, 10mg is given by intramuscular injection.

To differentiate between 'myasthenic' and 'cholinergic' crises:

In a myasthenic patient who is suffering from marked muscle weakness, in spite of taking large doses of Mestinon or Prostigmin, a test dose of 2mg Edrophonium Injection BP is given intravenously one hour after the last dose of the cholinergic compound. If therapy has been inadequate, there is a rapid, transient increase in muscle strength; if the patient has been overtreated, Edrophonium Injection BP causes a transient increase of muscle weakness.

Diagnosis of suspected 'dual block':

Edrophonium Injection BP 10mg intravenously. If the block is due to depolarisation, it is briefly potentiated, whereas in a 'dual block', it is reversed.

Children: Diagnostic tests:

A total dose of 100micrograms/kg body-weight may be given intravenously. One fifth of this dose should be injected initially; if no reaction occurs, the remainder of the dose is administered 30 seconds later.

Antagonist to non-depolarising neuromuscular blockade:

Generally, reversal of neuromuscular block with Edrophonium Injection BP should not be attempted until there is evidence of spontaneous recovery from paralysis. It is recommended that the patient be well ventilated and a patent airway maintained until complete recovery of normal respiration is assured.

Adults and children:

Edrophonium Injection BP 500 - 700micrograms/kg body-weight and atropine 7micrograms/kg body-weight, by slow intravenous injection over several minutes, is usually adequate for reversal of non-depolarising muscle relaxants within 5 - 15 minutes. The two drugs are usually given simultaneously, but in patients who show bradycardia the pulse rate should be increased to about 80/minute with atropine before administering Edrophonium Injection BP.

The speed of recovery from neuromuscular blockade is primarily determined by the intensity of the block at the time of antagonism but it is also subject to other factors, including the presence of drugs (eg. anaesthetic agents, antibiotics, antiarrhythmic drugs) and physiological changes (electrolyte and acid-base imbalance, renal impairment). These factors may prevent successful reversal with Edrophonium Injection BP or lead to recurarisation after apparently successful reversal. Therefore it is imperative that patients should not be left unattended until these possibilities have been excluded.

Elderly:

There are no specific dosage recommendations for Edrophonium Injection BP in elderly patients.

4.3 Contraindications

Edrophonium Injection BP should not be given to patients with mechanical intestinal or urinary obstruction.

Edrophonium Injection BP is contra-indicated in patients with known hypersensitivity to the drug.

4.4 Special warnings and precautions for use

Extreme caution is required when administering Edrophonium Injection BP to patients with bronchial asthma.

Care should also be taken in patients with bradycardia, recent coronary occlusion, vagotonia, hypotension, peptic ulcer, epilepsy or Parkinsonism.

In diagnostic uses of Edrophonium Injection BP, a syringe containing 1mg of atropine should be kept at hand to counteract severe cholinergic reactions, should they occur. In view of the possibility of provoking a cholinergic crisis it is recommended that facilities for resuscitation should always be available.

When Edrophonium Injection BP is used as an antagonist to neuromuscular blockade bradycardia may occur, to a possibly dangerous level, unless atropine is given simultaneously. In this indication, Edrophonium Injection BP should not be given during cyclopropane or halothane anaesthesia; however, it may be used after withdrawal of these agents.

There is no evidence to suggest that Edrophonium Injection BP has any special effects in the elderly. However, elderly patients may be more susceptible to dysrhythmias than younger adults.

4.5 Interaction with other medicinal products and other forms of interaction

With doses above 10mg, especially the higher dosage employed to antagonise neuromuscular blockade, Edrophonium Injection BP should not be used in conjunction with depolarising muscle relaxants such as suxamethonium as neuromuscular blockade may be potentiated and prolonged apnoea may result.

4.6 Pregnancy and lactation

The safety of Edrophonium Injection BP during pregnancy or lactation has not been established. Although the possible hazards to mother and child must be weighed against the potential benefits in every case, experience with Edrophonium Injection BP in pregnant patients with myasthenia gravis has revealed no untoward effect of the drug on the course of pregnancy.

There is no information on the excretion of Edrophonium Injection BP into breast milk. Although only negligible amounts would be expected to be present, due regard should be paid to possible effects on the breast-feeding infant.

4.7 Effects on ability to drive and use machines

None.

4.8 Undesirable effects

These may include nausea and vomiting, increased salivation, diarrhoea and abdominal cramps.

4.9 Overdose

Edrophonium Injection BP overdosage may give rise to bradycardia, arrhythmias, hypotension and bronchiolar spasm. Perspiration, gastro-intestinal hypermotility and visual disturbances may also occur.

Artificial ventilation should be instituted if respiration is severely depressed. Atropine sulphate 1 - 2mg intravenously is an antidote to the muscarinic effects.

5. PHARMACOLOGICAL PROPERTIES

5.1 Pharmacodynamic properties

Edrophonium Injection BP is an antagonist to cholinesterase, the enzyme which normally destroys acetylcholine. The action of Edrophonium Injection BP can briefly be described, therefore, as the potentiation of naturally occurring acetylcholine. It differs from Prostigmin (neostigmine) and Mestinon (pyridostigmine) in the rapidity and brevity of its action.

5.2 Pharmacokinetic properties

Following intravenous injection of Edrophonium Injection BP an initial rapid phase of elimination (0.5 - 2 minutes) precedes a much slower decline (24 - 45 minutes). It is suggested that the rapid fall in plasma concentration of edrophonium is not primarily due to metabolism and excretion but to the rapid uptake of the drug by other tissues.

5.3 Preclinical safety data

There are no pre-clinical data of relevance to the prescriber which are additional to that already included in other sections of the SPC.

6. PHARMACEUTICAL PARTICULARS

6.1 List of excipients

Sodium Sulphite anhydrous

Sodium Citrate BP

Citric Acid BP

Water for Injections BP

6.2 Incompatibilities

None known.

6.3 Shelf life

Five years.

6.4 Special precautions for storage

Protect from light.

6.5 Nature and contents of container

Colourless glass ampoules coded with orange and emerald green colour rings, each containing 1ml of solution, in packs of 10 ampoules. The ampoule solution is almost colourless.

6.6 Special precautions for disposal and other handling

None.

Administrative Data

7. MARKETING AUTHORISATION HOLDER

Cambridge Laboratories Limited

Deltic House

Kingfisher Way

Silverlink Business Park

Wallsend

Tyne & Wear

NE28 9NX

8. MARKETING AUTHORISATION NUMBER(S)

PL 12070/0008

9. DATE OF FIRST AUTHORISATION/RENEWAL OF THE AUTHORISATION

15 April 2002

10. DATE OF REVISION OF THE TEXT

May 2002

Efexor

(Wyeth Pharmaceuticals)

1. NAME OF THE MEDICINAL PRODUCT

Efexor*

2. QUALITATIVE AND QUANTITATIVE COMPOSITION

Efexor tablets contain 37.5mg or 75mg of venlafaxine as hydrochloride.

3. PHARMACEUTICAL FORM

Tablet

Efexor are peach coloured, shield-shaped tablets impressed with the tablet strength and embossed with a "W" on one side, and plain on the other.

4. CLINICAL PARTICULARS

4.1 Therapeutic indications

Major depressive disorder

Efexor is indicated for the treatment of major depressive disorder including depression accompanied by anxiety. All patients should be evaluated for the risk of suicidality and monitored for clinical worsening (see sections 4.2 and 4.4).

Following an initial response Efexor is indicated for the prevention of relapses of the initial episode of depression or for the prevention of the recurrence of new episodes.

4.2 Posology and method of administration

Treatment with Efexor should not be started until 14 days after discontinuing a monoamine oxidase inhibitor (MAOI).

Depression:

The recommended dose is 75mg per day given in two divided doses (37.5mg twice daily). Most patients respond to this dose. It is recommended that Efexor be taken with food.

If, after an adequate trial and evaluation, further clinical improvement is required, the dose may be increased to 150mg per day given in two divided doses (75mg twice daily). There may be an increased risk of side effects at higher doses and dose increments should be made only after a clinical evaluation and after at least 3-4 weeks of therapy (see section 4.4). The lowest effective dose should be maintained.

In more severely depressed or hospitalised patients, and under close supervision of a physician, the daily dose may then be increased by up to 75mg every two or three days until the desired response is achieved. In those more severely depressed or hospitalised patients who require daily doses of 300 mg or more, treatment should be initiated under specialist supervision including shared care arrangements. The maximum recommended dose is 375mg per day.

The dose should then be gradually reduced, to the minimum effective dose consistent with patient response and tolerance. A limited amount of venlafaxine should be provided to reduce the risk from overdose (see section 4.4).

Usually, the dosage for prevention of relapse or for prevention of recurrence of a new episode is similar to that used during the index episode. Patients should be re-assessed regularly in order to evaluate the benefit of long-term therapy.

Patients at increased risk for suicide (see also sections 4.4 and 4.9):

Patients with increased risk factors for suicide should be carefully evaluated for the presence or worsening of suicide-related behaviour (see sections 4.4 and 4.9) and a limited number of tablets should be provided to reduce the risk from overdose. A maximum of two weeks supply should be considered in these patients at initiation of treatment, during any dosage adjustment and until improvement occurs.

Patients with Renal or Hepatic Impairment:

For patients with mild renal impairment (GFR >30ml/minute) or mild hepatic impairment (PT <14 seconds), no change in dosage is necessary.

For patients with moderate renal impairment (GFR 10-30ml/minute) or moderate hepatic impairment (PT 14-18 seconds), the dose should be reduced by 50%. This dose may be given once daily due to the longer half-lives of venlafaxine and O-desmethylvenlafaxine (ODV) in these patients.

Insufficient data are available to support the use of Efexor in patients with severe renal impairment (GFR < 10ml/minute) or severe hepatic impairment (PT >18 seconds).

Elderly Patients:

No adjustment in the usual dosage is recommended for elderly patients. However, as with any therapy, caution should be exercised in treating the elderly (e.g. due to the possibility of renal impairment. See also dosage recommendations for renal impairment). The lowest effective dose should always be used and patients should be carefully monitored when an increase in the dose is required.

Children/Adolescents:

Controlled clinical studies in children and adolescents with Major Depressive Disorder failed to demonstrate efficacy and do not support the use of Efexor in these patients *(see sections 4.3 Contra-indications and 4.8 Undesirable Effects).*

The efficacy and safety of Efexor for other indications in children and adolescents under the age of 18 have not yet been established.

Maintenance/Continuation/Extended Treatment:

The physician should periodically re-evaluate the usefulness of long-term treatment with Efexor for the individual patient. It is generally agreed that acute episodes of major depression require several months or longer of sustained therapy. Efexor has been shown to be efficacious during long-term (up to 12 months) treatment.

In clinical trials venlafaxine was demonstrated to be effective for preventing relapse, or recurrence of new episodes, in patients responding to venlafaxine treatment during the index episode.

Withdrawal symptoms seen on discontinuation of venlafaxine

Abrupt discontinuation should be avoided (see section 4.4 Special Warnings and Special Precautions for Use and section 4.8 Undesirable Effects). Following treatment with daily doses of venlafaxine greater than 75mg for more than one week, it is recommended that when discontinuing treatment the dose should be gradually reduced over at least a further week. If high doses have been used for more than 6 weeks tapering over at least a 2 week period is recommended. If intolerable symptoms occur following a decrease in the dose or upon discontinuation of treatment, then resuming the previously prescribed dose may be considered. Subsequently, the physician may continue decreasing the dose, but at a more gradual rate.

4.3 Contraindications

1. Known hypersensitivity to venlafaxine or any other component of the product.

2. Concomitant use of venlafaxine with monoamine oxidase inhibitors (*See Interactions with other Medicaments and Other Forms of Interactions*).

3. Venlafaxine should not be used in patients with an identified very high risk of a serious cardiac ventricular arrhythmia (e.g. those with a significant left ventricular dysfunction, NYHA Class III/IV) or uncontrolled hypertension (see section 4.4).

4. Efexor should not be used in children and adolescents under the age of 18 years with Major Depressive Disorder (*see section 4.8 Undesirable Effects*).

4.4 Special warnings and precautions for use

1. Suicide/suicidal thoughts or clinical worsening

Depression is associated with an increased risk of suicidal thoughts, self harm and suicide (suicide-related events). This risk persists until significant remission occurs. As improvement may not occur during the first few weeks or more of treatment, patients should be closely monitored until such improvement occurs. It is general clinical experience that the risk of suicide may increase in the early stages of recovery.

Other psychiatric conditions for which venlafaxine is prescribed can also be associated with an increased risk of suicide-related events. In addition, these conditions may be co-morbid with major depressive disorder. The same precautions observed when treating patients with major depressive disorder should therefore be observed when treating patients with other psychiatric disorders.

Patients with a history of suicide-related events, or those exhibiting a significant degree of suicidal ideation prior to commencement of treatment are known to be at greater risk of suicidal thoughts or suicide attempts, and should receive careful monitoring during treatment. A meta-analysis of placebo-controlled clinical trials of antidepressant drugs in adult patients with psychiatric disorders showed an increased risk of suicidal behaviour with antidepressants compared to placebo in patients less than 25 years old.

Close supervision of patients and in particular those at high risk should accompany drug therapy especially in early treatment and following dose changes. Patients (and caregivers of patients) should be alerted about the need to monitor for any clinical worsening, suicidal behaviour or thoughts and unusual changes in behaviour and to seek medical advice immediately if these symptoms present.

2. Withdrawal symptoms seen on discontinuation of venlafaxine treatment

Withdrawal symptoms when treatment is discontinued are common, particularly if discontinuation is abrupt (see section 4.8 Undesirable effects). In clinical trials adverse events seen on treatment discontinuation occurred in approximately 31% of patients treated with venlafaxine and in approximately 17% of placebo patients. The risk of withdrawal symptoms may be dependent on several factors including the duration and dose of therapy and the rate of dose reduction.

Dizziness, sensory disturbances (including paraesthesia and electric shock sensations), sleep disturbances (including insomnia and abnormal dreams), agitation or anxiety, nausea and/or vomiting, tremor, sweating, headache, diarrhoea, palpitations and emotional instability are the most commonly reported withdrawal reactions. Generally these symptoms are mild to moderate, however, in some patients they may be severe in intensity. They usually occur within the first few days of discontinuing treatment, but there have been very rare reports of such symptoms in patients who have inadvertently missed a dose. Generally these symptoms are self-limiting and usually resolve within 2 weeks, though in some individuals they may be prolonged (2-3 months or more). It is therefore advised that venlafaxine should be gradually tapered when discontinuing treatment over a period of several weeks or months, according to the patient's needs (see "Withdrawal Symptoms Seen on Discontinuation of Venlafaxine", Section 4.2 Posology and Method of Administration).

3. Activation of mania or hypomania has been reported rarely in patients who have received antidepressants, including venlafaxine. As with all antidepressants, Efexor should be used with caution in patients with a history of mania.

4. Treatment with venlafaxine (especially starting and discontinuing treatment) has been associated with reports of aggression.

5. Psychomotor restlessness: The use of venlafaxine has been associated with the development of psychomotor restlessness, which clinically may be very similar to akathisia, characterised by a subjectively unpleasant or distressing restlessness and need to move often accompanied by an inability to sit or stand still. This is most likely to occur within the first few weeks of treatment. In patients who develop these symptoms, increasing the dose may be detrimental and it may be necessary to review the use of venlafaxine.

6. Patients with cardiac disease. Venlafaxine should be used with caution in patients with established cardiac disease that may increase the risk of ventricular arrhythmias (e.g. recent myocardial infarction) (see also sections 4.3 and 4.8). People with a recent history of myocardial infarction or unstable heart disease were excluded from all clinical trials. However, patients with other pre-existing heart disease were not excluded, although they were neither separately analysed nor systematically evaluated.

7. Significant electrocardiogram findings were observed in 0.8% of venlafaxine-treated patients compared with 0.7% of placebo-treated patients. Significant changes in PR, QRS or QTc intervals were rarely observed in patients treated with venlafaxine during clinical trials.

8. Dose-related increases in blood pressure have been reported commonly from clinical trials, particularly in patients receiving daily doses greater than 200mg (see section 4.8). Sustained increases of blood pressure could have adverse consequences. Measurement of blood pressure is therefore recommended for patients receiving venlafaxine. For patients who experience a sustained increase in blood pressure while receiving venlafaxine, either dose reduction or discontinuation should be considered. Pre-existing hypertension should be controlled before treatment with venlafaxine (see section 4.3). Cases of elevated blood pressure requiring immediate treatment have been reported in post-marketing experience.

9. Seizures are a potential risk with antidepressant drugs, especially in overdose. Efexor should be introduced with caution in patients with a history of seizure and should be discontinued in any patient developing a seizure or if there is an increase in seizure frequency Efexor should be avoided in patients with unstable epilepsy and patients with controlled epilepsy should be carefully monitored (see section 4.8).

10. Due to the possibility of drug abuse with CNS-active drugs, physicians should evaluate patients for a history of drug abuse, and follow such patients closely. Clinical studies have shown no evidence of drug-seeking behaviour, development of tolerance, or dose escalation over time among patients taking venlafaxine.

11. Increases in heart rate can occur, particularly at high doses. In clinical trials the mean heart rate was increased by approximately 4 beats/minute in patients treated with venlafaxine. Caution should be exercised in patients whose underlying conditions might be compromised by increases in heart rate.

12. Dosage should be reduced in patients with moderate-severe renal impairment or hepatic cirrhosis (see sections 4.2 and 4.5).

13. Postural hypotension has been observed occasionally during venlafaxine treatment. Patients, especially the elderly, should be alerted to the possibility of dizziness or unsteadiness.

14. Hyponatraemia (usually in the elderly and possibly due to inappropriate secretion of antidiuretic hormone) has been associated with all types of antidepressants and should be considered in all patients who develop drowsiness, confusion or convulsions while taking an antidepressant.

15. Mydriasis has been reported in association with venlafaxine; therefore patients with raised intra-ocular pressure or at a risk of narrow angle glaucoma should be monitored closely.

16. There have been reports of cutaneous bleeding abnormalities, such as ecchymosis and purpura, with serotonin-reuptake inhibitors (SSRIs). Other bleeding manifestations (e.g. gastrointestinal bleeding and mucous membrane bleeding) have been reported. Caution is advised in patients predisposed to bleeding due to factors such as age, underlying medical conditions or concomitant medications.

17. Clinically relevant increases in serum cholesterol were recorded in 5.3% of venlafaxine-treated patients and 0.0% of placebo-treated patients treated for at least 3 months in placebo-controlled trials. Measurement of serum cholesterol levels should be considered during long-term treatment.

18. The safety and efficacy of venlafaxine therapy in combination with weight loss agents, including phentermine, have not been established. Co-administration of venlafaxine and weight loss agents is not recommended. Venlafaxine is not indicated for weight loss alone or in combination with other products.

19. As with SSRIs, venlafaxine should be used with caution in patients already receiving neuroleptics, since symptoms suggestive of Neuroleptic Malignant Syndrome cases have been reported with this combination.

20. Serotonin syndrome has been rarely reported in association with concomitant use with SSRIs. Therefore venlafaxine should not be used in combination with SSRIs unless clinically indicated and on the advice of a specialist.

4.5 Interaction with other medicinal products and other forms of interaction

MAOIs: Adverse reactions, some serious, have been reported when venlafaxine therapy is initiated soon after discontinuation of an MAOI, and when an MAOI is initiated soon after discontinuation of venlafaxine. These reactions have included tremor, myoclonus, diaphoresis, nausea, vomiting, flushing, dizziness, and hyperthermia with features resembling neuroleptic malignant syndrome, seizures and death. Do not use Efexor in combination with a MAOI, or within at least 14 days of discontinuing MAOI treatment. Allow at least 7 days after stopping Efexor before starting an MAOI (see also Contra-indications).

Serotonergic drugs: Based on the known mechanism of action of venlafaxine and the potential for serotonergic syndrome, caution is advised when venlafaxine is co-administered with drugs that may affect the serotonergic neurotransmitter systems (such as triptans, SSRIs or lithium). (see section 4.4)

Lithium: Reports have been received of an interaction between lithium and venlafaxine leading to increased lithium levels.

Imipramine/desipramine: The metabolism of imipramine and its metabolite 2-OH-imipramine were unaffected by venlafaxine although the total renal clearance of 2-hydroxydesipramine was reduced and desipramine AUC and C_{max} were increased by approximately 35%.

Haloperidol: In a pharmacokinetic study co-administration of venlafaxine with a single 2mg oral dose of haloperidol resulted in a 42% decrease in renal clearance, a 70% increase in AUC and an 88% increase in C_{max} for haloperidol. The elimination half-life remained unchanged.

Diazepam: The pharmacokinetic profiles of venlafaxine and ODV were not significantly altered by the administration of diazepam. Venlafaxine has no effect on the pharmacokinetic profile of diazepam or on the psychomotor or psychometric effects induced by diazepam.

Clozapine: Increased levels of clozapine, that were temporally associated with adverse events, including seizures, have been reported following the addition of venlafaxine.

Alcohol: Venlafaxine has been shown not to increase the impairment of mental or motor skills caused by ethanol. However, as with all CNS-active drugs, patients should be advised to avoid alcohol consumption while taking Efexor.

ECT: There is little clinical experience of the concurrent use of venlafaxine with ECT. As prolonged seizure activity has been reported with concomitant SSRI antidepressants, caution is advised.

Drugs metabolised by Cytochrome P450 isoenzymes: The major elimination pathways for venlafaxine are through CYP2D6 and CYP3A4. Venlafaxine is primarily metabolised to its active metabolite, ODV, by the cytochrome P450 enzyme CYP2D6. Although CYP3A4 is a minor pathway relative to CYP2D6 in the metabolism of venlafaxine, there is potential for a clinically significant drug interaction between inhibitors of CYP3A4 mediated metabolism and venlafaxine as this could result in increased venlafaxine plasma levels in poor CYP2D6 metabolisers. Therefore, potent CYP3A4 inhibitors (e.g. ketoconazole, erythromycin) or drug combinations that inhibit both CYP3A4 and CYP2D6 should only be co-administered with venlafaxine if strictly indicated.

Effect of venlafaxine on the metabolism of other drugs metabolised by cytochrome P450: Studies indicate that venlafaxine is a relatively weak inhibitor of CYP2D6. Venlafaxine did not inhibit CYP1A2, CYP2C9 or CYP3A4. This was confirmed by in vivo studies with the following drugs: alprazolam (CYP3A4), caffeine (CYP1A2), carbamazepine (CYP3A4) and diazepam (CYP3A4 and CYP2C19).

Cimetidine: Cimetidine inhibited the first-pass metabolism of venlafaxine but had no significant effect on the formation or elimination of ODV, which is present in much greater quantities in the systemic circulation. No dosage adjustment therefore seems necessary when Efexor is co-administered with cimetidine. For elderly patients, or patients with hepatic dysfunction the interaction could potentially be more pronounced, and for such patients clinical monitoring is indicated when Efexor is administered with cimetidine.

Warfarin: Potentiation of anticoagulant effects including increases in PT or INR have been reported in patients taking warfarin following the addition of venlafaxine.

Indinavir: A pharmacokinetic study with indinavir has shown a 28% decrease in AUC and a 36% decrease in C_{max} for indinavir. Indinavir did not affect the pharmacokinetics of venlafaxine and ODV. The clinical significance of this interaction is not known.

4.6 Pregnancy and lactation

There are no adequate data from the use of venlafaxine in pregnant women. Animal studies are insufficient with respect to effects on pregnancy. The potential risk for humans is unknown. Efexor should not be used during pregnancy unless clearly necessary. If venlafaxine is used until or shortly before birth, discontinuation effects in the newborn should be considered.

There is evidence to suggest that venlafaxine and its metabolite, ODV, transfers into breast milk. Therefore, a decision should be made whether or not to breast-feed or to discontinue venlafaxine.

4.7 Effects on ability to drive and use machines

Although venlafaxine has been shown not to affect psychomotor, cognitive, or complex behaviour performance in healthy volunteers, any psychoactive drug may impair judgement, thinking or motor skills. Therefore patients should be cautioned about their ability to drive or operate hazardous machinery.

4.8 Undesirable effects

See also Special Warnings and Special Precautions for Use.

The most commonly observed adverse events associated with the use of venlafaxine in clinical trials, and which occurred more frequently than those which were associated with placebo were: nausea, insomnia, dry mouth, somnolence, dizziness, constipation, sweating, nervousness, asthenia and abnormal ejaculation/orgasm.

The occurrence of most of these adverse events was dose-related, and the majority of them decreased in intensity and frequency over time. They generally did not lead to cessation of treatment.

Adverse events observed with venlafaxine, from both spontaneous and clinical trials reports, are classified in body systems and listed below as very common (>1/10); common (<1/10 and >1/100); uncommon (<1/100 and >1/1000); rare (<1/1000); very rare (<1/10,000):

Blood and lymphatic system disorders - Uncommon: ecchymosis, mucous membrane bleeding; Rare: prolonged bleeding time, haemorrhage, thrombocytopenia; Very rare: blood dyscrasias (including agranulocytosis, aplastic anaemia, neutropenia and pancytopenia).

Cardiovascular and vascular disorders (see Special Warnings and Special Precautions for Use) - Common: hypertension, palpitation, vasodilatation; Uncommon: hypotension/postural hypotension, syncope, arrhythmias (including tachycardia); Very rare: Torsade de Pointes, QT prolongation, ventricular tachycardia, ventricular fibrillation.

Gastrointestinal disorders - Very common: constipation, nausea (see below); Common: anorexia, appetite decreased, diarrhoea, dyspepsia, vomiting; Uncommon: bruxism; Rare: gastrointestinal bleeding; Very rare: pancreatitis.

General disorders - Very common: asthenia, headache; Common: abdominal pain, chills, pyrexia; Rare: anaphylaxis

Metabolic and nutritional disorders - Common: serum cholesterol increased (particularly with prolonged administration and possibly with higher doses *(see Special Warnings and Special Precautions for Use)*, weight gain or loss; Uncommon: hyponatraemia including SIADH *(see Special Warnings and Special Precautions for Use)*, increased liver enzymes *(see below)*; Rare: hepatitis; Very rare: prolactin increased.

Musculo-skeletal disorders - Common: arthralgia, myalgia; Uncommon: muscle spasm; Very rare: rhabdomyolysis.

Neurological disorders - Very common: dizziness, dry mouth, insomnia, nervousness, somnolence; Common: abnormal dreams, agitation, anxiety, confusion, hypertonia, paraesthesia, tremor; Uncommon: apathy, hallucinations, myoclonus; Rare: ataxia and disorders of balance and co-ordination, speech disorders including dysarthria, mania or hypomania (*see Special Warnings and Special Precautions for Use*), neuroleptic malignant syndrome-like effects, seizures (*see below and Special Warnings and Special Precautions for Use*), serotonergic syndrome; Very rare: delirium, extrapyramidal disorders including dyskinesia and dystonia, tardive dyskinesia, psychomotor restlessness/akathisia (see section 4.4 Special Warnings and Special Precautions for Use).

Renal and urinary disorders - Common: urinary frequency; Uncommon: urinary retention.

Reproductive and breast disorders - Very common: anorgasmia, erectile dysfunction, abnormal ejaculation/orgasm; Common: decreased libido, impotence, menstrual cycle disorders; *Uncommon*: menorrhagia; Rare: galactorrhoea.

Respiratory system disorders - Common: dyspnoea, yawning; Very rare: pulmonary eosinophilia.

Skin and subcutaneous tissue disorders - Very common: sweating (including night sweats); Common: pruritus, rash; Uncommon: angioedema, maculopapular eruptions, urticaria, photosensitivity reactions, alopecia; Rare: erythema multiforme, Stevens Johnson syndrome.

Special senses - Common: abnormal vision/ accommodation, mydriasis, tinnitus; Uncommon: altered taste sensation.

Adverse events from paediatric clinical trials

In paediatric MDD clinical trials the following adverse events were reported at a frequency of at least 2% of patients and occurred at a rate of at least twice that of placebo: abdominal pain, chest pain, tachycardia, anorexia, weight loss, constipation, dyspepsia, nausea, ecchymosis, epistaxis, mydriasis, myalgia, dizziness, emotional lability, tremor, hostility and suicidal ideation.

Withdrawal symptoms seen on discontinuation of venlafaxine treatment

Discontinuation of venlafaxine (particularly when abrupt) commonly leads to withdrawal symptoms. Dizziness, sensory disturbances (including paraesthesia and electric shock sensations), sleep disturbances (including insomnia and abnormal dreams), agitation or anxiety, nausea and/or vomiting, tremor, sweating, headache, diarrhoea, palpitations and emotional instability are the most commonly reported withdrawal reactions. Additional withdrawal reactions include hypomania, nervousness, confusion, fatigue, somnolence, convulsion, vertigo, tinnitus, dry mouth and anorexia. Generally these events are mild to moderate and are self-limiting, however, in some patients they may be severe and/or prolonged. It is therefore advised that when venlafaxine treatment is no longer required, gradual discontinuation by dose tapering should be carried out (see section 4.2 Posology and Method of Administration and section 4.4 Special Warnings and Special Precautions for use).

Special Notes:

In all premarketing depression trials with venlafaxine tablets, seizures were reported in 0.3% of all venlafaxine-treated patients. All patients recovered. No seizures occurred in Efexor XL-treated patients in clinical trials for depression and GAD. No seizures occurred in placebo-treated patients in depression studies. Seizures were reported in 0.2% of placebo-treated patients in GAD studies (see section 4.4).

Nausea is most common at the start of treatment with the incidence decreasing over the first few weeks. The nausea experienced with Efexor is usually mild to moderate, and infrequently results in vomiting or withdrawal. The incidence increases with higher doses particularly when the dose is increased rapidly.

Reversible increases in liver enzymes are seen in a small number of patients treated with venlafaxine. These generally resolve on discontinuation of therapy.

Cases of suicidal ideation and suicidal behaviours have been reported during venlafaxine therapy or early after treatment discontinuation (see section 4.4).

4.9 Overdose

Electrocardiogram changes (e.g. prolongation of QT interval, bundle branch block, QRS prolongation), sinus and ventricular tachycardia, bradycardia and seizures, hypotension, vertigo, serotonin syndrome and changes in level of consciousness have been reported in association with overdosage of venlafaxine usually when in combination with alcohol and/or other CNS drugs.

Management of Overdosage - Ensure an adequate airway, oxygenation and ventilation. Monitoring of cardiac rhythm and vital signs is recommended, as are general supportive and symptomatic measures. Use of activated charcoal or gastric lavage should be considered. Induction of emesis is not recommended. No specific antidotes for venlafaxine are known. In managing overdose, consider the possibility of multiple drug involvement (e.g. concomitant intake with SSRIs or other psychotropic drugs).

The haemodialysis clearance of venlafaxine and its main active metabolite, are low. Therefore, they are not considered dialysable.

Retrospective analyses from the United Kingdom (UK) report the rate of antidepressant overdose deaths per million prescriptions. In these analyses, the rate for venlafaxine is higher than that for SSRIs, but lower than that for tricyclic antidepressants. These analyses did not adjust for suicide risk factors. An epidemiological study in patients prescribed antidepressants in the UK showed that venlafaxine is prescribed to patients with a higher pre-existing burden of suicide risk factors than patients prescribed SSRIs. As such these patients should be carefully evaluated for the presence or worsening of suicide-related behaviour (see sections 4.2 and 4.4).

5. PHARMACOLOGICAL PROPERTIES

5.1 Pharmacodynamic properties

Efexor is a structurally novel antidepressant which is chemically unrelated to tricyclic, tetracyclic, or other available antidepressant agents. It is a racemate with two active enantiomers.

The mechanism of Efexor's antidepressant action in humans is believed to be associated with its potentiation of neurotransmitter activity in the central nervous system. Preclinical studies have shown that venlafaxine and its major metabolite, O-desmethylvenlafaxine, are potent neuronal serotonin and noradrenaline re-uptake inhibitors (SNRI) and weak inhibitors of dopamine reuptake. In addition, venlafaxine and O-desmethylvenlafaxine reduce β-adrenergic responsiveness in animals after both acute (single dose) and chronic administration. Venlafaxine and its major metabolite appear to be equipotent with respect to their overall action on neurotransmitter re-uptake.

Venlafaxine has virtually no affinity for rat brain muscarinic, histaminergic or adrenergic receptors *in vitro*. Pharmacologic activity at these receptors may be related to various side effects seen with other antidepressant drugs, such as anticholinergic, sedative and cardiovascular effects.

5.2 Pharmacokinetic properties

Venlafaxine is well absorbed and undergoes extensive first-pass metabolism. Mean peak plasma concentrations of venlafaxine range from approximately 33 to 172ng/ml after 25 to 150mg single doses, and are reached in approximately 2.4 hours. Venlafaxine is extensively metabolised in the liver. O-desmethylvenlafaxine is the major active metabolite of venlafaxine. The mean disposition half-life of venlafaxine and O-desmethylvenlafaxine is approximately 5 and 11 hours, respectively. Mean peak O-desmethylvenlafaxine plasma concentrations range from approximately 61 to 325ng/ml and are reached in approximately 4.3 hours. Plasma concentrations of venlafaxine and O-desmethylvenlafaxine generally correlated well with dose levels. Venlafaxine and O-desmethylvenlafaxine are 27% and 30% bound to plasma proteins respectively. O-desmethylvenlafaxine, other minor venlafaxine metabolites, and non-metabolised venlafaxine are excreted primarily through the kidneys.

5.3 Preclinical safety data

Studies with venlafaxine in rats and mice revealed no evidence of carcinogenesis. Venlafaxine was not mutagenic in a wide range of in vitro and in vivo tests.

Reduced fertility was observed in a study in which both male and female rats were exposed to the major metabolite of venlafaxine (ODV). This exposure was approximately 2 to 3 times that of a human dose of 225mg/day.

6. PHARMACEUTICAL PARTICULARS

6.1 List of excipients

The active constituent is venlafaxine as hydrochloride. Other constituents are microcrystalline cellulose, lactose, sodium starch glycollate, magnesium stearate, yellow and brown iron oxide.

6.2 Incompatibilities

Not applicable

6.3 Shelf life

Three years

6.4 Special precautions for storage

Store in a dry place at room temperature (at or below 30°C)

6.5 Nature and contents of container

PVC/PVdC/aluminium foil blisters of 28 or 56 tablets

6.6 Special precautions for disposal and other handling

None

7. MARKETING AUTHORISATION HOLDER

John Wyeth and Brother Limited

Huntercombe Lane South

Taplow, Maidenhead, Berks SL6 0PH

UK

8. MARKETING AUTHORISATION NUMBER(S)

Efexor 37.5mg: 00011/0199

Efexor 75mg: 00011/0201

9. DATE OF FIRST AUTHORISATION/RENEWAL OF THE AUTHORISATION

22 November 1994

10. DATE OF REVISION OF THE TEXT

7 March 2008

* Trade Mark

Efexor XL

(Wyeth Pharmaceuticals)

1. NAME OF THE MEDICINAL PRODUCT

Efexor * XL

2. QUALITATIVE AND QUANTITATIVE COMPOSITION

Efexor XL 75mg capsules contain 84.8mg of venlafaxine hydrochloride, equivalent to 75mg of venlafaxine free base, in an extended release formulation.

Efexor XL 150mg capsules contain 169.7mg of venlafaxine hydrochloride, equivalent to 150mg of venlafaxine free base, in an extended release formulation.

Venlafaxine is chemically defined as (R/S)-1-[(2-dimethylamino)-1-(4-methoxy phenyl)ethyl]cyclohexanol hydrochloride.

3. PHARMACEUTICAL FORM

Efexor XL 75mg capsules are opaque peach modified release capsules printed in red with "W" and "75".

Efexor XL 150mg capsules are opaque dark orange modified release capsules printed in white with "W" and "150".

4. CLINICAL PARTICULARS

4.1 Therapeutic indications

Major depressive disorder

Efexor XL is indicated for the treatment of major depressive disorder including depression accompanied by anxiety. All patients should be evaluated for the risk of suicidality and monitored for clinical worsening (see section 4.2 and 4.4).

Following an initial response Efexor XL is indicated for the prevention of relapses of the initial episode of depression or for the prevention of the recurrence of new episodes.

Moderate to severe Generalised Anxiety Disorder

Efexor XL is also indicated for the treatment of moderate to severe Generalised Anxiety Disorder (GAD). This is primarily characterised by chronic and excessive worry and anxiety, sufficient to cause impairment in everyday functioning, for at least 6 months.

Moderate to severe generalised social anxiety disorder/social phobia:

Efexor XL is indicated for the treatment of moderate to severe generalised social anxiety disorder/social phobia in adults.

4.2 Posology and method of administration

Treatment with Efexor XL should not be started until 14 days after discontinuing a monoamine oxidase inhibitor (MAOI).

Efexor XL should be taken with food. Each capsule should be swallowed whole with fluid. Do not divide, crush, chew, or place the capsule in water. Efexor XL should be taken once daily, at approximately the same time, either in the morning or in the evening.

Depression:

The recommended dose is 75mg per day given once daily. Most patients respond to this dose.

If, after an adequate trial and evaluation, further clinical improvement is required, the dose may be increased to 150mg per day given once daily. There may be an increased risk of side effects at higher doses and dose increments should be made only after a clinical evaluation and after at least 3-4 weeks of therapy (see section 4.4). The lowest effective dose should be maintained.

In more severely depressed or hospitalised patients, and under close supervision of a physician, the daily dose may then be increased to the maximum recommended dose of Efexor XL capsules, 225mg given once daily. In those more severely depressed or hospitalised patients who require daily venlafaxine doses of 300 mg or more, treatment with Efexor tablets should be initiated under specialist supervision including shared care arrangements.

The dose should then be gradually reduced, to the minimum effective dose consistent with patient response and tolerance. A limited amount of venlafaxine should be provided to reduce the risk from overdose (see section 4.4).

Usually, the dosage for prevention of relapse or for prevention of recurrence of a new episode is similar to that used during the index episode. Patients should be re-assessed regularly in order to evaluate the benefit of long-term therapy.

Depressed patients who are currently being treated with Efexor Tablets may be switched to Efexor XL. For example, a patient receiving Efexor Tablets 37.5mg b.d. would receive Efexor XL 75mg o.d. When switching, individual dosage adjustments may be necessary.

Generalised Anxiety Disorder (GAD):

The recommended dose for GAD for Efexor XL is 75mg, given once daily.

Patients should be reviewed at regular intervals and treatment should be discontinued after 8 weeks if there is no evidence of clinical response.

Usually, the dosage for prevention of relapse or for prevention of recurrence of a new episode is similar to that used during the index episode. Patients should be re-assessed regularly in order to evaluate the benefit of long-term therapy.

Social Phobia (Social Anxiety Disorder):

The recommended dose for social phobia for Efexor XL is 75mg, given once daily.

Patients at increased risk for suicide (see also sections 4.4 and 4.9):

Patients with increased risk factors for suicide should be carefully evaluated for the presence or worsening of suicide-related behaviour (see sections 4.4 and 4.9) and a limited number of capsules should be provided to reduce the risk from overdose. A maximum of two weeks supply should be considered in these patients at initiation of treatment, during any dosage adjustment and until improvement occurs.

Patients with Renal or Hepatic Impairment:

For patients with mild renal impairment (GFR > 30ml/minute) or mild hepatic impairment (PT < 14 seconds), no change in dosage is necessary.

For patients with moderate renal impairment (GFR 10-30ml/minute) or moderate hepatic impairment (PT 14-18 seconds), the dose should be reduced by 50%. This dose may be given once daily due to the longer half-lives of venlafaxine and O-desmethylvenlafaxine (ODV) in these patients.

Insufficient data are available to support the use of Efexor XL in patients with severe renal impairment (GFR < 10ml/minute) or severe hepatic impairment (PT > 18 seconds).

Elderly Patients:

No adjustment in the usual dosage is recommended for elderly patients. However, as with any therapy, caution should be exercised in treating the elderly (e.g. due to the possibility of renal impairment. See also dosage recommendations for renal impairment). The lowest effective dose should always be used and patients should be carefully monitored when an increase in the dose is required.

Children/Adolescents:

Controlled clinical studies in children and adolescents with Major Depressive Disorder failed to demonstrate efficacy and do not support the use of Efexor XL in these patients *(see sections 4.3 Contra-indications and 4.8 Undesirable Effects)*.

The efficacy and safety of Efexor XL for other indications in children and adolescents under the age of 18 have not yet been established.

Maintenance/Continuation/Extended Treatment:

Depression: The physician should periodically re-evaluate the usefulness of long-term treatment with Efexor XL for the individual patient. It is generally agreed that acute episodes of major depression require several months or longer of sustained therapy. Efexor XL has been shown to be efficacious during long-term (up to 12 months) treatment.

In clinical trials venlafaxine was demonstrated to be effective for preventing relapse, or recurrence of new episodes, in patients responding to venlafaxine treatment during the index episode.

Generalised Anxiety Disorder: There is no evidence of efficacy for Efexor XL in GAD beyond 6 months. However, patients with GAD often suffer over many years and such patients may require long-term treatment.

Social Anxiety Disorder/social phobia: Social anxiety disorder is a disease with a chronic course, and treatment for 12 weeks is recommended to consolidate response. There is no evidence of benefit at doses higher than 75mg once daily, but side effects may be dose-related. If a patient fails to respond to 75mg after 12 weeks, alternative therapy should be considered. Continuation of treatment for a responding patient can be considered on an individual patient basis; treatment benefits should be re-evaluated at regular intervals. There is no evidence of efficacy of venlafaxine ER beyond six months.

Withdrawal symptoms seen on discontinuation of venlafaxine

Abrupt discontinuation should be avoided (see section 4.4 Special Warnings and Special Precautions for Use and section 4.8 Undesirable Effects). Following treatment with daily doses of venlafaxine greater than 75mg for more than one week, it is recommended that when discontinuing treatment the dose should be gradually reduced over at least a further week. If high doses have been used for more than 6 weeks tapering over at least a 2 week period is recommended. If intolerable symptoms occur following a decrease in the dose or upon discontinuation of treatment, then resuming the previously prescribed dose may be considered. Subsequently, the physician may continue decreasing the dose, but at a more gradual rate.

4.3 Contraindications

1. Known hypersensitivity to venlafaxine or any other component of the product.

2. Concomitant use of venlafaxine with monoamine oxidase inhibitors *(See Interactions with other Medicaments and Other Forms of Interactions)*.

3. Venlafaxine should not be used in patients with an identified very high risk of a serious cardiac ventricular arrhythmia (e.g. those with a significant left ventricular dysfunction, NYHA Class III/IV) or uncontrolled hypertension (see section 4.4).

4. Efexor XL should not be used in children and adolescents under the age of 18 years with Major Depressive Disorder *(see section 4.8 Undesirable Effects)*.

4.4 Special warnings and precautions for use

1. Suicide/suicidal thoughts or clinical worsening

Depression is associated with an increased risk of suicidal thoughts, self harm and suicide (suicide-related events). This risk persists until significant remission occurs. As improvement may not occur during the first few weeks or more of treatment, patients should be closely monitored until such improvement occurs. It is general clinical experience that the risk of suicide may increase in the early stages of recovery.

Other psychiatric conditions for which venlafaxine is prescribed can also be associated with an increased risk of suicide-related events. In addition, these conditions may be co-morbid with major depressive disorder. The same precautions observed when treating patients with major depressive disorder should therefore be observed when treating patients with other psychiatric disorders.

Patients with a history of suicide-related events, or those exhibiting a significant degree of suicidal ideation prior to commencement of treatment are known to be at greater risk of suicidal thoughts or suicide attempts, and should receive careful monitoring during treatment. A meta-analysis of placebo-controlled clinical trials of antidepressant drugs in adult patients with psychiatric disorders showed an increased risk of suicidal behaviour with antidepressants compared to placebo in patients less than 25 years old.

Close supervision of patients and in particular those at high risk should accompany drug therapy especially in early treatment and following dose changes. Patients (and caregivers of patients) should be alerted about the need to monitor for any clinical worsening, suicidal behaviour or thoughts and unusual changes in behaviour and to seek medical advice immediately if these symptoms present.

2. Withdrawal symptoms seen on discontinuation of venlafaxine treatment

Withdrawal symptoms when treatment is discontinued are common, particularly if discontinuation is abrupt (see section 4.8 Undesirable effects). In clinical trials adverse events seen on treatment discontinuation occurred in approximately 31% of patients treated with venlafaxine and in approximately 17% of placebo patients. The risk of withdrawal symptoms may be dependent on several factors including the duration and dose of therapy and the rate of dose reduction.

Dizziness, sensory disturbances (including paraesthesia and electric shock sensations), sleep disturbances (including insomnia and abnormal dreams), agitation or anxiety, nausea and/or vomiting, tremor, sweating, headache, diarrhoea, palpitations and emotional instability are the most commonly reported withdrawal reactions. Generally these symptoms are mild to moderate, however, in some patients they may be severe in intensity. They usually occur within the first few days of discontinuing treatment, but there have been very rare reports of such symptoms in patients who have inadvertently missed a dose. Generally these symptoms are self-limiting and usually resolve within 2 weeks, though in some individuals they may be prolonged (2-3 months or more). It is therefore advised that venlafaxine should be gradually tapered when discontinuing treatment over a period of several weeks or months, according to the patient's needs (see "Withdrawal Symptoms Seen on Discontinuation of Venlafaxine", Section 4.2 Posology and Method of Administration).

3. Activation of mania or hypomania has been reported rarely in patients who have received antidepressants, including venlafaxine. As with all antidepressants, Efexor XL should be used with caution in patients with a history of mania.

4. Treatment with venlafaxine (especially starting and discontinuing treatment) has been associated with reports of aggression.

5. **Psychomotor restlessness**: The use of venlafaxine has been associated with the development of psychomotor restlessness, which clinically may be very similar to akathisia, characterised by a subjectively unpleasant or distressing restlessness and need to move often accompanied by an inability to sit or stand still. This is most likely to occur within the first few weeks of treatment. In patients who develop these symptoms, increasing the dose may be detrimental and it may be necessary to review the use of venlafaxine.

6. Patients with cardiac disease. Venlafaxine should be used with caution in patients with established cardiac disease that may increase the risk of ventricular arrhythmias (e.g. recent myocardial infarction) (see also sections 4.3 and 4.8). People with a recent history of myocardial infarction or unstable heart disease were excluded from all clinical trials. However, patients with other pre-existing heart disease were not excluded, although they were neither separately analysed nor systematically evaluated.

7. Significant electrocardiogram findings were observed in 0.8% of venlafaxine-treated patients compared with 0.7% of placebo-treated patients. Significant changes in PR, QRS or QTc intervals were rarely observed in patients treated with venlafaxine during clinical trials.

8. Dose-related increases in blood pressure have been reported commonly from clinical trials, particularly in patients receiving daily doses greater than 200mg (see section 4.8). Sustained increases of blood pressure could have adverse consequences. Measurement of blood pressure is therefore recommended for patients receiving venlafaxine. For patients who experience a sustained increase in blood pressure while receiving venlafaxine, either dose reduction or discontinuation should be considered. Pre-existing hypertension should be controlled before treatment with venlafaxine (see section 4.3). Cases of elevated blood pressure requiring immediate treatment have been reported in post-marketing experience.

9. Seizures are a potential risk with antidepressant drugs, especially in overdose. Efexor XL should be introduced with caution in patients with a history of seizure and should be discontinued in any patient developing a seizure or if there is an increase in seizure frequency Efexor XL should be avoided in patients with unstable epilepsy and patients with controlled epilepsy should be carefully monitored (see section 4.8).

10. Due to the possibility of drug abuse with CNS-active drugs, physicians should evaluate patients for a history of drug abuse, and follow such patients closely. Clinical studies have shown no evidence of drug-seeking behaviour, development of tolerance, or dose escalation over time among patients taking venlafaxine.

11. Increases in heart rate can occur, particularly at high doses. In clinical trials the mean heart rate was increased by approximately 4 beats/minute in patients treated with venlafaxine. Caution should be exercised in patients whose underlying conditions might be compromised by increases in heart rate.

12. Dosage should be reduced in patients with moderate-severe renal impairment or hepatic cirrhosis (see sections 4.2 and 4.5).

13. Postural hypotension has been observed occasionally during venlafaxine treatment. Patients, especially the elderly, should be alerted to the possibility of dizziness or unsteadiness.

14. Hyponatraemia (usually in the elderly and possibly due to inappropriate secretion of antidiuretic hormone) has been associated with all types of antidepressants and should be considered in all patients who develop drowsiness, confusion or convulsions while taking an antidepressant.

15. Mydriasis has been reported in association with venlafaxine; therefore patients with raised intra-ocular pressure or at a risk of narrow angle glaucoma should be monitored closely.

16. There have been reports of cutaneous bleeding abnormalities, such as ecchymosis and purpura, with serotonin-reuptake inhibitors (SSRIs). Other bleeding manifestations (e.g. gastrointestinal bleeding and mucous membrane bleeding) have been reported. Caution is advised in patients predisposed to bleeding due to factors such as age, underlying medical conditions or concomitant medications.

17. Clinically relevant increases in serum cholesterol were recorded in 5.3% of venlafaxine-treated patients and 0.0% of placebo-treated patients treated for at least 3 months in placebo-controlled trials. Measurement of serum cholesterol levels should be considered during long-term treatment.

18. The safety and efficacy of venlafaxine therapy in combination with weight loss agents, including phentermine, have not been established. Co-administration of venlafaxine and weight loss agents is not recommended. Venlafaxine is not indicated for weight loss alone or in combination with other products.

19. As with SSRIs, venlafaxine should be used with caution in patients already receiving neuroleptics, since symptoms suggestive of Neuroleptic Malignant Syndrome cases have been reported with this combination.

20. Serotonin syndrome has been rarely reported in association with concomitant use with SSRIs. Therefore venlafaxine should not be used in combination with SSRIs unless clinically indicated and on the advice of a specialist.

4.5 Interaction with other medicinal products and other forms of interaction

MAOIs: Adverse reactions, some serious, have been reported when venlafaxine therapy is initiated soon after discontinuation of an MAOI, and when an MAOI is initiated soon after discontinuation of venlafaxine. These reactions have included tremor, myoclonus, diaphoresis, nausea, vomiting, flushing, dizziness, and hyperthermia with features resembling neuroleptic malignant syndrome, seizures and death. Do not use Efexor XL in combination with a MAOI, or within at least 14 days of discontinuing MAOI treatment. Allow at least 7 days after stopping Efexor XL before starting an MAOI (see also Contra-indications).

Serotonergic drugs: Based on the known mechanism of action of venlafaxine and the potential for serotonergic syndrome, caution is advised when venlafaxine is co-administered with drugs that may affect the serotonergic neurotransmitter systems (such as triptans, SSRIs or lithium). (see section 4.4)

Lithium: Reports have been received of an interaction between lithium and venlafaxine leading to increased lithium levels.

Imipramine/desipramine: The metabolism of imipramine and its metabolite 2-OH-imipramine were unaffected by venlafaxine although the total renal clearance of 2-hydroxydesipramine was reduced and desipramine AUC and C_{max} were increased by approximately 35%.

Haloperidol: In a pharmacokinetic study co-administration of venlafaxine with a single 2mg oral dose of haloperidol resulted in a 42% decrease in renal clearance, a 70% increase in AUC and an 88% increase in C_{max} for haloperidol. The elimination half-life remained unchanged.

Diazepam: The pharmacokinetic profiles of venlafaxine and ODV were not significantly altered by the administration of diazepam. Venlafaxine has no effect on the pharmacokinetic profile of diazepam or on the psychomotor or psychometric effects induced by diazepam.

Clozapine: Increased levels of clozapine, that were temporally associated with adverse events, including seizures, have been reported following the addition of venlafaxine.

Alcohol: Venlafaxine has been shown not to increase the impairment of mental or motor skills caused by ethanol. However, as with all CNS-active drugs, patients should be advised to avoid alcohol consumption while taking Efexor XL.

ECT: There is little clinical experience of the concurrent use of venlafaxine with ECT. As prolonged seizure activity has been reported with concomitant SSRI antidepressants, caution is advised.

Drugs metabolised by Cytochrome P450 isoenzymes: The major elimination pathways for venlafaxine are through CYP2D6 and CYP3A4. Venlafaxine is primarily metabolised to its active metabolite, ODV, by the cytochrome P450 enzyme CYP2D6. Although CYP3A4 is a minor pathway relative to CYP2D6 in the metabolism of venlafaxine, there is potential for a clinically significant drug interaction between inhibitors of CYP3A4 mediated metabolism and venlafaxine as this could result in increased venlafaxine plasma levels in poor CYP2D6 metabolisers. Therefore, potent CYP3A4 inhibitors (e.g. ketoconazole, erythromycin) or drug combinations that inhibit both CYP3A4 and CYP2D6 should only be co-administered with venlafaxine if strictly indicated.

Effect of venlafaxine on the metabolism of other drugs metabolised by cytochrome P450: Studies indicate that venlafaxine is a relatively weak inhibitor of CYP2D6. Venlafaxine did not inhibit CYP1A2, CYP2C9 or CYP3A4. This was confirmed by in vivo studies with the following drugs: alprazolam (CYP3A4), caffeine (CYP1A2), carbamazepine (CYP3A4) and diazepam (CYP3A4 and CYP2C19).

Cimetidine: Cimetidine inhibited the first-pass metabolism of venlafaxine but had no significant effect on the formation or elimination of ODV, which is present in much greater quantities in the systemic circulation. No dosage adjustment therefore seems necessary when Efexor XL is co-administered with cimetidine. For elderly patients, or patients with hepatic dysfunction the interaction could potentially be more pronounced, and for such patients clinical monitoring is indicated when Efexor XL is administered with cimetidine.

Warfarin: Potentiation of anticoagulant effects including increases in PT or INR have been reported in patients taking warfarin following the addition of venlafaxine.

Indinavir: A pharmacokinetic study with indinavir has shown a 28% decrease in AUC and a 36% decrease in C_{max} for indinavir. Indinavir did not affect the pharmacokinetics of venlafaxine and ODV. The clinical significance of this interaction is not known.

4.6 Pregnancy and lactation

There are no adequate data from the use of venlafaxine in pregnant women. Animal studies are insufficient with respect to effects on pregnancy. The potential risk for humans is unknown. Efexor XL should not be used during pregnancy unless clearly necessary. If venlafaxine is used until or shortly before birth, discontinuation effects in the newborn should be considered.

There is evidence to suggest that venlafaxine and its metabolite, ODV, transfers into breast milk. Therefore, a decision should be made whether or not to breast-feed or to discontinue venlafaxine.

4.7 Effects on ability to drive and use machines

Although venlafaxine has been shown not to affect psychomotor, cognitive, or complex behaviour performance in healthy volunteers, any psychoactive drug may impair judgement, thinking or motor skills. Therefore patients should be cautioned about their ability to drive or operate hazardous machinery.

4.8 Undesirable effects

See also Special Warnings and Special Precautions for Use.

The most commonly observed adverse events associated with the use of venlafaxine in clinical trials, and which occurred more frequently than those which were associated with placebo were: nausea, insomnia, dry mouth, somnolence, dizziness, constipation, sweating, nervousness, asthenia and abnormal ejaculation/orgasm.

The occurrence of most of these adverse events was dose-related, and the majority of them decreased in intensity and frequency over time. They generally did not lead to cessation of treatment.

Adverse events observed with venlafaxine, from both spontaneous and clinical trials reports, are classified in body systems and listed below as very common (>1/10); common (<1/10 and >1/100); uncommon (<1/100 and >1/1000); rare (<1/1000); very rare (<1/10,000):

Blood and lymphatic system disorders - Uncommon: ecchymosis, mucous membrane bleeding; Rare: prolonged bleeding time, haemorrhage, thrombocytopenia; Very rare: blood dyscrasias (including agranulocytosis, aplastic anaemia, neutropenia and pancytopenia).

Cardiovascular and vascular disorders (see Special Warnings and Special Precautions for Use) - Common: hypertension, palpitation, vasodilatation; Uncommon: hypotension/postural hypotension, syncope, arrhythmias (including tachycardia); Very rare: Torsade de Pointes, QT prolongation, ventricular tachycardia, ventricular fibrillation.

Gastrointestinal disorders - Very common: constipation, nausea (see below); Common: anorexia, appetite decreased, diarrhoea, dyspepsia, vomiting; Uncommon: bruxism; Rare: gastrointestinal bleeding; Very rare: pancreatitis.

General disorders - Very common: asthenia, headache; Common: abdominal pain, chills, pyrexia; Rare: anaphylaxis

Metabolic and nutritional disorders - Common: serum cholesterol increased (particularly with prolonged administration and possibly with higher doses *(see Special Warnings and Special Precautions for Use)*, weight gain or loss; Uncommon: hyponatraemia including SIADH *(see Special Warnings and Special Precautions for Use)*, increased liver enzymes *(see below);* Rare: hepatitis; Very rare: prolactin increased.

Musculo-skeletal disorders - Common: arthralgia, myalgia; Uncommon: muscle spasm; Very rare: rhabdomyolysis.

Neurological disorders - Very common: dizziness, dry mouth, insomnia, nervousness, somnolence; Common: abnormal dreams, agitation, anxiety, confusion, hypertonia, paraesthesia, tremor; Uncommon: apathy, hallucinations, myoclonus; Rare: ataxia and disorders of balance and co-ordination, speech disorders including dysarthria, mania or hypomania *(see Special Warnings and Special Precautions for Use)*, neuroleptic malignant syndrome-like effects, seizures *(see below and Special Warnings and Special Precautions for Use)*, serotonergic syndrome; Very rare: delirium, extrapyramidal disorders including dyskinesia and dystonia, tardive dyskinesia, psychomotor restlessness/akathisia (see section 4.4 Special Warnings and Special Precautions for Use).

Renal and urinary disorders - Common: urinary frequency; Uncommon: urinary retention.

Reproductive and breast disorders - Very common: anorgasmia, erectile dysfunction, abnormal ejaculation/orgasm; Common: decreased libido, impotence, menstrual cycle disorders; Uncommon: menorrhagia; Rare: galactorrhoea.

Respiratory system disorders - Common: dyspnoea, yawning; Very rare: pulmonary eosinophilia.

Skin and subcutaneous tissue disorders - Very common: sweating (including night sweats); Common: pruritus, rash; Uncommon: angioedema, maculopapular eruptions, urticaria, photosensitivity reactions, alopecia; Rare: erythema multiforme, Stevens Johnson syndrome.

Special senses - Common: abnormal vision/ accommodation, mydriasis, tinnitus; Uncommon: altered taste sensation.

Adverse events from paediatric clinical trials

In paediatric MDD clinical trials the following adverse events were reported at a frequency of at least 2% of patients and occurred at a rate of at least twice that of placebo: abdominal pain, chest pain, tachycardia, anorexia, weight loss, constipation, dyspepsia, nausea, ecchymosis, epistaxis, mydriasis, myalgia, dizziness, emotional lability, tremor, hostility and suicidal ideation.

Withdrawal symptoms seen on discontinuation of venlafaxine treatment

Discontinuation of venlafaxine (particularly when abrupt) commonly leads to withdrawal symptoms. Dizziness, sensory disturbances (including paraesthesia and electric shock sensations), sleep disturbances (including insomnia and abnormal dreams), agitation or anxiety, nausea and/or vomiting, tremor, sweating, headache, diarrhoea, palpitations and emotional instability are the most commonly reported withdrawal reactions. Additional withdrawal reactions include hypomania, nervousness, confusion, fatigue, somnolence, convulsion, vertigo, tinnitus, dry mouth and anorexia. Generally these events are mild to moderate and are self-limiting, however, in some patients they may be severe and/or prolonged. It is therefore advised that when venlafaxine treatment is no longer required, gradual discontinuation by dose tapering should be carried out (see section 4.2 Posology and Method of Administration and section 4.4 Special Warnings and Special Precautions for use).

Special Notes:

In all premarketing depression trials with venlafaxine tablets, seizures were reported in 0.3% of all venlafaxine-treated patients. All patients recovered. No seizures occurred in Efexor XL-treated patients in clinical trials for depression and GAD. No seizures occurred in placebo-treated patients in depression studies. Seizures were reported in 0.2% of placebo-treated patients in GAD studies (see section 4.4).

Nausea is most common at the start of treatment with the incidence decreasing over the first few weeks. The nausea experienced with Efexor XL is usually mild to moderate, and infrequently results in vomiting or withdrawal. The incidence increases with higher doses particularly when the dose is increased rapidly.

Reversible increases in liver enzymes are seen in a small number of patients treated with venlafaxine. These generally resolve on discontinuation of therapy.

Cases of suicidal ideation and suicidal behaviours have been reported during venlafaxine therapy or early after treatment discontinuation (see section 4.4).

4.9 Overdose

Electrocardiogram changes (e.g. prolongation of QT interval, bundle branch block, QRS prolongation), sinus and ventricular tachycardia, bradycardia and seizures, hypotension, vertigo, serotonin syndromeand changes in level of consciousness have been reported in association with overdosage of venlafaxine usually when in combination with alcohol and/or other CNS drugs.

Management of Overdosage - Ensure an adequate airway, oxygenation and ventilation. Monitoring of cardiac rhythm and vital signs is recommended, as are general supportive and symptomatic measures. Use of activated charcoal or gastric lavage should be considered. Induction of emesis is not recommended. No specific antidotes for venlafaxine are known. In managing overdose, consider the possibility of multiple drug involvement (e.g. concomitant intake with SSRIs or other psychotropic drugs).

The haemodialysis clearance of venlafaxine and its main active metabolite, are low. Therefore, they are not considered dialysable.

Retrospective analyses from the United Kingdom (UK) report the rate of antidepressant overdose deaths per million prescriptions. In these analyses, the rate for venlafaxine is higher than that for SSRIs, but lower than that for tricyclic antidepressants. These analyses did not adjust for suicide risk factors. An epidemiological study in patients prescribed antidepressants in the UK showed that venlafaxine is prescribed to patients with a higher pre-existing burden of suicide risk factors than patients prescribed SSRIs. As such these patients should be carefully evaluated for the presence or worsening of suicide-related behaviour (see sections 4.2 and 4.4).

5. PHARMACOLOGICAL PROPERTIES

Venlafaxine is a structurally novel antidepressant that is chemically unrelated to tricyclic, tetracyclic, or other available antidepressants. It is a racemate with two active enantiomers.

5.1 Pharmacodynamic properties

The mechanism of venlafaxine's antidepressant action in humans is believed to be associated with its potentiation of neurotransmitter activity in the central nervous system. Preclinical studies have shown that venlafaxine and its major metabolite, O-desmethylvenlafaxine (ODV), are potent inhibitors of serotonin and noradrenaline reuptake. Venlafaxine also weakly inhibits dopamine uptake. Studies in animals show that tricyclic antidepressants may reduce β-adrenergic responsiveness following chronic administration. In contrast, venlafaxine and its active metabolite reduced β-adrenergic responsiveness after both acute (single dose) and chronic administration. Venlafaxine and ODV are very similar with respect to their overall action on neurotransmitter reuptake.

Venlafaxine has virtually no affinity for rat brain muscarinic cholinergic, H_1-histaminergic or α_1-adrenergic receptors *in vitro*. Pharmacological activity at these receptors may be related to various side effects seen with other antidepressant drugs, such as anticholinergic, sedative and cardiovascular side effects.

Venlafaxine does not possess monoamine oxidase (MAO) inhibitory activity.

In vitro studies revealed that venlafaxine has virtually no affinity for opiate, benzodiazepine, phencyclidine (PCP), or N-methyl-d-aspartic acid (NMDA) receptors. It has no significant central nervous system (CNS) stimulant activity in rodents. In primate drug discrimination studies, venlafaxine showed no significant or depressant abuse liability.

5.2 Pharmacokinetic properties

At least 92% of a single oral dose of venlafaxine is absorbed. After administration of Efexor XL, the peak plasma concentrations of venlafaxine and ODV are attained within 6.0±1.5 and 8.8±2.2 hours, respectively. The rate of absorption of venlafaxine from the Efexor XL capsule is slower than its rate of elimination. Therefore, the apparent elimination half-life of venlafaxine following administration of Efexor XL (15±6 hours) is actually the absorption half-life instead of the true disposition half-life (5±2 hours) observed following administration of an immediate release tablet.

When equal daily doses of venlafaxine were administered as either the immediate release tablet, or the extended release capsule, the exposure (AUC, area under the concentration curve) to both venlafaxine and ODV was similar for the two treatments, and the fluctuation in plasma concentrations was slightly lower following treatment with the Efexor XL capsule. Therefore, the Efexor XL capsule provides a slower rate of absorption, but the same extent of absorption (i.e. AUC), as the Efexor immediate release tablet.

Venlafaxine undergoes extensive first-pass metabolism in the liver, primarily by CYP2D6, to the major metabolite ODV. Venlafaxine is also metabolised to N-desmethylvenlafaxine, catalysed by CYP3A3/4, and to other minor metabolites.

Venlafaxine and its metabolites are excreted primarily through the kidneys. Approximately 87% of a venlafaxine dose is recovered in the urine within 48 hours as either unchanged venlafaxine, unconjugated ODV, conjugated ODV, or other minor metabolites.

The half-lives of venlafaxine and its active metabolite O-desmethylvenlafaxine (ODV) are increased in patients with renal and hepatic impairment.

Administration of Efexor XL with food has no effect on the absorption of venlafaxine, or on the subsequent formation of ODV.

Subject age and sex do not significantly affect the pharmacokinetics of venlafaxine. No accumulation of venlafaxine or ODV has been observed during chronic administration in healthy subjects.

The extended release formulation of venlafaxine contains spheroids which release the drug slowly into the digestive tract. The insoluble portion of these spheroids is eliminated and may be seen in the stools.

5.3 Preclinical safety data

Studies with venlafaxine in rats and mice revealed no evidence of carcinogenesis. Venlafaxine was not mutagenic in a wide range of *in vitro* and *in vivo* tests.

Reduced fertility was observed in a study in which both male and female rats were exposed to the major metabolite of venlafaxine (ODV). This exposure was approximately 2 to 3 times that of a human dose of 225mg/day.

6. PHARMACEUTICAL PARTICULARS

6.1 List of excipients

Microcrystalline cellulose, ethylcellulose, hydroxypropyl methylcellulose, gelatin, red and yellow iron oxides (E172), titanium dioxide (E171) and printing ink.

6.2 Incompatibilities

Not applicable.

6.3 Shelf life

Three years.

6.4 Special precautions for storage

Store in a dry place at room temperature (at or below 25°C).

6.5 Nature and contents of container

PVC/ACLAR/aluminium foil blister packs of 14, 28 or 30 capsules.

High-density polyethylene (HDPE) bottles of 50 or 100 capsules.

6.6 Special precautions for disposal and other handling

Not applicable

7. MARKETING AUTHORISATION HOLDER

John Wyeth and Brother Limited

trading as: Wyeth Laboratories

Huntercombe Lane South, Taplow, Maidenhead,

Berks SL6 0PH

8. MARKETING AUTHORISATION NUMBER(S)

Efexor XL 75mg: PL 00011/0223

Efexor XL 150mg: PL 00011/0224

9. DATE OF FIRST AUTHORISATION/RENEWAL OF THE AUTHORISATION

5 August 1997

10. DATE OF REVISION OF THE TEXT

7 March 2008

* Trade mark

Further information may be obtained from:

Wyeth Pharmaceuticals, Huntercombe Lane South,

Taplow, Maidenhead, Berkshire, SL6 0PH

Telephone: 01628 415330

Effentora 100, 200, 400, 600 and 800 micrograms buccal tablets

(Cephalon (UK) Limited)

1. NAME OF THE MEDICINAL PRODUCT

Effentora®▼ 100, 200, 400, 600 and 800 micrograms buccal tablets

2. QUALITATIVE AND QUANTITATIVE COMPOSITION

Each buccal tablet contains 100, 200, 400, 600 and 800 micrograms fentanyl (as citrate).

Excipient(s): Each 100 micrograms tablet contains 8 mg of sodium. Each 200 micrograms tablet contains 16 mg of sodium. Each 400 micrograms tablet contains 16 mg of sodium. Each 600 micrograms tablet contains 16 mg of sodium. Each 800 micrograms tablet contains 16 mg of sodium.

For a full list of excipients, see section 6.1.

3. PHARMACEUTICAL FORM

Buccal tablet.

Flat-faced, white, round bevelled-edge tablet, embossed on one side with a "C" and on the other side with "1" for 100 micrograms tablet, "2" for 200 micrograms tablet, "4" for 400 micrograms tablet, "6" for 600 micrograms tablet and "8" for 800 micrograms tablet.

4. CLINICAL PARTICULARS

4.1 Therapeutic indications

Effentora is indicated for the treatment of breakthrough pain (BTP) in adults with cancer who are already receiving maintenance opioid therapy for chronic cancer pain.

BTP is a transitory exacerbation of pain that occurs on a background of otherwise controlled persistent pain.

Patients receiving maintenance opioid therapy are those who are taking at least 60 mg of oral morphine daily, at least 25 micrograms of transdermal fentanyl per hour, at least 30 mg of oxycodone daily, at least 8 mg of oral hydromorphone daily or an equianalgesic dose of another opioid for a week or longer.

4.2 Posology and method of administration

Treatment should be initiated by and remain under the guidance of a physician experienced in the management of opioid therapy in cancer patients. Physicians should keep in mind the potential of abuse of fentanyl.

Dose titration

Effentora should be individually titrated to an "effective" dose that provides adequate analgesia and minimises undesirable effects. In clinical studies, the effective dose of Effentora for BTP was not predictable from the daily maintenance dose of opioid.

Patients should be carefully monitored until an effective dose is reached.

Titration in patients not switching from other fentanyl containing products

The initial dose of Effentora should be 100 micrograms, titrating upwards as necessary through the range of available tablets strengths (100, 200, 400, 600, 800 micrograms).

Titration in patients switching from other fentanyl containing products

Due to different absorption profiles, switching must not be done at a 1:1 ratio. If switching from another oral fentanyl citrate product, independent dose titration with Effentora is required as bioavailability between products differs significantly. However, in these patients, a starting dose higher than 100 micrograms may be considered.

Method of titration

During titration, if adequate analgesia is not obtained within 30 minutes after the start of administration of a single tablet, a second Effentora tablet of the same strength may be used.

If treatment of a BTP episode requires more than one tablet, an increase in dose to the next higher available strength should be considered to treat the next BTP episode.

During titration, multiple tablets may be used: up to four 100 micrograms or up to four 200 micrograms tablets may be used to treat a single episode of BTP during dose titration according to the following schedule:

- If the initial 100 micrograms tablet is not efficacious, the patient can be instructed to treat the next episode of BTP with two 100 micrograms tablets. It is recommended that one tablet should be placed in each side of the mouth. If this dose is considered to be the effective dose, treatment of successive episodes of BTP may be continued with a single 200 micrograms tablet of Effentora.
- If a single 200 micrograms tablet of Effentora (or two 100 micrograms tablets) is not considered to be efficacious the patient can be instructed to use two 200 micrograms tablets (or four 100 micrograms tablets) to treat the next episode of BTP. It is recommended that two tablets should be placed in each side of the mouth. If this dose is considered to be the effective dose, treatment of successive episodes of BTP may be continued with a single 400 micrograms tablet of Effentora.
- For titration to 600 micrograms and 800 micrograms, tablets of 200 micrograms should be used.

Doses above 800 micrograms were not evaluated in clinical studies.

No more than two tablets should be used to treat any individual BTP episode, except when titrating using up to four tablets as described above.

Patients should wait at least 4 hours before treating another BTP episode with Effentora during titration.

Maintenance therapy

Once an effective dose has been established during titration, patients should continue to take this dose as a single tablet of that given strength.

Patients should wait at least 4 hours before treating another BTP episode with Effentora during maintenance therapy.

Dose readjustment

Generally, the maintenance dose of Effentora should be increased when a patient requires more than one dose per BTP episode for several consecutive BTP episodes.

Dose readjustment of Effentora and/or of the background opioid therapy may be required if patients consistently present with more than four BTP episodes per 24 hours.

Discontinuation of therapy

Effentora should be immediately discontinued if no longer required.

Use in children and adolescents:

Effentora is not recommended for use in children and adolescents below 18 years due to a lack of data on safety and efficacy.

Use in the elderly (older than 65 years):

In clinical studies patients older than 65 years tended to titrate to a lower effective dose than younger patients. It is recommended that increased caution should be exercised in titrating the dose of Effentora in elderly patients.

Hepatic or renal impairment:

Effentora should be administered with caution to patients with moderate or severe hepatic or renal impairment (see section 4.4).

Patients with xerostomia:

Patients experiencing xerostomia are advised to drink water to moisten the buccal cavity prior to administration of Effentora. If this recommendation does not result in an appropriate effervescence, then a switch of therapy may be advised.

Method of administration:

Effentora tablet once exposed to moisture utilises an effervescent reaction to deliver the active substance. Therefore patients should be instructed not to open the blister until ready to place the tablet in the buccal cavity.

Opening the blister package

Patients should be instructed NOT to attempt to push the tablet through the blister because this could damage the buccal tablet. The correct method of releasing the tablet from the blister is:

One of the blister units should be separated from the blister card by tearing it apart at the perforations. The blister unit should then be flexed along the line printed on the backing foil where indicated. The backing foil should be peeled back to expose the tablet.

Patients should be instructed not to attempt to crush or split the tablet.

The tablet should not be stored once removed from the blister package as the tablet integrity can not be guaranteed and a risk of accidental exposure to a tablet can occur.

Tablet administration

Patients should remove the tablet from the blister unit and immediately place the entire Effentora tablet in the upper portion of the buccal cavity (above an upper rear molar between the cheek and gum).

Effentora should be placed and retained within the buccal cavity for a period sufficient to allow disintegration of the tablet which usually takes approximately 14-25 minutes.

The Effentora tablet should not be sucked, chewed or swallowed, as this will result in lower plasma concentrations than when taken as directed.

After 30 minutes, if remnants from the Effentora tablet remain, they may be swallowed with a glass of water.

The length of time that the tablet takes to fully disintegrate following oromucosal administration does not appear to affect early systemic exposure to fentanyl.

Patients should not consume any food and drink when a tablet is in the buccal cavity.

In case of buccal mucosa irritation, a change in tablet placement within the buccal cavity should be recommended.

4.3 Contraindications

Hypersensitivity to the active substance or to any of the excipients.

Patients without maintenance opioid therapy (see section 4.1) as there is an increased risk of respiratory depression.

Severe respiratory depression or severe obstructive lung conditions.

4.4 Special warnings and precautions for use

Patients and their carers must be instructed that Effentora contains an active substance in an amount that can be fatal to a child, and therefore to keep all tablets out of the reach and sight of children.

In order to minimise the risks of opioid-related undesirable effects and to identify the effective dose, it is imperative that patients be monitored closely by health professionals during the titration process.

It is important that the long acting opioid treatment used to treat the patient's persistent pain has been stabilised before Effentora therapy begins.

As with all opioids, there is a risk of clinically significant respiratory depression associated with the use of fentanyl. Particular caution should be used when titrating Effentora in patients with non-severe chronic obstructive pulmonary disease or other medical conditions predisposing them to respiratory depression, as even normally therapeutic doses of Effentora may further decrease respiratory drive to the point of respiratory failure.

Effentora should only be administered with extreme caution in patients who may be particularly susceptible to the intracranial effects of CO_2 retention, such as those with evidence of increased intracranial pressure or impaired consciousness. Opioids may obscure the clinical course of a patient with a head injury and should be used only if clinically warranted.

Intravenous fentanyl may produce bradycardia. In clinical trials with Effentora, no clear evidence for bradycardia was observed. However, Effentora should be used with caution in patients with pre-existing bradyarrhythmias.

In addition, Effentora should be administered with caution to patients with hepatic or renal impairment. The influence of hepatic and renal impairment on the pharmacokinetics of the medicinal product has not been evaluated, however, when administered intravenously the clearance of fentanyl has been shown to be altered in hepatic and renal impairment due to alterations in metabolic clearance and plasma proteins. After administration of Effentora, impaired hepatic and renal function may both increase the bioavailability of swallowed fentanyl and decrease its systemic clearance, which could lead to increased and prolonged opioid effects. Therefore, special care should be taken during the titration process in patients with moderate or severe hepatic or renal impairment.

Figure 1

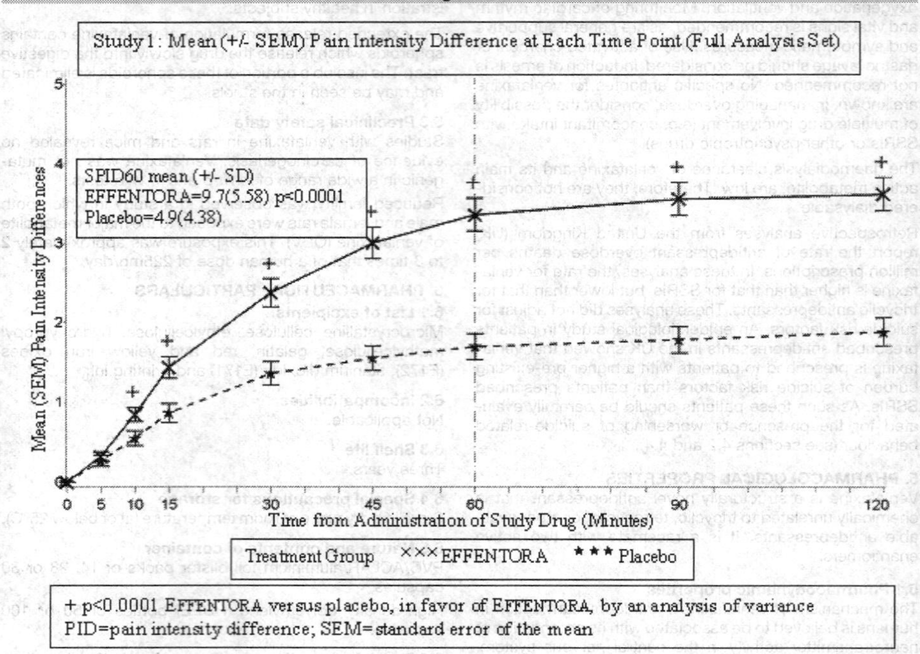

Careful consideration should be given to patients with hypovolaemia and hypotension.

Tolerance and physical and/or psychological dependence may develop upon repeated administration of opioids such as fentanyl. However, iatrogenic addiction following therapeutic use of opioids is rare.

This medicinal product contains

8 mg sodium per 100 micrograms tablet. 16 mg sodium per 200 micrograms tablet. 16 mg sodium per 400 micrograms tablet. 16 mg sodium per 600 micrograms tablet. 16 mg sodium per 800 micrograms tablet. To be taken into consideration by patients on a controlled sodium diet.

4.5 Interaction with other medicinal products and other forms of interaction

Fentanyl is metabolised mainly via the human cytochrome P450 3A4 isoenzyme system (CYP3A4), therefore potential interactions may occur when Effentora is given concurrently with agents that affect CYP3A4 activity. Coadministration with agents that induce 3A4 activity may reduce the efficacy of Effentora. The concomitant use of Effentora with strong CYP3A4 inhibitors (e.g., ritonavir, ketoconazole, itraconazole, troleandomycin, clarithromycin, and nelfinavir) or moderate CYP3A4 inhibitors (e.g., amprenavir, aprepitant, diltiazem, erythromycin, fluconazole, fosamprenavir, grapefruit juice, and verapamil) may result in increased fentanyl plasma concentrations, potentially causing serious adverse drug reactions including fatal respiratory depression. Patients receiving Effentora concomitantly with moderate or strong CYP3A4 inhibitors should be carefully monitored for an extended period of time. Dosage increase should be done with caution.

The concomitant use of other central nervous system depressants, including other opioids, sedatives or hypnotics, general anaesthetics, phenothiazines, tranquillisers, skeletal muscle relaxants, sedating antihistamines and alcohol may produce additive depressant effects.

Effentora is not recommended for use in patients who have received monoamine oxidase (MAO) inhibitors within 14 days because severe and unpredictable potentiation by MAO inhibitors has been reported with opioid analgesics.

The concomitant use of partial opioid agonists/antagonists (e.g. buprenorphine, nalbuphine, pentazocine) is not recommended. They have high affinity to opioid receptors with relatively low intrinsic activity and therefore partially antagonise the analgesic effect of fentanyl and may induce withdrawal symptoms in opioid dependant patients.

4.6 Pregnancy and lactation

There are no adequate data from the use of fentanyl in pregnant women. Studies in animals have shown reproductive toxicity (see section 5.3). The potential risk for humans is unknown. Effentora should not be used in pregnancy unless clearly necessary.

Following long-term treatment, fentanyl may cause withdrawal in the new-born infant.

It is advised not to use fentanyl during labour and delivery (including caesarean section) because fentanyl passes through the placenta and may cause respiratory depression in the foetus. If Effentora is administered, an antidote for the child should be readily available.

Fentanyl passes into breast milk and may cause sedation and respiratory depression in the breast-fed child. Fentanyl should only be used by breastfeeding women if the benefits outweigh the potential risks for both mother and child.

4.7 Effects on ability to drive and use machines

No studies of the effects on the ability to drive and use machines have been performed. However, opioid analgesics impair the mental and/or physical ability required for the performance of potentially dangerous tasks (e.g., driving a car or operating machinery). Patients should be advised not to drive or operate machinery if they experience somnolence, dizziness, or visual disturbance while taking Effentora and not to drive or operate machinery until they know how they react.

4.8 Undesirable effects

Typical opioid undesirable effects are to be expected with Effentora. Frequently, these will cease or decrease in intensity with continued use of the medicinal product, as the patient is titrated to the most appropriate dose. However, the most serious adverse reactions are respiratory depression (potentially leading to apnoea or respiratory arrest), circulatory depression, hypotension and shock and all patients should be closely monitored for these.

The clinical studies of Effentora were designed to evaluate safety and efficacy in treating BTP and all patients were also taking concomitant opioids, such as sustained-release morphine or transdermal fentanyl, for their persistent pain. Therefore it is not possible to definitively separate the effects of Effentora alone.

The adverse reactions considered to be at least possibly-related to treatment from clinical studies were as follows (frequencies defined as: very common ⩾1/10, common ⩾1/100 to <1/10, uncommon ⩾ 1/1,000 to < 1/100; within each frequency grouping, undesirable effects are presented in order of decreasing seriousness):

(see Table 1 on next page)

4.9 Overdose

The symptoms of fentanyl overdose are expected to be similar in nature to those of intravenous fentanyl and other opioids, and are an extension of its pharmacological actions, with the most serious significant effect being respiratory depression.

Immediate management of opioid overdose includes removal of the Effentora buccal tablet, if still in the mouth, ensuring a patent airway, physical and verbal stimulation of the patient, assessment of the level of consciousness, ventilatory and circulatory status, and assisted ventilation (ventilatory support) if necessary.

For treatment of overdose (accidental ingestion) in the opioid-naive person, intravenous access should be obtained and naloxone or other opioid antagonists should be employed as clinically indicated. The duration of respiratory depression following overdose may be longer than the effects of the opioid antagonist's action (e.g., the half-life of naloxone ranges from 30 to 81 minutes) and repeated administration may be necessary. Consult the Summary of Product Characteristics of the individual opioid antagonist for details about such use.

For treatment of overdose in opioid-maintained patients, intravenous access should be obtained. The judicious use of naloxone or another opioid antagonist may be warranted in some instances, but it is associated with the risk of precipitating an acute withdrawal syndrome.

Although muscle rigidity interfering with respiration has not been seen following the use of Effentora, this is possible with fentanyl and other opioids. If it occurs, it should be managed by the use of assisted ventilation, by an opioid antagonist, and as a final alternative, by a neuromuscular blocking agent.

5. PHARMACOLOGICAL PROPERTIES

5.1 Pharmacodynamic properties

Pharmacotherapeutic group: analgesics; opioids; phenylpiperidine derivatives; ATC code N02AB03.

Fentanyl is an opioid analgesic, interacting predominantly with the opioid μ-receptor. Its primary therapeutic actions are analgesia and sedation. Secondary pharmacological effects are respiratory depression, bradycardia, hypothermia, constipation, miosis, physical dependence and euphoria.

The analgesic effects of fentanyl are related to its plasma level. In general, the effective concentration and the concentration at which toxicity occurs increase with increasing tolerance to opioids. The rate of development of tolerance varies widely among individuals. As a result, the dose of Effentora should be individually titrated to achieve the desired effect (see section 4.2).

All opioid μ-receptor agonists, including fentanyl, produce dose dependent respiratory depression. The risk of respiratory depression is less in patients receiving chronic opioid therapy as these patients will develop tolerance to respiratory depressant effects.

The safety and efficacy of Effentora have been evaluated in patients taking the drug at the onset of the breakthrough pain episode. Pre-emptive use of Effentora for predictable pain episodes was not investigated in the clinical trials. Two double-blind, randomized, placebo-controlled crossover studies have been conducted involving a total of 248 patients with BTP and cancer who experienced on average 1 to 4 episodes of BTP per day while taking maintenance opioid therapy. During an initial open-label phase, patients were titrated to an effective dose of Effentora. Patients who identified an effective dose entered the double-blind phase of the study. The primary efficacy variable was the patient's assessment of pain intensity. Patients assessed pain intensity on a 11-point scale. For each BTP episode, pain intensity was assessed prior to and at several time points after treatment.

Sixty-seven percent of the patients were able to be titrated to an effective dose.

In the pivotal clinical study (study 1), the primary endpoint was the average sum of differences in pain intensity scores from dosing to 60 minutes, inclusive (SPID60), which was statistically significant compared to placebo ($p < 0.0001$).

(see Figure 1 on previous page)

(see Figure 2 on next page)

In the second pivotal study (study 2), the primary endpoint was SPID30, which was also statistically significant compared to placebo ($p < 0.0001$).

Statistically significant improvement in pain intensity difference was seen with Effentora versus placebo as early as 10 minutes in Study 1 and as early as 15 minutes (earliest time point measured) in Study 2. These differences continued to be significant at each subsequent time point in each individual study.

5.2 Pharmacokinetic properties

General introduction

Fentanyl is highly lipophilic and can be absorbed very rapidly through the oral mucosa and more slowly by the conventional gastrointestinal route. It is subject to first-pass hepatic and intestinal metabolism and the metabolites do not contribute to fentanyl's therapeutic effects.

Effentora employs a delivery technology which utilises an effervescent reaction which enhances the rate and extent of fentanyl absorbed through the buccal mucosa. Transient pH changes accompanying the effervescent reaction may optimise dissolution (at a lower pH) and membrane permeation (at a higher pH).

Dwell time (defined as the length of time that the tablet takes to fully disintegrate following buccal administration), does not affect early systemic exposure to fentanyl.

The effect of renal or hepatic impairment on the pharmacokinetics of Effentora has not been studied.

Absorption:

Following oromucosal administration of Effentora, fentanyl is readily absorbed with an absolute bioavailability of 65%. The absorption profile of Effentora is largely the result of an initial rapid absorption from the buccal mucosa, with peak plasma concentrations following venous sampling generally attained within an hour after oromucosal administration. Approximately 50% of the total dose administered is rapidly absorbed transmucosally and becomes systemically available. The remaining half of the total dose is swallowed and slowly absorbed from the gastrointestinal tract. About 30% of the amount swallowed (50% of the total dose) escapes hepatic and intestinal first-pass elimination and becomes systemically available.

The main pharmacokinetic parameters are shown in the following table.

Table 1

	Very common	Common	Uncommon
Investigations			Platelet count decreased Heart rate increased Haematocrit decreased Haemoglobin decreased
Cardiac disorders			Tachycardia, Bradycardia
Blood and lymphatic system disorders			Anaemia Neutropenia Thrombocytopenia
Nervous system disorders	Dizziness	Dysgeusia Somnolence Lethargy Headache Tremor Sedation	Depressed level of consciousness Disturbance in attention Cognitive disorder Hypoaesthesia Balance disorder Migraine Motor dysfunction Dysarthria
Eye disorders			Visual disturbance Ocular hyperaemia Abnormal sensation in eye Photopsia Blurred vision Visual acuity reduced
Ear and labyrinth disorders			Vertigo Tinnitus Ear discomfort
Respiratory, thoracic and mediastinal disorders			Dyspnoea Pharyngolaryngeal pain
Gastrointestinal disorders	Nausea	Vomiting Constipation Stomatitis Dry mouth Diarrhoea	Mouth ulceration Oral hypoaesthesia Oral discomfort Oral mucosal blistering Oral mucosal discolouration Oral soft tissue disorder Glossodynia Tongue blistering Gingival pain Stomach discomfort Tongue ulceration Tongue disorder Dyspepsia Abdominal pain Oesophagitis Gastrooesophagal reflux disease Chapped lips Dry lip Tooth disorder Toothache
Renal and urinary disorders			Urinary retention
Skin and subcutaneous tissue disorders		Pruritis Hyperhydrosis	Cold sweat Facial swelling Rash Generalised pruritus Alopecia Onychorrhexis
Musculoskeletal and connective tissue disorders			Myalgia Muscle twitching Muscular weakness Back pain
Metabolism and nutrition disorders			Anorexia
Infections and infestations			Oral candidiasis Pharyngitis Oral pustule
Injury, poisoning and procedural complications			Fall
Neoplasms benign, malignant and unspecified (including cysts and polyps)			Multiple myeloma
Vascular disorders			Flushing Hypertension Hot flush
General disorders and administration site conditions	Application site reactions including pain, ulcer, irritation, paraesthesia, anaesthesia, erythema, oedema, swelling and vesicles	Fatigue	Asthenia Malaise Sluggishness Chest discomfort Feeling abnormal Feeling jittery Thirst Feeling cold Chills Feeling hot Drug withdrawal syndrome
Psychiatric disorders		Disorientation Euphoric mood	Anxiety Nervousness Hallucination Visual hallucination Insomnia Confusional state

Figure 2

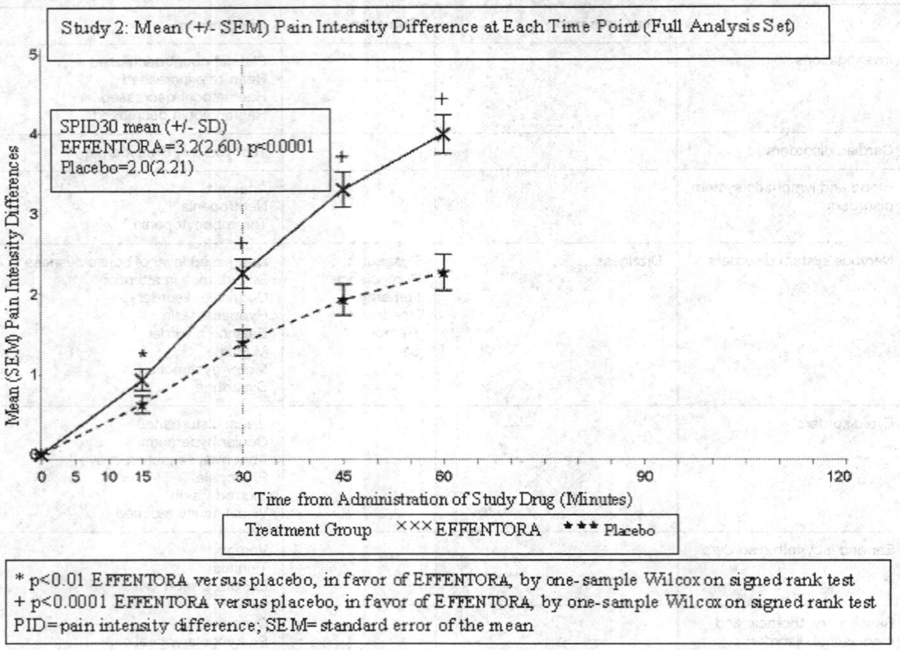

Figure 3

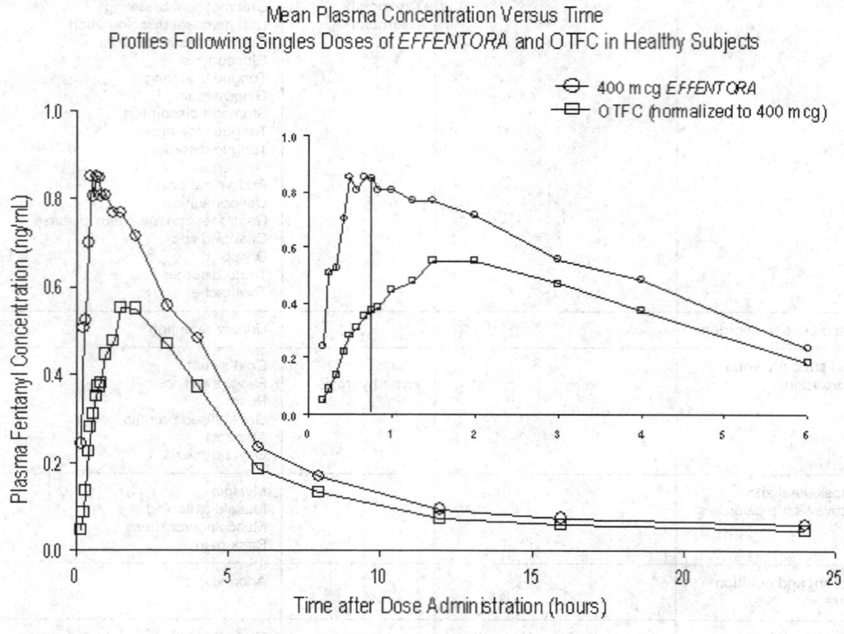

OTFC data was dose adjusted (800 mcg to 400 mcg)

<u>Pharmacokinetic Parameters* in Adult Subjects Receiving Effentora</u>

Pharmacokinetic parameter (mean)	Effentora 400 micrograms
Absolute bioavailability	65% (± 20%)
Fraction absorbed transmucosally	48% (± 31.8%)
T_{max} (minute) **	46.8 (20-240)
C_{max} (ng/ml)	1.02 (± 0.42)
$AUC_{0\text{-}tmax}$ (ng.hr/ml)	0.40 (± 0.18)
$AUC_{0\text{-}inf}$ (ng.hr/ml)	6.48 (± 2.98)

* Based on venous blood samples (plasma). Fentanyl citrate concentrations obtained in serum were higher than in plasma: Serum AUC and Cmax were approximately 20% and 30% higher than plasma AUC and Cmax, respectively. The reason of this difference is unknown.

** Data for T_{max} presented as median (range).

In pharmacokinetic studies that compared the absolute and relative bioavailability of Effentora and oral transmucosal fentanyl citrate (OTFC), the rate and extent of fentanyl absorption in Effentora demonstrated exposure that was between 30% to 50% greater than that for oral transmucosal fentanyl citrate. If switching from another oral fentanyl citrate product, independent dose titration with Effentora is required as bioavailability between products differs significantly. However, in these patients, a starting dose higher than 100 micrograms may be considered.

(see Figure 3 above)

Differences in exposure with Effentora were observed in a clinical study with patients with grade 1 mucositis. C_{max} and $AUC_{0\text{-}8}$ were 1% and 25% higher in patients with mucositis compared to those without mucositis, respectively. The differences observed were not clinically significant.

<u>Distribution</u>

Fentanyl is highly lipophilic and is well distributed beyond the vascular system, with a large apparent volume of distribution. After buccal administration of Effentora, fentanyl undergoes initial rapid distribution that represents an equilibration of fentanyl between plasma and the highly perfused tissues (brain, heart and lungs). Subsequently, fentanyl is redistributed between the deep tissue compartment (muscle and fat) and the plasma.

The plasma protein binding of fentanyl is 80% to 85%. The main binding protein is alpha-1-acid glycoprotein, but both albumin and lipoproteins contribute to some extent. The free fraction of fentanyl increases with acidosis.

<u>Biotransformation</u>

The metabolic pathways following buccal administration of Effentora have not been characterised in clinical studies. Fentanyl is metabolised in the liver and in the intestinal mucosa to norfentanyl by CYP3A4 isoform. Norfentanyl is not pharmacologically active in animal studies. More than 90% of the administered dose of fentanyl is eliminated by biotransformation to N-dealkylated and hydroxylated inactive metabolites.

<u>Elimination</u>

Following the intravenous administration of fentanyl, less than 7% of the administered dose is excreted unchanged in the urine, and only about 1% is excreted unchanged in the faeces. The metabolites are mainly excreted in the urine, while faecal excretion is less important.

Following the administration of Effentora, the terminal elimination phase of fentanyl is the result of the redistribution between plasma and a deep tissue compartment. This phase of elimination is slow, resulting in a median terminal elimination half-life $t_{1/2}$ of approximately 22 hours following buccal administration of the effervescent formulation and approximately 18 hours following intravenous administration. The total plasma clearance of fentanyl following intravenous administration is approximately 42 L/h.

<u>Linearity/non-linearity</u>

Dose proportionality from 100 micrograms to 1000 micrograms has been demonstrated.

5.3 Preclinical safety data

Non-clinical data reveal no special hazard for humans based on conventional studies of safety pharmacology, repeated dose toxicity and genotoxicity.

Studies with female rats revealed reduced fertility and enhanced embryonal mortality. More recent studies showed that effects on the embryo were due to maternal toxicity and not to direct effects of the substance on the developing embryo. In a study on pre- and postnatal development the survival rate of offspring was significantly reduced at doses which slightly reduced maternal weight. This effect could either be due to altered maternal care or a direct effect of fentanyl on the pups. Effects on somatic development and behaviour of the offspring were not observed. Teratogenic effects have not been demonstrated.

Long term carcinogenicity studies have not been performed.

6. PHARMACEUTICAL PARTICULARS

6.1 List of excipients

Mannitol

Sodium starch glycolate type A

Sodium hydrogen carbonate

Sodium carbonate anhydrous

Citric acid anhydrous

Magnesium stearate

6.2 Incompatibilities

Not applicable.

6.3 Shelf life

2 years

6.4 Special precautions for storage

Store in the original package in order to protect from moisture.

6.5 Nature and contents of container

Aluminium laminated blister of PVC/Al foil/Polyamide/PVC with paper/polyester lidding.

Blister packs are supplied in cartons of 4 or 28 tablets. Not all pack-sizes may be marketed.

6.6 Special precautions for disposal and other handling

Patients and carers must be advised to dispose of any unopened tablets remaining from a prescription as soon as they are no longer needed.

Any used or unused but no longer required product or waste material should be disposed of in accordance with local requirements.

7. MARKETING AUTHORISATION HOLDER

Cephalon Europe

5 rue Charles Martigny

F-94700 Maisons-Alfort

France

8. MARKETING AUTHORISATION NUMBER(S)

EU/1/08/441/001-010

9. DATE OF FIRST AUTHORISATION/RENEWAL OF THE AUTHORISATION

04 April 2008

10. DATE OF REVISION OF THE TEXT

Detailed information on this product is available on the website of the European Medicines Agency (EMEA) http://www.emea.europa.eu.

Effico Tonic

(Forest Laboratories UK Limited)

1. NAME OF THE MEDICINAL PRODUCT
EFFICO TONIC

2. QUALITATIVE AND QUANTITATIVE COMPOSITION
Each 5ml oral liquid contains:

Vitamin B_1 (Thiamine Hydrochloride)	0.18mg
Nicotinamide	2.10mg
Caffeine	20.20mg

3. PHARMACEUTICAL FORM
Clear colourless to pale straw coloured slightly viscous liquid

4. CLINICAL PARTICULARS

4.1 Therapeutic indications
A gentle pick-me-up and appetite promoter to combat the depressing effects that occur when tired, listless, run down, after a weakening illness or hospitalisation and due to too little nicotinamide and B_1.

4.2 Posology and method of administration
Adults and elderly:
10ml immediately before meals, three times a day.
Children (over 6 years):
2.5 to 5 ml taken as for adults.
Method of administration - oral use

4.3 Contraindications
Use in patients with known hypersensitivity to the product.

4.4 Special warnings and precautions for use
None stated

4.5 Interaction with other medicinal products and other forms of interaction
None stated

4.6 Pregnancy and lactation
Contra-indicated in pregnancy and lactation unless considered essential by the physician.

4.7 Effects on ability to drive and use machines
None stated

4.8 Undesirable effects
None stated

4.9 Overdose
None stated

5. PHARMACOLOGICAL PROPERTIES

5.1 Pharmacodynamic properties
Caffeine is a mild CNS stimulant and its inclusion in the formulation helps counteract symptoms of tiredness and listlessness after a weakening illness or hospitalisation.

Thiamine and nicotinamide are present as vitamin supplements. Deficiencies of these two vitamins produce symptoms including fatigue and lethargy with anorexia or loss of appetite.

5.2 Pharmacokinetic properties
Nicotinamide is readily absorbed from the gastrointestinal tract. It has a short half-life and after low doses, the principle metabolites are the N-methyl, 2- and 4- pyridone derivatives.

Thiamine is absorbed from the gastrointestinal tract and widely distributed to most body tissues. It is not stored in the body and amounts in excess of the body's requirements are excreted in the urine as unchanged thiamine or as metabolites.

Caffeine is absorbed readily after oral administration. The average half-life is reported to be 3.5 hours. Peak plasma concentrations of 1.5 to 1.8 mg/litre have been measured after a 100mg oral dose.

5.3 Preclinical safety data
There are no preclinical data of relevance to the prescriber which are additional to that already included in other sections of the SPC.

6. PHARMACEUTICAL PARTICULARS

6.1 List of excipients
Ethanol 96%
Sodium Benzoate
Citric acid
Concentrated Hydrochloric Acid
Sucrose
Compound Gentian Infusion
H & R Summer Fruit flavour 288234
Purified Water

6.2 Incompatibilities
None stated

6.3 Shelf life
Clear colourless or amber glass – 3 years
Clear colourless polyethene terephthalate (PET) or orange coloured PET – 2 years

6.4 Special precautions for storage
Store away from direct sunlight below 25°C

6.5 Nature and contents of container
Clear colourless or amber glass bottle, or clear colourless polyethene terephthalate (PET) or orange coloured PET bottle with food-grade polypropylene tamper-evident cap pigmented with titanium dioxide containing 300ml or 500ml.

6.6 Special precautions for disposal and other handling
None stated

7. MARKETING AUTHORISATION HOLDER
Forest Laboratories UK Limited
Bourne Road
Bexley
Kent DA5 1NX

8. MARKETING AUTHORISATION NUMBER(S)
PL 0108/5013

9. DATE OF FIRST AUTHORISATION/RENEWAL OF THE AUTHORISATION
24th November 1988 / 24 November 2003

10. DATE OF REVISION OF THE TEXT
March 2009

11. Legal Category
GSL

Efient 5mg & 10mg film-coated tablets (Eli Lilly and Company Ltd Daiichi Sankyo UK Limited)

(Eli Lilly and Company Limited)

1. NAME OF THE MEDICINAL PRODUCT
Efient*▼ 5 mg film-coated tablets.
Efient ▼10 mg film-coated tablets.

2. QUALITATIVE AND QUANTITATIVE COMPOSITION
Each tablet contains 5 mg prasugrel (as hydrochloride).
Excipient: Each tablet contains 2.7 mg lactose.
Each tablet contains 10 mg prasugrel (as hydrochloride).
Excipient: Each tablet contains 2.1 mg lactose.
For a full list of excipients, see section 6.1.

3. PHARMACEUTICAL FORM
Film-coated tablet (tablet).
Yellow and double-arrow-shaped tablets, debossed with "5 MG" on one side and "4760" on the other.
Film-coated tablet (tablet).
Beige and double-arrow-shaped tablets, debossed with "10 MG"on one side and "4759" on the other.

4. CLINICAL PARTICULARS

4.1 Therapeutic indications
Efient, co-administered with acetylsalicylic acid (ASA), is indicated for the prevention of atherothrombotic events in patients with acute coronary syndrome (i.e., unstable angina, non-ST segment elevation myocardial infarction [UA/NSTEMI] or ST segment elevation myocardial infarction [STEMI]) undergoing primary or delayed percutaneous coronary intervention (PCI).

For further information please refer to section 5.1.

4.2 Posology and method of administration
Posology
Adults
Efient should be initiated with a single 60 mg loading dose and then continued at 10 mg once a day. Patients taking Efient should also take ASA daily (75 mg to 325 mg).

In patients with acute coronary syndrome (ACS) who are managed with PCI, premature discontinuation of any antiplatelet agent, including Efient, could result in an increased risk of thrombosis, myocardial infarction or death due to the patient's underlying disease. A treatment of up to 12 months is recommended, unless the discontinuation of Efient is clinically indicated (see sections 4.4 and 5.1).

Patients ⩾ 75 years old
The use of Efient in patients ⩾ 75 years of age is generally not recommended. If, after a careful individual benefit/risk evaluation by the prescribing physician (see section 4.4), treatment is deemed necessary in the patients age group ⩾ 75 years, then following a 60 mg loading dose a reduced maintenance dose of 5 mg should be prescribed. Patients ⩾ 75 years of age have greater sensitivity to bleeding and higher exposure to the active metabolite of prasugrel (see sections 4.4, 4.8, 5.1 and 5.2). The evidence for the 5 mg dose is based only on pharmacodynamic/pharmacokinetic analyses and no clinical data currently exist on the safety of this dose in the patients age group ⩾ 75 years.

Patients weighing <60 kg
Efient should be given as a single 60 mg loading dose and then continued at a 5 mg once-daily dose. The 10 mg maintenance dose is not recommended. This is due to an increase in exposure to the active metabolite of prasugrel, and an increased risk of bleeding in patients with body weight <60 kg when given a 10 mg once-daily dose, compared with patients ⩾60 kg. Efficacy and safety of the 5 mg dose have not been prospectively assessed (see sections 4.4, 4.8 and 5.2).

Renal impairment
No dose adjustment is necessary for patients with renal impairment, including patients with end-stage renal disease (see section 5.2). There is limited therapeutic experience in patients with renal impairment (see section 4.4).

Hepatic impairment
No dose adjustment is necessary in subjects with mild to moderate hepatic impairment (Child-Pugh class A and B) (see section 5.2). There is limited therapeutic experience in patients with mild and moderate hepatic dysfunction (see section 4.4).

Children and adolescents
Efient is not recommended for use in children below age 18 due to a lack of data on safety and efficacy.

Method of administration
For oral use. Efient may be administered with or without food. Administration of the 60 mg prasugrel loading dose in the fasted state may provide most rapid onset of action (see section 5.2). Do not crush or break the tablet.

4.3 Contraindications
Hypersensitivity to the active substance or to any of the excipients.
Active pathological bleeding.
History of stroke or transient ischaemic attack (TIA).
Severe hepatic impairment (Child-Pugh class C).

4.4 Special warnings and precautions for use
Bleeding risk
In the phase 3 clinical trial, key exclusion criteria included an increased risk of bleeding; anaemia; thrombocytopenia; a history of pathological intracranial findings. Patients with acute coronary syndromes undergoing PCI treated with Efient and ASA showed an increased risk of major and minor bleeding according to the TIMI classification system. Therefore, the use of Efient in patients at increased risk of bleeding should only be considered when the benefits in terms of prevention of ischaemic events are deemed to outweigh the risk of serious bleedings. This concern applies especially to patients:

- ⩾75 years of age (see below).
- with a propensity to bleed (e.g., due to recent trauma, recent surgery, recent or recurrent gastrointestinal bleeding, or active peptic ulcer disease).
- with body weight <60 kg (see sections 4.2 and 4.8). In these patients the 10 mg maintenance dose is not recommended. A 5 mg maintenance dose should be used.
- with concomitant administration of medicinal products that may increase the risk of bleeding, including oral anticoagulants, clopidogrel, non-steroidal anti-inflammatory drugs (NSAIDs), and fibrinolytics.

The use of Efient in patients ⩾75 years of age is generally not recommended, and should only be undertaken with caution after a careful individual benefit/risk evaluation by the prescribing physician indicates that benefits in terms of prevention of ischaemic events outweigh the risk of serious bleedings. In the phase 3 clinical trial these patients were at greater risk of bleeding, including fatal bleeding, compared to patients <75 years of age. If prescribed, a lower maintenance dose of 5 mg should be used; the 10 mg maintenance dose is not recommended (see sections 4.2 and 4.8).

Therapeutic experience with prasugrel is limited in patients with renal impairment (including ESRD) and in patients with moderate hepatic impairment. These patients may have an increased bleeding risk. Therefore, prasugrel should be used with caution in these patients.

Therapeutic experience with prasugrel is limited in Asian patients. Therefore, prasugrel should be used with caution in these patients.

For patients with active bleeding for whom reversal of the pharmacological effects of Efient is required, platelet transfusion may be appropriate.

Patients should be told that it might take longer than usual to stop bleeding when they take prasugrel (in combination with ASA), and that they should report any unusual bleeding (site or duration) to their physician.

Surgery
Patients should be advised to inform physicians and dentists that they are taking prasugrel before any surgery is scheduled, and before any new medicinal product is taken. If a patient is to undergo elective surgery, and an antiplatelet effect is not desired, Efient should be discontinued at least 7 days prior to surgery. Increased frequency (3-fold) and severity of bleeding may occur in patients undergoing CABG surgery within 7 days of discontinuation of prasugrel (see section 4.8). The benefits and risks of prasugrel should be carefully considered in patients in whom the coronary anatomy has not been defined, and urgent CABG is a possibility.

Thrombotic Thrombocytopenic Purpura (TTP)
TTP has been reported with the use of other thienopyridines. TTP is a serious condition and requires prompt treatment. Efient was not associated with TTP in clinical trials supporting registration.

Lactose

Patients with rare hereditary problems of galactose intolerance, the Lapp lactase deficiency or glucose-galactose malabsorption should not take Efient.

4.5 Interaction with other medicinal products and other forms of interaction

Warfarin: Concomitant administration of Efient with coumarin derivatives other than warfarin has not been studied. Because of the potential for increased risk of bleeding, warfarin (or other coumarin derivatives) and prasugrel should be co-administered with caution (see section 4.4).

Non-steroidal anti-inflammatory drugs (NSAIDs): Concomitant administration with chronic NSAIDs has not been studied. Because of the potential for increased risk of bleeding, chronic NSAIDs (including COX-2 inhibitors) and Efient should be co-administered with caution (see section 4.4).

Efient can be concomitantly administered with medicinal products metabolised by cytochrome P450 enzymes (including statins), or medicinal products that are inducers or inhibitors of cytochrome P450 enzymes. Efient can also be concomitantly administered with ASA, heparin, digoxin, and medicinal products that elevate gastric pH, including proton pump inhibitors and H_2 blockers. Although not studied in specific interaction studies, Efient has been co-administered in the phase 3 clinical trial with low molecular weight heparin, bivalirudin, and GP IIb/IIIa inhibitors (no information available regarding the type of GP IIb/IIIa inhibitor used) without evidence of clinically significant adverse interactions.

Effects of other medicinal products on Efient:

Acetylsalicylic acid: Efient is to be administered concomitantly with acetylsalicylic acid (ASA). Although a pharmacodynamic interaction with ASA leading to an increased risk of bleeding is possible, the demonstration of the efficacy and safety of prasugrel comes from patients concomitantly treated with ASA.

Heparin: A single intravenous bolus dose of unfractionated heparin (100 U/kg) did not significantly alter the prasugrel-mediated inhibition of platelet aggregation. Likewise, prasugrel did not significantly alter the effect of heparin on measures of coagulation. Therefore, both medicinal products can be administered concomitantly. An increased risk of bleeding is possible when Efient is co-administered with heparin.

Statins: Atorvastatin (80 mg daily) did not alter the pharmacokinetics of prasugrel and its inhibition of platelet aggregation. Therefore, statins that are substrates of CYP3A are not anticipated to have an effect on the pharmacokinetics of prasugrel or its inhibition of platelet aggregation.

Medicinal products that elevate gastric pH: Daily co-administration of ranitidine (an H_2 blocker) or lansoprazole (a proton pump inhibitor) did not change the prasugrel active metabolite's AUC and T_{max}, but decreased the C_{max} by 14% and 29%, respectively. In the phase 3 clinical trial, Efient was administered without regard to co-administration of a proton pump inhibitor or H_2 blocker. Administration of the 60 mg prasugrel loading dose without concomitant use of proton pump inhibitors may provide most rapid onset of action.

Inhibitors of CYP3A: Ketoconazole (400 mg daily), a selective and potent inhibitor of CYP3A4 and CYP3A5, did not affect prasugrel-mediated inhibition of platelet aggregation or the prasugrel active metabolite's AUC and T_{max}, but decreased the C_{max} by 34% to 46%. Therefore, CYP3A inhibitors such as azol antifungals, HIV protease inhibitors, clarithromycin, telithromycin, verapamil, diltiazem, indinavir, ciprofloxacin, and grapefruit juice are not anticipated to have a significant effect on the pharmacokinetics of the active metabolite.

Inducers of cytochromes P450: Rifampicin (600 mg daily), a potent inducer of CYP3A and CYP2B6, and an inducer of CYP2C9, CYP2C19, and CYP2C8, did not significantly change the pharmacokinetics of prasugrel. Therefore, known CYP3A inducers such as rifampicin, carbamazepine, and other inducers of cytochromes P450 are not anticipated to have significant effect on the pharmacokinetics of the active metabolite.

Effects of Efient on other medicinal products:

Digoxin: Prasugrel has no clinically significant effect on the pharmacokinetics of digoxin.

Medicinal products metabolised by CYP2C9: Prasugrel did not inhibit CYP2C9, as it did not affect the pharmacokinetics of S-warfarin. Because of the potential for increased risk of bleeding, warfarin and Efient should be co-administered with caution (see section 4.4).

Medicinal products metabolised by CYP2B6: Prasugrel is a weak inhibitor of CYP2B6. In healthy subjects, prasugrel decreased exposure to hydroxybupropion, a CYP2B6-mediated metabolite of bupropion, by 23%. This effect is likely to be of clinical concern only when prasugrel is co-administered with medicinal products for which CYP2B6 is the only metabolic pathway, and have a narrow therapeutic window (e.g., cyclophosphamide, efavirenz).

4.6 Pregnancy and lactation

No clinical study has been conducted in pregnant or lactating women.

Table 1: Incidence of Non-CABG-related bleeding [a] (% Patients)

Event	All ACS		UA/NSTEMI		STEMI	
	Prasugrel[b] +ASA (N=6741)	Clopidogrel[b] +ASA (N=6716)	Prasugrel[b] +ASA (N=5001)	Clopidogrel[b] +ASA (N=4980)	Prasugrel[b] +ASA (N=1740)	Clopidogrel[b] +ASA (N=1736)
TIMI major bleeding[c]	2.2	1.7	2.2	1.6	2.2	2.0
Life-threatening[d]	1.3	0.8	1.3	0.8	1.2	1.0
Fatal	0.3	0.1	0.3	0.1	0.4	0.1
Symptomatic ICH[e]	0.3	0.3	0.3	0.3	0.2	0.2
Requiring inotropes	0.3	0.1	0.3	0.1	0.3	0.2
Requiring surgical intervention	0.3	0.3	0.3	0.3	0.1	0.2
Requiring transfusion (⩾4 units)	0.7	0.5	0.6	0.3	0.8	0.8
TIMI minor bleeding[f]	2.4	1.9	2.3	1.6	2.7	2.6

a Centrally adjudicated events defined by the Thrombolysis in Myocardial Infarction (TIMI) Study Group criteria.

b Other standard therapies were used as appropriate.

c Any intracranial haemorrhage or any clinically overt bleeding associated with a fall in haemoglobin ⩾5 g/dL.

d Life-threatening bleeding is a subset of TIMI major bleeding and includes the types indented below. Patients may be counted in more than one row.

e ICH=intracranial haemorrhage.

f Clinically overt bleeding associated with a fall in haemoglobin of ⩾3 g/dL but <5 g/dL.

Animal studies do not indicate direct harmful effects with respect to pregnancy, embryonal/foetal development, parturition or postnatal development (see section 5.3). Because animal reproduction studies are not always predictive of a human response, Efient should be used during pregnancy only if the potential benefit to the mother justifies the potential risk to the foetus.

It is unknown whether prasugrel is excreted in human breast milk. Animal studies have shown excretion of prasugrel in breast milk. The use of prasugrel during breast-feeding is not recommended.

Prasugrel had no effect on fertility of male and female rats at oral doses up to an exposure 240-times the recommended daily human maintenance dose (based on mg/m²).

4.7 Effects on ability to drive and use machines

No studies on the effects on ability to drive and use machines have been performed. Prasugrel is expected to have no or negligible influence on the ability to drive and use machines.

4.8 Undesirable effects

Safety in patients with acute coronary syndrome undergoing PCI was evaluated in one clopidogrel-controlled study (TRITON) in which 6741 patients were treated with prasugrel (60 mg loading dose and 10 mg once daily maintenance dose) for a median of 14.5 months (5802 patients were treated for over 6 months, 4136 patients were treated for more than 1 year). The rate of study drug discontinuation due to adverse events was 7.2% for prasugrel and 6.3% for clopidogrel. Of these, bleeding was the most common adverse reaction for both drugs leading to study drug discontinuation (2.5% for prasugrel and 1.4% for clopidogrel).

Bleeding

Non-Coronary Artery Bypass Graft (CABG) related bleeding

In TRITON, the frequency of patients experiencing a Non-CABG-related bleeding event is shown in Table 1. The incidence of Non-CABG-related TIMI major bleeding, including life-threatening and fatal, as well as TIMI minor bleeding, was statistically significantly higher in subjects treated with prasugrel compared to clopidogrel in the UA/NSTEMI and all ACS populations. No significant difference was seen in the STEMI population. The most common site of spontaneous bleeding was the gastrointestinal tract (1.7% rate with prasugrel and 1.3% rate with clopidogrel); the most frequent site of provoked bleeding was the arterial puncture site (1.3% rate with prasugrel and 1.2% with clopidogrel).

Table 1: Incidence of Non-CABG-related bleeding [a] (% Patients)

(see Table 1 above)

Patients ⩾ 75 years old

In the phase 3 clinical trial, Non-CABG-related TIMI major or minor bleeding rates for patients in two age groups were as follows:

Age	Prasugrel	Clopidogrel
⩾75 years (N=1785)	9.0% (1.0% fatal)	6.9% (0.1% fatal)
<75 years (N=11672)	3.8% (0.2% fatal)	2.9% (0.1% fatal)

Patients < 60 kg

In the phase 3 clinical trial, Non-CABG-related TIMI major or minor bleeding rates for patients in two weight groups were as follows:

Weight	Prasugrel	Clopidogrel
<60 kg (N=664)	10.1% (0% fatal)	6.5% (0.3% fatal)
⩾60 kg (N=12672)	4.2% (0.3% fatal)	3.3% (0.1% fatal)

In patients ⩾60 kg *and* age <75 years, Non-CABG-related TIMI major or minor bleeding rates were 3.6% for prasugrel and 2.8% for clopidogrel; rates for fatal bleeding were 0.2% for prasugrel and 0.1% for clopidogrel.

CABG-related bleeding

In the phase 3 clinical trial, 437 patients underwent CABG during the course of the study. Of those patients, the rate of CABG-related TIMI major or minor bleeding was 14.1% for the prasugrel group and 4.5% in the clopidogrel group. The higher risk for bleeding events in subjects treated with prasugrel persisted up to 7 days from the most recent dose of study drug. For patients who received their thienopyridine within 3 days prior to CABG, the frequencies of TIMI major or minor bleeding were 26.7% (12 of 45 patients) in the prasugrel group, compared with 5.0% (3 of 60 patients) in the clopidogrel group. For patients who received their last dose of thienopyridine within 4 to 7 days prior to CABG, the frequencies decreased to 11.3% (9 of 80 patients) in the prasugrel group and 3.3% (3 of 90 patients) in the clopidogrel group. Beyond 7 days after drug discontinuation, the observed rates of CABG-related bleeding were similar between treatment groups (see section 4.4).

Adverse Reactions

Table 2 summarises haemorrhagic and non-haemorrhagic adverse reactions in TRITON classified by frequency and system organ class. Frequencies are defined as follows: Very common (⩾ 1/10); common (⩾ 1/100 to < 1/10); uncommon (⩾ 1/1000 to < 1/100);

rare (⩾ 1/10,000 to <1/1,000); very rare (< 1/10,000); not known (cannot be estimated from the available data).

Table 2: Haemorrhagic and Non-haemorrhagic adverse reactions

(see Table 2 on next page)

In patients with or without a history of TIA or stroke, the incidence of stroke in the phase 3 clinical trial was as follows (see section 4.4):

History of TIA or stroke	Prasugrel	Clopidogrel
Yes (N=518)	6.5% (2.3% ICH*)	1.2% (0% ICH*)
No (N=13090)	0.9% (0.2% ICH*)	1.0% (0.3% ICH*)

* *ICH=intracranial haemorrhage.*

4.9 Overdose

Overdose of Efient may lead to prolonged bleeding time and subsequent bleeding complications. No data are

Table 2: Haemorrhagic and Non-haemorrhagic adverse reactions

System Organ Class	Common	Uncommon	Rare
Blood and Lymphatic System disorders	Anaemia		
Eye disorders		Eye haemorrhage	
Vascular disorders	Haematoma		
Respiratory, thoracic and mediastinal disorders	Epistaxis	Haemoptysis	
Gastrointestinal disorders	Gastrointestinal haemorrhage	Retroperitoneal haemorrhage Rectal haemorrhage Haematochezia Gingival bleeding	
Skin and subcutaneous tissue disorders	Rash Ecchymosis		
Renal and urinary disorders	Haematuria		
General disorders and administration site conditions	Vessel puncture site haematoma Puncture site haemorrhage		
Injury, poisoning and procedural complications	Contusion	Post-procedural haemorrhage	Subcutaneous haematoma

available on the reversal of the pharmacological effect of prasugrel; however, if prompt correction of prolonged bleeding time is required, platelet transfusion and/or other blood products may be considered.

5. PHARMACOLOGICAL PROPERTIES

5.1 Pharmacodynamic properties

Pharmacotherapeutic group: Platelet aggregation inhibitors excluding heparin, ATC code: B01AC22.

Pharmacodynamics

Prasugrel is an inhibitor of platelet activation and aggregation through the irreversible binding of its active metabolite to the $P2Y_{12}$ class of ADP receptors on platelets. Since platelets participate in the initiation and/or evolution of thrombotic complications of atherosclerotic disease, inhibition of platelet function can result in the reduction of the rate of cardiovascular events such as death, myocardial infarction, or stroke.

Following a 60 mg loading dose of prasugrel, inhibition of ADP-induced platelet aggregation occurs at 15 minutes with 5 μM ADP and 30 minutes with 20 μM ADP. The maximum inhibition by prasugrel of ADP-induced platelet aggregation is 83% with 5 μM ADP and 79% with 20 μM ADP, in both cases with 89% of healthy subjects and patients with stable atherosclerosis achieving at least 50% inhibition of platelet aggregation by 1 hour. Prasugrel-mediated inhibition of platelet aggregation exhibits low between-subject (12%) and within-subject (9%) variability with both 5 μM and 20 μM ADP. Mean steady-state inhibition of platelet aggregation was 74% and 69% respectively for 5 μM ADP and 20 μM ADP, and was achieved following 3 to 5 days of administration of the 10 mg prasugrel maintenance dose preceded by a 60 mg loading dose. More than 98% of subjects had $\geq$20% inhibition of platelet aggregation during maintenance dosing.

Platelet aggregation gradually returned to baseline values after treatment in 7 to 9 days after administration of a single 60 mg loading dose of prasugrel, and in 5 days following discontinuation of maintenance dosing at steady-state.

Clopidogrel: Following administration of 75 mg clopidogrel once daily for 10 days, 40 healthy subjects were switched to prasugrel 10 mg once daily with or without a loading dose of 60 mg. Similar or higher inhibition of platelet aggregation was observed with prasugrel. Switching directly to prasugrel 60 mg loading dose resulted in the most rapid onset of higher platelet inhibition. Following administration of a 900 mg loading dose of clopidogrel (with ASA), 56 subjects with ACS were treated for 14 days with either prasugrel 10 mg once daily or clopidogrel 150 mg once daily, and then switched to either clopidogrel 150 mg or prasugrel 10 mg for another 14 days. Higher inhibition of platelet aggregation was observed in patients switched to prasugrel 10 mg compared with those treated with clopidogrel 150 mg. No data are available on switching from a clopidogrel loading dose directly to a prasugrel loading dose.

Efficacy and Safety in Acute Coronary Syndrome (ACS)

The phase 3 TRITON study compared Efient (prasugrel) with clopidogrel, both co-administered with ASA and other standard therapy. TRITON was a 13,608 patient, multicentre international, randomised, double-blind, parallel group study. Patients had ACS with moderate to high risk UA, NSTEMI, or STEMI and were managed with PCI.

Patients with UA/NSTEMI within 72 hours of symptoms or STEMI between 12 hours to 14 days of symptoms were randomised after knowledge of coronary anatomy. Patients with STEMI within 12 hours of symptoms and planned for primary PCI could be randomised without knowledge of coronary anatomy. For all patients, the loading dose could be administered any time between randomisation and 1 hour after the patient left the catheterisation lab.

Patients randomised to receive prasugrel (60 mg loading dose followed by 10 mg once daily) or clopidogrel (300 mg loading dose followed by 75 mg once daily) were treated for a median of 14.5 months (maximum of 15 months with a minimum of 6 months follow-up). Patients also received ASA (75 mg to 325 mg once daily). Use of any thienopyridine within 5 days before enrolment was an exclusion criterion. Other therapies, such as heparin and GPIIb/IIIa inhibitors, were administered at the discretion of the physician. Approximately 40% of patients (in each of the treatment groups) received GPIIb/IIIa inhibitors in support of PCI (no information available regarding the type of GPIIb/IIIa inhibitor used). Approximately 98% of patients (in each of the treatment groups) received antithrombins (heparin, low molecular weight heparin, bivalirudin, or other agent) directly in support of PCI.

The trial's primary outcome measure was the time to first occurrence of cardiovascular (CV) death, non-fatal myocardial infarction (MI), or non-fatal stroke. Analysis of the composite endpoint in the All ACS population (combined UA/NSTEMI and STEMI cohorts) was contingent on showing statistical superiority of prasugrel versus clopidogrel in the UA/NSTEMI cohort ($p<0.05$).

All ACS population: Efient showed superior efficacy compared to clopidogrel in reducing the primary composite outcome events as well as the pre-specified secondary outcome events, including stent thrombosis (see Table 3). The benefit of prasugrel was apparent within the first 3 days and it persisted to the end of study. The superior efficacy was accompanied by an increase in major bleeding (see sections 4.4 and 4.8). The patient population was 92% Caucasian, 26% female, and 39% $\geq$65 years of age. The benefits associated with prasugrel were independent of the use of other acute and long-term cardiovascular therapies, including heparin/low molecular weight heparin, bivalirudin, intravenous GPIIb/IIIa inhibitors, lipid-lowering medicinal products, beta-blockers, and angiotensin converting enzyme inhibitors. The efficacy of prasugrel was independent of the ASA dose (75 mg to 325 mg once daily). The use of oral anticoagulants, non-study antiplatelet medicinal products and chronic NSAIDs was not allowed in TRITON. In the All ACS population, prasugrel was associated with a lower incidence of CV death, non-fatal MI, or non-fatal stroke compared to clopidogrel, regardless of baseline characteristics such as age, sex, body weight, geographical region, use of GPIIb/IIIa inhibitors, and stent type. The benefit was primarily due to a significant decrease in non-fatal MI (see Table 3). Subjects with diabetes had significant reductions in the primary, and all secondary composite endpoints.

The observed benefit of prasugrel in patients $\geq$ 75 years was less than that observed in patients $<$75 years. Patients $\geq$ 75 years were at increased risk of bleeding, including fatal (see sections 4.2, 4.4, and 4.8). Patients $\geq$ 75 years in whom the benefit with prasugrel was more evident included those with diabetes, STEMI, higher risk of stent thrombosis, or recurrent events.

Patients with a history of TIA or a history of ischaemic stroke more than 3 months prior to prasugrel therapy had no reduction in the primary composite endpoint.

Table 3: Patients with Outcome Events in TRITON Primary Analysis

(see Table 3 below)

In the All ACS population, analysis of each of the secondary endpoints showed a significant benefit ($p<0.001$) for prasugrel versus clopidogrel. These included definite or probable stent thrombosis at study end (0.9% vs 1.8%; HR 0.498; CI 0.364, 0.683); CV death, non-fatal MI, or urgent target vessel revascularisation through 30 days (5.9% vs 7.4%; HR 0.784; CI 0.688,0.894); all cause death, non-fatal MI, or non-fatal stroke through study end (10.2% vs 12.1%; HR 0.831; CI 0.751, 0.919); CV death, non-fatal MI, non-fatal stroke or rehospitalisation for cardiac ischaemic event through study end (11.7 % vs 13.8%; HR 0.838; CI 0.762, 0.921). Analysis of all cause death did not show any significant difference between prasugrel and clopidogrel in the All ACS population (2.76% vs 2.90%), in the UA/NSTEMI population (2.58% vs 2.41%), and in the STEMI population (3.28% vs 4.31%).

Prasugrel was associated with a 50% reduction in stent thrombosis through the 15-month follow-up period. The reduction in stent thrombosis with Efient was observed both early and beyond 30 days for both bare metal and drug eluting stents.

In an analysis of patients who survived an ischaemic event, prasugrel was associated with a reduction in the incidence

Table 3: Patients with Outcome Events in TRITON Primary Analysis

Outcome Events	Prasugrel + ASA	Clopidogrel +ASA	Hazard Ratio (HR) (95% CI)	p-value
All ACS	**(N=6813)** %	**(N=6795)** %		
Primary Composite Outcome Events Cardiovascular (CV) death, non-fatal MI, or non-fatal stroke	9.4	11.5	0.812 (0.732, 0.902)	<0.001
Primary Individual Outcome Events				
CV death	2.0	2.2	0.886 (0.701, 1.118)	0.307
Non-fatal MI	7.0	9.1	0.757 (0.672, 0.853)	<0.001
Non-fatal stroke	0.9	0.9	1.016 (0.712, 1.451)	0.930
UA/NSTEMI Primary Composite Outcome Events	**(N= 5044)** %	**(N=5030)** %		
CV death, non-fatal MI, or non-fatal stroke	9.3	11.2	0.820 (0.726, 0.927)	0.002
CV death	1.8	1.8	0.979 (0.732,1.309)	0.885
Non-fatal MI	7.1	9.2	0.761 (0.663,0.873)	<0.001
Non-fatal stroke	0.8	0.8	0.979 (0.633,1.513)	0.922
STEMI Primary Composite Outcome Events	**(N= 1769)** %	**(N=1765)** %		
CV death, non-fatal MI, or non-fatal stroke	9.8	12.2	0.793 (0.649, 0.968)	0.019
CV death	2.4	3.3	0.738 (0.497,1.094)	0.129
Non-fatal MI	6.7	8.8	0.746 (0.588,0.948)	0.016
Non-fatal stroke	1.2	1.1	1.097 (0.590,2.040)	0.770

of subsequent primary endpoint events (7.8% for prasugrel vs 11.9% for clopidogrel).

Although bleeding was increased with prasugrel, an analysis of the composite endpoint of death from any cause, non-fatal myocardial infarction, non-fatal stroke, and Non-CABG-related TIMI major haemorrhage favoured Efient compared to clopidogrel (Hazard Ratio, 0.87; 95% CI, 0.79 to 0.95; p=0.004). In TRITON, for every 1000 patients treated with Efient, there were 22 fewer patients with myocardial infarction, and 5 more with Non–CABG-related TIMI major haemorrhages, compared with patients treated with clopidogrel.

5.2 Pharmacokinetic properties

Prasugrel is a prodrug and is rapidly metabolised *in vivo* to an active metabolite and inactive metabolites. The active metabolite's exposure (AUC) has moderate to low between-subject (27%) and within-subject (19%) variability. Prasugrel's pharmacokinetics are similar in healthy subjects, patients with stable atherosclerosis, and patients undergoing percutaneous coronary intervention.

Absorption

The absorption and metabolism of prasugrel are rapid, with peak plasma concentration (C_{max}) of the active metabolite occurring in approximately 30 minutes. The active metabolite's exposure (AUC) increases proportionally over the therapeutic dose range. In a study of healthy subjects, AUC of the active metabolite was unaffected by a high fat, high calorie meal, but C_{max} was decreased by 49% and the time to reach C_{max} (T_{max}) was increased from 0.5 to 1.5 hours. Efient was administered without regard to food in TRITON. Therefore, Efient can be administered without regard to food; however, the administration of prasugrel loading dose in the fasted state may provide most rapid onset of action (see section 4.2).

Distribution

Active metabolite binding to human serum albumin (4% buffered solution) was 98%.

Metabolism

Prasugrel is not detected in plasma following oral administration. It is rapidly hydrolysed in the intestine to a thiolactone, which is then converted to the active metabolite by a single step of cytochrome P450 metabolism, primarily by CYP3A4 and CYP2B6, and to a lesser extent by CYP2C9 and CYP2C19. The active metabolite is further metabolised to two inactive compounds by S- methylation, or conjugation with cysteine.

In healthy subjects, patients with stable atherosclerosis, and patients with ACS receiving Efient, there was no relevant effect of genetic variation in CYP3A5, CYP2B6, CYP2C9, or CYP2C19 on the pharmacokinetics of prasugrel or its inhibition of platelet aggregation.

Elimination

Approximately 68% of the prasugrel dose is excreted in the urine and 27% in the faeces, as inactive metabolites. The active metabolite has an elimination half-life of about 7.4 hours (range 2 to 15 hours).

Special Populations:

Elderly: In a study of healthy subjects between the ages of 20 and 80 years, age had no significant effect on pharmacokinetics of prasugrel or its inhibition of platelet aggregation. In the large phase 3 clinical trial, the mean estimated exposure (AUC) of the active metabolite was 19% higher in very elderly patients (⩾75 years of age) compared to subjects <75 years of age. Prasugrel should be used with caution in patients ⩾ 75 years of age due to the potential risk of bleeding in this population (see sections 4.2 and 4.4).

Hepatic impairment: No dose adjustment is necessary for patients with mild to moderate impaired hepatic function (Child-Pugh class A and B). Pharmacokinetics of prasugrel and its inhibition of platelet aggregation were similar in subjects with mild to moderate hepatic impairment compared to healthy subjects. Pharmacokinetics and pharmacodynamics of prasugrel in patients with severe hepatic impairment have not been studied. Prasugrel must not be used in patients with severe hepatic impairment (see section 4.3).

Renal impairment: No dosage adjustment is necessary for patients with renal impairment, including patients with end stage renal disease (ESRD). Pharmacokinetics of prasugrel and its inhibition of platelet aggregation are similar in patients with moderate renal impairment (GFR 30-<50 ml/min/1.73m^2) and healthy subjects. Prasugrel-mediated inhibition of platelet aggregation was also similar in patients with ESRD who required haemodialysis compared to healthy subjects, although C_{max} and AUC of the active metabolite decreased 51% and 42%, respectively, in ESRD patients.

Body weight: The mean exposure (AUC) of the active metabolite of prasugrel is approximately 30 to 40% higher in healthy subjects and patients with a body weight of <60 kg compared to those weighing ⩾60 kg. Prasugrel should be used with caution in patients with a body weight of <60 kg due to the potential risk of bleeding in this population (see section 4.4).

Ethnicity: In clinical pharmacology studies, after adjusting for body weight, the AUC of the active metabolite was approximately 19% higher in Chinese, Japanese, and Korean subjects compared to that of Caucasians, predominantly related to higher exposure in Asian subjects <60 kg. There is no difference in exposure among Chinese, Japanese, and Korean subjects. Exposure in subjects of African and Hispanic descent is comparable to that of Caucasians. No dose adjustment is recommended based on ethnicity alone.

Gender: In healthy subjects and patients, the pharmacokinetics of prasugrel are similar in men and women.

Children and adolescents: Pharmacokinetics and pharmacodynamics of prasugrel have not been evaluated in a paediatric population (see section 4.2).

5.3 Preclinical safety data

Non-clinical data reveal no special hazard for humans based on conventional studies of safety pharmacology, repeat-dose toxicity, genotoxicity, carcinogenic potential, or toxicity to reproduction. Effects in non-clinical studies were observed only at exposures considered sufficiently in excess of the maximum human exposure indicating little relevance to clinical use.

Embryo-foetal developmental toxicology studies in rats and rabbits showed no evidence of malformations due to prasugrel. At a very high dose >240-times the recommended daily human maintenance dose on a mg/m^2 basis) that caused effects on maternal body weight and/or food consumption, there was a slight decrease in offspring body weight (relative to controls). In pre- and post-natal rat studies, maternal treatment had no effect on the behavioural or reproductive development of the offspring at doses up to an exposure 240-times the recommended daily human maintenance dose (based on mg/m^2).

No compound-related tumours were observed in a 2-year rat study with prasugrel exposures ranging to greater than 75-times the recommended therapeutic exposures in humans (based on plasma exposures to the active and major circulating human metabolites). There was an increased incidence of tumours (hepatocellular adenomas) in mice exposed for 2 years to high doses (>75-times human exposure), but this was considered secondary to prasugrel-induced enzyme induction. The rodent-specific association of liver tumours and drug-induced enzyme induction is well documented in the literature. The increase in liver tumours with prasugrel administration in mice is not considered a relevant human risk.

6. PHARMACEUTICAL PARTICULARS

6.1 List of excipients

Tablet Core:

Microcrystalline cellulose

Mannitol (E421)

Croscarmellose sodium

Hypromellose (E464)

Magnesium stearate

Film-Coat:

Lactose monohydrate

Hypromellose (E464)

Titanium dioxide (E171)

Triacetin (E1518)

Iron oxide red (E172) *[10 mg tablets only]*

Iron oxide yellow (E172)

Talc

6.2 Incompatibilities

Not applicable.

6.3 Shelf life

2 years.

6.4 Special precautions for storage

This medicinal product does not require any special temperature storage conditions. Store in the original package to protect from air and moisture.

6.5 Nature and contents of container

Aluminium foil blisters in cartons of 14, 28, 30 (x1), 56, 84, 90 (x1) and 98 tablets.

Not all pack sizes may be marketed.

6.6 Special precautions for disposal and other handling

No special requirements.

7. MARKETING AUTHORISATION HOLDER

Eli Lilly Nederland BV, Grootslag 1-5, NL-3991 RA Houten, The Netherlands.

8. MARKETING AUTHORISATION NUMBER(S)

EU/1/08/503/001 Efient 5mg - 14 film-coated tablets

EU/1/08/503/002 Efient 5mg - 28 film-coated tablets

EU/1/08/503/003 Efient 5mg - 30x1 film-coated tablet

EU/1/08/503/004 Efient 5mg - 56 film-coated tablets

EU/1/08/503/005 Efient 5mg - 84 film-coated tablets

EU/1/08/503/006 Efient 5mg - 90x1 film-coated tablet

EU/1/08/503/007 Efient 5mg - 98 film-coated tablets

EU/1/08/503/008 Efient 10mg - 14 film-coated tablets

EU/1/08/503/009 Efient 10mg - 28 film-coated tablets

EU/1/08/503/010 Efient 10mg - 30x1 film-coated tablet

EU/1/08/503/011 Efient 10mg - 56 film-coated tablets

EU/1/08/503/012 Efient 10mg - 84 film-coated tablets

EU/1/08/503/013 Efient 10mg - 90x1 film-coated tablet

EU/1/08/503/014 Efient 10mg - 98 film-coated tablets

9. DATE OF FIRST AUTHORISATION/RENEWAL OF THE AUTHORISATION

Date of first authorisation: 25 February 2009

10. DATE OF REVISION OF THE TEXT

18 May 2009

*EFIENT (prasugrel) is a trademark of Eli Lilly and Company. EF2M

Efracea 40mg Modified Release Hard Capsules

(Galderma (U.K) Ltd)

1. NAME OF THE MEDICINAL PRODUCT

EFRACEA 40 mg modified-release hard capsules

2. QUALITATIVE AND QUANTITATIVE COMPOSITION

Each capsule contains 40 mg doxycycline (as monohydrate).

Excipient: Each hard capsule contains 102 – 150 mg of sucrose and 26.6 - 29.4 μg of Allura red AC aluminium lake (E129).

For a full list of excipients, see section 6.1.

3. PHARMACEUTICAL FORM

Modified-release hard capsule

Beige capsule, No. 2 size, bear the marking "CGPI 40".

4. CLINICAL PARTICULARS

4.1 Therapeutic indications

EFRACEA is indicated to reduce papulopustular lesions in adult patients with facial rosacea.

4.2 Posology and method of administration

Adults, including the elderly:

The daily dose is 40 mg (1 capsule). The capsule should be taken in the morning with adequate amounts of water in order to reduce the risk of oesophageal irritation and ulceration (see section 4.4).

Patients should be evaluated after 6 weeks and, if no effect is seen, consideration should be given to stopping treatment. In clinical trials patients were treated for 16 weeks. Upon discontinuation, lesions tended to reappear at 4 weeks follow-up. Therefore it is recommended that patients should be assessed 4 weeks after stopping treatment.

Renal impairment

No dosage adjustment is necessary in patients with renal impairment.

Hepatic impairment

EFRACEA should be administered with caution to patients with hepatic impairment or to those receiving potentially hepatotoxic medicinal products (see section 4.4)

Children and adolescents

Doxycycline is contraindicated in children below age 12 (see section 4.3).

4.3 Contraindications

Hypersensitivity to the active substance, to other tetracyclines or to any of the excipients.

Infants and children up to 12 years of age.

Second and third trimesters of pregnancy (see section 4.6).

Patients known to have, or suspected to have, achlorhydria or who have had surgery that bypasses or excludes the duodenum must not be prescribed doxycycline.

4.4 Special warnings and precautions for use

EFRACEA contains doxycycline in a formulation designed to yield plasma levels below the antimicrobial threshold. EFRACEA must not be used to treat infections caused by organisms susceptible (or suspected to be susceptible) to doxycycline.

Solid dosage forms of the tetracyclines may cause oesophageal irritation and ulceration. To avoid oesophageal irritation and ulceration, adequate fluids (water) should be taken with this medicinal product (see section 4.2). EFRACEA should be swallowed whilst in an upright sitting or standing posture.

Whilst no overgrowth by opportunistic microorganisms such as yeasts were noted during the clinical studies with EFRACEA, therapy with tetracyclines at higher doses may result in overgrowth of non-susceptible microorganisms including fungi. Although not observed in clinical trials with EFRACEA, the use of tetracyclines at higher doses may increase the incidence of vaginal candidiasis. EFRACEA should be used with caution in patients with a history of predisposition to candidiasis overgrowth. If superinfection is suspected, appropriate measures should be taken, including consideration of discontinuing EFRACEA.

Treatment with higher doses of tetracyclines is associated with emergence of resistant intestinal bacteria, such as enterococci and enterobacteria. Although not observed during clinical studies with low dose doxycycline (40 mg/day), the risk for development of resistance in the normal microflora cannot be excluded in patients treated with EFRACEA.

Doxycycline blood levels in patients treated with EFRACEA are lower than in those treated with conventional antimicrobial formulations of doxycycline. However, as there are no data to support safety in hepatic impairment at this lower dose, EFRACEA should be administered with caution to patients with hepatic impairment or to those receiving potentially hepatotoxic medicinal products. The antianabolic action of tetracyclines may cause an increase in BUN. Studies to date indicate that this does not occur with the use of doxycycline in patients with impaired renal function.

Caution should be observed in the treatment of patients with myasthenia gravis who may be at risk of worsening of the condition.

All patients receiving doxycycline, including EFRACEA, should be advised to avoid excessive sunlight or artificial ultraviolet light whilst receiving doxycycline and to discontinue therapy if phototoxicity (eg skin eruption etc) occurs. Use of sunscreen or sunblock should be considered. Treatment should cease at the first sign of photosensitivity.

In common with the use of antimicrobial medicinal products in general, there is a risk of the development of pseudomembranous colitis with doxycycline treatment. In the event of the development of diarrhoea during treatment with EFRACEA, the possibility of pseudomembranous colitis should be considered and appropriate therapy instituted. This may include the discontinuation of doxycycline and the institution of specific antibiotic therapy. Agents inhibiting peristalsis should not be employed in this situation.

EFRACEA should not be used in patients with ocular manifestations of rosacea (such as ocular rosacea and/or blepharitis/meibomianitis) as there are limited efficacy and safety data in this population. If these manifestations appear during the course of the treatment Efracea should be discontinued and the patient should be referred to an ophthalmologist.

In humans, the use of tetracyclines during tooth development may cause permanent discolouration of the teeth (yellow-grey-brown). This reaction is more common during long-term use of the medicinal product but has been observed following repeated short-term courses. Enamel hypoplasia has also been reported. As for other tetracyclines, doxycycline forms a stable calcium complex in any bone-forming tissue. A decrease in fibula growth has been observed in premature infants given oral tetracycline in doses of 25 mg/kg every 6 hours. This reaction was shown to be reversible when the medicinal product was discontinued.

In the event of a severe acute hypersensitivity reaction (eg anaphylaxis), treatment with EFRACEA must be stopped at once and the usual emergency measures taken (eg administration of antihistamines, corticosteroids, sympathomimetics and, if necessary, artificial respiration).

Patients with rare hereditary problems of fructose intolerance, glucose-galactose malabsorption or sucrase-isomaltase insufficiency should not take this medicinal product.

Capsule printing ink contains Allura red AC aluminium lake (E129) which may cause allergic reactions.

4.5 Interaction with other medicinal products and other forms of interaction

The recommendations below regarding the potential interactions between doxycycline and other medicinal products are based upon experience with the larger doses generally used in antimicrobial formulations of doxycycline rather than with EFRACEA. However, at the present time, insufficient data exist for reassurance that the interactions described with higher doses of doxycycline will not occur with EFRACEA.

<u>*Interactions affecting doxycycline:*</u>

The absorption of doxycycline from the gastro-intestinal tract may be inhibited by bi- or tri-valent ions such as aluminium, zinc, calcium (found for example in milk, dairy products and calcium-containing fruit juices), by magnesium (found for example in antacids) or by iron preparations, activated charcoal, cholestyramine, bismuth chelates and sucralfate. Therefore such medicinal products or foodstuffs should be taken after a period of 2 to 3 hours following ingestion of doxycycline.

Medicinal products which increase gastric pH may reduce the absorption of doxycycline, and should be taken at least 2 hours after doxycycline.

Quinapril may reduce the absorption of doxycycline due to the high magnesium content in quinapril tablets.

Rifampicin, barbiturates, carbamazepine, diphenylhydantoin, primidone, phenytoin and chronic alcohol abuse may accelerate the decomposition of doxycycline due to enzyme induction in the liver thereby decreasing its half-life. Sub-therapeutic doxycycline concentrations may result.

Concurrent use of cyclosporin has been reported to decrease the half-life of doxycycline.

<u>*Interactions affecting other medicinal products:*</u>

Concomitant use not recommended:

When doxycycline is administered shortly before, during or after courses of isotretinoin, there is the possibility of potentiation between the medicinal products to cause reversible pressure increase in the intracranial cavity (pseudotumour cerebri). Concomitant administration should therefore be avoided.

Bacteriostatic medicinal products including doxycycline may interfere with the bacteriocidal action of penicillin and beta-lactam antibiotics. It is advisable that doxycycline and beta-lactam antibiotics should not therefore be used in combination.

Other interactions:

Tetracyclines and methoxyflurane used in combination have been reported to result in fatal renal toxicity.

Doxycycline has been shown to potentiate the hypoglycaemic effect of sulphonylurea oral antidiabetic agents. If administered in combination with these medicinal products, blood glucose levels should be monitored and, if necessary, the doses of the sulphonylureas should be reduced.

Doxycycline has been shown to depress plasma prothrombin activity thereby potentiating the effect of anticoagulants of the dicoumarol type. If administered in combination with these agents, coagulation parameters including INR should be monitored and, if necessary, the doses of the anticoagulant medicinal products reduced. The possibility of an increased risk of bleeding events should be borne in mind.

Tetracyclines used concurrently with oral contraceptives have in a few cases resulted in either breakthrough bleeding or pregnancy.

4.6 Pregnancy and lactation

Studies in animals have not demonstrated a teratogenic effect. In humans, the use of tetracyclines during a limited number of pregnancies has not revealed any specific malformation to date.

The administration of tetracyclines during the second and the third trimesters results in permanent discolouration of the deciduous teeth in the offspring. As a consequence, doxycycline is contraindicated during the second and third trimesters of pregnancy (see section 4.3).

Low levels of tetracyclines are secreted into the milk of lactating women. Doxycycline can be used by breast-feeding mothers for short term use only. Long term use of doxycycline may result in significant absorption by the suckling infant and is therefore not recommended because of a theoretical risk of dental discolouration and decreased bone growth of the suckling child.

4.7 Effects on ability to drive and use machines

Doxycycline has no or negligible influence on the ability to drive and use machines.

4.8 Undesirable effects

In the pivotal placebo-controlled studies with EFRACEA in rosacea, 269 patients were treated with EFRACEA 40 mg once daily and 268 patients were treated with placebo for 16 weeks. Gastrointestinal adverse reactions overall occurred in a higher proportion of patients on EFRACEA (13.4%) than on placebo (8.6%). The most commonly reported adverse reactions in patients treated with EFRACEA, ie those which occurred with ⩾ 3% frequency on EFRACEA and with a frequency at least 1% higher than on placebo, were nasopharyngitis, diarrhoea and hypertension.

The table below lists adverse reactions on EFRACEA in the pivotal clinical trials, ie adverse reactions for which the frequency on EFRACEA was greater than the frequency on placebo (by ⩾ 1%).

Adverse reactions reported for tetracycline antibiotics as a class are listed following the table. The frequency categories used are:

Common:	⩾ 1/100 to < 1/10
Uncommon:	⩾ 1/1,000 to < 1/100
Rare:	⩾ 1/10,000 to < 1/1,000
Very rare:	< 1/10,000

Adverse reactions[a] on EFRACEA in pivotal placebo-controlled studies in rosacea:

MedDRA system organ class	Common: Frequency ⩾ 1/100, < 1/10
Infections and infestations	Nasopharyngitis Sinusitis Fungal infection
Psychiatric disorders	Anxiety
Nervous system disorders	Sinus headache
Vascular disorders	Hypertension
Gastrointestinal disorders	Diarrhoea Abdominal pain, upper Dry mouth
Musculoskeletal, connective tissue and bone disorders	Back pain
General disorders and administration site conditions	Pain
Investigations	ASAT increased Blood pressure increased Blood LDH increased Blood glucose increased

[a] Defined as adverse events for which the frequency on EFRACEA was higher than on placebo (by at least 1%)

The following adverse reactions have been observed in patients receiving tetracyclines:-

Infections and infestations:

Very rare:	Anogenital candidiasis

Blood and lymphatic system disorders:

Rare:	Thrombocytopenia, neutropenia, eosinophilia
Very rare:	Haemolytic anaemia

Immune system disorders:

Rare:	Hypersensitivity reactions including anaphylaxis

There have also been reports of: Anaphylactoid purpura

Endocrine disorders:

Very rare:	Brown-black microscopic discolouration of thyroid tissue has been reported with long-term use of tetracyclines. Thyroid function is normal.

Nervous system disorders:

Rare:	Benign intracranial hypertension
Very rare:	Bulging fontanelle in infants

Treatment should cease if evidence of raised intracranial pressure develops. These conditions disappeared rapidly when the drug was discontinued.

Cardiac disorders:

Rare:	Pericarditis

Gastrointestinal disorders:

Rare:	Nausea, vomiting, diarrhoea, anorexia
Very rare:	Glossitis, dysphagia, enterocolitis. Oesophagitis and oesophageal ulceration have been reported most often in patients administered the hyclate salt in capsule form. Most of these patients took medication just prior to going to bed.

Hepatobiliary disorders:

Rare:	Hepatotoxicity

Skin and subcutaneous tissue disorders:

Rare:	Maculopapular and erythematous rashes, skin photosensitivity, urticaria
Very rare:	Exfoliative dermatitis, angioneurotic oedema

Musculoskeletal, connective tissue and bone disorders:

Very rare:	Exacerbation of systemic lupus erythematosus

Renal and urinary disorders:

Rare:	Increased blood urea.

Adverse reactions typical of the tetracycline class of medicinal products are less likely to occur during medication with EFRACEA, due to the reduced dosage and the relatively low plasma levels involved. However, the clinician should always be aware of the possibility of adverse events occurring and should monitor patients accordingly.

4.9 Overdose

<u>*Symptoms:*</u>

To date no significant acute toxicity has been described in the case of a single oral intake of a multiple of therapeutic doses of doxycycline. In case of overdose there is, however, a risk of parenchymatous hepatic and renal damage and of pancreatitis.

<u>Treatment:</u>

The usual dose of EFRACEA is less than half the usual doses of doxycycline used for antimicrobial therapy. Therefore clinicians should bear in mind that in many cases overdose is likely to produce blood concentrations of doxycycline within the therapeutic range for antimicrobial treatment, for which there is a large quantity of data supporting the safety of the medicinal product. In these cases observation is recommended. In cases of significant overdose, doxycycline therapy should be stopped immediately and symptomatic measures undertaken as required.

Intestinal absorption of unabsorbed doxycycline should be minimised by administering magnesium or calcium salt-containing antacids to produce non-absorbable chelate complexes with doxycycline. Gastric lavage should be considered.

Dialysis does not alter serum doxycycline half-life and thus would not be of benefit in treating cases of overdose.

5. PHARMACOLOGICAL PROPERTIES

5.1 Pharmacodynamic properties

Pharmacotherapeutic group: Antibacterials for systemic use, Tetracyclines. ATC code: J01AA02.

Mechanism of Action: The pathophysiology of the inflammatory lesions of rosacea is, in part, a manifestation of a neutrophil-mediated process. Doxycycline has been shown to inhibit neutrophil activity and several pro-inflammatory reactions including those associated with phospholipase A_2, endogenous nitric oxide and interleukin-6. The clinical significance of these findings is not known.

The plasma concentration of doxycycline following administration of EFRACEA is well below the level required to

Table 1 Mean change from baseline to Week 16 in total inflammatory lesion count

	Study 1		Study 2	
	EFRACEA 40 mg (N = 127)	Placebo (N = 124)	EFRACEA 40 mg (N = 142)	Placebo (N = 144)
Mean (SD) change from baseline	-11.8 (9.8)	-5.9 (13.9)	-9.5 (9.6)	-4.3 (11.6)
Mean between-group difference	-5.9		-5.2	
(95% confidence limits)	(-8.9, -2.9)		(-7.7, -2.7)	
p-Value[a]	0.0001		< 0.0001	

[a] p-Value for treatment difference in change from baseline (ANOVA)

inhibit mircoorganisms commonly associated with bacterial diseases.

In vivo microbiological studies using similar exposure to the active substance for 6 to 18 months could not demonstrate any effect on the dominating bacterial flora sampled from the oral cavity, skin, intestinal tract and vagina. However, it can not be excluded that long-term use of Efracea can lead to emergence of resistant intestinal bacteria such as Enterobacteriaceae and enterococci, as well as to enrichment of resistance genes.

EFRACEA has been evaluated in two pivotal randomised, double-blind, placebo-controlled, 16-week studies in 537 patients with rosacea (10 to 40 papules and pustules, and two or fewer nodules). In both studies, the mean reduction in the total inflammatory lesion count was significantly greater in the EFRACEA group than in the placebo group:

Mean change from baseline to Week 16 in total inflammatory lesion count:

(see Table 1 above)

5.2 Pharmacokinetic properties

Absorption:

Doxycycline is almost completely absorbed after oral administration. Following oral administration of EFRACEA, mean peak plasma concentrations were 510 ng/mL after a single dose and 600 ng/mL at steady state (Day 7). Peak plasma levels were generally achieved at 2 to 3 hours after administration. Coadministration with a high-fat, high-protein meal that included dairy products reduced the bioavailability (AUC) of doxycycline from EFRACEA by about 20% and reduced the peak plasma level by 43%.

Distribution, metabolism and elimination:

Doxycycline is greater than 90% bound to plasma proteins and has an apparent volume of distribution of 50 L. Major metabolic pathways of doxycycline have not been identified but enzyme inducers decrease the half-life of doxycycline.

Doxycycline is excreted in the urine and faeces as unchanged active substance. Between 40% and 60% of an administered dose can be accounted for in the urine by 92 hours, and approximately 30% in the faeces. The terminal elimination half-life of doxycycline after administration of EFRACEA was approximately 21 h after a single dose and approximately 23 h at steady state.

Pharmacokinetics in special populations:

The half-life of doxycycline is not significantly altered in patients with severely impaired renal function. Doxycycline is not eliminated to any great extent during haemodialysis.

There is no information on the pharmacokinetics of doxycycline in patients with hepatic impairment.

5.3 Preclinical safety data

Adverse reactions seen in repeat dose studies in animals include hyperpigmentation of the thyroid and tubular degeneration in the kidney. These effects were seen at exposure levels of 1.5 to 2 times those seen in humans administered EFRACEA at the proposed dose. The clinical relevance of these findings remains unknown.

Doxycycline showed no mutagenic activity and no convincing evidence of clastogenic activity. In a rat carcinogenicity study increases in benign tumours of the mammary gland (fibroadenoma), uterus (polyp) and thyroid (C-cell adenoma) were noted in females.

In rats, doses of 50 mg/kg/day doxycycline caused a decrease in the straight-line velocity of sperm but did not affect male or female fertility or sperm morphology. At this dose systemic exposure experienced by rats is likely to have been approximately 4 times that seen in humans taking the recommended dose of EFRACEA. At doses greater than 50 mg/kg/day fertility and reproductive performance were adversely affected in rats. A peri/postnatal toxicity study in rats revealed no significant effects at therapeutically relevant doses. Doxycycline is known to cross the placenta and literature data indicate that tetracyclines can have toxic effects on the developing foetus.

6. PHARMACEUTICAL PARTICULARS

6.1 List of excipients

Capsule shell

Gelatin

Black iron oxide

Red iron oxide

Yellow iron oxide

Titanium dioxide

Printing inks

Shellac

Propylene glycol

Black iron oxide

Indigo Carmine aluminium lake

Allura Red AC aluminium lake (E129)

Brilliant Blue FCF aluminium lake

D & C Yellow No. 10 aluminium lake

Capsule contents

Hypromellose

Methacrylic acid-ethyl acrylate copolymer (1:1)

Triethyl citrate

Talc

Hypromellose 3cP/6cP, Titanium dioxide, Macrogol 400, Yellow iron oxide, Red iron oxide, Polysorbate 80

Sugar spheres (Maize starch, Sucrose)

6.2 Incompatibilities

Not applicable.

6.3 Shelf life

2 years

6.4 Special precautions for storage

Store in the original package in order to protect from light.

6.5 Nature and contents of container

Aluminium/PVC/Aclar blister

Pack size: 56 capsules in 4 strips of 14 each

28 capsules in 2 strips of 14 each

6.6 Special precautions for disposal and other handling

No special requirements

7. MARKETING AUTHORISATION HOLDER

Galderma (UK) Ltd

Meridien House

69-71 Clarendon Road

Watford

Herts

WD17 1DS

UK

8. MARKETING AUTHORISATION NUMBER(S)

PL 10590/0056

9. DATE OF FIRST AUTHORISATION/RENEWAL OF THE AUTHORISATION

2nd April 2009

10. DATE OF REVISION OF THE TEXT

April 2009

Elantan 10

(UCB Pharma Limited)

1. NAME OF THE MEDICINAL PRODUCT

Elantan 10

2. QUALITATIVE AND QUANTITATIVE COMPOSITION

Isosorbide-5-mononitrate-lactose trituration 90%, 11.10 mg equivalent to isosorbide-5-mononitrate, 10.00 mg.

(The lactose complies with Ph.Eur.).

For excipients see 6.1.

3. PHARMACEUTICAL FORM

Tablets

White, upperside flat with bevelled edge and score engraving (E/10), underside rounded.

4. CLINICAL PARTICULARS

4.1 Therapeutic indications

For the prophylaxis of angina pectoris

4.2 Posology and method of administration

For oral administration

Adults

One tablet to be taken asymmetrically (to allow a nitrate low period) two or three times a day. For patients not already receiving prophylactic nitrate therapy it is recommended that the initial dose be one tablet of Elantan 10 twice a day.

The dosage may be increased up to 120 mg per day.

The lowest effective dose should be used.

Elderly

There is no evidence to suggest that an adjustment of the dosage is necessary.

Children

The safety and efficacy of Elantan 10 has yet to be established in children.

Treatment with Elantan, as with any other nitrate, should not be stopped suddenly. Both the dosage and frequency should be tapered gradually (see section 4.4)

4.3 Contraindications

Elantan 10 should not be used in cases of acute myocardial infarction with low filling pressure, acute circulatory failure (shock, vascular collapse), or very low blood pressure, hypertrophic obstructive cardiomyopathy (HOCM), constrictive pericarditis, cardiac tamponade, low cardiac filling pressures, aortic/mitral valve stenosis and diseases associated with a raised intra-cranial pressure e.g. following a head trauma and including cerebral haemorrhage.

This product should not be given to patients with a known sensitivity to isosorbide mononitrate, the listed ingredients or other nitrates.

Elantan 10 should not be used in patients with marked anaemia, severe hypotension, closed angle glaucoma or hypovolaemia.

Phosphodiesterase type-5 inhibitors (e.g. sildenafil, tadalafil and vardenafil) have been shown to potentiate the hypotensive effects of nitrates, and their co-administration with nitrates or nitric oxide donors is therefore contraindicated (see section 4.5).

4.4 Special warnings and precautions for use

Elantan 10 should be used with caution in patients who have a recent history of myocardial infarction, or who are suffering from hypothyroidism, hypothermia, malnutrition and severe liver or renal disease.

Symptoms of circulatory collapse may arise after first dose, particularly in patients with labile circulation.

This product may give rise to postural hypotension and syncope in some patients. Severe postural hypotension with light-headedness and dizziness is frequently observed after the consumption of alcohol.

Hypotension induced by nitrates may be accompanied by paradoxical bradycardia and increased angina.

Elantan tablets contain lactose and therefore should not be used in patients with rare hereditary problems of galactose intolerance, the Lapp lactase deficiency or glucose-galactose malabsorption.

In the event of an acute angina attack, a sublingual treatment such as a GTN spray or tablet should be used instead of Elantan tablets.

If the tablets are not taken as indicated (see section 4.2.) tolerance to the medication could develop. The lowest effective dose should be used.

Treatment with Elantan, as with any other nitrate, should not be stopped suddenly. Both the dosage and frequency should be tapered gradually (see section 4.2)

4.5 Interaction with other medicinal products and other forms of interaction

Concurrent administration of drugs with blood pressure lowering properties, e.g. beta-blockers, calcium channel blockers, vasodilators, alprostadil, aldesleukin, angiotensin II receptor antagonists etc and/or alcohol may potentiate the hypotensive effect of Elantan. This may also occur with neuroleptics and tricyclic antidepressants.

Any blood pressure lowering effect of Elantan will be increased if used together with phosphodiesterase type-5 inhibitors which are used for erectile dysfunction (see special warnings and contraindications). This might lead to life threatening cardiovascular complications. Patients who are on Elantan therapy therefore must not use phosphodiesterase type-5 inhibitors

Reports suggest that concomitant administration of Elantan may increase the blood level of dihydroergotamine and its hypertensive effect.

4.6 Pregnancy and lactation

No data have been reported which would indicate the possibility of adverse effects resulting from the use of isosorbide mononitrate in pregnancy. Safety in pregnancy, however, has not been established. It is not known whether nitrates are excreted in human milk and therefore caution should be exercised when administered to nursing women.

Isosorbide mononitrate should only be used in pregnancy and during lactation if, in the opinion of the physician, the possible benefits of treatment outweigh the hazards.

4.7 Effects on ability to drive and use machines

Dizziness, tiredness or blurred vision might occur at the start of treatment. The patient should therefore be advised that if affected, they should not drive or operate machinery. This effect may be increased by alcohol.

4.8 Undesirable effects

A very common (>10% of patients) adverse reaction to Elantan is throbbing headache. The incidence of headache diminishes gradually with time and continued use.

At the start of therapy or when the dosage is increased, hypotension and/or light headedness in the upright position are commonly observed (i.e in 1 – 10% of patients). These symptoms may be associated with dizziness, drowsiness, reflex tachychardia and a feeling of weakness.

Infrequently (i.e. in less than 1% of patients) nausea, vomiting, flushing and allergic skin reaction (e.g. rash) may occur sometimes severely. In single cases exfoliative dermatitis may occur.

Severe hypotensive responses have been reported for organic nitrates and include nausea, vomiting, restlessness pallor and excessive perspiration. Uncommonly collapse may occur (sometimes accompanied by bradyarrhythmia and syncope). Uncommonly severe hypotension may lead to enhanced angina symptoms.

A few reports of heartburn most likely due to a nitrate induced sphincter relaxation have been recorded.

Tachycardia and paroxysmal bradycardia have been reported.

4.9 Overdose

Symptoms and signs:

Headache, hypotension, nausea, vomiting, sweating, tachycardia, vertigo, restlessness, warm flushed skin, blurred vision and syncope. A rise in intracranial pressure with confusion and neurological deficits can sometimes occur. Methaemoglobinaemia (cyanosis, hypoxaemia, restlessness, respiratory depression, convulsions, cardiac arrhythmias, circulatory failure, raised intracranial pressure) occurs rarely.

Management:

Consider oral activated charcoal if ingestion of a potentially toxic amount has occurred within 1 hour. Observe for at least 12 hours after the overdose. Monitor blood pressure and pulse. Correct hypotension by raising the foot of the bed and/or by expanding the intravascular volume. Other measures as indicated by the patient's clinical condition. If severe hypotension persists despite the above measures consider use of inotropes.

If methaemoglobinaemia (symptoms or > 30% methaemoglobin), IV administration of methylene blue 1-2 mg/kg body weight. If therapy fails with second dose after 1 hour or contraindicated, consider red blood cell concentrates or exchange transfusion. In case of cerebral convulsions, diazepam or clonazepam IV, or if therapy fails, phenobarbital, phenytoin or propofol anaesthesia.

5. PHARMACOLOGICAL PROPERTIES

5.1 Pharmacodynamic properties

ATC Code: C01D A14 Vasodilator used in cardiac diseases

Isosorbide mononitrate is an organic nitrate which, in common with other cardioactive nitrates, is a vasodilator. It produces decreased left and right ventricular end-diastolic pressures to a greater extent than the decrease in systemic arterial pressure, thereby reducing afterload and especially the preload of the heart.

Isosorbide mononitrate influences the oxygen supply to ischaemic myocardium by causing the redistribution of blood flow along collateral channels and from epicardial to endocardial regions by selective dilation of large epicardial vessels.

It reduces the requirement of the myocardium for oxygen by increasing venous capacitance, causing a pooling of blood in peripheral veins, thereby reducing ventricular volume and heart wall distension.

5.2 Pharmacokinetic properties

Isosorbide-5-mononitrate is rapidly absorbed and peak plasma levels occur approx. 1 hour following oral dosing.

Isosorbide-5-mononitrate is completely bioavailable after oral doses and is not subject to pre-systemic elimination processes.

Isosorbide-5-mononitrate is eliminated from the plasma with a half-life of about 5.1 hours. It is metabolised to Isosorbide-5-MN-2-glucoronide, which has a half-life of approximately 2.5 hours. As well as being excreted unchanged in the urine.

After multiple oral dosing plasma concentrations are similar to those that can be predicted from single dose kinetic parameters.

5.3 Preclinical safety data

Preclinical data reveal no special hazard for humans based on conventional studies of single and repeated dose toxicity, genotoxicity, oncogenicity and toxicity to reproduction.

6. PHARMACEUTICAL PARTICULARS

6.1 List of excipients

Lactose monohydrate

Microcrystalline cellulose

Potato starch

Purified talc

Colloidal silicon dioxide

Aluminium stearate.

6.2 Incompatibilities

None Known

6.3 Shelf life

5 years

6.4 Special precautions for storage

None

6.5 Nature and contents of container

Cartons of blister strips of PP/aluminium or of PP/PP.

Aluminium foil thickness 16μm or 20μm.

Pack sizes: 14, 50,56,60,84 and 90 tablets.

6.6 Special precautions for disposal and other handling

None

7. MARKETING AUTHORISATION HOLDER

UCB Pharma Limited

208 Bath Road

Slough

Berkshire

SL1 3WE

United Kingdom

8. MARKETING AUTHORISATION NUMBER(S)

PL 00039/0738

9. DATE OF FIRST AUTHORISATION/RENEWAL OF THE AUTHORISATION

30th September 2008

10. DATE OF REVISION OF THE TEXT

Elantan 20

(UCB Pharma Limited)

1. NAME OF THE MEDICINAL PRODUCT

Elantan 20

2. QUALITATIVE AND QUANTITATIVE COMPOSITION

Isosorbide-5-mononitrate-lactose trituration 90%, 22.20 mg equivalent to Isosorbide-5-mononitrate, 20.00 mg.

(The lactose complies with Ph.Eur.).

For excipients see 6.1.

3. PHARMACEUTICAL FORM

Tablets

White tablets with breakscore and marked 'E20'.

4. CLINICAL PARTICULARS

4.1 Therapeutic indications

For the prophylaxis of angina pectoris

As adjunctive therapy in congestive heart failure not responding to cardiac glycosides or diuretics.

4.2 Posology and method of administration

For oral administration

Adults

One tablet to be taken asymmetrically (to allow a nitrate low period) two or three times a day. For patients not already receiving prophylactic nitrate therapy it is recommended that the initial dose be one tablet of Elantan 20 twice a day.

The dosage may be increased up to 120 mg per day.

The lowest effective dose should be used.

Elderly

There is no evidence to suggest that an adjustment of the dosage is necessary.

Children

The safety and efficacy of Elantan 20 has yet to be established in children.

Treatment with Elantan, as with any other nitrate, should not be stopped suddenly. Both the dosage and frequency should be tapered gradually (see section 4.4)

4.3 Contraindications

Elantan 20 should not be used in cases of acute myocardial infarction with low filling pressure, acute circulatory failure (shock, vascular collapse), or very low blood pressure, hypertrophic obstructive cardiomyopathy (HOCM), constrictive pericarditis, cardiac tamponade, low cardiac filling pressures, aortic/mitral valve stenosis and diseases associated with a raised intra-cranial pressure e.g. following a head trauma and including cerebral haemorrhage.

This product should not be given to patients with a known sensitivity to isosorbide mononitrate, the listed ingredients or other nitrates.

Elantan 20 should not be used in patients with marked anaemia, severe hypotension, closed angle glaucoma or hypovolaemia.

Phosphodiesterase type-5 inhibitors (e.g. sildenafil, tadalafil and vardenafil) have been shown to potentiate the hypotensive effects of nitrates, and their co-administration with nitrates or nitric oxide donors is therefore contraindicated (see section 4.5)

4.4 Special warnings and precautions for use

Elantan 20 should be used with caution in patients who have a recent history of myocardial infarction, or who are suffering from hypothyroidism, hypothermia, malnutrition and severe liver or renal disease.

Symptoms of circulatory collapse may arise after first dose, particularly in patients with labile circulation.

This product may give rise to postural hypotension and syncope in some patients. Severe postural hypotension with light-headedness and dizziness is frequently observed after the consumption of alcohol.

Hypotension induced by nitrates may be accompanied by paradoxical bradycardia and increased angina.

Elantan tablets contain lactose and therefore should not be used in patients with rare hereditary problems of galactose intolerance, the Lapp lactase deficiency or glucose-galactose malabsorption.

In the event of an acute angina attack, a sublingual treatment such as a GTN spray or tablet should be used instead of Elantan tablets.

If the tablets are not taken as indicated (see section 4.2.) tolerance to the medication could develop. The lowest effective dose should be used.

Treatment with Elantan, as with any other nitrate, should not be stopped suddenly. Both the dosage and frequency should be tapered gradually (see section 4.2)

4.5 Interaction with other medicinal products and other forms of interaction

Concurrent administration of drugs with blood pressure lowering properties, e.g. beta-blockers, calcium channel blockers, vasodilators, alprostadil, aldesleukin, angiotensin II receptor antagonists etc and/or alcohol may potentiate the hypotensive effect of Elantan. This may also occur with neuroleptics and tricyclic antidepressants.

Any blood pressure lowering effect of Elantan will be increased if used together with phosphodiesterase type-5 inhibitors which are used for erectile dysfunction (see special warnings and contraindications). This might lead to life threatening cardiovascular complications. Patients who are on Elantan therapy therefore must not use phosphodiesterase type-5 inhibitors.

Reports suggest that concomitant administration of Elantan may increase the blood level of dihydroergotamine and its hypertensive effect.

4.6 Pregnancy and lactation

No data have been reported which would indicate the possibility of adverse effects resulting from the use of isosorbide mononitrate in pregnancy. Safety in pregnancy, however, has not been established. It is not known whether nitrates are excreted in human milk and therefore caution should be exercised when administered to nursing women.

Isosorbide mononitrate should only be used in pregnancy and during lactation if, in the opinion of the physician, the possible benefits of treatment outweigh the hazards.

4.7 Effects on ability to drive and use machines

Dizziness, tiredness or blurred vision might occur at the start of treatment. The patient should therefore be advised that if affected, they should not drive or operate machinery. This effect may be increased by alcohol.

4.8 Undesirable effects

A very common (>10% of patients) adverse reaction to Elantan is throbbing headache. The incidence of headache diminishes gradually with time and continued use.

At the start of therapy or when the dosage is increased, hypotension and/or light headedness in the upright position are commonly observed (i.e. in 1 – 10% of patients). These symptoms may be associated with dizziness, drowsiness, reflex tachychardia and a feeling of weakness.

Infrequently (i.e. in less than 1% of patients) nausea, vomiting, flushing and allergic skin reaction (e.g. rash) may occur sometimes severely. In single cases exfoliative dermatitis may occur.

Severe hypotensive responses have been reported for organic nitrates and include nausea, vomiting, restlessness pallor and excessive perspiration. Uncommonly collapse may occur (sometimes accompanied by bradyarrhythmia and syncope). Uncommonly severe hypotension may lead to enhanced angina symptoms.

A few reports of heartburn most likely due to a nitrate induced sphincter relaxation have been recorded.

Tachycardia and paroxysmal bradycardia have been reported.

4.9 Overdose

Symptoms and signs:

Headache, hypotension, nausea, vomiting, sweating, tachycardia, vertigo, restlessness, warm flushed skin, blurred vision and syncope. A rise in intracranial pressure with confusion and neurological deficits can sometimes occur. Methaemoglobinaemia (cyanosis, hypoxaemia, restlessness, respiratory depression, convulsions, cardiac arrhythmias, circulatory failure, raised intracranial pressure) occurs rarely.

Management:

Consider oral activated charcoal if ingestion of a potentially toxic amount has occurred within 1 hour. Observe for at least 12 hours after the overdose. Monitor blood pressure and pulse. Correct hypotension by raising the foot of the bed and/or by expanding the intravascular volume. Other measures as indicated by the patient's clinical condition. If severe hypotension persists despite the above measures consider use of inotropes.

If methaemoglobinaemia (symptoms or > 30% methaemoglobin), IV administration of methylene blue 1-2 mg/kg body weight. If therapy fails with second dose after 1 hour or contraindicated, consider red blood cell concentrates or exchange transfusion. In case of cerebral convulsions, diazepam or clonazepam IV, or if therapy fails, phenobarbital, phenytoin or propofol anaesthesia.

5. PHARMACOLOGICAL PROPERTIES

5.1 Pharmacodynamic properties

ATC Code: C01D A14 Vasodilator used in cardiac diseases

Isosorbide mononitrate is an organic nitrate which, in common with other cardioactive nitrates, is a vasodilator. It produces decreased left and right ventricular end-diastolic pressures to a greater extent than the decrease in systemic arterial pressure, thereby reducing afterload and especially the preload of the heart.

Isosorbide mononitrate influences the oxygen supply to ischaemic myocardium by causing the redistribution of blood flow along collateral channels and from epicardial to endocardial regions by selective dilation of large epicardial vessels.

It reduces the requirement of the myocardium for oxygen by increasing venous capacitance, causing a pooling of blood in peripheral veins, thereby reducing ventricular volume and heart wall distension.

5.2 Pharmacokinetic properties

Isosorbide-5-mononitrate is rapidly absorbed and peak plasma levels occur approx. 1 hour following oral dosing.

Isosorbide-5-mononitrate is completely bioavailable after oral doses and is not subject to pre-systemic elimination processes.

Isosorbide-5-mononitrate is eliminated from the plasma with a half-life of about 5.1 hours. It is metabolised to Isosorbide-5-MN-2-glucoronide, which has a half-life of approximately 2.5 hours. As well as being excreted unchanged in the urine.

After multiple oral dosing plasma concentrations are similar to those that can be predicted from single dose kinetic parameters.

5.3 Preclinical safety data

Preclinical data reveal no special hazard for humans based on conventional studies of single and repeated dose toxicity, genotoxicity, oncogenicity and toxicity to reproduction.

6. PHARMACEUTICAL PARTICULARS

6.1 List of excipients

Lactose monohydrate

Purified talc

Colloidal silicon dioxide

Potato starch

Microcrystalline cellulose

Aluminium stearate

6.2 Incompatibilities

None Known

6.3 Shelf life

5 years

6.4 Special precautions for storage

None

6.5 Nature and contents of container

Cartons of blister strips of PP/aluminium or of PP/PP.

Aluminium foil thickness 16μm or 20μm.

Pack sizes: 50,56,60,84,90 and 100 tablets.

6.6 Special precautions for disposal and other handling

None

7. MARKETING AUTHORISATION HOLDER

UCB Pharma Limited

208 Bath Road

Slough

Berkshire

SL1 3WE

United Kingdom

8. MARKETING AUTHORISATION NUMBER(S)

PL 00039/0739

9. DATE OF FIRST AUTHORISATION/RENEWAL OF THE AUTHORISATION

28 February 2008

10. DATE OF REVISION OF THE TEXT

Elantan 40

(UCB Pharma Limited)

1. NAME OF THE MEDICINAL PRODUCT

Elantan 40

2. QUALITATIVE AND QUANTITATIVE COMPOSITION

Isosorbide-5-mononitrate-lactose trituration 90%, 44.40 mg equivalent to Isosorbide-5-mononitrate, 40.00 mg.

(The lactose complies with Ph.Eur.).

For excipients see 6.1.

3. PHARMACEUTICAL FORM

Tablets

White tablets upperside flat with facet and breakscore; underside arc-shaped marked 'E40'.

4. CLINICAL PARTICULARS

4.1 Therapeutic indications

For the prophylaxis of angina pectoris

As adjunctive therapy in congestive heart failure not responding to cardiac glycosides or diuretics.

4.2 Posology and method of administration

For oral administration

<u>Adults</u>

One tablet to be taken asymmetrically (to allow a nitrate low period) two or three times a day. For patients not already receiving prophylactic nitrate therapy it is recommended that the initial dose be one tablet of Elantan 40 twice a day.

The dosage may be increased up to 120 mg per day.

The lowest effective dose should be used.

<u>Elderly</u>

There is no evidence to suggest that an adjustment of the dosage is necessary.

<u>Children</u>

The safety and efficacy of Elantan 40 has yet to be established in children.

Treatment with Elantan, as with any other nitrate, should not be stopped suddenly. Both the dosage and frequency should be tapered gradually (see section 4.4)

4.3 Contraindications

Elantan 40 should not be used in cases of acute myocardial infarction with low filling pressure, acute circulatory failure (shock, vascular collapse), or very low blood pressure, hypertrophic obstructive cardiomyopathy (HOCM), constrictive pericarditis, cardiac tamponade, low cardiac filling pressures, aortic/mitral valve stenosis and diseases associated with a raised intra-cranial pressure e.g. following a head trauma and including cerebral haemorrhage.

This product should not be given to patients with a known sensitivity to isosorbide mononitrate, the listed ingredients or other nitrates.

Elantan 40 should not be used in patients with marked anaemia, severe hypotension, closed angle glaucoma or hypovolaemia.

Phosphodiesterase type-5 inhibitors (e.g. sildenafil, tadalafil and vardenafil) have been shown to potentiate the hypotensive effects of nitrates, and their co-administration with nitrates or nitric oxide donors is therefore contraindicated (see section 4.5)

4.4 Special warnings and precautions for use

Elantan 40 should be used with caution in patients who have a recent history of myocardial infarction, or who are suffering from hypothyroidism, hypothermia, malnutrition and severe liver or renal disease.

Symptoms of circulatory collapse may arise after first dose, particularly in patients with labile circulation.

This product may give rise to postural hypotension and syncope in some patients. Severe postural hypotension with light-headedness and dizziness is frequently observed after the consumption of alcohol.

Hypotension induced by nitrates may be accompanied by paradoxical bradycardia and increased angina.

Elantan tablets contain lactose and therefore should not be used in patients with rare hereditary problems of galactose intolerance, the Lapp lactase deficiency or glucose-galactose malabsorption.

In the event of an acute angina attack, a sublingual treatment such as a GTN spray or tablet should be used instead of Elantan tablets.

If the tablets are not taken as indicated (see section 4.2.) tolerance to the medication could develop. The lowest effective dose should be used.

Treatment with Elantan, as with any other nitrate, should not be stopped suddenly. Both the dosage and frequency should be tapered gradually (see section 4.2)

4.5 Interaction with other medicinal products and other forms of interaction

Concurrent administration of drugs with blood pressure lowering properties, e.g. beta-blockers, calcium channel blockers, vasodilators, alprostadil, aldesleukin, angiotensin II receptor antagonists etc and/or alcohol may potentiate the hypotensive effect of Elantan. This may also occur with neuroleptics and tricyclic antidepressants.

Any blood pressure lowering effect of Elantan will be increased if used together with phosphodiesterase type-5 inhibitors which are used for erectile dysfunction (see special warnings and contraindications). This might lead to life threatening cardiovascular complications. Patients who are on Elantan therapy therefore must not use phosphodiesterase type-5 inhibitors.

Reports suggest that concomitant administration of Elantan may increase the blood level of dihydroergotamine and its hypertensive effect.

4.6 Pregnancy and lactation

No data have been reported which would indicate the possibility of adverse effects resulting from the use of isosorbide mononitrate in pregnancy. Safety in pregnancy, however, has not been established. It is not known whether nitrates are excreted in human milk and therefore caution should be exercised when administered to nursing women.

Isosorbide mononitrate should only be used in pregnancy and during lactation if, in the opinion of the physician, the possible benefits of treatment outweigh the hazards.

4.7 Effects on ability to drive and use machines

Dizziness, tiredness or blurred vision might occur at the start of treatment. The patient should therefore be advised that if affected, they should not drive or operate machinery. This effect may be increased by alcohol.

4.8 Undesirable effects

A very common (>10% of patients) adverse reaction to Elantan is throbbing headache. The incidence of headache diminishes gradually with time and continued use.

At the start of therapy or when the dosage is increased, hypotension and/or light headedness in the upright position are commonly observed (i.e. in 1 – 10% of patients). These symptoms may be associated with dizziness, drowsiness, reflex tachychardia and a feeling of weakness.

Infrequently (i.e. in less than 1% of patients) nausea, vomiting, flushing and allergic skin reaction (e.g. rash) may occur sometimes severely. In single cases exfoliative dermatitis may occur.

Severe hypotensive responses have been reported for organic nitrates and include nausea, vomiting, restlessness pallor and excessive perspiration. Uncommonly collapse may occur (sometimes accompanied by bradyarrhythmia and syncope). Uncommonly severe hypotension may lead to enhanced angina symptoms.

A few reports of heartburn most likely due to a nitrate induced sphincter relaxation have been recorded.

Tachycardia and paroxysmal bradycardia have been reported.

4.9 Overdose

Symptoms and signs:

Headache, hypotension, nausea, vomiting, sweating, tachycardia, vertigo, restlessness, warm flushed skin, blurred vision and syncope. A rise in intracranial pressure with confusion and neurological deficits can sometimes occur. Methaemoglobinaemia (cyanosis, hypoxaemia, restlessness, respiratory depression, convulsions, cardiac arrhythmias, circulatory failure, raised intracranial pressure) occurs rarely.

Management:

Consider oral activated charcoal if ingestion of a potentially toxic amount has occurred within 1 hour. Observe for at least 12 hours after the overdose. Monitor blood pressure and pulse. Correct hypotension by raising the foot of the bed and/or by expanding the intravascular volume. Other measures as indicated by the patient's clinical condition. If severe hypotension persists despite the above measures consider use of inotropes.

If methaemoglobinaemia (symptoms or > 30% methaemoglobin), IV administration of methylene blue 1-2 mg/kg body weight. If therapy fails with second dose after 1 hour or contraindicated, consider red blood cell concentrates or exchange transfusion. In case of cerebral convulsions, diazepam or clonazepam IV, or if therapy fails, phenobarbital, phenytoin or propofol anaesthesia.

5. PHARMACOLOGICAL PROPERTIES

5.1 Pharmacodynamic properties

ATC Code: C01D A14 Vasodilator used in cardiac diseases

Isosorbide mononitrate is an organic nitrate which, in common with other cardioactive nitrates, is a vasodilator. It produces decreased left and right ventricular end-diastolic pressures to a greater extent than the decrease in systemic arterial pressure, thereby reducing afterload and especially the preload of the heart.

Isosorbide mononitrate influences the oxygen supply to ischaemic myocardium by causing the redistribution of blood flow along collateral channels and from epicardial to endocardial regions by selective dilation of large epicardial vessels.

It reduces the requirement of the myocardium for oxygen by increasing venous capacitance, causing a pooling of blood in peripheral veins, thereby reducing ventricular volume and heart wall distension.

5.2 Pharmacokinetic properties

Isosorbide-5-mononitrate is rapidly absorbed and peak plasma levels occur approx. 1 hour following oral dosing.

Isosorbide-5-mononitrate is completely bioavailable after oral doses and is not subject to pre-systemic elimination processes.

Isosorbide-5-mononitrate is eliminated from the plasma with a half-life of about 5.1 hours. It is metabolised to Isosorbide-5-mn-2-glucoronide which has a half-life of approximately 2.5 hours. As well as being excreted unchanged in the urine.

After multiple oral dosing plasma concentrations are similar to those that can be predicted from single dose kinetic parameters.

5.3 Preclinical safety data

Preclinical data reveal no special hazard for humans based on conventional studies of single and repeated dose toxicity, genotoxicity, oncogenicity and toxicity to reproduction.

6. PHARMACEUTICAL PARTICULARS

6.1 List of excipients

Lactose monohydrate

Purified talc

Colloidal silicon dioxide

Potato starch

Microcrystalline cellulose

Aluminium stearate

6.2 Incompatibilities

None Known

6.3 Shelf life

5 years

6.4 Special precautions for storage

None

6.5 Nature and contents of container

Cartons of blister strips of PP/aluminium or of PP/PP.

Aluminium foil thickness 16μm or 20μm.

Pack sizes: 50, 56, 60, 84, 90 and 100 tablets.

6.6 Special precautions for disposal and other handling

None

7. MARKETING AUTHORISATION HOLDER

UCB Pharma Limited

208 Bath Road

Slough

Berkshire

SL1 3WE

United Kingdom

8. MARKETING AUTHORISATION NUMBER(S)

PL 00039/0740

9. DATE OF FIRST AUTHORISATION/RENEWAL OF THE AUTHORISATION

27th March 2009

10. DATE OF REVISION OF THE TEXT

Elantan LA25

(UCB Pharma Limited)

1. NAME OF THE MEDICINAL PRODUCT

Elantan LA25

2. QUALITATIVE AND QUANTITATIVE COMPOSITION

Isosorbide mononitrate 25 mg

For excipients see 6.1.

3. PHARMACEUTICAL FORM

Prolonged release capsules

4. CLINICAL PARTICULARS

4.1 Therapeutic indications

For the prophylaxis of angina pectoris

4.2 Posology and method of administration

For oral administration

Adults

One capsule to be taken in the morning.

For patients with higher nitrate requirements the dose may be increased to two capsules taken simultaneously. The lowest effective dose should be used.

Elderly

There is no evidence to suggest an adjustment of dosage is necessary.

Children

The safety and efficacy of these capsules has yet to be established in children.

Attenuation of effect has occurred in some patients being treated with prolonged release preparations. In such patients intermittent therapy may be more appropriate (see section 4.4).

Treatment with Elantan LA, as with any other nitrate, should not be stopped suddenly. Both dosage and frequency should be tapered gradually (see section 4.4).

4.3 Contraindications

The capsules should not be used in cases of acute myocardial infarction with low filling pressure, acute circulatory failure, shock, vascular collapse, or very low blood pressure, hypertrophic obstructive cardiomyopathy (HOCM), constrictive pericarditis, cardiac tamponade, low cardiac filling pressures, aortic/mitral valve stenosis, and diseases associated with a raised intra-cranial pressure e.g. following a head trauma and including a cerebral haemorrhage.

This product should not be given to patients with a known sensitivity to Isosorbide mononitrate, the listed ingredients or other nitrates.

Elantan LA should not be used in patients with marked anaemia, closed angle glaucoma, severe hypotension or hypovolaemia.

Phosphodiesterase type-5 inhibitors (e.g. sildenafil, tadalafil and vardenafil) have been shown to potentiate the hypotensive effects of nitrates, and their co-administration with nitrates or nitric oxide donors is therefore contraindicated (see section 4.5).

4.4 Special warnings and precautions for use

The capsules should be used with caution in patients who have a recent history of myocardial infarction or who are suffering from hypothyroidism, hypothermia, malnutrition, severe liver or renal disease.

Symptoms of circulatory collapse may arise after first dose, particularly in patients with labile circulation.

This product may give rise to symptoms of postural hypotension and syncope in some patients. Severe postural hypotension with light-headedness and dizziness is frequently observed after the consumption of alcohol.

Hypotension induced by nitrates may be accompanied by paradoxical bradycardia and increased angina.

Elantan LA capsules contain lactose and therefore should not be used in patients with rare hereditary problems of galactose intolerance, the Lapp lactase deficiency or glucose-galactose malabsorption.

In the event of an acute angina attack, a sublingual treatment such as a GTN spray or tablet should be used instead of Elantan LA capsules.

If these capsules are not taken as indicated (see section 4.2.) tolerance to the medication could develop. In some patients being treated with prolonged release preparations, attenuation of effect is observed. In such patients, intermittent therapy may be more appropriate. The lowest effective dose should be used.

Treatment of Elantan LA, as with any other nitrate, should not be stopped suddenly. Both the dosage and frequency should be tapered gradually (See section 4.2).

4.5 Interaction with other medicinal products and other forms of interaction

Concurrent administration of drugs with blood pressure lowering properties, e.g. beta-blockers, calcium channel blockers, vasodilators, alprostadil, aldesleukin, angiotensin II receptor antagonists etc and/or alcohol may potentiate the hypotensive effect of Elantan LA. This may also occur with neuroleptics and tricyclic antidepressants.

Any blood pressure lowering effect of Elantan LA will be increased if used together with phosphodiesterase type-5 inhibitors which are used for erectile dysfunction (see special warnings and contraindications). This might lead to life threatening cardiovascular complications. Patients who are on Elantan LA therapy therefore must not use phosphodiesterase type-5 inhibitors.

Reports suggest that concomitant administration of Elantan LA may increase the blood level of dihydroergotamine and its hypertensive effect.

4.6 Pregnancy and lactation

No data have been reported which would indicate the possibility of adverse effects resulting from the use of isosorbide mononitrate in pregnancy. Safety in pregnancy, however, has not been established. It is not known whether nitrates are excreted in human milk and therefore caution should be exercised when administered to nursing women.

Isosorbide mononitrate should only be used in pregnancy and during lactation if, in the opinion of the physician, the possible benefits outweigh the possible hazards.

4.7 Effects on ability to drive and use machines

Dizziness, tiredness or blurred vision may occur at the start of treatment. The patient should therefore be advised that if affected, they should not drive or operate machinery. This effect may be increased by alcohol.

4.8 Undesirable effects

A very common (>10% of patients) adverse reaction to Elantan is throbbing headache. The incidence of headache diminishes gradually with time and continued use.

At the start of therapy or when the dosage is increased, hypotension and/or light headedness in the upright position are commonly observed (i.e. in 1 – 10% of patients). These symptoms may be associated with dizziness, drowsiness, reflex tachychardia and a feeling of weakness.

Infrequently (i.e. in less than 1% of patients) nausea, vomiting, flushing and allergic skin reaction (e.g. rash) may occur sometimes severely. In single cases exfoliative dermatitis may occur.

Severe hypotensive responses have been reported for organic nitrates and include nausea, vomiting, restlessness pallor and excessive perspiration. Uncommonly collapse may occur (sometimes accompanied by bradyarrhythmia and syncope). Uncommonly severe hypotension may lead to enhanced angina symptoms.

A few reports of heartburn most likely due to a nitrate induced sphincter relaxation have been recorded.

Tachycardia and paroxysmal bradycardia have been reported.

4.9 Overdose

Symptoms and signs:

Headache, hypotension, nausea, vomiting, sweating, tachycardia, vertigo, warm flushed skin, blurred vision and syncope. A rise in intracranial pressure with confusion and neurological deficits can sometimes occur. Methaemoglobinaemia (cyanosis, hypoxaemia, restlessness, respiratory depression, convulsions, cardiac arrhythmias, circulatory failure, raised intracranial pressure) occurs rarely.

Management:

Consider oral activated charcoal if ingestion of a potentially toxic amount has occurred within 1 hour. Observe for at least 12 hours after the overdose. Monitor blood pressure and pulse. Correct hypotension by raising the foot of the bed and/or by expanding the intravascular volume. Other measures as indicated by the patient's clinical condition. If severe hypotension persists despite the above measures consider the use of inotropes.

If methaemoglobinaemia (symptoms or > 30% methaemoglobin), IV administration of methylene blue 1-2 mg/kg body weight. If therapy fails with second dose after 1 hour or contraindicated, consider red blood cell concentrates or exchange transfusion. In case of cerebral convulsions, diazepam or clonazepam IV, or if therapy fails, phenobarbital, phenytoin or propofol anaesthesia.

5. PHARMACOLOGICAL PROPERTIES

5.1 Pharmacodynamic properties

ATC Code: C01D A14 Vasodilator used in cardiac diseases.

Isosorbide mononitrate is an organic nitrate which, in common with other cardioactive nitrates, is a vasodilator. It produces decreased left and right ventricular end-diastolic pressures to a greater extent than the decrease in systemic arterial pressure, thereby reducing afterload and especially preload of the heart.

Isosorbide mononitrate influences the oxygen supply to the ischaemic myocardium by causing the redistribution of blood flow along collateral channels and from epicardial to endocardial regions by selective dilation of large epicardial vessels.

It reduces the requirement of the myocardium for oxygen by increasing venous capacitance, causing a pooling of blood in peripheral veins, thereby reducing ventricular volume and heart wall distension.

5.2 Pharmacokinetic properties

Isosorbide mononitrate is a vasodilator, which is rapidly absorbed following oral administration. These capsules have a bioavailability of 84 (±7)% when compared to the immediate release isosorbide mononitrate tablets. There is no effect of food on bioavailability.

The capsules contain pellets which are formulated to release 30% of the dose immediately whilst 70% of the dose is released slowly.

Time to peak plasma levels (T_{max}) is 5.0 (±3) hrs; with a half life ($T_{½}$) of 5.02 (±0.68) hrs.

Isosorbide mononitrate is extensively metabolised to nitric oxide (NO-which is the active ingredient) and isosorbide (inactive). In patients with cirrhotic disease or cardiac failure or renal failure, parameters were similar to those obtained in healthy volunteers.

5.3 Preclinical safety data

Preclinical data reveal no special hazard for humans based on conventional studies of single and repeated dose toxicity, genotoxicity, oncogenicity and toxicity to reproduction.

6. PHARMACEUTICAL PARTICULARS

6.1 List of excipients

Lactose monohydrate

Purified Talc

Ethyl cellulose

Macrogol 20000

Hydroxypropyl cellulose

Sucrose

Corn starch

Gelatin

Titanium dioxide

Iron oxide red (E172)

Iron oxide black (E172)

6.2 Incompatibilities

None Known

6.3 Shelf life

5 years

6.4 Special precautions for storage

None

6.5 Nature and contents of container

Cartons of blister strips of PVC and aluminium or of PP and aluminium.

Aluminium foil thickness 20 μm or 16 μm.

Pack size: 28 capsules.

6.6 Special precautions for disposal and other handling

None

7. MARKETING AUTHORISATION HOLDER

UCB Pharma Limited

208 Bath Road

Slough

Berkshire

SL1 3WE

United Kingdom

8. MARKETING AUTHORISATION NUMBER(S)
PL 00039/0741

9. DATE OF FIRST AUTHORISATION/RENEWAL OF THE AUTHORISATION
28 February 2008

10. DATE OF REVISION OF THE TEXT

Elantan LA50

(UCB Pharma Limited)

1. NAME OF THE MEDICINAL PRODUCT
Elantan LA50

2. QUALITATIVE AND QUANTITATIVE COMPOSITION
Isosorbide mononitrate 50 mg

For excipients see 6.1.

3. PHARMACEUTICAL FORM
Prolonged release capsules, hard.

Hard capsule, upper half brown opaque and lower half flesh opaque. Contains white to off-white pellets.

4. CLINICAL PARTICULARS

4.1 Therapeutic indications
For the prophylaxis of angina pectoris

4.2 Posology and method of administration
For oral administration

Adults

One capsule to be taken in the morning.

For patients with higher nitrate requirements the dose may be increased to two capsules taken simultaneously. The lowest effective dose should be used.

Elderly

There is no evidence to suggest an adjustment of dosage is necessary.

Children

The safety and efficacy of these capsules has yet to be established in children.

Attenuation of effect has occurred in some patients being treated with prolonged release preparations. In such patients intermittent therapy may be more appropriate (see section 4.4).

Treatment with Elantan LA, as with any other nitrate, should not be stopped suddenly. Both dosage and frequency should be tapered gradually (see section 4.4).

4.3 Contraindications
The capsules should not be used in cases of acute myocardial infarction with low filling pressure, acute circulatory failure, (shock, vascular collapse), or very low blood pressure, hypertrophic obstructive cardiomyopathy (HOCM), constrictive pericarditis, cardiac tamponade, low cardiac filling pressures, aortic/mitral valve stenosis, and diseases associated with a raised intra-cranial pressure e.g. following a head trauma and including a cerebral haemorrhage.

This product should not be given to patients with a known sensitivity to Isosorbide mononitrate, the listed ingredients or other nitrates.

Elantan LA should not be used in patients with marked anaemia, closed angle glaucoma, severe hypotension or hypovolaemia.

Phosphodiesterase type-5 inhibitors (e.g. sildenafil, tadalafil and vardenafil) have been shown to potentiate the hypotensive effects of nitrates, and their co-administration with nitrates or nitric oxide donors is therefore contraindicated (see section 4.5)

4.4 Special warnings and precautions for use
The capsules should be used with caution in patients who have a recent history of myocardial infarction or who are suffering from hypothyroidism, hypothermia, malnutrition, severe liver disease or severe renal disease.

Symptoms of circulatory collapse may arise after first dose, particularly in patients with labile circulation.

This product may give rise to symptoms of postural hypotension and syncope in some patients. Severe postural hypotension with light-headedness and dizziness is frequently observed after the consumption of alcohol.

Hypotension induced by nitrates may be accompanied by paradoxical bradycardia and increased angina.

Elantan LA capsules contain lactose and therefore should not be used in patients with rare hereditary problems of galactose intolerance, the Lapp lactase deficiency or glucose-galactose malabsorption.

In the event of an acute angina attack, a sublingual treatment such as a GTN spray or tablet should be used instead of Elantan LA capsules.

If the capsules are not taken as indicated (see section 4.2.) tolerance to the medication could develop. In some patients being treated with prolonged release preparations, attenuation of effect is observed. In such patients, intermittent therapy may be more appropriate. The lowest effective dose should be used.

Treatment of Elantan LA, as with any other nitrate, should not be stopped suddenly. Both the dosage and frequency should be tapered gradually (See section 4.2).

4.5 Interaction with other medicinal products and other forms of interaction
Concurrent administration of drugs with blood pressure lowering properties, e.g. beta-blockers, calcium channel blockers, vasodilators, alprostadil, aldesleukin, angiotensin II receptor antagonists etc and/or alcohol may potentiate the hypotensive effect of Elantan LA. This may also occur with neuroleptics and tricyclic antidepressants.

Any blood pressure lowering effect of Elantan LA will be increased, if used together with phosphodiesterase type-5 inhibitors which are used for erectile dysfunction (see special warnings and contraindications). This might lead to life threatening cardiovascular complications. Patients who are on Elantan LA therapy therefore must not use phosphodiesterase type-5 inhibitors.

Reports suggest that concomitant administration of Elantan LA may increase the blood level of dihydroergotamine and its hypertensive effect.

4.6 Pregnancy and lactation
No data have been reported which would indicate the possibility of adverse effects resulting from the use of isosorbide mononitrate in pregnancy. Safety in pregnancy, however, has not been established. It is not known whether nitrates are excreted in human milk and therefore caution should be exercised when administered to nursing women.

Isosorbide mononitrate should only be used in pregnancy and during lactation if, in the opinion of the physician, the possible benefits outweigh the possible hazards.

4.7 Effects on ability to drive and use machines
Dizziness, tiredness or blurred vision may occur at the start of treatment. The patient should therefore be advised that if affected, they should not drive or operate machinery. This effect may be increased by alcohol.

4.8 Undesirable effects
A very common (>10% of patients) adverse reaction to Elantan is throbbing headache. The incidence of headache diminishes gradually with time and continued use.

At the start of therapy or when the dosage is increased, hypotension and/or light headedness in the upright position are commonly observed (i.e. in 1 – 10% of patients).

These symptoms may be associated with dizziness, drowsiness, reflex tachycardia and a feeling of weakness.

Uncommonly (i.e. in less than 1% of patients) nausea, vomiting, flushing and allergic skin reaction (e.g. rash) may occur sometimes severely. In single cases exfoliative dermatitis may occur.

Severe hypotensive responses have been reported for organic nitrates and include nausea, vomiting, restlessness pallor and excessive perspiration. Uncommonly collapse may occur (sometimes accompanied by bradyarrhythmia and syncope). Uncommonly severe hypotension may lead to enhanced angina symptoms.

A few reports of heartburn most likely due to a nitrate-induced sphincter relaxation have been reported.

Tachycardia and paroxysmal bradycardia have been reported.

4.9 Overdose
Symptoms and signs:

Headache, hypotension, nausea, vomiting, sweating, tachycardia, vertigo, warm flushed skin, blurred vision and syncope. A rise in intracranial pressure with confusion and neurological deficits can sometimes occur. Methaemoglobinaemia (cyanosis, hypoxaemia, restlessness, respiratory depression, convulsions, cardiac arrhythmias, circulatory failure, raised intracranial pressure) occurs rarely.

Management:

Consider oral activated charcoal if ingestion of a potentially toxic amount has occurred within 1 hour. Observe for at least 12 hours after the overdose. Monitor blood pressure and pulse. Correct hypotension by raising the foot of the bed and/or by expanding the intravascular volume. Other measures as indicated by the patient's clinical condition. If severe hypotension persists despite the above measures consider the use of inotropes.

If methaemoglobinaemia (symptoms or > 30% methaemoglobin), IV administration of methylene blue 1-2 mg/kg body weight. If therapy fails with second dose after 1 hour or contraindicated, consider red blood cell concentrates or exchange transfusion. In case of cerebral convulsions, diazepam or clonazepam IV, or if therapy fails, phenobarbital, phenytoin or propofol anaesthesia.

5. PHARMACOLOGICAL PROPERTIES

5.1 Pharmacodynamic properties
ATC Code: C01D A14 Vasodilator used in cardiac diseases.

Isosorbide mononitrate is an organic nitrate which, in common with other cardioactive nitrates, is a vasodilator. It produces decreased left and right ventricular end-diastolic pressures to a greater extent than the decrease in systemic arterial pressure, thereby reducing afterload and especially the preload of the heart.

Isosorbide mononitrate influences the oxygen supply to the ischaemic myocardium by causing the redistribution of blood flow along collateral channels and from epicardial to endocardial regions by selective dilation of large epicardial vessels.

It reduces the requirement of the myocardium for oxygen by increasing venous capacitance, causing a pooling of blood in peripheral veins, thereby reducing ventricular volume and heart wall distension.

5.2 Pharmacokinetic properties
Isosorbide mononitrate is a vasodilator, which is rapidly absorbed following oral administration. These capsules have a bioavailability of 84 (±7)% when compared to the immediate release isosorbide mononitrate tablets. There is no effect of food on bioavailability.

The capsules contain pellets which are formulated to release 30% of the dose immediately whilst 70% of the dose is released slowly.

Time to peak plasma levels (T_{max}) is 5.0 (±3) hrs; with a half life ($T_{½}$) of 5.02 (±0.68) hrs.

Isosorbide mononitrate is extensively metabolised to nitric oxide (NO-which is the active ingredient) and isosorbide (inactive). In patients with cirrhotic disease or cardiac failure or renal failure, parameters were similar to those obtained in healthy volunteers.

5.3 Preclinical safety data
Preclinical data reveal no special hazard for humans based on conventional studies of single and repeated dose toxicity, genotoxicity, oncogenicity and toxicity to reproduction.

6. PHARMACEUTICAL PARTICULARS

6.1 List of excipients
Lactose monohydrate

Purified talc

Ethyl cellulose

Macrogol 20,000

Hydroxypropyl cellulose

Sucrose

Corn starch

Gelatin

Titanium dioxide (E171)

Iron oxide red (E172)

Iron oxide black (E172)

6.2 Incompatibilities
None Known

6.3 Shelf life
5 years

6.4 Special precautions for storage
None

6.5 Nature and contents of container
Cartons of blister strips of PVC and aluminium or of PP and aluminium.

Aluminium foil thickness 20 µm or 16 µm.

Pack size: 28 capsules.

6.6 Special precautions for disposal and other handling
None

7. MARKETING AUTHORISATION HOLDER
UCB Pharma Limited

208 Bath Road

Slough

Berkshire

SL1 3WE

United Kingdom

8. MARKETING AUTHORISATION NUMBER(S)
PL 00039/0742

9. DATE OF FIRST AUTHORISATION/RENEWAL OF THE AUTHORISATION
23 June 2008

10. DATE OF REVISION OF THE TEXT

Elaprase 2 mg/ml concentrate for solution for infusion

(Shire Human Genetic Therapies)

1. NAME OF THE MEDICINAL PRODUCT
Elaprase ▼ 2 mg/ml concentrate for solution for infusion.

2. QUALITATIVE AND QUANTITATIVE COMPOSITION
Each vial of 3 ml contains 6 mg of idursulfase. Each ml contains 2 mg of idursulfase.

Idursulfase is produced by recombinant DNA technology in a continuous human cell line.

For a full list of excipients, see section 6.1.

3. PHARMACEUTICAL FORM
Concentrate for solution for infusion.

A clear to slightly opalescent, colourless solution.

4. CLINICAL PARTICULARS

4.1 Therapeutic indications
Elaprase is indicated for the long-term treatment of patients with Hunter syndrome (Mucopolysaccharidosis II, MPS II).

Heterozygous females were not studied in the clinical trials.

4.2 Posology and method of administration

Elaprase treatment should be supervised by a physician or other healthcare professional experienced in the management of patients with MPS II disease or other inherited metabolic disorders.

Elaprase is administered at a dose of 0.5 mg/kg body weight every week by intravenous infusion over a 3 hour period, which may be gradually reduced to 1 hour if no infusion-associated reactions are observed (see section 4.4).

For preparation and administration instructions see section 6.6.

Patients with renal or hepatic impairment

There is no clinical experience in patients with renal or hepatic insufficiency. See section 5.2.

Elderly patients

There is no clinical experience in patients over 65 years of age.

Paediatric patients

The dose for children and adolescents is 0.5 mg/kg body weight weekly.

For preparation and administration instructions see section 6.6.

There is no clinical experience in children under the age of 5.

4.3 Contraindications

Hypersensitivity to the active substance or to any of the excipients.

4.4 Special warnings and precautions for use

Patients treated with idursulfase may develop infusion-related reactions (see section 4.8). During clinical trials, the most common infusion-related reactions included cutaneous reactions (rash, pruritus, urticaria), pyrexia, headache, hypertension, and flushing. Infusion-related reactions were treated or ameliorated by slowing the infusion rate, interrupting the infusion, or by administration of medicines, such as antihistamines, antipyretics, low-dose corticosteroids (prednisone and methylprednisolone), or beta-agonist nebulization. No patient discontinued treatment due to an infusion reaction during clinical studies.

Special care should be taken when administering an infusion in patients with severe underlying airway disease. These patients should be closely monitored and infused in an appropriate clinical setting. Caution must be exercised in the management and treatment of such patients by limitation or careful monitoring of antihistamine and other sedative medicinal product use. Institution of positive-airway pressure may be necessary in some cases.

Consider delaying the infusion in patients who present with an acute febrile respiratory illness. Patients using supplemental oxygen should have this treatment readily available during infusion in the event of an infusion-related reaction.

Patients who develop IgM or IgG antibodies are at a higher risk of infusion reactions and other adverse reactions, however, IgE antibodies have not been observed.

Anaphylactoid reactions, which have the potential to be life threatening, have been observed in some patients treated with Elaprase, as with any intravenous protein product. Late emergent symptoms and signs of anaphylactoid reactions have been observed as long as 24 hours after an initial reaction. If an anaphylactoid reaction occurs the infusion should be immediately suspended and appropriate treatment and observation initiated. The current medical standards for emergency treatment are to be observed. Patients experiencing severe or refractory anaphylactoid reactions may require prolonged clinical monitoring. Patients who have experienced anaphylactoid reactions should be treated with caution when re-administering Elaprase.

4.5 Interaction with other medicinal products and other forms of interaction

No formal drug interaction studies have been conducted with Elaprase.

Based on its metabolism in cellular lysosomes, idursulfase would not be a candidate for cytochrome P450 mediated interactions.

4.6 Pregnancy and lactation

Elaprase is not indicated for use in women of child-bearing potential. No reproductive studies in female animals have been performed. No effects on male fertility were seen in reproductive studies in male rats.

Excretion of idursulfase in milk has not been studied.

4.7 Effects on ability to drive and use machines

No studies on the effects on the ability to drive and use machines have been performed.

4.8 Undesirable effects

Adverse drug reactions that were reported for the 32 patients treated with 0.5 mg/kg Elaprase weekly in the Phase II/III 52-week placebo-controlled study were almost all mild to moderate in severity. The most common were infusion-related reactions, 202 of which were reported in 22 out of 32 patients following administration of a total of 1580 infusions. In the placebo treatment group 128 infusion-related reactions were reported in 21 out of 32 patients following administration of a total of 1612 infusions. Since more than one infusion-related reaction may have occurred during any single infusion, the above numbers are likely to over estimate the true incidence of infusion reactions. Related reactions in the placebo group were similar in nature and severity to those in the treated group. The most common of these infusion-related reactions included cutaneous reactions (rash, pruritus, urticaria), pyrexia, headache, and hypertension. The frequency of infusion-related reactions decreased over time with continued treatment.

Adverse drug reactions are listed in the table below with information presented by system organ class and frequency. Frequency is given as very common (>1/10) or common (>1/100, <1/10). The occurrence of an event in a single patient is defined as common in view of the number of patients treated. Within each frequency grouping, undesirable effects are presented in order of decreasing seriousness.

Adverse drug reactions were defined as treatment-emergent events with suspected causality and excluded non-serious events that were reported only once in a single patient; treatment emergent events with an excess incidence of at least 9% compared with placebo were also considered as adverse drug reactions.

System Organ Class	Adverse Drug Reaction (Preferred Term)
Nervous system disorders	
Very common:	headache
Common:	dizziness, tremor
Eye disorders	
Common:	lacrimation increased
Cardiac disorders	
Common:	arrhythmia*, cyanosis
Vascular disorders	
Very common:	hypertension
Common:	hypotension, flushing
Respiratory, thoracic and mediastinal disorders	
Common:	bronchospasm, pulmonary embolism*, cough, wheezing, tachypnoea, dyspnoea
Gastrointestinal disorders	
Very common	dyspepsia
Common:	abdominal pain, nausea, diarrhoea, swollen tongue
Skin and subcutaneous tissue disorders	
Very common:	urticaria, rash, pruritus
Common:	face oedema, erythema, eczema
Musculoskeletal and connective tissue disorders	
Very common:	chest pain
Common:	arthralgia
General disorders and administration site conditions	
Very common:	pyrexia, infusion site swelling
Common:	oedema peripheral

* see serious adverse reactions below

Across studies, serious adverse reactions were reported in a total of 5 patients who received 0.5 mg/kg weekly or every other week. Four patients experienced a hypoxic episode during one or several infusions, which necessitated oxygen therapy in 3 patients with severe underlying obstructive airway disease (2 with a pre-existing tracheostomy). The most severe episode, which was associated with a short seizure, occurred in a patient who received his infusion while he had a febrile respiratory exacerbation. In the fourth patient, who had less severe underlying disease, spontaneous resolution occurred shortly after the infusion was interrupted. These events did not recur with subsequent infusions using a slower infusion rate and administration of pre-infusion medicinal products, usually low-dose steroids, antihistamine, and beta-agonist nebulization. The fifth patient, who had pre-existing cardiopathy, was diagnosed with ventricular premature complexes and pulmonary embolism during the study.

There have been post-marketing reports of anaphylactoid reactions. Please see section 4.4 for further information.

Across all studies, 53/108 patients (49%) developed anti-idursulfase IgG antibodies at some point. Six of the IgG positive patients also tested positive for IgM antibodies, and 1 patient tested positive for IgA antibodies. No patient developed IgE antibodies during any study. The overall neutralizing antibody rate was 11/108 patients (10%). In the 52-week study, rates of seropositivity peaked by Weeks 18 to 27 and steadily declined thereafter for the remainder of this study.

In general, patients who tested positive for IgG antibodies were more likely to have infusion-related events than those who did not test positive. However, overall rates of infusion-related adverse events declined over time, regardless of antibody status. The reduction of urinary GAG excretion was somewhat less in patients for whom circulating anti-idursulfase antibodies were detected.

4.9 Overdose

There is no experience with overdoses of Elaprase.

5. PHARMACOLOGICAL PROPERTIES

5.1 Pharmacodynamic properties

Pharmacotherapeutic group: Alimentary tract and metabolism products – enzymes, ATC code: A16AB09.

Hunter syndrome is an X-linked disease caused by insufficient levels of the lysosomal enzyme iduronate-2-sulfatase. Iduronate-2-sulfatase functions to catabolize the glycosaminoglycans (GAG) dermatan sulfate and heparan sulfate by cleavage of oligosaccharide-linked sulfate moieties. Due to the missing or defective iduronate-2-sulfatase enzyme in patients with Hunter syndrome, glycosaminoglycans progressively accumulate in the cells, leading to cellular engorgement, organomegaly, tissue destruction, and organ system dysfunction.

Idursulfase is a purified form of the lysosomal enzyme iduronate-2-sulfatase, produced in a human cell line providing a human glycosylation profile, which is analogous to the naturally occurring enzyme. Idursulfase is secreted as a 525 amino acid glycoprotein and contains 8 N-linked glycosylation sites that are occupied by complex, hybrid, and high-mannose type oligosaccharide chains. Idursulfase has a molecular weight of approximately 76 kD.

Treatment of Hunter syndrome patients with intravenous Elaprase provides exogenous enzyme for uptake into cellular lysosomes. Mannose-6-phosphate (M6P) residues on the oligosaccharide chains allow specific binding of the enzyme to the M6P receptors on the cell surface, leading to cellular internalization of the enzyme, targeting to intracellular lysosomes and subsequent catabolism of accumulated GAG.

A total of 108 male Hunter syndrome patients with a broad spectrum of symptoms were enrolled in two randomized, placebo-controlled clinical studies, 106 continued treatment in two open-label, extension studies.

In a 52-week, randomized, double-blind, placebo-controlled clinical study, 96 patients between the ages of 5 and 31 years received Elaprase 0.5 mg/kg every week (n=32) or 0.5 mg/kg every other week (n=32), or placebo (n=32). The study included patients with a documented deficiency in iduronate-2-sulfatase enzyme activity, a percent predicted FVC <80%, and a broad spectrum of disease severity.

The primary efficacy endpoint was a two-component composite score based on the sum of the ranks of the change from baseline to the end of the study in the distance walked during six minutes (6-minute walk test or 6MWT) as a measure of endurance, and % predicted forced vital capacity (FVC) as a measure of pulmonary function. This endpoint differed significantly from placebo for patients treated weekly (p=0.0049).

Additional clinical benefit analyses were performed on individual components of the primary endpoint composite score, absolute changes in FVC, changes in urine GAG levels, liver and spleen volumes, measurement of forced expiratory volume in 1 second (FEV_1), and changes in left ventricular mass (LVM).

(see Table 1 on next page)

A total of 11 of 31 (36%) patients in the weekly treatment group versus 5 of 31 (16%) patients in the placebo group had an increase in FEV_1 of at least 200 cc at or before the end of the study, indicating a dose-related improvement in airway obstruction. The patients in the weekly treatment group experienced a clinically significant 15% mean improvement in FEV_1 at the end of the study.

Urine GAG levels were normalized below the upper limit of normal (defined as 126.6 μg GAG/mg creatinine) in 50% of the patients receiving weekly treatment.

Of the 25 patients with abnormally large livers at baseline in the weekly treatment group, 80% (20 patients) had reductions in liver volume to within the normal range by the end of the study.

Of the 9 patients in the weekly treatment group with abnormally large spleens at baseline, 3 had spleen volumes that normalized by the end of the study.

Approximately half of the patients in the weekly treatment group (15 of 32; 47%) had left ventricular hypertrophy at baseline, defined as LVM index >103 g/m^2. Of these 6 (40%) had normalised LVM by the end of the study.

No clinical data exist demonstrating a benefit on the neurological manifestations of the disorder.

This medicinal product has been authorised under "Exceptional Circumstances".

This means that due to the rarity of the disease it has not been possible to obtain complete information on this medicinal product.

Table 1

Endpoint	52 Weeks of Treatment 0.5 mg/kg Weekly			
	Marginally Weighted (OM) Mean (SE)		Mean Treatment Difference Compared with Placebo (SE)	P-value (Compared with Placebo)
	Idursulfase	Placebo		
Composite (6MWT and %FVC)	74.5 (4.5)	55.5 (4.5)	19.0 (6.5)	0.0049
6MWT (m)	43.3 (9.6)	8.2 (9.6)	35.1 (13.7)	0.0131
% Predicted FVC	4.2 (1.6)	-0.04 (1.6)	4.3 (2.3)	0.0650
FVC Absolute Volume (cc)	230.0 (40.0)	50.0 (40.0)	190.0 (60.0)	0.0011
Urine GAG Levels (μg GAG/mg creatinine)	-223.3 (20.7)	52.23 (20.7)	-275.5 (30.1)	<0.0001
% Change in Liver Volume	-25.7 (1.5)	-0.5 (1.6)	-25.2 (2.2)	<0.0001
% Change in Spleen Volume	-25.5 (3.3)	7.7 (3.4)	-33.2 (4.8)	<0.0001

The European Medicines Agency (EMEA) will review any new information which may become available every year and this SPC will be updated as necessary.

5.2 Pharmacokinetic properties

Idursulfase is taken up by selective receptor-mediated mechanisms involving binding to mannose 6-phosphate receptors. Upon internalization by cells, it is localized within cellular lysosomes, thereby limiting distribution of the protein. Degradation of idursulfase is achieved by generally well understood protein hydrolysis mechanisms to produce small peptides and amino acids, consequently renal and liver function impairment is not expected to affect the pharmacokinetics of idursulfase.

Pharmacokinetics was evaluated in 10 patients at Week 1 and Week 27 following administration of 0.5 mg/kg weekly as a 3-hour infusion. There were no differences in pharmacokinetic parameters following 27 weeks of treatment.

Parameter	Week 1 (SD)	Week 27 (SD)
C_{max} (μg/ml)	1.5 (0.6)	1.1 (0.3)
AUC (min* μg/ml)	206 (87)	169 (55)
$T_{1/2}$ (min)	44 (19)	48 (21)
Cl (ml/min/kg)	3.0 (1.2)	3.40 (1.0)
V_{ss} (% BW)	21 (8)	25 (9)

5.3 Preclinical safety data

Nonclinical data reveal no special hazard for humans based on conventional studies of safety pharmacology, single dose toxicity, repeated dose toxicity and male fertility. No reproductive toxicity studies in female animals have been performed.

6. PHARMACEUTICAL PARTICULARS

6.1 List of excipients

Polysorbate 20

Sodium chloride

Sodium phosphate dibasic, heptahydrate

Sodium phosphate monobasic, monohydrate

Water for Injections

6.2 Incompatibilities

In the absence of compatibility studies, this medicinal product must not be mixed with other medicinal products except those mentioned in section 6.6.

6.3 Shelf life

2 years

Chemical and physical in-use stability has been demonstrated for 8 hours at 25°C.

From a microbiological safety point of view, the diluted product should be used immediately. If not used immediately, in-use storage times and conditions prior to use are the responsibility of the user and should not be longer than 24 hours at 2 to 8°C.

6.4 Special precautions for storage

Store in a refrigerator (2°C – 8°C).

Do not freeze.

For storage conditions of the diluted medicinal product, see section 6.3.

6.5 Nature and contents of container

3 ml of concentrate for solution for infusion in a 5 ml vial (type I glass) with a stopper (fluoro-resin coated butyl rubber), one piece seal and blue flip-off cap.

Pack sizes of 1, 4 and 10 vials.

Not all pack sizes may be marketed.

6.6 Special precautions for disposal and other handling

Each vial of Elaprase is intended for single use only and contains 6 mg of idursulfase in 3 ml of solution. Elaprase is for intravenous infusion and must be diluted in sodium chloride 9 mg/ml (0.9%) solution for infusion prior to use.

- Determine the number of vials to be diluted based on the individual patient's weight and the recommended dose of 0.5 mg/kg.

- Do not use if the solution in the vials is discoloured or if particulate matter is present. Do not shake.

- Withdraw the calculated volume of Elaprase from the appropriate number of vials.

- Dilute the total volume required of Elaprase in 100 ml of 9 mg/ml (0.9%) sodium chloride solution for infusion. Care must be taken to ensure the sterility of the prepared solutions since Elaprase does not contain any preservative or bacteriostatic agent; aseptic technique must be observed. Once diluted, the solution should be mixed gently, but not shaken.

Any unused product or waste material should be disposed of in accordance with local requirements.

7. MARKETING AUTHORISATION HOLDER

Shire Human Genetic Therapies AB, Svärdvägen 11D, 182 33 Danderyd, Sweden

8. MARKETING AUTHORISATION NUMBER(S)

EU/1/06/365/001-003

9. DATE OF FIRST AUTHORISATION/RENEWAL OF THE AUTHORISATION

08.01.2007

10. DATE OF REVISION OF THE TEXT

30.10.2008

11. LEGAL CATEGORY

POM

Eldepryl Syrup 10 mg / 5 ml

(Orion Pharma (UK) Limited)

1. NAME OF THE MEDICINAL PRODUCT

Eldepryl syrup 10 mg / 5ml

2. QUALITATIVE AND QUANTITATIVE COMPOSITION

Selegiline hydrochloride 10 mg /5 ml

For full list of excipients, see section 6.1

3. PHARMACEUTICAL FORM

Syrup for oral administration.

4. CLINICAL PARTICULARS

4.1 Therapeutic indications

Selegiline is indicated for the treatment of Parkinson's disease, or symptomatic parkinsonism. It may be used alone to delay the need for levodopa (with or without decarboxylase inhibitor) or as an adjunct to levodopa (with or without decarboxylase inhibitor).

4.2 Posology and method of administration

10 mg daily either alone or as an adjunct to levodopa or levodopa/peripheral decarboxylase inhibitor. Selegiline may be administered either as a single dose in the morning or in two divided doses of 5 mg, taken at breakfast and lunch. When selegiline is added to a levodopa regimen it is possible to reduce the levodopa dosage by an average of 30%.

4.3 Contraindications

Known hypersensitivity to selegiline or other components of the formulation.

4.4 Special warnings and precautions for use

Selegiline should be administered cautiously to patients with peptic or duodenal ulcer, labile hypertension, cardiac arrhythmias, severe angina pectoris, severe liver or kidney dysfunction or psychosis. In higher doses (more than 30 mg daily) the selectivity of selegiline begins to diminish resulting in increased inhibition of MAO-A. Thus in higher doses there is a risk of hypertension after ingestion of food rich in tyramine.

4.5 Interaction with other medicinal products and other forms of interaction

Foods containing tyramine have not been reported to induce hypertensive reactions during selegiline treatment at doses used in the treatment of Parkinson's disease.

A concomitant use of nonselective MAO-inhibitors may cause severe hypotension.

No tolerability problems have been reported when a combination of selegiline and moclobemide, an inhibitor of MAO-A, has been used. However, when they are used together, the tyramine sensitivity factor may increase up to 8-9 (being 1 for selegiline alone and 2-3 for moclobemide alone). Although tyramine induced hypertensive reactions are unlikely when selegiline and moclobemide are used together, dietary restrictions (excluding foods with large amounts of tyramine such as aged cheese and yeast products) are recommended when using this combination.

Interactions between nonselective MAO-inhibitors and pethidine, as well as selegiline and pethidine have been described. The mechanism of this interaction is not fully understood and therefore, use of pethidine concomitantly with selegiline should be avoided. Tramadol may also potentially interact with Selegiline.

Dopamine should be used with caution in patients receiving Selegiline.

Serious reactions with signs and symptoms that may include diaphoresis, flushing, ataxia, tremor, hyperthermia, hyper/hypotension, seizures, palpitation, dizziness and mental changes that include agitation, confusion and hallucinations progressing to delirium and coma have been reported in some patients receiving a combination of selegiline and fluoxetine. Similar experience has been reported in patients receiving selegiline and four serotonin reuptake inhibitors, fluvoxamine, sertraline, paroxetine or venlafaxine. Since the mechanisms of these reactions are not fully understood, it is recommended to avoid the combination of selegiline with fluoxetine, sertraline, paroxetine or venlafaxine. A minimum period of five weeks should be allowed between discontinuation of fluoxetine and initiation of selegiline treatment, due to the long half-lives of fluoxetine and its active metabolite. As the half-lives of selegiline and its metabolites are short, a wash-out period of 14 days after selegiline treatment would be sufficient before starting fluoxetine. The concomitant use of selegiline and citalopram has been investigated in healthy volunteers. No signs of clinically relevant pharmacokinetic or pharmacodynamic interactions between the two drugs were observed.

Severe CNS toxicity has been reported in patients with the combination of tricyclic antidepressants and selegiline. In one patient receiving amitriptyline and selegiline this included hyperpyrexia and death, and another patient receiving protriptyline and selegiline experienced tremor, agitation, and restlessness followed by unresponsiveness and death two weeks after selegiline was added. Other adverse reactions occasionally reported in patients receiving a combination of selegiline with various tricyclic antidepressants include hyper/hypotension, dizziness, diaphoresis, tremor, seizures, and changes in behavioural and mental status. Since the mechanisms of these reactions are not fully understood, it is recommended to be cautious when using selegiline together with tricyclic antidepressants.

Concomitant use of oral contraceptives (tablets containing the combination of gestodene/ethinyl estradiol or levonorgestrel/ethinyl estradiol) and selegiline may cause an increase in the oral bioavailability of selegiline. Thus appropriate caution during the concomitant administration of selegiline and oral contraceptives should be applied.

4.6 Pregnancy and lactation

The available safety data concerning the use during pregnancy and lactation is insufficient to justify the use of selegiline in these patient groups.

4.7 Effects on ability to drive and use machines

No effects on ability to drive or operate machines.

4.8 Undesirable effects

In monotherapy, selegiline has been found to be well tolerated. Dry mouth, transient rise of serum alanine aminotransferase (ALAT) values and sleeping disorders have been reported more frequently than in patients receiving placebo. Because selegiline potentiates the effects of levodopa, the adverse reactions of levodopa, e.g. abnormal movements (such as dyskinesias), nausea, agitation, confusion, hallucinations, headache, postural hypotension, cardiac arrhythmias and vertigo, may be emphasised, particularly if the dose of levodopa is too high. Such adverse reactions usually disappear when the levodopa dosage is decreased. Levodopa dosage can be reduced by an average of 30% when selegiline is added to the treatment. Micturition difficulties and skin reactions have also been reported during selegiline treatment. Follow-up of these possible adverse reactions is important. Hypersexuality has been very rarely reported in association with selegiline use, either as monotherapy or in combination with other dopaminergic antiparkinsonian medication.

A summary of the undesirable effects in terms of frequency of occurrence is shown below.

Psychiatric disorders	**Common (>1/100, <1/10)**	**Sleeping disorders, confusion, hallucinations**
	Very rare (<1/10,000)	**Hypersexuality**
Nervous system disorders	**Common (>1/100, <1/10)**	**Dry mouth, abnormal movements (such as dyskinesias), vertigo**
	Rare (>1/10,000, <1/1,000)	**Agitation, headache**
Cardiac disorders	**Rare (>1/10,000, <1/1,000)**	**Cardiac arrhythmias**
Vascular disorders	**Common (>1/100, <1/10)**	**Postural hypotension**
Gastrointestinal disorders	**Common (>1/100, <1/10)**	**Nausea**
Hepato-biliary disordrers	**Common (>1/100, <1/10)**	**Transient rise of serum alanine aminotransferase (ALAT)**
Skin and subcutaneous tissue	**Rare (>1/10,000, <1/1,000)**	**Skin reactions**
Renal and urinary disorders	**Rare (>1/10,000, <1/1,000)**	**Micturition difficulties**

4.9 Overdose

No overdosage cases are known. However, experience gained during selegiline's development reveals that some individuals exposed to doses of 600 mg/day selegiline suffered severe hypotension and psychomotor agitation.

Theoretically, overdosage causes significant inhibition of both MAO-A and MAO-B and thus, symptoms of overdosage may resemble those observed with non-selective MAO-inhibitors, such as different central nervous and cardiovascular system disorders (e.g. drowsiness, dizziness, faintness, irritability, hyperactivity, agitation, severe headache, hallucination, hypertension, hypotension, vascular collapse, rapid and irregular pulse, precordial pain, respiratory depression and failure, hyperpyrexia, diaphoresis). There is no specific antidote and the treatment is symptomatic.

5. PHARMACOLOGICAL PROPERTIES

5.1 Pharmacodynamic properties

Selegiline is a selective MAO-B-inhibitor which prevents dopamine breakdown in the brain. It also inhibits the reuptake of dopamine at the presynaptic dopamine receptor. These effects potentiate dopaminergic function in the brain and help to even out and prolong the effect of exogenous and endogenous dopamine. Thus, selegiline potentiates and prolongs the effect of levodopa in the treatment of parkinsonism.

Double-blind studies on early phase Parkinsonian patients showed that patients receiving selegiline monotherapy manage significantly longer without levodopa therapy than controls receiving placebo. These patients could also maintain their ability to work longer.

The addition of selegiline to levodopa (with or without decarboxylase inhibitor) therapy helps to alleviate dose related fluctuations and end of dose deterioration.

When selegiline is added to such a regimen it is possible to reduce the levodopa dosage by an average of 30%. Unlike conventional MAO-inhibitors, which inhibit both the MAO-A and MAO-B enzyme, selegiline is a specific MAO-B inhibitor and can be given safely with levodopa.

Selegiline HCl does not cause the so called "cheese effect" either when used alone as monotherapy, or when used with other drugs, except for moclobemide or nonselective MAO-inhibitors.

5.2 Pharmacokinetic properties

Selegiline HCl is readily absorbed from the gastrointestinal tract. The maximal concentrations are reached in half an hour after oral administration. The bioavailability is low; 10% (on the average; interindividual variation is large) of unchanged selegiline can reach the systemic circulation.

Selegiline is a lipophilic, slightly basic compound which quickly penetrates into tissues, also into brain. Selegiline HCl inhibits MAO irreversibly and enzyme activity only increases again after new enzyme is synthesised. The inhibitory effect of a single 10 mg dose lasts for 24 hours. Selegiline is rapidly distributed throughout the body, the apparent volume of distribution being 500 liters after an intravenous 10 mg dose. 75-85 % of selegiline is bound to plasma proteins at therapeutic concentrations.

Selegiline is rapidly metabolized, mainly in the liver, into desmethylselegiline, l-methamphetamine and to l-amphetamine. In humans, the three metabolites have been identified in plasma and urine after single and multiple doses of selegiline. The mean elimination half-life is 1.6 hours for selegiline. The total body clearance of selegiline is about 240 L/hour. Metabolites of selegiline are excreted mainly via the urine with about 15% occurring in the faeces.

5.3 Preclinical safety data

No mutagenicity or carcinogenicity due to selegiline have emerged in routine studies.

6. PHARMACEUTICAL PARTICULARS

6.1 List of excipients

Methyl parahydroxybenzoate, propyl parahydroxybenzoate, butyl parahydroxybenzoate, sucrose, xanthan gum T, saccharin sodium, flavour mango, purified water.

6.2 Incompatibilities

No other incompatibilities noted.

6.3 Shelf life

36 months

6.4 Special precautions for storage

No special precautions.

6.5 Nature and contents of container

Amber glass bottle (200 ml) sealed with a pilfer-proof type EPE/Aluminium Melinex screw cap. The container is packed in a cardboard box with a graduated dose dispenser.

6.6 Special precautions for disposal and other handling

None.

7. MARKETING AUTHORISATION HOLDER

Orion Corporation, Orionintie 1, FIN-02200 Espoo, Finland

8. MARKETING AUTHORISATION NUMBER(S)

PL 27925/0006

9. DATE OF FIRST AUTHORISATION/RENEWAL OF THE AUTHORISATION

1.7.1993/Renewal July 2007

10. DATE OF REVISION OF THE TEXT

June 2009

Eldepryl tablets 10mg

(Orion Pharma (UK) Limited)

1. NAME OF THE MEDICINAL PRODUCT

Eldepryl Tablets 10 mg

2. QUALITATIVE AND QUANTITATIVE COMPOSITION

Selegiline hydrochloride 10 mg

Full list of excipients, see section 6.1.

3. PHARMACEUTICAL FORM

Tablets for oral administration.

4. CLINICAL PARTICULARS

4.1 Therapeutic indications

Selegiline is indicated for the treatment of Parkinson's disease, or symptomatic parkinsonism. It may be used alone to delay the need for levodopa (with or without decarboxylase inhibitor) or as an adjunct to levodopa (with or without decarboxylase inhibitor).

4.2 Posology and method of administration

10 mg daily either alone or as an adjunct to levodopa or levodopa/peripheral decarboxylase inhibitor. Selegiline may be administered either as a single dose in the morning or in two divided doses of 5 mg, taken at breakfast and lunch. When selegiline is added to a levodopa regimen it is possible to reduce the levodopa dosage by an average of 30%.

4.3 Contraindications

Known hypersensitivity to selegiline or other components of the formulation.

4.4 Special warnings and precautions for use

Selegiline should be administered cautiously to patients with peptic or duodenal ulcer, labile hypertension, cardiac arrhythmias, severe angina pectoris, severe liver or kidney dysfunction or psychosis. In higher doses (more than 30 mg daily) the selectivity of selegiline begins to diminish resulting in increased inhibition of MAO-A. Thus in higher doses there is a risk of hypertension after ingestion of food rich in tyramine.

4.5 Interaction with other medicinal products and other forms of interaction

Foods containing tyramine have not been reported to induce hypertensive reactions during selegiline treatment at doses used in the treatment of Parkinson's disease.

A concomitant use of nonselective MAO-inhibitors may cause severe hypotension.

No tolerability problems have been reported when a combination of selegiline and moclobemide, an inhibitor of MAO-A, has been used. However, when they are used together, the tyramine sensitivity factor may increase up to 8-9 (being 1 for selegiline alone and 2-3 for moclobemide alone). Although tyramine induced hypertensive reactions are unlikely when selegiline and moclobemide are used together, dietary restrictions (excluding foods with large amounts of tyramine such as aged cheese and yeast products) are recommended when using this combination.

Interactions between nonselective MAO-inhibitors and pethidine, as well as selegiline and pethidine have been described. The mechanism of this interaction is not fully understood and therefore, use of pethidine concomitantly with selegiline should be avoided. Tramadol may also potentially interact with Selegiline.

Dopamine should be used with caution in patients receiving Selegiline.

Serious reactions with signs and symptoms that may include diaphoresis, flushing, ataxia, tremor, hyperthermia, hyper/hypotension, seizures, palpitation, dizziness and mental changes that include agitation, confusion and hallucinations progressing to delirium and coma have been reported in some patients receiving a combination of selegiline and fluoxetine. Similar experience has been reported in patients receiving selegiline and four serotonin reuptake inhibitors, fluvoxamine, sertraline, paroxetine or venlafaxine. Since the mechanisms of these reactions are not fully understood, it is recommended to avoid the combination of selegiline with fluoxetine, sertraline, paroxetine or venlafaxine. A minimum period of five weeks should be allowed between discontinuation of fluoxetine and initiation of selegiline treatment, due to the long half-lives of fluoxetine and its active metabolite. As the half-lives of selegiline and its metabolites are short, a wash-out period of 14 days after selegiline treatment would be sufficient before starting fluoxetine. The concomitant use of selegiline and citalopram has been investigated in healthy volunteers. No signs of clinically relevant pharmacokinetic or pharmacodynamic interactions between the two drugs were observed.

Severe CNS toxicity has been reported in patients with the combination of tricyclic antidepressants and selegiline. In one patient receiving amitriptyline and selegiline this included hyperpyrexia and death, and another patient receiving protriptyline and selegiline experienced tremor, agitation, and restlessness followed by unresponsiveness and death two weeks after selegiline was added. Other adverse reactions occasionally reported in patients receiving a combination of selegiline with various tricyclic antidepressants include hyper/hypotension, dizziness, diaphoresis, tremor, seizures, and changes in behavioural and mental status. Since the mechanisms of these reactions are not fully understood, it is recommended to be cautious when using selegiline together with tricyclic antidepressants.

Concomitant use of oral contraceptives (tablets containing the combination of gestodene/ethinyl estradiol or levonorgestrel/ethinyl estradiol) and selegiline may cause an increase in the oral bioavailability of selegiline. Thus appropriate caution during the concomitant administration of selegiline and oral contraceptives should be applied.

4.6 Pregnancy and lactation

The available safety data concerning the use during pregnancy and lactation is insufficient to justify the use of selegiline in these patient groups.

4.7 Effects on ability to drive and use machines

No effects on ability to drive or operate machines.

4.8 Undesirable effects

In monotherapy, selegiline has been found to be well tolerated. Dry mouth, transient rise of serum alanine aminotransferase (ALAT) values and sleeping disorders have been reported more frequently than in patients receiving placebo. Because selegiline potentiates the effects of levodopa, the adverse reactions of levodopa, e.g. abnormal movements (such as dyskinesias), nausea, agitation, confusion, hallucinations, headache, postural hypotension, cardiac arrhythmias and vertigo, may be emphasised, particularly if the dose of levodopa is too high. Such adverse reactions usually disappear when the levodopa dosage is decreased. Levodopa dosage can be reduced by an average of 30% when selegiline is added to the treatment. Micturition difficulties and skin reactions have also been reported during selegiline treatment. Follow-up of these possible adverse reactions is important.

Hypersexuality has been very rarely reported in association with selegiline use, either as monotherapy or in combination with other dopaminergic antiparkinsonian medication.

A summary of the undesirable effects in terms of frequency of occurrence is shown below.

Psychiatric disorders	**Common (>1/100, <1/10)**	**Sleeping disorders, confusion, hallucinations**
	Very rare (<1/10,000)	**Hypersexuality**
Nervous system disorders	**Common (>1/100, <1/10)**	**Dry mouth, abnormal movements (such as dyskinesias), vertigo**
	Rare (>1/10,000, <1/1,000)	**Agitation, headache**
Cardiac disorders	**Rare (>1/10,000, <1/1,000)**	**Cardiac arrhythmias**

Vascular disorders	**Common (>1/100, <1/10)**	**Postural hypotension**
Gastrointestinal disorders	**Common (>1/100, <1/10)**	**Nausea**
Hepato-biliary disorders	**Common (>1/100, <1/10)**	**Transient rise of serum alanine aminotransferase (ALAT)**
Skin and subcutaneous tissue	**Rare (>1/10,000, <1/1,000)**	**Skin reactions**
Renal and urinary disorders	**Rare (>1/10,000, <1/1,000)**	**Micturition difficulties**

4.9 Overdose

No overdosage cases are known. However, experience gained during selegiline's development reveals that some individuals exposed to doses of 600 mg/day selegiline suffered severe hypotension and psychomotor agitation.

Theoretically, overdosage causes significant inhibition of both MAO-A and MAO-B and thus, symptoms of overdosage may resemble those observed with non-selective MAO-inhibitors, such as different central nervous and cardiovascular system disorders (e.g. drowsiness, dizziness, faintness, irritability, hyperactivity, agitation, severe headache, hallucination, hypertension, hypotension, vascular collapse, rapid and irregular pulse, precordial pain, respiratory depression and failure, hyperpyrexia, diaphoresis). There is no specific antidote and the treatment is symptomatic.

5. PHARMACOLOGICAL PROPERTIES

5.1 Pharmacodynamic properties

Selegiline is a selective MAO-B-inhibitor which prevents dopamine breakdown in the brain. It also inhibits the reuptake of dopamine at the presynaptic dopamine receptor. These effects potentiate dopaminergic function in the brain and help to even out and prolong the effect of exogenous and endogenous dopamine. Thus, selegiline potentiates and prolongs the effect of levodopa in the treatment of parkinsonism.

Double-blind studies on early phase Parkinsonian patients showed that patients receiving selegiline monotherapy manage significantly longer without levodopa therapy than controls receiving placebo. These patients could also maintain their ability to work longer.

The addition of selegiline to levodopa (with or without decarboxylase inhibitor) therapy helps to alleviate dose related fluctuations and end of dose deterioration.

When selegiline is added to such a regimen it is possible to reduce the levodopa dosage by an average of 30%. Unlike conventional MAO-inhibitors, which inhibit both the MAO-A and MAO-B enzyme, selegiline is a specific MAO-B inhibitor and can be given safely with levodopa.

Selegiline HCl does not cause the so called "cheese effect" either when used alone as monotherapy, or when used with other drugs, except for moclobemide or nonselective MAO-inhibitors.

5.2 Pharmacokinetic properties

Selegiline HCl is readily absorbed from the gastrointestinal tract. The maximal concentrations are reached in half an hour after oral administration. The bioavailability is low; 10% (on the average; interindividual variation is large) of unchanged selegiline can reach the systemic circulation.

Selegiline is a lipophilic, slightly basic compound which quickly penetrates into tissues, also into brain. Selegiline HCl inhibits MAO irreversibly and enzyme activity only increases again after new enzyme is synthesised. The inhibitory effect of a single 10 mg dose lasts for 24 hours. Selegiline is rapidly distributed throughout the body, the apparent volume of distribution being 500 litres after an intravenous 10 mg dose. 75-85 % of selegiline is bound to plasma proteins at therapeutic concentrations.

Selegiline is rapidly metabolised, mainly in the liver, into desmethylselegiline, l-methamphetamine and to l-amphetamine. In humans, the three metabolites have been identified in plasma and urine after single and multiple doses of selegiline. The mean elimination half-life is 1.6 hours for selegiline. The total body clearance of selegiline is about 240 L/hour. Metabolites of selegiline are excreted mainly via the urine with about 15% occurring in the faeces.

5.3 Preclinical safety data

No mutagenicity or carcinogenicity due to selegiline have emerged in routine studies.

6. PHARMACEUTICAL PARTICULARS

6.1 List of excipients

Mannitol, maize starch, microcrystalline cellulose, povidone, and magnesium stearate.

6.2 Incompatibilities

No other incompatibilities noted.

6.3 Shelf life

36 months: Bottle

36 months: Blister

6.4 Special precautions for storage

HDPE bottle; Do not store above 25 °C. Keep the container tightly closed.

Al/Al blister; Do not store above 25 °C. Store in the original package.

6.5 Nature and contents of container

White polyethylene bottle with polyethylene closure; 50, 100 tablets

Al/Al blister; 30, 50, 60, 100 tablets

White HDPE bottle with HDPE screw cap: 50, 100 tablets

6.6 Special precautions for disposal and other handling

None.

7. MARKETING AUTHORISATION HOLDER

Orion Corporation, Orionintie 1, FIN-02200 Espoo, Finland

8. MARKETING AUTHORISATION NUMBER(S)

PL 27925/0005

9. DATE OF FIRST AUTHORISATION/RENEWAL OF THE AUTHORISATION

1.7.1993/Renewal July 2007

10. DATE OF REVISION OF THE TEXT

June 2009

Eldepryl tablets 5mg

(Orion Pharma (UK) Limited)

1. NAME OF THE MEDICINAL PRODUCT

Eldepryl Tablets 5 mg

2. QUALITATIVE AND QUANTITATIVE COMPOSITION

Selegiline hydrochloride 5 mg

For full list of excipients, see section 6.1

3. PHARMACEUTICAL FORM

Tablets for oral administration.

4. CLINICAL PARTICULARS

4.1 Therapeutic indications

Selegiline is indicated for the treatment of Parkinson's disease, or symptomatic parkinsonism. It may be used alone to delay the need for levodopa (with or without decarboxylase inhibitor) or as an adjunct to levodopa (with or without decarboxylase inhibitor).

4.2 Posology and method of administration

10 mg daily either alone or as an adjunct to levodopa or levodopa/peripheral decarboxylase inhibitor. Selegiline may be administered either as a single dose in the morning or in two divided doses of 5 mg, taken at breakfast and lunch. When selegiline is added to a levodopa regimen it is possible to reduce the levodopa dosage by an average of 30%.

4.3 Contraindications

Known hypersensitivity to selegiline or other components of the formulation.

4.4 Special warnings and precautions for use

Selegiline should be administered cautiously to patients with peptic or duodenal ulcer, labile hypertension, cardiac arrhythmias, severe angina pectoris, severe liver or kidney dysfunction or psychosis. In higher doses (more than 30 mg daily) the selectivity of selegiline begins to diminish resulting in increased inhibition of MAO-A. Thus in higher doses there is a risk of hypertension after ingestion of food rich in tyramine.

4.5 Interaction with other medicinal products and other forms of interaction

Foods containing tyramine have not been reported to induce hypertensive reactions during selegiline treatment at doses used in the treatment of Parkinson's disease.

A concomitant use of nonselective MAO-inhibitors may cause severe hypotension.

No tolerability problems have been reported when a combination of selegiline and moclobemide, an inhibitor of MAO-A, has been used. However, when they are used together, the tyramine sensitivity factor may increase up to 8-9 (being 1 for selegiline alone and 2-3 for moclobemide alone). Although tyramine induced hypertensive reactions are unlikely when selegiline and moclobemide are used together, dietary restrictions (excluding foods with large amounts of tyramine such as aged cheese and yeast products) are recommended when using this combination.

Interactions between nonselective MAO-inhibitors and pethidine, as well as selegiline and pethidine have been described. The mechanism of this interaction is not fully understood and therefore, use of pethidine concomitantly with selegiline should be avoided. Tramadol may also potentially interact with Selegiline.

Dopamine should be used with caution in patients receiving Selegiline.

Serious reactions with signs and symptoms that may include diaphoresis, flushing, ataxia, tremor, hyperthermia, hyper/hypotension, seizures, palpitation, dizziness and mental changes that include agitation, confusion and hallucinations progressing to delirium and coma have been reported in some patients receiving a combination of selegiline and fluoxetine. Similar experience has been reported in patients receiving selegiline and four serotonin reuptake inhibitors, fluvoxamine, sertraline, paroxetine or venlafaxine. Since the mechanisms of these reactions are not fully understood, it is recommended to avoid the combination of selegiline with fluoxetine, sertraline, paroxetine or venlafaxine. A minimum period of five weeks should be allowed between discontinuation of fluoxetine and initiation of selegiline treatment, due to the long half-lives of fluoxetine and its active metabolite. As the half-lives of selegiline and its metabolites are short, a wash-out period of 14 days after selegiline treatment would be sufficient before starting fluoxetine. The concomitant use of selegiline and citalopram has been investigated in healthy volunteers. No signs of clinically relevant pharmacokinetic or pharmacodynamic interactions between the two drugs were observed.

Severe CNS toxicity has been reported in patients with the combination of tricyclic antidepressants and selegiline. In one patient receiving amitriptyline and selegiline this included hyperpyrexia and death, and another patient receiving protriptyline and selegiline experienced tremor, agitation, and restlessness followed by unresponsiveness and death two weeks after selegiline was added. Other adverse reactions occasionally reported in patients receiving a combination of selegiline with various tricyclic antidepressants include hyper/hypotension, dizziness, diaphoresis, tremor, seizures, and changes in behavioural and mental status. Since the mechanisms of these reactions are not fully understood, it is recommended to be cautious when using selegiline together with tricyclic antidepressants.

Concomitant use of oral contraceptives (tablets containing the combination of gestodene/ethinyl estradiol or levonorgestrel/ethinyl estradiol) and selegiline may cause an increase in the oral bioavailability of selegiline. Thus appropriate caution during the concomitant administration of selegiline and oral contraceptives should be applied.

4.6 Pregnancy and lactation

The available safety data concerning the use during pregnancy and lactation is insufficient to justify the use of selegiline in these patient groups.

4.7 Effects on ability to drive and use machines

No effects on ability to drive or operate machines.

4.8 Undesirable effects

In monotherapy, selegiline has been found to be well tolerated. Dry mouth, transient rise of serum alanine aminotransferase (ALAT) values and sleeping disorders have been reported more frequently than in patients receiving placebo. Because selegiline potentiates the effects of levodopa, the adverse reactions of levodopa, e.g. abnormal movements (such as dyskinesias), nausea, agitation, confusion, hallucinations, headache, postural hypotension, cardiac arrhythmias and vertigo, may be emphasised, particularly if the dose of levodopa is too high. Such adverse reactions usually disappear when the levodopa dosage is decreased. Levodopa dosage can be reduced by an average of 30% when selegiline is added to the treatment. Micturition difficulties and skin reactions have also been reported during selegiline treatment. Follow-up of these possible adverse reactions is important.

Hypersexuality has been very rarely reported in association with selegiline use, either as monotherapy or in combination with other dopaminergic antiparkinsonian medication.

A summary of the undesirable effects in terms of frequency of occurrence is shown below.

Psychiatric disorders	**Common (>1/100, <1/10)**	**Sleeping disorders, confusion, hallucinations**
	Very rare (<1/10,000)	**Hypersexuality**
Nervous system disorders	**Common (>1/100, <1/10)**	**Dry mouth, abnormal movements (such as dyskinesias), vertigo**
	Rare (>1/10,000, <1/1,000)	**Agitation, headache**
Cardiac disorders	**Rare (>1/10,000, <1/1,000)**	**Cardiac arrhythmias**
Vascular disorders	**Common (>1/100, <1/10)**	**Postural hypotension**
Gastrointestinal disorders	**Common (>1/100, <1/10)**	**Nausea**
Hepato-biliary disorders	**Common (>1/100, <1/10)**	**Transient rise of serum alanine aminotransferase (ALAT)**
Skin and subcutaneous tissue	**Rare (>1/10,000, <1/1,000)**	**Skin reactions**
Renal and urinary disorders	**Rare (>1/10,000, <1/1,000)**	**Micturition difficulties**

4.9 Overdose

No overdosage cases are known. However, experience gained during selegiline's development reveals that some individuals exposed to doses of 600 mg/day selegiline suffered severe hypotension and psychomotor agitation.

Theoretically, overdosage causes significant inhibition of both MAO-A and MAO-B and thus, symptoms of overdosage may resemble those observed with non-selective MAO-inhibitors, such as different central nervous and cardiovascular system disorders (e.g. drowsiness, dizziness, faintness, irritability, hyperactivity, agitation, severe headache, hallucination, hypertension, hypotension, vascular collapse, rapid and irregular pulse, precordial pain, respiratory depression and failure, hyperpyrexia, diaphoresis). There is no specific antidote and the treatment is symptomatic.

5. PHARMACOLOGICAL PROPERTIES

5.1 Pharmacodynamic properties

Selegiline is a selective MAO-B-inhibitor which prevents dopamine breakdown in the brain. It also inhibits the reuptake of dopamine at the presynaptic dopamine receptor. These effects potentiate dopaminergic function in the brain and help to even out and prolong the effect of exogenous and endogenous dopamine. Thus, selegiline potentiates and prolongs the effect of levodopa in the treatment of parkinsonism.

Double-blind studies on early phase Parkinsonian patients showed that patients receiving selegiline monotherapy manage significantly longer without levodopa therapy than controls receiving placebo. These patients could also maintain their ability to work longer.

The addition of selegiline to levodopa (with or without decarboxylase inhibitor) therapy helps to alleviate dose related fluctuations and end of dose deterioration.

When selegiline is added to such a regimen it is possible to reduce the levodopa dosage by an average of 30%. Unlike conventional MAO-inhibitors, which inhibit both the MAO-A and MAO-B enzyme, selegiline is a specific MAO-B inhibitor and can be given safely with levodopa.

Selegiline HCl does not cause the so called "cheese effect" either when used alone as monotherapy, or when used with other drugs, except for moclobemide or nonselective MAO-inhibitors.

5.2 Pharmacokinetic properties

Selegiline HCl is readily absorbed from the gastrointestinal tract. The maximal concentrations are reached in half an hour after oral administration. The bioavailability is low; 10% (on the average; interindividual variation is large) of unchanged selegiline can reach the systemic circulation.

Selegiline is a lipophilic, slightly basic compound which quickly penetrates into tissues, also into brain. Selegiline HCl inhibits MAO irreversibly and enzyme activity only increases again after new enzyme is synthesised. The inhibitory effect of a single 10 mg dose lasts for 24 hours. Selegiline is rapidly distributed throughout the body, the apparent volume of distribution being 500 litres after an intravenous 10 mg dose. 75-85 % of selegiline is bound to plasma proteins at therapeutic concentrations.

Selegiline is rapidly metabolised, mainly in the liver, into desmethylselegiline, l-methamphetamine and to l-amphetamine. In humans, the three metabolites have been identified in plasma and urine after single and multiple doses of selegiline. The mean elimination half-life is 1.6 hours for selegiline. The total body clearance of selegiline is about 240 L/hour. Metabolites of selegiline are excreted mainly via the urine with about 15% occurring in the faeces.

5.3 Preclinical safety data

No mutagenicity or carcinogenicity due to selegiline have emerged in routine studies.

6. PHARMACEUTICAL PARTICULARS

6.1 List of excipients

Mannitol, maize starch, microcrystalline cellulose, povidone, and magnesium stearate.

6.2 Incompatibilities

No other incompatibilities noted.

6.3 Shelf life

36 months: bottle

36 months: blister

6.4 Special precautions for storage

HDPE bottle: Do not store above 25°C. Keep the container tightly closed.

Blister Pack: Do not store above 25°C. Store in the original package.

6.5 Nature and contents of container

a) White HDPE bottle with LDPE snap cap: 100 tablets

b) Al/Al blister packs: 30, 50, 60 and 100 tablets

c) White HDPE bottle with HDPE screw cap: 100 tablets

6.6 Special precautions for disposal and other handling

None.

7. MARKETING AUTHORISATION HOLDER

Orion Corporation, Orionintie 1, FIN-02200 Espoo, Finland

8. MARKETING AUTHORISATION NUMBER(S)

PL 27925/0004

9. DATE OF FIRST AUTHORISATION/RENEWAL OF THE AUTHORISATION

1.7.1993/Renewal July 2007

10. DATE OF REVISION OF THE TEXT

June 2009

Electrolade (Banana)

(Actavis UK Ltd)

1. NAME OF THE MEDICINAL PRODUCT

Electrolade (Banana).

2. QUALITATIVE AND QUANTITATIVE COMPOSITION

Each sachet contains 5.09 powder	per/sachet
Sodium Chloride Ph.Eur.	0.236 g
Potassium Chloride Ph.Eur.	0.300 g
Sodium Bicarbonate Ph.Eur.	0.500 g
Anhydrous Dextrose Ph.Eur.	4.000 g

The reconstituted solution contains Sodium 50 mmol/L, Potassium 20 mmol/L, Chloride 40 mmol/L, Bicarbonate 30 mmol/L, Dextrose 111 mmol/L.

3. PHARMACEUTICAL FORM

Oral powder in sachet.

4. CLINICAL PARTICULARS

4.1 Therapeutic indications

Oral replacement therapy of electrolyte and fluid loss in children and adults arising from dehydration associated with acute diarrhoea.

4.2 Posology and method of administration

Reconstitution: Only with water and at the volume stated.

Adults and children: The content of each sachet should be dissolved in approximately 200 ml of cool, fresh, clean drinking water. The resulting solution is both clear and colourless with an aroma of Banana.

Infants: The water should be boiled then cooled before reconstitution as above.

The reconstituted cooled solution should be used immediately and the unused remainder discarded, or stored in a refrigerator for no longer than 24 hours. Do not boil after reconstitution. The product must only be used at the recommended dilution.

Dosage: Oral fluid replacement and maintenance therapy must be tailored to individual patients needs. The volume of solution used will depend on the weight and age of the patient, using the basic principle of firstly rehydrating the patient by replacing lost fluid and thereafter maintaining fluid replacement in line with the volume of fluid lost from stools or vomiting plus normal daily requirements. As a basic guide, a daily intake of 150 ml/kg bodyweight for infants (under 2 years of age) or 100-120 ml/kg for adults and children is needed.

Replacement of fluid losses with Electrolade solution:

Infants (under 2 years of age): See special warnings and precautions for use. Reconstitute sachets according to directions and administer at 1-1.5 times usual feed volume. No milk (other than breast milk) or solids should be given during the first 24 hours. In breast-fed infants, Electrolade should be given before the feed. The re-introduction of normal feeding should only take place when symptoms of diarrhoea are abating and should be added gradually to make up the total daily fluid requirements.

Children: One sachet after every loose motion, up to 12 sachets in 24 hours.

Adults: 1-2 sachets after every loose motion, up to 16 sachets in 24 hours.

Elderly person: As for adults but care must be taken not to over-hydrate.

In adults and children Electrolade can be given in amounts necessary to satisfy thirst. As with infants, solids should be avoided during the first day, but may be gradually resumed as necessary during day 2.

It is extremely difficult to over-hydrate by mouth, thus when there is normal renal function, it is better to give more Electrolade than less.

4.3 Contraindications

Hypersensitivity to any of the ingredients.

Oral treatment is inappropriate in such conditions as severe dehydration, which requires parenteral fluid therapy or intestinal obstruction.

It is necessary for medical supervision in the presence of renal disease, including anuria or prolonged oliguaria, severe and persistent diarrhoea and vomiting, inability to drink or retain oral fluids.

4.4 Special warnings and precautions for use

Infants under the age of 2 years with severe diarrhoea/vomiting should be seen by a doctor as soon as possible.

If symptoms persist for longer than 24-48 hours, a doctor should be consulted.

The solution must be made up without adding extra sugar or salt. In treating diabetics with gastro-enteritis, the sugar content must be noted.

Solutions of greater concentration may result in hypernatraemia. Those of greater dilution may result in inadequate replacement.

4.5 Interaction with other medicinal products and other forms of interaction

None known.

4.6 Pregnancy and lactation

The dose is the same as adult dose. Breast feeding can be continued as normal. If vomiting is a problem then Electrolade solution should be taken in frequent small volumes.

Electrolade is not contraindicated in pregnancy or lactation but should be used on medical advice.

4.7 Effects on ability to drive and use machines

None known.

4.8 Undesirable effects

None.

4.9 Overdose

In oral electrolyte replacement therapy, toxicity is rare in previously healthy people. In subjects with renal impairment, hypernatraemia and hyperkalaemia might occur.

In the event of significant overdose serum electrolytes should be evaluated.

5. PHARMACOLOGICAL PROPERTIES

5.1 Pharmacodynamic properties

Sodium Chloride } Potassium Chloride }	Salts/Electrolytes
Sodium Bicarbonate	Acid Neutraliser
Dextrose Anhydrous	Carbohydrate Electrolyte carrier

5.2 Pharmacokinetic properties

The Electrolade formulation is based upon the well accepted WHO oral rehydration solution (ORS).

Dextrose has been shown to greatly enhance the absorption of salts and water. The concentration used in Electrolade is very effective and has been demonstrated as giving a twenty five-fold enhancement of absorption compared with isotonic saline.

The level of sodium in Electrolade reflects the stool concentration in most cases of severe diarrhoea. Also, as the solution is more palatable, patient compliance is increased.

Potassium and Chloride are included to replace these electrolytes lost in the stool.

Bicarbonate combats metabolic acidosis.

Saccharin sodium is used as the sweetening agent, which also improves the general flavour.

5.3 Preclinical safety data

Not available.

6. PHARMACEUTICAL PARTICULARS

6.1 List of excipients

Saccharin Sodium

Banana Flavour

6.2 Incompatibilities

None known.

6.3 Shelf life

3 years in the sealed sachet, not more than 24 hours after reconstitution.

6.4 Special precautions for storage

Electrolade should be stored in a dry place below 25°C.

6.5 Nature and contents of container

The powder is available in cartons containing 4, 6 or 20 individual sachets of powder and in multiflavour pack of Banana, Orange, Blackcurrant and Lemon/Lime.

6.6 Special precautions for disposal and other handling

Keep this medicine out of the reach and sight of children. This medicine must not be used after the date (Exp) printed on the pack. Return any left over medicine to your pharmacist.

7. MARKETING AUTHORISATION HOLDER

Actavis Group PTC ehf

Reykjavíkurvegi 76-78

220 Hafnarfjordur

Iceland.

8. MARKETING AUTHORISATION NUMBER(S)

PL 30306/0069

9. DATE OF FIRST AUTHORISATION/RENEWAL OF THE AUTHORISATION

14th April 2003

10. DATE OF REVISION OF THE TEXT

Electrolade (Blackcurrent)

(Actavis UK Ltd)

1. NAME OF THE MEDICINAL PRODUCT

Electrolade (Blackcurrent)

2. QUALITATIVE AND QUANTITATIVE COMPOSITION

Each sachet contains 5.09 powder	per/sachet
Sodium Chloride Ph.Eur.	0.236 g
Potassium Chloride Ph.Eur.	0.300 g
Sodium Bicarbonate Ph.Eur.	0.500 g
Anhydrous Dextrose Ph.Eur.	4.000 g

The reconstituted solution contains Sodium 50 mmol/L, Potassium 20 mmol/L, Chloride 40 mmol/L, Bicarbonate 30 mmol/L, Dextrose 111 mmol/L.

3. PHARMACEUTICAL FORM
Free flowing powder.

4. CLINICAL PARTICULARS

4.1 Therapeutic indications
Oral replacement therapy of electrolyte and fluid loss in children and adults arising from dehydration associated with acute diarrhoea.

4.2 Posology and method of administration
Reconstitution: Only with water and at the volume stated.

Adults and children: The content of each sachet should be dissolved in approximately 200 ml of cool, fresh, clean drinking water. The resulting solution is both clear and colourless with an aroma of Blackcurrant.

Infants: The water should be boiled then cooled before reconstitution as above.

The reconstituted cooled solution should be used immediately and the unused remainder discarded, or stored in a refrigerator for no longer than 24 hours. Do not boil after reconstitution. The product must only be used at the recommended dilution.

Dosage: Oral fluid replacement and maintenance therapy must be tailored to individual patients needs. The volume of solution used will depend on the weight and age of the patient, using the basic principle of firstly rehydrating the patient by replacing lost fluid and thereafter maintaining fluid replacement in line with the volume of fluid lost from stools or vomiting plus normal daily requirements. As a basic guide, a daily intake of 150 ml/kg bodyweight for infants (under 2 years of age) or 100-120 ml/kg for adults and children is needed.

Replacement of fluid losses with Electrolade solution:

Infants (under 2 years of age): See special warnings and precautions for use. Reconstitute sachets according to directions and administer at 1-1.5 times usual feed volume. No milk (other than breast milk) or solids should be given during the first 24 hours. In breast-fed infants, Electrolade should be given before the feed. The re-introduction of normal feeding should only take place when symptoms of diarrhoea are abating and should be added gradually to make up the total daily fluid requirements.

Children: One sachet after every loose motion, up to 12 sachets in 24 hours.

Adults: 1-2 sachets after every loose motion, up to 16 sachets in 24 hours.

Elderly person: As for adults but care must be taken not to over-hydrate.

In adults and children Electrolade can be given in amounts necessary to satisfy thirst. As with infants, solids should be avoided during the first day, but may be gradually resumed as necessary during day 2.

It is extremely difficult to over-hydrate by mouth, thus when there is normal renal function, it is better to give more Electrolade than less.

4.3 Contraindications
There are no absolute contra-indications to using Electrolade. However, it is necessary for medical supervision in the presence of renal disease, including anuria or prolonged oliguria, severe and persistent diarrhoea and vomiting, inability to drink or retain oral fluids.

4.4 Special warnings and precautions for use
Infants under the age of 2 years with severe diarrhoea/vomiting should be seen by a doctor as soon as possible.

If symptoms persist for longer than 24-48 hours, a doctor should be consulted.

The solution must be made up without adding extra sugar or salt. In treating diabetics with gastro-enteritis, the sugar content must be noted.

Solutions of greater concentration may result in hypernatraemia. Those of greater dilution may result in inadequate replacement.

4.5 Interaction with other medicinal products and other forms of interaction
None known.

4.6 Pregnancy and lactation
The dose is the same as adult dose. Breast feeding can be continued as normal. If vomiting is a problem then Electrolade solution should be taken in frequent small volumes.

4.7 Effects on ability to drive and use machines
None known.

4.8 Undesirable effects
None.

4.9 Overdose
In oral electrolyte replacement therapy, toxicity is rare in previously healthy people. In subjects with renal impairment, hypernatraemia and hyperkalaemia might occur. If these conditions occur, full biochemical profile under hospital conditions will be needed and the physician should take the appropriate measures.

5. PHARMACOLOGICAL PROPERTIES

5.1 Pharmacodynamic properties

Sodium Chloride } Potassium Chloride }	Salts/Electrolytes
Sodium Bicarbonate	Acid Neutraliser
Dextrose Anhydrous	Carbohydrate Electrolyte carrier

5.2 Pharmacokinetic properties
The Electrolade formulation is based upon the well accepted WHO oral rehydration solution (ORS).

Dextrose has been shown to greatly enhance the absorption of salts and water. The concentration used in Electrolade is very effective and has been demonstrated as giving a twenty five-fold enhancement of absorption compared with isotonic saline.

The level of sodium in Electrolade reflects the stool concentration in most cases of severe diarrhoea. Also, as the solution is more palatable, patient compliance is increased.

Potassium and Chloride are included to replace these electrolytes lost in the stool.

Bicarbonate combats metabolic acidosis.

Saccharin sodium is used as the sweetening agent, which also improves the general flavour.

5.3 Preclinical safety data
Not available.

6. PHARMACEUTICAL PARTICULARS

6.1 List of excipients
Saccharin Sodium

Blackcurrant Flavour

6.2 Incompatibilities
None known.

6.3 Shelf life
3 years in the sealed sachet, not more than 24 hours after reconstitution.

6.4 Special precautions for storage
Electrolade should be stored in a dry place below 25°C.

6.5 Nature and contents of container
The powder is available in cartons containing 4, 6 or 20 individual sachets of powder.

6.6 Special precautions for disposal and other handling
Keep this medicine out of the reach and sight of children. This medicine must not be used after the date (Exp) printed on the pack. Return any left over medicine to your pharmacist.

7. MARKETING AUTHORISATION HOLDER
Actavis Group PTC ehf

Reykjavíkurvegi 76-78

220 Hafnarfjordur

Iceland.

8. MARKETING AUTHORISATION NUMBER(S)
PL30306/0070

9. DATE OF FIRST AUTHORISATION/RENEWAL OF THE AUTHORISATION
14th April 2003

10. DATE OF REVISION OF THE TEXT

11. DOSIMETRY
Not applicable

12. INSTRUCTIONS FOR PREPARATION OF RADIOPHARMACEUTICALS
Not applicable

Electrolade (Lemon & Lime)

(Actavis UK Ltd)

1. NAME OF THE MEDICINAL PRODUCT
Electrolade (Lemon & Lime)

2. QUALITATIVE AND QUANTITATIVE COMPOSITION

Each sachet contains 5.09 powder	per/sachet
Sodium Chloride Ph.Eur.	0.236 g
Potassium Chloride Ph.Eur.	0.300 g
Sodium Bicarbonate Ph.Eur.	0.500 g
Anhydrous Dextrose Ph.Eur.	4.000 g

The reconstituted solution contains Sodium 50 mmol/L, Potassium 20 mmol/L, Chloride 40 mmol/L, Bicarbonate 30 mmol/L, Dextrose 111 mmol/L.

3. PHARMACEUTICAL FORM
Powder for oral solution.

4. CLINICAL PARTICULARS

4.1 Therapeutic indications
Oral replacement therapy of electrolyte and fluid loss in children and adults arising from dehydration associated with acute diarrhoea.

4.2 Posology and method of administration

Reconstitution:	Only with water and at the volume stated.
Adults and children:	The content of each sachet should be dissolved in approximately 200 ml of cool, fresh, clean drinking water. The resulting solution is both clear and colourless and odourless.
Infants:	The water should be boiled then cooled before reconstitution as above.

The reconstituted cooled solution should be used immediately and the unused remainder discarded, or stored in a refrigerator for no longer than 24 hours. Do not boil after reconstitution. The product must only be used at the recommended dilution.

Dosage: Oral fluid replacement and maintenance therapy must be tailored to individual patients needs. The volume of solution used will depend on the weight and age of the patient, using the basic principle of firstly rehydrating the patient by replacing lost fluid and thereafter maintaining fluid replacement in line with the volume of fluid lost from stools or vomiting plus normal daily requirements. As a basic guide, a daily intake of 150 ml/kg bodyweight for infants (under 2 years of age) or 100-120 ml/kg for adults and children is needed.

Replacement of fluid losses with Electrolade solution:

Infants (under 2 years of age):	See special warnings and precautions for use. Reconstitute sachets according to directions and administer at 1-1.5 times usual feed volume. No milk (other than breast milk) or solids should be given during the first 24 hours. In breast-fed infants, Electrolade should be given before the feed. The re-introduction of normal feeding should only take place when symptoms of diarrhoea are abating and should be added gradually to make up the total daily fluid requirements.
Children:	One sachet after every loose motion, up to 12 sachets in 24 hours.
Adults:	1-2 sachets after every loose motion, up to 16 sachets in 24 hours. Elderly person: As for adults but care must be taken not to over-hydrate.

In adults and children Electrolade can be given in amounts necessary to satisfy thirst. As with infants, solids should be avoided during the first day, but may be gradually resumed as necessary during day 2.

It is extremely difficult to over-hydrate by mouth, thus when there is normal renal function, it is better to give more Electrolade than less.

4.3 Contraindications
There are no absolute contra-indications to using Electrolade. However, it is necessary for medical supervision in the presence of renal disease, including anuria or prolonged oliguaria, severe and persistent diarrhoea and vomiting, inability to drink or retain oral fluids.

4.4 Special warnings and precautions for use
Infants under the age of 2 years with severe diarrhoea/vomiting should be seen by a doctor as soon as possible.

If symptoms persist for longer than 24-48 hours, a doctor should be consulted.

The solution must be made up without adding extra sugar or salt. In treating diabetics with gastro-enteritis, the sugar content must be noted.

Solutions of greater concentration may result in hypernatraemia. Those of greater dilution may result in inadequate replacement.

If there is no improvement within 24 hours to 48 hours the physician should be contacted.

4.5 Interaction with other medicinal products and other forms of interaction
None known.

4.6 Pregnancy and lactation
The dose is the same as adult dose. Breast feeding can be continued as normal. If vomiting is a problem then Electrolade solution should be taken in frequent small volumes.

Electrolade is not contraindicated in pregnancy or lactation but should be used on medical advice.

4.7 Effects on ability to drive and use machines
None known.

4.8 Undesirable effects
None.

4.9 Overdose
In oral electrolyte replacement therapy, toxicity is rare in previously healthy people. In subjects with renal impairment, hypernatraemia and hyperkalaemia might occur. If

these conditions occur, full biochemical profile under hospital conditions will be needed and the physician should take the appropriate measures.

5. PHARMACOLOGICAL PROPERTIES

5.1 Pharmacodynamic properties

Sodium Chloride } Potassium Chloride }	Salts/Electrolytes
Sodium Bicarbonate	Acid Neutraliser
Dextrose Anhydrous	Carbohydrate Electrolyte carrier

5.2 Pharmacokinetic properties

The Electrolade formulation is based upon the well accepted WHO oral rehydration solution (ORS).

Dextrose has been shown to greatly enhance the absorption of salts and water. The concentration used in Electrolade is very effective and has been demonstrated as giving a twenty five-fold enhancement of absorption compared with isotonic saline.

The level of sodium in Electrolade reflects the stool concentration in most cases of severe diarrhoea. Also, as the solution is more palatable, patient compliance is increased.

Potassium and Chloride are included to replace these electrolytes lost in the stool.

Bicarbonate combats metabolic acidosis.

Saccharin sodium is used as the sweetening agent, which also improves the general flavour.

5.3 Preclinical safety data

Not available.

6. PHARMACEUTICAL PARTICULARS

6.1 List of excipients

Saccharin Sodium

Lemon & Lime Flavour

6.2 Incompatibilities

None known.

6.3 Shelf life

3 years in the sealed sachet, not more than 24 hours after reconstitution.

6.4 Special precautions for storage

Electrolade should be stored in a dry place below 25°C.

6.5 Nature and contents of container

The powder is available in cartons containing 4, 6 or 20 individual sachets of powder and in Multiflavour pack of Banana, Orange, Blackcurrant and Lemon/Lime.

6.6 Special precautions for disposal and other handling

Keep this medicine out of the reach and sight of children. This medicine must not be used after the date (Exp) printed on the pack. Return any left over medicine to your pharmacist.

7. MARKETING AUTHORISATION HOLDER

Actavis Group PTC ehf

Reykjavíkurvegi 76-78

220 Hafnarfjordur

Iceland.

8. MARKETING AUTHORISATION NUMBER(S)

PL30306/0145

9. DATE OF FIRST AUTHORISATION/RENEWAL OF THE AUTHORISATION

14th April 2003

10. DATE OF REVISION OF THE TEXT

Electrolade Orange

(Actavis UK Ltd)

1. NAME OF THE MEDICINAL PRODUCT

Electrolade (Orange)

2. QUALITATIVE AND QUANTITATIVE COMPOSITION

Each sachet contains 5.09 powder	per/sachet
Sodium Chloride Ph.Eur.	0.236 g
Potassium Chloride Ph.Eur.	0.300 g
Sodium Bicarbonate Ph.Eur.	0.500 g
Anhydrous Dextrose Ph.Eur.	4.000 g

3. PHARMACEUTICAL FORM

The reconstituted solution contains Sodium 50 mmol/L, Potassium 20 mmol/L, Chloride 40 mmol/L, Bicarbonate 30 mmol/L, Dextrose 111 mmol/L.

4. CLINICAL PARTICULARS

4.1 Therapeutic indications

Oral replacement therapy of electrolyte and fluid loss in children and adults arising from dehydration associated with acute diarrhoea.

4.2 Posology and method of administration

Reconstitution: Only with water and at the volume stated.

Adults and children: The content of each sachet should be dissolved in approximately 200 ml of cool, fresh, clean drinking water. The resulting solution is both clear and colourless with an aroma of Orange.

Infants: The water should be boiled then cooled before reconstitution as above.

The reconstituted cooled solution should be used immediately and the unused remainder discarded, or stored in a refrigerator for no longer than 24 hours. Do not boil after reconstitution. The product must only be used at the recommended dilution.

Dosage: Oral fluid replacement and maintenance therapy must be tailored to individual patients needs. The volume of solution used will depend on the weight and age of the patient, using the basic principle of firstly rehydrating the patient by replacing lost fluid and thereafter maintaining fluid replacement in line with the volume of fluid lost from stools or vomiting plus normal daily requirements. As a basic guide, a daily intake of 150 ml/kg bodyweight for infants (under 2 years of age) or 100-120 ml/kg for adults and children is needed.

Replacement of fluid losses with Electrolade solution:

Infants (under 2 years of age): See special warnings and precautions for use. Reconstitute sachets according to directions and administer at 1-1.5 times usual feed volume. No milk (other than breast milk) or solids should be given during the first 24 hours. In breast-fed infants, Electrolade should be given before the feed. The re-introduction of normal feeding should only take place when symptoms of diarrhoea are abating and should be added gradually to make up the total daily fluid requirements.

Children: One sachet after every loose motion, up to 12 sachets in 24 hours.

Adults: 1-2 sachets after every loose motion, up to 16 sachets in 24 hours.

Elderly person: As for adults but care must be taken not to over-hydrate.

In adults and children Electrolade can be given in amounts necessary to satisfy thirst. As with infants, solids should be avoided during the first day, but may be gradually resumed as necessary during day 2.

It is extremely difficult to over-hydrate by mouth, thus when there is normal renal function, it is better to give more Electrolade than less.

4.3 Contraindications

There are no absolute contra-indications to using Electrolade. However, it is necessary for medical supervision in the presence of renal disease, including anuria or prolonged oliguaria, severe and persistent diarrhoea and vomiting, inability to drink or retain oral fluids.

4.4 Special warnings and precautions for use

Infants under the age of 2 years with severe diarrhoea/vomiting should be seen by a doctor as soon as possible.

If symptoms persist for longer than 24-48 hours, a doctor should be consulted.

The solution must be made up without adding extra sugar or salt. In treating diabetics with gastro-enteritis, the sugar content must be noted.

Solutions of greater concentration may result in hypernatraemia. Those of greater dilution may result in inadequate replacement.

4.5 Interaction with other medicinal products and other forms of interaction

None known.

4.6 Pregnancy and lactation

The dose is the same as adult dose. Breast feeding can be continued as normal. If vomiting is a problem then Electrolade solution should be taken in frequent small volumes.

4.7 Effects on ability to drive and use machines

None known.

4.8 Undesirable effects

None.

4.9 Overdose

In oral electrolyte replacement therapy, toxicity is rare in previously healthy people. In subjects with renal impairment, hypernatraemia and hyperkalaemia might occur.

5. PHARMACOLOGICAL PROPERTIES

5.1 Pharmacodynamic properties

Sodium Chloride } Potassium Chloride }	Salts/Electrolytes
Sodium Bicarbonate	Acid Neutraliser
Dextrose Anhydrous	Carbohydrate Electrolyte carrier

5.2 Pharmacokinetic properties

The Electrolade formulation is based upon the well accepted WHO oral rehydration solution (ORS).

Dextrose has been shown to greatly enhance the absorption of salts and water. The concentration used in Electrolade is very effective and has been demonstrated as giving a twenty five-fold enhancement of absorption compared with isotonic saline.

The level of sodium in Electrolade reflects the stool concentration in most cases of severe diarrhoea. Also, as the solution is more palatable, patient compliance is increased.

Potassium and Chloride are included to replace these electrolytes lost in the stool.

Bicarbonate combats metabolic acidosis.

Saccharin sodium is used as the sweetening agent, which also improves the general flavour.

5.3 Preclinical safety data

Not available.

6. PHARMACEUTICAL PARTICULARS

6.1 List of excipients

Saccharin Sodium

Orange Flavour

6.2 Incompatibilities

None known.

6.3 Shelf life

3 years in the sealed sachet, not more than 24 hours after reconstitution.

6.4 Special precautions for storage

Electrolade should be stored in a dry place below 25°C.

6.5 Nature and contents of container

The powder is available in cartons containing 4, 6 or 20 individual sachets of powder.

6.6 Special precautions for disposal and other handling

Keep this medicine out of the reach and sight of children. This medicine must not be used after the date (Exp) printed on the pack. Return any left over medicine to your pharmacist.

7. MARKETING AUTHORISATION HOLDER

Actavis Group PTC ehf

Reykjavíkurvegi 76-78

220 Hafnarfjordur

Iceland.

8. MARKETING AUTHORISATION NUMBER(S)

PL30306/0071

9. DATE OF FIRST AUTHORISATION/RENEWAL OF THE AUTHORISATION

14th April 2003

10. DATE OF REVISION OF THE TEXT

11. DOSIMETRY

(IF APPLICABLE)

12. INSTRUCTIONS FOR PREPARATION OF RADIOPHARMACEUTICALS

(IF APPLICABLE)

Ellimans Universal Muscle Rub Lotion

(Actavis UK Ltd)

1. NAME OF THE MEDICINAL PRODUCT

Ellimans Universal Muscle Rub Lotion

2. QUALITATIVE AND QUANTITATIVE COMPOSITION

Ellimans Universal Muscle Rub Lotion contains:

Turpentine oil BP 35.41%

Glacial acetic acid EP 3.562%

For excipients, see 6.1

3. PHARMACEUTICAL FORM

Cutaneous emulsion

A creamy, white liniment having an odour of turpentine and acetic acid

4. CLINICAL PARTICULARS

4.1 Therapeutic indications

Symptomatic relief of muscular pain and stiffness including backache, sciatica, lumbago, fibrositis, and rheumatic pain and the massage by athletes of arm or leg muscles.

4.2 Posology and method of administration

Shake the bottle immediately before use.

Adults and children aged 12 years and over.

Rub lotion freely onto affected part until thoroughly absorbed.

For the first 24 hours, apply every three hours, then twice daily.

Athletes: Massage of arm and leg muscles before and after activity.

Not to be used on children under 12 years of age.

The elderly

The adult directions for use apply.

4.3 Contraindications

Hypersensitivity to any of the ingredients.

4.4 Special warnings and precautions for use

Do not apply when skin is broken or inflammed

Keep away from the eyes and other sensitive areas.

Keep out of reach and sight of children.

If symptoms persist, consult your doctor.

For external use only.

4.5 Interaction with other medicinal products and other forms of interaction

None known.

4.6 Pregnancy and lactation
Use in pregnancy and lactation is not contra-indicated, however, as with all medicines, care should be exercised.

4.7 Effects on ability to drive and use machines
None known.

4.8 Undesirable effects
There have been reports that application to the skin of liniments containing Turpentine Oil may cause vesicular eruption, urticaria and vomiting in susceptible persons.

4.9 Overdose
Excessive percutaneous absorption as a result of over-application may rarely lead to reversible toxic nephritis.

Products containing turpentine, if ingested, could cause burning pain in the mouth and throat, abdominal pain, nausea, vomiting and occasionally diarrhoea.

This may be followed by painful urination, respiratory distress and convulsions. In high overdose, death may follow due to respiratory failure.

Treatment on Ingestion

The stomach should be emptied by aspiration and lavage, after which treatment is symptomatic.

5. PHARMACOLOGICAL PROPERTIES

5.1 Pharmacodynamic properties
MA02A X – Other topical products for joint and muscular pain

Turpentine oil is a rubefacient and counter-irritant.

Acetic acid is a counter irritant.

5.2 Pharmacokinetic properties
Not applicable.

5.3 Preclinical safety data
No data of relevance which is additional to that already included in other sections of the SPC.

6. PHARMACEUTICAL PARTICULARS

6.1 List of excipients
Dried whole egg powder (melange)

Purified Water

6.2 Incompatibilities
None known.

6.3 Shelf life
3 years

6.4 Special precautions for storage
None.

6.5 Nature and contents of container
Clear, white flint glass oval section bottles, with a screw-on wadless plastic cap fitted with an internal gasket contained in printed boxboard cartons, containing 100 ml of product

6.6 Special precautions for disposal and other handling
Shake the bottle before each use.

7. MARKETING AUTHORISATION HOLDER
Actavis Group PTC ehf

Reykjavíkurvegi 76-78

220 Hafnarfjordur

Iceland.

8. MARKETING AUTHORISATION NUMBER(S)
PL 30306/0075

9. DATE OF FIRST AUTHORISATION/RENEWAL OF THE AUTHORISATION
15 January 2003

10. DATE OF REVISION OF THE TEXT
4 February 2009

Eloxatin 5 mg/ml concentrate for solution for infusion

(sanofi-aventis)

1. NAME OF THE MEDICINAL PRODUCT
Eloxatin 5 mg/ml concentrate for solution for infusion

2. QUALITATIVE AND QUANTITATIVE COMPOSITION
1 ml concentrate for solution for infusion contains 5 mg oxaliplatin.

10 ml of concentrate for solution for infusion contains 50 mg of oxaliplatin

20 ml of concentrate for solution for infusion contains 100 mg of oxaliplatin

40 ml of concentrate for solution for infusion contains 200 mg of oxaliplatin

For excipients, see section 6.1.

3. PHARMACEUTICAL FORM
Concentrate for solution for infusion

Clear, colourless liquid

4. CLINICAL PARTICULARS

4.1 Therapeutic indications
Oxaliplatin in combination with 5-fluorouracil (5-FU) and folinic acid (FA) is indicated for:

• Adjuvant treatment of stage III (Duke's C) colon cancer after complete resection of primary tumor.

• Treatment of metastatic colorectal cancer.

4.2 Posology and method of administration
FOR ADULTS ONLY

The recommended dose for oxaliplatin in adjuvant setting is 85 mg/m^2 intravenously repeated every two weeks for 12 cycles (6 months).

The recommended dose for oxaliplatin in treatment of metastatic colorectal cancer is 85 mg/m^2 intravenously repeated every 2 weeks.

Dosage given should be adjusted according to tolerability (see section 4.4).

Oxaliplatin should always be administered before fluoropyrimidines – i.e. 5-fluorouracil.

Oxaliplatin is administered as a 2- to 6-hour intravenous infusion in 250 to 500 ml of 5% glucose solution to give a concentration between 0.2 mg/ml and 0.70 mg/ml; 0.70 mg/ml is the highest concentration in clinical practice for an oxaliplatin dose of 85 mg/m^2.

Oxaliplatin was mainly used in combination with continuous infusion 5-fluorouracil based regimens. For the two-weekly treatment schedule 5-fluorouracil regimens combining bolus and continuous infusion were used.

- Special Populations

- Renal impairment:

Oxaliplatin has not been studied in patients with severe renal impairment (see section 4.3).

In patients with moderate renal impairment, treatment may be initiated at the normally recommended dose (see section 4.4). There is no need for dose adjustment in patients with mild renal dysfunction.

- Hepatic insufficiency:

In a phase I study including patients with several levels of hepatic impairment, frequency and severity of hepato-biliary disorders appeared to be related to progressive disease and impaired liver function tests at baseline. No specific dose adjustment for patients with abnormal liver function tests was performed during clinical development.

- Elderly patients:

No increase in severe toxicities was observed when oxaliplatin was used as a single agent or in combination with 5-fluorouracil in patients over the age of 65. In consequence no specific dose adaptation is required for elderly patients.

Method of administration

Oxaliplatin is administered by intravenous infusion.

The administration of oxaliplatin does not require hyperhydration.

Oxaliplatin diluted in 250 to 500 ml of 5% glucose solution to give a concentration not less than 0.2 mg/ml must be infused via a central venous line or peripheral vein over 2 to 6 hours. Oxaliplatin infusion must always precede the administration of 5-fluorouracil.

In the event of extravasation, administration must be discontinued immediately.

Instructions for use:

Oxaliplatin must be diluted before use. Only 5% glucose diluent is to be used to dilute the concentrate for solution for infusion product. (see section 6.6).

4.3 Contraindications
Oxaliplatin is contraindicated in patients who

- have a known history of hypersensitivity to oxaliplatin.

- are breast feeding.

- have myelosuppression prior to starting first course, as evidenced by baseline neutrophils $<2x10^9$/l and/or platelet count of $<100x10^9$/l.

- have a peripheral sensitive neuropathy with functional impairment prior to first course.

- have a severely impaired renal function (creatinine clearance less than 30 ml/min).

4.4 Special warnings and precautions for use

Oxaliplatin should only be used in specialised departments of oncology and should be administered under the supervision of an experienced oncologist.

Due to limited information on safety in patients with moderatelyimpaired renal function, administration should only be considered after suitable appraisal of the benefit/risk for the patient.

In this situation, renal function should be closely monitored and dose adjusted according to toxicity.

Patients with a history of allergic reaction to platinum compounds should be monitored for allergic symptoms. In case of an anaphylactic-like reaction to oxaliplatin, the infusion should be immediately discontinued and appropriate symptomatic treatment initiated. Oxaliplatin rechallenge is contra-indicated.

In case of oxaliplatin extravasation, the infusion must be stopped immediately and usual local symptomatic treatment initiated.

Neurological toxicity of oxaliplatin should be carefully monitored, especially if co-administered with other medications with specific neurological toxicity.

A neurological examination should be performed before each administration and periodically thereafter.

For patients who develop acute laryngopharyngeal dysaesthesia (see section 4.8), during or within the hours following the 2-hour infusion, the next oxaliplatin infusion should be administered over 6 hours.

If neurological symptoms (paraesthesia, dysaesthesia) occur, the following recommended oxaliplatin dosage adjustment should be based on the duration and severity of these symptoms:

- If symptoms last longer than seven days and are troublesome, the subsequent oxaliplatin dose should be reduced from 85 to 65 mg/m^2 (metastatic setting) or 75 mg/m^2 (adjuvant setting).

- If paraesthesia without functional impairment persists until the next cycle, the subsequent oxaliplatin dose should be reduced from 85 to 65 mg/m^2 (metastatic setting) or 75 mg/m^2 (adjuvant setting).

- If paraesthesia with functional impairment persists until the next cycle, oxaliplatin should be discontinued.

- If these symptoms improve following discontinuation of oxaliplatin therapy, resumption of therapy may be considered.

Patients should be informed of the possibility of persistent symptoms of peripheral sensory neuropathy after the end of the treatment. Localized moderate paresthesias or paresthesias that may interfere with functional activities can persist after up to 3 years following treatment cessation in the adjuvant setting.

Gastrointestinal toxicity, which manifests as nausea and vomiting, warrants prophylactic and/or therapeutic anti-emetic therapy (see section 4.8).

Dehydration, paralytic ileus, intestinal obstruction, hypokalemia, metabolic acidosis and renal impairment may be caused by severe diarrhoea/emesis particularly when combining oxaliplatin with 5-fluorouracil.

If haematological toxicity occurs (neutrophils $< 1.5x10^9$/l or platelets $< 50x10^9$/l), administration of the next course of therapy should be postponed until haematological values return to acceptable levels. A full blood count with white cell differential should be performed prior to start of therapy and before each subsequent course.

Patients must be adequately informed of the risk of diarrhoea/emesis, mucositis/stomatitis and neutropenia after oxaliplatin and 5-fluorouracil administration so that they can urgently contact their treating physician for appropriate management.

If mucositis/stomatitis occurs with or without neutropenia, the next treatment should be delayed until recovery from mucositis/stomatitis to grade 1 or less and/or until the neutrophil count is $\geqslant 1.5 \times 10^9$/l.

For oxaliplatin combined with 5-fluorouracil (with or without folinic acid), the usual dose adjustments for 5-fluorouracil associated toxicities should apply.

If grade 4 diarrhoea, grade 3-4 neutropenia (neutrophils $< 1.0x10^9$/l), grade 3-4 thrombocytopenia (platelets $< 50x10^9$/l) occur, the dose of oxaliplatin should be reduced from 85 to 65 mg/m^2 (metastatic setting) or 75 mg/m^2 (adjuvant setting), in addition to any 5-fluorouracil dose reductions required.

In the case of unexplained respiratory symptoms such as non-productive cough, dyspnoea, crackles or radiological pulmonary infiltrates, oxaliplatin should be discontinued until further pulmonary investigations exclude an interstitial lung disease (see section 4.8).

In case of abnormal liver function test results or portal hypertension which does not obviously result from liver metastases, very rare cases of drug-induced hepatic vascular disorders should be considered.

For use in pregnant women, see section 4.6.

Genotoxic effects were observed with oxaliplatin in the preclinical studies. Therefore male patients treated with oxaliplatin are advised not to father a child during and up to 6 months after treatment and to seek advice on conservation of sperm prior to treatment because oxaliplatin may have an anti-fertility effect which could be irreversible.

Women should not become pregnant during treatment with oxaliplatin and should use an effective method of contraception (see section 4.6).

4.5 Interaction with other medicinal products and other forms of interaction
In patients who have received a single dose of 85 mg/m^2 of oxaliplatin, immediately before administration of 5-fluorouracil, no change in the level of exposure to 5-fluorouracil has been observed. *In vitro*, no significant displacement of oxaliplatin binding to plasma proteins has been observed with the following agents: erythromycin, salicylates, granisetron, paclitaxel, and sodium valproate.

4.6 Pregnancy and lactation
To date there is no available information on safety of use in pregnant women. In animal studies, reproductive toxicity

Table 1

MedDRA Organ system classes	Very common	Common	Uncommon	Rare
Investigations	- Hepatic enzyme increase - Blood alkaline phosphatase increase - Blood bilirubin increase - Blood lactate dehydrogenase increase - Weight increase (adjuvant setting)	- Blood creatinine increase - Weight decrease (metastatic setting)		
Blood and lymphatic system disorders*	- Anaemia - Neutropenia - Thrombocytopenia - Leukopenia - Lymphopenia			- Immunoallergic thrombocytopenia - Haemolytic anaemia
Nervous system disorders*	- Peripheral sensory neuropathy - ***Sensory disturbance*** - Dysgeusia - Headache	- ***Dizziness*** - Motor neuritis - Meningism		- Dysarthria
Eye disorders		- ***Conjunctivitis*** - Visual disturbance		- Visual acuity reduced transiently - Visual field disturbances - Optic neuritis - Transient vision loss, reversible following therapy discontinuation
Ear and labyrinth disorders			- Ototoxicity	- Deafness
Respiratory, thoracic and mediastinal disorders	- Dyspnoea - Cough	- Hiccups		- Interstitial lung disease - Pulmonary fibrosis**
Gastrointestinal disorders*	- ***Nausea*** - Diarrhoea - ***Vomiting*** - ***Stomatitis /Mucositis*** - ***Abdominal pain*** - Constipation	- ***Dyspepsia*** - ***Gastroesophageal reflux*** - Gastrointestinal hemorrhage - Rectal haemorrhage	- Ileus - Intestinal obstruction	- Colitis including clostridium difficile diarrhea
Renal and urinary disorders		- Haematuria - Dysuria - Micturition frequency abnormal		
Skin and subcutaneous tissue disorders	- Skin disorder - Alopecia	- Skin exfoliation (i.e. Hand & Foot syndrome) - Rash erythematous - Rash - Hyperhidrosis - Nail disorder		
Musculoskeletal and connective tissue disorders	- Back pain	- ***Arthralgia*** - Bone pain		
Metabolism and nutrition disorders	- Anorexia - Glycemia abnormalities - Hypokalaemia - Natraemia abnormalities	- ***Dehydration***	- Metabolic acidosis	
Infections and infestations *	- Infection	- Rhinitis - Upper respiratory tract infection - ***Febrile neutropenia / Neutropenic sepsis***		
Vascular disorders	- Epistaxis	- ***Haemorrhage*** - ***Flushing*** - ***Deep vein thrombosis*** - ***Pulmonary embolism*** - Hypertension		
General disorders and administration site conditions	- ***Fatigue*** - ***Fever++*** - ***Asthenia*** - ***Pain*** - Injection site reaction+++			
Immune system disorders*	- Allergy/ allergic reaction+			
Psychiatric disorders		- ***Depression*** - ***Insomnia***	- Nervousness	

* See detailed section below

** See section 4.4.

+ Common allergic reactions such as skin rash (particularly urticaria), conjunctivitis, rhinitis.

Common anaphylactic reactions, including bronchospasm, sensation of chest pain, angioedema, hypotension and anaphylactic shock.

++ Very common fever, rigors (tremors), either from infection (with or without febrile neutropenia) or possibly from immunological mechanism.

+++ Injection site reactions including local pain, redness, swelling and thrombosis have been reported. Extravasation may also result in local pain and inflammation which may be severe and lead to complications including necrosis, especially when oxaliplatin is infused through a peripheral vein (see section 4.4).

was observed. Consequently, oxaliplatin is not recommended during pregnancy and in women of childbearing potential not using contraceptive measures.

The use of oxaliplatin should only be considered after suitably appraising the patient of the risk to the foetus and with the patient's consent.

Appropriate contraceptive measures must be taken during and after cessation of therapy during 4 months for women and 6 months for men.

Excretion in breast milk has not been studied. Breast-feeding is contra-indicated during oxaliplatin therapy.

Oxaliplatin may have an anti-fertility effect (see section 4.4).

4.7 Effects on ability to drive and use machines

No studies on the effects on the ability to drive and use machines have been performed. However oxaliplatin treatment resulting in an increase risk of dizziness, nausea and vomiting, and other neurologic symptoms that affect gait and balance may lead to a minor or moderate influence on the ability to drive and use machines.

Vision abnormalities, in particular transient vision loss (reversible following therapy discontinuation), may affect patient's ability to drive and use machines. Therefore, patients should be warned of the potential effect of these events on the ability to drive or use machines.

4.8 Undesirable effects

The most frequent adverse events of oxaliplatin in combination with 5-fluorouracil/folinic acid (5-FU/FA) were gastrointestinal (diarrhea, nausea, vomiting and mucositis), haematological (neutropenia, thrombocytopenia) and neurological (acute and dose cumulative peripheral sensory neurophathy). Overall, these adverse events were more frequent and severe with oxaliplatin and 5-FU/FA combination than with 5-FU/FA alone.

The frequencies reported in the table below are derived from clinical trials in the metastatic and adjuvant settings (having included 416 and 1108 patients respectively in the oxaliplatin + 5-FU/FA treatment arms) and from post marketing experience.

Frequencies in this table are defined using the following convention: very common (⩾1/10) common (⩾1/100, <1/10), uncommon (⩾1/1000, <1/100), rare (⩾1/10000, <1/1000), very rare (<1/10000), not known (cannot be estimated from the available data).

Further details are given after the table.

(see Table 1 above)

Blood and lymphatic system disorders

Incidence by patient (%), by grade

(see Table 2 on next page)

Postmarketing experience with frequency unknown

Hemolytic uremic syndrome

Immune system disorders

Incidence of allergic reactions by patient (%), by grade

(see Table 3 on next page)

Table 2 Blood and lymphatic system disorders
Incidence by patient (%), by grade

Oxaliplatin and 5-FU/FA 85 mg/m^2	Metastatic Setting			Adjuvant Setting		
every 2 weeks	All grades	Gr 3	Gr 4	All grades	Gr 3	Gr 4
Anemia	82.2	3	<1	75.6	0.7	0.1
Neutropenia	71.4	28	14	78.9	28.8	12.3
Thrombocytopenia	71.6	4	<1	77.4	1.5	0.2
Febrile neutropenia	5.0	3.6	1.4	0.7	0.7	0.0
Neutropenic sepsis	1.1	0.7	0.4	1.1	0.6	0.4

Table 3 Immune system disorders
Incidence of allergic reactions by patient (%), by grade

Oxaliplatin and 5-FU/FA 85 mg/m^2	Metastatic Setting			Adjuvant Setting		
every 2 weeks	All grades	Gr 3	Gr 4	All grades	Gr 3	Gr 4
Allergic reactions / Allergy	9.1	1	<1	10.3	2.3	0.6

Nervous system disorders

The dose limiting toxicity of oxaliplatin is neurological. It involves a sensory peripheral neuropathy characterised by dysaesthesia and/or paraesthesia of the extremities with or without cramps, often triggered by the cold. These symptoms occur in up to 95% of patients treated. The duration of these symptoms, which usually regress between courses of treatment, increases with the number of treatment cycles.

The onset of pain and/or a functional disorder are indications, depending on the duration of the symptoms, for dose adjustment, or even treatment discontinuation (see section 4.4).

This functional disorder includes difficulties in executing delicate movements and is a possible consequence of sensory impairment. The risk of occurrence of persistent symptoms for a cumulative dose of 850 mg/m^2 (10 cycles) is approximately 10% and 20% for a cumulative dose of 1020 mg/m^2 (12 cycles).

In the majority of the cases, the neurological signs and symptoms improve or totally recover when treatment is discontinued. In the adjuvant setting of colon cancer, 6 months after treatment cessation, 87 % of patients had no or mild symptoms. After up to 3 years of follow up, about 3 % of patients presented either with persisting localized paresthesias of moderate intensity (2.3%) or with paresthesias that may interfere with functional activities (0.5%).

Acute neurosensory manifestations (see section 5.3) have been reported. They start within hours of administration and often occur on exposure to cold. They usually present as transient paresthesia, dysesthesia and hypoesthesia. An acute syndrome of pharyngolaryngeal dysesthesia occurs in 1% - 2% of patients and is characterised by subjective sensations of dysphagia or dyspnoea/feeling of suffocation, without any objective evidence of respiratory distress (no cyanosis or hypoxia) or of laryngospasm or bronchospasm (no stridor or wheezing); Although antihistamines and bronchodilators have been administered in such cases, the symptoms are rapidly reversible even in the absence of treatment. Prolongation of the infusion helps to reduce the incidence of this syndrome (see section 4.4). Occasionally other symptoms that have been observed include jaw spasm/muscle spasms/muscle contractions-involuntary/muscle twitching/myoclonus, coordination abnormal/gait abnormal/ ataxia/ balance disorders, throat or chest tightness/ pressure/ discomfort/ pain. In addition, cranial nerve dysfunctions may be associated, or also occur as an isolated event such as ptosis, diplopia, aphonia/ dysphonia/ hoarseness, sometimes described as vocal cord paralysis, abnormal tongue sensation or dysarthria, sometimes described as aphasia, trigeminal neuralgia/ facial pain/ eye pain, decrease in visual acuity, visual field disorders.

Other neurological symptoms such as dysarthria, loss of deep tendon reflex and Lhermitte's sign were reported during treatment with oxaliplatin. Isolated cases of optic neuritis have been reported.

Post marketing experience with frequency unknown

Convulsion

Gastrointestinal disorders

Incidence by patient (%), by grade

(see Table 4)

Prophylaxis and/or treatment with potent antiemetic agents is indicated.

Dehydration, paralytic ileus, intestinal obstruction, hypokalemia, metabolic acidosis and renal impairment may be caused by severe diarrhoea/emesis particularly when combining oxaliplatin with 5 fluorouracil (5 FU) (see section 4.4).

Hepato-biliary disorders

Very rare (< 1/10,000):

Liver sinusoidal obstruction syndrome, also known as veno-occlusive disease of liver, or pathological manifestations related to such liver disorder, including peliosis hepatis, nodular regenerative hyperplasia, perisinusoidal fibrosis. Clinical manifestations may be portal hypertension and/or increased transaminases.

Renal and urinary disorders

Very rare (< 1/10,000):

Acute tubular necrosis, acute interstitial nephritis and acute renal failure.

4.9 Overdose

There is no known antidote to oxaliplatin. In cases of overdose, exacerbation of adverse events can be expected. Monitoring of haematological parameters should be initiated and symptomatic treatment given.

5. PHARMACOLOGICAL PROPERTIES

5.1 Pharmacodynamic properties

Pharmacotherapeutic group: other antineoplastic agents, platinum compounds

ATC code: L01XA 03

Oxaliplatin is an antineoplastic drug belonging to a new class of platinum-based compounds in which the platinum atom is complexed with 1,2-diaminocyclohexane ("DACH") and an oxalate group.

Oxaliplatin is a single enantiomer, (*SP*-4-2)-[(1*R*,2*R*)-Cyclohexane-1,2-diamine-k*N*, k*N'*] [ethanedioato(2-)-kO^1, kO^2] platinum.

Oxaliplatin exhibits a wide spectrum of both *in vitro* cytotoxicity and *in vivo* antitumour activity in a variety of tumour model systems including human colorectal cancer models. Oxaliplatin also demonstrates *in vitro* and *in vivo* activity in various cisplatin resistant models.

A synergistic cytotoxic action has been observed in combination with 5-fluorouracil both *in vitro* and *in vivo*.

Studies on the mechanism of action of oxaliplatin, although not completely elucidated, show that the aqua-derivatives resulting from the biotransformation of oxaliplatin, interact with DNA to form both inter and intra-strand cross-links, resulting in the disruption of DNA synthesis leading to cytotoxic and antitumour effects.

In patients with metastatic colorectal cancer, the efficacy of oxaliplatin (85mg/m^2 repeated every two weeks) combined with 5-fluorouracil/folinic acid (5-FU/FA) is reported in three clinical studies:

- In front-line treatment, the 2-arm comparative phase III EFC2962 study randomised 420 patients either to 5-FU/FA alone (LV5FU2, N=210) or the combination of oxaliplatin with 5-FU/FA (FOLFOX4, N=210)

- In pretreated patients, the comparative three arms phase III study EFC4584 randomised 821 patients refractory to an irinotecan (CPT-11) + 5-FU/FA combination either to 5-FU/FA alone (LV5FU2, N=275), oxaliplatin single agent (N=275), or combination of oxaliplatin with 5-FU/FA (FOLFOX4, N=271).

- Finally, the uncontrolled phase II EFC2964 study included patients refractory to 5-FU/FA alone, that were treated with the oxaliplatin and 5-FU/FA combination (FOLFOX4, N=57)

The two randomised clinical trials, EFC2962 in front-line therapy and EFC4584 in pretreated patients, demonstrated a significantly higher response rate and a prolonged progression free survival (PFS)/time to progression (TTP) as compared to treatment with 5-FU/FA alone. In EFC4584 performed in refractory pretreated patients, the difference in median overall survival (OS) between the combination of oxaliplatin and 5-FU/FA did not reach statistical significance.

Response rate under FOLFOX4 versus LV5FU2

(see Table 5 below)

Median Progression Free Survival (PFS) / Median Time to Progression (TTP) FOLFOX4 versus LV5FU2

(see Table 6 on next page)

Median Overall Survival (OS) under FOLFOX4 versus LV5FU2

(see Table 7 on next page)

In pretreated patients (EFC4584), who were symptomatic at baseline, a higher proportion of those treated with oxaliplatin and 5-FU/FA experienced a significant improvement of their disease-related symptoms compared to those treated with 5-FU/FA alone (27.7% vs 14.6% p = 0.0033). In non-pretreated patients (EFC2962), no

Table 4 Gastrointestinal disorders
Incidence by patient (%), by grade

Oxaliplatin and 5-FU/FA 85 mg/m^2	Metastatic Setting			Adjuvant Setting		
every 2 weeks	All grades	Gr 3	Gr 4	All grades	Gr 3	Gr 4
Nausea	69.9	8	<1	73.7	4.8	0.3
Diarrhoea	60.8	9	2	56.3	8.3	2.5
Vomiting	49.0	6	1	47.2	5.3	0.5
Mucositis/Stomatitis	39.9	4	<1	42.1	2.8	0.1

Table 5 Response rate under FOLFOX4 versus LV5FU2

Response rate, % (95% CI) independent radiological review ITT analysis	LV5FU2	FOLFOX4	Oxaliplatin Single agent
Front-line treatment EFC2962	22 (16-27)	49 (42-46)	NA*
Response assessment every 8weeks	P value = 0.0001		
Pretreated patients EFC4584 (refractory to CPT-11 + 5-FU/FA)	0.7 (0.0-2.7)	11.1 (7.6-15.5)	1.1 (0.2-3.2))
Response assessment every 6 weeks	P value < 0.0001		
Pretreated patients EFC2964 (refractory to 5-FU/FA)	NA*	23 (13-36)	NA*
Response assessment every 12weeks			

* NA: Not Applicable

Table 6 Median Progression Free Survival (PFS) / Median Time to Progression (TTP) FOLFOX4 versus LV5FU2

Median PFS/TTP, Months (95% CI) independent radiological review ITT analysis	LV5FU2	FOLFOX4	Oxaliplatin Single agent
Front-line treatment EFC2962 (PFS)	6.0 (5.5-6.5)	8.2 (7.2-8.8)	NA*
	Log-rank P value = 0.0003		
Pretreated patients EFC4584 (TTP) **(refractory to** CPT-11 + 5-FU/FA)	2.6 (1.8-2.9)	5.3 (4.7-6.1)	2.1 (1.6-2.7)
	Log-rank P value < 0.0001		
Pretreated patients **EFC2964** (refractory to 5-FU/FA)	NA*	5.1 (3.1-5.7)	NA*

* NA: Not Applicable

Table 7 Median Overall Survival (OS) under FOLFOX4 versus LV5FU2

Median OS, months (95% CI) **ITT analysis**	LV5FU2	FOLFOX 4	Oxaliplatin Single agent
Front-line treatment EFC2962	14.7 (13.0-18.2)	16.2 (14.7-18.2)	NA*
	Log-rank P value = 0.12		
Pretreated patients **EFC4584** **(refractory to** CPT-11 + 5-FU/FA)	8.8 (7.3 - 9.3)	9.9 (9.1-10.5)	8.1 (7.2-8.7)
	Log-rank P value = 0.09		
Pretreated patients **EFC2964** (refractory to 5-FU/FA)	NA*	10.8 (9.3-12.8)	NA*

*NA: Not Applicable

statistically significant difference between the two treatment groups was found for any of the quality of life dimensions. However, the quality of life scores were generally better in the control arm for measurement of global health status and pain and worse in the oxaliplatin arm for nausea and vomiting. In the adjuvant setting, the MOSAÏC comparative phase III study (EFC3313) randomised 2246 patients (899 stage II/Duke's B2 and 1347 stage III/Duke's C) further to complete resection of the primary tumor of colon cancer either to 5-FU/FA alone (LV5FU2, N=1123 (B2/C = 448/675) or to combination of oxaliplatin and 5-FU/FA (FOLFOX4, N=1123 (B2/C) = 451/672).

EFC 3313 3-year disease free survival (ITT analysis)* for the overall population.

Treatment arm	LV5FU2	FOLFOX4
Percent 3-year disease free survival (95% CI)	73.3 (70.6-75.9)	78.7 (76.2-81.1)
Hazard ratio (95% CI)	0.76 (0.64-0.89)	
Stratified log rank test	P=0.0008	

* median follow up 44.2 months (all patients followed for at least 3 years)

The study demonstrated an overall significant advantage in 3-year disease free survival for the oxaliplatin and 5-FU/FA combination (FOLFOX4) over 5-FU/FA alone (LV5FU2).

EFC 3313 3-year Disease Free Survival (ITT analysis)* according to Stage of disease

(see Table 8 opposite)

Overall Survival (ITT analysis): At time of the analysis of the 3-year disease free survival, which was the primary endpoint of the MOSAIC trial, 85.1% of the patients were still alive in the FOLFOX4 arm versus 83.8% in the LV5FU2 arm. This translated into an overall reduction in mortality risk of 10% in favour of FOLFOX4 not reaching statistical significance (hazard ratio = 0.90). The figures were 92.2% versus 92.4% in the stage II (Duke's B2) sub-population (hazard ratio = 1.01) and 80.4% versus 78.1% in the stage III (Duke's C) sub-population (hazard ratio = 0.87), for FOLFOX4 and LV5FU2, respectively.

5.2 Pharmacokinetic properties

The pharmacokinetics of individual active compounds have not been determined. The pharmacokinetics of ultrafiltrable platinum, representing a mixture of all unbound, active and inactive platinum species, following a two-hour infusion of oxaliplatin at 130 mg /m^2 every three weeks for 1 to 5 cycles and oxaliplatin at 85 mg/m^2 every two weeks for 1 to 3 cycles are as follows:

Summary of Platinum Pharmacokinetic Parameter Estimates in Ultrafiltrate Following Multiple Doses of Oxaliplatin at 85 mg/m^2 Every Two Weeks or at 130 mg/m^2 Every Three Weeks

(see Table 9 on next page)

At the end of a 2-hour infusion, 15% of the administered platinum is present in the systemic circulation, the remaining 85% being rapidly distributed into tissues or eliminated in the urine. Irreversible binding to red blood cells and plasma, results in half-lives in these matrices that are close to the natural turnover of red blood cells and serum albumin. No accumulation was observed in plasma ultrafiltrate following 85 mg/m^2 every two weeks or 130mg/m^2 every three weeks and steady state was attained by cycle one in this matrix. Inter- and intra-subject variability is generally low.

Biotransformation *in vitro* is considered to be the result of non-enzymatic degradation and there is no evidence of cytochrome P450-mediated metabolism of the diaminocyclohexane (DACH) ring. Oxaliplatin undergoes extensive biotransformation in patients, and no intact drug was detectable in plasma ultrafiltrate at the end of a 2h-infusion. Several cytotoxic biotransformation products including the monochloro-, dichloro- and diaquo-DACH platinum species have been identified in the systemic circulation together with a number of inactive conjugates at later time points. Platinum is predominantly excreted in urine, with clearance mainly in the 48 hours following administration. By day 5, approximately 54% of the total dose was recovered in the urine and < 3% in the faeces.

A significant decrease in clearance from 17.6 ± 2.18 l/h to 9.95 ± 1.91 l/h in renal impairment was observed together with a statistically significant decrease in distribution volume from 330 ± 40.9 to 241 ± 36.1 l. The effect of severe renal impairment on platinum clearance has not been evaluated.

5.3 Preclinical safety data

The target organs identified in preclinical species (mice, rats, dogs, and/or monkeys) in single- and multiple-dose studies included the bone marrow, the gastrointestinal system, the kidney, the testes, the nervous system, and the heart. The target organ toxicities observed in animals are consistent with those produced by other platinum-containing drugs and DNA-damaging, cytotoxic drugs used in the treatment of human cancers with the exception of the effects produced on the heart. Effects on the heart were observed only in the dog and included electrophysiological disturbances with lethal ventricular fibrillation. Cardiotoxicity is considered specific to the dog not only because it was observed in the dog alone but also because doses similar to those producing lethal cardiotoxicity in dogs (150 mg/m^2) were well-tolerated by humans. Preclinical studies using rat sensory neurons suggest that the acute neurosensory symptoms related to Oxaliplatin may involve an interaction with voltage-gated Na^+ channels.

Oxaliplatin was mutagenic and clastogenic in mammalian test systems and produced embryo-fetal toxicity in rats. Oxaliplatin is considered a probable carcinogen, although carcinogenic studies have not been conducted.

6. PHARMACEUTICAL PARTICULARS

6.1 List of excipients

Water for injections

6.2 Incompatibilities

The diluted medicinal product should not be mixed with other medications in the same infusion bag or infusion line. Under instructions for use described in section 6.6, oxaliplatin can be co-administered with folinic acid via a Y-line.

- DO NOT mix with alkaline drugs or solutions, in particular 5-fluorouracil, folinic acid preparations containing trometamol as an excipient and trometamol salts of others drugs. Alkaline drugs or solutions will adversely affect the stability of oxaliplatin (see section 6.6).

- DO NOTdilute oxaliplatin with saline or other solutions containing chloride ions (including calcium, potassium or sodium chlorides).

- DO NOT mix with other drugs in the same infusion bag or infusion line (see section 6.6 for instructions concerning simultaneous administration with folinic acid).

- DO NOT use injection equipment containing aluminium.

6.3 Shelf life

3 years

After dilution in 5% glucose, chemical and physical in-use stability has been demonstrated for 48 hours at +2°C to +8°C and for 24 hours at +25°C.

From a microbiological point of view, the infusion preparation should be used immediately.

If not used immediately, in-use storage times and conditions prior to use are the responsibility of the user and would normally not be longer than 24 hours at 2°C to 8°C unless dilution has taken place in controlled and validated aseptic conditions.

6.4 Special precautions for storage

Keep the vial in the outer carton in order to protect from light.

Do not freeze.

Table 8 EFC 3313 3-year Disease Free Survival (ITT analysis)* according to Stage of disease

Patient stage	Stage II (Duke's B2)		Stage III (Duke's C)	
Treatment arm	LV5FU2	FOLFOX4	LV5FU2	FOLFOX4
Percent 3-year disease free survival (95% CI)	84.3 (80.9-87.7)	87.4 (84.3-90.5)	65.8 (62.2-69.5)	72.8 (69.4-76.2)
Hazard ratio (95% CI)	0.79 (0.57-1.09)		0.75 (0.62-0.90)	
Log-rank test	P=0.151		P=0.002	

* median follow up 44.2 months (all patients followed for at least 3 years)

Table 9 Summary of Platinum Pharmacokinetic Parameter Estimates in Ultrafiltrate Following Multiple Doses of Oxaliplatin at 85 mg/m² Every Two Weeks or at 130 mg/m² Every Three Weeks

Dose	Cmaxμg/mL	AUC0-48μg.h/mL	AUC μg.h/mL	t1/2αh	t1/2βh	t1/2γh	VssL	CL L/h
85 mg/m²								
Mean	0.814	4.19	4.68	0.43	16.8	391	440	17.4
SD	0.193	0.647	1.40	0.35	5.74	406	199	6.35
130 mg/m²								
Mean	1.21	8.20	11.9	0.28	16.3	273	582	10.1
SD	0.10	2.40	4.60	0.06	2.90	19.0	261	3.07

Mean AUC0-48, and Cmax values were determined on Cycle 3 (85 mg/m²) or cycle 5 (130 mg/m2).

Mean AUC, Vss, CL, and CLR0-48 values were determined on Cycle 1.

Cend, Cmax, AUC, AUC0-48, Vss and CL values were determinedby non-compartmental analysis.

t1/2α, t1/2β, and t1/2γ, were determined by compartmental analysis (Cycles 1-3 combined).

6.5 Nature and contents of container

1 vial with 10 ml concentrate (Type I clear glass) with bromobutyl elastomer stopper

1 vial with 20 ml concentrate (Type I clear glass) with bromobutyl elastomer stopper

1 vial with 40 ml concentrate (Type I clear glass) with bromobutyl elastomer stopper

6.6 Special precautions for disposal and other handling

As with other potentially toxic compounds, caution should be exercised when handling and preparing oxaliplatin solutions.

Instructions for Handling The handling of this cytotoxic agent by nursing or medical personnel requires every precaution to guarantee the protection of the handler and his surroundings.

The preparation of injectable solutions of cytotoxic agents must be carried out by trained specialist personnel with knowledge of the medicines used, in conditions that guarantee the integrity of the product, the protection of the environment and in particular the protection of the personnel handling the medicines, in accordance with the hospital policy. It requires a preparation area reserved for this purpose. It is forbidden to smoke, eat or drink in this area.

Personnel must be provided with appropriate handling materials, notably long sleeved gowns, protection masks, caps, protective goggles, sterile single-use gloves, protective covers for the work area, containers and collection bags for waste.

Excreta and vomit must be handled with care.

Pregnant women must be warned to avoid handling cytotoxic agents.

Any broken container must be treated with the same precautions and considered as contaminatedwaste. Contaminated waste should be incinerated in suitably labelled rigid containers. See below section "Disposal". If oxaliplatin concentrate or infusion solution, should come into contact with skin, wash immediately and thoroughly with water.

If oxaliplatin concentrate or infusion solution, should come into contact with mucous membranes, wash immediately and thoroughly with water.

Special precautions for administration

- DO NOT use injection equipment containing aluminium.
- DO NOT administer undiluted.
- Only glucose 5% infusion solution is to be used as a diluent. DO NOT dilute for infusion with sodium chloride or chloride containing solutions.
- DO NOT mix with any other medication in the same infusion bag or administer simultaneously by the same infusion line.
- DO NOT mix with alkaline drugs or solutions, in particular 5-fluorouracil, folinic acid preparations containing trometamol as an excipient and trometamol salts of others drugs. Alkaline drugs or solutions will adversely affect the stability of oxaliplatin.

Instruction for use with folinic acid (as calcium folinate or disodium folinate)

Oxaliplatin 85mg/m² IV infusion in 250 to 500 ml of 5% glucose solution is given at the same time as folinic acid IV infusion in 5% glucose solution, over 2 to 6 hours, using a Y-line placed immediately before the site of infusion. These two drugs should not be combined in the same infusion bag. Folinic acid must not contain trometamol as an excipient and must only be diluted using isotonic 5% glucose solution, never in alkaline solutions or sodium chloride or chloride containing solutions.

Instruction for use with 5-fluorouracil

Oxaliplatin should always be administered before fluoropyrimidines – i.e. 5-fluorouracil.

After oxaliplatin administration, flush the line and then administer 5-fluorouracil.

For additional information on drugs combined with oxaliplatin, see the corresponding manufacturer's summary of product characteristics.

Concentrate for solution for infusion

Inspect visually prior to use. Only clear solutions without particles should be used.

The medicinal product is for single use only. Any unused concentrate should be discarded.

Dilution before infusion

Withdraw the required amount of concentrate from the vial(s) and then dilute with 250 ml to 500 ml of a 5% glucose solution to give an oxaliplatin concentration between 0.2 mg/ml and 2 mg/ml; concentration range for which the physico-chemical stability of oxaliplatin has been demonstrated.

Administer by IV infusion.

After dilution in 5% glucose, chemical and physical in-use stability has been demonstrated for 48 hours at +2°C to +8°C and for 24 hours at +25°C. From a microbiological point of view, this infusion preparation should be used immediately. If not used immediately, in-use storage times and conditions prior to use are the responsibility of the user and would normally not be longer than 24 hours at 2°C to 8°C unless dilution has taken place in controlled and validated aseptic conditions.

Inspect visually prior to use. Only clear solutions without particles should be used.

The medicinal product is for single use only. Any unused infusion solution should be discarded.

NEVER use sodium chloride or chloride containing solutions for dilution.

The compatibility of Oxaliplatin solution for infusion has been tested with representative, PVC-based, administration sets.

Infusion

The administration of oxaliplatin does not require prehydration.

Oxaliplatin diluted in 250 to 500 ml of a 5% glucose solution to give a concentration not less than 0.2 mg/ml must be infused either by peripheral vein or central venous line over 2 to 6 hours. When oxaliplatin is administered with 5-fluorouracil, the oxaliplatin infusion must precede the administration of 5-fluorouracil.

Disposal

Remnants of the medicinal product as well as all materials that have been used for dilution and administration must be destroyed according to hospital standard procedures applicable to cytotoxic agents and with due regard to current laws related to the disposal of hazardous waste.

7. MARKETING AUTHORISATION HOLDER

Sanofi-aventis
One Onslow Street
Guildford
Surrey
GU1 4YS
UK

8. MARKETING AUTHORISATION NUMBER(S)

PL 11723/0423

9. DATE OF FIRST AUTHORISATION/RENEWAL OF THE AUTHORISATION

15th December 2005

10. DATE OF REVISION OF THE TEXT

August 2009

Legal Classification: POM

Emcor, Emcor LS

(Merck Serono)

1. NAME OF THE MEDICINAL PRODUCT

Emcor LS 5 mg film-coated tablets

Emcor 10 mg film coated tablets

2. QUALITATIVE AND QUANTITATIVE COMPOSITION

Emcor 5 mg: Each tablet contains 5 mg Bisoprolol hemifumarate (equivalent to 4.2mg bisoprolol).

Emcor 10 mg: Each tablet contains 10 mg Bisoprolol hemifumarate (equivalent to 8.4mg bisoprolol).

For excipients, see section 6.1.

3. PHARMACEUTICAL FORM

5mg Tablet:

Film-coated tablet

Yellowish-white, heart-shaped, scored and film-coated tablets

10mg Tablet:

Film-coated tablet

Pale orange-light orange, heart-shaped, scored and film-coated tablets

4. CLINICAL PARTICULARS

4.1 Therapeutic indications

(i) Management of hypertension

(ii) Management of angina pectoris

4.2 Posology and method of administration

Adults: The usual dose is 10 mg once daily with a maximum recommended dose of 20 mg per day. In some patients 5 mg per day may be adequate.

Administration

Emcor tablets should be taken in the morning and can be taken with food. They should be swallowed with liquid and should not be chewed.

Special populations

Elderly: No dosage adjustment is normally required, but 5 mg per day may be adequate in some patients; as for other adults, dosage may have to be reduced in cases of severe renal or hepatic dysfunction.

Children: There is no paediatric experience with bisoprolol, therefore its use cannot be recommended for children.

Renal or hepatic impairment: In patients with final stage impairment of renal function (creatinine clearance < 20 ml/min) or liver function, the dose should not exceed 10 mg bisoprolol once daily.

4.3 Contraindications

Bisoprolol is contra-indicated in patients with:

- acute heart failure or during episodes of heart failure decompensation requiring i.v. inotropic therapy
- cardiogenic shock
- second or third degree AV block (without a pacemaker)
- sick sinus syndrome
- sinoatrial block
- bradycardia (heart rate less than 60 beats/min prior to start of therapy)
- hypotension (systolic blood pressure < 100mmHg)
- severe bronchial asthma or severe chronic obstructive pulmonary disease
- severe forms of peripheral arterial occlusive disease and Raynaud's syndrome
- untreated phaeochromocytoma (see section 4.4)
- metabolic acidosis
- hypersensitivity to bisoprolol or to any of the excipients

4.4 Special warnings and precautions for use

Bisoprolol must be used with caution in:

- heart failure

The treatment of stable chronic heart failure with bisoprolol has to be initiated with a special titration phase (for details, see SPC for bisoprolol indicated for the treatment of stable chronic heart failure).

- bronchospasm (bronchial asthma, obstructive airways diseases).

In bronchial asthma or other chronic obstructive lung diseases, which may cause symptoms, bronchodilating therapy should be given concomitantly. Occasionally an increase of the airway resistance may occur in patients with asthma, therefore the dose of $beta_2$-stimulants may have to be increased.

- For patients with severe renal impairment and patients with severe liver function disorders please refer to section 4.2.
- diabetes mellitus with large fluctuations in blood glucose values; symptoms of hypoglycaemia can be masked.
- strict fasting.
- ongoing desensitisation therapy.
- first degree AV block.
- Prinzmetal's angina.
- peripheral arterial occlusive disease (intensification of complaints might happen especially during the start of therapy)
- general anaesthesia.

In patients undergoing general anaesthesia beta-blockade reduces the incidence of arrhythmias and myocardial ischemia during induction and intubation, and the post-operative period. It is currently recommended that maintenance of beta-blockade be continued peri-operatively. The anaesthesist must be aware of beta-blockade because of the potential for interactions with other drugs, resulting in bradyarrhythmias, attenuation of the reflex tachycardia and the decreased reflex ability to compensate for blood loss. If it is thought necessary to withdraw beta-blocker therapy before surgery, this should be done gradually and completed about 48 hours before anaesthesia.

Combination of bisoprolol with calcium antagonists of the verapamil or diltiazem type or with centrally acting antihypertensive drugs is generally not recommended, for details please refer to section 4.5.

As with other beta-blockers, bisoprolol may increase both the sensitivity towards allergens and the severity of anaphylactic reactions. Adrenaline treatment does not always give the expected therapeutic effect.

Patients with psoriasis or with a history of psoriasis should only be given beta-blockers (e.g. bisoprolol) after carefully balancing the benefits against the risks.

In patients with phaeochromocytoma bisoprolol must not be administered until after alpha-receptor blockade.

Under treatment with bisoprolol the symptoms of a thyrotoxicosis may be masked.

Treatment with bisoprolol should not be stopped abruptly unless clearly indicated, especially in patients with ischaemic heart disease.

4.5 Interaction with other medicinal products and other forms of interaction

Combinations not recommended

• Calcium antagonists of the verapamil type and to a lesser extent of the diltiazem type: Negative influence on contractility and atrio-ventricular conduction. Intravenous administration of verapamil in patients on beta-blocker treatment may lead to profound hypotension and atrioventricular block.

• Centrally acting antihypertensive drugs such as clonidine and others (e.g. methyldopa, moxonodine, rilmenidine): Concomitant use of centrally acting antihypertensive drugs may further decrease the central sympathetic tonus (reduction of heart rate and cardiac output, vasodilation). Abrupt withdrawal, particularly if prior to beta-blocker discontinuation, may increase risk of "rebound hypertension".

Combinations to be used with caution

• Calcium antagonists of the dihydropyridine type such as nifedipine: Concomitant use may increase the risk of hypotension, and an increase in the risk of a further deterioration of the ventricular pump function in patients with heart failure cannot be excluded.

• Class-I antiarrhythmic drugs (e.g. disopyramide, quinidine): Effect on atrio-ventricular conduction time may be potentiated and negative inotropic effect increased

• Class-III antiarrhythmic drugs (e.g. amiodarone): Effect on atrio-ventricular conduction time may be potentiated.

• Topical beta-blockers (e.g. eye drops for glaucoma treatment) may add to the systemic effects of bisoprolol.

• Parasympathomimetic drugs: Concomitant use may increase atrio-ventricular conduction time and the risk of bradycardia.

• Insulin and oral antidiabetic drugs: Intensification of blood sugar lowering effect. Blockade of beta-adrenoreceptors may mask symptoms of hypoglycaemia.

• Anaesthetic agents: Attenuation of the reflex tachycardia and increase of the risk of hypotension (for further information on general anaesthesia see also section 4.4).

• Digitalis glycosides: Reduction of heart rate, increase of atrio-ventricular conduction time.

• Non-steroidal anti-inflammatory drugs (NSAIDs): NSAIDs may reduce the hypotensive effect of bisoprolol.

• Beta-sympathomimetic agents (e.g. isoprenaline, dobutamine): Combination with bisoprolol may reduce the effect of both agents.

• Sympathomimetics that activate both beta- and alpha-adrenoceptors (e.g. noradrenaline, adrenaline): Combination with bisoprolol may unmask the alpha-adrenoceptor-mediated vasoconstrictor effects of these agents leading to blood pressure increase and exacerbated intermittent claudication. Such interactions are considered to be more likely with nonselective beta-blockers. Higher doses of adrenaline may be necessary for treatment of allergic reactions.

• Concomitant use with antihypertensive agents as well as with other drugs with blood pressure lowering potential (e.g. tricyclic antidepressants, barbiturates, phenothiazines) may increase the risk of hypotension.

• Moxisylyte: Possibly causes severe postural hypotension.

Combinations to be considered

• Mefloquine: increased risk of bradycardia

• Monoamine oxidase inhibitors (except MAO-B inhibitors): Enhanced hypotensive effect of the beta-blockers but also risk for hypertensive crisis.

4.6 Pregnancy and lactation

Pregnancy

Bisoprolol has pharmacological effects that may cause harmful effects on pregnancy and/or the foetus/newborn. In general, β-adrenoceptor blockers reduce placental perfusion, which has been associated with growth retardation, intrauterine death, abortion or early labour. Adverse effects (e.g. hypoglycaemia and bradycardia) may occur in the foetus and newborn infant. If treatment with β-adrenoceptor blockers is necessary, β_1-selective adrenoceptor blockers are preferable.

Bisoprolol should not be used during pregnancy unless clearly necessary. If treatment with bisoprolol is considered necessary, the uteroplacental blood flow and the foetal growth should be monitored. In case of harmful effects on pregnancy or the foetus alternative treatment should be considered. The newborn infant must be closely monitored. Symptoms of hypoglycaemia and bradycardia are generally to be expected within the first 3 days.

Lactation

It is not known whether this drug is excreted in human milk. Therefore, breastfeeding is not recommended during administration of bisoprolol.

4.7 Effects on ability to drive and use machines

In a study of coronary heart disease patients, bisoprolol did not impair driving performance. However, due to individual variations in reactions to the drug, the ability to drive a vehicle or to operate machinery may be impaired. This should be considered particularly at the start of treatment and upon change of medication as well as in conjunction with alcohol.

4.8 Undesirable effects

The following definitions apply to the frequency terminology used hereafter:

Very common (⩾ 1/10)

Common (⩾ 1/100, < 1/10)

Uncommon (⩾ 1/1,000, < 1/100)

Rare (⩾ 1/10,000, < 1/1,000)

Very rare (< 1/10,000)

Cardiac disorders:

Uncommon: AV-conduction disturbances, worsening of pre-existing heart failure, bradycardia.

Vascular disorders:

Common: feeling of coldness or numbness in the extremities, hypotension.

Uncommon: Orthostatic hypotension.

Metabolism and nutrition disorders:

Rare: Increased triglycerides.

Psychiatric disorders:

Uncommon: sleep disorders, depression.

Rare: nightmares, hallucinations.

Nervous system disorders:

Common: dizziness*, headache*.

Rare: syncope

Eye disorders:

Rare: reduced tear flow (to be considered if the patient uses lenses).

Very rare: conjunctivitis.

Ear and labyrinth disorders:

Rare: hearing disorders.

Respiratory, thoracic and mediastinal disorders:

Uncommon: bronchospasm in patients with bronchial asthma or a history of obstructive airways disease.

Rare: allergic rhinitis.

Gastrointestinal disorders:

Common: gastrointestinal complaints such as nausea, vomiting, diarrhoea, constipation.

Hepatobiliary disorders:

Rare: increased liver enzymes (ALAT, ASAT), hepatitis.

Skin and subcutaneous tissue disorders:

Rare: hypersensitivity reactions (itching, flush, rash).

Very rare: beta-blockers may provoke or worsen psoriasis or induce psoriasis-like rash, alopecia.

Musculoskeletal and connective tissue disorders:

Uncommon: muscular weakness and cramps.

Reproductive system and breast disorders:

Rare: potency disorders.

General disorders:

Common: fatigue*.

Uncommon: asthenia.

*These symptoms especially occur at the beginning of the therapy. They are generally mild and often disappear within 1-2 weeks.

4.9 Overdose

The most common signs expected with overdosage of a β-blocker are bradycardia, hypotension, bronchospasm, acute cardiac insufficiency and hypoglycaemia. To date a few cases of overdose (maximum: 2000 mg) with bisoprolol have been reported. Bradycardia and/or hypotension were noted. All patients recovered. There is a wide inter-individual variation in sensitivity to one single high dose of bisoprolol.

In general, if overdose occurs, bisoprolol treatment should be stopped and supportive and symptomatic treatment should be provided. Limited data suggest that bisoprolol is hardly dialysable. Based on the expected pharmacological actions and recommendations for other β-blockers, the following general measures should be considered when clinically warranted.

Bradycardia: Administer intravenous atropine. If the response is inadequate, isoprenaline or another agent with positive chronotropic properties may be given cautiously. Under some circumstances, transvenous pacemaker insertion may be necessary.

Hypotension: Intravenous fluids and vasopressors should be administered. Intravenous glucagon may be useful.

AV block (second or third degree): Patients should be carefully monitored and treated with isoprenaline infusion or transvenous cardiac pacemaker insertion.

Acute worsening of heart failure: Administer i.v. diuretics, inotropic agents, vasodilating agents.

Bronchospasm: Administer bronchodilator therapy such as isoprenaline, β_2-sympathomimetic drugs and/or aminophylline.

Hypoglycaemia: Administer i.v. glucose.

5. PHARMACOLOGICAL PROPERTIES

5.1 Pharmacodynamic properties

Bisoprolol is a potent, highly β1-selective adrenoreceptor blocking agent devoid of intrinsic sympathomimetic activity and without relevant membrane stabilising activity.

As with other β1-blocking agents, the mode of action in hypertension is not clear but it is known that bisoprolol markedly depresses plasma renin levels.

In patients with angina, the blockade of β1-receptors reduces heart action and thus reduces oxygen demand. Hence bisoprolol is effective in eliminating or reducing the symptoms.

5.2 Pharmacokinetic properties

Bisoprolol is absorbed almost completely from the gastro-intestinal tract. Together with the very small first pass effect in the liver, this results in a high bioavailability of approximately 90%. The drug is cleared equally by the liver and kidney.

The plasma elimination half-life (10-12 hours) provides 24 hours efficacy following a once daily dosage. About 95% of the drug substance is excreted through the kidney, half of this is as unchanged bisoprolol. There are no active metabolites in man.

5.3 Preclinical safety data

Not applicable

6. PHARMACEUTICAL PARTICULARS

6.1 List of excipients

Tablet core: silica, colloidal anhydrous; magnesium stearate; crospovidone; cellulose, microcrystalline; maize starch; calcium hydrogen phosphate, anhydrous.

Film coating: iron oxide red (E172); iron oxide yellow (E172); dimeticone; macrogol 400; titanium dioxide (E171); hypromellose.

6.2 Incompatibilities

None

6.3 Shelf life

4 years

6.4 Special precautions for storage

This product does not require any special storage conditions.

6.5 Nature and contents of container

Cartons containing blister packs of 4, 14 or 28 tablets.

6.6 Special precautions for disposal and other handling

None

7. MARKETING AUTHORISATION HOLDER

E. Merck Ltd

Bedfont Cross, Stanwell Road

Feltham, Middlesex,

TW14 8NX, UK

8. MARKETING AUTHORISATION NUMBER(S)

PL 0493/0126

PL 0493/0127

9. DATE OF FIRST AUTHORISATION/RENEWAL OF THE AUTHORISATION

27 July 2004

10. DATE OF REVISION OF THE TEXT

03 April 2009

Legal category

POM

EMEND 80mg, 125mg hard Capsules

(Merck Sharp & Dohme Limited)

1. NAME OF THE MEDICINAL PRODUCT

EMEND 125 mg hard capsules

EMEND 80 mg hard capsules

2. QUALITATIVE AND QUANTITATIVE COMPOSITION

Each 125 mg capsule contains 125 mg of aprepitant. Each 80 mg capsule contains 80 mg of aprepitant.

Excipient: 125 mg sucrose (in the 125 mg capsule).

Excipient: 80 mg sucrose (in the 80 mg capsule).

For a full list of excipients, see section 6.1.

3. PHARMACEUTICAL FORM

Hard capsule

The 125 mg capsule is opaque with a white body and pink cap with "462" and "125 mg" printed radially in black ink on the body. The 80 mg capsules are opaque with a white body and cap with "461" and "80 mg" printed radially in black ink on the body.

4. CLINICAL PARTICULARS

4.1 Therapeutic indications

Prevention of acute and delayed nausea and vomiting associated with highly emetogenic cisplatin-based cancer chemotherapy in adults

Prevention of nausea and vomiting associated with moderately emetogenic cancer chemotherapy.

EMEND 125/80mg is given as part of combination therapy (see section 4.2).

4.2 Posology and method of administration

Posology

EMEND is given for 3 days as part of a regimen that includes a corticosteroid and a 5-HT_3 antagonist. The recommended posology of EMEND is 125 mg orally (PO) once daily one hour before start of chemotherapy on Day 1 and 80 mg PO once daily on Days 2 and 3. Fosaprepitant 115mg, a lyophilized prodrug of aprepitant may be substituted for oral EMEND (125mg), 30 minutes prior to chemotherapy, on Day 1 only of the chemotherapy – induced nausea and vomiting (CINV) regimen as an intravenous infusion administered over 15 minutes. Please refer to the Summary of Product Characteristics for fosaprepitant.

In clinical studies with EMEND, the following regimens were used for the prevention of nausea and vomiting associated with emetogenic cancer chemotherapy:

Highly Emetogenic Chemotherapy Regimen

(see Table 1 below)

EMEND was administered orally 1 hour prior to chemotherapy treatment on Day 1 and in the morning on Days 2 and 3.

Dexamethasone was administered 30 minutes prior to chemotherapy treatment on Day 1 and in the morning on Days 2 to 4. The dose of dexamethasone was chosen to account for active substance interactions.

Ondansetron was administered intravenously 30 minutes prior to chemotherapy treatment on Day 1.

Moderately Emetogenic Chemotherapy Regimen

(see Table 2 below)

EMEND was administered orally 1 hour prior to chemotherapy treatment on Day 1 and in the morning on Days 2 and 3.

Dexamethasone was administered 30 minutes prior to chemotherapy treatment on Day 1. The dose of dexamethasone was chosen to account for active substance interactions.

One 8 mg capsule of ondansetron was administered 30 to 60 minutes prior to chemotherapy treatment and one 8 mg capsule was administered 8 hours after first dose on Day 1.

Efficacy data on combination with other corticosteroids and 5-HT_3 antagonists are limited. For additional information on the co-administration with corticosteroids, see section 4.5.

Please refer to the Summary of Product Characterisitics of coadministered antiemetics.

Elderly (≥65 years)

No dosage adjustment is necessary for the elderly. (see Section 5.2)

Gender

No dosage adjustment is necessary based on gender (see Section 5.2).

Renal impairment

No dosage adjustment is necessary for patients with renal impairment or for patients with end stage renal disease undergoing haemodialysis (see section 5.2).

Hepatic impairment

No dosage adjustment is necessary for patients with mild hepatic impairment. There are limited data in patients with moderate hepatic impairment and no data in patients with severe hepatic impairment. (see sections 4.4 and 5.2).

Children and adolescents

EMEND is not recommended for use in children below 18 years due to insufficient data on safety and efficacy (see section 5.2).

Method of administration

The hard capsule should be swallowed whole.

EMEND may be taken with or without food.

4.3 Contraindications

Hypersensitivity to the active substance or to any of the excipients.

Co-administration with pimozide, terfenadine, astemizole or cisapride (see section 4.5).

4.4 Special warnings and precautions for use

There are limited data in patients with moderate hepatic insufficiency and no data in patients with severe hepatic impairment. EMEND should be used with caution in these patients (see section 5.2).

EMEND should be used with caution in patients receiving concomitant orally administered active substances that are metabolised primarily through CYP3A4 and with a narrow therapeutic range, such as ciclosporin, tacrolimus, sirolimus, everolimus, alfentanil, diergotamine, ergotamine, fentanyl and quinidine (see section 4.5). Additionally, concomitant administration with irinotecan should be approached with particular caution as the combination might result in increased toxicity.

Co-administration of EMEND with ergot alkaloid derivatives, which are CYP3A4 substrates, may result in elevated plasma concentrations of these active substances. Therefore, caution is advised due to the potential risk of ergot-related toxicity.

Co-administration of EMEND with warfarin results in decreased prothrombin time, reported as International Normalised Ratio (INR). In patients on chronic warfarin therapy, the INR should be monitored closely during treatment with EMEND and for 2 weeks following each 3-day course of EMEND for chemotherapy induced nausea and vomiting (see section 4.5).

The efficacy of hormonal contraceptives may be reduced during and for 28 days after administration of EMEND. Alternative or back-up methods of contraception should be used during treatment with EMEND and for 2 months following the last dose of EMEND (see section 4.5).

Concomitant administration of EMEND with active substances that strongly induce CYP3A4 activity (e.g. rifampicin, phenytoin, carbamazepine, phenobarbital) should be avoided as the combination results in reductions of the plasma concentrations of aprepitant (see section 4.5). Concomitant administration of EMEND with herbal preparations containing St. John's Wort (*Hypericum perforatum*) is not recommended.

Concomitant administration of EMEND with active substances that inhibit CYP3A4 activity (e.g. ketoconazole, itraconazole, voriconazole, posaconazole, clarithromycin, telithromycin, nefazodone, and protease inhibitors) should be approached cautiously as the combination is expected to result in increased plasma concentrations of aprepitant (see section 4.5).

EMEND contains sucrose. Patients with rare hereditary problems of fructose intolerance, glucose-galactose malabsorption or sucrase-isomaltase insufficiency should not take this medicine.

4.5 Interaction with other medicinal products and other forms of interaction

Aprepitant (125 mg/80 mg) is a substrate, a moderate inhibitor, and an inducer of CYP3A4. Aprepitant is also an inducer of CYP2C9. During treatment with EMEND, CYP3A4 is inhibited. After the end of treatment, EMEND causes a transient mild induction of CYP2C9, CYP3A4 and glucuronidation. Aprepitant does not seem to interact with the P-glycoprotein transporter, as suggested by the lack of interaction of aprepitant with digoxin.

Effect aprepitant on the pharmacokinetics of other active substances

CYP3A4 Inhibition

As a moderate inhibitor of CYP3A4, aprepitant (125 mg/80 mg) can increase plasma concentrations of co-administered active substances that are metabolised through CYP3A4. The total exposure of orally administered CYP3A4 substrates may increase up to approximately 3-fold during the 3-day treatment with EMEND; the effect of aprepitant on the plasma concentrations of intravenously administered CYP3A4 substrates is expected to be smaller. Emend must not be used concurrently with pimozide, terfanadine, astemizole, or cisapride (see section 4.3). Inhibition of CYP3A4 by aprepitant could result in elevatated plasma concentrations of these active substances potentially causing serious or life-threatening reactions. Caution is advised during concomitant administration of EMEND and orally administered active substances that are metabolized primarily through CYP3A4 and with a narrow therapeutic range, such as ciclosporin, tacrolimus, sirolimus, everolimus, aflentanil, diergotamine, ergotamine, fentanyl, and quinidine (see section 4.4)

Corticosteroids:

Dexamethasone: The usual oral dexamethasone dose should be reduced by approximately 50 % when co-administered with EMEND 125 mg/80 mg regimen. The dose of dexamethasone in chemotherapy induced nausea and vomiting clinical trials was chosen to account for active substance interactions (see section 4.2). EMEND, when given as a regimen of 125 mg with dexamethasone co-administered orally as 20 mg on Day 1, and EMEND when given as 80 mg/day with dexamethasone coadministered orally as 8 mg on Days 2 through 5, increased the AUC of dexamethasone, a CYP3A4 substrate, 2.2-fold on Days 1 and 5.

Methylprednisolone: The usual intravenously administered methylprednisolone dose should be reduced approximately 25 %, and the usual oral methylprednisolone dose should be reduced approximately 50 % when coadministered with EMEND 125 mg/80 mg regimen. EMEND, when given as a regimen of 125 mg on Day 1 and 80 mg/day on Days 2 and 3, increased the AUC of methylprednisolone, a CYP3A4 substrate, by 1.3-fold on Day 1 and by 2.5-fold on Day 3, when methylprednisolone was co-administered intravenously as 125 mg on Day 1 and orally as 40 mg on Days 2 and 3.

During continuous treatment with methylprednisolone, the AUC of methylprednisolone may decrease at later time points within 2 weeks following initiation of dosing with EMEND, due to the inducing effect of aprepitant on CYP3A4. This effect may be expected to be more pronounced for orally administered methylprednisolone.

Chemotherapeutic agents: In pharmacokinetic studies, EMEND, when given as a regimen of 125 mg on Day 1 and 80 mg/day on Days 2 and 3, did not influence the pharmacokinetics of docetaxel administered intravenously on Day 1 or vinorelbine administered intravenously on Day 1 or Day 8. Because the effect of EMEND on the pharmacokinetics of orally administered CYP3A4 substrates is greater than the effect of EMEND on the pharmacokinetics of intravenously administered CYP3A4 substrates, an interaction with orally administered chemotherapeutic agents metabolised primarily or in part by CYP3A4 (e.g. etoposide, vinorelbine) cannot be excluded. Caution is advised and additional monitoring may be appropriate in patients receiving such agents orally (see section 4.4).

Immunosuppressants:

During the 3 day CINV regimen, a transient moderate increase followed by a mild decrease in exposure of immunosuppressants metabolised by CYP3A4 (e.g. cyclosporine, tacrolimus, everolimus and sirolimus) is expected. Given the short duration of the 3-day regimen and the time-dependent limited changes in exposure, dose reduction of the immunosuppressants is not recommended during the 3 days of co-administration with EMEND.

Midazolam: The potential effects of increased plasma concentrations of midazolam or other benzodiazepines metabolised via CYP3A4 (alprazolam, triazolam) should be considered when coadministering these agents with EMEND (125 mg/80 mg).

EMEND increased the AUC of midazolam, a sensitive CYP3A4 substrate, 2.3-fold on Day 1 and 3.3-fold on Day 5, when a single oral dose of 2mg midazolam was co-administered on Days 1 and 5 of a regimen of EMEND 125 mg on Day 1 and 80 mg/day on Days 2 to 5.

In another study with intravenous administration of midazolam, EMEND was given as 125 mg on Day 1 and 80 mg/day on Days 2 and 3, and 2mg midazolam was given intravenously prior to the administration of the 3-day regimen of EMEND and on Days 4, 8, and 15. EMEND increased the AUC of midazolam 25 % on Day 4 and decreased the AUC of midazolam 19 % on Day 8 and 4 % on Day 15. These effects were not considered clinically important.

Table 1 Highly Emetogenic Chemotherapy Regimen

	Day 1	Day 2	Day 3	Day 4
EMEND	125 mg PO	80 mg PO	80 mg PO	none
Dexamethasone	12 mg PO	8 mg PO	8 mg PO	8 mg PO
Ondansetron	32 mg IV	none	none	none

Table 2 Moderately Emetogenic Chemotherapy Regimen

	Day 1	Day 2	Day 3
EMEND	125 mg PO	80 mg PO	80 mg PO
Dexamethasone	12 mg PO	none	none
Ondansetron	2 × 8 mg PO	none	none

Induction

As a mild inducer of CYP2C9, CYP3A4 and glucuronidation, aprepitant can decrease plasma concentrations of substrates eliminated by these routes. This effect may become apparent only after the end of treatment with EMEND. For CYP2C9 and CYP3A4 substrates, the induction is transient with a maximum effect reached 3-5 days after end of the EMEND 3-day treatment. The effect is maintained for a few days, thereafter slowly declines and is clinically insignificant by two weeks after end of EMEND treatment. Mild induction of glucuronidation is also seen with 80 mg oral aprepitant given for 7 days. Data are lacking regarding effects on CYP2C8 and CYP2C19. Caution is advised when warfarin, acenocoumarol, tolbutamide, phenytoin or other active substances that are known to be metabolised by CYP2C9 are administered during this time period.

In a third study with intravenous and oral administration of midazolam, EMEND was given as 125 mg on Day 1 and 80 mg/day on Days 2 and 3, together with ondansetron 32 mg Day 1, dexamethasone 12 mg Day 1 and 8 mg Days 2-4. This combination (i.e. EMEND, ondansetron and dexamethasone) decreased the AUC of oral midazolam 16 % on Day 6, 9 % on Day 8, 7 % on Day 15 and 17 % on Day 22. These effects were not considered clinically important.

An additional study was completed with intravenous administration of midazolam and EMEND. Intravenous 2mg midazolam was given 1 hour after oral administration of a single dose of EMEND 125 mg. The plasma AUC of midazolam was increased by 1.5-fold. This effect was not considered clinically important.

Warfarin: In patients on chronic warfarin therapy, the prothrombin time (INR) should be monitored closely during treatment with EMEND and for 2 weeks following each 3-day course of EMEND for chemotherapy induced nausea and vomiting (see section 4.4). When a single 125-mg dose of EMEND was administered on Day 1 and 80 mg/day on Days 2 and 3 to healthy subjects who were stabilised on chronic warfarin therapy, there was no effect of EMEND on the plasma AUC of R(+) or S(-) warfarin determined on Day 3; however, there was a 34 % decrease in S(-) warfarin (a CYP2C9 substrate) trough concentration accompanied by a 14 % decrease in INR 5 days after completion of dosing with EMEND.

Tolbutamide: EMEND, when given as 125 mg on Day 1 and 80 mg/day on Days 2 and 3, decreased the AUC of tolbutamide (a CYP2C9 substrate) by 23 % on Day 4, 28 % on Day 8, and 15 % on Day 15, when a single dose of tolbutamide 500 mg was administered orally prior to the administration of the 3-day regimen of EMEND and on Days 4, 8, and 15.

Hormonal contraceptives: The efficacy of hormonal contraceptives may be reduced during and for 28 days after administration of EMEND. Alternative or back-up methods of contraception should be used during treatment with EMEND and for 2 months following the last dose of EMEND.

In a clinical study, single doses of an oral contraceptive containing ethinyl estradiol and norethindrone were administered on Days 1 through 21 with EMEND, given as a regimen of 125 mg on Day 8 and 80 mg/day on Days 9 and 10 with ondansetron 32 mg intravenously on Day 8 and oral dexamethasone given as 12 mg on Day 8 and 8 mg/day on Days 9, 10, and 11. During days 9 through 21 in this study, there was as much as a 64% decrease in ethinyl estradiol trough concentrations and as much as a 60% decrease in norethindrone trough concentrations.

5-HT_3 antagonists: In clinical interaction studies, aprepitant did not have clinically important effects on the pharmacokinetics of ondansetron, granisetron, or hydrodolasetron (the active metabolite of dolasetron).

Effect of other agents on the pharmacokinetics of aprepitant

Concomitant administration of EMEND with active substances that inhibit CYP3A4 activity (e.g., ketoconazole, itraconazole, voriconazole, posaconazole, clarithromycin, telithromycin nefazodone, and protease inhibitors)) should be approached cautiously, as the combination is expected to result in increased plasma concentrations of aprepitant (see section 4.4)

Concomitant administration of EMEND with active substances that strongly induce CYP3A4 activity (e.g. rifampicin, phenytoin, carbamazepine, phenobarbital) should be avoided as the combination results in reductions of the plasma concentrations of aprepitant that may result in decreased efficacy of EMEND. Concomitant administration of EMEND with herbal prepartions containing St. John's Wort (*Hypericum perforatum*) is not recommended.

Ketoconazole: When a single 125-mg dose of aprepitant was administered on Day 5 of a 10-day regimen of 400 mg/day of ketoconazole, a strong CYP3A4 inhibitor, the AUC of aprepitant increased approximately 5-fold and the mean terminal half-life of aprepitant increased approximately 3-fold.

Rifampicin: When a single 375-mg dose of aprepitant was administered on Day 9 of a 14-day regimen of 600 mg/day of rifampicin, a strong CYP3A4 inducer, the AUC of aprepitant decreased 91 % and the mean terminal half-life decreased 68 %.

4.6 Pregnancy and lactation

The potential for reproductive toxicity of aprepitant has not been fully characterized, since exposure levels above the therapeutic exposure in humans at the 125 mg/80 mg dose were not attained in animal studies. These studies did not indicate direct or indirect harmful effects with respect to pregnancy, embryonal/foetal development, parturition or postnatal development (see section 5.3). The potential effects on reproduction of alterations in neurokinin regulation are unknown. EMEND should not be used during pregnancy unless clearly necessary.

Aprepitant is excreted in the milk of lactating rats. It is not known whether aprepitant is excreted in human milk; therefore, breast-feeding is not recommended during treatment with EMEND.

4.7 Effects on ability to drive and use machines

No studies on the effects of EMEND on the ability to drive and use machines have been performed. However, when driving vehicles or operating machines, it should be taken into account that dizziness and fatigue have been reported after taking EMEND (see section 4.8).

4.8 Undesirable effects

The safety profile of aprepitant was evaluated in approximately 4,900 individuals.

Adverse reactions considered as drug-related by the investigator were reported in approximately 17 % of patients treated with the aprepitant regimen compared with approximately 13 % of patients treated with standard therapy in patients receiving highly emetogenic chemotherapy. Aprepitant was discontinued due to adverse reactions in 0.6 % of patients treated with the aprepitant regimen compared with 0.4 % of patients treated with standard therapy. In a clinical study of patients receiving moderately emetogenic chemotherapy, clinical adverse reactions were reported in approximately 21% of patients treated with the aprepitant regimen compared with approximately 20% of patients treated with standard therapy. Aprepitant was discontinued due to adverse reactions in 1.1% of patients treated with the aprepitant regimen compared with 0.5% of patients treated with standard therapy.

The most common adverse reactions reported at a greater incidence in patients treated with the aprepitant regimen than with standard therapy in patients receiving highly emetogenic chemotherapy were: hiccups (4.6 % versus 2.9%), asthenia/fatigue (2.9 % versus 1.6%), alanine aminotransferase (ALT) increased (2.8 % versus 1.5%), constipation (2.2 % versus 2.0%), headache (2.2 % versus 1.8%), and anorexia (2.0 % versus 0.5%). The most common adverse reaction reported at a greater incidence in patients treated with the aprepitant regimen than with standard therapy in patients receiving moderately emetogenic chemotherapy was fatigue (2.5 % versus 1.6%).

The following adverse reactions were observed in patients treated with the aprepitant regimen and at a greater incidence than with standard therapy:

Frequencies are defined as: very common (≥1/10); common (≥1/100 to <1/10); uncommon (≥1/1,000 to <1/100); rare (≥1/10,000 to <1/1,000) and very rare (<1/10,000), not known (cannot be estimated from the available data).

(see Table 3 below)

The adverse reactions profiles in the Multiple-Cycle extension for up to 5 additional cycles of chemotherapy were generally similar to those observed in Cycle 1.

Additional adverse reactions were observed in patients treated with aprepitant (40 mg) for postoperative nausea and vomiting and a greater incidence than with ondansetron: abdominal pain upper, bowel sounds abnormal, dysarthria, dyspnoea, hypoaesthesia, insomnia, miosis, nausea, sensory disturbance, stomach discomfort, visual acuity reduced, wheezing.

In addition, two serious adverse experiences were reported in postoperative nausea and vomiting (PONV) clinical studies in patients taking a higher dose of aprepitant: one case of constipation, and one case of sub-ileus.

One case of Stevens-Johnson syndrome was reported as a serious adverse event in a patient receiving aprepitant with cancer chemotherapy.

One case of angioedema and urticaria was reported as a serious adverse event in a patient receiving aprepitant in a non-CINV/non-PONV study.

Post-marketing experience

During post-marketing experience the following side effects have been reported (frequency not known):

Skin and subcutaneous tissue disorders: pruritus, rash, urticaria

Immune system disorders: hypersensitivity reactions including anaphylactic reactions

4.9 Overdose

No specific information is available on the treatment of overdose with EMEND.

Table 3

System Organ Class	Adverse reaction	Frequency
Investigations	ALT increased, AST increased	common
	alkaline phosphatase increased, hyperglycaemia, microscopic haematuria, hyponatraemia, weight decreased	uncommon
Cardiac disorders	bradycardia	uncommon
Blood and lymphatic system disorders	febrile neutropenia, anaemia	uncommon
Nervous system disorders	headache, dizziness	common
	dream abnormality, cognitive disorder	uncommon
Eye disorders	conjunctivitis	uncommon
Ear and labyrinth disorders	tinnitus	uncommon
Respiratory, thoracic and mediastinal disorders	hiccups	common
	pharyngitis, sneezing, cough, postnasal drip, throat irritation	uncommon
Gastrointestinal disorders	constipation, diarrhoea, dyspepsia, eructation	common
	perforating duodenal ulcer, nausea*, vomiting*, acid reflux, dysgeusia, epigastric discomfort, obstipation, gastroesophageal reflux disease, abdominal pain, dry mouth, enterocolitis, flatulence, stomatitis	uncommon
Renal and urinary disorders	polyuria, dysuria, pollakiuria	uncommon
Skin and subcutaneous tissue disorders	rash, acne, photosensitivity, hyperhidrosis, oily skin, pruritus, skin lesion	uncommon
Musculoskeletal and connective tissue disorders	muscle cramp, myalgia	uncommon
Metabolism and nutrition disorders	anorexia	common
	weight gain, polydipsia	uncommon
Infection and infestations	candidiasis, staphylococcal infection	uncommon
Vascular disorders	flushing/hot flush	uncommon
General disorders and administration site conditions	asthaenia/fatigue	common
	oedema, chest discomfort, lethargy, thirst	uncommon
Psychiatric disorders	disorientation, euphoria, anxiety	uncommon

*Nausea and vomiting were efficacy parameters in the first 5 days of post-chemotherapy treatment and were reported as adverse reactions only thereafter.

Drowsiness and headache were reported in one patient who ingested 1,440 mg of aprepitant.

In the event of overdose, EMEND should be discontinued and general supportive treatment and monitoring should be provided. Because of the antiemetic activity of aprepitant, drug-induced emesis may not be effective.

Aprepitant cannot be removed by haemodialysis.

5. PHARMACOLOGICAL PROPERTIES

5.1 Pharmacodynamic properties

Pharmacotherapeutic group: Antiemetics and antinauseants, ATC code: A04A D12

Aprepitant is a selective high-affinity antagonist at human substance P neurokinin 1 (NK_1) receptors.

In 2 randomised, double-blind studies encompassing a total of 1,094 patients receiving chemotherapy that included cisplatin ⩾70 mg/m^2, aprepitant in combination with an ondansetron/dexamethasone regimen (see section 4.2) was compared with a standard regimen (placebo plus ondansetron 32 mg intravenously administered on Day 1 plus dexamethasone 20 mg orally on Day 1 and 8 mg orally twice daily on Days 2 to 4).

Efficacy was based on evaluation of the following composite measure: complete response (defined as no emetic episodes and no use of rescue therapy) primarily during Cycle 1. The results were evaluated for each individual study and for the 2 studies combined.

A summary of the key study results from the combined analysis is shown in Table 4.

Table 4

Percent of Patients Receiving Highly Emetogenic Chemotherapy Responding by Treatment Group and Phase — Cycle 1

(see Table 4 above)

• The confidence intervals were calculated with no adjustment for gender and concomitant chemotherapy, which were included in the primary analysis of odds ratios and logistic models.

• † One patient in the Aprepitant Regimen only had data in the acute phase and was excluded from the overall and delayed phase analyses; one patient in the Standard Regimen only had data in the delayed phase and was excluded from the overall and acute phase analyses.

The estimated time to first emesis in the combined analysis is depicted by the Kaplan-Meier plot in Figure 1.

Figure 1

Percent of Patients Receiving Highly Emetogenic Chemotherapy

Who Remain Emesis Free Over Time – Cycle 1

(see Figure 1 on next page)

Statistically significant differences in efficacy were also observed in each of the 2 individual studies.

In the same 2 clinical studies, 851 patients continued into the Multiple-Cycle extension for up to 5 additional cycles of chemotherapy. The efficacy of the aprepitant regimen was apparently maintained during all cycles.

In a randomised, double-blind study in a total of 866 patients (864 females, 2 males) receiving chemotherapy that included cyclophosphamide 750-1500 mg/m^2; or cyclophosphamide 500-1500 mg/m^2 and doxorubicin (⩽ 60 mg/m^2) or epirubicin (⩽ 100 mg/m^2), aprepitant in combination with an ondansetron/dexamethasone regimen (see section 4.2) was compared with standard therapy (placebo plus ondansetron 8 mg orally (twice on Day 1, and every 12 hours on Days 2 and 3) plus dexamethasone 20 mg orally on Day 1).

Efficacy was based on evaluation of the composite measure: complete response (defined as no emetic episodes and no use of rescue therapy) primarily during Cycle 1.

A summary of the key study results is shown in Table 5.

Table 5

Percent of Patients Responding by Treatment Group and Phase — Cycle 1

Moderately Emetogenic Chemotherapy

(see Table 5 above)

• The confidence intervals were calculated with no adjustment for age category (<55 years, ⩾ 55 years) and investigator group, which were included in the primary analysis of odds ratios and logistic models.

• † One patient in the Aprepitant Regiment only had data in the acute phase and was excluded from the overall and delayed phase analyses.

The estimated time to first emesis in the study is depicted by the Kaplan-Meier plot in Figure 2.

Figure 2

Percent of Patients Receiving Moderately Emetogenic Chemotherapy

Who Remain Emesis Free Over Time – Cycle 1

(see Figure 2 on next page)

In the same clinical study, 744 patients continued into the Multiple-Cycle extension for up to 3 additional cycles of chemotherapy. The efficacy of the aprepitant regimen was apparently maintained during all cycles.

Table 4 Percent of Patients Receiving Highly Emetogenic Chemotherapy Responding by Treatment Group and Phase — Cycle 1

COMPOSITE MEASURES	Aprepitant Regimen (N= 521)† %	Standard Therapy (N= 524)† %	Differences* %	(95 % CI)
Complete Response (no emesis and no rescue therapy)				
Overall (0-120 hours)	67.7	47.8	19.9	(14.0, 25.8)
0-24 hours	86.0	73.2	12.7	(7.9, 17.6)
25-120 hours	71.5	51.2	20.3	(14.5, 26.1)
INDIVIDUAL MEASURES				
No Emesis (no emetic episodes regardless of use of rescue therapy)				
Overall (0-120 hours)	71.9	49.7	22.2	(16.4, 28.0)
0-24 hours	86.8	74.0	12.7	(8.0, 17.5)
25-120 hours	76.2	53.5	22.6	(17.0, 28.2)
No Significant Nausea (maximum VAS <25 mm on a scale of 0-100 mm)				
Overall (0-120 hours)	72.1	64.9	7.2	(1.6, 12.8)
25-120 hours	74.0	66.9	7.1	(1.5, 12.6)

Table 5 Percent of Patients Responding by Treatment Group and Phase — Cycle 1 Moderately Emetogenic Chemotherapy

COMPOSITE MEASURES	Aprepitant Regimen (N= 433)† %	Standard Therapy (N= 424) %	Differences* %	(95 % CI)
Complete Response (no emesis and no rescue therapy)				
Overall (0-120 hours)	50.8	42.5	8.3	(1.6, 15.0)
0-24 hours	75.7	69.0	6.7	(0.7, 12.7)
25-120 hours	55.4	49.1	6.3	(-0.4, 13.0)
INDIVIDUAL MEASURES				
No Emesis (no emetic episodes regardless of use of rescue therapy)				
Overall (0-120 hours)	75.7	58.7	17.0	(10.8, 23.2)
0-24 hours	87.5	77.3	10.2	(5.1, 15.3)
25-120 hours	80.8	69.1	11.7	(5.9, 17.5)
No Significant Nausea (maximum VAS <25 mm on a scale of 0-100 mm)				
Overall (0-120 hours)	60.9	55.7	5.3	(-1.3, 11.9)
0-24 hours	79.5	78.3	1.3	(-4.2, 6.8)
25-120 hours	65.3	61.5	3.9	(-2.6, 10.3)

5.2 Pharmacokinetic properties

Aprepitant displays non-linear pharmacokinetics. Both clearance and absolute bioavailability decrease with increasing dose.

Absorption

The mean absolute oral bioavailability of aprepitant is 67 % for the 80-mg capsule and 59 % for the 125-mg capsule. The mean peak plasma concentration (C_{max}) of aprepitant occurred at approximately 4 hours (t_{max}). Oral administration of the capsule with an approximately 800 Kcal standard breakfast resulted in an up to 40 % increase in AUC of aprepitant. This increase is not considered clinically relevant.

The pharmacokinetics of aprepitant is non-linear across the clinical dose range. In healthy young adults, the increase in $AUC_{0-\infty}$ was 26 % greater than dose proportional between 80-mg and 125-mg single doses administered in the fed state.

Following oral administration of a single 125 mg dose of EMEND on Day 1 and 80 mg once daily on Days 2 and 3, the AUC_{0-24hr} (mean±SD) was 19.6±2.5 microgram × hr/ml and 21.2±6.3 microgram × hr/ml on Days 1 and 3, respectively. C_{max} was 1.6±0.36 microgram/ml and 1.4±0.22 microgram/ml on Days 1 and 3, respectively.

Distribution

Aprepitant is highly protein bound, with a mean of 97 %. The geometric mean apparent volume of distribution at steady state (Vd_{ss}) is approximately 66 l in humans.

Metabolism

Aprepitant undergoes extensive metabolism. In healthy young adults, aprepitant accounts for approximately 19 % of the radioactivity in plasma over 72 hours following a single intravenous administration 100-mg dose of [^{14}C]-fosaprepitant, a prodrug for aprepitant indicating a substantial presence of metabolites in the plasma. Twelve metabolites of aprepitant have been identified in human plasma. The metabolism of aprepitant occurs largely via oxidation at the morpholine ring and its side chains and the resultant metabolites were only weakly active. *In vitro* studies using human liver microsomes indicate that aprepitant is metabolised primarily by CYP3A4 and potentially with minor contribution by CYP1A2 and CYP2C19.

Elimination

Aprepitant is not excreted unchanged in urine. Metabolites are excreted in urine and via biliary excretion in faeces. Following a single intravenously administered 100-mg dose of [^{14}C]- fosaprepitant a prodrug for aprepitant to healthy subjects, 57 % of the radioactivity was recovered in urine and 45 % in faeces.

The plasma clearance of aprepitant is dose-dependent, decreasing with increased dose and ranged from approximately 60 to 72 ml/min in the therapeutic dose range. The terminal half-life ranged from approximately 9 to 13 hours.

Pharmacokinetics in special populations

Elderly: Following oral administration of a single 125-mg dose of aprepitant on Day 1 and 80 mg once daily on Days 2 through 5, the AUC_{0-24hr} of aprepitant was 21 % higher on Day 1 and 36 % higher on Day 5 in elderly (⩾65 years) relative to younger adults. The C_{max} was 10 % higher on Day 1 and 24 % higher on Day 5 in elderly relative to younger adults. These differences are not considered clinically meaningful. No dosage adjustment for EMEND is necessary in elderly patients.

Gender: Following oral administration of a single 125-mg dose of aprepitant, the C_{max} for aprepitant is 16 % higher in females as compared with males. The half-life of aprepitant is 25 % lower in females as compared with males and its t_{max} occurs at approximately the same time. These differences are not considered clinically meaningful. No dosage adjustment for EMEND is necessary based on gender.

Hepatic insufficiency: Mild hepatic impairment (Child-Pugh class A) does not affect the pharmacokinetics of aprepitant to a clinically relevant extent. No dose adjustment is necessary for patients with mild hepatic impairment. Conclusions regarding the influence of moderate hepatic impairment (Child-Pugh class B) on aprepitant pharmacokinetics cannot be drawn from available data. There are no clinical or pharmacokinetic data in patients with severe hepatic impairment (Child-Pugh class C).

Renal impairment: A single 240-mg dose of aprepitant was administered to patients with severe renal impairment (CrCl< 30 ml/min) and to patients with end stage renal disease (ESRD) requiring haemodialysis.

In patients with severe renal impairment, the $AUC_{0-\infty}$ of total aprepitant (unbound and protein bound) decreased by 21 % and C_{max} decreased by 32 %, relative to healthy subjects. In patients with ESRD undergoing haemodialysis, the $AUC_{0-\infty}$ of total aprepitant decreased by 42 % and C_{max} decreased by 32 %. Due to modest decreases in protein binding of aprepitant in patients with renal disease, the

Figure 1 Percent of Patients Receiving Highly Emetogenic Chemotherapy Who Remain Emesis Free Over Time – Cycle 1

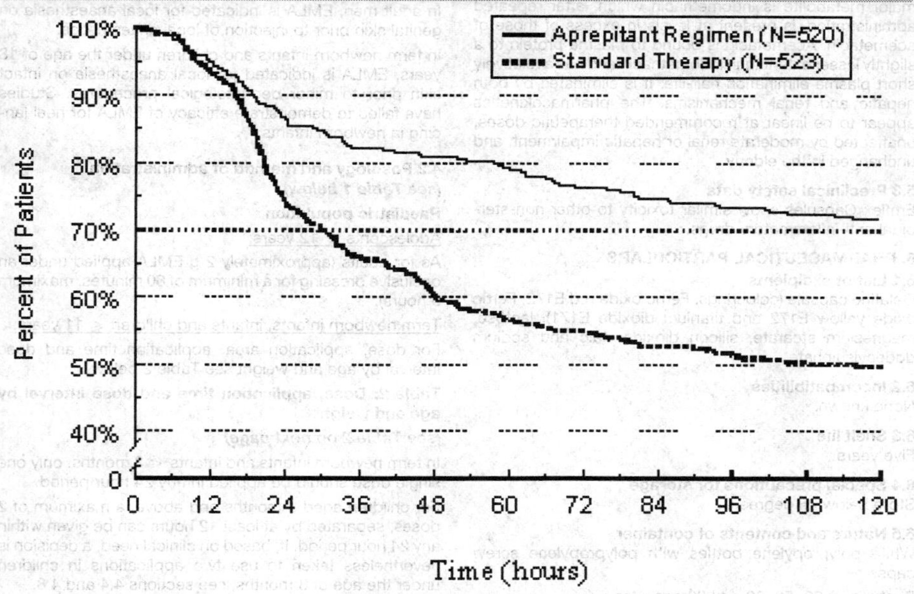

Figure 2 Percent of Patients Receiving Moderately Emetogenic Chemotherapy Who Remain Emesis Free Over Time – Cycle 1

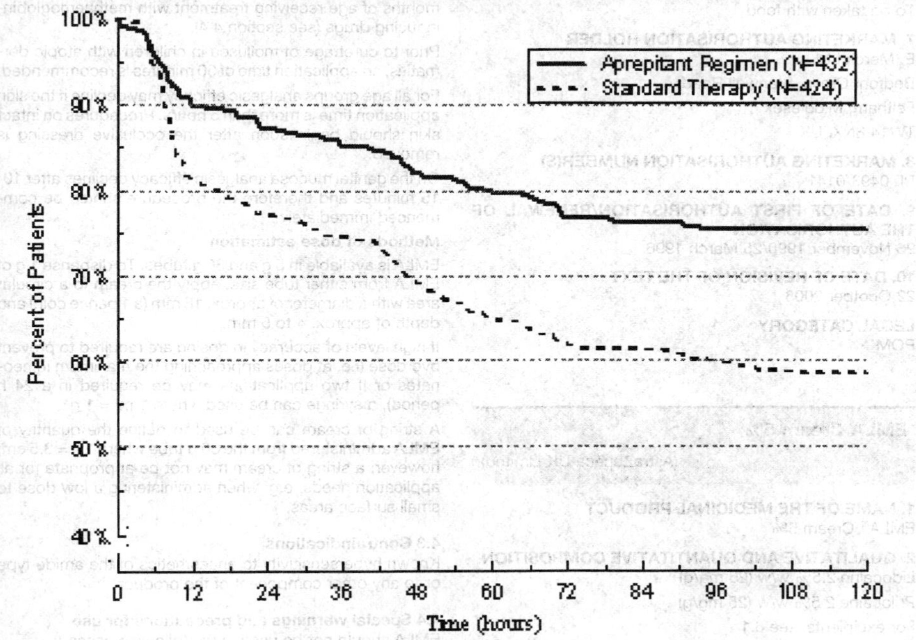

AUC of pharmacologically active unbound aprepitant was not significantly affected in patients with renal impairment compared with healthy subjects. Haemodialysis conducted 4 or 48 hours after dosing had no significant effect on the pharmacokinetics of aprepitant; less than 0.2 % of the dose was recovered in the dialysate.

No dose adjustment for EMEND is necessary for patients with renal impairment or for patients with ESRD undergoing haemodialysis.

Relationship between concentration and effect: Using a highly specific NK_1-receptor tracer, positron emission tomography (PET) studies in healthy young men have shown that aprepitant penetrates into the brain and occupies NK_1 receptors in a dose- and plasma- concentration-dependent manner. Aprepitant plasma concentrations achieved with the 3-day regimen of EMEND are predicted to provide greater than 95 % occupancy of brain NK_1 receptors.

5.3 Preclinical safety data

Pre-clinical data reveal no special hazard for humans based on conventional studies of single and repeated dose toxicity, genotoxicity, carcinogenic potential, and toxicity to reproduction. However, it should be noted that systemic exposure in rodents was similar or even lower than therapeutic exposure in humans at the 125 mg/80 mg dose. In particular, although no adverse effects were noted in reproduction studies at human exposure levels, the animal exposures are not sufficient to make an adequate risk assessment in man.

6. PHARMACEUTICAL PARTICULARS

6.1 List of excipients

Capsule content

Sucrose

Microcrystalline cellulose (E 460)

Hydroxypropyl cellulose (E 463)

Sodium laurilsulfate

Capsule shell (125 mg)

Gelatin

Sodium laurilsulfate and silica colloidal anhydrous may be used

Titanium dioxide (E 171)

Red iron oxide (E 172)

Yellow iron oxide (E 172)

Capsule shell (80 mg)

Gelatin

Sodium laurilsulfate and silica colloidal anhydrous may be used

Titanium dioxide (E 171)

Printing ink

Shellac

Potassium hydroxide

Black iron oxide (E 172)

6.2 Incompatibilities

Not applicable.

6.3 Shelf life

4 years

6.4 Special precautions for storage

Store in the original package in order to protect from moisture.

6.5 Nature and contents of container

Different pack sizes including different strengths are available.

Alminium blister containing one 125 mg capsule.

Aluminium blister containing one 80 mg capsule.

Aluminium blister containing two 80 mg capsules.

5 Aluminium blisters each containing one 80 mg capsule.

5 Aluminium blisters each containing one 125mg capsule.

Aluminium blister containing one 125 mg capsule and two 80 mg capsules.

Not all pack sizes may be marketed.

6.6 Special precautions for disposal and other handling

No special requirements.

7. MARKETING AUTHORISATION HOLDER

Merck Sharp & Dohme Ltd.

Hertford Road, Hoddesdon

Hertfordshire EN 11 9BU

United Kingdom

8. MARKETING AUTHORISATION NUMBER(S)

125 mg x1: EU/1/03/262/004

125 mg × 5: EU/1/03/262/005

80 mg x1: EU/1/03/262/001

80 mg x2: EU/1/03/262/002

80 mg x5: EU/1/03/262/003

80 mg x2 and 125 mg x1: EU/1/03/262/006

9. DATE OF FIRST AUTHORISATION/RENEWAL OF THE AUTHORISATION

Date of first authorization: 11th November 2003

Date of latest renewal: 22 September 2008

10. DATE OF REVISION OF THE TEXT

31 July 2009

Detailed information on this medicinal product is available on the website of the European Medicines Agency (EMEA) website: http://www.emea.europa.eu/.

SPC.EMD.09.UK.3116 (022+023)

® denotes registered trademark of Merck & Co. Inc., Whitehouse Station, NJ, USA.

Emflex Capsules

(Merck Serono)

1. NAME OF THE MEDICINAL PRODUCT

Emflex Capsules

2. QUALITATIVE AND QUANTITATIVE COMPOSITION

Each capsule contains Acemetacin 60mg

3. PHARMACEUTICAL FORM

Gelatine capsule

4. CLINICAL PARTICULARS

4.1 Therapeutic indications

Rheumatoid arthritis, osteoarthritis, low back pain, and post-operative pain and inflammation.

4.2 Posology and method of administration

The recommended starting dose is 120mg/day in divided doses, increasing to 180mg/day in divided doses, depending on patient response.

For the treatment of elderly patients, adjustment of dosage is not normally required. However, non-steroidal anti-inflammatory drugs should be used with particular care in older patients who may be more prone to adverse reactions.

Emflex should be taken with food, milk or an antacid to reduce the possibility of gastro-intestinal disturbance.

4.3 Contraindications

Active peptic ulcer; history of recurrent ulceration; known hypersensitivity to acemetacin or indomethacin. Patients who have experienced asthma attacks, urticaria or acute rhinitis resulting from treatment with aspirin or non-steroidal anti-inflammatory drugs. Patients with nasal polyps associated with angioneurotic oedema. Safety in children is not established.

4.4 Special warnings and precautions for use

As rare instances of peptic ulceration have been reported administration should be closely supervised in patients with a history of upper gastrointestinal disease. Treatment should be discontinued if peptic ulceration or gastrointestinal bleeding occurs.

Inhibition of platelet aggregation may occur.

Aggravation of psychiatric disorders, epilepsy or parkinsonism may occur.

Signs and symptoms of infection may be masked.

Emflex should be used with caution in patients with reduced renal blood flow where renal perfusion may be maintained by prostaglandins. In patients at particular risk - renal or hepatic dysfunction, congestive heart failure, electrolyte or fluid imbalance, sepsis, concomitant use of nephrotoxic drugs, the dose should be kept as low as possible and renal function should be monitored.

Patients receiving long-term treatment should be periodically screened for renal and hepatic function and blood counts. Borderline elevation of renal and hepatic function test parameters may occur. If this persists or worsens, treatment should be stopped.

Eye changes may occur in chronic rheumatoid disease and patients should receive periodic ophthalmological examinations and therapy discontinued if changes occur.

Hyperkalaemia has been reported with use of indomethacin and this should be considered when administration with potassium sparing diuretics is proposed.

4.5 Interaction with other medicinal products and other forms of interaction
Emflex is highly protein bound and it may therefore be necessary to modify the dosage of other highly protein bound drugs e.g. anti-coagulants. As there is a possibility of either a pharmacokinetic or pharmacodynamic interaction with aspirin or other salicylates, diflusinal, probenecid, lithium, triamterene, ACE inhibitors, haloperidol and methotrexate, patients receiving such combinations should be carefully monitored and dosages adjusted as necessary. Non-steroidal anti-inflammatory drugs may reduce the anti-hypertensive effects of beta-blockers, although clinical studies showed no propensity for Emflex to antagonise the effects of propranolol. Likewise the reduction of diuretic effects of thiazides and frusemide may occur with non-steroidal anti-inflammatory drugs and this should be borne in mind when treating patients with compromised cardiac function or hypertension.

4.6 Pregnancy and lactation
The safety of this product for use in human pregnancy and lactation has not been established. Animal reproduction studies do not provide reassurance regarding the lack of reproductive toxicity/ teratogenicity. Due to maternal toxicity, the studies were conducted at doses below the therapeutic dose or a very low multiple of the therapeutic dose. It should not therefore be used in pregnancy or lactation in women of childbearing age unless they are taking adequate contraceptive precautions.

4.7 Effects on ability to drive and use machines
The ability to drive a car or operate machinery may be affected.

4.8 Undesirable effects
The following side effects have been either reported with Emflex or could possibly occur as they are common to a number of NSAIDs:

Gastro-intestinal: Gastro-intestinal discomfort/pain, anorexia, nausea, vomiting, indigestion, diarrhoea and constipation, peptic ulceration, gastrointestinal perforation and haemorrhage.

Central Nervous System: Symptoms most frequently encountered are headache, dizziness, vertigo and insomnia. Rarely, confusion, depressed mood, irritability.

Hepatic: Occasional elevation of liver function test parameters without overt clinical symptomatology. Very rarely, symptoms of cholestasis.

Cardiovascular/renal: Rarely, oedema, chest pain, palpitations, blood urea elevation. NSAIDs have been reported to cause nephrotoxicity in various forms and their use can lead to interstitial nephritis, nephrotic syndrome and renal failure.

Dermatological/hypersensitivity: Pruritus, urticaria, erythema, skin rash, alopecia, angio-neurotic oedema and excessive sweating have been reported.

Haematological: Rarely, thrombocytopenia, leucopenia and reduced haemoglobin levels. Very rarely, reversible agranulocytosis, bone marrow depression.

Ocular/auditory: Infrequently, tinnitus, blurred vision and rarely, eye pain.

4.9 Overdose
Symptomatic and supportive therapy is indicated. If ingestion is recent, vomiting should be induced or gastric lavage should be performed. Progress should be followed for several days as gastrointestinal ulceration and haemorrhage have been reported with overdosage of other NSAIDs. Antacids may be helpful.

5. PHARMACOLOGICAL PROPERTIES
5.1 Pharmacodynamic properties
Acemetacin is a glycolic acid ester of indomethacin and the pharmacological activity resulting from acemetacin administration in man is derived from the presence of both acemetacin and indomethacin. The precise pharmacological mode of action of acemetacin is not known. However, unlike other NSAIDs, acemetacin is only a relatively weak inhibitor of prostaglandin synthetase.

Prostaglandins are known to have an antisecretory and cytoprotective effect on the gastric mucosa. Acemetacin shows activity in many of the established in vitro tests of anti-inflammatory activity, including inhibition of the release of a number of mediators of inflammation.

5.2 Pharmacokinetic properties
Acemetacin is well absorbed after oral administration. Its major metabolite is indomethacin which, after repeated administration, is present at levels in excess of those of acemetacin. Acemetacin is bound to plasma protein to a slightly lesser extent than indomethacin and has a relatively short plasma elimination half-life. It is eliminated by both hepatic and renal mechanisms. The pharmacokinetics appear to be linear at recommended therapeutic doses, unaffected by moderate renal or hepatic impairment, and unchanged in the elderly.

5.3 Preclinical safety data
Emflex Capsules show similar toxicity to other non-steroidal anti-inflammatory drugs.

6. PHARMACEUTICAL PARTICULARS
6.1 List of excipients
Gelatine capsule (colourings: Ferric oxide red E172, Ferric oxide yellow E172 and titanium dioxide E171), lactose, magnesium stearate, silicon dioxide, talc and sodium dodecylsulphate.

6.2 Incompatibilities
None known.

6.3 Shelf life
Five years

6.4 Special precautions for storage
Store below 25 degree C.

6.5 Nature and contents of container
White polypropylene bottles with polypropylene screw caps.

Pack sizes: 90, 56, 60 and 30 capsules.

PVC/PVDC foil blister packs in cartons:

Pack sizes: 90, 60, 56, 30, 10, and 6 capsules

6.6 Special precautions for disposal and other handling
To be taken with food.

7. MARKETING AUTHORISATION HOLDER
E. Merck Ltd.
Bedfont Cross, Stanwell Road
Feltham, Middlesex
TW14 8NX, UK

8. MARKETING AUTHORISATION NUMBER(S)
PL 0493/0141

9. DATE OF FIRST AUTHORISATION/RENEWAL OF THE AUTHORISATION
26 November 1990/25 March 1996

10. DATE OF REVISION OF THE TEXT
22 Ocotber 2008

LEGAL CATEGORY
POM

EMLA Cream 5%

(AstraZeneca UK Limited)

1. NAME OF THE MEDICINAL PRODUCT
EMLA® Cream 5%

2. QUALITATIVE AND QUANTITATIVE COMPOSITION
Lidocaine 2.5% w/w (25 mg/g)
Prilocaine 2.5% w/w (25 mg/g)
For excipients, see 6.1

3. PHARMACEUTICAL FORM
White soft cream.

4. CLINICAL PARTICULARS
4.1 Therapeutic indications
In adults, EMLA is indicated for local anaesthesia

- on intact skin prior to minor dermatological procedures (e.g. needle insertion and surgical treatment of localised lesions) and prior to dermal procedures on larger areas e.g. split skin grafting.
- on genital mucosa prior to surgical treatment of localised lesions.

In adult men, EMLA is indicated for local anaesthesia on genital skin prior to injection of local anaesthetics.

In term newborn infants and children under the age of 18 years, EMLA is indicated for local anaesthesia on intact skin prior to minor dermatological procedures. Studies have failed to demonstrate efficacy of EMLA for heel lancing in newborn infants.

4.2 Posology and method of administration
(see Table 1 below)

Paediatric population

Adolescents ⩾ 12 years:

As for adults (approximately 2 g EMLA applied under an occlusive dressing for a minimum of 60 minutes, maximum 5 hours).

Term newborn infants, infants and children ⩽ 11 years:

For dose, application area, application time and dose interval by age and weight see Table 2 below.

Table 2: Dose, application time and dose interval by age and weight

(see Table 2 on next page)

In term newborn infants and infants < 3 months, only one single dose should be applied in any 24 hour period.

For children aged 3 months and above, a maximum of 2 doses, separated by at least 12 hours can be given within any 24 hour period. If, based on clinical need, a decision is nevertheless taken to use two applications in children under the age of 3 months, see sections 4.4 and 4.8.

The safety of EMLA in pre-term newborn infants has not been established. Use of EMLA is not recommended in pre-term infants.

Use of EMLA is not recommended in infants less than 12 months of age receiving treatment with methaemoglobin-inducing drugs (see section 4.4).

Prior to curettage of mollusca in children with atopic dermatitis, an application time of 30 minutes is recommended.

For all age groups analgesic efficacy may decline if the skin application time is more than 5 hours. Procedures on intact skin should begin soon after the occlusive dressing is removed.

On the genital mucosa analgesic efficacy declines after 10-15 minutes and therefore the procedure should be commenced immediately.

Methods of dose estimation

EMLA is available in 5 g and 30 g tubes. To dispense 1 g of EMLA from either tube size, apply the cream to a circular area with a diameter of approx. 18 mm (a 1 pence coin) and depth of approx. 4 to 5 mm.

If high levels of accuracy in dosing are required to prevent overdose (i.e. at doses approaching the maximum in neonates or if two applications may be required in a 24 h period), a syringe can be used where 1 ml = 1 g.

A string of cream can be used to define the quantity of EMLA administered from the 30 g tube where 1 g = 3.5 cm; however, a string of cream may not be appropriate for all application needs, e.g. when administering a low dose to small surface areas.

4.3 Contraindications
Known hypersensitivity to anaesthetics of the amide type or to any other component of the product.

4.4 Special warnings and precautions for use
EMLA should not be used in the following cases:

(a) in pre-term neonates i.e. gestational age less than 37 weeks.

(b) in infants/neonates between 0 and 12 months of age receiving treatment with methaemoglobin-inducing agents due to the possible additive effects.

In infants/neonates younger than 12 months a transient, clinically insignificant increase in methaemoglobin level is commonly observed up to 12 hours after an application of EMLA.

Table 1

Age	Surface	Procedure	Application
Adults (including elderly)	Skin	Minor dermatological procedures e.g. needle insertion and surgical treatment of localised lesions.	Approximately 2 g EMLA applied under an occlusive dressing for a minimum of 60 minutes, maximum 5 hours.
		Dermal procedures on larger areas e.g. split skin grafting.	Approximately 1.5-2 g/10 cm^2 EMLA applied under an occlusive dressing for a minimum of 2 hours, maximum 5 hours.
	Male genital skin	Prior to injection of local anaesthetics	Approximately 1g/10cm^2 EMLA under an occlusive dressing applied for 15 minutes.
	Genital mucosa	Surgical treatment of localised lesions.	Apply up to 10 g EMLA for 5-10 minutes (no occlusive dressing required). Commence procedure immediately thereafter.

Table 2: Dose, application time and dose interval by age and weight

Age and body Weight Requirements	Max. total dose of EMLA Cream	Max. application area	Max. application time	Minimum dose interval
Term newborn infants to 3 months or < 5 kg	1 g	10 cm^2	1 hour	24 hours
3 up to 12 months and > 5 kg	2 g	20 cm^2	4 hours	12 hours
1 to 6 years and > 10 kg	10 g	100 cm^2	5 hours	12 hours
7 to 11 years and > 20 kg	20 g	200 cm^2	5 hours	12 hours

Patients with glucose-6-phosphate dehydrogenase deficiency or congenital or idiopathic methaemoglobinaemia are more susceptible to drug induced methaemoglobinaemia.

In term newborn infants, infants and children, EMLA should only be used on intact skin and should not be applied to genital mucosa.

In term neonates and infants < 3 months, only one single dose should be applied in any 24 hour period. If, based on clinical need, a decision is nevertheless taken to use two applications in children under the age of 3 months, the child should be clinically monitored for systemic adverse reactions (see sections 4.8 and 4.9).

Consideration should be given to the fact that pulse oximeter values may overestimate the actual oxygen saturation in case of increased methaemoglobin fraction; therefore, in cases of suspected methaemoglobinaemia, it may be more helpful to monitor oxygen saturation by co-oximetry.

Care must be taken to limit the dose and area of application and to prevent accidental ingestion.

Due to insufficient data on absorption, EMLA should not be applied to open wounds.

Care should be taken when applying EMLA to patients with atopic dermatitis. A shorter application time, 15-30 minutes, may be sufficient (see section 5.1 Pharmacodynamic properties). Prior to curettage of mollusca in children with atopic dermatitis, an application time of 30 minutes is recommended.

Care should be taken not to allow EMLA to come in contact with the eyes as it may cause eye irritation. Also the loss of protective reflexes may allow corneal irritation and potential abrasion. If contact with the eye occurs, immediately rinse the eye with water or sodium chloride solution and protect it until sensation returns.

EMLA, like other local anaesthetics may be ototoxic and should not be instilled in the middle ear nor should it be used for procedures which might allow penetration into the middle ear.

Although the systemic availability of prilocaine by percutaneous absorption of EMLA is low, caution should be exercised in patients with anaemia, congenital or acquired methaemoglobinaemia or patients on concomitant therapy known to produce such conditions.

Patients treated with anti-arrhythmic drugs class III (eg, amiodarone) should be under close surveillance and ECG monitoring considered, since cardiac effects may be additive.

Lidocaine and prilocaine have bactericidal and antiviral properties in concentrations above 0.5 – 2%. For this reason, although one clinical study suggests that the immunization response is not affected when EMLA Cream is used prior to BCG vaccination, the results of intracutaneous injections of live vaccines should be monitored.

4.5 Interaction with other medicinal products and other forms of interaction

Methaemoglobinaemia may be accentuated in patients already taking drugs known to induce the condition, e.g. sulphonamides, acetanilid, aniline dyes, benzocaine, chloroquine, dapsone, metoclopramide, naphthalene, nitrates and nitrites, nitrofurantoin, nitroglycerin, nitroprusside, pamaquine, para-aminosalicylic acid, phenacetin, phenobarbital, phenytoin, primaquine, quinine.

The risk of additional systemic toxicity should be considered when large doses of EMLA are applied to patients already using other local anaesthetics or structurally related drugs e.g. class I anti-arrhythmics such as mexiletine.

Specific interaction studies with lidocaine/prilocaine and anti-arrhythmic drugs class III (eg, amiodarone) have not been performed, but caution is advised (see also section 4.4).

4.6 Pregnancy and lactation

For EMLA Cream no adequate clinical data on exposed pregnancies are available. Animal studies do not indicate direct or indirect harmful effects with respect to pregnancy, embryonal/foetal development, parturition or postnatal development. In both animals and humans, lidocaine and prilocaine cross the placental barrier and may be absorbed by the foetal tissues. Caution should be exercised when used in pregnant women.

Lidocaine and prilocaine are excreted in breast milk, but in such small quantities that there is generally no risk of the child being affected at therapeutic dose levels.

4.7 Effects on ability to drive and use machines

None known.

4.8 Undesirable effects

Transient local reactions at the application site, most commonly erythema, paleness and/or oedema, may occur in >1% of patients treated with EMLA. Other types of reactions, such as allergic reactions or methaemoglobinaemia, occur in <0.1% of patients.

Intact skin

Blood and Lymphatic System Disorders:	Rare events (< 0.1%)	Methaemoglobinaemia in children (see sections 4.5 and 4.9)
Immune System Disorders:	Rare events (< 0.1%)	In rare cases, local anaesthetic preparations have been associated with allergic reactions (in the most severe instances anaphylactic shock).
Eye Disorders:	Rare events (< 0.1%)	Corneal irritation after accidental eye exposure
General Disorders and Administration Site Conditions:	Common events (>1%)	Transient local reactions at the application site such as paleness, erythema (redness) and oedema.
	Uncommon events (>0.1% and <1%)	Skin sensations (an initial mild burning or itching sensation at the application site).
	Rare events (< 0.1%)	Rare cases of discrete local lesions at the application site, described as purpuric or petechial, have been reported, especially after longer application times in children with atopic dermatitis or mollusca contagiosa

Genital mucosa

Immune System Disorders	Rare events (< 0.1%)	In rare cases, local anaesthetic preparations have been associated with allergic reactions (in the most severe instances anaphylactic shock).
General Disorders and Administration Site Conditions	Common events (>1%)	Application site: Transient local reactions such as erythema (redness), oedema and paleness. Local sensations (an initial, usually mild, burning sensation, itch or warmth at the application site).
	Uncommon events (>0.1% and <1%)	Application site: Local paraesthesia such as tingling.

Paediatric population

In clinical trials 298 neonates and infants aged up to 12 months were treated with EMLA (Table 3). A large number of infants and children aged 1 year and older have been treated with EMLA in clinical trials and in clinical practice since 1984.

Table 3. Number of paediatric patients, up to 12 months old, included in clinical studies with EMLA, by age group

Group	Number of patients
Pre-term neonates	21
Age 0–1 months	148
Age 1–3 months	55
Age 3–12 months	74
Total number	**298**

Frequency, type and severity of adverse reactions are similar in the paediatric and adult age groups, except for methaemoglobinaemia, which is more frequently observed, often in connection with overdose, in neonates and infants aged 0 to 12 months.

Rare cases of clinically significant methaemoglobinaemia in children have been reported in literature. Prilocaine, one of the components of EMLA, may in high doses cause an increase in the methaemoglobin level, particularly in susceptible individuals (Section 4.4) and in conjunction with other methaemoglobin-inducing agents. Clinically significant methaemoglobinaemia should be treated with a slow intravenous injection of methylthioninium chloride (Section 4.9).

4.9 Overdose

Rare cases of clinically significant methaemoglobinaemia have been reported in children. Prilocaine in high doses may cause an increase in the methaemoglobin level particularly in conjunction with methaemoglobin-inducing agents (e.g. sulphonamides). Clinically significant methaemoglobinaemia should be treated with a slow intravenous injection of methylthioninium chloride.

Should other symptoms of systemic toxicity occur, the signs are anticipated to be similar in nature to those following the administration of local anaesthetics by other routes. Local anaesthetic toxicity is manifested by symptoms of nervous system excitation and, in severe cases, central nervous and cardiovascular depression.

Severe neurological symptoms (convulsions, CNS depression) must be treated symptomatically by respiratory support and the administration of anticonvulsive drugs.

5. PHARMACOLOGICAL PROPERTIES

5.1 Pharmacodynamic properties

Pharmacotherapeutic group: Local anaesthetics

ATC Code: N01B B20

EMLA Cream provides dermal analgesia. The depth of analgesia depends upon the application time and the dose. EMLA causes transient local peripheral vasoconstriction or vasodilation at the treated area.

In patients with atopic dermatitis, a similar but shorter vascular reaction is seen, with erythema occurring after 30-60 minutes, indicating more rapid absorption through the skin (see section 4.5 Special precautions and special warnings for use).

Paediatric population

Clinical safety studies

Methaemoglobin formation after the use of EMLA in term infants was studied with the aim to establish the safety of 1 g EMLA Cream 5%. Forty-seven neonates and infants, aged 0-3 months, with a post conceptual age of ⩾37 weeks were included in a double blind, randomized, placebo-controlled study. Methaemoglobin concentrations before treatment with EMLA and placebo were in the range 0.67-1.57% and 0.50-1.53%, respectively. After treatment with 1 g EMLA/placebo for 60-70 min methaemoglobin concentrations were 0.50-2.53% for EMLA and 0.50-1.53% for placebo. From 3.5 to 13 h after application the concentrations were significantly higher with EMLA than with placebo, but were clinically insignificant. One sample, in the EMLA group (2.53%), had a methaemoglobin concentration above the reference value of 2%.

Altogether, data from eleven clinical studies in neonates and infants showed that peak methaemoglobin concentrations occur about 8 hours after epicutaneous EMLA administration, are clinically insignificant with recommended dosage, and return to normal values after about 12-13 hours. Methaemoglobin formation is related to the cumulative amount of prilocaine percutaneously absorbed, and may therefore increase with prolonged application times of EMLA.

Physiological methaemoglobin concentrations in both paediatric patients and adults are normally maintained below 2%. A major increase in methaemoglobin (to a concentration of 25-30%) will cause signs and symptoms of hypoxaemia. In neonates elevated methaemoglobin levels up to 5–6% are not regarded as clinically significant.

Circumcision

In two randomized, double-blind, placebo-controlled studies in full-term neonates aged 1 to 4 days EMLA Cream (0.5 or 1 g) was applied on the prepuce for one hour before circumcision, covered with an occlusive dressing. In the study using 0.5 g EMLA there was no significant differences with placebo in assessment of pain performed by evaluating facial expressions or heart rate, respiratory rate, oxygen saturation, nor in general skin colour.

EMLA Cream (1 g) significantly reduced the pain during parts of the circumcision procedure, as demonstrated by less facial activity, reduction in duration of cry and lower heart rates. No differences were found for oxygen saturation, respiratory rate and Neonatal Infant Pain Scale (NIPS) – which includes facial expression, cry, breathing pattern and state of arousal.

Vaccination

Two randomized double-blind, placebo-controlled studies in infants and neonates looked at anaesthetic efficacy of EMLA Cream in vaccinations and the effect on the immunogenicity of live vaccines.

The first study used EMLA Cream prior to subcutaneous measles-mumps-rubella vaccine, in patients aged 12-15 months, where 1g of cream was applied for 60-180 minutes. EMLA significantly reduced vaccination pain versus placebo, demonstrated by difference between the pre- and post-vaccination total score on the Modified Behavioural Pain Scale (MBPS - includes measurement of facial expression, cry and body movement). No difference versus placebo was seen with the separate assessment of proportion of patients that cry and duration of cry.

The second used EMLA Cream prior to intramuscular diptheria-pertussis-tetanus-inactivated poliovirus-*Haemophilus influenzae b* or Hepatitis B vaccines in patients aged 0-6 months, where 1 or 2g of cream was applied to patients aged 0-4 and 6 months respectively, for 60-180 minutes. EMLA significantly reduced vaccination pain versus placebo, demonstrated as above, for the 6 month-old group, however in the 0-4 month old group there was high variation in treatment response. In the 2 and 4 month-old groups, EMLA gave reduced pain versus placebo, however statistical significance was not shown (p=0.120 and 0.225 respectively).

Within both studies, the use of EMLA did not affect mean antibody titres, rate of seroconversion, or the proportion of patients achieving protective or positive antibody titres post immunization, as compared to placebo treated patients.

5.2 Pharmacokinetic properties

Systemic absorption of lidocaine and prilocaine from EMLA Cream is dependent upon the dose, application time, and the thickness of the skin, which varies between different areas of the body.

Intact skin: In order to provide reliable dermal analgesia, EMLA Cream should be applied under an occlusive dressing for at least 1 hour. The duration of analgesia after an application time of 1-2 hours is at least 2 hours after removal of the dressing.

After the application of EMLA Cream to intact male genital skin for 15 minutes (median 1g), plasma concentrations of lidocaine and prilocaine (mean 6.6 nanogram/ml and 4.1 nanogram/ml) were reached after approximately 1.5 hours.

After application to the thigh in adults (60 g cream/400 cm^2 for 3 hours) the extent of absorption was approximately 5% of lidocaine and prilocaine. Maximum plasma concentrations (mean 0.12 and 0.07 μg/ml) were reached approximately 2-6 hours after the application.

The extent of systemic absorption was approximately 10% following application to the face (10 g/100 cm^2 for 2 hours). Maximum plasma levels (mean 0.16 and 0.06 μg/ml) were reached after approximately 1.5-3 hours.

Genital mucosa: Absorption from the genital mucosa is more rapid than after application to the skin. After the application of 10 g EMLA Cream for 10 minutes to vaginal mucosa maximum plasma concentrations of lidocaine and prilocaine (mean 0.18 micrograms/ml and 0.15 micrograms/ml respectively) were reached after 20-45 minutes.

Paediatric population

Following the application of 1 g EMLA Cream in infants/neonates below 3 months of age, to approx 10 cm^2 for one hour, the maximum plasma concentrations of lidocaine and prilocaine were 0.135 micrograms/ml and 0.107 micrograms/ml respectively.

Following the application of 2 g EMLA Cream in infants between 3 and 12 months of age, to approx 16 cm^2 for four hours, the maximum plasma concentrations of lidocaine and prilocaine were 0.155 micrograms/ml and 0.131 micrograms/ml respectively.

Following the application of 10 g of EMLA Cream in children between 2 and 3 years of age, to approx 100 cm^2 for two hours, the maximum plasma concentrations of lidocaine and prilocaine were 0.315 micrograms/ml and 0.215 micrograms/ml respectively.

Following the application of 10-16 g EMLA Cream in children between 6 and 8 years of age, to approx 100-160 cm^2 for two hours, the maximum plasma concentrations of lidocaine and prilocaine were 0.299 micrograms/ml and 0.110 micrograms/ml respectively.

5.3 Preclinical safety data

Lidocaine and prilocaine are well established active ingredients.

6. PHARMACEUTICAL PARTICULARS

6.1 List of excipients

Polyoxyethylene hydrogenated castor oil, Carbomer 974P, sodium hydroxide and water purified.

6.2 Incompatibilities

None known.

6.3 Shelf life

3 years.

6.4 Special precautions for storage

Do not store above 30°C, do not freeze.

6.5 Nature and contents of container

"Pre-medication pack" containing 5 × 5 g tubes EMLA and 12 occlusive dressings.

Pack containing 1 × 5 g tube of EMLA and 2 occlusive dressings.

1 × 30 g tube with enclosed spatula

1 × 5 g tube

6.6 Special precautions for disposal and other handling

Not applicable.

7. MARKETING AUTHORISATION HOLDER

AstraZeneca UK Limited

600 Capability Green

Luton

LU1 3LU, UK

8. MARKETING AUTHORISATION NUMBER(S)

PL 17901/0120

9. DATE OF FIRST AUTHORISATION/RENEWAL OF THE AUTHORISATION

16th May 1996

10. DATE OF REVISION OF THE TEXT

19th November 2008

Emtriva 10 mg/ml oral solution

(Gilead Sciences Ltd)

1. NAME OF THE MEDICINAL PRODUCT

Emtriva 10 mg/ml oral solution

2. QUALITATIVE AND QUANTITATIVE COMPOSITION

Each ml of Emtriva oral solution contains 10 mg emtricitabine.

Excipient(s):

Each dose (24 ml) contains 36 mg methyl parahydroxybenzoate (E218), 3.6 mg propyl parahydroxybenzoate (E216), 1.2 mg Sunset Yellow (E110) and has a sodium content of 254 mg. For a full list of excipients, see section 6.1.

3. PHARMACEUTICAL FORM

Oral solution.

The clear solution is orange to dark orange in colour.

4. CLINICAL PARTICULARS

4.1 Therapeutic indications

Emtriva is indicated for the treatment of HIV-1 infected adults and children in combination with other antiretroviral agents.

This indication is based on studies in treatment-naïve patients and treatment-experienced patients with stable virological control. There is no experience of the use of Emtriva in patients who are failing their current regimen or who have failed multiple regimens (see section 5.1).

When deciding on a new regimen for patients who have failed an antiretroviral regimen, careful consideration should be given to the patterns of mutations associated with different medicinal products and the treatment history of the individual patient. Where available, resistance testing may be appropriate.

4.2 Posology and method of administration

Therapy should be initiated by a physician experienced in the management of HIV infection.

Emtriva 10 mg/ml oral solution may be taken with or without food. A measuring cup is provided (see section 6.5).

Adults: The recommended dose of Emtriva 10 mg/ml oral solution is 240 mg (24 ml) once daily.

Infants, children and adolescents up to 18 years of age: The recommended dose of Emtriva 10 mg/ml oral solution is 6 mg/kg up to a maximum of 240 mg (24 ml) once daily.

Children who weigh at least 33 kg may either take one 200 mg hard capsule daily or may take emtricitabine as the oral solution up to a maximum of 240 mg once daily.

There are no data regarding the efficacy and only very limited data regarding the safety of emtricitabine in infants below 4 months of age. Therefore Emtriva is not recommended for use in those aged less than 4 months. (For pharmacokinetic data in this age group, see section 5.2).

Emtriva 200 mg hard capsules are available for adults, adolescents and children who weigh at least 33 kg and can swallow hard capsules. Please refer to the Summary of Product Characteristics for Emtriva 200 mg hard capsules. Due to a difference in the bioavailability of emtricitabine between the hard capsule and oral solution presentations, 240 mg emtricitabine administered as the oral solution (24 ml) should provide similar plasma levels to those observed after administration of one 200 mg emtricitabine hard capsule (see section 5.2).

Elderly: There are no safety and efficacy data available in patients over the age of 65 years. However, no adjustment in the recommended daily dose for adults should be required unless there is evidence of renal insufficiency.

Renal insufficiency: Emtricitabine is eliminated by renal excretion and exposure to emtricitabine was significantly increased in patients with renal insufficiency (see section 5.2). Dose or dose interval adjustment is required in all patients with creatinine clearance < 50 ml/min (see section 4.4).

The table below provides daily doses of Emtriva 10 mg/ml oral solution according to the degree of renal insufficiency. The safety and efficacy of these doses have not been clinically evaluated. Therefore, clinical response to treatment and renal function should be closely monitored in these patients (see section 4.4).

Patients with renal insufficiency can also be managed by administration of Emtriva 200 mg hard capsules at modified dose intervals. Please refer to the Summary of Product Characteristics for Emtriva 200 mg hard capsules.

(see Table 1 on next page)

Patients with end-stage renal disease (ESRD) managed with other forms of dialysis such as ambulatory peritoneal dialysis have not been studied and no dose recommendations can be made.

No data are available on which to make a dosage recommendation in paediatric patients with renal insufficiency.

Hepatic insufficiency: No data are available on which to make a dose recommendation for patients with hepatic insufficiency. However, based on the minimal metabolism of emtricitabine and the renal route of elimination it is unlikely that a dose adjustment would be required in patients with hepatic insufficiency (see section 5.2).

If Emtriva is discontinued in patients co-infected with HIV and HBV, these patients should be closely monitored for evidence of exacerbation of hepatitis (see section 4.4).

4.3 Contraindications

Hypersensitivity to the active substance or to any of the excipients.

4.4 Special warnings and precautions for use

Emtriva should not be taken with any other medicinal products containing emtricitabine or medicinal products containing lamivudine.

General: Emtricitabine is not recommended as monotherapy for the treatment of HIV infection. It must be used in combination with other antiretrovirals. Please also refer to the Summaries of Product Characteristics of the other antiretroviral medicinal products used in the combination regimen.

Patients receiving emtricitabine or any other antiretroviral therapy may continue to develop opportunistic infections and other complications of HIV infection, and therefore should remain under close clinical observation by physicians experienced in the treatment of patients with HIV associated diseases.

Patients should be advised that antiretroviral therapies, including emtricitabine, have not been proven to prevent the risk of transmission of HIV to others through sexual contact or blood contamination. Appropriate precautions should continue to be used. Patients should also be informed that emtricitabine is not a cure for HIV infection.

Renal function: Emtricitabine is principally eliminated by the kidney via glomerular filtration and active tubular secretion. Emtricitabine exposure may be markedly increased in patients with moderate or severe renal insufficiency (creatinine clearance < 50 ml/min) receiving daily doses of 200 mg emtricitabine as hard capsules or 240 mg as the oral solution. Consequently, either a dose interval adjustment (using Emtriva 200 mg hard capsules) or a reduction in the daily dose of emtricitabine (using Emtriva 10 mg/ml oral solution) is required in all patients with creatinine clearance < 50 ml/min. The safety and efficacy of the reduced doses provided in section 4.2 are based on single dose pharmacokinetic data and modelling and have not been clinically evaluated. Therefore, clinical response to treatment and renal function should be closely monitored in patients treated with a reduced dose of emtricitabine (see sections 4.2 and 5.2).

Caution should be exercised when emtricitabine is co-administered with medicinal products that are eliminated by active tubular secretion as such co-administration may lead to an increase in serum concentrations of either emtricitabine or a co-administered medicinal product, due to competition for this elimination pathway (see section 4.5).

Lactic acidosis: Lactic acidosis, usually associated with hepatic steatosis, has been reported with the use of nucleoside analogues. Early symptoms (symptomatic hyperlactataemia) include benign digestive symptoms (nausea, vomiting and abdominal pain), non-specific malaise, loss of appetite, weight loss, respiratory symptoms (rapid and/or deep breathing) or neurological symptoms (including motor weakness). Lactic acidosis has a high mortality and may be associated with pancreatitis, liver failure or renal failure. Lactic acidosis generally occurred after a few or several months of treatment.

Treatment with nucleoside analogues should be discontinued in the setting of symptomatic hyperlactataemia and metabolic/lactic acidosis, progressive hepatomegaly, or rapidly elevating aminotransferase levels.

Caution should be exercised when administering nucleoside analogues to any patient (particularly obese women) with hepatomegaly, hepatitis or other known risk factors for liver disease and hepatic steatosis (including certain medicinal products and alcohol). Patients co-infected with hepatitis C and treated with alpha interferon and ribavirin may constitute a special risk.

Patients at increased risk should be followed closely.

Table 1

	Creatinine Clearance (CL_{cr}) (ml/min)			
	≥ 50	30-49	15-29	< 15 (functionally anephric, requiring intermittent haemodialysis)*
Recommended dose of Emtriva 10 mg/ml oral solution every 24 hours	240 mg (24 ml)	120 mg (12 ml)	80 mg (8 ml)	60 mg (6 ml)

* Assumes a 3 h haemodialysis session three times a week commencing at least 12 h after administration of the last dose of emtricitabine.

Lipodystrophy: Combination antiretroviral therapy has been associated with the redistribution of body fat (lipodystrophy) in HIV patients. The long-term consequences of these events are currently unknown. Knowledge about the mechanism is incomplete. A connection between visceral lipomatosis and protease inhibitors, and lipoatrophy and nucleoside reverse transcriptase inhibitors has been hypothesised. A higher risk of lipodystrophy has been associated with individual factors such as older age, and with drug related factors such as longer duration of antiretroviral treatment and associated metabolic disturbances. Clinical examination should include evaluation for physical signs of fat redistribution. Consideration should be given to the measurement of fasting serum lipids and blood glucose. Lipid disorders should be managed as clinically appropriate.

Liver function: Patients with pre-existing liver dysfunction including chronic active hepatitis have an increased frequency of liver function abnormalities during combination antiretroviral therapy and should be monitored according to standard practice. Patients with chronic hepatitis B or C infection treated with combination antiretroviral therapy are at increased risk of experiencing severe, and potentially fatal, hepatic adverse events. In case of concomitant antiviral therapy for hepatitis B or C, please also refer to the relevant Summary of Product Characteristics for these medicinal products.

If there is evidence of exacerbations of liver disease in such patients, interruption or discontinuation of treatment must be considered.

Patients co-infected with hepatitis B virus (HBV): Emtricitabine is active *in vitro* against HBV. However, limited data are available on the efficacy and safety of emtricitabine (as a 200 mg hard capsule once daily) in patients who are co-infected with HIV and HBV. The use of emtricitabine in patient with chronic HBV induces the same mutation pattern in the YMDD motif observed with lamivudine therapy. The YMDD mutation confers resistance to both emtricitabine and lamivudine.

Patients co-infected with HIV and HBV should be closely monitored with both clinical and laboratory follow-up for at least several months after stopping treatment with emtricitabine for evidence of exacerbations of hepatitis. Such exacerbations have been seen following discontinuation of emtricitabine treatment in HBV infected patients without concomitant HIV infection and have been detected primarily by serum alanine aminotransferase (ALT) elevations in addition to re-emergence of HBV DNA. In some of these patients, HBV reactivation was associated with more severe liver disease, including decompensation and liver failure. There is insufficient evidence to determine whether re-initiation of emtricitabine alters the course of post-treatment exacerbations of hepatitis.

Mitochondrial dysfunction: Nucleoside and nucleotide analogues have been demonstrated *in vitro* and *in vivo* to cause a variable degree of mitochondrial damage. There have been reports of mitochondrial dysfunction in HIV negative infants exposed *in utero* and/or postnatally to nucleoside analogues. The main adverse events reported are haematological disorders (anaemia, neutropenia), metabolic disorders (hyperlactataemia, hyperlipasaemia). These events are often transitory. Some late-onset neurological disorders have been reported (hypertonia, convulsion, abnormal behaviour). Whether the neurological disorders are transient or permanent is currently unknown. Any child exposed *in utero* to nucleoside and nucleotide analogues, even HIV negative children, should have clinical and laboratory follow-up and should be fully investigated for possible mitochondrial dysfunction in case of relevant signs or symptoms. These findings do not affect current national recommendations to use antiretroviral therapy in pregnant women to prevent vertical transmission of HIV.

Immune Reactivation Syndrome: In HIV infected patients with severe immune deficiency at the time of institution of combination antiretroviral therapy (CART), an inflammatory reaction to asymptomatic or residual opportunistic pathogens may arise and cause serious clinical conditions, or aggravation of symptoms. Typically, such reactions have been observed within the first few weeks or months of initiation of CART. Relevant examples are cytomegalovirus retinitis, generalised and/or focal mycobacterium infections, and *Pneumocystis carinii* pneumonia. Any inflammatory symptoms should be evaluated and treatment instituted when necessary.

Osteonecrosis: Although the etiology is considered to be multifactorial (including corticosteroid use, alcohol consumption, severe immunosuppression, higher body mass index), cases of osteonecrosis have been reported particularly in patients with advanced HIV-disease and/or long-term exposure to combination antiretroviral therapy (CART). Patients should be advised to seek medical advice if they experience joint aches and pain, joint stiffness or difficulty in movement.

Emtriva oral solution contains Sunset Yellow (E110) which may cause allergic reactions, methyl parahydroxybenzoate (E218) and propyl parahydroxybenzoate (E216) which may cause allergic reactions (possibly delayed). This medicinal product contains 254 mg of sodium per dose which should be taken into consideration by patients on a controlled sodium diet.

4.5 Interaction with other medicinal products and other forms of interaction

In vitro, emtricitabine did not inhibit metabolism mediated by any of the following human CYP450 isoforms: 1A2, 2A6, 2B6, 2C9, 2C19, 2D6 and 3A4. Emtricitabine did not inhibit the enzyme responsible for glucuronidation. Based on the results of these *in vitro* experiments and the known elimination pathways of emtricitabine, the potential for CYP450 mediated interactions involving emtricitabine with other medicinal products is low.

There are no clinically significant interactions when emtricitabine is co-administered with indinavir, zidovudine, stavudine, famciclovir or tenofovir disoproxil fumarate.

Emtricitabine is primarily excreted via glomerular filtration and active tubular secretion. With the exception of famciclovir and tenofovir disoproxil fumarate, the effect of co-administration of emtricitabine with medicinal products that are excreted by the renal route, or other medicinal products known to affect renal function, has not been evaluated. Co-administration of emtricitabine with medicinal products that are eliminated by active tubular secretion may lead to an increase in serum concentrations of either emtricitabine or a co-administered medicinal product due to competition for this elimination pathway.

There is no clinical experience as yet on the co-administration of cytidine analogues. Consequently, the use of emtricitabine in combination with lamivudine or zalcitabine for the treatment of HIV infection cannot be recommended at this time.

4.6 Pregnancy and lactation

The safety of emtricitabine in human pregnancy has not been established.

Animal studies do not indicate direct or indirect harmful effects of emtricitabine with respect to pregnancy, foetal development, parturition or postnatal development (see section 5.3).

Emtricitabine should be used during pregnancy only if necessary.

Given that the potential risks to developing human foetuses are unknown, the use of emtricitabine in women of childbearing potential must be accompanied by the use of effective contraception.

It is not known if emtricitabine is excreted in human milk.

It is recommended that HIV infected women do not breastfeed their infants under any circumstances in order to avoid transmission of HIV.

4.7 Effects on ability to drive and use machines

No studies on the effects on the ability to drive and use machines have been performed. However, patients should be informed that dizziness has been reported during treatment with emtricitabine.

4.8 Undesirable effects

Assessment of adverse reactions is based on data from three studies in adults (n=1,479) and three paediatric studies (n=169). In the adult studies, 1,039 treatment-naïve and 440 treatment-experienced patients received emtricitabine (n=814) or comparator medicinal product (n=665) for 48 weeks in combination with other antiretroviral medicinal products. In three paediatric studies, treatment-naïve (n=123) and treatment-experienced (n=46) paediatric patients aged 4 months to 18 years were treated with emtricitabine in combination with other antiretroviral agents.

The adverse reactions with suspected (at least possible) relationship to treatment in adults are listed below by body system organ class and absolute frequency. Within each frequency grouping, undesirable effects are presented in order of decreasing seriousness. Frequencies are defined as very common (≥ 1/10), common (≥ 1/100, < 1/10) or uncommon (≥ 1/1,000, < 1/100).

Blood and lymphatic system disorders:

Common: neutropenia

Uncommon: anaemia

Metabolism and nutrition disorders:

Common: hypertriglyceridaemia, hyperglycaemia

Lactic acidosis, usually associated with hepatic steatosis, has been reported with the use of nucleoside analogues (see section 4.4).

Psychiatric disorders:

Common: insomnia, abnormal dreams

Nervous system disorders:

Very common: headache

Common: dizziness

Gastrointestinal disorders:

Very common: diarrhoea, nausea

Common: vomiting, abdominal pain, elevated amylase including elevated pancreatic amylase, elevated serum lipase, dyspepsia

Hepatobiliary disorders:

Common: hyperbilirubinaemia, elevated serum aspartate aminotransferase (AST) and/or elevated serum alanine aminotransferase (ALT)

Skin and subcutaneous tissue disorders:

Common: allergic reaction, urticaria, vesiculobullous rash, pustular rash, maculopapular rash, pruritus, rash, and skin discolouration (hyper-pigmentation)

Musculoskeletal and connective tissue disorders:

Very common: elevated creatine kinase

General disorders and administration site conditions:

Common: asthenia, pain

In addition to the adverse reactions reported in adults, anaemia was common and skin discolouration (hyper-pigmentation) was very common in paediatric patients.

The adverse reaction profile in patients co-infected with HBV is similar to that observed in patients infected with HIV without co-infection with HBV. However, as would be expected in this patient population, elevations in AST and ALT occurred more frequently than in the general HIV infected population.

Combination antiretroviral therapy has been associated with metabolic abnormalities such as hypertriglyceridaemia, hypercholesterolaemia, insulin resistance, hyperglycaemia and hyperlactataemia (see section 4.4).

Combination antiretroviral therapy has been associated with redistribution of body fat (lipodystrophy) in HIV patients including the loss of peripheral and facial subcutaneous fat, increased intra-abdominal and visceral fat, breast hypertrophy and dorsocervical fat accumulation (buffalo hump) (see section 4.4).

In HIV infected patients with severe immune deficiency at the time of initiation of combination antiretroviral therapy (CART), an inflammatory reaction to asymptomatic or residual opportunistic infections may arise (see section 4.4).

Cases of osteonecrosis have been reported, particularly in patients with generally acknowledged risk factors, advanced HIV disease or long-term exposure to combination antiretroviral therapy (CART). The frequency of this is unknown (see section 4.4).

4.9 Overdose

Administration of up to 1,200 mg emtricitabine has been associated with the adverse reactions listed above (see section 4.8).

If overdose occurs, the patient should be monitored for signs of toxicity and standard supportive treatment applied as necessary.

Up to 30% of the emtricitabine dose can be removed by haemodialysis. It is not known whether emtricitabine can be removed by peritoneal dialysis.

5. PHARMACOLOGICAL PROPERTIES

5.1 Pharmacodynamic properties

Pharmacotherapeutic group: Nucleoside and nucleotide reverse transcriptase inhibitors, ATC code: J05AF09.

Mechanism of action: Emtricitabine is a synthetic nucleoside analogue of cytidine with activity that is specific to human immunodeficiency virus (HIV-1 and HIV-2) and hepatitis B virus (HBV).

Emtricitabine is phosphorylated by cellular enzymes to form emtricitabine 5'-triphosphate, which competitively inhibits HIV-1 reverse transcriptase, resulting in DNA chain termination. Emtricitabine is a weak inhibitor of mammalian DNA polymerase α, β and ε and mitochondrial DNA polymerase γ.

Emtricitabine did not exhibit cytotoxicity to peripheral blood mononuclear cells (PBMCs), established lymphocyte and monocyte-macrophage cell lines or bone marrow progenitor cells *in vitro*. There was no evidence of toxicity to mitochondria *in vitro* or *in vivo*.

Antiviral activity in vitro: The 50% inhibitory concentration (IC_{50}) value for emtricitabine against laboratory and clinical isolates of HIV-1 was in the range of 0.0013 to 0.5 μmol/l. In combination studies of emtricitabine with protease inhibitors, nucleoside, nucleotide and non-nucleoside analogue inhibitors of HIV reverse transcriptase, additive to synergistic effects were observed. Most of these combinations have not been studied in humans.

When tested for activity against laboratory strains of HBV, the 50% inhibitory concentration (IC_{50}) value for emtricitabine was in the range of 0.01 to 0.04 μmol/l.

Resistance: HIV-1 resistance to emtricitabine develops as the result of changes at codon 184 causing the methionine to be changed to a valine (an isoleucine intermediate has also been observed) of the HIV reverse transcriptase. This HIV-1 mutation was observed *in vitro* and in HIV-1 infected patients.

Emtricitabine-resistant viruses were cross-resistant to lamivudine, but retained sensitivity to other nucleoside reverse transcriptase inhibitors (NRTIs) (zidovudine, stavudine, tenofovir, abacavir, didanosine and zalcitabine), all non-nucleoside reverse transcriptase inhibitors (NNRTIs) and all protease inhibitors (PIs). Viruses resistant to zidovudine, zalcitabine, didanosine and NNRTIs retained their sensitivity to emtricitabine (IC_{50}=0.002 μmol/l to 0.08 μmol/l).

Clinical experience: Emtricitabine in combination with other antiretroviral agents, including nucleoside analogues, non-nucleoside analogues and protease inhibitors, has been shown to be effective in the treatment of HIV infection in treatment-naïve patients and treatment-experienced patients with stable virological control. There is no experience of the use of emtricitabine in patients who are failing their current regimen or who have failed multiple regimens. There is no clinical experience of the use of emtricitabine in infants less than 4 months of age.

In antiretroviral treatment-naïve adults, emtricitabine was significantly superior to stavudine when both medicinal products were taken in combination with didanosine and efavirenz through 48 weeks of treatment. Phenotypic analysis showed no significant changes in emtricitabine susceptibility unless the M184V/I mutation had developed.

In virologically stable treatment-experienced adults, emtricitabine, in combination with an NRTI (either stavudine or zidovudine) and a protease inhibitor (PI) or an NNRTI was shown to be non-inferior to lamivudine with respect to the proportion of responders (< 400 copies/ml) through 48 weeks (77% emtricitabine, 82% lamivudine). Additionally, in a second study, treatment-experienced adults on a stable PI based highly active antiretroviral therapy (HAART) regimen were randomised to a once daily regimen containing emtricitabine or to continue with their PI-HAART regimen. At 48 weeks of treatment the emtricitabine-containing regimen demonstrated an equivalent proportion of patients with HIV RNA < 400 copies/ml (94% emtricitabine *versus* 92%) and a greater proportion of patients with HIV RNA < 50 copies/ml (95% emtricitabine *versus* 87%) compared with the patients continuing with their PI-HAART regimen.

In infants and children older than 4 months, the majority of patients achieved or maintained complete suppression of plasma HIV-1 RNA through 48 weeks (89% achieved ⩽ 400 copies/ml and 77% achieved ⩽ 50 copies/ml).

5.2 Pharmacokinetic properties

Absorption: Emtricitabine is rapidly and extensively absorbed following oral administration with peak plasma concentrations occurring at 1 to 2 hours post-dose. In 20 HIV infected subjects receiving 200 mg emtricitabine daily as hard capsules, steady-state plasma emtricitabine peak concentrations (C_{max}), trough concentrations (C_{min}) and area under the plasma concentration time curve over a 24-hour dosing interval (AUC) were 1.8±0.7 μg/ml, 0.09±0.07 μg/ml and 10.0±3.1 μg·h/ml, respectively. Steady-state trough plasma concentrations reached levels approximately 4-fold above the *in vitro* IC_{90} values for anti-HIV activity.

The absolute bioavailability of emtricitabine from Emtriva 200 mg hard capsules was estimated to be 93% and the absolute bioavailability from Emtriva 10 mg/ml oral solution was estimated to be 75%.

In a pilot study in children and a definitive bioequivalence study in adults, the Emtriva 10 mg/ml oral solution was shown to have approximately 80% of the bioavailability of the Emtriva 200 mg hard capsules. The reason for this difference is unknown. Due to this difference in bioavailability, 240 mg emtricitabine administered as the oral solution should provide similar plasma levels to those observed after administration of one 200 mg emtricitabine hard capsule. Therefore, children who weigh at least 33 kg may take either one 200 mg hard capsule daily or the oral solution up to a maximum dose of 240 mg (24 ml), once daily.

Administration of Emtriva 200 mg hard capsules with a high-fat meal or administration of Emtriva 10 mg/ml oral solution with a low-fat or high-fat meal did not affect systemic exposure ($AUC_{0-\infty}$) of emtricitabine; therefore Emtriva 200 mg hard capsules and Emtriva 10 mg/ml oral solution may be administered with or without food.

Distribution: In vitro binding of emtricitabine to human plasma proteins was < 4% and independent of concentration over the range of 0.02-200 μg/ml. The mean plasma to blood concentration ratio was approximately 1.0 and the mean semen to plasma concentration ratio was approximately 4.0.

The apparent volume of distribution after intravenous administration of emtricitabine was 1.4±0.3 l/kg, indicating that emtricitabine is widely distributed throughout the body to both intracellular and extracellular fluid spaces.

Biotransformation: There is limited metabolism of emtricitabine. The biotransformation of emtricitabine includes oxidation of the thiol moiety to form the 3'-sulphoxide diastereomers (approximately 9% of dose) and conjugation with glucuronic acid to form 2'-O-glucuronide (approximately 4% of dose).

Emtricitabine did not inhibit *in vitro* drug metabolism mediated by the following human CYP450 isoenzymes: 1A2, 2A6, 2B6, 2C9, 2C19, 2D6 and 3A4.

Also, emtricitabine did not inhibit uridine-5'-diphosphoglucuronyl transferase, the enzyme responsible for glucuronidation.

Elimination: Emtricitabine is primarily excreted by the kidneys with complete recovery of the dose achieved in urine (approximately 86%) and faeces (approximately 14%). Thirteen percent of the emtricitabine dose was recovered in urine as three metabolites. The systemic clearance of emtricitabine averaged 307 ml/min (4.03 ml/min/kg). Following oral administration, the elimination half-life of emtricitabine is approximately 10 hours.

Linearity/non-linearity: The pharmacokinetics of emtricitabine are proportional to dose over the dose range of 25-200 mg following single or repeated administration.

Intracellular pharmacokinetics: In a clinical study, the intracellular half-life of emtricitabine-triphosphate in peripheral blood mononuclear cells was 39 hours. Intracellular triphosphate levels increased with dose, but reached a plateau at doses of 200 mg or greater.

Adults with renal insufficiency: Pharmacokinetic parameters were determined following administration of a single dose of 200 mg emtricitabine hard capsules to 30 non-HIV infected subjects with varying degrees of renal insufficiency. Subjects were grouped according to baseline creatinine clearance (> 80 ml/min as normal function; 50-80 ml/min as mild impairment; 30-49 ml/min as moderate impairment; < 30 ml/min as severe impairment; < 15 ml/min as functionally anephric requiring haemodialysis).

The systemic emtricitabine exposure (mean ± standard deviation) increased from 11.8±2.9 μg·h/ml in subjects with normal renal function to 19.9±1.1, 25.0±5.7 and 34.0±2.1 μg·h/ml, in patients with mild, moderate and severe renal impairment, respectively.

In patients with ESRD on haemodialysis, approximately 30% of the emtricitabine dose was recovered in dialysate over a 3 hour dialysis period which had been started within 1.5 hours of emtricitabine dosing (blood flow rate of 400 ml/min and dialysate flow rate of approximately 600 ml/min).

Hepatic insufficiency: The pharmacokinetics of emtricitabine have not been studied in non-HBV infected subjects with varying degrees of hepatic insufficiency. In general, emtricitabine pharmacokinetics in HBV infected subjects were similar to those in healthy subjects and in HIV infected subjects.

Age, gender and ethnicity: In general, the pharmacokinetics of emtricitabine in infants, children and adolescents (aged 4 months up to 18 years) are similar to those seen in adults.

The mean AUC in 77 infants, children and adolescents receiving 6 mg/kg emtricitabine once daily as oral solution or 200 mg emtricitabine as hard capsules once daily was similar to the mean AUC of 10.0 μg·h/ml in 20 adults receiving 200 mg hard capsules once daily.

In an open-label, non-comparative study, pharmacokinetic data were obtained from 20 neonates of HIV infected mothers who received two 4-day courses of emtricitabine oral solution between the first week of life and 3 months of age at a dose level of 3 mg/kg once daily. This dose is half of that approved for infants aged 4 months and over (6 mg/kg). The apparent total body clearance at steady state (CL/F) increased with age over the 3-month period with a corresponding decrease in AUC. Plasma emtricitabine exposure (AUC) in infants up to 3 months of age who received 3 mg/kg emtricitabine once daily was similar to that observed using 6 mg/kg daily doses in HIV infected adults and children aged 4 months and over.

Pharmacokinetic data are not available in the elderly.

Although the mean C_{max} and C_{min} were approximately 20% higher and mean AUC was 16% higher in females compared to males, this difference was not considered clinically significant. No clinically important pharmacokinetic difference due to race has been identified.

5.3 Preclinical safety data

Non-clinical data reveal no special hazard for humans based on conventional studies of safety pharmacology, repeated dose toxicity, genotoxicity and reproductive/developmental toxicity. Emtricitabine did not show any carcinogenic potential in long-term oral carcinogenicity studies in mice and rats.

6. PHARMACEUTICAL PARTICULARS

6.1 List of excipients

Cotton candy flavouring

Disodium edetate

Hydrochloric acid

Methyl parahydroxybenzoate (E218)

Propylene glycol

Propyl parahydroxybenzoate (E216)

Sodium hydroxide

Sodium phosphate monobasic hydrate

Sunset yellow (E110)

Purified water

Xylitol (E967)

6.2 Incompatibilities

Not applicable.

6.3 Shelf life

3 years.

After first opening: 45 days.

6.4 Special precautions for storage

Store in a refrigerator (2°C – 8°C).

After opening: Do not store above 25°C.

6.5 Nature and contents of container

Amber-coloured polyethylene terephthalate (PET) bottle with a child-resistant closure. The pack also contains a 30 ml polypropylene measuring cup with 1.0 ml graduations. The bottle contains 170 ml of solution.

6.6 Special precautions for disposal and other handling

Patients should be instructed that any solution left in the bottle 45 days after opening should be discarded according to local requirements or returned to the pharmacy.

7. MARKETING AUTHORISATION HOLDER

Gilead Sciences International Limited

Cambridge

CB21 6GT

United Kingdom

8. MARKETING AUTHORISATION NUMBER(S)

EU/1/03/261/003

9. DATE OF FIRST AUTHORISATION/RENEWAL OF THE AUTHORISATION

Date of first authorisation: 24 October 2003

Date of last renewal: 22 September 2008

10. DATE OF REVISION OF THE TEXT

09/2008

Detailed information on this medicinal product is available on the website of the European Medicines Agency (EMEA) http://www.emea.europa.eu/.

Emtriva 200 mg hard capsules

(Gilead Sciences Ltd)

1. NAME OF THE MEDICINAL PRODUCT

Emtriva 200 mg hard capsules

2. QUALITATIVE AND QUANTITATIVE COMPOSITION

Each hard capsule contains 200 mg emtricitabine.

For a full list of excipients, see section 6.1.

3. PHARMACEUTICAL FORM

Hard capsule.

Each capsule has a white opaque body with a light blue opaque cap. Each capsule is printed with "200 mg" on the cap and "GILEAD" and [Gilead logo] on the body in black ink.

4. CLINICAL PARTICULARS

4.1 Therapeutic indications

Emtriva is indicated for the treatment of HIV-1 infected adults and children in combination with other antiretroviral agents.

This indication is based on studies in treatment-naïve patients and treatment-experienced patients with stable virological control. There is no experience of the use of Emtriva in patients who are failing their current regimen or who have failed multiple regimens (see section 5.1).

When deciding on a new regimen for patients who have failed an antiretroviral regimen, careful consideration should be given to the patterns of mutations associated with different medicinal products and the treatment history of the individual patient. Where available, resistance testing may be appropriate.

4.2 Posology and method of administration

Therapy should be initiated by a physician experienced in the management of HIV infection.

Emtriva 200 mg hard capsules may be taken with or without food.

Adults: The recommended dose of Emtriva is one 200 mg hard capsule, taken orally, once daily.

Children and adolescents up to 18 years of age: The recommended dose of Emtriva for children and adolescents weighing at least 33 kg who are able to swallow hard capsules is one 200 mg hard capsule, taken orally, once daily.

There are no data regarding the efficacy and only very limited data regarding the safety of emtricitabine in infants below 4 months of age. Therefore Emtriva is not recommended for use in those aged less than 4 months. (For pharmacokinetic data in this age group, see section 5.2).

Emtriva is also available as a 10 mg/ml oral solution for use in infants older than 4 months of age, children and patients who are unable to swallow hard capsules and patients with renal insufficiency. Please refer to the Summary of Product Characteristics for Emtriva 10 mg/ml oral solution. Due to a difference in the bioavailability of emtricitabine between the hard capsule and oral solution presentations, 240 mg emtricitabine administered as the oral solution should provide similar plasma levels to those observed after administration of one 200 mg emtricitabine hard capsule (see section 5.2).

Elderly: There are no safety and efficacy data available in patients over the age of 65 years. However, no adjustment in the recommended daily dose for adults should be required unless there is evidence of renal insufficiency.

Renal insufficiency: Emtricitabine is eliminated by renal excretion and exposure to emtricitabine was significantly increased in patients with renal insufficiency (see section 5.2). Dose or dose interval adjustment is required in all patients with creatinine clearance < 50 ml/min (see section 4.4).

The table below provides dose interval adjustment guidelines for the 200 mg hard capsules according to the degree of renal insufficiency. The safety and efficacy of these dose interval adjustment guidelines have not been clinically evaluated. Therefore, clinical response to treatment and renal function should be closely monitored in these patients (see section 4.4).

Patients with renal insufficiency can also be managed by administration of Emtriva 10 mg/ml oral solution to provide a reduced daily dose of emtricitabine. Please refer to the Summary of Product Characteristics for Emtriva 10 mg/ml oral solution.

(see Table 1 below)

Patients with end-stage renal disease (ESRD) managed with other forms of dialysis such as ambulatory peritoneal dialysis have not been studied and no dose recommendations can be made.

No data are available on which to make a dosage recommendation in paediatric patients with renal insufficiency.

Hepatic insufficiency: No data are available on which to make a dose recommendation for patients with hepatic insufficiency. However, based on the minimal metabolism of emtricitabine and the renal route of elimination it is unlikely that a dose adjustment would be required in patients with hepatic insufficiency (see section 5.2).

If Emtriva is discontinued in patients co-infected with HIV and HBV, these patients should be closely monitored for evidence of exacerbation of hepatitis (see section 4.4).

4.3 Contraindications

Hypersensitivity to the active substance or to any of the excipients.

4.4 Special warnings and precautions for use

Emtriva should not be taken with any other medicinal products containing emtricitabine or medicinal products containing lamivudine.

General: Emtricitabine is not recommended as monotherapy for the treatment of HIV infection. It must be used in combination with other antiretrovirals. Please also refer to the Summaries of Product Characteristics of the other antiretroviral medicinal products used in the combination regimen.

Patients receiving emtricitabine or any other antiretroviral therapy may continue to develop opportunistic infections and other complications of HIV infection, and therefore should remain under close clinical observation by physicians experienced in the treatment of patients with HIV associated diseases.

Patients should be advised that antiretroviral therapies, including emtricitabine, have not been proven to prevent the risk of transmission of HIV to others through sexual contact or blood contamination. Appropriate precautions should continue to be used. Patients should also be informed that emtricitabine is not a cure for HIV infection.

Renal function: Emtricitabine is principally eliminated by the kidney via glomerular filtration and active tubular secretion. Emtricitabine exposure may be markedly increased in patients with moderate or severe renal insufficiency (creatinine clearance < 50 ml/min) receiving daily doses of 200 mg emtricitabine as hard capsules or 240 mg as the oral solution. Consequently, either a dose interval adjustment (using Emtriva 200 mg hard capsules) or a reduction in the daily dose of emtricitabine (using Emtriva 10 mg/ml oral solution) is required in all patients with creatinine clearance < 50 ml/min. The safety and efficacy of the dose interval adjustment guidelines provided in section 4.2 are based on single dose pharmacokinetic data and modelling and have not been clinically evaluated. Therefore, clinical response to treatment and renal function should be closely monitored in patients treated with emtricitabine at prolonged dosing intervals (see sections 4.2 and 5.2).

Caution should be exercised when emtricitabine is co-administered with medicinal products that are eliminated by active tubular secretion as such co-administration may lead to an increase in serum concentrations of either emtricitabine or a co-administered medicinal product, due to competition for this elimination pathway (see section 4.5).

Lactic acidosis: Lactic acidosis, usually associated with hepatic steatosis, has been reported with the use of nucleoside analogues. Early symptoms (symptomatic hyperlactataemia) include benign digestive symptoms (nausea, vomiting and abdominal pain), non-specific malaise, loss of appetite, weight loss, respiratory symptoms (rapid and/or deep breathing) or neurological symptoms (including motor weakness). Lactic acidosis has a high mortality and may be associated with pancreatitis, liver failure or renal failure. Lactic acidosis generally occurred after a few or several months of treatment.

Treatment with nucleoside analogues should be discontinued in the setting of symptomatic hyperlactataemia and metabolic/lactic acidosis, progressive hepatomegaly, or rapidly elevating aminotransferase levels.

Caution should be exercised when administering nucleoside analogues to any patient (particularly obese women) with hepatomegaly, hepatitis or other known risk factors for liver disease and hepatic steatosis (including certain medicinal products and alcohol). Patients co-infected with hepatitis C and treated with alpha interferon and ribavirin may constitute a special risk.

Patients at increased risk should be followed closely.

Lipodystrophy: Combination antiretroviral therapy has been associated with the redistribution of body fat (lipodystrophy) in HIV patients. The long-term consequences of these events are currently unknown. Knowledge about the mechanism is incomplete. A connection between visceral lipomatosis and protease inhibitors, and lipoatrophy and nucleoside reverse transcriptase inhibitors has been hypothesised. A higher risk of lipodystrophy has been associated with individual factors such as older age, and with drug related factors such as longer duration of antiretroviral treatment and associated metabolic disturbances. Clinical examination should include evaluation for physical signs of fat redistribution. Consideration should be given to the measurement of fasting serum lipids and blood glucose. Lipid disorders should be managed as clinically appropriate.

Liver function: Patients with pre-existing liver dysfunction including chronic active hepatitis have an increased frequency of liver function abnormalities during combination antiretroviral therapy and should be monitored according to standard practice. Patients with chronic hepatitis B or C infection treated with combination antiretroviral therapy are at increased risk of experiencing severe, and potentially fatal, hepatic adverse events. In case of concomitant antiviral therapy for hepatitis B or C, please also refer to the relevant Summary of Product Characteristics for these medicinal products.

If there is evidence of exacerbations of liver disease in such patients, interruption or discontinuation of treatment must be considered.

Patients co-infected with hepatitis B virus (HBV): Emtricitabine is active *in vitro* against HBV. However, limited data are available on the efficacy and safety of emtricitabine (as a 200 mg hard capsule once daily) in patients who are co-infected with HIV and HBV. The use of emtricitabine in patient with chronic HBV induces the same mutation pattern in the YMDD motif observed with lamivudine therapy. The YMDD mutation confers resistance to both emtricitabine and lamivudine.

Patients co-infected with HIV and HBV should be closely monitored with both clinical and laboratory follow-up for at least several months after stopping treatment with emtricitabine for evidence of exacerbations of hepatitis. Such exacerbations have been seen following discontinuation of emtricitabine treatment in HBV infected patients without concomitant HIV infection and have been detected primarily by serum alanine aminotransferase (ALT) elevations in addition to re-emergence of HBV DNA. In some of these patients, HBV reactivation was associated with more severe liver disease, including decompensation and liver failure. There is insufficient evidence to determine whether re-initiation of emtricitabine alters the course of post-treatment exacerbations of hepatitis.

Mitochondrial dysfunction: Nucleoside and nucleotide analogues have been demonstrated *in vitro* and *in vivo* to cause a variable degree of mitochondrial damage. There have been reports of mitochondrial dysfunction in HIV negative infants exposed *in utero* and/or postnatally to nucleoside analogues. The main adverse events reported are haematological disorders (anaemia, neutropenia), metabolic disorders (hyperlactataemia, hyperlipasaemia). These events are often transitory. Some late-onset neurological disorders have been reported (hypertonia, convulsion, abnormal behaviour). Whether the neurological disorders are transient or permanent is currently unknown. Any child exposed *in utero* to nucleoside and nucleotide analogues, even HIV negative children, should have clinical and laboratory follow-up and should be fully investigated for possible mitochondrial dysfunction in case of relevant signs or symptoms. These findings do not affect current national recommendations to use antiretroviral therapy in pregnant women to prevent vertical transmission of HIV.

Immune Reactivation Syndrome: In HIV infected patients with severe immune deficiency at the time of institution of combination antiretroviral therapy (CART), an inflammatory reaction to asymptomatic or residual opportunistic pathogens may arise and cause serious clinical conditions, or aggravation of symptoms. Typically, such reactions have been observed within the first few weeks or months of initiation of CART. Relevant examples are cytomegalovirus retinitis, generalised and/or focal mycobacterium infections, and *Pneumocystis carinii* pneumonia. Any inflammatory symptoms should be evaluated and treatment instituted when necessary.

Osteonecrosis: Although the etiology is considered to be multifactorial (including corticosteroid use, alcohol consumption, severe immunosuppression, higher body mass index), cases of osteonecrosis have been reported particularly in patients with advanced HIV-disease and/or long-term exposure to combination antiretroviral therapy (CART). Patients should be advised to seek medical advice if they experience joint aches and pain, joint stiffness or difficulty in movement.

4.5 Interaction with other medicinal products and other forms of interaction

In vitro, emtricitabine did not inhibit metabolism mediated by any of the following human CYP450 isoforms: 1A2, 2A6, 2B6, 2C9, 2C19, 2D6 and 3A4. Emtricitabine did not inhibit the enzyme responsible for glucuronidation. Based on the results of these *in vitro* experiments and the known elimination pathways of emtricitabine, the potential for CYP450 mediated interactions involving emtricitabine with other medicinal products is low.

There are no clinically significant interactions when emtricitabine is co-administered with indinavir, zidovudine, stavudine, famciclovir or tenofovir disoproxil fumarate.

Emtricitabine is primarily excreted via glomerular filtration and active tubular secretion. With the exception of famciclovir and tenofovir disoproxil fumarate, the effect of co-administration of emtricitabine with medicinal products that are excreted by the renal route, or other medicinal products known to affect renal function, has not been evaluated. Co-administration of emtricitabine with medicinal products that are eliminated by active tubular secretion may lead to an increase in serum concentrations of either emtricitabine or a co-administered medicinal product due to competition for this elimination pathway.

There is no clinical experience as yet on the co-administration of cytidine analogues. Consequently, the use of emtricitabine in combination with lamivudine or zalcitabine for the treatment of HIV infection cannot be recommended at this time.

4.6 Pregnancy and lactation

The safety of emtricitabine in human pregnancy has not been established.

Animal studies do not indicate direct or indirect harmful effects of emtricitabine with respect to pregnancy, foetal development, parturition or postnatal development (see section 5.3).

Emtricitabine should be used during pregnancy only if necessary.

Given that the potential risks to developing human foetuses are unknown, the use of emtricitabine in women of child-bearing potential must be accompanied by the use of effective contraception.

It is not known if emtricitabine is excreted in human milk.

It is recommended that HIV infected women do not breast-feed their infants under any circumstances in order to avoid transmission of HIV.

4.7 Effects on ability to drive and use machines

No studies on the effects on the ability to drive and use machines have been performed. However, patients should be informed that dizziness has been reported during treatment with emtricitabine.

4.8 Undesirable effects

Assessment of adverse reactions is based on data from three studies in adults (n=1,479) and three paediatric studies (n=169). In the adult studies, 1,039 treatment-naïve and 440 treatment-experienced patients received

Table 1

	Creatinine Clearance (CL_{cr}) (ml/min)			
	⩾ 50	**30-49**	**15-29**	**< 15 (functionally anephric, requiring intermittent haemodialysis) ***
Recommended dose interval for 200 mg hard capsules	One 200 mg hard capsule every 24 hours	One 200 mg hard capsule every 48 hours	One 200 mg hard capsule every 72 hours	One 200 mg hard capsule every 96 hours

* Assumes a 3 h haemodialysis session three times a week commencing at least 12 h after administration of the last dose of emtricitabine.

emtricitabine (n=814) or comparator medicinal product (n=665) for 48 weeks in combination with other antiretroviral medicinal products. In three paediatric studies, treatment-naïve (n=123) and treatment-experienced (n=46) paediatric patients aged 4 months to 18 years were treated with emtricitabine in combination with other antiretroviral agents.

The adverse reactions with suspected (at least possible) relationship to treatment in adults are listed below by body system organ class and absolute frequency. Within each frequency grouping, undesirable effects are presented in order of decreasing seriousness. Frequencies are defined as very common ($\geq$ 1/10), common ($\geq$ 1/100, $<$ 1/10) or uncommon ($\geq$ 1/1,000, $<$ 1/100).

Blood and lymphatic system disorders:

Common: neutropenia

Uncommon: anaemia

Metabolism and nutrition disorders:

Common: hypertriglyceridaemia, hyperglycaemia

Lactic acidosis, usually associated with hepatic steatosis, has been reported with the use of nucleoside analogues (see section 4.4).

Psychiatric disorders:

Common: insomnia, abnormal dreams

Nervous system disorders:

Very common: headache

Common: dizziness

Gastrointestinal disorders:

Very common: diarrhoea, nausea

Common: vomiting, abdominal pain, elevated amylase including elevated pancreatic amylase, elevated serum lipase, dyspepsia

Hepatobiliary disorders:

Common: hyperbilirubinaemia, elevated serum aspartate aminotransferase (AST) and/or elevated serum alanine aminotransferase (ALT)

Skin and subcutaneous tissue disorders:

Common: allergic reaction, urticaria, vesiculobullous rash, pustular rash, maculopapular rash, pruritus, rash, and skin discolouration (hyper-pigmentation)

Musculoskeletal and connective tissue disorders:

Very common: elevated creatine kinase

General disorders and administration site conditions:

Common: asthenia, pain

In addition to the adverse reactions reported in adults, anaemia was common and skin discolouration (hyper-pigmentation) was very common in paediatric patients.

The adverse reaction profile in patients co-infected with HBV is similar to that observed in patients infected with HIV without co-infection with HBV. However, as would be expected in this patient population, elevations in AST and ALT occurred more frequently than in the general HIV infected population.

Combination antiretroviral therapy has been associated with metabolic abnormalities such as hypertriglyceridaemia, hypercholesterolaemia, insulin resistance, hyperglycaemia and hyperlactataemia (see section 4.4).

Combination antiretroviral therapy has been associated with redistribution of body fat (lipodystrophy) in HIV patients including the loss of peripheral and facial subcutaneous fat, increased intra-abdominal and visceral fat, breast hypertrophy and dorsocervical fat accumulation (buffalo hump) (see section 4.4).

In HIV infected patients with severe immune deficiency at the time of initiation of combination antiretroviral therapy (CART), an inflammatory reaction to asymptomatic or residual opportunistic infections may arise (see section 4.4).

Cases of osteonecrosis have been reported, particularly in patients with generally acknowledged risk factors, advanced HIV disease or long-term exposure to combination antiretroviral therapy (CART). The frequency of this is unknown (see section 4.4).

4.9 Overdose

Administration of up to 1,200 mg emtricitabine has been associated with the adverse reactions listed above (see section 4.8).

If overdose occurs, the patient should be monitored for signs of toxicity and standard supportive treatment applied as necessary.

Up to 30% of the emtricitabine dose can be removed by haemodialysis. It is not known whether emtricitabine can be removed by peritoneal dialysis.

5. PHARMACOLOGICAL PROPERTIES

5.1 Pharmacodynamic properties

Pharmacotherapeutic group: Nucleoside and nucleotide reverse transcriptase inhibitors, ATC code: J05AF09.

Mechanism of action: Emtricitabine is a synthetic nucleoside analogue of cytidine with activity that is specific to human immunodeficiency virus (HIV-1 and HIV-2) and hepatitis B virus (HBV).

Emtricitabine is phosphorylated by cellular enzymes to form emtricitabine 5'-triphosphate, which competitively inhibits HIV-1 reverse transcriptase, resulting in DNA chain termination. Emtricitabine is a weak inhibitor of mammalian DNA polymerase α, β and ε and mitochondrial DNA polymerase γ.

Emtricitabine did not exhibit cytotoxicity to peripheral blood mononuclear cells (PBMCs), established lymphocyte and monocyte-macrophage cell lines or bone marrow progenitor cells *in vitro*. There was no evidence of toxicity to mitochondria *in vitro* or *in vivo*.

Antiviral activity in vitro: The 50% inhibitory concentration (IC_{50}) value for emtricitabine against laboratory and clinical isolates of HIV-1 was in the range of 0.0013 to 0.5 µmol/l. In combination studies of emtricitabine with protease inhibitors, nucleoside, nucleotide and non-nucleoside analogue inhibitors of HIV reverse transcriptase, additive to synergistic effects were observed. Most of these combinations have not been studied in humans.

When tested for activity against laboratory strains of HBV, the 50% inhibitory concentration (IC_{50}) value for emtricitabine was in the range of 0.01 to 0.04 µmol/l.

Resistance: HIV-1 resistance to emtricitabine develops as the result of changes at codon 184 causing the methionine to be changed to a valine (an isoleucine intermediate has also been observed) of the HIV reverse transcriptase. This HIV-1 mutation was observed *in vitro* and in HIV-1 infected patients.

Emtricitabine-resistant viruses were cross-resistant to lamivudine, but retained sensitivity to other nucleoside reverse transcriptase inhibitors (NRTIs) (zidovudine, stavudine, tenofovir, abacavir, didanosine and zalcitabine), all non-nucleoside reverse transcriptase inhibitors (NNRTIs) and all protease inhibitors (PIs). Viruses resistant to zidovudine, zalcitabine, didanosine and NNRTIs retained their sensitivity to emtricitabine (IC_{50}=0.002 µmol/l to 0.08 µmol/l).

Clinical experience: Emtricitabine in combination with other antiretroviral agents, including nucleoside analogues, non-nucleoside analogues and protease inhibitors, has been shown to be effective in the treatment of HIV infection in treatment-naïve patients and treatment-experienced patients with stable virological control. There is no experience of the use of emtricitabine in patients who are failing their current regimen or who have failed multiple regimens. There is no clinical experience of the use of emtricitabine in infants less than 4 months of age.

In antiretroviral treatment-naïve adults, emtricitabine was significantly superior to stavudine when both medicinal products were taken in combination with didanosine and efavirenz through 48 weeks of treatment. Phenotypic analysis showed no significant changes in emtricitabine susceptibility unless the M184V/I mutation had developed.

In virologically stable treatment-experienced adults, emtricitabine, in combination with an NRTI (either stavudine or zidovudine) and a protease inhibitor (PI) or an NNRTI was shown to be non-inferior to lamivudine with respect to the proportion of responders ($<$ 400 copies/ml) through 48 weeks (77% emtricitabine, 82% lamivudine). Additionally, in a second study, treatment-experienced adults on a stable PI based highly active antiretroviral therapy (HAART) regimen were randomised to a once daily regimen containing emtricitabine or to continue with their PI-HAART regimen. At 48 weeks of treatment the emtricitabine-containing regimen demonstrated an equivalent proportion of patients with HIV RNA $<$ 400 copies/ml (94% emtricitabine *versus* 92%) and a greater proportion of patients with HIV RNA $<$ 50 copies/ml (95% emtricitabine *versus* 87%) compared with the patients continuing with their PI-HAART regimen.

In infants and children older than 4 months, the majority of patients achieved or maintained complete suppression of plasma HIV-1 RNA through 48 weeks (89% achieved $\leq$ 400 copies/ml and 77% achieved $\leq$ 50 copies/ml).

5.2 Pharmacokinetic properties

Absorption: Emtricitabine is rapidly and extensively absorbed following oral administration with peak plasma concentrations occurring at 1 to 2 hours post-dose. In 20 HIV infected subjects receiving 200 mg emtricitabine daily as hard capsules, steady-state plasma emtricitabine peak concentrations (C_{max}), trough concentrations (C_{min}) and area under the plasma concentration time curve over a 24-hour dosing interval (AUC) were 1.8±0.7 µg/ml, 0.09±0.07 µg/ml and 10.0±3.1 µg·h/ml, respectively. Steady-state trough plasma concentrations reached levels approximately 4-fold above the *in vitro* IC_{90} values for anti-HIV activity.

The absolute bioavailability of emtricitabine from Emtriva 200 mg hard capsules was estimated to be 93% and the absolute bioavailability from Emtriva 10 mg/ml oral solution was estimated to be 75%.

In a pilot study in children and a definitive bioequivalence study in adults, the Emtriva 10 mg/ml oral solution was shown to have approximately 80% of the bioavailability of the Emtriva 200 mg hard capsules. The reason for this difference is unknown. Due to this difference in bioavailability, 240 mg emtricitabine administered as the oral solution should provide similar plasma levels to those observed after administration of one 200 mg emtricitabine hard capsule. Therefore, children who weigh at least 33 kg may take either one 200 mg hard capsule daily or the oral solution up to a maximum dose of 240 mg (24 ml), once daily.

Administration of Emtriva 200 mg hard capsules with a high-fat meal or administration of Emtriva 10 mg/ml oral solution with a low-fat or high-fat meal did not affect systemic exposure ($AUC_{0-\infty}$) of emtricitabine; therefore Emtriva 200 mg hard capsules and Emtriva 10 mg/ml oral solution may be administered with or without food.

Distribution: In vitro binding of emtricitabine to human plasma proteins was $<$ 4% and independent of concentration over the range of 0.02-200 µg/ml. The mean plasma to blood concentration ratio was approximately 1.0 and the mean semen to plasma concentration ratio was approximately 4.0.

The apparent volume of distribution after intravenous administration of emtricitabine was 1.4±0.3 l/kg, indicating that emtricitabine is widely distributed throughout the body to both intracellular and extracellular fluid spaces.

Biotransformation: There is limited metabolism of emtricitabine. The biotransformation of emtricitabine includes oxidation of the thiol moiety to form the 3'-sulphoxide diastereomers (approximately 9% of dose) and conjugation with glucuronic acid to form 2'-O-glucuronide (approximately 4% of dose).

Emtricitabine did not inhibit *in vitro* drug metabolism mediated by the following human CYP450 isoenzymes: 1A2, 2A6, 2B6, 2C9, 2C19, 2D6 and 3A4.

Also, emtricitabine did not inhibit uridine-5'-diphosphoglucuronyl transferase, the enzyme responsible for glucuronidation.

Elimination: Emtricitabine is primarily excreted by the kidneys with complete recovery of the dose achieved in urine (approximately 86%) and faeces (approximately 14%). Thirteen percent of the emtricitabine dose was recovered in urine as three metabolites. The systemic clearance of emtricitabine averaged 307 ml/min (4.03 ml/min/kg). Following oral administration, the elimination half-life of emtricitabine is approximately 10 hours.

Linearity/non-linearity: The pharmacokinetics of emtricitabine are proportional to dose over the dose range of 25-200 mg following single or repeated administration.

Intracellular pharmacokinetics: In a clinical study, the intracellular half-life of emtricitabine-triphosphate in peripheral blood mononuclear cells was 39 hours. Intracellular triphosphate levels increased with dose, but reached a plateau at doses of 200 mg or greater.

Adults with renal insufficiency: Pharmacokinetic parameters were determined following administration of a single dose of 200 mg emtricitabine hard capsules to 30 non-HIV infected subjects with varying degrees of renal insufficiency. Subjects were grouped according to baseline creatinine clearance ($>$ 80 ml/min as normal function; 50-80 ml/min as mild impairment; 30-49 ml/min as moderate impairment; $<$ 30 ml/min as severe impairment; $<$ 15 ml/min as functionally anephric requiring haemodialysis).

The systemic emtricitabine exposure (mean ± standard deviation) increased from 11.8±2.9 µg·h/ml in subjects with normal renal function to 19.9±1.1, 25.0±5.7 and 34.0±2.1 µg·h/ml, in patients with mild, moderate and severe renal impairment, respectively.

In patients with ESRD on haemodialysis, approximately 30% of the emtricitabine dose was recovered in dialysate over a 3 hour dialysis period which had been started within 1.5 hours of emtricitabine dosing (blood flow rate of 400 ml/min and dialysate flow rate of approximately 600 ml/min).

Hepatic insufficiency: The pharmacokinetics of emtricitabine have not been studied in non-HBV infected subjects with varying degrees of hepatic insufficiency. In general, emtricitabine pharmacokinetics in HBV infected subjects were similar to those in healthy subjects and in HIV infected subjects.

Age, gender and ethnicity: In general, the pharmacokinetics of emtricitabine in infants, children and adolescents (aged 4 months up to 18 years) are similar to those seen in adults.

The mean AUC in 77 infants, children and adolescents receiving 6 mg/kg emtricitabine once daily as oral solution or 200 mg emtricitabine as hard capsules once daily was similar to the mean AUC of 10.0 µg·h/ml in 20 adults receiving 200 mg hard capsules once daily.

In an open-label, non-comparative study, pharmacokinetic data were obtained from 20 neonates of HIV infected mothers who received two 4-day courses of emtricitabine oral solution between the first week of life and 3 months of age at a dose level of 3 mg/kg once daily. This dose is half of that approved for infants aged 4 months and over (6 mg/kg). The apparent total body clearance at steady state (CL/F) increased with age over the 3-month period with a corresponding decrease in AUC. Plasma emtricitabine exposure (AUC) in infants up to 3 months of age who received 3 mg/kg emtricitabine once daily was similar to that observed using 6 mg/kg daily doses in HIV infected adults and children aged 4 months and over.

Pharmacokinetic data are not available in the elderly.

Although the mean C_{max} and C_{min} were approximately 20% higher and mean AUC was 16% higher in females compared to males, this difference was not considered clinically significant. No clinically important pharmacokinetic difference due to race has been identified.

5.3 Preclinical safety data

Non-clinical data reveal no special hazard for humans based on conventional studies of safety pharmacology, repeated dose toxicity, genotoxicity and reproductive/developmental toxicity. Emtricitabine did not show any carcinogenic potential in long-term oral carcinogenicity studies in mice and rats.

6. PHARMACEUTICAL PARTICULARS

6.1 List of excipients

Capsule contents:

Cellulose, microcrystalline (E460)

Crospovidone

Magnesium stearate (E572)

Povidone (E1201)

Capsule shell:

Gelatin

Indigotine (E132)

Titanium dioxide (E171)

Printing ink containing:

Black iron oxide (E172)

Shellac (E904)

6.2 Incompatibilities

Not applicable.

6.3 Shelf life

3 years.

6.4 Special precautions for storage

This medicinal product does not require any special storage conditions.

6.5 Nature and contents of container

White high-density polyethylene (HDPE) bottle fitted with a child-resistant closure, containing 30 hard capsules.

Blisters made of polychlorotrifluorethylene (PCTFE) / polyethylene (PE) / polyvinylchloride (PVC) / aluminium. Each blister pack contains 30 hard capsules.

Pack size: 30 hard capsules.

6.6 Special precautions for disposal and other handling

Any unused product or waste material should be disposed of in accordance with local requirements.

7. MARKETING AUTHORISATION HOLDER

Gilead Sciences International Limited

Cambridge

CB21 6GT

United Kingdom

8. MARKETING AUTHORISATION NUMBER(S)

EU/1/03/261/001

EU/1/03/261/002

9. DATE OF FIRST AUTHORISATION/RENEWAL OF THE AUTHORISATION

Date of first authorisation: 24 October 2003

Date of last renewal: 22 September 2008

10. DATE OF REVISION OF THE TEXT

09/2008

Detailed information on this medicinal product is available on the website of the European Medicines Agency (EMEA) http://www.emea.europa.eu/.

Emulsiderm Emollient

(Dermal Laboratories Limited)

1. NAME OF THE MEDICINAL PRODUCT

EMULSIDERM™ EMOLLIENT

2. QUALITATIVE AND QUANTITATIVE COMPOSITION

Liquid Paraffin 25.0% w/w; Isopropyl Myristate 25.0% w/w; Benzalkonium Chloride 0.5% w/w.

3. PHARMACEUTICAL FORM

Pale blue bath additive and cutaneous emulsion.

4. CLINICAL PARTICULARS

4.1 Therapeutic indications

An antimicrobial bath emollient for use as an aid in the treatment of dry and pruritic skin conditions, especially eczema, dermatitis, ichthyosis or xeroderma. It permits the rehydration of the keratin by replacing lost lipids, and its antiseptic properties assist in overcoming secondary infection.

4.2 Posology and method of administration

For adults, children and the elderly:

For use in the bath Add 7 - 30 ml Emulsiderm to a bath of warm water (more or less according to the size of the bath and individual patient requirements). 1 litre bottle - use graduated measuring cup provided; 300 ml bottle - use ½ to 2 capfuls. Soak for 5 - 10 minutes. Pat dry.

For application to the skin Rub a small amount of undiluted emollient into the dry areas of skin until absorbed.

4.3 Contraindications

Sensitivity to any of the ingredients.

4.4 Special warnings and precautions for use

Keep away from the eyes. For external use only. Keep out of the reach and sight of children. Take care to avoid slipping in the bath.

4.5 Interaction with other medicinal products and other forms of interaction

None known.

4.6 Pregnancy and lactation

No known side effects.

4.7 Effects on ability to drive and use machines

None known.

4.8 Undesirable effects

Although the emollient has been specially formulated for use on dry or problem skin, in the unlikely event of a reaction discontinue treatment. These reactions are very rare (<1/10,000, based on spontaneous reporting) and may be irritant or allergic in nature. Reactions have been observed occasionally when used excessively as a leave-on application in areas of folded skin such as the anogenital area.

4.9 Overdose

Not applicable.

5. PHARMACOLOGICAL PROPERTIES

5.1 Pharmacodynamic properties

For dry skin conditions it is important to add an emollient to the bath water. Emulsiderm contains 50% of oils emulsified in water as well as the well-known antiseptic, benzalkonium chloride which assists in overcoming secondary infection.

5.2 Pharmacokinetic properties

Emulsiderm contains 0.5% of the quaternary ammonium antiseptic, benzalkonium chloride. The large positively charged cation is readily adsorbed from the formulation onto negatively charged bacterial cell surfaces, thereby conferring substantial antimicrobial activity. Even at extended dilution, it is particularly effective against *Staphylococcus aureus*, a bacterium which is known to colonise the skin in large numbers in patients with eczema, especially atopic eczema. Apart from its emollient properties, Emulsiderm therefore also helps to prevent and overcome secondary infection which may exacerbate the eczematous condition.

5.3 Preclinical safety data

The safety and efficacy of the emollients (liquid paraffin and isopropyl myristate) and the antiseptic (benzalkonium chloride) in topical dosage forms have been well established over many years of widespread clinical usage.

6. PHARMACEUTICAL PARTICULARS

6.1 List of excipients

Sorbitan Stearate; Polysorbate 60; Industrial Methylated Spirit 95%; Methylthioninium Chloride; Purified Water.

6.2 Incompatibilities

None known.

6.3 Shelf life

36 months.

6.4 Special precautions for storage

Do not store above 25°C. Always replace the cap after use.

6.5 Nature and contents of container

Supplied in plastic bottles; a 300 ml bottle with a measuring cap, and a 1 litre bottle with a measuring cup.

6.6 Special precautions for disposal and other handling

Not applicable.

7. MARKETING AUTHORISATION HOLDER

Dermal Laboratories

Tatmore Place, Gosmore

Hitchin, Herts SG4 7QR, UK.

8. MARKETING AUTHORISATION NUMBER(S)

00173/0036.

9. DATE OF FIRST AUTHORISATION/RENEWAL OF THE AUTHORISATION

13 July 2009.

10. DATE OF REVISION OF THE TEXT

July 2009.

Enbrel 25 mg powder and solvent for solution for injection

(Wyeth Pharmaceuticals)

1. NAME OF THE MEDICINAL PRODUCT

Enbrel®▼ 25 mg powder and solvent for solution for injection.

2. QUALITATIVE AND QUANTITATIVE COMPOSITION

Each vial contains 25 mg of etanercept.

Etanercept is a human tumour necrosis factor receptor p75 Fc fusion protein produced by recombinant DNA technology in a Chinese hamster ovary (CHO) mammalian expression system. Etanercept is a dimer of a chimeric protein genetically engineered by fusing the extracellular ligand binding domain of human tumour necrosis factor receptor-2 (TNFR2/p75) to the Fc domain of human IgG1. This Fc component contains the hinge, CH_2 and CH_3 regions but not the CH_1 region of IgG1. Etanercept contains 934 amino acids and has an apparent molecular weight of approximately 150 kilodaltons. The potency is determined by measuring the ability of etanercept to neutralise the TNFα-mediated growth inhibition of A375 cells. The specific activity of etanercept is 1.7×10^6 units/mg.

For a full list of excipients, see section 6.1.

3. PHARMACEUTICAL FORM

Powder and solvent for solution for injection.

The powder is white. The solvent is a clear, colourless liquid.

4. CLINICAL PARTICULARS

4.1 Therapeutic indications

Rheumatoid arthritis

Enbrel in combination with methotrexate is indicated for the treatment of moderate to severe active rheumatoid arthritis in adults when the response to disease-modifying antirheumatic drugs, including methotrexate (unless contraindicated), has been inadequate.

Enbrel can be given as monotherapy in case of intolerance to methotrexate or when continued treatment with methotrexate is inappropriate.

Enbrel is also indicated in the treatment of severe, active and progressive rheumatoid arthritis in adults not previously treated with methotrexate.

Enbrel, alone or in combination with methotrexate, has been shown to reduce the rate of progression of joint damage as measured by X-ray and to improve physical function.

Polyarticular juvenile idiopathic arthritis

Treatment of active polyarticular juvenile idiopathic arthritis in children and adolescents from the age of 4 years who have had an inadequate response to, or who have proved intolerant of, methotrexate. Enbrel has not been studied in children aged less than 4 years.

Psoriatic arthritis

Treatment of active and progressive psoriatic arthritis in adults when the response to previous disease-modifying antirheumatic drug therapy has been inadequate. Enbrel has been shown to improve physical function in patients with psoriatic arthritis, and to reduce the rate of progression of peripheral joint damage as measured by X-ray in patients with polyarticular symmetrical subtypes of the disease.

Ankylosing spondylitis

Treatment of adults with severe active ankylosing spondylitis who have had an inadequate response to conventional therapy.

Plaque psoriasis

Treatment of adults with moderate to severe plaque psoriasis who failed to respond to, or who have a contraindication to, or are intolerant to other systemic therapy including ciclosporin, methotrexate or PUVA (see section 5.1).

Paediatric plaque psoriasis

Treatment of chronic severe plaque psoriasis in children and adolescents from the age of 8 years who are inadequately controlled by, or are intolerant to, other systemic therapies or phototherapies.

4.2 Posology and method of administration

Enbrel treatment should be initiated and supervised by specialist physicians experienced in the diagnosis and treatment of rheumatoid arthritis, juvenile idiopathic arthritis, psoriatic arthritis, ankylosing spondylitis, plaque psoriasis or paediatric plaque psoriasis. Patients treated with Enbrel should be given the Patient Alert Card.

Enbrel is available in strengths of 25 and 50 mg.

Posology

Rheumatoid arthritis

25 mg Enbrel administered twice weekly is the recommended dose. Alternatively, 50 mg administered once weekly has been shown to be safe and effective (see section 5.1).

Psoriatic arthritis and ankylosing spondylitis

The recommended dose is 25 mg Enbrel administered twice weekly, or 50 mg administered once weekly.

Plaque psoriasis

The recommended dose of Enbrel is 25 mg administered twice weekly or 50 mg administered once weekly. Alternatively, 50 mg given twice weekly may be used for up to 12 weeks followed, if necessary, by a dose of 25 mg twice weekly or 50 mg once weekly. Treatment with Enbrel should continue until remission is achieved, for up to 24 weeks. Continuous therapy beyond 24 weeks may be appropriate for some adult patients (see section 5.1). Treatment should be discontinued in patients who show no response after 12 weeks. If re-treatment with Enbrel is indicated, the same guidance on treatment duration should be followed. The dose should be 25 mg twice weekly or 50 mg once weekly.

Special populations

Elderly patients (≥ 65 years)

No dose adjustment is required. Posology and administration are the same as for adults 18-64 years of age.

Paediatric use

Juvenile idiopathic arthritis (age 4 years and above)

0.4 mg/kg (up to a maximum of 25 mg per dose) after reconstitution of 25 mg Enbrel in 1 ml of solvent, given twice weekly as a subcutaneous injection with an interval of 3-4 days between doses.

Paediatric plaque psoriasis (age 8 years and above)

0.8 mg/kg (up to a maximum of 50 mg per dose) once weekly for up to 24 weeks. Treatment should be discontinued in patients who show no response after 12 weeks.

If re-treatment with Enbrel is indicated, the above guidance on treatment duration should be followed. The dose should be 0.8 mg/kg (up to a maximum of 50 mg per dose) once weekly.

Renal and hepatic impairment

No dose adjustment is required.

Method of administration

Comprehensive instructions for the preparation and administration of the reconstituted Enbrel vial are given in the package leaflet, section 7, "Instructions for preparation and giving an injection of Enbrel."

4.3 Contraindications

Hypersensitivity to the active substance or to any of the excipients.

Sepsis or risk of sepsis.

Treatment with Enbrel should not be initiated in patients with active infections including chronic or localised infections.

4.4 Special warnings and precautions for use

Infections

Patients should be evaluated for infections before, during, and after treatment with Enbrel, taking into consideration that the mean elimination half-life of etanercept is approximately 70 hours (range 7 to 300 hours).

Serious infections, sepsis, tuberculosis, and opportunistic infections, including invasive fungal infections, have been reported with the use of Enbrel (see section 4.8). These infections were due to bacteria, mycobacteria, fungi and viruses. In some cases, particular fungal and other opportunistic infections have not been recognised, resulting in delay of appropriate treatment and sometimes death. In evaluating patients for infections, the patient's risk for relevant opportunistic infections (e.g., exposure to endemic mycoses) should be considered.

Patients who develop a new infection while undergoing treatment with Enbrel should be monitored closely. **Administration of Enbrel should be discontinued if a patient develops a serious infection.** Physicians should exercise caution when considering the use of Enbrel in patients with a history of recurring or chronic infections or with underlying conditions that may predispose patients to infections such as advanced or poorly controlled diabetes.

Tuberculosis

Cases of active tuberculosis including miliary tuberculosis and tuberculosis with extra-pulmonary location have been reported in patients treated with Enbrel.

Before starting treatment with Enbrel, all patients must be evaluated for both active and inactive ('latent') tuberculosis. This evaluation should include a detailed medical history with personal history of tuberculosis or possible previous contact with tuberculosis and previous and/or current immunosuppressive therapy. Appropriate screening tests, i.e. tuberculin skin test and chest x-ray, should be performed in all patients (local recommendations may apply). It is recommended that the conduct of these tests should be recorded in the patient's alert card. Prescribers are reminded of the risk of false negative tuberculin skin test results, especially in patients who are severely ill or immunocompromised.

If active tuberculosis is diagnosed, Enbrel therapy must not be initiated. If inactive ('latent') tuberculosis is diagnosed, treatment for latent tuberculosis must be started with anti-tuberculosis therapy before the initiation of Enbrel, and in accordance with local recommendations. In this situation, the benefit/risk balance of Enbrel therapy should be very carefully considered.

All patients should be informed to seek medical advice if signs/symptoms suggestive of tuberculosis (e.g., persistent cough, wasting/weight loss, low-grade fever) appear during or after Enbrel treatment.

Hepatitis B virus reactivation

Reactivation of hepatitis B virus (HBV) in patients who are chronic carriers of this virus who are receiving TNF-antagonists including Enbrel has been reported. Patients at risk for HBV infection should be evaluated for prior evidence of HBV infection before initiating Enbrel therapy. Caution should be exercised when administering Enbrel to patients identified as carriers of HBV. If Enbrel is used in carriers of HBV, the patients should be monitored for signs and symptoms of active HBV infection and, if necessary, appropriate treatment should be initiated.

Worsening of hepatitis C

There have been reports of worsening of hepatitis C in patients receiving Enbrel.

Concurrent treatment with anakinra

Concurrent administration of Enbrel and anakinra has been associated with an increased risk of serious infections and neutropenia compared to Enbrel alone. This combination has not demonstrated increased clinical benefit. Thus the combined use of Enbrel and anakinra is not recommended (see sections 4.5 and 4.8).

Concurrent treatment with abatacept

In clinical studies, concurrent administration of abatacept and Enbrel resulted in increased incidences of serious adverse events. This combination has not demonstrated increased clinical benefit; such use is not recommended (see section 4.5).

Allergic reactions

Allergic reactions associated with Enbrel administration have been reported commonly. Allergic reactions have included angioedema and urticaria; serious reactions have occurred. If any serious allergic or anaphylactic reaction occurs, Enbrel therapy should be discontinued immediately and appropriate therapy initiated.

Immunosuppression

The possibility exists for TNF-antagonists, including Enbrel, to affect host defences against infections and malignancies since TNF mediates inflammation and modulates cellular immune responses. In a study of 49 adult patients with rheumatoid arthritis treated with Enbrel, there was no evidence of depression of delayed-type hypersensitivity, depression of immunoglobulin levels, or change in enumeration of effector cell populations.

Two juvenile idiopathic arthritis patients developed varicella infection and signs and symptoms of aseptic meningitis, which resolved without sequelae. Patients with a significant exposure to varicella virus should temporarily discontinue Enbrel therapy and be considered for prophylactic treatment with Varicella Zoster Immune Globulin.

The safety and efficacy of Enbrel in patients with immunosuppression or chronic infections have not been evaluated.

Malignancies and lymphoproliferative disorders

Solid and haematopoietic malignancies

Reports of various malignancies (including breast and lung carcinoma and lymphoma) have been received in the postmarketing period (see section 4.8).

In the controlled portions of clinical trials of TNF-antagonists, more cases of lymphoma have been observed among patients receiving a TNF-antagonist compared with control patients. However, the occurrence was rare, and the follow-up period of placebo patients was shorter than for patients receiving TNF-antagonist therapy. Furthermore, there is an increased background lymphoma risk in rheumatoid arthritis patients with long-standing, highly active, inflammatory disease, which complicates the risk estimation. With the current knowledge, a possible risk for the development of lymphomas or other malignancies in patients treated with a TNF-antagonist cannot be excluded.

Non-melanoma skin cancer (NMSC)

Non-melanoma skin cancer has been reported in patients treated with TNF-antagonists, including Enbrel. Combining the results of placebo- and active comparator-controlled clinical trials of Enbrel, more cases of NMSC were observed in patients receiving Enbrel compared with control patients, particularly in patients with psoriasis. Periodic skin examination is recommended for all patients who are at increased risk for NMSC (including patients with psoriasis or a history of PUVA therapy).

Vaccinations

Live vaccines should not be given concurrently with Enbrel. No data are available on the secondary transmission of infection by live vaccines in patients receiving Enbrel. It is recommended that juvenile idiopathic arthritis patients, if possible, be brought up to date with all immunisations in agreement with current immunisation guidelines prior to initiating Enbrel therapy. In a double blind, placebo controlled, randomised clinical study in adult patients with psoriatic arthritis 184 patients also received a multivalent pneumococcal polysaccharide vaccine at week 4. In this study most psoriatic arthritis patients receiving Enbrel were able to mount effective B-cell immune response to pneumococcal polysaccharide vaccine, but titers in aggregate were moderately lower and few patients had two-fold rises in titers compared to patients not receiving Enbrel. The clinical significance of this is unknown.

Autoantibody formation

Treatment with Enbrel may result in the formation of autoimmune antibodies (see section 4.8).

Haematologic reactions

Rare cases of pancytopenia and very rare cases of aplastic anaemia, some with fatal outcome, have been reported in patients treated with Enbrel. Caution should be exercised in patients being treated with Enbrel who have a previous history of blood dyscrasias. All patients and parents/caregivers should be advised that if the patient develops signs and symptoms suggestive of blood dyscrasias or infections (e.g., persistent fever, sore throat, bruising, bleeding, paleness) whilst on Enbrel, they should seek immediate medical advice. Such patients should be investigated urgently, including full blood count; if blood dyscrasias are confirmed, Enbrel should be discontinued.

CNS disorders

There have been rare reports of CNS demyelinating disorders in patients treated with Enbrel (see section 4.8). Although no clinical trials have been performed evaluating Enbrel therapy in patients with multiple sclerosis, clinical trials of other TNF antagonists in patients with multiple sclerosis have shown increases in disease activity. A careful risk/benefit evaluation, including a neurological assessment, is recommended when prescribing Enbrel to patients with pre-existing or recent onset of CNS demyelinating disease, or to those who are considered to have an increased risk of developing demyelinating disease.

Combination therapy

In a controlled clinical trial of two years duration in rheumatoid arthritis patients, the combination of Enbrel and methotrexate did not result in unexpected safety findings, and the safety profile of Enbrel when given in combination with methotrexate was similar to the profiles reported in studies of Enbrel and methotrexate alone. Long-term studies to assess the safety of the combination are ongoing. The long-term safety of Enbrel in combination with other disease-modifying antirheumatic drugs (DMARD) has not been established.

The use of Enbrel in combination with other systemic therapies or phototherapy for the treatment of psoriasis has not been studied.

Renal and hepatic impairment

Based on pharmacokinetic data (see section 5.2), no dose adjustment is needed in patients with renal or hepatic impairment; clinical experience in such patients is limited.

Congestive heart failure

Physicians should use caution when using Enbrel in patients who have congestive heart failure (CHF). There have been postmarketing reports of worsening of CHF, with and without identifiable precipitating factors, in patients taking Enbrel. Two large clinical trials evaluating the use of Enbrel in the treatment of CHF were terminated early due to lack of efficacy. Although not conclusive, data from one of these trials suggest a possible tendency toward worsening CHF in those patients assigned to Enbrel treatment.

Alcoholic hepatitis

In a phase II randomised placebo-controlled study of 48 hospitalised patients treated with Enbrel or placebo for moderate to severe alcoholic hepatitis, Enbrel was not efficacious, and the mortality rate in patients treated with Enbrel was significantly higher after 6 months. Consequently, Enbrel should not be used in patients for the treatment of alcoholic hepatitis. Physicians should use caution when using Enbrel in patients who also have moderate to severe alcoholic hepatitis.

Wegener's granulomatosis

A placebo-controlled trial, in which 89 adult patients were treated with Enbrel in addition to standard therapy (including cyclophosphamide or methotrexate, and glucocorticoids) for a median duration of 25 months, has not shown Enbrel to be an effective treatment for Wegener's granulomatosis. The incidence of non-cutaneous malignancies of various types was significantly higher in patients treated with Enbrel than in the control group. Enbrel is not recommended for the treatment of Wegener's granulomatosis.

4.5 Interaction with other medicinal products and other forms of interaction

Concurrent treatment with anakinra

Adult patients treated with Enbrel and anakinra were observed to have a higher rate of serious infection when compared with patients treated with either Enbrel or anakinra alone (historical data).

In addition, in a double-blind placebo-controlled trial in adult patients receiving background methotrexate, patients treated with Enbrel and anakinra were observed to have a higher rate of serious infections (7%) and neutropenia than patients treated with Enbrel (see sections 4.4 and 4.8). The combination Enbrel and anakinra has not demonstrated increased clinical benefit and is therefore not recommended.

Concurrent treatment with abatacept

In clinical studies, concurrent administration of abatacept and Enbrel resulted in increased incidences of serious adverse events. This combination has not demonstrated increased clinical benefit; such use is not recommended (see section 4.4).

Concurrent treatment with sulfasalazine

In a clinical study of adult patients who were receiving established doses of sulfasalazine, to which Enbrel was added, patients in the combination group experienced a statistically significant decrease in mean white blood cell counts in comparison to groups treated with Enbrel or sulfasalazine alone. The clinical significance of this interaction is unknown.

Non-interactions

In clinical trials, no interactions have been observed when Enbrel was administered with glucocorticoids, salicylates (except sulfasalazine), nonsteroidal anti-inflammatory drugs (NSAIDs), analgesics, or methotrexate. See section 4.4 for vaccination advice.

No clinically significant pharmacokinetic drug-drug interactions were observed in studies with digoxin or warfarin.

4.6 Pregnancy and lactation

Pregnancy

There are no studies of Enbrel in pregnant women. Developmental toxicity studies performed in rats and rabbits have revealed no evidence of harm to the foetus or neonatal rat due to etanercept. Preclinical data about peri- and postnatal toxicity of etanercept and of effects of etanercept on fertility and general reproductive performance are not available. Thus, the use of Enbrel in pregnant women is not recommended, and women of child-bearing potential should be advised not to get pregnant during Enbrel therapy.

Lactation

It is not known whether etanercept is excreted in human milk. Following subcutaneous administration to lactacting rats, etanercept was excreted in the milk and detected in the serum of pups. Because immunoglobulins, in common with many medicinal products, can be excreted in human milk, a decision should be made whether to discontinue breast-feeding or to discontinue Enbrel while breast-feeding.

4.7 Effects on ability to drive and use machines

No studies on the effects on the ability to drive and use machines have been performed.

4.8 Undesirable effects

Undesirable effects in adults

Enbrel has been studied in 2,680 patients with rheumatoid arthritis in double-blind and open-label trials. This experience includes 2 placebo-controlled studies (349 Enbrel patients and 152 placebo patients) and 2 active-controlled trials, one active-controlled trial comparing Enbrel to methotrexate (415 Enbrel patients and 217 methotrexate patients) and another active-controlled trial comparing Enbrel (223 patients), methotrexate (228 patients) and Enbrel in combination with methotrexate (231 patients). The proportion of patients who discontinued treatment due to adverse events was the same in both the Enbrel and placebo treatment groups; in the first active-controlled trial, the dropout rate was significantly higher for methotrexate (10%) than for Enbrel (5%). In the second active-controlled trial, the rate of discontinuation for adverse events after 2 years of treatment was similar among all three treatment groups, Enbrel (16%), methotrexate (21%) and Enbrel in combination with methotrexate (17%). Additionally, Enbrel has been studied in 240 psoriatic arthritis patients who participated in 2 double-blind placebo-controlled studies and an open-label extension study. Five hundred and eight (508) ankylosing spondylitis patients were treated with Enbrel in 4 double-blind placebo-controlled studies. Enbrel has also been studied in 1,492 patients with plaque psoriasis for up to 6 months in 5 double-blind placebo-controlled studies.

In double-blind clinical trials comparing Enbrel to placebo, injection site reactions were the most frequent adverse events among Enbrel-treated patients. Among patients with rheumatoid arthritis treated in placebo-controlled trials, serious adverse events occurred at a frequency of 4% in 349 patients treated with Enbrel compared with 5% of 152 placebo-treated patients. In the first active-controlled trial, serious adverse events occurred at a frequency of 6% in 415 patients treated with Enbrel compared with 8% of 217 methotrexate-treated patients. In the second active-controlled trial the rate of serious adverse events after 2 years of treatment was similar among the three treatment groups (Enbrel 16%, methotrexate 15% and Enbrel in combination with methotrexate 17%). Among patients with plaque psoriasis treated in placebo-controlled trials, the frequency of serious adverse events was about 1.4% of 1,341 patients treated with Enbrel compared with 1.4% of 766 placebo-treated patients.

The following list of adverse reactions is based on experience from clinical trials in adults and on postmarketing experience.

Within the organ system classes, adverse reactions are listed under headings of frequency (number of patients expected to experience the reaction), using the following categories: very common (⩾1/10); common (⩾1/100, <1/10); uncommon (⩾1/1000, <1/100); rare (⩾1/10,000, <1/1000); very rare (<1/10,000); not known (cannot be estimated from the available data).

Infections and infestations:

Very common:	Infections (including upper respiratory tract infections, bronchitis, cystitis, skin infections)*
Uncommon:	Serious infections (including pneumonia, cellulitis, septic arthritis, sepsis)*
Rare:	Tuberculosis, opportunistic infections (including invasive fungal, protozoal, bacterial and atypical mycobacterial infections)*

Blood and lymphatic system disorders:

Uncommon:	Thrombocytopenia
Rare:	Anaemia, leukopenia, neutropenia, pancytopenia*
Very rare:	Aplastic anaemia*

Immune system disorders:

Common:	Allergic reactions (see Skin and subcutaneous tissue disorders), autoantibody formation*
Rare:	Serious allergic/anaphylactic reactions (including angioedema, bronchospasm)
Not known:	Macrophage activation syndrome*, anti-neutrophilic cytoplasmic antibody positive vasculitis

Nervous system disorders:

Rare:	Seizures CNS demyelinating events suggestive of multiple sclerosis or localised demyelinating conditions such as optic neuritis and transverse myelitis (see section 4.4)

Respiratory, thoracic and mediastinal disorders:

Uncommon:	Interstitial lung disease (including pneumonitis and pulmonary fibrosis)*

Hepatobiliary disorders:

Rare:	Elevated liver enzymes

Skin and subcutaneous tissue disorders:

Common:	Pruritus
Uncommon:	Non-melanoma skin cancers (see section 4.4), angioedema, urticaria, rash, psoriasiform rash, psoriasis (including new onset and pustular, primarily palms and soles)
Rare:	Cutaneous vasculitis (including leukocytoclastic vasculitis), Stevens-Johnson syndrome, erythema multiforme
Very rare:	Toxic epidermal necrolysis

Musculoskeletal and connective tissue disorders:

Rare:	Subacute cutaneous lupus erythematosus, discoid lupus erythematosus, lupus like syndrome

General disorders and administration site conditions:

Very common:	Injection site reactions (including bleeding, bruising, erythema, itching, pain, swelling)*
Common:	Fever

Cardiac disorders:

There have been reports of worsening of congestive heart failure (see section 4.4).

*see Additional information, below.

Additional information

Serious adverse events reported in clinical trials

Among rheumatoid arthritis, psoriatic arthritis, ankylosing spondylitis and plaque psoriasis patients in placebo-controlled, active-controlled, and open-label trials of Enbrel, serious adverse events reported included malignancies (see below), asthma, infections (see below), heart failure, myocardial infarction, myocardial ischaemia, chest pain, syncope, cerebral ischaemia, hypertension, hypotension, cholecystitis, pancreatitis, gastrointestinal haemorrhage, bursitis, confusion, depression, dyspnoea, abnormal healing, renal insufficiency, kidney calculus, deep vein thrombosis, pulmonary embolism, membranous glomerulonephropathy, polymyositis, thrombophlebitis, liver damage, leucopenia, paresis, paresthesia, vertigo, allergic alveolitis, angioedema, scleritis, bone fracture, lymphadenopathy, ulcerative colitis, intestinal obstruction, eosinophilia, haematuria, and sarcoidosis.

Malignancies and lymphoproliferative disorders

One hundred and twenty-nine new malignancies of various types were observed in 4,114 rheumatoid arthritis patients treated in clinical trials with Enbrel for up to approximately 6 years, including 231 patients treated with Enbrel in combination with methotrexate in the 2-year active-controlled study. The observed rates and incidences in these clinical trials were similar to those expected for the population studied. A total of 2 malignancies were reported in clinical studies of approximately 2 years duration involving 240 Enbrel-treated psoriatic arthritis patients. In clinical studies conducted for more than 2 years with 351 ankylosing spondylitis patients, 6 malignancies were reported in Enbrel-treated patients. In a group of 2,711 plaque psoriasis patients treated with Enbrel in double-blind and open-label studies of up to 2.5 years, 30 malignancies and 43 nonmelanoma skin cancers were reported.

In a group of 7,416 patients treated with Enbrel in rheumatoid arthritis, psoriatic arthritis, ankylosing spondylitis and psoriasis clinical trials, 18 lymphomas were reported.

Reports of various malignancies (including breast and lung carcinoma and lymphoma) have also been received in the postmarketing period (see section 4.4).

Injection site reactions

Compared to placebo, patients with rheumatic diseases treated with Enbrel had a significantly higher incidence of injection site reactions (36% vs. 9%). Injection site reactions usually occurred in the first month. Mean duration was approximately 3 to 5 days. No treatment was given for the majority of injection site reactions in the Enbrel treatment groups, and the majority of patients who were given treatment received topical preparations such as corticosteroids, or oral antihistamines. Additionally, some patients developed recall injection site reactions characterised by a skin reaction at the most recent site of injection along with the simultaneous appearance of injection site reactions at previous injection sites. These reactions were generally transient and did not recur with treatment.

In controlled trials in patients with plaque psoriasis, approximately 13.6% of patients treated with Enbrel developed injection site reactions compared with 3.4% of placebo-treated patients during the first 12 weeks of treatment.

Serious infections

In placebo-controlled trials, no increase in the incidence of serious infections (fatal, life threatening, or requiring hospitalisation or intravenous antibiotics) was observed. Serious infections occurred in 6.3% of rheumatoid arthritis patients treated with Enbrel for up to 48 months. These included abscess (at various sites), bacteraemia, bronchitis, bursitis, cellulitis, cholecystitis, diarrhoea, diverticulitis, endocarditis (suspected), gastroenteritis, hepatitis B, herpes zoster, leg ulcer, mouth infection, osteomyelitis, otitis, peritonitis, pneumonia, pyelonephritis, sepsis, septic arthritis, sinusitis, skin infection, skin ulcer, urinary tract infection, vasculitis, and wound infection. In the 2-year active-controlled study where patients were treated with either Enbrel alone, methotrexate alone or Enbrel in combination with methotrexate, the rates of serious infections were similar among the treatment groups. However, it cannot be excluded that the combination of Enbrel with methotrexate could be associated with an increase in the rate of infections.

There were no differences in rates of infection among patients treated with Enbrel and those treated with placebo for plaque psoriasis in placebo controlled trials of up to 24 weeks duration. Serious infections experienced by Enbrel-treated patients included cellulitis, gastroenteritis, pneumonia, cholecystitis, osteomyelitis, gastritis, appendicitis, Streptococcal fasciitis, myositis, septic shock, diverticulitis and abscess. In the double-blind and open-label psoriatic arthritis trials, 1 patient reported a serious infection (pneumonia).

Serious and fatal infections have been reported during use of Enbrel; reported pathogens include bacteria, mycobacteria (including tuberculosis), viruses and fungi. Some have occurred within a few weeks after initiating treatment with Enbrel in patients who have underlying conditions (e.g. diabetes, congestive heart failure, history of active or chronic infections) in addition to their rheumatoid arthritis (see section 4.4). Enbrel treatment may increase mortality in patients with established sepsis.

Opportunistic infections have been reported in association with Enbrel including invasive fungal, protozoal, bacterial (including *Listeria* and *Legionella*), and atypical mycobacterial infections. In a pooled data set of clinical trials, the overall incidence of opportunistic infections was 0.09% for the 15,402 subjects who received Enbrel. The exposure-adjusted rate was 0.06 events per 100 patient-years. In postmarketing experience, approximately half of all of the case reports of opportunistic infections worldwide were invasive fungal infections. The most commonly reported invasive fungal infections were *Pneumocystis* and *Aspergillus*. Invasive fungal infections accounted for more than half of the fatalities amongst patients who developed opportunistic infections. The majority of the reports with a fatal outcome were in patients with *Pneumocystis* pneumonia, unspecified systemic fungal infections, and aspergillosis (see section 4.4).

Autoantibodies

Adult patients had serum samples tested for autoantibodies at multiple timepoints. Of the rheumatoid arthritis patients evaluated for antinuclear antibodies (ANA), the percentage of patients who developed new positive ANA (⩾1:40) was higher in patients treated with Enbrel (11%) than in placebo-treated patients (5%). The percentage of patients who developed new positive anti-double-stranded DNA antibodies was also higher by radioimmunoassay (15% of patients treated with Enbrel compared to 4% of placebo-treated patients) and by *Crithidia luciliae* assay (3% of patients treated with Enbrel compared to none of placebo-treated patients). The proportion of patients treated with Enbrel who developed anticardiolipin antibodies was similarly increased compared to placebo-treated patients. The impact of long-term treatment with Enbrel on the development of autoimmune diseases is unknown.

There have been rare reports of patients, including rheumatoid factor positive patients, who have developed other autoantibodies in conjunction with a lupus-like syndrome or rashes that are compatible with subacute cutaneous lupus or discoid lupus by clinical presentation and biopsy.

Pancytopenia and aplastic anaemia

There have been postmarketing reports of pancytopenia and aplastic anaemia, some of which had fatal outcomes (see section 4.4).

Interstitial lung disease

There have been postmarketing reports of interstitial lung disease (including pneumonitis and pulmonary fibrosis), some of which had fatal outcomes.

Laboratory evaluations

Based on the results of clinical studies, normally no special laboratory evaluations are necessary in addition to careful medical management and supervision of patients.

Concurrent treatment with anakinra

In studies when adult patients received concurrent treatment with Enbrel plus anakinra, a higher rate of serious infections compared to Enbrel alone was observed and 2% of patients (3/139) developed neutropenia (absolute neutrophil count < 1000 / mm^3). While neutropenic, one patient developed cellulitis that resolved after hospitalisation (see sections 4.4 and 4.5).

Undesirable effects in paediatric patients with polyarticular juvenile idiopathic arthritis

In general, the adverse events in paediatric patients with juvenile idiopathic arthritis were similar in frequency and type to those seen in adult patients. Differences from adults and other special considerations are discussed in the following paragraphs.

The types of infections seen in clinical trials in juvenile idiopathic arthritis patients aged 2 to 18 years were generally mild to moderate and consistent with those commonly seen in outpatient paediatric populations. Severe adverse events reported included varicella with signs and symptoms of aseptic meningitis, which resolved without sequelae (see also section 4.4), appendicitis, gastroenteritis, depression/personality disorder, cutaneous ulcer, oesophagitis/gastritis, group A streptococcal septic shock, type I diabetes mellitus, and soft tissue and post-operative wound infection.

In one study in children with juvenile idiopathic arthritis aged 4 to 17 years, 43 of 69 (62%) children experienced an infection while receiving Enbrel during 3 months of the study (part 1 open-label), and the frequency and severity of infections was similar in 58 patients completing 12 months of open-label extension therapy. The types and proportion of adverse events in juvenile idiopathic arthritis patients were similar to those seen in trials of Enbrel in adult patients with rheumatoid arthritis, and the majority were mild. Several adverse events were reported more commonly in 69 juvenile idiopathic arthritis patients receiving 3 months of Enbrel compared to the 349 adult rheumatoid arthritis patients. These included headache (19% of patients, 1.7 events per patient year), nausea (9%, 1.0 event per patient year), abdominal pain (19%, 0.74 events per patient year), and vomiting (13%, 0.74 events per patient year).

There were 4 reports of macrophage activation syndrome in juvenile idiopathic arthritis clinical trials.

Undesirable effects in paediatric patients with plaque psoriasis

In a 48-week study in 211 children aged 4 to 17 years with paediatric plaque psoriasis, the adverse events reported were similar to those seen in previous studies in adults with plaque psoriasis.

4.9 Overdose

No dose-limiting toxicities were observed during clinical trials of rheumatoid arthritis patients. The highest dose level evaluated has been an intravenous loading dose of 32 mg/m^2 followed by subcutaneous doses of 16 mg/m^2 administered twice weekly. One rheumatoid arthritis patient mistakenly self-administered 62 mg Enbrel subcutaneously twice weekly for 3 weeks without experiencing undesirable effects. There is no known antidote to Enbrel.

5. PHARMACOLOGICAL PROPERTIES

5.1 Pharmacodynamic properties

Pharmacotherapeutic group: Tumor Necrosis Factor alpha (TNF-α) inhibitors, ATC code: L04AB01

Tumour necrosis factor (TNF) is a dominant cytokine in the inflammatory process of rheumatoid arthritis. Elevated levels of TNF are also found in the synovium and psoriatic plaques of patients with psoriatic arthritis and in serum and synovial tissue of patients with ankylosing spondylitis. In plaque psoriasis, infiltration by inflammatory cells including T-cells leads to increased TNF levels in psoriatic lesions compared with levels in uninvolved skin. Etanercept is a competitive inhibitor of TNF-binding to its cell surface receptors and thereby inhibits the biological activity of TNF. TNF and lymphotoxin are pro-inflammatory cytokines that bind to two distinct cell surface receptors: the 55-kilodalton (p55) and 75-kilodalton (p75) tumour necrosis factor receptors (TNFRs). Both TNFRs exist naturally in membrane-bound and soluble forms. Soluble TNFRs are thought to regulate TNF biological activity.

TNF and lymphotoxin exist predominantly as homotrimers, with their biological activity dependent on cross-linking of cell surface TNFRs. Dimeric soluble receptors such as etanercept possess a higher affinity for TNF than monomeric receptors and are considerably more potent competitive inhibitors of TNF binding to its cellular receptors. In addition, use of an immunoglobulin Fc region as a fusion element in the construction of a dimeric receptor imparts a longer serum half-life.

Mechanism of action

Much of the joint pathology in rheumatoid arthritis and ankylosing spondylitis and skin pathology in plaque psoriasis is mediated by pro-inflammatory molecules that are linked in a network controlled by TNF. The mechanism of action of etanercept is thought to be its competitive inhibition of TNF binding to cell surface TNFR, preventing TNF-mediated cellular responses by rendering TNF biologically inactive. Etanercept may also modulate biologic responses controlled by additional downstream molecules (e.g., cytokines, adhesion molecules, or proteinases) that are induced or regulated by TNF.

Figure 1 RADIOGRAPHIC PROGRESSION: COMPARISON OF ENBREL vs METHOTREXATE IN PATIENTS WITH RA OF <3 YEARS DURATION

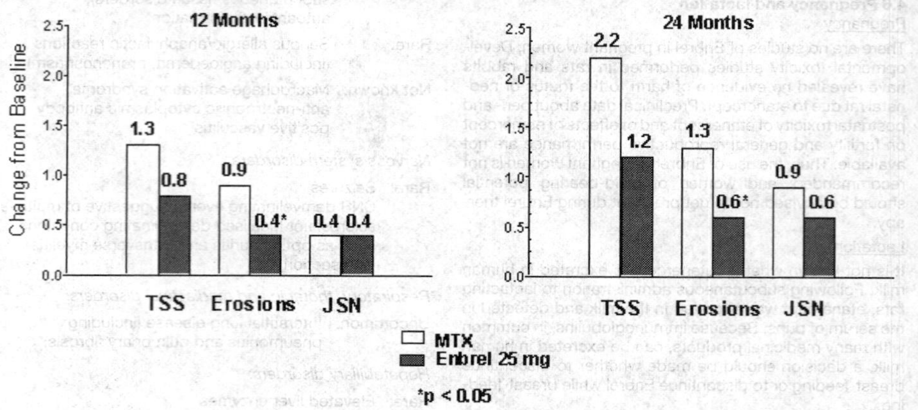

Clinical trials

This section presents data from four randomised controlled trials in adults with rheumatoid arthritis, one study in polyarticular juvenile idiopathic arthritis, one study in adults with psoriatic arthritis, one study in adults with ankylosing spondylitis, one study in paediatric patients with plaque psoriasis, and four studies in adults with plaque psoriasis.

Adult patients with rheumatoid arthritis

The efficacy of Enbrel was assessed in a randomised, double-blind, placebo-controlled study. The study evaluated 234 adult patients with active rheumatoid arthritis who had failed therapy with at least one but no more than four disease-modifying antirheumatic drugs (DMARDs). Doses of 10 mg or 25 mg Enbrel or placebo were administered subcutaneously twice a week for 6 consecutive months. The results of this controlled trial were expressed in percentage improvement in rheumatoid arthritis using AmericanCollege of Rheumatology (ACR) response criteria.

ACR 20 and 50 responses were higher in patients treated with Enbrel at 3 and 6 months than in patients treated with placebo (ACR 20: Enbrel 62% and 59%, placebo 23% and 11% at 3 and 6 months respectively; ACR 50: Enbrel 41% and 40%, placebo 8% and 5% at months 3 and 6 respectively; $p<0.01$ Enbrel vs Placebo at all time points for both ACR 20 and ACR 50 responses).

Approximately 15% of subjects who received Enbrel achieved an ACR 70 response at month 3 and month 6 compared to fewer than 5% of subjects in the placebo arm. Among patients receiving Enbrel, the clinical responses generally appeared within 1 to 2 weeks after initiation of therapy and nearly always occurred by 3 months. A dose response was seen; results with 10 mg were intermediate between placebo and 25 mg. Enbrel was significantly better than placebo in all components of the ACR criteria as well as other measures of rheumatoid arthritis disease activity not included in the ACR response criteria, such as morning stiffness. A Health Assessment Questionnaire (HAQ), which included disability, vitality, mental health, general health status, and arthritis-associated health status subdomains, was administered every 3 months during the trial. All subdomains of the HAQ were improved in patients treated with Enbrel compared to controls at 3 and 6 months.

After discontinuation of Enbrel, symptoms of arthritis generally returned within a month. Re-introduction of treatment with Enbrel after discontinuations of up to 24 months resulted in the same magnitudes of responses as patients who received Enbrel without interruption of therapy based on results of open-label studies. Continued durable responses have been seen for up to 48 months in open-label extension treatment trials when patients received Enbrel without interruption; longer-term experience is not available.

The efficacy of Enbrel was compared to methotrexate in a third randomised, active-controlled study with blinded radiographic evaluations as a primary endpoint in 632 adult patients with active rheumatoid arthritis (<3 years duration) who had never received treatment with methotrexate. Doses of 10 mg or 25 mg Enbrel were administered SC twice a week for up to 24 months. Methotrexate doses were escalated from 7.5 mg/week to a maximum of 20 mg/week over the first 8 weeks of the trial and continued for up to 24 months. Clinical improvement including onset of action within 2 weeks with Enbrel 25 mg was similar to that seen in the previous trials, and was maintained for up to 24 months. At baseline, patients had a moderate degree of disability, with mean HAQ scores of 1.4 to 1.5. Treatment with Enbrel 25 mg resulted in substantial improvement at 12 months, with about 44% of patients achieving a normal HAQ score (less than 0.5). This benefit was maintained in Year 2 of this study.

In this study, structural joint damage was assessed radiographically and expressed as change in Total Sharp Score (TSS) and its components, the erosion score and joint space narrowing score (JSN). Radiographs of hands/wrists and feet were read at baseline and 6, 12, and 24 months. The 10 mg Enbrel dose had consistently less effect on structural damage than the 25 mg dose. Enbrel 25 mg was significantly superior to methotrexate for erosion scores at both 12 and 24 months. The differences in TSS and JSN were not statistically significant between methotrexate and Enbrel 25 mg. The results are shown in the figure below.

RADIOGRAPHIC PROGRESSION: COMPARISON OF ENBREL vs METHOTREXATE IN PATIENTS WITH RA OF <3 YEARS DURATION

(see Figure 1 above)

In another active-controlled, double-blind, randomised study, clinical efficacy, safety, and radiographic progression in RA patients treated with Enbrel alone (25 mg twice weekly), methotrexate alone (7.5 to 20 mg weekly, median dose 20 mg), and of the combination of Enbrel and methotrexate initiated concurrently were compared in 682 adult patients with active rheumatoid arthritis of 6 months to 20 years duration (median 5 years) who had a less than satisfactory response to at least 1 disease-modifying antirheumatic drug (DMARD) other than methotrexate.

Patients in the Enbrel in combination with methotrexate therapy group had significantly higher ACR 20, ACR 50, ACR 70 responses and improvement for DAS and HAQ scores at both 24 and 52 weeks than patients in either of the single therapy groups (results shown in table below). Significant advantages for Enbrel in combination with methotrexate compared with Enbrel monotherapy and methotrexate monotherapy were also observed after 24 months.

(see Table 1 on next page)

Radiographic progression at 12 months was significantly less in the Enbrel group than in the methotrexate group, while the combination was significantly better than either monotherapy at slowing radiographic progression (see figure below).

RADIOGRAPHIC PROGRESSION: COMPARISON OF ENBREL vs METHOTREXATE vs ENBREL IN COMBINATION WITH METHOTREXATE IN PATIENTS WITH RA OF 6 MONTHS TO 20 YEARS DURATION (12 MONTH RESULTS)

(see Figure 2 on next page)

Significant advantages for Enbrel in combination with methotrexate compared with Enbrel monotherapy and methotrexate monotherapy were also observed after 24 months. Similarly, the significant advantages for Enbrel monotherapy compared with methotrexate monotherapy were also observed after 24 months.

In an analysis in which all patients who dropped out of the study for any reason were considered to have progressed, the percentage of patients without progression (TSS change ⩽ 0.5) at 24 months was higher in the Enbrel in combination with methotrexate group compared with the Enbrel alone and methotrexate alone groups (62%, 50%, and 36%, respectively; $p<0.05$). The difference between Enbrel alone and methotrexate alone was also significant ($p<0.05$). Among patients who completed a full 24 months of therapy in the study, the non-progression rates were 78%, 70%, and 61%, respectively.

The safety and efficacy of 50 mg Enbrel (two 25 mg SC injections) administered once weekly were evaluated in a double-blind, placebo-controlled study of 420 patients with active RA. In this study, 53 patients received placebo, 214 patients received 50 mg Enbrel once weekly and 153 patients received 25 mg Enbrel twice weekly. The safety and efficacy profiles of the two Enbrel treatment regimens were comparable at week 8 in their effect on signs and symptoms of RA; data at week 16 did not show comparability (non-inferiority) between the two regimens.

Table 1

CLINICAL EFFICACY RESULTS AT 12 MONTHS: COMPARISON OF ENBREL vs METHOTREXATE vs ENBREL IN COMBINATION WITH METHOTREXATE IN PATIENTS WITH RA OF 6 MONTHS TO 20 YEARS DURATION			
Endpoint	Methotrexate (n = 228)	Enbrel (n = 223)	Enbrel + Methotrexate (n = 231)
ACR Responses[a]			
ACR 20	58.8%	65.5%	74.5% †,ϕ
ACR 50	36.4%	43.0%	63.2% †,ϕ
ACR 70	16.7%	22.0%	39.8% †,ϕ
DAS			
Baseline score[b]	5.5	5.7	5.5
Week 52 score[b]	3.0	3.0	2.3†,ϕ
Remission[c]	14%	18%	37%†,ϕ
HAQ			
Baseline	1.7	1.7	1.8
Week 52	1.1	1.0	0.8†,ϕ

a: Patients who did not complete 12 months in the study were considered to be non-responders.

b: Values for Disease Activity Score (DAS) are means.

c: Remission is defined as DAS <1.6

Pairwise comparison p-values: † = $p < 0.05$ for comparisons of Enbrel + methotrexate vs methotrexate and ϕ = $p < 0.05$ for comparisons of Enbrel + methotrexate vs Enbrel

Figure 2 RADIOGRAPHIC PROGRESSION: COMPARISON OF ENBREL vs METHOTREXATE vs ENBREL IN COMBINATION WITH METHOTREXATE IN PATIENTS WITH RA OF 6 MONTHS TO 20 YEARS DURATION (12 MONTH RESULTS)

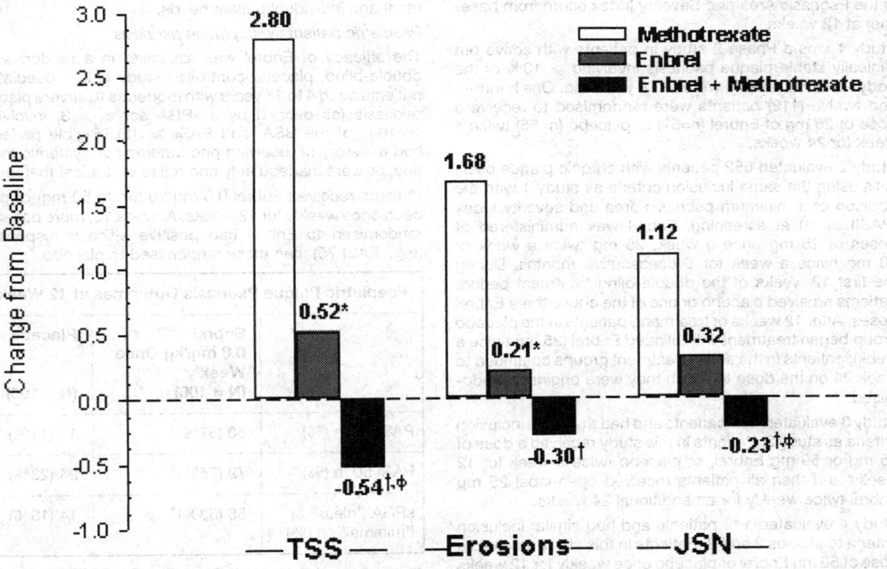

Pairwise comparison p-values: * = $p < 0.05$ for comparisons of Enbrel vs methotrexate, † = $p < 0.05$ for comparisons of Enbrel + methotrexate vs methotrexate and ϕ = $p < 0.05$ for comparisons of Enbrel + methotrexate vs Enbrel

Paediatric patients with polyarticular juvenile idiopathic arthritis

The safety and efficacy of Enbrel were assessed in a two-part study in 69 children with polyarticular juvenile idiopathic arthritis who had a variety of juvenile idiopathic arthritis onset types. Patients aged 4 to 17 years with moderately to severely active polyarticular juvenile idiopathic arthritis refractory to or intolerant of methotrexate were enrolled; patients remained on a stable dose of a single nonsteroidal anti-inflammatory drug and/or prednisone (< 0.2 mg/kg/day or 10 mg maximum). In part 1, all patients received 0.4 mg/kg (maximum 25 mg per dose) Enbrel subcutaneously twice weekly. In part 2, patients with a clinical response at day 90 were randomised to remain on Enbrel or receive placebo for four months and assessed for disease flare. Responses were measured using the JRA Definition of Improvement (DOI), defined as ⩾ 30% improvement in at least three of six and ⩾ 30% worsening in no more than one of six JRA core set criteria, including active joint count, limitation of motion, physician and patient/parent global assessments, functional assessment, and erythrocyte sedimentation rate (ESR). Disease flare was defined as a ⩾ 30% worsening in three of six JRA core set criteria and ⩾ 30% improvement in not more than one of the six JRA core set criteria and a minimum of two active joints.

In part 1 of the study, 51 of 69 (74%) patients demonstrated a clinical response and entered part 2. In part 2, 6 of 25 (24%) patients remaining on Enbrel experienced a disease flare compared to 20 of 26 (77%) patients receiving placebo (p=0.007). From the start of part 2, the median time to flare was ⩾ 116 days for patients who received Enbrel and 28 days for patients who received placebo. Of patients who demonstrated a clinical response at 90 days and entered part 2 of the study, some of the patients remaining on Enbrel continued to improve from month 3 through month 7, while those who received placebo did not improve.

Studies have not been done in patients with polyarticular juvenile idiopathic arthritis to assess the effects of continued Enbrel therapy in patients who do not respond within 3 months of initiating Enbrel therapy or to assess the combination of Enbrel with methotrexate.

Adult patients with psoriatic arthritis

The efficacy of Enbrel was assessed in a randomised, double-blind, placebo-controlled study in 205 patients with psoriatic arthritis. Patients were between 18 and 70 years of age and had active psoriatic arthritis (⩾ 3 swollen joints and ⩾ 3 tender joints) in at least one of the following forms: (1) distal interphalangeal (DIP) involvement; (2) polyarticular arthritis (absence of rheumatoid nodules and presence of psoriasis); (3) arthritis mutilans; (4) asymmetric psoriatic arthritis; or (5) spondylitis-like ankylosis. Patients also had plaque psoriasis with a qualifying target lesion ⩾ 2 cm in diameter. Patients had previously been treated with NSAIDs (86%), DMARDs (80%), and corticosteroids (24%). Patients currently on methotrexate therapy (stable for ⩾ 2 months) could continue at a stable dose of ⩽ 25 mg/week methotrexate. Doses of 25 mg Enbrel (based on dose-finding studies in patients with rheumatoid arthritis) or placebo were administered SC twice a week for 6 months. At the end of the double-blind study, patients could enter a long-term open-label extension study for a total duration of up to 2 years.

Clinical responses were expressed as percentages of patients achieving the ACR 20, 50, and 70 response and percentages with improvement in Psoriatic Arthritis Response Criteria (PsARC). Results are summarised in the Table below.

RESPONSES OF PATIENTS WITH PSORIATIC ARTHRITIS IN PLACEBO-CONTROLLED TRIAL		
	Percent of Patients	
	Placebo	Enbrel[a]
Psoriatic Arthritis Response	n = 104	n = 101
ACR 20		
Month 3	15	59[b]
Month 6	13	50[b]
ACR 50		
Month 3	4	38[b]
Month 6	4	37[b]
ACR 70		
Month 3	0	11[b]
Month 6	1	9[c]
PsARC		
Month 3	31	72[b]
Month 6	23	70[b]

a: 25 mg Enbrel SC twice weekly

b: $p < 0.001$, Enbrel vs. placebo

c: $p < 0.01$, Enbrel vs. placebo

Among patients with psoriatic arthritis who received Enbrel, the clinical responses were apparent at the time of the first visit (4 weeks) and were maintained through 6 months of therapy. Enbrel was significantly better than placebo in all measures of disease activity ($p < 0.001$), and responses were similar with and without concomitant methotrexate therapy. Quality of life in psoriatic arthritis patients was assessed at every timepoint using the disability index of the HAQ. The disability index score was significantly improved at all timepoints in psoriatic arthritis patients treated with Enbrel, relative to placebo ($p < 0.001$).

Radiographic changes were assessed in the psoriatic arthritis study. Radiographs of hands and wrists were obtained at baseline and months 6, 12, and 24. The modified TSS at 12 months is presented in the Table below. In an analysis in which all patients who dropped out of the study for any reason were considered to have progressed, the percentage of patients without progression (TSS change ⩽ 0.5) at 12 months was higher in the Enbrel group compared with the placebo group (73% vs. 47%, respectively, $p \leqslant 0.001$). The effect of Enbrel on radiographic progression was maintained in patients who continued on treatment during the second year. The slowing of peripheral joint damage was observed in patients with polyarticular symmetrical joint involvement.

MEAN (SE) ANNUALIZED CHANGE FROM BASELINE IN TOTAL SHARP SCORE		
	Placebo	Etanercept
Time	(n = 104)	(n = 101)
Month 12	1.00 (0.29)	-0.03 (0.09)[a]

SE = standard error.

a. p = 0.0001.

Enbrel treatment resulted in improvement in physical function during the double-blind period, and this benefit was maintained during the longer-term exposure of up to 2 years.

There is insufficient evidence of the efficacy of Enbrel in patients with ankylosing spondylitis-like and arthritis mutilans psoriatic arthropathies due to the small number of patients studied.

No study has been performed in patients with psoriatic arthritis using the 50mg once weekly dosing regimen. Evidence of efficacy for the once weekly dosing regimen

Table 2 RESPONSE OF PATIENTS WITH PSORIASIS IN STUDIES 2, 3 AND 4

Response (%)	Study 2					Study 3			Study 4		
	Placebo	Enbrel				Placebo	Enbrel		Placebo	Enbrel	
		25 mg BIW		50 mg BIW			25 mg BIW	50 mg BIW		50 mg QW	50 mg QW
	n = 166 wk 12	n = 162 wk 12	n = 162 wk 24[a]	n = 164 wk 12	n = 164 wk 24[a]	n = 193 wk 12	n = 196 wk 12	n = 196 wk 12	n = 46 wk 12	n = 96 wk 12	n = 90 wk 24[a]
PASI 50	14	58*	70	74*	77	9	64*	77*	9	69*	83
PASI 75	4	34*	44	49*	59	3	34*	49*	2	38*	71
DSGA [b], clear or almost clear	5	34*	39	49*	55	4	39*	57*	4	39*	64

*p ⩽ 0.0001 compared with placebo

a. No statistical comparisons to placebo were made at week 24 in studies 2 and 4 because the original placebo group began receiving Enbrel 25 mg BIW or 50 mg once weekly from week 13 to week 24.

b. Dermatologist Static Global Assessment. Clear or almost clear defined as 0 or 1 on a 0 to 5 scale.

in this patient population has been based on data from the study in patients with ankylosing spondylitis.

Adult patients with ankylosing spondylitis

The efficacy of Enbrel in ankylosing spondylitis was assessed in 3 randomised, double-blind studies comparing twice weekly administration of 25 mg Enbrel with placebo. A total of 401 patients were enrolled from which 203 were treated with Enbrel. The largest of these trials (n=277) enrolled patients who were between 18 and 70 years of age and had active ankylosing spondylitis defined as visual analog scale (VAS) scores of ⩾ 30 for average of duration and intensity of morning stiffness plus VAS scores of ⩾ 30 for at least 2 of the following 3 parameters: patient global assessment; average of VAS values for nocturnal back pain and total back pain; average of 10 questions on the Bath Ankylosing Spondylitis Functional Index (BASFI). Patients receiving DMARDs, NSAIDS, or corticosteroids could continue them on stable doses. Patients with complete ankylosis of the spine were not included in the study. Doses of 25 mg of Enbrel (based on dose-finding studies in patients with rheumatoid arthritis) or placebo were administered subcutaneously twice a week for 6 months in 138 patients.

The primary measure of efficacy (ASAS 20) was a ⩾20% improvement in at least 3 of the 4 Assessment in Ankylosing Spondylitis (ASAS) domains (patient global assessments, back pain, BASFI, and inflammation) and absence of deterioration in the remaining domain. ASAS 50 and 70 responses used the same criteria with a 50% improvement or a 70% improvement, respectively.

Compared to placebo, treatment with Enbrel resulted in significant improvements in the ASAS 20, ASAS 50 and ASAS 70 as early as 2 weeks after the initiation of therapy.

RESPONSES OF PATIENTS WITH ANKYLOSING SPONDYLITIS IN A PLACEBO-CONTROLLED TRIAL

	Percent of Patients	
Ankylosing Spondylitis Response	Placebo N = 139	Enbrel N = 138
ASAS 20		
2 weeks	22	46[a]
3 months	27	60[a]
6 months	23	58[a]
ASAS 50		
2 weeks	7	24[a]
3 months	13	45[a]
6 months	10	42[a]
ASAS 70:		
2 weeks	2	12[b]
3 months	7	29[b]
6 months	5	28[b]

a: p<0.001, Enbrel vs. Placebo

b: p = 0.002, Enbrel vs. placebo

Among patients with ankylosing spondylitis who received Enbrel, the clinical responses were apparent at the time of the first visit (2 weeks) and were maintained through 6 months of therapy. Responses were similar in patients who were or were not receiving concomitant therapies at baseline.

Similar results were obtained in the 2 smaller ankylosing spondylitis trials.

In a fourth study, the safety and efficacy of 50 mg Enbrel (two 25 mg SC injections) administered once weekly vs 25 mg Enbrel administered twice weekly were evaluated in a double-blind, placebo-controlled study of 356 patients with active ankylosing spondylitis. The safety and efficacy profiles of the 50 mg once weekly and 25 mg twice weekly regimens were similar.

Adult patients with plaque psoriasis

Enbrel is recommended for use in patients as defined in section 4.1. Patients who "failed to respond to" in the target population is defined by insufficient response (PASI<50 or PGA less than good), or worsening of the disease while on treatment, and who were adequately dosed for a sufficiently long duration to assess response with at least each of the three major systemic therapies as available.

The efficacy of Enbrel versus other systemic therapies in patients with moderate to severe psoriasis (responsive to other systemic therapies) has not been evaluated in studies directly comparing Enbrel with other systemic therapies. Instead, the safety and efficacy of Enbrel were assessed in four randomised, double-blind, placebo-controlled studies. The primary efficacy endpoint in all four studies was the proportion of patients in each treatment group who achieved the PASI 75 (i.e. at least a 75% improvement in the Psoriasis Area and Severity Index score from baseline) at 12 weeks.

Study 1 was a Phase 2 study in patients with active but clinically stable plaque psoriasis involving ⩾ 10% of the body surface area that were ⩾ 18 years old. One hundred and twelve (112) patients were randomised to receive a dose of 25 mg of Enbrel (n=57) or placebo (n=55) twice a week for 24 weeks.

Study 2 evaluated 652 patients with chronic plaque psoriasis using the same inclusion criteria as study 1 with the addition of a minimum psoriasis area and severity index (PASI) of 10 at screening. Enbrel was administered at doses of 25 mg once a week, 25 mg twice a week or 50 mg twice a week for 6 consecutive months. During the first 12 weeks of the double-blind treatment period, patients received placebo or one of the above three Enbrel doses. After 12 weeks of treatment, patients in the placebo group began treatment with blinded Enbrel (25 mg twice a week); patients in the active treatment groups continued to week 24 on the dose to which they were originally randomised.

Study 3 evaluated 583 patients and had the same inclusion criteria as study 2. Patients in this study received a dose of 25 mg or 50 mg Enbrel, or placebo twice a week for 12 weeks and then all patients received open-label 25 mg Enbrel twice weekly for an additional 24 weeks.

Study 4 evaluated 142 patients and had similar inclusion criteria to studies 2 and 3. Patients in this study received a dose of 50 mg Enbrel or placebo once weekly for 12 weeks and then all patients received open-label 50 mg Enbrel once weekly for an additional 12 weeks.

In study 1, the Enbrel-treated group had a significantly higher proportion of patients with a PASI 75 response at week 12 (30%) compared to the placebo-treated group (2%) (p<0.0001). At 24 weeks, 56% of patients in the Enbrel-treated group had achieved the PASI 75 compared to 5% of placebo-treated patients. Key results of studies 2, 3 and 4 are shown below.

(see Table 2 above)

Among patients with plaque psoriasis who received Enbrel, significant responses relative to placebo were apparent at the time of the first visit (2 weeks) and were maintained through 24 weeks of therapy.

Study 2 also had a drug withdrawal period during which patients who achieved a PASI improvement of at least 50% at week 24 had treatment stopped. Patients were observed off treatment for the occurrence of rebound (PASI ⩾150% of baseline) and for the time to relapse (defined as a loss of at least half of the improvement achieved between baseline and week 24). During the withdrawal period, symptoms of psoriasis gradually returned with a median time to disease relapse of 3 months. No rebound flare of disease and no psoriasis-related serious adverse events were observed. There was some evidence to support a benefit of re-treatment with Enbrel in patients initially responding to treatment.

In study 3, the majority of patients (77%) who were initially randomised to 50 mg twice weekly and had their Enbrel dose decreased at week 12 to 25 mg twice weekly maintained their PASI 75 response through week 36. For patients who received 25 mg twice weekly throughout the study, the PASI 75 response continued to improve between weeks 12 and 36.

In study 4, the Enbrel-treated group had a higher proportion of patients with PASI 75 at week 12 (38%) compared to the placebo-treated group (2%) (p<0.0001). For patients who received 50 mg once weekly throughout the study, the efficacy responses continued to improve with 71% achieving PASI 75 at week 24.

In long-term (up to 34 months) open-label studies where Enbrel was given without interruption, clinical responses were sustained and safety was comparable to shorter-term studies.

An analysis of clinical trial data did not reveal any baseline disease characteristics that would assist clinicians in selecting the most appropriate dosing option (intermittent or continuous). Consequently, the choice of intermittent or continuous therapy should be based upon physician judgment and individual patient needs.

Paediatric patients with plaque psoriasis

The efficacy of Enbrel was assessed in a randomised, double-blind, placebo-controlled study in 211 paediatric patients aged 4 to 17 years with moderate to severe plaque psoriasis (as defined by a sPGA score ⩾ 3, involving ⩾ 10% of the BSA, and PASI ⩾ 12). Eligible patients had a history of receiving phototherapy or systemic therapy, or were inadequately controlled on topical therapy.

Patients received Enbrel 0.8 mg/kg (up to 50 mg) or placebo once weekly for 12 weeks. At week 12, more patients randomised to Enbrel had positive efficacy responses (e.g., PASI 75) than those randomised to placebo.

Paediatric Plaque Psoriasis Outcomes at 12 Weeks

	Enbrel 0.8 mg/kg Once Weekly (N = 106)	Placebo (N = 105)
PASI 75, n (%)	60 (57%)[a]	12 (11%)
PASI 50, n (%)	79 (75%)[a]	24 (23%)
sPGA "clear" or "minimal", n (%)	56 (53%)[a]	14 (13%)

Abbreviation: sPGA-static Physician Global Assessment.

a. p < 0.0001 compared with placebo.

After the 12-week double-blind treatment period, all patients received Enbrel 0.8 mg/kg (up to 50 mg) once weekly for additional 24 weeks. Responses observed during the open-label period were similar to those observed in the double-blind period.

During a randomised withdrawal period, significantly more patients re-randomised to placebo experienced disease relapse (loss of PASI 75 response) compared with patients re-randomised to Enbrel. With continued therapy, responses were maintained up to 48 weeks.

Antibodies to Enbrel

Antibodies to etanercept have been detected in the sera of some subjects treated with etanercept. These antibodies have all been non-neutralising and are generally transient. There appears to be no correlation between antibody development and clinical response or adverse events.

In subjects treated with approved doses of etanercept in clinical trials for up to 12 months, cumulative rates of anti-etanercept antibodies were approximately 6% of subjects with rheumatoid arthritis, 7.5% of subjects with psoriatic arthritis, 2% of subjects with ankylosing spondylitis, 7% of subjects with psoriasis, 9.7% of subjects with paediatric psoriasis, and 3% of subjects with juvenile idiopathic arthritis.

The proportion of subjects who developed antibodies to etanercept in longer-term trials (of up to 3.5 years) increases over time, as expected. However, due to their transient nature, the incidence of antibodies detected at each assessment point was typically less than 7% in rheumatoid arthritis subjects and psoriasis subjects.

In a long-term psoriasis study in which patients received 50 mg twice weekly for 96 weeks, the incidence of antibodies observed at each assessment point was up to approximately 9%.

5.2 Pharmacokinetic properties

Etanercept serum values were determined by an ELISA method, which may detect ELISA-reactive degradation products as well as the parent compound.

Etanercept is slowly absorbed from the site of subcutaneous injection, reaching maximum concentration approximately 48 hours after a single dose. The absolute bioavailability is 76%. With twice weekly doses, it is anticipated that steady-state concentrations are approximately twice as high as those observed after single doses. After a single subcutaneous dose of 25 mg Enbrel, the average maximum serum concentration observed in healthy volunteers was 1.65 ± 0.66 μg/ml, and the area under the curve was 235 ± 96.6 μg•hr/ml. Dose proportionality has not been formally evaluated, but there is no apparent saturation of clearance across the dosing range.

A biexponential curve is required to describe the concentration time curve of etanercept. The central volume of distribution of etanercept is 7.6 l, while the volume of distribution at steady-state is 10.4 l. Etanercept is cleared slowly from the body. The half-life is long, approximately 70 hours. Clearance is approximately 0.066 l/hr in patients with rheumatoid arthritis, somewhat lower than the value of 0.11 l/hr observed in healthy volunteers. Additionally, the pharmacokinetics of Enbrel in rheumatoid arthritis patients, ankylosing spondylitis and plaque psoriasis patients are similar.

Mean serum concentration profiles at steady state in treated RA patients were Cmax of 2.4 mg/l vs 2.6 mg/l, Cmin of 1.2 mg/l vs 1.4 mg/l and partial AUC of 297 mgh/l vs 316 mgh/l for 50 mg Enbrel once weekly (n=21) vs 25 mg Enbrel twice weekly (n=16), respectively. In an open-label, single-dose, two-treatment, crossover study in healthy volunteers, etanercept administered as a single 50 mg/ml injection was found to be bioequivalent to two simultaneous injections of 25 mg/ml.

In a population pharmacokinetics analysis in ankylosing spondylitis patients the etanercept steady state AUCs were 466 μg•hr/ml and 474 μg•hr/ml for 50 mg Enbrel once weekly (N= 154) and 25 mg twice weekly (N = 148), respectively.

Although there is elimination of radioactivity in urine after administration of radiolabelled etanercept to patients and volunteers, increased etanercept concentrations were not observed in patients with acute renal or hepatic failure. The presence of renal and hepatic impairment should not require a change in dosage. There is no apparent pharmacokinetic difference between males and females.

Methotrexate has no effect on the pharmacokinetics of etanercept. The effect of Enbrel on the human pharmacokinetics of methotrexate has not been investigated.

Special populations

Elderly patients

The impact of advanced age was studied in the population pharmacokinetic analysis of etanercept serum concentrations. Clearance and volume estimates in patients aged 65 to 87 years were similar to estimates in patients less than 65 years of age.

Paediatric patients with polyarticular juvenile idiopathic arthritis

In a polyarticular juvenile idiopathic arthritis trial with Enbrel, 69 patients (aged 4 to 17 years) were administered 0.4 mg Enbrel/kg twice weekly for three months. Serum concentration profiles were similar to those seen in adult rheumatoid arthritis patients. The youngest children (4 years of age) had reduced clearance (increased clearance when normalised by weight) compared with older children (12 years of age) and adults. Simulation of dosing suggests that while older children (10-17 years of age) will have serum levels close to those seen in adults, younger children will have appreciably lower levels.

Paediatric patients with plaque psoriasis

Patients with paediatric plaque psoriasis (aged 4 to 17 years) were administered 0.8 mg/kg (up to a maximum dose of 50 mg per week) of etanercept once weekly for up to 48 weeks. The mean serum steady state trough concentrations ranged from 1.6 to 2.1 mcg/ml at weeks 12, 24, and 48. These mean concentrations in patients with paediatric plaque psoriasis were similar to the concentrations observed in patients with juvenile idiopathic arthritis (treated with 0.4 mg/kg etanercept twice weekly, up to maximum dose of 50 mg per week). These mean concentrations were similar to those seen in adult patients with plaque psoriasis treated with 25 mg etanercept twice weekly.

5.3 Preclinical safety data

In the toxicological studies with Enbrel, no dose-limiting or target organ toxicity was evident. Enbrel was considered to be non-genotoxic from a battery of *in vitro* and *in vivo* studies. Carcinogenicity studies, and standard assessments of fertility and postnatal toxicity, were not performed with Enbrel due to the development of neutralising antibodies in rodents.

Enbrel did not induce lethality or notable signs of toxicity in mice or rats following a single subcutaneous dose of 2000 mg/kg or a single intravenous dose of 1000 mg/kg. Enbrel did not elicit dose-limiting or target organ toxicity in cynomolgus monkeys following twice weekly subcutaneous administration for 4 or 26 consecutive weeks at a dose (15 mg/kg) that resulted in AUC-based serum drug concentrations that were over 27-fold higher than that obtained in humans at the recommended dose of 25 mg.

6. PHARMACEUTICAL PARTICULARS

6.1 List of excipients

Powder:

Mannitol

Sucrose

Trometamol.

Solvent:

Water for injections

6.2 Incompatibilities

In the absence of compatibility studies, this medicinal product must not be mixed with other medicinal products.

6.3 Shelf life

3 years.

After reconstitution, immediate use is recommended. Chemical and physical stability has been demonstrated for 48 hours at 2°– 8°C. From a microbiological point of view, the product should be used immediately. If not used immediately, storage times are the responsibility of the user and should normally not be longer than 6 hours at 2°– 8°C, unless reconstitution has taken place in controlled and validated aseptic conditions.

6.4 Special precautions for storage

Store in a refrigerator (2°C – 8°C). Do not freeze.

For storage conditions of the reconstituted medicinal product see section 6.3.

6.5 Nature and contents of container

Clear glass vial (4 ml, type I glass) with rubber stoppers, aluminium seals, and flip-off plastic caps. Enbrel is supplied with pre-filled syringes containing water for injections. The syringes are type I glass.

Cartons contain 4, 8 or 24 vials of Enbrel with 4, 8 or 24 pre-filled solvent syringes, 4, 8 or 24 needles, 4, 8 or 24 vial adaptors and 8, 16 or 48 alcohol swabs. Not all pack sizes may be marketed.

6.6 Special precautions for disposal and other handling

Any unused product or waste material should be disposed of in accordance with local requirements.

Instructions for use and handling

Enbrel is reconstituted with 1 ml water for injections before use, and administered by subcutaneous injection. Enbrel contains no antibacterial preservative, and therefore, solutions prepared with water for injections should be administered as soon as possible and within 6 hours following reconstitution. The solution should be clear and colourless to pale yellow with no lumps, flakes or particles. Some white foam may remain in the vial – this is normal. Enbrel should not be used if all the powder in the vial is not dissolved within 10 minutes. Start again with another vial.

Comprehensive instructions for the preparation and administration of the reconstituted Enbrel vial are given in the package leaflet, section 7, "Instructions for preparation and giving an injection of Enbrel."

7. MARKETING AUTHORISATION HOLDER

Wyeth Europa Ltd.

Huntercombe Lane South

Taplow, Maidenhead

Berkshire, SL6 0PH

United Kingdom

8. MARKETING AUTHORISATION NUMBER(S)

EU/1/99/126/003

9. DATE OF FIRST AUTHORISATION/RENEWAL OF THE AUTHORISATION

Date of first authorisation: 3 February 2000

Date of last renewal: 3 February 2005

10. DATE OF REVISION OF THE TEXT

16 July 2009

Detailed information on this product is available on the website of the European Medicines Agency (EMEA) http://www.emea.europa.eu

Enbrel 25mg solution for injection in pre-filled syringe

(Wyeth Pharmaceuticals)

1. NAME OF THE MEDICINAL PRODUCT

Enbrel®▼25 mg solution for injection in pre-filled syringe.

2. QUALITATIVE AND QUANTITATIVE COMPOSITION

Each pre-filled syringe contains 25 mg of etanercept.

Etanercept is a human tumour necrosis factor receptor p75 Fc fusion protein produced by recombinant DNA technology in a Chinese hamster ovary (CHO) mammalian expression system. Etanercept is a dimer of a chimeric protein genetically engineered by fusing the extracellular ligand binding domain of human tumour necrosis factor receptor-2 (TNFR2/p75) to the Fc domain of human IgG1. This Fc component contains the hinge, CH_2 and CH_3 regions but not the CH_1 region of IgG1. Etanercept contains 934 amino acids and has an apparent molecular weight of approximately 150 kilodaltons. The potency is determined by measuring the ability of etanercept to neutralise the TNFα-mediated growth inhibition of A375 cells. The specific activity of etanercept is 1.7×10^6 units/mg.

For a full list of excipients, see section 6.1.

3. PHARMACEUTICAL FORM

Solution for injection.

The solution is clear, and colourless or pale yellow.

4. CLINICAL PARTICULARS

4.1 Therapeutic indications

Rheumatoid arthritis

Enbrel in combination with methotrexate is indicated for the treatment of moderate to severe active rheumatoid arthritis in adults when the response to disease-modifying antirheumatic drugs, including methotrexate (unless contraindicated), has been inadequate.

Enbrel can be given as monotherapy in case of intolerance to methotrexate or when continued treatment with methotrexate is inappropriate.

Enbrel is also indicated in the treatment of severe, active and progressive rheumatoid arthritis in adults not previously treated with methotrexate.

Enbrel, alone or in combination with methotrexate, has been shown to reduce the rate of progression of joint damage as measured by X-ray and to improve physical function.

Polyarticular juvenile idiopathic arthritis

Treatment of active polyarticular juvenile idiopathic arthritis in children and adolescents from the age of 4 years who have had an inadequate response to, or who have proved intolerant of, methotrexate. Enbrel has not been studied in children aged less than 4 years.

Psoriatic arthritis

Treatment of active and progressive psoriatic arthritis in adults when the response to previous disease-modifying antirheumatic drug therapy has been inadequate. Enbrel has been shown to improve physical function in patients with psoriatic arthritis, and to reduce the rate of progression of peripheral joint damage as measured by X-ray in patients with polyarticular symmetrical subtypes of the disease.

Ankylosing spondylitis

Treatment of adults with severe active ankylosing spondylitis who have had an inadequate response to conventional therapy.

Plaque psoriasis

Treatment of adults with moderate to severe plaque psoriasis who failed to respond to, or who have a contraindication to, or are intolerant to other systemic therapy including ciclosporin, methotrexate or PUVA (see section 5.1).

Paediatric plaque psoriasis

Treatment of chronic severe plaque psoriasis in children and adolescents from the age of 8 years who are inadequately controlled by, or are intolerant to, other systemic therapies or phototherapies.

4.2 Posology and method of administration

Enbrel treatment should be initiated and supervised by specialist physicians experienced in the diagnosis and treatment of rheumatoid arthritis, juvenile idiopathic arthritis, psoriatic arthritis, ankylosing spondylitis, plaque psoriasis or paediatric plaque psoriasis. Patients treated with Enbrel should be given the Patient Alert Card.

Enbrel is available in strengths of 25 and 50 mg.

Posology

Rheumatoid arthritis

25 mg Enbrel administered twice weekly is the recommended dose. Alternatively, 50 mg administered once weekly has been shown to be safe and effective (see section 5.1).

Psoriatic arthritis and ankylosing spondylitis

The recommended dose is 25 mg Enbrel administered twice weekly, or 50 mg administered once weekly.

Plaque psoriasis

The recommended dose of Enbrel is 25 mg administered twice weekly or 50 mg administered once weekly. Alternatively, 50 mg given twice weekly may be used for up to 12 weeks followed, if necessary, by a dose of 25 mg twice weekly or 50 mg once weekly. Treatment with Enbrel should continue until remission is achieved, for up to 24 weeks. Continuous therapy beyond 24 weeks may be appropriate for some adult patients (see section 5.1). Treatment should be discontinued in patients who show no response after 12 weeks. If re-treatment with Enbrel is indicated, the same guidance on treatment duration should be followed. The dose should be 25 mg twice weekly or 50 mg once weekly.

Special populations

Elderly patients (⩾ 65 years)

No dose adjustment is required. Posology and administration are the same as for adults 18-64 years of age.

Paediatric use

Enbrel is available as a single use syringe for patients weighing 62.5 kg or more. Lyophilized vials containing a reconstituted dose of 25 mg/ml are available from which doses less than 25 mg can be administered.

Juvenile idiopathic arthritis (age 4 years and above)

0.4 mg/kg (up to a maximum of 25 mg per dose) given twice weekly as a subcutaneous injection with an interval of 3-4 days between doses.

Paediatric plaque psoriasis (age 8 years and above)

0.8 mg/kg (up to a maximum of 50 mg per dose) once weekly for up to 24 weeks. Treatment should be discontinued in patients who show no response after 12 weeks.

If re-treatment with Enbrel is indicated, the above guidance on treatment duration should be followed. The dose should be 0.8 mg/kg (up to a maximum of 50 mg per dose) once weekly.

Renal and hepatic impairment

No dose adjustment is required.

Method of administration

Comprehensive instructions for administration are given in the package leaflet, section 7, "Instructions for preparation and giving an injection of Enbrel."

4.3 Contraindications

Hypersensitivity to the active substance or to any of the excipients.

Sepsis or risk of sepsis.

Treatment with Enbrel should not be initiated in patients with active infections including chronic or localised infections.

4.4 Special warnings and precautions for use

Infections

Patients should be evaluated for infections before, during, and after treatment with Enbrel, taking into consideration that the mean elimination half-life of etanercept is approximately 70 hours (range 7 to 300 hours).

Serious infections, sepsis, tuberculosis, and opportunistic infections, including invasive fungal infections, have been reported with the use of Enbrel (see section 4.8). These infections were due to bacteria, mycobacteria, fungi and viruses. In some cases, particular fungal and other opportunistic infections have not been recognised, resulting in delay of appropriate treatment and sometimes death. In evaluating patients for infections, the patient's risk for relevant opportunistic infections (e.g., exposure to endemic mycoses) should be considered.

Patients who develop a new infection while undergoing treatment with Enbrel should be monitored closely. **Administration of Enbrel should be discontinued if a patient develops a serious infection.** Physicians should exercise caution when considering the use of Enbrel in patients with a history of recurring or chronic infections or with underlying conditions that may predispose patients to infections such as advanced or poorly controlled diabetes.

Tuberculosis

Cases of active tuberculosis including miliary tuberculosis and tuberculosis with extra-pulmonary location have been reported in patients treated with Enbrel.

Before starting treatment with Enbrel, all patients must be evaluated for both active and inactive ('latent') tuberculosis. This evaluation should include a detailed medical history with personal history of tuberculosis or possible previous contact with tuberculosis and previous and/or current immunosuppressive therapy. Appropriate screening tests, i.e. tuberculin skin test and chest x-ray, should be performed in all patients (local recommendations may apply). It is recommended that the conduct of these tests should be recorded in the patient's alert card. Prescribers are reminded of the risk of false negative tuberculin skin test results, especially in patients who are severely ill or immunocompromised.

If active tuberculosis is diagnosed, Enbrel therapy must not be initiated. If inactive ('latent') tuberculosis is diagnosed, treatment for latent tuberculosis must be started with anti-tuberculosis therapy before the initiation of Enbrel, and in accordance with local recommendations. In this situation, the benefit/risk balance of Enbrel therapy should be very carefully considered.

All patients should be informed to seek medical advice if signs/symptoms suggestive of tuberculosis (e.g., persistent cough, wasting/weight loss, low-grade fever) appear during or after Enbrel treatment.

Hepatitis B virus reactivation

Reactivation of hepatitis B virus (HBV) in patients who are chronic carriers of this virus who are receiving TNF-antagonists including Enbrel has been reported. Patients at risk for HBV infection should be evaluated for prior evidence of HBV infection before initiating Enbrel therapy. Caution should be exercised when administering Enbrel to patients identified as carriers of HBV. If Enbrel is used in carriers of HBV, the patients should be monitored for signs and symptoms of active HBV infection and, if necessary, appropriate treatment should be initiated.

Worsening of hepatitis C

There have been reports of worsening of hepatitis C in patients receiving Enbrel.

Concurrent treatment with anakinra

Concurrent administration of Enbrel and anakinra has been associated with an increased risk of serious infections and neutropenia compared to Enbrel alone. This combination has not demonstrated increased clinical benefit. Thus the combined use of Enbrel and anakinra is not recommended (see sections 4.5 and 4.8).

Concurrent treatment with abatacept

In clinical studies, concurrent administration of abatacept and Enbrel resulted in increased incidences of serious adverse events. This combination has not demonstrated increased clinical benefit; such use is not recommended (see section 4.5).

Allergic reactions

Allergic reactions associated with Enbrel administration have been reported commonly. Allergic reactions have included angioedema and urticaria; serious reactions have occurred. If any serious allergic or anaphylactic reaction occurs, Enbrel therapy should be discontinued immediately and appropriate therapy initiated.

The needle cover of the pre-filled syringe contains latex (dry natural rubber) that may cause hypersensitivity reactions when handled by or when Enbrel is administered to persons with known or possible latex sensitivity.

Immunosuppression

The possibility exists for TNF-antagonists, including Enbrel, to affect host defences against infections and malignancies since TNF mediates inflammation and modulates cellular immune responses. In a study of 49 adult patients with rheumatoid arthritis treated with Enbrel, there was no evidence of depression of delayed-type hypersensitivity, depression of immunoglobulin levels, or change in enumeration of effector cell populations.

Two juvenile idiopathic arthritis patients developed varicella infection and signs and symptoms of aseptic meningitis, which resolved without sequelae. Patients with a significant exposure to varicella virus should temporarily discontinue Enbrel therapy and be considered for prophylactic treatment with Varicella Zoster Immune Globulin.

The safety and efficacy of Enbrel in patients with immunosuppression or chronic infections have not been evaluated.

Malignancies and lymphoproliferative disorders

Solid and haematopoietic malignancies

Reports of various malignancies (including breast and lung carcinoma and lymphoma) have been received in the post-marketing period (see section 4.8).

In the controlled portions of clinical trials of TNF-antagonists, more cases of lymphoma have been observed among patients receiving a TNF-antagonist compared with control patients. However, the occurrence was rare, and the follow-up period of placebo patients was shorter than for patients receiving TNF-antagonist therapy. Furthermore, there is an increased background lymphoma risk in rheumatoid arthritis patients with long-standing, highly active, inflammatory disease, which complicates the risk estimation. With the current knowledge, a possible risk for the development of lymphomas or other malignancies in patients treated with a TNF-antagonist cannot be excluded.

Non-melanoma skin cancer (NMSC)

Non-melanoma skin cancer has been reported in patients treated with TNF-antagonists, including Enbrel. Combining the results of placebo- and active comparator-controlled clinical trials of Enbrel, more cases of NMSC were observed in patients receiving Enbrel compared with control patients, particularly in patients with psoriasis. Periodic skin examination is recommended for all patients who are at increased risk for NMSC (including patients with psoriasis or a history of PUVA therapy).

Vaccinations

Live vaccines should not be given concurrently with Enbrel. No data are available on the secondary transmission of infection by live vaccines in patients receiving Enbrel. It is recommended that juvenile idiopathic arthritis patients, if possible, be brought up to date with all immunisations in agreement with current immunisation guidelines prior to initiating Enbrel therapy. In a double blind, placebo controlled, randomised clinical study in adult patients with psoriatic arthritis 184 patients also received a multivalent pneumococcal polysaccharide vaccine at week 4. In this study most psoriatic arthritis patients receiving Enbrel were able to mount effective B-cell immune response to pneumococcal polysaccharide vaccine, but titers in aggregate were moderately lower and few patients had two-fold rises in titers compared to patients not receiving Enbrel. The clinical significance of this is unknown.

Autoantibody formation

Treatment with Enbrel may result in the formation of autoimmune antibodies (see section 4.8).

Haematologic reactions

Rare cases of pancytopenia and very rare cases of aplastic anaemia, some with fatal outcome, have been reported in patients treated with Enbrel. Caution should be exercised in patients being treated with Enbrel who have a previous history of blood dyscrasias. All patients and parents/caregivers should be advised that if the patient develops signs and symptoms suggestive of blood dyscrasias or infections (e.g. persistent fever, sore throat, bruising, bleeding, paleness) whilst on Enbrel, they should seek immediate medical advice. Such patients should be investigated urgently, including full blood count; if blood dyscrasias are confirmed, Enbrel should be discontinued.

CNS disorders

There have been rare reports of CNS demyelinating disorders in patients treated with Enbrel (see section 4.8). Although no clinical trials have been performed evaluating Enbrel therapy in patients with multiple sclerosis, clinical trials of other TNF antagonists in patients with multiple sclerosis have shown increases in disease activity. A careful risk/benefit evaluation, including a neurological assessment, is recommended when prescribing Enbrel to patients with pre-existing or recent onset of CNS demyelinating disease, or to those who are considered to have an increased risk of developing demyelinating disease.

Combination therapy

In a controlled clinical trial of two years duration in rheumatoid arthritis patients, the combination of Enbrel and methotrexate did not result in unexpected safety findings, and the safety profile of Enbrel when given in combination with methotrexate was similar to the profiles reported in studies of Enbrel and methotrexate alone. Long-term studies to assess the safety of the combination are ongoing. The long-term safety of Enbrel in combination with other disease-modifying antirheumatic drugs (DMARD) has not been established.

The use of Enbrel in combination with other systemic therapies or phototherapy for the treatment of psoriasis has not been studied.

Renal and hepatic impairment

Based on pharmacokinetic data (see section 5.2), no dose adjustment is needed in patients with renal or hepatic impairment; clinical experience in such patients is limited.

Congestive heart failure

Physicians should use caution when using Enbrel in patients who have congestive heart failure (CHF). There have been postmarketing reports of worsening of CHF, with and without identifiable precipitating factors, in patients taking Enbrel. Two large clinical trials evaluating the use of Enbrel in the treatment of CHF were terminated early due to lack of efficacy. Although not conclusive, data from one of these trials suggest a possible tendency toward worsening CHF in those patients assigned to Enbrel treatment.

Alcoholic hepatitis

In a phase II randomised placebo-controlled study of 48 hospitalised patients treated with Enbrel or placebo for moderate to severe alcoholic hepatitis, Enbrel was not efficacious, and the mortality rate in patients treated with Enbrel was significantly higher after 6 months. Consequently, Enbrel should not be used in patients for the treatment of alcoholic hepatitis. Physicians should use caution when using Enbrel in patients who also have moderate to severe alcoholic hepatitis.

Wegener's granulomatosis

A placebo-controlled trial, in which 89 adult patients were treated with Enbrel in addition to standard therapy (including cyclophosphamide or methotrexate, and glucocorticoids) for a median duration of 25 months, has not shown Enbrel to be an effective treatment for Wegener's granulomatosis. The incidence of non-cutaneous malignancies of various types was significantly higher in patients treated with Enbrel than in the control group. Enbrel is not recommended for the treatment of Wegener's granulomatosis.

4.5 Interaction with other medicinal products and other forms of interaction

Concurrent treatment with anakinra

Adult patients treated with Enbrel and anakinra were observed to have a higher rate of serious infection when compared with patients treated with either Enbrel or anakinra alone (historical data).

In addition, in a double-blind placebo-controlled trial in adult patients receiving background methotrexate, patients treated with Enbrel and anakinra were observed to have a higher rate of serious infections (7%) and neutropenia than patients treated with Enbrel (see sections 4.4 and 4.8). The combination Enbrel and anakinra has not demonstrated increased clinical benefit and is therefore not recommended.

Concurrent treatment with abatacept

In clinical studies, concurrent administration of abatacept and Enbrel resulted in increased incidences of serious adverse events. This combination has not demonstrated increased clinical benefit; such use is not recommended (see section 4.4).

Concurrent treatment with sulfasalazine

In a clinical study of adult patients who were receiving established doses of sulfasalazine, to which Enbrel was added, patients in the combination group experienced a statistically significant decrease in mean white blood cell counts in comparison to groups treated with Enbrel or sulfasalazine alone. The clinical significance of this interaction is unknown.

Non-interactions

In clinical trials, no interactions have been observed when Enbrel was administered with glucocorticoids, salicylates (except sulfasalazine), nonsteroidal anti-inflammatory drugs (NSAIDs), analgesics, or methotrexate. See section 4.4 for vaccination advice.

No clinically significant pharmacokinetic drug-drug interactions were observed in studies with digoxin or warfarin.

4.6 Pregnancy and lactation

Pregnancy

There are no studies of Enbrel in pregnant women. Developmental toxicity studies performed in rats and rabbits have revealed no evidence of harm to the foetus or neonatal rat due to etanercept. Preclinical data about peri- and postnatal toxicity of etanercept and of effects of etanercept on fertility and general reproductive performance are not available. Thus, the use of Enbrel in pregnant women is not recommended, and women of child-bearing potential should be advised not to get pregnant during Enbrel therapy.

Lactation

It is not known whether etanercept is excreted in human milk. Following subcutaneous administration to lactating rats, etanercept was excreted in the milk and detected in the serum of pups. Because immunoglobulins, in common with many medicinal products, can be excreted in human milk, a decision should be made whether to discontinue breast-feeding or to discontinue Enbrel while breast-feeding.

4.7 Effects on ability to drive and use machines

No studies on the effects on the ability to drive and use machines have been performed.

4.8 Undesirable effects

Undesirable effects in adults

Enbrel has been studied in 2,680 patients with rheumatoid arthritis in double-blind and open-label trials. This experience includes 2 placebo-controlled studies (349 Enbrel patients and 152 placebo patients) and 2 active-controlled trials, one active-controlled trial comparing Enbrel to methotrexate (415 Enbrel patients and 217 methotrexate patients) and another active-controlled trial comparing Enbrel (223 patients), methotrexate (228 patients) and Enbrel in combination with methotrexate (231 patients). The proportion of patients who discontinued treatment due to adverse events was the same in both the Enbrel and placebo treatment groups; in the first active-controlled trial, the dropout rate was significantly higher for methotrexate (10%) than for Enbrel (5%). In the second active-controlled trial, the rate of discontinuation for adverse events after 2 years of treatment was similar among all three treatment groups, Enbrel (16%), methotrexate (21%) and Enbrel in combination with methotrexate (17%). Additionally, Enbrel has been studied in 240 psoriatic arthritis patients who participated in 2 double-blind placebo-controlled studies and an open-label extension study. Five hundred and eight (508) ankylosing spondylitis patients were treated with Enbrel in 4 double-blind placebo-controlled studies. Enbrel has also been studied in 1,492 patients with plaque psoriasis for up to 6 months in 5 double-blind placebo-controlled studies.

In double-blind clinical trials comparing Enbrel to placebo, injection site reactions were the most frequent adverse events among Enbrel-treated patients. Among patients with rheumatoid arthritis treated in placebo-controlled trials, serious adverse events occurred at a frequency of 4% in 349 patients treated with Enbrel compared with 5% of 152 placebo-treated patients. In the first active-controlled trial, serious adverse events occurred at a frequency of 6% in 415 patients treated with Enbrel compared with 8% of 217 methotrexate-treated patients. In the second active-controlled trial the rate of serious adverse events after 2 years of treatment was similar among the three treatment groups (Enbrel 16%, methotrexate 15% and Enbrel in combination with methotrexate 17%). Among patients with plaque psoriasis treated in placebo-controlled trials, the frequency of serious adverse events was about 1.4% of 1,341 patients treated with Enbrel compared with 1.4% of 766 placebo-treated patients.

The following list of adverse reactions is based on experience from clinical trials in adults and on postmarketing experience.

Within the organ system classes, adverse reactions are listed under headings of frequency (number of patients expected to experience the reaction), using the following categories: very common (⩾1/10); common (⩾1/100, <1/10); uncommon (⩾1/1000, <1/100); rare (⩾1/10,000, <1/1000); very rare (<1/10,000); not known (cannot be estimated from the available data).

Infections and infestations:

Very common: Infections (including upper respiratory tract infections, bronchitis, cystitis, skin infections)*

Uncommon: Serious infections (including pneumonia, cellulitis, septic arthritis, sepsis)*

Rare: Tuberculosis, opportunistic infections (including invasive fungal, protozoal, bacterial and atypical mycobacterial infections)*

Blood and lymphatic system disorders:

Uncommon: Thrombocytopenia

Rare: Anaemia, leukopenia, neutropenia, pancytopenia*

Very rare: Aplastic anaemia*

Immune system disorders:

Common: Allergic reactions (see Skin and subcutaneous tissue disorders), autoantibody formation*

Rare: Serious allergic/anaphylactic reactions (including angioedema, bronchospasm)

Not known: Macrophage activation syndrome*, anti-neutrophilic cytoplasmic antibody positive vasculitis

Nervous system disorders:

Rare: Seizures
CNS demyelinating events suggestive of multiple sclerosis or localised demyelinating conditions such as optic neuritis and transverse myelitis (see section 4.4)

Respiratory, thoracic and mediastinal disorders:

Uncommon: Interstitial lung disease (including pneumonitis and pulmonary fibrosis)*

Hepatobiliary disorders:

Rare: Elevated liver enzymes

Skin and subcutaneous tissue disorders:

Common: Pruritus

Uncommon: Non-melanoma skin cancers (see section 4.4), angioedema, urticaria, rash, psoriasiform rash, psoriasis (including new onset and pustular, primarily palms and soles)

Rare: Cutaneous vasculitis (including leukocytoclastic vasculitis), Stevens-Johnson syndrome, erythema multiforme

Very rare: Toxic epidermal necrolysis

Musculoskeletal and connective tissue disorders:

Rare: Subacute cutaneous lupus erythematosus, discoid lupus erythematosus, lupus-like syndrome

General disorders and administration site conditions:

Very common: Injection site reactions (including bleeding, bruising, erythema, itching, pain, swelling)*

Common: Fever

Cardiac disorders:

There have been reports of worsening of congestive heart failure (see section 4.4).

*see Additional information, below.

Additional information

Serious adverse events reported in clinical trials

Among rheumatoid arthritis, psoriatic arthritis, ankylosing spondylitis and plaque psoriasis patients in placebo-controlled, active-controlled, and open-label trials of Enbrel, serious adverse events reported included malignancies (see below), asthma, infections (see below), heart failure, myocardial infarction, myocardial ischaemia, chest pain, syncope, cerebral ischaemia, hypertension, hypotension, cholecystitis, pancreatitis, gastrointestinal haemorrhage, bursitis, confusion, depression, dyspnoea, abnormal healing, renal insufficiency, kidney calculus, deep vein thrombosis, pulmonary embolism, membranous glomerulonephropathy, polymyositis, thrombophlebitis, liver damage, leucopenia, paresis, paresthesia, vertigo, allergic alveolitis, angioedema, scleritis, bone fracture, lymphadenopathy, ulcerative colitis, intestinal obstruction, eosinophilia, haematuria, and sarcoidosis.

Malignancies and lymphoproliferative disorders

One hundred and twenty-nine new malignancies of various types were observed in 4,114 rheumatoid arthritis patients treated in clinical trials with Enbrel for up to approximately 6 years, including 231 patients treated with Enbrel in combination with methotrexate in the 2-year active-controlled study. The observed rates and incidences in these clinical trials were similar to those expected for the population studied. A total of 2 malignancies were reported in clinical studies of approximately 2 years duration involving 240 Enbrel-treated psoriatic arthritis patients. In clinical studies conducted for more than 2 years with 351 ankylosing spondylitis patients, 6 malignancies were reported in Enbrel-treated patients. In a group of 2,711 plaque psoriasis patients treated with Enbrel in double-blind and open-label studies of up to 2.5 years, 30 malignancies and 43 nonmelanoma skin cancers were reported.

In a group of 7,416 patients treated with Enbrel in rheumatoid arthritis, psoriatic arthritis, ankylosing spondylitis and psoriasis clinical trials, 18 lymphomas were reported.

Reports of various malignancies (including breast and lung carcinoma and lymphoma) have also been received in the postmarketing period (see section 4.4).

Injection site reactions

Compared to placebo, patients with rheumatic diseases treated with Enbrel had a significantly higher incidence of injection site reactions (36% vs. 9%). Injection site reactions usually occurred in the first month. Mean duration was approximately 3 to 5 days. No treatment was given for the majority of injection site reactions in the Enbrel treatment groups, and the majority of patients who were given treatment received topical preparations such as corticosteroids, or oral antihistamines. Additionally, some patients developed recall injection site reactions characterised by a skin reaction at the most recent site of injection along with the simultaneous appearance of injection site reactions at previous injection sites. These reactions were generally transient and did not recur with treatment.

In controlled trials in patients with plaque psoriasis, approximately 13.6% of patients treated with Enbrel developed injection site reactions compared with 3.4% of placebo-treated patients during the first 12 weeks of treatment.

Serious infections

In placebo-controlled trials, no increase in the incidence of serious infections (fatal, life threatening, or requiring hospitalisation or intravenous antibiotics) was observed. Serious infections occurred in 6.3% of rheumatoid arthritis patients treated with Enbrel for up to 48 months. These included abscess (at various sites), bacteraemia, bronchitis, bursitis, cellulitis, cholecystitis, diarrhoea, diverticulitis, endocarditis (suspected), gastroenteritis, hepatitis B, herpes zoster, leg ulcer, mouth infection, osteomyelitis, otitis, peritonitis, pneumonia, pyelonephritis, sepsis, septic arthritis, sinusitis, skin infection, skin ulcer, urinary tract infection, vasculitis, and wound infection. In the 2-year active-controlled study where patients were treated with either Enbrel alone, methotrexate alone or Enbrel in combination with methotrexate, the rates of serious infections were similar among the treatment groups. However, it cannot be excluded that the combination of Enbrel with methotrexate could be associated with an increase in the rate of infections.

There were no differences in rates of infection among patients treated with Enbrel and those treated with placebo for plaque psoriasis in placebo controlled trials of up to 24 weeks duration. Serious infections experienced by Enbrel-treated patients included cellulitis, gastroenteritis, pneumonia, cholecystitis, osteomyelitis, gastritis, appendicitis, Streptococcal fasciitis, myositis, septic shock, diverticulitis and abscess. In the double-blind and open-label psoriatic arthritis trials, 1 patient reported a serious infection (pneumonia).

Serious and fatal infections have been reported during use of Enbrel; reported pathogens include bacteria, mycobacteria (including tuberculosis), viruses and fungi. Some have occurred within a few weeks after initiating treatment with Enbrel in patients who have underlying conditions (e.g. diabetes, congestive heart failure, history of active or chronic infections) in addition to their rheumatoid arthritis (see section 4.4). Enbrel treatment may increase mortality in patients with established sepsis.

Opportunistic infections have been reported in association with Enbrel including invasive fungal, protozoal, bacterial (including *Listeria* and *Legionella*), and atypical mycobacterial infections. In a pooled data set of clinical trials, the overall incidence of opportunistic infections was 0.09% for the 15,402 subjects who received Enbrel. The exposure-adjusted rate was 0.06 events per 100 patient-years. In postmarketing experience, approximately half of all of the case reports of opportunistic infections worldwide were invasive fungal infections. The most commonly reported invasive fungal infections were *Pneumocystis* and *Aspergillus*. Invasive fungal infections accounted for more than half of the fatalities amongst patients who developed opportunistic infections. The majority of the reports with a fatal outcome were in patients with *Pneumocystis* pneumonia, unspecified systemic fungal infections, and aspergillosis (see section 4.4).

Autoantibodies

Adult patients had serum samples tested for autoantibodies at multiple timepoints. Of the rheumatoid arthritis patients evaluated for antinuclear antibodies (ANA), the percentage of patients who developed new positive ANA (⩾1:40) was higher in patients treated with Enbrel (11%) than in placebo-treated patients (5%). The percentage of patients who developed new positive anti-double-stranded DNA antibodies was also higher by radioimmunoassay (15% of patients treated with Enbrel compared to 4% of placebo-treated patients) and by *Crithidia luciliae* assay (3% of patients treated with Enbrel compared to

For additional & updated information visit www.emc.medicines.org.uk

none of placebo-treated patients). The proportion of patients treated with Enbrel who developed anticardiolipin antibodies was similarly increased compared to placebo-treated patients. The impact of long-term treatment with Enbrel on the development of autoimmune diseases is unknown.

There have been rare reports of patients, including rheumatoid factor positive patients, who have developed other autoantibodies in conjunction with a lupus-like syndrome or rashes that are compatible with subacute cutaneous lupus or discoid lupus by clinical presentation and biopsy.

Pancytopenia and aplastic anaemia

There have been postmarketing reports of pancytopenia and aplastic anaemia, some of which had fatal outcomes (see section 4.4).

Interstitial lung disease

There have been postmarketing reports of interstitial lung disease (including pneumonitis and pulmonary fibrosis), some of which had fatal outcomes.

Laboratory evaluations

Based on the results of clinical studies, normally no special laboratory evaluations are necessary in addition to careful medical management and supervision of patients.

Concurrent treatment with anakinra

In studies when adult patients received concurrent treatment with Enbrel plus anakinra, a higher rate of serious infections compared to Enbrel alone was observed and 2% of patients (3/139) developed neutropenia (absolute neutrophil count < 1000 / mm3). While neutropenic, one patient developed cellulitis that resolved after hospitalisation (see sections 4.4 and 4.5).

Undesirable effects in paediatric patients with polyarticular juvenile idiopathic arthritis

In general, the adverse events in paediatric patients with juvenile idiopathic arthritis were similar in frequency and type to those seen in adult patients. Differences from adults and other special considerations are discussed in the following paragraphs.

The types of infections seen in clinical trials in juvenile idiopathic arthritis patients aged 2 to 18 years were generally mild to moderate and consistent with those commonly seen in outpatient paediatric populations. Severe adverse events reported included varicella with signs and symptoms of aseptic meningitis, which resolved without sequelae (see also section 4.4), appendicitis, gastroenteritis, depression/personality disorder, cutaneous ulcer, oesophagitis/gastritis, group A streptococcal septic shock, type I diabetes mellitus, and soft tissue and post-operative wound infection.

In one study in children with juvenile idiopathic arthritis aged 4 to 17 years, 43 of 69 (62%) children experienced an infection while receiving Enbrel during 3 months of the study (part 1 open-label), and the frequency and severity of infections was similar in 58 patients completing 12 months of open-label extension therapy. The types and proportion of adverse events in juvenile idiopathic arthritis patients were similar to those seen in trials of Enbrel in adult patients with rheumatoid arthritis, and the majority were mild. Several adverse events were reported more commonly in 69 juvenile idiopathic arthritis patients receiving 3 months of Enbrel compared to the 349 adult rheumatoid arthritis patients. These included headache (19% of patients, 1.7 events per patient year), nausea (9%, 1.0 event per patient year), abdominal pain (19%, 0.74 events per patient year), and vomiting (13%, 0.74 events per patient year).

There were 4 reports of macrophage activation syndrome in juvenile idiopathic arthritis clinical trials.

Undesirable effects in paediatric patients with plaque psoriasis

In a 48-week study in 211 children aged 4 to 17 years with paediatric plaque psoriasis, the adverse events reported were similar to those seen in previous studies in adults with plaque psoriasis.

4.9 Overdose

No dose-limiting toxicities were observed during clinical trials of rheumatoid arthritis patients. The highest dose level evaluated has been an intravenous loading dose of 32 mg/m^2 followed by subcutaneous doses of 16 mg/m^2 administered twice weekly. One rheumatoid arthritis patient mistakenly self-administered 62 mg Enbrel subcutaneously twice weekly for 3 weeks without experiencing undesirable effects. There is no known antidote to Enbrel.

5. PHARMACOLOGICAL PROPERTIES

5.1 Pharmacodynamic properties

Pharmacotherapeutic group: Tumor Necrosis Factor alpha (TNF-α) inhibitors, ATC code: L04AB01

Tumour necrosis factor (TNF) is a dominant cytokine in the inflammatory process of rheumatoid arthritis. Elevated levels of TNF are also found in the synovium and psoriatic plaques of patients with psoriatic arthritis and in serum and synovial tissue of patients with ankylosing spondylitis. In plaque psoriasis, infiltration by inflammatory cells including T-cells leads to increased TNF levels in psoriatic lesions compared with levels in uninvolved skin. Etanercept is a competitive inhibitor of TNF-binding to its cell surface receptors and thereby inhibits the biological activity of TNF. TNF and lymphotoxin are pro-inflammatory cytokines that bind to two distinct cell surface receptors: the 55-kilodalton (p55) and 75-kilodalton (p75) tumour necrosis factor receptors (TNFRs). Both TNFRs exist naturally in membrane-bound and soluble forms. Soluble TNFRs are thought to regulate TNF biological activity.

TNF and lymphotoxin exist predominantly as homotrimers, with their biological activity dependent on cross-linking of cell surface TNFRs. Dimeric soluble receptors such as etanercept possess a higher affinity for TNF than monomeric receptors and are considerably more potent competitive inhibitors of TNF binding to its cellular receptors. In addition, use of an immunoglobulin Fc region as a fusion element in the construction of a dimeric receptor imparts a longer serum half-life.

Mechanism of action

Much of the joint pathology in rheumatoid arthritis and ankylosing spondylitis and skin pathology in plaque psoriasis is mediated by pro-inflammatory molecules that are linked in a network controlled by TNF. The mechanism of action of etanercept is thought to be its competitive inhibition of TNF binding to cell surface TNFR, preventing TNF-mediated cellular responses by rendering TNF biologically inactive. Etanercept may also modulate biologic responses controlled by additional downstream molecules (e.g., cytokines, adhesion molecules, or proteinases) that are induced or regulated by TNF.

Clinical trials

This section presents data from four randomised controlled trials in adults with rheumatoid arthritis, one study in polyarticular juvenile idiopathic arthritis, one study in adults with psoriatic arthritis, one study in adults with ankylosing spondylitis, one study in paediatric patients with plaque psoriasis, and four studies in adults with plaque psoriasis.

Adult patients with rheumatoid arthritis

The efficacy of Enbrel was assessed in a randomised, double-blind, placebo-controlled study. The study evaluated 234 adult patients with active rheumatoid arthritis who had failed therapy with at least one but no more than four disease-modifying antirheumatic drugs (DMARDs). Doses of 10 mg or 25 mg Enbrel or placebo were administered subcutaneously twice a week for 6 consecutive months. The results of this controlled trial were expressed in percentage improvement in rheumatoid arthritis using American College of Rheumatology (ACR) response criteria.

ACR 20 and 50 responses were higher in patients treated with Enbrel at 3 and 6 months than in patients treated with placebo (ACR 20: Enbrel 62% and 59%, placebo 23% and 11% at 3 and 6 months respectively; ACR 50: Enbrel 41% and 40%, placebo 8% and 5% at months 3 and 6 respectively; $p<0.01$ Enbrel vs Placebo at all time points for both ACR 20 and ACR 50 responses).

Approximately 15% of subjects who received Enbrel achieved an ACR 70 response at month 3 and month 6 compared to fewer than 5% of subjects in the placebo arm. Among patients receiving Enbrel, the clinical responses generally appeared within 1 to 2 weeks after initiation of therapy and nearly always occurred by 3 months. A dose response was seen; results with 10 mg were intermediate between placebo and 25 mg. Enbrel was significantly better than placebo in all components of the ACR criteria as well as other measures of rheumatoid arthritis disease activity not included in the ACR response criteria, such as morning stiffness. A Health Assessment Questionnaire (HAQ), which included disability, vitality, mental health, general health status, and arthritis-associated health status subdomains, was administered every 3 months during the trial. All subdomains of the HAQ were improved in patients treated with Enbrel compared to controls at 3 and 6 months.

After discontinuation of Enbrel, symptoms of arthritis generally returned within a month. Re-introduction of treatment with Enbrel after discontinuations of up to 24 months resulted in the same magnitudes of responses as patients who received Enbrel without interruption of therapy based on results of open-label studies. Continued durable responses have been seen for up to 48 months in open-label extension treatment trials when patients received Enbrel without interruption; longer-term experience is not available.

The efficacy of Enbrel was compared to methotrexate in a third randomised, active-controlled study with blinded radiographic evaluations as a primary endpoint in 632 adult patients with active rheumatoid arthritis (<3 years duration) who had never received treatment with methotrexate. Doses of 10 mg or 25 mg Enbrel were administered SC twice a week for up to 24 months. Methotrexate doses were escalated from 7.5 mg/week to a maximum of 20 mg/week over the first 8 weeks of the trial and continued for up to 24 months. Clinical improvement including onset of action within 2 weeks with Enbrel 25 mg was similar to that seen in the previous trials, and was maintained for up to 24 months. At baseline, patients had a moderate degree of disability, with mean HAQ scores of 1.4 to 1.5. Treatment with Enbrel 25 mg resulted in substantial improvement at 12 months, with about 44% of patients achieving a normal HAQ score (less than 0.5). This benefit was maintained in Year 2 of this study.

In this study, structural joint damage was assessed radiographically and expressed as change in Total Sharp Score (TSS) and its components, the erosion score and joint space narrowing score (JSN). Radiographs of hands/wrists and feet were read at baseline and 6, 12, and 24 months. The 10 mg Enbrel dose had consistently less effect on structural damage than the 25 mg dose. Enbrel 25 mg was significantly superior to methotrexate for erosion scores at both 12 and 24 months. The differences in TSS and JSN were not statistically significant between methotrexate and Enbrel 25 mg. The results are shown in the figure below.

RADIOGRAPHIC PROGRESSION: COMPARISON OF ENBREL vs METHOTREXATE IN PATIENTS WITH RA OF <3 YEARS DURATION

(see Figure 1 above)

Figure 1 RADIOGRAPHIC PROGRESSION: COMPARISON OF ENBREL vs METHOTREXATE IN PATIENTS WITH RA OF <3 YEARS DURATION

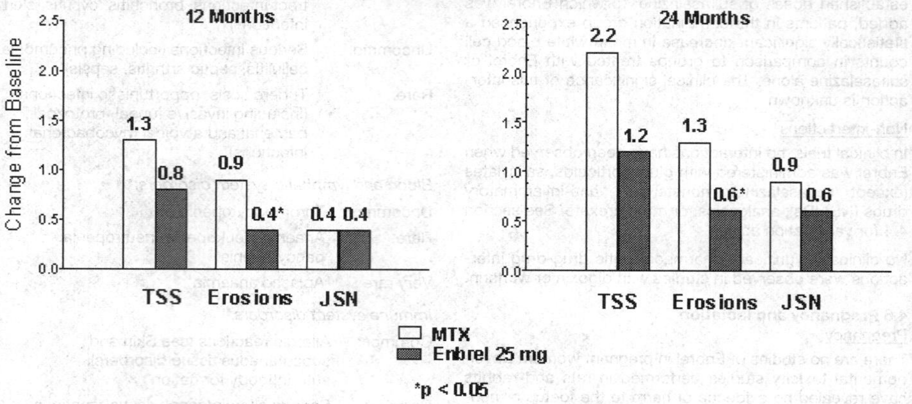

In another active-controlled, double-blind, randomised study, clinical efficacy, safety, and radiographic progression in RA patients treated with Enbrel alone (25 mg twice weekly), methotrexate alone (7.5 to 20 mg weekly, median dose 20 mg), and of the combination of Enbrel and methotrexate initiated concurrently were compared in 682 adult patients with active rheumatoid arthritis of 6 months to 20 years duration (median 5 years) who had a less than satisfactory response to at least 1 disease-modifying antirheumatic drug (DMARD) other than methotrexate.

Patients in the Enbrel in combination with methotrexate therapy group had significantly higher ACR 20, ACR 50, ACR 70 responses and improvement for DAS and HAQ scores at both 24 and 52 weeks than patients in either of the single therapy groups (results shown in table below). Significant advantages for Enbrel in combination with methotrexate compared with Enbrel monotherapy and methotrexate monotherapy were also observed after 24 months.

(see Table 1 on next page)

Radiographic progression at 12 months was significantly less in the Enbrel group than in the methotrexate group, while the combination was significantly better than either monotherapy at slowing radiographic progression (see figure below).

RADIOGRAPHIC PROGRESSION: COMPARISON OF ENBREL vs METHOTREXATE vs ENBREL IN COMBINATION WITH METHOTREXATE IN PATIENTS WITH RA OF 6 MONTHS TO 20 YEARS DURATION (12 MONTH RESULTS)

(see Figure 2 on next page)

Significant advantages for Enbrel in combination with methotrexate compared with Enbrel monotherapy and methotrexate monotherapy were also observed after 24 months. Similarly, the significant advantages for Enbrel monotherapy compared with methotrexate monotherapy were also observed after 24 months.

Table 1

CLINICAL EFFICACY RESULTS AT 12 MONTHS: COMPARISON OF ENBREL vs METHOTREXATE vs ENBREL IN COMBINATION WITH METHOTREXATE IN PATIENTS WITH RA OF 6 MONTHS TO 20 YEARS DURATION

Endpoint	Methotrexate (n = 228)	Enbrel (n = 223)	Enbrel + Methotrexate (n = 231)
ACR Responses[a]			
ACR 20	58.8%	65.5%	74.5% †,ϕ
ACR 50	36.4%	43.0%	63.2% †,ϕ
ACR 70	16.7%	22.0%	39.8% †,ϕ
DAS			
Baseline score[b]	5.5	5.7	5.5
Week 52 score[b]	3.0	3.0	2.3†,ϕ
Remission[c]	14%	18%	37%†,ϕ
HAQ			
Baseline	1.7	1.7	1.8
Week 52	1.1	1.0	0.8†,ϕ

a: Patients who did not complete 12 months in the study were considered to be non-responders.

b: Values for Disease Activity Score (DAS) are means.

c: Remission is defined as DAS <1.6

Pairwise comparison p-values: † = $p < 0.05$ for comparisons of Enbrel + methotrexate vs methotrexate and ϕ = $p < 0.05$ for comparisons of Enbrel + methotrexate vs Enbrel

Figure 2 RADIOGRAPHIC PROGRESSION: COMPARISON OF ENBREL vs METHOTREXATE vs ENBREL IN COMBINATION WITH METHOTREXATE IN PATIENTS WITH RA OF 6 MONTHS TO 20 YEARS DURATION (12 MONTH RESULTS)

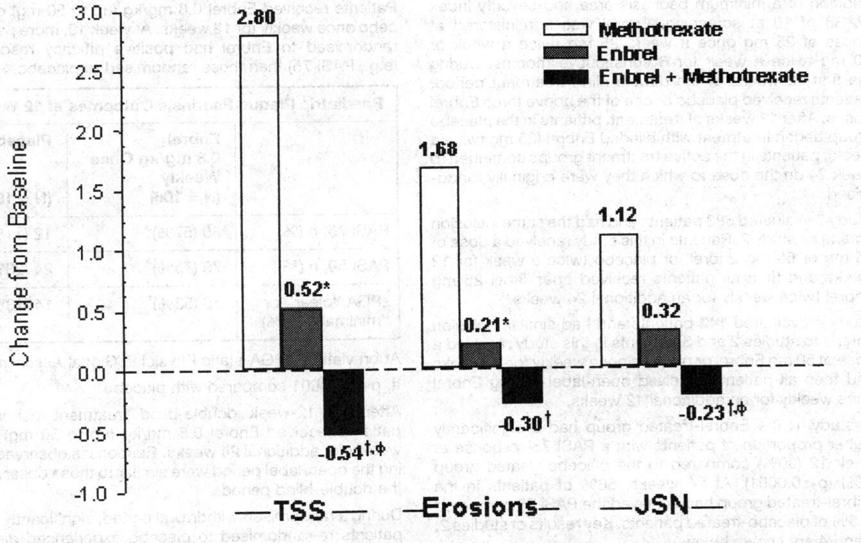

Pairwise comparison p-values: * = $p < 0.05$ for comparisons of Enbrel vs methotrexate, † = $p < 0.05$ for comparisons of Enbrel + methotrexate vs methotrexate and ϕ = $p < 0.05$ for comparisons of Enbrel + methotrexate vs Enbrel

In an analysis in which all patients who dropped out of the study for any reason were considered to have progressed, the percentage of patients without progression (TSS change ⩽ 0.5) at 24 months was higher in the Enbrel in combination with methotrexate group compared with the Enbrel alone and methotrexate alone groups (62%, 50%, and 36%, respectively; p<0.05). The difference between Enbrel alone and methotrexate alone was also significant (p<0.05). Among patients who completed a full 24 months of therapy in the study, the non-progression rates were 78%, 70%, and 61%, respectively.

The safety and efficacy of 50 mg Enbrel (two 25 mg SC injections) administered once weekly were evaluated in a double-blind, placebo-controlled study of 420 patients with active RA. In this study, 53 patients received placebo, 214 patients received 50 mg Enbrel once weekly and 153 patients received 25 mg Enbrel twice weekly. The safety and efficacy profiles of the two Enbrel treatment regimens were comparable at week 8 in their effect on signs and symptoms of RA; data at week 16 did not show comparability (non-inferiority) between the two regimens.

Paediatric patients with polyarticular juvenile idiopathic arthritis

The safety and efficacy of Enbrel were assessed in a two-part study in 69 children with polyarticular juvenile idiopathic arthritis who had a variety of juvenile idiopathic arthritis onset types. Patients aged 4 to 17 years with moderately to severely active polyarticular juvenile idiopathic arthritis refractory to or intolerant of methotrexate were enrolled; patients remained on a stable dose of a single nonsteroidal anti-inflammatory drug and/or prednisone (< 0.2 mg/kg/day or 10 mg maximum). In part 1, all patients received 0.4 mg/kg (maximum 25 mg per dose) Enbrel subcutaneously twice weekly. In part 2, patients with a clinical response at day 90 were randomised to remain on Enbrel or receive placebo for four months and assessed for disease flare. Responses were measured using the JRA Definition of Improvement (DOI), defined as ⩾ 30% improvement in at least three of six and ⩾ 30% worsening in no more than one of six JRA core set criteria, including active joint count, limitation of motion, physician and patient/parent global assessments, functional assessment, and erythrocyte sedimentation rate (ESR). Disease flare was defined as a ⩾ 30% worsening in three of six JRA core set criteria and ⩾ 30% improvement in not more than one of the six JRA core set criteria and a minimum of two active joints.

In part 1 of the study, 51 of 69 (74%) patients demonstrated a clinical response and entered part 2. In part 2, 6 of 25 (24%) patients remaining on Enbrel experienced a disease flare compared to 20 of 26 (77%) patients receiving placebo (p=0.007). From the start of part 2, the median time to flare was ⩾ 116 days for patients who received Enbrel and 28 days for patients who received placebo. Of patients who demonstrated a clinical response at 90 days and entered part 2 of the study, some of the patients remaining on Enbrel continued to improve from month 3 through month 7, while those who received placebo did not improve.

Studies have not been done in patients with polyarticular juvenile idiopathic arthritis to assess the effects of continued Enbrel therapy in patients who do not respond within 3 months of initiating Enbrel therapy or to assess the combination of Enbrel with methotrexate.

Adult patients with psoriatic arthritis

The efficacy of Enbrel was assessed in a randomised, double-blind, placebo-controlled study in 205 patients with psoriatic arthritis. Patients were between 18 and 70 years of age and had active psoriatic arthritis (⩾ 3 swollen joints and ⩾ 3 tender joints) in at least one of the following forms: (1) distal interphalangeal (DIP) involvement; (2) polyarticular arthritis (absence of rheumatoid nodules and presence of psoriasis); (3) arthritis mutilans; (4) asymmetric psoriatic arthritis; or (5) spondylitis-like ankylosis. Patients also had plaque psoriasis with a qualifying target lesion ⩾ 2 cm in diameter. Patients had previously been treated with NSAIDs (86%), DMARDs (80%), and corticosteroids (24%). Patients currently on methotrexate therapy (stable for ⩾ 2 months) could continue at a stable dose of ⩽ 25 mg/week methotrexate. Doses of 25 mg Enbrel (based on dose-finding studies in patients with rheumatoid arthritis) or placebo were administered SC twice a week for 6 months. At the end of the double-blind study, patients could enter a long-term open-label extension study for a total duration of up to 2 years.

Clinical responses were expressed as percentages of patients achieving the ACR 20, 50, and 70 response and percentages with improvement in Psoriatic Arthritis Response Criteria (PsARC). Results are summarised in the Table below.

RESPONSES OF PATIENTS WITH PSORIATIC ARTHRITIS IN PLACEBO-CONTROLLED TRIAL

	Percent of Patients	
	Placebo	Enbrel[a]
Psoriatic Arthritis Response	n = 104	n = 101
ACR 20		
Month 3	15	59[b]
Month 6	13	50[b]
ACR 50		
Month 3	4	38[b]
Month 6	4	37[b]
ACR 70		
Month 3	0	11[b]
Month 6	1	9[c]
PsARC		
Month 3	31	72[b]
Month 6	23	70[b]

a: 25 mg Enbrel SC twice weekly

b: $p < 0.001$, Enbrel vs. placebo

c: $p < 0.01$, Enbrel vs. placebo

Among patients with psoriatic arthritis who received Enbrel, the clinical responses were apparent at the time of the first visit (4 weeks) and were maintained through 6 months of therapy. Enbrel was significantly better than placebo in all measures of disease activity ($p < 0.001$), and responses were similar with and without concomitant methotrexate therapy. Quality of life in psoriatic arthritis patients was assessed at every timepoint using the disability index of the HAQ. The disability index score was significantly improved at all timepoints in psoriatic arthritis patients treated with Enbrel, relative to placebo ($p < 0.001$).

Radiographic changes were assessed in the psoriatic arthritis study. Radiographs of hands and wrists were obtained at baseline and months 6, 12, and 24. The modified TSS at 12 months is presented in the Table below. In an analysis in which all patients who dropped out of the study for any reason were considered to have progressed, the percentage of patients without progression (TSS change ⩽ 0.5) at 12 months was higher in the Enbrel group compared with the placebo group (73% vs. 47%, respectively, p ⩽ 0.001). The effect of Enbrel on radiographic progression was maintained in patients who continued on treatment during the second year. The slowing of peripheral joint damage was observed in patients with polyarticular symmetrical joint involvement.

MEAN (SE) ANNUALIZED CHANGE FROM BASELINE IN TOTAL SHARP SCORE

	Placebo	Etanercept
Time	(n = 104)	(n = 101)
Month 12	1.00 (0.29)	-0.03 (0.09)[a]

SE = standard error.

a. p = 0.0001.

Enbrel treatment resulted in improvement in physical function during the double-blind period, and this benefit was maintained during the longer-term exposure of up to 2 years.

There is insufficient evidence of the efficacy of Enbrel in patients with ankylosing spondylitis-like and arthritis mutilans psoriatic arthropathies due to the small number of patients studied.

No study has been performed in patients with psoriatic arthritis using the 50mg once weekly dosing regimen. Evidence of efficacy for the once weekly dosing regimen in this patient population has been based on data from the study in patients with ankylosing spondylitis.

Adult patients with ankylosing spondylitis

The efficacy of Enbrel in ankylosing spondylitis was assessed in 3 randomised, double-blind studies comparing twice weekly administration of 25 mg Enbrel with placebo. A total of 401 patients were enrolled from which 203 were treated with Enbrel. The largest of these trials (n=277) enrolled patients who were between 18 and 70 years of age and had active ankylosing spondylitis defined as visual analog scale (VAS) scores of ⩾ 30 for average of duration and intensity of morning stiffness plus VAS scores of ⩾ 30 for at least 2 of the following 3 parameters: patient global assessment; average of VAS values for nocturnal back pain and total back pain; average of 10 questions on the Bath Ankylosing Spondylitis Functional Index (BASFI). Patients receiving DMARDs, NSAIDS, or corticosteroids could continue them on stable doses. Patients with complete ankylosis of the spine were not included in the study. Doses of 25 mg of Enbrel (based on dose-finding studies in patients with rheumatoid arthritis) or placebo were administered subcutaneously twice a week for 6 months in 138 patients.

The primary measure of efficacy (ASAS 20) was a ⩾20% improvement in at least 3 of the 4 Assessment in Ankylosing Spondylitis (ASAS) domains (patient global assessments, back pain, BASFI, and inflammation) and absence of deterioration in the remaining domain. ASAS 50 and 70 responses used the same criteria with a 50% improvement or a 70% improvement, respectively.

Compared to placebo, treatment with Enbrel resulted in significant improvements in the ASAS 20, ASAS 50 and ASAS 70 as early as 2 weeks after the initiation of therapy.

RESPONSES OF PATIENTS WITH ANKYLOSING SPONDYLITIS IN A PLACEBO-CONTROLLED TRIAL

	Percent of Patients	
Ankylosing Spondylitis Response	Placebo N = 139	Enbrel N = 138
ASAS 20		
2 weeks	22	46[a]
3 months	27	60[a]
6 months	23	58[a]
ASAS 50		
2 weeks	7	24[a]
3 months	13	45[a]
6 months	10	42[a]
ASAS 70:		
2 weeks	2	12[b]
3 months	7	29[b]
6 months	5	28[b]

a: p<0.001, Enbrel vs. Placebo

b: p = 0.002, Enbrel vs. placebo

Among patients with ankylosing spondylitis who received Enbrel, the clinical responses were apparent at the time of the first visit (2 weeks) and were maintained through 6 months of therapy. Responses were similar in patients who were or were not receiving concomitant therapies at baseline.

Similar results were obtained in the 2 smaller ankylosing spondylitis trials.

In a fourth study, the safety and efficacy of 50 mg Enbrel (two 25 mg SC injections) administered once weekly vs 25 mg Enbrel administered twice weekly were evaluated in a double-blind, placebo-controlled study of 356 patients with active ankylosing spondylitis. The safety and efficacy profiles of the 50 mg once weekly and 25 mg twice weekly regimens were similar.

Adult patients with plaque psoriasis

Enbrel is recommended for use in patients as defined in section 4.1. Patients who "failed to respond to" in the target population is defined by insufficient response (PASI<50 or PGA less than good), or worsening of the disease while on treatment, and who were adequately dosed for a sufficiently long duration to assess response with at least each of the three major systemic therapies as available.

The efficacy of Enbrel versus other systemic therapies in patients with moderate to severe psoriasis (responsive to other systemic therapies) has not been evaluated in studies directly comparing Enbrel with other systemic therapies. Instead, the safety and efficacy of Enbrel were assessed in four randomised, double-blind, placebo-controlled studies. The primary efficacy endpoint in all four studies was the proportion of patients in each treatment group who achieved the PASI 75 (i.e. at least a 75% improvement in the Psoriasis Area and Severity Index score from baseline) at 12 weeks.

Study 1 was a Phase 2 study in patients with active but clinically stable plaque psoriasis involving ⩾ 10% of the body surface area that were ⩾ 18 years old. One hundred and twelve (112) patients were randomised to receive a dose of 25 mg of Enbrel (n=57) or placebo (n=55) twice a week for 24 weeks.

Study 2 evaluated 652 patients with chronic plaque psoriasis using the same inclusion criteria as study 1 with the addition of a minimum psoriasis area and severity index (PASI) of 10 at screening. Enbrel was administered at doses of 25 mg once a week, 25 mg twice a week or 50 mg twice a week for 6 consecutive months. During the first 12 weeks of the double-blind treatment period, patients received placebo or one of the above three Enbrel doses. After 12 weeks of treatment, patients in the placebo group began treatment with blinded Enbrel (25 mg twice a week); patients in the active treatment groups continued to week 24 on the dose to which they were originally randomised.

Study 3 evaluated 583 patients and had the same inclusion criteria as study 2. Patients in this study received a dose of 25 mg or 50 mg Enbrel, or placebo twice a week for 12 weeks and then all patients received open-label 25 mg Enbrel twice weekly for an additional 24 weeks.

Study 4 evaluated 142 patients and had similar inclusion criteria to studies 2 and 3. Patients in this study received a dose of 50 mg Enbrel or placebo once weekly for 12 weeks and then all patients received open-label 50 mg Enbrel once weekly for an additional 12 weeks.

In study 1, the Enbrel-treated group had a significantly higher proportion of patients with a PASI 75 response at week 12 (30%) compared to the placebo-treated group (2%) (p<0.0001). At 24 weeks, 56% of patients in the Enbrel-treated group had achieved the PASI 75 compared to 5% of placebo-treated patients. Key results of studies 2, 3 and 4 are shown below.

(see Table 2 below)

Among patients with plaque psoriasis who received Enbrel, significant responses relative to placebo were apparent at the time of the first visit (2 weeks) and were maintained through 24 weeks of therapy.

Study 2 also had a drug withdrawal period during which patients who achieved a PASI improvement of at least 50% at week 24 had treatment stopped. Patients were observed off treatment for the occurrence of rebound (PASI ⩾150% of baseline) and for the time to relapse (defined as a loss of at least half of the improvement achieved between baseline and week 24). During the withdrawal period, symptoms of psoriasis gradually returned with a median time to disease relapse of 3 months. No rebound flare of disease and no psoriasis-related serious adverse events were observed. There was some evidence to support a benefit of re-treatment with Enbrel in patients initially responding to treatment.

In study 3, the majority of patients (77%) who were initially randomised to 50 mg twice weekly and had their Enbrel dose decreased at week 12 to 25 mg twice weekly maintained their PASI 75 response through week 36. For patients who received 25 mg twice weekly throughout the study, the PASI 75 response continued to improve between weeks 12 and 36.

In study 4, the Enbrel-treated group had a higher proportion of patients with PASI 75 at week 12 (38%) compared to the placebo-treated group (2%) (p<0.0001). For patients who received 50 mg once weekly throughout the study, the efficacy responses continued to improve with 71% achieving PASI 75 at week 24.

In long-term (up to 34 months) open-label studies where Enbrel was given without interruption, clinical responses were sustained and safety was comparable to shorter-term studies.

An analysis of clinical trial data did not reveal any baseline disease characteristics that would assist clinicians in selecting the most appropriate dosing option (intermittent or continuous). Consequently, the choice of intermittent or continuous therapy should be based upon physician judgment and individual patient needs.

Paediatric patients with plaque psoriasis

The efficacy of Enbrel was assessed in a randomised, double-blind, placebo-controlled study in 211 paediatric patients aged 4 to 17 years with moderate to severe plaque psoriasis (as defined by a sPGA score ⩾ 3, involving ⩾ 10% of the BSA, and PASI ⩾ 12). Eligible patients had a history of receiving phototherapy or systemic therapy, or were inadequately controlled on topical therapy.

Patients received Enbrel 0.8 mg/kg (up to 50 mg) or placebo once weekly for 12 weeks. At week 12, more patients randomised to Enbrel had positive efficacy responses (e.g., PASI 75) than those randomised to placebo.

Paediatric Plaque Psoriasis Outcomes at 12 Weeks

	Enbrel 0.8 mg/kg Once Weekly (N = 106)	Placebo (N = 105)
PASI 75, n (%)	60 (57%)[a]	12 (11%)
PASI 50, n (%)	79 (75%)[a]	24 (23%)
sPGA "clear" or "minimal", n (%)	56 (53%)[a]	14 (13%)

Abbreviation: sPGA-static Physician Global Assessment.

a. p < 0.0001 compared with placebo.

After the 12-week double-blind treatment period, all patients received Enbrel 0.8 mg/kg (up to 50 mg) once weekly for additional 24 weeks. Responses observed during the open-label period were similar to those observed in the double-blind period.

During a randomised withdrawal period, significantly more patients re-randomised to placebo experienced disease relapse (loss of PASI 75 response) compared with patients re-randomised to Enbrel. With continued therapy, responses were maintained up to 48 weeks.

Antibodies to Enbrel

Antibodies to etanercept have been detected in the sera of some subjects treated with etanercept. These antibodies have all been non-neutralising and are generally transient. There appears to be no correlation between antibody development and clinical response or adverse events.

Table 2 RESPONSES OF PATIENTS WITH PSORIASIS IN STUDIES 2, 3 AND 4

Response (%)	Study 2					Study 3			Study 4		
	Placebo	Enbrel				Placebo	Enbrel		Placebo	Enbrel	
		25 mg BIW		50 mg BIW			25 mg BIW	50 mg BIW		50 mg QW	50 mg QW
	n = 166 wk 12	n = 162 wk 12	n = 162 wk 24[a]	n = 164 wk 12	n = 164 wk 24[a]	n = 193 wk 12	n = 196 wk 12	n = 196 wk 12	n = 46 wk 12	n = 96 wk 12	n = 90 wk 24[a]
PASI 50	14	58*	70	74*	77	9	64*	77*	9	69*	83
PASI 75	4	34*	44	49*	59	3	34*	49*	2	38*	71
DSGA [b], clear or almost clear	5	34*	39	49*	55	4	39*	57*	4	39*	64

*p ⩽ 0.0001 compared with placebo

a. No statistical comparisons to placebo were made at week 24 in studies 2 and 4 because the original placebo group began receiving Enbrel 25 mg BIW or 50 mg once weekly from week 13 to week 24.

b. Dermatologist Static Global Assessment. Clear or almost clear defined as 0 or 1 on a 0 to 5 scale.

In subjects treated with approved doses of etanercept in clinical trials for up to 12 months, cumulative rates of anti-etanercept antibodies were approximately 6% of subjects with rheumatoid arthritis, 7.5% of subjects with psoriatic arthritis, 2% of subjects with ankylosing spondylitis, 7% of subjects with psoriasis, 9.7% of subjects with paediatric psoriasis, and 3% of subjects with juvenile idiopathic arthritis.

The proportion of subjects who developed antibodies to etanercept in longer-term trials (of up to 3.5 years) increases over time, as expected. However, due to their transient nature, the incidence of antibodies detected at each assessment point was typically less than 7% in rheumatoid arthritis subjects and psoriasis subjects.

In a long-term psoriasis study in which patients received 50 mg twice weekly for 96 weeks, the incidence of antibodies observed at each assessment point was up to approximately 9%.

5.2 Pharmacokinetic properties

Etanercept serum values were determined by an ELISA method, which may detect ELISA-reactive degradation products as well as the parent compound.

Etanercept is slowly absorbed from the site of subcutaneous injection, reaching maximum concentration approximately 48 hours after a single dose. The absolute bioavailability is 76%. With twice weekly doses, it is anticipated that steady-state concentrations are approximately twice as high as those observed after single doses. After a single subcutaneous dose of 25 mg Enbrel, the average maximum serum concentration observed in healthy volunteers was 1.65 ± 0.66 μg/ml, and the area under the curve was 235 ± 96.6 μg•hr/ml. Dose proportionality has not been formally evaluated, but there is no apparent saturation of clearance across the dosing range.

A biexponential curve is required to describe the concentration time curve of etanercept. The central volume of distribution of etanercept is 7.6 l, while the volume of distribution at steady-state is 10.4 l. Etanercept is cleared slowly from the body. The half-life is long, approximately 70 hours. Clearance is approximately 0.066 l/hr in patients with rheumatoid arthritis, somewhat lower than the value of 0.11 l/hr observed in healthy volunteers. Additionally, the pharmacokinetics of Enbrel in rheumatoid arthritis patients, ankylosing spondylitis and plaque psoriasis patients are similar.

Mean serum concentration profiles at steady state in treated RA patients were Cmax of 2.4 mg/l vs 2.6 mg/l, Cmin of 1.2 mg/l vs 1.4 mg/l and partial AUC of 297 mgh/l vs 316 mgh/l for 50 mg Enbrel once weekly (n=21) vs 25 mg Enbrel twice weekly (n=16), respectively. In an open-label, single-dose, two-treatment, crossover study in healthy volunteers, etanercept administered as a single 50 mg/ml injection was found to be bioequivalent to two simultaneous injections of 25 mg/ml.

In a population pharmacokinetics analysis in ankylosing spondylitis patients the etanercept steady state AUCs were 466 μg•hr/ml and 474 μg•hr/ml for 50 mg Enbrel once weekly (N= 154) and 25 mg twice weekly (N = 148), respectively.

Although there is elimination of radioactivity in urine after administration of radiolabelled etanercept to patients and volunteers, increased etanercept concentrations were not observed in patients with acute renal or hepatic failure. The presence of renal and hepatic impairment should not require a change in dosage. There is no apparent pharmacokinetic difference between males and females.

Methotrexate has no effect on the pharmacokinetics of etanercept. The effect of Enbrel on the human pharmacokinetics of methotrexate has not been investigated.

Special populations

Elderly patients

The impact of advanced age was studied in the population pharmacokinetic analysis of etanercept serum concentrations. Clearance and volume estimates in patients aged 65 to 87 years were similar to estimates in patients less than 65 years of age.

Paediatric patients with polyarticular juvenile idiopathic arthritis

In a polyarticular juvenile idiopathic arthritis trial with Enbrel, 69 patients (aged 4 to 17 years) were administered 0.4 mg Enbrel/kg twice weekly for three months. Serum concentration profiles were similar to those seen in adult rheumatoid arthritis patients. The youngest children (4 years of age) had reduced clearance (increased clearance when normalised by weight) compared with older children (12 years of age) and adults. Simulation of dosing suggests that while older children (10-17 years of age) will have serum levels close to those seen in adults, younger children will have appreciably lower levels.

Paediatric patients with plaque psoriasis

Patients with paediatric plaque psoriasis (aged 4 to 17 years) were administered 0.8 mg/kg (up to a maximum dose of 50 mg per week) of etanercept once weekly for up to 48 weeks. The mean serum steady state trough concentrations ranged from 1.6 to 2.1 mcg/ml at weeks 12, 24, and 48. These mean concentrations in patients with paediatric plaque psoriasis were similar to the concentrations observed in patients with juvenile idiopathic arthritis (treated with 0.4 mg/kg etanercept twice weekly, up to maximum dose of 50 mg per week). These mean concentrations were similar to those seen in adult patients with plaque psoriasis treated with 25 mg etanercept twice weekly.

5.3 Preclinical safety data

In the toxicological studies with Enbrel, no dose-limiting or target organ toxicity was evident. Enbrel was considered to be non-genotoxic from a battery of *in vitro* and *in vivo* studies. Carcinogenicity studies, and standard assessments of fertility and postnatal toxicity, were not performed with Enbrel due to the development of neutralising antibodies in rodents.

Enbrel did not induce lethality or notable signs of toxicity in mice or rats following a single subcutaneous dose of 2000 mg/kg or a single intravenous dose of 1000 mg/kg. Enbrel did not elicit dose-limiting or target organ toxicity in cynomolgus monkeys following twice weekly subcutaneous administration for 4 or 26 consecutive weeks at a dose (15 mg/kg) that resulted in AUC-based serum drug concentrations that were over 27-fold higher than that obtained in humans at the recommended dose of 25 mg.

6. PHARMACEUTICAL PARTICULARS

6.1 List of excipients

Sucrose

Sodium chloride

L-Arginine hydrochloride

Sodium phosphate monobasic dihydrate

Sodium phosphate dibasic dihydrate

Water for injections

6.2 Incompatibilities

In the absence of compatibility studies, this medicinal product must not be mixed with other medicinal products.

6.3 Shelf life

2 years.

6.4 Special precautions for storage

Store in a refrigerator (2°C – 8°C).

Do not freeze.

Keep the pre-filled syringes in the outer carton in order to protect from light.

6.5 Nature and contents of container

Clear glass syringe (type I glass) with stainless steel needle, rubber needle cover and plastic plunger. Cartons contain 4, 8 or 24 pre-filled syringes of Enbrel and 8, 16, or 48 alcohol swabs. The needle cover contains dry natural rubber (latex) (see section 4.4). Not all pack sizes may be marketed.

6.6 Special precautions for disposal and other handling

Any unused product or waste material should be disposed of in accordance with local requirements.

Instructions for use and handling

Before injection, Enbrel single-use pre-filled syringe should be allowed to reach room temperature (approximately 15 to 30 minutes). The needle cover should not be removed while allowing the pre-filled syringe to reach room temperature. The solution should be clear and colourless or pale yellow and practically free from visible particles.

Comprehensive instructions for administration are given in the package leaflet, section 7, "Instructions for preparation and giving an injection of Enbrel."

7. MARKETING AUTHORISATION HOLDER

Wyeth Europa Ltd.
Huntercombe Lane South
Taplow, Maidenhead
Berkshire, SL6 0PH
United Kingdom

8. MARKETING AUTHORISATION NUMBER(S)

EU/1/99/126/013

9. DATE OF FIRST AUTHORISATION/RENEWAL OF THE AUTHORISATION

Date of first authorisation: 3 February 2000

Date of last renewal: 3 February 2005

10. DATE OF REVISION OF THE TEXT

16 July 2009

Detailed information on this product is available on the website of the European Medicines Agency (EMEA) http://www.emea.europa.eu

Enbrel 25mg/ml powder and solvent for solution for injection for paediatric use

(Wyeth Pharmaceuticals)

1. NAME OF THE MEDICINAL PRODUCT

Enbrel®▼ 25 mg/ml powder and solvent for solution for injection for paediatric use.

2. QUALITATIVE AND QUANTITATIVE COMPOSITION

Each vial contains 25 mg of etanercept. When reconstituted, the solution contains 25 mg/ml of etanercept.

Etanercept is a human tumour necrosis factor receptor p75 Fc fusion protein produced by recombinant DNA technology in a Chinese hamster ovary (CHO) mammalian expression system. Etanercept is a dimer of a chimeric protein genetically engineered by fusing the extracellular ligand binding domain of human tumour necrosis factor receptor-2 (TNFR2/p75) to the Fc domain of human IgG1. This Fc component contains the hinge, CH_2 and CH_3 regions but not the CH_1 region of IgG1. Etanercept contains 934 amino acids and has an apparent molecular weight of approximately 150 kilodaltons. The potency is determined by measuring the ability of etanercept to neutralise the TNFα-mediated growth inhibition of A375 cells. The specific activity of etanercept is 1.7×10^6 units/mg.

The solution contains benzyl alcohol 9 mg/ml as a preservative (see section 4.4). For a full list of excipients, see section 6.1.

3. PHARMACEUTICAL FORM

Powder and solvent for solution for injection.

The powder is white. The solvent is a clear, colourless liquid.

4. CLINICAL PARTICULARS

4.1 Therapeutic indications

Polyarticular juvenile idiopathic arthritis

Treatment of active polyarticular juvenile idiopathic arthritis in children and adolescents from the age of 4 years who have had an inadequate response to, or who have proved intolerant of, methotrexate. Enbrel has not been studied in children aged less than 4 years.

Paediatric plaque psoriasis

Treatment of chronic severe plaque psoriasis in children and adolescents from the age of 8 years who are inadequately controlled by, or are intolerant to, other systemic therapies or phototherapies.

4.2 Posology and method of administration

Enbrel treatment should be initiated and supervised by specialist physicians experienced in the diagnosis and treatment of juvenile idiopathic arthritis or paediatric plaque psoriasis. Patients treated with Enbrel should be given the Patient Alert Card.

Each vial of Enbrel 25 mg/ml should be used for a maximum of 2 doses administered to the same patient.

Posology

Special populations

Paediatric use

Juvenile idiopathic arthritis (age 4 years and above)

0.4 mg/kg (up to a maximum of 25 mg per dose) after reconstitution of 25 mg Enbrel in 1 ml of solvent, given twice weekly as a subcutaneous injection with an interval of 3-4 days between doses.

Paediatric plaque psoriasis (age 8 years and above)

0.8 mg/kg (up to a maximum of 50 mg per dose) once weekly for up to 24 weeks. Treatment should be discontinued in patients who show no response after 12 weeks.

If re-treatment with Enbrel is indicated, the above guidance on treatment duration should be followed. The dose should be 0.8 mg/kg (up to a maximum of 50 mg per dose) once weekly.

Renal and hepatic impairment

No dose adjustment is required.

Method of administration

Comprehensive instructions for the preparation, administration and re-use of the reconstituted Enbrel vial are given in the package leaflet, section 7, "Instructions for preparation and giving an injection of Enbrel."

4.3 Contraindications

Hypersensitivity to the active substance or to any of the excipients.

Sepsis or risk of sepsis.

Treatment with Enbrel should not be initiated in patients with active infections including chronic or localised infections.

Enbrel must not be given to premature babies or neonates as the solvent contains benzyl alcohol.

4.4 Special warnings and precautions for use

Infections

Patients should be evaluated for infections before, during, and after treatment with Enbrel, taking into consideration that the mean elimination half-life of etanercept is approximately 70 hours (range 7 to 300 hours).

Serious infections, sepsis, tuberculosis, and opportunistic infections, including invasive fungal infections, have been reported with the use of Enbrel (see section 4.8). These infections were due to bacteria, mycobacteria, fungi and viruses. In some cases, particular fungal and other opportunistic infections have not been recognised, resulting in delay of appropriate treatment and sometimes death. In evaluating patients for infections, the patient's risk for relevant opportunistic infections (e.g., exposure to endemic mycoses) should be considered.

Patients who develop a new infection while undergoing treatment with Enbrel should be monitored closely. **Administration of Enbrel should be discontinued if a patient develops a serious infection.** Physicians should exercise caution when considering the use of Enbrel in patients with a history of recurring or chronic infections or with underlying conditions that may predispose patients to infections such as advanced or poorly controlled diabetes.

Tuberculosis

Cases of active tuberculosis including miliary tuberculosis and tuberculosis with extra-pulmonary location have been reported in patients treated with Enbrel.

Before starting treatment with Enbrel, all patients must be evaluated for both active and inactive ('latent') tuberculosis. This evaluation should include a detailed medical history with personal history of tuberculosis or possible previous contact with tuberculosis and previous and/or current immunosuppressive therapy. Appropriate screening tests, i.e. tuberculin skin test and chest x-ray, should be performed in all patients (local recommendations may apply). It is recommended that the conduct of these tests should be recorded in the patient's alert card. Prescribers are reminded of the risk of false negative tuberculin skin test results, especially in patients who are severely ill or immunocompromised.

If active tuberculosis is diagnosed, Enbrel therapy must not be initiated. If inactive ('latent') tuberculosis is diagnosed, treatment for latent tuberculosis must be started with anti-tuberculosis therapy before the initiation of Enbrel, and in accordance with local recommendations. In this situation, the benefit/risk balance of Enbrel therapy should be very carefully considered.

All patients should be informed to seek medical advice if signs/symptoms suggestive of tuberculosis (e.g., persistent cough, wasting/weight loss, low-grade fever) appear during or after Enbrel treatment.

Hepatitis B virus reactivation

Reactivation of hepatitis B virus (HBV) in patients who are chronic carriers of this virus who are receiving TNF-antagonists including Enbrel has been reported. Patients at risk for HBV infection should be evaluated for prior evidence of HBV infection before initiating Enbrel therapy. Caution should be exercised when administering Enbrel to patients identified as carriers of HBV. If Enbrel is used in carriers of HBV, the patients should be monitored for signs and symptoms of active HBV infection and, if necessary, appropriate treatment should be initiated.

Worsening of hepatitis C

There have been reports of worsening of hepatitis C in patients receiving Enbrel.

Concurrent treatment with anakinra

Concurrent administration of Enbrel and anakinra has been associated with an increased risk of serious infections and neutropenia compared to Enbrel alone. This combination has not demonstrated increased clinical benefit. Thus the combined use of Enbrel and anakinra is not recommended (see sections 4.5 and 4.8).

Concurrent treatment with abatacept

In clinical studies, concurrent administration of abatacept and Enbrel resulted in increased incidences of serious adverse events. This combination has not demonstrated increased clinical benefit; such use is not recommended (see section 4.5).

Allergic reactions

Allergic reactions associated with Enbrel administration have been reported commonly. Allergic reactions have included angioedema and urticaria; serious reactions have occurred. If any serious allergic or anaphylactic reaction occurs, Enbrel therapy should be discontinued immediately and appropriate therapy initiated.

Immunosuppression

The possibility exists for TNF-antagonists, including Enbrel, to affect host defences against infections and malignancies since TNF mediates inflammation and modulates cellular immune responses. In a study of 49 adult patients with rheumatoid arthritis treated with Enbrel, there was no evidence of depression of delayed-type hypersensitivity, depression of immunoglobulin levels, or change in enumeration of effector cell populations.

Two juvenile idiopathic arthritis patients developed varicella infection and signs and symptoms of aseptic meningitis, which resolved without sequelae. Patients with a significant exposure to varicella virus should temporarily discontinue Enbrel therapy and be considered for prophylactic treatment with Varicella Zoster Immune Globulin.

The safety and efficacy of Enbrel in patients with immunosuppression or chronic infections have not been evaluated.

Malignancies and lymphoproliferative disorders

Solid and haematopoietic malignancies

Reports of various malignancies (including breast and lung carcinoma and lymphoma) have been received in the post-marketing period (see section 4.8).

In the controlled portions of clinical trials of TNF-antagonists, more cases of lymphoma have been observed among patients receiving a TNF-antagonist compared with control patients. However, the occurrence was rare, and the follow-up period of placebo patients was shorter than for patients receiving TNF-antagonist therapy. Furthermore, there is an increased background lymphoma risk in rheumatoid arthritis patients with long-standing, highly active, inflammatory disease, which complicates the risk estimation. With the current knowledge, a possible risk for the development of lymphomas or other malignancies in patients treated with a TNF-antagonist cannot be excluded.

Non-melanoma skin cancer (NMSC)

Non-melanoma skin cancer has been reported in patients treated with TNF-antagonists, including Enbrel. Combining the results of placebo- and active comparator-controlled clinical trials of Enbrel, more cases of NMSC were observed in patients receiving Enbrel compared with control patients, particularly in patients with psoriasis. Periodic skin examination is recommended for all patients who are at increased risk for NMSC (including patients with psoriasis or a history of PUVA therapy).

Vaccinations

Live vaccines should not be given concurrently with Enbrel. No data are available on the secondary transmission of infection by live vaccines in patients receiving Enbrel. It is recommended that juvenile idiopathic arthritis patients, if possible, be brought up to date with all immunisations in agreement with current immunisation guidelines prior to initiating Enbrel therapy. In a double blind, placebo controlled, randomised clinical study in adult patients with psoriatic arthritis 184 patients also received a multivalent pneumococcal polysaccharide vaccine at week 4. In this study most psoriatic arthritis patients receiving Enbrel were able to mount effective B-cell immune response to pneumococcal polysaccharide vaccine, but titers in aggregate were moderately lower and few patients had two-fold rises in titers compared to patients not receiving Enbrel. The clinical significance of this is unknown.

Autoantibody formation

Treatment with Enbrel may result in the formation of autoimmune antibodies (see section 4.8).

Haematologic reactions

Rare cases of pancytopenia and very rare cases of aplastic anaemia, some with fatal outcome, have been reported in patients treated with Enbrel. Caution should be exercised in patients being treated with Enbrel who have a previous history of blood dyscrasias. All patients and parents/caregivers should be advised that if the patient develops signs and symptoms suggestive of blood dyscrasias or infections (e.g. persistent fever, sore throat, bruising, bleeding, paleness) whilst on Enbrel, they should seek immediate medical advice. Such patients should be investigated urgently, including full blood count; if blood dyscrasias are confirmed, Enbrel should be discontinued.

CNS disorders

There have been rare reports of CNS demyelinating disorders in patients treated with Enbrel (see section 4.8). Although no clinical trials have been performed evaluating Enbrel therapy in patients with multiple sclerosis, clinical trials of other TNF antagonists in patients with multiple sclerosis have shown increases in disease activity. A careful risk/benefit evaluation, including a neurologic assessment, is recommended when prescribing Enbrel to patients with pre-existing or recent onset of CNS demyelinating disease, or to those who are considered to have an increased risk of developing demyelinating disease.

Combination therapy

In a controlled clinical trial of two years duration in adult rheumatoid arthritis patients, the combination of Enbrel and methotrexate did not result in unexpected safety findings, and the safety profile of Enbrel when given in combination with methotrexate was similar to the profiles reported in studies of Enbrel and methotrexate alone. Long-term studies to assess the safety of the combination are ongoing. The long-term safety of Enbrel in combination with other disease-modifying antirheumatic drugs (DMARD) has not been established.

Renal and hepatic impairment

Based on pharmacokinetic data (see section 5.2), no dose adjustment is needed in patients with renal or hepatic impairment; clinical experience in such patients is limited.

Congestive heart failure

Physicians should use caution when using Enbrel in patients who have congestive heart failure (CHF). There have been postmarketing reports of worsening of CHF, with and without identifiable precipitating factors, in patients taking Enbrel. Two large clinical trials evaluating the use of Enbrel in the treatment of CHF were terminated early due to lack of efficacy. Although not conclusive, data from one of these trials suggest a possible tendency toward worsening CHF in those patients assigned to Enbrel treatment.

Alcoholic hepatitis

In a phase II randomised placebo-controlled study of 48 hospitalised patients treated with Enbrel or placebo for moderate to severe alcoholic hepatitis, Enbrel was not efficacious, and the mortality rate in patients treated with Enbrel was significantly higher after 6 months. Consequently, Enbrel should not be used in patients for the treatment of alcoholic hepatitis. Physicians should use caution when using Enbrel in patients who also have moderate to severe alcoholic hepatitis.

Wegener's granulomatosis

A placebo-controlled trial, in which 89 adult patients were treated with Enbrel in addition to standard therapy (including cyclophosphamide or methotrexate, and glucocorticoids) for a median duration of 25 months, has not shown Enbrel to be an effective treatment for Wegener's granulomatosis. The incidence of non-cutaneous malignancies of various types was significantly higher in patients treated with Enbrel than in the control group. Enbrel is not recommended for the treatment of Wegener's granulomatosis.

Benzyl alcohol

Enbrel contains benzyl alcohol as an excipient, which may cause toxic reactions and anaphylactoid reactions in infants and children up to 3 years old and must not be given to premature babies or neonates.

4.5 Interaction with other medicinal products and other forms of interaction

Concurrent treatment with anakinra

Adult patients treated with Enbrel and anakinra were observed to have a higher rate of serious infection when compared with patients treated with either Enbrel or anakinra alone (historical data).

In addition, in a double-blind placebo-controlled trial in adult patients receiving background methotrexate, patients treated with Enbrel and anakinra were observed to have a higher rate of serious infections (7%) and neutropenia than patients treated with Enbrel (see sections 4.4 and 4.8). The combination Enbrel and anakinra has not demonstrated increased clinical benefit and is therefore not recommended.

Concurrent treatment with abatacept

In clinical studies, concurrent administration of abatacept and Enbrel resulted in increased incidences of serious adverse events. This combination has not demonstrated increased clinical benefit; such use is not recommended (see section 4.4).

Concurrent treatment with sulfasalazine

In a clinical study of adult patients who were receiving established doses of sulfasalazine, to which Enbrel was added, patients in the combination group experienced a statistically significant decrease in mean white blood cell counts in comparison to groups treated with Enbrel or sulfasalazine alone. The clinical significance of this interaction is unknown.

Non-interactions

In clinical trials, no interactions have been observed when Enbrel was administered with glucocorticoids, salicylates (except sulfasalazine), nonsteroidal anti-inflammatory drugs (NSAIDs), analgesics, or methotrexate. See section 4.4 for vaccination advice.

No clinically significant pharmacokinetic drug-drug interactions were observed in studies with digoxin or warfarin.

4.6 Pregnancy and lactation

Pregnancy

There are no studies of Enbrel in pregnant women. Developmental toxicity studies performed in rats and rabbits have revealed no evidence of harm to the foetus or neonatal rat due to etanercept. Preclinical data about peri- and postnatal toxicity of etanercept and of effects of etanercept on fertility and general reproductive performance are not available. Thus, the use of Enbrel in pregnant women is not recommended, and women of child-bearing potential should be advised not to get pregnant during Enbrel therapy.

Lactation

It is not known whether etanercept is excreted in human milk. Following subcutaneous administration to lactating rats, etanercept was excreted in the milk and detected in the serum of pups. Because immunoglobulins, in common with many medicinal products, can be excreted in human milk, a decision should be made whether to discontinue breast-feeding or to discontinue Enbrel while breast-feeding.

4.7 Effects on ability to drive and use machines

No studies on the effects on the ability to drive and use machines have been performed.

4.8 Undesirable effects

Undesirable effects in paediatric patients with polyarticular juvenile idiopathic arthritis

In general, the adverse events in paediatric patients with juvenile idiopathic arthritis were similar in frequency and type to those seen in adult patients (see below, Undesirable effects in adults). Differences from adults and other special considerations are discussed in the following paragraphs.

The types of infections seen in clinical trials in juvenile idiopathic arthritis patients aged 2 to 18 years were generally mild to moderate and consistent with those commonly seen in outpatient paediatric populations. Severe adverse events reported included varicella with signs and symptoms of aseptic meningitis, which resolved without sequelae (see also section 4.4), appendicitis, gastroenteritis, depression/personality disorder, cutaneous ulcer, oesophagitis/gastritis, group A streptococcal septic shock, type I diabetes mellitus, and soft tissue and post-operative wound infection.

In one study in children with juvenile idiopathic arthritis aged 4 to 17 years, 43 of 69 (62%) children experienced an infection while receiving Enbrel during 3 months of the study (part 1 open-label), and the frequency and severity of infections was similar in 58 patients completing 12 months of open-label extension therapy. The types and proportion of adverse events in juvenile idiopathic arthritis patients were similar to those seen in trials of Enbrel in adult patients with rheumatoid arthritis, and the majority were mild. Several adverse events were reported more commonly in 69 juvenile idiopathic arthritis patients receiving 3 months of Enbrel compared to the 349 adult rheumatoid arthritis patients. These included headache (19% of patients, 1.7 events per patient year), nausea (9%, 1.0 event per patient year), abdominal pain (19%, 0.74 events per patient year), and vomiting (13%, 0.74 events per patient year).

There were 4 reports of macrophage activation syndrome in juvenile idiopathic arthritis clinical trials.

Undesirable effects in paediatric patients with plaque psoriasis

In a 48-week study in 211 children aged 4 to 17 years with paediatric plaque psoriasis, the adverse events reported were similar to those seen in previous studies in adults with plaque psoriasis.

Undesirable effects in adults

Enbrel has been studied in 2,680 patients with rheumatoid arthritis in double-blind and open-label trials. This experience includes 2 placebo-controlled studies (349 Enbrel patients and 152 placebo patients) and 2 active-controlled trials, one active-controlled trial comparing Enbrel to methotrexate (415 Enbrel patients and 217 methotrexate patients) and another active-controlled trial comparing Enbrel (223 patients), methotrexate (228 patients) and Enbrel in combination with methotrexate (231 patients). The proportion of patients who discontinued treatment due to adverse events was the same in both the Enbrel and placebo treatment groups; in the first active-controlled trial, the dropout rate was significantly higher for methotrexate (10%) than for Enbrel (5%). In the second active-controlled trial, the rate of discontinuation for adverse events after 2 years of treatment was similar among all three treatment groups, Enbrel (16%), methotrexate (21%) and Enbrel in combination with methotrexate (17%). Additionally, Enbrel has been studied in 240 psoriatic arthritis patients who participated in 2 double-blind placebo-controlled studies and an open-label extension study. Five hundred and eight (508) ankylosing spondylitis patients were treated with Enbrel in 4 double-blind placebo-controlled studies. Enbrel has also been studied in 1,492 patients with plaque psoriasis for up to 6 months in 5 double-blind placebo-controlled studies.

In double-blind clinical trials comparing Enbrel to placebo, injection site reactions were the most frequent adverse events among Enbrel-treated patients. Among patients with rheumatoid arthritis treated in placebo-controlled trials, serious adverse events occurred at a frequency of 4% in 349 patients treated with Enbrel compared with 5% of 152 placebo-treated patients. In the first active-controlled trial, serious adverse events occurred at a frequency of 6% in 415 patients treated with Enbrel compared with 8% of 217 methotrexate-treated patients. In the second active-controlled trial the rate of serious adverse events after 2 years treatment was similar among the three treatment groups (Enbrel 16%, methotrexate 15% and Enbrel in combination with methotrexate 17%). Among patients with plaque psoriasis treated in placebo-controlled trials, the frequency of serious adverse events was about 1.4% of 1,341 patients treated with Enbrel compared with 1.4% of 766 placebo-treated patients.

The following list of adverse reactions is based on experience from clinical trials in adults and on postmarketing experience.

Within the organ system classes, adverse reactions are listed under headings of frequency (number of patients expected to experience the reaction), using the following categories: very common (⩾1/10); common (⩾1/100, <1/10); uncommon (⩾1/1000, <1/100); rare (⩾1/10,000, <1/1000); very rare (<1/10,000); not known (cannot be estimated from the available data).

Infections and infestations:

Very common: Infections (including upper respiratory tract infections, bronchitis, cystitis, skin infections)*

Uncommon: Serious infections (including pneumonia, cellulitis, septic arthritis, sepsis)*

Rare: Tuberculosis, opportunistic infections (including invasive fungal, protozoal, bacterial and atypical mycobacterial infections)*

Blood and lymphatic system disorders:

Uncommon: Thrombocytopenia

Rare: Anaemia, leukopenia, neutropenia, pancytopenia*

Very rare: Aplastic anaemia*

Immune system disorders:

Common: Allergic reactions (see Skin and subcutaneous tissue disorders), autoantibody formation*

Rare: Serious allergic/anaphylactic reactions (including angioedema, bronchospasm)

Not known: Macrophage activation syndrome†, anti-neutrophilic cytoplasmic antibody positive vasculitis

Nervous system disorders:

Rare: Seizures
CNS demyelinating events suggestive of multiple sclerosis or localised demyelinating conditions such as optic neuritis and transverse myelitis (see section 4.4)

Respiratory, thoracic and mediastinal disorders:

Uncommon: Interstitial lung disease (including pneumonitis and pulmonary fibrosis)*

Hepatobiliary disorders:

Rare: Elevated liver enzymes

Skin and subcutaneous tissue disorders:

Common: Pruritus

Uncommon: Non-melanoma skin cancers (see section 4.4), angioedema, urticaria, rash, psoriasiform rash, psoriasis (including new onset and pustular, primarily palms and soles)

Rare: Cutaneous vasculitis (including leukocytoclastic vasculitis), Stevens-Johnson syndrome, erythema multiforme

Very rare: Toxic epidermal necrolysis

Musculoskeletal and connective tissue disorders:

Rare: Subacute cutaneous lupus erythematosus, discoid lupus erythematosus, lupus like syndrome

General disorders and administration site conditions:

Very common: Injection site reactions (including bleeding, bruising, erythema, itching, pain, swelling)*

Common: Fever

Cardiac disorders:

There have been reports of worsening of congestive heart failure (see section 4.4).

*see Additional information, below.

† Please see sub-section 'Undesirable effects in paediatric patients with polyarticular juvenile idiopathic arthritis' above.

Additional information

Serious adverse events reported in clinical trials

Among rheumatoid arthritis, psoriatic arthritis, ankylosing spondylitis and plaque psoriasis patients in placebo-controlled, active-controlled, and open-label trials of Enbrel, serious adverse events reported included malignancies (see below), asthma, infections (see below), heart failure, myocardial infarction, myocardial ischaemia, chest pain, syncope, cerebral ischaemia, hypertension, hypotension, cholecystitis, pancreatitis, gastrointestinal haemorrhage, bursitis, confusion, depression, dyspnoea, abnormal healing, renal insufficiency, kidney calculus, deep vein thrombosis, pulmonary embolism, membranous glomerulonephropathy, polymyositis, thrombophlebitis, liver damage, leucopenia, paresis, paresthesia, vertigo, allergic alveolitis, angioedema, scleritis, bone fracture, lymphadenopathy, ulcerative colitis, intestinal obstruction, eosinophilia, haematuria, and sarcoidosis.

Malignancies and lymphoproliferative disorders

One hundred and twenty-nine new malignancies of various types were observed in 4,114 rheumatoid arthritis patients treated in clinical trials with Enbrel for up to approximately 6 years, including 231 patients treated with Enbrel in combination with methotrexate in the 2-year active-controlled study. The observed rates and incidences in these clinical trials were similar to those expected for the population studied. A total of 2 malignancies were reported in clinical studies of approximately 2 years duration involving 240 Enbrel-treated psoriatic arthritis patients. In clinical studies conducted for more than 2 years with 351 ankylosing spondylitis patients, 6 malignancies were reported in Enbrel-treated patients. In a group of 2,711 plaque psoriasis patients treated with Enbrel in double-blind and open-label studies of up to 2.5 years, 30 malignancies and 43 nonmelanoma skin cancers were reported.

In a group of 7,416 patients treated with Enbrel in rheumatoid arthritis, psoriatic arthritis, ankylosing spondylitis and psoriasis clinical trials, 18 lymphomas were reported.

Reports of various malignancies (including breast and lung carcinoma and lymphoma) have also been received in the postmarketing period (see section 4.4).

Injection site reactions

Compared to placebo, patients with rheumatic diseases treated with Enbrel had a significantly higher incidence of injection site reactions (36% vs. 9%). Injection site reactions usually occurred in the first month. Mean duration was approximately 3 to 5 days. No treatment was given for the majority of injection site reactions in the Enbrel treatment groups, and the majority of patients who were given treatment received topical preparations such as corticosteroids, or oral antihistamines. Additionally, some patients developed recall injection site reactions characterised by a skin reaction at the most recent site of injection along with the simultaneous appearance of injection site reactions at previous injection sites. These reactions were generally transient and did not recur with treatment.

In controlled trials in patients with plaque psoriasis, approximately 13.6% of patients treated with Enbrel developed injection site reactions compared with 3.4% of placebo-treated patients during the first 12 weeks of treatment.

Serious infections

In placebo-controlled trials, no increase in the incidence of serious infections (fatal, life threatening, or requiring hospitalisation or intravenous antibiotics) was observed. Serious infections occurred in 6.3% of rheumatoid arthritis patients treated with Enbrel for up to 48 months. These included abscess (at various sites), bacteraemia, bronchitis, bursitis, cellulitis, cholecystitis, diarrhoea, diverticulitis, endocarditis (suspected), gastroenteritis, hepatitis B, herpes zoster, leg ulcer, mouth infection, osteomyelitis, otitis, peritonitis, pneumonia, pyelonephritis, sepsis, septic arthritis, sinusitis, skin infection, skin ulcer, urinary tract infection, vasculitis, and wound infection. In the 2-year active-controlled study where patients were treated with either Enbrel alone, methotrexate alone or Enbrel in combination with methotrexate, the rates of serious infections were similar among the treatment groups. However, it cannot be excluded that the combination of Enbrel with methotrexate could be associated with an increase in the rate of infections.

There were no differences in rates of infection among patients treated with Enbrel and those treated with placebo for plaque psoriasis in placebo controlled trials of up to 24 weeks duration. Serious infections experienced by Enbrel-treated patients included cellulitis, gastroenteritis, pneumonia, cholecystitis, osteomyelitis, gastritis, appendicitis, Streptococcal fasciitis, myositis, septic shock, diverticulitis and abscess. In the double-blind and open-label psoriatic arthritis trials, 1 patient reported a serious infection (pneumonia).

Serious and fatal infections have been reported during use of Enbrel; reported pathogens include bacteria, mycobacteria (including tuberculosis), viruses and fungi. Some have occurred within a few weeks after initiating treatment with Enbrel in patients who have underlying conditions (e.g. diabetes, congestive heart failure, history of active or chronic infections) in addition to their rheumatoid arthritis (see section 4.4). Enbrel treatment may increase mortality in patients with established sepsis.

Opportunistic infections have been reported in association with Enbrel including invasive fungal, protozoal, bacterial (including *Listeria* and *Legionella*), and atypical mycobacterial infections. In a pooled data set of clinical trials, the overall incidence of opportunistic infections was 0.09% for the 15,402 subjects who received Enbrel. The exposure-adjusted rate was 0.06 events per 100 patient-years. In postmarketing experience, approximately half of all of the case reports of opportunistic infections worldwide were invasive fungal infections. The most commonly reported invasive fungal infections were *Pneumocystis* and *Aspergillus*. Invasive fungal infections accounted for more than half of the fatalities amongst patients who developed opportunistic infections. The majority of the reports with a fatal outcome were in patients with *Pneumocystis* pneumonia, unspecified systemic fungal infections, and aspergillosis (see section 4.4).

Autoantibodies

Adult patients had serum samples tested for autoantibodies at multiple timepoints. Of the rheumatoid arthritis patients evaluated for antinuclear antibodies (ANA), the percentage of patients who developed new positive ANA (⩾1:40) was higher in patients treated with Enbrel (11%) than in placebo-treated patients (5%). The percentage of patients who developed new positive anti-double-stranded DNA antibodies was also higher by radioimmunoassay (15% of patients treated with Enbrel compared to 4% of placebo-treated patients) and by *Crithidia luciliae* assay (3% of patients treated with Enbrel compared to none of placebo-treated patients). The proportion of patients treated with Enbrel who developed anticardiolipin antibodies was similarly increased compared to placebo-treated patients. The impact of long-term treatment with Enbrel on the development of autoimmune diseases is unknown.

There have been rare reports of patients, including rheumatoid factor positive patients, who have developed other autoantibodies in conjunction with a lupus-like syndrome or rashes that are compatible with subacute cutaneous lupus or discoid lupus by clinical presentation and biopsy.

Pancytopenia and aplastic anaemia

There have been postmarketing reports of pancytopenia and aplastic anaemia, some of which had fatal outcomes (see section 4.4)

Interstitial lung disease

There have been postmarketing reports of interstitial lung disease (including pneumonitis and pulmonary fibrosis), some of which had fatal outcomes.

Laboratory evaluations

Based on the results of clinical studies, normally no special laboratory evaluations are necessary in addition to careful medical management and supervision of patients.

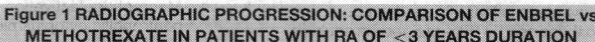

Concurrent treatment with anakinra

In studies when adult patients received concurrent treatment with Enbrel plus anakinra, a higher rate of serious infections compared to Enbrel alone was observed and 2% of patients (3/139) developed neutropenia (absolute neutrophil count < 1000 / mm3). While neutropenic, one patient developed cellulitis that resolved after hospitalisation (see sections 4.4 and 4.5).

4.9 Overdose

No dose-limiting toxicities were observed during clinical trials of rheumatoid arthritis patients. The highest dose level evaluated has been an intravenous loading dose of 32 mg/m^2 followed by subcutaneous doses of 16 mg/m^2 administered twice weekly. One rheumatoid arthritis patient mistakenly self-administered 62 mg Enbrel subcutaneously twice weekly for 3 weeks without experiencing undesirable effects. There is no known antidote to Enbrel.

5. PHARMACOLOGICAL PROPERTIES

5.1 Pharmacodynamic properties

Pharmacotherapeutic group: Tumor Necrosis Factor alpha (TNF-α) inhibitors, ATC code: L04AB01

Tumour necrosis factor (TNF) is a dominant cytokine in the inflammatory process of rheumatoid arthritis. Elevated levels of TNF are also found in the synovium and psoriatic plaques of patients with psoriatic arthritis and in serum and synovial tissue of patients with ankylosing spondylitis. In plaque psoriasis, infiltration by inflammatory cells including T-cells leads to increased TNF levels in psoriatic lesions compared with levels in uninvolved skin. Etanercept is a competitive inhibitor of TNF-binding to its cell surface receptors and thereby inhibits the biological activity of TNF. TNF and lymphotoxin are pro-inflammatory cytokines that bind to two distinct cell surface receptors: the 55-kilodalton (p55) and 75-kilodalton (p75) tumour necrosis factor receptors (TNFRs). Both TNFRs exist naturally in membrane-bound and soluble forms. Soluble TNFRs are thought to regulate TNF biological activity.

TNF and lymphotoxin exist predominantly as homotrimers, with their biological activity dependent on cross-linking of cell surface TNFRs. Dimeric soluble receptors such as etanercept possess a higher affinity for TNF than monomeric receptors and are considerably more potent competitive inhibitors of TNF binding to its cellular receptors. In addition, use of an immunoglobulin Fc region as a fusion element in the construction of a dimeric receptor imparts a longer serum half-life.

Mechanism of action

Much of the joint pathology in rheumatoid arthritis and ankylosing spondylitis and skin pathology in plaque psoriasis is mediated by pro-inflammatory molecules that are linked in a network controlled by TNF. The mechanism of action of etanercept is thought to be its competitive inhibition of TNF binding to cell surface TNFR, preventing TNF-mediated cellular responses by rendering TNF biologically inactive. Etanercept may also modulate biologic responses controlled by additional downstream molecules (e.g., cytokines, adhesion molecules, or proteinases) that are induced or regulated by TNF.

Clinical trials

This section presents data from one study in polyarticular juvenile idiopathic arthritis, four studies in adults with rheumatoid arthritis, one study in paediatric patients with plaque psoriasis, and four studies in adults with plaque psoriasis.

Paediatric patients with polyarticular juvenile idiopathic arthritis

The safety and efficacy of Enbrel were assessed in a two-part study in 69 children with polyarticular juvenile idiopathic arthritis who had a variety of juvenile idiopathic arthritis onset types. Patients aged 4 to 17 years with moderately to severely active polyarticular juvenile idiopathic arthritis refractory to or intolerant of methotrexate were enrolled; patients remained on a stable dose of a single nonsteroidal anti-inflammatory drug and/or prednisone (< 0.2 mg/kg/day or 10 mg maximum). In part 1, all patients received 0.4 mg/kg (maximum 25 mg per dose) Enbrel subcutaneously twice weekly. In part 2, patients with a clinical response at day 90 were randomised to remain on Enbrel or receive placebo for four months and assessed for disease flare. Responses were measured using the JRA Definition of Improvement (DOI), defined as ≥ 30% improvement in at least three of six and ≥ 30% worsening in no more than one of six JRA core set criteria, including active joint count, limitation of motion, physician and patient/parent global assessments, functional assessment, and erythrocyte sedimentation rate (ESR). Disease flare was defined as a ≥ 30% worsening in three of six JRA core set criteria and ≥ 30% improvement in not more than one of the six JRA core set criteria and a minimum of two active joints.

In part 1 of the study, 51 of 69 (74%) patients demonstrated a clinical response and entered part 2. In part 2, 6 of 25 (24%) patients remaining on Enbrel experienced a disease flare compared to 20 of 26 (77%) patients receiving placebo (p=0.007). From the start of part 2, the median time to flare was ≥ 116 days for patients who received Enbrel and 28 days for patients who received placebo. Of patients who demonstrated a clinical response at 90 days and entered part 2 of the study, some of the patients remaining on Enbrel continued to improve from month 3 through month 7, while those who received placebo did not improve.

Studies have not been done in patients with polyarticular juvenile idiopathic arthritis to assess the effects of continued Enbrel therapy in patients who do not respond within 3 months of initiating Enbrel therapy or to assess the combination of Enbrel with methotrexate.

Adult patients with rheumatoid arthritis

The efficacy of Enbrel was assessed in a randomised, double-blind, placebo-controlled study. The study evaluated 234 adult patients with active rheumatoid arthritis who had failed therapy with at least one but no more than four disease-modifying antirheumatic drugs (DMARDs). Doses of 10 mg or 25 mg Enbrel or placebo were administered subcutaneously twice a week for 6 consecutive months. The results of this controlled trial were expressed in percentage improvement in rheumatoid arthritis using American College of Rheumatology (ACR) response criteria.

ACR 20 and 50 responses were higher in patients treated with Enbrel at 3 and 6 months than in patients treated with placebo (ACR 20: Enbrel 62% and 59%, placebo 23% and 11% at 3 and 6 months respectively: ACR 50: Enbrel 41% and 40%, placebo 8% and 5% at months 3 and 6 respectively; p < 0.01 Enbrel vs placebo at all time points for both ACR 20 and ACR 50 responses).

Approximately 15% of subjects who received Enbrel achieved an ACR 70 response at month 3 and month 6 compared to fewer than 5% of subjects in the placebo arm. Among patients receiving Enbrel, the clinical responses generally appeared within 1 to 2 weeks after initiation of therapy and nearly always occurred by 3 months. A dose response was seen; results with 10 mg were intermediate between placebo and 25 mg. Enbrel was significantly better than placebo in all components of the ACR criteria as well as other measures of rheumatoid arthritis disease activity not included in the ACR response criteria, such as morning stiffness. A Health Assessment Questionnaire (HAQ), which included disability, vitality, mental health, general health status, and arthritis-associated health status subdomains, was administered every 3 months during the trial. All subdomains of the HAQ were improved in patients treated with Enbrel compared to controls at 3 and 6 months.

After discontinuation of Enbrel, symptoms of arthritis generally returned within a month. Re-introduction of treatment with Enbrel after discontinuation of up to 24 months resulted in the same magnitudes of responses as patients who received Enbrel without interruption of therapy based on results of open-label studies. Continued durable responses have been seen for up to 48 months in open-label extension treatment trials when patients received Enbrel without interruption; longer-term experience in not available.

The efficacy of Enbrel was compared to methotrexate in a randomised, active-controlled study with blinded radiographic evaluations as a primary endpoint in 632 adult patients with active rheumatoid arthritis (<3 years duration) who had never received treatment with methotrexate. Doses of 10 mg or 25 mg Enbrel were administered SC twice a week for up to 24 months. Methotrexate doses were escalated from 7.5 mg/week to a maximum of 20 mg/week over the first 8 weeks of the trial and continued for up to 24 months. Clinical improvement including onset of action within 2 weeks with Enbrel 25 mg was similar to that seen in the previous trials, and was maintained for up to 24 months. At baseline, patients had a moderate degree of disability, with mean HAQ scores of 1.4 to 1.5. Treatment with Enbrel 25 mg resulted in substantial improvement at 12 months, with about 44% of patients achieving a normal HAQ score (less than 0.5). This benefit was maintained in Year 2 of this study.

In this study, structural joint damage was assessed radiographically and expressed as change in Total Sharp Score (TSS) and its components, the erosion score and joint space narrowing score (JSN). Radiographs of hands/wrists and feet were read at baseline and 6, 12, and 24 months. The 10 mg Enbrel dose had consistently less effect on structural damage than the 25 mg dose. Enbrel 25 mg was significantly superior to methotrexate for erosion scores at both 12 and 24 months. The differences in TSS and JSN were not statistically significant between methotrexate and Enbrel 25 mg. The results are shown in the figure below.

RADIOGRAPHIC PROGRESSION: COMPARISON OF ENBREL vs METHOTREXATE IN PATIENTS WITH RA OF <3 YEARS DURATION

(see Figure 1 above)

Figure 1 RADIOGRAPHIC PROGRESSION: COMPARISON OF ENBREL vs METHOTREXATE IN PATIENTS WITH RA OF <3 YEARS DURATION

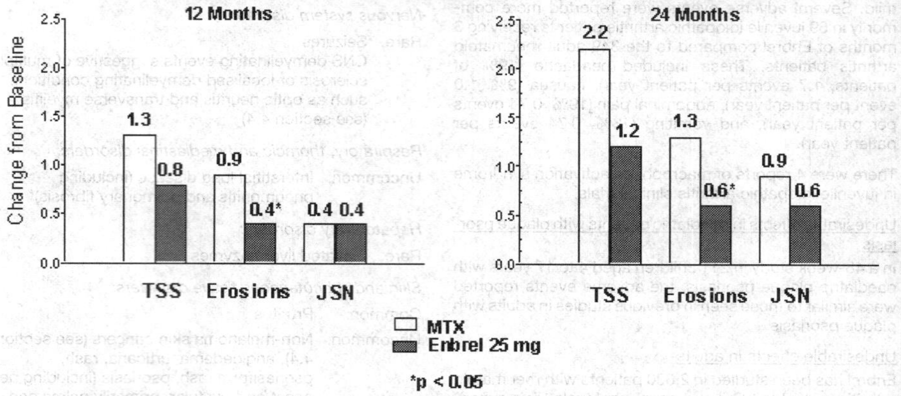

In another active-controlled, double-blind, randomised study, clinical efficacy, safety, and radiographic progression in RA patients treated with Enbrel alone (25 mg twice weekly), methotrexate alone (7.5 to 20 mg weekly, median dose 20 mg), and of the combination of Enbrel and methotrexate initiated concurrently were compared in 682 adult patients with active rheumatoid arthritis of 6 months to 20 years duration (median 5 years) who had a less than satisfactory response to at least 1 disease-modifying antirheumatic drug (DMARD) other than methotrexate.

Patients in the Enbrel in combination with methotrexate therapy group had significantly higher ACR 20, ACR 50, ACR 70 responses and improvement for DAS and HAQ scores at both 24 and 52 weeks than patients in either of the single therapy groups (results shown in table below). Significant advantages for Enbrel in combination with methotrexate compared with Enbrel monotherapy and methotrexate monotherapy were also observed after 24 months.

CLINICAL EFFICACY RESULTS AT 12 MONTHS: COMPARISON OF ENBREL vs METHOTREXATE vs ENBREL IN COMBINATION WITH METHOTREXATE IN PATIENTS WITH RA OF 6 MONTHS TO 20 YEARS DURATION

Endpoint	Methotrexate (n = 228)	Enbrel (n = 223)	Enbrel + Methotrexate (n = 231)
ACR Responses[a]			
ACR 20	58.8%	65.5%	74.5% †,φ
ACR 50	36.4%	43.0%	63.2% †,φ
ACR 70	16.7%	22.0%	39.8% †,φ
DAS			
Baseline score[b]	5.5	5.7	5.5
Week 52 score[b]	3.0	3.0	2.3[†,φ]
Remission[c]	14%	18%	37%[†,φ]
HAQ			
Baseline	1.7	1.7	1.8
Week 52	1.1	1.0	0.8[†,φ]

a: Patients who did not complete 12 months in the study were considered to be non-responders.

b: Values for Disease Activity Score (DAS) are means.

c: Remission is defined as DAS <1.6

Pairwise comparison p-values: † = p < 0.05 for comparisons of Enbrel + methotrexate vs methotrexate and φ = p < 0.05 for comparisons of Enbrel + methotrexate vs Enbrel

Radiographic progression at 12 months was significantly less in the Enbrel group than in the methotrexate group, while the combination was significantly better than either monotherapy at slowing radiographic progression (see figure below).

Figure 2 RADIOGRAPHIC PROGRESSION: COMPARISON OF ENBREL vs METHOTREXATE vs ENBREL IN COMBINATION WITH METHOTREXATE IN PATIENTS WITH RA OF 6 MONTHS TO 20 YEARS DURATION (12 MONTH RESULTS)

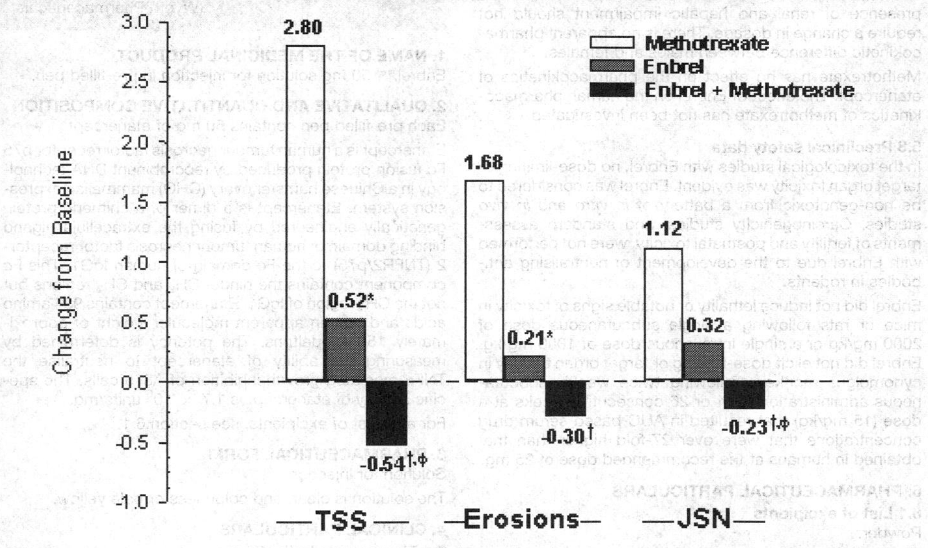

Pairwise comparison p-values: * = $p < 0.05$ for comparisons of Enbrel vs methotrexate, † = $p < 0.05$ for comparisons of Enbrel + methotrexate vs methotrexate and ϕ = $p < 0.05$ for comparisons of Enbrel + methotrexate vs Enbrel

RADIOGRAPHIC PROGRESSION: COMPARISON OF ENBREL vs METHOTREXATE vs ENBREL IN COMBINATION WITH METHOTREXATE IN PATIENTS WITH RA OF 6 MONTHS TO 20 YEARS DURATION (12 MONTH RESULTS)

(see Figure 2 above)

Significant advantages for Enbrel in combination with methotrexate compared with Enbrel monotherapy and methotrexate monotherapy were also observed after 24 months. Similarly, the significant advantages for Enbrel monotherapy compared with methotrexate monotherapy were also observed after 24 months.

In an analysis in which all patients who dropped out of the study for any reason were considered to have progressed, the percentage of patients without progression (TSS change ⩽ 0.5) at 24 months was higher in the Enbrel in combination with methotrexate group compared with the Enbrel alone and methotrexate alone groups (62%, 50%, and 36%, respectively; p<0.05). The difference between Enbrel alone and methotrexate alone was also significant (p<0.05). Among patients who completed a full 24 months of therapy in the study, the non-progression rates were 78%, 70%, and 61%, respectively.

The safety and efficacy of 50mg Enbrel (two 25 mg SC injections) administered once weekly were evaluated in a double-blind, placebo-controlled study of 420 patients with active RA. In this study, 53 patients received placebo, 214 patients received 50 mg Enbrel once weekly and 153 patients received 25 mg Enbrel twice weekly. The safety and efficacy profiles of the two Enbrel treatment regimens were comparable at week 8 in their effect on signs and symptoms of RA; data at week 16 did not show comparability (non-inferiority) between the two regimens.

Adult patients with plaque psoriasis

Enbrel is recommended for use in patients as defined in section 4.1. Patients who "failed to respond to" in the target population is defined by insufficient response (PASI < 50 or PGA less than good), or worsening of the disease while on treatment, and who were adequately dosed for a sufficiently long duration to assess response with at least each of the three major systemic therapies as available.

The efficacy of Enbrel versus other systemic therapies in patients with moderate to severe psoriasis (responsive to other systemic therapies) has not been evaluated in studies directly comparing Enbrel with other systemic therapies. Instead, the safety and efficacy of Enbrel were assessed in four randomised, double-blind, placebo-controlled studies. The primary efficacy endpoint in all four studies was the proportion of patients in each treatment group who achieved the PASI 75 (i.e., at least a 75% improvement in the Psoriasis Area and Severity Index score from baseline) at 12 weeks.

Study 1 was a Phase 2 study in patients with active but clinically stable plaque psoriasis involving ⩾ 10% of the body surface area that were ⩾ 18 years old. One hundred and twelve (112) patients were randomised to receive a dose of 25 mg of Enbrel (n=57) or placebo (n=55) twice a week for 24 weeks.

Study 2 evaluated 652 patients with chronic plaque psoriasis using the same inclusion criteria as study 1 with the addition of a minimum psoriasis area and severity index (PASI) of 10 at screening. Enbrel was administered at doses of 25 mg once a week, 25 mg twice a week or 50 mg twice a week for 6 consecutive months. During the first 12 weeks of the double-blind treatment period, patients received placebo or one of the above three Enbrel doses. After 12 weeks of treatment, patients in the placebo group began treatment with blinded Enbrel (25 mg twice a week); patients in the active treatment groups continued to week 24 on the dose to which they were originally randomised.

Study 3 evaluated 583 patients and had the same inclusion criteria as study 2. Patients in this study received a dose of 25 mg or 50 mg Enbrel, or placebo twice a week for 12 weeks and then all patients received open-label 25 mg Enbrel twice weekly for an additional 24 weeks.

Study 4 evaluated 142 patients and had similar inclusion criteria to studies 2 and 3. Patients in this study received a dose of 50 mg Enbrel or placebo once weekly for 12 weeks and then all patients received open-label 50 mg Enbrel once weekly for an additional 12 weeks.

In study 1, the Enbrel-treated group had a significantly higher proportion of patients with a PASI 75 response at week 12 (30%) compared to the placebo-treated group (2%) (p<0.0001). At 24 weeks, 56% of patients in the Enbrel-treated group had achieved the PASI 75 compared to 5% of placebo-treated patients. Key results of studies 2, 3 and 4 are shown below.

(see Table 1 below)

Among patients with plaque psoriasis who received Enbrel, significant responses relative to placebo were apparent at the time of the first visit (2 weeks) and were maintained through 24 weeks of therapy.

Study 2 also had a drug withdrawal period during which patients who achieved a PASI improvement of at least 50% at week 24 had treatment stopped. Patients were observed off treatment for the occurrence of rebound (PASI ⩾150% of baseline) and for the time to relapse (defined as a loss of at least half of the improvement achieved between baseline and week 24). During the withdrawal period, symptoms of psoriasis gradually returned with a median time to disease relapse of 3 months. No rebound flare of disease and no psoriasis-related serious adverse events were observed. There was some evidence to support a benefit of re-treatment with Enbrel in patients initially responding to treatment.

In study 3, the majority of patients (77%) who were initially randomised to 50 mg twice weekly and had their Enbrel dose decreased at week 12 to 25 mg twice weekly maintained their PASI 75 response through week 36. For patients who received 25 mg twice weekly throughout the study, the PASI 75 response continued to improve between weeks 12 and 36.

In study 4, the Enbrel-treated group had a higher proportion of patients with PASI 75 at week 12 (38%) compared to the placebo-treated group (2%) (p<0.0001). For patients who received 50 mg once weekly throughout the study, the efficacy responses continued to improve with 71% achieving PASI 75 at week 24.

In long-term (up to 34 months) open-label studies where Enbrel was given without interruption, clinical responses were sustained and safety was comparable to shorter-term studies.

An analysis of clinical trial data did not reveal any baseline disease characteristics that would assist clinicians in selecting the most appropriate dosing option (intermittent or continuous). Consequently, the choice of intermittent or continuous therapy should be based upon physician judgment and individual patient needs.

Paediatric patients with plaque psoriasis

The efficacy of Enbrel was assessed in a randomised, double-blind, placebo-controlled study in 211 paediatric patients aged 4 to 17 years with moderate to severe plaque psoriasis (as defined by a sPGA score ⩾ 3, involving ⩾ 10% of the BSA, and PASI ⩾ 12). Eligible patients had a history of receiving phototherapy or systemic therapy, or were inadequately controlled on topical therapy.

Patients received Enbrel 0.8 mg/kg (up to 50 mg) or placebo once weekly for 12 weeks. At week 12, more patients randomised to Enbrel had positive efficacy responses (e.g., PASI 75) than those randomised to placebo.

Paediatric Plaque Psoriasis Outcomes at 12 Weeks		
	Enbrel 0.8 mg/kg Once Weekly (N = 106)	**Placebo (N = 105)**
PASI 75, n (%)	60 (57%)[a]	12 (11%)
PASI 50, n (%)	79 (75%)[a]	24 (23%)
sPGA "clear" or "minimal", n (%)	56 (53%)[a]	14 (13%)

Abbreviation: sPGA-static Physician Global Assessment.

a. p < 0.0001 compared with placebo.

After the 12-week double-blind treatment period, all patients received Enbrel 0.8 mg/kg (up to 50 mg) once weekly for additional 24 weeks. Responses observed during the open-label period were similar to those observed in the double-blind period.

Table 1 RESPONSES OF PATIENTS WITH PSORIASIS IN STUDIES 2, 3 AND 4

Response (%)	Study 2					Study 3			Study 4		
	Placebo	Enbrel				Placebo	Enbrel		Placebo	Enbrel	
		25 mg BIW		50 mg BIW			25 mg BIW	50 mg BIW		50 mg QW	50 mg QW
	n = 166 wk 12	n = 162 wk 12	n = 162 wk 24[a]	n = 164 wk 12	n = 164 wk 24[a]	n = 193 wk 12	n = 196 wk 12	n = 196 wk 12	n = 46 wk 12	n = 96 wk 12	n = 90 wk 24[a]
PASI 50	14	58*	70	74*	77	9	64*	77*	9	69*	83
PASI 75	4	34*	44	49*	59	3	34*	49*	2	38*	71
DSGA [b], clear or almost clear	5	34*	39	49*	55	4	39*	57*	4	39*	64

*p ⩽ 0.0001 compared with placebo

a. No statistical comparisons to placebo were made at week 24 in studies 2 and 4 because the original placebo group began receiving Enbrel 25 mg BIW or 50 mg once weekly from week 13 to week 24.

b. Dermatologist Static Global Assessment. Clear or almost clear defined as 0 or 1 on a 0 to 5 scale.

During a randomised withdrawal period, significantly more patients re-randomised to placebo experienced disease relapse (loss of PASI 75 response) compared with patients re-randomised to Enbrel. With continued therapy, responses were maintained up to 48 weeks.

Antibodies to Enbrel

Antibodies to etanercept have been detected in the sera of some subjects treated with etanercept. These antibodies have all been non-neutralising and are generally transient. There appears to be no correlation between antibody development and clinical response or adverse events.

In subjects treated with approved doses of etanercept in clinical trials for up to 12 months, cumulative rates of anti-etanercept antibodies were approximately 6% of subjects with rheumatoid arthritis, 7.5% of subjects with psoriatic arthritis, 2% of subjects with ankylosing spondylitis, 7% of subjects with psoriasis, 9.7% of subjects with paediatric psoriasis, and 3% of subjects with juvenile idiopathic arthritis.

The proportion of subjects who developed antibodies to etanercept in longer-term trials (of up to 3.5 years) increases over time, as expected. However, due to their transient nature, the incidence of antibodies detected at each assessment point was typically less than 7% in rheumatoid arthritis subjects and psoriasis subjects.

In a long-term psoriasis study in which patients received 50 mg twice weekly for 96 weeks, the incidence of antibodies observed at each assessment point was up to approximately 9%.

5.2 Pharmacokinetic properties

Etanercept serum values were determined by an ELISA method, which may detect ELISA-reactive degradation products as well as the parent compound.

<u>Special populations</u>

Paediatric patients with polyarticular juvenile idiopathic arthritis

In a polyarticular juvenile idiopathic arthritis trial with Enbrel, 69 patients (aged 4 to 17 years) were administered 0.4 mg Enbrel/kg twice weekly for three months. Serum concentration profiles were similar to those seen in adult rheumatoid arthritis patients. The youngest children (4 years of age) had reduced clearance (increased clearance when normalised by weight) compared with older children (12 years of age) and adults. Simulation of dosing suggests that while older children (10-17 years of age) will have serum levels close to those seen in adults, younger children will have appreciably lower levels.

Paediatric patients with plaque psoriasis

Patients with paediatric plaque psoriasis (aged 4 to 17 years) were administered 0.8 mg/kg (up to a maximum dose of 50 mg per week) of etanercept once weekly for up to 48 weeks. The mean serum steady state trough concentrations ranged from 1.6 to 2.1 mcg/ml at weeks 12, 24, and 48. These mean concentrations in patients with paediatric plaque psoriasis were similar to the concentrations observed in patients with juvenile idiopathic arthritis (treated with 0.4 mg/kg etanercept twice weekly, up to maximum dose of 50 mg per week). These mean concentrations were similar to those seen in adult patients with plaque psoriasis treated with 25 mg etanercept twice weekly.

Adults

Etanercept is slowly absorbed from the site of subcutaneous injection, reaching maximum concentration approximately 48 hours after a single dose. The absolute bioavailability is 76%. With twice weekly doses, it is anticipated that steady-state concentrations are approximately twice as high as those observed after single doses. After a single subcutaneous dose of 25 mg Enbrel, the average maximum serum concentration observed in healthy volunteers was 1.65 ± 0.66 μg/ml, and the area under the curve was 235 ± 96.6 μg•hr/ml. Dose proportionality has not been formally evaluated, but there is no apparent saturation of clearance across the dosing range.

A biexponential curve is required to describe the concentration time curve of etanercept. The central volume of distribution of etanercept is 7.6 l, while the volume of distribution at steady-state is 10.4 l. Etanercept is cleared slowly from the body. The half-life is long, approximately 70 hours. Clearance is approximately 0.066 l/hr in patients with rheumatoid arthritis, somewhat lower than the value of 0.11 l/hr observed in healthy volunteers. Additionally, the pharmacokinetics of Enbrel in rheumatoid arthritis patients, ankylosing spondylitis and plaque psoriasis patients are similar.

Mean serum concentration profiles at steady state in treated RA patients were Cmax of 2.4 mg/l vs 2.6 mg/l, Cmin of 1.2 mg/l vs 1.4 mg/l, and partial AUC of 297 mgh/l vs 316 mgh/l for 50 mg Enbrel once weekly (n=21) vs 25 mg Enbrel twice weekly (n=16), respectively. In an open-label, single-dose, two-treatment, crossover study in healthy volunteers, etanercept administered as a single 50 mg/ml injection was found to be bioequivalent to two simultaneous injections of 25 mg/ml.

In a population pharmacokinetics analysis in ankylosing spondylitis patients the etanercept steady state AUCs were 466 μg•hr/ml and 474 μg•hr/ml for 50 mg Enbrel once weekly (N= 154) and 25 mg twice weekly (N = 148), respectively.

Although there is elimination of radioactivity in urine after administration of radiolabelled etanercept to patients and volunteers, increased etanercept concentrations were not observed in patients with acute renal or hepatic failure. The presence of renal and hepatic impairment should not require a change in dosage. There is no apparent pharmacokinetic difference between males and females.

Methotrexate has no effect on the pharmacokinetics of etanercept. The effect of Enbrel on the human pharmacokinetics of methotrexate has not been investigated.

5.3 Preclinical safety data

In the toxicological studies with Enbrel, no dose-limiting or target organ toxicity was evident. Enbrel was considered to be non-genotoxic from a battery of *in vitro* and *in vivo* studies. Carcinogenicity studies, and standard assessments of fertility and postnatal toxicity, were not performed with Enbrel due to the development of neutralising antibodies in rodents.

Enbrel did not induce lethality or notable signs of toxicity in mice or rats following a single subcutaneous dose of 2000 mg/kg or a single intravenous dose of 1000 mg/kg. Enbrel did not elicit dose-limiting or target organ toxicity in cynomolgus monkeys following twice weekly subcutaneous administration for 4 or 26 consecutive weeks at a dose (15 mg/kg) that resulted in AUC-based serum drug concentrations that were over 27-fold higher than that obtained in humans at the recommended dose of 25 mg.

6. PHARMACEUTICAL PARTICULARS

6.1 List of excipients

Powder:

Mannitol

Sucrose

Trometamol.

Solvent:

Water for injections

Benzyl alcohol.

6.2 Incompatibilities

In the absence of compatibility studies, this medicinal product must not be mixed with other medicinal products.

6.3 Shelf life

3 years.

After reconstitution, chemical and physical stability has been demonstrated for 14 days at 2°C – 8°C. From a microbiological point of view, once reconstituted, the product may be stored for a maximum of 14 days at 2°C – 8°C. Other storage times and conditions are the responsibility of the user.

6.4 Special precautions for storage

Store in a refrigerator (2°C – 8°C). Do not freeze

For storage conditions of the reconstituted medicinal product see section 6.3.

6.5 Nature and contents of container

Clear glass vial (4 ml, type I glass) with rubber stoppers, aluminium seals, and flip-off plastic caps. Enbrel is supplied with pre-filled syringes containing bacteriostatic water for injections. The syringes are type I glass-fitted with stainless steel needles. Cartons contain 4 vials of Enbrel with 4 pre-filled solvent syringes, 8 empty plastic syringes, 20 stainless steel needles and 24 alcohol swabs.

6.6 Special precautions for disposal and other handling

Any unused product or waste material should be disposed of in accordance with local requirements.

<u>Instructions for use and handling</u>

Enbrel is reconstituted with 1 ml bacteriostatic water for injections before use, and administered by subcutaneous injection. The solution should be clear and colourless to pale yellow, with no lumps, flakes or particles. Some white foam may remain in the vial – this is normal. Enbrel should not be used if all the powder in the vial is not dissolved within 10 minutes. Start again with another vial.

Comprehensive instructions for the preparation, administration and re-use of the reconstituted Enbrel vial are given in the package leaflet, section 7, "Instructions for preparation and giving an injection of Enbrel.

7. MARKETING AUTHORISATION HOLDER

Wyeth Europa Ltd.

Huntercombe Lane South

Taplow, Maidenhead

Berkshire, SL6 0PH

United Kingdom

8. MARKETING AUTHORISATION NUMBER(S)

EU/1/99/126/012

9. DATE OF FIRST AUTHORISATION/RENEWAL OF THE AUTHORISATION

Date of first authorisation: 3 February 2000

Date of last renewal: 3 February 2005

10. DATE OF REVISION OF THE TEXT

16 July 2009

Detailed information on this product is available on the website of the European Medicines Agency (EMEA) http://www.emea.europa.eu

Enbrel 50 mg solution for injection in pre-filled pen

(Wyeth Pharmaceuticals)

1. NAME OF THE MEDICINAL PRODUCT

Enbrel®▼50 mg solution for injection in pre-filled pen.

2. QUALITATIVE AND QUANTITATIVE COMPOSITION

Each pre-filled pen contains 50 mg of etanercept.

Etanercept is a human tumour necrosis factor receptor p75 Fc fusion protein produced by recombinant DNA technology in a Chinese hamster ovary (CHO) mammalian expression system. Etanercept is a dimer of a chimeric protein genetically engineered by fusing the extracellular ligand binding domain of human tumour necrosis factor receptor-2 (TNFR2/p75) to the Fc domain of human IgG1. This Fc component contains the hinge, CH_2 and CH_3 regions but not the CH_1 region of IgG1. Etanercept contains 934 amino acids and has an apparent molecular weight of approximately 150 kilodaltons. The potency is determined by measuring the ability of etanercept to neutralise the TNFα-mediated growth inhibition of A375 cells. The specific activity of etanercept is 1.7×10^6 units/mg.

For a full list of excipients, see section 6.1.

3. PHARMACEUTICAL FORM

Solution for injection.

The solution is clear, and colourless or pale yellow.

4. CLINICAL PARTICULARS

4.1 Therapeutic indications

<u>Rheumatoid arthritis</u>

Enbrel in combination with methotrexate is indicated for the treatment of moderate to severe active rheumatoid arthritis in adults when the response to disease-modifying antirheumatic drugs, including methotrexate (unless contraindicated), has been inadequate.

Enbrel can be given as monotherapy in case of intolerance to methotrexate or when continued treatment with methotrexate is inappropriate.

Enbrel is also indicated in the treatment of severe, active and progressive rheumatoid arthritis in adults not previously treated with methotrexate.

Enbrel, alone or in combination with methotrexate, has been shown to reduce the rate of progression of joint damage as measured by X-ray and to improve physical function.

<u>Psoriatic arthritis</u>

Treatment of active and progressive psoriatic arthritis in adults when the response to previous disease-modifying antirheumatic drug therapy has been inadequate. Enbrel has been shown to improve physical function in patients with psoriatic arthritis, and to reduce the rate of progression of peripheral joint damage as measured by X-ray in patients with polyarticular symmetrical subtypes of the disease.

<u>Ankylosing spondylitis</u>

Treatment of adults with severe active ankylosing spondylitis who have had an inadequate response to conventional therapy.

<u>Plaque psoriasis</u>

Treatment of adults with moderate to severe plaque psoriasis who failed to respond to, or who have a contraindication to, or are intolerant to other systemic therapy including ciclosporin, methotrexate or PUVA (see section 5.1).

<u>Paediatric plaque psoriasis</u>

Treatment of chronic severe plaque psoriasis in children and adolescents from the age of 8 years who are inadequately controlled by, or are intolerant to, other systemic therapies or phototherapies.

4.2 Posology and method of administration

Enbrel treatment should be initiated and supervised by specialist physicians experienced in the diagnosis and treatment of rheumatoid arthritis, psoriatic arthritis, ankylosing spondylitis, plaque psoriasis or paediatric plaque psoriasis. Patients treated with Enbrel should be given the Patient Alert Card.

The Enbrel pre-filled pen is available in a 50 mg strength. Other presentations of Enbrel are available in strengths of 25 mg and 50 mg.

<u>Posology</u>

Rheumatoid arthritis

25 mg Enbrel administered twice weekly is the recommended dose. Alternatively, 50 mg Enbrel administered once weekly has been shown to be safe and effective (see section 5.1).

Psoriatic arthritis and ankylosing spondylitis

The recommended dose is 25 mg Enbrel administered twice weekly, or 50 mg Enbrel administered once weekly.

Plaque psoriasis

The recommended dose of Enbrel is 25 mg administered twice weekly or 50 mg administered once weekly. Alternatively, 50 mg given twice weekly may be used for up to 12 weeks followed, if necessary, by a dose of 25 mg twice weekly or 50 mg once weekly. Treatment with Enbrel should continue until remission is achieved, for up to 24 weeks. Continuous therapy beyond 24 weeks may be appropriate for some adult patients (see section 5.1). Treatment should be discontinued in patients who show no response after 12 weeks. If re-treatment with Enbrel is indicated, the same guidance on treatment duration should be followed. The dose should be 25 mg twice weekly or 50 mg once weekly.

Special populations

Paediatric use

Enbrel is available as a single use syringe for patients weighing 62.5 kg or more. Lyophilized vials containing a reconstituted dose of 25 mg/ml are available from which doses less than 25 mg can be administered.

Paediatric plaque psoriasis (age 8 years and above)

0.8 mg/kg (up to a maximum of 50 mg per dose) once weekly for up to 24 weeks. Treatment should be discontinued in patients who show no response after 12 weeks.

If re-treatment with Enbrel is indicated, the above guidance on treatment duration should be followed. The dose should be 0.8 mg/kg (up to a maximum of 50 mg per dose) once weekly.

Elderly patients (⩾ 65 years)

No dose adjustment is required. Posology and administration are the same as for adults 18-64 years of age.

Renal and hepatic impairment

No dose adjustment is required.

Method of administration

Comprehensive instructions for administration are given in the package leaflet, section 7, "Using the MYCLIC pre-filled pen to inject Enbrel."

4.3 Contraindications

Hypersensitivity to the active substance or to any of the excipients.

Sepsis or risk of sepsis.

Treatment with Enbrel should not be initiated in patients with active infections including chronic or localised infections.

4.4 Special warnings and precautions for use

Infections

Patients should be evaluated for infections before, during, and after treatment with Enbrel, taking into consideration that the mean elimination half-life of etanercept is approximately 70 hours (range 7 to 300 hours).

Serious infections, sepsis, tuberculosis, and opportunistic infections, including invasive fungal infections, have been reported with the use of Enbrel (see section 4.8). These infections were due to bacteria, mycobacteria, fungi and viruses. In some cases, particular fungal and other opportunistic infections have not been recognised, resulting in delay of appropriate treatment and sometimes death. In evaluating patients for infections, the patient's risk for relevant opportunistic infections (e.g., exposure to endemic mycoses) should be considered.

Patients who develop a new infection while undergoing treatment with Enbrel should be monitored closely. **Administration of Enbrel should be discontinued if a patient develops a serious infection.** Physicians should exercise caution when considering the use of Enbrel in patients with a history of recurring or chronic infections or with underlying conditions that may predispose patients to infections such as advanced or poorly controlled diabetes.

Tuberculosis

Cases of active tuberculosis including miliary tuberculosis and tuberculosis with extra-pulmonary location have been reported in patients treated with Enbrel.

Before starting treatment with Enbrel, all patients must be evaluated for both active and inactive ('latent') tuberculosis. This evaluation should include a detailed medical history with personal history of tuberculosis or possible previous contact with tuberculosis and previous and/or current immunosuppressive therapy. Appropriate screening tests, i.e. tuberculin skin test and chest x-ray, should be performed in all patients (local recommendations may apply). It is recommended that the conduct of these tests should be recorded in the patient's alert card. Prescribers are reminded of the risk of false negative tuberculin skin test results, especially in patients who are severely ill or immunocompromised.

If active tuberculosis is diagnosed, Enbrel therapy must not be initiated. If inactive ('latent') tuberculosis is diagnosed, treatment for latent tuberculosis must be started with anti-tuberculosis therapy before the initiation of Enbrel, and in accordance with local recommendations. In this situation, the benefit/risk balance of Enbrel therapy should be very carefully considered.

All patients should be informed to seek medical advice if signs/symptoms suggestive of tuberculosis (e.g., persistent cough, wasting/weight loss, low-grade fever) appear during or after Enbrel treatment.

Hepatitis B virus reactivation

Reactivation of hepatitis B virus (HBV) in patients who are chronic carriers of this virus who are receiving TNF-antagonists including Enbrel has been reported. Patients at risk for HBV infection should be evaluated for prior evidence of HBV infection before initiating Enbrel therapy. Caution should be exercised when administering Enbrel to patients identified as carriers of HBV. If Enbrel is used in carriers of HBV, the patients should be monitored for signs and symptoms of active HBV infection and, if necessary, appropriate treatment should be initiated.

Worsening of hepatitis C

There have been reports of worsening of hepatitis C in patients receiving Enbrel.

Concurrent treatment with anakinra

Concurrent administration of Enbrel and anakinra has been associated with an increased risk of serious infections and neutropenia compared to Enbrel alone. This combination has not demonstrated increased clinical benefit. Thus the combined use of Enbrel and anakinra is not recommended (see sections 4.5 and 4.8).

Concurrent treatment with abatacept

In clinical studies, concurrent administration of abatacept and Enbrel resulted in increased incidences of serious adverse events. This combination has not demonstrated increased clinical benefit; such use is not recommended (see section 4.5).

Allergic reactions

Allergic reactions associated with Enbrel administration have been reported commonly. Allergic reactions have included angioedema and urticaria; serious reactions have occurred. If any serious allergic or anaphylactic reaction occurs, Enbrel therapy should be discontinued immediately and appropriate therapy initiated.

The needle cap of the pre-filled pen contains latex (dry natural rubber) that may cause hypersensitivity reactions when handled by or when Enbrel is administered to persons with known or possible latex sensitivity.

Immunosuppression

The possibility exists for TNF-antagonists, including Enbrel, to affect host defences against infections and malignancies since TNF mediates inflammation and modulates cellular immune responses. In a study of 49 adult patients with rheumatoid arthritis treated with Enbrel, there was no evidence of depression of delayed-type hypersensitivity, depression of immunoglobulin levels, or change in enumeration of effector cell populations.

Two juvenile idiopathic arthritis patients developed varicella infection and signs and symptoms of aseptic meningitis, which resolved without sequelae. Patients with a significant exposure to varicella virus should temporarily discontinue Enbrel therapy and be considered for prophylactic treatment with Varicella Zoster Immune Globulin.

The safety and efficacy of Enbrel in patients with immunosuppression or chronic infections have not been evaluated.

Malignancies and lymphoproliferative disorders

Solid and haematopoietic malignancies

Reports of various malignancies (including breast and lung carcinoma and lymphoma) have been received in the post-marketing period (see section 4.8).

In the controlled portions of clinical trials of TNF-antagonists, more cases of lymphoma have been observed among patients receiving a TNF-antagonist compared with control patients. However, the occurrence was rare, and the follow-up period of placebo patients was shorter than for patients receiving TNF-antagonist therapy. Furthermore, there is an increased background lymphoma risk in rheumatoid arthritis patients with long-standing, highly active, inflammatory disease, which complicates the risk estimation. With the current knowledge, a possible risk for the development of lymphomas or other malignancies in patients treated with a TNF-antagonist cannot be excluded.

Non-melanoma skin cancer (NMSC)

Non-melanoma skin cancer has been reported in patients treated with TNF-antagonists, including Enbrel. Combining the results of placebo- and active comparator-controlled clinical trials of Enbrel, more cases of NMSC were observed in patients receiving Enbrel compared with control patients, particularly in patients with psoriasis. Periodic skin examination is recommended for all patients who are at increased risk for NMSC (including patients with psoriasis or a history of PUVA therapy).

Vaccinations

Live vaccines should not be given concurrently with Enbrel. No data are available on the secondary transmission of infection by live vaccines in patients receiving Enbrel. In a double blind, placebo controlled, randomised clinical study in adult patients with psoriatic arthritis 184 patients also received a multivalent pneumococcal polysaccharide vaccine at week 4. In this study most psoriatic arthritis patients receiving Enbrel were able to mount effective B-cell immune response to pneumococcal polysaccharide vaccine, but titers in aggregate were moderately lower and few patients had two-fold rises in titers compared to patients not receiving Enbrel. The clinical significance of this is unknown.

Autoantibody formation

Treatment with Enbrel may result in the formation of autoimmune antibodies (see section 4.8).

Haematologic reactions

Rare cases of pancytopenia and very rare cases of aplastic anaemia, some with fatal outcome, have been reported in patients treated with Enbrel. Caution should be exercised in patients being treated with Enbrel who have a previous history of blood dyscrasias. All patients and parents/caregivers should be advised that if the patient develops signs and symptoms suggestive of blood dyscrasias or infections (e.g. persistent fever, sore throat, bruising, bleeding, paleness) whilst on Enbrel, they should seek immediate medical advice. Such patients should be investigated urgently, including full blood count; if blood dyscrasias are confirmed, Enbrel should be discontinued.

CNS disorders

There have been rare reports of CNS demyelinating disorders in patients treated with Enbrel (see section 4.8). Although no clinical trials have been performed evaluating Enbrel therapy in patients with multiple sclerosis, clinical trials of other TNF antagonists in patients with multiple sclerosis have shown increases in disease activity. A careful risk/benefit evaluation, including a neurological assessment, is recommended when prescribing Enbrel to patients with pre-existing or recent onset of CNS demyelinating disease, or to those who are considered to have an increased risk of developing demyelinating disease.

Combination therapy

In a controlled clinical trial of two years duration in rheumatoid arthritis patients, the combination of Enbrel and methotrexate did not result in unexpected safety findings, and the safety profile of Enbrel when given in combination with methotrexate was similar to the profiles reported in studies of Enbrel and methotrexate alone. Long-term studies to assess the safety of the combination are ongoing. The long-term safety of Enbrel in combination with other disease-modifying antirheumatic drugs (DMARD) has not been established.

The use of Enbrel in combination with other systemic therapies or phototherapy for the treatment of psoriasis has not been studied.

Renal and hepatic impairment

Based on pharmacokinetic data (see section 5.2), no dose adjustment is needed in patients with renal or hepatic impairment; clinical experience in such patients is limited.

Congestive heart failure

Physicians should use caution when using Enbrel in patients who have congestive heart failure (CHF). There have been postmarketing reports of worsening of CHF, with and without identifiable precipitating factors, in patients taking Enbrel. Two large clinical trials evaluating the use of Enbrel in the treatment of CHF were terminated early due to lack of efficacy. Although not conclusive, data from one of these trials suggest a possible tendency toward worsening CHF in those patients assigned to Enbrel treatment.

Alcoholic hepatitis

In a phase II randomised placebo-controlled study of 48 hospitalised patients treated with Enbrel or placebo for moderate to severe alcoholic hepatitis, Enbrel was not efficacious, and the mortality rate in patients treated with Enbrel was significantly higher after 6 months. Consequently, Enbrel should not be used in patients for the treatment of alcoholic hepatitis. Physicians should use caution when using Enbrel in patients who also have moderate to severe alcoholic hepatitis.

Wegener's granulomatosis

A placebo-controlled trial, in which 89 adult patients were treated with Enbrel in addition to standard therapy (including cyclophosphamide or methotrexate, and glucocorticoids) for a median duration of 25 months, has not shown Enbrel to be an effective treatment for Wegener's granulomatosis. The incidence of non-cutaneous malignancies of various types was significantly higher in patients treated with Enbrel than in the control group. Enbrel is not recommended for the treatment of Wegener's granulomatosis.

4.5 Interaction with other medicinal products and other forms of interaction

Concurrent treatment with anakinra

Adult patients treated with Enbrel and anakinra were observed to have a higher rate of serious infection when compared with patients treated with either Enbrel or anakinra alone (historical data).

In addition, in a double-blind placebo-controlled trial in adult patients receiving background methotrexate, patients treated with Enbrel and anakinra were observed to have a higher rate of serious infections (7%) and neutropenia than patients treated with Enbrel (see sections 4.4 and 4.8). The combination Enbrel and anakinra has not demonstrated increased clinical benefit and is therefore not recommended.

Concurrent treatment with abatacept

In clinical studies, concurrent administration of abatacept and Enbrel resulted in increased incidences of serious adverse events. This combination has not demonstrated increased clinical benefit; such use is not recommended (see section 4.4).

Concurrent treatment with sulfasalazine

In a clinical study of adult patients who were receiving established doses of sulfasalazine, to which Enbrel was added, patients in the combination group experienced a statistically significant decrease in mean white blood cell counts in comparison to groups treated with Enbrel or sulfasalazine alone. The clinical significance of this interaction is unknown.

Non-interactions

In clinical trials, no interactions have been observed when Enbrel was administered with glucocorticoids, salicylates (except sulfasalazine), nonsteroidal anti-inflammatory drugs (NSAIDs), analgesics, or methotrexate. See section 4.4 for vaccination advice.

No clinically significant pharmacokinetic drug-drug interactions were observed in studies with digoxin or warfarin.

4.6 Pregnancy and lactation

Pregnancy

There are no studies of Enbrel in pregnant women. Developmental toxicity studies performed in rats and rabbits have revealed no evidence of harm to the foetus or neonatal rat due to etanercept. Preclinical data about peri- and postnatal toxicity of etanercept and of effects of etanercept on fertility and general reproductive performance are not available. Thus, the use of Enbrel in pregnant women is not recommended, and women of child-bearing potential should be advised not to get pregnant during Enbrel therapy.

Lactation

It is not known whether etanercept is excreted in human milk. Following subcutaneous administration to lactacting rats, etanercept was excreted in the milk and detected in the serum of pups. Because immunoglobulins, in common with many medicinal products, can be excreted in human milk, a decision should be made whether to discontinue breast-feeding or to discontinue Enbrel while breast-feeding.

4.7 Effects on ability to drive and use machines

No studies on the effects on the ability to drive and use machines have been performed.

4.8 Undesirable effects

Undesirable effects in adults

Enbrel has been studied in 2,680 patients with rheumatoid arthritis in double-blind and open-label trials. This experience includes 2 placebo-controlled studies (349 Enbrel patients and 152 placebo patients) and 2 active-controlled trials, one active-controlled trial comparing Enbrel to methotrexate (415 Enbrel patients and 217 methotrexate patients) and another active-controlled trial comparing Enbrel (223 patients), methotrexate (228 patients) and Enbrel in combination with methotrexate (231 patients). The proportion of patients who discontinued treatment due to adverse events was the same in both the Enbrel and placebo treatment groups; in the first active-controlled trial, the dropout rate was significantly higher for methotrexate (10%) than for Enbrel (5%). In the second active-controlled trial, the rate of discontinuation for adverse events after 2 years of treatment was similar among all three treatment groups, Enbrel (16%), methotrexate (21%) and Enbrel in combination with methotrexate (17%). Additionally, Enbrel has been studied in 240 psoriatic arthritis patients who participated in 2 double-blind placebo-controlled studies and an open-label extension study. Five hundred and eight (508) ankylosing spondylitis patients were treated with Enbrel in 4 double-blind placebo-controlled studies. Enbrel has also been studied in 1,492 patients with plaque psoriasis for up to 6 months in 5 double-blind placebo-controlled studies.

In double-blind clinical trials comparing Enbrel to placebo, injection site reactions were the most frequent adverse events among Enbrel-treated patients. Among patients with rheumatoid arthritis treated in placebo-controlled trials, serious adverse events occurred at a frequency of 4% in 349 patients treated with Enbrel compared with 5% of 152 placebo-treated patients. In the first active-controlled trial, serious adverse events occurred at a frequency of 6% in 415 patients treated with Enbrel compared with 8% of 217 methotrexate-treated patients. In the second active-controlled trial the rate of serious adverse events after 2 years of treatment was similar among the three treatment groups (Enbrel 16%, methotrexate 15% and Enbrel in combination with methotrexate 17%). Among patients with plaque psoriasis treated in placebo-controlled trials, the frequency of serious adverse events was about 1.4% of 1,341 patients treated with Enbrel compared with 1.4% of 766 placebo-treated patients.

The following list of adverse reactions is based on experience from clinical trials in adults and on postmarketing experience.

Within the organ system classes, adverse reactions are listed under headings of frequency (number of patients expected to experience the reaction), using the following categories: very common (≥1/10); common (≥1/100, <1/10); uncommon (≥1/1000, <1/100); rare (≥1/10,000, <1/1000); very rare (<1/10,000); not known (cannot be estimated from the available data).

Infections and infestations:

Very common: Infections (including upper respiratory tract infections, bronchitis, cystitis, skin infections)*

Uncommon: Serious infections (including pneumonia, cellulitis, septic arthritis, sepsis)*

Rare: Tuberculosis, opportunistic infections (including invasive fungal, protozoal, bacterial and atypical mycobacterial infections)*

Blood and lymphatic system disorders:

Uncommon: Thrombocytopenia

Rare: Anaemia, leukopenia, neutropenia, pancytopenia*

Very rare: Aplastic anaemia*

Immune system disorders:

Common: Allergic reactions (see Skin and subcutaneous tissue disorders), autoantibody formation*

Rare: Serious allergic/anaphylactic reactions (including angioedema, bronchospasm)

Not known: Macrophage activation syndrome*, anti-neutrophilic cytoplasmic antibody positive vasculitis

Nervous system disorders:

Rare: Seizures
CNS demyelinating events suggestive of multiple sclerosis or localised demyelinating conditions such as optic neuritis and transverse myelitis (see section 4.4)

Respiratory, thoracic and mediastinal disorders:

Uncommon: Interstitial lung disease (including pneumonitis and pulmonary fibrosis)*

Hepatobiliary disorders:

Rare: Elevated liver enzymes

Skin and subcutaneous tissue disorders:

Common: Pruritus

Uncommon: Non-melanoma skin cancers (see section 4.4), angioedema, urticaria, rash, psoriasiform rash, psoriasis (including new onset and pustular, primarily palms and soles)

Rare: Cutaneous vasculitis (including leukocytoclastic vasculitis), Stevens-Johnson syndrome, erythema multiforme

Very rare: Toxic epidermal necrolysis

Musculoskeletal and connective tissue disorders:

Rare: Subacute cutaneous lupus erythematosus, discoid lupus erythematosus, lupus like syndrome

General disorders and administration site conditions:

Very common: Injection site reactions (including bleeding, bruising, erythema, itching, pain, swelling)*

Common: Fever

Cardiac disorders:

There have been reports of worsening of congestive heart failure (see section 4.4).

*see Additional information, below.

Additional information

Serious adverse events reported in clinical trials

Among rheumatoid arthritis, psoriatic arthritis, ankylosing spondylitis and plaque psoriasis patients in placebo-controlled, active-controlled, and open-label trials of Enbrel, serious adverse events reported included malignancies (see below), asthma, infections (see below), heart failure, myocardial infarction, myocardial ischaemia, chest pain, syncope, cerebral ischaemia, hypertension, hypotension, cholecystitis, pancreatitis, gastrointestinal haemorrhage, bursitis, confusion, depression, dyspnoea, abnormal healing, renal insufficiency, kidney calculus, deep vein thrombosis, pulmonary embolism, membranous glomerulonephropathy, polymyositis, thrombophlebitis, liver damage, leucopenia, paresis, paresthesia, vertigo, allergic alveolitis, angioedema, scleritis, bone fracture, lymphadenopathy, ulcerative colitis, intestinal obstruction, eosinophilia, haematuria, and sarcoidosis.

Malignancies and lymphoproliferative disorders

One hundred and twenty-nine new malignancies of various types were observed in 4,114 rheumatoid arthritis patients treated in clinical trials with Enbrel for up to approximately 6 years, including 231 patients treated with Enbrel in combination with methotrexate in the 2-year active-controlled study. The observed rates and incidences in these clinical trials were similar to those expected for the population studied. A total of 2 malignancies were reported in clinical studies of approximately 2 years duration involving 240 Enbrel-treated psoriatic arthritis patients. In clinical studies conducted for more than 2 years with 351 ankylosing spondylitis patients, 6 malignancies were reported in Enbrel-treated patients. In a group of 2,711 plaque psoriasis patients treated with Enbrel in double-blind and open-label studies of up to 2.5 years, 30 malignancies and 43 nonmelanoma skin cancers were reported.

In a group of 7,416 patients treated with Enbrel in rheumatoid arthritis, psoriatic arthritis, ankylosing spondylitis and psoriasis clinical trials, 18 lymphomas were reported.

Reports of various malignancies (including breast and lung carcinoma and lymphoma) have also been received in the postmarketing period (see section 4.4).

Injection site reactions

Compared to placebo, patients with rheumatic diseases treated with Enbrel had a significantly higher incidence of injection site reactions (36% vs. 9%). Injection site reactions usually occurred in the first month. Mean duration was approximately 3 to 5 days. No treatment was given for the majority of injection site reactions in the Enbrel treatment groups, and the majority of patients who were given treatment received topical preparations such as corticosteroids, or oral antihistamines. Additionally, some patients developed recall injection site reactions characterised by a skin reaction at the most recent site of injection along with the simultaneous appearance of injection site reactions at previous injection sites. These reactions were generally transient and did not recur with treatment.

In controlled trials in patients with plaque psoriasis, approximately 13.6% of patients treated with Enbrel developed injection site reactions compared with 3.4 % of placebo-treated patients during the first 12 weeks of treatment.

Serious infections

In placebo-controlled trials, no increase in the incidence of serious infections (fatal, life threatening, or requiring hospitalisation or intravenous antibiotics) was observed. Serious infections occurred in 6.3% of rheumatoid arthritis patients treated with Enbrel for up to 48 months. These included abscess (at various sites), bacteraemia, bronchitis, bursitis, cellulitis, cholecystitis, diarrhoea, diverticulitis, endocarditis (suspected), gastroenteritis, hepatitis B, herpes zoster, leg ulcer, mouth infection, osteomyelitis, otitis, peritonitis, pneumonia, pyelonephritis, sepsis, septic arthritis, sinusitis, skin infection, skin ulcer, urinary tract infection, vasculitis, and wound infection. In the 2-year active-controlled study where patients were treated with either Enbrel alone, methotrexate alone or Enbrel in combination with methotrexate, the rates of serious infections were similar among the treatment groups. However, it cannot be excluded that the combination of Enbrel with methotrexate could be associated with an increase in the rate of infections.

There were no differences in rates of infection among patients treated with Enbrel and those treated with placebo for plaque psoriasis in placebo controlled trials of up to 24 weeks duration. Serious infections experienced by Enbrel-treated patients included cellulitis, gastroenteritis, pneumonia, cholecystitis, osteomyelitis, gastritis, appendicitis, Streptococcal fasciitis, myositis, septic shock, diverticulitis and abscess. In the double-blind and open-label psoriatic arthritis trials, 1 patient reported a serious infection (pneumonia).

Serious and fatal infections have been reported during use of Enbrel; reported pathogens include bacteria, mycobacteria (including tuberculosis), viruses and fungi. Some have occurred within a few weeks after initiating treatment with Enbrel in patients who have underlying conditions (e.g. diabetes, congestive heart failure, history of active or chronic infections) in addition to their rheumatoid arthritis (see section 4.4). Enbrel treatment may increase mortality in patients with established sepsis.

Opportunistic infections have been reported in association with Enbrel including invasive fungal, protozoal, bacterial (including *Listeria* and *Legionella*), and atypical mycobacterial infections. In a pooled data set of clinical trials, the overall incidence of opportunistic infections was 0.09% for the 15,402 subjects who received Enbrel. The exposure-adjusted rate was 0.06 events per 100 patient-years. In postmarketing experience, approximately half of all of the case reports of opportunistic infections worldwide were invasive fungal infections. The most commonly reported invasive fungal infections were *Pneumocystis* and *Aspergillus*. Invasive fungal infections accounted for more than half of the fatalities amongst patients who developed opportunistic infections. The majority of the reports with a fatal outcome were in patients with *Pneumocystis* pneumonia, unspecified systemic fungal infections, and aspergillosis (see section 4.4).

Autoantibodies

Adult patients had serum samples tested for autoantibodies at multiple timepoints. Of the rheumatoid arthritis patients evaluated for antinuclear antibodies (ANA), the percentage of patients who developed new positive ANA (≥1:40) was higher in patients treated with Enbrel (11%) than in placebo-treated patients (5%). The percentage of patients who developed new positive anti-double-stranded DNA antibodies was also higher by radioimmunoassay (15% of patients treated with Enbrel compared to 4% of placebo-treated patients) and by *Crithidia luciliae* assay (3% of patients treated with Enbrel compared to none of placebo-treated patients). The proportion of patients treated with Enbrel who developed anticardiolipin antibodies was similarly increased compared to placebo-treated patients. The impact of long-term treatment with Enbrel on the development of autoimmune diseases is unknown.

There have been rare reports of patients, including rheumatoid factor positive patients, who have developed other autoantibodies in conjunction with a lupus-like syndrome or rashes that are compatible with subacute cutaneous lupus or discoid lupus by clinical presentation and biopsy.

Pancytopenia and aplastic anaemia

There have been postmarketing reports of pancytopenia and aplastic anaemia, some of which had fatal outcomes (see section 4.4).

Interstitial lung disease

There have been postmarketing reports of interstitial lung disease (including pneumonitis and pulmonary fibrosis), some of which had fatal outcomes.

Laboratory evaluations

Based on the results of clinical studies, normally no special laboratory evaluations are necessary in addition to careful medical management and supervision of patients.

Concurrent treatment with anakinra

In studies when adult patients received concurrent treatment with Enbrel plus anakinra, a higher rate of serious infections compared to Enbrel alone was observed and 2% of patients (3/139) developed neutropenia (absolute neutrophil count < 1000 / mm^3). While neutropenic, one patient developed cellulitis that resolved after hospitalisation (see sections 4.4 and 4.5).

Undesirable effects in paediatric patients with plaque psoriasis

In a 48-week study in 211 children aged 4 to 17 years with paediatric plaque psoriasis, the adverse events reported were similar to those seen in previous studies in adults with plaque psoriasis.

There were 4 reports of macrophage activation syndrome in juvenile idiopathic arthritis clinical trials.

4.9 Overdose

No dose-limiting toxicities were observed during clinical trials of rheumatoid arthritis patients. The highest dose level evaluated has been an intravenous loading dose of 32 mg/m^2 followed by subcutaneous doses of 16 mg/m^2 administered twice weekly. One rheumatoid arthritis patient mistakenly self-administered 62 mg Enbrel subcutaneously twice weekly for 3 weeks without experiencing undesirable effects. There is no known antidote to Enbrel.

5. PHARMACOLOGICAL PROPERTIES

5.1 Pharmacodynamic properties

Pharmacotherapeutic group: Tumor Necrosis Factor alpha (TNF-α) inhibitors, *ATC code:* L04AB01.

Tumour necrosis factor (TNF) is a dominant cytokine in the inflammatory process of rheumatoid arthritis. Elevated levels of TNF are also found in the synovium and psoriatic plaques of patients with psoriatic arthritis and in serum and synovial tissue of patients with ankylosing spondylitis. In plaque psoriasis, infiltration by inflammatory cells including T-cells leads to increased TNF levels in psoriatic lesions compared with levels in uninvolved skin. Etanercept is a competitive inhibitor of TNF-binding to its cell surface receptors and thereby inhibits the biological activity of TNF. TNF and lymphotoxin are pro-inflammatory cytokines that bind to two distinct cell surface receptors: the 55-kilodalton (p55) and 75-kilodalton (p75) tumour necrosis factor receptors (TNFRs). Both TNFRs exist naturally in membrane-bound and soluble forms. Soluble TNFRs are thought to regulate TNF biological activity.

TNF and lymphotoxin exist predominantly as homotrimers, with their biological activity dependent on cross-linking of cell surface TNFRs. Dimeric soluble receptors such as etanercept possess a higher affinity for TNF than monomeric receptors and are considerably more potent competitive inhibitors of TNF binding to its cellular receptors. In addition, use of an immunoglobulin Fc region as a fusion element in the construction of a dimeric receptor imparts a longer serum half-life.

Mechanism of action

Much of the joint pathology in rheumatoid arthritis and ankylosing spondylitis and skin pathology in plaque psoriasis is mediated by pro-inflammatory molecules that are linked in a network controlled by TNF. The mechanism of action of etanercept is thought to be its competitive inhibition of TNF binding to cell surface TNFR, preventing TNF-mediated cellular responses by rendering TNF biologically inactive. Etanercept may also modulate biologic responses controlled by additional downstream molecules (e.g., cytokines, adhesion molecules, or proteinases) that are induced or regulated by TNF.

Clinical trials

This section presents data from four randomised controlled trials in adults with rheumatoid arthritis, one study in polyarticular juvenile idiopathic arthritis, one study in adults with psoriatic arthritis, one study in adults with ankylosing spondylitis, one study in paediatric patients with plaque psoriasis, and four studies in adults with plaque psoriasis.

Adult patients with rheumatoid arthritis

The efficacy of Enbrel was assessed in a randomised, double-blind, placebo-controlled study. The study evaluated 234 adult patients with active rheumatoid arthritis who had failed therapy with at least one but no more than four disease-modifying antirheumatic drugs (DMARDs). Doses of 10 mg or 25 mg Enbrel or placebo were administered subcutaneously twice a week for 6 consecutive months. The results of this controlled trial were expressed in percentage improvement in rheumatoid arthritis using American College of Rheumatology (ACR) response criteria. ACR 20 and 50 responses were higher in patients treated with Enbrel at 3 and 6 months than in patients treated with placebo (ACR 20: Enbrel 62% and 59%, placebo 23% and 11% at 3 and 6 months respectively; ACR 50: Enbrel 41% and 40%, placebo 8% and 5% at months 3 and 6 respectively; $p<0.01$ Enbrel vs Placebo at all time points for both ACR 20 and ACR 50 responses).

Approximately 15% of subjects who received Enbrel achieved an ACR 70 response at month 3 and month 6 compared to fewer than 5% of subjects in the placebo arm. Among patients receiving Enbrel, the clinical responses generally appeared within 1 to 2 weeks after initiation of therapy and nearly always occurred by 3 months. A dose response was seen; results with 10 mg were intermediate between placebo and 25 mg. Enbrel was significantly better than placebo in all components of the ACR criteria as well as other measures of rheumatoid arthritis disease activity not included in the ACR response criteria, such as morning stiffness. A Health Assessment Questionnaire (HAQ), which included disability, vitality, mental health, general health status, and arthritis-associated health status subdomains, was administered every 3 months during the trial. All subdomains of the HAQ were improved in patients treated with Enbrel compared to controls at 3 and 6 months.

After discontinuation of Enbrel, symptoms of arthritis generally returned within a month. Re-introduction of treatment with Enbrel after discontinuations of up to 24 months resulted in the same magnitudes of responses as patients who received Enbrel without interruption of therapy based on results of open-label studies. Continued durable responses have been seen for up to 48 months in open-label extension treatment trials when patients received Enbrel without interruption; longer-term experience is not available.

The efficacy of Enbrel was compared to methotrexate in a third randomised, active-controlled study with blinded radiographic evaluations as a primary endpoint in 632 adult patients with active rheumatoid arthritis (<3 years duration) who had never received treatment with methotrexate. Doses of 10 mg or 25 mg Enbrel were administered SC twice a week for up to 24 months. Methotrexate doses were escalated from 7.5 mg/week to a maximum of 20 mg/week over the first 8 weeks of the trial and continued for up to 24 months. Clinical improvement including onset of action within 2 weeks with Enbrel 25 mg was similar to that seen in the previous trials, and was maintained for up to 24 months. At baseline, patients had a moderate degree of disability, with mean HAQ scores of 1.4 to 1.5. Treatment with Enbrel 25 mg resulted in substantial improvement at 12 months, with about 44% of patients achieving a normal HAQ score (less than 0.5). This benefit was maintained in Year 2 of this study.

In this study, structural joint damage was assessed radiographically and expressed as change in Total Sharp Score (TSS) and its components, the erosion score and joint space narrowing score (JSN). Radiographs of hands/wrists and feet were read at baseline and 6, 12, and 24 months. The 10 mg Enbrel dose had consistently less effect on structural damage than the 25 mg dose. Enbrel 25 mg was significantly superior to methotrexate for erosion scores at both 12 and 24 months. The differences in TSS and JSN were not statistically significant between methotrexate and Enbrel 25 mg. The results are shown in the figure below.

RADIOGRAPHIC PROGRESSION: COMPARISON OF ENBREL vs METHOTREXATE IN PATIENTS WITH RA OF <3 YEARS DURATION

(see Figure 1 above)

Figure 1 RADIOGRAPHIC PROGRESSION: COMPARISON OF ENBREL vs METHOTREXATE IN PATIENTS WITH RA OF <3 YEARS DURATION

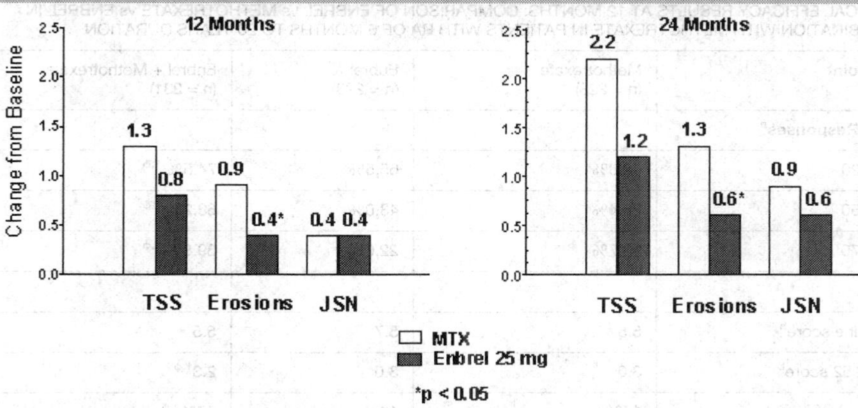

In another active-controlled, double-blind, randomised study, clinical efficacy, safety, and radiographic progression in RA patients treated with Enbrel alone (25 mg twice weekly), methotrexate alone (7.5 to 20 mg weekly, median dose 20 mg), and of the combination of Enbrel and methotrexate initiated concurrently were compared in 682 adult patients with active rheumatoid arthritis of 6 months to 20 years duration (median 5 years) who had a less than satisfactory response to at least 1 disease-modifying anti-rheumatic drug (DMARD) other than methotrexate.

Patients in the Enbrel in combination with methotrexate therapy group had significantly higher ACR 20, ACR 50, ACR 70 responses and improvement for DAS and HAQ scores at both 24 and 52 weeks than patients in either of the single therapy groups (results shown in table below). Significant advantages for Enbrel in combination with methotrexate compared with Enbrel monotherapy and methotrexate monotherapy were also observed after 24 months.

(see Table 1 on next page)

Radiographic progression at 12 months was significantly less in the Enbrel group than in the methotrexate group, while the combination was significantly better than either monotherapy at slowing radiographic progression (see figure below).

RADIOGRAPHIC PROGRESSION: COMPARISON OF ENBREL vs METHOTREXATE vs ENBREL IN COMBINATION WITH METHOTREXATE IN PATIENTS WITH RA OF 6 MONTHS TO 20 YEARS DURATION (12 MONTH RESULTS)

(see Figure 2 on next page)

Significant advantages for Enbrel in combination with methotrexate compared with Enbrel monotherapy and methotrexate monotherapy were also observed after 24 months. Similarly, the significant advantages for Enbrel monotherapy compared with methotrexate monotherapy were also observed after 24 months.

In an analysis in which all patients who dropped out of the study for any reason were considered to have progressed, the percentage of patients without progression (TSS change $\leqslant$ 0.5) at 24 months was higher in the Enbrel in combination with methotrexate group compared with the Enbrel alone and methotrexate alone groups (62%, 50%, and 36%, respectively; $p<0.05$). The difference between Enbrel alone and methotrexate alone was also significant ($p<0.05$). Among patients who completed a full 24 months of therapy in the study, the non-progression rates were 78%, 70%, and 61%, respectively.

The safety and efficacy of 50 mg Enbrel (two 25 mg SC injections) administered once weekly were evaluated in a double-blind, placebo-controlled study of 420 patients with active RA. In this study, 53 patients received placebo, 214 patients received 50 mg Enbrel once weekly and 153 patients received 25 mg Enbrel twice weekly. The safety and efficacy profiles of the two Enbrel treatment regimens were comparable at week 8 in their effect on signs and symptoms of RA; data at week 16 did not show comparability (non-inferiority) between the two regimens. A single 50 mg/ml injection of Enbrel was found to be bioequivalent to two simultaneous injections of 25 mg/ml.

Adult patients with psoriatic arthritis

The efficacy of Enbrel was assessed in a randomised, double-blind, placebo-controlled study in 205 patients with psoriatic arthritis. Patients were between 18 and 70 years of age and had active psoriatic arthritis ($\geqslant$ 3 swollen joints and $\geqslant$ 3 tender joints) in at least one of the following forms: (1) distal interphalangeal (DIP) involvement; (2) polyarticular arthritis (absence of rheumatoid nodules and presence of psoriasis); (3) arthritis mutilans; (4) asymmetric psoriatic arthritis; or (5) spondylitis-like ankylosis. Patients also had plaque psoriasis with a qualifying target lesion $\geqslant$ 2 cm in diameter. Patients had previously been treated with NSAIDs (86%), DMARDs (80%), and corticosteroids (24%). Patients currently on methotrexate therapy (stable for $\geqslant$ 2 months) could continue at a stable dose of $\leqslant$ 25 mg/week methotrexate. Doses of 25 mg of Enbrel (based on dose-finding studies in patients with rheumatoid arthritis) or placebo were administered SC twice a week for 6 months. At the end of the double-blind study, patients could enter a long-term open-label extension study for a total duration of up to 2 years.

Clinical responses were expressed as percentages of patients achieving the ACR 20, 50, and 70 response and

Table 1

CLINICAL EFFICACY RESULTS AT 12 MONTHS: COMPARISON OF ENBREL vs METHOTREXATE vs ENBREL IN COMBINATION WITH METHOTREXATE IN PATIENTS WITH RA OF 6 MONTHS TO 20 YEARS DURATION

Endpoint	Methotrexate (n = 228)	Enbrel (n = 223)	Enbrel + Methotrexate (n = 231)
ACR Responses[a]			
ACR 20	58.8%	65.5%	74.5% †,ϕ
ACR 50	36.4%	43.0%	63.2% †,ϕ
ACR 70	16.7%	22.0%	39.8% †,ϕ
DAS			
Baseline score[b]	5.5	5.7	5.5
Week 52 score[b]	3.0	3.0	2.3†,ϕ
Remission[c]	14%	18%	37%†,ϕ
HAQ			
Baseline	1.7	1.7	1.8
Week 52	1.1	1.0	0.8†,ϕ

a: Patients who did not complete 12 months in the study were considered to be non-responders.
b: Values for Disease Activity Score (DAS) are means.
c: Remission is defined as DAS <1.6
Pairwise comparison p-values: † = $p < 0.05$ for comparisons of Enbrel + methotrexate vs methotrexate and ϕ = $p < 0.05$ for comparisons of Enbrel + methotrexate vs Enbrel

percentages with improvement in Psoriatic Arthritis Response Criteria (PsARC). Results are summarised in the Table below.

RESPONSES OF PATIENTS WITH PSORIATIC ARTHRITIS IN PLACEBO-CONTROLLED TRIAL

	Percent of Patients	
	Placebo	Enbrel[a]
Psoriatic Arthritis Response	n = 104	n = 101
ACR 20		
Month 3	15	59[b]
Month 6	13	50[b]
ACR 50		
Month 3	4	38[b]
Month 6	4	37[b]
ACR 70		
Month 3	0	11[b]
Month 6	1	9[c]
PsARC		
Month 3	31	72[b]
Month 6	23	70[b]

a: 25 mg Enbrel SC twice weekly
b: $p < 0.001$, Enbrel vs. placebo
c: $p < 0.01$, Enbrel vs. placebo

Among patients with psoriatic arthritis who received Enbrel, the clinical responses were apparent at the time of the first visit (4 weeks) and were maintained through 6 months of therapy. Enbrel was significantly better than placebo in all measures of disease activity ($p < 0.001$), and responses were similar with and without concomitant methotrexate therapy. Quality of life in psoriatic arthritis patients was assessed at every timepoint using the disability index of the HAQ. The disability index score was significantly improved at all timepoints in psoriatic arthritis patients treated with Enbrel, relative to placebo ($p < 0.001$).

Radiographic changes were assessed in the psoriatic arthritis study. Radiographs of hands and wrists were obtained at baseline and months 6, 12, and 24. The modified TSS at 12 months is presented in the Table below. In an analysis in which all patients who dropped out of the study for any reason were considered to have progressed, the percentage of patients without progression (TSS change ⩽ 0.5) at 12 months was higher in the Enbrel group compared with the placebo group (73% vs. 47%, respectively, $p \leqslant 0.001$). The effect of Enbrel on radiographic progression was maintained in patients who continued on treatment during the second year. The slowing of peripheral joint damage was observed in patients with polyarticular symmetrical joint involvement.

MEAN (SE) ANNUALIZED CHANGE FROM BASELINE IN TOTAL SHARP SCORE

	Placebo	Etanercept
Time	(n = 104)	(n = 101)
Month 12	1.00 (0.29)	-0.03 (0.09)[a]

SE = standard error.
a. p = 0.0001.

Enbrel treatment resulted in improvement in physical function during the double-blind period, and this benefit was maintained during the longer-term exposure of up to 2 years.

There is insufficient evidence of the efficacy of Enbrel in patients with ankylosing spondylitis-like and arthritis mutilans psoriatic arthropathies due to the small number of patients studied.

No study has been performed in patients with psoriatic arthritis using the 50 mg once weekly dosing regimen. Evidence of efficacy for the once weekly dosing regimen in this patient population has been based on data from the study in patients with ankylosing spondylitis.

Adult patients with ankylosing spondylitis

The efficacy of Enbrel in ankylosing spondylitis was assessed in 3 randomised, double-blind studies comparing twice weekly administration of 25 mg Enbrel with placebo. A total of 401 patients were enrolled from which 203 were treated with Enbrel. The largest of these trials (n= 277) enrolled patients who were between 18 and 70 years of age and had active ankylosing spondylitis defined as visual analog scale (VAS) scores of ⩾ 30 for average of duration and intensity of morning stiffness plus VAS scores of ⩾ 30 for at least 2 of the following 3 parameters: patient global assessment; average of VAS values for nocturnal back pain and total back pain; average of 10 questions on the Bath Ankylosing Spondylitis Functional Index (BASFI). Patients receiving DMARDs, NSAIDS, or corticosteroids could continue them on stable doses. Patients with complete ankylosis of the spine were not included in the study. Doses of 25 mg of Enbrel (based on dose-finding studies in patients with rheumatoid arthritis) or placebo were administered subcutaneously twice a week for 6 months in 138 patients.

The primary measure of efficacy (ASAS 20) was a ⩾20% improvement in at least 3 of the 4 Assessment in Ankylosing Spondylitis (ASAS) domains (patient global assessments, back pain, BASFI, and inflammation) and absence of deterioration in the remaining domain. ASAS 50 and 70 responses used the same criteria with a 50% improvement or a 70% improvement, respectively.

Compared to placebo, treatment with Enbrel resulted in significant improvements in the ASAS 20, ASAS 50 and ASAS 70 as early as 2 weeks after the initiation of therapy.

RESPONSES OF PATIENTS WITH ANKYLOSING SPONDYLITIS IN A PLACEBO-CONTROLLED TRIAL

	Percent of Patients	
Ankylosing Spondylitis Response	Placebo N = 139	Enbrel N = 138
ASAS 20		
2 weeks	22	46[a]
3 months	27	60[a]
6 months	23	58[a]
ASAS 50		
2 weeks	7	24[a]
3 months	13	45[a]
6 months	10	42[a]
ASAS 70:		
2 weeks	2	12[b]
3 months	7	29[b]
6 months	5	28[b]

a: $p < 0.001$, Enbrel vs. Placebo
b: p = 0.002, Enbrel vs. placebo

Figure 2 RADIOGRAPHIC PROGRESSION: COMPARISON OF ENBREL vs METHOTREXATE vs ENBREL IN COMBINATION WITH METHOTREXATE IN PATIENTS WITH RA OF 6 MONTHS TO 20 YEARS DURATION (12 MONTH RESULTS)

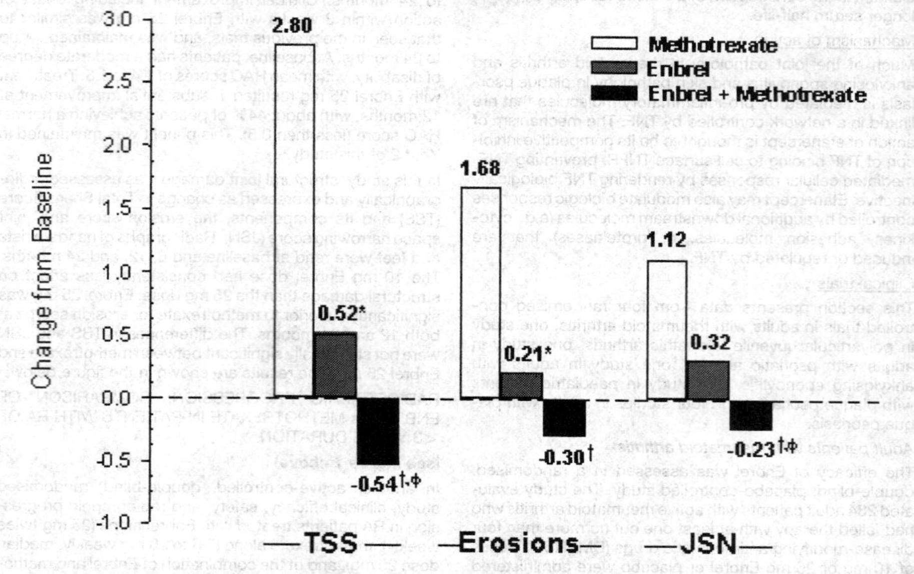

Pairwise comparison p-values: * = $p < 0.05$ for comparisons of Enbrel vs methotrexate, † = $p < 0.05$ for comparisons of Enbrel + methotrexate vs methotrexate and ϕ = $p < 0.05$ for comparisons of Enbrel + methotrexate vs Enbrel

Among patients with ankylosing spondylitis who received Enbrel, the clinical responses were apparent at the time of the first visit (2 weeks) and were maintained through 6 months of therapy. Responses were similar in patients who were or were not receiving concomitant therapies at baseline.

Similar results were obtained in the 2 smaller ankylosing spondylitis trials.

In a fourth study, the safety and efficacy of 50 mg Enbrel (two 25 mg SC injections) administered once weekly vs 25 mg Enbrel administered twice weekly were evaluated in a double-blind, placebo-controlled study of 356 patients with active ankylosing spondylitis. The safety and efficacy profiles of the 50 mg once weekly and 25 mg twice weekly regimens were similar.

Adult patients with plaque psoriasis

Enbrel is recommended for use in patients as defined in section 4.1. Patients who "failed to respond to" in the target population is defined by insufficient response (PASI $<$ 50 or PGA less than good), or worsening of the disease while on treatment, and who were adequately dosed for a sufficiently long duration to assess response with at least each of the three major systemic therapies as available.

The efficacy of Enbrel versus other systemic therapies in patients with moderate to severe psoriasis (responsive to other systemic therapies) has not been evaluated in studies directly comparing Enbrel with other systemic therapies. Instead, the safety and efficacy of Enbrel were assessed in four randomised, double-blind, placebo-controlled studies. The primary efficacy endpoint in all four studies was the proportion of patients in each treatment group who achieved the PASI 75 (i.e. at least a 75% improvement in the Psoriasis Area and Severity Index score from baseline) at 12 weeks.

Study 1 was a Phase 2 study in patients with active but clinically stable plaque psoriasis involving $\geqslant$ 10% of the body surface area that were $\geqslant$ 18 years old. One hundred and twelve (112) patients were randomised to receive a dose of 25 mg of Enbrel (n=57) or placebo (n=55) twice a week for 24 weeks.

Study 2 evaluated 652 patients with chronic plaque psoriasis using the same inclusion criteria as study 1 with the addition of a minimum psoriasis area and severity index (PASI) of 10 at screening. Enbrel was administered at doses of 25 mg once a week, 25 mg twice a week or 50 mg twice a week for 6 consecutive months. During the first 12 weeks of the double-blind treatment period, patients received placebo or one of the above three Enbrel doses. After 12 weeks of treatment, patients in the placebo group began treatment with blinded Enbrel (25 mg twice a week); patients in the active treatment groups continued to week 24 on the dose to which they were originally randomised.

Study 3 evaluated 583 patients and had the same inclusion criteria as study 2. Patients in this study received a dose of 25 mg or 50 mg Enbrel, or placebo twice a week for 12 weeks and then all patients received open-label 25 mg Enbrel twice weekly for an additional 24 weeks.

Study 4 evaluated 142 patients and had similar inclusion criteria to studies 2 and 3. Patients in this study received a dose of 50 mg Enbrel or placebo once weekly for 12 weeks and then all patients received open-label 50 mg Enbrel once weekly for an additional 12 weeks.

In study 1, the Enbrel-treated group had a significantly higher proportion of patients with a PASI 75 response at week 12 (30%) compared to the placebo-treated group (2%) ($p < 0.0001$). At 24 weeks, 56% of patients in the Enbrel-treated group had achieved the PASI 75 compared to 5% of placebo-treated patients. Key results of studies 2, 3 and 4 are shown below.

(see Table 2 below)

Among patients with plaque psoriasis who received Enbrel, significant responses relative to placebo were apparent at the time of the first visit (2 weeks) and were maintained through 24 weeks of therapy.

Study 2 also had a drug withdrawal period during which patients who achieved a PASI improvement of at least 50% at week 24 had treatment stopped. Patients were observed off treatment for the occurrence of rebound (PASI $\geqslant$150% of baseline) and for the time to relapse (defined as a loss of at least half of the improvement achieved between baseline and week 24). During the withdrawal period, symptoms of psoriasis gradually returned with a median time to disease relapse of 3 months. No rebound flare of disease and no psoriasis-related serious adverse events were observed. There was some evidence to support a benefit of re-treatment with Enbrel in patients initially responding to treatment.

In study 3, the majority of patients (77%) who were initially randomised to 50 mg twice weekly and had their Enbrel dose decreased at week 12 to 25 mg twice weekly maintained their PASI 75 response through week 36. For patients who received 25 mg twice weekly throughout the study, the PASI 75 response continued to improve between weeks 12 and 36.

In study 4, the Enbrel-treated group had a higher proportion of patients with PASI 75 at week 12 (38%) compared to the placebo-treated group (2%) ($p < 0.0001$). For patients who received 50 mg once weekly throughout the study, the efficacy responses continued to improve with 71% achieving PASI 75 at week 24.

In long-term (up to 34 months) open-label studies where Enbrel was given without interruption, clinical responses were sustained and safety was comparable to shorter-term studies.

An analysis of clinical trial data did not reveal any baseline disease characteristics that would assist clinicians in selecting the most appropriate dosing option (intermittent or continuous). Consequently, the choice of intermittent or continuous therapy should be based upon physician judgment and individual patient needs.

Paediatric patients with plaque psoriasis

The efficacy of Enbrel was assessed in a randomised, double-blind, placebo-controlled study in 211 paediatric patients aged 4 to 17 years with moderate to severe plaque psoriasis (as defined by a sPGA score $\geqslant$ 3, involving $\geqslant$ 10% of the BSA, and PASI $\geqslant$ 12). Eligible patients had a history of receiving phototherapy or systemic therapy, or were inadequately controlled on topical therapy.

Patients received Enbrel 0.8 mg/kg (up to 50 mg) or placebo once weekly for 12 weeks. At week 12, more patients randomised to Enbrel had positive efficacy responses (e.g., PASI 75) than those randomised to placebo.

Paediatric Plaque Psoriasis Outcomes at 12 Weeks

	Enbrel 0.8 mg/kg Once Weekly (N = 106)	**Placebo (N = 105)**
PASI 75, n (%)	60 (57%)[a]	12 (11%)
PASI 50, n (%)	79 (75%)[a]	24 (23%)
sPGA "clear" or "minimal", n (%)	56 (53%)[a]	14 (13%)

Abbreviation: sPGA-static Physician Global Assessment.

a. $p < 0.0001$ compared with placebo.

After the 12-week double-blind treatment period, all patients received Enbrel 0.8 mg/kg (up to 50 mg) once weekly for additional 24 weeks. Responses observed during the open-label period were similar to those observed in the double-blind period.

During a randomised withdrawal period, significantly more patients re-randomised to placebo experienced disease relapse (loss of PASI 75 response) compared with patients re-randomised to Enbrel. With continued therapy, responses were maintained up to 48 weeks.

Antibodies to Enbrel

Antibodies to etanercept have been detected in the sera of some subjects treated with etanercept. These antibodies have all been non-neutralising and are generally transient. There appears to be no correlation between antibody development and clinical response or adverse events.

In subjects treated with approved doses of etanercept in clinical trials for up to 12 months, cumulative rates of anti-etanercept antibodies were approximately 6% of subjects with rheumatoid arthritis, 7.5% of subjects with psoriatic arthritis, 2% of subjects with ankylosing spondylitis, 7% of subjects with psoriasis, 9.7% of subjects with paediatric psoriasis, and 3% of subjects with juvenile idiopathic arthritis.

The proportion of subjects who developed antibodies to etanercept in longer-term trials (of up to 3.5 years) increases over time, as expected. However, due to their transient nature, the incidence of antibodies detected at each assessment point was typically less than 7% in rheumatoid arthritis subjects and psoriasis subjects.

In a long-term psoriasis study in which patients received 50 mg twice weekly for 96 weeks, the incidence of antibodies observed at each assessment point was up to approximately 9%.

5.2 Pharmacokinetic properties

Etanercept serum values were determined by an ELISA method, which may detect ELISA-reactive degradation products as well as the parent compound.

Etanercept is slowly absorbed from the site of subcutaneous injection, reaching maximum concentration approximately 48 hours after a single dose. The absolute bioavailability is 76%. With twice weekly doses, it is anticipated that steady-state concentrations are approximately twice as high as those observed after single doses. After a single subcutaneous dose of 25 mg Enbrel, the average maximum serum concentration observed in healthy volunteers was 1.65 ± 0.66 μg/ml, and the area under the curve was 235 ± 96.6 μg•hr/ml. Dose proportionality has not been formally evaluated, but there is no apparent saturation of clearance across the dosing range.

A biexponential curve is required to describe the concentration time curve of etanercept. The central volume of distribution of etanercept is 7.6 l, while the volume of distribution at steady-state is 10.4 l. Etanercept is cleared slowly from the body. The half-life is long, approximately 70 hours. Clearance is approximately 0.066 l/hr in patients with rheumatoid arthritis, somewhat lower than the value of 0.11 l/hr observed in healthy volunteers. Additionally, the pharmacokinetics of Enbrel in rheumatoid arthritis patients, ankylosing spondylitis and plaque psoriasis patients are similar.

Mean serum concentration profiles at steady state i.e. Cmax (2.4 mg/l vs 2.6 mg/l), Cmin (1.2 mg/l vs 1.4 mg/l), and partial AUC (297 mgh/l vs 316 mgh/l), were shown to be comparable in RA patients treated with 50 mg etanercept once weekly (n=21) and 25 mg etanercept twice weekly (n=16), respectively. In an open-label, single-dose, two-treatment, crossover study in healthy volunteers, etanercept administered as a single 50 mg/ml injection was found to be bioequivalent to two simultaneous injections of 25 mg/ml.

In a population pharmacokinetics analysis in ankylosing spondylitis patients, the etanercept steady state AUCs were 466 μg•hr/ml and 474 μg•hr/ml for 50 mg Enbrel once weekly (N= 154) and 25 mg twice weekly (N = 148), respectively.

Although there is elimination of radioactivity in urine after administration of radiolabelled etanercept to patients and volunteers, increased etanercept concentrations were not observed in patients with acute renal or hepatic failure. The presence of renal and hepatic impairment should not require a change in dosage. There is no apparent pharmacokinetic difference between males and females.

Methotrexate has no effect on the pharmacokinetics of etanercept. The effect of Enbrel on the human pharmacokinetics of methotrexate has not been investigated.

Special populations

Elderly patients

The impact of advanced age was studied in the population pharmacokinetic analysis of etanercept serum

Table 2 RESPONSES OF PATIENTS WITH PSORIASIS IN STUDIES 2, 3 AND 4

Response (%)	Study 2					Study 3			Study 4		
	Placebo	Enbrel				Placebo	Enbrel		Placebo	Enbrel	
		25 mg BIW		50 mg BIW			25 mg BIW	50 mg BIW		50 mg QW	50 mg QW
	n = 166 wk 12	n = 162 wk 12	n = 162 wk 24[a]	n = 164 wk 12	n = 164 wk 24[a]	n = 193 wk 12	n = 196 wk 12	n = 196 wk 12	n = 46 wk 12	n = 96 wk 12	n = 90 wk 24[a]
PASI 50	14	58*	70	74*	77	9	64*	77*	9	69*	83
PASI 75	4	34*	44	49*	59	3	34*	49*	2	38*	71
DSGA [b], clear or almost clear	5	34*	39	49*	55	4	39*	57*	4	39*	64

*p $\leqslant$ 0.0001 compared with placebo

a. No statistical comparisons to placebo were made at week 24 in studies 2 and 4 because the original placebo group began receiving Enbrel 25 mg BIW or 50 mg once weekly from week 13 to week 24.

b. Dermatologist Static Global Assessment. Clear or almost clear defined as 0 or 1 on a 0 to 5 scale.

concentrations. Clearance and volume estimates in patients aged 65 to 87 years were similar to estimates in patients less than 65 years of age.

Paediatric patients with plaque psoriasis

Patients with paediatric plaque psoriasis (aged 4 to 17 years) were administered 0.8 mg/kg (up to a maximum dose of 50 mg per week) of etanercept once weekly for up to 48 weeks. The mean serum steady state trough concentrations ranged from 1.6 to 2.1 mcg/ml at weeks 12, 24, and 48. These mean concentrations in patients with paediatric plaque psoriasis were similar to the concentrations observed in patients with juvenile idiopathic arthritis (treated with 0.4 mg/kg etanercept twice weekly, up to maximum dose of 50 mg per week). These mean concentrations were similar to those seen in adult patients with plaque psoriasis treated with 25 mg etanercept twice weekly.

5.3 Preclinical safety data

In the toxicological studies with Enbrel, no dose-limiting or target organ toxicity was evident. Enbrel was considered to be non-genotoxic from a battery of *in vitro* and *in vivo* studies. Carcinogenicity studies, and standard assessments of fertility and postnatal toxicity, were not performed with Enbrel due to the development of neutralising antibodies in rodents.

Enbrel did not induce lethality or notable signs of toxicity in mice or rats following a single subcutaneous dose of 2000 mg/kg or a single intravenous dose of 1000 mg/kg. Enbrel did not elicit dose-limiting or target organ toxicity in cynomolgus monkeys following twice weekly subcutaneous administration for 4 or 26 consecutive weeks at a dose (15 mg/kg) that resulted in AUC-based serum drug concentrations that were over 27-fold higher than that obtained in humans at the recommended dose of 25 mg.

6. PHARMACEUTICAL PARTICULARS

6.1 List of excipients

Sucrose

Sodium chloride

L-Arginine hydrochloride

Sodium phosphate monobasic dihydrate

Sodium phosphate dibasic dihydrate

Water for injections

6.2 Incompatibilities

In the absence of compatibility studies, this medicinal product must not be mixed with other medicinal products.

6.3 Shelf life

2 years.

6.4 Special precautions for storage

Store in a refrigerator (2°C – 8°C).

Do not freeze.

Keep the pre-filled pens in the outer carton in order to protect from light.

6.5 Nature and contents of container

Pre-filled pen (MYCLIC) containing a pre-filled syringe of Enbrel. The syringe inside the pen is made from clear type 1 glass with a stainless steel 27 gauge needle, rubber needle cover, and plastic plunger. The needle cap of the pre-filled pen contains dry natural rubber (a derivative of latex). See section 4.4.

Cartons contain 2, 4 or 12 pre-filled pens of Enbrel with 4, 8 or 24 alcohol swabs. Not all pack sizes may be marketed.

6.6 Special precautions for disposal and other handling

Any unused product or waste material should be disposed of in accordance with local requirements.

Instructions for use and handling

Before injection, Enbrel single-use pre-filled pens should be allowed to reach room temperature (approximately 15 to 30 minutes). The needle cover should not be removed while allowing the pre-filled pen to reach room temperature. By looking though the inspection window, the solution should be clear and colourless or pale yellow and practically free from visible particles.

Comprehensive instructions for administration are given in the package leaflet, section 7, "Using the MYCLIC pre-filled pen to inject Enbrel."

7. MARKETING AUTHORISATION HOLDER

Wyeth Europa Ltd.

Huntercombe Lane South

Taplow, Maidenhead

Berkshire, SL6 0PH

United Kingdom

8. MARKETING AUTHORISATION NUMBER(S)

EU/1/99/126/020

9. DATE OF FIRST AUTHORISATION/RENEWAL OF THE AUTHORISATION

Date of first authorisation: 3 February 2000

Date of last renewal: 3 February 2005

10. DATE OF REVISION OF THE TEXT

16 July 2009

Detailed information on this product is available on the website of the European Medicines Agency (EMEA) http://www.emea.europa.eu

Enbrel 50mg solution for injection in pre-filled syringe

(Wyeth Pharmaceuticals)

1. NAME OF THE MEDICINAL PRODUCT

Enbrel®▼50 mg solution for injection in pre-filled syringe.

2. QUALITATIVE AND QUANTITATIVE COMPOSITION

Each pre-filled syringe contains 50 mg of etanercept.

Etanercept is a human tumour necrosis factor receptor p75 Fc fusion protein produced by recombinant DNA technology in a Chinese hamster ovary (CHO) mammalian expression system. Etanercept is a dimer of a chimeric protein genetically engineered by fusing the extracellular ligand binding domain of human tumour necrosis factor receptor-2 (TNFR2/p75) to the Fc domain of human IgG1. This Fc component contains the hinge, CH_2 and CH_3 regions but not the CH_1 region of IgG1. Etanercept contains 934 amino acids and has an apparent molecular weight of approximately 150 kilodaltons. The potency is determined by measuring the ability of etanercept to neutralise the TNFα-mediated growth inhibition of A375 cells. The specific activity of etanercept is 1.7×10^6 units/mg.

For a full list of excipients, see section 6.1.

3. PHARMACEUTICAL FORM

Solution for injection.

The solution is clear, and colourless or pale yellow.

4. CLINICAL PARTICULARS

4.1 Therapeutic indications

Rheumatoid arthritis

Enbrel in combination with methotrexate is indicated for the treatment of moderate to severe active rheumatoid arthritis in adults when the response to disease-modifying antirheumatic drugs, including methotrexate (unless contraindicated), has been inadequate.

Enbrel can be given as monotherapy in case of intolerance to methotrexate or when continued treatment with methotrexate is inappropriate.

Enbrel is also indicated in the treatment of severe, active and progressive rheumatoid arthritis in adults not previously treated with methotrexate.

Enbrel, alone or in combination with methotrexate, has been shown to reduce the rate of progression of joint damage as measured by X-ray and to improve physical function.

Psoriatic arthritis

Treatment of active and progressive psoriatic arthritis in adults when the response to previous disease-modifying antirheumatic drug therapy has been inadequate. Enbrel has been shown to improve physical function in patients with psoriatic arthritis, and to reduce the rate of progression of peripheral joint damage as measured by X-ray in patients with polyarticular symmetrical subtypes of the disease.

Ankylosing spondylitis

Treatment of adults with severe active ankylosing spondylitis who have had an inadequate response to conventional therapy.

Plaque psoriasis

Treatment of adults with moderate to severe plaque psoriasis who failed to respond to, or who have a contraindication to, or are intolerant to other systemic therapy including ciclosporin, methotrexate or PUVA (see section 5.1).

Paediatric plaque psoriasis

Treatment of chronic severe plaque psoriasis in children and adolescents from the age of 8 years who are inadequately controlled by, or are intolerant to, other systemic therapies or phototherapies.

4.2 Posology and method of administration

Enbrel treatment should be initiated and supervised by specialist physicians experienced in the diagnosis and treatment of rheumatoid arthritis, psoriatic arthritis, ankylosing spondylitis, plaque psoriasis or paediatric plaque psoriasis. Patients treated with Enbrel should be given the Patient Alert Card.

Enbrel is available in strengths of 25 and 50 mg.

Posology

Rheumatoid arthritis

25 mg Enbrel administered twice weekly is the recommended dose. Alternatively, 50 mg Enbrel administered once weekly has been shown to be safe and effective (see section 5.1).

Psoriatic arthritis and ankylosing spondylitis

The recommended dose is 25 mg Enbrel administered twice weekly, or 50 mg Enbrel administered once weekly.

Plaque psoriasis

The recommended dose of Enbrel is 25 mg administered twice weekly or 50 mg administered once weekly. Alternatively, 50 mg given twice weekly may be used for up to 12 weeks followed, if necessary, by a dose of 25 mg twice weekly or 50 mg once weekly. Treatment with Enbrel should continue until remission is achieved, for up to 24 weeks. Continuous therapy beyond 24 weeks may be appropriate for some adult patients (see section 5.1). Treatment should be discontinued in patients who show no response after 12 weeks. If re-treatment with Enbrel is indicated, the same guidance on treatment duration should be followed. The dose should be 25 mg twice weekly or 50 mg once weekly.

Special populations

Paediatric use

Enbrel is available as a single use syringe for patients weighing 62.5 kg or more. Lyophilized vials containing a reconstituted dose of 25 mg/ml are available from which doses less than 25 mg can be administered.

Paediatric plaque psoriasis (age 8 years and above)

0.8 mg/kg (up to a maximum of 50 mg per dose) once weekly for up to 24 weeks. Treatment should be discontinued in patients who show no response after 12 weeks.

If re-treatment with Enbrel is indicated, the above guidance on treatment duration should be followed. The dose should be 0.8 mg/kg (up to a maximum of 50 mg per dose) once weekly.

Elderly patients (⩾ 65 years)

No dose adjustment is required. Posology and administration are the same as for adults 18-64 years of age.

Renal and hepatic impairment

No dose adjustment is required.

Method of administration

Comprehensive instructions for administration are given in the package leaflet, section 7, "Instructions for preparation and giving an injection of Enbrel."

4.3 Contraindications

Hypersensitivity to the active substance or to any of the excipients.

Sepsis or risk of sepsis.

Treatment with Enbrel should not be initiated in patients with active infections including chronic or localised infections.

4.4 Special warnings and precautions for use

Infections

Patients should be evaluated for infections before, during, and after treatment with Enbrel, taking into consideration that the mean elimination half-life of etanercept is approximately 70 hours (range 7 to 300 hours).

Serious infections, sepsis, tuberculosis, and opportunistic infections, including invasive fungal infections, have been reported with the use of Enbrel (see section 4.8). These infections were due to bacteria, mycobacteria, fungi and viruses. In some cases, particular fungal and other opportunistic infections have not been recognised, resulting in delay of appropriate treatment and sometimes death. In evaluating patients for infections, the patient's risk for relevant opportunistic infections (e.g., exposure to endemic mycoses) should be considered.

Patients who develop a new infection while undergoing treatment with Enbrel should be monitored closely. **Administration of Enbrel should be discontinued if a patient develops a serious infection.** Physicians should exercise caution when considering the use of Enbrel in patients with a history of recurring or chronic infections or with underlying conditions that may predispose patients to infections such as advanced or poorly controlled diabetes.

Tuberculosis

Cases of active tuberculosis including miliary tuberculosis and tuberculosis with extra-pulmonary location have been reported in patients treated with Enbrel.

Before starting treatment with Enbrel, all patients must be evaluated for both active and inactive ('latent') tuberculosis. This evaluation should include a detailed medical history with personal history of tuberculosis or possible previous contact with tuberculosis and previous and/or current immunosuppressive therapy. Appropriate screening tests, i.e. tuberculin skin test and chest x-ray, should be performed in all patients (local recommendations may apply). It is recommended that the conduct of these tests should be recorded in the patient's alert card. Prescribers are reminded of the risk of false negative tuberculin skin test results, especially in patients who are severely ill or immunocompromised.

If active tuberculosis is diagnosed, Enbrel therapy must not be initiated. If inactive ('latent') tuberculosis is diagnosed, treatment for latent tuberculosis must be started with anti-tuberculosis therapy before the initiation of Enbrel, and in accordance with local recommendations. In this situation, the benefit/risk balance of Enbrel therapy should be very carefully considered.

All patients should be informed to seek medical advice if signs/symptoms suggestive of tuberculosis (e.g., persistent cough, wasting/weight loss, low-grade fever) appear during or after Enbrel treatment.

Hepatitis B virus reactivation

Reactivation of hepatitis B virus (HBV) in patients who are chronic carriers of this virus who are receiving TNF-antagonists including Enbrel has been reported. Patients at risk for HBV infection should be evaluated for prior evidence of HBV infection before initiating Enbrel therapy. Caution should be exercised when administering Enbrel to patients identified as carriers of HBV. If Enbrel is used in carriers of HBV, the patients should be monitored for signs and symptoms of active HBV infection and, if necessary, appropriate treatment should be initiated.

Worsening of hepatitis C

There have been reports of worsening of hepatitis C in patients receiving Enbrel.

Concurrent treatment with anakinra

Concurrent administration of Enbrel and anakinra has been associated with an increased risk of serious infections and neutropenia compared to Enbrel alone. This combination has not demonstrated increased clinical benefit. Thus the combined use of Enbrel and anakinra is not recommended (see sections 4.5 and 4.8).

Concurrent treatment with abatacept

In clinical studies, concurrent administration of abatacept and Enbrel resulted in increased incidences of serious adverse events. This combination has not demonstrated increased clinical benefit; such use is not recommended (see section 4.5).

Allergic reactions

Allergic reactions associated with Enbrel administration have been reported commonly. Allergic reactions have included angioedema and urticaria; serious reactions have occurred. If any serious allergic or anaphylactic reaction occurs, Enbrel therapy should be discontinued immediately and appropriate therapy initiated.

The needle cover of the pre-filled syringe contains latex (dry natural rubber) that may cause hypersensitivity reactions when handled by or when Enbrel is administered to persons with known or possible latex sensitivity.

Immunosuppression

The possibility exists for TNF-antagonists, including Enbrel, to affect host defences against infections and malignancies since TNF mediates inflammation and modulates cellular immune responses. In a study of 49 adult patients with rheumatoid arthritis treated with Enbrel, there was no evidence of depression of delayed-type hypersensitivity, depression of immunoglobulin levels, or change in enumeration of effector cell populations.

Two juvenile idiopathic arthritis patients developed varicella infection and signs and symptoms of aseptic meningitis, which resolved without sequelae. Patients with a significant exposure to varicella virus should temporarily discontinue Enbrel therapy and be considered for prophylactic treatment with Varicella Zoster Immune Globulin.

The safety and efficacy of Enbrel in patients with immunosuppression or chronic infections have not been evaluated.

Malignancies and lymphoproliferative disorders

Solid and haematopoietic malignancies

Reports of various malignancies (including breast and lung carcinoma and lymphoma) have been received in the post-marketing period (see section 4.8).

In the controlled portions of clinical trials of TNF-antagonists, more cases of lymphoma have been observed among patients receiving a TNF-antagonist compared with control patients. However, the occurrence was rare, and the follow-up period of placebo patients was shorter than for patients receiving TNF-antagonist therapy. Furthermore, there is an increased background lymphoma risk in rheumatoid arthritis patients with long-standing, highly active, inflammatory disease, which complicates the risk estimation. With the current knowledge, a possible risk for the development of lymphomas or other malignancies in patients treated with a TNF-antagonist cannot be excluded.

Non-melanoma skin cancer (NMSC)

Non-melanoma skin cancer has been reported in patients treated with TNF-antagonists, including Enbrel. Combining the results of placebo- and active comparator-controlled clinical trials of Enbrel, more cases of NMSC were observed in patients receiving Enbrel compared with control patients, particularly in patients with psoriasis. Periodic skin examination is recommended for all patients who are at increased risk for NMSC (including patients with psoriasis or a history of PUVA therapy).

Vaccinations

Live vaccines should not be given concurrently with Enbrel. No data are available on the secondary transmission of infection by live vaccines in patients receiving Enbrel. In a double blind, placebo controlled, randomised clinical study in adult patients with psoriatic arthritis 184 patients also received a multivalent pneumococcal polysaccharide vaccine at week 4. In this study most psoriatic arthritis patients receiving Enbrel were able to mount effective B-cell immune response to pneumococcal polysaccharide vaccine, but titers in aggregate were moderately lower and few patients had two-fold rises in titers compared to patients not receiving Enbrel. The clinical significance of this is unknown.

Autoantibody formation

Treatment with Enbrel may result in the formation of autoimmune antibodies (see section 4.8).

Haematologic reactions

Rare cases of pancytopenia and very rare cases of aplastic anaemia, some with fatal outcome, have been reported in patients treated with Enbrel. Caution should be exercised in patients being treated with Enbrel who have a previous history of blood dyscrasias. All patients and parents/caregivers should be advised that if the patient develops signs and symptoms suggestive of blood dyscrasias or infections (e.g. persistent fever, sore throat, bruising, bleeding, paleness) whilst on Enbrel, they should seek immediate medical advice. Such patients should be investigated urgently, including full blood count; if blood dyscrasias are confirmed, Enbrel should be discontinued.

CNS disorders

There have been rare reports of CNS demyelinating disorders in patients treated with Enbrel (see section 4.8). Although no clinical trials have been performed evaluating Enbrel therapy in patients with multiple sclerosis, clinical trials of other TNF antagonists in patients with multiple sclerosis have shown increases in disease activity. A careful risk/benefit evaluation, including a neurological assessment, is recommended when prescribing Enbrel to patients with pre-existing or recent onset of CNS demyelinating disease, or to those who are considered to have an increased risk of developing demyelinating disease.

Combination therapy

In a controlled clinical trial of two years duration in rheumatoid arthritis patients, the combination of Enbrel and methotrexate did not result in unexpected safety findings, and the safety profile of Enbrel when given in combination with methotrexate was similar to the profiles reported in studies of Enbrel and methotrexate alone. Long-term studies to assess the safety of the combination are ongoing. The long-term safety of Enbrel in combination with other disease-modifying antirheumatic drugs (DMARD) has not been established.

The use of Enbrel in combination with other systemic therapies or phototherapy for the treatment of psoriasis has not been studied.

Renal and hepatic impairment

Based on pharmacokinetic data (see section 5.2), no dose adjustment is needed in patients with renal or hepatic impairment; clinical experience in such patients is limited.

Congestive heart failure

Physicians should use caution when using Enbrel in patients who have congestive heart failure (CHF). There have been postmarketing reports of worsening of CHF, with and without identifiable precipitating factors, in patients taking Enbrel. Two large clinical trials evaluating the use of Enbrel in the treatment of CHF were terminated early due to lack of efficacy. Although not conclusive, data from one of these trials suggest a possible tendency toward worsening CHF in those patients assigned to Enbrel treatment.

Alcoholic hepatitis

In a phase II randomised placebo-controlled study of 48 hospitalised patients treated with Enbrel or placebo for moderate to severe alcoholic hepatitis, Enbrel was not efficacious, and the mortality rate in patients treated with Enbrel was significantly higher after 6 months. Consequently, Enbrel should not be used in patients for the treatment of alcoholic hepatitis. Physicians should use caution when using Enbrel in patients who also have moderate to severe alcoholic hepatitis.

Wegener's granulomatosis

A placebo-controlled trial, in which 89 adult patients were treated with Enbrel in addition to standard therapy (including cyclophosphamide or methotrexate, and glucocorticoids) for a median duration of 25 months, has not shown Enbrel to be an effective treatment for Wegener's granulomatosis. The incidence of non-cutaneous malignancies of various types was significantly higher in patients treated with Enbrel than in the control group. Enbrel is not recommended for the treatment of Wegener's granulomatosis.

4.5 Interaction with other medicinal products and other forms of interaction

Concurrent treatment with anakinra

Adult patients treated with Enbrel and anakinra were observed to have a higher rate of serious infection when compared with patients treated with either Enbrel or anakinra alone (historical data).

In addition, in a double-blind placebo-controlled trial in adult patients receiving background methotrexate, patients treated with Enbrel and anakinra were observed to have a higher rate of serious infections (7%) and neutropenia than patients treated with Enbrel (see sections 4.4 and 4.8). The combination Enbrel and anakinra has not demonstrated increased clinical benefit and is therefore not recommended.

Concurrent treatment with abatacept

In clinical studies, concurrent administration of abatacept and Enbrel resulted in increased incidences of serious adverse events. This combination has not demonstrated increased clinical benefit; such use is not recommended (see section 4.4).

Concurrent treatment with sulfasalazine

In a clinical study of adult patients who were receiving established doses of sulfasalazine, to which Enbrel was added, patients in the combination group experienced a statistically significant decrease in mean white blood cell counts in comparison to groups treated with Enbrel or sulfasalazine alone. The clinical significance of this interaction is unknown.

Non-interactions

In clinical trials, no interactions have been observed when Enbrel was administered with glucocorticoids, salicylates (except sulfasalazine), nonsteroidal anti-inflammatory drugs (NSAIDs), analgesics, or methotrexate. See section 4.4 for vaccination advice.

No clinically significant pharmacokinetic drug-drug interactions were observed in studies with digoxin or warfarin.

4.6 Pregnancy and lactation

Pregnancy

There are no studies of Enbrel in pregnant women. Developmental toxicity studies performed in rats and rabbits have revealed no evidence of harm to the foetus or neonatal rat due to etanercept. Preclinical data about peri- and postnatal toxicity of etanercept and of effects of etanercept on fertility and general reproductive performance are not available. Thus, the use of Enbrel in pregnant women is not recommended, and women of child-bearing potential should be advised not to get pregnant during Enbrel therapy.

Lactation

It is not known whether etanercept is excreted in human milk. Following subcutaneous administration to lactacting rats, etanercept was excreted in the milk and detected in the serum of pups. Because immunoglobulins, in common with many medicinal products, can be excreted in human milk, a decision should be made whether to discontinue breast-feeding or to discontinue Enbrel while breast-feeding.

4.7 Effects on ability to drive and use machines

No studies on the effects on the ability to drive and use machines have been performed.

4.8 Undesirable effects

Undesirable effects in adults

Enbrel has been studied in 2,680 patients with rheumatoid arthritis in double-blind and open-label trials. This experience includes 2 placebo-controlled studies (349 Enbrel patients and 152 placebo patients) and 2 active-controlled trials, one active-controlled trial comparing Enbrel to methotrexate (415 Enbrel patients and 217 methotrexate patients) and another active-controlled trial comparing Enbrel (223 patients), methotrexate (228 patients) and Enbrel in combination with methotrexate (231 patients). The proportion of patients who discontinued treatment due to adverse events was the same in both the Enbrel and placebo treatment groups; in the first active-controlled trial, the dropout rate was significantly higher for methotrexate (10%) than for Enbrel (5%). In the second active-controlled trial, the rate of discontinuation for adverse events after 2 years of treatment was similar among all three treatment groups, Enbrel (16%), methotrexate (21%) and Enbrel in combination with methotrexate (17%). Additionally, Enbrel has been studied in 240 psoriatic arthritis patients who participated in 2 double-blind placebo-controlled studies and an open-label extension study. Five hundred and eight (508) ankylosing spondylitis patients were treated with Enbrel in 4 double-blind placebo-controlled studies. Enbrel has also been studied in 1,492 patients with plaque psoriasis for up to 6 months in 5 double-blind placebo-controlled studies.

In double-blind clinical trials comparing Enbrel to placebo, injection site reactions were the most frequent adverse events among Enbrel-treated patients. Among patients with rheumatoid arthritis treated in placebo-controlled trials, serious adverse events occurred at a frequency of 4% in 349 patients treated with Enbrel compared with 5% of 152 placebo-treated patients. In the first active-controlled trial, serious adverse events occurred at a frequency of 6% in 415 patients treated with Enbrel compared with 8% of 217 methotrexate-treated patients. In the second active-controlled trial the rate of serious adverse events after 2 years of treatment was similar among the three treatment groups (Enbrel 16%, methotrexate 15% and Enbrel in combination with methotrexate 17%). Among patients with plaque psoriasis treated in placebo-controlled trials, the frequency of serious adverse events was about 1.4% of 1,341 patients treated with Enbrel compared with 1.4% of 766 placebo-treated patients.

The following list of adverse reactions is based on experience from clinical trials in adults and on postmarketing experience.

Within the organ system classes, adverse reactions are listed under headings of frequency (number of patients expected to experience the reaction), using the following categories: very common (≥1/10); common (≥1/100, <1/10); uncommon (≥1/1000, <1/100); rare (≥1/10,000, <1/1000); very rare (<1/10,000); not known (cannot be estimated from the available data).

Infections and infestations:

Very common:	Infections (including upper respiratory tract infections, bronchitis, cystitis, skin infections)*
Uncommon:	Serious infections (including pneumonia, cellulitis, septic arthritis, sepsis)*
Rare:	Tuberculosis, opportunistic infections (including invasive fungal, protozoal, bacterial and atypical mycobacterial infections)*

Blood and lymphatic system disorders:

Uncommon: Thrombocytopenia

Rare: Anaemia, leukopenia, neutropenia, pancytopenia*

Very rare: Aplastic anaemia*

Immune system disorders:

Common: Allergic reactions (see Skin and subcutaneous tissue disorders), autoantibody formation*

Rare: Serious allergic/anaphylactic reactions (including angioedema, bronchospasm)

Not known: Macrophage activation syndrome*, anti-neutrophilic cytoplasmic antibody positive vasculitis

Nervous system disorders:

Rare: Seizures

CNS demyelinating events suggestive of multiple sclerosis or localised demyelinating conditions such as optic neuritis and transverse myelitis (see section 4.4)

Respiratory, thoracic and mediastinal disorders:

Uncommon: Interstitial lung disease (including pneumonitis and pulmonary fibrosis)*

Hepatobiliary disorders:

Rare: Elevated liver enzymes

Skin and subcutaneous tissue disorders:

Common: Pruritus

Uncommon: Non-melanoma skin cancers (see section 4.4), angioedema, urticaria, rash, psoriasiform rash, psoriasis (including new onset and pustular, primarily palms and soles)

Rare: Cutaneous vasculitis (including leukocytoclastic vasculitis), Stevens-Johnson syndrome, erythema multiforme

Very rare: Toxic epidermal necrolysis

Musculoskeletal and connective tissue disorders:

Rare: Subacute cutaneous lupus erythematosus, discoid lupus erythematosus, lupus like syndrome

General disorders and administration site conditions:

Very common: Injection site reactions (including bleeding, bruising, erythema, itching, pain, swelling)*

Common: Fever

Cardiac disorders:

There have been reports of worsening of congestive heart failure (see section 4.4).

*see Additional information, below.

Additional information

Serious adverse events reported in clinical trials

Among rheumatoid arthritis, psoriatic arthritis, ankylosing spondylitis and plaque psoriasis patients in placebo-controlled, active-controlled, and open-label trials of Enbrel, serious adverse events reported included malignancies (see below), asthma, infections (see below), heart failure, myocardial infarction, myocardial ischaemia, chest pain, syncope, cerebral ischaemia, hypertension, hypotension, cholecystitis, pancreatitis, gastrointestinal haemorrhage, bursitis, confusion, depression, dyspnoea, abnormal healing, renal insufficiency, kidney calculus, deep vein thrombosis, pulmonary embolism, membranous glomerulonephropathy, polymyositis, thrombophlebitis, liver damage, leucopenia, paresis, paresthesia, vertigo, allergic alveolitis, angioedema, scleritis, bone fracture, lymphadenopathy, ulcerative colitis, intestinal obstruction, eosinophilia, haematuria, and sarcoidosis.

Malignancies and lymphoproliferative disorders

One hundred and twenty-nine new malignancies of various types were observed in 4,114 rheumatoid arthritis patients treated in clinical trials with Enbrel for up to approximately 6 years, including 231 patients treated with Enbrel in combination with methotrexate in the 2-year active-controlled study. The observed rates and incidences in these clinical trials were similar to those expected for the population studied. A total of 2 malignancies were reported in clinical studies of approximately 2 years duration involving 240 Enbrel-treated psoriatic arthritis patients. In clinical studies conducted for more than 2 years with 351 ankylosing spondylitis patients, 6 malignancies were reported in Enbrel-treated patients. In a group of 2,711 plaque psoriasis patients treated with Enbrel in double-blind and open-label studies of up to 2.5 years, 30 malignancies and 43 nonmelanoma skin cancers were reported.

In a group of 7,416 patients treated with Enbrel in rheumatoid arthritis, psoriatic arthritis, ankylosing spondylitis and psoriasis clinical trials, 18 lymphomas were reported.

Reports of various malignancies (including breast and lung carcinoma and lymphoma) have also been received in the postmarketing period (see section 4.4).

Injection site reactions

Compared to placebo, patients with rheumatic diseases treated with Enbrel had a significantly higher incidence of injection site reactions (36% vs. 9%). Injection site reactions usually occurred in the first month. Mean duration was approximately 3 to 5 days. No treatment was given for the majority of injection site reactions in the Enbrel treatment groups, and the majority of patients who were given treatment received topical preparations such as corticosteroids, or oral antihistamines. Additionally, some patients developed recall injection site reactions characterised by a skin reaction at the most recent site of injection along with the simultaneous appearance of injection site reactions at previous injection sites. These reactions were generally transient and did not recur with treatment.

In controlled trials in patients with plaque psoriasis, approximately 13.6% of patients treated with Enbrel developed injection site reactions compared with 3.4% of placebo-treated patients during the first 12 weeks of treatment.

Serious infections

In placebo-controlled trials, no increase in the incidence of serious infections (fatal, life threatening, or requiring hospitalisation or intravenous antibiotics) was observed. Serious infections occurred in 6.3% of rheumatoid arthritis patients treated with Enbrel for up to 48 months. These included abscess (at various sites), bacteraemia, bronchitis, bursitis, cellulitis, cholecystitis, diarrhoea, diverticulitis, endocarditis (suspected), gastroenteritis, hepatitis B, herpes zoster, leg ulcer, mouth infection, osteomyelitis, otitis, peritonitis, pneumonia, pyelonephritis, sepsis, septic arthritis, sinusitis, skin infection, skin ulcer, urinary tract infection, vasculitis, and wound infection. In the 2-year active-controlled study where patients were treated with either Enbrel alone, methotrexate alone or Enbrel in combination with methotrexate, the rates of serious infections were similar among the treatment groups. However, it cannot be excluded that the combination of Enbrel with methotrexate could be associated with an increase in the rate of infections.

There were no differences in rates of infection among patients treated with Enbrel and those treated with placebo for plaque psoriasis in placebo controlled trials of up to 24 weeks duration. Serious infections experienced by Enbrel-treated patients included cellulitis, gastroenteritis, pneumonia, cholecystitis, osteomyelitis, gastritis, appendicitis, Streptococcal fasciitis, myositis, septic shock, diverticulitis and abscess. In the double-blind and open-label psoriatic arthritis trials, 1 patient reported a serious infection (pneumonia).

Serious and fatal infections have been reported during use of Enbrel; reported pathogens include bacteria, mycobacteria (including tuberculosis), viruses and fungi. Some have occurred within a few weeks after initiating treatment with Enbrel in patients who have underlying conditions (e.g. diabetes, congestive heart failure, history of active or chronic infections) in addition to their rheumatoid arthritis (see section 4.4). Enbrel treatment may increase mortality in patients with established sepsis.

Opportunistic infections have been reported in association with Enbrel including invasive fungal, protozoal, bacterial (including *Listeria* and *Legionella*), and atypical mycobacterial infections. In a pooled data set of clinical trials, the overall incidence of opportunistic infections was 0.09% for the 15,402 subjects who received Enbrel. The exposure-adjusted rate was 0.06 events per 100 patient-years. In postmarketing experience, approximately half of all of the case reports of opportunistic infections worldwide were invasive fungal infections. The most commonly reported invasive fungal infections were *Pneumocystis* and *Aspergillus*. Invasive fungal infections accounted for more than half of the fatalities amongst patients who developed opportunistic infections. The majority of the reports with a fatal outcome were in patients with *Pneumocystis* pneumonia, unspecified systemic fungal infections, and aspergillosis (see section 4.4).

Autoantibodies

Adult patients had serum samples tested for autoantibodies at multiple timepoints. Of the rheumatoid arthritis patients evaluated for antinuclear antibodies (ANA), the percentage of patients who developed new positive ANA (⩾1:40) was higher in patients treated with Enbrel (11%) than in placebo-treated patients (5%). The percentage of patients who developed new positive anti-double-stranded DNA antibodies was also higher by radioimmunoassay (15% of patients treated with Enbrel compared to 4% of placebo-treated patients) and by *Crithidia luciliae* assay (3% of patients treated with Enbrel compared to none of placebo-treated patients). The proportion of patients treated with Enbrel who developed anticardiolipin antibodies was similarly increased compared to placebo-treated patients. The impact of long-term treatment with Enbrel on the development of autoimmune diseases is unknown.

There have been rare reports of patients, including rheumatoid factor positive patients, who have developed other autoantibodies in conjunction with a lupus-like syndrome or rashes that are compatible with subacute cutaneous lupus or discoid lupus by clinical presentation and biopsy.

Pancytopenia and aplastic anaemia

There have been postmarketing reports of pancytopenia and aplastic anaemia, some of which had fatal outcomes (see section 4.4).

Interstitial lung disease

There have been postmarketing reports of interstitial lung disease (including pneumonitis and pulmonary fibrosis), some of which had fatal outcomes.

Laboratory evaluations

Based on the results of clinical studies, normally no special laboratory evaluations are necessary in addition to careful medical management and supervision of patients.

Concurrent treatment with anakinra

In studies when adult patients received concurrent treatment with Enbrel plus anakinra, a higher rate of serious infections compared to Enbrel alone was observed and 2% of patients (3/139) developed neutropenia (absolute neutrophil count < 1000 / mm^3). While neutropenic, one patient developed cellulitis that resolved after hospitalisation (see sections 4.4 and 4.5).

Undesirable effects in paediatric patients with plaque psoriasis

In a 48-week study in 211 children aged 4 to 17 years with paediatric plaque psoriasis, the adverse events reported were similar to those seen in previous studies in adults with plaque psoriasis.

There were 4 reports of macrophage activation syndrome in juvenile idiopathic arthritis clinical trials.

4.9 Overdose

No dose-limiting toxicities were observed during clinical trials of rheumatoid arthritis patients. The highest dose level evaluated has been an intravenous loading dose of 32 mg/m^2 followed by subcutaneous doses of 16 mg/m^2 administered twice weekly. One rheumatoid arthritis patient mistakenly self-administered 62 mg Enbrel subcutaneously twice weekly for 3 weeks without experiencing undesirable effects. There is no known antidote to Enbrel.

5. PHARMACOLOGICAL PROPERTIES

5.1 Pharmacodynamic properties

Pharmacotherapeutic group: Tumor Necrosis Factor alpha (TNF-α) inhibitors, ATC code: L04AB01

Tumour necrosis factor (TNF) is a dominant cytokine in the inflammatory process of rheumatoid arthritis. Elevated levels of TNF are also found in the synovium and psoriatic plaques of patients with psoriatic arthritis and in serum and synovial tissue of patients with ankylosing spondylitis. In plaque psoriasis, infiltration by inflammatory cells including T-cells leads to increased TNF levels in psoriatic lesions compared with levels in uninvolved skin. Etanercept is a competitive inhibitor of TNF-binding to its cell surface receptors and thereby inhibits the biological activity of TNF. TNF and lymphotoxin are pro-inflammatory cytokines that bind to two distinct cell surface receptors: the 55-kilodalton (p55) and 75-kilodalton (p75) tumour necrosis factor receptors (TNFRs). Both TNFRs exist naturally in membrane-bound and soluble forms. Soluble TNFRs are thought to regulate TNF biological activity.

TNF and lymphotoxin exist predominantly as homotrimers, with their biological activity dependent on cross-linking of cell surface TNFRs. Dimeric soluble receptors such as etanercept possess a higher affinity for TNF than monomeric receptors and are considerably more potent competitive inhibitors of TNF binding to its cellular receptors. In addition, use of an immunoglobulin Fc region as a fusion element in the construction of a dimeric receptor imparts a longer serum half-life.

Mechanism of action

Much of the joint pathology in rheumatoid arthritis and ankylosing spondylitis and skin pathology in plaque psoriasis is mediated by pro-inflammatory molecules that are linked in a network controlled by TNF. The mechanism of action of etanercept is thought to be its competitive inhibition of TNF binding to cell surface TNFR, preventing TNF-mediated cellular responses by rendering TNF biologically inactive. Etanercept may also modulate biologic responses controlled by additional downstream molecules (e.g., cytokines, adhesion molecules, or proteinases) that are induced or regulated by TNF.

Clinical trials

This section presents data from four randomised controlled trials in adults with rheumatoid arthritis, one study in polyarticular juvenile idiopathic arthritis, one study in adults with psoriatic arthritis, one study in adults with ankylosing spondylitis, one study in paediatric patients with plaque psoriasis, and four studies in adults with plaque psoriasis.

Adult patients with rheumatoid arthritis

The efficacy of Enbrel was assessed in a randomised, double-blind, placebo-controlled study. The study evaluated 234 adult patients with active rheumatoid arthritis who had failed therapy with at least one but no more than four disease-modifying antirheumatic drugs (DMARDs). Doses of 10 mg or 25 mg Enbrel or placebo were administered subcutaneously twice a week for 6 consecutive months. The results of this controlled trial were expressed in percentage improvement in rheumatoid arthritis using AmericanCollege of Rheumatology (ACR) response criteria. ACR 20 and 50 responses were higher in patients treated

Figure 1 RADIOGRAPHIC PROGRESSION: COMPARISON OF ENBREL vs METHOTREXATE IN PATIENTS WITH RA OF <3 YEARS DURATION

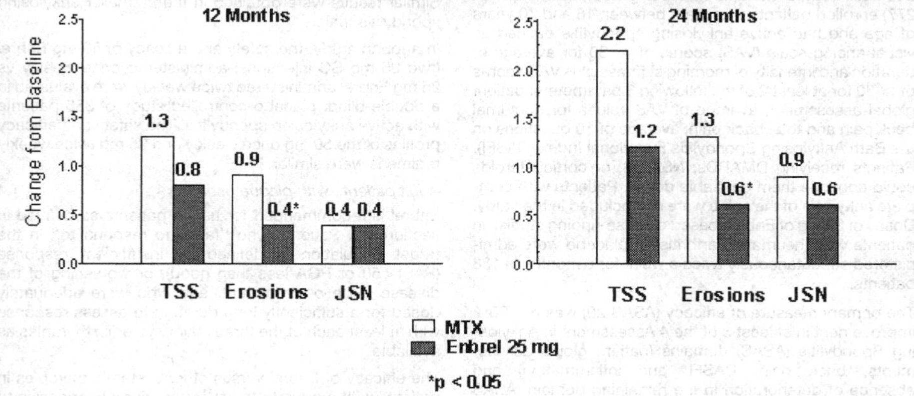

with Enbrel at 3 and 6 months than in patients treated with placebo (ACR 20: Enbrel 62% and 59%, placebo 23% and 11% at 3 and 6 months respectively; ACR 50: Enbrel 41% and 40%, placebo 8% and 5% at months 3 and 6 respectively; p<0.01 Enbrel vs Placebo at all time points for both ACR 20 and ACR 50 responses).

Approximately 15% of subjects who received Enbrel achieved an ACR 70 response at month 3 and month 6 compared to fewer than 5% of subjects in the placebo arm. Among patients receiving Enbrel, the clinical responses generally appeared within 1 to 2 weeks after initiation of therapy and nearly always occurred by 3 months. A dose response was seen; results with 10 mg were intermediate between placebo and 25 mg. Enbrel was significantly better than placebo in all components of the ACR criteria as well as other measures of rheumatoid arthritis disease activity not included in the ACR response criteria, such as morning stiffness. A Health Assessment Questionnaire (HAQ), which included disability, vitality, mental health, general health status, and arthritis-associated health status subdomains, was administered every 3 months during the trial. All subdomains of the HAQ were improved in patients treated with Enbrel compared to controls at 3 and 6 months.

After discontinuation of Enbrel, symptoms of arthritis generally returned within a month. Re-introduction of treatment with Enbrel after discontinuations of up to 24 months resulted in the same magnitudes of responses as patients who received Enbrel without interruption of therapy based on results of open-label studies. Continued durable responses have been seen for up to 48 months in open-label extension treatment trials when patients received Enbrel without interruption; longer-term experience is not available.

The efficacy of Enbrel was compared to methotrexate in a third randomised, active-controlled study with blinded radiographic evaluations as a primary endpoint in 632 adult patients with active rheumatoid arthritis (<3 years duration) who had never received treatment with methotrexate.

Doses of 10 mg or 25 mg Enbrel were administered SC twice a week for up to 24 months. Methotrexate doses were escalated from 7.5 mg/week to a maximum of 20 mg/week over the first 8 weeks of the trial and continued for up to 24 months. Clinical improvement including onset of action within 2 weeks with Enbrel 25 mg was similar to that seen in the previous trials, and was maintained for up to 24 months. At baseline, patients had a moderate degree of disability, with mean HAQ scores of 1.4 to 1.5. Treatment with Enbrel 25 mg resulted in substantial improvement at 12 months, with about 44% of patients achieving a normal HAQ score (less than 0.5). This benefit was maintained in Year 2 of this study.

In this study, structural joint damage was assessed radiographically and expressed as change in Total Sharp Score (TSS) and its components, the erosion score and joint space narrowing score (JSN). Radiographs of hands/wrists and feet were read at baseline and 6, 12, and 24 months. The 10 mg Enbrel dose had consistently less effect on structural damage than the 25 mg dose. Enbrel 25 mg was significantly superior to methotrexate for erosion scores at both 12 and 24 months. The differences in TSS and JSN were not statistically significant between methotrexate and Enbrel 25 mg. The results are shown in the figure below.

RADIOGRAPHIC PROGRESSION: COMPARISON OF ENBREL vs METHOTREXATE IN PATIENTS WITH RA OF <3 YEARS DURATION

(see Figure 1 above)

In another active-controlled, double-blind, randomised study, clinical efficacy, safety, and radiographic progression in RA patients treated with Enbrel alone (25 mg twice weekly), methotrexate alone (7.5 to 20 mg weekly, median dose 20 mg), and of the combination of Enbrel and methotrexate initiated concurrently were compared in 682 adult patients with active rheumatoid arthritis of 6 months to 20 years duration (median 5 years) who had a less than satisfactory response to at least 1 disease-modifying antirheumatic drug (DMARD) other than methotrexate.

Table 1

CLINICAL EFFICACY RESULTS AT 12 MONTHS: COMPARISON OF ENBREL vs METHOTREXATE vs ENBREL IN COMBINATION WITH METHOTREXATE IN PATIENTS WITH RA OF 6 MONTHS TO 20 YEARS DURATION

Endpoint	Methotrexate (n = 228)	Enbrel (n = 223)	Enbrel + Methotrexate (n = 231)
ACR Responses[a]			
ACR 20	58.8%	65.5%	74.5% †,ϕ
ACR 50	36.4%	43.0%	63.2% †,ϕ
ACR 70	16.7%	22.0%	39.8% †,ϕ
DAS			
Baseline score[b]	5.5	5.7	5.5
Week 52 score[b]	3.0	3.0	2.3†,ϕ
Remission[c]	14%	18%	37%†,ϕ
HAQ			
Baseline	1.7	1.7	1.8
Week 52	1.1	1.0	0.8†,ϕ

a: Patients who did not complete 12 months in the study were considered to be non-responders.

b: Values for Disease Activity Score (DAS) are means.

c: Remission is defined as DAS <1.6

Pairwise comparison p-values: † = $p < 0.05$ for comparisons of Enbrel + methotrexate vs methotrexate and ϕ = $p < 0.05$ for comparisons of Enbrel + methotrexate vs Enbrel

Patients in the Enbrel in combination with methotrexate therapy group had significantly higher ACR 20, ACR 50, ACR 70 responses and improvement for DAS and HAQ scores at both 24 and 52 weeks than patients in either of the single therapy groups (results shown in table below). Significant advantages for Enbrel in combination with methotrexate compared with Enbrel monotherapy and methotrexate monotherapy were also observed after 24 months.

(see Table 1 below)

Radiographic progression at 12 months was significantly less in the Enbrel group than in the methotrexate group, while the combination was significantly better than either monotherapy at slowing radiographic progression (see figure below).

RADIOGRAPHIC PROGRESSION: COMPARISON OF ENBREL vs METHOTREXATE vs ENBREL IN COMBINATION WITH METHOTREXATE IN PATIENTS WITH RA OF 6 MONTHS TO 20 YEARS DURATION (12 MONTH RESULTS)

(see Figure 2 on next page)

Significant advantages for Enbrel in combination with methotrexate compared with Enbrel monotherapy and methotrexate monotherapy were also observed after 24 months. Similarly, the significant advantages for Enbrel monotherapy compared with methotrexate monotherapy were also observed after 24 months.

In an analysis in which all patients who dropped out of the study for any reason were considered to have progressed, the percentage of patients without progression (TSS change ⩽ 0.5) at 24 months was higher in the Enbrel in combination with methotrexate group compared with the Enbrel alone and methotrexate alone groups (62%, 50%, and 36%, respectively; $p<0.05$). The difference between Enbrel alone and methotrexate alone was also significant ($p<0.05$). Among patients who completed a full 24 months of therapy in the study, the non-progression rates were 78%, 70%, and 61%, respectively.

The safety and efficacy of 50 mg Enbrel (two 25 mg SC injections) administered once weekly were evaluated in a double-blind, placebo-controlled study of 420 patients with active RA. In this study, 53 patients received placebo, 214 patients received 50 mg Enbrel once weekly and 153 patients received 25 mg Enbrel twice weekly. The safety and efficacy profiles of the two Enbrel treatment regimens were comparable at week 8 in their effect on signs and symptoms of RA; data at week 16 did not show comparability (non-inferiority) between the two regimens. A single 50 mg/ml injection of Enbrel was found to be bioequivalent to two simultaneous injections of 25 mg/ml.

Adult patients with psoriatic arthritis

The efficacy of Enbrel was assessed in a randomised, double-blind, placebo-controlled study in 205 patients with psoriatic arthritis. Patients were between 18 and 70 years of age and had active psoriatic arthritis (⩾ 3 swollen joints and ⩾ 3 tender joints) in at least one of the following forms: (1) distal interphalangeal (DIP) involvement; (2) polyarticular arthritis (absence of rheumatoid nodules and presence of psoriasis); (3) arthritis mutilans; (4) asymmetric psoriatic arthritis; or (5) spondylitis-like ankylosis. Patients also had plaque psoriasis with a qualifying target lesion ⩾ 2 cm in diameter. Patients had previously been treated with NSAIDs (86%), DMARDs (80%), and corticosteroids (24%). Patients currently on methotrexate therapy (stable for ⩾ 2 months) could continue at a stable dose of ⩽ 25 mg/week methotrexate. Doses of 25 mg of Enbrel (based on dose-finding studies in patients with rheumatoid arthritis) or placebo were administered SC twice a week for 6 months. At the end of the double-blind study, patients could enter a long-term open-label extension study for a total duration of up to 2 years.

Clinical responses were expressed as percentages of patients achieving the ACR 20, 50, and 70 response and percentages with improvement in Psoriatic Arthritis Response Criteria (PsARC). Results are summarised in the Table below.

RESPONSES OF PATIENTS WITH PSORIATIC ARTHRITIS IN PLACEBO-CONTROLLED TRIAL

	Percent of Patients	
	Placebo	Enbrel[a]
Psoriatic Arthritis Response	n = 104	n = 101
ACR 20		
Month 3	15	59[b]
Month 6	13	50[b]
ACR 50		
Month 3	4	38[b]
Month 6	4	37[b]
ACR 70		
Month 3	0	11[b]

Month 6	1	9[c]
PsARC		
Month 3	31	72[b]
Month 6	23	70[b]

a: 25 mg Enbrel SC twice weekly

b: $p < 0.001$, Enbrel vs. placebo

c: $p < 0.01$, Enbrel vs. placebo

Among patients with psoriatic arthritis who received Enbrel, the clinical responses were apparent at the time of the first visit (4 weeks) and were maintained through 6 months of therapy. Enbrel was significantly better than placebo in all measures of disease activity ($p < 0.001$), and responses were similar with and without concomitant methotrexate therapy. Quality of life in psoriatic arthritis patients was assessed at every timepoint using the disability index of the HAQ. The disability index score was significantly improved at all timepoints in psoriatic arthritis patients treated with Enbrel, relative to placebo ($p < 0.001$).

Radiographic changes were assessed in the psoriatic arthritis study. Radiographs of hands and wrists were obtained at baseline and months 6, 12, and 24. The modified TSS at 12 months is presented in the Table below. In an analysis in which all patients who dropped out of the study for any reason were considered to have progressed, the percentage of patients without progression (TSS change ⩽ 0.5) at 12 months was higher in the Enbrel group compared with the placebo group (73% vs. 47%, respectively, $p \leqslant 0.001$). The effect of Enbrel on radiographic progression was maintained in patients who continued on treatment during the second year. The slowing of peripheral joint damage was observed in patients with polyarticular symmetrical joint involvement.

MEAN (SE) ANNUALIZED CHANGE FROM BASELINE IN TOTAL SHARP SCORE		
	Placebo	Etanercept
Time	(n = 104)	(n = 101)
Month 12	1.00 (0.29)	-0.03 (0.09)[a]

SE = standard error.

a. p = 0.0001.

Enbrel treatment resulted in improvement in physical function during the double-blind period, and this benefit was maintained during the longer-term exposure of up to 2 years.

There is insufficient evidence of the efficacy of Enbrel in patients with ankylosing spondylitis-like and arthritis mutilans psoriatic arthropathies due to the small number of patients studied.

No study has been performed in patients with psoriatic arthritis using the 50mg once weekly dosing regimen. Evidence of efficacy for the once weekly dosing regimen in this patient population has been based on data from the study in patients with ankylosing spondylitis.

Adult patients with ankylosing spondylitis

The efficacy of Enbrel in ankylosing spondylitis was assessed in 3 randomised, double-blind studies comparing twice weekly administration of 25 mg Enbrel with placebo. A total of 401 patients were enrolled from which 203 were treated with Enbrel. The largest of these trials (n= 277) enrolled patients who were between 18 and 70 years of age and had active ankylosing spondylitis defined as visual analog scale (VAS) scores of ⩾ 30 for average of duration and intensity of morning stiffness plus VAS scores of ⩾ 30 for at least 2 of the following 3 parameters: patient global assessment; average of VAS values for nocturnal back pain and total back pain; average of 10 questions on the Bath Ankylosing Spondylitis Functional Index (BASFI). Patients receiving DMARDs, NSAIDS, or corticosteroids could continue them on stable doses. Patients with complete ankylosis of the spine were not included in the study. Doses of 25 mg of Enbrel (based on dose-finding studies in patients with rheumatoid arthritis) or placebo were administered subcutaneously twice a week for 6 months in 138 patients.

The primary measure of efficacy (ASAS 20) was a ⩾20% improvement in at least 3 of the 4 Assessment in Ankylosing Spondylitis (ASAS) domains (patient global assessments, back pain, BASFI, and inflammation) and absence of deterioration in the remaining domain. ASAS 50 and 70 responses used the same criteria with a 50% improvement or a 70% improvement, respectively.

Compared to placebo, treatment with Enbrel resulted in significant improvements in the ASAS 20, ASAS 50 and ASAS 70 as early as 2 weeks after the initiation of therapy.

RESPONSES OF PATIENTS WITH ANKYLOSING SPONDYLITIS IN A PLACEBO-CONTROLLED TRIAL		
	Percent of Patients	
Ankylosing Spondylitis Response	Placebo N = 139	Enbrel N = 138
ASAS 20		
2 weeks	22	46[a]
3 months	27	60[a]
6 months	23	58[a]
ASAS 50		
2 weeks	7	24[a]
3 months	13	45[a]
6 months	10	42[a]
ASAS 70:		
2 weeks	2	12[b]
3 months	7	29[b]
6 months	5	28[b]

a: p<0.001, Enbrel vs. Placebo

b: p = 0.002, Enbrel vs. placebo

Among patients with ankylosing spondylitis who received Enbrel, the clinical responses were apparent at the time of the first visit (2 weeks) and were maintained through 6 months of therapy. Responses were similar in patients who were or were not receiving concomitant therapies at baseline.

Similar results were obtained in the 2 smaller ankylosing spondylitis trials.

In a fourth study, the safety and efficacy of 50 mg Enbrel (two 25 mg SC injections) administered once weekly vs 25 mg Enbrel administered twice weekly were evaluated in a double-blind, placebo-controlled study of 356 patients with active ankylosing spondylitis. The safety and efficacy profiles of the 50 mg once weekly and 25 mg twice weekly regimens were similar.

Adult patients with plaque psoriasis

Enbrel is recommended for use in patients as defined in section 4.1. Patients who "failed to respond to" in the target population is defined by insufficient response (PASI<50 or PGA less than good), or worsening of the disease while on treatment, and who were adequately dosed for a sufficiently long duration to assess response with at least each of the three major systemic therapies as available.

The efficacy of Enbrel versus other systemic therapies in patients with moderate to severe psoriasis (responsive to other systemic therapies) has not been evaluated in studies directly comparing Enbrel with other systemic therapies. Instead, the safety and efficacy of Enbrel were assessed in four randomised, double-blind, placebo-controlled studies. The primary efficacy endpoint in all four studies was the proportion of patients in each treatment group who achieved the PASI 75 (i.e. at least a 75% improvement in the Psoriasis Area and Severity Index score from baseline) at 12 weeks.

Study 1 was a Phase 2 study in patients with active but clinically stable plaque psoriasis involving ⩾ 10% of the body surface area that were ⩾ 18 years old. One hundred and twelve (112) patients were randomised to receive a dose of 25 mg of Enbrel (n=57) or placebo (n=55) twice a week for 24 weeks.

Study 2 evaluated 652 patients with chronic plaque psoriasis using the same inclusion criteria as study 1 with the addition of a minimum psoriasis area and severity index (PASI) of 10 at screening. Enbrel was administered at doses of 25 mg once a week, 25 mg twice a week or 50 mg twice a week for 6 consecutive months. During the first 12 weeks of the double-blind treatment period, patients received placebo or one of the above three Enbrel doses. After 12 weeks of treatment, patients in the placebo group began treatment with blinded Enbrel (25 mg twice a week); patients in the active treatment groups continued to week 24 on the dose to which they were originally randomised.

Study 3 evaluated 583 patients and had the same inclusion criteria as study 2. Patients in this study received a dose of 25 mg or 50 mg Enbrel, or placebo twice a week for 12 weeks and then all patients received open-label 25 mg Enbrel twice weekly for an additional 24 weeks.

Study 4 evaluated 142 patients and had similar inclusion criteria to studies 2 and 3. Patients in this study received a dose of 50 mg Enbrel or placebo once weekly for 12 weeks and then all patients received open-label 50 mg Enbrel once weekly for an additional 12 weeks.

In study 1, the Enbrel-treated group had a significantly higher proportion of patients with a PASI 75 response at week 12 (30%) compared to the placebo-treated group (2%) (p<0.0001). At 24 weeks, 56% of patients in the Enbrel-treated group had achieved the PASI 75 compared to 5% of placebo-treated patients. Key results of studies 2, 3 and 4 are shown below.

(see Table 2 on next page)

Among patients with plaque psoriasis who received Enbrel, significant responses relative to placebo were apparent at the time of the first visit (2 weeks) and were maintained through 24 weeks of therapy.

Study 2 also had a drug withdrawal period during which patients who achieved a PASI improvement of at least 50% at week 24 had treatment stopped. Patients were observed off treatment for the occurrence of rebound (PASI ⩾150% of baseline) and for the time to relapse (defined as a loss of at least half of the improvement achieved between baseline and week 24). During the withdrawal period, symptoms of psoriasis gradually returned with a median time to disease relapse of 3 months. No rebound flare of disease and no psoriasis-related serious adverse events were observed. There was some evidence to support a benefit of re-treatment with Enbrel in patients initially responding to treatment.

In study 3, the majority of patients (77%) who were initially randomised to 50 mg twice weekly and had their Enbrel dose decreased at week 12 to 25 mg twice weekly maintained their PASI 75 response through week 36. For patients who received 25 mg twice weekly throughout the study, the PASI 75 response continued to improve between weeks 12 and 36.

In study 4, the Enbrel-treated group had a higher proportion of patients with PASI 75 at week 12 (38%) compared to the placebo-treated group (2%) (p<0.0001). For patients who received 50 mg once weekly throughout the study, the efficacy responses continued to improve with 71% achieving PASI 75 at week 24.

Figure 2 RADIOGRAPHIC PROGRESSION: COMPARISON OF ENBREL vs METHOTREXATE vs ENBREL IN COMBINATION WITH METHOTREXATE IN PATIENTS WITH RA OF 6 MONTHS TO 20 YEARS DURATION (12 MONTH RESULTS)

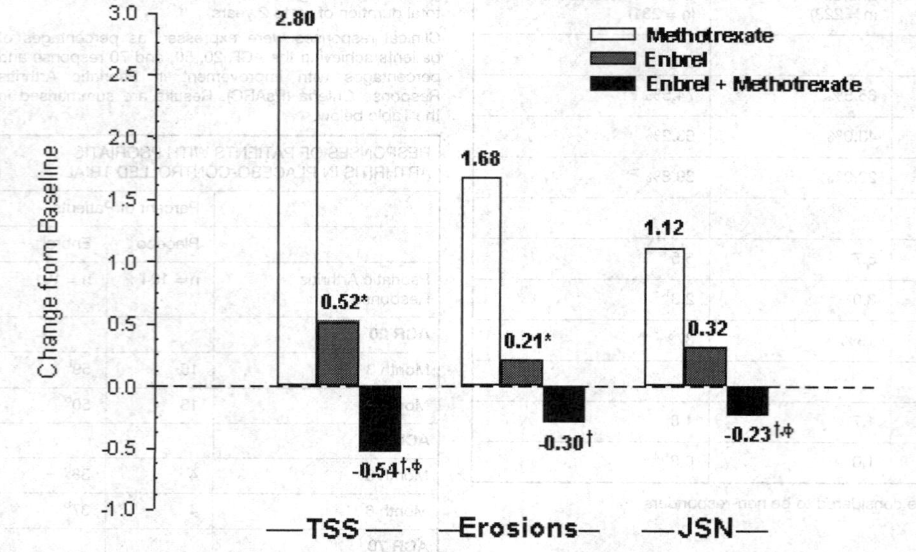

Pairwise comparison p-values: * = $p < 0.05$ for comparisons of Enbrel vs methotrexate, † = $p < 0.05$ for comparisons of Enbrel + methotrexate vs methotrexate and ϕ = $p < 0.05$ for comparisons of Enbrel + methotrexate vs Enbrel

Table 2 RESPONSES OF PATIENTS WITH PSORIASIS IN STUDIES 2, 3 AND 4

Response (%)	Study 2					Study 3			Study 4		
	Placebo	Enbrel				Placebo	Enbrel		Placebo	Enbrel	
		25 mg BIW		50 mg BIW			25 mg BIW	50 mg BIW		50 mg QW	50 mg QW
	n = 166 wk 12	n = 162 wk 12	n = 162 wk 24[a]	n = 164 wk 12	n = 164 wk 24[a]	n = 193 wk 12	n = 196 wk 12	n = 196 wk 12	n = 46 wk 12	n = 96 wk 12	n = 90 wk 24[a]
PASI 50	14	58*	70	74*	77	9	64*	77*	9	69*	83
PASI 75	4	34*	44	49*	59	3	34*	49*	2	38*	71
DSGA [b], clear or almost clear	5	34*	39	49*	55	4	39*	57*	4	39*	64

*$p \leqslant 0.0001$ compared with placebo

a. No statistical comparisons to placebo were made at week 24 in studies 2 and 4 because the original placebo group began receiving Enbrel 25 mg BIW or 50 mg once weekly from week 13 to week 24.

b. Dermatologist Static Global Assessment. Clear or almost clear defined as 0 or 1 on a 0 to 5 scale.

In long-term (up to 34 months) open-label studies where Enbrel was given without interruption, clinical responses were sustained and safety was comparable to shorter-term studies.

An analysis of clinical trial data did not reveal any baseline disease characteristics that would assist clinicians in selecting the most appropriate dosing option (intermittent or continuous). Consequently, the choice of intermittent or continuous therapy should be based upon physician judgment and individual patient needs.

Paediatric patients with plaque psoriasis

The efficacy of Enbrel was assessed in a randomised, double-blind, placebo-controlled study in 211 paediatric patients aged 4 to 17 years with moderate to severe plaque psoriasis (as defined by a sPGA score $\geqslant 3$, involving $\geqslant 10\%$ of the BSA, and PASI $\geqslant 12$). Eligible patients had a history of receiving phototherapy or systemic therapy, or were inadequately controlled on topical therapy.

Patients received Enbrel 0.8 mg/kg (up to 50 mg) or placebo once weekly for 12 weeks. At week 12, more patients randomised to Enbrel had positive efficacy responses (e.g., PASI 75) than those randomised to placebo.

Paediatric Plaque Psoriasis Outcomes at 12 Weeks

	Enbrel 0.8 mg/kg Once Weekly (N = 106)	Placebo (N = 105)
PASI 75, n (%)	60 (57%)[a]	12 (11%)
PASI 50, n (%)	79 (75%)[a]	24 (23%)
sPGA "clear" or "minimal", n (%)	56 (53%)[a]	14 (13%)

Abbreviation: sPGA-static Physician Global Assessment.

a. $p < 0.0001$ compared with placebo.

After the 12-week double-blind treatment period, all patients received Enbrel 0.8 mg/kg (up to 50 mg) once weekly for additional 24 weeks. Responses observed during the open-label period were similar to those observed in the double-blind period.

During a randomised withdrawal period, significantly more patients re-randomised to placebo experienced disease relapse (loss of PASI 75 response) compared with patients re-randomised to Enbrel. With continued therapy, responses were maintained up to 48 weeks.

Antibodies to Enbrel

Antibodies to etanercept have been detected in the sera of some subjects treated with etanercept. These antibodies have all been non-neutralising and are generally transient. There appears to be no correlation between antibody development and clinical response or adverse events.

In subjects treated with approved doses of etanercept in clinical trials for up to 12 months, cumulative rates of anti-etanercept antibodies were approximately 6% of subjects with rheumatoid arthritis, 7.5% of subjects with psoriatic arthritis, 2% of subjects with ankylosing spondylitis, 7% of subjects with psoriasis, 9.7% of subjects with paediatric psoriasis, and 3% of subjects with juvenile idiopathic arthritis.

The proportion of subjects who developed antibodies to etanercept in longer-term trials (of up to 3.5 years) increases over time, as expected. However, due to their transient nature, the incidence of antibodies detected at each assessment point was typically less than 7% in rheumatoid arthritis subjects and psoriasis subjects.

In a long-term psoriasis study in which patients received 50 mg twice weekly for 96 weeks, the incidence of antibodies observed at each assessment point was up to approximately 9%.

5.2 Pharmacokinetic properties

Etanercept serum values were determined by an ELISA method, which may detect ELISA-reactive degradation products as well as the parent compound.

Etanercept is slowly absorbed from the site of subcutaneous injection, reaching maximum concentration approximately 48 hours after a single dose. The absolute bioavailability is 76%. With twice weekly doses, it is anticipated that steady-state concentrations are approximately twice as high as those observed after single doses. After a single subcutaneous dose of 25 mg Enbrel, the average maximum serum concentration observed in healthy volunteers was 1.65 ± 0.66 μg/ml, and the area under the curve was 235 ± 96.6 μg•hr/ml. Dose proportionality has not been formally evaluated, but there is no apparent saturation of clearance across the dosing range.

A biexponential curve is required to describe the concentration time curve of etanercept. The central volume of distribution of etanercept is 7.6 l, while the volume of distribution at steady-state is 10.4 l. Etanercept is cleared slowly from the body. The half-life is long, approximately 70 hours. Clearance is approximately 0.066 l/hr in patients with rheumatoid arthritis, somewhat lower than the value of 0.11 l/hr observed in healthy volunteers. Additionally, the pharmacokinetics of Enbrel in rheumatoid arthritis patients, ankylosing spondylitis and plaque psoriasis patients are similar.

Mean serum concentration profiles at steady state i.e. Cmax (2.4 mg/l vs 2.6 mg/l), Cmin (1.2 mg/l vs 1.4 mg/l), and partial AUC (297 mgh/l vs 316 mgh/l), were shown to be comparable in RA patients treated with 50 mg etanercept once weekly (n=21) and 25 mg etanercept twice weekly (n=16), respectively. In an open-label, single-dose, two-treatment, crossover study in healthy volunteers, etanercept administered as a single 50 mg/ml injection was found to be bioequivalent to two simultaneous injections of 25 mg/ml.

In a population pharmacokinetics analysis in ankylosing spondylitis patients, the etanercept steady state AUCs were 466 μg•hr/ml and 474 μg•hr/ml for 50 mg Enbrel once weekly (N= 154) and 25 mg twice weekly (N = 148), respectively.

Although there is elimination of radioactivity in urine after administration of radiolabelled etanercept to patients and volunteers, increased etanercept concentrations were not observed in patients with acute renal or hepatic failure. The presence of renal and hepatic impairment should not require a change in dosage. There is no apparent pharmacokinetic difference between males and females.

Methotrexate has no effect on the pharmacokinetics of etanercept. The effect of Enbrel on the human pharmacokinetics of methotrexate has not been investigated.

Special populations

Elderly patients

The impact of advanced age was studied in the population pharmacokinetic analysis of etanercept serum concentrations. Clearance and volume estimates in patients aged 65 to 87 years were similar to estimates in patients less than 65 years of age.

Paediatric patients with plaque psoriasis

Patients with paediatric plaque psoriasis (aged 4 to 17 years) were administered 0.8 mg/kg (up to a maximum dose of 50 mg per week) of etanercept once weekly for up to 48 weeks. The mean serum steady state trough concentrations ranged from 1.6 to 2.1 mcg/ml at weeks 12, 24, and 48. These mean concentrations in patients with paediatric plaque psoriasis were similar to the concentrations observed in patients with juvenile idiopathic arthritis (treated with 0.4 mg/kg etanercept twice weekly, up to maximum dose of 50 mg per week). These mean concentrations were similar to those seen in adult patients with plaque psoriasis treated with 25 mg etanercept twice weekly.

5.3 Preclinical safety data

In the toxicological studies with Enbrel, no dose-limiting or target organ toxicity was evident. Enbrel was considered to be non-genotoxic from a battery of *in vitro* and *in vivo* studies. Carcinogenicity studies, and standard assessments of fertility and postnatal toxicity, were not performed with Enbrel due to the development of neutralising antibodies in rodents.

Enbrel did not induce lethality or notable signs of toxicity in mice or rats following a single subcutaneous dose of 2000 mg/kg or a single intravenous dose of 1000 mg/kg. Enbrel did not elicit dose-limiting or target organ toxicity in cynomolgus monkeys following twice weekly subcutaneous administration for 4 or 26 consecutive weeks at a dose (15 mg/kg) that resulted in AUC-based serum drug concentrations that were over 27-fold higher than that obtained in humans at the recommended dose of 25 mg.

6. PHARMACEUTICAL PARTICULARS

6.1 List of excipients

Sucrose

Sodium chloride

L-Arginine hydrochloride

Sodium phosphate monobasic dihydrate

Sodium phosphate dibasic dihydrate

Water for injections

6.2 Incompatibilities

In the absence of compatibility studies, this medicinal product must not be mixed with other medicinal products.

6.3 Shelf life

2 years.

6.4 Special precautions for storage

Store in a refrigerator (2°C – 8°C).

Do not freeze.

Keep the pre-filled syringes in the outer carton in order to protect from light.

6.5 Nature and contents of container

Clear glass syringe (type I glass) with stainless steel needle, rubber needle cover and plastic plunger.

Cartons contain 2, 4 or 12 pre-filled syringes of Enbrel with 4, 8 or 24 alcohol swabs. The needle cover contains dry natural rubber (latex) (see section 4.4). Not all pack sizes may be marketed.

6.6 Special precautions for disposal and other handling

Any unused product or waste material should be disposed of in accordance with local requirements.

Instructions for use and handling

Before injection, Enbrel single-use pre-filled syringe should be allowed to reach room temperature (approximately 15 to 30 minutes). The needle cover should not be removed while allowing the pre-filled syringe to reach room temperature. The solution should be clear and colourless or pale yellow and practically free from visible particles.

Comprehensive instructions for administration are given in the package leaflet, section 7, "Instructions for preparation and giving an injection of Enbrel."

7. MARKETING AUTHORISATION HOLDER

Wyeth Europa Ltd.

Huntercombe Lane South

Taplow, Maidenhead

Berkshire, SL6 0PH

United Kingdom

8. MARKETING AUTHORISATION NUMBER(S)

EU/1/99/126/017

9. DATE OF FIRST AUTHORISATION/RENEWAL OF THE AUTHORISATION

Date of first authorisation: 3 February 2000

Date of last renewal: 3 February 2005

10. DATE OF REVISION OF THE TEXT

16 July 2009

Detailed information on this product is available on the website of the European Medicines Agency (EMEA) http://www.emea.europa.eu

Engerix B 20 micrograms/1 ml Suspension for injection, Hepatitis B recombinant vaccine, adsorbed

(GlaxoSmithKline UK)

1. NAME OF THE MEDICINAL PRODUCT

Engerix B® 20 micrograms/1 ml

Suspension for injection

Hepatitis B recombinant vaccine, adsorbed

2. QUALITATIVE AND QUANTITATIVE COMPOSITION

1 dose (0.5 ml) contains:

Hepatitis B surface antigen[1,2], 10 micrograms

[1]Adsorbed on aluminium hydroxide, hydrated Total: 0.25 milligrams Al^{3+}

[2]Produced in yeast cells (*Saccharomyces cerevisiae*) by recombinant DNA technology

1 dose (1 ml) contains:

Hepatitis B surface antigen [1,2], 20 micrograms

[1]Adsorbed on aluminium hydroxide, hydrated Total: 0.50 milligrams Al^{3+}

[2]Produced in yeast cells (*Saccharomyces cerevisiae*) by recombinant DNA technology

For excipients, see section 6.1

3. PHARMACEUTICAL FORM

Suspension for injection.

4. CLINICAL PARTICULARS

4.1 Therapeutic indications

Engerix B is indicated for active immunisation against hepatitis B virus infection (HBV) caused by all known subtypes in non immune subjects. The categories within the population to be immunised are determined on the basis of official recommendations.

It can be expected that hepatitis D will also be prevented by immunisation with Engerix B as hepatitis D (caused by the delta agent) does not occur in the absence of hepatitis B infection.

4.2 Posology and method of administration

Posology

Dosage

The 20 μg dose vaccine in 1.0 ml suspension is intended for use in subjects 16 years of age and above.

The 10 μg dose vaccine in 0.5 ml suspension is intended for use in subjects up to and including 15 years of age, including neonates.

However, the 20 μg vaccine can also be used in subjects from 11 years up to and including 15 years of age as a 2-dose schedule in situations when there is a low risk of hepatitis B infection during the vaccination course, and when compliance with the complete vaccination course can be assured (see below and section 5.1).

Primary Immunisation schedules

Subjects up to and including 15 years of age:

Two primary immunisation schedules can be recommended:

A 0, 1, 6 months schedule which gives optimal protection at month 7 and produces high antibody titres.

An accelerated schedule, with immunisation at 0, 1 and 2 months, which will confer protection more quickly and is expected to provide better patient compliance. With this schedule, a fourth dose should be administered at 12 months to assure long term protection as titres after the third dose are lower than those obtained after the 0, 1, 6 months schedule. In infants this schedule will allow for simultaneous administration of hepatitis B with other childhood vaccines.

- Patients with renal insufficiency including patients undergoing haemodialysis:

Patients with renal insufficiency, including patients undergoing haemodialysis, have a reduced immune response to hepatitis B vaccines. Either the 0, 1, 2 and 12 months or the 0, 1, 6 months schedule of Engerix B (10 μg) can be used. Based on adult experience, vaccination with a higher dosage of antigen may improve the immune response. Consideration should be given to serological testing following vaccination. Additional doses of vaccine may be needed to ensure a protective anti-HBs level of ≥ 10 IU/l.

- Neonates born of mothers who are HBV carriers:

The immunisation with Engerix B (10 μg) of these neonates should start at birth, and two immunisation schedules have been followed. Either the 0, 1, 2 and 12 months or the 0, 1 and 6 months schedule can be used; however, the former schedule provides a more rapid immune response. When available, hepatitis B immune globulins (HBIg) should be given simultaneously with Engerix B at a separate injection site as this may increase the protective efficacy.

Subjects from 11 years up to and including 15 years of age:

The 20 μg vaccine may be administered in subjects from 11 years up to and including 15 years of age according to a 0, 6 months schedule. However, in this case, protection against hepatitis B infections may not be obtained until after the second dose (see section 5.1). Therefore, this schedule should be used only when there is a low risk of hepatitis B infection during the vaccination course and when completion of the two-dose vaccination course can be assured. If both conditions cannot be assured (for instance patients undergoing haemodialysis, travellers to endemic regions and close contacts of infected subjects), the three dose or the accelerated schedule of the 10 μg vaccine should be used.

Subjects 16 years of age and above:

Two primary immunisation schedules can be recommended:

A 0, 1, 6 months schedule which gives optimal protection at month 7 and produces high antibody titres.

An accelerated schedule, with immunisation at 0, 1 and 2 months, which will confer protection more quickly and is expected to provide better patient compliance. With this schedule, a fourth dose should be administered at 12 months to assure long term protection as titres after the third dose are lower than those obtained with the 0, 1, 6 months schedule.

Subjects 18 years of age and above:

In exceptional circumstances in adults, where an even more rapid induction of protection is required, e.g. persons travelling to areas of high endemicity and who commence a course of vaccination against hepatitis B within one month prior to departure, a schedule of three intramuscular injections given at 0, 7 and 21 days may be used. When this schedule is applied, a fourth dose is recommended 12 months after the first dose.

- Patients with renal insufficiency including patients undergoing haemodialysis, 16 years of age and above:

The primary immunisation schedule for patients, with renal insufficiency including patients undergoing haemodialysis is four double doses (2 × 20 μg) at elected date, 1 month, 2 months and 6 months from the date of the first dose. The immunisation schedule should be adapted in order to ensure that the anti-HBs antibody titre remains equal to or higher than the accepted protective level of 10 IU/l.

- Known or presumed exposure to HBV:

In circumstances where exposure to HBV has recently occurred (eg needlestick with contaminated needle) the first dose of Engerix B can be administered simultaneously with HBIg which, however, must be given at a separate injection site (see section 4.5). The 0, 1, 2-12 months immunisation schedule should be advised.

These immunisation schedules may be adjusted to accommodate local immunisation practices.

Booster dose

Current data do not support the need for booster vaccination among immunocompetent subjects who have responded to a full primary vaccination course (Lancet 2000, 355:561).

However, in immunocompromised subjects (eg subjects with chronic renal failure, haemodialysis patients, HIV positive subjects), boosters should be administered to maintain anti-HBs antibody titre equal or higher than the accepted protective level of 10 IU/l. For these immunocompromised subjects, post-vaccination testing every 6-12 months is advised.

National recommendations on booster vaccination should be considered.

Interchangeability of hepatitis B vaccines

See section 4.5. Interaction with other medicaments and other forms of interaction.

Method of Administration

Engerix B should be injected intramuscularly in the deltoid region in adults and children or in the anterolateral thigh in neonates, infants and young children.

Exceptionally the vaccine may be administered subcutaneously in patients with thrombocytopenia or bleeding disorders.

4.3 Contraindications

Engerix B should not be administered to subjects with known hypersensitivity to any component of the vaccine, or to subjects having shown signs of hypersensitivity after previous Engerix B administration.

As with other vaccines, the administration of Engerix B should be postponed in subjects suffering from acute severe febrile illness. The presence of a minor infection, however, is not a contra-indication for immunisation.

4.4 Special warnings and precautions for use

Because of the long incubation period of hepatitis B it is possible for unrecognised infection to be present at the time of immunisation. The vaccine may not prevent hepatitis B infection in such cases.

The vaccine will not prevent infection caused by other pathogens known to infect the liver such as hepatitis A, hepatitis C and hepatitis E viruses.

As with any vaccine, a protective immune response may not be elicited in all vaccinees.

A number of factors have been observed to reduce the immune response to hepatitis B vaccines. These factors include older age, male gender, obesity, smoking, route of administration and some chronic underlying diseases. Consideration should be given to serological testing of those subjects who may be at risk of not achieving seroprotection following a complete course of Engerix B. Additional doses may need to be considered for persons who do not respond or have a sub-optimal response to a course of vaccinations.

Patients with chronic liver disease or with HIV infection or hepatitis C carriers should not be precluded from vaccination against hepatitis B. The vaccine could be advised since HBV infection can be severe in these patients: the HB vaccination should thus be considered on a case by case basis by the physician. In HIV infected patients, as also in patients with renal insufficiency including patients undergoing haemodialysis and persons with an impaired immune system, adequate anti-HBs antibody titres may not be obtained after the primary immunisation course and such patients may therefore require administration of additional doses of vaccine.

Engerix B should not be administered in the buttock or intradermally since this may result in a lower immune response.

Engerix B should under no circumstances be administered intravenously.

As with all injectable vaccines, appropriate medical treatment should always be readily available in case of rare anaphylactic reactions following the administration of the vaccine.

4.5 Interaction with other medicinal products and other forms of interaction

The simultaneous administration of Engerix B and a standard dose of HBIg does not result in lower anti-HBs antibody titres provided that they are administered at separate injection sites.

Engerix B can be given concomitantly with *Haemophilus influenzae* b, BCG, hepatitis A, polio, measles, mumps, rubella, diphtheria, tetanus and pertussis vaccines.

Different injectable vaccines should always be administered at different injection sites.

Engerix B may be used to complete a primary immunisation course started either with plasma-derived or with other genetically-engineered hepatitis B vaccines, or, if it is desired to administer a booster dose, it may be administered to subjects who have previously received a primary immunisation course with plasma-derived or with other genetically-engineered hepatitis B vaccines.

4.6 Pregnancy and lactation

Pregnancy

The effect of the HBsAg on foetal development has not been assessed.

However, as with all inactivated viral vaccines one does not expect harm for the foetus. Engerix B should be used during pregnancy only when clearly needed, and the possible advantages outweigh the possible risks for the foetus.

Lactation

The effect on breastfed infants of the administration of Engerix B to their mothers has not been evaluated in clinical studies, as information concerning the excretion into the breast milk is not available.

No contra-indication has been established.

4.7 Effects on ability to drive and use machines

Some of the effects mentioned under section 4.8 "Undesirable Effects" may affect the ability to drive or operate machinery.

4.8 Undesirable effects

Engerix B is generally well tolerated.

The current formulation of Engerix B does not contain thiomersal (an organomercuric compound).

In one clinical study conducted in adults, the incidence of pain, redness, swelling, fatigue, gastroenteritis, headache and fever was comparable to the incidence observed with former thiomersal containing vaccine formulation.

In one clinical study conducted in children, the incidence of pain, redness, swelling, drowsiness, irritability, loss of appetite and fever was comparable to the incidence observed with the former thiomersal containing vaccine formulation.

The following undesirable events have been reported following the widespread use of former thiomersal containing vaccine formulations. As with other hepatitis B vaccines, in many instances the causal relationship to the vaccine has not been established.

Very common: ≥1/10

Common: ≥1/100, <1/10

Uncommon: ≥1/1000, <1/100

Rare; ≥1/10,000, <1/1000

Very rare: <1/10,000

Blood and lymphatic system disorders

Very rare: thrombocytopenia

Immune system disorders

Very rare: anaphylaxis, serum sickness, lymphadenopathy

Nervous system disorders

Rare: dizziness, headache, paraesthesia

Very rare: syncope, paralysis, neuropathy, neuritis (including Guillain-Barré syndrome, optic neuritis and multiple sclerosis), encephalitis, encephalophy, meningitis, convulsions

Vascular disorders

Very rare: hypotension, vasculitis

Respiratory, thoracic and mediastinal disorders

Very rare: bronchospasm

Gastrointestinal disorders

Rare: nausea, vomiting, diarrhoea, abdominal pain

Hepatobiliary disorders

Rare: hepatic function abnormal

Skin and subcutaneous tissue disorders

Rare: rash, pruritus, urticaria

Very rare: angioneurotic oedema, erythema multiforme

Musculoskeletal and connective tissue disorders

Rare: athralgia, myalgia

Very rare: arthritis

General disorders and administration site conditions

Common: injection site pain, injection site erythema, injection site induration

Rare: fatigue, fever, malaise, influenza-like symptoms

The booster dose is as well tolerated as the primary vaccination.

In a comparative trial in subjects from 11 years up to and including 15 years of age, the incidence of local and general solicited symptoms reported after a two-dose regimen of Engerix B 20 µg was similar overall to that reported after the standard three-dose regimen of Engerix B 10 µg.

4.9 Overdose

Not applicable.

5. PHARMACOLOGICAL PROPERTIES

5.1 Pharmacodynamic properties

Engerix B, hepatitis B vaccine is a sterile suspension containing the purified major surface antigen of the virus manufactured by recombinant DNA technology, adsorbed onto aluminium oxide hydrated.

The antigen is produced by culture of genetically-engineered yeast cells (*Saccharomyces cerevisiae*) which carry the gene which codes for the major surface antigen of the hepatitis B virus (HBV). This hepatitis B surface antigen (HBsAg) expressed in yeast cells is purified by several physico-chemical steps.

The HBsAg assembles spontaneously, in the absence of chemical treatment, into spherical particles of 20 nm in average diameter containing non-glycosylated HBsAg polypeptides and a lipid matrix consisting mainly of phospholipids. Extensive tests have demonstrated that these particles display the characteristic properties of natural HBsAg.

The HBV component is formulated in phosphate buffered saline.

The vaccine is highly purified, and meets the WHO requirements for recombinant hepatitis B vaccines. No substances of human origin are used in its manufacture.

Engerix B induces specific humoral antibodies against HBsAg (anti-HBs antibodies). An anti-HBs antibody titre ≥ 10 IU/l correlates with protection to HBV infection.

Protective efficacy

- In risk groups:

In field studies, a protective efficacy between 95% and 100% was demonstrated in neonates, children and adults at risk.

A 95% protective efficacy was demonstrated in neonates of HBeAg positive mothers, immunised according to the 0, 1, 2 and 12 or 0, 1 and 6 schedules without the concomitant administration of HBIg at birth. However, simultaneous administration of HBIg and vaccine at birth increased the protective efficacy to 98%.

- In healthy subjects up to and including 15 years of age:

When the 0, 1 and 6 month schedule is followed, ≥ 96 % of vaccinees have seroprotective levels of antibody 7 months after the first dose.

When the 0, 1, 2 and 12 month schedule is followed, 15% and 89% of vaccinees have seroprotective levels of antibody one month after first dose and one month after the third dose respectively. One month after the fourth dose 95.8 % of vaccinees achieved seroprotective levels of antibody.

- The table below summarizes seroprotection rates (i.e. percentages of subjects with anti-HBs antibody titre ≥ 10 IU/l) obtained in clinical studies with Engerix B 20µg, given according to the different schedules mentioned in Section 4.2:

Population	Schedule	Seroprotection rate
Healthy subjects 16 years of age and above	0, 1, 6 months	at month 7: ≥ 96 %
	0, 1, 2 – 12 months	at month 1: 15 % at month 3: 89 % at month 13: 95.8 %
Healthy subjects 18 years of age and above	0, 7, 21 days – 12 months	at day 28: 65.2 % at month 2: 76 % at month 13: 98.6 %
Healthy subjects from 11 years up to and including 15 years of age*	0, 6 months	at month 2: 11.3 % at month 6: 26.4 % at month 7: 96.7 %**
Patients with renal insufficiency including patients undergoing haemodialysis 16 years of age and above	0, 1, 2, 6 months (2 × 20 µg)	at month 3: 55.4 % at month 7: 87.1 %

The data in the table were generated with thiomersal containing vaccines. Two additional clinical studies conducted with the current formulation of Engerix B, which contains no thiomersal, among healthy infants and adults, elicit similar seroprotection rates as compared to former thiomersal containing formulations of Engerix B.

*Seroprotection rates obtained with the Engerix B 10µg (0, 1, 6 months schedule) in subjects from 11 years up to and including 15 years of age were respectively of 55.8% at month 2, 87.6% at month 6 and 98.2% at month 7.

** At month 7, 88.8% and 97.3% of subjects aged 11 to 15 years vaccinated with Engerix B 20 µg (0, 6 months schedule) or Engerix B 10 µg (0, 1, 6 months schedule respectively developed anti-HBs antibody titres ≥100mIU/ml. Geometric Mean Titres were 2739 mIU/ml and 7238 mIU/ml respectively.

Reduction in the incidence of hepatocellular carcinoma in children:

A clear link has been demonstrated between hepatitis B infection and the occurrence of hepatocellular carcinoma (HCC). The prevention of hepatitis B by vaccination results in a reduction of the incidence of HCC, as has been observed in Taiwan in children aged 6-14 years.

5.2 Pharmacokinetic properties

Not applicable.

5.3 Preclinical safety data

The preclinical safety data satisfy the requirements of the WHO.

6. PHARMACEUTICAL PARTICULARS

6.1 List of excipients

Sodium chloride,

Disodium phosphate dihydrate,

Sodium dihydrogen phosphate,

Water for injections.

For adsorbent, see section 2

6.2 Incompatibilities

Engerix B should not be mixed with other medicinal products.

6.3 Shelf life

3 years.

6.4 Special precautions for storage

Store at 2°C to 8°C (in a refrigerator).

Do not freeze; discard if vaccine has been frozen.

6.5 Nature and contents of container

0.5 ml or 1.0 ml of suspension in a vial (type I glass) with a stopper (rubber butyl). Pack of 1, 10, 25 & 100

0.5 ml or 1.0 ml of suspension in a pre-filled syringe (type I glass). Pack of 1, 10, 25 & 50.

Disposable syringe(s) may be supplied.

Not all pack sizes may be marketed.

6.6 Special precautions for disposal and other handling

Upon storage, the content may present a fine white deposit with a clear colourless supernatant. Once shaken the vaccine is slightly opaque.

The vaccine should be inspected visually for any foreign particulate matter and/or coloration prior to administration. Discard if the content appears otherwise.

The entire contents of a mono-dose container must be withdrawn and should be used immediately.

Administrative Data

7. MARKETING AUTHORISATION HOLDER

SmithKline Beecham plc

Trading as: GlaxoSmithKline UK,

Stockley Park West,

Uxbridge, Middlesex, UB11 1BT

8. MARKETING AUTHORISATION NUMBER(S)

Vial: PL 10592/0165

Pre-filled syringe: PL 10592/0166

9. DATE OF FIRST AUTHORISATION/RENEWAL OF THE AUTHORISATION

5 February 2001

10. DATE OF REVISION OF THE TEXT

1 March 2007

11. Legal Category

POM

Entocort CR 3mg Capsules

(AstraZeneca UK Limited)

1. NAME OF THE MEDICINAL PRODUCT

Entocort® CR 3 mg Capsules

2. QUALITATIVE AND QUANTITATIVE COMPOSITION

Each capsule contains budesonide 3 mg

For excipients, see section 6.1.

3. PHARMACEUTICAL FORM

Entocort CR 3 mg Capsules: Hard gelatin capsules for oral administration with an opaque, light grey body and opaque, pink cap marked **CIR 3mg** in black radial print. Each capsule contains budesonide 3 mg as gastro-resistant, prolonged-release granules.

4. CLINICAL PARTICULARS

4.1 Therapeutic indications

Entocort CR Capsules are indicated for the induction of remission in patients with mild to moderate Crohn's disease affecting the ileum and/or the ascending colon.

4.2 Posology and method of administration

Adults

Active Crohn's disease: The recommended daily dose for induction of remission is 9 mg once daily in the morning, for up to eight weeks. The full effect is usually achieved within 2–4 weeks.

When treatment is to be discontinued, the dose should normally be reduced for the last 2 to 4 weeks of therapy.

Children

There are limited data on the use of Entocort CR Capsules in children (see Sections 5.1 and 5.2). The available data are insufficient to support safety and efficacy in the paediatric population, therefore such use cannot be recommended until further data become available.

Elderly

No special dose adjustment is recommended. However, experience with Entocort CR Capsules in the elderly is limited.

The capsules should be swallowed whole with water. The capsules must not be chewed.

4.3 Contraindications

Known hypersensitivity to any of the ingredients.

4.4 Special warnings and precautions for use

Use with caution in patients with infections, hypertension, diabetes mellitus, osteoporosis, peptic ulcer, glaucoma or cataracts or with a family history of diabetes or glaucoma or with any other condition where the use of glucocorticosteroids may have unwanted effects.

Particular care is required when considering the use of systemic corticosteroids in patients with existing or previous history of severe affective disorders in themselves or in their first degree relatives. These would include depressive or manic-depressive illness and previous steroid psychosis.

Systemic effects of steroids may occur, particularly when prescribed at high doses and for prolonged periods. Such effects may include Cushing's syndrome, adrenal suppression, growth retardation, decreased bone mineral density, cataract, glaucoma and very rarely a wide range of psychiatric/behavioural effects (see Section 4.8).

Treatment with Entocort CR Capsules results in lower systemic steroid levels than conventional oral glucocorticosteroid therapy. When patients are transferred from systemic glucocorticosteroid treatment with higher systemic effect to Entocort CR Capsules, they may have adrenocortical suppression. Therefore, monitoring of adrenocortical function may be considered in these patients and their dose of systemic steroid should be reduced cautiously.

Replacement of systemic glucocorticosteroid treatment with higher systemic effect with Entocort CR Capsules, sometimes unmasks allergies, e.g. rhinitis and eczema, which were previously controlled by the systemic drug.

Chicken pox and measles may follow a more serious course in patients on oral glucocorticosteroids. Particular care should be taken to avoid exposure in patients who have not previously had these diseases. If patients are infected or suspected of being infected, consider reduction or discontinuation of glucocorticosteroids treatment and immediately consult a physician. Glucocorticosteroids may cause suppression of the HPA axis and reduce the stress response. Where patients are subject to surgery or other stresses, supplementary systemic glucocorticoid treatment is recommended.

Reduced liver function may affect the elimination of glucocorticosteroids. The pharmacokinetics after oral ingestion of budesonide was affected by compromised liver function as evidenced by increased systemic availability in patients with moderately severe hepatic cirrhosis.

When treatment is to be discontinued, the dose should normally be reduced for the last 2 to 4 weeks of therapy. Some patients may feel unwell in a non-specific way during the withdrawal phase, e.g. pain in muscles and joints. A general insufficient glucocorticosteroid effect should be suspected if, in rare cases, symptoms such as tiredness, headache, nausea and vomiting should occur. In these cases a temporary increase in the dose of systemic glucocorticosteroids is sometimes necessary.

In vivo studies have shown that oral administration of ketoconazole (a known inhibitor of CYP3A activity in the liver and in the intestinal mucosa), caused a several fold increase of the systemic exposure to oral budesonide. If treatment with ketoconazole together with budesonide is indicated, reduction of the budesonide dose should be considered if side effects typical of systemic glucocorticosteroids occur.

After extensive intake of grapefruit juice (which inhibits CYP3A activity predominantly in the intestinal mucosa), the systemic exposure for oral budesonide increased about two times. As with other drugs primarily being metabolised through CYP3A, regular ingestion of grapefruit or juice of it, should be avoided in connection with budesonide administration (other juices such as orange juice or apple juice do not inhibit CYP3A). See also Section 4.5.

When Entocort CR Capsules are used chronically in excessive doses, systemic glucocorticosteroid effects such as hypercorticism and adrenal suppression may appear.

4.5 Interaction with other medicinal products and other forms of interaction

Although not studied, concomitant administration of colestyramine may reduce Entocort uptake, in common with other drugs.

Elevated plasma levels and enhanced effects of corticosteroids have been reported in women also receiving oestrogens or oral contraceptives. However, a low-dose combination oral contraceptive that more than doubled the plasma concentration of oral prednisolone, had no significant effect on the plasma concentration of oral budesonide.

At recommended doses, omeprazole was without effect on the pharmacokinetics of oral budesonide, whereas cimetidine had a slight but clinically insignificant effect.

The metabolism of budesonide is primarily mediated by CYP3A4, one of the cytochrome p450 enzymes. Inhibitors of this enzyme, e.g. ketoconazole, itraconazole and grapefruit juice, can therefore increase systemic exposure to budesonide (see Sections 4.4 and 5.2). Other potent inhibitors of CYP3A4 are also likely to markedly increase plasma levels of budesonide. Inhibition by budesonide on other drugs metabolism via CYP3A4 is unlikely, since budesonide has low affinity to the enzyme.

4.6 Pregnancy and lactation

Pregnancy

The ability of corticosteroids to cross the placenta varies between individual drugs, however, in mice, budesonide and/or its metabolites have been shown to cross the placenta.

Administration of corticosteroids to pregnant animals can cause abnormalities of foetal development including cleft palate, intra-uterine growth retardation and effects on brain growth and development. There is no evidence that corticosteroids result in an increased incidence of congenital abnormalities, such as cleft palate/lip in man. However, when administered for prolonged periods or repeatedly during pregnancy, corticosteroids may increase the risk of intra-uterine growth retardation.

Hypoadrenalism may, in theory, occur in the neonate following prenatal exposure to corticosteroids but usually resolves spontaneously following birth and is rarely clinically important. As with all drugs, corticosteroids should only be prescribed when the benefits to the mother and child outweigh the risks. When corticosteroids are essential however, patients with normal pregnancies may be treated as though they were in the non-gravid state.

Lactation

Corticosteroids are secreted in small amounts in breast milk, however, budesonide given at the clinically recommended dose is unlikely to cause systematic effects in the infant. Infants of mothers taking higher than recommended doses of budesonide may have a degree of adrenal suppression but the benefits of breast-feeding are likely to outweigh any theoretical risk.

4.7 Effects on ability to drive and use machines

No effects are known.

4.8 Undesirable effects

In clinical studies most adverse events were of mild to moderate intensity and of a non-serious character.

Undesirable effects characteristic of systemic corticosteroid therapy, such as Cushingoid features and reduced growth velocity, may occur.

In clinical trials other adverse events: dyspepsia, muscle cramps, tremor, palpitations, blurred vision, skin reactions (urticaria, exanthema), menstrual disorders, hypokalemia and behavioural changes such as nervousness, insomnia and mood swings have been reported.

In clinical studies, at recommended doses, the incidence of adverse events was comparable to placebo.

Clinical studies showed the frequency of steroid associated side effects for Entocort CR Capsules to be approximately half that of conventional prednisolone treatment, at equipotent doses. In studies of patients with active disease, receiving Entocort 9 mg daily, the incidence of adverse events was comparable to placebo. Very rarely a wide range of psychiatric/ behavioural effects may occur, when systemic steroids are prescribed at high doses and for prolonged periods (See section 4.4).

4.9 Overdose

Acute overdosage with Entocort CR Capsules even at very high doses, is not expected to lead to an acute clinical crisis. In the event of acute overdosage, no specific antidote is available. Treatment consists of supportive and symptomatic therapy.

Chronic overdosage may lead to systemic corticosteroid effects, such as Cushingoid features. If such changes occur, the dose of Entocort CR Capsules should be gradually reduced until treatment is discontinued, in accordance with normal procedures for the discontinuation of prolonged oral glucocorticosteroid therapy.

5. PHARMACOLOGICAL PROPERTIES

5.1 Pharmacodynamic properties

Budesonide is a glucocorticosteroid with a high local anti-inflammatory effect.

ATC-code: A07E A06

The exact mechanism of budesonide in the treatment of Crohn's disease is not fully understood.

Data from clinical pharmacology studies and controlled clinical trials strongly indicate that the mode of action of Entocort CR Capsules is based, at least partly, on a local action in the gut. Budesonide is a glucocorticosteroid with a high local anti-inflammatory effect. At doses clinically equivalent to prednisolone, budesonide gives significantly less HPA axis suppression and has a lower impact on inflammatory markers.

At recommended doses, Entocort CR Capsules caused significantly less effect than prednisolone 20–40 mg daily on morning plasma cortisols; on 24 hour plasma cortisol (AUC 0–24 h) and on 24 hour urine cortisol levels.

ACTH tests have shown Entocort CR Capsules to have significantly less effect than prednisolone on adrenal functions.

In a study assessing cortisol suppression of Entocort CR Capsules in 8 children (mean age 12.4 years [range 9–14 years]; mean weight 40 kg [range 33–50 kg]) and 6 adults (mean weight 64 kg [range 50–81 kg]), administered 9 mg Entocort CR orally for 7 days, mean (± SD) cortisol suppression compared to baseline was 64% (±18%) in children and 50% (±27%) in adults. A study of children with mild to moderate Crohn's disease (CDAI ⩾ 200) compared 9 mg Entocort CR once daily with a reducing dose of prednisolone, which commenced at 1 mg/kg. The study was discontinued prematurely; however, data are available for 22 patients who received Entocort CR Capsules and 26 who received the comparator prednisolone regimen. After 8 weeks of treatment, 70.8% of patients who received prednisolone reached the endpoint (CDAI ⩽ 150) compared with 54.5% of those who received Entocort CR Capsules. This difference was not significant (p=0.13). At 8 weeks, 11.1% of patients who received prednisolone were judged to have normal function on a short ACTH test compared with 37.5% of those who received Entocort CR Capsules. This difference was not statistically significant (p=0.07). After 8 weeks, 29% of patients who received prednisolone and 58% of those who received Entocort CR Capsules had a normal morning P-cortisol value. This difference was not statistically significant (p=0.052). The mean morning P-cortisol after 8 weeks was 98 nmol/L in the patients who received prednisolone and 200 nmol/L in those who received Entocort CR Capsules. This difference was statistically significant (P=0.0028). Adverse events were reported in 96% of patients who received prednisolone compared with 91% of those who received Entocort CR Capsules.

5.2 Pharmacokinetic properties

Absorption

After oral dosing of plain micronised compound, absorption is rapid and seems to be complete. A large proportion of the drug is absorbed from the ileum and ascending colon. Systemic availability in healthy subjects is approximately 9–12% for Entocort CR Capsules. This is similar to the systemic availability of plain micronised budesonide, indicating complete absorption. In patients with active Crohn's disease systemic availability is approximately 12–20% at the start of treatment.

Distribution

Budesonide has a high volume of distribution (about 3 L/kg). Plasma protein binding averages 85–90%. In healthy volunteers mean maximal plasma concentrations of 5–10 nmol/L were seen at 3–5 hours following a single oral dose of Entocort CR Capsules 9 mg.

Biotransformation

Budesonide then undergoes extensive biotransformation in the liver to metabolites of low glucocorticosteroid activity. The glucocorticosteroid activity of the major metabolites, 6β-hydroxybudesonide and 16α-hydroxyprednisolone, is less than 1% of that of budesonide. The metabolism of budesonide is primarily mediated by CYP3A, a subfamily of cytochrome P450.

Elimination

Elimination is rate limited by absorption. The average terminal half-life is 4 hours. Budesonide has a high systemic clearance (about 1.2 L/min).

Information in children

In a study comparing the pharmacokinetics of Entocort CR Capsules in 8 children (mean age 12.4 years [range 9–14 years]; mean weight 40 kg [range 33–50 kg]) and 6 adults (mean weight 64 kg [range 50–81 kg]), administered 9 mg Entocort CR orally for 7 days, systemic exposure (AUC) was 17% higher in children than adults and maximum concentration (C_{max}) was 50% higher in children than in adults. (Mean AUC ± SD: children = 41.3 nmol/L.h ± 21.2; adults = 35.0 nmol/L.h ± 19.8. Mean C_{max}± SD: children = 5.99 nmo/L ± 3.45; adults = 3.97 nmo/L ± 2.11.)

5.3 Preclinical safety data

Results from acute, subacute and chronic toxicity studies show that the systemic effects of budesonide are less severe or similar to those observed after administration of other glucocorticosteroids, e.g. decreased body-weight gain and atrophy of lymphoid tissues and adrenal cortex.

Budesonide, evaluated in six different test systems, did not show any mutagenic or clastogenic effects.

An increased incidence of brain gliomas in male rats in a carcinogenicity study could not be verified in a repeat study, in which the incidence of gliomas did not differ between any of the groups on active treatment (budesonide, prednisolone, triamcinolone acetonide) and the control groups.

Liver changes (primary hepatocellular neoplasms) found in male rats in the original carcinogenicity study were noted again in the repeat study with budesonide as well as the reference glucocorticosteroids. These effects are most probably related to a receptor effect and thus represent a class effect.

Available clinical experience shows that there are no indications that budesonide or other glucocorticosteroids induce brain gliomas or primary hepatocellular neoplasms in man.

The toxicity of Entocort CR Capsules, with focus on the gastro-intestinal tract, has been studied in cynomolgus monkeys in doses up to 5 mg/kg after repeated oral administration for up to 6 months. No effects were observed in the gastrointestinal tract, neither at gross pathology nor in the histopathological examination.

6. PHARMACEUTICAL PARTICULARS

6.1 List of excipients

Ethylcellulose, Tributyl acetylcitrate, Methacrylic acid copolymer, Triethylcitrate, Antifoam M, Polysorbate 80, Talc, Sucrose, Maize starch, Gelatine, Titanium dioxide (E171), Iron-oxide (E172).

6.2 Incompatibilities

No known incompatibilities.

6.3 Shelf life

Entocort CR Capsules have a shelf-life of 3 years when stored not above 30°C in the original container.

6.4 Special precautions for storage

Do not store above 30°C. Store in the original container. Replace cap firmly after use. Store out of reach and sight of children.

6.5 Nature and contents of container

White polyethylene bottles of 100 capsules, having either a tamper-evident or child-resistant polypropylene screw cap, with an integral desiccant.

6.6 Special precautions for disposal and other handling

No special requirements. See Section 4.2.

7. MARKETING AUTHORISATION HOLDER

AstraZeneca UK Limited,

600 Capability Green,

Luton,

LU1 3LU,

UK.

8. MARKETING AUTHORISATION NUMBER(S)

PL 17901/0122

9. DATE OF FIRST AUTHORISATION/RENEWAL OF THE AUTHORISATION

4th June 2002

10. DATE OF REVISION OF THE TEXT

2nd July 2009

Entocort Enema

(AstraZeneca UK Limited)

1. NAME OF THE MEDICINAL PRODUCT

Entocort®Enema.

2. QUALITATIVE AND QUANTITATIVE COMPOSITION

0.02 mg/ml budesonide (2 mg budesonide/100 ml).

For excipients, see section 6.1.

3. PHARMACEUTICAL FORM

Dispersible tablet and solution for rectal suspension.

Each Entocort enema consists of 2 components

- A 2.3 mg faintly yellow, circular biconvex tablet with the engraving B^A1 on one side. On the other side 2.3 is engraved.
- A 115 ml clear colourless solution.

4. CLINICAL PARTICULARS

4.1 Therapeutic indications

Ulcerative colitis involving rectal and recto-sigmoid disease.

4.2 Posology and method of administration

Adults: One Entocort Enema nightly for 4 weeks. Full effect is usually achieved within 2–4 weeks. If the patient is not in remission after 4 weeks, the treatment period may be prolonged to 8 weeks.

Children: Not recommended.

Elderly: Dosage as for adults.

No dosage reduction is necessary in patients with reduced liver function.

The route of administration is rectal.

Instructions for correct use of Entocort enema.

Entocort enema consists of two components: a dispersible tablet and a vehicle.

Note: it is important to instruct the patient

- To carefully read the instructions for use in the patient information leaflet which are packed together with each product.
- To reconstitute the enema immediately before use, ensuring that the tablet is completely dissolved.
- To administer in the evening before going to bed.

4.3 Contraindications

Hypersensitivity to any of the ingredients.

4.4 Special warnings and precautions for use

When patients are transferred from systemic glucocorticosteroid treatment with higher systemic effect to Entocort enema, they may have adrenocortical suppression. Therefore, monitoring of adrenocortical function may be considered in these patients and their dose of systemic steroid should be reduced cautiously.

Replacement of systemic glucocorticosteroid treatment with higher systemic effect with Entocort enema sometimes unmasks allergies, e.g. rhinitis and eczema, which were previously controlled by the systemic drug.

Reduced liver function may affect the elimination of glucocorticosteroids. The pharmacokinetics after oral ingestion of budesonide was affected by compromised liver function as evidenced by increased systemic availability in patients with moderately severe hepatic cirrhosis.

Particular care is required when considering the use of systemic corticosteroids in patients with existing or previous history of severe affective disorders in themselves or their first degree relatives. These would include depressive or manic-depressive illness and previous steroid psychosis (See section 4.8). Systemic effects of steroids may occur, particularly when prescribed at high doses and for prolonged periods. Such effects may include Cushing's syndrome, adrenal suppression, growth retardation, decreased bone mineral density, cataract, glaucoma and very rarely a wide range of psychiatric/ behavioural effects (see Section 4.8).

In vivo studies have shown that oral administration of ketoconazole (a known inhibitor of CYP3A activity in the liver and the intestinal mucosa), caused a several fold increase of the systemic exposure to oral budesonide. Therefore, it cannot be excluded that concomitant intake of Entocort Enema and ketoconazole may also result in increase systemic availability of budesonide. (See section 4.5)

Entocort enema contains the excipients lactose and methyl-, propyl-parahydroxybenzoate, therefore caution should be taken in patients with hypersensitivity to these excipients.

Some patients may feel unwell in a non-specific way during the withdrawal phase, e.g. pain in muscles and joints. A general insufficient glucocorticosteroid effect should be suspected if, in rare cases, symptoms such as tiredness, headache, nausea and vomiting should occur. In these cases a temporary increase in the dose of systemic glucocorticosteroids is sometimes necessary.

4.5 Interaction with other medicinal products and other forms of interaction

Elevated plasma levels and enhanced effects of corticosteroids have been reported in women also receiving oestrogens or oral contraceptives. However, a low-dose combination oral contraceptive that more than doubled the plasma concentration of prednisolone, had no significant effect on the plasma concentration of oral budesonide.

The metabolism of budesonide is primarily mediated by CYP3A4, one of the cytochrome p450 enzymes. Inhibitors of this enzyme, e.g. ketoconazole and itraconazole, can therefore increase systemic exposure to budesonide (see Sections 4.4 and 5.2). Other potent inhibitors of CYP3A4 are also likely to markedly increase plasma levels of budesonide. Inhibition by budesonide on other drugs metabolism via CYP3A4 is unlikely, since budesonide has low affinity to the enzyme.

4.6 Pregnancy and lactation

Pregnancy

The ability of corticosteroids to cross the placenta varies between individual drugs, however, in mice, budesonide and/or its metabolites have been shown to cross the placenta.

Administration of corticosteroids to pregnant animals can cause abnormalities of foetal development including cleft palate, intra-uterine growth retardation and affects on brain growth and development. There is no evidence that corticosteroids result in an increased incidence of congenital abnormalities, such as cleft palate/lip in man. However, when administered for prolonged periods or repeatedly during pregnancy, corticosteroids may increase the risk of intra-uterine growth retardation. Hypoadrenalism may, in theory, occur in the neonate following prenatal exposure to corticosteroids but usually resolves spontaneously following birth and is rarely clinically important. As with all drugs, corticosteroids should only be prescribed when the benefits to the mother and child outweigh the risks. When corticosteroids are essential however, patients with normal pregnancies may be treated as though they were in the non-gravid state.

Lactation

Corticosteroids are secreted in small amounts in breast milk, however, budesonide given at the clinically recommended dose is unlikely to cause systematic effects in the infant. Infants of mothers taking higher than recommended doses of budesonide may have a degree of adrenal suppression but the benefits of breast feeding are likely to outweigh any theoretical risk.

4.7 Effects on ability to drive and use machines

Entocort Enema does not affect the ability to drive and operate machinery.

4.8 Undesirable effects

The most common adverse reactions are gastrointestinal disturbances e.g. flatulence, nausea, diarrhoea. Skin reactions (e.g. urticaria, exanthema) may occur. Less common adverse reactions include agitation and insomnia.

In rare cases signs or symptoms of systemic glucocorticosteroid effects, including hypofunction of the adrenal gland, may occur with rectally administered glucocorticosteroids, probably depending on dose, treatment time, concomitant and previous glucocorticosteroid intake, and individual sensitivity.

Very rarely a wide range of psychiatric/ behavioural effects may occur, when systemic steroids are prescribed at high doses and for prolonged periods. (See section 4.4)

4.9 Overdose

Reports of acute toxicity and/or death following overdosage of glucocorticosteroids are rare. Thus, acute overdosage with Entocort Enema, even in excessive doses, is not expected to be a clinical problem. In the event of acute overdosage, no specific antidote is available. If, by mistake, high doses of Entocort dispersible tablet have been taken orally, treatment consists of immediate gastric lavage or emesis followed by supportive and symptomatic therapy.

5. PHARMACOLOGICAL PROPERTIES

5.1 Pharmacodynamic properties

Budesonide is a glucocorticosteroid with a high local anti-inflammatory effect.

ATC Code A07E AO6.

5.2 Pharmacokinetic properties

Budesonide undergoes an extensive degree (~90%) of biotransformation in the liver to metabolites of low glucocorticosteroid activity. The glucocorticosteroid activity of the major metabolites, 6β-hydroxybudesonide and 16α-hydroxyprednisolone, is less than 1% of that of budesonide.

The metabolism of budesonide is primarily mediated by CYP3A4, a subfamily of cytochrome P450.

At recommended doses, budesonide causes no or small suppression of plasma cortisol.

The mean maximal plasma concentration after rectal administration of 2 mg budesonide is 3 nmol/L (range 1-9 nmol/L), reached within 1.5 hours.

5.3 Preclinical safety data

Results from acute, subacute and chronic toxicity studies show that the systemic effects of budesonide, e.g. decreased body-weight gain and atrophy of lymphoid tissues and adrenal cortex, are less severe or similar to those observed after administration of other glucocorticosteroids.

Budesonide evaluated in six different test systems did not show any mutagenic or clastogenic effects.

An increased incidence of brain gliomas in male rats in a carcinogenicity study could not be verified in a repeat study, in which the incidence of gliomas did not differ between any of the groups with active treatment (budesonide, prednisolone, triamcinolone acetonide) and the control groups.

Liver changes (primary hepatocellular neoplasms) found in male rats in the original carcinogenicity study were noted again in a repeat study with budesonide as well as with the reference glucocorticosteroids. These effects are most probably related to a receptor effect and thus represent a class-effect.

Available clinical experience shows that there are no indications that budesonide or other glucocorticosteroids induce brain gliomas or primary hepatocellular neoplasms in man.

6. PHARMACEUTICAL PARTICULARS

6.1 List of excipients

Tablet

Lactose anhydrous, riboflavine sodium phosphate (E101), lactose monohydrate, polyvidone, colloidal anhydrous silica and magnesium stearate.

Vehicle

Sodium chloride, methyl parahydroxybenzoate (E218), propyl parahydroxybenzoate (E216) and water purified.

6.2 Incompatibilities

None stated.

6.3 Shelf life

24 months.

6.4 Special precautions for storage

Do not store above 30°C

6.5 Nature and contents of container

Entocort Enema 0.02 mg/ml consists of 2 components: A dispersible tablet and a vehicle.

The primary package for the tablets is an aluminium blister package consisting of polyamide 25 μm/ Al 43 μm/ polyvinylchloride 60 μm/ A1 20 μm.

The primary package for the vehicle is a polyethylene bottle equipped with a combined seal gasket and non-return valve, a rectal nozzle and a protective cap for the nozzle.

The bottle, the nozzle and the protective cap are made of LD-polyethylene. The combined seal gasket and non-return valve is made of thermoplastic rubber.

Pack Size: 7 tablets

6.6 Special precautions for disposal and other handling

See section 4.2

7. MARKETING AUTHORISATION HOLDER

AstraZeneca UK Ltd.,
600 Capability Green,
Luton, LU1 3LU, UK.

8. MARKETING AUTHORISATION NUMBER(S)

PL 17901/0123

9. DATE OF FIRST AUTHORISATION/RENEWAL OF THE AUTHORISATION

4th June 2002

10. DATE OF REVISION OF THE TEXT

2nd July 2009

Enzira Suspension for injection, pre-filled syringe/Influenza vaccine (split virion, inactivated) PH. Eur.

(Wyeth Pharmaceuticals)

1. NAME OF THE MEDICINAL PRODUCT

Enzira® Suspension for injection, pre-filled syringe

Influenza vaccine (split virion, inactivated) Ph. Eur.

2. QUALITATIVE AND QUANTITATIVE COMPOSITION

Split influenza virus*, inactivated with β-Propiolactone, containing antigens equivalent to:

A/Brisbane/59/2007 (H1N1)-like strain (A/Brisbane/59/2007 IVR-148)	15 micrograms HA**
A/Brisbane/10/2007 (H3N2)-like strain (A/Uruguay/716/2007NYMC X-175C)	15 micrograms HA**
B/Brisbane/60/2008-like strain (B/Brisbane/60/2008)	15 micrograms HA**

per 0.5 ml dose.

* propagated in fertilised hens' eggs from healthy chicken flocks

** haemagglutinin

This vaccine complies with the WHO recommendation (Northern Hemisphere) and EU decision for the 2009/ 2010 season.

For a full list of excipients, see section 6.1.

3. PHARMACEUTICAL FORM

Suspension for injection in a pre-filled syringe.

Clear to slightly opaque liquid with some sediment that resuspends upon shaking.

4. CLINICAL PARTICULARS

4.1 Therapeutic indications

Prophylaxis of influenza, especially in those who run an increased risk of associated complications.

The use of Enzira should be based on official recommendations.

4.2 Posology and method of administration

Posology

Adults and children from 36 months:	0.5 ml
Children from 6 months to 35 months:	Clinical data are limited. Dosages of 0.25 ml or 0.5 ml have been used.

For children who have not previously been vaccinated, a second dose should be given after an interval of at least 4 weeks.

Method of administration

Immunisation should be carried out by intramuscular or deep subcutaneous injection.

For instructions for preparation, see section 6.6.

4.3 Contraindications
Hypersensitivity to the active substances, to any of the excipients (see section 6.1), to eggs and/or chicken proteins.

Enzira does not contain more than 1 μg ovalbumin per dose.

The vaccine may contain residues of the following substances: neomycin, polymyxin.

Immunisation shall be postponed in patients with febrile illness or acute infection.

4.4 Special warnings and precautions for use
As with all injectable vaccines, appropriate medical treatment and supervision should always be readily available in case of an anaphylactic event following administration of the vaccine.

Enzira should under no circumstances be administered intravascularly.

Antibody response in patients with endogenous or iatrogenic immunosuppression may be insufficient.

4.5 Interaction with other medicinal products and other forms of interaction
Enzira may be given at the same time as other vaccines. Immunisation should be carried out on separate limbs. It should be noted that the adverse reactions may be intensified.

The immunological response may be diminished if the patient is undergoing immunosuppressant treatment.

Following influenza vaccination, false positive results in serological tests using the ELISA method to detect antibodies against HIV1, Hepatitis C and especially HTLV1 have been observed. The Western Blot technique disproves the false-positive ELISA test results. The transient false positive reactions could be due to the IgM response to the vaccine.

4.6 Pregnancy and lactation
Pregnancy

The limited data from vaccination in pregnant women do not indicate that adverse foetal and maternal outcomes were attributable to the vaccine. The use of this vaccine may be considered from the second trimester of pregnancy. For pregnant women with medical conditions that increase their risk of complications from influenza, administration of the vaccine is recommended, irrespective of their stage of pregnancy.

Lactation

Enzira may be used during lactation.

4.7 Effects on ability to drive and use machines
The vaccine is unlikely to produce an effect on the ability to drive and use machines.

4.8 Undesirable effects
Adverse reactions observed from clinical trials

The safety of trivalent inactivated influenza vaccines is assessed in open label, uncontrolled clinical trials performed as annual update requirements, including at least 50 adults aged 18 – 60 years of age and at least 50 elderly aged 61 years or older. Safety evaluation is performed during the first three days following vaccination.

The following undesirable effects have been observed during clinical trials with the following frequencies: Very common (>1/10), common (≥1/100, <1/10), uncommon (≥1/1,000, <1/100), rare (≥1/10,000, <1/1,000), very rare (<1/10,000), including isolated reports.

(see Table 1 below)

Adverse reactions reported from post-marketing surveillance

Adverse reactions reported from post marketing surveillance for trivalent influenza vaccines are, next to the reactions which have also been observed during the clinical trials, the following:

Blood and lymphatic system disorders

Transient thrombocytopenia, transient lymphadenopathy

Immune system disorders

Allergic reactions, in rare cases leading to anaphylactic shock, angioedema

Nervous system disorders

Neuralgia, paraesthesia, convulsions

Neurological disorders, such as encephalomyelitis, neuritis and Guillain-Barré syndrome

Vascular disorders

Vasculitis associated in very rare cases with transient renal involvement

Skin and subcutaneous tissue disorders

Generalised skin reactions including pruritus, urticaria or non-specific rash

4.9 Overdose
Overdosage is unlikely to have any untoward effects.

5. PHARMACOLOGICAL PROPERTIES
5.1 Pharmacodynamic properties
Pharmacotherapeutic group: Influenza vaccine, ATC Code: J07B B02

Seroprotection is generally obtained within 2 to 3 weeks. The duration of postvaccinal immunity to homologous strains or to strains closely related to the vaccine strains varies but is usually 6 to 12 months.

5.2 Pharmacokinetic properties
Not applicable.

5.3 Preclinical safety data
Not applicable.

6. PHARMACEUTICAL PARTICULARS
6.1 List of excipients
Sodium chloride

Anhydrous disodium phosphate

Sodium dihydrogen phosphate dihydrate

Potassium chloride

Potassium dihydrogen phosphate

Calcium chloride

Water for injection

6.2 Incompatibilities
In the absence of compatibility studies, this medicinal product must not be mixed with other medicinal products.

6.3 Shelf life
1 year.

6.4 Special precautions for storage
Store in a refrigerator (2°C to 8°C). Do not freeze.

Keep the syringe in the outer carton in order to protect from light.

6.5 Nature and contents of container
0.5 ml suspension in pre-filled syringe (Type I glass) with plunger stopper (chlorobutyl rubber) with attached needle in pack sizes of 1 or 10.

Not all pack sizes may be marketed.

6.6 Special precautions for disposal and other handling
The vaccine should be allowed to reach room temperature before use. Shake before use. After shaking, the vaccine should appear as a homogenous suspension. The vaccine must be inspected visually prior to administration and should not be used if there is any variation of physical appearance (see section 3).

Enzira is presented as a single use syringe and any remaining contents should be disposed of in compliance with local rules for the disposal of products of this nature.

When a 0.25 ml dose is indicated, the pre-filled syringe should be held in an upright position and half the volume should be eliminated. To do so, depress the plunger to the half dose marking on the glass syringe barrel, the remaining volume should be injected.

7. MARKETING AUTHORISATION HOLDER
CSL Biotherapies GmbH

Emil-von-Behring-Strasse 76

35041 Marburg

Germany

8. MARKETING AUTHORISATION NUMBER(S)
PL 22236/0001

9. DATE OF FIRST AUTHORISATION/RENEWAL OF THE AUTHORISATION
19 April 2005 / 29 March 2009

Table 1

Organ class	Very common >1/10	Common ≥1/100, <1/10	Uncommon ≥1/1,000, <1/100	Rare ≥1/10,000, <1/1,000	Very rare <1/10,000
Nervous system disorders		Headache*			
Skin and subcutaneous tissue disorders		Sweating*			
Musculoskeletal and connective tissue disorders		Myalgia, arthralgia*			
General disorders and administration site conditions		Fever, malaise, shivering, fatigue. Local reactions: redness, swelling, pain, ecchymosis, induration*			

* These reactions usually disappear within 1-2 days without treatment

10. DATE OF REVISION OF THE TEXT
11 August 2009

Epanutin 30mg/5ml oral Suspension
(Pfizer Limited)

1. NAME OF THE MEDICINAL PRODUCT
EPANUTIN 30MG/5ML ORAL SUSPENSION

2. QUALITATIVE AND QUANTITATIVE COMPOSITION
Each 5ml of suspension contains 30mg Phenytoin

For excipients see 6.1.

3. PHARMACEUTICAL FORM
Oral suspension.

Viscous Cherry red coloured oral suspension.

4. CLINICAL PARTICULARS
4.1 Therapeutic indications
Control of tonic-clonic seizures (grand mal epilepsy), partial seizures (focal including temporal lobe) or a combination of these, and the prevention and treatment of seizures occurring during or following neurosurgery and/or severe head injury. Epanutin has also been employed in the treatment of trigeminal neuralgia but it should only be used as second line therapy if carbamazepine is ineffective or patients are intolerant to carbamazepine.

4.2 Posology and method of administration
For oral administration only.

Dosage:

Dosage should be individualised as there may be wide interpatient variability in phenytoin serum levels with equivalent dosage. Epanutin should be introduced in small dosages with gradual increments until control is achieved or until toxic effects appear. In some cases serum level determinations may be necessary for optimal dosage adjustments - the clinically effective level is usually 10-20mg/l (40-80 micromoles/l) although some cases of tonic-clonic seizures may be controlled with lower serum levels of phenytoin. With recommended dosage a period of seven to ten days may be required to achieve steady state serum levels with Epanutin and changes in dosage should not be carried out at intervals shorter than seven to ten days. Maintenance of treatment should be the lowest dose of anticonvulsant consistent with control of seizures.

Epanutin Capsules, Suspension and Infatabs:

Epanutin Capsules contain phenytoin sodium whereas Epanutin Suspension and Epanutin Infatabs contain phenytoin. Although 100mg of phenytoin sodium is equivalent to 92mg of phenytoin on a molecular weight basis, these molecular equivalents are not necessarily biologically equivalent. Physicians should therefore exercise care in those situations where it is necessary to change the dosage form and serum level monitoring is advised.

Adults:

Initially 3 to 4mg/kg/day with subsequent dosage adjustment if necessary. For most adults a satisfactory maintenance dose will be 200 to 500mg daily in single or divided doses. Exceptionally, a daily dose outside this range may be indicated. Dosage should normally be adjusted according to serum levels where assay facilities exist.

Elderly:

Elderly (over 65 years): As with adults the dosage of Epanutin should be titrated to the patient's individual requirements using the same guidelines. As elderly patients tend to receive multiple drug therapies, the possibility of drug interactions should be borne in mind.

Infants and Children:

Initially, 5mg/kg/day in two divided doses, with subsequent dosage individualised to a maximum of 300mg daily. A recommended daily maintenance dosage is usually 4-8mg/kg.

Neonates:

The absorption of phenytoin following oral administration in neonates is unpredictable. Furthermore, the metabolism of phenytoin may be depressed. It is therefore especially important to monitor serum levels in the neonate.

4.3 Contraindications
Hypersensitivity to hydantoins.

4.4 Special warnings and precautions for use
Suicidal ideation and behaviour have been reported in patients treated with anti-epileptic agents in several indications. A meta-analysis of randomised placebo controlled trials of anti-epileptic drugs has also shown a small increased risk of suicidal ideation and behaviour. The mechanism of this risk is not known and the available data do not exclude the possibility of an increased risk for Phenytoin.

Therefore patients should be monitored for signs of suicidal ideation and behaviours and appropriate treatment should be considered. Patients (and caregivers of patients) should be advised to seek medical advice should signs of suicidal ideation or behaviour emerge.

Abrupt withdrawal of phenytoin in epileptic patients may precipitate status epilepticus. When, in the judgement of the clinician, the need for dosage reduction, discontinuation, or substitution of alternative anti-epileptic medication arises, this should be done gradually. However, in the event of an allergic or hypersensitivity reaction, rapid substitution of alternative therapy may be necessary. In this case, alternative therapy should be an anti-epileptic drug not belonging to the hydantoin chemical class.

Phenytoin is highly protein bound and extensively metabolised by the liver. Reduced dosage to prevent accumulation and toxicity may therefore be required in patients with impaired liver function. Where protein binding is reduced, as in uraemia, total serum phenytoin levels will be reduced accordingly. However, the pharmacologically active free drug concentration is unlikely to be altered. Therefore, under these circumstances therapeutic control may be achieved with total phenytoin levels below the normal range of 10-20 mg/l (40-80 micromoles/l). Patients with impaired liver function, elderly patients or those who are gravely ill may show early signs of toxicity.

Phenytoin should be discontinued if a skin rash appears. If the rash is exfoliative, purpuric, or bullous or if lupus erythematosus or Stevens-Johnson syndrome or toxic epidermal necrolysis is suspected, use of the drug should not be resumed (see Adverse Reactions). If the rash is of a milder type (measles-like or scarlatiniform), therapy may be resumed after the rash has completely disappeared. If the rash recurs upon reinstitution of therapy, further phenytoin medication is contra-indicated.

Phenytoin is not effective for absence (petit mal) seizures. If tonic-clonic (grand mal) and absence seizures are present together, combined drug therapy is needed.

Phenytoin may affect glucose metabolism and inhibit insulin release. Hyperglycaemia has been reported in association with toxic levels. Phenytoin is not indicated for seizures due to hypoglycaemia or other metabolic causes.

Serum levels of phenytoin sustained above the optimal range may produce confusional states referred to as "delirium", "psychosis", or "encephalopathy", or rarely irreversible cerebellar dysfunction. Accordingly, at the first sign of acute toxicity, serum drug level determinations are recommended. Dose reduction of phenytoin therapy is indicated if serum levels are excessive; if symptoms persist, termination of therapy with phenytoin is recommended.

Herbal preparations containing St John's wort (*Hypericum perforatum*) should not be used while taking phenytoin due to the risk of decreased plasma concentrations and reduced clinical effects of phenytoin (see Section 4.5).

Phenytoin therapy may interfere with Vitamin D metabolism. In the absence of an adequate dietary intake of Vitamin D or exposure to sunlight, osteomalacia, hypocalcaemia or rickets may develop.

In view of isolated reports associating phenytoin with exacerbation of porphyria, caution should be exercised in using the medication in patients suffering from this disease.

4.5 Interaction with other medicinal products and other forms of interaction

1. Drugs which may increase phenytoin serum levels include:

Amiodarone, antifungal agents (such as, but not limited to, amphotericin B, fluconazole, ketoconazole, miconazole and itraconazole), chloramphenicol, chlordiazepoxide, diazepam, dicoumarol, diltiazem, disulfiram, fluoxetine, H_2-antagonists, halothane, isoniazid, methylphenidate, nifedipine, omeprazole, oestrogens, phenothiazines, phenylbutazone, salicylates, succinimides, sulphonamides, tolbutamide, trazodone and viloxazine.

2. Drugs which may decrease phenytoin serum levels include:

Folic acid, reserpine, rifampicin, sucralfate, theophylline and vigabatrin.

Serum levels of phenytoin can be reduced by concomitant use of the herbal preparations containing St John's wort (*Hypericum perforatum*). This is due to induction of drug metabolising enzymes by St John's wort. Herbal preparations containing St John's wort should therefore not be combined with phenytoin. The inducing effect may persist for at least 2 weeks after cessation of treatment with St John's wort. If a patient is already taking St John's wort check the anticonvulsant levels and stop St John's wort. Anticonvulsant levels may increase on stopping St John's wort. The dose of anticonvulsant may need adjusting.

3. Drugs which may either increase or decrease phenytoin serum levels include:

Carbamazepine, phenobarbital, valproic acid, sodium valproate, antineoplastic agents, certain antacids and ciprofloxacin. Similarly, the effect of phenytoin on carbamazepine, phenobarbitone, valproic acid and sodium valproate serum levels is unpredictable.

Acute alcohol intake may increase phenytoin serum levels while chronic alcoholism may decrease serum levels.

4. Although not a true pharmacokinetic interaction, tricylic antidepressants and phenothiazines may precipitate seizures in susceptible patients and phenytoin dosage may need to be adjusted.

5. Drugs whose effect is impaired by phenytoin include:

Antifungal agents, antineoplastic agents, calcium channel blockers, clozapine, corticosteroids, ciclosporin, dicoumarol, digitoxin, doxycycline, furosemide, lamotrigine, methadone, neuromuscular blockers, oestrogens, oral contraceptives, paroxetine, quinidine, rifampicin, theophylline and vitamin D.

6. Drugs whose effect is altered by phenytoin include:

Warfarin. The effect of phenytoin on warfarin is variable and prothrombin times should be determined when these agents are combined.

Serum level determinations are especially helpful when possible drug interactions are suspected.

Drug-Enteral Feeding/Nutritional Preparations Interaction:

Literature reports suggest that patients who have received enteral feeding preparations and/or related nutritional supplements have lower than expected phenytoin plasma levels. It is therefore suggested that phenytoin should not be administered concomitantly with an enteral feeding preparation.

More frequent serum phenytoin level monitoring may be necessary in these patients.

There is some evidence that this effect is reduced if continuous feeding is stopped 2 hours before, and for 2 hours after, phenytoin suspension administration. However, it may still be necessary to monitor the serum phenytoin level and increase the dose of phenytoin.

Drug/Laboratory Test Interactions:

Phenytoin may cause a slight decrease in serum levels of total and free thyroxine, possibly as a result of enhanced peripheral metabolism. These changes do not lead to clinical hypothyroidism and do not affect the levels of circulating TSH. The latter can therefore be used for diagnosing hypothyroidism in the patient on phenytoin. Phenytoin does not interfere with uptake and suppression tests used in the diagnosis of hypothyroidism. It may, however, produce lower than normal values for dexamethasone or metapyrone tests. Phenytoin may cause raised serum levels of glucose, alkaline phosphatase, and gamma glutamyl transpeptidase and lowered serum levels of calcium and folic acid. It is recommended that serum folate concentrations be measured at least once every 6 months, and folic acid supplements given if necessary. Phenytoin may affect blood sugar metabolism tests.

4.6 Pregnancy and lactation

There are intrinsic methodologic problems in obtaining adequate data on drug teratogenicity in humans. Genetic factors or the epileptic condition itself may be more important than drug therapy in leading to birth defects. The great majority of mothers on anticonvulsant medication deliver normal infants. It is important to note that anticonvulsant drugs should not be discontinued in patients in whom the drug is administered to prevent major seizures because of the strong possibility of precipitating status epilepticus with attendant hypoxia and threat to life. In individual cases where the severity and frequency of the seizure disorder are such that the removal of medication does not pose a serious threat to the patient, discontinuation of the drug may be considered prior to and during pregnancy although it cannot be said with any confidence that even minor seizures do not pose some hazard to the developing embryo or foetus.

Anticonvulsants including phenytoin may produce congenital abnormalities in the offspring of a small number of epileptic patients. The exact role of drug therapy in these abnormalities is unclear and genetic factors, in some studies, have also been shown to be important. Epanutin should only be used during pregnancy, especially early pregnancy, if in the judgement of the physician the potential benefits clearly outweigh the risk.

In addition to the reports of increased incidence of congenital malformations, such as cleft lip/palate and heart malformations in children of women receiving phenytoin and other antiepileptic drugs, there have more recently been reports of a foetal hydantoin syndrome. This consists of prenatal growth deficiency, micro-encephaly and mental deficiency in children born to mothers who have received phenytoin, barbiturates, alcohol, or trimethadione. However, these features are all interrelated and are frequently associated with intrauterine growth retardation from other causes.

There have been isolated reports of malignancies, including neuroblastoma, in children whose mothers received phenytoin during pregnancy.

An increase in seizure frequency during pregnancy occurs in a proportion of patients, and this may be due to altered phenytoin absorption or metabolism. Periodic measurement of serum phenytoin levels is particularly valuable in the management of a pregnant epileptic patient as a guide to an appropriate adjustment of dosage. However, postpartum restoration of the original dosage will probably be indicated.

Neonatal coagulation defects have been reported within the first 24 hours in babies born to epileptic mothers receiving phenytoin. Vitamin K_1 has been shown to prevent or correct this defect and may be given to the mother before delivery and to the neonate after birth.

Infant breast-feeding is not recommended for women taking phenytoin because phenytoin appears to be secreted in low concentrations in human milk.

4.7 Effects on ability to drive and use machines

None known

4.8 Undesirable effects

Central Nervous System:

The most common manifestations encountered with phenytoin therapy are referable to this system and are usually dose-related. These include nystagmus, ataxia, slurred speech, decreased coordination, mental confusion, paraesthesia, drowsiness and vertigo. Dizziness, insomnia, transient nervousness, motor twitchings, and headaches have also been observed. There have also been rare reports of phenytoin induced dyskinesias, including chorea, dystonia, tremor and asterixis, similar to those induced by phenothiazine and other neuroleptic drugs. There are occasional reports of irreversible cerebellar dysfunction associated with severe phenytoin overdosage. A predominantly sensory peripheral polyneuropathy has been observed in patients receiving long-term phenytoin therapy.

Gastrointestinal:

Nausea, vomiting and constipation, toxic hepatitis, and liver damage.

Dermatological:

Dermatological manifestations sometimes accompanied by fever have included scarlatiniform or morbilliform rashes. A morbilliform rash is the most common; dermatitis is seen more rarely. Other more serious and rare forms have included bullous, exfoliative or purpuric dermatitis, lupus erythematosus, Stevens-Johnson syndrome and toxic epidermal necrolysis (see Section 4.4).

Connective Tissue:

Coarsening of the facial features, enlargement of the lips, gingival hyperplasia, hirsutism, hypertrichosis, Peyronie's Disease and Dupuytren's contracture may occur rarely.

Haemopoietic:

Haemopoietic complications, some fatal, have occasionally been reported in association with administration of phenytoin. These have included thrombocytopenia, leucopenia, granulocytopenia, agranulocytosis, pancytopenia with or without bone marrow suppression, and aplastic anaemia. While macrocytosis and megaloblastic anaemia have occurred, these conditions usually respond to folic acid therapy.

There have been a number of reports suggesting a relationship between phenytoin and the development of lymphadenopathy (local and generalised) including benign lymph node hyperplasia, pseudolymphoma, lymphoma, and Hodgkin's Disease. Although a cause and effect relationship has not been established, the occurrence of lymphadenopathy indicates the need to differentiate such a condition from other types of lymph node pathology. Lymph node involvement may occur with or without symptoms and signs resembling serum sickness, eg fever, rash and liver involvement. In all cases of lymphadenopathy, follow-up observation for an extended period is indicated and every effort should be made to achieve seizure control using alternative antiepileptic drugs.

Frequent blood counts should be carried out during treatment with phenytoin.

Immune System:

Hypersensitivity syndrome has been reported and may in rare cases be fatal (the syndrome may include, but is not limited to, symptoms such as arthralgias, eosinophilia, fever, liver dysfunction, lymphadenopathy or rash), systemic lupus erythematosus, polyarteritis nodosa, and immunoglobulin abnormalities may occur. Several individual case reports have suggested that there may be an increased, although still rare, incidence of hypersensitivity reactions, including skin rash and hepatotoxicity, in black patients.

Other:

Polyarthropathy, interstitial nephritis, pneumonitis.

4.9 Overdose

The lethal dose in children is not known. The mean lethal dose for adults is estimated to be 2 to 5g. The initial symptoms are nystagmus, ataxia and dysarthria. The patient then becomes comatose, the pupils are unresponsive and hypotension occurs followed by respiratory depression and apnoea. Death is due to respiratory and circulatory depression.

There are marked variations among individuals with respect to phenytoin serum levels where toxicity may occur. Nystagmus on lateral gaze usually appears at 20mg/l, and ataxia at 30mg/l, dysarthria and lethargy appear when the serum concentration is greater than 40mg/l, but a concentration as high as 50mg/l has been reported without evidence of toxicity.

As much as 25 times therapeutic dose has been taken to result in serum concentration over 100mg/l (400 micromoles/l) with complete recovery.

Treatment:

Treatment is non-specific since there is no known antidote. If ingested within the previous 4 hours the stomach should be emptied. If the gag reflex is absent, the airway should be supported. Oxygen, and assisted ventilation may be necessary for central nervous system, respiratory and cardiovascular depression. Haemodialysis can be considered since phenytoin is not completely bound to plasma proteins. Total exchange transfusion has been utilised in the treatment of severe intoxication in children.

In acute overdosage the possibility of the presence of other CNS depressants, including alcohol, should be borne in mind.

5. PHARMACOLOGICAL PROPERTIES

5.1 Pharmacodynamic properties

Phenytoin is effective in various animal models of generalised convulsive disorders, reasonably effective in models of partial seizures but relatively ineffective in models of myoclonic seizures.

It appears to stabilise rather than raise the seizure threshold and prevents spread of seizure activity rather than abolish the primary focus of seizure discharge.

The mechanism by which phenytoin exerts its anticonvulsant action has not been fully elucidated however, possible contributory effects include:

1. Non-synaptic effects to reduce sodium conductance, enhance active sodium extrusion, block repetitive firing and reduce post-tetanic potentiation

2. Post-synaptic action to enhance gaba-mediated inhibition and reduce excitatory synaptic transmission

3. Pre-synaptic actions to reduce calcium entry and block release of neurotransmitter.

5.2 Pharmacokinetic properties

Phenytoin is absorbed from the small intestine after oral administration. Various formulation factors may affect the bioavailability of phenytoin, however, non-linear techniques have estimated absorption to be essentially complete. After absorption it is distributed into body fluid including CSF. Its volume of distribution has been estimated to be between 0.52 and 1.19 litres/kg, and it is highly protein bound (usually 90% in adults).

The plasma half-life of phenytoin in man averages 22 hours with a range of 7 to 42 hours. Steady state therapeutic drug levels are achieved at least 7 to 10 days after initiation of therapy.

Phenytoin is hydroxylated in the liver by an enzyme system which is saturable. Small incremental doses may produce very substantial increases in serum levels when these are in the upper range of therapeutic concentrations.

The parameters controlling elimination are also subject to wide interpatient variation. The serum level achieved by a given dose is therefore also subject to wide variation.

5.3 Preclinical safety data

Pre-clinical safety data do not add anything of further significance to the prescriber.

6. PHARMACEUTICAL PARTICULARS

6.1 List of excipients

Aluminium magnesium silicate, sodium benzoate (E211), citric acid monohydrate, carmellose sodium, glycerol, polysorbate 40, sucrose, ethanol, vanillin, banana flavour, orange oil, carmoisine (E122), sunset yellow (E110), water.

6.2 Incompatibilities

Refer to Enteral feeding/Nutritional Preparations Interaction in section 4.5.

6.3 Shelf life

3 years

6.4 Special precautions for storage

Do not store above 25°C

6.5 Nature and contents of container

Amber glass bottle with 3 piece tamper evident child resistant closure fitted with a polyethylene faced liner containing 500ml. Finished pack will either have a label/leaflet or be enclosed in a carton with a separate PIL.

6.6 Special precautions for disposal and other handling

Shake well before use

7. MARKETING AUTHORISATION HOLDER

Pfizer Limited

Sandwich

Kent, CT13 9NJ

United Kingdom

8. MARKETING AUTHORISATION NUMBER(S)

PL 00057/0528

9. DATE OF FIRST AUTHORISATION/RENEWAL OF THE AUTHORISATION

1 April 2003

10. DATE OF REVISION OF THE TEXT

18th November 2008

Ref: EPF 5_0 UK

Epanutin Capsules 25, 50, 100 and 300mg

(Pfizer Limited)

1. NAME OF THE MEDICINAL PRODUCT

Epanutin 25 mg Hard Capsules

Epanutin 50 mg Hard Capsules

Epanutin 100 mg Hard Capsules

Epanutin 300 mg Hard Capsules

2. QUALITATIVE AND QUANTITATIVE COMPOSITION

Each capsule contains 25 mg phenytoin sodium.

Each capsule also contains 66.857 mg lactose monohydrate

Each capsule contains 50mg phenytoin sodium

Each capsule also contains 90.71 mg lactose monohydrate

Each capsule contains 100mg phenytoin sodium

Each capsule also contains 96.15 mg lactose monohydrate

Each capsule contains 300mg phenytoin sodium

Each capsule also contains 61.88 mg lactose monohydrate

For full list of excipients, see Section 6.1

3. PHARMACEUTICAL FORM

Capsules, hard

Epanutin Capsules 25mg: A white powder in a No 4 hard gelatin capsule with a white opaque body and blue-violet cap, radially printed 'EPANUTIN 25'.

Epanutin Capsules 50mg: A white powder in a No 4 hard gelatin capsule with a white opaque body and a flesh-coloured transparent cap, radially printed 'EPANUTIN 50'.

Epanutin Capsules 100mg: A white powder in a No 3 hard gelatin capsule with a white opaque body and orange cap, radially printed 'EPANUTIN 100'.

Epanutin Capsules 300mg: A white powder in a No 1 hard gelatin capsule with a white opaque body and green cap, radially printed 'EPANUTIN 300'.

4. CLINICAL PARTICULARS

4.1 Therapeutic indications

Control of tonic-clonic seizures (grand mal epilepsy), partial seizures (focal including temporal lobe) or a combination of these, and the prevention and treatment of seizures occurring during or following neurosurgery and/or severe head injury. Epanutin has also been employed in the treatment of trigeminal neuralgia but it should only be used as second line therapy if carbamazepine is ineffective or patients are intolerant to carbamazepine.

4.2 Posology and method of administration

For oral administration only.

Dosage:

Dosage should be individualised as there may be wide interpatient variability in phenytoin serum levels with equivalent dosage. Epanutin should be introduced in small dosages with gradual increments until control is achieved or until toxic effects appear. In some cases serum level determinations may be necessary for optimal dosage adjustments - the clinically effective level is usually 10-20mg/l (40-80 micromoles/l) although some cases of tonic-clonic seizures may be controlled with lower serum levels of phenytoin. With recommended dosage a period of seven to ten days may be required to achieve steady state serum levels with Epanutin and changes in dosage should not be carried out at intervals shorter than seven to ten days. Maintenance of treatment should be the lowest dose of anticonvulsant consistent with control of seizures.

Epanutin Capsules, Suspension and Infatabs:

Epanutin Capsules contain phenytoin sodium whereas Epanutin Suspension and Epanutin Infatabs contain phenytoin. Although 100mg of phenytoin sodium is equivalent to 92mg of phenytoin on a molecular weight basis, these molecular equivalents are not necessarily biologically equivalent. Physicians should therefore exercise care in those situations where it is necessary to change the dosage form and serum level monitoring is advised.

Adults:

Initially 3 to 4mg/kg/day with subsequent dosage adjustment if necessary. For most adults a satisfactory maintenance dose will be 200 to 500mg daily in single or divided doses. Exceptionally, a daily dose outside this range may be indicated. Dosage should normally be adjusted according to serum levels where assay facilities exist.

Elderly:

Elderly (over 65 years): As with adults the dosage of Epanutin should be titrated to the patient's individual requirements using the same guidelines. As elderly patients tend to receive multiple drug therapies, the possibility of drug interactions should be borne in mind.

Infants and Children:

Initially, 5mg/kg/day in two divided doses, with subsequent dosage individualised to a maximum of 300mg daily. A recommended daily maintenance dosage is usually 4-8mg/kg.

Neonates:

The absorption of phenytoin following oral administration in neonates is unpredictable. Furthermore, the metabolism of phenytoin may be depressed. It is therefore especially important to monitor serum levels in the neonate.

4.3 Contraindications

Hypersensitivity to hydantoins.

4.4 Special warnings and precautions for use

Suicidal ideation and behaviour have been reported in patients treated with anti-epileptic agents in several indications. A meta-analysis of randomised placebo controlled trials of anti-epileptic drugs has also shown a small increased risk of suicidal ideation and behaviour. The mechanism of this risk is not known and the available data do not exclude the possibility of an increased risk for Phenytoin Sodium.

Therefore patients should be monitored for signs of suicidal ideation and behaviours and appropriate treatment should be considered. Patients (and caregivers of patients) should be advised to seek medical advice should signs of suicidal ideation or behaviour emerge.

Abrupt withdrawal of phenytoin in epileptic patients may precipitate status epilepticus. When, in the judgement of the clinician, the need for dosage reduction, discontinuation, or substitution of alternative anti-epileptic medication arises, this should be done gradually. However, in the event of an allergic or hypersensitivity reaction, rapid substitution of alternative therapy may be necessary. In this case, alternative therapy should be an anti-epileptic drug not belonging to the hydantoin chemical class.

Phenytoin is highly protein bound and extensively metabolised by the liver. Reduced dosage to prevent accumulation and toxicity may therefore be required in patients with impaired liver function. Where protein binding is reduced, as in uraemia, total serum phenytoin levels will be reduced accordingly. However, the pharmacologically active free drug concentration is unlikely to be altered. Therefore, under these circumstances therapeutic control may be achieved with total phenytoin levels below the normal range of 10-20mg/l (40-80 micromoles/l). Patients with impaired liver function, elderly patients or those who are gravely ill may show early signs of toxicity.

Phenytoin should be discontinued if a skin rash appears. If the rash is exfoliative, purpuric, or bullous or if lupus erythematosus or Stevens-Johnson syndrome or toxic epidermal necrolysis is suspected, use of the drug should not be resumed (see Adverse Reactions). If the rash is of a milder type (measles-like or scarlatiniform), therapy may be resumed after the rash has completely disappeared. If the rash recurs upon reinstitution of therapy, further phenytoin medication is contra-indicated.

Phenytoin is not effective for absence (petit mal) seizures. If tonic-clonic (grand mal) and absence seizures are present together, combined drug therapy is needed.

Phenytoin may affect glucose metabolism and inhibit insulin release. Hyperglycaemia has been reported in association with toxic levels. Phenytoin is not indicated for seizures due to hypoglycaemia or other metabolic causes.

Serum levels of phenytoin sustained above the optimal range may produce confusional states referred to as "delirium", "psychosis", or "encephalopathy", or rarely irreversible cerebellar dysfunction. Accordingly, at the first sign of acute toxicity, serum drug level determinations are recommended. Dose reduction of phenytoin therapy is indicated if serum levels are excessive; if symptoms persist, termination of therapy with phenytoin is recommended.

Herbal preparations containing St John's wort (*Hypericum perforatum*) should not be used while taking phenytoin due to the risk of decreased plasma concentrations and reduced clinical effects of phenytoin (see Section 4.5).

Phenytoin therapy may interfere with Vitamin D metabolism. In the absence of an adequate dietary intake of Vitamin D or exposure to sunlight, osteomalacia, hypocalcaemia or rickets may develop.

In view of isolated reports associating phenytoin with exacerbation of porphyria, caution should be exercised in using the medication in patients suffering from this disease.

Patients with rare hereditary problems of galactose intolerance, the Lapp lactase deficiency or glucose-galactose metabolism should not take this medicine

4.5 Interaction with other medicinal products and other forms of interaction

1. Drugs which may increase phenytoin serum levels include:

Amiodarone, antifungal agents (such as, but not limited to, amphotericin B, fluconazole, ketoconazole, miconazole and itraconazole), chloramphenicol, chlordiazepoxide, diazepam, dicoumarol, diltiazem, disulfiram, fluoxetine, H_2-antagonists, halothane, isoniazid, methylphenidate, nifedipine, omeprazole, oestrogens, phenothiazines, phenylbutazone, salicylates, succinimides, sulphonamides, tolbutamide, trazodone and viloxazine.

2. Drugs which may decrease phenytoin serum levels include:

Folic acid, reserpine, rifampicin, sucralfate, theophylline and vigabatrin.

Serum levels of phenytoin can be reduced by concomitant use of the herbal preparations containing St John's wort (*Hypericum perforatum*). This is due to induction of drug metabolising enzymes by St John's wort. Herbal preparations containing St John's wort should therefore not be combined with phenytoin. The inducing effect may persist for at least 2 weeks after cessation of treatment with St John's wort. If a patient is already taking St John's wort check the anticonvulsant levels and stop St John's wort. Anticonvulsant levels may increase on stopping St John's wort. The dose of anticonvulsant may need adjusting.

3. Drugs which may either increase or decrease phenytoin serum levels include:

Carbamazepine, phenobarbital, valproic acid, sodium valproate, antineoplastic agents, certain antacids and ciprofloxacin. Similarly, the effect of phenytoin on carbamazepine, phenobarbital, valproic acid and sodium valproate serum levels is unpredictable.

Acute alcohol intake may increase phenytoin serum levels while chronic alcoholism may decrease serum levels.

4. Although not a true pharmacokinetic interaction, tricyclic antidepressants and phenothiazines may precipitate seizures in susceptible patients and phenytoin dosage may need to be adjusted.

5. Drugs whose effect is impaired by phenytoin include:

Antifungal agents, antineoplastic agents, calcium channel blockers, clozapine, corticosteroids, ciclosporin, dicoumarol, digitoxin, doxycycline, furosemide, lamotrigine, methadone, neuromuscular blockers, oestrogens, oral contraceptives, paroxetine, quinidine, rifampicin, theophylline and vitamin D.

6. Drugs whose effect is altered by phenytoin include:

Warfarin. The effect of phenytoin on warfarin is variable and prothrombin times should be determined when these agents are combined.

Serum level determinations are especially helpful when possible drug interactions are suspected.

Drug/Laboratory Test Interactions:

Phenytoin may cause a slight decrease in serum levels of total and free thyroxine, possibly as a result of enhanced peripheral metabolism. These changes do not lead to clinical hypothyroidism and do not affect the levels of circulating TSH. The latter can therefore be used for diagnosing hypothyroidism in the patient on phenytoin. Phenytoin does not interfere with uptake and suppression tests used in the diagnosis of hypothyroidism. It may, however, produce lower than normal values for dexamethasone or metapyrone tests. Phenytoin may cause raised serum levels of glucose, alkaline phosphatase, and gamma glutamyl transpeptidase and lowered serum levels of calcium and folic acid. It is recommended that serum folate concentrations be measured at least once every 6 months, and folic acid supplements given if necessary. Phenytoin may affect blood sugar metabolism tests.

4.6 Pregnancy and lactation

There are intrinsic methodologic problems in obtaining adequate data on drug teratogenicity in humans. Genetic factors or the epileptic condition itself may be more important than drug therapy in leading to birth defects. The great majority of mothers on anticonvulsant medication deliver normal infants. It is important to note that anticonvulsant drugs should not be discontinued in patients in whom the drug is administered to prevent major seizures because of the strong possibility of precipitating status epilepticus with attendant hypoxia and threat to life. In individual cases where the severity and frequency of the seizure disorder are such that the removal of medication does not pose a serious threat to the patient, discontinuation of the drug may be considered prior to and during pregnancy although it cannot be said with any confidence that even minor seizures do not pose some hazard to the developing embryo or foetus.

Anticonvulsants including phenytoin may produce congenital abnormalities in the offspring of a small number of epileptic patients. The exact role of drug therapy in these abnormalities is unclear and genetic factors, in some studies, have also been shown to be important. Epanutin should only be used during pregnancy, especially early pregnancy, if in the judgement of the physician the potential benefits clearly outweigh the risk.

In addition to the reports of increased incidence of congenital malformations, such as cleft lip/palate and heart malformations in children of women receiving phenytoin and other antiepileptic drugs, there have more recently been reports of a foetal hydantoin syndrome. This consists of prenatal growth deficiency, micro-encephaly and mental deficiency in children born to mothers who have received phenytoin, barbiturates, alcohol, or trimethadione. However, these features are all interrelated and are frequently associated with intrauterine growth retardation from other causes.

There have been isolated reports of malignancies, including neuroblastoma, in children whose mothers received phenytoin during pregnancy.

An increase in seizure frequency during pregnancy occurs in a proportion of patients, and this may be due to altered phenytoin absorption or metabolism. Periodic measurement of serum phenytoin levels is particularly valuable in the management of a pregnant epileptic patient as a guide to an appropriate adjustment of dosage. However, postpartum restoration of the original dosage will probably be indicated.

Neonatal coagulation defects have been reported within the first 24 hours in babies born to epileptic mothers receiving phenytoin. Vitamin K_1 has been shown to prevent or correct this defect and may be given to the mother before delivery and to the neonate after birth.

Infant breast-feeding is not recommended for women taking phenytoin because phenytoin appears to be secreted in low concentrations in human milk.

4.7 Effects on ability to drive and use machines

None known.

4.8 Undesirable effects

Central Nervous System:

The most common manifestations encountered with phenytoin therapy are referable to this system and are usually dose-related. These include nystagmus, ataxia, slurred speech, decreased co-ordination, mental confusion, paraesthesia, drowsiness and vertigo. Dizziness, insomnia, transient nervousness, motor twitchings, and headaches have also been observed. There have also been rare reports of phenytoin induced dyskinesias, including chorea, dystonia, tremor and asterixis, similar to those induced by phenothiazine and other neuroleptic drugs. There are occasional reports of irreversible cerebellar dysfunction associated with severe phenytoin overdosage. A predominantly sensory peripheral polyneuropathy has been observed in patients receiving long-term phenytoin therapy.

Gastrointestinal:

Nausea, vomiting and constipation, toxic hepatitis, and liver damage.

Dermatological:

Dermatological manifestations sometimes accompanied by fever have included scarlatiniform or morbilliform rashes. A morbilliform rash is the most common; dermatitis is seen more rarely. Other more serious and rare forms have included bullous, exfoliative or purpuric dermatitis, lupus erythematosus, Stevens-Johnson syndrome and toxic epidermal necrolysis (see Section 4.4).

Connective Tissue:

Coarsening of the facial features, enlargement of the lips, gingival hyperplasia, hirsutism, hypertrichosis, Peyronie's Disease and Dupuytren's contracture may occur rarely.

Haemopoietic:

Haemopoietic complications, some fatal, have occasionally been reported in association with administration of phenytoin. These have included thrombocytopenia, leucopenia, granulocytopenia, agranulocytosis, pancytopenia with or without bone marrow suppression, and aplastic anaemia. While macrocytosis and megaloblastic anaemia have occurred, these conditions usually respond to folic acid therapy.

There have been a number of reports suggesting a relationship between phenytoin and the development of lymphadenopathy (local and generalised) including benign lymph node hyperplasia, pseudolymphoma, lymphoma, and Hodgkin's Disease. Although a cause and effect relationship has not been established, the occurrence of lymphadenopathy indicates the need to differentiate such a condition from other types of lymph node pathology. Lymph node involvement may occur with or without symptoms and signs resembling serum sickness, eg fever, rash and liver involvement. In all cases of lymphadenopathy, follow-up observation for an extended period is indicated and every effort should be made to achieve seizure control using alternative antiepileptic drugs.

Frequent blood counts should be carried out during treatment with phenytoin.

Immune System:

Hypersensitivity syndrome has been reported and may in rare cases be fatal (the syndrome may include, but is not limited to, symptoms such as arthralgias, eosinophilia, fever, liver dysfunction, lymphadenopathy or rash), systemic lupus erythematosus, polyarteritis nodosa, and immunoglobulin abnormalities may occur. Several individual case reports have suggested that there may be an increased, although still rare, incidence of hypersensitivity reactions, including skin rash and hepatotoxicity, in black patients.

Other:

Polyarthropathy, interstitial nephritis, pneumonitis.

4.9 Overdose

The lethal dose in children is not known. The mean lethal dose for adults is estimated to be 2 to 5g. The initial symptoms are nystagmus, ataxia and dysarthria. The patient then becomes comatose, the pupils are unresponsive and hypotension occurs followed by respiratory depression and apnoea. Death is due to respiratory and circulatory depression.

There are marked variations among individuals with respect to phenytoin serum levels where toxicity may occur. Nystagmus on lateral gaze usually appears at 20mg/l, and ataxia at 30mg/l, dysarthria and lethargy appear when the serum concentration is greater than 40mg/l, but a concentration as high as 50mg/l has been reported without evidence of toxicity.

As much as 25 times therapeutic dose has been taken to result in serum concentration over 100mg/l (400 micromoles/l) with complete recovery.

Treatment:

Treatment is non-specific since there is no known antidote. If ingested within the previous 4 hours the stomach should be emptied. If the gag reflex is absent, the airway should be supported. Oxygen, and assisted ventilation may be necessary for central nervous system, respiratory and cardiovascular depression. Haemodialysis can be considered since phenytoin is not completely bound to plasma proteins. Total exchange transfusion has been utilised in the treatment of severe intoxication in children.

In acute overdosage the possibility of the presence of other CNS depressants, including alcohol, should be borne in mind.

5. PHARMACOLOGICAL PROPERTIES

5.1 Pharmacodynamic properties

Phenytoin is effective in various animal models of generalised convulsive disorders, reasonably effective in models of partial seizures but relatively ineffective in models of myoclonic seizures.

It appears to stabilise rather than raise the seizure threshold and prevents spread of seizure activity rather than abolish the primary focus of seizure discharge.

The mechanism by which phenytoin exerts its anticonvulsant action has not been fully elucidated however, possible contributory effects include:

1. Non-synaptic effects to reduce sodium conductance, enhance active sodium extrusion, block repetitive firing and reduce post-tetanic potentiation
2. Post-synaptic action to enhance gaba-mediated inhibition and reduce excitatory synaptic transmission
3. Pre-synaptic actions to reduce calcium entry and block release of neurotransmitter.

5.2 Pharmacokinetic properties

Phenytoin is absorbed from the small intestine after oral administration. Various formulation factors may affect the bioavailability of phenytoin, however, non-linear techniques have estimated absorption to be essentially complete. After absorption it is distributed into body fluid including CSF. Its volume of distribution has been estimated to be between 0.52 and 1.19 litres/kg, and it is highly protein bound (usually 90% in adults).

The plasma half-life of phenytoin in man averages 22 hours with a range of 7 to 42 hours. Steady state therapeutic drug levels are achieved at least 7 to 10 days after initiation of therapy.

Phenytoin is hydroxylated in the liver by an enzyme system which is saturable. Small incremental doses may produce very substantial increases in serum levels when these are in the upper range of therapeutic concentrations.

The parameters controlling elimination are also subject to wide interpatient variation. The serum level achieved by a given dose is therefore also subject to wide variation.

5.3 Preclinical safety data

Pre-clinical safety data do not add anything of further significance to the prescriber.

6. PHARMACEUTICAL PARTICULARS

6.1 List of excipients

25 mg

Core:

Lactose monohydrate
Magnesium stearate

Shell:

Gelatin
Erythrosine (E127)
Patent blue V (E131)
Titanium dioxide (E171)
Sodium laurilsulfate

Printing Ink:

Shellac
Black iron oxide (E172)
Propylene glycol

50 mg

Core:

Lactose monohydrate
Magnesium stearate

Shell:

Gelatin
Erythrosine (E127)
Quinoline yellow (E104)
Titanium dioxide (E171)
Sodium laurilsulfate

Printing ink:

Shellac
Black iron oxide (E172)
Propylene glycol

100 mg

Core:

Lactose monohydrate
Magnesium stearate

Shell:

Gelatin
Erythrosine (E127)
Quinoline yellow (E104)
Titanium dioxide (E171)
Sodium laurilsulfate

Printing ink:

Shellac
Black iron oxide (E172)
Propylene glycol

300 mg
Core:
Lactose monohydrate
Magnesium stearate
Silica
Shell:
Gelatin
Patent blue V (E131)
Quinoline yellow (E104)
Titanium dioxide (E171)
Sodium laurilsulfate
Printing ink:
Shellac
Black iron oxide (E172)
Propylene glycol

6.2 Incompatibilities
None known

6.3 Shelf life
18 months (25mg)
36 months (50mg)
36 months (100mg)
24 months (300mg)

6.4 Special precautions for storage
Do not store above 25°C. Store in the original package in order to protect from light.

6.5 Nature and contents of container
Epanutin Capsules, 25mg and 50mg:
White HDPE container with white LDPE cap, containing 28 capsules
Epanutin Capsules 100mg:
White HDPE container with white LDPE cap, containing 84 capsules
Epanutin Capsules 300mg:
PVC/PVdC blister pack containing 28 capsules
Not all pack sizes may be marketed

6.6 Special precautions for disposal and other handling
No special requirements.

7. MARKETING AUTHORISATION HOLDER
Pfizer Limited
Ramsgate Road
Sandwich
Kent
CT13 9NJ
United Kingdom

8. MARKETING AUTHORISATION NUMBER(S)
PL 00057/0522 (25mg)
PL 00057/0523 (50mg)
PL 00057/0524 (100mg)
PL 00057/0525 (300mg)

9. DATE OF FIRST AUTHORISATION/RENEWAL OF THE AUTHORISATION
1st March 2004 (25mg)
1st March 2004 (50mg)
1st March 2004 (100mg)
1st February 2004 (300mg)

10. DATE OF REVISION OF THE TEXT
18 November 2008
Ref: EP_13_0

Epanutin Infatabs

(Pfizer Limited)

1. NAME OF THE MEDICINAL PRODUCT
EPANUTIN INFATABS 50MG CHEWABLE TABLETS

2. QUALITATIVE AND QUANTITATIVE COMPOSITION
Each tablet contains Phenytoin 50mg
For excipients see 6.1

3. PHARMACEUTICAL FORM
Chewable tablet
A yellow triangular chewable tablet with a breaking line on one side.

4. CLINICAL PARTICULARS

4.1 Therapeutic indications
Control of tonic-clonic seizures (grand mal epilepsy), partial seizures (focal including temporal lobe) or a combination of these, and the prevention and treatment of seizures occurring during or following neurosurgery and/or severe head injury. Epanutin has also been employed in the treatment of trigeminal neuralgia but it should only be used as second line therapy if carbamazepine is ineffective or patients are intolerant to carbamazepine.

4.2 Posology and method of administration
For oral administration only.

Dosage:
Dosage should be individualised as there may be wide interpatient variability in phenytoin serum levels with equivalent dosage. Epanutin should be introduced in small dosages with gradual increments until control is achieved or until toxic effects appear. In some cases serum level determinations may be necessary for optimal dosage adjustments - the clinically effective level is usually 10-20mg/l (40-80 micromoles/l) although some cases of tonic-clonic seizures may be controlled with lower serum levels of phenytoin. With recommended dosage a period of seven to ten days may be required to achieve steady state serum levels with Epanutin and changes in dosage should not be carried out at intervals shorter than seven to ten days. Maintenance of treatment should be the lowest dose of anticonvulsant consistent with control of seizures.

Epanutin Capsules, Suspension and Infatabs:
Epanutin Capsules contain phenytoin sodium whereas Epanutin Suspension and Epanutin Infatabs contain phenytoin. Although 100mg of phenytoin sodium is equivalent to 92mg of phenytoin on a molecular weight basis, these molecular equivalents are not necessarily biologically equivalent. Physicians should therefore exercise care in those situations where it is necessary to change the dosage form and serum level monitoring is advised.

Adults:
Initially 3 to 4mg/kg/day with subsequent dosage adjustment if necessary. For most adults a satisfactory maintenance dose will be 200 to 500mg daily in single or divided doses. Exceptionally, a daily dose outside this range may be indicated. Dosage should normally be adjusted according to serum levels where assay facilities exist.

Elderly:
Elderly (over 65 years): As with adults the dosage of Epanutin should be titrated to the patient's individual requirements using the same guidelines. As elderly patients tend to receive multiple drug therapies, the possibility of drug interactions should be borne in mind.

Infants and Children:
Initially, 5mg/kg/day in two divided doses, with subsequent dosage individualised to a maximum of 300mg daily. A recommended daily maintenance dosage is usually 4-8mg/kg.
Epanutin Infatabs may be chewed.

Neonates:
The absorption of phenytoin following oral administration in neonates is unpredictable. Furthermore, the metabolism of phenytoin may be depressed. It is therefore especially important to monitor serum levels in the neonate.

4.3 Contraindications
Hypersensitivity to hydantoins.

4.4 Special warnings and precautions for use
Suicidal ideation and behaviour have been reported in patients treated with anti-epileptic agents in several indications. A meta-analysis of randomised placebo controlled trials of anti-epileptic drugs has also shown a small increased risk of suicidal ideation and behaviour. The mechanism of this risk is not known and the available data do not exclude the possibility of an increased risk for Phenytoin.

Therefore patients should be monitored for signs of suicidal ideation and behaviours and appropriate treatment should be considered. Patients (and caregivers of patients) should be advised to seek medical advice should signs of suicidal ideation or behaviour emerge.

Abrupt withdrawal of phenytoin in epileptic patients may precipitate status epilepticus. When, in the judgement of the clinician, the need for dosage reduction, discontinuation, or substitution of alternative anti-epileptic medication arises, this should be done gradually. However, in the event of an allergic or hypersensitivity reaction, rapid substitution of alternative therapy may be necessary. In this case, alternative therapy should be an anti-epileptic drug not belonging to the hydantoin chemical class.

Phenytoin is highly protein bound and extensively metabolised by the liver. Reduced dosage to prevent accumulation and toxicity may therefore be required in patients with impaired liver function. Where protein binding is reduced, as in uraemia, total serum phenytoin levels will be reduced accordingly. However, the pharmacologically active free drug concentration is unlikely to be altered. Therefore, under these circumstances therapeutic control may be achieved with total phenytoin levels below the normal range of 10-20 mg/l (40-80 micromoles/l). Patients with impaired liver function, elderly patients or those who are gravely ill may show early signs of toxicity.

Phenytoin should be discontinued if a skin rash appears. If the rash is exfoliative, purpuric, or bullous or if lupus erythematosus or Stevens-Johnson syndrome or toxic epidermal necrolysis is suspected, use of the drug should not be resumed (see Adverse Reactions). If the rash is of a milder type (measles-like or scarlatiniform), therapy may be resumed after the rash has completely disappeared. If the rash recurs upon reinstitution of therapy, further phenytoin medication is contra-indicated.

Phenytoin is not effective for absence (petit mal) seizures. If tonic-clonic (grand mal) and absence seizures are present together, combined drug therapy is needed.

Phenytoin may affect glucose metabolism and inhibit insulin release. Hyperglycaemia has been reported in association with toxic levels. Phenytoin is not indicated for seizures due to hypoglycaemia or other metabolic causes.

Serum levels of phenytoin sustained above the optimal range may produce confusional states referred to as "delirium", "psychosis", or "encephalopathy", or rarely irreversible cerebellar dysfunction. Accordingly, at the first sign of acute toxicity, serum drug level determinations are recommended. Dose reduction of phenytoin therapy is indicated if serum levels are excessive; if symptoms persist, termination of therapy with phenytoin is recommended.

Herbal preparations containing St John's wort (*Hypericum perforatum*) should not be used while taking phenytoin due to the risk of decreased plasma concentrations and reduced clinical effects of phenytoin (see Section 4.5).

Phenytoin therapy may interfere with Vitamin D metabolism. In the absence of an adequate dietary intake of Vitamin D or exposure to sunlight, osteomalacia, hypocalcaemia or rickets may develop.

In view of isolated reports associating phenytoin with exacerbation of porphyria, caution should be exercised in using the medication in patients suffering from this disease.

Patients with rare hereditary problems of fructose intolerance, glucose-galactose malabsorption or sucrase-isomaltase insufficiency should not take this medicine.

This product contains sucrose and may be harmful to the teeth when used over an extended period.

4.5 Interaction with other medicinal products and other forms of interaction
1. Drugs which may increase phenytoin serum levels include:

Amiodarone, antifungal agents (such as, but not limited to, amphotericin B, fluconazole, ketoconazole, miconazole and itraconazole), chloramphenicol, chlordiazepoxide, diazepam, dicoumarol, diltiazem, disulfiram, fluoxetine, H_2-antagonists, halothane, isoniazid, methylphenidate, nifedipine, omeprazole, oestrogens, phenothiazines, phenylbutazone, salicylates, succinimides, sulphonamides, tolbutamide, trazodone and viloxazine.

2. Drugs which may decrease phenytoin serum levels include:

Folic acid, reserpine, rifampicin, sucralfate, theophylline and vigabatrin.

Serum levels of phenytoin can be reduced by concomitant use of the herbal preparations containing St John's wort (*Hypericum perforatum*). This is due to induction of drug metabolising enzymes by St John's wort. Herbal preparations containing St John's wort should therefore not be combined with phenytoin. The inducing effect may persist for at least 2 weeks after cessation of treatment with St John's wort. If a patient is already taking St John's wort check the anticonvulsant levels and stop St John's wort. Anticonvulsant levels may increase on stopping St John's wort. The dose of anticonvulsant may need adjusting.

3. Drugs which may either increase or decrease phenytoin serum levels include:

Carbamazepine, phenobarbital, valproic acid, sodium valproate, antineoplastic agents, certain antacids and ciprofloxacin. Similarly, the effect of phenytoin on carbamazepine, phenobarbital, valproic acid and sodium valproate serum levels is unpredictable.

Acute alcohol intake may increase phenytoin serum levels while chronic alcoholism may decrease serum levels.

4. Although not a true pharmacokinetic interaction, tricyclic antidepressants and phenothiazines may precipitate seizures in susceptible patients and phenytoin dosage may need to be adjusted.

5. Drugs whose effect is impaired by phenytoin include:

Antifungal agents, antineoplastic agents, calcium channel blockers, clozapine, corticosteroids, ciclosporin, dicoumarol, digitoxin, doxycycline, furosemide, lamotrigine, methadone, neuromuscular blockers, oestrogens, oral contraceptives, paroxetine, quinidine, rifampicin, theophylline and vitamin D.

6. Drugs whose effect is altered by phenytoin include:

Warfarin. The effect of phenytoin on warfarin is variable and prothrombin times should be determined when these agents are combined.

Serum level determinations are especially helpful when possible drug interactions are suspected.

Drug/Laboratory Test Interactions:
Phenytoin may cause a slight decrease in serum levels of total and free thyroxine, possibly as a result of enhanced peripheral metabolism. These changes do not lead to clinical hypothyroidism and do not affect the levels of circulating TSH. The latter can therefore be used for diagnosing hypothyroidism in the patient on phenytoin. Phenytoin does not interfere with uptake and suppression tests used in the diagnosis of hypothyroidism. It may, however, produce lower than normal values for dexamethasone or metapyrone tests. Phenytoin may cause raised serum levels of glucose, alkaline phosphatase, and gamma glutamyl transpeptidase and lowered serum levels of calcium and folic acid. It is recommended that serum folate concentrations be measured at least once every 6 months, and

folic acid supplements given if necessary. Phenytoin may affect blood sugar metabolism tests.

4.6 Pregnancy and lactation

There are intrinsic methodologic problems in obtaining adequate data on drug teratogenicity in humans. Genetic factors or the epileptic condition itself may be more important than drug therapy in leading to birth defects. The great majority of mothers on anticonvulsant medication deliver normal infants. It is important to note that anticonvulsant drugs should not be discontinued in patients in whom the drug is administered to prevent major seizures because of the strong possibility of precipitating status epilepticus with attendant hypoxia and threat to life. In individual cases where the severity and frequency of the seizure disorder are such that the removal of medication does not pose a serious threat to the patient, discontinuation of the drug may be considered prior to and during pregnancy although it cannot be said with any confidence that even minor seizures do not pose some hazard to the developing embryo or foetus.

Anticonvulsants including phenytoin may produce congenital abnormalities in the offspring of a small number of epileptic patients. The exact role of drug therapy in these abnormalities is unclear and genetic factors, in some studies, have also been shown to be important. Epanutin should only be used during pregnancy, especially early pregnancy, if in the judgement of the physician the potential benefits clearly outweigh the risk.

In addition to the reports of increased incidence of congenital malformations, such as cleft lip/palate and heart malformations in children of women receiving phenytoin and other antiepileptic drugs, there have more recently been reports of a foetal hydantoin syndrome. This consists of prenatal growth deficiency, micro-encephaly and mental deficiency in children born to mothers who have received phenytoin, barbiturates, alcohol, or trimethadione. However, these features are all interrelated and are frequently associated with intrauterine growth retardation from other causes.

There have been isolated reports of malignancies, including neuroblastoma, in children whose mothers received phenytoin during pregnancy.

An increase in seizure frequency during pregnancy occurs in a proportion of patients, and this may be due to altered phenytoin absorption or metabolism. Periodic measurement of serum phenytoin levels is particularly valuable in the management of a pregnant epileptic patient as a guide to an appropriate adjustment of dosage. However, postpartum restoration of the original dosage will probably be indicated.

Neonatal coagulation defects have been reported within the first 24 hours in babies born to epileptic mothers receiving phenytoin. Vitamin K_1 has been shown to prevent or correct this defect and may be given to the mother before delivery and to the neonate after birth.

Infant breast-feeding is not recommended for women taking phenytoin because phenytoin appears to be secreted in low concentrations in human milk.

4.7 Effects on ability to drive and use machines

None known

4.8 Undesirable effects

Central Nervous System:

The most common manifestations encountered with phenytoin therapy are referable to this system and are usually dose-related. These include nystagmus, ataxia, slurred speech, decreased coordination, mental confusion, paraesthesia, drowsiness and vertigo. Dizziness, insomnia, transient nervousness, motor twitchings, and headaches have also been observed. There have also been rare reports of phenytoin induced dyskinesias, including chorea, dystonia, tremor and asterixis, similar to those induced by phenothiazine and other neuroleptic drugs. There are occasional reports of irreversible cerebellar dysfunction associated with severe phenytoin overdosage. A predominantly sensory peripheral polyneuropathy has been observed in patients receiving long-term phenytoin therapy.

Gastrointestinal:

Nausea, vomiting and constipation, toxic hepatitis, and liver damage.

Dermatological:

Dermatological manifestations sometimes accompanied by fever have included scarlatiniform or morbilliform rashes. A morbilliform rash is the most common; dermatitis is seen more rarely. Other more serious and rare forms have included bullous, exfoliative or purpuric dermatitis, lupus erythematosus, Stevens-Johnson syndrome and toxic epidermal necrolysis (see Section 4.4).

Connective Tissue:

Coarsening of the facial features, enlargement of the lips, gingival hyperplasia, hirsutism, hypertrichosis, Peyronie's Disease and Dupuytren's contracture may occur rarely.

Haemopoietic:

Haemopoietic complications, some fatal, have occasionally been reported in association with administration of phenytoin. These have included thrombocytopenia, leucopenia, granulocytopenia, agranulocytosis, pancytopenia with or without bone marrow suppression, and aplastic anaemia. While macrocytosis and megaloblastic anaemia have occurred, these conditions usually respond to folic acid therapy.

There have been a number of reports suggesting a relationship between phenytoin and the development of lymphadenopathy (local and generalised) including benign lymph node hyperplasia, pseudolymphoma, lymphoma, and Hodgkin's Disease. Although a cause and effect relationship has not been established, the occurrence of lymphadenopathy indicates the need to differentiate such a condition from other types of lymph node pathology. Lymph node involvement may occur with or without symptoms and signs resembling serum sickness, eg fever, rash and liver involvement. In all cases of lymphadenopathy, follow-up observation for an extended period is indicated and every effort should be made to achieve seizure control using alternative antiepileptic drugs.

Frequent blood counts should be carried out during treatment with phenytoin.

Immune System:

Hypersensitivity syndrome has been reported and may in rare cases be fatal (the syndrome may include, but is not limited to, symptoms such as arthralgias, eosinophilia, fever, liver dysfunction, lymphadenopathy or rash), systemic lupus erythematosus, polyarteritis nodosa, and immunoglobulin abnormalities may occur. Several individual case reports have suggested that there may be an increased, although still rare, incidence of hypersensitivity reactions, including skin rash and hepatotoxicity, in black patients.

Other:

Polyarthropathy, interstitial nephritis, pneumonitis.

4.9 Overdose

The lethal dose in children is not known. The mean lethal dose for adults is estimated to be 2 to 5g. The initial symptoms are nystagmus, ataxia and dysarthria. The patient then becomes comatose, the pupils are unresponsive and hypotension occurs followed by respiratory depression and apnoea. Death is due to respiratory and circulatory depression.

There are marked variations among individuals with respect to phenytoin serum levels where toxicity may occur. Nystagmus on lateral gaze usually appears at 20mg/l, and ataxia at 30mg/l, dysarthria and lethargy appear when the serum concentration is greater than 40mg/l, but a concentration as high as 50mg/l has been reported without evidence of toxicity.

As much as 25 times therapeutic dose has been taken to result in serum concentration over 100mg/l (400 micromoles/l) with complete recovery.

Treatment:

Treatment is non-specific since there is no known antidote. If ingested within the previous 4 hours the stomach should be emptied. If the gag reflex is absent, the airway should be supported. Oxygen, and assisted ventilation may be necessary for central nervous system, respiratory and cardiovascular depression. Haemodialysis can be considered since phenytoin is not completely bound to plasma proteins. Total exchange transfusion has been utilised in the treat-ment of severe intoxication in children.

In acute overdosage the possibility of the presence of other CNS depressants, including alcohol, should be borne in mind.

5. PHARMACOLOGICAL PROPERTIES

5.1 Pharmacodynamic properties

Phenytoin is effective in various animal models of generalised convulsive disorders, reasonably effective in models of partial seizures but relatively ineffective in models of myoclonic seizures.

It appears to stabilise rather than raise the seizure threshold and prevents spread of seizure activity rather than abolish the primary focus of seizure discharge.

The mechanism by which phenytoin exerts its anticonvulsant action has not been fully elucidated however, possible contributory effects include:

1. Non-synaptic effects to reduce sodium conductance, enhance active sodium extrusion, block repetitive firing and reduce post-tetanic potentiation
2. Post-synaptic action to enhance gaba-mediated inhibition and reduce excitatory synaptic transmission
3. Pre-synaptic actions to reduce calcium entry and block release of neurotransmitter.

5.2 Pharmacokinetic properties

Phenytoin is absorbed from the small intestine after oral administration. Various formulation factors may affect the bioavailability of phenytoin, however, non-linear techniques have estimated absorption to be essentially complete. After absorption it is distributed into body fluid including CSF. Its volume of distribution has been estimated to be between 0.52 and 1.19 litres/kg, and it is highly protein bound (usually 90% in adults).

The plasma half-life of phenytoin in man averages 22 hours with a range of 7 to 42 hours. Steady state therapeutic drug levels are achieved at least 7 to 10 days after initiation of therapy.

Phenytoin is hydroxylated in the liver by an enzyme system which is saturable. Small incremental doses may produce very substantial increases in serum levels when these are in the upper range of therapeutic concentrations.

The parameters controlling elimination are also subject to wide interpatient variation. The serum level achieved by a given dose is therefore also subject to wide variation.

5.3 Preclinical safety data

Pre-clinical safety data do not add anything of further significance to the prescriber.

6. PHARMACEUTICAL PARTICULARS

6.1 List of excipients

Sucrose (icing sugar),

Maize starch,

Saccharin sodium,

Spearmint flavour,

Sucrose solution (66.6% w/w),

Magnesium stearate,

Purified talc

E104 (quinoline yellow).

6.2 Incompatibilities

Not applicable

6.3 Shelf life

3years

6.4 Special precautions for storage

Do not store above 30°C

6.5 Nature and contents of container

White HDPE container with white LDPE cap, containing 112 tablets

6.6 Special precautions for disposal and other handling

No special requirements.

7. MARKETING AUTHORISATION HOLDER

Pfizer Limited

Sandwich

Kent

CT13 9NJ

United Kingdom

8. MARKETING AUTHORISATION NUMBER(S)

PL 00057/0526

9. DATE OF FIRST AUTHORISATION/RENEWAL OF THE AUTHORISATION

01 September 2003

10. DATE OF REVISION OF THE TEXT

18 November 2008

Ref: EPE 5_0

Epanutin Ready Mixed Parenteral

(Pfizer Limited)

1. NAME OF THE MEDICINAL PRODUCT

Epanutin® Ready Mixed Parenteral 250 mg/5 ml Solution for Injection or infusion

2. QUALITATIVE AND QUANTITATIVE COMPOSITION

Each 5 ml ampoule contains phenytoin sodium 250 mg (50 mg/ml)

For excipients see 6.1.

3. PHARMACEUTICAL FORM

Solution for Injection or Infusion.

Clear, colourless, sterile solution.

4. CLINICAL PARTICULARS

4.1 Therapeutic indications

Parenteral Epanutin is indicated for the control of status epilepticus of the tonic-clonic (grand mal) type and prevention and treatment of seizures occurring during or following neurosurgery and/or severe head injury.

It is of use in the treatment of cardiac arrhythmias where first line therapy is not effective. It is of particular value when these are digitalis induced.

4.2 Posology and method of administration

For parenteral administration.

Parenteral drug products should be inspected visually for particulate matter and discolouration prior to administration, whenever solution and container permit. Parenteral Epanutin is suitable for use as long as it remains free of haziness and precipitate. Upon refrigeration or freezing a precipitate might form; this will dissolve again after the solution is allowed to stand at room temperature. The product is still suitable for use. Only a clear solution should be used. A faint yellow colouration may develop, however, this has no effect on the potency of this solution.

There is a relatively small margin between full therapeutic effect and minimally toxic doses of this drug. Optimum control without clinical signs of toxicity occurs most often with serum levels between 10 and 20 mg/l (40-80 micromoles/l).

Parenteral Epanutin should be injected slowly directly into a large vein through a large-gauge needle or intravenous catheter.

Each injection or infusion of intravenous Epanutin should be preceded and followed by an injection of sterile saline through the same needle or catheter to avoid local venous irritation due to alkalinity of the solution.

(See section 4.4)

For infusion administration the parenteral phenytoin should be diluted in 50-100 ml of normal saline, with the final concentration of phenytoin in the solution not exceeding 10 mg/ml. Administration should commence immediately after the mixture has been prepared and must be completed within one hour (the infusion mixture should not be refrigerated). An in-line filter (0.22-0.50 microns) should be used.

The diluted form is suitable for use as long as it remains free of haziness and precipitate.

Continuous monitoring of the electrocardiogram and blood pressure is essential. Cardiac resuscitative equipment should be available. The patient should be observed for signs of respiratory depression. If administration of intravenous Epanutin does not terminate seizures, the use of other measures, including general anaesthesia, should be considered.

Epanutin Ready Mixed Parenteral contains phenytoin sodium whereas Epanutin Suspension and Epanutin Infatabs contain phenytoin. Although 100 mg of phenytoin sodium is equivalent to 92 mg of phenytoin on a molecular weight basis, these molecular equivalents are not necessarily biologically equivalent. Physicians should therefore exercise care in those situations where it is necessary to change the dosage form and serum level monitoring is advised.

Status Epilepticus:

In a patient having continuous seizure activity, as compared to the more common rapidly recurring seizures, i.e. serial epilepsy, injection of intravenous diazepam or a short acting barbiturate is recommended because of their rapid onset of action, prior to administration of Epanutin.

Following the use of diazepam in patients having continuous seizures and in the initial management of serial epilepsy a loading dose of Epanutin 10-15 mg/kg should be injected slowly intravenously, at a rate not exceeding 50 mg per minute in adults (this will require approximately 20 minutes in a 70 kg patient). The loading dose should be followed by maintenance doses of 100 mg orally or intravenously every 6 to 8 hours.

Recent work in neonates has shown that absorption of phenytoin is unreliable after oral administration, but a loading dose of 15-20 mg/kg of Epanutin intravenously will usually produce serum concentrations of phenytoin within the generally accepted therapeutic range (10-20 mg/l).

The drug should be injected slowly intravenously at a rate of 1-3 mg/kg/min.

Determination of phenytoin serum levels is advised when using Epanutin in the management of status epilepticus and in the subsequent establishing of maintenance dosage. The clinically effective level is usually 10-20 mg/l although some cases of tonic-clonic seizures may be controlled with lower serum levels of phenytoin.

Intramuscular administration should not be used in the treatment of status epilepticus because the attainment of peak plasma levels may require up to 24 hours.

Use in Cardiac Arrhythmias:

3.5-5 mg per kg of bodyweight intravenously initially, repeated once if necessary. The solution should be injected slowly, intravenously and at a uniform rate which should not exceed 1ml (50 mg) per minute.

Other clinical conditions:

It is not possible to set forth a universally applicable dosage schedule.

The intravenous route of administration is preferred. Dosage and dosing interval will, of necessity, be determined by the needs of the individual patient. Factors such as previous antiepileptic therapy, seizure control, age and general medical condition must be considered. Notwithstanding the slow absorption of Epanutin, when given intramuscularly, its use in certain conditions may be appropriate.

When short-term intramuscular administration is necessary for a patient previously stabilised orally, compensating dosage adjustments are essential to maintain therapeutic serum levels. An intramuscular dose 50% greater than the oral dose is necessary to maintain these levels. When returned to oral administration, the dose should be reduced by 50% of the original oral dose, for the same period of time the patient received Epanutin intramuscularly, to prevent excessive serum levels due to continued release from intramuscular tissue sites.

Neurosurgery:

In a patient who has not previously received the drug, Parenteral Epanutin 100-200 mg (2-4 ml) may be given intramuscularly at approximately 4-hour intervals prophylactically during neurosurgery and continued during the postoperative period for 48-72 hrs. The dosage should then be reduced to a maintenance dose of 300 mg and adjusted according to serum level estimations.

If the patient requires more than a week of intramuscular Epanutin, alternative routes should be explored such as gastric intubation. For time periods less than one week, the patient switched from intramuscular administration should receive one half the original oral dose for the same period of time the patient received Epanutin intramuscularly.

Measurement of serum levels is of value as a guide to an appropriate adjustment of dosage.

Elderly (over 65 years):

As for adults. However, complications may occur more readily in elderly patients.

Neonates:

Recent work in neonates has shown that absorption of phenytoin is unreliable after oral administration, but a loading dose of 15-20 mg/kg of Epanutin intravenously will usually produce serum concentrations of phenytoin within the generally accepted therapeutic range (10-20 mg/l).

The drug should be injected slowly intravenously at a rate of 1-3 mg/kg/min.

Infants and children:

As for adults, however, it has been shown that children tend to metabolise phenytoin more rapidly than adults. This should be borne in mind when determining dosage regimens; the use of serum level monitoring being particularly beneficial in such cases.

4.3 Contraindications

Phenytoin is contra-indicated in patients who are hypersensitive to phenytoin or other hydantoins. Intra-arterial administration must be avoided in view of the high pH of the preparation.

Because of its effect on ventricular automaticity, phenytoin is contra-indicated in sinus bradycardia, sino-atrial block, and second and third degree A-V block, and patients with Adams-Stokes syndrome.

4.4 Special warnings and precautions for use

Suicidal ideation and behaviour have been reported in patients treated with anti-epileptic agents in several indications. A meta-analysis of randomised placebo controlled trials of anti-epileptic drugs has also shown a small increased risk of suicidal ideation and behaviour. The mechanism of this risk is not known and the available data do not exclude the possibility of an increased risk for Phenytoin Sodium.

Therefore patients should be monitored for signs of suicidal ideation and behaviours and appropriate treatment should be considered. Patients (and caregivers of patients) should be advised to seek medical advice should signs of suicidal ideation or behaviour emerge.

In adults, intravenous administration should not exceed 50 mg per minute.

In neonates, the drug should be administered at a rate of 1-3 mg/kg/min.

The most notable signs of toxicity associated with the intravenous use of this drug are cardiovascular collapse and/or central nervous system depression. Severe cardiotoxic reactions and fatalities due to depression of atrial and ventricular conduction and ventricular fibrillation, respiratory arrest and tonic seizures have been reported particularly in elderly or gravely ill patients, if the preparation is given too rapidly or in excess.

Hypotension usually occurs when the drug is administered rapidly by the intravenous route. Soft tissue irritation and inflammation has occurred at the site of injection with and without extravasation of intravenous phenytoin. Soft tissue irritation may vary from slight tenderness to extensive necrosis, sloughing and in rare instances has led to amputation. Subcutaneous or perivascular injection should be avoided because of the highly alkaline nature of the solution.

The intramuscular route is not recommended for the treatment of status epilepticus because of slow absorption. Serum levels of phenytoin in the therapeutic range cannot be rapidly achieved by this method.

General:

Intravenous Epanutin should be used with caution in patients with hypotension and severe myocardial insufficiency.

Phenytoin should be discontinued if a skin rash appears. If the rash is exfoliative, purpuric, or bullous or if lupus erythematosus, Stevens-Johnson syndrome, or toxic epidermal necrolysis is suspected, use of this drug should not be resumed and alternative therapy should be considered. If the rash is of a milder type (measles-like or scarlatiniform), therapy may be resumed after the rash has completely disappeared. If the rash recurs upon reinstitution of therapy, further phenytoin medication is contra-indicated.

Phenytoin is not effective for absence (petit mal) seizures. If tonic-clonic (grand mal) and absence (petit mal) seizures are present together, combined drug therapy is needed.

Serum levels of phenytoin sustained above the optimal range may produce confusional states referred to as "delirium", "psychosis", or "encephalopathy", or rarely irreversible cerebellar dysfunction. Accordingly, at the first sign of acute toxicity, serum drug level determinations are recommended. Dose reduction of phenytoin therapy is indicated if serum levels are excessive; if symptoms persist, termination of therapy with phenytoin is recommended.

Herbal preparations containing St John's Wort (Hypericum perforatum) should not be used while taking phenytoin due to the risk of decreased plasma concentrations and reduced clinical effects of phenytoin (see Section 4.5).

Phenytoin is highly protein bound and extensively metabolised by the liver.

Reduced maintenance dosage to prevent accumulation and toxicity may therefore be required in patients with impaired liver function. Where protein binding is reduced, as in uraemia, total serum phenytoin levels will be reduced accordingly. However, the pharmacologically active free drug concentration is unlikely to be altered. Therefore, under these circumstances therapeutic control may be achieved with total phenytoin levels below the normal range of 10-20 mg/l. Dosage should not exceed the minimum necessary to control convulsions.

The liver is the chief site of biotransformation of phenytoin. Patients with impaired liver function, elderly patients, or those who are gravely ill may show early signs of toxicity.

Phenytoin may affect glucose metabolism and inhibit insulin release.

Hyperglycaemia has been reported. Phenytoin is not indicated for seizures due to hypoglycaemia or other metabolic causes. Caution is advised when treating diabetic patients.

In view of isolated reports associating phenytoin with exacerbation of porphyria, caution should be exercised in using this medication in patients suffering from this disease.

Laboratory Tests:

Phenytoin serum level determinations may be necessary to achieve optimal dosage adjustments.

This product contains a number of excipients known to have a recognised action or effect. These are:

Propylene glycol (may cause alcohol-like symptoms)

Sodium (1.1 mmol per 5 ml ampoule)

Ethanol (440.4 mg per 5 ml ampoule). This may be harmful for those suffering from alcoholism and should be taken into account in pregnant or breast-feeding women, children and high-risk groups such as patients with liver disease.

4.5 Interaction with other medicinal products and other forms of interaction

Drugs which may increase phenytoin serum levels include: amiodarone, antifungal agents (such as, but not limited to, amphotericin B, fluconazole, ketoconazole, miconazole and itraconazole), chloramphenicol, chlordiazepoxide, diazepam, dicoumarol, diltiazem, disulfiram, oestrogens, fluoxetine, H2-antagonists, halothane, isoniazid, methylphenidate, nifedipine, omeprazole, phenothiazines, phenylbutazone, salicylates, succinimides, sulphonamides, tolbutamide, trazodone, and viloxazine.

Drugs which may decrease phenytoin serum levels include: folic acid, reserpine, rifampicin, sucralfate, theophylline and vigabatrin.

Serum levels of phenytoin can be reduced by concomitant use of the herbal preparations containing St John's wort (Hypericum perforatum).

This is due to induction of drug metabolising enzymes by St John's wort. Herbal preparations containing St John's wort should therefore not be combined with phenytoin. The inducing effect may persist for at least 2 weeks after cessation of treatment with St John's wort. If a patient is already taking St John's wort check the anticonvulsant levels and stop St John's wort. Anticonvulsant levels may increase on stopping St John's wort. The dose of anticonvulsant may need adjusting.

Drugs which may either increase or decrease phenytoin serum levels include: carbamazepine, phenobarbital, valproic acid, sodium valproate, antineoplastic agents, certain antacids and ciprofloxacin. Similarly the effect of phenytoin on carbamazepine, phenobarbital, valproic acid and sodium valproate serum levels is unpredictable.

Acute alcoholic intake may increase phenytoin serum levels while chronic alcoholic use may decrease serum levels.

Although not a true pharmacokinetic interaction, tricyclic antidepressants and phenothiazines may precipitate seizures in susceptible patients and phenytoin dosage may need to be adjusted.

Drugs whose effect is impaired by phenytoin include: antifungal agents, antineoplastic agents, calcium channel blockers, clozapine, corticosteroids, ciclosporin, dicoumarol, digitoxin, doxycycline, furosemide, lamotrigine, methadone, neuromuscular blockers, oestrogens, oral contraceptives, paroxetine, quinidine, rifampicin, theophylline and vitamin D.

Drugs whose effect is enhanced by phenytoin include: warfarin.

The effect of phenytoin on warfarin is variable and prothrombin times should be determined when these agents are combined.

Serum level determinations are especially helpful when possible drug interactions are suspected.

Drug/Laboratory Test Interactions:

Phenytoin may cause a slight decrease in serum levels of total and free thyroxine, possibly as a result of enhanced peripheral metabolism.

These changes do not lead to clinical hypothyroidism and do not affect the levels of circulating TSH. The latter can therefore be used for diagnosing hypothyroidism in the patient on phenytoin. Phenytoin does not interfere with uptake and suppression tests used in the diagnosis of hypothyroidism.

It may, however, produce lower than normal values for dexamethasone or metapyrone tests. Phenytoin may cause raised serum levels of glucose, alkaline phosphatase, gamma glutamyl transpeptidase and lowered serum levels of calcium and folic acid. It is recommended that serum folate concentrations be measured at least every 6 months, and folic acid supplements given if necessary. Phenytoin may affect blood sugar metabolism tests.

4.6 Pregnancy and lactation

In considering the use of Epanutin intravenously in the management of status epilepticus in pregnancy, the following information should be weighed in assessing the risks and the benefits. The potential adverse effects upon the foetus of status epilepticus, specifically hypoxia, make it imperative to control the condition in the shortest possible time.

There are intrinsic methodologic problems in obtaining adequate data on drug teratogenicity in humans. Genetic factors or the epileptic condition itself may be more important than drug therapy in leading to birth defects.

The great majority of mothers on anticonvulsant medication deliver normal infants. It is important to note that anticonvulsant drugs should not be discontinued in patients in whom the drug is administered to prevent major seizures because of the strong possibility of precipitating status epilepticus and attendant hypoxia and threat to life. In individual cases where the severity and frequency of the seizure disorder are such that the removal of medication does not pose a serious threat to the patient, discontinuation of the drug may be considered prior to and during pregnancy although it cannot be said with any confidence that even minor seizures do not pose some hazard to the developing embryo or foetus.

There is some evidence that phenytoin may produce congenital abnormalities in the offspring of a small number of epileptic patients, therefore it should not be used as the first drug during pregnancy, especially early pregnancy, unless in the judgement of the physician the potential benefits outweigh the risk.

In addition to the reports of increased incidence of congenital malformations, such as cleft lip/palate and heart malformations in children of women receiving phenytoin and other antiepileptic drugs, there have been recent reports of a foetal hydantoin syndrome. This consists of prenatal growth deficiency, microencephaly and mental deficiency in children born to mothers who have received phenytoin, barbiturates, alcohol, or trimethadione. However, these features are all interrelated and are frequently associated with intrauterine growth retardation from other causes.

There have been isolated reports of malignancies, including neuroblastoma, in children whose mothers received phenytoin during pregnancy.

An increase in seizure frequency during pregnancy occurs in a proportion of patients, because of altered phenytoin absorption or metabolism.

Periodic measurement of serum phenytoin levels is particularly valuable in the management of a pregnant epileptic patient as a guide to an appropriate adjustment of dosage. However, post partum restoration of the original dosage will probably be indicated. Neonatal coagulation defects have been reported within the first 24 hours in babies born to epileptic mothers receiving phenytoin. Vitamin K has been shown to prevent or correct this defect and may be given to the mother before delivery and to the neonate after birth.

Infant breast-feeding is not recommended for women taking this drug because phenytoin appears to be secreted in low concentrations in human milk.

4.7 Effects on ability to drive and use machines

None known.

4.8 Undesirable effects

Signs of toxicity are associated with cardiovascular and central nervous system depression.

Central Nervous System:

The most common manifestations encountered with phenytoin therapy are referable to this system and are usually dose-related. These include nystagmus, ataxia, slurred speech, decreased coordination, mental confusion, paraesthesia, drowsiness and vertigo. Dizziness, insomnia, transient nervousness, motor twitching, and headache have also been observed.

There have also been rare reports of phenytoin-induced dyskinesia, including chorea, dystonia, tremor, and asterixis, similar to those induced by phenothiazine and other neuroleptic drugs. A predominantly sensory peripheral polyneuropathy has been observed in patients receiving longterm phenytoin therapy. Tonic seizures have also been reported.

Cardiovascular:

Severe cardiotoxic reactions and fatalities have been reported with atrial and ventricular conduction depression and ventricular fibrillation. Severe complications are most commonly encountered in elderly or gravely ill patients.

Respiratory:

Alterations in respiratory function including respiratory arrest may occur.

Injection Site:

Local irritation, inflammation and tenderness. Necrosis and sloughing have been reported after subcutaneous or perivascular injection. Subcutaneous or perivascular injection should be avoided. Soft tissue irritation and inflammation have occurred at the site of injection with and without extravasation of intravenous phenytoin.

Dermatological System:

Dermatological manifestations sometimes accompanied by fever have included scarlatiniform or morbilliform rashes. A morbilliform rash (measles-like) is the most common. Other types of dermatitis are seen more rarely. Other more serious forms which may be fatal have included bullous, exfoliative or purpuric dermatitis, lupus erythematosus, Stevens-Johnson syndrome, and toxic epidermal necrolysis.

Haemopoietic System:

Haemopoietic complications, some fatal, have occasionally been reported in association with administration of phenytoin. These have included thrombocytopenia, leucopenia, granulocytopenia, agranulocytosis, and pancytopenia with or without bone marrow suppression and aplastic anaemia. While macrocytosis and megaloblastic anaemia have occurred, these conditions usually respond to folic acid therapy. There have been a number of reports suggesting a relationship between phenytoin and the development of lymphadenopathy (local or generalised) including benign lymph node hyperplasia, pseudolymphoma, lymphoma, and Hodgkin's Disease. Although a cause and effect relationship has not been established, the occurrence of lymphadenopathy indicates the need to differentiate such a condition from other types of lymph node pathology. Lymph node involvement may occur with or without symptoms and signs resembling serum sickness, e.g. fever, rash and liver involvement.

In all cases of lymphadenopathy, follow-up observation for an extended period is indicated and every effort should be made to achieve seizure control using alternative antiepileptic drugs.

Gastrointestinal System:

Nausea, vomiting, constipation, toxic hepatitis, and liver damage.

Connective Tissue System:

Coarsening of the facial features, enlargement of the lips, gingival hyperplasia, hirsutism, hypertrichosis, Peyronie's disease and Dupuytren's contracture may occur rarely.

Immune System:

Hypersensitivity syndrome has been reported and may in rare cases be fatal (the syndrome may include, but is not limited to, symptoms such as arthralgias, eosinophilia, fever, liver dysfunction, lymphadenopathy or rash), systemic lupus erythematosus, periarteritis nodosa, and immunoglobulin abnormalities may occur. Several individual case reports have suggested that there may be an increased, although still rare, incidence of hypersensitivity reactions, including skin rash and hepatotoxicity, in black patients.

Other:

Polyarthropathy, interstitial nephritis, pneumonitis.

4.9 Overdose

The lethal dose in children is not known. The mean lethal dose in adults is estimated to be 2 to 5 grams. The initial symptoms are nystagmus, ataxia and dysarthria. Other signs are tremor, hyperflexia, lethargy, nausea, vomiting. The patient may become comatose and hypotensive. Death is due to respiratory and circulatory depression.

Attempts to relate serum levels of the drug to toxic effects have shown wide interpatient variation. Nystagmus on lateral gaze usually appears at 20 mg/l, and ataxia at 30 mg/l, dysarthria and lethargy appear when the serum concentration is >40 mg/l, but a concentration as high as 50 mg/l has been reported without evidence of toxicity.

As much as 25 times the therapeutic dose, which resulted in a serum concentration of 100 mg/l, was taken with complete recovery.

Treatment:

Treatment is non-specific since there is no known antidote.

The adequacy of the respiratory and circulatory systems should be carefully observed and appropriate supportive measures employed.

Haemodialysis can be considered since phenytoin is not completely bound to plasma proteins. Total exchange transfusion has been used in the treatment of severe intoxication in children.

In acute overdosage the possibility of the presence of other CNS depressants, including alcohol, should be borne in mind.

5. PHARMACOLOGICAL PROPERTIES

5.1 Pharmacodynamic properties

Phenytoin is effective in various animal models of generalised convulsive disorders and reasonably effective in models of partial seizures but relatively ineffective in models of myoclonic seizures.

It appears to stabilize rather than raise the seizure threshold and prevents spread of seizure activity rather than abolish the primary focus of seizure discharge.

The mechanism by which phenytoin exerts its anticonvulsant action has not been fully elucidated, however, possible contributory effects include:

1. Non-synaptic effects to reduce sodium conductance, enhance active sodium extrusion, block repetitive firing and reduce post-tetanic potentiation.

2. Post-synaptic action to enhance GABA-mediated inhibition and reduce excitory synaptic transmission.

3. Pre-synaptic actions to reduce calcium entry and block release of neurotransmitter.

5.2 Pharmacokinetic properties

After injection phenytoin is distributed into body fluids including CSF.

Its volume of distribution has been estimated to be between 0.52 and 1.19 litres/kg, and it is highly protein bound (usually 90% in adults).

In serum, phenytoin binds rapidly and reversibly to proteins. About 90% of phenytoin in plasma is bound to albumin. The plasma half-life of phenytoin in man averages 22 hours with a range of 7 to 42 hours.

Phenytoin is hydroxylated in the liver by an enzyme system which is saturable. Small incremental doses may produce very substantial increases in serum levels when these are in the upper range of therapeutic concentrations.

The parameters controlling elimination are also subject to wide interpatient variation. The serum level achieved by a given dose is therefore also subject to wide variation.

5.3 Preclinical safety data

Pre-clinical safety data do not add anything of further significance to the prescriber.

6. PHARMACEUTICAL PARTICULARS

6.1 List of excipients

Each 5 ml contains: Propylene glycol, Ethanol 96%, Water for injection, Sodium hydroxide.

6.2 Incompatibilities

Epanutin Ready Mixed Parenteral should not be mixed with other drugs because of precipitation of phenytoin acid.

6.3 Shelf life

Unopened: 30 months

Once opened, use immediately and discard any unused contents.

6.4 Special precautions for storage

Do not store above 25°C. Keep the ampoule in the outer carton.

6.5 Nature and contents of container

5 ml, colourless neutral glass, Type 1, Ph Eur, with a white colour break band. Each pack contains 10 ampoules.

6.6 Special precautions for disposal and other handling

For single use only.

Epanutin Ready Mixed Parenteral should be used immediately after opening. Discard any unused product once opened. See sections 4.2 and 6.2 for further information.

The product should not be used if a precipitate or haziness develops in the solution in the ampoule.

7. MARKETING AUTHORISATION HOLDER

United Kingdom: Pfizer Limited, Sandwich, Kent CT13 9NJ

8. MARKETING AUTHORISATION NUMBER(S)

PL 00057/0527

9. DATE OF FIRST AUTHORISATION/RENEWAL OF THE AUTHORISATION

1st March 2004

10. DATE OF REVISION OF THE TEXT

18 November 2008

Ref: EPG8_0

Epilim

(sanofi-aventis)

1. NAME OF THE MEDICINAL PRODUCT

Epilim 100mg Crushable Tablets

Epilim 200 Enteric Coated Tablets

Epilim 500 Enteric Coated Tablets

Epilim Liquid

Epilim Syrup

2. QUALITATIVE AND QUANTITATIVE COMPOSITION

Epilim 100mg Crushable: Each tablet contains 100mg of Sodium Valproate.

Epilim 200 Enteric Coated: 200mg Sodium Valproate

Epilim 500 Enteric Coated: 500mg Sodium Valproate

Epilim Syrup and Liquid: 200mg Sodium Valproate per 5ml

3. PHARMACEUTICAL FORM

Epilim 100mg Crushable: Tablet

Epilim 200 Enteric Coated: Enteric coated tablets

Epilim 500 Enteric Coated: Enteric coated tablets

Epilim Syrup: Syrup

Epilim Liquid: Liquid

4. CLINICAL PARTICULARS

4.1 Therapeutic indications

In the treatment of generalized, partial or other epilepsy.

4.2 Posology and method of administration

Epilim tablets, syrup & liquid are for oral administration.

Daily dosage requirements vary according to age and body weight.

Epilim tablets, syrup and liquid may be given twice daily. Uncoated tablets may be crushed if necessary.

Epilim Liquid should not be diluted.

In patients where adequate control has been achieved Epilim Chrono formulations are interchangeable with other conventional or prolonged release formulations on an equivalent daily dosage basis.

Dosage

Usual requirements are as follows:

Adults

Dosage should start at 600mg daily increasing by 200mg at three-day intervals until control is achieved. This is generally within the dosage range 1000mg to 2000mg per day, ie 20-30mg/kg/day body weight. Where adequate control is not achieved within this range the dose may be further increased to 2500mg per day.

Children over 20kg

Initial dosage should be 400mg/day (irrespective of weight) with spaced increases until control is achieved; this is usually within the range 20-30mg/kg body weight per day. Where adequate control is not achieved within this range the dose may be increased to 35mg/kg body weight per day.

Children under 20kg

20mg/kg of body weight per day; in severe cases this may be increased but only in patients in whom plasma valproic acid levels can be monitored. Above 40mg/kg/day, clinical chemistry and haematological parameters should be monitored.

Use in elderly

Although the pharmacokinetics of Epilim are modified in the elderly, they have limited clinical significance and dosage should be determined by seizure control. The volume of distribution is increased in the elderly and because of decreased binding to serum albumin, the proportion of free drug is increased. This will affect the clinical interpretation of plasma valproic acid levels.

In patients with renal insufficiency

It may be necessary to decrease the dosage. Dosage should be adjusted according to clinical monitoring since monitoring of plasma concentrations may be misleading (see section 5.2 Pharmacokinetic Properties).

In patients with hepatic insufficiency

Salicylates should not be used concomitantly with Epilim since they employ the same metabolic pathway (see also sections 4.4 Special Warnings and Precautions for Use and 4.8 Undesirable Effects).

Liver dysfunction, including hepatic failure resulting in fatalities, has occurred in patients whose treatment included valproic acid (see sections 4.3 Contraindications and 4.4 Special Warnings and Precautions for Use).

Salicylates should not be used in children under 16 years (see aspirin/salicylate product information on Reye's syndrome). In addition in conjunction with Epilim, concomitant use in children under 3 years can increase the risk of liver toxicity (see section 4.4.1 Special warnings).

Combined Therapy

When starting Epilim in patients already on other anticonvulsants, these should be tapered slowly: initiation of Epilim therapy should then be gradual, with target dose being reached after about 2 weeks. In certain cases it may be necessary to raise the dose by 5 to 10mg/kg/day when used in combination with anticonvulsants which induce liver enzyme activity, e.g. phenytoin, phenobarbital and carbamazepine. Once known enzyme inducers have been withdrawn it may be possible to maintain seizure control on a reduced dose of Epilim. When barbiturates are being administered concomitantly and particularly if sedation is observed (particularly in children) the dosage of barbiturate should be reduced.

NB: In children requiring doses higher than 40mg/kg/day clinical chemistry and haematological parameters should be monitored.

Optimum dosage is mainly determined by seizure control and routine measurement of plasma levels is unnecessary. However, a method for measurement of plasma levels is available and may be helpful where there is poor control or side effects are suspected (see section 5.2 Pharmacokinetic Properties).

4.3 Contraindications

- Active liver disease
- Personal or family history of severe hepatic dysfunction, especially drug related
- Hypersensitivity to sodium valproate
- Porphyria

4.4 Special warnings and precautions for use

Although there is no specific evidence of sudden recurrence of underlying symptoms following withdrawal of valproate, discontinuation should normally only be done under the supervision of a specialist in a gradual manner. This is due to the possibility of sudden alterations in plasma concentrations giving rise to a recurrence of symptoms. NICE has advised that generic switching of valproate preparations is not normally recommended due to the clinical implications of possible variations in plasma concentrations.

4.4.1 Special warnings

Liver dysfunction:

Conditions of occurrence:

Severe liver damage, including hepatic failure sometimes resulting in fatalities, has been very rarely reported. Experience in epilepsy has indicated that patients most at risk, especially in cases of multiple anticonvulsant therapy, are infants and in particular young children under the age of 3 and those with severe seizure disorders, organic brain disease, and (or) congenital metabolic or degenerative disease associated with mental retardation.

After the age of 3, the incidence of occurrence is significantly reduced and progressively decreases with age.

The concomitant use of salicylates should be avoided in children under 3 due to the risk of liver toxicity. Additionally, salicylates should not be used in children under 16 years (see aspirin/salicylate product information on Reye's syndrome).

Monotherapy is recommended in children under the age of 3 years when prescribing Epilim, but the potential benefit of Epilim should be weighed against the risk of liver damage or pancreatitis in such patients prior to initiation of therapy

In most cases, such liver damage occurred during the first 6 months of therapy, the period of maximum risk being 2-12 weeks.

Suggestive signs:

Clinical symptoms are essential for early diagnosis. In particular the following conditions, which may precede jaundice, should be taken into consideration, especially in patients at risk (see above: 'Conditions of occurrence'):

- non specific symptoms, usually of sudden onset, such as asthenia, malaise, anorexia, lethargy, oedema and drowsiness, which are sometimes associated with repeated vomiting and abdominal pain.
- in patients with epilepsy, recurrence of seizures.

These are an indication for immediate withdrawal of the drug.

Patients (or their family for children) should be instructed to report immediately any such signs to a physician should they occur. Investigations including clinical examination and biological assessment of liver function should be undertaken immediately.

Detection:

Liver function should be measured before and then periodically monitored during the first 6 months of therapy, especially in those who seem most at risk, and those with a prior history of liver disease.

Amongst usual investigations, tests which reflect protein synthesis, particularly prothrombin rate, are most relevant.

Confirmation of an abnormally low prothrombin rate, particularly in association with other biological abnormalities (significant decrease in fibrinogen and coagulation factors; increased bilirubin level and raised transaminases) requires cessation of Epilim therapy.

As a matter of precaution and in case they are taken concomitantly salicylates should also be discontinued since they employ the same metabolic pathway.

As with most antiepileptic drugs, increased liver enzymes are common, particularly at the beginning of therapy; they are also transient.

More extensive biological investigations (including prothrombin rate) are recommended in these patients; a reduction in dosage may be considered when appropriate and tests should be repeated as necessary.

Pancreatitis: Pancreatitis, which may be severe and result in fatalities, has been very rarely reported. Patients experiencing nausea, vomiting or acute abdominal pain should have a prompt medical evaluation (including measurement of serum amylase). Young children are at particular risk; this risk decreases with increasing age. Severe seizures and severe neurological impairment with combination anticonvulsant therapy may be risk factors. Hepatic failure with pancreatitis increases the risk of fatal outcome. In case of pancreatitis, Epilim should be discontinued.

Suicidal ideation and behaviour:

Suicidal ideation and behaviour have been reported in patients treated with anti-epileptic agents in several indications. A meta-analysis of randomised placebo controlled trials of anti-epileptic drugs has also shown a small increased risk of suicidal ideation and behaviour. The mechanism of this risk is not known and the available data do not exclude the possibility of an increased risk for sodium valproate.

Therefore patients should be monitored for signs of suicidal ideation and behaviours and appropriate treatment should be considered. Patients (and caregivers of patients) should be advised to seek medical advice should signs of suicidal ideation or behaviour emerge.

4.4.2 Precautions

Haematological: Blood tests (blood cell count, including platelet count, bleeding time and coagulation tests) are recommended prior to initiation of therapy or before surgery, and in case of spontaneous bruising or bleeding (see section 4.8 Undesirable Effects).

Renal insufficiency:

In patients with renal insufficiency, it may be necessary to decrease dosage. As monitoring of plasma concentrations may be misleading, dosage should be adjusted according to clinical monitoring (see sections 4.2 Posology and Method of Adminstration and 5.2. Pharmacokinetic Properties).

Systemic lupus erythematosus: Although immune disorders have only rarely been noted during the use of Epilim, the potential benefit of Epilim should be weighed against its potential risk in patients with systemic lupus erythematosus (see also section 4.8 Undesirable Effects).

Hyperammonaemia: When a urea cycle enzymatic deficiency is suspected, metabolic investigations should be performed prior to treatment because of the risk of hyperammonaemia with Epilim.

Weight gain: Epilim very commonly causes weight gain, which may be marked and progressive. Patients should be warned of the risk of weight gain at the initiation of therapy and appropriate strategies should be adopted to minimise it (see section 4.8 Undesirable Effects).

Pregnancy: Women of childbearing potential should not be started on Epilim without specialist neurological advice. Adequate councelling should be made available to all women with epilepsy of childbearing potential regarding the risks associated with pregnancy - because of the potential teratogenic risk to the foetus (see also section 4.6 Pregnancy and Lactation).

Diabetic patients: Epilim is eliminated mainly through the kidneys, partly in the form of ketone bodies; this may give false positives in the urine testing of possible diabetics.

4.5 Interaction with other medicinal products and other forms of interaction

4.5.1 Effects of Epilim on other drugs

- Antipsychotics, MAO inhibitors, antidepressants and benzodiazepines

Epilim may potentiate the effect of other psychotropics such as antipsychotics, MAO inhibitors, antidepressants and benzodiazepines; therefore, clinical monitoring is advised and the dosage of the other psychotropics should be adjusted when appropriate.

In particular, a clinical study has suggested that adding olanzapine to valproate or lithium therapy may significantly increase the risk of certain adverse events associated with olanzapine e.g. neutropenia, tremor, dry mouth, increased appetite and weight gain, speech disorder and somnolence.

- Phenobarbital

Epilim increases phenobarbital plasma concentrations (due to inhibition of hepatic catabolism) and sedation may occur, particularly in children. Therefore, clinical monitoring is recommended throughout the first 15 days of combined treatment with immediate reduction of phenobarbital doses if sedation occurs and determination of phenobarbital plasma levels when appropriate.

- Primidone

Epilim increases primidone plasma levels with exacerbation of its adverse effects (such as sedation); these signs cease with long term treatment. Clinical monitoring is recommended especially at the beginning of combined therapy with dosage adjustment when appropriate.

- Phenytoin

Epilim decreases phenytoin total plasma concentration. Moreover Epilim increases phenytoin free form with possible overdosage symptoms (valproic acid displaces phenytoin from its plasma protein binding sites and reduces its hepatic catabolism). Therefore clinical monitoring is recommended; when phenytoin plasma levels are determined, the free form should be evaluated.

- Carbamazepine

Clinical toxicity has been reported when Epilim was administered with carbamazepine as Epilim may potentiate toxic effects of carbamazepine. Clinical monitoring is recommended especially at the beginning of combined therapy with dosage adjustment when appropriate.

- Lamotrigine

Epilim may reduce lamotrigine metabolism and increase its mean half-life, dosages should be adjusted (lamotrigine dosage decreased) when appropriate. Co-administration of lamotrigine and Epilim might increase the risk of rash.

- Zidovudine

Epilim may raise zidovudine plasma concentration leading to increased zidovudine toxicity.

- Vitamin K-dependent anticoagulants

The anticoagulant effect of warfarin and other coumarin anticoagulants may be increased following displacement from plasma protein binding sites by valproic acid. The prothrombin time should be closely monitored.

- Temozolomide

Co-administration of temozolomide and Epilim may cause a small decrease in the clearance of temozolomide that is not thought to be clinically relevant.

4.5.2 Effects of other drugs on Epilim

Antiepileptics with enzyme inducing effect (including ***phenytoin, phenobarbital, carbamazepine***) decrease valproic acid plasma concentrations. Dosages should be adjusted according to blood levels in case of combined therapy.

On the other hand, combination of ***felbamate*** and Epilim may increase valproic acid plasma concentration. Epilim dosage should be monitored.

Mefloquine and ***chloroquine*** increase valproic acid metabolism and may lower the seizure threshold; therefore epileptic seizures may occur in cases of combined therapy. Accordingly, the dosage of Epilim may need adjustment.

In case of concomitant use of Epilim and ***highly protein bound agents (e.g. aspirin)***, free valproic acid plasma levels may be increased.

Valproic acid plasma levels may be increased (as a result of reduced hepatic metabolism) in case of concomitant use with ***cimetidine*** or ***erythromycin***.

Carbapenem antibiotics such as ***imipenem, panipenem*** and ***meropenem***: Decrease in valproic acid blood level, sometimes associated with convulsions, has been observed when imipenem or meropenem were combined. If these antibiotics have to be administered, close monitoring of valproic acid blood levels is recommended.

Colestyramine may decrease the absorption of Epilim.

4.5.3 Other Interactions

Caution is advised when using Epilim in combination with newer anti-epileptics whose pharmacodynamics may not be well established.

Epilim usually has no enzyme-inducing effect; as a consequence, Epilim does not reduce efficacy of oestroprogestative agents in women receiving hormonal contraception, including the oral contraceptive pill.

4.6 Pregnancy and lactation

Women of childbearing potential should not be started on Epilim without specialist neurological advice.

Adequate counselling should be made available to all women with epilepsy of childbearing potential regarding the risks associated with pregnancy because of the potential teratogenic risk to the foetus (See also section 4.6.1). Women who are taking Epilim and who may become pregnant should receive specialist neurological advice and the benefits of its use should be weighed against the risks.

Epilim is the antiepileptic of choice in patients with certain types of epilepsy such as generalised epilepsy ± myoclonus/photosensitivity. For partial epilepsy, Epilim should be used only in patients resistant to other treatment.

If pregnancy is planned, consideration should be given to cessation of Epilim treatment, if appropriate.

When Epilim treatment is deemed necessary, precautions to minimize the potential teratogenic risk should be followed. (See also section 4.6.1 paragraph entitled "In view of the above")

4.6.1 Pregnancy

From experience in treating mothers with epilepsy, the risk associated with the use of Epilim during pregnancy has been described as follows:

- Risk associated with epilepsy and antiepileptics

In offspring born to mothers with epilepsy receiving any anti-epileptic treatment, the overall rate of malformations has been demonstrated to be 2 to 3 times higher than the rate (approximately 3 %) reported in the general population. An increased number of children with malformations have been reported in cases of multiple drug therapy. Malformations most frequently encountered are cleft lip and cardio-vascular malformations.

Epidemiological studies have suggested an association between in-utero exposure to Epilim and a risk of developmental delay. Developmental delay has been reported in children born to mothers with epilepsy. It is not possible to differentiate what may be due to genetic, social, environmental factors, maternal epilepsy or antiepileptic treatment. Notwithstanding those potential risks, no sudden discontinuation in the anti-epileptic therapy should be undertaken as this may lead to breakthrough seizures which could have serious consequences for both the mother and the foetus.

- Risk associated with valproate

In animals: teratogenic effects have been demonstrated in the mouse, rat and rabbit.

There is animal experimental evidence that high plasma peak levels and the size of an individual dose are associated with neural tube defects.

In humans: Valproate use is associated with neural tube defects such as myelomeningocele and spina bifida. The frequency of this effect is estimated to be 1 to 2%. An increased incidence of minor or major malformations including neural tube defects, craniofacial defects, malformations of the limbs, cardiovascular malformations, hypospadias and multiple anomalies involving various body systems has been reported in offspring born to mothers with epilepsy treated with valproate.

Some data from studies, of women with epilepsy, have suggested an association between in-utero exposure to valproate and the risk of developmental delay (frequently associated with craniofacial abnormalities), particularly of verbal IQ.

- In view of the above data

When a woman is planning pregnancy, this provides an opportunity to review the need for anti-epileptic treatment. Women of childbearing age should be informed of the risks and benefits of continuing anti-epileptic treatment throughout pregnancy.

Folate supplementation, **prior** to pregnancy, has been demonstrated to reduce the incidence of neural tube defects in the offspring of women at high risk. Although no direct evidence exists of such effects in women receiving anti-epileptic drugs, women should be advised to start taking folic acid supplementation (5mg) as soon as contraception is discontinued.

The available evidence suggests that anticonvulsant monotherapy is preferred. Dosage should be reviewed before conception and the lowest effective dose used, in divided doses, as abnormal pregnancy outcome tends to be associated with higher total daily dosage and with the size of an individual dose. The incidence of neural tube defects rises with increasing dosage, particularly above 1000mg daily. The administration in several divided doses over the day and the use of a prolonged release formulation is preferable in order to avoid high peak plasma levels.

During pregnancy, Epilim anti-epileptic treatment should not be discontinued if it has been effective.

Nevertheless, specialised prenatal monitoring should be instituted in order to detect the possible occurrence of a neural tube defect or any other malformation. Pregnancies should be carefully screened by ultrasound, and other techniques if appropriate (see Section 4.4 Special Warnings and Special Precautions for use).

- Risk in the neonate

Very rare cases of haemorrhagic syndrome have been reported in neonates whose mothers have taken Epilim during pregnancy. This haemorrhagic syndrome is related to hypofibrinogenemia; afibrinogenemia has also been reported and may be fatal. These are possibly associated with a decrease of coagulation factors. However, this syndrome has to be distinguished from the decrease of the vitamin-K factors induced by phenobarbital and other anti-epileptic enzyme inducing drugs.

Therefore, platelet count, fibrinogen plasma level, coagulation tests and coagulation factors should be investigated in neonates.

4.6.2 Lactation

Excretion of Epilim in breast milk is low, with a concentration between 1 % to 10 % of total maternal serum levels; up to now children breast fed that have been monitored during the neonatal period have not experienced clinical effects. There appears to be no contra-indication to breast feeding by patients on Epilim.

4.7 Effects on ability to drive and use machines

Use of Epilim may provide seizure control such that the patient may be eligible to hold a driving licence.

Patients should be warned of the risk of transient drowsiness, especially in cases of anticonvulsant polytherapy or association with benzodiazepines (see section 4.5 Interactions with Other Medicaments and Other Forms of Interaction).

4.8 Undesirable effects

Congenital and familial/genetic disorders: (see section 4.6 Pregnancy and Lactation)

Hepato-biliary disorders:

Rare cases of liver dysfunction (see section 4.4.1 Warnings) Severe liver damage, including hepatic failure sometimes resulting in death, has been reported (see also sections 4.2, 4.3 and 4.4.1). Increased liver enzymes are common, particularly early in treatment, and may be transient (see section 4.4.1).

Gastrointestinal disorders: (nausea, gastralgia, diarrhoea) Frequently occur at the start of treatment, but they usually disappear after a few days without discontinuing treatment. These problems can usually be overcome by taking Epilim with or after food or by using Enteric Coated Epilim.

Very rare cases of pancreatitis, sometimes lethal, have been reported (see section 4.4 Special Warnings and Special Precautions for Use).

Nervous system disorders:

Sedation has been reported occasionally, usually when in combination with other anticonvulsants. In monotherapy it occurred early in treatment on rare occasions and is usually transient. Rare cases of lethargy and confusion occasionally progressing to stupor, sometimes with associated hallucinations or convulsions have been reported. Encephalopathy and coma have very rarely been observed. These cases have often been associated with too high a starting dose or too rapid a dose escalation or concomitant use of other anticonvulsants, notably phenobarbital. They have usually been reversible on withdrawal of treatment or reduction of dosage.

Very rare cases of reversible extrapyramidal symptoms including parkinsonism, or reversible dementia associated with reversible cerebral atrophy have been reported. Dose-related ataxia and fine postural tremor have occasionally been reported.

An increase in alertness may occur; this is generally beneficial but occasionally aggression, hyperactivity and behavioural deterioration have been reported.

Metabolic disorders:

Cases of isolated and moderate hyperammonaemia without change in liver function tests may occur frequently, are usually transient and should not cause treatment discontinuation. However, they may present clinically as vomiting, ataxia, and increasing clouding of consciousness. Should these symptoms occur Epilim should be discontinued. Very rare cases of hyponatraemia have been reported.

Hyperammonaemia associated with neurological symptoms has also been reported (see section 4.4.2 Precautions). In such cases further investigations should be considered.

Blood and lymphatic system disorders:

Frequent occurrence of thrombocytopenia, rare cases of anaemia, leucopenia or pancytopenia. The blood picture returned to normal when the drug was discontinued.

Isolated reduction of fibrinogen or reversible increase in bleeding time have been reported, usually without associated clinical signs and particularly with high doses (Epilim has an inhibitory effect on the second phase of platelet aggregation). Spontaneous bruising or bleeding is an indication for withdrawal of medication pending investigations (see also section 4.6 Pregnancy and Lactation).

Skin and subcutaneous tissue disorders:

Cutaneous reactions such as exanthematous rash rarely occur with valproate. In very rare cases toxic epidermal necrolysis, Stevens-Johnson syndrome and erythema multiforme have been reported.

Transient hair loss, which may sometimes be dose-related, has often been reported. Regrowth normally begins within six months, although the hair may become more curly than previously. Hirsutism and acne have been very rarely reported.

Reproductive system and breast disorders:

Amenorrhoea and irregular periods have been reported. Very rarely gynaecomastia has occurred.

Vascular disorders:

The occurrence of vasculitis has occasionally been reported.

Ear disorders:

Hearing loss, either reversible or irreversible has been reported rarely; however a cause and effect relationship has not been established.

Renal and urinary disorders:

There have been isolated reports of a reversible Fanconi's syndrome (a defect in proximal renal tubular function giving rise to glycosuria, amino aciduria, phosphaturia, and uricosuria) associated with Epilim therapy, but the mode of action is as yet unclear.

Very rare cases of enuresis have been reported.

Immune system disorders:

Allergic reactions (ranging from rash to hypersensitivity reactions) have been reported.

General disorders:

Very rare cases of non-severe peripheral oedema have been reported.

Increase in weight may also occur. Weight gain being a risk factor for polycystic ovary syndrome, it should be carefully monitored (see section 4.4 Special Warnings and Special Precautions for Use).

4.9 Overdose

Cases of accidental and deliberate Epilim overdosage have been reported. At plasma concentrations of up to 5 to 6 times the maximum therapeutic levels, there are unlikely to be any symptoms other than nausea, vomiting and dizziness.

Signs of massive overdose, i.e. plasma concentration 10 to 20 times maximum therapeutic levels, usually include CNS depression or coma with muscular hypotonia, hyporeflexia, miosis, impaired respiratory function, metabolic acidosis.

Symptoms may however be variable and seizures have been reported in the presence of very high plasma levels (see also section 5.2 Pharmacokinetic Properties).

Cases of intracranial hypertension related to cerebral oedema have been reported.

Hospital management of overdose should be symptomatic, including cardio-respiratory monitoring. Gastric lavage may be useful up to 10 to 12 hours following ingestion.

Haemodialysis and haemoperfusion have been used successfully.

Naloxone has been successfully used in a few isolated cases, sometimes in association with activated charcoal given orally. Deaths have occurred following massive overdose; nevertheless, a favourable outcome is usual.

5. PHARMACOLOGICAL PROPERTIES

5.1 Pharmacodynamic properties

Sodium valproate is an anticonvulsant.

The most likely mode of action for Epilim is potentiation of the inhibitory action of gamma amino-butyric acid (GABA) through an action on the further synthesis or further metabolism of GABA.

In certain *in-vitro* studies it was reported that Epilim could stimulate HIV replication but studies on peripheral blood mononuclear cells from HIV-infected subjects show that Epilim does not have a mitogen-like effect on inducing HIV replication. Indeed the effect of Epilim on HIV replication *ex-vivo* is highly variable, modest in quantity, appears to be unrelated to the dose and has not been documented in man.

5.2 Pharmacokinetic properties

The half-life of Epilim is usually reported to be within the range 8-20 hours. It is usually shorter in children.

In patients with severe renal insufficiency it may be necessary to alter dosage in accordance with free plasma valproic acid levels.

The reported effective therapeutic range for plasma valproic acid levels is 40-100mg/litre (278-694 micromol/litre). This reported range may depend on time of sampling and presence of co-medication. The percentage of free (unbound) drug is usually between 6% and 15% of the total plasma levels. An increased incidence of adverse effects may occur with plasma levels above the effective therapeutic range.

The pharmacological (or therapeutic) effects of Epilim may not be clearly correlated with the total or free (unbound) plasma valproic acid levels.

5.3 Preclinical safety data

Not applicable.

6. PHARMACEUTICAL PARTICULARS

6.1 List of excipients

Epilim Crushable Tablets; Maize Starch, Kaolin light (natural), Silica colloidal hydrated, Magnesium stearate and Purified water*. (* not detected in final formulation).

Epilim Liquid: Hydroxyethyl cellulose, Sorbitol, Sodium methyl hydroxybenzoate, Sodium propyl hydroxybenzoate, Saccharin sodium, Ponceau 4R (E124), Flavour IFF cherry 740, Citric acid anhydrous and Purified water.

Epilim Enteric Coated Tablets; Povidone, talc, calcium silicate, magnesium stearate, hypromellose 6, citric acid anhydrous, macrogel 6000, polyvinyl acetate phthalate, diethyl phthalate, stearic acid, violet lake solids (containing titanium dioxide, amaranth lake, indigo carmine lake and hydroxypropyl cellulose), industrial methylated spirits, purified water.

Epilim Syrup: Sorbitol powder, Sodium methyl hydroxybenzoate, Sodium propyl hydroxybenzoate, Sodium saccharin, Sucrose, Flavour IFF cherry 740, Ponceau 4R (E124) and Purified water.

6.2 Incompatibilities

None.

6.3 Shelf life

36 months.

6.4 Special precautions for storage

Epilim is hygroscopic. The tablets should not be removed from their foil until immediately before they are taken. Where possible, blister strips should not be cut. Store in a dry place below 30°C.

6.5 Nature and contents of container

Epilim 100mg Crushable Tablets are supplied in blister packs further packed into a cardboard carton. Pack size of 100 tablets.

Epilim Enteric Coated tablets are supplied in blister packs further packed into a cardboard carton. Pack size of 100 tablets.

Epilim Syrup and Liquid is supplied in amber glass bottles with polypropylene J-cap or aluminium tamper evident cap with expanded polyethylene seal and amber polyethylene tetraphthalate bottles with polypropylene tamper evident closure. Bottle size of 300ml.

6.6 Special precautions for disposal and other handling

None.

7. MARKETING AUTHORISATION HOLDER

Sanofi-Aventis Limited

One Onslow Street

Guildford

Surrey GU1 4YS

8. MARKETING AUTHORISATION NUMBER(S)

Epilim Crushable: PL 11723/0017

Epilim 200 Enteric Coated: PL 11723/0018

Epilim 500 Enteric Coated: PL 11723/0020

Epilim Syrup: PL 11723/0025

Epilim Liquid: PL 11723/0024

9. DATE OF FIRST AUTHORISATION/RENEWAL OF THE AUTHORISATION

Epilim Crushable: 18 August 1993

Epilim 200 Enteric Coated: 17 July 2000

Epilim 500 Enteric Coated: 9 March 1998

Epilim Syrup: 17th August 2001

Epilim Liquid: 14 June 1999

10. DATE OF REVISION OF THE TEXT

7 November 2008

Legal category: POM

Epilim Chrono

(sanofi-aventis)

1. NAME OF THE MEDICINAL PRODUCT

Epilim Chrono 200 Controlled Release

Epilim Chrono 300 Controlled Release

Epilim Chrono 500 Controlled Release

2. QUALITATIVE AND QUANTITATIVE COMPOSITION

Active Constituents

Epilim Chrono 200 Controlled Release tablets contain 133.2mg Sodium Valproate and 58.0mg Valproic Acid equivalent to 200mg sodium valproate.

Epilim Chrono 300 Controlled Release tablets contain 199.8mg Sodium Valproate and 87.0mg Valproic Acid equivalent to 300mg sodium valproate.

Epilim Chrono 500 Controlled Release tablets contain 333mg Sodium Valproate and 145mg Valproic Acid equivalent to 500mg sodium valproate.

3. PHARMACEUTICAL FORM

Prolonged Release Tablet

4. CLINICAL PARTICULARS

4.1 Therapeutic indications

Treatment of generalised, partial or other epilepsy.

4.2 Posology and method of administration

Epilim Chrono Controlled Release Tablets are for oral administration.

Epilim Chrono is a prolonged release formulation of Epilim which reduces peak concentration and ensures more even plasma concentrations throughout the day.

Epilim Chrono may be given once or twice daily. The tablets should be swallowed whole and not crushed or chewed.

Daily dosage requirements vary according to age and body weight.

In patients where adequate control has been achieved Epilim Chrono formulations are interchangeable with other conventional or prolonged release formulations on an equivalent daily dosage basis.

Dosage

Usual requirements are as follows:

Adults

Dosage should start at 600mg daily increasing by 200mg at three-day intervals until control is achieved. This is generally within the dosage range 1000mg to 2000mg per day, ie 20-30mg/kg/day body weight. Where adequate control is not achieved within this range the dose may be further increased to 2500mg per day.

Children over 20kg

Initial dosage should be 400mg/day (irrespective of weight) with spaced increases until control is achieved; this is usually within the range 20-30mg/kg body weight per day. Where adequate control is not achieved within this range the dose may be increased to 35mg/kg body weight per day.

Children under 20kg

An alternative formulation of Epilim should be used in this group of patients, due to the tablet size and need for dose titration. Epilim Liquid (sugar-free) or Epilim Syrup are alternatives.

Elderly

Although the pharmacokinetics of Epilim are modified in the elderly, they have limited clinical significance and dosage should be determined by seizure control. The volume of distribution is increased in the elderly and because of decreased binding to serum albumin, the proportion of free drug is increased. This will affect the clinical interpretation of plasma valproic acid levels.

In patients with renal insufficiency

It may be necessary to decrease the dosage. Dosage should be adjusted according to clinical monitoring since monitoring of plasma concentrations may be misleading (see section 5.2 Pharmacokinetic Properties).

In patients with hepatic insufficiency

Salicylates should not be used concomitantly with Epilim since they employ the same metabolic pathway (see also sections 4.4 Special Warnings and Precautions for Use and 4.8 Undesirable Effects).

Liver dysfunction, including hepatic failure resulting in fatalities, has occurred in patients whose treatment included valproic acid (see sections 4.3 Contraindications and 4.4 Special Warnings and Precautions for Use).

Salicylates should not be used in children under 16 years (see aspirin/salicylate product information on Reye's syndrome). In addition in conjunction with Epilim, concomitant use in children under 3 years can increase the risk of liver toxicity (see section 4.4.1 Special warnings).

Combined Therapy

When starting Epilim in patients already on other anticonvulsants, these should be tapered slowly; initiation of Epilim therapy should then be gradual, with target dose being reached after about 2 weeks. In certain cases it may be necessary to raise the dose by 5 to 10mg/kg/day when used in combination with anticonvulsants which induce liver enzyme activity, e.g. phenytoin, phenobarbital and carbamazepine. Once known enzyme inducers have been withdrawn it may be possible to maintain seizure control on a reduced dose of Epilim. When barbiturates are being administered concomitantly and particularly if sedation is observed (particularly in children) the dosage of barbiturate should be reduced.

NB: In children requiring doses higher than 40mg/kg/day clinical chemistry and haematological parameters should be monitored.

Optimum dosage is mainly determined by seizure control and routine measurement of plasma levels is unnecessary. However, a method for measurement of plasma levels is available and may be helpful where there is poor control or side effects are suspected (see section 5.2 Pharmacokinetic Properties).

4.3 Contraindications

- Active liver disease
- Personal or family history of severe hepatic dysfunction, especially drug related
- Hypersensitivity to sodium valproate
- Porphyria

4.4 Special warnings and precautions for use

Although there is no specific evidence of sudden recurrence of underlying symptoms following withdrawal of valproate, discontinuation should normally only be done under the supervision of a specialist in a gradual manner. This is due to the possibility of sudden alterations in plasma concentrations giving rise to a recurrence of symptoms. NICE has advised that generic switching of valproate preparations is not normally recommended due to the clinical implications of possible variations in plasma concentrations.

4.4.1 Special warnings

Liver dysfunction:

Conditions of occurrence:

Severe liver damage, including hepatic failure sometimes resulting in fatalities, has been very rarely reported. Experience in epilepsy has indicated that patients most at risk, especially in cases of multiple anticonvulsant therapy, are infants and in particular young children under the age of 3 and those with severe seizure disorders, organic brain disease, and (or) congenital metabolic or degenerative disease associated with mental retardation.

After the age of 3, the incidence of occurrence is significantly reduced and progressively decreases with age.

The concomitant use of salicylates should be avoided in children under 3 due to the risk of liver toxicity. Additionally, salicylates should not be used in children under 16 years (see aspirin/salicylate product information on Reye's syndrome).

Monotherapy is recommended in children under the age of 3 years when prescribing Epilim, but the potential benefit of Epilim should be weighed against the risk of liver damage or pancreatitis in such patients prior to initiation of therapy

In most cases, such liver damage occurred during the first 6 months of therapy, the period of maximum risk being 2-12 weeks.

Suggestive signs:

Clinical symptoms are essential for early diagnosis. In particular the following conditions, which may precede jaundice, should be taken into consideration, especially in patients at risk (see above: 'Conditions of occurrence'):

- non specific symptoms, usually of sudden onset, such as asthenia, malaise, anorexia, lethargy, oedema and drowsiness, which are sometimes associated with repeated vomiting and abdominal pain.
- in patients with epilepsy, recurrence of seizures.

These are an indication for immediate withdrawal of the drug.

Patients (or their family for children) should be instructed to report immediately any such signs to a physician should they occur. Investigations including clinical examination and biological assessment of liver function should be undertaken immediately.

Detection:

Liver function should be measured before and then periodically monitored during the first 6 months of therapy, especially in those who seem most at risk, and those with a prior history of liver disease.

Amongst usual investigations, tests which reflect protein synthesis, particularly prothrombin rate, are most relevant.

Confirmation of an abnormally low prothrombin rate, particularly in association with other biological abnormalities (significant decrease in fibrinogen and coagulation factors;

increased bilirubin level and raised transaminases) requires cessation of Epilim therapy.

As a matter of precaution and in case they are taken concomitantly salicylates should also be discontinued since they employ the same metabolic pathway.

As with most antiepileptic drugs, increased liver enzymes are common, particularly at the beginning of therapy; they are also transient.

More extensive biological investigations (including prothrombin rate) are recommended in these patients; a reduction in dosage may be considered when appropriate and tests should be repeated as necessary.

Pancreatitis: Pancreatitis, which may be severe and result in fatalities, has been very rarely reported. Patients experiencing nausea, vomiting or acute abdominal pain should have a prompt medical evaluation (including measurement of serum amylase). Young children are at particular risk; this risk decreases with increasing age. Severe seizures and severe neurological impairment with combination anticonvulsant therapy may be risk factors. Hepatic failure with pancreatitis increases the risk of fatal outcome. In case of pancreatitis, Epilim should be discontinued.

Suicidal ideation and behaviour:

Suicidal ideation and behaviour have been reported in patients treated with anti-epileptic agents in several indications. A meta-analysis of randomised placebo controlled trials of anti-epileptic drugs has also shown a small increased risk of suicidal ideation and behaviour. The mechanism of this risk is not known and the available data do not exclude the possibility of an increased risk for sodium valproate.

Therefore patients should be monitored for signs of suicidal ideation and behaviours and appropriate treatment should be considered. Patients (and caregivers of patients) should be advised to seek medical advice should signs of suicidal ideation or behaviour emerge.

4.4.2 Precautions

Haematological: Blood tests (blood cell count, including platelet count, bleeding time and coagulation tests) are recommended prior to initiation of therapy or before surgery, and in case of spontaneous bruising or bleeding (see section 4.8 Undesirable Effects).

Renal insufficiency:

In patients with renal insufficiency, it may be necessary to decrease dosage. As monitoring of plasma concentrations may be misleading, dosage should be adjusted according to clinical monitoring (see sections 4.2 Posology and Method of Administration and 5.2. Pharmacokinetic Properties).

Systemic lupus erythematosus: Although immune disorders have only rarely been noted during the use of Epilim, the potential benefit of Epilim should be weighed against its potential risk in patients with systemic lupus erythematosus (see also section 4.8 Undesirable Effects).

Hyperammonaemia: When a urea cycle enzymatic deficiency is suspected, metabolic investigations should be performed prior to treatment because of the risk of hyperammonaemia with Epilim.

Weight gain: Epilim very commonly causes weight gain, which may be marked and progressive. Patients should be warned of the risk of weight gain at the initiation of therapy and appropriate strategies should be adopted to minimise it (see section 4.8 Undesirable Effects).

Pregnancy: Women of childbearing potential should not be started on Epilim without specialist neurological advice. Adequate councelling should be made available to all women with epilepsy of childbearing potential regarding the risks associated with pregnancy because of the potential teratogenic risk to the foetus (see also section 4.6 Pregnancy and Lactation).

Diabetic patients: Epilim is eliminated mainly through the kidneys, partly in the form of ketone bodies; this may give false positives in the urine testing of possible diabetics.

4.5 Interaction with other medicinal products and other forms of interaction

4.5.1 Effects of Epilim on other drugs

- Antipsychotics, MAO inhibitors, antidepressants and benzodiazepines

Epilim may potentiate the effect of other psychotropics such as antipsychotics, MAO inhibitors, antidepressants and benzodiazepines; therefore, clinical monitoring is advised and the dosage of the other psychotropics should be adjusted when appropriate.

In particular, a clinical study has suggested that adding olanzapine to valproate or lithium therapy may significantly increase the risk of certain adverse events associated with olanzapine e.g. neutropenia, tremor, dry mouth, increased appetite and weight gain, speech disorder and somnolence.

- Phenobarbital

Epilim increases phenobarbital plasma concentrations (due to inhibition of hepatic catabolism) and sedation may occur, particularly in children. Therefore, clinical monitoring is recommended throughout the first 15 days of combined treatment with immediate reduction of phenobarbital doses if sedation occurs and determination of phenobarbital plasma levels when appropriate.

- Primidone

Epilim increases primidone plasma levels with exacerbation of its adverse effects (such as sedation); these signs cease with long term treatment. Clinical monitoring is recommended especially at the beginning of combined therapy with dosage adjustment when appropriate.

- Phenytoin

Epilim decreases phenytoin total plasma concentration. Moreover Epilim increases phenytoin free form with possible overdosage symptoms (valproic acid displaces phenytoin from its plasma protein binding sites and reduces its hepatic catabolism). Therefore clinical monitoring is recommended; when phenytoin plasma levels are determined, the free form should be evaluated.

- Carbamazepine

Clinical toxicity has been reported when Epilim was administered with carbamazepine as Epilim may potentiate toxic effects of carbamazepine. Clinical monitoring is recommended especially at the beginning of combined therapy with dosage adjustment when appropriate.

- Lamotrigine

Epilim may reduce lamotrigine metabolism and increase its mean half-life, dosages should be adjusted (lamotrigine dosage decreased) when appropriate. Co-administration of lamotrigine and Epilim might increase the risk of rash.

- Zidovudine

Epilim may raise zidovudine plasma concentration leading to increased zidovudine toxicity.

- Vitamin K-dependent anticoagulants

The anticoagulant effect of warfarin and other coumarin anticoagulants may be increased following displacement from plasma protein binding sites by valproic acid. The prothrombin time should be closely monitored.

- Temozolomide

Co-administration of temozolomide and Epilim may cause a small decrease in the clearance of temozolomide that is not thought to be clinically relevant.

4.5.2 Effects of other drugs on Epilim

Antiepileptics with enzyme inducing effect (including ***phenytoin, phenobarbital, carbamazepine***) decrease valproic acid plasma concentrations. Dosages should be adjusted according to blood levels in case of combined therapy.

On the other hand, combination of ***felbamate*** and Epilim may increase valproic acid plasma concentration. Epilim dosage should be monitored.

Mefloquine and ***chloroquine*** increase valproic acid metabolism and may lower the seizure threshold; therefore epileptic seizures may occur in cases of combined therapy. Accordingly, the dosage of Epilim may need adjustment.

In case of concomitant use of Epilim and ***highly protein bound agents (e.g. aspirin)***, free valproic acid plasma levels may be increased.

Valproic acid plasma levels may be increased (as a result of reduced hepatic metabolism) in case of concomitant use with ***cimetidine*** or ***erythromycin***.

Carbapenem antibiotics such as ***imipenem, panipenem*** and ***meropenem***: Decrease in valproic acid blood level, sometimes associated with convulsions, has been observed when imipenem or meropenem were combined. If these antibiotics have to be administered, close monitoring of valproic acid blood levels is recommended.

Colestyramine may decrease the absorption of Epilim.

4.5.3 Other Interactions

Caution is advised when using Epilim in combination with newer anti-epileptics whose pharmacodynamics may not be well established.

Epilim usually has no enzyme-inducing effect; as a consequence, Epilim does not reduce efficacy of oestroprogestative agents in women receiving hormonal contraception, including the oral contraceptive pill.

4.6 Pregnancy and lactation

Women of childbearing potential should not be started on Epilim without specialist nurological advice.

Adequate counselling should be made available to all women with epilepsy of childbearing potential regarding the risks associated with pregnancy because of the potential teratogenic risk to the foetus (See also section 4.6.1). Women who are taking Epilim and who may become pregnant should receive specialist neurological advice and the benefits of its use should be weighed against the risks.

Epilim is the antiepileptic of choice in patients with certain types of epilepsy such as generalised epilepsy ± myoclonus/photosensitivity. For partial epilepsy, Epilim should be used only in patients resistant to other treatment.

If pregnancy is planned, consideration should be given to cessation of Epilim treatment, if appropriate.

When Epilim treatment is deemed necessary, precautions to minimize the potential teratogenic risk should be followed. (See also section 4.6.1 paragraph entitled "In view of the above")

4.6.1 Pregnancy

From experience in treating mothers with epilepsy, the risk associated with the use of Epilim during pregnancy has been described as follows:

- Risk associated with epilepsy and antiepileptics

In offspring born to mothers with epilepsy receiving any anti-epileptic treatment, the overall rate of malformations has been demonstrated to be 2 to 3 times higher than the rate (approximately 3 %) reported in the general population. An increased number of children with malformations have been reported in cases of multiple drug therapy. Malformations most frequently encountered are cleft lip and cardio-vascular malformations.

Epidemiological studies have suggested an association between in-utero exposure to Epilim and a risk of developmental delay. Developmental delay has been reported in children born to mothers with epilepsy. It is not possible to differentiate what may be due to genetic, social, environmental factors, maternal epilepsy or antiepileptic treatment. Notwithstanding those potential risks, no sudden discontinuation in the anti-epileptic therapy should be undertaken as this may lead to breakthrough seizures which could have serious consequences for both the mother and the foetus.

- Risk associated with valproate

In animals: teratogenic effects have been demonstrated in the mouse, rat and rabbit.

There is animal experimental evidence that high plasma peak levels and the size of an individual dose are associated with neural tube defects.

In humans: Valproate use is associated with neural tube defects such as myelomeningocele and spina bifida. The frequency of this effect is estimated to be 1 to 2%. An increased incidence of minor or major malformations including neural tube defects, craniofacial defects, malformation of the limbs, cardiovascular malformations, hypospadias and multiple anomalies involving various body systems has been reported in offspring born to mothers with epilepsy treated with valproate.

Some data from studies, of women with epilepsy, have suggested an association between in-utero exposure to valproate and the risk of developmental delay (frequently associated with craniofacial abnormalities), particularly of verbal IQ.

- In view of the above data

When a woman is planning pregnancy, this provides an opportunity to review the need for anti-epileptic treatment. Women of childbearing age should be informed of the risks and benefits of continuing anti-epileptic treatment throughout pregnancy.

Folate supplementation, **prior** to pregnancy, has been demonstrated to reduce the incidence of neural tube defects in the offspring of women at high risk. Although no direct evidence exists of such effects in women receiving anti-epileptic drugs, women should be advised to start taking folic acid supplementation (5mg) as soon as contraception is discontinued.

The available evidence suggests that anticonvulsant monotherapy is preferred. Dosage should be reviewed before conception and the lowest effective dose used, in divided doses, as abnormal pregnancy outcome tends to be associated with higher total daily dosage and with the size of an individual dose. The incidence of neural tube defects rises with increasing dosage, particularly above 1000mg daily. The administration in several divided doses over the day and the use of a prolonged release formulation is preferable in order to avoid high peak plasma levels.

During pregnancy, Epilim anti-epileptic treatment should not be discontinued if it has been effective.

Nevertheless, specialised prenatal monitoring should be instituted in order to detect the possible occurrence of a neural tube defect or any other malformation. Pregnancies should be carefully screened by ultrasound, and other techniques if appropriate (see Section 4.4 Special Warnings and Special Precautions for use).

- Risk in the neonate

Very rare cases of haemorrhagic syndrome have been reported in neonates whose mothers have taken Epilim during pregnancy. This haemorrhagic syndrome is related to hypofibrinogenemia; afibrinogenemia has also been reported and may be fatal. These are possibly associated with a decrease of coagulation factors. However, this syndrome has to be distinguished from the decrease of the vitamin-K factors induced by phenobarbital and other anti-epileptic enzyme inducing drugs.

Therefore, platelet count, fibrinogen plasma level, coagulation tests and coagulation factors should be investigated in neonates.

4.6.2 Lactation

Excretion of Epilim in breast milk is low, with a concentration between 1 % to 10 % of total maternal serum levels; up to now children breast fed that have been monitored during the neonatal period have not experienced clinical effects. There appears to be no contra-indication to breast feeding by patients on Epilim.

4.7 Effects on ability to drive and use machines
Use of Epilim may provide seizure control such that the patient may be eligible to hold a driving licence.

Patients should be warned of the risk of transient drowsiness, especially in cases of anticonvulsant polytherapy or association with benzodiazepines (see section 4.5 Interactions with Other Medicaments and Other Forms of Interaction).

4.8 Undesirable effects
Congenital and familial/genetic disorders: (see section 4.6 Pregnancy and Lactation)

Hepato-biliary disorders:

Rare cases of liver dysfunction (see section 4.4.1 Warnings) Severe liver damage, including hepatic failure sometimes resulting in death, has been reported (see also sections 4.2, 4.3 and 4.4.1). Increased liver enzymes are common, particularly early in treatment, and may be transient (see section 4.4.1).

Gastrointestinal disorders: (nausea, gastralgia, diarrhoea)

Frequently occur at the start of treatment, but they usually disappear after a few days without discontinuing treatment. These problems can usually be overcome by taking Epilim with or after food or by using Enteric Coated Epilim.

Very rare cases of pancreatitis, sometimes lethal, have been reported (see section 4.4 Special Warnings and Special Precautions for Use).

Nervous system disorders:

Sedation has been reported occasionally, usually when in combination with other anticonvulsants. In monotherapy it occurred early in treatment on rare occasions and is usually transient. Rare cases of lethargy and confusion occasionally progressing to stupor, sometimes with associated hallucinations or convulsions have been reported. Encephalopathy and coma have very rarely been observed. These cases have often been associated with too high a starting dose or too rapid a dose escalation or concomitant use of other anticonvulsants, notably phenobarbital. They have usually been reversible on withdrawal of treatment or reduction of dosage.

Very rare cases of reversible extrapyramidal symptoms including parkinsonism, or reversible dementia associated with reversible cerebral atrophy have been reported. Dose-related ataxia and fine postural tremor have occasionally been reported.

An increase in alertness may occur; this is generally beneficial but occasionally aggression, hyperactivity and behavioural deterioration have been reported.

Metabolic disorders:

Cases of isolated and moderate hyperammonaemia without change in liver function tests may occur frequently, are usually transient and should not cause treatment discontinuation. However, they may present clinically as vomiting, ataxia, and increasing clouding of consciousness. Should these symptoms occur Epilim should be discontinued. Very rare cases of hyponatraemia have been reported.

Hyperammonaemia associated with neurological symptoms has also been reported (see section 4.4.2 Precautions). In such cases further investigations should be considered.

Blood and lymphatic system disorders:

Frequent occurrence of thrombocytopenia, rare cases of anaemia, leucopenia or pancytopenia. The blood picture returned to normal when the drug was discontinued.

Isolated reduction of fibrinogen or reversible increase in bleeding time have been reported, usually without associated clinical signs and particularly with high doses (Epilim has an inhibitory effect on the second phase of platelet aggregation). Spontaneous bruising or bleeding is an indication for withdrawal of medication pending investigations (see also section 4.6 Pregnancy and Lactation).

Skin and subcutaneous tissue disorders:

Cutaneous reactions such as exanthematous rash rarely occur with Epilim. In very rare cases toxic epidermal necrolysis, Stevens-Johnson syndrome and erythema multiforme have been reported.

Transient hair loss, which may sometimes be dose-related, has often been reported. Regrowth normally begins within six months, although the hair may become more curly than previously. Hirsutism and acne have been very rarely reported.

Reproductive system and breast disorders:

Amenorrhoea and irregular periods have been reported. Very rarely gynaecomastia has occurred.

Vascular disorders:

The occurrence of vasculitis has occasionally been reported.

Ear disorders:

Hearing loss, either reversible or irreversible has been reported rarely; however a cause and effect relationship has not been established.

Renal and urinary disorders:

There have been isolated reports of a reversible Fanconi's syndrome (a defect in proximal renal tubular function giving rise to glycosuria, amino aciduria, phosphaturia, and uricosuria) associated with Epilim therapy, but the mode of action is as yet unclear.

Very rare cases of enuresis have been reported.

Immune system disorders:

Allergic reactions (ranging from rash to hypersensitivity reactions) have been reported.

General disorders:

Very rare cases of non-severe peripheral oedema have been reported.

Increase in weight may also occur. Weight gain being a risk factor for polycystic ovary syndrome, it should be carefully monitored (see section 4.4 Special Warnings and Special Precautions for Use).

4.9 Overdose
Cases of accidental and deliberate Epilim overdosage have been reported. At plasma concentrations of up to 5 to 6 times the maximum therapeutic levels, there are unlikely to be any symptoms other than nausea, vomiting and dizziness.

Signs of massive overdose, i.e. plasma concentration 10 to 20 times maximum therapeutic levels, usually include CNS depression or coma with muscular hypotonia, hyporeflexia, miosis, impaired respiratory function, metabolic acidosis.

Symptoms may however be variable and seizures have been reported in the presence of very high plasma levels (see also section 5.2 Pharmacokinetic Properties). Cases of intracranial hypertension related to cerebral oedema have been reported.

Hospital management of overdose should be symptomatic, including cardio-respiratory monitoring. Gastric lavage may be useful up to 10 to 12 hours following ingestion.

Haemodialysis and haemoperfusion have been used successfully.

Naloxone has been successfully used in a few isolated cases, sometimes in association with activated charcoal given orally. Deaths have occurred following massive overdose; nevertheless, a favourable outcome is usual.

5. PHARMACOLOGICAL PROPERTIES

5.1 Pharmacodynamic properties
Sodium valproate and valproic acid are anticonvulsants.

The most likely mode of action for Epilim is potentiation of the inhibitory action of gamma amino butyric acid (GABA) through an action on the further synthesis or further metabolism of GABA.

In certain *in-vitro* studies it was reported that Epilim could stimulate HIV replication but studies on peripheral blood mononuclear cells from HIV-infected subjects show that Epilim does not have a mitogen-like effect on inducing HIV replication. Indeed the effect of Epilim on HIV replication *ex-vivo* is highly variable, modest in quantity, appears to be unrelated to the dose and has not been documented in man.

5.2 Pharmacokinetic properties
The half-life of Epilim is usually reported to be within the range of 8-20 hours. It is usually shorter in children.

In patients with severe renal insufficiency it may be necessary to alter dosage in accordance with free plasma valproic acid levels.

The reported effective therapeutic range for plasma valproic acid levels is 40-100mg/litre (278-694 micromol/litre). This reported range may depend on time of sampling and presence of co-medication. The percentage of free (unbound) drug is usually between 6% and 15% of total plasma levels. An increased incidence of adverse effects may occur with plasma levels above the effective therapeutic range.

The pharmacological (or therapeutic) effects of Epilim Chrono may not be clearly correlated with the total or free (unbound) plasma valproic acid levels.

Epilim Chrono formulations are prolonged release formulations which demonstrate in pharmacokinetic studies less fluctuation in plasma concentration compared with other established conventional and modified release Epilim formulations.

In cases where measurement of plasma levels is considered necessary, the pharmacokinetics of Epilim Chrono make the measurement of plasma levels less dependent upon time of sampling.

The Epilim Chrono formulations are bioequivalent to Epilim Liquid and enteric coated (EC) formulations with respect to the mean areas under the plasma concentration time curves. Steady-state pharmacokinetic data indicate that the peak concentration (Cmax) and trough concentration (Cmin) of Epilim Chrono lie within the effective therapeutic range of plasma levels found in pharmacokinetic studies with Epilim EC.

5.3 Preclinical safety data
There are no preclinical data of relevance to the prescriber which are additional to that already included in other sections of the SPC.

6. PHARMACEUTICAL PARTICULARS

6.1 List of excipients
Hypromellose, Ethylcellulose, Hydrated Silica.

Film Coat

Violet coat (Opadry 04-S-6705), containing: Titanium dioxide (E171), Erythrosine BS aluminium lake (E127), Indigo Carmine aluminium lake (E132), Iron Oxide Black (E172), Hypromellose (E464), Macrogel 400, Purified water*.

* Not detected in final formulation.

6.2 Incompatibilities
None.

6.3 Shelf life
36 months.

6.4 Special precautions for storage
Epilim is hygroscopic. The tablets should not be removed from their foil until immediately before they are taken. Where possible, blister strips should not be cut. Store in a dry place below 30°C.

6.5 Nature and contents of container
Epilim Chrono Controlled Release tablets are supplied in blister packs further packed into a cardboard carton. Pack size 100 tablets.

6.6 Special precautions for disposal and other handling
Not applicable.

7. MARKETING AUTHORISATION HOLDER
Sanofi-aventis Limited

One Onslow Street

Guildford

Surrey GU1 4YS

8. MARKETING AUTHORISATION NUMBER(S)
Epilim Chrono 200 Controlled Release - PL 11723/0078

Epilim Chrono 300 Controlled Release - PL 11723/0021

Epilim Chrono 500 Controlled Release - PL 11723/0079

9. DATE OF FIRST AUTHORISATION/RENEWAL OF THE AUTHORISATION
Epilim Chrono 200 Controlled Release - 25 November 1998

Epilim Chrono 300 Controlled Release - 28 January 2002

Epilim Chrono 500 Controlled Release - 25 November 1998

10. DATE OF REVISION OF THE TEXT
7 November 2008

Legal category: POM

Epilim Chronosphere
(sanofi-aventis)

1. NAME OF THE MEDICINAL PRODUCT
Epilim Chronosphere MR 50mg modified release granules

Epilim Chronosphere MR 100mg modified release granules

Epilim Chronosphere MR 250mg modified release granules

Epilim Chronosphere MR 500mg modified release granules

Epilim Chronosphere MR 750mg modified release granules

Epilim Chronosphere MR 1000mg modified release granules

2. QUALITATIVE AND QUANTITATIVE COMPOSITION
Epilim Chronosphere MR 50mg modified release granules sachet of 152mg modified-release granules contains: Sodium valproate 33.33mg and Valproic acid 14.51mg equivalent to 50mg sodium valproate

Epilim Chronosphere MR 100mg modified release granules sachet of 303mg modified-release granules contains: Sodium valproate 66.66mg and Valproic acid 29.03mg equivalent to 100mg sodium valproate

Epilim Chronosphere MR 250mg modified release granules sachet of 758mg modified-release granules contains: Sodium valproate 166.76mg and Valproic acid 72.61mg equivalent to 250mg sodium valproate

Epilim Chronosphere MR 500mg modified release granules sachet of 1515mg modified-release granules contains: Sodium valproate 333.30mg and valproic acid 145.14mg equivalent to 500mg sodium valproate

Epilim Chronosphere MR 750mg modified release granules sachet of 2273mg modified-release granules contains: Sodium valproate 500.06mg and valproic acid 217.75mg equivalent to 750mg sodium valproate

Epilim Chronosphere MR 750mg modified release granules sachet of 3030mg modified-release granules contains: Sodium valproate 666.60mg and valproic acid 290.27mg equivalent to 1000mg sodium valproate

For a full list of excipients, see section 6.1.

3. PHARMACEUTICAL FORM
Modified release granules

Sachets containing small, off-white to slightly yellow, waxy microgranules.

4. CLINICAL PARTICULARS

4.1 Therapeutic indications
Treatment of generalised, partial or other epilepsy.

4.2 Posology and method of administration
Epilim Chronosphere is a pharmaceutical form for oral administration, particularly suitable for children (when they are able to swallow soft food) and adults with swallowing difficulties).

Epilim Chronosphere is a controlled release formulation of Epilim, which reduces peak concentration and ensures more even plasma concentration throughout the day.

Epilim Chronosphere may be given once or twice daily.

In patients where adequate control has been achieved, Epilim Chronosphere formulations are interchangeable with other conventional or prolonged release formulations of Epilim on an equivalent daily dosage basis.

Daily dosage should be established according to age and body weight and should be given to the nearest whole 50mg sachet. Partial sachets should not be used. However, the wide individual sensitivity to valproate should also be considered.

Dosage Usual requirements are as follows:

Adults

Dosage should start at 600mg daily increasing by 200mg at three-day intervals until control is achieved. This is generally within the dosage range 1000mg to 2000mg per day, ie 20-30mg/kg/day body weight (to the nearest whole 50mg sachet). Where adequate control is not achieved within this range the dose may be further increased to 2500mg per day.

Children over 20kg

Initial dosage should be 400mg/day (irrespective of weight) with spaced increases until control is achieved; this is usually within the range 20-30mg/kg body weight per day (to the nearest whole 50mg sachet. Where adequate control is not achieved within this range the dose may be increased to 35mg/kg body weight per day. Above 40mg/kg/day, clinical chemistry and haematological parameters should be monitored.

Children under 20kg

20mg/kg of body weight per day (to the nearest whole 50mg sachet); in severe cases this may be increased but only in patients in whom plasma valproic acid levels can be monitored. Above 40mg/kg/day, clinical chemistry and haemotological parameters should be monitored.

Elderly

Although the pharmacokinetics of Epilim are modified in the elderly, they have limited clinical significance and dosage should be determined by seizure control. The volume of distribution is increased in the elderly and because of decreased binding to serum albumin, the proportion of free drug is increased. This will affect the clinical interpretation of plasma valproic acid levels.

In patients with renal insufficiency

It may be necessary to decrease the dosage. Dosage should be adjusted according to clinical monitoring since monitoring of plasma concentrations may be misleading (see section 5.2 Pharmacokinetic Properties).

In patients with hepatic insufficiency

Salicylates should not be used concomitantly with Epilim since they employ the same metabolic pathway (see also sections 4.4 Special warnings and Precautions for Use and 4.8 Undesirable Effects).

Liver dysfunction, including hepatic failures resulting in fatalities, has occurred in patients whose treatment included valproic acid (see Sections 4.3 Contraindications and 4.4. Special Warnings and Precautions for Use).

Salicylates should not be used in children under 16 years (see aspirin/salicylate product information on Reye's syndrome). In addition in conjunction with Epilim, concomitant use in children under 3 years can increase the risk of liver toxicity (see section 4.4.1 Special Warnings).

Combined Therapy

When starting Epilim Chronosphere in patients already on other anticonvulsants, these should be tapered slowly; initiation of Epilim therapy should then be gradual, with target dose being reached after about 2 weeks. In certain cases it may be necessary to raise the dose by 5 to 10mg/kg/day when used in combination with anticonvulsants which induce liver enzyme activity, e.g. phenytoin, phenobarbital and carbamazepine. Once known enzyme inducers have been withdrawn it may be possible to maintain seizure control on a reduced dose of Epilim Chronosphere. When barbiturates are being administered concomitantly and particularly if sedation is observed (particularly in children) the dosage of barbiturate should be reduced.

Optimum dosage is mainly determined by seizure control and routine measurement of plasma levels is unnecessary. However, a method for measurement of plasma levels is available and may be helpful where there is poor control or side effects are suspected (see section 5.2 Pharmacokinetic Properties).

Administration

Epilim Chronosphere modified release granules should be sprinkled on a small amount of soft food or in drinks, which should be cold or at room temperature, for example yoghurt, mousse, jam, ice-cream, milk shake, orange juice or something similar.

If the granules are taken in a drink, after the drink has been finished the glass should be rinsed with a small amount of water and this water should be taken as well, as some granules may stick to the glass.

The mixture of food or drink and granules should be swallowed immediately; the granules should not be crushed or chewed.

A mixture of the granules with liquid or soft food should not be stored for future use.

Epilim Chronosphere modified release granules should not be sprinkled on warm or hot foods and drinks, for example soup, coffee, tea, or something similar.

If preferred the granules can be poured directly into the mouth and washed down with a cold drink.

Epilim Chronosphere modified release granules should not be given in babies' bottles as they can block the nipple.

4.3 Contraindications

- Active liver disease
- Personal or family history of severe hepatitis, especially drug related
- Hypersensitivity to sodium valproate
- Porphyria

4.4 Special warnings and precautions for use

Although there is no specific evidence of sudden recurrence of underlying symptoms following withdrawal of valproate, discontinuation should normally only be done under the supervision of a specialist in a gradual manner. This is due to the possibility of sudden alterations in plasma concentrations giving rise to a recurrence of symptoms. NICE has advised that generic switching of valproate preparations is not normally recommended due to the clinical implications of possible variations in plasma concentrations.

4.4.1 Special warnings

Liver dysfunction:

Conditions of occurrence:

Severe liver damage, including hepatic failure sometimes resulting in fatalities, has been very rarely reported.

Experience in epilepsy has indicated that patients most at risk, especially in cases of multiple anticonvulsant therapy, are infants and in particular young children under the age of 3 and those with severe seizure disorders, organic brain disease, and (or) congenital metabolic or degenerative disease associated with mental retardation.

After the age of 3, the incidence of occurrence is significantly reduced and progressively decreases with age.

The concomitant use of salicylates should be avoided in children under 3 due to the risk of liver toxicity. Additionally, salicylates should not be used in children under 16 years (see aspirin/salicylate product information on Reye's syndrome).

Monotherapy is recommended in children under the age of 3 years when prescribing Epilim, but the potential benefit of Epilim should be weighed against the risk of liver damage or pancreatitis in such patients prior to initiation of therapy

In most cases, such liver damage occurred during the first 6 months of therapy, the period of maximum risk being 2-12 weeks.

Suggestive signs:

Clinical symptoms are essential for early diagnosis. In particular the following conditions, which may precede jaundice, should be taken into consideration, especially in patients at risk (see above: 'Conditions of occurrence'):

- non specific symptoms, usually of sudden onset, such as asthenia, malaise, anorexia, lethargy, oedema and drowsiness, which are sometimes associated with repeated vomiting and abdominal pain.

- in patients with epilepsy, recurrence of seizures.

These are an indication for immediate withdrawal of the drug.

Patients (or their family for children) should be instructed to report immediately any such signs to a physician should they occur. Investigations including clinical examination and biological assessment of liver function should be undertaken immediately.

Detection:

Liver function should be measured before and then periodically monitored during the first 6 months of therapy, especially in those who seem most at risk, and those with a prior history of liver disease.

Amongst usual investigations, tests which reflect protein synthesis, particularly prothrombin rate, are most relevant.

Confirmation of an abnormally low prothrombin rate, particularly in association with other biological abnormalities (significant decrease in fibrinogen and coagulation factors; increased bilirubin level and raised transaminases) requires cessation of Epilim therapy.

As a matter of precaution and in case they are taken concomitantly salicylates should also be discontinued since they employ the same metabolic pathway.

As with most antiepileptic drugs, increased liver enzymes are common, particularly at the beginning of therapy; they are also transient.

More extensive biological investigations (including prothrombin rate) are recommended in these patients; a reduction in dosage may be considered when appropriate and tests should be repeated as necessary.

Pancreatitis: Pancreatitis, which may be severe and result in fatalities, has been very rarely reported. Patients experiencing nausea, vomiting or acute abdominal pain should have a prompt medical evaluation (including measurement of serum amylase). Young children are at particular risk; this risk decreases with increasing age. Severe seizures and severe neurological impairment with combination anticonvulsant therapy may be risk factors. Hepatic failure with pancreatitis increases the risk of fatal outcome. In case of pancreatitis, Epilim should be discontinued.

Suicidal ideation and behaviour:

Suicidal ideation and behaviour have been reported in patients treated with anti-epileptic agents in several indications. A meta-analysis of randomised placebo controlled trials of anti-epileptic drugs has also shown a small increased risk of suicidal ideation and behaviour. The mechanism of this risk is not known and the available data do not exclude the possibility of an increased risk for sodium valproate.

Therefore patients should be monitored for signs of suicidal ideation and behaviours and appropriate treatment should be considered. Patients (and caregivers of patients) should be advised to seek medical advice should signs of suicidal ideation or behaviour emerge.

4.4.2 Precautions

Haematological: Blood tests (blood cell count, including platelet count, bleeding time and coagulation tests) are recommended prior to initiation of therapy or before surgery, and in case of spontaneous bruising or bleeding (see section 4.8 Undesirable Effects).

Renal insufficiency: In patients with renal insufficiency, it may be necessary to decrease dosage. As monitoring of plasma concentrations may be misleading, dosage should be adjusted according to clinical monitoring (see sections 4.2 Posology and Method of Administration and 5.2. Pharmacokinetic Properties).

Systemic lupus erythematosus: Although immune disorders have only rarely been noted during the use of Epilim, the potential benefit of Epilim should be weighed against its potential risk in patients with systemic lupus erythematosus(see also section 4.8 Undesirable Effects).

Hyperammonaemia: When a urea cycle enzymatic deficiency is suspected, metabolic investigations should be performed prior to treatment because of the risk of hyperammonaemia with Epilim.

Weight gain: Epilim very commonly causes weight gain, which may be marked and progressive. Patients should be warned of the risk at the initiation of therapy and appropriate strategies should be adopted to minimise it (see section 4.8 Undesirable Effects).

Pregnancy: Women of childbearing potential should not be started on Epilim without specialist neurological advice. Adequate counselling should be made available to all women with epilepsy of childbearing potential regarding the risks associated with pregnancy because of the potential teratogenic risk to the foetus (see also section 4.6 Pregnancy and Lactation).

Diabetic patients: Epilim is eliminated mainly through the kidneys, partly in the form of ketone bodies; this may give false positives in the urine testing of possible diabetics.

4.5 Interaction with other medicinal products and other forms of interaction

4.5.1 Effects of Epilim on other drugs

- Antipsychotics, MAO inhibitors, antidepressants and benzodiazepines

Epilim may potentiate the effect of other psychotropics such as antipsychotics, MAO inhibitors, antidepressants and benzodiazepines; therefore, clinical monitoring is advised and the dosage of the other psychotropics should be adjusted when appropriate.

In particular, a clinical study has suggested that adding olanzapine to valproate or lithium therapy may significantly increase the risk of certain adverse events associated with olanzapine e.g. neutropenia, tremor, dry mouth, increased appetite and weight gain, speech disorder and somnolence.

- Phenobarbital

Epilim increases phenobarbital plasma concentrations (due to inhibition of hepatic catabolism) and sedation may occur, particularly in children. Therefore, clinical monitoring is recommended throughout the first 15 days of combined treatment with immediate reduction of phenobarbital doses if sedation occurs and determination of phenobarbital plasma levels when appropriate.

- Primidone

Epilim increases primidone plasma levels with exacerbation of its adverse effects (such as sedation); these signs cease with long term treatment. Clinical monitoring is recommended especially at the beginning of combined therapy with dosage adjustment when appropriate.

- Phenytoin

Epilim decreases phenytoin total plasma concentration. Moreover Epilim increases phenytoin free form with possible overdosage symptoms (valproic acid displaces phenytoin from its plasma protein binding sites and reduces its hepatic catabolism). Therefore clinical monitoring is recommended; when phenytoin plasma levels are determined, the free form should be evaluated.

- Carbamazepine

Clinical toxicity has been reported when Epilim was administered with carbamazepine as Epilim may potentiate toxic effects of carbamazepine. Clinical monitoring is recommended especially at the beginning of combined therapy with dosage adjustment when appropriate.

- Lamotrigine

Epilim may reduce lamotrigine metabolism and increase its mean half-life, dosages should be adjusted (lamotrigine dosage decreased) when appropriate. Co-administration of lamotrigine and Epilim might increase the risk of rash.

- Zidovudine

Epilim may raise zidovudine plasma concentration leading to increased zidovudine toxicity.

- Vitamin K-dependent anticoagulants

The anticoagulant effect of warfarin and other coumarin anticoagulants may be increased following displacement from plasma protein binding sites by valproic acid. The prothrombin time should be closely monitored.

- Temozolomide

Co-administration of temozolomide and Epilim may cause a small decrease in the clearance of temozolomide that is not thought to be clinically relevant.

4.5.2 Effects of other drugs on Epilim

Antiepileptics with enzyme inducing effect (including *phenytoin, phenobarbital, carbamazepine*) decrease valproic acid plasma concentrations. Dosages should be adjusted according to blood levels in case of combined therapy.

On the other hand, combination of *felbamate* and Epilim may increase valproic acid plasma concentration. Epilim dosage should be monitored.

Mefloquine and *chloroquine* increase valproic acid metabolism and may lower the seizure threshold; therefore epileptic seizures may occur in cases of combined therapy. Accordingly, the dosage of Epilim may need adjustment.

In case of concomitant use of Epilim and *highly protein bound agents (e.g. aspirin)*, free valproic acid plasma levels may be increased.

Valproic acid plasma levels may be increased (as a result of reduced hepatic metabolism) in case of concomitant use with *cimetidine or erythromycin*.

Carbapenem antibiotics such as imipenem, panipenem and meropenem: Decrease in valproic acid blood level, sometimes associated with convulsions, has been observed when imipenem or meropenem were combined. If these antibiotics have to be administered, close monitoring of valproic acid blood levels is recommended.

Colestyramine may decrease the absorption of Epilim.

4.5.3 Other Interactions

Caution is advised when using Epilim in combination with newer anti-epileptics whose pharmacodynamics may not be well established.

Epilim usually has no enzyme-inducing effect; as a consequence, Epilim does not reduce efficacy of oestroprogestative agents in women receiving hormonal contraception, including the oral contraceptive pill.

Concomitant food intake does not significantly influence the bioavailability of sodium valproate when administered as the Chronosphere formulation.

4.6 Pregnancy and lactation

Women of childbearing potential should not be started on Epilim without specialist neurological advice.

Adequate counselling should be made available to all women with epilepsy of childbearing potential regarding the risks associated with pregnancy because of the potential teratogenic risk to the foetus (see also section 4.6.1). Women who are taking Epilim and who may become pregnant should receive specialist neurological advice and the benefits of its use should be weighed against the risks.

Epilim is the antiepileptic of choice in patients with certain types of epilepsy such as generalised epilepsy ± myoclonus/photosensitivity. For partial epilepsy, Epilim should be used only in patients resistant to other treatment.

If pregnancy is planned, consideration should be given to the cessation of Epilim treatment, if appropriate.

When Epilim treatment is deemed necessary, precautions to minimise the potential teratogenic risk should be followed. (See also section 4.6.1 paragraph entitled "In view of the above data".)

4.6.1 Pregnancy

From experience in treating mothers with epilepsy, the risk associated with the use of Epilim during pregnancy has been described as follows:

- Risk associated with epilepsy and antiepileptics

In offspring born to mothers with epilepsy receiving any anti-epileptic treatment, the overall rate of malformations has been demonstrated to be 2 to 3 times higher than the rate (approximately 3%) reported in the general population. An increased number of children with malformations have been reported in cases of multiple drug therapy. Malformations most frequently encountered are cleft lip and cardio-vascular malformations.

Epidemiological studies have suggested an association between in-utero exposure to Epilim and a risk of developmental delay. Developmental delay has been reported in children born to mothers with epilepsy. It is not possible to differentiate what may be due to genetic, social, environmental factors, maternal epilepsy or antiepileptic treatment. Notwithstanding those potential risks, no sudden discontinuation in the anti-epileptic therapy should be undertaken as this may lead to breakthrough seizures which could have serious consequences for both the mother and the foetus.

- Risk associated with valproate

In animals: teratogenic effects have been demonstrated in the mouse, rat and rabbit.

There is animal experimental evidence that high plasma peak levels and the size of an individual dose are associated with neural tube defects.

In humans:.

Valproate use is associated with neural tube defects such as myelomeningocele and spina bifida. The frequency of this effect is estimated to be 1 to 2%. An increased incidence of minor or major malformations including neural tube defects, craniofacial defects, malformations of the limbs, cardiovascular malformations, hypospadias and multiple anomalies involving various body systems has been reported in offspring born to mothers with epilepsy treated with valproate.

Some data from studies, of women with epilepsy, have suggested an association between in-utero exposure to valproate and the risk of developmental delay (frequently associated with craniofacial abnormalities), particularly of verbal IQ.

- In view of the above data

When a woman is planning pregnancy, this provides an opportunity to review the need for anti-epileptic treatment. Women of childbearing age should be informed of the risks and benefits of continuing anti-epileptic treatment throughout pregnancy.

Folate supplementation, **prior** to pregnancy, has been demonstrated to reduce the incidence of neural tube defects in the offspring of women at high risk. Although no direct evidence exists of such effects in women receiving anti-epileptic drugs, women should be advised to start taking folic acid supplementation (5mg) as soon as contraception is discontinued.

The available evidence suggests that anticonvulsant monotherapy is preferred. Dosage should be reviewed before conception and the lowest effective dose used, in divided doses, as abnormal pregnancy outcome tends to be associated with higher total daily dosage and with the size of an individual dose. The incidence of neural tube defects rises with increasing dosage, particularly above 1000mg daily. The administration in several divided doses over the day and the use of a prolonged release formulation is preferable in order to avoid high peak plasma levels.

During pregnancy, Epilim anti-epileptic treatment should not be discontinued if it has been effective.

Nevertheless, specialised prenatal monitoring should be instituted in order to detect the possible occurrence of a neural tube defect or any other malformation. Pregnancies should be carefully screened by ultrasound, and other techniques if appropriate (see Section 4.4 Special Warnings and Special Precautions for use).

- Risk in the neonate

Very rare cases of haemorrhagic syndrome have been reported in neonates whose mothers have taken Epilim during pregnancy. This haemorrhagic syndrome is related to hypofibrinogenemia; afibrinogenemia has also been reported and may be fatal. These are possibly associated with a decrease of coagulation factors. However, this syndrome has to be distinguished from the decrease of the vitamin-K factors induced by phenobarbital and other anti-epileptic enzyme inducing drugs.

Therefore, platelet count, fibrinogen plasma level, coagulation tests and coagulation factors should be investigated in neonates.

4.6.2 Lactation

Excretion of Epilim in breast milk is low, with a concentration between 1% to 10% of total maternal serum levels; up to now children breast fed that have been monitored during the neonatal period have not experienced clinical effects. There appears to be no contra-indication to breast feeding by patients on Epilim.

4.7 Effects on ability to drive and use machines

Use of Epilim may provide seizure control such that the patient may be eligible to hold a driving licence.

However, patients should be warned of the risk of transient drowsiness, especially in cases of anticonvulsant polytherapy or association with benzodiazepines (see section 4.5 Interactions with Other Medicaments and Other Forms of Interaction).

4.8 Undesirable effects

Congenital and familial/genetic disorders: (see section 4.6 Pregnancy and Lactation)

Hepato-biliary disorders: rare cases of liver dysfunction (see section 4.4.1 Warnings)

Severe liver damage, including hepatic failure sometimes resulting in death, has been reported (see also sections 4.2, 4.3 and 4.4.1). Increased liver enzymes are common, particularly early in treatment, and may be transient (see section 4.4.1).

Gastrointestinal disorders (nausea, gastralgia, diarrhoea) frequently occur at the start of treatment, but they usually disappear after a few days without discontinuing treatment. These problems can usually be overcome by taking Epilim with or after food, or by using Enteric Coated Epilim tablets.

Very rare cases of pancreatitis, sometimes lethal, have been reported (see section 4.4 Special Warnings and Special Precautions for Use).

Nervous system disorders:

Sedation has been reported occasionally, usually when in combination with other anticonvulsants. In monotherapy it occurred early in treatment on rare occasions, and is usually transient. Rare cases of lethargy and confusion, occasionally progressing to stupor, sometimes with associated hallucinations or convulsions, have been reported. Encephalopathy and coma have very rarely been observed. These cases have often been associated with too high a starting dose or too rapid a dose escalation, or concomitant use of other anticonvulsants, notably phenobarbital. They have usually been reversible on withdrawal of treatment or reduction of dosage.

Very rare cases of reversible extrapyramidal symptoms including parkinsonism, or reversible dementia associated with reversible cerebral atrophy, have been reported.

An increase in alertness may occur; this is generally beneficial, but occasionally aggression, hyperactivity and behavioural deterioration have been reported.

Metabolic disorders:

Cases of isolated and moderate hyperammonaemia without change in liver function tests may occur frequently, are usually transient and should not cause treatment discontinuation. However, they may present clinically as vomiting, ataxia, and increasing clouding of consciousness. Should these symptoms occur Epilim should be discontinued. Very rare cases of hyponatraemia have been reported.

Hyperammonaemia associated with neurological symptoms has also been reported (see section 4.4.2 Precautions). In such cases further investigations should be considered.

Blood and lymphatic system disorders:

Frequent occurrence of thrombocytopenia, rare cases of anaemia, leucopenia or pancytopenia. The blood picture returned to normal when the drug was discontinued. Isolated reduction of fibrinogen may also occur.

Isolated reduction of fibrinogen or reversible increase in bleeding time have been reported, usually without associated clinical signs and particularly with high doses (Epilim has an inhibitory effects on the second phase of platelet aggregation). Spontaneous bruising or bleeding is an indication for withdrawal of medication pending investigations (see also section 4.6 Pregnancy and Lactation).

Skin and subcutaneous tissue disorders:

Cutaneous reactions such as exanthematous rash rarely occur with Epilim. In very rare cases toxic epidermal necrolysis, Stevens-Johnson syndrome and erythema multiforme have been reported.

Transient hair loss, which may sometimes be dose-related, has often been reported. Regrowth normally begins within six months, although the hair may become more curly than previously. Hirsutism and acne have been very rarely reported.

Reproductive system and breast disorders:

Amenorrhoea and irregular periods have been reported. Very rarely gynaecomastia has occurred.

Vascular disorders:

The occurrence of vasculitis has occasionally been reported.

Ear disorders:

Hearing loss, either reversible or irreversible, has been reported rarely; however a cause and effect relationship has not been established.

Renal and urinary disorders:

There have been isolated reports of a reversible Fanconi's syndrome (a defect in proximal renal tubular function giving rise to glycosuria, amino aciduria, phosphaturia, and uricosuria) associated with Epilim therapy, but the mode of action is as yet unclear.

Very rare cases of enuresis have been reported.

Immune system disorders:

Allergic reactions (ranging from rash to hypersensitivity reactions) have been reported.

General disorders:

Very rare cases of non-severe peripheral oedema have been reported.

Increase in weight may also occur. Weight gain being a risk factor for polycystic ovary syndrome, it should be carefully monitored (see section 4.4 Special warnings and Special Precautions for Use).

4.9 Overdose

Cases of accidental and deliberate Epilim overdosage have been reported. At plasma concentrations of up to 5 to 6 times the maximum therapeutic levels, there are unlikely to be any symptoms other than nausea, vomiting and dizziness.

Signs of massive overdose, i.e. plasma concentration 10 to 20 times maximum therapeutic levels, usually include CNS depression or coma with muscular hypotonia, miosis, impaired respiratory function, metabolic acidosis.

Symptoms may however be variable and seizures have been reported in the presence of very high plasma levels (see also section 5.2 Pharmacokinetic Properties). Cases of intracranial hypertension related to cerebral oedema have been reported.

Hospital management of overdose should be symptomatic including cardio-respiratory monitoring. Gastric lavage may be useful up to 10 to 12 hours following ingestion.

Haemodialysis and haemoperfusion have been used successfully.

Naloxone has been successfully used in a few isolated cases, sometimes in association with activated charcoal given orally. Deaths have occurred following massive overdose; nevertheless a favourable outcome is usual.

5. PHARMACOLOGICAL PROPERTIES

5.1 Pharmacodynamic properties

Valproic acid pharmacotherapeutic group: Antiepileptics, Fatty acid derivatives.

ATC code N03A G01.

Sodium valproate and valproic acid are anticonvulsants.

The most likely mode of action for Epilim is potentiation of the inhibitory action of gamma amino butyric acid (GABA) through an action on the further synthesis or further metabolism of GABA.

In certain *in-vitro* studies it was reported that Epilim could stimulate HIV replication but studies on peripheral blood mononuclear cells from HIV-infected subjects show that Epilim does not have a mitogen-like effect on inducing HIV replication. Indeed the effect of Epilim on HIV replication *ex-vivo* is highly variable, modest in quantity, appears to be unrelated to the dose and has not been documented in man.

5.2 Pharmacokinetic properties

The half-life of Epilim is usually reported to be within the range of 8-20 hours. It is usually shorter in children.

In patients with severe renal insufficiency it may be necessary to alter dosage in accordance with free plasma valproic acid levels (see also section 4.2 Posology and Method of Administration).

The reported effective therapeutic range for plasma valproic acid levels is 40-100mg/litre (278-694 micromol/litre). This reported range may depend on time of sampling and presence of co-medication. The percentage of free (unbound) drug is usually between 6% and 15% of total plasma levels. An increased incidence of adverse effects may occur with plasma levels above the effective therapeutic range.

The pharmacological (or therapeutic) effects of Epilim Chronosphere may not be clearly correlated with the total or free (unbound) plasma valproic acid levels.

Epilim Chronosphere is a prolonged (or modified) release formulation of Epilim which reduces peak concentration and ensures more even plasma concentrations throughout the day, comparable with other modified release Epilim formulations.

Epilim Chronosphere has been shown to be bioequivalent to Epilim Chrono tablets. Compared with immediate release forms of Epilim, Epilim Chrono is characterized at an equivalent dose by:

- a similar bioavailability,
- a lower Cmax (decrease of approximately 25%),
- a relatively stable plateau between 4 and 14 hours after administration.
- Following twice daily administration, the range of plasma fluctuations is approximately reduced by half.

Steady-state pharmacokinetic data indicate that the peak concentration (Cmax) and trough concentration (Cmin) of Epilim Chronosphere lie within the effective therapeutic range of plasma levels found in pharmacokinetic studies with Epilim Enteric Coated tablets.

In cases where measurement of plasma levels is considered necessary, the pharmacokinetics of Epilim Chronosphere make the measurement of plasma levels less dependent upon time of sampling.

The peak plasma level is achieved approximately 7 hours after administration, with an elimination half life of approximately 16 hours.

This pharmacokinetic profile is not affected by taking the drug with food.

5.3 Preclinical safety data

There are no preclinical data of relevance to the prescriber which are additional to that already included in other sections of the SPC.

6. PHARMACEUTICAL PARTICULARS

6.1 List of excipients

Paraffin hard, glycerol dibehenate, silica colloidal hydrated.

6.2 Incompatibilities

This medicinal product must not be administered with hot meals or drinks.

6.3 Shelf life

24 months

6.4 Special precautions for storage

Do not store above 25°C. Store in the original packaging. Do not refrigerate of freeze.

6.5 Nature and contents of container

Epilim Chronosphere MR modified release granules are filled into sachets of a paper/aluminium/ionomer resin complex.

Epilim Chronosphere sachets are available in cartons of 30 sachets.

6.6 Special precautions for disposal and other handling

See 4.2. Posology and Method of Administration.

This medicinal product must not be administered with hot meals or drinks.

7. MARKETING AUTHORISATION HOLDER

Sanofi-aventis Limited

One Onslow Street

Guildford

Surrey GU1 4YS

8. MARKETING AUTHORISATION NUMBER(S)

Epilim Chronosphere MR 50mg modified release granules - PL 04425/0310

Epilim Chronosphere MR 100mg modified release granules - PL 04425/0312

Epilim Chronosphere MR 250mg modified release granules - PL 04425/0313

Epilim Chronosphere MR 500mg modified release granules - PL 04425/0314

Epilim Chronosphere MR 750mg modified release granules - PL 04425/0315

Epilim Chronosphere MR 1000mg modified release granules - PL 04425/0316

9. DATE OF FIRST AUTHORISATION/RENEWAL OF THE AUTHORISATION

5 February 2009

10. DATE OF REVISION OF THE TEXT

5 February 2009

Legal category: POM

Epilim Intravenous

(sanofi-aventis)

1. NAME OF THE MEDICINAL PRODUCT

Epilim Intravenous

2. QUALITATIVE AND QUANTITATIVE COMPOSITION

Each vial contains 400mg of Sodium Valproate freeze-dried powder.

3. PHARMACEUTICAL FORM

Powder for Injection or Intravenous Infusions

4. CLINICAL PARTICULARS

4.1 Therapeutic indications

The treatment of epileptic patients who would normally be maintained on oral sodium valproate, and for whom oral therapy is temporarily not possible.

4.2 Posology and method of administration

Epilim Intravenous may be given by direct slow intravenous injection or by infusion using a separate intravenous line in normal saline, dextrose 5%, or dextrose saline.

Dosage

Daily dosage requirements vary according to age and body weight.

To reconstitute, inject the solvent provided (4ml) into the vial, allow to dissolve and extract the appropriate dose. Due to displacement of solvent by sodium valproate the concentration of reconstituted sodium valproate is 95mg/ml.

Each vial of Epilim Intravenous is for single dose injection only. It should be reconstituted immediately prior to use and infusion solutions containing it used within 24 hours. Any unused portion should be discarded. (See section 6.6).

Epilim Intravenous should not be administered via the same IV line as other IV additives. The intravenous solution is suitable for infusion by PVC, polyethylene or glass containers.

Patients already satisfactorily treated with Epilim may be continued at their current dosage using continuous or repeated infusion. Other patients may be given a slow intravenous injection over 3-5 minutes, usually 400-800mg depending on body weight (up to 10mg/kg) followed by continuous or repeated infusion up to a maximum of 2500mg/day.

Epilim Intravenous should be replaced by oral Epilim therapy as soon as practicable.

Use with children

Daily requirement for children is usually in the range 20-30mg/kg/day and method of administration is as above. Where adequate control is not achieved within this range the dose may be increased up to 40mg/kg/day but only in patients in whom plasma valproic acid levels can be monitored. Above 40mg/kg/day clinical chemistry and haematological parameters should be monitored.

Use in the elderly

Although the pharmacokinetics of Epilim are modified in the elderly, they have limited clinical significance and dosage should be determined by seizure control. The volume of distribution is increased in the elderly and because of decreased binding to serum albumin, the proportion of free drug is increased. This will affect the clinical interpretation of plasma valproic acid levels.

In patients with renal insufficiency

It may be necessary to decrease the dosage. Dosage should be adjusted according to clinical monitoring since monitoring of plasma concentrations may be misleading (see section 5.2 Pharmacokinetic Properties).

In patients with hepatic insufficiency

Salicylates should not be used concomitantly with Epilim since they employ the same metabolic pathway (see also sections 4.4 Special Warnings and Precautions for Use and 4.8 Undesirable Effects).

Liver dysfunction, including hepatic failure resulting in fatalities, has occurred in patients whose treatment included valproic acid (see sections 4.3 Containdications and 4.4 Special Warnings and Precautions for Use).

Salicylates should not be used in children under 16 years (see aspirin/salicylate product information on Reye's syndrome). In addition in conjunction with Epilim, concomitant use in children under 3 years can increase the risk of liver toxicity (see section 4.4.1 Special warnings).

Combined Therapy

When starting Epilim in patients already on other anticonvulsants, these should be tapered slowly: initiation of Epilim therapy should then be gradual, with target dose being reached after about 2 weeks. In certain cases it may be necessary to raise the dose by 5 to 10mg/kg/day when used in combination with anticonvulsants which induce liver enzyme activity, e.g. phenytoin, phenobarbital and carbamazepine. Once known enzyme inducers have been withdrawn it may be possible to maintain seizure control on a reduced dose of Epilim. When barbiturates are being administered concomitantly and particularly if sedation is observed (particularly in children) the dosage of barbiturate should be reduced.

NB: In children requiring doses higher than 40mg/kg/day clinical chemistry and haematological parameters should be monitored.

Optimum dosage is mainly determined by seizure control and routine measurement of plasma levels is unnecessary. However, a method for measurement of plasma levels is available and may be helpful where there is poor control or side effects are suspected (see section 5.2 Pharmacokinetic Properties).

4.3 Contraindications

- Active liver disease
- Personal or family history of severe hepatic dysfunction, especially drug related
- Hypersensitivity to sodium valproate
- Porphyria

4.4 Special warnings and precautions for use

Although there is no specific evidence of sudden recurrence of underlying symptoms following withdrawal of valproate, discontinuation should normally only be done under the supervision of a specialist in a gradual manner. This is due to the possibility of sudden alterations in plasma concentrations giving rise to a recurrence of symptoms. NICE has advised that generic switching of valproate preparations is not normally recommended due to the clinical implications of possible variations in plasma concentrations.

4.4.1 Special warnings

Liver dysfunction:

Conditions of occurrence:

Severe liver damage, including hepatic failure sometimes resulting in fatalities, has been very rarely reported. Experience in epilepsy has indicated that patients most at risk, especially in cases of multiple anticonvulsant therapy, are infants and in particular young children under the age of 3 and those with severe seizure disorders, organic brain disease, and (or) congenital metabolic or degenerative disease associated with mental retardation.

After the age of 3, the incidence of occurrence is significantly reduced and progressively decreases with age.

The concomitant use of salicylates should be avoided in children under 3 due to the risk of liver toxicity. Additionally, salicylates should not be used in children under 16 years (see aspirin/salicylate product information on Reye's syndrome).

Monotherapy is recommended in children under the age of 3 years when prescribing Epilim, but the potential benefit of Epilim should be weighed against the risk of liver damage or pancreatitis in such patients prior to initiation of therapy.

In most cases, such liver damage occurred during the first 6 months of therapy, the period of maximum risk being 2-12 weeks.

Suggestive signs:

Clinical symptoms are essential for early diagnosis. In particular the following conditions, which may precede jaundice, should be taken into consideration, especially in patients at risk (see above: 'Conditions of occurrence'):

- non specific symptoms, usually of sudden onset, such as asthenia, malaise, anorexia, lethargy, oedema and drowsiness, which are sometimes associated with repeated vomiting and abdominal pain.

- in patients with epilepsy, recurrence of seizures.

These are an indication for immediate withdrawal of the drug.

Patients (or their family for children) should be instructed to report immediately any such signs to a physician should they occur. Investigations including clinical examination and biological assessment of liver function should be undertaken immediately.

Detection:

Liver function should be measured before and then periodically monitored during the first 6 months of therapy, especially in those who seem most at risk, and those with a prior history of liver disease.

Amongst usual investigations, tests which reflect protein synthesis, particularly prothrombin rate, are most relevant.

Confirmation of an abnormally low prothrombin rate, particularly in association with other biological abnormalities (significant decrease in fibrinogen and coagulation factors; increased bilirubin level and raised transaminases) requires cessation of Epilim therapy.

As a matter of precaution and in case they are taken concomitantly salicylates should also be discontinued since they employ the same metabolic pathway.

As with most antiepileptic drugs, increased liver enzymes are common, particularly at the beginning of therapy; they are also transient.

More extensive biological investigations (including prothrombin rate) are recommended in these patients; a reduction in dosage may be considered when appropriate and tests should be repeated as necessary.

Pancreatitis: Pancreatitis, which may be severe and result in fatalities, has been very rarely reported. Patients experiencing nausea, vomiting or acute abdominal pain should have a prompt medical evaluation (including measurement of serum amylase). Young children are at particular risk; this risk decreases with increasing age. Severe seizures and severe neurological impairment with combination anticonvulsant therapy may be risk factors. Hepatic failure with pancreatitis increases the risk of fatal outcome. In case of pancreatitis, Epilim should be discontinued.

4.4.2 Precautions

Haematological: Blood tests (blood cell count, including platelet count, bleeding time and coagulation tests) are recommended prior to initiation of therapy or before surgery, and in case of spontaneous bruising or bleeding (see section 4.8 Undesirable Effects).

Renal insufficiency: In patients with renal insufficiency, it may be necessary to decrease dosage. As monitoring of plasma concentrations may be misleading, dosage should be adjusted according to clinical monitoring (see sections 4.2 Posology and Method of Adminstration and 5.2. Pharmacokinetic Properties).

Systemic lupus erythematosus: Although immune disorders have only rarely been noted during the use of Epilim, the potential benefit of Epilim should be weighed against its potential risk in patients with systemic lupus erythematosus (see also section 4.8 Undesirable Effects).

Hyperammonaemia: When a urea cycle enzymatic deficiency is suspected, metabolic investigations should be performed prior to treatment because of the risk of hyperammonaemia with Epilim.

Weight gain: Epilim very commonly causes weight gain, which may be marked and progressive. Patients should be warned of the risk of weight gain at the initiation of therapy and appropriate strategies should be adopted to minimise it (see section 4.8 Undesirable Effects).

Pregnancy: Women of childbearing potential should not be started on Epilim without specialist neurological advice. Adequate counselling should be made available to all women with epilepsy of childbearing potential regarding the risks associated with pregnancy because of the potential teratogenic risk to the foetus (see also section 4.6 Pregnancy and Lactation).

Diabetic patients: Epilim is eliminated mainly through the kidneys, partly in the form of ketone bodies; this may give false positives in the urine testing of possible diabetics.

4.5 Interaction with other medicinal products and other forms of interaction

4.5.1 Effects of Epilim on other drugs

- Antipsychotics, MAO inhibitors, antidepressants and benzodiazepines

Epilim may potentiate the effect of other psychotropics such as antipsychotics, MAO inhibitors, antidepressants and benzodiazepines; therefore, clinical monitoring is advised and the dosage of the other psychotropics should be adjusted when appropriate.

In particular, a clinical study has suggested that adding olanzapine to valproate or lithium therapy may significantly increase the risk of certain adverse events associated with olanzapine e.g. neutropenia, tremor, dry mouth, increased appetite and weight gain, speech disorder and somnolence.

- Phenobarbital

Epilim increases phenobarbital plasma concentrations (due to inhibition of hepatic catabolism) and sedation may occur, particularly in children. Therefore, clinical monitoring is recommended throughout the first 15 days of combined treatment with immediate reduction of phenobarbital doses if sedation occurs and determination of phenobarbital plasma levels when appropriate.

- Primidone

Epilim increases primidone plasma levels with exacerbation of its adverse effects (such as sedation); these signs cease with long term treatment. Clinical monitoring is recommended especially at the beginning of combined therapy with dosage adjustment when appropriate.

- Phenytoin

Epilim decreases phenytoin total plasma concentration. Moreover Epilim increases phenytoin free form with possible overdosage symptoms (valproic acid displaces phenytoin from its plasma protein binding sites and reduces its hepatic catabolism). Therefore clinical monitoring is recommended; when phenytoin plasma levels are determined, the free form should be evaluated.

- Carbamazepine

Clinical toxicity has been reported when Epilim was administered with carbamazepine as Epilim may potentiate toxic effects of carbamazepine. Clinical monitoring is recommended especially at the beginning of combined therapy with dosage adjustment when appropriate.

- Lamotrigine

Epilim may reduce lamotrigine metabolism and increase its mean half-life, dosages should be adjusted (lamotrigine dosage decreased) when appropriate. Co-administration of lamotrigine and Epilim might increase the risk of rash.

- Zidovudine

Epilim may raise zidovudine plasma concentration leading to increased zidovudine toxicity.

- Vitamin K-dependent anticoagulants

The anticoagulant effect of warfarin and other coumarin anticoagulants may be increased following displacement from plasma protein binding sites by valproic acid. The prothrombin time should be closely monitored.

- Temozolomide

Co-administration of temozolomide and Epilim may cause a small decrease in the clearance of temozolomide that is not thought to be clinically relevant.

4.5.2 Effects of other drugs on Epilim

Antiepileptics with enzyme inducing effect (including ***phenytoin, phenobarbital, carbamazepine***) decrease valproic acid plasma concentrations. Dosages should be adjusted according to blood levels in case of combined therapy.

On the other hand, combination of ***felbamate*** and Epilim may increase valproic acid plasma concentration. Epilim dosage should be monitored.

Mefloquine and ***chloroquine*** increase valproic acid metabolism and may lower the seizure threshold; therefore epileptic seizures may occur in cases of combined therapy. Accordingly, the dosage of Epilim may need adjustment.

In case of concomitant use of Epilim and ***highly protein bound agents (e.g. aspirin)***, free valproic acid plasma levels may be increased.

Valproic acid plasma levels may be increased (as a result of reduced hepatic metabolism) in case of concomitant use with ***cimetidine*** or ***erythromycin***.

Carbapenem antibiotics such as ***imipenem, panipenem*** and ***meropenem***: Decrease in valproic acid blood level, sometimes associated with convulsions, has been observed when imipenem or meropenem were combined. If these antibiotics have to be administered, close monitoring of valproic acid blood levels is recommended.

Colestyramine may decrease the absorption of Epilim.

4.5.3 Other Interactions

Caution is advised when using Epilim in combination with newer anti-epileptics whose pharmacodynamics may not be well established.

Epilim usually has no enzyme-inducing effect; as a consequence, Epilim does not reduce efficacy of oestroprogestative agents in women receiving hormonal contraception, including the oral contraceptive pill.

4.6 Pregnancy and lactation

Women of childbearing potential should not be started on Epilim without specialist neurological advice.

Adequate counselling should be made available to all women with epilepsy of childbearing potential regarding the risks associated with pregnancy because of the potential teratogenic risk to the foetus (See also section 4.6.1). Women who are taking Epilim and who may become pregnant should receive specialist neurological advice and the benefits of its use should be weighed against the risks.

Epilim is the antiepileptic of choice in patients with certain types of epilepsy such as generalised epilepsy ± myoclonus/photosensitivity. For partial epilepsy, Epilim should be used only in patients resistant to other treatment.

If pregnancy is planned, consideration should be given to cessation of Epilim treatment, if appropriate.

When Epilim treatment is deemed necessary, precautions to minimize the potential teratogenic risk should be followed. (See also section 4.6.1 paragraph entitled "In view of the above")

4.6.1 Pregnancy

From experience in treating mothers with epilepsy, the risk associated with the use of Epilim during pregnancy has been described as follows:

- Risk associated with epilepsy and antiepileptics

In offspring born to mothers with epilepsy receiving any anti-epileptic treatment, the overall rate of malformations has been demonstrated to be 2 to 3 times higher than the rate (approximately 3 %) reported in the general population. An increased number of children with malformations have been reported in cases of multiple drug therapy. Malformations most frequently encountered are cleft lip and cardio-vascular malformations.

Epidemiological studies have suggested an association between in-utero exposure to Epilim and a risk of developmental delay. Developmental delay has been reported in children born to mothers with epilepsy. It is not possible to differentiate what may be due to genetic, social, environmental factors, maternal epilepsy or antiepileptic treatment. Notwithstanding those potential risks, no sudden discontinuation in the anti-epileptic therapy should be undertaken as this may lead to breakthrough seizures which could have serious consequences for both the mother and the foetus.

- Risk associated with valproate

In animals: teratogenic effects have been demonstrated in the mouse, rat and rabbit.

There is animal experimental evidence that high plasma peak levels and the size of an individual dose are associated with neural tube defects.

In humans: Valproate use is associated with neural tube defects such as myelomeningocele and spina bifida. The frequency of this effect is estimated to be 1 to 2%. An increased incidence of minor or major malformations including neural tube defects, craniofacial defects, malformation of the limbs, cardiovascular malformations, hypospadias and multiple anomalies involving various body systems has been reported in offspring born to mothers with epilepsy treated with valproate. Some data from studies, of women with epilepsy, have suggested an association between in-utero exposure to valproate and the risk of developmental delay (frequently associated with craniofacial abnormalities), particularly of verbal IQ.

- In view of the above data

When a woman is planning pregnancy, this provides an opportunity to review the need for anti-epileptic treatment. Women of childbearing age should be informed of the risks and benefits of continuing anti-epileptic treatment throughout pregnancy.

Folate supplementation, **prior** to pregnancy, has been demonstrated to reduce the incidence of neural tube defects in the offspring of women at high risk. Although no direct evidence exists of such effects in women receiving anti-epileptic drugs, women should be advised to start taking folic acid supplementation (5mg) as soon as contraception is discontinued.

The available evidence suggests that anticonvulsant monotherapy is preferred. Dosage should be reviewed before conception and the lowest effective dose used, in divided doses, as abnormal pregnancy outcome tends to be associated with higher total daily dosage and with the size of an individual dose. The incidence of neural tube defects rises with increasing dosage, particularly above 1000mg daily. The administration in several divided doses over the day and the use of a prolonged release formulation is preferable in order to avoid high peak plasma levels.

During pregnancy, Epilim anti-epileptic treatment should not be discontinued if it has been effective.

Nevertheless, specialised prenatal monitoring should be instituted in order to detect the possible occurrence of a neural tube defect or any other malformation. Pregnancies should be carefully screened by ultrasound, and other techniques if appropriate (see Section 4.4 Special Warnings and Special Precautions for use).

- Risk in the neonate

Very rare cases of haemorrhagic syndrome have been reported in neonates whose mothers have taken Epilim during pregnancy. This haemorrhagic syndrome is related to hypofibrinogenemia; afibrinogenemia has also been reported and may be fatal. These are possibly associated with a decrease of coagulation factors. However, this syndrome has to be distinguished from the decrease of the vitamin-K factors induced by phenobarbital and other anti-epileptic enzyme inducing drugs.

Therefore, platelet count, fibrinogen plasma level, coagulation tests and coagulation factors should be investigated in neonates.

4.6.2 Lactation

Excretion of Epilim in breast milk is low, with a concentration between 1 % to 10 % of total maternal serum levels; up to now children breast fed that have been monitored during the neonatal period have not experienced clinical effects. There appears to be no contra-indication to breast feeding by patients on Epilim.

4.7 Effects on ability to drive and use machines

Not applicable - use of intravenous formulation restricted to patients unable to take oral therapy. However, note use of Epilim may provide seizure control such that the patient may again be eligible to hold a driving licence.

Patients should be warned of the risk of transient drowsiness, especially in cases of anticonvulsant polytherapy or association with benzodiazepines (see section 4.5 Interactions with Other Medicaments and Other Forms of Interaction).

4.8 Undesirable effects

Congenital and familial/genetic disorders: (see section 4.6 Pregnancy and Lactation)

Hepato-biliary disorders:

Rare cases of liver dysfunction (see section 4.4.1 Warnings) Severe liver damage, including hepatic failure sometimes resulting in death, has been reported (see also sections 4.2, 4.3 and 4.4.1). Increased liver enzymes are common, particularly early in treatment, and may be transient (see section 4.4.1).

Gastrointestinal disorders: (nausea, gastralgia, diarrhoea)

Frequently occur at the start of treatment, but they usually disappear after a few days without discontinuing treatment. These problems can usually be overcome by taking Epilim with or after food or by using Enteric Coated Epilim.

Very rare cases of pancreatitis, sometimes lethal, have been reported (see section 4.4 Special Warnings and Special Precautions for Use).

Nervous system disorders:

Sedation has been reported occasionally, usually when in combination with other anticonvulsants. In monotherapy it occurred early in treatment on rare occasions and is usually transient. Rare cases of lethargy and confusion occasionally progressing to stupor, sometimes with associated hallucinations or convulsions have been reported. Encephalopathy and coma have very rarely been observed. These cases have often been associated with too high a starting dose or too rapid a dose escalation or concomitant use of other anticonvulsants, notably phenobarbital. They have usually been reversible on withdrawal of treatment or reduction of dosage.

Very rare cases of reversible extrapyramidal symptoms including parkinsonism, or reversible dementia associated with reversible cerebral atrophy have been reported. Dose-related ataxia and fine postural tremor have occasionally been reported.

An increase in alertness may occur; this is generally beneficial but occasionally aggression, hyperactivity and behavioural deterioration have been reported.

Metabolic disorders:

Cases of isolated and moderate hyperammonaemia without change in liver function tests may occur frequently, are usually transient and should not cause treatment discontinuation. However, they may present clinically as vomiting, ataxia, and increasing clouding of consciousness. Should these symptoms occur Epilim should be discontinued. Very rare cases of hyponatraemia have been reported.

Hyperammonaemia associated with neurological symptoms has also been reported (see section 4.4.2 Precautions). In such cases further investigations should be considered.

Blood and lymphatic system disorders:

Frequent occurrence of thrombocytopenia, rare cases of anaemia, leucopenia or pancytopenia. The blood picture returned to normal when the drug was discontinued.

Isolated reduction of fibrinogen or reversible increase in bleeding time have been reported, usually without associated clinical signs and particularly with high doses (Epilim has an inhibitory effect on the second phase of platelet aggregation). Spontaneous bruising or bleeding is an indication for withdrawal of medication pending investigations (see also section 4.6 Pregnancy and Lactation).

Skin and subcutaneous tissue disorders:

Cutaneous reactions such as exanthematous rash rarely occur with Epilim. In very rare cases toxic epidermal necrolysis, Stevens-Johnson syndrome and erythema multiforme have been reported.

Transient hair loss, which may sometimes be dose-related, has often been reported. Regrowth normally begins within six months, although the hair may become more curly than previously. Hirsutism and acne have been very rarely reported.

Reproductive system and breast disorders:

Amenorrhoea and irregular periods have been reported. Very rarely gynaecomastia has occurred.

Vascular disorders:

The occurrence of vasculitis has occasionally been reported.

Ear disorders:

Hearing loss, either reversible or irreversible has been reported rarely; however a cause and effect relationship has not been established.

Renal and urinary disorders:

There have been isolated reports of a reversible Fanconi's syndrome (a defect in proximal renal tubular function giving rise to glycosuria, amino aciduria, phosphaturia, and uricosuria) associated with Epilim therapy, but the mode of action is as yet unclear.

Very rare cases of enuresis have been reported

Immune system disorders:

Allergic reactions (ranging from rash to hypersensitivity reactions) have been reported.

General disorders and administration site conditions:

Very rare cases of non-severe peripheral oedema have been reported.

Increase in weight may also occur. Weight gain being a risk factor for polycystic ovary syndrome, it should be carefully monitored (see section 4.4 Special Warnings and Special Precautions for Use).

When using Epilim intravenously, nausea or dizziness may occur a few minutes after injection; they disappear spontaneously within a few minutes.

4.9 Overdose

Cases of accidental and deliberate Epilim overdosage have been reported. At plasma concentrations of up to 5 to 6 times the maximum therapeutic levels, there are unlikely to be any symptoms other than nausea, vomiting and dizziness.

Signs of massive overdose, i.e. plasma concentration 10 to 20 times maximum therapeutic levels, usually include CNS depression or coma with muscular hypotonia, hyporeflexia, miosis, impaired respiratory function, metabolic acidosis.

Symptoms may however be variable and seizures have been reported in the presence of very high plasma levels (see also section 5.2 Pharmacokinetic Properties).

Cases of intracranial hypertension related to cerebral oedema have been reported.

Hospital management of overdose should be symptomatic, including cardio-respiratory monitoring. Gastric lavage may be useful up to 10 to 12 hours following ingestion.

Haemodialysis and haemoperfusion have been used successfully.

Naloxone has been successfully used in a few isolated cases, sometimes in association with activated charcoal given orally. Deaths have occurred following massive overdose; nevertheless, a favourable outcome is usual.

5. PHARMACOLOGICAL PROPERTIES

5.1 Pharmacodynamic properties

Sodium valproate is an anticonvulsant.

In certain *in-vitro* studies it was reported that Epilim could stimulate HIV replication but studies on peripheral blood mononuclear cells from HIV-infected subjects show that Epilim does not have a mitogen-like effect on inducing HIV replication. Indeed the effect of Epilim on HIV replication *ex-vivo* is highly variable, modest in quantity, appears to be unrelated to the dose and has not been documented in man.

5.2 Pharmacokinetic properties

The half-life of Epilim is usually reported to be within the range 8-20 hours. It is usually shorter in children.

In patients with severe renal insufficiency it may be necessary to alter dosage in accordance with free plasma valproic acid levels.

The reported effective therapeutic range for plasma valproic acid levels is 40-100mg/litre (278-694 micromol/litre). This reported range may depend on time of sampling and presence of co-medication. The percentage of free (unbound) drug is usually between 6% and 15% of the total plasma levels. An increased incidence of adverse effects may occur with plasma levels above the effective therapeutic range.

The pharmacological (or therapeutic) effects of Epilim may not be clearly correlated with the total or free (unbound) plasma valproic acid levels.

5.3 Preclinical safety data

There are no pre-clinical data of relevance to the prescriber which are additional to that already included in other sections of the SPC.

6. PHARMACEUTICAL PARTICULARS

6.1 List of excipients

None.

6.2 Incompatibilities

Epilim Intravenous should not be administered via the same line as other IV additives.

6.3 Shelf life

60 months as unopened vial of freeze-dried powder. 24 hours after reconstitution and dilution for use as infusion solution (See Section 6.4 and 6.6).

6.4 Special precautions for storage

Epilim freeze-dried powder: No specific storage conditions.

Reconstituted infusion solutions: at 2-8°C if stored before use, discarding any remaining solution after 24 hours.

6.5 Nature and contents of container

Colourless glass vial (Type I) with chlorobutyl rubber closure and crimped with an aluminium cap. The vial is supplied packed in a carbord carton along with one ampoule containing 4ml of solvent (Water for Injection).

6.6 Special precautions for disposal and other handling

For intravenous use, the reconstituted solution should be used immediately and any unused portion discarded.

If the reconstituted solution is further diluted for use as an infusion solution, the dilute solution may be stored for up to 24 hours if kept at 2 to 8°C before use, discarding any remaining after 24 hours.

7. MARKETING AUTHORISATION HOLDER

sanofi-aventis

One Onslow Street

Guildford

Surrey

GU1 4YS

8. MARKETING AUTHORISATION NUMBER(S)

PL 11723/0022

9. DATE OF FIRST AUTHORISATION/RENEWAL OF THE AUTHORISATION

18 August 1993

10. DATE OF REVISION OF THE TEXT

16 January 2009

Legal Status

POM

Epinephrine (Adrenaline) Injection 1:10,000

(International Medication Systems (UK) Ltd)

1. NAME OF THE MEDICINAL PRODUCT

Adrenaline (Epinephrine) 1:10,000 Sterile Solution Minijet®.

2. QUALITATIVE AND QUANTITATIVE COMPOSITION

Adrenaline (Epinephrine) USP 0.1mg per ml.

3. PHARMACEUTICAL FORM

Sterile aqueous solution for parenteral administration.

4. CLINICAL PARTICULARS

4.1 Therapeutic indications

Adjunctive use in the management of cardiac arrest.

In cardiopulmonary resuscitation. Intracardiac puncture and intramyocardial injection of adrenaline may be effective when external cardiac compression and attempts to restore the circulation by electrical defibrillation or use of a pacemaker fail.

4.2 Posology and method of administration

Ventricular fibrillation (pulseless ventricular tachycardia)

Adults:

Intravenous injection: 10ml (1mg) by intravenous injection repeated every 2-3 minutes as necessary.

Endotracheal: 20-30ml (2-3mg) via an endotracheal tube, repeated as necessary.

Intracardiac injection: 1 to 10ml (0.1 to 1mg), direct into the atrium of the heart.

Intracardiac injection should only be considered if there is no other access available. It should be undertaken by personnel trained in the technique.

Children:

Intravenous injection: Initially 0.1ml/kg body weight (10mcg/kg); e.g. 2kg infant would receive 0.2ml of Adrenaline 1:10,000. Subsequent doses should be 1ml/kg (100mcg/kg).

Intraosseous: 0.1ml/kg body weight (10mcg/kg).

Endotracheal: A dose has not been established; 10 times the intravenous dose may be appropriate.

Asystole

Adults:

Intravenous: 10ml (1mg) by intravenous injection repeated every 2-3 minutes as necessary. If there is no response after three cycles, consider injections of adrenaline 5mg.

Endotracheal: 20-30 ml (2-3mg) via an endotracheal tube, repeated as necessary.

Children:

Intravenous: 0.1ml/kg initially (10mcg/kg). If no response give 1ml/kg (100mcg/kg). After 3 cycles consider alkalising or antiarrhythmic agents.

Intraosseus: 0.1 ml/kg initially (10mcg/kg). If no response give 1ml/kg (100mcg/kg). After 3 cycles consider alkalising or antiarrhythmic agents.

Electromechanical Dissociation (EMD)

Adults:

Intravenous: 10ml (1mg) by intravenous injection repeated every 2-3 minutes as necessary. If normal rhythm does not return after standard measures, consider adrenaline 5mg intravenous.

Children:

Intravenous: 0.1ml/kg initially (10mcg/kg) every 3 minutes, until underlying cause identified. Subsequent doses should be 1ml/kg (100mcg/kg).

4.3 Contraindications

Contraindications are relative as this product is intended for use in life-threatening emergencies.

Other than in the emergency situation, the following contraindications should be considered: hyperthyroidism, hypertension, ischaemic heart disease, diabetes mellitus and closed angle glaucoma.

4.4 Special warnings and precautions for use

These special warnings and precautions are relative as this product is intended for use in life-threatening situations.

Administer slowly with caution to elderly patients and to patients with ischaemic heart disease, hypertension, diabetes mellitus, hyperthyroidism or psychoneurosis. Use with extreme caution in patients with long-standing bronchial asthma and emphysema who have developed degenerative heart disease. Anginal pain may be induced when coronary insufficiency is present.

4.5 Interaction with other medicinal products and other forms of interaction

The effects of adrenaline may be potentiated by tricyclic antidepressants. Volatile liquid anaesthetics such as halothane increase the risk of adrenaline-induced ventricular arrhythmias and acute pulmonary oedema if hypoxia is present. Severe hypertension and bradycardia may occur with non-selective beta-blocking drugs such as propranolol. Propranolol also inhibits the bronchodilator effect of adrenaline. The risk of cardiac arrhythmias is higher when adrenaline is given to patients receiving digoxin or quinidine. Adrenaline -induced hyperglycaemia may lead to loss of blood-sugar control in diabetic patients treated with hypoglycaemic agents.

The vasoconstrictor and pressor effects of adrenaline, mediated by its alpha-adrenergic action, may be enhanced by concomitant administration of drugs with similar effects, such as ergot alkaloids or oxytocin. Adrenaline specifically reverses the antihypertensive effects of adrenergic neurone blockers such as guanethidine with the risk of severe hypertension.

4.6 Pregnancy and lactation

Adrenaline crosses the placenta. There is some evidence of a slightly increased incidence of congenital abnormalities. Injection of adrenaline may cause foetal tachycardia, cardiac irregularities, extrasystoles and louder heart sounds. In labour, adrenaline may delay the second stage. Adrenaline should only be used in pregnancy if the potential benefits outweigh the risks to the foetus.

Adrenaline is excreted in breast milk, but as pharmacologically active plasma concentrations are not achieved by the oral route, the use of adrenaline in breast feeding mothers is presumed to be safe.

4.7 Effects on ability to drive and use machines

Not applicable; this preparation is intended for use only in emergencies.

4.8 Undesirable effects

The potentially severe adverse effects of adrenaline arise from its effect upon blood pressure and cardiac rhythm. Ventricular fibrillation may occur and severe hypertension may lead to cerebral haemorrhage and pulmonary oedema. Symptomatic adverse effects are anxiety, dyspnoea, restlessness, palpitations, tachycardia, anginal pain, tremor, weakness, dizziness, headache and cold extremities. Biochemical effects include inhibition of insulin secretion, stimulation of growth hormone secretion, hyperglycaemia (even with low doses), gluconeogenesis, glycolysis, lipolysis and ketogenesis.

4.9 Overdose

Symptoms: cardiac arrhythmias leading to ventricular fibrillation and death; severe hypertension leading to pulmonary oedema and cerebral haemorrhage.

Treatment: combined alpha- and beta-adrenergic blocking agents such as labetalol may counteract the effects of adrenaline, or a beta-blocking agent may be used to treat any supraventricular arrhythmias and phentolamine to control the alpha-mediated effects on the peripheral circulation. Rapidly acting vasodilators such as nitrates and sodium nitroprusside may also be helpful.

Immediate resuscitation support must be available.

5. PHARMACOLOGICAL PROPERTIES

5.1 Pharmacodynamic properties

Adrenaline is a direct-acting sympathomimetic agent exerting its effect on alpha- and beta-adrenoceptors. The overall effect of adrenaline depends on the dose used, and may be complicated by the homeostatic reflex responses. In resuscitation procedures it is used to increase the efficacy of basic life support. It is a positive cardiac inotrope. Major effects are increased systolic blood pressure, reduced diastolic pressure(increased at higher doses), tachycardia, hyperglycaemia and hypokalaemia.

5.2 Pharmacokinetic properties

Adrenaline is rapid in onset and of short duration. After i.v. infusion the half-life is approximately 5-10 minutes. It is rapidly distributed to the heart, spleen, several glandular tissues and adrenergic nerves. It crosses the placenta and is excreted in breast milk. It is approximately 50% bound to plasma proteins.

Adrenaline is rapidly metabolised in the liver and tissues by oxidative deamination and O-methylation followed by reduction or by conjugation with glucuronic acid or sulphate. Up to 90% of the i.v. dose is excreted in the urine as metabolites.

5.3 Preclinical safety data

Not applicable since Adrenaline (Epinephrine) Injection has been used in clinical practice for many years and its effects in man are well known.

6. PHARMACEUTICAL PARTICULARS

6.1 List of excipients

Citric Acid Monohydrate

Sodium Citrate Dihydrate

Sodium Chloride

Sodium Bisulphite

Hydrochloric Acid 10%w/v

Water for Injection

6.2 Incompatibilities

Adrenaline should not be mixed with sodium bicarbonate; the solution is oxidised to adrenochrome and then forms polymers.

6.3 Shelf life

3ml - 18 months.

10ml - 24 months.

6.4 Special precautions for storage

Do not store above 25°C. Keep container in outer carton.

6.5 Nature and contents of container

The solution is contained in a USP type I glass vial with an elastomeric closure which meets all the relevant USP specifications. The product is available either as 3ml or 10ml.

6.6 Special precautions for disposal and other handling

The container is specially designed for use with the IMS Minijet injector.

7. MARKETING AUTHORISATION HOLDER

International Medication Systems (UK) Ltd

208 Bath Road

Slough

Berkshire

SL1 3WE

UK

8. MARKETING AUTHORISATION NUMBER(S)

PL 03265/0011R

9. DATE OF FIRST AUTHORISATION/RENEWAL OF THE AUTHORISATION

21 March 1991 / 30 August 2001

10. DATE OF REVISION OF THE TEXT

14 October 2005

POM

Epinephrine (Adrenaline) Injection 1:1000 Minijet

(International Medication Systems (UK) Ltd)

1. NAME OF THE MEDICINAL PRODUCT

Adrenaline (Epinephrine) Injection 1:1,000 Minijet.

2. QUALITATIVE AND QUANTITATIVE COMPOSITION

Adrenaline (Epinephrine) 1mg per ml.

3. PHARMACEUTICAL FORM

Sterile aqueous solution for intramuscular or subcutaneous administration.

4. CLINICAL PARTICULARS

4.1 Therapeutic indications

Emergency treatment of anaphylaxis or acute angioneurotic oedema with airways obstruction, or acute allergic reactions.

4.2 Posology and method of administration

For the relief of life-threatening angioneurotic oedema and anaphylactic shock, adrenaline should be administered by intramuscular injection.

For acute allergic reactions due to insect stings etc.: Intramuscular or subcutaneous injection.

The presentation with the 0.25" integral needle is intended for self-administration by the subcutaneous route and the presentation with the 1.5" integral needle is for paramedic use by subcutaneous or intramuscular injection.

Adults and children over 12 years: 0.5 ml (0.5 mg), administered slowly. The dose may be repeated every 5 to 15 minutes as needed.

This presentation may not be suitable for small or prepubertal patients over 12 years of age who require a smaller dose.

Elderly: as for adults, use with caution.

Children (up to age of 12): not recommended

4.3 Contraindications

Contraindications are relative as this product is intended for use in life-threatening emergencies.

Other than in the emergency situation, the following contraindications should be considered: hyperthyroidism, hypertension, ischaemic heart disease, diabetes mellitus, and closed angle glaucoma.

4.4 Special warnings and precautions for use

These special warnings and precautions are relative as this product is intended for use in life-threatening situations.

Administer slowly with caution to elderly patients and to patients with ischaemic heart disease, hypertension, diabetes mellitus, hyperthyroidism or psychoneurosis. Use with extreme caution in patients with long-standing bronchial asthma and emphysema who have developed degenerative heart disease. Anginal pain may be induced when coronary insufficiency is present.

4.5 Interaction with other medicinal products and other forms of interaction

The effects of adrenaline may be potentiated by tricyclic antidepressants. Volatile liquid anaesthetics such as halothane increase the risk of adrenaline-induced ventricular arrhythmias and acute pulmonary oedema if hypoxia is present. Severe hypertension and bradycardia may occur with non-selective beta-blocking drugs such as propranolol. Propranolol also inhibits the bronchodilator effect of adrenaline. The risk of cardiac arrhythmias is higher when adrenaline is given to patients receiving digoxin, quinidine, fluorohydrocarbons or cocaine. Adrenaline -induced hyperglycaemia may lead to loss of blood-sugar control in diabetic patients treated with hypoglycaemic agents.

The vasoconstrictor and pressor effects of adrenaline, mediated by its alpha-adrenergic action, may be enhanced by concomitant administration of drugs with similar effects, such as ergot alkaloids or oxytocin. Adrenaline specifically reverses the antihypertensive effects of adrenergic neurone blockers such as guanethidine with the risk of severe hypertension.

4.6 Pregnancy and lactation

Adrenaline crosses the placenta. There is some evidence of a slightly increased incidence of congenital abnormalities. Injection of adrenaline may cause foetal tachycardia, cardiac irregularities, extrasystoles and louder heart sounds. In labour, adrenaline may delay the second stage. Adrenaline should only be used in pregnancy if the potential benefits outweigh the risks to the foetus.

Adrenaline is excreted in breast milk, but as pharmacologically active plasma concentrations are not achieved by the oral route, the use of adrenaline in breast-feeding mothers is presumed to be safe.

4.7 Effects on ability to drive and use machines

Not applicable; this preparation is intended for use only in emergencies.

4.8 Undesirable effects

The potentially severe adverse effects of adrenaline arise from its effect upon blood pressure and cardiac rhythm. Ventricular fibrillation may occur and severe hypertension may lead to cerebral haemorrhage and pulmonary oedema. Symptomatic adverse effects are anxiety, dyspnoea, restlessness, palpitations, tachycardia, anginal pain, tremor, weakness, dizziness, headache, cold extremities, nausea, vomiting, sweating, local ischaemic necrosis. Biochemical effects include inhibition of insulin secretion and hyperglycaemia even with low doses, gluconeogenesis, glycolysis, lipolysis and ketogenesis.

4.9 Overdose

Symptoms: cardiac arrhythmias leading to ventricular fibrillation and death, severe hypertension leading to pulmonary oedema and cerebral haemorrhage.

Treatment: combined alpha- and beta-adrenergic blocking agents such as labetalol may counteract the effects of adrenaline, or a beta-blocking agent may be used to treat any supraventricular arrhythmias and phentolamine to control the alpha-mediated effects on the peripheral circulation. Rapidly acting vasodilators such as nitrates and sodium nitroprusside may also be helpful.

Immediate resuscitation support must be available.

5. PHARMACOLOGICAL PROPERTIES

5.1 Pharmacodynamic properties

Adrenaline is a direct-acting sympathomimetic agent exerting its effect on alpha- and beta-adrenoceptors. Major effects are increased systolic blood pressure, reduced diastolic pressure, tachycardia, hyperglycaemia and hypokalaemia. It is a powerful cardiac stimulant. It has vasopressor properties and is a bronchodilator.

5.2 Pharmacokinetic properties

Adrenaline is rapid in onset and of short duration and is rapidly distributed to the heart, spleen, several glandular tissues and adrenergic nerves. It crosses the placenta and is excreted in breast milk. It is approximately 50% bound to plasma proteins. The onset of action is rapid and after i.v. infusion the half-life is approximately 5-10 minutes.

Adrenaline is rapidly metabolised in the liver and tissues by oxidative deamination and O-methylation followed by reduction or by conjugation with glucuronic acid or sulphate. Up to 90% of the i.v. dose is excreted in the urine as metabolites.

5.3 Preclinical safety data
Not applicable since Adrenaline (Epinephrine) Injection has been used in clinical practice for many years and its effects in man are well known.

6. PHARMACEUTICAL PARTICULARS

6.1 List of excipients
Citric Acid Monohydrate USP
Sodium Citrate Dihydrate USP
Sodium Chloride USP
Sodium Bisulphite USP
Hydrochloric Acid 10% w/v USP
Water for Injection USP

6.2 Incompatibilities
Adrenaline should not be mixed with sodium bicarbonate; the solution is oxidised to adrenochrome and then forms polymers.

6.3 Shelf life
9 months.

6.4 Special precautions for storage
Store below 25°C. Protect from light.

6.5 Nature and contents of container
The solution is contained in a USP type I glass vial with an elastomeric closure which meets all the relevant USP specifications. Two presentations are available; one for patient self-administration with a 0.25″ integral needle and one for paramedic use with a 1.5″ integral needle. Both are 1ml presentations.

6.6 Special precautions for disposal and other handling
The container is specially designed for use with the IMS Minijet injector.

7. MARKETING AUTHORISATION HOLDER
International Medication Systems (UK) Limited
208 Bath Road
Slough
Berkshire
SL1 3WE
UK

8. MARKETING AUTHORISATION NUMBER(S)
PL 03265/0030

9. DATE OF FIRST AUTHORISATION/RENEWAL OF THE AUTHORISATION
Date first granted: 8 February 1978
Date renewed: 31 August 2000

10. DATE OF REVISION OF THE TEXT
14 October 2005
POM

EpiPen Auto-Injector 0.3mg
(ALK-Abello Ltd)

1. NAME OF THE MEDICINAL PRODUCT
EpiPen Adrenaline (Epinephrine) Auto-Injector 0.3mg

2. QUALITATIVE AND QUANTITATIVE COMPOSITION
Per 1 ml:

Active ingredient	Quantity / Unit	Reference Standards
Adrenaline (Epinephrine)	1.0 mg	BP/USP

3. PHARMACEUTICAL FORM
Solution for injection in an Auto-Injector (prefilled, disposable automatic injection device) for intramuscular use.

4. CLINICAL PARTICULARS

4.1 Therapeutic indications
EpiPen Auto-Injectors are automatic injection devices containing adrenaline for allergic emergencies. The Auto-Injectors should be used only by a person with a history or an acknowledged risk of an anaphylactic reaction. The Auto-Injectors are indicated in the emergency treatment of allergic reactions (anaphylaxis) to insect stings or bites, foods, drugs and other allergens as well as idiopathic or exercise induced anaphylaxis. Such reactions may occur within minutes after exposure and consist of flushing, apprehension, syncope, tachycardia, thready or unobtainable pulse associated with a fall in blood pressure, convulsions, vomiting, diarrhoea and abdominal cramps, involuntary voiding, wheezing, dyspnea due to laryngeal spasm, pruritis, rashes, urticaria or angioedema.

For these reasons Auto-Injectors should always be carried by such persons in situations of potential risks.

Adrenaline is considered the first line drug of choice for allergic emergencies. Adrenaline effectively reverses the symptoms of rhinitis, urticaria, bronchospasm and hypotension because it is a pharmacological antagonist to the effects of the chemical mediators on smooth muscles, blood vessels and other tissues. Adrenaline is recommended as the initial and primary therapeutic agent in the treatment of anaphylaxis by every recognised authority in allergy, and its appropriate use in these circumstances is widely documented in the medical literature.

4.2 Posology and method of administration
The EpiPen Auto-Injector is for adult intramuscular administration. It is designed for easy use by the lay person and has to be considered as first aid. EpiPen Auto-Injector delivers a single dose 0.3 ml injection equal to 0.3 mg adrenaline when activated. Usual adrenaline adult dose for allergic emergencies is 0.3 mg. For paediatric use the appropriate dosage may be 0.15 mg or 0.30 mg depending upon the body weight of the patient (0.01 mg/kg body weight). However, the prescribing physician has the option of prescribing more or less than these amounts based on careful assessment of each individual patient and recognising the life-threatening nature of reactions for which this is being described.

The physician should consider using other forms of injectable adrenaline if lower doses are felt to be necessary for small children.

In the absence of clinical improvement or if deterioration occurs after the initial treatment, a second injection with an additional EpiPen Auto-Injector may be necessary. The repeated injection may be administered after about 5 – 15 minutes.

As EpiPen is designed as emergency treatment only, the patient should be advised always to seek medical help immediately.

A physician who prescribes EpiPen Auto-Injector should take appropriate steps to ensure that the patient understands the indications and use of this device thoroughly. The physician should review with the patient or any other person who might be in a position to administer EpiPen Auto-Injector to a patient experiencing anaphylaxis, in detail, the patient instructions and operation of the EpiPen Auto-Injector.

Administration:

Inject the delivered dose of the EpiPen Auto-Injector (0.3 ml equal to 0.3 mg) into the anterolateral aspect of the thigh, through clothing if necessary. See detailed instructions for use, point 6.6.

4.3 Contraindications
There are no known absolute contraindications to the use of EpiPen Auto-Injector during an allergic emergency. Clinical conditions where special precautions are advised and drug interactions are prescribed in sections 4.4 and 4.5.

4.4 Special warnings and precautions for use
Patients must be instructed in the proper use of EpiPen Auto-Injectors. See section 6.6.

Adrenaline is ordinarily administered with extreme caution to patients who have a heart disease. Use of adrenaline with drugs that may sensitise the heart to arrhythmias, e.g., digitalis, mercurial diuretics, or quinidine, ordinarily is not recommended. Anginal pain may be induced by adrenaline in patients with coronary insufficiency.

Hyperthyroid individuals (hyperfunction of the thyroid gland), individuals with cardiovascular disease, hypertension (raised blood pressure), or diabetes, elderly individuals, pregnant women, and children under 30 kg body weight using EpiPen Auto-Injector may theoretically be at greater risk of developing adverse reactions after adrenaline administration.

Accidental injection into the hands or feet may result in loss of blood flow to the affected area and should be avoided. If there is an accidental injection into these areas, advise the patient to go immediately to the nearest emergency room or hospital casualty department for treatment.

The patient should be instructed to check the contents of the glass cartridge in the Auto-Injector periodically through the viewing window of the unit to make sure the solution is clear and colourless. The Auto-Injector should be discarded if discoloured or contains a precipitate. For emergency treatment use of an EpiPen Auto-Injector with discoloured contents may be recommended rather than to postpone the treatment.

The Auto-Injectors should ONLY be injected into the anterolateral aspect of the thigh. Patients should be advised NOT to inject into the buttock. Large doses or accidental intravenous injection of adrenaline may result in cerebral haemorrhage due to sharp rise in blood pressure. Directions for proper use of the Auto-injectors must be followed in order to avoid intravenous injection. Rapidly acting vasodilators can counteract the marked pressor effects of adrenaline.

The adrenaline solution contains sodium metabisulfite, a sulfite that may in other products cause allergic-type reactions including anaphylactic symptoms or life-threatening or less severe asthmatic episodes in certain susceptible persons. The alternatives to using adrenaline in a life-threatening situation may not be satisfactory. The presence of a sulfite in this product should not deter administration of the drug for treatment of serious allergic or other emergency situations.

Despite these concerns, adrenaline is essentially for the treatment of anaphylaxis. Therefore, patients with these conditions, and/or any other person who might be in a position to administer EpiPen Auto-Injector to a patient experiencing anaphylaxis should be carefully instructed in regard to the circumstances under which this life-saving medication should be used.

4.5 Interaction with other medicinal products and other forms of interaction
Caution is indicated in patients receiving drugs that may sensitise the heart to arrhythmias, including digitalis, mercurial diuretics or quinidine. The effects of adrenaline may be potentiated by tricyclic antidepressants and mono amine oxidase inhibitors.

Pressor effects of adrenaline may be counteracted by rapidly acting vasodilators or alpha-adrenergic blocking drugs. If prolonged hypotension follows such measures, it may be necessary to administer another pressor drug, such as levarterenol.

Adrenaline inhibits the secretion of insulin, thus increasing the blood glucose level. It may be necessary for diabetic patients receiving adrenaline to increase their dosage of insulin or oral hypoglycaemic drugs.

4.6 Pregnancy and lactation
Adrenaline has been used for years in the treatment of allergic emergencies and its use is well documented in the literature. No clinical trials were performed in conjunction with this application. As adrenaline is a substance that naturally occurs in the body, it is unlikely that this drug would have any detrimental effects on fertility.

Adrenaline should be used during pregnancy only if the potential benefit justifies the potential risk to fetus.

4.7 Effects on ability to drive and use machines
The patients' ability to drive and use machines may be affected by the anaphylactic reaction, as well as by possible adverse reactions to adrenaline.

4.8 Undesirable effects
Repeated dose toxicity studies were not performed in conjunction with this application. Side effects associated with adrenaline's alpha and beta receptor activity may include palpitations, tachycardia, sweating, nausea and vomiting, respiratory difficulty, pallor, dizziness, weakness, tremor, headache, apprehension, nervousness and anxiety. Cardiac arrhythmias may follow administration of adrenaline.

Accidental injection into hands or fingers resulting in peripheral ischaemia has been reported. Patients may need treatment following accidental injection. See section 4.4.

4.9 Overdose
Overdose or inadvertent intravascular injection of adrenaline may cause cerebral haemorrhage resulting from a sharp rise in blood pressure. Fatalities may also result from pulmonary edema because of peripheral vascular constriction together with cardiac stimulation.

Pressor effects of adrenaline may be counteracted by rapidly acting vasodilators or alpha-adrenergic blocking drugs. If prolonged hypotension follows such measures, it may be necessary to administer another pressor drug, such as levarterenol.

If an adrenaline overdose induces pulmonary edema that interferes with respiration, treatment consists of a rapidly acting alpha-adrenergic blocking drug such as phentolamine and/or intermittent positive-pressure respiration.

Adrenaline overdose can also cause transient bradycardia followed by tachycardia, and these may be accompanied by potentially fatal cardiac arrhythmias. Treatment of arrhythmias may consist of administration of beta-adrenergic blocking drugs.

5. PHARMACOLOGICAL PROPERTIES

5.1 Pharmacodynamic properties
Adrenaline is one of the catecholamines which are a group of sympathomimetic amines containing a catechol moiety. Adrenaline activates an adrenergic receptive mechanism on effector cells and imitates all actions of the sympathetic nervous system except those on the arteries of the face and sweat glands. Adrenaline acts on both alpha and beta receptors and is the most potent alpha receptor activator.

The strong vasoconstrictor action of adrenaline through its effect on alpha adrenergic receptors acts quickly to counter vasodilation and increased vascular permeability which can lead to loss of intravascular fluid volume and hypotension during anaphylactic reactions. Adrenaline through its action on beta receptors on bronchial smooth muscles causes bronchial smooth muscle relaxation which alleviates wheezing and dyspnea. Adrenaline also alleviates pruritis, urticaria, and angioedema and may be effective in relieving gastrointestinal and genitourinary symptoms associated with anaphylaxis.

5.2 Pharmacokinetic properties
Adrenaline is a naturally occurring substance produced by the adrenal medulla and secreted in response to exertion or stress. It is rapidly inactivated in the body mostly by the enzymes

COMT and MAO. The liver is rich in these enzymes and is an important, although not essential, tissue in the degradation process. Much of the dose of adrenaline is accounted for by excretion of metabolites in the urine.

According to Remington's Pharmaceutical Sciences, the plasma half-life of adrenaline is about 2.5 min. However, by subcutaneous or intramuscular routes, local vasoconstriction retards absorption, so that the effects occur insidiously and last much longer than the half-life would predict. Massage around the injection area is advised.

5.3 Preclinical safety data

Adrenaline has been utilised in the treatment of allergic emergencies for many years. No preclinical studies have been performed in connection with this application.

6. PHARMACEUTICAL PARTICULARS

6.1 List of excipients

Sodium Chloride

Sodium Metabisulfite

Hydrochloric Acid

Water for Injection

6.2 Incompatibilities

Adrenaline and its salts are rapidly destroyed in solution with oxidising agents. The solution darkens in colour upon exposure to air or light.

6.3 Shelf life

The expiration period for the EpiPen Auto-Injector is 18 months from the date of manufacture.

The expiry date is indicated on the label, and EpiPen Auto-Injector should not be used after this date. Replace the Auto-Injector by expiration date or earlier if the solution is discoloured or contains a precipitate. Check the solution periodically through the viewing window of the unit to make sure the solution is clear and colourless.

Shelf life after opening: The Auto-Injectors must be discarded immediately after use.

6.4 Special precautions for storage

Adrenaline is sensitive to light. Keep the auto-injector in the outer carton. Do not store above 25 °C. Do not refrigerate or freeze.

6.5 Nature and contents of container

The immediate container/closure system consists of a glass cartridge sealed by a rubber plunger at one end and by rubber diaphragm which has been inserted into an aluminium hub with attached stainless steel needle at the other end. The glass cartridge contains the product.

The Auto-Injector administration device:

Glass cartridge container:

Type I, Borosilicate Glass - complies with USP and Ph. Eur

Diaphragm - Stopper:

PH 701/50/Black (butyl rubber plunger) - complies with USP and Ph. Eur.

Needle - Hub - Sheath:

Materials compatible with adrenaline injection

Needle: Siliconised Type 304 stainless steel

Hub: Anodized 3003 aluminium alloy

Sheath: Synthetic polyisoprene

The EpiPen Auto-Injector contains 2 ml of Adrenaline injection 1 mg/ml in a prefilled disposable automatic injection device which is designed to deliver a single dose (0.3 ml) of 0.3 mg adrenaline when activated. After activation of the Auto-Injector 1.7 ml remains in the Auto-Injector.

Pack sizes: 1 Auto-injector and 2 Auto-Injectors

6.6 Special precautions for disposal and other handling

Do not remove grey safety cap until ready for use.

Under no circumstances place the black end of the EpiPen Auto-Injector on or near your thumbs, fingers or hands. Accidental injection into hands or fingers resulting in peripheral ischaemia has been reported. See section 4.4. The EpiPen Auto-Injector should be used on the outer thigh. The injection is activated immediately the black end of the EpiPen Auto-Injector comes into contact with any skin or other surface.

The EpiPen Auto-Injectors are designed for easy use by the lay person and has to be considered as a first aid. The Auto-Injector should simply be jabbed firmly against the outer portion of the thigh from a distance of approximately 10 cm. There is no need for more precise placement on the outer portion of the thigh. When EpiPen Auto-Injector is jabbed against the thigh, it releases a spring activated plunger, pushing the concealed needle into the thigh muscle and expelling a dose of adrenaline:

1. Grasp EpiPen Auto-Injector in dominant hand, with thumb closest to grey safety cap.
2. With the other hand pull off grey safety cap.
3. Hold the EpiPen Auto-Injector in a distance of approximately 10 cm away from the outer thigh. The black tip should point towards the outer thigh.
4. Jab firmly into the outer thigh so that the EpiPen Auto-Injector is at a right angle to (at a 90 degree angle) the outer thigh.
5. Hold in place for 10 seconds. The EpiPen Auto-Injector should be removed and safely discarded.
6. Massage the injection area for 10 seconds.

A small air bubble may occur in the EpiPen Auto-Injector. It has no influence on either the use or the efficacy of the product.

Administrative Data

7. MARKETING AUTHORISATION HOLDER

ALK-Abelló A/S,
Bøge Allé 6-8,
DK 2970 Hørsholm,
Denmark

8. MARKETING AUTHORISATION NUMBER(S)

PL 10085/0012

9. DATE OF FIRST AUTHORISATION/RENEWAL OF THE AUTHORISATION

28th of March 1996

10. DATE OF REVISION OF THE TEXT

25th July 2008

EpiPen Jr. Auto-Injector 0.15mg

(ALK-Abello Ltd)

1. NAME OF THE MEDICINAL PRODUCT

EpiPen® Jr. Adrenaline (Epinephrine) Auto-Injector 0.15mg

2. QUALITATIVE AND QUANTITATIVE COMPOSITION

Per 1 ml:

Active ingredient	Quantity / Unit	Reference Standards
Adrenaline (Epinephrine)	0.5 mg	BP/USP

3. PHARMACEUTICAL FORM

Solution for injection in an Auto-Injector (prefilled, disposable automatic injection device) for intramuscular use.

4. CLINICAL PARTICULARS

4.1 Therapeutic indications

EpiPen Jr. Auto-Injectors are automatic injection devices containing adrenaline for allergic emergencies. The Auto-Injector is intended for children at a body weight of 15-30 kg. The Auto-Injectors should be used only by a person with a history or an acknowledged risk of an anaphylactic reaction. The Auto-Injectors are indicated in the emergency treatment of allergic reactions (anaphylaxis) to insect stings or bites, foods, drugs and other allergens as well as idiopathic or exercise induced anaphylaxis. Such reactions may occur within minutes after exposure and consist of flushing, apprehension, syncope, tachycardia, thready or unobtainable pulse associated with a fall in blood pressure, convulsions, vomiting, diarrhoea and abdominal cramps, involuntary voiding, wheezing, dyspnea due to laryngeal spasm, pruritis, rashes, urticaria or angioedema.

For these reasons Auto-Injectors should always be carried by such persons in situations of potential risks.

Adrenaline is considered the first line drug of choice for allergic emergencies. Adrenaline effectively reverses the symptoms of rhinitis, urticaria, bronchospasm and hypotension because it is a pharmacological antagonist to the effects of the chemical mediators on smooth muscles, blood vessels and other tissues. Adrenaline is recommended as the initial and primary therapeutic agent in the treatment of anaphylaxis by every recognised authority in allergy, and its appropriate use in these circumstances is widely documented in the medical literature.

4.2 Posology and method of administration

The EpiPen Jr. Auto-Injector is for paediatric intramuscular administration. It is designed for easy use by the lay person and has to be considered as first aid. EpiPen Jr. Auto-Injector delivers a single dose 0.3 ml injection equal to 0.15 mg adrenaline when activated. For paediatric use, the appropriate dosage may be 0.15 mg or 0.30 mg depending upon the body weight of the patient (0.01 mg/kg body weight).

EpiPen Jr. Auto-Injector 0.15 mg is recommended for children weighing 15 - 30 kg. For children weighing more than 30 kg, EpiPen Auto-Injector 0.3 mg (adult formulation) is recommended.

The prescribing physician has the option of prescribing more or less than these amounts based on careful assessment of each individual patient and recognising the life-threatening nature of reactions for which this is being described.

The physician should consider using other forms of injectable adrenaline if lower doses are felt to be necessary for small children.

In the absence of clinical improvement or if deterioration occurs after the initial treatment a second injection with an additional EpiPen Auto-Injector may be necessary. The repeated injection may be administered after about 5 - 15 minutes.

As EpiPen Jr. is designed as emergency treatment only, the patient should be advised always to seek medical help immediately.

A physician who prescribes EpiPen Jr. Auto-Injector should take appropriate steps to ensure that the patient understands the indications and use of this device thoroughly. The physician should review with the patient or any other person who might be in a position to administer EpiPen Jr. Auto-Injector to a patient experiencing anaphylaxis, in detail, the patient instructions and operation of the EpiPen Jr. Auto-Injector.

Administration:

Inject the delivered dose of the EpiPen Jr. Auto-Injector (0.3 ml equal to 0.15 mg) into the anterolateral aspect of the thigh, through clothing if necessary. See detailed instructions for use, point 6.6.

4.3 Contraindications

There are no known absolute contraindications to the use of EpiPen Jr. Auto-Injector during an allergic emergency. Clinical conditions where special precautions are advised and drug interactions are prescribed in sections 4.4 and 4.5.

4.4 Special warnings and precautions for use

Patients must be instructed in the proper use of EpiPen Jr. Auto-Injectors. See section 6.6.

Adrenaline is ordinarily administered with extreme caution to patients who have a heart disease. Use of adrenaline with drugs that may sensitise the heart to arrhythmias, e.g., digitalis, mercurial diuretics, or quinidine, ordinarily is not recommended. Anginal pain may be induced by adrenaline in patients with coronary insufficiency.

Hyperthyroid individuals (hyperfunction of the thyroid gland), individuals with cardiovascular disease, hypertension (raised blood pressure), or diabetes, elderly individuals, pregnant women, and children under 15 kg body weight using EpiPen Jr. Auto-Injector may theoretically be at greater risk of developing adverse reactions after adrenaline administration.

Accidental injection into the hands or feet may result in loss of blood flow to the affected area and should be avoided. If there is an accidental injection into these areas, advise the patient to go immediately to the nearest emergency room or hospital casualty department for treatment.

The patient should be instructed to check the contents of the glass cartridge in the Auto-Injector periodically through the viewing window of the unit to make sure the solution is clear and colourless. The Auto-Injector should be discarded if discoloured or contains a precipitate. For emergency treatment use of an EpiPen Jr. Auto-Injector with discoloured contents may be recommended rather than to postpone the treatment.

The Auto-Injectors should ONLY be injected into the anterolateral aspect of the thigh. Patients should be advised NOT to inject into the buttock. Large doses or accidental intravenous injection of adrenaline may result in cerebral haemorrhage due to sharp rise in blood pressure. Directions for proper use of the Auto-injectors must be followed in order to avoid intravenous injection. Rapidly acting vasodilators can counteract the marked pressor effects of adrenaline.

The adrenaline solution contains sodium metabisulfite, a sulfite that may in other products cause allergic-type reactions including anaphylactic symptoms or life-threatening or less severe asthmatic episodes in certain susceptible persons. The alternatives to using adrenaline in a life-threatening situation may not be satisfactory. The presence of a sulfite in this product should not deter administration of the drug for treatment of serious allergic or other emergency situations.

Despite these concerns, adrenaline is essentially for the treatment of anaphylaxis. Therefore, patients with these conditions, and/or any other person who might be in a position to administer EpiPen Jr. Auto-Injector to a patient experiencing anaphylaxis should be carefully instructed in regard to the circumstances under which this life-saving medication should be used.

4.5 Interaction with other medicinal products and other forms of interaction

Caution is indicated in patients receiving drugs that may sensitise the heart to arrhythmias, including digitalis, mercurial diuretics or quinidine. The effects of adrenaline may be potentiated by tricyclic antidepressants and mono amine oxidase inhibitors.

Pressor effects of adrenaline may be counteracted by rapidly acting vasodilators or alpha-adrenergic blocking drugs. If prolonged hypotension follows such measures, it may be necessary to administer another pressor drug, such as levarterenol.

Adrenaline inhibits the secretion of insulin, thus increasing the blood glucose level. It may be necessary for diabetic patients receiving adrenaline to increase their dosage of insulin or oral hypoglycaemic drugs.

4.6 Pregnancy and lactation

Adrenaline has been used for years in the treatment of allergic emergencies and its use is well documented in the literature. No clinical trials were performed in conjunction with this application. As adrenaline is a substance that naturally occurs in the body, it is unlikely that this drug would have any detrimental effects on fertility.

Adrenaline should be used during pregnancy only if the potential benefit justifies the potential risk to foetus.

4.7 Effects on ability to drive and use machines

The patients' ability to drive and use machines may be affected by the anaphylactic reaction, as well as by possible adverse reactions to adrenaline.

4.8 Undesirable effects

Repeated dose toxicity studies were not performed in conjunction with this application. Side effects associated with adrenaline's alpha and beta receptor activity may include palpitations, tachycardia, sweating, nausea and vomiting, respiratory difficulty, pallor, dizziness, weakness, tremor, headache, apprehension, nervousness and anxiety. Cardiac arrhythmias may follow administration of adrenaline.

Accidental injection into hands or fingers resulting in peripheral ischaemia has been reported. Patients may need treatment following accidental injection. See section 4.4.

4.9 Overdose

Overdose or inadvertent intravascular injection of adrenaline may cause cerebral haemorrhage resulting from a sharp rise in blood pressure. Fatalities may also result from pulmonary edema because of peripheral vascular constriction together with cardiac stimulation.

Pressor effects of adrenaline may be counteracted by rapidly acting vasodilators or alpha-adrenergic blocking drugs. If prolonged hypotension follows such measures, it may be necessary to administer another pressor drug, such as levarterenol.

If an adrenaline overdose induces pulmonary edema that interferes with respiration, treatment consists of a rapidly acting alpha-adrenergic blocking drug such as phentolamine and/or intermittent positive-pressure respiration.

Adrenaline overdose can also cause transient bradycardia followed by tachycardia, and these may be accompanied by potentially fatal cardiac arrhythmias. Treatment of arrhythmias may consist of administration of beta-adrenergic blocking agents.

5. PHARMACOLOGICAL PROPERTIES

5.1 Pharmacodynamic properties

Adrenaline is one of the catecholamines which are a group of sympathomimetic amines containing a catechol moiety. Adrenaline activates an adrenergic receptive mechanism on effector cells and imitates all actions of the sympathetic nervous system except those on the arteries of the face and sweat glands. Adrenaline acts on both alpha and beta receptors and is the most potent alpha receptor activator.

The strong vasoconstrictor action of adrenaline through its effect on alpha adrenergic receptors acts quickly to counter vasodilatation and increased vascular permeability which can lead to loss of intravascular fluid volume and hypotension during anaphylactic reactions. Adrenaline through its action on beta receptors on bronchial smooth muscles causes bronchial smooth muscle relaxation which alleviates wheezing and dyspnea. Adrenaline also alleviates pruritis, urticaria, and angioedema and may be effective in relieving gastrointestinal and genitourinary symptoms associated with anaphylaxis.

5.2 Pharmacokinetic properties

Adrenaline is a naturally occurring substance produced by the adrenal medulla and secreted in response to exertion or stress. It is rapidly inactivated in the body mostly by the enzymes COMT and MAO. The liver is rich in these enzymes and is an important, although not essential, tissue in the degradation process. Much of the dose of adrenaline is accounted for by excretion of metabolites in the urine.

According to Remington's Pharmaceutical Sciences, the plasma half-life of adrenaline is about 2.5 min. However, by subcutaneous or intramuscular routes, local vasoconstriction retards absorption, so that the effects occur insidiously and last much longer than the half-life would predict. Massage around the injection area is advised.

5.3 Preclinical safety data

Adrenaline has been utilised in the treatment of allergic emergencies for many years. No preclinical studies have been performed in connection with this application.

6. PHARMACEUTICAL PARTICULARS

6.1 List of excipients

Sodium Chloride

Sodium Metabisulfite

Hydrochloric Acid

Water for Injection

6.2 Incompatibilities

Adrenaline and its salts are rapidly destroyed in solution with oxidising agents. The solution darkens in colour upon exposure to air or light.

6.3 Shelf life

The expiration period for the EpiPen Jr. Auto-Injector is 18 months from the date of manufacture. The expiry date is indicated on the label, and EpiPen Jr. Auto-Injector should not be used after this date. Replace the Auto-Injector by expiration date or earlier if the solution is discoloured or contains a precipitate. Check the solution periodically through the viewing window of the unit to make sure the solution is clear and colourless.

Shelf life after opening: The Auto-Injectors must be discarded immediately after use.

6.4 Special precautions for storage

Adrenaline is light sensitive and the Auto-Injectors should be stored in the tube provided. Store in dark place at below 25°C. Do not refrigerate.

6.5 Nature and contents of container

The immediate container/closure system consists of a glass cartridge sealed by a rubber plunger at one end and by rubber diaphragm which has been inserted into an aluminium hub with attached stainless steel needle at the other end. The glass cartridge contains the product.

The Auto-Injector administration device:

Glass cartridge container:

Type I, Borosilicate Glass - complies with USP and Ph. Eur

Diaphragm - Stopper:

PH 701/50/Black (butyl rubber plunger) - complies with USP and Ph. Eur.

Needle - Hub - Sheath:

Materials compatible with adrenaline injection

Needle: Siliconised Type 304 stainless steel

Hub: Anodized 3003 aluminium alloy

Sheath: Synthetic polyisoprene

The EpiPen Jr. Auto-Injector contains 2 ml of Adrenaline injection 0.5 mg/ml in a prefilled disposable automatic injection device which is designed to deliver a single dose (0.3 ml) of 0.15 mg adrenaline when activated. After activation of the Auto-Injector 1.7 ml remains in the Auto-Injector.

Pack-sizes: 1 Auto-Injector and 2 Auto-Injectors

6.6 Special precautions for disposal and other handling

Do not remove grey safety cap until ready for use.

Under no circumstances place the black end of the EpiPen Auto-Injector on or near your thumbs, fingers or hands. Accidental injection into hands or fingers resulting in peripheral ischaemia has been reported. See section 4.4. The EpiPen Auto-Injector should be used on the outer thigh. The injection is activated immediately the black end of the EpiPen Auto-Injector comes into contact with any skin or other surface.

The EpiPen Jr. Auto-Injectors are designed for easy use by the lay person and has to be considered as a first aid. The Auto-Injector should simply be jabbed firmly against the outer portion of the thigh from a distance of approximately 10 cm. There is no need for more precise placement on the outer portion of the thigh. When EpiPen Jr. Auto-Injector is jabbed against the thigh, it releases a spring activated plunger, pushing the concealed needle into the thigh muscle and expelling a dose of adrenaline:

1. Grasp EpiPen Jr. Auto-Injector in dominant hand, with thumb closest to grey safety cap.
2. With the other hand pull of grey safety cap.
3. Hold the EpiPen Auto-Injector in a distance of approximately 10 cm away from the outer thigh. The black tip should point towards the outer thigh.
4. Jab firmly into the outer thigh so that the EpiPen Auto-Injector is at a right angle to (at a 90 degree angle) the outer thigh.
5. Hold in place for 10 seconds. The EpiPen Auto-Injector should be removed and safely discarded.
6. Massage the injection area for 10 seconds.

A small air bubble may occur in the EpiPen Auto-Injector. It has no influence on either the use or the efficacy of the product.

Administrative Data

7. MARKETING AUTHORISATION HOLDER

ALK-Abelló A/S,
Bøge Allé 6-8,
DK 2970 Hørsholm,
Denmark

8. MARKETING AUTHORISATION NUMBER(S)

PL 10085/0013

9. DATE OF FIRST AUTHORISATION/RENEWAL OF THE AUTHORISATION

28th March 1996

10. DATE OF REVISION OF THE TEXT

25th July 2008

Epirubicin hydrochloride 2 mg/ml solution for injection (medac UK)

(medac GmbH)

1. NAME OF THE MEDICINAL PRODUCT

Epirubicin hydrochloride 2 mg/ml solution for injection

2. QUALITATIVE AND QUANTITATIVE COMPOSITION

1 ml of solution contains 2 mg epirubicin hydrochloride.

One 5 ml / 10 ml / 25 ml / 50 ml / 100 ml vial contains 10 mg / 20 mg / 50 mg / 100 mg / 200 mg epirubicin hydrochloride.

For a full list of excipients, see section 6.1.

3. PHARMACEUTICAL FORM

Solution for Injection

A clear red solution.

4. CLINICAL PARTICULARS

4.1 Therapeutic indications

Epirubicin is used in the treatment of a range of neoplastic conditions including:

- Carcinoma of the breast
- Advanced ovarian cancer
- Gastric cancer
- Small cell lung cancer

When administered intravesically, epirubicin has been shown to be beneficial in the treatment of:

- Papillary transitional cell carcinoma of the bladder
- Carcinoma-in-situ of the bladder

Intravesical prophylaxis of recurrences of superficial bladder carcinoma following transurethral resection.

4.2 Posology and method of administration

Epirubicin is for intravenous or intravesical use only.

The safety and efficacy of epirubicin in children has not been established.

Intravenous administration

It is advisable to administer epirubicin via the tubing of a free-running intravenous saline infusion after checking that the needle is properly placed in the vein. Care should be taken to avoid extravasation (see section 4.4). In case of extravasation, administration should be stopped immediately.

Dosage

In order to avoid cardiac toxicity, a total cumulative dose of 900 – 1000 mg/m^2 epirubicin should not be exceeded (see section 4.4).

Conventional dose

When epirubicin is used as a single agent, the recommended dosage in adults is 60 – 90 mg/m^2 body surface area. Epirubicin should be injected intravenously over 3 – 5 minutes. The dose should be repeated at 21 - day intervals, depending upon the patient's haematological status and bone marrow function.

If signs of toxicity, including severe neutropenia/neutropenic fever and thrombocytopenia occur (which could persist at day 21), dose modification or postponement of the subsequent dose may be required.

High dose

Epirubicin as a single agent for the high dose treatment of lung cancer should be administered according to the following regimens:

– Small cell lung cancer (previously untreated): 120 mg/m^2 day 1, every 3 weeks.

For high dose treatment, epirubicin may be given as an intravenous bolus over 3 – 5 minutes or as an infusion of up to 30 minutes duration.

Breast Cancer

In the adjuvant treatment of early breast cancer patients with positive lymph nodes, intravenous doses of epirubicin ranging from 100 mg/m^2 (as a single dose on day 1) to 120 mg/m^2 (in two divided doses on days 1 and 8) every 3 – 4 weeks, in combination with intravenous cyclophosphamide and 5-fluorouracil and oral tamoxifen, are recommended.

Lower doses (60 – 75 mg/m^2 for conventional treatment and 105 – 120 mg/m^2 for high dose treatment) are recommended for patients whose bone marrow function has been impaired by previous chemotherapy or radiotherapy, by age, or neoplastic bone marrow infiltration. The total dose per cycle may be divided over 2 – 3 successive days.

The following doses of epirubicin are commonly used in monotherapy and combination chemotherapy for various other tumours, as shown:

	Epirubicin Dose (mg/m^2)[a]	
Cancer Indication	**Monotherapy**	**Combination Therapy**
Advanced ovarian cancer	60 – 90	50 – 100
Gastric cancer	60 – 90	50
SCLC	120	120
Bladder cancer	Intravesical administration of 50 mg/ 50 ml or 80 mg/ 50 ml (carcinoma in situ) Prophylaxis: 50 mg/ 50 ml weekly for 4 weeks then monthly for 11 months	

[a] Doses generally given Day 1 or Day 1, 2 and 3 at 21-day intervals

Combination therapy

If epirubicin is used in combination with other cytotoxic products, the dose should be reduced accordingly. Commonly used doses are shown in the table above.

Impaired liver function

The major route of elimination of epirubicin is the hepatobiliary system. In patients with impaired liver function the dose should be reduced based on serum bilirubin levels as follows:

Serum Bilirubin	SGOT	Dose Reduction
1.4 – 3 mg/100 ml		50 %
> 3 mg/100 ml	> 4 times upper normal limit	75 %

Table 1 DILUTION TABLE FOR BLADDER INSTILLATION SOLUTIONS

Dose epirubicin required	Volume of 2 mg/ ml epirubicin injection	Volume of diluent water for injection or 0.9 % sterile saline	Total volume for bladder installation
30 mg	15 ml	35 ml	50 ml
50 mg	25 ml	25 ml	50 ml
80 mg	40 ml	10 ml	50 ml

Impaired renal function

Moderate renal impairment does not appear to require a dose reduction in view of the limited amount of epirubicin excreted by this route. However, dosage adjustment may be necessary in patients with serum creatinine > 5 mg/dl.

Intravesical administration

Epirubicin can be given by intravesical administration for the treatment of superficial bladder cancer and carcinoma - in-situ. It should not be given intravesically for the treatment of invasive tumours that have penetrated the bladder wall, systemic therapy or surgery is more appropriate in these situations (see section 4.3). Epirubicin has also been successfully used intravesically as a prophylactic agent after transurethral resection of superficial tumours to prevent recurrence.

For the treatment of superficial bladder cancer the following regimen is recommended, using the dilution table below:

8 weekly instillations of 50 mg/ 50 ml (diluted with saline or water for injection).

If local toxicity is observed: A dose reduction to 30 mg/ 50 ml is advised.

Carcinoma-in-situ: Up to 80 mg/ 50 ml (depending on individual tolerability of the patient)

For prophylaxis: 4 weekly administrations of 50 mg/ 50 ml followed by 11 monthly instillations at the same dose.

DILUTION TABLE FOR BLADDER INSTILLATION SOLUTIONS

(see Table 1 above)

The solution should be retained intravesically for 1 – 2 hours. To avoid undue dilution with urine, the patient should be instructed not to drink any fluid in the 12 hours prior to instillation. During the instillation, the patient should be rotated occasionally and should be instructed to void urine at the end of the instillation time.

4.3 Contraindications

Epirubicin is contraindicated in:

– Patients who have demonstrated hypersensitivity to the active substance or to any of the excipients.

– Patients with marked myelosuppression induced by previous treatment with either other anti-neoplastic agents or radiotherapy.

– Patients treated with maximal cumulative doses of other anthracyclines such as doxorubicin or daunorubicin.

– Patients with current or previous history of cardiac impairment (including 4th degree heart failure, acute heart attack and previous heart attack which led to 3rd and 4th degree heart failure, acute inflammatory heart diseases, arrhythmia with serious haemodynamic consequences).

– Patients with acute systemic infections

– Lactation (see section 4.6).

For intravesical administration, epirubicin is contraindicated in:

– Urinary tract infections

– Invasive tumours penetrating the bladder

– Catheterisation problems

– Vesical inflammation

– Large volume of residual urine

Contracted bladder.

4.4 Special warnings and precautions for use

Epirubicin should only be administered under the supervision of a qualified physician who is experienced in the use of chemotherapeutic agents. Diagnostic and treatment facilities should be readily available for management of therapy and possible complications due to myelosuppression, especially following treatment with higher doses of epirubicin.

Extravasation of epirubicin from the vein during injection may cause severe tissue lesions and necrosis. Venous sclerosis may result from injection into small vessels or repeated injections into the same vein.

Careful baseline monitoring of various laboratory parameters and cardiac function should precede initial treatment with epirubicin.

During treatment with epirubicin, red blood cell, white blood cell, neutrophil and platelet counts should be carefully monitored both before and during each cycle of therapy. Leucopenia and neutropenia are usually transient with conventional and high-dose schedules reaching a nadir between the 10th and 14th day, values should return to normal by the 21st day; they are more severe with high dose schedules. Thrombocytopenia (< 100,000 platelets/mm^3) is experienced in very few patients, even following high doses of epirubicin.

Patients must have adequately recovered from severe stomatitis or mucositis before starting treatment with epirubicin.

In establishing the maximal cumulative dose of epirubicin, consideration should be given to any concomitant therapy with potentially cardiotoxic medicinal products. A cumulative dose of 900 – 1000 mg/m^2 should only be exceeded with extreme caution with both conventional and high doses of epirubicin. Above this level the risk of irreversible congestive heart failure increases greatly. An ECG is recommended before and after each treatment cycle. Alterations in the ECG tracing, such as flattening or inversion of the T - wave, depression of the S - T segment, or the onset of arrhythmias, generally transient and reversible, need not necessarily be taken as indications to discontinue treatment. With cumulative doses < 900 mg/m^2, there is evidence that cardiac toxicity rarely occurs. However, cardiac function must be carefully monitored during treatment to minimise the risk of heart failure of the type described for other anthracyclines. In case of cardiac insufficiency, treatment with epirubicin should be discontinued.

Cardiomyopathy induced by anthracyclines is associated with persistent reduction of the QRS voltage, prolongation beyond normal limits of the systolic interval (PEP/ LVET) and a reduction of the ejection fraction. Cardiac monitoring of patients receiving epirubicin treatment is highly important and it is advisable to assess cardiac function by non-invasive techniques. Electrocardiogram (ECG) changes may be indicative of anthracycline-induced cardiomyopathy, but ECG is not a sensitive or specific method for following anthracycline-related cardiotoxicity. The risk of serious cardiac impairment may be decreased through regular monitoring of left ventricular ejection fraction (LVEF) during the course of treatment with prompt discontinuation of epirubicin at the first sign of impaired function. The preferred method for repeated assessment of cardiac function is evaluation of LVEF measure by multi-gated radionuclide angiography (MUGA) or echocardiography (ECHO). A baseline cardiac evaluation with an ECG and a MUGA scan or an ECHO is recommended, especially in patients with risk factors for increased cardiac toxicity. Repeated MUGA or ECHO determinations of LVEF should be performed, particularly with higher, cumulative anthracycline doses. The technique used for assessment should be consistent through follow-up. In patients with risk factors, particularly prior anthracycline or anthracenedione use, the monitoring of cardiac function must be particularly strict.

As with other cytotoxic agents, epirubicin may induce hyperuricaemia as a result of rapid lysis of neoplastic cells. Blood uric acid levels should therefore be checked so that this phenomenon may be recognised and properly managed. Hydration, urine alkalinisation and prophylaxis with allopurinol to prevent hyperuricaemia may minimize potential complications of tumor-lysis syndrome.

Epirubicin may impart a red colour to the urine for one or two days after administration.

Heart failure may appear several weeks after discontinuing therapy with epirubicin and may be unresponsive to specific medical treatment. The potential risk of cardiotoxicity may increase in patients who have received concomitant, or prior, radiotherapy to the mediastinal pericardial area and/or who are under medical treatment with potentially cardiotoxic medicinal products (see section 4.5).

Epirubicin is mainly eliminated via the liver. Before commencing therapy with epirubicin, and if possible during treatment, liver function should be evaluated (SGOT, SGT, alkaline phosphatase, bilirubin), (see section 4.2). In patients with decreased liver function, epirubicin clearance can be reduced. For these patients a dose reduction is recommended (see section 4.2).

Serum creatinine levels should be checked regularly prior to and during treatment. For patients with increased serum creatinine (> 5 mg/dl) a dose reduction is proposed (see section 4.2).

Concurrent administration of attenuated live vaccines is not recommended, due to the risk of a potentially fatal generalised vaccine disease. The risk is increased in patients who are already immunocompromised by the primary disease. If available, inactivated vaccines should be used (e.g. inactivated poliomyelitis vaccine).

4.5 Interaction with other medicinal products and other forms of interaction

Epirubicin can be used in combination with other anti-cancer agents but patients should be monitored for additive toxicity, especially myelotoxicity and gastrointestinal toxicity.

Drug interactions with epirubicin have been observed with cimetidine, dexverapamil, dexrazoxane, docetaxel, interferon α_{2b}, paclitaxel and quinine.

Dexverapamil may alter the pharmacokinetics of epirubicin and possibly increase its bone marrow depressant effects.

Prior administration of higher doses (900 mg/m^2 and 1200 mg/m^2) of dexrazoxane may increase the systemic clearance of epirubicin and result in a decrease in AUC.

One study found that docetaxel may increase the plasma concentrations of epirubicin metabolites when administered immediately after epirubicin.

The co-administration of interferon α_{2b} may cause a reduction in both the terminal elimination half-life and the total clearance of epirubicin.

Paclitaxel has been shown to increase plasma concentrations of epirubicin when paclitaxel is administered before epirubicin. When paclitaxel is administered after epirubicin no detectable changes in epirubicin plasma concentrations have been observed. With concomitant use, the latter administration schedule is therefore recommended.

Quinine may accelerate the initial distribution of epirubicin from blood into the tissues and may have an influence on the red blood cells partitioning of epirubicin.

Cimetidine 400 mg b.i.d given prior to epirubicin 100 mg/m^2 every 3 weeks led to a 50 % increase in epirubicin AUC and a 41 % increase in epirubicinol AUC (latter $p < 0.05$). The AUC of the 7-deoxy-doxorubicinol aglycone and liver blood flow were not reduced, so results are not explained by reduced cytochrome P - 450 activity.

The possibility of a marked disturbance of haematopoiesis needs to be kept in mind with a (pre-) treatment with medications which influence the bone marrow (i.e. cytostatic agents, sulphonamide, chloramphenicol, diphenylhydantoin, amidopyrine-derivate, antiretroviral agents).

The potential risk of cardiotoxicity may increase in patients who have received concomitant cardiotoxic agents (e.g. 5-fluorouracil, cyclophosphamide, cisplatin, taxanes), or concomitant (or prior) radiotherapy to the mediastinal area.

The combination of Epirubicin and monoclonal antibodies like Trastuzumab can have a higher risk of cardiac dysfunction.

If epirubicin is used concomitantly with other medicinal products that may cause heart failure, e.g. calcium channel blockers, then cardiac function must be monitored throughout the course of treatment.

Epirubicin is mainly metabolised in the liver; each concomitant medication which affects hepatic function can also affect the metabolism or the pharmacokinetics of epirubicin and, consequently, its efficacy and/or toxicity.

4.6 Pregnancy and lactation

There is no conclusive information as to whether epirubicin may adversely affect human fertility or cause teratogenesis. Experimental data, however, suggest that epirubicin may harm the foetus (see section 5.3). Like most other anti-cancer agents, epirubicin has shown mutagenic and carcinogenic properties in animals. Both men and women receiving epirubicin should be informed of the potential risk of adverse effects on reproduction and should use an effective method of contraception during treatment and for six months thereafter.

Male patients treated with epirubicin are advised not to father a child during and up to 6 months after treatment and to seek advice on conservation of sperm prior to treatment because of the possibility of infertility due to therapy with epirubicin.

Women of childbearing potential should be fully informed of the potential hazard to the foetus and the possibility of genetic counselling should be considered if they become pregnant during epirubicin therapy. In cancer chemotherapy, epirubicin should not be used in pregnant women or women of childbearing potential who might become pregnant unless the potential benefits to the mother outweigh the possible risks to the foetus.

Epirubicin has been shown to be excreted into the milk of rats. It is not known whether epirubicin is excreted into human breast milk. Breastfeeding must be discontinued before and during therapy with epirubicin.

4.7 Effects on ability to drive and use machines

There have been no reports of particular adverse events relating to the effects on ability to drive and to use machines.

Epirubicin may cause episodes of nausea and vomiting, which can temporarily lead to an impairment of ability to drive or operate machines.

4.8 Undesirable effects

Adverse event frequencies have been categorised as follows:

Frequencies:

Very common (⩾ 1/10)

Common (⩾ 1/100, < 1/10)

Uncommon (⩾ 1/1,000, < 1/100)

Rare (⩾ 1/10,000, < 1/1,000)

Very rare (< 1/10,000), not known (cannot be estimated from the available data)

Infections and infestations:

Very common: Infections as a result of myelosuppression may occur with fever.

Very rare, not known: Pneumonia, sepsis and septic shock may occur as a result of myelosuppression.

Neoplasms benign, malignant and unspecified (including cysts and polyps):

Rare: Secondary acute myeloid leukaemia with or without a pre-leukaemic phase, in patients treated with epirubicin in combination with DNA-damaging antineoplastic agents.

These leukaemias have a short (1-3 year) latency.

Blood and the lymphatic system disorders:

Very common: Myelosuppression (leukocytopenia, granulocytopenia, neutropenia, febrile neutropenia, thrombocytopenia, anaemia).

Very rare, not known: Haemorrhage and tissue hypoxia may occur as a result of myelosuppression.

High doses of epirubicin have been safely administered in a large number of untreated patients having various solid tumours and have caused adverse events which are not different from those seen at conventional doses with the exception of reversible severe neutropenia (< 500 neutrophils/mm^3 for < 7 days) which occurred in the majority of patients. Only few patients required hospitalisation and supportive therapy for severe infectious complications at high doses.

Immune system disorders:

Common: Allergic reactions following intravesical administration.

Uncommon: Sensitivity to light or hypersensitivity in case of radiotherapy ("recall phenomenon").

Rare: Anaphylaxis (anaphylactic/anaphylactoid reactions with or without shock including skin rash, pruritus, fever and chills).

Cardiac disorders:

Rare: Cardiotoxicity (ECG changes, tachycardia, arrhythmia, cardiomyopathy, congestive heart failure (dyspnoea, oedema, enlargement of the liver, ascites, pulmonary oedema, pleural effusions, gallop rhythm), ventricular tachycardia, bradycardia, AV block, bundle-branch block (see section 4.4)).

Vascular disorders:

Uncommon: Thrombophlebitis

Coincidental cases of thromboembolic events (including pulmonary embolism [in isolated cases with fatal outcome]) have occurred.

Gastrointestinal disorders:

Common: Nausea, vomiting, diarrhoea, which can result in dehydration, loss of appetite and abdominal pain. Oesophagitis and hyperpigmentation of the oral mucosa may also occur.

Skin and subcutaneous tissue disorders:

Very common: Alopecia, normally reversible, appears in 60 – 90 % of treated cases; it is accompanied by lack of beard growth in males.

Common: Hot flushes

Uncommon: Hyperpigmentation of skin and nails. Skin reddening.

Rare: Urticaria.

General disorders and administration site conditions:

Common: Mucositis – may appear 5 – 10 days after the start of treatment, and usually involves stomatitis with areas of painful erosions, ulceration and bleeding, mainly along the side of the tongue and the sublingual mucosa.

Redness along the infusion vein. Local phlebitis, phlebosclerosis. Local pain and tissue necrosis (following accidental paravenous injection) may occur.

Uncommon: Headache

Rare: Fever, chills, dizziness, amenorrhea, azoospermia, hyperuricaemia (as a result of rapid lysis of neoplastic cells). Hyperpyrexia, malaise, weakness and increased transaminase levels have also been reported.

Injury, poisoning and procedural complications:

Common: Chemical cystitis, sometimes haemorrhagic, has been observed following intravesical administration.

4.9 Overdose

Very high single doses of epirubicin may be expected to cause acute myocardial degeneration within 24 hours and severe myelosuppression within 10 – 14 days. Treatment should aim to support the patient during this period and should utilise such measures as antibiotics, blood transfusion and reverse barrier nursing. Delayed cardiac failure has been seen with the anthracyclines up to 6 months after the overdose. Patients should be observed carefully and should, if signs of cardiac failure arise, be treated along conventional lines. Epirubicin is not dialyzable.

5. PHARMACOLOGICAL PROPERTIES

5.1 Pharmacodynamic properties

Pharmacotherapeutic group: Antineoplastic agent. ATC code: L01D B03

Epirubicin is a cytotoxic active antibiotic from the anthracycline group.

The mechanism of action of epirubicin is related to its ability to bind to DNA. Cell culture studies have shown rapid cell penetration, localisation in the nucleus and inhibition of nucleic acid synthesis and mitosis. Epirubicin has proved to be active on a wide spectrum of experimental tumours including L1210 and P388 leukaemias, sarcomas SA180 (solid and ascitic forms), B16 melanoma, mammary carcinoma, Lewis lung carcinoma and colon carcinoma 38. It has also shown activity against human tumours transplanted into athymic nude mice (melanoma, mammary, lung, prostatic and ovarian carcinomas).

5.2 Pharmacokinetic properties

In patients with normal hepatic and renal function, plasma levels after intravenous injection of 60-150 mg/m^2 of the medicinal product follow a tri-exponential decreasing pattern with a very fast first phase and a slow terminal phase with a mean half-life of about 40 hours. These doses are within the limits of pharmacokinetic linearity both in terms of plasma clearance values and metabolic pathway. Between 60 and 120 mg/m^2 there is an extensive linear pharmacokinetic, 150 mg/m^2 is at the margin of dose linearity. The major metabolites that have been identified are epirubicinol (13 - OH epirubicin) and glucuronides of epirubicin and epirubicinol.

In pharmacokinetic studies of patients with carcinoma in situ of the bladder the plasma levels of epirubicin after intravesical instillation are typically low (< 10 ng/ml). A significant systemic resorption can therefore not be assumed. In patients with lesions of the mucosa of the bladder (e.g. tumour, cystitis, operations), a higher resorption rate can be expected.

The 4' – O - glucuronidation distinguishes epirubicin from doxorubicin and may account for the faster elimination of epirubicin and its reduced toxicity. Plasma levels of the main metabolite, the 13 - OH derivative (epirubicinol) are consistently lower and virtually parallel those of the unchanged active substance.

Epirubicin is eliminated mainly through the liver; high plasma clearance values (0.9 l/min) indicate that this slow elimination is due to extensive tissue distribution. Urinary excretion accounts for approximately 9 – 10 % of the administered dose in 48 hours.

Biliary excretion represents the major route of elimination, about 40 % of the administered dose being recovered in the bile in 72 hours. The active substance does not cross the blood brain barrier.

5.3 Preclinical safety data

Following repeated dosing with epirubicin, the target organs in rat, rabbit and dog were the haemolymphopoietic system, GI tract, kidney, liver and reproductive organs. Epirubicin was also cardiotoxic in the rat, rabbit and dog.

Epirubicin, like other anthracyclines, was mutagenic, genotoxic and carcinogenic in rats. Embryotoxicity was seen in rats at clinically relevant doses.

No malformations were seen in rats or rabbits, but like other anthracyclines and cytotoxic active substances, epirubicin must be considered potentially teratogenic.

A local tolerance study in rats and mice showed extravasation of epirubicin causes tissue necrosis.

6. PHARMACEUTICAL PARTICULARS

6.1 List of excipients

sodium chloride

hydrochloric acid (for pH adjustment)

water for injections

6.2 Incompatibilities

Prolonged contact of the medicinal product with any solution of an alkaline pH (including sodium bicarbonate solutions) should be avoided; this will result in hydrolysis (degradation) of the active substance. Only the diluents detailed in section 6.3 should be used.

A physical incompatibility of the medicinal product with heparin has been reported.

This medicinal product must not be mixed with other medicinal products except those mentioned in Section 6.6.

6.3 Shelf life

2 years

In use:

Epirubicin hydrochloride may be further diluted, under aseptic conditions, in glucose 5 % solution or sodium chloride 0.9 % solution and administered as an intravenous infusion. The chemical and physical in-use stability has been demonstrated for 48 hours at 25 °C in the absence of light.

However, from a microbiological point of view, the product should be used immediately. If not used immediately, in-use storage times and conditions prior to use are the responsibility of the user and would normally not be longer than 24 hours at 2 to 8 °C, unless dilution has taken place in controlled and validated aseptic conditions.

6.4 Special precautions for storage

Store in a refrigerator (2 °C – 8 °C).

Keep the vial in the outer carton in order to protect from light.

For storage after dilution see section 6.3.

6.5 Nature and contents of container

Clear glass vials Type I with fluoropolymer-coated chlorobutyl rubber stoppers containing 5 ml, 10 ml, 25 ml, 50 ml or 100 ml solution of epirubicin hydrochloride 2 mg/ml.

Pack size: 1 vial.

6.6 Special precautions for disposal and other handling

Epirubicin hydrochloride may be further diluted in glucose 5 % solution or sodium chloride 0.9 % solution and administered as an intravenous infusion. For information on the stability of the infusion solutions please refer to section 6.3.

The injection solution contains no preservative and any unused portion of the vial should be disposed of immediately in accordance with local requirements.

Guidelines for the safe handling and disposal of antineoplastic agents:

1. If an infusion solution is to be prepared, this should be performed by trained personnel under aseptic conditions.

2. Preparation of an infusion solution should be performed in a designated aseptic area.

3. Adequate protective disposable gloves, goggles, gown and mask should be worn.

4. Precautions should be taken to avoid the medicinal product accidentally coming into contact with the eyes. In the event of contact with the eyes, irrigate with large amounts of water and/or 0.9 % sodium chloride solution. Then seek medical evaluation by a physician.

5. In case of skin contact, thoroughly wash the affected area with soap and water or sodium bicarbonate solution. However, do not abrade the skin by using a scrub brush. Always wash hands after removing gloves.

6. Spillage or leakage should be treated with dilute sodium hypochlorite (1 % available chlorine) solution, preferably by soaking, and then water. All cleaning materials should be disposed of as detailed below.

7. Pregnant staff should not handle the cytotoxic preparation.

8. Adequate care and precautions should be taken in the disposal of items (syringes, needles etc.) used to reconstitute and/or dilute cytotoxic medicinal products. Any unused product or waste material should be disposed of in accordance with local requirements.

7. MARKETING AUTHORISATION HOLDER

medac

Gesellschaft für klinische Spezialpräparate mbH

Fehlandtstr. 3

D-20354 Hamburg

Tel.: +49 / 4103 / 8006-0

Fax: +49 / 4103 / 8006-100

8. MARKETING AUTHORISATION NUMBER(S)

PL 11587/0043

9. DATE OF FIRST AUTHORISATION/RENEWAL OF THE AUTHORISATION

16/04/2008

10. DATE OF REVISION OF THE TEXT

05/2008

Episenta 150mg and 300mg Prolonged Release Capsules

(Beacon Pharmaceuticals)

1. NAME OF THE MEDICINAL PRODUCT

Episenta® 150 mg Prolonged-release Capsule and Episenta® 300 mg Prolonged-release Capsule

2. QUALITATIVE AND QUANTITATIVE COMPOSITION

Each prolonged-release capsule contains sodium valproate 150 mg

For excipients see 6.1

3. PHARMACEUTICAL FORM

Prolonged-release capsule, hard.

150 mg - Blue and transparent capsule containing white or almost white, round, film-coated prolonged-release granules.

300 mg - Green and transparent capsule containing white or almost white, round, film-coated prolonged-release granules.

4. CLINICAL PARTICULARS

4.1 Therapeutic indications

Sodium valproate is used in the treatment of all forms of epilepsy.

4.2 Posology and method of administration

Dosage requirements vary according to age and body weight and should be adjusted individually to achieve adequate seizure control. The daily dosage should be given in 1 – 2 single doses.

Monotherapy: usual requirements are as follows:

Adults: Dosage should start at 600mg daily increasing by 150-300mg at three day intervals until control is achieved. This is generally within the dosage range of 1000mg to 2000mg per day i.e. 20-30mg/kg body weight daily. Where adequate control is not achieved within this range the dose may be further increased to a maximum of 2500mg per day.

Children over 20kg: Initial dosage should be 300mg/day increasing until control is achieved. This is usually within the range 20-30mg/kg body weight per day. Where adequate control is not achieved within this range, the dose may be increased to 35 mg/kg body weight per day.

Children under 20kg: 20mg/kg body weight per day; in severe cases this may be increased up to 40mg/kg/day.

Use in the elderly: Care should be taken when adjusting dosage in the elderly since the pharmacokinetics of sodium valproate are modified. The volume of distribution is increased in the elderly and because of decreased binding to serum albumin, the proportion of free drug is increased. This will affect the clinical interpretation of plasma valproic acid levels. Dosage should be determined by seizure control.

In patients with renal insufficiency: It may be necessary to decrease dosage. Dosage should be adjusted according to clinical monitoring since monitoring of plasma concentrations may be misleading.

Combined Therapy: In certain cases it may be necessary to raise the dose by 5 to 10mg/kg/day when used in combination with liver enzyme inducing drugs such as phenytoin, phenobarbital and carbamazepine.

When barbiturates are being administered concomitantly and particularly if sedation is observed (particularly in children) the dosage of barbiturate should be reduced.

Method of administration

For oral administration.

The capsules should be swallowed whole without chewing, with plenty of liquid, such as a full glass of water. For patients with swallowing difficulties, the contents of the capsule may be sprinkled or stirred into soft food or drinks and swallowed immediately without chewing or crushing the prolonged-release granules. The food or drink should be cold or at room temperature. A mixture of granules of the granules with liquid or soft food should not be stored for future use. If the contents of the capsule are taken in a drink, as some granules may stick to the glass after the drink has been finished, the glass should be rinsed with a small amount of water and this water swallowed as well. The prolonged-release granules should not be given in babies' bottles as they can block the teat.

When changing from sodium valproate enteric coated tablets to Episenta® it is recommended to keep the same daily dose.

4.3 Contraindications

Active liver disease.

Personal or family history of severe hepatic dysfunction, especially drug related.

Porphyria.

Hypersensitivity to valproate or any of the excipients.

4.4 Special warnings and precautions for use

Suicidal ideation and behaviour have been reported in patients treated with antiepileptic agents in several indications. A meta-analysis of randomised placebo controlled trials of antiepileptic drugs has also shown a small increased risk of suicidal ideation and behaviour. The mechanism of this risk is not known and the available data do not exclude the possibility of an increased risk for sodium valproate.

Therefore patients should be monitored for signs of suicidal ideation and behaviours and appropriate treatment should be considered. Patients (and caregivers of patients) should be advised to seek medical advice should signs of suicidal ideation or behaviour emerge.

Hepatic dysfunction:

Conditions of occurrence:

Severe liver damage, including hepatic failure sometimes resulting in fatalities, has been very rarely reported. Experience in epilepsy has indicated that patients most at risk, especially in cases of multiple anticonvulsants therapy, are infants and in particular young children under the age of 3 and those with severe seizure disorders, organic brain disease, and (or) congenital metabolic or degenerative disease associated with mental retardation. After the age of 3, the incidence of occurrence is significantly reduced and progressively decreases with age. The concomitant use of salicylates should be avoided in children under 3 due to the risk liver toxicity. Additionally, salicylates should not be used in children under 16 years of age (see aspirin/salicylate product information on Reye's syndrome).

Monotherapy is recommended in children under the age of 3 years when prescribing Episenta®, but the potential benefit of Episenta® should be weighed against the risk of liver damage or pancreatitis in such patients prior to initiation of therapy.

In most cases, such liver damage occurred during the first 6 months of therapy, the period of maximum risk being 2 – 12 weeks.

Suggestive signs:

Clinical symptoms are essential for early diagnosis. In particular the following conditions, which may precede jaundice, should be taken into consideration, especially in patients at risk (see above: Conditions of occurrence):

- non-specific symptoms, usually of sudden onset, such as asthenia, malaise, anorexia, lethargy, oedema and drowsiness, which are sometimes associated with repeated vomiting and abdominal pain.

- in patients with epilepsy, recurrence of seizures

These are an indication for immediate withdrawal of the drug.

Patients (or their carers), should be instructed to report immediately any such signs to a physician should they occur. Investigations including clinical examination and biological assessment of liver function should be undertaken immediately.

Detection:

Liver function should be measured before and then periodically monitored during the first 6 months of therapy, especially in those who seem at risk, and those with a prior history of liver disease. Amongst usual investigations, tests which reflect protein synthesis, particularly prothrombin rate, are most relevant. Confirmation of an abnormally low prothrombin rate, particularly in association with other biological abnormalities (significant decreases in fibrinogen and coagulation factors; increased bilirubin level and raised transaminases) require cessation of Episenta® therapy.

As a matter of precaution and in case they are taken concomitantly salicylates should also be discontinued since they employ the same metabolic pathway.

As with most antiepileptic drugs, increased liver enzymes are common, particularly at the beginning of therapy; they are also transient.

More extensive biological investigations (including prothrombin rate) are recommended in these patients; a reduction in dosage may be considered when appropriate and tests should be repeated as necessary.

Pancreatitis:

Pancreatitis, which may be severe and result in fatalities, has been very rarely reported. Patients experiencing nausea, vomiting or acute abdominal pain should have a prompt medical evaluation (including measurement of serum amylase). Young children are at particular risk; this risk decreases with increasing age. Severe seizures and severe neurological impairment with combination anticonvulsant therapy may be risk factors. Hepatic failure with pancreatitis increases the risk of fatal outcome. In case of pancreatitis, Episenta® should be discontinued.

Haematological:

Blood tests (blood cell count, including platelet count, bleeding time and coagulation tests) are recommended prior to initiation of therapy or before surgery, and in case of spontaneous bruising or bleeding. (see section 4.8 Undesirable effects).

Renal insufficiency:

In patients with renal insufficiency, it may be necessary to decrease dosage. As monitoring of plasma concentrations may be misleading, dosage should be adjusted according to clinical monitoring (see sections 4.2 Posology and method of administration and 5.2 Pharmacokinetic properties).

Systemic lupus erythematosus:

Although immune disorders have only rarely been noted during the use of sodium valproate, the potential benefit of Episenta® should be weighed against its potential risk in patients with systemic lupus erythematosus (see section 4.8 Undesirable effects).

Hyperammonaemia:

When urea cycle enzymatic deficiency is suspected, metabolic investigations should be performed prior to treatment because of risk of hyperammonaemia with sodium valproate.

Weight gain:

Sodium valproate very commonly causes weight gain, which may be marked and progressive. Patients should be warned of the risk of weight gain at the initiation of therapy and appropriate strategies should be adopted to minimise it (see section 4.8 Undesirable effects)

Pregnancy:

Women of childbearing potential should not be started on Episenta® without specialist neurological advice. Adequate counselling should be made available to all women with epilepsy of childbearing potential regarding the risks associated with pregnancy because of the potential teratogenic risk to the foetus (see section 4.6 Pregnancy and lactation).

Diabetic Patients:

Sodium valproate is eliminated mainly through the kidneys, partly in the form of ketone bodies: this may give false positive in the urine testing of possible diabetics.

Granules in Stools:

The prolonged-release granules are surrounded by an indigestible cellulose shell through which the sodium valproate is released and these shells will be seen as white residues in the stools of the patient. There are no safety issues concerning such residues.

4.5 Interaction with other medicinal products and other forms of interaction

4.5.1 Effects of Episenta® on other drugs

Like many other drugs, Episenta® may potentiate the effect of other psychotropics, such as antipsychotics, monoamine oxidase inhibitors, antidepressants and benzodiazepines. Therefore, clinical monitoring and the dosage of other psychotropics should be adjusted when appropriate.

Sodium valproate increases phenobarbital plasma concentrations and sedation may occur, particularly in children. Clinical monitoring is recommended throughout the first 15 days of combined treatment with an immediate reduction of phenobarbital doses if sedation occurs and determination of phenobarbital levels when appropriate.

Sodium valproate increases primidone plasma levels causing an exacerbation of side effects, e.g. sedation. Clinical monitoring is recommended especially when initiating combined therapy with dosage adjustment as necessary.

Phenytoin total plasma levels are decreased by sodium valproate acid; the free form of phenytoin is increased leading to possible overdosage symptoms. Therefore, clinical monitoring is recommended with the free form of phenytoin being measured.

The toxic effects of carbamazepine may be potentiated by sodium valproate requiring clinical monitoring and dosage adjustment particularly at initiation of combined therapy.

Sodium valproate may reduce lamotrigine metabolism and increase its mean half-life. The dosage of lamotrigine should be decreased as necessary. The risk of rash is increased in combined therapy with lamotrigine.

Sodium valproate may raise zidovudine plasma concentrations leading to increased zidovudine toxicity.

The anticoagulant effect of warfarin and other coumarin anticoagulants may be increased following displacement from the plasma protein binding site by valproate. The prothombin time should be closely monitored.

4.5.2 Effects of other drugs on Episenta®

Antiepileptics with enzyme inducing effects e.g. phenytoin, phenobarbital, carbamazepine, decrease valproate plasma levels. Plasma levels should be monitored and dosage adjusted accordingly.

Mefloquine and chloroquine increases valproate metabolism and therefore epileptic seizures may occur in combined therapy. The dosage of sodium valproate may need adjustment.

Free valproate levels may be increased in the case of concomitant use with highly protein bound agents e.g. acetylsalicylic acid. Valproate plasma levels may also be increased when used concomitantly with cimetidine or erythromycin as a result of reduced hepatic metabolism.

Carbapenem antibiotics such as imipenem and meropenem decrease plasma valproate levels. If administering these antibiotics with sodium valproate close monitoring of valproate plasma levels is recommended.

Colestyramine may decrease the absorption of valproate.

The effect of hormonal contraceptives ("the pill") is not reduced by sodium valproate.

Caution is advised when using Episenta® in combination with newer antiepileptics whose pharmacodynamics may not be well established.

4.6 Pregnancy and lactation

4.6.1 Pregnancy

From experience in treating mothers with epilepsy, the risk associated with the use of valproate during pregnancy has been described as follows:

Risk associated with epilepsy and antiepileptics

In offspring born to mothers with epilepsy receiving any antiepileptic treatment, the overall rate of malformations has been demonstrated to be 2 to 3 times higher than the rate (approximately 3%) reported in the general population. Although an increased number of children with malformations have been reported in cases of multiple drug therapy, the respective role of treatments and disease in causing the malformations has not been formally established. Malformations most frequently encountered are cleft lip and cardiovascular malformations.

Epidemiological studies have suggested an association between in-utero exposure to sodium valproate and a risk of developmental delay. Developmental delay has been reported in children born to mothers with epilepsy. It is not possible to differentiate what may be due to genetic, social, environmental factors, maternal epilepsy or antiepileptic treatment. Many factors including maternal epilepsy may also contribute to this risk but it is difficulty to quantify the relative contributions of these or of maternal anti-epileptic treatment. Notwithstanding those potential risks, no sudden discontinuation in the anti-epileptic therapy should be undertaken as this may lead to breakthrough seizures which could have serious consequences for both the mother and the foetus.

Risks associated with valproate

In animals: teratogenic effects have been demonstrated in the mouse, rat and rabbit. There is animal experimental evidence that high plasma peak levels and the size of an individual dose are associated with neural tube defects.

In humans: valproate is associated with neural tube defects such as myelomeningocele and spina bifida. The frequency of this effect is estimated to be 1 to 2%. An increased incidence of major malformations including neural tube defects, craniofacial defects, malformation of the limbs, cardiovascular malformations, hypospadias and multiple anomalies involving various body systems has been reported in offspring born to mothers with epilepsy treated with valproate. Some data from studies, of women with epilepsy, have suggested an association between in-utero exposure to valproate and the risk of developmental delay (frequently associated with craniofacial abnormalities), particularly of verbal IQ.

In view of the above data

When a woman is planning pregnancy, this provides an opportunity to review the need for antiepileptic treatment. Women of childbearing age should be informed of the risks and benefits of continuing anti-epileptic treatment throughout pregnancy.

Folate supplementation, **prior** to pregnancy, has been demonstrated to reduce the incidence of neural tube defects in the offspring of women at high risk. Although no direct evidence exists of such effects in women receiving anti-epileptic drugs, woman should be advised to start taking folic acid supplementation (5 mg) as soon as contraception is discontinued.

The available evidence suggests that anticonvulsants monotherapy is preferred. Dosage should be reviewed before conception and the lowest effective dose used, in divided doses, as abnormal pregnancy outcome tends to be associated with higher total daily dosage and with the size of an individual dose. The incidence of neural tube defects rises with increasing dosage, particularly above 1000 mg daily. The administration in several divided doses over the day and the use of a prolonged release formulation is preferable in order to avoid high peak plasma levels.

During pregnancy, Episenta® antiepileptic treatment should not be discontinued if it has been effective. Nevertheless, specialist prenatal monitoring should be instituted in order to detect the possible occurrence of a neural tube defect or any other malformation. Pregnancies should be carefully screened by ultrasound, and other techniques if appropriate (see Section 4.4 Special warnings and special precautions for use).

Risk in the neonate

Very rare cases of haemorrhagic syndrome have been reported in neonates whose mothers have taken valproate during pregnancy. This haemorrhagic syndrome is related to hypofibrinogenaemia; afibrinogenaemia has also been reported and may be fatal. These are possibly associated with a decrease of coagulation factors. However, this syndrome has to be distinguished from the decrease of the vitamin-K factors induced by phenobarbital and other antiepileptic enzyme inducing drugs. Therefore platelet count, fibrinogen plasma level, coagulation tests and coagulation factors should be investigated in neonates.

4.6.2 Lactation

Excretion of valproate in breast milk is low, with a concentration between 1% to 10% of total maternal serum levels; up to now children breast fed that have been monitored during the neonatal period have not experienced clinical effects. There appears to be no contraindications to breast feeding by patients on Episenta®.

4.7 Effects on ability to drive and use machines

Use of Episenta® may provide seizure control such that the patient may be eligible to hold a driving licence.

At the start of treatment with sodium valproate, at higher dosages or with a combination of other centrally acting drugs, reaction time may be altered to an extent that affects the ability to drive or to operate machinery, irrespective of the effect on the primary disease being treated. Patients should be warned of the risk of transient drowsiness. This is especially the case when taken during anticonvulsant polytherapy, concomitant use of benzodiazepines or in combination with alcohol.

4.8 Undesirable effects

Congenital and familial/genetic disorders: (see section 4.6 Pregnancy and lactation)

Hepato-biliary disorders:

Rare cases of hepatic dysfunction (see section 4.4 Special warnings and precautions for use). Severe liver damage, including hepatic failure sometimes resulting in fatalities, has been reported (see sections 4.2 (Posology and method of administration, 4.3 Contraindications and 4.4 Special warnings and precautions for use). Increased liver enzymes are common, particularly early in treatment, and may be transient (see section 4.4 Special warnings and precautions for use).

Gastro-intestinal disorders: (nausea, gastralgia, diarrhoea)

Frequently occur at the start of the treatment, but they usually disappear after a few days without discontinuing treatment. These problems can usually be overcome by taking Episenta® with or after food.

Very rare cases of pancreatitis, sometimes fatal, have been reported (see section 4.4 Special warnings and precautions for use).

Nervous system disorders:

Sedation has been reported occasionally, usually when in combination with other anticonvulsants. In monotherapy it occurred early in treatment on rare occasions and is usually transient. Rare cases of lethargy and confusion occasionally progressing to stupor, sometimes with associated hallucinations or convulsions have been reported. Encephalopathy and coma have very rarely been observed. These cases have often been associated with a too high starting dose or a too rapid dose escalation or concomitant use of other anticonvulsants, notably phenobarbital. They have usually been reversible on withdrawal of treatment or reduction of dosage.

Very rare cases of reversible extrapyramidal symptoms including parkinsonism, or reversible dementia associated with reversible cerebral atrophy have been reported. Dose related ataxia and fine postural tremor have occasionally been reported.

An increase in alertness may occur, this is generally beneficial but occasionally aggression, hyperactivity and behavioural deterioration have been reported.

Metabolic disorders:

Cases of isolated and moderate hyperammonaemia without change in liver function tests may occur frequently, are usually transient and should not cause treatment discontinuation. However, they may present clinically as vomiting, ataxia, and increasing clouding of consciousness. Should these symptoms occur Episenta® should be discontinued. Very rare cases of hyponatraemia have been reported. Hyperammonaemia associated with neurological symptoms have also been reported (see section 4.4 Special warnings and precautions for use). In such cases further investigation should be considered.

Blood and lymphatic system disorders:

Frequent occurrence of thrombocytopenia, rare cases of anaemia, leucopenia or panocytopenia. The blood picture returned to normal when the drug was discontinued. Isolated reduction of fibrinogen or reversible increase in bleeding time have been reported, usually without associated clinical signs and particularly with high doses (sodium valproate has an inhibitory effect on the second phase of platelet aggregation). Spontaneous bruising or bleeding is an indication of withdrawal of medication pending investigations (see section 4.6 Pregnancy and lactation).

Skin and subcutaneous disorders:

Cutaneous reactions such as exanthematous rash rarely occur with sodium valproate. In very rare cases, toxic epidermal necrolysis, Stevens-Johnson syndrome and erythema multiforme have been reported. Transient hair loss, which may sometimes be dose-related, has often been reported. Regrowth normally begins within 6 months, although the hair may become more curly than previously. Hirsutism and acne have been very rarely reported.

Reproductive system and breast disorders:

Amenorrhoea and irregular periods have been reported. Very rarely gynaecomastia has occurred

Vascular disorders:

The occurrence of vasculitis has occasionally been reported.

Ear disorders:

Hearing loss, either reversible or irreversible has been reported rarely; however a cause and effect relationship has not been established.

Renal and urinary disorders:

There have been isolated reports of reversible Fanconi's syndrome (a defect in proximal renal tubular function giving rise to glycosuria, amino aciduria, phospaturia, and uricosuria) associated with sodium valproate therapy, but the mode of action is as yet unclear. Very rare cases of enuresis have been reported.

Immune system disorders:

Allergic reactions (ranging from rash to hypersensitivity reactions) have been reported.

General disorders:

Very rare cases of non-severe peripheral oedema have been reported.

Increase in weight may also occur. Weight gain being a risk factor for polycystic ovary syndrome, it should be carefully monitored (see section 4.4 Special warnings and precautions for use).

4.9 Overdose

Cases of accidental and deliberate overdosage with oral therapy have been reported. At plasma concentrations of up to 5 to 6 times the maximum therapeutic levels, there are unlikely to be any symptoms other than nausea, vomiting and dizziness. In massive overdose, 10 to 20 times the maximum therapeutic levels, there may be serious CNS depression or coma with muscular hypotonia, hyperflexia, miosis, impaired respiratory function, metabolic acidosis. The symptoms may however be variable and seizures have been reported in the presence of very high plasma levels. Cases of intracranial hypertension related to cerebral oedema have been reported. A number of deaths have occurred following large overdoses. Hospital management of overdose includes induced vomiting, gastric lavage, assisted ventilation and other supportive measures. Haemodialysis and haemoperfusion have been used successfully. Intravenous naloxone has also been used sometimes in association with activated charcoal given orally.

5. PHARMACOLOGICAL PROPERTIES

5.1 Pharmacodynamic properties

Pharmacotherapeutic Group: Fatty acid derivatives

ATC no: N03AG01

The mode of action of valproic acid is not fully understood but may involve an elevation of gamma-amino butyric acid levels in the brain.

In certain in-vitro studies, it was reported that sodium valproate could stimulate HIV replication, but studies on peripheral blood mononuclear cells from HIV-infected subjects show that sodium valproate does not have a mitogen-like effect on inducing HIV replication. Indeed, the effect of sodium valproate on HIV replication ex-vivo is highly variable, modest in quantity, appears to be unrelated to the dose and has not been documented in man.

5.2 Pharmacokinetic properties

With peroral administration 90-100% of the dose is rapidly absorbed.

Maximal plasma concentration is achieved with Episenta® within 6.5 ±3.3 hours. The half-life is 12-16 h in most patients but can in exceptional cases be considerably lower. Impaired renal function prolongs the half-life. In infants under 2 months the half-life can be prolonged up to 60 hours but in older children it is the same as in adults.

Steady-state concentration is normally achieved after treatment in 3-5 days. A satisfactory effect is most often achieved at 50 – 100 µg/ml, but the patient's overall situation must be considered.

The relation between the dose and effect, and between plasma concentrations and effect, has not been fully clarified. The CSF concentration is up to 10% of the plasma concentration. About 90% of sodium valproate is bound to plasma protein, which may entail a risk of clinically significant interactions with other antiepileptics, primarily phenytoin. Sodium valproate is metabolised to a great extent and is excreted in the urine as conjugated metabolites. Sodium valproate crosses the placental barrier and concentrations of foetal plasma are comparable to those in the mother.

Valproic acid passes into breast milk but is not likely to influence the child when therapeutic doses are used.

5.3 Preclinical safety data

There are no preclinical data of relevance t to the prescriber which are additional to that already included in other sections of the SPC.

6. PHARMACEUTICAL PARTICULARS

6.1 List of excipients

Prolonged –release granule:

calcium stearate

silicon dioxide (methylated)

ammonio methacrylate copolymer type B

sodium lauryl sulfate

polysorbate 80

Granule coating:

ethylcellulose

dibutylsebacate

oleic acid

150 mg Capsule shell:

gelatine

indigo carmine (E132)

sodium lauryl sulfate

300 mg Capsule shell:

gelatine

indigo carmine (E132)

quinoline yellow (E104)

sodium lauryl sulphate

6.2 Incompatibilities

None known

6.3 Shelf life

36 months

6.4 Special precautions for storage

Do not store above 30°C. Store in the original container. Keep the container tightly closed.

6.5 Nature and contents of container

Polypropylene container with polyethylene stopper or polyethylene container with polypropylene screw cap containing 50, 100 or 200 prolonged-release capsules

6.6 Special precautions for disposal and other handling

None.

7. MARKETING AUTHORISATION HOLDER

Beacon Pharmaceuticals Limited

85 High Street

Tunbridge Wells

Kent

TN1 1YG

UK

8. MARKETING AUTHORISATION NUMBER(S)

Episenta 150 mg prolonged-release capsule PL18157/0021

Episenta 300mg prolonged-release capsule PL18157/0022

9. DATE OF FIRST AUTHORISATION/RENEWAL OF THE AUTHORISATION

6th October 2006

10. DATE OF REVISION OF THE TEXT

6th July 2009

Episenta 500mg and 1000mg Prolonged Release Granules

(Beacon Pharmaceuticals)

1. NAME OF THE MEDICINAL PRODUCT

Episenta® 500 mg Prolonged-release Granules and Episenta® 1000mg Prolonged-release Granules

2. QUALITATIVE AND QUANTITATIVE COMPOSITION

Each sachet of prolonged-release granules contains sodium valproate 500 mg

For excipients see 6.1

3. PHARMACEUTICAL FORM

Prolonged-release granules.

White or almost white, round, film-coated prolonged-release granules.

4. CLINICAL PARTICULARS

4.1 Therapeutic indications

Sodium valproate is used in the treatment of all forms of epilepsy.

4.2 Posology and method of administration

Dosage requirements vary according to age and body weight and should be adjusted individually to achieve adequate seizure control. The daily dosage should be given in 1 – 2 single doses.

Monotherapy: usual requirements are as follows:

Adults: Dosage should start at 600mg daily increasing by 150-300mg at three day intervals until control is achieved. This is generally within the dosage range of 1000mg to 2000mg per day i.e. 20-30mg/kg body weight daily. Where adequate control is not achieved within this range the dose may be further increased to a maximum of 2500mg per day.

Children over 20kg: Initial dosage should be 300mg/day increasing until control is achieved. This is usually within the range 20-30mg/kg body weight per day. Where adequate control is not achieved within this range, the dose may be increased to 35 mg/kg body weight per day.

Children under 20kg: 20mg/kg body weight per day; in severe cases this may be increased up to 40mg/kg/day.

Use in the elderly: Care should be taken when adjusting dosage in the elderly since the pharmacokinetics of sodium valproate are modified. The volume of distribution is increased in the elderly and because of decreased binding to serum albumin, the proportion of free drug is increased. This will affect the clinical interpretation of plasma valproic acid levels. Dosage should be determined by seizure control.

In patients with renal insufficiency: It may be necessary to decrease dosage. Dosage should be adjusted according to clinical monitoring since monitoring of plasma concentrations may be misleading.

Combined Therapy: In certain cases it may be necessary to raise the dose by 5 to 10mg/kg/day when used in combination with liver enzyme inducing drugs such as phenytoin, phenobarbital and carbamazepine.

When barbiturates are being administered concomitantly and particularly if sedation is observed (particularly in children) the dosage of barbiturate should be reduced.

Method of administration

For oral administration.

The contents of the sachet may be sprinkled or stirred into soft food or drinks and swallowed immediately without chewing, or crushing the prolonged-release granules. The food or drink should be cold or at room temperature. A mixture of the granules with liquid or soft food should not be stored for future use. If the contents of the sachet are taken in a drink, as some granules may stick to the glass after the drink has been finished, the glass should be rinsed with a small amount of water and this water swallowed as well. The prolonged-release granules should not be given in babies' bottles as they can block the teat.

When changing from sodium valproate enteric coated tablets to Episenta® it is recommended to keep the same daily dose.

4.3 Contraindications

Active liver disease.

Personal or family history of severe hepatic dysfunction, especially drug related.

Porphyria.

Hypersensitivity to valproate or any of the excipients.

4.4 Special warnings and precautions for use

Suicidal ideation and behaviour have been reported in patients treated with antiepileptic agents in several indications. A meta-analysis of randomised placebo controlled trials of antiepileptic drugs has also shown a small increased risk of suicidal ideation and behaviour. The mechanism of this risk is not known and the available data do not exclude the possibility of an increased risk for sodium valproate.

Therefore patients should be monitored for signs of suicidal ideation and behaviours and appropriate treatment should be considered. Patients (and caregivers of patients) should be advised to seek medical advice should signs of suicidal ideation or behaviour emerge.

Hepatic dysfunction:

Conditions of occurrence:

Severe liver damage, including hepatic failure sometimes resulting in fatalities, has been very rarely reported. Experience in epilepsy has indicated that patients most at risk, especially in cases of multiple anticonvulsants therapy, are infants and in particular young children under the age of 3 and those with severe seizure disorders, organic brain disease, and (or) congenital metabolic or degenerative disease associated with mental retardation. After the age of 3, the incidence of occurrence is significantly reduced and progressively decreases with age. The concomitant use of salicylates should be avoided in children under 3 due to the risk liver toxicity. Additionally, salicylates should not be used in children under 16 years of age (see aspirin/salicylate product information on Reye's syndrome).

Monotherapy is recommended in children under the age of 3 years when prescribing Episenta®, but the potential benefit of Episenta® should be weighed against the risk of liver damage or pancreatitis in such patients prior to initiation of therapy.

In most cases, such liver damage occurred during the first 6 months of therapy, the period of maximum risk being 2 – 12 weeks.

Suggestive signs:

Clinical symptoms are essential for early diagnosis. In particular the following conditions, which may precede jaundice, should be taken into consideration, especially in patients at risk (see above: Conditions of occurrence):

- non-specific symptoms, usually of sudden onset, such as asthenia, malaise, anorexia, lethargy, oedema and drowsiness, which are sometimes associated with repeated vomiting and abdominal pain.

- in patients with epilepsy, recurrence of seizures

These are an indication for immediate withdrawal of the drug.

Patients (or their carers), should be instructed to report immediately any such signs to a physician should they occur. Investigations including clinical examination and biological assessment of liver function should be undertaken immediately.

Detection:

Liver function should be measured before and then periodically monitored during the first 6 months of therapy, especially in those who seem at risk, and those with a prior history of liver disease. Amongst usual investigations, tests which reflect protein synthesis, particularly prothrombin rate, are most relevant. Confirmation of an abnormally low prothrombin rate, particularly in association with other biological abnormalities (significant decreases in fibrinogen and coagulation factors; increased bilirubin level and raised transaminases) require cessation of Episenta® therapy.

As a matter of precaution and in case they are taken concomitantly salicylates should also be discontinued since they employ the same metabolic pathway.

As with most antiepileptic drugs, increased liver enzymes are common, particularly at the beginning of therapy; they are also transient.

More extensive biological investigations (including prothrombin rate) are recommended in these patients; a reduction in dosage may be considered when appropriate and tests should be repeated as necessary.

Pancreatitis:

Pancreatitis, which may be severe and result in fatalities, has been very rarely reported. Patients experiencing nausea, vomiting or acute abdominal pain should have a prompt medical evaluation (including measurement of serum amylase). Young children are at particular risk; this risk decreases with increasing age. Severe seizures and severe neurological impairment with combination anticonvulsant therapy may be risk factors. Hepatic failure with pancreatitis increases the risk of fatal outcome. In case of pancreatitis, Episenta® should be discontinued.

Haematological:

Blood tests (blood cell count, including platelet count, bleeding time and coagulation tests) are recommended prior to initiation of therapy or before surgery, and in case of spontaneous bruising or bleeding. (see section 4.8 Undesirable effects).

Renal insufficiency:

In patients with renal insufficiency, it may be necessary to decrease dosage. As monitoring of plasma concentrations may be misleading, dosage should be adjusted according to clinical monitoring (see sections 4.2 Posology and method of administration and 5.2 Pharmacokinetic properties).

Systemic lupus erythematosus:

Although immune disorders have only rarely been noted during the use of sodium valproate, the potential benefit of Episenta® should be weighed against its potential risk in patients with systemic lupus erythematosus (see section 4.8 Undesirable effects).

Hyperammonaemia:

When urea cycle enzymatic deficiency is suspected, metabolic investigations should be performed prior to treatment because of risk of hyperammonaemia with sodium valproate.

Weight gain:

Sodium valproate very commonly causes weight gain, which may be marked and progressive. Patients should be warned of the risk of weight gain at the initiation of therapy and appropriate strategies should be adopted to minimise it (see section 4.8 Undesirable effects)

Pregnancy:

Women of childbearing potential should not be started on Episenta® without specialist neurological advice. Adequate counselling should be made available to all women with epilepsy of childbearing potential regarding the risks associated with pregnancy because of the potential teratogenic risk to the foetus (see section 4.6 Pregnancy and lactation).

Diabetic Patients:

Sodium valproate is eliminated mainly through the kidneys, partly in the form of ketone bodies: this may give false positive in the urine testing of possible diabetics.

Granules in Stools:

The prolonged-release granules are surrounded by an indigestible cellulose shell through which the sodium valproate is released and these shells will be seen as white residues in the stools of the patient. There are no safety issues concerning such residues.

4.5 Interaction with other medicinal products and other forms of interaction

4.5.1 Effects of Episenta® on other drugs

Like many other drugs, Episenta® may potentiate the effect of other psychotropics, such as antipsychotics, monoamine oxidase inhibitors, antidepressants and benzodiazepines. Therefore, clinical monitoring and the dosage of other psychotropics should be adjusted when appropriate.

Sodium valproate increases phenobarbital plasma concentrations and sedation may occur, particularly in children. Clinical monitoring is recommended throughout the first 15 days of combined treatment with an immediate reduction of phenobarbital doses if sedation occurs and determination of phenobarbital levels when appropriate.

Sodium valproate increases primidone plasma levels causing an exacerbation of side effects, e.g. sedation. Clinical monitoring is recommended especially when initiating combined therapy with dosage adjustment as necessary.

Phenytoin total plasma levels are decreased by sodium valproate acid; the free form of phenytoin is increased leading to possible overdosage symptoms. Therefore, clinical monitoring is recommended with the free form of phenytoin being measured.

The toxic effects of carbamazepine may be potentiated by sodium valproate requiring clinical monitoring and dosage adjustment particularly at initiation of combined therapy.

Sodium valproate may reduce lamotrigine metabolism and increase its mean half-life. The dosage of lamotrigine should be decreased as necessary. The risk of rash is increased in combined therapy with lamotrigine.

Sodium valproate may raise zidovudine plasma concentrations leading to increased zidovudine toxicity.

The anticoagulant effect of warfarin and other coumarin anticoagulants may be increased following displacement from the plasma protein binding site by valproate. The prothombin time should be closely monitored.

4.5.2 Effects of other drugs on Episenta®

Antiepileptics with enzyme inducing effects e.g. phenytoin, phenobarbital, carbamazepine, decrease valproate plasma levels. Plasma levels should be monitored and dosage adjusted accordingly.

Mefloquine and chloroquine increases valproate metabolism and therefore epileptic seizures may occur in combined therapy. The dosage of sodium valproate may need adjustment.

Free valproate levels may be increased in the case of concomitant use with highly protein bound agents e.g. acetylsalicylic acid. Valproate plasma levels may also be increased when used concomitantly with cimetidine or erythromycin as a result of reduced hepatic metabolism.

Carbapenem antibiotics such as imipenem and meropenem decrease plasma valproate levels. If administering these antibiotics with sodium valproate close monitoring of valproate plasma levels is recommended.

Colestyramine may decrease the absorption of valproate.

The effect of hormonal contraceptives ("the pill") is not reduced by sodium valproate.

Caution is advised when using Episenta® in combination with newer antiepileptics whose pharmacodynamics may not be well established.

4.6 Pregnancy and lactation

4.6.1 Pregnancy

From experience in treating mothers with epilepsy, the risk associated with the use of valproate during pregnancy has been described as follows:

Risk associated with epilepsy and antiepileptics

In offspring born to mothers with epilepsy receiving any antiepileptic treatment, the overall rate of malformations has been demonstrated to be 2 to 3 times higher than the rate (approximately 3%) reported in the general population. Although an increased number of children with malformations have been reported in cases of multiple drug therapy, the respective role of treatments and disease in causing the malformations has not been formally established. Malformations most frequently encountered are cleft lip and cardiovascular malformations.

Epidemiological studies have suggested an association between in-utero exposure to sodium valproate and a risk of developmental delay. Developmental delay has been reported in children born to mothers with epilepsy. It is not possible to differentiate what may be due to genetic, social, environmental factors, maternal epilepsy or antiepileptic treatment. Many factors including maternal epilepsy may also contribute to this risk but it is difficulty to quantify the relative contributions of these or of maternal anti-epileptic treatment. Notwithstanding those potential risks, no sudden discontinuation in the anti-epileptic therapy should be undertaken as this may lead to breakthrough seizures which could have serious consequences for both the mother and the foetus.

Risks associated with valproate

In animals: teratogenic effects have been demonstrated in the mouse, rat and rabbit. There is animal experimental evidence that high plasma peak levels and the size of an individual dose are associated with neural tube defects.

In humans: valproate is associated with neural tube defects such as myelomeningocele and spina bifida. The frequency of this effect is estimated to be 1 to 2%. An increased incidence of major malformations including neural tube defects, craniofacial defects, malformation of the limbs, cardiovascular malformations, hypospadias and multiple anomalies involving various body systems has been reported in offspring born to mothers with epilepsy treated with valproate. Some data from studies, of women with epilepsy, have suggested an association between in-utero exposure to valproate and the risk of developmental delay (frequently associated with craniofacial abnormalities), particularly of verbal IQ.

In view of the above data

When a woman is planning pregnancy, this provides an opportunity to review the need for antiepileptic treatment. Women of childbearing age should be informed of the risks and benefits of continuing anti-epileptic treatment throughout pregnancy.

Folate supplementation, **prior** to pregnancy, has been demonstrated to reduce the incidence of neural tube defects in the offspring of women at high risk. Although no direct evidence exists of such effects in women receiving anti-epileptic drugs, woman should be advised to start taking folic acid supplementation (5 mg) as soon as contraception is discontinued.

The available evidence suggests that anticonvulsants monotherapy is preferred. Dosage should be reviewed before conception and the lowest effective dose used, in divided doses, as abnormal pregnancy outcome tends to be associated with higher total daily dosage and with the size of an individual dose. The incidence of neural tube defects rises with increasing dosage, particularly above 1000 mg daily. The administration in several divided doses over the day and the use of a prolonged release formulation is preferable in order to avoid high peak plasma levels.

During pregnancy, Episenta® antiepileptic treatment should not be discontinued if it has been effective. Nevertheless, specialist prenatal monitoring should be instituted in order to detect the possible occurrence of a neural tube defect or any other malformation. Pregnancies should be carefully screened by ultrasound, and other techniques if appropriate (see Section 4.4 Special warnings and special precautions for use).

Risk in the neonate

Very rare cases of haemorrhagic syndrome have been reported in neonates whose mothers have taken valproate during pregnancy. This haemorrhagic syndrome is related to hypofibrinogenaemia; afibrinogenaemia has also been reported and may be fatal. These are possibly associated with a decrease of coagulation factors. However, this syndrome has to be distinguished from the decrease of the vitamin-K factors induced by phenobarbital and other antiepileptic enzyme inducing drugs. Therefore platelet count, fibrinogen plasma level, coagulation tests and coagulation factors should be investigated in neonates.

4.6.2 Lactation

Excretion of valproate in breast milk is low, with a concentration between 1% to 10% of total maternal serum levels; up to now children breast fed that have been monitored during the neonatal period have not experienced clinical effects. There appears to be no contraindications to breast feeding by patients on Episenta®.

4.7 Effects on ability to drive and use machines

Use of Episenta® may provide seizure control such that the patient may be eligible to hold a driving licence.

At the start of treatment with sodium valproate, at higher dosages or with a combination of other centrally acting drugs, reaction time may be altered to an extent that affects the ability to drive or to operate machinery, irrespective of the effect on the primary disease being treated. Patients should be warned of the risk of transient drowsiness. This is especially the case when taken during anticonvulsant polytherapy, concomitant use of benzodiazepines or in combination with alcohol.

4.8 Undesirable effects

Congenital and familial/genetic disorders: (see section 4.6 Pregnancy and lactation)

Hepato-biliary disorders:

Rare cases of hepatic dysfunction (see section 4.4 Special warnings and precautions for use). Severe liver damage, including hepatic failure sometimes resulting in fatalities, has been reported (see sections 4.2 (Posology and method of administration, 4.3 Contraindications and 4.4 Special warnings and precautions for use). Increased liver enzymes are common, particularly early in treatment, and may be transient (see section 4.4 Special warnings and precautions for use).

Gastro-intestinal disorders: (nausea, gastralgia, diarrhoea)

Frequently occur at the start of the treatment, but they usually disappear after a few days without discontinuing treatment. These problems can usually be overcome by taking Episenta® with or after food.

Very rare cases of pancreatitis, sometimes fatal, have been reported (see section 4.4 Special warnings and precautions for use).

Nervous system disorders:

Sedation has been reported occasionally, usually when in combination with other anticonvulsants. In monotherapy it occurred early in treatment on rare occasions and is usually transient. Rare cases of lethargy and confusion occasionally progressing to stupor, sometimes with associated hallucinations or convulsions have been reported. Encephalopathy and coma have very rarely been observed. These cases have often been associated with a too high starting dose or a too rapid dose escalation or concomitant use of other anticonvulsants, notably phenobarbital. They have usually been reversible on withdrawal of treatment or reduction of dosage.

Very rare cases of reversible extrapyramidal symptoms including parkinsonism, or reversible dementia associated with reversible cerebral atrophy have been reported. Dose related ataxia and fine postural tremor have occasionally been reported.

An increase in alertness may occur, this is generally beneficial but occasionally aggression, hyperactivity and behavioural deterioration have been reported.

Metabolic disorders:

Cases of isolated and moderate hyperammonaemia without change in liver function tests may occur frequently, are usually transient and should not cause treatment discontinuation. However, they may present clinically as vomiting, ataxia, and increasing clouding of consciousness. Should these symptoms occur Episenta® should be discontinued. Very rare cases of hyponatraemia have been reported. Hyperammonaemia associated with neurological symptoms have also been reported (see section 4.4 Special warnings and precautions for use). In such cases further investigation should be considered.

Blood and lymphatic system disorders:

Frequent occurrence of thrombocytopenia, rare cases of anaemia, leucopenia or panocytopenia. The blood picture returned to normal when the drug was discontinued. Isolated reduction of fibrinogen or reversible increase in bleeding time have been reported, usually without associated clinical signs and particularly with high doses (sodium valproate has an inhibitory effect on the second phase of platelet aggregation). Spontaneous bruising or bleeding is an indication of withdrawal of medication pending investigations (see section 4.6 Pregnancy and lactation).

Skin and subcutaneous disorders:

Cutaneous reactions such as exanthematous rash rarely occur with sodium valproate. In very rare cases, toxic epidermal necrolysis, Stevens-Johnson syndrome and erythema multiforme have been reported. Transient hair loss, which may sometimes be dose-related, has often been reported. Regrowth normally begins within 6 months, although the hair may become more curly than previously. Hirsutism and acne have been very rarely reported.

Reproductive system and breast disorders:

Amenorrhoea and irregular periods have been reported. Very rarely gynaecomastia has occurred.

Vascular disorders:

The occurrence of vasculitis has occasionally been reported.

Ear disorders:

Hearing loss, either reversible or irreversible has been reported rarely; however a cause and effect relationship has not been established.

Renal and urinary disorders:

There have been isolated reports of reversible Fanconi's syndrome (a defect in proximal renal tubular function giving rise to glycosuria, amino aciduria, phospaturia, and uricosuria) associated with sodium valproate therapy, but the mode of action is as yet unclear. Very rare cases of enuresis have been reported.

Immune system disorders:

Allergic reactions (ranging from rash to hypersensitivity reactions) have been reported.

General disorders:

Very rare cases of non-severe peripheral oedema have been reported.

Increase in weight may also occur. Weight gain being a risk factor for polycystic ovary syndrome, it should be carefully monitored (see section 4.4 Special warnings and precautions for use).

4.9 Overdose

Cases of accidental and deliberate overdosage with oral therapy have been reported. At plasma concentrations of up to 5 to 6 times the maximum therapeutic levels, there are unlikely to be any symptoms other than nausea, vomiting and dizziness. In massive overdose, 10 to 20 times the maximum therapeutic levels, there may be serious CNS depression or coma with muscular hypotonia, hyperflexia, miosis, impaired respiratory function, metabolic acidosis. The symptoms may however be variable and seizures have been reported in the presence of very high plasma levels. Cases of intracranial hypertension related to cerebral oedema have been reported. A number of deaths have occurred following large overdoses. Hospital management of overdose includes induced vomiting, gastric lavage, assisted ventilation and other supportive measures. Haemodialysis and haemoperfusion have been used successfully. Intravenous naloxone has also been used sometimes in association with activated charcoal given orally.

5. PHARMACOLOGICAL PROPERTIES

5.1 Pharmacodynamic properties

Pharmacotherapeutic Group: Fatty acid derivatives

ATC no: N03AG01

The mode of action of valproic acid is not fully understood but may involve an elevation of gamma-amino butyric acid levels in the brain.

In certain in-vitro studies, it was reported that sodium valproate could stimulate HIV replication, but studies on peripheral blood mononuclear cells from HIV-infected subjects show that sodium valproate does not have a mitogen-like effect on inducing HIV replication. Indeed, the effect of sodium valproate on HIV replication ex-vivo is highly variable, modest in quantity, appears to be unrelated to the dose and has not been documented in man.

5.2 Pharmacokinetic properties

With peroral administration 90-100% of the dose is rapidly absorbed.

Maximal plasma concentration is achieved with Episenta® within 6.5 ±3.3 hours. The half-life is 12-16 h in most patients but can in exceptional cases be considerably lower. Impaired renal function prolongs the half-life. In infants under 2 months the half-life can be prolonged up to 60 hours but in older children it is the same as in adults.

Steady-state concentration is normally achieved after treatment in 3-5 days. A satisfactory effect is most often achieved at 50 – 100 μg/ml, but the patient's overall situation must be considered.

The relation between the dose and effect, and between plasma concentrations and effect, has not been fully clarified. The CSF concentration is up to 10% of the plasma concentration. About 90% of sodium valproate is bound to plasma protein, which may entail a risk of clinically significant interactions with other antiepileptics, primarily phenytoin. Sodium valproate is metabolised to a great extent and is excreted in the urine as conjugated metabolites. Sodium valproate crosses the placental barrier and concentrations of foetal plasma are comparable to those in the mother.

Valproic acid passes into breast milk but is not likely to influence the child when therapeutic doses are used.

5.3 Preclinical safety data

There are no preclinical data of relevance t to the prescriber which are additional to that already included in other sections of the SPC.

6. PHARMACEUTICAL PARTICULARS

6.1 List of excipients

Prolonged–release granule:

calcium stearate

silicon dioxide (methylated)

ammonio methacrylate copolymer type B

sodium lauryl sulfate

polysorbate 80

Granule coating:

ethylcellulose

dibutylsebacate

oleic acid

6.2 Incompatibilities

None known

6.3 Shelf life

36 months

6.4 Special precautions for storage

Do not store above 30°C. Store in the original container. Keep the container tightly closed.

6.5 Nature and contents of container

50, 100 or 200 Clay coated kraftpaper/Aluminium/PE sachets.

6.6 Special precautions for disposal and other handling
None.

7. MARKETING AUTHORISATION HOLDER
Beacon Pharmaceuticals Limited
85 High Street
Tunbridge Wells
Kent
TN1 1YG
UK

8. MARKETING AUTHORISATION NUMBER(S)
Episenta® 500 mg Prolonged-release granules PL18157/0023
Episenta® 1000 mg Prolonged-release granules PL18157/0024

9. DATE OF FIRST AUTHORISATION/RENEWAL OF THE AUTHORISATION
6th October 2006

10. DATE OF REVISION OF THE TEXT
7th July 2009

Episenta solution for injection (sodium valproate)

(Beacon Pharmaceuticals)

1. NAME OF THE MEDICINAL PRODUCT
Episenta® solution for injection

2. QUALITATIVE AND QUANTITATIVE COMPOSITION
Sodium valproate 100mg/ml

3. PHARMACEUTICAL FORM
Solution for injection

4. CLINICAL PARTICULARS

4.1 Therapeutic indications
Episenta®solution for injection may be used for epileptic patients who would normally be maintained on oral sodium valproate but for whom oral therapy is temporarily not possible.

4.2 Posology and method of administration
Dosage requirements vary according to age and body weight and should be adjusted individually to achieve adequate seizure control. Patients already satisfactorily treated with oral sodium valproate may be continued at their current dosage. Episenta®solution for injection is ready to use by intravenous infusion.

The total daily dose should be divided in three to four single slow intravenous injections or should be given by continuous or repeated infusion.

Monotherapy:

Adults: Dosage should start at 400 – 800mg daily increasing by 150 – 300mg at three day intervals until control is achieved. This is generally within the dosage range of 1000mg to 2000mg per day i.e. 20 – 30mg/kg body weight per daily. Where adequate control is not achieved within this range the dose may be further increased to a maximum of 2500mg per day.

Children: Initial dosage should be 300mg/day increasing until control is achieved. This is usually within the range 20 – 30mg/kg body weight per day. Where adequate control is not achieved within this range, the dose may be increased to 40 mg/kg bodyweight per day but only in patients in whom plasma valproic acid levels can be monitored. Above 40 mg/kg body weight per day clinical chemistry and haematological parameters should be monitored.

Use in elderly: Care should be taken when adjusting dosage in the elderly since the pharmacokinetics of sodium valproate are modified. The volume of distribution is increased in the elderly and because of decreasing binding to serum albumin, the proportion of free drug is increased. This will affect the clinical interpretation of plasma valproic acid levels. Dosage should be determined by seizure control.

In patients with renal insufficiency: It may be necessary to decrease dosage. Dosage should be adjusted according to clinical monitoring of plasma concentration may be misleading.

Combined Therapy: When starting Episenta®in patients already on other anticonvulsants these should be tapered slowly. Initiation of Episenta®therapy should then be gradual, with target dose reached after about two weeks. In certain cases it may be necessary to raise the dose by 5 to 10mg/kg/day when used in combination with liver enzymes inducing drugs such as phenytoin, phenobarbital and carbamazepine. Once known enzyme inducers have been withdrawn it may be possible to maintain seizure control on a reduced dose of Episenta®.

When barbiturates are being administered concomitantly and particularly if sedation is observed (particularly in children) the dosage of barbiturates should be reduced.

Method of administration

Episenta®solution for injection may be given by slow intravenous injection over 3 – 5 minutes or by infusion in 0.9% saline or 5% dextrose.

Episenta®solution for injection should not be administered via the same intravenous line with other drugs.

The intravenous administration of Episenta®solution for injection should be replaced by oral therapy as soon as practicable.

Close monitoring of plasma levels and – if necessary – dosage adjustments have to be performed during the change-over to a parenteral therapy, during parenteral therapy and during the switch back to oral therapy, in particular in such patients receiving higher doses of valproate or in patients receiving drugs potentially influencing the metabolism of valproate.

For instructions on preparation and dilution of Episenta® solution for injection before administration see section 6.6 Special Precautions for Disposal.

4.3 Contraindications
Active liver disease.

Personal or family history of severe hepatic dysfunction, especially drug related.

Porphyria.

Hypersensitivity to valproate or any of the excipents.

4.4 Special warnings and precautions for use
Suicidal ideation and behaviour have been reported in patients treated with antiepileptic agents in several indications. A meta-analysis of randomised placebo controlled trials of antiepileptic drugs has also shown a small increased risk of suicidal ideation and behaviour. The mechanism of this risk is not known and the available data do not exclude the possibility of an increased risk for sodium valproate.

Therefore patients should be monitored for signs of suicidal ideation and behaviours and appropriate treatment should be considered. Patients (and caregivers of patients) should be advised to seek medical advice should signs of suicidal ideation or behaviour emerge.

Hepatic dysfunction:

Conditions of occurrence:

Severe liver damage, including hepatic failure sometimes resulting in fatalities, has been very rarely reported. Experience in epilepsy has indicated that patients most at risk, especially in cases of multiple anticonvulsants therapy, are infants and in particular young children under the age of 3 and those with severe seizure disorders, organic brain disease, and (or) congenital metabolic or degenerative disease associated with mental retardation. After the age of 3, the incidence of occurrence is significantly reduced and progressively decreases with age. The concomitant use of salicylates should be avoided in children under 3 due to the risk liver toxicity. Additionally, salicylates should not be used in children under 16 years of age (see aspirin/salicylate product information on Reye's syndrome).

Monotherapy is recommended in children under the age of 3 years when prescribing Episenta®, but the potential benefit of Episenta® should be weighed against the risk of liver damage or pancreatitis in such patients prior to initiation of therapy.

In most cases, such liver damage occurred during the first 6 months of therapy, the period of maximum risk being 2 – 12 weeks.

Suggestive signs:

Clinical symptoms are essential for early diagnosis. In particular the following conditions, which may precede jaundice, should be taken into consideration, especially in patients at risk (see above: Conditions of occurrence):

- non-specific symptoms, usually of sudden onset, such as asthenia, malaise, anorexia, lethargy, oedema and drowsiness, which are sometimes associated with repeated vomiting and abdominal pain.

- in patients with epilepsy, recurrence of seizures

These are an indication for immediate withdrawal of the drug.

Patients (or their carers), should be instructed to report immediately any such signs to a physician should they occur. Investigations including clinical examination and biological assessment of liver function should be undertaken immediately.

Detection:

Liver function should be measured before and then periodically monitored during the first 6 months of therapy, especially in those who seem at risk, and those with a prior history of liver disease. Amongst usual investigations, tests which reflect protein synthesis, particularly prothrombin rate, are most relevant. Confirmation of an abnormally low prothrombin rate, particularly in association with other biological abnormalities (significant decreases in fibrinogen and coagulation factors; increased bilirubin level and raised transaminases) require cessation of Episenta® therapy.

As a matter of precaution and in case they are taken concomitantly salicylates should also be discontinued since they employ the same metabolic pathway.

As with most antiepileptic drugs, increased liver enzymes are common, particularly at the beginning of therapy; they are also transient.

More extensive biological investigations (including prothrombin rate) are recommended in these patients; a reduction in dosage may be considered when appropriate and tests should be repeated as necessary.

Pancreatitis:

Pancreatitis, which may be severe and result in fatalities, has been very rarely reported. Patients experiencing nausea, vomiting or acute abdominal pain should have a prompt medical evaluation (including measurement of serum amylase). Young children are at particular risk; this risk decreases with increasing age. Severe seizures and severe neurological impairment with combination anticonvulsant therapy may be risk factors. Hepatic failure with pancreatitis increases the risk of fatal outcome. In case of pancreatitis, Episenta® should be discontinued.

Haematological:

Blood tests (blood cell count, including platelet count, bleeding time and coagulation tests) are recommended prior to initiation of therapy or before surgery, and in case of spontaneous bruising or bleeding. (see section 4.8 Undesirable effects).

Renal insufficiency:

In patients with renal insufficiency, it may be necessary to decrease dosage. As monitoring of plasma concentrations may be misleading, dosage should be adjusted according to clinical monitoring (see sections 4.2 Posology and method of administration and 5.2 Pharmacokinetic properties).

Systemic lupus erythematosus:

Although immune disorders have only rarely been noted during the use of sodium valproate, the potential benefit of Episenta® should be weighed against its potential risk in patients with systemic lupus erythematosus (see section 4.8 Undesirable effects).

Hyperammonaemia:

When urea cycle enzymatic deficiency is suspected, metabolic investigations should be performed prior to treatment because of risk of hyperammonaemia with sodium valproate.

Weight gain:

Sodium valproate very commonly causes weight gain, which may be marked and progressive. Patients should be warned of the risk of weight gain at the initiation of therapy and appropriate strategies should be adopted to minimise it (see section 4.8 Undesirable effects)

Pregnancy:

Women of childbearing potential should not be started on Episenta® without specialist neurological advice. Adequate counselling should be made available to all women with epilepsy of childbearing potential regarding the risks associated with pregnancy because of the potential teratogenic risk to the foetus (see section 4.6 Pregnancy and lactation).

Diabetic Patients:

Sodium valproate is eliminated mainly through the kidneys, partly in the form of ketone bodies: this may give false positive in the urine testing of possible diabetics.

4.5 Interaction with other medicinal products and other forms of interaction

4.5.1 Effects of Episenta® on other drugs

Like many other drugs, Episenta®may potentiate the effect of other psychotropics, such as antipsychotics, monoamine oxidase inhibitors, antidepressants and benzodiazepines. Therefore, clinical monitoring and the dosage of other psychotropics should be adjusted when appropriate.

Sodium valproate increases phenobarbital plasma concentrations and sedation may occur, particularly in children. Clinical monitoring is recommended throughout the first 15 days of combined treatment with an immediate reduction of phenobarbital doses if sedation occurs and determination of phenobarbital levels when appropriate.

Sodium valproate increases primidone plasma levels causing an exacerbation of side effects, e.g. sedation. Clinical monitoring is recommended especially when initiating combined therapy with dosage adjustment as necessary.

Phenytoin total plasma levels are decreased by sodium valproate acid; the free form of phenytoin is increased leading to possible overdosage symptoms. Therefore, clinical monitoring is recommended with the free form of phenytoin being measured.

The toxic effects of carbamazepine may be potentiated by sodium valproate requiring clinical monitoring and dosage adjustment particularly at initiation of combined therapy.

Sodium valproate may reduce lamotrigine metabolism and increase its mean half-life. The dosage of lamotrigine should be decreased as necessary. The risk of rash is increased in combined therapy with lamotrigine.

Sodium valproate may raise zidovudine plasma concentrations leading to increased zidovudine toxicity.

The anticoagulant effect of warfarin and other coumarin anticoagulants may be increased following displacement from the plasma protein binding site by valproate. The prothombin time should be closely monitored.

4.5.2 Effects of other drugs on Episenta®

Antiepileptics with enzyme inducing effects e.g. phenytoin, phenobarbital, carbamazepine, decrease valproate plasma levels. Plasma levels should be monitored and dosage adjusted accordingly.

Mefloquine and chloroquine increases valproate metabolism and therefore epileptic seizures may occur in combined therapy. The dosage of sodium valproate may need adjustment.

Free valproate levels may be increased in the case of concomitant use with highly protein bound agents e.g. acetylsalicylic acid. Valproate plasma levels may also be increased when used concomitantly with cimetidine or erythromycin as a result of reduced hepatic metabolism.

Carbapenem antibiotics such as imipenem and meropenem decrease plasma valproate levels. If administering these antibiotics with sodium valproate close monitoring of valproate plasma levels is recommended.

Colestyramine may decrease the absorption of valproate.

The effect of hormonal contraceptives ("the pill") is not reduced by sodium valproate.

Caution is advised when using Episenta® in combination with newer antiepileptics whose pharmacodynamics may not be well established

4.6 Pregnancy and lactation

4.6.1 Pregnancy

From experience in treating mothers with epilepsy, the risk associated with the use of valproate during pregnancy has been described as follows:

Risk associated with epilepsy and antiepileptics

In offspring born to mothers with epilepsy receiving any antiepileptic treatment, the overall rate of malformations has been demonstrated to be 2 to 3 times higher than the rate (approximately 3%) reported in the general population. Although an increased number of children with malformations have been reported in cases of multiple drug therapy, the respective role of treatments and disease in causing the malformations has not been formally established. Malformations most frequently encountered are cleft lip and cardiovascular malformations.

Epidemiological studies have suggested an association between in-utero exposure to sodium valproate and a risk of developmental delay. Developmental delay has been reported in children born to mothers with epilepsy. It is not possible to differentiate what may be due to genetic, social, environmental factors, maternal epilepsy or antiepileptic treatment. Many factors including maternal epilepsy may also contribute to this risk but it is difficulty to quantify the relative contributions of these or of maternal anti-epileptic treatment. Notwithstanding those potential risks, no sudden discontinuation in the anti-epileptic therapy should be undertaken as this may lead to breakthrough seizures which could have serious consequences for both the mother and the foetus.

Risks associated with valproate

In animals: teratogenic effects have been demonstrated in the mouse, rat and rabbit. There is animal experimental evidence that high plasma peak levels and the size of an individual dose are associated with neural tube defects.

In humans: valproate is associated with neural tube defects such as myelomeningocele and spina bifida. The frequency of this effect is estimated to be 1 to 2%. An increased incidence of major malformations including neural tube defects, craniofacial defects, malformation of the limbs, cardiovascular malformations, hypospadias and multiple anomalies involving various body systems has been reported in offspring born to mothers with epilepsy treated with valproate. Some data from studies, of women with epilepsy, have suggested an association between in-utero exposure to valproate and the risk of developmental delay (frequently associated with craniofacial abnormalities), particularly of verbal IQ.

In view of the above data

When a woman is planning pregnancy, this provides an opportunity to review the need for antiepileptic treatment. Women of childbearing age should be informed of the risks and benefits of continuing anti-epileptic treatment throughout pregnancy.

Folate supplementation, **prior** to pregnancy, has been demonstrated to reduce the incidence of neural tube defects in the offspring of women at high risk. Although no direct evidence exists of such effects in women receiving anti-epileptic drugs, woman should be advised to start taking folic acid supplementation (5 mg) as soon as contraception is discontinued.

The available evidence suggests that anticonvulsants monotherapy is preferred. Dosage should be reviewed before conception and the lowest effective dose used, in divided doses, as abnormal pregnancy outcome tends to be associated with higher total daily dosage and with the size of an individual dose. The incidence of neural tube defects rises with increasing dosage, particularly above 1000 mg daily. The administration in several divided doses over the day and the use of a prolonged release formulation is preferable in order to avoid high peak plasma levels.

During pregnancy, Episenta® antiepileptic treatment should not be discontinued if it has been effective. Nevertheless, specialist prenatal monitoring should be instituted in order to detect the possible occurrence of a neural tube defect or any other malformation. Pregnancies should be carefully screened by ultrasound, and other techniques if appropriate (see Section 4.4 Special warnings and special precautions for use).

Risk in the neonate

Very rare cases of haemorrhagic syndrome have been reported in neonates whose mothers have taken valproate during pregnancy. This haemorrhagic syndrome is related to hypofibrinogenaemia; afibrinogenaemia has also been reported and may be fatal. These are possibly associated with a decrease of coagulation factors. However, this syndrome has to be distinguished from the decrease of the vitamin-K factors induced by phenobarbital and other antiepileptic enzyme inducing drugs. Therefore platelet count, fibrinogen plasma level, coagulation tests and coagulation factors should be investigated in neonates.

4.6.2 Lactation

Excretion of valproate in breast milk is low, with a concentration between 1% to 10% of total maternal serum levels; up to now children breast fed that have been monitored during the neonatal period have not experienced clinical effects. There appears to be no contraindications to breast feeding by patients on Episenta®.

4.7 Effects on ability to drive and use machines

Use of Episenta® may provide seizure control such that the patient may be eligible to hold a driving licence.

At the start of treatment with sodium valproate, at higher dosages or with a combination of other centrally acting drugs, reaction time may be altered to an extent that affects the ability to drive or to operate machinery, irrespective of the effect on the primary disease being treated. Patients should be warned of the risk of transient drowsiness. This is especially the case when taken during anticonvulsant polytherapy, concomitant use of benzodiazepines or in combination with alcohol.

4.8 Undesirable effects

Congenital and familial/genetic disorders: (see section 4.6 Pregnancy and lactation)

Hepato-biliary disorders:

Rare cases of hepatic dysfunction (see section 4.4 Special warnings and precautions for use). Severe liver damage, including hepatic failure sometimes resulting in fatalities, has been reported (see sections 4.2 (Posology and method of administration, 4.3 Contraindications and 4.4 Special warnings and precautions for use). Increased liver enzymes are common, particularly early in treatment, and may be transient (see section 4.4 Special warnings and precautions for use).

Gastro-intestinal disorders: (nausea, gastralgia, diarrhoea)

Frequently occur at the start of the treatment, but they usually disappear after a few days without discontinuing treatment. These problems can usually be overcome by taking Episenta® with or after food.

Very rare cases of pancreatitis, sometimes fatal, have been reported (see section 4.4 Special warnings and precautions for use).

Nervous system disorders:

Sedation has been reported occasionally, usually when in combination with other anticonvulsants. In monotherapy it occurred early in treatment on rare occasions and is usually transient. Rare cases of lethargy and confusion occasionally progressing to stupor, sometimes with associated hallucinations or convulsions have been reported. Encephalopathy and coma have very rarely been observed. These cases have often been associated with a too high starting dose or a too rapid dose escalation or concomitant use of other anticonvulsants, notably phenobarbital. They have usually been reversible on withdrawal of treatment or reduction of dosage.

Very rare cases of reversible extrapyramidal symptoms including parkinsonism, or reversible dementia associated with reversible cerebral atrophy have been reported. Dose related ataxia and fine postural tremor have occasionally been reported.

An increase in alertness may occur, this is generally beneficial but occasionally aggression, hyperactivity and behavioural deterioration have been reported.

Metabolic disorders:

Cases of isolated and moderate hyperammonaemia without change in liver function tests may occur frequently, are usually transient and should not cause treatment discontinuation. However, they may present clinically as vomiting, ataxia, and increasing clouding of consciousness. Should these symptoms occur Episenta® should be discontinued. Very rare cases of hyponatraemia have been reported. Hyperammonaemia associated with neurological symptoms have also been reported (see section 4.4 Special warnings and precautions for use). In such cases further investigation should be considered.

Blood and lymphatic system disorders:

Frequent occurrence of thrombocytopenia, rare cases of anaemia, leucopenia or panocytopenia. The blood picture returned to normal when the drug was discontinued. Isolated reduction of fibrinogen or reversible increase in bleeding time have been reported, usually without associated clinical signs and particularly with high doses (sodium valproate has an inhibitory effect on the second phase of platelet aggregation). Spontaneous bruising or bleeding is an indication of withdrawal of medication pending investigations (see section 4.6 Pregnancy and lactation).

Skin and subcutaneous disorders:

Cutaneous reactions such as exanthematous rash rarely occur with sodium valproate. In very rare cases, toxic epidermal necrolysis, Stevens-Johnson syndrome and erythema multiforme have been reported. Transient hair loss, which may sometimes be dose-related, has often been reported. Regrowth normally begins within 6 months, although the hair may become more curly than previously. Hirsutism and acne have been very rarely reported.

Reproductive system and breast disorders:

Amenorrhoea and irregular periods have been reported. Very rarely gynaecomastia has occurred

Vascular disorders:

The occurrence of vasculitis has occasionally been reported.

Ear disorders:

Hearing loss, either reversible or irreversible has been reported rarely; however a cause and effect relationship has not been established.

Renal and urinary disorders:

There have been isolated reports of reversible Fanconi's syndrome (a defect in proximal renal tubular function giving rise to glycosuria, amino aciduria, phospaturia, and uricosuria) associated with sodium valproate therapy, but the mode of action is as yet unclear. Very rare cases of enuresis have been reported.

Immune system disorders:

Allergic reactions (ranging from rash to hypersensitivity reactions) have been reported.

General disorders:

Very rare cases of non-severe peripheral oedema have been reported.

Increase in weight may also occur. Weight gain being a risk factor for polycystic ovary syndrome, it should be carefully monitored (see section 4.4 Special warnings and precautions for use).

When using Episenta® intravenously, transient nausea or dizziness may occur.

4.9 Overdose

Cases of accidental and deliberate overdosage with oral therapy have been reported. At plasma concentrations of up to 5 to 6 times the maximum therapeutic levels, there are unlikely to be any symptoms other than nausea, vomiting and dizziness. In massive overdose, 10 to 20 times the maximum therapeutic levels, there may be serious CNS depression or coma with muscular hypotonia, hyperflexia, miosis, impaired respiratory function, metabolic acidosis. The symptoms may however be variable and seizures have been reported in the presence of very high plasma levels. Cases of intracranial hypertension related to cerebral oedema have been reported. A number of deaths have occurred following large overdoses. Hospital management of overdose includes induced vomiting, gastric lavage, assisted ventilation and other supportive measures. Haemodialysis and haemoperfusion have been used successfully. Intravenous naloxone has also been used sometimes in association with activated charcoal given orally.

5. PHARMACOLOGICAL PROPERTIES

5.1 Pharmacodynamic properties

ATC no: N03AG01

The mode of action of valproic acid in epilepsy is not fully understood but may involve an elevation of gamma-amino butyric acid levels in the brain.

In certain in-vitro studies, it was reported that sodium valproate could stimulate HIV replication but studies on peripheral blood mononuclear cells from HIV-infected subjects show that sodium valproate does not have a mitogen-like effect on inducing HIV replication. Indeed, the effect of sodium valproate on HIV replication ex-vivo is highly variable, modest in quantity, appears to be unrelated to the dose and has not been documented in man.

5.2 Pharmacokinetic properties

Per definition, with intravenous injection the bioavailability amounts to 100. The half-life is 8 – 20 h in most patients but can in exceptional cases be considerable lower. It is usually shorter in children. In infants under 2 months the half-life can be prolonged up to 60 hours. In patients with severe renal insufficiency it may be necessary to alter dosage in accordance with free serum valproic acid levels.

Steady-state concentration is normally achieved after treatment in 3 - 5 days. A satisfactory effect is most often achieved at 40 – 100mg/litre (278 – 694 micromol/litre), but the patient's overall situation must be considered. The reported range may depend on time of sampling and presence of co-medication. An increased incidence of adverse effects may occur with plasma levels above the effective therapeutic range.

The pharmacological (or therapeutic) effects of Episenta®-may not be clearly correlated with the total or free (unbound) plasma valproic acid levels. The CFS concentration is up to 10% of the plasma concentration. The percentage of free (unbound) drug is usually between 6 and 15% of the total plasma levels. Sodium valproate is metabolised to a great extent and is excreted in the urine as conjugated metabolites. Sodium valproate crosses the placental barrier and concentrations in foetal plasma are comparable to those in the mother.

Valproic acid passes into breast milk but is not likely to influence the child when therapeutic doses are used.

5.3 Preclinical safety data

Acute toxicity

Depending on the species of the animal and mode of administration the LD_{50} is between 0.5 – 1.5g/kg body weight. The symptoms observed included, for example, ataxia, sedation, hypothermia, catalepsy, co-ordination disorders and vomiting.

Chronic toxicity

Testicular atrophy, degeneration of the vas deferens and insufficient spermatogenesis as well as lung and prostate gland changes have been observed in chronic toxicity studies at dosages of more than 250 mg/kg in rats and 90 mg/kg in the dog. In rats, at 200 mg/kg p.o., morphological hepatocytes changes were seen. At 750 mg/kg i.p., functional liver disorders and, among other things, hyperammonaemia, occurred.

Carcinogenic and mutagenic potential

Carcinogenic studies have been conducted in the rat and mouse. At very high doses, increased subcutaneous fibrosarcoma was observed in male rats.

Studies of mutagenic potential have shown no mutagenic effect.

Reproduction toxicology

Valproic acid has been found to be teratogenic in mice, rats, hamsters, monkeys and rabbits. The effects occur primarily as skeletal (palatal cleft, costal and vertebral fusion) and renal malformations, in mice also as encephalocele and malformation of the neural tube. Malformations have also been observed in neurulation studies in chicken embryo in vitro.

6. PHARMACEUTICAL PARTICULARS

6.1 List of excipients

Disodium edetate

Water for injections

6.2 Incompatibilities

Episenta®solution for injection should not be administered via the same intravenous line with other drugs.

6.3 Shelf life

Shelf life of the medicinal product as packaged for sale: 24 months.

Shelf life after dilution or reconstitution according to the directions: Chemical and physical in-use stability has been demonstrated for 3 days at 20 - 22°C.

6.4 Special precautions for storage

Do not freeze.

6.5 Nature and contents of container

Glass ampoule containing 3 ml or 10 ml solution for injection.

6.6 Special precautions for disposal and other handling

From a microbiological point of view, the product should be used immediately after opening. If not used immediately, in-use storage times and conditions prior to use are the responsibility of the user and would normally be not longer than 24 hours at 2 to 8°C, unless dilution has taken place in controlled and validated aseptic conditions.

For infusion of Episenta®solution for injection it may be diluted in 0.9% saline or 5% dextrose. Tests with the recommended infusion solutions over three days at 20 - 22°C show compatibility.

Prior to use Episenta®solution for injection and the diluted solution should be visually inspected. Only clear solutions without particles should be used.

7. MARKETING AUTHORISATION HOLDER

Beacon Pharmaceuticals Ltd

85, High Street

Tunbridge Wells

Kent TN1 1YG

UK

8. MARKETING AUTHORISATION NUMBER(S)

PL 18157/0027.

9. DATE OF FIRST AUTHORISATION/RENEWAL OF THE AUTHORISATION

28th July 2006.

10. DATE OF REVISION OF THE TEXT

14th October 2008

Epivir 150 mg film-coated tablets

(GlaxoSmithKline UK)

1. NAME OF THE MEDICINAL PRODUCT

Epivir 150 mg film-coated tablets

2. QUALITATIVE AND QUANTITATIVE COMPOSITION

Each film-coated tablet contains 150 mg lamivudine.

For a full list of excipients, see section 6.1.

3. PHARMACEUTICAL FORM

Film-coated tablet

White, diamond shaped scored tablets engraved with "GX CJ7" on both faces.

4. CLINICAL PARTICULARS

4.1 Therapeutic indications

Epivir is indicated as part of antiretroviral combination therapy for the treatment of Human Immunodeficiency Virus (HIV) infected adults and children.

4.2 Posology and method of administration

The therapy should be initiated by a physician experienced in the management of HIV infection.

Epivir may be administered with or without food.

To ensure administration of the entire dose, the tablet(s) should ideally be swallowed without crushing. For patients who are unable to swallow tablets, lamivudine is available as an oral solution. Alternatively, the tablets may be crushed and added to a small amount of semi-solid food or liquid, all of which should be consumed immediately (see section 5.2).

Adults and adolescents (over 12 years of age): the recommended dose of Epivir is 300 mg daily. This may be administered as either 150 mg twice daily or 300 mg once daily (see section 4.4). The 300 mg tablet is only suitable for the once a day regimen.

Patients changing to the once daily regimen should take 150 mg twice a day and switch to 300 mg once a day the following morning. Where an evening once daily regimen is preferred, 150 mg of Epivir should be taken on the first morning only, followed by 300 mg in the evening. When changing back to a twice daily regimen patients should complete the days treatment and start 150 mg twice a day the following morning.

Children (under 12 years of age):

Since an accurate dosing can not be achieved with this formulation, dosing according to weight bands is recommended for Epivir tablets. This dosing regimen for paediatric patients weighing 14-30 kg is based primarily on pharmacokinetic modelling, with supporting data from clinical studies.

For children weighing at least 30 kg: the adult dosage of 150 mg twice daily should be taken.

For children weighing between 21 kg to 30 kg: the recommended oral dose of Epivir (150 mg) is one-half tablet taken in the morning and one whole tablet taken in the evening.

For children weighing 14 to 21 kg: the recommended oral dose of Epivir (150 mg) is one half of a scored tablet taken twice daily.

Epivir is also available as an oral solution for children over three months of age and who weigh less than 14 kg or for patients who are unable to swallow tablets.

Less than three months of age: the limited data available are insufficient to propose specific dosage recommendations (see section 5.2).

Renal impairment: Lamivudine concentrations are increased in patients with moderate - severe renal impairment due to decreased clearance. The dose should therefore be adjusted, using oral solution presentation of Epivir for patients whose creatinine clearance falls below 30 ml/min (see tables).

Dosing recommendations – Adults and adolescents weighing at least 30 kg:

Creatinine clearance (ml/min)	First dose	Maintenance dose
⩾50	150 mg	150 mg twice daily
30-<50	150 mg	150 mg once daily
<30	As doses below 150 mg are needed the use of the oral solution is recommended	

There are no data available on the use of lamivudine in children with renal impairment. Based on the assumption that creatinine clearance and lamivudine clearance are correlated similarly in children as in adults it is recommended that the dosage in children with renal impairment be reduced according to their creatinine clearance by the same proportion as in adults.

Dosing recommendations – Children aged at least 3 months and weighing less than 30 kg:

Creatinine clearance (ml/min)	First dose	Maintenance dose
⩾50	4 mg/kg	4 mg/kg twice daily
30 to <50	4 mg/kg	4 mg/kg once daily
15 to <30	4 mg/kg	2.6 mg/kg once daily
5 to <15	4 mg/kg	1.3 mg/kg once daily
<5	1.3 mg/kg	0.7 mg/kg once daily

Hepatic impairment: Data obtained in patients with moderate to severe hepatic impairment shows that lamivudine pharmacokinetics are not significantly affected by hepatic dysfunction. Based on these data, no dose adjustment is necessary in patients with moderate or severe hepatic impairment unless accompanied by renal impairment.

4.3 Contraindications

Hypersensitivity to the active substance or to any of the excipients.

4.4 Special warnings and precautions for use

Epivir is not recommended for use as monotherapy.

Renal impairment: In patients with moderate to severe renal impairment, the terminal plasma half-life of lamivudine is increased due to decreased clearance, therefore the dose should be adjusted (see section 4.2).

Triple nucleoside therapy: There have been reports of a high rate of virological failure and of emergence of resistance at an early stage when lamivudine was combined with tenofovir disoproxil fumarate and abacavir as well as with tenofovir disoproxil fumarate and didanosine as a once daily regimen.

Opportunistic infections: Patients receiving Epivir or any other antiretroviral therapy may continue to develop opportunistic infections and other complications of HIV infection, and therefore should remain under close clinical observation by physicians experienced in the treatment of patients with associated HIV diseases.

Transmission of HIV: Patients should be advised that current antiretroviral therapy, including Epivir, has not been proven to prevent the risk of transmission of HIV to others through sexual contact or contamination with blood. Appropriate precautions should continue to be taken.

Pancreatitis: Cases of pancreatitis have occurred rarely. However it is not clear whether these cases were due to the antiretroviral treatment or to the underlying HIV disease. Treatment with Epivir should be stopped immediately if clinical signs, symptoms or laboratory abnormalities suggestive of pancreatitis occur.

Lactic acidosis: lactic acidosis, usually associated with hepatomegaly and hepatic steatosis, has been reported with the use of nucleoside analogues. Early symptoms (symptomatic hyperlactatemia) include benign digestive symptoms (nausea, vomiting and abdominal pain), non-specific malaise, loss of appetite, weight loss, respiratory symptoms (rapid and/or deep breathing) or neurological symptoms (including motor weakness).

Lactic acidosis has a high mortality and may be associated with pancreatitis, liver failure, or renal failure.

Lactic acidosis generally occurred after a few or several months of treatment.

Treatment with nucleoside analogues should be discontinued in the setting of symptomatic hyperlactatemia and metabolic/lactic acidosis, progressive hepatomegaly, or rapidly elevating aminotransferase levels.

Caution should be exercised when administering nucleoside analogues to any patient (particularly obese women) with hepatomegaly, hepatitis or other known risk factors for liver disease and hepatic steatosis (including certain medicinal products and alcohol).

Patients co-infected with hepatitis C and treated with alpha interferon and ribavirin may constitute a special risk.

Patients at increased risk should be followed closely.

Mitochondrial dysfunction: Nucleoside and nucleotide analogues have been demonstrated *in vitro* and *in vivo* to cause a variable degree of mitochondrial damage. There have been reports of mitochondrial dysfunction in HIV-negative infants exposed *in utero* and/or post-natally to nucleoside analogues. The main adverse events reported are haematological disorders (anaemia, neutropenia), metabolic disorders (hyperlactatemia, hyperlipasemia). These events are often transitory. Some late-onset neurological disorders have been reported (hypertonia, convulsion, abnormal behaviour). Whether the neurological disorders are transient or permanent is currently unknown. Any child exposed *in utero* to nucleoside and nucleotide analogues, even HIV-negative children, should have clinical and laboratory follow-up and should be fully investigated for possible mitochondrial dysfunction in case of relevant signs or symptoms. These findings do not affect current national recommendations to use antiretroviral therapy in pregnant women to prevent vertical transmission of HIV.

Lipodystrophy: Combination antiretroviral therapy has been associated with the redistribution of body fat (lipodystrophy) in HIV patients. The long-term consequences of these events are currently unknown. Knowledge about the mechanism is incomplete. A connection between visceral lipomatosis and protease inhibitors (PIs) and lipoatrophy and nucleoside reverse transcriptase inhibitors (NRTIs) has been hypothesised. A higher risk of lipodystrophy has been associated with individual factors such as older age, and with drug related factors such as longer duration of antiretroviral treatment and associated metabolic disturbances. Clinical examination should include evaluation for physical signs of fat redistribution. Consideration should be given to the measurement of fasting serum lipids and blood glucose. Lipid disorders should be managed as clinically appropriate (see section 4.8).

Immune Reactivation Syndrome: In HIV-infected patients with severe immune deficiency at the time of institution of combination antiretroviral therapy (CART), an inflammatory reaction to asymptomatic or residual opportunistic pathogens may arise and cause serious clinical conditions, or aggravation of symptoms. Typically, such reactions have been observed within the first few weeks or months of initiation of CART. Relevant examples are cytomegalovirus retinitis, generalised and/or focal mycobacterium infections, and *Pneumocystis carinii* pneumonia. Any inflammatory symptoms should be evaluated and treatment instituted when necessary.

Liver disease: If lamivudine is being used concomitantly for the treatment of HIV and HBV, additional information relating to the use of lamivudine in the treatment of hepatitis B infection is available in the Zeffix SPC.

Patients with chronic hepatitis B or C and treated with combination antiretroviral therapy are at an increased risk of severe and potentially fatal hepatic adverse events. In case of concomitant antiviral therapy for hepatitis B or C, please refer also to the relevant product information for these medicinal products.

If Epivir is discontinued in patients co-infected with hepatitis B virus, periodic monitoring of liver function tests and markers of HBV replication is recommended, as withdrawal of lamivudine may result in an acute exacerbation of hepatitis (see Zeffix SPC).

Patients with pre-existing liver dysfunction, including chronic active hepatitis, have an increased frequency of liver function abnormalities during combination antiretroviral therapy, and should be monitored according to standard practice. If there is evidence of worsening liver disease in such patients, interruption or discontinuation of treatment must be considered (see section 4.8).

Osteonecrosis: Although the etiology is considered to be multifactorial (including corticosteroid use, alcohol consumption, severe immunosuppression, higher body mass index), cases of osteonecrosis have been reported particularly in patients with advanced HIV-disease and/or long-term exposure to combination antiretroviral therapy (CART). Patients should be advised to seek medical advice if they experience joint aches and pain, joint stiffness or difficulty in movement.

4.5 Interaction with other medicinal products and other forms of interaction

Interaction studies have only been performed in adults

Lamivudine may inhibit the intracellular phosphorylation of zalcitabine when the two medicinal products are used concurrently. Epivir is therefore not recommended to be used in combination with zalcitabine.

Co-administration of lamivudine with intravenous ganciclovir or foscarnet is not recommended.

The likelihood of metabolic interactions is low due to limited metabolism and plasma protein binding and almost complete renal clearance.

Administration of trimethoprim/sulfamethoxazole 160 mg/800 mg results in a 40 % increase in lamivudine exposure, because of the trimethoprim component; the sulfamethoxazole component did not interact. However, unless the patient has renal impairment, no dosage adjustment of lamivudine is necessary (see section 4.2). Lamivudine has no effect on the pharmacokinetics of trimethoprim or sulfamethoxazole. When concomitant administration is warranted, patients should be monitored clinically. Co-administration of lamivudine with high doses of co-trimoxazole for the treatment of *Pneumocystis carinii* pneumonia (PCP) and toxoplasmosis should be avoided.

The possibility of interactions with other medicinal products administered concurrently should be considered, particularly when the main route of elimination is active renal secretion via the organic cationic transport system e.g. trimethoprim. Other medicinal products (e.g. ranitidine, cimetidine) are eliminated only in part by this mechanism and were shown not to interact with lamivudine. The nucleoside analogues (e.g. didanosine and zalcitabine) like zidovudine, are not eliminated by this mechanism and are unlikely to interact with lamivudine.

A modest increase in C_{max} (28 %) was observed for zidovudine when administered with lamivudine, however overall exposure (AUC) is not significantly altered. Zidovudine has no effect on the pharmacokinetics of lamivudine (see section 5.2).

Lamivudine metabolism does not involve CYP3A, making interactions with medicinal products metabolised by this system (e.g. PIs) unlikely.

4.6 Pregnancy and lactation

Pregnancy: The safety of lamivudine in human pregnancy has not been established. Reproductive studies in animals have not shown evidence of teratogenicity, and showed no effect on male or female fertility. Lamivudine induces early embryonic death when administered to pregnant rabbits at exposure levels comparable to those achieved in man. In humans, consistent with passive transmission of lamivudine across the placenta, lamivudine concentrations in infant serum at birth were similar to those in maternal and cord serum at delivery.

Although animal reproductive studies are not always predictive of the human response, administration is not recommended during the first three months of pregnancy.

Lactation: Following oral administration lamivudine was excreted in breast milk at similar concentrations to those found in serum. Since lamivudine and the virus pass into breast milk, it is recommended that mothers taking Epivir do not breast-feed their infants. It is recommended that HIV infected women do not breast-feed their infants under any circumstances in order to avoid transmission of HIV.

4.7 Effects on ability to drive and use machines

No studies on the effects on the ability to drive and use machines have been performed.

4.8 Undesirable effects

The following adverse reactions have been reported during therapy for HIV disease with Epivir.

The adverse reactions considered at least possibly related to the treatment are listed below by body system, organ class and absolute frequency. Frequencies are defined as very common (> 1/10), common (> 1/100, < 1/10), uncommon (> 1/1,000, < 1/100), rare (> 1/10,000, < 1/1,000), very rare (< 1/10,000). Within each frequency grouping, undesirable effects are presented in order of decreasing seriousness.

Blood and lymphatic systems disorders

Uncommon: Neutropenia and anaemia (both occasionally severe), thrombocytopenia

Very rare: Pure red cell aplasia

Nervous system disorders

Common: Headache, insomnia

Very rare: peripheral neuropathy (or paraesthesia)

Respiratory, thoracic and mediastinal disorders

Common: Cough, nasal symptoms

Gastrointestinal disorders

Common: Nausea, vomiting, abdominal pain or cramps, diarrhoea

Rare: Pancreatitis. elevations in serum amylase.

Hepatobiliary disorders

Uncommon: Transient elevations in liver enzymes (AST, ALT).

Rare: Hepatitis

Skin and subcutaneous tissue disorders

Common: Rash, alopecia

Musculoskeletal and connective tissue disorders

Common: Arthralgia, muscle disorders

Rare: Rhabdomyolysis

General disorders and administration site conditions

Common: Fatigue, malaise, fever.

Cases of lactic acidosis, sometimes fatal, usually associated with severe hepatomegaly and hepatic steatosis, have been reported with the use of nucleoside analogues (see section 4.4).

Combination antiretroviral therapy has been associated with redistribution of body fat (lipodystrophy) in HIV patients including the loss of peripheral and facial subcutaneous fat, increased intra-abdominal and visceral fat, breast hypertrophy and dorsocervical fat accumulation (buffalo hump).

Combination antiretroviral therapy has been associated with metabolic abnormalities such as hypertriglyceridaemia, hypercholesterolaemia, insulin resistance, hyperglycaemia and hyperlactataemia (see section 4.4).

In HIV-infected patients with severe immune deficiency at the time of initiation of combination antiretroviral therapy (CART), an inflammatory reaction to asymptomatic or residual opportunistic infections may arise (see section 4.4).

Cases of osteonecrosis have been reported, particularly in patients with generally acknowledged risk factors, advanced HIV disease or long-term combined antiretroviral exposure (cART). The frequency of which is unknown (see section 4.4).

4.9 Overdose

Administration of lamivudine at very high dose levels in acute animal studies did not result in any organ toxicity. Limited data are available on the consequences of ingestion of acute overdoses in humans. No fatalities occurred, and the patients recovered. No specific signs or symptoms have been identified following such overdose.

If overdosage occurs the patient should be monitored, and standard supportive treatment applied as required. Since lamivudine is dialysable, continuous haemodialysis could be used in the treatment of overdosage, although this has not been studied.

5. PHARMACOLOGICAL PROPERTIES

5.1 Pharmacodynamic properties

Pharmacotherapeutic group: nucleoside analogue, ATC Code: J05AF05.

Lamivudine is a nucleoside analogue which has activity against human immunodeficiency virus (HIV) and hepatitis B virus (HBV). It is metabolised intracellularly to the active moiety, lamivudine 5'-triphosphate. Its main mode of action is as a chain terminator of viral reverse transcription. The triphosphate has selective inhibitory activity against HIV-1 and HIV-2 replication *in vitro*, it is also active against zidovudine-resistant clinical isolates of HIV. Lamivudine in combination with zidovudine exhibits synergistic anti-HIV activity against clinical isolates in cell culture.

HIV-1 resistance to lamivudine involves the development of a M184V amino acid change close to the active site of the viral reverse transcriptase (RT). This variant arises both *in vitro* and in HIV-1 infected patients treated with lamivudine-containing antiretroviral therapy. M184V mutants display greatly reduced susceptibility to lamivudine and show diminished viral replicative capacity *in vitro*. *In vitro* studies indicate that zidovudine-resistant virus isolates can become zidovudine sensitive when they simultaneously acquire resistance to lamivudine. The clinical relevance of such findings remains, however, not well defined.

In vitro data tend to suggest that the continuation of lamivudine in anti-retroviral regimen despite the development of M184V might provide residual anti-retroviral activity (likely through impaired viral fitness). The clinical relevance of these findings is not established. Indeed, the available clinical data are very limited and preclude any reliable conclusion in the field. In any case, initiation of susceptible NRTI's should always be preferred to maintenance of lamivudine therapy. Therefore, maintaining lamivudine therapy despite emergence of M184V mutation should only be considered in cases where no other active NRTI's are available.

Cross-resistance conferred by the M184V RT is limited within the nucleoside inhibitor class of antiretroviral agents. Zidovudine and stavudine maintain their antiretroviral activities against lamivudine-resistant HIV-1. Abacavir maintains its antiretroviral activities against lamivudine-resistant HIV-1 harbouring only the M184V mutation. The M184V RT mutant shows a <4-fold decrease in susceptibility to didanosine and zalcitabine; the clinical significance of these findings is unknown. *In vitro* susceptibility testing has not been standardised and results may vary according to methodological factors.

Lamivudine demonstrates low cytotoxicity to peripheral blood lymphocytes, to established lymphocyte and monocyte-macrophage cell lines, and to a variety of bone marrow progenitor cells *in vitro*.

Clinical experience:

In clinical trials, lamivudine in combination with zidovudine has been shown to reduce HIV-1 viral load and increase CD4 cell count. Clinical end-point data indicate that lamivudine in combination with zidovudine, results in a significant reduction in the risk of disease progression and mortality.

Evidence from clinical studies shows that lamivudine plus zidovudine delays the emergence of zidovudine resistant isolates in individuals with no prior antiretroviral therapy.

Lamivudine has been widely used as a component of antiretroviral combination therapy with other antiretroviral agents of the same class (NRTIs) or different classes (PIs, non-nucleoside reverse transcriptase inhibitors).

Multiple drug antiretroviral therapy containing lamivudine has been shown to be effective in antiretrovirally-naive patients as well as in patients presenting with viruses containing the M184V mutations.

The relationship between *in vitro* susceptibility of HIV to lamivudine and clinical response to lamivudine-containing therapy remains under investigation.

Lamivudine at a dose of 100 mg once daily has also been shown to be effective for the treatment of adult patients with chronic HBV infection (for details of clinical studies, see the prescribing information for Zeffix). However, for the treatment of HIV infection only a 300 mg daily dose of lamivudine (in combination with other antiretroviral agents) has been shown to be efficacious.

Lamivudine has not been specifically investigated in HIV patients co-infected with HBV.

Once daily dosing (300 mg once a day): a clinical study has demonstrated the non inferiority between Epivir once a day and Epivir twice a day containing regimens. These results were obtained in an antiretroviral naïve-population, primarily consisting of asymptomatic HIV infected patients (CDC stage A).

5.2 Pharmacokinetic properties

Absorption: Lamivudine is well absorbed from the gastrointestinal tract, and the bioavailability of oral lamivudine in adults is normally between 80 and 85%. Following oral administration, the mean time (t_{max}) to maximal serum concentrations (C_{max}) is about an hour. Based on data derived from a study in healthy volunteers, at a therapeutic dose of 150mg twice daily, mean (CV) steady-state C_{max} and C_{min} of lamivudine in plasma are 1.2 μg/ml (24%) and 0.09 μg/ml (27%), respectively. The mean (CV) AUC over a dosing interval of 12 hours is 4.7 μg.h/ml (18%). At a therapeutic dose of 300mg once daily, the mean (CV) steady-state C_{max}, C_{min} and 24h AUC are 2.0 μg/ml (26%), 0.04 μg/ml (34%) and 8.9 μg.h/ml (21%), respectively.

The 150 mg tablet is bioequivalent and dose proportional to the 300 mg tablet with respect to AUC_{∞}, C_{max}, and t_{max}.

Co-administration of lamivudine with food results in a delay of t_{max} and a lower C_{max} (decreased by 47%). However, the extent (based on the AUC) of lamivudine absorbed is not influenced.

Administration of crushed tablets with a small amount of semi-solid food or liquid would not be expected to have an impact on the pharmaceutical quality, and would therefore not be expected to alter the clinical effect. This conclusion is based on the physiochemical and pharmacokinetic data assuming that the patient crushes and transfers 100% of the tablet and ingests immediately.

Co-administration of zidovudine results in a 13% increase in zidovudine exposure and a 28 % increase in peak plasma levels. This is not considered to be of significance to patient safety and therefore no dosage adjustments are necessary.

Distribution: From intravenous studies, the mean volume of distribution is 1.3 l/kg. The observed half-life of elimination is 5 to 7 hours. The mean systemic clearance of lamivudine is approximately 0.32 l/h/kg, with predominantly renal clearance (> 70%) via the organic cationic transport system.

Lamivudine exhibits linear pharmacokinetics over the therapeutic dose range and displays limited binding to the major plasma protein albumin (< 16% - 36% to serum albumin in *in vitro* studies).

Limited data show that lamivudine penetrates the central nervous system and reaches the cerebro-spinal fluid (CSF). The mean ratio CSF/serum lamivudine concentration 2-4 hours after oral administration was approximately 0.12. The true extent of penetration or relationship with any clinical efficacy is unknown.

Metabolism: The active moiety, intracellular lamivudine triphosphate, has a prolonged terminal half-life in the cell (16 to 19 hours) compared to the plasma lamivudine half-life (5 to 7 hours). In 60 healthy adult volunteers, Epivir 300 mg once daily has been demonstrated to be pharmacokinetically equivalent at steady-state to Epivir 150 mg twice daily with respect to intracellular triphosphate AUC_{24} and C_{max}.

Lamivudine is predominately cleared unchanged by renal excretion. The likelihood of metabolic interactions of lamivudine with other medicinal products is low due to the small extent of hepatic metabolism (5-10%) and low plasma protein binding.

Elimination: Studies in patients with renal impairment show lamivudine elimination is affected by renal dysfunction. A recommended dosage regimen for patients with creatinine clearance below 50 ml/min is shown in the dosage section (see section 4.2).

An interaction with trimethoprim, a constituent of co-trimoxazole, causes a 40% increase in lamivudine exposure at therapeutic doses. This does not require dose adjustment unless the patient also has renal impairment (see sections 4.5 and 4.2). Administration of co-trimoxazole with lamivudine in patients with renal impairment should be carefully assessed.

Pharmacokinetics in children: In general, lamivudine pharmacokinetics in paediatric patients is similar to adults. However, absolute bioavailability (approximately 55-65%) was reduced in paediatric patients below 12 years of age. In addition, systemic clearance values were greater in younger paediatric patients and decreased with age, approaching adult values around 12 years of age. Due to these differences, the recommended dose for lamivudine in children (aged more than three months and weighing less than 30 kg) is 4 mg/kg twice daily. This dose will achieve an average AUC_{0-12} ranging from approximately 3,800 to 5,300 ng.h/ml. Recent findings indicate that exposure in children < 6 years of age may be reduced by about 30% compared with other age groups. Further data addressing this issue are currently awaited. At present, the available data do not suggest that lamivudine is less efficacious in this age group.

There are limited pharmacokinetic data for patients less than three months of age. In neonates one week of age, lamivudine oral clearance was reduced when compared to paediatric patients and is likely to be due to immature renal function and variable absorption. Therefore to achieve similar adult and paediatric exposure, the recommended dose for neonates is 4 mg/kg/day. Glomerular filtration estimates suggests that to achieve similar adult and paediatric exposure, the recommended dose for children aged six weeks and older could be 8 mg/kg/day.

Pharmacokinetics in pregnancy: Following oral administration, lamivudine pharmacokinetics in late-pregnancy were similar to non-pregnant women.

5.3 Preclinical safety data

Administration of lamivudine in animal toxicity studies at high doses was not associated with any major organ toxicity. At the highest dosage levels, minor effects on indicators of liver and kidney function were seen together with occasional reductions in liver weight. The clinically relevant effects noted were a reduction in red blood cell count and neutropenia.

Lamivudine was not mutagenic in bacterial tests but, like many nucleoside analogues, showed activity in an *in vitro* cytogenetic assay and the mouse lymphoma assay. Lamivudine was not genotoxic *in vivo* at doses that gave plasma concentrations around 40-50 times higher than the anticipated clinical plasma levels. As the *in vitro* mutagenic activity of lamivudine could not be confirmed in *in vivo* tests, it is concluded that lamivudine should not represent a genotoxic hazard to patients undergoing treatment.

A transplacental genotoxicity study conducted in monkeys compared zidovudine alone with the combination of zidovudine and lamivudine at human-equivalent exposures. The study demonstrated that foetuses exposed *in utero* to the combination sustained a higher level of nucleoside analogue-DNA incorporation into multiple foetal organs, and showed evidence of more telomere shortening than in those exposed to zidovudine alone. The clinical significance of these findings is unknown.

The results of long-term carcinogenicity studies in rats and mice did not show any carcinogenic potential relevant for humans.

6. PHARMACEUTICAL PARTICULARS

6.1 List of excipients

Tablet core:

Microcrystalline cellulose (E460),

Sodium starch glycollate

Magnesium stearate

Tablet film-coat:

Hypromellose (E464)

Titanium dioxide (E171),

Macrogol,

Polysorbate 80

6.2 Incompatibilities

Not applicable.

6.3 Shelf life

HDPE bottles: 5 years

PVC/aluminium foil blister packs: 2 years

6.4 Special precautions for storage

Do not store above 30°C

6.5 Nature and contents of container

Child resistant HDPE bottles or PVC/aluminium foil blister packs each containing 60 tablets.

6.6 Special precautions for disposal and other handling

No special requirements

7. MARKETING AUTHORISATION HOLDER

Glaxo Group Ltd

Greenford Road

Greenford

Middlesex UB6 0NN

United Kingdom

8. MARKETING AUTHORISATION NUMBER(S)

EU/1/96/015/001 (Bottle)

EU/1/96/015/004 (Blister pack)

9. DATE OF FIRST AUTHORISATION/RENEWAL OF THE AUTHORISATION

Date of first authorisation: 8 August 1996

Date of last renewal: 28 July 2006

10. DATE OF REVISION OF THE TEXT

05 September 2008

Detailed information on this medicinal product is available on the website of the European Medicines Agency (EMEA) http://www.emea.europa.eu

Epivir 300mg Tablets

(GlaxoSmithKline UK)

1. NAME OF THE MEDICINAL PRODUCT

Epivir 300 mg film-coated tablets

2. QUALITATIVE AND QUANTITATIVE COMPOSITION

Each film-coated tablet contains 300 mg lamivudine.

For a full list of excipients, see section 6.1.

3. PHARMACEUTICAL FORM

Film-coated tablet

Grey, diamond shaped and engraved with "GX EJ7" on one face.

4. CLINICAL PARTICULARS

4.1 Therapeutic indications

Epivir is indicated as part of antiretroviral combination therapy for the treatment of Human Immunodeficiency Virus (HIV) infected adults and children.

4.2 Posology and method of administration

The therapy should be initiated by a physician experienced in the management of HIV infection.

Epivir may be administered with or without food.

To ensure administration of the entire dose, the tablet(s) should ideally be swallowed without crushing. For patients who are unable to swallow tablets, lamivudine is available as an oral solution. Alternatively, the tablets may be crushed and added to a small amount of semi-solid food or liquid, all of which should be consumed immediately (see section 5.2).

Adults and adolescents over 12 years of age: the recommended dose of Epivir is 300 mg daily. This may be administered as either 150 mg twice daily or 300 mg once daily (see section 4.4). The 300 mg tablet is only suitable for the once a day regimen.

Patients changing to the once daily regimen should take 150 mg twice a day and switch to 300 mg once a day the following morning. Where an evening once daily regimen is preferred, 150 mg of Epivir should be taken on the first morning only, followed by 300 mg in the evening. When changing back to a twice daily regimen patients should complete the days treatment and start 150 mg twice a day the following morning.

Children:

Three months to 12 years of age: the recommended dose is 4 mg/kg twice daily up to a maximum of 300 mg daily.

Less than three months of age: the limited data available are insufficient to propose specific dosage recommendations (see section 5.2)

Renal impairment: Lamivudine concentrations are increased in patients with moderate - severe renal impairment due to decreased clearance. The dose should therefore be adjusted, using oral solution presentation of Epivir for patients whose creatinine clearance falls below 30 ml/min (see tables).

Dosing recommendations – Adults and adolescents over 12 years:

Creatinine clearance (ml/min)	First dose	Maintenance dose
≥50	150 mg	150 mg twice daily
30-<50	150 mg	150 mg once daily
<30	As doses below 150 mg are needed the use of the oral solution is recommended	

There are no data available on the use of lamivudine in children with renal impairment. Based on the assumption that creatinine clearance and lamivudine clearance are correlated similarly in children as in adults it is recommended that the dosage in children with renal impairment be reduced according to their creatinine clearance by the same proportion as in adults.

Dosing recommendations – Children from 3 months to 12 years:

Creatinine clearance (ml/min)	First dose	Maintenance dose
≥50	4 mg/kg	4 mg/kg twice daily
30 to <50	4 mg/kg	4 mg/kg once daily
15 to <30	4 mg/kg	2.6 mg/kg once daily
5 to <15	4 mg/kg	1.3 mg/kg once daily
<5	1.3 mg/kg	0.7 mg/kg once daily

Hepatic Impairment: Data obtained in patients with moderate to severe hepatic impairment shows that lamivudine pharmacokinetics are not significantly affected by hepatic dysfunction. Based on these data, no dose adjustment is necessary in patients with moderate or severe hepatic impairment unless accompanied by renal impairment.

4.3 Contraindications

Hypersensitivity to the active substance or to any of the excipients.

4.4 Special warnings and precautions for use

Epivir is not recommended for use as monotherapy.

Renal impairment: In patients with moderate to severe renal impairment, the terminal plasma half-life of lamivudine is increased due to decreased clearance, therefore the dose should be adjusted (see section 4.2).

Triple nucleoside therapy: There have been reports of a high rate of virological failure and of emergence of resistance at an early stage when lamivudine was combined with tenofovir disoproxil fumarate and abacavir as well as with tenofovir disoproxil fumarate and didanosine as a once daily regimen.

Opportunistic infections: Patients receiving Epivir or any other antiretroviral therapy may continue to develop opportunistic infections and other complications of HIV infection, and therefore should remain under close clinical observation by physicians experienced in the treatment of patients with associated HIV diseases.

Transmission of HIV: Patients should be advised that current antiretroviral therapy, including Epivir, has not been proven to prevent the risk of transmission of HIV to others through sexual contact or contamination with blood. Appropriate precautions should continue to be taken.

Pancreatitis: Cases of pancreatitis have occurred rarely. However it is not clear whether these cases were due to the antiretroviral treatment or to the underlying HIV disease. Treatment with Epivir should be stopped immediately if clinical signs, symptoms or laboratory abnormalities suggestive of pancreatitis occur.

Lactic acidosis: lactic acidosis, usually associated with hepatomegaly and hepatic steatosis, has been reported with the use of nucleoside analogues. Early symptoms (symptomatic hyperlactatemia) include benign digestive symptoms (nausea, vomiting and abdominal pain), non-specific malaise, loss of appetite, weight loss, respiratory symptoms (rapid and/or deep breathing) or neurological symptoms (including motor weakness).

Lactic acidosis has a high mortality and may be associated with pancreatitis, liver failure, or renal failure.

Lactic acidosis generally occurred after a few or several months of treatment.

Treatment with nucleoside analogues should be discontinued in the setting of symptomatic hyperlactatemia and metabolic/lactic acidosis, progressive hepatomegaly, or rapidly elevating aminotransferase levels.

Caution should be exercised when administering nucleoside analogues to any patient (particularly obese women) with hepatomegaly, hepatitis or other known risk factors for liver disease and hepatic steatosis (including certain medicinal products and alcohol). Patients co-infected with hepatitis C and treated with alpha interferon and ribavirin may constitute a special risk.

Patients at increased risk should be followed closely.

Mitochondrial dysfunction: Nucleoside and nucleotide analogues have been demonstrated *in vitro* and *in vivo* to cause a variable degree of mitochondrial damage. There have been reports of mitochondrial dysfunction in HIV-negative infants exposed *in utero* and/or post-natally to nucleoside analogues. The main adverse events reported are haematological disorders (anaemia, neutropenia), metabolic disorders (hyperlactatemia, hyperlipasemia). These events are often transitory. Some late-onset neurological disorders have been reported (hypertonia, convulsion, abnormal behaviour). Whether the neurological disorders are transient or permanent is currently unknown. Any child exposed *in utero* to nucleoside and nucleotide analogues, even HIV-negative children, should have clinical and laboratory follow-up and should be fully investigated for possible mitochondrial dysfunction in case of relevant signs or symptoms. These findings do not affect current national recommendations to use antiretroviral therapy in pregnant women to prevent vertical transmission of HIV.

Lipodystrophy: Combination antiretroviral therapy has been associated with the redistribution of body fat (lipodystrophy) in HIV patients. The long-term consequences of these events are currently unknown. Knowledge about the mechanism is incomplete. A connection between visceral lipomatosis and protease inhibitors (PIs) and lipoatrophy and nucleoside reverse transcriptase inhibitors (NRTIs) has been hypothesised. A higher risk of lipodystrophy has been associated with individual factors such as older age, and with drug related factors such as longer duration of antiretroviral treatment and associated metabolic disturbances. Clinical examination should include evaluation for physical signs of fat redistribution. Consideration should be given to the measurement of fasting serum lipids and blood glucose. Lipid disorders should be managed as clinically appropriate (see section 4.8).

Immune Reactivation Syndrome: In HIV-infected patients with severe immune deficiency at the time of institution of combination antiretroviral therapy (CART), an inflammatory reaction to asymptomatic or residual opportunistic pathogens may arise and cause serious clinical conditions, or aggravation of symptoms. Typically, such reactions have been observed within the first few weeks or months of initiation of CART. Relevant examples are cytomegalovirus retinitis, generalised and/or focal mycobacterium infections, and *Pneumocystis carinii* pneumonia. Any inflammatory symptoms should be evaluated and treatment instituted when necessary.

Liver disease: If lamivudine is being used concomitantly for the treatment of HIV and HBV, additional information relating to the use of lamivudine in the treatment of hepatitis B infection is available in the Zeffix SPC.

Patients with chronic hepatitis B or C and treated with combination antiretroviral therapy are at an increased risk of severe and potentially fatal hepatic adverse events. In case of concomitant antiviral therapy for hepatitis B or C, please refer also to the relevant product information for these medicinal products.

If Epivir is discontinued in patients co-infected with hepatitis B virus, periodic monitoring of liver function tests and markers of HBV replication is recommended, as withdrawal of lamivudine may result in an acute exacerbation of hepatitis (see Zeffix SPC).

Patients with pre-existing liver dysfunction, including chronic active hepatitis, have an increased frequency of liver function abnormalities during combination antiretroviral therapy, and should be monitored according to standard practice. If there is evidence of worsening liver disease in such patients, interruption or discontinuation of treatment must be considered (see section 4.8).

Osteonecrosis: Although the etiology is considered to be multifactorial (including corticosteroid use, alcohol consumption, severe immunosuppression, higher body mass index), cases of osteonecrosis have been reported particularly in patients with advanced HIV-disease and/or long-term exposure to combination antiretroviral therapy (CART). Patients should be advised to seek medical advice if they experience joint aches and pain, joint stiffness or difficulty in movement.

4.5 Interaction with other medicinal products and other forms of interaction

Interaction studies have only been performed in adults

Lamivudine may inhibit the intracellular phosphorylation of zalcitabine when the two medicinal products are used concurrently. Epivir is therefore not recommended to be used in combination with zalcitabine.

Co-administration of lamivudine with intravenous ganciclovir or foscarnet is not recommended.

The likelihood of metabolic interactions is low due to limited metabolism and plasma protein binding and almost complete renal clearance.

Administration of trimethoprim/sulfamethoxazole 160 mg/800 mg results in a 40 % increase in lamivudine exposure, because of the trimethoprim component; the sulfamethoxazole component did not interact. However, unless the patient has renal impairment, no dosage adjustment of lamivudine is necessary (see section 4.2). Lamivudine has no effect on the pharmacokinetics of trimethoprim or sulfamethoxazole. When concomitant administration is warranted, patients should be monitored clinically. Co-administration of lamivudine with high doses of co-trimoxazole for the treatment of *Pneumocystis carinii* pneumonia (PCP) and toxoplasmosis should be avoided.

The possibility of interactions with other medicinal products administered concurrently should be considered, particularly when the main route of elimination is active renal secretion via the organic cationic transport system e.g. trimethoprim. Other medicinal products (e.g. ranitidine, cimetidine) are eliminated only in part by this mechanism and were shown not to interact with lamivudine. The nucleoside analogues (e.g. didanosine and zalcitabine) like zidovudine, are not eliminated by this mechanism and are unlikely to interact with lamivudine.

A modest increase in C_{max} (28 %) was observed for zidovudine when administered with lamivudine, however overall exposure (AUC) is not significantly altered. Zidovudine has no effect on the pharmacokinetics of lamivudine (see section 5.2).

Lamivudine metabolism does not involve CYP3A, making interactions with medicinal products metabolised by this system (e.g. PIs) unlikely.

4.6 Pregnancy and lactation

Pregnancy: The safety of lamivudine in human pregnancy has not been established. Reproductive studies in animals have not shown evidence of teratogenicity, and showed no effect on male or female fertility. Lamivudine induces early embryonic death when administered to pregnant rabbits at exposure levels comparable to those achieved in man. In humans, consistent with passive transmission of lamivudine across the placenta, lamivudine concentrations in infant serum at birth were similar to those in maternal and cord serum at delivery.

Although animal reproductive studies are not always predictive of the human response, administration is not recommended during the first three months of pregnancy.

Lactation: Following oral administration lamivudine was excreted in breast milk at similar concentrations to those found in serum. Since lamivudine and the virus pass into breast milk, it is recommended that mothers taking Epivir do not breast-feed their infants. It is recommended that HIV infected women do not breast-feed their infants under any circumstances in order to avoid transmission of HIV.

4.7 Effects on ability to drive and use machines

No studies on the effects on the ability to drive and use machines have been performed.

4.8 Undesirable effects

The following adverse reactions have been reported during therapy for HIV disease with Epivir.

The adverse reactions considered at least possibly related to the treatment are listed below by body system, organ class and absolute frequency. Frequencies are defined as very common (> 1/10), common (> 1/100, < 1/10), uncommon (> 1/1,000, < 1/100), rare (> 1/10,000, < 1/1,000), very rare (< 1/10,000). Within each frequency grouping, undesirable effects are presented in order of decreasing seriousness.

Blood and lymphatic systems disorders

Uncommon: Neutropenia and anaemia (both occasionally severe), thrombocytopenia

Very rare: Pure red cell aplasia

Nervous system disorders

Common: Headache, insomnia

Very rare: Peripheral neuropathy (or paraesthesia)

Respiratory, thoracic and mediastinal disorders

Common: Cough, nasal symptoms

Gastrointestinal disorders

Common: Nausea, vomiting, abdominal pain or cramps, diarrhoea

Rare: Pancreatitis. Elevations in serum amylase.

Hepatobiliary disorders

Uncommon: Transient elevations in liver enzymes (AST, ALT).

Rare: Hepatitis

Skin and subcutaneous tissue disorders

Common: Rash, alopecia

Musculoskeletal and connective tissue disorders

Common: Arthralgia, muscle disorders

Rare: Rhabdomyolysis

General disorders and administration site conditions

Common: Fatigue, malaise, fever.

Cases of lactic acidosis, sometimes fatal, usually associated with severe hepatomegaly and hepatic steatosis, have been reported with the use of nucleoside analogues (see section 4.4).

Combination antiretroviral therapy has been associated with redistribution of body fat (lipodystrophy) in HIV patients including the loss of peripheral and facial subcutaneous fat, increased intra-abdominal and visceral fat, breast hypertrophy and dorsocervical fat accumulation (buffalo hump).

Combination antiretroviral therapy has been associated with metabolic abnormalities such as hypertriglyceridaemia, hypercholesterolaemia, insulin resistance, hyperglycaemia and hyperlactataemia (see section 4.4).

In HIV-infected patients with severe immune deficiency at the time of initiation of combination antiretroviral therapy (CART), an inflammatory reaction to asymptomatic or residual opportunistic infections may arise (see section 4.4).

Cases of osteonecrosis have been reported, particularly in patients with generally acknowledged risk factors, advanced HIV disease or long-term combined antiretroviral exposure (CART). The frequency of which is unknown (see section 4.4).

4.9 Overdose

Administration of lamivudine at very high dose levels in acute animal studies did not result in any organ toxicity. Limited data are available on the consequences of ingestion of acute overdoses in humans. No fatalities occurred, and the patients recovered. No specific signs or symptoms have been identified following such overdose.

If overdosage occurs the patient should be monitored, and standard supportive treatment applied as required. Since lamivudine is dialysable, continuous haemodialysis could be used in the treatment of overdosage, although this has not been studied.

5. PHARMACOLOGICAL PROPERTIES

5.1 Pharmacodynamic properties

Pharmacotherapeutic group: nucleoside analogue, ATC Code: J05AF05.

Lamivudine is a nucleoside analogue which has activity against human immunodeficiency virus (HIV) and hepatitis B virus (HBV). It is metabolised intracellularly to the active moiety, lamivudine 5'-triphosphate. Its main mode of action is as a chain terminator of viral reverse transcription. The triphosphate has selective inhibitory activity against HIV-1 and HIV-2 replication *in vitro*; it is also active against zidovudine-resistant clinical isolates of HIV. Lamivudine in combination with zidovudine exhibits synergistic anti-HIV activity against clinical isolates in cell culture.

HIV-1 resistance to lamivudine involves the development of a M184V amino acid change close to the active site of the viral reverse transcriptase (RT). This variant arises both *in vitro* and in HIV-1 infected patients treated with lamivudine-containing antiretroviral therapy. M184V mutants display greatly reduced susceptibility to lamivudine and show diminished viral replicative capacity *in vitro*. *In vitro* studies indicate that zidovudine-resistant virus isolates can become zidovudine sensitive when they simultaneously acquire resistance to lamivudine. The clinical relevance of such findings remains, however, not well defined.

In vitro data tend to suggest that the continuation of lamivudine in anti-retroviral regimen despite the development of M184V might provide residual anti-retroviral activity (likely through impaired viral fitness). The clinical relevance of these findings is not established. Indeed, the available clinical data are very limited and preclude any reliable conclusion in the field. In any case, initiation of susceptible NRTI's should always be preferred to maintenance of lamivudine therapy. Therefore, maintaining lamivudine therapy despite emergence of M184V mutation should only be considered in cases where no other active NRTI's are available.

Cross-resistance conferred by the M184V RT is limited within the nucleoside inhibitor class of antiretroviral agents. Zidovudine and stavudine maintain their antiretroviral activities against lamivudine-resistant HIV-1. Abacavir maintains its antiretroviral activities against lamivudine-resistant HIV-1 harbouring only the M184V mutation. The M184V RT mutant shows a < 4-fold decrease in susceptibility to didanosine and zalcitabine; the clinical significance of these findings is unknown. *In vitro* susceptibility testing has not been standardised and results may vary according to methodological factors.

Lamivudine demonstrates low cytotoxicity to peripheral blood lymphocytes, to established lymphocyte and monocyte-macrophage cell lines, and to a variety of bone marrow progenitor cells *in vitro*.

Clinical experience:

In clinical trials, lamivudine in combination with zidovudine has been shown to reduce HIV-1 viral load and increase CD4 cell count. Clinical end-point data indicate that lamivudine in combination with zidovudine, results in a significant reduction in the risk of disease progression and mortality.

Evidence from clinical studies shows that lamivudine plus zidovudine delays the emergence of zidovudine resistant isolates in individuals with no prior antiretroviral therapy.

Lamivudine has been widely used as a component of antiretroviral combination therapy with other antiretroviral agents of the same class (NRTIs) or different classes (PIs, non-nucleoside reverse transcriptase inhibitors).

Multiple drug antiretroviral therapy containing lamivudine has been shown to be effective in antiretrovirally-naive patients as well as in patients presenting with viruses containing the M184V mutations.

The relationship between *in vitro* susceptibility of HIV to lamivudine and clinical response to lamivudine-containing therapy remains under investigation.

Lamivudine at a dose of 100 mg once daily has also been shown to be effective for the treatment of adult patients with chronic HBV infection (for details of clinical studies, see the prescribing information for Zeffix). However, for the treatment of HIV infection, only a 300 mg daily dose of lamivudine (in combination with other antiretroviral agents) has been shown to be efficacious.

Lamivudine has not been specifically investigated in HIV patients co-infected with HBV.

Once daily dosing (300 mg once a day): a clinical study has demonstrated the non inferiority between Epivir once a day and Epivir twice a day containing regimens. These results were obtained in an antiretroviral naïve-population, primarily consisting of asymptomatic HIV infected patients (CDC stage A).

5.2 Pharmacokinetic properties

Absorption: Lamivudine is well absorbed from the gastro-intestinal tract, and the bioavailability of oral lamivudine in adults is normally between 80 and 85%. Following oral administration, the mean time (t_{max}) to maximal serum concentrations (C_{max}) is about an hour. Based on data derived from a study in healthy volunteers, at a therapeutic dose of 150mg twice daily, mean (CV) steady-state C_{max} and C_{min} of lamivudine in plasma are 1.2 μg/ml (24%) and 0.09 μg/ml (27%), respectively. The mean (CV) AUC over a dosing interval of 12 hours is 4.7 μg.h/ml (18%). At a therapeutic dose of 300mg once daily, the mean (CV) steady-state C_{max}, C_{min} and 24h AUC are 2.0 μg/ml (26%), 0.04 μg/ml (34%) and 8.9 μg.h/ml (21%), respectively.

The 150 mg tablet is bioequivalent and dose proportional to the 300 mg tablet with respect to AUC_{∞}, C_{max}, and t_{max}.

Co-administration of lamivudine with food results in a delay of t_{max} and a lower C_{max} (decreased by 47%). However, the extent (based on the AUC) of lamivudine absorbed is not influenced.

Administration of crushed tablets with a small amount of semi-solid food or liquid would not be expected to have an impact on the pharmaceutical quality, and would therefore not be expected to alter the clinical effect. This conclusion is based on the physiochemical and pharmacokinetic data assuming that the patient crushes and transfers 100% of the tablet and ingests immediately.

Co-administration of zidovudine results in a 13 % increase in zidovudine exposure and a 28 % increase in peak plasma levels. This is not considered to be of significance to patient safety and therefore no dosage adjustments are necessary.

Distribution: From intravenous studies, the mean volume of distribution is 1.3 l/kg. The observed half-life of elimination is 5 to 7 hours. The mean systemic clearance of lamivudine is approximately 0.32 l/h/kg, with predominantly renal clearance (> 70%) via the organic cationic transport system.

Lamivudine exhibits linear pharmacokinetics over the therapeutic dose range and displays limited binding to the major plasma protein albumin (< 16% - 36% to serum albumin in *in vitro* studies).

Limited data show that lamivudine penetrates the central nervous system and reaches the cerebro-spinal fluid (CSF). The mean ratio CSF/serum lamivudine concentration 2-4 hours after oral administration was approximately 0.12. The true extent of penetration or relationship with any clinical efficacy is unknown.

Metabolism: The active moiety, intracellular lamivudine triphosphate, has a prolonged terminal half-life in the cell (16 to 19 hours) compared to the plasma lamivudine half-life (5 to 7 hours). In 60 healthy adult volunteers, Epivir 300 mg once daily has been demonstrated to be pharmacokinetically equivalent at steady-state to Epivir 150 mg twice daily with respect to intracellular triphosphate AUC_{24} and C_{max}.

Lamivudine is predominately cleared unchanged by renal excretion. The likelihood of metabolic interactions of lamivudine with other medicinal products is low due to the small extent of hepatic metabolism (5-10%) and low plasma protein binding.

Elimination: Studies in patients with renal impairment show lamivudine elimination is affected by renal dysfunction. A recommended dosage regimen for patients with creatinine clearance below 50 ml/min is shown in the dosage section (see section 4.2).

An interaction with trimethoprim, a constituent of co-trimoxazole, causes a 40% increase in lamivudine exposure at therapeutic doses. This does not require dose adjustment unless the patient also has renal impairment (see sections 4.5 and 4.2). Administration of co-trimoxazole with lamivudine in patients with renal impairment should be carefully assessed.

Pharmacokinetics in children: In general, lamivudine pharmacokinetics in paediatric patients is similar to adults. However, absolute bioavailability (approximately 55-65%) was reduced in paediatric patients below 12 years of age. In addition, systemic clearance values were greater in younger paediatric patients and decreased with age, approaching adult values around 12 years of age. Due to these differences, the recommended dose for lamivudine in children (aged more than three months and weighing less than 30 kg) is 4 mg/kg twice daily. This dose will achieve an average AUC_{0-12} ranging from approximately 3,800 to 5,300 ng.h/ml. Recent findings indicate that exposure in children < 6 years of age may be reduced by about 30% compared with other age groups. Further data addressing this issue are currently awaited. At present, the available data do not suggest that lamivudine is less efficacious in this age group.

There are limited pharmacokinetic data for patients less than three months of age. In neonates one week of age, lamivudine oral clearance was reduced when compared to paediatric patients and is likely to be due to immature renal function and variable absorption. Therefore to achieve similar adult and paediatric exposure, the recommended dose for neonates is 4 mg/kg/day. Glomerular filtration estimates suggests that to achieve similar adult and paediatric exposure, the recommended dose for children aged six weeks and older could be 8 mg/kg/day.

Pharmacokinetics in pregnancy: Following oral administration, lamivudine pharmacokinetics in late-pregnancy were similar to non-pregnant women.

5.3 Preclinical safety data

Administration of lamivudine in animal toxicity studies at high doses was not associated with any major organ toxicity. At the highest dosage levels, minor effects on indicators of liver and kidney function were seen together with occasional reductions in liver weight. The clinically relevant effects noted were a reduction in red blood cell count and neutropenia.

Lamivudine was not mutagenic in bacterial tests but, like many nucleoside analogues, showed activity in an *in vitro* cytogenetic assay and the mouse lymphoma assay. Lamivudine was not genotoxic *in vivo* at doses that gave plasma concentrations around 40-50 times higher than the anticipated clinical plasma levels. As the *in vitro* mutagenic activity of lamivudine could not be confirmed in *in vivo* tests, it is concluded that lamivudine should not represent a genotoxic hazard to patients undergoing treatment.

A transplacental genotoxicity study conducted in monkeys compared zidovudine alone with the combination of zidovudine and lamivudine at human-equivalent exposures. The study demonstrated that foetuses exposed *in utero* to the combination sustained a higher level of nucleoside analogue-DNA incorporation into multiple foetal organs, and showed evidence of more telomere shortening than in those exposed to zidovudine alone. The clinical significance of these findings is unknown.

The results of long-term carcinogenicity studies in rats and mice did not show any carcinogenic potential relevant for humans.

6. PHARMACEUTICAL PARTICULARS

6.1 List of excipients

Tablet core:

Microcrystalline cellulose (E460),

Sodium starch glycollate

Magnesium stearate

Tablet film-coat:

Hypromellose (E464),

Titanium dioxide (E171),

Black iron oxide (E172),

Macrogol, Polysorbate 80

6.2 Incompatibilities

Not applicable

6.3 Shelf life

HDPE bottles: 3 years

PVC/aluminium foil blister packs: 2 years

6.4 Special precautions for storage

Do not store above 30°C

6.5 Nature and contents of container

Child resistant HDPE bottles or PVC/aluminium foil blister packs each containing 30 tablets.

6.6 Special precautions for disposal and other handling

No special requirements

7. MARKETING AUTHORISATION HOLDER

Glaxo Group Ltd

Greenford Road

Greenford

Middlesex UB6 0NN

United Kingdom

8. MARKETING AUTHORISATION NUMBER(S)

EU/1/96/015/003 (Bottle)

EU/1/96/015/005 (Blister pack)

9. DATE OF FIRST AUTHORISATION/RENEWAL OF THE AUTHORISATION

Date of first authorisation: 15 November 2001

Date of last renewal: 28 July 2006

10. DATE OF REVISION OF THE TEXT

05 September 2008

Detailed information on this medicinal product is available on the website of the European Medicines Agency (EMEA) http://www.emea.europa.eu

Epivir Oral Solution

(GlaxoSmithKline UK)

1. NAME OF THE MEDICINAL PRODUCT

Epivir 10 mg/ml oral solution

2. QUALITATIVE AND QUANTITATIVE COMPOSITION

Each ml of oral solution contains 10 mg of lamivudine.

Excipients:

Sucrose 20% (3 g/15 ml)

Methyl parahydroxybenzoate

Propyl parahydroxybenzoate

For a full list of excipients, see section 6.1.

3. PHARMACEUTICAL FORM

Oral solution

Clear, colourless to pale yellow solution.

4. CLINICAL PARTICULARS

4.1 Therapeutic indications

Epivir is indicated as part of antiretroviral combination therapy for the treatment of Human Immunodeficiency Virus (HIV) infected adults and children.

4.2 Posology and method of administration

The therapy should be initiated by a physician experienced in the management of HIV infection.

Adults and adolescents over 12 years of age: the recommended dose of Epivir is 300 mg daily. This may be administered as either 150 mg (15 ml) twice daily or 300 mg (30 ml) once daily (see section 4.4).

Patients changing to the once daily regimen should take 150 mg (15 ml) twice a day and switch to 300 mg (30 ml) once a day the following morning. Where an evening once daily regimen is preferred, 150 mg (15 ml) of Epivir should be taken on the first morning only, followed by 300 mg (30 ml) in the evening. When changing back to a twice daily regimen, patients should complete the days treatment and start 150 mg (15 ml) twice a day the following morning.

Children

Three months to 12 years of age: the recommended dose is 4 mg/kg twice daily up to a maximum of 300 mg daily.

Less than three months of age: the limited data available are insufficient to propose specific dosage recommendations (see section 5.2).

Epivir is also available as a tablet formulation.

Epivir may be administered with or without food.

Renal impairment: Lamivudine concentrations are increased in patients with moderate - severe renal impairment due to decreased clearance. The dose should therefore be adjusted (see tables).

Dosing recommendations – Adults and adolescents over 12 years:

Creatinine clearance (ml/min)	First dose	Maintenance dose
≥50	150 mg (15 ml)	150 mg (15 ml) twice daily
30 to <50	150 mg (15 ml)	150 mg (15 ml) once daily
15 to <30	150 mg (15 ml)	100 mg (10 ml) once daily
5 to <15	150 mg (15 ml)	50 mg (5 ml) once daily
<5	50 mg (5 ml)	25 mg (2.5 ml) once daily

There are no data available on the use of lamivudine in children with renal impairment. Based on the assumption that creatinine clearance and lamivudine clearance are correlated similarly in children as in adults it is recommended that the dosage in children with renal impairment be reduced according to their creatinine clearance by the same proportion as in adults.

Dosing recommendations – Children from 3 months to 12 years:

Creatinine clearance (ml/min)	First dose	Maintenance dose
⩾50	4 mg/kg	4 mg/kg twice daily
30 to <50	4 mg/kg	4 mg/kg once daily
15 to <30	4 mg/kg	2.6 mg/kg once daily
5 to <15	4 mg/kg	1.3 mg/kg once daily
<5	1.3 mg/kg	0.7 mg/kg once daily

Hepatic impairment: Data obtained in patients with moderate to severe hepatic impairment shows that lamivudine pharmacokinetics are not significantly affected by hepatic dysfunction. Based on these data, no dose adjustment is necessary in patients with moderate or severe hepatic impairment unless accompanied by renal impairment.

4.3 Contraindications

Hypersensitivity to the active substance or to any of the excipients.

4.4 Special warnings and precautions for use

Epivir is not recommended for use as monotherapy.

Renal impairment: In patients with moderate –to- severe renal impairment, the terminal plasma half-life of lamivudine is increased due to decreased clearance, therefore the dose should be adjusted (see section 4.2).

Triple nucleoside therapy: There have been reports of a high rate of virological failure and of emergence of resistance at an early stage when lamivudine was combined with tenofovir disoproxil fumarate and abacavir as well as with tenofovir disoproxil fumarate and didanosine as a once daily regimen.

Opportunistic infections: Patients receiving Epivir or any other antiretroviral therapy may continue to develop opportunistic infections and other complications of HIV infection, and therefore should remain under close clinical observation by physicians experienced in the treatment of patients with associated HIV diseases.

Transmission of HIV: Patients should be advised that current antiretroviral therapy, including Epivir, has not been proven to prevent the risk of transmission of HIV to others through sexual contact or contamination with blood. Appropriate precautions should continue to be taken.

Pancreatitis: Cases of pancreatitis have occurred rarely. However it is not clear whether these cases were due to the antiretroviral treatment or to the underlying HIV disease. Treatment with Epivir should be stopped immediately if clinical signs, symptoms or laboratory abnormalities suggestive of pancreatitis occur.

Lactic acidosis: lactic acidosis, usually associated with hepatomegaly and hepatic steatosis, has been reported with the use of nucleoside analogues. Early symptoms (symptomatic hyperlactatemia) include benign digestive symptoms (nausea, vomiting and abdominal pain), non-specific malaise, loss of appetite, weight loss, respiratory symptoms (rapid and/or deep breathing) or neurological symptoms (including motor weakness).
Lactic acidosis has a high mortality and may be associated with pancreatitis, liver failure, or renal failure.
Lactic acidosis generally occurred after a few or several months of treatment.
Treatment with nucleoside analogues should be discontinued in the setting of symptomatic hyperlactatemia and metabolic/lactic acidosis, progressive hepatomegaly, or rapidly elevating aminotransferase levels.
Caution should be exercised when administering nucleoside analogues to any patient (particularly obese women) with hepatomegaly, hepatitis or other known risk factors for liver disease and hepatic steatosis (including certain medicinal products and alcohol). Patients co-infected with hepatitis C and treated with alpha interferon and ribavirin may constitute a special risk.
Patients at increased risk should be followed closely.

Mitochondrial dysfunction: Nucleoside and nucleotide analogues have been demonstrated *in vitro* and *in vivo* to cause a variable degree of mitochondrial damage. There have been reports of mitochondrial dysfunction in HIV-negative infants exposed *in utero* and/or post-natally to nucleoside analogues. The main adverse events reported are haematological disorders (anaemia, neutropenia), metabolic disorders (hyperlactatemia, hyperlipasemia). These events are often transitory. Some late-onset neurological disorders have been reported (hypertonia, convulsion, abnormal behaviour). Whether the neurological disorders are transient or permanent is currently unknown. Any child exposed *in utero* to nucleoside and nucleotide analogues, even HIV-negative children, should have clinical and laboratory follow-up and should be fully investigated for possible mitochondrial dysfunction in case of relevant signs or symptoms. These findings do not affect current national recommendations to use antiretroviral therapy in pregnant women to prevent vertical transmission of HIV.

Lipodystrophy: Combination antiretroviral therapy has been associated with the redistribution of body fat (lipodystrophy) in HIV patients. The long-term consequences of these events are currently unknown. Knowledge about the mechanism is incomplete. A connection between visceral lipomatosis and protease inhibitors (PIs) and lipoatrophy and nucleoside analogue reverse transcriptase inhibitors (NRTIs) has been hypothesised. A higher risk of lipodystrophy has been associated with individual factors such as older age, and with drug related factors such as longer duration of antiretroviral treatment and associated metabolic disturbances. Clinical examination should include evaluation for physical signs of fat redistribution. Consideration should be given to the measurement of fasting serum lipids and blood glucose. Lipid disorders should be managed as clinically appropriate (see section 4.8).

Immune Reactivation Syndrome: In HIV-infected patients with severe immune deficiency at the time of institution of combination antiretroviral therapy (CART), an inflammatory reaction to asymptomatic or residual opportunistic pathogens may arise and cause serious clinical conditions, or aggravation of symptoms. Typically, such reactions have been observed within the first few weeks or months of initiation of CART. Relevant examples are cytomegalovirus retinitis, generalised and/or focal mycobacterium infections, and *Pneumocystis carinii* pneumonia. Any inflammatory symptoms should be evaluated and treatment instituted when necessary.

Liver disease: If lamivudine is being used concomitantly for the treatment of HIV and HBV, additional information relating to the use of lamivudine in the treatment of hepatitis B infection is available in the Zeffix SPC.

Patients with chronic hepatitis B or C and treated with combination antiretroviral therapy are at an increased risk of severe and potentially fatal hepatic adverse events. In case of concomitant antiviral therapy for hepatitis B or C, please refer also to the relevant product information for these medicinal products.

If Epivir is discontinued in patients co-infected with hepatitis B virus, periodic monitoring of liver function tests and markers of HBV replication is recommended, as withdrawal of lamivudine may result in an acute exacerbation of hepatitis (see Zeffix SPC).

Patients with pre-existing liver dysfunction, including chronic active hepatitis, have an increased frequency of liver function abnormalities during combination antiretroviral therapy, and should be monitored according to standard practice. If there is evidence of worsening liver disease in such patients, interruption or discontinuation of treatment must be considered (see section 4.8).

Diabetic patients should be advised that each dose (150 mg = 15 ml) contains 3 g of sucrose.

Patients with rare hereditary problems of fructose intolerance, glucose-galactose malabsorption or sucrase-isomaltase insufficiency should not take this medicine.

Epivir contains methyl parahydroxybenzoate and propyl parahydroxybenzoate. These may cause allergic reactions (possibly delayed).

Osteonecrosis: Although the etiology is considered to be multifactorial (including corticosteroid use, alcohol consumption, severe immunosuppression, higher body mass index), cases of osteonecrosis have been reported particularly in patients with advanced HIV-disease and/or long-term exposure to combination antiretroviral therapy (CART). Patients should be advised to seek medical advice if they experience joint aches and pain, joint stiffness or difficulty in movement.

4.5 Interaction with other medicinal products and other forms of interaction

Interaction studies have only been performed in adults

Lamivudine may inhibit the intracellular phosphorylation of zalcitabine when the two medicinal products are used concurrently. Epivir is therefore not recommended to be used in combination with zalcitabine.

Co-administration of lamivudine with intravenous ganciclovir or foscarnet is not recommended.

The likelihood of metabolic interactions is low due to limited metabolism and plasma protein binding and almost complete renal clearance.

Administration of trimethoprim/sulfamethoxazole 160 mg/800 mg results in a 40 % increase in lamivudine exposure, because of the trimethoprim component; the sulfamethoxazole component did not interact. However, unless the patient has renal impairment, no dosage adjustment of lamivudine is necessary (see section 4.2). Lamivudine has no effect on the pharmacokinetics of trimethoprim or sulfamethoxazole. When concomitant administration is warranted, patients should be monitored clinically. Co-administration of lamivudine with high doses of co-trimoxazole for the treatment of *Pneumocystis carinii* pneumonia (PCP) and toxoplasmosis should be avoided.

The possibility of interactions with other medicinal products administered concurrently should be considered, particularly when the main route of elimination is active renal secretion via the organic cationic transport system e.g. trimethoprim. Other medicinal products (e.g. ranitidine, cimetidine) are eliminated only in part by this mechanism and were shown not to interact with lamivudine. The nucleoside analogues (e.g. didanosine and zalcitabine) like zidovudine, are not eliminated by this mechanism and are unlikely to interact with lamivudine.

A modest increase in C_{max} (28 %) was observed for zidovudine when administered with lamivudine, however overall exposure (AUC) is not significantly altered. Zidovudine has no effect on the pharmacokinetics of lamivudine (see section 5.2).

Lamivudine metabolism does not involve CYP3A, making interactions with medicinal products metabolised by this system (e.g. PIs) unlikely.

4.6 Pregnancy and lactation

Pregnancy: The safety of lamivudine in human pregnancy has not been established. Reproductive studies in animals have not shown evidence of teratogenicity, and showed no effect on male or female fertility. Lamivudine induces early embryonic death when administered to pregnant rabbits at exposure levels comparable to those achieved in man. In humans, consistent with passive transmission of lamivudine across the placenta, lamivudine concentrations in infant serum at birth were similar to those in maternal and cord serum at delivery.

Although animal reproductive studies are not always predictive of the human response, administration is not recommended during the first three months of pregnancy.

Lactation: Following oral administration lamivudine was excreted in breast milk at similar concentrations to those found in serum. Since lamivudine and the virus pass into breast milk, it is recommended that mothers taking Epivir do not breast-feed their infants. It is recommended that HIV infected women do not breast-feed their infants under any circumstances in order to avoid transmission of HIV.

4.7 Effects on ability to drive and use machines

No studies on the effects on the ability to drive and use machines have been performed.

4.8 Undesirable effects

The following adverse reactions have been reported during therapy for HIV disease with Epivir.

The adverse reactions considered at least possibly related to the treatment are listed below by body system, organ class and absolute frequency. Frequencies are defined as very common (>1/10), common (>1/100, <1/10), uncommon (>1/1,000, <1/100), rare (>1/10,000, <1/1,000), very rare (<1/10,000). Within each frequency grouping, undesirable effects are presented in order of decreasing seriousness.

Blood and lymphatic systems disorders

Uncommon: Neutropenia and anaemia (both occasionally severe), thrombocytopenia

Very rare: Pure red cell aplasia

Nervous system disorders

Common: Headache, insomnia

Very rare: Peripheral neuropathy (or paraesthesia)

Respiratory, thoracic and mediastinal disorders

Common: Cough, nasal symptoms

Gastrointestinal disorders

Common: Nausea, vomiting, abdominal pain or cramps, diarrhoea

Rare: Pancreatitis elevations in serum amylase.

Hepatobiliary disorders

Uncommon: Transient elevations in liver enzymes (AST, ALT).

Rare: Hepatitis

Skin and subcutaneous tissue disorders

Common: Rash, alopecia

Musculoskeletal and connective tissue disorders

Common: Arthralgia, muscle disorders

Rare: Rhabdomyolysis

General disorders and administration site conditions

Common: Fatigue, malaise, fever.

Cases of lactic acidosis, sometimes fatal, usually associated with severe hepatomegaly and hepatic steatosis, have been reported with the use of nucleoside analogues (see section 4.4).

Combination antiretroviral therapy has been associated with redistribution of body fat (lipodystrophy) in HIV patients including the loss of peripheral and facial subcutaneous fat, increased intra-abdominal and visceral fat, breast hypertrophy and dorsocervical fat accumulation (buffalo hump).

Combination antiretroviral therapy has been associated with metabolic abnormalities such as hypertriglyceridaemia, hypercholesterolaemia, insulin resistance, hyperglycaemia and hyperlactataemia (see section 4.4).

In HIV-infected patients with severe immune deficiency at the time of initiation of combination antiretroviral therapy (CART), an inflammatory reaction to asymptomatic or residual opportunistic infections may arise (see section 4.4).

Cases of osteonecrosis have been reported, particularly in patients with generally acknowledged risk factors, advanced HIV disease or long-term combined antiretroviral exposure (CART). The frequency of which is unknown (see section 4.4).

4.9 Overdose

Administration of lamivudine at very high dose levels in acute animal studies did not result in any organ toxicity. Limited data are available on the consequences of ingestion of acute overdoses in humans. No fatalities occurred, and the patients recovered. No specific signs or symptoms have been identified following such overdose.

If overdosage occurs the patient should be monitored, and standard supportive treatment applied as required. Since lamivudine is dialysable, continuous haemodialysis could be used in the treatment of overdosage, although this has not been studied.

5. PHARMACOLOGICAL PROPERTIES

5.1 Pharmacodynamic properties

Pharmacotherapeutic group: nucleoside analogue, ATC Code: J05AF05.

Lamivudine is a nucleoside analogue which has activity against human immunodeficiency virus (HIV) and hepatitis B virus (HBV). It is metabolised intracellularly to the active moiety, lamivudine 5'- triphosphate. Its main mode of action is as a chain terminator of viral reverse transcription. The triphosphate has selective inhibitory activity against HIV-1 and HIV-2 replication *in vitro*; it is also active against zidovudine-resistant clinical isolates of HIV. Lamivudine in combination with zidovudine exhibits synergistic anti-HIV activity against clinical isolates in cell culture.

HIV-1 resistance to lamivudine involves the development of a M184V amino acid change close to the active site of the viral reverse transcriptase (RT). This variant arises both *in vitro* and in HIV-1 infected patients treated with lamivudine-containing antiretroviral therapy. M184V mutants display greatly reduced susceptibility to lamivudine and show diminished viral replicative capacity *in vitro*. *In vitro* studies indicate that zidovudine-resistant virus isolates can become zidovudine sensitive when they simultaneously acquire resistance to lamivudine. The clinical relevance of such findings remains, however, not well defined.

In vitro data tend to suggest that the continuation of lamivudine in anti-retroviral regimen despite the development of M184V might provide residual anti-retroviral activity (likely through impaired viral fitness). The clinical relevance of these findings is not established. Indeed, the available clinical data are very limited and preclude any reliable conclusion in the field. In any case, initiation of susceptible NRTI's should always be preferred to maintenance of lamivudine therapy. Therefore, maintaining lamivudine therapy despite emergence of M184V mutation should only be considered in cases where no other active NRTI's are available.

Cross-resistance conferred by the M184V RT is limited within the nucleoside inhibitor class of antiretroviral agents. Zidovudine and stavudine maintain their antiretroviral activities against lamivudine-resistant HIV-1. Abacavir maintains its antiretroviral activities against lamivudine-resistant HIV-1 harbouring only the M184V mutation. The M184V RT mutant shows a <4-fold decrease in susceptibility to didanosine and zalcitabine; the clinical significance of these findings is unknown. *In vitro* susceptibility testing has not been standardised and results may vary according to methodological factors.

Lamivudine demonstrates low cytotoxicity to peripheral blood lymphocytes, to established lymphocyte and monocyte-macrophage cell lines, and to a variety of bone marrow progenitor cells *in vitro*.

Clinical experience:

In clinical trials, lamivudine in combination with zidovudine has been shown to reduce HIV-1 viral load and increase CD4 cell count. Clinical end-point data indicate that lamivudine in combination with zidovudine, results in a significant reduction in the risk of disease progression and mortality.

Evidence from clinical studies shows that lamivudine plus zidovudine delays the emergence of zidovudine resistant isolates in individuals with no prior antiretroviral therapy.

Lamivudine has been widely used as a component of antiretroviral combination therapy with other antiretroviral agents of the same class (NRTIs) or different classes (PIs, non-nucleoside reverse transcriptase inhibitors).

Multiple drug antiretroviral therapy containing lamivudine has been shown to be effective in antiretrovirally-naive patients as well as in patients presenting with viruses containing the M184V mutations.

The relationship between *in vitro* susceptibility of HIV to lamivudine and clinical response to lamivudine-containing therapy remains under investigation.

Lamivudine at a dose of 100 mg once daily has also been shown to be effective for the treatment of adult patients with chronic HBV infection (for details of clinical studies, see the prescribing information for Zeffix). However, for the treatment of HIV infection, only a 300 mg daily dose of lamivudine (in combination with other antiretroviral agents) has been shown to be efficacious.

Lamivudine has not been specifically investigated in HIV patients co-infected with HBV.

Once daily dosing (300 mg once a day): a clinical study has demonstrated the non inferiority between Epivir once a day and Epivir twice a day containing regimens. These results were obtained in an antiretroviral naïve-population, primarily consisting of asymptomatic HIV infected patients (CDC stage A).

5.2 Pharmacokinetic properties

Absorption: Lamivudine is well absorbed from the gastrointestinal tract, and the bioavailability of oral lamivudine in adults is normally between 80 and 85 %. Following oral administration, the mean time (t_{max}) to maximal serum concentrations (C_{max}) is about an hour. Based on data derived from a study in healthy volunteers, at a therapeutic dose of 150mg twice daily, mean (CV) steady-state C_{max} and C_{min} of lamivudine in plasma are 1.2 μg/ml (24%) and 0.09 μg/ml (27%), respectively. The mean (CV) AUC over a dosing interval of 12 hours is 4.7 μg.h/ml (18%). At a therapeutic dose of 300mg once daily, the mean (CV) steady-state C_{max}, C_{min} and 24h AUC are 2.0 μg/ml (26%), 0.04 μg/ml (34%) and 8.9 μg.h/ml (21%), respectively.

Co-administration of lamivudine with food results in a delay of t_{max} and a lower C_{max} (decreased by 47 %). However, the extent (based on the AUC) of lamivudine absorbed is not influenced.

Co-administration of zidovudine results in a 13 % increase in zidovudine exposure and a 28 % increase in peak plasma levels. This is not considered to be of significance to patient safety and therefore no dosage adjustments are necessary.

Distribution: From intravenous studies, the mean volume of distribution is 1.3 l/kg. The observed half-life of elimination is 5 to 7 hours. The mean systemic clearance of lamivudine is approximately 0.32 l/h/kg, with predominantly renal clearance (> 70 %) via the organic cationic transport system.

Lamivudine exhibits linear pharmacokinetics over the therapeutic dose range and displays limited binding to the major plasma protein albumin (< 16 % - 36 % to serum albumin in *in vitro* studies).

Limited data show that lamivudine penetrates the central nervous system and reaches the cerebro-spinal fluid (CSF). The mean ratio CSF/serum lamivudine concentration 2-4 hours after oral administration was approximately 0.12. The true extent of penetration or relationship with any clinical efficacy is unknown.

Metabolism: The active moiety, intracellular lamivudine triphosphate, has a prolonged terminal half-life in the cell (16 to 19 hours) compared to the plasma lamivudine half-life (5 to 7 hours). In 60 healthy adult volunteers, Epivir 300 mg once daily has been demonstrated to be pharmacokinetically equivalent at steady-state to Epivir 150 mg twice daily with respect to intracellular triphosphate AUC_{24} and C_{max}.

Lamivudine is predominately cleared unchanged by renal excretion. The likelihood of metabolic interactions of lamivudine with other medicinal products is low due to the small extent of hepatic metabolism (5-10 %) and low plasma protein binding.

Elimination: Studies in patients with renal impairment show lamivudine elimination is affected by renal dysfunction. A recommended dosage regimen for patients with creatinine clearance below 50 ml/min is shown in the dosage section (see section 4.2).

An interaction with trimethoprim, a constituent of co-trimoxazole, causes a 40 % increase in lamivudine exposure at therapeutic doses. This does not require dose adjustment unless the patient also has renal impairment (see sections 4.5 and 4.2). Administration of co-trimoxazole with lamivudine in patients with renal impairment should be carefully assessed.

Pharmacokinetics in children: In general, lamivudine pharmacokinetics in paediatric patients is similar to adults. However, absolute bioavailability (approximately 55-65 %) was reduced in paediatric patients below 12 years of age. In addition, systemic clearance values were greater in younger paediatric patients and decreased with age approaching adult values around 12 years of age. Due to these differences, the recommended dose for children from three months to 12 years is 8 mg/kg/day, which will achieve similar adult and paediatric exposure (average AUC approximately 5,000 ng.h/ml). Recent findings indicate that exposure in children < 6 years of age may be reduced by about 30% compared to that of other age groups. Further data addressing this issue are currently awaited. However, presently available data does not suggest that lamivudine is less efficacious in this age group.

There are limited pharmacokinetic data for patients less than three months of age. In neonates one week of age, lamivudine oral clearance was reduced when compared to paediatric patients and is likely to be due to immature renal function and variable absorption. Therefore to achieve similar adult and paediatric exposure, the recommended dose for neonates is 4 mg/kg/day. Glomerular filtration estimates suggests that to achieve similar adult and paediatric exposure, the recommended dose for children aged six weeks and older could be 8 mg/kg/day.

Pharmacokinetics in pregnancy: Following oral administration, lamivudine pharmacokinetics in late-pregnancy were similar to non-pregnant women.

5.3 Preclinical safety data

Administration of lamivudine in animal toxicity studies at high doses was not associated with any major organ toxicity. At the highest dosage levels, minor effects on indicators of liver and kidney function were seen together with occasional reductions in liver weight. The clinically relevant effects noted were a reduction in red blood cell count and neutropenia.

Lamivudine was not mutagenic in bacterial tests but, like many nucleoside analogues, showed activity in an *in vitro* cytogenetic assay and the mouse lymphoma assay. Lamivudine was not genotoxic *in vivo* at doses that gave plasma concentrations around 40-50 times higher than the anticipated clinical plasma levels. As the *in vitro* mutagenic activity of lamivudine could not be confirmed in *in vivo* tests, it is concluded that lamivudine should not represent a genotoxic hazard to patients undergoing treatment.

A transplacental genotoxicity study conducted in monkeys compared zidovudine alone with the combination of zidovudine and lamivudine at human-equivalent exposures. The study demonstrated that foetuses exposed *in utero* to the combination sustained a higher level of nucleoside analogue-DNA incorporation into multiple foetal organs, and showed evidence of more telomere shortening than in those exposed to zidovudine alone. The clinical significance of these findings is unknown.

The results of long-term carcinogenicity studies in rats and mice did not show any carcinogenic potential relevant for humans.

6. PHARMACEUTICAL PARTICULARS

6.1 List of excipients

Sucrose 20 % (3 g/15 ml)

Methyl parahydroxybenzoate

Propyl parahydroxybenzoate

Citric acid Anhydrous

Propylene glycol

Sodium citrate

Artificial strawberry flavour

Artificial banana flavour

Purified water

6.2 Incompatibilities

Not applicable

6.3 Shelf life

2 years

Discard the oral solution one month after first opening.

6.4 Special precautions for storage

Do not store above 25°C.

6.5 Nature and contents of container

Cartons containing 240 ml oral solution in a white high density polyethylene (HDPE) bottle, with a child resistant closure. A 10 ml polypropylene oral dosing syringe and a polyethylene adapter are also included in the pack.

The oral dosing syringe is provided for accurate measurement of the prescribed dose of the oral solution. Instructions for use are included in the pack.

6.6 Special precautions for disposal and other handling

No special requirements.

7. MARKETING AUTHORISATION HOLDER

Glaxo Group Ltd

Greenford Road

Greenford

Middlesex UB6 0NN

United Kingdom

8. MARKETING AUTHORISATION NUMBER(S)

EU/1/96/015/002

9. DATE OF FIRST AUTHORISATION/RENEWAL OF THE AUTHORISATION

Date of first authorisation: 8 August 1996

Date of last renewal: 28 July 2006

10. DATE OF REVISION OF THE TEXT

31 August 2007

Detailed information on this medicinal product is available on the website of the European Medicines Agency (EMEA) http://www.emea.europa.eu

Eposin

(medac GmbH)

1. NAME OF THE MEDICINAL PRODUCT

Eposin

2. QUALITATIVE AND QUANTITATIVE COMPOSITION

1 vial with 5 ml concentrate for solution for infusion contains 100 mg etoposide, Ph.Eur.

1 vial with 25 ml concentrate for solution for infusion contains 500 mg etoposide, Ph.Eur.

1 ml concentrate for solution for infusion contains 20 mg etoposide.

3. PHARMACEUTICAL FORM

Concentrate for solution for infusion (to dilute).

4. CLINICAL PARTICULARS

4.1 Therapeutic indications

Etoposide is indicated for the management of:

- testicular tumours in combination with other chemotherapeutic agents

- small cell lung cancer, in combination with other chemotherapeutic agents

- monoblastic leukaemia (AML M5) and acute myelomonoblastic leukaemia (AML M4) when standard therapy has failed (in combination with other chemotherapeutic agents).

4.2 Posology and method of administration

Eposin, concentrate for solution for infusion 20 mg/ml must be diluted immediately prior to use with either 5 % dextrose in water, or 0.9 % sodium chloride solution to give a final concentration of 0.2 to 0.4 mg/ml. At higher concentrations precipitation of etoposide may occur.

The usual dose of etoposide, in combination with other approved chemotherapeutic agents, ranges from 100-120 mg/m^2/day via continuous infusion over 30 minutes for 3-5 days, followed by a resting period of 10-20 days.

Generally 3 to 4 chemotherapy cycles are administered. Dose and amount of cycles should be adjusted to the level of bone marrow suppression and the reaction of the tumour.

In patients with renal function impairment the dose should be adjusted.

Etoposide is intended for intravenous administration only.

To prevent the occurrence of hypotension, the infusion should be given over at least 30 minutes.

Dosage adjustment in case of renal function impairment.

In patients with a measured creatinine clearance of greater than 50 mL/minute, no initial dose modification is required. In patients with a measured creatinine clearance of 15-50 mL/minute, 75% of the initial recommended etoposide dose should be administered. Although specific data are not available in patients with a measured creatinine clearance less than 15 mL/minute, further dose reduction should be considered. Subsequent etoposide dosing should be based on patient tolerance and clinical effect.

4.3 Contraindications

Severe myelosuppression, unless when this is caused by the underlying disease.

Liver impairment.

Hypersensitivity to etoposide or one of the other constituents.

Breastfeeding.

Patients with severe renal impairment (creatinine clearance < 15 ml/min).

Eposin must not be used in neonates because of the excipient benzyl alcohol.

4.4 Special warnings and precautions for use

If Eposin is to be used as part of a chemotherapy regimen, the physician should weigh the necessity to use the drug against the potential risk and side effects (see "Undesirable effects").

Etoposide should only be administered under strict observation by a doctor specialised in oncology, preferable in institutions specialised in such therapies. It should not be injected intraarterially, intrapleurally, or intraperitoneally. Etoposide vials are intended for intravenous administration only. Extravasation should be strictly avoided. If extravasation occurs, the administration should be terminated immediately and restarted in another vein. Cooling, flooding with normal saline and local infiltration with corticosteroids have been reported as therapeutic measures.

Etoposide should be given by slow intravenous infusion over a period of 30-60 minutes; rapid intravenous administration may cause hypotension.

One should be aware of the possible occurrence of an anaphylactic reaction manifested by flushing, tachycardia, bronchospasm, and hypotension (see "Undesirable effects" section).

The substance etoposide can have genotoxic effects. Therefore, men being treated with etoposide are advised not to father a child during and up to 6 months after treatment and to seek advice on cryo-conservation of sperm prior to treatment because of the possibility of irreversible infertility due to therapy with etoposide. Women should not become pregnant during treatment with etoposide.

The occurrence of a leucopenia with a leucocyte count below 2,000/mm^3 is an indication to withhold further therapy until the blood counts have sufficiently recovered (usually after 10 days).

The administration of etoposide should be terminated at the occurrence of thrombocytopenia.

Bacterial infections should be treated before the start of the therapy with etoposide. Great care should be taken on giving etoposide to patients who have, or have been exposed to infection with herpes zoster.

The occurrence of bone marrow depression, caused by radiotherapy or chemotherapy, necessitates a resting period. It is advised not to restart treatment with etoposide until the platelet count has reached at least 100,000/mm^3.

Peripheral blood counts and liver function should be monitored.

Patients with a low serum albumin concentration may have an increased risk of etoposide toxicity.

The occurrence of acute leukemia, which can occur with or without myelodysplastic syndrome, has been described in patients that were treated with etoposide containing chemotherapeutic regimens.

This product contains 24% m/v of ethanol. Each 5 ml vial contains up to 1.2 g of alcohol, each 25 ml vial contains up to 6 g of alcohol. This can be harmful for those suffering from liver disease, alcoholism, epilepsy, brain injury or disease as well as for children and pregnant women. Alcohol also may modify or increase the effect of other medicines.

Handling precautions: see "Instructions for Use/Handling" section.

4.5 Interaction with other medicinal products and other forms of interaction

The action of oral anticoagulants can be increased.

Phenylbutazone, sodium salicylate and salicylic acid can affect protein binding of etoposide.

Etoposide may potentiate the cytotoxic and myelosuppressive action of other drugs.

The coadministration of etoposide and high-dose cyclosporine may greatly increase etoposide serum concentrations and risk of adverse reactions. This is probably a result of decreased clearance and increased volume of distribution of etoposide when cyclosporine serum concentration exceeds 2000 ng/mL. The dose of etoposide should be reduced by 50% with concurrent use of high-dose cyclosporine infusion.

Co-administration of myelosuppressive drugs (such as cyclophosphamide, BCNU, CCNU, 5-fluorouracil, vinblastine, doxorubicin and cisplatin) may increase the effect of etoposide and/or co-administered drug on the bone marrow.

Experimentally confirmed cross-resistance between anthracyclines and etoposide has been reported.

The occurrence of acute leukemia, which can occur with or without preleukemic phase has been reported in patients treated with etoposide in association with other anti-neoplastic drugs, e.g. bleomycin, cisplatin, ifosfamide, methotrexate.

4.6 Pregnancy and lactation

Pregnancy

There is no experience with the use of etoposide during the first trimester of human pregnancy and very limited experience (isolated case reports) during the second and third trimester. Etoposide was teratogenic in animals (see section 5.3). On the basis of the results from animal studies and the mechanism of action of the substance, the use of etoposide during pregnancy, in particular during the first trimester, is advised against. In every individual case, the expected advantages of the treatment should be weighed against the possible risk for the embryo/foetus.

Lactation

Etoposide is excreted into human breast milk. Breast feeding is contraindicated during treatment with Eposin.

4.7 Effects on ability to drive and use machines

Due to the frequent occurrence of nausea and vomiting, driving and operation of machinery should be discouraged.

4.8 Undesirable effects

The following frequencies have been used:

- Very common (>1/10)
- Common (>1/100, <1/10)
- Uncommon (>1/1,000, <1/100)
- Rare (>1/10,000, <1/1,000)
- Very rare (<1/10,000) including isolated reports

Neoplasms benign and malignant

The risk of secondary leukemia among patients with germ-cell tumours after treatment with etoposide is about 1%. This leukemia is characterised with a relatively short latency period (mean 35 months), monocytic or myelomonocytic FAB subtype, chromosomal abnormalities at 11q23 in about 50% and a good response to chemotherapy. A total cumulative dose (etoposide > 2 g/m^2) is associated with increased risk.

Etoposide is also associated with development of acute promyelocytic leukemia (APL). High doses of etoposide (> 4,000 mg/m^2) appear to increase the risk of APL.

Blood and lymphatic systems disorders

Very common: The dose limiting toxicity of etoposide is myelosuppression, predominantly leucopenia and thrombocytopenia (leucopenia in 60 - 91%, severe leucopenia [<1000/µl] in 7 - 17%, thrombocytopenia in 28 - 41%, severe thrombocytopenia [< 50,000/µl] in 4 -20% of patients). Anaemia occurs in approx. 40% of patients.

Myelosuppression is dose limiting, with granulocyte nadirs occurring 5 to 15 days after drug administration and platelet nadirs occurring 9 to 16 days after drug administration. Bone marrow recovery is usually complete by day 21, and no cumulative toxicity has been reported.

Fatal cases of myelosuppression have been reported.

Infections have been reported in patients with bone marrow depression.

Common: Haemorrhage (in patients with severe myelosuppression)

Immune system disorders

Common: Anaphylactic-like reactions characterised by fever, flushing, tachycardia, bronchospasm, and hypotension have been reported (incidence 0.7-2%), also apnoea followed by spontaneous recurrence of breathing after withdrawal of etoposide infusion, increase in blood pressure. The reactions can be managed by cessation of the infusion and administration of pressor agents, corticosteroids, antihistamines and/or volume expanders as appropriate.

Anaphylactoid - like reactions may occur after the first intravenous administration of etoposide.

In children receiving dosages higher than recommended, anaphylactoid-like reactions have been reported more frequently.

Erythema, facial and tongue oedema, coughing, sweating, cyanosis, convulsions, laryngospasm and hypertension have also been observed. The blood pressure usually returns to normal within few hours following cessation of therapy.

Seldom hypersensitivity reactions caused by benzyl alcohol may occur.

Nervous system disorders

Common: Central nervous system disorders (fatigue, drowsiness) were observed in 0 - 3% of patients.

Uncommon: Peripheral neuropathies were observed in 0.7% of patients.

Rare: Insults have been reported, occasionally in association with hypersensitivity reactions. Asthenia has been reported, as well as paresthesiae.

Eye disorders

Rare: Reversible loss of vision. Optic neuritis and transient cortical blindness have been reported.

Cardiac disorders

Uncommon: Cases of arrhythmia and myocardial infarction have been reported.

Vascular disorders

Common: Transient hypotension following rapid intravenous administration has been reported in 1% to 2% of patients. It has not been associated with cardiac toxicity or electrocardiographic changes. To prevent this rare occurrence, it is recommended that etoposide be administered by slow intravenous infusion over a 30- to 60-minute period. If hypotension occurs, it usually responds to supportive therapy after cessation of the administration. When restarting the infusion, a slower administration rate should be used.

Respiratory, thoracic and mediastinal disorders

Uncommon: Bronchospasm, coughing, cyanosis, laryngospasm.

Rare: Apnoea, Interstitial pneumonitis or pulmonary fibrosis.

Gastrointestinal disorders

Very common: Nausea and vomiting are the major gastrointestinal toxicities (30-40%). The severity of such nausea and vomiting is generally mild to moderate with treatment discontinuation required in 1% of patients. Anorexia (10-13%).

Common: Abdominal pain and diarrhoea (1-13%) are commonly observed. Stomatitis has been observed in approx. 1 - 6 % of patients.

Uncommon: Mucositis and oesophagitis may occur.

Rare: Constipation and swallowing disorders have been observed rarely. Dysphagia and taste impairment have been reported.

Hepato-biliary disorder

Common: Hepatic dysfunction has been observed in 0 - 3% of patients. High dosages of etoposide may cause an increase in bilirubin, SGOT and alkaline phosphatases.

Skin and subcutaneous tissue disorders

Very common: Reversible alopecia, sometimes progressing to total baldness was observed in up to 70% of patients.

Uncommon: Rash, urticaria, pigmentation and pruritus have also been reported following the administration of etoposide.

Very Rare: toxic epidermal necrolysis (1 fatal case). Stevens Johnson syndrome has also been reported, however, a causal relationship with etoposide has not been established. Radiation "recall" dermatitis, hand-foot syndrome.

Renal and urinary disorders

Etoposide has been shown to reach high concentrations in the liver and kidney, thus presenting a potential for accumulation in cases of functional impairment.

General disorders and administration site conditions

Etoposide has been shown to reach high concentrations in the liver and kidney, thus presenting a potential for accumulation in cases of functional impairment.

Rare: In rare cases, phlebitis has been observed following bolus injection of etoposide.

This adverse reaction can be avoided by I.V. infusion over 30 to 60 minutes. After extravasation, irritation of soft tissue and inflammation occur occasionally. Hyperuricaemia due to rapid destruction of malignant cells.

4.9 Overdose

Acute overdosage results in severe forms of normally occurring adverse reactions, in particular leucopenia and thrombopenia.

Severe mucositis and elevated values of serum bilirubin, SGOT and alkaline phosphatase have been reported after administration of high doses of etoposide. Metabolic acidosis and severe hepatic toxicity have been reported after administration of dosages higher than recommended.

The management of bone marrow depression is symptomatic, including antibiotics and transfusions.

If hypersensitivity to etoposide occurs, antihistamines and intravenously administered corticosteroids are appropriate.

5. PHARMACOLOGICAL PROPERTIES

5.1 Pharmacodynamic properties

Pharmacotherapeutic classification: podophyllotoxine derivatives (ATC: L01CB01)

Etoposide is a semisynthetic derivative of podophyllotoxin used in the treatment of certain neoplastic diseases. Podophyllotoxins inhibit mitosis by blocking microtubular assembly. Etoposide inhibits cell cycle progression at a premitotic phase (late S and G2).

It does not interfere with the synthesis of nucleinic acids.

5.2 Pharmacokinetic properties

The concentration of etoposide in blood and organs is low with maximum values in the liver and the kidneys. Protein binding could be as high as 98%.

On intravenous administration, the disposition of etoposide is best described as a biphasic process with an initial half-life of about 1.5 hours. After distribution, half-life is about 40 hours. The terminal half-life is 6-8 hours.

Following a single intravenous dose etoposide is excreted in the urine for about 63% and in the faeces for about 31% after 80 hours.

Etoposide is cleared by both renal and nonrenal processes i.e. metabolism and biliary excretion. In patients with renal dysfunction plasma etoposide clearance is decreased.

In adults, the total body clearance of etoposide is correlated with creatinine clearance, serum albumin concentration and nonrenal clearance. In children, elevated serum ALT levels are associated with reduced drug total body clearance. Prior use of cisplatin may result in a decrease of etoposide total body clearance.

5.3 Preclinical safety data

Etoposide has been shown to be embryotoxic and teratogenic in animal experiments with rats and mice.

There are positive results from in vitro and in vivo test with regard to gene and chromosome mutations induced by etoposide. The results justify the suspicion of a mutagenic effect in humans.

No animal tests with regard to carcinogenicity were performed. Based on the DNA-damaging effect and the mutagenic properties, etoposide is potentially carcinogenic.

6. PHARMACEUTICAL PARTICULARS

6.1 List of excipients

Macrogol 300, polysorbate 80, benzyl alcohol, ethanol, citric acid, anhydrous.

6.2 Incompatibilities

Plastic devices made of acrylic or ABS polymers have been reported to crack when used with undiluted Eposin, concentrate for solution for infusion 20 mg/ml. This effect has not been reported with etoposide after dilution of the concentrate for solution for infusion according to instructions.

6.3 Shelf life

Vial before opening

3 years.

After dilution

Chemical and physical in-use stability of the solution diluted to a concentration of 0.2 mg/ml or 0.4 mg/ml has been demonstrated for 24 hours at 15 – 25 °C. From a microbiological point of view, the diluted product should be used immediately. If not used immediately, in-use storage times and conditions prior to use are the responsibility of the user and would normally not be longer than 12 hours at 15 – 25 °C, unless dilution has taken place in controlled and validated aseptic conditions.

6.4 Special precautions for storage

Store below 25° C, protected from light (keep vials in the outer carton). Do not freeze.

Diluted solutions: see section 6.3

Do not store the diluted product in a refrigerator (2 – 8 °C) as this might cause precipitation.

Solutions showing any sign of precipitation should not be used.

6.5 Nature and contents of container

Each injection vial contains 100 mg (5 ml) of etoposide.

Each injection vial contains 500 mg (25 ml) of etoposide.

One package contains 1 vial or 10 vials of Eposin.

6.6 Special precautions for disposal and other handling

Eposin should not be used without diluting! Dilute with 0.9 % sodium chloride or 5 % dextrose. Solutions showing any signs of precipitation should not be used.

For waste-disposal and safety information guidelines on safe-handling of antineoplastic drugs should be followed. Any contact with the fluid should be avoided. During preparation and reconstitution a strictly aseptic working technique should be used; protective measures should include the use of gloves, mask, safety goggles and protective clothing. Use of a vertical laminar airflow (LAF) hood is recommended.

Gloves should be worn during administration. Waste-disposal procedures should take into account the cytotoxic nature of this substance.

If etoposide contacts skin, mucosae or eyes, immediately wash thoroughly with water. Soap may be used for skin cleansing.

7. MARKETING AUTHORISATION HOLDER

Pharmachemie B.V.
P.O. Box 552
2003 RN Haarlem
The Netherlands.

8. MARKETING AUTHORISATION NUMBER(S)

PL 04946/0018.

9. DATE OF FIRST AUTHORISATION/RENEWAL OF THE AUTHORISATION

17 December 1996 / 10 January 2005

10. DATE OF REVISION OF THE TEXT

10/01/2005

Eprex 2000, 4000 and 10000 IU/ml solution for injection in pre-filled syringe

(Janssen-Cilag Ltd)

1. NAME OF THE MEDICINAL PRODUCT

EPREX®

2. QUALITATIVE AND QUANTITATIVE COMPOSITION

• Epoetin alfa*..........2000 IU/ml (16.8 micrograms per ml)

A pre-filled syringe of 0.5 ml contains 1000 IU (8.4 micrograms) of epoetin alfa

• Epoetin alfa*..........4000 IU/ml (33.6 micrograms per ml)

A pre-filled syringe of 0.5 ml contains 2000 IU (16.8 micrograms) of epoetin alfa

• Epoetin alfa*.......10,000 IU/ml (84.0 micrograms per ml)

A pre-filled syringe of 0.3 ml contains 3000 IU (25.2 micrograms) of epoetin alfa

A pre-filled syringe of 0.4 ml contains 4000 IU (33.6 micrograms) of epoetin alfa

A pre-filled syringe of 0.5 ml contains 5000 IU (42.0 micrograms) of epoetin alfa

A pre-filled syringe of 0.6 ml contains 6000 IU (50.4 micrograms) of epoetin alfa

A pre-filled syringe of 0.8 ml contains 8000 IU (67.2 micrograms) of epoetin alfa

A pre-filled syringe of 1.0 ml contains 10,000 IU (84.0 micrograms) of epoetin alfa

*produced in Chinese Hamster Ovary (CHO) cells by recombinant DNA technology

For a full list of excipients, see section 6.1.

3. PHARMACEUTICAL FORM

Solution for injection in pre-filled syringe.

Clear, colourless solution.

4. CLINICAL PARTICULARS

4.1 Therapeutic indications

Treatment of symptomatic anaemia associated with chronic renal failure (CRF) in adult and paediatric patients:

• Treatment of anaemia associated with chronic renal failure in paediatric and adult patients on haemodialysis and adult patients on peritoneal dialysis.

• Treatment of severe anaemia of renal origin accompanied by clinical symptoms in adult patients with renal insufficiency not yet undergoing dialysis.

Treatment of anaemia and reduction of transfusion requirements in adult patients receiving chemotherapy for solid tumours, malignant lymphoma or multiple myeloma, and at risk of transfusion as assessed by the patient's general status (e.g. cardiovascular status, pre-existing anaemia at the start of chemotherapy).

EPREX can be used to increase the yield of autologous blood from patients in a predonation programme. Its use in this indication must be balanced against the reported risk of thromboembolic events. Treatment should only be given to patients with moderate anaemia (Hb 10-13 g/dl [6.2-8.1 mmol/l], no iron deficiency) if blood saving procedures are not available or insufficient when the scheduled major elective surgery requires a large volume of blood (4 or more units of blood for females or 5 or more units for males).

EPREX can be used to reduce exposure to allogeneic blood transfusions in adult non-iron deficient patients prior to major elective orthopaedic surgery, having a high perceived risk for transfusion complications. Use should be restricted to patients with moderate anaemia (e.g. Hb 10-13 g/dl) who do not have an autologous predonation programme available and with expected moderate blood loss (900 to 1800 ml).

Good blood management practices should always be used in the perisurgical setting.

4.2 Posology and method of administration

Method of administration

As with any other injectable product, check that there are no particles in the solution or change in colour.

a) intravenous injection: over at least one to five minutes, depending on the total dose. In haemodialysed patients, a bolus injection may be given during the dialysis session through a suitable venous port in the dialysis line. Alternatively, the injection can be given at the end of the dialysis session via the fistula needle tubing, followed by 10 ml of isotonic saline to rinse the tubing and ensure satisfactory injection of the product into the circulation.

A slower injection is preferable in patients who react to the treatment with "flu-like" symptoms.

Do not administer by intravenous infusion or mixed with other drugs.

b) subcutaneous injection: a maximum volume of 1 ml at one injection site should generally not be exceeded. In case of larger volumes, more than one site should be chosen for the injection.

The injections are given in the limbs or the anterior abdominal wall.

In those situations in which the physician determines that a patient or caregiver can safely and effectively administer EPREX subcutaneously, instruction as to the proper dosage and administration should be provided.

Refer to section 3. How to use EPREX (instructions on how to inject EPREX) of the package leaflet.

Treatment of symptomatic anaemia in adult and paediatric chronic renal failure patients:

In patients with chronic renal failure where intravenous access is routinely available (haemodialysis patients) administration by the intravenous route is preferable. Where intravenous access is not readily available (patients not yet undergoing dialysis and peritoneal dialysis patients) EPREX may be administered subcutaneously.

Anaemia symptoms and sequelae may vary with age, gender, and co-morbid medical conditions; a physician's evaluation of the individual patient's clinical course and condition is necessary.

EPREX should be administered in order to increase haemoglobin to not greater than 12 g/dl (7.5 mmol/l). A rise in haemoglobin of greater than 2g/dl (1.25 mmol/l) over a four week period should be avoided. If it occurs, appropriate dose adjustment should be made as provided.

Due to intra-patient variability, occasional individual haemoglobin values for a patient above and below the desired haemoglobin level may be observed. Haemoglobin variability should be addressed through dose management, with consideration for the haemoglobin target range of 10g/dl (6.2 mmol/l) to 12g/dl (7.5mmol/l). In paediatric patients the recommended target haemoglobin range is between 9.5 and 11 g/dl (5.9-6.8 mmol/l).

A sustained haemoglobin level of greater than 12g/dl (7.5mmol/l) should be avoided. If the haemoglobin is rising by more than 2 g/dl (1.25 mmol/l) per month, or if the sustained haemoglobin exceeds 12g/dl (7.5mmol/l) reduce the epoetin alfa dose by 25%. If the haemoglobin exceeds 13 g/dl (8.1 mmol/l), discontinue therapy until it falls below 12 g/dl (7.5 mmol/l) and then reinstitute epoetin alfa therapy at a dose 25% below the previous dose.

Patients should be monitored closely to ensure that the lowest approved dose of EPREX is used to provide adequate control of anaemia and of the symptoms of anaemia.

Iron status should be evaluated prior to and during treatment and iron supplementation administered if necessary. In addition, other causes of anaemia, such as B_{12} or folate deficiency, should be excluded before instituting therapy with epoetin alfa. Non response to epoetin alfa therapy should prompt a search for causative factors. These include: iron, folate, or Vitamin B_{12} deficiency; aluminium intoxication; intercurrent infections; inflammatory or traumatic episodes; occult blood loss; haemolysis; and bone marrow fibrosis of any origin.

Adult haemodialysis patients:

In patients on haemodialysis where intravenous access is readily available, administration by the intravenous route is preferable.

The treatment is divided into two stages:

Correction phase:

50 IU/kg, 3 times per week.

When a dose adjustment is necessary, this should be done in steps of at least four weeks. At each step, the increase or reduction in dose should be of 25 IU/kg, 3 times per week.

Maintenance phase:

Dosage adjustment in order to maintain haemoglobin values at the desired level: Hb between 10 and 12 g/dl (6.2 - 7.5 mmol/l).

The recommended total weekly dose is between 75 and 300 IU/kg.

The clinical data available suggest that those patients whose initial haemoglobin is very low (<6 g/dl or <3.75 mmol/l) may require higher maintenance doses than those whose initial anaemia is less severe (>8 g/dl or >5 mmol/l).

Paediatric haemodialysis patients:

The treatment is divided into two stages:

Correction phase:

50 IU/kg, 3 times per week by the intravenous route. When a dose adjustment is necessary, this should be done in steps of 25 IU/kg, 3 times per week at intervals of at least 4 weeks until the desired goal is achieved.

Maintenance phase:

Dosage adjustment in order to maintain haemoglobin values at the desired level: Hb between 9.5 and 11 g/dl (5.9 - 6.8 mmol/l).

Generally, children under 30 kg require higher maintenance doses than children over 30 kg and adults. For example, the following maintenance doses were observed in clinical trials after 6 months of treatment.

	Dose (IU/kg given 3x week)	
Weight (kg)	Median	Usual maintenance dose
< 10	100	75-150
10-30	75	60-150
> 30	33	30-100

The clinical data available suggest that those patients whose initial haemoglobin is very low (<6.8 g/dl or <4.25 mmol/l) may require higher maintenance doses than those whose initial haemoglobin is higher (>6.8 g/dl or >4.25 mmol/l).

Adult patients with renal insufficiency not yet undergoing dialysis:

Where intravenous access is not readily available EPREX may be administered subcutaneously.

The treatment is divided into two stages:

Correction phase

Starting dose of 50 IU/kg, 3 times per week, followed if necessary by a dosage increase with 25 IU/kg increments (3 times per week) until the desired goal is achieved (this should be done in steps of at least four weeks).

Maintenance phase

Dosage adjustment in order to maintain haemoglobin values at the desired level: Hb between 10 and 12 g/dl (6.2 - 7.5 mmol/l) (maintenance dose between 17 and 33 IU/kg, 3 times per week).

The maximum dosage should not exceed 200 IU/kg, 3 times per week.

Adult peritoneal dialysis patients:

Where intravenous access is not readily available EPREX may be administered subcutaneously.

The treatment is divided into two stages:

Correction phase

Starting dose of 50 IU/kg, 2 times per week.

Maintenance phase

Dosage adjustment in order to maintain haemoglobin values at the desired level: (Hb between 10 and 12 g/dl (6.2 - 7.5 mmol/l) (maintenance dose between 25 and 50 IU/kg 2 times per week into 2 equal injections).

Treatment of patients with chemotherapy induced anaemia:

EPREX should be administered by the subcutaneous route to patients with anaemia (e.g. haemoglobin concentration ≤ 10g/dl (6.2 mmol/l)). Anaemia symptoms and sequelae may vary with age, gender, and overall burden of disease; a physician's evaluation of the individual patient's clinical course and condition is necessary.

Due to intra-patient variability, occasional individual haemoglobin values for a patient above and below the desired haemoglobin level may be observed. Haemoglobin variability should be addressed through dose management, with consideration for the haemoglobin target range of 10g/dl (6.2 mmol/l) to 12g/dl (7.5mmol/l). A sustained haemoglobin level of greater than 12g/dl (7.5mmol/l) should be avoided; guidance for appropriate dose adjustment for when haemoglobin values exceed 12g/dl (7.5mmol/l) are described below.

Epoetin alfa therapy should continue until one month after the end of chemotherapy.

The initial dose is 150 IU/kg given subcutaneously 3 times per week. Alternatively, EPREX can be administered at an initial dose of 450 IU/kg subcutaneously once weekly. If the haemoglobin has increased by at least 1 g/dl (0.62 mmol/l) or the reticulocyte count has increased ≥40,000 cells/µl above baseline after 4 weeks of treatment, the dose should remain at 150 IU/kg 3 times per week or 450 IU/kg once weekly. If the haemoglobin increase is <1 g/dl (<0.62 mmol/l) and the reticulocyte count has increased <40,000 cells/µl above baseline, increase the dose to 300 IU/kg 3 times per week. If after an additional 4 weeks of

Figure 1

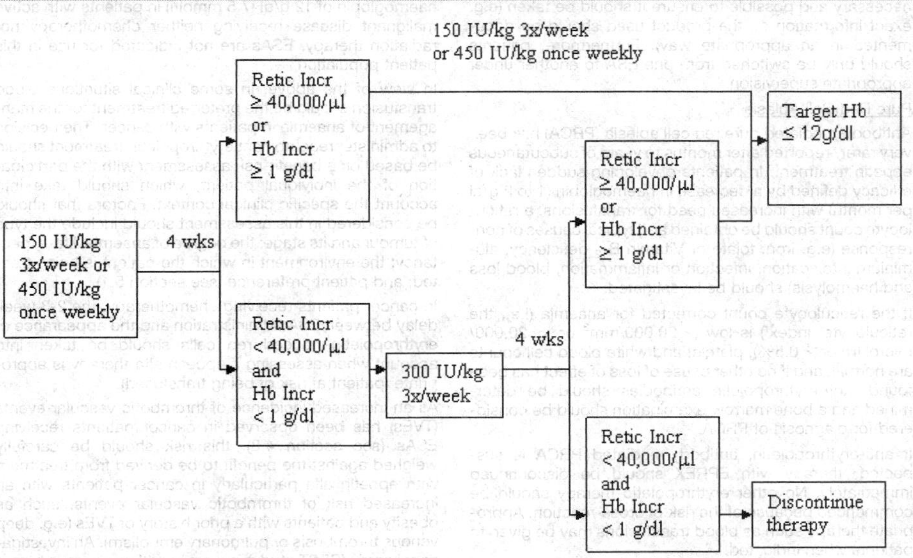

therapy at 300 IU/kg 3 times per week, the haemoglobin has increased ≥1 g/dl (≥0.62 mmol/l) or the reticulocyte count has increased ≥40,000 cells/µl, the dose should remain at 300 IU/kg 3 times per week. However, if the haemoglobin has increased <1 g/dl (<0.62 mmol/l) and the reticulocyte count has increased <40,000 cells/µl above baseline, response is unlikely and treatment should be discontinued. The recommended dosing regimen is described in the following diagram:

(see Figure 1 above)

Patients should be monitored closely to ensure that the lowest approved dose of erythropoiesis-stimulating agent (ESA) is used to provide adequate control of the symptoms of anaemia.

Dose adjustment to maintain haemoglobin concentrations between 10g/dl – 12 g/dl:

If the haemoglobin is rising by more than 2 g/dl (1.25 mmol/l) per month, or if the haemoglobin exceeds 12 g/dl (7.5 mmol/l), reduce the epoetin alfa dose by about 25 - 50%. If the haemoglobin exceeds 13 g/dl (8.1 mmol/l), discontinue therapy until it falls below 12 g/dl (7.5 mmol/l) and then reinstitute epoetin alfa therapy at a dose 25% below the previous dose.

Adult surgery patients in an autologous predonation programme:

The intravenous route of administration should be used. At the time of donating blood, epoetin alfa should be administered after the completion of the blood donation procedure.

Mildly anaemic patients (haematocrit of 33-39%) requiring predeposit of ≥4 units of blood should be treated with epoetin alfa at 600 IU/kg, 2 times weekly for 3 weeks prior to surgery. Using this regimen, it was possible to withdraw ≥4 units of blood from 81% of epoetin alfa-treated patients compared to 37% of placebo-treated patients. Epoetin alfa therapy reduced the risk of exposure to homologous blood by 50% compared to patients not receiving epoetin alfa.

All patients being treated with epoetin alfa should receive adequate iron supplementation (e.g. 200 mg oral elemental iron daily) throughout the course of epoetin alfa treatment. Iron supplementation should be started as soon as possible, even several weeks prior to initiating the autologous predeposit, in order to achieve high iron stores prior to starting epoetin alfa therapy.

Adult patients scheduled for major elective orthopaedic surgery:

The subcutaneous route of administration should be used.

The recommended dose regimen is 600 IU/kg of epoetin alfa, given weekly for three weeks (days -21, -14 and -7) prior to surgery and on the day of surgery. In cases where there is a medical need to shorten the lead time before surgery to less than three weeks, 300 IU/kg epoetin alfa should be given daily for 10 consecutive days prior to surgery, on the day of surgery and for four days immediately thereafter. When performing haematologic assessments during the preoperative period, if the haemoglobin level reaches 15 g/dl, or higher, administration of epoetin alfa should be stopped and further dosages should not be given.

Care should be taken to ensure that at the outset of the treatment patients are not iron deficient. All patients being treated with epoetin alfa should receive adequate iron supplementation (e.g. 200 mg oral elemental iron daily) throughout the course of epoetin alfa treatment. If possible, iron supplementation should be started prior to epoetin alfa therapy, to achieve adequate iron stores.

4.3 Contraindications

Patients who develop pure red cell aplasia (PRCA) following treatment with erythropoietin should not receive EPREX or any other erythropoietin (see Section 4.4 - Pure Red Cell Aplasia).

Uncontrolled hypertension.

All contraindications associated with autologous blood predonation programmes should be respected in patients being supplemented with epoetin alfa.

Hypersensitivity to the active substance or to any of the excipients.

The use of epoetin alfa in patients scheduled for major elective orthopaedic surgery and not participating in an autologous blood predonation programme is contraindicated in patients with severe coronary, peripheral arterial, carotid or cerebral vascular disease, including patients with recent myocardial infarction or cerebral vascular accident.

Surgery patients who for any reason cannot receive adequate antithrombotic prophylaxis.

4.4 Special warnings and precautions for use

General

In all patients receiving epoetin alfa, blood pressure should be closely monitored and controlled as necessary. Epoetin alfa should be used with caution in the presence of untreated, inadequately treated or poorly controllable hypertension. It may be necessary to add or increase anti-hypertensive treatment. If blood pressure cannot be controlled, epoetin alfa treatment should be discontinued.

Epoetin alfa should also be used with caution in the presence of epilepsy and chronic liver failure.

Chronic renal failure and cancer patients on epoetin alfa should have haemoglobin levels measured on a regular basis until a stable level is achieved, and periodically thereafter.

In all patients, haemoglobin levels should be closely monitored due to a potential increased risk of thromboembolic events and fatal outcomes when patients are treated at haemoglobin levels above the target for the indication of use.

There may be a moderate dose-dependent rise in the platelet count within the normal range during treatment with epoetin alfa. This regresses during the course of continued therapy. In addition, thrombocythaemia above the normal range has been reported. It is recommended that the platelet count is regularly monitored during the first 8 weeks of therapy.

All other causes of anaemia (iron deficiency, haemolysis, blood loss, vitamin B_{12} or folate deficiencies) should be considered and treated prior to initiating therapy with epoetin alfa. In most cases, the ferritin values in the serum fall simultaneously with the rise in packed cell volume. In order to ensure optimum response to epoetin alfa, adequate iron stores should be assured:

- iron supplementation, e.g. 200-300 mg/day orally (100-200 mg/day for paediatric patients) is recommended for chronic renal failure patients whose serum ferritin levels are below 100 ng/ml.
- oral iron substitution of 200-300 mg/day is recommended for all cancer patients whose transferrin saturation is below 20%.

All of these additive factors of anaemia should also be carefully considered when deciding to increase the dose of epoetin alfa in cancer patients.

Very rarely, development of or exacerbation of porphyria has been observed in epoetin alfa-treated patients. Epoetin alfa should be used with caution in patients with porphyria.

In order to improve the traceability of the ESA all measures necessary and possible to ensure it should be taken (e.g. exact information on the product used should be documented in an appropriate way). Furthermore, patients should only be switched from one ESA to another under appropriate supervision.

Pure Red Cell Aplasia

Antibody-mediated pure red cell aplasia (PRCA) has been very rarely reported after months to years of subcutaneous epoetin treatment. In patients developing sudden lack of efficacy defined by a decrease in haemoglobin (1 to 2 g/dl per month) with increased need for transfusions, a reticulocyte count should be obtained and typical causes of non-response (e.g. iron, folate or Vitamin B_{12} deficiency, aluminium intoxication, infection or inflammation, blood loss and haemolysis) should be investigated.

If the reticulocyte count corrected for anaemia (i.e., the reticulocyte 'index') is low (<20,000/mm^3 or < 20,000/microlitre or <0.5%), platelet and white blood cell counts are normal, and if no other cause of loss of effect has been found, anti-erythropoietin antibodies should be determined and a bone marrow examination should be considered for diagnosis of PRCA.

If anti-erythropoietin, antibody-mediated PRCA is suspected, therapy with EPREX should be discontinued immediately. No other erythropoietic therapy should be commenced because of the risk of cross-reaction. Appropriate therapy such as blood transfusions may be given to patients when indicated.

Treatment of symptomatic anaemia in adult and paediatric chronic renal failure patients

In chronic renal failure patients therate of increase in haemoglobin should be approximately 1 g/dl (0.62 mmol/l) per month and should not exceed 2 g/dl (1.25 mmol/l) per month to minimise risks of an increase in hypertension.

In patients with chronic renal failure maintenance haemoglobin concentration should not exceed the upper limit of the target haemoglobin concentration as recommended in section 4.2. In clinical trials, an increased risk of death and serious cardiovascular events was observed when ESAs were administered to target a haemoglobin of greater than 12g/dl (7.5 mmol/l).

Controlled clinical trials have not shown significant benefits attributable to the administration of epoetins when haemoglobin concentration is increased beyond the level necessary to control symptoms of anaemia and to avoid blood transfusion.

Chronic renal failure patients treated with EPREX by the subcutaneous route should be monitored regularly for loss of efficacy, defined as absent or decreased response to EPREX treatment in patients who previously responded to such therapy. This is characterised by a sustained decrease in haemoglobin despite an increase in EPREX dosage.

Shunt thromboses have occurred in haemodialysis patients, especially in those who have a tendency to hypotension or whose arteriovenous fistulae exhibit complications (e.g. stenoses, aneurysms, etc.). Early shunt revision and thrombosis prophylaxis by administration of acetylsalicylic acid, for example, is recommended in these patients.

Hyperkalaemia has been observed in isolated cases though causality has not been established. Serum electrolytes should be monitored in chronic renal failure patients. If an elevated or rising serum potassium level is detected, then in addition to appropriate treatment of the hyperkalaemia, consideration should be given to ceasing epoetin alfa administration until the serum potassium level has been corrected.

An increase in heparin dose during haemodialysis is frequently required during the course of therapy with epoetin alfa as a result of the increased packed cell volume. Occlusion of the dialysis system is possible if heparinisation is not optimum.

Based on information available to date, correction of anaemia with epoetin alfa in adult patients with renal insufficiency not yet undergoing dialysis does not accelerate the rate of progression of renal insufficiency.

Treatment of patients with chemotherapy induced anaemia:

Epoetins are growth factors that primarily stimulate red blood cell production. Erythropoietin receptors may be expressed on the surface of a variety of tumour cells. As with all growth factors, there is a concern that epoetins could stimulate the growth of tumours. In several controlled studies, epoetins have not been shown to improve overall survival or decrease the risk of tumour progression in patients with anaemia associated with cancer.

In controlled clinical studies, use of EPREX and other ESAs have shown:

- decreased locoregional control in patients with advanced head and neck cancer receiving radiation therapy when administered to target a haemoglobin of greater than 14 g/dl (8.7 mmol/l),
- shortened overall survival and increased deaths attributed to disease progression at 4 months in patients with metastatic breast cancer receiving chemotherapy when administered to target a haemoglobin of 12-14 g/dl (7.5-8.7 mmol/l),
- increased risk of death when administered to target a haemoglobin of 12 g/dl (7.5 mmol/l) in patients with active malignant disease receiving neither chemotherapy nor radiation therapy. ESAs are not indicated for use in this patient population.

In view of the above, in some clinical situations blood transfusion should be the preferred treatment for the management of anaemia in patients with cancer. The decision to administer recombinant erythropoietin treatment should be based on a benefit-risk assessment with the participation of the individual patient, which should take into account the specific clinical context. Factors that should be considered in this assessment should include the type of tumour and its stage; the degree of anaemia; life-expectancy; the environment in which the patient is being treated; and patient preference (see section 5.1).

In cancer patients receiving chemotherapy, the 2-3 week delay between ESA administration and the appearance of erythropoietin-induced red cells should be taken into account when assessing if epoetin alfa therapy is appropriate (patient at risk of being transfused).

As an increased incidence of thrombotic vascular events (TVEs) has been observed in cancer patients receiving ESAs (see section 4.8), this risk should be carefully weighed against the benefit to be derived from treatment with epoetin alfa particularly in cancer patients with an increased risk of thrombotic vascular events, such as obesity and patients with a prior history of TVEs (e.g. deep venous thrombosis or pulmonary embolism). An investigational study (BEST study) in women with metastatic breast cancer was designed to determine whether epoetin alfa treatment that extended beyond the correction of anaemia could improve treatment outcomes. In that study the incidence of fatal thromboembolic events was higher in patients receiving epoetin alfa than in those receiving placebo.

Surgery patients in autologous predonation programmes

All special warnings and special precautions associated with autologous predonation programmes, especially routine volume replacement, should be respected.

Patients scheduled for major elective orthopaedic surgery

In patients scheduled for major elective orthopaedic surgery the cause of anaemia should be established and treated, if possible, before the start of epoetin alfa treatment. Thrombotic events can be a risk in this population and this possibility should be carefully weighed against the benefit to be derived from the treatment in this patient group.

Patients scheduled for major elective orthopaedic surgery should receive adequate antithrombotic prophylaxis, as thrombotic and vascular events may occur in surgical patients, especially in those with underlying cardiovascular disease. In addition, special precaution should be taken in patients with predisposition for development of DVTs. Moreover, in patients with a baseline haemoglobin of >13 g/dl, the possibility that epoetin alfa treatment may be associated with an increased risk of postoperative thrombotic/vascular events cannot be excluded. Therefore, it should not be used in patients with baseline haemoglobin >13 g/dl.

This medicinal product contains less than 1 mmol sodium (23 mg) per dose i.e. essentially "sodium free".

4.5 Interaction with other medicinal products and other forms of interaction

No evidence exists that indicates that treatment with epoetin alfa alters the metabolism of other drugs. However, since cyclosporin is bound by RBCs there is potential for a drug interaction. If epoetin alfa is given concomitantly with cyclosporin, blood levels of cyclosporin should be monitored and the dose of cyclosporin adjusted as the haematocrit rises.

No evidence exists that indicates an interaction between epoetin alfa and G-CSF or GM-CSF with regard to haematological differentiation or proliferation of tumour biopsy specimens in vitro.

4.6 Pregnancy and lactation

There are no adequate and well-controlled studies in pregnant women. Studies in animals have shown reproduction toxicology (see section 5.3). Consequently:

- In chronic renal failure patients, epoetin alfa should be used in pregnancy only if the potential benefit outweighs the potential risk to the foetus.
- In pregnant or lactating surgical patients participating in an autologous blood predonation programme, the use of epoetin alfa is not recommended.

It is not known whether exogenous epoetin alfa is excreted in human milk. Epoetin alfa should be used with caution in nursing women. A decision on whether to continue/discontinue breast-feeding or to continue/discontinue therapy with epoetin alfa should be made taking into account the benefit of breast-feeding to the child and the benefit of epoetin alfa therapy to the woman.

4.7 Effects on ability to drive and use machines

None.

4.8 Undesirable effects

General

In cancer patients and in chronic renal failure patients the most frequent adverse drug reaction during treatment with epoetin alfa is a dose-dependent increase in blood pressure or aggravation of existing hypertension. Monitoring of the blood pressure should be performed, particularly at the start of therapy (see section 4.4). Other common adverse drug reactions observed in clinical trials of epoetin alfa are deep vein thrombosis, pulmonary embolism, seizures, diarrhoea, nausea, headache, influenza-like illness, pyrexia, rash, and vomiting. Influenza-like illness including headaches, arthralgia, myalgia, and pyrexia may occur especially at the start of treatment. Frequencies may vary depending on the indication (see table below).

Serious adverse drug reactions include venous and arterial thromboses and embolism (including some with fatal outcomes), such as deep venous thrombosis, pulmonary emboli, arterial thrombosis (including myocardial infarction and myocardial ischaemia), retinal thrombosis, and shunt thrombosis (including dialysis equipment). Additionally, cerebrovascular accidents (including cerebral infarction and cerebral haemorrhage) and transient ischaemic attacks have been reported in clinical trials of epoetin alfa.

Aneurysms have been reported.

Hypersensitivity reactions, including cases of rash, urticaria, anaphylactic reaction, and angioneurotic oedema have been reported.

Hypertensive crisis with encephalopathy and seizures, requiring the immediate attention of a physician and intensive medical care, have occurred also during epoetin alfa treatment in patients with previously normal or low blood pressure. Particular attention should be paid to sudden stabbing migraine-like headaches as a possible warning signal.

Antibody-mediated pure red cell aplasia has been very rarely reported in < 1/10,000 cases per patient year after months to years of treatment with EPREX (see section 4.4).

The overall safety profile of EPREX was evaluated in 142 subjects with chronic renal failure and in 765 subjects with cancer who participated in placebo-controlled, double-blind clinical registration trials. Adverse drug reactions reported by ≥0.2% of EPREX -treated subjects from these trials, additional clinical trials and from post-marketing experience are listed below by system organ class and frequency.

Frequencies are defined as: Very common (≥1/10); common (≥1/100, <1/10); uncommon (≥1/1,000, <1/100); rare (≥1/10,000, <1/1,000); very rare (<1/10,000). A frequency is defined as not known if the adverse drug reaction was not reported in the placebo-controlled, double-blind clinical registration trials or when the frequency cannot be estimated from other available data.

Within each frequency grouping, adverse drug reactions are presented in order of decreasing seriousness.

System Organ Class	Frequency	Adverse Drug Reaction
Blood & Lymphatic System Disorders	Uncommon	Thrombocythaemia (cancer patients)
	Frequency not known	Erythropoeitin antibody-mediated pure red cell aplasia[1] Thrombocythaemia (chronic renal failure patients)
Immune System Disorders	Frequency not known	Anaphylactic reaction Hypersensitivity
Nervous System Disorders	Very common	Headache (cancer patients)
	Common	Seizures (chronic renal failure patients) Headache (chronic renal failure patients)
	Uncommon	Cerebral haemorrhage[2] Seizures (cancer patients)
	Frequency not known	Cerebrovascular accident[2] Hypertensive encephalopathy Transient ischaemic attacks
Eye Disorders	Frequency not known	Retinal thrombosis
Vascular Disorders	Common	Deep vein thrombosis[2] (cancer patients) Hypertension
	Frequency not known	Deep vein thrombosis[2] (chronic renal failure patients) Arterial thrombosis Hypertensive crisis

Respiratory, Thoracic, and Mediastinal Disorders	Common	Pulmonary embolism[2] (cancer patients)
	Frequency not known	Pulmonary embolism[2] (chronic renal failure patients)
Gastrointestinal Disorders	Very common	Nausea
	Common	Diarrhoea (cancer patients) Vomiting
	Uncommon	Diarrhoea (chronic renal failure patients)
Skin and Subcutaneous Tissue Disorders	Common	Rash
	Frequency not known	Angioneurotic oedema Urticaria
Musculoskeletal, Connective Tissue, and Bone Disorders	Very common	Arthralgia (chronic renal failure patients)
	Common	Arthralgia (cancer patients)
	Uncommon	Myalgia (cancer patients)
	Frequency not known	Myalgia (chronic renal failure patients)
Congenital and Familial/Genetic Disorders	Frequency not known	Porphyria
General Disorders and Administration Site Conditions	Very common	Pyrexia (cancer patients) Influenza-like illness (chronic renal failure patients)
	Common	Influenza-like illness (cancer patients)
	Frequency not known	Drug ineffective Peripheral oedema Pyrexia (chronic renal failure patients) Injection site reaction
Investigations	Frequency not known	Anti-erythropoietin antibody positive[1]
Injury, Poisoning, and Procedural Complications	Common	Shunt thromboses including dialysis equipment (chronic renal failure patients)

[1] The frequency cannot be estimated from clinical trials

[2] Including cases with a fatal outcome.

Chronic renal failure patients

In chronic renal failure patients, haemoglobin levels greater than 12 g/dl may be associated with a higher risk of cardiovascular events, including death (see section 4.4).

Shunt thromboses have occurred in haemodialysis patients, especially in those who have a tendency to hypotension or whose arteriovenous fistulae exhibit complications (e.g. stenoses, aneurysms, etc) (see section 4.4).

Cancer patients

An increased incidence of thromboembolic events has been reported in cancer patients receiving ESAs, including epoetin alfa (see section 4.4).

Surgery patients

In patients scheduled for major elective orthopaedic surgery, with a baseline haemoglobin of 10 to 13 g/dl, the incidence of thrombotic/vascular events (most of which were deep vein thrombosis) in the overall patient population of the clinical trials appeared to be similar across the different epoetin alfa dosing groups and placebo group, although the clinical experience is limited.

Moreover, in patients with a baseline haemoglobin of >13 g/dl, the possibility that epoetin alfa treatment may be associated with an increased risk of postoperative thrombotic/vascular events cannot be excluded.

4.9 Overdose

The therapeutic margin of epoetin alfa is very wide. Overdosage of epoetin alfa may produce effects that are extensions of the pharmacological effects of the hormone. Phlebotomy may be performed if excessively high haemoglobin levels occur. Additional supportive care should be provided as necessary.

5. PHARMACOLOGICAL PROPERTIES

5.1 Pharmacodynamic properties

ATC Classification: B03XA01

Erythropoietin is a glycoprotein that stimulates, as a mitosis-stimulating factor and differentiating hormone, the formation of erythrocytes from precursors of the stem cell compartment.

The apparent molecular weight of erythropoietin is 32,000 to 40,000 dalton. The protein fraction of the molecule contributes about 58% and consists of 165 amino acids. The four carbohydrate chains are attached via three N-glycosidic bonds and one O-glycosidic bond to the protein. Epoetin alfa obtained by gene technology is glycosylated and is identical in its amino acid and carbohydrate composition to endogenous human erythropoietin that has been isolated from the urine of anaemic patients.

Epoetin alfa has the highest possible purity according to the present state of the art. In particular, no residues of the cell line used for the production are detectable at the concentrations of the active ingredient that are used in humans.

The biological efficacy of epoetin alfa has been demonstrated in various animal models in vivo (normal and anaemic rats, polycythaemic mice). After administration of epoetin alfa, the number of erythrocytes, the Hb values and reticulocyte counts increase as well as the 59Fe-incorporation rate.

An increased 3H-thymidine incorporation in the erythroid nucleated spleen cells has been found in vitro (mouse spleen cell culture) after incubation with epoetin alfa.

It could be shown with the aid of cell cultures of human bone marrow cells that epoetin alfa stimulates erythropoiesis specifically and does not affect leucopoiesis. Cytotoxic actions of epoetin alfa on bone marrow cells could not be detected.

721 cancer patients receiving non-platinum chemotherapy were included in three placebo-controlled studies, 389 patients with haematological malignancies (221 multiple myeloma, 144 non-Hodgkin's lymphoma and 24 other haematological malignancies) and 332 with solid tumours (172 breast, 64 gynaecological, 23 lung, 22 prostate, 21 gastrointestinal, and 30 other tumour types). In two large, open-label studies, 2697 cancer patients receiving non-platinum chemotherapy were included, 1895 with solid tumours (683 breast, 260 lung, 174 gynaecological, 300 gastrointestinal, and 478 other tumour types) and 802 with haematological malignancies.

In a prospective, randomised, double-blind, placebo-controlled trial conducted in 375 anaemic patients with various non-myeloid malignancies receiving non-platinum chemotherapy, there was a significant reduction of anaemia-related sequelae (e.g. fatigue, decreased energy, and activity reduction), as measured by the following instruments and scales: Functional Assessment of Cancer Therapy-Anaemia (FACT-An) general scale, FACT-An fatigue scale, and Cancer Linear Analogue Scale (CLAS). Two other smaller, randomised, placebo-controlled trials failed to show a significant improvement in quality of life parameters on the EORTC-QLQ-C30 scale or CLAS, respectively.

Erythropoietin is a growth factor that primarily stimulates red cell production. Erythropoietin receptors may be expressed on the surface of a variety of tumour cells.

Survival and tumour progression have been examined in five large controlled studies involving a total of 2833 patients, of which four were double-blind placebo-controlled studies and one was an open-label study. The studies either recruited patients who were being treated with chemotherapy (two studies) or used patient populations in which ESAs are not indicated: anaemia in patients with cancer not receiving chemotherapy, and head and neck cancer patients receiving radiotherapy. The target haemoglobin concentration in two studies was >13 g/dl; in the remaining three studies it was 12-14 g/dl. In the open-label study there was no difference in overall survival between patients treated with recombinant human erythropoietin and controls. In the four placebo-controlled studies the hazard ratios for overall survival ranged between 1.25 and 2.47 in favour of controls. These studies have shown a consistent unexplained statistically significant excess mortality in patients who have anaemia associated with various common cancers who received recombinant human erythropoietin compared to controls. Overall survival outcome in the trials could not be satisfactorily explained by differences in the incidence of thrombosis and related complications between those given recombinant human erythropoietin and those in the control group.

A systematic review has also been performed involving more than 9000 cancer patients participating in 57 clinical trials. Meta-analysis of overall survival data produced a hazard ratio point estimate of 1.08 in favour of controls (95% CI: 0.99, 1.18; 42 trials and 8167 patients). An increased relative risk of thromboembolic events (RR 1.67, 95% CI: 1.35, 2.06, 35 trials and 6769 patients) was observed in patients treated with recombinant human erythropoietin. There is an increased risk for thromboembolic events in patients with cancer treated with recombinant human erythropoietin and a negative overall impact on survival cannot be excluded. The extent to which these outcomes might apply to the administration of recombinant human erythropoietin to patients with cancer, treated with chemotherapy to achieve haemoglobin concentrations less than 13 g/dl, is unclear because few patients with these characteristics were included in the data reviewed.

5.2 Pharmacokinetic properties

I.V. route

Measurement of epoetin alfa following multiple dose intravenous administration revealed a half-life of approximately 4 hours in normal volunteers and a somewhat more prolonged half-life in renal failure patients, approximately 5 hours. A half-life of approximately 6 hours has been reported in children.

S.C. route

Following subcutaneous injection, serum levels of epoetin alfa are much lower than the levels achieved following i.v. injection, the levels increase slowly and reach a peak between 12 and 18 hours postdose. The peak is always well below the peak achieved using the i.v. route (approximately 1/20th of the value).

There is no accumulation: the levels remain the same, whether they are determined 24 hours after the first injection or 24 hours after the last injection.

The half-life is difficult to evaluate for the subcutaneous route and is estimated about 24 hours.

The bioavailability of subcutaneous injectable epoetin alfa is much lower than that of the intravenous drug: approximately 20%.

5.3 Preclinical safety data

In some pre-clinical toxicological studies in dogs and rats, but not in monkeys, epoetin alfa therapy was associated with subclinical bone marrow fibrosis (bone marrow fibrosis is a known complication of chronic renal failure in humans and may be related to secondary hyperparathyroidism or unknown factors. The incidence of bone marrow fibrosis was not increased in a study of haemodialysis patients who were treated with epoetin alfa for 3 years compared to a matched control group of dialysis patients who had not been treated with epoetin alfa).

In animal studies, epoetin alfa has been shown to decrease foetal body weight, delay ossification and increase foetal mortality when given in weekly doses of approximately 20 times the recommended human weekly dose. These changes are interpreted as being secondary to decreased maternal body weight gain.

Epoetin alfa did not show any changes in bacterial and mammalian cell culture mutagenicity tests and an in vivo micronucleus test in mice.

Long-term carcinogenicity studies have not been carried out. There are conflicting reports in the literature regarding whether erythropoietins may play a role as tumour proliferators. These reports are based on in vitro findings from human tumour samples, but are of uncertain significance in the clinical situation.

6. PHARMACEUTICAL PARTICULARS

6.1 List of excipients

Polysorbate 80

Glycine

Water for injections

Excipients known to have a recognised action or effect (present in this product at <1 mmol):

Sodium dihydrogen phosphate dihydrate

Disodium phosphate dihydrate

Sodium chloride

6.2 Incompatibilities

In the absence of compatibility studies, this medicinal product must not be mixed with other medicinal products.

6.3 Shelf life

18 months.

6.4 Special precautions for storage

Store in a refrigerator (2°C-8°C). This temperature range should be closely maintained until administration to the patient. Store in the original package in order to protect from light. Do not freeze or shake.

For the purpose of ambulatory use, the patient may remove EPREX from the refrigerator and store it not above 25°C for one single period of up to 3 days.

6.5 Nature and contents of container

0.5 ml (1000 IU) of solution for injection in a pre-filled syringe (type I glass) with plunger (Teflon-faced rubber) and needle with a needle shield (rubber with polypropylene cover) and a needle safety device (copolyester and polycarbonate) attached to the syringe – pack size of 6.

0.5 ml (2000 IU) of solution for injection in a pre-filled syringe (type I glass) with plunger (Teflon-faced rubber) and needle with a needle shield (rubber with polypropylene cover) and a needle safety device (copolyester and polycarbonate) attached to the syringe - pack size of 6.

0.3 ml (3000 IU) of solution for injection in a pre-filled syringe (type I glass) with plunger (Teflon-faced rubber) and needle with a needle shield (rubber with polypropylene cover) and a needle safety device (copolyester and polycarbonate) attached to the syringe - pack size of 6.

0.4 ml (4000 IU) of solution for injection in a pre-filled syringe (type I glass) with plunger (Teflon-faced rubber) and needle with a needle shield (rubber with polypropylene cover) and a needle safety device (copolyester and polycarbonate) attached to the syringe - pack size of 6.

0.5 ml (5000 IU) of solution for injection in a pre-filled syringe (type I glass) with plunger (Teflon-faced rubber) and needle with a needle shield (rubber with polypropylene cover) and a needle safety device (copolyester and polycarbonate) attached to the syringe - pack size of 6.

0.6 ml (6000 IU) of solution for injection in a pre-filled syringe (type I glass) with plunger (Teflon-faced rubber) and needle with a needle shield (rubber with polypropylene cover) and a needle safety device (copolyester and polycarbonate) attached to the syringe - pack size of 6.

0.8 ml (8000 IU) of solution for injection in a pre-filled syringe (type I glass) with plunger (Teflon-faced rubber) and needle with a needle shield (rubber with polypropylene cover) and a needle safety device (copolyester and polycarbonate) attached to the syringe - pack size of 6.

1.0 ml (10,000 IU) of solution for injection in a pre-filled syringe (type I glass) with plunger (Teflon-faced rubber) and needle with a needle shield (rubber with polypropylene cover) and a needle safety device (copolyester and polycarbonate) attached to the syringe - pack size of 6

6.6 Special precautions for disposal and other handling

Do not administer by intravenous infusion or in conjunction with other drug solutions.

Before use, leave the EPREX syringe to stand until it reaches room temperature. This usually takes between 15 and 30 minutes.

The product should not be used, and discarded

- if the seal is broken,
- if the liquid is coloured or you can see particles floating in it,
- if you know, or think that it may have been accidentally frozen, or
- if there has been a refrigerator failure.

The product is for single use only. Only take one dose of EPREX from each syringe removing unwanted solution before injection. Refer to section 3. How to use EPREX (instructions on how to inject EPREX) of the package leaflet.

The pre-filled syringes are fitted with a needle safety device to help prevent needle stick injuries after use. The package leaflet includes full instructions for the use and handling of pre-filled syringes.

Any unused product or waste material should be disposed of in accordance with local requirements.

7. MARKETING AUTHORISATION HOLDER

Janssen-Cilag Ltd

50-100 Holmers Farm Way

High Wycombe

Buckinghamshire

HP12 4EG

UK

8. MARKETING AUTHORISATION NUMBER(S)

PL 0242/0297

PL 0242/0298

PL 0242/0299

9. DATE OF FIRST AUTHORISATION/RENEWAL OF THE AUTHORISATION

Renewal of Authorisation: 04 August 2008

10. DATE OF REVISION OF THE TEXT

29th April 2009

Eprex 40,000 IU/ml solution for injection in pre-filled syringe

(Janssen-Cilag Ltd)

1. NAME OF THE MEDICINAL PRODUCT

EPREX 40,000 IU/ml, solution for injection in pre-filled syringe.

2. QUALITATIVE AND QUANTITATIVE COMPOSITION

Epoetin alfa* ....40,000 IU/ml (336.0 micrograms per ml)

A pre-filled syringe of 0.5 ml contains 20 000 IU (168.0 micrograms) of epoetin alfa

A pre-filled syringe of 0.75 ml contains 30 000 IU (252.0 micrograms) of epoetin alfa

A pre-filled syringe of 1.0 ml contains 40,000 IU (336.0 micrograms) of epoetin alfa

*produced in Chinese Hamster Ovary cells by recombinant DNA technology.

For a full list of excipients, see section 6.1.

3. PHARMACEUTICAL FORM

Solution for injection in pre-filled syringe.

Clear, colourless solution.

4. CLINICAL PARTICULARS

4.1 Therapeutic indications

Treatment of anaemia and reduction of transfusion requirements in adult patients receiving chemotherapy for solid tumours, malignant lymphoma or multiple myeloma, and at risk of transfusion as assessed by the patient's general status (e.g. cardiovascular status, pre-existing anaemia at the start of chemotherapy).

Figure 1

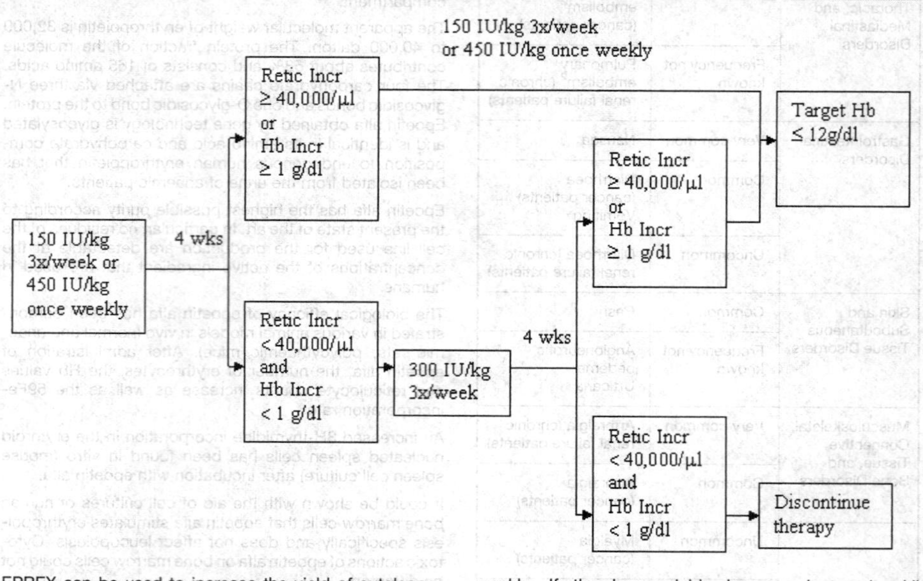

EPREX can be used to increase the yield of autologous blood from patients in a predonation programme. Its use in this indication must be balanced against the reported risk of thromboembolic events. Treatment should only be given to patients with moderate anaemia (Hb 10-13 g/dl [6.2-8.1 mmol/l], no iron deficiency) if blood saving procedures are not available or insufficient when the scheduled major elective surgery requires a large volume of blood (4 or more units of blood for females or 5 or more units for males).

EPREX can be used to reduce exposure to allogeneic blood transfusions in adult non-iron deficient patients prior to major elective orthopaedic surgery, having a high perceived risk for transfusion complications. Use should be restricted to patients with moderate anaemia (e.g. Hb 10-13 g/dl) who do not have an autologous predonation programmeme available and with expected moderate blood loss (900 to 1800 ml).

Good blood management practices should always be used in the perisurgical setting.

4.2 Posology and method of administration

Method of administration

As with any other injectable product, check that there are no particles in the solution or change in colour.

a) intravenous injection: over at least one to five minutes, depending on the total dose.

A slower injection is preferable in patients who react to the treatment with "flu-like" symptoms.

Do not administer by intravenous infusion or mixed with other drugs.

b) subcutaneous injection: a maximum volume of 1 ml at one injection site should generally not be exceeded. In case of larger volumes, more than one site should be chosen for the injection.

The injections are given in the limbs or the anterior abdominal wall.

In those situations in which the physician determines that a patient or caregiver can safely and effectively administer EPREX subcutaneously, instruction as to the proper dosage and administration should be provided.

Refer to section 3. How to use EPREX (instructions on how to inject EPREX) of the package leaflet.

Treatment of patients with chemotherapy induced anaemia:

EPREX should be administered by the subcutaneous route to patients with anaemia (e.g. haemoglobin concentration ⩽ 10g/dl (6.2 mmol/l)). Anaemia symptoms and sequelae may vary with age, gender, and overall burden of disease; a physician's evaluation of the individual patient's clinical course and condition is necessary.

Due to intra-patient variability, occasional individual haemoglobin values for a patient above and below the desired haemoglobin level may be observed. Haemoglobin variability should be addressed through dose management, with consideration for the haemoglobin target range of 10g/dl (6.2 mmol/l) to 12g/dl (7.5mmol/l). A sustained haemoglobin level of greater than 12g/dl (7.5mmol/l) should be avoided; guidance for appropriate dose adjustment for when haemoglobin values exceed 12g/dl (7.5mmol/l) are described below.

Epoetin alfa therapy should continue until one month after the end of chemotherapy.

The initial dose is 150 IU/kg given subcutaneously 3 times per week. Alternatively, EPREX can be administered at an initial dose of 450 IU/kg subcutaneously once weekly. If the haemoglobin has increased by at least 1 g/dl (0.62 mmol/l) or the reticulocyte count has increased ⩾ 40,000 cells/µl above baseline after 4 weeks of treatment, the dose should remain at 150 IU/kg 3 times per week or 450 IU/kg once weekly. If the haemoglobin increase is < 1 g/dl (< 0.62 mmol/l) and the reticulocyte count has increased < 40,000 cells/µl above baseline, increase the dose to 300 IU/kg 3 times per week. If after an additional 4 weeks of therapy at 300 IU/kg 3 times per week, the haemoglobin has increased ⩾ 1 g/dl (⩾ 0.62 mmol/l) or the reticulocyte count has increased ⩾ 40,000 cells/µl, the dose should remain at 300 IU/kg 3 times per week. However, if the haemoglobin has increased < 1 g/dl (< 0.62 mmol/l) and the reticulocyte count has increased < 40,000 cells/µl above baseline, response is unlikely and treatment should be discontinued. The recommended dosing regimen is described in the following diagram:

(see Figure 1 above)

Patients should be monitored closely to ensure that the lowest approved dose of erythropoiesis-stimulating agent (ESA) is used to provide adequate control of the symptoms of anaemia.

Dose adjustment to maintain haemoglobin concentrations between 10g/dl – 12 g/dl:

If the haemoglobin is rising by more than 2 g/dl (1.25 mmol/l) per month, or if the haemoglobin exceeds 12 g/dl (7.5 mmol/l), reduce the epoetin alfa dose by about 25 - 50%. If the haemoglobin exceeds 13 g/dl (8.1 mmol/l), discontinue therapy until it falls below 12 g/dl (7.5 mmol/l) and then reinstitute epoetin alfa therapy at a dose 25% below the previous dose.

Adult surgery patients in an autologous predonation programme:

The intravenous route of administration should be used. At the time of donating blood, epoetin alfa should be administered after the completion of the blood donation procedure.

Mildly anaemic patients (haematocrit of 33-39%) requiring predeposit of ⩾ 4 units of blood should be treated with epoetin alfa at 600 IU/kg, 2 times weekly for 3 weeks prior to surgery. Using this regimen, it was possible to withdraw ⩾ 4 units of blood from 81% of epoetin alfa-treated patients compared to 37% of placebo-treated patients. Epoetin alfa therapy reduced the risk of exposure to homologous blood by 50% compared to patients not receiving epoetin alfa.

All patients being treated with epoetin alfa should receive adequate iron supplementation (e.g. 200 mg oral elemental iron daily) throughout the course of epoetin alfa treatment. Iron supplementation should be started as soon as possible, even several weeks prior to initiating the autologous predeposit, in order to achieve high iron stores prior to starting epoetin alfa therapy.

Adult patients scheduled for major elective orthopaedic surgery:

The subcutaneous route of administration should be used. The recommended dose regimen is 600 IU/kg of epoetin alfa, given weekly for three weeks (days -21, -14 and -7) prior to surgery and on the day of surgery. In cases where there is a medical need to shorten the lead time before surgery to less than three weeks, 300 IU/kg epoetin alfa should be given daily for 10 consecutive days prior to surgery, on the day of surgery and for four days immediately thereafter. When performing haematologic assessments during the preoperative period, if the haemoglobin level reaches 15 g/dl, or higher, administration of epoetin alfa should be stopped and further dosages should not be given.

Care should be taken to ensure that at the outset of the treatment patients are not iron deficient. All patients being treated with epoetin alfa should receive adequate iron supplementation (e.g. 200 mg oral elemental iron daily) throughout the course of epoetin alfa treatment. If possible, iron supplementation should be started prior to epoetin alfa therapy, to achieve adequate iron stores.

4.3 Contraindications

Patients who develop pure red cell aplasia (PRCA) following treatment with any erythropoietin should not receive EPREX or any other erythropoietin (see Section 4.4 - Pure Red Cell Aplasia).

Uncontrolled hypertension.

All contraindications associated with autologous blood predonation programmes should be respected in patients being supplemented with epoetin alfa.

Hypersensitivity to the active substance or to any of the excipients.

The use of epoetin alfa in patients scheduled for major elective orthopaedic surgery and not participating in an autologous blood predonation programme is contraindicated in patients with severe coronary, peripheral arterial, carotid or cerebral vascular disease, including patients with recent myocardial infarction or cerebral vascular accident.

Surgery patients who for any reason cannot receive adequate antithrombotic prophylaxis.

4.4 Special warnings and precautions for use

General

In all patients receiving epoetin alfa, blood pressure should be closely monitored and controlled as necessary. Epoetin alfa should be used with caution in the presence of untreated, inadequately treated or poorly controllable hypertension. It may be necessary to add or increase anti-hypertensive treatment. If blood pressure cannot be controlled, epoetin alfa treatment should be discontinued.

Epoetin alfa should also be used with caution in the presence of epilepsy and chronic liver failure.

Chronic renal failure and cancer patients on epoetin alfa should have haemoglobin levels measured on a regular basis until a stable level is achieved, and periodically thereafter.

In all patients, haemoglobin levels should be closely monitored due to a potential increased risk of thromboembolic events and fatal outcomes when patients are treated at haemoglobin levels above the target for the indication of use.

There may be a moderate dose-dependent rise in the platelet count within the normal range during treatment with epoetin alfa. This regresses during the course of continued therapy. In addition, thrombocythaemia above the normal range has been reported. It is recommended that the platelet count is regularly monitored during the first 8 weeks of therapy.

All other causes of anaemia (iron deficiency, haemolysis, blood loss, vitamin B12 or folate deficiencies) should be considered and treated prior to initiating therapy with epoetin alfa. In most cases, the ferritin values in the serum fall simultaneously with the rise in packed cell volume. In order to ensure optimum response to epoetin alfa, adequate iron stores should be assured:

- oral iron substitution of 200-300 mg/day is recommended for all cancer patients whose transferrin saturation is below 20%.

All of these additive factors of anaemia should also be carefully considered when deciding to increase the dose of epoetin alfa in cancer patients.

Very rarely, development of or exacerbation of porphyria has been observed in epoetin alfa-treated patients. Epoetin alfa should be used with caution in patients with porphyria.

In order to improve the traceability of the ESA all measures necessary and possible to ensure it should be taken (e.g. exact information on the product used should be documented in an appropriate way). Furthermore, patients should only be switched from one ESA to another under appropriate supervision.

Pure Red Cell Aplasia

Antibody-mediated pure red cell aplasia (PRCA) has been very rarely reported after months to years of subcutaneous epoetin treatment. In patients developing sudden lack of efficacy defined by a decrease in haemoglobin (1 to 2 g/dl per month) with increased need for transfusions, a reticulocyte count should be obtained and typical causes of non-response (e.g. iron, folate or Vitamin B12 deficiency, aluminium intoxication, infection or inflammation, blood loss and haemolysis) should be investigated.

If the reticulocyte count corrected for anaemia (i.e. the reticulocyte 'index') is low (<20,000/mm3 or < 20,000/microlitre or <0.5%), platelet and white blood cell counts are normal, and if no other cause of loss of effect has been found, anti-erythropoietin antibodies should be determined and a bone marrow examination should be considered for diagnosis of PRCA.

If anti-erythropoietin, antibody-mediated PRCA is suspected, therapy with EPREX should be discontinued immediately. No other erythropoietic therapy should be commenced because of the risk of cross-reaction. Appropriate therapy such as blood transfusions may be given to patients when indicated.

Treatment of patients with chemotherapy induced anaemia

Epoetins are growth factors that primarily stimulate red blood cell production. Erythropoietin receptors may be expressed on the surface of a variety of tumour cells. As with all growth factors, there is a concern that epoetins could stimulate the growth of tumours. In several controlled studies, epoetins have not been shown to improve overall survival or decrease the risk of tumour progression in patients with anaemia associated with cancer.

In controlled clinical studies, use of EPREX and other ESAs have shown:

- decreased locoregional control in patients with advanced head and neck cancer receiving radiation therapy when administered to target a haemoglobin of greater than 14 g/dl (8.7 mmol/l),
- shortened overall survival and increased deaths attributed to disease progression at 4 months in patients with metastatic breast cancer receiving chemotherapy when administered to target a haemoglobin of 12-14 g/dl (7.5-8.7 mmol/l),
- increased risk of death when administered to target a haemoglobin of 12 g/dl (7.5 mmol/l) in patients with active malignant disease receiving neither chemotherapy nor radiation therapy. ESAs are not indicated for use in this patient population.

In view of the above, in some clinical situations blood transfusion should be the preferred treatment for the management of anaemia in patients with cancer. The decision to administer recombinant erythropoietin treatment should be based on a benefit-risk assessment with the participation of the individual patient, which should take into account the specific clinical context. Factors that should be considered in this assessment should include the type of tumour and its stage; the degree of anaemia; life-expectancy; the environment in which the patient is being treated; and patient preference (see section 5.1).

In cancer patients receiving chemotherapy, the 2-3 week delay between ESA administration and the appearance of erythropoietin-induced red cells should be taken into account when assessing if epoetin alfa therapy is appropriate (patient at risk of being transfused).

As an increased incidence of thrombotic vascular events (TVEs) has been observed in cancer patients receiving ESAs (see section 4.8), this risk should be carefully weighed against the benefit to be derived from treatment with epoetin alfa particularly in cancer patients with an increased risk of thrombotic vascular events, such as obesity and patients with a prior history of TVEs (e.g. deep venous thrombosis or pulmonary embolism). An investigational study (BEST study) in women with metastatic breast cancer was designed to determine whether epoetin alfa treatment that extended beyond the correction of anaemia could improve treatment outcomes. In that study the incidence of fatal thromboembolic events was higher in patients receiving epoetin alfa than in those receiving placebo.

Surgery patients in autologous predonation programmes

All special warnings and special precautions associated with autologous predonation programmes, especially routine volume replacement, should be respected.

Patients scheduled for major elective orthopaedic surgery

In patients scheduled for major elective orthopaedic surgery the cause of anaemia should be established and treated, if possible, before the start of epoetin alfa treatment. Thrombotic events can be a risk in this population and this possibility should be carefully weighed against the benefit to be derived from the treatment in this patient group. Patients scheduled for major elective orthopaedic surgery should receive adequate antithrombotic prophylaxis, as thrombotic and vascular events may occur in surgical patients, especially in those with underlying cardiovascular disease. In addition, special precaution should be taken in patients with predisposition for development of deep vein thrombosis (DVTs). Moreover, in patients with a baseline haemoglobin of >13 g/dl, the possibility that epoetin alfa treatment may be associated with an increased risk of postoperative thrombotic/vascular events cannot be excluded. Therefore, it should not be used in patients with baseline haemoglobin >13 g/dl.

Chronic renal failure patients

Chronic renal failure patients treated with EPREX by the subcutaneous route should be monitored regularly for loss of efficacy, defined as absent or decreased response to EPREX treatment in patients who previously responded to such therapy. This is characterised by a sustained decrease in haemoglobin despite an increase in EPREX dosage.

This medicinal product contains less than 1 mmol sodium (23 mg) per dose i.e. essentially "sodium free".

4.5 Interaction with other medicinal products and other forms of interaction

No evidence exists that indicates that treatment with epoetin alfa alters the metabolism of other drugs. However, since cyclosporin is bound by RBCs there is potential for a drug interaction. If epoetin alfa is given concomitantly with cyclosporin, blood levels of cyclosporin should be monitored and the dose of cyclosporin adjusted as the haematocrit rises.

No evidence exists that indicates an interaction between epoetin alfa and G-CSF or GM-CSF with regard to haematological differentiation or proliferation of tumour biopsy specimens in vitro.

4.6 Pregnancy and lactation

There are no adequate and well-controlled studies in pregnant women. Studies in animals have shown reproduction toxicology (see section 5.3). Consequently, in pregnant or lactating surgical patients participating in an autologous blood predonation programme, the use of epoetin alfa is not recommended.

It is not known whether exogenous epoetin alfa is excreted in human milk. Epoetin alfa should be used with caution in nursing women. A decision on whether to continue/discontinue breast-feeding or to continue/discontinue therapy with epoetin alfa should be made taking into account the benefit of breast-feeding to the child and the benefit of epoetin alfa therapy to the woman.

4.7 Effects on ability to drive and use machines

None.

4.8 Undesirable effects

General

In cancer patients and in chronic renal failure patients the most frequent adverse drug reaction during treatment with epoetin alfa is a dose-dependent increase in blood pressure or aggravation of existing hypertension. Monitoring of the blood pressure should be performed, particularly at the start of therapy (see section 4.4). Other common adverse drug reactions observed in clinical trials of epoetin alfa are deep vein thrombosis, pulmonary embolism, seizures, diarrhoea, nausea, headache, influenza-like illness, pyrexia, rash, and vomiting. Influenza-like illness including headaches, arthralgia, myalgia, and pyrexia may occur especially at the start of treatment. Frequencies may vary depending on the indication (see table below).

Serious adverse drug reactions include venous and arterial thromboses and embolism (including some with fatal outcomes), such as deep venous thrombosis, pulmonary emboli, arterial thrombosis (including myocardial infarction and myocardial ischaemia), retinal thrombosis, and shunt thrombosis (including dialysis equipment). Additionally, cerebrovascular accidents (including cerebral infarction and cerebral haemorrhage) and transient ischaemic attacks have been reported in clinical trials of epoetin alfa.

Aneurysms have been reported.

Hypersensitivity reactions, including cases of rash, urticaria, anaphylactic reaction, and angioneurotic oedema have been reported.

Hypertensive crisis with encephalopathy and seizures, requiring the immediate attention of a physician and intensive medical care, have occurred also during epoetin alfa treatment in patients with previously normal or low blood pressure. Particular attention should be paid to sudden stabbing migraine-like headaches as a possible warning signal.

Antibody-mediated pure red cell aplasia has been very rarely reported in < 1/10,000 cases per patient year after months to years of treatment with EPREX (see section 4.4).

The overall safety profile of EPREX was evaluated in 142 subjects with chronic renal failure and in 765 subjects with cancer who participated in placebo-controlled, double-blind clinical registration trials. Adverse drug reactions reported by ⩾0.2% of EPREX-treated subjects from these trials, additional clinical trials and from post-marketing experience are listed below by system organ class and frequency.

Frequencies are defined as: Very common (⩾1/10); common (⩾1/100, <1/10); uncommon (⩾1/1,000, <1/100); rare (⩾1/10,000, <1/1,000); very rare (<1/10,000). A frequency is defined as not known if the adverse drug reaction was not reported in the placebo-controlled, double-blind clinical registration trials or when the frequency cannot be estimated from other available data.

Within each frequency grouping, adverse drug reactions are presented in order of decreasing seriousness.

System Organ Class	Frequency	Adverse Drug Reaction
Blood & Lymphatic System Disorders	Uncommon	Thrombocythaemia (cancer patients)
	Frequency not known	Erythropoeitin antibody-mediated pure red cell aplasia[1] Thrombocythaemia (chronic renal failure patients)
Immune System Disorders	Frequency not known	Anaphylactic reaction Hypersensitivity
Nervous System Disorders	Very common	Headache (cancer patients)

	Common	Seizures (chronic renal failure patients) Headache (chronic renal failure patients)
	Uncommon	Cerebral haemorrhage[2] Seizures (cancer patients)
	Frequency not known	Cerebrovascular accident[2] Hypertensive encephalopathy Transient ischaemic attacks
Eye Disorders	Frequency not known	Retinal thrombosis
Vascular Disorders	Common	Deep vein thrombosis[2] (cancer patients) Hypertension
	Frequency not known	Deep vein thrombosis[2] (chronic renal failure patients) Arterial thrombosis Hypertensive crisis
Respiratory, Thoracic, and Mediastinal Disorders	Common	Pulmonary embolism[2] (cancer patients)
	Frequency not known	Pulmonary embolism[2] (chronic renal failure patients)
Gastrointestinal Disorders	Very common	Nausea
	Common	Diarrhoea (cancer patients) Vomiting
	Uncommon	Diarrhoea (chronic renal failure patients)
Skin and Subcutaneous Tissue Disorders	Common	Rash
	Frequency not known	Angioneurotic oedema Urticaria
Musculoskeletal, Connective Tissue, and Bone Disorders	Very common	Arthralgia (chronic renal failure patients)
	Common	Arthralgia (cancer patients)
	Uncommon	Myalgia (cancer patients)
	Frequency not known	Myalgia (chronic renal failure patients)
Congenital and Familial/Genetic Disorders	Frequency not known	Porphyria
General Disorders and Administration Site Conditions	Very common	Pyrexia (cancer patients) Influenza-like illness (chronic renal failure patients)
	Common	Influenza-like illness (cancer patients)
	Frequency not known	Drug ineffective Peripheral oedema Pyrexia (chronic renal failure patients) Injection site reaction
Investigations	Frequency not known	Anti-erythropoietin antibody positive[1]
Injury, Poisoning, and Procedural Complications	Common	Shunt thromboses including dialysis equipment (chronic renal failure patients)

[1] The frequency cannot be estimated from clinical trials.

[2] Including cases with a fatal outcome.

Chronic renal failure patients

In chronic renal failure patients, haemoglobin levels greater than 12 g/dl may be associated with a higher risk of cardiovascular events, including death (see section 4.4).

Shunt thromboses have occurred in haemodialysis patients, especially in those who have a tendency to hypotension or whose arteriovenous fistulae exhibit complications (e.g. stenoses, aneurysms, etc).

Cancer patients

An increased incidence of thromboembolic events has been reported in cancer patients receiving ESAs, including epoetin alfa (see section 4.4).

Surgery patients

In patients scheduled for major elective orthopaedic surgery, with a baseline haemoglobin of 10 to 13 g/dl, the incidence of thrombotic/vascular events (most of which were deep vein thrombosis) in the overall patient population of the clinical trials appeared to be similar across the different epoetin alfa dosing groups and placebo group, although the clinical experience is limited.

Moreover, in patients with a baseline haemoglobin of >13 g/dl, the possibility that epoetin alfa treatment may be associated with an increased risk of postoperative thrombotic/vascular events cannot be excluded.

4.9 Overdose

The therapeutic margin of epoetin alfa is very wide. Overdosage of epoetin alfa may produce effects that are extensions of the pharmacological effects of the hormone. Phlebotomy may be performed if excessively high haemoglobin levels occur. Additional supportive care should be provided as necessary.

5. PHARMACOLOGICAL PROPERTIES

5.1 Pharmacodynamic properties

ATC Classification: B03XA01

Erythropoietin is a glycoprotein that stimulates, as a mitosis-stimulating factor and differentiating hormone, the formation of erythrocytes from precursors of the stem cell compartment.

The apparent molecular weight of erythropoietin is 32,000 to 40,000 dalton. The protein fraction of the molecule contributes about 58% and consists of 165 amino acids. The four carbohydrate chains are attached via three N-glycosidic bonds and one O-glycosidic bond to the protein. Epoetin alfa obtained by gene technology is glycosylated and is identical in its amino acid and carbohydrate composition to endogenous human erythropoietin that has been isolated from the urine of anaemic patients.

Epoetin alfa has the highest possible purity according to the present state of the art. In particular, no residues of the cell line used for the production are detectable at the concentrations of the active ingredient that are used in humans.

The biological efficacy of epoetin alfa has been demonstrated in various animal models in vivo (normal and anaemic rats, polycythaemic mice). After administration of epoetin alfa, the number of erythrocytes, the Hb values and reticulocyte counts increase as well as the 59Fe-incorporation rate.

An increased 3H-thymidine incorporation in the erythroid nucleated spleen cells has been found in vitro (mouse spleen cell culture) after incubation with epoetin alfa.

It could be shown with the aid of cell cultures of human bone marrow cells that epoetin alfa stimulates erythropoiesis specifically and does not affect leucopoiesis. Cytotoxic actions of epoetin alfa on bone marrow cells could not be detected.

721 cancer patients receiving non-platinum chemotherapy were included in three placebo-controlled studies, 389 patients with haematological malignancies (221 multiple myeloma, 144 non-Hodgkin's lymphoma and 24 other haematological malignancies) and 332 with solid tumours (172 breast, 64 gynaecological, 23 lung, 22 prostate, 21 gastrointestinal, and 30 other tumour types). In two large, open-label studies, 2697 cancer patients receiving non-platinum chemotherapy were included, 1895 with solid tumours (683 breast, 260 lung, 174 gynaecological, 300 gastrointestinal, and 478 other tumour types) and 802 with haematological malignancies.

In a prospective, randomised, double-blind, placebo-controlled trial conducted in 375 anaemic patients with various non-myeloid malignancies receiving non-platinum chemotherapy, there was a significant reduction of anaemia-related sequelae (e.g. fatigue, decreased energy, and activity reduction), as measured by the following instruments and scales: Functional Assessment of Cancer Therapy-Anaemia (FACT-An) general scale, FACT-An fatigue scale, and Cancer Linear Analogue Scale (CLAS). Two other smaller, randomised, placebo-controlled trials failed to show a significant improvement in quality of life parameters on the EORTC-QLQ-C30 scale or CLAS, respectively.

Erythropoietin is a growth factor that primarily stimulates red cell production. Erythropoietin receptors may be expressed on the surface of a variety of tumour cells.

Survival and tumour progression have been examined in five large controlled studies involving a total of 2833 patients, of which four were double-blind placebo-controlled studies and one was an open-label study. The studies either recruited patients who were being treated with chemotherapy (two studies) or used patient populations in which ESAs are not indicated: anaemia in patients with cancer not receiving chemotherapy, and head and neck cancer patients receiving radiotherapy. The target haemoglobin concentration in two studies was >13 g/dl; in the remaining three studies it was 12-14 g/dl. In the open-label study there was no difference in overall survival between patients treated with recombinant human erythropoietin and controls. In the four placebo-controlled studies the hazard ratios for overall survival ranged between 1.25 and 2.47 in favour of controls. These studies have shown a consistent unexplained statistically significant excess mortality in patients who have anaemia associated with various common cancers who received recombinant human erythropoietin compared to controls. Overall survival outcome in the trials could not be satisfactorily explained by differences in the incidence of thrombosis and related complications between those given recombinant human erythropoietin and those in the control group.

A systematic review has also been performed involving more than 9000 cancer patients participating in 57 clinical trials. Meta-analysis of overall survival data produced a hazard ratio point estimate of 1.08 in favour of controls (95% CI: 0.99, 1.18; 42 trials and 8167 patients). An increased relative risk of thromboembolic events (RR 1.67, 95% CI: 1.35, 2.06, 35 trials and 6769 patients) was observed in patients treated with recombinant human erythropoietin. There is an increased risk for thromboembolic events in patients with cancer treated with recombinant human erythropoietin and a negative overall impact on survival cannot be excluded. The extent to which these outcomes might apply to the administration of recombinant human erythropoietin to patients with cancer, treated with chemotherapy to achieve haemoglobin concentrations less than 13 g/dl, is unclear because few patients with these characteristics were included in the data reviewed.

5.2 Pharmacokinetic properties

I.V. route

Measurement of epoetin alfa following multiple dose intravenous administration revealed a half-life of approximately 4 hours in normal volunteers and a somewhat more prolonged half life in renal failure patients, approximately 5 hours. A half-life of approximately 6 hours has been reported in children.

S.C. route

Following subcutaneous injection, serum levels of epoetin alfa are much lower than the levels achieved following i.v. injection, the levels increase slowly and reach a peak between 12 and 18 hours postdose. The peak is always well below the peak achieved using the i.v. route (approximately 1/20th of the value).

There is no accumulation: the levels remain the same, whether they are determined 24 hours after the first injection or 24 hours after the last injection.

The half-life is difficult to evaluate for the subcutaneous route and is estimated about 24 hours.

The bioavailability of subcutaneous injectable epoetin alfa is much lower than that of the intravenous drug: approximately 20%.

5.3 Preclinical safety data

In some pre-clinical toxicological studies in dogs and rats, but not in monkeys, epoetin alfa therapy was associated with subclinical bone marrow fibrosis (bone marrow fibrosis is a known complication of chronic renal failure in humans and may be related to secondary hyperparathyroidism or unknown factors. The incidence of bone marrow fibrosis was not increased in a study of haemodialysis patients who were treated with epoetin alfa for 3 years compared to a matched control group of dialysis patients who had not been treated with epoetin alfa).

In animal studies, epoetin alfa has been shown to decrease foetal body weight, delay ossification and increase foetal mortality when given in weekly doses of approximately 20 times the recommended human weekly dose. These changes are interpreted as being secondary to decreased maternal body weight gain.

Epoetin alfa did not show any changes in bacterial and mammalian cell culture mutagenicity tests and an in vivo micronucleus test in mice.

Long-term carcinogenicity studies have not been carried out. There are conflicting reports in the literature regarding whether erythropoietins may play a role as tumour proliferators. These reports are based on in vitro findings from human tumour samples, but are of uncertain significance in the clinical situation.

6. PHARMACEUTICAL PARTICULARS

6.1 List of excipients

Polysorbate 80

Glycine

Water for injections

Excipients known to have recognised action or effect (present in this product at < 1 mmol):

Sodium dihydrogen phosphate dihydrate

Disodium phosphate dihydrate

Sodium chloride

6.2 Incompatibilities

In the absence of compatibility studies, this medicinal product must not be mixed with other medicinal products.

6.3 Shelf life

18 months.

6.4 Special precautions for storage
Store in a refrigerator (2°C-8°C). This temperature range should be closely maintained until administration to the patient. Store in the original package in order to protect from light. Do not freeze or shake.

For the purpose of ambulatory use, the patient may remove EPREX from the refrigerator and store it not above 25°C for one single period of up to 3 days.

6.5 Nature and contents of container
0.5 ml (20 000 IU) of solution for injection in a pre-filled syringe (type I glass) with plunger (Teflon-faced rubber) and needle with a needle shield (rubber with polypropylene cover) and a needle safety device (copolyester and polycarbonate) attached to the syringe - pack sizes of 1, 4 or 6.

0.75 ml (30,000 IU) of solution for injection in a pre-filled syringe (type I glass) with plunger (Teflon-faced rubber) and needle with a needle shield (rubber with polypropylene cover) and a needle safety device (copolyester and polycarbonate) attached to the syringe - pack sizes of 1, 4 or 6.

1.0 ml (40,000 IU) of solution for injection in a pre-filled syringe (type I glass) with plunger (Teflon-faced rubber) and needle with a needle shield (rubber with polypropylene cover) and a needle safety device (copolyester and polycarbonate) attached to the syringe - pack sizes of 1, 4 or 6.

6.6 Special precautions for disposal and other handling
Do not administer by intravenous infusion or in conjunction with other drug solutions.

Before use, leave the EPREX syringe to stand until it reaches room temperature. This usually takes between 15 and 30 minutes.

The product should not be used, and discarded

- if the seal is broken,
- if the liquid is coloured or you can see particles floating in it,
- if you know, or think that it may have been accidentally frozen, or
- if there has been a refrigerator failure.

The product is for single use only. Only take one dose of EPREX from each syringe removing unwanted solution before injection. Refer to section 3. How to use EPREX (instructions on how to inject EPREX) of the package leaflet.

The pre-filled syringes are fitted with a needle safety device to help prevent needle stick injuries after use. The package leaflet includes full instructions for the use and handling of pre-filled syringes.

Any unused product or waste material should be disposed of in accordance with local requirements.

7. MARKETING AUTHORISATION HOLDER
Janssen-Cilag Ltd
50-100 Holmers Farm Way
High Wycombe
Buckinghamshire
HP12 4EG
UK

8. MARKETING AUTHORISATION NUMBER(S)
PL 0242/0618

9. DATE OF FIRST AUTHORISATION/RENEWAL OF THE AUTHORISATION
Renewal of Authorisation: 04 August 2008

10. DATE OF REVISION OF THE TEXT
29th April 2009

Equasym 5mg, 10mg and 20mg Tablets

(Shire Pharmaceuticals Limited)

1. NAME OF THE MEDICINAL PRODUCT
Equasym® 5 mg, 10 mg, 20 mg tablets

2. QUALITATIVE AND QUANTITATIVE COMPOSITION
One tablet contains 5 mg, 10 mg, 20 mg of methylphenidate hydrochloride

For excipients, see section 6.1.

3. PHARMACEUTICAL FORM
Tablet.

Tablet with breakline, 'Medeva' and strength embossed on one side.

4. CLINICAL PARTICULARS

4.1 Therapeutic indications
Methylphenidate is indicated as part of a comprehensive treatment programme for attention-deficit hyperactivity disorder (ADHD) in children over 6 years of age when remedial measures alone prove insufficient. The decision to treat as well as follow-up must be under supervision of a specialist in childhood behavioural disorders. Diagnosis should be made according to DSM-IV criteria or the guidelines in ICD-10.

Additional information on the safe use of the product:

ADHD is also known as attention-deficit disorder (ADD).

A comprehensive treatment programme typically includes psychological, educational and social measures and is aimed at stabilising children with a behavioural syndrome characterised by symptoms which may include chronic history of short attention span, distractibility, emotional lability, impulsivity, moderate to severe hyperactivity, minor neurological signs and abnormal EEG. Learning may or may not be impaired.

Methylphenidate treatment is not indicated in all children with this syndrome and the decision to use the drug must be based on a very thorough assessment of the severity of the child's symptoms in relation to the child's age and the persistence of the symptoms.

4.2 Posology and method of administration
Adults: Not applicable.

Elderly: Not applicable

Children: *(less than 6 years of age). Equasym is not indicated in children less than 6 years of age.*

Children: (over 6 years). Begin with 5 mg once or twice daily (e.g. at breakfast and lunch), increasing the dose and frequency of administration if necessary by weekly increments of 5-10 mg in the daily dose. Doses above 60 mg daily are not recommended. The total daily dose should be administered in divided doses.

The last doses should, in general, not be given within 4 hours before bedtime in order to prevent disturbances in falling asleep. However, if the effect of the drug wears off too early in the evening, disturbed behaviour and/or inability to go to sleep may recur. A small evening dose may help to solve this problem. The pros and cons of a small evening dose versus disturbances in falling asleep should be considered.

Note: If improvement of symptoms is not observed after appropriate dosage adjustment over a one-month period, the drug should be discontinued. Methylphenidate should be discontinued periodically to assess the child's condition. Drug treatment is usually discontinued during or after puberty.

4.3 Contraindications
The presence of marked anxiety, agitation or tension is a contra-indication to the use of Equasym as it may aggravate these symptoms. Equasym is also contra-indicated in patients with diagnosis or a family history of motor tics, Tourette's syndrome or other movement disorders.

Methylphenidate is contra-indicated in patients with known drug dependence or history of drug dependence or alcoholism, severe depression, schizophrenic symptoms, anorexia nervosa, psychopathological personality structure, history of aggression, or suicidal tendency.

It is also contra-indicated in patients with severe hypertension, hyperthyroidism, angina pectoris, cardiac arrhythmia, glaucoma, thyrotoxicosis, or known hypersensitivity to the active substance or to any of the excipients.

Methylphenidate is contraindicated in concomitant use, or use within the last two weeks, of MAO inhibitors.

4.4 Special warnings and precautions for use
Warnings: Equasym should not be used in children under 6 years of age, since safety and efficacy in this age group have not been established.

Clinical experience suggests that Equasym may exacerbate symptoms of behavioural disturbance and thought disorder in psychotic children.

Chronic abuse of Equasym can lead to marked tolerance and psychological dependence with varying degrees of abnormal behaviour. Frank psychotic episodes can occur, especially in response to parenteral abuse.

Whether treatment with methylphenidate during childhood does increase the likelihood of addiction for substances in later life is debated.

Precautions: Treatment with Equasym is not indicated in all cases of Attention-Deficit-Hyperactivity disorders, and should be considered only after detailed history taking and evaluation. The decision to prescribe Equasym should depend on an assessment of the severity and persistence of symptoms and their appropriateness to the child's age and not simply on the presence of one or more abnormal behavioural characteristics. Where these symptoms are associated with acute stress reactions, treatment with Equasym is usually not indicated.

Reduced weight gain and growth retardation have been reported with the long term use of stimulants in children. Careful monitoring of growth is recommended during extended treatment with methylphenidate. Usually patients catch up when treatment is discontinued. Whether drug holidays are beneficial in this respect is debated by experts.

Blood pressure should be monitored at appropriate intervals in all patients taking Equasym.

Caution is called for in emotionally unstable patients, such as those with a history of drug dependence or alcoholism, because such patients may increase the dosage on their own initiative.

Equasym should be used with caution in patients with epilepsy as clinical experience has shown that it can cause an increase in seizure frequency in a small number of patients. If seizure frequency rises, methylphenidate should be discontinued.

The long term safety and efficacy profiles of methylphenidate are not fully known. Patients requiring long term therapy should therefore be carefully monitored and complete and differential blood counts and a platelet count performed periodically.

Careful supervision is required during drug withdrawal, since this may unmask depression as well as chronic over-activity. Some patients may require long term follow up.

In theory, there is a possibility that the clearance of methylphenidate might be affected by urinary pH, either being increased with acidifying agents or decreased with alkalising agents. This should be considered when methylphenidate is given in combination with agents that alter urinary pH.

This medicinal product contains lactose. Therefore, patients with rare hereditary problems of galactose intolerance, the Lapp lactase deficiency or glucose-galactose malabsorption should not take this medicine.

Females of child-bearing potential should not use methylphenidate unless clearly necessary (see section 4.6, Pregnancy and Lactation,- (Section 5.3, Preclinical Safety Data).

4.5 Interaction with other medicinal products and other forms of interaction
Human pharmacological studies have shown that methylphenidate may inhibit the metabolism of coumarin anticoagulants, some anticonvulsants (phenobarbitone, phenytoin, primidone), phenylbutazone and tricyclic antidepressants. The dosage of these drugs may have to be reduced. Equasym should be used cautiously in patients being treated with pressor agents. Equasym should not be used in patients being treated (currently or within the last 2 weeks) with MAO inhibitors.

Methylphenidate may also decrease the antihypertensive effect of guanethidine.

Alcohol may exacerbate the CNS adverse reactions of psychoactive drugs, including methylphenidate. It is therefore advisable for patients to abstain from alcohol during treatment.

4.6 Pregnancy and lactation
There are no adequate data from the use of methylphenidate in pregnant women.

Studies in animals have shown reproductive toxicity (teratogenic effects) of methylphenidate (see Section 5.3 Preclinical Safety Data). The potential risk for humans is unknown.

Methylphenidate should not be used during pregnancy unless clearly necessary.

It is not known whether methylphenidate or its metabolites pass into breast milk but for safety reasons breast-feeding mothers should not use Equasym.

4.7 Effects on ability to drive and use machines
Equasym may cause dizziness and drowsiness. It is therefore advisable to exercise caution when driving, operating machinery or engaging in other potentially hazardous activities.

4.8 Undesirable effects
Frequency estimate: very common $\geqslant$ 10%; common $\geqslant$ 1% to $<$10%; uncommon $\geqslant$ 0.1% to $<$1%; rare $\geqslant$0.01% to $<$0.1%; very rare $<$0.01%.

Nervousness and insomnia are very common adverse reactions occurring at the beginning of treatment but can usually be controlled by reducing the dosage and/or omitting the afternoon or evening dose.

Decreased appetite is also common but usually transient.

Central and peripheral nervous system:

Common: Headache, drowsiness, dizziness, dyskinesia, irritability.

Rare: Difficulties in visual accommodation, and blurred vision.

Very rare: Hyperactivity, convulsions, muscle cramps, choreo-athetoid movements, tics or exacerbation of pre-existing tics, and Tourette's syndrome have been reported. Isolated cases of toxic psychosis (some with visual and tactile hallucinations), transient depressed mood, cerebral arteritis and/or occlusion.

Very rare reports of poorly documented neuroleptic malignant syndrome (NMS) have been received. In most of these reports patients were also receiving other medications. It is uncertain what role methylphenidate played in these cases.

Gastro-intestinal tract:

Common: Abdominal pain, nausea and vomiting. These usually occur at the beginning of treatment and may be alleviated by concomitant food intake. Dry mouth.

Very rare: Abnormal liver function, ranging from transaminase elevation to hepatic coma.

Cardiovascular system:

Common: Tachycardia, palpitations, arrhythmias, changes in blood pressure and heart rate (usually an increase).

Rare: Angina pectoris.

Skin and appendages

Common: Rash, pruritus, urticaria, fever, arthralgia, scalp hair loss.

Very rare: Thrombocytopenic purpura, exfoliative dermatitis and erythema multiforme.

Blood:

Very rare: Leucopenia, thrombocytopenia, anaemia.

Miscellaneous:

Rare: Reduced weight gain and growth retardation during prolonged use with stimulants in children have been observed.

4.9 Overdose

Signs and symptoms: Acute overdose, mainly due to overstimulation of the central and sympathetic nervous systems, may result in vomiting, agitation, tremors, hyperreflexia, muscle twitching, convulsions (may be followed by coma), euphoria, confusion, hallucinations, delirium, sweating, flushing, headache, hyperpyrexia, tachycardia, palpitations, cardiac arrhythmias, hypertension, mydriasis and dryness of mucous membranes.

Treatment: There is no specific antidote to Equasym overdosage.

Management consists of appropriate supportive measures, preventing self-injury and protecting the patient from external stimuli that would aggravate over-stimulation already present. If the signs and symptoms are not too severe and the patient is conscious, gastric contents may be evacuated by induction of vomiting or gastric lavage. In the presence of severe intoxication, a carefully titrated dose of a short-acting barbiturate should be given before performing gastric lavage.

Intensive care must be provided to maintain adequate circulation and respiratory exchange; external cooling procedures may be required for hyperpyrexia.

Efficacy of peritoneal dialysis or extracorporeal haemodialysis for overdose of Equasym has not been established.

5. PHARMACOLOGICAL PROPERTIES

5.1 Pharmacodynamic properties

Pharmacotherapeutic group: Psychoanaleptics, Psychostimulants and Nootropics, Centrally acting Sympathomimetics, ATC code: N06B A04.

Mode of action: Methylphenidate is a CNS stimulant. The mode of action is not completely understood. Methylphenidate is an indirect sympatheticomimetic. The pharmacological properties are amphetamine-like.

MAO-enzyme inhibition may result in an increased catecholamine concentration.

5.2 Pharmacokinetic properties

Absorption: The active substance methylphenidate hydrochloride is rapidly and almost completely absorbed from the tablets. Owing to extensive first-pass metabolism its systemic availability amounts to only 30% (11-51%) of the dose. Ingestion together with food accelerates its absorption, but has no influence on the amount absorbed. Peak plasma concentrations of approximately 40 nmol/litre (11 ng/ml) are attained, on average, 1-2 hours after administration of 0.30 mg/kg. The peak plasma concentrations, however, show considerable intersubject variability. The area under the plasma concentration curve (AUC), as well as the peak plasma concentration, is proportional to the dose.

Distribution: In the blood, methylphenidate and its metabolites become distributed in the plasma (57%) and the erythrocytes (43%). Methylphenidate and its metabolites have a low plasma protein-building rate (10-33%). The apparent distribution volume has been calculated as 13.1 litres/kg.

Biotransformation: Biotransformation of methylphenidate is rapid and extensive. Peak plasma concentrations of 2-phenyl -2-piperidyl acetic acid (PPAA) are attained approximately 2 hours after administration of methylphenidate and are 30 - 50 times higher than those of the unchanged substance. The half-life of PPAA is roughly twice as long as that of methylphenidate, and the mean systemic clearance is 0.17 litres/h/kg. Only small amounts of hydroxylated metabolites (e.g. hydroxymethylphenidate and hydroxyritalinic acid) are detectable. Therapeutic activity seems to be principally due to the parent compound.

Elimination: Methylphenidate is eliminated from the plasma with a mean half-life of 2 hours, and the calculated mean systemic clearance is 10 litres/h/kg. Within 48-96 hours 78-97% of the dose administered is excreted in the urine and 1-3% in the faeces in the form of metabolites. Unchanged methylphenidate appears in the urine only in small quantities (<1%). The bulk of the dose is excreted in the urine as 2-phenyl-2-piperidyl acetic acid (PPAA, 60-86%).

Characteristics in patients: There are no apparent differences in the pharmacokinetic behaviour of methylphenidate in hyperactive children and healthy adult volunteers.

Elimination data from patients with normal renal function suggest that renal excretion of the unchanged methylphenidate would hardly be diminished at all in the presence of impaired renal function. However, renal excretion of PPAA may be reduced.

5.3 Preclinical safety data

There is evidence that methylphenidate may be a teratogen in two species. Spina bifida and limb malformations have been reported in rabbits whilst in the rat, equivocal evidence of induction of abnormalities of the vertebrae was found.

Methylphenidate did not affect reproductive performance or fertility at low multiples of the clinical dose.

In life-time rat and mouse carcinogenicity studies, increased numbers of malignant liver tumours were noted in male mice only. The significance of this finding to humans is unknown.

6. PHARMACEUTICAL PARTICULARS

6.1 List of excipients

Anhydrous Lactose

Magnesium Stearate

Microcrystalline Cellulose

Sodium Starch Glycollate

6.2 Incompatibilities

Not applicable.

6.3 Shelf life

3 years

6.4 Special precautions for storage

Do not store above 25°C. Store in the original package

6.5 Nature and contents of container

PVC/Aluminium blisters of 30 tablets.

PVC/Aluminium blisters of 20 and 50 tablets.

Not all pack sizes may be marketed.

6.6 Special precautions for disposal and other handling

No special requirements.

7. MARKETING AUTHORISATION HOLDER

Shire Pharmaceuticals Ireland Limited

5 Riverwalk

Citywest Business Campus

Dublin 24

Ireland

8. MARKETING AUTHORISATION NUMBER(S)

5 mg: 27303/001, 10 mg: 27303/002, 20 mg: 27303/003

9. DATE OF FIRST AUTHORISATION/RENEWAL OF THE AUTHORISATION

22 February 2000 / 15 June 2009

10. DATE OF REVISION OF THE TEXT

17 June 2009

Equasym XL 10 mg, 20 mg or 30 mg Capsules

(Shire Pharmaceuticals Limited)

1. NAME OF THE MEDICINAL PRODUCT

Equasym XL 10 mg modified-release capsules, hard

Equasym XL 20 mg modified-release capsules, hard

Equasym XL 30 mg modified-release capsules, hard

2. QUALITATIVE AND QUANTITATIVE COMPOSITION

Each capsule contains 10 mg methylphenidate hydrochloride corresponding to 8.65 mg methylphenidate.

Each capsule contains 20 mg methylphenidate hydrochloride corresponding to 17.30 mg methylphenidate.

Each capsule contains 30 mg methylphenidate hydrochloride corresponding to 25.94 mg methylphenidate.

Excipient: 45 mg sucrose/capsule for Equasym XL 10mg

Excipient: 90 mg sucrose/capsule for Equasym XL 20mg

Excipient: 135 mg sucrose/capsule for Equasym XL 30mg

For a full list excipients, see Section 6.1

3. PHARMACEUTICAL FORM

Modified release capsule, hard.

Equasym XL 10mg capsule: The capsule has a dark green opaque cap imprinted with "UCB 579" in white and a white opaque body imprinted with "10mg" in black.

Equasym XL 20mg capsule: The capsule has a blue opaque cap imprinted with "UCB 580" in white and a white opaque body imprinted with "20mg" in black.

Equasym XL 30mg capsule: The capsule has a reddish-brown opaque cap imprinted with "UCB 581" in white and a white opaque body imprinted with "30mg" in black.

4. CLINICAL PARTICULARS

4.1 Therapeutic indications

Equasym XL is indicated as part of a comprehensive treatment programme for attention-deficit/hyperactivity disorder (ADHD) in children over 6 years of age when remedial measures alone prove insufficient. Treatment must be under the supervision of a specialist in childhood behavioural disorders. Diagnosis should be made according to DSM-IV criteria or the guidelines in ICD-10.

Additional information on the safe use of the medicinal product:

The specific aetiology of this syndrome is unknown, and there is no single diagnostic test. Adequate diagnosis requires the use of medical and special psychological, educational, and social resources.

A comprehensive treatment programme typically includes psychological, educational and social measures and is aimed at stabilising children with a behavioural syndrome characterised by symptoms which may include chronic history of short attention span, distractibility, emotional lability, impulsivity, moderate to severe hyperactivity, minor neurological signs and abnormal EEG. Learning may or may not be impaired. Equasym XL treatment is not indicated in all children with this syndrome and the decision to use the medicinal product must be based on a very thorough assessment of the severity of the child's symptoms.

4.2 Posology and method of administration

Equasym XL consists of an immediate release component (30% of the dose) and a modified release component (70% of the dose). Hence Equasym XL 10mg yields an immediate-release dose of 3mg and an extended release dose of 7mg methylphenidate hydrochloride. The extended-release portion of each dose is designed to maintain a treatment response through the afternoon without the need for a midday dose. It is designed to deliver therapeutic plasma levels for a period of approximately 8 hours, which is consistent with the school day rather than the whole day (see section 5.2 "Pharmacokinetic properties"). For example, 20mg of Equasym XL is intended to take the place of 10mg at breakfast and 10mg at lunchtime of immediate release methylphenidate hydrochloride.

Adults: Not applicable.

Elderly: Not applicable.

Children (over 6 years) and adolescents.

Dose titration:

Careful dose titration is necessary at the start of treatment with methylphenidate. This is normally achieved using an immediate release formulation taken in divided doses. The recommended starting daily dose is 5mg once daily or twice daily (e.g. at breakfast and lunch), increasing if necessary by weekly increments of 5-10mg in the daily dose according to tolerability and degree of efficacy observed. Equasym XL 10mg once daily may be used in place of immediate release methylphenidate hydrochloride 5mg twice daily from the beginning of treatment where the treating physician considers that twice daily dosing is appropriate from the outset and twice daily treatment administration is impracticable.

For doses not realisable/practicable with this strength, other strengths of this medicinal product and other methylphenidate containing products are available.

Patients Currently Using Methylphenidate: Patients established on an immediate release methylphenidate hydrochloride formulation may be switched to the milligram equivalent daily dose of Equasym XL.

If the effect of the medicinal product wears off too early in the late afternoon or evening, disturbed behaviour and/or inability to go to sleep may recur. A small dose of an immediate-release methylphenidate hydrochloride tablet late in the day may help to solve this problem. In that case, it could be considered that adequate symptom control might be achieved with a twice daily immediate release methylphenidate regimen. Treatment should not continue with Equasym XL if an additional late dose of immediate-release methylphenidate is required, unless it is known that the same extra dose was also required for a conventional immediate-release regimen at equivalent breakfast/lunchtime dose. The regimen that achieves satisfactory symptom control with the lowest total daily dose should be employed.

The maximum daily dose of methylphenidate hydrochloride is 60mg.

Equasym XL should not be used in children less than 6 years due to a lack of data on safety and efficacy.

Equasym XL should be given in the morning before breakfast.

The capsules may be swallowed whole with the aid of liquids, or alternatively, the capsule may be opened and the capsule contents sprinkled onto a small amount (tablespoon) of applesauce and given immediately, and not stored for future use. Drinking some fluids, e.g. water, should follow the intake of the sprinkles with applesauce. The capsules and the capsule contents must not be crushed or chewed.

Maintenance/Extended treatment:

The long term use of methylphenidate has not been systematically evaluated in controlled trials. The physician who elects to use Equasym for extended periods in patients with ADHD should periodically re-evaluate the long term usefulness of the drug for the individual patient with trial periods off medication to assess the patient's functioning without pharmacotherapy. Improvement may be sustained when the drug is either temporarily or permanently discontinued.

Note: If improvement of symptoms is not observed after appropriate dosage adjustment over a one-month period, the medicinal product should be discontinued. Methylphenidate should be discontinued periodically to assess the child's condition. Medicinal product treatment is usually discontinued during or after puberty.

4.3 Contraindications

Equasym XL is contra-indicated:

- in patients known to be hypersensitive to methylphenidate or to any of the excipients.

- in patients with marked anxiety, agitation or tension as the use of Equasym XL may aggravate these symptoms

- in patients with glaucoma
- in patients with hyperthyroidism
- in patients with thyrotoxicosis
- in patients with severe angina pectoris
- in patients with cardiac arrhythmia,
- in patients with severe hypertension
- in patients with heart failure
- in patients with myocardial infarction
- in patients who currently exhibit severe depression, psychotic symptoms, psychopathological personality structure, history of aggression or suicidal tendency, since methylphenidate might worsen these conditions
- in patients with known drug dependence or alcoholism
- in combination with non-selective, irreversible monoamine oxydase inhibitors, and also within a minimum of 14 days following discontinuation of a non-selective irreversible MAO inhibitor (hypertensive crises and hyperthermia may result) (see Section 4.5).
- in patients with motor tics, tics in siblings, or a family history or diagnosis of Tourette's syndrome.
- during pregnancy (see Section 5.3).

4.4 Special warnings and precautions for use

Warnings: Equasym XL should not be used in children less than 6 years of age due to a lack of data on safety and efficacy.

Equasym XL should not be used to treat severe exogenous or endogenous depression.

Clinical experience suggests that Equasym XL may exacerbate symptoms of behavioural disturbance and thought disorder in psychotic children.

Available clinical evidence suggests that treatment with methylphenidate during childhood does not increase the likelihood of addiction in later life, though this should always be carefully monitored in each individual case.

Chronic abuse of methylphenidate can lead to marked tolerance and psychological dependence with varying degrees of abnormal behaviour. Frank psychotic episodes can occur, especially in response to parenteral abuse.

The choice between treatment with either Equasym XL or an immediate release methylphenidate formulation should be determined on an individual basis with particular consideration of the requirement for symptom control in the latter part of the day (see also section 4.2).

Methylphenidate should not be used for the prevention or treatment of normal fatigue states.

Precautions: Treatment with methylphenidate is not indicated in all cases of ADHD, and should be considered only after detailed history taking and evaluation. The decision to prescribe methylphenidate should depend on an assessment of the severity of symptoms and their appropriateness to the child's age and not simply on the presence of one or more abnormal behavioural characteristics. Where these symptoms are associated with acute stress reactions, treatment with methylphenidate is usually not indicated.

Reduced weight gain and slight growth retardation have been reported with the long term use of stimulants in children. Careful monitoring of growth is recommended during extended treatment with methylphenidate. Patients who are not growing or gaining weight as expected should have their treatment interrupted temporarily.

Blood pressure should be monitored at appropriate intervals in all patients taking methylphenidate, especially those with hypertension.

Exacerbation of motor and phonic tics and Tourette's syndrome has been reported. Therefore, clinical evaluation for tics and Tourette's syndrome should precede use of stimulant medications (see Section 4.3 Contraindications).

Due to the potential decreased appetite associated with methylphenidate use, caution is advised in the presence of anorexia nervosa.

Caution is called for in emotionally unstable patients, such as those with a history of drug dependence or alcoholism, because such patients may increase the dosage on their own initiative.

There is some clinical evidence that methylphenidate may lower the convulsive threshold in patients with prior history of seizures, in patients with prior EEG abnormalities in absence of seizures, and, very rarely, in absence of history of seizures and no prior EEG evidence of seizures. In the presence of seizures, the drug should be discontinued.

The long term safety and efficacy profiles of methylphenidate are not fully known. Patients requiring long term therapy should therefore be carefully monitored and complete and differential blood counts and a platelet count performed periodically.

Careful supervision is required during drug withdrawal, since this may unmask depression as well as chronic over-activity. Some patients may require long-term follow up.

There is no experience with the use of Equasym XL in patients with renal insufficiency or hepatic insufficiency.

Women of childbearing potential should use effective contraceptive measures (see Section 4.3, Section 4.6 and Section 5.3).

This medicinal product contains sucrose. Patients with rare hereditary problems of fructose intolerance, glucosegalactose malabsorption or sucrase-isomaltase insufficiency should not take this medicine.

Sport: This medicinal product contains methylphenidate which results in a positive result during drug testing.

4.5 Interaction with other medicinal products and other forms of interaction

Because of possible hypertensive crisis Equasym XL is contraindicated in patients being treated (currently or within the preceding 2 weeks) with non-selective, irreversible MAO-inhibitors (see Section 4.3).

Because of possible increases in blood pressure, Equasym XL should be used cautiously with vasopressor agents.

It is not known how methylphenidate may affect plasma concentrations of concomitantly administered drugs. Caution is recommended at combination of methylphenidate with other drugs, especially those with a narrow therapeutic window. Case reports have indicated that methylphenidate may inhibit the metabolism of coumarin anticoagulants, anticonvulsants (eg, phenobarbital, phenytoin, primidone), and some antidepressants (tricyclics and selective serotonin reuptake inhibitors). Downward dose adjustment of these drugs may be required when given concomitantly with methylphenidate. It may be necessary to adjust the dosage and monitor plasma drug concentrations (or, in the case of coumarin, coagulation times), when initiating or discontinuing concomitant methylphenidate.

Serious adverse events, including sudden death, have been reported in concomitant use with clonidine, although no causality for the combination has been established. The safety of using methylphenidate in combination with clonidine or other centrally acting alpha-2 agonists has not been systematically evaluated. Possible interactions with antipsychotics (haloperidol and thioridazine) have also been reported.

Methylphenidate may also decrease the antihypertensive effect of guanethidine.

Alcohol may exacerbate the CNS adverse reactions of psychoactive drugs, including methylphenidate. It is therefore advisable for patients to abstain from alcohol during treatment.

Halogenated anaesthetics: There is a risk of sudden blood pressure increase during surgery. If surgery is planned, methylphenidate treatment should not be used on the day of surgery.

4.6 Pregnancy and lactation

Experience on the use of methylphenidate in pregnant women is limited.

Studies in animals have shown reproductive toxicity of methylphenidate (see Section 5.3). The potential risk for humans is unknown.

Methylphenidate is contraindicated during pregnancy (see Section 4.3 and 4.4).

It is not known whether methylphenidate or its metabolites pass into breast milk but for safety reasons a decision should be made whether to discontinue breastfeeding or discontinue the treatment taking into account the importance of the medicinal product to breast feeding mothers.

4.7 Effects on ability to drive and use machines

Equasym XL may cause dizziness and drowsiness. It has a major influence on the ability to drive and use machines. It is therefore advisable to exercise caution when driving, operating machinery or engaging in other potentially hazardous activities.

4.8 Undesirable effects

Frequency estimate: very common ($\geqslant$ 1/10); common ($\geqslant$ 1/100 to $<$ 1/10); uncommon ($\geqslant$ 1/1000 to $<$ 1/100); rare ($\geqslant$ 1/10000 to $<$ 1/1000); very rare ($<$ 1/10000), not known (cannot be estimated from the available data).

Nervousness and insomnia are very common adverse reactions occurring at the beginning of treatment but can usually be controlled by reducing the dosage.

Decreased appetite is also common but usually transient.

Blood and lymphatic system disorders:

Very rare: Anaemia, leucopenia, thrombocytopenia, thrombocytopenic purpura

Cardiac disorders:

Common: Arrhythmia, palpitations, tachycardia

Rare: Angina pectoris,

Very rare: Cardiac arrest

Congenital, familial and genetic disorders:

Very rare: Tourette's syndrome

Eye disorders:

Rare: Difficulties in visual accommodation, blurred vision

Gastrointestinal disorders:

Common: Abdominal pain, nausea, and vomiting. These usually occur at the beginning of treatment and may be alleviated by concomitant food intake. Dry mouth.

General disorders and administration site conditions:

Rare: Growth retardation during prolonged use in children

Very rare: Sudden death

Hepatobiliary disorders:

Very rare: Abnormal liver function, ranging from transaminase elevation to hepatic coma

Investigations:

Common: Changes in blood pressure and heart rate (usually an increase)

Metabolism and nutrition disorders:

Common: Decreased appetite, reduced weight gain during prolonged use in children

Musculoskeletal and connective tissue disorders:

Common: Arthralgia

Very rare: Muscle spasms

Nervous system disorders:

Common: Dizziness, drowsiness, dyskinesia, headache, hyperactivity

Very rare: Convulsions, choreo-athetoid movements

Very rare reports of poorly documented neuroleptic malignant syndrome (NMS) have been received. In most of these reports patients were also receiving other medications. It is uncertain what role methylphenidate played in these cases.

Psychiatric disorders:

Very common: Insomnia, nervousness

Common: Abnormal behaviour, aggression, agitation, anorexia, anxiety, depression, irritability

Very rare: Hallucinations, psychotic disorder, suicidal behaviour (including completed suicide), tics or exacerbation of pre-existing tics, transient depressed mood

Skin and subcutaneous tissue disorders:

Common: Alopecia, pruritus, rash, urticaria

Very rare: Erythema multiforme, exfoliative dermatitis, fixed drug eruption

Vascular disorders:

Very rare: Cerebral arteritis and/or occlusion

4.9 Overdose

The prolonged release of methylphenidate form Equasym XL should be considered when treating patients with overdose.

Signs and symptoms: Acute overdose, mainly due to overstimulation of the central and sympathetic nervous systems, may result in vomiting, agitation, tremors, hyperreflexia, muscle twitching, convulsions (may be followed by coma), euphoria, confusion, hallucinations, delirium, sweating, flushing, headache, hyperpyrexia, tachycardia, palpitations, cardiac arrhythmias, hypertension, mydriasis and dryness of mucous membranes.

Treatment: There is no specific antidote to Equasym XL overdose.

Management consists of appropriate supportive measures, preventing selfinjury and protecting the patient from external stimuli that would aggravate over-stimulation already present. If the signs and symptoms are not too severe and the patient is conscious, gastric contents may be evacuated by induction of vomiting or gastric lavage. In the presence of severe intoxication, a carefully titrated dose of a short-acting barbiturate should be given before performing gastric lavage.

Intensive care must be provided to maintain adequate circulation and respiratory exchange; external cooling procedures may be required for hyperpyrexia.

Efficacy of peritoneal dialysis or extracorporeal haemodialysis for overdose of Equasym XL has not been established.

5. PHARMACOLOGICAL PROPERTIES

5.1 Pharmacodynamic properties

Pharmacotherapeutic group: Psychoanaleptics, Psychostimulants and agents used for ADHD and nootropics, Centrally acting Sympathomimetics, ATC code: N06BA04

Mechanism of action: Equasym XL is a mild CNS stimulant with more prominent effects on mental than on motor activities. Its mode of action in man is not completely understood but its effects are thought to be due to cortical stimulation and possibly to stimulation of the reticular activating system.

In a pivotal study 318 subjects aged between 6 and 12 years received at least one dose of study medication out of 327 subjects randomized. Scores for the IOWA Conner's rating, the primary efficacy endpoint assessed by teachers during the school day, showed the following results for the per protocol population (279 patients treated for 21 days):

(see Table 1 on next page)

In contrast to these results for the primary efficacy measure, differences between the Equasym XL and immediate release methylphenidate groups were observed for the Parent IOWA Conner's secondary efficacy variable. This was based on assessments later in the evening, suggesting that there is some loss of efficacy of Equasym XL late in the day relative to twice daily immediate release methylphenidate. See also section 5.2. (Pharmacokinetic properties) and section 4.2 (Posology and method of administration).

The mechanism by which Equasym XL exerts its mental and behavioural effects in children is not clearly established, nor is there conclusive evidence showing how these

Table 1

	Placebo (N=39) [a]	Immediate Release Methylphenidate (N=120) [b]	Equasym XL (N=120)
Baseline Mean **(SD)**	6.0 (3.64)	6.1 (3.74)	5.8 (3.59)
Day 21/Withdrawal			
LS Mean (SE)	7.7 (0.50)	4.3 (0.29)	4.5 (0.29)
95% CI	6.69, 8.66	3.71, 4.84	3.98, 51.0
Difference from Placebo	-	-3.4	-3.1
95% CI for the difference	-	-4.53, -2.26	-4.26, -2.00
P-value[c]	-	<0.001	<0.001
Difference from MIR	-	-	**-0.3**
97.5% lower CI bound for the difference	-	-	**-1.06**

a N=38 at Day 7

b N=118 at Day 7

c Treatment groups have been compared using ANCOVA, with effects for treatment and baseline as covariates

effects relate to the condition of the central nervous system. It is thought to block the re-uptake of norepinephrine and dopamine into the presynaptic neurone and increase the release of these monoamines into the extraneuronal space. Equasym XL is a racemic mixture of the *d*- and *l*threo enantiomers of methylphenidate. The *d*-enantiomer is more pharmacologically active than the *l*-enantiomer.

5.2 Pharmacokinetic properties

Absorption: Equasym XL has a plasma profile showing two phases of active substance release, with a sharp, initial, upward slope similar to a methylphenidate immediate-release tablet, and a second rising portion approximately three hours later, followed by a gradual decline.

Peak plasma concentrations of approximately 40 nmol/litre (11 ng/ml) are attained, on average, 1-2 hours after administration of 0.30 mg/kg. The peak plasma concentrations, however, show considerable intersubject variability.

The range of concentrations at 1.5 hours was 3.2 – 13.3 ng/ml with a mean of 7.7 ng/ml. The second phase of release resulted in a second maximum observed concentration in most subjects at 4.5 hours after dosing, with the observed concentrations ranging from 4.9 – 15.5 ng/ml with a mean of 8.2 ng/ml. Administration of an extended release formulation at breakfast instead of two immediate release formulation tablets (breakfast and lunch) may reduce the pre-lunch trough and post lunch peak of methylphenidate, and plasma levels may be lower after the end of the school day. Clinical trial data suggest that the different pharmacokinetic profiles may result in a different pattern of behaviour and symptom control during the day for some patients compared with a conventional immediate release methylphenidate regimen. In particular there may be some reduction of symptom control in the late afternoon and early evening (see section 5.1 Pharmacodynamic properties). These differences should be taken into consideration when assessing their individual requirements.

The area under the plasma concentration curve (AUC), as well as the peak plasma concentration, is proportional to the dose.

Food Effects: Ingestion together with food with a high fat content delays its absorption (T_{max}) by approximately one hour and increases the maximum concentration (C_{max}) by approximately 30% and the amount absorbed (AUC) by approximately 17%.

Sprinkle Administration: The $C_{max}T_{max}$ and AUC of the sprinkled contents of the Equasym XL capsule are similar (bioequivalent) to the intact capsule. Equasym XL may, therefore, be administered either as an intact capsule, or the capsule may be opened and the contents swallowed, without chewing, immediately after sprinkling onto apple-sauce or other similar soft food.

Age: the Pharmacokinetics of Equasym XL have not been studied in children younger than 7 years of age.

Availability, systemic: Owing to extensive first-pass metabolism its systemic availability amounts to approximately 30% (11-51%) of the dose.

Distribution: In the blood, methylphenidate and its metabolites become distributed in the plasma (57%) and the erythrocytes (43%). Methylphenidate and its metabolites have a low plasma protein-building rate (10-33%). The apparent distribution has been calculated as 13.1 litres/kg.

Elimination: Methylphenidate is eliminated from the plasma with a mean half-life 2 hours, and the calculated mean systemic clearance is 10 litres/h/kg.

Within 48-96 hours 78-97% of the dose administered is excreted in the urine and 1-3% in the faeces in the form of metabolites.

The bulk of the dose is excreted in the urine as 2-phenyl-2-piperidyl acetic acid (PPAA, 60-86%).

5.3 Preclinical safety data

There is evidence that methylphenidate may be a teratogen in two species. Spina bifida and limb malformations have been reported in rabbits whilst in the rat, equivocal evidence of induction of abnormalities of the vertebrae was found.

Methylphenidate did not affect reproductive performance or fertility at low multiples (2-5 times) of the clinical dose.

In life-time rat and mouse carcinogenicity studies, increased numbers of malignant liver tumours were noted in male mice only. The significance of this finding to humans is unknown.

The weight of evidence from the genotoxicity studies reveals no special hazard for humans.

6. PHARMACEUTICAL PARTICULARS

6.1 List of excipients

Capsule content

Sugar Spheres:

Sucrose

Maize starch

Povidone K29 to K32

Opadry Clear YS-1-7006 (hypromellose, macrogol 400 and macrogol 8000)

Ethylcellulose Aqueous Dispersion

Dibutyl Sebacate

Capsule shell

Gelatin

Titanium dioxide (E171)

Indigo carmine aluminium salt (E132)

Yellow iron oxide (E172)

White printing ink:

Shellac

Propylene glycol

Sodium hydroxide

Povidone K16

Titanium dioxide (E171)

Black printing ink:

Shellac glaze 45% (20% esterified) in ethanol

Propylene glycol

Ammonium hydroxide 28%

Iron oxide black

6.2 Incompatibilities

Not applicable.

6.3 Shelf life

36 months

6.4 Special precautions for storage

Store below 30°C.

6.5 Nature and contents of container

Clear or opaque PVC/Aclar blister with aluminum foil backing and vinyl seal coating.

Pack sizes: 10 modified-release capsules, hard.

30 modified-release capsules, hard.

60 modified-release capsules, hard.

100 modified-release capsules, hard

Not all pack sizes may be marketed.

6.6 Special precautions for disposal and other handling

No special requirements.

7. MARKETING AUTHORISATION HOLDER

Shire Pharmaceuticals Ireland Limited

5 Riverwalk

Citywest Business Campus

Dublin 24

Ireland

8. MARKETING AUTHORISATION NUMBER(S)

Equasym XL 10mg: PL 27303/0004

Equasym XL 20mg: PL 27303/0005

Equasym XL 30mg: PL 27303/0006

9. DATE OF FIRST AUTHORISATION/RENEWAL OF THE AUTHORISATION

11 February 2005

10. DATE OF REVISION OF THE TEXT

18 June 2009

Erbitux 5mg/ml solution for infusion

(Merck Serono)

1. NAME OF THE MEDICINAL PRODUCT

Erbitux ▼ 5 mg/ml solution for infusion

2. QUALITATIVE AND QUANTITATIVE COMPOSITION

Each ml of solution for infusion contains 5 mg cetuximab.

Each vial contains 10 ml, 20 ml, 50 ml or 100 ml.

Cetuximab is a chimeric monoclonal IgG_1 antibody produced in a mammalian cell line (Sp2/0) by recombinant DNA technology.

For a full list of excipients, see section 6.1.

3. PHARMACEUTICAL FORM

Solution for infusion.

Colourless solution.

4. CLINICAL PARTICULARS

4.1 Therapeutic indications

Erbitux is indicated for the treatment of patients with epidermal growth factor receptor (EGFR)-expressing, KRAS wild-type metastatic colorectal cancer

- in combination with chemotherapy
- as a single agent in patients who have failed oxaliplatin- and irinotecan-based therapy and who are intolerant to irinotecan.

Erbitux is indicated for the treatment of patients with squamous cell cancer of the head and neck

- in combination with radiation therapy for locally advanced disease
- in combination with platinum-based chemotherapy for recurrent and/or metastatic disease.

4.2 Posology and method of administration

Erbitux must be administered under the supervision of a physician experienced in the use of antineoplastic medicinal products. Close monitoring is required during the infusion and for at least 1 hour after the end of the infusion. Availability of resuscitation equipment must be ensured.

Posology

Prior to the first infusion, patients must receive premedication with an antihistamine and a corticosteroid. This premedication is recommended prior to all subsequent infusions.

In all indications, Erbitux is administered once a week. The very first dose is 400 mg cetuximab per m^2 body surface area. All subsequent weekly doses are 250 mg cetuximab per m^2 each.

Colorectal cancer

In patients with metastatic colorectal cancer, cetuximab is used in combination with chemotherapy or as a single agent (see section 5.1). It is recommended that the detection of KRAS mutational status be performed by an experienced laboratory using a validated test method.

For the dosage or recommended dose modifications of concomitantly used chemotherapeutic agents, refer to the product information for these medicinal products. They must not be administered earlier than 1 hour after the end of the cetuximab infusion.

It is recommended that cetuximab treatment be continued until progression of the underlying disease.

Squamous cell cancer of the head and neck

In patients with locally advanced squamous cell cancer of the head and neck, cetuximab is used concomitantly with radiation therapy. It is recommended to start cetuximab therapy one week before radiation therapy and to continue cetuximab therapy until the end of the radiation therapy period.

In patients with recurrent and/or metastatic squamous cell cancer of the head and neck, cetuximab is used in combination with platinum-based chemotherapy followed by cetuximab as maintenance therapy until disease progression (see section 5.1). Chemotherapy must not be administered earlier than 1 hour after the end of the cetuximab infusion.

Method of administration

Erbitux 5 mg/ml is administered intravenously with an infusion pump, gravity drip or a syringe pump (for handling instructions, see section 6.6).

For the initial dose, the recommended infusion period is 120 minutes. For the subsequent weekly doses, the recommended infusion period is 60 minutes. The maximum infusion rate must not exceed 10 mg/min.

Special populations

Only patients with adequate renal and hepatic function have been investigated to date (see section 4.4).

Cetuximab has not been studied in patients with pre-existing haematological disorders (see section 4.4).

No dose adjustment is required in the elderly, but the experience is limited in patients 75 years of age and above.

Paediatric population

There is no experience in children (see section 4.4).

4.3 Contraindications

Erbitux is contraindicated in patients with known severe (grade 3 or 4) hypersensitivity reactions to cetuximab.

Before initiation of combination treatment, contraindications for concomitantly used chemotherapeutic agents or radiation therapy must be considered.

4.4 Special warnings and precautions for use

Infusion-related reactions

If the patient experiences a mild or moderate infusion-related reaction, the infusion rate may be decreased. It is recommended to maintain this lower infusion rate in all subsequent infusions.

Severe infusion-related reactions have been reported in patients treated with cetuximab (see section 4.8). Symptoms usually occurred during the first infusion and up to 1 hour after the end of infusion, but may occur after several hours or with subsequent infusions. It is recommended to warn patients of the possibility of such a late onset and instruct them to contact their physician if symptoms of an infusion-related reaction occur. Occurrence of a severe infusion-related reaction requires immediate and permanent discontinuation of cetuximab therapy and may necessitate emergency treatment.

Special attention is recommended for patients with reduced performance status and pre-existing cardio-pulmonary disease.

Respiratory disorders

Individual cases of interstitial lung disorders of unknown causal relationship to cetuximab have been reported. If interstitial lung disease is diagnosed, cetuximab must be discontinued and the patient be treated appropriately.

Skin reactions

If a patient experiences a severe skin reaction (⩾ grade 3; US National Cancer Institute - Common Toxicity Criteria, NCI-CTC), cetuximab therapy must be interrupted. Treatment may only be resumed, if the reaction has resolved to grade 2 (see section 4.8).

If the severe skin reaction occurred for the first time, treatment may be resumed without any change in dose level.

With the second and third occurrences of severe skin reactions, cetuximab therapy must again be interrupted. Treatment may only be resumed at a lower dose level (200 mg/m^2 body surface area after the second occurrence and 150 mg/m^2 after the third occurrence), if the reaction has resolved to grade 2.

If severe skin reactions occur a fourth time or do not resolve to grade 2 during interruption of treatment, permanent discontinuation of cetuximab treatment is required.

Electrolyte disturbances

Progressively decreasing serum magnesium levels occur frequently and may lead to severe hypomagnesaemia. Hypomagnesaemia is reversible following discontinuation of cetuximab. In addition, hypokalaemia may develop as a consequence of diarrhoea. Hypocalcaemia may also occur; in particular in combination with platinum-based chemotherapy the frequency of severe hypocalcaemia may be increased.

Determination of serum electrolyte levels is recommended prior to and periodically during cetuximab treatment. Electrolyte repletion is recommended, as appropriate.

Neutropenia and related infectious complications

Patients who receive cetuximab in combination with platinum-based chemotherapy are at an increased risk for the occurrence of severe neutropenia, which may lead to subsequent infectious complications such as febrile neutropenia, pneumonia or sepsis. Careful monitoring is recommended in such patients, in particular in those who experience skin lesions, mucositis or diarrhoea that may facilitate the occurrence of infections (see section 4.8).

Special populations

Only patients with adequate renal and hepatic function have been investigated to date (serum creatinine ⩽ 1.5fold, transaminases ⩽ 5fold and bilirubin ⩽ 1.5fold the upper limit of normal).

Cetuximab has not been studied in patients presenting with one or more of the following laboratory parameters:

- haemoglobin < 9 g/dl
- leukocyte count < 3000/mm^3
- absolute neutrophil count < 1500/mm^3
- platelet count < 100000/mm^3

There is limited experience in the use of cetuximab in combination with radiation therapy in colorectal cancer.

Paediatric population

The safety and effectiveness of cetuximab in paediatric patients have not been established.

4.5 Interaction with other medicinal products and other forms of interaction

In combination with platinum-based chemotherapy, the frequency of severe leukopenia or severe neutropenia may be increased, and thus may lead to a higher rate of infectious complications such as febrile neutropenia, pneumonia and sepsis compared to platinum-based chemotherapy alone (see section 4.4).

In combination with infusional 5-fluorouracil, the frequency of cardiac ischaemia including myocardial infarction and congestive heart failure as well as the frequency of hand-foot syndrome (palmar-plantar erythrodysaesthesia) were increased compared to that with infusional 5-fluorouracil.

A formal interaction study showed that the pharmacokinetic characteristics of cetuximab remain unaltered after co-administration of a single dose of irinotecan (350 mg/m^2 body surface area). Similarly, the pharmacokinetics of irinotecan were unchanged when cetuximab was co-administered.

No other formal interaction studies with cetuximab have been performed in humans.

4.6 Pregnancy and lactation

EGFR is involved in foetal development. Limited observations in animals are indicative of a placental transfer of cetuximab, and other IgG_1 antibodies have been found to cross the placental barrier. Animal data revealed no evidence of teratogenicity. However, dependent on the dose, an increased incidence of abortion was observed (see section 5.3). Sufficient data from pregnant or lactating women are not available.

It is strongly recommended that Erbitux be given during pregnancy or to any woman not employing adequate contraception only if the potential benefit justifies a potential risk to the foetus.

It is recommended that women do not breast-feed during treatment with Erbitux and for 2 months after the last dose, because it is not known whether cetuximab is excreted in breast milk.

4.7 Effects on ability to drive and use machines

No studies on the effects on the ability to drive and use machines have been performed. If patients experience treatment-related symptoms affecting their ability to concentrate and react, it is recommended that they do not drive or use machines until the effect subsides.

4.8 Undesirable effects

The primary undesirable effects of cetuximab are skin reactions, which occur in more than 80% of patients, hypomagnesaemia which occurs in more than 10% of patients and infusion-related reactions, which occur with mild to moderate symptoms in more than 10% of patients and with severe symptoms in more than 1% of patients.

The following definitions apply to the frequency terminology used hereafter:

Very common (⩾ 1/10)

Common (⩾ 1/100 to < 1/10)

Uncommon (⩾ 1/1,000 to < 1/100)

Rare (⩾ 1/10,000 to < 1/1,000)

Very rare (< 1/10,000)

Frequency not known (cannot be estimated from the available data)

An asterisk (*) indicates that additional information on the respective undesirable effect is provided below the table.

Metabolism and nutrition disorders

Very common:	Hypomagnesaemia (see section 4.4).
Common:	Dehydration, in particular secondary to diarrhoea or mucositis; hypocalcaemia (see section 4.4); anorexia which may lead to weight decrease.

Nervous system disorders

Common:	Headache.

Eye disorders

Common:	Conjunctivitis.
Uncommon:	Blepharitis, keratitis.

Vascular disorders

Uncommon:	Deep vein thrombosis.

Respiratory, thoracic and mediastinal disorders

Uncommon:	Pulmonary embolism.

Gastrointestinal disorders

Common:	Diarrhoea, nausea, vomiting.

Hepatobiliary disorders

Very common:	Increase in liver enzyme levels (ASAT, ALAT, AP).

Skin and subcutaneous tissue disorders

Very common:	Skin reactions*.
Frequency not known:	Superinfection of skin lesions*

General disorders and administration site conditions

Very common:	Mild or moderate infusion related reactions*; mild to moderate mucositis which may lead to epistaxis.
Common:	Severe infusion related reactions*, fatigue.

Additional information

Overall, no clinically relevant difference between genders was observed.

Infusion-related reactions

Mild or moderate infusion-related reactions are very common comprising symptoms such as fever, chills, dizziness, or dyspnoea that occur in a close temporal relationship mainly to the first cetuximab infusion.

Severe infusion-related reactions may commonly occur, in rare cases with fatal outcome. They usually develop during or within 1 hour of the initial cetuximab infusion, but may occur after several hours or with subsequent infusions. Although the underlying mechanism has not been identified, some of these reactions may be anaphylactoid/anaphylactic in nature and may include symptoms such as bronchospasm, urticaria, increase or decrease in blood pressure, loss of consciousness or shock. In rare cases, angina pectoris, myocardial infarction or cardiac arrest have been observed.

For clinical management of infusion-related reactions, see section 4.4.

Skin reactions

Skin reactions may develop in more than 80% of patients and mainly present as acne-like rash and/or, less frequently, as pruritus, dry skin, desquamation, hypertrichosis, or nail disorders (e.g. paronychia). Approximately 15% of the skin reactions are severe, including single cases of skin necrosis. The majority of skin reactions develop within the first three weeks of therapy. They generally resolve, without sequelae, over time following cessation of treatment if the recommended adjustments in dose regimen are followed (see section 4.4). According to NCI-CTC, grade 2 skin reactions are characterised by rash up to 50% of body surface area, while grade 3 reactions affect equal or more than 50% of body surface area.

Skin lesions induced by cetuximab may predispose patients to superinfections (e.g. with *S. aureus*), which may lead to subsequent complications, e.g. cellulitis, erysipelas, or, potentially with fatal outcome, staphylococcal scalded skin syndrome or sepsis.

Combination treatment

When cetuximab is used in combination with chemotherapeutic agents, also refer to their respective product information.

In combination with platinum-based chemotherapy, the frequency of severe leukopenia or severe neutropenia may be increased, and thus may lead to a higher rate of infectious complications such as febrile neutropenia, pneumonia and sepsis compared to platinum-based chemotherapy alone (see section 4.4).

In combination with infusional 5-fluorouracil, the frequency of cardiac ischaemia including myocardial infarction and congestive heart failure as well as the frequency of hand-foot syndrome (palmar-plantar erythrodysaesthesia) were increased compared to that with infusional 5-fluorouracil.

In combination with local radiation therapy of the head and neck area, additional undesirable effects were those typical of radiation therapy (such as mucositis, radiation dermatitis, dysphagia or leukopenia, mainly presenting as lymphocytopenia). In a randomised controlled clinical study with 424 patients, reporting rates of severe acute radiation dermatitis and mucositis as well as of late radiation-therapy-related events were slightly higher in patients receiving radiation therapy in combination with cetuximab than in those receiving radiation therapy alone.

4.9 Overdose

There is limited experience with single doses higher than 400 mg/m^2 body surface area to date or weekly administrations of doses higher than 250 mg/m^2 body surface area. In clinical studies with doses up to 700 mg/m^2 given every 2 weeks the safety profile was consistent with that described in section 4.8.

5. PHARMACOLOGICAL PROPERTIES

5.1 Pharmacodynamic properties

Pharmacotherapeutic group: Antineoplastic agents, monoclonal antibodies, ATC code: L01XC06

Mechanism of action

Cetuximab is a chimeric monoclonal IgG_1 antibody that is specifically directed against the epidermal growth factor receptor (EGFR).

EGFR signalling pathways are involved in the control of cell survival, cell cycle progression, angiogenesis, cell migration and cellular invasion/metastasis.

Cetuximab binds to the EGFR with an affinity that is approximately 5- to 10fold higher than that of endogenous ligands. Cetuximab blocks binding of endogenous EGFR ligands resulting in inhibition of the function of the receptor. It further induces the internalisation of EGFR, which can lead to down-regulation of EGFR. Cetuximab also targets cytotoxic immune effector cells towards EGFR-expressing tumour cells (antibody dependent cell-mediated cytotoxicity, ADCC).

Cetuximab does not bind to other receptors belonging to the HER family.

Table 1

Variable/ statistic	Overall population				KRAS wild-type population			
	Cetuximab plus FOLFIRI		FOLFIRI		Cetuximab plus FOLFIRI		FOLFIRI	
	(N=599)		(N=599)		(N=172)		(N=176)	
ORR								
% (95% CI)	46.9	(42.9, 51.0)	38.7	(34.8, 42.8)	59.3	(51.6, 66.7)	43.2	(35.8, 50.9)
p-value	0.0038				0.0025			
PFS								
Hazard Ratio (95% CI)	0.85 (0.726, 0.998)				0.68 (0.501, 0.934)			
p-value	0.0479				0.0167			

CI = confidence interval, FOLFIRI = irinotecan plus infusional 5-FU/FA, ORR = objective response rate (patients with complete response or partial response), PFS = progression-free survival time

The protein product of the proto-oncogene KRAS (Kirsten rat sarcoma 2 viral oncogene homologue) is a central down-stream signal-transducer of EGFR. In tumours, activation of KRAS by EGFR contributes to EGFR-mediated increased proliferation, survival and the production of pro-angiogenic factors.

KRAS is one of the most frequently activated oncogenes in human cancers. Mutations of the KRAS gene at certain hot-spots (mainly codons 12 and 13) result in constitutive activation of the KRAS protein independently of EGFR signalling.

Pharmacodynamic effects

In both *in vitro* and *in vivo* assays, cetuximab inhibits the proliferation and induces apoptosis of human tumour cells that express EGFR. *In vitro* cetuximab inhibits the production of angiogenic factors by tumour cells and blocks endothelial cell migration. *In vivo* cetuximab inhibits expression of angiogenic factors by tumour cells and causes a reduction in tumour neo-vascularisation and metastasis.

Immunogenicity

The development of human anti-chimeric antibodies (HACA) is a class effect of monoclonal chimeric antibodies. Current data on the development of HACAs is limited. Overall, measurable HACA titres were noted in 3.4% of the patients studied, with incidences ranging from 0% to 9.6% in the target indication studies. No conclusive data on the neutralising effect of HACAs on cetuximab is available to date. The appearance of HACA did not correlate with the occurrence of hypersensitivity reactions or any other undesirable effect to cetuximab.

Colorectal cancer

A diagnostic assay (EGFR pharmDx) was used for immunohistochemical detection of EGFR expression in tumour material. A tumour was considered to be EGFR-expressing, if one stained cell could be identified. Approximately 75% of the patients with metastatic colorectal cancer screened for clinical studies had an EGFR-expressing tumour and were therefore considered eligible for cetuximab treatment. The efficacy and safety of cetuximab have not been documented in patients with tumours where EGFR was not detected.

In metastatic colorectal cancer, the incidence of KRAS mutations is in the range of 30 - 50%. Recent data demonstrate that patients with KRAS wild-type metastatic colorectal cancer have a significantly higher chance to benefit from treatment with cetuximab or a combination of cetuximab and chemotherapy.

Cetuximab as a single agent or in combination with chemotherapy was investigated in 5 randomised controlled clinical studies and several supportive studies. The 5 randomised studies investigated a total of 3734 patients with metastatic colorectal cancer, in whom EGFR expression was detectable and who had an ECOG performance status of ⩽ 2. The majority of patients included had an ECOG performance status of ⩽ 1. In all studies, cetuximab was administered as described in section 4.2.

The KRAS status was recognised as predictive factor for the treatment with cetuximab in 4 of the randomised controlled studies. KRAS mutational status was available for 1261 patients. Only in study EMR 62 202-007, an analysis was not possible.

Cetuximab in combination with chemotherapy

• EMR 62 202-013: This randomised study in patients with metastatic colorectal cancer who had not received prior treatment for metastatic disease compared the combination of cetuximab and irinotecan plus infusional 5-fluorouracil/folinic acid (5-FU/FA) (599 patients) to the same chemotherapy alone (599 patients). The proportion of patients with KRAS wild-type tumours from the patient population evaluable for KRAS status comprised 64%.

The efficacy data generated in this study are summarised in the table above:

(see Table 1 above)

• EMR 62 202-047: This randomised study in patients with metastatic colorectal cancer who had not received prior treatment for metastatic disease compared the combination of cetuximab and oxaliplatin plus infusional 5-fluorouracil/folinic acid (5-FU/FA) (169 patients) to the same chemotherapy alone (168 patients). The proportion of patients with KRAS wild-type tumours from the patient population evaluable for KRAS status comprised 58%.

The efficacy data generated in this study are summarised in the table below:

(see Table 2 below)

• CA225006: This randomised study in patients with metastatic colorectal cancer who had received initial combination treatment with oxaliplatin plus fluoropyrimidine for metastatic disease compared the combination of cetuximab and irinotecan (648 patients) with irinotecan alone (650 patients). The proportion of patients with KRAS wild-type tumours from the patient population evaluable for KRAS status comprised 64%.

A significant difference in overall survival time could not be shown in this study. Following disease progression, treatment with EGFR-targeting agents was initiated in 50% of patients in the irinotecan-alone arm, which most likely impacted survival results. Objective response rate and progression free survival time were significantly improved with cetuximab. However, as no independent review of imaging data was conducted, these results have to be interpreted with caution.

• EMR 62 202-007: This randomised study in patients with metastatic colorectal cancer after failure of irinotecan-based treatment for metastatic disease as the last treatment before study entry compared the combination of cetuximab and irinotecan (218 patients) with cetuximab monotherapy (111 patients).

The combination of cetuximab with irinotecan compared to cetuximab alone reduced the overall risk of disease progression by 46% and significantly increased objective response rate. In the randomised trial, the improvement in overall survival time did not reach statistical significance; however, in the follow-up treatment, nearly 50% of the patients of the cetuximab alone arm received a combination of cetuximab and irinotecan after progression of disease, which may have influenced overall survival time.

Cetuximab as a single agent

• CA225025: This randomised study in patients with metastatic colorectal cancer who had received prior oxaliplatin-, irinotecan- and fluoropyrimidine-based treatment for metastatic disease compared the addition of cetuximab as a single agent to best supportive care (BSC) (287 patients) with best supportive care (285 patients). The proportion of patients with KRAS wild-type tumours from the patient population evaluable for KRAS status comprised 59%.

Addition of cetuximab to best supportive care reduced the overall risk of death in the overall study population by 23% and the overall risk of disease progression by 32%. Preliminary data from patients with KRAS wild-type tumours showed a more pronounced beneficial effect of cetuximab on overall survival time and progression free survival time.

Squamous cell cancer of the head and neck

Immunohistochemical detection of EGFR expression was not performed since more than 90% of patients with squamous cell cancer of the head and neck have tumours that express EGFR.

Cetuximab in combination with radiation therapy for locally advanced disease

• EMR 62 202-006: This randomised study compared the combination of cetuximab and radiation therapy (211 patients) with radiation therapy alone (213 patients) in patients with locally advanced squamous cell cancer of the head and neck. Cetuximab was started one week before radiation therapy and administered at the doses described in section 4.2 until the end of the radiation therapy period.

The efficacy data generated in this study are summarised in the table below:

(see Table 3 below)

Patients with a good prognosis as indicated by tumour stage, Karnofsky performance status (KPS) and age had a more pronounced benefit, when cetuximab was added to radiation therapy. No clinical benefit could be demonstrated in patients with KPS ⩽ 80 who were 65 years of age or older.

The use of cetuximab in combination with chemo-radiotherapy has so far not been adequately investigated. Thus, a benefit-risk ratio for this combination has not yet been established.

Table 2

Variable/ statistic	Overall population				KRAS wild-type population			
	Cetuximab plus FOLFOX		FOLFOX		Cetuximab plus FOLFOX		FOLFOX	
	(N=169)		(N=168)		(N=61)		(N=73)	
ORR								
% (95% CI)	45.6	(37.9, 53.4)	35.7	(28.5, 43.5)	60.7	(47.3, 72.9)	37.0	(26.0, 49.1)
p-value	0.064				0.011			
PFS								
Hazard Ratio (95% CI)	0.93 (0.70, 1.23)				0.57 (0.35, 0.91)			
p-value	0.6170				0.0163			

CI = confidence interval, FOLFOX = oxaliplatin plus infusional 5-FU/FA, ORR = objective response rate (patients with complete response or partial response), PFS = progression-free survival time

Table 3

Variable/ statistic	Radiation therapy + cetuximab		Radiation therapy alone	
	(N=211)		(N=213)	
Locoregional control				
months, median (95% CI)	24.4	(15.7, 45.1)	14.9	(11.8, 19.9)
Hazard Ratio (95% CI)	0.68 (0.52, 0.89)			
p-value	0.005			
OS				
months, median (95% CI)	49.0	(32.8, 62.6+)	29.3	(20.6, 42.8)
Hazard Ratio (95% CI)	0.74 (0.56, 0.97)			
p-value	0.032			

CI = confidence interval, OS = overall survival time, a '+' denotes that the upper bound limit had not been reached at cut-off

Cetuximab in combination with platinum-based chemotherapy in recurrent and/or metastatic disease

• EMR 62 202-002: This randomised study in patients with recurrent and/or metastatic squamous cell cancer of the head and neck who had not received prior chemotherapy for this disease compared the combination of cetuximab and cisplatin or carboplatin plus infusional 5-fluorouracil (222 patients) to the same chemotherapy alone (220 patients). Treatment in the cetuximab arm consisted of up to 6 cycles of platinum-based chemotherapy in combination with cetuximab followed by cetuximab as maintenance therapy until disease progression.

The efficacy data generated in this study are summarised in the table below:

Variable/ statistic	Cetuximab + CTX (N=222)	CTX (N=220)
OS		
months, median (95% CI)	10.1 (8.6, 11.2)	7.4 (6.4, 8.3)
Hazard Ratio (95% CI)	0.797 (0.644, 0.986)	
p-value	0.0362	
PFS		
months, median (95% CI)	5.6 (5.0, 6.0)	3.3 (2.9, 4.3)
Hazard Ratio (95% CI)	0.538 (0.431, 0.672)	
p-value	<0.0001	
ORR		
% (95% CI)	35.6 (29.3, 42.3)	19.5 (14.5, 25.4)
p-value	0.0001	

CI = confidence interval, CTX = platinum-based chemotherapy, ORR = objective response rate, OS = overall survival time, PFS = progression-free survival time

Patients with a good prognosis as indicated by tumour stage, Karnofsky performance status (KPS) and age had a more pronounced benefit, when cetuximab was added to platinum-based chemotherapy. In contrast to progression free survival time, no benefit in overall survival time could be demonstrated in patients with KPS ⩽ 80 who were 65 years of age or older.

5.2 Pharmacokinetic properties

Cetuximab pharmacokinetics were studied when cetuximab was administered as monotherapy or in combination with concomitant chemotherapy or radiation therapy in clinical studies. Intravenous infusions of cetuximab exhibited dose-dependent pharmacokinetics at weekly doses ranging from 5 to 500 mg/m^2 body surface area.

When cetuximab was administered at an initial dose of 400 mg/m^2 body surface area, the mean volume of distribution was approximately equivalent to the vascular space (2.9 l/m^2 with a range of 1.5 to 6.2 l/m^2). The mean C_{max} (± standard deviation) was 185±55 microgram per ml. The mean clearance was 0.022 l/h per m^2 body surface area. Cetuximab has a long elimination half-life with values ranging from 70 to 100 hours at the target dose.

Cetuximab serum concentrations reached stable levels after three weeks of cetuximab monotherapy. Mean peak cetuximab concentrations were 155.8 microgram per ml in week 3 and 151.6 microgram per ml in week 8, whereas the corresponding mean trough concentrations were 41.3 and 55.4 microgram per ml, respectively. In a study of cetuximab administered in combination with irinotecan, the mean cetuximab trough levels were 50.0 microgram per ml in week 12 and 49.4 microgram per ml in week 36.

Several pathways have been described that may contribute to the metabolism of antibodies. All of these pathways involve the biodegradation of the antibody to smaller molecules, i.e. small peptides or amino acids.

Pharmacokinetics in special populations

An integrated analysis across all clinical studies showed that the pharmacokinetic characteristics of cetuximab are not influenced by race, age, gender, renal or hepatic status.

Only patients with adequate renal and hepatic function have been investigated to date (serum creatinine ⩽ 1.5fold, transaminases ⩽ 5fold and bilirubin ⩽ 1.5fold the upper limit of normal).

5.3 Preclinical safety data

Dose-dependent skin alterations, starting at dose levels equivalent to those used in humans, were the major findings observed in toxicity studies with Cynomolgus monkeys (a chronic repeat-dose toxicity study and an embryo-foetal development study).

An embryo-foetal toxicity study in Cynomolgus monkeys revealed no signs of teratogenicity. However, dependent on the dose, an increased incidence of abortion was observed.

Non-clinical data on genotoxicity and local tolerance including accidental administration by routes other than the intended infusion revealed no special hazard for humans.

No formal animal studies have been performed to establish the carcinogenic potential of cetuximab or to determine its effects on male and female fertility.

Toxicity studies with co-administration of cetuximab and chemotherapeutic agents have not been performed.

No non-clinical data on the effect of cetuximab on wound healing are available to date. However, in preclinical wound healing models EGFR selective tyrosine kinase inhibitors were shown to retard wound healing.

6. PHARMACEUTICAL PARTICULARS

6.1 List of excipients

Sodium chloride

Glycine

Polysorbate 80

Citric acid monohydrate

Sodium hydroxide

Water for injections

6.2 Incompatibilities

This medicinal product must not be mixed with other medicinal products except those mentioned in section 6.6.

A separate infusion line must be used.

6.3 Shelf life

3 years.

Chemical and physical in-use stability of Erbitux 5 mg/ml has been demonstrated for 48 hours at 25°C, if the solution is prepared as described in section 6.6.

Erbitux does not contain any antimicrobial preservative or bacteriostatic agent. From a microbiological point of view, the product shall be used immediately after opening. If not used immediately, in-use storage times and conditions prior to use are the responsibility of the user and would normally not be longer than 24 hours at 2 to 8°C, unless opening has taken place in controlled and validated aseptic conditions.

6.4 Special precautions for storage

Store in a refrigerator (2°C - 8°C). Do not freeze.

For storage conditions after opening, see section 6.3.

6.5 Nature and contents of container

10 ml, 20 ml, 50 ml or 100 ml of solution in a vial (Type I glass) with a stopper (flurotec-coated bromobutyl rubber) and a seal (aluminium/polypropylen).

Pack size of 1.

Not all vial sizes may be marketed.

6.6 Special precautions for disposal and other handling

Erbitux may be administered via a gravity drip, an infusion pump or a syringe pump. A separate infusion line must be used for the infusion, and the line must be flushed with sterile sodium chloride 9 mg/ml (0.9%) solution for injection at the end of infusion.

Erbitux 5 mg/ml is compatible

• with polyethylene (PE), ethyl vinyl acetate (EVA) or polyvinyl chloride (PVC) bags,

• with polyethylene (PE), polyurethane (PUR), ethyl vinyl acetate (EVA), polyolefine thermoplastic (TP) or polyvinyl chloride (PVC) infusion sets,

• with polypropylene (PP) syringes for syringe pump.

Care must be taken to ensure aseptic handling when preparing the infusion.

Erbitux 5 mg/ml must be prepared as follows:

• For administration with infusion pump or gravity drip (diluted with sterile sodium chloride 9 mg/ml (0.9%) solution): Take an infusion bag of adequate size of sterile sodium chloride 9 mg/ml (0.9%) solution. Calculate the required volume of Erbitux. Remove an adequate volume of the sodium chloride solution from the infusion bag, using an appropriate sterile syringe with a suitable needle. Take an appropriate sterile syringe and attach a suitable needle. Draw up the required volume of Erbitux from a vial. Transfer the Erbitux into the prepared infusion bag. Repeat this procedure until the calculated volume has been reached. Connect the infusion line and prime it with the diluted Erbitux before starting the infusion. Use a gravity drip or an infusion pump for administration. Set and control the rate as explained in section 4.2.

• For administration with infusion pump or gravity drip (undiluted): Calculate the required volume of Erbitux. Take an appropriate sterile syringe (minimum 50 ml) and attach a suitable needle. Draw up the required volume of Erbitux from a vial. Transfer the Erbitux into a sterile evacuated container or bag. Repeat this procedure until the calculated volume has been reached. Connect the infusion line and prime it with Erbitux before starting the infusion. Set and control the rate as explained in section 4.2.

• For administration with a syringe pump: Calculate the required volume of Erbitux. Take an appropriate sterile syringe and attach a suitable needle. Draw up the required volume of Erbitux from a vial. Remove the needle and put the syringe into the syringe pump. Connect the infusion line to the syringe, set and control the rate as explained in section 4.2 and start the infusion after priming the line with Erbitux or sterile sodium chloride 9 mg/ml (0.9%) solution. If necessary, repeat this procedure until the calculated volume has been infused.

7. MARKETING AUTHORISATION HOLDER

Merck KGaA

64271 Darmstadt

Germany

8. MARKETING AUTHORISATION NUMBER(S)

EU/1/04/281/002

EU/1/04/281/003

EU/1/04/281/004

EU/1/04/281/005

9. DATE OF FIRST AUTHORISATION/RENEWAL OF THE AUTHORISATION

Date of first authorisation: 29/06/2004

Date of renewal: 01/07/2009

10. DATE OF REVISION OF THE TEXT

Detailed information on this medicinal product is available on the website of the European Medicines Agency (EMEA) http://www.emea.europa.eu/.

Erdotin 300mg capsules

(Galen Limited)

1. NAME OF THE MEDICINAL PRODUCT

Erdotin▼ 300 mg capsules

2. QUALITATIVE AND QUANTITATIVE COMPOSITION

Each capsule contains 300 mg of erdosteine

For full list of excipients, see section 6.1.

3. PHARMACEUTICAL FORM

Capsules, hard. The product appears as a capsule with a green cap and a yellow body

4. CLINICAL PARTICULARS

4.1 Therapeutic indications

As an expectorant. For the symptomatic treatment of acute exacerbations of chronic bronchitis in adults.

4.2 Posology and method of administration

Elderly and adults above 18 years:

300 mg twice daily for maximum 10 days.

The capsules must be swallowed whole with a glass of water.

4.3 Contraindications

Hypersensitivity to the active substance or to any of the other excipients.

Since there are no data in patients with creatinine clearance <25ml/min, or with severe liver failure, the use of erdosteine is not recommended in these patients.

Patients with active peptic ulcer.

4.4 Special warnings and precautions for use

No increase in adverse events has been observed with erdosteine in patients with mild liver failure; however these patients should not exceed a dose of 300 mg per day.

4.5 Interaction with other medicinal products and other forms of interaction

No adverse interactions have been reported.

4.6 Pregnancy and lactation

Pregnancy:

There is no experience for the use of erdosteine in pregnant women.

Lactation:

Experience is missing.

Therefore, the use of erdosteine in pregnant or breast-feeding women is not recommended.

4.7 Effects on ability to drive and use machines

Erdotin has minor or negligible influence on the ability to drive and use machines.

4.8 Undesirable effects

Less than 1 in 1,000 can expect to get gastrointestinal undesirable effects.

Nervous system disorders Very rare (<1/10,000)	Headache
Respiratory, thoracic and mediastinal disorders Very rare (<1/10,000)	Cold, dyspnoea
Gastrointestinal disorders Very rare (<1/10,000)	Taste alterations, nausea, vomiting, diarrhoea, epigastric pain
Dermatological disorders Very rare (<1/10,000)	Urticaria, erythema, eczema

4.9 Overdose

No experience of acute overdosage is available.

Symptomatic treatment and general supportive measures should be followed in all cases of overdosage.

Gastric lavage may be beneficial, followed by observation.

5. PHARMACOLOGICAL PROPERTIES
ATC Code: R 05 CB 15

Pharmacotherapeutic Group: Mucolytic Agent

5.1 Pharmacodynamic properties
Mucolytic agent reducing the viscosity of mucus and purulent sputum.

Erdosteine is a prodrug, becoming active after metabolism whereby free thiol groups are formed.

This effect is due to the opening of the disulfide bonds of the bronchial mucoproteins.

It has also been demonstrated that erdosteine inhibits bacterial adhesion to epithelial cells.

Due to the presence of a free thiol group in its active metabolite, erdosteine has a significant antioxidant action, demonstrated by both 'in vitro' and 'in vivo' studies.

5.2 Pharmacokinetic properties
Absorption

Erdosteine is quickly absorbed after oral administration and rapidly transformed through a first-pass metabolism to its biologically active metabolite – N-thiodiglycolyl-homocysteine (M1).

After administration of 300 mg, the peak plasma concentration of erdosteine (Cmax) - 1.26 ± 0.23 μg/ml - was reached 1.18 ± 0.26 hour after administration (Tmax), while M1 showed a Cmax of 3.46 μg/ml and a Tmax of 1.48 h.

The plasma concentrations of erdosteine increase in a dose-dependent manner. Plasma concentrations of M1 increased also with the dose, but not as proportionally as in the case of unchanged erdosteine.

The absorption is independent from food intake.

Distribution

In animal models, erdosteine was distributed mainly to kidneys, bone, spinal cord and liver.

Pharmacologically active concentrations of both erdosteine and M1 were found in Broncho Alveolar Lavage.

Elimination

The elimination T½ is 1.46 ± 0.60 h and 1.62 ± 0.59 h, respectively, for erdosteine and M1. In urine, only M1 and sulphates were found, faecal elimination is negligible.

No accumulation or change in the metabolism of erdosteine and M1 has been observed after oral administration of 600 to 900 mg daily for 8 days.

Influence of age

Age does not change the pharmacokinetics of erdosteine.

Binding to plasma proteins

The drug binding of erdosteine to plasma proteins is 64.5% (range: 50-86%).

5.3 Preclinical safety data
Preclinical safety data reveal no special hazard for humans based on conventional studies of safety pharmacology, repeated dose toxicity, genotoxicity and toxicity to reproduction.

6. PHARMACEUTICAL PARTICULARS
6.1 List of excipients
Capsule content:

Microcrystalline cellulose

Povidone

Magnesium stearate

Capsule shell:

Gelatin

Titanium dioxide (E171)

Iron oxide, yellow (E172)

Indigotine (E132)

6.2 Incompatibilities
Not applicable.

6.3 Shelf life
3 years

6.4 Special precautions for storage
Do not store above 25 °C.

6.5 Nature and contents of container
Each PVC/PVdC/Aluminium blister pack contains 10 capsules.

Pack-sizes of 20 or 60 capsules per carton.

Not all pack sizes may be marketed.

6.6 Special precautions for disposal and other handling
No special requirements

7. MARKETING AUTHORISATION HOLDER
Edmond Pharma S.r.l.

Via G. B. Grassi 15

20157 Milano

Italy

Representative in the United Kingdom and Ireland:

koGEN Limited

Seagoe Industrial Estate

Craigavon

BT63 5UA

UK

8. MARKETING AUTHORISATION NUMBER(S)
PL 14682/0012

PA 1325/1/1

9. DATE OF FIRST AUTHORISATION/RENEWAL OF THE AUTHORISATION
UK: 31st October 2006

ROI: 13th October 2006

10. DATE OF REVISION OF THE TEXT
UK: 31st October 2006

ROI: 13th October 2006

Ergocalciferol Injection BP 300,000U and 600,000U (UCB Pharma Ltd)

(UCB Pharma Limited)

1. NAME OF THE MEDICINAL PRODUCT
Ergocalciferol Injection BP 300,000U

Ergocalciferol Injection BP 600,000U

2. QUALITATIVE AND QUANTITATIVE COMPOSITION
Ergocalciferol BP 0.75% W/V

For a full list of excipients see section 6.1

3. PHARMACEUTICAL FORM
Solution for Injection

4. CLINICAL PARTICULARS
4.1 Therapeutic indications
Intramuscular therapy with Ergocalciferol Injection is used in patients with gastrointestinal, liver or biliary disease associated with malabsorption of Vitamin D, resulting in hypophosphataemia, rickets, and osteomalacia.

4.2 Posology and method of administration
Route of Administration: IM injection

Adults, Children and Elderly:

Dosage should be individualised by the clinician for each patient. Serum and urinary calcium concentrations, phosphate and BUN should be monitored at regular intervals, initially weekly, in order to achieve optimum clinical response and to avoid hypercalcaemia.

Doses should not normally exceed 40,000 units/day (1.0mg/day) for adults and 10,000 units/day (0.25mg/day) for children.

Ergocalciferol Injection may be administered as a single dose or repeated daily, dependent upon clinical response and requirements. Calcium and phosphorous supplements should be administered where necessary.

4.3 Contraindications
Hypercalcaemia, evidence of vitamin D toxicity, hypervitaminosis D, decreased renal function, metastatic calcification.

4.4 Special warnings and precautions for use
Adequate dietary calcium is necessary for clinical response to Ergocalciferol therapy.

Caution should be used when the injectable forms are used in patients with vitamin D resistant rickets as the range between the toxic and therapeutic dosage is narrow.

Vitamin D should be administered with caution to infants and patients who may have an increased sensitivity to its effects. Use with care in patients with renal impairment, renal calculi or heart disease or arteriosclerosis who might be at increased risk of organ damage if hypercalcaemia were to occur.

Ergocalciferol is not recommended for use in hypoparathyroidism. In the event of hypoparathyroidism when Ergocalciferol is used, calcium, parathyroid hormone or dihydrotachysterol may be required.

Dosage should be individualised. Frequent serum and urinary calcium, phosphate and urea nitrogen determinations should be carried out. Adequate fluid intake should be maintained.

Should hyperglycaemia develop, Ergocalciferol should be discontinued immediately.

Because of the effect on serum calcium, Ergocalciferol should only be administered to patients with renal stones when potential benefits outweigh possible hazards.

4.5 Interaction with other medicinal products and other forms of interaction
Ergocalciferol and:-

i) Magnesium-containing antacids: hypermagnesaemia may develop in patients on chronic renal dialysis.

ii) Digitalis glycosides: hypercalcaemia in patients on digitalis may precipitate cardiac arrhythmias.

iii) Verapamil atrial fibrillation has recurred when supplemental calcium and Ergocalciferol have induced hypercalcaemia.

iv) Anti-convulsants: vitamin D requirements may be increased in patients taking anti-convulsants (e.g. carbamazepine, phenobarbital, phenytoin and primidone).

v) Thiazide diuretics: hypoparathyroid patients on Ergocalciferol may develop hypercalcaemia due to increased Ergocalciferol (although Ergocalciferol is not recommended for use in hypoparathyroidism).

4.6 Pregnancy and lactation
Pregnancy: There are no adequate data on the use of Ergocalciferol in pregnant women. Ergocalciferol Injection should not be used in pregnancy unless the potential benefit outweighs the potential hazards to the foetus.

Animal studies have shown foetal abnormalities associated with hypervitaminosis D. Calcifediol and calcitriol are teratogenic in animals when given in doses several times the human dose. The offspring of a woman administered 17-144 times the recommended dose of calcitriol during pregnancy manifested mild hypercalcaemia in the first 2 days of life, which returned to normal at day 3.

Lactation: Ergocalciferol is excreted in breast milk in limited amounts. In a mother given large doses of Ergocalciferol, 25-hydroxycholecalciferol appeared in the milk and caused hypercalcaemia in the child. Monitoring of the infants serum calcium is required in such cases. Ergocalciferol should not be administered to breast-feeding mothers.

4.7 Effects on ability to drive and use machines
Ergocalciferol may cause drowsiness and, if affected, patients should not drive or operate machinery.

4.8 Undesirable effects
Adverse events are generally associated with excessive intake of ergocalciferol leading to the development of hypercalcaemia. The symptoms of hypercalcaemia can include:

Early: weakness; headache; somnolence; nausea; vomiting; dry mouth; constipation; diarrhoea; abdominal pain; fatigue; muscle weakness or pain; bone pain; metallic taste.

Late: polyuria; polydipsia; anorexia; irritability; weight loss; nocturia; mild acidosis; reversible azotaemia; generalised vascular calcification; nephrocalcinosis; conjunctivitis (calcific); pancreatitis; photophobia; rhinorrhoea; pruritis; hyperthermia; decreased libido; elevated BUN; albuminuria; hypercholesterolaemia; elevated AST and ALT; ectopic calcification; hypertension; cardiac arrhythmias; overt psychosis (rare).

In clinical studies on hypoparathyroidism and pseudohypopathyroidism, hypercalcaemia was noted on at least one occasion in about 1 in 3 patients and hypercalciuria in about 1 in 7. Elevated serum creatinine levels were observed in about 1 in 6 patients (approximately one half of whom had normal levels at baseline).

4.9 Overdose
Administration to patients in excess of their daily requirement can cause hypercalcaemia (see Section 4.8 Undesirable Effects), hypercalciuria and hyperphosphataemia. Concomitant high intake of calcium and phosphate may lead to similar abnormalities.

Treatment of chronic overdose with resulting hypercalcaemia consists of immediate withdrawal of the vitamin, a low calcium diet and generous fluid intake. Severe cases may require hydration with intravenous saline together with symptomatic and supportive treatment as indicated by the patient's clinical condition. Plasma calcium U & E's should be monitored.

5. PHARMACOLOGICAL PROPERTIES
5.1 Pharmacodynamic properties
Ergocalciferol (vitamin D) is a fat soluble vitamin. In conjunction with parathyroid hormone and calcitonin, it regulates calcium haemostasis. Ergocalciferol metabolites promote active absorption of calcium and phosphorous by the small intestine, increase rate of excretion and resorption of minerals in bone and promote resorption of minerals in bone and promote resorption of phosphate by renal tubules.

Ergocalciferol deficiency leads to rickets in children and osteomalacia in adults. Ergocalciferol reverses symptoms of nutritional rickets or osteomalacia unless permanent deformities have occurred.

5.2 Pharmacokinetic properties
Distribution - Stored chiefly in the liver, Ergocalciferol is also found in fat, muscle, skin and bones. In plasma, it is bound to alpha globulins and albumin.

Metabolism - There is a lag of 10 to 24 hours between administration of Ergocalciferol and initiation of its action in the body. Maximal hypercalcaemic effects occur about 4 weeks daily administration of a fixed dose and the duration of action can be ⩾ 2 months. Ergocalciferol is hydroxylated in the liver and further metabolism occurs in the kidney.

Excretion - The primary route of excretion of Ergocalciferol is in the bile. Additionally, some is excreted in the urine and faeces. There is also enterohepatic re-cycling.

5.3 Preclinical safety data
None stated.

6. PHARMACEUTICAL PARTICULARS
6.1 List of excipients
Ethyl oleate

6.2 Incompatibilities
None stated

6.3 Shelf life
36 months

6.4 Special precautions for storage
Store below 25°C

Protect from light

6.5 Nature and contents of container
Ergocalciferol Injection BP 300,000U - 1ml neutral glass (Type 1) ampoules

Ergocalciferol Injection BP 600,000U - 2ml neutral glass (Type 1) ampoules

6.6 Special precautions for disposal and other handling
Plastic syringes should not be used to administer Ergocalciferol Injection

7. MARKETING AUTHORISATION HOLDER
UCB Pharma Limited

208 Bath Road

Slough

Berkshire

SL1 3WE

UK

8. MARKETING AUTHORISATION NUMBER(S)
PL 00039/5655R - Ergocalciferol Injection BP 300,000U

PL 00039/5656R - Ergocalciferol Injection BP 600,000U

9. DATE OF FIRST AUTHORISATION/RENEWAL OF THE AUTHORISATION
25 July 1988 / 13 December 1994 / 04 August 2000

10. DATE OF REVISION OF THE TEXT
Approved: April 2009

Ergocalciferol Tablets BP 0.25mg (UCB Pharma Ltd)

(UCB Pharma Limited)

1. NAME OF THE MEDICINAL PRODUCT
Ergocalciferol Tablets BP 0.25 mg

2. QUALITATIVE AND QUANTITATIVE COMPOSITION
Vitamin D_2 11.8 mg equivalent to 10,000 iu of Vitamin D. ≡ Ergocalciferol 0.25 mg.

For excipients, see 6.1.

3. PHARMACEUTICAL FORM
White biconvex sugar coated tablets with white cores.

4. CLINICAL PARTICULARS

4.1 Therapeutic indications
Simple Vitamin D deficiency

Vitamin D deficiency caused by intestinal malabsorption or chronic liver disease.

Hypocalcaemia of hypoparathyroidism.

4.2 Posology and method of administration
In the treatment of Vitamin D deficiency conditions 0.25 mg (10 000 units or one tablet) daily.

Vitamin D deficiency caused by intestinal malabsorption or chronic liver disease usually requires doses of up to 1 mg (40,000 iu or 4 tablets) daily in divided doses.

In the treatment of hypoparathyroidism 1.25 mg to 5 mg (50 000 to 200 000 units or 5 to 20 tablets) daily.

The hypocalcaemia of hypoparathyroidism often requires doses of up to 5 mg (200,000 iu or 20 tablets) daily in divided doses.

Patients with renal osteodystrophy may require as much as 5 mg (200 000 units or 20 tablets) daily.

For children and the elderly the adult dosage may require adjustment according to the severity of the condition.

This medicine is taken by mouth.

4.3 Contraindications
Renal insufficiency, Hypercalcaemia, evidence of vitamin D toxicity and metastatic calcification.

4.4 Special warnings and precautions for use
Vitamin D should be administered with caution to infants and patients who may have an increased sensitivity to its effects. Use with care in patients with renal impairment, renal calculi or heart disease or arteriosclerosis who might be at increased risk of organ damage if hypercalcaemia were to occur.

All patients receiving pharmacological doses of vitamin D should have their plasma calcium concentration checked at intervals and whenever nausea and vomiting are present.

Patients with rare hereditary problems of galactose intolerance, fructose intolerance, glucose-galactose malabsorption, the Lapp-lactase deficiency or sucrase-isomaltase insufficiency should not take this medicine.

Adequate fluid intake should be maintained.

4.5 Interaction with other medicinal products and other forms of interaction
Phosphate infusions should not be administered to lower hypercalcaemia of hypervitaminosis D because of the dangers of metastatic calcification.

Vitamin D requirements may be increased in patients taking anti-convulsants (e.g. carbamazepine, phenobarbital, phenytoin, and primidone).

Absorption of calcium may be reduced by oral sodium sulphate or parenteral magnesium sulphate.

Concurrent use of Vitamin D analogues and cardiac glycosides may result in cardiac arrhythmias due to hypercalcaemia.

There is an increased risk of hypercalcaemia if vitamin D is administered with thiazide diuretics and calcium.

4.6 Pregnancy and lactation
Pregnancy: There are no adequate data on the use of Ergocalciferol in pregnant women. Ergocalciferol should not be used in pregnancy unless the potential benefit outweighs the potential hazards to the foetus.

Animal studies have shown foetal abnormalities associated with hypervitaminosis D. Calcifediol and calcitriol are teratogenic in animals when given in doses several times the human dose. The offspring of a woman administered 17-144 times the recommended dose of calcitriol during pregnancy manifested mild hypercalcaemia in the first 2 days of life, which returned to normal at day 3.

Lactation: Ergocalciferol is excreted in breast milk in limited amounts. In a mother given large doses of Ergocalciferol, 25-hydroxycholecalciferol appeared in the milk and caused hypercalcaemia in the child. Monitoring of the infants serum calcium is required in such cases. Ergocalciferol should not be administered to breast-feeding mothers.

4.7 Effects on ability to drive and use machines
None documented.

4.8 Undesirable effects
Adverse events are generally associated with excessive intake of ergocalciferol leading to the development of hypercalcaemia. The symptoms of hypercalcaemia can include; anorexia, nausea, vomiting, diarrhoea, loss of weight, headache, polyuria, thirst, vertigo, constipation, fatigue, bone pain, muscle weakness, abdominal pain, mental disturbances, impaired renal function, kidney stones and cardiac arrhythmias.

4.9 Overdose
A single acute overdose is virtually non-toxic and requires supportive treatment liberal fluids only.

Chronic administration to patients in excess of their daily requirement can cause hypercalcaemia (see Section 4.8 undesirable effects), hypercalciuria and hyperphosphataemia. Concomitant high intake of calcium and phosphate may lead to similar abnormalities.

Treatment of chronic overdose with resulting hypercalcaemia consists of immediate withdrawal of the vitamin, a low calcium diet, and generous fluid intake. Severe cases may require hydration with intravenous saline together with symptomatic and supportive treatment as indicated by the patient's clinical condition. Plasma calcium and U&E's should be monitored.

5. PHARMACOLOGICAL PROPERTIES

5.1 Pharmacodynamic properties
Vitamin D_2 is a steroid derivative which controls the calcification of bones in both the young and old.

Although naturally produced under normal conditions, pharmacological doses are often required in disease states.

5.2 Pharmacokinetic properties
Vitamin D_2 is partly esterified during its absorption and is blood borne bound to α_2-globulins and albumin. About ½ of the ingested oral dose is excreted into the bile and lost with the faeces.

5.3 Preclinical safety data
Not applicable since ergocalciferol has been used in clinical practice for many years and its effects in man are well known.

6. PHARMACEUTICAL PARTICULARS

6.1 List of excipients
Avicel PH 101 (microcrystalline cellulose),

Magnesium Stearate,

Lactose DCL 11,

Acacia,

Sugar,

Talc,

Gelatin,

Titanium Dioxide,

Opaglos AG 7350.

6.2 Incompatibilities
None stated.

6.3 Shelf life
36 months.

6.4 Special precautions for storage
Store below 25°C in a well closed container protected from light.

6.5 Nature and contents of container
1.) Containers having snap-on Polythene lids, with integral tear-off security seals eg Jaycare "securitainer" or Wragby "snap-secure" container containing 100 tablets.

2.) Blister packs of 28 or 50 tablets in cartons which are white folding box board printed on white, the blister comprises 250 micron white rigid UPVC backed by 20 micron hard tempered aluminium foil, bearing a 6-8 gm^{-2} vinyl heat seal coating on the inner surface and printed / over lacquered on the reverse.

6.6 Special precautions for disposal and other handling
No special precautions are required.

7. MARKETING AUTHORISATION HOLDER
UCB Pharma Ltd

208 Bath Road

Slough

Berkshire

SL1 3WE

8. MARKETING AUTHORISATION NUMBER(S)
PL 00039/0545

9. DATE OF FIRST AUTHORISATION/RENEWAL OF THE AUTHORISATION
April 2007

10. DATE OF REVISION OF THE TEXT
November 2007

Ergocalciferol Tablets BP 1.25mg (UCB Pharma Ltd)

(UCB Pharma Limited)

1. NAME OF THE MEDICINAL PRODUCT
Ergocalciferol Tablets BP 1.25mg

2. QUALITATIVE AND QUANTITATIVE COMPOSITION
Ergocalciferol 1.25 mg as Vitamin D_2 (gelatin coated) 62 mg

3. PHARMACEUTICAL FORM
White biconvex sugar coated tablets

4. CLINICAL PARTICULARS

4.1 Therapeutic indications
For the treatment of hypocalcaemia caused by of hypoparathyroidism or in patients with renal osteodystrophy.

4.2 Posology and method of administration
Adults, Children and Elderly

A dose of 1.25 to 5mg daily is recommended. The dose should be adjusted according to the severity of the condition.

This medicine is delivered by oral administration

4.3 Contraindications
Renal insufficiency, Hypercalcaemia, evidence of vitamin D toxicity and metastatic calcification.

Ergocalciferol Tablets BP 1.25mg are unsuitable for use in vitamin D deficiency diseases such as rickets.

4.4 Special warnings and precautions for use
Vitamin D should be administered with caution to infants and patients who may have an increased sensitivity to its effects. Use with care in patients with renal impairment, renal calculi or heart disease or arteriosclerosis who might be at increased risk of organ damage if hypercalcaemia were to occur.

All patients receiving pharmacological doses of vitamin D should have their plasma calcium concentration checked at intervals and whenever nausea and vomiting are present.

Patients with rare hereditary problems of galactose intolerance, fructose intolerance, glucose-galactose malabsorption, the Lapp-lactase deficiency or sucrase-isomaltase insufficiency should not take this medicine.

Adequate fluid intake should be maintained.

4.5 Interaction with other medicinal products and other forms of interaction
Phosphate infusions should not be administered to lower hypercalcaemia of hypervitaminosis D because of the dangers of metastatic calcification.

Vitamin D requirements may be increased in patients taking anti-convulsants (e.g. carbamazepine, phenobarbital, phenytoin, and primidone).

Absorption of calcium may be reduced by oral sodium sulphate or parenteral magnesium sulphate.

Concurrent use of Vitamin D analogues and cardiac glycosides may result in cardiac arrhythmias due to hypercalcaemia.

There is an increased risk of hypercalcaemia if vitamin D is administered with thiazide diuretics and calcium.

4.6 Pregnancy and lactation
Pregnancy: There are no adequate data on the use of Ergocalciferol in pregnant women. Ergocalciferol should not be used in pregnancy unless the potential benefit outweighs the potential hazards to the foetus.

Animal studies have shown foetal abnormalities associated with hypervitaminosis D. Calcifediol and calcitriol are teratogenic in animals when given in doses several times the human dose. The offspring of a woman administered 17-144 times the recommended dose of calcitriol during pregnancy manifested mild hypercalcaemia in the first 2 days of life, which returned to normal at day 3.

Lactation: Ergocalciferol is excreted in breast milk in limited amounts. In a mother given large doses of Ergocalciferol, 25-hydroxycholecalciferol appeared in the milk and caused hypercalcaemia in the child. Monitoring of the infants serum calcium is required in such cases. Ergocalciferol should not be administered to breast-feeding mothers.

4.7 Effects on ability to drive and use machines
None documented.

4.8 Undesirable effects
Adverse events are generally associated with excessive intake of ergocalciferol leading to the development of hypercalcaemia. The symptoms of hypercalcaemia can include; anorexia, nausea, vomiting, diarrhoea, loss of weight, headache, polyuria, thirst, vertigo, constipation, fatigue, bone pain, muscle weakness, abdominal pain, mental disturbances, impaired renal function, kidney stones and cardiac arrhythmias.

4.9 Overdose
A single acute overdose is virtually non-toxic and requires supportive treatment with liberal fluids only.

Chronic administration to patients in excess of their daily requirement can cause hypercalcaemia (see Section 4.8 undesirable effects), hypercalciuria and hyperphosphataemia. Concomitant high intake of calcium and phosphate may lead to similar abnormalities.

Treatment of chronic overdose with resulting hypercalcaemia consists of immediate withdrawal of the vitamin, a low calcium diet, and generous fluid intake. Severe cases may require hydration with intravenous saline together with symptomatic and supportive treatment as indicated by the patient's clinical condition. Plasma calcium and U&E's should be monitored.

5. PHARMACOLOGICAL PROPERTIES

5.1 Pharmacodynamic properties
ATC code: A11CC01.

Ergocalciferol, an oil soluble vitamin, increases the intestinal absorption of dietary calcium and increases the release of calcium from bone. These effects combine to raise the plasma calcium concentration.

Hyperparathyroidism causes a fall in plasma calcium concentration. Large doses of ergocalciferol control plasma calcium levels and is the preferred maintenance therapy of this disease.

5.2 Pharmacokinetic properties
Ergocalciferol is well absorbed after oral administration. The half-life is about 960 hours, with protein binding in the blood to alpha and beta-lipoproteins. It is secreted in milk and stored in the liver. Metabolism is by 25 hydroxylation in the liver, followed by hydroxylation at positions 12 or 24 by the kidney. The rate of kidney metabolism is controlled by parathyroid hormone. There is possible conjugation with sulphate or glucuronic acid and decreased absorption may result from impaired liver or biliary function.

5.3 Preclinical safety data
Not applicable.

6. PHARMACEUTICAL PARTICULARS

6.1 List of excipients
Tablet core:

Avicel PH 101 (microcrystalline cellulose)

Magnesium Stearate

Lactose monohydrate

Tablet coats:

Acacia

Sugar

Talc

Gelatin

Titanium Dioxide

Opaglos AG-7350 (containing: purified water, beeswax, carnuaba wax, polysorbate 20, sorbic acid (E200)).

6.2 Incompatibilities
None stated.

6.3 Shelf life
36 months

6.4 Special precautions for storage
Store below 25° C in a well closed container.

6.5 Nature and contents of container
Containers of pigmented polypropylene having snap secure closure of pigmented low density polyethylene, containing 100 tablets.

6.6 Special precautions for disposal and other handling
No special precautions are required.

7. MARKETING AUTHORISATION HOLDER
UCB Pharma Ltd

208 Bath Road

Slough

Berkshire

SL1 3WE

8. MARKETING AUTHORISATION NUMBER(S)
PL 00039/0546

9. DATE OF FIRST AUTHORISATION/RENEWAL OF THE AUTHORISATION
April 2007

10. DATE OF REVISION OF THE TEXT
November 2007.

Erwinase

(EUSA Pharma (Europe) Limited)

1. NAME OF THE MEDICINAL PRODUCT
ERWINASE®, 10,000 Units/vial, Lyophilisate for solution for injection.

2. QUALITATIVE AND QUANTITATIVE COMPOSITION
Crisantaspase (Asparaginase from *Erwinia chrysanthemi*; *Erwinia* L-asparaginase), 10,000 Units/vial.

For a full list of excipients, see section 6.1.

3. PHARMACEUTICAL FORM
Lyophilisate for solution for injection.

White lyophilised powder in a vial.

4. CLINICAL PARTICULARS

4.1 Therapeutic indications
Erwinase is used in combination with other anti-neoplastic agents to treat acute lymphoblastic leukaemia. It may also be used in other neoplastic conditions where depletion of asparagine might be expected to have a useful effect. Patients receiving treatment with L-asparaginase from *Escherichia coli*, and who develop hypersensitivity to that enzyme may be able to continue treatment with Erwinase as the enzymes are immunologically distinct.

4.2 Posology and method of administration
Erwinase solution can be given by intravenous injection or by intramuscular or subcutaneous injection.

For all patients the usual dose is 6,000 Units/m^2 body surface area (200 Units/kg of body weight), three times a week for three weeks.

Therapy may be further intensified according to protocol.

Reference to current Medical Research Council protocols on leukaemia therapy should be made for information on dose, route and frequency of treatment.

4.3 Contraindications
Previous allergic reaction to *Erwinia* asparaginase.

Previous episode of acute pancreatitis related to L-asparaginase therapy.

Breast-feeding (see section 4.6).

4.4 Special warnings and precautions for use
Warnings: Anaphylactic reactions have been observed after the use of Erwinase. Facilities should be made available for management of an anaphylactic reaction, should it occur, during administration.

Careful observation is required on re-exposure to L-asparaginase after any time interval (e.g. between induction and consolidation), which may increase the risk of anaphylactic reactions occurring.

Careful monitoring before and during therapy is necessary:

• Serum amylase, lipase and/or insulin levels should be monitored to exclude hyperglycaemia and severe pancreatitis. Hyperglycaemia may be treated with insulin, if needed.

• Routine clotting screening may be performed before treatment initiation. If significant symptomatic coagulopathy occurs withhold L-asparaginase treatment until resolved then continue according to protocol.

• Hepatic function tests should be monitored regularly during therapy.

4.5 Interaction with other medicinal products and other forms of interaction
Asparaginase must not be mixed with any other drugs prior to administration.

Concomitant use of L-asparaginase and drugs affecting liver function may increase the risk of a change in liver parameters (e.g. increase of ASAT, ALAT, bilirubin).

L-asparaginase may diminish or abolish methotrexate's effect on malignant cells; this effect persists as long as plasma asparagine levels are suppressed. Do not use methotrexate with, or following L-asparaginase, while asparagine levels are below normal.

Concomitant use of prednisone and L-asparaginase may increase the risk of a change in clotting parameters (e.g. a decrease in fibrinogen and ATIII levels).

Administration of vincristine concurrently with or immediately before treatment with L-asparaginase may be associated with increased toxicity and increased risk of anaphylaxis.

4.6 Pregnancy and lactation
Pregnancy: there are no adequate data from the use of Crisantaspase (*Erwinia* L-asparaginase) in pregnant women.

Limited reports in humans of the use of *E.coli* asparaginase in combination with other antineoplastics during pregnancy did not provide sufficient data to conclude.

However, based on effects on embryonal/foetal development shown in pre-clinical studies (see section 5.3), Erwinase should not be used during pregnancy unless clearly necessary.

Lactation: it is not known whether Crisantaspase (*Erwinia* L-asparaginase) is excreted in human breast milk. The excretion of Crisantaspase (*Erwinia* L-asparaginase) has not been studied in animals. Because potential serious adverse reactions may occur in nursing infants, breast-feeding is contra-indicated.

4.7 Effects on ability to drive and use machines
None known.

4.8 Undesirable effects
Adverse effects reported spontaneously and in the literature, from patients treated with L-asparaginase as part of their chemotherapy regime, are listed in the table below. Adverse effects are categorised by system organ class and frequency.

The two most frequent adverse reactions are:

- Hypersensitivity, including urticaria, laryngeal oedema, bronchospasm, hypotension or even anaphylactic shock. In case of systemic hypersensitivity reaction, treatment should be discontinued immediately and withdrawn.

- Coagulation abnormalities (e.g. thromboses), due to protein synthesis impairment, are the second most frequent class of adverse reactions. Thromboses of peripheral, pulmonary or central nervous system blood vessels have been reported, potentially fatal or with residual delayed affects dependent upon the location of the occlusion. Other risk factors contributing to coagulation abnormalities include the disease itself, concomitant steroid therapy and central venous catheters.

Pancreatic disorders – acute pancreatitis occurs in < 10% of cases. There have been isolated reports of pseudocyst formation up to four months after last treatment, so appropriate testing (e.g. ultrasound) may need to be considered beyond last treatment. In very rare cases, haemorrhagic or necrotising pancreatitis occurs, with fatal consequences. L-asparaginase can affect endocrine pancreatic function. Hyperglycaemia is the most commonly reported undesired effect and is readily controlled with administration of insulin. Isolated cases of diabetic ketoacidosis have been reported.

Nervous system and cardiac disorders are often secondary to other adverse effects (e.g. thrombo-embolism) or synergistic to the effects of other chemotherapy drugs (e.g. delayed methotrexate clearance).

Undesirable effects are generally reversible.

Frequency definitions: very common (≥1/10), common (≥1/100 to < 1/10), uncommon (≥1/1000 to < 1/100), rare (≥1/10000 to < 1/1000) and very rare (< 1/10000).

When no valid estimate of the incidence rate for an adverse event from available data can be calculated, the frequency of such ADR has been classified as "Not known".

Isolated cases reported in the literature or spontaneously have been classified as "Rare" or "Very Rare".

(see Table 1 on next page)

4.9 Overdose
No specific measures are recommended.

5. PHARMACOLOGICAL PROPERTIES

5.1 Pharmacodynamic properties
Pharmacotherapeutic group: other antineoplastic agents

ATC code: L01XX02

Asparagine is found incorporated into most proteins, and protein synthesis is halted in its absence, thereby inhibiting RNA and DNA synthesis with a resulting halt to cellular proliferation.

Neoplastic cells associated with Acute Lymphoblastic Leukaemia (ALL), Acute Myeloid Leukaemia (AML) and Non-Hodgkin's Lymphoma (especially the lymphoblastic form) are lacking asparagine synthetase activity and are dependent upon exogenous asparagine.

The anti-tumour activity of L-asparaginase is a result of the sustained depletion of exogenous asparagine. L-asparaginase catalyses the deamination of asparagine to aspartic acid with the release of ammonia. The biochemical reaction may be depicted schematically as follows:

$$\text{Asparagine} \xrightarrow{\textit{Erwinia}\ \text{L-asparaginase}} \text{Aspartate} + NH_3$$

It has also been noted that asparaginase, in addition to its asparaginase activity, has significant glutaminase activity. It catalyses the deamination of glutamine in glutamic acid with the release of ammonia as follows:

$$\text{Glutamine} \xrightarrow{\textit{Erwinia}\ \text{L-asparaginase}} \text{Glutamate} + NH_3$$

Glutamine may lead to alternative asparagine synthesis and therefore glutamine depletion may complement asparagine depletion. However, exact potential of this glutaminase activity remains unknown.

Table 1

Infections and infestations:	
Very rare:	Infections and life-threatening sepsis.
Blood and lymphatic system disorders:	
Very Common:	Coagulation abnormalities - decreased levels of clotting factor, antithrombin III, protein C, protein S and fibrinogen[1].
Common:	Coagulation abnormalities associated with bleeding or thrombotic complications, hypofibrinogenemia, asymptomatic coagulopathy.
Very Rare:	Neutropenia, febrile neutropenia and thrombocytopenia.
Not known:	Haemorrhage.
Immune system disorders:	
Common:	Hypersensitivity or systemic allergic reactions.
Uncommon:	Anaphylaxis.
Metabolic and nutrition disorders:	
Common:	Elevation of serum amylases and lipase.
Uncommon:	Hyperlipidaemia[1] and hyperglycaemia.
Rare:	Diabetic ketoacidosis.
Not known:	Hyperammonaemia[3]
Nervous system disorders:	
Common:	Lethargy, somnolence, confusion, dizziness, neurotoxicity, convulsions (grand mal, partial seizures)[2], headache.
Rare:	Dysphasia, dysphagia, paresis and encephalopathy[3], CNS depression and coma.
Cardiac disorders:	
Rare:	Myocardial infarction – secondary to other adverse events (e.g. thrombosis, pancreatitis).
Vascular disorders:	
Common:	Thrombosis of peripheral, pulmonary or central nervous system blood vessels and pallor.
Not known:	Hypertension, flushing[4] and hypotension[4].
Respiratory, thoracic and mediastinal disorders:	
Common:	Dyspnoea[4].
Uncommon:	Laryngeal oedema[4], respiratory arrest, hypoxia, rhinitis and bronchospasm[4]
Gastrointestinal system disorders:	
Common:	Diarrhoea and acute pancreatitis.
Very rare:	Haemorrhagic or necrotising pancreatitis.
Not known:	Nausea, vomiting and abdominal pain.
Hepato-biliary disorders:	
Common:	Elevation of bilirubin, ALT, AST, alkaline phosphatase and cholesterol levels, liver toxicity.
Rare:	Hepatic failure.
Not known:	Hepatomegaly, jaundice (cholestatic), increased BSP retention.
Skin and sub-cutaneous tissue disorders:	
Common:	Rashes, urticaria, pruritis, erythema, facial oedema and swelling lips[4].
Musculoskeletal and connective tissue disorders:	
Very rare:	Myalgia and reactive arthritis.
Not known:	Pain in extremities.
General disorders:	
Common:	Pyrexia, chills, swelling of limbs and injection site reactions (including pain, erythema, purpura and swelling at injection site), generalised pain.

1 As a consequence of inhibition of protein synthesis.

2 Convulsions may be associated with cases of thrombosis or metabolic encephalopathy.

3 As a consequence of excessive ammonia production induced by the action of L-asparaginase on endogenous asparagine and glutamine.

4 These symptoms are commonly associated with hypersensitivity reactions.

5.2 Pharmacokinetic properties

Peak levels of Erwinase are achieved in blood in 1 to 2 hours. The fall in enzyme levels follows first order kinetics with a half-life of 7 to 13 hours.

5.3 Preclinical safety data

Embryotoxicity studies with *Erwinia* L-asparaginase have given evidence of teratogenic potential in rabbits. In addition, pre-clinical experience with other asparaginase preparations has shown teratogenic potential in rats, mice and rabbits with doses in the therapeutic ranges.

6. PHARMACEUTICAL PARTICULARS

6.1 List of excipients

Sodium Chloride

Glucose Monohydrate

6.2 Incompatibilities

See section 4.5 "Interactions with other medicinal products and other forms of interaction".

6.3 Shelf life

Shelf-life of product as packed for sale: 3 years.

Shelf-life following reconstitution according to directions: 15 minutes in the original container, 8 hours in a glass or polypropylene syringe. (See section 6.6 "Instructions for use/handling").

6.4 Special precautions for storage

Store in a refrigerator (+2°C to +8°C).

6.5 Nature and contents of container

Type 1 clear neutral glass vials of 3 ml nominal capacity, closed with 13 mm halobutyl freeze-drying stoppers and aluminium overseals, containing a white lyophilised solid.

Pack size: 5 vials.

6.6 Special precautions for disposal and other handling

The contents of each vial should be reconstituted in 1 ml to 2 ml of sodium chloride (0.9%) solution for injection. Slowly add the reconstitution solution against the inner vial wall, do not squirt directly onto or into the powder. Allow the contents to dissolve by gentle mixing or swirling maintaining the vial in an upright position. Avoid froth formation due to excessive or vigorous shaking.

The solution should be clear without any visible particles. Fine crystalline or thread-like wisps of protein aggregates may be visible if shaking is excessive. If there are any visible particles or protein aggregates present the reconstituted solution should be rejected.

The solution should be administered within 15 minutes of reconstitution. If a delay of more than 15 minutes between reconstitution and administration is unavoidable, the solution should be withdrawn into a glass or polypropylene syringe for the period of the delay. The solution should be used within 8 hours.

Erwinase is not a cytotoxic drug (such as vincristine or methotrexate) and does not require the special precautions needed for manipulating such agents.

It should be handled in the same way as other therapeutic enzymes such as hyaluronidase.

Any unused product or waste material should be disposed of in accordance with local requirements.

7. MARKETING AUTHORISATION HOLDER

Health Protection Agency

Centre for Emergency Preparedness and Response

Porton Down, Salisbury, SP4 0JG

United Kingdom

8. MARKETING AUTHORISATION NUMBER(S)

PL 20170/0001

9. DATE OF FIRST AUTHORISATION/RENEWAL OF THE AUTHORISATION

First authorisation: 19 July 1985

Latest renewal: 25 May 2006

10. DATE OF REVISION OF THE TEXT

March 2009

Local representative:

EUSA Pharma (Europe) Limited

Pharmacovigilance and medical information

Tel: +44 (0)14 38 740 720

Fax: +44 (0)14 38 735 740

e-mail: medinfo-uk@eusapharma.com

Erwinase is a registered trademark of the Health Protection Agency.

Eryacne 4

(Galderma (U.K) Ltd)

1. NAME OF THE MEDICINAL PRODUCT

Eryacne 4

2. QUALITATIVE AND QUANTITATIVE COMPOSITION

Eryacne 4 contains 4% w/w erythromycin Ph. Eur, expressed as erythromycin base with a potency of 1,000 IU/mg.

3. PHARMACEUTICAL FORM

Eryacne 4 is an alcohol-based gel for topical (cutaneous) use.

4. CLINICAL PARTICULARS

4.1 Therapeutic indications

Eryacne 4 is intended for the topical (cutaneous) treatment of *acne vulgaris*.

4.2 Posology and method of administration

Eryacne 4 is recommended for the first four weeks of treatment. If the condition has improved after four weeks, Eryacne 2 (containing 2% w/w erythromycin) may be substituted.

A thin film of Eryacne should be applied to the affected areas twice daily, morning and evening. These areas should be washed and dried before the product is used.

As a rule, treatment is continued for eight weeks, although this period may be extended to obtain a satisfactory response.

4.3 Contraindications
Eryacne 4 is contra-indicated in persons known to be sensitive to any of the ingredients.

4.4 Special warnings and precautions for use
Eryacne 4 is for external use only and should be kept away from the eyes, nose, mouth and other mucous membranes. If accidental contact does occur, the area should be washed with lukewarm water.

If a reaction suggesting sensitivity or a severe reaction occurs, use of the product should be discontinued. Depending upon the degree of irritation, the patient should be advised to use the product less frequently, to discontinue its use temporarily or to discontinue its use altogether.

Cross-resistance could occur with other antibiotics of the macrolide group.

4.5 Interaction with other medicinal products and other forms of interaction
Concurrent topical acne therapy should be used with caution because a cumulative irritant effect could occur.

Concurrent use of exfoliants or medicated soaps or cosmetics containing alcohol could also cause a cumulative irritant or drying effect in patients using Eryacne 4.

Erythromycin and clindamycin topical preparations should not be used concurrently.

4.6 Pregnancy and lactation
There is no evidence of risk from using erythromycin in human pregnancy. It has been in wide use for many years without apparent ill consequence. Animal reproduction studies have shown no risk.

If Eryacne 4 is used during lactation, it should not be applied on the chest to avoid accidental ingestion by the infant.

4.7 Effects on ability to drive and use machines
Performance related to driving and using machines should not be affected by the use of Eryacne 4.

4.8 Undesirable effects
Adverse reactions reported to date with topical erythromycin therapy include dryness, irritation, pruritis, erythema, desquamation, oiliness and a burning sensation.

Most of these reactions appear to be caused by alcohol or other excipients rather than by erythromycin and are reversible when the frequency of application is reduced or treatment is discontinued.

4.9 Overdose
Eryacne 4 is for cutaneous use only. If the product is applied excessively, no more rapid or better results will be obtained, and marked redness, peeling or discomfort could occur. If these effects should occur, the frequency of application could be reduced or treatment discontinued and appropriate symptomatic therapy instituted.

The acute oral toxicity in mice and rats is greater than 10ml.kg^{-1}. Unless the amount accidentally ingested is small, an appropriate method of gastric emptying should be considered provided that this is carried out soon after ingestion. One unopened 30g tube of Eryacne 4 contains about 30ml of alcohol.

5. PHARMACOLOGICAL PROPERTIES

5.1 Pharmacodynamic properties
Erythromycin is a macrolide antibiotic active *in vivo* and *in vitro* against most aerobic and anaerobic gram-positive bacteria as well as some gram-negative bacilli.

Erythromycin is usually bacteriostatic in action, but may be bacteriocidal in high concentrations or against highly susceptible organisms.

Erythromycin appears to inhibit protein synthesis in susceptible organisms by reversible binding to 50S ribosomal subunits. Following application to the skin, the drug inhibits the growth of susceptible organisms (principally *Propionibacterium acnes*) on the surface of the skin and reduces the concentration of free fatty acids in the sebum. The reduction of free fatty acids in sebum may be an indirect result of the inhibition of lipase-producing organisms that convert triglycerides into free fatty acids. It may also be a direct result of interference with lipase production in these organisms.

Free fatty acids are comedogenic and are believed to be a positive cause of the inflammatory lesions of acne, e.g. papules, pustules, nodules and cysts. However, other mechanisms may be involved in the clinical improvement of *acne* as a direct result of the anti-inflammatory action of erythromycin applied topically to the skin.

5.2 Pharmacokinetic properties
Erythromycin does not appear to be absorbed systemically following application of Eryacne 4 to the skin, although it is not known whether it is absorbed from denuded or broken skin, wounds or mucous membranes.

5.3 Preclinical safety data
There is no evidence from toxicological studies that cutaneous application of the proposed clinical dose of erythromycin would be associated with the risk of significant adverse reactions in humans. Published data and information on the toxicity of erythromycin applied to the skin support this conclusion.

6. PHARMACEUTICAL PARTICULARS

6.1 List of excipients
Butylhydroxytoluene

Hydroxypropylcellulose

Alcohol

6.2 Incompatibilities
None known.

6.3 Shelf life
Twenty-four (24) months.

6.4 Special precautions for storage
Store below 25°C, and out of the sight and the reach of children.

6.5 Nature and contents of container
Eryacne 4 is presented in a collapsible aluminium tube. The tube has an internal coating of an epoxy-phenolic resin. It is closed with a polypropylene screw cap. This cap is used to pierce the tube before its first use. A tube of Eryacne 4 contains 30g of product.

6.6 Special precautions for disposal and other handling
On first use, the screw cap is removed and is used to pierce the neck of the tube. Unscrew the cap, remove the plastic collar and screw the cap back onto the tube.

7. MARKETING AUTHORISATION HOLDER
Galderma (UK) Limited,

Meridien House

69-71 Clarendon Road

Watford

Herts.

WD17 1DS

UK

8. MARKETING AUTHORISATION NUMBER(S)
PL 10590/0022

9. DATE OF FIRST AUTHORISATION/RENEWAL OF THE AUTHORISATION
29 November 1996

10. DATE OF REVISION OF THE TEXT
February 2006

Erymax Capsules

(Cephalon Limited)

1. NAME OF THE MEDICINAL PRODUCT
Erymax 250mg Gastro-resistant Hard Capsules

2. QUALITATIVE AND QUANTITATIVE COMPOSITION
Each capsule contains 250mg of erythromycin.

For excipients, see 6.1.

3. PHARMACEUTICAL FORM
Gastro-resistant capsule, hard.

Hard gelatin capsule with opaque orange cap and clear orange body, imprinted with "Erymax 250mg", and containing white and orange enteric coated pellets of erythromycin base.

4. CLINICAL PARTICULARS

4.1 Therapeutic indications
Erythromycin is an antibiotic effective in the treatment of bacterial disease caused by susceptible organisms.

Examples of its use are in the treatment of upper and lower respiratory tract infections of mild to moderate severity; skin and soft tissue infections including pustular acne.

Erythromycin is usually active against the following organisms *in vitro* and in clinical infection: *Streptococcus pyogenes*; Alpha haemolytic streptococci; *Staphylococcus aureus*; *Streptococcus pneumoniae*; *Haemophilus influenzae*; *Mycoplasma pneumoniae*; *Treponema pallidum*; *Corynebacterium diphtheriae*; *Corynebacterium minutissimum*; *Entamoeba histolytica*; *Listeria monocytogenes*; *Neisseria gonorrhoeae*; *Bordetella pertussis*; *Legionella pneumophila*; *Chlamydia trachomatis*; *Propionibacterium acnes*.

4.2 Posology and method of administration
Oral use.

Adults and elderly

250 mg every six hours - before or with meals. 500 mg every twelve hours may be given if desired; b.i.d. dosage should not be used if dosage exceeds one gram.

Children

The usual dose is 30-50 mg/kg/day erythromycin, in divided doses given twice daily or every six hours. In severe infections, this dose may be doubled; elevated doses should be given every six hours. The drug should be given before or with meals.

Note: Erymax Capsules may be given to children of any age who can swallow the capsules whole.

The capsules should be swallowed whole either before or with food; they should not be chewed.

Streptococcal Infections:

For active infection - a full therapeutic dose is given for at least ten days.

For continuous prophylaxis against recurrences of streptococcal infections in patients with evidence of rheumatic fever or heart disease, the dose is 250 mg b.i.d.

For the prevention of bacterial endocarditis in patients with valvular disease scheduled for dental or surgical procedures of the upper respiratory tract, the adult dose is 1 gram (children 20 mg/kg) 2 hours before surgery. Following surgery, the dose is 500 mg for adults (children 10mg/kg) orally every six hours for 8 doses.

Primary Syphilis: 30-40 grams given in divided doses over a period of 10-15 days.

Intestinal Amoebiasis: 250 mg four times daily for 10 to 14 days for adults: 30 to 50 mg/kg/day in divided doses for 10 to 14 days for children.

Legionnaires' Disease: 1-4 g daily until clinical signs and symptoms indicate a clinical cure. Treatment may be prolonged.

Pertussis: 30-50 mg/kg/day given in divided doses for 5 - 14 days, depending upon eradication of a positive culture.

Acne: initially, 250 mg twice daily, which may be reduced to a maintenance dose of 250 mg once daily after one month according to response.

4.3 Contraindications
Use in patients hypersensitive to erythromycin or to any of the excipients, and in patients taking astemizole, terfenadine, cisapride, pimozide, ergotamine, dihydroergotamine, simvastatin, tolterodine, mizolastine, amisulpride or sertindole.

4.4 Special warnings and precautions for use
In patients with impaired hepatic function, liver function should be monitored, since a few reports of hepatic dysfunction have been received in patients taking erythromycin as the estolate, base or stearate. Extended administration requires regular evaluation particularly of liver function. Therapy should be discontinued if significant hepatic dysfunction occurs.

Prolonged use of erythromycin has caused overgrowth of nonsusceptible bacteria or fungi; this is a rare occurrence.

It has been reported that erythromycin may aggravate the weakness of patients with myasthenia gravis.

Patients receiving erythromycin concurrently with drugs which can cause prolongation of the QT interval should be carefully monitored; the concomitant use of erythromycin with some of these drugs is contraindicated (see sections 4.3 and 4.5).

Owing to the presence of lactose, patients with rare hereditary problems of galactose intolerance, the Lapp lactase deficiency or glucose-galactose malabsorption should not take this medicine.

4.5 Interaction with other medicinal products and other forms of interaction
Concomitant use of erythromycin with certain drugs metabolised by the cytochrome P450 system is likely to result in an increased frequency or seriousness of adverse effects associated with these drugs. The concomitant use of erythromycin with mizolastine, amisulpride, astemizole, cisapride, pimozide, sertindole and terfenadine is contraindicated due to the risk of QT prolongation and cardiac arrhythmias including ventricular tachycardia, ventricular fibrillation and Torsades de pointes. The concomitant use of erythromycin with ergotamine and dihydroergotamine is contraindicated due to the risk of ergot toxicity. Concomitant use with simvastatin is contraindicated due to the risk of myopathy and rhabdomyolysis whilst concomitant use with tolterodine is contraindicated due to increased risk of overdose.

Other drugs metabolised by the cytochrome P450 system, such as acenocoumarol, atorvastatin, bromocriptine, buspirone, cabergoline, carbamazepine, ciclosporin, cilostazol, clozapine, digoxin, disopyramide, eletriptan, felodipine, hexobarbital, midazolam, phenytoin, quetiapine, quinidine, rifabutin, sildenafil, tacrolimus, tadalafil, theophylline, triazolam, valproate, warfarin and zopiclone, may be associated with elevated serum levels if administered concomitantly with erythromycin. Because of the risk of toxicity, appropriate monitoring should be undertaken, and dosage should be adjusted as necessary.

When oral erythromycin is given concurrently with theophylline, there is also a significant decrease in erythromycin serum concentrations, which could result in subtherapeutic concentrations of erythromycin.

Erythromycin should be used with caution if administered concomitantly with lincomycin, clindamycin or chloramphenicol, as competitive inhibition may occur.

The concomitant use of erythromycin with alfentanil can significantly inhibit the clearance of alfentanil and may increase the risk of prolonged or delayed respiratory depression.

Patients receiving concomitant lovastatin and erythromycin should be carefully monitored as cases of rhabdomyolysis have been reported in seriously ill patients. Rhabdomyolysis has also been reported with concomitant simvastatin and erythromycin, and caution is therefore recommended when erythromycin is used concurrently with other HMG-CoA reductase inhibitors. It is recommended that therapy with simvastatin is suspended during the course of treatment.

An increased plasma concentration of erythromycin has been reported with concomitant cimetidine treatment, leading to increased risk of toxicity, including reversible deafness.

Erythromycin may interfere with the determination of urinary catecholamines and 17-hydroxycorticosteroids.

4.6 Pregnancy and lactation

Like all drugs erythromycin should be used in pregnancy only when clearly indicated. Erythromycin crosses the placental barrier.

Nursing mothers: erythromycin is excreted in human milk and should be used in lactating women only if clearly needed.

4.7 Effects on ability to drive and use machines

None known.

4.8 Undesirable effects

Serious allergic reaction, including anaphylaxis, has been reported.

There have been rare reports of skin rashes, including pruritus, urticaria and, very rarely, Stevens-Johnson syndrome.

Nausea and abdominal discomfort can occur at elevated doses; diarrhoea and vomiting are less common.

Hepatotoxicity: There have been reports of hepatic dysfunction, with or without jaundice, occurring in patients receiving erythromycin products and due to combined cholestatic and hepatocellular injury although less commonly than with erythromycin estolate.

Pancreatitis has been reported rarely.

Superinfections including pseudomembranous colitis have been occasionally reported to occur in association with erythromycin therapy.

Transient hearing disturbances and deafness have been reported with doses of erythromycin usually greater than 4g daily, and usually given intravenously.

There have been isolated reports of transient central nervous system side effects including confusion, hallucinations, seizures, and vertigo; however, a cause and effect relationship has not been established.

Cardiac arrhythmias have been reported rarely in patients receiving erythromycin.

4.9 Overdose

Nausea, vomiting and diarrhoea have been reported.

Treatment

Gastric lavage and general supportive therapy. Erythromycin is not removed by peritoneal dialysis or haemodialysis.

5. PHARMACOLOGICAL PROPERTIES

5.1 Pharmacodynamic properties

Erythromycin base and its salts are readily absorbed in the microbiologically active form. Erythromycin is largely bound to plasma proteins and after absorption erythromycin diffuses readily into most body fluids.

Erythromycin acts by inhibition of protein synthesis by binding 50s ribosomal subunits of susceptible organisms. It does not affect nucleic acid synthesis.

5.2 Pharmacokinetic properties

After administration of a single dose of Erymax 250 mg, peak serum levels are attained in approximately 3 hours. In the presence of normal hepatic function, erythromycin is concentrated in the liver and is excreted in the bile. After oral administration, less than 5% of the administered dose can be recovered in the active form in the urine.

5.3 Preclinical safety data

Pre-clinical safety data does not add anything of further significance to the prescriber.

6. PHARMACEUTICAL PARTICULARS

6.1 List of excipients

Cellulose acetate phthalate, lactose, potassium phosphate monobasic, povidone, diethyl phthalate, purified water, sunset yellow, titanium dioxide, gelatin, erythrosine, quinoline yellow.

The printing ink contains:

Black iron oxide (E172), shellac, potassium hydroxide and propylene glycol.

6.2 Incompatibilities

None known.

6.3 Shelf life

18 months.

6.4 Special precautions for storage

Do not store above 25°C. Store in the original package. Protect from moisture and light.

6.5 Nature and contents of container

PVdC/ PVC/ Aluminium Blister packs containing 4, 8, 28, 30, 100, 112 capsules.

6.6 Special precautions for disposal and other handling

No special requirements.

7. MARKETING AUTHORISATION HOLDER

Cephalon Limited

1 Albany Place

Hyde Way

Welwyn Garden City

Hertfordshire

AL7 3BT

8. MARKETING AUTHORISATION NUMBER(S)

PL 21799/0010

9. DATE OF FIRST AUTHORISATION/RENEWAL OF THE AUTHORISATION

May 2006

10. DATE OF REVISION OF THE TEXT

January 2009

11. LEGAL CATEGORY

POM

Estracyt Capsules

(Pharmacia Limited)

1. NAME OF THE MEDICINAL PRODUCT

Estracyt Capsules.

2. QUALITATIVE AND QUANTITATIVE COMPOSITION

Estramustine phosphate 140 mg as estramustine sodium phosphate.

3. PHARMACEUTICAL FORM

White, hard, gelatin capsules.

4. CLINICAL PARTICULARS

4.1 Therapeutic indications

Carcinoma of the prostate, especially in cases unresponsive to, or relapsing after, treatment by conventional oestrogens (stilboestrol, polyoestradiol phosphate etc.) or by orchidectomy.

4.2 Posology and method of administration

Adult and the elderly

Dosage range may be from 1 to 10 capsules a day by mouth. The capsules should be taken not less than 1 hour before or 2 hours after meals. The capsules should not be taken with milk or milk products. Standard starting dosage is 4-6 capsules a day in divided doses with later adjustment according to response and gastrointestinal tolerance.

Children

Estracyt should not be administered to children.

4.3 Contraindications

Use in patients with peptic ulceration, or those with severe liver dysfunction or myocardial insufficiency.

Use in children.

Use in patients hypersensitive to oestradiol or nitrogen mustard.

4.4 Special warnings and precautions for use

Use with caution in patients with moderate to severe bone marrow depression, thrombophlebitis, thrombosis, thromboembolic disorders, cardiovascular disease, coronary artery disease and congestive heart failure.

Caution should also be exercised in patients with diabetes, hypertension, epilepsy, hepatic and renal impairment and diseases associated with hypercalcaemia. Blood counts, liver function tests and serum calcium in hypercalcaemia should be performed at regular intervals. Patients with prostate cancer and osteoblastic metastases are at risk of hypocalcaemia and should have calcium levels closely monitored.

Immunosuppreant Effects/Increased Susceptibility to Infections - Administration of live or live-attenuated vaccines in patients immunocompromised by chemotherapeutic agents including estramustine, may result in serious or fatal infections. Vaccination with a live vaccine should be avoided in patients receiving estramustine. Killed or inactivated vaccines may be administered; however, the response to such vaccines may be diminished

4.5 Interaction with other medicinal products and other forms of interaction

Milk, milk products or drugs containing calcium may impair the absorption of Estracyt and should not be taken simultaneously with Estracyt.

An interaction between Estracyt and ACE-inhibitors, possibly leading to an increased risk of angioneurotic oedema cannot be excluded.

4.6 Pregnancy and lactation

Not applicable.

4.7 Effects on ability to drive and use machines

No adverse effects on a patient's ability to drive or operate heavy machinery have been reported.

4.8 Undesirable effects

The most common adverse reactions include gynaecomastia and impotence, nausea/vomiting and fluid retention/oedema.

The most serious reactions are thromboembolism, ischaemic heart disease, congestive heart failure and, rarely and angioneurotic oedema.

Reported reactions arranged according to MedDRA System Organ System are the following:

Blood and lymphatic system disorders: Anemia, leukopenia, thrombocytopenia rarely occur.

Immune system disorders: Hypersensitivity reaction

Metabolism and nutrition disorders: Fluid retention

Psychiatric disorders: Confusion and depression rarely occur.

Nervous system disorders: Headache and lethargy rarely occur

Cardiac disorders: Congestive heart failure, ischemic heart disease, myocardial infarction

Vascular disorders: Hypertension, thromboembolism

Gastrointestinal disorders: Nausea and vomiting, diarrhea (particularly during the first two weeks of treatment)

Hepato-biliary disorders: Impairment of liver function

Skin and subcutaneous tissue disorders: Allergic skin rash.

Angioneurotic edema (Quincke edema, larynx edema) can rarely occur. In many reported cases, including a fatal one, patients were concomitantly receiving ACE-inhibitors. Therapy with Estracyt is to be immediately discontinued should angioneurotic edema occur.

Musculoskeletal and connective tissue disorders: Muscular weakness rarely occurs.

Reproductive system and breast disorders: Gynecomastia, impotence

4.9 Overdose

There is no specific antidote. Treatment is symptomatic and supportive and in the event of dangerously low red cell, white cell or platelet count, whole blood should be given as necessary. Liver function should be monitored.

5. PHARMACOLOGICAL PROPERTIES

5.1 Pharmacodynamic properties

ATC Code: L01XX11

Estracyt is a chemical compound of oestradiol and nitrogen mustard. It is effective in the treatment of advanced prostatic carcinoma.

Estracyt has a dual mode of action. The intact molecule acts as an anti-miotic agent; after hydrolysis of the carbamate ester, the metabolites act to bridge the released oestrogens and exert an anti-gonadotrophic effect. The low level of clinical side effects may be due to the fact that estramustine binds to a protein present in the tumour tissue, so resulting in accumulation of the drug at the target site. Estracyt also has weak oestrogenic and anti-gonadotrophic properties.

Estracyt causes little or no bone marrow depression at usual therapeutic dosage. Estracyt is effective in patients who have not previously received drug therapy, as well as in those who have shown no response to conventional hormone treatment.

5.2 Pharmacokinetic properties

Estramustine phosphate sodium is rapidly dephosphorylated in the intestine and prostate to estramustine and estromustine, which accumulate in the prostatic tissue. The plasma half-lives of these metabolites are 10 - 20 hours. Estramustine and estromustine are further metabolised before excretion.

5.3 Preclinical safety data

No particular information is presented given the experience gained with the use of estramustine phosphate sodium in humans over the past several years.

6. PHARMACEUTICAL PARTICULARS

6.1 List of excipients

Talcum, sodium lauryl sulphate, colloidal silicon dioxide, magnesium stearate, titanium dioxide (E171), hard gelatin capsule, black ink (containing black iron oxide (E172), propylene glycol (E1520) and shellac).

6.2 Incompatibilities

None that are relevant.

6.3 Shelf life

60 months in brown glass bottles.

6.4 Special precautions for storage

Store out of the sight and reach of children.

The product is stable at storage conditions of 25°C ± 2°C/ 60%RH (long term) and 40°C ± 2°C/75%RH (short term). Therefore the product does not require any special storage precautions within EU countries (Climactic zone 2).

6.5 Nature and contents of container

Brown glass bottle containing 100 capsules.

6.6 Special precautions for disposal and other handling

No special instructions.

7. MARKETING AUTHORISATION HOLDER

Pharmacia Limited

Ramsgate Road, Sandwich, Kent

CT13 9NJ

UK

8. MARKETING AUTHORISATION NUMBER(S)
PL 00032/0316

9. DATE OF FIRST AUTHORISATION/RENEWAL OF THE AUTHORISATION
25 May 2002/13 Nov 2008

10. DATE OF REVISION OF THE TEXT
13 November 2008

Legal Category: POM
Ref: ES 4_0

Estring

(Pharmacia Limited)

1. NAME OF THE MEDICINAL PRODUCT
ESTRING vaginal ring

2. QUALITATIVE AND QUANTITATIVE COMPOSITION
Each vaginal ring contains:

Active ingredient

Estradiol Hemihydrate Ph.Eur. 2.0 mg

For excipients, see 6.1

3. PHARMACEUTICAL FORM
Estradiol vaginal ring is a slightly opaque ring, made of a silicone elastomer, with a whitish core, containing a drug reservoir of Estradiol Hemihydrate. The product has the following dimensions. Outer diameter - 55 mm; cross sectional diameter - 9 mm; core diameter - 2 mm.

4. CLINICAL PARTICULARS

4.1 Therapeutic indications
Hormone replacement therapy (HRT) for atrophic vaginitis, (due to estrogen deficiency) in postmenopausal women.

4.2 Posology and method of administration
Estring vaginal ring is an estrogen-only product for vaginal use.

Adults including the elderly

One ring to be inserted into the upper third of the vagina, to be worn continuously for 3 months, then replaced by a new ring as appropriate. For initiation and continuation of treatment of postmenopausal symptoms, the lowest effective dose for the shortest duration (See also Section 4.4) should be used. The maximum recommended duration of continuous therapy is two years.

Therapy may start at any time in women with established amenorrhoea or who are experiencing long intervals between spontaneous menses. Patients changing from a cyclical or continuous sequential preparation should complete the cycle, after a withdrawal bleed, and then change to Estring vaginal ring. Patients changing from a continuous combined preparation may start therapy at any time.

Estring vaginal ring is a local therapy and in women with an intact uterus, progestogen treatment is *not* necessary, (But see Section 4.4, Special Warnings and Precautions for Use, Endometrial Hyperplasia).

To put Estring into the vagina:

- A relaxed position must be found
- With one hand, the folds of skin around the vagina are opened.
- With the other hand, the ring is pressed into an oval.
- The ring is pushed into the vagina as far as it will go, upwards and backwards towards the small of the back.

To take out Estring

- A relaxed position must be found
- A finger is placed into the vagina and hooked around the ring.
- The ring is gently pulled out - downwards and forwards.

Comprehensive advice for removal and reinsertion of the ring are provided in the Patient Information Leaflet, which is included in every pack.

Children

Estring vaginal ring is not recommended for use in children.

4.3 Contraindications
Active or recent arterial thromboembolic disease (e.g. angina, myocardial infarction);

Known or suspected estrogen-dependent malignancy, (e.g. endometrial carcinoma)

Undiagnosed genital bleeding;

Untreated endometrial hyperplasia:

Acute liver disease, or a history of liver disease as long as liver function tests have failed to return to normal;

Porphyria;

Previous idiopathic or current venous thromboembolism (deep vein thrombosis, pulmonary embolism);

Known, past or suspected breast cancer.

Known hypersensitivity to the active substances or to any of the excipients.

4.4 Special warnings and precautions for use
For the treatment of postmenopausal symptoms, HRT should only be initiated for symptoms that adversely affect quality of life. In all cases, a careful appraisal of the risks and benefits should be undertaken at least annually and HRT should only be continued as long as the benefit outweighs the risk

Assessment of each woman prior to taking hormone replacement therapy (and at regular intervals thereafter) should include a personal and family medical history. Physical examination should be guided by this and by the contraindications (see Section 4.3) and warnings (see Section 4.4) for this product. During assessment of each individual woman, clinical examination of the breasts and pelvic examination should be performed where clinically indicated rather than as a routine procedure. Women should be encouraged to participate in the national cervical cancer screening programme (cervical cytology) and the national breast cancer screening programme (mammography) as appropriate for their age. Breast awareness should also be encouraged and women advised to report any changes in their breasts to their doctor or nurse.

Patients on long-term corticosteroid treatment or those with conditions causing poor skin integrity, e.g Cushing's Disease, may be unsuitable for treatment as they may have vaginal atrophy unresponsive to estrogen therapy.

The pharmacokinetic profile shows that there is low systemic absorption of estradiol (see Section 5.2 Pharmacokinetic Properties), however, being a HRT product the following need to be considered, especially for long term or repeated use of this product.

Conditions which need supervision:

If any of the following conditions are present, have occurred previously, and/or have been aggravated during pregnancy or previous hormone treatment, the patient should be closely supervised. It should be taken into account that these conditions may recur or be aggravated during treatment with Estring vaginal ring, in particular:

Risk factors for estrogen dependent tumours, e.g. 1st degree heredity for breast cancer (see below)

Diabetes mellitus with or without vascular involvement

Migraine or (severe) headache

Epilepsy

A history of, or risk of factors for, thromboembolic disorders (see below)

Systemic lupus erythematosus

Liver disorders (e.g. liver adenoma)

Otosclerosis

Cholelithiasis

Leiomyoma (uterine fibroids)

Endometriosis

A history of endometrial hyperplasia (see below);

Hypertension;

Asthma.

Reasons for immediate withdrawal of therapy:

Therapy should be discontinued in case a contra-indication is discovered and in the following situations:

- Jaundice or deterioration in liver function
- Significant increase in blood pressure
- New onset of migraine-type headache
- Pregnancy

Endometrial Hyperplasia

The risk of endometrial hyperplasia and carcinoma is increased when systemic estrogens are administered alone for prolonged periods of time, (See Section 4.8). The endometrial safety of long-term or repeated use of topical vaginal estrogens is uncertain. Therefore, if repeated, treatment should be reviewed at least annually, with special consideration given to any symptoms of endometrial hyperplasia or carcinoma.

If breakthrough bleeding or spotting appears at any time on therapy, the reason should be investigated, which may include endometrial biopsy to exclude endometrial malignancy.

Unopposed estrogen stimulation may lead to premalignant or malignant transformation in the residual foci of endometriosis. Therefore, caution is advised when using this product in women who have undergone hysterectomy, because of endometriosis, especially if they are known to have residual endometriosis.

Breast Cancer

A randomised placebo-controlled trials, the Women's Health Initiative study (WHI), and epidemiological studies, including the Million Women Study (MWS), have reported an increased risk of breast cancer in women taking estrogens, estrogen-progestogen combinations or tibolone for HRT for several years (see Section 4.8). For all HRT, an excess risk becomes apparent within a few years of use and increases with duration of intake but returns to within a few (at most five) years after stopping treatment.

In the MWS, the relative risk of breast cancer with conjugated equine estrogens (CEE) or estradiol (E2) was greater when a progestogen was added, either sequentially or continuously, and regardless of type of progestogen. There was no evidence of a difference in risk between the different routes of administration.

In the WHI study, the continuous combined conjugated equine estrogen and medroxyprogesterone acetate (CEE + MPA) product used was associated with breast cancers that were slightly larger in size and more frequently had local lymph node metastases compared to placebo.

HRT, especially estrogen-progestogen combined treatment, increases the density of mammographic images which may adversely affect the radiological detection of breast cancer.

Venous Thromboembolism

HRT is associated with a higher relative risk of developing venous thromboembolism (VTE), i.e. deep vein thrombosis or pulmonary embolism. One randomised controlled trial and epidemiological studies found a two to threefold higher risk for users compared with non-users. For non-users, it is estimated that the number of cases of VTE that will occur over a 5 year period is about 3 per 1000 women aged 50-59 years and 8 per 1000 women aged between 60-69 years. It is estimated that in healthy women who use HRT for 5 years, the number of additional cases of VTE over a 5 year period will be between 2 and 6 (best estimate = 4) per 1000 women aged 50-59 years and between 5 and 15 (best estimate = 9) per 1000 women aged 60-69 years. The occurrence of such an event is more likely in the first year of HRT than later.

Generally recognised risk factors for VTE include a personal history or family history, severe obesity (BM > 30 kg/m^2) and systemic lupus erythematosus (SLE). There is no consensus about the possible role of varicose veins in VTE.

Patients with a history of VTE or known thrombophilic states have an increased risk of VTE. HRT may add to this risk. Personal or strong family history of thromboembolism or recurrent spontaneous abortion should be investigated in order to exclude a thrombophilic predisposition. Until a thorough evaluation of thrombophilic factors has been made or anticoagulant treatment initiated, use of HRT in such patients should be viewed as contraindicated. Those women already on anticoagulant treatment require careful consideration of the benefit-risk of use of HRT.

The risk of VTE may be temporarily increased with prolonged immobilisation, major trauma or major surgery. As in all postoperative patients, scrupulous attention should be given to prophylactic measures to prevent VTE following surgery. Where prolonged immobilisation is liable to follow elective surgery, particularly abdominal or orthopaedic surgery to the lower limbs, consideration should be given to temporarily stopping HRT 4 to 6 weeks earlier, if possible. Treatment should not be restarted until the woman is completely mobilised.

If VTE develops after initiating therapy, the drug should be discontinued. Patients should be told to contact their doctor immediately when they are aware of a potential thromboembolic symptom (e.g. painful swelling of a leg, sudden pain in the chest, dyspnea).

Coronary Artery Disease

There is no evidence from randomised controlled trials of cardiovasular benefit with continuous combined conjugated estrogens and medroxyprogesterone acetate (MPA). Twp large clinical trials (WHI and HERS, i.e. Heart and Estrogen/progestin Replacement Study) showed a possible increased risk of cardiovascular morbidity in the first year of use and no overall benefit. For other HRT products there are only limited data from randomised controlled trials to date examining effects in cardiovascular morbidity or mortality. Therefore, it is uncertain whether these findings also extend to other HRT products.

Stroke

One large randomised clinical trial (WHI-trial) found, as a secondary outcome, an increased risk of ischaemic stroke in healthy women during treatment with continuous combined conjugated estrogens and medroxyprogesterone acetate. For women who do not use HRT, it is estimated that the number of cases of stroke that will occur over a 5 year period is about 3 per 1000 women aged 50-59 years and 11 per 1000 women aged 60-69 years. It is estimated that for women who use conjugated estrogens and medroxyprogesterone acetate for 5 years, the number of additional cases will be between 0 and 3 (best estimate = 1) per 1000 users aged 50-59 years and between 1 and 9 (best estimate = 4) per 1000 users aged 60-69 years. It is unknown whether the increased risk also extends to other HRT products.

Ovarian Cancer

Long-term (at least 5 to 10 years) use of estrogen-only HRT products in hysterectomised women has been associated with an increased risk of ovarian cancer in some epidemiological studies. It is uncertain whether long-term use of combined HRT confers a different risk than estrogen-only products.

Other Conditions

Some women may be unsuitable for treatment with Estring vaginal ring, in particular those with short narrow vaginas due to previous surgery or the effect of atrophy, or those with a degree of uterovaginal prolapse severe enough to prevent retention of the ring.

In addition, any woman with symptoms/signs of abnormal vaginal discharge, vaginal discomfort, or any vaginal bleeding should be examined fully, to exclude ulceration, infection, or unresponsive atrophic vaginitis. Minor signs of irritation are often transient.

Any woman experiencing persistent or severe discomfort due to the presence of the ring or excessive movement of the ring should be withdrawn from treatment. Patients with signs of ulceration or severe inflammation due to unresponsive atrophic vaginitis should also be withdrawn from treatment.

Patients with vaginal infection should be treated appropriately. In the case of systemic therapy, Estring vaginal ring treatment may continue without interruption. However, removal of Estring vaginal ring should be considered while using other vaginal preparations.

There have been incidences of both the ring falling out and movement of the ring, generally at defaecation. Therefore, if the woman is constipated she should remove the ring before defaecation. There may also be other instances when some women wish to remove the ring, e.g. prior to sexual intercourse.

Estrogens may cause fluid retention and therefore patients with cardiac or renal dysfunction should be carefully observed. Patients with terminal renal insufficiency should be closely observed, since it is expected that the level of circulating active ingredients in Estring vaginal ring are increased.

Women with pre-existing hypertriglyceridaemia should be followed closely during estrogen replacement or hormone replacement therapy, since rare cases of large increases of plasma triglycerides leading to pancreatitis have been reported with estrogen therapy in this condition.

Estrogens increase thyroid binding globulin (TBG), leading to increased circulating total thyroid hormone, as measured by protein-bound iodine (PBI), T4 levels (by column or by radio-immunoassay) or T3 levels (by radio-immunoassay). T3 resin uptake is decreased, reflecting the elevated TBG. Free T4 and free T3 concentrations are unaltered. Other binding proteins may be elevated in serum, i.e. corticoid binding globulin (CBG), sex-hormone-binding globulin (SHGB) leading to increased circulating corticosteroids and sex steroids, respectively. Free or biologically active hormone concentrations are unchanged. Other plasma proteins may be increased (angiotensinogen/renin substrate, alpha-1-antitrypsin, ceruloplasmin). The low systemic absorption of estradiol with vaginal administration (see Section 5.2 Pharmacokinetic Properties) may result in less pronounced effects on plasma binding proteins than with oral hormones.

There is no conclusive evidence for improvement of cognitive function. There is some evidence from the WHI trial of increased risk of probable dementia in women who start using continuous combined CEE and MPA after the age of 65. It is unknown whether the findings apply to younger post-menopausal women or other HRT products.

In rare cases benign, and in even rarer cases malignant liver tumours leading in isolated cases to life-threatening intra-abdominal haemorrhage have been observed after the use of hormonal substances such as those contained in Estring. If severe upper abdominal complaints, enlarged liver or signs of intra-abdominal haemorrhage occur, a liver tumour should be considered in the differential diagnosis.

Women who may be at risk of pregnancy should be advised to adhere to non-hormonal contraceptive methods.

The requirement for oral anti-diabetics or insulin can change as a result of the effect on glucose tolerance.

4.5 Interaction with other medicinal products and other forms of interaction

As the estrogen is administered vaginally and due to the low levels released, it is unlikely that any clinically relevant drug interactions will occur with Estring vaginal ring.

However, the prescriber should be aware that the metabolism of estrogens may be increased by concomitant use of substances known to induce drug-metabolising enzymes, specifically cytochrome P450 enzymes, such as anticonvulsants (e.g. phenobarbital, phenytoin, carbamazepine) and anti-infectives (e.g. rifampicin, rifabutin, nevirapine, efavirenz).

Ritonavir and nelfinavir, although known as strong inhibitors, by contrast exhibit inducing properties when used concomitantly with steroid hormones. Herbal preparations containing St John's wort (Hypericum Perforatum) may induce the metabolism of estrogens.

Clinically, an increased metabolism of estrogens may lead to decreased effect and changes in the uterine bleeding profile.

Removal of Estring vaginal ring should be considered when using other vaginal preparations (See Section 4.4 Special Warnings and Precautions for Use).

4.6 Pregnancy and lactation

Pregnancy

Estring vaginal ring is not indicated during pregnancy. If pregnancy occurs during medication with Estring vaginal ring treatment should be withdrawn immediately. The results of most epidemiological studies to date relevant to inadvertent foetal exposure to estrogens indicate no teratogenic or foetotoxic effects

Lactation

Estring vaginal ring is not indicated during lactation.

4.7 Effects on ability to drive and use machines

Estring vaginal ring is unlikely to have any effect on alertness or coordination.

4.8 Undesirable effects

Adverse reactions with Estring vaginal ring are rare. Adverse reactions reported with a frequency of 1% or more in clinical trials, in order of decreasing frequency, were vaginal irritation, abdominal pain/lower abdominal pain/ abdominal discomfort, vulvovaginal infection, urogenital pruritus, pressure symptoms in vagina/on bladder/on rectum, generalised pruritus, urinary tract infection and increased sweating (See Section 4.4 Special Warnings and Precautions for Use). However, some of these symptoms occur more frequently in untreated post-menopausal women, e.g. vaginal irritation, urinary tract infection, urogenital pruritus, vulvovaginal infection and increased sweating.

The following adverse reactions have been reported with estrogen therapy:

1. *Genito-urinary tract:* Endometrial neoplasia*, intermenstrual bleeding, increase in the size of uterine fibromyomata, endometrial proliferation or aggravation of endometriosis, changes in cervical eversion and excessive production of cervical mucus, thrush, vaginal ulceration;

2. *Breast:* Tenderness, pain, enlargement or secretion,; breast cancer* ‡ (uncommon)

3. *Gastro-intestinal tract*: Nausea, vomiting, abdominal cramp, bloating;

4. *Cardiovascular system*: Hypertension, thrombosis, thrombophlebitis, venous thromboembolism*, myocardial infarction* and stroke*;

5. *Liver/biliary system*: In rare cases benign, and in even rarer cases malignant liver tumours, gall bladder disease, cholelithiasis, cholestatic jaundice; aggravation of porphyria;

6. *Skin*: Chloasma which may persist when the drug is discontinued, erythema multiforme, erythema nodosum, candidal infections, vascular purpura, rash, loss of scalp hair, hirsutism;

7. *Eyes*: Steepening of corneal curvature, intolerance to contact lenses;

8. *CNS*: Headache, migraine, dizziness, mood changes (elation or depression), chorea;

9. *Miscellaneous:* Sodium and water retention, reduced glucose tolerance, change in body weight, changes in libido, muscle cramps.

* See sections 4.3, Contraindications and Section 4.4 Special Warnings and Special Precautions for Use.

Breast cancer

According to evidence from a large number of epidemiological studies and one randomised placebo-controlled trial, the Women's Health Initiative (WHI), the overall risk of breast cancer increases with increasing duration of HRT use in current or recent HRT users.

For *estrogen-only* HRT, estimates of relative risk (RR) from a reanalysis of original data from 51 epidemiological studies (in which >80% of HRT use was estrogen-only HRT) and from the epidemiological Million Women Study (MWS) are similar at 1.35 (95% CI 1.21 – 1.49) and 1.30 (95% CI 1.21 - 1.40), respectively.

For *estrogen plus progestogen* combined HRT, several epidemiological studies have reported an overall higher risk for breast cancer than with estrogens alone.

The MWS reported that, compared to never users, the use of various types of estrogen-progestogen combined HRT was associated with a higher risk of breast cancer (RR = 2.00, 95% CI: 1.88 – 2.12) than use of estrogens alone (RR = 1.30, 95% CI: 1.21 - 1.40) or use of tibolone (RR=1.45; 95%CI 1.25-1.68).

The WHI trial reported a risk estimate of 1.24 (95% CI 1.01 – 1.54) after 5.6 years of use of estrogen-progestogen combined HRT (CEE + MPA) in all users compared with placebo.

The absolute risks calculated from the MWS and the WHI trial are presented below:

The MWS has estimated, from the known average incidence of breast cancer in developed countries, that:

- *For women not using HRT, about 32 in every 1000 are expected to have breast cancer diagnosed between the ages of 50 and 64 years.*
- For 1000 current or recent users of HRT, the number of *additional* cases during the corresponding period will be
  - For users of *estrogen-only* replacement therapy
    - between 0 and 3 (best estimate = 1.5) for 5 years' use
    - between 3 and 7 (best estimate = 5) for 10 years' use.
  - For users of *estrogen plus progestogen* combined HRT,
    - between 5 and 7 (best estimate = 6) for 5 years' use
    - between 18 and 20 (best estimate = 19) for 10 years' use.

The WHI trial estimated that after 5.6 years of follow-up of women between the ages of 50 and 79 years, an *additional* 8 cases of invasive breast cancer would be due to *estrogen-progestogen combined* HRT (CEE + MPA) per 10,000 women years.

According to calculations from the trial data, it is estimated that:

- For 1000 women in the placebo group, about 16 cases of invasive breast cancer would be diagnosed in 5 years.
- For 1000 women who used estrogen + progestogen combined HRT (CEE + MPA), the number of *additional* cases would be between 0 and 9 (best estimate = 4) for 5 years' use.

The number of additional cases of breast cancer in women who use HRT is broadly similar for women who start HRT irrespective of age at start of use (between the ages of 45-65) (see section 4.4).

4.9 Overdose

This is not relevant due to the mode of administration.

5. PHARMACOLOGICAL PROPERTIES

5.1 Pharmacodynamic properties

Pharmacotherapeutic group: Natural and semisynthetic estrogens, plain.

ATC Code G03C A

Estring vaginal ringis a vaginal ring, which delivers approximately 7.5 μg/24 hours of 17 β-estradiol for 3 months. Estring vaginal ring is only suitable for the treatment of urogenital complaints due to estrogen deficiency. Its pharmacokinetic profile shows that it is not suitable for post-menopausal complaints which require a systemically active dose of estrogen (eg vasomotor symptoms), neither is it suitable for osteoporosis prevention.

The active ingredient, synthetic 17β-estradiol, is chemically and biologically identical to endogenous human estradiol. The estradiol from the vaginal ring substitutes for the loss of estrogen production in menopausal women, and alleviates menopausal symptoms. It acts locally to restore vaginal pH and to eliminate or reduce symptoms and signs of post-menopausal urogenital estrogen deficiency

Estring vaginal ring presumably increases local estradiol target concentrations, while maintaining very low and stable systemic plasma concentrations. The maximum duration of use during clinical trials was 2 years and, therefore, the maximum recommended duration of continuous therapy is 2 years.

5.2 Pharmacokinetic properties

After a brief initial peak, the release of estradiol from Estring vaginal ring is constant (7.5 μg/24 h), according to Fick's law, for at least 90 days. As a consequence of the initial release peak, plasma levels of estradiol reach about 200 pmol/l within 3 hours.

After this initial peak, plasma estradiol concentrations decline rapidly and constant levels are achieved after 2-3 days. These levels are maintained at, or near, the quantification limit (20-30 pmol/l) throughout the rest of the treatment period. The levels are considerably lower than the lowest levels commonly detected in pre-menopausal women, i.e during the early follicular phase.

Estradiol is mainly metabolized in the liver. Its main metabolites are estriol, estrone, and their conjugates. The plasma half life of estradiol is 1-2 hours. Metabolic plasma clearance varies between 450-625 ml/min/m^2. The metabolites are mainly excreted via the kidneys as glucuronides and sulphates. Estrogens also undergo enterohepatic circulation.

5.3 Preclinical safety data

Silicone elastomer in Estring vaginal ring

The biological safety of the silicone elastomer has been studied in various in-vitro and in-vivo test models.

The results show that the silicone elastomer was non-toxic in in-vitro studies, and non-pyrogenic, non-irritant, and non-sensitizing in short term in-vivo tests. Long-term implantation induced encapsulation equal to or less than the negative control (polyethylene) used in the prescribed USP test. No toxic reaction or further formation was observed with the silicone elastomer.

6. PHARMACEUTICAL PARTICULARS

6.1 List of excipients

Silicone elastomer Q7-4735 A, Silicone elastomer Q7-4735 B

Silicone Fluid, Barium sulphate

6.2 Incompatibilities

No incompatibilities are known.

6.3 Shelf life

Results from stability studies indicate that Estring vaginal ring is stable for at least 24 months when stored at room temperature (below 30°C).

6.4 Special precautions for storage

Keep out of the reach of children.

Do not store above 30°C.

6.5 Nature and contents of container

One ring is individually packed in a heat-sealed rectangular pouch consisting of, from outside to inside: Polyester/ Aluminium foil/Low density Poly-ethylene. Each pouch is provided with a tear-off notch on one side and is packed into a cardboard carton. Each carton contains a Patient Information Leaflet.

6.6 Special precautions for disposal and other handling
Comprehensive details are provided in the Patient Information Leaflet.

Administrative Details

7. MARKETING AUTHORISATION HOLDER
Pharmacia Limited
Ramsgate Road,
Sandwich,
Kent CT13 9NJ, UK

8. MARKETING AUTHORISATION NUMBER(S)
PL 00032/0340

9. DATE OF FIRST AUTHORISATION/RENEWAL OF THE AUTHORISATION
12/02/2009

10. DATE OF REVISION OF THE TEXT
12/02/2009

11. Legal Category
POM

Ref: ET 4_0

Ethanolamine Oleate Injection BP
(UCB Pharma Limited)

1. NAME OF THE MEDICINAL PRODUCT
Ethanolamine Oleate Injection (monoethanolamine oleate). Solution for injection.

2. QUALITATIVE AND QUANTITATIVE COMPOSITION
Oleic acid 4.23% w/v
Ethanolamine 0.910% w/v
For excipients see 6.1.

3. PHARMACEUTICAL FORM
Solution for injection.
5 ml neutral glass ampoule containing a clear solution.

4. CLINICAL PARTICULARS

4.1 Therapeutic indications
The injection is recommended for use as a sclerosing agent in the treatment of small, uncomplicated varicose veins in the lower extremities.

4.2 Posology and method of administration
Ethanolamine Oleate is administered by slow intravenous injection.

Adults Including The Elderly

The product is used only as a sclerosant and injected directly into the varicose vein. A dose of 2 to 5ml, divided between 3 or 4 sites, administered by slow injection into empty isolated segments of vein.

Children

The product is not recommended for use in children.

4.3 Contraindications
Inability to walk, acute phlebitis, oral contraceptive use, obese legs, known hypersensitivity to Ethanolamine Oleate or benzyl alcohol. Superficial thrombophlebitis and deep vein thrombosis in the region of the varicose veins. Marked arterial, cardiac or renal disease. Uncontrolled metabolic disorders such as diabetes mellitus. Patients with local or systemic infections.

4.4 Special warnings and precautions for use
Care should be taken to ensure that the injection does not leak into perivenous tissue which could cause sloughing, ulceration and in severe cases, necrosis.

4.5 Interaction with other medicinal products and other forms of interaction
None known.

4.6 Pregnancy and lactation
Safety during pregnancy has not been established. Use in pregnancy is not recommended.

4.7 Effects on ability to drive and use machines
None known.

4.8 Undesirable effects
Burning, cramping sensation, urticaria. Allergic reactions and anaphylaxis have been reported following use of sclerosing agents.

4.9 Overdose
Acute nephrotoxicity has been reported in two patients given 15-20ml of a solution containing 5% Ethanolamine with 2% Benzl Alcohol.

5. PHARMACOLOGICAL PROPERTIES

5.1 Pharmacodynamic properties
ATC Code: C05B B 01; sclerosing agent for local injection.

Ethanolamine Oleate is an irritant. An injection of Ethanolamine Oleate into a vein irritates the intimal endothelium resulting in the formation of a thrombus. The thrombus occludes the vein and fibrous tissue develops resulting in a permanent obliteration of the vein.

5.2 Pharmacokinetic properties
Ethanolamine Oleate is a locally acting agent. Absorption from the site of administration is not anticipated as its mode of action is to cause a permanent obstruction in the vein.

5.3 Preclinical safety data
None.

6. PHARMACEUTICAL PARTICULARS

6.1 List of excipients
Benzyl alcohol
Water for Injection

6.2 Incompatibilities
Not applicable.

6.3 Shelf life
36 months.

6.4 Special precautions for storage
Do not store above 25°C. Keep the ampoule in the outer carton.

6.5 Nature and contents of container
5 ml Neutral Glass (Type 1) Ampoules.

6.6 Special precautions for disposal and other handling
The product is used only as a sclerosant and injected directly into the varicose vein.

7. MARKETING AUTHORISATION HOLDER
UCB Pharma Limited
208 Bath Road
Slough
Berkshire
SL1 3WE
UK

8. MARKETING AUTHORISATION NUMBER(S)
PL 0039/5671R

9. DATE OF FIRST AUTHORISATION/RENEWAL OF THE AUTHORISATION
27 March 1987 / 26 May 1994 / 27 May 1999

10. DATE OF REVISION OF THE TEXT
June 2005

Ethinyloestradiol Tablets BP 10 mcg, 50 mcg, 1 mg
(UCB Pharma Limited)

1. NAME OF THE MEDICINAL PRODUCT
Ethinyloestradiol Tablets BP 10 mcg, 50mcg and 1mg

2. QUALITATIVE AND QUANTITATIVE COMPOSITION
Ethinylestradiol 10.5 mcg, 52.5mcg or 1.048mg
For excipients see 6.1.

3. PHARMACEUTICAL FORM
White uncoated tablets for oral administration

4. CLINICAL PARTICULARS

4.1 Therapeutic indications
Post menopausal symptoms due to oestrogen deficiency.

Second line therapy for prevention of osteoporosis in postmenopausal women at high risk of future fractures who are intolerant of, or contraindicated for, other medicinal products approved for the prevention of osteoporosis.

Palliative treatment of prostatic cancer.

Hormone replacement therapy for failure of ovarian development e.g. in patients with gonadal dysgenesis where initial oestrogen therapy is later followed by combined oestrogen/progestogen therapy.

Disorders of menstruation, given in conjunction with a progestogen.

4.2 Posology and method of administration
Ethinyloestradiol Tablets is an oestrogen-only preparation of hormone replacement therapy (HRT) for oral administration.

Post menopausal symptoms due to oestrogen deficiency including prevention of postmenopausal osteoporosis: the lowest dose that will control symptoms should be chosen. The usual dose range is 10 to 50 micrograms daily, usually on a cyclical basis (e.g., 3 weeks on and 1 week off).

For women without a uterus, who did not have endometriosis diagnosed, it is not recommended to add a progestogen.

In women with an intact uterus (or in endometriosis when endometrial foci may be present despite hysterectomy), where a progestogen is necessary, it should be added for at least 12-14 days every month/28 day cycle to reduce the risk to the endometrium.

The benefits of the lower risk of endometrial hyperplasia and endometrial cancer due to adding progestogen should be weighed against the increased risk of breast cancer (see sections 4.4 and 4.8).

Therapy with Ethinyloestradiol Tablets may start at any time in women with established amenorrhoea or who are experiencing long intervals between spontaneous menses. In women who are menstruating, it is advised that therapy starts on the first day of bleeding. As Ethinyloestradiol Tablets are usually taken on a cyclical basis direct switching from other oestrogen-only HRT preparations taken cyclically is possible.

HRT should only be continued as long as the benefit in alleviation of severe symptoms outweighs the risks of HRT.

Palliative treatment of prostatic cancer: 150 micrograms to 1.5 mg daily. Larger dose Ethinyloestradiol Tablets are available.

Hormone replacement therapy for failure of ovarian development e.g. in patients with gonadal dysgenesis: 10 to 50 micrograms daily, usually on a cyclical basis. Initial oestrogen therapy should be followed by combined oestrogen/progestogen therapy.

Disorders of menstruation: 20 to 50 micrograms daily from day 5 to day 25 of each cycle. A progestogen is given daily in addition, either throughout the cycle or from days 15 to 25 of the cycle.

If a dose is forgotten it should be taken as soon as it is remembered. If it is nearly time for the next dose then the patient should wait until then. Two doses should not be taken together. Forgetting a dose may increase the likelihood of break-through bleeding and spotting.

4.3 Contraindications
Active or recent arterial thromboembolic disease, e.g. angina, myocardial infarction

Current or previous idiopathic venous thromboembolism (deep venous thrombosis, pulmonary embolism)

Known, past or suspected breast cancer or other known or suspected oestrogen dependent tumours (e.g. endometrial cancer)

Untreated endometrial hyperplasia

Undiagnosed genital bleeding

Acute liver disease or a history of liver disease as long as liver function tests have failed to return to normal

Porphyria

Known hypersensitivity to the active substance or to any of the excipients

4.4 Special warnings and precautions for use
Medical examination/follow-up

Before initiating or reinstituting HRT, a complete personal and family medical history should be taken. Physical (including pelvic and breast) examination should be guided by this and by the contraindications and warnings for use. During treatment, periodic check-ups are recommended of a frequency and nature adapted to the individual woman. Women should be advised what changes in their breasts should be reported to their doctor or nurse (see 'Breast cancer' below). Investigation, including mammography, should be carried out in accordance with currently accepted screening practices, modified to the clinical needs of the individual. A careful appraisal of the risks and benefits should be undertaken at least annually in women treated with hormone replacement therapy.

In women with an intact uterus, the benefits of the lower risk of endometrial hyperplasia and endometrial cancer due to adding a progestogen should be weighed against the increased risk of breast cancer (see below and Section 4.8).

Conditions which need supervision

If any of the following conditions are present, have occurred previously, and/or have been aggravated during pregnancy or previous hormone treatment, the patient should be closely supervised. It should be taken into account that these conditions may recur or be aggravated during treatment with ethinyloestradiol tablets, in particular:

Risk factors for oestrogen dependent tumours e.g. 1st degree heredity for breast cancer

Leimyoma (uterine fibroids) or endometriosis

A history of, or risk factors for, thromboembolic disorders (see below)

Hypertension

Liver disorders (e.g. liver adenoma)

Diabetes Mellitus with or without vascular involvement

Cholelithiasis

Otosclerosis

Asthma

Migraine or (severe) headache and epilepsy

Systemic Lupus erythematosis

Hyperplasia of the endometrium (see below)

Reasons for immediate withdrawal of therapy

Jaundice or deterioration in liver function

Significant increase in blood pressure

New onset of migraine-type headache

Pregnancy

Endometrial hyperplasia

The risk of endometrial hyperplasia and carcinoma is increased when oestrogens are administered alone for prolonged periods. The addition of a progestogen for at least 12 days of the cycle in non-hysterectomised women reduces, but may not eliminate, this risk (see section 4.8).

The reduction in risk to the endometrium should be weighed against the increase in the risk of breast cancer of added progestogen (see 'Breast cancer' below and in Section 4.8)

Break-through bleeding and spotting may occur during the first months of treatment. If break-through bleeding or spotting appears after some time on therapy, or continues after treatment has been discontinued, the reason should be investigated, which may include endometrial biopsy to exclude endometrial malignancy.

Unopposed oestrogen stimulation may lead to premalignant or malignant transformation in the residual foci of endometriosis. Therefore, the addition of progestogens to oestrogen replacement therapy should be considered in women who have undergone hysterectomy because of endometriosis, especially if they are known to have residual endometriosis (but see above).

Breast cancer

Randomised controlled trials and epidemiological studies have reported an increased risk of breast cancer in women taking oestrogens or oestrogen-progestogen combinations for HRT for several years (see section 4.8). An observational study of almost 829,000 women has shown that, compared to never-users, use of oestrogen-progestogen combined HRT is associated with a higher risk of breast cancer (RR = 2.00, 95%CI: 1.88 – 2.12) than use of oestrogens alone (RR = 1.30, 95%CI: 1.21 – 1.40). In this study the magnitude of the increase in breast cancer risk was similar for all oestrogen-only preparations, irrespective of the type, dose or route of administration of the oestrogen (oral, transdermal and implanted). Likewise the magnitude of the increased risk was similar for all oestrogen plus progestogen preparations, irrespective of the type of progestogen or the number of days of addition per cycle. For all HRT, an excess risk becomes apparent within 1-2 years of starting treatment and increases with duration of use of HRT but begins to decline when HRT is stopped and by 5 years reaches the same level as in women who have never taken HRT.

The increase in risk applies to all women studied, although the relative risk was significantly higher in those with a lean or normal body build (body mass index or BMI of < 25kg/m2) compared to those with a BMI of ⩾25kg/m2.

At present the effect of HRT on the diagnosis of breast tumours remains unclear – all women should be encouraged to report any changes in their breasts to their doctor or nurse.

Ovarian Cancer

Long-term (at least 5 to 10 years) use of oestrogen-only HRT products in hysterectomised women has been associated with an increased risk of ovarian cancer in some epidemiological studies. It is uncertain whether long-term use of combined HRT confers a different risk than oestrogen-only products.

Venous thromboembolism

HRT is associated with a higher relative risk of developing venous thromboembolism (VTE), i.e. deep vein thrombosis or pulmonary embolism. One randomised controlled trial and epidemiological studies found a two- to three fold higher risk for users compared with non-users. For non-users, it is estimated that the number of cases of VTE that will occur over a 5 year period is about 3 per 1000 women aged 50 – 59 years and 8 per 1000 women aged between 60 – 69 years. It is estimated that in healthy women who use HRT for 5 years, the number of additional cases of VTE over a 5 year period will be between 2 and 6 (best estimate = 4) per 1000 women aged 50 – 59 years and between 5 and 15 (best estimate = 9) per 1000 women aged 60 – 69 years. The occurrence of such an event is more likely in the first year of HRT than later.

Generally recognised risk factors for VTE include a personal history or family history, severe obesity (BMI> 30 kg/m2) and systemic lupus erythematosus (SLE). There is no consensus about the possible role of varicose veins in VTE.

Patients with a history of VTE or known thrombophilic states have an increased risk of VTE. HRT may add further to this risk. Personal or strong family history of recurrent thromboembolism or recurrent spontaneous abortion, should be investigated in order to exclude a thrombophilic predisposition. Until a thorough evaluation of thrombophilic factors has been made or anticoagulant treatment initiated, use of HRT in such patients should be viewed as contraindicated. Those women already on anticoagulant treatment require careful consideration of the benefit-risk of use of HRT.

The risk of VTE may be temporarily increased with prolonged immobilisation, major trauma or major surgery. As in all postoperative patients, scrupulous attention should be given to prophylactic measures to prevent VTE following surgery. Where prolonged immobilisation is liable to follow elective surgery, particularly abdominal or orthopaedic surgery to the lower limbs, consideration should be given to temporarily stopping HRT 4 to 6 weeks earlier, if possible. Treatment should not be restarted until the woman is completely mobilised.

If VTE develops after initiating therapy, the drug should be discontinued. Patients should be told to contact their doctors immediately when they are aware of a potential thromboembolic symptom (e.g., painful swelling of a leg, sudden pain in the chest, dyspnoea).

Stroke

One large randomised clinical trial (WHI-trial) found, as a secondary outcome, an increased risk of stroke in healthy women during treatment with continuous combined conjugated oestrogens and medroxyprogesterone acetate (MPA). For women who do not use HRT, it is estimated that the number of cases of stroke that will occur over a 5 year period is about 3 per 1000 women aged 50 – 59 years and 11 per 1000 women aged 60 – 69 years. It is estimated that for women who use conjugated oestrogens and MPA for 5 years, the number of additional cases will be between 0 and 3 (best estimate = 1) per 1000 users aged 50 – 59 years and between 1 and 9 (best estimate = 4) per 1000 users aged 60 – 69 years. It is unknown whether the increased risk also extends to other HRT products.

Coronary Artery Disease (CAD)

There is no evidence from randomised controlled trials of cardiovascular benefit with continuous combined conjugated oestrogens and MPA. Large clinical trials showed a possible increased risk of cardiovascular morbidity in the first year of use and no benefit thereafter. For other HRT products there are as yet no randomised controlled trials to date examining benefit in cardiovascular morbidity or mortality. Therefore, it is uncertain whether these findings also extend to other HRT products.

Other conditions

Oestrogens may cause fluid retention, and therefore patients with cardiac or renal dysfunction should be carefully observed. Patients with terminal renal insufficiency should be closely observed, since it is expected that the level of circulating active ingredients in Ethinyloestradiol Tablets is increased.

Women with pre-existing hypertriglyceridemia should be followed closely during oestrogen replacement or hormone replacement therapy, since rare cases of large increases of plasma triglycerides leading to pancreatitis have been reported with oestrogen therapy in this condition.

Oestrogens increase thyroid binding globulin (TBG), leading to increased circulating total thyroid hormone, as measured by protein-bound iodine (PBI), T4 levels (by column or by radio-immunoassay) or T3 levels (by radio-immunoassay). T3 resin uptake is decreased, reflecting the elevated TBG. Free T4 and free T3 concentrations are unaltered. Other binding proteins may be elevated in serum, i.e. corticoid binding globulin (CBG), sex-hormone-binding globulin (SHBG) leading to increased circulating corticosteroids and sex steroids, respectively. Free or biological active hormone concentrations are unchanged. Other plasma proteins may be increased (angiotensinogen/renin substrate, alpha-I-antitrypsin, ceruloplasmin).

Patients with rare hereditary problems of galactose intolerance, the Lapp-lactose deficiency, or glucose-galactose malabsorption should not take this medicine.

4.5 Interaction with other medicinal products and other forms of interaction

The metabolism of oestrogens may be increased by concomitant use of substances known to induce drug metabolising enzymes, specifically cytochrome P450 enzymes, such as anti-convulsants (e.g. phenobarbitol, phenytoin, carbamazepine) and anti-infectives (e.g. rifampicin, rifabutin, nevirapine, efavirenz).

Ritonavir and nelfinavir, although known as strong inhibitors, by contrast exhibit inducing properties when used concomitantly with steroid hormones. Herbal preparations containing St Johns Wort (Hypericum Perforatum) may induce the metabolism of oestrogens.

Clinically, an increased metabolism of oestrogens may lead to decreased effect and changes in the uterine bleeding profile.

Ethinyloestradiol doses greater than 50 micrograms per day may cause imipramine toxicity in patients on concomitant therapy.

Through its effects on the coagulation system, ethinyloestradiol may reduce the effects of anticoagulants such as warfarin, phenindione or nicoumalone.

The doses of insulin or hypoglycaemic drugs may need to be adjusted due to the mild diabetogenic effect of ethinyloestradiol.

Ethinyloestradiol may inhibit the metabolism of theophylline and reduce its clearance.

4.6 Pregnancy and lactation

Ethinyloestradiol Tablets are not indicated during pregnancy. If pregnancy occurs during medication with Ethinyloestradiol Tablets treatment should be withdrawn immediately. The results of most epidemiological studies to date relevant to inadvertent fetal exposure to oestrogens indicate no teratogenic or fetotoxic effects.

Ethinyloestradiol Tablets are not indicated during lactation.

4.7 Effects on ability to drive and use machines

None stated

4.8 Undesirable effects

Breast cancer

The risk of breast cancer increases with the number of years of HRT usage. According to data from a recent epidemiological study in about 829,000 postmenopausal women, the best estimate of the risk is that for women not using HRT, in total about 32 in every 1000 are expected to have breast cancer diagnosed between the ages of 50 and 65 years. Among those with current or recent use of oestrogen-only replacement therapy, it is estimated that the total number of additional cases during the corresponding period will be between 0 and 3 (best estimate = 1.5) per 1000 for 5 years' use and between 3 and 7 (best estimate = 5) per 1000 for 10 years' use (see table) Among those with current or recent use of oestrogen plus progestogen combined HRT, it is estimated that the total number of additional cases will be between 5 and 7 (best estimate = 6) per 1000 for 5 years' use and between 18 and 20 (best estimate = 19) per 1000 for 10 years' use (see section 4.4). The number of additional cases of breast cancer is broadly similar for women who start HRT irrespective of age at start of HRT use (between the ages of 45 and 65).

	No of additional cases of breast cancer diagnosed per 1000 users (95% confidence intervals)	
Type of HRT	5 years of use	10 years of use
Oestrogen-only	1.5 (0 – 3)	5 (3 – 7)
Combined	6 (5 – 7)	19 (18 – 20)

Endometrial cancer

In women with an intact uterus, the risk of endometrial hyperplasia and endometrial cancer increases with increasing duration of use of unopposed oestrogens and is substantially reduced by the addition of a progestogen (see section 4.4). According to the data from epidemiological studies, the best estimate of the risk of endometrial cancer is that for women not using HRT, about 5 in every 1000 are expected to have endometrial cancer diagnosed between the ages of 50 and 65. It is estimated that, among those who use oestrogen-only replacement therapy, there will be 4 additional cases per 1000 after 5 years' use and 10 additional cases per 1000 after 10 years' use. Adding a progestogen to oestrogen-only therapy substantially reduces, but may not eliminate, this increased risk.

Other adverse reactions have been reported in association with oestrogen treatment;

Genito-urinary tract: endometrial neoplasia, endometrial cancer, intermenstrual bleeding, increase in the size of uterine fibromyomata, endometrial proliferation or aggravation of endometriosis, excessive production of cervical mucus.

Breast: tenderness, pain, enlargement, secretion.

Gastro-intestinal tract: nausea, vomiting, cholelithiasis, cholestatic jaundice.

Cardiovascular system: hypertension, thrombosis, thrombophlebitis, thromboembolism, myocardial infarction, stroke.

Venous thromboembolism, i.e. deep leg or pelvic venous thrombosis and pulmonary embolism, is more frequent among hormone replacement therapy users than among non-users. For further information, see section 4.3 Contra-indications and 4.4 Special warnings and precautions for use.

Skin: erythema nodosum, erythema multiforme, vascular purpura, rash, chloasma.

Eyes: corneal discomfort if contact lenses are used.

CNS: headache, migraine, mood changes (elation or depression).

Metabolic: sodium and water retention, reduced glucose tolerance and change in body weight, hypercalcaemia.

In men: feminisation, gynaecomastia, testicular atrophy and impotence.

4.9 Overdose

Acute overdose of ethinyloestradiol may cause nausea and vomiting and may result in withdrawal bleeding in females.

5. PHARMACOLOGICAL PROPERTIES

5.1 Pharmacodynamic properties

Oestrogen deficiency at menopause is associated with an increasing bone turnover and decline in bone mass. Therefore, if possible, treatment for prevention of osteoporosis should start as soon as possible after the onset of menopause in women with increased risk for future osteoporotic fractures. The effect of oestrogens on the bone mineral density is dose-dependent. Protection appears to be effective for as long as treatment is continued.

The active ingredient, ethinyloestradiol, is chemically and biologically identical to endogenous human oestradiol. It substitutes for the loss of oestrogen production in menopausal women, and alleviates menopausal symptoms. Oestrogens prevent bone loss following menopause or ovariectomy.

The main therapeutic use of exogenous oestrogens is replacement in deficiency states.

5.2 Pharmacokinetic properties

Ethinyloestradiol is rapidly and completely absorbed from the gut but it undergoes some first pass metabolism in the gut wall.

Ethinyloestradiol is rapidly distributed throughout most body tissues with the largest concentration found in adipose tissue. It distributes into breast milk in low concentrations. More than 80% of ethinyloestradiol in serum is conjugated as the sulphate and almost all the conjugated form is bound to albumin.

Ethinyloestradiol is metabolised in the liver. Hydroxylation appears to be the main metabolic pathway. 60% of a dose is excreted in the urine and 40% in the faeces. About 30% is excreted in the urine and bile as the glucuronide or sulphate conjugate.

The rate of metabolism of ethinyloestradiol is affected by several factors, including enzyme-inducing agents, antibiotics and cigarette smoking.

After oral administration, an initial peak occurs in plasma at 2 to 3 hours, with a secondary peak at about 12 hours after dosing; the second peak is interpreted as evidence for extensive enterohepatic circulation of ethinyloestradiol.

The elimination half-life of ethinyloestradiol ranges from 5 to 16 hours.

5.3 Preclinical safety data
None stated

6. PHARMACEUTICAL PARTICULARS
6.1 List of excipients
Lactose
Starch Maize
Magnesium Stearate
IMS 99%
Purified water

6.2 Incompatibilities
None stated

6.3 Shelf life
36 months

6.4 Special precautions for storage
Store below 25° C

6.5 Nature and contents of container
Pigmented polypropylene container fitted with a tamper evident closure containing 21, 28, 100, or 500 tablets. All pack sizes may not be marketed.

6.6 Special precautions for disposal and other handling
Not applicable

7. MARKETING AUTHORISATION HOLDER
UCB Pharma Ltd
208 Bath Road
Slough
Berkshire
SL1 3WE

8. MARKETING AUTHORISATION NUMBER(S)
10mcg: PL 00039/0548
50mcg: PL 00039/0549
1mg: PL 00039/0550

9. DATE OF FIRST AUTHORISATION/RENEWAL OF THE AUTHORISATION
4 July 2005

10. DATE OF REVISION OF THE TEXT
July 2005

Etrivex 500 micrograms/g Shampoo
(Galderma (U.K) Ltd)

1. NAME OF THE MEDICINAL PRODUCT
Etrivex500 micrograms/g shampoo

2. QUALITATIVE AND QUANTITATIVE COMPOSITION
One gram of shampoo contains 500 micrograms of clobetasol propionate.

For a full list of excipients, see section 6.1.

3. PHARMACEUTICAL FORM
Shampoo.

Viscous, translucent, colourless to pale yellow liquid shampoo with alcoholic odour.

4. CLINICAL PARTICULARS
4.1 Therapeutic indications
Topical treatment of moderate scalp psoriasis in adults.

4.2 Posology and method of administration
For cutaneous use on the scalp only.

Etrivex 500 micrograms/g shampoo should be applied directly on dry scalp once daily taking care to well cover and massage the lesions. An amount equivalent to around a half tablespoon (around 7.5 ml) per application is sufficient to cover all the scalp. Etrivex 500 micrograms/g shampoo should be then kept in place without covering for 15 minutes before rinsing. Hands should be washed carefully after application. After 15 minutes, the product must be rinsed with water and / or hair can be washed by using an additional amount of regular shampoo if needed to facilitate washing. Then, hair can be dried as usual.

The treatment duration should be limited to a maximum of 4 weeks. As soon as clinical results are observed, applications should be spaced out or replaced, if needed, by an alternative treatment. If no improvement is seen within four weeks, reassessment of the diagnosis may be necessary.

Repeated courses of Etrivex 500 micrograms/g shampoo may be used to control exacerbations provided the patient is under regular medical supervision.

Paediatric population
The experience in the paediatric population is limited. Etrivex 500 micrograms/g shampoo is not recommended for use in children and adolescents below 18 years of age. It is contraindicated in children under 2 years of age (see sections 4.3 and 4.4).

4.3 Contraindications
- Hypersensitivity to the active substance or to any of the excipients
- Skin areas affected by bacterial, viral (varicella, herpes simplex, herpes zoster), fungal or parasitic infections and specific skin diseases (skin tuberculosis, skin diseases caused by lues).
- Etrivex 500 micrograms/g shampoo must not be applied to the eye (risk of glaucoma) or to ulcerous wounds.
- Children under 2 years of age

4.4 Special warnings and precautions for use
Topical corticosteroids should be used with caution for a number of reasons including post treatment rebound relapses, development of tolerance (tachyphylaxis) and development of local or systemic toxicity. In rare instances, treatment of psoriasis with corticosteroids (or its withdrawal) is thought to have provoked generalised pustular psoriasis in case of intensive and prolonged topical use. In very rare cases, hypersensitivity to corticosteroids can be observed. This can be suspected in case of resistance to treatment.

In general, long-term continuous therapy with corticosteroids, use of occlusive mobcaps or treatment of children can lead to a higher risk of systemic effects. In such cases, medical supervision should be increased and patients may be evaluated periodically for evidence of HPA axis suppression. Such systemic effects disappear when treatment is stopped. However, abrupt discontinuation can lead to acute adrenal insufficiency, especially in children. If Etrivex 500 micrograms/g shampoo is required for use in children and adolescents below 18 years of age, it is recommended that the treatment should be reviewed weekly.

Etrivex 500 micrograms/g shampoo is only intended for the treatment of scalp psoriasis and should not be used to treat other skin areas. In particular, Etrivex 500 micrograms/g shampoo is not recommended for use in the face, eyelids, intertriginous areas (axillae and genitoanal regions) and on other erosive skin surfaces as this could increase the risk of topical adverse events such as atrophic changes, telangectasia or cortico-induced dermatitis.

If Etrivex 500 micrograms/g shampoo does enter the eye, the affected eye should be rinsed with copious amounts of water.

4.5 Interaction with other medicinal products and other forms of interaction
No interaction studies have been performed

4.6 Pregnancy and lactation
Pregnancy
There are no adequate data from the use of topical clobetasol propionate in pregnant women. Studies in animals have shown reproductive toxicity (see section 5.3). The potential risk for humans is unknown.

Etrivex 500 micrograms/g shampoo should not be used during pregnancy unless clearly necessary.

Lactation
Systemically administered corticosteroids pass into breast milk. Damage to the infant is not reported to date. Nevertheless, as there are no adequate data on the possible milk transfer of topical clobetasol propionate and its biological or clinical repercussions, Etrivex 500 micrograms/g shampoo should not be prescribed to breastfeeding women unless clearly indicated.

4.7 Effects on ability to drive and use machines
As a topical corticosteroid, Etrivex 500 micrograms/g shampoo has no or negligible influence on the ability to drive and use machines.

4.8 Undesirable effects
During clinical development of Etrivex 500 micrograms/g shampoo, in a total of 558 patients receiving Etrivex 500 micrograms/g shampoo, the most commonly reported adverse drug reaction was skin discomfort. Its incidence was about 5%. Most adverse events were rated as mild to moderate and they were not affected by race or gender. Clinical signs of irritation wereuncommon (0.5%). No serious drug-related adverse events were reported during any of the clinical trials.

If signs of local intolerance appear, application should be suspended until they disappear. If signs of hypersensitivity appear, application should be stopped immediately.

The table below reports the adverse reactions related to treatment by body system and by absolute frequency:

Body System	Incidence	Adverse reactions
Skin and subcutaneous tissue disorders	Common (≥ 1/100, < 1/10)	Skin discomfort Acne/folliculitis
	Uncommon (≥ 1/1000, < 1/100)	Local signs of irritation Pruritus Urticaria Telangiectasia Skin atrophy
Eye disorders	Common (≥ 1/100, < 1/10)	Eye stinging/burning

As a class attribution, prolonged use of topical corticosteroids, treatment of extensive areas or use of large amounts can result in sufficient systemic absorption to produce the features of hypercortisolism (Cushing syndrome) or of Hypothalamus-Pituitary-Adrenal (HPA) axis suppression. Should HPA axis suppression occur, it is likely to be transient with a rapid return to normal values. However, as Etrivex 500 micrograms/g shampoo is to be kept in place for only 15 minutes before rinsing, systemic absorption is seldom observed (see section 5.2) and therefore, the risk of appearance of HPA axis suppression is very low compared to non rinsed potent corticosteroids products. No HPA axis suppression has been observed during clinical trials with Etrivex 500 micrograms/g shampoo.

Prolonged and/or intensive treatment with potent corticosteroid preparations may cause local atrophic changes, such as local skin atrophy, striae, telangiectasia, erythema, purpura, contact dermatitis. When applied to the face, very potent corticosteroids can induce perioral dermatitis, skin atrophy or worsen rosacea. During development of Etrivex 500 micrograms/g shampoo, skin atrophy was assessed using ultrasound measurement of skin thickness in a specific clinical trial involving 13 patients. After 4 weeks of treatment with Etrivex 500 micrograms/g shampoo, no skin thinning was observed.

There are reports of pigmentation changes, acne, pustular eruptions and hypertrichosis with topical corticosteroids.

4.9 Overdose
Acute overdose is very unlikely to occur, however, in the case of chronic overdose or misuse, the features of hypercortisolism may appear and in this situation, treatment should be discontinued gradually. However, because of the risk of acute adrenal suppression, this should be done under medical supervision.

5. PHARMACOLOGICAL PROPERTIES
5.1 Pharmacodynamic properties
Pharmacotherapeutic group: Corticosteroids, Very Potent (Group IV)

ATC code: D07AD01

Like other topical corticosteroids, clobetasol propionate has anti-inflammatory, antipruritic, and vasoconstrictive properties. The mechanism of the anti-inflammatory activity of topical corticosteroids in general is unclear. However, corticosteroids are thought to act by induction of phospholipase A_2 inhibitory proteins, collectively called lipocortins. It is postulated that these proteins control the biosynthesis of potent mediators of inflammation such as prostaglandins and leukotrienes by inhibiting the release of their common precursor, arachidonic acid. Arachidonic acid is released from membrane phospholipids by phospholipase A_2.

5.2 Pharmacokinetic properties
In vitro liberation –penetration studies on human skin showed that only a small percentage (0.1 %) of the applied dose of Etrivex Shampoo can be found in the epidermis (including the stratum corneum) when applied for 15 minutes and then rinsed. The very low topical absorption of clobetasol propionate from Etrivex Shampoo when applied according to the recommended clinical use (15 minutes before rinse off) resulted in negligible systemic exposure in animal studies and in clinical trials. Available clinical data revealed that only 1 of 141 subjects had a quantifiable clobetasol propionate plasma concentration (0.43 ng/ml). The present pharmacokinetic data indicate that systemic effects following clinical treatment with Etrivex Shampoo are highly unlikely due to the low systemic bioavailability of clobetasol propionate.

5.3 Preclinical safety data
Non clinical data reveal no special hazard for humans based on conventional studies of safety pharmacology, single, repeated dose toxicity and genotoxicity. The carcinogenicity of clobetasol has not been studied.

In rabbits, Etrivex Shampoo was slightly irritating to the skin and eyes, but no delayed-type hypersensitivity was seen on guinea pigs' skin.

In developmental toxicity studies in the rabbit and the mouse, clobetasol propionate was shown to be teratogenic when administered subcutaneously at low doses. In a topical embryotoxicity study of clobetasol in the rat, foetal immaturity and skeletal and visceral malformations were observed at relatively low dosage levels. In addition to malformations, studies in animals exposed to high systemic levels of glucocorticoids during pregnancy have also shown other effects on the offspring, such as intrauterine growth retardation.

The clinical relevance of the effects of clobetasol and other corticosteroids in developmental animal studies is unknown.

6. PHARMACEUTICAL PARTICULARS

6.1 List of excipients

Ethanol

Coco alkyl dimethyl betaine

Sodium laurethsulfate

Polyquaternium-10

Sodium citrate

Citric acid monohydrate

Purified water

6.2 Incompatibilities

Not applicable

6.3 Shelf life

3 years

Shelf life after first opening: 4 weeks

6.4 Special precautions for storage

Store in the original container

6.5 Nature and contents of container

The product is packaged in high density polyethylene (HDPE) bottles of 60 ml or 125 ml fitted with polypropylene snap closures. The HDPE bottle of 30 ml is fitted with polypropylene screw closure.

Bottles contain 30 ml, 60 ml or 125 ml of shampoo.

1 g of shampoo corresponds to 1 millilitre of shampoo.

Not all pack sizes may be marketed.

6.6 Special precautions for disposal and other handling

No special requirements.

7. MARKETING AUTHORISATION HOLDER

Galderma (UK) Limited

Meridien House

69-71 Clarendon Road

Watford

Herts

WD17 1DS

UK

8. MARKETING AUTHORISATION NUMBER(S)

PL 10590/0052

9. DATE OF FIRST AUTHORISATION/RENEWAL OF THE AUTHORISATION

10. DATE OF REVISION OF THE TEXT

January 2007

Eucardic

(Roche Products Limited)

1. NAME OF THE MEDICINAL PRODUCT

Eucardic 25mg Tablets

2. QUALITATIVE AND QUANTITATIVE COMPOSITION

Each tablet contains 25mg carvedilol.

Excipients: lactose, sucrose.

Each tablet contains 10mg lactose and 25mg sucrose.

For a full list of excipients, see section 6.1.

3. PHARMACEUTICAL FORM

Tablet.

Round white to pale yellowish beige tablet, scored on both sides, marked BM on one side and D5 on the other.

4. CLINICAL PARTICULARS

4.1 Therapeutic indications

Symptomatic chronic heart failure (CHF)

Eucardic is indicated for the treatment of stable mild, moderate and severe chronic heart failure as adjunct to standard therapies e.g. diuretics, digoxin, and ACE inhibitors in patients with euvolemia.

Hypertension

Eucardic is indicated for the treatment of hypertension.

Angina

Eucardic is indicated for the prophylactic treatment of stable angina.

4.2 Posology and method of administration

The tablets should be taken with fluid. For CHF patients Eucardic should be given with food.

Symptomatic chronic heart failure

Initiation of therapy with Eucardic should only be under the supervision of a hospital physician, following a thorough assessment of the patient's condition.

Prior to any subsequent titration of the dose, the patient must be clinically evaluated on the day of up-titration by a health-care professional experienced in the management of heart failure to ensure that the clinical status has remained stable. The dose of carvedilol should not be increased in any patient with deteriorating heart failure since last visit or with signs of decompensated or unstable chronic heart failure.

The dosage must be titrated to individual requirements.

For those patients receiving diuretics and/or digoxin and/or ACE inhibitors, dosing of these other drugs should be stabilised prior to initiation of Eucardic treatment.

Adults

The recommended dose for the initiation of therapy is 3.125mg twice a day for two weeks. If this dose is tolerated, the dosage should be increased subsequently, at intervals of not less than two weeks, to 6.25mg twice daily, followed by 12.5mg twice daily and thereafter 25mg twice daily. Dosing should be increased to the highest level tolerated by the patient.

The recommended maximum daily dose is 25mg given twice daily for all patients with severe CHF and for patients with mild to moderate CHF weighing less than 85kg (187lbs). In patients with mild or moderate CHF weighing more than 85kg, the recommended maximum dose is 50mg twice daily.

During up-titration of the dose in patients with systolic blood pressure < 100mmHg, deterioration of renal and/or cardiac functions may occur. Therefore, before each dose increase these patients should be evaluated by the physician for renal function and symptoms of worsening heart failure or vasodilation. Transient worsening of heart failure, vasodilation or fluid retention may be treated by adjusting doses of diuretics or ACE inhibitors or by modifying or temporarily discontinuing Eucardic treatment. Under these circumstances, the dose of Eucardic should not be increased until symptoms of worsening heart failure or vasodilation have been stabilised.

If Eucardic is discontinued for more than two weeks, therapy should be recommenced at 3.125mg twice daily and up-titrated in line with the above dosing recommendation.

Elderly

As for adults.

Children

Safety and efficacy in children (under 18 years) has not been established.

Hypertension

Once daily dosing is recommended.

Adults

The recommended dose for initiation of therapy is 12.5mg once a day for the first two days. Thereafter the recommended dosage is 25mg once a day. Although this is an adequate dose in most patients, if necessary the dose may be titrated up to a recommended daily maximum dose of 50mg given once a day or in divided doses.

Dose titration should occur at intervals of at least two weeks.

Elderly

An initial dose of 12.5mg daily is recommended. This has provided satisfactory control in some cases. If the response is inadequate the dose may be titrated up to the recommended daily maximum dose of 50mg given once a day or in divided doses.

Children

Safety and efficacy in children (under 18 years) has not been established.

Angina

Adults

The recommended dose for initiation of therapy is 12.5mg twice a day for the first two days. Thereafter, the recommended dosage is 25mg twice a day.

Elderly

The recommended maximum daily dose is 50mg given in divided doses.

Children

Safety and efficacy in children (under 18 years) has not been established.

Patients with co-existing hepatic disease

Eucardic is contraindicated in patients with hepatic dysfunction (see sections *4.3 Contraindications* and *5.2 Pharmacokinetic properties*).

Patients with co-existing renal dysfunction

No dose adjustment is anticipated as long as systolic blood pressure is above 100mmHg (see also sections *4.4 Special warnings and precautions for use* and *5.2 Pharmacokinetic properties*).

4.3 Contraindications

Hypersensitivity to the active substance or to any of the excipients.

Eucardic is contraindicated in patients with marked fluid retention or overload requiring intravenous inotropic support.

Patients with obstructive airways disease, liver dysfunction.

As with other beta-blocking agents: History of bronchospasm or asthma, 2nd and 3rd degree A-V heart block, (unless a permanent pacemaker is in place), severe bradycardia (< 50 bpm), cardiogenic shock, sick sinus syndrome (including sino-atrial block), severe hypotension (systolic blood pressure < 85mmHg), metabolic acidosis and phaeochromocytoma (unless adequately controlled by alpha blockade).

4.4 Special warnings and precautions for use

This medicinal product contains lactose, therefore patients with rare hereditary problems of galactose intolerance, the Lapp lactase deficiency, or glucose-galactose malabsorption should not take this medicine.

This medicinal product contains sucrose, therefore patients with rare hereditary problems of fructose intolerance, glucose-galactose malabsorption or sucrase-isomaltase insufficiency should not take this medicine.

In chronic heart failure patients, worsening cardiac failure or fluid retention may occur during up-titration of Eucardic. If such symptoms occur, the dose of diuretic should be adjusted and the Eucardic dose should not be advanced until clinical stability resumes. Occasionally it may be necessary to lower the Eucardic dose or temporarily discontinue it. Such episodes do not preclude subsequent successful titration of Eucardic.

In hypertensive patients who have chronic heart failure controlled with digoxin, diuretics and/or an ACE inhibitor, Eucardic should be used with caution since both digoxin and Eucardic may slow A-V conduction.

As with other drugs with beta-blocking activity, Eucardic may mask the early signs of acute hypoglycaemia in patients with diabetes mellitus. Alternatives to beta-blocking agents are generally preferred in insulin-dependent patients. In patients with diabetes, the use of Eucardic may be associated with worsening control of blood glucose. Therefore, regular monitoring of blood glucose is required in diabetics when Eucardic is initiated or up-titrated and hypoglycaemic therapy adjusted accordingly.

Reversible deterioration of renal function has been observed with Eucardic therapy in chronic heart failure patients with low blood pressure (systolic BP < 100mmHg), ischaemic heart disease and diffuse vascular disease, and/or underlying renal insufficiency. In CHF patients with these risk factors, renal function should be monitored during up-titration of Eucardic and the drug discontinued or dosage reduced if worsening of renal failure occurs.

Wearers of contact lenses should be advised of the possibility of reduced lacrimation.

Although angina has not been reported on stopping treatment, discontinuation should be gradual (1 - 2 weeks) particularly in patients with ischaemic heart disease, as Eucardic has beta-blocking activity.

Eucardic may be used in patients with peripheral vascular disease. Pure beta-blockers can precipitate or aggravate symptoms of arterial insufficiency. However as Eucardic also has alpha-blocking properties this effect is largely counterbalanced.

Eucardic, as with other agents with beta-blocking activity, may mask the symptoms of thyrotoxicosis.

If Eucardic induces bradycardia, with a decrease in pulse rate to less than 55 beats per minute, the dosage of Eucardic should be reduced.

Care should be taken in administering Eucardic to patients with a history of serious hypersensitivity reactions and in those undergoing desensitisation therapy as beta-blockers may increase both the sensitivity towards allergens and the seriousness of anaphylactic reactions.

In patients suffering from the peripheral circulatory disorder Raynaud's phenomenon, there may be exacerbation of symptoms.

Patients with a history of psoriasis associated with beta-blocker therapy should be given Eucardic only after consideration of the risk-benefit ratio.

In patients with phaeochromocytoma, an alpha-blocking agent should be initiated prior to the use of any beta-blocking agent. There is no experience of the use of carvedilol in this condition. Therefore, caution should be taken in the administration of Eucardic to patients suspected of having phaeochromocytoma.

Agents with non-selective beta-blocking activity may provoke chest pain in patients with Prinzmetal's variant angina. There is no clinical experience with Eucardic in these patients, although the alpha-blocking activity of Eucardic may prevent such symptoms. However, caution should be taken in the administration of Eucardic to patients suspected of having Prinzmetal's variant angina.

In patients with a tendency to bronchospastic reactions, respiratory distress can occur as a result of a possible increase in airway resistance. The following warnings will be included on the outer packaging and leaflet:

Packaging

Do not take this medicine if you have a history of wheezing due to asthma or other lung diseases.

Leaflet

Do not take this medicine if you have a history of wheezing due to asthma or other lung diseases. Consult your doctor or pharmacist first.

4.5 Interaction with other medicinal products and other forms of interaction

As with other agents with beta-blocking activity, Eucardic may potentiate the effect of other concomitantly administered drugs that are anti-hypertensive in action (e.g. alpha$_1$-receptor antagonists) or have hypotension as part of their adverse effect profile.

Patients taking an agent with β-blocking properties and a drug that can deplete catecholamines (e.g. reserpine and monoamine oxidase inhibitors) should be observed closely for signs of hypotension and/or severe bradycardia.

Isolated cases of conduction disturbance (rarely with haemodynamic disruption) have been observed when Eucardic and diltiazem were given concomitantly. Therefore, as with other drugs with beta-blocking activity, careful monitoring of ECG and blood pressure should be undertaken when co-administering calcium channel blockers of the verapamil or diltiazem type, or class I antiarrhythmic drugs. These types of drugs should not be co-administered intravenously in patients receiving Eucardic.

The effects of insulin or oral hypoglycaemics may be intensified. Regular monitoring of blood glucose is therefore recommended.

Trough plasma digoxin levels may be increased by approximately 16% in hypertensive patients co-administered Eucardic and digoxin. Increased monitoring of digoxin levels is recommended when initiating, adjusting or discontinuing Eucardic. Concomitant administration of Eucardic and cardiac glycosides may prolong AV conduction time.

When treatment with Eucardic and clonidine together is to be terminated, Eucardic should be withdrawn first, several days before gradually decreasing the dosage of clonidine.

Care may be required in those receiving inducers of mixed function oxidases e.g. rifampicin, as serum levels of carvedilol may be reduced or inhibitors of mixed function oxidases e.g. cimetidine, as serum levels may be increased.

During general anaesthesia, attention should be paid to the potential synergistic negative inotropic effects of carvedilol and anaesthetic drugs.

Modest increases in mean trough cyclosporin concentrations were observed following initiation of carvedilol treatment in 21 renal transplant patients suffering from chronic vascular rejection. In about 30% of patients, the dose of cyclosporin had to be reduced in order to maintain cyclosporin concentrations within the therapeutic range, while in the remainder no adjustment was needed. On average, the dose of cyclosporin was reduced about 20% in these patients. Due to wide interindividual variability in the dose adjustment required, it is recommended that cyclosporin concentrations be monitored closely after initiation of carvedilol therapy and that the dose of cyclosporin be adjusted as appropriate.

4.6 Pregnancy and lactation

Pregnancy

There are no adequate data from the use of carvedilol in pregnant women.

Animal studies are insufficient with respect to effects on pregnancy, embryonal/foetal development, parturition and postnatal development (see section 5.3). The potential risk for humans is unknown.

Eucardic should not be used during pregnancy unless clearly necessary (i.e. unless the anticipated benefits outweigh the potential risks).

Lactation

It is unknown whether carvedilol is excreted in human breast milk. Animal studies have shown excretion of carvedilol or its metabolites in breast milk. A decision on whether to continue/discontinue breast-feeding or to continue/discontinue therapy with Eucardic should be made taking into account the benefit of breast-feeding to the child and the benefit of Eucardic therapy to the woman.

4.7 Effects on ability to drive and use machines

No studies of the effects on ability to drive and use machines have been performed.

As for other drugs which produce changes in blood pressure, patients taking Eucardic should be warned not to drive or operate machinery if they experience dizziness or related symptoms. This applies particularly when starting or changing treatment and in conjunction with alcohol.

4.8 Undesirable effects

Clinical Trials

Adverse events are listed separately for CHF because of differences in the background diseases.

In chronic heart failure:

Haematological

Rare: thrombocytopenia.

Leucopenia has been reported in isolated cases.

Metabolic

Common: weight increase and hypercholesterolaemia. Hyperglycaemia, hypoglycaemia and worsening control of blood glucose are also common in patients with pre-existing diabetes mellitus (see section *4.5 Interaction with other medicinal products and other forms of interaction*).

Central nervous system

Very common: dizziness, headache are usually mild and occur particularly at the start of treatment. Asthenia (including fatigue).

Cardiovascular system

Common: bradycardia, postural hypotension, hypotension, oedema (including generalised, peripheral, dependent and genital oedema, oedema of the legs, hypervolaemia and fluid overload).

Uncommon: syncope (including presyncope), AV-block and cardiac failure during up-titration.

Gastro-intestinal system

Common: nausea, diarrhoea, and vomiting.

Skin and appendages

Dermatitis, and increased sweating.

Others

Common: vision abnormalities.

Rare: acute renal failure and renal function abnormalities in patients with diffuse vascular disease and/or impaired renal function (see section *4.4 Special warnings and precautions for use*).

The frequency of adverse experiences is not dose dependent, with the exception of dizziness, abnormal vision and bradycardia.

In hypertension and angina:

The profile is similar to that observed in chronic heart failure although the incidence of events is generally lower in patients with hypertension or angina treated with Eucardic.

Blood chemistry and haematological

Isolated cases of changes in serum transaminases, thrombocytopenia and leucopenia have been reported.

Central nervous system

Common: dizziness, headaches and fatigue, which are usually mild and occur particularly at the beginning of treatment.

Uncommon: depressed mood, sleep disturbance, paraesthesia, asthenia.

Metabolic

Due to the beta-blocking properties it is also possible for latent diabetes mellitus to become manifest, manifest diabetes to be aggravated, and blood glucose counter-regulation to be inhibited.

Cardiovascular system

Common: bradycardia, postural hypotension, especially at the beginning of treatment.

Uncommon: syncope, hypotension, disturbances of peripheral circulation (cold extremities, PVD, exacerbation of intermittent claudication and Raynauds phenomenon). AV-block, angina pectoris (including chest pain), symptoms of heart failure and peripheral oedema.

Respiratory system

Common: asthma and dyspnoea in predisposed patients.

Rare: stuffy nose. Wheezing and flu-like symptoms.

Gastro-intestinal system

Common: gastro-intestinal upset (with symptoms such as nausea, abdominal pain, diarrhoea).

Uncommon: constipation and vomiting.

Skin and appendages

Uncommon: skin reactions (e.g. allergic exanthema, dermatitis, urticaria, pruritus, lichen planus-like reactions, and increased sweating). Psoriatic skin lesions may occur or existing lesions exacerbated.

Others

Common: pain in the extremities, reduced lacrimation.

Uncommon: cases of sexual impotence and disturbed vision.

Rare: dryness of the mouth and disturbances of micturition and eye irritation.

Isolated cases of allergic reactions have been reported.

Post-marketing experience

Isolated cases of urinary incontinence in women, which resolved upon discontinuation of the medication, have been reported.

4.9 Overdose

Symptoms and signs

Profound cardiovascular effects such as hypotension and bradycardia would be expected after massive overdose. Heart failure, cardiogenic shock and cardiac arrest may follow. There may also be respiratory problems, bronchospasm, vomiting, disturbed consciousness and generalised seizures.

Treatment

Gastric lavage or induced emesis may be useful in the first few hours after ingestion.

In addition to general procedures, vital signs must be monitored and corrected, if necessary under intensive care conditions.

Patients should be placed in the supine position. Atropine, 0.5mg to 2mg i.v. and/or glucagon 1 to 10mg i.v. (followed by a slow i.v. infusion of 2 to 5mg/hour if necessary) may be given when bradycardia is present. Pacemaker therapy may be necessary. For excessive hypotension, intravenous fluids may be administered. In addition, norepinephrine may be given, either 5 to 10 micrograms i.v., repeated according to blood pressure response, or 5 micrograms per minute by infusion titrated to blood pressure. Bronchospasm may be treated using salbutamol or other beta$_2$-agonists given as aerosol or, if necessary, by the intravenous route. In the event of seizures, slow i.v. injection of diazepam or clonazepam is recommended.

In cases of severe overdose with symptoms of shock, supportive treatment as described should be continued for a sufficiently long period of time, i.e. until the patient stabilises, since prolonged elimination half life and redistribution of carvedilol from deeper compartments can be expected.

5. PHARMACOLOGICAL PROPERTIES

5.1 Pharmacodynamic properties

Pharmacotherapeutic group: Alpha and beta blocking agents. ATC code: C07AG02.

Carvedilol is a vasodilating non-selective beta-blocking agent with antioxidant properties. Vasodilation is predominantly mediated through alpha$_1$ receptor antagonism.

Carvedilol reduces the peripheral vascular resistance through vasodilation and suppresses the renin-angiotensin-aldosterone system through beta-blockade. The activity of plasma renin is reduced and fluid retention is rare.

Carvedilol has no intrinsic sympathomimetic activity and like propranolol, it has membrane stabilising properties.

Carvedilol is a racemate of two stereoisomers. Beta-blockade is attributed to the S(-) enantiomer; in contrast, both enantiomers exhibit the same α_1-blocking activity.

Carvedilol is a potent antioxidant, a scavenger of reactive oxygen radicals and an anti-proliferative agent. The properties of carvedilol and its metabolites have been demonstrated in *in vitro* and *in vivo* animal studies and *in vitro* in a number of human cell types.

Clinical studies have shown that the balance of vasodilation and beta-blockade provided by carvedilol results in the following effects:

– In hypertensive patients, a reduction in blood pressure is not associated with a concomitant increase in total peripheral resistance, as observed with pure beta-blocking agents. Heart rate is slightly decreased. Renal blood flow and renal function are maintained. Peripheral blood flow is maintained, therefore, cold extremities, often observed with drugs possessing beta-blocking activity, are rarely seen.

– In patients with stable angina, Eucardic has demonstrated anti-ischaemic and anti-anginal properties. Acute haemodynamic studies demonstrated that Eucardic reduces ventricular pre- and after-load.

– In patients with left ventricular dysfunction or chronic heart failure, carvedilol has demonstrated favourable effects on haemodynamics and improvements in left ventricular ejection fraction and dimensions.

– In a large, multi-centre, double-blind, placebo-controlled mortality trial (COPERNICUS), 2289 patients with severe stable CHF of ischaemic or non-ischaemic origin, on standard therapy, were randomised to either carvedilol (1156 patients) or placebo (1133 patients). Patients had left ventricular systolic dysfunction with a mean ejection fraction of < 20%. All-cause mortality was reduced by 35% from 19.7% in the placebo group to 12.8% in the carvedilol group (Cox proportional hazards, $p = 0.00013$).

Combined secondary endpoints of mortality or hospitalisation for heart failure, mortality or cardiovascular hospitalisation and mortality or all-cause hospitalisation were all significantly lower in the carvedilol group than placebo (31%, 27% and 24% reductions, respectively, all $p < 0.00004$).

The incidence of serious adverse events during the study was lower in the carvedilol group (39.0% *vs* 45.4%). During initiation of treatment, the incidence of worsening heart failure was similar in both carvedilol and placebo groups. The incidence of serious worsening heart failure during the study was lower in the carvedilol group (14.6% *vs* 21.6%).

Serum lipid profile and electrolytes are not affected.

5.2 Pharmacokinetic properties

The absolute bioavailability of carvedilol is approximately 25% in humans. Bioavailability is stereo-selective, 30% for the R-form and 15% for the S-form. Serum levels peak at approximately 1 hour after an oral dose. There is a linear relationship between the dose and serum concentrations. Food does not affect bioavailability or the maximum serum concentration although the time to reach maximum serum concentration is delayed. Carvedilol is highly lipophilic, approximately 98% to 99% is bound to plasma proteins. The distribution volume is approximately 2 l/kg and increased in patients with liver cirrhosis. The first pass effect after oral administration is approximately 60 - 75%; enterohepatic circulation of the parent substance has been shown in animals.

Carvedilol exhibits a considerable first pass effect. The metabolite pattern reveals intensive metabolism with glucuronidation as one of the major steps. Demethylation and hydroxylation at the phenol ring produce 3 metabolites with beta-receptor blocking activity.

The average elimination half-life ranges from 6 to 10 hours. Plasma clearance is approximately 590ml/min. Elimination is mainly biliary. The primary route of excretion is via the faeces. A minor portion is eliminated via the kidneys in the form of various metabolites.

The pharmacokinetics of carvedilol are affected by age; plasma levels of carvedilol are approximately 50% higher in the elderly compared to young subjects. In a study in patients with cirrhotic liver disease, the bioavailability of carvedilol was four times greater and the peak plasma level five times higher than in healthy subjects. Since carvedilol is primarily excreted via the faeces, significant accumulation in patients with renal impairment is unlikely. In patients with impaired liver function, bioavailability is raised to as much as 80% due to a reduced first pass effect.

5.3 Preclinical safety data

There is no evidence from animal studies that Eucardic has any teratogenic effects. Embryotoxicity was observed only after large doses in rabbits. The relevance of these findings for humans is uncertain. Beta-blockers reduce placental perfusion which may result in intrauterine foetal death and immature and premature deliveries. In addition, animal studies have shown that carvedilol crosses the placental barrier and therefore the possible consequences of alpha and beta-blockade in the human foetus and neonate should also be borne in mind. With other alpha and beta-blocking agents, effects have included perinatal and neonatal distress (bradycardia, hypotension, respiratory depression, hypoglycaemia, hypothermia). There is an increased risk of cardiac and pulmonary complications in the neonate in the postnatal period.

6. PHARMACEUTICAL PARTICULARS

6.1 List of excipients

Lactose

Sucrose

Povidone

Crospovidone

Colloidal silicon dioxide

Magnesium stearate

6.2 Incompatibilities

Not applicable.

6.3 Shelf life

5 years.

6.4 Special precautions for storage

Store below 25°C.

Store in the original package in order to protect from moisture.

Keep the blister strips in the outer carton in order to protect from light.

6.5 Nature and contents of container

Blister packs, PVC/Aluminium of 14, 28, 30, 56 or 100 tablets. Standard polypropylene tube packs of 100 tablets.

Not all pack sizes may be marketed.

6.6 Special precautions for disposal and other handling

No special requirements.

7. MARKETING AUTHORISATION HOLDER

Roche Products Limited, 6 Falcon Way, Shire Park, Welwyn Garden City, AL7 1TW, United Kingdom.

8. MARKETING AUTHORISATION NUMBER(S)

PL 00031/0553

9. DATE OF FIRST AUTHORISATION/RENEWAL OF THE AUTHORISATION

7 September 2001

10. DATE OF REVISION OF THE TEXT

23 July 2007

LEGAL STATUS

POM

Eucardic is a registered trade mark.

Item Code

Eucardic 12.5mg Tablets

(Roche Products Limited)

1. NAME OF THE MEDICINAL PRODUCT

Eucardic 12.5mg Tablets

2. QUALITATIVE AND QUANTITATIVE COMPOSITION

Each tablet contains 12.5mg carvedilol.

Excipients: lactose, sucrose.

Each tablet contains 59.1mg lactose and 12.5mg sucrose.

For a full list of excipients, see section 6.1.

3. PHARMACEUTICAL FORM

Tablet.

Round light brown tablet, scored on both sides, marked BM on one side and H3 on the other.

4. CLINICAL PARTICULARS

4.1 Therapeutic indications

Symptomatic chronic heart failure (CHF)

Eucardic is indicated for the treatment of stable mild, moderate and severe chronic heart failure as adjunct to standard therapies e.g. diuretics, digoxin, and ACE inhibitors in patients with euvolemia.

Hypertension

Eucardic is indicated for the treatment of hypertension.

Angina

Eucardic is indicated for the prophylactic treatment of stable angina.

4.2 Posology and method of administration

The tablets should be taken with fluid. For CHF patients Eucardic should be given with food.

Symptomatic chronic heart failure

Initiation of therapy with Eucardic should only be under the supervision of a hospital physician, following a thorough assessment of the patient's condition.

Prior to any subsequent titration of the dose, the patient must be clinically evaluated on the day of up-titration by a health-care professional experienced in the management of heart failure to ensure that the clinical status has remained stable. The dose of carvedilol should not be increased in any patient with deteriorating heart failure since last visit or with signs of decompensated or unstable chronic heart failure.

The dosage must be titrated to individual requirements.

For those patients receiving diuretics and/or digoxin and/or ACE inhibitors, dosing of these other drugs should be stabilised prior to initiation of Eucardic treatment.

Adults

The recommended dose for the initiation of therapy is 3.125mg twice a day for two weeks. If this dose is tolerated, the dosage should be increased subsequently, at intervals of not less than two weeks, to 6.25mg twice daily, followed by 12.5mg twice daily and thereafter 25mg twice daily. Dosing should be increased to the highest level tolerated by the patient.

The recommended maximum daily dose is 25mg given twice daily for all patients with severe CHF and for patients with mild to moderate CHF weighing less than 85kg (187lbs). In patients with mild or moderate CHF weighing more than 85kg, the recommended maximum dose is 50mg twice daily.

During up-titration of the dose in patients with systolic blood pressure < 100mmHg, deterioration of renal and/or cardiac functions may occur. Therefore, before each dose increase these patients should be evaluated by the physician for renal function and symptoms of worsening heart failure or vasodilation. Transient worsening of heart failure, vasodilation or fluid retention may be treated by adjusting doses of diuretics or ACE inhibitors or by modifying or temporarily discontinuing Eucardic treatment. Under these circumstances, the dose of Eucardic should not be increased until symptoms of worsening heart failure or vasodilation have been stabilised.

If Eucardic is discontinued for more than two weeks, therapy should be recommenced at 3.125mg twice daily and up-titrated in line with the above dosing recommendation.

Elderly

As for adults.

Children

Safety and efficacy in children (under 18 years) has not been established.

Hypertension

Once daily dosing is recommended.

Adults

The recommended dose for initiation of therapy is 12.5mg once a day for the first two days. Thereafter the recommended dosage is 25mg once a day. Although this is an adequate dose in most patients, if necessary the dose may be titrated up to a recommended daily maximum dose of 50mg given once a day or in divided doses.

Dose titration should occur at intervals of at least two weeks.

Elderly

An initial dose of 12.5mg daily is recommended. This has provided satisfactory control in some cases. If the response is inadequate the dose may be titrated up to the recommended daily maximum dose of 50mg given once a day or in divided doses.

Children

Safety and efficacy in children (under 18 years) has not been established.

Angina

Adults

The recommended dose for initiation of therapy is 12.5mg twice a day for the first two days. Thereafter, the recommended dosage is 25mg twice a day.

Elderly

The recommended maximum daily dose is 50mg given in divided doses.

Children

Safety and efficacy in children (under 18 years) has not been established.

Patients with co-existing hepatic disease

Eucardic is contraindicated in patients with hepatic dysfunction (see sections *4.3 Contraindications* and *5.2 Pharmacokinetic properties*).

Patients with co-existing renal dysfunction

No dose adjustment is anticipated as long as systolic blood pressure is above 100mmHg (see also sections *4.4 Special warnings and precautions for use* and *5.2 Pharmacokinetic properties*).

4.3 Contraindications

Hypersensitivity to the active substance or to any of the excipients.

Eucardic is contraindicated in patients with marked fluid retention or overload requiring intravenous inotropic support.

Patients with obstructive airways disease, liver dysfunction.

As with other beta-blocking agents: History of bronchospasm or asthma, 2nd and 3rd degree A-V heart block, (unless a permanent pacemaker is in place), severe bradycardia (< 50 bpm), cardiogenic shock, sick sinus syndrome (including sino-atrial block), severe hypotension (systolic blood pressure < 85mmHg), metabolic acidosis and phaeochromocytoma (unless adequately controlled by alpha blockade).

4.4 Special warnings and precautions for use

This medicinal product contains lactose, therefore patients with rare hereditary problems of galactose intolerance, the Lapp lactase deficiency, or glucose-galactose malabsorption should not take this medicine.

This medicinal product contains sucrose, therefore patients with rare hereditary problems of fructose intolerance, glucose-galactose malabsorption or sucrase-isomaltase insufficiency should not take this medicine.

In chronic heart failure patients, worsening cardiac failure or fluid retention may occur during up-titration of Eucardic. If such symptoms occur, the dose of diuretic should be adjusted and the Eucardic dose should not be advanced until clinical stability resumes. Occasionally it may be necessary to lower the Eucardic dose or temporarily discontinue it. Such episodes do not preclude subsequent successful titration of Eucardic.

In hypertensive patients who have chronic heart failure controlled with digoxin, diuretics and/or an ACE inhibitor, Eucardic should be used with caution since both digoxin and Eucardic may slow A-V conduction.

As with other drugs with beta-blocking activity, Eucardic may mask the early signs of acute hypoglycaemia in patients with diabetes mellitus. Alternatives to beta-blocking agents are generally preferred in insulin-dependent patients. In patients with diabetes, the use of Eucardic may be associated with worsening control of blood glucose. Therefore, regular monitoring of blood glucose is required in diabetics when Eucardic is initiated or up-titrated and hypoglycaemic therapy adjusted accordingly.

Reversible deterioration of renal function has been observed with Eucardic therapy in chronic heart failure patients with low blood pressure (systolic BP < 100mmHg), ischaemic heart disease and diffuse vascular disease, and/or underlying renal insufficiency. In CHF patients with these risk factors, renal function should be monitored during up-titration of Eucardic and the drug discontinued or dosage reduced if worsening of renal failure occurs.

Wearers of contact lenses should be advised of the possibility of reduced lacrimation.

Although angina has not been reported on stopping treatment, discontinuation should be gradual (1 - 2 weeks) particularly in patients with ischaemic heart disease, as Eucardic has beta-blocking activity.

Eucardic may be used in patients with peripheral vascular disease. Pure beta-blockers can precipitate or aggravate symptoms of arterial insufficiency. However as Eucardic also has alpha-blocking properties this effect is largely counterbalanced.

Eucardic, as with other agents with beta-blocking activity, may mask the symptoms of thyrotoxicosis.

If Eucardic induces bradycardia, with a decrease in pulse rate to less than 55 beats per minute, the dosage of Eucardic should be reduced.

Care should be taken in administering Eucardic to patients with a history of serious hypersensitivity reactions and in those undergoing desensitisation therapy as beta-blockers may increase both the sensitivity towards allergens and the seriousness of anaphylactic reactions.

In patients suffering from the peripheral circulatory disorder Raynaud's phenomenon, there may be exacerbation of symptoms.

Patients with a history of psoriasis associated with beta-blocker therapy should be given Eucardic only after consideration of the risk-benefit ratio.

In patients with phaeochromocytoma, an alpha-blocking agent should be initiated prior to the use of any beta-blocking agent. There is no experience of the use of carvedilol in this condition. Therefore, caution should be taken in the administration of Eucardic to patients suspected of having phaeochromocytoma.

Agents with non-selective beta-blocking activity may provoke chest pain in patients with Prinzmetal's variant angina. There is no clinical experience with Eucardic in these patients, although the alpha-blocking activity of

Eucardic may prevent such symptoms. However, caution should be taken in the administration of Eucardic to patients suspected of having Prinzmetal's variant angina.

In patients with a tendency to bronchospastic reactions, respiratory distress can occur as a result of a possible increase in airway resistance. The following warnings will be included on the outer packaging and leaflet:

Packaging

Do not take this medicine if you have a history of wheezing due to asthma or other lung diseases.

Leaflet

Do not take this medicine if you have a history of wheezing due to asthma or other lung diseases. Consult your doctor or pharmacist first.

4.5 Interaction with other medicinal products and other forms of interaction

As with other agents with beta-blocking activity, Eucardic may potentiate the effect of other concomitantly administered drugs that are anti-hypertensive in action (e.g. $alpha_1$-receptor antagonists) or have hypotension as part of their adverse effect profile.

Patients taking an agent with β-blocking properties and a drug that can deplete catecholamines (e.g. reserpine and monoamine oxidase inhibitors) should be observed closely for signs of hypotension and/or severe bradycardia.

Isolated cases of conduction disturbance (rarely with haemodynamic disruption) have been observed when Eucardic and diltiazem were given concomitantly. Therefore, as with other drugs with beta-blocking activity, careful monitoring of ECG and blood pressure should be undertaken when co-administering calcium channel blockers of the verapamil or diltiazem type, or class I antiarrhythmic drugs. These types of drugs should not be co-administered intravenously in patients receiving Eucardic.

The effects of insulin or oral hypoglycaemics may be intensified. Regular monitoring of blood glucose is therefore recommended.

Trough plasma digoxin levels may be increased by approximately 16% in hypertensive patients co-administered Eucardic and digoxin. Increased monitoring of digoxin levels is recommended when initiating, adjusting or discontinuing Eucardic. Concomitant administration of Eucardic and cardiac glycosides may prolong AV conduction time.

When treatment with Eucardic and clonidine together is to be terminated, Eucardic should be withdrawn first, several days before gradually decreasing the dosage of clonidine.

Care may be required in those receiving inducers of mixed function oxidases e.g. rifampicin, as serum levels of carvedilol may be reduced or inhibitors of mixed function oxidases e.g. cimetidine, as serum levels may be increased.

During general anaesthesia, attention should be paid to the potential synergistic negative inotropic effects of carvedilol and anaesthetic drugs.

Modest increases in mean trough cyclosporin concentrations were observed following initiation of carvedilol treatment in 21 renal transplant patients suffering from chronic vascular rejection. In about 30% of patients, the dose of cyclosporin had to be reduced in order to maintain cyclosporin concentrations within the therapeutic range, while in the remainder no adjustment was needed. On average, the dose of cyclosporin was reduced about 20% in these patients. Due to wide interindividual variability in the dose adjustment required, it is recommended that cyclosporin concentrations be monitored closely after initiation of carvedilol therapy and that the dose of cyclosporin be adjusted as appropriate.

4.6 Pregnancy and lactation

Pregnancy

There are no adequate data from the use of carvedilol in pregnant women.

Animal studies are insufficient with respect to effects on pregnancy, embryonal/foetal development, parturition and postnatal development (see section 5.3). The potential risk for humans is unknown.

Eucardic should not be used during pregnancy unless clearly necessary (i.e. unless the anticipated benefits outweigh the potential risks).

Lactation

It is unknown whether carvedilol is excreted in human breast milk. Animal studies have shown excretion of carvedilol or its metabolites in breast milk. A decision on whether to continue/discontinue breast-feeding or to continue/discontinue therapy with Eucardic should be made taking into account the benefit of breast-feeding to the child and the benefit of Eucardic therapy to the woman.

4.7 Effects on ability to drive and use machines

No studies of the effects on ability to drive and use machines have been performed.

As for other drugs which produce changes in blood pressure, patients taking Eucardic should be warned not to drive or operate machinery if they experience dizziness or related symptoms. This applies particularly when starting or changing treatment and in conjunction with alcohol.

4.8 Undesirable effects

Clinical Trials

Adverse events are listed separately for CHF because of differences in the background diseases.

In chronic heart failure:

Haematological

Rare: thrombocytopenia.

Leucopenia has been reported in isolated cases.

Metabolic

Common: weight increase and hypercholesterolaemia. Hyperglycaemia, hypoglycaemia and worsening control of blood glucose are also common in patients with preexisting diabetes mellitus (see section *4.5 Interaction with other medicinal products and other forms of interaction*).

Central nervous system

Very common: dizziness, headache are usually mild and occur particularly at the start of treatment. Asthenia (including fatigue).

Cardiovascular system

Common: bradycardia, postural hypotension, hypotension, oedema (including generalised, peripheral, dependent and genital oedema, oedema of the legs, hypervolaemia and fluid overload).

Uncommon: syncope (including presyncope), AV-block and cardiac failure during up-titration.

Gastro-intestinal system

Common: nausea, diarrhoea, and vomiting.

Skin and appendages

Dermatitis, and increased sweating.

Others

Common: vision abnormalities.

Rare: acute renal failure and renal function abnormalities in patients with diffuse vascular disease and/or impaired renal function (see section *4.4 Special warnings and precautions for use*).

The frequency of adverse experiences is not dose dependent, with the exception of dizziness, abnormal vision and bradycardia.

In hypertension and angina:

The profile is similar to that observed in chronic heart failure although the incidence of events is generally lower in patients with hypertension or angina treated with Eucardic.

Blood chemistry and haematological

Isolated cases of changes in serum transaminases, thrombocytopenia and leucopenia have been reported.

Central nervous system

Common: dizziness, headaches and fatigue, which are usually mild and occur particularly at the beginning of treatment.

Uncommon: depressed mood, sleep disturbance, paraesthesia, asthenia.

Metabolic

Due to the beta-blocking properties it is also possible for latent diabetes mellitus to become manifest, manifest diabetes to be aggravated, and blood glucose counter-regulation to be inhibited.

Cardiovascular system

Common: bradycardia, postural hypotension, especially at the beginning of treatment.

Uncommon: syncope, hypotension, disturbances of peripheral circulation (cold extremities, PVD, exacerbation of intermittent claudication and Raynauds phenomenon). AV-block, angina pectoris (including chest pain), symptoms of heart failure and peripheral oedema.

Respiratory system

Common: asthma and dyspnoea in predisposed patients.

Rare: stuffy nose. Wheezing and flu-like symptoms.

Gastro-intestinal system

Common: gastro-intestinal upset (with symptoms such as nausea, abdominal pain, diarrhoea).

Uncommon: constipation and vomiting.

Skin and appendages

Uncommon: skin reactions (e.g. allergic exanthema, dermatitis, urticaria, pruritus, lichen planus-like reactions, and increased sweating). Psoriatic skin lesions may occur or existing lesions exacerbated.

Others

Common: pain in the extremities, reduced lacrimation.

Uncommon: cases of sexual impotence and disturbed vision.

Rare: dryness of the mouth and disturbances of micturition and eye irritation.

Isolated cases of allergic reactions have been reported.

Post-marketing experience

Isolated cases of urinary incontinence in women, which resolved upon discontinuation of the medication, have been reported.

4.9 Overdose

Symptoms and signs

Profound cardiovascular effects such as hypotension and bradycardia would be expected after massive overdose. Heart failure, cardiogenic shock and cardiac arrest may follow. There may also be respiratory problems, bronchospasm, vomiting, disturbed consciousness and generalised seizures.

Treatment

Gastric lavage or induced emesis may be useful in the first few hours after ingestion.

In addition to general procedures, vital signs must be monitored and corrected, if necessary under intensive care conditions.

Patients should be placed in the supine position. Atropine, 0.5mg to 2mg i.v. and/or glucagon 1 to 10mg i.v. (followed by a slow i.v. infusion of 2 to 5mg/hour if necessary) may be given when bradycardia is present. Pacemaker therapy may be necessary. For excessive hypotension, intravenous fluids may be administered. In addition, norepinephrine may be given, either 5 to 10 micrograms i.v., repeated according to blood pressure response, or 5 micrograms per minute by infusion titrated to blood pressure. Bronchospasm may be treated using salbutamol or other $beta_2$-agonists given as aerosol or, if necessary, by the intravenous route. In the event of seizures, slow i.v. injection of diazepam or clonazepam is recommended.

In cases of severe overdose with symptoms of shock, supportive treatment as described should be continued for a sufficiently long period of time, i.e. until the patient stabilises, since prolonged elimination half life and redistribution of carvedilol from deeper compartments can be expected.

5. PHARMACOLOGICAL PROPERTIES

5.1 Pharmacodynamic properties

Pharmacotherapeutic group: Alpha and beta blocking agents. ATC code C07AG02.

Carvedilol is a vasodilating non-selective beta-blocking agent with antioxidant properties. Vasodilation is predominantly mediated through $alpha_1$ receptor antagonism.

Carvedilol reduces the peripheral vascular resistance through vasodilation and suppresses the renin-angiotensin-aldosterone system through beta-blockade. The activity of plasma renin is reduced and fluid retention is rare.

Carvedilol has no intrinsic sympathomimetic activity and like propranolol, it has membrane stabilising properties.

Carvedilol is a racemate of two stereoisomers. Beta-blockade is attributed to the S(-) enantiomer; in contrast, both enantiomers exhibit the same α_1-blocking activity.

Carvedilol is a potent antioxidant, a scavenger of reactive oxygen radicals and an anti-proliferative agent. The properties of carvedilol and its metabolites have been demonstrated in *in vitro* and *in vivo* animal studies and *in vitro* in a number of human cell types.

Clinical studies have shown that the balance of vasodilation and beta-blockade provided by carvedilol results in the following effects:

– In hypertensive patients, a reduction in blood pressure is not associated with a concomitant increase in total peripheral resistance, as observed with pure beta-blocking agents. Heart rate is slightly decreased. Renal blood flow and renal function are maintained. Peripheral blood flow is maintained, therefore, cold extremities, often observed with drugs possessing beta-blocking activity, are rarely seen.

– In patients with stable angina, Eucardic has demonstrated anti-ischaemic and anti-anginal properties. Acute haemodynamic studies demonstrated that Eucardic reduces ventricular pre- and after-load.

– In patients with left ventricular dysfunction or chronic heart failure, carvedilol has demonstrated favourable effects on haemodynamics and improvements in left ventricular ejection fraction and dimensions.

– In a large, multi-centre, double-blind, placebo-controlled mortality trial (COPERNICUS), 2289 patients with severe stable CHF of ischaemic or non-ischaemic origin, on standard therapy, were randomised to either carvedilol (1156 patients) or placebo (1133 patients). Patients had left ventricular systolic dysfunction with a mean ejection fraction of $< 20\%$. All-cause mortality was reduced by 35% from 19.7% in the placebo group to 12.8% in the carvedilol group (Cox proportional hazards, $p = 0.00013$).

Combined secondary endpoints of mortality or hospitalisation for heart failure, mortality or cardiovascular hospitalisation and mortality or all-cause hospitalisation were all significantly lower in the carvedilol group than placebo (31%, 27% and 24% reductions, respectively, all $p < 0.00004$).

The incidence of serious adverse events during the study was lower in the carvedilol group (39.0% *vs* 45.4%). During initiation of treatment, the incidence of worsening heart failure was similar in both carvedilol and placebo groups. The incidence of serious worsening heart failure during the study was lower in the carvedilol group (14.6% *vs* 21.6%).

Serum lipid profile and electrolytes are not affected.

5.2 Pharmacokinetic properties

The absolute bioavailability of carvedilol is approximately 25% in humans. Bioavailability is stereo-selective, 30% for the R-form and 15% for the S-form. Serum levels peak at approximately 1 hour after an oral dose. There is a linear relationship between the dose and serum concentrations. Food does not affect bioavailability or the maximum serum concentration although the time to reach maximum serum concentration is delayed. Carvedilol is highly lipophilic, approximately 98% to 99% is bound to plasma proteins. The distribution volume is approximately 2 l/kg and increased in patients with liver cirrhosis. The first pass effect after oral administration is approximately 60 - 75%; enterohepatic circulation of the parent substance has been shown in animals.

Carvedilol exhibits a considerable first pass effect. The metabolite pattern reveals intensive metabolism with glucuronidation as one of the major steps. Demethylation and hydroxylation at the phenol ring produce 3 metabolites with beta-receptor blocking activity.

The average elimination half-life ranges from 6 to 10 hours. Plasma clearance is approximately 590ml/min. Elimination is mainly biliary. The primary route of excretion is via the faeces. A minor portion is eliminated via the kidneys in the form of various metabolites.

The pharmacokinetics of carvedilol are affected by age; plasma levels of carvedilol are approximately 50% higher in the elderly compared to young subjects. In a study in patients with cirrhotic liver disease, the bioavailability of carvedilol was four times greater and the peak plasma level five times higher than in healthy subjects. Since carvedilol is primarily excreted via the faeces, significant accumulation in patients with renal impairment is unlikely. In patients with impaired liver function, bioavailability is raised to as much as 80% due to a reduced first pass effect.

5.3 Preclinical safety data

There is no evidence from animal studies that Eucardic has any teratogenic effects. Embryotoxicity was observed only after large doses in rabbits. The relevance of these findings for humans is uncertain. Beta-blockers reduce placental perfusion which may result in intrauterine foetal death and immature and premature deliveries. In addition, animal studies have shown that carvedilol crosses the placental barrier and therefore the possible consequences of alpha and beta-blockade in the human foetus and neonate should also be borne in mind. With other alpha and beta-blocking agents, effects have included perinatal and neonatal distress (bradycardia, hypotension, respiratory depression, hypoglycaemia, hypothermia). There is an increased risk of cardiac and pulmonary complications in the neonate in the postnatal period.

6. PHARMACEUTICAL PARTICULARS

6.1 List of excipients

Lactose

Sucrose

Povidone

Crospovidone

Colloidal silicon dioxide

Magnesium stearate

Yellow iron oxide E172

Red iron oxide E172

6.2 Incompatibilities

Not applicable.

6.3 Shelf life

4 years.

6.4 Special precautions for storage

Store below 25°C.

Store in the original package in order to protect from moisture.

Keep the blister strips in the outer carton in order to protect from light.

6.5 Nature and contents of container

Blister packs, PVC/Aluminium of 14, 28, 30, 56 or 100 tablets. Standard polypropylene tube packs of 100 tablets.

Not all pack sizes may be marketed.

6.6 Special precautions for disposal and other handling

No special requirements.

7. MARKETING AUTHORISATION HOLDER

Roche Products Limited, 6 Falcon Way, Shire Park, Welwyn Garden City, AL7 1TW, United Kingdom.

8. MARKETING AUTHORISATION NUMBER(S)

PL 00031/0552

9. DATE OF FIRST AUTHORISATION/RENEWAL OF THE AUTHORISATION

7 September 2001

10. DATE OF REVISION OF THE TEXT

13 August 07

LEGAL CATEGORY

POM

Eucardic is a registered trade mark.

Item Code

Eucardic 3.125mg Tablets

(Roche Products Limited)

1. NAME OF THE MEDICINAL PRODUCT

Eucardic 3.125mg Tablets

2. QUALITATIVE AND QUANTITATIVE COMPOSITION

Each tablet contains 3.125mg carvedilol.

Excipients: lactose, sucrose.

Each tablet contains 55.98mg lactose and 20.625mg sucrose.

For a full list of excipients, see section 6.1.

3. PHARMACEUTICAL FORM

Tablet.

Round pale pink tablet, scored on both sides, marked BM on one side and K1 on the other.

4. CLINICAL PARTICULARS

4.1 Therapeutic indications

Symptomatic chronic heart failure (CHF)

Eucardic is indicated for the treatment of stable mild, moderate and severe chronic heart failure as adjunct to standard therapies e.g. diuretics, digoxin, and ACE inhibitors in patients with euvolemia.

Hypertension

Eucardic is indicated for the treatment of hypertension.

Angina

Eucardic is indicated for the prophylactic treatment of stable angina.

4.2 Posology and method of administration

The tablets should be taken with fluid. For CHF patients Eucardic should be given with food.

Symptomatic chronic heart failure

Initiation of therapy with Eucardic should only be under the supervision of a hospital physician, following a thorough assessment of the patient's condition.

Prior to any subsequent titration of the dose, the patient must be clinically evaluated on the day of up-titration by a health-care professional experienced in the management of heart failure to ensure that the clinical status has remained stable. The dose of carvedilol should not be increased in any patient with deteriorating heart failure since last visit or with signs of decompensated or unstable chronic heart failure.

The dosage must be titrated to individual requirements.

For those patients receiving diuretics and/or digoxin and/or ACE inhibitors, dosing of these other drugs should be stabilised prior to initiation of Eucardic treatment.

Adults

The recommended dose for the initiation of therapy is 3.125mg twice a day for two weeks. If this dose is tolerated, the dosage should be increased subsequently, at intervals of not less than two weeks, to 6.25mg twice daily, followed by 12.5mg twice daily and thereafter 25mg twice daily. Dosing should be increased to the highest level tolerated by the patient.

The recommended maximum daily dose is 25mg given twice daily for all patients with severe CHF and for patients with mild to moderate CHF weighing less than 85kg (187lbs). In patients with mild or moderate CHF weighing more than 85kg, the recommended maximum dose is 50mg twice daily.

During up-titration of the dose in patients with systolic blood pressure < 100mmHg, deterioration of renal and/ or cardiac functions may occur. Therefore, before each dose increase these patients should be evaluated by the physician for renal function and symptoms of worsening heart failure or vasodilation. Transient worsening of heart failure, vasodilation or fluid retention may be treated by adjusting doses of diuretics or ACE inhibitors or by modifying or temporarily discontinuing Eucardic treatment. Under these circumstances, the dose of Eucardic should not be increased until symptoms of worsening heart failure or vasodilation have been stabilised.

If Eucardic is discontinued for more than two weeks, therapy should be recommenced at 3.125mg twice daily and up-titrated in line with the above dosing recommendation.

Elderly

As for adults.

Children

Safety and efficacy in children (under 18 years) has not been established.

Hypertension

Once daily dosing is recommended.

Adults

The recommended dose for initiation of therapy is 12.5mg once a day for the first two days. Thereafter the recommended dosage is 25mg once a day. Although this is an adequate dose in most patients, if necessary the dose may be titrated up to a recommended daily maximum dose of 50mg given once a day or in divided doses.

Dose titration should occur at intervals of at least two weeks.

Elderly

An initial dose of 12.5mg daily is recommended. This has provided satisfactory control in some cases. If the response is inadequate the dose may be titrated up to the recommended daily maximum dose of 50mg given once a day or in divided doses.

Children

Safety and efficacy in children (under 18 years) has not been established.

Angina

Adults

The recommended dose for initiation of therapy is 12.5mg twice a day for the first two days. Thereafter, the recommended dosage is 25mg twice a day.

Elderly

The recommended maximum daily dose is 50mg given in divided doses.

Children

Safety and efficacy in children (under 18 years) has not been established.

Patients with co-existing hepatic disease

Eucardic is contraindicated in patients with hepatic dysfunction (see sections *4.3 Contraindications* and *5.2 Pharmacokinetic properties*).

Patients with co-existing renal dysfunction

No dose adjustment is anticipated as long as systolic blood pressure is above 100mmHg (see also sections *4.4 Special warnings and precautions for use* and *5.2 Pharmacokinetic properties*).

4.3 Contraindications

Hypersensitivity to the active substance or to any of the excipients.

Eucardic is contraindicated in patients with marked fluid retention or overload requiring intravenous inotropic support.

Patients with obstructive airways disease, liver dysfunction.

As with other beta-blocking agents: History of bronchospasm or asthma, 2nd and 3rd degree A-V heart block, (unless a permanent pacemaker is in place), severe bradycardia (< 50 bpm), cardiogenic shock, sick sinus syndrome (including sino-atrial block), severe hypotension (systolic blood pressure < 85mmHg), metabolic acidosis and phaeochromocytoma (unless adequately controlled by alpha blockade).

4.4 Special warnings and precautions for use

This medicinal product contains lactose, therefore patients with rare hereditary problems of galactose intolerance, the Lapp lactase deficiency, or glucose-galactose malabsorption should not take this medicine.

This medicinal product contains sucrose, therefore patients with rare hereditary problems of fructose intolerance, glucose-galactose malabsorption or sucrase-isomaltase insufficiency should not take this medicine.

In chronic heart failure patients, worsening cardiac failure or fluid retention may occur during up-titration of Eucardic. If such symptoms occur, the dose of diuretic should be adjusted and the Eucardic dose should not be advanced until clinical stability resumes. Occasionally it may be necessary to lower the Eucardic dose or temporarily discontinue it. Such episodes do not preclude subsequent successful titration of Eucardic.

In hypertensive patients who have chronic heart failure controlled with digoxin, diuretics and/or an ACE inhibitor, Eucardic should be used with caution since both digoxin and Eucardic may slow A-V conduction.

As with other drugs with beta-blocking activity, Eucardic may mask the early signs of acute hypoglycaemia in patients with diabetes mellitus. Alternatives to beta-blocking agents are generally preferred in insulin-dependent patients. In patients with diabetes, the use of Eucardic may be associated with worsening control of blood glucose. Therefore, regular monitoring of blood glucose is required in diabetics when Eucardic is initiated or up-titrated and hypoglycaemic therapy adjusted accordingly.

Reversible deterioration of renal function has been observed with Eucardic therapy in chronic heart failure patients with low blood pressure (systolic BP < 100mmHg), ischaemic heart disease and diffuse vascular disease, and/or underlying renal insufficiency. In CHF patients with these risk factors, renal function should be monitored during up-titration of Eucardic and the drug discontinued or dosage reduced if worsening of renal failure occurs.

Wearers of contact lenses should be advised of the possibility of reduced lacrimation.

Although angina has not been reported on stopping treatment, discontinuation should be gradual (1 - 2 weeks) particularly in patients with ischaemic heart disease, as Eucardic has beta-blocking activity.

Eucardic may be used in patients with peripheral vascular disease. Pure beta-blockers can precipitate or aggravate symptoms of arterial insufficiency. However as Eucardic also has alpha-blocking properties this effect is largely counterbalanced.

Eucardic, as with other agents with beta-blocking activity, may mask the symptoms of thyrotoxicosis.

If Eucardic induces bradycardia, with a decrease in pulse rate to less than 55 beats per minute, the dosage of Eucardic should be reduced.

Care should be taken in administering Eucardic to patients with a history of serious hypersensitivity reactions and in those undergoing desensitisation therapy as beta-blockers may increase both the sensitivity towards allergens and the seriousness of anaphylactic reactions.

In patients suffering from the peripheral circulatory disorder Raynaud's phenomenon, there may be exacerbation of symptoms.

Patients with a history of psoriasis associated with beta-blocker therapy should be given Eucardic only after consideration of the risk-benefit ratio.

In patients with phaeochromocytoma, an alpha-blocking agent should be initiated prior to the use of any beta-blocking agent. There is no experience of the use of carvedilol in this condition. Therefore, caution should be taken in the administration of Eucardic to patients suspected of having phaeochromocytoma.

Agents with non-selective beta-blocking activity may provoke chest pain in patients with Prinzmetal's variant angina. There is no clinical experience with Eucardic in these patients, although the alpha-blocking activity of Eucardic may prevent such symptoms. However, caution should be taken in the administration of Eucardic to patients suspected of having Prinzmetal's variant angina.

In patients with a tendency to bronchospastic reactions, respiratory distress can occur as a result of a possible increase in airway resistance. The following warnings will be included on the outer packaging and leaflet:

Packaging

Do not take this medicine if you have a history of wheezing due to asthma or other lung diseases.

Leaflet

Do not take this medicine if you have a history of wheezing due to asthma or other lung diseases. Consult your doctor or pharmacist first.

4.5 Interaction with other medicinal products and other forms of interaction

As with other agents with beta-blocking activity, Eucardic may potentiate the effect of other concomitantly administered drugs that are anti-hypertensive in action (e.g. $alpha_1$-receptor antagonists) or have hypotension as part of their adverse effect profile.

Patients taking an agent with β-blocking properties and a drug that can deplete catecholamines (e.g. reserpine and monoamine oxidase inhibitors) should be observed closely for signs of hypotension and/or severe bradycardia.

Isolated cases of conduction disturbance (rarely with haemodynamic disruption) have been observed when Eucardic and diltiazem were given concomitantly. Therefore, as with other drugs with beta-blocking activity, careful monitoring of ECG and blood pressure should be undertaken when co-administering calcium channel blockers of the verapamil or diltiazem type, or class I antiarrhythmic drugs. These types of drugs should not be co-administered intravenously in patients receiving Eucardic.

The effects of insulin or oral hypoglycaemics may be intensified. Regular monitoring of blood glucose is therefore recommended.

Trough plasma digoxin levels may be increased by approximately 16% in hypertensive patients co-administered Eucardic and digoxin. Increased monitoring of digoxin levels is recommended when initiating, adjusting or discontinuing Eucardic. Concomitant administration of Eucardic and cardiac glycosides may prolong AV conduction time.

When treatment with Eucardic and clonidine together is to be terminated, Eucardic should be withdrawn first, several days before gradually decreasing the dosage of clonidine.

Care may be required in those receiving inducers of mixed function oxidases e.g. rifampicin, as serum levels of carvedilol may be reduced or inhibitors of mixed function oxidases e.g. cimetidine, as serum levels may be increased.

During general anaesthesia, attention should be paid to the potential synergistic negative inotropic effects of carvedilol and anaesthetic drugs.

Modest increases in mean trough cyclosporin concentrations were observed following initiation of carvedilol treatment in 21 renal transplant patients suffering from chronic vascular rejection. In about 30% of patients, the dose of cyclosporin had to be reduced in order to maintain cyclosporin concentrations within the therapeutic range, while in the remainder no adjustment was needed. On average, the dose of cyclosporin was reduced about 20% in these patients. Due to wide interindividual variability in the dose adjustment required, it is recommended that cyclosporin concentrations be monitored closely after initiation of carvedilol therapy and that the dose of cyclosporin be adjusted as appropriate.

4.6 Pregnancy and lactation

Pregnancy

There are no adequate data from the use of carvedilol in pregnant women.

Animal studies are insufficient with respect to effects on pregnancy, embryonal/foetal development, parturition and postnatal development (see section 5.3). The potential risk for humans is unknown.

Eucardic should not be used during pregnancy unless clearly necessary (i.e. unless the anticipated benefits outweigh the potential risks).

Lactation

It is unknown whether carvedilol is excreted in human breast milk. Animal studies have shown excretion of carvedilol or its metabolites in breast milk. A decision on whether to continue/discontinue breast-feeding or to continue/discontinue therapy with Eucardic should be made taking into account the benefit of breast-feeding to the child and the benefit of Eucardic therapy to the woman.

4.7 Effects on ability to drive and use machines

No studies of the effects on ability to drive and use machines have been performed.

As for other drugs which produce changes in blood pressure, patients taking Eucardic should be warned not to drive or operate machinery if they experience dizziness or related symptoms. This applies particularly when starting or changing treatment and in conjunction with alcohol.

4.8 Undesirable effects

Clinical Trials

Adverse events are listed separately for CHF because of differences in the background diseases.

In chronic heart failure:

Haematological

Rare: thrombocytopenia.

Leucopenia has been reported in isolated cases.

Metabolic

Common: weight increase and hypercholesterolaemia. Hyperglycaemia, hypoglycaemia and worsening control of blood glucose are also common in patients with pre-existing diabetes mellitus (see section *4.5 Interaction with other medicinal products and other forms of interaction*).

Central nervous system

Very common: dizziness, headache are usually mild and occur particularly at the start of treatment. Asthenia (including fatigue).

Cardiovascular system

Common: bradycardia, postural hypotension, hypotension, oedema (including generalised, peripheral, dependent and genital oedema, oedema of the legs, hypervolaemia and fluid overload).

Uncommon: syncope (including presyncope), AV-block and cardiac failure during up-titration.

Gastro-intestinal system

Common: nausea, diarrhoea, and vomiting.

Skin and appendages

Dermatitis, and increased sweating.

Others

Common: vision abnormalities.

Rare: acute renal failure and renal function abnormalities in patients with diffuse vascular disease and/or impaired renal function (see section *4.4 Special warnings and precautions for use*).

The frequency of adverse experiences is not dose dependent, with the exception of dizziness, abnormal vision and bradycardia.

In hypertension and angina:

The profile is similar to that observed in chronic heart failure although the incidence of events is generally lower in patients with hypertension or angina treated with Eucardic.

Blood chemistry and haematological

Isolated cases of changes in serum transaminases, thrombocytopenia and leucopenia have been reported.

Central nervous system

Common: dizziness, headaches and fatigue, which are usually mild and occur particularly at the beginning of treatment.

Uncommon: depressed mood, sleep disturbance, paraesthesia, asthenia.

Metabolic

Due to the beta-blocking properties it is also possible for latent diabetes mellitus to become manifest, manifest diabetes to be aggravated, and blood glucose counter-regulation to be inhibited.

Cardiovascular system

Common: bradycardia, postural hypotension, especially at the beginning of treatment.

Uncommon: syncope, hypotension, disturbances of peripheral circulation (cold extremities, PVD, exacerbation of intermittent claudication and Raynauds phenomenon). AV-block, angina pectoris (including chest pain), symptoms of heart failure and peripheral oedema.

Respiratory system

Common: asthma and dyspnoea in predisposed patients.

Rare: stuffy nose. Wheezing and flu-like symptoms.

Gastro-intestinal system

Common: gastro-intestinal upset (with symptoms such as nausea, abdominal pain, diarrhoea).

Uncommon: constipation and vomiting.

Skin and appendages

Uncommon: skin reactions (e.g. allergic exanthema, dermatitis, urticaria, pruritus, lichen planus-like reactions, and increased sweating). Psoriatic skin lesions may occur or existing lesions exacerbated.

Others

Common: pain in the extremities, reduced lacrimation.

Uncommon: cases of sexual impotence and disturbed vision.

Rare: dryness of the mouth and disturbances of micturition and eye irritation.

Isolated cases of allergic reactions have been reported.

Post-marketing experience

Isolated cases of urinary incontinence in women, which resolved upon discontinuation of the medication, have been reported.

4.9 Overdose

Symptoms and signs

Profound cardiovascular effects such as hypotension and bradycardia would be expected after massive overdose. Heart failure, cardiogenic shock and cardiac arrest may follow. There may also be respiratory problems, bronchospasm, vomiting, disturbed consciousness and generalised seizures.

Treatment

Gastric lavage or induced emesis may be useful in the first few hours after ingestion.

In addition to general procedures, vital signs must be monitored and corrected, if necessary under intensive care conditions.

Patients should be placed in the supine position. Atropine, 0.5mg to 2mg i.v. and/or glucagon 1 to 10mg i.v. (followed by a slow i.v. infusion of 2 to 5mg/hour if necessary) may be given when bradycardia is present. Pacemaker therapy may be necessary. For excessive hypotension, intravenous fluids may be administered. In addition, norepinephrine may be given, either 5 to 10 micrograms i.v., repeated according to blood pressure response, or 5 micrograms per minute by infusion titrated to blood pressure. Bronchospasm may be treated using salbutamol or other $beta_2$-agonists given as aerosol or, if necessary, by the intravenous route. In the event of seizures, slow i.v. injection of diazepam or clonazepam is recommended.

In cases of severe overdose with symptoms of shock, supportive treatment as described should be continued for a sufficiently long period of time, i.e. until the patient stabilises, since prolonged elimination half life and redistribution of carvedilol from deeper compartments can be expected.

5. PHARMACOLOGICAL PROPERTIES

5.1 Pharmacodynamic properties

Pharmacotherapeutic group: Alpha and beta blocking agents. ATC code: C07AG02.

Carvedilol is a vasodilating non-selective beta-blocking agent with antioxidant properties. Vasodilation is predominantly mediated through $alpha_1$ receptor antagonism.

Carvedilol reduces the peripheral vascular resistance through vasodilation and suppresses the renin-angiotensin-aldosterone system through beta-blockade. The activity of plasma renin is reduced and fluid retention is rare.

Carvedilol has no intrinsic sympathomimetic activity and like propranolol, it has membrane stabilising properties.

Carvedilol is a racemate of two stereoisomers. Beta-blockade is attributed to the S(-) enantiomer; in contrast, both enantiomers exhibit the same α_1-blocking activity.

Carvedilol is a potent antioxidant, a scavenger of reactive oxygen radicals and an anti-proliferative agent. The properties of carvedilol and its metabolites have been demonstrated in *in vitro* and *in vivo* animal studies and *in vitro* in a number of human cell types.

Clinical studies have shown that the balance of vasodilation and beta-blockade provided by carvedilol results in the following effects:

– In hypertensive patients, a reduction in blood pressure is not associated with a concomitant increase in total peripheral resistance, as observed with pure beta-blocking agents. Heart rate is slightly decreased. Renal blood flow and renal function are maintained. Peripheral blood flow is maintained, therefore, cold extremities, often observed with drugs possessing beta-blocking activity, are rarely seen.

– In patients with stable angina, Eucardic has demonstrated anti-ischaemic and anti-anginal properties. Acute haemodynamic studies demonstrated that Eucardic reduces ventricular pre- and after-load.

– In patients with left ventricular dysfunction or chronic heart failure, carvedilol has demonstrated favourable effects on haemodynamics and improvements in left ventricular ejection fraction and dimensions.

– In a large, multi-centre, double-blind, placebo-controlled mortality trial (COPERNICUS), 2289 patients with severe stable CHF of ischaemic or non-ischaemic origin, on standard therapy, were randomised to either carvedilol (1156 patients) or placebo (1133 patients). Patients had left ventricular systolic dysfunction with a mean ejection fraction of < 20%. All-cause mortality was reduced by 35% from 19.7% in the placebo group to 12.8% in the carvedilol group (Cox proportional hazards, p = 0.00013).

Combined secondary endpoints of mortality or hospitalisation for heart failure, mortality or cardiovascular hospitalisation and mortality or all-cause hospitalisation were all significantly lower in the carvedilol group than placebo (31%, 27% and 24% reductions, respectively, all p < 0.00004).

The incidence of serious adverse events during the study was lower in the carvedilol group (39.0% *vs* 45.4%). During initiation of treatment, the incidence of worsening heart failure was similar in both carvedilol and placebo groups. The incidence of serious worsening heart failure during the study was lower in the carvedilol group (14.6% *vs* 21.6%).

Serum lipid profile and electrolytes are not affected.

5.2 Pharmacokinetic properties

The absolute bioavailability of carvedilol is approximately 25% in humans. Bioavailability is stereo-selective, 30% for the R-form and 15% for the S-form. Serum levels peak at approximately 1 hour after an oral dose. There is a linear relationship between the dose and serum concentrations. Food does not affect bioavailability or the maximum serum concentration although the time to reach maximum serum concentration is delayed. Carvedilol is highly lipophilic, approximately 98% to 99% is bound to plasma proteins. The distribution volume is approximately 2 l/kg and increased in patients with liver cirrhosis. The first pass effect after oral administration is approximately 60 - 75%; enterohepatic circulation of the parent substance has been shown in animals.

Carvedilol exhibits a considerable first pass effect. The metabolite pattern reveals intensive metabolism with glucuronidation as one of the major steps. Demethylation and hydroxylation at the phenol ring produce 3 metabolites with beta-receptor blocking activity.

The average elimination half-life ranges from 6 to 10 hours. Plasma clearance is approximately 590ml/min. Elimination is mainly biliary. The primary route of excretion is via the faeces. A minor portion is eliminated via the kidneys in the form of various metabolites.

The pharmacokinetics of carvedilol are affected by age; plasma levels of carvedilol are approximately 50% higher in the elderly compared to young subjects. In a study in patients with cirrhotic liver disease, the bioavailability of carvedilol was four times greater and the peak plasma level five times higher than in healthy subjects. Since carvedilol is primarily excreted via the faeces, significant accumulation in patients with renal impairment is unlikely. In patients with impaired liver function, bioavailability is raised to as much as 80% due to a reduced first pass effect.

5.3 Preclinical safety data

There is no evidence from animal studies that Eucardic has any teratogenic effects. Embryotoxicity was observed only after large doses in rabbits. The relevance of these findings for humans is uncertain. Beta-blockers reduce placental perfusion which may result in intrauterine foetal death and immature and premature deliveries. In addition, animal studies have shown that carvedilol crosses the placental barrier and therefore the possible consequences of alpha and beta-blockade in the human foetus and neonate should also be borne in mind. With other alpha and beta-blocking agents, effects have included perinatal and neonatal distress (bradycardia, hypotension, respiratory depression, hypoglycaemia, hypothermia). There is an increased risk of cardiac and pulmonary complications in the neonate in the postnatal period.

6. PHARMACEUTICAL PARTICULARS

6.1 List of excipients

Lactose

Sucrose

Povidone

Crospovidone

Colloidal silicon dioxide

Magnesium stearate

Red iron oxide E172

6.2 Incompatibilities

Not applicable.

6.3 Shelf life

3 years.

6.4 Special precautions for storage

Store below 25°C.

Store in the original package in order to protect from moisture.

Keep the blister strips in the outer carton in order to protect from light.

6.5 Nature and contents of container

Blister packs, PVC/Aluminium of 28 or 56 tablets.

Not all pack sizes may be marketed.

6.6 Special precautions for disposal and other handling

No special requirements.

7. MARKETING AUTHORISATION HOLDER

Roche Products Limited, 6 Falcon Way, Shire Park, Welwyn Garden City, AL7 1TW, United Kingdom.

8. MARKETING AUTHORISATION NUMBER(S)

PL 00031/0550

9. DATE OF FIRST AUTHORISATION/RENEWAL OF THE AUTHORISATION

20 July 2003

10. DATE OF REVISION OF THE TEXT

23 July 2007

LEGAL STATUS

POM

Eucardic is a registered trade mark.

Item Code

Eucardic 6.25mg Tablets

(Roche Products Limited)

1. NAME OF THE MEDICINAL PRODUCT

Eucardic 6.25mg Tablets

2. QUALITATIVE AND QUANTITATIVE COMPOSITION

Each tablet contains 6.25mg carvedilol.

Excipients: lactose, sucrose.

Each tablet contains 51.8mg lactose and 21.25mg sucrose.

For a full list of excipients, see section 6.1.

3. PHARMACEUTICAL FORM

Tablet.

Round yellow tablet, scored on both sides, marked BM on one side and F1 on the other.

4. CLINICAL PARTICULARS

4.1 Therapeutic indications

Symptomatic chronic heart failure (CHF)

Eucardic is indicated for the treatment of stable mild, moderate and severe chronic heart failure as adjunct to standard therapies e.g. diuretics, digoxin, and ACE inhibitors in patients with euvolemia.

Hypertension

Eucardic is indicated for the treatment of hypertension.

Angina

Eucardic is indicated for the prophylactic treatment of stable angina.

4.2 Posology and method of administration

The tablets should be taken with fluid. For CHF patients Eucardic should be given with food.

Symptomatic chronic heart failure

Initiation of therapy with Eucardic should only be under the supervision of a hospital physician, following a thorough assessment of the patient's condition.

Prior to any subsequent titration of the dose, the patient must be clinically evaluated on the day of up-titration by a health-care professional experienced in the management of heart failure to ensure that the clinical status has remained stable. The dose of carvedilol should not be increased in any patient with deteriorating heart failure since last visit or with signs of decompensated or unstable chronic heart failure.

The dosage must be titrated to individual requirements.

For those patients receiving diuretics and/or digoxin and/or ACE inhibitors, dosing of these other drugs should be stabilised prior to initiation of Eucardic treatment.

Adults

The recommended dose for the initiation of therapy is 3.125mg twice a day for two weeks. If this dose is tolerated, the dosage should be increased subsequently, at intervals of not less than two weeks, to 6.25mg twice daily, followed by 12.5mg twice daily and thereafter 25mg twice daily. Dosing should be increased to the highest level tolerated by the patient.

The recommended maximum daily dose is 25mg given twice daily for all patients with severe CHF and for patients with mild to moderate CHF weighing less than 85kg (187lbs). In patients with mild or moderate CHF weighing more than 85kg, the recommended maximum dose is 50mg twice daily.

During up-titration of the dose in patients with systolic blood pressure < 100mmHg, deterioration of renal and/or cardiac functions may occur. Therefore, before each dose increase these patients should be evaluated by the physician for renal function and symptoms of worsening heart failure or vasodilation. Transient worsening of heart failure, vasodilation or fluid retention may be treated by adjusting doses of diuretics or ACE inhibitors or by modifying or temporarily discontinuing Eucardic treatment. Under these circumstances, the dose of Eucardic should not be increased until symptoms of worsening heart failure or vasodilation have been stabilised.

If Eucardic is discontinued for more than two weeks, therapy should be recommenced at 3.125mg twice daily and up-titrated in line with the above dosing recommendation.

Elderly

As for adults.

Children

Safety and efficacy in children (under 18 years) has not been established.

Hypertension

Once daily dosing is recommended.

Adults

The recommended dose for initiation of therapy is 12.5mg once a day for the first two days. Thereafter the recommended dosage is 25mg once a day. Although this is an adequate dose in most patients, if necessary the dose may be titrated up to a recommended daily maximum dose of 50mg given once a day or in divided doses.

Dose titration should occur at intervals of at least two weeks.

Elderly

An initial dose of 12.5mg daily is recommended. This has provided satisfactory control in some cases. If the response is inadequate the dose may be titrated up to the recommended daily maximum dose of 50mg given once a day or in divided doses.

Children

Safety and efficacy in children (under 18 years) has not been established.

Angina

Adults

The recommended dose for initiation of therapy is 12.5mg twice a day for the first two days. Thereafter, the recommended dosage is 25mg twice a day.

Elderly

The recommended maximum daily dose is 50mg given in divided doses.

Children

Safety and efficacy in children (under 18 years) has not been established.

Patients with co-existing hepatic disease

Eucardic is contraindicated in patients with hepatic dysfunction (see sections *4.3 Contraindications* and *5.2 Pharmacokinetic properties*).

Patients with co-existing renal dysfunction

No dose adjustment is anticipated as long as systolic blood pressure is above 100mmHg (see also sections *4.4 Special warnings and precautions for use* and *5.2 Pharmacokinetic properties*).

4.3 Contraindications

Hypersensitivity to the active substance or to any of the excipients.

Eucardic is contraindicated in patients with marked fluid retention or overload requiring intravenous inotropic support.

Patients with obstructive airways disease, liver dysfunction.

As with other beta-blocking agents: History of bronchospasm or asthma, 2nd and 3rd degree A-V heart block, (unless a permanent pacemaker is in place), severe bradycardia (< 50 bpm), cardiogenic shock, sick sinus syndrome (including sino-atrial block), severe hypotension (systolic blood pressure < 85mmHg), metabolic acidosis and phaeochromocytoma (unless adequately controlled by alpha blockade).

4.4 Special warnings and precautions for use

This medicinal product contains lactose, therefore patients with rare hereditary problems of galactose intolerance, the Lapp lactase deficiency, or glucose-galactose malabsorption should not take this medicine.

This medicinal product contains sucrose, therefore patients with rare hereditary problems of fructose intolerance, glucose-galactose malabsorption or sucrase-isomaltase insufficiency should not take this medicine.

In chronic heart failure patients, worsening cardiac failure or fluid retention may occur during up-titration of Eucardic. If such symptoms occur, the dose of diuretic should be adjusted and the Eucardic dose should not be advanced until clinical stability resumes. Occasionally it may be necessary to lower the Eucardic dose or temporarily discontinue it. Such episodes do not preclude subsequent successful titration of Eucardic.

In hypertensive patients who have chronic heart failure controlled with digoxin, diuretics and/or an ACE inhibitor, Eucardic should be used with caution since both digoxin and Eucardic may slow A-V conduction.

As with other drugs with beta-blocking activity, Eucardic may mask the early signs of acute hypoglycaemia in patients with diabetes mellitus. Alternatives to beta-blocking agents are generally preferred in insulin-dependent patients. In patients with diabetes, the use of Eucardic may be associated with worsening control of blood glucose. Therefore, regular monitoring of blood glucose is required in diabetics when Eucardic is initiated or up-titrated and hypoglycaemic therapy adjusted accordingly.

Reversible deterioration of renal function has been observed with Eucardic therapy in chronic heart failure patients with low blood pressure (systolic BP < 100mmHg), ischaemic heart disease and diffuse vascular disease, and/or underlying renal insufficiency. In CHF patients with these risk factors, renal function should be monitored during up-titration of Eucardic and the drug discontinued or dosage reduced if worsening of renal failure occurs.

Wearers of contact lenses should be advised of the possibility of reduced lacrimation.

Although angina has not been reported on stopping treatment, discontinuation should be gradual (1 - 2 weeks) particularly in patients with ischaemic heart disease, as Eucardic has beta-blocking activity.

Eucardic may be used in patients with peripheral vascular disease. Pure beta-blockers can precipitate or aggravate symptoms of arterial insufficiency. However as Eucardic also has alpha-blocking properties this effect is largely counterbalanced.

Eucardic, as with other agents with beta-blocking activity, may mask the symptoms of thyrotoxicosis.

If Eucardic induces bradycardia, with a decrease in pulse rate to less than 55 beats per minute, the dosage of Eucardic should be reduced.

Care should be taken in administering Eucardic to patients with a history of serious hypersensitivity reactions and in those undergoing desensitisation therapy as beta-blockers may increase both the sensitivity towards allergens and the seriousness of anaphylactic reactions.

In patients suffering from the peripheral circulatory disorder Raynaud's phenomenon, there may be exacerbation of symptoms.

Patients with a history of psoriasis associated with beta-blocker therapy should be given Eucardic only after consideration of the risk-benefit ratio.

In patients with phaeochromocytoma, an alpha-blocking agent should be initiated prior to the use of any beta-blocking agent. There is no experience of the use of carvedilol in this condition. Therefore, caution should be taken in the administration of Eucardic to patients suspected of having phaeochromocytoma.

Agents with non-selective beta-blocking activity may provoke chest pain in patients with Prinzmetal's variant angina. There is no clinical experience with Eucardic in these patients, although the alpha-blocking activity of Eucardic may prevent such symptoms. However, caution should be taken in the administration of Eucardic to patients suspected of having Prinzmetal's variant angina.

In patients with a tendency to bronchospastic reactions, respiratory distress can occur as a result of a possible increase in airway resistance. The following warnings will be included on the outer packaging and leaflet:

Packaging

Do not take this medicine if you have a history of wheezing due to asthma or other lung diseases.

Leaflet

Do not take this medicine if you have a history of wheezing due to asthma or other lung diseases. Consult your doctor or pharmacist first.

4.5 Interaction with other medicinal products and other forms of interaction

As with other agents with beta-blocking activity, Eucardic may potentiate the effect of other concomitantly administered drugs that are anti-hypertensive in action (e.g. alpha$_1$-receptor antagonists) or have hypotension as part of their adverse effect profile.

Patients taking an agent with β-blocking properties and a drug that can deplete catecholamines (e.g. reserpine and monoamine oxidase inhibitors) should be observed closely for signs of hypotension and/or severe bradycardia.

Isolated cases of conduction disturbance (rarely with haemodynamic disruption) have been observed when Eucardic and diltiazem were given concomitantly. Therefore, as with other drugs with beta-blocking activity, careful monitoring of ECG and blood pressure should be undertaken when co-administering calcium channel blockers of the verapamil or diltiazem type, or class I antiarrhythmic drugs. These types of drugs should not be co-administered intravenously in patients receiving Eucardic.

The effects of insulin or oral hypoglycaemics may be intensified. Regular monitoring of blood glucose is therefore recommended.

Trough plasma digoxin levels may be increased by approximately 16% in hypertensive patients co-administered Eucardic and digoxin. Increased monitoring of digoxin levels is recommended when initiating, adjusting or discontinuing Eucardic. Concomitant administration of Eucardic and cardiac glycosides may prolong AV conduction time.

When treatment with Eucardic and clonidine together is to be terminated, Eucardic should be withdrawn first, several days before gradually decreasing the dosage of clonidine.

Care may be required in those receiving inducers of mixed function oxidases e.g. rifampicin, as serum levels of carvedilol may be reduced or inhibitors of mixed function oxidases e.g. cimetidine, as serum levels may be increased.

During general anaesthesia, attention should be paid to the potential synergistic negative inotropic effects of carvedilol and anaesthetic drugs.

Modest increases in mean trough cyclosporin concentrations were observed following initiation of carvedilol treatment in 21 renal transplant patients suffering from chronic vascular rejection. In about 30% of patients, the dose of cyclosporin had to be reduced in order to maintain cyclosporin concentrations within the therapeutic range, while in the remainder no adjustment was needed. On average, the dose of cyclosporin was reduced about 20% in these patients. Due to wide interindividual variability in the dose adjustment required, it is recommended that cyclosporin concentrations be monitored closely after initiation of carvedilol therapy and that the dose of cyclosporin be adjusted as appropriate.

4.6 Pregnancy and lactation

Pregnancy

There are no adequate data from the use of carvedilol in pregnant women.

Animal studies are insufficient with respect to effects on pregnancy, embryonal/foetal development, parturition and postnatal development (see section 5.3). The potential risk for humans is unknown.

Eucardic should not be used during pregnancy unless clearly necessary (i.e. unless the anticipated benefits outweigh the potential risks).

Lactation

It is unknown whether carvedilol is excreted in human breast milk. Animal studies have shown excretion of carvedilol or its metabolites in breast milk. A decision on whether to continue/discontinue breast-feeding or to continue/discontinue therapy with Eucardic should be made taking into account the benefit of breast-feeding to the child and the benefit of Eucardic therapy to the woman.

4.7 Effects on ability to drive and use machines

No studies of the effects on ability to drive and use machines have been performed.

As for other drugs which produce changes in blood pressure, patients taking Eucardic should be warned not to drive or operate machinery if they experience dizziness or related symptoms. This applies particularly when starting or changing treatment and in conjunction with alcohol.

4.8 Undesirable effects

Clinical Trials

Adverse events are listed separately for CHF because of differences in the background diseases.

In chronic heart failure:

Haematological

Rare: thrombocytopenia.

Leucopenia has been reported in isolated cases.

Metabolic

Common: weight increase and hypercholesterolaemia. Hyperglycaemia, hypoglycaemia and worsening control of blood glucose are also common in patients with pre-existing diabetes mellitus (see section *4.5 Interaction with other medicinal products and other forms of interaction*).

Central nervous system

Very common: dizziness, headache are usually mild and occur particularly at the start of treatment. Asthenia (including fatigue).

Cardiovascular system

Common: bradycardia, postural hypotension, hypotension, oedema (including generalised, peripheral, dependent and genital oedema, oedema of the legs, hypervolaemia and fluid overload).

Uncommon: syncope (including presyncope), AV-block and cardiac failure during up-titration.

Gastro-intestinal system

Common: nausea, diarrhoea, and vomiting.

Skin and appendages

Dermatitis, and increased sweating.

Others

Common: vision abnormalities.

Rare: acute renal failure and renal function abnormalities in patients with diffuse vascular disease and/or impaired renal function (see section *4.4 Special warnings and precautions for use*).

The frequency of adverse experiences is not dose dependent, with the exception of dizziness, abnormal vision and bradycardia.

In hypertension and angina:

The profile is similar to that observed in chronic heart failure although the incidence of events is generally lower in patients with hypertension or angina treated with Eucardic.

Blood chemistry and haematological

Isolated cases of changes in serum transaminases, thrombocytopenia and leucopenia have been reported.

Central nervous system

Common: dizziness, headaches and fatigue, which are usually mild and occur particularly at the beginning of treatment.

Uncommon: depressed mood, sleep disturbance, paraesthesia, asthenia.

Metabolic

Due to the beta-blocking properties it is also possible for latent diabetes mellitus to become manifest, manifest diabetes to be aggravated, and blood glucose counter-regulation to be inhibited.

Cardiovascular system

Common: bradycardia, postural hypotension, especially at the beginning of treatment.

Uncommon: syncope, hypotension, disturbances of peripheral circulation (cold extremities, PVD, exacerbation of intermittent claudication and Raynauds phenomenon). AV-block, angina pectoris (including chest pain), symptoms of heart failure and peripheral oedema.

Respiratory system

Common: asthma and dyspnoea in predisposed patients.

Rare: stuffy nose. Wheezing and flu-like symptoms.

Gastro-intestinal system

Common: gastro-intestinal upset (with symptoms such as nausea, abdominal pain, diarrhoea).

Uncommon: constipation and vomiting.

Skin and appendages

Uncommon: skin reactions (e.g. allergic exanthema, dermatitis, urticaria, pruritus, lichen planus-like reactions, and increased sweating). Psoriatic skin lesions may occur or existing lesions exacerbated.

Others

Common: pain in the extremities, reduced lacrimation.

Uncommon: cases of sexual impotence and disturbed vision.

Rare: dryness of the mouth and disturbances of micturition and eye irritation.

Isolated cases of allergic reactions have been reported.

Post-marketing experience

Isolated cases of urinary incontinence in women, which resolved upon discontinuation of the medication, have been reported.

4.9 Overdose

Symptoms and signs

Profound cardiovascular effects such as hypotension and bradycardia would be expected after massive overdose. Heart failure, cardiogenic shock and cardiac arrest may follow. There may also be respiratory problems, bronchospasm, vomiting, disturbed consciousness and generalised seizures.

Treatment

Gastric lavage or induced emesis may be useful in the first few hours after ingestion.

In addition to general procedures, vital signs must be monitored and corrected, if necessary under intensive care conditions.

Patients should be placed in the supine position. Atropine, 0.5mg to 2mg i.v. and/or glucagon 1 to 10mg i.v. (followed by a slow i.v. infusion of 2 to 5mg/hour if necessary) may be given when bradycardia is present. Pacemaker therapy may be necessary. For excessive hypotension, intravenous fluids may be administered. In addition, norepinephrine may be given, either 5 to 10 micrograms i.v., repeated according to blood pressure response, or 5 micrograms per minute by infusion titrated to blood pressure. Bronchospasm may be treated using salbutamol or other beta$_2$-agonists given as aerosol or, if necessary, by the intravenous route. In the event of seizures, slow i.v. injection of diazepam or clonazepam is recommended.

In cases of severe overdose with symptoms of shock, supportive treatment as described should be continued for a sufficiently long period of time, i.e. until the patient stabilises, since prolonged elimination half life and redistribution of carvedilol from deeper compartments can be expected.

5. PHARMACOLOGICAL PROPERTIES

5.1 Pharmacodynamic properties

Pharmacotherapeutic group: Alpha and beta blocking agents. ATC code: C07AG02.

Carvedilol is a vasodilating non-selective beta-blocking agent with antioxidant properties. Vasodilation is predominantly mediated through alpha$_1$ receptor antagonism.

Carvedilol reduces the peripheral vascular resistance through vasodilation and suppresses the renin-angiotensin-aldosterone system through beta-blockade. The activity of plasma renin is reduced and fluid retention is rare.

Carvedilol has no intrinsic sympathomimetic activity and like propranolol, it has membrane stabilising properties.

Carvedilol is a racemate of two stereoisomers. Beta-blockade is attributed to the S(-) enantiomer; in contrast, both enantiomers exhibit the same α_1-blocking activity.

Carvedilol is a potent antioxidant, a scavenger of reactive oxygen radicals and an anti-proliferative agent. The properties of carvedilol and its metabolites have been demonstrated in *in vitro* and *in vivo* animal studies and *in vitro* in a number of human cell types.

Clinical studies have shown that the balance of vasodilation and beta-blockade provided by carvedilol results in the following effects:

– In hypertensive patients, a reduction in blood pressure is not associated with a concomitant increase in total peripheral resistance, as observed with pure beta-blocking agents. Heart rate is slightly decreased. Renal blood flow and renal function are maintained. Peripheral blood flow is maintained, therefore, cold extremities, often observed with drugs possessing beta-blocking activity, are rarely seen.

– In patients with stable angina, Eucardic has demonstrated anti-ischaemic and anti-anginal properties. Acute haemodynamic studies demonstrated that Eucardic reduces ventricular pre- and after-load.

– In patients with left ventricular dysfunction or chronic heart failure, carvedilol has demonstrated favourable effects on haemodynamics and improvements in left ventricular ejection fraction and dimensions.

– In a large, multi-centre, double-blind, placebo-controlled mortality trial (COPERNICUS), 2289 patients with severe stable CHF of ischaemic or non-ischaemic origin, on standard therapy, were randomised to either carvedilol (1156 patients) or placebo (1133 patients). Patients had left ventricular systolic dysfunction with a mean ejection fraction of < 20%. All-cause mortality was reduced by 35% from 19.7% in the placebo group to 12.8% in the carvedilol group (Cox proportional hazards, p = 0.00013).

Combined secondary endpoints of mortality or hospitalisation for heart failure, mortality or cardiovascular hospitalisation and mortality or all-cause hospitalisation were all significantly lower in the carvedilol group than placebo (31%, 27% and 24% reductions, respectively, all p < 0.00004).

The incidence of serious adverse events during the study was lower in the carvedilol group (39.0% *vs* 45.4%). During initiation of treatment, the incidence of worsening heart failure was similar in both carvedilol and placebo groups. The incidence of serious worsening heart failure during the study was lower in the carvedilol group (14.6% *vs* 21.6%).

Serum lipid profile and electrolytes are not affected.

5.2 Pharmacokinetic properties

The absolute bioavailability of carvedilol is approximately 25% in humans. Bioavailability is stereo-selective, 30% for the R-form and 15% for the S-form. Serum levels peak at approximately 1 hour after an oral dose. There is a linear relationship between the dose and serum concentrations. Food does not affect bioavailability or the maximum serum concentration although the time to reach maximum serum concentration is delayed. Carvedilol is highly lipophilic, approximately 98% to 99% is bound to plasma proteins. The distribution volume is approximately 2 l/kg and increased in patients with liver cirrhosis. The first pass effect after oral administration is approximately 60 - 75%; enterohepatic circulation of the parent substance has been shown in animals.

Carvedilol exhibits a considerable first pass effect. The metabolite pattern reveals intensive metabolism with glucuronidation as one of the major steps. Demethylation and hydroxylation at the phenol ring produce 3 metabolites with beta-receptor blocking activity.

The average elimination half-life ranges from 6 to 10 hours. Plasma clearance is approximately 590ml/min. Elimination is mainly biliary. The primary route of excretion is via the faeces. A minor portion is eliminated via the kidneys in the form of various metabolites.

The pharmacokinetics of carvedilol are affected by age; plasma levels of carvedilol are approximately 50% higher in the elderly compared to young subjects. In a study in patients with cirrhotic liver disease, the bioavailability of carvedilol was four times greater and the peak plasma level five times higher than in healthy subjects. Since carvedilol is primarily excreted via the faeces, significant accumulation in patients with renal impairment is unlikely. In patients with impaired liver function, bioavailability is raised to as much as 80% due to a reduced first pass effect.

5.3 Preclinical safety data

There is no evidence from animal studies that Eucardic has any teratogenic effects. Embryotoxicity was observed only after large doses in rabbits. The relevance of these findings for humans is uncertain. Beta-blockers reduce placental perfusion which may result in intrauterine foetal death and immature and premature deliveries. In addition, animal studies have shown that carvedilol crosses the placental barrier and therefore the possible consequences of alpha and beta-blockade in the human foetus and neonate should also be borne in mind. With other alpha and beta-blocking agents, effects have included perinatal and neonatal distress (bradycardia, hypotension, respiratory depression, hypoglycaemia, hypothermia). There is an increased risk of cardiac and pulmonary complications in the neonate in the postnatal period.

6. PHARMACEUTICAL PARTICULARS

6.1 List of excipients

Lactose

Sucrose

Povidone

Crospovidone

Colloidal silicon dioxide

Magnesium stearate

Yellow iron oxide E172

6.2 Incompatibilities

Not applicable.

6.3 Shelf life

3 years.

6.4 Special precautions for storage

Store below 25°C.

Store in the original package in order to protect from moisture.

Keep the blister strips in the outer carton in order to protect from light.

6.5 Nature and contents of container

Blister packs, PVC/Aluminium of 28 or 56 tablets.

Not all pack sizes may be marketed.

6.6 Special precautions for disposal and other handling

No special requirements.

7. MARKETING AUTHORISATION HOLDER

Roche Products Limited, 6 Falcon Way, Shire Park, Welwyn Garden City, AL7 1TW, United Kingdom.

8. MARKETING AUTHORISATION NUMBER(S)

PL 00031/0551

9. DATE OF FIRST AUTHORISATION/RENEWAL OF THE AUTHORISATION

20 July 2003

10. DATE OF REVISION OF THE TEXT

23 July 2007

LEGAL STATUS

POM

Eucardic is a registered trade mark.

Item Code

Eudemine Tablets

(UCB Pharma Limited)

1. NAME OF THE MEDICINAL PRODUCT

Eudemine Tablets

2. QUALITATIVE AND QUANTITATIVE COMPOSITION

Diazoxide 50mg

3. PHARMACEUTICAL FORM

White, sugar coated tablet

4. CLINICAL PARTICULARS

4.1 Therapeutic indications

Eudemine Tablets are used orally in the treatment of intractable hypoglycaemia.

Diazoxide also causes salt and water retention.

Hypoglycaemia: Eudemine administered orally is indicated for the treatment of intractable hypoglycaemia with severe symptoms from a variety of causes including: idiopathic hypoglycaemia in infancy, leucine-sensitive or unclassified; functional islet cell tumours both malignant and benign if inoperable, extra-pancreatic neoplasms producing hypoglycaemia; glycogen storage disease; hypoglycaemia of unknown origin.

4.2 Posology and method of administration

Hypoglycaemia: In hypoglycaemia, the dosage schedule of Eudemine tablets is determined according to the clinical needs and the response of the individual patient. For both adults and children a starting oral dose of 5mg/kg body weight divided into 2 or 3 equal doses per 24 hours will establish the patient's response and thereafter the dose can be increased until the symptoms and blood glucose level respond satisfactorily. Regular determinations of the blood glucose in the initial days of treatment are essential. The usual maintenance dose is 3 - 8mg/kg/day given in two or three divided doses.

Reduced doses may be required in patients with impaired renal function.

In children with leucine-sensitive hypoglycaemia, a dosage range of 15-20mg/kg/day is suggested.

In adults with benign or malignant islet-cell tumours producing large quantities of insulin, high dosages of up to 1,000mg per day have been used.

4.3 Contraindications

In the treatment of hypoglycaemia, Eudemine is contra-indicated in all cases which are amenable to surgery or other specific therapy.

Hypersensitivity to any component of the preparation or other thiazides.

4.4 Special warnings and precautions for use

In the treatment of hypoglycaemia it is necessary that the blood pressure be monitored regularly.

Retention of sodium and water is likely to necessitate therapy with an oral diuretic such as frusemide or ethacrynic acid. The dosage of either of the diuretics mentioned may be up to 1g daily. It must be appreciated that if diuretics are employed then both the hypotensive and hyperglycaemic activities of diazoxide will be potentiated and it is likely that the dosage of diazoxide will require adjustment downwards. In patients with severe renal failure it is desirable to maintain, with diuretic therapy, urinary volumes in excess of 1 litre daily. Hypokalaemia should be avoided by adequate potassium replacement.

Diazoxide should be used with caution in patients with cardiac failure or impaired cardiac reserve in whom sodium and water retention may worsen or precipitate congestive heart failure. A direct effect on myocardium and cardiac function cannot be excluded.

Diazoxide should be used with care in patients with impaired cardiac or cerebral circulation and in patients with aortic coarctation, aortic stenosis, arteriovenous shunt, heart failure or other cardiovascular disorders in which an increase in cardiac output could be detrimental.

Diazoxide should be administered with caution to patients with hyperuricaemia or a history of gout, and it is advisable to monitor serum uric acid concentration.

Whenever Eudemine is given over a prolonged period regular haematological examinations are indicated to exclude changes in white blood cell and platelet counts.

Also in children there should be regular assessment of growth, bone and psychological maturation.

The very rapid, almost complete protein binding of diazoxide requires cautious dosage to be used in patients whose plasma proteins may be lower than normal.

4.5 Interaction with other medicinal products and other forms of interaction

Drugs potentiated by diazoxide therapy include: oral diuretics, anti-hypertensive agents and anticoagulants.

Phenytoin levels should be monitored as increased dosage may be needed if administered concurrently with diazoxide.

The risk of hyperglycaemia may be increased by concurrent administration of corticosteroids or oestrogen-progestogen combinations.

4.6 Pregnancy and lactation

Eudemine Tablets are only to be used in pregnant women when the indicated condition is deemed to put the mother's life at risk.

Side Effects

Prolonged oral therapy of Eudemine during pregnancy has been reported to cause alopecia in the newborn.

Eudemine should not be given to nursing mothers as the safety of diazoxide during lactation has not been established.

4.7 Effects on ability to drive and use machines

None known.

4.8 Undesirable effects

With oral therapy, nausea is common in the first two or three weeks and may require relief with an anti-nauseant. Prolonged therapy has given rise to reports of hypertrichosis lanuginosa, anorexia and hyperuricaemia.

Extra-pyramidal side-effects have been reported with oral diazoxide. It was found that extra-pyramidal effects such as parkinsonian tremor, cogwheel rigidity and oculogyric crisis could be easily suppressed by intravenous injection of an antiparkinsonian drug such as procyclidine and that they could be prevented by maintenance therapy with such a drug given orally.

Other adverse effects of Eudemine which have been reported are listed below.

Blood and lymphatic system disorders

Leucopenia, thrombocytopenia, decreased haemoglobin and / or haematocrit, eosinophilia, bleeding

Immune system disorders

Hypogammaglobulinaemia, hypersensitivity reactions such as rash, fever and leucopenia, decreased immunoglobulins (IgG) in infants,

Endocrine disorder

Hirsutism, galactorrhoea, pancreatitis, increased serum androgens

Metabolism and nutrition disorders

Hyperuricaemia (after prolonged therapy), hyperosmolar non-ketotic coma, inappropriate hyperglycaemia including ketoacidosis

Psychiatric disorders

Anorexia (after prolonged therapy), decreased libido

Nervous system disorders

Extra-pyramidal side-effects such as parkinsonian tremor, cogwheel rigidity and oculogyric crisis, headache, dizziness

Eye disorders

Blurred vision, transient cataracts, subconjunctival haemorrhage, ring scotoma, diplopia, lacrimation.

Ear and labyrinth disorders

Tinnitus

Cardiac disorders

Cardiomegaly, cardiac failure, arrhythmias

Vascular disorders

Inappropriate hypotension

Respiratory, thoracic and mediastinal disorders

Dysponea, pulmonary hypertension

Gastrointestinal disorders

Nausea, vomiting, abdominal pain, diarrhoea, ileus, constipation, dysgeusia

Hepatobiliary disorders

Increased AST and alkaline phosphate

Skin and subcutaneous tissue disorders
Pruritis, dermatitis, lichenoid eruption
Musculoskeletal and connective tissue disorders
Musculoskeletal pain
Renal and urinary disorders
Azotemia, decreased creatinine clearance, reversible nephritic syndrome, haematuria and albuminuria.
Congenital, familial and genetic disorders
Hypertrichosis lanuginose (after prolonged therapy)
General disorders and administration site disorders
Voice changes and abnormal faces in children (on long term therapy), sodium retention, fluids retention

4.9 Overdose
Excessive dosage of Eudemine can result in hyperglycaemia. Severe hyperglycaemia may be corrected by giving insulin and less severe hyperglycaemia may respond to oral hypoglycaemics. Hypotension may be managed with intravenous fluids and in severe cases may require sympathomimetics.

5. PHARMACOLOGICAL PROPERTIES
5.1 Pharmacodynamic properties
None stated

5.2 Pharmacokinetic properties
None stated

5.3 Preclinical safety data
None stated

6. PHARMACEUTICAL PARTICULARS
6.1 List of excipients
The tablet core consists of:
Lactose
Maize starch
Maize starch, pre-gelatinised
Magnesium stearate
Purified water
The tablet coating consists of:
Sugar (mineral water grade)
Gelatin coarse powder 200 bloom
Purified water
Opaglos AG-7350
Opaglos AG-7350 consists of:
Purified water
Carnauba wax (E903)
Beeswax, white (E901)
Polysorbate 20 (E432)
Sorbic acid (E200)

6.2 Incompatibilities
None stated

6.3 Shelf life
36 months

6.4 Special precautions for storage
None

6.5 Nature and contents of container
Plastic containers with tamper evident closure containing 100 tablets.

6.6 Special precautions for disposal and other handling
None stated

7. MARKETING AUTHORISATION HOLDER
UCB Pharma Limited
208 Bath Road
Slough
Berkshire
SL1 3WE
UK

8. MARKETING AUTHORISATION NUMBER(S)
PL 00039/0412

9. DATE OF FIRST AUTHORISATION/RENEWAL OF THE AUTHORISATION
17 December 1992 / 17 December 1997

10. DATE OF REVISION OF THE TEXT
Drafted 24 March 2009

Eumovate Cream

(GlaxoSmithKline UK)

1. NAME OF THE MEDICINAL PRODUCT
Eumovate Cream

2. QUALITATIVE AND QUANTITATIVE COMPOSITION
0.05% w/w clobetasone butyrate.

3. PHARMACEUTICAL FORM
Water miscible cream.

4. CLINICAL PARTICULARS
4.1 Therapeutic indications
Eumovate is suitable for the treatment of eczema and dermatitis of all types including atopic eczema, photodermatitis, otitis externa, primary irritant and allergic dermatitis (including napkin rash), intertrigo, prurigo nodularis, seborrhoeic dermatitis and insect bite reactions.

Eumovate may be used as maintenance therapy between courses of one of the more active topical steroids.

4.2 Posology and method of administration
Route of administration: Topical application

For all ages:

Eumovate should be applied to the affected area up to four times a day until improvement occurs, when the frequency of application may be reduced.

4.3 Contraindications
Skin lesions caused by infection with viruses (e.g. herpes simplex, chickenpox), fungi (e.g. candidiasis, tinea) or bacteria (e.g. impetigo).

4.4 Special warnings and precautions for use
Hypersensitivity to the preparations.

Although generally regarded as safe, even for long-term administration in adults, there is a potential for overdosage, and in infants and children this may result in adrenal suppression. Extreme caution is required in dermatoses in such patients and treatment should not normally exceed seven days. In infants, the napkin may act as an occlusive dressing, and increase absorption.

Appropriate antimicrobial therapy should be used whenever treating inflammatory lesions which have become infected. Any spread of infection requires withdrawal of topical corticosteroid therapy, and systemic administration of antimicrobial agents.

As with all corticosteroids, prolonged application to the face is undesirable.

Topical corticosteroids may be hazardous in psoriasis for a number of reasons including rebound relapses, development of tolerance, risk of generalised pustular psoriasis and development of local or systemic toxicity due to impaired barrier function of the skin. If used in psoriasis, careful patient supervision is important.

If applied to the eyelids, care is needed to ensure that the preparation does not enter the eye as glaucoma might result.

4.5 Interaction with other medicinal products and other forms of interaction
None stated.

4.6 Pregnancy and lactation
There is inadequate evidence of safety in human pregnancy. Topical administration of corticosteroids to pregnant animals can cause abnormalities of foetal development including cleft palate and intra-uterine growth retardation. There may therefore be a very small risk of such effects in the human foetus.

4.7 Effects on ability to drive and use machines
None stated.

4.8 Undesirable effects
Adverse events are listed below by system organ class and frequency. Frequencies are defined as: very common ($\geq 1/10$), common ($\geq 1/100$ and $< 1/10$), uncommon ($\geq 1/1000$ and $< 1/100$), rare ($\geq 1/10,000$ and $< 1/1000$) and very rare ($< 1/10,000$) including isolated reports. Very common, common and uncommon events were generally determined from clinical trial data. The background rates in placebo and comparator groups were not taken into account when assigning frequency categories to adverse events derived from clinical trial data, since these rates were generally comparable to those in the active treatment group. Rare and very rare events were generally derived from spontaneous data.

Immune System Disorders
Very rare: Hypersensitivity

Local hypersensitivity reactions such as erythema, rash, pruritus, urticaria, local skin burning and allergic contact dermatitis may occur at the site of application and may resemble symptoms of the condition under treatment.

In the unlikely event of signs of hypersensitivity appearing, application should stop immediately.

Endocrine Disorders
Very rare: Adrenal suppression

When large areas of the body are being treated with clobetasone 17-butyrate, it is possible that some patients will absorb sufficient steroid to cause transient adrenal suppression despite the low degree of systemic activity associated with clobetasone 17-butyrate.

Skin and Subcutaneous Tissue Disorders
Very rare: Skin atrophy, pigmentation changes, hypertrichosis

Local atrophic changes could possibly occur in situations where moisture increases absorption of clobetasone 17-butyrate, but only after prolonged use.

General Disorders and Administration Site Conditions
Very rare: Exacerbation of underlying symptoms

4.9 Overdose
Acute overdosage is very unlikely to occur, however, in the case of chronic overdosage or misuse the features of hypercortisol may appear and in this situation topical steroids should be reduced or discontinued gradually under medical supervision because of the risk of adrenal insufficiency.

5. PHARMACOLOGICAL PROPERTIES
5.1 Pharmacodynamic properties
Clobetasone butyrate is a topically active corticosteroid.

Clobetasone butyrate has little effect on hypothalamo-pituitary-adrenal function. This was so even when Eumovate was applied to adults in large amounts under whole body occlusion.

Clobetasone butyrate is less potent than other available corticosteroid preparations and has been shown not to suppress the hypothalamo-pituitary-adrenal axis in patients treated for psoriasis or eczema.

Pharmacological studies in man and animals have shown that clobetasone butyrate has a relatively high level of topical activity accompanied by a low level of systemic activity.

5.2 Pharmacokinetic properties
A single application of 30g clobetasone butyrate 0.05% ointment to eight patients resulted in a measurable rise in plasma clobetasone butyrate levels during the first three hours but then the levels gradually decreased. The maximum plasma level reached in the first three hours was 0.6ng/ml. This rise in levels was followed by a more gradual decline with plasma levels of clobetasone butyrate falling below 0.1ng/ml (the lower limit of the assay) after 72 hours. The normal diurnal variation in plasma cortisol levels was not affected by the application of clobetasone butyrate ointment.

5.3 Preclinical safety data
No additional data included.

6. PHARMACEUTICAL PARTICULARS
6.1 List of excipients
Glycerol
Glycerol monostearate
Cetostearyl alcohol
Beeswax substitute 6621
Arlacel 165
Dimeticone 20
Chlorocresol
Sodium citrate
Citric acid monohydrate
Purified water

6.2 Incompatibilities
None stated.

6.3 Shelf life
36 months

6.4 Special precautions for storage
Store below 25°C.

6.5 Nature and contents of container
Internally lacquered aluminium tubes with latex band and wadless polypropylene cap.

30 and 100gm tubes are available (25gm pack is also registered).

6.6 Special precautions for disposal and other handling
Patients should be advised to wash their hands after applying Eumovate, unless it is the hands that are being treated.

Administrative Data
7. MARKETING AUTHORISATION HOLDER
Glaxo Wellcome UK Limited
trading as GlaxoSmithKline UK
Stockley Park West
Uxbridge
Middlesex UB11 1BT

8. MARKETING AUTHORISATION NUMBER(S)
PL 10949/0035

9. DATE OF FIRST AUTHORISATION/RENEWAL OF THE AUTHORISATION
30 April 1999

10. DATE OF REVISION OF THE TEXT
14 February 2007

Eumovate Ointment

(GlaxoSmithKline UK)

1. NAME OF THE MEDICINAL PRODUCT
Eumovate Ointment

2. QUALITATIVE AND QUANTITATIVE COMPOSITION
0.05% w/w clobetasone butyrate.

3. PHARMACEUTICAL FORM
Paraffin based ointment.

4. CLINICAL PARTICULARS
4.1 Therapeutic indications
Eumovate is suitable for the treatment of eczema and dermatitis of all types including atopic eczema, photodermatitis, otitis externa, primary irritant and allergic dermatitis (including napkin rash), intertrigo, prurigo nodularis, seborrhoeic dermatitis and insect bite reactions.

Eumovate may be used as maintenance therapy between courses of one of the more active topical steroids.

4.2 Posology and method of administration
Route of administration: Topical application

For all ages:

Eumovate should be applied to the affected area up to four times a day until improvement occurs, when the frequency of application may be reduced.

4.3 Contraindications
Skin lesions caused by infection with viruses (e.g. herpes simplex, chickenpox), fungi (e.g. candidiasis, tinea) or bacteria (e.g. impetigo).

Hypersensitivity to the preparation.

4.4 Special warnings and precautions for use
Although generally regarded as safe, even for long-term administration in adults, there is a potential for overdosage, and in infants and children this may result in adrenal suppression. Extreme caution is required in dermatoses in such patients and treatment should not normally exceed seven days. In infants, the napkin may act as an occlusive dressing, and increase absorption.

Appropriate antimicrobial therapy should be used whenever treating inflammatory lesions which have become infected. Any spread of infection requires withdrawal of topical corticosteroid therapy, and systemic administration of antimicrobial agents.

As with all corticosteroids, prolonged application to the face is undesirable.

Topical corticosteroids may be hazardous in psoriasis for a number of reasons including rebound relapses, development of tolerance, risk of generalised pustular psoriasis and development of local or systemic toxicity due to impaired barrier function of the skin. If used in psoriasis, careful patient supervision is important.

If applied to the eyelids, care is needed to ensure that the preparation does not enter the eye as glaucoma might result.

4.5 Interaction with other medicinal products and other forms of interaction
None stated.

4.6 Pregnancy and lactation
There is inadequate evidence of safety in human pregnancy. Topical administration of corticosteroids to pregnant animals can cause abnormalities of foetal development including cleft palate and intra-uterine growth retardation. There may therefore be a very small risk of such effects in the human foetus.

4.7 Effects on ability to drive and use machines
None stated.

4.8 Undesirable effects
Adverse events are listed below by system organ class and frequency. Frequencies are defined as: very common ($\geq$1/10), common ($\geq$1/100 and <1/10), uncommon ($\geq$1/1000 and <1/100), rare ($\geq$1/10,000 and <1/1000) and very rare (<1/10,000) including isolated reports. Very common, common and uncommon events were generally determined from clinical trial data. The background rates in placebo and comparator groups were not taken into account when assigning frequency categories to adverse events derived from clinical trial data, since these rates were generally comparable to those in the active treatment group. Rare and very rare events were generally derived from spontaneous data.

Immune System Disorders

Very rare: Hypersensitivity

Local hypersensitivity reactions such as erythema, rash, pruritus, urticaria, local skin burning and allergic contact dermatitis may occur at the site of application and may resemble symptoms of the condition under treatment.

In the unlikely event of signs of hypersensitivity appearing, application should stop immediately.

Endocrine Disorders

Very rare: Adrenal suppression

When large areas of the body are being treated with clobetasone 17-butyrate, it is possible that some patients will absorb sufficient steroid to cause transient adrenal suppression despite the low degree of systemic activity associated with clobetasone 17-butyrate.

Skin and Subcutaneous Tissue Disorders

Very rare: Skin atrophy, pigmentation changes, hypertrichosis

Local atrophic changes could possibly occur in situations where moisture increases absorption of clobetasone 17-butyrate, but only after prolonged use.

General Disorders and Administration Site Conditions

Very rare: Exacerbation of underlying symptoms

4.9 Overdose
Acute overdosage is very unlikely to occur, however, in the case of chronic overdosage or misuse the features of hypercortisol may appear and in this situation topical steroids should be reduced or discontinued gradually under medical supervision because of the risk of adrenal insufficiency.

5. PHARMACOLOGICAL PROPERTIES
5.1 Pharmacodynamic properties
Clobetasone butyrate is a topically active corticosteroid.

Clobetasone butyrate has little effect on hypothalamo-pituitary-adrenal function. This was so even when Eumovate was applied to adults in large amounts under whole body occlusion.

Clobetasone butyrate is less potent than other available corticosteroid preparations and has been shown not to suppress the hypothalamo-pituitary-adrenal axis in patients treated for psoriasis or eczema.

Pharmacological studies in man and animals have shown that clobetasone butyrate has a relatively high level of topical activity accompanied by a low level of systemic activity.

5.2 Pharmacokinetic properties
A single application of 30g clobetasone butyrate 0.05% ointment to eight patients resulted in a measurable rise in plasma clobetasone butyrate levels during the first three hours but then the levels gradually decreased. The maximum plasma level reached in the first three hours was 0.6ng/ml. This rise in levels was followed by a more gradual decline with plasma levels of clobetasone butyrate falling below 0.1ng/ml (the lower limit of the assay) after 72 hours. The normal diurnal variation in plasma cortisol levels was not affected by the application of clobetasone butyrate ointment.

5.3 Preclinical safety data
No additional data included.

6. PHARMACEUTICAL PARTICULARS
6.1 List of excipients
Liquid paraffin

White soft paraffin

6.2 Incompatibilities
None stated.

6.3 Shelf life
36 months

6.4 Special precautions for storage
Store below 25°C.

6.5 Nature and contents of container
Collapsible aluminium tube and wadless polypropylene cap.

30 and 100gm tubes are available (25gm pack is also registered).

6.6 Special precautions for disposal and other handling
Patients should be advised to wash their hands after applying Eumovate, unless it is the hands that are being treated.

Administrative Data
7. MARKETING AUTHORISATION HOLDER
Glaxo Wellcome UK Limited

Trading as GlaxoSmithKline UK

Stockley Park West

Uxbridge

Middlesex UB11 1BT

8. MARKETING AUTHORISATION NUMBER(S)
PL 10949/0037

9. DATE OF FIRST AUTHORISATION/RENEWAL OF THE AUTHORISATION
15 March 2001

10. DATE OF REVISION OF THE TEXT
14 February 2007

Eurax Cream

(Novartis Consumer Health)

1. NAME OF THE MEDICINAL PRODUCT
Eurax® Cream

2. QUALITATIVE AND QUANTITATIVE COMPOSITION
Crotamiton 10%

For excipients, see Section 6.1.

3. PHARMACEUTICAL FORM
Cream

A white to cream coloured cream.

4. CLINICAL PARTICULARS
4.1 Therapeutic indications
For the relief of itching and skin irritation caused by, for example, sunburn, dry eczema, itchy dermatitis, allergic rashes, hives, nettle rash, chickenpox, insect bites and stings, heat rashes and personal itching.

The treatment of scabies.

4.2 Posology and method of administration
Pruritus

Apply to the affected area 2-3 times daily. Eurax will provide relief from irritation for 6-10 hours after each application. Eurax can be used in children. There are no special dosage recommendations in the elderly.

Scabies

Adults (including the elderly):

After the patient has taken a warm bath, the skin should be well dried and Eurax rubbed into the entire body surface (excluding the face and scalp) until no traces of the preparation remain visible on the surface. The application should be repeated once daily, preferably in the evening, for a total of 3-5 days. Depending on the response, special attention should be paid to sites that are particularly susceptible to infestation by the mites (eg interdigital spaces, wrists, axillae and genitalia). Areas where there is pus formation should be covered with a dressing impregnated with Eurax. While the treatment is in progress the patient may take a bath shortly before the next application. After completion of the treatment, a cleansing bath should be taken followed by a change of bed linen and underclothing.

In children under three years of age Eurax should not be applied more than once a day. There are no special dosage recommendations in the elderly.

Method of administration: Cutaneous use.

4.3 Contraindications
Acute exudative dermatoses. Hypersensitivity to any of the ingredients. Eurax should not be used in or around the eyes since contact with the eyelids may give rise to conjunctival inflammation.

4.4 Special warnings and precautions for use
Eurax can be used for children; consult your doctor before use on children under 3 years of age.

For external use only.

Do not use in or around the eyes, on broken skin, for weeping skin conditions or if you are sensitive to any of the ingredients.

Consult your doctor or pharmacist before using Eurax if you are pregnant or breast feeding, or suffering from genital itching.

If symptoms persist consult your doctor.

4.5 Interaction with other medicinal products and other forms of interaction
None.

4.6 Pregnancy and lactation
There is no experience to judge the safety of Eurax in pregnancy, therefore Eurax is not recommended during pregnancy, especially in the first three months. It is not known whether the active substance passes into the breast milk. Nursing mothers should avoid applying Eurax in the area of the nipples.

4.7 Effects on ability to drive and use machines
None.

4.8 Undesirable effects
Occasionally irritation of the skin or contact allergy may occur. In such cases the preparation should be discontinued.

4.9 Overdose
Eurax is for application to the skin only. Following accidental ingestion, nausea, vomiting and irritation of the buccal, oesophageal and gastric mucosa have been reported. If accidental ingestion of large quantities occurs, there is no specific antidote and general measures to eliminate the drug and reduce its absorption should be undertaken. Symptomatic treatment should be administered as appropriate. A risk of methaemoglobinaemia exists, which may be treated with methylene blue.

5. PHARMACOLOGICAL PROPERTIES
5.1 Pharmacodynamic properties
Eurax has a symptomatic action on pruritus and is an acaricide.

5.2 Pharmacokinetic properties
Eurax penetrates rapidly into human skin. Low but measurable concentrations of crotamiton are found in plasma, with a maximum level after 4-10 hours, declining rapidly thereafter.

5.3 Preclinical safety data
Eurax cream administered dermally once daily under occlusive dressing for 3 months to rabbits was tolerated at doses of up to 250mg/kg without signs of toxicity, apart from transient skin irritation. No sensitising or photo-sensitising potential has been observed in animal studies.

Crotamiton does not induce mutations in bacteria nor chromosomal damage in mammalian cells. Studies to detect a possible effect on fertility and reproductive behaviour also gave negative results.

6. PHARMACEUTICAL PARTICULARS

6.1 List of excipients

Methyl hydroxybenzoate

Phenylethyl alcohol

Glycerol

Triethanolamine

Sodium lauryl sulphate

Ethylene glycol monostearate

Stearyl alcohol

Strong ammonia solution 25%

Stearic acid

Hard paraffin

White beeswax

Perfume Givaudan No 45

Purified water

6.2 Incompatibilities

None.

6.3 Shelf life

60 months.

6.4 Special precautions for storage

Protect from heat.

6.5 Nature and contents of container

Internally lacquered aluminium tube, with a screw cap, in a cardboard carton.

Pack sizes: 20, 30 and 100g

6.6 Special precautions for disposal and other handling

None.

7. MARKETING AUTHORISATION HOLDER

Novartis Consumer Health UK Ltd

Wimblehurst Road

Horsham

West Sussex

RH12 5AB

Trading as: Novartis Consumer Health

8. MARKETING AUTHORISATION NUMBER(S)

PL 00030/0092

9. DATE OF FIRST AUTHORISATION/RENEWAL OF THE AUTHORISATION

Granted: 1 September 1997 (transferred from PL 0001/5008R)

10. DATE OF REVISION OF THE TEXT

27 April 2004

Legal category: GSL

Eurax Hydrocortisone Cream

(Novartis Consumer Health)

1. NAME OF THE MEDICINAL PRODUCT

Eurax® Hydrocortisone Cream

2. QUALITATIVE AND QUANTITATIVE COMPOSITION

Active ingredients: Crotamiton 10.0% w/w

Hydrocortisone BP 0.25% w/w

For excipients see section 6.1

3. PHARMACEUTICAL FORM

Cream

A white to cream coloured, giving a homogenous smear, apart from trapped air bubbles

4. CLINICAL PARTICULARS

4.1 Therapeutic indications

Eczema and dermatitis of all types including atopic eczema, photodermatitis, otitis externa, primary irritant and allergic dermatitis, intertrigo, prurigo nodularis, seborrhoeic dermatitis and insect bite reactions.

Route of Administration: Cutaneous use.

4.2 Posology and method of administration

Adults

A thin layer of Eurax Hydrocortisone Cream should be applied to the affected area 2-3 times a day. Occlusive dressings should not be used. Treatment should be limited to 10-14 days or up to 7 days if applied to the face.

Use in the Elderly

Clinical evidence would indicate that no special dosage regime is necessary.

Use in Children

Eurax Hydrocortisone should be used with caution in infants and for not more than 7 days. Eurax Hydrocortisone should not be applied more than once a day to large areas of the body surface in young children.

4.3 Contraindications

Hypersensitivity to any component of the formulation. Bacterial, viral or fungal infections of the skin. Acute exudative dermatoses. Application to ulcerated areas.

4.4 Special warnings and precautions for use

Eurax Hydrocortisone should be used with caution in infants and for not more than 7 days; long-term continuous topical therapy should be avoided since this can lead to adrenal suppression even without occlusion.

Eurax Hydrocortisone should not be allowed to come into contact with the conjunctiva and mucous membranes.

4.5 Interaction with other medicinal products and other forms of interaction

None known.

4.6 Pregnancy and lactation

There is inadequate evidence of safety in human pregnancy. Topical administration of corticosteroids to pregnant animals can cause abnormalities of foetal development, including cleft palate and intra-uterine growth retardation. There may therefore be a very small risk of such effects in the human foetus.

It is not known whether the active substances of Eurax Hydrocortisone and/or their metabolites pass into the breast milk after topical administration. Use in lactating mothers should only be at the doctor's discretion.

4.7 Effects on ability to drive and use machines

None known.

4.8 Undesirable effects

Occasionally at the site of application signs of irritation such as a burning sensation, itching, contact dermatitis/contact allergy may occur. Treatment should be discontinued if patients experience severe irritation or sensitisation.

4.9 Overdose

Eurax Hydrocortisone is for application to the skin only. If accidental ingestion of large quantities occurs, there is no specific antidote and general measures to eliminate the drug and reduce its absorption should be undertaken. Symptomatic treatment should be administered as appropriate.

5. PHARMACOLOGICAL PROPERTIES

5.1 Pharmacodynamic properties

Eurax Hydrocortisone combines the antipruritic action of crotamiton with the anti-inflammatory and anti-allergic properties of hydrocortisone.

5.2 Pharmacokinetic properties

No pharmacokinetic data on Eurax Hydrocortisone Cream are available.

5.3 Preclinical safety data

Not applicable.

6. PHARMACEUTICAL PARTICULARS

6.1 List of excipients

Stearyl alcohol

White soft paraffin

Polyoxy 40 stearate

Propyl hydroxybenzoate

Propylene glycol

Methyl hydroxybenzoate

Perfume Givaudan no 45

Purified water

6.2 Incompatibilities

None known

6.3 Shelf life

60 months

6.4 Special precautions for storage

Do not store above 25°C

6.5 Nature and contents of container

Collapsible aluminium tube

Pack Size: 30g

6.6 Special precautions for disposal and other handling

Medicines should be kept out of the reach and sight of children.

Administrative Data

7. MARKETING AUTHORISATION HOLDER

Novartis Consumer Health UK Ltd

Trading as

Novartis Consumer Health

Wimblehurst Road

Horsham

West Sussex

RH12 5AB

8. MARKETING AUTHORISATION NUMBER(S)

PL 00030/0094

9. DATE OF FIRST AUTHORISATION/RENEWAL OF THE AUTHORISATION

Original grant date: 17 January 1991

Date of renewal: 17 January 1996

10. DATE OF REVISION OF THE TEXT

24 July 2006

Legal category

POM

Evista 60mg film coated tablets

(Daiichi Sankyo UK Limited)

1. NAME OF THE MEDICINAL PRODUCT

Evista 60mg film coated tablets

2. QUALITATIVE AND QUANTITATIVE COMPOSITION

Each film coated tablet contains 60 mg raloxifene hydrochloride, equivalent to 56 mg raloxifene free base.

Excipient: each tablet contains lactose (149.40 mg).

For a full list of excipients, see section 6.1.

3. PHARMACEUTICAL FORM

Film coated tablet.

Elliptically shaped, white tablets imprinted with the code '4165'.

4. CLINICAL PARTICULARS

4.1 Therapeutic indications

EVISTA is indicated for the treatment and prevention of osteoporosis in postmenopausal women. A significant reduction in the incidence of vertebral, but not hip fractures has been demonstrated.

When determining the choice of EVISTA or other therapies, including oestrogens, for an individual postmenopausal woman, consideration should be given to menopausal symptoms, effects on uterine and breast tissues, and cardiovascular risks and benefits (see section 5.1).

4.2 Posology and method of administration

The recommended dose is one tablet daily by oral administration, which may be taken at any time of the day without regard to meals. No dose adjustment is necessary for the elderly. Due to the nature of this disease process, EVISTA is intended for long term use.

Generally calcium and vitamin D supplements are advised in women with a low dietary intake.

Use in renal impairment:

EVISTA should not be used in patients with severe renal impairment (see section 4.3). In patients with moderate and mild renal impairment, EVISTA should be used with caution.

Use in hepatic impairment:

EVISTA should not be used in patients with hepatic impairment (see section 4.3).

4.3 Contraindications

Hypersensitivity to the active substance or to any of the excipients.

Must not be used in women with child bearing potential.

Active or past history of venous thromboembolic events (VTE), including deep vein thrombosis, pulmonary embolism and retinal vein thrombosis.

Hepatic impairment including cholestasis.

Severe renal impairment.

Unexplained uterine bleeding.

EVISTA should not be used in patients with signs or symptoms of endometrial cancer as safety in this patient group has not been adequately studied.

4.4 Special warnings and precautions for use

Raloxifene is associated with an increased risk for venous thromboembolic events that is similar to the reported risk associated with current use of hormone replacement therapy. The risk-benefit balance should be considered in patients at risk of venous thromboembolic events of any aetiology. EVISTA should be discontinued in the event of an illness or a condition leading to a prolonged period of immobilisation. Discontinuation should happen as soon as possible in case of the illness, or from 3 days before the immobilisation occurs. Therapy should not be restarted until the initiating condition has resolved and the patient is fully mobile.

In a study of postmenopausal women with documented coronary heart disease or at increased risk for coronary events, raloxifene did not affect the incidence of myocardial infarction, hospitalized acute coronary syndrome, overall mortality, including overall cardiovascular mortality, or stroke, compared to placebo. However, there was an increase in death due to stroke in women assigned to raloxifene. The incidence of stroke mortality was 1.5 per 1000 women per year for placebo versus 2.2 per 1000 women per year for raloxifene. This finding should be considered when prescribing raloxifene for postmenopausal women with a history of stroke or other significant stroke risk factors, such as transient ischemic attack or atrial fibrillation.

There is no evidence of endometrial proliferation. Any uterine bleeding during EVISTA therapy is unexpected and should be fully investigated by a specialist. The two most frequent diagnoses associated with uterine bleeding during raloxifene treatment were endometrial atrophy and benign endometrial polyps. In postmenopausal women who received raloxifene treatment for 4 years, benign endometrial polyps were reported in 0.9 % compared to 0.3 % in women who received placebo treatment.

Raloxifene is metabolised primarily in the liver. Single doses of raloxifene given to patients with cirrhosis and mild hepatic impairment (Child-Pugh class A) produced plasma concentrations of raloxifene which were approximately 2.5 times the controls. The increase correlated with total bilirubin concentrations. Until safety and efficacy have been evaluated further in patients with hepatic insufficiency, the use of EVISTA is not recommended in this patient population. Serum total bilirubin, gamma-glutamyl transferase, alkaline phosphatase, ALT and AST should be closely monitored during treatment if elevated values are observed.

Limited clinical data suggest that in patients with a history of oral oestrogen-induced hypertriglyceridemia (>5.6 mmol/l), raloxifene may be associated with a marked increase in serum triglycerides. Patients with this medical history should have serum triglycerides monitored when taking raloxifene.

The safety of EVISTA in patients with breast cancer has not been adequately studied. No data are available on the concomitant use of EVISTA and agents used in the treatment of early or advanced breast cancer. Therefore, EVISTA should be used for osteoporosis treatment and prevention only after the treatment of breast cancer, including adjuvant therapy, has been completed.

As safety information regarding co-administration of raloxifene with systemic oestrogens is limited, such use is not recommended.

EVISTA is not effective in reducing vasodilatation (hot flushes), or other symptoms of the menopause associated with oestrogen deficiency.

EVISTA contains lactose. Patients with rare hereditary problems of galactose intolerance, the Lapp lactase deficiency or glucose-galactose malabsorption should not take this medicine.

4.5 Interaction with other medicinal products and other forms of interaction

Concurrent administration of either calcium carbonate or aluminium and magnesium-hydroxide containing antacids do not affect the systemic exposure of raloxifene.

Co-administration of raloxifene and warfarin does not alter the pharmacokinetics of either compound. However, modest decreases in the prothrombin time have been observed, and if raloxifene is given concurrently with warfarin or other coumarin derivatives, the prothrombin time should be monitored. Effects on prothrombin time may develop over several weeks if EVISTA treatment is started in patients who are already on coumarin anticoagulant therapy.

Raloxifene has no effect on the pharmacokinetics of methylprednisolone given as a single dose.

Raloxifene does not affect the steady-state AUC of digoxin. The C_{max} of digoxin increased by less than 5%.

The influence of concomitant medication on raloxifene plasma concentrations was evaluated in the prevention and treatment trials. Frequently co-administered medicinal products included: paracetamol, non-steroidal anti-inflammatory drugs (such as acetylsalicylic acid, ibuprofen, and naproxen), oral antibiotics, H1 antagonists, H2 antagonists, and benzodiazepines. No clinically relevant effects of the co-administration of the agents on raloxifene plasma concentrations were identified.

Concomitant use of vaginal oestrogen preparations was allowed in the clinical trial programme, if necessary to treat atrophic vaginal symptoms. Compared to placebo there was no increased use in EVISTA treated patients.

In vitro, raloxifene did not interact with the binding of warfarin, phenytoin, or tamoxifen.

Raloxifene should not be co-administered with cholestyramine (or other anion exchange resins), which significantly reduces the absorption and enterohepatic cycling of raloxifene.

Peak concentrations of raloxifene are reduced with co-administration with ampicillin. However, since the overall extent of absorption and the elimination rate of raloxifene are not affected, raloxifene can be concurrently administered with ampicillin.

Raloxifene modestly increases hormone-binding globulin concentrations, including sex steroid binding globulins (SHBG), thyroxine binding globulin (TBG), and corticosteroid binding globulin (CBG), with corresponding increases in total hormone concentrations. These changes do not affect concentrations of free hormones.

4.6 Pregnancy and lactation

EVISTA is only for use in postmenopausal women.

EVISTA must not be taken by women of child bearing potential. Raloxifene may cause foetal harm when administered to a pregnant woman. If this medicinal product is used mistakenly during pregnancy or the patient becomes pregnant while taking it, the patient should be informed of the potential hazard to the foetus (see section 5.3).

It is not known whether raloxifene is excreted in human milk. Its clinical use, therefore, cannot be recommended in breast-feeding women. EVISTA may affect the development of the baby.

4.7 Effects on ability to drive and use machines

Raloxifene has no known influence on the ability to drive and use machines.

4.8 Undesirable effects

In osteoporosis treatment and prevention studies involving over 13,000 postmenopausal women all adverse reactions were recorded. The duration of treatment in these studies ranged from 6 to 60 months. The majority of adverse reactions have not usually required cessation of therapy.

In the prevention population discontinuations of therapy due to any adverse reaction occurred in 10.7 % of 581 EVISTA treated patients and 11.1 % of 584 placebo-treated patients. In the treatment population discontinuations of therapy due to any clinical adverse event occurred in 12.8 % of 2,557 EVISTA treated patients and 11.1 % of 2,576 placebo treated patients.

The adverse reactions associated with the use of raloxifene in osteoporosis clinical trials are summarised in the table below. The following convention has been used for the classification of the adverse reactions: very common (≥1/10), common (≥1/100 to <1/10), uncommon (≥1/1,000 to <1/100), rare (≥1/10,000 to <1/1,000) very rare (<1/10,000), not known (cannot be estimated from the available data).

Vascular disorders *Very common:* Vasodilation (hot flushes) *Uncommon:* Venous thromboembolic events, including deep vein thrombosis, pulmonary embolism, retinal vein thrombosis Superficial vein thrombophlebitis
Musculoskeletal and connective tissue disorders *Common:* Leg cramps
General disorders and administration site conditions *Very common:* Flu syndrome *Common:* Peripheral oedema

Compared with placebo-treated patients the occurrence of vasodilatation (hot flushes) was modestly increased in EVISTA patients (clinical trials for the prevention of osteoporosis, 2 to 8 years postmenopausal, 24.3 % EVISTA and 18.2 % placebo; clinical trials for the treatment of osteoporosis, mean age 66, 10.6 % for EVISTA and 7.1 % placebo). This adverse reaction was most common in the first 6 months of treatment, and seldom occurred de novo after that time.

In a study of 10,101 postmenopausal women with documented coronary heart disease or at increased risk for coronary events (RUTH), the occurrence of vasodilatation (hot flushes) was 7.8 % in the raloxifene-treated patients and 4.7 % in the placebo-treated patients.

Across all placebo-controlled clinical trials of raloxifene in osteoporosis, venous thromboembolic events, including deep vein thrombosis, pulmonary embolism, and retinal vein thrombosis occurred at a frequency of approximately 0.8 % or 3.22 cases per 1,000 patient years. A relative risk of 1.60 (CI 0.95, 2.71) was observed in EVISTA treated patients compared to placebo. The risk of a thromboembolic event was greatest in the first four months of therapy. Superficial vein thrombophlebitis occurred in a frequency of less than 1 %.

In the RUTH study, venous thromboembolic events occurred at a frequency of approximately 2.0 % or 3.88 cases per 1000 patient-years in the raloxifene group and 1.4 % or 2.70 cases per 1000 patient-years in the placebo group. The hazard ratio for all VTE events in the RUTH study was HR = 1.44 (1.06 – 1.95). Superficial vein thrombophlebitis occurred in a frequency of 1 % in the raloxifene group and 0.6 % in the placebo group.

Another adverse reaction observed was leg cramps (5.5 % for EVISTA, 1.9 % for placebo in the prevention population and 9.2 % for EVISTA, 6.0 % for placebo in the treatment population).

In the RUTH study, leg cramps were observed in 12.1 % of raloxifene-treated patients and 8.3 % of placebo-treated patients.

Flu syndrome was reported by 16.2 % of EVISTA treated patients and 14.0 % of placebo treated patients.

One further change was seen which was not statistically significant ($p > 0.05$), but which did show a significant dose trend. This was peripheral oedema, which occurred in the prevention population at an incidence of 3.1 % for EVISTA and 1.9 % for placebo; and in the treatment population occurred at an incidence of 7.1 % for EVISTA and 6.1 % for placebo.

In the RUTH study, peripheral oedema occurred in 14.1 % of the raloxifene-treated patients and 11.7 % of the placebo-treated patients, which was statistically significant.

Slightly decreased (6-10 %) platelet counts have been reported during raloxifene treatment in placebo-controlled clinical trials of raloxifene in osteoporosis.

Rare cases of moderate increases in AST and/or ALT have been reported where a causal relationship to raloxifene can not be excluded. A similar frequency of increases was noted among placebo patients.

In a study (RUTH) of postmenopausal women with documented coronary heart disease or at increased risk for coronary events, an additional adverse reaction of cholelithiasis occurred in 3.3 % of patients treated with raloxifene and 2.6 % of patients treated with placebo. Cholecystectomy rates for raloxifene (2.3 %) were not statistically significantly different from placebo (2.0 %).

EVISTA (n = 317) was compared with continuous combined (n = 110) hormone replacement therapy (HRT) or cyclic (n = 205) HRT patients in some clinical trials. The incidence of breast symptoms and uterine bleeding in raloxifene treated women was significantly lower than in women treated with either form of HRT.

The adverse reactions reported in post-marketing experience and are presented in the table below.

Blood and lymphatic system disorders *Very rare:* thrombocytopenia
Gastrointestinal disorders *Very rare:* Gastrointestinal symptoms such as nausea, vomiting, abdominal pain, dyspepsia
General disorders and administration site conditions *Rare:* peripheral oedema
Investigations *Very rare:* Increased blood pressure
Nervous system disorders *Very rare:* Headache, including migraine
Skin and subcutaneous tissue disorders *Very rare:* Rash
Reproductive system and breast disorders *Very rare:* Mild breast symptoms such as pain, enlargement and tenderness
Vascular disorders *Rare:* venous thromboembolic reaction *Very rare:* arterial thromboembolic reaction

4.9 Overdose

In some clinical trials, daily doses were given up to 600 mg for 8 weeks and 120 mg, for 3 years. No cases of raloxifene overdose were reported during clinical trials.

In adults, symptoms of leg cramps and dizziness have been reported in patients who took more than 120 mg as a single ingestion.

In accidental overdose in children younger than 2 years of age, the maximum reported dose has been 180 mg. In children, symptoms of accidental overdose included ataxia, dizziness, vomiting, rash, diarrhea, tremor, and flushing, and elevation in alkaline phosphatase.

The highest overdose has been approximately 1.5 grams. No fatalities associated with overdose have been reported.

There is no specific antidote for raloxifene hydrochloride.

5. PHARMACOLOGICAL PROPERTIES

5.1 Pharmacodynamic properties

Pharmaco-therapeutic group: Selective Oestrogen Receptor Modulator, ATC code: G03XC01.

As a selective oestrogen receptor modulator (SERM), raloxifene has selective agonist or antagonist activities on tissues responsive to oestrogen. It acts as an agonist on bone and partially on cholesterol metabolism (decrease in total and LDL-cholesterol), but not in the hypothalamus or in the uterine or breast tissues.

Raloxifene's biological actions, like those of oestrogen, are mediated through high affinity binding to oestrogen receptors and regulation of gene expression. This binding results in differential expression of multiple oestrogen-regulated genes in different tissues. Recent data suggests that the oestrogen receptor can regulate gene expression by at least two distinct pathways which are ligand-, tissue-, and/or gene-specific.

a) Skeletal Effects

The decrease in oestrogen availability which occurs at menopause, leads to marked increases in bone resorption, bone loss and risk of fracture. Bone loss is particularly rapid for the first 10 years after menopause when the compensatory increase in bone formation is inadequate to keep up with resorptive losses. Other risk factors which may lead to the development of osteoporosis include early menopause; osteopenia (at least 1 SD below peak bone mass); thin body build; Caucasian or Asian ethnic origin; and a family history of osteoporosis. Replacement therapies generally reverse the excessive resorption of bone. In postmenopausal women with osteoporosis, EVISTA reduces the incidence of vertebral fractures, preserves bone mass and increases bone mineral density (BMD).

Based on these risk factors, prevention of osteoporosis with EVISTA is indicated for women within ten years of menopause, with BMD of the spine between 1.0 and 2.5 SD below the mean value of a normal young population, taking into account their high lifetime risk for osteoporotic fractures. Likewise, EVISTA is indicated for the treatment of osteoporosis or established osteoporosis in women with BMD of the spine 2.5 SD below the mean value of a normal young population and/or with vertebral fractures, irrespective of BMD.

i) Incidence of fractures. In a study of 7,705 postmenopausal women with a mean age of 66 years and with osteoporosis or osteoporosis with an existing fracture, EVISTA treatment for 3 years reduced the incidence of vertebral fractures by 47 % (RR 0.53, CI 0.35, 0.79; $p < 0.001$) and 31 % (RR 0.69, CI 0.56, 0.86; $p < 0.001$) respectively. Forty five women with osteoporosis or 15 women with osteoporosis with an existing fracture would need to be treated with EVISTA for 3 years to prevent one or more vertebral fractures. EVISTA treatment for 4 years reduced the incidence of vertebral fractures by 46 % (RR 0.54, CI 0.38, 0.75) and 32 % (RR 0.68, CI 0.56, 0.83) in patients with osteoporosis or osteopenia with an existing fracture respectively. In the 4th year alone, EVISTA reduced the new vertebral fracture risk by 39 % (RR 0.61, CI 0.43, 0.88). An effect on non-vertebral fractures has not been demonstrated. From the 4th to the 8th year, patients were permitted the concomitant use of bisphosphonates, calcitonin and fluorides and all patients in this study received calcium and vitamin D supplementation.

In the RUTH study overall clinical fractures were collected as a secondary endpoint. EVISTA reduced the incidence of clinical vertebral fractures by 35% compared with placebo (HR 0.65, CI 0.47 0.89). These results may have been confounded by baseline differences in BMD and vertebral fractures. There was no difference between treatment groups in the incidence of new nonvertebral fractures. During the whole length of the study concomitant use of other bone-active medications was permitted.

ii) Bone Mineral Density (BMD): The efficacy of EVISTA once daily in postmenopausal women aged up to 60 years and with or without a uterus was established over a two-year treatment period. The women were 2 to 8 years postmenopausal. Three trials included 1,764 postmenopausal women who were treated with EVISTA and calcium or calcium supplemented placebo. In one of these trials the women had previously undergone hysterectomy. EVISTA produced significant increases in bone density of hip and spine as well as total body mineral mass compared to placebo. This increase was generally a 2 % increase in BMD compared to placebo. A similar increase in BMD was seen in the treatment population who received EVISTA for up to 7 years. In the prevention trials, the percentage of subjects experiencing an increase or decrease in BMD during raloxifene therapy was: for the spine 37 % decreased and 63 % increased; and for the total hip 29 % decreased and 71 % increased.

iii) Calcium kinetics. EVISTA and oestrogen affect bone remodelling and calcium metabolism similarly. EVISTA was associated with reduced bone resorption and a mean positive shift in calcium balance of 60 mg per day, due primarily to decreased urinary calcium losses.

iv) Histomorphometry (bone quality). In a study comparing EVISTA with oestrogen, bone from patients treated with either medicinal product was histologically normal, with no evidence of mineralisation defects, woven bone or marrow fibrosis.

Raloxifene decreases resorption of bone; this effect on bone is manifested as reductions in the serum and urine levels of bone turnover markers, decreases in bone resorption based on radiocalcium kinetics studies, increases in BMD and decreases in the incidence of fractures.

b) Effects on lipid metabolism and cardiovascular risk

Clinical trials showed that a 60 mg daily dose of EVISTA significantly decreased total cholesterol (3 to 6 %), and LDL cholesterol (4 to 10 %). Women with the highest baseline cholesterol levels had the greatest decreases. HDL cholesterol and triglyceride concentrations did not change significantly. After 3 years therapy EVISTA decreased fibrinogen (6.71 %). In the osteoporosis treatment study, significantly fewer EVISTA-treated patients required initiation of hypolipidaemic therapy compared to placebo.

EVISTA therapy for 8 years did not significantly affect the risk of cardiovascular events in patients enrolled in the osteoporosis treatment study. Similarly, in the RUTH study, raloxifene did not affect the incidence of myocardial infarction, hospitalized acute coronary syndrome, stroke or overall mortality, including overall cardiovascular mortality, compared to placebo (for the increase in risk of fatal stroke see section 4.4).

The relative risk of venous thromboembolic events observed during raloxifene treatment was 1.60 (CI 0.95, 2.71) when compared to placebo, and was 1.0 (CI 0.3, 6.2) when compared to oestrogen or hormonal replacement therapy. The risk of a thromboembolic event was greatest in the first four months of therapy.

c) Effects on the endometrium and on the pelvic floor

In clinical trials, EVISTA did not stimulate the postmenopausal uterine endometrium. Compared to placebo, raloxifene was not associated with spotting or bleeding or endometrial hyperplasia. Nearly 3,000 transvaginal ultrasound (TVUs) examinations were evaluated from 831 women in all dose groups. Raloxifene treated women consistently had an endometrial thickness which was indistinguishable from placebo. After 3 years of treatment, at least a 5 mm increase in endometrial thickness, assessed with transvaginal ultrasound, was observed in 1.9 % of the 211 women treated with raloxifene 60 mg/day compared to 1.8 % of the 219 women who received placebo. There were no differences between the raloxifene and placebo groups with respect to the incidence of reported uterine bleeding.

Endometrial biopsies taken after six months therapy with EVISTA 60 mg daily demonstrated non-proliferative endometrium in all patients. In addition, in a study with 2.5 × the recommended daily dose of EVISTA there was no evidence of endometrial proliferation and no increase in uterine volume.

In the osteoporosis treatment trial, endometrial thickness was evaluated annually in a subset of the study population (1,644 patients) for 4 years. Endometrial thickness measurements in EVISTA treated women were not different from baseline after 4 years of therapy. There was no difference between EVISTA and placebo treated women in the incidences of vaginal bleeding (spotting) or vaginal discharge. Fewer EVISTA treated women than placebo treated women required surgical intervention for uterine prolapse. Safety information following 3 years of raloxifene treatment suggests that raloxifene treatment does not increase pelvic floor relaxation and pelvic floor surgery.

After 4 years, raloxifene did not increase the risk of endometrial or ovarian cancer. In postmenopausal women who received raloxifene treatment for 4 years, benign endometrial polyps were reported in 0.9 % compared to 0.3 % in women who received placebo treatment.

d) Effects on breast tissue

EVISTA does not stimulate breast tissue. Across all placebo-controlled trials, EVISTA was indistinguishable from placebo with regard to frequency and severity of breast symptoms (no swelling, tenderness and breast pain).

Over the 4 years of the osteoporosis treatment trial (involving 7705 patients), EVISTA treatment compared to placebo reduced the risk of total breast cancer by 62 % (RR 0.38; CI 0.21, 0.69), the risk of invasive breast cancer by 71 % (RR 0.29, CI 0.13, 0.58) and the risk of invasive oestrogen receptor (ER) positive breast cancer by 79 % (RR 0.21, CI 0.07, 0.50). EVISTA has no effect on the risk of ER negative breast cancers. These observations support the conclusion that raloxifene has no intrinsic oestrogen agonist activity in breast tissue.

e) Effects on cognitive function

No adverse effects on cognitive function have been seen.

5.2 Pharmacokinetic properties

Absorption

Raloxifene is absorbed rapidly after oral administration. Approximately 60 % of an oral dose is absorbed. Presystemic glucuronidation is extensive. Absolute bioavailability of raloxifene is 2 %. The time to reach average maximum plasma concentration and bioavailability are functions of systemic interconversion and enterohepatic cycling of raloxifene and its glucuronide metabolites.

Distribution

Raloxifene is distributed extensively in the body. The volume of distribution is not dose dependent. Raloxifene is strongly bound to plasma proteins (98-99%).

Metabolism

Raloxifene undergoes extensive first pass metabolism to the glucuronide conjugates: raloxifene-4'-glucuronide, raloxifene-6-glucuronide, and raloxifene-6, 4'-diglucuronide. No other metabolites have been detected. Raloxifene comprises less than 1 % of the combined concentrations of raloxifene and the glucuronide metabolites. Raloxifene levels are maintained by enterohepatic recycling, giving a plasma half-life of 27.7 hours.

Results from single oral doses of raloxifene predict multiple dose pharmacokinetics. Increasing doses of raloxifene result in slightly less than proportional increase in the area under the plasma time concentration curve (AUC).

Excretion

The majority of a dose of raloxifene and glucuronide metabolites are excreted within 5 days and are found primarily in the faeces, with less than 6 % excreted in urine.

Special populations

Renal insufficiency - Less than 6 % of the total dose is eliminated in urine. In a population pharmacokinetic study, a 47 % decrease in lean body mass adjusted creatinine clearance resulted in a 17 % decrease in raloxifene clearance and a 15 % decrease in the clearance of raloxifene conjugates.

Hepatic insufficiency - The pharmacokinetics of a single dose of raloxifene in patients with cirrhosis and mild hepatic impairment (Child-Pugh class A) have been compared to that in healthy individuals. Plasma raloxifene concentrations were approximately 2.5-fold higher than in controls and correlated with bilirubin concentrations.

5.3 Preclinical safety data

In a 2-year carcinogenicity study in rats, an increase in ovarian tumors of granulosa/theca cell origin was observed in high-dose females (279 mg/kg/day). Systemic exposure (AUC) of raloxifene in this group was approximately 400 times that in postmenopausal women administered a 60 mg dose. In a 21-month carcinogenicity study in mice, there was an increased incidence of testicular interstitial cell tumours and prostatic adenomas and adenocarcinomas in males given 41 or 210 mg/kg, and prostatic leiomyoblastoma in males given 210 mg/kg. In female mice, an increased incidence of ovarian tumours in animals given 9 to 242 mg/kg (0.3 to 32 times the AUC in humans) included benign and malignant tumours of granulosa/theca cell origin and benign tumours of epithelial cell origin. The female rodents in these studies were treated during their reproductive lives, when their ovaries were functional and highly responsive to hormonal stimulation. In contrast to the highly responsive ovaries in this rodent model, the human ovary after menopause is relatively unresponsive to reproductive hormonal stimulation.

Raloxifene was not genotoxic in any of the extensive battery of test systems applied.

The reproductive and developmental effects observed in animals are consistent with the known pharmacological profile of raloxifene. At doses of 0.1 to 10 mg/kg/day in female rats, raloxifene disrupted estrous cycles of female rats during treatment, but did not delay fertile matings after treatment termination and only marginally reduced litter size, increased gestation length, and altered the timing of events in neonatal development. When given during the preimplantation period, raloxifene delayed and disrupted embryo implantation resulting in prolonged gestation and reduced litter size but development of offspring to weaning was not affected. Teratology studies were conducted in rabbits and rats. In rabbits, abortion and a low rate of ventricular septal defects (≥ 0.1 mg/kg) and hydrocephaly (≥ 10 mg/kg) were seen. In rats retardation of foetal development, wavy ribs and kidney cavitation occurred (≥ 1 mg/kg).

Raloxifene is a potent antioestrogen in the rat uterus and prevented growth of oestrogen-dependent mammary tumours in rats and mice.

6. PHARMACEUTICAL PARTICULARS

6.1 List of excipients

Tablet core:

Povidone

Polysorbate 80

Anhydrous lactose

Lactose monohydrate

Crospovidone

Magnesium stearate

Tablet coating:

Titanium dioxide (E 171)

Polysorbate 80

Hypromellose

Macrogol 400

Carnauba wax

Ink:

Shellac

Propylene glycol

Indigo carmine (E 132)

6.2 Incompatibilities

Not applicable.

6.3 Shelf life

3 years.

6.4 Special precautions for storage

Store in the original package. Do not freeze.

6.5 Nature and contents of container

EVISTA tablets are packed either in PVC/PE/PCTFE blisters or in high density polyethylene bottles. Blister boxes contain 14, 28, or 84 tablets. Bottles contain 100 tablets.

Not all pack sizes may be marketed in all countries.

6.6 Special precautions for disposal and other handling

No special requirements.

7. MARKETING AUTHORISATION HOLDER

Daiichi Sankyo Europe GmbH

Zielstattstrasse 48

D-81379 Munich

Germany

8. MARKETING AUTHORISATION NUMBER(S)

EU/1/98/073/001

EU/1/98/073/002

EU/1/98/073/003

EU/1/98/073/004

9. DATE OF FIRST AUTHORISATION/RENEWAL OF THE AUTHORISATION

Date of first authorisation: 5 August 1998

Date of last renewal: 5 August 2003

10. DATE OF REVISION OF THE TEXT

Evorel 25, 50, 75 & 100 patches

(Janssen-Cilag Ltd)

1. NAME OF THE MEDICINAL PRODUCT

Evorel® 25 Patch, Evorel 50 Patch, Evorel 75 Patch and Evorel 100 Patch.

2. QUALITATIVE AND QUANTITATIVE COMPOSITION

- Evorel 25: 1.6 mg estradiol/patch
- Evorel 50: 3.2 mg estradiol/patch
- Evorel 75: 4.8 mg estradiol/patch
- Evorel 100: 6.4 mg estradiol/patch

3. PHARMACEUTICAL FORM

Evorel is a square shaped, transparent, self-adhesive transdermal delivery system (patch) of 0.2 mm thickness for application to the skin surface. It consists of a monolayered adhesive matrix throughout which 17β estradiol is uniformly distributed. The adhesive matrix is protected on the outside surface (from clothes etc) by a polyethylene teraphthalate backing foil, while the adhesive surface of the patch is covered by a polyester sheet (the release liner) which is removed before placing the patch on the body surface. This release liner has an S-shaped incision which facilitates easy removal from the patch.

- Evorel is available in four sizes corresponding to the four different concentrations:
- Evorel 25 is marked 'CE25', has a surface area of 8 sq cm and contains 1.6 mg estradiol corresponding to a release rate of 25 micrograms of estradiol in 24 hours.
- Evorel 50 is marked 'CE50', has a surface area of 16 sq cm and contains 3.2 mg estradiol corresponding to a release rate of 50 micrograms of estradiol in 24 hours.
- Evorel 75 is marked 'CE75', has a surface area of 24 sq cm. and contains 4.8 mg estradiol corresponding to a release rate of 75 micrograms of estradiol in 24 hours.
- Evorel 100 is marked 'CE100', has a surface area of 32 sq cm. and contains 6.4 mg estradiol corresponding to a release rate of 100 micrograms of estradiol in 24 hours.

4. CLINICAL PARTICULARS

4.1 Therapeutic indications

Hormone Replacement Therapy (HRT) for oestrogen deficiency symptoms in peri- and post-menopausal women.

Evorel 50, 75 and 100 only:

Prevention of osteoporosis in post-menopausal women at high risk of future fractures who are intolerant of, or contra-indicated for, other medicinal products approved for the prevention of osteoporosis. (See Section 4.4)

The experience of treating women older than 65 years is limited.

4.2 Posology and method of administration

Adults

Evorel is an oestrogen-only HRT patch applied to the skin twice weekly.

For initiation and continuation of treatment of menopausal symptoms, the lowest effective dose for the shortest duration (see also Section 4.4) should be used.

Treatment of oestrogen deficiency symptoms

Therapy should be started with one Evorel 50 patch (delivering 50 micrograms of estradiol/24 hours) and the dose adjusted after the first month if necessary depending on efficacy and signs of over-oestrogenisation (eg breast tenderness). For maintenance therapy the lowest effective dose should be used; a maximum dose of 100 micrograms of estradiol/24 hours should not be exceeded.

Evorel 50, 75, 100

Prevention of post-menopausal osteoporosis

Therapy should be started with Evorel 50. The dose may be adjusted depending on efficacy and signs of over-oestrogenisation (eg breast tenderness). Note, however, that the efficacy of Evorel 25 for the prevention of post-menopausal osteoporosis has not been demonstrated. For maintenance therapy, the lowest effective dose should be used. A dose of 100micrograms of estradiol/24 hours should not be exceeded.

Progestogen use

For women with an intact uterus progestogen should normally be added to Evorel for the prevention of adverse endometrial effects, eg hyperplasia and cancer. The regimen may be either cyclic or continuous sequential.

Only progestogens approved for addition to oestrogen treatment may be prescribed (eg oral norethisterone, 1mg/day or medroxyprogesterone acetate, 2.5mg/day) and should be added for at least 12-14 days every month/28 day cycle.

Unless there is a previous diagnosis of endometriosis, it is not recommended to add a progestogen in hysterectomised women.

Guidance on how to start therapy:

Post-menopausal women currently not on HRT may start Evorel at any time.

Peri-menopausal women who are still having regular menstrual cycles and are not currently on HRT should start Evorel within 5 days of the start of bleeding. Peri-menopausal women with irregular menstrual cycles, for whom pregnancy has been excluded, can start Evorel at any time.

Switching from other HRT

The switch from another oestrogen-only therapy in post-menopausal women to Evorel may occur at any time.

Women on a continuous combined regimen wishing to switch from another oestrogen to Evorel may do so at any time.

Women on a cyclic or continuous sequential regimen wishing to switch from a sequential combined HRT preparation to Evorel may do so at the end of a cycle of the current therapy or after a 7 day hormone free interval.

Method of Administration

Evorel should be applied to the skin as soon as it is removed from the wrapper. Recommended application sites are on clean, dry, healthy, intact skin and each application should be made to a slightly different area of skin on the trunk below waistline. **Evorel should not be applied on or near the breasts.**

Evorel should remain in place during bathing and showering. Should it fall off during bathing or showering the patient should wait until cutaneous vasodilation ceases before applying a replacement patch to avoid potential excessive absorption. Should a patch fall off at other times it should be replaced immediately.

Patients can be advised to use baby oil to help remove any gum/glue which may remain on their skin after patch removal.

Missed dose

If the patient forgets to change their patch, they should change it as soon as possible and apply the next one at the normal time. However, if it is almost time for the next patch, the patient should skip the missed one and go back to their regular schedule. Only one patch should be applied at a time.

There is an increased likelihood of break-through bleeding and spotting when a patch is not replaced at the normal time.

Children

Evorel is not indicated in children.

Elderly

Data are insufficient in regard to the use of Evorel in the elderly (> 65 years old).

Route of administration

Transdermal use.

4.3 Contraindications

Known, past or suspected breast cancer

Known or suspected oestrogen-dependent malignant tumours (eg endometrial cancer)

Undiagnosed genital bleeding

Untreated endometrial hyperplasia

Previous idiopathic or current venous thrombo-embolism (deep venous thrombosis, pulmonary embolism),

Active or recent arterial thrombo-embolic disease (eg angina, myocardial infarction)

Acute liver disease, or a history of liver disease as long as liver function tests have failed to return to normal

Known hypersensitivity to the active substances or to any of the excipients

Porphyria

4.4 Special warnings and precautions for use

For the treatment of menopausal symptoms, HRT should only be initiated for symptoms that adversely affect quality of life. In all cases, a careful appraisal of the risks and benefits should be undertaken at least annually and HRT should only be continued as long as the benefit outweighs the risk.

Medical examination/follow-up

Before initiating or re-instituting HRT, a complete personal and family medical history should be taken. Physical (including pelvic and breast) examination should be guided by this and by the contraindications and warnings for use. During treatment, periodic check-ups are recommended of a frequency and nature adapted to the individual woman. Women should be advised what changes in their breasts should be reported to their doctor or nurse (see 'Breast cancer' below). Investigations, including mammography, should be carried out in accordance with currently accepted screening practices, modified to the clinical needs of the individual.

Conditions which need supervision

If any of the following conditions are present, have occurred previously, and/or have been aggravated during pregnancy or previous hormone treatment, the patient should be closely supervised. It should be taken into account that these conditions may recur or be aggravated during treatment with Evorel, in particular:

Leiomyoma (uterine fibroids) or endometriosis

A history of, or risk factors for, thrombo-embolic disorders (see below)

Risk factors for oestrogen dependent tumours, eg 1st degree heredity for breast cancer

Hypertension

Liver disorders (eg liver adenoma)

Diabetes mellitus with or without vascular involvement

Cholelithiasis

Migraine or (severe) headache

Systemic lupus erythematosus.

A history of endometrial hyperplasia (see below)

Epilepsy

Asthma

Otosclerosis.

Reasons for immediate withdrawal of therapy:

Therapy should be discontinued in case a contra-indication is discovered and in the following situations:

Jaundice or deterioration in liver function

Significant increase in blood pressure

New onset of migraine-type headache

Pregnancy.

Endometrial hyperplasia

The risk of endometrial hyperplasia and carcinoma is increased when oestrogens are administered alone for prolonged periods (see Section 4.8). The addition of a progestogen for at least 12 days per cycle in non-hysterectomised women greatly reduces this risk.

For Evorel 75 and 100 the endometrial safety of added progestogens has not been studied.

Break-through bleeding and spotting may occur during the first months of treatment. If break-through bleeding or spotting appears after some time on therapy, or continues after treatment has been discontinued, the reason should be investigated, which may include endometrial biopsy to exclude endometrial malignancy.

Unopposed oestrogen stimulation may lead to premalignant or malignant transformation in the residual foci of endometriosis. Therefore, the addition of a progestogen to oestrogen replacement therapy should be considered in women who have undergone hysterectomy because of endometriosis if they are known to have residual endometriosis.

Breast cancer

A randomised placebo- controlled trial, the Women's Health Initiative study (WHI), and epidemiological studies, including the Million Women Study (MWS) have reported an increased risk of breast cancer in women taking oestrogens, oestrogen-progestogen combinations or tibolone for HRT for several years (see Section 4.8, Undesirable Effects). For all HRT, an excess risk becomes apparent within a few years of use and increases with duration of intake but returns to baseline within a few (at most five) years after stopping treatment.

In the MWS, the relative risk of breast cancer with conjugated equine oestrogens (CEE) or estradiol (E2) was greater when a progestogen was added, whether sequentially or continuously, and regardless of type of progestogen. There was no evidence of a difference in risk between the different routes of administration.

In the WHI study, the continuous combined conjugated equine oestrogen and medroxyprogesterone acetate (CEE +MPA) product used was associated with breast cancers that were slightly larger in size and more frequently had local lymph node metastases compared to placebo.

HRT, especially oestrogen-progestogen combined treatment, increases the density of mammographic images which may adversely affect the radiological detection of breast cancer.

Ovarian cancer

Long-term (at least 5-10 years) use of oestrogen-only HRT products in hysterectomised women has been associated with an increased risk of ovarian cancer in some epidemiological studies. It is uncertain whether long-term use of combined HRT confers a different risk than oestrogen-only products.

Venous thrombo-embolism

HRT is associated with a higher relative risk of developing venous thrombo-embolism (VTE), ie deep vein thrombosis or pulmonary embolism. One randomised controlled trial and epidemiological studies found a two- to threefold higher risk for users compared with non-users. For non-users, it is estimated that the number of cases of VTE that will occur over a 5 year period is about 3 per 1000 women aged 50-59 years and 8 per 1000 women aged 60-69 years. It is estimated that in healthy women who use HRT for 5 years, the number of additional cases of VTE over a 5 year period will be between 2 and 6 (best estimate = 4) per 1000 women aged 50-59 years and between 5 and 15 (best estimate = 9) per 1000 women aged 60-69 years. The occurrence of such an event is more likely in the first year of HRT than later.

Generally recognised risk factors for VTE include a personal history or family history, severe obesity (BMI > 30 kg/m^2) and systemic lupus erythematosus (SLE). There is no consensus about the possible role of varicose veins in VTE.

Patients with a history of VTE or known thrombophilic states have an increased risk of VTE. HRT may add to this risk. Personal or strong family history of thrombo-embolism or recurrent spontaneous abortion should be investigated in order to exclude a thrombophilic predisposition. Until a thorough evaluation of thrombophilic factors has been made or anticoagulant treatment initiated, use of HRT in such patients should be viewed as contraindicated. Women already on anticoagulant treatment require careful consideration of the benefit-risk of use of HRT.

The risk of VTE may be temporarily increased with prolonged immobilisation, major trauma or major surgery. As in all postoperative patients, scrupulous attention should be given to prophylactic measures to prevent VTE following surgery. Where prolonged immobilisation is liable to follow elective surgery, particularly abdominal or orthopaedic surgery to the lower limbs, consideration should be given to temporarily stopping HRT 4 to 6 weeks earlier, if possible. Treatment should not be restarted until the woman is completely mobilised.

If VTE develops after initiating therapy, the drug should be discontinued. Patients should be told to contact their doctors immediately when they are aware of a potential thrombo-embolic symptom (eg, painful swelling of a leg, sudden pain in the chest, dyspnoea).

Coronary artery disease (CAD)

There is no evidence from randomised controlled trials of cardiovascular benefit with continuous combined conjugated oestrogens and medroxyprogesterone acetate (MPA). Two large clinical trials (WHI and HERS i.e. Heart and Oestrogen/progestin Replacement Study) showed a possible increased risk of cardiovascular morbidity in the first year of use and no overall benefit. For other HRT products there are only limited data from randomised controlled trials examining effects in cardiovascular morbidity or mortality. Therefore, it is uncertain whether these findings also extend to other HRT products.

Stroke

One large randomised clinical trial (WHI-trial) found, as a secondary outcome, an increased risk of ischaemic stroke in healthy women during treatment with continuous combined conjugated oestrogens and MPA. For women who do not use HRT, it is estimated that the number of cases of stroke that will occur over a 5 year period is about 3 per 1000 women aged 50-59 years and 11 per 1000 women aged 60-69 years. It is estimated that for women who use conjugated oestrogens and MPA for 5 years, the number of additional cases will be between 0 and 3 (best estimate = 1) per 1000 users aged 50-59 years and between 1 and 9 (best estimate = 4) per 1000 users aged 60-69 years. It is unknown whether the increased risk also extends to other HRT products.

Other conditions

Oestrogens may cause fluid retention, and therefore patients with cardiac or renal dysfunction should be carefully observed. Patients with terminal renal insufficiency should be closely observed, since it is expected that the level of circulating active ingredients in Evorel is increased.

Women with pre-existing hypertriglyceridaemia should be followed closely during oestrogen replacement or hormone replacement therapy, since rare cases of large increases of plasma triglycerides leading to pancreatitis have been reported with oestrogen therapy in this condition.

Oestrogens increase thyroid binding globulin (TBG), leading to increased circulating total thyroid hormone, as measured by protein-bound iodine (PBI), T4 levels (by column or by radio-immunoassay) or T3 levels (by radio-immunoassay). T3 resin uptake is decreased, reflecting the elevated TBG. Free T4 and free T3 concentrations are unchanged. Other binding proteins may be elevated in serum, i.e. corticoid binding globulin (CBG), sex-hormone binding globulin (SHBG) leading to increased circulating corticosteroids and sex steroids, respectively. Free or biological active hormone concentrations are unchanged. Other plasma proteins may be increased (angiotensinogen/renin substrate, alpha-I-antitrypsin, ceruloplasmin).

There is no conclusive evidence for improvement of cognitive function. There is some evidence from the WHI trial of increased risk of probable dementia in women who start using continuous combined CEE and MPA after the age of 65. It is unknown whether the findings apply to younger post-menopausal women or other HRT products.

Evorel is not to be used for contraception. Women of childbearing potential should be advised to use non-hormonal contraceptive methods to avoid pregnancy.

4.5 Interaction with other medicinal products and other forms of interaction

The metabolism of oestrogens (and progestogens) may be increased by concomitant use of substances known to induce drug-metabolising enzymes, specifically cytochrome P450 enzymes, such as anticonvulsants (eg, phenobarbital, phenytoin, carbamazepine) and anti-infectives (eg, rifampicin, rifabutin, nevirapine, efavirenz) and also bosentan.

Ritonavir and nelfinavir, although known as strong inhibitors, by contrast exhibit inducing properties when used concomitantly with steroid hormones. Herbal preparations containing St. John's Wort (*Hypericum perforatum*) may raise the metabolism of oestrogens (and progestogens).

With transdermal administration, the first-pass effect in the liver is avoided and thus, transdermal oestrogens (and progestogens) might be less affected by enzyme inducers than oral hormones.

Clinically, an increased metabolism of oestrogens (and progestogens) may lead to decreased effect and changes in the uterine bleeding profile.

Estrogen-containing oral contraceptives have been shown to significantly decrease plasma concentrations of lamotrigine when co-administered due to induction of lamotrigine glucuronidation. This may reduce seizure control. Although the potential interaction between estrogen-containing hormone replacement therapy and lamotrigine has not been studied, it is expected that a similar interaction exists, which may lead to a reduction in seizure control among women taking both drugs together. Therefore, dose adjustment of lamotrigine may be necessary.

4.6 Pregnancy and lactation

Pregnancy

Evorel is not indicated during pregnancy. If pregnancy occurs during use of Evorel, treatment should be withdrawn immediately.

There are no clinical data on exposed pregnancies.

Studies in animals have not shown reproductive toxicity.

The results of most epidemiological studies to date relevant to inadvertent fetal exposure to combinations of oestrogens (and progestogens) indicate no teratogenic or foetotoxic effect.

Lactation

Evorel is not indicated during lactation.

4.7 Effects on ability to drive and use machines

In normal use, Evorel would not be expected to have any effect on the ability to drive or use machinery.

4.8 Undesirable effects

Information on undesirable effects was obtained in two clinical trials comparing Evorel 100 and Evorel 50 to placebo. Of the just over 100 women in each group, one half (with an intact uterus) were followed for up to three years, the other half (hysterectomised) for up to 24 months. 21 % of women on Evorel 100 followed for up to three months reported at least one drug related adverse event. During follow-up for up to 25 months, the proportion was 26%. Of women on Evorel 50, 18% of those followed for up to three months and 27% of those followed for up to 24 months reported at least one drug related adverse event. Breast pain, reported by 17% of women on Evorel 100 was the most frequent adverse event. In two clinical trials with Evorel Sequi (which contains Evorel 50 patches), the most frequent adverse event was irritation at the application site reported in ~13% of subjects. This was not severe enough to cause discontinuation of therapy,

Other side effects reported in the clinical trials with a frequency below 10% are listed in the table below.

(see Table 1 below)

The frequency of oestrogen-related adverse events (eg breast pain) is expected to increase with the dosage of estradiol transdermal systems.

The adverse event profile, their frequencies and severity in women with an intact uterus, treated with Evorel 25 or 50 in conjunction with a progestogen, is expected to vary with the nature and the dose of the progestogen used concomitantly with Evorel.

Breast Cancer

According to evidence from a large number of epidemiological studies and one randomised placebo-controlled trial, the Women's Health Initiative (WHI), the overall risk of breast cancer increases with increasing duration of HRT use in current or recent HRT users.

For *oestrogen-only* HRT, estimates of relative risk (RR) from a reanalysis of original data from 51 epidemiological studies (in which >80% of HRT use was oestrogen-only HRT) and from the epidemiological Million Women Study (MWS) are similar at 1.35 (95% CI 1.21-1.49) and 1.30 (95% CI 1.21-1.40), respectively.

For *oestrogen plus progestogen* combined HRT, several epidemiological studies have reported an overall higher risk for breast cancer than with oestrogens alone.

The MWS reported that, compared to never users, the use of various types of *oestrogen-progestogen* combined HRT was associated with a higher risk of breast cancer (RR = 2.00, 95%CI: 1.88-2.12) than use oestrogens alone (RR = 1.30, 95% CI: 1.21-1.40) or use of tibolone (RR = 1.45; 95% CI 1.25-1.68).

The WHI trial reported a risk estimate of 1.24 (95% CI: 1.01-1.54) after 5.6 years of use of oestrogen-*progestogen* combined HRT (CEE +MPA) in all users compared with placebo.

The absolute risks calculated from the MWS and the WHI trial are presented below:

The MWS has estimated, from the known average incidence of breast cancer in developed countries, that:

For women not using HRT, about 32 in every 1000 are expected to have breast cancer diagnosed between the ages of 50 and 64 years.

For 1000 current or recent users of HRT, the number of additional cases during the corresponding period will be

For users of *oestrogen-only* replacement therapy

between 0 and 3 (best estimate = 1.5) for 5 years' use

between 3 and 7 (best estimate = 5) for 10 years' use.

For users of *oestrogen plus progestogen* combined HRT,

between 5 and 7 (best estimate = 6) for 5 years' use

between 18 and 20 (best estimate = 19) for 10 years' use.

The WHI trial estimated that after 5.6 years of follow-up of women between the ages of 50 and 79 years, an *additional* 8 cases of invasive breast cancer would be due to *oestrogen-progestogen combined* HRT (CEE + MPA) per 10 000 women years.

According to calculations from the trial data, it is estimated that:

For 1000 women in the placebo group,

about 16 cases of invasive breast cancer would be diagnosed in 5 years.

For 1000 women who used oestrogen + *progestogen* combined HRT (CEE + MPA) the number of additional cases would be

between 0 and 9 (best estimate = 4) for 5 years' use.

The number of additional cases of breast cancer in women who use HRT is broadly similar for women who start HRT irrespective of age at start of use (between the ages of 45-65) (see section 4.4).

Endometrial Cancer

In women with an intact uterus, the risk of endometrial hyperplasia and endometrial cancer increases with increasing duration of use of unopposed oestrogens. According to data from epidemiological studies, the best estimate of the risk is that for women not using HRT, about 5 in every 1000 are expected to have endometrial cancer diagnosed between the ages of 50 and 65. Depending on the duration of treatment and oestrogen dose, the reported increase in endometrial cancer risk among unopposed oestrogen users varies from 2- to 12-fold greater compared with non-users. Adding a progestogen to oestrogen-only therapy greatly reduces this increased risk.

Adverse events which have been reported in association with oestrogen/ progestogen treatment are:

Neoplasms benign and malignant; endometrial cancer

Venous thrombo-embolism, ie deep leg or pelvic venous thrombosis and pulmonary embolism, is more frequent among hormone HRT users than among non-users. For further information see Section 4.3 Contra-indications and 4.4 Special warnings and precautions for use.

Myocardial infarction and stroke

Gall bladder disease

Skin and subcutaneous disorder: chloasma, erythema multiforme, erythema nodosum, vascular purpura.

Probable dementia (see Section 4.4).

4.9 Overdose

By virtue of the mode of administration of Evorel, overdosage is unlikely, but effects can if necessary be reversed by removal of the patch. The most commonly observed symptoms of overdose with oestrogen therapy are breast tenderness, nausea and breakthrough bleeding.

5. PHARMACOLOGICAL PROPERTIES

5.1 Pharmacodynamic properties

ATC code: G03CA03

Table 1

Body System	Common ADRs ≥1/100 to <1/10	Rare ADRs ≥1/10,000 to <1/1000	Very rare ≤1/10,000
Vascular disorders		deep vein thrombosis, pulmonary embolism	
Metabolism and nutrition disorders	weight increase		
Cardiac disorders	palpitations		
Gastro-intestinal disorders	nausea	bloating	
Skin and subcutaneous tissue disorders	rash		urticaria, angioedema
Musculoskeletal, connective tissue and bone disorders	generalised and local pain	leg cramps	
Nervous system disorders		dizziness	
Reproductive system and breast disorders	breast pain, genital candidiasis, uterine bleeding		
General disorders and administration site conditions	application site erythema and irritation, oedema		

Table 2 Pharmacokinetic parameters for the four sizes of Evorel patches

	Evorel 25		Evorel 50		Evorel 75		Evorel 100	
	Serum estradiol (pmol/L; mean+/-SD)							
Cmax	151±	69	277±	121	473±	286	655±	447
C96h	64±	27	113±	47	176±	112	226±	125
Cavg	96±	35	173±	68	271±	161	382±	232

Estradiol hemihydrate:

The active ingredient, synthetic estradiol, is chemically and biologically identical to endogenous human estradiol. It substitutes for the loss of oestrogen production in menopausal women, and alleviates menopausal symptoms.

For Evorel 50, 75 and 100:

Oestrogens prevent bone loss following menopause or ovariectomy.

Clinical trial information:

Relief of menopausal symptoms was achieved to a similar degree during the first few weeks of treatment with Evorel 50 and Evorel 100.

Prevention of osteoporosis

For Evorel 50, 75 and 100:

Oestrogen deficiency at menopause is associated with increasing bone turnover and decline in bone mass. The effect of oestrogens on the bone mineral density (BMD) is dose-dependent; the relationship is not linear, however. Protection appears to be effective as long as treatment is continued. After discontinuation of HRT, bone mass is lost at a rate similar to that in untreated women.

Evidence from the WHI trial and meta-analysed trials shows that current use of HRT, alone or in combination with a progestogen – given to predominantly healthy women – reduces the risk of hip, vertebral, and other osteoporotic fractures. HRT may also prevent fractures in women with low bone density and/ or established osteoporosis, but the evidence for that is limited.

In a clinical trial of two years duration comparing Evorel 50 and 100 to placebo, the increase in lumbar spine bone mineral density (BMD) with Evorel 50 was 4.46 ± 4.04 % (mean±SD). With Evorel 100, the gain in lumbar spine bone density was 5.93 ± 4.34 %.

The percentage of women who maintained or gained BMD in the lumbar spine with Evorel 50 was 84% and with Evorel 100, 92.5%.

Evorel also had an effect on hip BMD. The increase in BMD in the femoral neck with Evorel 50 was 1.26 ± 2.86 % and with Evorel 100, 1.61±0.53 %. The percentage of women maintaining or gaining BMD in the femoral neck was 65 and 63.5 %, respectively. In the total hip, the increase in BMD was 2.17 ± 2.33 % with Evorel 50 and 2.82±0.51 % with Evorel 100. The percentage of women maintaining or gaining BMD in the total hip was 93 and 82.5 %, respectively.

5.2 Pharmacokinetic properties

The estradiol hemihydrate of the patch is taken up through the skin as estradiol. Estradiol is metabolised primarily in the liver to estrone, which has weak estrogenic activity. Estrone is either conjugated with glucuronic or sulphuric acid or reconverted to estradiol. Conjugates are excreted mainly by the kidneys. In contrast to oral preparations, the estradiol / estrone ratio on use of Evorel is in the physiological range below 2, similar to that in pre-menopausal women. Estradiol circulates in the blood bound to sex hormone binding globulin (35-45%) and albumin (60-65%).

Estradiol is metabolised mainly in the liver by the P450 enzyme system. (see Section 4.5 Interactions).

Due to the transdermal administration, there is no noticeable first-pass effect.

Pharmacokinetic parameters for the four sizes of Evorel patches are shown in the following table.

(see Table 2 above)

5.3 Preclinical safety data

Preclinical effects were observed at exposures considered sufficiently in excess of the maximum human exposure, or were related to an exaggerated pharmacological effect, or were related to differences between species regarding hormonal regulation/metabolism and indicate little relevance to clinical use.

Subchronic skin irritation studies in rabbits and dermal sensitisation tests in guinea pigs have been performed. The studies show that the estradiol transdermal patch is an irritant and that estradiol contributes to the irritancy. It is recognised that test studies on rabbits over-predict skin irritation which occurs in humans.

The dermal sensitisation test shows that Evorel is not a skin sensitiser.

6. PHARMACEUTICAL PARTICULARS

6.1 List of excipients

Adhesive acrylic polymer (Duro-Tak 387-2287)

Guar gum (meyprogat 90)

Hostaphan MN19 (polyester film - removed before application)

6.2 Incompatibilities

None known

6.3 Shelf life

36 months for the product as packed for sale.

6.4 Special precautions for storage

Do not store above 25°C.

Evorel should be kept away from children and pets.

6.5 Nature and contents of container

Each Evorel patch size is presented in a sealed protective pouch. The pouches are packed in a cardboard carton.

6.6 Special precautions for disposal and other handling

None.

7. MARKETING AUTHORISATION HOLDER

Janssen-Cilag Ltd

50 -100 Holmers Farm Way

High Wycombe

Buckinghamshire

HP12 4EG

UK

8. MARKETING AUTHORISATION NUMBER(S)

Evorel 25 PL 00242/0293

Evorel 50 PL 00242/0223

Evorel 75 PL 00242/0294

Evorel 100 PL 00242/0295

9. DATE OF FIRST AUTHORISATION/RENEWAL OF THE AUTHORISATION

1 November 1995

10. DATE OF REVISION OF THE TEXT

2 June 2009

Legal category POM

Evorel Conti

(Janssen-Cilag Ltd)

1. NAME OF THE MEDICINAL PRODUCT

Trademark

EVOREL® CONTI

International non-proprietary name

estradiol

norethisterone acetate

2. QUALITATIVE AND QUANTITATIVE COMPOSITION

EVOREL®CONTI

3.2 mg of estradiol hemihydrate

11.2 mg of norethisterone acetate

3. PHARMACEUTICAL FORM

The EVOREL® CONTI Transdermal Delivery System (TDS), or transdermal patch, is a flat two-layer laminate which is 0.1 mm in thickness. The first layer is a flexible, translucent, and nearly colourless backing film. The second layer is a monolayer adhesive film (matrix) composed of acrylic adhesive and guar gum and contains the hormones. This system is protected by a polyester foil release liner, which is affixed to the adhesive matrix and is removed prior to application of the patch to the skin. The polyester foil used is coated with silicone on both sides. The release liner has a S-shaped opening to facilitate its removal prior to use. Each TDS is enclosed in a protective, hermetically-sealed sachet.

EVOREL®CONTI has a surface area of 16 sq cm and contains 3.2 mg of estradiol corresponding to a nominal release of 50 micrograms of estradiol per 24 hours and 11.2 mg of norethisterone acetate corresponding to a nominal release of 170 micrograms of norethisterone acetate per 24 hours. Each TDS is marked in the centre of the lower margin on the outside of the backing film: CEN1

4. CLINICAL PARTICULARS

4.1 Therapeutic indications

Hormone replacement therapy (HRT) for oestrogen deficiency symptoms in peri- and post-menopausal women more than 6 months post-menopause (or 18 months since last period).

Prevention of osteoporosis in postmenopausal women at high risk of future fractures who are intolerant of, or contra-indicated for, other medicinal products approved for the prevention of osteoporosis. (See also Section 4.4)

The experience treating women older than 65 years is limited.

4.2 Posology and method of administration

Adults

Evorel Conti is a continuous combined HRT preparation. Patches are applied to the skin twice weekly.

One Evorel Conti patch should be worn at all times, without interruptions. For initiation and continuation of treatment of menopausal symptoms, the lowest effective dose for the shortest duration (see also Section 4.4) should be used.

Guidance on how to start therapy:

Post-menopausal women currently not on HRT may start Evorel Conti at any time.

Switching from other HRT

Women on a continuous combined regimen wishing to switch from another oestrogen to Evorel Conti may do so at any time.

Women on a cyclic or continuous sequential regimen wishing to switch from a sequential combined HRT preparation to Evorel Conti may do so at the end of a cycle of the current therapy or after a 7 day hormone free interval.

Unless there is a previous diagnosis of endometriosis, it is not recommended to add a progestogen in hysterectomised women.

Method of Administration

The sachet containing one Evorel Conti patch should be opened and one part of the protective foil removed at the S-shaped incision. The patch should be applied to clean, dry, healthy, intact skin as soon as it is removed from the sachet.

The patient should avoid contact between fingers and the adhesive part of the patch during application. Each application should be made to a different area of the skin, on the trunk below the waist. The patch should not be applied on or near the breasts.

Evorel Conti patch should remain in place during bathing and showering.

Should a patch fall off, it should be replaced immediately with a new patch. However the usual day of changing Evorel Conti patches should be maintained.

Missed dose

If the patient forgets to change their patch, they should change it as soon as possible and apply the next one at the normal time. However, if it is almost time for the next patch, the patient should skip the missed one and go back to their regular schedule. Only one patch should be applied at a time.

Wearing a patch for more than 4 days by mistake or any period without a patch may increase the likelihood of breakthrough bleeding or spotting.

Children

Evorel Conti is not indicated in children.

Elderly

Data are insufficient in regard to the use of Evorel Conti in the elderly (>65 years old).

Route of administration

Transdermal use.

4.3 Contraindications

Known, past or suspected breast cancer

Known or suspected estrogen-dependent malignant tumours (eg endometrial cancer)

Undiagnosed genital bleeding

Untreated endometrial hyperplasia

Previous idiopathic or current venous thrombo-embolism (deep venous thrombosis, pulmonary embolism)

Active or recent arterial thrombo-embolic disease (eg angina, myocardial infarction)

Acute liver disease, or a history of liver disease as long as liver function tests have failed to return to normal

Known hypersensitivity to the active substances or to any of the excipients

Porphyria

4.4 Special warnings and precautions for use

For the treatment of menopausal symptoms, HRT should only be initiated for symptoms that adversely affect quality of life. In all cases, a careful appraisal of the risks and benefits should be undertaken at least annually and HRT should only be continued as long as the benefit outweighs the risk

Medical examination/follow-up

Before initiating or re-instituting HRT, a complete personal and family medical history should be taken. Physical (including pelvic and breast) examination should be guided by this and by the contra-indications and warnings for use. During treatment, periodic check-ups are recommended of a frequency and nature adapted to the individual woman. Women should be advised what changes in their breasts should be reported to their doctor or nurse (see 'Breast cancer' below). Investigations, including mammography, should be carried out in accordance with currently accepted screening practices, modified to the clinical needs of the individual.

Conditions which need supervision

If any of the following conditions are present, have occurred previously, and/or have been aggravated during pregnancy or previous hormone treatment, the patient should be closely supervised. It should be taken into account that these conditions may recur or be aggravated during treatment with Evorel Conti, in particular:

Leiomyoma (uterine fibroids) or endometriosis

A history of, or risk factors for, thrombo-embolic disorders (see below)

Risk factors for oestrogen dependent tumours, eg 1st degree heredity for breast cancer

Hypertension

Liver disorders (eg liver adenoma)

Diabetes mellitus with or without vascular involvement

Cholelithiasis

Migraine or (severe) headache

Systemic lupus erythematosus

A history of endometrial hyperplasia (see below)

Epilepsy

Asthma

Otosclerosis

Reasons for immediate withdrawal of therapy:

Therapy should be discontinued if a contra-indication is discovered and in the following situations:

Jaundice or deterioration in liver function

Significant increase in blood pressure

New onset of migraine-type headache

Pregnancy

Endometrial hyperplasia

The risk of endometrial hyperplasia and carcinoma is increased when oestrogens are administered alone for prolonged periods (see Section 4.8). The addition of a progestogen for at least 12 days per cycle in non-hysterectomised women greatly reduces this risk.

Break-through bleeding and spotting may occur during the first months of treatment. If break-through bleeding or spotting appears after some time on therapy, or continues after treatment has been discontinued, the reason should be investigated, which may include endometrial biopsy to exclude endometrial malignancy.

Breast cancer

A randomised placebo-controlled trial, the Women's Health Initiative (WHI) and epidemiological studies, including the Million Women Study (MWS) have reported an increased risk of breast cancer in women taking oestrogens or oestrogen-progestogen combinations or tibolone for HRT for several years (see Section 4.8 For all HRT, an excess risk becomes apparent within a few years of use and increases with duration of intake but returns to baseline within a few (at most five) years after stopping treatment.

In the MWS, the relative risk of breast cancer with conjugated equine oestrogens (CEE) or estradiol (E2) was greater when a progestogen was added, either sequentially or continuously, and regardless of type of progestogen. There was no evidence of a difference in risk between the different routes of administration.

In the WHI study, the continuous combined conjugated equine estrogen and medroxyprogesterone acetate (CEE + MPA) product used was associated with breast cancers that were slightly larger in size and more frequently had local lymph node metastases compared to placebo.

HRT, especially oestrogen-progestogen combined treatment, increases the density of mammographic images which may adversely affect the radiological detection of breast cancer.

Venous thrombo-embolism

HRT is associated with a higher relative risk of developing venous thrombo-embolism (VTE), i.e. deep vein thrombosis or pulmonary embolism. One randomised controlled trial and epidemiological studies found a two- to threefold higher risk for users compared with non-users. For non-users it is estimated that the number of cases of VTE that will occur over a 5 year period is about 3 per 1000 women aged 50-59 years and 8 per 1000 women aged 60-69 years. It is estimated that in healthy women who use HRT for 5 years, the number of additional cases of VTE over a 5 year period will be between 2 and 6 (best estimate =4) per 1000 women aged 50-59 years and between 5 and 15 (best estimate =9) per 1000 women aged 60-69 years. The occurrence of such an event is more likely in the first year of HRT than later.

Generally recognised risk factors for VTE include a personal history or family history, severe obesity (BMI > 30 kg/m^2) and systemic lupus erythematosus (SLE). There is no consensus about the possible role of varicose veins in VTE.

Patients with a history of VTE or known thrombophilic states have an increased risk of VTE. HRT may add to this risk. Personal or strong family history of thrombo-embolism or recurrent spontaneous abortion should be investigated in order to exclude a thrombophilic predisposition. Until a thorough evaluation of thrombophilic factors has been made or anticoagulant treatment initiated, use of HRT in such patients should be viewed as contra-indicated. The women already on anticoagulant treatment require careful consideration of the benefit-risk of use of HRT.

Table 1

Body System	Very common ADRs ≥1/10	Common ADRs ≥1/100 to <1/10	Uncommon ADRs ≥1/1,000 to <1/100	Rare ADRs ≥1/10,000 to <1/1,000	Very Rare ADRs ≤1/10,000
Metabolism and nutrition disorders		weight increase			
Psychiatric disorders		decreased libido	depression, emotional lability, anti-social feelings, tenseness, irritability, insomnia		
Nervous system disorders		migraine, paraesthesia		aggravation of epilepsy	
Cardiac disorders		hypertension			
Vascular disorders			varicose veins anaemia aggravated	thrombo-embolism (see below)	
Respiratory, thoracic and mediastinal disorders			dyspnoea		
Gastro-intestinal disorders		nausea	upper abdominal pain		
Hepato-biliary disorders			liver function tests elevated		
Skin and subcutaneous tissue disorders		pruritus	rash, psoriasis aggravated, hirsutism		urticaria, angioedema
Musculoskeletal, connective tissue and bone disorders		generalised and local pain			
Reproductive system and breast disorders	uterine bleeding episodes	breast pain, dysmenorrhoea (including lower abdominal pain), leukorrhoea	premenstrual tension syndrome, uterine fluid retention, uterine fibromyomia, endometrial polyps	galactorrhoea	
General disorders and administration site conditions		application site erythema and irritation, oedema	allergic reaction		

The risk of VTE may be temporarily increased with prolonged immobilisation, major trauma or major surgery. As in all postoperative patients, scrupulous attention should be given to prophylactic measures to prevent VTE following surgery. Where prolonged immobilisation is liable to follow elective surgery, particularly abdominal or orthopaedic surgery to the lower limbs, consideration should be given to temporarily stopping HRT 4 to 6 weeks earlier, if possible. Treatment should not be restarted until the woman is completely mobilised.

If VTE develops after initiating therapy, the drug should be discontinued. Patients should be told to contact their doctors immediately when they are aware of a potential thrombo-embolic symptom (eg, painful swelling of a leg, sudden pain in the chest, dyspnoea).

Coronary artery disease (CAD)

There is no evidence from randomised controlled trials of cardiovascular benefit with continuous combined conjugated estrogens and medroxyprogesterone acetate MPA. Two large clinical trials (WHI and HERS i.e. Heart and Oestrogen/progestin Replacement Study) showed a possible increased risk of cardiovascular morbidity in the first year of use and no overall benefit. For other HRT products there are only limited data from randomised controlled trials examining effects in cardiovascular morbidity or mortality. Therefore, it is uncertain whether these findings also extend to other HRT products.

Stroke

One large randomised clinical trial (WHI-trial) found, as a secondary outcome, an increased risk of ischaemic stroke in healthy women during treatment with continuous combined conjugated oestrogens and MPA. For women who do not use HRT, it is estimated that the number of cases of stroke that will occur over a 5 year period is about 3 per 1000 women aged 50-59 years and 11 per 1000 women aged 60-69 years. It is estimated that for women who use conjugated oestrogens and MPA for 5 years, the number of additional cases will be between 0 and 3 (best estimate = 1) per 1000 users aged 50-59 years and between 1 and 9 (best estimate = 4) per 1000 users aged 60-69 years. It is unknown whether the increased risk also extends to other HRT products.

Ovarian cancer

Long-term (at least 5-10 years) use of oestrogen-only HRT products in hysterectomised women has been associated with an increased risk of ovarian cancer in some epidemiological studies. It is uncertain whether long-term use of combined HRT confers a different risk than oestrogen-only products.

Other conditions

Oestrogens may cause fluid retention, and therefore patients with cardiac or renal dysfunction should be carefully observed. Patients with terminal renal insufficiency should be closely observed, since it is expected that the level of circulating active ingredients in Evorel Conti is increased.

Women with pre-existing hypertriglyceridaemia should be followed closely during oestrogen replacement or hormone replacement therapy, since rare cases of large increases of plasma triglycerides leading to pancreatitis have been reported with oestrogen therapy in this condition.

Oestrogens increase thyroid binding globulin (TBG), leading to increased circulating total thyroid hormone, as measured by protein-bound iodine (PBI), T4 levels (by column or radio-immunoassay) or T3 levels (by radio-immunoassay). T3 resin uptake is decreased, reflecting the elevated TBG. Free T4 and free T3 concentrations are unaltered. Other binding proteins may be elevated in serum, i.e. corticoid binding globulin (CBG), sex-hormone-binding globulin (SHBG) leading to increased circulating corticosteroids and sex steroids, respectively. Free or biological active hormone concentrations are unchanged. Other plasma proteins may be increased (angiotensinogen/renin substrate, alpha-I-antitrypsin, ceruloplasmin).

There is no conclusive evidence for improvement of cognitive function. There is some evidence from the WHI trial of increased risk of probable dementia in women who start using continuous combined CEE and MPA after the age of 65. It is unknown whether the findings apply to younger post-menopausal women or other HRT products.

Evorel Conti is not to be used for contraception. Women of child-bearing potential should be advised to use non-hormonal contraceptive methods to avoid pregnancy.

4.5 Interaction with other medicinal products and other forms of interaction

The metabolism of oestrogens and progestogens may be increased by concomitant use of substances known to induce drug-metabolising enzymes, specifically cytochrome P450 enzymes, such as anticonvulsants (e.g., phenobarbital, phenytoin, carbamazepine) and anti-infectives (e.g., rifampicin, rifabutin, nevirapine, efavirenz) and also bosentan.

Ritonavir and nelfinavir, although known as strong inhibitors, by contrast exhibit inducing properties when used concomitantly with steroid hormones. Herbal preparations containing St. John's Wort *(Hypericum perforatum)* may raise the metabolism of oestrogens and progestogens.

With transdermal administration, the first-pass effect in the liver is avoided and thus, transdermally applied oestrogens and progestogens might be less affected by enzyme inducers than oral hormones.

Clinically, an increased metabolism of oestrogens and progestogens may lead to decreased effect and changes in the uterine bleeding profile.

Estrogen-containing oral contraceptives have been shown to significantly decrease plasma concentrations of lamotrigine when co-administered due to induction of lamotrigine glucuronidation. This may reduce seizure control. Although the potential interaction between estrogen-containing hormone replacement therapy and lamotrigine has not been studied, it is expected that a similar interaction exists, which may lead to a reduction in seizure control among women taking both drugs together. Therefore, dose adjustment of lamotrigine may be necessary.

4.6 Pregnancy and lactation

Pregnancy

Evorel Conti is not indicated during pregnancy. If pregnancy occurs during use of Evorel Conti, treatment should be withdrawn immediately.

Data on a limited number of exposed pregnancies indicate adverse effects of norethisterone on the foetus. At doses higher than normally used in oral contraceptives and HRT formulations masculinisation of female foetuses was observed.

The results of most epidemiological studies to date relevant to inadvertent foetal exposure to combinations of oestrogens and progestogens indicate no teratogenic or foetotoxic effect.

Lactation

Evorel Conti is not indicated during lactation.

4.7 Effects on ability to drive and use machines

There are no known data on the effects of Evorel Conti on the ability to drive or use machinery.

4.8 Undesirable effects

In three clinical trials of one year's duration, the most commonly reported side effect was uterine bleeding occurring in 16% women (53 of 344). Overall 46% of the 344 women followed for up to one year reported at least one other adverse event possibly related to study therapy. Each of these adverse events are listed below.

(see Table 1 on previous page)

Breast Cancer

According to evidence from a large number of epidemiological studies and one randomised placebo-controlled trial, the Women's Health Initiative (WHI), the overall risk of breast cancer increases with increasing duration of HRT use in current or recent HRT users.

For *oestrogen-only* HRT, estimates of relative risk (RR) from a reanalysis of original data from 51 epidemiological studies (in which >80% of HRT use was oestrogen-only HRT) and from the epidemiological Million Women Study (MWS) are similar at 1.35 (95% CI 1.21-1.49) and 1.30 (95% CI 1.21-1.40), respectively.

For *oestrogen plus progestogen* combined HRT, several epidemiological studies have reported an overall higher risk for breast cancer than with oestrogens alone.

The MWS reported that, compared to never users, the use of various types of *oestrogen-progestogen* combined HRT was associated with a higher risk of breast cancer (RR = 2.00, 95%CI: 1.88-2.12) than use oestrogens alone (RR = 1.30, 95% CI: 1.21-1.40) or use of tibolone (RR = 1.45; 95% CI 1.25-1.68).

The WHI trial reported a risk estimate of 1.24 (95% CI: 1.01-1.54) after 5.6 years of use of oestrogen-*progestogen* combined HRT (CEE +MPA) in all users compared with placebo.

The absolute risks calculated from the MWS and the WHI trial are presented below:

The MWS has estimated, from the known average incidence of breast cancer in developed countries, that:

For women not using HRT, about 32 in every 1000 are expected to have breast cancer diagnosed between the ages of 50 and 64 years.

For 1000 current or recent users of HRT, the number of additional cases during the corresponding period will be

For users of *oestrogen-only* replacement therapy

- between 0 and 3 (best estimate = 1.5) for 5 year's use
- between 3 and 7 (best estimate = 5) for 10 year's use.

For users of *oestrogen plus progestogen* combined HRT,

- between 5 and 7 (best estimate = 6) for 5 year's use
- between 18 and 20 (best estimate = 19) for 10 years' use.

The WHI trial estimated that after 5.6 years of follow-up of women between the ages of 50 and 79 years, an *additional* 8 cases of invasive breast cancer would be due to *oestrogen-progestogen combined* HRT (CEE + MPA) per 10 000 women years.

According to calculations from the trial data, it is estimated that:

For 1000 women in the placebo group,

- about 16 cases of invasive breast cancer would be diagnosed in 5 years.

For 1000 women who used oestrogen + progestogen combined HRT (CEE + MPA) the number of additional cases would be

- between 0 and 9 (best estimate = 4) for 5 year's use.

The number of additional cases of breast cancer in women who use HRT is broadly similar for women who start HRT irrespective of age at start of use (between the ages of 45-65) (see section 4.4).

Endometrial Cancer

In women with an intact uterus, the risk of endometrial hyperplasia and endometrial cancer increases with increasing duration of use of unopposed oestrogens. According to data from epidemiological studies, the best estimate of the risk is that for women not using HRT, about 5 in every 1000 are expected to have endometrial cancer diagnosed between the ages of 50 and 65. Depending on the duration of treatment and oestrogen dose, the reported increase in endometrial cancer risk among unopposed oestrogen users varies from 2- to 12-fold greater compared with non-users. Adding a progestogen to oestrogen-only therapy greatly reduces this increased risk.

Adverse events which have been reported in association with oestrogen/ progestogen treatment are:

Neoplasms benign and malignant; endometrial cancer

Venous thrombo-embolism, ie deep leg or pelvic venous thrombosis and pulmonary embolism, is more frequent among hormone HRT users than among non-users. For further information see Section 4.3 Contra-indications and 4.4 Special warnings and precautions for use.

Myocardial infarction and stroke

Gall bladder disease

Skin and subcutaneous disorder: chloasma, erythema multiforme, erythema nodosum, vascular purpura.

Probable dementia (see Section 4.4).

4.9 Overdose

Symptoms of overdose of oestrogen and progestogen therapy may include nausea, break-through bleeding, breast tenderness, abdominal cramps and/or bloating. These symptoms can be reversed by removing the patch.

5. PHARMACOLOGICAL PROPERTIES

5.1 Pharmacodynamic properties

ATC code: G03F A01

Estradiol hemihydrate:

The active ingredient, synthetic estradiol, is chemically and biologically identical to endogenous human estradiol. It substitutes for the loss of oestrogen production in menopausal women, and alleviates menopausal symptoms. Oestrogens prevent bone loss following menopause or ovariectomy.

Norethisterone:

As oestrogens promote the growth of the endometrium, unopposed oestrogens increase the risk of endometrial hyperplasia and cancer. The addition of a progestogen reduces the oestrogen-induced risk of endometrial hyperplasia in non-hysterectomised women.

Clinical trial information:

Relief of oestrogen-deficiency symptoms and bleeding patterns:

Relief of menopausal symptoms was achieved during the first few weeks of treatment.

When starting Evorel Conti, bleeding episodes occur mostly during the first month of treatment, with a quick improvement of the bleeding profile. In first users of HRT, or after a hormone free period of at least 2 weeks, absence of bleeding was seen in 33 % of women during the first three months of treatment and 54 % were bleed-free during months 2 and 3. When Evorel Conti was started directly after a cycle of sequential HRT, only 7.5 % of the women were bleed-free during the first three months, 47 % reported no bleeding for months 2 and 3. Over time, bleeding stops in the majority of women so that 63% of women from either group were bleed-free during the last 3 months of 12 months therapy with Evorel Conti. In women with well established menopause (mean 7 years since the last natural menstrual period), 56% were bleed-free during the first three months of treatment and 92% were bleed free during months 10-12.

Bleeding lasted five or less days in not more than 2 episodes per quarter year in >95% of subjects.

Starting Evorel Conti after a hormone free period may reduce the likelihood of uterine bleeding during the initial period of use of Evorel Conti.

In three clinical trials of one year duration, uterine bleeding episodes were reported as an adverse event by 53 of 344 (16%) women - the most frequently reported undesirable effect.

Prevention of osteoporosis

Oestrogen deficiency at menopause is associated with increasing bone turnover and decline in bone mass. The effect of oestrogens on the bone mineral density (BMD) is dose-dependent. Protection appears to be effective as long as treatment is continued. After discontinuation of HRT, bone mass is lost at a rate similar to that in untreated women.

Evidence from the WHI trial and meta-analysed trials shows that current use of HRT, alone or in combination with a progestogen – given to predominantly healthy women – reduces the risk of hip, vertebral, and other osteoporotic fractures. HRT may also prevent fractures in women with low bone density and/ or established osteoporosis, but the evidence for that is limited.

After one year of treatment with Evorel Conti, the increase in lumbar spine bone mineral density (BMD) was 2.94 ± 2.62 % (mean±SD). The percentage of women who maintained or gained BMD in the lumbar zone during treatment was 90%.

Evorel Conti also had an effect on hip BMD. The increase in BMD in the femoral neck was 2.42 ± 3.04 % and the percentage of women maintaining or gaining BMD in the femoral neck was 82%. In the total hip, the increase in BMD was 1.73 ± 2.55 % (mean±SD) with 74% women maintaining or gaining in BMD.

5.2 Pharmacokinetic properties

The estradiol hemihydrate of the patch is taken up through the skin as estradiol. Estradiol is metabolised primarily in the liver to estrone, which has weak estrogenic activity. Estrone is either conjugated with glucuronic or sulphuric acid or reconverted to estradiol. Conjugates are excreted mainly by the kidneys. The estradiol / estrone ratio on use of Evorel Conti is close to one, similar to pre-menopausal women. Estradiol circulates in the blood bound to sex hormone binding globulin (35-45%) and albumin (60-65%).

Norethisterone acetate is cleaved immediately on resorption to yield norethisterone. Norethisterone distributes widely in the body and circulates bound to sex hormone binding globulin (about 36%) and albumin (about 61%). It is metabolised mainly in the liver. Metabolites are conjugated with glucuronic or sulfuric acid. Conjugates are excreted in faeces and urine.

The hepatic metabolism of both estradiol and norethisterone is mediated primarily by the P450 enzyme system. (see Section 4.5, Interactions with other medicinal products and other forms of interaction).

Due to the transdermal administration, there is no noticeable first-pass effect.

Estradiol pharmacokinetics

Following first use of an Evorel Conti patch by post-menopausal women, serum estradiol levels rise within 23 hours (T_{max}, single application) from, on average, ~ 18 pmol/L (~5 pg/ml) by an average of 150 pmol/L (41 pg/mL) (C_{max}, single application). Levels decrease over 3.5 days to an average of 66 pmol/L (18 pg/mL). During continued use of Evorel Conti, estradiol levels rise over 21 hours from patch change (T_{max}, multiple application) by an average of 121 pmol/L (33 pg/mL) (C_{max}, multiple applications). The 95% confidence interval for C_{max} ranges from 77 to 165 pmol/L (21 to 45 pg/mL). When patch use is discontinued, serum estradiol levels decrease with a half-life of 6.6 hours. After 24 hours, baseline levels are again observed.

Norethisterone pharmacokinetics

Following first use of Evorel Conti by post-menopausal women, serum norethisterone levels rise over 37 hours (T_{max}, single application) to 706 pmol/L (240 pg/mL)(C_{max}, single application) and then decrease to 420 pmol/L (143 pg/mL) at day 3.5. On patch change, levels rise again over 22 hours (T_{max}, multiple applications) to 756 pmol/L (257 pg/mL)(C_{max}, multiple applications). When patch use is discontinued, norethisterone levels decrease with a half-life of ~15 hours.

5.3 Preclinical safety data

Preclinical effects were observed at exposures considered sufficiently in excess of the maximum human exposure, or were related to an exaggerated pharmacological effect, or were related to differences between species regarding hormonal regulation/metabolism and indicate little relevance to clinical use.

Norethisterone, like other progestogens, caused virilisation of female foetuses in rats and monkeys. After high doses of norethisterone embryolethal effects were observed.

Local tolerance studies with Evorel Conti were conducted in rabbits. In this model, Evorel Conti showed a mild irritation potential. It is recognised that the rabbit model is over-predictive of irritation of human skin.

Sensitisation studies with Evorel Conti in guinea pigs showed a weak sensitisation potential. Clinical trial experience with Evorel Conti use for up to two years gave no evidence of a clinically relevant sensitisation potential in humans.

6. PHARMACEUTICAL PARTICULARS

6.1 List of excipients

EVOREL® CONTI TDS

Adhesive: acrylate-vinylacetate copolymer (Duro-Tak 387-2287)

Guar gum

Backing film: polyethylene terephthalate foil (Hostaphan MN 19)

Release liner: siliconised polyethylene terephthalate foil, is removed before application

6.2 Incompatibilities

No creams, lotions, or powders should be applied to the skin area where the TDS is to be applied to prevent interference with the adhesive properties of EVOREL®CONTI TDS.

6.3 Shelf life

EVOREL®CONTI has a shelf-life of 24 months, when stored at or below 25degrees Celsius. The product can be used until the expiration date mentioned on the container.

6.4 Special precautions for storage

Store at room temperature, at or below 25 degrees Celsius, within the original sachet and box.

Keep out of reach of children. This also applies to used and disposed TDSs.

6.5 Nature and contents of container

Each carton box has 2, 8 or 24 TDSs in individual foil-lined sachets. The sachet comprises a 4 layer laminate including:

- surlyn-ionomer film on the inside
- then aluminium foil
- then polyethylene
- with a layer of bleached reinforced paper on the outside

6.6 Special precautions for disposal and other handling

The EVOREL®CONTI TDS should be placed on a clean, dry area of skin on the trunk of the body below the waist. Creams, lotions, or powders may interfere with the adhesive properties of the EVOREL®CONTI TDS. The TDS should not be applied on or near to the breasts. The area of application should be changed, with an interval of at least one week allowed between applications to a particular site. The skin area selected should not be damaged or irritated. The waistline should not be used because excessive rubbing of the TDS may occur.

The TDS should be used immediately after opening the sachet. Remove one part of the protecting foil. Apply the exposed part of adhesive to the application site from the edge to the middle; avoid wrinkling of the TDS. The second part of the protective foil should now be removed and the freshly exposed adhesive applied. Wrinkling should again be avoided and the palm of the hand used to press the TDS onto the skin and to bring the TDS to skin temperature, at which the adhesive effect is optimised. Do not touch the adhesive part of the TDS.

To remove the EVOREL® TDS, peel away an edge of the patch and pull smoothly away from the skin.

Any gum that remains on the skin after removal of EVOREL® TDS may be removed by rubbing it off with the fingers or washing with soap and water.

The TDSs should be disposed of in household waste (do not flush down the toilet).

7. MARKETING AUTHORISATION HOLDER

Janssen-Cilag Ltd
50 -100 Holmers Farm Way
High Wycombe
Buckinghamshire
HP12 4EG
UK

8. MARKETING AUTHORISATION NUMBER(S)

PL 00242/0319

9. DATE OF FIRST AUTHORISATION/RENEWAL OF THE AUTHORISATION

03/06/2008

10. DATE OF REVISION OF THE TEXT

2 June 2009

Evorel Sequi

(Janssen-Cilag Ltd)

1. NAME OF THE MEDICINAL PRODUCT

EVOREL® SEQUI

International non-proprietary names

estradiol
norethisterone acetate

2. QUALITATIVE AND QUANTITATIVE COMPOSITION

EVOREL® SEQUI is a transdermal therapy comprising

a) 4 EVOREL® 50 TDSs, each containing:
 3.2 mg of estradiol hemihydrate

b) 4 EVOREL® CONTI TDSs, each containing:
 3.2 mg of estradiol hemihydrate
 11.2 mg of norethisterone acetate

3. PHARMACEUTICAL FORM

EVOREL® SEQUI is composed of EVOREL® 50 and EVOREL® CONTI. Both EVOREL® 50 and EVOREL® CONTI are a Transdermal Delivery System (TDS), or transdermal patch, composed of a flat two-layer laminate which is 0.1 mm in thickness. The first layer is a flexible, translucent, and nearly colourless backing film. The second layer is a monolayer adhesive film (matrix) composed of acrylic adhesive and guar gum and contains the hormones. This system is protected by a polyester foil release liner, which is affixed to the adhesive matrix and is removed prior to application of the patch to the skin. The polyester foil used is coated with silicone on both sides. The release liner has an S-shaped opening to facilitate its removal prior to use. Each TDS is enclosed in a protective, hermetically-sealed sachet.

EVOREL® CONTI has a surface area of 16 sq cm and contains 3.2 mg of estradiol corresponding to a nominal release of 50 micrograms of estradiol per 24 hours and 11.2 mg of norethisterone acetate corresponding to a nominal release of 170 micrograms of norethisterone acetate per 24 hours. Each EVOREL Conti patch is marked in the centre of the lower margin on the outside of the backing film: CENI.

EVOREL® 50 has a surface area of 16 sq cm and contains 3.2 mg of estradiol corresponding to a nominal release of 50 micrograms of estradiol per 24 hours. The release liner of EVOREL® 50 is aluminised on one side. Each EVOREL 50 patch is marked in the centre of the lower margin of the outside of the backing film: CE50.

4. CLINICAL PARTICULARS

4.1 Therapeutic indications

Hormone replacement therapy (HRT) for oestrogen deficiency symptoms in peri- and post-menopausal women.

Prevention of osteoporosis in postmenopausal women at high risk of future fractures who are intolerant of, or contraindicated for, other medicinal products approved for the prevention of osteoporosis. (See also Section 4.4)

The experience treating women older than 65 years is limited.

4.2 Posology and method of administration

Adults

Evorel Sequi is a continuous sequential HRT preparation. Patches are applied to the skin twice weekly.

One Evorel Sequi patch should be worn at all times, without interruptions. For initiation and continuation of treatment of menopausal symptoms, the lowest effective dose for the shortest duration (see also Section 4.4) should be used.

Guidance on how to start therapy:

Any previous therapy with HRT must be stopped prior to starting Evorel Sequi.

Post-menopausal women currently not on HRT may start Evorel Sequi at any time.

Peri-menopausal women who are still having regular menstrual cycles and are not currently on HRT should start Evorel Sequi within 5 days of the start of bleeding. Peri-menopausal women with irregular menstrual cycles, for whom pregnancy has been excluded, can start Evorel Sequi at any time.

Switching from other HRT

Women on a continuous combined regimen wishing to switch from another oestrogen to Evorel Sequi may do so at any time.

Women on a cyclic or continuous sequential regimen wishing to switch from a sequential combined HRT preparation to Evorel Sequi may do so at the end of a cycle of the current therapy or after a 7 day hormone free interval.

Unless there is a previous diagnosis of endometriosis, it is not recommended to add a progestogen in hysterectomised women.

Method of Administration

A treatment cycle with Evorel Sequi is 28 days. During the first 14 days, one estradiol-only (Evorel 50) patch should be worn at all times, without interruption. During days 15-28, one estradiol + norethisterone (Evorel Conti) patch should be worn at all times, without interruption. A subsequent treatment cycle should follow immediately, without a treatment free interval.

Patches should be applied to the trunk, below the waist. Patches should be changed twice a week, i.e. every three to four days. Application of a new patch should be to a site different from the previous application site. The patch should not be applied on or near the breasts.

Evorel should remain in place during bathing and showering. Should it fall off during bathing or showering the patient should wait until cutaneous vasodilation ceases before applying a replacement patch to avoid potential excessive absorption. Should a patch fall off at other times it should be replaced immediately.

Missed dose

If the patient forgets to change their patch, they should change it as soon as possible and apply the next one at the normal time. However, if it is almost time for the next patch, the patient should skip the missed one and go back to their regular schedule. Only one patch should be applied at a time.

Wearing a patch for more than 4 days by mistake or any period without a patch may increase the likelihood of breakthrough bleeding or spotting.

Children

Evorel Sequi is not indicated in children.

Elderly

Data are insufficient in regard to the use of Evorel Sequi in the elderly (>65 years old).

Route of administration

Transdermal use.

4.3 Contraindications

Known, past or suspected breast cancer

Known or suspected estrogen-dependent malignant tumours (eg endometrial cancer)

Undiagnosed genital bleeding

Untreated endometrial hyperplasia

Previous idiopathic or current venous thrombo-embolism (deep venous thrombosis, pulmonary embolism)

Active or recent arterial thrombo-embolic disease (eg angina, myocardial infarction)

Acute liver disease, or a history of liver disease as long as liver function tests have failed to return to normal

Known hypersensitivity to the active substances or to any of the excipients

Porphyria

4.4 Special warnings and precautions for use

For the treatment of menopausal symptoms, HRT should only be initiated for symptoms that adversely affect quality of life. In all cases, a careful appraisal of the risks and benefits should be undertaken at least annually and HRT should only be continued as long as the benefit outweighs the risk

Medical examination/follow-up

Before initiating or re-instituting HRT, a complete personal and family medical history should be taken. Physical (including pelvic and breast) examination should be guided by this and by the contra-indications and warnings for use. During treatment, periodic check-ups are recommended of a frequency and nature adapted to the individual woman. Women should be advised what changes in their breasts should be reported to their doctor or nurse (see 'Breast cancer' below). Investigations, including mammography, should be carried out in accordance with currently accepted screening practices, modified to the clinical needs of the individual.

Conditions which need supervision

If any of the following conditions are present, have occurred previously, and/or have been aggravated during pregnancy or previous hormone treatment, the patient should be closely supervised. It should be taken into account that these conditions may recur or be aggravated during treatment with Evorel Sequi, in particular:

Leiomyoma (uterine fibroids) or endometriosis

A history of, or risk factors for, thrombo-embolic disorders (see below)

Risk factors for oestrogen dependent tumours, eg 1st degree heredity for breast cancer

Hypertension

Liver disorders (eg liver adenoma)

Diabetes mellitus with or without vascular involvement

Cholelithiasis

Migraine or (severe) headache

Systemic lupus erythematosus

A history of endometrial hyperplasia (see below)

Epilepsy

Asthma

Otosclerosis

Reasons for immediate withdrawal of therapy:

Therapy should be discontinued if a contra-indication is discovered and in the following situations:

Jaundice or deterioration in liver function

Significant increase in blood pressure

New onset of migraine-type headache

Pregnancy

Endometrial hyperplasia

The risk of endometrial hyperplasia and carcinoma is increased when oestrogens are administered alone for prolonged periods (see Section 4.8). The addition of a progestogen for at least 12 days per cycle in non-hysterectomised women greatly reduces this risk.

Break-through bleeding and spotting may occur during the first months of treatment. If break-through bleeding or spotting appears after some time on therapy, or continues after treatment has been discontinued, the reason should be investigated, which may include endometrial biopsy to exclude endometrial malignancy.

Breast cancer

A randomised placebo-controlled trial, the Women's Health Initiative (WHI) and epidemiological studies, including the Million Women Study (MWS) have reported an increased risk of breast cancer in women taking oestrogens or oestrogen-progestogen combinations or tibolone for HRT for several years (see Section 4.8). For all HRT, an excess risk becomes apparent within a few years of use and increases with duration of intake but returns to baseline within a few (at most five) years after stopping treatment.

In the MWS, the relative risk of breast cancer with conjugated equine oestrogens (CEE) or estradiol (E2) was greater when a progestogen was added, either sequentially or continuously, and regardless of type of progestogen. There was no evidence of a difference in risk between the different routes of administration.

In the WHI study, the continuous combined conjugated equine estrogen and medroxyprogesterone acetate (CEE + MPA) product used was associated with breast cancers that were slightly larger in size and more frequently had local lymph node metastases compared to placebo.

HRT, especially oestrogen-progestogen combined treatment, increases the density of mammographic images which may adversely affect the radiological detection of breast cancer.

Venous thrombo-embolism

HRT is associated with a higher relative risk of developing venous thrombo-embolism (VTE), i.e. deep vein thrombosis or pulmonary embolism. One randomised controlled trial and epidemiological studies found a two- to threefold higher risk for users compared with non-users. For non-users it is estimated that the number of cases of VTE that will occur over a 5 year period is about 3 per 1000 women aged 50-59 years and 8 per 1000 women aged 60-69 years. It is estimated that in healthy women who use HRT for 5 years, the number of additional cases of VTE over a 5 year period will be between 2 and 6 (best estimate =4) per 1000 women aged 50-59 years and between 5 and 15 (best estimate =9) per 1000 women aged 60-69 years. The occurrence of such an event is more likely in the first year of HRT than later.

Generally recognised risk factors for VTE include a personal history or family history, severe obesity (BMI > 30 kg/m^2) and systemic lupus erythematosus (SLE). There is no consensus about the possible role of varicose veins in VTE.

Patients with a history of VTE or known thrombophilic states have an increased risk of VTE. HRT may add to this risk. Personal or strong family history of thrombo-embolism or recurrent spontaneous abortion should be investigated in order to exclude a thrombophilic predisposition. Until a thorough evaluation of thrombophilic factors has been made or anticoagulant treatment initiated, use of HRT in such patients should be viewed as contra-indicated. The women already on anticoagulant treatment require careful consideration of the benefit-risk of use of HRT.

The risk of VTE may be temporarily increased with prolonged immobilisation, major trauma or major surgery. As in all postoperative patients, scrupulous attention should be given to prophylactic measures to prevent VTE following surgery. Where prolonged immobilisation is liable to follow elective surgery, particularly abdominal or orthopaedic surgery to the lower limbs, consideration should be given to temporarily stopping HRT 4 to 6 weeks earlier, if possible. Treatment should not be restarted until the woman is completely mobilised.

If VTE develops after initiating therapy, the drug should be discontinued. Patients should be told to contact their doctors immediately when they are aware of a potential thrombo-embolic symptom (eg, painful swelling of a leg, sudden pain in the chest, dyspnoea).

Coronary artery disease (CAD)

There is no evidence from randomised controlled trials of cardiovascular benefit with continuous combined conjugated estrogens and medroxyprogesterone acetate MPA. Two large clinical trials (WHI and HERS i.e. Heart and Oestrogen/progestin Replacement Study) showed a possible increased risk of cardiovascular morbidity in the first year of use and no overall benefit. For other HRT products there are only limited data from randomised controlled trials examining effects in cardiovascular morbidity or mortality. Therefore, it is uncertain whether these findings also extend to other HRT products.

Stroke

One large randomised clinical trial (WHI-trial) found, as a secondary outcome, an increased risk of ischaemic stroke in healthy women during treatment with continuous combined conjugated oestrogens and MPA. For women who do not use HRT, it is estimated that the number of cases of stroke that will occur over a 5 year period is about 3 per 1000 women aged 50-59 years and 11 per 1000 women aged 60-69 years. It is estimated that for women who use conjugated oestrogens and MPA for 5 years, the number of additional cases will be between 0 and 3 (best estimate = 1) per 1000 users aged 50-59 years and between 1 and 9 (best estimate = 4) per 1000 users aged 60-69 years. It is unknown whether the increased risk also extends to other HRT products.

Ovarian cancer

Long-term (at least 5-10 years) use of oestrogen-only HRT products in hysterectomised women has been associated with an increased risk of ovarian cancer in some epidemiological studies. It is uncertain whether long-term use of combined HRT confers a different risk than oestrogen-only products.

Other conditions

Oestrogens may cause fluid retention, and therefore patients with cardiac or renal dysfunction should be carefully observed. Patients with terminal renal insufficiency should be closely observed, since it is expected that the level of circulating active ingredients in Evorel Sequi is increased.

Women with pre-existing hypertriglyceridaemia should be followed closely during oestrogen replacement or hormone replacement therapy, since rare cases of large increases of plasma triglycerides leading to pancreatitis have been reported with oestrogen therapy in this condition.

Oestrogens increase thyroid binding globulin (TBG), leading to increased circulating total thyroid hormone, as measured by protein-bound iodine (PBI), T4 levels (by column or radio-immunoassay) or T3 levels (by radio-immunoassay). T3 resin uptake is decreased, reflecting the elevated TBG. Free T4 and free T3 concentrations are unaltered. Other binding proteins may be elevated in serum, i.e. corticoid binding globulin (CBG), sex-hormone-binding globulin (SHBG) leading to increased circulating corticosteroids and sex steroids, respectively. Free or biological active hormone concentrations are unchanged. Other plasma proteins may be increased (angiotensinogen/renin substrate, alpha-I-antitrypsin, ceruloplasmin).

There is no conclusive evidence for improvement of cognitive function. There is some evidence from the WHI trial of increased risk of probable dementia in women who start using continuous combined CEE and MPA after the age of 65. It is unknown whether the findings apply to younger post-menopausal women or other HRT products.

Evorel Sequi is not to be used for contraception. Women of child-bearing potential should be advised to use non-hormonal contraceptive methods to avoid pregnancy.

4.5 Interaction with other medicinal products and other forms of interaction

The metabolism of oestrogens and progestogens may be increased by concomitant use of substances known to induce drug-metabolising enzymes, specifically cytochrome P450 enzymes, such as anticonvulsants (e.g. phenobarbital, phenytoin, carbamazepine) and anti-infectives (e.g. rifampicin, rifabutin, nevirapine, efavirenz) and also bosentan.

Ritonavir and nelfinavir, although known as strong inhibitors, by contrast exhibit inducing properties when used concomitantly with steroid hormones. Herbal preparations containing St. John's Wort *(Hypericum perforatum)* may raise the metabolism of oestrogens and progestogens.

With transdermal administration, the first-pass effect in the liver is avoided and thus, transdermally applied oestrogens and progestogens might be less affected by enzyme inducers than oral hormones.

Clinically, an increased metabolism of oestrogens and progestogens may lead to decreased effect and changes in the uterine bleeding profile.

Estrogen-containing oral contraceptives have been shown to significantly decrease plasma concentrations of lamotrigine when co-administered due to induction of lamotrigine glucuronidation. This may reduce seizure control. Although the potential interaction between estrogen-containing hormone replacement therapy and lamotrigine has not been studied, it is expected that a similar interaction exists, which may lead to a reduction in seizure control among women taking both drugs together. Therefore, dose adjustment of lamotrigine may be necessary.

4.6 Pregnancy and lactation

Pregnancy

Evorel Sequi is not indicated during pregnancy. If pregnancy occurs during use of Evorel Sequi, treatment should be withdrawn immediately.

Data on a limited number of exposed pregnancies indicate adverse effects of norethisterone on the foetus. At doses higher than normally used in oral contraceptives and HRT formulations masculinisation of female foetuses was observed.

The results of most epidemiological studies to date relevant to inadvertent foetal exposure to combinations of oestrogens and progestogens indicate no teratogenic or foetotoxic effect.

Lactation

Evorel Sequi is not indicated during lactation.

4.7 Effects on ability to drive and use machines

There are no known data on the effects of Evorel Sequi on the ability to drive or use machinery.

4.8 Undesirable effects

From two clinical trials of one year duration and involving a total of 240 women, adverse events considered at least possibly related to Evorel Sequi may be expected in about half the treated women over a year. The most prominent is likely to be some irritation at the application site in ~13% of subjects, not severe enough to cause discontinuation of therapy, and breast pain, expected in ~12 % of users of Evorel Sequi.

Other undesirable effects observed in clinical trials, which were thought to be at least possibly related to the use of Evorel Sequi, are listed below.

(see Table 1 below)

Breast Cancer

According to evidence from a large number of epidemiological studies and one randomised placebo-controlled trial, the Women's Health Initiative (WHI), the overall risk of breast cancer increases with increasing duration of HRT use in current or recent HRT users.

For *oestrogen-only* HRT, estimates of relative risk (RR) from a reanalysis of original data from 51 epidemiological studies (in which >80% of HRT use was oestrogen-only HRT) and from the epidemiological Million Women Study (MWS) are similar at 1.35 (95% CI 1.21-1.49) and 1.30 (95% CI 1.21-1.40), respectively.

For *oestrogen plus progestogen* combined HRT, several epidemiological studies have reported an overall higher risk for breast cancer than with oestrogens alone.

The MWS reported that, compared to never users, the use of various types of *oestrogen-progestogen* combined HRT was associated with a higher risk of breast cancer (RR = 2.00, 95%CI: 1.88-2.12) than use oestrogens alone (RR = 1.30, 95% CI: 1.21-1.40) or use of tibolone (RR =1.45; 95% CI 1.25-1.68).

Table 1

Body System	Common ADRs ≥1/100 to <1/10	Uncommon ADRs ≥1/1,000 to <1/100	Rare ADRs ≥1/10,000 to <1,000	Very rare <1/10,000
Psychiatric disorders	depression, tiredness;	concentration problems, emotional lability, libido decreased or increased, irritability, insomnia, panic attack		
Nervous system disorders	dizziness	paraesthesia, hypoesthesia	aggravation of epilepsy	
Vascular disorders	hypertension	Raynaud's Syndrome aggravated	deep vein thrombosis, pulmonary embolism (see below)	
Gastro-intestinal disorders	nausea, abdominal pain, abdominal bloating, stomach pain			
Hepato-biliary disorders		liver function tests elevated		
Skin and subcutaneous tissue disorder		rash, erythema, pruritus, hirsutism, acne		urticaria, angioedema
Musculoskeletal, connective tissue and bone disorders	arthralgia			
Reproductive system and breast disorders	uterine bleeding, dysmenorrhoea, PMS-syndrome, vaginal candidiasis	breast fibroadenoma, breast cysts, uterine fibroids	galactorrhoea	
General disorders and administration site conditions	oedema, weight increase			

The WHI trial reported a risk estimate of 1.24 (95% CI: 1.01-1.54) after 5.6 years of use of oestrogen-*progestogen* combined HRT (CEE +MPA) in all users compared with placebo.

The absolute risks calculated from the MWS and the WHI trial are presented below:

The MWS has estimated, from the known average incidence of breast cancer in developed countries, that:

For women not using HRT, about 32 in every 1000 are expected to have breast cancer diagnosed between the ages of 50 and 64 years.

For 1000 current or recent users of HRT, the number of additional cases during the corresponding period will be

For users of *oestrogen-only* replacement therapy

between 0 and 3 (best estimate = 1.5) for 5 year's use
between 3 and 7 (best estimate = 5) for 10 year's use.

For users of *oestrogen plus progestogen* combined HRT,

between 5 and 7 (best estimate = 6) for 5 year's use
between 18 and 20 (best estimate = 19) for 10 years' use.

The WHI trial estimated that after 5.6 years of follow-up of women between the ages of 50 and 79 years, an *additional* 8 cases of invasive breast cancer would be due to *oestrogen-progestogen combined* HRT (CEE + MPA) per 10 000 women years.

According to calculations from the trial data, it is estimated that:

For 1000 current or recent users of HRT, the number of additional cases during the corresponding period will be

For 1000 women in the placebo group,

about 16 cases of invasive breast cancer would be diagnosed in 5 years.

For 1000 women who used oestrogen + progestogen combined HRT (CEE + MPA) the number of additional cases would be

between 0 and 9 (best estimate = 4) for 5 year's use.

The number of additional cases of breast cancer in women who use HRT is broadly similar for women who start HRT irrespective of age at start of use (between the ages of 45-65) (see section 4.4).

Endometrial Cancer

In women with an intact uterus, the risk of endometrial hyperplasia and endometrial cancer increases with increasing duration of use of unopposed oestrogens. According to data from epidemiological studies, the best estimate of the risk is that for women not using HRT, about 5 in every 1000 are expected to have endometrial cancer diagnosed between the ages of 50 and 65. Depending on the duration of treatment and oestrogen dose, the reported increase in endometrial cancer risk among unopposed oestrogen users varies from 2- to 12-fold greater compared with non-users. Adding a progestogen to oestrogen-only therapy greatly reduces this increased risk.

Other adverse events have been reported in association with oestrogen/progestogen treatment:

Oestrogen-dependent neoplasms benign and malignant; endometrial cancer

Venous thrombo-embolism, ie deep leg or pelvic venous thrombosis and pulmonary embolism, is more frequent among hormone HRT users than among non-users. For further information see Sections 4.3 Contraindications and 4.4 Special Warnings and Special Precautions for use.

Myocardial infarction and stroke

Gall bladder disease

Skin and subcutaneous disorder: chloasma, erythema multiforme, erythema nodosum, vascular purpura

Probable dementia (see section 4.4).

4.9 Overdose

Symptoms of overdose of oestrogen and progestogen therapy may include nausea, break-through bleeding, breast tenderness, abdominal cramps and/or bloating. These symptoms can be reversed by removing the patch.

5. PHARMACOLOGICAL PROPERTIES

5.1 Pharmacodynamic properties

ATC code: G03F B05

Estradiol hemihydrate:

The active ingredient, synthetic estradiol, is chemically and biologically identical to endogenous human estradiol. It substitutes for the loss of oestrogen production in menopausal women, and alleviates menopausal symptoms. Oestrogens prevent bone loss following menopause or ovariectomy.

Norethisterone:

As oestrogens promote the growth of the endometrium, unopposed oestrogens increase the risk of endometrial hyperplasia and cancer. The addition of a progestogen reduces the oestrogen-induced risk of endometrial hyperplasia in non-hysterectomised women.

Clinical trial information:

Relief of oestrogen-deficiency symptoms and bleeding patterns:

Relief of menopausal symptoms was achieved during the first few weeks of treatment with Evorel Sequi.

Regular withdrawal bleeding occurs in over 95% of women using Evorel Sequi. Two thirds of treatment cycles have only one bleeding episode of a median duration of five days. Where secondary bleeding episodes occurred, they were shorter with a median duration of 1.5 days.

Prevention of osteoporosis

Oestrogen deficiency at menopause is associated with increasing bone turnover and decline in bone mass. The effect of oestrogens on the bone mineral density (BMD) is dose-dependent. Protection appears to be effective as long as treatment is continued. After discontinuation of HRT, bone mass is lost at a rate similar to that in untreated women.

Evidence from the WHI trial and meta-analysed trials shows that current use of HRT, alone or in combination with a progestogen – given to predominantly healthy women – reduces the risk of hip, vertebral, and other osteoporotic fractures. HRT may also prevent fractures in women with low bone density and/ or established osteoporosis, but the evidence for that is limited.

Evorel Sequi was not tested for effects on bone mineral density (BMD). However, information is available on the efficacy of the two constituents of Evorel Sequi (Evorel 50 and Evorel Conti).

After two years of treatment with Evorel 50, the increase in lumbar spine bone mineral density (BMD) was 4.46 ± 4.04 % (mean±SD). The percentage of women who maintained or gained BMD in the lumbar zone during treatment was 84%.

Evorel 50 also had an effect on hip BMD. The increase in BMD in the femoral neck was 1.26 ± 2.86 % and the percentage of women maintaining or gaining BMD in the femoral neck was 65%. In the total hip, the increase in BMD was 2.17 ± 2.33 % (mean±SD) with 93% women maintaining or gaining BMD.

After one year of treatment with Evorel Conti, the increase in lumbar spine bone mineral density (BMD) was 2.94 ± 2.62 % (mean±SD). The percentage of women who maintained or gained BMD in the lumbar zone during treatment was 90%.

Evorel Conti also had an effect on hip BMD. The increase in BMD in the femoral neck was 2.42 ± 3.04 % and the percentage of women maintaining or gaining BMD in the femoral neck was 82%. In the total hip, the increase in BMD was 1.73 ± 2.55 % (mean±SD) with 74% women maintaining or gaining in BMD.

5.2 Pharmacokinetic properties

The estradiol hemihydrate of the patch is taken up through the skin as estradiol. Estradiol is metabolised primarily in the liver to estrone, which has weak estrogenic activity. Estrone is either conjugated with glucuronic or sulphuric acid or reconverted to estradiol. Conjugates are excreted mainly by the kidneys. The estradiol / estrone ratio on use of Evorel 50 and Evorel Conti is close to one, similar to pre-menopausal women. Estradiol circulates in the blood bound to sex hormone binding globulin (35-45%) and albumin (60-65%).

Norethisterone acetate is cleaved immediately on resorption to yield norethisterone. Norethisterone distributes widely in the body and circulates bound to sex hormone binding globulin (about 36%) and albumin (about 61%). It is metabolised mainly in the liver. Metabolites are conjugated with glucuronic or sulfuric acid. Conjugates are excreted in faeces and urine.

The metabolism of both estradiol and norethisterone in the liver is mediated primarily by the P450 enzyme system. See Section 4.5, Interactions with other medicinal products and other forms of interaction.

Due to the transdermal administration, there is no noticeable first-pass effect.

Estradiol pharmacokinetics

Upon use of an estradiol-only patch (Evorel 50), serum estradiol levels rise within 11 hours (T_{max}, multiple application) from pre-treatment levels by an average of 316 pmol/L (86 pg/mL) (C_{max}, multiple application). The 95% confidence interval ranges from 150 to 484 pmol/L (42-132 pg/mL). Levels decrease over 3.5 days to an average of 77 pmol/L (21 pg/mL). When patch use is discontinued, serum estradiol levels decrease with a half-life of 6.6 hours. 24 hours after patch removal, pre-treatment levels are again observed.

On use of an estradiol+norethisterone patch (Evorel Conti), serum estradiol levels rise from pre-treatment levels within 21 hours from patch change (T_{max}, multiple application) by an average of 121 pmol/L (33 pg/mL) (C_{max}, multiple applications). The 95% confidence interval for C_{max} ranges from 77 to 165 pmol/L (21 to 45 pg/mL). 24 hours after patch removal, baseline levels are again observed.

Norethisterone pharmacokinetics

On first use of Evorel Conti by post-menopausal women, serum norethisterone levels rise over 37 hours (T_{max}, single application) to 706 pmol/L (240 pg/mL)(C_{max}, single application) and then decrease to 420 pmol/L (143 pg/mL) at day 3.5. On patch change, levels rise again over 22 hours (T_{max}, multiple applications) to 756 pmol/L (257 pg/mL)(C_{max}, multiple applications). When patch use is discontinued, norethisterone levels decrease with a half-life of ~15 hours.

5.3 Preclinical safety data

Preclinical effects were observed at exposures considered sufficiently in excess of the maximum human exposure, or were related to an exaggerated pharmacological effect, or were related to differences between species regarding hormonal regulation/metabolism and indicate little relevance to clinical use.

Norethisterone, like other progestogens, caused virilisation of female foetuses in rats and monkeys. After high doses of norethisterone embryolethal effects were observed.

Local tolerance studies with Evorel Conti were conducted in rabbits. In this model, Evorel Conti showed a mild irritation potential. It is recognised that the rabbit model is over-predictive of irritation of human skin.

Sensitisation studies with Evorel Conti in guinea pigs showed a weak sensitisation potential. Clinical trial experience with Evorel Conti use for up to two years gave no evidence of a clinically relevant sensitisation potential in humans.

6. PHARMACEUTICAL PARTICULARS

6.1 List of excipients

EVOREL® 50

Adhesive: acrylate-vinylacetate copolymer (Duro-Tak 387-2287)

Guar gum

Backing film: polyethylene terephthalate foil (Hostaphan MN19)

Release liner: siliconised polyethylene terephthalate foil, is removed before application

EVOREL® CONTI

Adhesive: acrylate-vinylacetate copolymer (Duro-Tak 387-2287)

Guar gum

Backing film: polyethylene terephthalate foil (Hostaphan MN19)

Release liner: siliconised polyethylene terephthalate foil, is removed before application

6.2 Incompatibilities

No creams, lotions or powders should be applied to the skin area where the TDS is to be applied to prevent interference with the adhesive properties of EVOREL® 50 TDS and EVOREL® CONTI TDS.

6.3 Shelf life

EVOREL® SEQUI has a shelf-life of 24 months, when stored at or below 25°C. The product can be used until the expiration date mentioned on the container.

6.4 Special precautions for storage

Do not store above 25°C. Store within the original sachet and box.

Keep out of reach and sight of children. This also applies to used and disposed TDSs.

6.5 Nature and contents of container

Each carton box has 8 TDSs in individual foil-lined sachets. The sachet comprises a 4 layer laminate including:

- surlyn-ionomer film on the inside,
- then aluminium foil,
- then polyethylene film,
- with a layer of bleached reinforced paper on the outside.

One EVOREL® SEQUI box contains 4 EVOREL® 50 TDS and 4 EVOREL® CONTI TDSs.

6.6 Special precautions for disposal and other handling

The EVOREL® SEQUI TDS should be placed on a clean, dry area of skin on the trunk of the body below the waist. Creams, lotions or powders may interfere with the adhesive properties of the EVOREL® SEQUI TDS. The TDS should not be applied on or near to the breasts. The area of application should be changed, with an interval of at least one week allowed between applications to a particular site. The skin area selected should not be damaged or irritated. The waistline should not be used because excessive rubbing of the TDS may occur.

The TDS should be used immediately after opening the sachet. Remove one part of the protecting foil. Apply the exposed part of adhesive to the application site from the edge to the middle; avoid wrinkling of the TDS. The second part of the protective foil should now be removed and the freshly exposed adhesive applied. Wrinkling should again be avoided and the palm of the hand used to press the TDS onto the skin and to bring the TDS to skin temperature at which the adhesive effect is optimised. Do not touch the adhesive part of the TDS.

When using EVOREL® SEQUI for the first two weeks, one of the EVOREL® 50 TDSs should be applied and changed twice weekly. During the following two weeks of EVOREL® SEQUI, one of the EVOREL® CONTI TDSs should be applied, also to be changed twice weekly. The patient then starts again with a new box of EVOREL® SEQUI.

To remove the EVOREL® TDS, peel away an edge of the patch and pull smoothly away from the skin.

Any gum that remains on the skin after removal of EVOREL® TDS may be removed by rubbing it off with the fingers, washing with soap and water or by using baby oil.

The EVOREL® TDS should be disposed of in household waste (do not flush down the toilet).

7. MARKETING AUTHORISATION HOLDER
Janssen-Cilag Ltd
50 -100 Holmers Farm Way
High Wycombe
Buckinghamshire
HP12 4EG UK

8. MARKETING AUTHORISATION NUMBER(S)
PL 00242/0320

9. DATE OF FIRST AUTHORISATION/RENEWAL OF THE AUTHORISATION
25/09/2006

10. DATE OF REVISION OF THE TEXT
2 June 2009

Evra transdermal patch

(Janssen-Cilag Ltd)

1. NAME OF THE MEDICINAL PRODUCT
EVRA transdermal patch

2. QUALITATIVE AND QUANTITATIVE COMPOSITION
Each 20 cm^2 transdermal patch contains 6 mg norelgestromin (NGMN) and 600 micrograms ethinyl estradiol (EE).

Each transdermal patch releases an average of 203 micrograms of NGMN and 33.9 micrograms of EE per 24 hours. Medicinal product exposure is more appropriately characterized by the pharmacokinetic profile (see section 5.2).

For a full list of excipients, see section 6.1.

3. PHARMACEUTICAL FORM
Transdermal patch.

EVRA is a thin, matrix-type transdermal patch consisting of three layers.

The outside of the backing layer is beige and heat-stamped "EVRA".

4. CLINICAL PARTICULARS

4.1 Therapeutic indications
Female contraception

EVRA is intended for women of fertile age. The safety and efficacy has been established in women aged 18 to 45 years.

4.2 Posology and method of administration
Posology

To achieve maximum contraceptive effectiveness, patients must be advised to use EVRA exactly as directed. For initiation instructions see 'How to start EVRA' below.

Only one patch is to be worn at a time.

Each used patch is removed and immediately replaced with a new one on the same day of the week (Change Day) on Day 8 and Day 15 of the cycle. Patch changes may occur at any time on the scheduled Change Day. The fourth week is patch-free starting on Day 22.

A new contraceptive cycle begins on the next day following patch-free week; the next EVRA patch should be applied even if there has been no bleeding or if bleeding has not yet stopped.

Under no circumstances should there be more than a 7-day patch-free interval between dosing cycles. If there are more than 7 patch-free days, the user may not be protected against pregnancy. A non-hormonal contraceptive must then be used concurrently for 7 days. As with combined oral contraceptives, the risk of ovulation increases with each day beyond the recommended contraceptive-free period. If intercourse has occurred during such an extended patch-free interval, the possibility of fertilisation should be considered.

Method of administration

EVRA should be applied to clean, dry, hairless, intact healthy skin on the buttock, abdomen, upper outer arm or upper torso, in a place where it will not be rubbed by tight clothing. EVRA should not be placed on the breasts or on skin that is red, irritated or cut. Each consecutive patch should be applied to a different place on the skin to help avoid potential irritation, although they may be kept within the same anatomic site.

The patch should be pressed down firmly until the edges stick well.

To prevent interference with the adhesive properties of the patch, no make-up, creams, lotions, powders or other topical products should be applied to the skin area where the patch is placed or where it will be applied shortly.

It is recommended that users visually check their patch daily to ensure continued proper adhesion.

Used patches should be discarded carefully in accordance with the instructions given in section 6.6.

How to start EVRA

When there has been no hormonal contraceptive use in the preceding cycle

Contraception with EVRA begins on the first day of menses. A single patch is applied and worn for one full week (7 days). The day the first patch is applied (Day 1/Start Day) determines the subsequent Change Days. The patch Change Day will be on this day every week (cycle Days 8, 15, 22 and Day 1 of the next cycle) The fourth week is patch-free starting on Day 22.

If Cycle 1 therapy starts after first day of the menstrual cycle, a non-hormonal contraceptive should be used concurrently for the first 7 consecutive days of the first treatment cycle only.

When switching from an oral combined contraceptive

Treatment with EVRA should begin on the first day of withdrawal bleeding. If there is no withdrawal bleeding within 5 days of the last active (hormone containing) tablet, pregnancy must be ruled out prior to the start of treatment with EVRA. If therapy starts after the first day of withdrawal bleeding, a non-hormonal contraceptive must be used concurrently for 7 days.

If more than 7 days elapse after taking the last active oral contraceptive tablet, the woman may have ovulated and should, therefore, be advised to consult a physician before initiating treatment with EVRA. If intercourse has occurred during such an extended pill-free interval, the possibility of pregnancy should be considered.

When changing from a progestogen-only-method

The woman may switch any day from the minipill (from an implant on the day of its removal, from an injectable when the next injection would be due), but a back-up barrier method of birth control must be used during the first 7 days.

Following abortion or miscarriage

After an abortion or miscarriage that occurs before 20 weeks gestation, EVRA may be started immediately. An additional method of contraception is not needed if EVRA is started immediately. Be advised that ovulation may occur within 10 days of an abortion or miscarriage.

After an abortion or miscarriage that occurs at or after 20 weeks gestation, EVRA may be started either on Day 21 post-abortion or on the first day of the first spontaneous menstruation, whichever comes first. The incidence of ovulation on Day 21 post abortion (at 20 weeks gestation) is not known.

Following delivery

Users who choose not to breast-feed should start contraceptive therapy with EVRA no sooner than 4 weeks after child-birth. When starting later, the woman should be advised to additionally use a barrier method for the first 7 days. However, if intercourse has already occurred, pregnancy should be excluded before the actual start of EVRA or the woman has to wait for her first menstrual period.

For breast-feeding women, see section 4.6.

What to do if the patch comes off or partly detaches

If the EVRA patch partly or completely detaches and remains detached, insufficient medicinal product delivery occurs.

If EVRA remains even partly detached:

- for less than one day (up to 24 hours): it should be re-applied to the same place or replaced with a new EVRA patch immediately. No additional contraceptive is needed. The next EVRA patch should be applied on the usual "Change Day".

- for more than one day (24 hours or more) or if the user is not aware when the patch has lifted or become detached: the user may not be protected from pregnancy: The user should stop the current contraceptive cycle and start a new cycle immediately by applying a new EVRA patch. There is now a new "Day 1" and a new "Change Day". A non-hormonal contraceptive must be used concurrently for the first 7 days of the new cycle only.

A patch should not be reapplied if it is no longer sticky; a new patch should be applied immediately. Supplemental adhesives or bandages should not be used to hold the EVRA patch in place.

If subsequent EVRA patch change days are delayed

At the start of any patch cycle (Week One/Day 1):

The user may not be protected from pregnancy. The user should apply the first patch of the new cycle as soon as remembered. There is now a new patch "Change Day" and a new "Day 1". A non-hormonal contraceptive must be used concurrently for the first 7 days of the new cycle. If intercourse has occurred during such an extended patch-free interval, the possibility of fertilisation should be considered.

In the middle of the cycle (Week Two/Day 8 or Week Three/ Day 15):

- for one or two days (up to 48 hours): The user should apply a new EVRA patch immediately. The next EVRA patch should be applied on the usual "Change Day". If during the 7 days preceding the first skipped day of patch application, the patch was worn correctly, no additional contraceptive use is required.

- for more than two days (48 hours or more): The user may not be protected from pregnancy. The user should stop the current contraceptive cycle and start a new four-week cycle immediately by putting on a new EVRA patch. There is now a new "Day 1" and a new "Change Day". A non-hormonal contraceptive must be used concurrently for the first 7 days of the new cycle.

- at the end of the cycle (Week Four/Day 22): If the EVRA patch is not removed at the beginning of Week 4 (Day 22), it should be removed as soon as possible. The next cycle should begin on the usual "Change Day", which is the day after Day 28. No additional contraceptive use is required.

Change Day adjustment

In order to postpone a menstrual period for one cycle, the woman must apply another patch at the beginning of Week 4 (Day 22) thus not observing the patch free interval. Breakthrough bleeding or spotting may occur. After 6 consecutive weeks of patch wear, there should be a patch free interval of 7 days. Following this, the regular application of EVRA is resumed.

If the user wishes to move the Change Day the current cycle should be completed, removing the third EVRA patch on the correct day. During the patch-free week a new Change Day may be selected by applying the first EVRA patch of the next cycle on the first occurrence of the desired day. In no case should there be more than 7 consecutive patch-free days. The shorter the patch-free interval, the higher the risk that the user does not have a withdrawal bleed and may experience breakthrough bleeding and spotting during the subsequent treatment cycle.

In case of minor skin irritation

If patch use results in uncomfortable irritation, a new patch may be applied to a new location until the next Change Day. Only one patch should be worn at a time.

Special populations

Body weight equal or greater than 90 kg: contraceptive efficacy may be decreased in women weighing equal or greater than 90 kg.

Renal impairment: EVRA has not been studied in women with renal impairment. No dose adjustment is necessary but as there is a suggestion in the literature that the unbound fraction of ethinyl estradiol is higher, EVRA should be used with supervision in this population.

Hepatic impairment: EVRA has not been studied in women with hepatic impairment. EVRA is contraindicated in women with hepatic impairment (see section 4.3).

Post-menopausal women: EVRA is not intended for use as hormonal replacement therapy.

Children and adolescents: EVRA is not recommended for use in children and adolescents under age 18 due to insufficient data on safety and efficacy.

4.3 Contraindications
EVRA should not be used in the presence of one of the following disorders. If one of these disorders occurs during the use of EVRA, EVRA must be discontinued immediately.

- Hypersensitivity to the active substances or to any of the excipients

- Presence or history of venous thrombosis, with or without the involvement of pulmonary embolism

- Presence or history of arterial thrombosis (e.g., cerebrovascular accident, myocardial infarction, retinal thrombosis) or prodrome of a thrombosis (e.g., angina pectoris or transient ischaemic attack)

- Migraine with focal aura

- The presence of serious or multiple risk factor(s) for the occurrence of arterial thrombosis:

- Severe hypertension (Persistent blood pressure values of ⩾160 mm Hg systolic or ⩾100 mm Hg diastolic)

- Diabetes Mellitus with vascular involvement

- Hereditary dyslipoproteinemia

- Possible hereditary predisposition for venous or arterial thrombosis, such as activated protein C (APC-) resistance, antithrombin-III deficiency, protein C deficiency, protein S deficiency, hyperhomocysteinemia, and antiphospholipid antibodies (anticardiolipin antibodies, lupus anticoagulant)

- Known or suspected carcinoma of the breast

- Carcinoma of the endometrium or other known or suspected estrogen-dependent neoplasia

- Abnormal liver function related to acute or chronic hepatocellular disease

- Hepatic adenomas or carcinomas

- Undiagnosed abnormal genital bleeding

4.4 Special warnings and precautions for use
There is no clinical evidence indicating that a transdermal patch is, in any aspect, safer than combined oral contraceptives.

EVRA is not indicated during pregnancy (see section 4.6).

If any of the conditions/risk factors mentioned below is present, the benefits of the use of EVRA should be weighed against the possible risks for each individual woman and discussed with the woman before she decides to start using EVRA. In the event of aggravation, exacerbation or first appearance of any of these conditions or risk factors, the woman should be emphatically told to contact her physician who will decide on whether its use should be discontinued.

Thromboembolic and other vascular disorders

The use of any combined hormonal contraceptive, including EVRA, carries an increased risk of venous thromboembolism (deep vein thrombosis, pulmonary embolism) compared to no use. Epidemiological studies have shown that the incidence of venous thromboembolism (VTE) in women with no other risk factors for VTE who use low dose oestrogen (<50 micrograms ethinyl estradiol) combined contraceptives ranges from about 20 to 40 cases per 100,000 women-years, but this risk estimate varies according to the type of progestagen. This compares with 5 to 10 cases per 100,000 women-years for non-users and 60 cases per 100,000 pregnancies. VTE is fatal in 1%-2% of cases.

Data from a retrospective cohort study in women aged 15 to 44 years have suggested that the incidence of VTE in women who used EVRA is increased in comparison with users of a levonorgestrel-containing OC (so-called "second generation" OC).

The incidence was 1.4 fold (95% CI 0.9-2.3) increased in women with or without other risk factors for VTE and 1.5 fold (95% CI 0.8-2.7) increased in women with no other risk factors for VTE.

Epidemiological studies have also associated the use of combined oral contraceptives (COCs) with an increased risk for arterial (myocardial infarction, transient ischaemic attack, stroke) thromboembolism.

Extremely rarely, thrombosis has been reported to occur in other blood vessels e.g., hepatic, mesenteric, renal, cerebral or retinal veins and arteries, in COC users. There is no consensus as to whether the occurrence of these events is associated with the use of COCs.

Symptoms of venous or arterial thrombosis can include:

- Unilateral leg pain, and/or swelling
- Sudden severe pain in the chest with possible radiation to the left arm
- Sudden breathlessness, sudden onset of coughing without a clear cause
- Any unusual, severe, prolonged headache
- Sudden partial or complete loss of vision
- Diplopia
- Slurred speech or aphasia
- Vertigo; collapse with or without focal seizure
- Weakness or very marked numbness suddenly affecting one side or one part of the body
- Motor disturbances
- 'Acute' abdominal pain

The risk of venous thromboembolism in combined contraceptives users increases with:

- Increasing age
- A positive family history (i.e. venous thromboembolism ever in a sibling or parent at relatively early age). If a hereditary predisposition is suspected, the woman should be referred to a specialist for advice before deciding about any hormonal contraceptive use
- Prolonged immobilisation, major surgery to the legs, or major trauma. In these situations it is advisable to discontinue use (in the case of elective surgery at least 4 weeks in advance) and not to resume until two weeks after complete remobilisation
- Obesity (body mass index over 30 kg/m^2)
- Possibly also with superficial thrombophlebitis and varicose veins. There is no consensus about the possible role of these conditions in the aetiology of venous thrombosis.

The risk of arterial thromboembolic complications in combined contraceptives users increases with:

- Increasing age;
- Smoking (with heavier smoking and increasing age the risk further increases, especially in women over 35 years of age);
- Dyslipoproteiniaemia;
- Obesity (body mass index over 30 kg/m^2);
- Hypertension;
- Valvular heart disease;
- Atrial fibrillation;
- A positive family history (arterial thrombosis ever in a sibling or parent at a relatively early age). If a hereditary predisposition is suspected, the woman should be referred to a specialist for advice before deciding about any hormonal contraceptive use.

Biochemical factors that may be indicative of hereditary or acquired predisposition for venous or arterial thrombosis include Activated Protein C (APC) resistance, hyper homocysteinaemia, antithrombin-III deficiency, protein C deficiency, protein S deficiency, antiphospholipid antibodies (anticardiolipin antibodies, lupus anticoagulant).

Other medical conditions, which have been associated with adverse circulatory events, included diabetes mellitus, systemic lupus erythematosus, haemolytic uraemic syndrome, chronic inflammatory bowel disease (e.g., Crohn's disease or ulcerative colitis).

The increased risk for thromboembolism in the puerperium must be considered (see section 4.6).

An increase in frequency or severity of headache (which may be prodromal of a cerebrovascular event) may be a reason for immediate discontinuation of combination contraceptives.

Women using combined contraceptives should be emphatically advised to contact their physician in case of possible symptoms of thrombosis. In case of suspected or confirmed thrombosis, hormonal contraceptive use should be discontinued. Adequate contraception should be initiated because of the teratogenicity of anti-coagulant therapy (coumarins).

Tumours

An increased risk of cervical cancer in long-term users of COCs has been reported in some epidemiological studies, but there continues to be controversy about the extent to which this finding is attributable to the compounding effects of sexual behaviour and other factors such as human papilloma virus (HPV).

A meta-analysis of 54 epidemiological studies reported that there is a slightly increased risk (RR = 1.24) of having breast cancer diagnosed in women who are currently using COCs. The excess risk gradually disappears during the course of the 10 years after cessation of COC use. Because breast cancer is rare in women under 40 years of age, the excess number of breast cancer diagnoses in current and recent COC users is small in relation to the overall risk of breast cancer. The breast cancers diagnosed in ever-users tend to be less advanced clinically than the cancers diagnosed in never-users. The observed pattern of increased risk may be due to an earlier diagnosis of breast cancer in COC users, the biological effects of COCs or a combination of both.

In rare cases, benign liver tumours, and even more rarely, malignant liver tumours have been reported in users of COCs. In isolated cases, these tumours have led to life-threatening intra-abdominal haemorrhages. Therefore a hepatic tumour should be considered in the differential diagnosis when severe upper abdominal pain, liver enlargement or signs of intra-abdominal haemorrhage occur in women using EVRA.

Other conditions

- Contraceptive efficacy may be reduced in women weighing equal or greater than 90 kg (see sections 4.2 and 5.1).
- Women with hypertriglyceridaemia, or a family history thereof, may be at an increased risk of pancreatitis when using combination hormonal contraceptives.
- Although small increases of blood pressure have been reported in many women using hormonal contraceptives, clinically relevant increases are rare. A definitive relationship between hormonal contraceptive use and clinical hypertension has not been established. If, during the use of a combination hormonal contraceptive in pre-existing hypertension, constantly elevated blood pressure values or a significant increase in blood pressure do not respond adequately to antihypertensive treatment, the combination hormonal contraceptive must be withdrawn. Combination hormonal contraceptive use may be resumed if normotensive values can be achieved with antihypertensive therapy.
- The following conditions have been reported to occur or deteriorate with both pregnancy and COC use, but the evidence of an association with COC use is inconclusive: Jaundice and/or pruritus related to cholestasis; gallstones; porphyria; systemic erythematosus; haemolytic uraemic syndrome; Sydenham's chorea; herpes gestationis; otosclerosis-related hearing loss.
- Acute or chronic disturbances of liver function may necessitate the discontinuation of combination hormonal contraceptives until markers of liver function return to normal. Recurrence of cholestatic-related pruritus, which occurred during a previous pregnancy or previous use of sex steroids necessitates the discontinuation of combination hormonal contraceptives.
- Although combined hormonal contraceptives may have an effect on peripheral insulin resistance and glucose tolerance there is no evidence for a need to alter the therapeutic regimen in diabetes during use of combined hormonal contraception. However, diabetic women should be carefully observed, particularly in the early stage of EVRA use.
- Worsening of endogenous depression, of epilepsy, of Crohn's disease and of ulcerative colitis has been reported during COC use.
- Chloasma may occasionally occur with the use of hormonal contraception, especially in users with a history of chloasma gravidarum. Users with a tendency to chloasma should avoid exposure to the sun or ultraviolet radiation while using EVRA. Chloasma is often not fully reversible.

Medical examination/consultation

Prior to the initiation or reinstitution of EVRA a complete medical history (including family history) should be taken and pregnancy should be ruled out. Blood pressure should be measured and a physical examination should be performed guided by the contraindications (see section 4.3) and warnings (see section 4.4). The woman should also be instructed to carefully read the package leaflet and to adhere to the advice given.

The frequency and nature of subsequent examinations should be based on established guidelines and be adapted to the individual woman on the basis of clinical impression.

Women should be advised that hormonal contraceptives do not protect against HIV infections (AIDS) and other sexually transmissible diseases.

Bleeding irregularities

With all combination hormonal contraceptives, irregular blood loss (spotting or breakthrough bleeding) can occur, especially during the initial months of usage. For this reason, a medical opinion on irregular blood loss will only be useful after an adjustment period of approximately three cycles. If breakthrough bleeding persists, or breakthrough bleeding occurs after previously regular cycles, while EVRA has been used according the recommended regimen, a cause other than EVRA should be considered. Non-hormonal causes should be considered and, if necessary, adequate diagnostic measures taken to rule out organic disease or pregnancy. This may include curettage. In some women withdrawal bleeding may not occur during this patch free period. If EVRA has been taken according to the directions described in section 4.2, it is unlikely that the woman is pregnant. However, if EVRA has not been taken according to these directions prior to the first missed withdrawal bleed or if two withdrawal bleeds are missed, pregnancy must be ruled out before EVRA use is continued.

Some users may experience amenorrhoea or oligomenorrhoea after discontinuing hormonal contraception, especially when such a condition was pre-existent.

Herbal preparations containing St John's Wort (*Hypericum perforatum*) should not be used while taking EVRA (see section 4.5)

4.5 Interaction with other medicinal products and other forms of interaction

Influence of other medicinal products on EVRA

Medicinal product interactions, which result in an increased clearance of sex hormones can lead to breakthrough bleeding and hormonal contraceptive failure. This has been established with hydantoins, barbiturates, primidone, carbamazepine and rifampicin; bosentan, oxcarbazepine, topiramate, felbamate, ritonavir, griseofulvin, modafinil and phenyl butazone are also suspected. The mechanism of these interactions appears to be based on the hepatic enzyme inducing properties of these medicinal products. Maximal enzyme induction is generally not seen for 2-3 weeks but may be sustained for at least 4 weeks after cessation of therapy.

The herbal preparation of St John's Wort (*Hypericum perforatum*) should not be taken concomitantly with this medicinal product as this could potentially lead to a loss of contraceptive effect. Breakthrough bleeding and unintended pregnancies have been reported. This is due to induction of metabolising enzymes by St John's Wort. The inducing effect may persist for at least 2 weeks after cessation of treatment with St John's Wort.

Contraceptive failures have also been reported with antibiotics, such as ampicillin and tetracyclines. The mechanism of this effect has not been elucidated. In a pharmacokinetic interaction study, oral administration of tetracycline hydrochloride, 500 mg four times daily for 3 days prior to and 7 days during wear of EVRA, did not significantly affect the pharmacokinetics of norelgestromin or EE.

Women on treatment with any of these medicinal products should temporarily use a barrier method in addition to EVRA or choose another method of contraception. With microsomal enzyme-inducing medicinal products, the barrier method should be used during the time of concomitant administration of these medicinal products and for 28 days after their discontinuation. Women on treatment with antibiotics (except tetracycline) should use the barrier method until 7 days after discontinuation. If concomitant medicinal product administration runs beyond the 3 weeks of patch treatment, a new treatment cycle should be started immediately without having the usual patch-free interval.

For women on long-term therapy with hepatic enzyme inducers, another method of contraception should be considered.

Influence of EVRA on other medications

Progestogens and estrogens inhibit a variety of P450 enzymes (e.g., CYP 3A4, CYP 2C19) in human liver microsomes. However, under the recommended dosing regimen, the *in vivo* concentrations of norelgestromin and its metabolites, even at the peak serum levels, are relatively low compared to the inhibitory constant (Ki), indicating a low potential for clinical interaction. Nevertheless, physicians are advised to refer to prescribing information for recommendations regarding management of concomitant therapy, especially for agents with a narrow therapeutic index metabolised by these enzymes (e.g. cyclosporin).

Combined hormonal contraceptives have been shown to significantly decrease plasma concentrations of lamotrigine when co-administered due to induction of lamotrigine glucuronidation. This may reduce seizure control; therefore, dosage adjustments of lamotrigine may be necessary.

Laboratory tests

Certain endocrine and liver function tests and blood components may be affected by hormonal contraceptives:

– Increased prothrombin and factors VII, VIII, IX and X; decreased anti-thrombin III; decreased protein S; increased norepinephrine (noradrenaline)-induced platelet aggregability.

– Increased thyroid binding globulin (TBG) leading to increased circulating total thyroid hormone, as measured by protein-bound iodine (PBI), T4 by column or by radio-immunoassay. Free T3 resin uptake is decreased, reflecting the elevated TBG, free T4 concentration is unaltered.

Table 1

System Organ Class	Adverse Drug Reactions in Clinical Trials				
	Frequency				
	Very common	Common	Uncommon	Rare	Very rare
Infections and infestations		Fungal infection (vaginal only), Vaginal candidiasis, Vulvovaginal mycotic infection			
Metabolism and nutrition disorders			Fluid retention, Hypercholesterolemia		
Psychiatric disorders		Depression, Mood altered, Mood swings	Affect lability, Anxiety, Insomnia, Libido decreased	Crying, Libido increased, Tearfulness	Aggression
Nervous system disorders	Headache	Dizziness, Migraine			
Respiratory, thoracic and mediastinal disorders				Pulmonary embolism	
Gastrointestinal disorders	Nausea	Abdominal distension, Abdominal pain, Abdominal pain lower, Abdominal pain upper, Vomiting, Diarrhoea			
Hepatobiliary disorders				Cholecystitis	
Skin and subcutaneous tissue disorders		Acne, Pruritus, Skin irritation	Dermatitis contact, Erythema	Chloasma	
Musculoskeletal and connective tissue disorders		Muscle spasms			
Reproductive system and breast disorders	Breast tenderness	Breast discomfort, Breast enlargement, Breast pain, Dysmenorrhoea, Menorrhagia, Metrorrhagia, Uterine spasm, Vaginal discharge	Breast disorder, Breast engorgement, Breast swelling, Fibrocystic breast disease, Galactorrhoea, Premenstrual syndrome, Vaginal haemorrhage, Vulvovaginal dryness	Genital discharge, Menstrual disorder, Menstruation irregular	Polymenorrhoea
General disorders and administration site conditions		Application site erythema, Application site irritation, Application site pruritus, Application site rash, Application site reaction, Fatigue, Malaise	Application site dermatitis, Application site discolouration, Application site hypersensitivity, Application site pain, Application site papules, Application site vesicles, Generalized oedema	Application site urticaria, Swelling	Application site oedema
Investigations		Weight increased	Blood pressure increased, Blood triglycerides increased	Blood cholesterol increased	

Other binding proteins may be elevated in serum.

Sex hormone-binding globulins (SHBG) are increased and result in elevated levels of total circulating endogenous sex steroids. However, the free or biologically active levels of sex steroids either decrease or remain the same.

High-density lipoprotein (HDL-C), total cholesterol (Total-C), low-density lipoprotein (LDL-C) and triglycerides may all increase slightly with EVRA, while LDL-C/HDL-C ratio may remain unchanged.

Glucose tolerance may be decreased.

Serum folate levels may be depressed by hormonal contraceptive therapy. This has potential to be of clinical significance if a woman becomes pregnant shortly after discontinuing hormonal contraceptives. All women are now advised to take supplemental folic acid peri-conceptionally.

4.6 Pregnancy and lactation

EVRA is not indicated during pregnancy.

Epidemiological studies indicate no increased risk of birth defects in children born to women who used hormonal contraceptives prior to pregnancy. The majority of recent studies also do not indicate a teratogenic effect when hormonal contraceptives are used inadvertently during early pregnancy.

For EVRA there are no clinical data on exposed pregnancies, which allow conclusions about its safety during pregnancy.

Studies in animals have shown reproductive toxicity (see section 5.3). On the basis of available data, a potential risk of masculinisation as a consequence of an exaggerated hormonal action cannot be excluded.

If pregnancy occurs during use of EVRA, EVRA should be stopped immediately.

Lactation may be influenced by combination hormonal contraceptives as they may reduce the quantity and change the composition of breast milk. Therefore, the use of EVRA is not to be recommended until the breast-feeding mother has completely weaned her child.

4.7 Effects on ability to drive and use machines

EVRA has no or negligible influence on the ability to drive and use machines.

4.8 Undesirable effects

4.8.1 Clinical Trial Data

The most commonly reported adverse drug reactions (ADRs) in clinical trials were headache, nausea, and breast tenderness, occurring in approximately 21.0%, 16.6%, and 15.9% of patients, respectively.

Frequency estimate: very common (⩾ 1/10); common (⩾ 1/100 to < 1/10); uncommon (⩾ 1/1,000 to < 1/100); rare (⩾ 1/10,000 to < 1/1,000); very rare (< 1/10,000); not known (cannot be estimated from the available data).

(see Table 1 above)

4.8.2 Postmarketing Data

Additional adverse drug reactions first identified during postmarketing experience with EVRA are listed below:

Infections and infestations	Application site pustules, Rash pustular
Neoplasms benign, malignant and unspecified (incl cysts and polyps)	Breast cancer, Breast cancer stage IV, Cervix carcinoma, Fibroadenoma of breast, Hepatic adenoma, Hepatic neoplasm, Uterine leiomyoma
Immune system disorders	Hypersensitivity
Metabolism and nutrition disorders	Hyperglycaemia, Insulin resistance
Psychiatric disorders	Anger, Emotional disorder, Frustration
Nervous system disorders	Basilar artery thrombosis, Brain stem infarction, Carotid artery occlusion, Cerebral artery embolism, Cerebral artery occlusion, Cerebral artery thrombosis, Cerebral haemorrhage, Cerebral infarction, Cerebral thrombosis, Cerebral venous thrombosis, Cerebrovascular accident, Embolic stroke, Haemorrhage intracranial, Haemorrhagic stroke, Intracranial venous sinus thrombosis, Ischaemic cerebral infarction, Ischaemic stroke, Lacunar infarction, Migraine with aura, Subarachnoid haemorrhage, Superior sagittal sinus thrombosis, Thromboembolic stroke, Thrombotic stroke, Transient ischaemic attack, Transverse sinus thrombosis
Eye disorders	Contact lens intolerance
Cardiac disorders	Acute myocardial infarction, Myocardial infarction
Vascular disorders	Arterial thrombosis, Arterial thrombosis limb, Axillary vein thrombosis, Budd-Chiari syndrome, Coronary artery thrombosis, Deep vein thrombosis, Embolism, Hepatic vein thrombosis, Hypertension, Hypertensive crisis, Iliac artery thrombosis, Intracardiac thrombus, Jugular vein thrombosis, Mesenteric vein thrombosis, Pelvic venous thrombosis, Peripheral embolism, Portal vein thrombosis, Renal embolism, Renal vein thrombosis, Retinal artery occlusion, Retinal vascular thrombosis, Retinal vein occlusion, Splenic vein thrombosis, Superficial thrombophlebitis, Thrombophlebitis, Thrombosis, Vena cava thrombosis, Venous thrombosis, Venous thrombosis limb
Respiratory, thoracic and mediastinal disorders	Pulmonary artery thrombosis, Pulmonary thrombosis
Gastrointestinal disorders	Colitis
Hepatobiliary disorders	Cholelithiasis, Cholestasis, Hepatic lesion, Jaundice cholestatic
Skin and subcutaneous tissues disorders	Alopecia, Angioedema, Dermatitis allergic, Eczema, Erythema multiforme, Erythema nodosum, Exfoliative rash, Photosensitivity reaction, Pruritus generalised, Rash, Rash erythematous, Rash pruritic, Seborrhoeic dermatitis, Skin reaction, Urticaria
Reproductive system and breast disorders	Amenorrhoea, Breast mass, Cervical dysplasia, Hypomenorrhoea, Menometrorrhagia, Oligomenorrhoea, Suppressed lactation
General disorders and administration site conditions	Application site abscess, Application site anaesthesia, Application site atrophy, Application site bleeding, Application site bruising, Application site burn, Application site discharge, Application site discomfort, Application site dryness, Application site eczema, Application site erosion, Application site excoriation, Application site exfoliation, Application site induration, Application site infection, Application site inflammation, Application site mass, Application site nodule, Application site odour, Application site paraesthesia, Application site photosensitivity reaction, Application site scab, Application site scar, Application site swelling, Application site ulcer, Application site warmth, Face oedema, Irritability, Localised oedema, Oedema peripheral, Pitting oedema
Investigations	Blood cholesterol abnormal, Blood glucose abnormal, Blood glucose decreased, Low density lipoprotein increased
Injury, poisoning and procedural complications	Contact lens complication

4.9 Overdose

Serious ill effects have not been reported following accidental ingestion of large doses of oral contraceptives. Overdosage may cause nausea or vomiting. Vaginal bleeding may occur in some females. In cases of suspected overdose, all transdermal contraceptive systems should be removed and symptomatic treatment given.

5. PHARMACOLOGICAL PROPERTIES

5.1 Pharmacodynamic properties

Pharmacotherapeutic group: Norelgestromin and estrogen; ATC-code: G03AA13.

EVRA acts through the mechanism of gonadotropin suppression by the estrogenic and progestational actions of ethinyl estradiol and norelgestromin. The primary mechanism of action is inhibition of the ovulation, but the alterations of the cervical mucus, and to the endometrium may also contribute to the efficacy of the product.

Pearl Indices (see table):

(see Table 2 on next page)

Table 2 Pearl Indices

Study Group	CONT-002 EVRA	CONT-003 EVRA	CONT-003 COC*	CONT-004 EVRA	CONT-004 COC**	All EVRA Subjects
# of cycles	10,743	5831	4592	5095	4005	21,669
Overall Pearl Index (95% CI)	0.73 (0.15,1.31)	0.89 (0.02,1.76)	0.57 (0,1.35)	1.28 (0.16,2.39)	2.27 (0.59,3.96)	0.90 (0.44,1.35)
Method Failure Pearl Index (95% CI)	0.61 (0.0,1.14)	0.67 (0,1.42)	0.28 (0,0.84)	1.02 (0.02,2.02)	1.30 (0.03,2.57)	0.72 (0.31,1.13)

*: DSG 150 µg + 20 µg EE

**: 50 µg LNG + 30 µg for days 1 – 6, 75 µg LNG + 40 µg EE for days 7 – 11, 125 µg LNG + 30 µg EE for 12 – 21 days

Exploratory analyses were performed to determine whether in the Phase III studies (n=3319) the population characteristics of age, race and weight were associated with pregnancy. The analyses indicated no association of age and race with pregnancy. With respect to weight, 5 of the 15 pregnancies reported with EVRA were among women with baseline body weight equal or greater than 90 kg, which constituted < 3 % of the study population. Below 90 kg there was no association between body weight and pregnancy. Although only 10-20 % of the variability in pharmacokinetic data can be explained by weight (see Pharmacokinetic Properties, Special Populations), the greater proportions of pregnancies among women at or above 90 kg was statistically significant and indicates the EVRA is less effective in these women.

With the use of higher dosed COCs (50 microgram ethinyl estradiol) the risk of endometrial and ovarian cancer is reduced. Whether this is also applies to the lower dosed combined hormonal contraceptives remains to be confirmed.

5.2 Pharmacokinetic properties

Absorption

Following application of EVRA, norelgestromin and ethinyl estradiol levels in serum reach a plateau by approximately 48 hours. Steady state concentrations of norelgestromin and EE during one week of patch wear are approximately 0.8 ng/ml and 50 pg/ml, respectively. In multiple-dose studies, serum concentrations and AUC for norelgestromin and EE were found to increase only slightly over time when compared to week 1 cycle 1.

The absorption of norelgestromin and ethinyl estradiol following application of EVRA was studied under conditions encountered in a health club (sauna, whirlpool, treadmill and other aerobic exercise) and in a cold water bath. The results indicated that for norelgestromin there were no significant treatment effects on C_{ss} or AUC when compared to normal wear. For EE, slight increases were observed due to treadmill and other aerobic exercise; however, the C_{ss} values following these treatments were within the reference range. There was no significant effect of cool water on these parameters.

Results from an EVRA study of extended wear of single contraceptive patch for 7 days and 10 days indicated that target C_{ss} of norelgestromin and ethinyl estradiol were maintained during a 3-day period of extended wear of EVRA (10 days). These findings suggest that clinical efficacy would be maintained even if a scheduled change is missed for as long as 2 full days.

Distribution

Norelgestromin and norgestrel (a serum metabolite of norelgestromin) are highly bound (> 97 %) to serum proteins. Norelgestromin is bound to albumin and not to SHBG, while norgestrel is bound primarily to SHBG, which limits its biological activity. Ethinyl estradiol is extensively bound to serum albumin.

Biotransformation

Hepatic metabolism of norelgestromin occurs and metabolites include norgestrel, which is largely bound to SHBG, and various hydroxylated and conjugated metabolites. Ethinyl estradiol is also metabolised to various hydroxylated products and their glucuronide and sulfate conjugates.

Elimination

Following removal of a patch, the mean elimination half-lives of norelgestromin and ethinyl estradiol were approximately 28 hours and 17 hours, respectively. The metabolites of norelgestromin and ethinyl estradiol are eliminated by renal and fecal pathways.

Transdermal versus Oral Contraceptives

The pharmacokinetic profiles of transdermal and oral combined hormonal contraceptives are different and caution should be exercised when making a direct comparison of these PK parameters.

In a study comparing EVRA to an oral contraceptive containing norgestimate (parent drug of norelgestromin) 250 µg/ethinyl estradiol 35 µg, C_{max} values were 2-fold higher for NGMN and EE in subjects administered the oral contraceptive compared to EVRA, while overall exposure (AUC and C_{ss}) was comparable in subjects treated with EVRA. Inter-subject variability (%CV) for the PK parameters following delivery from EVRA was higher relative to the variability determined from the oral contraceptive.

Effects of age, body weight, and body surface area

The effects of age, body weight, and body surface area on the pharmacokinetics of norelgestromin and ethinyl estradiol were evaluated in 230 healthy women from nine pharmacokinetic studies of single 7-day applications of EVRA. For both norelgestromin and EE, increasing age, body weight and body surface area each were associated with slight decreases in C_{ss} and AUC values. However, only a small fraction (10 –20 %) of the overall variability in the pharmacokinetics of the norelgestromin and EE following application of EVRA may be associated with any or all of the above demographic parameters.

5.3 Preclinical safety data

Preclinical data reveal no special hazard for humans based on conventional studies of safety pharmacology, repeated dose toxicity, genotoxicity and carcinogenic potential. With respect to the reproductive toxicity norelgestromin showed foetal toxicity in rabbits, but the safety margin for this effect was sufficiently high. Data on reproductive toxicity of the combination of norelgestromin with ethinyl estradiol are not available. Data for combination of norgestimate (precursor of norelgestromin) with ethinyl estradiol indicate for female animals a decrease in fertility and implantation efficiency (rat), an increase in foetal resorption (rat, rabbit) and, with high dosages, a decrease in viability and fertility of female offspring (rat). The relevance of these data for human exposure is unknown as these effects have been seen as related to well-known pharmacodynamic or species-specific actions.

Studies conducted to examine the dermal effect of EVRA indicate this system has no potential to produce sensitisation and results in only mild irritation when applied to rabbits skin.

6. PHARMACEUTICAL PARTICULARS

6.1 List of excipients

Backing layer:

low-density pigmented polyethylene outer layer,

polyester inner layer.

Middle layer:

polyisobutylene/polybutene adhesive,

crospovidone,

non-woven polyester fabric,

lauryl lactate.

Third layer:

polyethylene terephthalate (PET) film,

polydimethylsiloxane coating.

6.2 Incompatibilities

To prevent interference with the adhesive properties of EVRA, no creams, lotions or powders should be applied to the skin area where the EVRA transdermal patch is to be applied.

6.3 Shelf life

2 years

6.4 Special precautions for storage

Store in the original package in order to protect from light and moisture.

Do not refrigerate or freeze.

6.5 Nature and contents of container

Primary packaging material

A sachet is composed of four layers: a low-density polyethylene film (innermost layer), an aluminium foil, a low-density polyethylene film, and an outer layer of bleached paper.

Secondary packaging material

Sachets are packaged in a cardboard carton.

Every carton has 3, 9 or 18 EVRA transdermal patches in individual foil-lined sachets.

Sachets are wrapped per three in a transparent perforated plastic film and packed in a cardboard carton.

6.6 Special precautions for disposal and other handling

Apply immediately upon removal from the protective sachet. After use the patch still contains substantial quantities of active ingredients. Remaining hormonal active ingredients of the patch may have harmful effects if reaching the aquatic environment. Therefore, the used patch should be discarded carefully. The disposal label from the outside of the sachet should be peeled open. The used patch should be placed within the open disposal label so that the sticky surface covers the shaded area on the sachet. The disposal label should then be closed sealing the used patch within. Any used or unused patches should be discarded according to local requirements or returned to the pharmacy. Used patches should not be flushed down the toilet nor placed in liquid waste disposal systems.

7. MARKETING AUTHORISATION HOLDER

JANSSEN-CILAG INTERNATIONAL N.V.

Turnhoutseweg, 30

B-2340 Beerse

Belgium

8. MARKETING AUTHORISATION NUMBER(S)

EU/1/02/223/001

EU/1/02/223/002

EU/1/02/223/003

9. DATE OF FIRST AUTHORISATION/RENEWAL OF THE AUTHORISATION

Date of first authorization: 22 August 2002.

Date of latest renewal: 22 August 2007.

10. DATE OF REVISION OF THE TEXT

22 December 2008

Detailed information on this medicinal product is available on the website of the European Medicines Agency (EMEA) http://www.emea.europa.eu/

Exocin

(Allergan Ltd)

1. NAME OF THE MEDICINAL PRODUCT

EXOCIN.

2. QUALITATIVE AND QUANTITATIVE COMPOSITION

Ofloxacin 0.3% w/v.

3. PHARMACEUTICAL FORM

Eye drops.

4. CLINICAL PARTICULARS

4.1 Therapeutic indications

Exocin is indicated for the topical treatment of external ocular infections (such as conjunctivitis and keratoconjunctivitis) in adults and children caused by ofloxacin - sensitive organisms. Safety and efficacy in the treatment of ophthalmia neonatorum has not been established.

4.2 Posology and method of administration

Topical ocular instillation.

For all ages: one to two drops in the affected eye(s) every two to four hours for the first two days and then four times daily. The length of treatment should not exceed ten days.

4.3 Contraindications

Exocin is contra-indicated in patients sensitive to ofloxacin or any of its other components.

4.4 Special warnings and precautions for use

When using Exocin eye drops the risk of rhinopharyngeal passage which can contribute to the occurrence and the diffusion of bacterial resistance should be considered. As with other anti-infectives, prolonged use may result in overgrowth of non-susceptible organisms.

If worsening infection occurs, or if clinical improvement is not noted within a reasonable period, discontinue use and institute alternative therapy.

Use Exocin with caution in patients who have exhibited sensitivities to other quinolone antibacterial agents.

Data are very limited to establish efficacy and safety of ofloxacin eye drops 0.3% in the treatment of conjunctivitis in neonates.

The use of ofloxacin eye drops in neonates with ophthalmia neonatorum caused by Neisseria gonorrhoeae or Chlamydia trachomatis is not recommended as it has not been evaluated in such patients. Neonates with ophthalmia neonatorum should receive appropriate treatment for their condition, e.g. systemic treatment in cases caused by Chlamydia trachomatis or Neisseria gonorrhoeae.

Use in elderly: No comparative data are available with topical dosing in elderly versus other age groups.

Clinical and non-clinical publications have reported the occurrence of corneal perforation in patients with pre-existing corneal epithelial defect or corneal ulcer, when treated with topical fluoroquinolone antibiotics. However, significant confounding factors were involved in many of these reports, including advanced age, presence of large ulcers, concomitant ocular conditions (e.g. severe dry eye), systemic inflammatory diseases (e.g. rheumatoid arthritis), and concomitant use of ocular steroids or non-steroidal anti-inflammatory drugs. Nevertheless, it is necessary to advise caution regarding the risk of corneal perforation when using product to treat patients with corneal epithelial defects or corneal ulcers.

The multidose eye drop presentation contains the preservative benzalkonium chloride, which may cause eye irritation. Exocin contains the preservative benzalkonium chloride, which may be absorbed by soft contact lenses and discolour them. Contact lenses should be removed prior to instillation and may be reinserted 15 minutes following administration.

4.5 Interaction with other medicinal products and other forms of interaction
None known

4.6 Pregnancy and lactation
Use in pregnancy: There have been no adequate and well-controlled studies performed in pregnant women. Since systemic quinolones have been shown to cause arthropathy in immature animals, it is recommended that Exocin be used in pregnant women only if the potential benefit justifies the potential risk to the foetus.

Use during lactation: Because ofloxacin and other quinolones taken systemically are excreted in breast milk, and there is potential for harm to nursing infants, a decision should be made whether to temporarily discontinue nursing or not to administer the drug, taking into account the importance of the drug to the mother.

4.7 Effects on ability to drive and use machines
None known.

4.8 Undesirable effects
Adverse reactions: Transient ocular irritation (burning, stinging, redness, itching or photophobia) has been reported. Extremely low incidence of dizziness, with numbness and nausea and of headache were reported from clinical trials. Since ofloxacin is systemically absorbed after topical administration, side-effects reported with systemic use could possibly occur.

4.9 Overdose
In the event of a topical overdosage, flush the eye with water.

5. PHARMACOLOGICAL PROPERTIES

5.1 Pharmacodynamic properties
Ofloxacin is a synthetic fluorinated 4-quinolone antibacterial agent with activity against a broad spectrum of Gram negative and to a lesser degree Gram positive organisms.

Ofloxacin has been shown to be active against most strains of the following organisms both in vitro and clinically in ophthalmic infections. Clinical trial evidence of the efficacy of Exocin against S. pneumoniae was based on a limited number of isolates.

Gram-negative bacteria: Acinetobacter calcoaceticus var. anitratum, and A. calcoaceticus var. iwoffi; Enterobacter Sp. including E. cloacae; Haemophilis Sp. including H. influenza and H. aegyptius; Klebsiella Sp., including K. Pneumoniae; Moraxella Sp., Morganella morganii; Proteus Sp., including P. Mirabilis; Pseudomonas Sp.; including P. Aeruginosa, P. cepacia, and P. fluoroscens; and Serratia Sp., including S. marcescens.

Gram-positive bacteria: Bacillus Sp.; Corynebacterium Sp.; Micrococcus Sp.; Staphylococcus Sp., including S. aureus and S. epidermidis; Streptococcus Sp., including S. Pneumoniae (see above), S. viridans and Beta-haemolytic.

The primary mechanisms of action is through inhibition of bacterial DNA gyrase, the enzyme responsible for maintaining the structure of DNA.

Ofloxacin is not subject to degradation by beta-lactamase enzymes nor is it modified by enzymes such as aminoglycoside adenylases or phosphorylases, or chloramphenicol acetyltransferase.

5.2 Pharmacokinetic properties
After ophthalmic instillation, ofloxacin is well maintained in the tear-film.

In a healthy volunteer study, mean tear film concentrations of ofloxacin measured four hours after topical dosing (9.2 μg/g) were higher than the 2μg/ml minimum concentration of ofloxacin necessary to inhibit 90% of most ocular bacterial strains (MIC_{90}) in-vitro.

Maximum serum ofloxacin concentrations after ten days of topical dosing were about 1000 times lower than those reported after standard oral doses of ofloxacin, and no systemic side-effects attributable to topical ofloxacin were observed.

5.3 Preclinical safety data
There are no toxicological safety issues with this product in man as the level of systemic absorption from topical ocular administration of ofloxacin is minimal.

Animal studies in the dog have found cases of arthropathy in weight bearing joints of juvenile animals after high oral doses of certain quinolones. However, these findings have not been seen in clinical studies and their relevance to man is unknown.

6. PHARMACEUTICAL PARTICULARS

6.1 List of excipients
Benzalkonium chloride (EP) 0.005% w/v

Sodium chloride (EP) 0.9% w/v

Purified water (EP)

6.2 Incompatibilities
None known.

6.3 Shelf life
24 months.

6.4 Special precautions for storage
Do not store above 25°C.

6.5 Nature and contents of container
5 ml or 10 ml low density polyethylene (LDPE) bottles with LDPE tip and medium or high impact polystyrene cap.

6.6 Special precautions for disposal and other handling
Discard bottle 28 days after opening.

7. MARKETING AUTHORISATION HOLDER
Allergan Ltd

Marlow International

The Parkway

Marlow

Bucks SL7 1YL

United Kingdom

8. MARKETING AUTHORISATION NUMBER(S)
PL 00426/0070

9. DATE OF FIRST AUTHORISATION/RENEWAL OF THE AUTHORISATION
26th October 1992 / 8th November 2004

10. DATE OF REVISION OF THE TEXT
4th August 2008

Exorex Lotion

(Forest Laboratories UK Limited)

1. NAME OF THE MEDICINAL PRODUCT
Exorex Lotion 5% v/w Cutaneous Emulsion

2. QUALITATIVE AND QUANTITATIVE COMPOSITION
Coal Tar Solution 5% v/w.

For a full list of excipients, see 6.1.

3. PHARMACEUTICAL FORM
Cutaneous emulsion

A smooth mustard coloured emulsion.

4. CLINICAL PARTICULARS

4.1 Therapeutic indications
Exorex is for the treatment of psoriasis of the skin and scalp.

4.2 Posology and method of administration
Adults and children over 12 years of age:

Ensure that the lesions are clean. Apply a thin layer of Exorex two or three times per day to the affected areas. Massage gently and leave to dry.

For young children under 12 years of age and the elderly:

The emulsion may be diluted by mixing with a few drops of freshly boiled and cooled water in the palm of the hand.

4.3 Contraindications
Do not use if sensitive to any of the ingredients.

Presence of folliculitis and acne vulgaris.

Exorex should not be used on patients who have disease characterised by photosensitivity such as lupus erythematosus or allergy to sunlight.

Exorex should not be applied to inflamed or broken skin (open exuding wounds or infection of the skin).

4.4 Special warnings and precautions for use
Coal tar may cause skin irritation. If irritation occurs, the treatment should be reviewed and discontinued if necessary.

Coal tar enhances photosensitivity of the skin, and exposure to direct sunlight after application of Exorex should be avoided.

Use with care near the eyes and mucous membranes. If any emulsion should accidentally enter the eye, flush with normal saline solution or water.

Do not apply to genital and rectal areas.

Apply with caution to the face.

4.5 Interaction with other medicinal products and other forms of interaction
None known.

4.6 Pregnancy and lactation
There is inadequate evidence of safety in pregnant and lactating women but coal tar preparations have been in use for many years without apparent ill-consequence and no harmful effects on the health of the child is anticipated with the proper use of this product. However it is recommended that the use of coal tar in pregnancy and lactation be restricted to intermittent use, in a low concentration on a relatively small percentage of body surface and that use during the first trimester be avoided.

4.7 Effects on ability to drive and use machines
None known.

4.8 Undesirable effects
Skin irritation, photosensitivity of the skin. In addition coal tar may cause acne-like eruptions of the skin.

An increased risk of skin cancer in psoriatic patients treated with a combination of coal tar and UVB radiation has been reported. However epidemiological studies of patients treated with coal tar alone are inconclusive. The risk of toxicity should be taken into account when considering the suitability of this product for the patient (see also Section 5.3).

4.9 Overdose
There is no evidence that overdose of topical Exorex would be harmful other than possibly inducing a hypersensitivity to coal tar. Ingestion of Exorex may require gastric lavage depending on the quantity taken and should be treated symptomatically.

5. PHARMACOLOGICAL PROPERTIES

5.1 Pharmacodynamic properties
Exorex contains coal tar, an antipruritic and keratoplastic. It is used in eczema, psoriasis and other skin conditions. Tar acids have also been shown to have disinfectant properties. Exorex may be used alone, or as part of a more extensive treatment regimen.

5.2 Pharmacokinetic properties
Not applicable.

5.3 Preclinical safety data
In animal studies coal tar has been shown to increase the incidence of epidermal carcinomas and self-limiting keratoacanthomas.

While the ingredients of coal tar have been shown to express genotoxic properties, epidemiological studies with patients have been shown to be inconclusive concerning the potential carcinogenic risks of coal tar products in human long term treatment. Nevertheless the possible risk of prolonged treatment should be taken into account when considering the usage of the product.

6. PHARMACEUTICAL PARTICULARS

6.1 List of excipients
Polysorbate 80

Ethanol

DL-alpha tocopherol

Complex of esterified essential fatty acids

Xanthan gum

Propyl hydroxybenzoate (E216)

Methyl hydroxybenzoate (E218)

Hydrogenated polyoxyl castor oil

Water

6.2 Incompatibilities
None known

6.3 Shelf life
2 years

6.4 Special precautions for storage
Do not store above 25°C.

6.5 Nature and contents of container
High density polyethylene bottle containing titanium dioxide.

Polypropylene green flip-top caps.

Pack sizes: 100 and 250ml

A professional sales pack of 30ml is also available.

6.6 Special precautions for disposal and other handling
No special requirements.

7. MARKETING AUTHORISATION HOLDER
Forest Tosara Limited

Baldoyle Industrial Estate

Grange Road

Dublin 13

Ireland

8. MARKETING AUTHORISATION NUMBER(S)
PL 06166/0001

9. DATE OF FIRST AUTHORISATION/RENEWAL OF THE AUTHORISATION
3 November 1999 / 16 October 2003

10. DATE OF REVISION OF THE TEXT
August 2009

11. Legal Category
GSL

Exterol 5% w/w Ear Drops, Solution

(Dermal Laboratories Limited)

1. NAME OF THE MEDICINAL PRODUCT
EXTEROL™ 5% w/w EAR DROPS, SOLUTION

2. QUALITATIVE AND QUANTITATIVE COMPOSITION
Urea Hydrogen Peroxide 5.0% w/w.

3. PHARMACEUTICAL FORM
Ear drops, solution.

Clear, straw-coloured, viscous ear drops.

4. CLINICAL PARTICULARS

4.1 Therapeutic indications
As an aid in the removal of hardened ear wax.

4.2 Posology and method of administration
For adults, children and the elderly: Instil up to 5 drops into the ear. Retain drops in ear for several minutes by keeping

the head tilted and then wipe away any surplus. Repeat once or twice daily for at least 3 to 4 days, or as required.

4.3 Contraindications
Do not use if the eardrum is known or suspected to be damaged, in cases of dizziness, or if there is any other ear disorder (such as pain, discharge, inflammation, infection or tinnitus). Do not use after ill-advised attempts to dislodge wax using fingernails, cotton buds or similar implements, as such mechanical efforts can cause the ear's delicate inner lining to become damaged, inflamed or infected, whereupon the use of ear drops can be painful. For similar reasons, it is inadvisable to use Exterol within 2 to 3 days of syringing. Do not use where there is a history of ear problems, unless under close medical supervision. Do not use if sensitive to any of the ingredients.

4.4 Special warnings and precautions for use
Keep Exterol away from the eyes. For external use only. Replace cap after use, and return bottle to carton.

4.5 Interaction with other medicinal products and other forms of interaction
Exterol should not be used at the same time as anything else in the ear.

4.6 Pregnancy and lactation
No known side-effects.

4.7 Effects on ability to drive and use machines
None known.

4.8 Undesirable effects
Due to the release of oxygen, patients may experience a mild, temporary effervescence in the ear. Stop usage if irritation or pain occurs. Instillation of ear drops can aggravate the painful symptoms of excessive ear wax, including some loss of hearing, dizziness and tinnitus. Very rarely, unpleasant taste has been reported. If patients encounter any of these problems, or if their symptoms persist or worsen, they should discontinue treatment and consult a doctor.

4.9 Overdose
No adverse effects.

5. PHARMACOLOGICAL PROPERTIES

5.1 Pharmacodynamic properties
After insertion of the drops into the ear, the urea hydrogen peroxide complex liberates oxygen which acts to break up the hardened wax. The hydrogen peroxide component is also an antiseptic, especially in sites with relative anaerobiosis. The glycerol assists in softening the wax, so that it may more easily be removed from the ear, either with or without syringing. The urea acts as a mild keratolytic, helping to reduce the keratin-load in the wax debris, thereby assisting penetration of the other components.

5.2 Pharmacokinetic properties
Exterol is intended only for the treatment of impacted wax in the external auditory canal. The ingredients of the formulation are therefore readily available for intimate contact with the affected area, as the drops are instilled into the ear and retained therein for several minutes by tilting the head.

5.3 Preclinical safety data
No special information.

6. PHARMACEUTICAL PARTICULARS

6.1 List of excipients
8-Hydroxyquinoline; Glycerol.

6.2 Incompatibilities
None known.

6.3 Shelf life
24 months.

6.4 Special precautions for storage
Store upright. Do not store above 25°C. Replace cap after use.

6.5 Nature and contents of container
8 ml easy squeeze plastic dropper bottle with screw cap. This is supplied as an original pack (OP).

6.6 Special precautions for disposal and other handling
Not applicable.

7. MARKETING AUTHORISATION HOLDER
Dermal Laboratories
Tatmore Place, Gosmore
Hitchin, Herts SG4 7QR, UK.

8. MARKETING AUTHORISATION NUMBER(S)
00173/0037.

9. DATE OF FIRST AUTHORISATION/RENEWAL OF THE AUTHORISATION
10 January 2007.

10. DATE OF REVISION OF THE TEXT
September 2007.

Ezetrol 10mg Tablets

(MSD-SP LTD)

1. NAME OF THE MEDICINAL PRODUCT
EZETROL® 10 mg Tablets

2. QUALITATIVE AND QUANTITATIVE COMPOSITION
Each tablet contains 10 mg of ezetimibe.

Excipients(s):

Each tablet contains 55 mg of lactose monohydrate.

For a full list of excipients see section 6.1.

3. PHARMACEUTICAL FORM
Tablet.

White to off-white, capsule-shaped tablets debossed with '414' on one side.

4. CLINICAL PARTICULARS

4.1 Therapeutic indications
Primary hypercholesterolaemia

'Ezetrol', co-administered with an HMG-CoA reductase inhibitor (statin) is indicated as adjunctive therapy to diet for use in patients with primary (heterozygous familial and non-familial) hypercholesterolaemia who are not appropriately controlled with a statin alone.

'Ezetrol' monotherapy is indicated as adjunctive therapy to diet for use in patients with primary (heterozygous familial and non-familial) hypercholesterolaemia in whom a statin is considered inappropriate or is not tolerated.

Homozygous Familial Hypercholesterolaemia (HoFH)

'Ezetrol' co-administered with a statin, is indicated as adjunctive therapy to diet for use in patients with HoFH. Patients may also receive adjunctive treatments (e.g. LDL apheresis).

Homozygous sitosterolaemia (phytosterolaemia)

'Ezetrol' is indicated as adjunctive therapy to diet for use in patients with homozygous familial sitosterolaemia.

A beneficial effect of Ezetrol on cardiovascular morbidity and mortality has not yet been demonstrated.

4.2 Posology and method of administration
The patient should be on an appropriate lipid-lowering diet and should continue on this diet during treatment with 'Ezetrol'.

Route of administration is oral. The recommended dose is one 'Ezetrol' 10 mg tablet daily. 'Ezetrol' can be administered at any time of the day, with or without food.

When 'Ezetrol' is added to a statin, either the indicated usual initial dose of that particular statin or the already established higher statin dose should be continued. In this setting, the dosage instructions for that particular statin should be consulted.

Co-administration with bile acid sequestrants

Dosing of 'Ezetrol' should occur either ⩾2 hours before or ⩾4 hours after administration of a bile acid sequestrant.

Use in the elderly

No dosage adjustment is required for elderly patients (see section 5.2).

Use in paediatric patients

Children and adolescents ⩾10 years: No dosage adjustment is required (see section 5.2). However, clinical experience in paediatric and adolescent patients (ages 9 to 17) is limited.

Children <10 years: 'Ezetrol' is not recommended for use in children below age 10 due to insufficient data on safety and efficacy (see section 5.2).

Use in hepatic impairment

No dosage adjustment is required in patients with mild hepatic insufficiency (Child Pugh score 5 to 6). Treatment with 'Ezetrol' is not recommended in patients with moderate (Child Pugh score 7 to 9) or severe (Child Pugh score >9) liver dysfunction. (See sections 4.4 and 5.2.)

Use in renal impairment

No dosage adjustment is required for renally impaired patients (see section 5.2).

4.3 Contraindications
Hypersensitivity to the active substance or to any of the excipients.

When 'Ezetrol' is co-administered with a statin, please refer to the SPC for that particular medicinal product.

Therapy with 'Ezetrol' co-administered with a statin is contraindicated during pregnancy and lactation.

'Ezetrol' co-administered with a statin is contraindicated in patients with active liver disease or unexplained persistent elevations in serum transaminases.

4.4 Special warnings and precautions for use
When 'Ezetrol' is co-administered with a statin, please refer to the SPC for that particular medicinal product.

Liver enzymes

In controlled co-administration trials in patients receiving 'Ezetrol' with a statin, consecutive transaminase elevations (⩾3 X the upper limit of normal [ULN]) have been observed. When 'Ezetrol' is co-administered with a statin, liver function tests should be performed at initiation of therapy and according to the recommendations of the statin. (See section 4.8.)

Skeletal muscle

In post-marketing experience with 'Ezetrol', cases of myopathy and rhabdomyolysis have been reported. Most patients who developed rhabdomyolysis were taking a statin concomitantly with 'Ezetrol'. However, rhabdomyolysis has been reported very rarely with 'Ezetrol' monotherapy and very rarely with the addition of 'Ezetrol' to other agents known to be associated with increased risk of rhabdomyolysis. If myopathy is suspected based on muscle symptoms or is confirmed by a creatine phosphokinase (CPK) level >10 times the ULN, 'Ezetrol', any statin, and any of these other agents that the patient is taking concomitantly should be immediately discontinued. All patients starting therapy with 'Ezetrol' should be advised of the risk of myopathy and told to report promptly any unexplained muscle pain, tenderness or weakness (see section 4.8).

Hepatic insufficiency

Due to the unknown effects of the increased exposure to ezetimibe in patients with moderate or severe hepatic insufficiency, 'Ezetrol' is not recommended (see section 5.2).

Fibrates

The safety and efficacy of 'Ezetrol' administered with fibrates have not been established.

If cholelithiasis is suspected in a patient receiving 'Ezetrol' and fenofibrate, gallbladder investigations are indicated and this therapy should be discontinued (see sections 4.5 and 4.8).

Ciclosporin

Caution should be exercised when initiating 'Ezetrol' in the setting of ciclosporin. Ciclosporin concentrations should be monitored in patients receiving 'Ezetrol' and ciclosporin (see section 4.5).

Anticoagulants

If 'Ezetrol' is added to warfarin, another coumarin anticoagulant, or fluindione, the International Normalised Ratio (INR) should be appropriately monitored (see section 4.5).

Excipient

Patients with rare hereditary problems of galactose intolerance, the Lapp lactase deficiency or glucose-galactose malabsorption should not take this medicine.

4.5 Interaction with other medicinal products and other forms of interaction
Interaction studies have only been performed in adults.

In preclinical studies, it has been shown that ezetimibe does not induce cytochrome P450 drug metabolising enzymes. No clinically significant pharmacokinetic interactions have been observed between ezetimibe and drugs known to be metabolised by cytochromes P450 1A2, 2D6, 2C8, 2C9, and 3A4, or N-acetyltransferase.

In clinical interaction studies, ezetimibe had no effect on the pharmacokinetics of dapsone, dextromethorphan, digoxin, oral contraceptives (ethinyl estradiol and levonorgestrel), glipizide, tolbutamide, or midazolam, during co-administration. Cimetidine, co-administered with ezetimibe, had no effect on the bioavailability of ezetimibe.

Antacids: Concomitant antacid administration decreased the rate of absorption of ezetimibe but had no effect on the bioavailability of ezetimibe. This decreased rate of absorption is not considered clinically significant.

Colestyramine: Concomitant colestyramine administration decreased the mean area under the curve (AUC) of total ezetimibe (ezetimibe + ezetimibe glucuronide) approximately 55%. The incremental low-density lipoprotein cholesterol (LDL-C) reduction due to adding 'Ezetrol' to colestyramine may be lessened by this interaction (see section 4.2).

Fibrates: In patients receiving fenofibrate and 'Ezetrol', physicians should be aware of the possible risk of cholelithiasis and gallbladder disease (see section 4.4 and 4.8).

If cholelithiasis is suspected in a patient receiving 'Ezetrol' and fenofibrate, gallbladder investigations are indicated and this therapy should be discontinued (see section 4.8).

Concomitant fenofibrate or gemfibrozil administration modestly increased total ezetimibe concentrations (approximately 1.5- and 1.7-fold respectively).

Co-administration of 'Ezetrol' with other fibrates has not been studied.

Fibrates may increase cholesterol excretion into the bile, leading to cholelithiasis. In animal studies, ezetimibe sometimes increased cholesterol in the gallbladder bile, but not in all species (see section 5.3). A lithogenic risk associated with the therapeutic use of 'Ezetrol' cannot be ruled out.

Statins: No clinically significant pharmacokinetic interactions were seen when ezetimibe was co-administered with atorvastatin, simvastatin, pravastatin, lovastatin, fluvastatin or rosuvastatin.

Ciclosporin: In a study of eight post-renal transplant patients with creatinine clearance of >50 ml/min on a stable dose of ciclosporin, a single 10-mg dose of 'Ezetrol' resulted in a 3.4-fold (range 2.3 to 7.9-fold) increase in the mean AUC for total ezetimibe compared to a healthy control population, receiving ezetimibe alone, from another study (n=17). In a different study, a renal transplant patient with severe renal insufficiency who was receiving ciclosporin and multiple other medications, demonstrated a 12-fold greater exposure to total ezetimibe compared to concurrent controls receiving ezetimibe alone. In a two-period crossover study in 12 healthy subjects, daily administration of 20 mg ezetimibe for 8 days with a single 100-mg dose of ciclosporin on Day 7 resulted in a mean 15 % increase in ciclosporin AUC (range 10 % decrease to 51 % increase) compared to a single 100-mg dose of ciclosporin alone. A controlled study on the effect of co-administered ezetimibe on ciclosporin exposure in renal transplant patients has not been conducted. Caution should be exercised when initiating Ezetrol in the setting of ciclosporin. Ciclosporin concentrations should be monitored in patients receiving Ezetrol and ciclosporin (see section 4.4).

Anticoagulants: Concomitant administration of ezetimibe (10 mg once daily) had no significant effect on bioavailability of warfarin and prothrombin time in a study of twelve healthy adult males. However, there have been post-marketing reports of increased International Normalised Ratio (INR) in patients who had 'Ezetrol' added to warfarin or fluindione. If 'Ezetrol' is added to warfarin, another coumarin anticoagulant, or fluindione, INR should be appropriately monitored (see Section 4.4).

4.6 Pregnancy and lactation

'Ezetrol' co-administered with a statin is contraindicated during pregnancy and lactation (see section 4.3), please refer to the SPC for that particular statin.

Pregnancy:

'Ezetrol' should be given to pregnant women only if clearly necessary. No clinical data are available on the use of 'Ezetrol' during pregnancy. Animal studies on the use of ezetimibe in monotherapy have shown no evidence of direct or indirect harmful effects on pregnancy, embryofoetal development, birth or postnatal development (see section 5.3).

Lactation:

'Ezetrol' should not be used during lactation. Studies on rats have shown that ezetimibe is secreted into breast milk. It is not known if ezetimibe is secreted into human breast milk.

4.7 Effects on ability to drive and use machines

No studies on the effects on the ability to drive and use machines have been performed. However, when driving vehicles or operating machines, it should be taken into account that dizziness has been reported.

4.8 Undesirable effects

Clinical Studies

In clinical studies of up to 112 weeks duration, 'Ezetrol' 10 mg daily was administered alone in 2396 patients, or with a statin in 11,308 patients or with fenofibrate in 185 patients. Adverse reactions were usually mild and transient. The overall incidence of side effects was similar between 'Ezetrol' and placebo. Similarly, the discontinuation rate due to adverse experiences was comparable between 'Ezetrol' and placebo.

'Ezetrol' administered alone or co-administered with a statin:

The following adverse reactions were observed in patients treated with 'Ezetrol' (N=2396) and at a greater incidence than placebo (N=1159) or in patients treated with 'Ezetrol' co-administered with a statin (N=11308) and at a greater incidence than statin administered alone (N=9361):

Frequencies are defined as: very common (≥1/10); common (≥1/100 to <1/10); uncommon (≥1/1,000 to <1/100); rare (≥1/10,000 to <1/1,000) and very rare (<1/10,000)

'Ezetrol' monotherapy

System organ class	Adverse reactions	Frequency
Investigations	ALT and/or AST increased; blood CPK increased; gamma-glutamyltransferase increased; liver function test abnormal	Uncommon
Respiratory, Thoracic and Mediastinal Disorders	cough	Uncommon
Gastrointestinal Disorders	abdominal pain; diarrhoea; flatulence	Common
	dyspepsia; gastrooesophageal reflux disease; nausea	Uncommon
Musculoskeletal and Connective Tissue Disorders	arthralgia; muscle spasms; neck pain	Uncommon
Metabolism and Nutrition Disorders	decreased appetite	Uncommon
Vascular Disorders	hot flush; hypertension	Uncommon
General Disorders and Administration Site Condition	fatigue	Common
	chest pain, pain	Uncommon

Additional adverse reactions with 'Ezetrol' co-administered with a statin

System organ class	Adverse reactions	Frequency
Investigations	ALT and/or AST increased	Common
Nervous System Disorders	headache	Common
	paraesthesia	Uncommon
Gastrointestinal Disorders	dry mouth; gastritis	Uncommon
Skin and Subcutaneous Tissue Disorders	pruritus; rash; urticaria	Uncommon
Musculoskeletal and Connective Tissue Disorders	myalgia	Common
	back pain; muscular weakness; pain in extremity	Uncommon
General Disorders and Administration Site Condition	asthenia; oedema peripheral	Uncommon

'Ezetrol' co-administered with fenofibrate:

Gastrointestinal disorders: abdominal pain.

In a multicentre, double-blind, placebo-controlled, clinical study in patients with mixed hyperlipidaemia, 625 patients were treated for up to 12 weeks and 576 patients for up to 1 year. In this study, 172 patients treated with 'Ezetrol' and fenofibrate completed 12 weeks of therapy, and 230 patients treated with 'Ezetrol' and fenofibrate (including 109 who received 'Ezetrol' alone for the first 12 weeks) completed 1 year of therapy. This study was not designed to compare treatment groups for infrequent events. Incidence rates (95% CI) for clinically important elevations (>3 X ULN, consecutive) in serum transaminases were 4.5% (1.9, 8.8) and 2.7% (1.2, 5.4) for fenofibrate monotherapy and 'Ezetrol' co-administered with fenofibrate, respectively, adjusted for treatment exposure. Corresponding incidence rates for cholecystectomy were 0.6% (0.0, 3.1) and 1.7% (0.6, 4.0) for fenofibrate monotherapy and 'Ezetrol' co-administered with fenofibrate, respectively (see sections 4.4 and 4.5).

Laboratory values

In controlled clinical monotherapy trials, the incidence of clinically important elevations in serum transaminases (ALT and/or AST ≥3 X ULN, consecutive) was similar between 'Ezetrol' (0.5%) and placebo (0.3%). In co-administration trials, the incidence was 1.3% for patients treated with 'Ezetrol' co-administered with a statin and 0.4% for patients treated with a statin alone. These elevations were generally asymptomatic, not associated with cholestasis, and returned to baseline after discontinuation of therapy or with continued treatment. (See section 4.4.)

In clinical trials, CPK >10 X ULN was reported for 4 of 1,674 (0.2%) patients administered 'Ezetrol' alone vs 1 of 786 (0.1%) patients administered placebo, and for 1 of 917 (0.1%) patients co-administered 'Ezetrol' and a statin vs 4 of 929 (0.4%) patients administered a statin alone. There was no excess of myopathy or rhabdomyolysis associated with 'Ezetrol' compared with the relevant control arm (placebo or statin alone). (See section 4.4.)

Post-marketing Experience

The following additional adverse reactions have been reported in post-marketing experience. Because these adverse experiences have been identified from spontaneous reports, their true frequencies are not known and cannot be estimated.

Blood and lymphatic system disorders: thrombocytopenia

Nervous system disorders: dizziness; paraesthesia

Respiratory, thoracic and mediastinal disorders: dyspnoea

Gastro-intestinal disorders: pancreatitis; constipation

Musculoskeletal and connective tissue disorders: myalgia; myopathy/rhabdomyolysis (see section 4.4).

General disorders and administration site conditions: asthenia

Immune system disorders: hypersensitivity, including rash, urticaria, anaphylaxis and angioedema

Hepatobiliary disorders: hepatitis, cholelithiasis, cholecystitis

Psychiatric disorders: depression.

4.9 Overdose

In clinical studies, administration of ezetimibe, 50 mg/day, to 15 healthy subjects for up to 14 days, or 40 mg/day to 18 patients with primary hypercholesterolaemia for up to 56 days, was generally well tolerated. In animals, no toxicity was observed after single oral doses of 5,000 mg/kg of ezetimibe in rats and mice and 3,000 mg/kg in dogs.

A few cases of overdosage with 'Ezetrol' have been reported: most have not been associated with adverse experiences. Reported adverse experiences have not been serious. In the event of an overdose, symptomatic and supportive measures should be employed.

5. PHARMACOLOGICAL PROPERTIES

5.1 Pharmacodynamic properties

Pharmacotherapeutic group: Other lipid modifying agents. ATC code: C10A X09

'Ezetrol' is in a new class of lipid-lowering compounds that selectively inhibit the intestinal absorption of cholesterol and related plant sterols. 'Ezetrol' is orally active, and has a mechanism of action that differs from other classes of cholesterol-reducing compounds (e.g. statins, bile acid sequestrants [resins], fibric acid derivatives, and plant stanols). The molecular target of ezetimibe is the sterol transporter, Niemann-Pick C1-Like 1 (NPC1L1), which is responsible for the intestinal uptake of cholesterol and phytosterols.

Ezetimibe localises at the brush border of the small intestine and inhibits the absorption of cholesterol, leading to a decrease in the delivery of intestinal cholesterol to the liver; statins reduce cholesterol synthesis in the liver and together these distinct mechanisms provide complementary cholesterol reduction. In a 2-week clinical study in 18 hypercholesterolaemic patients, 'Ezetrol' inhibited intestinal cholesterol absorption by 54%, compared with placebo.

A series of preclinical studies was performed to determine the selectivity of ezetimibe for inhibiting cholesterol absorption. Ezetimibe inhibited the absorption of [^{14}C]-cholesterol with no effect on the absorption of triglycerides, fatty acids, bile acids, progesterone, ethinyl estradiol, or fat soluble vitamins A and D.

Epidemiologic studies have established that cardiovascular morbidity and mortality vary directly with the level of total-C and LDL-C and inversely with the level of HDL-C. A beneficial effect of 'Ezetrol' on cardiovascular morbidity and mortality has not yet been demonstrated.

CLINICAL TRIALS

In controlled clinical studies, 'Ezetrol', either as monotherapy or co-administered with a statin significantly reduced total cholesterol (total-C), low-density lipoprotein cholesterol (LDL-C), apolipoprotein B (Apo B), and trigylcerides (TG) and increased high-density lipoprotein cholesterol (HDL-C) in patients with hypercholesterolaemia.

Primary hypercholesterolaemia

In a double-blind, placebo-controlled, 8-week study, 769 patients with hypercholesterolaemia already receiving statin monotherapy and not at National Cholesterol Education Program (NCEP) LDL-C goal (2.6 to 4.1 mmol/l [100 to 160 mg/dl], depending on baseline characteristics) were randomised to receive either 'Ezetrol' 10 mg or placebo in addition to their on-going statin therapy.

Among statin-treated patients not at LDL-C goal at baseline (~82%), significantly more patients randomised to 'Ezetrol' achieved their LDL-C goal at study endpoint compared to patients randomised to placebo, 72% and 19% respectively. The corresponding LDL-C reductions were significantly different (25% and 4% for 'Ezetrol' versus placebo, respectively). In addition, 'Ezetrol', added to on-going statin therapy, significantly decreased total-C, Apo B, TG and increased HDL-C, compared with placebo. 'Ezetrol' or placebo added to statin therapy reduced median C-reactive protein by 10% or 0% from baseline, respectively.

In two, double-blind, randomised placebo-controlled, 12-week studies in 1,719 patients with primary hypercholesterolaemia, 'Ezetrol' 10 mg significantly lowered total-C (13%), LDL-C (19%), Apo B (14%), and TG (8%) and increased HDL-C (3%) compared to placebo. In addition, 'Ezetrol' had no effect on the plasma concentrations of the fat-soluble vitamins A, D, and E, no effect on prothrombin time, and, like other lipid-lowering agents, did not impair adrenocortical steroid hormone production.

Homozygous Familial Hypercholesterolaemia (HoFH)

A double-blind, randomised, 12-week study enrolled 50 patients with a clinical and/or genotypic diagnosis of HoFH, who were receiving atorvastatin or simvastatin (40 mg) with or without concomitant LDL apheresis. 'Ezetrol' co-administered with atorvastatin (40 or 80 mg) or simvastatin (40 or 80 mg), significantly reduced LDL-C by 15% compared with increasing the dose of simvastatin or atorvastatin monotherapy from 40 to 80 mg.

Homozygous sitosterolaemia (phytosterolaemia)

In a double-blind, placebo-controlled, 8-week trial, 37 patients with homozygous sitosterolaemia were randomised to receive 'Ezetrol' 10 mg (n=30) or placebo (n=7). Some patients were receiving other treatments (e.g. statins, resins). 'Ezetrol' significantly lowered the two major plant sterols, sitosterol and campesterol, by 21% and 24% from baseline, respectively. The effects of decreasing sitosterol on morbidity and mortality in this population are not known.

5.2 Pharmacokinetic properties

Absorption: After oral administration, ezetimibe is rapidly absorbed and extensively conjugated to a pharmacologically-active phenolic glucuronide (ezetimibe-glucuronide). Mean maximum plasma concentrations (C_{max}) occur within 1 to 2 hours for ezetimibe-glucuronide and 4 to 12 hours for ezetimibe. The absolute bioavailability of ezetimibe cannot be determined as the compound is virtually insoluble in aqueous media suitable for injection.

Concomitant food administration (high fat or non-fat meals) had no effect on the oral bioavailability of ezetimibe when administered as 'Ezetrol' 10-mg tablets. 'Ezetrol' can be administered with or without food.

Distribution: Ezetimibe and ezetimibe-glucuronide are bound 99.7% and 88 to 92% to human plasma proteins, respectively.

Biotransformation: Ezetimibe is metabolised primarily in the small intestine and liver via glucuronide conjugation (a phase II reaction) with subsequent biliary excretion. Minimal oxidative metabolism (a phase I reaction) has been observed in all species evaluated. Ezetimibe and ezetimibe-glucuronide are the major drug-derived compounds detected in plasma, constituting approximately 10 to 20 % and 80 to 90 % of the total drug in plasma, respectively. Both ezetimibe and ezetimibe-glucuronide are slowly eliminated from plasma with evidence of significant enterohepatic recycling. The half-life for ezetimibe and ezetimibe-glucuronide is approximately 22 hours.

Elimination: Following oral administration of ^{14}C-ezetimibe (20 mg) to human subjects, total ezetimibe accounted for approximately 93% of the total radioactivity in plasma. Approximately 78% and 11% of the administered radioactivity were recovered in the faeces and urine, respectively, over a 10-day collection period. After 48 hours, there were no detectable levels of radioactivity in the plasma.

Special populations:

Paediatric patients

The absorption and metabolism of ezetimibe are similar between children and adolescents (10 to 18 years) and adults. Based on total ezetimibe, there are no pharmacokinetic differences between adolescents and adults. Pharmacokinetic data in the paediatric population < 10 years of age are not available. Clinical experience in paediatric and adolescent patients (ages 9 to 17) has been limited to patients with HoFH or sitosterolaemia.

Geriatric patients

Plasma concentrations for total ezetimibe are about 2-fold higher in the elderly (≥65 years) than in the young (18 to 45 years). LDL-C reduction and safety profile are comparable between elderly and young subjects treated with 'Ezetrol'. Therefore, no dosage adjustment is necessary in the elderly.

Hepatic insufficiency

After a single 10-mg dose of ezetimibe, the mean AUC for total ezetimibe was increased approximately 1.7-fold in patients with mild hepatic insufficiency (Child Pugh score 5 or 6), compared to healthy subjects. In a 14-day, multiple-dose study (10 mg daily) in patients with moderate hepatic insufficiency (Child Pugh score 7 to 9), the mean AUC for total ezetimibe was increased approximately 4-fold on Day 1 and Day 14 compared to healthy subjects. No dosage adjustment is necessary for patients with mild hepatic insufficiency. Due to the unknown effects of the increased exposure to ezetimibe in patients with moderate or severe (Child Pugh score > 9) hepatic insufficiency, 'Ezetrol' is not recommended in these patients (see section 4.4).

Renal insufficiency

After a single 10-mg dose of ezetimibe in patients with severe renal disease (n=8; mean CrCl ≤30 ml/min/1.73m^2), the mean AUC for total ezetimibe was increased approximately 1.5-fold, compared to healthy subjects (n=9). This result is not considered clinically significant. No dosage adjustment is necessary for renally impaired patients.

An additional patient in this study (post-renal transplant and receiving multiple medications, including ciclosporin) had a 12-fold greater exposure to total ezetimibe.

Gender

Plasma concentrations for total ezetimibe are slightly higher (approximately 20%) in women than in men. LDL-C reduction and safety profile are comparable between men and women treated with 'Ezetrol'. Therefore, no dosage adjustment is necessary on the basis of gender.

5.3 Preclinical safety data

Animal studies on the chronic toxicity of ezetimibe identified no target organs for toxic effects. In dogs treated for four weeks with ezetimibe (≥0.03 mg/kg/day) the cholesterol concentration in the cystic bile was increased by a factor of 2.5 to 3.5. However, in a one-year study on dogs given doses of up to 300 mg/kg/day no increased incidence of cholelithiasis or other hepatobiliary effects were observed. The significance of these data for humans is not known. A lithogenic risk associated with the therapeutic use of 'Ezetrol' cannot be ruled out.

In co-administration studies with ezetimibe and statins the toxic effects observed were essentially those typically associated with statins. Some of the toxic effects were more pronounced than observed during treatment with statins alone. This is attributed to pharmacokinetic and pharmacodynamic interactions in co-administration therapy. No such interactions occurred in the clinical studies. Myopathies occurred in rats only after exposure to doses that were several times higher than the human therapeutic dose (approximately 20 times the AUC level for statins and 500 to 2,000 times the AUC level for the active metabolites).

In a series of *in vivo* and *in vitro* assays ezetimibe, given alone or co-administered with statins, exhibited no genotoxic potential. Long-term carcinogenicity tests on ezetimibe were negative.

Ezetimibe had no effect on the fertility of male or female rats, nor was it found to be teratogenic in rats or rabbits, nor did it affect prenatal or postnatal development. Ezetimibe crossed the placental barrier in pregnant rats and rabbits given multiple doses of 1,000 mg/kg/day. The co-administration of ezetimibe and statins was not teratogenic in rats. In pregnant rabbits a small number of skeletal deformities (fused thoracic and caudal vertebrae, reduced number of caudal vertebrae) were observed. The co-administration of ezetimibe with lovastatin resulted in embryolethal effects.

6. PHARMACEUTICAL PARTICULARS

6.1 List of excipients

Croscarmellose sodium

Lactose monohydrate

Magnesium stearate

Microcrystalline cellulose

Povidone (K29-32)

Sodium laurilsulphate

6.2 Incompatibilities

Not applicable.

6.3 Shelf life

3 years.

6.4 Special precautions for storage

Do not store above 30°C.

Blisters: Store in the original package in order to protect from moisture.

Bottles: Keep the bottle tightly closed in order to protect from moisture.

6.5 Nature and contents of container

Unit Dose peelable blisters of clear polychlorotrifluoroethylene/PVC sealed to vinyl coated aluminium backed with paper and polyester in packs of 7, 10, 14, 20, 28, 30, 50, 98, 100, or 300 tablets.

Push through blisters of clear polychlorotrifluoroethylene/PVC sealed to vinyl coated aluminium in packs of 7, 10, 14, 20, 28, 30, 50, 84, 90, 98, 100, or 300 tablets.

Unit dose push through blisters of clear polychlorotrifluoroethylene/PVC coated aluminium in packs of 50, 100, or 300 tablets.

HDPE bottles with polypropylene cap, containing 100 tablets.

Not all pack sizes may be marketed.

6.6 Special precautions for disposal and other handling

No special requirements.

7. MARKETING AUTHORISATION HOLDER

MSD-SP Limited

Hertford Road, Hoddesdon, Hertfordshire EN11 9BU, UK

8. MARKETING AUTHORISATION NUMBER(S)

PL 19945/0001

9. DATE OF FIRST AUTHORISATION/RENEWAL OF THE AUTHORISATION

3 April 2003/ 17 October 2007

10. DATE OF REVISION OF THE TEXT

31 July 2009

LEGAL CATEGORY

POM

® denotes registered trademark of MSP Singapore Company, LLC

SPC.EZE.09.UK.3136

Fareston 60mg Tablets

(Orion Pharma (UK) Limited)

1. NAME OF THE MEDICINAL PRODUCT

Fareston 60 mg tablets

2. QUALITATIVE AND QUANTITATIVE COMPOSITION

Each tablet contains 60 mg toremifene (as citrate).

Excipients: 30 mg lactose per tablet.

For a full list of excipients, see section 6.1.

3. PHARMACEUTICAL FORM

Tablet.

White, round, flat, bevelled edge tablet with TO 60 on one side.

4. CLINICAL PARTICULARS

4.1 Therapeutic indications

First line hormone treatment of hormone-dependent metastatic breast cancer in postmenopausal patients.

Fareston is not recommended for patients with estrogen receptor negative tumours.

4.2 Posology and method of administration

Posology

The recommended dose is 60 mg daily.

Renal impairment

No dose adjustment is needed in patients with renal insufficiency.

Hepatic impairment

Toremifene should be used cautiously in patients with liver impairment(see section 5.2).

Pediatric use

There is no relevant indication for use of Fareston in children.

Method of administration

Toremifene is administered orally. Toremifene can be taken with or without food.

4.3 Contraindications

- Pre-existing endometrial hyperplasia and severe hepatic failure are contra-indications in long-term use of toremifene.

- Hypersensitivity to toremifene or to any of the excipients.

- Both in preclinical investigations and in humans, changes in cardiac electrophysiology have been observed following exposure to toremifene, in the form of QT prolongation. For reasons of drug safety, toremifene is therefore contraindicated in patients with:

- Congenital or documented acquired QT prolongation
- Electrolyte disturbances, particularly in uncorrected hypokalaemia
- Clinically relevant bradycardia
- Clinically relevant heart failure with reduced left-ventricular ejection fraction
- Previous history of symptomatic arrhythmias.

Toremifene should not be used concurrently with other drugs that prolong the QT interval (see also section 4.5).

4.4 Special warnings and precautions for use

Gynaecological examination should be performed before treatment administration, closely looking at pre-existing endometrial abnormality. Afterwards gynaecological examination should be repeated at least once a year. Patients with additional risk of endometrial cancer, e.g. patients suffering from hypertension or diabetes, having high BMI (>30) or history of hormone replacement therapy should be closely monitored (see also section 4.8).

Patients with a history of severe thromboembolic disease should generally not be treated with toremifene(see also section 4.8).

Fareston has been shown to prolong the QTc interval on the electrocardiogram in some patients in a dose-related manner. The following information regarding QT-prolongation is of special importance (for contraindications see section 4.3).

A QT clinical study with a 5-arm parallel design (placebo, moxifloxacin 400 mg, toremifene 20 mg, 80 mg, and 300 mg) has been performed in 250 male patients to characterize the effects of toremifene on the QTc interval duration. The results of this study show a clear positive effect of toremifine in the 80 mg group with mean prolongations of 21 – 26 ms. Regarding the 20 mg group, this effect is significant as well, according to ICH guidelines, with upper confidence interval of 10 – 12 ms. These results strongly suggest an important dose-dependent effect. As women tend to have a longer baseline QTc interval compared with men, they may be more sensitive to QTc-prolonging medications. Elderly patients may also be more susceptible to drug-associated effects on the QT interval.

Fareston should be used with caution in patients with ongoing proarrhythmic conditions (especially elderly patients) such as acute myocardial ischaemia or QT prolongation as this may lead to an increased risk for ventricular arrhythmias (incl. Torsade de pointes) and cardiac arrest (see also section 4.3). If signs or symptoms that may be associated with cardiac arrhythmia occur during treatment with Fareston, treatment should be stopped and an ECG should be performed.

If the QTc interval is >500 ms, Fareston should not be used.

Hypercalcemia may occur at the beginning of toremifene treatment in patients with bone metastasis and thus these patients should be closely monitored.

There are no systematic data available from patients with labile diabetes, from patients with severely altered performance status or from patients with cardiac failure.

Fareston tablets contain lactose (30 mg/tablet). Patients with rare hereditary problems of galactose intolerance, the Lapp lactase deficiency or glucose-galactose malabsorption should not take this medicine.

4.5 Interaction with other medicinal products and other forms of interaction

An additive effect on QT interval prolongation between Fareston and the following drugs and other medicinal products that may prolong the QTc interval cannot be excluded. This might lead to an increased risk of ventricular arrhythmias, including Torsade de points. Therefore co-administration of Fareston with any of the following medicinal products is contraindicated (see also section 4.3):

- antiarrhythmics class 1A (e.g. quinidine, hydroquinidine, disopyramide) or

- antiarrhythmics class III (e.g. amiodarone, sotalol, dofetilide, ibutilide).

- neuroleptics (e.g. phenothiazines, pimozide, sertindole, haloperidol, sultopride).

- certain antimimicrobials agents (moxifloxacin, erythromycin IV, pentamidine, antimalarials particularly halofantrine).

- certain antihistaminics (terfenadine, astemizole, mizolastine).

- others (cisapride, vincamine IV, bepridil, diphemanil).

Drugs which decrease renal calcium excretion, e.g. thiazide, diuretics, may increase the risk of hypercalcaemia.

Enzyme inducers, like phenobarbital, phenytoin and carbamazepine, may increase the rate of toremifene metabolism thus lowering the steady-state concentration in serum. In such cases doubling of the daily dose may be necessary.

There is a known interaction between anti-estrogens and warfarin-type anticoagulants leading to a seriously increased bleeding time. Therefore, the concomitant use of toremifene with such drugs should be avoided.

Theoretically the metabolism of toremifene is inhibited by drugs known to inhibit the CYP 3A enzyme system which is reported to be responsible for its main metabolic pathways. Examples of such drugs are ketoconazole and similar antimycotics, erythromycin and troleandomycin. Concomitant use of those drugs with toremifene should be carefully considered.

4.6 Pregnancy and lactation

Toremifene is recommended for postmenopausal patients.

There are no adequate data from the use of Fareston in pregnant women. Studies in animals have shown reproductive toxicity (see section 5.3). The potential risk for humans is unknown.

Fareston should not be used during pregnancy.

In rats, decreased body weight gain of the offspring during lactation was observed.

Fareston should not be used during lactation.

4.7 Effects on ability to drive and use machines

Toremifene has no influence on the ability to drive and use machines.

4.8 Undesirable effects

The most frequent adverse reactions are hot flushes, sweating, uterine bleeding, leukorrhea, fatigue, nausea, rash, itching, dizziness and depression. The reactions are usually mild and mostly due to the hormonal action of toremifene.

The frequencies of the adverse reactions are classified as follows:

Very common (⩾ 1/10)

Common (⩾1/100 to <1/10)

Uncommon (⩾1/1,000 to <1/100)

Rare (⩾1/10,000 to <1/1,000)

Very rare (<1/10,000), not known (cannot be estimated from the available data).

(see Table 1 below)

Thromboembolic events include deep venous thrombosis, thrombophlebitis and pulmonary embolism (see also section 4.4).

Toremifene treatment has been associated with changes in liver enzyme levels (increases of transaminases) and in very rare occasions with more severe liver function abnormalities (jaundice).

A few cases of hypercalcaemia have been reported in patients with bone metastases at the beginning of toremifene treatment.

Endometrial hypertrophy may develop during the treatment due to the partial estrogenic effect of toremifene. There is a risk of increased endometrial changes including hyperplasia, polyps and cancer. This may be due to the underlying mechanism/estrogenic stimulation (see also section 4.4).

Fareston increases the QT interval in a dose-related manner (see also section 4.4).

Table 1

System organ class	Very Common	Common	Uncommon	Rare	Very rare
Neoplasms benign, malignant and unspecified (including cysts and polyps)					endometrial cancer
Metabolism and nutrition disorders			loss of appetite		
Psychiatric disorders		depression	Insomnia		
Nervous system disorders		dizziness	headache		
Eye disorders					transient corneal opacity
Ear and labyrinth disorders				vertigo	
Vascular disorders	hot flushes		thromboembolic events		
Respiratory, thoracic and mediastinal disorders			dyspnoea		
Gastrointestinal disorders		nausea, vomiting	constipation		
Hepatobiliary disorders				increase of transaminases	jaundice
Skin and subcutaneous tissue disorders	sweating	rash, itching			alopecia
Reproductive system and breast disorders		uterine bleeding leukorrhea	endometrial hypertrophy	endometrial polyps	endometrial hyperplasia.
General disorders and administration site conditions		fatigue oedema	weight increase		

4.9 Overdose
Vertigo, headache and dizziness were observed in healthy volunteer studies at daily dose of 680 mg. The dose-related QTc interval prolongation potential of Fareston should also be taken into account in cases of overdose. There is no specific antidote and the treatment is symptomatic

5. PHARMACOLOGICAL PROPERTIES

5.1 Pharmacodynamic properties
Pharmacotherapeutic group: Anti-estrogens, ATC code: L02BA02

Toremifene is a nonsteroidal triphenylethylene derivative. As other members of this class, e.g. tamoxifen and clomifene, toremifene binds to estrogen receptors and may produce estrogenic, anti-estrogenic or both effects, depending upon the duration of treatment, animal species, gender, target organ and variable selected. In general, however, nonsteroidal triphenylethylene derivatives are predominantly anti-estrogenic in rats and man and estrogenic in mice.

In post-menopausal breast cancer patients, toremifene treatment is associated with modest reductions in both total serum cholesterol and low density lipoprotein (LDL).

Toremifene binds specifically to estrogen receptors, competitively with estradiol, and inhibits oestrogen-induced stimulation of DNA synthesis and cell replication. In some experimental cancers and/or using high-dose, toremifene displays anti-tumour effects which are not estrogen-dependent.

The anti-tumour effect of toremifene in breast cancer is mainly due to the anti-estrogenic effect, although other mechanisms (changes in oncogene expression, growth factor secretion, induction of apoptosis and influence on cell cycle kinetics) may also be involved in the anti-tumour effect.

5.2 Pharmacokinetic properties

Absorption

Toremifene is readily absorbed after oral administration. Peak concentrations in serum are obtained within 3 (range 2 - 5) hours. Food intake has no effect on the extent of absorption but may delay the peak concentrations by 1.5 - 2 hours. The changes due to food intake are not clinically significant.

Distribution

The serum concentration curve can be described by a biexponential equation. The half-life of the first (distribution) phase is 4 (range 2 - 12) hours, and of the second (elimination) phase 5 (range 2 - 10) days. The basal disposition parameters (CL and V) could not be estimated due to the lack of intravenous study. Toremifene binds extensively (> 99.5 %) to serum proteins, mainly to albumin. Toremifene obeys linear serum kinetics at oral daily doses between 11 and 680 mg. The mean concentration of toremifene at steady-state is 0.9 (range 0.6 - 1.3) μg/ml at the recommended dose of 60 mg per day.

Metabolism

Toremifene is extensively metabolised. In human serum the main metabolite is N-demethyltoremifene with mean half-life of 11 (range 4 - 20) days. Its steady-state concentrations are about twice compared to those of the parent compound. It has similar anti-estrogenic, albeit weaker anti-tumour activity than the parent compound.

It is bound to plasma proteins even more extensively than toremifene, the protein bound fraction being > 99.9 %. Three minor metabolites have been detected in human serum: (deaminohydroxy)toremifene, 4-hydroxytoremifene, and N,N-didemethyltoremifene. Although they have theoretically interesting hormonal effects, their concentrations during toremifene treatment are too low to have any major biological importance.

Elimination

Toremifene is eliminated mainly as metabolites to the faeces. Enterohepatic circulation can be expected. About 10 % of the administered dose is eliminated via urine as metabolites. Owing to the slow elimination, steady-state concentrations in serum are reached in 4 to 6 weeks.

Characteristics in patients

Clinical anti-tumour efficacy and serum concentrations have no positive correlation at the recommended daily dose of 60 mg.

No information is available concerning polymorphic metabolism. Enzyme complex, known to be responsible for the metabolism of toremifene in humans, is cytochrome P450-dependent hepatic mixed function oxidase. The main metabolic pathway, N-demethylation, is mediated mainly by CYP 3A.

Pharmacokinetics of toremifene were investigated in an open study with four parallel groups of ten subjects: normal subjects, patients with impaired (mean AST 57 U/L - mean ALT 76 U/L - mean gamma GT 329 U/L) or activated liver function (mean AST 25 U/L - mean ALT 30 U/L - mean gamma GT 91 U/L - patients treated with antiepileptics) and patients with impaired renal function (creatinine: 176 μmol/L). In this study the kinetics of toremifene in patients with impaired renal function were not significantly altered as compared to normal subjects. The elimination of toremifene and its metabolites was significantly increased in patients with activated liver function and decreased in patients with impaired liver function.

5.3 Preclinical safety data
The acute toxicity of toremifene is low with LD-50 in rats and mice of more than 2000 mg/kg. In repeated toxicity studies the cause of death in rats is gastric dilatation. In the acute and chronic toxicity studies most of the findings are related to the hormonal effects of toremifene. The other findings are not toxicologically significant. Toremifene has not shown any genotoxicity and has not been found to be carcinogenic in rats. In mice, estrogens induce ovarian and testicular tumours as well as hyperostosis and osteosarcomas. Toremifene has a species-specific estrogen-like effect in mice and causes similar tumours. These findings are postulated to be of little relevance for the safety in man, where toremifene acts mainly as an anti-estrogen.

Non-clinical *in vitro* and *in vivo* studies have evidenced the potential of toremifene and its metabolite to prolong cardiac repolarisation and this can be attributed to the blockade of hERG channels.

In vivo, high plasma concentrations in monkeys caused a 24% prolongation in QTc, which is in line with QTc findings in humans.

It is also to be noted that the C_{max} observed in the monkeys (1800 ng/ml) is two-fold compared to the mean C_{max} observed in humans at a daily dose of 60 mg.

Action potential studies in isoloated rabbit heart have shown that toremifene induce cardiac electrophysiological changes which start to develop at concentrations approximately 10 fold compared to the calculated free therapeutic plasma concentration in human.

6. PHARMACEUTICAL PARTICULARS

6.1 List of excipients
Maize starch

Lactose

Povidone

Sodium starch glycolate

Magnesium stearate

Cellulose, microcrystalline

Silica, colloidal anhydrous

6.2 Incompatibilities
Not applicable.

6.3 Shelf life
5 years.

6.4 Special precautions for storage
This medicinal product does not require any special storage conditions.

6.5 Nature and contents of container
Green PVC foil and aluminium foil blister in a cardboard box.

Package sizes: 30 and 100 tablets.

Not all pack sizes may be marketed.

6.6 Special precautions for disposal and other handling
No special requirements.

7. MARKETING AUTHORISATION HOLDER
Orion Corporation
Orionintie 1
FIN-02200 Espoo
Finland

8. MARKETING AUTHORISATION NUMBER(S)
EU/1/96/004/001
EU/1/96/004/002

9. DATE OF FIRST AUTHORISATION/RENEWAL OF THE AUTHORISATION
14 February 1996/2 February 2006

10. DATE OF REVISION OF THE TEXT
January 2009

Detailed information on this medicinal product is available on the website of the European Medicines Agency (EMEA) http://www.emea.europa.eu/

Fasigyn

(Pfizer Limited)

1. NAME OF THE MEDICINAL PRODUCT
FASIGYN

2. QUALITATIVE AND QUANTITATIVE COMPOSITION
Tinidazole 500mg

3. PHARMACEUTICAL FORM
Film-coated tablets

White, round, biconvex film-coated tablet embossed on one side with "FAS 500"

4. CLINICAL PARTICULARS

4.1 Therapeutic indications
Treatment of the following infections:

• Eradication of *Helicobacter pylori* associated with duodenal ulcers, in the presence of antibiotic and acid suppressant therapy. (See 'Posology and method of administration'.)

• Anaerobic infections such as:

Intraperitoneal infections: peritonitis, abscess.

Gynaecological infections: endometritis, endomyometritis, tube-ovarian abscess.

Bacterial septicaemia.

Post-operative wound infections.

Skin and soft tissue infections.

Upper and lower respiratory tract infections: pneumonia, empyema, lung abscess.

• Non-specific vaginitis.

• Acute ulcerative gingivitis.

• Urogenital trichomoniasis in both male and female patients.

• Giardiasis.

• Intestinal amoebiasis.

• Amoebic involvement of the liver.

Prophylaxis

The prevention of post-operative infections caused by anaerobic bacteria, especially those associated with colonic, gastro-intestinal and gynaecological surgery.

4.2 Posology and method of administration
Oral administration during or after a meal.

•Eradication of H.pylori associated with duodenal ulcers

Adults The usual dose of Fasigyn is 500mg twice daily coadministered with omeprazole 20mg twice daily and clarithromycin 250mg twice daily for 7 days. Clinical studies using this 7 day regimen have shown similar *H.pylori* eradication rates when omeprazole 20mg once daily was used. For further information on the dosage for omeprazole see Astra data sheet.

•Anaerobic infections

Adults An initial dose of 2g the first day followed by 1g daily given as a single dose or as 500mg twice daily. Treatment for 5 to 6 days will generally be adequate but clinical judgement must be used in determining the duration of therapy, particularly when eradication of infection from certain sites may be difficult. Routine clinical and laboratory observation is recommended if it is considered necessary to continue therapy for more than 7 days.

Children < 12 years – there is no data available.

•Non-specific vaginitis

Adults Non-specific vaginitis has been successfully treated with a single oral dose of 2g. Higher cure rates have been achieved with 2g single doses on 2 consecutive days (total dose 4g).

•Acute ulcerative gingivitis

Adults A single oral dose of 2g.

•Urogenital trichomoniasis

(When infection with *Trichomonas vaginalis* is confirmed, simultaneous treatment of the consort is recommended).

Adults A single dose of 2g.

Children A single dose of 50 to 75mg/kg of body weight. It may be necessary to repeat this dose.

• Giardiasis

Adults A single dose of 2g.

Children A single dose of 50 to 75mg/kg of body weight. It may be necessary to repeat this dose.

•Intestinal amoebiasis

Adults A single daily dose of 2g for 2 to 3 days.

Children A single daily dose of 50 to 60mg/kg of body weight on each of 3 successive days.

•Amoebic involvement in the liver

Adults Total dosage varies from 4.5 to 12g, depending on the virulence of the *Entamoeba histolytica*.

For amoebic involvement of the liver, the aspiration of pus may be required in addition to therapy with Fasigyn.

Initiate treatment with 1.5 to 2g as a single oral daily dose for three days. Occasionally when a three-day course is ineffective, treatment may be continued for up to six days.

Children A single dose of 50 to 60 mg/kg of body weight per day for five successive days.

•Use in Renal Impairment

Dosage adjustments in patients with impaired renal function are generally not necessary. However because tinidazole is easily removed by haemodialysis, patients may require additional doses of tinidazole to compensate.

•Prevention of post-operative infection

Adults A single dose of 2g approximately 12 hours before surgery.

Children < 12 years – there is no data available.

Use in the elderly There are no special recommendations for this age group.

4.3 Contraindications
As with other drugs of similar structure, tinidazole is contraindicated in patients having, or with a history of, blood dyscrasia, although no persistent haematological abnormalities have been noted in clinical or animal studies.

Tinidazole should be avoided in patients with organic neurological disorders.

Tinidazole, other 5-nitroimidazole derivatives or any of the components of this product should not be administered to patients with known hypersensitivity to the drug.

Use of tinidazole is contraindicated during the first trimester of pregnancy and in nursing mothers. See Section 4.6 'Pregnancy and lactation'.

4.4 Special warnings and precautions for use

As with related compounds, alcoholic beverages should be avoided during Fasigyn therapy because of the possibility of a disulfiram-like reaction (flushing, abdominal cramps, vomiting, tachycardia). Alcohol should be avoided until 72 hours after discontinuing Fasigyn.

Drugs of similar chemical structure have also produced various neurological disturbances such as dizziness, vertigo, in-coordination and ataxia. If during therapy with Fasigyn abnormal neurological signs develop, therapy should be discontinued.

4.5 Interaction with other medicinal products and other forms of interaction

Alcohol: Concurrent use of tinidazole and alcohol may produce a disulfiram-like reaction and should be avoided. (See Section 4.4 – Special Warnings and Special Precautions for Use).

Anticoagulants: Drugs of similar chemical structure have been shown to potentiate the effects of oral anticoagulants. Prothrombin times should be closely monitored and adjustments to the dose of the anticoagulant should be made as necessary.

4.6 Pregnancy and lactation

Use in pregnancy: Fertility studies in rats receiving 100mg and 300mg tinidazole/kg had no effect on fertility, adult and pup weights, gestation, viability or lactation. There was a slight, not significant, increase in resorption rate at the 300mg/kg dose.

Tinidazole crosses the placental barrier. Since the effects of compounds of this class on foetal development are unknown, the use of tinidazole during the first trimester is contraindicated. There is no evidence that Fasigyn is harmful during the latter stages of pregnancy, but its use during the second and third trimesters requires that the potential benefits be weighed against possible hazards to mother or foetus.

Use in lactation: Tinidazole is excreted in breast milk. Tinidazole may continue to appear in breast milk for more than 72 hours after administration. Women should not nurse until at least 3 days after having discontinued taking Fasigyn.

4.7 Effects on ability to drive and use machines

No special precautions should be necessary. However, drugs of similar chemical structure, including Fasigyn, have been associated with various neurological disturbances such as dizziness, vertigo, ataxia, peripheral neuropathy (paraesthesia, sensory disturbances, hypoaesthesia) and rarely convulsions. If any abnormal neurological signs develop during Fasigyn therapy, the drug should be discontinued.

4.8 Undesirable effects

Reported side effects have generally been infrequent, mild and self-limiting.

Blood and lymphatic system disorders: transient leukopenia

Nervous System: ataxia, convulsions (rarely), dizziness, headache, hypesthesia, parathesia, peripheral neuropathy, sensory disturbances, vertigo, metallic taste, flushing.

Gastrointestinal disorders: abdominal pain, anorexia, diarrhoea, furry tongue, glossitis, nausea, stomatitis, vomiting

Skin and subcutaneous tissue disorders: hypersensitivity reactions, occasionally severe, may occur in rare cases in the form of skin rash, puritus, urticaria and angioneurotic edema

Renal and Urinary disorders: dark urine

General disoders and administration site conditions: fever, tiredness

4.9 Overdose

In acute animal studies with mice and rats, the LD50 for mice was >3600mg/kg and >2300mg/kg for oral and intraperitoneal administration respectively. For rats, the LD50 was >2000mg/kg for both oral and intraperitoneal administration.

Signs and symptoms of overdosage There are no reported overdoses in humans with Fasigyn.

Treatment for overdosage There is no specific antidote for treatment of overdosage with tinidazole. Treatment is symptomatic and supportive. Gastric lavage may be useful. Tinidazole is easily dialysable.

5. PHARMACOLOGICAL PROPERTIES

5.1 Pharmacodynamic properties

Fasigyn is active against both protozoa and obligate anaerobic bacteria. The activity against protozoa involves *Trichomonas vaginalis, Entamoeba histolytica* and *Giardia lamblia.*

The mode of action of Fasigyn against anaerobic bacteria and protozoa involves penetration of the drug into the cell of the micro-organism and subsequent damage of DNA strands or inhibition of their synthesis.

Fasigyn is active against *Helicobacter pylori, Gardnerella vaginalis* and most anaerobic bacteria including *Bacteroides fragilis, Bacteroides melaninogenicus, Bacteroides* spp., *Clostridium* spp., *Eubacterium* spp., *Fusobacterium* spp., *Peptococcus* spp., *Peptostreptococcus* spp. and *Veillonella* spp.

Helicobacter pylori (H. pylori) is associated with acid peptic disease including duodenal ulcer and gastric ulcer in which about 95% and 80% of patients respectively are infected with this agent. *H. pylori* is also implicated as a major contributing factor in the development of gastritis and ulcer recurrence in such patients. Evidence suggests a causative link between *H. pylori* and gastric carcinoma.

Clinical evidence has shown that the combination of Fasigyn with omeprazole and clarithromycin eradicates 91-96% of *H. pylori* isolates.

Various different *H. pylori* eradication regimens have shown that eradication of *H. pylori* heals duodenal ulcers and reduces the risk of ulcer recurrence.

5.2 Pharmacokinetic properties

Fasigyn is rapidly and completely absorbed following oral administration. In studies with healthy volunteers receiving 2g tinidazole orally, peak serum levels of 40-51 micrograms/ml were achieved within two hours and decreased to between 11-19 micrograms/ml at 24 hours. Healthy volunteers who received 800mg and 1.6g tinidazole IV over 10-15 minutes achieved peak plasma concentrations that ranged from 14 to 21mcg/ml for the 800mg dose and averaged 32mcg/ml for the 1.6g dose. At 24 hours post-infusion, plasma levels of tinidazole decreased to 4-5mcg/ml and 8.6mcg/ml respectively, justifying once daily dosing. Plasma levels decline slowly and tinidazole can be detected in plasma at concentrations of up to 1 microgram/ml at 72 hours after oral administration. The plasma elimination half-life for tinidazole is between 12-14 hours.

Tinidazole is widely distributed in all body tissues and also crosses the blood brain barrier, obtaining clinically effective concentrations in all tissues. The apparent volume of distribution is about 50 litres. About 12% of plasma tinidazole is bound to plasma protein.

Tinidazole is excreted by the liver and kidneys. Studies in healthy patients have shown that over 5 days, 60-65% of an administered dose is excreted by the kidneys with 20-25% of the administered dose excreted as unchanged tinidazole. Up to 5% of the administered dose is excreted in the faeces.

Studies in patients with renal failure (creatinine clearance <22ml/min) indicate that there is no statistically significant change in tinidazole pharmacokinetic parameters in these patients. (See section 4.2 – Posology and Method of Administration).

5.3 Preclinical safety data

None.

6. PHARMACEUTICAL PARTICULARS

6.1 List of excipients

Fasigyn tablets contain the following ingredients:

Tablet core: microcrystalline cellulose (Avicel PH 101), alginic acid, maize starch, magnesium stearate and sodium lauryl sulphate.

Film coating: hydroxypropyl methyl cellulose, propylene glycol, titanium dioxide (E171).

6.2 Incompatibilities

No major incompatibilities have been noted.

6.3 Shelf life

3 years.

6.4 Special precautions for storage

Store below 25°C in a dry place in the absence of light.

6.5 Nature and contents of container

Fasigyn tablets will be supplied in aluminium foil backed blister packs of 16 500mg tablets consisting of:

a) 250 micron PVC blister coated with 40gsm of PVdC

b) 20 micron aluminium foil backing coated with 20gsm PVdC.

6.6 Special precautions for disposal and other handling

Fasigyn tablets should be swallowed whole.

7. MARKETING AUTHORISATION HOLDER

Pfizer Limited

Ramsgate Road

Sandwich

Kent CT13 9NJ

United Kingdom

8. MARKETING AUTHORISATION NUMBER(S)

PL 00057/0150

9. DATE OF FIRST AUTHORISATION/RENEWAL OF THE AUTHORISATION

22 December 1994

10. DATE OF REVISION OF THE TEXT

December 2008

Legal Category

POM

FAS3_0

Faslodex 250 mg/5 ml solution for injection

(AstraZeneca UK Limited)

1. NAME OF THE MEDICINAL PRODUCT

Faslodex 250 mg/5 ml solution for injection.

2. QUALITATIVE AND QUANTITATIVE COMPOSITION

One pre-filled syringe contains 250 mg fulvestrant in 5 ml solution.

For excipients, see 6.1.

3. PHARMACEUTICAL FORM

Solution for injection.

Clear, colourless to yellow, viscous liquid.

4. CLINICAL PARTICULARS

4.1 Therapeutic indications

Faslodex is indicated for the treatment of postmenopausal women with oestrogen receptor positive, locally advanced or metastatic breast cancer for disease relapse on or after adjuvant antioestrogen therapy or disease progression on therapy with an antioestrogen.

4.2 Posology and method of administration

Adult females (including the elderly):

The recommended dose is 250 mg at intervals of 1 month.

Children and adolescents:

Faslodex is not recommended for use in children or adolescents, as safety and efficacy have not been established in this age group.

Patients with renal impairment:

No dose adjustments are recommended for patients with mild to moderate renal impairment (creatinine clearance ≥ 30 ml/min). Safety and efficacy have not been evaluated in patients with severe renal impairment (creatinine clearance < 30 ml/min) (see 4.4).

Patients with hepatic impairment:

No dose adjustments are recommended for patients with mild to moderate hepatic impairment. However, as fulvestrant exposure may be increased, Faslodex should be used with caution in these patients. There are no data in patients with severe hepatic impairment (see 4.3, 4.4 and 5.2).

Method of administration:

Administer intramuscularly slowly into the buttock. For full administration instructions see 6.6.

4.3 Contraindications

Faslodex is contraindicated in:

- patients with known hypersensitivity to the active substance or to any of the excipients
- pregnancy and in breast-feeding (see 4.6)
- severe hepatic impairment

4.4 Special warnings and precautions for use

Use Faslodex with caution in patients with mild to moderate, hepatic impairment (see 4.2, 4.3 and 5.2).

Use Faslodex with caution in patients with severe renal impairment (creatinine clearance less than 30 ml/min) (see 5.2).

Due to the route of administration, use Faslodex with caution if treating patients with bleeding diatheses, thrombocytopenia or those taking anticoagulant treatment.

Thromboembolic events are commonly observed in women with advanced breast cancer and have been observed in clinical trials (see 4.8). This should be taken into consideration when prescribing Faslodex to patients at risk.

There are no long-term data on the effect of fulvestrant on bone. Due to the mode of action of fulvestrant, there is a potential risk of osteoporosis.

4.5 Interaction with other medicinal products and other forms of interaction

A clinical interaction study with midazolam demonstrated that fulvestrant does not inhibit CYP 3A4.

Clinical interaction studies with rifampicin (inducer of CYP 3A4) and ketoconazole (inhibitor of CYP 3A4) showed no clinically relevant change in fulvestrant clearance. Dosage adjustment is therefore not necessary in patients who are co-prescribed fulvestrant and CYP 3A4 inhibitors or inducers.

4.6 Pregnancy and lactation

Faslodex is contraindicated in pregnancy (see 4.3). Fulvestrant has been shown to cross the placenta after single intramuscular doses in rat and rabbit. Studies in animals have shown reproductive toxicity including an increased incidence of foetal abnormalities and deaths (see 5.3). If pregnancy occurs while taking Faslodex the patient must be informed of the potential hazard to the foetus and potential risk for loss of pregnancy.

Fulvestrant is excreted in milk in lactating rats. It is not known whether fulvestrant is excreted in human milk. Considering the potential for serious adverse reactions due to fulvestrant in breast-fed infants, breast-feeding is contra-indicated (see 4.3).

4.7 Effects on ability to drive and use machines

Faslodex has no or negligible influence on the ability to drive or use machines. However, during treatment with

Faslodex, asthenia has been reported. Therefore caution must be observed by those patients who experience this symptom when driving or operating machinery.

4.8 Undesirable effects

Approximately 47% of patients experienced adverse reactions in the clinical trial programme. However, only 0.9% of patients stopped therapy because of an adverse reaction. The most commonly reported adverse reactions are hot flushes, nausea, and injection site reactions.

The adverse reactions are summarised as follows:

(see Table 1 below)

4.9 Overdose

There is no human experience of overdosage. Animal studies suggest that no effects other than those related directly or indirectly to anti-oestrogenic activity were evident with higher doses of fulvestrant. If overdose occurs, manage symptomatically.

5. PHARMACOLOGICAL PROPERTIES

5.1 Pharmacodynamic properties

Pharmacotherapeutic group: anti-oestrogen, ATC code: L02BA03

Fulvestrant is an oestrogen receptor antagonist and binds to oestrogen receptors in a competitive manner with an affinity comparable with that of oestradiol. Fulvestrant blocks the trophic actions of oestrogens without itself having any partial agonist (oestrogen-like) activity. The mode of action is associated with down-regulation of oestrogen receptor (ER) protein.

Clinical trials in postmenopausal women with primary breast cancer have shown that fulvestrant significantly down-regulates ER protein in ER positive tumours compared with placebo. There was also a significant decrease in progesterone receptor expression consistent with a lack of intrinsic oestrogen agonist effects.

Effects on advanced breast cancer

Two Phase III clinical trials were completed in a total of 851 postmenopausal women with advanced breast cancer who had disease recurrence on or after adjuvant endocrine therapy or progression following endocrine therapy for advanced disease. 77% of the study population had oestrogen receptor positive breast cancer. These trials compared the safety and efficacy of monthly administration of 250 mg fulvestrant with a third-generation aromatase inhibitor, anastrozole, at a daily dose of 1 mg.

Overall, fulvestrant at the 250 mg monthly dose was at least as effective as anastrozole in terms of time to progression, objective response, and time to death. There were no statistically significant differences in any of these endpoints between the two treatment groups. Time to progression was the primary endpoint. Combined analysis of both trials showed that 83% of patients who received fulvestrant progressed, compared with 85% of patients who received anastrozole. The hazard ratio of fulvestrant to anastrozole for time to progression was 0.95 (95% CI 0.82 to 1.10). The objective response rate for fulvestrant was 19.2% compared with 16.5% for anastrozole. The median time to death was 27.4 months for patients treated with fulvestrant and 27.6 months for patients treated with anastrozole. The hazard ratio of fulvestrant to anastrozole for time to death was 1.01 (95% CI 0.86 to 1.19). Analysis of results by ER status showed that the use of fulvestrant should be restricted to patients with ER positive breast cancer.

Effects on the postmenopausal endometrium

Preclinical data suggest that fulvestrant will not have a stimulatory effect on the postmenopausal endometrium. A 2-week study in healthy postmenopausal volunteers showed that compared to placebo, pre-treatment with 250 mg fulvestrant resulted in significantly reduced stimulation of the postmenopausal endometrium, as judged by ultrasound measurement of endometrium thickness, in volunteers treated with 20 micrograms per day ethinyl oestradiol.

There are no data on the long-term effects of fulvestrant on the postmenopausal endometrium. No data are available regarding endometrial morphology.

In two studies with premenopausal patients with benign gynaecologic disease, no significant differences in endometrial thickness were observed (measured with ultrasound) between fulvestrant and placebo. However, the duration of treatment was short (1, and 12 weeks, respectively).

Effects on bone

There are no long-term data on the effect of fulvestrant on bone.

5.2 Pharmacokinetic properties

Absorption:

After administration of Faslodex long-acting intramuscular injection, fulvestrant is slowly absorbed and maximum plasma concentrations are reached after about 7 days. Absorption continues for over one month and monthly administration results in an approximate 2-fold accumulation. Steady-state levels are reached after about 6 doses during monthly injections with the major part of the accumulation achieved after 3-4 doses. The terminal half-life is governed by the absorption rate and was estimated to be 50 days. At steady state, fulvestrant plasma concentrations are maintained within a relatively narrow range with approximately 2- to 3-fold difference between maximum and trough concentrations.

After intramuscular administration, the exposure is approximately dose proportional in the dose range 50 to 250 mg.

Distribution:

Fulvestrant is subject to extensive and rapid distribution. The apparent volume of distribution at steady state is large (approximately 3 to 5 l/kg), which suggests that the compound distribution is largely extravascular. Fulvestrant is highly (99%) bound to plasma proteins. Very low density lipoprotein (VLDL), low density lipoprotein (LDL), and high density lipoprotein (HDL) fractions are the major binding components. Therefore no drug interaction studies were conducted on competitive protein binding. The role of sex hormone-binding globulin has not been determined.

Metabolism:

The metabolism of fulvestrant has not been fully evaluated, but involves combinations of a number of possible biotransformation pathways analogous to those of endogenous steroids (includes 17-ketone, sulphone, 3-sulphate, 3- and 17-glucuronide metabolites). Identified metabolites are either less active or exhibit similar activity to fulvestrant in anti-oestrogen models. Studies using human liver preparations and recombinant human enzymes indicate that CYP 3A4 is the only P450 isoenzyme involved in the oxidation of fulvestrant, however non-P450 routes appear to be more predominant *in vivo*. *In vitro* data suggest that fulvestrant does not inhibit CYP450 isoenzymes.

Table 1

Body System/ Frequency	Very Common (>1/10)	Common (>1/100, <1/10)	Uncommon (>1/1000, <1/100)
Cardiovascular	• Hot flushes		
Gastrointestinal		• Gastrointestinal disturbance including nausea, vomiting, diarrhoea and anorexia.	
Hepatobiliary disorders		• Elevated liver enzymes, the vast majority <2xULN	
Reproductive and breast			• Vaginal haemorrhage • Vaginal moniliasis • Leukorrhea
Skin		• Rash	• Hypersensitivity reactions, including angioedema and urticaria
Urogenital		• Urinary tract infections	
Vascular		• Venous thromboembolism	
Whole body		• Injection site reactions including transient pain and inflammation in 7% of patients (1% of injections) when given as a single 5 ml injection. • Headache • Asthenia • Back pain	

Elimination:

Fulvestrant is eliminated mainly by metabolism. The major route of excretion is via the faeces with less than 1% being excreted in the urine. Fulvestrant has a high clearance, 11±1.7 ml/min/kg, suggesting a high hepatic extraction ratio.

Special populations:

In a population pharmacokinetic analysis of data from Phase III studies, no difference in fulvestrant pharmacokinetic profile was detected with regard to age (range 33 to 89 years), weight (40-127 kg) or race.

Renal impairment

Mild to moderate impairment of renal function did not influence the pharmacokinetics of fulvestrant to any clinically relevant extent.

Hepatic impairment

The pharmacokinetics of fulvestrant has been evaluated in a single-dose clinical trial conducted in subjects with Child-Pugh category A and B hepatic impairment due to cirrhosis. A high dose of a shorter duration intramuscular injection formulation was used. There was up to about 2.5-fold increase in AUC in subjects with hepatic impairment compared to healthy subjects. In patients administered Faslodex, an increase in exposure of this magnitude is expected to be well tolerated. Child-Pugh category C subjects were not evaluated.

5.3 Preclinical safety data

The acute toxicity of fulvestrant is low.

Faslodex and other formulations of fulvestrant were well tolerated in animal species used in multiple dose studies. Local reactions, including myositis and granulomatoma at the injection site were attributed to the vehicle but the severity of myositis in rabbits increased with fulvestrant, compared to the saline control. In toxicity studies with multiple intramuscular doses of fulvestrant in rats and dogs, the anti-oestrogenic activity of fulvestrant was responsible for most of the effects seen, particularly in the female reproductive system, but also in other organs sensitive to hormones in both sexes.

In dog studies following oral and intravenous administration, effects on the cardiovascular system (slight elevations of the S-T segment of the ECG [oral], and sinus arrest in one dog [intravenous]) were seen. These occurred at exposure levels higher than in patients (C_{max} >40 times) and are likely to be of limited significance for human safety at the clinical dose.

Fulvestrant showed no genotoxic potential.

Fulvestrant showed effects upon reproduction and embryo/foetal development consistent with its anti-oestrogenic activity, at doses similar to the clinical dose. In rats a reversible reduction in female fertility and embryonic survival, dystocia and an increased incidence of foetal abnormalities including tarsal flexure were observed. Rabbits given fulvestrant failed to maintain pregnancy. Increases in placental weight and post-implantation loss of foetuses were seen. There was an increased incidence of foetal variations in rabbits (backwards displacement of the pelvic girdle and 27 pre-sacral vertebrae).

A two-year oncogenicity study in rats (intramuscular administration of Faslodex) showed increased incidence of ovarian benign granulosa cell tumours in female rats at the high dose, 10 mg/rat/15 days and an increased incidence of testicular Leydig cell tumours in males. Induction of such tumours is consistent with pharmacology-related endocrine feedback alterations. These findings are not of clinical relevance for the use of fulvestrant in postmenopausal women with advanced breast cancer.

6. PHARMACEUTICAL PARTICULARS

6.1 List of excipients

Ethanol 96%

Benzyl alcohol

Benzyl benzoate

Castor oil

6.2 Incompatibilities

In the absence of incompatibility studies, this medicinal product must not be mixed with other medicinal products.

6.3 Shelf life

4 years.

6.4 Special precautions for storage

Store at 2°C-8°C (in a refrigerator).

Store in the original package in order to protect from light.

6.5 Nature and contents of container

One 5 ml clear neutral glass (Type 1) pre-filled syringe with polystyrene plunger rod. The syringe has a nominal content of 5 ml solution and is fitted with a tamper evident closure.

A safety needle (SafetyGlide) for connection to the barrel is also provided.

6.6 Special precautions for disposal and other handling

Remove glass syringe barrel from tray and check that it is not damaged.

Peel open the safety needle (SafetyGlide) outer packaging. (For safety needle instructions see below).

Break the seal of the white plastic cover on the syringe Luer connector to remove the cover with the attached rubber tip

Figure 1

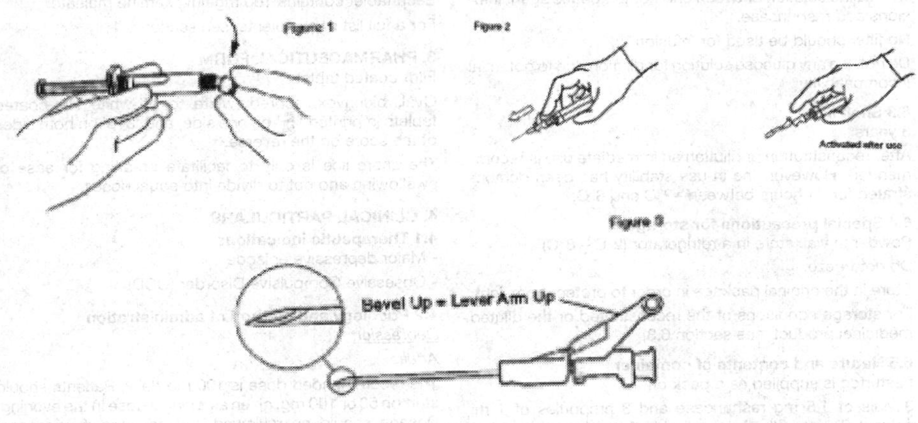

cap (see Figure 1). Twist to lock the needle to the Luer connector.

Remove needle sheath.

Parenteral solutions must be inspected visually for particulate matter and discolouration prior to administration.

Remove excess gas from the syringe (a small gas bubble may remain). Administer intramuscularly slowly into the buttock.

Immediately activate needle protection device upon withdrawal of the needle from patient by pushing lever arm completely forward until needle tip is fully covered (see Figure 2).

Visually confirm that the lever arm has fully advanced and the needle tip is covered. If unable to activate the safety needle, discard immediately into an approved sharps collector.

SafetyGlide Information from Becton Dickinson

WARNING: - Do not autoclave safety needle before use. Hands must remain behind the needle at all times during use and disposal.

Directions for Use of safety needle

Peel apart packaging of the safety needle, break the seal of the white plastic cover on the syringe Luer connector and attach the safety needle to the Luer Lock of the syringe by twisting.

Transport filled syringe to point of administration.

Pull shield straight off needle to avoid damaging needle point.

Administer injection following package instruction.

For user convenience, the needle 'bevel up' position is orientated to the lever arm, as shown in Figure 3.

Immediately activate needle protection device upon withdrawal from patient by pushing lever arm completely forward until needle tip is fully covered (Figure 2).

Visually confirm that the lever arm has fully advanced and the needle tip is covered. If unable to activate, discard immediately into an approved sharps collector.

Activation of the protective mechanism may cause minimal splatter of fluid that may remain on the needle after injection.

For greatest safety, use a one-handed technique and activate away from self and others.

After single use, discard in an approved sharps collector in accordance with applicable regulations and institutional policy.

(see Figure 1 above)

7. MARKETING AUTHORISATION HOLDER

AstraZeneca UK Limited

Alderley Park

Macclesfield

Cheshire

SK10 4TG

United Kingdom

8. MARKETING AUTHORISATION NUMBER(S)

EU/1/03/269/001

9. DATE OF FIRST AUTHORISATION/RENEWAL OF THE AUTHORISATION

10th March 2004

10. DATE OF REVISION OF THE TEXT

9th November 2006

Fasturtec

(sanofi-aventis)

1. NAME OF THE MEDICINAL PRODUCT

Fasturtec 1.5 mg/ml powder and solvent for concentrate for solution for infusion.

2. QUALITATIVE AND QUANTITATIVE COMPOSITION

After reconstitution, 1 ml of Fasturtec concentrate contains 1.5 mg rasburicase.

Fasturtec is a recombinant urate-oxidase enzyme produced by genetically modified *Saccharomyces cerevisiae* strain. Rasburicase is a tetrameric protein with identical subunits of a molecular mass of about 34 kDa.

1 mg corresponds to 18.2 EAU*.

*One enzyme activity unit (EAU) corresponds to the enzyme activity that converts 1μmol of uric acid into allantoin per minute under the operating conditions described: +30°C±1°C TEA pH8.9 buffer.

For a full list of excipients, see section 6.1.

3. PHARMACEUTICAL FORM

Powder and solvent for concentrate for solution for infusion.

The powder is an entire or broken white to off white pellet.

The solvent is a colourless and clear liquid.

4. CLINICAL PARTICULARS

4.1 Therapeutic indications

Treatment and prophylaxis of acute hyperuricaemia, in order to prevent acute renal failure, in patients with haematological malignancy with a high tumour burden and at risk of a rapid tumour lysis or shrinkage at initiation of chemotherapy.

4.2 Posology and method of administration

Fasturtec should be administered under the supervision of a physician trained in chemotherapy of haematological malignancies.

Fasturtec is to be used immediately prior to and during the initiation of chemotherapy only, as at the present, there is insufficient data to recommend multiple treatment courses.

The recommended dose for Fasturtec is 0.20 mg/kg/day. Fasturtec is administered as a once daily 30 minute intravenous infusion in 50 ml of a sodium chloride 9 mg/ml (0.9%) solution (see section 6.6).

The duration of treatment with Fasturtec may be up to 7 days, the exact duration should be based upon adequate monitoring of uric acid levels in plasma and clinical judgment.

Administration of rasburicase does not require any change in the timing or schedule of initiation of cytoreductive chemotherapy.

Rasburicase solution should be infused over 30 minutes. Rasburicase solution should be infused through a different line than that used for infusion of chemotherapeutic agents to prevent any possible drug incompatibility. If use of a separate line is not possible, the line should be flushed out with saline solution between infusion of chemotherapeutic agents and rasburicase. For instruction on use, see section 6.6.

Because rasburicase may degrade uric acid in vitro, special precautions must be used during sample handling for plasma uric acid measurements, see section 6.6.

<u>Additional information on special populations</u>

Renally or hepatically impaired patients: No dose adjustment is necessary.

Paediatric patients: As no dose adjustment is necessary, the recommended dose is 0.20 mg/kg/day.

4.3 Contraindications

Hypersensitivity to the active substance or to any of the excipients.

G6PD deficiency and other cellular metabolic disorders known to cause haemolytic anaemia. Hydrogen peroxide is a by-product of the conversion of uric acid to allantoin. In order to prevent possible haemolytic anaemia induced by hydrogen peroxide, rasburicase is contraindicated in patients with these disorders.

4.4 Special warnings and precautions for use

Rasburicase like other proteins, has the potential to induce allergic responses in humans. Clinical experience with Fasturtec demonstrates that patients should be closely monitored for the onset of allergic-type undesirable effects, especially severe hypersensitivity reactions including anaphylaxis (see section 4.8). In such cases, treatment should immediately and permanently be discontinued and appropriate therapy initiated.

Caution should be used in patients with a history of atopic allergies.

At present, there is insufficient data available on patients being retreated to recommend multiple treatment courses. Anti-rasburicase antibodies have been detected in treated patients and healthy volunteers administered rasburicase.

Methaemoglobinaemia has been reported in patients receiving Fasturtec. Fasturtec should immediately and permanently be discontinued in patients having developed methaemoglobinaemia, and appropriate measures initiated (see section 4.8).

Haemolysis has been reported in patients receiving Fasturtec. In such case, treatment should immediately and permanently be discontinued and appropriate measures initiated (see section 4.8).

Administration of Fasturtec reduces the uric acid levels to below normal levels and by this mechanism reduces the chance of development of renal failure due to precipitation of uric acid crystals in renal tubules as a consequence of hyperuricaemia. Tumour lysis can also result in hyperphosphataemia, hyperkalaemia and hypocalcaemia. Fasturtec is not directly effective in the treatment of these abnormalities. Therefore, patients must be monitored closely.

Fasturtec has not been investigated in the patients with hyperuricemia in the context of myeloproliferative disorders.

There is no data available to recommend the sequential use of Fasturtec and allopurinol.

To ensure accurate measurement of uric acid plasma level during treatment with Fasturtec, a strict sample handling procedure must be followed (see section 6.6).

4.5 Interaction with other medicinal products and other forms of interaction

No metabolism studies have been performed. Rasburicase being an enzyme itself, it would be an unlikely candidate for drug-drug interactions.

4.6 Pregnancy and lactation

For rasburicase no clinical data on exposed pregnancies are available. Animal studies with respect to effects on parturition and postnatal development have not been performed (see section 5.3.). The potential risk for humans is unknown. Fasturtec should not be used during pregnancy or breast-feeding women.

It is unknown whether rasburicase is excreted in human milk.

4.7 Effects on ability to drive and use machines

No studies on the effects on the ability to drive and use machines have been performed.

4.8 Undesirable effects

Fasturtec is concomitantly administered as supportive care to cytoreductive chemotherapy of advanced malignancies, the causality of adverse events is therefore difficult to assess due to the significant burden of adverse events expected from the underlying disease and its treatment.

The most significant drug-related adverse events were common allergic reactions, mainly rashes and urticaria. Cases of hypotension (< 1%), bronchospasm (< 1%), rhinitis (< 0.1%) and severe hypersensitivity reactions (< 1%), including anaphylaxis (< 0.1%) have also been attributed to Fasturtec.

In clinical trials, haematological disorders such as haemolysis, haemolytic anaemia and methaemoglobinaemia are uncommonly caused by Fasturtec. The enzymatic digestion of uric acid to allantoin by rasburicase produces hydrogen peroxide and haemolytic anaemia or methaemoglobinaemia have been observed in certain at risk populations such as those with G6PD deficiency.

In addition, grade 3 or 4 adverse reactions possibly attributable to Fasturtec and reported in the clinical trials, are listed below, by system organ class and by frequency. Frequencies are defined as: common (⩾1/100, <1/10), uncommon (⩾ 1/1,000, <1/100).

	Common	Uncommon
Nervous system disorders		Headache
Gastrointestinal disorders		Diarrhoea Vomiting Nausea
General disorders and administration site conditions	Fever	

Within each frequency grouping, undesirable effects are presented in order of decreasing seriousness.

4.9 Overdose

In view of the mechanism of action of Fasturtec, an overdose will lead to low or undetectable plasma uric acid concentrations and increased production of hydrogen peroxide. Thus patients suspected of receiving an overdose should be monitored for haemolysis, and general supportive measures should be initiated as no specific antidote for Fasturtec has been identified.

5. PHARMACOLOGICAL PROPERTIES

5.1 Pharmacodynamic properties

Pharmacotherapeutic group: Detoxifying agents for antineoplastic treatment, ATC code: V03AF07.

In humans, uric acid is the final step in the catabolic pathway of purines. The acute increase in plasma levels of uric acid subsequent to the lysis of large numbers of malignant cells and during cytoreductive chemotherapy may lead to impairment of renal function and renal failure resulting from the precipitation of crystals of uric acid in renal tubules. Rasburicase is a highly potent uricolytic agent that catalyses enzymatic oxidation of uric acid into allantoin, a water soluble product, easily excreted by the kidneys in the urine.

The enzymatic oxidation of uric acid leads to stoichiometric formation of hydrogen peroxide. The increased of hydrogen peroxide over ambient levels can be eliminated by endogenous antioxidants and the only increased risk is for haemolysis in G6PD deficient and inherited anaemia patients.

In healthy volunteers, a marked dose-related decrease in plasma uric acid levels was observed across the dose range 0.05 mg/kg to 0.20 mg/kg of Fasturtec.

A randomised comparative phase III study, using the recommended dose, showed a significantly more rapid onset of action of Fasturtec in comparison with allopurinol. At 4 hours post first dose, there was a significant difference in the mean percentage change from baseline plasma uric acid concentration ($p<0.0001$) in the Fasturtec group (-86.0%) compared to that for the allopurinol group (-12.1%).

Time to first confirmation of normal levels of uric acid in hyperuricaemic patients is four hours for Fasturtec and 24 hours for allopurinol. In addition this rapid control of uric acid in this population is accompanied by improvements in renal function. In turn, this allows efficient excretion of the serum phosphate load preventing further deterioration of renal function from calcium/phosphorus precipitation.

Paediatric patients

In pivotal clinical studies, 246 patients (<18 years) were treated with rasburicase at doses of 0.15 mg/kg/day or 0.20 mg/kg/day for 1 to 8 days (mainly 5 to 7 days). Efficacy results on 229 evaluable patients showed an overall response rate (normalization of plasma uric acid levels) of 96.1%. Safety results on 246 patients were consistent with the adverse events profile in the overall population.

In long term safety studies, an analysis of data from 867 patients (< 18 years) treated with rasburicase at 0.20 mg/kg/day for 1 to 24 days (mainly 1 to 4 days) showed consistent findings with pivotal clinical studies in terms of efficacy and safety.

5.2 Pharmacokinetic properties

After infusion of rasburicase at a dose of 0.20 mg/kg/day, steady state is achieved at day 2-3. No unexpected accumulation of rasburicase was observed. In patients, the volume of distribution ranged from 110 - 127 ml/kg, which is comparable to the physiological vascular volume. Clearance of rasburicase was ca. 3.5 ml/h/kg and the elimination half-life ca. 19 hours. The patients included in the pharmacokinetic studies were mainly children and adolescents. Based upon these limited data, it seems that clearance is increased (ca. 35%) in children and adolescents compared to adults, resulting in a lower systemic exposure.

Rasburicase is a protein, and therefore: 1) not expected to bind to proteins, 2) expected that metabolic degradation will follow the pathways of other proteins, i.e. peptide hydrolysis, 3) unlikely to be candidate for drug-drug interactions.

Renal elimination of rasburicase is considered to be a minor pathway for rasburicase clearance. As metabolism is expected to occur by peptide hydrolysis, an impaired liver function is not expected to affect the pharmacokinetics.

5.3 Preclinical safety data

Non-clinical data reveal no special hazard for humans based on conventional studies of safety pharmacology, repeated dose toxicity and genotoxicity. The interpretation of the non-clinical studies is hampered due to the presence of endogenous urate oxidase in standard animal models.

6. PHARMACEUTICAL PARTICULARS

6.1 List of excipients

Powder:

alanine

mannitol

disodium phosphate dodecahydrate

disodium phosphate dihydrate

sodium dihydrogen phosphate dihydrate

Solvent:

poloxamer 188

water for injection

6.2 Incompatibilities

This medicinal product must not be mixed with other medicinal products except those mentioned in section 6.6.

Rasburicase solution should be infused through a different line than that used for infusion of chemotherapeutic agents to prevent any possible drug incompatibility. If use of a separate line is not possible, the line should be flushed out with saline solution between chemotherapeutic agent infusions and rasburicase.

No filter should be used for infusion.

Do not use any glucose solution for dilution due to potential incompatibility.

6.3 Shelf life

3 years

After reconstitution or dilution an immediate use is recommended. However, the in-use stability has been demonstrated for 24 hours between +2°C and 8°C.

6.4 Special precautions for storage

Powder in vial: store in a refrigerator (2°C – 8°C).

Do not freeze.

Store in the original package in order to protect from light.

For storage conditions of the reconstituted or the diluted medicinal product, see section 6.3.

6.5 Nature and contents of container

Fasturtec is supplied as a pack of:

3 vials of 1.5 mg rasburicase and 3 ampoules of 1 ml solvent. The powder is supplied in 3 ml clear glass (type I) vial with a rubber stopper and the solvent in a 2 ml clear glass (type I) ampoule.

1 vial of 7.5 mg rasburicase and 1 ampoule of 5 ml solvent. The powder is supplied in 10 ml clear glass (type I) vial with a rubber stopper and the solvent in a 5 ml clear glass (type I) ampoule.

6.6 Special precautions for disposal and other handling

Rasburicase must be reconstituted with the entire volume of the supplied solvent ampoule (1.5 mg rasburicase vial to be reconstituted with the 1 ml solvent ampoule; 7.5 mg rasburicase vial to be reconstituted with the 5 ml solvent ampoule). Reconstitution results in a solution with a concentration of 1.5 mg/ml rasburicase to be further diluted with sodium chloride 9 mg/ml (0.9%) intravenous solution.

Reconstitution of the solution:

Add the content of one ampoule of solvent to one vial containing rasburicase and mix by swirling very gently under controlled and validated aseptic conditions.

Do not shake.

Inspect visually prior to use. Only clear and colourless solutions without particles should be used.

For single-use only, any unused solution should be discarded.

The solvent contains no preservative. Therefore the reconstituted solution should be diluted under controlled and validated aseptic conditions.

Dilution before infusion:

The required volume of the reconstituted solution depends on the patient's body weight. The use of several vials may be necessary to obtain the quantity of rasburicase required for one administration. The required volume of the reconstituted solution, taken from one or more vials, is to be further diluted with sodium chloride 9 mg/ml (0.9%) solution to make a total volume of 50 ml. The concentration of rasburicase in the final solution for infusion depends on the patient's body weight.

The reconstituted solution contains no preservative. Therefore the diluted solution should be infused immediately.

Infusion:

The final solution should be infused over 30 minutes.

Sample handling:

If it is necessary to monitor a patient's uric acid level, a strict sample-handling procedure must be followed to minimise *ex vivo* degradation of the analyte. Blood must be collected into pre-chilled tubes containing heparin anticoagulant. Samples must be immersed in an ice/water bath. Plasma samples should immediately be prepared by centrifugation in a pre-cooled centrifuge (4°C). Finally, plasma must be maintained in an ice/water bath and analysed for uric acid within 4 hours.

7. MARKETING AUTHORISATION HOLDER

sanofi-aventis

174, avenue de France

F - 75013 Paris, France

8. MARKETING AUTHORISATION NUMBER(S)

EU/1/00/170/001-002

9. DATE OF FIRST AUTHORISATION/RENEWAL OF THE AUTHORISATION

Date of first authorisation: 23 February 2001

Date of last renewal: 23 February 2006

10. DATE OF REVISION OF THE TEXT

February 2009

Legal category: POM

Faverin 100 mg film-coated tablets

(Solvay Healthcare Limited)

1. NAME OF THE MEDICINAL PRODUCT

Faverin® 100 mg film-coated tablets

2. QUALITATIVE AND QUANTITATIVE COMPOSITION

Each tablet contains 100 mg fluvoxamine maleate.

For a full list of excipients, see section 6.1

3. PHARMACEUTICAL FORM

Film-coated tablet

Oval, biconvex, scored, white to off-white film-coated tablets imprinted '$' on one side, and '313' on both sides of the score on the reverse.

The score line is only to facilitate breaking for ease of swallowing and not to divide into equal doses.

4. CLINICAL PARTICULARS

4.1 Therapeutic indications

- Major depressive episode
- Obsessive Compulsive Disorder (OCD)

4.2 Posology and method of administration

Depression

Adults

The recommended dose is 100 mg daily. Patients should start on 50 or 100 mg, given as a single dose in the evening. Dosage should be reviewed and adjusted if necessary within 3 to 4 weeks of initiation of therapy and thereafter as judged clinically appropriate. Although there may be an increased potential for undesirable effects at higher doses, if after some weeks on the recommended dose insufficient response is seen some patients may benefit from having their dose increased gradually up to a maximum of 300 mg a day (see section 5.1). Doses up to 150 mg can be given as a single dose, preferably in the evening. It is advisable that a total daily dose of more than 150 mg is given in 2 or 3 divided doses. Dosage adjustments should be made carefully on an individual patient basis, to maintain the patients at the lowest effective dose.

Patients with depression should be treated for a sufficient period of at least 6 months to ensure that they are free from symptoms.

Children/adolescents

Faverin should not be used in children and adolescents under the age of 18 years for the treatment of major depressive episode. The efficacy and safety of Faverin have not been established in the treatment of paediatric major depressive episode (see 4.4).

Obsessive Compulsive Disorder

Adults

The recommended dose is between 100-300 mg daily. Patients should start at 50 mg per day. Although there may be an increased potential for undesirable effects at higher doses, if after some weeks on the recommended dose insufficient response is seen some patients may benefit from having their dose increased gradually up to maximum of 300 mg a day (see section 5.1). Doses up to 150 mg can be given as a single dose, preferably in the evening. It is advisable that a total daily dose of more than 150 mg is given in 2 or 3 divided doses. If a good therapeutic response has been obtained, treatment can be continued at a dosage adjusted on an individual basis.

While there are no systematic studies to answer the question of how long to continue fluvoxamine treatment, OCD is a chronic condition and it is reasonable to consider continuation beyond 10 weeks in responding patients. Dosage adjustments should be made carefully on an individual patient basis, to maintain the patients at the lowest effective dose. The need for treatment should be reassessed periodically. Some clinicians advocate concomitant behavioural psychotherapy for patients who have done well on pharmacotherapy. Long-term efficacy (more than 24 weeks) has not been demonstrated in OCD.

Children/adolescents

In children over 8 years and adolescents there is limited data on a dose of up to 100 mg b.i.d for 10 weeks. The starting dose is 25 mg per day. Increase every 4-7 days in 25 mg increments as tolerated until an effective dose is achieved. The maximum dose in children should not exceed 200 mg/day. (For further details see 5.1 and 5.2). It is advisable that a total daily dose of more than 50 mg should be given in two divided doses. If the two divided doses are not equal, the larger dose should be given at bedtime.

Withdrawal symptoms seen on discontinuation of fluvoxamine

Abrupt discontinuation should be avoided. When stopping treatment with fluvoxamine the dose should be gradually reduced over a period of at least one or two weeks in order to reduce the risk of withdrawal reactions. (see section 4.4 Special warnings and special precautions for use and section 4.8 Undesirable effects). If intolerable symptoms occur following a decrease in the dose or upon discontinuation of treatment, then resuming the previously prescribed dose may be considered. Subsequently, the physician may continue decreasing the dose, but at a more gradual rate.

Hepatic or renal insufficiency

Patients suffering from hepatic or renal insufficiency should start on a low dose and be carefully monitored.

Method of administration

Fluvoxamine tablets should be swallowed with water and without chewing.

4.3 Contraindications

Faverin tablets are contraindicated in combination with monoamine oxidase inhibitors (MAOIs). Treatment with fluvoxamine can be initiated:

- two weeks after discontinuation of an irreversible MAOI, or

- the following day after discontinuation of a reversible MAOI (e.g. moclobemide).

At least one week should elapse between discontinuation of fluvoxamine and initiation of therapy with any MAOI.

Hypersensitivity to the active substance or to any of the excipients.

4.4 Special warnings and precautions for use

Suicide/suicidal thoughts or clinical worsening

Depression is associated with an increased risk of suicidal thoughts, self harm and suicide (suicide-related events). This risk persists until significant remission occurs. As improvement may not occur during the first few weeks or more of treatment, patients should be closely monitored until such improvement occurs. It is general clinical experience that the risk of suicide may increase in the early stages of recovery.

Other psychiatric conditions for which Faverin is prescribed can also be associated with an increased risk of suicide-related events. In addition, these conditions may be co-morbid with major depressive disorder. The same precautions observed when treating patients with major depressive disorder should therefore be observed when treating patients with other psychiatric disorders.

Patients with a history of suicide-related events, or those exhibiting a significant degree of suicidal ideation prior to commencement of treatment are known to be at greater risk of suicidal thoughts or suicide attempts, and should receive careful monitoring during treatment. A meta-analysis of placebo-controlled clinical trials of antidepressant drugs in adult patients with psychiatric disorders showed an increased risk of suicidal behaviour with antidepressants compared to placebo in patients less than 25 years old.

Close supervision of patients and in particular those at high risk should accompany drug therapy especially in early treatment and following dose changes.

Patients (and caregivers of patients) should be alerted about the need to monitor for any clinical worsening, suicidal behaviour or thoughts and unusual changes in behaviour and to seek medical advice immediately if these symptoms present.

Akathisia/ Psychomotor restlessness

The use of fluvoxamine has been associated with the development of akathisia, characterised by a subjectively unpleasant or distressing restlessness and need to move, often accompanied by an inability to sit or stand still. This is most likely to occur within the first few weeks of treatment. In patients who develop these symptoms, increasing the dose may be detrimental.

Withdrawal symptoms seen on discontinuation of fluvoxamine treatment

Withdrawal symptoms when treatment is discontinued are common, particularly if discontinuation is abrupt (see section 4.8 Undesirable effects). In clinical trials adverse events seen on treatment discontinuation occurred in approximately 12% of patients treated with fluvoxamine, which is similar to the incidence seen in patients taking placebo. The risk of withdrawal symptoms may be dependent on several factors including the duration and dose of therapy and the rate of dose reduction.

Dizziness, sleep disturbances (including insomnia and intense dreams), nausea, headache and asthenia are the most commonly reported reactions. Generally these symptoms are mild to moderate, however, in some patients they may be severe in intensity. They usually occur within the first few days of discontinuing treatment, but there have been very rare reports of such symptoms in patients who have inadvertently missed a dose. Generally these symptoms are self-limiting and usually resolve within 2 weeks, though in some individuals they may be prolonged (2-3 months or more). It is therefore advised that fluvoxamine should be gradually tapered when discontinuing treatment over a period of several weeks or months, according tothe patient's needs (see "Withdrawal Symptoms Seen on Discontinuation of Fluvoxamine", Section 4.2 Posology and method of administration).

Patients suffering from hepatic or renal insufficiency should start on a low dose and be carefully monitored.

Treatment with fluvoxamine has rarely been associated with an increase in hepatic enzymes, generally accompanied by clinical symptoms. In such cases treatment should be discontinued.

Glycaemic control may be disturbed, especially in the early stages of treatment. The dosage of anti-diabetic drugs may need to be adjusted.

Although in animal studies fluvoxamine has no pro-convulsive properties, caution is recommended when the drug is administered to patients with a history of convulsive disorders. Fluvoxamine should be avoided in patients with unstable epilepsy and patients with controlled epilepsy should be carefully monitored. Treatment with fluvoxamine should be discontinued if seizures occur or if seizure frequency increases.

On rare occasions development of a serotonin syndrome or neuroleptic malignant syndrome-like events have been reported in association with treatment of fluvoxamine, particularly when given in combination with other serotonergic and/or neuroleptic drugs. As these syndromes may result in potentially life-threatening conditions, treatment with fluvoxamine should be discontinued if such events (characterised by clusters of symptoms such as hyperthermia, rigidity, myoclonus, autonomic instability with possible rapid fluctuations of vital signs, mental status changes including confusion, irritability, extreme agitation progressing to delirium and coma) occur and supportive symptomatic treatment should be initiated.

As with other SSRIs, hyponatremia has been rarely reported, and appears to be reversible when fluvoxamine is discontinued. Some cases were possibly due to the syndrome of inappropriate antidiuretic hormone secretion. The majority of reports were associated with older patients.

There have been reports of cutaneous bleeding abnormalities such as ecchymoses and purpura with SSRIs. Caution is advised in patients taking SSRIs particularly in concomitant use with drugs known to affect platelet function (e.g. atypical antipsychotics and phenothiazines, most TCAs, aspirin NSAIDs) as well as in patients with a history of bleeding disorders.

Fluvoxamine should be used with caution in patients with a history of mania/hypomania. Fluvoxamine should be discontinued in any patient entering a manic phase.

When combined with fluvoxamine plasma concentrations of terfenadine, astemizole or cisapride may be increased resulting in an increased risk for QT-prolongation/Torsade de Pointes. Therefore, fluvoxamine should not be co-administered with these drugs.

Due to lack of clinical experience special attention is advised in the situation of post-acute myocardial infarction.

There is limited clinical experience of concomitant administration of fluvoxamine and ECT therefore caution is advisable.

Data in elderly subjects give no indication of clinically significant differences in normal daily dosages compared to younger subjects. However upward dose titration should be done slower in the elderly, and dosing should always be done with caution.

Use in children and adolescents under 18 years of age

Fluvoxamine should not be used in the treatment of children and adolescents under the age of 18 years, except for patients with Obsessive Compulsive Disorder. Suicide-related behaviours (suicide attempt and suicidal thoughts), and hostility (predominantly aggression, oppositional behaviour and anger) were more frequently observed in clinical trials among children and adolescents treated with antidepressants compared to those treated with placebo. If, based on clinical need, a decision to treat is nevertheless taken; the patient should be carefully monitored for the appearance of suicidal symptoms. In addition, long-term safety data in children and adolescents concerning growth, maturation and cognitive and behavioural development are lacking.

4.5 Interaction with other medicinal products and other forms of interaction

Fluvoxamine should not be used in combination with MAOIs (see also 4.4 Contraindications).

Fluvoxamine is a potent inhibitor of CYP1A2, and to a lesser extent of CYP2C and CYP3A4. Drugs which are largely metabolised via these isoenzymes are eliminated slower and may have higher plasma concentrations when co-administered with fluvoxamine. This is particularly relevant for drugs with a narrow therapeutic index. Patients should be carefully monitored and, if necessary, dose adjustment of these drugs is recommended.

Fluvoxamine has marginal inhibitory effects on CYP2D6 and seems not to affect non-oxidative metabolism or renal excretion.

CYP1A2

An increase in previously stable plasma levels of those tricyclic antidepressants (e.g., clomipramine, imipramine, amitriptyline) and neuroleptics (e.g., clozapine, olanzapine) which are largely metabolised through cytochrome P450 1A2 when given together with fluvoxamine, has been reported. A decrease in the dose of these products should be considered if treatment with fluvoxamine is initiated.

Patients co-administered fluvoxamine and CYP1A2 metabolised drugs with a narrow therapeutic index (such as tacrine, theophylline, methadone, mexiletine) should be carefully monitored and, if necessary, dose adjustment of these drugs is recommended.

When given with fluvoxamine, warfarin plasma concentrations were significantly increased and prothrombin times prolonged.

Isolated cases of cardiac toxicity have been reported when fluvoxamine was combined with thioridazine.

As plasma concentrations of propranolol are increased in combination with fluvoxamine, the propranolol dose may need to be lowered.

Caffeine plasma levels are likely to be increased during co-administration with fluvoxamine. Thus, patients who consume high quantities of caffeine-containing beverages should lower their intake when fluvoxamine is administered and adverse caffeine effects (like tremor, palpitations, nausea, restlessness, insomnia) are observed.

As plasma concentrations of ropinirole may be increased in combination with Fluvoxamine thus increasing the risk of overdose, surveillance and reduction in the posology of ropinirole during Fluvoxamine treatment and after its withdrawal may be required.

CYP2C

Patients co-administered fluvoxamine and CYP2C metabolised drugs with a narrow therapeutic index (such as phenytoin) should be carefully monitored and, if necessary, dose adjustment of these drugs is recommended.

CYP3A4

Terfenadine, astemizole, cisapride (see also 4.4 Special Warnings and Special Precautions for Use).

Patients co-administered fluvoxamine and CYP3A4 metabolised drugs with a narrow therapeutic index (such as carbamazepine, ciclosporin) should be carefully monitored and, if necessary, dose adjustment of these drugs is recommended.

The plasma levels of oxidatively metabolised benzodiazepines (e.g. triazolam, midazolam, alprazolam, and diazepam) are likely to be increased when co-administered with fluvoxamine. The dosage of these benzodiazepines should be reduced during co-administration with fluvoxamine.

Glucuronidation

Fluvoxamine does not influence plasma concentrations of digoxin.

Renal excretion

Fluvoxamine does not influence plasma concentrations of atenolol.

Pharmacodynamic interactions

The serotonergic effects of fluvoxamine may be enhanced when used in combination with other serotonergic agents (including triptans, SSRIs and St. John's Wort preparations). (See also 4.4 Special Warnings and Special Precautions for Use).

Fluvoxamine has been used in combination with lithium in the treatment of severely ill, drug-resistant patients. However, lithium (and possibly also tryptophan) enhances the serotonergic effects of fluvoxamine. The combination should be used with caution in patients with severe, drug-resistant depression.

In patients on oral anticoagulants and fluvoxamine, the risk for haemorrhage may increase and these patients should therefore be closely monitored.

As with other psychotropic drugs patients should be advised to avoid alcohol use while taking fluvoxamine.

4.6 Pregnancy and lactation

Data on a limited number of exposed pregnancies indicate no adverse effects of fluvoxamine on pregnancy. To date, no other relevant epidemiological data are available.

Reproduction studies in animals at high doses revealed no evidence of impaired fertility, reproductive performance or teratogenic effects in the offspring. Caution should be exercised when prescribing to pregnant women.

Isolated cases of withdrawal symptoms in the newborn child have been described after the use of fluvoxamine at the end of pregnancy.

Fluvoxamine is excreted via human milk in small quantities. Therefore, the drug should not be used by women who breast feed.

4.7 Effects on ability to drive and use machines

Fluvoxamine up to 150 mg has no or negligible influence on the ability to drive and use machines. It showed no effect on psychomotor skills associated with driving and operating machinery in healthy volunteers. However, somnolence has been reported during treatment with fluvoxamine. Therefore, caution is recommended until the individual response to the drug has been determined.

4.8 Undesirable effects

Nausea, sometimes accompanied by vomiting is the most frequently observed symptom associated with fluvoxamine treatment. This side effect usually diminishes within the first two weeks of treatment. Other adverse events, observed in clinical studies at frequencies listed below, are often associated with the illness and are not necessarily related to treatment.

Common (Frequency 1-10%):

Body: Asthenia, headache, malaise

Cardiovascular: Palpitations/tachycardia

Digestive system: Abdominal pain, anorexia, constipation, diarrhoea, dry mouth, dyspepsia

Nervous system: Agitation, anxiety, dizziness, insomnia, nervousness, somnolence, tremor

Skin: Sweating

Uncommon (Frequency $<1\%$):

Cardiovascular: (Postural) hypotension

Musculoskeletal: Arthralgia, myalgia

Nervous System: Ataxia, confusion, extrapyramidal symptoms, hallucinations

Urogenital: Abnormal (delayed) ejaculation

Skin: Cutaneous hypersensitivity reactions (incl. rash, pruritus, angioedema)

Rare (Frequency <0.1%):

Digestive system: Liver function abnormality

Nervous system: Convulsions, mania

Urogenital: Galactorrhoea

Skin: Photosensitivity

Psychomotor restlessness/akathisia (see section 4.4 Special warnings and special precautions for use)

Other adverse events observed during marketing:

Weight gain and loss have been reported.

Rarely, serotonin syndrome, neuroleptic malignant syndrome-like events, hyponatremia and SIADH have been reported (see also 4.4 Special Warnings and Special Precautions for Use).

It is possible that withdrawal reactions may occur on stopping therapy with fluvoxamine although the available preclinical and clinical evidence does not suggest that this treatment causes dependence. The following symptoms have been reported in association with withdrawal of the product: dizziness, paresthesia, headache, nausea and anxiety. The majority of the withdrawal reactions are mild and self-limiting.

When stopping, a gradual dose reduction may be considered.

Haemorrhage (see also 4.4 Special warnings and special precautions for use)

Very rarely, paresthesia, anorgasmy and taste perversion have been reported.

Cases of suicidal ideation and suicidal behaviours have been reported during Fluvoxamine therapy or early after treatment discontinuation (see section 4.4)

In one 10-week placebo-controlled trial in children and adolescents with OCD, frequently reported adverse events with a higher incidence than placebo, were: insomnia, asthenia, agitation, hyperkinesia, somnolence and dyspepsia. Serious adverse events in this study included: agitation and hypomania. Convulsions in children and adolescents have been reported during use outside clinical trials.

Withdrawal symptoms seen on discontinuation of fluvoxamine treatment

Discontinuation of fluvoxamine (particularly when abrupt) commonly leads to withdrawal symptoms. Dizziness, sensory disturbance (including paraesthesia, visual disturbance and electric shock sensations), sleep disturbances (including insomnia and intense dreams), agitation and anxiety, irritability, confusion, emotional instability, nausea and/or vomiting, diarrhoea, sweating, palpitations, headache and tremor are the most commonly reported reactions. Generally these events are mild to moderate and are self-limiting, however, in some patients they may be severe and/or prolonged. It is therefore advised that when fluvoxamine treatment is no longer required, gradual discontinuation by dose tapering should be carried out (see section 4.2 Posology and method of administration and section 4.4 Special warnings and special precautions for use).

4.9 Overdose

Symptoms

Symptoms include gastro-intestinal complaints (nausea, vomiting and diarrhoea), somnolence and dizziness. Cardiac events (tachycardia, bradycardia, hypotension), liver function disturbances, convulsions and coma have also been reported.

Fluvoxamine has a wide margin of safety in overdose. Since market introduction, reports of deaths attributed to overdose of fluvoxamine alone have been extremely rare. The highest documented dose of fluvoxamine ingested by a patient is 12 grams. This patient recovered completely. Occasionally, more serious complications were observed in cases of deliberate overdose of fluvoxamine in combination with other drugs.

Treatment

There is no specific antidote to fluvoxamine. In case of overdose the stomach should be emptied as soon as possible after tablet ingestion and symptomatic treatment should be given. The repeated use of medicinal charcoal, if necessary accompanied by an osmotic laxative, is also recommended. Forced diuresis or dialysis are unlikely to be of benefit.

5. PHARMACOLOGICAL PROPERTIES

5.1 Pharmacodynamic properties

Pharmacotherapeutic group: Antidepressants, Selective serotonin reuptake inhibitors, ATC code: N06AB08.

The mechanism of action of fluvoxamine is thought to be related to selective serotonin re-uptake inhibition in brain neurones. There is minimum interference with noradrenergic processes. Receptor binding studies have demonstrated that fluvoxamine has negligible binding capacity to alpha adrenergic, beta adrenergic, histaminergic, muscarine cholinergic, dopaminergic or serotonergic receptors.

In a placebo controlled trial in 120 patients with OCD, aged between 8 and 17 years, a statistically significant improvement was seen in the total population in favour of fluvoxamine at 10 weeks. A further subgroup analysis showed improvement on the C-YBOCS rating scale in children whereas no effect was seen in adolescents. The mean dose was respectively 158 mg and 168 mg/day.

Dose response

No formal clinical trials were conducted investigating the dose response of fluvoxamine. However, it is clinical experience that up-titrating the dose might be beneficial for some patients.

5.2 Pharmacokinetic properties

Absorption

Fluvoxamine is completely absorbed following oral administration. Maximum plasma concentrations occur within 3-8 hours of dosing. The mean absolute bioavailability is 53% due to first-pass metabolism.

The pharmacokinetics of Faverin is not influenced by concomitant food intake.

Distribution

In vitro plasma protein binding of fluvoxamine is 80%. Volume of distribution in humans is 25 l/kg.

Metabolism

Fluvoxamine undergoes extensive metabolism in the liver. Although CYP2D6 is *in vitro* the main isoenzyme involved in fluvoxamine's metabolism, plasma concentrations in poor metabolisers for CYP2D6 are not much higher than those in extensive metabolisers.

The mean plasma half-life is approximately 13-15 hours after a single dose and slightly longer (17-22 hours) during repeated dosing, when steady-state plasma levels are usually achieved within 10-14 days.

Fluvoxamine undergoes extensive hepatic transformation, mainly via oxidative demethylation, into at least nine metabolites, which are excreted by the kidneys. The two major metabolites showed negligible pharmacological activity. The other metabolites are not expected to be pharmacologically active. Fluvoxamine is a potent inhibitor of CYP1A2 and a moderate inhibitor of CYP2C and CYP3A4, with only marginal inhibitory effects on CYP2D6.

Fluvoxamine displays linear single-dose pharmacokinetics. Steady-state concentrations are higher than calculated from single-dose data, and are disproportionably higher at higher daily doses.

Special Patients groups

The pharmacokinetics of fluvoxamine is similar in healthy adults, elderly patients, and patients with renal insufficiency. The metabolism of fluvoxamine is impaired in patients with liver disease.

Steady-state plasma concentrations of fluvoxamine were twice as high in children (aged 6-11) as in adolescents (aged 12-17). Plasma concentrations in adolescents are similar to those in adults.

5.3 Preclinical safety data

There is no evidence of carcinogenicity, mutagenicity or impairment of fertility with fluvoxamine.

Reproduction studies in animals at high doses revealed no evidence of impaired fertility, reproductive performance or teratogenic effects in the offspring.

The potential for abuse, tolerance and physical dependence has been studied in a non-human primate model. No evidence of dependency phenomena was found.

6. PHARMACEUTICAL PARTICULARS

6.1 List of excipients

Tablet cores:

Mannitol

Maize starch

Pregelatinised starch

Sodium stearyl fumarate

Colloidal anhydrous silica

Film-coat:

Hypromellose

Macrogol 6000

Talc

Titanium Dioxide E171

6.2 Incompatibilities

Not applicable.

6.3 Shelf life

3 years.

6.4 Special precautions for storage

Do not store above 25°C.

Store in the original package.

6.5 Nature and contents of container

PVC/PVdC/Aluminium press-through blisters.

Packs contain 15, 30, 50, 60, 90, 100, 120 or 250 tablets.

Not all pack sizes may be marketed.

6.6 Special precautions for disposal and other handling

No special requirements

7. MARKETING AUTHORISATION HOLDER

Solvay Healthcare Limited

Mansbridge Road

West End

Southampton

SO18 3JD

8. MARKETING AUTHORISATION NUMBER(S)

PL 00512/0072

9. DATE OF FIRST AUTHORISATION/RENEWAL OF THE AUTHORISATION

22/06/2004

10. DATE OF REVISION OF THE TEXT

04/06/2009

Faverin 50mg film-coated tablets

(Solvay Healthcare Limited)

1. NAME OF THE MEDICINAL PRODUCT

Faverin® 50 mg film-coated tablets

2. QUALITATIVE AND QUANTITATIVE COMPOSITION

Each tablet contains 50 mg fluvoxamine maleate.

For a full list of excipients, see section 6.1

3. PHARMACEUTICAL FORM

Film-coated tablet

Round, biconvex, scored, white to off-white film coated tablets imprinted '$' on one side, and '291' on both sides of the score on the reverse.

The score line is only to facilitate breaking for ease of swallowing and not to divide into equal doses.

4. CLINICAL PARTICULARS

4.1 Therapeutic indications

- Major depressive episode
- Obsessive Compulsive Disorder (OCD)

4.2 Posology and method of administration

Depression

Adults

The recommended dose is 100 mg daily. Patients should start on 50 or 100 mg, given as a single dose in the evening. Dosage should be reviewed and adjusted if necessary within 3 to 4 weeks of initiation of therapy and thereafter as judged clinically appropriate. Although there may be an increased potential for undesirable effects at higher doses, if after some weeks on the recommended dose insufficient response is seen some patients may benefit from having their dose increased gradually up to a maximum of 300 mg a day (see section 5.1). Doses up to 150 mg can be given as a single dose, preferably in the evening. It is advisable that a total daily dose of more than 150 mg is given in 2 or 3 divided doses. Dosage adjustments should be made carefully on an individual patient basis, to maintain the patients at the lowest effective dose.

Patients with depression should be treated for a sufficient period of at least 6 months to ensure that they are free from symptoms.

Children/adolescents

Faverin should not be used in children and adolescents under the age of 18 years for the treatment of major depressive episode. The efficacy and safety of Faverin have not been established in the treatment of paediatric major depressive episode (see 4.4).

Obsessive Compulsive Disorder

Adults

The recommended dose is between 100-300 mg daily. Patients should start at 50 mg per day. Although there may be an increased potential for undesirable effects at higher doses, if after some weeks on the recommended dose insufficient response is seen some patients may benefit from having their dose increased gradually up to maximum of 300 mg a day (see section 5.1). Doses up to 150 mg can be given as a single dose, preferably in the evening. It is advisable that a total daily dose of more than 150 mg is given in 2 or 3 divided doses. If a good therapeutic response has been obtained, treatment can be continued at a dosage adjusted on an individual basis.

While there are no systematic studies to answer the question of how long to continue fluvoxamine treatment, OCD is a chronic condition and it is reasonable to consider continuation beyond 10 weeks in responding patients. Dosage adjustments should be made carefully on an individual patient basis, to maintain the patients at the lowest effective dose. The need for treatment should be reassessed periodically. Some clinicians advocate concomitant behavioural psychotherapy for patients who have done well on pharmacotherapy. Long-term efficacy (more than 24 weeks) has not been demonstrated in OCD.

Children/adolescents

In children over 8 years and adolescents there is limited data on a dose of up to 100 mg b.i.d for 10 weeks. The starting dose is 25 mg per day. Increase every 4-7 days in 25 mg increments as tolerated until an effective dose is achieved. The maximum dose in children should not exceed 200 mg/day. (For further details see 5.1 and 5.2). It is advisable that a total daily dose of more than 50 mg should be given in two divided doses. If the two divided doses are not equal, the larger dose should be given at bedtime.

Withdrawal symptoms seen on discontinuation of fluvoxamine

Abrupt discontinuation should be avoided. When stopping treatment with fluvoxamine the dose should be gradually reduced over a period of at least one or two weeks in order to reduce the risk of withdrawal reactions. (see section 4.4 Special warnings and special precautions for use and section 4.8 Undesirable effects). If intolerable symptoms occur following a decrease in the dose or upon discontinuation of treatment, then resuming the previously prescribed dose may be considered. Subsequently, the physician may continue decreasing the dose, but at a more gradual rate.

Hepatic or renal insufficiency

Patients suffering from hepatic or renal insufficiency should start on a low dose and be carefully monitored.

Method of administration

Fluvoxamine tablets should be swallowed with water and without chewing.

4.3 Contraindications

Faverin tablets are contraindicated in combination with monoamine oxidase inhibitors (MAOIs). Treatment with fluvoxamine can be initiated:

- two weeks after discontinuation of an irreversible MAOI, or

- the following day after discontinuation of a reversible MAOI (e.g. moclobemide).

At least one week should elapse between discontinuation of fluvoxamine and initiation of therapy with any MAOI.

Hypersensitivity to the active substance or to any of the excipients.

4.4 Special warnings and precautions for use

Suicide/suicidal thoughts or clinical worsening

Depression is associated with an increased risk of suicidal thoughts, self harm and suicide (suicide-related events). This risk persists until significant remission occurs. As improvement may not occur during the first few weeks or more of treatment, patients should be closely monitored until such improvement occurs. It is general clinical experience that the risk of suicide may increase in the early stages of recovery.

Other psychiatric conditions for which Faverin is prescribed can also be associated with an increased risk of suicide-related events. In addition, these conditions may be co-morbid with major depressive disorder. The same precautions observed when treating patients with major depressive disorder should therefore be observed when treating patients with other psychiatric disorders.

Patients with a history of suicide-related events, or those exhibiting a significant degree of suicidal ideation prior to commencement of treatment are known to be at greater risk of suicidal thoughts or suicide attempts, and should receive careful monitoring during treatment. A meta-analysis of placebo-controlled clinical trials of antidepressant drugs in adult patients with psychiatric disorders showed an increased risk of suicidal behaviour with antidepressants compared to placebo in patients less than 25 years old.

Close supervision of patients and in particular those at high risk should accompany drug therapy especially in early treatment and following dose changes.

Patients (and caregivers of patients) should be alerted about the need to monitor for any clinical worsening, suicidal behaviour or thoughts and unusual changes in behaviour and to seek medical advice immediately if these symptoms present.

Akathisia/ Psychomotor restlessness

The use of fluvoxamine has been associated with the development of akathisia, characterised by a subjectively unpleasant or distressing restlessness and need to move, often accompanied by an inability to sit or stand still. This is most likely to occur within the first few weeks of treatment. In patients who develop these symptoms, increasing the dose may be detrimental.

Withdrawal symptoms seen on discontinuation of fluvoxamine treatment

Withdrawal symptoms when treatment is discontinued are common, particularly if discontinuation is abrupt (see section 4.8 Undesirable effects). In clinical trials adverse events seen on treatment discontinuation occurred in approximately 12% of patients treated with fluvoxamine, which is similar to the incidence seen in patients taking placebo. The risk of withdrawal symptoms may be dependent on several factors including the duration and dose of therapy and the rate of dose reduction.

Dizziness, sleep disturbances (including insomnia and intense dreams), nausea, headache and asthenia are the most commonly reported reactions. Generally these symptoms are mild to moderate, however, in some patients they may be severe in intensity. They usually occur within the first few days of discontinuing treatment, but there have been very rare reports of such symptoms in patients who have inadvertently missed a dose. Generally these symptoms are self-limiting and usually resolve within 2 weeks, though in some individuals they may be prolonged (2-3 months or more). It is therefore advised that fluvoxamine should be gradually tapered when discontinuing treatment over a period of several weeks or months, according to the patient's needs (see "Withdrawal Symptoms Seen on Discontinuation of Fluvoxamine", Section 4.2 Posology and method of administration).

Patients suffering from hepatic or renal insufficiency should start on a low dose and be carefully monitored.

Treatment with fluvoxamine has rarely been associated with an increase in hepatic enzymes, generally accompanied by clinical symptoms. In such cases treatment should be discontinued.

Glycaemic control may be disturbed, especially in the early stages of treatment. The dosage of anti-diabetic drugs may need to be adjusted.

Although in animal studies fluvoxamine has no pro-convulsive properties, caution is recommended when the drug is administered to patients with a history of convulsive disorders. Fluvoxamine should be avoided in patients with unstable epilepsy and patients with controlled epilepsy should be carefully monitored. Treatment with fluvoxamine should be discontinued if seizures occur or if seizure frequency increases.

On rare occasions development of a serotonin syndrome or neuroleptic malignant syndrome-like events have been reported in association with treatment of fluvoxamine, particularly when given in combination with other serotonergic and/or neuroleptic drugs. As these syndromes may result in potentially life-threatening conditions, treatment with fluvoxamine should be discontinued if such events (characterised by clusters of symptoms such as hyperthermia, rigidity, myoclonus, autonomic instability with possible rapid fluctuations of vital signs, mental status changes including confusion, irritability, extreme agitation progressing to delirium and coma) occur and supportive symptomatic treatment should be initiated.

As with other SSRIs, hyponatremia has been rarely reported, and appears to be reversible when fluvoxamine is discontinued. Some cases were possibly due to the syndrome of inappropriate antidiuretic hormone secretion. The majority of reports were associated with older patients.

There have been reports of cutaneous bleeding abnormalities such as ecchymoses and purpura with SSRIs. Caution is advised in patients taking SSRIs particularly in concomitant use with drugs known to affect platelet function (e.g. atypical antipsychotics and phenothiazines, most TCAs, aspirin NSAIDs) as well as in patients with a history of bleeding disorders.

Fluvoxamine should be used with caution in patients with a history of mania/hypomania. Fluvoxamine should be discontinued in any patient entering a manic phase.

When combined with fluvoxamine plasma concentrations of terfenadine, astemizole or cisapride may be increased resulting in an increased risk for QT-prolongation/Torsade de Pointes. Therefore, fluvoxamine should not be co-administered with these drugs.

Due to lack of clinical experience special attention is advised in the situation of post-acute myocardial infarction.

There is limited clinical experience of concomitant administration of fluvoxamine and ECT therefore caution is advisable.

Data in elderly subjects give no indication of clinically significant differences in normal daily dosages compared to younger subjects. However upward dose titration should be done slower in the elderly, and dosing should always be done with caution.

Use in children and adolescents under 18 years of age

Fluvoxamine should not be used in the treatment of children and adolescents under the age of 18 years, except for patients with Obsessive Compulsive Disorder. Suicide-related behaviours (suicide attempt and suicidal thoughts), and hostility (predominantly aggression, oppositional behaviour and anger) were more frequently observed in clinical trials among children and adolescents treated with antidepressants compared to those treated with placebo. If, based on clinical need, a decision to treat is nevertheless taken; the patient should be carefully monitored for the appearance of suicidal symptoms. In addition, long-term safety data in children and adolescents concerning growth, maturation and cognitive and behavioural development are lacking.

4.5 Interaction with other medicinal products and other forms of interaction

Fluvoxamine should not be used in combination with MAOIs (see also 4.4 Contraindications).

Fluvoxamine is a potent inhibitor of CYP1A2, and to a lesser extent of CYP2C and CYP3A4. Drugs which are largely metabolised via these isoenzymes are eliminated slower and may have higher plasma concentrations when co-administered with fluvoxamine. This is particularly relevant for drugs with a narrow therapeutic index. Patients should be carefully monitored and, if necessary, dose adjustment of these drugs is recommended.

Fluvoxamine has marginal inhibitory effects on CYP2D6 and seems not to affect non-oxidative metabolism or renal excretion.

CYP1A2

An increase in previously stable plasma levels of those tricyclic antidepressants (e.g., clomipramine, imipramine, amitriptyline) and neuroleptics (e.g., clozapine, olanzapine) which are largely metabolised through cytochrome P450 1A2 when given together with fluvoxamine, has been reported. A decrease in the dose of these products should be considered if treatment with fluvoxamine is initiated.

Patients co-administered fluvoxamine and CYP1A2 metabolised drugs with a narrow therapeutic index (such as tacrine, theophylline, methadone, mexiletine) should be carefully monitored and, if necessary, dose adjustment of these drugs is recommended.

When given with fluvoxamine, warfarin plasma concentrations were significantly increased and prothrombin times prolonged.

Isolated cases of cardiac toxicity have been reported when fluvoxamine was combined with thioridazine.

As plasma concentrations of propranolol are increased in combination with fluvoxamine, the propranolol dose may need to be lowered.

Caffeine plasma levels are likely to be increased during co-administration with fluvoxamine. Thus, patients who consume high quantities of caffeine-containing beverages should lower their intake when fluvoxamine is administered and adverse caffeine effects (like tremor, palpitations, nausea, restlessness, insomnia) are observed.

As plasma concentrations of ropinirole may be increased in combination with Fluvoxamine thus increasing the risk of overdose, surveillance and reduction in the posology of ropinirole during fluvoxamine treatment and after its withdrawal may be required.

CYP2C

Patients co-administered fluvoxamine and CYP2C metabolised drugs with a narrow therapeutic index (such as phenytoin) should be carefully monitored and, if necessary, dose adjustment of these drugs is recommended.

CYP3A4

Terfenadine, astemizole, cisapride (see also 4.4 Special Warnings and Special Precautions for Use).

Patients co-administered fluvoxamine and CYP3A4 metabolised drugs with a narrow therapeutic index (such as carbamazepine, ciclosporin) should be carefully monitored and, if necessary, dose adjustment of these drugs is recommended.

The plasma levels of oxidatively metabolised benzodiazepines (e.g. triazolam, midazolam, alprazolam, and diazepam) are likely to be increased when co-administered with fluvoxamine. The dosage of these benzodiazepines should be reduced during co-administration with fluvoxamine.

Glucuronidation

Fluvoxamine does not influence plasma concentrations of digoxin.

Renal excretion

Fluvoxamine does not influence plasma concentrations of atenolol.

Pharmacodynamic interactions

The serotonergic effects of fluvoxamine may be enhanced when used in combination with other serotonergic agents (including triptans, SSRIs and St. John's Wort preparations). (See also 4.4 Special Warnings and Special Precautions for Use).

Fluvoxamine has been used in combination with lithium in the treatment of severely ill, drug-resistant patients. However, lithium (and possibly also tryptophan) enhances the serotonergic effects of fluvoxamine. The combination should be used with caution in patients with severe, drug-resistant depression.

In patients on oral anticoagulants and fluvoxamine, the risk for haemorrhage may increase and these patients should therefore be closely monitored.

As with other psychotropic drugs patients should be advised to avoid alcohol use while taking fluvoxamine.

4.6 Pregnancy and lactation

Data on a limited number of exposed pregnancies indicate no adverse effects of fluvoxamine on pregnancy. To date, no other relevant epidemiological data are available.

Reproduction studies in animals at high doses revealed no evidence of impaired fertility, reproductive performance or teratogenic effects in the offspring. Caution should be exercised when prescribing to pregnant women.

Isolated cases of withdrawal symptoms in the newborn child have been described after the use of fluvoxamine at the end of pregnancy.

Fluvoxamine is excreted via human milk in small quantities. Therefore, the drug should not be used by women who breast feed.

4.7 Effects on ability to drive and use machines

Fluvoxamine up to 150 mg has no or negligible influence on the ability to drive and use machines. It showed no effect on psychomotor skills associated with driving and operating machinery in healthy volunteers. However, somnolence has been reported during treatment with fluvoxamine. Therefore, caution is recommended until the individual response to the drug has been determined.

4.8 Undesirable effects

Nausea, sometimes accompanied by vomiting is the most frequently observed symptom associated with fluvoxamine treatment. This side effect usually diminishes within the first two weeks of treatment. Other adverse events, observed in clinical studies at frequencies listed below, are often associated with the illness and are not necessarily related to treatment.

Common (Frequency 1-10%):

Body: Asthenia, headache, malaise

Cardiovascular: Palpitations/tachycardia

Digestive system: Abdominal pain, anorexia, constipation, diarrhoea, dry mouth, dyspepsia

Nervous system: Agitation, anxiety, dizziness, insomnia, nervousness, somnolence, tremor

Skin: Sweating

Uncommon (Frequency <1%):

Cardiovascular: (Postural) hypotension

Musculoskeletal: Arthralgia, myalgia

Nervous System: Ataxia, confusion, extrapyramidal symptoms, hallucinations

Urogenital: Abnormal (delayed) ejaculation

Skin: Cutaneous hypersensitivity reactions (incl. rash, pruritus, angioedema)

Rare (Frequency <0.1%):

Digestive system: Liver function abnormality

Nervous system: Convulsions, mania

Urogenital: Galactorrhoea

Skin: Photosensitivity

Psychomotor restlessness/akathisia (see section 4.4 Special warnings and special precautions for use)

Other adverse events observed during marketing:

Weight gain and loss have been reported.

Rarely, serotonin syndrome, neuroleptic malignant syndrome-like events, hyponatremia and SIADH have been reported (see also 4.4 Special Warnings and Special Precautions for Use).

It is possible that withdrawal reactions may occur on stopping therapy with fluvoxamine although the available preclinical and clinical evidence does not suggest that this treatment causes dependence. The following symptoms have been reported in association with withdrawal of the product: dizziness, paresthesia, headache, nausea and anxiety. The majority of the withdrawal reactions are mild and self-limiting.

When stopping, a gradual dose reduction may be considered.

Haemorrhage (see also 4.4 Special warnings and special precautions for use)

Very rarely, paresthesia, anorgasmy and taste perversion have been reported.

Cases of suicidal ideation and suicidal behaviours have been reported during Fluvoxamine therapy or early after treatment discontinuation (see section 4.4)

In one 10-week placebo-controlled trial in children and adolescents with OCD, frequently reported adverse events with a higher incidence than placebo, were: insomnia, asthenia, agitation, hyperkinesia, somnolence and dyspepsia. Serious adverse events in this study included: agitation and hypomania. Convulsions in children and adolescents have been reported during use outside clinical trials.

Withdrawal symptoms seen on discontinuation of fluvoxamine treatment

Discontinuation of fluvoxamine (particularly when abrupt) commonly leads to withdrawal symptoms. Dizziness, sensory disturbance (including paraesthesia, visual disturbance and electric shock sensations), sleep disturbances (including insomnia and intense dreams), agitation and anxiety, irritability, confusion, emotional instability, nausea and/or vomiting, diarrhoea, sweating, palpitations, headache and tremor are the most commonly reported reactions. Generally these events are mild to moderate and are self-limiting, however, in some patients they may be severe and/or prolonged. It is therefore advised that when fluvoxamine treatment is no longer required, gradual discontinuation by dose tapering should be carried out (see section 4.2 Posology and method of administration and section 4.4 Special warnings and special precautions for use).

4.9 Overdose

Symptoms

Symptoms include gastro-intestinal complaints (nausea, vomiting and diarrhoea), somnolence and dizziness. Cardiac events (tachycardia, bradycardia, hypotension), liver function disturbances, convulsions and coma have also been reported.

Fluvoxamine has a wide margin of safety in overdose. Since market introduction, reports of deaths attributed to overdose of fluvoxamine alone have been extremely rare. The highest documented dose of fluvoxamine ingested by a patient is 12 grams. This patient recovered completely. Occasionally, more serious complications were observed in cases of deliberate overdose of fluvoxamine in combination with other drugs.

Treatment

There is no specific antidote to fluvoxamine. In case of overdose the stomach should be emptied as soon as possible after tablet ingestion and symptomatic treatment should be given. The repeated use of medicinal charcoal, if necessary accompanied by an osmotic laxative, is also recommended. Forced diuresis or dialysis are unlikely to be of benefit.

5. PHARMACOLOGICAL PROPERTIES

5.1 Pharmacodynamic properties

Pharmacotherapeutic group: Antidepressants, Selective serotonin reuptake inhibitors, ATC code: N06AB08.

The mechanism of action of fluvoxamine is thought to be related to selective serotonin re-uptake inhibition in brain neurones. There is minimum interference with noradrenergic processes. Receptor binding studies have demonstrated that fluvoxamine has negligible binding capacity to alpha adrenergic, beta adrenergic, histaminergic, muscarine cholinergic, dopaminergic or serotonergic receptors.

In a placebo controlled trial in 120 patients with OCD, aged between 8 and 17 years, a statistically significant improvement was seen in the total population in favour of fluvoxamine at 10 weeks. A further subgroup analysis showed improvement on the C-YBOCS rating scale in children whereas no effect was seen in adolescents. The mean dose was respectively 158 mg and 168 mg/day.

Dose response

No formal clinical trials were conducted investigating the dose response of fluvoxamine. However, it is clinical experience that up-titrating the dose might be beneficial for some patients.

5.2 Pharmacokinetic properties

Absorption

Fluvoxamine is completely absorbed following oral administration. Maximum plasma concentrations occur within 3-8 hours of dosing. The mean absolute bioavailability is 53% due to first-pass metabolism.

The pharmacokinetics of Faverin is not influenced by concomitant food intake.

Distribution

In vitro plasma protein binding of fluvoxamine is 80%. Volume of distribution in humans is 25 l/kg.

Metabolism

Fluvoxamine undergoes extensive metabolism in the liver. Although CYP2D6 is *in vitro* the main isoenzyme involved in fluvoxamine's metabolism, plasma concentrations in poor metabolisers for CYP2D6 are not much higher than those in extensive metabolisers.

The mean plasma half-life is approximately 13-15 hours after a single dose and slightly longer (17-22 hours) during repeated dosing, when steady-state plasma levels are usually achieved within 10-14 days.

Fluvoxamine undergoes extensive hepatic transformation, mainly via oxidative demethylation, into at least nine metabolites, which are excreted by the kidneys. The two major metabolites showed negligible pharmacological activity. The other metabolites are not expected to be pharmacologically active. Fluvoxamine is a potent inhibitor of CYP1A2 and a moderate inhibitor of CYP2C and CYP3A4, with only marginal inhibitory effects on CYP2D6.

Fluvoxamine displays linear single-dose pharmacokinetics. Steady-state concentrations are higher than calculated from single-dose data, and are disproportionably higher at higher daily doses.

Special Patients groups

The pharmacokinetics of fluvoxamine is similar in healthy adults, elderly patients, and patients with renal insufficiency. The metabolism of fluvoxamine is impaired in patients with liver disease.

Steady-state plasma concentrations of fluvoxamine were twice as high in children (aged 6-11) as in adolescents (aged 12-17). Plasma concentrations in adolescents are similar to those in adults.

5.3 Preclinical safety data

There is no evidence of carcinogenicity, mutagenicity or impairment of fertility with fluvoxamine.

Reproduction studies in animals at high doses revealed no evidence of impaired fertility, reproductive performance or teratogenic effects in the offspring.

The potential for abuse, tolerance and physical dependence has been studied in a non-human primate model. No evidence of dependency phenomena was found.

6. PHARMACEUTICAL PARTICULARS

6.1 List of excipients

Tablet cores:

Mannitol

Maize starch

Pregelatinised starch

Sodium stearyl fumarate

Colloidal anhydrous silica

Film-coat:

Hypromellose

Macrogol 6000

Talc

Titanium Dioxide E171

6.2 Incompatibilities

Not applicable.

6.3 Shelf life

3 years.

6.4 Special precautions for storage

Do not store above 25°C.

Store in the original package.

6.5 Nature and contents of container

PVC/PVdC/Aluminium press-through blister.

Pack sizes: 5, 10, 20, 30, 50, 60, 90, 100 and 250 tablets.

Not all pack sizes may be marketed.

6.6 Special precautions for disposal and other handling

No special requirements.

7. MARKETING AUTHORISATION HOLDER

Solvay Healthcare Limited

Mansbridge Road

West End

Southampton

SO18 3JD

8. MARKETING AUTHORISATION NUMBER(S)

PL 00512/0070

9. DATE OF FIRST AUTHORISATION/RENEWAL OF THE AUTHORISATION

22/06/2004

10. DATE OF REVISION OF THE TEXT

04/06/2009

Feldene Capsules, Feldene I.M. Intramuscular Injection, Feldene MELT

(Pfizer Limited)

1. NAME OF THE MEDICINAL PRODUCT

FELDENE™ 10mg CAPSULES

FELDENE™ 20mg CAPSULES

FELDENE™ 20mg/ml INTRAMUSCULAR INJECTION

Feldene® Melt 20mg

2. QUALITATIVE AND QUANTITATIVE COMPOSITION

Active Ingredient: piroxicam

Capsules: piroxicam 10mg or 20mg (anhydrous)

I.M.: the intramuscular injection contains 1ml of piroxicam solution (20mg/ml) in ampoules of 1ml

Melt tablets: piroxicam 20mg

For a full list of excipients, see section 6.1.

3. PHARMACEUTICAL FORM

Capsules (10mg and 20mg): Capsules for oral administration.

I.M.: Solution for intramuscular injection.

Melt tablets: Fast Dissolving Dosage Form (Tablet).

4. CLINICAL PARTICULARS

4.1 Therapeutic indications

Capsules, Melt tablets, IM: Feldene is indicated for symptomatic relief of osteoarthritis, rheumatoid arthritis or ankylosing spondylitis.

Due to its safety profile (see sections 4.2, 4.3 and 4.4), Feldene is not a first line option should an NSAID be indicated. The decision to prescribe Feldene should be based on an assessment of the individual patient's overall risks (see sections 4.3 and 4.4).

4.2 Posology and method of administration

IM only: Feldene I.M. is for intramuscular administration only

The prescription of Feldene should be initiated by physicians with experience in the diagnostic evaluation and treatment of patients with inflammatory or degenerative rheumatic diseases.

The maximum recommended daily dose is 20 mg.

Undesirable effects may be minimised by using the minimum effective dose for the shortest duration necessary to control symptoms. The benefit and tolerability of treatment should be reviewed within 14 days. If continued treatment is considered necessary, this should be accompanied by frequent review.

Given that piroxicam has been shown to be associated with an increased risk of gastrointestinal complications, the need for possible combination therapy with gastro-protective agents (e.g. misoprostol or proton pump inhibitors) should be carefully considered, in particular for elderly patients.

Use in the elderly

Elderly, frail or debilitated patients may tolerate side-effects less well and such patients should be carefully supervised. As with other NSAIDs, caution should be used in the treatment of elderly patients who are more likely to be suffering from impaired renal, hepatic or cardiac function.

I.M. only:

The dosage of Feldene I.M. intramuscular injection is identical to the dosage of oral Feldene. For continuation of treatment, oral (capsules or FDDF tablets) dose forms should be used. Feldene I.M. intramuscular injection should be administered by deep intramuscular injection into the upper, outer quadrant of the buttock. Feldene I.M. intramuscular injection should not be administered intravenously.

Melt tablets and capsules only: For oral administration. To be taken preferably with or after food.

Melt tablets only:

The fast dissolving dosage form may be swallowed with water, or placed on the tongue to disperse and then swallowed with the saliva. The fast dissolving dosage form dissolves almost instantly in the mouth in the presence of water or saliva.

Undesirable effects may be minimised by using the lowest effective dose for the shortest duration necessary to control symptoms (see section 4.4).

4.3 Contraindications

History of gastro-intestinal ulceration, bleeding or perforation.

Patient history of gastrointestinal disorders that predispose to bleeding disorders such as ulcerative colitis, Crohn's disease, gastrointestinal cancers or diverticulitis.

Patients with active peptic ulcer, inflammatory gastrointestinal disorder or gastrointestinal bleeding.

Concomitant use with other NSAIDs, including COX-2 selective NSAIDs and acetylsalicylic acid at analgesic doses.

Concomitant use with anticoagulants.

History of previous serious allergic drug reaction of any type, especially cutaneous reactions such as erythema multiforme, Stevens-Johnson syndrome, toxic epidermal necrolysis.

Hypersensitivity to the active substance or excipients, previous skin reaction (regardless of severity) to piroxicam, other NSAIDs and other medications.

Patients in whom aspirin and other non-steroidal anti-inflammatory drugs induce the symptoms of asthma, nasal polyps, angioedema or urticaria.

Severe heart failure.

During the last trimester of pregnancy.

4.4 Special warnings and precautions for use

Undesirable effects may be minimised by using the minimum effective dose for the shortest duration necessary to control symptoms (see section 4.2, and GI and cardiovascular risks below).

The clinical benefit and tolerability should be re-evaluated periodically and treatment should be immediately discontinued at the first appearance of cutaneous reactions or relevant gastrointestinal events.

Gastrointestinal (GI) Effects, Risk of GI Ulceration, Bleeding, and Perforation

NSAIDs, including piroxicam, can cause serious gastrointestinal events including bleeding, ulceration, and perforation of the stomach, small intestine or large intestine, which can be fatal. These serious adverse events can occur at any time, with or without warning symptoms, in patients treated with NSAIDs.

NSAID exposures of both short and long duration have an increased risk of serious GI event. Evidence from observational studies suggests that piroxicam may be associated with a high risk of serious gastrointestinal toxicity, relative to other NSAIDs.

Patients with significant risk factors for serious GI events should be treated with piroxicam only after careful consideration (see sections 4.3 and below).

The possible need for combination therapy with gastroprotective agents (e.g. misoprostol or proton pump inhibitors) should be carefully considered (see section 4.2).

Serious GI Complications

Identification of at-risk subjects

The risk for developing serious GI complications increases with age. Age over 70 years is associated with high risk of complications. The administration to patients over 80 years should be avoided.

Patients taking concomitant oral corticosteroids, selective serotonin reuptake inhibitors (SSRIs) or anti-platelet agents such as low-dose acetylsalicylic acid are at increased risk of serious GI complications (see below and section 4.5). As with other NSAIDs, the use of piroxicam in combination with protective agents (e.g. misoprostol or proton pump inhibitors) must be considered for these at-risk patients.

Patients and physicians should remain alerted for signs and symptoms of GI ulceration and/or bleeding during piroxicam treatment. Patients should be asked to report any new or unusual abdominal symptom during treatment. If a gastrointestinal complication is suspected during treatment, piroxicam should be discontinued immediately and additional clinical evaluation and treatment should be considered.

Appropriate monitoring and advice are required for patients with a history of hypertension and/or mild to moderate congestive heart failure as fluid retention and oedema have been reported in association with NSAID therapy.

Patients with uncontrolled hypertension, congestive heart failure, established ischaemic heart disease, peripheral arterial disease, and/or cerebrovascular disease should only be treated with piroxicam after careful consideration. Similar consideration should be made before initiating longer-term treatment of patients with risk factors for cardiovascular events (e.g. hypertension, hyperlipidaemia, diabetes mellitus, smoking).

Clinical trial and epidemiological data suggest that use of some NSAIDs (particularly at high doses and in long term treatment) may be associated with a small increased risk of arterial thrombotic events (for example myocardial infarction or stroke). There are insufficient data to exclude such a risk for Feldene.

Feldene should be used with caution in patients with a history of bronchial asthma (see also section 4.3).

Skin reactions

Serious skin reactions, some of them fatal, including exfoliative dermatitis, Stevens-Johnson syndrome, and toxic epidermal necrolysis, have been reported very rarely in association with the use of NSAIDs (see section 4.8). Evidence from observational studies suggests that piroxicam may be associated with a higher risk of serious skin reaction than other non-oxicam NSAIDs. Patients appear to be at highest risk of these reactions early in the course of therapy, the onset of the reaction occurring in the majority of cases within the first month of treatment. Piroxicam should be discontinued at the first appearance of skin rash, mucosal lesions, or any other sign of hypersensitivity.

Feldene should be used with caution in patients with renal, hepatic and cardiac impairment. In rare cases, non-steroidal anti-inflammatory drugs may cause interstitial nephritis, glomerulitis, papillary necrosis and the nephrotic syndrome. Such agents inhibit the synthesis of the prostaglandin which plays a supportive role in the maintenance of renal perfusion in patients whose renal blood flow and blood volume are decreased. In these patients, administration of a non-steroidal anti-inflammatory drug may precipitate overt renal decompensation, which is typically followed by recovery to pretreatment state upon discontinuation of non-steroidal anti-inflammatory therapy. Patients at greatest risk of such a reaction are those with congestive heart failure, liver cirrhosis, nephrotic syndrome and overt renal disease, such patients should be carefully monitored whilst receiving NSAID therapy. Because of reports of adverse eye findings with non-steroidal anti-inflammatory drugs, it is recommended that patients who develop visual complaints during treatment with Feldene have ophthalmic evaluation.

Impaired female fertility

The use of Feldene may impair female fertility and is not recommended in women attempting to conceive. In women who have difficulties conceiving or who are undergoing investigation of infertility, withdrawal of Feldene should be considered.

Melt tablets only:

Patients with phenylketonuria:

Due to aspartame content of Feldene Melt, each 20mg tablet contains 0.14mg phenylalanine.

4.5 Interaction with other medicinal products and other forms of interaction

Antacids: Concomitant administration of antacids had no effect on piroxicam plasma levels.

Anticoagulants: NSAIDs, including piroxicam, may enhance the effects of anticoagulants, such as warfarin. Therefore the use of piroxicam with concomitant anticoagulant such as warfarin should be avoided (see section 4.3).

Anti-platelet agents and selective serotonin reuptake inhibitors (SSRIs): increased risk of gastrointestinal bleeding (see section 4.4).

Aspirin and other Non-Steroidal Anti-Inflammatory Drugs: Feldene, like other non-steroidal anti-inflammatory drugs decreases platelet aggregation and prolongs bleeding time. This effect should be kept in mind when bleeding times are determined.

As with other NSAIDs, the use of piroxicam together with acetylsalicylic acid or concomitant use with other NSAIDs, including other piroxicam formulations, must be avoided, since data are inadequate to show that combinations produce greater improvement that that achieved with piroxicam alone; moreover, the potential for adverse reactions is enhanced (see section 4.4). Human studies have shown that concomitant use of piroxicam and acetylsalicylic acid reduces the plasma piroxicam concentration to about 80% of the usual value.

Cardiac glycosides: NSAIDs may exacerbate cardiac failure, reduce GFR and increase plasma glycoside levels.

Ciclosporin, Tacrolimus: possible increased risk of nephrotoxicity when NSAIDs are given with ciclosporin or tacrolimus.

Cimetidine: Results of two separate studies indicate a slight but significant increase in absorption of piroxicam following cimetidine administration but no significant changes in elimination rate constants or half-life. The small increase in absorption is unlikely to be clinically significant.

Corticosteroids: increased risk of gastrointestinal ulceration or bleeding (see section 4.4).

Digoxin, Digitoxin: Concurrent therapy with Feldene and digoxin, or Feldene and digitoxin, did not affect the plasma levels of either drug.

Diuretics: Non-steroidal anti-inflammatory drugs may cause sodium, potassium and fluid retention and may interfere with the natriuretic action of diuretic agents. These properties should be kept in mind when treating patients with compromised cardiac function or hypertension since they may be responsible for the worsening of those conditions.

Highly protein-bound drugs: Feldene is highly protein-bound and therefore might be expected to displace other protein-bound drugs. The physician should closely monitor patients for change when administering Feldene to patients on highly protein-bound drugs.

Lithium: Non-steroidal anti-inflammatory drugs, including Feldene, have been reported to increase steady state plasma lithium levels. It is recommended that these levels are monitored when initiating, adjusting and discontinuing Feldene.

Feldene, like other non-steroidal anti-inflammatory drugs, may interact with the following drugs / classes of therapeutic agents:

Antihypertensives - antagonism of the hypotensive effect

Methotrexate - reduced excretion of methotrexate, possibly leading to acute toxicity

Quinolone antibiotics - possible increased risk of convulsions

Mifepristone - NSAIDs could interfere with mifepristone-mediated termination of pregnancy

4.6 Pregnancy and lactation

Use in pregnancy: Although no teratogenic effects were seen in animal testing, the safety of Feldene during pregnancy or during lactation has not yet been established. Feldene inhibits prostaglandin synthesis and release through a reversible inhibition of the cyclo-oxygenase enzyme. This effect, as with other non-steroidal anti-inflammatory drugs, has been associated with an increased incidence of dystocia and delayed parturition in pregnant animals when drug administration was continued in late pregnancy. In view of the known effects of NSAIDs on the foetal cardiovascular system (risk of closure of the ductus arteriosus), use in the last trimester of pregnancy is contraindicated. The onset of labour may be delayed and the duration increased with an increased bleeding tendency in both mother and child (see section 4.3). NSAIDs should not be used during the first two trimesters of pregnancy or labour unless the potential benefit to the patient outweighs the potential risk to the foetus.

Nursing mothers: A study indicates that piroxicam appears in the breast milk at about 1% to 3% of the maternal plasma concentrations. No accumulation of piroxicam occurred in milk relative to that in plasma during treatment for up to 52 days. Feldene is not recommended for use in nursing mothers as clinical safety has not been established.

4.7 Effects on ability to drive and use machines

Undesirable effects such as dizziness, drowsiness, fatigue and visual disturbances are possible after taking NSAIDs. If affected, patients should not drive or operate machinery.

4.8 Undesirable effects

Gastro-intestinal: These are the most commonly encountered side-effects but in most instances do not interfere with the course of therapy. They include stomatitis, anorexia, epigastric distress, gastritis, nausea, vomiting, constipation, abdominal discomfort, flatulance, diarrhoea, abdominal pain and indigestion, rare cases of pancreatitis have been reported.

Objective evaluations of gastric mucosa appearances and intestinal blood loss show that 20mg/day of Feldene administered either in single or divided doses is significantly less irritating to the gastro-intestinal tract than aspirin. Peptic ulceration, perforation and gastro-intestinal bleeding (including haematemesis and melaena) in rare cases fatal, have been reported with Feldene.

Some epidemiological studies have suggested that piroxicam is associated with higher risk of gastro-intestinal adverse reactions compared with some NSAIDs, but this has not been confirmed in all studies. Administration of doses exceeding 20mg daily (of more than several days duration) carries an increased risk of gastro-intestinal side-effects, but they may also occur with lower doses. See section 4.2 Posology and method of administration.

Oedema, hypertension, and cardiac failure, have been reported in association with NSAID treatment. The possibility of precipitating congestive heart failure in elderly patients or those with compromised cardiac function should therefore be borne in mind.

CNS: Dizziness, headache, somnolence, insomnia, depression, nervousness, hallucinations, mood alterations, dream abnormalities, mental confusion, paraesthesiae and vertigo have been reported rarely.

Dermal hypersensitivity: Rash and pruritis. Onycholysis and analopoecia have rarely been reported. Photosensitivity reactions occur infrequently. As with other non-steroidal anti-inflammatory drugs, toxic epidermal necrolysis (Lyell's disease) and Stevens-Johnson syndrome may develop in rare cases. Vesiculo bullous reactions have been reported rarely.

Hypersensitivity reactions: Hypersensitivity reactions such as anaphylaxis, bronchospasm, urticaria/angioneurotic oedema, vasculitis and serum sickness have been reported rarely.

Renal function: Interstitial nephritis, nephrotic syndrome, renal failure and renal papillary necrosis have been reported rarely.

Haematological: Decreases in haemoglobin and haematocrit, unassociated with obvious gastro-intestinal bleeding have occurred. Anaemia, thrombocytopenia and non-thrombocytopenia purpura (Henoch-Schoenlein), leucopenia and eosinophilia have been reported. Cases of aplastic anaemia, haemolytic anaemia and epistaxis have rarely been reported.

Liver function: Changes in various liver function parameters have been observed. As with most other non-steroidal anti-inflammatory drugs, some patients may develop increased serum transaminase levels during treatment with Feldene. Severe hepatic reactions including jaundice and cases of fatal hepatitis have been reported with Feldene. Although such reactions are rare, if abnormal liver function tests persist or worsen, if clinical symptoms consistent with liver disease develop, or if systemic manifestations occur e.g. eosinophilia, rash etc., Feldene should be discontinued.

Other: The following have been reported rarely, palpitations and dyspnoea, anecdotal cases of positive ANA, anecdotal cases of hearing abnormalities, metabolic abnormalities such as hypoglycaemia, hyperglycaemia, weight increase or decrease. Swollen eyes, blurred vision and eye irritations have been reported. Routine ophthalmoscopy and slit-lamp examination have revealed no evidence of ocular changes. Malaise and tinnitus may occur.

Clinical trial and epidemiological data suggest that use of some NSAIDs (particularly at high doses and in long term treatment) may be associated with a small increased risk of arterial thrombotic events (for example myocardial infarction or stroke) (see section 4.4).

I.M. only:

Intramuscular: Transient pain upon injection has occasionally been reported. Local adverse reactions (burning sensations) or tissue damage (sterile abscess formation, fatty tissue necrosis) may occasionally occur at the site of injection.

4.9 Overdose

In the event of overdosage with Feldene, supportive and symptomatic therapy is indicated. Studies indicate that administration of activated charcoal may result in reduced re-absorption of piroxicam, thus reducing the total amount of active drug available.

Although there are no studies to date, haemodialysis is probably not useful in enhancing elimination of piroxicam since the drug is highly protein bound.

5. PHARMACOLOGICAL PROPERTIES

5.1 Pharmacodynamic properties

Capsules and Melt tablets:

Piroxicam is a non-steroidal anti-inflammatory agent which also possesses analgesic and antipyretic properties. Oedema, erythema, tissue proliferation, fever and pain can all be inhibited in laboratory animals by the administration of piroxicam. It is effective regardless of the aetiology of the inflammation. While its mode of action is not fully understood, independent studies *in vitro* as well as *in vivo* have shown that piroxicam interacts at several steps in the immune and inflammation responses through:

Inhibition of prostanoid synthesis, including prostaglandins, through a reversible inhibition of the cyclo-oxygenase enzyme.

Inhibition of neutrophil aggregation.

Inhibition of polymorphonuclear cell and monocyte migration to the area of inflammation.

Inhibition of lyosomal enzyme release from stimulated leucocytes.

Reduction of both systemic and synovial fluid rheumatoid factor production in patients with seropositive rheumatoid arthritis.

It is established that piroxicam does not act by pituitary-adrenal axis stimulation. In-vitro studies have not revealed any negative effects on cartilage metabolism.

I.M. only:

Feldene is a non-steroidal anti-inflammatory agent useful in the treatment of inflammatory conditions. Although the mode of action for this agent is not precisely understood, Feldene inhibits prostaglandin synthesis and release through a reversible inhibition of the cyclo-oxygenase enzyme.

Transient pain upon injection has occasionally been reported. Local adverse reactions (burning sensations) or tissue damage (sterile abscess formation, fatty tissue necrosis) may occasionally occur at the site of injection.

5.2 Pharmacokinetic properties

Capsules and Melt tablets:

Piroxicam is well absorbed following oral administration. With food there is a slight delay in the rate but not the extent of absorption following administration. The plasma half-life is approximately 50 hours in man and stable plasma concentrations are maintained throughout the day on once-daily dosage. Continuous treatment with 20mg/day for periods of 1 year produces similar blood levels to those seen once steady state is first achieved.

Drug plasma concentrations are proportional for 10 and 20mg doses and generally peak within 3 to 5 hours after medication. A single 20mg dose generally produces peak piroxicam plasma levels of 1.5 to 2 microgram/ml while maximum plasma concentrations, after repeated daily ingestion of 20mg piroxicam, usually stabilise at 3 to 8 microgram/ml. Most patients approximate steady state plasma levels within 7 to 12 days.

Treatment with a loading dose regimen of 40mg daily for the first 2 days followed by 20mg daily thereafter allows a high percentage (approximately 76%) of steady state levels to be achieved immediately following the second dose. Steady state levels, area under the curves and elimination half-life are similar to that following a 20mg daily dose regimen.

A multiple dose comparative study of the bioavailability of the injectable forms with the oral capsule has shown that after intramuscular administration of piroxicam, plasma levels are significantly higher than those obtained after ingestion of capsules during the 45 minutes following administration the first day, during 30 minutes the second day and 15 minutes the seventh day. Bioequivalence exists between the two dosage forms.

A multiple dose comparative study of the pharmacokinetics and the bioavailability of Feldene FDDF with the oral capsule has shown that after once daily administration for 14 days, the mean plasma piroxicam concentration time profiles for capsules and Feldene FDDF were nearly superimposable. There were no significant differences between the mean steady state C_{max} values, C_{min} values, T½, or T_{max} values. This study concluded that Feldene FDDF (Fast Dissolving Dosage Form) is bioequivalent to the capsule after once daily dosing. Single dose studies have demonstrated bioequivalence as well when the tablet is taken with or without water.

Piroxicam is extensively metabolised and less than 5% of the daily dose is excreted unchanged in urine and faeces. One important metabolic pathway is hydroxylation of the pyridyl ring of the piroxicam side-chain, followed by conjugation with glucuronic acid and urinary elimination.

I.M. only:

Feldene I.M. and Feldene capsules are bioequivalent. However, Feldene I.M. provides significantly higher plasma levels of piroxicam during the first 45 minutes on the first day and 30 minutes on the second day.

The plasma half-life is approximately 50 hours in man and stable plasma concentrations are maintained throughout the day on once-daily dosage.

Feldene is extensively metabolised and less than 5% of the daily dose is excreted unchanged in urine and faeces. One important metabolic pathway is hydroxyiation of the pyridyl ring of the piroxicam side chain followed by conjugation with glucaronic acid and urinary elimination.

6. PHARMACEUTICAL PARTICULARS

6.1 List of excipients

Capsules 10mg and 20mg:

Lactose

Corn starch

Vegetable magnesium stearate

Sodium lauryl sulphate

10mg capsule shell cap (red) contains:

Gelatin

Titanium dioxide (E171)

Red iron oxide (E172)

The body of the capsule shell (blue) contains:

Gelatin

Titanium dioxide (E171)

Indigotin (E132)

20mg capsule shell (white opaque) and body (white opaque) contain gelatin and titanium dioxide (E171).

I.M. Intramuscular Injection:

Sodium dihydrogen phosphate

Nicotinamide

Propylene glycol

Ethanol

Benzyl alcohol

Sodium hydroxide

Hydrochloric acid

Water for injection

Melt tablets:

Gelatin USNF

Mannitol Ph.Eur

Aspartame USNF

Citric acid Ph.Eur

Purified water Ph.Eur

6.2 Incompatibilities

None stated.

6.3 Shelf life

Capsules	36 months
I.M. Intramuscular Injection	48 months
Melt tablets	5 years

6.4 Special precautions for storage

Capsules:

Store below 30°C.

I.M., Melt tablets:

Store below 25°C.

6.5 Nature and contents of container

Capsules 10mg: original pack of 56 capsules contained in a white HDPE bottle with a blue round ribbed cap.

Capsules 20mg: original pack of 28 capsules contained in a white HDPE bottle with a blue round ribbed cap.

I.M.: Type I, 2ml amber glass ampoules containing 1ml.

Melt tablets 20mg: blister strip PVC/PVdC and paper foil laminate containing 10 units. Each pack contains 30 units (3 × strips of 10 tablets).

6.6 Special precautions for disposal and other handling

No special requirements.

7. MARKETING AUTHORISATION HOLDER

Pfizer Limited

Ramsgate Road

Sandwich

Kent

CT13 9NJ

United Kingdom

8. MARKETING AUTHORISATION NUMBER(S)

Capsules 10mg	PL 00057/0145
Capsules 20mg	PL 00057/0146
I.M. intramuscular injection 20mg/ml	PL 00057/0320
Melt tablets 20mg	PL 00057/0352

9. DATE OF FIRST AUTHORISATION/RENEWAL OF THE AUTHORISATION

Capsules 10mg	08 August 1979/20 July 2009
Capsules 20mg	08 August 1979/20 July 2009
I.M. intramuscular injection 20mg/ml	29 May 1991/20 July 2009
Melt tablets 20mg	14 September 1992/31 March 2009

10. DATE OF REVISION OF THE TEXT

Capsules: 20/07/2009

IM: 20/07/2009

Melt tablets: 05/06/2009

LEGAL CATEGORY

POM

Ref: FE 7_0

Feldene Gel

(Pfizer Limited)

1. NAME OF THE MEDICINAL PRODUCT

FELDENE GEL

FELDENE SPORTS GEL

FELDENE GEL STARTER PACK.

2. QUALITATIVE AND QUANTITATIVE COMPOSITION

Active ingredient: Piroxicam

The Gel contains 5mg piroxicam in each gram in tubes of 7.5g - Feldene Gel starter Pack, 30g - Feldene Sports Gel, 60g and 112g - Feldene Gel.

3. PHARMACEUTICAL FORM

Gel for topical application.

4. CLINICAL PARTICULARS

4.1 Therapeutic indications

Feldene Gel is a non-steroidal anti-inflammatory agent indicated for a variety of conditions characterised by pain and inflammation, or stiffness. It is effective in the treatment of osteoarthritis of superficial joints such as the knee, acute musculoskeletal injuries, periarthritis, epicondylitis, tendinitis, and tenosynovitis.

4.2 Posology and method of administration

Dosage

Adults Feldene Gel, Feldene Sports Gel and Feldene Gel Starter Pack are for external use only. No occlusive dressings should be employed. Apply 1g of Gel, corresponding to 3cms, and rub into the affected site three to four times daily leaving no residual material on the skin. Therapy should be reviewed after 4 weeks.

Use in Children (See under 'Special warnings and special precautions for use').

Use in the Elderly (See under 'Special warnings and special precautions for use').

4.3 Contraindications

Feldene Gel, Feldene Sports Gel and Feldene Gel Starter Pack should not be used in those patients who have previously shown a hypersensitivity to the Gel or piroxicam in any of its forms. The potential exists for cross sensitivity to aspirin and other non-steroidal anti-inflammatory agents. Feldene Gel, Feldene Sports Gel and Feldene Gel Starter Pack should not be given to patients in whom aspirin and other non-steroidal anti-inflammatory agents induce the symptoms of asthma, nasal polyps, angioneurotic oedema or urticaria.

4.4 Special warnings and precautions for use

If local irritation develops, the use of the Gel should be discontinued and appropriate therapy instituted as necessary.

Keep away from the eyes and mucosal surfaces. Do not apply to any sites affected by open skin lesions, dermatoses or infection.

Use in patients with impaired hepatic function

Use in patients with renal impairment

Use in the Elderly No special precautions are required.

Use in Children Dosage recommendations and indications for the use of Feldene Gel, Feldene Sports Gel and Feldene Gel Starter Pack in children under 12 years have not been established.

4.5 Interaction with other medicinal products and other forms of interaction

None known.

4.6 Pregnancy and lactation

Use in pregnancy Although no teratogenic effects were seen when piroxicam was orally administered in animal testing, the use of Feldene Gel, Feldene Sports Gel and Feldene Gel Starter Pack during pregnancy or during lactation is not recommended.

Nursing mothers Feldene Gel, Feldene Sports Gel and Feldene Gel Starter Pack are not recommended for use in nursing mothers as clinical safety has not been established.

4.7 Effects on ability to drive and use machines

None known.

4.8 Undesirable effects

Feldene Gel is well tolerated. Mild to moderate local irritation, erythema, pruritus and dermatitis may occur at the application site. The systemic absorption of Feldene Gel, is very low. In common with other topical non-steroidal anti-inflammatory agents, systemic reactions occur infrequently and have included minor gastro-intestinal side-effects such as nausea and dyspepsia. Cases of abdominal pain and gastritis have been reported rarely. There have been isolated reports of bronchospasm and dyspnoea (see also Contra-indications).

Contact dermatitis, eczema and photosensitivity skin reaction have also been observed from post-marketing experience.

4.9 Overdose

Overdosage is unlikely to occur with this topical preparation.

5. PHARMACOLOGICAL PROPERTIES

5.1 Pharmacodynamic properties

Piroxicam is a non-steroidal anti-inflammatory agent useful in the treatment of inflammatory conditions. Although the mode of action for this agent is not precisely understood, piroxicam inhibits prostaglandin synthesis and release through a reversible inhibition of the cyclo-oxygenase enzyme. New data are presented on the anti-inflammatory and analgesic effects of Feldene Gel compared with its vehicle and indomethacin 1% Gel in rats and guinea pigs. Using established animal models of pain and inflammation, Feldene Gel was as effective as oral Feldene and indomethacin 1% Gel and significantly more effective than its vehicle.

5.2 Pharmacokinetic properties

On the basis of various pharmacokinetic and tissue distribution studies in animals, with piroxicam gel 0.5%, the highest concentrations of piroxicam were achieved in the tissues below the site of application with low concentrations being reached in the plasma. Piroxicam gel 0.5% was continuously and gradually released from the skin to underlying tissues, equilibrium between skin, and muscle or synovial fluid appeared to be reached rapidly, within a few hours of application.

From a pharmacokinetic study in man, 2g of the Gel was applied to the shoulders of normal volunteers twice daily (corresponding to 20mg piroxicam/day) for 14 days, plasma levels of piroxicam rose slowly, reaching steady state after about 11 days. The plasma levels at this time were between 300-400 ng/ml, or one-twentieth of those observed in subjects receiving 20mg orally.

The serum half-life of piroxicam is approximately 50 hours.

6. PHARMACEUTICAL PARTICULARS

6.1 List of excipients

Propylene Glycol EP, Carbopol 980 EP, Ethyl Alcohol EP, Benzyl Alcohol EP, di-isopropanolamine NF, Hydroxyethyl Cellulose EP, Purified Water EP.

6.2 Incompatibilities

None known.

6.3 Shelf life

3 years.

6.4 Special precautions for storage

Store below 30°C.

6.5 Nature and contents of container

Aluminium blind-ended tube incorporating epoxy-phenol internal lacquer with a white vinyl pressure sensitive polyethylene end seal, fitted with a polypropylene cap containing either 7.5g, 30g, 60g or 112g of Feldene Gel

6.6 Special precautions for disposal and other handling

No special requirements

7. MARKETING AUTHORISATION HOLDER

Pfizer Limited

Ramsgate Road

Sandwich

Kent

CT 13 9NJ

United Kingdom

8. MARKETING AUTHORISATION NUMBER(S)

Feldene Gel, Feldene Sports Gel and Feldene Gel Starter Pack PL 0057/0284

9. DATE OF FIRST AUTHORISATION/RENEWAL OF THE AUTHORISATION

13 January 2000

10. DATE OF REVISION OF THE TEXT

February 2003

11. LEGAL CATEGORY

POM

Ref (UK): FE 3_1

Felotens XL 10mg Prolonged Release Tablets

(Genus Pharmaceuticals)

1. NAME OF THE MEDICINAL PRODUCT

Felotens XL 10 mg Prolonged Release Tablets

2. QUALITATIVE AND QUANTITATIVE COMPOSITION

Felotens XL 10 mg Prolonged Release Tablets contain 10mg of felodipine.

3. PHARMACEUTICAL FORM

Reddish brown, round, biconvex, film coated prolonged-release tablets with imprint 10.

4. CLINICAL PARTICULARS

4.1 Therapeutic indications

In the management of hypertension and prophylaxis of chronic stable angina pectoris.

4.2 Posology and method of administration

For oral administration

Hypertension:

Adults (including elderly): The dose should be adjusted to the individual requirements of the patient. The recommended starting dose is 5 mg once daily. If necessary the dose may be further increased or another antihypertensive agent added. The usual maintenance dose is 5-10 mg once daily. Doses higher than 20 mg daily are not usually needed. For dose titration purposes a 2.5 mg tablet is available. In elderly patients an initial treatment with 2.5 mg daily should be considered.

Angina pectoris:

Adults: The dose should be adjusted individually. Treatment should be started with 5 mg once daily and if needed be increased to 10 mg once daily.

Administration: The tablets should regularly be taken in the morning without food or with a light meal. Felotens XL 10 mg Prolonged Release Tablets must not be chewed or crushed. They should be swallowed whole with half a glass of water.

Children: The safety and efficacy of Felotens XL 10 mg Prolonged Release Tablets in children has not been established.

Felotens XL 10 mg Prolonged Release Tablets can be used in combination with β-blockers, ACE inhibitors or diuretics. The effects on blood pressure are likely to be additive and combination therapy will usually enhance the antihypertensive effect. Care should be taken to avoid hypotension. In patients with severely impaired liver function the dose of felodipine should be low. The pharmacokinetics are not significantly affected in patients with impaired renal function.

4.3 Contraindications

Unstable angina pectoris.

Pregnancy.

Patient with a previous allergic reaction to Felotens XL 10 mg Prolonged Release Tablets or other dihydropyridines because of the theoretical risk of cross-reactivity.

Felotens XL 10 mg Prolonged Release Tablets should not be used in patients with clinically significant aortic stenosis, and during or within one month of a myocardial infarction.

As with other calcium channel blockers, Felotens XL 10 mg Prolonged Release Tablets should be discontinued in patients who develop cardiogenic shock.

4.4 Special warnings and precautions for use

As with other vasodilators, Felotens XL 10 mg Prolonged Release Tablets may, in rare cases, precipitate significant hypotension with tachycardia which in susceptible individuals may result in myocardial ischaemia.

There is no evidence that Felotens XL 10 mg Prolonged Release Tablets are useful for secondary prevention of myocardial infarction.

The efficacy and safety of Felotens XL 10 mg Prolonged Release Tablets in the treatment of malignant hypertension has not been studied.

Felotens XL 10 mg Prolonged Release Tablets should be used with caution in patients with severe left ventricular dysfunction.

4.5 Interaction with other medicinal products and other forms of interaction

Concomitant administration of substances which interfere with the cytochrome P450 system may affect plasma concentrations of felodipine. Enzyme inhibitors such as cimetidine, erythromycin and itraconazole impair the elimination of felodipine, and Felotens XL 10 mg Prolonged Release Tablets dosage may need to be reduced when drugs are given concomitantly. Conversely, powerful enzyme inducing agents such as some anticonvulsants (phenytoin, carbamazepine, phenobarbitone) can increase felodipine elimination and higher than normal Felotens XL 10 mg Prolonged Release Tablets doses may be required in patients taking the drugs.

No dosage adjustment is required when Felotens XL 10 mg Prolonged Release Tablets are given concomitantly with digoxin.

Felodipine does not appear to affect the unbound fraction of other extensively plasma protein bound drugs such as warfarin.

Grapefruit juice results in increased peak plasma levels and bioavailability possibly due to an interaction with flavonoids in the fruit juice. This interaction has been seen with other dihydropyridine calcium antagonists and represents a class effect. Therefore grapefruit juice should not be taken together with Felotens XL 10 mg Prolonged Release Tablets.

4.6 Pregnancy and lactation

Felodipine should not be given during pregnancy.

In a study on fertility and general reproductive performance in rats, a prolongation of parturition resulting in difficult labour, increased foetal deaths and early postnatal deaths were observed in the medium- and high-dose groups. Reproductive studies in rabbits have shown a dose-related reversible enlargement of the mammary glands of the parent animals and dose-related digital abnormalities in the foetuses when felodipine was administered during stages of early foetal development.

Felodipine has been detected in breast milk, but it is unknown whether it has harmful effects on the new-born.

4.7 Effects on ability to drive and use machines

None.

4.8 Undesirable effects

As with other calcium antagonists, flushing, headache, palpitations, dizziness and fatigue may occur. These reactions are usually transient and are most likely to occur at the start of treatment or after an increase in dosage.

As with other calcium antagonists ankle swelling, resulting from precapillary vasodilation, may occur. The degree of ankle swelling is dose related.

In patients with gingivitis/periodontitis, mild gingival enlargement has been reported with Felotens XL 10 mg Prolonged Release Tablets, as with other calcium antagonists. The enlargement can be avoided or reversed by careful dental hygiene.

As with other dihydropyridines, aggravation of angina has been reported in a small number of individuals especially after starting treatment. This is more likely to happen in patients with symptomatic ischaemic heart disease.

The following adverse events have been reported from clinical trials and from Post Marketing Surveillance. In the great majority of cases a causal relationship between these events and treatment with felodipine has not been established.

Skin: rarely - rash and/or pruritus, and isolated cases of photosensitivity.

Musculoskeletal: in isolated cases arthralgia and myalgia.

Central and peripheral nervous system: headache, dizziness. In isolated cases paraesthesia.

Gastrointestinal: in isolated cases nausea, gum hyperplasia.

Hepatic: in isolated cases increased liver enzymes.

Cardiovascular: rarely - tachycardia, palpitations and syncope.

Vascular (extracardiac): peripheral oedema, flush.

Other: rarely - fatigue, in isolated cases hypersensitivity reactions e.g. urticaria, angiooedema.

4.9 Overdose

Symptoms: Overdosage may cause excessive peripheral vasodilatation with marked hypotension which may sometimes be accompanied by bradycardia.

Management: Severe hypotension should be treated symptomatically, with the patient placed supine and the legs elevated. Bradycardia, if present, should be treated with atropine 0.5-1 mg i.v. If this is not sufficient, plasma volume should be increased by infusion of e.g. glucose, saline or dextran. Sympathomimetic drugs with predominant effect on the α_1-adrenoceptor may be given e.g. metaraminol or phenylephrine.

5. PHARMACOLOGICAL PROPERTIES

5.1 Pharmacodynamic properties

Felodipine is a vascular selective calcium antagonist, which lowers arterial blood pressure by decreasing peripheral vascular residence. Due to the high degree of selectivity for smooth muscle in the arterioles, felodipine in therapeutic doses has no direct effect on cardiac contractility or conduction.

It can be used as monotherapy or in combination with other antihypertensive drugs, e.g. β-receptor blockers, diuretics or ACE-inhibitors, in order to achieve an increased antihypertensive effect. Felodipine reduces both systolic and diastolic blood pressure and can be used in isolated systolic hypertension. In a study of 12 patients, felodipine maintained its antihypertensive effect during concomitant therapy with indomethacin.

Because there is no effect on venous smooth muscle or adrenergic vasomotor control, felodipine is not associated with orthostatic hypotension.

Felodipine has anti-anginal and anti-ischaemic effects due to improved myocardial oxygen supply/ demand balance. Coronary vascular resistance is decreased and coronary blood flow as well as myocardial oxygen supply are increased by felodipine due to dilation of both epicardial arteries and arterioles. Felodipine effectively counteracts coronary vasospasm. The reduction in systemic blood pressure caused by felodipine leads to decreased left ventricular afterload.

Felodipine improves exercise tolerance and reduces anginal attacks in patients with stable effort induced angina pectoris. Both symptomatic and silent myocardial ischaemia are reduced by felodipine in patients with vasospastic angina. Felodipine can be used as monotherapy or in combination with β-receptor blockers in patients with stable angina pectoris.

Felodipine possesses a mild natriuretic/diuretic effect and generalised fluid retention does not occur.

Felodipine is well tolerated in patients with concomitant disease such as congestive heart failure well controlled on appropriate therapy, asthma and other obstructive pulmonary diseases, diabetes, gout, hyperlipidemia impaired renal function, renal transplant recipients and Raynaud's disease. Felodipine has no significant effect on bland glucose levels or lipid profiles.

Haemodynamic effects: The primary haemodynamic effect of felodipine is a reduction of total peripheral vascular resistance which leads to a decrease in blood pressure. These effects are dose- dependent. In patients with mild to moderate essential hypertension, a reduction in blood pressure usually occurs 2 hours after the first oral dose and lasts for at least 24 hours with a trough/peak ratio usually above 50%.

Plasma concentration of felodipine and decrease in total peripheral resistance and blood pressure are positively correlated.

Electrophysiological and other cardiac effects: Felodipine in therapeutic doses has no effect on cardiac contractility or atrioventricular conduction or refractoriness.

Renal effects: Felodipine has a natriuretic and diuretic effect. Studies have shown that the tubular reabsorption of filtered sodium is reduced. This counteracts the salt and water retention observed for other vasodilators. Felodipine does not affect the daily potassium excretion. The renal vascular resistance is decreased by felodipine. Normal glomerular filtration rate is unchanged. In patients with impaired renal function glomerular filtration rate may increase.

Felodipine is well tolerated in renal transplant recipients.

Site and mechanism of action: The predominant pharmacodynamic feature of felodipine is its pronounced vascular versus myocardial selectivity. Myogenically active smooth muscles in arterial resistance vessels are particularly sensitive to felodipine.

Felodipine inhibits electrical and contractile activity of vascular smooth muscle cells via an effect on the calcium channels in the cell membrane.

5.2 Pharmacokinetic properties

Absorption and distribution: Felodipine is completely absorbed from the gastrointestinal tract after administration of felodipine extended release tablets.

The systemic availability of felodipine is approximately 15% in man and is independent of dose in the therapeutic dose range.

With the extended-release tablets the absorption phase is prolonged. This results in even felodipine plasma concentrations within the therapeutic range for 24 hours.

The plasma protein binding of felodipine is approximately 99%. It is bound predominantly to the albumin fraction.

Elimination and metabolism: The average half-life of felodipine in the terminal phase is 25 hours. There is no significant accumulation during long-term treatment. Felodipine is extensively metabolised by the liver and all identified metabolites are inactive. Elderly patients and patients with reduced liver function have an average higher plasma concentration of felodipine than younger patients.

About 70% of a given dose is excreted as metabolites in the urine; the remaining fraction is excreted in the faeces. Less than 0.5% of a dose is recovered unchanged in the urine.

The kinetics of felodipine are not changed in patients with renal impairment.

5.3 Preclinical safety data

Felodipine is a calcium antagonist and lowers arterial blood pressure by decreasing vascular resistance. In general a reduction in blood pressure is evident 2 hours after the first oral dose and at steady state lasts for at least 24 hours after dose.

Felodipine exhibits a high degree of selectivity for smooth muscles in the arterioles and in therapeutic doses has no direct effect on cardiac contractility. Felodipine does not affect venous smooth muscle and adrenergic vasomotor control.

Electrophysiological studies have shown that felodipine has no direct effect on conduction in the specialised conducting system of the heart and no effect on the AV nodal refractories.

Felotens XL 10 mg Prolonged Release Tablets possess a mild natriuretic/diuretic effect and does not produce general fluid retention, nor affect daily potassium excretion. Felotens XL 10 mg Prolonged Release Tablets are well tolerated in patients with congestive heart failure.

6. PHARMACEUTICAL PARTICULARS

6.1 List of excipients

Lactose monohydrate, Cellulose microcristalline, Hypromellose, Povidone, Propyl gallate, Silica colloidal anhydrous, Magnesium stearate, Ferric oxide yellow (E172), Ferric oxide red (E172), Titanium dioxide (E171), Talc, Propylene glycol.

6.2 Incompatibilities

None stated.

6.3 Shelf life

48 months.

6.4 Special precautions for storage

Do not store above 25 °C. Store in the original package.

6.5 Nature and contents of container

PVC/PE/PVDC Aluminium Blisters.

A single pack contains 10, 20, 28, 30, 50, 56 or 100 tablets.

6.6 Special precautions for disposal and other handling

None stated.

7. MARKETING AUTHORISATION HOLDER

Genus Pharmaceuticals Limited

T/A Genus Pharmaceuticals

Park View House

65 London Road

Newbury

Berkshire

RG14 1JN

8. MARKETING AUTHORISATION NUMBER(S)

PL06831/0227

9. DATE OF FIRST AUTHORISATION/RENEWAL OF THE AUTHORISATION

11 May 2009

10. DATE OF REVISION OF THE TEXT

11 May 2009

Felotens XL 2.5mg Prolonged Release Tablets

(Genus Pharmaceuticals)

1. NAME OF THE MEDICINAL PRODUCT

Felotens XL 2.5 mg Prolonged Release Tablets

2. QUALITATIVE AND QUANTITATIVE COMPOSITION

Felotens XL 2.5 mg Prolonged Release Tablets contain 2.5mg of felodipine.

3. PHARMACEUTICAL FORM

Yellow, round, biconvex, film coated prolonged-release tablets with imprint 2.5.

4. CLINICAL PARTICULARS

4.1 Therapeutic indications

In the management of hypertension and prophylaxis of chronic stable angina pectoris.

4.2 Posology and method of administration

For oral administration

Hypertension:

Adults (including elderly): The dose should be adjusted to the individual requirements of the patient. The recommended starting dose is 5 mg once daily. If necessary the dose may be further increased or another antihypertensive agent added. The usual maintenance dose is 5-10 mg once daily. Doses higher than 20 mg daily are not usually needed. In elderly patients an initial treatment with 2.5 mg daily should be considered.

Angina pectoris:

Adults: The dose should be adjusted individually. Treatment should be started with 5 mg once daily and if needed be increased to 10 mg once daily.

Administration: The tablets should regularly be taken in the morning without food or with a light meal. Felotens XL 2.5 mg Prolonged Release Tablets must not be chewed or crushed. They should be swallowed whole with half a glass of water.

Children: The safety and efficacy of Felotens XL 2.5 mg Prolonged Release Tablets in children has not been established.

Felotens XL 2.5 mg Prolonged Release Tablets can be used in combination with β-blockers, ACE inhibitors or diuretics. The effects on blood pressure are likely to be additive and combination therapy will usually enhance the antihypertensive effect. Care should be taken to avoid hypotension. In patients with severely impaired liver function the dose of felodipine should be low. The pharmacokinetics are not significantly affected in patients with impaired renal function.

4.3 Contraindications

Unstable angina pectoris.

Pregnancy.

Patient with a previous allergic reaction to Felotens XL 2.5 mg Prolonged Release Tablets or other dihydropyridines because of the theoretical risk of cross-reactivity.

Felotens XL 2.5 mg Prolonged Release Tablets should not be used in patients with clinically significant aortic stenosis, and during or within one month of a myocardial infarction.

As with other calcium channel blockers, Felotens XL 2.5 mg Prolonged Release Tablets should be discontinued in patients who develop cardiogenic shock.

4.4 Special warnings and precautions for use

As with other vasodilators, Felotens XL 2.5 mg Prolonged Release Tablets may, in rare cases, precipitate significant hypotension with tachycardia which in susceptible individuals may result in myocardial ischaemia.

There is no evidence that Felotens XL 2.5 mg Prolonged Release Tablets are useful for secondary prevention of myocardial infarction.

The efficacy and safety of Felotens XL 2.5 mg Prolonged Release Tablets in the treatment of malignant hypertension has not been studied.

Felotens XL 2.5 mg Prolonged Release Tablets should be used with caution in patients with severe left ventricular dysfunction.

4.5 Interaction with other medicinal products and other forms of interaction

Concomitant administration of substances which interfere with the cytochrome P450 system may affect plasma concentrations of felodipine. Enzyme inhibitors such as cimetidine, erythromycin and itraconazole impair the elimination of felodipine, and Felotens XL 2.5 mg Prolonged Release Tablets dosage may need to be reduced when drugs are given concomitantly. Conversely, powerful enzyme inducing agents such as some anticonvulsants (phenytoin, carbamazepine, phenobarbitone) can increase felodipine elimination and higher than normal Felotens XL 2.5 mg Prolonged Release Tablets doses may be required in patients taking the drugs.

No dosage adjustment is required when Felotens XL 2.5 mg Prolonged Release Tablets are given concomitantly with digoxin.

Felodipine does not appear to affect the unbound fraction of other extensively plasma protein bound drugs such as warfarin.

Grapefruit juice results in increased peak plasma levels and bioavailability possibly due to an interaction with flavonoids in the fruit juice. This interaction has been seen with other dihydropyridine calcium antagonists and represents a class effect. Therefore grapefruit juice should not be taken together with Felotens XL 2.5 mg Prolonged Release Tablets.

4.6 Pregnancy and lactation

Felodipine should not be given during pregnancy.

In a study on fertility and general reproductive performance in rats, a prolongation of parturition resulting in difficult labour, increased foetal deaths and early postnatal deaths were observed in the medium- and high-dose groups. Reproductive studies in rabbits have shown a dose-related reversible enlargement of the mammary glands of the parent animals and dose-related digital abnormalities in the foetuses when felodipine was administered during stages of early foetal development.

Felodipine has been detected in breast milk, but it is unknown whether it has harmful effects on the new-born.

4.7 Effects on ability to drive and use machines

None.

4.8 Undesirable effects

As with other calcium antagonists, flushing, headache, palpitations, dizziness and fatigue may occur. These reactions are usually transient and are most likely to occur at the start of treatment or after an increase in dosage.

As with other calcium antagonists ankle swelling, resulting from precapillary vasodilation, may occur. The degree of ankle swelling is dose related.

In patients with gingivitis/periodontitis, mild gingival enlargement has been reported with Felotens XL 2.5 mg Prolonged Release Tablets, as with other calcium antagonists. The enlargement can be avoided or reversed by careful dental hygiene.

As with other dihydropyridines, aggravation of angina has been reported in a small number of individuals especially after starting treatment. This is more likely to happen in patients with symptomatic ischaemic heart disease.

The following adverse events have been reported from clinical trials and from Post Marketing Surveillance. In the great majority of cases a causal relationship between these events and treatment with felodipine has not been established.

Skin: rarely - rash and/or pruritus, and isolated cases of photosensitivity.

Musculoskeletal: in isolated cases arthralgia and myalgia.

Central and peripheral nervous system: headache, dizziness. In isolated cases paraesthesia.

Gastrointestinal: in isolated cases nausea, gum hyperplasia.

Hepatic: in isolated cases increased liver enzymes.

Cardiovascular: rarely - tachycardia, palpitations and syncope.

Vascular (extracardiac): peripheral oedema, flush.

Other: rarely - fatigue, in isolated cases hypersensitivity reactions e.g. urticaria, angiooedema.

4.9 Overdose

Symptoms: Overdosage may cause excessive peripheral vasodilatation with marked hypotension which may sometimes be accompanied by bradycardia.

Management: Severe hypotension should be treated symptomatically, with the patient placed supine and the legs elevated. Bradycardia, if present, should be treated with atropine 0.5-1 mg i.v. If this is not sufficient, plasma volume should be increased by infusion of e.g. glucose, saline or dextran. Sympathomimetic drugs with predominant effect on the (α_1-adrenoceptor may be given e.g. metaraminol or phenylephrine.

5. PHARMACOLOGICAL PROPERTIES

5.1 Pharmacodynamic properties

Felodipine is a vascular selective calcium antagonist, which lowers arterial blood pressure by decreasing peripheral vascular residence. Due to the high degree of selectivity for smooth muscle in the arterioles, felodipine in therapeutic doses has no direct effect on cardiac contractility or conduction.

It can be used as monotherapy or in combination with other antihypertensive drugs, e.g. β-receptor blockers, diuretics or ACE-inhibitors, in order to achieve an increased antihypertensive effect. Felodipine reduces both systolic and diastolic blood pressure and can be used in isolated systolic hypertension. In a study of 12 patients, felodipine maintained its antihypertensive effect during concomitant therapy with indomethacin.

Because there is no effect on venous smooth muscle or adrenergic vasomotor control, felodipine is not associated with orthostatic hypotension.

Felodipine has anti-anginal and anti-ischaemic effects due to improved myocardial oxygen supply/ demand balance. Coronary vascular resistance is decreased and coronary blood flow as well as myocardial oxygen supply are increased by felodipine due to dilation of both epicardial arteries and arterioles. Felodipine effectively counteracts coronary vasospasm. The reduction in systemic blood pressure caused by felodipine leads to decreased left ventricular afterload.

Felodipine improves exercise tolerance and reduces anginal attacks in patients with stable effort induced angina pectoris. Both symptomatic and silent myocardial ischaemia are reduced by felodipine in patients with vasospastic angina. Felodipine can be used as monotherapy or in combination with β-receptor blockers in patients with stable angina pectoris.

Felodipine possesses a mild natriuretic/diuretic effect and generalised fluid retention does not occur.

Felodipine is well tolerated in patients with concomitant disease such as congestive heart failure well controlled on appropriate therapy, asthma and other obstructive pulmonary diseases, diabetes, gout, hyperlipidemia impaired renal function, renal transplant recipients and Raynaud's disease. Felodipine has no significant effect on bland glucose levels or lipid profiles.

Haemodynamic effects: The primary haemodynamic effect of felodipine is a reduction of total peripheral vascular resistance which leads to a decrease in blood pressure. These effects are dose- dependent. In patients with mild to moderate essential hypertension, a reduction in blood pressure usually occurs 2 hours after the first oral dose and lasts for at least 24 hours with a trough/peak ratio usually above 50%.

Plasma concentration of felodipine and decrease in total peripheral resistance and blood pressure are positively correlated.

Electrophysiological and other cardiac effects: Felodipine in therapeutic doses has no effect on cardiac contractility or atrioventricular conduction or refractoriness.

Renal effects: Felodipine has a natriuretic and diuretic effect. Studies have shown that the tubular reabsorption of filtered sodium is reduced. This counteracts the salt and water retention observed for other vasodilators. Felodipine does not affect the daily potassium excretion. The renal vascular resistance is decreased by felodipine. Normal glomerular filtration rate is unchanged. In patients with impaired renal function glomerular filtration rate may increase.

Felodipine is well tolerated in renal transplant recipients.

Site and mechanism of action: The predominant pharmacodynamic feature of felodipine is its pronounced vascular versus myocardial selectivity. Myogenically active smooth muscles in arterial resistance vessels are particularly sensitive to felodipine.

Felodipine inhibits electrical and contractile activity of vascular smooth muscle cells via an effect on the calcium channels in the cell membrane.

5.2 Pharmacokinetic properties

Absorption and distribution: Felodipine is completely absorbed from the gastrointestinal tract after administration of felodipine extended release tablets.

The systemic availability of felodipine is approximately 15% in man and is independent of dose in the therapeutic dose range.

With the extended-release tablets the absorption phase is prolonged. This results in even felodipine plasma concentrations within the therapeutic range for 24 hours.

The plasma protein binding of felodipine is approximately 99%. It is bound predominantly to the albumin fraction.

Elimination and metabolism: The average half-life of felodipine in the terminal phase is 25 hours. There is no significant accumulation during long-term treatment. Felodipine is extensively metabolised by the liver and all identified metabolites are inactive. Elderly patients and patients with reduced liver function have an average higher plasma concentration of felodipine than younger patients.

About 70% of a given dose is excreted as metabolites in the urine; the remaining fraction is excreted in the faeces. Less than 0.5% of a dose is recovered unchanged in the urine.

The kinetics of felodipine are not changed in patients with renal impairment.

5.3 Preclinical safety data

Felodipine is a calcium antagonist and lowers arterial blood pressure by decreasing vascular resistance. In general a reduction in blood pressure is evident 2 hours after the first oral dose and at steady state lasts for at least 24 hours after dose.

Felodipine exhibits a high degree of selectivity for smooth muscles in the arterioles and in therapeutic doses has no direct effect on cardiac contractility. Felodipine does not affect venous smooth muscle and adrenergic vasomotor control.

Electrophysiological studies have shown that felodipine has no direct effect on conduction in the specialised conducting system of the heart and no effect on the AV nodal refractories.

Felotens XL 2.5 mg Prolonged Release Tablets possess a mild natriuretic/diuretic effect and does not produce general fluid retention, nor affect daily potassium excretion. Felotens XL 2.5 mg Prolonged Release Tablets are well tolerated in patients with congestive heart failure.

6. PHARMACEUTICAL PARTICULARS

6.1 List of excipients

Lactose monohydrate, Cellulose microcristalline, Hypromellose, Povidone, Propyl gallate, Silica colloidal anhydrous, Magnesium stearate, Ferric oxide yellow (E172), Titanium dioxide (E171), Talc, Propylene glycol.

6.2 Incompatibilities

None stated.

6.3 Shelf life

48 months.

6.4 Special precautions for storage

Do not store above 25°C. Store in the original package.

6.5 Nature and contents of container

PVC/PE/PVDC Aluminium Blisters.

A single pack contains 10, 20, 28, 30, 50, 56 or 100 tablets.

6.6 Special precautions for disposal and other handling

None stated.

7. MARKETING AUTHORISATION HOLDER

Genus Pharmaceuticals Limited

T/A Genus Pharmaceuticals

Park View House

65 London Road

Newbury

Berkshire

RG14 1JN

8. MARKETING AUTHORISATION NUMBER(S)

PL06831/0225

9. DATE OF FIRST AUTHORISATION/RENEWAL OF THE AUTHORISATION

11 May 2009

10. DATE OF REVISION OF THE TEXT

11 May 2009

Felotens XL 5mg Prolonged Release Tablets

(Genus Pharmaceuticals)

1. NAME OF THE MEDICINAL PRODUCT

Felotens XL 5 mg Prolonged Release Tablets

2. QUALITATIVE AND QUANTITATIVE COMPOSITION

Felotens XL 5 mg Prolonged Release Tablets contain 5mg of felodipine.

3. PHARMACEUTICAL FORM

Light pink, round, biconvex, film coated prolonged-release tablets with imprint 5.

4. CLINICAL PARTICULARS

4.1 Therapeutic indications

In the management of hypertension and prophylaxis of chronic stable angina pectoris.

4.2 Posology and method of administration

For oral administration

Hypertension:

Adults (including elderly): The dose should be adjusted to the individual requirements of the patient. The recommended starting dose is 5 mg once daily. If necessary the dose may be further increased or another antihypertensive agent added. The usual maintenance dose is 5-10 mg once daily. Doses higher than 20 mg daily are not usually needed. For dose titration purposes a 2.5 mg tablet is available. In elderly patients an initial treatment with 2.5 mg daily should be considered.

Angina pectoris:

Adults: The dose should be adjusted individually. Treatment should be started with 5 mg once daily and if needed be increased to 10 mg once daily.

Administration: The tablets should regularly be taken in the morning without food or with a light meal. Felotens XL 5 mg Prolonged Release Tablets must not be chewed or crushed. They should be swallowed whole with half a glass of water.

Children: The safety and efficacy of Felotens XL 5 mg Prolonged Release Tablets in children has not been established.

Felotens XL 5 mg Prolonged Release Tablets can be used in combination with β-blockers, ACE inhibitors or diuretics. The effects on blood pressure are likely to be additive and combination therapy will usually enhance the antihypertensive effect. Care should be taken to avoid hypotension. In patients with severely impaired liver function the dose of felodipine should be low. The pharmacokinetics are not significantly affected in patients with impaired renal function.

4.3 Contraindications

Unstable angina pectoris.

Pregnancy.

Patient with a previous allergic reaction to Felotens XL 5 mg Prolonged Release Tablets or other dihydropyridines because of the theoretical risk of cross-reactivity.

Felotens XL 5 mg Prolonged Release Tablets should not be used in patients with clinically significant aortic stenosis, and during or within one month of a myocardial infarction.

As with other calcium channel blockers, Felotens XL 5 mg Prolonged Release Tablets should be discontinued in patients who develop cardiogenic shock.

4.4 Special warnings and precautions for use

As with other vasodilators, Felotens XL 5 mg Prolonged Release Tablets may, in rare cases, precipitate significant hypotension with tachycardia which in susceptible individuals may result in myocardial ischaemia.

There is no evidence that Felotens XL 5 mg Prolonged Release Tablets are useful for secondary prevention of myocardial infarction.

The efficacy and safety of Felotens XL 5 mg Prolonged Release Tablets in the treatment of malignant hypertension has not been studied.

Felotens XL 5 mg Prolonged Release Tablets should be used with caution in patients with severe left ventricular dysfunction.

4.5 Interaction with other medicinal products and other forms of interaction

Concomitant administration of substances which interfere with the cytochrome P450 system may affect plasma concentrations of felodipine. Enzyme inhibitors such as cimetidine, erythromycin and itraconazole impair the elimination of felodipine, and Felotens XL 5 mg Prolonged Release Tablets dosage may need to be reduced when drugs are given concomitantly. Conversely, powerful enzyme inducing agents such as some anticonvulsants (phenytoin, carbamazepine, phenobarbitone) can increase felodipine elimination and higher than normal Felotens XL 5 mg

Prolonged Release Tablets doses may be required in patients taking the drugs.

No dosage adjustment is required when Felotens XL 5 mg Prolonged Release Tablets are given concomitantly with digoxin.

Felodipine does not appear to affect the unbound fraction of other extensively plasma protein bound drugs such as warfarin.

Grapefruit juice results in increased peak plasma levels and bioavailability possibly due to an interaction with flavonoids in the fruit juice. This interaction has been seen with other dihydropyridine calcium antagonists and represents a class effect. Therefore grapefruit juice should not be taken together with Felotens XL 5 mg Prolonged Release Tablets.

4.6 Pregnancy and lactation
Felodipine should not be given during pregnancy.

In a study on fertility and general reproductive performance in rats, a prolongation of parturition resulting in difficult labour, increased foetal deaths and early postnatal deaths were observed in the medium- and high-dose groups. Reproductive studies in rabbits have shown a dose-related reversible enlargement of the mammary glands of the parent animals and dose-related digital abnormalities in the foetuses when felodipine was administered during stages of early foetal development.

Felodipine has been detected in breast milk, but it is unknown whether it has harmful effects on the new-born.

4.7 Effects on ability to drive and use machines
None.

4.8 Undesirable effects
As with other calcium antagonists, flushing, headache, palpitations, dizziness and fatigue may occur. These reactions are usually transient and are most likely to occur at the start of treatment or after an increase in dosage.

As with other calcium antagonists ankle swelling, resulting from precapillary vasodilation, may occur. The degree of ankle swelling is dose related.

In patients with gingivitis/periodontitis, mild gingival enlargement has been reported with Felotens XL 5 mg Prolonged Release Tablets, as with other calcium antagonists. The enlargement can be avoided or reversed by careful dental hygiene.

As with other dihydropyridines, aggravation of angina has been reported in a small number of individuals especially after starting treatment. This is more likely to happen in patients with symptomatic ischaemic heart disease.

The following adverse events have been reported from clinical trials and from Post Marketing Surveillance. In the great majority of cases a causal relationship between these events and treatment with felodipine has not been established.

Skin: rarely - rash and/or pruritus, and isolated cases of photosensitivity.

Musculoskeletal: in isolated cases arthralgia and myalgia.

Central and peripheral nervous system: headache, dizziness. In isolated cases paraesthesia.

Gastrointestinal: in isolated cases nausea, gum hyperplasia.

Hepatic: in isolated cases increased liver enzymes.

Cardiovascular: rarely - tachycardia, palpitations and syncope.

Vascular (extracardiac): peripheral oedema, flush.

Other: rarely - fatigue, in isolated cases hypersensitivity reactions e.g. urticaria, angiooedema.

4.9 Overdose
Symptoms: Overdosage may cause excessive peripheral vasodilatation with marked hypotension which may sometimes be accompanied by bradycardia.

Management: Severe hypotension should be treated symptomatically, with the patient placed supine and the legs elevated. Bradycardia, if present, should be treated with atropine 0.5-1 mg i.v. If this is not sufficient, plasma volume should be increased by infusion of e.g. glucose, saline or dextran. Sympathomimetic drugs with predominant effect on the (α_1-adrenoceptor may be given e.g. metaraminol or phenylephrine.

5. PHARMACOLOGICAL PROPERTIES

5.1 Pharmacodynamic properties
Felodipine is a vascular selective calcium antagonist, which lowers arterial blood pressure by decreasing peripheral vascular residence. Due to the high degree of selectivity for smooth muscle in the arterioles, felodipine in therapeutic doses has no direct effect on cardiac contractility or conduction.

It can be used as monotherapy or in combination with other antihypertensive drugs, e.g. β-receptor blockers, diuretics or ACE-inhibitors, in order to achieve an increased antihypertensive effect. Felodipine reduces both systolic and diastolic blood pressure and can be used in isolated systolic hypertension. In a study of 12 patients, felodipine maintained its antihypertensive effect during concomitant therapy with indomethacin.

Because there is no effect on venous smooth muscle or adrenergic vasomotor control, felodipine is not associated with orthostatic hypotension.

Felodipine has anti-anginal and anti-ischaemic effects due to improved myocardial oxygen supply/ demand balance. Coronary vascular resistance is decreased and coronary blood flow as well as myocardial oxygen supply are increased by felodipine due to dilation of both epicardial arteries and arterioles. Felodipine effectively counteracts coronary vasospasm. The reduction in systemic blood pressure caused by felodipine leads to decreased left ventricular afterload.

Felodipine improves exercise tolerance and reduces anginal attacks in patients with stable effort induced angina pectoris. Both symptomatic and silent myocardial ischaemia are reduced by felodipine in patients with vasospastic angina. Felodipine can be used as monotherapy or in combination with β-receptor blockers in patients with stable angina pectoris.

Felodipine possesses a mild natriuretic/diuretic effect and generalised fluid retention does not occur.

Felodipine is well tolerated in patients with concomitant disease such as congestive heart failure well controlled on appropriate therapy, asthma and other obstructive pulmonary diseases, diabetes, gout, hyperlipidemia impaired renal function, renal transplant recipients and Raynaud's disease. Felodipine has no significant effect on bland glucose levels or lipid profiles.

Haemodynamic effects: The primary haemodynamic effect of felodipine is a reduction of total peripheral vascular resistance which leads to a decrease in blood pressure. These effects are dose- dependent. In patients with mild to moderate essential hypertension, a reduction in blood pressure usually occurs 2 hours after the first oral dose and lasts for at least 24 hours with a trough/peak ratio usually above 50%.

Plasma concentration of felodipine and decrease in total peripheral resistance and blood pressure are positively correlated.

Electrophysiological and other cardiac effects: Felodipine in therapeutic doses has no effect on cardiac contractility or atrioventricular conduction or refractoriness.

Renal effects: Felodipine has a natriuretic and diuretic effect. Studies have shown that the tubular reabsorption of filtered sodium is reduced. This counteracts the salt and water retention observed for other vasodilators. Felodipine does not affect the daily potassium excretion. The renal vascular resistance is decreased by felodipine. Normal glomerular filtration rate is unchanged. In patients with impaired renal function glomerular filtration rate may increase.

Felodipine is well tolerated in renal transplant recipients.

Site and mechanism of action: The predominant pharmacodynamic feature of felodipine is its pronounced vascular versus myocardial selectivity. Myogenically active smooth muscles in arterial resistance vessels are particularly sensitive to felodipine.

Felodipine inhibits electrical and contractile activity of vascular smooth muscle cells via an effect on the calcium channels in the cell membrane.

5.2 Pharmacokinetic properties
Absorption and distribution: Felodipine is completely absorbed from the gastrointestinal tract after administration of felodipine extended release tablets.

The systemic availability of felodipine is approximately 15% in man and is independent of dose in the therapeutic dose range.

With the extended-release tablets the absorption phase is prolonged. This results in even felodipine plasma concentrations within the therapeutic range for 24 hours.

The plasma protein binding of felodipine is approximately 99%. It is bound predominantly to the albumin fraction.

Elimination and metabolism: The average half-life of felodipine in the terminal phase is 25 hours. There is no significant accumulation during long-term treatment. Felodipine is extensively metabolised by the liver and all identified metabolites are inactive. Elderly patients and patients with reduced liver function have an average higher plasma concentration of felodipine than younger patients.

About 70% of a given dose is excreted as metabolites in the urine; the remaining fraction is excreted in the faeces. Less than 0.5% of a dose is recovered unchanged in the urine.

The kinetics of felodipine are not changed in patients with renal impairment.

5.3 Preclinical safety data
Felodipine is a calcium antagonist and lowers arterial blood pressure by decreasing vascular resistance. In general a reduction in blood pressure is evident 2 hours after the first oral dose and at steady state lasts for at least 24 hours after dose.

Felodipine exhibits a high degree of selectivity for smooth muscles in the arterioles and in therapeutic doses has no direct effect on cardiac contractility. Felodipine does not affect venous smooth muscle and adrenergic vasomotor control.

Electrophysiological studies have shown that felodipine has no direct effect on conduction in the specialised conducting system of the heart and no effect on the AV nodal refractories.

Felotens XL 5 mg Prolonged Release Tablets possess a mild natriuretic/diuretic effect and does not produce general fluid retention, nor affect daily potassium excretion. Felotens XL 5 mg Prolonged Release Tablets are well tolerated in patients with congestive heart failure.

6. PHARMACEUTICAL PARTICULARS

6.1 List of excipients
Lactose monohydrate, Cellulose microcristalline, Hypromellose, Povidone, Propyl gallate, Silica colloidal anhydrous, Magnesium stearate, Ferric oxide yellow (E172), Ferric oxide red (E172), Titanium dioxide (E171), Talc, Propylene glycol.

6.2 Incompatibilities
None stated.

6.3 Shelf life
48 months.

6.4 Special precautions for storage
Do not store above 25 °C. Store in the original package.

6.5 Nature and contents of container
PVC/PE/PVDC Aluminium Blisters.

A single pack contains 10, 20, 28, 30, 50, 56 or 100 tablets.

6.6 Special precautions for disposal and other handling
None stated.

7. MARKETING AUTHORISATION HOLDER
Genus Pharmaceuticals Limited

T/A Genus Pharmaceuticals

Park View House

65 London Road

Newbury

Berkshire

RG14 1JN

8. MARKETING AUTHORISATION NUMBER(S)
PL06831/0226

9. DATE OF FIRST AUTHORISATION/RENEWAL OF THE AUTHORISATION
11 May 2009

10. DATE OF REVISION OF THE TEXT
11 May 2009

Femapak 40

(Solvay Healthcare Limited)

1. NAME OF THE MEDICINAL PRODUCT
Femapak 40

2. QUALITATIVE AND QUANTITATIVE COMPOSITION
Femapak 40 consists of a pack containing eight Fematrix 40 transdermal patches and a blister strip of 14 Duphaston tablets. Each Fematrix 40 patch contains 1.25 mg estradiol (each patch delivers approximately 40 micrograms of estradiol per 24 hours).

Each Duphaston tablet contains 10 mg Dydrogesterone.

For excipient, see 6.1

3. PHARMACEUTICAL FORM
Trandermal patch

Fematrix 40 self adhesive, flexible transdermal delivery system comprising a layer of clear adhesive sandwiched between a translucent patch and a metallised polyester backing. Fematrix 40 is a rectangular shape with rounded corners and has an active surface area of 14.25 cm^2.

Duphaston film-coated tablets: Round, white tablet, scored on one side with the inscriptions '155' on each half of the tablet and '§' on the reverse.

4. CLINICAL PARTICULARS

4.1 Therapeutic indications
Hormone replacement therapy (HRT) for estrogen deficiency symptoms in peri and postmenopausal women.

The experience of treating women older than 65 years is limited.

4.2 Posology and method of administration
Femapak 40 is a continuous sequential hormone replacement therapy. Unless there is previous diagnosis of endometriosis, it is not recommended to add a progestagen in hysterectomised women.

For initiation and continuation of treatment of postmenopausal symptoms, the lowest effective dose for the shortest duration (see also section 4.4) should be used.

In general, treatment should start with Femapak 40. Depending on the clinical response, the dosage can afterwards be adjusted to individual need. If the complaints linked to estrogen deficiency are not ameliorated the dosage can be increased by using Femapak 80.

Starting Femapak 40

In women who are not taking hormone replacement therapy and who are amenorrhoeic or women who switch from a continuous combined hormone replacement therapy, treatment may be started on any convenient day. In women transferring from a cyclic or continuous sequential HRT regimen, treatment should begin the day following completion of the prior regimen. If the patient has regular menstruation periods, treatment is started within five days of the start of bleeding.

Administration

One Fematrix 40 transdermal patch should be applied twice weekly on a continuous basis. Each patch should be removed after 3 to 4 days and replaced with a new patch applied to a slightly different site. Patches should be applied to clean, dry and intact areas of skin below the waist on the lower back or buttocks. Patches should not be applied on or near the breasts. During the second two weeks of the cycle, that is from the 15th day after applying the first patch, one Duphaston tablet should be taken each day for the next 14 days. Most patients will commence bleeding towards the end of the Duphaston therapy.

If a tablet has been forgotten, it should be taken as soon as possible. When more than 12 hours have elapsed, it is recommended to continue with the next dose without taking the forgotten tablet. The likelihood of breakthrough bleeding or spotting may have increased. If a patch has been forgotten, it should be changed as soon as possible. The next patch should be applied on the usual day.

4.3 Contraindications

Known, past or suspected breast cancer;

Known or suspected estrogen-dependent malignant tumours (e.g. endometrial cancer);

Undiagnosed genital bleeding;

Untreated endometrial hyperplasia;

Previous idiopathic or current venous thromboembolism (deep vein thrombosis, pulmonary embolism);

Active or recent arterial thromboembolic disease (e.g. angina, myocardial infarction);

Acute liver disease, or a history of liver disease as long as liver function tests have failed to return to normal;

Known hypersensitivity to the active substance or to any of the excipients;

Porphyria.

4.4 Special warnings and precautions for use

For the treatment of postmenopausal symptoms, HRT should only be initiated for symptoms that adversely affect quality of life. In all cases, a careful appraisal of the risks and benefits should be undertaken at least annually and HRT should only be continued as long as the benefit outweighs the risk.

Medical examination/follow up

Before initiating or reinstituting HRT, a complete personal and family medical history should be taken. Physical (including pelvic and breast) examination should be guided by this and by the contraindications and warnings for use. During treatment, periodic check-ups are recommended of a frequency and nature adapted to the individual woman. Women should be advised what changes in their breasts should be reported to their doctor or nurse (See 'breast cancer' below). Investigations, including mammography, should be carried out in accordance with currently accepted screening practices, modified to the clinical needs of the individual.

Conditions which need supervision

If any of the following conditions are present, have occurred previously, and/or have been aggravated during pregnancy or previous hormone treatment, the patient should be closely supervised. It should be taken into account that these conditions may recur or be aggravated during treatment with Femapak, in particular:

- Leiomyoma (uterine fibroids) or endometriosis
- A history of, or risk factors for, thromboembolic disorders (see below)
- Risk factors for estrogen dependent tumours, e.g. 1st degree heredity for breast cancer
- Hypertension
- Liver disorders (e.g. liver adenoma)
- Diabetes mellitus with or without vascular involvement
- Cholelithiasis
- Migraine or (severe) headache
- Systemic lupus erythematosus
- A history of endometrial hyperplasia (see below)
- Epilepsy
- Asthma
- Otosclerosis

Reasons for immediate withdrawal of therapy:

- Therapy should be discontinued in cases where a contra-indication is discovered and in the following situations:

- Jaundice or deterioration in liver function
- Significant increase in blood pressure
- New onset of migraine-type headache
- Pregnancy

Endometrial hyperplasia

The risk of endometrial hyperplasia and carcinoma is increased when estrogens are administered alone for prolonged periods (see section 4.8). The addition of a progestagen for at least 12 days of the cycle in non-hysterectomised women greatly reduces this risk.

Break-through bleeding and spotting may occur during the first few months of treatment. If break-through bleeding or spotting appears after some time on therapy, or continues after treatment has been discontinued, the reason should be investigated, which may include endometrial biopsy to exclude endometrial malignancy.

Breast cancer

A randomised placebo-controlled trial, the Womens Health Initiative study (WHI) and epidemiological studies, including the Million Women Study (MWS), have reported an increased risk of breast cancer in women taking estrogens, estrogen-progestagen combinations or tibolone for HRT for several years (see Section 4.8).

For all HRT, an excess risk becomes apparent within a few years of use and increases with duration of intake but returns to baseline within a few (at most five) years after stopping treatment.

In the MWS, the relative risk of breast cancer with conjugated equine estrogens (CEE) or estradiol (E2) was greater when a progestagen was added, either sequentially or continuously, and regardless of type of progestagen. There was no evidence of a difference in risk between the different routes of administration.

In the WHI study, the continuous combined conjugated equine estrogen and medroxyprogesterone acetate (CEE + MPA) product used was associated with breast cancers that were slightly larger in size and more frequently had local lymph node metastases compared to placebo.

HRT, especially estrogen-progestagen combined treatment, increases the density of mammographic images which may adversely affect the radiological detection of breast cancer.

Venous thromboembolism

HRT is associated with a higher relative risk of developing venous thromboembolism (VTE), i.e. deep vein thrombosis or pulmonary embolism. One randomised controlled trial and epidermiological studies found a two-to threefold higher risk for users compared with non-users. For non-users, it is estimated that the number of cases of VTE that will occur over a 5 year period is about 3 per 1000 women aged 50-59 years and 8 per 1000 women aged between 60-69 years. It is estimated that in healthy women who use HRT for 5 years, the number of additional cases of VTE over a 5 year period will be between 2 and 6 (best estimate=4) per 1000 women aged 50-59 years and between 5 and 15 (best estimate = 9) per 1000 women aged 60-69 years. The occurrence of such an event is more likely in the first year of HRT than later.

- Generally recognised risk factors for VTE include a personal or family history, severe obesity (BMI >30 kg/m^2) and systemic lupus erythematosus (SLE). There is no consensus about the possible role of varicose veins in VTE.

- Patients with a history of VTE or known thrombophilic states have an increased risk of VTE. HRT may add to this risk. Personal or strong family history of thromboembolism or recurrent spontaneous abortion should be investigated in order to exclude a thrombophilic predisposition. Until a thorough evaluation of thrombophilic factors has been made or anticoagulant treatment initiated, use of HRT in such patients should be viewed as contraindicated. Those women already on anticoagulant treatment require careful consideration of the benefit-risk of use of HRT.

- The risk of VTE may be temporarily increased with prolonged immobilisation, major trauma or major surgery. As in all postoperative patients, scrupulous attention should be given to prophylactic measures to prevent VTE following surgery. Where prolonged immobilisation is liable to follow elective surgery, particularly abdominal or orthopaedic surgery to the lower limbs, consideration should be given to temporarily stopping HRT 4 to 6 weeks earlier, if possible. Treatment should not be restarted until the woman is completely mobilised.

- If VTE develops after initiating therapy, the drug should be discontinued. Patients should be told to contact their doctors immediately when they are aware of a potential thromboembolic symptom (e.g. painful swelling of a leg, sudden pain in the chest, dyspnea).

Coronary artery disease (CAD)

There is no evidence from randomised controlled trials of cardiovascular benefit with continuous combined conjugated estrogens and medroxyprogesterone acetate (MPA). Two large clinical trials (WHI and HERS i.e. Heart and Estrogen/progestin Replacement Study) showed a possible increased risk of cardiovascular morbidity in the first year of use and no overall benefit. For other HRT products there are only limited data from randomised controlled trials examining effects in cardiovascular morbidity or mortality. Therefore, it is uncertain whether these findings also extend to other HRT products.

Stroke

One large randomised clinical trial (WHI-trial) found, as a secondary outcome, an increased risk of ischaemic stroke in healthy women during treatment with continuous combined conjugated estrogens and MPA. For women who do not use HRT, it is estimated that the number of cases of stroke that will occur over a 5 year period is about 3 per 1000 women aged 50-59 and 11 per 1000 women aged 60-69 years. It is estimated that for women who use conjugated estrogens and MPA for 5 years, the number of additional cases will be between 0 and 3 (best estimate = 1) per 1000 users aged 50-59 years and between 1 and 9 (best estimate = 4) per 1000 users aged 60-69 years. It is unknown whether the increased risk also extends to other HRT products.

Ovarian cancer

Long-term (at least 5 to 10 years) use of estrogen-only HRT products in hysterectomised women has been associated with an increased risk of ovarian cancer in some epidemiological studies. It is uncertain whether long term use of combined HRT confers a different risk than estrogen-only products.

Other conditions

- Estrogens may cause fluid retention, and therefore patients with cardiac or renal dysfunction should be carefully observed. Patients with terminal renal insufficiency should be closely observed, since it is expected that the level of circulating active ingredients in Femapak is increased.

- Women with pre-existing hypertriglyceridemia should be followed closely during estrogen replacement or hormone replacement therapy, since rare cases of large increases of plasma triglycerides leading to pancreatitis have been reported with estrogen therapy in this condition.

- Estrogens increase thyroid binding globulin (TBG), leading to increased circulating total thyroid hormone, as measured by protein-bound iodine (PBI), T4 levels (by column or by radio-immunoassay) or T3 levels (by radio-immunoassay). T3 resin uptake is decreased, reflecting the elevated TBG. Free T4 and free T3 concentrations are unaltered. Other binding proteins may be elevated in serum, i.e. corticoid binding globulin (CBG), sex-hormone-binding globulin (SHBG) leading to increased circulating corticosteroids and sex steroids, respectively. Free or biological active hormone concentrations are unchanged. Other plasma proteins may be increased (angiotensinogen/renin substrate, alpha-1-antitrypsin, ceruloplasmin).

- There is no conclusive evidence for improvement of cognitive function. There is some evidence from the WHI trial of increased risk of probable dementia in women who start using continuous combined CEE and MPA after the age of 65. It is unknown whether the findings apply to younger post-menopausal women or other HRT products.

- Patients with rare hereditary problems of galactose intolerance, the Lapp lactase deficiency or glucose-galactose malabsorption should not take this medicine.

- Women who may be at risk of pregnancy should be advised to adhere to non-hormonal contraceptive methods.

4.5 Interaction with other medicinal products and other forms of interaction

- The metabolism of estrogens and progestagens may be increased by concomitant use of substances known to induce drug-metabolising enzymes, specifically cytochrome P450 enzymes, such as anticonvulsants (eg. phenobarbital, phenytoin, carbamezapine) and anti-infectives (e.g. rifampicin, rifabutin, nevirapine, efavirenz).

- Ritonavir and nelfinavir, although known as strong inhibitors, by contrast exhibit inducing properties when used concomitantly with steroid hormones.

- Herbal preparations containing St John's wort (Hypericum perforatum) may induce the metabolism of estrogens and progestagens.

- Clinically an increased metabolism of estrogens and progestagens may lead to decreased effect and changes in the uterine bleeding profile.

- At transdermal administration, the first-pass effect of the liver is avoided and, thus, transdermally applied estrogens might be less affected than oral hormones by enzyme inducers.

4.6 Pregnancy and lactation

Pregnancy

Femapak is not indicated during pregnancy. If pregnancy occurs during medication with Femapak, treatment should be withdrawn immediately. Clinically, data on a large number of exposed pregnancies indicate no adverse effects of dydrogesterone on the foetus.

The results of most epidemiological studies to date relevant to inadvertant foetal exposure to estrogens indicate no teratogenic or foetotoxic effects.

Lactation

Femapak is not indicated during lactation.

4.7 Effects on ability to drive and use machines

Fempak does not affect the ability to drive or use machines.

4.8 Undesirable effects

Application site reactions to patches

Some patients experience mild and transient local erythema at the site of application with or without itching; this usually disappears rapidly on removal of the patch. The overall incidence of general patch irritation in clinical studies is less than 5%. In a clinical study 3% of 102 patients showed well defined erythema (Draize scale) 30 minutes after patch removal. No instances of permanent skin damage have been reported. If unacceptable topical side

Table 1

MedDRA system organ class	Common >1/100, <1/10	Uncommon >1/1,000, <1/100	Rare >1/10,000, <1/1,000	Very rare <1/10,000 incl. isolated reports
Infections and infestations		Cystitis-like syndrome, Vaginal candidiasis		
Neoplasms benign, malignant and unspecified		Increase in size of leiomyoma		
Blood and the lymphatic system disorders				Haemolytic anaemia
Psychiatric disorders		Depression, Change in libido, Nervousness		
Nervous system disorders	Headache, Migraine	Dizziness		Chorea
Eye disorders			Intolerance to contact lenses, Steepening of corneal curvature	
Cardiac disorders				Myocardial infarction
Vascular disorders		Hypertension, Peripheral vascular disease, Varicose vein, Venous thromboembolism		Stroke
Gastrointestinal disorders	Nausea, Abdominal pain, Flatulence	Dyspepsia		Vomiting
Hepatobiliary disorders		Gall bladder disease	Alterations in liver function, sometimes with Asthenia or Malaise, Jaundice and Abdominal pain	
Skin and subcutaneous tissue disorders		Allergic skin reactions, Rash, Urticaria, Pruritus		Chloasma or melasma, which may persist when drug is discontinued, Erythema multiforme, Erythema nodosum, Vascular purpura, Angioedema
Musculoskeletal and connective tissue disorders	Leg cramps	Back pain		
Reproductive system and breast disorders	Breast pain/ tenderness, Breakthrough bleeding and spotting, Pelvic pain	Change in cervical erosion, Change in cervical secretion, Dysmenorrhoea, Menorrhagia, Metrorrhagia	Breast enlargement, Premenstrual-like symptoms	
Congenital and familial/genetic disorders				Aggravation of porphyria
General disorders and administration site reactions	Asthenia	Peripheral oedema		
Investigations	Increase/decrease in weight			

effects do occur discontinuation of treatment should be considered.

The following undesirable effects have been reported with Femapak 40 and /or with other estrogen/progestagen therapy:

(see Table 1 above)

Breast Cancer

According to evidence from a large number of epidemiological studies and one randomised placebo-controlled trial, the Women's Health Initiative (WHI), the overall risk of breast cancer increases with increasing duration of HRT use in current or recent HRT users.

For *estrogen-only* HRT, estimates of relative risk (RR) from a reanalysis of original data from 51 epidemiological studies (in which >80% of HRT use was estrogen-only HRT) and from the epidemiological Million Women Study (MWS) are similar at 1.35 (95%CI 1.21 – 1.49) and 1.30 (95%CI 1.21 – 1.40), respectively.

For *estrogen plus progestagen* combined HRT, several epidemiological studies have reported an overall higher risk for breast cancer than with estrogens alone.

The MWS reported that, compared to never users, the use of various types of estrogen-progestagen combined HRT was associated with a higher risk of breast cancer (RR = 2.00, 95%CI: 1.88 – 2.12) than use of estrogens alone (RR = 1.30, 95%CI: 1.21 – 1.40) or use of tibolone (RR=1.45; 95%CI 1.25-1.68).

The WHI trial reported a risk estimate of 1.24 (95%CI 1.01 – 1.54) after 5.6 years of use of estrogen-progestagen combined HRT (CEE + MPA) in all users compared with placebo.

The absolute risks calculated from the MWS and the WHI trials are presented below:

The MWS has estimated, from the known average incidence of breast cancer in developed countries, that:

- For women not using HRT, about 32 in every 1000 are expected to have breast cancer diagnosed between the ages of 50 and 64 years.

- For 1000 current or recent users of HRT, the number of *additional* cases during the corresponding period will be

- For users of *estrogen-only* replacement therapy

• between 0 and 3 (best estimate = 1.5) for 5 years' use

• between 3 and 7 (best estimate = 5) for 10 years' use.

- For users of *estrogen plus progestagen* combined HRT,

• between 5 and 7 (best estimate = 6) for 5 years' use

• between 18 and 20 (best estimate = 19) for 10 years' use.

The WHI trial estimated that after 5.6 years of follow-up of women between the ages of 50 and 79 years, an *additional* 8 cases of invasive breast cancer would be due to *estrogen-progestagen combined* HRT (CEE + MPA) per 10,000 women years.

According to calculations from the trial data, it is estimated that:

- For 1000 women in the placebo group,

• about 16 cases of invasive breast cancer would be diagnosed in 5 years.

- For 1000 women who used estrogen + progestagen combined HRT (CEE + MPA), the number of *additional* cases would be

• between 0 and 9 (best estimate = 4) for 5 years' use.

The number of additional cases of breast cancer in women who use HRT is broadly similar for women who start HRT irrespective of age at start of use (between the ages of 45-65) (see section 4.4).

Endometrial cancer

In women with an intact uterus, the risk of endometrial hyperplasia and endometrial cancer increases with increasing duration of use of unopposed estrogens. According to data from epidemiological studies, the best estimate of the risk is that for women not using HRT, about 5 in every 1000 are expected to have endometrial cancer diagnosed between the ages of 50 and 65. Depending on the duration of treatment and estrogen dose, the reported increase in endometrial cancer risk among unopposed estrogen users varies from 2-to 12-fold greater compared with non-users. Adding a progestagen to estrogen-only therapy greatly reduces this increased risk.

Other adverse reactions have been reported in association with estrogen/progestagen treatment:

- Estrogen-dependent neoplasms benign and malignant, e.g. endometrial cancer.

- Venous thromboembolism, i.e. deep leg or pelvic venous thrombosis and pulmonary embolism, is more frequent among hormone replacement therapy users than among non-users. For further information, see section 4.3 Contra-indications and 4.4 Special warnings and precautions for use.

- Probable dementia (see section 4.4)

4.9 Overdose

Fematrix 40 Patches

This is not likely due to the mode of administration. If it is necessary to stop delivery then the patch can be removed and plasma oestradiol levels will fall rapidly.

Duphaston Tablets

If overdosage is discovered within two or three hours and is so large that treatment seems desirable, gastric lavage can safely be used. There is no specific antidote and further treatment should be symptomatic.

5. PHARMACOLOGICAL PROPERTIES

5.1 Pharmacodynamic properties

Estradiol

The active ingredient, synthetic 17β-estradiol, is chemically and biologically identical to endogenous human estradiol. It substitutes for the loss of estrogen production in menopausal women, and alleviates menopausal symptoms.

Dydrogesterone

Dydrogesterone is an orally-active progestagen. The addition of a progestagen greatly reduces the estrogen-induced risk of endometrial hyperplasia and cancer in non-hysterectomised women, by reducing the growth of the endometrium.

Clinical trial information

• Relief of estrogen-deficiency symptoms and bleeding patterns.

- Relief of menopausal symptoms was achieved during the first few weeks of treatment.

5.2 Pharmacokinetic properties

Estradiol

Absorption

Estradiol is absorbed from the patch across the stratum corneum and is delivered systemically at a low but constant rate throughout the period of application (3 to 4 days). The estimated delivery of estradiol is around 40 µg/day.

The primary unconjugated and conjugated metabolites are estrone and estrone sulphate. These metabolites can contribute to the estrogen effect, both directly and after conversion to estradiol. Estrogens are excreted in the bile and reabsorbed from the intestine. During this enterohepatic cycle the estrogens are broken down. Estrogens are excreted in the urine as biologically inactive glucuronide and sulphate compounds (90 to 95%), or in the faeces (5 to 10%), mostly unconjugated. Estrogens are excreted in mothers' milk.

Steady state plasma estradiol concentrations have been demonstrated in the range of C_{min} is 26 pg/ml and the C_{max} is 34 pg/ml for the Fematrix 40 patch and C_{min} is 34 pg/ml and the C_{max} is 62 pg/ml for the Fematrix 80 patch (including baseline levels) and these are maintained throughout the dose interval (for up to four days). Absorption rate may vary between individual patients. After removal of the last patch plasma estradiol and estrone concentrations return to baseline values in less than 24 hours. The median terminal half-life for estradiol following patch removal has been determined as 5.24h.

Dydrogesterone

After oral administration of labelled dydrogesterone, on average 63% of the dose is excreted into the urine. Within 72 hours, excretion is complete.

In man, dydrogesterone is completely metabolised. The main metabolite of dydrogesterone is 20α-dihydrodydrogesterone (DHD) and is present in the urine predominantly as the glucuronic acid conjugate. A common feature of all metabolites characterised is the retention of the 4,6 diene-3-one configuration of the parent compound and the absence of 17α-hydroxylation. This explains the absence of estrogenic and androgenic activity.

After oral administration of dydrogesterone, plasma concentrations of DHD are substantially higher as compared to the parent drug. The AUC and C_{max} ratios of DHD to dydrogesterone are in the order of 40 and 25, respectively. Dydrogesterone is rapidly absorbed. The T_{max} values of dydrogesterone and DHD vary between 0.5 and 2.5 hours.

Mean terminal half lives of dydrogesterone and DHD vary between 5 to 7 and 14 to 17 hours, respectively.

The dihydrodydrogesterone $C_{average}$ is 13 ng/ml, the C_{min} is 4.1 ng/ml and the C_{max} is 63 ng/ml. The dydrogesterone $C_{average}$ is 0.38 ng/ml the C_{min} is <0.1 ng/ml and the C_{max} is 2.5 ng/ml.

Dydrogesterone is not excreted in urine as pregnanediol, like progesterone. Analysis of endogenous progesterone production based on pregnanediol excretion therefore remains possible.

5.3 Preclinical safety data

Supraphysiological doses (prolonged overdoses) of estradiol have been associated with the induction of tumours in estrogen-dependent target organs for all rodent species tested.

The changes observed with dydrogesterone in animal toxicity studies are characteristic for progesterone-like compounds. *In-vitro* and *in-vivo* data gave no indications of mutagenic effects of dydrogesterone. In long-term studies, doses administered to rats and mice were sufficient to produce hormone-mediated changes, but did not provide tumorogenic potential.

6. PHARMACEUTICAL PARTICULARS

6.1 List of excipients

Fematrix

Diethyltoluamide

Acrylic adhesive (Dow Corning MG-0560)

Acrylic thickener (Acrysol 33)

Backing: Polyester film

Release liner: Aluminised/Polyester film.

Duphaston

Tablet core: Lactose

Hypromellose

Maize starch

Colloidal anhydrous silica

Magnesium stearate

Film-coat: Hypromellose

Macrogol 400

Titanium dioxide (E171)

6.2 Incompatibilities

None known.

6.3 Shelf life

3 years.

6.4 Special precautions for storage

Do not store above 25°C.

Store in original package.

6.5 Nature and contents of container

Fematrix: Sealed laminated sachet (paper/polyethylene/aluminium foil/polyethylene) containing one transdermal patch. Duphaston: Blister strip containing 14 tablets. Each carton contains eight Fematrix patches and 14 Duphaston HRT tablets sufficient for one 28 day cycle.

6.6 Special precautions for disposal and other handling

After use, fold the Fematrix patch in two with the adhesive surface to the inside and dispose with the normal household waste.

7. MARKETING AUTHORISATION HOLDER

Solvay Healthcare Ltd

Mansbridge Road

West End

Southampton

SO18 3JD

United Kingdom

8. MARKETING AUTHORISATION NUMBER(S)

PL 00512/0175

9. DATE OF FIRST AUTHORISATION/RENEWAL OF THE AUTHORISATION

01 February 2002

10. DATE OF REVISION OF THE TEXT

January 2006

Legal category

POM

Femapak 80

(Solvay Healthcare Limited)

1. NAME OF THE MEDICINAL PRODUCT

Femapak 80

2. QUALITATIVE AND QUANTITATIVE COMPOSITION

Femapak 80 consists of a pack containing eight Fematrix 80 transdermal patches and a blister strip of 14 Duphaston tablets. Each Fematrix 80 patch contains 2.5 mg estradiol (each patch delivers approximately 80 micrograms of estradiol per 24 hours).

Each Duphaston tablet contains 10 mg Dydrogesterone.

For excipient, see 6.1

3. PHARMACEUTICAL FORM

Transdermal patch

Fematrix 80 self adhesive, flexible transdermal delivery system comprising a layer of clear adhesive sandwiched between a translucent patch and a metallised polyester backing. Fematrix 80 is a rectangular shape with rounded corners and has an active surface area of 28.5 cm^2.

Duphaston film-coated tablets: Round, white tablet, scored on one side with the inscriptions '155' on each half of the tablet and '**S̲**' on the reverse.

4. CLINICAL PARTICULARS

4.1 Therapeutic indications

Hormone replacement therapy (HRT) for estrogen deficiency symptoms in peri and postmenopausal women.

Prevention of osteoporosis in postmenopausal women at high risk of future fractures who are intolerant of, or contra-indicated for, other medicinal products approved for the prevention of osteoporosis.

(See also section 4.4)

The experience of treating women older than 65 years is limited.

4.2 Posology and method of administration

Femapak 80 is a continuous sequential hormone replacement therapy. Unless there is previous diagnosis of endometriosis, it is not recommended to add a progestagen in hysterectomised women.

For initiation and continuation of treatment of postmenopausal symptoms, the lowest effective dose for the shortest duration (see also section 4.4) should be used.

In general, treatment should start with Femapak 40. Depending on the clinical response, the dosage can afterwards be adjusted to individual need. If the complaints linked to estrogen deficiency are not ameliorated the dosage can be increased by using Femapak 80.

For the prevention of osteoporosis Femapak 80 should be used.

Starting Femapak 80

In women who are not taking hormone replacement therapy and who are amenorrhoeic or women who switch from a continuous combined hormone replacement therapy, treatment may be started on any convenient day. In women transferring from a cyclic or continuous sequential HRT regimen, treatment should begin the day following completion of the prior regimen. If the patient has regular menstruation periods, treatment is started within five days of the start of bleeding.

Administration

One Fematrix 80 transdermal patch should be applied twice weekly on a continuous basis. Each patch should be removed after 3 to 4 days and replaced with a new patch applied to a slightly different site. Patches should be applied to clean, dry and intact areas of skin below the waist on the lower back or buttocks. Patches should not be applied on or near the breasts. During the second two weeks of the cycle, that is from the 15th day after applying the first patch, one Duphaston tablet should be taken each day for the next 14 days. Most patients will commence bleeding towards the end of the Duphaston therapy.

If a tablet has been forgotten, it should be taken as soon as possible. When more than 12 hours have elapsed, it is recommended to continue with the next dose without taking the forgotten tablet. The likelihood of breakthrough bleeding or spotting may have increased. If a patch has been forgotten, it should be changed as soon as possible. The next patch should be applied on the usual day.

4.3 Contraindications

Known, past or suspected breast cancer;

Known or suspected estrogen-dependent malignant tumours (e.g. endometrial cancer);

Undiagnosed genital bleeding;

Untreated endometrial hyperplasia;

Previous idiopathic or current venous thromboembolism (deep vein thrombosis, pulmonary embolism);

Active or recent arterial thromboembolic disease (e.g. angina, myocardial infarction);

Acute liver disease, or a history of liver disease as long as liver function tests have failed to return to normal;

Known hypersensitivity to the active substance or to any of the excipients;

Porphyria.

4.4 Special warnings and precautions for use

For the treatment of postmenopausal symptoms, HRT should only be initiated for symptoms that adversely affect quality of life. In all cases, a careful appraisal of the risks and benefits should be undertaken at least annually and HRT should only be continued as long as the benefit outweighs the risk.

Medical examination/follow up

Before initiating or reinstituting HRT, a complete personal and family medical history should be taken. Physical (including pelvic and breast) examination should be guided by this and by the contraindications and warnings for use. During treatment, periodic check-ups are recommended of a frequency and nature adapted to the individual woman.

Women should be advised what changes in their breasts should be reported to their doctor or nurse (see 'breast cancer' below). Investigations, including mammography, should be carried out in accordance with currently accepted screening practices, modified to the clinical needs of the individual.

Conditions which need supervision

If any of the following conditions are present, have occurred previously, and/or have been aggravated during pregnancy or previous hormone treatment, the patient should be closely supervised. It should be taken into account that these conditions may recur or be aggravated during treatment with Femapak, in particular:

- Leiomyoma (uterine fibroids) or endometriosis
- A history of, or risk factors for, thromboembolic disorders (see below)
- Risk factors for estrogen dependent tumours, e.g. 1st degree heredity for breast cancer
- Hypertension
- Liver disorders (e.g. liver adenoma)
- Diabetes mellitus with or without vascular involvement
- Cholelithiasis
- Migraine or (severe) headache
- Systemic lupus erythematosus
- A history of endometrial hyperplasia (see below)
- Epilepsy
- Asthma
- Otosclerosis

Reasons for immediate withdrawal of therapy:

Therapy should be discontinued in cases where a contra-indication is discovered and in the following situations:

- Jaundice or deterioration in liver function
- Significant increase in blood pressure
- New onset of migraine-type headache
- Pregnancy

Endometrial hyperplasia

The risk of endometrial hyperplasia and carcinoma is increased when estrogens are administered alone for prolonged periods (see section 4.8). The addition of a progestagen for at least 12 days of the cycle in non-hysterectomised women greatly reduces this risk.

Break-through bleeding and spotting may occur during the first few months of treatment. If break-through bleeding or spotting appears after some time on therapy, or continues after treatment has been discontinued, the reason should be investigated, which may include endometrial biopsy to exclude endometrial malignancy.

Breast cancer

A randomised placebo-controlled trial, the Womens Health Initiative study (WHI) and epidemiological studies, including the Million Women Study (MWS), have reported an increased risk of breast cancer in women taking estrogens, estrogen-progestagen combinations or tibolone for HRT for several years (see Section 4.8).

For all HRT, an excess risk becomes apparent within a few years of use and increases with duration of intake but returns to baseline within a few (at most five) years after stopping treatment.

In the MWS, the relative risk of breast cancer with conjugated equine estrogens (CEE) or estradiol (E2) was greater when a progestagen was added, either sequentially or continuously, and regardless of type of progestagen. There was no evidence of a difference in risk between the different routes of administration.

In the WHI study, the continuous combined conjugated equine estrogen and medroxyprogesterone acetate (CEE + MPA) product used was associated with breast cancers that were slightly larger in size and more frequently had local lymph node metastases compared to placebo.

HRT, especially estrogen-progestagen combined treatment, increases the density of mammographic images which may adversely affect the radiological detection of breast cancer.

Venous thromboembolism

HRT is associated with a higher relative risk of developing venous thromboembolism (VTE), i.e. deep vein thrombosis or pulmonary embolism. One randomised controlled trial and epidermiological studies found a two-to threefold higher risk for users compared with non-users. For non-users, it is estimated that the number of cases of VTE that will occur over a 5 year period is about 3 per 1000 women aged 50-59 years and 8 per 1000 women aged between 60-69 years. It is estimated that in healthy women who use HRT for 5 years, the number of additional cases of VTE over a 5 year period will be between 2 and 6 (best estimate=4) per 1000 women aged 50-59 years and between 5 and 15 (best estimate = 9) per 1000 women aged 60-69 years. The occurrence of such an event is more likely in the first year of HRT than later.

• Generally recognised risk factors for VTE include a personal or family history, severe obesity (BMI >30 kg/m^2) and systemic lupus erythematosus (SLE). There is no consensus about the possible role of varicose veins in VTE.

• Patients with a history of VTE or known thrombophilic states have an increased risk of VTE. HRT may add to this risk. Personal or strong family history of thromboembolism or recurrent spontaneous abortion should be investigated in order to exclude a thrombophilic predisposition. Until a thorough evaluation of thrombophilic factors has been made or anticoagulant treatment initiated, use of HRT in such patients should be viewed as contraindicated. Those women already on anticoagulant treatment require careful consideration of the benefit-risk of use of HRT.

• The risk of VTE may be temporarily increased with prolonged immobilisation, major trauma or major surgery. As in all postoperative patients, scrupulous attention should be given to prophylactic measures to prevent VTE following surgery. Where prolonged immobilisation is liable to follow elective surgery, particularly abdominal or orthopaedic surgery to the lower limbs, consideration should be given to temporarily stopping HRT 4 to 6 weeks earlier, if possible. Treatment should not be restarted until the woman is completely mobilised.

• If VTE develops after initiating therapy, the drug should be discontinued. Patients should be told to contact their doctors immediately when they are aware of a potential thromboembolic symptom (e.g. painful swelling of a leg, sudden pain in the chest, dyspnea).

Coronary artery disease (CAD)

There is no evidence from randomised controlled trials of cardiovascular benefit with continuous combined conjugated estrogens and medroxyprogesterone acetate (MPA). Two large clinical trials (WHI and HERS i.e. Heart and Estrogen/progestin Replacement Study) showed a possible increased risk of cardiovascular morbidity in the first year of use and no overall benefit. For other HRT products there are only limited data from randomised controlled trials examining effects in cardiovascular morbidity or mortality. Therefore, it is uncertain whether these findings also extend to other HRT products.

Stroke

One large randomised clinical trial (WHI-trial) found, as a secondary outcome, an increased risk of ischaemic stroke in healthy women during treatment with continuous combined conjugated estrogens and MPA. For women who do not use HRT, it is estimated that the number of cases of stroke that will occur over a 5 year period is about 3 per 1000 women aged 50-59 and 11 per 1000 women aged 60-69 years. It is estimated that for women who use conjugated estrogens and MPA for 5 years, the number of additional cases will be between 0 and 3 (best estimate = 1) per 1000 users aged 50-59 years and between 1 and 9 (best estimate = 4) per 1000 users aged 60-69 years. It is unknown whether the increased risk also extends to other HRT products.

Ovarian cancer

Long-term (at least 5 to 10 years) use of estrogen-only HRT products in hysterectomised women has been associated with an increased risk of ovarian cancer in some epidemiological studies. It is uncertain whether long term use of combined HRT confers a different risk than estrogen-only products.

Other conditions

• Estrogens may cause fluid retention, and therefore patients with cardiac or renal dysfunction should be carefully observed. Patients with terminal renal insufficiency should be closely observed, since it is expected that the level of circulating active ingredients in Femapak is increased.

• Women with pre-existing hypertriglyceridemia should be followed closely during estrogen replacement or hormone replacement therapy, since rare cases of large increases of plasma triglycerides leading to pancreatitis have been reported with estrogen therapy in this condition.

• Estrogens increase thyroid binding globulin (TBG), leading to increased circulating total thyroid hormone, as measured by protein-bound iodine (PBI), T4 levels (by column or by radio-immunoassay) or T3 levels (by radio-immunoassay). T3 resin uptake is decreased, reflecting the elevated TBG. Free T4 and free T3 concentrations are unaltered. Other binding proteins may be elevated in serum, i.e. corticoid binding globulin (CBG), sex-hormone-binding globulin (SHBG) leading to increased circulating corticosteroids and sex steroids, respectively. Free or biological active hormone concentrations are unchanged. Other plasma proteins may be increased (angiotensinogen/renin substrate, alpha-1-antitrypsin, ceruloplasmin).

• There is no conclusive evidence for improvement of cognitive function. There is some evidence from the WHI trial of increased risk of probable dementia in women who start using continuous combined CEE and MPA after the age of 65. It is unknown whether the findings apply to younger post-menopausal women or other HRT products.

Table 1

MedDRA system organ class	Common >1/100, <1/10	Uncommon >1/1,000, <1/100	Rare >1/10,000, <1/1,000	Very rare <1/10,000 incl. isolated reports
Infections and infestations		Cystitis-like syndrome, Vaginal candidiasis		
Neoplasms benign, malignant and unspecified		Increase in size of leiomyoma		
Blood and the lymphatic system disorders				Haemolytic anaemia
Psychiatric disorders		Depression, Change in libido, Nervousness		
Nervous system disorders	Headache, Migraine	Dizziness		Chorea
Eye disorders			Intolerance to contact lenses, Steepening of corneal curvature	
Cardiac disorders				Myocardial infarction
Vascular disorders		Hypertension, Peripheral vascular disease, Varicose vein, Venous thromboembolism		Stroke
Gastrointestinal disorders	Nausea, Abdominal pain, Flatulence	Dyspepsia		Vomiting
Hepatobiliary disorders		Gall bladder disease	Alterations in liver function, sometimes with Asthenia or Malaise, Jaundice and Abdominal pain	
Skin and subcutaneous tissue disorders		Allergic skin reactions, Rash, Urticaria, Pruritus		Chloasma or melasma, which may persist when drug is discontinued, Erythema multiforme, Erythema nodosum, Vascular purpura, Angioedema
Musculoskeletal and connective tissue disorders	Leg cramps	Back pain		
Reproductive system and breast disorders	Breast pain/tenderness, Breakthrough bleeding and spotting, Pelvic pain	Change in cervical erosion, Change in cervical secretion, Dysmenorrhoea, Menorrhagia, Metrorrhagia	Breast enlargement, Premenstrual-like symptoms	
Congenital and familial/genetic disorders				Aggravation of porphyria
General disorders and administration site reactions	Asthenia	Peripheral oedema		
Investigations	Increase/decrease in weight			

• Patients with rare hereditary problems of galactose intolerance, the Lapp lactase deficiency or glucose-galactose malabsorption should not take this medicine.

• Women who may be at risk of pregnancy should be advised to adhere to non-hormonal contraceptive methods.

4.5 Interaction with other medicinal products and other forms of interaction

- The metabolism of estrogens and progestagens may be increased by concomitant use of substances known to induce drug-metabolising enzymes, specifically cytochrome P450 enzymes, such as anticonvulsants (eg. phenobarbital, phenytoin, carbamazepine) and anti-infectives (e.g. rifampicin, rifabutin, nevirapine, efavirenz).

- Ritonavir and nelfinavir, although known as strong inhibitors, by contrast exhibit inducing properties when used concomitantly with steroid hormones.

- Herbal preparations containing St John's wort (Hypericum perforatum) may induce the metabolism of estrogens and progestagens.

- Clinically an increased metabolism of estrogens and progestagens may lead to decreased effect and changes in the uterine bleeding profile.

- At transdermal administration, the first-pass effect of the liver is avoided and, thus, transdermally applied estrogens might be less affected than oral hormones by enzyme inducers.

4.6 Pregnancy and lactation

Pregnancy

Femapak is not indicated during pregnancy. If pregnancy occurs during medication with Femapak, treatment should be withdrawn immediately.

Clinically, data on a large number of exposed pregnancies indicate no adverse effects of dydrogesterone on the foetus.

The results of most epidemiological studies to date relevant to inadvertant foetal exposure to estrogens indicate no teratogenic or foetotoxic effects.

Lactation:

Femapak is not indicated during lactation.

4.7 Effects on ability to drive and use machines

Femapak does not affect the ability to drive or use machines.

4.8 Undesirable effects

Application site reactions to patches

Some patients experience mild and transient local erythema at the site of application with or without itching; this usually disappears rapidly on removal of the patch. The overall incidence of general patch irritation in clinical studies is less than 5%. In a clinical study 3% of 102 patients showed well defined erythema (Draize scale) 30 minutes after patch removal. No instances of permanent skin damage have been reported. If unacceptable topical side effects do occur discontinuation of treatment should be considered.

The following undesirable effects have been reported with Femapak 80 and/or with other estrogen/progestagen therapy:

(see Table 1 above)

Breast Cancer

According to evidence from a large number of epidemiological studies and one randomised placebo-controlled trial, the Women's Health Initiative (WHI), the overall risk of breast cancer increases with increasing duration of HRT use in current or recent HRT users.

For *estrogen-only* HRT, estimates of relative risk (RR) from a reanalysis of original data from 51 epidemiological studies (in which >80% of HRT use was estrogen-only HRT) and from the epidemiological Million Women Study (MWS) are similar at 1.35 (95%CI 1.21 – 1.49) and 1.30 (95%CI 1.21 – 1.40), respectively.

For *estrogen plus progestagen* combined HRT, several epidemiological studies have reported an overall higher risk for breast cancer than with estrogens alone.

The MWS reported that, compared to never users, the use of various types of estrogen-progestagen combined HRT was associated with a higher risk of breast cancer (RR = 2.00, 95%CI: 1.88 – 2.12) than use of estrogens alone (RR = 1.30, 95%CI: 1.21 – 1.40) or use of tibolone (RR=1.45; 95%CI 1.25-1.68).

The WHI trial reported a risk estimate of 1.24 (95%CI 1.01 – 1.54) after 5.6 years of use of estrogen-progestagen combined HRT (CEE + MPA) in all users compared with placebo.

The absolute risks calculated from the MWS and the WHI trials are presented below:

The MWS has estimated, from the known average incidence of breast cancer in developed countries, that:

- For women not using HRT, about 32 in every 1000 are expected to have breast cancer diagnosed between the ages of 50 and 64 years.

- For 1000 current or recent users of HRT, the number of *additional* cases during the corresponding period will be

- For users of *estrogen-only* replacement therapy

• between 0 and 3 (best estimate = 1.5) for 5 years' use

• between 3 and 7 (best estimate = 5) for 10 years' use.

- For users of *estrogen plus progestagen* combined HRT,

• between 5 and 7 (best estimate = 6) for 5 years' use

• between 18 and 20 (best estimate = 19) for 10 years' use.

The WHI trial estimated that after 5.6 years of follow-up of women between the ages of 50 and 79 years, an *additional* 8 cases of invasive breast cancer would be due to *estrogen-progestagen combined* HRT (CEE + MPA) per 10,000 women years.

According to calculations from the trial data, it is estimated that:

- For 1000 women in the placebo group,

• about 16 cases of invasive breast cancer would be diagnosed in 5 years.

- For 1000 women who used estrogen + progestagen combined HRT (CEE + MPA), the number of *additional* cases would be

• between 0 and 9 (best estimate = 4) for 5 years' use.

The number of additional cases of breast cancer in women who use HRT is broadly similar for women who start HRT irrespective of age at start of use (between the ages of 45-65) (see section 4.4).'

Endometrial cancer

In women with an intact uterus, the risk of endometrial hyperplasia and endometrial cancer increases with increasing duration of use of unopposed estrogens. According to data from epidemiological studies, the best estimate of the risk is that for women not using HRT, about 5 in every 1000 are expected to have endometrial cancer diagnosed between the ages of 50 and 65. Depending on the duration of treatment and estrogen dose, the reported increase in endometrial cancer risk among unopposed estrogen users varies from 2-to 12-fold greater compared with non-users. Adding a progestagen to estrogen-only therapy greatly reduces this increased risk.

Other adverse reactions have been reported in association with estrogen/progestagen treatment:

- Estrogen-dependent neoplasms benign and malignant, e.g. endometrial cancer.

- Venous thromboembolism, i.e. deep leg or pelvic venous thrombosis and pulmonary embolism, is more frequent among hormone replacement therapy users than among non-users. For further information, see section 4.3 Contra-indications and 4.4 Special warnings and precautions for use.

- Probable dementia (see section 4.4)

4.9 Overdose

Fematrix 80 Patches

This is not likely due to the mode of administration. If it is necessary to stop delivery then the patch can be removed and plasma oestradiol levels will fall rapidly.

Duphaston Tablets

If overdosage is discovered within two or three hours and is so large that treatment seems desirable, gastric lavage can safely be used. There is no specific antidote and further treatment should be symptomatic.

5. PHARMACOLOGICAL PROPERTIES

5.1 Pharmacodynamic properties

Estradiol

The active ingredient, synthetic 17β-estradiol, is chemically and biologically identical to endogenous human estradiol. It substitutes for the loss of estrogen production in menopausal women, and alleviates menopausal symptoms. Estrogens prevent bone loss following menopause or ovariectomy.

Dydrogesterone

Dydrogesterone is an orally-active progesterone. The addition of a progesterone greatly reduces the estrogen induced risk of endometrial hyperplasia and cancer in non-hysterectomised woman, by reducing the growth of the endometrium.

Clinical trial information

• Relief of estrogen-deficiency symptoms and bleeding patterns.

- Relief of menopausal symptoms was achieved during the first few weeks of treatment.

- In women treated with Fematrix 80 patches and progesterone tablets, regular withdrawal bleeding occurred in approximately 90% with a mean duration of 6.8 days. Withdrawal bleeding usually started on the day of the last pill of the progestagen phase. Break-through bleeding and/or spotting appeared in 3% of the women. Amenorrhoea (no bleeding or spotting) occurred in about 5 % of patients in month 6 of treatment.

• Prevention of osteoporosis

- Estrogen deficiency at menopause is associated with an increasing bone turnover and decline in bone mass. The effect of estrogens on the bone mineral density is dose-dependent. Protection appears to be effective for as long as treatment is continued. After discontinuation of HRT, bone mass is lost at a rate similar to that in untreated women.

- Evidence from the WHI trial and meta-analysed trials shows that current use of HRT, alone or in combination with a progestagen – given to predominantly healthy women – reduces the risk of hip, vertebral, and other osteoporotic fractures. HRT may also prevent fractures in women with low bone density and/or established osteoporosis, but the evidence for that is limited.

- After two years of treatment with Fematrix 80 patches, the increase in lumbar spine bone mineral density (BMD) was 6.54%. The percentage of women who maintained or gained BMD in lumbar zone during treatment was 96%.

5.2 Pharmacokinetic properties

Estradiol

Absorption

Estradiol is absorbed from the patch across the stratum corneum and is delivered systemically at a low but constant rate throughout the period of application (3 to 4 days). The estimated delivery of estradiol is around 40 μg/day.

The primary unconjugated and conjugated metabolites are estrone and estrone sulphate. These metabolites can contribute to the estrogen effect, both directly and after conversion to estradiol. Estrogens are excreted in the bile and reabsorbed from the intestine. During this enterohepatic cycle the estrogens are broken down. Estrogens are excreted in the urine as biologically inactive glucuronide and sulphate compounds (90 to 95%), or in the faeces (5 to 10%), mostly unconjugated. Estrogens are excreted in mothers' milk.

Steady state plasma estradiol concentrations have been demonstrated in the range of C_{min} is 26 pg/ml and the C_{max} is 34 pg/ml for the Fematrix 40 patch and C_{min} is 34 pg/ml and the C_{max} is 62 pg/ml for the Fematrix 80 patch (including baseline levels) and these are maintained throughout the dose interval (for up to four days). Absorption rate may vary between individual patients. After removal of the last patch plasma estradiol and oestrone concentrations return to baseline values in less than 24 hours. The median terminal half-life for estradiol following patch removal has been determined as 5.24h.

Dydrogesterone

After oral administration of labelled dydrogesterone, on average 63% of the dose is excreted into the urine. Within 72 hours, excretion is complete.

In man, dydrogesterone is completely metabolised. The main metabolite of dydrogesterone is 20α-dihydrodydrogesterone (DHD) and is present in the urine predominantly as the glucoronic acid conjugate. A common feature of all metabolites characterised is the retention of the 4,6 diene-3-one configuration of the parent compound and the absence of 17α-hydroxylation. This explains the absence of estrogenic and androgenic activity.

After oral administration of dydrogesterone, plasma concentrations of DHD are substantially higher as compared to the parent drug. The AUC and C_{max} ratios of DHD to dydrogesterone are in the order of 40 and 25, respectively. Dydrogesterone is rapidly absorbed. The T_{max} values of dydrogesterone and DHD vary between 0.5 and 2.5 hours.

Mean terminal half lives of dydrogesterone and DHD vary between 5 to 7 and 14 to 17 hours, respectively.

The dihydrodydrogesterone $C_{average}$ is 13 ng/ml, the C_{min} is 4.1 ng/ml and the C_{max} is 63 ng/ml. The dydrogesterone $C_{average}$ is 0.38 ng/ml the C_{min} is <0.1 ng/ml and the C_{max} is 2.5 ng/ml.

Dydrogesterone is not excreted in urine as pregnanediol, like progesterone. Analysis of endogenous progesterone production based on pregnanediol excretion therefore remains possible

5.3 Preclinical safety data

Supraphysiological doses (prolonged overdoses) of estradiol have been associated with the induction of tumours in estrogen-dependent target organs for all rodent species tested.

The changes observed with dydrogesterone in animal toxicity studies are characteristic for progesterone-like compounds. *In-vitro* and *in-vivo* data gave no indications of mutagenic effects of dydrogesterone. In long-term studies, doses administered to rats and mice were sufficient to produce hormone-mediated changes, but did not provide tumorogenic potential.

6. PHARMACEUTICAL PARTICULARS

6.1 List of excipients

Fematrix

Diethyltoluamide

Acrylic adhesive (Dow Corning MG-0560)

Acrylic thickener (Acrysol 33)

Backing: Polyester film

Release liner: Aluminised/Polyester film.

Duphaston

Tablet core: Lactose

Hypromellose

Maize starch

Colloidal anhydrous silica

Magnesium stearate

Film-coat: Hypromellose

Macrogol 400

Titanium dioxide (E171)

6.2 Incompatibilities

None known.

6.3 Shelf life

3 years

6.4 Special precautions for storage

Do not store above 25°C.

Store in original packaging

6.5 Nature and contents of container

Fematrix: Sealed laminated sachet (paper/polyethylene/aluminium foil/polyethylene) containing one transdermal patch.

Duphaston: Blister strip containing 14 tablets. Each carton contains eight Fematrix patches and 14 Duphaston HRT tablets sufficient for one 28 day cycle.

6.6 Special precautions for disposal and other handling

After use, fold the Fematrix patch in two with the adhesive surface to the inside and dispose with the normal household waste.

7. MARKETING AUTHORISATION HOLDER

Solvay Healthcare Ltd

Mansbridge Road

West End

Southampton

SO18 3JD

United Kingdom

8. MARKETING AUTHORISATION NUMBER(S)

PL 00512/0174

9. DATE OF FIRST AUTHORISATION/RENEWAL OF THE AUTHORISATION

01 February 2002

10. DATE OF REVISION OF THE TEXT

January 2006

Legal category

POM

Fematrix 40 transdermal patch

(Solvay Healthcare Limited)

1. NAME OF THE MEDICINAL PRODUCT

Fematrix 40 Transdermal Patch.

2. QUALITATIVE AND QUANTITATIVE COMPOSITION

Fematrix 40 contains 1.25 mg of estradiol and each patch delivers approximately 40 micrograms of estradiol per 24 hours.

For excipients, see 6.1.

3. PHARMACEUTICAL FORM

Transdermal patch.

Self adhesive, flexible transdermal patch comprising a layer of clear adhesive sandwiched between a translucent patch and a metallised polyester backing. Fematrix 40 is a rectangular shape with rounded corners and has an active surface area of 14.25 cm^2.

4. CLINICAL PARTICULARS

4.1 Therapeutic indications

Hormone replacement therapy (HRT) for estrogen deficiency symptoms in peri and postmenopausal women.

The experience treating women older than 65 years is limited.

4.2 Posology and method of administration

Fematrix 40 is an estrogen-only continuous hormone replacement therapy for women with or without a uterus. In women with a uterus, a progestagen such as Dydrogesterone 10mg, should be added to Fematrix 40 for 12-14 days each month to reduce the risk to the endometrium. Unless there is a previous diagnosis of endometriosis, it is not recommended to add a progestagen in hysterectomised women.

For initiation and continuation of treatment of postmenopausal symptoms, the lowest effective dose for the shortest duration (see also section 4.4) should be used.

In general, treatment should start with Fematrix 40. Depending on the clinical response, the dosage can afterwards be adjusted to individual need. If the complaints linked to estrogen deficiency are not ameliorated the dosage can be increased by using Fematrix 80.

Starting Fematrix 40

In women who are not taking hormone replacement therapy and who are amenorrhoeic, are hysterectomised, or women who switch from a continuous combined hormone replacement therapy, treatment may be started on any convenient day. In women transferring from a cyclic or continuous sequential HRT regimen, treatment should begin the day following completion of the prior regimen. If the patient has regular menstruation periods, treatment is started within five days of the start of bleeding.

Administration

One Fematrix 40 transdermal patch should be applied twice weekly on a continuous basis. Each patch should be removed after 3 to 4 days and replaced with a new patch applied to a slightly different site. Patches should be applied to clean, dry and intact areas of skin below the waist on the lower back or buttocks. Fematrix should not be applied on or near the breasts.

If a patch has been forgotten or falls off, it should be changed as soon as possible. The next patch should be applied on the usual day. In the case of a missed or delayed dose the likelihood of breakthrough bleeding or spotting may be increased.

4.3 Contraindications

Known, past or suspected breast cancer;

Known or suspected estrogen-dependent malignant tumours (e.g. endometrial cancer);

Undiagnosed genital bleeding;

Untreated endometrial hyperplasia;

Previous idiopathic or current venous thromboembolism (deep vein thrombosis, pulmonary embolism);

Active or recent arterial thromboembolic disease (e.g. angina, myocardial infarction);

Acute liver disease, or a history of liver disease as long as liver function tests have failed to return to normal;

Known hypersensitivity to the active substance or to any of the excipients;

Porphyria.

4.4 Special warnings and precautions for use

For the treatment of postmenopausal symptoms, HRT should only be initiated for symptoms that adversely affect quality of life. In all cases, a careful appraisal of the risks and benefits should be undertaken at least annually and HRT should only be continued as long as the benefit outweighs the risk.

Medical examination/follow up

Before initiating or reinstituting HRT, a complete personal and family medical history should be taken. Physical (including pelvic and breast) examination should be guided by this and by the contraindications and warnings for use. During treatment, periodic check-ups are recommended of a frequency and nature adapted to the individual woman. Women should be advised what changes in their breasts should be reported to their doctor or nurse (See 'breast cancer' below). Investigations, including mammography, should be carried out in accordance with currently accepted screening practices, modified to the clinical needs of the individual.

Conditions which need supervision

If any of the following conditions are present, have occurred previously, and/or have been aggravated during pregnancy or previous hormone treatment, the patient should be closely supervised. It should be taken into account that these conditions may recur or be aggravated during treatment with Fematrix, in particular:

- Leiomyoma (uterine fibroids) or endometriosis
- A history of, or risk factors for, thromboembolic disorders (see below)
- Risk factors for estrogen dependent tumours, e.g. 1st degree heredity for breast cancer
- Hypertension
- Liver disorders (e.g. liver adenoma)
- Diabetes mellitus with or without vascular involvement
- Cholelithiasis
- Migraine or (severe) headache
- Systemic lupus erythematosus
- A history of endometrial hyperplasia (see below)
- Epilepsy
- Asthma
- Otosclerosis

Reasons for immediate withdrawal of therapy:

- Therapy should be discontinued in cases where a contraindication is discovered and in the following situations:

- Jaundice or deterioration in liver function
- Significant increase in blood pressure
- New onset of migraine-type headache
- Pregnancy

Endometrial hyperplasia

The risk of endometrial hyperplasia and carcinoma is increased when estrogens are administered alone for prolonged periods (see section 4.8). The addition of a progestagen for at least 12 days of the cycle in non-hysterctomised women greatly reduces this risk.

Break-through bleeding and spotting may occur during the first few months of treatment. If break-through bleeding or spotting appears after some time on therapy, or continues after treatment has been discontinued, the reason should be investigated, which may include endometrial biopsy to exclude endometrial malignancy.

Unopposed estrogen stimulation may lead to premalignant or malignant transformation in the residual foci of endometriosis. Therefore, the addition of progestagens to estrogen replacement therapy should be considered in women who have undergone hysterectomy because of endometriosis, if they are known to have residual endometriosis.

Breast cancer

A randomised placebo-controlled trial, the Womens Health Initiative study (WHI) and epidemiological studies, including the Million Women Study (MWS), have reported an increased risk of breast cancer in women taking estrogens, estrogen-progestagen combinations or tibolone for HRT for several years (see Section 4.8).

For all HRT, an excess risk becomes apparent within a few years of use and increases with duration of intake but returns to baseline within a few (at most five) years after stopping treatment.

In the MWS, the relative risk of breast cancer with conjugated equine estrogens (CEE) or estradiol (E2) was greater when a progestagen was added, either sequentially or continuously, and regardless of type of progestagen. There was no evidence of a difference in risk between the different routes of administration.

In the WHI study, the continuous combined conjugated equine estrogen and medroxyprogesterone acetate (CEE + MPA) product used was associated with breast cancers that were slightly larger in size and more frequently had local lymph node metastases compared to placebo.

HRT, especially estrogen-progestagen combined treatment, increases the density of mammographic images which may adversely affect the radiological detection of breast cancer.

Venous thromboembolism

HRT is associated with a higher relative risk of developing venous thromboembolism (VTE), i.e. deep vein thrombosis or pulmonary embolism. One randomised controlled trial and epidermiological studies found a two-to threefold higher risk for users compared with non-users. For non-users, it is estimated that the number of cases of VTE that will occur over a 5 year period is about 3 per 1000 women aged 50-59 years and 8 per 1000 women aged between 60-69 years. It is estimated that in healthy women who use HRT for 5 years, the number of additional cases of VTE over a 5 year period will be between 2 and 6 (best estimate=4) per 1000 women aged 50-59 years and between 5 and 15 (best estimate = 9) per 1000 women aged 60-69 years. The occurrence of such an event is more likely in the first year of HRT than later.

• Generally recognised risk factors for VTE include a personal or family history, severe obesity (BMI >30 kg/m^2) and systemic lupus erythematosus (SLE). There is no consensus about the possible role of varicose veins in VTE.

• Patients with a history of VTE or known thrombophilic states have an increased risk of VTE. HRT may add to this risk. Personal or strong family history of thromboembolism or recurrent spontaneous abortion should be investigated in order to exclude a thrombophilic predisposition. Until a thorough evaluation of thrombophilic factors has been made or anticoagulant treatment initiated, use of HRT in such patients should be viewed as contraindicated. Those women already on anticoagulant treatment require careful consideration of the benefit-risk of use of HRT.

• The risk of VTE may be temporarily increased with prolonged immobilisation, major trauma or major surgery. As in all postoperative patients, scrupulous attention should be given to prophylactic measures to prevent VTE following surgery. Where prolonged immobilisation is liable to follow elective surgery, particularly abdominal or orthopaedic surgery to the lower limbs, consideration should be given to temporarily stopping HRT 4 to 6 weeks earlier, if possible. Treatment should not be restarted until the woman is completely mobilised.

• If VTE develops after initiating therapy, the drug should be discontinued. Patients should be told to contact their doctors immediately when they are aware of a potential thromboembolic symptom (e.g. painful swelling of a leg, sudden pain in the chest, dyspnea).

Coronary artery disease (CAD)

There is no evidence from randomised controlled trials of cardiovascular benefit with continuous combined conjugated estrogens and medroxyprogesterone acetate (MPA). Two large clinical trials (WHI and HERS i.e. Heart and Estrogen/progestin Replacement Study) showed a possible increased risk of cardiovascular morbidity in the first year of use and no overall benefit. For other HRT products there are only limited data from randomised controlled trials examining effects in cardiovascular morbidity or mortality. Therefore, it is uncertain whether these findings also extend to other HRT products.

Stroke

One large randomised clinical trial (WHI-trial) found, as a secondary outcome, an increased risk of ischaemic stroke in healthy women during treatment with continuous combined conjugated estrogens and MPA. For women who do not use HRT, it is estimated that the number of cases of stroke that will occur over a 5 year period is about 3 per 1000 women aged 50-59 and 11 per 1000 women aged 60-69 years. It is estimated that for women who use conjugated estrogens and MPA for 5 years, the number of additional cases will be between 0 and 3 (best estimate = 1) per 1000 users aged 50-59 years and between 1 and 9 (best estimate = 4) per 1000 users aged 60-69 years. It is unknown whether the increased risk also extends to other HRT products.

Ovarian cancer

Long-term (at least 5 to 10 years) use of estrogen-only HRT products in hysterectomised women has been associated with an increased risk of ovarian cancer in some epidemiological studies. It is uncertain whether long term use of combined HRT confers a different risk than estrogen-only products.

Other conditions

• Estrogens may cause fluid retention, and therefore patients with cardiac or renal dysfunction should be carefully observed. Patients with terminal renal insufficiency should be closely observed, since it is expected that the level of circulating active ingredients in Fematrix is increased.

• Women with pre-existing hypertriglyceridemia should be followed closely during estrogen replacement or hormone replacement therapy, since rare cases of large increases of plasma triglycerides leading to pancreatitis have been reported with estrogen therapy in this condition.

• Estrogens increase thyroid binding globulin (TBG), leading to increased circulating total thyroid hormone, as measured by protein-bound iodine (PBI), T4 levels (by column or by radio-immunoassay) or T3 levels (by radio-immunoassay). T3 resin uptake is decreased, reflecting the elevated TBG. Free T4 and free T3 concentrations are unaltered. Other binding proteins may be elevated in serum, i.e. corticoid binding globulin (CBG), sex-hormone-binding globulin (SHBG) leading to increased circulating corticosteroids and sex steroids, respectively. Free or biological active hormone concentrations are unchanged. Other plasma proteins may be increased (angiotensinogen/renin substrate, alpha-1-antitrypsin, ceruloplasmin).

• There is no conclusive evidence for improvement of cognitive function. There is some evidence from the WHI trial of increased risk of probable dementia in women who start using continuous combined CEE and MPA after the age of 65. It is unknown whether the findings apply to younger post-menopausal women or other HRT products.

• Women who may be at risk of pregnancy should be advised to adhere to non-hormonal contraceptive methods.

4.5 Interaction with other medicinal products and other forms of interaction

- The metabolism of estrogens may be increased by concomitant use of substances known to induce drug-metabolising enzymes, specifically cytochrome P450 enzymes, such as anticonvulsants (eg. phenobarbital, phenytoin, carbamezapine) and anti-infectives (e.g. rifampicin, rifabutin, nevirapine, efavirenz).

- Ritonavir and nelfinavir, although known as strong inhibitors, by contrast exhibit inducing properties when used concomitantly with steroid hormones.

- Herbal preparations containing St John's wort (Hypericum perforatum) may induce the metabolism of estrogens and progestagens.

- Clinically an increased metabolism of estrogens and progestagens may lead to decreased effect and changes in the uterine bleeding profile.

- At transdermal administration, the first-pass effect of the liver is avoided and, thus, transdermally applied estrogens might be less affected than oral hormones by enzyme inducers.

4.6 Pregnancy and lactation

Pregnancy

Fematrix is not indicated during pregnancy. If pregnancy occurs during medication with Fematrix, treatment should be withdrawn immediately.

The results of most epidemiological studies to date relevant to inadvertant foetal exposure to estrogens indicate no teratogenic or foetotoxic effects.

Lactation:

Fematrix is not indicated during lactation.

4.7 Effects on ability to drive and use machines

Fematrix does not affect the abilitiy to drive or use machines.

4.8 Undesirable effects

Application site reactions to patches

Some patients experience mild and transient local erythema at the site of application with or without itching; this usually disappears rapidly on removal of the patch. The overall incidence of general patch irritation in clinical studies is less than 5%. In a clinical study 3% of 102 patients showed well defined erythema (Draize scale) 30 minutes after patch removal. No instances of permanent skin damage have been reported. If unacceptable topical side effects do occur discontinuation of treatment should be considered.

The following undesirable effects have been reported with Fematrix 40 and /or with other estrogen/progestagen therapy:

(see Table 1 below)

Breast Cancer

According to evidence from a large number of epidemiological studies and one randomised placebo-controlled trial, the Women's Health Initiative (WHI), the overall risk of breast cancer increases with increasing duration of HRT use in current or recent HRT users.

For *estrogen-only* HRT, estimates of relative risk (RR) from a reanalysis of original data from 51 epidemiological studies (in which >80% of HRT use was estrogen-only HRT) and from the epidemiological Million Women Study (MWS) are similar at 1.35 (95%CI 1.21 – 1.49) and 1.30 (95%CI 1.21 – 1.40), respectively.

For *estrogen plus progestagen* combined HRT, several epidemiological studies have reported an overall higher risk for breast cancer than with estrogens alone.

The MWS reported that, compared to never users, the use of various types of estrogen-progestagen combined HRT was associated with a higher risk of breast cancer (RR = 2.00, 95%CI: 1.88 – 2.12) than use of estrogens alone (RR = 1.30, 95%CI: 1.21 – 1.40) or use of tibolone (RR=1.45; 95%CI 1.25-1.68).

The WHI trial reported a risk estimate of 1.24 (95%CI 1.01 – 1.54) after 5.6 years of use of estrogen-progestagen combined HRT (CEE + MPA) in all users compared with placebo.

The absolute risks calculated from the MWS and the WHI trials are presented below:

The MWS has estimated, from the known average incidence of breast cancer in developed countries, that:

- For women not using HRT, about 32 in every 1000 are expected to have breast cancer diagnosed between the ages of 50 and 64 years.

- For 1000 current or recent users of HRT, the number of *additional* cases during the corresponding period will be

- For users of *estrogen-only* replacement therapy

• between 0 and 3 (best estimate = 1.5) for 5 years' use

• between 3 and 7 (best estimate = 5) for 10 years' use.

- For users of *estrogen plus progestagen* combined HRT,

• between 5 and 7 (best estimate = 6) for 5 years' use

• between 18 and 20 (best estimate = 19) for 10 years' use.

The WHI trial estimated that after 5.6 years of follow-up of women between the ages of 50 and 79 years, an *additional* 8 cases of invasive breast cancer would be due to *estrogen-progestagen combined* HRT (CEE + MPA) per 10,000 women years.

According to calculations from the trial data, it is estimated that:

- For 1000 women in the placebo group,

• about 16 cases of invasive breast cancer would be diagnosed in 5 years.

- For 1000 women who used estrogen + progestagen combined HRT (CEE + MPA), the number of *additional* cases would be

• between 0 and 9 (best estimate = 4) for 5 years' use.

The number of additional cases of breast cancer in women who use HRT is broadly similar for women who start HRT irrespective of age at start of use (between the ages of 45-65) (see section 4.4).

Endometrial cancer

In women with an intact uterus, the risk of endometrial hyperplasia and endometrial cancer increases with increasing duration of use of unopposed estrogens. According to data from epidemiological studies, the best estimate of the risk is that for women not using HRT, about 5 in every 1000 are expected to have endometrial cancer diagnosed between the ages of 50 and 65. Depending on the duration of treatment and estrogen dose, the reported increase in endometrial cancer risk among unopposed estrogen users varies from 2-to 12-fold greater compared with non-users. Adding a progestagen to estrogen-only therapy greatly reduces this increased risk.

Other adverse reactions have been reported in association with estrogen/progestagen treatment:

- Estrogen-dependent neoplasms benign and malignant, e.g. endometrial cancer.

- Venous thromboembolism, i.e. deep leg or pelvic venous thrombosis and pulmonary embolism, is more frequent among hormone replacement therapy users than among non-users. For further information, see section 4.3 Contra-indications and 4.4 Special warnings and precautions for use.

- Probable dementia (see section 4.4).

Table 1

MedDRA system organ class	Common >1/100, <1/10	Uncommon >1/1,000, <1/100	Rare >1/10,000, <1/1,000	Very rare <1/10,000 incl. isolated reports
Infections and infestations		Cystitis-like syndrome, Vaginal candidiasis		
Neoplasms benign, malignant and unspecified		Increase in size of leiomyoma		
Blood and the lymphatic system disorders				Haemolytic anaemia
Psychiatric disorders		Depression, Change in libido, Nervousness		
Nervous system disorders	Headache, Migraine	Dizziness		Chorea
Eye disorders		Intolerance to contact lenses, Steepening of corneal curvature		
Cardiac disorders				Myocardial infarction
Vascular disorders		Hypertension, Peripheral vascular disease, Varicose vein, Venous thromboembolism		Stroke
Gastrointestinal disorders	Nausea, Abdominal pain, Flatulence	Dyspepsia		Vomiting
Hepatobiliary disorders		Gall bladder disease	Alterations in liver function, sometimes with Asthenia or Malaise, Jaundice and Abdominal pain	
Skin and subcutaneous tissue disorders		Allergic skin reactions, Rash, Urticaria, Pruritus		Chloasma or melasma, which may persist when drug is discontinued, Erythema multiforme, Erythema nodosum, Vascular purpura, Angioedema
Musculoskeletal and connective tissue disorders	Leg cramps	Back pain		
Reproductive system and breast disorders	Breast pain/ tenderness, Breakthrough bleeding and spotting, Pelvic pain	Change in cervical erosion, Change in cervical secretion, Dysmenorrhoea, Menorrhagia, Metrorrhagia	Breast enlargement, Premenstrual-like symptoms	
Congenital and familial/genetic disorders				Aggravation of porphyria
General disorders and administration site reactions	Asthenia	Peripheral oedema		
Investigations	Increase/decrease in weight			

4.9 Overdose

This is not likely due to the mode of administration. If it is necessary to stop delivery then the patch can be removed and plasma oestradiol levels will fall rapidly.

5. PHARMACOLOGICAL PROPERTIES

5.1 Pharmacodynamic properties

The active ingredient, synthetic 17β-estradiol, is chemically and biologically identical to endogenous human estradiol. It substitutes for the loss of estrogen production in menopausal women, and alleviates menopausal symptoms.

Clinical trial information

• Relief of estrogen-deficiency symptoms and bleeding patterns.

- Relief of menopausal symptoms was achieved during the first few weeks of treatment.

5.2 Pharmacokinetic properties

General characteristics of the active substance

Absorption

Estradiol is absorbed from the patch across the stratum corneum and is delivered systemically at a low but constant rate throughout the period of application (3 to 4 days). The estimated delivery of estradiol is approximately 40 µg/day for Fematrix 40.

The primary unconjugated and conjugated metabolites are estrone and estrone sulphate. These metabolites can contribute to the estrogen effect, both directly and after conversion to estradiol. Estrogens are excreted in the bile and reabsorbed from the intestine. During this enterohepatic cycle the estrogens are broken down. Estrogens are excreted in the urine as biologically inactive glucuronide and sulphate compounds (90 to 95%), or in the faeces (5 to 10%), mostly unconjugated. Estrogens are excreted in mothers' milk.

Steady state plasma estradiol concentrations have been demonstrated in the range of C_{min} is 26 pg/ml and the C_{max} is 34 pg/ml for the Fematrix 40 patch (including baseline levels) and these are maintained throughout the dose interval (for up to four days). Absorption rate may vary between individual patients. After removal of the last patch plasma estradiol and oestrone concentrations return to baseline values in less than 24 hours.

The median terminal half-life for estradiol following patch removal has been determined as 5.24h.

5.3 Preclinical safety data

Supraphysiological doses (prolonged overdoses) of estradiol have been associated with the induction of tumours in estrogen-dependent target organs for all rodent species tested.

In long-term studies, doses administered to rats and mice were sufficient to produce hormone-mediated changes, but did not provide tumorogenic potential.

6. PHARMACEUTICAL PARTICULARS

6.1 List of excipients

Diethyltoluamide

Acrylic adhesive (Dow Corning MG-0560)

Acrylic thickener (Acrysol 33)

Backing: Polyester

Release liner: Siliconised/Aluminised/Polyester

6.2 Incompatibilities

Not applicable.

6.3 Shelf life

3 years.

6.4 Special precautions for storage

Do not store above 25°C.

Store in the original container.

6.5 Nature and contents of container

Sealed laminated sachet (paper/polyethylene/aluminium foil/polyethylene) containing one transdermal patch. Each carton contains eight patches, sufficient for one 28 day cycle and a patient leaflet.

6.6 Special precautions for disposal and other handling

Detailed instructions for use are provided in the patient information leaflet.

7. MARKETING AUTHORISATION HOLDER

Solvay Healthcare Ltd

Mansbridge Road

West End

Southampton

SO18 3JD

United Kingdom

8. MARKETING AUTHORISATION NUMBER(S)

PL 00512/0173

9. DATE OF FIRST AUTHORISATION/RENEWAL OF THE AUTHORISATION

12 November 2001/1 September 2006

10. DATE OF REVISION OF THE TEXT

1 September 2006

Legal category

POM

Fematrix 80 transdermal patch

(Solvay Healthcare Limited)

1. NAME OF THE MEDICINAL PRODUCT

Fematrix 80 Transdermal Patch

2. QUALITATIVE AND QUANTITATIVE COMPOSITION

Fematrix 80 contains 2.5 mg of estradiol and each patch delivers approximately 80 micrograms of estradiol per 24 hours.

For excipients, see 6.1

3. PHARMACEUTICAL FORM

Transdermal patch

Self adhesive, flexible transdermal patch comprising a layer of clear adhesive sandwiched between a translucent patch and a metallised polyester backing. Fematrix 80 is a rectangular shape with rounded corners and has an active surface area of 28.5 cm^2.

4. CLINICAL PARTICULARS

4.1 Therapeutic indications

Hormone replacement therapy (HRT) for estrogen deficiency symptoms in peri and postmenopausal women.

Prevention of osteoporosis in postmenopausal women at high risk of future fractures who are intolerant of, or contraindicated for, other medicinal products approved for the prevention of osteoporosis.

(See also section 4.4)

The experience treating women older than 65 years is limited.

4.2 Posology and method of administration

Fematrix 80 is an estrogen-only continuous HRT for women with or without a uterus.

In women with a uterus, a progestagen such as Dydrogesterone 10mg, should be added to Fematrix 80 for 12-14 days each month to reduce the risk to the endometrium. Unless there is a previous diagnosis of endometriosis, it is not recommended to add a progestagen in hysterectomised women.

For initiation and continuation of treatment of postmenopausal symptoms, the lowest effective dose for the shortest duration (see also section 4.4) should be used.

In general, treatment should start with Fematrix 40. Depending on the clinical response, the dosage can afterwards be adjusted to individual need. If the complaints linked to estrogen deficiency are not ameliorated the dosage can be increased by using Fematrix 80.

For the prevention of osteoporosis Fematrix 80 should be used.

Starting Fematrix 80

In women who are not taking hormone replacement therapy and who are amenorrhoeic, are hysterectomised, or women who switch from a continuous combined hormone replacement therapy, treatment may be started on any convenient day. In women transferring from a cyclic or continuous sequential HRT regimen, treatment should begin the day following completion of the prior regimen. If the patient has regular menstruation periods, treatment is started within five days of the start of bleeding.

Administation

One Fematrix 80 transdermal patch should be applied twice weekly on a continuous basis. Each patch should be removed after 3 to 4 days and replaced with a new patch applied to a slightly different site. Patches should be applied to clean, dry and intact areas of skin below the waist on the lower back or buttocks. Fematrix should not be applied on or near the breasts.

If a patch has been forgotten or falls off, it should be changed as soon as possible. The next patch should be applied on the usual day. In the case of a missed or delayed dose the likelihood of breakthrough bleeding or spotting may be increased.

4.3 Contraindications

Known, past or suspected breast cancer;

Known or suspected estrogen-dependent malignant tumours (e.g. endometrial cancer);

Undiagnosed genital bleeding;

Untreated endometrial hyperplasia;

Previous idiopathic or current venous thromboembolism (deep vein thrombosis, pulmonary embolism);

Active or recent arterial thromboembolic disease (e.g. angina, myocardial infarction);

Acute liver disease, or a history of liver disease as long as liver function tests have failed to return to normal;

Known hypersensitivity to the active substance or to any of the excipients;

Porphyria.

4.4 Special warnings and precautions for use

For the treatment of postmenopausal symptoms, HRT should only be initiated for symptoms that adversely affect quality of life. In all cases, a careful appraisal of the risks and benefits should be undertaken at least annually and HRT should only be continued as long as the benefit outweighs the risk.

Medical examination/follow up

Before initiating or reinstituting HRT, a complete personal and family medical history should be taken. Physical (including pelvic and breast) examination should be guided by this and by the contraindications and warnings for use. During treatment, periodic check-ups are recommended of a frequency and nature adapted to the individual woman. Women should be advised what changes in their breasts should be reported to their doctor or nurse (see Breast Cancer below). Investigations, including mammography, should be carried out in accordance with currently accepted screening practices, modified to the clinical needs of the individual.

Conditions which need supervision

If any of the following conditions are present, have occurred previously, and/or have been aggravated during pregnancy or previous hormone treatment, the patient should be closely supervised. It should be taken into account that these conditions may recur or be aggravated during treatment with Fematrix, in particular:

- Leiomyoma (uterine fibroids) or endometriosis
- A history of, or risk factors for, thromboembolic disorders (see below)
- Risk factors for estrogen dependent tumours, e.g. 1st degree heredity for breast cancer
- Hypertension
- Liver disorders (e.g. liver adenoma)
- Diabetes mellitus with or without vascular involvement
- Cholelithiasis
- Migraine or (severe) headache
- Systemic lupus erythematosus
- A history of endometrial hyperplasia (see below)
- Epilepsy
- Asthma
- Otosclerosis

Reasons for immediate withdrawal of therapy:

- Therapy should be discontinued in cases where a contra-indication is discovered and in the following situations:

- Jaundice or deterioration in liver function
- Significant increase in blood pressure
- New onset of migraine-type headache
- Pregnancy

Endometrial hyperplasia

The risk of endometrial hyperplasia and carcinoma is increased when estrogens are administered alone for prolonged periods (see section 4.8). The addition of a progestagen for at least 12 days of the cycle in non-hysterectomised women greatly reduces this risk.

For Fematrix 80, the endometrial safety of added progesterone has not been studied.

Break-through bleeding and spotting may occur during the first few months of treatment. If break-through bleeding or spotting appears after some time on therapy, or continues after treatment has been discontinued, the reason should be investigated, which may include endometrial biopsy to exclude endometrial malignancy.

Unopposed estrogen stimulation may lead to premalignant or malignant transformation in the residual foci of endometriosis. Therefore, the addition of progestagens to estrogen replacement therapy should be considered in women who have undergone hysterectomy because of endometriosis, if they are known to have residual endometriosis.

Breast cancer

A randomised placebo-controlled trial, the Womens Health Initiative study (WHI) and epidemiological studies, including the Million Women Study (MWS), have reported an increased risk of breast cancer in women taking estrogens, estrogen-progestagen combinations or tibolone for HRT for several years (see Section 4.8).

For all HRT, an excess risk becomes apparent within a few years of use and increases with duration of intake but returns to baseline within a few (at most five) years after stopping treatment.

In the MWS, the relative risk of breast cancer with conjugated equine estrogens (CEE) or estradiol (E2) was greater when a progestagen was added, either sequentially or continuously, and regardless of type of progestagen. There was no evidence of a difference in risk between the different routes of administration.

In the WHI study, the continuous combined conjugated equine estrogen and medroxyprogesterone acetate (CEE + MPA) product used was associated with breast cancers that were slightly larger in size and more frequently had local lymph node metastases compared to placebo.

HRT, especially estrogen-progestagen combined treatment, increases the density of mammographic images which may adversely affect the radiological detection of breast cancer.

Venous thromboembolism

HRT is associated with a higher relative risk of developing venous thromboembolism (VTE), i.e. deep vein thrombosis or pulmonary embolism. One randomised controlled trial and epidemiological studies found a two-to threefold higher risk for users compared with non-users. For non-users, it is estimated that the number of cases of VTE that will occur over a 5 year period is about 3 per 1000 women aged 50-59 years and 8 per 1000 women aged between 60-69 years. It is estimated that in healthy women who use HRT for 5 years, the number of additional cases of VTE over a 5 year period will be between 2 and 6 (best estimate=4) per 1000 women aged 50-59 years and between 5 and 15 (best estimate = 9) per 1000 women aged 60-69 years. The occurrence of such an event is more likely in the first year of HRT than later.

• Generally recognised risk factors for VTE include a personal or family history, severe obesity (BMI >30 kg/m^2) and systemic lupus erythematosus (SLE). There is no consensus about the possible role of varicose veins in VTE.

• Patients with a history of VTE or known thrombophilic states have an increased risk of VTE. HRT may add to this risk. Personal or strong family history of thromboembolism or recurrent spontaneous abortion should be investigated in order to exclude a thrombophilic predisposition. Until a thorough evaluation of thrombophilic factors has been made or anticoagulant treatment initiated, use of HRT in such patients should be viewed as contraindicated. Those women already on anticoagulant treatment require careful consideration of the benefit-risk of use of HRT.

• The risk of VTE may be temporarily increased with prolonged immobilisation, major trauma or major surgery. As in all postoperative patients, scrupulous attention should be given to prophylactic measures to prevent VTE following surgery. Where prolonged immobilisation is liable to follow elective surgery, particularly abdominal or orthopaedic surgery to the lower limbs, consideration should be given to temporarily stopping HRT 4 to 6 weeks earlier, if possible. Treatment should not be restarted until the woman is completely mobilised.

• If VTE develops after initiating therapy, the drug should be discontinued. Patients should be told to contact their doctors immediately when they are aware of a potential thromboembolic symptom (e.g. painful swelling of a leg, sudden pain in the chest, dyspnea).

Coronary artery disease (CAD)

There is no evidence from randomised controlled trials of cardiovascular benefit with continuous combined conjugated estrogens and medroxyprogesterone acetate (MPA). Two large clinical trials (WHI and HERS i.e. Heart and Estrogen/progestin Replacement Study) showed a possible increased risk of cardiovascular morbidity in the first year of use and no overall benefit. For other HRT products there are only limited data from randomised controlled trials examining effects in cardiovascular morbidity or mortality. Therefore, it is uncertain whether these findings also extend to other HRT products.

Stroke

One large randomised clinical trial (WHI-trial) found, as a secondary outcome, an increased risk of ischaemic stroke in healthy women during treatment with continuous combined conjugated estrogens and MPA. For women who do not use HRT, it is estimated that the number of cases of stroke that will occur over a 5 year period is about 3 per 1000 women aged 50-59 and 11 per 1000 women aged 60-69 years. It is estimated that for women who use conjugated estrogens and MPA for 5 years, the number of additional cases will be between 0 and 3 (best estimate = 1) per 1000 users aged 50-59 years and between 1 and 9 (best estimate = 4) per 1000 users aged 60-69 years. It is unknown whether the increased risk also extends to other HRT products.

Ovarian cancer

Long-term (at least 5 to 10 years) use of estrogen-only HRT products in hysterectomised women has been associated with an increased risk of ovarian cancer in some epidemiological studies. It is uncertain whether long term use of combined HRT confers a different risk than estrogen-only products.

Other conditions

• Estrogens may cause fluid retention, and therefore patients with cardiac or renal dysfunction should be carefully observed. Patients with terminal renal insufficiency should be closely observed, since it is expected that the level of circulating active ingredients in Fematrix is increased.

• Women with pre-existing hypertriglyceridemia should be followed closely during estrogen replacement or hormone replacement therapy, since rare cases of large increases of plasma triglycerides leading to pancreatitis have been reported with estrogen therapy in this condition.

• Estrogens increase thyroid binding globulin (TBG), leading to increased circulating total thyroid hormone, as measured by protein-bound iodine (PBI), T4 levels (by column or by radio-immunoassay) or T3 levels (by radio-immunoassay). T3 resin uptake is decreased, reflecting the elevated TBG. Free T4 and free T3 concentrations are unaltered. Other binding proteins may be elevated in serum, i.e. corticoid binding globulin (CBG), sex-hormone-binding globulin (SHBG) leading to increased circulating corticosteroids and sex steroids, respectively. Free or biological active hormone concentrations are unchanged. Other plasma proteins may be increased (angiotensinogen/renin substrate, alpha-1-antitrypsin, ceruloplasmin).

• There is no conclusive evidence for improvement of cognitive function. There is some evidence from the WHI trial of increased risk of probable dementia in women who start using continuous combined CEE and MPA after the age of 65. It is unknown whether the findings apply to younger post-menopausal women or other HRT products.

• Women who may be at risk of pregnancy should be advised to adhere to non-hormonal contraceptive methods.

4.5 Interaction with other medicinal products and other forms of interaction

The metabolism of estrogens may be increased by concomitant use of substances known to induce drug-metabolising enzymes, specifically cytochrome P450 enzymes, such as anticonvulsants (eg. phenobarbital, phenytoin, carbamezapine) and anti-infectives (e.g. rifampicin, rifabutin, nevirapine, efavirenz).

- Ritonavir and nelfinavir, although known as strong inhibitors, by contrast exhibit inducing properties when used concomitantly with steroid hormones.

- Herbal preparations containing St John's wort (Hypericum perforatum) may induce the metabolism of estrogens and progestagens.

- Clinically an increased metabolism of estrogens and progestagens may lead to decreased effect and changes in the uterine bleeding profile.

- At transdermal administration, the first-pass effect of the liver is avoided and, thus, transdermally applied estrogens might be less affected than oral hormones by enzyme inducers.

4.6 Pregnancy and lactation

Pregnancy

Fematrix is not indicated during pregnancy. If pregnancy occurs during medication with Fematrix, treatment should be withdrawn immediately.

The results of most epidemiological studies to date relevant to inadvertant foetal exposure to estrogens indicate no teratogenic or foetotoxic effects.

Lactation:

Fematrix is not indicated during lactation

4.7 Effects on ability to drive and use machines

Fematrix does not affect the ability to drive or use machines.

4.8 Undesirable effects

Application site reactions to patches

Some patients experience mild and transient local erythema at the site of application with or without itching; this usually disappears rapidly on removal of the patch. The overall incidence of general patch irritation in clinical studies is less than 5%. In a clinical study 3% of 102 patients showed well defined erythema (Draize scale) 30 minutes after patch removal. No instances of permanent skin damage have been reported. If unacceptable topical side effects do occur discontinuation of treatment should be considered.

The following undesirable effects have been reported with Fematrix 80 and/or other estrogen/progestagen therapy:

(see Table 1 below)

Breast Cancer

According to evidence from a large number of epidemiological studies and one randomised placebo-controlled trial, the Women's Health Initiative (WHI), the overall risk of breast cancer increases with increasing duration of HRT use in current or recent HRT users.

For *estrogen-only* HRT, estimates of relative risk (RR) from a reanalysis of original data from 51 epidemiological studies (in which >80% of HRT use was estrogen-only HRT) and from the epidemiological Million Women Study (MWS) are similar at 1.35 (95%CI 1.21 – 1.49) and 1.30 (95%CI 1.21 – 1.40), respectively.

For *estrogen plus progestagen* combined HRT, several epidemiological studies have reported an overall higher risk for breast cancer than with estrogens alone.

The MWS reported that, compared to never users, the use of various types of estrogen-progestagen combined HRT was associated with a higher risk of breast cancer (RR = 2.00, 95%CI: 1.88 – 2.12) than use of estrogens alone (RR = 1.30, 95%CI: 1.21 – 1.40) or use of tibolone (RR=1.45; 95%CI 1.25-1.68).

The WHI trial reported a risk estimate of 1.24 (95%CI 1.01 – 1.54) after 5.6 years of use of estrogen-progestagen combined HRT (CEE + MPA) in all users compared with placebo.

The absolute risks calculated from the MWS and the WHI trials are presented below:

The MWS has estimated, from the known average incidence of breast cancer in developed countries, that:

- For women not using HRT, about 32 in every 1000 are expected to have breast cancer diagnosed between the ages of 50 and 64 years.

- For 1000 current or recent users of HRT, the number of *additional* cases during the corresponding period will be

- For users of *estrogen-only* replacement therapy

• between 0 and 3 (best estimate = 1.5) for 5 years' use

• between 3 and 7 (best estimate = 5) for 10 years' use.

- For users of *estrogen plus progestagen* combined HRT,

• between 5 and 7 (best estimate = 6) for 5 years' use

• between 18 and 20 (best estimate = 19) for 10 years' use.

The WHI trial estimated that after 5.6 years of follow-up of women between the ages of 50 and 79 years, an *additional* 8 cases of invasive breast cancer would be due to *estrogen-progestagen combined* HRT (CEE + MPA) per 10,000 women years.

According to calculations from the trial data, it is estimated that:

- For 1000 women in the placebo group,

• about 16 cases of invasive breast cancer would be diagnosed in 5 years.

Table 1

MedDRA system organ class	Common >1/100, <1/10	Uncommon >1/1,000, <1/100	Rare >1/10,000, <1/1,000	Very rare <1/10,000 incl. isolated reports
Infections and infestations		Cystitis-like syndrome, Vaginal candidiasis		
Neoplasms benign, malignant and unspecified		Increase in size of leiomyoma		
Blood and the lymphatic system disorders				Haemolytic anaemia
Psychiatric disorders		Depression, Change in libido, Nervousness		
Nervous system disorders	Headache, Migraine	Dizziness		Chorea
Eye disorders			Intolerance to contact lenses, Steepening of corneal curvature	
Cardiac disorders				Myocardial infarction
Vascular disorders		Hypertension, Peripheral vascular disease, Varicose vein, Venous thromboembolism		Stroke
Gastrointestinal disorders	Nausea, Abdominal pain, Flatulence	Dyspepsia		Vomiting
Hepatobiliary disorders		Gall bladder disease	Alterations in liver function, sometimes with Asthenia or Malaise, Jaundice and Abdominal pain	
Skin and subcutaneous tissue disorders		Allergic skin reactions, Rash, Urticaria, Pruritus		Chloasma or melasma, which may persist when drug is discontinued, Erythema multiforme, Erythema nodosum, Vascular purpura, Angioedema
Musculoskeletal and connective tissue disorders	Leg cramps	Back pain		
Reproductive system and breast disorders	Breast pain/ tenderness, Breakthrough bleeding and spotting, Pelvic pain	Change in cervical erosion, Change in cervical secretion, Dysmenorrhoea, Menorrhagia, Metrorrhagia	Breast enlargement, Premenstrual-like symptoms	
Congenital and familial/genetic disorders				Aggravation of porphyria
General disorders and administration site reactions	Asthenia	Peripheral oedema		
Investigations	Increase/decrease in weight			

- For 1000 women who used estrogen + progestagen combined HRT (CEE + MPA), the number of *additional* cases would be

- between 0 and 9 (best estimate = 4) for 5 years' use.

The number of additional cases of breast cancer in women who use HRT is broadly similar for women who start HRT irrespective of age at start of use (between the ages of 45-65) (see section 4.4).

Endometrial cancer

In women with an intact uterus, the risk of endometrial hyperplasia and endometrial cancer increases with increasing duration of use of unopposed estrogens. According to data from epidemiological studies, the best estimate of the risk is that for women not using HRT, about 5 in every 1000 are expected to have endometrial cancer diagnosed between the ages of 50 and 65. Depending on the duration of treatment and estrogen dose, the reported increase in endometrial cancer risk among unopposed estrogen users varies from 2-to 12-fold greater compared with non-users. Adding a progestagen to estrogen-only therapy greatly reduces this increased risk.

Other adverse reactions have been reported in association with estrogen/progestagen treatment:

- Estrogen-dependent neoplasms benign and malignant, e.g. endometrial cancer.

- Venous thromboembolism, i.e. deep leg or pelvic venous thrombosis and pulmonary embolism, is more frequent among hormone replacement therapy users than among non-users. For further information, see section 4.3 Contra-indications and 4.4 Special warnings and precautions for use.

- Probable dementia (see section 4.4)

4.9 Overdose

This is not likely due to the mode of administration. If it is necessary to stop delivery then the patch can be removed and plasma estradiol levels will fall rapidly.

5. PHARMACOLOGICAL PROPERTIES

5.1 Pharmacodynamic properties

The active ingredient, synthetic 17β-estradiol, is chemically and biologically identical to endogenous human estradiol. It substitutes for the loss of estrogen production in menopausal women, and alleviates menopausal symptoms. Estrogens prevent bone loss following menopause or ovariectomy.

Clinical trial information

- Relief of estrogen-deficiency symptoms and bleeding patterns

- Relief of menopausal symptoms was achieved during the first few weeks of treatment.

- In women treated with Fematrix 80 patches and progestagen tablets, regular withdrawal bleeding occurred in approximately 90% with a mean duration of 6.8 days. Withdrawal bleeding usually started on the day of the last pill of the progestagen phase. Break-through bleeding and/or spotting appeared in 3% of the women. Amenorrhoea (no bleeding or spotting) occurred in about 5 % of patients in month 6 of treatment.

Prevention of osteoporosis

- Estrogen deficiency at menopause is associated with an increasing bone turnover and decline in bone mass. The effect of estrogens on the bone mineral density is dose-dependent. Protection appears to be effective for as long as treatment is continued. After discontinuation of HRT, bone mass is lost at a rate similar to that in untreated women.

- Evidence from the WHI trial and meta-analysed trials shows that current use of HRT, alone or in combination with a progestagen – given to predominantly healthy women – reduces the risk of hip, vertebral, and other osteoporotic fractures. HRT may also prevent fractures in women with low bone density and/or established osteoporosis, but the evidence for that is limited.

- After two years of treatment with Fematrix 80, the increase in lumbar spine bone mineral density (BMD) was 6.54%. The percentage of women who maintained or gained BMD in lumbar zone during treatment was 96%.

5.2 Pharmacokinetic properties

General characteristics of the active substance:

Absorption

Estradiol is absorbed from the patch across the stratum corneum and is delivered systemically at a low but constant rate throughout the period of application (3 to 4 days). The estimated delivery of estradiol is approximately 80 micrograms per day for Fematrix 80.

The primary unconjugated and conjugated metabolites are estrone and estrone sulphate. These metabolites can contribute to the estrogen effect, both directly and after conversion to estradiol. Estrogens are excreted in the bile and reabsorbed from the intestine. During this enterohepatic cycle the estrogens are broken down. Estrogens are excreted in the urine as biologically inactive glucuronide and sulphate compounds (90 to 95%), or in the faeces (5 to 10%), mostly unconjugated. Estrogens are excreted in mothers' milk.

Steady state plasma estradiol concentrations have been demonstrated in the range of C_{min} is 34 pg/ml and the C_{max} is 62 pg/ml for the Fematrix 80 patch (including baseline levels) and these are maintained throughout the dose interval (for up to four days). Absorption rate may vary between individual patients. After removal of the last patch plasma estradiol and oestrone concentrations return to baseline values in less than 24 hours. The median terminal half-life for estradiol following patch removal has been determined as 5.24h.

5.3 Preclinical safety data

Supraphysiological doses (prolonged overdoses) of estradiol have been associated with the induction of tumours in estrogen-dependent target organs for all rodent species tested.

In long-term studies, doses administered to rats and mice were sufficient to produce hormone-mediated changes, but did not provide tumorogenic potential.

6. PHARMACEUTICAL PARTICULARS

6.1 List of excipients

Diethyltoluamide

Acrylic adhesive (Dow Corning MG-0560)

Acrylic thickener (Acrysol 33)

Backing: Polyester

Release liner: Siliconised/Aluminised/Polyester

6.2 Incompatibilities

Not applicable.

6.3 Shelf life

3 years.

6.4 Special precautions for storage

Do not store above 25°C.

Store in original package.

6.5 Nature and contents of container

Sealed laminated sachet (paper/polyethylene/aluminium foil/polyethylene) containing one transdermal patch. Each carton contains eight patches, sufficient for one 28 day cycle and a patient leaflet. An additional pack containing two patches may also be available.

6.6 Special precautions for disposal and other handling

Detailed instructions for use are provided in the patient information leaflet.

7. MARKETING AUTHORISATION HOLDER

Solvay Healthcare Limited

Mansbridge Road

West End

Southampton

SO18 3JD

United Kingdom

8. MARKETING AUTHORISATION NUMBER(S)

PL 00512/0172

9. DATE OF FIRST AUTHORISATION/RENEWAL OF THE AUTHORISATION

12 November 2001/01 September 2006

10. DATE OF REVISION OF THE TEXT

1 September 2006

Legal category

POM

Femoston 1/10mg

(Solvay Healthcare Limited)

1. NAME OF THE MEDICINAL PRODUCT

Femoston® 1/10 mg Film-coated Tablets

2. QUALITATIVE AND QUANTITATIVE COMPOSITION

Each tablet contains 1 mg estradiol (as hemihydrate) or a combination of 1 mg estradiol (as hemihydrate) and 10 mg dydrogesterone.

For excipients see 6.1

3. PHARMACEUTICAL FORM

Film-coated tablets

Estradiol only tablets: Round, biconvex, white film-coated tablets with inscriptions '$' and '379'.

Estradiol/dydrogesterone combination tablets: Round, biconvex, grey film-coated tablets with inscriptions '$' and '379'.

4. CLINICAL PARTICULARS

4.1 Therapeutic indications

Hormone replacement therapy (HRT) for estrogen deficiency symptoms in peri and postmenopausal women.

Prevention of osteoporosis in postmenopausal women at high risk of future fractures who are intolerant of, or contra-indicated for, other medicinal products approved for the prevention of osteoporosis.

(See also section 4.4)

The experience in treating women older than 65 years is limited.

4.2 Posology and method of administration

Femoston 1/10 and Femoston 2/10, are continuous sequential hormone replacement therapies. Unless there is a previous diagnosis of endometriosis, it is not recommended to add a progestagen in hysterectomised women.

For initiation and continuation of treatment of postmenopausal symptoms, the lowest effective dose for the shortest duration (see also section 4.4) should be used.

In general, treatment should start with Femoston 1/10. Depending on the clinical response, the dosage can afterwards be adjusted to individual need. If the complaints linked to estrogen deficiency are not ameliorated the dosage can be increased by using Femoston 2/10.

Starting Femoston

In women who are not taking hormone replacement therapy and who are amenorrhoeic, or women who switch from a continuous combined hormone replacement therapy, treatment may be started on any convenient day. In women transferring from a cyclic or continuous sequential HRT regimen, treatment should begin the day following completion of the prior regimen. If the patient has regular menstruation periods, treatment is started within five days of the start of bleeding.

Administration

For the first 14 days during a 28-cycle, one tablet containing estradiol is taken daily; during the following 14 days one tablet containing estradiol and dydrogesterone is taken.

After a cycle of 28 days, on the 29th day, a new 28-day cycle begins. This means that the treatment should be taken continuously without a break between packs. Femoston can be taken with or without food.

The days of the week are printed on the back of the blister strips. Firstly, the tablets from the part marked with arrow 1 should be taken, then all the tablets from the part marked with arrow 2 should be taken.

If a dose has been forgotten, it should be taken as soon as possible. When more than 12 hours have elapsed, it is recommended to continue with the next dose without taking the forgotten tablet. The likelihood of breakthrough bleeding or spotting may be increased.

4.3 Contraindications

Known, past or suspected breast cancer;

Known or suspected estrogen-dependent malignant tumours (e.g. endometrial cancer);

Undiagnosed genital bleeding;

Untreated endometrial hyperplasia;

Previous idiopathic or current venous thromboembolism (deep vein thrombosis, pulmonary embolism);

Active or recent arterial thromboembolic disease (e.g. angina, myocardial infarction);

Acute liver disease or a history of liver disease as long as liver function tests have failed to return to normal;

Known hypersensitivity to the active substances or to any of the excipients;

Porphyria.

4.4 Special warnings and precautions for use

For the treatment of postmenopausal symptoms, HRT should only be initiated for symptoms that adversely affect quality of life. In all cases, a careful appraisal of the risks and benefits should be undertaken at least annually and HRT should only be continued as long as the benefit outweighs the risk.

Medical examination/follow up

Before initiating or reinstituting HRT, a complete personal and family medical history should be taken. Physical (including pelvic and breast) examination should be guided by this and by the contraindications and warnings for use. During treatment, periodic check-ups are recommended of a frequency and nature adapted to the individual woman. Women should be advised what changes in their breasts should be reported to their doctor or nurse (see 'breast cancer' below). Investigations, including mammography, should be carried out in accordance with currently accepted screening practices, modified to the clinical needs of the individual.

Conditions which need supervision

If any of the following conditions are present, have occurred previously, and/or have been aggravated during pregnancy or previous hormone treatment, the patient should be closely supervised. It should be taken into account that these conditions may recur or be aggravated during treatment with Femoston, in particular:

- Leiomyoma (uterine fibroids) or endometriosis
- A history of, or risk factors for, thromboembolic disorders (see below)
- Risk factors for estrogen dependent tumours, e.g. 1st degree heredity for breast cancer
- Hypertension
- Liver disorders (e.g. liver adenoma)
- Diabetes mellitus with or without vascular involvement
- Cholelithiasis
- Migraine or (severe) headache
- Systemic lupus erythematosus
- A history of endometrial hyperplasia (see below)
- Epilepsy
- Asthma
- Otosclerosis

Reasons for immediate withdrawal of therapy:

-Therapy should be discontinued in cases where a contra-indication is discovered and in the following situations:

- Jaundice or deterioration in liver function
- Significant increase in blood pressure
- New onset of migraine-type headache
- Pregnancy

Endometrial hyperplasia

The risk of endometrial hyperplasia and carcinoma is increased when estrogens are administered alone for prolonged periods (see section 4.8). The addition of a progestagen for at least 12 days of the cycle in non-hysterectomised women greatly reduces this risk.

Break-through bleeding and spotting may occur during the first months of treatment. If break-through bleeding or spotting appears after some time on therapy, or continues after treatment has been discontinued, the reason should be investigated, which may include endometrial biopsy to exclude endometrial malignancy.

Breast cancer

A randomised placebo-controlled trial, the Womens Health Initiative study (WHI) and epidemiological studies, including the Million Women Study (MWS), have reported an increased risk of breast cancer in women taking estrogens, estrogen-progestagen combinations or tibolone for HRT for several years (see Section 4.8).

For all HRT, an excess risk becomes apparent within a few years of use and increases with duration of intake but returns to baseline within a few (at most five) years after stopping treatment.

In the MWS, the relative risk of breast cancer with conjugated equine estrogens (CEE) or estradiol (E2) was greater when a progestagen was added, either sequentially or continuously, and regardless of type of progestagen. There was no evidence of a difference in risk between the different routes of administration.

In the WHI study, the continuous combined conjugated equine estrogen and medroxyprogesterone acetate (CEE + MPA) product used was associated with breast cancers that were slightly larger in size and more frequently had local lymph node metastases compared to placebo.

HRT, especially estrogen-progestagen combined treatment, increases the density of mammographic images which may adversely affect the radiological detection of breast cancer.

Venous thromboembolism

HRT is associated with a higher relative risk of developing venous thromboembolism (VTE), i.e. deep vein thrombosis or pulmonary embolism. One randomised controlled trial and epidemiological studies found a two-to threefold higher risk for users compared with non-users. For non-users, it is estimated that the number of cases of VTE that will occur over a 5 year period is about 3 per 1000 women aged 50-59 years and 8 per 1000 women aged between 60-69 years. It is estimated that in healthy women who use HRT for 5 years, the number of additional cases of VTE over a 5 year period will be between 2 and 6 (best estimate = 4) per 1000 women aged 50-59 years and between 5 and 15 (best estimate = 9) per 1000 women aged 60-69 years. The occurrence of such an event is more likely in the first year of HRT than later.

Generally recognised risk factors for VTE include a personal or family history,

• severe obesity (BMI >30 kg/m^2) and systemic lupus erythematosus (SLE). There is no consensus about the possible role of varicose veins in VTE.

• Patients with a history of VTE or known thrombophilic states have an increased risk of VTE. HRT may add to this risk. Personal or strong family history of thromboembolism or recurrent spontaneous abortion should be investigated in order to exclude a thrombophilic predisposition. Until a thorough evaluation of thrombophilic factors has been made or anticoagulant treatment initiated, use of HRT in such patients should be viewed as contraindicated.

Those women already on anticoagulant treatment require careful consideration of the benefit-risk of use of HRT.

• The risk of VTE may be temporarily increased with prolonged immobilisation, major trauma or major surgery. As in all postoperative patients, scrupulous attention should be given to prophylactic measures to prevent VTE following surgery. Where prolonged immobilisation is liable to follow elective surgery, particularly abdominal or orthopaedic surgery to the lower limbs, consideration should be given to temporarily stopping HRT 4 to 6 weeks earlier, if possible. Treatment should not be restarted until the woman is completely mobilised.

If VTE develops after initiating therapy, the drug should be discontinued. Patients should be told to contact their doctors immediately when they are aware of a potential thromboembolic symptom (e.g. painful swelling of a leg, sudden pain in the chest, dyspnea).

Coronary artery disease (CAD)

There is no evidence from randomised controlled trials of cardiovascular benefit with continuous combined conjugated estrogens and medroxyprogesterone acetate (MPA). Two large clinical trials (WHI and HERS i.e. Heart and Estrogen/progestin Replacement Study) showed a possible increased risk of cardiovascular morbidity in the first year of use and no overall benefit. For other HRT products there are only limited data from randomised controlled trials examining effects in cardiovascular morbidity or mortality. Therefore, it is uncertain whether these findings also extend to other HRT products.

Stroke

One large randomised clinical trial (WHI-trial) found, as a secondary outcome, an increased risk of ischaemic stroke in healthy women during treatment with continuous combined conjugated estrogens and MPA. For women who do not use HRT, it is estimated that the number of cases of stroke that will occur over a 5 year period is about 3 per 1000 women aged 50-59 and 11 per 1000 women aged 60-69 years. It is estimated that for women who use conjugated estrogens and MPA for 5 years, the number of additional cases will be between 0 and 3 (best estimate = 1) per 1000 users aged 50-59 years and between 1 and 9 (best estimate = 4) per 1000 users aged 60-69 years. It is unknown whether the increased risk also extends to other HRT products.

Ovarian cancer

Long-term (at least 5 to 10 years) use of estrogen-only HRT products in hysterectomised women has been associated with an increased risk of ovarian cancer in some epidemiological studies. It is uncertain whether long term use of combined HRT confers a different risk than estrogen-only products.

Other conditions

• Estrogens may cause fluid retention, and therefore patients with cardiac or renal dysfunction should be carefully observed. Patients with terminal renal insufficiency should be closely observed, since it is expected that the level of circulating active ingredients in Femoston is increased.

• Women with pre-existing hypertriglyceridemia should be followed closely during estrogen replacement or hormone replacement therapy, since rare cases of large increases of plasma triglycerides leading to pancreatitis have been reported with estrogen therapy in this condition.

• Estrogens increase thyroid binding globulin (TBG), leading to increased circulating total thyroid hormone, as measured by protein-bound iodine (PBI), T4 levels (by column or by radio-immunoassay) or T3 levels (by radio-immunoassay). T3 resin uptake is decreased, reflecting the elevated TBG. Free T4 and free T3 concentrations are unaltered. Other binding proteins may be elevated in serum, i.e. corticoid binding globulin (CBG), sex-hormone-binding globulin (SHBG) leading to increased circulating corticosteroids and sex steroids, respectively. Free or biological active hormone concentrations are unchanged. Other plasma proteins may be increased (angiotensinogen/renin substrate, alpha-1-antitrypsin, ceruloplasmin).

• There is no conclusive evidence for improvement of cognitive function. There is some evidence from the WHI trial of increased risk of probable dementia in women who start using continuous combined CEE and MPA after the age of 65. It is unknown whether the findings apply to younger post-menopausal women or other HRT products.

• Patients with rare hereditary problems of galactose intolerance, the Lapp lactase deficiency or glucose-galactose malabsorption should not take this medicine.

• Women who may be at risk of pregnancy should be advised to adhere to non-hormonal contraceptive methods.

4.5 Interaction with other medicinal products and other forms of interaction

- The metabolism of estrogens and progestagens may be increased by concomitant use of substances known to induce drug-metabolising enzymes, specifically cytochrome P450 enzymes, such as anticonvulsants (eg. phenobarbital, phenytoin, carbamezapine) and anti-infectives (e.g. rifampicin, rifabutin, nevirapine, efavirenz).

- Ritonavir and nelfinavir, although known as strong inhibitors, by contrast exhibit inducing properties when used concomitantly with steroid hormones.

- Herbal preparations containing St John's wort (Hypericum perforatum) may induce the metabolism of estrogens and progestagens.

- Clinically an increased metabolism of estrogens and progestagens may lead to decreased effect and changes in the uterine bleeding profile.

4.6 Pregnancy and lactation

Pregnancy:

Femoston is not indicated during pregnancy. If pregnancy occurs during medication with Femoston, treatment should be withdrawn immediately.

Clinically, data based on an assumed large number of exposed pregnancies indicate no adverse effects of dydrogesterone on the foetus.

The results of most epidemiological studies to date relevant to inadvertent foetal exposure to combinations of estrogens and progestagens indicate no teratogenic or foetotoxic effect.

Lactation:

Femoston is not indicated during lactation.

4.7 Effects on ability to drive and use machines

Femoston does not affect the ability to drive or use machines.

4.8 Undesirable effects

Undesirable effects reported in clinical trials and in post-marketing experience are the following:

(see Table 1 on next page)

Breast Cancer

According to evidence from a large number of epidemiological studies and one randomised placebo-controlled trial, the Women's Health Initiative (WHI), the overall risk of breast cancer increases with increasing duration of HRT use in current or recent HRT users.

For *estrogen-only* HRT, estimates of relative risk (RR) from a reanalysis of original data from 51 epidemiological studies (in which $>80\%$ of HRT use was estrogen-only HRT) and from the epidemiological Million Women Study (MWS) are similar at 1.35 (95%CI 1.21 – 1.49) and 1.30 (95%CI 1.21 – 1.40), respectively.

For *estrogen plus progestagen* combined HRT, several epidemiological studies have reported an overall higher risk for breast cancer than with estrogens alone.

The MWS reported that, compared to never users, the use of various types of estrogen-progestagen combined HRT was associated with a higher risk of breast cancer (RR = 2.00, 95%CI: 1.88 – 2.12) than use of estrogens alone (RR = 1.30, 95%CI: 1.21 – 1.40) or use of tibolone (RR=1.45; 95%CI 1.25-1.68).

The WHI trial reported a risk estimate of 1.24 (95%CI 1.01 – 1.54) after 5.6 years of use of estrogen-progestagen combined HRT (CEE + MPA) in all users compared with placebo.

The absolute risks calculated from the MWS and the WHI trials are presented below:

The MWS has estimated, from the known average incidence of breast cancer in developed countries, that:

– For women not using HRT, about 32 in every 1000 are expected to have breast cancer diagnosed between the ages of 50 and 64 years.

- For 1000 current or recent users of HRT, the number of *additional* cases during the corresponding period will be

- For users of *estrogen-only* replacement therapy

• between 0 and 3 (best estimate = 1.5) for 5 years' use

• between 3 and 7 (best estimate = 5) for 10 years' use.

- For users of *estrogen plus progestagen* combined HRT,

• between 5 and 7 (best estimate = 6) for 5 years' use

• between 18 and 20 (best estimate = 19) for 10 years' use.

The WHI trial estimated that after 5.6 years of follow-up of women between the ages of 50 and 79 years, an *additional* 8 cases of invasive breast cancer would be due to *estrogen-progestagen combined* HRT (CEE + MPA) per 10,000 women years.

According to calculations from the trial data, it is estimated that:

- For 1000 women in the placebo group,

• about 16 cases of invasive breast cancer would be diagnosed in 5 years.

- For 1000 women who used estrogen + progestagen combined HRT (CEE + MPA), the number of *additional* cases would be

• between 0 and 9 (best estimate = 4) for 5 years' use.

The number of additional cases of breast cancer in women who use HRT is broadly similar for women who start HRT irrespective of age at start of use (between the ages of 45-65) (see section 4.4).

Endometrial cancer

In women with an intact uterus, the risk of endometrial hyperplasia and endometrial cancer increases with increasing duration of use of unopposed estrogens. According to data from epidemiological studies, the best estimate of the risk is that for women not using HRT, about 5 in every 1000 are expected to have endometrial cancer diagnosed between the ages of 50 and 65. Depending on the duration of treatment and estrogen dose, the reported increase in endometrial cancer risk among unopposed estrogen users varies from 2-to 12-fold greater compared with non-users. Adding a progestagen to estrogen-only therapy greatly reduces this increased risk.

Other adverse reactions have been reported in association with estrogen/progestagen treatment:

- Estrogen-dependent neoplasms benign and malignant, e.g. endometrial cancer.

- Venous thromboembolism, i.e. deep leg or pelvic venous thrombosis and pulmonary embolism, is more frequent among hormone replacement therapy users than among non-users. For further information, see section 4.3 Contra-indications and 4.4 Special warnings and precautions for use.

- Probable dementia (see section 4.4).

4.9 Overdose

Both estradiol and dydrogesterone are substances with low toxicity. Theoretically, symptoms such as nausea, vomiting, sleepiness and dizziness could occur in cases of overdosing. It is unlikely that any specific or symptomatic treatment will be necessary.

Table 1

MedDRA system organ class	Common >1/100, <1/10	Uncommon >1/1,000, <1/100	Rare >1/10,000, <1/1,000	Very rare <1/10,000 incl. isolated reports
Infections and infestations		Cystitis-like syndrome, Vaginal candidiasis		
Neoplasms benign, malignant and unspecified		Increase in size of leiomyoma		
Blood and the lymphatic system disorders				Haemolytic anaemia
Psychiatric disorders		Depression, Change in libido, Nervousness		
Nervous system disorders	Headache, Migraine	Dizziness		Chorea
Eye disorders			Intolerance to contact lenses, Steepening of corneal curvature	
Cardiac disorders				Myocardial infarction
Vascular disorders		Hypertension, Peripheral vascular disease, Varicose vein, Venous thromboembolism		Stroke
Gastrointestinal disorders	Nausea, Abdominal pain, Flatulence	Dyspepsia		Vomiting
Hepatobiliary disorders		Gall bladder disease	Alterations in liver function, sometimes with Asthenia or Malaise, Jaundice and Abdominal pain	
Skin and subcutaneous tissue disorders		Allergic skin reactions, Rash, Urticaria, Pruritus		Chloasma or melasma, which may persist when drug is discontinued, Erythema multiforme, Erythema nodosum, Vascular purpura, Angioedema
Musculoskeletal and connective tissue disorders	Leg cramps	Back pain		
Reproductive system and breast disorders	Breast pain/ tenderness, Breakthrough bleeding and spotting, Pelvic pain	Change in cervical erosion, Change in cervical secretion, Dysmenorrhoea, Menorrhagia, Metrorrhagia	Breast enlargement, Premenstrual-like symptoms	
Congenital and familial/genetic disorders				Aggravation of porphyria
General disorders and administration site reactions	Asthenia	Peripheral oedema		
Investigations	Increase/decrease in weight			

Aforementioned information is applicable for overdosing by children also.

5. PHARMACOLOGICAL PROPERTIES

5.1 Pharmacodynamic properties

The ATC code is G03FB08. (Estrogens: urogenital system and sex hormones)

Sequential hormone replacement therapy (combined estradiol and dydrogesterone).

Estradiol

The active ingredient, synthetic 17β-estradiol, is chemically and biologically identical to endogenous human estradiol. It substitutes for the loss of estrogen production in menopausal women, and alleviates menopausal symptoms. Estrogens prevent bone loss following menopause or ovariectomy.

Dydrogesterone

Dydrogesterone is an orally-active progestagen. The addition of a progestagen greatly reduces the estrogen-induced risk of endometrial hyperplasia and cancer in non-hysterectomised women, by reducing the growth of the endometrium.

Clinical trial Information

- Relief of estrogen-deficiency symptoms and bleeding patterns.

- Relief of menopausal symptoms was achieved during the first few weeks of treatment.

- Regular withdrawal bleeding with Femoston 1/10 occurred in approximately 75-80% of women with a mean duration of 5 days. Withdrawal bleeding usually started on the day of the last pill of the progestagen phase. Breakthrough bleeding and/or spotting occurred in approximately 10% of the women; amenorrhoea (no bleeding or spotting) occurred in 21-25% of the women for months 10 to 12 of treatment.

- With Femoston 2/10, approximately 90% of women had regular withdrawal bleeding. The start day and duration of bleeding, and the number of women with intermittent bleeding was the same as with Femoston 1/10, amenorrhoea occurred in 7-11% of the women for months 10 to 12 of treatment.

- Prevention of osteoporosis

- Estrogen deficiency at menopause is associated with an increasing bone turnover and decline in bone mass. The effect of estrogens on the bone mineral density is dose-dependent. Protection appears to be effective for as long as treatment is continued. After discontinuation of HRT, bone mass is lost at a rate similar to that in untreated women.

- Evidence from the WHI trial and meta-analysed trials shows that current use of HRT, alone or in combination with a progestagen – given to predominantly healthy women – reduces the risk of hip, vertebral, and other osteoporotic fractures. HRT may also prevent fractures in women with low bone density and/or established osteoporosis, but the evidence for that is limited.

- After two years of treatment with Femoston 2/10, the increase in lumbar spine bone mineral density (BMD) was 6.7% ± 3.9% (mean ± SD). The percentage of women who maintained or gained BMD in lumbar zone during treatment was 94.5%. For Femoston 1/10 the increase in lumbar spine BMD was 5.2% ± 3.8% (mean ± SD), and the percentage of women with no change or an increase in lumbar spine BMD was 93%.

- Femoston also had an effect on hip BMD. The increase after two years of treatment with 1mg estradiol was 2.7% ± 4.2% (mean ± SD) at femoral neck, 3.5% ± 5.0% (mean ± SD) at trochanter and 2.7%± 6.7% (mean ± SD) at Wards triangle. After two years of treatment with 2mg estradiol these figures were respectively, 2.6% ± 5.0%; 4.6% ± 5.0% and 4.1% ± 7.4%. The percentage of women who maintained or gained BMD in the 3 hip areas after treatment with 1mg estradiol was 67-78% and 71-88% after treatment with 2mg estradiol.

5.2 Pharmacokinetic properties

Estradiol

Orally administered estradiol, comprising particles whose size has been reduced to less than 5 μm, is quickly and efficiently absorbed from the gastrointestinal tract. The primary unconjugated and conjugated metabolites are estrone and estrone sulphate. These metabolites can contribute to the estrogen effect, both directly and after conversion to estradiol. Estrogens are excreted in the bile and reabsorbed from the intestine. During this enterohepatic cycle the estrogens are broken down. Estrogens are excreted in the urine as biologically inactive glucuronide and sulphate compounds (90 to 95%), or in the faeces (5 to 10%), mostly unconjugated. Estrogens are excreted in mothers' milk.

During the administration of oral estradiol to post-menopausal women at 1 mg once a day, the $C_{average}$ is 28 pg/ml, the C_{min} is 20 pg/ml and the C_{max} is 54 pg/ml. The E1/E2 (Estrone/Estradiol) ratio is 7.0.

Dydrogesterone

After oral administration of labelled dydrogesterone, on average 63% of the dose is excreted into the urine. Within 72 hours, excretion is complete.

In man, dydrogesterone is completely metabolised. The main metabolite of dydrogesterone is 20α-dihydrodydrogesterone (DHD) and is present in the urine predominantly as the glucoronic acid conjugate. A common feature of all metabolites characterised is the retention of the 4,6 diene-3-one configuration of the parent compound and the absence of 17α-hydroxylation. This explains the absence of estrogenic and androgenic activity.

After oral administration of dydrogesterone, plasma concentrations of DHD are substantially higher as compared to the parent drug. The AUC and C_{max} ratios of DHD to dydrogesterone are in the order of 40 and 25, respectively. Dydrogesterone is rapidly absorbed. The T_{max} values of dydrogesterone and DHD vary between 0.5 and 2.5 hours.

Mean terminal half lives of dydrogesterone and DHD vary between 5 to 7 and 14 to 17 hours, respectively.

The dihydrodydrogesterone $C_{average}$ is 13 ng/ml, the C_{min} is 4.1 ng/ml and the C_{max} is 63 ng/ml. The dydrogesterone $C_{average}$ is 0.38 ng/ml the C_{min} is <0.1 ng/ml and the C_{max} is 2.5 ng/ml.

Dydrogesterone is not excreted in urine as pregnanediol, like progesterone. Analysis of endogenous progesterone production based on pregnanediol excretion therefore remains possible.

5.3 Preclinical safety data

Supraphysiologically high doses (prolonged overdoses) of estradiol have been associated with the induction of tumours in estrogen-dependent target organs for all rodent species tested. The changes observed with dydrogesterone in animal toxicity studies are characteristic for progesterone-like compounds. *In-vitro* and *in-vivo* data gave no indications of mutagenic effects of dydrogesterone. In long-term studies, doses administered to rats and mice were sufficient to produce hormone-mediated changes, but did not provide tumorogenic potential.

6. PHARMACEUTICAL PARTICULARS

6.1 List of excipients

Estradiol only tablets (white):

Tablet core: Lactose

Hypromellose

Maize starch

Colloidal anhydrous silica

Magnesium stearate

Film coat: Hypromellose

Macrogol 400

Titanium dioxide (E171)

Estradiol/Dydrogesterone tablets (Grey):

Tablet core: Lactose

Hypromellose

Maize starch

Colloidal anhydrous silica

Magnesium stearate

Film coat: Hypromellose

Macrogol 400

Titanium dioxide (E171)

Iron oxide black (E172)

6.2 Incompatibilities

Not applicable.

6.3 Shelf life
3 years.

6.4 Special precautions for storage
Do not store above 30°C.

6.5 Nature and contents of container
The tablets are packed in blister strips of 28. The blister strips are made of PVC film with a covering aluminium foil. Each carton contains 84 tablets.

6.6 Special precautions for disposal and other handling
Not applicable.

7. MARKETING AUTHORISATION HOLDER
Solvay Healthcare Limited

Mansbridge Road

West End

Southampton

SO18 3JD

8. MARKETING AUTHORISATION NUMBER(S)
PL 00512/0121

9. DATE OF FIRST AUTHORISATION/RENEWAL OF THE AUTHORISATION
27 September 1995

10. DATE OF REVISION OF THE TEXT
January 2006

Legal category
POM

Femoston 2/10mg

(Solvay Healthcare Limited)

1. NAME OF THE MEDICINAL PRODUCT
Femoston® 2/10 mg Film-coated tablets

2. QUALITATIVE AND QUANTITATIVE COMPOSITION
Each tablet contains 2 mg estradiol (as hemihydrate) or a combination of 2 mg estradiol (as hemihydrate) and 10 mg dydrogesterone.

For excipients see 6.1

3. PHARMACEUTICAL FORM
Film-coated tablets

Estradiol only tablets: Round, biconvex, brick-red film-coated tablets with inscriptions '$' and '379'.

Estradiol/dydrogesterone combination tablets: Round, biconvex, yellow film-coated tablets with inscriptions '$' and '379'.

4. CLINICAL PARTICULARS

4.1 Therapeutic indications
Hormone replacement therapy (HRT) for estrogen deficiency symptoms in peri and postmenopausal women.

Prevention of osteoporosis in postmenopausal women at high risk of future fractures who are intolerant of, or contra-indicated for, other medicinal products approved for the prevention of osteoporosis.

(See also section 4.4)

The experience in treating women older than 65 years is limited.

4.2 Posology and method of administration
Femoston 1/10, and Femoston 2/10, are continuous sequential hormone replacement therapy. Unless there is a previous diagnosis of endometriosis, it is not recommended to add a progestagen in hysterectomised women.

For initiation and continuation of treatment of postmenopausal symptoms, the lowest effective dose for the shortest duration (see also section 4.4) should be used.

In general, treatment should start with Femoston 1/10. Depending on the clinical response, the dosage can afterwards be adjusted to individual need. If the complaints linked to estrogen deficiency are not ameliorated the dosage can be increased by using Femoston 2/10.

Starting Femoston

In women who are not taking hormone replacement therapy and who are amenorrhoeic, or women who switch from a continuous combined hormone replacement therapy, treatment may be started on any convenient day. In women transferring from a cyclic or continuous sequential HRT regimen, treatment should begin the day following completion of the prior regimen. If the patient has regular menstruation periods, treatment is started within five days of the start of bleeding.

Administration

For the first 14 days during a 28-cycle, one tablet containing estradiol is taken daily; during the following 14 days one tablet containing estradiol and dydrogesterone is taken.

After a cycle of 28 days, on the 29th day, a new 28-day cycle begins. This means that the treatment should be taken continuously without a break between packs. Femoston can be taken with or without food.

The days of the week are printed on the back of the blister strips. Firstly the tablets from the part marked with arrow 1 should be taken, then all the tablets from the part marked with arrow 2 should be taken.

If a dose has been forgotten, it should be taken as soon as possible. When more than 12 hours have elapsed, it is recommended to continue with the next dose without taking the forgotten tablet. The likelihood of breakthrough bleeding or spotting may be increased.

4.3 Contraindications
Known, past or suspected breast cancer;

Known or suspected estrogen-dependent malignant tumours (e.g. endometrial cancer);

Undiagnosed genital bleeding;

Untreated endometrial hyperplasia;

Previous idiopathic or current venous thromboembolism (deep vein thrombosis, pulmonary embolism);

Active or recent arterial thromboembolic disease (e.g. angina, myocardial infarction);

Acute liver disease or a history of liver disease as long as liver function tests have failed to return to normal;

Known hypersensitivity to the active substances or to any of the excipients;

Porphyria.

4.4 Special warnings and precautions for use
For the treatment of postmenopausal symptoms, HRT should only be initiated for symptoms that adversely affect quality of life. In all cases, a careful appraisal of the risks and benefits should be undertaken at least annually and HRT should only be continued as long as the benefit outweighs the risk.

Medical examination/follow up

Before initiating or reinstituting HRT, a complete personal and family medical history should be taken. Physical (including pelvic and breast) examination should be guided by this and by the contraindications and warnings for use. During treatment, periodic check-ups are recommended of a frequency and nature adapted to the individual woman. Women should be advised what changes in their breasts should be reported to their doctor or nurse (see 'breast cancer' below). Investigations, including mammography, should be carried out in accordance with currently accepted screening practices, modified to the clinical needs of the individual.

Conditions which need supervision

If any of the following conditions are present, have occurred previously, and/or have been aggravated during pregnancy or previous hormone treatment, the patient should be closely supervised. It should be taken into account that these conditions may recur or be aggravated during treatment with Femoston, in particular:

- Leiomyoma (uterine fibroids) or endometriosis
- A history of, or risk factors for, thromboembolic disorders (see below)
- Risk factors for estrogen dependent tumours, e.g. 1st degree heredity for breast cancer
- Hypertension
- Liver disorders (e.g. liver adenoma)
- Diabetes mellitus with or without vascular involvement
- Cholelithiasis
- Migraine or (severe) headache
- Systemic lupus erythematosus
- A history of endometrial hyperplasia (see below)
- Epilepsy
- Asthma
- Otosclerosis

Reasons for immediate withdrawal of therapy:

Therapy should be discontinued in cases where a contra-indication is discovered and in the following situations:

- Jaundice or deterioration in liver function
- Significant increase in blood pressure
- New onset of migraine-type headache
- Pregnancy

Endometrial hyperplasia

The risk of endometrial hyperplasia and carcinoma is increased when estrogens are administered alone for prolonged periods (see section 4.8). The addition of a progestagen for at least 12 days of the cycle in non-hysterectomised women greatly reduces this risk.

Break-through bleeding and spotting may occur during the first months of treatment. If break-through bleeding or spotting appears after some time on therapy, or continues after treatment has been discontinued, the reason should be investigated, which may include endometrial biopsy to exclude endometrial malignancy.

Breast cancer

A randomised placebo-controlled trial, the Womens Health Initiative study (WHI) and epidemiological studies, including the Million Women Study (MWS), have reported an increased risk of breast cancer in women taking estrogens, estrogen-progestagen combinations or tibolone for HRT for several years (see Section 4.8).

For all HRT, an excess risk becomes apparent within a few years of use and increases with duration of intake but returns to baseline within a few (at most five) years after stopping treatment.

In the MWS, the relative risk of breast cancer with conjugated equine estrogens (CEE) or estradiol (E2) was greater when a progestagen was added, either sequentially or continuously, and regardless of type of progestagen. There was no evidence of a difference in risk between the different routes of administration.

In the WHI study, the continuous combined conjugated equine estrogen and medroxyprogesterone acetate (CEE + MPA) product used was associated with breast cancers that were slightly larger in size and more frequently had local lymph node metastases compared to placebo.

HRT, especially estrogen-progestagen combined treatment, increases the density of mammographic images which may adversely affect the radiological detection of breast cancer.

Venous thromboembolism

HRT is associated with a higher relative risk of developing venous thromboembolism (VTE), i.e. deep vein thrombosis or pulmonary embolism. One randomised controlled trial and epidemiological studies found a two-to threefold higher risk for users compared with non-users. For non-users, it is estimated that the number of cases of VTE that will occur over a 5 year period is about 3 per 1000 women aged 50-59 years and 8 per 1000 women aged between 60-69 years. It is estimated that in healthy women who use HRT for 5 years, the number of additional cases of VTE over a 5 year period will be between 2 and 6 (best estimate = 4) per 1000 women aged 50-59 years and between 5 and 15 (best estimate = 9) per 1000 women aged 60-69 years. The occurrence of such an event is more likely in the first year of HRT than later.

- Generally recognised risk factors for VTE include a personal or family history, severe obesity (BM > 30 kg/m2) and systemic lupus erythematosus (SLE). There is no consensus about the possible role of varicose veins in VTE.
- Patients with a history of VTE or known thrombophilic states have an increased risk of VTE. HRT may add to this risk. Personal or strong family history of thromboembolism or recurrent spontaneous abortion should be investigated in order to exclude a thrombophilic predisposition. Until a thorough evaluation of thrombophilic factors has been made or anticoagulant treatment initiated, use of HRT in such patients should be viewed as contraindicated. Those women already on anticoagulant treatment require careful consideration of the benefit-risk of use of HRT.
- The risk of VTE may be temporarily increased with prolonged immobilisation, major trauma or major surgery. As in all postoperative patients, scrupulous attention should be given to prophylactic measures to prevent VTE following surgery. Where prolonged immobilisation is liable to follow elective surgery, particularly abdominal or orthopaedic surgery to the lower limbs, consideration should be given to temporarily stopping HRT 4 to 6 weeks earlier, if possible. Treatment should not be restarted until the woman is completely mobilised.
- If VTE develops after initiating therapy, the drug should be discontinued. Patients should be told to contact their doctors immediately when they are aware of a potential thromboembolic symptom (e.g. painful swelling of a leg, sudden pain in the chest, dyspnea).

Coronary artery disease (CAD)

There is no evidence from randomised controlled trials of cardiovascular benefit with continuous combined conjugated estrogens and medroxyprogesterone acetate (MPA). Two large clinical trials (WHI and HERS i.e. Heart and Estrogen/progestin Replacement Study) showed a possible increased risk of cardiovascular morbidity in the first year of use and no overall benefit. For other HRT products there are only limited data from randomised controlled trials to date examining effects in cardiovascular morbidity or mortality. Therefore, it is uncertain whether these findings also extend to other HRT products.

Stroke

One large randomised clinical trial (WHI-trial) found, as a secondary outcome, an increased risk of ischaemic stroke in healthy women during treatment with continuous combined conjugated estrogens and MPA. For women who do not use HRT, it is estimated that the number of cases of stroke that will occur over a 5 year period is about 3 per 1000 women aged 50-59 and 11 per 1000 women aged 60-69 years. It is estimated that for women who use conjugated estrogens and MPA for 5 years, the number of additional cases will be between 0 and 3 (best estimate = 1) per 1000 users aged 50-59 years and between 1 and 9 (best estimate = 4) per 1000 users aged 60-69 years. It is unknown whether the increased risk also extends to other HRT products.

Ovarian cancer

Long-term (at least 5 to 10 years) use of estrogen-only HRT products in hysterectomised women has been associated with an increased risk of ovarian cancer in some epidemiological studies. It is uncertain whether long term use of combined HRT confers a different risk than estrogen-only products.

Other conditions

- Estrogens may cause fluid retention, and therefore patients with cardiac or renal dysfunction should be carefully observed. Patients with terminal renal insufficiency should be closely observed, since it is expected that the level of circulating active ingredients in Femoston is increased.

• Women with pre-existing hypertriglyceridemia should be followed closely during estrogen replacement or hormone replacement therapy, since rare cases of large increases of plasma triglycerides leading to pancreatitis have been reported with estrogen therapy in this condition.

• Estrogens increase thyroid binding globulin (TBG), leading to increased circulating total thyroid hormone, as measured by protein-bound iodine (PBI), T4 levels (by column or by radio-immunoassay) or T3 levels (by radio-immunoassay). T3 resin uptake is decreased, reflecting the elevated TBG. Free T4 and free T3 concentrations are unaltered. Other binding proteins may be elevated in serum, i.e. corticoid binding globulin (CBG), sex-hormone-binding globulin (SHBG) leading to increased circulating corticosteroids and sex steroids, respectively. Free or biological active hormone concentrations are unchanged. Other plasma proteins may be increased (angiotensinogen/renin substrate, alpha-1-antitrypsin, ceruloplasmin).

• There is no conclusive evidence for improvement of cognitive function. There is some evidence from the WHI trial of increased risk of probable dementia in women who start using continuous combined CEE and MPA after the age of 65. It is unknown whether the findings apply to younger post-menopausal women or other HRT products.

• Patients with rare hereditary problems of galactose intolerance, the Lapp lactase deficiency or glucose-galactose malabsorption should not take this medicine.

• Women who may be at risk of pregnancy should be advised to adhere to non-hormonal contraceptive methods.

4.5 Interaction with other medicinal products and other forms of interaction

- The metabolism of estrogens and progestagens may be increased by concomitant use of substances known to induce drug-metabolising enzymes, specifically cytochrome P450 enzymes, such as anticonvulsants (eg. phenobarbital, phenytoin, carbamezapine) and anti-infectives (e.g. rifampicin, rifabutin, nevirapine, efavirenz).

- Ritonavir and nelfinavir, although known as strong inhibitors, by contrast exhibit inducing properties when used concomitantly with steroid hormones.

- Herbal preparations containing St John's wort (Hypericum perforatum) may induce the metabolism of estrogens and progestagens.

- Clinically an increased metabolism of estrogens and progestagens may lead to decreased effect and changes in the uterine bleeding profile.

4.6 Pregnancy and lactation

Pregnancy:

Femoston is not indicated during pregnancy. If pregnancy occurs during medication with Femoston, treatment should be withdrawn immediately.

Clinically, data based on a large number of exposed pregnancies indicate no adverse effects of dydrogesterone on the foetus.

The results of most epidemiological studies to date relevant to inadvertent foetal exposure to combinations of estrogens and progestagens indicate no teratogenic or foetotoxic effect.

Lactation:

Femoston is not indicated during lactation.

4.7 Effects on ability to drive and use machines

Femoston does not affect the ability to drive or use machines.

4.8 Undesirable effects

Undesirable effects reported in clinical trials and in post-marketing experience are the following:

(see Table 1 above)

Table 1

MedDRA system organ class	Common >1/100, <1/10	Uncommon >1/1,000, <1/100	Rare >1/10,000, <1/1,000	Very rare <1/10,000 incl. isolated reports
Infections and infestations		Cystitis-like syndrome, Vaginal candidiasis		
Neoplasms benign, malignant and unspecified		Increase in size of leiomyoma		
Blood and the lymphatic system disorders				Haemolytic anaemia
Psychiatric disorders		Depression, Change in libido, Nervousness		
Nervous system disorders	Headache, Migraine	Dizziness		Chorea
Eye disorders			Intolerance to contact lenses, Steepening of corneal curvature	
Cardiac disorders				Myocardial infarction
Vascular disorders		Hypertension, Peripheral vascular disease, Varicose vein, Venous thromboembolism		Stroke
Gastrointestinal disorders	Nausea, Abdominal pain, Flatulence	Dyspepsia		Vomiting
Hepatobiliary disorders		Gall bladder disease	Alterations in liver function, sometimes with Asthenia or Malaise, Jaundice and Abdominal pain	
Skin and subcutaneous tissue disorders		Allergic skin reactions, Rash, Urticaria, Pruritus		Chloasma or melasma, which may persist when drug is discontinued, Erythema multiforme, Erythema nodosum, Vascular purpura, Angioedema
Musculoskeletal and connective tissue disorders	Leg cramps	Back pain		
Reproductive system and breast disorders	Breast pain/ tenderness, Breakthrough bleeding and spotting, Pelvic pain	Change in cervical erosion, Change in cervical secretion, Dysmenorrhoea, Menorrhagia, Metrorrhagia	Breast enlargement, Premenstrual-like symptoms	
Congenital and familial/genetic disorders				Aggravation of porphyria
General disorders and administration site reactions	Asthenia	Peripheral oedema		
Investigations	Increase/decrease in weight			

Breast Cancer

According to evidence from a large number of epidemiological studies and one randomised placebo-controlled trial, the Women's Health Initiative (WHI), the overall risk of breast cancer increases with increasing duration of HRT use in current or recent HRT users.

For *estrogen-only* HRT, estimates of relative risk (RR) from a reanalysis of original data from 51 epidemiological studies (in which >80% of HRT use was estrogen-only HRT) and from the epidemiological Million Women Study (MWS) are similar at 1.35 (95%CI 1.21 – 1.49) and 1.30 (95%CI 1.21 – 1.40), respectively.

For *estrogen plus progestagen* combined HRT, several epidemiological studies have reported an overall higher risk for breast cancer than with estrogens alone.

The MWS reported that, compared to never users, the use of various types of estrogen-progestagen combined HRT was associated with a higher risk of breast cancer (RR = 2.00, 95%CI: 1.88 – 2.12) than use of estrogens alone (RR = 1.30, 95%CI: 1.21 – 1.40) or use of tibolone (RR=1.45; 95%CI 1.25-1.68).

The WHI trial reported a risk estimate of 1.24 (95%CI 1.01 – 1.54) after 5.6 years of use of estrogen-progestagen combined HRT (CEE + MPA) in all users compared with placebo.

The absolute risks calculated from the MWS and the WHI trials are presented below:

The MWS has estimated, from the known average incidence of breast cancer in developed countries, that:

– For women not using HRT, about 32 in every 1000 are expected to have breast cancer diagnosed between the ages of 50 and 64 years.

- For 1000 current or recent users of HRT, the number of *additional* cases during the corresponding period will be

- For users of *estrogen-only* replacement therapy

• between 0 and 3 (best estimate = 1.5) for 5 years' use

• between 3 and 7 (best estimate = 5) for 10 years' use.

- For users of *estrogen plus progestagen* combined HRT,

• between 5 and 7 (best estimate = 6) for 5 years' use

• between 18 and 20 (best estimate = 19) for 10 years' use.

The WHI trial estimated that after 5.6 years of follow-up of women between the ages of 50 and 79 years, an *additional* 8 cases of invasive breast cancer would be due to *estrogen-progestagen combined* HRT (CEE + MPA) per 10,000 women years.

According to calculations from the trial data, it is estimated that:

- For 1000 women in the placebo group,

• about 16 cases of invasive breast cancer would be diagnosed in 5 years.

- For 1000 women who used estrogen + progestagen combined HRT (CEE + MPA), the number of *additional* cases would be

• between 0 and 9 (best estimate = 4) for 5 years' use.

The number of additional cases of breast cancer in women who use HRT is broadly similar for women who start HRT irrespective of age at start of use (between the ages of 45-65) (see section 4.4).

Endometrial cancer

In women with an intact uterus, the risk of endometrial hyperplasia and endometrial cancer increases with increasing duration of use of unopposed estrogens. According to data from epidemiological studies, the best estimate of the risk is that for women not using HRT, about 5 in every 1000 are expected to have endometrial cancer diagnosed between the ages of 50 and 65. Depending on the duration of treatment and estrogen dose, the reported increase in endometrial cancer risk among unopposed estrogen users varies from 2-to 12-fold greater compared with non-users. Adding a progestagen to estrogen-only therapy greatly reduces this increased risk.

Other adverse reactions have been reported in association with estrogen/progestagen treatment:

- Estrogen-dependent neoplasms benign and malignant, e.g. endometrial cancer.

- Venous thromboembolism, i.e. deep leg or pelvic venous thrombosis and pulmonary embolism, is more frequent among hormone replacement therapy users than among non-users. For further information, see section 4.3 Contra-indications and 4.4 Special warnings and precautions for use.

- Probable dementia (see section 4.4).

4.9 Overdose

Both estradiol and dydrogesterone are substances with low toxicity. Theoretically, symptoms such as nausea, vomiting, sleepiness and dizziness could occur in cases of overdosing. It is unlikely that any specific or symptomatic treatment will be necessary.

Aforementioned information is applicable for overdosing by children also.

5. PHARMACOLOGICAL PROPERTIES

5.1 Pharmacodynamic properties

The ATC code is G03FB08. (Estrogens: urogenital system and sex hormones)

Sequential hormone replacement therapy (combined estradiol and dydrogesterone).

Estradiol

The active ingredient, synthetic 17β-estradiol, is chemically and biologically identical to endogenous human estradiol. It substitutes for the loss of estrogen production in menopausal women, and alleviates menopausal symptoms. Estrogens prevent bone loss following menopause or ovariectomy.

Dydrogesterone

Dydrogesterone is an orally-active progestagen. The addition of a progestagen greatly reduces the estrogen-induced risk of endometrial hyperplasia and cancer in non-hysterectomised women, by reducing the growth of the endometrium.

Clinical trial Information

- Relief of estrogen-deficiency symptoms and bleeding patterns.

- Relief of menopausal symptoms was achieved during the first few weeks of treatment.

- Regular withdrawal bleeding with Femoston 1/10 occurred in approximately 75-80% of women with a mean duration of 5 days. Withdrawal bleeding usually started on the day of the last pill of the progestagen phase. Breakthrough bleeding and/or spotting occurred in approximately 10% of the women; amenorrhoea (no bleeding or spotting) occurred in 21-25% of the women for months 10 to 12 of treatment.

- With Femoston 2/10, approximately 90% of women had regular withdrawal bleeding. The start day and duration of bleeding, and the number of women with intermittent bleeding was the same as with Femoston 1/10, amenorrhoea occurred in 7-11% of the women for months 10 to 12 of treatments.

- Prevention of osteoporosis

- Estrogen deficiency at menopause is associated with an increasing bone turnover and decline in bone mass. The effect of estrogens on the bone mineral density is dose-dependent. Protection appears to be effective for as long as treatment is continued. After discontinuation of HRT, bone mass is lost at a rate similar to that in untreated women.

- Evidence from the WHI trial and meta-analysed trials shows that current use of HRT, alone or in combination with a progestagen – given to predominantly healthy women – reduces the risk of hip, vertebral, and other osteoporotic fractures. HRT may also prevent fractures in women with low bone density and/or established osteoporosis, but the evidence for that is limited.

- After two years of treatment with Femoston 2/10, the increase in lumbar spine bone mineral density (BMD) was 6.7% ± 3.9% (mean ± SD). The percentage of women who maintained or gained BMD in lumbar zone during treatment was 94.5%. For Femoston 1/10 the increase in lumbar spine BMD was 5.2% ± 3.8% (mean ± SD), and the percentage of women with no change or an increase in lumbar spine BMD was 93%.

- Femoston also had an effect on hip BMD. The increase after two years of treatment with 1mg estradiol was 2.7% ± 4.2% (mean ± SD) at femoral neck, 3.5% ± 5.0% (mean ± SD) at trochanter and 2.7%± 6.7% (mean ± SD) at Wards triangle. After two years of treatment with 2mg estradiol these figures were respectively, 2.6% ± 5.0%; 4.6% ± 5.0% and 4.1% ± 7.4%. The percentage of women who maintained or gained BMD in the 3 hip areas after treatment with 1mg estradiol was 67-78% and 71-88% after treatment with 2mg estradiol.

5.2 Pharmacokinetic properties

Estradiol

Orally administered estradiol, comprising particles whose size has been reduced to less than 5 μm, is quickly and efficiently absorbed from the gastrointestinal tract. The primary unconjugated and conjugated metabolites are estrone and estrone sulphate. These metabolites can contribute to the estrogen effect, both directly and after conversion to estradiol. Estrogens are excreted in the bile and reabsorbed from the intestine. During this enterohepatic cycle the estrogens are broken down. Estrogens are excreted in the urine as biologically inactive glucuronide and sulphate compounds (90 to 95%), or in the faeces (5 to 10%), mostly unconjugated. Estrogens are excreted in mothers' milk.

During the administration of oral estradiol to post-menopausal women at 2 mg once a day the $C_{average}$ is 58 pg/ml, the C_{min} is 44 pg/ml and the C_{max} is 93 pg/ml. The E1/E2 (Estrone/Estradiol) ratio is 5.8.

Dydrogesterone

After oral administration of labelled dydrogesterone, on average 63% of the dose is excreted into the urine. Within 72 hours, excretion is complete.

In man, dydrogesterone is completely metabolised. The main metabolite of dydrogesterone is 20α-dihydrodydrogesterone (DHD) and is present in the urine predominantly as the glucoronic acid conjugate. A common feature of all metabolites characterised is the retention of the 4,6 diene-3-one configuration of the parent compound and the absence of 17α-hydroxylation. This explains the absence of estrogenic and androgenic activity.

After oral administration of dydrogesterone, plasma concentrations of DHD are substantially higher as compared to the parent drug. The AUC and C_{max} ratios of DHD to dydrogesterone are in the order of 40 and 25, respectively. Dydrogesterone is rapidly absorbed. The T_{max} values of dydrogesterone and DHD vary between 0.5 and 2.5 hours.

Mean terminal half lives of dydrogesterone and DHD vary between 5 to 7 and 14 to 17 hours, respectively.

The dihydrodydrogesterone $C_{average}$ is 13 ng/ml, the C_{min} is 4.1 ng/ml and the C_{max} is 63 ng/ml. The dydrogesterone $C_{average}$ is 0.38 ng/ml the C_{min} is <0.1 ng/ml and the C_{max} is 2.5 ng/ml.

Dydrogesterone is not excreted in urine as pregnanediol, like progesterone. Analysis of endogenous progesterone production based on pregnanediol excretion therefore remains possible.

5.3 Preclinical safety data

Supraphysiologically high doses (prolonged overdoses) of estradiol have been associated with the induction of tumours in estrogen-dependent target organs for all rodent species tested. The changes observed with dydrogesterone in animal toxicity studies are characteristic for progesterone-like compounds. *In-vitro* and *in-vivo* data gave no indications of mutagenic effects of dydrogesterone. In long-term studies, doses administered to rats and mice were sufficient to produce hormone-mediated changes, but did not provide tumorogenic potential.

6. PHARMACEUTICAL PARTICULARS

6.1 List of excipients

Estradiol only tablets (brick-red):

Tablet core: Lactose

Hypromellose

Maize starch

Colloidal anhydrous silica

Magnesium stearate

Film coat: Hypromellose

Talc

Macrogol 400

Titanium dioxide E171

Iron oxide red E171

Iron oxide black E172

Iron oxides yellow E172

Estradiol/Dydrogesterone tablets (yellow):

Tablet core: Lactose

Hypromellose

Maize starch

Colloidal anhydrous silica

Magnesium stearate

Film coat: Hypromellose

Talc

Macrogol 400

Titanium dioxide (E171)

Iron oxide yellow (E172)

6.2 Incompatibilities

Not applicable.

6.3 Shelf life

3 years.

6.4 Special precautions for storage

Do not store above 30°C.

6.5 Nature and contents of container

The tablets are packed in blister strips of 28. The blister packs are made of PVC/PVdC or PVC film with a covering aluminium foil. Each carton contains 28 or 84 tablets.

6.6 Special precautions for disposal and other handling

Not applicable.

7. MARKETING AUTHORISATION HOLDER

Solvay Healthcare Limited

Mansbridge Road

West End

Southampton

SO18 3JD

8. MARKETING AUTHORISATION NUMBER(S)

PL 00512/0113

9. DATE OF FIRST AUTHORISATION/RENEWAL OF THE AUTHORISATION

17 January 1995

10. DATE OF REVISION OF THE TEXT

January 2006

Legal category

POM

Femoston-conti

(Solvay Healthcare Limited)

1. NAME OF THE MEDICINAL PRODUCT

Femoston-conti ® 1 mg/5 mg film-coated tablets

2. QUALITATIVE AND QUANTITATIVE COMPOSITION

Each film-coated tablet contains 1 mg estradiol as estradiol hemihydrate and 5 mg dydrogesterone.

For excipients, see 6.1.

3. PHARMACEUTICAL FORM

Film-coated tablet.

Salmon-coloured, round, biconvex, film-coated tablets imprinted '$' on one side and '379' on the other.

4. CLINICAL PARTICULARS

4.1 Therapeutic indications

Hormone replacement therapy (HRT) for estrogen deficiency symptoms in postmenopausal women. Femoston-conti should be used only in postmenopausal women more than 12 months after menopause.

Prevention of osteoporosis in postmenopausal women at high risk of future fractures who are intolerant of, or contra-indicated for, other medicinal products approved for the prevention of osteoporosis.

(See also section 4.4)

The experience in treating women older than 65 years is limited.

4.2 Posology and method of administration

Femoston-conti is a continuous combined HRT.

The dosage is one tablet per day. Femoston-conti should be taken continuously without a break between packs.

Femoston-conti can be taken with or without food.

Starting Femoston-conti:

Women experiencing a natural menopause should commence treatment with Femoston-conti 12 months after their last natural menstrual bleed. For surgically induced menopause, treatment may start immediately.

In women who are not taking hormone replacement therapy or women, who switch from a continuous combined hormone replacement therapy, treatment may be started on any convenient day. In women transferring from a cyclic or continuous sequential HRT regimen, treatment should begin the day following completion of the prior regimen.

If a dose has been forgotten, it should be taken as soon as possible. When more than 12 hours have elapsed, it is recommended to continue with the next dose without taking the forgotten tablet. The likelihood of breakthrough bleeding or spotting may be increased.

For initiation and continuation of treatment of postmenopausal symptoms, the lowest effective dose for the shortest duration (see also section 4.4) should be used.

4.3 Contraindications

Known, past or suspected breast cancer;

Known or suspected estrogen-dependent malignant tumours (e.g. endometrial cancer);

Undiagnosed genital bleeding;

Untreated endometrial hyperplasia;

Previous idiopathic or current venous thromboembolism (deep vein thrombosis, pulmonary embolism);

Active or recent arterial thromboembolic disease (e.g. angina, myocardial infarction);

Acute liver disease or a history of liver disease as long as liver function tests have failed to return to normal;

Known hypersensitivity to the active substances or to any of the excipients;

Porphyria.

4.4 Special warnings and precautions for use

For the treatment of postmenopausal symptoms, HRT should only be initiated for symptoms that adversely affect quality of life. In all cases, a careful appraisal of the risks and benefits should be undertaken at least annually and HRT should only be continued as long as the benefit outweighs the risk.

Medical examination/follow up

Before initiating or reinstituting HRT, a complete personal and family medical history should be taken. Physical (including pelvic and breast) examination should be guided by this and by the contraindications and warnings for use. During treatment, periodic check-ups are recommended of a frequency and nature adapted to the individual woman. Women should be advised what changes in their breasts should be reported to their doctor or nurse. Investigations, including mammography, should be carried out in accordance with currently accepted screening practices, modified to the clinical needs of the individual.

Conditions which need supervision

If any of the following conditions are present, have occurred previously, and/or have been aggravated during pregnancy or previous hormone treatment, the patient should be closely supervised. It should be taken into account that these conditions may recur or be aggravated during treatment with Femoston-conti in particular:

- Leiomyoma (uterine fibroids) or endometriosis

- A history of, or risk factors for, thromboembolic disorders (see below)
- Risk factors for estrogen dependent tumours, e.g. 1st degree heredity for breast cancer
- Hypertension
- Liver disorders (e.g. liver adenoma)
- Diabetes mellitus with or without vascular involvement
- Cholelithiasis
- Migraine or (severe) headache
- Systemic lupus erythematosus
- A history of endometrial hyperplasia (see below)
- Epilepsy
- Asthma
- Otosclerosis

Reasons for immediate withdrawal of therapy:

Therapy should be discontinued in cases where a contra-indication is discovered and in the following situations:

- Jaundice or deterioration in liver function
- Significant increase in blood pressure
- New onset of migraine-type headache
- Pregnancy

Endometrial hyperplasia

The risk of endometrial hyperplasia and carcinoma is increased when estrogens are administered alone for prolonged periods (see section 4.8). The addition of a progestagen for at least 12 days per cycle in non-hysterectomised women greatly reduces this risk.

Break-through bleeding and spotting may occur during the first months of treatment. If break-through bleeding or spotting appears after some time on therapy, or continues after treatment has been discontinued, the reason should be investigated, which may include endometrial biopsy to exclude endometrial malignancy.

Breast cancer

A randomised placebo-controlled trial, the Womens Health Initiative study (WHI) and epidemiological studies, including the Million Women Study (MWS), have reported an increased risk of breast cancer in women taking estrogens, estrogen-progestagen combinations or tibolone for HRT for several years (see Section 4.8).

For all HRT, an excess risk becomes apparent within a few years of use and increases with duration of intake but returns to baseline within a few (at most five) years after stopping treatment.

In the MWS, the relative risk of breast cancer with conjugated equine estrogens (CEE) or estradiol (E2) was greater when a progestagen was added, either sequentially or continuously, and regardless of type of progestagen. There was no evidence of a difference in risk between the different routes of administration.

In the WHI study, the continuous combined conjugated equine estrogen and medroxyprogesterone acetate (CEE + MPA) product used was associated with breast cancers that were slightly larger in size and more frequently had local lymph node metastases compared to placebo.

HRT, especially estrogen-progestagen combined treatment, increases the density of mammographic images which may adversely affect the radiological detection of breast cancer.

Venous thromboembolism

HRT is associated with a higher relative risk of developing venous thromboembolism (VTE), i.e. deep vein thrombosis or pulmonary embolism. One randomised controlled trial and epidemiological studies found a two-to threefold higher risk for users compared with non-users. For non-users, it is estimated that the number of cases of VTE that will occur over a 5 year period is about 3 per 1000 women aged 50-59 years and 8 per 1000 women aged between 60-69 years. It is estimated that in healthy women who use HRT for 5 years, the number of additional cases of VTE over a 5 year period will be between 2 and 6 (best estimate = 4) per 1000 women aged 50-59 years and between 5 and 15 (best estimate = 9) per 1000 women aged 60-69 years. The occurrence of such an event is more likely in the first year of HRT than later.

- Generally recognised risk factors for VTE include a personal or family history; severe obesity (BMI > 30 kg/m^2) and systemic lupus erythematosus (SLE). There is no consensus about the possible role of varicose veins in VTE.
- Patients with a history of VTE or known thrombophilic states have an increased risk of VTE. HRT may add to this risk. Personal or strong family history of thromboembolism or recurrent spontaneous abortion should be investigated in order to exclude a thrombophilic predisposition. Until a thorough evaluation of thrombophilic factors has been made or anticoagulant treatment initiated, use of HRT in such patients should be viewed as contraindicated. Those women already on anticoagulant treatment require careful consideration of the benefit-risk of use of HRT.
- The risk of VTE may be temporarily increased with prolonged immobilisation, major trauma or major surgery. As in all postoperative patients, scrupulous attention should be given to prophylactic measures to prevent VTE following surgery. Where prolonged immobilisation is liable to follow elective surgery, particularly abdominal or orthopaedic surgery to the lower limbs, consideration should be given to temporarily stopping HRT 4 to 6 weeks earlier, if possible. Treatment should not be restarted until the women is completely mobilised.
- If VTE develops after initiating therapy, the drug should be discontinued. Patients should be told to contact their doctors immediately when they are aware of a potential thromboembolic symptom (e.g. painful swelling of a leg, sudden pain in the chest, dyspnea).

Table 1

MedDRA system organ class	Common >1/100, <1/10	Uncommon >1/1,000, <1/100	Rare >1/10,000, <1/1,000	Very rare <1/10,000 incl. isolated reports
Infections and infestations		Cystitis-like syndrome, Vaginal candidiasis		
Neoplasms benign, Malignant and unspecified		Increase in size of leiomyoma		
Blood and the lymphatic system disorders				Haemolytic anaemia
Psychiatric disorders		Depression, Change in libido, Nervousness		
Nervous system disorders	Headache, Migraine	Dizziness		Chorea
Eye disorders			Intolerance to contact lenses, Steepening of corneal curvature	
Cardiac disorders				Myocardial infarction
Vascular disorders		Hypertension, Peripheral vascular disease, Varicose vein, Venous thromboembolism		Stroke
Gastrointestinal disorders	Nausea, Abdominal pain, Flatulence	Dyspepsia		Vomiting
Hepatobiliary disorders		Gall bladder disease	Alterations in liver function, sometimes with asthenia or malaise, jaundice and abdominal pain	
Skin and subcutaneous tissue disorders		Allergic skin reactions, Rash, Urticaria, Pruritus		Chloasma or melasma, which may persist when drug is discontinued, Erythema multiforme, Erythema nodosum, Vascular purpura, Angioedema
Musculoskeletal and connective tissue disorders	Leg cramps	Back pain		
Reproductive system and breast disorders	Breast pain/ tenderness, Breakthrough bleeding and spotting Pelvic pain	Change in cervical erosion, Change in cervical secretion, Dysmenorrhoea, Menorrhagia, Metrorrhagia	Breast enlargement, Premenstrual-like symptoms	
Congenital and familial/genetic disorders				Aggravation of porphyria
General disorders and administration site reactions	Asthenia	Peripheral oedema		
Investigations	Increase/decrease in weight			

Coronary artery disease (CAD)

There is no evidence from randomised controlled trials of cardiovascular benefit with continuous combined conjugated estrogens and medroxyprogesterone acetate (MPA). Two large clinical trials (WHI and HERS i.e. Heart and Estrogen/progestin Replacement Study) showed a possible increased risk of cardiovascular morbidity in the first year of use and no overall benefit. For other HRT products there are only limited data from randomised controlled trials examining effects in cardiovascular morbidity or mortality. Therefore, it is uncertain whether these findings also extend to other HRT products.

Stroke

One large randomised clinical trial (WHI-trial) found, as a secondary outcome, an increased risk of ischaemic stroke in healthy women during treatment with continuous combined conjugated estrogens and MPA. For women who do not use HRT, it is estimated that the number of cases of stroke that will occur over a 5 year period is about 3 per 1000 women aged 50-59 and 11 per 1000 women aged 60-69 years. It is estimated that for women who use conjugated estrogens and MPA for 5 years, the number of additional cases will be between 0 and 3 (best estimate = 1) per 1000 users aged 50-59 years and between 1 and 9 (best estimate = 4) per 1000 users aged 60-69 years. It is unknown whether the increased risk also extends to other HRT products.

Ovarian cancer

Long-term (at least 5 to 10 years) use of estrogen-only HRT products in hysterectomised women has been associated with an increased risk of ovarian cancer in some epidemiological studies. It is uncertain whether long term use of combined HRT confers a different risk than estrogen-only products

Other conditions

– Estrogens may cause fluid retention and therefore patients with cardiac or renal dysfunction should be carefully observed. Patients with terminal renal insufficiency should be closely observed, since it is expected that the level of circulating active ingredients in Femoston-conti is increased.

– Women with pre-existing hypertriglyceridemia should be followed closely during estrogen replacement or hormone replacement therapy, since rare cases of large increases of plasma triglycerides leading to pancreatitis have been reported with estrogen therapy in this condition.

– Estrogens increase thyroid binding globulin (TBG), leading to increased circulating total thyroid hormone, as measured by protein-bound iodine (PBI), T4 levels (by column or by radio-immunoassay) or T3 levels (by radio-immunoassay). T3 resin uptake is decreased, reflecting the elevated TBG. Free T4 and free T3 concentrations are unaltered. Other binding proteins may be elevated in serum, i.e. corticoid binding globulin (CBG), sex-hormone—binding globulin (SHBG) leading to increased circulating corticosteroids and sex steroids, respectively. Free or biological active hormone concentrations are unchanged. Other plasma proteins may be increased (angiotensinogen/renin substrate, alpha-1-antitrypsin, ceruloplasmin).

– There is no conclusive evidence for improvement of cognitive function. There is some evidence from the WHI trial of increased risk of probable dementia in women who start using continuous combined CEE and MPA after the age of 65. It is unknown whether the findings apply to younger post-menopausal women or other HRT products.

This medicinal product contains lactose monohydrate and therefore should not be used by patients with rare hereditary problems of galactose intolerance, the Lapp lactase deficiency or glucose-galactose malabsorption.

4.5 Interaction with other medicinal products and other forms of interaction

- The metabolism of estrogens and progestagens may be increased by concomitant use of substances known to induce drug-metabolising enzymes, specifically cytochrome P450 enzymes, such as anticonvulsants (eg. phenobarbital, phenytoin, carbamazepine) and anti-infectives (e.g. rifampicin, rifabutin, nevirapine, efavirenz).

- Ritonavir and nelfinavir, although known as strong inhibitors, by contrast exhibit inducing properties when used concomitantly with steroid hormones.

- Herbal preparations containing St John's wort (Hypericum perforatum) may induce the metabolism of estrogens and progestagens.

- Clinically an increased metabolism of estrogens and progestagens may lead to decreased effect and changes in the uterine bleeding profile.

4.6 Pregnancy and lactation

Pregnancy:

Femoston-conti is not indicated during pregnancy. If pregnancy occurs during medication with Femoston-conti, treatment should be withdrawn immediately.

Clinically, data based on an assumed large number of exposed pregnancies indicate no adverse effects of dydrogesterone on the foetus.

The results of most epidemiological studies to date relevant to inadvertent foetal exposure to combinations of estrogens and progestagens indicate no teratogenic or foetotoxic effect.

Lactation:

Femoston-conti is not indicated during lactation.

4.7 Effects on ability to drive and use machines

Femoston-conti does not affect the ability to drive or use machines.

4.8 Undesirable effects

Undesirable effects reported in clinical trials and in post-marketing experience are the following:

(see Table 1 on previous page)

Breast cancer

According to evidence from a large number of epidemiological studies and one randomised placebo-controlled trial, the Women's Health Initiative (WHI), the overall risk of breast cancer increases with increasing duration of HRT use in current or recent HRT users.

For *estrogen-only* HRT, estimates of relative risk (RR) from a reanalysis of original data from 51 epidemiological studies (in which >80% of HRT use was estrogen-only HRT) and from the epidemiological Million Women Study (MWS) are similar at 1.35 (95%CI 1.21 – 1.49) and 1.30 (95%CI 1.21 – 1.40), respectively.

For *estrogen plus progestagen* combined HRT, several epidemiological studies have reported an overall higher risk for breast cancer than with estrogens alone.

The MWS reported that, compared to never users, the use of various types of estrogen-progestagen combined HRT was associated with a higher risk of breast cancer (RR = 2.00, 95%CI: 1.88 – 2.12) than use of estrogens alone (RR = 1.30, 95%CI: 1.21 – 1.40) or use of tibolone (RR=1.45; 95%CI 1.25-1.68).

The WHI trial reported a risk estimate of 1.24 (95%CI 1.01 – 1.54) after 5.6 years of use of estrogen-progestagen combined HRT (CEE + MPA) in all users compared with placebo.

The absolute risks calculated from the MWS and the WHI trials are presented below:

The MWS has estimated, from the known average incidence of breast cancer in developed countries, that:

– For women not using HRT, about 32 in every 1000 are expected to have breast cancer diagnosed between the ages of 50 and 64 years.

- For 1000 current or recent users of HRT, the number of *additional* cases during the corresponding period will be

- For users of *estrogen-only* replacement therapy

• between 0 and 3 (best estimate = 1.5) for 5 years' use

• between 3 and 7 (best estimate = 5) for 10 years' use.

- For users of *estrogen plus progestagen* combined HRT,

• between 5 and 7 (best estimate = 6) for 5 years' use

• between 18 and 20 (best estimate = 19) for 10 years' use.

The WHI trial estimated that after 5.6 years of follow-up of women between the ages of 50 and 79 years, an *additional* 8 cases of invasive breast cancer would be due to *estrogen-progestagen combined* HRT (CEE + MPA) per 10,000 women years.

According to calculations from the trial data, it is estimated that:

- For 1000 women in the placebo group,

• about 16 cases of invasive breast cancer would be diagnosed in 5 years.

- For 1000 women who used estrogen + progestagen combined HRT (CEE + MPA), the number of *additional* cases would be

• between 0 and 9 (best estimate = 4) for 5 years' use.

The number of additional cases of breast cancer in women who use HRT is broadly similar for women who start HRT irrespective of age at start of use (between the ages of 45-65) (see section 4.4).'

Endometrial cancer

In women with an intact uterus, the risk of endometrial hyperplasia and endometrial cancer increases with increasing duration of use of unopposed estrogens. According to data from epidemiological studies, the best estimate of the risk is that for women not using HRT, about 5 in every 1000 are expected to have endometrial cancer diagnosed between the ages of 50 and 65. Depending on the duration of treatment and estrogen dose, the reported increase in endometrial cancer risk among unopposed estrogen users varies from 2-to 12-fold greater compared with non-users. Adding a progestagen to estrogen-only therapy greatly reduces this increased risk.

Other adverse reactions have been reported in association with estrogen/progestagen treatment:

- Estrogen-dependent neoplasms benign and malignant, e.g. endometrial cancer.

- Venous thromboembolism, i.e. deep leg or pelvic venous thrombosis and pulmonary embolism, is more frequent among hormone replacement therapy users than among non-users. For further information, see section 4.3 Contra-indications and 4.4 Special warnings and precautions for use.

- Probable dementia (see section 4.4)

4.9 Overdose

Both estradiol and dydrogesterone are substances with low toxicity. Theoretically, symptoms such as nausea, vomiting, sleepiness and dizziness could occur in cases of overdosing. It is unlikely that any specific or symptomatic treatment will be necessary.

Aforementioned information is applicable for overdosing by children also.

5. PHARMACOLOGICAL PROPERTIES

5.1 Pharmacodynamic properties

The ATC code is G03 F A14. (Estrogens: urogenital system and sex hormones).

Hormone replacement therapy (combined estradiol and dydrogesterone).

Estradiol

The active ingredient, synthetic 17β-estradiol, is chemically and biologically identical to endogenous human estradiol. It substitutes for the loss of estrogen production in menopausal women, and alleviates menopausal symptoms. Estrogens prevent bone loss following menopause or ovariectomy.

Dydrogesterone

As estrogens promote the growth of the endometrium, unopposed estrogens increase the risk of endometrial hyperplasia and cancer. The addition of a progestagen greatly reduces the estrogen-induced risk of endometrial hyperplasia in non-hysterectomised women.

- Clinical trial Information

- Relief of estrogen-deficiency symptoms and bleeding patterns

Relief of menopausal symptoms was achieved during the first few weeks of treatment.

Amenorrhoea (no bleeding or spotting) was seen in 76% of women during months 10 -12 of treatment.

Bleeding and/or spotting appeared in 29 % of the women during the first three months of treatment and in 24% during months 10 -12 of treatment.

- Prevention of osteoporosis

- Estrogen deficiency at menopause is associated with an increasing bone turnover and decline in bone mass. The effect of estrogens on the bone mineral density is dose-dependent. Protection appears to be effective for as long as treatment is continued. After discontinuation of HRT, bone mass is lost at a rate similar to that in untreated women.

- Evidence from the WHI trial and meta-analysed trials shows that current use of HRT, alone or in combination with a progestagen – given to predominantly healthy women – reduces the risk of hip, vertebral, and other osteoporotic fractures. HRT may also prevent fractures in women with low bone density and/or established osteoporosis, but the evidence for that is limited.

After two years of treatment with Femoston-conti, the increase in lumbar spine bone mineral density (BMD) was 5.20% ± 3.76 % (mean ± SD). The percentage of women who maintained or gained BMD in lumbar zone during treatment was 95%.

Femoston-conti also had an effect on hip BMD. The increase after two years was 2.7% ± 4.2 % (mean ± SD) at femoral neck, 3.5% +/- 5.0% (mean ± SD) at trochanter and 2.7%±6.7% (mean ± SD) at Wards triangle. The percentage of women who maintained or gained BMD in the 3 hip areas during treatment was 67-78%.

5.2 Pharmacokinetic properties

Estradiol

Orally administered estradiol, comprising particles whose size has been reduced to less than 5 μm, is quickly and efficiently absorbed from the gastrointestinal tract. The primary unconjugated and conjugated metabolites are estrone and estrone sulphate. These metabolites can contribute to the estrogen effect, both directly and after conversion to estradiol. Estrogens are excreted in the bile and reabsorbed from the intestine. During this enterohepatic cycle the estrogens are broken down. Estrogens are excreted in the urine as biologically inactive glucuronide and sulphate compounds (90 to 95%), or in the faeces (5 to 10%), mostly unconjugated. Estrogens are secreted in the milk of nursing mothers.

The $C_{average}$ is 28 pg/ml, the C_{min} is 20 pg/ml and the C_{max} is 54 pg/ml. The E1/E2 (Estrone/Estradiol) ratio is 7.0.

Dydrogesterone

After oral administration of labelled dydrogesterone, on average 63% of the dose is excreted into the urine. Within 72 hours, excretion is complete.

In man, dydrogesterone is completely metabolised. The main metabolite of dydrogesterone is 20α-dihydrodydrogesterone (DHD) and is present in the urine predominantly as the glucoronic acid conjugate. A common feature of all metabolites characterised is the retention of the 4,6 diene-3-one configuration of the parent compound and the absence of 17α-hydroxylation. This explains the absence of estrogenic and androgenic activity.

After oral administration of dydrogesterone, plasma concentrations of DHD are higher as compared to the parent drug. The AUC and C_{max} ratios of DHD to dydrogesterone are in the order of 40 and 25, respectively. Dydrogesterone is rapidly absorbed. The T_{max} values of dydrogesterone and DHD vary between 0.5 and 2.5 hours.

Mean terminal half lives of dydrogesterone and DHD vary between 5 to 7 and 14 to 17 hours, respectively.

The dihydrodydrogesterone $C_{average}$ is 13 ng/ml, the C_{min} is 4.1 ng/ml and the C_{max} is 63 ng/ml. The dydrogesterone $C_{average}$ is 0.38 ng/ml the C_{min} is <0.1 ng/ml and the C_{max} is 2.5 ng/ml.

Dydrogesterone is not excreted in urine as pregnanediol, like progesterone. Analysis of endogenous progesterone production based on pregnanediol excretion therefore remains possible.

5.3 Preclinical safety data

Supraphysiologically high doses (prolonged application) of estradiol have been associated with the induction of tumours in estrogen-dependent target organs for all rodent species tested. Furthermore, inherent to its hormonal activity, estradiol displays untoward embryotoxic effects and feminisation of male fetuses was occasionally observed. The changes observed with dydrogesterone in animal toxicity studies are associated with the effects of progesterone-like compounds.

Doses administered to rats and mice sufficient to produce hormone mediated changes gave no evidence of carcinogenesis

6. PHARMACEUTICAL PARTICULARS

6.1 List of excipients

Tablet core: Lactose monohydrate

Hypromellose

Maize starch

Colloidal anhydrous silica

Magnesium stearate

Film coat: Hypromellose

Macrogol 400

Titanium dioxide (E171)

Iron oxides, yellow and red (E172)

6.2 Incompatibilities

Not applicable.

6.3 Shelf life

3 years.

6.4 Special precautions for storage

Do not store above 30°C. Keep blister in the outer carton.

6.5 Nature and contents of container

Calendar packs of 14, 28, 84 (3 × 28) or 280 (10 × 28) tablets in PVC-Aluminium blister strips.

Not all pack sizes may be marketed.

6.6 Special precautions for disposal and other handling

Not applicable.

7. MARKETING AUTHORISATION HOLDER
Solvay Healthcare Limited
Mansbridge Road
Southampton
SO18 3JD
United Kingdom

8. MARKETING AUTHORISATION NUMBER(S)
PL 00512/0157

9. DATE OF FIRST AUTHORISATION/RENEWAL OF THE AUTHORISATION
Date of First authorisation: 23 November 1999
Date of last renewal: December 2004

10. DATE OF REVISION OF THE TEXT
November 2004

Femseven 50, 75, 100

(Merck Serono)

1. NAME OF THE MEDICINAL PRODUCT
FemSeven 50, 50 microgram/24 hours, transdermal patch.
FemSeven 75, 75 microgram/24 hours, transdermal patch.
FemSeven 100, 100 microgram/24 hours, transdermal patch.

2. QUALITATIVE AND QUANTITATIVE COMPOSITION
One FemSeven 50 transdermal patch contains 1.5 mg estradiol hemihydrate delivering 50 microgram of estradiol in 24 hours. The area of the releasing surface is 15 cm^2.
One FemSeven 75 transdermal patch contains 2.25 mg estradiol hemihydrate delivering 75 microgram of estradiol in 24 hours. The area of the releasing surface is 22.5 cm^2.
One FemSeven 100 transdermal patch contains 3.00 mg estradiol hemihydrate delivering 100 microgram of estradiol in 24 hours. The area of the releasing surface is 30 cm^2.

3. PHARMACEUTICAL FORM
Transdermal patch.

4. CLINICAL PARTICULARS
4.1 Therapeutic indications
• Hormone replacement therapy for oestrogen deficiency symptoms in post-menopausal women.
• Prevention of osteoporosis in postmenopausal women at high risk of future fractures who are intolerant of, or contra-indicated for, other medicinal products approved for the prevention of osteoporosis.
(See also section 4.4)
The experience of treating women older than 65 years is limited.

4.2 Posology and method of administration
FemSeven is an oestrogen-only patch that should be applied to the skin once weekly on a continuous basis, i.e. each patch is replaced with a new one after 7 days.
In women with an intact uterus the addition of a progestogen for at least 12 to 14 days per cycle is essential to help prevent any endometrial hyperplasia induced by the oestrogen. For more detailed information, please refer to section 4.4. (Special warnings and precautions for use - "Endometrial hyperplasia").
Unless there is a previous diagnosis of endometriosis, the addition of a progestogen in hysterectomised women is not recommended.
For initiation and continuation of treatment of postmenopausal symptoms, the lowest effective dose for the shortest duration (see also section 4.4) should be used. Therefore, therapy should normally be started with one FemSeven 50 patch (delivering 50 micrograms of estradiol in 24 hours). If the prescribed dose does not eliminate the menopausal symptoms the dose should be adjusted stepwise after the first few months by using a transdermal patch delivering 75 or 100 micrograms estradiol per day. A maximum of 100 micrograms estradiol per day should not be exceeded. If there are persistent signs of overdose, such as breast tenderness, the dose should be reduced accordingly.
Hysterectomised women not taking HRT or transferring from another HRT product may start treatment with FemSeven on any convenient day. The same holds true for non-hysterectomised women not taking HRT or transferring from a continuous combined HRT product. In non-hysterectomised women switching from sequential HRT regimens, treatment with FemSeven should start after the previous treatment regimen has ended.
Consecutive new patches should be applied to different sites. It is recommended that sites are chosen below the waist where little wrinkling of the skin occurs e.g., buttocks, hip or abdomen. FemSeven must not be applied on or near the breasts. The patch should be applied to clean, dry, healthy and intact skin. The patch should be applied to the skin as soon as it is removed from its wrapping. The patch is applied by removing both parts of the protective liner and then holding it in contact with the skin for at least 30 seconds (warmth is essential to ensure maximal adhesive strength).
Should part or all of a patch detach prematurely (before 7 days) it should be removed and a new patch applied. To aid compliance it is recommended the patient then continues to change the patch on the usual day. This advice also applies if a patient forgets to change the patch on schedule. Forgetting a patch may increase the likelihood of break-through bleeding or spotting.

4.3 Contraindications
FemSeven is contra-indicated in:
- Known, past or suspected breast cancer;
- Known or suspected oestrogen-dependent malignant tumours (e.g. endometrial cancer);
- Undiagnosed genital bleeding;
- Untreated endometrial hyperplasia;
- Previous idiopathic or current venous thromboembolism (deep venous thrombosis, pulmonary embolism);
- Active or recent arterial thromboembolic disease (e.g. angina, myocardial infarction);
- Acute liver disease, or a history of liver disease as long as liver function tests have failed to return to normal;
- Known hypersensitivity to the active substances or to any of the excipients;
- Porphyria.

4.4 Special warnings and precautions for use
For the treatment of postmenopausal symptoms, HRT should only be initiated for symptoms that adversely affect quality of life. In all cases, a careful appraisal of the risks and benefits should be undertaken at least annually and HRT should only be continued as long as the benefit outweighs the risk.

Medical examination/follow up

Before initiating or reinstituting HRT, a complete personal and family medical history should be taken. Physical (including pelvic and breast) examination should be guided by this and by the contraindications and warnings for use. During treatment, periodic check-ups are recommended of a frequency and nature adapted to the individual woman.
Women should be advised what changes in their breasts should be reported to their doctor or nurse (see "Breast cancer" below). Investigations, including mammography, should be carried out in accordance with currently accepted screening practices, modified to the clinical needs of the individual.

Conditions which need supervision

If any of the following conditions are present, have occurred previously and/or have been aggravated during pregnancy or previous hormone treatment, the patient should be closely supervised. It should be taken into account that these conditions may recur or be aggravated during treatment with FemSeven:
- Leiomyoma (uterine fibroids) or endometriosis
- A history of, or risk factors for, thromboembolic disorders (see below)
- Risk factors for oestrogen dependent tumours, e.g. 1st degree heredity for breast cancer
- Hypertension
- Liver disorders (e.g. liver adenoma)
- Diabetes mellitus with or without vascular involvement
- Cholelithiasis
- Migraine or severe headache
- Systemic lupus erythematosus
- A history of endometrial hyperplasia (see below)
- Epilepsy
- Asthma
- Otosclerosis.

Reasons for immediate withdrawal of therapy

Therapy should be discontinued if a contra-indication is discovered and in the following situations:
- Jaundice or deterioration in liver function
- Significant increase in blood pressure
- New onset of migraine-type headache
- Pregnancy

Endometrial hyperplasia

• The risk of endometrial hyperplasia and carcinoma is increased when oestrogens are administered alone for prolonged periods (see section 4.8). The addition of a progestogen for at least 12 days per cycle in non-hysterectomised women greatly reduces this risk.
• For FemSeven 75 and 100, the endometrial safety of added progestogens has not been established.
• Break-through bleeding and spotting may occur during the first months of treatment. If break-through bleeding or spotting appears after some time on therapy, or continues after treatment has been discontinued, the reason should be investigated, which may include endometrial biopsy to exclude endometrial malignancy.
• Unopposed oestrogen stimulation may lead to premalignant or malignant transformation in the residual foci of endometriosis. Therefore, the addition of progestogens to oestrogen replacement therapy should be considered in women who have undergone hysterectomy because of endometriosis, if they are known to have residual endometriosis.

Breast cancer

A randomised placebo-controlled trial, the Women's Health Initative study (WHI), and epidemiological studies, including the Million Women Study (MWS), have reported an increased risk of breast cancer in women taking oestrogens, oestrogen-progestogen combinations or tibolone for HRT for several years (see section 4.8). For all HRT, an excess risk becomes apparent within a few years of use and increases with duration of intake but returns to baseline within a few (at most five) years after stopping treatment.
In the MWS, the relative risk of breast cancer with conjugated equine oestrogens (CEE) or estradiol (E2) was greater when a progestogen was added, either sequentially or continuously, and regardless of type of progestogen. There was no evidence of a difference in risk between the different routes of administration.
In the WHI study, the continuous combined conjugated equine oestrogen and medroxyprogesterone acetate (CEE + MPA) product used was associated with breast cancers that were slightly larger in size and more frequently had local lymph node metastases compared to placebo.
HRT, especially oestrogen-progestogen combined treatment, increases the density of mammographic images which may adversely affect the radiological detection of breast cancer.

Venous thromboembolism

• HRT is associated with a higher relative risk of developing venous thromboembolism (VTE), i.e. deep vein thrombosis or pulmonary embolism. One randomised controlled trial and epidemiological studies found a two to three fold higher risk for users compared with non-users. For non-users it is estimated that the number of cases of VTE that will occur over a 5 year period is about 3 per 1000 women aged 50-59 years and 8 per 1000 women aged between 60-69 years.

It is estimated that in healthy women who use HRT for 5 years the number of additional cases of VTE over a 5 year period will be between 2 and 6 (best estimate = 4) per 1000 women aged 50-59 years and between 5 and 15 (best estimate = 9) per 1000 women aged 60-69 years. The occurrence of such an event is more likely in the first year of HRT than later.

• Generally recognized risk factors for VTE include a personal history or family history, severe obesity (Body Mass Index 30 kg/m^2) and systemic lupus erythematosus (SLE). There is no consensus about the possible role of varicose veins in VTE.
• Patients with a history of VTE or known thrombophilic states have an increased risk of VTE. HRT may add to this risk. Personal or strong family history of thromboembolism or recurrent spontaneous abortion should be investigated in order to exclude a thrombophilic predisposition. Until a thorough evaluation of thrombophilic factors has been made or anticoagulant treatment initiated, use of HRT in such patients should be viewed as contraindicated. Those women already on anticoagulant treatment require careful consideration of the benefit-risk of use of HRT.
• The risk of VTE may be temporarily increased with prolonged immobilisation, major trauma or major surgery. As in all post-operative patients, scrupulous attention should be given to prophylactic measures to prevent VTE following surgery. Where prolonged immobilisation is liable to follow elective surgery, particularly abdominal or orthopaedic surgery to the lower limbs, consideration should be given to temporarily stopping HRT four to six weeks earlier, if possible. Treatment should not be restarted until the woman is completely mobilised.
• If VTE develops after initiating therapy, the drug should be discontinued.

Patients should be told to contact their doctors immediately when they are aware of a potential thromboembolic symptom (e.g. painful swelling of a leg, sudden pain in the chest, dyspnoea).

Coronary artery disease (CAD)

There is no evidence from randomised controlled trials of cardiovascular benefit with continuous combined conjugated oestrogens and medroxyprogesterone acetate (MPA). Two large clinical trials (WHI and HERS i.e. Heart and Estrogen/progestin Replacement Study) showed a possible increased risk of cardiovascular morbidity in the first year of use and no overall benefit. For other HRT products there are only limited data from randomised controlled trials examining effects in cardiovascular morbidity or mortality. Therefore, it is uncertain whether these findings also extend to other HRT products.

Stroke

One large randomised clinical trial (WHI-trial) found, as a secondary outcome, an increased risk of ischaemic stroke in healthy women during treatment with continuous combined conjugated oestrogens and MPA. For women who do not use HRT, it is estimated that the number of cases of stroke that will occur over a 5 year period is about 3 per 1000 women aged 50-59 years and 11 per 1000 women aged 60-69 years.

It is estimated that for women who use conjugated oestrogens and MPA for 5 years, the number of additional cases will be between 0 and 3 (best estimate = 1) per 1000 users aged 50-59 years and between 1 and 9 (best estimate = 4) per 1000 users aged 60-69 years. It is unknown whether the increased risk also extends to other HRT products.

Ovarian cancer

Long-term (at least 5-10 years) use of oestrogen-only HRT products in hysterectomised women has been associated with an increased risk of ovarian cancer in some epidemiological studies. It is uncertain whether long-term use of combined HRT confers a different risk than oestrogen-only products.

Other conditions

- Oestrogens may cause fluid retention, and therefore patients with cardiac or renal dysfunction should be carefully observed. Patients with terminal renal insufficiency should be closely observed, since it is expected that the level of circulating active ingredients in FemSeven is increased.
- Women with pre-existing hypertriglyceridemia should be followed closely during oestrogen replacement or hormone replacement therapy, since rare cases of large increases of plasma triglycerides leading to pancreatitis have been reported with oestrogen therapy in this condition.
- Oestrogens increase thyroid binding globulin (TBG), leading to increased circulating total thyroid hormone, as measured by protein-bound iodine (PBI), T4 levels (by column or by radio-immunoassay) or T3 levels (by radio-immunoassay). T3 resin uptake is decreased, reflecting the elevated TBG. Free T4 and free T3 concentrations are unaltered. Other binding proteins may be elevated in serum, i.e. corticoid binding globulin (CBG), sex-hormone-binding globulin (SHBG) leading to increased circulating corticosteroids and sex steroids, respectively. Free or biological active hormone concentrations are unchanged. Other plasma proteins may be increased (angiotensinogen/renin substrate, alpha-I-antitrypsin, ceruloplasmin).
- There is no conclusive evidence for improvement of cognitive function. There is some evidence from the WHI trial of increased risk of probable dementia in women who start using continuous combined CEE and MPA after the age of 65. It is unknown whether the findings apply to younger post-menopausal women or other HRT products.

4.5 Interaction with other medicinal products and other forms of interaction

The metabolism of oestrogens may be increased by concomitant use of substances known to induce drug-metabolising enzymes, specifically cytochrome P450 enzymes, such as anticonvulsants (e.g. phenobarbital, phenytoin, carbamazepine) and anti-infectives (e.g. rifampicin, rifabutin, nevirapine, efavirenz).

Ritonavir and nelfinavir, although known as strong inhibitors, by contrast exhibit inducing properties when used concomitantly with steroid hormones. Herbal preparations containing St John's wort (Hypericum Perforatum) may induce the metabolism of oestrogens.

With transdermal administration, the first-pass effect in the liver is avoided and, thus, transdermally applied oestrogens might be less affected than oral hormones by enzyme inducers.

Clinically, an increased metabolism of oestrogens may lead to decreased effect and changes in the uterine bleeding profile.

4.6 Pregnancy and lactation

- Pregnancy:

FemSeven is not indicated during pregnancy. If pregnancy occurs during medication with FemSeven, treatment should be withdrawn immediately.

The results of most epidemiological studies to date relevant to inadvertent fœtal exposure to oestrogens indicate no teratogenic or foetotoxic effects.

- Lactation:

FemSeven is not indicated during lactation.

4.7 Effects on ability to drive and use machines

There is no evidence from the clinical data available on oestrogen therapy to suggest that FemSeven should have any effect on a patient's ability to drive or operate machinery.

4.8 Undesirable effects

The most frequently reported undesirable effects (> 10 %) in clinical trials during treatment with FemSeven were application site reactions, e.g. pruritus, erythema, eczema, urticaria, oedema and changes in skin pigmentation. They were mostly mild skin reactions and usually disappeared 2 – 3 days after patch removal. These effects are usually observed with transdermal oestrogen replacement therapy.

All adverse events considered to be drug-related, which were observed during the Phase III (> 500 patients) and Phase IV (> 10,000 patients) clinical trials or from the spontaneous reporting system and literature, are summarised in the following table:

(see Table 1 below)

Breast cancer

According to evidence from a large number of epidemiological studies and one randomised placebo-controlled trial, the Women's Health Initiative (WHI), the overall risk of breast cancer increases with increasing duration of HRT use in current or recent HRT users.

For *oestrogen-only* HRT, estimates of relative risk (RR) from a reanalysis of original data from 51 epidemiological studies (in which >80% of HRT use was oestrogen-only HRT) and from the epidemiological Million Women Study (MWS) are similar at 1.35 (95%CI: 1.21 – 1.49) and 1.30 (95%CI: 1.21 – 1.40), respectively.

For *oestrogen plus progestogen* combined HRT, several epidemiological studies have reported an overall higher risk for breast cancer than with oestrogens alone.

The MWS reported that, compared to never users, the use of various types of oestrogen-progestogen combined HRT was associated with a higher risk of breast cancer (RR = 2.00, 95%CI: 1.88 – 2.12) than use of oestrogens alone (RR = 1.30, 95%CI: 1.21 – 1.40) or use of tibolone (RR = 1.45, 95%CI: 1.25-1.68).

The WHI trial reported a risk estimate of 1.24 (95%CI: 1.01 – 1.54) after 5.6 years of use of oestrogen-progestogen combined HRT (CEE + MPA) in all users compared with placebo.

The absolute risks calculated from the MWS and the WHI trial are presented below:

The MWS has estimated, from the known average incidence of breast cancer in developed countries, that:

◆ For women not using HRT, about 32 in every 1000 are expected to have breast cancer diagnosed between the ages of 50 and 64 years.

◆ For 1000 current or recent users of HRT, the number of *additional* cases during the corresponding period will be

- For users of *oestrogen-only* replacement therapy
- between 0 and 3 (best estimate = 1.5) for 5 years' use
- between 3 and 7 (best estimate = 5) for 10 years' use.
- For users of *oestrogen plus progestogen* combined HRT,
- between 5 and 7 (best estimate = 6) for 5 years' use
- between 18 and 20 (best estimate = 19) for 10 years' use.

The WHI trial estimated that after 5.6 years of follow-up of women between the ages of 50 and 79 years, an *additional* 8 cases of invasive breast cancer would be due to *oestrogen-progestogen combined* HRT (CEE + MPA) per 10,000 women years.

According to calculations from the trial data, it is estimated that:

◆ For 1000 women in the placebo group,

- about 16 cases of invasive breast cancer would be diagnosed in 5 years.

◆ For 1000 women who used oestrogen + progestogen combined HRT (CEE + MPA), the number of *additional* cases would be

- between 0 and 9 (best estimate = 4) for 5 years' use.

The number of additional cases of breast cancer in women who use HRT is broadly similar for women who start HRT irrespective of age at start of use (between the ages of 45-65) (see section 4.4).

Endometrial cancer

In women with an intact uterus, the risk of endometrial hyperplasia and endometrial cancer increases with increasing duration of use of unopposed oestrogens. According to data from epidemiological studies, the best estimate of the risk is that for women not using HRT, about 5 in every 1000 are expected to have endometrial cancer diagnosed between the ages of 50 and 65. Depending on the duration of treatment and oestrogen dose, the reported increase in endometrial cancer risk among unopposed oestrogen users varies from 2-to 12-fold greater compared with non-users. Adding a progestogen to oestrogen-only therapy greatly reduces this increased risk.

Other adverse reactions have been reported in association with oestrogen/progestogen treatment (class-effect):

- Oestrogen-dependent neoplasms benign and malignant, e.g. endometrial cancer.
- Venous thromboembolism, i.e. deep leg or pelvic venous thrombosis and pulmonary embolism, is more frequent among hormone replacement therapy users than among non-users. For further information, see section 4.3 Contraindications and 4.4 Special warnings and precautions for use.
- Myocardial infarction and stroke
- Gall bladder disease
- Skin and subcutaneous disorders: chloasma, erythema multiforme, erythema nodosum, vascular purpura
- Deterioration of liver function
- Probable dementia (see section 4.4).

4.9 Overdose

The mode of administration makes significant overdose unlikely; removal of the patches is all that is required should it occur.

5. PHARMACOLOGICAL PROPERTIES

5.1 Pharmacodynamic properties

ATC code: G03 A03

Oestrogens

The active ingredient, synthetic 17β-estradiol, is chemically and biologically identical to endogenous human estradiol. It substitutes for the loss of oestrogen production in menopausal women, and alleviates menopausal symptoms. Oestrogens prevent bone loss following menopause or ovariectomy.

Clinical Trial Information:

- Relief of menopausal symptoms was achieved during the first few weeks of the treatment.

In non-hysterectomised women the bleeding profile depends on the type and dose of the progestogen and duration used in combination with FemSeven.

- Prevention of osteoporosis

- Oestrogen deficiency at menopause is associated with an increasing bone turnover and decline in bone mass. The effect of oestrogens on the bone mineral density is dose-dependent. Protection appears to be effective for as long as treatment is continued. After discontinuation of HRT, bone mass is lost at a rate similar to that in untreated women.

- Evidence from the WHI trial and meta-analysed trials shows that current use of HRT, alone or in combination with a progestogen – given to predominantly healthy women – reduces the risk of hip, vertebral, and other osteoporotic fractures. HRT may also prevent fractures in women with low bone density and/or established osteoporosis, but the evidence for that is limited.

5.2 Pharmacokinetic properties

After application of the transdermal system containing estradiol, therapeutic concentrations of estradiol are achieved within 3 hours and maintained throughout the

Table 1

Organ system class	Common ADRs > 1/100; < 1/10	Uncommon ADRs >1/1000; < 1/100	Rare ADRs >1/10000; < 1/1000
Skin and sub-utaneous tissue		Hair changes, sweating increased	
Muscular and skeletal		Arthralgia, leg cramps	
Central & peri. nervous system	Headache	Dizziness, paresthesia, migraine	
Psychiatric disorders		Anxiety, appetite increase, depression, insomnia, nervousness	
Gastrointestinal system dis.		Nausea, dyspepsia, abdominal pain, vomiting	
Cardiovasc.		Blood pressure changes	
Myo-, endo-, pericards		Chest pain	
Vascular (extracardial)		Vein disorders	
Reproductive disease female	Breast discomfort (e.g. Mastalgia/ mastopathies, breast tenderness, breast enlargement)	Vaginal discharge, breakthrough bleeding	Worsening of uterine fibroids
Body as a whole/general dis.		Edema, fatigue, weight changes	

entire application period of the transdermal patch (7 days). Estradiol peak plasma concentrations (C_{max}) range from 59 to 155 pg/ml (baseline corrected geometric mean 92 pg/ml) and $AUC_{0\text{-}168h}$ values were between 2478 and 10694 h*pg/ml (baseline corrected geometric mean 5188 h*pg/ml). The mean average plasma concentration (C_{av}) is 42 pg/ml (range: 20 to 145 pg/ml) and mean C_{pre} (trough concentration before next patch application) is 29 pg/ml. After removal of the transdermal patch, estradiol concentrations return to pre-treatment values (below 10 pg/ml) within 12 hours.

By transdermal administration of FemSeven, there is no hepatic first-pass effect and the estradiol reaches the bloodstream directly in unchanged form and in physiological amounts. With the use of FemSeven the estradiol concentrations are raised to values similar to those of the early to middle follicular phase.

The liver is the major site for estradiol metabolism. The primary metabolites are estrone and estriol and their conjugates (glucuronide and sulfate). Estradiol is excreted into the urine mostly as glucuronide and sulfate. The urinary excretion approaches pretreatment levels within 24 hours after patch removal.

5.3 Preclinical safety data

No adverse effects can be predicted from animal toxicology studies other than those documented from human use of estradiol.

6. PHARMACEUTICAL PARTICULARS

6.1 List of excipients

Backing layer: Transparent polyethylene terephthalate (PET) foil.

Adhesive matrix: Styrene-isoprene block copolymer, glycerine esters of completely hydrogenated resins.

6.2 Incompatibilities

None known.

6.3 Shelf life

2 years.

6.4 Special precautions for storage

Do not store above 30°C.

6.5 Nature and contents of container

The container (primary packaging) consists of a sealed laminated sachet. This comprises layers of food grade paper/polyethylene/aluminium/ethylene copolymer.

Package sizes:

FemSeven 50: Cartons of 4 and 12 patches.

FemSeven 75 & FemSeven 100: Cartons of 1, 4, 8, 9 and 12 patches.

6.6 Special precautions for disposal and other handling

After removal from the laminated sachet, peel off the two part protective liner. Try to avoid touching the adhesive. Stick the adhesive side down to the upper left or right buttock on a clean and dry area of skin. Hold the applied patch to the skin with the palm of the hand for at least 30 seconds, in order to ensure optimal adhesion to the skin.

Recommended application sites are clean, dry and intact areas of skin on the trunk below the waistline. FemSeven should not be applied on or near the breasts. After removal the used patch should be folded and disposed of with the normal household solid waste.

7. MARKETING AUTHORISATION HOLDER

Merck Serono Ltd

Bedfont Cross

Stanwell Road

Feltham

Middlesex

TW14 8NX

UK

8. MARKETING AUTHORISATION NUMBER(S)

FemSeven 50, 50 microgram/24 hours, transdermal patch. - PL 11648/0021

FemSeven 75, 75 microgram/24 hours, transdermal patch. - PL 11648/0023

FemSeven 100, 100 microgram/24 hours, transdermal patch. - PL 11648/0024

9. DATE OF FIRST AUTHORISATION/RENEWAL OF THE AUTHORISATION

14 December 2000

10. DATE OF REVISION OF THE TEXT

18 April 2008

FemSeven Conti

(Merck Serono)

1. NAME OF THE MEDICINAL PRODUCT

Femseven Conti,

50 micrograms / 7 micrograms / 24 hours, transdermal patch

2. QUALITATIVE AND QUANTITATIVE COMPOSITION

Each patch contains 1.5 mg of estradiol hemihydrate and 0.525 mg levonorgestrel in a patch size of 15 cm^2, releasing 50 micrograms of estradiol and 7 micrograms of levonorgestrel per 24 hours.

For excipients, see 6.1.

3. PHARMACEUTICAL FORM

Transdermal patch

Octagonal, transparent, flexible, rounded-edge transdermal matrix patch located on an oversized removable protective liner.

4. CLINICAL PARTICULARS

4.1 Therapeutic indications

Hormone replacement therapy (HRT) for oestrogen deficiency symptoms in postmenopausal women more than one year after menopause.

Experience of treating women older than 65 years is limited.

4.2 Posology and method of administration

For transdermal use.

Femseven Conti has to be applied once a week, i.e. each patch is replaced every 7 days. Femseven Conti is a continuous combined hormone replacement therapy (HRT) treatment without a treatment-off phase: as one patch is removed, the next is applied immediately. Forgetting to change a patch on schedule may increase the likelihood of break-through bleeding or spotting.

In women with amenorrhoea and not taking HRT or women transferring from another continuous combined HRT product, treatment with Femseven Conti may be started on any convenient day.

In women transferring from sequential HRT regimens, treatment should start right after their withdrawal bleeding has ended.

For initiation and continuation of treatment of postmenopausal symptoms, the lowest effective dose for the shortest duration (see also section 4.4) should be used.

Method of administration

Femseven Conti should be applied to clean, dry, healthy skin (which is neither irritated nor grazed), free from any cream, lotion or other oily product.

Femseven Conti should be applied to an area of skin without major skin folds, i.e. the buttocks or hips, and not subject to chafing by clothing (avoid the waist and also avoid wearing tight clothing that could loosen the transdermal patch).

Femseven Conti must not be applied either on or near the breasts. It is advisable to avoid applying the patch to the same site twice running. At least one week should be allowed to elapse between applications to the same site.

After opening the sachet, one-half of the protective foil is peeled off, being careful not to touch the adhesive part of the transdermal patch with the fingers. Then the patch must be applied directly to the skin. After that the other half of the protective foil is peeled off, and the patch must be firmly pressed **with the palm of the hand for at least 30 seconds, concentrating on the edges. Pressure and the warmth of the hand are essential to ensure maximal adhesive strength of the patch.**

It is possible to take a shower or have a bath without removing the transdermal patch. In the event that the transdermal patch should become detached prematurely, i.e. before the seventh day (due to vigorous physical activity, excessive sweating, abnormal chafing of clothing), a new patch should be applied (to aid compliance it is recommended that the patient then continues to change the patch on the original scheduled day).

Once applied, the transdermal patch has to be covered by clothes to avoid direct exposure to sunlight.

Removal of the transdermal patch should be carried out slowly to avoid irritating the skin. In the event of some of the adhesive remaining on the skin, this can usually be removed by gently rubbing with a cream or an oily lotion.

After use, Femseven Conti is to be folded in two (with the adhesive surface to the inside) and disposed of with normal household solid waste.

4.3 Contraindications

- Known, past or suspected breast cancer;
- Known or suspected oestrogen-dependent malignant tumours (e.g. endometrial cancer);
- Undiagnosed genital bleeding;
- Untreated endometrial hyperplasia;
- Previous idiopathic or current venous thromboembolism (deep venous thrombosis, pulmonary embolism);
- Active or recent arterial thromboembolic disease, (e.g. angina, myocardial infarction);
- Acute liver disease, or a history of liver disease as long as liver function tests have failed to return to normal;
- Known hypersensitivity to the active substances or to any of the excipients;
- Porphyria.

4.4 Special warnings and precautions for use

For the treatment of postmenopausal symptoms, HRT should only be initiated for symptoms that adversely affect quality of life. In all cases, a careful appraisal of the risks and benefits should be undertaken at least annually and HRT should only be continued as long as the benefit outweighs the risk.

Medical examination/follow-up

Before initiating or reinstituting HRT, a complete personal and family medical history should be taken. Physical (including pelvic and breast) examination should be guided by this and by the contraindications and warnings for use. During treatment, periodic check-ups are recommended of a frequency and nature adapted to the individual woman. Women should be advised what changes in their breasts should be reported to their doctor or nurse (see "Breast cancer" below). Investigations, including mammography, should be carried out in accordance with currently accepted screening practices, modified to the clinical needs of the individual.

Conditions which need supervision

If any of the following conditions are present, have occurred previously, and/or have been aggravated during pregnancy or previous hormone treatment, the patient should be closely supervised. It should be taken into account that these conditions may recur or be aggravated during treatment with Femseven Conti, in particular:

- Leiomyoma (uterine fibroids) or endometriosis
- A history of, or risk factors for, thromboembolic disorders (see below)
- Risk factors for oestrogen-dependent tumours, e.g. 1st degree heredity for breast cancer
- Hypertension
- Liver disorders (e.g. liver adenoma)
- Diabetes mellitus with or without vascular involvement
- Cholelithiasis
- Migraine or (severe) headache
- Systemic lupus erythematosus
- A history of endometrial hyperplasia (see below)
- Epilepsy
- Asthma
- Otosclerosis

Reasons for immediate withdrawal of therapy:

Therapy should be discontinued in case a contra-indication is discovered and in the following situations:

- Jaundice or deterioration in liver function
- Significant increase in blood pressure
- New onset of migraine-type headache
- Pregnancy

Endometrial hyperplasia

• The risk of endometrial hyperplasia and carcinoma is increased when oestrogens are administered alone for prolonged periods (see section 4.8). The addition of a progestagen for at least 12 days per cycle in non-hysterectomised women greatly reduces this risk.

• Break-through bleeding and spotting may occur during the first months of treatment. If break-through bleeding or spotting appears after some time on therapy, or continues after treatment has been discontinued, the reason should be investigated, which may include an endometrial biopsy to exclude endometrial malignancy.

Breast cancer

A randomised placebo-controlled trial, the Women's Health Initiative study (WHI), and epidemiological studies, including the Million Women Study (MWS), have reported an increased risk of breast cancer in women taking oestrogens, oestrogen-progestagen combinations or tibolone for HRT for several years (see Section 4.8). For all HRT, an excess risk becomes apparent within a few years of use and increases with duration of intake but returns to baseline within a few (at most five) years after stopping treatment.

In the MWS, the relative risk of breast cancer with conjugated equine oestrogens (CEE) or estradiol (E2) was greater when a progestagen was added, either sequentially or continuously, and regardless of type of progestagen. There was no evidence of a difference in risk between the different routes of administration.

In the WHI study, the continuous combined conjugated equine oestrogen and medroxyprogesterone acetate (CEE + MPA) product used was associated with breast cancers that were slightly larger in size and more frequently had local lymph node metastases compared to placebo.

HRT, especially oestrogen-progestagen combined treatment, increases the density of mammographic images which may adversely affect the radiological detection of breast cancer.

Venous thromboembolism

• HRT is associated with a higher relative risk of developing venous thromboembolism (VTE), i.e. deep vein thrombosis or pulmonary embolism. One randomised controlled trial and epidemiological studies found a two- to threefold higher risk for users compared with non-users. For non-users it is estimated that the number of cases of VTE that will occur over a 5 year period is about 3 per 1000 women aged 50-59 years and 8 per 1000 women aged between 60-69 years. It is estimated that in healthy women who use HRT for 5 years, the number of additional cases of VTE over a 5 year period will be between 2 and 6 (best estimate = 4) per 1000 women aged 50-59 years and between 5 and 15 (best estimate = 9) per 1000 women aged 60-69 years. The occurrence of such an event is more likely in the first year of HRT than later.

• Generally recognised risk factors for VTE include a personal history or family history, severe obesity (BMI > 30 kg/m^2) and systemic lupus erythematosus (SLE). There is no consensus about the possible role of varicose veins in VTE.

• Patients with a history of VTE or known thrombophilic states have an increased risk of VTE. HRT may add to this risk. A personal or strong family history of thromboembolism or recurrent spontaneous abortion should be investigated in order to exclude a thrombophilic predisposition. Until a thorough evaluation of thrombophilic factors has been made or anticoagulant treatment initiated, use of HRT in such patients should be viewed as contraindicated. Those women already on anticoagulant treatment require careful consideration of the benefit-risk of use of HRT.

• The risk of VTE may be temporarily increased with prolonged immobilisation, major trauma or major surgery. As in all post-operative patients, scrupulous attention should be given to prophylactic measures to prevent VTE following surgery. Where prolonged immobilisation is liable to follow elective surgery, particularly abdominal or orthopaedic surgery to the lower limbs, consideration should be given to temporarily stopping HRT 4 to 6 weeks earlier, if possible. Treatment should not be restarted until the woman is completely mobilised.

• If VTE develops after initiating therapy, the drug should be discontinued. Patients should be told to contact their doctors immediately when they are aware of a potential thromboembolic symptom (e.g. painful swelling of a leg, sudden pain in the chest, dyspnea).

Coronary artery disease (CAD)

• There is no evidence from randomised controlled trials of cardiovascular benefit with continuous combined conjugated oestrogens and medroxyprogesterone acetate (MPA). Two large clinical trials (WHI and HERS i.e. Heart and Estrogen/progestin Replacement Study) showed a possible increased risk of cardiovascular morbidity in the first year of use and no overall benefit. For other HRT products there are only limited data from randomised controlled trials examining effects in cardiovascular morbidity or mortality. Therefore, it is uncertain whether these findings also extend to other HRT products.

Stroke

• One large randomised clinical trial (WHI-trial) found, as a secondary outcome, an increased risk of ischaemic stroke in healthy women during treatment with continuous combined conjugated oestrogens and MPA. For women who do not use HRT, it is estimated that the number of cases of stroke that will occur over a 5 year period is about 3 per 1000 women aged 50-59 years and 11 per 1000 women aged 60-69 years. It is estimated that for women who use conjugated oestrogens and MPA for 5 years, the number of additional cases will be between 0 and 3 (best estimate = 1) per 1000 users aged 50-59 years and between 1 and 9 (best estimate = 4) per 1000 users aged 60-69 years. It is unknown whether the increased risk also extends to other HRT products.

Ovarian cancer

• Long-term (at least 5-10 years) use of oestrogen-only HRT products in hysterectomised women has been associated with an increased risk of ovarian cancer in some epidemiological studies. It is uncertain whether long-term use of combined HRT confers a different risk than oestrogen-only products.

Other conditions

• Oestrogens may cause fluid retention, and therefore patients with cardiac or renal dysfunction should be carefully observed. Patients with terminal renal insufficiency should be closely observed, since it is expected that the level of circulating active ingredients in Femseven Conti is increased.

• Women with pre-existing hypertriglyceridemia should be followed closely during oestrogen replacement or hormone replacement therapy, since rare cases of large increases of plasma triglycerides leading to pancreatitis have been reported with oestrogen therapy in this condition.

• Oestrogens increase thyroid binding globulin (TBG), leading to increased circulating total thyroid hormone, as measured by protein-bound iodine (PBI), T4 levels (by column or by radio-immunoassay) or T3 levels (by radio-immunoassay). T3 resin uptake is decreased, reflecting the elevated TBG. Free T4 and free T3 concentrations are unaltered. Other binding proteins may be elevated in serum, i.e. corticoid binding globulin (CBG), sex hormone-binding globulin (SHBG) leading to increased circulating corticosteroids and sex steroids, respectively. Free or biological active hormone concentrations are unchanged. Other plasma proteins may be increased (angiotensinogen/renin substrate, alpha-I-antitrypsin, ceruloplasmin).

• There is no conclusive evidence for improvement of cognitive function. There is some evidence from the WHI trial of increased risk of probable dementia in women who start using continuous combined CEE and MPA after the age of 65. It is unknown whether the findings apply to younger post-menopausal women or other HRT products.

4.5 Interaction with other medicinal products and other forms of interaction

The metabolism of oestrogens and progestagens may be increased by concomitant use of substances known to induce drug-metabolising enzymes, specifically cytochrome P450 enzymes, such as anticonvulsants (e.g. phenobarbital, phenytoin, carbamazepine) and anti-infectives (e.g. rifampicin, rifabutin, nevirapine, efavirenz).

Ritonavir and nelfinavir, although known as strong inhibitors, by contrast exhibit inducing properties when used concomitantly with steroid hormones.

Herbal preparations containing St John's wort (Hypericum Perforatum) may induce the metabolism of oestrogens and progestagens.

With transdermal administration, the first-pass effect in the liver is avoided and, thus, transdermally applied oestrogens and progestagens might be less affected than oral hormones by enzyme inducers.

Clinically, an increased metabolism of oestrogens and progestagens may lead to decreased effect and changes in the uterine bleeding profile.

4.6 Pregnancy and lactation

Pregnancy

Femseven Conti is not indicated during pregnancy. If pregnancy occurs during treatment with Femseven Conti, treatment should be withdrawn immediately.

Clinically, data on a large number of exposed pregnancies indicate no adverse effects of levonorgestrel on the foetus.

The results of most epidemiological studies to date that are relevant to inadvertent foetal exposure to combinations of oestrogens and progestagens indicate no teratogenic or foetotoxic effect.

Lactation

Femseven Conti is not indicated during lactation.

4.7 Effects on ability to drive and use machines

No effects on ability to drive and use machines have been observed.

4.8 Undesirable effects

The most frequently reported undesirable effects (> 10 %) in clinical trials during treatment with Femseven Conti were application site reactions, breast tenderness and bleeding or spotting. The application site reactions were mostly mild skin reactions and usually disappeared 2 – 3 days after patch removal. In the majority of cases breast tenderness was reported as mild or moderate and tend to decrease during treatment time.

Other potential systemic undesirable effects are those commonly observed with oestrogen and progestin treatments.

(see Table 1 below)

Breast cancer

According to evidence from a large number of epidemiological studies and one randomised placebo-controlled trial, the Women's Health Initiative (WHI), the overall risk of breast cancer increases with increasing duration of HRT use in current or recent HRT users.

For *oestrogen-only* HRT, estimates of relative risk (RR) from a reanalysis of original data from 51 epidemiological studies (in which >80% of HRT use was oestrogen-only HRT) and from the epidemiological Million Women Study (MWS) are similar at 1.35 (95%CI: 1.21 – 1.49) and 1.30 (95%CI: 1.21 – 1.40), respectively.

For *oestrogen plus progestagen* combined HRT, several epidemiological studies have reported an overall higher risk for breast cancer than with oestrogens alone.

The MWS reported that, compared to never users, the use of various types of oestrogen-progestagen combined HRT was associated with a higher risk of breast cancer (RR = 2.00, 95%CI: 1.88 – 2.12) than use of oestrogens alone (RR = 1.30, 95%CI: 1.21 – 1.40) or use of tibolone (RR = 1.45, 95%CI: 1.25 - 1.68).

The WHI trial reported a risk estimate of 1.24 (95%CI: 1.01 – 1.54) after 5.6 years of use of oestrogen-progestagen combined HRT (CEE + MPA) in all users compared with placebo.

The absolute risks calculated from the MWS and the WHI trial are presented below:

The MWS has estimated, from the known average incidence of breast cancer in developed countries, that:

◆ For women not using HRT, about 32 in every 1000 are expected to have breast cancer diagnosed between the ages of 50 and 64 years.

◆ For 1000 current or recent users of HRT, the number of *additional* cases during the corresponding period will be

• For users of *oestrogen-only* replacement therapy

- between 0 and 3 (best estimate = 1.5) for 5 years' use
- between 3 and 7 (best estimate = 5) for 10 years' use.

• For users of *oestrogen plus progestogen* combined HRT,

- between 5 and 7 (best estimate = 6) for 5 years' use
- between 18 and 20 (best estimate = 19) for 10 years' use.

The WHI trial estimated that after 5.6 years of follow-up of women between the ages of 50 and 79 years, an *additional* 8 cases of invasive breast cancer would be due to *oestrogen-progestogen combined* HRT (CEE + MPA) per 10,000 women years.

According to calculations from the trial data, it is estimated that:

◆ For 1000 women in the placebo group,

• about 16 cases of invasive breast cancer would be diagnosed in 5 years.

◆ For 1000 women who used oestrogen + progestogen combined HRT (CEE + MPA), the number of *additional* cases would be

• between 0 and 9 (best estimate = 4) for 5 years' use.

The number of additional cases of breast cancer in women who use HRT is broadly similar for women who start HRT irrespective of age at start of use (between the ages of 45-65) (see section 4.4).

Endometrial cancer

In women with an intact uterus, the risk of endometrial hyperplasia and endometrial cancer increases with increasing duration of use of unopposed oestrogens. According to data from epidemiological studies, the best estimate of the risk is that for women not using HRT, about 5 in every 1000 are expected to have endometrial cancer diagnosed between the ages of 50 and 65. Depending on the duration of treatment and oestrogen dose, the reported increase in endometrial cancer risk among unopposed oestrogen users varies from 2-to 12-fold greater compared with non-users. Adding a progestagen to oestrogen-only therapy greatly reduces this increased risk.

Other adverse reactions have been reported in association with oestrogen/progestagen treatment:

- Oestrogen-dependent neoplasms benign and malignant, e.g. endometrial cancer.
- Venous thromboembolism, i.e. deep leg or pelvic venous thrombosis and pulmonary embolism, is more frequent among hormone replacement therapy users than among non-users. For further information, see section 4.3 Contra-indications and 4.4 Special warnings and precautions for use.
- Myocardial infarction and stroke.
- Gall bladder disease.
- Skin and subcutaneous disorders: chloasma, erythema multiforme, erythema nodosum, vascular purpura.
- Probable dementia (see section 4.4).

4.9 Overdose

The method of administration makes significant overdose unlikely. Signs of an overdose are generally breast tenderness, swelling of the abdomen/pelvis, anxiety, irritability, nausea and vomiting. Removal of the transdermal patches is all that is required should it occur.

Table 1

Organ system	Common ADRs > 1/100, < 1/10	Uncommon ADRs > 1/1000, < 1/100	Rare ADRs > 1/10,000, < 1/1000
General disorders		Fluid retention/ oedema/ weight increase/loss, fatigue, leg cramps	
Nervous system disorders	Headache	Dizziness, migraine	
Gastrointestinal disorders	Dyspepsia	Bloating, abdominal cramps, nausea	Cholelithiasis, cholestatic jaundice
Cardiovascular disorders		Hypertension	
Reproductive system and breast disorders	Mastodynia	Endometrial hyperplasia, benign breast tissue changes,	Increase in size of uterine fibrosis
Psychiatric disorders		Depression	

5. PHARMACOLOGICAL PROPERTIES

5.1 Pharmacodynamic properties

Pharmacotherapeutic group:

Progestagens and oestrogens, combinations, levonorgestrel and oestrogen

ATC code: G03F A11

Femseven Conti contains a continuous combined combination of oestrogen and progestagen for continuous use, combining estradiol hemihydrate and levonorgestrel.

Estradiol: The active substance, synthetic 17β-estradiol, is chemically and biologically identical to endogenous human estradiol. It substitutes for the loss of oestrogen production in menopausal women, and alleviates menopausal symptoms.

Levonorgestrel: As oestrogens promote the growth of the endometrium, unopposed oestrogens increase the risk of endometrial hyperplasia and cancer. The addition of levonorgestrel greatly reduces the oestrogen-induced risk of endometrial hyperplasia in non-hysterectomised women.

Clinical trial information

Relief of oestrogen-deficiency symptoms and bleeding patterns:

- Under treatment with Femseven Conti, relief of menopausal symptoms was achieved during the first weeks of treatment.
- Femseven Conti is a continuous-combined HRT given with the intent of avoiding the regular withdrawal bleeding associated with cyclic or sequential HRT.

Amenorrhoea (no bleeding or spotting) was seen in 59-68 % of the women during months 10-12 of treatment. Spottings were seen in 19-16 % of women within the same period. Break through bleeding and/or spotting appeared in 28-39 % of the women during the first three months of treatment and in 37 % during months 10-12 of treatment.

Women with longer-established menopause and with an atrophic endometrium will reach amenorrhoea earlier.

5.2 Pharmacokinetic properties

By transdermal administration there is no hepatic first-pass effect as observed with oral administration; estradiol reaches the bloodstream in unchanged form and in physiological amounts. Therapeutic estradiol concentrations are comparable to those observed in the follicular phase.

After continuous application of Femseven Conti, maximum plasma concentration of estradiol (C_{max}) reaches 82 pg/ml and average plasma concentration (C_{av}) is about 34 pg/ml. Trough plasma concentration (C_{trough}) at the end of a 7-day wearing period is 27 pg/ml. After removal of the transdermal patch, estradiol concentrations return to their baseline values within 12 to 24 hours.

The maximum plasma concentration of levonorgestrel is reached after three to four days and C_{max} is approximately 113 pg/ml at steady state. The average plasma concentration of levonorgestrel during a 7-day period is approximately 88 pg/ml and trough plasma concentration (C_{trough}) reaches 72 pg/ml.

After percutaneous absorption, levonorgestrel is bound to plasma proteins, i.e. albumin (50%), and sex hormone-binding globulin (SHBG) (47.5%). Affinity to SHBG is higher than for other commonly used progestagens.

5.3 Preclinical safety data

In experimental animals estradiol displayed an embryo-lethal effect already at relatively low doses; malformations of the urogenital tract and feminisation of male foetuses were observed. Levonorgestrel displayed an embryolethal effect in animal experiments and, in high doses, a virilising effect on female fetuses.

Because of marked differences between animal species and between animals and humans, preclinical results are of limited predictive value for the treatment of humans with oestrogens.

6. PHARMACEUTICAL PARTICULARS

6.1 List of excipients

Backing layer: Polyethylene terephthalate (PET) foil.

Adhesive matrix: Styrene-isoprene-styrene block copolymer, glycerine esters of completely hydrogenated resins.

Protective liner: Siliconized polyethylene terephthalate (PET) foil.

6.2 Incompatibilities

Not applicable.

6.3 Shelf life

2 years.

6.4 Special precautions for storage

Do not store above 30°C.

6.5 Nature and contents of container

Sachet (Paper/PE/aluminium/ethylene copolymer). Carton of 4 or 12 sachets.

6.6 Special precautions for disposal and other handling

See 4.2 Posology and method of administration.

No special requirements.

7. MARKETING AUTHORISATION HOLDER

Merck Serono Ltd
Bedfont Cross
Stanwell Road
Feltham
Middlesex
TW14 8NX
UK

8. MARKETING AUTHORISATION NUMBER(S)

PL 11648/0050

9. DATE OF FIRST AUTHORISATION/RENEWAL OF THE AUTHORISATION

5 November 2002

10. DATE OF REVISION OF THE TEXT

16 April 2008

FemSeven Sequi

(Merck Serono)

1. NAME OF THE MEDICINAL PRODUCT

FemSeven Sequi,
50 micrograms/10 micrograms/24 hours,
transdermal patch

2. QUALITATIVE AND QUANTITATIVE COMPOSITION

Phase 1:

Each patch contains 1.5 mg of estradiol hemihydrate in a patch size of 15 cm^2, releasing 50 micrograms of estradiol per 24 hours.

Phase 2:

Each patch contains 1.5 mg of estradiol hemihydrate and 1.5 mg of levonorgestrel in a patch size of 15 cm^2, releasing 50 micrograms of estradiol and 10 micrograms of levonorgestrel per 24 hours.

For excipients, see 6.1.

3. PHARMACEUTICAL FORM

Transdermal patch

Octagonal, transparent, flexible, rounded-edge transdermal matrix patch located on an oversized removable protective liner.

4. CLINICAL PARTICULARS

4.1 Therapeutic indications

Hormone replacement therapy (HRT) for oestrogen deficiency symptoms in post-menopausal women.

Experience of treating women older than 65 years is limited.

4.2 Posology and method of administration

For transdermal use.

Apply FemSeven Sequi once a week, i.e. replace each patch every 7 days. FemSeven Sequi is a continuous sequential hormone replacement therapy (HRT) without a treatment-off phase: as one patch is removed, the next is applied immediately.

Each treatment cycle with FemSeven Sequi consists of the successive application of two transdermal patches containing estradiol (phase 1) and then two transdermal patches containing estradiol and levonorgestrel (phase 2). Accordingly, the following treatment cycle should be observed:

- one phase 1 patch once a week for the first two weeks
- then one phase 2 patch once a week for the following two weeks.

In women who are not taking HRT or women who switch from a continuous combined HRT product, treatment may be started on any convenient day.

In women transferring from a sequential HRT regimen, treatment should begin the day following completion of the prior regimen.

For initiation and continuation of treatment of postmenopausal symptoms, the lowest effective dose for the shortest duration (see also section 4.4) should be used.

Method of administration

FemSeven Sequi should be applied to clean, dry, healthy skin (which is neither irritated nor grazed), free from any cream, lotion or other oily product.

FemSeven Sequi should be applied to an area of skin without major skin folds, e.g. the buttocks or hips, and not subject to chafing by clothing (avoid the waist and also avoid wearing tight clothing that could loosen the transdermal patch).

FemSeven Sequi must not be applied either on or near the breasts. It is advisable to avoid applying the patch to the same site twice. At least one week should be allowed to elapse between applications to the same site.

After opening the sachet, peel off one-half of the protective foil, being careful not to touch the adhesive part of the transdermal patch with the fingers. Apply directly to the skin. Now peel off the other half of the protective foil and press the patch on firmly with the palm of the hand for at least 30 seconds, concentrating on the edges. The pressure and the warmth of the hand are essential to ensure maximal adhesive strength of the patch.

It is possible to take a shower or have a bath without removing the transdermal patch.

Should a patch detach prematurely, before 7 days (due to vigorous physical activity, excessive sweating, abnormal chafing of clothing), it should be removed and a new patch of the same phase applied. To aid compliance it is recommended the patient then continues to change the patch on the usual day and according to the initial treatment cycle. This advice also applies if a patient forgets to change the patch on schedule. Forgetting a patch may increase the likelihood of break-through bleeding or spotting.

Once applied, the transdermal patch should not be exposed to sunlight.

Removal of the transdermal patch should be carried out slowly to avoid irritating the skin. In the event of some of the adhesive remaining on the skin, this can usually be removed by gently rubbing with a cream or an oily lotion.

After use, fold FemSeven Sequi in two (with the adhesive surface to the inside) and dispose of it with normal household solid waste.

4.3 Contraindications

- Known, past or suspected breast cancer;
- Known or suspected oestrogen-dependent malignant tumours (e.g. endometrial cancer);
- Undiagnosed genital bleeding;
- Untreated endometrial hyperplasia;
- Previous idiopathic or current venous thromboembolism (deep venous thrombosis, pulmonary embolism);
- Active or recent arterial thromboembolic disease (e.g. angina, myocardial infarction);
- Acute liver disease or a history of liver disease as long as liver function tests have failed to return to normal;
- Known hypersensitivity to the active substances or to any of the excipients;
- Porphyria.

4.4 Special warnings and precautions for use

For the treatment of postmenopausal symptoms, HRT should only be initiated for symptoms that adversely affect quality of life. In all cases, a careful appraisal of the risks and benefits should be undertaken at least annually and HRT should only be continued as long as the benefit outweighs the risk.

Medical examination/follow-up

Before initiating or reinstituting HRT, a complete personal and family medical history should be taken. Physical (including pelvic and breast) examination should be guided by this and by the contraindications and warnings for use. During treatment, periodic check-ups are recommended of a frequency and nature adapted to the individual woman.

Women should be advised what changes in their breasts should be reported to their doctor or nurse (see "Breast cancer" below). Investigations, including mammography, should be carried out in accordance with currently accepted screening practices, modified according to the clinical needs of the individual.

Conditions which need supervision

If any of the following conditions are present, have occurred previously and/or have been aggravated during pregnancy or previous hormone treatment, the patient should be closely supervised. It should be taken into account that these conditions may recur or be aggravated during treatment with FemSeven Sequi, in particular:

- Leiomyoma (uterine fibroids) or endometriosis
- A history of, or risk factors for, thromboembolic disorders (see below)
- Risk factors for oestrogen dependent tumours, e.g. 1st degree heredity for breast cancer
- Hypertension
- Liver disorders (e.g. liver adenoma)
- Diabetes mellitus with or without vascular involvement
- Cholelithiasis
- Migraine or (severe) headache
- Systemic lupus erythematosus
- A history of endometrial hyperplasia (see below)
- Epilepsy
- Asthma
- Otosclerosis.

Reasons for immediate withdrawal of therapy:

-Therapy should be discontinued if a contra-indication is discovered and in the following situations:

- Jaundice or deterioration in liver function
- Significant increase in blood pressure
- New onset of migraine-type headache
- Pregnancy.

Endometrial hyperplasia

- The risk of endometrial hyperplasia and carcinoma is increased when oestrogens are administered alone for prolonged periods (see section 4.8). The addition of a progestagen for at least 12 days per cycle in non-hysterectomised women greatly reduces this risk.

• Break-through bleeding and spotting may occur during the first months of treatment. If break-through bleeding or spotting appears after some time on therapy, or continues after treatment has been discontinued, the reason should be investigated, which may include endometrial biopsy to exclude endometrial malignancy.

Breast cancer

A randomised placebo-controlled trial, the Women's Health Initiative study (WHI), and epidemiological studies, including the Million Women Study (MWS), have reported an increased risk of breast cancer in women taking oestrogens, oestrogen-progestagen combinations or tibolone for HRT for several years (see section 4.8). For all HRT, an excess risk becomes apparent within a few years of use and increases with duration of intake but returns to baseline within a few (at most five) years after stopping treatment.

In the MWS, the relative risk of breast cancer with conjugated equine oestrogens (CEE) or estradiol (E2) was greater when a progestagen was added, eithersequentially or continuously, and regardless of type of progestagen. There was no evidence of a difference in risk between the different routes of administration.

In the WHI study, the continuous combined conjugated equine oestrogen and medroxyprogesterone acetate (CEE + MPA) product used was associated with breast cancers that were slightly larger in size and more frequently had local lymph node metastases compared to placebo.

HRT, especially oestrogen-progestagen combined treatment, increases the density of mammographic images which may adversely affect the radiological detection of breast cancer.

Venous thromboembolism

• HRT is associated with a higher relative risk of developing venous thromboembolism (VTE), i.e. deep vein thrombosis or pulmonary embolism. One randomised controlled trial and epidemiological studies found a two- to threefold higher risk for users compared with non-users. For non-users it is estimated that the number of cases of VTE that will occur over a 5 year period is about 3 per 1000 women aged 50-59 years and 8 per 1000 women aged between 60-69 years. It is estimated that in healthy women who use HRT for 5 years the number of additional cases of VTE over a 5 year period will be between 2 and 6 (best estimate = 4) per 1000 women aged 50-59 years and between 5 and 15 (best estimate = 9) per 1000 women aged 60-69 years. The occurrence of such an event is more likely in the first year of HRT than later.

• Generally recognized risk factors for VTE include a personal history or family history, severe obesity (BMI > 30 kg/m^2) and systemic lupus erythematosus (SLE). There is no consensus about the possible role of varicose veins in VTE.

• Patients with a history of VTE or known thrombophilic states have an increased risk of VTE. HRT may add to this risk. Personal or strong family history of thromboembolism or recurrent spontaneous abortion should be investigated in order to exclude a thrombophilic predisposition. Until a thorough evaluation of thrombophilic factors has been made or anticoagulant treatment initiated, use of HRT in such patients should be viewed as contra-indicated. Those women already on anticoagulant treatment require careful consideration of the benefit-risk of use of HRT.

• The risk of VTE may be temporarily increased with prolonged immobilisation, major trauma or major surgery. As in all postoperative patients, scrupulous attention should be given to prophylactic measures to prevent VTE following surgery. Where prolonged immobilisation is liable to follow elective surgery, particularly abdominal or orthopaedic surgery to the lower limbs, consideration should be given to temporarily stopping HRT four to six weeks earlier, if possible. Treatment should not be restarted until the woman is completely mobilised.

• If VTE develops after initiating therapy, the drug should be discontinued.

Patients should be told to contact their doctors immediately when they are aware of a potential thromboembolic symptom (e.g. painful swelling of a leg, sudden pain in the chest, dyspnea).

Coronary artery disease (CAD)

There is no evidence from randomised controlled trials of cardiovascular benefit with continuous combined conjugated oestrogens and medroxyprogesterone acetate (MPA). Two large clinical trials (WHI and HERS i.e. Heart and Estrogen/progestin Replacement Study) showed a possible increased risk of cardiovascular morbidity in the first year of use and no overall benefit. For other HRT products there are only limited data from randomised controlled trials examining effects in cardiovascular morbidity or mortality. Therefore, it is uncertain whether these findings also extend to other HRT products.

Stroke

One large randomised clinical trial (WHI-trial) found, as a secondary outcome, an increased risk of ischaemic stroke in healthy women during treatment with continuous combined conjugated oestrogens and MPA. For women who do not use HRT, it is estimated that the number of cases of stroke that will occur over a 5 year period is about 3 per 1000 women aged 50-59 years and 11 per 1000 women aged 60-69 years. It is estimated that for women who use conjugated oestrogens and MPA for 5 years, the number of additional cases will be between 0 and 3 (best estimate = 1) per 1000 users aged 50-59 years and between 1 and 9 (best estimate = 4) per 1000 users aged 60-69 years. It is unknown whether the increased risk also extends to other HRT products.

Ovarian cancer

Long-term (at least 5-10 years) use of oestrogen-only HRT products in hysterectomised women has been associated with an increased risk of ovarian cancer in some epidemiological studies. It is uncertain whether long-term use of combined HRT confers a different risk than oestrogen-only products.

Other conditions

Oestrogens may cause fluid retention, and therefore patients with cardiac or renal dysfunction should be carefully observed. Patients with terminal renal insufficiency should be closely observed, since it is expected that the level of circulating active ingredients in FemSeven Sequi transdermal patch is increased.

Women with pre-existing hypertriglyceridemia should be followed closely during oestrogen replacement or hormone replacement therapy, since rare cases of large increases of plasma triglycerides leading to pancreatitis have been reported with oestrogen therapy in this condition.

Oestrogens increase thyroid binding globulin (TBG), leading to increased circulating total thyroid hormone, as measured by protein-bound iodine (PBI), T4 levels (by column or by radio-immunoassay) or T3 levels (by radio-immunoassay). T3 resin uptake is decreased, reflecting the elevated TBG. Free T4 and free T3 concentrations are unaltered. Other binding proteins may be elevated in serum, i.e. corticoid binding globulin (CBG), sex-hormone-binding globulin (SHBG) leading to increased circulating corticosteroids and sex steroids, respectively. Free or biological active hormone concentrations are unchanged. Other plasma proteins may be increased (angiotensinogen/renin substrate, alpha-I-antitrypsin, ceruloplasmin).

There is no conclusive evidence for improvement of cognitive function. There is some evidence from the WHI trial of increased risk of probable dementia in women who start using continuous combined CEE and MPA after the age of 65. It is unknown whether the findings apply to younger post-menopausal women or other HRT products.

4.5 Interaction with other medicinal products and other forms of interaction

The metabolism of oestrogens and progestagens may be increased by concomitant use of substances known to induce drug-metabolising enzymes, specifically cytochrome P450 enzymes, such as anticonvulsants (e.g. phenobarbital, phenytoin, carbamazepine) and anti-infectives (e.g. rifampicin, rifabutin, nevirapine, efavirenz).

Ritonavir and nelfinavir, although known as strong inhibitors, by contrast exhibit inducing properties when used concomitantly with steroid hormones.

Herbal preparations containing St John's wort (*Hypericum Perforatum*) may induce the metabolism of oestrogens and progestagens.

At transdermal administration, the first-pass effect in the liver is avoided and, thus, transdermally applied oestrogens and progestagens might be less affected than oral hormones by enzyme inducers.

Clinically, an increased metabolism of oestrogens and progestagens may lead to decreased effect and changes in the uterine bleeding profile.

4.6 Pregnancy and lactation

Pregnancy:

FemSeven Sequi is not indicated during pregnancy. If pregnancy occurs during medication with FemSeven Sequi, treatment should be withdrawn immediately.

Clinically, data on a large number of exposed pregnancies indicate no adverse effects of levonorgestrel on the fœtus.

The results of most epidemiological studies to date relevant to inadvertent fœtal exposure to combinations of oestrogens and progestagens indicate no teratogenic or foetotoxic effects.

Lactation:

FemSeven Sequi is not indicated during lactation.

4.7 Effects on ability to drive and use machines

No effects on ability to drive and use machines have been observed.

4.8 Undesirable effects

The most frequently reported undesirable effects (> 10 %) in clinical trials during treatment with FemSeven Sequi were application site reactions. They usually disappeared 2 – 3 days after patch removal.

Other potential systemic undesirable effects are those commonly observed with oestrogen and progestin treatments.

(see Table 1 below)

Breast cancer

According to evidence from a large number of epidemiological studies and one randomised placebo-controlled trial, the Women's Health Initiative (WHI), the overall risk of breast cancer increases with increasing duration of HRT use in current or recent HRT users.

For *oestrogen-only* HRT, estimates of relative risk (RR) from a reanalysis of original data from 51 epidemiological studies (in which >80% of HRT use was oestrogen-only HRT) and from the epidemiological Million Women Study (MWS) are similar at 1.35 (95%CI: 1.21 – 1.49) and 1.30 (95%CI: 1.21 – 1.40), respectively.

For *oestrogen plus progestagen* combined HRT, several epidemiological studies have reported an overall higher risk for breast cancer than with oestrogens alone.

The MWS reported that, compared to never users, the use of various types of oestrogen-progestagen combined HRT was associated with a higher risk of breast cancer (RR = 2.00, 95%CI: 1.88 - 2.12) than use with oestrogens alone (RR = 1.30, 95%CI: 1.21 – 1.40) or use of tibolone (RR=1.45, 95%CI: 1.25 – 1.68).

The WHI trial reported a risk estimate of 1.24 (95%CI: 1.01 – 1.54) after 5.6 years of use of oestrogen-progestagen combined HRT (CEE + MPA) in all users compared with placebo.

The absolute risks calculated from the MWS and the WHI trial are presented below:

The MWS has estimated, from the known average incidence of breast cancer in developed countries that:

◆ For women not using HRT, about 32 in every 1000 are expected to have breast cancer diagnosed between the ages of 50 and 64 years.

◆ For 1000 current or recent users of HRT, the number of *additional* cases during the corresponding period will be

• For users of *oestrogen-only* replacement therapy

- between 0 and 3 (best estimate = 1.5) for 5 years' use
- between 3 and 7 (best estimate = 5) for 10 years' use.

• For users of *oestrogen plus progestogen* combined HRT,

- between 5 and 7 (best estimate = 6) for 5 years' use
- between 18 and 20 (best estimate = 19) for 10 years' use.

The WHI trial estimated that after 5.6 years of follow-up of women between the ages of 50 and 79 years, an *additional* 8 cases of invasive breast cancer would be due to *oestrogen-progestogen combined* HRT (CEE + MPA) per 10,000 women years.

According to calculations from the trial data, it is estimated that:

◆ For 1000 women in the placebo group,

• about 16 cases of invasive breast cancer would be diagnosed in 5 years.

◆ For 1000 women who used oestrogen + progestogen combined HRT (CEE + MPA), the number of *additional* cases would be

• between 0 and 9 (best estimate = 4) for 5 years' use.

The number of additional cases of breast cancer in women who use HRT is broadly similar for women who start HRT irrespective of age at start of use (between the ages of 45-65) (see section 4.4).

Endometrial cancer

In women with an intact uterus, the risk of endometrial hyperplasia and endometrial cancer increases with increasing duration of use of unopposed oestrogens.

Table 1

Organ system	Common ADRs > 1/100, < 1/10	Uncommon ADRs > 1/1000, < 1/100	Rare ADRs > 1/10,000, < 1/1000
Body as a whole	Headache, Mastodynia	Fluid retention/oedema/weight increase/loss, fatigue, dizziness, leg cramps, migraine	
Gastro-intestinal	Nausea, Vomiting	Bloating, abdominal cramps	Cholelithiasis, cholestatic jaundice
Cardio-vascular		Hypertension	
Reproductive	Breakthrough bleeding, spotting	Dysmenorrhoea, endometrial hyperplasia, benign breast tumours,	Increase in size of uterine fibrosis
Psychiatric	Increase/ decrease in libido		Depression

According to data from epidemiological studies, the best estimate of the risk is that for women not using HRT, about 5 in every 1000 are expected to have endometrial cancer diagnosed between the ages of 50 and 65. Depending on the duration of treatment and oestrogen dose, the reported increase in endometrial cancer risk among unopposed oestrogen users varies from 2-to 12-fold greater compared with non-users. Adding a progestagen to oestrogen-only therapy greatly reduces this increased risk.

Other adverse reactions have been reported in association with oestrogen/progestagen treatment:

- Oestrogen-dependent neoplasms benign and malignant: e.g. endometrial cancer.
- Venous thromboembolism, i.e. deep leg or pelvic venous thrombosis and pulmonary embolism, is more frequent among hormone replacement therapy users than among non-users. For further information see sections 4.3 Contra-indications and 4.4 Special warnings and precautions for use.
- Myocardial infarction and stroke.
- Gall bladder disease.
- Skin and subcutaneous disorders: chloasma, erythema multiforme, erythema nodosum, vascular purpura.
- Probable dementia (see section 4.4).

4.9 Overdose

The mode of administration makes significant overdose unlikely. Signs of an overdose are generally breast tenderness, swelling of the abdomen/pelvis, anxiety, irritability, nausea and vomiting. Removal of the transdermal patches is all that is required should it occur.

5. PHARMACOLOGICAL PROPERTIES

5.1 Pharmacodynamic properties

Pharmacotherapeutic group:

Progestogens and oestrogens for sequential administration

ATC code: G03FB 09

Transdermal route.

Estradiol: the active ingredient, synthetic 17β-estradiol is chemically and biologically identical to endogenous human estradiol. It substitutes for the loss of oestrogen production in postmenopausal women, and alleviates menopausal symptoms.

Levonorgestrel: as oestrogens promote the growth of the endometrium, unopposed oestrogens increase the risk of endometrial hyperplasia and cancer. The addition of levonorgestrel, a synthetic progestin, greatly reduces the oestrogen-induced risk of endometrial hyperplasia in non-hysterectomised women.

Under treatment with FemSeven Sequi, relief of menopausal symptoms was achieved during the first weeks of treatment.

At the end of one year treatment, 82.7% of women with bleeding reported regular withdrawal bleeding. The day of onset was rather constant 1 – 2 days before the end of the cycle with a mean duration of 4 - 5 days. The percentage of women with breakthrough bleeding and/or spotting was 17.3%. During the 13 cycles of therapy, 19.4% of women treated presented with amenorrhoea.

5.2 Pharmacokinetic properties

With transdermal administration there is no hepatic first-pass effect as observed with oral administration; estradiol reaches the bloodstream in unchanged form and in physiological amounts. Therapeutic estradiol concentrations are comparable to those observed in the follicular phase.

After application of the transdermal system containing estradiol alone (phase 1), therapeutic concentrations of estradiol are achieved within 4 hours; these concentrations are maintained throughout the entire application period of the transdermal patch (7 days). When estradiol is administered simultaneously with levonorgestrel (phase 2), the pharmacokinetics of estradiol are unaltered by levonorgestrel. Peak plasma concentrations of estradiol (C_{max}) range from 58 to 71 pg/ml, average plasma concentration (C_{av}) is between 29 to 33 pg/ml and trough plasma concentration (C_{pre}) is about 21 pg/ml during both treatment phases. After removal of the transdermal patch, estradiol concentrations return to their baseline values within 12 to 24 hours.

After application of the transdermal system containing estradiol and levonorgestrel at a dose of 10 μg/day (phase 2), the maximum plasma concentration of levonorgestrel (C_{max}) range from 156 to 189 pg/ml and is reached within 63 to 91 hours (t_{max}). The average plasma concentration of levonorgestrel (C_{av}) during a 7-day period is between 121 and 156 pg/ml and the trough plasma concentration (C_{pre}) levels are 118 pg/ml. The half-life of levonorgestrel after transdermal application is approximately 28 hours (minimum: 16 hours, maximum: 42 hours).

After percutaneous absorption, levonorgestrel is bound to plasma proteins, i.e. albumin (50%), and SHBG (47.5%). Affinity to SHBG is higher than for other commonly used progestogens.

5.3 Preclinical safety data

Animal studies with estradiol and levonorgestrel have shown expected estrogenic and gestagenic effects.

There are no preclinical data of relevance to the prescriber that are additional to those already included in other sections of the SPC (see notably section 4.6).

6. PHARMACEUTICAL PARTICULARS

6.1 List of excipients

Backing layer Transparent polyethylene terephthalate (PET) foil

Adhesive matrix: Styrene-isoprene-styrene block copolymer, glycerine esters of completely hydrogenated resins

Protective liner: Siliconized transparent polyethylene terephthalate (PET) foil.

6.2 Incompatibilities

Not applicable.

6.3 Shelf life

2 years

6.4 Special precautions for storage

Do not store above 30°C

6.5 Nature and contents of container

Each phase 1 or phase 2 transdermal patch is contained in an individual sachet (Paper/PE/aluminium/ethylene copolymer). Each carton contains 4 or 12 sachets consisting of 2 × phase 1 patches and 2 × phase 2 patches or 6 × phase 1 patches and 6 × phase 2 patches.

6.6 Special precautions for disposal and other handling

See 4.2 Posology and method of administration

7. MARKETING AUTHORISATION HOLDER

Merck Ltd. (t/a Merck Pharmaceuticals (A division of Merck Ltd.))

Harrier House

High Street

West Drayton

Middlesex

UB7 7QG

UK

8. MARKETING AUTHORISATION NUMBER(S)

PL 11648/0044

9. DATE OF FIRST AUTHORISATION/RENEWAL OF THE AUTHORISATION

27 September 2005

10. DATE OF REVISION OF THE TEXT

27 September 2005

Femulen Tablets

(Pharmacia Limited)

1. NAME OF THE MEDICINAL PRODUCT

Femulen.

2. QUALITATIVE AND QUANTITATIVE COMPOSITION

Each tablet contains 500 micrograms etynodiol diacetate.

3. PHARMACEUTICAL FORM

White tablet inscribed "SEARLE" on both sides.

4. CLINICAL PARTICULARS

4.1 Therapeutic indications

Oral contraception.

4.2 Posology and method of administration

Starting on the first day of menstruation, one pill every day without a break in medication for as long as contraception is required. Additional contraceptive precautions (such as a condom) should be used for the first 7 days of the first pack. Pills should be taken at the same time each day.

Missed Pills

If a pill is missed within 3 hours of the correct dosage time then the missed pill should be taken as soon as possible; this will ensure that contraceptive protection is maintained. If a pill is taken 3 or more hours late it is recommended that the woman takes the last missed pill as soon as possible and then continues to take the rest of the pills in the normal manner. However, to provide continued contraceptive protection it is recommended that an alternative method of contraception, such as a condom, is used for the next 7 days.

Changing from another oral contraceptive

In order to ensure that contraception is maintained it is advised that the first pill is taken on the day immediately after the patient has finished the previous pack.

Use after childbirth, miscarriage or abortion

The first pill should be taken on the 21st day after childbirth. This will ensure the patient is protected immediately. If there is any delay in taking the first pill, contraception may not be established until 7 days after the first pill has been taken. In these circumstances women should be advised that extra contraceptive methods will be necessary.

After a miscarriage or abortion patients can take the first pill on the next day; in this way they will be protected immediately.

Vomiting or diarrhoea

Gastrointestinal upsets, such as vomiting and diarrhoea, may interfere with the absorption of the pill leading to a reduction in contraceptive efficacy. Women should continue to take Femulen, but they should also be advised to use another contraceptive method during the period of gastrointestinal upset and for the next 7 days.

4.3 Contraindications

The contraindications for progestogen-only oral contraceptives are:

(i) Known, suspected, or a past history of breast, genital or hormone dependent cancer;

(ii) Acute or severe chronic liver diseases including past or present liver tumours, Dubin-Johnson or Rotor syndrome;

(iii) Active liver disease;

(iv) History during pregnancy of idiopathic jaundice or severe pruritus;

(v) Disorders of lipid metabolism;

(vi) Undiagnosed abnormal vaginal bleeding;

(vii) Known or suspected pregnancy;

(viii) Hypersensitivity to any component.

Combined oestrogen/progestogen preparations have been associated with an increase in the risk of thromboembolic and thrombotic disease. Risk has been reported to be related to both oestrogenic and progestogenic activity. In the absence of long term epidemiological studies with progestogen-only oral contraceptives, it is required that the existence, or history of thrombophlebitis, thromboembolic disorders, cerebral vascular disease, myocardial infarction, angina, coronary artery disease, or a haemoglobinopathy be described as a contraindication to Femulen as it is to oestrogen containing oral contraceptives.

4.4 Special warnings and precautions for use

Assessment of women prior to starting oral contraceptives (and at regular intervals thereafter) should include a personal and family medical history of each woman. Physical examination should be guided by this and by the contraindications (section 4.3) and warnings (section 4.4) for this product. The frequency and nature of these assessments should be based upon relevant guidelines and should be adapted to the individual woman, but should include measurement of blood pressure and, if judged appropriate by the clinician, breast, abdominal and pelvic examination including cervical cytology.

Femulen should be discontinued if there is a gradual or sudden, partial or complete loss of vision or any evidence of ocular changes, onset or aggravation of migraine or development of headache of a new kind which is recurrent, persistent or severe, suspicion of thrombosis or infarction, significant rise in blood pressure or if jaundice occurs.

Malignant hepatic tumours have been reported on rare occasions in long-term users of contraceptives. Benign hepatic tumours have also been associated with oral contraceptive usage. A hepatic tumour should be considered in the differential diagnosis when upper abdominal pain, enlarged liver or signs of intra-abdominal haemorrhage occur.

Progestogen-only oral contraceptives may offer less protection against ectopic pregnancy, than against intrauterine pregnancy.

Femulen should be discontinued at least 4 weeks before elective surgery or during periods of prolonged immobilisation. It would be reasonable to resume Femulen two weeks after surgery provided the woman is ambulant. However, every woman, should be considered individually with regard to the nature of the operation, the extent of immobilisation, the presence of additional risk factors and the chance of unwanted conception.

Caution should be exercised where there is the possibility of an interaction between a pre-existing disorder and a known or suspected side effect. The use of Femulen in women suffering from epilepsy, or with a history of migraine or cardiac or renal dysfunction may result in exacerbation of these disorders because of fluid retention. Caution should also be observed in women who wear contact lenses, women with impaired carbohydrate tolerance, depression, gallstones, a past history of liver disease, varicose veins, hypertension, asthma or any disease that is prone to worsen during pregnancy (eg. multiple sclerosis, porphyria, tetany and otosclerosis). Progestogen-only oral contraceptives may offer less protection against ectopic pregnancy, than against intrauterine pregnancy.

A meta-analysis from 54 epidemiological studies reported that there is a slightly increased relative risk of having breast cancer diagnosed in women who are currently using oral contraceptives (OC). The observed pattern of increased risk may be due to an earlier diagnosis of breast cancer in OC users, the biological effects of OCs or a combination of both. The additional breast cancers diagnosed in current users of OCs or in women who have used OCs in the last ten years are more likely to be localised to the breast than those in women who never used OCs.

Breast cancer is rare among women under 40 years of age whether or not they take OCs. Whilst the background risk increases with age, the excess number of breast cancer diagnoses in current and recent progesterone-only pill (POP) users is small in relation to the overall risk of breast cancer, possibly of similar magnitude to that associated with combined OCs. However, for POPs, the evidence is based on much smaller populations of users and so is less conclusive than that for combined OCs.

The most important risk factor for breast cancer in POP users is the age women discontinue the POP; the older the age at stopping, the more breast cancers are diagnosed. Duration of use is less important and the excess risk gradually disappears during the course of the 10 years after stopping POP use, such that by 10 years there appears to be no excess.

The evidence suggests that compared with never-users, among 10,000 women who use POPs for up to 5 years but stop by age 20, there would be much less than 1 extra case of breast cancer diagnosed up to 10 years afterwards. For those stopping by age 30 after 5 years use of the POP, there would be an estimated 2-3 extra cases (additional to the 44 cases of breast cancer per 10,000 women in this age group never exposed to oral contraceptives). For those stopping by age 40 after 5 years use, there would be an estimated 10 extra cases diagnosed up to 10 years afterwards (additional to the 160 cases of breast cancer per 10,000 never-exposed women in this age group).

It is important to inform patients that users of all contraceptive pills appear to have a small increase in the risk of being diagnosed with breast cancer, compared with non-users of oral contraceptives, but this has to be weighed against the known benefits.

4.5 Interaction with other medicinal products and other forms of interaction

Drug Interactions

The herbal remedy St John's wort (*Hypericum perforatum*) should not be taken concomitantly with this medicine as this could potentially lead to a loss of contraceptive effect.

Some drugs may modify the metabolism of Femulen reducing its effectiveness; these include certain sedatives, antibiotics, anti-epileptic and anti-arthritic drugs. During the time such agents are used concurrently, it is advised that mechanical contraceptives also be used.

4.6 Pregnancy and lactation

Pregnancy

Femulen is contraindicated in women with suspected pregnancy. Several reports suggest an association between foetal exposure to female sex hormones, including oral contraceptives, and congenital anomalies.

Lactation

There is no evidence that progestogen - only oral contraceptives diminish the yield of breast milk. In a study of nursing mothers taking Femulen, the median percentage of norethisterone, the principal metabolite of etynodiol diacetate given to the mother which was ingested by the infant was 0.02%. No adverse effect of the drug on the infants was noted.

4.7 Effects on ability to drive and use machines

None known.

4.8 Undesirable effects

Clinical investigations with Femulen indicate that side effects are infrequent and tend to decrease with time. Known or suspected side effects of progestogen-only oral contraceptives include gastrointestinal disorders such as nausea and vomiting, skin disorders including chloasma, breast changes, ocular changes, headache, migraine and depression, appetite and weight changes, changes in libido, increase in size of uterine myofibromata, and changes in carbohydrate, lipid or vitamin metabolism. Rarely dizziness, hirsutism and colitis have been reported in users of progestogen-only oral contraceptive.

The use of oral contraceptives has also been associated with a possible increased incidence of gallbladder disease.

Tests of endocrine, hepatic and thyroid function, as well as coagulation tests may be affected by Femulen.

Menstrual pattern: Women taking Femulen for the first time should be informed that they may initially experience menstrual irregularity. This may include amenorrhoea, prolonged bleeding and/or spotting but such irregularity tends to decrease with time. If a woman misses two consecutive periods, pregnancy should be ruled out before continuing the contraceptive regimen.

4.9 Overdose

Serious ill effects have not been reported following acute ingestion of large doses of oral contraceptives by young children. Nausea and vomiting may occur and vaginal withdrawal bleeding may present in pre-pubertal girls. There is no specific antidote and treatment should be symptomatic. Gastric lavage may be employed if the overdose is large and the patient is seen sufficiently early (within four hours).

5. PHARMACOLOGICAL PROPERTIES

5.1 Pharmacodynamic properties

Femulen does not necessarily inhibit ovulation but it is believed to discourage implantation of the fertilised ovum by altering the endometrium. Cervical mucus viscosity is also changed which may render the passage of sperm less likely.

5.2 Pharmacokinetic properties

Etynodiol diacetate is readily absorbed from the gastrointestinal tract and rapidly metabolised, largely to norethisterone. Following administration of a radiolabelled dose of etynodiol diacetate about 60% of the radioactivity is stated to be excreted in urine and about 30% in faeces; half life in plasma was about 25 hours.

5.3 Preclinical safety data

The toxicity of norethisterone is very low. Reports of teratogenic effects in animals are uncommon. No carcinogenic effects have been found even in long-term studies. In subacute and chronic studies only minimal differences between treated and control animals are observed.

6. PHARMACEUTICAL PARTICULARS

6.1 List of excipients

Calcium phosphate dibasic anhydrous, maize starch, polyvinyl pyrrolidine, sodium phosphate dibasic anhydrous, calcium acetate anhydrous, thixcin R (hydrogenated castor oil).

6.2 Incompatibilities

None known.

6.3 Shelf life

The shelf life of Femulen is 5 years.

6.4 Special precautions for storage

Store in a dry place below 30°C.

6.5 Nature and contents of container

Femulen tablets are stored in PVC/foil blister packs of 28 and 84 tablets.

6.6 Special precautions for disposal and other handling

None.

7. MARKETING AUTHORISATION HOLDER

Pharmacia Limited

Ramsgate Road

Sandwich

Kent CT13 9NJ, UK

8. MARKETING AUTHORISATION NUMBER(S)

PL 00032/0406

9. DATE OF FIRST AUTHORISATION/RENEWAL OF THE AUTHORISATION

1st September 2002

10. DATE OF REVISION OF THE TEXT

June 2007

FU 2_0

Fendrix

(GlaxoSmithKline UK)

1. NAME OF THE MEDICINAL PRODUCT

Fendrix suspension for injection.

Hepatitis B (rDNA) vaccine (adjuvanted, adsorbed).

2. QUALITATIVE AND QUANTITATIVE COMPOSITION

1 dose (0.5 ml) of Fendrix contains:

Hepatitis B surface antigen [1, 2, 3]

20 micrograms

[1]adjuvanted by AS04C containing:

- 3-*O*-desacyl-4'- monophosphoryl lipid A (MPL) [2]

50 micrograms

[2]adsorbed on aluminium phosphate (0.5 milligrams Al^{3+} in total)

[3]produced in yeast cells (*Saccharomyces cerevisiae*) by recombinant DNA technology.

For a full list of excipients, see section 6.1

3. PHARMACEUTICAL FORM

Suspension for injection.

Turbid white suspension. Upon storage, a fine white deposit with a clear colourless supernatant can be observed.

4. CLINICAL PARTICULARS

4.1 Therapeutic indications

Fendrix is indicated for active immunisation against hepatitis B virus infection (HBV) caused by all known subtypes for patients with renal insufficiency (including pre-haemodialysis and haemodialysis patients), from the age of 15 years onwards.

4.2 Posology and method of administration

Posology

Primary Immunisation schedule:

A four dose schedule, with immunisations at the elected date, 1 month, 2 months and 6 months from the date of the first dose is recommended.

Once initiated, the primary course of vaccination at 0, 1, 2 and 6 months should be completed with Fendrix, and not with other commercially available HBV vaccine.

Booster dose:

As pre-haemodialysis and haemodialysis patients are particularly exposed to HBV and have a higher risk to become chronically infected, a precautionary attitude should be considered i.e. giving a booster dose in order to ensure a protective antibody level as defined by national recommendations and guidelines.

Fendrix can be used as a booster dose after a primary vaccination course with either Fendrix or any other commercial recombinant hepatitis B vaccine.

Special dosage recommendation for known or presumed exposure to HBV:

Data on concomitant administration of Fendrix with specific hepatitis B immunoglobulin (HBIg) have not been generated. However, in circumstances where exposure to HBV has recently occurred (e.g. stick with contaminated needle) and where simultaneous administration of Fendrix and a standard dose of HBIg is necessary, these should be given at separate injection sites.

Method of administration

Fendrix should be injected intramuscularly in the deltoid region.

4.3 Contraindications

Hypersensitivity to the active substance or to any of the excipients.

Hypersensitivity after previous administration of other hepatitis B vaccines.

Subjects suffering from acute severe febrile illness. The presence of a minor infection such as a cold, is not a contraindication for immunisation.

4.4 Special warnings and precautions for use

Because of the long incubation period of hepatitis B, it is possible that patients could have been infected before the time of immunisation. The vaccine may not prevent hepatitis B infection in such cases.

The vaccine will not prevent infection caused by other agents such as hepatitis A, hepatitis C and hepatitis E or other pathogens known to infect the liver.

As with any vaccine, a protective immune response may not be elicited in all vaccinees.

A number of factors have been observed to reduce the immune response to hepatitis B vaccines. These factors include older age, male gender, obesity, smoking, route of administration, and some chronic underlying diseases. Consideration should be given to serological testing of those subjects who may be at risk of not achieving seroprotection following a complete course of Fendrix. Additional doses may need to be considered for persons who do not respond or have a sub-optimal response to a course of vaccinations.

Since intramuscular administration into the gluteal muscle could lead to a suboptimal response to the vaccine, this route should be avoided.

Fendrix should under no circumstances be administered intradermally or intravenously.

Patients with chronic liver disease or with HIV infection or hepatitis C carriers should not be precluded from vaccination against hepatitis B. The vaccine could be advised since HBV infection can be severe in these patients: the Hepatitis B vaccination should thus be considered on a casebycase basis by the physician.

Thiomersal (an organomercuric compound) has been used in the manufacturing process of this medicinal product and residues of it are present in the final product. Therefore, sensitisation reactions may occur.

Appropriate medical treatment should always be readily available in case of rare anaphylactic reactions following the administration of the vaccine.

4.5 Interaction with other medicinal products and other forms of interaction

No data on the concomitant administration of Fendrix and other vaccines or with specific hepatitis B immunoglobulin have been generated. If concomitant administration of specific hepatitis B immunoglobulin and Fendrix is required, these should be given at different injection sites. As no data are available for the concomitant administration of this particular vaccine with other vaccines, an interval of 2 to 3 weeks should be respected.

4.6 Pregnancy and lactation

No clinical data on use during pregnancies are available with Fendrix.

Animal studies do not indicate direct or indirect harmful effects with respect to pregnancy, embryonal/foetal development, parturition or postnatal development.

Vaccination during pregnancy should only be performed if the risk-benefit ratio at individual level outweighs possible risks for the foetus.

Adequate human data on use during lactation are not available. In a reproductive toxicity study in animals which included post-natal follow-up until weaning (see section 5.3), no effect on the development of the pups was observed. Vaccination should only be performed if the risk-benefit ratio at individual level outweighs possible risks for the infant.

4.7 Effects on ability to drive and use machines

Fendrix has a minor or moderate influence on the ability to drive and use machine.

Some of the undesirable effects mentioned under section 4.8 may affect the ability to drive or operate machinery.

4.8 Undesirable effects

- Clinical trials involving the administration of 2476 doses of Fendrix to 82 pre-haemodialysis and haemodialysis patients and to 713 healthy subjects ⩾ 15 years of age allowed to document the reactogenicity of the vaccine.

Pre-haemodialysis and haemodialysis patients

The reactogenicity profile of Fendrix in a total of 82 pre-haemodialysis and haemodialysis patients was generally comparable to that seen in healthy subjects.

Adverse reactions reported in a clinical trial following primary vaccination with Fendrix and considered as being related or possibly related to vaccination have been categorised by frequency.

Frequencies are reported as:

Very common: (⩾1/10)

Common: (⩾1/100 to <1/10)

Uncommon: (⩾1/1,000 to <1/100)

Rare: (⩾1/10,000 to <1/1,000)

Very rare: (<1/10,000)

Within each frequency grouping, undesirable effects are presented in order of decreasing seriousness.

Nervous system disorders:

Very common: headache

Gastrointestinal disorders:

Common: gastrointestinal disorder

General disorders and administration site conditions

Very common: fatigue, pain *Common:* fever, injection site swelling, redness

Unsolicited symptoms considered to be at least possibly related to vaccination were uncommonly reported and consisted of rigors, other injection site reaction and maculo-papular rash.

Healthy subjects

The reactogenicity profile of Fendrix in healthy subjects was generally comparable to that seen in pre-haemodialysis and haemodialysis patients.

In a large double-blind randomised comparative study, healthy subjects were enrolled to receive a three dose primary course of Fendrix (N= 713) or a commercially available hepatitis B vaccine (N= 238) at 0, 1, 2 months. Fendrix was generally well tolerated. The most common adverse events reported were local reactions at the injection site.

Vaccination with Fendrix induced more transient local symptoms as compared to the comparator vaccine, with pain at the injection site being the most frequently reported solicited local symptom. However, solicited general symptoms were observed with similar frequencies in both groups.

Adverse reactions reported in a clinical trial following primary vaccination with Fendrix and considered as being at least possibly related to vaccination have been categorised by frequency.

Nervous system disorders:

Common: headache

Ear and labyrinth disorders:

Rare: vertigo

Gastrointestinal disorders:

Common: gastrointestinal disorder

Muskuloskeletal and connective tissue disorders:

Rare: tendinitis, back pain

Infections and infestations:

Rare: viral infection

General disorders and administration site conditions

Very common: injection site swelling, fatigue, pain, redness

Common: fever

Uncommon: other injection site reaction

Rare: rigors, hot flushes, thirst, asthenia

Immune system disorders:

Rare: allergy

Psychiatric disorders:

Rare: nervousness

No increase in the incidence or severity of these undesirable events was seen with subsequent doses of the primary vaccination schedule.

No increase in the reactogenicity was observed after the booster vaccination with respect to the primary vaccination.

Allergic reactions, including anaphylactoid reactions, may occur very rarely.

• Experience with hepatitis B vaccine:

Following widespread use of hepatitis B vaccines, in very rare cases, syncope, paralysis, neuropathy, neuritis (including Guillain-Barré syndrome, optic neuritis and multiple sclerosis), encephalitis, encephalopathy, meningitis and convulsions have been reported. The causal relationship to the vaccine has not been established.

4.9 Overdose

No case of overdose has been reported.

5. PHARMACOLOGICAL PROPERTIES

5.1 Pharmacodynamic properties

Pharmacotherapeutic group: Hepatitis vaccines, ATC code J07BC01.

Fendrix induces specific humoral antibodies against HBsAg (anti-HBs antibodies). An anti-HBs antibody titre ⩾ 10 mIU/ml correlates with protection to HBV infection.

It can be expected that hepatitis D will also be prevented by immunisation with Fendrix as hepatitis D (caused by the delta agent) does not occur in the absence of hepatitis B infection.

Immunological data

In pre-haemodialysis and haemodialysis patients:

In a comparative clinical study in 165 pre-haemodialysis and haemodialysis patients (15 years and above), protective levels of specific humoral antibodies (anti-HBs titres ⩾ 10 mIU/ml) were observed in 74.4% of Fendrix recipients (N = 82) one month after the third dose (i.e at month 3), as compared to 52.4% of patients in the control group who received a double dose of a commercially available hepatitis B vaccine (N = 83) for this population.

At month 3, Geometric Mean Titres (GMT) were 223.0 mIU/ml and 50.1 mIU/ml in the Fendrix and control groups respectively, with 41.0% and 15.9% of subjects with anti-HBs antibody titres ⩾100 mIU/ml respectively.

After completion of a four dose primary course (i.e at month 7), 90.9% of Fendrix recipients were seroprotected (⩾ 10 mIU/ml) against hepatitis B, in comparison with 84.4% in a control group who received the commercially available hepatitis B vaccine.

At month 7, GMTs were 3559.2 mIU/ml and 933.0 mIU/ml in the Fendrix and control groups who received the commercially available hepatitis B vaccine respectively, with 83.1% and 67.5% of subjects with anti-HBs antibody titres ⩾100 mIU/ml respectively.

Antibody persistence

In pre-haemodialysis and haemodialysis patients:

Anti-HBs antibodies have been shown to persist for at least 36 months following a 0, 1, 2, 6 month primary course of Fendrix in pre-haemodialysis and haemodialysis patients. At month 36, 80.4% of these patients retained protective antibody levels (anti-HBs titres ⩾ 10mIU/ml), as compared to 51.3% of patients who received a commercially available hepatitis B vaccine.

At month 36, GMTs were 154.1 mIU/ml and 111.9 mIU/ml in the Fendrix and control groups respectively, with 58.7% and 38.5% of subjects with anti-HBs antibody titres ⩾100 mIU/ml respectively.

5.2 Pharmacokinetic properties

Pharmacokinetic properties of Fendrix or MPL alone has not been studied in humans.

5.3 Preclinical safety data

Non-clinical data reveal no special hazard for humans based on conventional animal studies consisting of acute and repeated dose toxicity, cardiovascular and respiratory safety pharmacology and reproductive toxicity including pregnancy and peri and postnatal development of the pups till weaning (see section 4.6).

6. PHARMACEUTICAL PARTICULARS

6.1 List of excipients

Sodium chloride

Water for injections

For adjuvants, see section 2.

6.2 Incompatibilities

In the absence of compatibility studies, this medicinal product must not be mixed with other medicinal products.

6.3 Shelf life

3 years.

6.4 Special precautions for storage

Store in a refrigerator (2°C – 8°C).

Do not freeze.

Store in the original package in order to protect from light.

6.5 Nature and contents of container

0.5 ml of suspension in pre-filled syringe (type I glass) with a plunger stopper (rubber butyl) with or without separate needle in a pack size of 1, or without needles in a pack size of 10.

Not all pack sizes may be marketed.

6.6 Special precautions for disposal and other handling

Upon storage, a fine white deposit with a clear colourless supernatant can be observed.

Before administration, the vaccine should be well shaken to obtain a slightly opaque, white suspension.

The vaccine should be visually inspected both before and after re-suspension for any foreign particulate matter and/or change in physical appearance. The vaccine must not be used if any change in the appearance of the vaccine has taken place.

Any unused vaccine or waste material should be disposed of in accordance with local requirements.

7. MARKETING AUTHORISATION HOLDER

GlaxoSmithKline Biologicals s.a.

Rue de l'Institut 89

B-1330 Rixensart, Belgium

8. MARKETING AUTHORISATION NUMBER(S)

EU/1/04/0299/001

EU/1/04/0299/002

EU/1/04/0299/003

9. DATE OF FIRST AUTHORISATION/RENEWAL OF THE AUTHORISATION

Date of first authorisation: 02 February 2005

10. DATE OF REVISION OF THE TEXT

02 March 2009

Detailed information on this product is available on the website of the European Medicines Agency (EMEA) http://www.emea.europa.eu

Fentalis Reservoir Transdermal Patches

(Sandoz Limited)

1. NAME OF THE MEDICINAL PRODUCT

Fentalis Reservoir 25 microgram/hour transdermal patches

Fentalis Reservoir 50 microgram/hour transdermal patches

Fentalis Reservoir 75 microgram/hour transdermal patches

Fentalis Reservoir 100 microgram/hour transdermal patches

2. QUALITATIVE AND QUANTITATIVE COMPOSITION

Fentalis Reservoir 25 microgram/hour transdermal patches:

Each transdermal patch (active surface area 10 cm^2) contains 2.5 mg fentanyl (corresponding to 25 microgram/hour fentanyl release rate).

Fentalis Reservoir 50 microgram/hour transdermal patches:

Each transdermal patch (active surface area 20 cm^2) contains 5.0 mg fentanyl (corresponding to 50 microgram/hour fentanyl release rate).

Fentalis Reservoir 75 microgram/hour transdermal patches:

Each transdermal patch (active surface area 30 cm^2) contains 7.5 mg fentanyl (corresponding to 75 microgram/hour fentanyl release rate).

Fentalis Reservoir 100 microgram/hour transdermal patches:

Each transdermal patch (active surface area 40 cm^2) contains 10.0 mg fentanyl (corresponding to 100 microgram/hour fentanyl release rate).

For excipients, see section 6.1.

3. PHARMACEUTICAL FORM

Transdermal patch

Transparent and oblong transdermal patch which consists of a protective layer (to be removed prior to application of the patch) and four functional layers: an occlusive backing, a drug reservoir, a release membrane and an adhesive surface.

Surface area of the transdermal patch:

Fentanyl 25 microgram/hour transdermal patches: 10 cm^2

Fentanyl 50 microgram/hour transdermal patches: 20 cm^2

Fentanyl 75 microgram/hour transdermal patches: 30 cm^2

Fentanyl 100 microgram/hour transdermal patches: 40 cm^2

4. CLINICAL PARTICULARS

4.1 Therapeutic indications

Chronic severe pain requiring treatment with opioid analgesics, e.g. cancer pain.

4.2 Posology and method of administration

Fentalis Reservoir 25 microgram/hour transdermal patches:

Fentalis Reservoir transdermal patches release the active substance over 72 hours. The fentanyl release rate is 25 microgram/hour and the corresponding active surface area is 10 cm^2.

Fentalis Reservoir 50 microgram/hour transdermal patches:

Fentalis Reservoir transdermal patches release the active substance over 72 hours. The fentanyl release rate is 50 microgram/hour and the corresponding active surface area is 20 cm^2.

Fentalis Reservoir 75 microgram/hour transdermal patches:

Fentalis Reservoir transdermal patches release the active substance over 72 hours. The fentanyl release rate is 75 microgram/hour and the corresponding active surface area is 30 cm^2.

Fentalis Reservoir 100 microgram/hour transdermal patches:

Fentalis Reservoir transdermal patches release the active substance over 72 hours. The fentanyl release rate is 100 microgram/hour and the corresponding active surface area is 40 cm^2.

The required fentanyl dosage is adjusted individually and should be assessed regularly after each administration.

Choice of initial dosage: The dosage level of fentanyl is based upon the previous use of opioids and takes into account the possible development of tolerance, concomitant medicinal treatment, the patient's general state of health and the degree of severity of the disorder.

In opioid-naive patients, who have not previously been treated with opioids, the initial dosage should not exceed 25 microgram/hour.

Changing from other opioid treatment

When changing over from oral or parenteral opioids to fentanyl treatment, the initial dosage should be calculated as follows:

1. The quantity of analgesics required over the last 24 hours should be determined.

2. The obtained sum should be converted to correspond the oral morphine dosage using Table 1.

3. The corresponding fentanyl dosage should be determined using Table 2.

Table 1: Equianalgesic efficacy of medicinal products

All i.m. and oral dosages given in the table are equivalent in analgesic effect to 10 mg morphine administered intramuscularly.

Name of medicinal product	Equianalgesic dosage (mg)	
	i.m.*	Oral
Morphine	10	30 (assuming repeated administration)**
		60 (assuming a single dose or occasional doses)
Hydromorphine	1.5	7.5
Methadone	10	20
Oxycodone	10-15	20-30
Levorphanol	2	4
Oxymorphine	1	10 (rectal)
Diamorphine	5	60
Pethidine	75	
Codeine	130	200
Buprenorphine	0.4	0.8 (sublingual)
Ketobemidone	10	30

[Ref.: Foley KM: The Treatment of Cancer Pain. NEJM 1985; 313 (2): 84-95.]

*Based on studies conducted with single doses, in which the i.m. dosage of each above-mentioned agent was compared with morphine in order to achieve an equivalent efficacy. Oral dosages are the recommended dosages when changing from parenteral to oral administration.

** The efficacy ratio of 3:1 for morphine i.m./oral dosage is based upon a study conducted in patients suffering from chronic pain.

*Table 2: Recommended dosage of Fentanyl transdermal patches based upon the oral daily morphine dosage**

Oral morphine (mg/24 h)	Dosage of Fentanyl transdermal patches (µg/h)
<135	25
135-224	50
225-314	75
315-404	100
405-494	125
495-584	150
585-674	175
675-764	200
765-854	225
855-944	250
945-1034	275
1035-1124	300

* These oral morphine dosages were used as a basis in clinical trials when changing medication to fentanyl transdermal patches. Other conversion schemes which have proved their usefulness in clinical practice are existing and may be applied.

Both in opioid-naive patients and in those who have previously used opioids, the maximum analgesic efficacy of Fentalis Reservoir transdermal patches cannot be evaluated until the transdermal patch has been in situ for 24 hours, since the serum concentration of fentanyl rises gradually over a period of 24 hours. Previous analgesic treatment should therefore not be discontinued before 12 hours after the application of the first transdermal patch, then administered as needed.

Determination of the dosage level, and the maintenance dosage: The Fentalis Reservoir transdermal patch is replaced at intervals of 72 hours. In patients who experience a marked decrease in analgesia in the period of 48-72 hours after application, replacement of the Fentalis Reservoir transdermal patch after 48 hours may be necessary. The dosage is titrated individually, until the analgesic effect is attained. If analgesia is inadequate at the end of the initial application period, the dosage may be increased at intervals of 3 days, until the desired effect is obtained for each patient. The dosage is normally raised in increments of 25 microgram/hour, but the need for additional medication and the pain experienced by the patient should be taken into account. When the required dosage exceeds 100 microgram/hour, several transdermal patches may be used at the same time. Patients may require a short-acting analgesic for so-called "breakthrough" pain. Additional or alternative methods of analgesia should be considered when the Fentalis Reservoir transdermal patch dose exceeds 300 microgram/hour.

Conversion or discontinuation of treatment

To convert patients to another opioid, Fentalis Reservoir transdermal patch is removed and the dose of the new analgesic titrated based upon the patient's report of pain until adequate analgesia has been attained. Opioid withdrawal symptoms (such as nausea, vomiting, diarrhaea, anxiety and muscular tremor) are possible in some patients after conversion or dose reduction. For patients requiring discontinuation of Fentalis Reservoir transdermal patches, a gradual downward titration is recommended since it is not known at what dose level the opioid may be discontinued without producing the signs and symptoms of abrupt withdrawal. Fentanyl levels fall gradually after Fentalis Reservoir transdermal patch is removed (see section 5.2).

Use in children

In children, the starting dose and titration schedule requires a fentanyl release rate of less than 25 microgram/hour. Due to the dosage strengths of this product, use in children is not recommended.

Use in elderly patients

Elderly patients should carefully be observed for symptoms of an overdosage and the dose possibly be reduced (see section 4.4).

Use in patients with hepatic or renal impairment

Patients with impaired hepatic or renal function should carefully be observed for symptoms of an overdosage and the dose possibly be reduced (see section 4.4).

Use in febrile patients

Dose adjustment may be necessary in patients during episodes of fever (see section 4.4).

Method of administration

For transdermal use.

Fentalis Reservoir transdermal patch should be applied to non-irritated and non-irradiated skin on a flat surface of the torso or upper arm. Hair at the application site (hairless area is preferred) should be clipped (not shaved) prior to system application. If the site requires to be cleansed prior to application of the patch, this should be done with water. Soaps, oils, lotions, alcohol or any other agent that might irritate the skin or alter its characteristics should not be used. The skin should be completely dry before application of the patch.

Since the transdermal patch is protected outwardly by a waterproof covering foil, it may also be worn when taking a shower.

Fentalis Reservoir transdermal patch is to be attached as soon as the pack has been opened. Following removal of the protective layer, the transdermal patch should be pressed firmly in place with the palm of the hand for approximately 30 seconds, making sure the contact is complete, especially around the edges. An additional fixing of the transdermal patch may be necessary. Fentalis Reservoir transdermal patch should be worn continuously for 72 hours after which the transdermal patch is replaced. A new transdermal patch should always be applied to a different site from the previous one. The same application site may be re-used only after an interval of at least 7 days.

4.3 Contraindications

- Known hypersensitivity to fentanyl, any of the excipients or to the transdermal patch adhesive
- Acute or post-operative pain, since dosage titration is not possible during short-term use
- Severly impaired central nervous system function
- Concomitant use of MAO-inhibitors or within 14 days after discontinuation of treatment with MAO-inhibitors

4.4 Special warnings and precautions for use

After exhibiting a serious adverse reaction a patient should be monitored for 24 hours following removal of a transdermal patch due to the half life of fentanyl (see section 5.2).

Both unused and used Fentalis Reservoir transdermal patches should be kept out of reach and sight of children.

Fentalis Reservoir transdermal patches should not be divided, cut or damaged in any other way, since this would result in the uncontrolled release of fentanyl.

Treatment with Fentalis Reservoir transdermal patches should only be initiated by an experienced physician familiar with the pharmacokinetics of fentanyl transdermal patches and the risk for severe hypoventilation.

Respiratory depression

Fentanyl may cause significant respiratory depression. Patients must be observed for this effect, the likelihood of which increases with increasing dosage (see also section 4.9) but is also dependent on the developed tolerance for this side effect. Respiratory depression may persist after removal of the transdermal patch, since the serum concentration of fentanyl falls slowly. The combined use of medicinal products that act upon the CNS together with fentanyl may increase the risk of respiratory depression (see section 4.5). Fentanyl should be used only with caution and at lower dose in patients with existing respiratory depression.

If a patient is to undergo measures that fully remove the sensation of pain (anaesthetisation of sympathetic nerves), it is advisable to prepare for the possibility of respiratory depression. Before such measures are carried out, the fentanyl dosage should be reduced or a changeover should be made to rapid- or short-acting opioid medication.

Chronic lung disease

In patients suffering from chronic obstructive pulmonary disease or some other diseases of the respiratory organs, fentanyl treatment may cause more serious undesirable effects such as a fall in respiration rate and an increase in airway resistance.

Drug dependence

As a result of repeated administration, tolerance and psychological and/or physical dependence on the agent may develop. Therapy-induced dependence is however rare.

Increased intracranial pressure

Caution should be exercised when using fentanyl for patients who are particularly susceptible to the effects of intracranial carbon dioxide retention, such as patients in whom an increase in cerebral pressure, an impaired level of consciousness or coma has been observed. Fentanyl should be used with caution in patients in whom a cerebral tumour has been detected.

Cardiac diseases

Fentanyl may cause bradycardia and for this reason caution should be exercised when treating patients with bradyarrhythmia.

Opioids can cause hypotension, especially in patients who are hypovolemic. For this reason caution should be exercised when treating patients with hypotension and/or who are hypovolemic.

Hepatic diseases

Fentanyl is metabolised to pharmacologically inactive metabolites in the liver. In patients with impaired liver function the elimination of fentanyl may be delayed. Therefore, patients with an impaired liver function may need a lower dose and should be closely monitored for undesirable effects.

Renal diseases

Less than 10% of fentanyl is excreted unchanged via the kidneys. Unlike morphine, fentanyl does not have known active metabolites that are eliminated through the kidneys. Data obtained with intravenous fentanyl in patients with renal failure suggest that the volume of distribution of fentanyl may be changed by dialysis. This may affect serum concentrations. If patients with renal impairment receive Fentalis Reservoir transdermal patches, they should be observed carefully for signs of possible undesirable effects and the dose reduced if necessary.

Fever / external heat sources

On the basis of a pharmacokinetic model, serum fentanyl levels may rise by approximately one third if the skin temperature rises to 40 °C. Consequently, patients with fever should be monitored very closely for opioid side effects and if necessary the fentanyl dosage should be adjusted (see section 4.2). Patients should also be advised to avoid exposing the Fentalis Reservoir transdermal patch application site to direct external heat sources such as heating pads, hot water bottles, electric blankets, heat lamps or hot whirlpool spa baths while wearing the patch, since there is potential for temperature dependent increases in release of fentanyl from the patch.

The transdermal patch must always be removed before taking a sauna. Sauna bathing is possible only when replacing a transdermal patch (at intervals of 72 hours). A new transdermal patch is to be applied to cool, very dry skin.

Elderly Patients

Data from intravenous studies with fentanyl suggest that elderly patients may have reduced clearance, a prolonged half-life and they may be more sensitive to the drug than younger patients. Studies of fentanyl transdermal patches in elderly patients demonstrated fentanyl pharmacokinetics which did not differ significantly from young patients although serum concentrations tended to be higher. Elderly, cachectic, or debilitated patients should be observed carefully for signs of fentanyl toxicity and the dose reduced if necessary.

Others

Non-epileptic (myo)clonic reactions can occur.

Caution should be exercised when treating patients with myasthenia gravis.

4.5 Interaction with other medicinal products and other forms of interaction

Central nervous system

Fentanyl exhibits an additive effect with other CNS depressants (e.g. opioids, sedatives, hypnotics, general anaesthetics, phenothiazines, anxiolytics, muscle relaxants, sedative antihistamines and alcoholic beverages). Combined use may result in hypoventilation, hypotension, intense sedation or coma. Patients using these agents should be observed very closely during fentanyl treatment.

Agents affecting Cytochrome P450 3A4

Fentanyl is a high-clearance drug and is mainly metabolised by the enzyme CYP3A4. Potent inhibitors of CYP3A4 such as ritonavir, ketoconazole, itraconazole and some of the macrolide antibiotics, may give rise to increased plasma concentrations of fentanyl.

Orally administered itraconazole (a potent inhibitor of CYP3A4 enzyme), 200 mg daily for 4 days, did not significantly affect the pharmacokinetics of intravenously administered fentanyl.

Orally administered ritonavir (one of the most potent CYP3A4 enzyme inhibitors) reduced the clearance of intravenously administered fentanyl by two thirds.

The interaction of transdermally administered fentanyl and potent CYP3A4 enzyme inhibitors could result in prolonged therapeutic effect and adverse reactions including respiratory depression. Concomitant treatment with potent CYP3A4 inhibitors and transdermal fentanyl is therefore not recommended unless the patient is under extensive monitoring for adverse reactions.

As pethidine and monoamine oxidase inhibitors (e.g. tranylcypromine) reciprocally potentiate their toxic effects, a similar interaction can be expected with fentanyl.

Although pentazocine or buprenorphine have an analgesic effect, they partially antagonise some effects of fentanyl (e.g. analgesia) and may induce withdrawal symptoms in opioid dependants.

4.6 Pregnancy and lactation

The safety of the use of fentanyl transdermal patches during pregnancy is not established. Experimental studies in animals have shown reproductive toxicity (see section 5.3). The potential risk for human is unknown. Consequently Fentalis Reservoir transdermal patches should not be used during pregnancy unless clearly necessary.

Long-term treatment during pregnancy may cause withdrawal symptoms in the neonate.

It is adviced not to use fentanyl during labor and delivery (including caesarean section) because fentanyl passes the placenta and may cause respiratory depression in the fetus/newborn child.

Fentanyl passes into breast milk and may cause sedation and respiratory depression in the suckling child. Therefore, breast-feeding should be stopped for at least 72 hours after the last administration of Fentalis Reservoir transdermal patch.

4.7 Effects on ability to drive and use machines

Fentalis Reservoir transdermal patches have major influence on the ability to drive and use machines. This has to be expected especially at the beginning of treatment, at any change of dosage as well as in connection with alcohol or tranquilizers. Patients stabilized on a specific dosage will not necessarily be restricted. Therefore, patients should consult their physician as to whether driving or use of machines is permitted.

4.8 Undesirable effects

The following frequency data is the basis for the description of adverse reactions:

Very common (> 1/10), common (>1/100, <1/10), uncommon (>1/1,000,< 1/100), rare (>1/10,000, <1/1,000), very rare (< 1/10,000).

The most serious undesirable effect of fentanyl is respiratory depression.

Psychiatric disorders

Very common: somnolence

Common: sedation, confusion, depression, anxiety, nervousness, hallucinations, diminished appetite

Uncommon: euphoria, amnesia, insomnia, agitation

Very rare: delusional idea, asthenia, disorder of sexual function

Nervous system disorders

Very common: drowsiness, headache

Uncommon: tremor, paraesthesia, speech disorder

Very rare: ataxia

Non-epileptic myoclonic reactions

Eye disorders

Rare: amblyopia

Cardiac disorders

Uncommon: bradycardia, tachycardia, hypotension, hypertension

Rare: arrhythmia, vasodilatation

Respiratory, thoracic and mediastinal disorders

Uncommon: dyspnea, hypoventilation

Very rare: respiratory depression, apnea

Haemoptysis, pulmonary congestion and pharyngitis

Gastrointestinal disorders

Very common: nausea, vomiting, constipation

Common: xerostomia, dyspespia

Uncommon: diarrhaea

Rare: hiccup

Very rare: ileus, painful flatulence

Hypersensitivity disorders

Anaphylactic reactions, laryngospasm

Skin and subcutaneous tissue disorders

Very common: sweating, pruritus

Common: skin reaction on application site

Uncommon: rash, erythema

Rash, erythema and pruritus generally disappear within 24 hours of removal of the transdermal patch.

Renal and urinary disorders

Uncommon: urinary retention

Very rare: oliguria, bladder pain

Body as a whole:

Rare: oedema, sensation of cold

Other undesirable effects

Tolerance, physical and psychological depencence may develop during administration of fentanyl over a longer period of time.

Opioid withdrawal symptoms (such as nausea, vomiting, diarrhoea, anxiety and muscular tremor) may occur in some patients after they change over from a previously prescribed opioid analgesic to Fentalis Reservoir transdermal patches.

4.9 Overdose

Symptoms of an overdose

The symptoms are exaggerations of the pharmacological effects of fentanyl, such as stupor, coma, respiratory depression with cheyne-stokes breathing and/or cyanosis. Other possible symptoms are hypothermia, loss of muscle tension, bradycardia and hypotension. Signs of toxication are deep sedation, ataxia, miosis, seizures and respiratory depression, which is the main symptom.

Therapy for an overdose

For management of respiratory depression, immediate countermeasures include removing Fentalis Reservoir transdermal patch and physically or verbally stimulating the patient. These actions can be followed by administration of a specific opioid antagonist such as naloxone.

An initial dose of 0.4-2 mg of naloxone hydrochloride i.v. in adults is recommended. If necessary, the initial dose is to be repeated every 2 or 3 minutes, or given as a continuous infusion of 2 mg in 500 ml of isotonic sodium chloride solution (0.9 %) or 5 % dextrose solution (0.004 mg/ml). The infusion rate should be adjusted to the previous bolus injections and the patient's individual response. If the intravenous route is unavailable, naloxone hydrochloride may be administered also i.m. or s.c. After i.m. and s.c. application, the onset of action is only slightly less rapid than after i.v. application. The i.m. route produces a more prolonged effect than i.v. administration. Respiratory depression resulting from overdosage may last longer than the effect of the opioid antagonist. Reversal of the narcotic effect may result in acute onset of pain and the release of catecholamines.

If required by the patient's clinical condition, intensive care unit treatment is essential.

If severe or persistent hypotension occurs, the possibility of hypovolaemia should be considered and the situation remedied with such parenteral fluid treatment as is considered appropriate.

5. PHARMACOLOGICAL PROPERTIES

5.1 Pharmacodynamic properties

Pharmacotherapeutic group: opioid analgesic

ATC Code: N02AB03

Fentanyl is an opioid analgesic with an affinity for the μ-receptors. Its principal therapeutic effects are analgesia and sedation. In patients who have not been previously treated with opioids, analgesic efficacy is achieved with serum fentanyl concentrations of 0.3-1.5 ng/ml. The incidence of adverse effects increases when serum concentrations exceed 2 ng/ml. During long-term therapy potential adverse effects may emerge with higher serum concentrations. The speed of tolerance development shows considerable inter-individual variety.

5.2 Pharmacokinetic properties

A release membrane controls the transdermal delivery of fentanyl. Transdermal diffusion occurs at a relatively even speed for 72 hours following the application of the transdermal patch.

Absorption: After the first application of Fentalis Reservoir transdermal patches, serum fentanyl concentrations increase gradually, generally levelling off between 12 and 24 hours, and remaining relatively constant for the remainder of the 72-hour application period. The serum fentanyl concentrations attained are dependant on the Fentalis Reservoir transdermal patch size. For all practical purposes by the second 72-hour application, a steady state serum concentration is reached and is maintained during subsequent applications of a patch of the same size.

Distribution: The plasma protein binding for fentanyl is 84 %.

Biotransformation: Fentanyl is metabolized primarily in the liver via CYP3A4. The major metabolite, norfentanyl, is inactive.

Elimination: When treatment with Fentalis Reservoir transdermal patches is withdrawn, serum fentanyl concentrations decline gradually, falling approximately 50% in 13-22 hours in adults or 22-25 hours in children, respectively.

Continued absorption of fentanyl from the skin accounts for a slower reduction in serum concentration than is seen after an intravenous infusion.

Around 75% of fentanyl is excreted into the urine, mostly as metabolites, with less than 10% as unchanged drug. About 9% of the dose is recovered in the faeces, primarily as metabolites.

Pharmacokinetics in special groups

Elderly and debilitated patients may have reduced clearance of fentanyl leading to prolonged terminal half life. In patients with renal or hepatic impairment, clearance of fentanyl may be altered because of changes of plasma proteins and metabolic clearance resulting in increased serum concentrations.

5.3 Preclinical safety data

Similar effects as previously described for other opioids were observed in repeated dose toxicity studies up to 4 weeks.

In a rat study fentanyl did not influence male fertility. Studies with female rats revealed reduced fertility and enhanced embryonal mortality. More recent studies showed that effects on the embryo were due to maternal toxicity and not to direct effects of the substance on the developing embryo. There were no indications for teratogenic effects in studies in two species. In a study on pre- and postnatal development the survival rate of offspring was significantly reduced at doses which slightly reduced maternal weight. This effect could either be due to altered maternal care or a direct effect of fentanyl on the pups. Effects on somatic development and behaviour of the offspring were not observed.

Mutagenicity testing in bacteria and in rodents yielded negative results. As well as other opioids fentanyl showed mutagenic effects in vitro in mammalian cells. A mutagenic risk in therapeutic condition seems unlikely since effects were induced only in very high concentrations.

Long term carcinogenicity studies have not been performed.

6. PHARMACEUTICAL PARTICULARS

6.1 List of excipients

Occlusive backing:	polyethylene-terephthalate/ ethylenvinylacetate-copolymer
Drug reservoir:	ethanol 96 %
	hydroxyethylcellulose
	purified water
Release membrane:	ethylenvinylacetate-copolymer
Adhesive surface:	silicone medical adhesive

Protective layer (remove before patch application): polyethylene-terephthalate, release coated

6.2 Incompatibilities

Not applicable.

6.3 Shelf life

3 years

6.4 Special precautions for storage

Store in the original package. Do not refrigerate or freeze.

6.5 Nature and contents of container

The transdermal patch is individually packaged in a protective sachet foil paper/PE/Al/PE.

Packages containing 3, 5, 7, 10, 14 and 20 transdermal patches

Not all pack sizes may be marketed.

6.6 Special precautions for disposal and other handling

Used transdermal patches are to be folded with the adhesive surfaces facing each other and disposed of in an appropriate manner. Unused packs are to be returned to the pharmacist.

7. MARKETING AUTHORISATION HOLDER

Sandoz Limited

37 Woolmer Way

Bordon

Hampshire

GU35 9QE

8. MARKETING AUTHORISATION NUMBER(S)

PL 04416/0744

PL 04416/0745

PL 04416/0746

PL 04416/0747

9. DATE OF FIRST AUTHORISATION/RENEWAL OF THE AUTHORISATION

14/06/2007

10. DATE OF REVISION OF THE TEXT

09/2007

Ferinject

(Syner-Med (Pharmaceutical Products) Ltd)

1. NAME OF THE MEDICINAL PRODUCT

Ferinject®▼ 50 mg iron/ml solution for injection/infusion.

2. QUALITATIVE AND QUANTITATIVE COMPOSITION

One millilitre of solution contains 50 mg of iron as ferric carboxymaltose.

Each 2 ml vial contains 100 mg of iron as ferric carboxymaltose.

Each 10 ml vial contains 500 mg of iron as ferric carboxymaltose.

Ferinject® contains sodium hydroxide. One millilitre of solution contains up to 0.24 mmol (5.5 mg) sodium, see section 4.2. For a full list of excipients, see section 6.1.

3. PHARMACEUTICAL FORM

Solution for injection/infusion. Dark brown, non-transparent, aqueous solution.

4. CLINICAL PARTICULARS

4.1 Therapeutic indications

Ferinject® is indicated for treatment of iron deficiency when oral iron preparations are ineffective or cannot be used.

The diagnosis must be based on laboratory tests.

4.2 Posology and method of administration

Calculation of the cumulative dose

The adequate cumulative dose of Ferinject® must be calculated for each patient individually and must not be exceeded. For overweight patients, a normal body weight/blood volume relation should be assumed when determining the iron requirement. The dose of Ferinject® is expressed in mg of elemental iron.

The cumulative dose required for Hb restoration and repletion of iron stores is calculated by the following Ganzoni formula:

Cumulative iron deficit [mg] =

body weight [kg] × (target Hb* - actual Hb) [g/dl] × 2.4*** + iron storage depot [mg]******

* *Target Hb for body weight below 35 kg = 13 g/dl respectively 8.1 mmol/l.*

Target Hb for body weight 35 kg and above = 15 g/dl respectively 9.3 mmol/l.

** *To convert Hb [mM] to Hb [g/dl]: multiply Hb [mM] by the factor 1.61145.*

*** *Factor 2.4 = 0.0034 × 0.07 × 10,000; 0.0034: iron content of haemoglobin ≌ 0.34%;0.07: blood volume ≌ 7% of body weight;10,000: conversion factor 1 g/dl =10,000 mg/l.*

**** *Depot iron for body weight below 35 kg = 15 mg/kg body weight.*
Depot iron for body weight 35 kg and above = 500 mg.

For patients ⩽ 66 kg: the calculated cumulative dose is to be rounded down to the nearest 100 mg.

For patients > 66 kg: the calculated cumulative dose is to be rounded up to the nearest 100 mg.

Patients may continue to require therapy with Ferinject® at the lowest dose necessary to maintain target levels of haemoglobin, and other laboratory values of iron storage parameters within acceptable limits.

Maximum tolerated single dose

The adequate cumulative dose of Ferinject® must be calculated for each patient individually and must not be exceeded.

Intravenous bolus injection

Ferinject® may be administered by intravenous injection up to a maximum single dose of 4 ml (200 mg of iron) per day but not more than three times a week.

Intravenous drip infusion

Ferinject® may be administered by intravenous infusion up to a maximum single dose of 20 ml of Ferinject® (1000 mg of iron) but not exceeding 0.3 ml of Ferinject® (15 mg of iron) per kg body weight or the calculated cumulative dose. Do not administer 20 ml (1000 mg of iron) as an infusion more than once a week.

The use of Ferinject® has not been studied in children, and therefore is not recommended in children under 14 years.

Method of administration

Ferinject® must be administered only by the intravenous route: by bolus injection, during a haemodialysis session undiluted directly into the venous limb of the dialyser, or by drip infusion. In case of drip infusion Ferinject® must be diluted only in sterile 0.9% sodium chloride solution as follows:

Dilution plan of Ferinject® for intravenous drip infusion ***(see Table 1 below)***

Note: For stability reasons, dilutions to concentrations less than 2 mg iron/ml are not permissible.

Ferinject® must not to be administered by the intramuscular route.

4.3 Contraindications

The use of Ferinject® is contraindicated in cases of:

- known hypersensitivity to Ferinject® or to any of its excipients
- anaemia not attributed to iron deficiency, e.g. other microcytic anaemia
- evidence of iron overload or disturbances in utilisation of iron
- pregnancy in the first trimester

4.4 Special warnings and precautions for use

Parenterally administered iron preparations can cause hypersensitivity reactions including anaphylactoid reactions, which may be potentially fatal (see section 5.3). Therefore, facilities for cardio-pulmonary resuscitation must be available.

In patients with liver dysfunction, parenteral iron should only be administered after careful risk/benefit assessment. Parenteral iron administration should be avoided in patients with hepatic dysfunction where iron overload is a precipitating factor, in particular Porphyria Cutanea Tarda (PCT). Careful monitoring of iron status is recommended to avoid iron overload.

Parenteral iron must be used with caution in cases of acute or chronic infection, asthma, eczema or atopic allergies. It is recommended that the administration of Ferinject® is stopped in patients with ongoing bacteraemia. In patients with chronic infection a risk/benefit evaluation has to be performed, taking into account the suppression of erythropoiesis.

Caution should be exercised to avoid paravenous leakage when administering Ferinject®. Paravenous leakage of Ferinject® at the injection site may lead to brown discolouration and irritation of the skin. In case of paravenous leakage, the administration of Ferinject® must be stopped immediately.

One millilitre of undiluted Ferinject® contains up to 0.24 mmol (5.5 mg) of sodium. This has to be taken into account in patients on a sodium-controlled diet.

The use of Ferinject® has not been studied in children.

4.5 Interaction with other medicinal products and other forms of interaction

As with all parenteral iron preparations the absorption of oral iron is reduced when administered concomitantly.

4.6 Pregnancy and lactation

Clinical data on pregnant women are not available. A careful risk/benefit evaluation is required before use during pregnancy.

Animal data suggest that iron released from Ferinject® can cross the placental barrier and that its use during pregnancy may influence skeletal development in the fetus.

Clinical studies showed that transfer of iron from Ferinject® to human milk was negligible (⩽ 1%). Based on limited data on nursing women it is unlikely that Ferinject® represents a risk to the nursing child.

4.7 Effects on ability to drive and use machines

Ferinject® is unlikely to impair the ability to drive or operate machines.

4.8 Undesirable effects

The most commonly reported ADR is headache, occurring in 3.3% of the patients.

Very common (>1/10)

Common (>1/100, <1/10)

Uncommon (>1/1,000, <1/100)

Rare (>1/10,000, <1/1,000)

Very rare (<1/10,000), including isolated reports

Immune system disorders:

Uncommon (>1/1,000, <1/100): Hypersensitivity including anaphylactoid reactions

Nervous system disorders:

Common (>1/100, <1/10): Headache, dizziness

Uncommon (>1/1,000, <1/100): Paraesthesia

Vascular disorders:

Uncommon (>1/1,000, <1/100): Hypotension, flushing

Respiratory, thoracic and mediastinal disorders:

Rare (>1/10,000, <1/1,000): Dyspnoea

Gastrointestinal disorders:

Common (>1/100, <1/10): Nausea, abdominal pain, constipation, diarrhoea

Uncommon (>1/1,000, <1/100): Dysgeusia, vomiting, dyspepsia, flatulence

Skin and subcutaneous tissue disorders:

Common (>1/100, <1/10): Rash

Uncommon >1/1,000, <1/100): Pruritus, urticaria

Musculoskeletal and connective tissue disorders:

Uncommon (>1/1,000, <1/100): Myalgia, back pain, arthralgia

General disorders and administration site conditions:

Common (>1/100, <1/10): Injection site reactions

Uncommon (>1/1,000, <1/100): Pyrexia, fatigue, chest pain, rigors, malaise, oedema peripheral

Investigations:

Common (>1/100, <1/10): Transient blood phosphorus decreased, alanine aminotransferase increased

Uncommon (>1/1,000, <1/100): Aspartate aminostransferase increased, gamma-glutamyltransferase increased, blood lactate dehydrogenase increased

4.9 Overdose

Administration of Ferinject® in quantities exceeding the amount needed to correct iron deficit at the time of administration may lead to accumulation of iron in storage sites eventually leading to haemosiderosis. Monitoring of iron parameters such as serum ferritin and transferrin saturation may assist in recognising iron accumulation.

5. PHARMACOLOGICAL PROPERTIES

5.1 Pharmacodynamic properties

Pharmacotherapeutic group: Iron trivalent, parenteral preparation.

ATC Code: B03A C01

Ferinject® solution for injection/infusion contains iron in a stable ferric state as a complex with a carbohydrate polymer designed to release utilisable iron to the iron transport and storage proteins in the body (ferritin and transferrin).

Clinical studies showed that the haematological response and the filling of the iron stores was faster after intravenous administration of Ferinject® than with orally administered comparators.

Using positron emission tomography (PET) it was demonstrated that red cell utilisation of ^{59}Fe and ^{52}Fe from Ferinject® ranged from 61% to 99%. Patients with iron deficiency showed utilisation of radio-labelled iron of 91% to 99% after 24 days, and patients with renal anaemia showed utilisation of radio-labelled iron of 61% to 84% after 24 days.

One millilitre of undiluted Ferinject® contains less than 75µg aluminium. This should be considered in the treatment of patients undergoing dialysis.

5.2 Pharmacokinetic properties

Using positron emission tomography (PET) it was demonstrated that ^{59}Fe and ^{52}Fe from Ferinject® was rapidly eliminated from the blood, transferred to the bone marrow, and deposited in the liver and spleen.

After administration of a single dose of Ferinject® of 100 to 1,000 mg of iron in iron deficient patients, maximum iron levels of 37 µg/ml up to 333 µg/ml after 15 minutes to 1.21 hours respectively are obtained. The volume of the central compartment corresponds well to the volume of the plasma (approximately 3 litres).

The iron injected or infused was rapidly cleared from the plasma, the terminal half-life ranged from 7 to 12 hours, the mean residence time (MRT) from 11 to 18 hours. Renal elimination of iron was negligible.

5.3 Preclinical safety data

Pre-clinical data revealed no special hazard for humans based on conventional studies of safety pharmacology, repeat dose toxicity and genotoxicity. Animal studies indicate that iron released from Ferinject® does cross the placental barrier and is excreted in milk. In reproductive toxicology studies using iron replete animals Ferinject® was associated with minor skeletal abnormalities in the fetus. No long-term studies in animals have been performed to evaluate the carcinogenic potential of Ferinject®. No evidence of allergic or immunotoxic potential has been observed. A controlled *in-vivo* test demonstrated no cross-reactivity of Ferinject® with anti-dextran antibodies. No local irritation or intolerance was observed after intravenous administration.

6. PHARMACEUTICAL PARTICULARS

6.1 List of excipients

Sodium hydroxide (for pH adjustment)

Hydrochloric acid (for pH adjustment)

Water for injection

6.2 Incompatibilities

This medicinal product must not be mixed with other medicinal products than those mentioned in section 6.6.

The compatibility with containers other than polyethylene and glass is not known.

6.3 Shelf life

Shelf-life of the product as packaged for sale:

3 years.

Table 1 Dilution plan of Ferinject® for intravenous drip infusion

Ferinject®			Iron			Maximum amount of sterile 0.9% sodium chloride solution	Minimum administration time
2	to	< 4 ml	100	to	< 200 mg	50 ml	-
4	to	< 10 ml	200	to	< 500 mg	100 ml	6 minutes
10	to	20 ml	500	to	1000 mg	250 ml	15 minutes

Shelf-life after first opening of the container:

From a microbiological point of view, preparations for parenteral administration should be used immediately.

Shelf-life after dilution with sterile 0.9% sodium chloride solution:

From a microbiological point of view, preparations for parenteral administration should be used immediately after dilution with sterile 0.9% sodium chloride solution.

6.4 Special precautions for storage

Store in the original package. Do not store above 30°C. Do not refrigerate or freeze.

6.5 Nature and contents of container

2 ml of solution in a vial (type I glass) with bromobutyl rubber stopper and aluminium cap.

10 ml of solution in a vial (type I glass) with bromobutyl rubber stopper and aluminium cap.

6.6 Special precautions for disposal and other handling

Inspect vials visually for sediment and damage before use. Use only those containing sediment-free, homogeneous solution.

Each vial of Ferinject® is intended for single use only. Any unused product or waste material should be disposed of in accordance with local requirements.

Ferinject® must only be mixed with sterile 0.9% sodium chloride solution. No other intravenous dilution solutions and therapeutic agents should be used, as there is the potential for precipitation and/or interaction. For dilution instructions, see section 4.2.

7. MARKETING AUTHORISATION HOLDER

Vifor France SA
7-13 Bd Paul Emile Victor
92200 Neuilly-sur-Seine
France
Tel. +33 (0) 1 41 06 58 90
Fax +33 (0) 1 41 06 58 99

8. MARKETING AUTHORISATION NUMBER(S)

UK: PL 15240/0002
Ireland: PA 0949/004/001

9. DATE OF FIRST AUTHORISATION/RENEWAL OF THE AUTHORISATION

19.07.2007

10. DATE OF REVISION OF THE TEXT

09.07.2009

Distributed by
Syner-Med (PP) Ltd
2nd Floor, Beech House
840 Brighton Road
Purley
Surrey
CR8 2 BH
Tel: 0845 634 2100
Fax: 0845 634 2101
Int Tel: +44 208 655 6380
Int Fax: +44 208 655 6398

Ferinject® is a registered trademark

Fibro-Vein 3.0%, 1.0%, 0.5%, 0.2%

(STD Pharmaceutical Products Ltd)

1. NAME OF THE MEDICINAL PRODUCT

Fibro-vein 3.0%, 1.0%, 0.5%, 0.2%

2. QUALITATIVE AND QUANTITATIVE COMPOSITION

Active ingredient

Fibro-vein 3% Sodium Tetradecyl Sulphate BP 3.0% w/v
Fibro-vein 1% Sodium Tetradecyl Sulphate BP 1.0% w/v
Fibro-vein 0.5% Sodium Tetradecyl Sulphate BP 0.5% w/v
Fibro-vein 0.2% Sodium Tetradecyl Sulphate BP 0.2% w/v

For excipients, see 6.1

3. PHARMACEUTICAL FORM

Intravenous injection

4. CLINICAL PARTICULARS

4.1 Therapeutic indications

Fibro-vein 3%

For the treatment of varicose veins of the leg by injection sclerotherapy.

Fibro-vein 1%

For the treatment of small varicose veins and the larger venules of the leg by injection sclerotherapy.

Fibro-vein 0.5%

For the treatment of minor venules and spider veins (venous flares) of the leg by injection sclerotherapy.

Fibro-vein 0.2%

For the treatment of minor venules and spider veins (venous flares) by injection sclerotherapy.

4.2 Posology and method of administration

Route of administration

For intravenous administration into the lumen of an isolated segment of emptied vein followed by immediate continuous compression.

Recommended doses and dosage schedules.

Adults

Fibro-vein 3%

0.5 to 1.0ml of 3.0% Fibro-vein injected intravenously at each of 4 sites (maximum 4ml).

Fibro-vein 1%

0.25 to 1.0ml of 1.0% Fibro-vein injected intravenously at each of 10 sites (maximum 10ml).

Fibro-vein 0.5%

0.25 to 1.0ml of 0.5% Fibro-vein injected intravenously at each of 10 sites (maximum 10ml).

Fibro-vein 0.2%

0.1 to 1.0ml of Fibro-vein 0.2% injected intravenously at each of 10 sites (maximum 10ml).

The smallest of needles (30 gauge) should be used to perform the injection which should be made slowly so that the blood content of these veins is expelled. In the treatment of spider veins an air block technique may be used.

Children

Not recommended in children

The elderly

As for adults

4.3 Contraindications

1. Allergy to sodium tetradecyl sulphate or to any component of the preparation.
2. Patients unable to walk due to any cause.
3. Patients currently taking oral contraceptives.
4. Significant obesity.
5. Acute superficial thrombophlebitis.
6. Local or systemic infection.
7. Varicosities caused by pelvic or abdominal tumours.
8. Uncontrolled systemic disease eg diabetes mellitus.
9. Surgical valvular incompetence requiring surgical treatment.

4.4 Special warnings and precautions for use

1. Fibro-vein should only be administered by practitioners familiar with an acceptable injection technique. Thorough pre-injection assessment for valvular competence and deep vein patency must be carried out.

Extreme care in needle placement and slow injection of the minimal effective volume at each injection site are essential for safe and efficient use.

2. A history of allergy should be taken from all patients prior to treatment. Where special caution is indicated a test dose of 0.25 to 0.5ml Fibro-vein should be given up to 24 hours before any further therapy.

3. Treatment of anaphylaxis may require, depending on the severity of attack, some or all of the following: injection of adrenaline, injection of hydrocortisone, injection of antihistamine, endotracheal intubation with use of a laryngoscope and suction.

The treatment of varicose veins by Fibro-vein should not be undertaken in clinics where these items are not readily available.

4. Extreme caution in use is required in patients with arterial disease such as severe peripheral atherosclerosis or thromboangiitis obliterans (Buerger's disease).

5. Special care is required when injecting above and posterior to the medial malleolus where the posterior tibial artery may be at risk.

6. Pigmentation may be more likely to result if blood is extravasated at the injection site (particularly when treating smaller surface veins) and compression is not used.

4.5 Interaction with other medicinal products and other forms of interaction

Do not use with heparin in the same syringe

4.6 Pregnancy and lactation

Safety for use in pregnancy has not been established. Use only when clearly needed for symptomatic relief and when the potential benefits outweigh the potential hazards to the foetus.

It is not known whether sodium tetradecyl sulphate is excreted in human milk. Caution should be exercised when used in nursing mothers.

4.7 Effects on ability to drive and use machines

None known

4.8 Undesirable effects

1. Local: Pain or burning. Skin pigmentation. Tissue necrosis and ulceration may occur with extravasation. Paraesthesia and anaesthesia may occur if an injection effects a cutaneous nerve.

2. Vascular: Superficial thrombophlebitis. Deep vein thrombosis and pulmonary embolism are very rare. Inadvertent intra-arterial injection is very rare but may lead to gangrene. Most cases have involved the posterior tibial artery above the medial malleolus.

3. Systemic reactions: Allergic reactions are rare, presenting as local or generalised rash, urticaria, nausea or vomiting, asthma, vascular collapse. Anaphylactic shock, which may potentially be fatal, is extremely rare.

4.9 Overdose

Not applicable.

5. PHARMACOLOGICAL PROPERTIES

5.1 Pharmacodynamic properties

Sodium tetradecyl sulphate damages the endothelium cells within the lumen of the injected vein. The object of compression sclerotherapy is then to compress the vein so that the resulting thrombus is kept to the minimum and the subsequent formation of scar tissue within the vein produces a fibrous cord and permanent obliteration. Non-compressed veins permit the formation of a large thrombus and produce less fibrosis within the vein.

5.2 Pharmacokinetic properties

Not applicable.

5.3 Preclinical safety data

Not applicable

6. PHARMACEUTICAL PARTICULARS

6.1 List of excipients

Benzyl Alcohol BP 2.0% w/v
Di-Sodium Hydrogen Phosphate BP 0.75% w/v
Potassium Di-Hydrogen Phosphate BP 0.1% w/v
Water For Injection BP to 100%
Potassium Di-Hydrogen Phosphate* BP qs
Sodium Carbonate (anhydrous)* BP qs
Sodium Hydroxide (5% soln)* BP qs

* Either sodium carbonate or sodium hydroxide is used for adjustment of pH

6.2 Incompatibilities

Do not use with heparin in the same syringe

6.3 Shelf life

36 months

6.4 Special precautions for storage

Store below 25°C away from direct sunlight

6.5 Nature and contents of container

2ml ampoules type 1 neutral hydrolytic glass conforming with EP requirements for injectable preparations. Five 2ml ampoules per pack.

5ml glass vials type 1 neutral hydrolytic glass conforming with EP requirements for injectable preparations. Sealed with a chlorobutyl rubber bung and silver aluminium "tear off" seal conforming with the European Pharmacopoeia requirements. Ten 5ml vials per pack.

Fibro-vein 3.0% available as 5 × 2ml ampoules and 10 × 5ml vials
Fibro-vein 1.0% available as 5 × 2ml ampoules
Fibro-vein 0.5% available as 5 × 2ml ampoules
Fibro-vein 0.2% available as 5 × 2ml ampoules and 10 × 5ml vials

6.6 Special precautions for disposal and other handling

The in use period of each 5ml multidose vial is a single session of therapy and for use in the treatment of a single patient. Unused vial contents should be discarded immediately afterwards.

7. MARKETING AUTHORISATION HOLDER

STD Pharmaceutical Products Ltd
Plough Lane
Hereford
HR4 0EL
United Kingdom

8. MARKETING AUTHORISATION NUMBER(S)

Fibro-vein 3.0% PL 0398/5000R
Fibro-vein 1.0% PL 0398/0003
Fibro-vein 0.5% PL 0398/0002
Fibro-vein 0.2% PL 0398/0004

9. DATE OF FIRST AUTHORISATION/RENEWAL OF THE AUTHORISATION

Fibro-vein 3.0% 23/02/2006
Fibro-vein 1.0% 26/03/2008
Fibro-vein 0.5% 26/03/2008
Fibro-vein 0.2% 26/03/2008

10. DATE OF REVISION OF THE TEXT

26/03/2008

Firazyr 30 mg solution for injection in pre-filled syringe

(Shire Human Genetic Therapies)

1. NAME OF THE MEDICINAL PRODUCT

Firazyr▼ 30 mg solution for injection in pre-filled syringe

2. QUALITATIVE AND QUANTITATIVE COMPOSITION

Each pre-filled syringe of 3 ml contains icatibant acetate equivalent to 30 mg icatibant.

Each ml of the solution contains 10 mg of icatibant.

For a full list of excipients see section 6.1.

3. PHARMACEUTICAL FORM

Solution for injection.

The solution is a clear and colourless liquid.

4. CLINICAL PARTICULARS

4.1 Therapeutic indications

Firazyr is indicated for symptomatic treatment of acute attacks of hereditary angioedema (HAE) in adults (with C1-esterase-inhibitor deficiency).

4.2 Posology and method of administration

The recommended dose of Firazyr is one subcutaneous injection of 30 mg administered by a health care professional, preferably in the abdominal area, for the treatment of a hereditary angioedema attack.

Firazyr is not for self-administration.

Firazyr is intended for subcutaneous use. For single use only.

Patients with laryngeal attacks need to be carefully managed in an appropriate medical institution after injection until the physician considers discharge to be safe.

Injection should be given slowly due to the large volume to be administered (3 ml).

In the majority of cases a single injection of Firazyr is sufficient to treat an attack. In case of insufficient relief or recurrence of symptoms, a second injection of Firazyr can be administered after 6 hours. If the second injection produces insufficient relief or a recurrence of symptoms is observed, a third injection of Firazyr can be administered after a further 6 hours. No more than 3 injections of Firazyr should be administered in a 24 hour period.

In the clinical trials, not more than 8 injections of Firazyr per month have been administered.

Children and adolescents

There is no experience in children.

Elderly patients

Limited information is available on patients older than 65 years of age.

Elderly patients have been shown to have increased systemic exposure to icatibant. The relevance of this to the safety of Firazyr is unknown (see section 5.2).

Hepatic impairment

No dosage adjustment is required in patients with hepatic impairment.

Renal impairment

No dosage adjustment is required in patients with renal impairment.

4.3 Contraindications

Hypersensitivity to the active substance or to any of the excipients.

4.4 Special warnings and precautions for use

Ischemic heart disease

Under ischemic conditions, a deterioration of cardiac function and a decrease in coronary blood flow could theoretically arise from antagonism of bradykinin receptor type 2. Caution should therefore be observed in the administration of Firazyr to patients with acute ischemic heart disease or unstable angina pectoris (see section 5.3).

Stroke

Although there is evidence to support a beneficial effect of B2 receptor blockade immediately following a stroke, there is a theoretical possibility that icatibant may attenuate the positive late phase neuroprotective effects of bradykinin. Accordingly, caution should be observed in the administration of icatibant to patients in the weeks following a stroke.

4.5 Interaction with other medicinal products and other forms of interaction

Pharmacokinetic drug interactions involving CYP450 are not expected (see section 5.2)

Co-administration of Firazyr with ACE inhibitors has not been studied. ACE inhibitors are contraindicated in HAE patients due to possible enhancement of bradykinin levels.

4.6 Pregnancy and lactation

For icatibant, no clinical data on exposed pregnancies are available. Animal studies showed effects on uterine implantation and parturition (see section 5.3), but the potential risk for humans is unknown.

Firazyr should be used during pregnancy only, if the potential benefit justifies the potential risk for the foetus, (e.g for treatment of potentially life threatening laryngeal attacks).

Icatibant is excreted in the milk of lactating rats at concentrations similar to those in maternal blood. No effects were detected in the post-natal development of rat pups.

It is unknown whether icatibant is excreted in human breast milk but it is recommended that breastfeeding women, who wish to take Firazyr, should not breastfeed for 12 hours after treatment.

In immature animals repeated use of icatibant reversibly delayed sexual maturation (see section 5.3).

4.7 Effects on ability to drive and use machines

Firazyr has minor or moderate influence on the ability to drive and use machines. Fatigue, lethargy, tiredeness, somnolence, and dizziness have been reported uncommonly following the use of Firazyr. These symptoms may occur as a result of an attack of HAE. However, a causal relationship to the use of Firazyr cannot be excluded. Patients should be advised not to drive and use machines if they feel tired or dizzy.

4.8 Undesirable effects

The safety of icatibant has been established in 1022 subjects treated with various doses, regimens and routes of administration during Phase I-III studies in various indications.

Sixty three (HAE) patients received icatibant in two Phase III trials for treatment of an attack in the controlled phase and 118 patients were treated in the open label phase.

Almost all subjects who were treated with subcutaneous icatibant in clinical trials developed reactions at the site of injection including erythema, swelling, warm sensation, burning, itching and/or cutaneous pain. These reactions were generally mild in severity, transient, and resolved without further intervention.

The frequency of adverse reactions listed in Table 1 is defined using the following convention:

Very common (⩾1/10); common (⩾1/100, <1/10); uncommon (⩾1/1,000, <1/100); rare (⩾1/10,000, <1/1,000); very rare (<1/10,000).

Note: Due to the low number of patients, each of the uncommon events has only been reported in a single patient.

Table 1: Adverse reactions reported with icatibant in the phase III clinical trials.

(see Table 1 below)

4.9 Overdose

No clinical information on overdose is available.

A dose of 3.2 mg/kg intravenously (approximately 8 times the therapeutic dose) caused transient erythema, itching or hypotension in healthy subjects. No therapeutic intervention was necessary.

5. PHARMACOLOGICAL PROPERTIES

5.1 Pharmacodynamic properties

Pharmacotherapeutic group: other cardiac preparations ATC code: C01EB19.

HAE (an autosomal dominant disease) is caused by an absence or dysfunction of C1-esterase-inhibitor. HAE attacks are accompanied by an increased release of bradykinin, which is the key mediator in the development of the clinical symptoms.

HAE manifests as intermittent attacks of subcutaneous and/or sub mucosal oedema involving the upper respiratory tract, the skin and the gastrointestinal tract. An attack usually lasts between 2 to 5 days.

Icatibant is a selective competitive antagonist at the bradykinin type 2 (B2) receptor. It is a synthetic decapeptide with a structure similar to bradykinin, but with 5 non-proteinogenic amino acids. In HAE increased bradykinin concentrations are the key mediator in the development of the clinical symptoms.

In healthy young subjects, icatibant administered in doses of 0.8 mg/kg over 4 hours; 1.5 mg/kg/day or 0.15 mg/kg/day for 3 days, development of bradykinin-induced hypotension, vasodilatation and reflex tachycardia was prevented. Icatibant was shown to be a competitive antagonist when the bradykinin challenge dose was increased 4-fold.

Efficacy data were obtained from an initial open-label Phase II study and from two randomised, double blind controlled multi centre Phase III studies (one with oral tranexamic acid as the comparator and one placebo controlled). The pivotal Phase III studies were otherwise identical in design. A total of 130 patients were randomized to receive either a 30 mg dose of icatibant (63 patients) or comparator (either tranexamic acid, - 38 or placebo - 29 patients). Subsequent episodes of HAE were treated in an open label extension. Patients with symptoms of laryngeal angioedema received open label treatment with icatibant.

In the Phase III trials, the primary efficacy endpoint was time to onset of symptom relief using a visual analogue scale (VAS). In both studies, patients on icatibant had a faster median time to onset of symptom relief (2.0 and 2.5 hours, respectively) compared to tranexamic acid (12.0 hours) and placebo (4.6 hours). The treatment effect of icatibant was confirmed by secondary efficacy endpoints.

The following table shows the results for the two pivotal trials

(see Table 2 on next page)

One hundred and eighteen patients were treated in the open label extension (OLE) phase for a total of 597 separate attacks. The efficacy results were similar to those seen in the controlled phase of the studies. The majority of attacks (89.3% and 90.9%, respectively) in both studies required only a single dose of icatibant.

A total of 36 patients were treated for a total of 61 attacks of HAE affecting the larynx. The results were again similar to patients with non-laryngeal attacks of HAE with a median time to start of regression of symptoms of 0.6 - 1.0 hours (controlled phase).

5.2 Pharmacokinetic properties

The pharmacokinetics of icatibant has been extensively characterized by studies using both intravenous and subcutaneous administration to healthy volunteers and patients. The pharmacokinetic profile of icatibant in patients with HAE is similar to that in healthy volunteers.

Absorption

Following subcutaneous administration, the absolute bioavailability of icatibant is 97%. The time to maximum concentration is approximately 0.5 hours.

Distribution

Icatibant volume of distribution (Vss) is about 20-25 L. Plasma protein binding is 44%.

Elimination

Icatibant is mainly eliminated by metabolism with less than 10% of the dose eliminated in the urine as unchanged drug.

Table 1 : Adverse reactions reported with icatibant in the phase III clinical trials

	Adverse reactions Very common	Common	Uncommon
Congenital, familial and genetic disorders		Hereditary angioedema*	
Gastrointestinal disorders		Nausea, abdominal pain	Vomiting
General disorders and administration site conditions	Erythema, swelling, warm sensation, burning, itching, cutaneous pain	Asthenia	Fatigue, pyrexia
Infections and infestations			Pharyngitis
Injury, poisoning and procedural complications			Contusion
Investigations		Blood creatinine phosphokinase increased, liver function test abnormal	Weight increased, prothrombin time prolonged
Metabolism and nutrition disorders			Hyperuricaemia
Nervous system disorders		Dizziness, headache	
Renal and urinary disorders			Proteinuria
Respiratory, thoracic and mediastinal disorders		Nasal congestion	Asthma, cough
Skin and subcutaneous tissue disorders		Rash	Pruritus, erythema,
Vascular disorders			Hot flush

* HAE attacks were reported as adverse reactions, however based on time of occurrence, the majority were recurrent attacks and not related to treatment with Firazyr.

Table 2

Controlled Clinical Study of FIRAZYR vs Tranexamic acid or Placebo: Efficacy Results

STUDY 1	Icatibant	Tranexamic acid	STUDY 2	Icatibant	Placebo
Number of subjects in ITT Population	36	38	Number of subjects in ITT Population	27	29
Baseline VAS(mm)	63.7	61.5	Baseline VAS(mm)	69.3	67.7
Change from baseline to 4 hours	-41.6	-14.6	Change from baseline to 4 hours	-44.6	-23.5
Difference between treatments (95% CI, p-value)	-27.8 (-39.4, -16.2) p < 0.001		Difference between treatments (95% CI, p-value)	-22.3 (-36.1, -9.3) p = 0.002	
Change from baseline to 12 hours	-54.0	-30.3	Change from baseline to 12 hours	-53.9	-41.0
Difference between treatments (95% CI, p-value)	-24.1 (-33.6, -14.6) p < 0.001		Difference between treatments (95% CI, p-value)	-14.0 (-27.7, -0.3) p = 0.046	
Median time to onset of symptom relief (hours)			Median time to onset of symptom relief (hours)		
All episodes (N = 74)	2.0	12.0	All episodes (N = 56)	2.5	4.6
Response rate (%, CI) at 4 hours after start of treatment			Response rate (%, CI) at 4 hours after start of treatment		
All episodes (N = 74)	80.0 (63.1, 91.6)	30.6 (16.3, 48.1)	All episodes (N = 56)	66.7 (46.0, 83.5)	46.4 (27.5, 66.1)
Median time to onset of symptom relief: all symptoms (hours):			Median time to onset of symptom relief: all symptoms (hours):		
Abdominal pain Skin swelling Skin pain	1.6 2.6 1.5	3.5 18.1 12.0	Abdominal pain Skin swelling Skin pain	2.0 3.1 1.6	3.3 10.2 9.0
Median time to almost complete symptom relief (hours)			Median time to almost complete symptom relief (hours)		
All episodes (N = 74)	10.0	51.0	All episodes (N = 56)	8.5	23.3
Median time to regression of symptoms, by patient (hours)			Median time to regression of symptoms, by patient (hours)		
All episodes (N = 74)	0.8	7.9	All episodes (N = 56)	0.8	16.9
Median time to overall patient improvement, by physician (hours)			Median time to overall patient improvement, by physician (hours)		
All episodes (N = 74)	1.5	6.9	All episodes (N = 56)	1.0	5.7

Clearance is about 15-20 l/h and independent of dose. The terminal half-life is about 1-2 hours.

Metabolism

Icatibant is extensively metabolized by proteolytic enzymes to inactive metabolites that are primarily excreted in the urine.

In vitro studies have confirmed that icatibant is not degraded by oxidative metabolic pathways and is not an inhibitor of major cytochrome P450 (CYP) isoenzymes (CYP 1A2, 2A6, 2B6, 2C8, 2C9, 2C19, 2D6, 2E1, and 3A4) and is not an inducer of CYP 1A2 and 3A4.

Special populations

Data suggest an age-related decline in clearance resulting in about 50-60% higher exposure in the elderly (75-80 years) compared to a patient aged 40 years. Data suggests that gender and weight do not have a significant influence on icatibant pharmacokinetics.

Limited data suggest that icatibant exposure is not influenced by hepatic or renal impairment. The influence of race on icatibant pharmacokinetics has not been evaluated. There are no pharmacokinetic data in children.

5.3 Preclinical safety data

Repeated-dose studies of up to 3-months duration have been conducted in rat and dog. Maximum daily exposures (AUC) at the No Observed Adverse Effect Levels in the 3-month study in rat were 3.6 times and in the 4 week study in dog were 9.4 times the AUC in humans after a subcutaneous dose of 30 mg.

Long-term studies to determine the carcinogenic potential of icatibant have not been conducted to date.

In a standard battery of *in vitro* and *in vivo* tests icatibant was not genotoxic.

Icatibant was not teratogenic when administered by s.c. injection during early embryonic and fetal development in rat (top dose 25 mg/kg/day) and rabbit (top dose 10 mg/kg/day). Icatibant is a potent antagonist of bradykinin and therefore, at high dose levels, treatment can have effects on the uterine implantation process and subsequent uterine stability in early pregnancy. These uterine effects also manifest in late stage pregnancy where icatibant exhibits a tocolytic effect resulting in delayed parturition in the rat, with increased fetal distress and perinatal death at high doses (10 mg/kg/day).

In immature rats and dogs, repeated use of icatibant reversibly delayed sexual maturation. The effects appeared to be secondary to icatibant-induced changes in gonadotrophin levels, and were reversible. Similar effects of icatibant on gonadotrophins also occurred in sexually mature dogs.

Icatibant had no effect on the fertility of male mice and rats.

Icatibant did not elicit any cardiac conduction change *in vitro* (hERG channel) or *in vivo* in normal dogs or in various dog models (ventricular pacing, physical exertion and coronary ligation) where no associated hemodynamic changes were observed. Icatibant has been shown to aggravate induced cardiac ischemia in several non-clinical models, although a detrimental effect has not consistently been shown in acute ischemia.

6. PHARMACEUTICAL PARTICULARS

6.1 List of excipients

Sodium chloride

Acetic acid, glacial (for pH adjustment)

Sodium hydroxide (for pH adjustment)

Water for injections

6.2 Incompatibilities

Not applicable.

6.3 Shelf life

24 months.

6.4 Special precautions for storage

Do not store above 25°C.

Do not freeze.

6.5 Nature and contents of container

One pre-filled syringe (type I glass) with plunger stopper (bromobutyl coated with fluorocarbon polymer). 3 ml of solution filled in a 3 ml syringe.

A hypodermic needle (25 G; 16 mm) is included in the package.

6.6 Special precautions for disposal and other handling

The solution should be clear and colourless and free from visible particles. For single use only.

Any unused product or waste material should be disposed of in accordance with local requirements.

7. MARKETING AUTHORISATION HOLDER

Jerini AG

Invalidenstr. 130

D-10115 Berlin

Germany

8. MARKETING AUTHORISATION NUMBER(S)

EU/1/08/461/001

9. DATE OF FIRST AUTHORISATION/RENEWAL OF THE AUTHORISATION

11/07/2008

10. DATE OF REVISION OF THE TEXT

26/06/2009

Detailed information on this product is available on the website of the European Medicines Agency (EMEA) http://www.emea.europa.eu

Firmagon 120mg Injection

(Ferring Pharmaceuticals Ltd)

1. NAME OF THE MEDICINAL PRODUCT

FIRMAGON ▼ 120 mg powder and solvent for solution for injection

2. QUALITATIVE AND QUANTITATIVE COMPOSITION

Each vial contains 120 mg degarelix (as acetate). After reconstitution, each ml solution contains 40 mg of degarelix.

For a full list of excipients, see section 6.1.

3. PHARMACEUTICAL FORM

Powder and solvent for solution for injection (Powder for injection and solvent)

Powder: White to off-white powder

Solvent: Clear, colourless solution

4. CLINICAL PARTICULARS

4.1 Therapeutic indications

FIRMAGON is a gonadotrophin releasing hormone (GnRH) antagonist indicated for treatment of adult male patients with advanced hormone-dependent prostate cancer.

4.2 Posology and method of administration

Posology

Starting dose	Maintenance dose – monthly administration
240 mg administered as two subcutaneous injections of 120 mg each	80 mg administered as one subcutaneous injection

The first maintenance dose should be given one month after the starting dose.

The therapeutic effect of degarelix should be monitored by clinical parameters and prostate specific antigen (PSA) serum levels. Clinical studies have shown that testosterone (T) suppression occurs immediately after administration of the starting dose with 96% of the patients having plasma testosterone levels corresponding to medical castration ($T \leqslant 0.5$ ng/ml) after three days and 100% after one month. Long term treatment with the maintenance dose up to 1 year shows that 97% of the patients have sustained suppressed testosterone levels ($T \leqslant 0.5$ ng/ml).

In case the patient's clinical response appears to be sub-optimal, it should be confirmed that serum testosterone levels are remaining sufficiently suppressed.

Since degarelix does not induce a testosterone surge it is not necessary to add an anti-androgen as surge protection at initiation of therapy.

Method of administration

FIRMAGON must be reconstituted prior to administration. For instructions on reconstitution and administration, please see section 6.6.

Subcutaneous use ONLY, not to be administered intravenously.

Intramuscular administration is not recommended as it has not been studied.

FIRMAGON is administered as a subcutaneous injection in the abdominal region. As with other medicinal products administered by subcutaneous injection, the injection site should vary periodically. Injections should be given in areas where the patient will not be exposed to pressure e.g. not close to waistband or belt and not close to the ribs.

Special patient populations

Elderly, hepatically or renally impaired patients:

There is no need to adjust the dose for the elderly or in patients with mild or moderate liver or kidney function impairment (see section 5.2). Patients with severe liver or kidney impairment have not been studied and caution is therefore warranted (see section 4.4).

There is no relevant indication for use of FIRMAGON in women, children and adolescents.

4.3 Contraindications

Hypersensitivity to the active substance or to any of the excipients.

4.4 Special warnings and precautions for use

The data available on efficacy and safety experience with degarelix is limited to a one year treatment.

Effect on QT/QTc interval

Long-term androgen deprivation therapy may prolong the QT interval. In the confirmatory study comparing FIRMAGON to leuprorelin periodic (monthly) ECGs were performed; both therapies showed QT/QTc intervals exceeding 450 msec in approximately 20% of the patients, and 500 msec in 1% and 2% of the degarelix and leuprorelin patients, respectively (see section 5.1). FIRMAGON has not been studied in patients with a history of a corrected QT interval over 450 msec, in patients with a history of or risk factors for torsades de pointes and in patients receiving concomitant medicinal products that might prolong the QT interval. Therefore in such patients, the benefit/risk ratio of FIRMAGON must be thoroughly appraised (see sections 4.5 and 4.8).

Hepatic impairment

Patients with known or suspected hepatic disorder have not been included in long-term clinical trials with degarelix. Mild, transient increases in ALT and AST have been seen, these were not accompanied by a rise in bilirubin or clinical symptoms. Monitoring of liver function in patients with known or suspected hepatic disorder is advised during treatment. The pharmacokinetics of degarelix has been investigated after single intravenous administration in subjects with mild to moderate hepatic impairment (see section 5.2).

Renal impairment

Degarelix has not been studied in patients with severe renal impairment and caution is therefore warranted.

Hypersensitivity

Degarelix has not been studied in patients with a history of severe untreated asthma, anaphylactic reactions or severe urticaria or angioedema.

Changes in bone density

Decreased bone density has been reported in the medical literature in men who have had orchiectomy or who have been treated with a GnRH agonist. It can be anticipated that long periods of testosterone suppression in men will have effects on bone density. Bone density has not been measured during treatment with degarelix.

Glucose tolerance

A reduction in glucose tolerance has been observed in men who have had orchiectomy or who have been treated with a GnRH agonist. Development or aggravation of diabetes may occur; therefore diabetic patients may require more frequent monitoring of blood glucose when receiving androgen deprivation therapy. The effect of degarelix on insulin and glucose levels has not been studied.

4.5 Interaction with other medicinal products and other forms of interaction

No formal drug-drug interaction studies have been performed.

Since androgen deprivation treatment may prolong the QTc interval, the concomitant use of degarelix with medicinal products known to prolong the QTc interval or medicinal products able to induce torsades de pointes such as class IA (e.g. quinidine, disopyramide) or class III (e.g. amiodarone, sotalol, dofetilide, ibutilide) antiarrhythmic medicinal products, methadone, cisapride, moxifloxacine, antipsychotics, etc. should be carefully evaluated (see section 4.4).

Degarelix is not a substrate for the human CYP450 system and has not been shown to induce or inhibit CYP1A2, CYP2C8, CYP2C9, CYP2C19, CYP2D6, CYP2E1, or CYP3A4/5 to any great extent *in vitro*. Therefore, clinically significant pharmacokinetic drug-drug interactions in metabolism related to these isoenzymes are unlikely.

4.6 Pregnancy and lactation

There is no relevant indication for use of FIRMAGON in women.

4.7 Effects on ability to drive and use machines

No studies on the effects of degarelix on the ability to drive and use machines have been performed. However, fatigue and dizziness are common adverse reactions that might influence the ability to drive and use machines.

4.8 Undesirable effects

The most commonly observed adverse reactions during degarelix therapy in the confirmatory phase III study (N=409) were due to the expected physiological effects of testosterone suppression, including hot flushes and weight increase (reported in 25% and 7%, respectively, of patients receiving treatment for one year), or injection site adverse events. Transient chills, fever or influenza like illness were reported to occur hours after dosing (in 3%, 2% and 1% of patients, respectively).

The injection site adverse events reported were mainly pain and erythema, reported in 28% and 17% of patients, respectively, less frequently reported were swelling (6%), induration (4%) and nodule (3%). These events occurred primarily with the starting dose whereas during maintenance therapy with the 80 mg dose, the incidence of these events pr 100 injections was: 3 for pain and <1 for erythema, swelling, nodule and induration. The reported events were mostly transient, of mild to moderate intensity and led to very few discontinuations (<1%).

The frequency of undesirable effects listed below is defined using the following convention:

Very common (≥ 1/10); common (≥ 1/100 to < 1/10); uncommon (≥ 1/1,000 to < 1/100). Within each frequency grouping, undesirable effects are presented in order of decreasing seriousness.

Table 1: Frequency of adverse drug reactions reported in 1259 patients treated for a total of 1781 patient years (phase II and III studies).

(see Table 1 below)

The following events have been reported as being related to treatment in single patients: Febrile neutropenia, myocardial infarction and congestive heart failure.

Changes in laboratory parameters

Changes in laboratory values seen during one year of treatment in the confirmatory phase III study (N=409) were in the same range for degarelix and a GnRH-agonist (leuprorelin) used as comparator. Markedly abnormal (>3*ULN) liver transaminase values (ALT, AST and GGT) were seen in 2-6% of patients with normal values prior to treatment, following treatment with both medicinal products. Marked decrease in haematological values, hematocrit (≤0.37) and hemoglobin (≤115 g/l) were seen in 40% and 13-15%, respectively, of patients with normal values prior to treatment, following treatment with both medicinal products. It is unknown to what extent this decrease in haematological values was caused by the underlying prostate cancer and to what extent it was a consequence of androgen deprivation therapy. Markedly abnormal values of potassium (≥5.8 mmol/l), creatinine (≥177 μmol/l) and BUN (≥10.7 mmol/l) in patients with normal values prior to treatment, were seen in 6%, 2% and 15% of degarelix treated patients and 3%, 2% and 14% of leuprorelin treated patients, respectively.

Changes in ECG measurements

Changes in ECG measurements seen during one year of treatment in the confirmatory phase III study (N=409) were in the same range for degarelix and a GnRH-agonist (leuprorelin) used as comparator. Three (<1%) out of 409 patients in the degarelix group and four (2%) out of 201 patients in the leuprorelin 7.5 mg group, had a QTcF ≥ 500 msec. From baseline to end of study the median change in QTcF for degarelix was 12.0 msec and for leuprorelin was 16.7 msec.

4.9 Overdose

There is no clinical experience with the effects of an acute overdose with degarelix. In the event of an overdose the patient should be monitored and appropriate supportive treatment should be given, if considered necessary.

5. PHARMACOLOGICAL PROPERTIES

5.1 Pharmacodynamic properties

Pharmacotherapeutic group: Other hormone antagonists and related agents, ATC code: L02BX02

Degarelix is a selective gonadotrophin releasing-hormone (GnRH) antagonist that competitively and reversibly binds to the pituitary GnRH receptors, thereby rapidly reducing the release of the gonadotrophins, luteinizing hormone (LH) and follicle stimulating hormone (FSH), and thereby reducing the secretion of testosterone (T) by the testes. Prostatic carcinoma is known to be androgen sensitive and responds to treatment that removes the source of androgen. Unlike GnRH agonists, GnRH antagonists do not induce a LH surge with subsequent testosterone surge/tumour stimulation and potential symptomatic flare after the initiation of treatment.

A single dose of 240 mg degarelix, followed by a monthly maintenance dose of 80 mg, rapidly causes a decrease in the concentrations of LH, FSH and subsequently testosterone. The plasma concentration of dihydrotestosterone (DHT) decreases in a similar manner to testosterone.

Degarelix is effective in achieving and maintaining testosterone suppression well below medical castration level of 0.5 ng/ml. Maintenance monthly dosing of 80 mg resulted in sustained testosterone suppression in 97% of patients for at least one year. Median testosterone levels after one

Table 1: Frequency of adverse drug reactions reported in 1259 patients treated for a total of 1781 patient years (phase II and III studies)

MedDRA System Organ Class (SOC)	Very common	Common	Uncommon
Blood and lymphatic system disorders		Anaemia*	
Immune system disorders			Hypersensitivity
Metabolism and nutrition disorders		Weight increase*	Hyperglycemia/Diabetes mellitus, cholesterol increased, weight decreased, appetite decreased, changes in blood calcium
Psychiatric disorders		Insomnia	Depression, libido decreased*
Nervous system disorders		Dizziness, headache	Mental impairment, hypoaesthesia
Eye disorders			Vission blurred
Cardiac disorders			Cardiac arrhythmia (incl. atrial fibrillation), palpitations, QT prolongation*(see sections 4.4 and 4.5)
Vascular disorders	Hot flush*		Hypertension, vasovagal reaction (incl. hypotension)
Respiratory, thoracic and mediastinal disorders			Dyspnoea
Gastrointestinal disorders		Diarrhoea, nausea	Constipation, vomiting, abdominal pain, abdominal discomfort, dry mouth
Hepatobiliary disorders		Liver transaminases increased	Bilirubin increased, alkaline phosphatase increased
Skin and subcutaneous tissue disorders		Hyperhidrosis (incl. night sweats)*, rash	Urticaria, skin nodule, alopecia, pruritus, erythema
Musculoskeletal, connective tissue and bone disorders		Musculoskeletal pain and discomfort	Osteoporosis/osteopenia, arthralgia, muscular weakness, muscle spasms, joint swelling/stiffness
Renal and urinary disorders			Pollakiuria, micturition urgency, dysuria, nocturia, renal impairment, incontinence
Reproductive system and breast disorders		Gynaecomastia*, testicular atrophy*, erectile dysfunction*	Testicular pain, breast pain, pelvic pain, genital irritation, ejaculation failure
General disorders and administration site conditions	Injection site adverse events	Chills, pyrexia, fatigue*, Influenza-like illness	Malaise, peripheral oedema

* Known physiological consequence of testosterone suppression

Figure 1: Percentage change in testosterone from baseline by treatment group until day 28 (median with interquartile ranges)

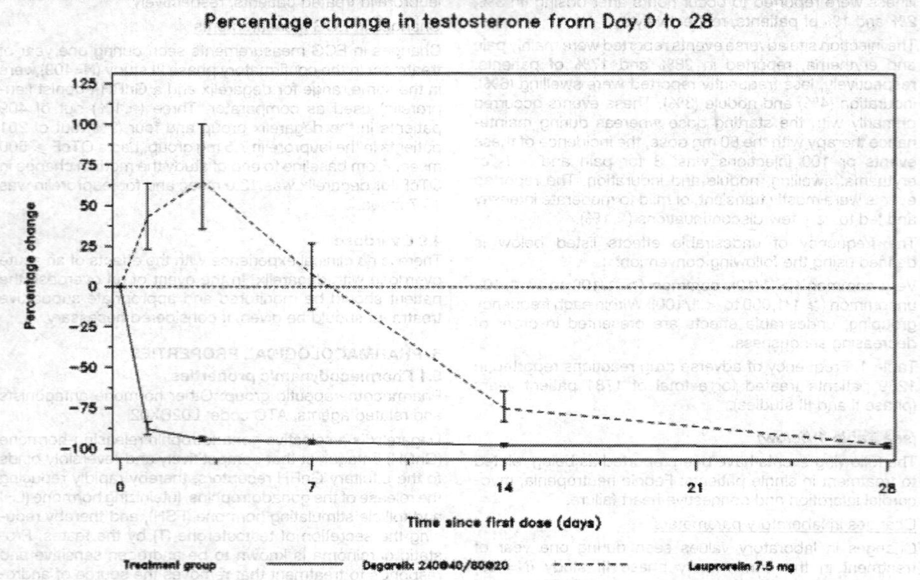

Figure 2: Percentage change in PSA from baseline by treatment group until day 56 (median with interquartile ranges)

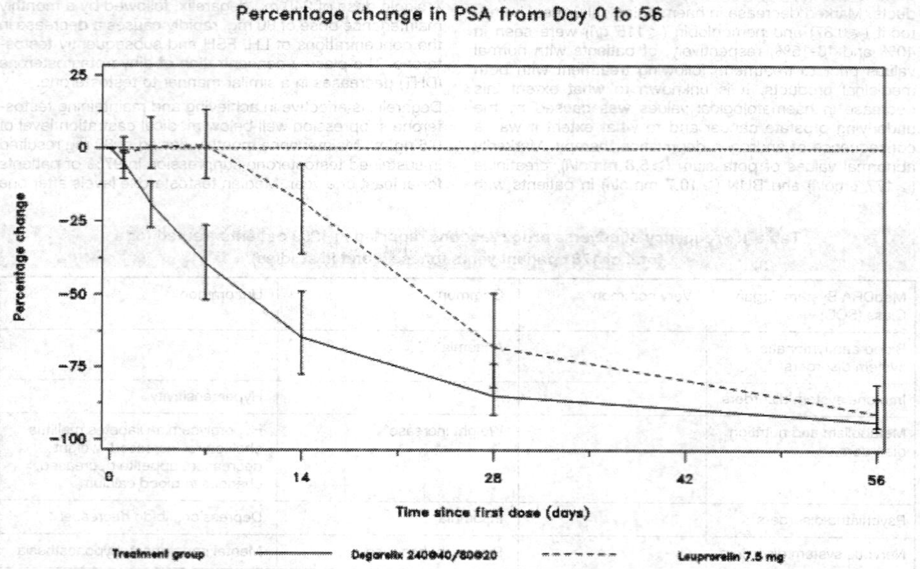

year of treatment were 0.087 ng/ml (interquartile range 0.06-0.15) N=167.

Results of the confirmatory Phase III study

The efficacy and safety of degarelix was evaluated in an open-label, multi-centre, randomised, active comparator controlled, parallel-group study. The study investigated the efficacy and safety of two different degarelix monthly dosing regimens with a starting dose of 240 mg (40 mg/ml) followed by monthly doses subcutaneous administration of 160 mg (40 mg/ml) or 80 mg (20 mg/ml), in comparison to monthly intramuscular administration of 7.5 mg leuprorelin in patients with prostate cancer requiring androgen deprivation therapy. In total 620 patients were randomised to one of the three treatment groups, of which 504 (81%) patients completed the study. In the degarelix 240/80 mg treatment group 41 (20%) patients discontinued the study, as compared to 32 (16%) patients in the leuprorelin group.

Of the 610 patients treated

- 31% had localised prostate cancer
- 29% had locally advanced prostate cancer
- 20% had metastatic prostate cancer
- 7% had an unknown metastatic status
- 13% had previous curative intent surgery or radiation and a rising PSA

Baseline demographics were similar between the arms. The median age was 74 years (range 47 to 98 years). The primary objective was to demonstrate that degarelix is effective with respect to achieving and maintaining testosterone suppression to below 0.5 ng/ml, during 12 months of treatment.

The lowest effective maintenance dose of 80 mg degarelix was chosen.

Attainment of serum testosterone (T) ≤0.5 ng/ml

FIRMAGON is effective in achieving fast testosterone suppression, see Table 2.

Table 2: Percentage of patients attaining T≤0.5 ng/ml after start of treatment.

Time	Degarelix 240/80 mg	Leuprorelin 7.5 mg
Day 1	52%	0%
Day 3	96%	0%
Day 7	99%	1%
Day 14	100%	18%
Day 28	100%	100%

Avoidance of testosterone surge

Surge was defined as testosterone exceeding baseline by ≥15% within the first 2 weeks.

None of the degarelix-treated patients experienced a testosterone surge; there was an average decrease of 94% in testosterone at day 3. Most of the leuprorelin-treated patients experienced testosterone surge; there was an average increase of 65% in testosterone at day 3. This difference was statistically significant (p<0.001).

Figure 1: Percentage change in testosterone from baseline by treatment group until day 28 (median with interquartile ranges).

(see Figure 1 above)

The primary end-point in the study was testosterone suppression rates after one year of treatment with degarelix or leuprorelin. The clinical benefit for degarelix compared to leuprorelin plus anti-androgen in the initial phase of treatment has not been demonstrated.

Long-term effect

Successful response in the study was defined as attainment of medical castration at day 28 and maintenance through day 364 where no single testosterone concentration was greater than 0.5 ng/ml.

Table 3: Cumulative probability of testosterone ≤0.5 ng/ml from Day 28 to Day 364.

	Degarelix 240/ 80 mg N=207	Leuprorelin 7.5 mg N=201
No. of responders	202	194
Response Rate (confidence intervals)*	97.2% (93.5; 98.8%)	96.4% (92.5; 98.2%)

* Kaplan Meier estimates within group

Attainment of prostate specific antigen (PSA) reduction

Tumour size was not measured directly during the clinical trial programme, but there was an indirect beneficial tumour response as shown by a 95% reduction after 12 months in median PSA for degarelix.

The median PSA in the study at baseline was:

- for the degarelix 240/80 mg treatment group 19.8 ng/ml (interquartile range: P25 9.4 ng/ml, P75 46.4 ng/ml)
- for the leuprorelin 7.5 mg treatment group 17.4 ng/ml (interquartile range: P25 8.4 ng/ml, P75 56.5 ng/ml)

Figure 2: Percentage change in PSA from baseline by treatment group until day 56 (median with interquartile ranges).

(see Figure 2 opposite)

This difference was statistically significant (p<0.001) for the pre-specified analysis at day 14 and day 28.

Prostate specific antigen (PSA) levels are lowered by 64% two weeks after administration of degarelix, 85% after one month, 95% after three months, and remained suppressed (approximately 97%) throughout the one year of treatment.

From day 56 to day 364 there were no significant differences between degarelix and the comparator in the percentage change from baseline.

In the confirmatory study comparing FIRMAGON to leuprorelin periodic electrocardiograms were performed. Both therapies showed QT/QTc intervals exceeding 450 msec in approximately 20% of the patients. From baseline to end of study the median change for FIRMAGON was 12.0 msec and for leuprorelin it was 16.7 msec.

Anti-degarelix antibody development has been observed in 10% of patients after treatment with FIRMAGON for one year. There is no indication that the efficacy or safety of FIRMAGON treatment is affected by antibody formation after one year of treatment. Efficacy and safety data in relation to antibody development beyond one year is not available.

5.2 Pharmacokinetic properties

Absorption

Following subcutaneous administration of 240 mg degarelix at a concentration of 40 mg/ml to prostate cancer patients in the pivotal study CS21, $AUC_{0\text{-}28\ days}$ was 635 (602-668) day*ng/ml, C_{max} was 66.0 (61.0-71.0) ng/ml and occurred at t_{max} at 40 (37-42) hours. Mean trough values were approximately 11-12 ng/ml after the starting dose and 11-16 ng/ml after maintenance dosing of 80 mg at a concentration of 20 mg/ml. Degarelix is eliminated in a biphasic fashion, with a median terminal half-life ($t_{½}$) of approximately 43 days for the starting dose or 28 days for the maintenance dose, as estimated based on population pharmacokinetics modelling. The long half-life after subcutaneous administration is a consequence of a very slow release of degarelix from the depot formed at the injection site(s). The pharmacokinetic behavior of the medicinal product is influenced by its concentration in the solution for injection. Thus, C_{max} and bioavailability tend to decrease with increasing dose concentration while the half-life is increased. Therefore, no other dose concentrations than the recommended should be used.

Distribution

The distribution volume in healthy elderly men is approximately 1 l/kg. Plasma protein binding is estimated to be approximately 90%.

Metabolism

Degarelix is subject to common peptidic degradation during the passage of the hepato-biliary system and is mainly excreted as peptide fragments in the faeces. No significant metabolites were detected in plasma samples after subcutaneous administration. *In vitro* studies have shown that degarelix is not a substrate for the human CYP450 system.

Excretion

In healthy men, approximately 20-30% of a single intravenously administered dose is excreted in the urine, suggesting that 70-80% is excreted via the hepato-biliary system. The clearance of degarelix when administered as single intravenous doses (0.864-49.4 µg/kg) in healthy elderly men was found to be 35-50 ml/h/kg.

Special populations:

Patients with renal impairment

No pharmacokinetic studies in renally impaired patients have been conducted. Only about 20-30% of a given dose of degarelix is excreted unchanged by the kidneys. A population pharmacokinetics analysis of the data from the confirmatory Phase III study has demonstrated that the clearance of degarelix in patients with mild to moderate renal impairment is reduced by approximately 23%; therefore, dose adjustment in patients with mild or moderate renal impairment is not recommended. Data on patients with severe renal impairment is scarce and caution is therefore warranted in this patient population.

Patients with hepatic impairment

Degarelix has been investigated in a pharmacokinetic study in patients with mild to moderate hepatic impairment. No signs of increased exposure in the hepatically impaired subjects were observed compared to healthy subjects. Dose adjustment is not necessary in patients with mild or moderate hepatic impairment. Patients with severe hepatic dysfunction have not been studied and caution is therefore warranted in this group.

5.3 Preclinical safety data

Animal reproduction studies showed that degarelix caused infertility in male animals. This is due to the pharmacological effect; and the effect was reversible.

In female reproduction toxicity studies degarelix revealed findings expected from the pharmacological properties. It caused a dosage dependent prolongation of the time to mating and to pregnancy, a reduced number of *corpora lutea*, and an increase in the number of pre- and post-implantation losses, abortions, early embryo/foetal deaths, premature deliveries and in the duration of parturition.

Preclinical studies on safety pharmacology, repeated dose toxicity, genotoxicity, and carcinogenic potential revealed no special hazard for humans. Both *in vitro* and *in vivo* studies showed no signs of QT prolongation.

No target organ toxicity was observed from acute, subacute and chronic toxicity studies in rats and monkeys following subcutaneous administration of degarelix. Drug-related local irritation was noted in animals when degarelix was administered subcutaneously in high doses.

6. PHARMACEUTICAL PARTICULARS

6.1 List of excipients

Powder

Mannitol (E421)

Solvent

Water for injections

6.2 Incompatibilities

In the absence of compatibility studies, this medicinal product must not be mixed with other medicinal products.

6.3 Shelf life

3 years.

After reconstitution

Chemical and physical in-use stability has been demonstrated for 2 hours at 25°C. From a microbiological point of view, unless the method of reconstitution precludes the risk of microbial contamination, the product should be used immediately. If not used immediately, in-use storage times and conditions are the responsibility of the user.

6.4 Special precautions for storage

This medicinal product does not require any special storage conditions.

For storage conditions of the reconstituted medicinal product, see section 6.3.

6.5 Nature and contents of container

Vials of glass Type I with bromobutyl rubber stopper and aluminium flip-off seal.

2 vials containing 120 mg powder for solution for injection

2 vials containing 6 ml solvent

2 syringes (5 ml)

2 reconstitution needles (21G 0.8 × 50 mm)

2 injection needles (27G 0.4 × 25 mm)

6.6 Special precautions for disposal and other handling

No special requirements for disposal.

Instructions for use:

The instructions for reconstitution must be followed carefully.

Administration of other concentrations is not recommended because the gel depot formation is influenced by the concentration. The reconstituted solution should be a clear liquid, free of undissolved matter.

NOTE:

• THE VIALS SHOULD BE KEPT VERTICAL AT ALL TIMES

• THE VIALS SHOULD NOT BE SHAKEN

The pack contains 2 sets of powder and solvent that must be prepared for subcutaneous injection. Hence, the instructions here below need to be repeated a second time.

1. Draw up 3.0 ml solvent for injection with the reconstitution needle (green needle, 21G / 0.8 × 50 mm). Discard the vial with the remaining solvent.

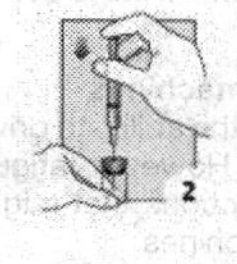

2. Inject the solvent slowly into the vial with powder. DO NOT REMOVE THE SYRINGE AND THE NEEDLE, to keep the medicinal product and syringe sterile.

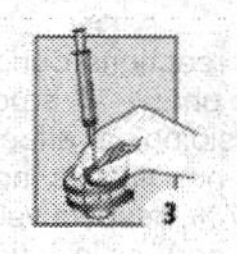

3. KEEP THE VIAL IN AN UPRIGHT POSITION. Swirl very gently until the liquid looks clear and without undissolved powder or particles. In case the powder adheres to the vial over the liquid surface, the vial can be tilted slightly. **AVOID SHAKING TO PREVENT FOAM FORMATION.** A ring of small air bubbles on the surface of the liquid is acceptable. The reconstitution procedure may take, in some cases, up to 15 minutes, but usually takes a few minutes.

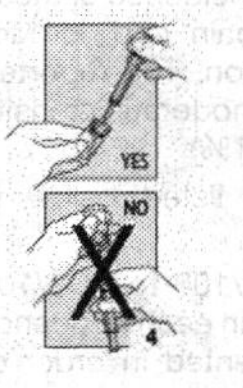

4. Tilt the vial slightly and keep the needle in the lowest part of the vial. Withdraw **3.0 ml** of the solution **without turning the vial upside down.**

5. Exchange the green needle with the white needle for deep subcutaneous injection (27G / 0.4 × 25 mm). Remove any air bubbles.

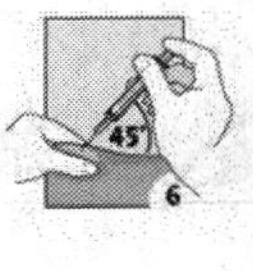

6. Grasp the skin of the abdomen, elevate the subcutaneous tissue. Perform a profound subcutaneous injection. To do so, insert the needle deeply at an angle of not less than **45 degrees.**

7. Inject **3.0 ml of FIRMAGON 120 mg** immediately after reconstitution.*

8. Do not inject directly into a vein. Gently pull back the plunger to check if blood is aspirated. If blood appears in the syringe, the medicinal product can no longer be used. Discontinue the procedure and discard the syringe and the needle (reconstitute a new dose for the patient).

9. Repeat the reconstitution procedure for the second dose. Choose a different injection site **and inject 3.0 ml.**

Please be aware:

• No injections should be given in areas where the patient will be exposed to pressure, e.g. around the belt or waistband or close to the ribs.

* Chemical and physical in-use stability has been demonstrated for 2 hours at 25°C. From a microbiological point of view, unless the method of reconstitution precludes the risk of microbial contamination, the product should be used immediately. If not used immediately, in-use storage times and conditions are the responsibility of the user.

7. MARKETING AUTHORISATION HOLDER

Ferring Pharmaceuticals A/S

Kay Fiskers Plads 11

DK-2300 Copenhagen S

Denmark

Tel: +45 88 33 88 34

8. MARKETING AUTHORISATION NUMBER(S)

EU/1/08/504/002

9. DATE OF FIRST AUTHORISATION/RENEWAL OF THE AUTHORISATION

17/02/2009

10. DATE OF REVISION OF THE TEXT

30/07/2009

Detailed information on this medicinal product is available on the website of the European Medicines Agency (EMEA) http://www.emea.europa.eu/.

Firmagon 80mg Injection

(Ferring Pharmaceuticals Ltd)

1. NAME OF THE MEDICINAL PRODUCT

FIRMAGON ▼ 80 mg powder and solvent for solution for injection

2. QUALITATIVE AND QUANTITATIVE COMPOSITION

Each vial contains 80 mg degarelix (as acetate). After reconstitution, each ml of solution contains 20 mg of degarelix.

For a full list of excipients, see section 6.1.

3. PHARMACEUTICAL FORM

Powder and solvent for solution for injection (Powder for injection and solvent)

Powder: White to off-white powder

Solvent: Clear, colourless solution

4. CLINICAL PARTICULARS

4.1 Therapeutic indications

FIRMAGON is a gonadotrophin releasing hormone (GnRH) antagonist indicated for treatment of adult male patients with advanced hormone-dependent prostate cancer.

4.2 Posology and method of administration

Posology

Starting dose	Maintenance dose – monthly administration
240 mg administered as two subcutaneous injections of 120 mg each	80 mg administered as one subcutaneous injection

The first maintenance dose should be given one month after the starting dose.

The therapeutic effect of degarelix should be monitored by clinical parameters and prostate specific antigen (PSA) serum levels. Clinical studies have shown that testosterone (T) suppression occurs immediately after administration of the starting dose with 96% of the patients having plasma testosterone levels corresponding to medical castration (T ≤ 0.5 ng/ml) after three days and 100% after one month. Long term treatment with the maintenance dose up to 1 year shows that 97% of the patients have sustained suppressed testosterone levels (T ≤ 0.5 ng/ml).

In case the patient's clinical response appears to be sub-optimal, it should be confirmed that serum testosterone levels are remaining sufficiently suppressed.

Since degarelix does not induce a testosterone surge it is not necessary to add an anti-androgen as surge protection at initiation of therapy.

Method of administration

FIRMAGON must be reconstituted prior to administration. For instructions on reconstitution and administration, please see section 6.6.

Subcutaneous use ONLY, not to be administered intravenously.

Intramuscular administration is not recommended as it has not been studied.

FIRMAGON is administered as a subcutaneous injection in the abdominal region. As with other medicinal products administered by subcutaneous injection, the injection site should vary periodically. Injections should be given in areas where the patient will not be exposed to pressure e.g. not close to waistband or belt and not close to the ribs.

Special patient populations

Elderly, hepatically or renally impaired patients:

There is no need to adjust the dose for the elderly or in patients with mild or moderate liver or kidney function impairment (see section 5.2). Patients with severe liver or kidney impairment have not been studied and caution is therefore warranted (see section 4.4).

There is no relevant indication for use of FIRMAGON in women, children and adolescents.

4.3 Contraindications

Hypersensitivity to the active substance or to any of the excipients.

4.4 Special warnings and precautions for use

The data available on efficacy and safety experience with degarelix is limited to a one year treatment.

Effect on QT/QTc interval

Long-term androgen deprivation therapy may prolong the QT interval. In the confirmatory study comparing FIRMAGON to leuprorelin periodic (monthly) ECGs were performed; both therapies showed QT/QTc intervals exceeding 450 msec in approximately 20% of the patients, and 500 msec in 1% and 2% of the degarelix and leuprorelin patients, respectively (see section 5.1). FIRMAGON has not been studied in patients with a history of a corrected QT interval over 450 msec, in patients with a history of or risk factors for torsades de pointes and in patients receiving concomitant medicinal products that might prolong the QT interval. Therefore in such patients, the benefit/risk ratio of FIRMAGON must be thoroughly appraised (see sections 4.5 and 4.8).

Hepatic impairment

Patients with known or suspected hepatic disorder have not been included in long-term clinical trials with degarelix. Mild, transient increases in ALT and AST have been seen, these were not accompanied by a rise in bilirubin or clinical symptoms. Monitoring of liver function in patients with known or suspected hepatic disorder is advised during treatment. The pharmacokinetics of degarelix has been investigated after single intravenous administration in subjects with mild to moderate hepatic impairment (see section 5.2).

Renal impairment

Degarelix has not been studied in patients with severe renal impairment and caution is therefore warranted.

Hypersensitivity

Degarelix has not been studied in patients with a history of severe untreated asthma, anaphylactic reactions or severe urticaria or angioedema.

Changes in bone density

Decreased bone density has been reported in the medical literature in men who have had orchiectomy or who have been treated with a GnRH agonist. It can be anticipated that long periods of testosterone suppression in men will have effects on bone density. Bone density has not been measured during treatment with degarelix.

Glucose tolerance

A reduction in glucose tolerance has been observed in men who have had orchiectomy or who have been treated with a GnRH agonist. Development or aggravation of diabetes may occur; therefore diabetic patients may require more frequent monitoring of blood glucose when receiving androgen deprivation therapy. The effect of degarelix on insulin and glucose levels has not been studied.

4.5 Interaction with other medicinal products and other forms of interaction

No formal drug-drug interaction studies have been performed.

Since androgen deprivation treatment may prolong the QTc interval, the concomitant use of degarelix with medicinal products known to prolong the QTc interval or medicinal products able to induce torsades de pointes such as class IA (e.g. quinidine, disopyramide) or class III (e.g. amiodarone, sotalol, dofetilide, ibutilide) antiarrhythmic medicinal products, methadone, cisapride, moxifloxacine, antipsychotics, etc. should be carefully evaluated (see section 4.4).

Degarelix is not a substrate for the human CYP450 system and has not been shown to induce or inhibit CYP1A2, CYP2C8, CYP2C9, CYP2C19, CYP2D6, CYP2E1, or CYP3A4/5 to any great extent *in vitro*. Therefore, clinically significant pharmacokinetic drug-drug interactions in metabolism related to these isoenzymes are unlikely.

4.6 Pregnancy and lactation

There is no relevant indication for use of FIRMAGON in women.

4.7 Effects on ability to drive and use machines

No studies on the effects of degarelix on the ability to drive and use machines have been performed. However, fatigue and dizziness are common adverse reactions that might influence the ability to drive and use machines.

4.8 Undesirable effects

The most commonly observed adverse reactions during degarelix therapy in the confirmatory phase III study (N=409) were due to the expected physiological effects of testosterone suppression, including hot flushes and weight increase (reported in 25% and 7%, respectively, of patients receiving treatment for one year), or injection site adverse events. Transient chills, fever or influenza like illness were reported to occur hours after dosing (in 3%, 2% and 1% of patients, respectively).

The injection site adverse events reported were mainly pain and erythema, reported in 28% and 17% of patients, respectively, less frequently reported were swelling (6%), induration (4%) and nodule (3%). These events occurred primarily with the starting dose whereas during maintenance therapy with the 80 mg dose, the incidence of these events pr 100 injections was: 3 for pain and <1 for erythema, swelling, nodule and induration. The reported events were mostly transient, of mild to moderate intensity and led to very few discontinuations (<1%).

The frequency of undesirable effects listed below is defined using the following convention:

Very common (≥ 1/10); common (≥ 1/100 to < 1/10); uncommon (≥ 1/1,000 to < 1/100). Within each frequency grouping, undesirable effects are presented in order of decreasing seriousness.

Table 1: Frequency of adverse drug reactions reported in 1259 patients treated for a total of 1781 patient years (phase II and III studies).

(see Table 1 below)

Table 1: Frequency of adverse drug reactions reported in 1259 patients treated for a total of 1781 patient years (phase II and III studies)

MedDRA System Organ Class (SOC)	Very common	Common	Uncommon
Blood and lymphatic system disorders		Anaemia*	
Immune system disorders			Hypersensitivity
Metabolism and nutrition disorders		Weight increase*	Hyperglycemia/Diabetes mellitus, cholesterol increased, weight decreased, appetite decreased, changes in blood calcium
Psychiatric disorders		Insomnia	Depression, libido decreased*
Nervous system disorders		Dizziness, headache	Mental impairment, hypoaesthesia
Eye disorders			Vision blurred
Cardiac disorders			Cardiac arrhythmia (incl. atrial fibrillation), palpitations, QT prolongation*(see sections 4.4 and 4.5)
Vascular disorders	Hot flush*		Hypertension, vasovagal reaction (incl. hypotension)
Respiratory, thoracic and mediastinal disorders			Dyspnoea
Gastrointestinal disorders		Diarrhoea, nausea	Constipation, vomiting, abdominal pain, abdominal discomfort, dry mouth
Hepatobiliary disorders		Liver transaminases increased	Bilirubin increased, alkaline phosphatase increased
Skin and subcutaneous tissue disorders		Hyperhidrosis (incl. night sweats)*, rash	Urticaria, skin nodule, alopecia, pruritus, erythema
Musculoskeletal, connective tissue and bone disorders		Musculoskeletal pain and discomfort	Osteoporosis/osteopenia, arthralgia muscular weakness, muscle spasms, joint swelling/stiffness
Renal and urinary disorders			Pollakiuria, micturition urgency, dysuria, nocturia, renal impairment, incontinence
Reproductive system and breast disorders		Gynaecomastia*, testicular atrophy*, erectile dysfunction*	Testicular pain, breast pain, pelvic pain, genital irritation, ejaculation failure
General disorders and administration site conditions	Injection site adverse events	Chills, pyrexia, fatigue*, Influenza-like illness	Malaise, peripheral oedema

* Known physiological consequence of testosterone suppression

The following events have been reported as being related to treatment in single patients: Febrile neutropenia, myocardial infarction and congestive heart failure.

Changes in laboratory parameters

Changes in laboratory values seen during one year of treatment in the confirmatory phase III study (N=409) were in the same range for degarelix and a GnRH-agonist (leuprorelin) used as comparator. Markedly abnormal (>3*ULN) liver transaminase values (ALT, AST and GGT) were seen in 2-6% of patients with normal values prior to treatment, following treatment with both medicinal products. Marked decrease in haematological values, hematocrit (≤0.37) and hemoglobin (≤115 g/l) were seen in 40% and 13-15%, respectively, of patients with normal values prior to treatment, following treatment with both medicinal products. It is unknown to what extent this decrease in haematological values was caused by the underlying prostate cancer and to what extent it was a consequence of androgen deprivation therapy. Markedly abnormal values of potassium (≥5.8 mmol/l), creatinine (≥177 μmol/l) and BUN (≥10.7 mmol/l) in patients with normal values prior to treatment, were seen in 6%, 2% and 15% of degarelix treated patients and 3%, 2% and 14% of leuprorelin treated patients, respectively.

Changes in ECG measurements

Changes in ECG measurements seen during one year of treatment in the confirmatory phase III study (N=409) were in the same range for degarelix and a GnRH-agonist (leuprorelin) used as comparator. Three (<1%) out of 409 patients in the degarelix group and four (2%) out of 201 patients in the leuprorelin 7.5 mg group, had a QTcF ≥ 500 msec. From baseline to end of study the median change in QTcF for degarelix was 12.0 msec and for leuprorelin was 16.7 msec.

4.9 Overdose

There is no clinical experience with the effects of an acute overdose with degarelix. In the event of an overdose the patient should be monitored and appropriate supportive treatment should be given, if considered necessary.

5. PHARMACOLOGICAL PROPERTIES

5.1 Pharmacodynamic properties

Pharmacotherapeutic group: Other hormone antagonists and related agents, ATC code: L02BX02

Degarelix is a selective gonadotrophin releasing-hormone (GnRH) antagonist that competitively and reversibly binds to the pituitary GnRH receptors, thereby rapidly reducing the release of the gonadotrophins, luteinizing hormone (LH) and follicle stimulating hormone (FSH), and thereby reducing the secretion of testosterone (T) by the testes. Prostatic carcinoma is known to be androgen sensitive and responds to treatment that removes the source of androgen. Unlike GnRH agonists, GnRH antagonists do not induce a LH surge with subsequent testosterone surge/tumour stimulation and potential symptomatic flare after the initiation of treatment.

A single dose of 240 mg degarelix, followed by a monthly maintenance dose of 80 mg, rapidly causes a decrease in the concentrations of LH, FSH and subsequently testosterone. The plasma concentration of dihydrotestosterone (DHT) decreases in a similar manner to testosterone.

Degarelix is effective in achieving and maintaining testosterone suppression well below medical castration level of 0.5 ng/ml. Maintenance monthly dosing of 80 mg resulted in sustained testosterone suppression in 97% of patients for at least one year. Median testosterone levels after one year of treatment were 0.087 ng/ml (interquartile range 0.06-0.15) N=167.

Results of the confirmatory Phase III study

The efficacy and safety of degarelix was evaluated in an open-label, multi-centre, randomised, active comparator controlled, parallel-group study. The study investigated the efficacy and safety of two different degarelix monthly dosing regimens with a starting dose of 240 mg (40 mg/ml) followed by monthly doses subcutaneous administration of 160 mg (40 mg/ml) or 80 mg (20 mg/ml), in comparison to monthly intramuscular administration of 7.5 mg leuprorelin in patients with prostate cancer requiring androgen deprivation therapy. In total 620 patients were randomised to one of the three treatment groups, of which 504 (81%) patients completed the study. In the degarelix 240/80 mg treatment group 41 (20%) patients discontinued the study, as compared to 32 (16%) patients in the leuprorelin group.

Of the 610 patients treated

- 31% had localised prostate cancer
- 29% had locally advanced prostate cancer
- 20% had metastatic prostate cancer
- 7% had an unknown metastatic status
- 13% had previous curative intent surgery or radiation and a rising PSA

Baseline demographics were similar between the arms. The median age was 74 years (range 47 to 98 years). The primary objective was to demonstrate that degarelix is effective with respect to achieving and maintaining testosterone suppression to below 0.5 ng/ml, during 12 months of treatment.

The lowest effective maintenance dose of 80 mg degarelix was chosen.

Figure 1: Percentage change in testosterone from baseline by treatment group until day 28 (median with interquartile ranges)

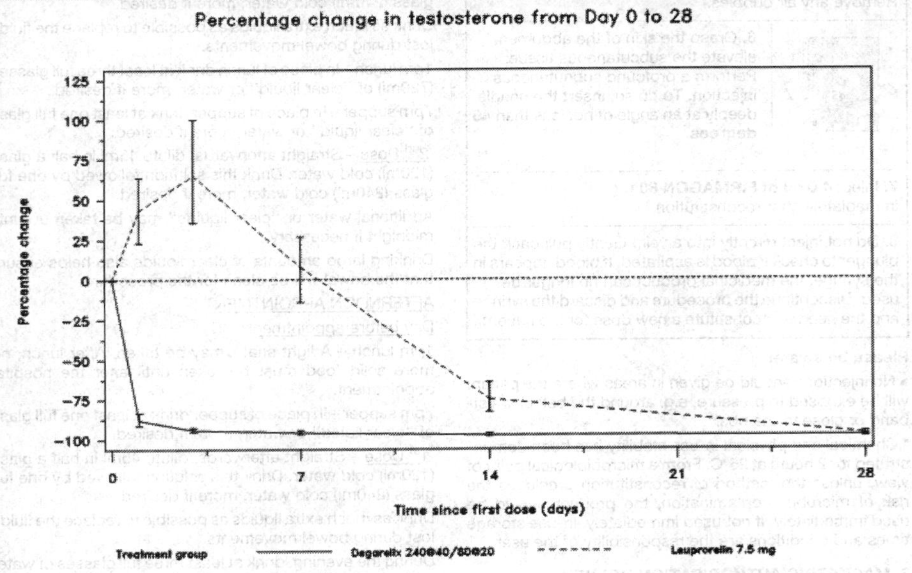

Figure 2: Percentage change in PSA from baseline by treatment group until day 56 (median with interquartile ranges)

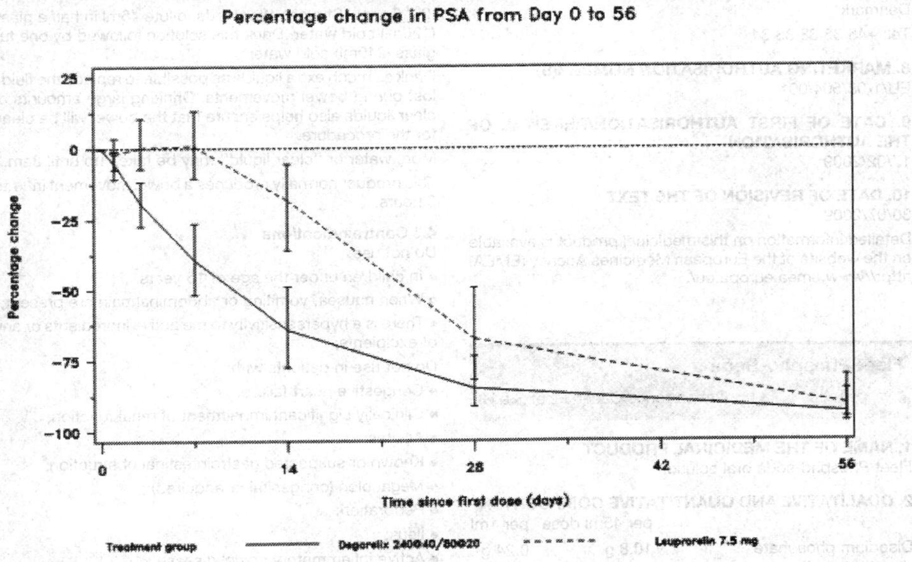

Attainment of serum testosterone (T) ≤0.5 ng/ml

FIRMAGON is effective in achieving fast testosterone suppression, see Table 2.

Table 2: Percentage of patients attaining T≤0.5 ng/ml after start of treatment.

Time	Degarelix 240/80 mg	Leuprorelin 7.5 mg
Day 1	52%	0%
Day 3	96%	0%
Day 7	99%	1%
Day 14	100%	18%
Day 28	100%	100%

Avoidance of testosterone surge

Surge was defined as testosterone exceeding baseline by ≥15% within the first 2 weeks.

None of the degarelix-treated patients experienced a testosterone surge; there was an average decrease of 94% in testosterone at day 3. Most of the leuprorelin-treated patients experienced testosterone surge; there was an average increase of 65% in testosterone at day 3. This difference was statistically significant ($p<0.001$).

Figure 1: Percentage change in testosterone from baseline by treatment group until day 28 (median with interquartile ranges).

(see Figure 1 above)

The primary end-point in the study was testosterone suppression rates after one year of treatment with degarelix or leuprorelin. The clinical benefit for degarelix compared to leuprorelin plus anti-androgen in the initial phase of treatment has not been demonstrated.

Long-term effect

Successful response in the study was defined as attainment of medical castration at day 28 and maintenance through day 364 where no single testosterone concentration was greater than 0.5 ng/ml.

Table 3: Cumulative probability of testosterone ≤0.5 ng/ml from Day 28 to Day 364.

	Degarelix 240/ 80 mg N=207	Leuprorelin 7.5 mg N=201
No. of responders	202	194
Response Rate (confidence intervals)*	97.2% (93.5; 98.8%)	96.4% (92.5; 98.2%)

* Kaplan Meier estimates within group

Attainment of prostate specific antigen (PSA) reduction

Tumour size was not measured directly during the clinical trial programme, but there was an indirect beneficial tumour response as shown by a 95% reduction after 12 months in median PSA for degarelix.

The median PSA in the study at baseline was:

- for the degarelix 240/80 mg treatment group 19.8 ng/ml (interquartile range: P25 9.4 ng/ml, P75 46.4 ng/ml)
- for the leuprorelin 7.5 mg treatment group 17.4 ng/ml (interquartile range: P25 8.4 ng/ml, P75 56.5 ng/ml)

Figure 2: Percentage change in PSA from baseline by treatment group until day 56 (median with interquartile ranges).

(see Figure 2 below)

This difference was statistically significant ($p<0.001$) for the pre-specified analysis at day 14 and day 28.

Prostate specific antigen (PSA) levels are lowered by 64% two weeks after administration of degarelix, 85% after one month, 95% after three months, and remained suppressed (approximately 97%) throughout the one year of treatment.

From day 56 to day 364 there were no significant differences between degarelix and the comparator in the percentage change from baseline.

In the confirmatory study comparing FIRMAGON to leuprorelin periodic electrocardiograms were performed. Both therapies showed QT/QTc intervals exceeding 450 msec in approximately 20% of the patients. From baseline to end of study the median change for FIRMAGON was 12.0 msec and for leuprorelin it was 16.7 msec.

Anti-degarelix antibody development has been observed in 10% of patients after treatment with FIRMAGON for one year. There is no indication that the efficacy or safety of FIRMAGON treatment is affected by antibody formation after one year of treatment. Efficacy and safety data in relation to antibody development beyond one year is not available.

5.2 Pharmacokinetic properties

Absorption

Following subcutaneous administration of 240 mg degarelix at a concentration of 40 mg/ml to prostate cancer patients in the pivotal study CS21, $AUC_{0\text{-}28\ days}$ was 635 (602-668) day*ng/ml, C_{max} was 66.0 (61.0-71.0) ng/ml and occurred at t_{max} at 40 (37-42) hours. Mean trough values were approximately 11-12 ng/ml after the starting dose and 11-16 ng/ml after maintenance dosing of 80 mg at a concentration of 20 mg/ml. Degarelix is eliminated in a biphasic fashion, with a median terminal half-life ($t_{½}$) of approximately 43 days for the starting dose or 28 days for the maintenance dose, as estimated based on population pharmacokinetics modelling. The long half-life after subcutaneous administration is a consequence of a very slow release of degarelix from the depot formed at the injection site(s). The pharmacokinetic behavior of the medicinal product is influenced by its concentration in the solution for injection. Thus, C_{max} and bioavailability tend to decrease with increasing dose concentration while the half-life is increased. Therefore, no other dose concentrations than the recommended should be used.

Distribution

The distribution volume in healthy elderly men is approximately 1 l/kg. Plasma protein binding is estimated to be approximately 90%.

Metabolism

Degarelix is subject to common peptidic degradation during the passage of the hepato-biliary system and is mainly excreted as peptide fragments in the faeces. No significant metabolites were detected in plasma samples after subcutaneous administration. *In vitro* studies have shown that degarelix is not a substrate for the human CYP450 system.

Excretion

In healthy men, approximately 20-30% of a single intravenously administered dose is excreted in the urine, suggesting that 70-80% is excreted via the hepato-biliary system. The clearance of degarelix when administered as single intravenous doses (0.864-49.4 μg/kg) in healthy elderly men was found to be 35-50 ml/h/kg.

Special populations:

Patients with renal impairment

No pharmacokinetic studies in renally impaired patients have been conducted. Only about 20-30% of a given dose of degarelix is excreted unchanged by the kidneys. A population pharmacokinetics analysis of the data from the confirmatory Phase III study has demonstrated that the clearance of degarelix in patients with mild to moderate renal impairment is reduced by approximately 23%; therefore, dose adjustment in patients with mild or moderate renal impairment is not recommended. Data on patients with severe renal impairment is scarce and caution is therefore warranted in this patient population.

Patients with hepatic impairment

Degarelix has been investigated in a pharmacokinetic study in patients with mild to moderate hepatic impairment. No signs of increased exposure in the hepatically impaired subjects were observed compared to healthy subjects. Dose adjustment is not necessary in patients with mild or moderate hepatic impairment. Patients with severe hepatic dysfunction have not been studied and caution is therefore warranted in this group.

5.3 Preclinical safety data

Animal reproduction studies showed that degarelix caused infertility in male animals. This is due to the pharmacological effect; and the effect was reversible.

In female reproduction toxicity studies degarelix revealed findings expected from the pharmacological properties. It caused a dosage dependent prolongation of the time to mating and to pregnancy, a reduced number of *corpora lutea*, and an increase in the number of pre- and post-implantation losses, abortions, early embryo/foetal deaths, premature deliveries and in the duration of parturition.

Preclinical studies on safety pharmacology, repeated dose toxicity, genotoxicity, and carcinogenic potential revealed no special hazard for humans. Both *in vitro* and *in vivo* studies showed no signs of QT prolongation.

No target organ toxicity was observed from acute, subacute and chronic toxicity studies in rats and monkeys following subcutaneous administration of degarelix. Drug-related local irritation was noted in animals when degarelix was administered subcutaneously in high doses.

6. PHARMACEUTICAL PARTICULARS

6.1 List of excipients

Powder

Mannitol (E421)

Solvent

Water for injections

6.2 Incompatibilities

In the absence of compatibility studies, this medicinal product must not be mixed with other medicinal products.

6.3 Shelf life

3 years.

After reconstitution

Chemical and physical in-use stability has been demonstrated for 2 hours at 25°C. From a microbiological point of view, unless the method of reconstitution precludes the risk of microbial contamination, the product should be used immediately. If not used immediately, in-use storage times and conditions are the responsibility of the user.

6.4 Special precautions for storage

This medicinal product does not require any special storage conditions.

For storage conditions of the reconstituted medicinal product, see section 6.3.

6.5 Nature and contents of container

Vials of glass Type I with bromobutyl rubber stopper and aluminium flip-off seal.

1 vial containing 80 mg powder for solution for injection

1 vial containing 6 ml solvent

1 syringe (5 ml)

1 reconstitution needle (21G 0.8 × 50 mm)

1 injection needle (27G 0.4 × 25 mm)

6.6 Special precautions for disposal and other handling

No special requirements for disposal.

Instructions for use:

The instructions for reconstitution must be followed carefully.

Administration of other concentrations is not recommended because the gel depot formation is influenced by the concentration. The reconstituted solution should be a clear liquid, free of undissolved matter.

NOTE:

- **THE VIALS SHOULD BE KEPT VERTICAL AT ALL TIMES**
- **THE VIALS SHOULD NOT BE SHAKEN**

The pack contains 1 set of powder and solvent that must be prepared for subcutaneous injection.

1. Draw up 4.2 ml solvent for injection with the reconstitution needle (green needle, 21G / 0.8 × 50 mm). Discard the vial with the remaining solvent.

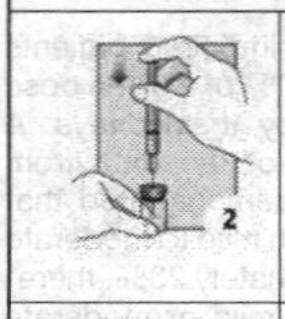

2. Inject the solvent slowly into the vial with powder. DO NOT REMOVE THE SYRINGE AND THE NEEDLE, to keep the medicinal product and syringe sterile.

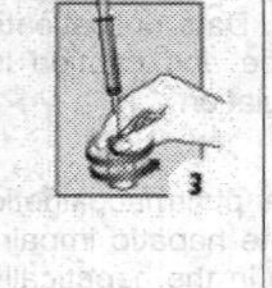

3. KEEP THE VIAL IN AN UPRIGHT POSITION. Swirl very gently until the liquid looks clear and without undissolved powder or particles. In case the powder adheres to the vial over the liquid surface, the vial can be tilted slightly. **AVOID SHAKING TO PREVENT FOAM FORMATION.** A ring of small air bubbles on the surface of the liquid is acceptable. The reconstitution procedure may take, in some cases, up to 15 minutes, but usually takes a few minutes.

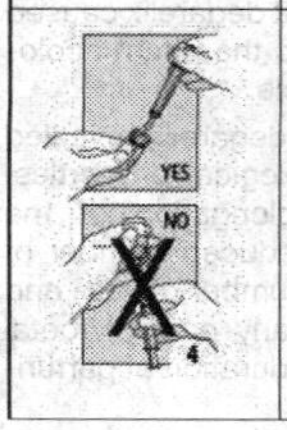

4. Tilt the vial slightly and keep the needle in the lowest part of the vial. Withdraw **4.0 ml** of the solution **without turning the vial upside down.**

5. Exchange the green needle with the white needle for deep subcutaneous injection (27G / 0.4 × 25 mm). Remove any air bubbles.

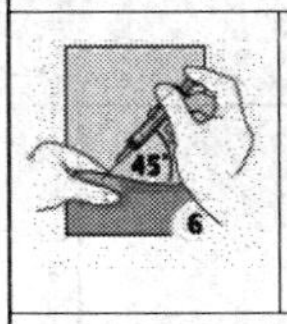

6. Grasp the skin of the abdomen, elevate the subcutaneous tissue. Perform a profound subcutaneous injection. To do so, insert the needle deeply at an angle of not less than **45 degrees.**

7. Inject **4.0 ml of FIRMAGON 80 mg** immediately after reconstitution.*

8. Do not inject directly into a vein. Gently pull back the plunger to check if blood is aspirated. If blood appears in the syringe, the medicinal product can no longer be used. Discontinue the procedure and discard the syringe and the needle (reconstitute a new dose for the patient).

Please be aware:

- No injections should be given in areas where the patient will be exposed to pressure, e.g. around the belt or waistband or close to the ribs.

* Chemical and physical in-use stability has been demonstrated for 2 hours at 25°C. From a microbiological point of view, unless the method of reconstitution precludes the risk of microbial contamination, the product should be used immediately. If not used immediately, in-use storage times and conditions are the responsibility of the user.

7. MARKETING AUTHORISATION HOLDER

Ferring Pharmaceuticals A/S

Kay Fiskers Plads 11

DK-2300 Copenhagen S

Denmark

Tel: +45 88 33 88 34

8. MARKETING AUTHORISATION NUMBER(S)

EU/1/08/504/001

9. DATE OF FIRST AUTHORISATION/RENEWAL OF THE AUTHORISATION

17/02/2009

10. DATE OF REVISION OF THE TEXT

30/07/2009

Detailed information on this medicinal product is available on the website of the European Medicines Agency (EMEA) http://www.emea.europa.eu/.

Fleet Phospho-Soda

(Laboratorios Casen Fleet S.L.U)

1. NAME OF THE MEDICINAL PRODUCT

Fleet Phospho-soda oral solution

2. QUALITATIVE AND QUANTITATIVE COMPOSITION

	per 45ml dose	per 1ml
Disodium phosphate dodecahydrate	10.8 g	0.24 g
Sodium dihydrogen phosphate dihydrate	24.4 g	0.542 g

Each 45ml bottle contains 5.0 g sodium.

For a full list of excipients, see Section 6.1

3. PHARMACEUTICAL FORM

Oral solution. Clear colourless solution with a ginger-lemon odour, free from precipitation and turbidity.

4. CLINICAL PARTICULARS

4.1 Therapeutic indications

As a bowel cleanser in preparing the patient for colon surgery, or for preparing the colon for x-ray or for endoscopic examination.

Bowel cleansing agents are not to be considered as treatments for constipation.

4.2 Posology and method of administration

Adults Only: Not to be given to children under the age of 15 years.

Elderly patients: As for Adults.

The taking of Fleet Phospho-soda should be started the day before the hospital appointment.

For hospital appointments before 12 noon the dosage instructions for morning appointments should be followed and for appointments after 12 noon the dosage instructions for an afternoon appointment should be followed.

MORNING APPOINTMENT:

Day before appointment

7am – In place of breakfast drink at least one full glass of "clear liquid" or water, more if desired.

"Clear liquids" include water, clear soup, strained fruit juices without pulp, black tea or black coffee, clear carbonated and non-carbonated soft drinks.

1st Dose – Straight afterwards, dilute 45ml in half a glass (120ml) cold water. Drink this solution followed by one full glass (240ml) cold water, more if desired.

Drink as much extra liquids as possible to replace the fluids lost during bowel movements.

1pm lunch – In place of lunch drink at least three full glasses (720ml) of "clear liquid" or water, more if desired.

7pm supper – In place of supper drink at least one full glass of "clear liquid" or water, more if desired.

2nd Dose – Straight afterwards, dilute 45ml in half a glass (120ml) cold water. Drink this solution followed by one full glass (240ml) cold water, more if desired.

Additional water or "clear liquids" may be taken up until midnight if necessary.

Drinking large amounts of clear liquids also helps ensure that the bowel will be clean for the procedure.

AFTERNOON APPOINTMENT:

Day before appointment

1pm lunch – A light snack may be taken. After lunch, no more solid food must be taken until after the hospital appointment.

7pm supper – In place of supper drink at least one full glass of "clear liquid" or water, more if desired.

1st Dose – Straight afterwards, dilute 45ml in half a glass (120ml) cold water. Drink this solution followed by one full glass (240ml) cold water, more if desired.

Drink as much extra liquids as possible to replace the fluids lost during bowel movements.

During the evening, drink at least three full glasses of water or "clear liquid" before going to bed.

Day of appointment

7am breakfast – In place of breakfast drink at least one full glass of "clear liquid" or water, more if desired.

2nd Dose – Straight afterwards, dilute 45ml in half a glass (120ml) cold water. Drink this solution followed by one full glass (240ml) cold water

Drink as much extra liquids as possible to replace the fluids lost during bowel movements. Drinking large amounts of clear liquids also helps ensure that the bowel will be clean for the procedure.

More water or "clear liquid" may be taken up until 8am.

This product normally produces a bowel movement in ½ to 6 hours.

4.3 Contraindications

Do not use:

- In children under the age of 15 years.
- When nausea, vomiting or abdominal pain are present;
- There is a hypersensitivity to the active ingredients or any of excipients;

Do not use in patients with:

- Congestive heart failure;
- Clinically significant impairment of renal function;
- Ascites;
- Known or suspected gastrointestinal obstruction;
- Megacolon (congenital or acquired);
- Perforation;
- Ileus;
- Active inflammatory bowel disease.

4.4 Special warnings and precautions for use

Fleet® Phospho-soda® has been rarely associated with severe and potentially fatal cases of electrolyte disorders in elderly patients. **The benefit/risk ratio of Fleet® Phospho-soda® needs to be carefully considered before initiating treatment in this at-risk population.**

Special attention should be taken when prescribing Fleet® Phospho-soda® to any patient with regard to known contraindications and the importance of adequate hydration and, in at-risk populations (see below and sections 4.2 and 4.3.), the importance of also obtaining baseline and post-treatment electrolyte levels.

Use with caution in patients with heart disease an increased risk for underlying renal impairment, acute myocardial infarction, unstable angina, pre-existing electrolyte disturbances, increased risk for electrolyte disturbances (e.g. dehydration, gastric retention, colitis, inability to take adequate oral fluid, hypertension or other conditions in which the patients are taking drug products that may result in dehydration, see below), or with debilitated or elderly patients. In these at-risk patients, consider obtaining baseline and post-treatment sodium, potassium, calcium, chloride, bicarbonate, phosphate, blood urea nitrogen and creatinine values.

There is a risk of elevated serum levels of sodium and phosphate and decreased levels of calcium and potassium; consequently hypernatraemia, hyperphosphataemia, hypocalcaemia, hypokalaemia, and acidosis may occur.

If the patient has had a colostomy or ileostomy, or must keep to a salt-free diet, the preparation must be used with caution, since a disturbance of electrolyte balance, dehydration or a disturbance of acid balance may arise.

Patients should be warned to expect frequent, liquid stools. Patients should be encouraged to drink as much liquid as possible to help prevent dehydration. Inadequate fluid intake when using any effective purgative may lead to excessive fluid loss possibly producing dehydration and hypovolemia. Dehydration and hypovolemia from purgation may be exacerbated by inadequate oral fluid intake, nausea, vomiting, loss of appetite, or use of diuretics, angiotensin converting enzyme inhibitors (ACE-Is), angiotensin receptor blockers (ARBS), and non-steroidal anti-inflammatory drugs (NSAIDs) and may be associated with acute renal failure. There have been rare reports of acute renal failure with purgatives, including sodium phosphates and PEG-3350.

Nephrocalcinosis associated with transient renal insufficiency and renal failure has been very rarely reported in patients using sodium phosphates for bowel cleansing; the majority of these reports occurred in elderly female patients taking drugs to treat hypertension or other drug products, such as diuretics or NSAIDs, that may result in dehydration. Patients with conditions that may predispose to dehydration or those taking medications which may decrease glomerular filtration rate, such as angiotensin converting enzyme inhibitors (ACE-I) or angiotensin receptor blockers (ARBs), should be assessed for hydration status prior to use of purgative preparations and managed appropriately. Care should be taken to prescribe Fleet Phospho-soda per recommendations with a particular attention to known contraindications and adequate hydration.

This product usually works within ½ to 6 hours. If there has been no bowel movement within 6 hours of taking Fleet Phospho-soda, instruct the patient to stop use and contact a doctor immediately as dehydration could occur.

Very rarely, single or multiple aphthoid-like punctiform lesions located in the rectosigmoid region have been observed by endoscopy. These were either lymphoid follicles or discrete inflammatory infiltrates or epithelial congestions/changes revealed by the colonic preparation. These abnormalities are not clinically significant and disappear spontaneously without any treatment.

Slight QT interval prolongation may rarely occur as a result of electrolyte imbalances such as hypocalcaemia or hypokalaemia. These changes are clinically insignificant.

4.5 Interaction with other medicinal products and other forms of interaction

Use with caution in patients taking calcium channel blockers, diuretics, lithium treatment or other medications that might affect electrolyte levels as hyperphosphataemia, hypocalcaemia, hypokalaemia, hypernatraemic dehydration and acidosis may occur.

During the intake of Fleet Phospho-soda the absorption of drugs from the gastrointestinal tract may be delayed or even completely prevented. The efficacy of regularly taken oral drugs (e.g. oral contraceptives, antiepileptic drugs, antidiabetics, antibiotics) may be reduced or completely absent. Caution is also advised when taking medicines known to prolong the QT interval.

No other sodium phosphate preparations should be given concomitantly.

4.6 Pregnancy and lactation

For Fleet Phospho-soda, no clinical data on exposed pregnancies and no data from animal studies with respect to effects on pregnancy, embryonal/fetal development, parturition and postnatal development are available. The potential risk for humans is unknown. Fleet Phospho-soda should not be used during pregnancy unless clearly necessary.

It is not known whether Fleet Phospho-soda is excreted in human milk. As sodium phosphate may pass into the breast milk, it is advised that breast milk is expressed and discarded from the first dose to 24 hours after the second dose of the bowel cleansing solution. Women should not breast-feed their infants until 24 hours after receiving the second dose of Fleet Phospho-soda.

4.7 Effects on ability to drive and use machines

Not applicable.

4.8 Undesirable effects

MedDRA 8.0

CARDIAC DISORDERS

Very rare (<1/10,000), including isolated reports

Myocardial infarction

Arrhythmia

GASTROINTESTINAL DISORDERS

Very common (>1/10)

Nausea

Abdominal pain

Abdominal distension

Diarrhoea

Common (>1/100, <1/10)

Vomiting

Colonoscopia abnormal (Single or multiple aphthoid-like punctiform lesions located in the rectosigmoid region that are not clinically significant and disappear spontaneously without any treatment)

GENERAL DISORDERS AND ADMINISTRATION SITE CONDITIONS

Very common (>1/10)

Chills

Asthenia

Common (>1/100, <1/10)

Chest pain

IMMUNE SYSTEM DISORDERS

Very rare (<1/10,000), including isolated reports

Hypersensitivity

METABOLISM AND NUTRITION DISORDERS

Uncommon (>1/1,000, <1/100)

Dehydration

Very rare (<1/10,000), including isolated reports

Hyperphosphataemia

Hypocalcaemia

Hypokalaemia

Hypernatraemia

Metabolic acidosis

Tetany

MUSCULOESKELETAL AND CONNECTIVE TISSUE DISORDERS

Very rare (<1/10,000), including isolated reports

Muscle cramp

NERVOUS SYSTEM DISORDERS

Very common (>1/10)

Dizziness

Common (>1/100, <1/10)

Headache

Very rare (<1/10,000), including isolated reports

Paraesthesia

Loss of consciousness

RENAL AND URINARY DISORDERS

Very rare (<1/10,000), including isolated reports

Renal failure acute

Renal failure chronic

Nephrocalcinosis

SKIN AND SUBCUTANEOUS TISSUE DISORDERS

Very rare (<1/10,000), including isolated reports

Dermatitis allergic

4.9 Overdose

There have been fatal cases of hyperphosphataemia with concomitant hypocalcaemia, hypernatraemia and acidosis when Fleet Phospho-soda has been used in excessive doses, given to children or to obstructed patients.

Patients experiencing overdose have presented the following symptoms: dehydration, hypotension, tachycardia, bradycardia, tachypnoea, cardiac arrest, shock, respiratory failure, dyspnoea, convulsions, ileus paralytic, anxiety, pain. Overdoses can lead to elevated serum levels of sodium and phosphate and decreased levels of calcium and potassium. In those cases, hypernatremia, hyperphosphatemia, hypocalcemia, hypokalemia, and acidosis may occur.

There are also documented cases of complete recovery from overdoses in both children accidentally given Fleet Phospho-soda, and also in patients with obstruction, one of whom received a six-fold overdose.

Recovery from the toxic effect of excess ingestion can normally be achieved by rehydration, though the intravenous administration of 10% calcium gluconate may be necessary.

5. PHARMACOLOGICAL PROPERTIES

5.1 Pharmacodynamic properties

A06AD – Osmotically acting laxative.

Fleet Phospho-soda is a saline laxative that acts by osmotic processes to increase fluid retention in the lumen of the small intestine. Fluid accumulation in the ileum produces distension and, in turn, promotes peristalsis and bowel evacuation.

5.2 Pharmacokinetic properties

Not applicable.

5.3 Preclinical safety data

No animal studies on reproduction toxicity have been conducted with Fleet Phospho-soda.

6. PHARMACEUTICAL PARTICULARS

6.1 List of excipients

Glycerol

Saccharin Sodium

Sodium Benzoate (E211)

Ginger Lemon Flavour*

Purified Water

*Ginger Lemon Flavour:

Oleoresin Ginger

Alcohol

Oil Lemon

Partially Deterpinated Oil Lemon

Citric Acid

Water

6.2 Incompatibilities

Not applicable.

6.3 Shelf life

3 years

6.4 Special precautions for storage

Do not store above 25°C.

6.5 Nature and contents of container

Fleet Phospho-soda is supplied in cartons containing 2 × 45ml or 100 × 45ml (hospital pack) polyethylene bottles with polypropylene, aluminium foil-lined screw caps.

Not all pack sizes may be marketed.

6.6 Special precautions for disposal and other handling

No special requirements.

7. MARKETING AUTHORISATION HOLDER

Laboratorios Casen-Fleet S.L.U.

Autovía de Logroño, Km. 13,300

50180 UTEBO. Zaragoza (Spain)

8. MARKETING AUTHORISATION NUMBER(S)

PL 12695/0001

9. DATE OF FIRST AUTHORISATION/RENEWAL OF THE AUTHORISATION

06 July 1995 / 06 July 2005

10. DATE OF REVISION OF THE TEXT

01 November 2007

Fleet Ready-to-Use Enema

(Laboratorios Casen Fleet S.L.U)

1. NAME OF THE MEDICINAL PRODUCT

Fleet Ready-to-Use 21.4g / 9.4g Enema

2. QUALITATIVE AND QUANTITATIVE COMPOSITION

	Per 118ml delivered dose
Sodium Dihydrogen Phosphate Dihydrate	18.1% w/v
Disodium Phosphate Dodecahydrate	8.0% w/v

The delivered dose contains 4.4 g of sodium

For a full list of excipients, see section 6.1.

3. PHARMACEUTICAL FORM

Rectal Solution (Enema)

Clear, colourless, odourless, solution, free from precipitation and turbidity.

4. CLINICAL PARTICULARS

4.1 Therapeutic indications

- For use in the relief of occasional constipation
- For use where bowel cleansing is required, such as before and after lower bowel surgery, delivery and post partum, before proctoscopy, sigmoidoscopy or colonoscopy and before radiological examinations of the lower bowel

4.2 Posology and method of administration

Posology

Adults, Elderly and Children over 12 years old: 1 bottle (118ml delivered dose) no more than once daily or as directed by a physician

Children aged 3 years to less than 12 years: As directed by a physician.

Do not administer to children under 3 years of age

Method of administration

For rectal use only:

Lie on left side with both knees bent, arms at rest.

Remove orange protective shield.

With steady pressure, gently insert enema Comfortip into anus with nozzle pointing towards navel.

Squeeze bottle until nearly all liquid is expelled.

Discontinue use if resistance is encountered. Forcing the enema can result in injury.

Return enema to carton for disposal.

Generally, 2 to 5 minutes are sufficient to obtain the desired effect. If delayed discontinue further use and consult a physician

For occasional constipation rectal enemas are to be used to provide short-term relief only.

4.3 Contraindications

Fleet Ready-to-Use Enema is contraindicated in patients with:

- hypersensitivity to active ingredients or to any of the excipients of the product.
- Conditions causing decreased gastric motility, e.g.,
  - o suspected intestinal obstruction
  - o paralytic ileus
  - o anorectal stenosis
  - o imperforate anus
  - o congenital or acquired megacolon
  - o Hirschsprung's Disease
- Undiagnosed gastrointestinal pathology, e.g.,
  - o symptoms of appendicitis, intestinal perforation or active inflammatory bowel disease
  - o undiagnosed rectal bleeding

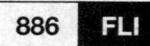

- congestive heart failure
- dehydration and generally in all cases where absorption capacity is increased or elimination capacity is decreased
- Children under 3 years of age

4.4 Special warnings and precautions for use
Do not use Fleet Ready-to-use enema when nausea, vomiting or abdominal pain is present unless directed by a physician.

Patients should be advised to expect liquid stools and should be encouraged to drink clear liquids to help prevent dehydration

Use with caution in: elderly or debilitated patients and in patients with uncontrolled arterial hypertension, ascites, heart disease, rectal mucosal changes (ulcers, fissures), colostomy or pre-existing electrolyte imbalance as hypocalcaemia, hypokalaemia, hyperphosphataemia, hypernatraemia and acidosis may occur. Where electrolyte disorders are suspected and in patients who may experience hyperphosphataemia, electrolyte levels should be monitored before and after administration of Fleet Ready-to-Use Enema.

The product should be used with caution in patients with abnormal renal function. Where the clinical benefit is expected to outweigh the risk of hyperphosphataemia

Repeated and prolonged use of Fleet Ready-to-Use Enema is not recommended as it may cause habituation. Unless directed by a physician, Fleet Ready-to-use enema should not be used for more than two weeks.

Rectal bleeding or failure in bowel evacuation after using Fleet Ready-to-Use Enema (evacuation occurs within 5 minutes of administration) may indicate a serious condition. No further administrations should be given and the condition of the patient should be assessed by a physician.

Fleet Ready-to-Use Enema should be administered following the instructions for use and handling (see section 4.2). Patients should be warned to stop administration if resistance is felt because forced administration may cause local damage.

Keep all medicines out of the reach and sight of children.

4.5 Interaction with other medicinal products and other forms of interaction
Use with caution in patients taking calcium channel blockers, diuretics, lithium treatment or other medications that might affect electrolyte levels as hyperphosphataemia, hypocalcaemia, hypokalaemia, hypernatraemic dehydration and acidosis may occur.

As hypernatraemia is associated with lower lithium levels, concomitant use of Fleet RTU Enema and lithium therapy could lead to a fall in serum lithium levels with a lessening of effectiveness.

4.6 Pregnancy and lactation
As there is no relevant data available to evaluate the potential for foetal malformation or other foetotoxic effects when administered during pregnancy Fleet Ready-to-Use Enema should only be used as directed by a physician at the time of delivery or postpartum.

As sodium phosphate may pass into the breast milk, it is advised that breast milk is expressed and discarded for up to 24 hours after receiving the Fleet Ready-to-Use Enema.

4.7 Effects on ability to drive and use machines
Not relevant.

4.8 Undesirable effects
The frequencies of adverse reactions to Fleet Ready-to-Use Enema are not known (cannot be estimated from the available data). Adverse reactions that have been reported are presented below by System Organ Class and Preferred term.

IMMUNE SYSTEM DISORDERS	Hypersensitivity e.g. urticria, pruritus
METABOLISM AND NUTRITION DISORDERS	Dehydration Hyperphosphataemia Hypocalcaemia Hypokalaemia Hypernatraemia Metabolic acidosis
GASTROINTESTINAL DISORDERS	Nausea Vomiting Abdominal pain Abdominal distension Diarrhoea Gastrointestinal pain Pruritis ani
GENERAL DISORDERS AND ADMINISTRATION SITE CONDITIONS	Chills Rectal irritation Blistering Stinging Pruritus Pain

4.9 Overdose
There have been fatalities when Fleet Ready-to-use Enema has been administered in excessive doses or retained, used in children or used in obstructed patients.

Hyperphosphataemia, hypocalcaemia, hypernatraemia, hypernatraemic dehydration, acidosis and tetany may occur in overdose or retention.

Recovery from the toxic effects can normally be achieved by rehydration. In severe cases correction of electrolyte changes by providing calcium and magnesium salts (10% calcium gluconate) while promoting elimination of exogenous phosphorus and the use of dialysis should be considered

5. PHARMACOLOGICAL PROPERTIES

5.1 Pharmacodynamic properties
ATC classification: A06AG01 Sodium phosphate enema

Fleet Ready-to-Use Enema will act as a saline laxative when administered by the rectal route. Fluid accumulation in the lower bowel produces distension and promotes peristalsis and bowel movement with only the rectum, sigmoid and part or all of the descending colon being evacuated.

5.2 Pharmacokinetic properties
Colonic absorption is probably minimal, but it has been reported that asymptomatic hyperphosphataemia up to 2–3 times above normal phosphorus levels occurs in nearly 25% of individuals with normal renal function after administration of ORAL sodium phosphate containing colonic preparations. Data for rectal solutions has been generated by a small, open-label, healthy volunteer company sponsored study which looked at both 250mL (high volume) and 133mL sodium phosphate enemas. This study confirmed a transient increase in serum phosphate above the upper limit of normal in 30% of subjects, with mean phosphorus levels falling after the 10-minute sample Under normal conditions the greatest phosphorus absorption occurs in the small bowel which is never reached from rectal administration.

5.3 Preclinical safety data
No preclinical safety studies have been performed.

6. PHARMACEUTICAL PARTICULARS

6.1 List of excipients
Disodium Edetate

Benzalkonium Chloride

Purified water

Nozzle lubricant: white soft paraffin

6.2 Incompatibilities
None reported or expected

6.3 Shelf life
3 years

6.4 Special precautions for storage
Do not store above 25°C.

Do not refrigerate

6.5 Nature and contents of container
Fleet Ready-to-Use Enema is supplied in a 133ml disposable LDPE squeeze bottle, fitted with a LDPE cap, neoprene/isoprene free-latex valve and a soft pre-lubricated Comfortip (ethylene vinyl acetate), which is covered by a protective LDPE shield until use.

The bottle contains 133ml of Fleet Ready-to-Use Enema, which gives a delivered dose of 118ml.

6.6 Special precautions for disposal and other handling
No special requirements.

7. MARKETING AUTHORISATION HOLDER
Laboratorios Casen-Fleet S.L.U.

Autovía de Logroño, Km 13,300

50180 UTEBO

Zaragoza

Spain

8. MARKETING AUTHORISATION NUMBER(S)
PL 12695/0003

9. DATE OF FIRST AUTHORISATION/RENEWAL OF THE AUTHORISATION
07th October 1993 / 09th February 1999 / 09th February 2004

10. DATE OF REVISION OF THE TEXT
October 2007

Flixonase Aqueous Nasal Spray

(Allen & Hanburys)

1. NAME OF THE MEDICINAL PRODUCT
Flixonase Aqueous Nasal Spray

2. QUALITATIVE AND QUANTITATIVE COMPOSITION
Aqueous suspension of 0.05% w/w micronised fluticasone propionate. Each metered dose contains 50 micrograms of fluticasone propionate.

3. PHARMACEUTICAL FORM
Aqueous suspension for intranasal inhalation via metered dose atomising pump.

4. CLINICAL PARTICULARS

4.1 Therapeutic indications
The prophylaxis and treatment of seasonal allergic rhinitis (including hay fever) and perennial rhinitis. Fluticasone propionate has potent anti-inflammatory activity but when used topically on the nasal mucosa has no detectable systemic activity.

4.2 Posology and method of administration
Flixonase Aqueous Nasal Spray is for administration by the intranasal route only.

Adults and children over 12 years of age:

For the prophylaxis and treatment of seasonal allergic rhinitis and perennial rhinitis. Two sprays into each nostril once a day, preferably in the morning. In some cases two sprays into each nostril twice daily may be required. Once symptoms are under control a maintenance dose of one spray per nostril once a day may be used. If symptoms recur the dosage may be increased accordingly. The minimum dose should be used at which effective control of symptoms is maintained. The maximum daily dose should not exceed four sprays into each nostril.

Elderly patients:

The normal adult dosage is applicable.

Children under 12 years of age:

For the prophylaxis and treatment of seasonal allergic rhinitis and perennal rhinitis in children aged 4-11 years a dose of one spray into each nostril once daily preferably in the morning is recommended. In some cases one spray into each nostril twice daily may be required. The maximum daily dose should not exceed two sprays into each nostril. The minimum dose should be used at which effective control of symptoms is maintained.

For full therapeutic benefit regular usage is essential. The absence of an immediate effect should be explained to the patient, as maximum relief may not be obtained until after 3 to 4 days of treatment.

4.3 Contraindications
Hypersensitivity to any of its ingredients.

4.4 Special warnings and precautions for use
Local infections: infections of the nasal airways should be appropriately treated but do not constitute a specific contra-indication to treatment with Flixonase Aqueous Nasal Spray.

The full benefit of Flixonase Aqueous Nasal Spray may not be achieved until treatment has been administered for several days.

Care must be taken while transferring patients from systemic steroid treatment to Flixonase Aqueous Nasal Spray if there is any reason to suppose that their adrenal function is impaired.

Although Flixonase Aqueous Nasal Spray will control seasonal allergic rhinitis in most cases, an abnormally heavy challenge of summer allergens may in certain instances necessitate appropriate additional therapy.

Systemic effects of nasal corticosteroids may occur particularly at high doses prescribed for prolonged periods. These effects vary between patients and different corticosteroids (please refer to Sections 5.1 and 5.2).

Growth retardation has been reported in children receiving some nasal corticosteroids at licensed doses. It is recommended that the height of children receiving prolonged treatment with nasal corticosteroids is regularly monitored. If growth is slowed, therapy should be reviewed with the aim of reducing the dose of nasal corticosteroid, if possible, to the lowest dose at which effective control of symptoms is maintained. In addition, consideration should be given to referring the patient to a paediatric specialist.

Treatment with higher than recommended doses of nasal corticosteroids may result in clinically significant adrenal suppression. If there is evidence for higher than recommended doses being used then additional systemic corticosteroid cover should be considered during periods of stress or elective surgery (see Section 5.1 for data on intranasal fluticasone propionate).

Ritonavir can greatly increase the concentration of fluticasone propionate in plasma. Therefore, concomitant use should be avoided, unless the potential benefit to the patient outweighs the risk of systemic corticosteroid side effects. There is also an increased risk of systemic side effects when combining fluticasone propionate with other potent CYP3A inhibitors (see 4.5 Interaction with Other Medicinal Products and Other Forms of Interaction).

4.5 Interaction with other medicinal products and other forms of interaction
Under normal circumstances, low plasma concentrations of fluticasone propionate are achieved after inhaled dosing, due to extensive first pass metabolism and high systemic clearance mediated by cytochrome P450 3A4 in the gut and liver. Hence, clinically significant drug interactions mediated by fluticasone propionate are unlikely.

In an interaction study in healthy subjects with intranasal fluticasone propionate, ritonavir (a highly potent cytochrome P450 3A4 inhibitor) 100 mg b.i.d. increased the fluticasone propionate plasma concentrations several hundred fold, resulting in markedly reduced serum cortisol concentrations. Cases of Cushing's syndrome and adrenal suppression have been reported. The combination should be avoided unless the benefit outweighs the increased risk of systemic glucocorticoid side-effects.

In a small study using inhaled fluticasone propionate in healthy volunteers, the slightly less potent CYP3A inhibitor ketoconazole increased the exposure of fluticasone propionate after a single inhalation by 150%. This resulted in a greater reduction of plasma cortisol as compared with fluticasone propionate alone. Co-treatment with other potent CYP3A inhibitors, such as itraconazole, is also expected to increase the systemic fluticasone propionate exposure and the risk of systemic side-effects. Caution is recommended and long-term treatment with such drugs should if possible be avoided.

4.6 Pregnancy and lactation

There is inadequate evidence of safety in human pregnancy. Administration of corticosteroids to pregnant animals can cause abnormalities of foetal development, including cleft palate and intra-uterine growth retardation. There may therefore be a very small risk of such effects in the human foetus. It should be noted, however, that the foetal changes in animals occur after relatively high systemic exposure; direct intranasal application ensures minimal systemic exposure.

As with other drugs the use of Flixonase Aqueous Nasal Spray during human pregnancy requires that the possible benefits of the drug be weighed against the possible hazards.

The secretion of fluticasone propionate in human breast milk has not been investigated. Subcutaneous administration of fluticasone propionate to lactating laboratory rats produced measurable plasma levels and evidence of fluticasone propionate in the milk. However, following intranasal administration to primates, no drug was detected in the plasma, and it is therefore unlikely that the drug would be detectable in milk. When Flixonase Aqueous Nasal Spray is used in breast feeding mothers the therapeutic benefits must be weighed against the potential hazards to mother and baby.

4.7 Effects on ability to drive and use machines

None reported.

4.8 Undesirable effects

Adverse events are listed below by system organ class and frequency. Frequencies are defined as: very common (≥1/10), common (≥1/100 and <1/10), uncommon (≥1/1000 and <1/100), rare (≥1/10,000 and <1/1000) and very rare (<1/10,000) including isolated reports. Very common, common and uncommon events were generally determined from clinical trial data. Rare and very rare events were generally determined from spontaneous data. In assigning adverse event frequencies, the background rates in placebo groups were not taken into account.

System Organ Class	Adverse Event	Frequency
Immune system disorders	Hypersensitivity reactions with the following manifestations:	
	Cutaneous hypersensitivity reactions	Very rare
	Angioedema (mainly facial and oropharyngeal oedema)	Very rare
	Respiratory symptoms (bronchospasm)	Very rare
	Anaphylactic reactions	Very rare
Nervous system disorders	Headache, unpleasant taste, unpleasant smell.	Common
Eye disorders	Glaucoma, raised intraocular pressure, cataract	Very rare
	These events have been identified from spontaneous reports following prolonged treatment.	
Respiratory, Thoracic & Mediastinal disorders	Epistaxis	Very common
	Nasal dryness, nasal irritation, throat dryness, throat irritation.	Common
	Nasal septal perforation.	Very rare

As with other nasal sprays, unpleasant taste and smell and headache have been reported.

As with other nasal sprays, dryness and irritation of the nose and throat, and epistaxis have been reported. Nasal septal perforation has also been reported following the use of intranasal corticosteroids.

Systemic effects of some nasal corticosteroids may occur, particularly when prescribed at high doses for prolonged periods.

4.9 Overdose

There are no data available on the effects of acute or chronic overdosage with Flixonase Aqueous Nasal Spray. Intranasal administration of 2 mg fluticasone propionate twice daily for seven days to healthy human volunteers has no effect on hypothalamo-pituitary-adrenal (HPA) axis function.

Inhalation or oral administration of high doses of corticosteroids over a long period may lead to suppression of HPA axis function.

5. PHARMACOLOGICAL PROPERTIES

5.1 Pharmacodynamic properties

Fluticasone propionate causes little or no hypothalamic-pituitary-adrenal axis suppression following intranasal administration.

Following intranasal dosing of fluticasone propionate, (200mcg/day) no significant change in 24h serum cortisol AUC was found compared to placebo (ratio1.01, 90%CI 0.9-1.14).

In a 1-year randomised, double-blind, placebo-controlled, parallel group growth study in pre-pubescent children aged 3 to 9 years (56 patients receiving intranasal fluticasone propionate and 52 receiving placebo,) no statistically significant difference in growth velocity was observed in patients receiving intranasal fluticasone propionate (200 micrograms per day nasal spray) compared to placebo. The estimated growth velocity over one year of treatment was 6.20 cm/year (SE=0.23) in the placebo group and 5.99 cm/year (SE=0.23) in the fluticasone propionate group; the mean difference between treatments in growth velocity after one year was 0.20 cm/year (SE=0.28, 95% CI= -0.35, 0.76). No evidence of clinically relevant changes in HPA axis function or bone mineral density was observed as assessed by 12-hour urinary cortisol excretion and dual-energy x-ray absorptiometry, respectively.

5.2 Pharmacokinetic properties

Absorption: Following intranasal dosing of fluticasone propionate, (200mcg/day) steady-state maximum plasma concentrations were not quantifiable in most subjects (<0.01ng/mL). The highest Cmax observed was 0.017ng/mL. Direct absorption in the nose is negligible due to the low aqueous solubility with the majority of the dose being eventually swallowed. When administered orally the systemic exposure is <1% due to poor absorption and pre-systemic metabolism. The total systemic absorption arising from both nasal and oral absorption of the swallowed dose is therefore negligible.

Distribution: Fluticasone propionate has a large volume of distribution at steady-state (approximately 318L). Plasma protein binding is moderately high (91%).

Metabolism: Fluticasone propionate is cleared rapidly from the systemic circulation, principally by hepatic metabolism to an inactive carboxylic acid metabolite, by the cytochrome P450 enzyme CYP3A4. Swallowed fluticasone propionate is also subject to extensive first pass metabolism. Care should be taken when co-administering potent CYP3A4 inhibitors such as ketoconazole and ritonavir as there is potential for increased systemic exposure to fluticasone propionate.

Elimination: The elimination rate of intravenous administered fluticasone propionate is linear over the 250-1000mcg dose range and are characterized by a high plasma clearance (CL=1.1L/min). Peak plasma concentrations are reduced by approximately 98% within 3-4 hours and only low plasma concentrations were associated with the 7.8h terminal half-life. The renal clearance of fluticasone propionate is negligible (<0.2%) and less than 5% as the carboxylic acid metabolite. The major route of elimination is the excretion of fluticasone propionate and its metabolites in the bile.

5.3 Preclinical safety data

There are no preclinical data of relevance to the prescriber which are additional to that already included in other sections of the SPC.

6. PHARMACEUTICAL PARTICULARS

6.1 List of excipients

Dextrose (Anhydrous) PhEur

Microcrystalline Celluose NF

Carboxymethylcellulose Sodium NF

Phenylethyl Alcohol USP

Benzalkonium Chloride PhEur

Polysorbate 80 PhEur

Purified Water PhEur

6.2 Incompatibilities

None reported.

6.3 Shelf life

24 months

6.4 Special precautions for storage

Flixonase Aqueous Nasal Spray should not be stored above 30°C

6.5 Nature and contents of container

Flixonase Aqueous Nasal Spray is supplied in an amber glass bottle fitted with a metering, atomising pump. Pack size of 120 and 150 metered sprays.

Not all pack sizes may be marketed.

6.6 Special precautions for disposal and other handling

Shake gently before use.

Administrative Data

7. MARKETING AUTHORISATION HOLDER

Glaxo Wellcome UK Limited trading as:

Allen & Hanburys

Stockley Park West

Uxbridge

Middlesex UB11 1BT

8. MARKETING AUTHORISATION NUMBER(S)

PL 10949/0036

9. DATE OF FIRST AUTHORISATION/RENEWAL OF THE AUTHORISATION

13 September 2005

10. DATE OF REVISION OF THE TEXT

19 April 2007

11. Legal Category

POM

Flixonase Nasule Drops

(Allen & Hanburys)

1. NAME OF THE MEDICINAL PRODUCT

Flixonase™ Nasule™ Drops 400 micrograms (1 mg/ml), nasal drops suspension.

2. QUALITATIVE AND QUANTITATIVE COMPOSITION

Each single dose of Flixonase Nasule Drops contain:

Fluticasone propionate 400 micrograms (1mg/ml).

For a full list of excipients see section 6.1.

3. PHARMACEUTICAL FORM

Nasal drops

Single dose aqueous suspension.

4. CLINICAL PARTICULARS

4.1 Therapeutic indications

Flixonase Nasule Drops are indicated for the regular treatment of nasal polyps and associated symptoms of nasal obstruction.

4.2 Posology and method of administration

Adults

The contents of one container (400 micrograms) to be instilled once or twice daily. The dose should be divided between the affected nostrils.

After shaking and opening the container, the patient should adopt one of the positions outlined in the patient information leaflet. The dose should be divided between the nostrils by either counting approximately 6 drops into each nostril or by holding the dimpled sides of the container and squeezing once into each nostril (one squeeze delivers approximately half the dose).

Full instructions for use are given in the patient information leaflet.

Elderly

The normal adult dosage is applicable.

Children

There are insufficient data at present to recommend the use of fluticasone propionate for the treatment of nasal polyps in children less than 16 years.

The dose should be titrated to the lowest dose at which effective control of disease is maintained.

For full therapeutic benefit regular usage is essential. The absence of an immediate effect should be explained to the patient as maximum relief may not be obtained until after several weeks of treatment. However, if no improvement in symptoms is seen after four to six weeks, alternative therapies should be considered.

4.3 Contraindications

Flixonase Nasule Drops are contra-indicated in patients with a history of hypersensitivity to the active substance or to any of the excipients.

4.4 Special warnings and precautions for use

Local infection: Infections of the nasal airways should be appropriately treated but do not constitute a specific contra-indication to treatment with Flixonase Nasule Drops.

Unilateral polyposis rarely occurs, and could be indicative of other conditions. Diagnosis should be confirmed by a specialist.

Nasal polyps require regular medical assessment to monitor severity of the condition.

Contact with the eyes and broken skin should be avoided.

Care must be taken when withdrawing patients from systemic steroid treatment, and commencing therapy with Flixonase Nasule Drops, particularly if there is any reason to suppose that their adrenal function is impaired.

Systemic effects of nasal corticosteroids may occur, particularly at high doses prescribed for prolonged periods.

It is possible that long term treatment with higher than recommended doses of nasal corticosteroids could result in clinically significant adrenal suppression. If there is evidence of higher than recommended doses being used then additional systemic corticosteroid cover should be considered during periods of stress or elective surgery.

Ritonavir can greatly increase the concentration of fluticasone propionate in plasma. Therefore, concomitant use should be avoided, unless the potential benefit to the patient outweighs the risk of systemic corticosteroid side-effects. There is also an increased risk of systemic side effects when combining fluticasone propionate with other potent CYP3A inhibitors (see 4.5 Interaction with Other Medicinal Products and Other Forms of Interaction).

4.5 Interaction with other medicinal products and other forms of interaction

Under normal circumstances, low plasma concentrations of fluticasone propionate are achieved after intranasal dosing, due to extensive first pass metabolism and high systemic clearance mediated by cytochrome P450 3A4 in the gut and liver. Hence, clinically significant drug interactions mediated by fluticasone propionate are unlikely.

In an interaction study in healthy subjects with intranasal fluticasone propionate, ritonavir (a highly potent cytochrome P450 3A4 inhibitor) 100 mg b.i.d. increased the fluticasone propionate plasma concentrations several hundred fold, resulting in markedly reduced serum cortisol concentrations. Cases of Cushing's syndrome and adrenal suppression have been reported. The combination should be avoided unless the benefit outweighs the increased risk of systemic glucocorticoid side-effects.

Other inhibitors of cytochrome P450 3A4 produce negligible (erythromycin) and minor (ketoconazole) increases in systemic exposure to fluticasone propionate without notable reductions in serum cortisol concentrations. Care is advised when co-administering cytochrome P450 3A4 inhibitors, especially in long-term use and in case of potent inhibitors, as there is potential for increased systemic exposure to fluticasone propionate.

4.6 Pregnancy and lactation

The use of Flixonase Nasule Drops during pregnancy and lactation requires that the benefits be weighed against possible risks associated with the product or with any alternative therapy.

Pregnancy

There is inadequate evidence of safety in human pregnancy. In animal reproduction studies adverse effects typical of potent corticosteroids are only seen at high systemic exposure levels; direct intranasal application ensures minimal systemic exposure.

Lactation

The excretion of fluticasone propionate into human breast milk has not been investigated. Following subcutaneous administration in lactating laboratory rats, there was evidence of fluticasone propionate in the breast milk, however plasma levels in patients following intranasal application of fluticasone propionate at recommended doses are low.

4.7 Effects on ability to drive and use machines

Not relevant.

4.8 Undesirable effects

Adverse events are listed below by system organ class and frequency. Frequencies are defined as: very common (≥1/10), common (≥1/100 and <1/10), uncommon (≥1/1000 and <1/100), rare (≥1/10,000 and <1/1000) very rare (<1/10,000) and not known (frequency cannot be estimated from available data). In assigning adverse event frequencies, the background rates in placebo groups in clinical trials were not taken into account, since these rates were generally comparable to or higher than those in the active treatment group.

Within each frequency grouping, undesirable effects are presented in order of decreasing seriousness.

(see Table 1 below)

4.9 Overdose

There are no data available from patients on the effects of acute or chronic overdosage with Flixonase Nasule Drops.

In healthy volunteers, intranasal administration of 2 milligrams fluticasone propionate twice daily for seven days had no effect on hypothalamic-pituitary-adrenal axis (HPA) function. Administration of doses higher than those recommended over a long period of time may lead to temporary suppression of the adrenal function. In these patients, treatment with fluticasone propionate should be continued at a dose sufficient to control symptoms; the adrenal function will recover in a few days and can be verified by measuring plasma cortisol.

5. PHARMACOLOGICAL PROPERTIES

5.1 Pharmacodynamic properties

Pharmacotherapeutic Group: Nasal preparations, Corticosteroids

ATC code: R01AD08

Fluticasone propionate has potent anti-inflammatory activity when used topically on the nasal mucosa.

Fluticasone propionate causes little or no HPA axis suppression following intranasal administration.

5.2 Pharmacokinetic properties

After recommended doses of intranasal fluticasone propionate plasma levels are low. Systemic bioavailability for the nasal drop formula is extremely low (mean value 0.06 %).

Following intravenous administration the pharmacokinetics of fluticasone propionate are proportional to the dose, and can be described by three exponentials.

Absolute oral bio-availability is negligible (<1 %) due to a combination of incomplete absorption from the gastro-intestinal tract and extensive first pass metabolism.

Fluticasone propionate is extensively distributed within the body (Vss is approximately 300 litre). Plasma protein binding is 91 %.

After intravenous administration, fluticasone propionate has a very high clearance (estimated Cl 1.1 litre/min) indicating extensive hepatic extraction. It is extensively metabolised by CYP3A4 enzyme to an inactive carboxylic derivative.

Peak plasma concentrations are reduced by approximately 98 % within 3-4 hours, and only low plasma concentrations are associated with the terminal half life, which is approximately 8 hours.

Following oral administration of fluticasone propionate, 87-100 % of the dose is excreted in the faeces as parent compoundor as metabolites.

5.3 Preclinical safety data

At doses in excess of those recommended for therapeutic use, only class effects typical of potent corticosteroids have been shown in repeat dose toxicity tests, reproductive toxicology and teratology studies. Fluticasone propionate has no mutagenic effect in vitro or in vivo, no tumorigenic potential in rodents and is non-irritant and non-sensitising in animals.

6. PHARMACEUTICAL PARTICULARS

6.1 List of excipients

Polysorbate 20, sorbitan laurate, sodium dihydrogenphosphate dihydrate, disodium phosphate anhydrous, sodium chloride, water for injections.

6.2 Incompatibilities

Not applicable.

6.3 Shelf life

3 years.

After removal of foil: 28 days.

6.4 Special precautions for storage

Do not freeze.

Keep the containers in the outer carton.

Store upright.

Do not store above 30°C.

6.5 Nature and contents of container

Strips of polyethylene single dose (400 micrograms) containers, within foil wrapping are available in the following pack sizes:

28 containers (4 strips of 7 Nasules)

84 containers (12 strips of 7 Nasules)

Not all pack sizes may be marketed.

6.6 Special precautions for disposal and other handling

No special requirements

7. MARKETING AUTHORISATION HOLDER

Glaxo Wellcome UK Limited trading as Allen & Hanburys

Stockley Park West

Uxbridge

Middlesex

UB11 1BT

8. MARKETING AUTHORISATION NUMBER(S)

PL 10949/0323

9. DATE OF FIRST AUTHORISATION/RENEWAL OF THE AUTHORISATION

27 January 1999 / 23 March 2009

10. DATE OF REVISION OF THE TEXT

23 March 2009

Table 1

	Very common (≥1/10)	Common (≥1/100 and <1/10)	Very rare (<1/10,000)
Immune system disorders			Hypersensitivity reactions, anaphylaxis/ anaphylactic reactions, bronchospasm, rash, oedema of the face and mouth
Eye disorders			***Glaucoma, raised intraocular pressure, cataract
Respiratory, thoracic and mediastinal disorders	Epistaxis	*Nasal dryness, nasal irritation, throat dryness, throat irritation	**Nasal septal perforation

*As with other intranasal products dryness and irritation of the nose and throat, and epistaxis may occur.

**There have also been cases of nasal septal perforation following the use of intranasal corticosteroids.

***These events have been identified from spontaneous reports following prolonged treatment.

Flixotide 50, 125, 250 micrograms Evohaler

(Allen & Hanburys)

1. NAME OF THE MEDICINAL PRODUCT

Flixotide™ 50 micrograms Evohaler™

Flixotide™ 125 micrograms Evohaler™

Flixotide™ 250 micrograms Evohaler™

2. QUALITATIVE AND QUANTITATIVE COMPOSITION

Flixotide 50 micrograms Evohaler, Flixotide 125 micrograms Evohaler and Flixotide 250 micrograms Evohaler are pressurised inhalation, suspensions, delivering either 50, 125 or 250 micrograms of fluticasone propionate per actuation, respectively.

3. PHARMACEUTICAL FORM

Pressurised inhalation, suspension

Flixotide Evohaler does not contain any chlorofluorocarbons (CFCs).

4. CLINICAL PARTICULARS

4.1 Therapeutic indications

Fluticasone propionate given by inhalation offers prophylactic treatment for asthma.

Adults:

Mild asthma: Patients requiring intermittent symptomatic bronchodilator asthma medication on a regular daily basis.

Moderate asthma: Patients with unstable or worsening asthma despite prophylactic therapy or bronchodilator alone.

Severe asthma: Patients with severe chronic asthma and those who are dependent on systemic corticosteroids for adequate control of symptoms. On introduction of inhaled fluticasone propionate many of these patients may be able to reduce significantly, or to eliminate, their requirement for oral corticosteroids.

Children:

Any child who requires prophylactic medication, including patients not controlled on currently available prophylactic medication.

4.2 Posology and method of administration

Flixotide Evohaler is for oral inhalation use only. Flixotide Evohaler may be used with a Volumatic® spacer device by patients who find it difficult to synchronise aerosol actuation with inspiration of breath.

Patients should be made aware of the prophylactic nature of therapy with Flixotide Evohaler and that it should be taken regularly even when they are asymptomatic. The onset of therapeutic effect is within 4 to 7 days.

Adults and children over 16 years:

100 to 1,000 micrograms twice daily, usually as two twice daily inhalations.

Prescribers should be aware that fluticasone propionate is as effective as other inhaled steroids approximately at half the microgram daily dose. For example, a 100mcg of fluticasone propionate is approximately equivalent to 200mcg dose of beclometasone dipropionate (CFC containing) or budesonide.

Due to the risk of systemic effects, doses above 500 micrograms twice daily should be prescribed only for adult patients with severe asthma where additional clinical benefit is expected, demonstrated by either an improvement in pulmonary function and/or symptom control, or by a reduction in oral corticosteroid therapy (see 4.4 Special Warnings and Precautions for Use and 4.8 Undesirable Effects).

Patients should be given a starting dose of inhaled fluticasone propionate which is appropriate to the severity of their disease.

Typical Adult Starting Doses:

For patients with mild asthma, a typical starting dose is 100 micrograms twice daily. In moderate and more severe asthma, starting doses may need to be 250 to 500 micrograms twice daily. Where additional clinical benefit is expected, doses of up to 1000 micrograms twice daily may be used. Initiation of such doses should be prescribed only by a specialist in the management of asthma (such as a consultant physician or general practitioner with appropriate experience).

The dose should be titrated down to the lowest dose at which effective control of asthma is maintained

Typical starting doses for children over 4years of age:

50 to 100 micrograms twice daily.

Many children's asthma will be well controlled using the 50 to 100 microgram twice daily dosing regime. For those patients whose asthma is not sufficiently controlled, additional benefit may be obtained by increasing the dose up to 200 micrograms twice daily. **The maximum licensed dose in children is 200 micrograms twice daily.**

The starting dose should be appropriate to the severity of the disease. The dose should be titrated down to the lowest dose at which effective control of asthma is maintained.

Should Flixotide 50 microgram Evohaler presentation not offer the exact paediatric dose prescribed by the physician, please see data sheets of alternative Flixotide presentation (Accuhaler, Diskhaler, Inhaler).

Administration of doses above 1000 micrograms (500 micrograms twice daily) should be via a spacer device to help reduce side-effects in the mouth and throat. (See section 4.4)

Special patient groups:

There is no need to adjust the dose in elderly patients or those with hepatic or renal impairment.

4.3 Contraindications

Hypersensitivity to any ingredient of the preparation.

4.4 Special warnings and precautions for use

Patients' inhaler technique should be checked regularly to make sure that inhaler actuation is synchronised with inspiration to ensure optimum delivery to the lungs. During inhalation, the patient should preferably sit or stand. The inhaler has been designed for use in a vertical position.

Flixotide Evohaler is not designed to relieve acute symptoms for which an inhaled short-acting bronchodilator is required. Patients should be advised to have such rescue medication available.

Severe asthma requires regular medical assessment, including lung-function testing, as patients are at risk of severe attacks and even death. Increasing use of short-acting inhaled β_2-agonists to relieve symptoms indicates deterioration of asthma control. If patients find that short-acting relief bronchodilator treatment becomes less effective, or they need more inhalations than usual, medical attention must be sought. In this situation patients should be reassessed and consideration given to the need for increased anti-inflammatory therapy (e.g. higher doses of inhaled corticosteroids or a course of oral corticosteroids). Severe exacerbations of asthma must be treated in the normal way.

There have been very rare reports of increases in blood glucose levels, in patients with or without a history of diabetes mellitus (See 4.8 'Undesirable Effects'). This should be considered in particular when prescribing to patients with a history of diabetes mellitus.

As with other inhalation therapy, paradoxical bronchospasm may occur with an immediate increase in wheezing after dosing. Flixotide Evohaler should be discontinued immediately, the patient assessed and alternative therapy instituted if necessary.

Systemic effects of inhaled corticosteroids may occur, particularly at high doses prescribed for prolonged periods. These effects are much less likely to occur than with oral corticosteroids. Possible systemic effects include Cushing's syndrome, Cushingoid features, adrenal suppression, growth retardation in children and adolescents, decrease in bone mineral density, cataract and glaucoma. **It is important therefore that the dose of inhaled corticosteroid is reviewed regularly and reduced to the lowest dose at which effective control of asthma is maintained.**

Prolonged treatment with high doses of inhaled corticosteroids may result in adrenal suppression and acute adrenal crisis. Children aged < 16 years taking higher than licensed doses of fluticasone (typically ⩾1000mcg/day) may be at particular risk. Situations, which could potentially trigger acute adrenal crisis, include trauma, surgery, infection or any rapid reduction in dosage. Presenting symptoms are typically vague and may include anorexia, abdominal pain, weight loss, tiredness, headache, nausea, vomiting, decreased level of consciousness, hypoglycaemia, and seizures. Additional systemic corticosteroid cover should be considered during periods of stress or elective surgery.

It is recommended that the height of children receiving prolonged treatment with inhaled corticosteroids is regularly monitored. If growth is slowed, therapy should be reviewed with the aim of reducing the dose of inhaled corticosteroid, if possible, to the lowest dose at which effective control of asthma is maintained. In addition, consideration should be given to referring the patient to a paediatric respiratory specialist.

Administration of high doses, above 1000 mcg daily is recommended through a spacer to reduce side effects in the mouth and throat. However, as systemic absorption is largely through the lungs, the use of a spacer plus metered dose inhaler may increase drug delivery to the lungs. It should be noted that this could potentially lead to an increase in the risk of systemic adverse effects. A lower dose may be required. (See section 4.2)

The benefits of inhaled fluticasone propionate should minimise the need for oral steroids. However, patients transferred from oral steroids, remain at risk of impaired adrenal reserve for a considerable time after transferring to inhaled fluticasone propionate. The possibility of adverse effects may persist for some time. These patients may require specialised advice to determine the extent of adrenal impairment before elective procedures. The possibility of residual impaired adrenal response should always be considered in emergency (medical or surgical) and elective situations likely to produce stress, and appropriate corticosteroid treatment considered.

Lack of response or severe exacerbations of asthma should be treated by increasing the dose of inhaled fluticasone propionate and, if necessary, by giving a systemic steroid and/or an antibiotic if there is an infection.

Replacement of systemic steroid treatment with inhaled therapy sometimes unmasks allergies such as allergic rhinitis or eczema previously controlled by the systemic drug. These allergies should be symptomatically treated with antihistamine and/or topical preparations, including topical steroids.

As with all inhaled corticosteroids, special care is necessary in patients with active or quiescent pulmonary tuberculosis.

Treatment with Flixotide Evohaler should not be stopped abruptly.

For the transfer of patients being treated with oral corticosteroids:

The transfer of oral steroid-dependent patients to Flixotide Evohaler and their subsequent management needs special care as recovery from impaired adrenocortical function, caused by prolonged systemic steroid therapy, may take a considerable time.

Patients who have been treated with systemic steroids for long periods of time or at a high dose may have adrenocortical suppression. With these patients adrenocortical function should be monitored regularly and their dose of systemic steroid reduced cautiously.

After approximately a week, gradual withdrawal of the systemic steroid is commenced. Decrements in dosages should be appropriate to the level of maintenance systemic steroid, and introduced at not less than weekly intervals. For maintenance doses of prednisolone (or equivalent) of 10mg daily or less, the decrements in dose should not be greater than 1mg per day, at not less than weekly intervals. For maintenance doses of prednisolone in excess of 10mg daily, it may be appropriate to employ cautiously, larger decrements in dose at weekly intervals.

Some patients feel unwell in a non-specific way during the withdrawal phase despite maintenance or even improvement of the respiratory function. They should be encouraged to persevere with inhaled fluticasone propionate and to continue withdrawal of systemic steroid, unless there are objective signs of adrenal insufficiency.

Patients weaned off oral steroids whose adrenocortical function is still impaired should carry a steroid warning card indicating that they need supplementary systemic steroid during periods of stress, e.g. worsening asthma attacks, chest infections, major intercurrent illness, surgery, trauma, etc.

Ritonavir can greatly increase the concentration of fluticasone propionate in plasma. Therefore, concomitant use should be avoided, unless the potential benefit to the patient outweighs the risk of systemic corticosteroid side-effects. There is also an increased risk of systemic side effects when combining fluticasone propionate with other potent CYP3A inhibitors (see 4.5 Interaction with Other Medicinal Products and Other Forms of Interaction).

4.5 Interaction with other medicinal products and other forms of interaction

Under normal circumstances, low plasma concentrations of fluticasone propionate are achieved after inhaled dosing, due to extensive first pass metabolism and high systemic clearance mediated by cytochrome P450 3A4 in the gut and liver. Hence, clinically significant drug interactions mediated by fluticasone propionate are unlikely.

In an interaction study in healthy subjects with intranasal fluticasone propionate, ritonavir (a highly potent cytochrome P450 3A4 inhibitor) 100 mg b.i.d. increased the fluticasone propionate plasma concentrations several hundred fold, resulting in markedly reduced serum cortisol concentrations. Information about this interaction is lacking for inhaled fluticasone propionate, but a marked increase in fluticasone propionate plasma levels is expected. Cases of Cushing's syndrome and adrenal suppression have been reported. The combination should be avoided unless the benefit outweighs the increased risk of systemic glucocorticoid side-effects.

In a small study in healthy volunteers, the slightly less potent CYP3A inhibitor ketoconazole increased the exposure of fluticasone propionate after a single inhalation by 150%. This resulted in a greater reduction of plasma cortisol as compared with fluticasone propionate alone. Co-treatment with other potent CYP3A inhibitors, such as itraconazole, is also expected to increase the systemic fluticasone propionate exposure and the risk of systemic side-effects. Caution is recommended and long-term treatment with such drugs should, if possible, be avoided.

4.6 Pregnancy and lactation

There is inadequate evidence of safety of fluticasone propionate in human pregnancy. Data on a limited number (200) of exposed pregnancies indicate no adverse effects of Flixotide Evohaler on pregnancy or the health of the foetus/new born child. To date no other relevant epidemological data are available. Administration of corticosteroids to pregnant animals can cause abnormalities of fetal development, including cleft palate and intra-uterine growth retardation. There may therefore be a very small risk of such effects in the human fetus. It should be noted, however, that the fetal changes in animals occur after relatively high systemic exposure. Because Flixotide Evohaler delivers fluticasone propionate directly to the lungs by the inhaled route it avoids the high level of exposure that occurs when corticosteroids are given by systemic routes. Administration of fluticasone propionate during pregnancy should only be considered if the expected benefit to the mother is greater than any possible risk to the fetus.

The secretion of fluticasone propionate in human breast milk has not been investigated. Subcutaneous administration of fluticasone propionate to lactating laboratory rats produced measurable plasma levels and evidence of fluticasone propionate in the milk. However, plasma levels in humans after inhalation at recommended doses are likely to be low. When fluticasone propionate is used in breast-feeding mothers the therapeutic benefits must be weighed against the potential hazards to mother and baby.

4.7 Effects on ability to drive and use machines

Fluticasone propionate is unlikely to produce an effect.

4.8 Undesirable effects

Adverse events are listed below by system organ class and frequency. Frequencies are defined as: very common (⩾1/10), common (⩾1/100 and <1/10), uncommon (⩾1/1000 and <1/100), rare (⩾1/10,000 and <1/1000) and very rare (<1/10,000) including isolated reports. Very common, common and uncommon events were generally determined from clinical trial data. Rare and very rare events were generally determined from spontaneous data.

System Organ Class	Adverse Event	Frequency
Infections & Infestations	Candidiasis of the mouth and throat	Very Common
	Pneumonia (in COPD patients)	Common
Immune System Disorders	Hypersensitivity reactions with the following manifestations:	
	Cutaneous hypersensitivity reactions	Uncommon
	Angioedema (mainly facial and oropharyngeal oedema)	Very Rare
	Respiratory symptoms (dyspnoea and/or bronchospasm)	Very Rare
	Anaphylactic reactions	Very Rare
Endocrine Disorders	Cushing's syndrome, Cushingoid features, adrenal suppression, growth retardation in children and adolescents, decreased bone mineral density, cataract, glaucoma	Very Rare
Metabolism & Nutrition Disorders	Hyperglycaemia (see 4.4 'Special Warnings and Precautions for Use')	Very Rare
Gastrointestinal Disorders	Dyspepsia	Very Rare

Musculoskeletal & Connective Tissue Disorders	Arthralgia	Very Rare
Psychiatric Disorders	Anxiety, sleep disorders, behavioural changes, including hyperactivity and irritability (predominantly in children)	Very Rare
Respiratory, Thoracic & Mediastinal Disorders	Hoarseness/ dysphonia	Common
	Paradoxical bronchospasm	Very Rare
Skin & Subcutaneous Tissue Disorders	Contusions	Common

Hoarseness and candidiasis of the mouth and throat (thrush) occurs in some patients. Such patients may find it helpful to rinse out their mouth with water after using the inhaler. Symptomatic candidiasis can be treated with topical anti-fungal therapy whilst still continuing with Flixotide Evohaler.

Possible systemic effects include Cushing's syndrome, Cushingoid features, adrenal suppression, growth retardation, decreased bone mineral density, cataract, glaucoma (see 4.4 Special Warning and Special Precautions for Use).

As with other inhalation therapy, paradoxical bronchospasm may occur (see 4.4 'Special Warnings and Precautions for Use'). This should be treated immediately with a fast-acting inhaled bronchodilator. Flixotide Evohaler should be discontinued immediately, the patient assessed, and if necessary alternative therapy instituted.

There was an increased reporting of pneumonia in studies of patients with COPD receiving FLIXOTIDE 500 micrograms. Physicians should remain vigilant for the possible development of pneumonia in patients with COPD as the clinical features of pneumonia and exacerbation frequently overlap.

4.9 Overdose

Acute:

Inhalation of the drug in doses in excess of those recommended may lead to temporary suppression of adrenal function. This does not necessitate emergency action being taken. In these patients treatment with fluticasone propionate by inhalation should be continued at a dose sufficient to control asthma adrenal function recovers in a few days and can be verified by measuring plasma cortisol.

Chronic:

refer to section 4.4: risk of adrenal suppression.

Monitoring of adrenal reserve may be indicated. Treatment with inhaled fluticasone propionate should be continued at a dose sufficient to control asthma.

5. PHARMACOLOGICAL PROPERTIES

5.1 Pharmacodynamic properties

Fluticasone propionate given by inhalation at recommended doses has a potent glucocorticoid anti-inflammatory action within the lungs, resulting in a reduction of both symptoms and exacerbations of asthma, with a lower incidence and severity of adverse effects than those observed when corticosteroids are administered systemically.

5.2 Pharmacokinetic properties

In healthy subjects the mean systemic bioavailability of Flixotide Evohaler is 28.6%. In patients with asthma (FEV $_1$ < 75% predicted) the mean systemic absolute bioavailability was reduced by 62%. Systemic absorption occurs mainly through the lungs and has been shown to be linearly related to dose over the dose range 500 to 2000 micrograms. Absorption is initially rapid then prolonged and the remainder of the dose may be swallowed.

Absolute oral bioavailability is negligible (<1%) due to a combination of incomplete absorption from the GI tract and extensive first-pass metabolism.

87-100% of an oral dose is excreted in the faeces, up to 75% as parent compound. There is also a non-active major metabolite.

After an intravenous dose, fluticasone propionate is extensively distributed in the body. The very high clearance rate indicates extensive hepatic clearance.

5.3 Preclinical safety data

Toxicology has shown only those class effects typical of potent corticosteroids, and these only at doses greatly in excess of that proposed for therapeutic use. No novel effects were identified in repeat dose toxicity tests, reproductive studies or teratology studies. Fluticasone propionate is devoid of mutagenic activity *in vitro* and *in vivo* and showed no tumorigenic potential in rodents. It is both non-irritant and non-sensitising in animal models.

The non-CFC propellant, HFA 134a, has been shown to have no toxic effect at very high vapour concentrations, far in excess of those likely to be experienced by patients, in a wide range of animal species exposed daily for periods of two years.

The use of HFA 134a as a propellant has not altered the toxicity profile of fluticasone propionate compared to that using the conventional CFC propellant.

6. PHARMACEUTICAL PARTICULARS

6.1 List of excipients

HFA 134a.

6.2 Incompatibilities

None reported.

6.3 Shelf life

24 months

6.4 Special precautions for storage

Do not store above 30°C (86°F). Do not refrigerate or freeze. Protect from frost and direct sunlight.

As with most medicines in pressurised canisters, the therapeutic effect of this medication may decrease when the canister is cold.

The canister should not be punctured, broken or burnt even when apparently empty.

Replace the mouthpiece cover firmly and snap into position.

6.5 Nature and contents of container

An inhaler comprising an aluminium alloy can sealed with a metering valve, actuator and dust cap. Each canister contains 120 metered actuations of either 50, 125 or 250 micrograms of fluticasone propionate. (60 metered actuation hospital packs are available in the 125 or 250 microgram products).

6.6 Special precautions for disposal and other handling

The aerosol spray is inhaled through the mouth into the lungs. After shaking the inhaler the patient should exhale, the mouthpiece should be placed in the mouth and the lips closed around it. The actuator is depressed to release a spray, which must coincide with inspiration of breath.

For detailed instructions for use refer to the Patient Information Leaflet in every pack.

Administrative Data

7. MARKETING AUTHORISATION HOLDER

Glaxo Wellcome UK Ltd, trading as

Allen & Hanburys, Stockley Park West, Uxbridge, Middlesex, UB11 1BT

8. MARKETING AUTHORISATION NUMBER(S)

Flixotide 50 micrograms Evohaler PL 10949/0324

Flixotide 125 micrograms Evohaler PL 10949/0265

Flixotide 250 micrograms Evohaler PL 10949/0266

9. DATE OF FIRST AUTHORISATION/RENEWAL OF THE AUTHORISATION

Flixotide Evohaler 50 micrograms 27 June 2000

Flixotide Evohaler 125/250 micrograms 14 March 2000

10. DATE OF REVISION OF THE TEXT

03 February 2009

Flixotide Accuhaler

(Allen & Hanburys)

1. NAME OF THE MEDICINAL PRODUCT

Flixotide$_{TM}$ Accuhaler$_{TM}$

2. QUALITATIVE AND QUANTITATIVE COMPOSITION

Flixotide Accuhaler is a moulded plastic device containing a foil strip with 28 or 60 regularly placed blisters each containing a mixture of microfine fluticasone propionate (50 micrograms, 100 micrograms, 250 micrograms or 500 micrograms) and larger particle size lactose.

3. PHARMACEUTICAL FORM

Multi-dose dry powder inhalation device.

4. CLINICAL PARTICULARS

4.1 Therapeutic indications

Fluticasone propionate given by inhalation offers preventative treatment for asthma. At recommended doses it has a potent glucocorticoid anti-inflammatory action within the lungs, with a lower incidence and severity of adverse effects than those observed when corticosteroids are administered systemically.

Adults:

Prophylactic management in:

Mild asthma: Patients requiring intermittent symptomatic bronchodilator asthma medication on a regular daily basis.

Moderate asthma: Patients with unstable or worsening asthma despite prophylactic therapy or bronchodilator alone.

Severe asthma: Patients with severe chronic asthma and those who are dependent on systemic corticosteroids for adequate control of symptoms. On introduction of inhaled fluticasone propionate many of these patients may be able to reduce significantly, or to eliminate, their requirement for oral corticosteroids.

Children:

Any child who requires prophylactic medication, including patients not controlled on currently available prophylactic medication.

4.2 Posology and method of administration

Flixotide Accuhaler is for oral inhalation use only. Flixotide Accuhaler is suitable for many patients, including those who cannot use a metered-dose inhaler successfully.

Patients should be made aware of the prophylactic nature of therapy with Flixotide Accuhaler and that it should be taken regularly even when they are asymptomatic. The onset of therapeutic effect is within 4 to 7 days.

Adults and children over 16 years:

100 to 1,000 micrograms twice daily.

Prescribers should be aware that fluticasone propionate is as effective as other inhaled steroids approximately at half the microgram daily dose. For example, a 100mcg of fluticasone propionate is approximately equivalent to 200mcg dose of beclometasone dipropionate (CFC containing) or budesonide.

Due to the risk of systemic effects, doses above 500 micrograms twice daily should be prescribed only for adult patients with severe asthma where additional clinical benefit is expected, demonstrated by either an improvement in pulmonary function and/or symptom control, or by a reduction in oral corticosteroid therapy (see 4.4 Special Warnings and Precautions for Use and 4.8 Undesirable Effects).

Patients should be given a starting dose of inhaled fluticasone propionate which is appropriate to the severity of their disease.

Typical Adult Starting Doses:

For patients with mild asthma, a typical starting dose is 100 micrograms twice daily. In moderate and more severe asthma, starting doses may need to be 250 to 500 micrograms twice daily. Where additional clinical benefit is expected, doses of up to 1000 micrograms twice daily may be used. Initiation of such doses should be prescribed only by a specialist in the management of asthma (such as a consultant physician or general practitioner with appropriate experience).

The dose should be titrated down to the lowest dose at which effective control of asthma is maintained.

Typical starting doses for children over 4 years of age:

50 to 100 micrograms twice daily.

Many children's asthma will be well controlled using the 50 to100 microgram twice daily dosing regime. For those patients whose asthma is not sufficiently controlled, additional benefit may be obtained by increasing the dose up to 200 micrograms twice daily. **The maximum licensed dose in children is 200 micrograms twice daily.**

The starting dose should be appropriate to the severity of the disease.

The dose should be titrated down to the lowest dose at which effective control of asthma is maintained.

Special patient groups:

There is no need to adjust the dose in elderly patients or in those with hepatic or renal impairment.

4.3 Contraindications

Hypersensitivity to any ingredient of the preparation. (See Pharmaceutical Particulars – List of Excipients).

4.4 Special warnings and precautions for use

Flixotide Accuhaler is not designed to relieve acute symptoms for which an inhaled short acting bronchodilator is required. Patients should be advised to have such rescue medication available.

Severe asthma requires regular medical assessment, including lung-function testing, as patients are at risk of severe attacks and even death. Increasing use of short-acting inhaled β_2-agonists to relieve symptoms indicates deterioration of asthma control. If patients find that short-acting relief bronchodilator treatment becomes less effective, or they need more inhalations than usual, medical attention must be sought. In this situation patients should be reassessed and consideration given to the need for increased anti-inflammatory therapy (e.g. higher doses of inhaled corticosteroids or a course of oral corticosteroids). Severe exacerbations of asthma must be treated in the normal way.

There have been very rare reports of increases in blood glucose levels, in patients with or without a history of diabetes mellitus (See 4.8 'Undesirable Effects'). This should be considered in particular when prescribing to patients with a history of diabetes mellitus.

As with other inhalation therapy, paradoxical bronchospasm may occur with an immediate increase in wheezing after dosing. Flixotide Accuhaler should be discontinued immediately, the patient assessed and alternative therapy instituted if necessary

Systemic effects of inhaled corticosteroids may occur, particularly at high doses prescribed for prolonged periods. These effects are much less likely to occur than with oral corticosteroids. Possible systemic effects include Cushing's syndrome, Cushingoid features, adrenal suppression, growth retardation in children and adolescents, decrease in bone mineral density, cataract and glaucoma. **It is important therefore that the dose of inhaled**

corticosteroid is reviewed regularly and reduced to the lowest dose at which effective control of asthma is maintained.

Prolonged treatment with high doses of inhaled corticosteroids may result in adrenal suppression and acute adrenal crisis. Children aged < 16 years taking higher than licensed doses of fluticasone (typically ≥ 1000mcg/day) may be at particular risk. Situations, which could potentially trigger acute adrenal crisis, include trauma, surgery, infection or any rapid reduction in dosage. Presenting symptoms are typically vague and may include anorexia, abdominal pain, weight loss, tiredness, headache, nausea, vomiting, decreased level of consciousness, hypoglycaemia, and seizures. Additional systemic corticosteroid cover should be considered during periods of stress or elective surgery.

It is recommended that the height of children receiving prolonged treatment with inhaled corticosteroids is regularly monitored. If growth is slowed, therapy should be reviewed with the aim of reducing the dose of inhaled corticosteroid, if possible, to the lowest dose at which effective control of asthma is maintained. In addition, consideration should be given to referring the patient to a paediatric respiratory specialist.

When changing from a dry powder inhaler to a metered dose inhaler, administration of high doses, above 1000 mcg daily, is recommended through a spacer to reduce side effects in the mouth and throat. However, this may increase drug delivery to the lungs. As systemic absorption is largely through the lungs, there may be an increase in the risk of systemic adverse effects. A lower dose may be required.

The benefits of inhaled fluticasone propionate should minimise the need for oral steroids. However, patients transferred from oral steroids, remain at risk of impaired adrenal reserve for a considerable time after transferring to inhaled fluticasone propionate. The possibility of adverse effects may persist for some time. These patients may require specialised advice to determine the extent of adrenal impairment before elective procedures. The possibility of residual impaired adrenal response should always be considered in emergency (medical or surgical) and elective situations likely to produce stress, and appropriate corticosteroid treatment considered.

Lack of response or severe exacerbations of asthma should be treated by increasing the dose of inhaled fluticasone propionate and, if necessary, by giving a systemic steroid and/or an antibiotic if there is an infection.

Replacement of systemic steroid treatment with inhaled therapy sometimes unmasks allergies such as allergic rhinitis or eczema previously controlled by the systemic drug. These allergies should be symptomatically treated with antihistamine and/or topical preparations, including topical steroids.

As with all inhaled corticosteroids, special care is necessary in patients with active or quiescent pulmonary tuberculosis.

Treatment with Flixotide Accuhaler should not be stopped abruptly.

For the transfer of patients being treated with oral corticosteroids:

The transfer of oral steroid-dependent patients to Flixotide Accuhaler and their subsequent management needs special care as recovery from impaired adrenocortical function, caused by prolonged systemic steroid therapy, may take a considerable time.

Patients who have been treated with systemic steroids for long periods of time or at a high dose may have adrenocortical suppression. With these patients adrenocortical function should be monitored regularly and their dose of systemic steroid reduced cautiously.

After approximately a week, gradual withdrawal of the systemic steroid is commenced. Decrements in dosages should be appropriate to the level of maintenance systemic steroid, and introduced at not less than weekly intervals. For maintenance doses of prednisolone (or equivalent) of 10mg daily or less, the decrements in dose should not be greater than 1mg per day, at not less than weekly intervals. For maintenance doses of prednisolone in excess of 10mg daily, it may be appropriate to employ cautiously, larger decrements in dose at weekly intervals.

Some patients feel unwell in a non-specific way during the withdrawal phase despite maintenance or even improvement of the respiratory function. They should be encouraged to persevere with inhaled fluticasone propionate and to continue withdrawal of systemic steroid, unless there are objective signs of adrenal insufficiency.

Patients weaned off oral steroids whose adrenocortical function is still impaired should carry a steroid warning card indicating that they need supplementary systemic steroid during periods of stress, e.g. worsening asthma attacks, chest infections, major intercurrent illness, surgery, trauma, etc.

Ritonavir can greatly increase the concentration of fluticasone propionate in plasma. Therefore, concomitant use should be avoided, unless the potential benefit to the patient outweighs the risk of systemic corticosteroid side-effects. There is also an increased risk of systemic side effects when combining fluticasone propionate with other potent CYP3A inhibitors (see 4.5 Interaction with Other Medicinal Products and Other Forms of Interaction).

4.5 Interaction with other medicinal products and other forms of interaction

Under normal circumstances, low plasma concentrations of fluticasone propionate are achieved after inhaled dosing, due to extensive first pass metabolism and high systemic clearance mediated by cytochrome P450 3A4 in the gut and liver. Hence, clinically significant drug interactions mediated by fluticasone propionate are unlikely.

In an interaction study in healthy subjects with intranasal fluticasone propionate, ritonavir (a highly potent cytochrome P450 3A4 inhibitor) 100 mg b.i.d. increased the fluticasone propionate plasma concentrations several hundred fold, resulting in markedly reduced serum cortisol concentrations. Information about this interaction is lacking for inhaled fluticasone propionate, but a marked increase in fluticasone propionate plasma levels is expected. Cases of Cushing's syndrome and adrenal suppression have been reported. The combination should be avoided unless the benefit outweighs the increased risk of systemic glucocorticoid side-effects.

In a small study in healthy volunteers, the slightly less potent CYP3A inhibitor ketoconazole increased the exposure of fluticasone propionate after a single inhalation by 150%. This resulted in a greater reduction of plasma cortisol as compared with fluticasone propionate alone. Co-treatment with other potent CYP3A inhibitors, such as itraconazole, is also expected to increase the systemic fluticasone propionate exposure and the risk of systemic side-effects. Caution is recommended and long-term treatment with such drugs should, if possible, be avoided.

4.6 Pregnancy and lactation

There is inadequate evidence of safety of fluticasone propionate in human pregnancy. Administration of corticosteroids to pregnant animals can cause abnormalities of fetal development, including cleft palate and intra-uterine growth retardation. There may therefore be a very small risk of such effects in the human fetus. It should be noted, however, that the fetal changes in animals occur after relatively high systemic exposure. Because Flixotide Accuhaler delivers fluticasone propionate directly to the lungs by the inhaled route it avoids the high level of exposure that occurs when corticosteroids are given by systemic routes. Administration of fluticasone propionate during pregnancy should only be considered if the expected benefit to the mother is greater than any possible risk to the fetus.

The secretion of fluticasone propionate in human breast milk has not been investigated. Subcutaneous administration of fluticasone propionate to lactating laboratory rats produced measurable plasma levels and evidence of fluticasone propionate in the milk. However, plasma levels in humans after inhalation at recommended doses are likely to be low.

When fluticasone propionate is used in breast feeding mothers the therapeutic benefits must be weighed against the potential hazards to mother and baby.

4.7 Effects on ability to drive and use machines

Fluticasone propionate is unlikely to produce an effect.

4.8 Undesirable effects

Adverse events are listed below by system organ class and frequency. Frequencies are defined as: very common (≥ 1/10), common (≥ 1/100 and < 1/10), uncommon (≥ 1/1000 and < 1/100), rare (≥ 1/10,000 and < 1/1000) and very rare (< 1/10,000) including isolated reports. Very common, common and uncommon events were generally determined from clinical trial data. Rare and very rare events were generally determined from spontaneous data.

System Organ Class	Adverse Event	Frequency
Infections & Infestations	Candidiasis of the mouth and throat	Very Common
	Pneumonia (in COPD patients)	Common
Immune System Disorders	Hypersensitivity reactions with the following manifestations:	
	Cutaneous hypersensitivity reactions	Uncommon
	Angioedema (mainly facial and oropharyngeal oedema)	Very Rare
	Respiratory symptoms (dyspnoea and/or bronchospasm)	Very Rare
	Anaphylactic reactions	Very Rare
Endocrine Disorders	Cushing's syndrome, Cushingoid features, adrenal suppression, growth retardation in children and adolescents, decreased bone mineral density, cataract, glaucoma	Very Rare
Metabolism & Nutrition Disorders	Hyperglycaemia (see 4.4 'Special Warnings and Precautions for Use')	Very Rare
Gastrointestinal Disorders	Dyspepsia	Very Rare
Musculoskeletal & Connective Tissue Disorders	Arthralgia	Very Rare
Psychiatric Disorders	Anxiety, sleep disorders, behavioural changes, including hyperactivity and irritability (predominantly in children)	Very Rare
Respiratory, Thoracic & Mediastinal Disorders	Hoarseness/ dysphonia	Common
	Paradoxical bronchospasm	Very Rare
Skin & Subcutaneous Tissue Disorders	Contusions	Common

Hoarseness and candidiasis of the mouth and throat (thrush) occurs in some patients. Such patients may find it helpful to rinse out their mouth with water after using the Accuhaler. Symptomatic candidiasis can be treated with topical anti-fungal therapy whilst still continuing with the Flixotide Accuhaler.

Possible systemic effects include Cushing's syndrome, Cushingoid features, adrenal suppression, growth retardation, decreased bone mineral density, cataract, glaucoma (see 4.4 Special Warnings and Special Precautions for Use).

As with other inhalation therapy, paradoxical bronchospasm may occur (see 4.4 'Special Warnings and Precautions for Use'). This should be treated immediately with a fast-acting inhaled bronchodilator. Flixotide Accuhaler should be discontinued immediately, the patient assessed, and if necessary alternative therapy instituted.

There was an increased reporting of pneumonia in studies of patients with COPD receiving FLIXOTIDE 500 micrograms. Physicians should remain vigilant for the possible development of pneumonia in patients with COPD as the clinical features of pneumonia and exacerbation frequently overlap.

4.9 Overdose

Acute:

Inhalation of the drug in doses in excess of those recommended may lead to temporary suppression of adrenal function. This does not necessitate emergency action being taken. In these patients treatment with fluticasone propionate by inhalation should be continued at a dose sufficient to control asthma; adrenal function recovers in a few days and can be verified by measuring plasma cortisol.

Chronic:

refer to section 4.4: risk of adrenal suppression.

Monitoring of adrenal reserve may be indicated. Treatment with inhaled fluticasone propionate should be continued at a dose sufficient to control asthma.

5. PHARMACOLOGICAL PROPERTIES

5.1 Pharmacodynamic properties

Fluticasone propionate given by inhalation at recommended doses has a potent glucocorticoid anti-inflammatory action within the lungs, resulting in reduced symptoms and exacerbations of asthma, with a lower incidence and severity of adverse effects than those observed when corticosteroids are administered systemically.

5.2 Pharmacokinetic properties

Systemic absolute bioavailability of fluticasone propionate is estimated at 12-26% of an inhaled dose, dependent on presentation. Systemic absorption occurs mainly through the lungs and is initially rapid then prolonged. The remainder of the dose may be swallowed.

Absolute oral bioavailability is negligible (<1%) due to a combination of incomplete absorption from the GI tract and extensive first-pass metabolism.

87-100% of an oral dose is excreted in the faeces, up to 75% as parent compound. There is also a non-active major metabolite.

After an intravenous dose, fluticasone propionate is extensively distributed in the body. The very high clearance rate indicates extensive hepatic clearance.

5.3 Preclinical safety data
Toxicology has shown only those class effects typical of potent corticosteroids, and these only at doses greatly in excess of that proposed for therapeutic use. No novel effects were identified in repeat dose toxicity tests, reproductive studies or teratology studies. Fluticasone propionate is devoid of mutagenic activity *in vitro* and *in vivo* and showed no tumorigenic potential in rodents. It is both non-irritant and non-sensitising in animal models.

6. PHARMACEUTICAL PARTICULARS
6.1 List of excipients
Lactose (which contains milk protein)

6.2 Incompatibilities
None reported.

6.3 Shelf life
Flixotide 50 Accuhaler 18 months when not stored above 30°C.

Flixotide 100 Accuhaler 24 months when not stored above 30°C.

Flixotide 250/500 Accuhaler 36 months when not stored above 30°C.

6.4 Special precautions for storage
Do not store above 30°C (86°F). Store in the original package.

6.5 Nature and contents of container
The powder mix of fluticasone propionate and lactose is filled into a blister strip consisting of a formed base foil with a peelable foil laminate lid. The foil strip is contained within the Accuhaler device.

6.6 Special precautions for disposal and other handling
The powdered medicine is inhaled through the mouth into the lungs.

The Accuhaler device contains the medicine in individual blisters which are opened as the device is manipulated.

For detailed instructions for use refer to the Patient Information Leaflet in every pack.

Administrative Data

7. MARKETING AUTHORISATION HOLDER
Glaxo Wellcome UK Ltd,
trading as Allen & Hanburys,
Stockley Park West,
Uxbridge,
Middlesex, UB11 1BT

8. MARKETING AUTHORISATION NUMBER(S)

Flixotide Accuhaler 50 micrograms	10949/0226
Flixotide Accuhaler 100 micrograms	10949/0227
Flixotide Accuhaler 250 micrograms	10949/0228
Flixotide Accuhaler 500 micrograms	10949/0229

9. DATE OF FIRST AUTHORISATION/RENEWAL OF THE AUTHORISATION
April 1995.

10. DATE OF REVISION OF THE TEXT
03 February 2009

Legal Status
POM.

Flixotide Diskhaler 100 mcg

(Allen & Hanburys)

1. NAME OF THE MEDICINAL PRODUCT
Flixotide$_{TM}$ Diskhaler$_{TM}$100 Micrograms

2. QUALITATIVE AND QUANTITATIVE COMPOSITION
Fluticasone Propionate (micronised) 100 micrograms

3. PHARMACEUTICAL FORM
Inhalation Powder.

4. CLINICAL PARTICULARS
4.1 Therapeutic indications
Fluticasone propionate given by inhalation offers preventative treatment for asthma. At recommended doses it has a potent glucocorticoid anti-inflammatory action within the lungs, with a lower incidence and severity of adverse effects than those observed when corticosteroids are administered systemically.

Prophylactic management in: -

Adults

Mild asthma:

Patients requiring intermittent symptomatic bronchodilator asthma medication on a regular daily basis.

Moderate asthma:

Patients with unstable or worsening asthma despite prophylactic therapy or bronchodilator alone.

Severe asthma:

Patients with severe chronic asthma and those who are dependent on systemic corticosteroids for adequate control of symptoms. On introduction of inhaled fluticasone propionate many of these patients may be able to reduce significantly, or to eliminate, their requirement for oral corticosteroids.

Children:

Any child who requires prophylactic medication, including patients not controlled on currently available prophylactic medication.

Route of administration: by inhalation.

4.2 Posology and method of administration
The onset of therapeutic effect is within 4 to 7 days.

Adults and children over 16 years: 100 to 1,000 micrograms twice daily.

Patients should be given a starting dose of inhaled fluticasone propionate, which is appropriate to the severity of their disease.

Prescribers should be aware that fluticasone propionate is as effective as other inhaled steroids approximately at half the microgram daily dose. For example, a 100mcg of fluticasone propionate is approximately equivalent to 200mcg dose of beclometasone dipropionate (CFC containing) or budesonide

Due to the risk of systemic effects, doses above 500 micrograms twice daily should be prescribed only for adult patients with severe asthma where additional clinical benefit is expected, demonstrated by either an improvement in pulmonary function and/or symptom control, or by a reduction in oral corticosteroid therapy (see 4.4 Special Warnings and Precautions for Use and 4.8 Undesirable Effects).

***Typical Adult Starting Doses*:**

For patients with mild asthma, a typical starting dose is 100 micrograms twice daily. In moderate and more severe asthma, starting doses may need to be 250 to 500 micrograms twice daily. Where additional clinical benefit is expected, doses of up to 1000 micrograms twice daily may be used. Initiation of such doses should be prescribed only by a specialist in the management of asthma (such as a consultant physician or general practitioner with appropriate experience).

The dose should be titrated down to the lowest dose at which effective control of asthma is maintained.

Typical starting doses for children over 4years of age:
50 to 100 micrograms twice daily.

Many children's asthma will be well controlled using the 50 to 100 microgram twice daily dosing regime. For those patients whose asthma is not sufficiently controlled, additional benefit may be obtained by increasing the dose up to 200 micrograms twice daily. **The maximum licensed dose in children is 200 micrograms twice daily.**

The starting dose should be appropriate to the severity of the disease. The dose should be titrated down to the lowest dose at which effective control of asthma is maintained.

Special patient groups:

There is no need to adjust the dose in elderly patients or those with hepatic or renal impairment.

4.3 Contraindications
Flixotide preparations are contra-indicated in patients with a history of hypersensitivity to any of their components.

4.4 Special warnings and precautions for use
Flixotide Diskhalers are not designed to relieve acute symptoms for which an inhaled short acting bronchodilator is required. Patients should be advised to have such rescue medication available.

Severe asthma requires regular medical assessment, including lung-function testing, as patients are at risk of severe attacks and even death. Increasing use of short-acting inhaled β_2-agonists to relieve symptoms indicates deterioration of asthma control. If patients find that short-acting relief bronchodilator treatment becomes less effective, or they need more inhalations than usual, medical attention must be sought.

In this situation patients should be reassessed and consideration given to the need for increased anti-inflammatory therapy (e.g. higher doses of inhaled corticosteroids or a course of oral corticosteroids). Severe exacerbations of asthma must be treated in the normal way.

There have been very rare reports of increases in blood glucose levels, in patients with or without a history of diabetes mellitus (See 4.8 'Undesirable Effects'). This should be considered in particular when prescribing to patients with a history of diabetes mellitus.

As with other inhalation therapy, paradoxical bronchospasm may occur with an immediate increase in wheezing after dosing. Flixotide Diskhaler should be discontinued immediately, the patient assessed and alternative therapy instituted if necessary.

Systemic effects of inhaled corticosteroids may occur, particularly at high doses prescribed for prolonged periods. These effects are much less likely to occur than with oral corticosteroids. Possible systemic effects include Cushing's syndrome, Cushingoid features, adrenal suppression, growth retardation in children and adolescents, decrease in bone mineral density, cataract and glaucoma. **It is important therefore that the dose of inhaled corticosteroid is reviewed regularly and reduced to the lowest dose at which effective control of asthma is maintained.**

Prolonged treatment with high doses of inhaled corticosteroids may result in adrenal suppression and acute adrenal crisis. Children aged < 16 years taking higher than licensed doses of fluticasone (typically ⩾1000mcg/day) may be at particular risk. Situations, which could potentially trigger acute adrenal crisis, include trauma, surgery, infection or any rapid reduction in dosage. Presenting symptoms are typically vague and may include anorexia, abdominal pain, weight loss, tiredness, headache, nausea, vomiting, decreased level of consciousness, hypoglycaemia, and seizures. Additional systemic corticosteroid cover should be considered during periods of stress or elective surgery.

It is recommended that the height of children receiving prolonged treatment with inhaled corticosteroids is regularly monitored. If growth is slowed, therapy should be reviewed with the aim of reducing the dose of inhaled corticosteroid, if possible, to the lowest dose at which effective control of asthma is maintained. In addition, consideration should be given to referring the patient to a paediatric respiratory specialist.

When changing from a dry powder inhaler to a metered dose inhaler, administration of high doses, above 1000 mcg daily, is recommended through a spacer to reduce side effects in the mouth and throat. However, this may increase drug delivery to the lungs. As systemic absorption is largely through the lungs, there may be an increase in the risk of systemic adverse effects. A lower dose may be required.

The benefits of inhaled fluticasone propionate should minimise the need for oral steroids. However, patients transferred from oral steroids, remain at risk of impaired adrenal reserve for a considerable time after transferring to inhaled fluticasone propionate. The possibility of adverse effects may persist for some time.

These patients may require specialised advice to determine the extent of adrenal impairment before elective procedures. The possibility of residual impaired adrenal response should always be considered in emergency (medical or surgical) and elective situations likely to produce stress, and appropriate corticosteroid treatment considered.

Lack of response or severe exacerbations of asthma should be treated by increasing the dose of inhaled fluticasone propionate and, if necessary, by giving a systemic steroid and/or an antibiotic if there is an infection.

For the transfer of patients being treated with oral corticosteroids:

The transfer of oral steroid-dependent patients to Flixotide and their subsequent management needs special care as recovery from impaired adrenocortical function, caused by prolonged systemic steroid therapy, may take a considerable time.

Patients who have been treated with systemic steroids for long periods of time or at a high dose may have adrenocortical suppression. With these patients adrenocortical function should be monitored regularly and their dose of systemic steroid reduced cautiously.

After approximately a week, gradual withdrawal of the systemic steroid is started by reducing the daily dose by one milligram prednisolone, or its equivalent. For maintenance doses of prednisolone in excess of 10mg daily, it may be appropriate to cautiously use larger reductions in dose at weekly intervals.

Some patients feel unwell in a non-specific way during the withdrawal phase despite maintenance or even improvement of the respiratory function. They should be encouraged to persevere with inhaled fluticasone propionate and to continue withdrawal of systemic steroid, unless there are objective signs of adrenal insufficiency.

Patients transferred from oral steroids whose adrenocortical function is still impaired should carry a steroid warning card indicating that they need supplementary systemic steroid during periods of stress, e.g. worsening asthma attacks, chest infections, major intercurrent illness, surgery, trauma, etc.

Replacement of systemic steroid treatment with inhaled therapy sometimes unmasks allergies such as allergic rhinitis or eczema previously controlled by the systemic drug. These allergies should be symptomatically treated with antihistamine and/or topical preparations, including topical steroids.

Treatment with Flixotide Diskhalers should not be stopped abruptly.

Special care is necessary in patients with active or quiescent pulmonary tuberculosis.

Ritonavir can greatly increase the concentration of fluticasone propionate in plasma. Therefore, concomitant use should be avoided, unless the potential benefit to the patient outweighs the risk of systemic corticosteroid side-effects. There is also an increased risk of systemic side effects when combining fluticasone propionate with other potent CYP3A inhibitors (see 4.5 Interaction with Other Medicinal Products and Other Forms of Interaction).

4.5 Interaction with other medicinal products and other forms of interaction
Under normal circumstances, low plasma concentrations of fluticasone propionate are achieved after inhaled

dosing, due to extensive first pass metabolism and high systemic clearance mediated by cytochrome P450 3A4 in the gut and liver. Hence, clinically significant drug interactions mediated by fluticasone propionate are unlikely.

In an interaction study in healthy subjects with intranasal fluticasone propionate, ritonavir (a highly potent cytochrome P450 3A4 inhibitor) 100 mg b.i.d. increased the fluticasone propionate plasma concentrations several hundred fold, resulting in markedly reduced serum cortisol concentrations. Information about this interaction is lacking for inhaled fluticasone propionate, but a marked increase in fluticasone propionate plasma levels is expected. Cases of Cushing's syndrome and adrenal suppression have been reported. The combination should be avoided unless the benefit outweighs the increased risk of systemic glucocorticoid side-effects.

In a small study in healthy volunteers, the slightly less potent CYP3A inhibitor ketoconazole increased the exposure of fluticasone propionate after a single inhalation by 150%. This resulted in a greater reduction of plasma cortisol as compared with fluticasone propionate alone. Co-treatment with other potent CYP3A inhibitors, such as itraconazole, is also expected to increase the systemic fluticasone propionate exposure and the risk of systemic side-effects. Caution is recommended and long-term treatment with such drugs should if possible be avoided.

4.6 Pregnancy and lactation

There is inadequate evidence of safety of fluticasone propionate in human pregnancy. Administration of corticosteroids to pregnant animals can cause abnormalities of fetal development, including cleft palate and intra-uterine growth retardation. There may therefore be a very small risk of such effects in the human fetus. It should be noted, however, that the fetal changes in animals occur after relatively high systemic exposure. Because fluticasone propionate is delivered directly to the lungs by the inhaled route it avoids the high level of exposure that occurs when corticosteroids are given by systemic routes.

Administration of fluticasone propionate during pregnancy should only be considered if the expected benefit to the mother is greater than any possible risk to the fetus.

The secretion of fluticasone propionate in human breast milk has not been investigated. Subcutaneous administration of fluticasone propionate to lactating laboratory rats produced measurable plasma levels and evidence of fluticasone propionate in the milk. However, plasma levels in humans after inhalation at recommended doses are likely to be low.

When fluticasone propionate is used in breast feeding mothers the therapeutic benefits must be weighed against the potential hazards to mother and baby.

4.7 Effects on ability to drive and use machines

Fluticasone propionate is unlikely to produce an effect.

4.8 Undesirable effects

Adverse events are listed below by system organ class and frequency. Frequencies are defined as: very common ($\geq$1/10), common ($\geq$1/100 and $<$1/10), uncommon ($\geq$1/1000 and $<$1/100), rare ($\geq$1/10,000 and $<$1/1000) and very rare ($<$1/10,000) including isolated reports. Very common, common and uncommon events were generally determined from spontaneous data.

System Organ Class	Adverse Event	Frequency
Infections & Infestations	Candidiasis of the mouth and throat	Very Common
	Pneumonia (in COPD patients)	Common
Immune System Disorders	Hypersensitivity reactions with the following manifestations:	
	Cutaneous hypersensitivity reactions	Uncommon
	Angioedema (mainly facial and oropharyngeal oedema),	Very Rare
	Respiratory symptoms (dyspnoea and/or bronchospasm),	Very Rare
	Anaphylactic reactions	Very Rare
Endocrine Disorders	Cushing's syndrome, Cushingoid features, adrenal suppression, growth retardation in children and adolescents, decreased bone mineral density, cataract, glaucoma	Very Rare
Metabolism & Nutrition Disorders	Hyperglycaemia (see 4.4 'Special Warnings and Precautions for Use')	Very Rare
Gastrointestinal Disorders	Dyspepsia	Very Rare
Musculoskeletal & Connective Tissue Disorders	Arthralgia	Very Rare
Psychiatric Disorders	Anxiety, sleep disorders, behavioural changes, including hyperactivity and irritability (predominantly in children)	Very Rare
Respiratory, Thoracic & Mediastinal Disorders	Hoarseness/ dysphonia	Common
	Paradoxical bronchospasm	Very Rare
Skin & Subcutaneous Tissue Disorders	Contusions	Common

Hoarseness and candidiasis of the mouth and throat (thrush) occurs in some patients. Such patients may find it helpful to rinse out their mouth with water after using the Diskhaler. Symptomatic candidiasis can be treated with topical anti-fungal therapy whilst still continuing with the Flixotide Diskhaler.

Possible systemic effects include Cushing's syndrome, Cushingoid features, adrenal suppression, growth retardation, decreased bone mineral density, cataract, glaucoma.(see 4.4 Special Warnings and Special Precautions for Use).

As with other inhalation therapy, paradoxical bronchospasm may occur (see 4.4 'Special Warnings and Precautions for Use'). This should be treated immediately with a fast-acting inhaled bronchodilator. Flixotide Diskhaler should be discontinued immediately, the patient assessed, and if necessary alternative therapy instituted.

There was an increased reporting of pneumonia in studies of patients with COPD receiving FLIXOTIDE 500 micrograms. Physicians should remain vigilant for the possible development of pneumonia in patients with COPD as the clinical features of pneumonia and exacerbation frequently overlap.

4.9 Overdose

Acute: Inhalation of the drug in doses in excess of those recommended may lead to temporary suppression of adrenal function. This does not necessitate emergency action being taken.

In these patients treatment with fluticasone propionate by inhalation should be continued at a dose sufficient to control asthma adrenal function recovers in a few days and can be verified by measuring plasma cortisol.

Chronic: refer to section 4.4: risk of adrenal suppression.

Monitoring of adrenal reserve may be indicated. Treatment with inhaled fluticasone propionate should be continued at a dose sufficient to control asthma.

5. PHARMACOLOGICAL PROPERTIES

5.1 Pharmacodynamic properties

Fluticasone propionate given by inhalation at recommended doses has a potent glucocorticoid anti-inflammatory action within the lungs, with a lower incidence and severity of adverse effects than those observed when corticosteroids are administered systemically.

5.2 Pharmacokinetic properties

Systemic absolute bioavailability of fluticasone propionate is estimated at 12-26% of an inhaled dose, dependent on presentation. Systemic absorption occurs mainly through the lungs and is initially rapid then prolonged. The remainder of the dose may be swallowed.

Absolute oral bioavailability is negligible ($<$1%) due to a combination of incomplete absorption from the GI tract and extensive first-pass metabolism.

87-100% of an oral dose is excreted in the faeces, up to 75% as parent compound. There is also a non-active major metabolite.

After an intravenous dose, fluticasone propionate is extensively distributed in the body. The very high clearance rate indicates extensive hepatic clearance.

5.3 Preclinical safety data

No clinically relevant findings were observed in preclinical studies.

6. PHARMACEUTICAL PARTICULARS

6.1 List of excipients

Lactose Ph Eur

6.2 Incompatibilities

None known

6.3 Shelf life

24 months

6.4 Special precautions for storage

Whilst the disks provide good protection to the blister contents from the effects of the atmosphere, they should not be exposed to extremes of temperature and should not be stored above 30°C. A disk may be kept in the diskhaler at all times but a blister should only be pierced immediately prior to use. Failure to observe this instruction will affect the operation of the diskhaler.

6.5 Nature and contents of container

A circular double-foil (PVC/Aluminium) disk with four blisters, containing a mixture of fluticasone propionate and lactose. The foil disk is inserted into the Diskhaler device.

The following packs are registered: 5, 7, 10, 14 or 15 disks with or without a diskhaler. Refill packs of 5, 7, 10, 14 or 15 disks. A starter pack consisting of diskhaler pre-loaded with one disk (with or without a peak flow meter and diary card). A starter pack plus a spare disk (with or without a peak flow meter and diary card).

The following packs are marketed: cartons containing 14 disks (14x4 blisters), together with a Diskhaler inhaler. Cartons containing 5 disks (5x4 blisters) together with a Diskhaler inhaler (250 micrograms and 500 micrograms hospital packs only). Refill packs containing 14 disks (14x4 blisters).

6.6 Special precautions for disposal and other handling

See Patient Information Leaflet for detailed instructions.

Administrative Data

7. MARKETING AUTHORISATION HOLDER

Glaxo Wellcome UK Ltd

trading as Allen & Hanburys

Stockley Park West

Uxbridge,

Middlesex

UB11 1BT

8. MARKETING AUTHORISATION NUMBER(S)

PL 10949/0006

9. DATE OF FIRST AUTHORISATION/RENEWAL OF THE AUTHORISATION

25 February 1993

10. DATE OF REVISION OF THE TEXT

03 February 2009

11. Legal Status

POM.

Flixotide Diskhaler 250 mcg

(Allen & Hanburys)

1. NAME OF THE MEDICINAL PRODUCT

Flixotide$_{TM}$ Diskhaler$_{TM}$ 250 Micrograms

2. QUALITATIVE AND QUANTITATIVE COMPOSITION

Fluticasone Propionate (micronised) 250 micrograms

3. PHARMACEUTICAL FORM

Inhalation Powder.

4. CLINICAL PARTICULARS

4.1 Therapeutic indications

Fluticasone propionate given by inhalation offers preventative treatment for asthma. At recommended doses it has a potent glucocorticoid anti-inflammatory action within the lungs, with a lower incidence and severity of adverse effects than those observed when corticosteroids are administered systemically.

Prophylactic management in:-

Adults

Mild asthma:

Patients requiring intermittent symptomatic bronchodilator asthma medication on a regular daily basis.

Moderate asthma:

Patients with unstable or worsening asthma despite prophylactic therapy or bronchodilator alone.

Severe asthma:

Patients with severe chronic asthma and those who are dependent on systemic corticosteroids for adequate control of symptoms. On introduction of inhaled fluticasone propionate many of these patients may be able to reduce significantly, or to eliminate, their requirement for oral corticosteroids.

Route of administration: by inhalation.

4.2 Posology and method of administration

The onset of therapeutic effect is within 4 to 7 days.

Adults and children over 16 years: 100 to 1,000 micrograms twice daily.

Patients should be given a starting dose of inhaled fluticasone propionate, which is appropriate to the severity of their disease.

Prescribers should be aware that fluticasone propionate is as effective as other inhaled steroids approximately at half the microgram daily dose. For example, a 100mcg of fluticasone propionate is approximately equivalent to

200mcg dose of beclometasone dipropionate (CFC containing) or budesonide.

Due to the risk of systemic effects, doses above 500 micrograms twice daily should be prescribed only for adult patients with severe asthma where additional clinical benefit is expected, demonstrated by either an improvement in pulmonary function and/or symptom control, or by a reduction in oral corticosteroid therapy (see 4.4 Special Warnings and Precautions for Use and 4.8 Undesirable Effects).

Typical Adult Starting Doses:

For patients with mild asthma, a typical starting dose is 100 micrograms twice daily. In moderate and more severe asthma, starting doses may need to be 250 to 500 micrograms twice daily. Where additional clinical benefit is expected, doses of up to 1000 micrograms twice daily may be used. Initiation of such doses should be prescribed only by a specialist in the management of asthma (such as a consultant physician or general practitioner with appropriate experience).

The dose should be titrated down to the lowest dose at which effective control of asthma is maintained.

Flixotide Diskhaler 250 micrograms is not suitable for use in children.

The maximum licensed dose in children is 200 micrograms twice daily.

Special patient groups:

There is no need to adjust the dose in elderly patients or those with hepatic or renal impairment.

4.3 Contraindications

Flixotide preparations are contra-indicated in patients with a history of hypersensitivity to any of their components.

4.4 Special warnings and precautions for use

Flixotide Diskhalers are not designed to relieve acute symptoms for which an inhaled short acting bronchodilator is required. Patients should be advised to have such rescue medication available.

Severe asthma requires regular medical assessment, including lung-function testing, as patients are at risk of severe attacks and even death. Increasing use of short-acting inhaled β_2-agonists to relieve symptoms indicates deterioration of asthma control. If patients find that short-acting relief bronchodilator treatment becomes less effective, or they need more inhalations than usual, medical attention must be sought.

In this situation patients should be reassessed and consideration given to the need for increased anti-inflammatory therapy (e.g. higher doses of inhaled corticosteroids or a course of oral corticosteroids). Severe exacerbations of asthma must be treated in the normal way.

There have been very rare reports of increases in blood glucose levels, in patients with or without a history of diabetes mellitus (See 4.8 'Undesirable Effects'). This should be considered in particular when prescribing to patients with a history of diabetes mellitus.

As with other inhalation therapy, paradoxical bronchospasm may occur with an immediate increase in wheezing after dosing. Flixotide Diskhaler should be discontinued immediately, the patient assessed and alternative therapy instituted if necessary.

Systemic effects of inhaled corticosteroids may occur, particularly at high doses prescribed for prolonged periods. These effects are much less likely to occur than with oral corticosteroids. Possible systemic effects include Cushing's syndrome, Cushingoid features, adrenal suppression, growth retardation in children and adolescents, decrease in bone mineral density, cataract and glaucoma. **It is important therefore that the dose of inhaled corticosteroid is reviewed regularly and reduced to the lowest dose at which effective control of asthma is maintained.**

Prolonged treatment with high doses of inhaled corticosteroids may result in adrenal suppression and acute adrenal crisis. Children aged < 16 years taking higher than licensed doses of fluticasone (typically ≥1000mcg/day) may be at particular risk. Situations, which could potentially trigger acute adrenal crisis, include trauma, surgery, infection or any rapid reduction in dosage. Presenting symptoms are typically vague and may include anorexia, abdominal pain, weight loss, tiredness, headache, nausea, vomiting, decreased level of consciousness, hypoglycaemia, and seizures. Additional systemic corticosteroid cover should be considered during periods of stress or elective surgery.

It is recommended that the height of children receiving prolonged treatment with inhaled corticosteroids is regularly monitored. If growth is slowed, therapy should be reviewed with the aim of reducing the dose of inhaled corticosteroid, if possible, to the lowest dose at which effective control of asthma is maintained. In addition, consideration should be given to referring the patient to a paediatric respiratory specialist.

When changing from a dry powder inhaler to a metered dose inhaler, administration of high doses, above 1000 mcg daily, is recommended through a spacer to reduce side effects in the mouth and throat. However, this may increase drug delivery to the lungs. As systemic absorption is largely through the lungs, there may be an increase in the risk of systemic adverse effects. A lower dose may be required.

The benefits of inhaled fluticasone propionate should minimise the need for oral steroids. However, patients transferred from oral steroids, remain at risk of impaired adrenal reserve for a considerable time after transferring to inhaled fluticasone propionate. The possibility of adverse effects may persist for some time.

These patients may require specialised advice to determine the extent of adrenal impairment before elective procedures. The possibility of residual impaired adrenal response should always be considered in emergency (medical or surgical) and elective situations likely to produce stress, and appropriate corticosteroid treatment considered.

Lack of response or severe exacerbations of asthma should be treated by increasing the dose of inhaled fluticasone propionate and, if necessary, by giving a systemic steroid and/or an antibiotic if there is an infection.

<u>For the transfer of patients being treated with oral corticosteroids:</u>

The transfer of oral steroid-dependent patients to Flixotide and their subsequent management needs special care as recovery from impaired adrenocortical function, caused by prolonged systemic steroid therapy, may take a considerable time.

Patients who have been treated with systemic steroids for long periods of time or at a high dose may have adrenocortical suppression. With these patients adrenocortical function should be monitored regularly and their dose of systemic steroid reduced cautiously.

After approximately a week, gradual withdrawal of the systemic steroid is started by reducing the daily dose by one milligram prednisolone, or its equivalent. For maintenance doses of prednisolone in excess of 10mg daily, it may be appropriate to cautiously use larger reductions in dose at weekly intervals.

Some patients feel unwell in a non-specific way during the withdrawal phase despite maintenance or even improvement of the respiratory function. They should be encouraged to persevere with inhaled fluticasone propionate and to continue withdrawal of systemic steroid, unless there are objective signs of adrenal insufficiency.

Patients transferred from oral steroids whose adrenocortical function is still impaired should carry a steroid warning card indicating that they need supplementary systemic steroid during periods of stress, e.g. worsening asthma attacks, chest infections, major intercurrent illness, surgery, trauma, etc.

Replacement of systemic steroid treatment with inhaled therapy sometimes unmasks allergies such as allergic rhinitis or eczema previously controlled by the systemic drug. These allergies should be symptomatically treated with antihistamine and/or topical preparations, including topical steroids.

Treatment with Flixotide Diskhalers should not be stopped abruptly.

Special care is necessary in patients with active or quiescent pulmonary tuberculosis.

Ritonavir can greatly increase the concentration of fluticasone propionate in plasma. Therefore, concomitant use should be avoided, unless the potential benefit to the patient outweighs the risk of systemic corticosteroid side-effects. There is also an increased risk of systemic side effects when combining fluticasone propionate with other potent CYP3A inhibitors (see 4.5 Interaction with Other Medicinal Products and Other Forms of Interaction).

4.5 Interaction with other medicinal products and other forms of interaction

Under normal circumstances, low plasma concentrations of fluticasone propionate are achieved after inhaled dosing, due to extensive first pass metabolism and high systemic clearance mediated by cytochrome P450 3A4 in the gut and liver. Hence, clinically significant drug interactions mediated by fluticasone propionate are unlikely.

In an interaction study in healthy subjects with intranasal fluticasone propionate, ritonavir (a highly potent cytochrome P450 3A4 inhibitor) 100 mg b.i.d. increased the fluticasone propionate plasma concentrations several hundred fold, resulting in markedly reduced serum cortisol concentrations. Information about this interaction is lacking for inhaled fluticasone propionate, but a marked increase in fluticasone propionate plasma levels is expected. Cases of Cushing's syndrome and adrenal suppression have been reported. The combination should be avoided unless the benefit outweighs the increased risk of systemic glucocorticoid side-effects.

In a small study in healthy volunteers, the slightly less potent CYP3A inhibitor ketoconazole increased the exposure of fluticasone propionate after a single inhalation by 150%. This resulted in a greater reduction of plasma cortisol as compared with fluticasone propionate alone. Co-treatment with other potent CYP3A inhibitors, such as itraconazole, is also expected to increase the systemic fluticasone propionate exposure and the risk of systemic side-effects. Caution is recommended and long-term treatment with such drugs should, if possible, be avoided.

4.6 Pregnancy and lactation

There is inadequate evidence of safety of fluticasone propionate in human pregnancy. Administration of corticosteroids to pregnant animals can cause abnormalities of fetal development, including cleft palate and intra-uterine growth retardation. There may therefore be a very small risk of such effects in the human fetus. It should be noted, however, that the fetal changes in animals occur after relatively high systemic exposure. Because fluticasone propionate is delivered directly to the lungs by the inhaled route it avoids the high level of exposure that occurs when corticosteroids are given by systemic routes.

Administration of fluticasone propionate during pregnancy should only be considered if the expected benefit to the mother is greater than any possible risk to the fetus.

The secretion of fluticasone propionate in human breast milk has not been investigated. Subcutaneous administration of fluticasone propionate to lactating laboratory rats produced measurable plasma levels and evidence of fluticasone propionate in the milk. However, plasma levels in humans after inhalation at recommended doses are likely to be low.

When fluticasone propionate is used in breast feeding mothers the therapeutic benefits must be weighed against the potential hazards to mother and baby.

4.7 Effects on ability to drive and use machines

Fluticasone propionate is unlikely to produce an effect.

4.8 Undesirable effects

Adverse events are listed below by system organ class and frequency. Frequencies are defined as: very common (≥1/10), common (≥1/100 and <1/10), uncommon (≥1/1000 and <1/100), rare (≥1/10,000 and <1/1000) and very rare (<1/10,000) including isolated reports. Very common, common and uncommon events were generally determined from spontaneous data.

System Organ Class	Adverse Event	Frequency
Infections & Infestations	Candidiasis of the mouth and throat	Very Common
	Pneumonia (in COPD patients)	Common
Immune System Disorders	Hypersensitivity reactions with the following manifestations:	
	Cutaneous hypersensitivity reactions	Uncommon
	Angioedema (mainly facial and oropharyngeal oedema),	Very Rare
	Respiratory symptoms (dyspnoea and/or bronchospasm),	Very Rare
	Anaphylactic reactions	Very Rare
Endocrine Disorders	Cushing's syndrome, Cushingoid features, adrenal suppression, growth retardation in children and adolescents, decreased bone mineral density, cataract, glaucoma	Very Rare
Metabolism & Nutrition Disorders	Hyperglycaemia (see 4.4 'Special Warnings and Precautions for Use')	Very Rare
Gastrointestinal Disorders	Dyspepsia	Very Rare
Musculoskeletal & Connective Tissue Disorders	Arthralgia	Very Rare
Psychiatric Disorders	Anxiety, sleep disorders, behavioural changes, including hyperactivity and irritability (predominantly in children)	Very Rare
Respiratory, Thoracic & Mediastinal Disorders	Hoarseness/ dysphonia	Common
	Paradoxical bronchospasm	Very Rare
Skin & Subcutaneous Tissue Disorders	Contusions	Common

Hoarseness and candidiasis of the mouth and throat (thrush) occurs in some patients. Such patients may find it helpful to rinse out their mouth with water after using the Diskhaler. Symptomatic candidiasis can be treated with topical anti-fungal therapy whilst still continuing with the Flixotide Diskhaler.

Possible systemic effects include Cushing's syndrome, Cushingoid features, adrenal suppression, growth retardation, decreased bone mineral density, cataract, glaucoma (see 4.4 Special Warnings and Special Precautions for Use).

As with other inhalation therapy, paradoxical bronchospasm may occur (see 4.4 'Special Warnings and Precautions for Use'). This should be treated immediately with a fast-acting inhaled bronchodilator. Flixotide Diskhaler should be discontinued immediately, the patient assessed, and if necessary alternative therapy instituted.

There was an increased reporting of pneumonia in studies of patients with COPD receiving FLIXOTIDE 500 micrograms. Physicians should remain vigilant for the possible development of pneumonia in patients with COPD as the clinical features of pneumonia and exacerbation frequently overlap.

4.9 Overdose

Acute: Inhalation of the drug in doses in excess of those recommended may lead to temporary suppression of adrenal function. This does not necessitate emergency action being taken.

In these patients treatment with fluticasone propionate by inhalation should be continued at a dose sufficient to control asthma adrenal function recovers in a few days and can be verified by measuring plasma cortisol.

Chronic: refer to section 4.4: risk of adrenal suppression.

Monitoring of adrenal reserve may be indicated. Treatment with inhaled fluticasonepropionate should be continued at a dose sufficient to control asthma.

5. PHARMACOLOGICAL PROPERTIES

5.1 Pharmacodynamic properties

Fluticasone propionate given by inhalation at recommended doses has a potent glucocorticoid anti-inflammatory action within the lungs, with a lower incidence and severity of adverse effects than those observed when corticosteroids are administered systemically.

5.2 Pharmacokinetic properties

Systemic absolute bioavailability of fluticasone propionate is estimated at 12-26% of an inhaled dose, dependent on presentation. Systemic absorption occurs mainly through the lungs and is initially rapid then prolonged. The remainder of the dose may be swallowed.

Absolute oral bioavailability is negligible (<1%) due to a combination of incomplete absorption from the GI tract and extensive first-pass metabolism.

87-100% of an oral dose is excreted in the faeces, up to 75% as parent compound. There is also a non-active major metabolite.

After an intravenous dose, fluticasone propionate is extensively distributed in the body. The very high clearance rate indicates extensive hepatic clearance.

5.3 Preclinical safety data

No clinically relevant findings were observed in preclinical studies.

6. PHARMACEUTICAL PARTICULARS

6.1 List of excipients

Lactose Ph Eur

6.2 Incompatibilities

None known

6.3 Shelf life

24 months

6.4 Special precautions for storage

Whilst the disks provide good protection to the blister contents from the effects of the atmosphere, they should not be exposed to extremes of temperature and should not be stored above 30°C. A disk may be kept in the diskhaler at all times but a blister should only be pierced immediately prior to use. Failure to observe this instruction will affect the operation of the diskhaler.

6.5 Nature and contents of container

A circular double-foil (PVC/Aluminium) disk with four blisters, containing a mixture of fluticasone propionate and lactose. The foil disk is inserted into the Diskhaler device.

The following packs are registered: 5, 7, 10, 14 or 15 disks with or without a diskhaler. Refill packs of 5, 7, 10, 14 or 15 disks. A starter pack consisting of diskhaler pre-loaded with one disk (with or without a peak flow meter and diary card). A starter pack plus a spare disk (with or without a peak flow meter and diary card).

The following packs are marketed: cartons containing 14 disks (14x4 blisters), together with a Diskhaler inhaler. Cartons containing 5 disks (5x4 blisters) together with a Diskhaler inhaler (250 micrograms and 500 micrograms hospital packs only). Refill packs containing 14 disks (14x4 blisters).

6.6 Special precautions for disposal and other handling

See Patient Information Leaflet for detailed instructions.

Administrative Data

7. MARKETING AUTHORISATION HOLDER

Glaxo Wellcome UK Ltd
trading as Allen & Hanburys
Stockley Park West
Uxbridge,
Middlesex
UB11 1BT

8. MARKETING AUTHORISATION NUMBER(S)

PL 10949/0007

9. DATE OF FIRST AUTHORISATION/RENEWAL OF THE AUTHORISATION

25 February 1993

10. DATE OF REVISION OF THE TEXT

03 February 2009

11. Legal Status

POM.

Flixotide Diskhaler 500 mcg

(Allen & Hanburys)

1. NAME OF THE MEDICINAL PRODUCT

Flixotide$_{TM}$ Diskhaler$_{TM}$500 Micrograms

2. QUALITATIVE AND QUANTITATIVE COMPOSITION

Fluticasone Propionate (micronised) 500 micrograms

3. PHARMACEUTICAL FORM

Inhalation Powder.

4. CLINICAL PARTICULARS

4.1 Therapeutic indications

Fluticasone propionate given by inhalation offers preventative treatment for asthma. At recommended doses it has a potent glucocorticoid anti-inflammatory action within the lungs, with a lower incidence and severity of adverse effects than those observed when corticosteroids are administered systemically.

Prophylactic management in: -

Adults

Moderate asthma:

Patients with unstable or worsening asthma despite prophylactic therapy or bronchodilator alone.

Severe asthma:

Patients with severe chronic asthma and those who are dependent on systemic corticosteroids for adequate control of symptoms. On introduction of inhaled fluticasone propionate many of these patients may be able to reduce significantly, or to eliminate, their requirement for oral corticosteroids.

Route of administration: by inhalation.

4.2 Posology and method of administration

The onset of therapeutic effect is within 4 to 7 days.

Adults and children over 16 years: 100 to 1,000 micrograms twice daily.

Patients should be given a starting dose of inhaled fluticasone propionate, which is appropriate to the severity of their disease.

Prescribers should be aware that fluticasone propionate is as effective as other inhaled steroids approximately at half the microgram daily dose. For example, a 100mcg of fluticasone propionate is approximately equivalent to 200mcg dose of beclometasone dipropionate (CFC containing) or budesonide.

Due to the risk of systemic effects, doses above 500 micrograms twice daily should be prescribed only for adult patients with severe asthma where additional clinical benefit is expected, demonstrated by either an improvement in pulmonary function and/or symptom control, or by a reduction in oral corticosteroid therapy (see 4.4 Special Warnings and Precautions for Use and 4.8 Undesirable Effects).

Typical Adult Starting Doses:

For patients with mild asthma, a typical starting dose is 100 micrograms twice daily. In moderate and more severe asthma, starting doses may need to be 250 to 500 micrograms twice daily. Where additional clinical benefit is expected, doses of up to 1000 micrograms twice daily may be used. Initiation of such doses should be prescribed only by a specialist in the management of asthma (such as a consultant physician or general practitioner with appropriate experience).

The dose should be titrated down to the lowest dose at which effective control of asthma is maintained.

Flixotide Diskhaler 500 micrograms is not suitable for use in children.

The maximum licensed dose in children is 200 micrograms twice daily.

Special patient groups:

There is no need to adjust the dose in elderly patients or those with hepatic or renal impairment.

4.3 Contraindications

Flixotide preparations are contra-indicated in patients with a history of hypersensitivity to any of their components.

4.4 Special warnings and precautions for use

Flixotide Diskhalers are not designed to relieve acute symptoms for which an inhaled short acting bronchodilator is required. Patients should be advised to have such rescue medication available.

Severe asthma requires regular medical assessment, including lung-function testing, as patients are at risk of severe attacks and even death. Increasing use of short-acting inhaled β_2-agonists to relieve symptoms indicates deterioration of asthma control. If patients find that short-acting relief bronchodilator treatment becomes less effective, or they need more inhalations than usual, medical attention must be sought.

In this situation patients should be reassessed and consideration given to the need for increased anti-inflammatory therapy (e.g. higher doses of inhaled corticosteroids or a course of oral corticosteroids). Severe exacerbations of asthma must be treated in the normal way.

There have been very rare reports of increases in blood glucose levels, in patients with or without a history of diabetes mellitus (See 4.8 'Undesirable Effects'). This should be considered in particular when prescribing to patients with a history of diabetes mellitus.

As with other inhalation therapy, paradoxical bronchospasm may occur with an immediate increase in wheezing after dosing. Flixotide Diskhaler should be discontinued immediately, the patient assessed and alternative therapy instituted if necessary.

Systemic effects of inhaled corticosteroids may occur, particularly at high doses prescribed for prolonged periods. These effects are much less likely to occur than with oral corticosteroids. Possible systemic effects include Cushing's syndrome, Cushingoid features, adrenal suppression, growth retardation in children and adolescents, decrease in bone mineral density, cataract and glaucoma. **It is important therefore that the dose of inhaled corticosteroid is reviewed regularly and reduced to the lowest dose at which effective control of asthma is maintained.**

Prolonged treatment with high doses of inhaled corticosteroids may result in adrenal suppression and acute adrenal crisis. Children aged < 16 years taking higher than licensed doses of fluticasone (typically ⩾1000mcg/day) may be at particular risk. Situations, which could potentially trigger acute adrenal crisis, include trauma, surgery, infection or any rapid reduction in dosage. Presenting symptoms are typically vague and may include anorexia, abdominal pain, weight loss, tiredness, headache, nausea, vomiting, decreased level of consciousness, hypoglycaemia, and seizures. Additional systemic corticosteroid cover should be considered during periods of stress or elective surgery.

It is recommended that the height of children receiving prolonged treatment with inhaled corticosteroids is regularly monitored. If growth is slowed, therapy should be reviewed with the aim of reducing the dose of inhaled corticosteroid, if possible, to the lowest dose at which effective control of asthma is maintained. In addition, consideration should be given to referring the patient to a paediatric respiratory specialist.

When changing from a dry powder inhaler to a metered dose inhaler, administration of high doses, above 1000 mcg daily, is recommended through a spacer to reduce side effects in the mouth and throat. However, this may increase drug delivery to the lungs. As systemic absorption is largely through the lungs, there may be an increase in the risk of systemic adverse effects. A lower dose may be required.

The benefits of inhaled fluticasone propionate should minimise the need for oral steroids. However, patients transferred from oral steroids, remain at risk of impaired adrenal reserve for a considerable time after transferring to inhaled fluticasone propionate. The possibility of adverse effects may persist for some time.

These patients may require specialised advice to determine the extent of adrenal impairment before elective procedures. The possibility of residual impaired adrenal response should always be considered in emergency (medical or surgical) and elective situations likely to produce stress, and appropriate corticosteroid treatment considered.

Lack of response or severe exacerbations of asthma should be treated by increasing the dose of inhaled fluticasone propionate and, if necessary, by giving a systemic steroid and/or an antibiotic if there is an infection.

For the transfer of patients being treated with oral corticosteroids:

The transfer of oral steroid-dependent patients to Flixotide and their subsequent management needs special care as recovery from impaired adrenocortical function, caused by prolonged systemic steroid therapy, may take a considerable time.

Patients who have been treated with systemic steroids for long periods of time or at a high dose may have adrenocortical suppression. With these patients adrenocortical function should be monitored regularly and their dose of systemic steroid reduced cautiously.

After approximately a week, gradual withdrawal of the systemic steroid is started by reducing the daily dose by one milligram prednisolone, or its equivalent. For maintenance doses of prednisolone in excess of 10mg daily, it may be appropriate to cautiously use larger reductions in dose at weekly intervals.

Some patients feel unwell in a non-specific way during the withdrawal phase despite maintenance or even improvement of the respiratory function. They should be encouraged to persevere with inhaled fluticasone propionate and to continue withdrawal of systemic steroid, unless there are objective signs of adrenal insufficiency.

Patients transferred from oral steroids whose adrenocortical function is still impaired should carry a steroid warning card indicating that they need supplementary systemic steroid during periods of stress, e.g. worsening asthma attacks, chest infections, major intercurrent illness, surgery, trauma, etc.

Replacement of systemic steroid treatment with inhaled therapy sometimes unmasks allergies such as allergic rhinitis or eczema previously controlled by the systemic drug. These allergies should be symptomatically treated with antihistamine and/or topical preparations, including topical steroids.

Treatment with Flixotide Diskhalers should not be stopped abruptly.

Special care is necessary in patients with active or quiescent pulmonary tuberculosis.

Ritonavir can greatly increase the concentration of fluticasone propionate in plasma. Therefore, concomitant use should be avoided, unless the potential benefit to the patient outweighs the risk of systemic corticosteroid side-effects. There is also an increased risk of systemic side effects when combining fluticasone propionate with other potent CYP3A inhibitors (see 4.5 Interaction with Other Medicinal Products and Other Forms of Interaction).

4.5 Interaction with other medicinal products and other forms of interaction

Under normal circumstances, low plasma concentrations of fluticasone propionate are achieved after inhaled dosing, due to extensive first pass metabolism and high systemic clearance mediated by cytochrome P450 3A4 in the gut and liver. Hence, clinically significant drug interactions mediated by fluticasone propionate are unlikely.

In an interaction study in healthy subjects with intranasal fluticasone propionate, ritonavir (a highly potent cytochrome P450 3A4 inhibitor) 100 mg b.i.d. increased the fluticasone propionate plasma concentrations several hundred fold, resulting in markedly reduced serum cortisol concentrations. Information about this interaction is lacking for inhaled fluticasone propionate, but a marked increase in fluticasone propionate plasma levels is expected. Cases of Cushing's syndrome and adrenal suppression have been reported. The combination should be avoided unless the benefit outweighs the increased risk of systemic glucocorticoid side-effects.

In a small study in healthy volunteers, the slightly less potent CYP3A inhibitor ketoconazole increased the exposure of fluticasone propionate after a single inhalation by 150%. This resulted in a greater reduction of plasma cortisol as compared with fluticasone propionate alone. Co-treatment with other potent CYP3A inhibitors, such as itraconazole, is also expected to increase the systemic fluticasone propionate exposure and the risk of systemic side-effects. Caution is recommended and long-term treatment with such drugs should if possible be avoided.

4.6 Pregnancy and lactation

There is inadequate evidence of safety of fluticasone propionate in human pregnancy. Administration of corticosteroids to pregnant animals can cause abnormalities of fetal development, including cleft palate and intra-uterine growth retardation. There may therefore be a very small risk of such effects in the human fetus. It should be noted, however, that the fetal changes in animals occur after relatively high systemic exposure. Because fluticasone propionate is delivered directly to the lungs by the inhaled route it avoids the high level of exposure that occurs when corticosteroids are given by systemic routes.

Administration of fluticasone propionate during pregnancy should only be considered if the expected benefit to the mother is greater than any possible risk to the fetus.

The secretion of fluticasone propionate in human breast milk has not been investigated. Subcutaneous administration of fluticasone propionate to lactating laboratory rats produced measurable plasma levels and evidence of fluticasone propionate in the milk. However, plasma levels in humans after inhalation at recommended doses are likely to be low.

When fluticasone propionate is used in breast feeding mothers the therapeutic benefits must be weighed against the potential hazards to mother and baby.

4.7 Effects on ability to drive and use machines

Fluticasone propionate is unlikely to produce an effect.

4.8 Undesirable effects

Adverse events are listed below by system organ class and frequency. Frequencies are defined as: very common (≥1/10), common (≥1/100 and <1/10), uncommon (≥1/1000 and <1/100), rare (≥1/10,000 and <1/1000) and very rare (<1/10,000) including isolated reports. Very common, common and uncommon events were generally determined from spontaneous data.

System Organ Class	Adverse Event	Frequency
Infections & Infestations	Candidiasis of the mouth and throat	Very Common
	Pneumonia (in COPD patients)	Common
Immune System Disorders	Hypersensitivity reactions with the following manifestations:	
	Cutaneous hypersensitivity reactions	Uncommon
	Angioedema (mainly facial and oropharyngeal oedema),	Very Rare
	Respiratory symptoms (dyspnoea and/or bronchospasm),	Very Rare
	Anaphylactic reactions	Very Rare
Endocrine Disorders	Cushing's syndrome, Cushingoid features, adrenal suppression, growth retardation in children and adolescents, decreased bone mineral density, cataract, glaucoma	Very Rare
Metabolism & Nutrition Disorders	Hyperglycaemia (see 4.4 'Special Warnings and Precautions for Use')	Very Rare
Gastrointestinal Disorders	Dyspepsia	Very Rare
Musculoskeletal & Connective Tissue Disorders	Arthralgia	Very Rare
Psychiatric Disorders	Anxiety, sleep disorders, behavioural changes, including hyperactivity and irritability (predominantly in children)	Very Rare
Respiratory, Thoracic & Mediastinal Disorders	Hoarseness/ dysphonia	Common
	Paradoxical bronchospasm	Very Rare
Skin & Subcutaneous Tissue Disorders	Contusions	Common

Hoarseness and candidiasis of the mouth and throat (thrush) occurs in some patients. Such patients may find it helpful to rinse out their mouth with water after using the Diskhaler. Symptomatic candidiasis can be treated with topical anti-fungal therapy whilst still continuing with the Flixotide Diskhaler.

Possible systemic effects include Cushing's syndrome, Cushingoid features, adrenal suppression, growth retardation, decreased bone mineral density, cataract, glaucoma. (see 4.4 Special Warnings and Special Precautions for Use).

As with other inhalation therapy, paradoxical bronchospasm may occur (see 4.4 'Special Warnings and Precautions for Use'). This should be treated immediately with a fast-acting inhaled bronchodilator. Flixotide Diskhaler should be discontinued immediately, the patient assessed, and if necessary alternative therapy instituted.

There was an increased reporting of pneumonia in studies of patients with COPD receiving FLIXOTIDE 500 micrograms. Physicians should remain vigilant for the possible development of pneumonia in patients with COPD as the clinical features of pneumonia and exacerbation frequently overlap.

4.9 Overdose

Acute: Inhalation of the drug in doses in excess of those recommended may lead to temporary suppression of adrenal function. This does not necessitate emergency action being taken.

In these patients treatment with fluticasone propionate by inhalation should be continued at a dose sufficient to control asthma adrenal function recovers in a few days and can be verified by measuring plasma cortisol.

Chronic: refer to section 4.4: risk of adrenal suppression.

Monitoring of adrenal reserve may be indicated. Treatment with inhaled fluticasone propionate should be continued at a dose sufficient to control asthma.

5. PHARMACOLOGICAL PROPERTIES

5.1 Pharmacodynamic properties

Fluticasone propionate given by inhalation at recommended doses has a potent glucocorticoid anti-inflammatory action within the lungs, with a lower incidence and severity of adverse effects than those observed when corticosteroids are administered systemically.

5.2 Pharmacokinetic properties

Systemic absolute bioavailability of fluticasone propionate is estimated at 12-26% of an inhaled dose, dependent on presentation. Systemic absorption occurs mainly through the lungs and is initially rapid then prolonged. The remainder of the dose may be swallowed.

Absolute oral bioavailability is negligible (<1%) due to a combination of incomplete absorption from the GI tract and extensive first-pass metabolism.

87-100% of an oral dose is excreted in the faeces, up to 75% as parent compound. There is also a non-active major metabolite.

After an intravenous dose, fluticasone propionate is extensively distributed in the body. The very high clearance rate indicates extensive hepatic clearance.

5.3 Preclinical safety data

No clinically relevant findings were observed in preclinical studies.

6. PHARMACEUTICAL PARTICULARS

6.1 List of excipients

Lactose Ph Eur

6.2 Incompatibilities

None known

6.3 Shelf life

24 months

6.4 Special precautions for storage

Whilst the disks provide good protection to the blister contents from the effects of the atmosphere, they should not be exposed to extremes of temperature and should not be stored above 30°C. A disk may be kept in the diskhaler at all times but a blister should only be pierced immediately prior to use. Failure to observe this instruction will affect the operation of the diskhaler.

6.5 Nature and contents of container

A circular double-foil (PVC/Aluminium) disk with four blisters, containing a mixture of fluticasone propionate and lactose. The foil disk is inserted into the Diskhaler device.

The following packs are registered: 5, 7, 10, 14 or 15 disks with or without a diskhaler. Refill packs of 5, 7, 10, 14 or 15 disks. A starter pack consisting of diskhaler pre-loaded with one disk (with or without a peak flow meter and diary card). A starter pack plus a spare disk (with or without a peak flow meter and diary card).

The following packs are marketed: cartons containing 14 disks (14x4 blisters), together with a Diskhaler inhaler. Cartons containing 5 disks (5x4 blisters) together with a Diskhaler inhaler (250 micrograms and 500 micrograms hospital packs only). Refill packs containing 14 disks (14x4 blisters).

6.6 Special precautions for disposal and other handling

See Patient Information Leaflet for detailed instructions.

Administrative Data

7. MARKETING AUTHORISATION HOLDER

Glaxo Wellcome UK Ltd
trading as Allen & Hanburys
Stockley Park West
Uxbridge,
Middlesex
UB11 1BT

8. MARKETING AUTHORISATION NUMBER(S)

PL 10949/0008

9. DATE OF FIRST AUTHORISATION/RENEWAL OF THE AUTHORISATION

25 February 1993

10. DATE OF REVISION OF THE TEXT

03 February 2009

11. Legal Status

POM.

Flixotide Nebules 0.5mg/2ml

(Allen & Hanburys)

1. NAME OF THE MEDICINAL PRODUCT

Flixotide Nebules 0.5mg/2ml.

2. QUALITATIVE AND QUANTITATIVE COMPOSITION

Plastic ampoules containing 2ml of a buffered, isotonic saline suspension containing 0.5mg fluticasone propionate

3. PHARMACEUTICAL FORM

Inhalation suspension for nebulisation.

4. CLINICAL PARTICULARS

4.1 Therapeutic indications

In adults and adolescents over 16 years Flixotide Nebules can be used:

For prophylactic management of severe chronic asthma in patients requiring high dose inhaled or oral corticosteroid therapy. On introduction of inhaled fluticasone propionate many patients currently treated with oral corticosteroids may be able to reduce significantly, or eliminate, their oral dose.

Children and adolescents from 4 to 16 years of age:

Treatment of acute exacerbations of asthma. Subsequent maintenance dosing may be more conveniently accomplished using a pressurised metered dose inhaler or powder formulation.

Fluticasone propionate given by inhalation has a potent glucocorticoid anti-inflammatory action within the lungs. It reduces symptoms and exacerbations of asthma in patients previously treated with bronchodilators alone or with other prophylactic therapy. Relatively brief symptomatic episodes can generally be relieved by the use of fast-acting bronchodilators, but longer-lasting exacerbations require, in addition, the use of corticosteroid therapy as soon as possible to control the inflammation.

4.2 Posology and method of administration

Adults and adolescents over 16 years: 500-2,000 micrograms twice daily.

Prescribers should be aware that fluticasone propionate is as effective as other inhaled steroids approximately at half the microgram daily dose. For example, a 100mcg of fluticasone propionate is approximately equivalent to 200mcg dose of beclometasone dipropionate (CFC containing) or budesonide

Prescribers should be aware of the risks of systemic effects when using high doses of corticosteroids (see 4.4 special warnings and precautions for use and 4.8 undesirable effects).

Patients should be given a starting dose of inhaled fluticasone propionate, which is appropriate to the severity of their disease.

The dose should be titrated down to the lowest dose at which effective control of asthma is maintained.

Children and adolescents from 4 to 16 years of age: 1000 mcg twice daily

Special patient groups: There is no need to adjust the dose in elderly patients or those with hepatic or renal impairment.

Flixotide Nebules are for inhalation use only. They should be administered as an aerosol produced by a jet nebuliser, as directed by a physician. As drug delivery from nebulisers is variable, the manufacturer's instructions for using the nebuliser must be followed.

Use of Flixotide Nebules with ultrasonic nebulisers is not generally recommended.

Flixotide Nebules should not be injected or administered orally.

Patients should be made aware of the prophylactic nature of therapy with inhaled fluticasone propionate and that it should be taken regularly.

It is advisable to administer Flixotide Nebules via a mouthpiece to avoid the possibility of atrophic changes to facial skin which may occur with prolonged use with a face-mask. When a face-mask is used, the exposed skin should be protected using a barrier cream, or the face should be thoroughly washed after treatment.

4.3 Contraindications

Hypersensitivity to any ingredient of the preparation.

4.4 Special warnings and precautions for use

Flixotide Nebules are not designed to relieve acute symptoms for which an inhaled short-acting bronchodilator is required. Patients should be advised to have such rescue medication available. Flixotide Nebules are intended for regular daily prophylactic treatment.

Flixotide Nebules are not a substitute for injectable or oral corticosteroids in an emergency (i.e. life threatening asthma).

Severe asthma requires regular medical assessment, including lung function testing, as patients are at risk of severe attacks and even death. Increasing use of short-acting inhaled β_2-agonists to relieve symptoms indicates deterioration of asthma control. If patients find that short-acting relief bronchodilator treatment becomes less effective, or they need more inhalations than usual, medical attention must be sought. In this situation patients should be reassessed and consideration given to the need for increased anti-inflammatory therapy (e.g. higher doses of inhaled corticosteroids or a course of oral corticosteroids). Severe exacerbations of asthma must be treated in the normal way.

There have been very rare reports of increases in blood glucose levels, in patients with or without a history of diabetes mellitus (See 4.8 'Undesirable Effects'). This should be considered in particular when prescribing to patients with a history of diabetes mellitus.

As with other inhalation therapy, paradoxical bronchospasm may occur with an immediate increase in wheezing after dosing. Flixotide Nebules should be discontinued immediately, the patient assessed and alternative therapy instituted if necessary.

Systemic effects of inhaled corticosteroids may occur, particularly at high doses prescribed for prolonged periods. These effects are much less likely to occur than with oral steroids. Possible systemic effects include Cushing's syndrome, Cushingoid features, adrenal suppression, growth retardation in children and adolescents, decrease in bone mineral density, cataract and glaucoma. **It is important therefore that the dose of inhaled corticosteroid is reviewed regularly and reduced to the lowest dose at which effective control of asthma is maintained.**

Prolonged treatment with high doses of inhaled corticosteroids may result in adrenal suppression and acute adrenal crisis. Children aged < 16 years taking higher than licensed doses of fluticasone (typically ≥1000mcg/day) may be at particular risk. Situations, which could potentially trigger acute adrenal crisis, include trauma, surgery, infection or any rapid reduction in dosage. Presenting symptoms are typically vague and may include anorexia, abdominal pain, weight loss, tiredness, headache, nausea, vomiting, decreased level of consciousness, hypoglycaemia, and seizures. Additional systemic corticosteroid cover should be considered during periods of stress or elective surgery.

It is recommended that the height of children receiving prolonged treatment with inhaled corticosteroids is regularly monitored. If growth is slowed, therapy should be reviewed with the aim of reducing the dose of inhaled corticosteroid, if possible to the lowest dose at which effective control of asthma is maintained. In addition, consideration should be given to referring the patient to a paediatric respiratory specialist.

The benefits of inhaled fluticasone propionate should minimise the need for oral steroids. However, patients transferred from oral steroids, remain at risk of impaired adrenal reserve for a considerable time after transferring to inhaled fluticasone propionate. The possibility of adverse effects may persist for some time. These patients may require specialised advice to determine the extent of adrenal impairment before elective procedures. The possibility of residual impaired adrenal response should always be considered in emergency (medical or surgical) and elective situations likely to produce stress, and appropriate corticosteroid treatment considered.

Patients should receive a dose appropriate to the severity of their disease; the dose should be titrated to the lowest dose at which effective control of asthma is maintained. If control cannot be maintained, the use of a systemic steroid and/or an antibiotic may be necessary.

Replacement of systemic steroid treatment with inhaled therapy sometimes unmasks allergies such as allergic rhinitis or eczema previously controlled by the systemic drug. These allergies should be symptomatically treated with antihistamine and/or topical preparations, including topical steroids.

As with all inhaled corticosteroids, special care is necessary in patients with active or quiescent pulmonary tuberculosis.

Treatment with Flixotide Nebules should not be stopped abruptly.

For the transfer of patients being treated with oral corticosteroids: The transfer of oral steroid-dependent patients to Flixotide Nebules and their subsequent management needs special care as recovery from impaired adrenocortical function, caused by prolonged systemic steroid therapy, may take a considerable time.

Patients who have been treated with systemic steroids for long periods of time or at a high dose may have adrenocortical suppression. With these patients adrenocortical function should be monitored regularly and their dose of systemic steroid reduced cautiously.

After approximately a week, gradual withdrawal of the systemic steroid is commenced. Dosage reductions should be appropriate to the level of maintenance systemic steroid, and introduced at not less than weekly intervals. In general, for maintenance doses of prednisolone (or equivalent) of 10mg daily or less, the dosage reductions should not be greater than 1mg per day, at not less than weekly intervals. For maintenance doses of prednisolone in excess of 10mg daily, it may be appropriate to employ cautiously, larger reductions in dose at weekly intervals.

Some patients feel unwell in a non-specific way during the withdrawal phase despite maintenance or even improvement of the respiratory function. They should be encouraged to persevere with inhaled fluticasone propionate and to continue withdrawal of systemic steroid, unless there are objective signs of adrenal insufficiency.

Patients weaned off oral steroids whose adrenocortical function is still impaired should carry a steroid warning card indicating that they need supplementary systemic steroid during periods of stress, e.g. worsening asthma attacks, chest infections, major intercurrent illness, surgery, trauma, etc.

Ritonavir can greatly increase the concentration of fluticasone propionate in plasma. Therefore, concomitant use should be avoided, unless the potential benefit to the patient outweighs the risk of systemic corticosteroid side-effects. There is also an increased risk of systemic side effects when combining fluticasone propionate with other potent CYP3A inhibitors (see 4.5 Interaction with Other Medicinal Products and Other Forms of Interaction).

4.5 Interaction with other medicinal products and other forms of interaction

Under normal circumstances, low plasma concentrations of fluticasone propionate are achieved after inhaled dosing, due to extensive first pass metabolism and high systemic clearance mediated by cytochrome P450 3A4 in the gut and liver. Hence, clinically significant drug interactions mediated by fluticasone propionate are unlikely.

In an interaction study in healthy subjects with intranasal fluticasone propionate, ritonavir (a highly potent cytochrome P450 3A4 inhibitor) 100 mg b.i.d. increased the fluticasone propionate plasma concentrations several hundred fold, resulting in markedly reduced serum cortisol concentrations. Information about this interaction is lacking for inhaled fluticasone propionate, but a marked increase in fluticasone propionate plasma levels is expected. Cases of Cushing's syndrome and adrenal suppression have been reported. The combination should be avoided unless the benefit outweighs the increased risk of systemic glucocorticoid side-effects.

In a small study in healthy volunteers, the slightly less potent CYP3A inhibitor ketoconazole increased the exposure of fluticasone propionate after a single inhalation by 150%. This resulted in a greater reduction of plasma cortisol as compared with fluticasone propionate alone. Co-treatment with other potent CYP3A inhibitors, such as itraconazole, is also expected to increase the systemic fluticasone propionate exposure and the risk of systemic side-effects. Caution is recommended and long-term treatment with such drugs should if possible be avoided.

4.6 Pregnancy and lactation

There is inadequate evidence of safety of fluticasone propionate in human pregnancy. Administration of corticosteroids to pregnant animals can cause abnormalities of fetal development, including cleft palate and intra-uterine growth retardation. There may therefore be a very small risk of such effects in the human fetus. It should be noted, however, that the fetal changes in animals occur after relatively high systemic exposure. Because Flixotide Nebules deliver fluticasone propionate directly to the lungs by the inhaled route the high level of exposure that occurs when corticosteroids are given by systemic routes is avoided. Administration of fluticasone propionate during pregnancy should only be considered if the expected benefit to the mother is greater than any possible risk to the fetus.

The secretion of fluticasone propionate in human breast milk has not been investigated. Subcutaneous administration of fluticasone propionate to lactating laboratory rats produced measurable plasma levels and evidence of fluticasone propionate in the milk. However, plasma levels in humans after inhalation at recommended doses are likely to be low. When fluticasone propionate is used in breast-feeding mothers the therapeutic benefits must be weighed against the potential hazards to mother and baby.

4.7 Effects on ability to drive and use machines

Fluticasone propionate is unlikely to produce an effect.

4.8 Undesirable effects

Adverse events are listed below by system organ class and frequency. Frequencies are defined as: very common (≥1/10), common (≥1/100 and <1/10), uncommon (≥1/1000 and <1/100), rare (≥1/10,000 and <1/1000) and very rare (<1/10,000) including isolated reports. Very common, common and uncommon events were generally determined from clinical trial data. Rare and very rare events were generally determined from spontaneous data.

System Organ Class	Adverse Event	Frequency
Infections and Infestations	Candidiasis of the mouth and throat	Very Common
	Pneumonia (in COPD Patients)	Common
Immune System Disorders	Hypersensitivity reactions with the following manifestations:	
	Cutaneous hypersensitivity reactions	Uncommon
	Angioedema (mainly facial and oropharyngeal oedema),	Very Rare

	Respiratory symptoms (dyspnoea and/or bronchospasm)	Very Rare
	Anaphylactic reactions	Very Rare
Endocrine Disorders	Cushing's syndrome, Cushingoid features, adrenal suppression, growth retardation in children and adolescents, decreased bone mineral density, cataract, glaucoma	Very Rare
Metabolism and Nutrition Disorders	Hyperglycaemia (see 4.4 'Special Warnings and Precautions for Use')	Very Rare
Gastrointestinal Disorders	Dyspepsia	Very Rare
Musculoskeletal and Connective Tissue Disorders	Arthralgia	Very Rare
Psychiatric Disorders	Anxiety, sleep disorders, behavioural changes, including hyperactivity and irritability (predominantly in children)	Very Rare
Respiratory, Thoracic and	Hoarseness/ dysphonia	Common
Mediastinal Disorders	Paradoxical bronchospasm	Very Rare
Skin & Subcutaneous Tissue Disorders	Contusions	Common

Hoarseness and candidiasis of the mouth and throat (thrush) occurs in some patients. Such patients may find it helpful to rinse out their mouth with water after inhalation from the nebuliser. Symptomatic candidiasis can be treated with topical anti-fungal therapy whilst still continuing with Flixotide Nebules.

Possible systemic effects include Cushing's syndrome, Cushingoid features, adrenal suppression, growth retardation, decreased bone mineral density, cataract, glaucoma (see 4.4 Special Warnings and Special Precautions for Use).

As with other inhalation therapy, paradoxical bronchospasm may occur (see 4.4 'Special Warnings and Precautions for Use'). This should be treated immediately with a fast acting inhaled bronchodilators. Flixotide Nebules should be discontinued immediately, the patient assessed, and if necessary alternative therapy instituted.

There was an increased reporting of pneumonia in studies of patients with COPD receiving FLIXOTIDE 500 micrograms. Physicians should remain vigilant for the possible development of pneumonia in patients with COPD as the clinical features of pneumonia and exacerbation frequently overlap.

4.9 Overdose

Acute: Inhalation of the drug in doses in excess of those recommended may lead to temporary suppression of adrenal function. This does not necessitate emergency action being taken. In these patients treatment with fluticasone propionate by inhalation should be continued at a dose sufficient to control asthma adrenal function recovers in a few days and can be verified by measuring plasma cortisol.

Chronic: refer to section 4.4: risk of adrenal suppression.

Monitoring of adrenal reserve may be indicated. Treatment with inhaled fluticasone propionate should be continued at a dose sufficient to control asthma.

5. PHARMACOLOGICAL PROPERTIES

5.1 Pharmacodynamic properties

Fluticasone propionate given by inhalation at recommended doses has a potent glucocorticoid anti-inflammatory action within the lungs, which results in reduced symptoms and exacerbations of asthma.

5.2 Pharmacokinetic properties

Following inhaled dosing, systemic availability of the nebulised fluticasone propionate in healthy volunteers is estimated at 8% as compared with up to 26% received from the metered dose inhaler presentation. Systemic absorption occurs mainly through the lungs and is initially rapid then prolonged. The remainder of the dose may be swallowed.

Absolute oral bioavailability is negligible ($<1\%$) due to a combination of incomplete absorption from the GI tract and extensive first-pass metabolism.

87-100% of an oral dose is excreted in the faeces, up to 75% as parent compound. There is also a non-active major metabolite.

After an intravenous dose, fluticasone propionate is extensively distributed in the body. The very high clearance rate indicates extensive hepatic clearance.

5.3 Preclinical safety data

Generally, toxicology has shown only those class effects typical of potent corticosteroids, and these only at doses greatly in excess of that proposed for therapeutic use. However, corticosteroid overdosage effects were produced in juvenile rats at systemic fluticasone propionate doses similar to the maximum paediatric dose. No novel effects were identified in repeat dose toxicity tests, reproductive studies or teratology studies. Fluticasone propionate is devoid of mutagenic activity *in vitro* and *in vivo* and showed no tumorigenic potential in rodents. It is both non-irritant and non-sensitising in animal models.

6. PHARMACEUTICAL PARTICULARS

6.1 List of excipients

Polysorbate 20

Sorbitan laurate

Monosodium phosphate dihydrate

Dibasic sodium phosphate anhydrous

Sodium Chloride

Water for Injection

6.2 Incompatibilities

None reported.

6.3 Shelf life

36 months unopened.

6.4 Special precautions for storage

Flixotide Nebules should not be stored above 30°C. Keep container in the outer carton. Protect from freezing. Store upright.

The blister pack should be opened immediately before use. Opened Nebules should be refrigerated and used within 12 hours of opening.

6.5 Nature and contents of container

2.5ml low density polyethylene ampoules wrapped in a double foil blister, in boxes of 10 or 20.

The foil blister pack consists of a base and lidding foil. The base foil of the blister consists of aluminium (60 microns) coated on the outside with polyamide and on the inside with polyvinylchloride. The lidding consists of paper bonded to polyethyleneterephthalate bonded to aluminium (20 microns), with a coating of vinyl/acrylate lacquer on the inner surface.

6.6 Special precautions for disposal and other handling

It is important to ensure that the contents of the Nebule are well mixed before use. While holding the Nebule horizontally by the labelled tab, 'flick' the other end a few times and shake. Repeat this process several times until the entire contents of the Nebule are completely mixed. To open the Nebule, twist off the tab.

Dilution: Flixotide Nebules may be diluted with Sodium Chloride Injection BP if required, to aid administration of small volumes or if a prolonged delivery time is desirable. Any unused suspension remaining in the nebuliser should be discarded.

For detailed instructions please refer to the Patient Information Leaflet in every pack.

The nebuliser must be used according to the manufacturer's instructions. It is advisable to administer Flixotide Nebules via a mouthpiece (see *Posology and method of administration*).

As many nebulisers operate on a continuous flow basis, it is likely that some nebulised drug will be released into the local environment. Flixotide Nebules should therefore be administered in a well-ventilated room, particularly in hospitals where several patients may be using nebulisers at the same time.

Administrative Data

7. MARKETING AUTHORISATION HOLDER

Glaxo Wellcome UK Ltd,

trading as Allen & Hanburys,

Stockley Park West,

Uxbridge,

Middlesex, UB11 1BT.

8. MARKETING AUTHORISATION NUMBER(S)

PL 10949/0297

9. DATE OF FIRST AUTHORISATION/RENEWAL OF THE AUTHORISATION

21 August 1998

10. DATE OF REVISION OF THE TEXT

03 February 2009

11. Legal Category

POM.

Flixotide Nebules 2mg/2ml

(Allen & Hanburys)

1. NAME OF THE MEDICINAL PRODUCT

Flixotide Nebules 2mg/2ml.

2. QUALITATIVE AND QUANTITATIVE COMPOSITION

Plastic ampoules containing 2ml of a buffered, isotonic saline suspension containing 2mg fluticasone propionate

3. PHARMACEUTICAL FORM

Inhalation suspension for nebulisation.

4. CLINICAL PARTICULARS

4.1 Therapeutic indications

In adults and adolescents over 16 years Flixotide Nebules can be used:

For prophylactic management of severe chronic asthma in patients requiring high dose inhaled or oral corticosteroid therapy. On introduction of inhaled fluticasone propionate many patients currently treated with oral corticosteroids may be able to reduce significantly, or eliminate, their oral dose.

Flixotide Nebules 2mg/2ml are not licensed for use in children under 16 years and therefore should not be used in this patient population. Current clinical data do not allow appropriate dosage recommendations to be made in this patient population.

Fluticasone propionate given by inhalation has a potent glucocorticoid anti-inflammatory action within the lungs. It reduces symptoms and exacerbations of asthma in patients previously treated with bronchodilators alone or with other prophylactic therapy. Relatively brief symptomatic episodes can generally be relieved by the use of fast-acting bronchodilators, but longer-lasting exacerbations require, in addition, the use of corticosteroid therapy as soon as possible to control the inflammation.

4.2 Posology and method of administration

Adults and adolescents over 16 years: 500-2,000 micrograms twice daily.

Prescribers should be aware that fluticasone propionate is as effective as other inhaled steroids approximately at half the microgram daily dose. For example, a 100mcg of fluticasone propionate is approximately equivalent to 200mcg dose of beclometasone dipropionate (CFC containing) or budesonide.

Prescribers should be aware of the risks of systemic effects when using high doses of corticosteroids (see 4.4 special warnings and precautions for use and 4.8 undesirable effects).

Patients should be given a starting dose of inhaled fluticasone propionate, which is appropriate to the severity of their disease.

The dose should be titrated down to the lowest dose at which effective control of asthma is maintained.

Children 16 years and under: Flixotide Nebules 2mg/2ml are not licensed for use in children under 16 years and therefore should not be used in this patient population. Current clinical data do not allow appropriate dosage recommendations to be made in this patient population.

Special patient groups: There is no need to adjust the dose in elderly patients or those with hepatic or renal impairment.

Flixotide Nebules are for inhalation use only. They should be administered as an aerosol produced by a jet nebuliser, as directed by a physician. As drug delivery from nebulisers is variable, the manufacturer's instructions for using the nebuliser must be followed.

Use of Flixotide Nebules with ultrasonic nebulisers is not generally recommended.

Flixotide Nebules should not be injected or administered orally.

Patients should be made aware of the prophylactic nature of therapy with inhaled fluticasone propionate and that it should be taken regularly.

It is advisable to administer Flixotide Nebules via a mouthpiece to avoid the possibility of atrophic changes to facial skin, which may occur with prolonged use with a facemask. When a face-mask is used, the exposed skin should be protected using a barrier cream, or the face should be thoroughly washed after treatment.

4.3 Contraindications

Hypersensitivity to any ingredient of the preparation.

4.4 Special warnings and precautions for use

Flixotide Nebules are not designed to relieve acute symptoms for which an inhaled short-acting bronchodilator is required. Patients should be advised to have such rescue medication available. Flixotide Nebules are intended for regular daily prophylactic treatment.

Flixotide Nebules are not a substitute for injectable or oral corticosteroids in an emergency (i.e. life threatening asthma).

Severe asthma requires regular medical assessment, including lung function testing, as patients are at risk of severe attacks and even death. Increasing use of short-acting inhaled β_2-agonists to relieve symptoms indicates deterioration of asthma control. If patients find that short-acting relief bronchodilator treatment becomes less effective, or they need more inhalations than usual, medical attention must be sought. In this situation patients should be reassessed and consideration given to the need for increased anti-inflammatory therapy (e.g. higher doses of inhaled corticosteroids or a course of oral corticosteroids).

Severe exacerbations of asthma must be treated in the normal way.

There have been very rare reports of increases in blood glucose levels, in patients with or without a history of diabetes mellitus (See 4.8 'Undesirable Effects'). This should be considered in particular when prescribing to patients with a history of diabetes mellitus.

As with other inhalation therapy, paradoxical bronchospasm may occur with an immediate increase in wheezing after dosing. Flixotide Nebules should be discontinued immediately, the patient assessed and alternative therapy instituted if necessary.

Systemic effects of inhaled corticosteroids may occur, particularly at high doses prescribed for prolonged periods. These effects are much less likely to occur than with oral steroids. Possible systemic effects include Cushing's syndrome, Cushingoid features, adrenal suppression, growth retardation in children and adolescents, decrease in bone mineral density, cataract and glaucoma. **It is important therefore that the dose of inhaled corticosteroid is reviewed regularly and reduced to the lowest dose at which effective control of asthma is maintained.**

Prolonged treatment with high doses of inhaled corticosteroids may result in adrenal suppression and acute adrenal crisis. Children aged $<$ 16 years taking higher than licensed doses of fluticasone (typically $\geqslant$1000mcg/day) may be at particular risk. Situations, which could potentially trigger acute adrenal crisis, include trauma, surgery, infection or any rapid reduction in dosage. Presenting symptoms are typically vague and may include anorexia, abdominal pain, weight loss, tiredness, headache, nausea, vomiting, decreased level of consciousness, hypoglycaemia, and seizures. Additional systemic corticosteroid cover should be considered during periods of stress or elective surgery.

It is recommended that the height of children receiving prolonged treatment with inhaled corticosteroids is regularly monitored. If growth is slowed, therapy should be reviewed with the aim of reducing the dose of inhaled corticosteroid, if possible to the lowest dose at which effective control of asthma is maintained. In addition, consideration should be given to referring the patient to a paediatric respiratory specialist.

The benefits of inhaled fluticasone propionate should minimise the need for oral steroids. However, patients transferred from oral steroids, remain at risk of impaired adrenal reserve for a considerable time after transferring to inhaled fluticasone propionate. The possibility of adverse effects may persist for some time. These patients may require specialised advice to determine the extent of adrenal impairment before elective procedures. The possibility of residual impaired adrenal response should always be considered in emergency (medical or surgical) and elective situations likely to produce stress, and appropriate corticosteroid treatment considered.

Patients should receive a dose appropriate to the severity of their disease; the dose should be titrated to the lowest dose at which effective control of asthma is maintained. If control cannot be maintained, the use of a systemic steroid and/or an antibiotic may be necessary.

Replacement of systemic steroid treatment with inhaled therapy sometimes unmasks allergies such as allergic rhinitis or eczema previously controlled by the systemic drug. These allergies should be symptomatically treated with antihistamine and/or topical preparations, including topical steroids.

As with all inhaled corticosteroids, special care is necessary in patients with active or quiescent pulmonary tuberculosis.

Treatment with Flixotide Nebules should not be stopped abruptly.

For the transfer of patients being treated with oral corticosteroids: The transfer of oral steroid-dependent patients to Flixotide Nebules and their subsequent management needs special care as recovery from impaired adrenocortical function, caused by prolonged systemic steroid therapy, may take a considerable time.

Patients who have been treated with systemic steroids for long periods of time or at a high dose may have adrenocortical suppression. With these patients adrenocortical function should be monitored regularly and their dose of systemic steroid reduced cautiously.

After approximately a week, gradual withdrawal of the systemic steroid is commenced. Dosage reductions should be appropriate to the level of maintenance systemic steroid, and introduced at not less than weekly intervals. In general, for maintenance doses of prednisolone (or equivalent) of 10mg daily or less, the dosage reductions should not be greater than 1mg per day, at not less than weekly intervals. For maintenance doses of prednisolone in excess of 10mg daily, it may be appropriate to employ cautiously, larger reductions in dose at weekly intervals.

Some patients feel unwell in a non-specific way during the withdrawal phase despite maintenance or even improvement of the respiratory function. They should be encouraged to persevere with inhaled fluticasone propionate and to continue withdrawal of systemic steroid, unless there are objective signs of adrenal insufficiency.

Patients weaned off oral steroids whose adrenocortical function is still impaired should carry a steroid warning card indicating that they need supplementary systemic steroid during periods of stress, e.g. worsening asthma attacks, chest infections, major intercurrent illness, surgery, trauma, etc.

Ritonavir can greatly increase the concentration of fluticasone propionate in plasma. Therefore, concomitant use should be avoided, unless the potential benefit to the patient outweighs the risk of systemic corticosteroid side-effects. There is also an increased risk of systemic side effects when combining fluticasone propionate with other potent CYP3A inhibitors (see 4.5 Interaction with Other Medicinal Products and Other Forms of Interaction).

4.5 Interaction with other medicinal products and other forms of interaction

Under normal circumstances, low plasma concentrations of fluticasone propionate are achieved after inhaled dosing, due to extensive first pass metabolism and high systemic clearance mediated by cytochrome P450 3A4 in the gut and liver. Hence, clinically significant drug interactions mediated by fluticasone propionate are unlikely.

In an interaction study in healthy subjects with intranasal fluticasone propionate, ritonavir (a highly potent cytochrome P450 3A4 inhibitor) 100 mg b.i.d. increased the fluticasone propionate plasma concentrations several hundred fold, resulting in markedly reduced serum cortisol concentrations. Information about this interaction is lacking for inhaled fluticasone propionate, but a marked increase in fluticasone propionate plasma levels is expected. Cases of Cushing's syndrome and adrenal suppression have been reported. The combination should be avoided unless the benefit outweighs the increased risk of systemic glucocorticoid side-effects.

In a small study in healthy volunteers, the slightly less potent CYP3A inhibitor ketoconazole increased the exposure of fluticasone propionate after a single inhalation by 150%. This resulted in a greater reduction of plasma cortisol as compared with fluticasone propionate alone. Co-treatment with other potent CYP3A inhibitors, such as itraconazole, is also expected to increase the systemic fluticasone propionate exposure and the risk of systemic side-effects. Caution is recommended and long-term treatment with such drugs should if possible be avoided.

4.6 Pregnancy and lactation

There is inadequate evidence of safety of fluticasone propionate in human pregnancy. Administration of corticosteroids to pregnant animals can cause abnormalities of fetal development, including cleft palate and intra-uterine growth retardation. There may therefore be a very small risk of such effects in the human fetus. It should be noted, however, that the fetal changes in animals occur after relatively high systemic exposure. Because Flixotide Nebules deliver fluticasone propionate directly to the lungs by the inhaled route the high level of exposure that occurs when corticosteroids are given by systemic routes is avoided. Administration of fluticasone propionate during pregnancy should only be considered if the expected benefit to the mother is greater than any possible risk to the fetus.

The secretion of fluticasone propionate in human breast milk has not been investigated. Subcutaneous administration of fluticasone propionate to lactating laboratory rats produced measurable plasma levels and evidence of fluticasone propionate in the milk. However, plasma levels in humans after inhalation at recommended doses are likely to be low. When fluticasone propionate is used in breast-feeding mothers the therapeutic benefits must be weighed against the potential hazards to mother and baby.

4.7 Effects on ability to drive and use machines

Fluticasone propionate is unlikely to produce an effect.

4.8 Undesirable effects

Adverse events are listed below by system organ class and frequency. Frequencies are defined as: very common ($\geqslant$1/10), common ($\geqslant$1/100 and $<$1/10), uncommon ($\geqslant$1/1000 and $<$1/100), rare ($\geqslant$1/10,000 and $<$1/1000) and very rare ($<$1/10,000) including isolated reports. Very common, common and uncommon events were generally determined from clinical trial data. Rare and very rare events were generally determined from spontaneous data.

System Organ Class	Adverse Event	Frequency
Infections & Infestations	Candidiasis of the mouth and throat	Very Common
	Pneumonia (in COPD Patients)	Common
Immune System Disorders	Hypersensitivity reactions with the following manifestations:	
	Cutaneous hypersensitivity reactions	Uncommon
	Angioedema (mainly facial and oropharyngeal oedema),	Very Rare
	Respiratory symptoms (dyspnoea and/or bronchospasm)	Very Rare
	Anaphylactic reactions	Very Rare
Endocrine Disorders	Cushing's syndrome, Cushingoid features, adrenal suppression, growth retardation in children and adolescents, decreased bone mineral density, cataract, glaucoma	Very Rare
Metabolism & Nutrition Disorders	Hyperglycaemia (see 4.4 'Special Warnings and Precautions for Use')	Very Rare
Gastrointestinal Disorders	Dyspepsia	Very Rare
Musculoskeletal & Connective Tissue Disorders	Arthralgia	Very Rare
Psychiatric Disorders	Anxiety, sleep disorders, behavioural changes, including hyperactivity and irritability (predominantly in children)	Very Rare
Respiratory, Thoracic & Mediastinal Disorders	Hoarseness/dysphonia	Common
	Paradoxical bronchospasm	Very Rare
Skin & Subcutaneous Tissue Disorders	Contusions	Common

Hoarseness and candidiasis of the mouth and throat (thrush) occurs in some patients. Such patients may find it helpful to rinse out their mouth with water after inhalation from the nebuliser. Symptomatic candidiasis can be treated with topical anti-fungal therapy whilst still continuing with Flixotide Nebules.

Possible systemic effects include Cushing's syndrome, Cushingoid features, adrenal suppression, growth retardation, decreased bone mineral density, cataract, glaucoma (see 4.4 Special Warnings and Special Precautions for Use).

As with other inhalation therapy, paradoxical bronchospasm may occur (see 4.4 'Special Warnings and Precautions for Use'). This should be treated immediately with a fast acting inhaled bronchodilators. Flixotide Nebules should be discontinued immediately, the patient assessed, and if necessary alternative therapy instituted.

There was an increased reporting of pneumonia in studies of patients with COPD receiving FLIXOTIDE 500 micrograms. Physicians should remain vigilant for the possible development of pneumonia in patients with COPD as the clinical features of pneumonia and exacerbation frequently overlap.

4.9 Overdose

Acute: Inhalation of the drug in doses in excess of those recommended may lead to temporary suppression of adrenal function. This does not necessitate emergency action being taken. In these patients treatment with fluticasone propionate by inhalation should be continued at a dose sufficient to control asthma adrenal function recovers in a few days and can be verified by measuring plasma cortisol.

Chronic: refer to section 4.4: risk of adrenal suppression.

Monitoring of adrenal reserve may be indicated. Treatment with inhaled fluticasone propionate should be continued at a dose sufficient to control asthma.

5. PHARMACOLOGICAL PROPERTIES

5.1 Pharmacodynamic properties

Fluticasone propionate given by inhalation at recommended doses has a potent glucocorticoid anti-inflammatory action within the lungs, which results in reduced symptoms and exacerbations of asthma.

5.2 Pharmacokinetic properties

Following inhaled dosing, systemic availability of the nebulised fluticasone propionate in healthy volunteers is estimated at 8% as compared with up to 26% received from the metered dose inhaler presentation. Systemic absorption occurs mainly through the lungs and is initially rapid then prolonged. The remainder of the dose may be swallowed.

Absolute oral bioavailability is negligible (<1%) due to a combination of incomplete absorption from the GI tract and extensive first-pass metabolism.

87-100% of an oral dose is excreted in the faeces, up to 75% as parent compound. There is also a non-active major metabolite.

After an intravenous dose, fluticasone propionate is extensively distributed in the body. The very high clearance rate indicates extensive hepatic clearance.

5.3 Preclinical safety data

Toxicology has shown only those class effects typical of potent corticosteroids, and these only at doses greatly in excess of that proposed for therapeutic use. No novel effects were identified in repeat dose toxicity tests, reproductive studies or teratology studies. Fluticasone propionate is devoid of mutagenic activity *in vitro* and *in vivo* and showed no tumorigenic potential in rodents. It is both non-irritant and non-sensitising in animal models.

6. PHARMACEUTICAL PARTICULARS

6.1 List of excipients

Polysorbate 20 Ph. Eur

Sorbitan laurate Ph. Eur

Monosodium phosphate dihydrate Ph. Eur

Dibasic sodium phosphate anhydrous USP

Sodium Chloride Ph. Eur

Water for Injection Ph. Eur

6.2 Incompatibilities

None reported.

6.3 Shelf life

36 months unopened.

6.4 Special precautions for storage

Flixotide Nebules should not be stored above 30°C. Keep container in the outer carton. Protect from freezing. Store upright.

The blister pack should be opened immediately before use. Opened Nebules should be refrigerated and used within 12 hours of opening.

6.5 Nature and contents of container

2.5ml low density polyethylene ampoules wrapped in a double foil blister, in boxes of 10 or 20.

The foil blister pack consists of a base and lidding foil. The base foil of the blister consists of aluminium (60 microns) coated on the outside with polyamide and on the inside with polyvinylchloride. The lidding consists of paper bonded to polyethyleneterephthalate bonded to aluminium (20 microns), with a coating of vinyl/acrylate lacquer on the inner surface.

6.6 Special precautions for disposal and other handling

It is important to ensure that the contents of the Nebule are well mixed before use. While holding the Nebule horizontally by the labelled tab, 'flick' the other end a few times and shake. Repeat this process several times until the entire contents of the Nebule are completely mixed. To open the Nebule, twist off the tab.

Dilution: Flixotide Nebules may be diluted with Sodium Chloride Injection BP if required, to aid administration of small volumes or if a prolonged delivery time is desirable. Any unused suspension remaining in the nebuliser should be discarded.

For detailed instructions please refer to the Patient Information Leaflet in every pack.

The nebuliser must be used according to the manufacturer's instructions. It is advisable to administer Flixotide Nebules via a mouthpiece (see *Posology and method of administration*).

As many nebulisers operate on a continuous flow basis, it is likely that some nebulised drug will be released into the local environment. Flixotide Nebules should therefore be administered in a well-ventilated room, particularly in hospitals where several patients may be using nebulisers at the same time.

Administrative Data

7. MARKETING AUTHORISATION HOLDER

Glaxo Wellcome UK Ltd,
trading as Allen & Hanburys,
Stockley Park West,
Uxbridge,
Middlesex, UB11 1BT.

8. MARKETING AUTHORISATION NUMBER(S)

PL 10949/0298

9. DATE OF FIRST AUTHORISATION/RENEWAL OF THE AUTHORISATION

21 August 1998

10. DATE OF REVISION OF THE TEXT

03 February 2009

11. Legal Status

POM.

Flolan 0.5mg Injection

(GlaxoSmithKline UK)

1. NAME OF THE MEDICINAL PRODUCT

Flolan 0.5mg Injection

2. QUALITATIVE AND QUANTITATIVE COMPOSITION

Epoprostenol Sodium 0.5mg

3. PHARMACEUTICAL FORM

Freeze-Dried Powder

4. CLINICAL PARTICULARS

4.1 Therapeutic indications

Flolan is indicated for use in renal dialysis when use of heparin carries a high risk of causing or exacerbating bleeding or when heparin is otherwise contra-indicated.

Route of administration

By continuous infusion, either intravascularly or into the blood supplying the dialyser.

4.2 Posology and method of administration

Flolan is suitable for continuous infusion only, either intravascularly or into the blood supplying the dialyser.

The following schedule of infusion has been found effective in adults:

Prior to dialysis: 4 nanogram/kg/min intravenously.

During dialysis: 4 nanogram/kg/min into the arterial inlet of the dialyser.

The infusion should be stopped at the end of dialysis.

The recommended doses should be exceeded only with careful monitoring of patient blood pressure.

Use in children: There is no specific information on the use of Flolan in children.

Use in the elderly: There is no specific information available on the use of Flolan in elderly patients.

Reconstitution: Only the GlaxoSmithKline Glycine Buffer Diluent provided for the purpose should be used. The enclosed filter unit must be used once only and then discarded after use.

To reconstitute Flolan, a strict aseptic technique must be used. Particular care should be taken in calculating dilutions, and in diluting Flolan the following procedure is recommended:

1. Withdraw approximately 10 ml of the sterile GlaxoSmithKline Glycine Buffer Diluent into a sterile syringe.

2. Inject the contents of the syringe into the vial containing Flolan and shake gently until the powder has dissolved.

3. Draw up all the Flolan solution into the syringe.

4. Re-inject the entire contents into the residue of the original 50 ml of sterile GlaxoSmithKline Glycine Buffer Diluent.

5. Mix well. This solution is now referred to as the *concentrated solution* and contains Flolan 10,000 nanograms per millilitre. When 0.5mg Flolan powder for intravenous infusion is reconstituted with 50 ml sterile GlaxoSmithKline Glycine Buffer Diluent solution, the final injection has a pH of approximately 10.5 and a sodium ion content of approximately 56mg. The *concentrated solution* is normally further diluted before use. It may be diluted with physiological saline (0.9%), provided a ratio of 6 volumes of saline to 1 volume of *concentrated solution* is not exceeded; e.g. 50 ml of *concentrated solution* further diluted with a maximum of 300 ml saline. Other common intravenous fluids are unsatisfactory for the dilution of the *concentrated solution* as the required pH is not attained. Flolan solutions are less stable at low pH. For administration using a pump capable of delivering small volume constant infusions, suitable aliquots of concentrated solution may be diluted with sterile physiological saline.

6. Before further dilution, draw up the *concentrated solution* into a larger syringe.

7. The filter provided should then be attached to the syringe and the *concentrated solution* is dispensed by filtration using firm but not excessive pressure. The typical time taken for filtration of 50 ml of of solution is 70 seconds.

When reconstituted and diluted as directed, Flolan infusion solutions have a pH of approximately 10 and will retain 90% of their initial potency for approximately 12 hours at 25°C.

Infusion rate guidance In general, the infusion rate may be calculated by the following formula:

$$\text{Infusion rate (ml/min)} = \frac{\text{Dosage (ng/kg/min)} \times \text{body weight (kg)}}{\text{Concentration of infusion (ng/ml)}}$$

Examples:

Flolan may be administered in diluted form (1) or as the *concentrated solution* (2)

1. *Diluted*: A commonly used dilution is:

10ml *concentrated solution* + 40 ml physiological saline (0.9%).

Resultant concentration = 2,000 nanogram/ml epoprostenol.

Body weight (kilograms)

(see Table 1 below)

2. Using *concentrated solution* ie 10,000 ng/ml epoprostenol.

Bodyweight (kilograms)

(see Table 2 below)

4.3 Contraindications

Flolan is contra-indicated in patients with known hypersensitivity to the drug.

4.4 Special warnings and precautions for use

Because of the high pH of the final infusion solutions, care should be taken to avoid extravasation during their administration and consequent risk of tissue damage.

Flolan is a potent vasodilator. The cardiovascular effects during infusion disappear within 30 minutes of the end of administration.

Flolan is not a conventional anticoagulant. Flolan has been successfully used instead of heparin in renal dialysis, but in a small proportion of dialyses clotting has developed in the dialysis circuit, requiring termination of dialysis.

Haemorrhagic complications have not been encountered with Flolan but the possibility should be considered when the drug is administered to patients with spontaneous or drug-induced haemorrhagic diatheses. When Flolan is used alone, measurements such as activated whole blood clotting time may not be reliable.

Blood pressure and heart rate should be monitored during administration of Flolan. Flolan may either decrease or increase heart rate. The change is thought to depend on the concentration of epoprostenol administered. Hypotension may occur during infusions of Flolan.

The effects of Flolan on heart-rate may be masked by concomitant use of drugs which affect cardiovascular reflexes.

If excessive hypotension occurs during administration of Flolan, the dose should be reduced or the infusion discontinued. Hypotension may be profound in overdose and may result in loss of consciousness. (See section 4.9, Overdose.)

The hypotensive effect of Flolan may be enhanced by the use of acetate buffer in the dialysis bath during renal dialysis.

Table 1 Body weight (kilograms)

		30	40	50	60	70	80	90	100
Dosage (ng/kg/min)	1	0.90	1.20	1.50	1.80	2.10	2.40	2.70	3.00
	2	1.80	2.40	3.00	3.60	4.20	4.80	5.40	6.00
	3	2.70	3.60	4.50	5.40	6.30	7.20	8.10	9.00
	4	3.60	4.80	6.00	7.20	8.40	9.60	10.80	12.00
	5	4.50	6.00	7.50	9.00	10.50	12.00	13.50	15.00

Flow rates in mls/hr

Table 2 Bodyweight (kilograms)

		30	40	50	60	70	80	90	100
Dosage (ng/kg/min)	1	0.18	0.24	0.30	0.36	0.42	0.48	0.54	0.60
	2	0.36	0.48	0.60	0.72	0.84	0.96	1.08	1.20
	3	0.54	0.72	0.90	1.08	1.26	1.44	1.62	1.80
	4	0.72	0.96	1.20	1.44	1.68	1.92	2.16	2.40
	5	0.90	1.20	1.50	1.80	2.10	2.40	2.70	3.00

Flow rates in mls/hr

During renal dialysis with Flolan there is a need for careful haematological monitoring and it should be ensured that cardiac output is adequately maintained so that delivery of oxygen to peripheral tissues is not diminished.

Elevated serum glucose levels have been reported during infusion of Flolan in man but these are not inevitable.

The pack for this product will contain the following statements:

Keep out reach of children

Store below 25°C

Do not freeze

Protect from light

Keep dry

Reconstitute only with the GlaxoSmithKline Glycine Buffer Diluent provided

Prepare immediately prior to use

Discard any unused solution after 12 hours

4.5 Interaction with other medicinal products and other forms of interaction

When Flolan is administered to patients receiving concomitant anticoagulants standard anticoagulant monitoring is advisable as there may be potentiation of effect.

The vasodilator effect of Flolan may augment or be augmented by concomitant use of other vasodilators.

Flolan may reduce the thrombolytic efficacy of tissue plasminogen activator (t-PA) by increasing hepatic clearance of t-PA.

4.6 Pregnancy and lactation

For epoprostenol sodium no clinical data on exposed pregnancies are available. Animal studies do not indicate direct or indirect harmful effects with respect to pregnancy, embryonal/foetal development, parturition or postnatal development. Caution should be exercised when prescribing to pregnant women.

Lactation:

There is no information on the use of Flolan during lactation.

4.7 Effects on ability to drive and use machines

Not applicable.

4.8 Undesirable effects

Adverse events are listed below by system organ class and frequency. Frequencies are defined as follows: very common 1/10 (10%); common 1/100 and <1/10 (1% and <10%); uncommon 1/1000 and <1/100 (0.1% and <1%); rare 1/10,000 and <1/1000 (0.01% and <0.1%); very rare <1/10,000 (< 0.01%).

The interpretation of adverse events during long term administration of Flolan is complicated by the clinical features of the underlying disease being treated.

Infections and Infestations

Very common Sepsis, septicaemia (mostly related to delivery system for Flolan)

Blood and Lymphatic System Disorders

Common Decreased platelet count

Psychiatric Disorders

Common Anxiety, nervousness

Very rare Agitation

Nervous System Disorders

Very common Headache

Cardiac Disorders

Common Tachycardia has been reported as a response to Flolan at doses of 5 nanograms/kg/min and below.]

Bradycardia, sometimes accompanied by orthostatic hypotension, has occurred in healthy volunteers at doses of Flolan greater than 5 nanograms/kg/min. Bradycardia associated with a considerable fall in systolic and diastolic blood pressure has followed i.v. administration of a dose of Flolan equivalent to 30 nanograms/kg/min in healthy conscious volunteers.

Vascular Disorders

Very common Facial flushing (seen even in the anaesthetised patient)

Very rare Pallor

Gastrointestinal Disorders

Very common Nausea, vomiting

Common Abdominal colic, sometimes reported as abdominal discomfort

Uncommon Dry mouth

Skin and Subcutaneous Tissue Disorders

Very rare Sweating

Musculoskeletal and Connective Tissue Disorders

Very common Jaw pain

General Disorders and Administration Site Conditions

Rare Local infection*, chest pain

Very rare Reddening over the infusion site*, occlusion of the long i.v. catheter*, pain at the injection site*, lassitude, chest tightness

* Associated with the delivery system for Flolan

4.9 Overdose

The main feature of overdosage is likely to be hypotension.

In general, events seen after overdose of epoprostenol represent exaggerated pharmacological effects of the drug. If overdose occurs reduce the dose or discontinue the infusion and initiate appropriate supportive measures as necessary; for example, plasma volume expansion and/or adjustment to pump flow.

5. PHARMACOLOGICAL PROPERTIES

5.1 Pharmacodynamic properties

Flolan is epoprostenol sodium, the monosodium salt of epoprostenol, a naturally occurring prostaglandin produced by the intima of blood vessels. Epoprostenol is the most potent inhibitor of platelet aggregation known. It is also a potent vasodilator.

Infusions of 4ng/kg/min for 30 minutes have been shown to have no significant effect on heart rate or blood pressure, although facial flushing may occur at these levels.

Many of the actions of epoprostenol are exerted via the stimulation of adenylate cyclase, which leads to increased intracellular levels of cyclic adenosine 3'5' monophosphate (cAMP). A sequential stimulation of adenylate cyclase, followed by activation of phosphodiesterase, has been described in human platelets. Elevated cAMP levels regulate intracellular calcium concentrations by stimulating calcium removal, and thus platelet aggregation is ultimately inhibited by the reduction of cytoplasmic calcium, upon which platelet shape change, aggregation and the release reaction depend.

The effect of epoprostenol on platelet aggregation is dose-related when between 2 and 16 ng/kg/min is administered intravenously, and significant inhibition of aggregation induced by adenosine diphosphate is observed at doses 4ng/kg/min and above.

Effects on platelets have been found to disappear within 2 hours of discontinuing the infusion, and haemodynamic changes due to epoprostenol to return to baseline within 10 minutes of termination of 60-minute infusions at 1-16 ng/kg/min.

Higher doses of epoprostenol sodium (20 nanograms/kg/min) disperse circulating platelet aggregates and increase by up to two fold the cutaneous bleeding time.

Epoprostenol potentiates the anticoagulant activty of heparin by approximately 50%, possibly reducing the release of heparin neutralising factor.

5.2 Pharmacokinetic properties

Intravenously administered epoprostenol sodium is rapidly distributed from blood to tissue. At normal physiological pH and temperature, it breaks down spontaneously to 6-oxo-prostaglandin F_1a, although there is some enzymatic degradation to other products. The half-life for this process in man is expected to be no more than 6 minutes, and may be as short as 2-3 minutes, as estimated from in vitro rates of degradation of epoprostenol in human whole blood.

Pharmacokinetic studies in animals have shown the whole body distribution to be 1015ml/kg, and the whole body clearance to be 4.27ml/kg/sec. Following intravenous injection of radiolabelled epoprostenol, the highest concentrations are found in the liver, kidneys and small intestine. Steady-state plasma concentrations are reached within 15 minutes and are proportional to infusion rates. Extensive clearance by the liver has been demonstrated, with approximately 80% being removed in a single pass. Urinary excretion of the metabolites of epoprostenol accounts for between 40% and 90% of the administered dose, with biliary excretion accounting for the remainder. Urinary excretion is greater than 95% complete within 25 hours of dosing. Tissue levels decline rapidly with no evidence of accumulation.

Following the administration of radiolabelled epoprostenol to humans, the urinary and faecal recoveries of radioactivity were 82% and 4% respectively. At least 16 compounds were found, 10 of which were structurally identified. Unlike many other prostaglandins, epoprostenol is not metabolised during passage through the pulmonary circulation.

Due to the chemical instability, high potency and short half-life of epoprostenol, no precise and accurate assay has been identified as appropriate for quantifying epoprostenol in biological fluids.

5.3 Preclinical safety data

Fertility:

A study in which male and female rats were dosed subcutaneously for 74 or 63 days respectively, with 0, 10, 30 or 100mg/kg/day, showed no effects on fertility.

6. PHARMACEUTICAL PARTICULARS

6.1 List of excipients

FREEZE-DRIED POWDER

Glycine BP 3.76 mg

Sodium chloride EP 2-932 mg

Mannitol BP 50.0 mg

Sodium hydroxide BP (quantity not fixed - used to adjust pH)

*Water for injections EP

*Water for injections is used during manufacture but is not present in the finished product, but removed during the freeze-drying process.

6.2 Incompatibilities

None known.

6.3 Shelf life

2 years - freeze dried powder

0.5 day - reconstituted solution for injection

6.4 Special precautions for storage

Freeze dried powder:

Keep dry

Protect from light

Store below 25°C

6.5 Nature and contents of container

0.5 mg freeze dried powder is contained in glass vials with synthetic butyl rubber plugs and aluminium collars.

6.6 Special precautions for disposal and other handling

No special instructions.

Administrative Data

7. MARKETING AUTHORISATION HOLDER

Glaxo Wellcome UK Ltd

Trading as GlaxoSmithKline UK

Stockley Park West

Uxbridge

Middlesex

UB11 1BT

United Kingdom

8. MARKETING AUTHORISATION NUMBER(S)

PL 10949/0310

9. DATE OF FIRST AUTHORISATION/RENEWAL OF THE AUTHORISATION

MAA 18.03.81

Renewal: 13.08.87, 23.04.91, 03.08.02

10. DATE OF REVISION OF THE TEXT

29 September 2006

11. Legal Status

POM

Flolan Injection 1.5mg

(GlaxoSmithKline UK)

1. NAME OF THE MEDICINAL PRODUCT

Flolan 1.5mg Injection ▼

2. QUALITATIVE AND QUANTITATIVE COMPOSITION

Epoprostenol sodium equivalent to 1.5 mg epoprostenol.

3. PHARMACEUTICAL FORM

Sterile freeze-dried powder for solution for infusion.

4. CLINICAL PARTICULARS

4.1 Therapeutic indications

Flolan is indicated for use in renal dialysis when use of heparin carries a high risk of causing or exacerbating bleeding or when heparin is otherwise contraindicated.

Flolan is also indicated for the intravenous treatment of primary pulmonary hypertension (PPH) in New York Heart Association (NYHA) functional Class III and Class IV patients who do not respond adequately to conventional therapy. There are limited data on long term use.

4.2 Posology and method of administration

Flolan is not to be used for bolus administration.

Flolan (epoprostenol sodium) must be reconstituted only with specific sterile diluent for Flolan. (*See section 6.6 Instructions for use/handling).*

Renal Dialysis:

Flolan is suitable for continuous infusion only, either intravascularly or into the blood supplying the dialyser.

The following general schedule of infusion has been found effective in adults:

Prior to dialysis: 4 nanogram/kg/min intravenously.

During dialysis: 4 nanogram/kg/min into the arterial inlet of the dialyser.

The infusion should be stopped at the end of dialysis.

The recommended dose for renal dialysis should be exceeded only with careful monitoring of patient blood pressure.

Children and the elderly:

There is no specific information available on the use of Flolan for renal dialysis in children or in elderly patients.

Primary Pulmonary Hypertension:

The following schedules have been found effective:

Adults

Short-term (acute) dose ranging:

A short-term dose-ranging procedure administered via either a peripheral or central venous line is required to determine the long-term infusion rate. The infusion rate is initiated at 2 nanogram/kg/min and increased by increments of 2 nanogram/kg/min every 15 minutes or longer until maximum haemodynamic benefit or dose-limiting pharmacological effects are elicited.

During acute dose ranging in clinical trials, the mean maximum tolerated dose was 8.6±0.3 nanogram/kg/min.

Long-term continuous infusion:

Long-term continuous infusion of Flolan should be administered through a central venous catheter. Temporary peripheral intravenous infusions may be used until central access is established. Long-term infusions should be initiated at 4 nanogram/kg/min less than the maximum tolerated infusion rate determined during short-term dose-ranging. If the maximum tolerated infusion rate is less than 5 nanogram/kg/min; the long-term infusion should be started at one-half the maximum tolerated infusion rate.

Dosage adjustments:

Changes in the long-term infusion rate should be based on persistence, recurrence or worsening of the patient's symptoms of PPH or the occurrence of adverse events due to excessive doses of Flolan.

In general, the need for increases in dose from the initial long-term dose should be expected over time. Increases in dose should be considered if symptoms of PPH persist, or recur after improving. The infusion rate should be increased by 1 to 2 nanogram/kg/min increments at intervals sufficient to allow assessment of clinical response; these intervals should be of at least 15 minutes. Following establishment of a new infusion rate, the patient should be observed, and erect and supine blood pressure and heart rate monitored for several hours to ensure that the new dose is tolerated.

During long-term infusion, the occurrence of dose-related pharmacological events similar to those observed during the dose-ranging period may necessitate a decrease in infusion rate, but the adverse event may occasionally resolve without dosage adjustment. Dosage decreases should be made gradually in 2 nanogram/kg/min decrements every 15 minutes or longer until the dose-limiting effects resolve. Abrupt withdrawal of Flolan or sudden large reductions in infusion rates should be avoided. Except in life-threatening situations (eg. unconsciousness, collapse, etc) infusion rates of Flolan should be adjusted only under the direction of a physician.

Oral anticoagulation was continued in the PPH clinical trial population in addition to continuous intravenous Flolan administration and was well tolerated. Concurrent oral anticoagulation is recommended.

Children

There is limited information on the use of Flolan for PPH in children.

Elderly

There is limited information on the use of Flolan in patients over 65. In general, dose selection for an elderly patient should be made carefully, reflecting the greater frequency of decreased hepatic, renal or cardiac function and of concomitant disease or other drug therapy.

4.3 Contraindications

Flolan is contraindicated in patients with known hypersensitivity to the drug.

Flolan is contraindicated in patients with congestive heart failure arising from severe left ventricular dysfunction.

Flolan should not be used chronically in patients who develop pulmonary oedema during dose-ranging.

4.4 Special warnings and precautions for use

Because of the high pH of the final infusion solutions, care should be taken to avoid extravasation during their administration and consequent risk of tissue damage

Flolan is a potent pulmonary and systemic vasodilator. The cardiovascular effects during infusion disappear within 30 minutes of the end of administration.

Blood pressure and heart rate should be monitored during administration of Flolan. Flolan may either decrease or increase heart rate. The change is thought to depend on the concentration of epoprostenol administered.

The effects of Flolan on heart-rate may be masked by concomitant use of drugs which affect cardiovascular reflexes.

If excessive hypotension occurs during administration of Flolan, the dose should be reduced or the infusion discontinued. Hypotension may be profound in overdose and may result in loss of consciousness. (See section 4.9, Overdose.)

Elevated serum glucose levels have been reported during infusion of Flolan in man but these are not inevitable.

Renal Dialysis:

The hypotensive effect of Flolan may be enhanced by the use of acetate buffer in the dialysis bath during renal dialysis.

Flolan is not a conventional anticoagulant. Flolan has been successfully used instead of heparin in renal dialysis, but in a small proportion of dialyses clotting has developed in the dialysis circuit, requiring termination of dialysis.

During renal dialysis with Flolan there is a need for careful haematological monitoring and it should be ensured that cardiac output is adequately maintained so that delivery of oxygen to peripheral tissues is not diminished.

Haemorrhagic complications have not been encountered with Flolan but the possibility should be considered when the drug is administered to patients with spontaneous or drug-induced haemorrhagic diatheses. When Flolan is used alone, measurements such as activated whole blood clotting time may not be reliable.

Primary Pulmonary Hypertension:

The hazards of Flolan treatment are considered to outweigh the risks of the disease in patients with functional capacity of New York Heart Association (NYHA) Class I and Class II. Flolan therapy should therefore not be initiated in these patients.

Flolan should be used only by clinicians experienced in the diagnosis and treatment of this disorder.

Short-term dose-ranging with Flolan must be performed in a hospital setting with adequate personnel and equipment for haemodynamic monitoring and emergency care.

Some patients with primary pulmonary hypertension have developed pulmonary oedema during dose-ranging, which may be associated with pulmonary veno-occlusive disease.

Flolan is infused continuously through a permanent indwelling central venous catheter via a small, portable infusion pump. Thus, therapy with Flolan requires commitment by the patient to sterile drug reconstitution, drug administration, care of the permanent central venous catheter, and access to intense and ongoing patient education.

Sterile technique must be adhered to in preparing the drug and in the care of the catheter. Even brief interruptions in the delivery of Flolan may result in rapid symptomatic deterioration. The decision to receive Flolan for PPH should be based upon the understanding that there is a high likelihood that therapy with Flolan will be needed for prolonged periods, possibly years, and the patient's ability to accept and care for a permanent intravenous catheter and infusion pump should be carefully considered.

GlaxoSmithKline Glycine Buffer Diluent contains no preservative, consequently a vial should be used once only and then discarded.

4.5 Interaction with other medicinal products and other forms of interaction

When Flolan is administered to patients receiving concomitant anticoagulants standard anticoagulant monitoring is advisable as there may be potentiation of effect.

The vasodilator effects of Flolan may augment or be augmented by concomitant use of vasodilators.

Flolan may reduce the thrombolytic efficacy of tissue plasminogen activator (t-PA) by increasing hepatic clearance of t-PA.

When NSAIDS or other drugs affecting platelets aggregation are used concomitantly, there is the potential for Flolan to increase the risk of bleeding.

4.6 Pregnancy and lactation

No teratogenic effects have been seen in rats or rabbits. However, as animal studies are not always predictive of human response, administration of this drug should only be considered if the expected benefit to the mother is greater than any risk to the foetus.

For epoprostenol sodium no clinical data on exposed pregnancies are available. Animal studies do not indicate direct or indirect harmful effects with respect to pregnancy, embryonal/foetal development, parturition or postnatal development. Caution should be exercised when prescribing to pregnant women.

It is not known whether epoprostenol is excreted in breast milk. Nursing mothers should be advised to discontinue breast feeding during treatment with Flolan.

4.7 Effects on ability to drive and use machines

There are no data regarding the effect of Flolan used in renal dialysis on the ability to drive or operate machinery.

PPH and its therapeutic management may affect the ability to drive and operate machinery.

4.8 Undesirable effects

Adverse events are listed below by system organ class and frequency. Frequencies are defined as follows: very common 1/10 (10%); common 1/100 and <1/10 (1% and <10%); uncommon 1/1000 and <1/100 (0.1% and <1%); rare 1/10,000 and <1/1000 (0.01% and <0.1%); very rare <1/10,000 (< 0.01%).

The interpretation of adverse events during long term administration of Flolan is complicated by the clinical features of the underlying disease being treated.

Infections and Infestations

Very common Sepsis, septicaemia (mostly related to delivery system for Flolan)

Blood and Lymphatic System Disorders

Common Decreased platelet count

Psychiatric Disorders

Common Anxiety, nervousness

Very rare Agitation

Nervous System Disorders

Very common Headache

Cardiac Disorders

Common Tachycardia has been reported as a response to Flolan at doses of 5 nanograms/kg/min and below.

Bradycardia, sometimes accompanied by orthostatic hypotension, has occurred in healthy volunteers at doses of Flolan greater than 5 nanograms/kg/min. Bradycardia associated with a considerable fall in systolic and diastolic blood pressure has followed i.v. administration of a dose of Flolan equivalent to 30 nanograms/kg/min in healthy conscious volunteers.

Vascular Disorders

Very common Facial flushing (seen even in the anaesthetised patient)

Very rare Pallor

Gastrointestinal Disorders

Very common Nausea, vomiting

Common Abdominal colic, sometimes reported as abdominal discomfort

Uncommon Dry mouth

Skin and Subcutaneous Tissue Disorders

Very rare Sweating

Musculoskeletal and Connective Tissue Disorders

Very common Jaw pain

General Disorders and Administration Site Conditions

Rare Local infection*, chest pain

Very rare Reddening over the infusion site*, occlusion of the long i.v. catheter*, pain at the injection site*, lassitude, chest tightness

* Associated with the delivery system for Flolan

4.9 Overdose

The main feature of overdosage is likely to be hypotension.

In general, events seen after overdose of epoprostenol represent exaggerated pharmacological effects of the drug. If overdose occurs reduce the dose or discontinue the infusion and initiate appropriate supportive measures as necessary; for example plasma volume expansion and/or adjustment to pump flow.

5. PHARMACOLOGICAL PROPERTIES

5.1 Pharmacodynamic properties

Flolan is epoprostenol sodium, the monosodium salt of epoprostenol, a naturally occurring prostaglandin produced by the intima of blood vessels. Epoprostenol is a potent inhibitor of platelet aggregation. It is also a potent vasodilator.

Infusions of 4 nanogram/kg/min for 30 minutes have been shown to have no significant effect on heart rate or blood pressure, although facial flushing may occur at these levels.

Renal Dialysis:

Many of the actions of epoprostenol are exerted via the stimulation of adenylate cyclase, which leads to increased intracellular levels of cyclic adenosine 3'5' monophosphate (cAMP). A sequential stimulation of adenylate cyclase, followed by activation of phosphodiesterase, has been described in human platelets. Elevated cAMP levels regulate intracellular calcium concentrations by stimulating calcium removal, and this platelet aggregation is ultimately inhibited by the reduction of cytoplasmic calcium, upon which platelet shape change, aggregation and the release reaction depend.

The effect of epoprostenol on platelet aggregation is dose-related when between 2 and 16 ng/kg/min is administered intravenously, and significant inhibition of aggregation induced by adenosine diphosphate is observed at doses 4ng/kg/min and above.

Effects on platelets have been found to disappear within 2 hours of discontinuing the infusion, and haemodynamic changes due to epoprostenol to return to baseline within 10 minutes of termination of 60-minute infusions at 1-16 ng/kg/min.

Higher doses of epoprostenol sodium (20 nanograms/kg/min) disperse circulating platelet aggregates and increase by up to two fold the cutaneous bleeding time.

Epoprostenol potentiates the anticoagulant activty of heparin by approximately 50%, possibly reducing the release of heparin neutralising factor.

Primary Pulmonary Hypertension:

Intravenous Flolan infusions of up to 15 minutes have been found to produce dose-related increases in cardiac index (CI) and stroke volume (SV), and dose-related decreases in pulmonary vascular resistance (PVR), total pulmonary resistance (TPR), and mean systemic arterial pressure (SAPm). The effects of Flolan on mean pulmonary artery pressure (PAPm) in patients with PPH were variable and minor.

Chronic haemodynamic effects are generally similar to acute effects. During chronic infusion cardiac index (CI), stroke volume (SV) and arterial oxygen saturation are increased and mean systemic arterial pressure (SAPm), right atrial pressure, total pulmonary resistance (TPR) and systemic vascular resistance are decreased.

5.2 Pharmacokinetic properties

Intravenously administered epoprostenol sodium is rapidly distributed from blood to tissue. At normal physiological pH and temperature, it breaks down spontaneously to 6-oxo-prostaglandin F_1a, although there is some enzymatic degradation to other products. The half-life for this process in man is expected to be no more than 6 minutes, and may be as short as 2-3 minutes, as estimated from in vitro rates of degradation of epoprostenol in human whole blood.

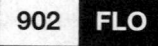

Pharmacokinetic studies in animals have shown the whole body distribution to be 1015ml/kg, and the whole body clearance to be 4.27ml/kg/sec. Following intravenous injection of radiolabelled epoprostenol, the highest concentrations are found in the liver, kidneys and small intestine. Steady-state plasma concentrations are reached within 15 minutes and are proportional to infusion rates. Extensive clearance by the liver has been demonstrated, with approximately 80% being removed in a single pass. Urinary excretion of the metabolites of epoprostenol accounts for between 40% and 90% of the administered dose, with biliary excretion accounting for the remainder. Urinary excretion is greater than 95% complete within 25 hours of dosing. Tissue levels decline rapidly with no evidence of accumulation.

Following the administration of radiolabelled epoprostenol to humans, the urinary and faecal recoveries of radioactivity were 82% and 4% respectively. At least 16 compounds were found, 10 of which were structurally identified. Unlike many other prostaglandins, epoprostenol is not metabolised during passage through the pulmonary circulation.

Due to the chemical instability, high potency and short half-life of epoprostenol, no precise and accurate assay has been identified as appropriate for quantifying epoprostenol in biological fluids.

5.3 Preclinical safety data

Fertility: A study in which male and female rats were dosed subcutaneously for 74 or 63 days respectively, with 0, 10, 30 or 100mg/kg/day, showed no effects on fertility.

There was no evidence of mutagenicity in the Ames test, micronucleus assay or DNA elution.

Carcinogenicity: Oncology studies have not been performed.

6. PHARMACEUTICAL PARTICULARS

6.1 List of excipients

Freeze-dried powder:

Glycine

Sodium Chloride

Mannitol

Sodium hydroxide

6.2 Incompatibilities

Flolan must be reconstituted using only the sterile buffer provided. Any further dilution must be performed using only the recommended solutions *(see 6.6, instructions for use/handling)*

6.3 Shelf life

FLOLAN freeze dried powder: 3 years.

Renal Dialysis: When reconstituted with GlaxoSmithKline Glycine Buffer Diluent and diluted with physiological saline as instructed (see 6.6, Instructions for Use/Handling, Renal Dialysis), freshly prepared Flolan solutions should be used within 12 hours at 25°C.

Primary Pulmonary Hypertension: When reconstituted and diluted with GlaxoSmithKline Glycine Buffer Diluent as instructed (see 6.6, Instructions for Use/Handling, Primary Pulmonary Hypertension), freshly prepared Flolan solutions should be infused immediately. If not used immediately, in-use storage times are the responsibilty of the user and should not be longer than 24 hours at 2-8°C.

Where the solution is held in an ambulatory infusion pump system, a cold pouch must be used to maintain the temperature of the solution at 2-8°C for the full administration period. Flolan solution may then be used over a 24 hour period provided that the cold pouch is changed as necessary throughout the day.

Where an ambulatory cold pouch system cannot be used the maximum administration time at 25°C is 12 hours for freshly prepared solutions and 8 hours for solutions that have been stored prior to use.

6.4 Special precautions for storage

Do not store above 25°C. Protect from light. Keep dry. Do not freeze. Keep container in the outer carton. Under these conditions, freeze-dried Flolan in an unopened vial should not be affected by moisture present in the atmosphere.

Any cold pouch used must be capable of maintaining the temperature of reconstituted Flolan between 2°C and 8°C for the full administration period.

The stability of solutions of Flolan is pH dependent. Only the diluent supplied should be used for reconstitution of freeze-dried Flolan and only the recommended infusion solutions, in the stated ratio, should be used for further dilution, otherwise the required pH may not be maintained.

Reconstitution and dilution should be carried out immediately prior to use *(see Posology and method of administration, and instructions for use/handling).*

GlaxoSmithKline Glycine Buffer Diluent contains no preservative, consequently a vial should be used once only and then discarded.

6.5 Nature and contents of container

Freeze dried powder in glass vials with synthetic butyl rubber plugs and aluminium collars.

Pack presentations:

Single 1.5 mg vial mg of freeze dried powder (Non-marketed)

Single 1.5 mg vial of freeze dried powder plus single vial of diluent

Single 1.5 mg vial of freeze dried powder plus two vials of diluent (Non-marketed)

6.6 Special precautions for disposal and other handling

Reconstitution and dilution:-

Particular care should be taken in the preparation of the infusion and in calculating the rate of infusion. The procedure given below should be closely followed.

Reconstitution and dilution of Flolan must be carried out using sterile techniques, immediately prior to clinical use.

Renal dialysis

Reconstitution:-

1. Use only the GlaxoSmithKline Glycine Buffer Diluent provided for reconstitution.

2. Withdraw approximately 10 ml of the GlaxoSmithKline Glycine Buffer Diluent into a sterile syringe, inject the contents of the syringe into the vial containing 1.5 mg freeze-dried Flolan and shake gently until the powder has dissolved.

3. Draw up the resulting Flolan solution into the syringe, re-inject it into the remaining volume of the GlaxoSmithKline Glycine Buffer Diluent solution and mix thoroughly.

This solution is now referred to as the concentrated solution and contains 30,000 nanograms per ml epoprostenol. Only this concentrated solution is suitable for further dilution prior to use.

When 0.5 mg Flolan powder is reconstituted with 50 ml of GlaxoSmithKline Glycine Buffer Diluent, the final injection has a pH of approximately 10.5 and a sodium ion content of approximately 56 mg.

Dilution:-

For administration using a pump capable of delivering small volume constant infusions, suitable aliquots of concentrated solution may be diluted with sterile physiological saline.

It may be diluted with physiological saline (0.9%), provided a ratio of 6 volumes of saline to 1 volume of concentrated solution is not exceeded; e.g. 50 ml of concentrated solution further diluted with a maximum of 300 ml saline.

Other common intravenous fluids are unsatisfactory for the dilution of the concentrated solution as the required pH is not attained. Flolan solutions are less stable at low pH.

Prior to using the concentrated solution, or the diluted form, a filtration step is needed. To filter, draw the reconstituted product into a large syringe and then attach the sterile filter provided to the syringe.

Dispense the concentrated solution directly into the chosen infusion solution using firm but not excessive pressure; the typical time taken for filtration of 50 ml of concentrated solution is 70 seconds. Mix well.

The filter unit must be used once only and then discarded.

When reconstituted and diluted as directed above, Flolan infusion solutions have a pH of approximately 10 and will retain 90% of their initial potency for approximately 12 hours at 25°C.

CALCULATION OF INFUSION RATE:-

The infusion rate may be calculated from the following formula:-

$$\text{Infusion rate (ml/min)} = \frac{\text{dosage (ng/kg/min) X bodyweight (kg)}}{\text{concentration of solution (ng/ml)}}$$

Infusion rate (ml/hr) = Infusion rate (ml/min) × 60

Infusion rate formulae - examples

When used in renal dialysis Flolan may be administered as the concentrated solution (a) or in diluted form (b).

a. Using concentrated solution, i.e. 30 000 nanogram/ml epoprostenol:

(see Table 1 below)

b. *Diluted*: A commonly used dilution is: -

10 ml concentrated solution plus50 ml physiological saline (0.9%). To give a final total volume of 60 ml.

Resultant concentration = 5000 nanogram/ml epoprostenol:

(see Table 2 below)

Primary Pulmonary Hypertension

The following packs are available for use in the treatment of primary pulmonary hypertension:

One vial containing sterile freeze-dried epoprostenol sodium equivalent to 1.5 mg epoprostenol supplied with one 50 ml vial of sterile GlaxoSmithKline Glycine Buffer Diluent solution.

One vial containing sterile freeze-dried epoprostenol sodium equivalent to 1.5 mg epoprostenol supplied with two 50 ml vials of sterile GlaxoSmithKline Glycine Buffer Diluent (Non-Marketed).

One vial containing sterile freeze-dried epoprostenol sodium equivalent to 1.5 mg epoprostenol supplied alone (Non-Marketed).

Initially a pack containing diluent buffer must be used. During chronic Flolan therapy the final concentration of solution may be increased by the addition of a 1.5 mg vial of freeze dried epoprostenol.

Only vials of the same amount as that included in the initial starter pack may be used to increase the final concentration of solution.

Reconstitution:

This should be carried out according to the instructions given for renal dialysis. Where a pack containing 1.5 mg epoprostenol is reconstituted with 50 ml sterile diluent the resultant concentration is 30,000 nanograms per ml.

Dilution:

Flolan may be used either as concentrated solution or in a diluted form for the treatment of PPH. Only GlaxoSmithKline Glycine Buffer Diluent provided may be used for the further dilution of reconstituted Flolan. Physiological saline must not be used when Flolan is to be used for the treatment of primary pulmonary hypertension.

Table 1

Concentration of solution = 30 000ng/ml epoprostenol

Dosage (ng/kg/min)	Bodyweight (kilograms)							
	30	40	50	60	70	80	90	100
1	n/a*	n/a*	n/a*	n/a*	n/a*	n/a*	0.18	0.20
2	n/a*	n/a*	0.20	0.24	0.28	0.32	0.36	0.40
3	0.18	0.24	0.30	0.36	0.42	0.48	0.54	0.60
4	0.24	0.32	0.40	0.48	0.56	0.64	0.72	0.80
5	0.30	0.40	0.50	0.60	0.70	0.80	0.90	1.00
	Flow rates in **ml/hr**							

* Very low flow rates required. Diluted solutions in physiological saline should be considered.

Table 2

Concentration of solution = 5000ng/ml epoprostenol

Dosage (ng/kg/ min)	Bodyweight (kilograms)							
	30	40	50	60	70	80	90	100
1	0.4	0.5	0.6	0.7	0.9	1.0	1.1	1.2
2	0.7	1.0	1.2	1.4	1.7	1.9	2.2	2.4
3	1.1	1.5	1.8	2.2	2.5	2.9	3.2	3.6
4	1.4	1.9	2.4	2.9	3.4	3.8	4.3	4.8
5	1.8	2.4	3.0	3.6	4.2	4.8	5.4	6.0
	Flow rates in **ml/hr**							

Table 3

Concentration of solution = 15 000ng/ml epoprostenol								
Dosage (ng/kg/ min)	Bodyweight (kilograms)							
	30	40	50	60	70	80	90	100
4				1.0	1.1	1.3	1.4	1.6
6		1.0	1.2	1.4	1.7	1.9	2.2	2.4
8	1.0	1.3	1.6	1.9	2.2	2.6	2.9	3.2
10	1.2	1.6	2.0	2.4	2.8	3.2	3.6	4.0
12	1.4	1.9	2.4	2.9	3.4	3.8	4.3	4.8
14	1.7	2.2	2.8	3.4	3.9	4.5	5.0	5.6
16	1.9	2.6	3.2	3.8	4.5	5.1	5.8	6.4
	Flow rates in **ml/hr**							

Concentrations commonly used in the treatment of primary pulmonary hypertension are as follows:

30,000ng/ml - 1.5mg epoprostenol reconstituted to a total volume of 50 ml in GlaxoSmithKline Glycine Buffer Diluent

15,000ng/ml – 1.5mg epoprostenol reconstituted and diluted to a total volume of 100ml in GlaxoSmithKline Glycine Buffer Diluent.

The maximum recommended concentration for administration in primary pulmonary hypertension is 60,000ng/ml.

Flolan must not be administered with other parenteral solutions or medications when used for primary pulmonary hypertension.

To dilute the concentrated solution, draw it up into a larger syringe and then attach the sterile filter provided to the syringe.

Dispense the concentrated solution directly into the pump cassette using firm but not excessive pressure; the typical time taken for filtration of 50 ml of concentrated solution is 70 seconds.

Remove the filter from the syringe and draw up the additional volume of GlaxoSmithKline Glycine Buffer Diluent required to achieve the desired dilution.

Refit the filter to the syringe and dispense the additional buffer through this into the concentrated Flolan solution in the cassette.

Mix well.

The filter unit must be used for the dilution of one pack only and then discarded.

The ambulatory pump used to administer Flolan should (1) be small and lightweight, (2) be able to adjust infusion rates in ng/kg/min increments, (3) have occlusion, end of infusion, and low battery alarms, (4) be accurate to ± 6% of the programmed rate (5) be positive pressure driven (continuous or pulsatile) with intervals between pulses not exceeding 3 minutes at infusion rates used to deliver Flolan, and (6) include a cold pouch system The reservoir should be made of polyvinyl chloride, polypropylene, or glass.

CALCULATION OF INFUSION RATE: -

The infusion rate may be calculated from the formula given above for renal dialysis. An example of a concentration commonly used in primary pulmonary hypertension is shown below.

Infusion rates for a concentration of 15,000 nanogram/ml ***(see Table 3 above)***

Administrative Data

7. MARKETING AUTHORISATION HOLDER

GlaxoWellcome UK Ltd

Trading as GlaxoSmithKline UK

Stockley Park West

Uxbridge

Middlesex

UB11 1BT

8. MARKETING AUTHORISATION NUMBER(S)

PL10949/0312

9. DATE OF FIRST AUTHORISATION/RENEWAL OF THE AUTHORISATION

7th March 2001

10. DATE OF REVISION OF THE TEXT

29 September 2006

11. Legal Status

POM

Flomaxtra XL, 400 micrograms, film-coated prolonged release tablet

(Astellas Pharma Ltd)

1. NAME OF THE MEDICINAL PRODUCT

Flomaxtra® XL, 400 micrograms, film-coated prolonged release tablet

2. QUALITATIVE AND QUANTITATIVE COMPOSITION

Each tablet contains as active ingredient tamsulosin hydrochloride 400 micrograms, equivalent to 367 micrograms tamsulosin.

For excipients, see section 6.1.

3. PHARMACEUTICAL FORM

Film coated, prolonged release tablet.

Approximately 9 mm, round, bi-convex, yellow, film-coated tablets debossed with the code '04'.

4. CLINICAL PARTICULARS

4.1 Therapeutic indications

Treatment of functional symptoms of benign prostatic hyperplasia (BPH).

4.2 Posology and method of administration

Posology

One tablet daily, to be taken with or without food.

Method of administration

For oral use.

The tablet should be swallowed whole and should not be crunched or chewed as this will interfere with the prolonged release of the active ingredient.

4.3 Contraindications

A history of orthostatic hypotension; severe hepatic insufficiency.

Hypersensitivity to tamsulosin hydrochloride or any other component of the product.

4.4 Special warnings and precautions for use

As with other alpha$_1$ blockers, a reduction in blood pressure can occur in individual cases during treatment with Flomaxtra XL, as a result of which, rarely, syncope can occur. At the first signs of orthostatic hypotension (dizziness, weakness), the patient should sit or lie down until the symptoms have disappeared.

Before therapy with Flomaxtra XL is initiated, the patient should be examined in order to exclude the presence of other conditions which can cause the same symptoms as benign prostatic hyperplasia. Digital rectal examination and, when necessary, determination of prostate specific antigen (PSA) should be performed before treatment and at regular intervals afterwards.

The treatment of severely renally impaired patients (creatinine clearance of less than 10 ml/min) should be approached with caution as these patients have not been studied.

The 'Intraoperative Floppy Iris Syndrome' (IFIS, a variant of small pupil syndrome) has been observed during cataract surgery in some patients on or previously treated with tamsulosin. IFIS may lead to increased procedural complications during the operation. The initiation of therapy with tamsulosin in patients for whom cataract surgery is scheduled is not recommended.

Discontinuing tamsulosin 1-2 weeks prior to cataract surgery is anecdotally considered helpful, but the benefit and duration of stopping of therapy prior to cataract surgery has not yet been established.

During pre-operative assessment, cataract surgeons and ophthalmic teams should consider whether patients scheduled for cataract surgery are being or have been treated with tamsulosin in order to ensure that appropriate measures will be in place to manage the IFIS during surgery.

4.5 Interaction with other medicinal products and other forms of interaction

No interactions have been seen when tamsulosin was given concomitantly with atenolol, enalapril, nifedipine or theophylline. Concomitant cimetidine brings about a rise in plasma levels of tamsulosin, and furosemide a fall, but as levels remain within the normal range, posology need not be changed.

In vitro, neither diazepam nor propranolol, trichlormethiazide, chlormadinon, amitryptyline, diclofenac, glibenclamide, simvastatin and warfarin change the free fraction of tamsulosin in human plasma. Neither does tamsulosin change the free fractions of diazepam, propranolol, trichlormethiazide, and chlormadinon.

No interactions at the level of hepatic metabolism have been seen during *in vitro* studies with liver microsomal fractions (representative of the cytochrome P_{450}-linked drug metabolising enzyme system), involving amitriptyline, salbutamol, glibenclamide and finasteride. Diclofenac and warfarin, however, may increase the elimination rate of tamsulosin.

There is a theoretical risk of enhanced hypotensive effect when given concomitantly with drugs which may reduce blood pressure, including anaesthetic agents and other α_1-adrenoceptor antagonists.

4.6 Pregnancy and lactation

Not applicable, as Flomaxtra XL is intended for male patients only.

4.7 Effects on ability to drive and use machines

No data is available on whether Flomaxtra XL adversely affects the ability to drive or operate machines. However, in this respect patients should be aware of the fact that drowsiness, blurred vision, dizziness and syncope can occur.

4.8 Undesirable effects

Flomaxtra XL was evaluated in two double - blind placebo controlled trials. Adverse events were mostly mild and their incidence was generally low. The most commonly reported ADR was abnormal ejaculation occurring in approximately 2% of patients.

Suspected adverse reactions reported with Flomaxtra XL or an alternative formulation of tamsulosin, were:-

Nervous systems disorders

Common: dizziness, headache

Uncommon: syncope

Cardiac disorders

Uncommon: palpitations

Vascular disorders

Uncommon: postural hypotension

Respiratory disorders

Uncommon: rhinitis

Gastrointestinal disorders

Uncommon: nausea, vomiting, constipation, diarrhoea

Skin and subcutaneous tissue disorders

Uncommon: rash, pruritus, urticaria

Very rare: angioedema

Reproductive system disorders

Common: abnormal ejaculation

Very rare: priapism

General disorders

Common: asthenia

As with other alpha-blockers, drowsiness, blurred vision, dry mouth or oedema can occur.

During cataract surgery a small pupil situation, known as Intraoperative Floppy Iris Syndrome (IFIS), has been associated with therapy of tamsulosin during post-marketing surveillance (see also section 4.4).

4.9 Overdose

Acute overdose with 5 mg tamsulosin hydrochloride has been reported. Acute hypotension (systolic blood pressure 70 mm Hg), vomiting and diarrhoea were observed, which were treated with fluid replacement and the patient was able to be discharged the same day. In case of acute hypotension occurring after overdose, cardiovascular support should be given. Blood pressure can be restored and heart rate brought back to normal by lying the patient down. If this does not help, then volume expanders, and when necessary, vasopressors could be employed. Renal function should be monitored and general supportive measures applied. Dialysis is unlikely to be of help, as tamsulosin is very highly bound to plasma proteins.

Measures, such as emesis, can be taken to impede absorption. When large quantities are involved, gastric lavage can be applied and activated charcoal and an osmotic laxative, such as sodium sulphate, can be administered.

5. PHARMACOLOGICAL PROPERTIES

5.1 Pharmacodynamic properties

Pharmacotherapeutic group:

Alpha$_1$-adrenoceptor antagonist.

ATC code: G04C A02. Preparations for the exclusive treatment of prostatic disease.

Mechanism of action:

Tamsulosin binds selectively and competitively to postsynaptic alpha$_1$-receptors, in particular to the subtype alpha$_{1A}$, which bring about relaxation of the smooth muscle of the prostate, whereby tension is reduced.

Pharmacodynamic effects:

Flomaxtra XL increases maximum urinary flow rate by reducing smooth muscle tension in the prostate and urethra, thereby relieving obstruction.

It also improves the complex of irritative and obstructive symptoms in which bladder instability and tension of the smooth muscles of the lower urinary tract play an important role. Alpha$_1$-blockers can reduce blood pressure by lowering peripheral resistance. No reduction in blood pressure of any clinical significance was observed during studies with Flomaxtra XL.

5.2 Pharmacokinetic properties

Absorption:

Flomaxtra XL is formulated as an Oral Controlled Absorption System (OCAS) and is a prolonged release tablet of the non-ionic gel matrix type.

Tamsulosin administered as Flomaxtra XL is absorbed from the intestine and is approximately 55 - 59% bioavailable. A consistent slow release of tamsulosin is maintained over the whole pH range encountered in the gastro-intestinal tract with little fluctuation over 24 hours. The rate and extent of absorption of tamsulosin administered as Flomaxtra XL is not affected by food.

Tamsulosin shows linear kinetics.

After a single dose of Flomaxtra in the fasted state, plasma levels of tamsulosin peak at a median time of 6 hours. In steady state, which is reached by day 4 of multiple dosing, plasma levels of tamsulosin peak at 4 to 6 hours in the fasted and fed state. Peak plasma levels increase from approximately 6 ng/ml after the first dose to 11 ng/ml in steady state.

As a result of the prolonged release characteristics of Flomaxtra XL, the trough concentration of tamsulosin in plasma amounts to 40% of the peak plasma concentration under fasted and fed conditions.

There is a considerable inter-patient variation in plasma levels, both after single and multiple dosing.

Distribution:

In man, tamsulosin is about 99% bound to plasma proteins and volume of distribution is small (about 0.2l/kg).

Metabolism:

Tamsulosin has a low first pass effect, being metabolised slowly. Most tamsulosin is present in plasma in the form of unchanged drug. It is metabolised in the liver.

In rats, hardly any induction of microsomal liver enzymes was seen to be caused by tamsulosin.

No dose adjustment is warranted in hepatic insufficiency.

None of the metabolites are more active than the original compound.

Elimination:

Tamsulosin and its metabolites are mainly excreted in the urine. The amount excreted as unchanged drug is estimated to be about 4 - 6% of the dose, administered as Flomaxtra XL.

After a single dose of Flomaxtra XL, and in steady state, elimination half-lives of about 19 and 15 hours, respectively, have been measured.

No dose adjustment is necessary in patients with renal impairment.

5.3 Preclinical safety data

Single and repeat dose toxicity studies were performed in mice, rats and dogs. In addition, reproduction toxicity studies were performed in rats, carcinogenicity in mice and rats, and *in vivo* and *in vitro* genotoxicity were examined. The general toxicity profile, as seen with high doses of tamsulosin, is consistent with the known pharmacological actions of the alpha-adrenergic blocking agents. At very high dose levels, the ECG was altered in dogs. This response is considered to be not clinically relevant. Tamsulosin showed no relevant genotoxic properties.

Increased incidences of proliferative changes of mammary glands of female rats and mice have been reported. These findings, which are probably mediated by hyperprolactinaemia and only occurred at high dose levels, are regarded as irrelevant.

6. PHARMACEUTICAL PARTICULARS

6.1 List of excipients

Core

Macrogol (containing butylhydroxytoluene)

Magnesium stearate

Film-coat

Hypromellose

Macrogol

Yellow iron oxide (E172)

6.2 Incompatibilities

None known.

6.3 Shelf life

2 years

6.4 Special precautions for storage

There are no special storage instructions

6.5 Nature and contents of container

Aluminium foil blister packs containing 30 tablets.

6.6 Special precautions for disposal and other handling

No special instructions.

7. MARKETING AUTHORISATION HOLDER

Astellas Pharma Ltd

Lovett House

Lovett Road

Staines

TW18 3AZ

United Kingdom

8. MARKETING AUTHORISATION NUMBER(S)

PL 00166/ 0199

9. DATE OF FIRST AUTHORISATION/RENEWAL OF THE AUTHORISATION

11th July 2005

10. DATE OF REVISION OF THE TEXT

10th October 2006

11. LEGAL CATEGORY

POM

Floxapen Capsules 250mg

(Actavis UK Ltd)

1. NAME OF THE MEDICINAL PRODUCT

FLOXAPEN® Capsules 250mg

2. QUALITATIVE AND QUANTITATIVE COMPOSITION

Floxapen Capsules (Flucloxacillin Capsules BP) containing 250 mg flucloxacillin as Flucloxacillin Sodium BP.

3. PHARMACEUTICAL FORM

Capsule, hard

Caramel coloured hard gelatin capsules printed with 'actavis 250', fitted with black caps

4. CLINICAL PARTICULARS

Flucloxacillin is an isoxazolyl penicillin of the β-lactam group of antibiotics which exerts a bactericidal effect upon many Gram-positive organisms including β-lactamase-producing staphylococci and streptococci.

4.1 Therapeutic indications

Floxapen is indicated for the treatment of infections due to sensitive Gram-positive organisms, including β-lactamase-producing staphylococci and streptococci. Typical indications include:

Skin and soft tissue infections:

Boils	Cellulitis	Infected burns
Abscesses	Infected skin conditions, e.g. ulcer, eczema, and acne	Protection for skin grafts
Carbuncles		
Furunculosis	Infected wounds	Impetigo

Respiratory tract infections:

Pneumonia	Lung abscess	Empyema
Sinusitis	Pharyngitis	Otitis media and externa
Tonsillitis	Quinsy	

Other infections caused by Floxapen-sensitive organisms:

Osteomyelitis	Urinary tract infection
Enteritis	Meningitis
Endocarditis	Septicaemia

Floxapen is also indicated for use as a prophylactic agent during major surgical procedures when appropriate; for example cardiothoracic and orthopaedic surgery.

Parenteral usage is indicated where oral dosage is inappropriate.

4.2 Posology and method of administration

Depends on the age, weight and renal function of the patient, as well as the severity of the infection.

Usual adult dosage (including elderly patients)

Oral - 250 mg four times a day.

Osteomyelitis, endocarditis - Up to 8 g daily, in divided doses six to eight hourly.

Surgical prophylaxis - 1 to 2 g IV at induction of anaesthesia followed by 500 mg six hourly IV, IM or orally for up to 72 hours.

Usual children's dosage

2-10 years: half adult dose.

Under 2 years: quarter adult dose.

Abnormal renal function: In common with other penicillins, Floxapen usage in patients with renal impairment does not usually require dosage reduction. However, in the presence of severe renal failure (creatinine clearance < 10 ml/min) a reduction in dose or an extension of dose interval should be considered. Floxapen is not significantly removed by dialysis and hence no supplementary dosages need to be administered either during, or at the end of the dialysis period.

Administration

Oral: Oral doses should be administered half to one hour before meals.

4.3 Contraindications

Flucloxacillin should not be given to patients with a history of hypersensitivity to β-lactam antibiotics (e.g. penicillins, cephalosporins) or excipients.

Flucloxacillin is contra-indicated in patients with a previous history of flucloxacillin-associated jaundice/hepatic dysfunction.

4.4 Special warnings and precautions for use

Before initiating therapy with flucloxacillin, careful enquiry should be made concerning previous hypersensitivity reactions to β-lactams.

Serious and occasionally fatal hypersensitivity reactions (anaphylaxis) have been reported in patients receiving β-lactam antibiotics. Although anaphylaxis is more frequent following parenteral therapy, it has occurred in patients on oral therapy. These reactions are more likely to occur in individuals with a history of β-lactam hypersensitivity.

Flucloxacillin should be used with caution in patients with evidence of hepatic dysfunction, patients ⩾ 50 years and those with serious underlying disease. In these patients, hepatic events may be severe, and in very rare circumstances, deaths have been reported (see section 4.8).

During prolonged treatments (e.g. osteomyelitis, endocarditis), regular monitoring of hepatic and renal functions is recommended.

Prolonged use may occasionally result in overgrowth of non-susceptible organisms.

Floxapen capsules contain approximately 51 mg sodium per g. This should be included in the daily allowance of patients on sodium restricted diets.

4.5 Interaction with other medicinal products and other forms of interaction

Probenecid decreases the renal tubular secretion of flucloxacillin. Concurrent administration of probenecid delays the renal excretion of flucloxacillin.

In common with other antibiotics, flucloxacillin may affect the gut flora, leading to lower oestrogen reabsorption and reduced efficacy of combined oral contraceptives

4.6 Pregnancy and lactation

Pregnancy: Animal studies with flucloxacillin have shown no teratogenic effects. The product has been in clinical use since 1970 and the limited number of reported cases of use in human pregnancy have shown no evidence of untoward effects. The decision to administer any drug during pregnancy should be taken with the utmost care. Therefore flucloxacillin should only be used in pregnancy when the potential benefits outweigh the potential risks associated with treatment.

Lactation: Trace quantities of flucloxacillin can be detected in breast milk. The possibility of hypersensitivity reactions must be considered in breast-feeding infants. Therefore flucloxacillin should only be administered to a breast-feeding mother when the potential benefits outweigh the potential risks associated with the treatment.

4.7 Effects on ability to drive and use machines

Adverse effects on the ability to drive or operate machinery have not been observed.

4.8 Undesirable effects

The following convention has been utilised for the classification of undesirable effects:- Very common (>1/10), common (>1/100, <1/10), uncommon (>1/1000, <1/100), rare (>1/10,000, <1/1,000), very rare (<1/10,000).

Unless otherwise stated, the frequency of the adverse events has been derived from more than 30 years of post-marketing reports.

Blood and lymphatic system disorders

Very rare: Neutropenia (including agranulocytosis) and thrombocytopenia. These are reversible when treatment is discontinued. Haemolytic anaemia.

Immune system disorders

Very rare: Anaphylactic shock (exceptional with oral administration) (see Section 4.4 Special warnings and special precautions for use), angioneurotic oedema.

If any hypersensitivity reaction occurs, the treatment should be discontinued. (See also Skin and subcutaneous tissue disorders).

Gastrointestinal disorders

***Common:** Minor gastrointestinal disturbances.

Very rare: Pseudomembranous colitis.

If pseudomembranous colitis develops, flucloxacillin treatment should be discontinued and appropriate therapy, e.g. oral vancomycin should be initiated.

Hepato-biliary disorders

Very rare: Hepatitis and cholestatic jaundice. (See Section 4.4 Special Warnings and Special Precautions for Use). Changes in liver function laboratory test results (reversible when treatment is discontinued).

These reactions are related neither to the dose nor to the route of administration. The onset of these effects may be delayed for up to two months post-treatment; in several cases the course of the reactions has been protracted and lasted for some months. Hepatic events may be severe and in very rare circumstances a fatal outcome has been reported. Most reports of deaths have been in patients ⩾ 50 years and in patients with serious underlying disease.

Skin and subcutaneous tissue disorders

***Uncommon:** Rash, urticaria and purpura.

Very rare: Erythema multiforme, Stevens-Johnson syndrome and toxic epidermal necrolysis.

(See also Immune system disorders).

Musculoskeletal and connective tissue disorders

Very rare: Arthralgia and myalgia sometimes develop more than 48 hours after the start of the treatment.

Renal and urinary disorders

Very rare: Interstitial nephritis.

This is reversible when treatment is discontinued.

General disorders and administration site conditions

Very rare: Fever sometimes develops more than 48 hours after the start of the treatment.

*The incidence of these AEs was derived from clinical studies involving a total of approximately 929 adult and paediatric patients taking flucloxacillin.

4.9 Overdose

Gastrointestinal effects such as nausea, vomiting and diarrhoea may be evident and should be treated symptomatically.

Flucloxacillin is not removed from the circulation by haemodialysis.

5. PHARMACOLOGICAL PROPERTIES

5.1 Pharmacodynamic properties

Properties: Flucloxacillin is a narrow-spectrum antibiotic of the group of isoxazolyl penicillins; it is not inactivated by staphylococcal β-lactamases.

Activity: Flucloxacillin, by its action on the synthesis of the bacterial wall, exerts a bactericidal effect on streptococci except those of group D (*Enterococcus faecalis*) staphylococci. It is not active against methicillin-resistant staphylococci.

5.2 Pharmacokinetic properties

Absorption: Flucloxacillin is stable in acid media and can therefore be administered either by the oral or parenteral route. The peak serum levels of flucloxacillin reached after one hour are as follows.

- After 250 mg by the oral route (in fasting subjects): Approximately 8.8 mg/l.

- After 500 mg by the oral route (in fasting subjects): Approximately 14.5mg/l.

- After 500 mg by the IM route: Approximately 16.5 mg/l.

The total quantity absorbed by the oral route represents approximately 79% of the quantity administered.

Distribution: Flucloxacillin diffuses well into most tissue. Specifically, active concentrations of flucloxacillin have been recovered in bones: 11.6 mg/l (compact bone) and 15.6 mg/l (spongy bone), with a mean serum level of 8.9 mg/l.

Crossing the meningeal barrier: Flucloxacillin diffuses in only small proportion into the cerebrospinal fluid of subjects whose meninges are not inflamed.

Crossing into mother's milk: Flucloxacillin is excreted in small quantities in mother's milk.

Metabolism: In normal subjects approximately 10% of the flucloxacillin administered is metabolised to penicilloic acid. The elimination half-life of flucloxacillin is in the order of 53 minutes.

Excretion: Excretion occurs mainly through the kidney. Between 65.5% (oral route) and 76.1% (parenteral route) of the dose administered is recovered in unaltered active form in the urine within 8 hours. A small portion of the dose administered is excreted in the bile. The excretion of flucloxacillin is slowed in cases of renal failure.

Protein binding: The serum protein-binding rate is 95%.

5.3 Preclinical safety data

No further information of relevance to add.

6. PHARMACEUTICAL PARTICULARS

6.1 List of excipients

Capsule content:

Magnesium stearate

Capsule shell:

Gelatin

Titanium dioxide (E171)

Black iron oxide (E172)

Yellow iron oxide (E172)

Red iron oxide (E172)

Printing ink:

Shellac (E904)

Propylene glycol (E1520)

Sodium hydroxide (E524)

Povidone

Titanium dioxide (E171)

6.2 Incompatibilities

None known.

6.3 Shelf life

Tray foil blister: 24 months

Fibreboard drums: 36 months

6.4 Special precautions for storage

Floxapen Capsules in Original Packs should be stored in a dry place. Floxapen Capsules in reclosable containers should be stored in a cool, dry place. Fibreboard drums should be kept tightly closed in a cool, dry place.

6.5 Nature and contents of container

Floxapen Capsules 250 mg: Aluminium canister - 20, 50, 100 and 500; Glass bottle with screwcap - 20, 50, 100 and 500; Polypropylene tube with polyethylene closure - 20, 50, 100 and 500; Aluminium foil – 12; Aluminium/PVC Blister with an aluminium overseal (tray foil blister pack) – 28; Fibreboard drum with metal or HDPE lid – 50,000

6.6 Special precautions for disposal and other handling

None stated.

7. MARKETING AUTHORISATION HOLDER

Actavis Group PTC ehf

Reykjavikurvegi 76-78

220 Hafnarfjordur

Iceland.

8. MARKETING AUTHORISATION NUMBER(S)

PL 30306/0015

9. DATE OF FIRST AUTHORISATION/RENEWAL OF THE AUTHORISATION

11th October 2007

10. DATE OF REVISION OF THE TEXT

27/02/09

11. DOSIMETRY

12. INSTRUCTIONS FOR PREPARATION OF RADIOPHARMACEUTICALS (IF APPLICABLE)

Floxapen Capsules 500mg

(Actavis UK Ltd)

1. NAME OF THE MEDICINAL PRODUCT

Floxapen Capsules 500mg

2. QUALITATIVE AND QUANTITATIVE COMPOSITION

Floxapen Capsules (Flucloxacillin Capsules BP) containing 500 mg flucloxacillin as Flucloxacillin Sodium BP.

3. PHARMACEUTICAL FORM

Capsule, hard

Caramel coloured hard gelatin capsules printed with 'actavis 500', fitted with black caps

4. CLINICAL PARTICULARS

Flucloxacillin is an isoxazolyl penicillin of the β-lactam group of antibiotics which exerts a bactericidal effect upon many Gram-positive organisms including β-lactamase-producing staphylococci and streptococci.

4.1 Therapeutic indications

Floxapen is indicated for the treatment of infections due to sensitive Gram-positive organisms, including β-lactamase-producing staphylococci and streptococci. Typical indications include:

Skin and soft tissue infections:

Boils	Cellulitis	Infected burns
Abscesses	Infected skin conditions	Protection for skin grafts
Carbuncles	e.g. ulcer, eczema, and acne	Impetigo
Furunculosis	Infected wounds	

Respiratory tract infections:

Pneumonia	Lung abscess	Empyema
Sinusitis	Pharyngitis	Otitis media and externa
Tonsillitis	Quinsy	

Other infections caused by Floxapen-sensitive organisms:

Osteomyelitis	Urinary tract infection
Enteritis	Meningitis
Endocarditis	Septicaemia

Floxapen is also indicated for use as a prophylactic agent during major surgical procedures when appropriate; for example cardiothoracic and orthopaedic surgery.

Parenteral usage is indicated where oral dosage is inappropriate.

4.2 Posology and method of administration

Depends on the age, weight and renal function of the patient, as well as the severity of the infection.

Usual adult dosage (including elderly patients)

Oral - 250 mg four times a day.

Osteomyelitis, endocarditis - Up to 8 g daily, in divided doses six to eight hourly.

Surgical prophylaxis - 1 to 2 g IV at induction of anaesthesia followed by

500 mg six hourly IV, IM or orally for up to 72 hours.

Usual children's dosage

2-10 years: half adult dose.

Under 2 years: quarter adult dose.

Abnormal renal function: In common with other penicillins, Floxapen usage in patients with renal impairment does not usually require dosage reduction. However, in the presence of severe renal failure (creatinine clearance < 10 ml/min) a reduction in dose or an extension of dose interval should be considered. Floxapen is not significantly removed by dialysis and hence no supplementary dosages need to be administered either during, or at the end of the dialysis period.

Administration

Oral: Oral doses should be administered half to one hour before meals.

4.3 Contraindications

Flucloxacillin should not be given to patients with a history of hypersensitivity to β-lactam antibiotics (e.g. penicillins, cephalosporins) or excipients.

Flucloxacillin is contra-indicated in patients with a previous history of flucloxacillin-associated jaundice/hepatic dysfunction.

4.4 Special warnings and precautions for use

Before initiating therapy with flucloxacillin, careful enquiry should be made concerning previous hypersensitivity reactions to β-lactams.

Serious and occasionally fatal hypersensitivity reactions (anaphylaxis) have been reported in patients receiving β-lactam antibiotics. Although anaphylaxis is more frequent following parenteral therapy, it has occurred in patients on oral therapy. These reactions are more likely to occur in individuals with a history of β-lactam hypersensitivity.

Flucloxacillin should be used with caution in patients with evidence of hepatic dysfunction, patients ≥ 50 years and those with serious underlying disease. In these patients, hepatic events may be severe, and in very rare circumstances, deaths have been reported (see section 4.8).

During prolonged treatments (e.g. osteomyelitis, endocarditis), regular monitoring of hepatic and renal functions is recommended.

Prolonged use may occasionally result in overgrowth of non-susceptible organisms.

Floxapen capsules contain 51 mg sodium per g. This should be included in the daily allowance of patients on sodium restricted diets.

4.5 Interaction with other medicinal products and other forms of interaction

Probenecid decreases the renal tubular secretion of flucloxacillin. Concurrent administration of probenecid delays the renal excretion of flucloxacillin.

In common with other antibiotics, flucloxacillin may affect the gut flora, leading to lower oestrogen reabsorption and reduced efficacy of combined oral contraceptives

4.6 Pregnancy and lactation

Pregnancy: Animal studies with flucloxacillin have shown no teratogenic effects. The product has been in clinical use since 1970 and the limited number of reported cases of use in human pregnancy have shown no evidence of untoward effects. The decision to administer any drug during pregnancy should be taken with the utmost care. Therefore flucloxacillin should only be used in pregnancy when the potential benefits outweigh the potential risks associated with treatment.

Lactation: Trace quantities of flucloxacillin can be detected in breast milk. The possibility of hypersensitivity reactions must be considered in breast-feeding infants. Therefore flucloxacillin should only be administered to a breast-feeding mother when the potential benefits outweigh the potential risks associated with the treatment.

4.7 Effects on ability to drive and use machines

Adverse effects on the ability to drive or operate machinery have not been observed.

4.8 Undesirable effects

The following convention has been utilised for the classification of undesirable effects:- Very common ($>1/10$), common ($>1/100$, $<1/10$), uncommon ($>1/1000$, $<1/100$), rare ($>1/10,000$, $<1/1000$), very rare ($<1/10,000$).

Unless otherwise stated, the frequency of the adverse events has been derived from more than 30 years of post-marketing reports.

Blood and lymphatic system disorders

Very rare: Neutropenia (including agranulocytosis) and thrombocytopenia. These are reversible when treatment is discontinued. Haemolytic anaemia.

Immune system disorders

Very rare: Anaphylactic shock (exceptional with oral administration) (see Item 4.4 Warnings), angioneurotic oedema.

If any hypersensitivity reaction occurs, the treatment should be discontinued. (See also Skin and subcutaneous tissue disorders).

Gastrointestinal disorders

*Common: Minor gastrointestinal disturbances.

Very rare: Pseudomembranous colitis.

If pseudomembranous colitis develops, flucloxacillin treatment should be discontinued and appropriate therapy, e.g. oral vancomycin should be initiated.

Hepato-biliary disorders

Very rare: Hepatitis and cholestatic jaundice. (See Section 4.4 Special Warnings and Special Precautions for Use). Changes in liver function laboratory test results (reversible when treatment is discontinued).

These reactions are related neither to the dose nor to the route of administration. The onset of these effects may be delayed for up to two months post-treatment; in several cases the course of the reactions has been protracted and lasted for some months. Hepatic events may be severe and in very rare circumstances a fatal outcome has been reported. Most reports of deaths have been in patients ⩾ 50 years and in patients with serious underlying disease.

Skin and subcutaneous tissue disorders

*Uncommon: Rash, urticaria and purpura.

Very rare: Erythema multiforme, Stevens-Johnson syndrome and toxic epidermal necrolysis.

(See also Immune system disorders).

Musculoskeletal and connective tissue disorders

Very rare: Arthralgia and myalgia sometimes develop more than 48 hours after the start of the treatment.

Renal and urinary disorders

Very rare: Interstitial nephritis.

This is reversible when treatment is discontinued.

General disorders and administration site conditions

Very rare: Fever sometimes develops more than 48 hours after the start of the treatment.

*The incidence of these AEs was derived from clinical studies involving a total of approximately 929 adult and paediatric patients taking flucloxacillin.

4.9 Overdose

Gastrointestinal effects such as nausea, vomiting and diarrhoea may be evident and should be treated symptomatically.

Flucloxacillin is not removed from the circulation by haemodialysis.

5. PHARMACOLOGICAL PROPERTIES

5.1 Pharmacodynamic properties

Properties: Flucloxacillin is a narrow-spectrum antibiotic of the group of isoxazolyl penicillins; it is not inactivated by staphylococcal β-lactamases.

Activity: Flucloxacillin, by its action on the synthesis of the bacterial wall, exerts a bactericidal effect on streptococci except those of group D (*Enterococcus faecalis*) staphylococci. It is not active against methicillin-resistant staphylococci.

5.2 Pharmacokinetic properties

Absorption: Flucloxacillin is stable in acid media and can therefore be administered either by the oral or parenteral route. The peak serum levels of flucloxacillin reached after one hour are as follows.

- After 250 mg by the oral route (in fasting subjects): Approximately 8.8 mg/l.
- After 500 mg by the oral route (in fasting subjects): Approximately 14.5mg/l.
- After 500 mg by the IM route: Approximately 16.5 mg/l.

The total quantity absorbed by the oral route represents approximately 79% of the quantity administered.

Distribution: Flucloxacillin diffuses well into most tissue. Specifically, active concentrations of flucloxacillin have been recovered in bones: 11.6 mg/l (compact bone) and 15.6 mg/l (spongy bone), with a mean serum level of 8.9 mg/l.

Crossing the meningeal barrier: Flucloxacillin diffuses in only small proportion into the cerebrospinal fluid of subjects whose meninges are not inflamed.

Crossing into mother's milk: Flucloxacillin is excreted in small quantities in mother's milk.

Metabolism: In normal subjects approximately 10% of the flucloxacillin administered is metabolised to penicilloic acid. The elimination half-life of flucloxacillin is in the order of 53 minutes.

Excretion: Excretion occurs mainly through the kidney. Between 65.5% (oral route) and 76.1% (parenteral route) of the dose administered is recovered in unaltered active form in the urine within 8 hours. A small portion of the dose administered is excreted in the bile. The excretion of flucloxacillin is slowed in cases of renal failure.

Protein binding: The serum protein-binding rate is 95%.

5.3 Preclinical safety data

No further information of relevance to add.

6. PHARMACEUTICAL PARTICULARS

6.1 List of excipients

Capsule content:

Magnesium stearate

Capsule shell:

Gelatin

Titanium dioxide (E171)

Black iron oxide (E172)

Yellow iron oxide (E172)

Red iron oxide (E172)

Printing ink:

Shellac (E904)

Propylene glycol (E1520)

Sodium hydroxide (E524)

Povidone

Titanium dioxide (E171)

6.2 Incompatibilities

None known.

6.3 Shelf life

Tray foil blister: 24 months

Other Packaging: 12 months

6.4 Special precautions for storage

Floxapen Capsules in Original Packs should be stored in a dry place. Floxapen Capsules in reclosable containers should be stored in a cool, dry place.

6.5 Nature and contents of container

Floxapen Capsules 500 mg: Aluminium canister - 50 and 100; Glass bottle with screwcap - 50 and 100; Polypropylene tube with polyethylene closure - 50 and 100; Aluminium foil - 12; Aluminium/PVC Blister with an aluminium overseal (tray foil blister pack) -28

6.6 Special precautions for disposal and other handling

None stated.

7. MARKETING AUTHORISATION HOLDER

Actavis Group PTC ehf

Reykjavíkurvegi 76-78

220 Hafnarfjordur

Iceland.

8. MARKETING AUTHORISATION NUMBER(S)

PL 30306/0016

9. DATE OF FIRST AUTHORISATION/RENEWAL OF THE AUTHORISATION

12th October 2007

10. DATE OF REVISION OF THE TEXT

27/02/09

11. DOSIMETRY

12 INSTRUCTIONS FOR PREPARATION OF RADIOPHARMACEUTICALS (IF APPLICABLE)

Floxapen Syrup 125mg/5ml

(Actavis UK Ltd)

1. NAME OF THE MEDICINAL PRODUCT

FLOXAPEN® Syrup 125mg/5 ml

2. QUALITATIVE AND QUANTITATIVE COMPOSITION

Floxapen Syrup (Flucloxacillin Oral Suspension BP) when reconstituted each 5 ml contains 125 mg flucloxacillin as Flucloxacillin Magnesium BP.

3. PHARMACEUTICAL FORM

Floxapen Syrups: Bottles containing powder for the preparation of suspension.

4. CLINICAL PARTICULARS

Flucloxacillin is an isoxazolyl penicillin of the β-lactam group of antibiotics which exerts a bactericidal effect upon many Gram-positive organisms including β-lactamase-producing staphylococci and streptococci.

4.1 Therapeutic indications

Floxapen is indicated for the treatment of infections due to sensitive Gram-positive organisms, including β-lactamase-producing staphylococci and streptococci. Typical indications include:

Skin and soft tissue infections:

Boils, Cellulitis, Infected burns, Abscesses, Infected skin conditions, e.g. ulcer, eczema, and acne, Protection for skin grafts, Carbuncles, Furunculosis, Infected wounds, Impetigo

Respiratory tract infections:

Pneumonia, Lung abscess, Empyema, Sinusitis, Pharyngitis, Otitis media and externa, Tonsillitis, Quinsy

Other infections caused by Floxapen-sensitive organisms:

Osteomyelitis, Urinary tract infection, Enteritis, Meningitis, Endocarditis, Septicaemia

Floxapen is also indicated for use as a prophylactic agent during major surgical procedures when appropriate; for example cardiothoracic and orthopaedic surgery.

Parenteral usage is indicated where oral dosage is inappropriate.

4.2 Posology and method of administration

Depends on the age, weight and renal function of the patient, as well as the severity of the infection.

Usual adult dosage (including elderly patients)

Oral - 250 mg four times a day.

Usual children's dosage

2-10 years: half adult dose

Under 2 years: quarter adult dose.

Abnormal renal function: In common with other penicillins, Floxapen usage in patients with renal impairment does not usually require dosage reduction. However, in the presence of severe renal failure (creatinine clearance < 10 ml/min) a reduction in dose or an extension of dose interval should be considered. Floxapen is not significantly removed by dialysis and hence no supplementary dosages need to be administered either during, or at the end of the dialysis period.

Administration

Oral: Oral doses should be administered half to one hour before meals.

4.3 Contraindications

Flucloxacillin should not be given to patients with a history of hypersensitivity to β-lactam antibiotics (e.g. penicillins, cephalosporins) or excipients.

Flucloxacillin is contra-indicated in patients with a previous history of flucloxacillin-associated jaundice/hepatic dysfunction.

4.4 Special warnings and precautions for use

Before initiating therapy with flucloxacillin, careful enquiry should be made concerning previous hypersensitivity reactions to β-lactams.

Serious and occasionally fatal hypersensitivity reactions (anaphylaxis) have been reported in patients receiving β-lactam antibiotics. Although anaphylaxis is more frequent following parenteral therapy, it has occurred in patients on oral therapy. These reactions are more likely to occur in individuals with a history of β-lactam hypersensitivity.

Flucloxacillin should be used with caution in patients with evidence of hepatic dysfunction, (patients ⩾ 50 years and those with serious underlying disease. In these patients, hepatic events may be severe, and in very rare circumstances, deaths have been reported (see section 4.8).

Special caution is essential in the newborn because of the risk of hyperbilirubinaemia. Studies have shown that, at high dose following parenteral administration, flucloxacillin can displace bilirubin from plasma protein binding sites, and may therefore predispose to kernicterus in a jaundiced baby. In addition, special caution is essential in the newborn because of the potential for high serum levels of flucloxacillin due to a reduced rate of renal excretion.

During prolonged treatments (e.g. osteomyelitis, endocarditis), regular monitoring of hepatic and renal functions is recommended.

Prolonged use may occasionally result in overgrowth of non-susceptible organisms.

4.5 Interaction with other medicinal products and other forms of interaction

Probenecid decreases the renal tubular secretion of flucloxacillin. Concurrent administration of probenecid delays the renal excretion of flucloxacillin.

In common with other antibiotics, flucloxacillin may affect the gut flora, leading to lower oestrogen reabsorption and reduced efficacy of combined oral contraceptives

4.6 Pregnancy and lactation

Pregnancy: Animal studies with flucloxacillin have shown no teratogenic effects. The product has been in clinical use since 1970 and the limited number of reported cases of use in human pregnancy have shown no evidence of untoward effects. The decision to administer any drug during pregnancy should be taken with the utmost care. Therefore flucloxacillin should only be used in pregnancy when the potential benefits outweigh the potential risks associated with treatment.

Lactation: Trace quantities of flucloxacillin can be detected in breast milk. The possibility of hypersensitivity reactions must be considered in breast-feeding infants. Therefore flucloxacillin should only be administered to a breast-feeding mother when the potential benefits outweigh the potential risks associated with the treatment.

4.7 Effects on ability to drive and use machines

Adverse effects on the ability to drive or operate machinery have not been observed.

4.8 Undesirable effects

The following convention has been utilised for the classification of undesirable effects:- Very common (>1/10), common (>1/100, <1/10), uncommon (>1/1000, <1/100), rare (>1/10,000, <1/1000), very rare (<1/10,000).

Unless otherwise stated, the frequency of the adverse events has been derived from more than 30 years of post-marketing reports.

Blood and lymphatic system disorders

Very rare: Neutropenia (including agranulocytosis) and thrombocytopenia. These are reversible when treatment is discontinued. Haemolytic anaemia.

Immune system disorders

Very rare: Anaphylactic shock (exceptional with oral administration) (see Item 4.4 Warnings), angioneurotic oedema.

If any hypersensitivity reaction occurs, the treatment should be discontinued. (See also Skin and subcutaneous tissue disorders).

Gastrointestinal disorders

*Common: Minor gastrointestinal disturbances.

Very rare: Pseudomembranous colitis.

If pseudomembranous colitis develops, flucloxacillin treatment should be discontinued and appropriate therapy, e.g. oral vancomycin should be initiated.

Hepato-biliary disorders

Very rare: Hepatitis and cholestatic jaundice. (See Section 4.4 Special Warnings and Special Precautions for Use). Changes in liver function laboratory test results (reversible when treatment is discontinued).

These reactions are related neither to the dose nor to the route of administration. The onset of these effects may be delayed for up to two months post-treatment; in several cases the course of the reactions has been protracted and lasted for some months. Hepatic events may be severe and in very rare circumstances a fatal outcome has been reported. Most reports of deaths have been in patients ⩾ 50 years and in patients with serious underlying disease.

Skin and subcutaneous tissue disorders

*Uncommon: Rash, urticaria and purpura.

Very rare: Erythema multiforme, Stevens-Johnson syndrome and toxic epidermal necrolysis.

(See also Immune system disorders).

Musculoskeletal and connective tissue disorders

Very rare: Arthralgia and myalgia sometimes develop more than 48 hours after the start of the treatment.

Renal and urinary disorders

Very rare: Interstitial nephritis.

This is reversible when treatment is discontinued.

General disorders and administration site conditions

Very rare: Fever sometimes develops more than 48 hours after the start of the treatment.

*The incidence of these AEs was derived from clinical studies involving a total of approximately 929 adult and paediatric patients taking flucloxacillin.

4.9 Overdose

Gastrointestinal effects such as nausea, vomiting and diarrhoea may be evident and should be treated symptomatically.

Flucloxacillin is not removed from the circulation by haemodialysis.

5. PHARMACOLOGICAL PROPERTIES

5.1 Pharmacodynamic properties

Properties: Flucloxacillin is a narrow-spectrum antibiotic of the group of isoxazolyl penicillins; it is not inactivated by staphylococcal β-lactamases.

Activity: Flucloxacillin, by its action on the synthesis of the bacterial wall, exerts a bactericidal effect on streptococci except those of group D (*Enterococcus faecalis*) staphylococci. It is not active against methicillin-resistant staphylococci.

5.2 Pharmacokinetic properties

Absorption: Flucloxacillin is stable in acid media and can therefore be administered either by the oral or parenteral route. The peak serum levels of flucloxacillin reached after one hour are as follows.

- After 250 mg by the oral route (in fasting subjects): Approximately 8.8 mg/l.

- After 500 mg by the oral route (in fasting subjects): Approximately 14.5 mg/l.

- After 500 mg by the IM route: Approximately 16.5 mg/l.

The total quantity absorbed by the oral route represents approximately 79% of the quantity administered.

Distribution: Flucloxacillin diffuses well into most tissue. Specifically, active concentrations of flucloxacillin have been recovered in bones: 11.6 mg/l (compact bone) and 15.6 mg/l (spongy bone), with a mean serum level of 8.9 mg/l.

Crossing the meningeal barrier: Flucloxacillin diffuses in only small proportion into the cerebrospinal fluid of subjects whose meninges are not inflamed.

Crossing into mothers' milk: Flucloxacillin is excreted in small quantities in mothers' milk.

Metabolism: In normal subjects approximately 10% of the flucloxacillin administered is metabolised to penicilloic acid. The elimination half-life of flucloxacillin is in the order of 53 minutes.

Excretion: Excretion occurs mainly through the kidney. Between 65.5% (oral route) and 76.1% (parenteral route) of the dose administered is recovered in unaltered active form in the urine within 8 hours. A small portion of the dose administered is excreted in the bile. The excretion of flucloxacillin is slowed in cases of renal failure.

Protein binding: The serum protein-binding rate is 95%.

5.3 Preclinical safety data

No further information of relevance to add.

6. PHARMACEUTICAL PARTICULARS

6.1 List of excipients

Floxapen Syrups: Saccharin sodium, xanthan gum, citric acid, sodium citrate, sodium benzoate, blood orange, tutti fruitti, menthol dry flavours and sucrose.

6.2 Incompatibilities

None known.

6.3 Shelf life

Floxapen Syrups: Two years (following reconstitution: 14 days).

6.4 Special precautions for storage

Floxapen Syrups: Do not store above 25°C.

Once dispensed, Floxapen Syrups (bottles) remain stable for 14 days stored in a refrigerator (5°C).

6.5 Nature and contents of container

Floxapen Syrup 125 mg/5 ml: Clear glass bottles, reconstituted volume of 61ml or 100 ml.

6.6 Special precautions for disposal and other handling

If a dilution of the reconstituted syrup is required, Syrup BP should be used.

7. MARKETING AUTHORISATION HOLDER

Actavis Group PTC ehf
Reykjavíkurvegi 76-78
220 Hafnarfjordur
Iceland.

8. MARKETING AUTHORISATION NUMBER(S)

PL 30306/0017

9. DATE OF FIRST AUTHORISATION/RENEWAL OF THE AUTHORISATION

12th October 2007

10. DATE OF REVISION OF THE TEXT

Floxapen Syrup 250mg/5ml

(Actavis UK Ltd)

1. NAME OF THE MEDICINAL PRODUCT

FLOXAPEN® Syrups

2. QUALITATIVE AND QUANTITATIVE COMPOSITION

Floxapen Syrups (Flucloxacillin Oral Suspension BP) when reconstituted each 5 ml contains 250 mg flucloxacillin as Flucloxacillin Magnesium BP.

3. PHARMACEUTICAL FORM

Floxapen Syrups: Bottles containing powder for the preparation of suspension.

4. CLINICAL PARTICULARS

Flucloxacillin is an isoxazolyl penicillin of the β-lactam group of antibiotics which exerts a bactericidal effect upon many Gram-positive organisms including β-lactamase-producing staphylococci and streptococci.

4.1 Therapeutic indications

Floxapen is indicated for the treatment of infections due to sensitive Gram-positive organisms, including β-lactamase producing staphylococci and streptococci. Typical indications include:

Skin and soft tissue infections:

Boils, Cellulitis, Infected burns, Abscesses, Infected skin conditions, e.g. ulcer, eczema, and acne, Protection for skin grafts, Carbuncles, Furunculosis, Infected wounds, Impetigo

Respiratory tract infections:

Pneumonia, Lung abscess, Empyema, Sinusitis, Pharyngitis, Otitis media and externa, Tonsillitis, Quinsy

Other infections caused by Floxapen-sensitive organisms:

Osteomyelitis, Urinary tract infection, Enteritis, Meningitis, Endocarditis, Septicaemia

Floxapen is also indicated for use as a prophylactic agent during major surgical procedures when appropriate; for example cardiothoracic and orthopaedic surgery.

Parenteral usage is indicated where oral dosage is inappropriate.

4.2 Posology and method of administration

Depends on the age, weight and renal function of the patient, as well as the severity of the infection.

Usual adult dosage (including elderly patients)

Oral - 250 mg four times a day.

Usual children's dosage

2-10 years: half adult dose

Under 2 years: quarter adult dose.

Abnormal renal function: In common with other penicillins, Floxapen usage in patients with renal impairment does not usually require dosage reduction. However, in the presence of severe renal failure (creatinine clearance < 10 ml/min) a reduction in dose or an extension of dose interval should be considered. Floxapen is not significantly removed by dialysis and hence no supplementary dosages need to be administered either during, or at the end of the dialysis period.

Administration

Oral: Oral doses should be administered half to one hour before meals.

4.3 Contraindications

Flucloxacillin should not be given to patients with a history of hypersensitivity to β-lactam antibiotics (e.g. penicillins, cephalosporins) or excipients.

Flucloxacillin is contra-indicated in patients with a previous history of flucloxacillin-associated jaundice/hepatic dysfunction.

4.4 Special warnings and precautions for use

Before initiating therapy with flucloxacillin, careful enquiry should be made concerning previous hypersensitivity reactions to β-lactams.

Serious and occasionally fatal hypersensitivity reactions (anaphylaxis) have been reported in patients receiving β-lactam antibiotics. Although anaphylaxis is more frequent following parenteral therapy, it has occurred in patients on oral therapy. These reactions are more likely to occur in individuals with a history of β-lactam hypersensitivity.

Flucloxacillin should be used with caution in patients with evidence of hepatic dysfunction, patients ⩾ 50 years and those with serious underlying disease. In these patients, hepatic events may be severe, and in very rare circumstances, deaths have been reported (see section 4.8).

Special caution is essential in the newborn because of the risk of hyperbilirubinaemia. Studies have shown that, at high dose following parenteral administration, flucloxacillin can displace bilirubin from plasma protein binding sites, and may therefore predispose to kernicterus in a jaundiced baby. In addition, special caution is essential in the newborn because of the potential for high serum levels of flucloxacillin due to a reduced rate of renal excretion.

During prolonged treatments (e.g. osteomyelitis, endocarditis), regular monitoring of hepatic and renal functions is recommended.

Prolonged use may occasionally result in overgrowth of non-susceptible organisms.

4.5 Interaction with other medicinal products and other forms of interaction

Probenecid decreases the renal tubular secretion of flucloxacillin. Concurrent administration of probenecid delays the renal excretion of flucloxacillin.

In common with other antibiotics, flucloxacillin may affect the gut flora, leading to lower oestrogen reabsorption and reduced efficacy of combined oral contraceptives

4.6 Pregnancy and lactation

Pregnancy: Animal studies with flucloxacillin have shown no teratogenic effects. The product has been in clinical use since 1970 and the limited number of reported cases of use in human pregnancy have shown no evidence of untoward effects. The decision to administer any drug during pregnancy should be taken with the utmost care. Therefore flucloxacillin should only be used in pregnancy when the potential benefits outweigh the potential risks associated with treatment.

Lactation: Trace quantities of flucloxacillin can be detected in breast milk. The possibility of hypersensitivity reactions must be considered in breast-feeding infants. Therefore flucloxacillin should only be administered to a breast-feeding mother when the potential benefits outweigh the potential risks associated with the treatment.

4.7 Effects on ability to drive and use machines

Adverse effects on the ability to drive or operate machinery have not been observed.

4.8 Undesirable effects

The following convention has been utilised for the classification of undesirable effects:- Very common (>1/10), common (>1/100, <1/10), uncommon (>1/1000, <1/100), rare (>1/10,000, <1/1000), very rare (<1/10,000).

Unless otherwise stated, the frequency of the adverse events has been derived from more than 30 years of post-marketing reports.

Blood and lymphatic system disorders

Very rare: Neutropenia (including agranulocytosis) and thrombocytopenia. These are reversible when treatment is discontinued. Haemolytic anaemia.

Immune system disorders

Very rare: Anaphylactic shock (exceptional with oral administration) (see Item 4.4 Warnings), angioneurotic oedema.

If any hypersensitivity reaction occurs, the treatment should be discontinued. (See also Skin and subcutaneous tissue disorders).

Gastrointestinal disorders

*Common: Minor gastrointestinal disturbances.

Very rare: Pseudomembranous colitis.

If pseudomembranous colitis develops, flucloxacillin treatment should be discontinued and appropriate therapy, e.g. oral vancomycin should be initiated.

Hepato-biliary disorders

Very rare: Hepatitis and cholestatic jaundice. (See Section 4.4 Special Warnings and Special Precautions for Use). Changes in liver function laboratory test results (reversible when treatment is discontinued).

These reactions are related neither to the dose nor to the route of administration. The onset of these effects may be delayed for up to two months post-treatment; in several cases the course of the reactions has been protracted and lasted for some months. Hepatic events may be severe and in very rare circumstances a fatal outcome has been reported. Most reports of deaths have been in patients ⩾ 50 years and in patients with serious underlying disease.

Skin and subcutaneous tissue disorders

*Uncommon: Rash, urticaria and purpura.

Very rare: Erythema multiforme, Stevens-Johnson syndrome and toxic epidermal necrolysis.

(See also Immune system disorders).

Musculoskeletal and connective tissue disorders

Very rare: Arthralgia and myalgia sometimes develop more than 48 hours after the start of the treatment.

Renal and urinary disorders

Very rare: Interstitial nephritis.

This is reversible when treatment is discontinued.

General disorders and administration site conditions

Very rare: Fever sometimes develops more than 48 hours after the start of the treatment.

*The incidence of these AEs was derived from clinical studies involving a total of approximately 929 adult and paediatric patients taking flucloxacillin.

4.9 Overdose

Gastrointestinal effects such as nausea, vomiting and diarrhoea may be evident and should be treated symptomatically.

Flucloxacillin is not removed from the circulation by haemodialysis.

5. PHARMACOLOGICAL PROPERTIES

5.1 Pharmacodynamic properties

Properties: Flucloxacillin is a narrow-spectrum antibiotic of the group of isoxazolyl penicillins; it is not inactivated by staphylococcal β-lactamases.

Activity: Flucloxacillin, by its action on the synthesis of the bacterial wall, exerts a bactericidal effect on streptococci except those of group D (*Enterococcus faecalis*) staphylococci. It is not active against methicillin-resistant staphylococci.

5.2 Pharmacokinetic properties

Absorption: Flucloxacillin is stable in acid media and can therefore be administered either by the oral or parenteral route. The peak serum levels of flucloxacillin reached after one hour are as follows:

- After 250 mg by the oral route (in fasting subjects): Approximately 8.8 mg/l.
- After 500 mg by the oral route (in fasting subjects): Approximately 14.5 mg/l.
- After 500 mg by the IM route: Approximately 16.5 mg/l.

The total quantity absorbed by the oral route represents approximately 79% of the quantity administered.

Distribution: Flucloxacillin diffuses well into most tissue. Specifically, active concentrations of flucloxacillin have been recovered in bones: 11.6 mg/l (compact bone) and 15.6 mg/l (spongy bone), with a mean serum level of 8.9 mg/l.

Crossing the meningeal barrier: Flucloxacillin diffuses in only small proportion into the cerebrospinal fluid of subjects whose meninges are not inflamed.

Crossing into mothers' milk: Flucloxacillin is excreted in small quantities in mothers' milk.

Metabolism: In normal subjects approximately 10% of the flucloxacillin administered is metabolised to penicilloic acid. The elimination half-life of flucloxacillin is in the order of 53 minutes.

Excretion: Excretion occurs mainly through the kidney. Between 65.5% (oral route) and 76.1% (parenteral route) of the dose administered is recovered in unaltered active form in the urine within 8 hours. A small portion of the dose administered is excreted in the bile. The excretion of flucloxacillin is slowed in cases of renal failure.

Protein binding: The serum protein-binding rate is 95%.

5.3 Preclinical safety data

No further information of relevance to add.

6. PHARMACEUTICAL PARTICULARS

6.1 List of excipients

Floxapen Syrups: Saccharin sodium, xanthan gum, citric acid, sodium citrate, sodium benzoate, blood orange, tutti fruitti, menthol dry flavours and sucrose.

6.2 Incompatibilities

None known.

6.3 Shelf life

Floxapen Syrups: Two years (following reconstitution: 14 days).

6.4 Special precautions for storage

Floxapen Syrups: Do not store above 25°C.

Once dispensed, Floxapen Syrups (bottles) remain stable for 14 days stored in a refrigerator (5°C).

6.5 Nature and contents of container

Floxapen Syrup 250 mg/5 ml: Clear glass bottles, reconstituted volume of 61 ml or 100 ml.

6.6 Special precautions for disposal and other handling

If a dilution of the reconstituted syrup is required, Syrup BP should be used.

7. MARKETING AUTHORISATION HOLDER

Actavis Group PTC ehf

Reykjavíkurvegi 76-78

220 Hafnarfjordur

Iceland.

8. MARKETING AUTHORISATION NUMBER(S)

PL 30306/0018

9. DATE OF FIRST AUTHORISATION/RENEWAL OF THE AUTHORISATION

12th October 2007

10. DATE OF REVISION OF THE TEXT

Fluanxol Tablets

(Lundbeck Limited)

1. NAME OF THE MEDICINAL PRODUCT

Fluanxol Tablets 0.5 mg

Fluanxol Tablets 1 mg

2. QUALITATIVE AND QUANTITATIVE COMPOSITION

0.5 mg tablets (containing 0.584 mg flupentixol dihydrochloride equivalent to 0.5 mg flupentixol base).

1 mg tablets (containing 1.168 mg flupentixol dihydrochloride equivalent to 1 mg flupentixol base).

3. PHARMACEUTICAL FORM

Round, biconvex, ochre-yellow, sugar-coated tablets.

4. CLINICAL PARTICULARS

4.1 Therapeutic indications

Symptomatic treatment of depression (with or without anxiety).

4.2 Posology and method of administration

Route of administration: Oral.

Adults: The standard initial dosage is 1 mg as a single morning dose. After one week the dose may be increased to 2 mg if there is inadequate clinical response. Daily dosage of more than 2 mg should be in divided doses up to a maximum of 3 mg daily.

Elderly: The standard initial dosage is 0.5 mg as a single morning dose. After one week, if response is inadequate, dosage may be increased to 1 mg once a day. Caution should be exercised in further increasing the dosage but occasional patients may require up to a maximum of 2 mg a day which should be given in divided doses.

Children: Not recommended for children.

Patients often respond within 2-3 days. If no effect has been observed within one week at maximum dosage the drug should be withdrawn.

4.3 Contraindications

Hypersensitivity to the active substance or to any of the excipients (see section 6.1).

Severe depression requiring ECT or hospitalisation, states of excitement or overactivity, including mania.

Circulatory collapse, depressed level of consciousness due to any cause (e.g. intoxication with alcohol, barbiturates or opiates), coma

Not recommended for excitable or agitated patients.

4.4 Special warnings and precautions for use

Caution should be exercised in patients having: liver disease; cardiac disease or arrhythmias; severe respiratory disease; renal failure; epilepsy (and conditions predisposing to epilepsy e.g. alcohol withdrawal or brain damage); Parkinson's disease; narrow angle glaucoma; prostatic hypertrophy; hypothyroidism; hyperthyroidism; myasthenia gravis; phaeochromocytoma and patients who have shown hypersensitivity to thioxanthenes or other antipsychotics.

The elderly require close supervision because they are specially prone to experience such adverse effects as sedation, hypotension, confusion and temperature changes.

Recurrence of depressive symptoms on abrupt withdrawal is rare.

Dependence has not been reported to date.

Suicide/suicidal thoughts or clinical worsening

Depression is associated with an increased risk of suicidal thoughts, self harm and suicide (suicide-related events). This risk persists until significant remission occurs. As improvement may not occur during the first few weeks or more of treatment, patients should be closely monitored until such improvement occurs.

It is general clinical experience that the risk of suicide may increase in the early stages of recovery. Other psychiatric conditions for which Flupentixol is prescribed can also be associated with an increased risk of suicide-related events. In addition, these conditions may be co-morbid with major depressive disorder. The same precautions observed when treating patients with major depressive disorder should therefore be observed when treating patients with other psychiatric disorders.

Patients with a history of suicide-related events, or those exhibiting a significant degree of suicidal ideation prior to commencement of treatment are known to be at greater risk of suicidal thoughts or suicide attempts, and should receive careful monitoring during treatment. A meta-analysis of placebo-controlled clinical trials of antidepressant drugs in adult patients with psychiatric disorders showed an increased risk of suicidal behaviour with antidepressants compared to placebo in patients less than 25 years old. Close supervision of patients and in particular those at high risk should accompany drug therapy especially in early treatment and following dose changes. Patients (and caregivers of patients) should be alerted about the need to monitor for any clinical worsening, suicidal behaviour or thoughts and unusual changes in behaviour and to seek medical advice immediately if these symptoms present.

As described for other psychotropics flupentixol may modify insulin and glucose responses calling for adjustment of the antidiabetic therapy in diabetic patients.

An approximately 3-fold increased risk of cerebrovascular adverse events have been seen in randomised placebo controlled clinical trials in the dementia population with some atypical antipsychotics. The mechanism for this increased risk is not known. An increased risk cannot be excluded for other antipsychotics or other patient populations.

Flupentixol should be used with caution in patients with risk factors for stroke.

As with other drugs belonging to the therapeutic class of antipsychotics, flupentixol may cause QT prolongation. Persistently prolonged QT intervals may increase the risk of malignant arrhythmias. Therefore, flupentixol should be used with caution in susceptible individuals (with hypokalemia, hypomagnesia or genetic predisposition) and in patients with a history of cardiovascular disorders, e.g. QT prolongation, significant bradycardia (<50 beats per minute), a recent acute myocardial infarction, uncompensated heart failure, or cardiac arrhythmia.

Concomitant treatment with other antipsychotics should be avoided (see section 4.5).

The possibility of development of neuroleptic malignant syndrome (hyperthermia, muscle rigidity, fluctuating consciousness, instability of the autonomous nervous system) exists with any neuroleptic. The risk is possibly greater with the more potent agents. Patients with pre-existing organic brain syndrome, mental retardation, and opiate and alcohol abuse are over-represented among fatal cases.

Treatment: Discontinuation of the neuroleptic. Symptomatic treatment and use of general supportive measures. Dantrolene and bromocriptine may be helpful. Symptoms may persist for more than a week after oral neuroleptics are discontinued and somewhat longer when associated with the depot forms of the drug.

Blood dyscrasias, including thrombocytopenia, have been reported rarely. Blood counts should be carried out if a patient develops signs of persistent infection.

Excipients

The tablets contain lactose monohydrate. Patients with rare hereditary problems of galactose intolerance, the Lapp lactase deficiency or glucose-galactose malabsorption should not receive this medicine.

The tablets also contain sucrose. Patients with rare hereditary problems of fructose intolerance, glucose-galactose malabsorption or sucrase-isomaltase insufficiency should not take this medicine.

4.5 Interaction with other medicinal products and other forms of interaction

In common with other similar drugs, flupentixol enhances the response to alcohol, the effects of barbiturates and other CNS depressants. Flupentixol may potentiate the effects of general anaesthetics and anticoagulants and prolong the action of neuromuscular blocking agents.

The anticholinergic effects of atropine or other drugs with anticholinergic properties may be increased. Concomitant use of drugs such as metoclopramide, piperazine or antiparkinson drugs may increase the risk of extrapyramidal effects such as tardive dyskinesia. Combined use of antipsychotics and lithium or sibutramine has been associated with an increased risk of neurotoxicity.

Antipsychotics may enhance the cardiac depressant effects of quinidine; the absorptiion of corticosteroids and digoxin. The hypotensive effect of vasodilator antihypertensive agents such as hydralazine and α-blockers (e.g. doxazosin), or methyl-dopa may be enhanced.

Increases in the QT interval related to antipsychotic treatment may be exacerbated by the co-administration of other drugs known to significantly increase the QT interval. Co-administration of such drugs should be avoided.

Relevant classes include:

class Ia and III antiarrhythmics (e.g. quinidine, amiodarone, sotalol, dofetilide)

some antipsychotics (e.g. thioridazine)

some macrolides (e.g. erythromycin)

some antihistamines

some quinolone antibiotics (e.g. moxifloxacin)

The above list is not exhaustive and other individual drugs known to significantly increase QT interval (e.g. cisapride, lithium) should be avoided.

Drugs known to cause electrolyte disturbances such as thiazide diuretics (hypokalaemia) and drugs known to increase the plasma concentration of flupentixol should also be used with caution as they may increase the risk of QT prolongation and malignant arrythmias (see section 4.4).

Antipsychotics may antagonise the effects of adrenaline and other sympathomimetic agents, and reverse the antihypertensive effects of guanethidine, possibily clonidine and similar adrenergic-blocking agents. Antipsychotics may also impair the effect of levodopa, adrenergic drugs and anticonvulsants.

The metabolism of tricyclic antidepressants may be inhibited and the control of diabetes may be impaired.

4.6 Pregnancy and lactation

As the safety of Fluanxol in human pregnancy has not been established, use during pregnancy, especially the first and last trimesters, should be avoided unless the expected benefit to the patient outweighs the potential risk to the foetus.

Flupentixol is excreted into the breast milk. If the use of Fluanxol is considered essential, nursing mothers should be advised to stop breast feeding.

The newborn of mothers treated with antipsychotics in late pregnancy, or labour, may show signs of intoxication such as lethargy, tremor and hyperexcitability, and have a low apgar score.

4.7 Effects on ability to drive and use machines

Alertness may be impaired, especially at the start of treatment, or following the consumption of alcohol; patients should be warned of this risk and advised not to drive or operate machinery until their susceptibility is known. Patients should not drive if they have blurred vision.

4.8 Undesirable effects

Cases of suicidal ideation and suicidal behaviours have been reported during Flupentixol therapy or early after treatment discontinuation (see section 4.4).

Undesirable effects are for the majority dose dependent. The frequency and severity are most pronounced in the early phase of treatment and decline during continued treatment.

Extrapyramidal reactions may occur, especially in the early phase of treatment. In most cases these side effects can be satisfactorily controlled by reduction of dosage and/or use of antiparkinson drugs. The routine prophylactic use of antiparkinson drugs is not recommended. Antiparkinson drugs do not alleviate tardive dyskinesia and may aggravate them. Reduction in dosage or, if possible, discontinuation of zuclopenthixol therapy is recommended. In persistent akathisia a benzodiazepine or propranolol may be useful.

Cardiac disorders

Tachycardia, palpitations. Electrocardiogram QT prolonged.

Blood and lymphatic system disorders

Thrombocytopenia, neutropenia, leukopenia, agranulocytosis

Nervous system disorders

Somnolence, akathisia, hyperkinesia, hypokinesia. Tremor, dystonia, dizziness, headache, disturbance in attention. Tardive dyskinesia, dyskinesia, parkinsonism, speech disorder, convulsion. Neuroleptic malignant syndrome.

Eye disorders

Accommodation disorder, vision abnormal. Oculogyration.

Respiratory, thoracic and mediastinal disorders

Dyspnoea.

Gastrointestinal disorders

Dry mouth. Salivary hypersecretion, constipation, vomiting, dyspepsia, diarrhoea. Abdominal pain, nausea, flatulence.

Renal and urinary disorders

Micturition disorder, urinary retention.

Skin and subcutaneous tissue disorders

Hyperhidrosis, pruritus. Rash, photosensitivity reaction, dermatitis.

Musculoskeletal and connective tissue disorder

Myalgia. Muscle rigidity.

Endocrine disorder

Hyperprolactinaemia.

Metabolism and nutrition disorders

Increased appetite, weight increased. Decreased appetite. Hyperglycaemia, glucose tolerance abnormal.

Vascular disorders

Hypotension, hot flush.

General disorders and administration site conditions

Asthenia, fatigue.

Immune system disorders

Hypersensitivity, anaphylactic reaction.

Hepatobiliary disorders

Liver function test abnormal. Jaundice.

Reproductive system and breast disorders

Ejaculation failure, erectile dysfunction. Gynaecomastia, galactorrhoea, amenorrhoea.

Psychiatric disorders

Insomnia, depression, nervousness, agitation, libido decreased. Confusional state.

As with other drugs belonging to the therapeutic class of antipsychotics, rare cases of QT prolongation, ventricular arrhythmias - ventricular fibrillation, ventricular tachycardia, Torsade de Pointes and sudden unexplained death have been reported for flupentixol (see section 4.4).

Abrupt discontinuation of flupentixol may be accompanied by withdrawal symptoms. The most common symptoms are nausea, vomiting, anorexia, diarrhoea, rhinorrhoea, sweating, myalgias, paraesthesias, insomnia, restlessness, anxiety, and agitation. Patients may also experience vertigo, alternate feelings of warmth and coldness, and tremor. Symptoms generally begin within 1 to 4 days of withdrawal and abate within 7 to 14 days.

4.9 Overdose

Overdosage may cause somnolence, or even coma, extrapyramidal symptoms, convulsions, hypotension, shock, hyper- or hypothermia. ECG changes, QT prolongation, Torsade de Pointes, cardiac arrest and ventricular arrhythmias have been reported when administered in overdose together with drugs known to affect the heart.

Treatment is symptomatic and supportive, with measures aimed at supporting the respiratory and cardiovascular systems. The following specific measures may be employed if required.

- anticholinergic antiparkinson drugs if extrapyramidal symptoms occur.
- sedation (with benzodiazepines) in the unlikely event of agitation or excitement or convulsions.
- noradrenaline in saline intravenous drip if the patient is in shock. Adrenaline must not be given.
- ingestion of activated charcoal and gastric lavage should be considered

5. PHARMACOLOGICAL PROPERTIES

5.1 Pharmacodynamic properties

The precise pharmacological mode of action of flupentixol has not been determined. It has been postulated that at low dosage flupentixol binds to presynaptic dopamine receptors causing increased neurotransmitter release. There is evidence that postsynaptic aminergic receptors become down regulated in response to increased levels of neurotransmitter and this is responsible for the observed improvement in depressive symptoms.

5.2 Pharmacokinetic properties

Mean oral bioavailability is about 55%. Maximum drug serum concentrations occur about 4 hours after dosing and the biological half-life is about 35 hours. Flupentixol is widely distributed in the body. Metabolism is by sulphoxidation, N-dealkylation and glucuronic acid conjugation. Excretion is via the urine and faeces.

5.3 Preclinical safety data

Nil of relevance

6. PHARMACEUTICAL PARTICULARS

6.1 List of excipients

Lactose monohydrate

Potato starch

Magnesium stearate

Gelatin

Sucrose

Yellow iron oxide (E 172)

Beeswax

White wax

Carnauba wax.

6.2 Incompatibilities

None known.

6.3 Shelf life

Fluanxol tablets are stable for 2 years. The box is labelled with an expiry date.

6.4 Special precautions for storage

Do not store above 25(C.

6.5 Nature and contents of container

PVC/PVdC blister strips of 60 tablets per box.

6.6 Special precautions for disposal and other handling

Nil

7. MARKETING AUTHORISATION HOLDER

Lundbeck Limited

Lundbeck House

Caldecotte Lake Business Park

Caldecotte

Milton Keynes

MK7 8LF

8. MARKETING AUTHORISATION NUMBER(S)

Fluanxol Tablets 0.5 mg:

PL 0458/0011R

Fluanxol Tablets 1 mg:

PL 0458/0037

9. DATE OF FIRST AUTHORISATION/RENEWAL OF THE AUTHORISATION

First Authorisation Fluanxol Tablets 0.5 mg:

25 November 1982

First Authorisation Fluanxol Tablets 1 mg:

23 September 1982

Renewal of Authorisations:

15 July 2008

10. DATE OF REVISION OF THE TEXT

28 January 2009

® Trademark

Fluarix

(GlaxoSmithKline UK)

1. NAME OF THE MEDICINAL PRODUCT

Fluarix, suspension for injection in a pre-filled syringe

Influenza vaccine (split virion, inactivated)

2. QUALITATIVE AND QUANTITATIVE COMPOSITION

Split Influenza virus, inactivated, containing antigens* equivalent to:

A/Brisbane/59/2007 (H1N1)-like strain:

A/Brisbane/59/2007 (IVR-148) 15 micrograms HA**

A/Brisbane/10/2007 (H3N2)-like strain:

A/Uruguay/716/2007 (NYMC X-175C) 15 micrograms HA**

B/Brisbane/60/2008-like strain:

B/Brisbane/60/2008 15 micrograms HA**

per 0.5 ml dose

* propagated in fertilized hens' eggs from healthy chicken flocks

** haemagglutinin

This vaccine complies with the WHO recommendation (northern hemisphere) and EU decision for the 2009/2010 season.

For a full list of excipients see section 6.1.

3. PHARMACEUTICAL FORM

Suspension for injection in a pre-filled syringe.

Fluarix is colourless to slightly opalescent.

4. CLINICAL PARTICULARS

4.1 Therapeutic indications

Prophylaxis of influenza, especially in those who run an increased risk of associated complications.

The use of Fluarix should be based on official recommendations.

4.2 Posology and method of administration

Adults and children from 36 months: 0.5 ml.

Children from 6 months to 35 months: Clinical data are limited. Dosages of 0.25 ml or 0.5 ml have been used.

For children aged < 9 years, who have not previously been vaccinated, a second dose should be given after an interval of at least 4 weeks.

Immunisation should be carried out by intramuscular or deep subcutaneous injection.

For instructions for preparation, see section 6.6.

4.3 Contraindications

Hypersensitivity to the active substances, to any of the excipients, to residues, to egg and to chicken protein. Fluarix does not contain more than 0.05 microgram ovalbumin per dose. The vaccine may contain residues of the following substances, e.g. formaldehyde, gentamicin sulphate and sodium deoxycholate.

Immunisation shall be postponed in patients with febrile illness or acute infection.

4.4 Special warnings and precautions for use

As with all injectable vaccines, appropriate medical treatment and supervision should always be readily available in case of an anaphylactic event following the administration of the vaccine.

Fluarix should under no circumstances be administered intravascularly.

Antibody response in patients with endogenous or iatrogenic immunosuppression may be insufficient.

4.5 Interaction with other medicinal products and other forms of interaction

Fluarix may be given at the same time as other vaccines. Immunisation should be carried out on separate limbs. It should be noted that the adverse reactions may be intensified.

The immunological response may be diminished if the patient is undergoing immunosuppressant treatment.

Following influenza vaccination, false positive results in serology tests using the ELISA method to detect antibodies against HIV1, hepatitis C and especially HTLV1 have been observed. The Western Blot technique disproves the false positive ELISA test results. The transient false positive reactions could be due to the IgM response by the vaccine.

4.6 Pregnancy and lactation

The limited data from vaccinations in pregnant women do not indicate that adverse fetal and maternal outcomes were attributable to the vaccine. The use of this vaccine may be considered from the second trimester of pregnancy. For pregnant women with medical conditions that increase their risk of complications from influenza, administration of the vaccine is recommended, irrespective of their stage of pregnancy.

Fluarix may be used during lactation.

Table 1

Organ class	Very common ≥1/10	Common ≥1/100, <1/10	Uncommon ≥1/1,000, <1/100	Rare ≥1/10,000, <1/1,000	Very rare <1/10,000
Nervous system disorders		Headache*			
Skin and subcutaneous tissue disorders		Sweating*			
Musculoskeletal and connective tissue disorders		Myalgia, arthralgia*			
General disorders and administration site conditions		fever, malaise, shivering, fatigue Local reactions: redness, swelling, pain, ecchymosis, induration*			

*These reactions usually disappear within 1-2 days without treatment.

4.7 Effects on ability to drive and use machines
The vaccine is unlikely to produce an effect on the ability to drive and use machines.

4.8 Undesirable effects

Adverse reactions observed from clinical trials

The safety of trivalent inactivated influenza vaccines is assessed in open label, uncontrolled clinical trials performed as annual update requirement, including at least 50 adults aged 18–60 years of age and at least 50 elderly aged 61 years or older. Safety evaluation is performed during the first 3 days following vaccination.

The following undesirable effects have been observed during clinical trials with the following frequencies:

Very common (≥1/10), Common (≥1/100, <1/10); Uncommon (≥1/1,000, <1/100); Rare (≥1/10,000, <1/1,000); Very rare (<1/10,000), including isolated reports.

(see Table 1 above)

Adverse reactions reported from post marketing surveillance

Adverse reactions reported from post marketing surveillance are, next to the reactions which have also been observed during the clinical trials, the following:

Blood and lymphatic system disorders:

Transient thrombocytopenia, transient Lymphadenopathy

Immune system disorders:

Allergic reactions, in rare cases leading to shock, angioedema

Nervous system disorders:

Neuralgia, paraesthesia, febril convulsions, neurological disorders, such as encephalomyelitis, neuritis and Guillain Barré syndrome

Vascular disorders:

Vasculitis associated in very rare cases with transient renal involvement

Skin and subcutaneous tissue disorders:

Generalised skin reactions including pruritus, urticaria or non-specific rash

4.9 Overdose
Overdosage is unlikely to have any untoward effect.

5. PHARMACOLOGICAL PROPERTIES

5.1 Pharmacodynamic properties
Pharmacotherapeutic group: Influenza vaccine, ATC Code: J07 BB 02

Seroprotection is generally obtained within 2 to 3 weeks. The duration of postvaccinal immunity to homologous strains or to strains closely related to the vaccine strains varies but is usually 6-12 months.

5.2 Pharmacokinetic properties
Not applicable.

5.3 Preclinical safety data
Not applicable.

6. PHARMACEUTICAL PARTICULARS

6.1 List of excipients
Sodium chloride, disodium phosphate dodecahydrate, potassium dihydrogen phosphate, potassium chloride, magnesium chloride hexahydrate, RRR-α-tocopheryl hydrogen succinate, polysorbate 80, octoxynol 10 and water for injections.

6.2 Incompatibilities
In the absence of compatibility studies, this medicinal product must not be mixed with other medicinal products.

6.3 Shelf life
1 year.

6.4 Special precautions for storage
Store in a refrigerator at (2°C–8°C).

Do not freeze.

Keep the syringe in the outer carton in order to protect from light.

6.5 Nature and contents of container
0.5 ml suspension for injection in prefilled syringe (Type I glass) with a plunger stopper (butyl) with or without needles – pack of 1, 10 or 20.

Not all pack sizes may be marketed

6.6 Special precautions for disposal and other handling
Unused vaccine and other waste material should be disposed of in compliance with local rules for the disposal of products of this nature.

The vaccine should be allowed to reach room temperature before use. Shake before use.

When a dose of 0.25 ml is indicated, the prefilled syringe should be held in upright position and half of the volume should be eliminated. The remaining volume should be injected.

7. MARKETING AUTHORISATION HOLDER
SmithKline Beecham plc
980 Great West Road
Brentford
Middlesex TW8 9GS
Trading as:
GlaxoSmithKline UK,
Stockley Park West
Uxbridge
Middlesex UB11 1BT

8. MARKETING AUTHORISATION NUMBER(S)
PL 10592/0118

9. DATE OF FIRST AUTHORISATION/RENEWAL OF THE AUTHORISATION
Date of first authorization: 27 February 1998
Renewal of the authorization: 30 December 2002

10. DATE OF REVISION OF THE TEXT
07/08/2009

Fluorouracil Injection, 25 mg / ml, solution for injection (Medac UK)

(medac GmbH)

1. NAME OF THE MEDICINAL PRODUCT
5-Fluorouracil injection, 25 mg / ml, solution for injection

2. QUALITATIVE AND QUANTITATIVE COMPOSITION
One vial of 5-Fluorouracil injection contains:

2500 mg Fluorouracil in 100 ml solution (25 mg/ml)

For excipients, see 6.1

3. PHARMACEUTICAL FORM
Solution for injection

5-Fluorouracil injection, 25 mg / ml, solution for injection is a clear, colourless or almost colourless solution.

4. CLINICAL PARTICULARS

4.1 Therapeutic indications
5-Fluorouracil injection 25 mg/ml, solution for injection, may be used alone or in combination, for its palliative action in the management of common malignancies particularly cancer of the colon and breast, either as single agent or in combination with other cytotoxic agents.

4.2 Posology and method of administration
Routes of administration:

Fluorouracil Injection can be given by intravenous injection or intravenous or intra-arterial infusion.

Adults:

Selection of an appropriate dose and treatment regime depends upon the condition of the patient, the type of carcinoma being treated and whether Fluorouracil is to be administered alone or in combination with other therapy. Initial treatment should be given in hospital and the total daily dose should not exceed 0.8 - 1 gram. It is customary to calculate the dose in accordance with the patient's actual bodyweight unless there is obesity, oedema or some other form of abnormal fluid retention such as ascites. In this case, ideal weight is used as the basis for calculation.

Reduction of the dose is advisable in patients with any of the following:

1. Cachexia.
2. Major surgery within preceding 30 days.
3. Reduced bone marrow function.
4. Impaired hepatic or renal function.

ADULT DOSE

The following regimen have been recommended for use as a single agent-

Initial Treatment:

this may be in the form of an infusion or an injection, the former usually being preferred because of lesser toxicity.

Intravenous Infusion:

15 mg/kg bodyweight but not more than 1 g per infusion, diluted in 300 - 500 ml of 5% glucose or 0.9% NaCl injection and given over 4 hours. Alternatively the daily dose may be infused over 30-60 minutes or may be given as a continuous infusion over 24 hours. The infusion may be repeated daily until there is evidence of toxicity or a total dose of 12-15 g has been reached.

Intravenous Injection:

12 mg/kg bodyweight may be given daily for 3 days and then, if there is no evidence of toxicity, 6 mg/kg on alternate days for 3 further doses. An alternative regime is 15 mg/kg as a single intravenous injection once a week throughout the course.

Intra-arterial Infusion:

5 - 7.5 mg/kg bodyweight daily may be given by 24 hour continuous intra-arterial infusion.

Maintenance Therapy:

An initial intensive course may be followed by maintenance therapy providing there are no significant toxic effects.

In all instances, toxic side effects must disappear before maintenance therapy is started.

The initial course of Fluorouracil can be repeated after an interval of 4 to 6 weeks from the last dose or, alternatively, treatment can be continued with intravenous injections of 5-15 mg/kg bodyweight at weekly intervals.

This sequence constitutes a course of therapy. Some patients have received up to 30 g at a maximum rate of 1 g daily. A more recent alternative method is to give 15 mg/kg IV once a week throughout the course of treatment. This obviates the need for an initial period of daily administration.

In combination with Irradiation:

Irradiation combined with 5-FU has been found to be useful in the treatment of certain types of metastatic lesions in the lungs and for the relief of pain caused by recurrent, inoperable growth. The standard dose of 5-FU should be used.

CHILDREN:

No recommendations are made regarding the use of Fluorouracil in children.

ELDERLY:

Fluorouracil should be used in the elderly with similar considerations as with normal adult doses.

4.3 Contraindications
Fluorouracil is contraindicated in seriously debilitated patients or those with bone marrow depression after radiotherapy or treatment with other antineoplastic agents.

Fluorouracil is strictly contraindicated in pregnant or breast feeding women.

Fluorouracil should not be used in the management of non-malignant disease.

4.4 Special warnings and precautions for use
It is recommended that Fluorouracil should only be given by, or under the strict supervision of, a qualified physician who is conversant with the use of potent antimetabolites.

All patients should be admitted to hospital for initial treatment.

Adequate treatment with Fluorouracil is usually followed by leucopenia, the lowest white blood cell (W.B.C.) count commonly being observed between the 7th and 14th day of the first course, but occasionally being delayed for as long as 20 days.

The count usually returns to normal by the 30th day. Daily monitoring of platelet and W.B.C. count is recommended and treatment should be stopped if platelets fall below 100,000 per mm^3 or the W.B.C. count falls below 3,500 per mm^3. If the total count is less than 2000 per mm^3, and especially if there is granulocytopenia, it is recommended that the patient be placed in protective isolation in the hospital and treated with appropriate measures to prevent systemic infection.

Treatment should also be stopped at the first sign of oral ulceration or if there is evidence of gastrointestinal side effects such as stomatitis, diarrhoea, bleeding from the G.I. tract or haemorrhage at any site. The ratio between effective and toxic dose is small and therapeutic response is unlikely without some degree of toxicity. Care must be taken therefore, in the selection of patients and adjustment of dosage.

Fluorouracil should be used with caution in patients with reduced renal or liver function or jaundice. Isolated cases of angina, ECG abnormalities and rarely, myocardial infarction have been reported following administration of Fluorouracil. Caution should therefore be exercised in treating patients who experience chest pain during courses of treatment, or patients with a history of heart disease.

4.5 Interaction with other medicinal products and other forms of interaction

Drug Interactions

Various agents have been reported to biochemically modulate the antitumour efficacy or toxicity of Fluorouracil, common drugs include Methotrexate, Metronidazole, Leucovorin as well as Allopurinol and Cimetidine which can affect the availability of the active drug.

4.6 Pregnancy and lactation

Fluorouracil is strictly contraindicated in pregnant and breast feeding women.

4.7 Effects on ability to drive and use machines

Not applicable

4.8 Undesirable effects

Diarrhoea, nausea and vomiting are observed quite commonly during therapy and may be treated symptomatically. An anti-emetic may be given for nausea and vomiting.

Alopecia may be seen in a substantial number of cases, particularly in females, but is reversible. Other side effects include dermatitis, pigmentation, changes in the nails, ataxia and fever.

There have been reports of chest pain, tachycardia, breathlessness and E.C.G. changes after administration of Fluorouracil. Special attention is therefore advisable in treating patients with a history of heart disease or those who develop chest pain during treatment.

Leucopenia is common and the precautions described above should be followed.

Systemic Fluorouracil treatment has been associated with various types of ocular toxicity.

Additionally several other reports have been noted including:

Incidences of excessive lacrimation, dacryostenosis, visual changes and photophobia.

A transient reversible cerebellar syndrome can occur after the use of 5-Fluorouracil. Rarely, a reversible confusional state may occur. Both neurological conditions usually respond to withdrawal of 5-fluorouracil.

Palmar-Plantar Erythrodysesthesia Syndrome has been reported as an unusual complication of high dose bolus or protracted continuous therapy with Fluorouracil.

Thrombophlebitis/Vein tracking.

4.9 Overdose

The symptoms and signs of overdosage are qualitatively similar to the adverse reactions and should be managed as indicated under *'Other Undesirable effects'* and *'Precautions and Special Warnings'*.

5. PHARMACOLOGICAL PROPERTIES

5.1 Pharmacodynamic properties

Fluorouracil is an analogue of uracil, a component of ribonucleic acid. The drug is believed to function as an antimetabolite. After intracellular conversion to the active deoxynucleotide, it interferes with the synthesis of DNA by blocking the conversion of deoxyuridylic acid to thymidylic acid by the cellular enzyme thymidylate synthetase. Fluorouracil may also interfere with RNA synthesis.

Pharmacotherapeutic group:	Antimetabolite
ATC code:	L01B C02

5.2 Pharmacokinetic properties

After intravenous administration, Fluorouracil is distributed through the body water and disappears from the blood within 3 hours. It is preferentially taken up by actively dividing tissues and tumours after conversion to its nucleotide. Fluorouracil readily enters the C.S.F. and brain tissue.

Following IV administration, the plasma elimination half-life averages about 16 minutes and is dose dependant. Following a single IV dose of Fluorouracil approximately 15 % of the dose is excreted unchanged in the urine within 6 hours; over 90% of this is excreted in the first hour. The remainder is mostly metabolised in the liver by the usual body mechanisms for uracil.

5.3 Preclinical safety data

not applicable

6. PHARMACEUTICAL PARTICULARS

6.1 List of excipients

Sodium hydroxide, water for injections

6.2 Incompatibilities

5-Fluorouracil is incompatible with Carboplatin, Cisplatin, Cytarabine, Diazepam, Doxorubicin, other Anthracyclines and possibly Methotrexate.

Formulated solutions are alkaline and it is recommended that admixture with acidic drug preparations should be avoided.

6.3 Shelf life

18 months

5-Fluorouracil injection 25 mg/ml, solution for injection, is intended for single use only.

The chemical and physical in-use stability of the solution diluted with glucose 5% or sodium chloride 0.9% injection has been demonstrated for 24 hours at a temperature not exceeding 25°C.

From a microbiological point of view, the product should be used immediately. If not used immediately, in use storage times and conditions prior to use are the responsibility of the user and would normally not be longer than 24 hours at 2 - 8°C, unless dilution has taken place in controlled and validated aseptic conditions.

6.4 Special precautions for storage

Do not store above 25°C.

Do not refrigerate or freeze.

Keep container in outer carton.

If a precipitate has formed as a result of exposure to low temperatures, redissolve by heating to 40°C accompanied by vigorous shaking. Allow to cool to body temperature prior to use.

6.5 Nature and contents of container

Type I conventional clear glass vials, rubber closures. The rubber stopper is protected by a flanged aluminium cap with a flip-off top.

2500 mg/ 100 ml: Pack Size: Singles, 10

6.6 Special precautions for disposal and other handling

5-Fluorouracil injection 25 mg/ml, solution for injection, should only be opened by trained staff and as with all cytotoxic agents, precautions should be taken to avoid exposing staff during pregnancy. Preparation of solution for administration should be carried out in a designated handling area and working over a washable tray or disposable plastic-backed absorbent paper.

Suitable eye protection, disposable gloves, face mask and disposable apron should be worn. Syringes and infusion sets should be assembled carefully to avoid leakage (use of Luer lock fittings is recommended).

On completion, any exposed surface should be thoroughly cleaned and hands and face washed.

Fluorouracil is an irritant, contact with skin and mucous membranes should be avoided.

In the event of spillage, operators should put on gloves, face masks, eye-protection and disposable apron and mop up the spilled material with an absorbent material tapped in the area for that purpose. The area should then be cleaned and all contaminated material transferred to a cytotoxic spillage bag or bin or sealed for incineration.

Disposal:

All materials that have been utilised for dilution and administration should be disposed of according to standard procedures (incineration).

Diluents:

5-Fluorouracil injection, 25 mg/ml, solution for injection may be diluted with 5% glucose or 0.9% sodium chloride intravenous infusions immediately before parenteral use. The remainder of solutions should be discarded after use; do not make up into multi-dose preparations.

First aid:

Eye contact: Irrigate immediately with water and seek medical advice

Skin contact: Wash thoroughly with soap and water and remove contaminated clothing.

Inhalation, Ingestion: Seek medical advice.

7. MARKETING AUTHORISATION HOLDER

medac

Gesellschaft für klinische Spezialpräparate mbH

Fehlandtstrasse 3

D-20354 Hamburg

8. MARKETING AUTHORISATION NUMBER(S)

PL 11587 / 0023

9. DATE OF FIRST AUTHORISATION/RENEWAL OF THE AUTHORISATION

30 July 2003

10. DATE OF REVISION OF THE TEXT

07 March 2003

Fluorouracil Injection, 50 mg / ml, solution for injection (Medac UK)

(medac GmbH)

1. NAME OF THE MEDICINAL PRODUCT

Fluorouracil Injection, 50 mg / ml, solution for injection

2. QUALITATIVE AND QUANTITATIVE COMPOSITION

One vial of Fluorouracil Injection contains:

500 mg fluorouracil in 10 ml solution (50 mg/ml)

1000 mg fluorouracil in 20 ml solution (50 mg/ml)

2500 mg fluorouracil in 50 ml solution (50 mg/ml)

5000 mg fluorouracil in 100 ml solution (50 mg/ml)

For a full list of excipients, see section 6.1.

3. PHARMACEUTICAL FORM

Solution for injection

Fluorouracil Injection, 50 mg / ml, solution for injection is a clear, colourless or almost colourless solution.

4. CLINICAL PARTICULARS

4.1 Therapeutic indications

Fluorouracil Injection, 50 mg/ml, solution for injection, may be used alone or in combination, for its palliative action in the management of common malignancies particularly cancer of the colon and breast, either as single agent or in combination with other cytotoxic agents.

4.2 Posology and method of administration

Routes of administration:

Fluorouracil Injection can be given by intravenous injection or intravenous or intra-arterial infusion.

Adults:

Selection of an appropriate dose and treatment regime depends upon the condition of the patient, the type of carcinoma being treated and whether fluorouracil is to be administered alone or in combination with other therapy. Initial treatment should be given in hospital and the total daily dose should not exceed 1 gram. It is customary to calculate the dose in accordance with the patient's actual bodyweight unless there is obesity, oedema or some other form of abnormal fluid retention such as ascites. In this case, ideal weight is used as the basis for calculation.

Reduction of the dose is advisable in patients with any of the following:

1. Cachexia.
2. Major surgery within preceding 30 days.
3. Reduced bone marrow function.
4. Impaired hepatic or renal function.

ADULT DOSE:

The following regimens have been recommended for use as a single agent:

Initial Treatment:

This may be in the form of an infusion or an injection, the former usually being preferred because of lesser toxicity.

Intravenous Infusion:

15 mg/kg bodyweight but not more than 1 g per infusion, diluted in 500 ml of 5 % glucose or 0.9 % NaCl injection and given by intravenous infusion at a rate of 40 drops per minute over 4 hours. Alternatively the daily dose may be infused over 30 – 60 minutes or may be given as a continuous infusion over 24 hours. The infusion may be repeated daily until there is evidence of toxicity or a total dose of 12 – 15 g has been reached.

Intravenous Injection:

12 mg/kg bodyweight may be given daily for 3 days and then, if there is no evidence of toxicity, 6 mg/kg on alternate days for 3 further doses. An alternative regime is 15 mg/kg as a single intravenous injection once a week throughout the course.

Intra-arterial Infusion:

5 – 7.5 mg/kg bodyweight daily may be given by 24 hour continuous intra-arterial infusion.

Maintenance Therapy:

An initial intensive course may be followed by maintenance therapy providing there are no significant toxic effects. In all instances, toxic side effects must disappear before maintenance therapy is started.

The initial course of fluorouracil can be repeated after an interval of 4 to 6 weeks from the last dose or, alternatively, treatment can be continued with intravenous injections of 5 – 15 mg/kg bodyweight at weekly intervals.

This sequence constitutes a course of therapy. Some patients have received up to 30 g at a maximum rate of 1 g daily. A more recent alternative method is to give 15 mg/kg IV once a week throughout the course of treatment. This obviates the need for an initial period of daily administration.

In combination with Irradiation: Irradiation combined with fluorouracil has been found to be useful in the treatment of certain types of metastatic lesions in the lungs and for the relief of pain caused by recurrent, inoperable growth. The standard dose of fluorouracil should be used.

CHILDREN:

No recommendations are made regarding the use of Fluorouracil in children.

ELDERLY:

Fluorouracil should be used in the elderly with similar considerations as with normal adult doses.

4.3 Contraindications

Fluorouracil is contraindicated in seriously debilitated patients or those with bone marrow depression after radiotherapy or treatment with other antineoplastic agents.

Fluorouracil is strictly contraindicated in pregnant or breast feeding women.

Fluorouracil should not be used in the management of non-malignant disease.

Fluorouracil is contraindicated in patients who have had a serious hypersensitivity reaction to previous doses of fluorouracil or any of its constituents.

Fluorouracil must not be taken or used concomitantly with brivudin, sorivudine and analogues. Brivudin, sorivudine and analogues are potent inhibitors of the enzyme dihydropyrimidine dehydrogenase (DPD) which degrades fluorouracil (see also sections 4.4 and 4.5).

4.4 Special warnings and precautions for use

It is recommended that fluorouracil should only be given by, or under the strict supervision of, a qualified physician who is conversant with the use of potent antimetabolites.

All patients should be admitted to hospital for initial treatment.

Adequate treatment with fluorouracil is usually followed by leukopenia, the lowest white blood cell (W.B.C.) count commonly being observed between the 7th and 14th day of the first course, but occasionally being delayed for as long as 20 days.

The count usually returns to normal by the 30th day. Daily monitoring of platelet and W.B.C. count is recommended and treatment should be stopped if platelets fall below 100,000 per mm^3 or the W.B.C. count falls below 3,500 per mm^3. If the total count is less than 2,000 per mm^3, and especially if there is granulocytopenia, it is recommended that the patient be placed in protective isolation in the hospital and treated with appropriate measures to prevent systemic infection.

Treatment should also be stopped at the first sign of oral ulceration or if there is evidence of gastrointestinal side effects such as stomatitis, diarrhoea, bleeding from the G.I. tract or haemorrhage at any site. The ratio between effective and toxic dose is small and therapeutic response is unlikely without some degree of toxicity. Care must be taken therefore, in the selection of patients and adjustment of dosage.

Fluorouracil should be used with caution in patients with reduced renal or liver function or jaundice. Isolated cases of angina, ECG abnormalities and rarely, myocardial infarction have been reported following administration of fluorouracil. Caution should therefore be exercised in treating patients who experience chest pain during courses of treatment, or patients with a history of heart disease.

There have been reports of increased toxicity in patients who have reduced activity/deficiency of the enzyme dihydropyrimidine dehydrogenase. The enzyme dihydropyrimidine dehydrogenase (DPD) plays an important role in the degradation of fluorouracil. The nucleoside analogues, such as brivudin and sorivudine, can cause a sharp rise in the plasma concentration of 5-fluorouracil or other fluoropyrimidines, with accompanying toxic reactions. For this reason, a period of at least 4 weeks should elapse between taking or using fluorouracil and taking or using brivudin, sorivudine and analogues.

Where applicable, determination of DPD enzyme activity is indicated before starting treatment with 5-fluorpyrimidines. In the event of accidental administration of brivudin to patients being treated with fluorouracil, effective measures should be taken to reduce the toxicity of fluorouracil. Immediate admission to hospital is recommended. All measures should be initiated to prevent systemic infections and dehydration.

Patients taking phenytoin concomitantly with fluorouracil should undergo regular testing because of the possibility of an elevated plasma level of phenytoin.

4.5 Interaction with other medicinal products and other forms of interaction

Various agents have been reported to biochemically modulate the antitumour efficacy or toxicity of fluorouracil, common drugs include methotrexate, metronidazole, leucovorin as well as allopurinol and cimetidine which can affect the availability of the active drug.

Marked elevations of prothrombin time and INR have been reported in a few patients stabilised on warfarin therapy following initiation of fluorouracil regimes.

The enzyme dihydropyrimidine dehydrogenase (DPD) plays an important role in the degradation of fluorouracil. The nucleoside analogues such as brivudin and sorivudine can cause a sharp rise in the plasma concentration of 5-fluorouracil or other fluoropyrimidines, with accompanying toxic reactions. For this reason, a period of at least 4 weeks should elapse between taking or using fluorouracil and taking or using brivudin, sorivudine and analogues. Where applicable, determination of DPD enzyme activity is indicated before starting treatment with 5-fluorpyrimidines.

Where phenytoin and fluorouracil have been administered concomitantly, there have been reports of elevated plasma levels of phenytoin, resulting in symptoms of phenytoin intoxication (see 4.4).

Fluorouracil should be avoided in combination with clozapine due to the increased risk of agranulocytosis.

4.6 Pregnancy and lactation

Fluorouracil is strictly contraindicated in pregnant and breast feeding women.

4.7 Effects on ability to drive and use machines

Fluorouracil may induce side effects such as nausea and vomiting which could interfere with driving or the use of heavy machinery.

4.8 Undesirable effects

The most commonly reported undesirable effects are diarrhoea, nausea. Leukopenia is also very common and the precautions described above should be followed.

Frequency assessment:

Very common (⩾ 1/10)

Common (⩾ 1/100, < 1/10)

Uncommon (⩾ 1/1,000, < 1/100)

Rare (⩾ 1/10,000, < 1/1,000)

Very rare (< 1/10,000), not known

Infections and infestations	Very common Infections Uncommon Sepsis
Blood and lymphatic system disorders	Very common Leukopenia, myelosuppression, neutropenia, granulocytopenia, thrombocytopenia, anemia, pancytopenia Rare Agranulocytosis
Immune system disorders	Very common Immunosuppression Very rare Anaphylactic reaction, anaphylactic shock
Endocrine disorders	Rare Increase of T4 (total thyroxin), increase of T3 (total trijodthyronin)
Metabolism and nutrition disorders	Uncommon Hyperuricemia
Psychiatric disorders	Rare Confusion
Nervous system disorders	Rare Ataxia, extrapyramidalmotoric disturbances, cerebellar disturbances, cortical disturbances, nystagmus, headache, vertigo, parkinson-like symptoms, pyramid signs, euphoria, leuko-encephalopathy, speech disorders, aphasia, convulsions, coma, opticus neuritis, peripheral neuropathy
Eye disorders	Common Conjunctivitis Uncommon Excessive lacrimation, dacryostenosis, visual changes, photophobia, diplopia, decreased visus, blepharitis, ectropion
Cardiac disorders	Common Chest pain, tachycardia, ECG-changes, angina pectoris Rare Arrhythmia, myocardial infarction, myocarditis, heart failure, dilatative cardiomyopathy, cardiac shock, heart arrest, sudden cardiac death
Vascular disorders	Rare Vasculitis, Raynaud's phenomenon, cerebral ischaemia, intestinal ischaemia, peripheral ischaemia, thromboembolism
Respiratory, thoracic and mediastinal disorders	Uncommon Epistaxis, dyspnea, bronchospasmus
Gastrointestinal disorders	Very common Diarrhoea, nausea, vomiting, mucositis, stomatitis Uncommon Gastrointestinal ulceration, gastrointestinal hemorrhage
Hepatobiliary disorders	Uncommon Liver cell damage Rare Liver necrosis
Skin and subcutaneous tissue disorders	Very common Alopecia, palmar-plantar erythrodysesthesia Uncommon Dermatitis, hyperpigmentation, hypopigmentation, nail discoloration, nail hyperpigmentation, nail dystrophy, nailbed pain, nailbed inflammation, onycholysis, exanthema, dry skin, urticaria, photosensitivity, recall phenomenon
General disorders and administration site conditions	Very common Fever, fatigue Uncommon Thrombophlebitis, vein tracking, dehydration

4.9 Overdose

Manifestations of overdosage of fluorouracil can be nausea, vomiting, diarrhoea, gastrointestinal ulceration and bleeding, bone marrow depression (including thrombocytopenia, leukopenia and agranulocytosis). No specific antidotal therapy exists. Patients who have been exposed to an overdose of fluorouracil should be monitored haematologically for at least four weeks. Should abnormalities appear, appropriate therapy should be utilised.

5. PHARMACOLOGICAL PROPERTIES

5.1 Pharmacodynamic properties

Fluorouracil is an analogue of uracil, a component of ribonucleic acid. The drug is believed to function as an antimetabolite. After intracellular conversion to the active deoxynucleotide, it interferes with the synthesis of DNA by blocking the conversion of deoxyuridylic acid to thymidylic acid by the cellular enzyme thymidylate synthetase. Fluorouracil may also interfere with RNA synthesis.

Pharmacotherapeutic group: Antimetabolite

ATC code: L01B C02

5.2 Pharmacokinetic properties

After intravenous administration, fluorouracil is distributed through the body water and disappears from the blood within 3 hours. It is preferentially taken up by actively dividing tissues and tumours after conversion to its nucleotide. Fluorouracil readily enters the C.S.F. and brain tissue.

Following IV administration, the plasma elimination half-life averages about 16 minutes and is dose dependant. Following a single IV dose of fluorouracil approximately 15 % of the dose is excreted unchanged in the urine within 6 hours; over 90 % of this is excreted in the first hour. The remainder is mostly metabolised in the liver by the usual body mechanisms for uracil.

5.3 Preclinical safety data

Not applicable

6. PHARMACEUTICAL PARTICULARS

6.1 List of excipients

Sodium hydroxide, water for injections

6.2 Incompatibilities

Fluorouracil is incompatible with calcium folinate, carboplatin, cisplatin, cytarabine, diazepam, doxorubicin, droperidol, filgrastim, gallium nitrate, methotrexate, metoclopramide, morphine, ondansetron, parenteral nutrition, vinorelbin, other anthracylines.

Formulated solutions are alkaline and it is recommended that admixture with acidic drug preparations should be avoided.

6.3 Shelf life

2 years

Fluorouracil Injection, 50 mg/ml, solution for injection, is intended for single use only.

The chemical and physical in-use stability of the solution diluted with glucose or sodium chloride injection has been demonstrated for 24 hours at a temperature not exceeding 25°C.

From a microbiological point of view, the product should be used immediately. If not used immediately, in-use storage times and conditions prior to use are the responsibility of the user and would normally not be longer than 24 hours at 2 – 8°C, unless dilution has taken place in controlled and validated aseptic conditions.

6.4 Special precautions for storage

Do not store Fluorouracil Injection, 50 mg/ml, solution for injection above 25°C.

Do not refrigerate or freeze.

Keep the container in the outer carton.

If a precipitate has formed as a result of exposure to low temperatures, redissolve by heating to 40 °C accompanied by vigorous shaking. Allow to cool to body temperature prior to use.

6.5 Nature and contents of container

Type I conventional clear glass vials, rubber closures. The rubber stopper is protected by a flanged aluminium cap with a flip-off top.

500 mg/ 10 ml: Pack Size: Singles, 10

1000 mg/ 20 ml: Pack Size: Singles, 10

2500 mg/ 50 ml: Pack Size: Singles, 10

5000 mg/100 ml: Pack Size: Singles, 10

6.6 Special precautions for disposal and other handling

Fluorouracil Injection, 50 mg/ml, solution for injection should be administered only by or under the direct supervision of a qualified physician who is experienced in the use of cancer chemotherapeutic agents.

Fluorouracil Injection should only be prepared for administration by professionals who have been trained in the safe use of the preparation. Preparation should only be carried out in an aseptic cabinet or suite dedicated for the assembly of cytotoxics.

In the event of spillage, operators should put on gloves, face mask, eye-protection and disposable apron and mop up the spilled material with an absorbent material kept in the area for that purpose. The area should then be cleaned and all contaminated material transferred to a cytotoxic spillage bag or bin and sealed for incineration.

Contamination

Fluorouracil is an irritant, contact with skin and mucous membranes should be avoided. In the event of contact with the skin or eyes, the affected area should be washed with copious amounts of water or normal saline. A bland cream may be used to treat the transient stinging of the skin. Medical advice should be sought if the eyes are affected or if the preparation is inhaled or ingested.

Preparation Guidelines

a) Chemotherapeutic agents should be prepared for administration only by professionals who have been trained in the safe use of the preparation.

b) Operations such as reconstitution of powder and transfer to syringes should be carried out only under aseptic conditions in a suite or cabinet dedicated for the assembly of cytotoxics.

c) The personnel carrying out these procedures should be adequately protected with clothing, gloves and eye shield.

d) Pregnant personnel are advised not to handle chemotherapeutic agents.

Disposal:

All materials that have been utilised for dilution and administration should be disposed of according to standard procedures (incineration).

Diluents:

Fluorouracil may be diluted with 5 % glucose or 0.9 % sodium chloride intravenous infusions immediately before parenteral use. The remainder of solutions should be discarded after use; do not make up into multi-dose preparations.

Administrative Data

7. MARKETING AUTHORISATION HOLDER

medac

Gesellschaft für klinische Spezialpräparate mbH

Fehlandtstr. 3

20354 Hamburg

Germany

8. MARKETING AUTHORISATION NUMBER(S)

PL 11587/0015

9. DATE OF FIRST AUTHORISATION/RENEWAL OF THE AUTHORISATION

6 July 2000 / 11 October 2006

10. DATE OF REVISION OF THE TEXT

November 2007

Fluvirin, suspension for injection in pre-filled syringe

(Novartis Vaccines)

1. NAME OF THE MEDICINAL PRODUCT

FLUVIRIN®, suspension for injection in pre-filled syringe. [Influenza Vaccine (Surface Antigen, Inactivated)]

2. QUALITATIVE AND QUANTITATIVE COMPOSITION

Influenza virus surface antigens (haemagglutinin and neuraminidase) of the following strains*:

A/Brisbane/59/2007 (H1N1)-like strain (A/Brisbane/59/2007, IVR-148) 15 micrograms HA**

A/Brisbane/10/2007 (H3N2)-like strain (A/Uruguay/716/2007, NYMC X-175C) 15 micrograms HA**

B/Brisbane/60/2008-like strain (B/Brisbane/60/2008) 15 micrograms HA**

per 0.5 ml dose.

* propagated in fertilised hens' eggs from healthy chicken flocks

** haemagglutinin

This vaccine complies with the WHO recommendation (Northern hemisphere) and EU decision for the 2009/2010 season.

For a full list of excipients see section 6.1.

3. PHARMACEUTICAL FORM

Suspension for injection in pre-filled syringe.

4. CLINICAL PARTICULARS

4.1 Therapeutic indications

Prophylaxis of influenza, especially in those who run an increased risk of associated complications.

The use of FLUVIRIN® should be based on official recommendations.

4.2 Posology and method of administration

Adults and children from 4 years: 0.5 ml.

For children, who have not previously been vaccinated, a second dose should be given after an interval of at least 4 weeks.

Immunisation should be carried out by intramuscular or deep subcutaneous injection.

For instructions for preparation, see section 6.6.

4.3 Contraindications

Hypersensitivity to the active substances, to any of the excipients and to eggs, or chicken proteins. FLUVIRIN® does not contain more than 1 microgram ovalbumin per dose. The vaccine may contain residues of the following substances, betapropriolactone, nonoxynol 9, neomycin, polymixin, formaldehyde or thiomersal.

Immunisation shall be postponed in patients with febrile illness or acute infection.

4.4 Special warnings and precautions for use

As with all injectable vaccines, appropriate medical treatment and supervision should always be readily available in case of a rare anaphylactic event following the administration of the vaccine.

FLUVIRIN® should under no circumstances be administered intravascularly.

Antibody response in patients with endogenous or iatrogenic immunosuppression may be insufficient.

Thiomersal (an organomercuric compound) has been used in the manufacturing process of this medicinal product and residues of it are present in the final product. Therefore, sensitisation reactions may occur (see section 4.3). The maximum thiomersal content in FLUVIRIN® is 0.002mg (0.0004% w/v).

4.5 Interaction with other medicinal products and other forms of interaction

FLUVIRIN® may be given at the same time as other vaccines. Immunisation should be carried out on separate limbs. It should be noted that the adverse reactions may be intensified.

The immunological response may be diminished if the patient is undergoing immunosuppressant treatment.

Following influenza vaccination, false positive results in serology tests using the ELISA method to detect antibodies against HIV1, Hepatitis C and especially HTLV1 have been observed. The Western Blot technique disproves the false-positive ELISA test results. The transient false positive reactions could be due to the IgM response by the vaccine.

4.6 Pregnancy and lactation

The limited data from vaccinations in pregnant women do not indicate that adverse foetal and maternal outcomes were attributable to the vaccine. The use of this vaccine may be considered from the second trimester of pregnancy. For pregnant women with medical conditions that increase their risk of complications from influenza, administration of the vaccine is recommended, irrespective of their stage of pregnancy.

FLUVIRIN® may be used during lactation.

4.7 Effects on ability to drive and use machines

The vaccine is unlikely to produce an effect on the ability to drive and use machines.

4.8 Undesirable effects

Adverse reactions observed from clinical trials

The safety of trivalent inactivated influenza vaccines is assessed in open label, uncontrolled clinical trials performed as annual update requirement, including at least 50 adults aged 18 – 60 years of age and at least 50 elderly aged 61 years or older. Safety evaluation is performed during the first 3 days following vaccination.

The following undesirable effects have been observed during clinical trials with the following frequencies:

very common (≥1/10); common (≥1/100, <1/10); uncommon (≥1/1000, <1/100); rare (≥1/10000, <1/1000); very rare (<1/10000), including isolated reports.

(see Table 1 below)

Adverse reactions reported from post-marketing surveillance

Adverse reactions reported from post marketing surveillance are, next to the reactions which have also been observed during the clinical trials, the following:

Blood and lymphatic system disorders:

Transient thrombocytopenia, transient lymphadenopathy

Immune system disorders:

Allergic reactions, in rare cases leading to shock, angioedema

Nervous system disorders:

Neuralgia, paraesthesia, febril convulsions, neurological disorders, such as encephalomyelitis, neuritis and Guillain Barré syndrome

Vascular disorders:

Vasculitis associated in very rare cases with transient renal involvement

Skin and subcutaneous tissue disorders:

Generalised skin reactions including pruritus, urticaria or non-specific rash

4.9 Overdose

Overdosage is unlikely to have any untoward effect.

5. PHARMACOLOGICAL PROPERTIES

5.1 Pharmacodynamic properties

Pharmacotherapeutic group: Influenza vaccine, ATC Code: J07BB02

Seroprotection is generally obtained within 2 to 3 weeks. The duration of postvaccinal immunity to homologous strains or to strains closely related to the vaccine strains varies but is usually 6-12 months.

5.2 Pharmacokinetic properties

Not applicable

5.3 Preclinical safety data

Not applicable

6. PHARMACEUTICAL PARTICULARS

6.1 List of excipients

Buffer solution:

Potassium dihydrogen phosphate

Disodium hydrogen phosphate

Sodium chloride

Water for injection.

6.2 Incompatibilities

In the absence of compatibility studies, this medicinal product must not be mixed with other medicinal products.

6.3 Shelf life

1 year.

6.4 Special precautions for storage

Store at +2°C to +8°C (in a refrigerator). Do not freeze. Keep container in the original carton.

6.5 Nature and contents of container

0.5 ml in pre-filled syringe (glass, type I) with stopper (rubber), fitted with a stainless steel needle, pack sizes of 1 and 10 syringes.

Not all pack sizes may be marketed.

6.6 Special precautions for disposal and other handling

Unused vaccine and other waste material should be disposed of in compliance with local rules for the disposal of products of this nature.

The vaccine should be allowed to reach room temperature before use.

Shake before use.

7. MARKETING AUTHORISATION HOLDER

Novartis Vaccines and Diagnostics Limited

Gaskill Road

Speke

Liverpool

L24 9GR

UK.

8. MARKETING AUTHORISATION NUMBER(S)

PL 18532/0038.

9. DATE OF FIRST AUTHORISATION/RENEWAL OF THE AUTHORISATION

Date of first authorisation: 7 June 2006

10. DATE OF REVISION OF THE TEXT

June 2009

Table 1

Organ class	Very common ≥ 1/10	Common ≥ 1/100, < 1/10	Uncommon ≥ 1/1000, < 1/100	Rare ≥ 1/10000, < 1/1000	Very rare < 1/10000
Nervous system disorders		Headache*			
Skin and subcutaneous tissue disorders		Sweating*			
Musculoskeletal and connective tissue disorders		Myalgia, arthralgia*			
General disorders and administration site conditions		Fever, malaise, shivering, fatigue. Local reactions: redness, swelling, pain, ecchymosis, induration*			

* these reactions usually disappear within 1-2 days without treatment

FML

(Allergan Ltd)

1. NAME OF THE MEDICINAL PRODUCT
FML Liquifilm Ophthalmic Suspension

2. QUALITATIVE AND QUANTITATIVE COMPOSITION
Fluorometholone 0.10% w/v

3. PHARMACEUTICAL FORM
Sterile Ophthalmic Suspension

4. CLINICAL PARTICULARS

4.1 Therapeutic indications
For steroid-responsive inflammation of the palpebral and bulbar conjunctiva, cornea and anterior segment of the globe.

4.2 Posology and method of administration
Route of administration: topical ophthalmic administration.

Adults: One to two drops instilled into the conjunctival sac two to four times daily. During the initial 24 to 48 hours the dosage may be safely increased to 2 drops every hour. Care should be taken not to discontinue therapy prematurely.

Children: Not recommended for children aged two and under.

4.3 Contraindications
Acute superficial herpes simplex (dendritic) keratitis, vaccinia, varicella and most other viral diseases of the conjunctiva and cornea. Ocular tuberculosis. Fungal diseases of the eye. Hypersensitivity to any of the constituents of the medication.

4.4 Special warnings and precautions for use
Steroid medication in the treatment of herpes simplex keratitis (involving the stroma) requires great caution: frequent slit-lamp microscopy is mandatory. Prolonged use may result in glaucoma, damage to the optic nerve, defects in visual acuity and fields of vision, posterior subcapsular cataract formation, or may aid in the establishment of secondary ocular infections from fungi or viruses liberated from ocular tissue.

In those diseases causing thinning of the cornea or sclera, perforation has been known to occur with use of topical steroids.

Safety and effectiveness have not been demonstrated in children of the age group two years or below.

This preparation contains benzalkonium chloride and should not be used by patients continuing to wear soft (hydrophilic) contact lenses.

As fungal infections of the cornea are particularly prone to develop coincidentally with long term local steroid applications, fungus invasion must be suspected in any persistent corneal ulceration where a steroid has been or is in use.

Intraocular pressure should be checked frequently.

4.5 Interaction with other medicinal products and other forms of interaction
None known.

4.6 Pregnancy and lactation
There is inadequate evidence of safety in human pregnancy. Administration of corticosteroids to pregnant animals can cause abnormalities of foetal development including cleft palate and intra-uterine growth retardation. There may therefore be a very small risk of such effects in the human foetus.

4.7 Effects on ability to drive and use machines
None known.

4.8 Undesirable effects
Glaucoma with optic nerve damage, visual acuity or field defects, posterior subcapsular cataract formation, secondary ocular infection from pathogens liberated from ocular tissues, perforation of the globe.

Local side-effects of steroid therapy, i.e. skin atrophy, striae and telangiectasia, are especially likely to affect facial skin.

4.9 Overdose
Not likely to occur.

5. PHARMACOLOGICAL PROPERTIES

5.1 Pharmacodynamic properties
FML is a synthetic adrenocorticosteroid (glucocorticoid), a derivative of desoxyprednisolone. It forms part of a well-known group of steroids used to treat ocular inflammation. Glucocorticosteroids complex with cytoplasmic receptors and subsequently stimulate synthesis of proteins with anti-inflammatory effects. They inhibit early phenomena of the inflammatory response (oedema, fibrin deposition, capillary dilation, phagocytic migration) as well as capillary proliferation, collagen deposition and scar formation.

Whilst topical corticosteroid therapy frequently increases intraocular pressure in normal eyes and in ocular hypertensive subjects, fluorometholone has a substantially lower propensity to elevate IOP than, for example, dexamethasone.

5.2 Pharmacokinetic properties
Topical application of a 0.1% tritium-labelled-fluorometholone suspension gave rise to peak radioactivity levels in the aqueous humour 30 minutes post-instillation. A high concentration of rapidly-produced metabolite was found both in aqueous humour and corneal extracts, indicating that fluorometholone undergoes metabolic change as it penetrates into the cornea and aqueous humour.

5.3 Preclinical safety data
No information.

6. PHARMACEUTICAL PARTICULARS

6.1 List of excipients
Polyvinyl alcohol
Benzalkonium chloride
Edetate Disodium
Sodium chloride
Sodium phosphate, dibasic, heptahydrate
Sodium phosphate, monobasic, monohydrate
Polysorbate 80
Sodium hydroxide to adjust pH
Purified water

6.2 Incompatibilities
None known.

6.3 Shelf life
36 months unopened.
28 days after first opening.

6.4 Special precautions for storage
Do not store above 25°C. Do not freeze.

6.5 Nature and contents of container
5 ml and 10 ml bottles and dropper tips composed of low density polyethylene. Caps are impact polystyrene.

6.6 Special precautions for disposal and other handling
No information.

7. MARKETING AUTHORISATION HOLDER
Allergan Ltd
The Parkway
Marlow International
Marlow
Bucks
SL7 1YL
UK

8. MARKETING AUTHORISATION NUMBER(S)
PL 00426/0028

9. DATE OF FIRST AUTHORISATION/RENEWAL OF THE AUTHORISATION
15th July 2003

10. DATE OF REVISION OF THE TEXT
20th December 2007

Forane, Isoflurane (Inhalation Anaesthetic)

(Abbott Laboratories Limited)

1. NAME OF THE MEDICINAL PRODUCT
Isoflurane or Forane

2. QUALITATIVE AND QUANTITATIVE COMPOSITION
Isoflurane 99.9% w/w

3. PHARMACEUTICAL FORM
Isoflurane is an inhalation anaesthetic with a mildly pungent ethereal odour. No additive or stabiliser present.

4. CLINICAL PARTICULARS

4.1 Therapeutic indications
Isoflurane is indicated as a general anaesthetic by inhalation.

4.2 Posology and method of administration
Vaporisers specially calibrated for Isoflurane should be used so that the concentration of anaesthetic delivered can be accurately controlled.

MAC values for Isoflurane vary with age. The table below indicates average MAC values for different age groups.

Age	Average MAC Value In 100% Oxygen	70% N_2O
0-1 month	1.60%	
1-6 months	1.87%	
6-12 months	1.80%	
1-5 years	1.60%	
26 ± 4 years	1.28%	0.56%
44 ± 7 years	1.15%	0.50%
64 ± 5 years	1.05%	0.37%

Premedication: Drugs used for premedication should be selected for the individual patient bearing in mind the respiratory depressant effect of Isoflurane. The use of anticholinergic drugs is a matter of choice, but may be advisable for inhalation induction in paediatrics.

Induction: A short-acting barbiturate or other intravenous induction agent is usually administered followed by inhalation of the Isoflurane mixture. Alternatively, Isoflurane with oxygen or with an oxygen/nitrous oxide mixture may be used.

It is recommended that induction with Isoflurane be initiated at a concentration of 0.5%. Concentrations of 1.5 to 3.0% usually produce surgical anaesthesia in 7 to 10 minutes.

Maintenance: Surgical levels of anaesthesia may be maintained with 1.0-2.5% Isoflurane in oxygen/nitrous oxide mixtures. An additional 0.5-1.0% Isoflurane may be required when given with oxygen alone.

For caesarean section, 0.5-0.75% Isoflurane in a mixture of oxygen/nitrous oxide is suitable to maintain anaesthesia for this procedure.

Arterial pressure levels during maintenance tend to be inversely related to alveolor Isoflurane concentrations in the absence of other complicating factors. Excessive falls in blood pressure may be due to depth of anaesthesia and in these circumstances, should be corrected by reducing the inspired Isoflurane concentration.

Elderly: As with other agents, lesser concentrations of Isoflurane are normally required to maintain surgical anaesthesia in elderly patients. See above for MAC values related to age.

4.3 Contraindications
Isoflurane is contra-indicated in patients with known sensitivity to Isoflurane or other halogenated anaesthetics. It is also contraindicated in patients with known or suspected genetic susceptibility to malignant hyperpyrexia.

4.4 Special warnings and precautions for use
Since levels of anaesthesia may be altered quickly and easily with Isoflurane, only vaporisers which deliver a predictable output with reasonable accuracy, or techniques during which inspired or expired concentrations can be monitored, should be used. The degree of hypotension and respiratory depression may provide some indication of anaesthetic depth.

Reports demonstrate that Isoflurane can produce hepatic injury ranging from mild transient increase in liver enzymes to fatal hepatic necrosis in very rare instances. It has been reported that previous exposure to halogenated hydrocarbon anaesthetics, especially if the interval is less than 3 months, may increase the potential for hepatic injury.

As with other halogenated agents, Isoflurane must be used with caution in patients with increased intracranial pressure. In such cases hyperventilation may be necessary.

Isoflurane has been reported to interact with dry carbon dioxide absorbents to form carbon monoxide. In order to minimise the risk of formation of carbon monoxide in rebreathing circuits and the possibility of elevated carboxyhaemoglobin levels, carbon dioxide absorbent should not be allowed to dry out.

Rare cases of extreme heat, smoke and/or spontaneous fire in the anesthesia machine have been reported during the administration of general anesthesia with drugs in this class when used in conjunction with desiccated CO_2 absorbents, specifically those containing potassium hydroxide (e.g. Baralyme). When a clinician suspects that the CO_2 absorbent may be desiccated, it should be replaced before administration of Isoflurane. The colour indicator of most CO_2 absorbents does not necessarily change as a result of desiccation.

Therefore, the lack of significant colour change should not be taken as an assurance of adequate hydration. CO_2 absorbents should be replaced routinely regardless of the state of the colour indicator.

Use of inhaled anaesthetic agents has been associated with very rare increases in serum potassium levels that have resulted in cardiac arrhythmias and death in children during the postoperative period. The condition has been described in patients with latent as well as overt neuromuscular disease, particularly Duchenne muscular dystrophy. Use of suxamethonium has been associated with most, but not all of these cases. These patients showed evidence of muscle damage with increased serum creatine kinase concentration and myoglobinuria. These patients did NOT have classical signs of malignant hyperthermia such as muscle rigidity, rapid increase in body temperature, or increased oxygen uptake and carbon dioxide production. Prompt and vigorous treatment for hyperkalaemia and arrhythmias is recommended. Subsequent evaluation for latent neuromuscular disease is indicated.

4.5 Interaction with other medicinal products and other forms of interaction
The actions of non-depolarising relaxants are markedly potentiated with Isoflurane, therefore, when administered with Isoflurane, dosage adjustments of these agents should be made.

4.6 Pregnancy and lactation
Reproduction studies have been carried out on animals after repeated exposures to anaesthetic concentrations of Isoflurane. Studies in the rat demonstrated no effect on the fertility, pregnancy or delivery or on the viability of offspring. No evidence of teratogenicity was revealed. Comparable experiments in rabbits produced similar negative results. The relevance of these studies to the human is not known. As there is insufficient experience in the use of Isoflurane in pregnant women safety in human pregnancy has not been established. Blood losses comparable with those found following anaesthesia with other inhalation

agents have been recorded with Isoflurane in patients undergoing induced abortion. Adequate data have not been developed to establish the safety of Isoflurane in obstetric anaesthesia other than for caesarean section.

4.7 Effects on ability to drive and use machines
Not applicable.

4.8 Undesirable effects
Arrhythmias, respiratory depression and hypotension have been occasionally reported.

Elevation of the white blood cell count has been observed, even in the absence of surgical stress.

Minimally raised levels of serum inorganic fluoride occur during and after Isoflurane anaesthesia, due to biodegradation of the agent. It is unlikely that the low levels of serum inorganic fluoride observed (mean 4.4 μmol/l in one study) could cause renal toxicity, as these are well below the proposed threshold levels for kidney toxicity.

Undesirable effects during recovery (shivering, nausea and vomiting) are minor in nature and comparable in incidence with those found with other anaesthetics.

Malignant hyperthermia has been reported.

Reports demonstrate that Isoflurane can produce hepatic injury ranging from mild transient increase of liver enzymes to fatal hepatic necrosis in very rare instances. It has been reported that previous exposure to halogenated hydrocarbon anaesthetics, especially if the interval is less than 3 months, may increase the potential for hepatic injury.

Rare reports of hypersensitivity (including dermatitis contact, rash, dyspnoea, wheezing, chest discomfort, swelling face, or anaphylactic reaction) have been received, especially in association with long-term occupational exposure to inhaled anaesthetic agents, including Isoflurane. These reactions have been confirmed by clinical testing (e.g., methancholine challenge). The cause of anaphylactic reactions experienced during inhalational anaesthetic exposure is, however, unclear because the exposure to multiple concomitant drugs, many of which are known to cause such reactions.

4.9 Overdose
As with other halogenated anaesthetics, hypotension and respiratory depression have been observed. Close monitoring of blood pressure and respiration is recommended. Supportive measures may be necessary to correct hypotension and respiratory depression resulting from excessively deep levels of anaesthesia.

5. PHARMACOLOGICAL PROPERTIES

5.1 Pharmacodynamic properties
Induction and particularly recovery are rapid. Although slight pungency may limit the rate of induction, excessive salivation and tracheo-bronchial secretions are not stimulated. Pharyngeal and laryngeal reflexes are diminished quickly. Levels of anaesthesia change rapidly with Isoflurane. Heart rhythm remains stable. Spontaneous respiration becomes depressed as depth of anaesthesia increases and should be closely monitored.

During induction there is a decrease in blood pressure which returns towards normal with surgical stimulation.

Blood pressure tends to fall during maintenance in direct relation to depth of anaesthesia, due to peripheral vasodilation, but cardiac rhythm remains stable. With controlled respiration and normal $PaCO_2$, cardiac output tends to be maintained despite increasing depth of anaesthesia, primarily through a rise in heart rate. With spontaneous respiration, the resulting hypercapnia may increase heart rate and cardiac output above awake levels.

Cerebral blood flow remains unchanged during light Isoflurane anaesthesia but tends to rise at deeper levels. Increases in cerebrospinal fluid pressure may be prevented or reversed by hyperventilating the patient before or during anaesthesia. Electro-encephalographic changes and convulsion are extremely rare with isoflurane.

Isoflurane appears to sensitise the myocardium to adrenaline to an even lesser extent than Enflurane. Limited data suggest that subcutaneous infiltration of up to 50ml of 1:200,000 solution adrenaline does not induce ventricular arrhythmias, in patients anaesthetised with isoflurane.

Muscular relaxation may be adequate for some intra-abdominal operations at normal levels of anaesthesia, but should greater relaxation be required small doses of intravenous muscle relaxants may be used. All commonly used muscle relaxants are markedly potentiated by Isoflurane, the effect being most profound with non-depolarising agents. Neostigmine reverses the effects of non-depolarising muscle relaxants but has no effect on the relaxant properties of Isoflurane itself. All commonly used muscle relaxants are compatible with Isoflurane.

Isoflurane may be used for the induction and maintenance of general anaesthesia. Adequate data are not available to establish its place in pregnancy or obstetric anaesthesia other than for caesarean section.

Relatively little metabolism of Isoflurane occurs in the human body. In the post operative period only 0.17% of the Isoflurane taken up can be recovered as urinary metabolites. Peak serum inorganic fluoride values usually average less than 5μmol/litre and occur about four hours after anaesthesia, returning to normal levels within 24 hours. No signs of renal injury have been reported after Isoflurane administration.

5.2 Pharmacokinetic properties
MAC (Minimum Alveolar Concentration in man):

Age	100% Oxygen	70% N_2O
26 ± 4	1.28	0.56
44 ± 7	1.15	0.50
64 ± 5	1.05	0.37

5.3 Preclinical safety data
None stated.

6. PHARMACEUTICAL PARTICULARS

6.1 List of excipients
None.

6.2 Incompatibilities
Isoflurane has been reported to interact with dry carbon dioxide absorbents to form carbon monoxide. In order to minimise the risk of formation of carbon monoxide in rebreathing circuits and the possibility of elevated carboxyhaemoglobin levels, carbon dioxide absorbents should not be allowed to dry out. (See also section 4.4).

6.3 Shelf life
The recommended shelf life is 5 years.

6.4 Special precautions for storage
Do not store above 25°C. Keep container well closed.

6.5 Nature and contents of container
100 ml and 250 ml glass bottles.

6.6 Special precautions for disposal and other handling
Vaporisers specially calibrated for Isoflurane should be used so that the concentration of anaesthetic delivered can be accurately controlled.

It is recommended that vapour from this and other inhalation agents be efficiently extracted from the area of use.

7. MARKETING AUTHORISATION HOLDER
Abbott Laboratories Limited
Queenborough
Kent
ME11 5EL

8. MARKETING AUTHORISATION NUMBER(S)
PL 00037/0115

9. DATE OF FIRST AUTHORISATION/RENEWAL OF THE AUTHORISATION
17 July 2001

10. DATE OF REVISION OF THE TEXT
21 July 2009

Forceval Capsules

(Alliance Pharmaceuticals)

1. NAME OF THE MEDICINAL PRODUCT
Forceval Capsules

2. QUALITATIVE AND QUANTITATIVE COMPOSITION
Each capsule contains:
Vitamin A (as β-Carotene) HSE 2,500.0 iu
Vitamin D2 (Ergocalciferol) HSE 400.0 iu
Vitamin B1 (Thiamine) USP 1.2 mg
Vitamin B2 (Riboflavin) BP 1.6 mg
Vitamin B6 (Pyridoxine) BP 2.0 mg
Vitamin B12 (Cyanocobalamin) PhEur 3.0 mcg
Vitamin C (Ascorbic Acid) BP 60.0 mg
Vitamin E (dl-α-Tocopheryl Acetate) USP 10.0 mg
d-Biotin (Vitamin H) FCC 100.0 mcg
Nicotinamide (Vitamin B3) BP 18.0 mg
Pantothenic Acid (Vitamin B5) USP 4.0 mg
Folic Acid (Vitamin B Complex) BP 400.0 mcg
Calcium FCC 100.0 mg
Iron BP 12.0 mg
Copper HSE 2.0 mg
Phosphorus HSE 77.0 mg
Magnesium BP 30.0 mg
Potassium HSE 4.0 mg
Zinc HSE 15.0 mg
Iodine BP 140.0 mcg
Manganese HSE 3.0 mg
Selenium BP 50.0 mcg
Chromium HSE 200.0 mcg
Molybdenum HSE 250.0 mcg

3. PHARMACEUTICAL FORM
Brown and maroon, oblong, soft gelatin capsule printed with **FORCEVAL** in white on one side and with **6377** in white on the other side.

4. CLINICAL PARTICULARS

4.1 Therapeutic indications
1. As a therapeutic nutritional adjunct where the intake of vitamins and minerals is suboptimal, e.g. in the presence of organic disease such as malignancy and immune deficiency syndromes, such as AIDS.

2. As a therapeutic nutritional adjunct in conditions where the absorption of vitamins and minerals is suboptimal, e.g. malabsorption, inflammatory bowel disease and fistulae, short bowel syndrome and Crohn's disease, and where concurrent medication decreases vitamin and mineral absorption.

3. As a therapeutic nutritional adjunct in convalescence from illness, e.g. where anorexia or cachexia exists and following chemo- or radio-therapy.

4. As a therapeutic nutritional adjunct in convalescence from surgery, e.g. where nutritional intake continues to be inadequate.

5. As a therapeutic nutritional adjunct for patients on special or restricted diets, e.g. in renal diets and where several food groups are restricted in therapeutic weight reducing diets.

6. As a therapeutic nutritional adjunct where food intolerance exists, e.g. exclusion diets.

7. As an adjunct in synthetic diets, e.g. in phenylketonuria, galactosaemia and ketogenic diets.

4.2 Posology and method of administration
Adults and the Elderly
One capsule daily, preferably taken one hour after meals. Do not exceed the stated dose. The capsule should be swallowed whole with water.

Children under 12 years of age
Forceval Capsules are not recommended for this age group.

4.3 Contraindications
Hypercalcaemia, haemochromatosis and other iron storage disorders.

4.4 Special warnings and precautions for use
Whilst taking Forceval Capsules both protein and energy are also required to provide complete nutrition in the daily diet. No other vitamins, minerals or supplements with or without vitamin A should be taken with this preparation except under medical supervision.

Do not take Forceval Capsules on an empty stomach. Do not exceed the stated dose. Keep out of the reach of children. If symptoms persist, consult your doctor.

Important warning: Contains iron. Keep out of the reach and sight of children, as overdose may be fatal.

This medicine contains E123 (amaranth) and E124 (ponceau 4R red) which may cause allergic reactions.

Evidence from Randomised Control Trials suggests that high doses (20-30 mg/day) b-carotene intake may increase the risk of lung cancer in current smokers and those previously exposed to asbestos. This high-risk population should consider the potential risks and benefits of Forceval Capsules, which contain 4.5mg per recommended daily dose, before use.

4.5 Interaction with other medicinal products and other forms of interaction
Folic acid can reduce the plasma concentration of phenytoin. Oral iron and zinc sulphate reduce the absorption of tetracyclines.

4.6 Pregnancy and lactation
Forceval Capsules may be administered during pregnancy and lactation at the recommendation of the physician.

4.7 Effects on ability to drive and use machines
None anticipated.

4.8 Undesirable effects
No undesirable effects due to Forceval therapy have been reported and none can be expected if the dosage schedule is adhered to.

4.9 Overdose
No cases of overdosage due to Forceval therapy have been reported. Any symptoms which may be observed due to the ingestion of large quantities of Forceval capsules will be due to the fat soluble vitamin content. If iron overdosage is suspected, symptoms may include nausea, vomiting, diarrhoea, abdominal pain, haematemesis, rectal bleeding, lethargy and circulatory collapse. Hyperglycaemia and metabolic acidosis may also occur. Treatment should be implemented immediately. In severe cases, after a latent phase, relapse may occur after 24 - 48 hours, manifest by hypotension coma and hepatocellular necrosis and renal failure.

Treatment
The following steps are recommended to minimise or prevent further absorption of the medication:

1. Administer an emetic.

2. Gastric lavage may be necessary to remove drug already released into the stomach. This should be undertaken using desferrioxamine solution (2 g/l). Desferrioxamine 5 g in 50 - 100 ml water should be introduced into the stomach following gastric emptying. Keep the patient under constant surveillance to detect possible aspiration of vomitus; maintain suction apparatus and standby emergency oxygen in case of need.

3. A drink of mannitol or sorbitol should be given to induce small bowel emptying.

4. Severe poisoning: in the presence of shock and/or coma with high serum iron levels > 142 μmol/l) immediate supportive measures plus i.v. infusion of desferrioxamine should be instituted. The recommended dose of desferrioxamine is 5 mg/kg/h by slow i.v. infusion up to a maximum of 80 mg/kg/24 hours. Warning: hypotension may occur if the infusion rate is too rapid.

5. Less severe poisoning: i.m. desferrioxamine 50 mg/kg up to a maximum dose of 4 g should be given.

6. Serum iron levels should be monitored throughout.

7. Any fluid or electrolyte imbalance should be corrected.

5. PHARMACOLOGICAL PROPERTIES

5.1 Pharmacodynamic properties

The following account summarises the pharmacological effects of the vitamins and minerals in Forceval Capsules and describes the conditions caused by deficiency of these.

Vitamin A

Vitamin A plays an important role in the visual process. It is isomerised to the 11-cis isomer and subsequently bound to the opsin to form the photoreceptor for vision under subdued light. One of the earliest symptoms of deficiency is night blindness which may develop into the more serious condition xerophthalmia. Vitamin A also participates in the formation and maintenance of the integrity of epithelial tissues and mucous membranes. Deficiency may cause skin changes resulting in a dry rough skin with lowered resistance to minor skin infections. Deficiency of Vitamin A, usually accompanied by protein-energy malnutrition, is linked with a frequency of infection and with defective immunological defence mechanisms.

Vitamin D

Vitamin D is required for the absorption of calcium and phosphate from the gastro-intestinal tract and for their transport. Its involvement in the control of calcium metabolism and hence the normal calcification of bones is well documented. Deficiency of Vitamin D in children may result in the development of rickets.

Vitamin B_1 (Thiamine)

Thiamine (as the coenzyme, thiamine pyrophosphate) is associated with carbohydrate metabolism. Thiamine pyrophosphate also acts as a co-enzyme in the direct oxidative pathway of glucose metabolism. In thiamine deficiency, pyruvic and lactic acids accumulate in the tissues. The pyruvate ion is involved in the biosynthesis of acetylcholine via its conversion to acetyl co-enzyme A through a thiamine-dependent process. In thiamine deficiency, therefore, there are effects on the central nervous system due either to the effect on acetylcholine synthesis or to the lactate and pyruvate accumulation. Deficiency of thiamine results in fatigue, anorexia, gastro-intestinal disturbances, tachycardia, irritability and neurological symptoms. Gross deficiency of thiamine (and other Vitamin B group factors) leads to the condition beri-beri.

Vitamin B_2 (Riboflavine)

Riboflavine is phosphorylated to flavine mononucleotide and flavine adenine dinucleotide which act as co-enzymes in the respiratory chain and in oxidative phosphorylation. Riboflavine deficiency presents with ocular symptoms, as well as lesions on the lips and at angles of the mouth.

Vitamin B_6 (Pyridoxine)

Pyridoxine, once absorbed, is rapidly converted to the co-enzymes pyridoxal phosphate and pyridoxamine phosphate which play an essential role in protein metabolism. Convulsions and hypochromic anaemia have occurred in infants deficient in pyridoxine.

Vitamin B_{12} (Cyanocobalamin)

Vitamin B_{12} is present in the body mainly as methylcobalamin and as adenosylcobalamin and hydroxocobalamin. These act as co-enzymes in the trans methylation of homocysteine to methionine; in the isomerisation of methylmalonyl co-enzyme to succinyl co-enzyme and with folate in several metabolic pathways respectively. Deficiency of Vitamin B_{12} interferes with haemopoiesis and produces megaloblastic anaemia.

Vitamin C (Ascorbic Acid)

Vitamin C cannot be synthesised by man therefore a dietary source is necessary. It acts as a cofactor in numerous biological processes including the hydroxylation of proline to hydroxyproline. In deficiency, the formation of collagen is, therefore, impaired. Ascorbic acid is important in the hydroxylation of dopamine to noradrenaline and in hydroxylations occurring in steroid synthesis in the adrenals. It is a reducing agent in tyrosine metabolism and by acting as an electron donor in the conversion of folic acid to tetrahydrofolic acid is indirectly involved in the synthesis of purine and thymine. Vitamin C is also necessary for the incorporation of iron into ferritin. Vitamin C increases the phagocytic function of leucocytes; it possesses anti-inflammatory activity and it promotes wound healing. Deficiency can produce scurvy. Features include swollen inflamed gums, petechial haemorrhages and subcutaneous bruising. The deficiency of collagen leads to development of thin watery ground substances in which blood vessels are insecurely fixed and readily ruptured. The supportive components of bone and cartilage are also deficient causing bones to fracture easily and teeth to become loose. Anaemia commonly occurs probably due to Vitamin C's role in iron metabolism.

Vitamin E

Vitamin E deficiency has been linked to disorders such as cystic fibrosis where fat absorption is impaired. It is essential for the normal function of the muscular system and the blood.

Nicotinamide

The biochemical functions of nicotinamide as NAD and NADP (nicotinamide adenine dinucleotide phosphate) include the degradation and synthesis of fatty acids, carbohydrates and amino acids as well as hydrogen transfer. Deficiency produces pellagra and mental neurological changes.

Calcium (Dicalcium Phosphate)

Calcium is an essential body electrolyte. It is involved in the maintenance of normal muscle and nerve function and essential for normal cardiac function and the clotting of blood. Calcium is mainly found in the bones and teeth. Deficiency of calcium leads to rickets, osteomalacia in children and osteoporosis in the elderly.

Phosphorus (Dicalcium Phosphate)

Phosphate plays important roles in the osteoblastic and osteoclastic reactions. It interacts with calcium to modify the balance between these two processes. Organic phosphate esters play a key role in the metabolism of carbohydrates, fats and proteins and in the formation of 'high energy phosphate' compounds. Phosphate also acts as a buffer and plays a role in the renal excretion of sodium and hydrogen ions.

Pantothenic Acid

Pantothenic acid is incorporated into co-enzyme A and is involved in metabolic pathways involving acetylation which includes detoxification of drug molecules and biosynthesis of cholesterol, steroid hormones, mucopolysaccharides and acetylcholine. CoA has an essential function in lipid metabolism.

Folic Acid

Folic acid is reduced in the body to tetrahydrofolate which is a co-enzyme for various metabolic processes, including the synthesis of purine and pyrimidine nucleotides and hence in the synthesis of DNA. It is also involved in some amino acid conversion and in the formation and utilisation of formate. Deficiency of folic acid leads to megaloblastic anaemia.

Vitamin H (d-Biotin)

Biotin is a co-enzyme for carboxylation during the metabolism of proteins and carbohydrates.

Selenium

Selenium is an essential trace element, deficiency of which has been reported in man. It is thought to be involved in the functioning of membranes and the synthesis of amino acids. Deficiency of selenium in the diet of experimental animals produces fatty liver followed by necrosis.

Iron

Iron, as a constituent of haemoglobin, plays an essential role in oxygen transport. It is also present in the muscle protein myoglobin and in the liver. Deficiency of iron leads to anaemia.

Copper (Copper Sulphate)

Traces of copper are essential to the body as constituents of enzyme systems involved in oxidation reactions.

Magnesium (Magnesium Oxide)

Magnesium is essential to the body as a constituent of skeletal structures and in maintaining cell integrity and fluid balance. It is utilised in many of the functions in which calcium is concerned but often exerts the opposite effect. Some enzymes require the magnesium ion as a co-factor.

Potassium (Potassium Sulphate)

Potassium is the principle cation of intracellular fluid and is intimately involved in the cell function and metabolism. It is essential for carbohydrate metabolism and glycogen storage and protein synthesis and is involved in transmembrane potential where it is necessary to maintain the resting potential in excitable cells. Potassium ions maintain intracellular pH and osmotic pressure. Prolonged or severe diarrhoea may lead to potassium deficiency.

Zinc (Zinc Sulphate)

Zinc is a constituent of many enzymes and is, therefore, essential to the body. It is present with insulin in the pancreas. It plays a role in DNA synthesis and cell division. Reported effects of deficiency include delayed puberty and hypogonadal dwarfism.

Manganese (Manganese Sulphate)

Manganese is a constituent of enzyme systems including those involved in lipid synthesis, the tricarboxylic acid cycle and purine and pyrimidine metabolism. It is bound to arginase of the liver and activates many enzymes.

Iodine (Potassium Iodide)

Iodine is an essential constituent of the thyroid hormones.

Chromium (Chromium Amino Acid Chelate 10%)

Chromium is an essential trace element involved in carbohydrate metabolism.

Molybdenum (Sodium Molybdate)

Molybdenum is an essential trace element although there have been no reports of deficiency states in man. Molybdenum salts have been used to treat copper poisoning in sheep.

5.2 Pharmacokinetic properties

The following account describes the absorption and fate of each of the active constituents of Forceval Capsules.

Vitamin A

Except when liver function is impaired, Vitamin A is readily absorbed. β-carotene (as in Forceval Capsules) is Provitamin A and is the biological precursor to Vitamin A. It is converted to Vitamin A (Retinol) in the liver; retinol is emulsified by bile salts and phospholipids and absorbed in a micellar form. Part is conjugated with glucuronic acid in the kidney and part is metabolised in the liver and kidney, leaving 30 to 50% of the dose for storage in the liver. It is bound to a globulin in the blood. Metabolites of Vitamin A are excreted in the faeces and the urine.

Vitamin D

The metabolism of ergocalciferol is similar to that of cholecalciferol. Cholecalciferol is absorbed from the gastro-intestinal tract into the circulation. In the liver, it is hydroxylated to 25-hydroxycholecalciferol, is subject to enterohepatic circulation and is further hydroxylated to 1,25-dihydroxycholecalciferol in the renal tubule cells. Vitamin D metabolites are bound to specific plasma proteins.

Vitamin B_1 (Thiamine)

Thiamine is absorbed from the gastro-intestinal tract and is widely distributed to most body tissues. Amounts in excess of the body's requirements are not stored but excreted in the urine as unchanged thiamine or its metabolites.

Vitamin B_2 (Riboflavine)

Riboflavine is absorbed from the gastro-intestinal tract and in the circulation is bound to plasma proteins. It is widely distributed. Little is stored and excess amounts are excreted in the urine. In the body riboflavine is converted to flavine mononucleotide (FMN) and then to flavine adenine dinucleotide (FAD).

Vitamin B_6 (Pyridoxine)

Pyridoxine is absorbed from the gastro-intestinal tract and converted to the active pyridoxal phosphate which is bound to plasma proteins. It is excreted in the urine as 4-pyridoxic acid.

Vitamin B_{12} (Cyanocobalamin)

Cyanocobalamin is absorbed from the gastro-intestinal tract and is extensively bound to specific plasma proteins. A study with labelled Vitamin B_{12} showed it was quickly taken up by the intestinal mucosa and held there for 2 - 3 hours. Peak concentrations in the blood and tissues did not occur until 8 - 12 hours after dosage with maximum concentrations in the liver within 24 hours. Cobalamins are stored in the liver, excreted in the bile and undergo enterohepatic recycling. Part of a dose is excreted in the urine, most of it in the first eight hours.

Vitamin C (Ascorbic Acid)

Ascorbic acid is readily absorbed from the gastro-intestinal tract and is widely distributed in the body tissues. Ascorbic acid in excess of the body's needs is rapidly eliminated in the urine and this elimination is usually accompanied by a mild diuresis.

Vitamin E

Vitamin E is absorbed from the gastro-intestinal tract. Most appears in the lymph and is then widely distributed to all tissues. Most of a dose is slowly excreted in the bile and the remainder is eliminated in the urine as glucuronides of tocopheronic acid or other metabolites.

Nicotinamide (Nicotinic Acid Amide)

Nicotinic acid is absorbed from the gastro-intestinal tract, is widely distributed in the body tissues and has a short half-life.

Calcium (Dicalcium Phosphate)

A third of ingested calcium is absorbed from the small intestine. Absorption of calcium decreases with age.

Phosphorus (Dicalcium Phosphate)

The body contains from 600 - 800 g of phosphorus, over 80% of which is present in the bone as phosphate salts, mainly hydroxyapatite crystals. The phosphate in these crystals is available for exchange with phosphate ions in the extra-cellular fluids.

Calcium Pantothenate

Pantothenic acid is readily absorbed from the gastro-intestinal tract and is widely distributed in the body tissues. About 70% of pantothenic acid is excreted unchanged in the urine and about 30% in the faeces.

Folic Acid

Folic acid is absorbed mainly from the proximal part of the small intestine. Folate polyglutamates are considered to be deconjugated to monoglutamates during absorption. Folic acid rapidly appears in the blood where it is extensively bound to plasma proteins. Some folic acid is distributed in body tissues, some is excreted as folate in the urine and some is stored in the liver as folate.

Vitamin H (d-Biotin)

Following absorption, biotin is stored in the liver, kidney and pancreas.

Selenium

Although it has been established that selenium is essential to human life, very little information is available on its function and metabolism.

Ferrous Fumarate (Iron)

Iron is absorbed chiefly in the duodenum and jejunum. Absorption is aided by the acid secretion of the stomach and if the iron is in the ferrous state as in ferrous fumarate. In conditions of iron deficiency, absorption is increased and, conversely, it is decreased in iron overload. Iron is stored as ferritin.

Copper Sulphate (Copper)

Copper is absorbed from the gastro-intestinal tract and its major route of excretion is in the bile.

Magnesium Oxide (Magnesium)

Magnesium salts are poorly absorbed from the gastro-intestinal tract; however, sufficient magnesium will normally be absorbed to replace deficiency states. Magnesium is excreted in both the urine and the faeces but excretion is reduced in deficiency states.

Potassium Sulphate (Potassium)

Potassium salts are absorbed from the gastro-intestinal tract. Potassium is excreted in the urine, the faeces and in perspiration. Urinary excretion of potassium continues even when intake is low.

Zinc Sulphate (Zinc)

Zinc is poorly absorbed from the gastro-intestinal tract. It is widely distributed throughout the body. It is excreted in the faeces with traces appearing in the urine.

Manganese Sulphate (Manganese)

Manganese salts are poorly absorbed.

Potassium Iodide (Iodine)

Iodides are absorbed and stored in the thyroid gland as thyroglobulin. Iodides are excreted in the urine with smaller amounts appearing in the faeces, saliva and sweat.

Chromium Amino Acid Chelate 10% (Chromium)

Although it has been established that chromium is essential to human life, little information is available on its function and metabolism.

Sodium Molybdate (Molybdenum)

Although it has been established that molybdenum is essential to human life, little information is available on its function and metabolism.

5.3 Preclinical safety data

There are no pre-clinical data of relevance to the prescriber which are additional to that already included in other sections of the SPC.

6. PHARMACEUTICAL PARTICULARS

6.1 List of excipients

Soya Bean Oil BP
Soya Lecithin HSE
Hard Vegetable Fat (Biscuitine 621) HSE
Yellow Beeswax BP
Purified Water PhEur
Gelatin BP
Glycerine BP
Ponceau 4R (E124) HSE
Amaranth (E123) HSE
Titanium Dioxide (E171) BP
Red Iron Oxide Paste (E172) HSE
Vegetable Black Paste (E153) HSE

6.2 Incompatibilities

No major incompatibilities are known.

6.3 Shelf life

24 months, as packaged for sale.

6.4 Special precautions for storage

Store in a cool dry place at a temperature not exceeding 25°C.

Protect from light.

6.5 Nature and contents of container

The product is presented in press-thru blister packs, each blister strip containing 15 Forceval capsules. The blister strip is composed of PVC/PVdC with a printed aluminium foil lidding. The foil is printed (red on gold) with the name and PL number of the product, the number of vitamins and minerals per capsule and the daily dose.

The product is available in packs of 30, 45 or 90 capsules.

6.6 Special precautions for disposal and other handling

Not applicable.

7. MARKETING AUTHORISATION HOLDER

Alliance Pharmaceuticals Ltd
Avonbridge House
2 Bath Road
Chippenham
Wiltshire
SN15 2BB
United Kingdom

8. MARKETING AUTHORISATION NUMBER(S)

PL 16853/0079

9. DATE OF FIRST AUTHORISATION/RENEWAL OF THE AUTHORISATION

30/11/2005

10. DATE OF REVISION OF THE TEXT

14/02/2007

Forceval Junior Capsules

(Alliance Pharmaceuticals)

1. NAME OF THE MEDICINAL PRODUCT

Forceval Junior Capsules

2. QUALITATIVE AND QUANTITATIVE COMPOSITION

Each capsule contains:

Vitamin A (as β-Carotene) HSE 1,250.0 iu
Vitamin D2 (Ergocalciferol) HSE 200.0 iu
Vitamin B1 (Thiamine) USP 1.5 mg
Vitamin B2 (Riboflavin) BP 1.0 mg
Vitamin B6 (Pyridoxine) BP 1.0 mg
Vitamin B12 (Cyanocobalamin) PhEur 2.0 mcg
Vitamin C (Ascorbic Acid) BP 25.0 mg
Vitamin E (dl-α-Tocopheryl Acetate) USP 5.0 mg
d-Biotin (Vitamin H) FCC 50.0 mcg
Nicotinamide (Vitamin B3) BP 7.5 mg
Pantothenic Acid (Vitamin B5) USP 2.0 mg
Vitamin K1 (Phytomenadione) BP 25.0 mcg
Folic Acid (Vitamin B Complex) BP 100.0 mcg
Iron BP 5.0 mg
Copper HSE 1.0 mg
Magnesium BP 1.0 mg
Zinc HSE 5.0 mg
Iodine BP 75.0 mcg
Manganese HSE 1.25 mg
Selenium BP 25.0 mcg
Chromium HSE 50.0 mcg
Molybdenum HSE 50.0 mcg

3. PHARMACEUTICAL FORM

Small, opaque, brown, oval, soft gelatin capsule printed in white with **571**.

4. CLINICAL PARTICULARS

4.1 Therapeutic indications

1. As a therapeutic nutritional adjunct where the intake of vitamins and minerals is suboptimal, e.g. in the presence of organic disease such as malignancy and immune deficiency syndromes, such as AIDS.

2. As a therapeutic nutritional adjunct in conditions where the absorption of vitamins and minerals is suboptimal, e.g. malabsorption, inflammatory bowel disease and fistulae, short bowel syndrome and Crohn's disease, and where concurrent medication decreases vitamin and mineral absorption.

3. As a therapeutic nutritional adjunct in convalescence from illness, e.g. where anorexia or cachexia exists and following chemo- or radio-therapy.

4. As a therapeutic nutritional adjunct in convalescence from surgery, e.g. where nutritional intake continues to be inadequate.

5. As a therapeutic nutritional adjunct for patients on special or restricted diets, e.g. in renal diets and where several food groups are restricted in therapeutic weight reducing diets.

6. As a therapeutic nutritional adjunct where food intolerance exists, e.g. exclusion diets.

7. As an adjunct in synthetic diets, e.g. in phenylketonuria, galactosaemia and ketogenic diets.

4.2 Posology and method of administration

Children over 5 years of age

2 capsules per day or as recommended by the doctor.

Do not exceed the stated dose.

Adults and the Elderly

Not recommended - use Forceval Capsules.

4.3 Contraindications

Haemochromatosis and other iron storage disorders.

4.4 Special warnings and precautions for use

Forceval Junior Capsules should be used as a vitamin and mineral source in conjunction with an energy-providing diet suitable for individual patient requirements. No other vitamins, minerals or supplements with or without vitamin A should be taken with this preparation except under medical supervision.

Do not exceed the stated dose. Keep out of the reach of children.

The label will state:

Important warning: Contains iron. Keep out of the reach and sight of children, as overdose may be fatal.

This warning will appear on the front of pack, enclosed in a rectangle, in which there is no other information of any kind.

This medicine contains sorbitol. Patients with rare hereditary problems of fructose intolerance should not take this medicine.

Evidence from Randomised Control Trials suggests that high doses (20-30 mg/day) b-carotene intake may increase the risk of lung cancer in current smokers and those previously exposed to asbestos. This high-risk population should consider the potential risks and benefits of Forceval Junior Capsules, which contain 4.5mg per recommended daily dose, before use.

4.5 Interaction with other medicinal products and other forms of interaction

Vitamin K may interact with anticoagulants such as phenindione, warfarin and nicoumalone inhibiting their effect. Folic acid can reduce the plasma concentration of phenytoin. Oral iron and zinc sulphate reduce the absorption of tetracyclines.

4.6 Pregnancy and lactation

Forceval Junior Capsules can be given to pregnant and lactating women, provided the product is administered with the approval of their clinician.

4.7 Effects on ability to drive and use machines

None anticipated.

4.8 Undesirable effects

No undesirable effects due to Forceval Junior therapy have been reported and none can be expected if the dosage schedule is adhered to.

4.9 Overdose

No cases of overdosage due to Forceval Junior therapy have been reported. Any symptoms which may be observed due to ingestion of large quantities of Forceval Junior capsules will be due to the fat soluble vitamin content. If iron overdosage is suspected, symptoms may include nausea, vomiting, diarrhoea, abdominal pain, haematemesis, rectal bleeding, lethargy and circulatory collapse. Hyperglycaemia and metabolic acidosis may also occur. Treatment should be implemented immediately. In severe cases, after a latent phase, relapse may occur after 24 - 48 hours, manifest by hypotension coma and hepatocellular necrosis and renal failure.

Treatment

The following steps are recommended to minimise or prevent further absorption of the medication:

1. Administer an emetic.

2. Gastric lavage may be necessary to remove drug already released into the stomach. This should be undertaken using desferrioxamine solution (2 g/l). Desferrioxamine 5 g in 50-100 ml water should be introduced into the stomach following gastric emptying. Keep the patient under constant surveillance to detect possible aspiration of vomitus; maintain suction apparatus and standby emergency oxygen in case of need.

3. A drink of mannitol or sorbitol should be given to induce small bowel emptying.

4. Severe poisoning: in the presence of shock and/or coma with high serum iron levels >142 μmol/l) immediate supportive measures plus i.v. infusion of desferrioxamine should be instituted. The recommended dose of desferrioxamine is 5 mg/kg/h by slow i.v. infusion up to a maximum of 80 mg/kg/24 hours. Warning: hypotension may occur if the infusion rate is too rapid.

5. Less severe poisoning: i.m. desferrioxamine 50 mg/kg up to a maximum dose of 4 g should be given.

6. Serum iron levels should be monitored throughout.

7. Any fluid or electrolyte imbalance should be corrected.

5. PHARMACOLOGICAL PROPERTIES

5.1 Pharmacodynamic properties

The following account summarises the pharmacological effects of the vitamins and minerals in Forceval Junior Capsules and describes the conditions caused by deficiency of these.

Vitamin A

Vitamin A plays an important role in the visual process. It is isomerised to the 11-cis isomer and subsequently bound to the opsin to form the photoreceptor for vision under subdued light. One of the earliest symptoms of deficiency is night blindness which may develop into the more serious condition xerophthalmia. Vitamin A also participates in the formation and maintenance of the integrity of epithelial tissues and mucous membranes. Deficiency may cause skin changes resulting in a dry rough skin with lowered resistance to minor skin infections. Deficiency of Vitamin A, usually accompanied by protein-energy malnutrition, is linked with a frequency of infection and with defective immunological defence mechanisms.

Vitamin D

Vitamin D is required for the absorption of calcium and phosphate from the gastro-intestinal tract and for their transport. Its involvement in the control of calcium metabolism and hence the normal calcification of bones is well documented. Deficiency of Vitamin D in children may result in the development of rickets.

Vitamin B_1 (Thiamine)

Thiamine (as the coenzyme, thiamine pyrophosphate) is associated with carbohydrate metabolism. Thiamine pyrophosphate also acts as a co-enzyme in the direct oxidative pathway of glucose metabolism. In thiamine deficiency, pyruvic and lactic acids accumulate in the tissues. The pyruvate ion is involved in the biosynthesis of acetylcholine via its conversion to acetyl co-enzyme A through a thiamine-dependent process. In thiamine deficiency, therefore, there are effects on the central nervous system due either to the effect on acetylcholine synthesis or to the lactate and pyruvate accumulation. Deficiency of thiamine results in fatigue, anorexia, gastro-intestinal disturbances, tachycardia, irritability and neurological symptoms. Gross deficiency of thiamine (and other Vitamin B group factors) leads to the condition beri-beri.

Vitamin B_2 (Riboflavine)

Riboflavine is phosphorylated to flavine mononucleotide and flavine adenine dinucleotide which act as co-enzymes in the respiratory chain and in oxidative phosphorylation. Riboflavine deficiency presents with ocular symptoms, as well as lesions on the lips and at angles of the mouth.

Vitamin B_6 (Pyridoxine)

Pyridoxine, once absorbed, is rapidly converted to the co-enzymes pyridoxal phosphate and pyridoxamine phosphate which play an essential role in protein metabolism. Convulsions and hypochromic anaemia have occurred in infants deficient in pyridoxine.

Vitamin B_{12} (Cyanocobalamin)

Vitamin B_{12} is present in the body mainly as methylcobalamin and as adenosylcobalamin and hydroxocobalamin. These act as co-enzymes in the trans methylation of homocysteine to methionine; in the isomerisation of methylmalonyl co-enzyme to succinyl co-enzyme and with folate in several metabolic pathways respectively. Deficiency of Vitamin B_{12} interferes with haemopoiesis and produces megaloblastic anaemia.

Vitamin C (Ascorbic Acid)

Vitamin C cannot be synthesised by man therefore a dietary source is necessary. It acts as a cofactor in numerous biological processes including the hydroxylation of proline to hydroxyproline. In deficiency, the formation of collagen is, therefore, impaired. Ascorbic acid is important in the hydroxylation of dopamine to noradrenaline and in hydroxylations occurring in steroid synthesis in the adrenals. It is a reducing agent in tyrosine metabolism and by acting as an electron donor in the conversion of folic acid to tetrahydrofolic acid is indirectly involved in the synthesis of purine and thymine. Vitamin C is also necessary for the incorporation of iron into ferritin. Vitamin C increases the phagocytic function of leucocytes; it possesses anti-inflammatory activity and it promotes wound healing. Deficiency can produce scurvy. Features include swollen inflamed gums, petechial haemorrhages and subcutaneous bruising. The deficiency of collagen leads to development of thin watery ground substances in which blood vessels are insecurely fixed and readily ruptured. The supportive components of bone and cartilage are also deficient causing bones to fracture easily and teeth to become loose. Anaemia commonly occurs probably due to Vitamin C's role in iron metabolism.

Vitamin E

Vitamin E deficiency has been linked to disorders such as cystic fibrosis where fat absorbtion is impaired. It is essential for the normal function of the muscular system and the blood.

Nicotinamide

The biochemical functions of nicotinamide as NAD and NADP (nicotinamide adenine dinucleotide phosphate) include the degradation and synthesis of fatty acids, carbohydrates and amino acids as well as hydrogen transfer. Deficiency produces pellagra and mental neurological changes.

Pantothenic Acid

Pantothenic acid is incorporated into co-enzyme A and is involved in metabolic pathways involving acetylation which includes detoxification of drug molecules and biosynthesis of cholesterol, steroid hormones, mucopolysaccharides and acetylcholine. CoA has an essential function in lipid metabolism.

Vitamin K1 (Phytomenadione)

Phytomenadione is a provitamin; following activation it exerts Vitamin K effects. Vitamin K is essential for the formation of prothrombin (Factor II) and other clotting factors (Factors VII, IX and X) in the liver. Deficiency of Vitamin K produces hypoprothrombinaemia, in which the clotting time of the blood is prolonged and spontaneous haemorrhage may occur.

Folic Acid

Folic acid is reduced in the body to tetrahydrofolate which is a co-enzyme for various metabolic processes, including the synthesis of purine and pyrimidine nucleotides and hence in the synthesis of DNA. It is also involved in some amino acid conversion and in the formation and utilisation of formate. Deficiency of folic acid leads to megaloblastic anaemia.

Vitamin H (d-Biotin)

Biotin is a co-enzyme for carboxylation during the metabolism of proteins and carbohydrates.

Selenium

Selenium is an essential trace element, deficiency of which has been reported in man. It is thought to be involved in the functioning of membranes and the synthesis of amino acids. Deficiency of selenium in the diet of experimental animals produces fatty liver followed by necrosis.

Iron

Iron, as a constituent of haemoglobin, plays an essential role in oxygen transport. It is also present in the muscle protein myoglobin and in the liver. Deficiency of iron leads to anaemia.

Copper (Copper Sulphate)

Traces of copper are essential to the body as constituents of enzyme systems involved in oxidation reactions.

Magnesium (Magnesium Sulphate)

Magnesium is essential to the body as a constituent of skeletal structures and in maintaining cell integrity and fluid balance. It is utilised in many of the functions in which calcium is concerned but often exerts the opposite effect. Some enzymes require the magnesium ion as a co-factor.

Zinc (Zinc Sulphate)

Zinc is a constituent of many enzymes and is, therefore, essential to the body. It is present with insulin in the pancreas. It plays a role in DNA synthesis and cell division. Reported effects of deficiency include delayed puberty and hypogonadal dwarfism.

Manganese (Manganese Sulphate)

Manganese is a constituent of enzyme systems including those involved in lipid synthesis, the tricarboxylic acid cycle and purine and pyrimidine metabolism. It is bound to arginase of the liver and activates many enzymes.

Iodine (Potassium Iodide)

Iodine is an essential constituent of the thyroid hormones.

Chromium (Chromium Amino Acid Chelate 10%)

Chromium is an essential trace element involved in carbohydrate metabolism.

Molybdenum (Sodium Molybdate)

Molybdenum is an essential trace element although there have been no reports of deficiency states in man. Molybdenum salts have been used to treat copper poisoning in sheep.

5.2 Pharmacokinetic properties

The following account describes the absorption and fate of each of the active constituents of Forceval Junior Capsules.

Vitamin A

Except when liver function is impaired, Vitamin A is readily absorbed. β-carotene (as in Forceval Junior Capsules) is Provitamin A and is the biological precursor to Vitamin A. It is converted to Vitamin A (Retinol) in the liver; retinol is emulsified by bile salts and phospholipids and absorbed in a micellar form. Part is conjugated with glucuronic acid in the kidney and part is metabolised in the liver and kidney, leaving 30 to 50% of the dose for storage in the liver. It is bound to a globulin in the blood. Metabolites of Vitamin A are excreted in the faeces and the urine.

Vitamin D

The metabolism of ergocalciferol is similar to that of cholecalciferol. Cholecalciferol is absorbed from the gastro-intestinal tract into the circulation. In the liver, it is hydroxylated to 25-hydroxycholecalciferol, is subject to entero-hepatic circulation and is further hydroxylated to 1,25-dihydroxycholecalciferol in the renal tubule cells. Vitamin D metabolites are bound to specific plasma proteins.

Vitamin B_1 (Thiamine)

Thiamine is absorbed from the gastro-intestinal tract and is widely distributed to most body tissues. Amounts in excess of the body's requirements are not stored but excreted in the urine as unchanged thiamine or its metabolites.

Vitamin B_2 (Riboflavine)

Riboflavine is absorbed from the gastro-intestinal tract and in the circulation is bound to plasma proteins. It is widely distributed. Little is stored and excess amounts are excreted in the urine. In the body riboflavine is converted to flavine mononucleotide (FMN) and then to flavine adenine dinucleotide (FAD).

Vitamin B_6 (Pyridoxine)

Pyridoxine is absorbed from the gastro-intestinal tract and converted to the active pyridoxal phosphate which is bound to plasma proteins. It is excreted in the urine as 4-pyridoxic acid.

Vitamin B_{12} (Cyanocobalamin)

Cyanocobalamin is absorbed from the gastro-intestinal tract and is extensively bound to specific plasma proteins. Vitamin B_{12} is taken up by the intestinal mucosa and held there for 2 - 3 hours. Peak concentrations in the blood and tissues occur 8 - 12 hours after dosage with maximum concentrations in the liver within 24 hours. Cobalamins are stored in the liver, excreted in the bile and undergo enterohepatic recycling. Part of a dose is excreted in the urine, most of it in the first eight hours.

Vitamin C (Ascorbic Acid)

Ascorbic acid is readily absorbed from the gastro-intestinal tract and is widely distributed in the body tissues. Ascorbic acid in excess of the body's needs is rapidly eliminated in the urine.

Vitamin E

Vitamin E is absorbed from the gastro-intestinal tract. Most appears in the lymph and is then widely distributed to all tissues. Most of a dose is slowly excreted in the bile and the remainder is eliminated in the urine as glucuronides of tocopheronic acid or other metabolites.

Nicotinamide (Nicotinic Acid Amide)

Nicotinamide is absorbed from the gastro-intestinal tract, is widely distributed in the body tissues and has a short half-life.

Calcium Pantothenate

Pantothenic acid is readily absorbed from the gastro-intestinal tract and is widely distributed in the body tissues. About 70% of pantothenic acid is excreted unchanged in the urine and about 30% in the faeces.

Vitamin K1 (Phytomenadione)

Phytomenadione is absorbed from the gastro-intestinal tract. It is rapidly metabolised and excreted and is not significantly stored in the body.

Folic Acid

Folic acid is absorbed mainly from the proximal part of the small intestine. Folate polyglutamates are considered to be deconjugated to monoglutamates during absorption. Folic acid rapidly appears in the blood where it is extensively bound to plasma proteins. Some folic acid is distributed in body tissues, some is excreted as folate in the urine and some is stored in the liver as folate.

Vitamin H (d-Biotin)

Following absorption, biotin is stored in the liver, kidney and pancreas.

Selenium

Although it has been established that selenium is essential to human life, very little information is available on its function and metabolism.

Ferrous Fumarate (Iron)

Iron is absorbed chiefly in the duodenum and jejunum. Absorption is aided by the acid secretion of the stomach and if the iron is in the ferrous state as in ferrous fumarate. In iron deficiency, absorption is increased and, conversely, it is decreased in iron overload. Iron is stored as ferritin.

Copper Sulphate (Copper)

Copper is absorbed from the gastro-intestinal tract and its major route of excretion is in the bile.

Magnesium Sulphate (Magnesium)

Magnesium salts are poorly absorbed from the gastro-intestinal tract; however, sufficient magnesium will normally be absorbed to replace deficiency states. It is excreted in both the urine and the faeces but excretion in the urine is reduced in deficiency states.

Zinc Sulphate (Zinc)

Zinc is poorly absorbed from the gastro-intestinal tract. It is widely distributed throughout the body. It is excreted in the faeces with traces appearing in the urine.

Manganese Sulphate (Manganese)

Manganese salts are poorly absorbed.

Potassium Iodide (Iodine)

Iodides are absorbed and stored in the thyroid gland as thyroglobulin. Iodides are excreted in the urine with smaller amounts appearing in the faeces, saliva and sweat.

Chromium Amino Acid Chelate 10% (Chromium)

Although it has been established that chromium is essential to human life, little information is available on its function and metabolism.

Sodium Molybdate (Molybdenum)

Although it has been established that molybdenum is essential to human life, little information is available on its function and metabolism.

5.3 Preclinical safety data

There are no pre-clinical data of relevance to the prescriber which are additional to that already included in other sections of the SPC.

6. PHARMACEUTICAL PARTICULARS

6.1 List of excipients

Soya Bean Oil BP

Soya Lecithin HSE

Fat Mix HSE

Purified Water PhEur

Gelatin BP

Glycerine BP

Black Iron Oxide Pigment (E172) HSE

Red Iron Oxide Pigment (E172) HSE

Sorbitol Solution 70% BP

6.2 Incompatibilities

No major incompatibilities are known.

6.3 Shelf life

24 months, as packaged for sale.

6.4 Special precautions for storage

Store in a cool dry place at a temperature not exceeding 25°C.

Protect from light.

6.5 Nature and contents of container

The product is presented in press-thru blister packs, each blister strip containing 10 Forceval Junior capsules. The blister strip is composed of PVC/PVdC with a printed aluminium foil lidding. The foil is printed (red on gold) with the name and PL number of the product, the number of vitamins and minerals per capsule and the daily dose.

The product is available in packs of 30, 60 or 120 capsules.

6.6 Special precautions for disposal and other handling

Not applicable.

7. MARKETING AUTHORISATION HOLDER

Alliance Pharmaceuticals Ltd

Avonbridge House

2 Bath Road

Chippenham

Wiltshire

SN15 2BB

United Kingdom

8. MARKETING AUTHORISATION NUMBER(S)

PL 16853/0080

9. DATE OF FIRST AUTHORISATION/RENEWAL OF THE AUTHORISATION

18th April 2005

10. DATE OF REVISION OF THE TEXT

April 2005

Formoterol Easyhaler 12 micrograms per inhalation powder

(Orion Pharma (UK) Limited)

1. NAME OF THE MEDICINAL PRODUCT

Formoterol Easyhaler® 12 micrograms per actuation Inhalation Powder

2. QUALITATIVE AND QUANTITATIVE COMPOSITION

One metered dose contains 12 micrograms of formoterol fumarate dihydrate.

With the Easyhaler device the delivered dose (ex-actuator) contains the same quantity of active substance as the metered dose (ex-reservoir).

For excipients, see Section 6.1.

3. PHARMACEUTICAL FORM

Inhalation powder.

White to yellowish white powder.

4. CLINICAL PARTICULARS

4.1 Therapeutic indications

Formoterol Easyhaler 12 micrograms per actuation Inhalation Powder is indicated for use in the treatment of asthma in patients treated with inhaled corticosteroids and who also require a long-acting beta2-agonist in accordance with current treatment guidelines.

Formoterol Easyhaler 12 micrograms per actuation Inhalation Powder is indicated also for the relief of reversible airways obstruction in patients with chronic obstructive pulmonary disease (COPD) and requiring long-term bronchodilator therapy.

4.2 Posology and method of administration

For inhalation use.

ADULTS (INCLUDING THE ELDERLY) AND ADOLESCENTS

Asthma

Regular maintenance therapy:

1 inhalation (12 micrograms) to be inhaled twice daily. For more severe disease this dose regimen can be increased to 2 inhalations (24 micrograms) to be inhaled twice daily.

The maximum daily dose is 4 inhalations (2 inhalations inhaled twice daily).

Chronic Obstructive Pulmonary Disease

Regular maintenance therapy:

1 inhalation (12 micrograms) to be inhaled twice daily.

The maximum daily dose is 2 inhalations (1 inhalation inhaled twice daily).

CHILDREN 6 YEARS AND OLDER

Asthma

Regular maintenance therapy:

1 inhalation (12 micrograms) to be inhaled twice daily. For more severe disease this dose regimen can be increased to 2 inhalations (24 micrograms) to be inhaled twice daily but only after assessment by a physician.

The maximum daily dose is 4 inhalations (2 inhalations inhaled twice daily).

Chronic Obstructive Pulmonary Disease

Not appropriate.

CHILDREN UNDER THE AGE OF 6 YEARS

Formoterol Easyhaler is not recommended for use in children under the age of 6 years.

Renal and hepatic impairment

There is no theoretical reason to suggest that Formoterol Easyhaler dosage requires adjustment in patients with renal or hepatic impairment, however no clinical data have been generated to support its use in these groups.

The duration of action of formoterol has been shown to last for about 12 hours. The treatment should always aim for the lowest effective dose.

Current asthma management guidelines recommend that long-acting inhaled beta2-agonists should be used for maintenance bronchodilator therapy. They further recommend that in the event of an acute attack, a short-acting beta2-agonist should be used.

In accordance with the current asthma management guidelines, long-acting beta2-agonists may be added to the treatment regimen in patients experiencing problems with high dose inhaled steroids. Patients should be advised not to stop or change their steroid therapy when treatment with formoterol is introduced.

If the symptoms persist or worsen, or if the recommended dose of Formoterol Easyhaler fails to control symptoms (maintain effective relief), this is usually an indication of a worsening of the underlying condition.

When transferring a patient to Formoterol Easyhaler from other inhalation devices, the treatment should be individualised. The previous active substance, dose regimen, and method of delivery should be considered.

Instructions for use and handling

Easyhaler is an inspiratory flow driven inhaler, which means that when the patient inhales through the mouthpiece, the substance will follow the inspired air into the airways.

Note: It is important to instruct the patient

- To carefully read the instructions for use in the patient information leaflet which is packed together with each inhaler.

- That it is recommended to keep the device in the protective cover after opening the laminate pouch to enhance the stability of the product during use and make the inhaler more tamper proof.

- To shake and actuate the device prior to each inhalation.

- To breathe in forcefully and deeply through the mouthpiece to ensure that an optimal dose is delivered to the lungs.

- Never to breathe out through the mouthpiece as this will result in a reduction in the delivered dose. Should this happen the patient is instructed to tap the mouthpiece onto a table top or the palm of a hand to empty the powder, and then to repeat the dosing procedure.

- Never to actuate the device more than once without inhalation of the powder. Should this happen the patient is instructed to tap the mouthpiece onto a table top or the palm of a hand to empty the powder, and then to repeat the dosing procedure.

- To always replace the dust cap and close the protective cover after use to prevent accidental actuation of the device (which could result in either overdosing or underdosing the patient when subsequently used).

- To clean the mouthpiece with a dry cloth at regular intervals. Water should never be used for cleaning because the powder is sensitive to moisture.

- To replace Formoterol Easyhaler when the counter reaches zero even though powder can still be observed within the device.

4.3 Contraindications

Hypersensitivity to formoterol fumarate dihydrate or to lactose monohydrate (which contains small amounts of milk proteins).

4.4 Special warnings and precautions for use

Patients with asthma who require regular treatment with a beta2-agonist should also be receiving regular and appropriate doses of an inhaled anti-inflammatory drug (e.g. corticosteroids and/or in children sodium cromoglycate) or oral corticosteroids. Formoterol Easyhaler should only be used in patients requiring long-term regular bronchodilator therapy and not as an alternative to short-acting beta2-agonists in the event of an acute asthma attack.

When treatment with formoterol is prescribed, patients should be assessed in respect of the appropriateness of the anti-inflammatory therapy they are receiving. Patients should be instructed to continue taking anti-inflammatory therapy and told that the dose of anti-inflammatory therapy should remain unchanged following the introduction of formoterol, even when symptoms improve. If there is no improvement in symptoms or the number of doses of formoterol required to control symptoms increases, this usually indicates deterioration of the underlying condition and the patients should be told to contact their doctor in order that their asthma and its treatment can be reassessed.

Therapy should not be initiated during an exacerbation. In the event of an acute asthma attack, a short-acting beta2-agonist should be used.

Special care and supervision, with particular emphasis on dosage limits, is required in patients receiving Formoterol Easyhaler when the following conditions may exist:

Severe hypertension, severe heart failure, ischaemic heart disease, cardiac arrhythmias, especially third degree atrioventricular block, idiopathic subvalvular aortic stenosis, hypertrophic obstructive cardiomyopathy, thyrotoxicosis, phaeochromocytoma, aneurysm, known or suspected prolongation of the QT interval (QT > 0.44 sec.; see Section 4.5 Interaction with other medicinal products and other forms of interaction) and in patients treated with drugs affecting the QT interval. Formoterol itself may induce prolongation of QT interval.

Caution should be used when co-administering theophylline and formoterol in patients with pre-existing cardiac conditions.

Due to the hyperglycaemic effect of beta2-stimulants, additional blood glucose controls are recommended in diabetic patients.

Potentially serious hypokalaemia may result from beta2-agonist therapy. Particular caution is recommended in acute severe asthma as the associated risk may be augmented by hypoxia. The hypokalaemic effect may be potentiated by concomitant treatment with other medicines, such as xanthine derivatives, steroids and diuretics (see Section 4.5 Interaction with other medicinal products and other forms of interaction). It is recommended that serum potassium levels are monitored in such situations.

As with other inhalation therapy there is a risk of paradoxical bronchospasm. If this occurs the patient will experience an immediate increase in wheezing and shortness of breath after dosing which should be treated straightaway with a fast-acting inhaled bronchodilator. Formoterol Easyhaler inhalation powder should be discontinued immediately, the patient should be assessed and, if necessary, alternative therapy instituted.

Formoterol Easyhaler contains approx. 8 mg of lactose per dose. Patients with rare hereditary problems of galactose intolerance, the Lapp lactase deficiency or glucose-galactose malabsorption should not take this medicine.

4.5 Interaction with other medicinal products and other forms of interaction

No specific interaction studies have been carried out with Formoterol Easyhaler.

Drugs such as quinidine, disopyramide, procainamide, phenothiazines, antihistamines and tricyclic antidepressants may be associated with QT interval prolongation and an increased risk of ventricular arrhythmia (see Section 4.4 Special warnings and precautions for use). In addition, levodopa, levothyroxine, oxytocin and alcohol can impair cardiac tolerance towards beta2-agonists.

Concomitant administration of other sympathomimetic agents has the potential to produce additive effects both in respect of the desirable effects and the undesirable effects of Formoterol Easyhaler.

Formoterol may interact with monoamine oxidase inhibitors and should not be given to patients receiving treatment with monoamine oxidase inhibitors or for up to 14 days after their discontinuation.

There may be an increased risk of arrhythmias in patients undergoing concomitant treatment with tricyclic antidepressants.

Concomitant administration of formoterol and corticosteroids may increase the hyperglycaemic effect seen with these drugs.

Concomitant treatment with xanthine derivatives, steroids, or potassium-depleting diuretics may potentiate a possible hypokalaemic effect of beta2-agonists. Hypokalaemia may increase susceptibility to cardiac arrhythmias in patients treated with digitalis (see Section 4.4 Special warnings and precautions for use).

There is an elevated risk of arrhythmias in patients receiving concomitant anaesthesia with halogenated hydrocarbons.

Beta-adrenergic blockers may weaken or antagonise the effect of Formoterol Easyhaler. Therefore Formoterol Easyhaler should not be given together with beta-adrenergic blockers (including eye drops) unless there are compelling reasons for their use.

4.6 Pregnancy and lactation

Clinical experience with formoterol in pregnant women is limited. No teratogenic effects have been revealed in animal tests. However, until further experience is gained, Formoterol Easyhaler is not recommended for use during pregnancy (particularly at the end of pregnancy or during labour) unless there is no other (safer) established alternative. As with any medicine, use during pregnancy should only be considered if the expected benefit to the mother is greater than any risk to the foetus. The substance has been detected in the milk of lactating rats, but it is not known whether formoterol passes into human breast milk, therefore mothers using Formoterol Easyhaler should refrain from breast-feeding their infants.

4.7 Effects on ability to drive and use machines

Formoterol has no or negligible influence on the ability to drive and use machines.

4.8 Undesirable effects

(see Table 1 on next page)

Treatment with $beta_2$-agonists may result in an increase in blood levels of insulin, free fatty acids, glycerol and ketone bodies.

Table 1 Undesirable effects

Metabolism and nutrition disorders	Rare >1/10,000, <1/1,000)	Hypokalaemia
	Very rare including isolated reports (<1/10,000)	Hyperglycaemia
Nervous system disorders	Common >1/100, <1/10)	Headache
	Uncommon >1/1,000, <1/100)	Agitation, dizziness, anxiety, nervousness, insomnia
Cardiac disorders	Common >1/100, <1/10)	Palpitations
	Uncommon >1/1,000, <1/100)	Tachycardia
	Rare >1/10,000, <1/1,000)	Atrial fibrillation, supraventricular tachycardia, extrasystoles
	Very rare including isolated reports (<1/10,000)	Angina pectoris, prolongation of QTc interval
Vascular disorders	Very rare including isolated reports (<1/10,000)	Variation in blood pressure
Respiratory, thoracic and mediastinal disorders	Rare >1/10,000, <1/1,000)	Aggravated bronchospasm, paradoxical bronchospasm (see Section 4.4 Special warnings and precautions for use), oropharyngeal irritation
Gastrointestinal disorders	Very rare including isolated reports (<1/10,000)	Taste disturbance, nausea
Musculoskeletal, connective tissue and bone disorders	Common >1/100, <1/10)	Tremor
	Uncommon >1/1,000, <1/100)	Muscle cramps, myalgia
General disorders and administration site conditions	Very rare including isolated reports (<1/10,000)	Hypersensitivity reactions such as severe hypotension, urticaria, angioedema, pruritus, exanthema, peripheral oedema

Lactose monohydrate contains small amounts of milk proteins and can therefore cause allergic reactions.

4.9 Overdose

Symptoms

There is no clinical experience to date on the management of overdose, however, an overdosage of Formoterol Easyhaler would be likely to lead to effects that are typical of beta2-adrenergic agonists: nausea, vomiting, headache, tremor, somnolence, palpitations, tachycardia, ventricular arrhythmias, metabolic acidosis, hypokalaemia, hyperglycaemia.

Treatment

Supportive and symptomatic treatment is indicated. Serious cases should be hospitalised.

Use of cardioselective beta-blockers may be considered, but only subject to extreme caution since the use of beta-adrenergic blocker medication may provoke bronchospasm.

Serum potassium should be monitored.

5. PHARMACOLOGICAL PROPERTIES

5.1 Pharmacodynamic properties

Pharmacotherapeutic group: Selective beta2-adrenoreceptor agonists.

ATC code: R03AC13.

Formoterol is a potent selective beta2-adrenergic stimulant. It exerts a bronchodilator effect in patients with reversible airways obstruction. The effect sets in rapidly (within 1–3 minutes) and is still significant 12 hours after inhalation.

In man, formoterol has been shown to be effective in preventing bronchospasm induced by exercise and methacholine.

Formoterol has been studied in the treatment of conditions associated with COPD, and has been shown to improve symptoms and pulmonary function. Formoterol acts on the reversible component of the disease.

5.2 Pharmacokinetic properties

Absorption

As reported for other inhaled drugs, it is likely that about 80% of formoterol administered from the Easyhaler inhaler will be swallowed and then absorbed from the gastrointestinal tract. This means that the pharmacokinetic characteristics of the oral formulation largely apply also to the inhalation powder. Following inhalation of therapeutic doses, formoterol cannot be detected in the plasma using current analytical methods.

Absorption is both rapid and extensive: At a higher than therapeutic dose (120 micrograms), the peak plasma concentration is observed at 5 minutes post inhalation whilst at least 65% of a radio-labelled 80 micrograms oral dose is absorbed, and oral doses of up to 300 micrograms are readily absorbed with the peak concentrations of unchanged formoterol at 0.5–1 hour. In COPD patients treated for 12 weeks with formoterol fumarate 12 or 24 micrograms b.i.d. the plasma concentrations of formoterol ranged between 11.5 and 25.7 pmol/L and 23.3 and 50.3 pmol/L respectively at 10 minutes, 2 hours and 6 hours post inhalation.

The pharmacokinetics of formoterol appear linear in the range of oral doses investigated, i.e. 20–300 micrograms. Repeated oral administration of 40–160 micrograms daily does not lead to significant accumulation of the drug. The maximum excretion rate after administration of 12–96 micrograms is reached within 1–2 hours of inhalation.

After 12 weeks administration of 12 micrograms or 24 micrograms formoterol powder b.i.d., the urinary excretion of unchanged formoterol increased by 63–73% in adult patients and by 18–84% in children, suggesting a modest and self-limiting accumulation of formoterol in plasma after repeated dosing.

Studies investigating the cumulative urinary excretion of formoterol and/or its (R,R) and (S,S)-enantiomers, after inhalation of dry powder (12–96 micrograms) or aerosol formulations (12-96 micrograms), showed that absorption increased linearly with the dose.

Distribution

The plasma protein binding of formoterol is 61–64% (34% primarily to albumin). There is no saturation of binding sites in the concentration range reached with therapeutic doses.

Biotransformation

Formoterol is eliminated primarily by metabolism, direct glucuronidation being the major pathway of biotransformation, with O-demethylation followed by further glucuronidation being another pathway. Multiple CYP450 isoenzymes (2D6, 2C19, 2C9, and 2A6) catalyze the transformation and so consequently the potential for metabolic drug-drug interaction is low. The kinetics of formoterol are similar after single and repeated administration, indicating no auto-induction or inhibition of metabolism.

Elimination

Elimination of formoterol from the circulation seems to be polyphasic; the apparent half-life depends on the time interval considered. On the basis of plasma or blood concentrations up to 6, 8 or 12 hours after oral administration, an elimination half-life of about 2–3 hours was determined. From urinary excretion rates between 3 and 16 hours after inhalation, a half-life of about 5 hours was calculated.

After inhalation, plasma formoterol kinetics and urinary excretion rate data in healthy volunteers indicate a biphasic elimination, with the terminal elimination half-lives of the (R,R)- and (S,S)-enantiomers being 13.9 and 12.3 hours, respectively. Approximately 6.4–8% of the dose was recovered in the urine as unchanged formoterol, with the (R,R) and (S,S)-enantiomers contributing 40% and 60% respectively.

After a single oral dose of 3H-formoterol, 59–62% of the dose was recovered in the urine and 32–34% in the faeces. Renal clearance of formoterol is 150 ml/min.

In adult asthmatics, approximately 10% and 15–18% of the dose was recovered in the urine as unchanged and conjugated formoterol, respectively, after multiple doses of 12 and 24 micrograms. In children, approximately 6% and 6.5–9% of the dose was recovered in the urine as unchanged and conjugated formoterol, respectively, after multiple doses of 12 and 24 micrograms. As in healthy volunteers, the (R,R) and (S,S)-enantiomers contributed approximately 40% and 60% of unchanged drug excreted in the urine of adults, respectively, and there was no relative accumulation of one enantiomer over the other after repeated dosing.

5.3 Preclinical safety data

Preclinical data reveal no special hazard for humans in the therapeutic dose range based on conventional studies of repeated dose toxicity, genotoxicity, carcinogenicity, and reproduction toxicity. A somewhat reduced fertility in male rats was observed at high systemic exposure to formoterol. In rats and mice a slight increase in the incidence of uterine leiomyomas has been observed. This effect is looked upon as a class-effect observed in rodents after long exposure to high doses of beta2-receptor agonists.

6. PHARMACEUTICAL PARTICULARS

6.1 List of excipients

Lactose monohydrate

6.2 Incompatibilities

Not applicable.

6.3 Shelf life

As packaged for sale: 2 years.

After first opening the laminate pouch: 4 months.

6.4 Special precautions for storage

After opening the pouch: Do not store above 30°C.

6.5 Nature and contents of container

The multi-dose powder inhaler consists of seven plastic parts and a stainless steel spring. The plastic materials of the inhaler are: polybutylene terepthalate, low density polyethylene, polycarbonate, styrenebutadiene, polypropylene. The inhaler is sealed in a laminate pouch and packed with or without a protective cover in a cardboard box.

Packages:

Formoterol Easyhaler 12 micrograms per actuation inhalation powder:

- 120 actuations + protective cover
- 120 actuations
- 2 × 120 actuations

(Protective cover is available separately)

6.6 Special precautions for disposal and other handling

No special requirements.

7. MARKETING AUTHORISATION HOLDER

Ranbaxy (UK) Ltd
20 Balderton St
London
W1K 6TL
UK

8. MARKETING AUTHORISATION NUMBER(S)

PL 14894/0415

9. DATE OF FIRST AUTHORISATION/RENEWAL OF THE AUTHORISATION

February 2007

10. DATE OF REVISION OF THE TEXT

February 2007

Forsteo 20 micrograms/80 microlitres, solution for injection, in pre-filled pen

(Eli Lilly and Company Limited)

1. NAME OF THE MEDICINAL PRODUCT

FORSTEO*▼ 20 micrograms/80 microlitres, solution for injection, in pre-filled pen.

2. QUALITATIVE AND QUANTITATIVE COMPOSITION

Each dose contains 20 micrograms of teriparatide.

One pre-filled pen of 3ml contains 750 micrograms of teriparatide (corresponding to 250 micrograms per ml).

or

One pre-filled pen of 2.4 ml contains 600 micrograms of teriparatide (corresponding to 250 micrograms per ml).

Teriparatide, rhPTH(1-34), produced in *E. coli*, using recombinant DNA technology, is identical to the 34 N-terminal amino acid sequence of endogenous human parathyroid hormone.

For a full list of excipients, see section 6.1.

3. PHARMACEUTICAL FORM

Solution for injection in a pre-filled pen.

Colourless, clear solution.

4. CLINICAL PARTICULARS

4.1 Therapeutic indications

Treatment of osteoporosis in postmenopausal women and in men at increased risk of fracture (see section 5.1). In postmenopausal women, a significant reduction in the incidence of vertebral and non-vertebral fractures but not hip fractures has been demonstrated.

Treatment of osteoporosis associated with sustained systemic glucocorticoid therapy in women and men at increased risk for fracture (see section 5.1).

4.2 Posology and method of administration

The recommended dose of FORSTEO is 20 micrograms administered once daily by subcutaneous injection in the thigh or abdomen.

Patients must be trained to use the proper injection techniques (see section 6.6). A User Manual is also available to instruct patients on the correct use of the pen.

The maximum total duration of treatment with FORSTEO should be 24 months (see section 4.4). The 24-month course of FORSTEO should not be repeated over a patient's lifetime.

Patients should receive supplemental calcium and vitamin D supplements if dietary intake is inadequate.

Following cessation of FORSTEO therapy, patients may be continued on other osteoporosis therapies.

Use in renal impairment: FORSTEO should not be used in patients with severe renal impairment (see section 4.3). In patients with moderate renal impairment, FORSTEO should be used with caution.

Use in hepatic impairment: No data are available in patients with impaired hepatic function (see section 5.3).

Paediatric population and young adults with open epiphyses: There is no experience in paediatric patients (less than 18 years). FORSTEO should not be used in paediatric patients (less than 18 years), or young adults with open epiphyses.

Elderly patients: Dosage adjustment based on age is not required (see section 5.2).

4.3 Contraindications

- Hypersensitivity to the active substance or to any of the excipients.
- Pregnancy and lactation (see sections 4.4 and 4.6).
- Pre-existing hypercalcaemia.
- Severe renal impairment.
- Metabolic bone diseases (including hyperparathyroidism and Paget's disease of the bone) other than primary osteoporosis or glucorticoid-induced osteoporosis.
- Unexplained elevations of alkaline phosphatase.
- Prior external beam or implant radiation therapy to the skeleton.
- Patients with skeletal malignancies or bone metastases should be excluded from treatment with teriparatide.

4.4 Special warnings and precautions for use

In normocalcaemic patients, slight and transient elevations of serum calcium concentrations have been observed following teriparatide injection. Serum calcium concentrations reach a maximum between 4 and 6 hours and return to baseline by 16 to 24 hours after each dose of teriparatide. Routine calcium monitoring during therapy is not required.

Therefore if any blood samples are taken from a patient, this should be done at least 16 hours after the most recent FORSTEO injection.

FORSTEO may cause small increases in urinary calcium excretion, but the incidence of hypercalciuria did not differ from that in the placebo-treated patients in clinical trials.

FORSTEO has not been studied in patients with active urolithiasis. FORSTEO should be used with caution in patients with active or recent urolithiasis because of the potential to exacerbate this condition.

In short-term clinical studies with FORSTEO, isolated episodes of transient orthostatic hypotension were observed. Typically, an event began within 4 hours of dosing and spontaneously resolved within a few minutes to a few hours. When transient orthostatic hypotension occurred, it happened within the first several doses, was relieved by placing subjects in a reclining position, and did not preclude continued treatment.

Caution should be exercised in patients with moderate renal impairment.

Experience in the younger adult population, including premenopausal women, is limited (see section 5.1). Treatment should only be initiated if the benefit clearly outweighs risks in this population.

Women of childbearing potential should use effective methods of contraception during use of FORSTEO. If pregnancy occurs, FORSTEO should be discontinued.

Studies in rats indicate an increased incidence of osteosarcoma with long-term administration of teriparatide (see section 5.3). Until further clinical data become available, the recommended treatment time of 24 months should not be exceeded.

4.5 Interaction with other medicinal products and other forms of interaction

FORSTEO has been evaluated in pharmacodynamic interaction studies with hydrochlorothiazide. No clinically significant interactions were noted.

Co-administration of raloxifene or hormone replacement therapy with FORSTEO did not alter the effects of FORSTEO on serum or urine calcium or on clinical adverse events.

In a study of 15 healthy subjects administered digoxin daily to steady state, a single FORSTEO dose did not alter the cardiac effect of digoxin. However, sporadic case reports have suggested that hypercalcaemia may predispose patients to digitalis toxicity. Because FORSTEO transiently increases serum calcium, FORSTEO should be used with caution in patients taking digitalis.

4.6 Pregnancy and lactation

General recommendation

Studies in rabbits have shown reproductive toxicity (see section 5.3). The effect of teriparatide on human foetal development has not been studied. The potential risk for humans is unknown.

It is not known whether teriparatide is excreted in human milk.

FORSTEO is contraindicated for use during pregnancy or breast-feeding.

Women of childbearing potential / Contraception in females

Women of childbearing potential should use effective methods of contraception during use of FORSTEO. If pregnancy occurs, FORSTEO should be discontinued.

4.7 Effects on ability to drive and use machines

No studies on the effects on the ability to drive and use machines have been performed. However, transient, orthostatic hypotension or dizziness was observed in some patients. These patients should refrain from driving or the use of machines until symptoms have subsided.

4.8 Undesirable effects

Of patients in the teriparatide trials, 82.8% of the FORSTEO patients and 84.5% of the placebo patients reported at least 1 adverse event.

The most commonly reported adverse reactions in patients treated with FORSTEO are nausea, pain in limb, headache and dizziness.

The undesirable reactions associated with the use of teriparatide in osteoporosis clinical trials and post-marketing exposure are summarised in the table below. The following convention has been used for the classification of the adverse reactions: very common (≥ 1/10), common (≥ 1/100 to < 1/10), uncommon (≥ 1/1,000 to < 1/100), rare (≥ 1/10,000 to < 1/1,000), very rare (< 1/10,000), not known (cannot be estimated from the available data).

Investigations *Uncommon*: Weight increased, Cardiac murmur, Alkaline phosphatase increase
Cardiac disorders *Common*: Palpitations *Uncommon*: Tachycardia
Blood and lymphatic system disorders *Common*: Anaemia
Nervous system disorders *Common*: Dizziness, Headache, Sciatica
Ear and labyrinth disorders *Common*: Vertigo
Respiratory, thoracic and mediastinal disorders *Common*: Dyspnoea *Uncommon*: Emphysema
Gastrointestinal disorders *Common*: Nausea, Vomiting, Hiatus hernia, Gastro-oesophageal reflux disease *Uncommon*: Haemorrhoids
Renal and urinary disorders *Uncommon*: Urinary incontinence, Polyuria, Micturition urgency *Not known*: Renal failure/impairment
Skin and subcutaneous tissue disorders *Common*: Sweating increased
Musculoskeletal and connective tissue disorders *Very common*: Pain in limb *Common*: Muscle cramps *Uncommon*: Myalgia, Arthralgia *Not known*: Back cramp/pain*
Metabolism and nutrition disorders *Common*: Hypercholesterolaemia *Uncommon*: Hypercalcaemia greater than 2.76 mmol/L, Hyperuricaemia *Rare*: Hypercalcaemia greater than 3.25 mmol/L
Vascular disorders *Common*: Hypotension
General disorders and administration site conditions *Common*: Fatigue, Chest pain, Asthenia, Mild and transient injection site events, including pain, swelling, erythema, localised bruising, pruritus and minor bleeding at injection site *Uncommon*: Injection site erythema, Injection site reaction *Rare*: Possible allergic events soon after injection: acute dyspnoea, oro/facial oedema, generalised urticaria, chest pain, oedema (mainly peripheral)
Psychiatric disorders *Common*: Depression

* Serious cases of back cramp or pain have been reported within minutes of the injection.

In clinical trials the following reactions were reported at a ≥ 1% difference in frequency from placebo: vertigo, nausea, pain in limb, dizziness, depression, dyspnoea.

FORSTEO increases serum uric acid concentrations. In clinical trials, 2.8% of FORSTEO patients had serum uric acid concentrations above the upper limit of normal compared with 0.7% of placebo patients. However, the hyperuricaemia did not result in an increase in gout, arthralgia, or urolithiasis.

In a large clinical trial, antibodies that cross-reacted with teriparatide were detected in 2.8% of women receiving FORSTEO. Generally, antibodies were first detected following 12 months of treatment and diminished after withdrawal of therapy. There was no evidence of hypersensitivity reactions, allergic reactions, effects on serum calcium, or effects on BMD response.

4.9 Overdose

Signs and symptoms: No cases of overdose were reported during clinical trials. FORSTEO has been administered in single doses of up to 100 micrograms and in repeated doses of up to 60 micrograms/day for 6 weeks.

The effects of overdose that might be expected include delayed hypercalcaemia and risk of orthostatic hypotension. Nausea, vomiting, dizziness, and headache can also occur.

Overdose experience based on post-marketing spontaneous reports: In post-marketing spontaneous reports, there have been cases of medication error where the entire contents (up to 800μg) of the teriparatide pen have been administered as a single dose. Transient events reported have included nausea, weakness/lethargy and hypotension. In some cases, no adverse events occurred as a result of the overdose. No fatalities associated with overdose have been reported.

Overdose management: There is no specific antidote for FORSTEO. Treatment of suspected overdose should include transitory discontinuation of FORSTEO, monitoring of serum calcium, and implementation of appropriate supportive measures, such as hydration.

5. PHARMACOLOGICAL PROPERTIES

5.1 Pharmacodynamic properties

Pharmacotherapeutic group: Parathyroid hormones and analogues. *ATC code:* H05 AA02.

Mechanism of action: Endogenous 84-amino-acid parathyroid hormone (PTH) is the primary regulator of calcium and phosphate metabolism in bone and kidney. FORSTEO (rhPTH[1-34]) is the active fragment (1-34) of endogenous human parathyroid hormone. Physiological actions of PTH include stimulation of bone formation by direct effects on bone-forming cells (osteoblasts) indirectly increasing the intestinal absorption of calcium and increasing the tubular re-absorption of calcium and excretion of phosphate by the kidney.

Pharmacodynamic effects: FORSTEO is a bone formation agent to treat osteoporosis. The skeletal effects of FORSTEO depend upon the pattern of systemic exposure. Once-daily administration of FORSTEO increases apposition of new bone on trabecular and cortical bone surfaces by preferential stimulation of osteoblastic activity over osteoclastic activity.

Clinical efficacy

Risk Factors

Independent risk factors, for example, low BMD, age, the existence of previous fracture, family history of hip fractures, high bone turnover and low body mass index should be considered in order to identify women and men at increased risk of osteoporotic fractures who could benefit from treatment.

Premenopausal women with glucocorticoid-induced osteoporosis should be considered at high risk for fracture if they have a prevalent fracture or a combination of risk factors that place them at high risk for fracture (e.g., low bone density [e.g., T-score ≤ −2], sustained high dose glucocorticoid therapy [e.g., ≥7.5 mg/day for at least 6 months], high underlying disease activity, low sex steroid levels).

Postmenopausal osteoporosis:

The pivotal study included 1,637 postmenopausal women (mean age 69.5 years). At baseline, ninety percent of the patients had one or more vertebral fractures and on average, vertebral BMD was 0.82 g/cm^2 (equivalent to a T-score = -2.6). All patients were offered 1000mg calcium per day and at least 400IU vitamin D per day. Results from up to 24 months (median: 19 months) treatment with FORSTEO demonstrate statistically significant fracture reduction (Table 4). To prevent one or more new vertebral fractures, 11 women had to be treated for a median of 19 months.

(see Table 1 on next page)

After 19 months (median) treatment, bone mineral density (BMD) had increased in the lumbar spine and total hip, respectively, by 9% and 4% compared with placebo (p < 0.001).

Post-treatment management: Following treatment with FORSTEO, 1,262 postmenopausal women from the pivotal trial enrolled in a post-treatment follow-up study. The primary objective of the study was to collect safety data on FORSTEO. During this observational period, other osteoporosis treatments were allowed and additional assessment of vertebral fractures was performed.

During a median of 18 months following discontinuation of FORSTEO, there was a 41% reduction (p = 0.004)

Table 1 Fracture Incidence in Postmenopausal Women

	Placebo (N = 544) (%)	FORSTEO (N = 541) (%)	Relative Risk (95% CI) vs placebo
New vertebral fracture (≥1)[a]	14.3	5.0 [b]	0.35 (0.22, 0.55)
Multiple vertebral fractures (≥2)[a]	4.9	1.1 [b]	0.23 (0.09, 0.60)
Non-vertebral fragility fractures [c]	5.5	2.6 [d]	0.47 (0.25, 0.87)
Major non-vertebral fragility fractures[c] (hip, radius, humerus, ribs and pelvis)	3.9	1.5 [d]	0.38 (0.17, 0.86)

Abbreviations: N = number of patients randomly assigned to each treatment group; CI = Confidence Interval.

[a] The incidence of vertebral fractures was assessed in 448 placebo and 444 FORSTEO patients who had baseline and follow-up spine radiographs.

[b] $p \leq 0.001$ compared with placebo.

[c] A significant reduction in the incidence of hip fractures has not been demonstrated.

[d] $p \leq 0.025$ compared with placebo.

compared with placebo in the number of patients with a minimum of one new vertebral fracture.

In an open-label study, 503 postmenopausal women with severe osteoporosis and a fragility fracture within the previous 3 years (83% had received previous osteoporosis therapy) were treated with FORSTEO for up to 24 months. At 24 months, the mean increase from baseline in lumbar spine, total hip and femoral neck BMD was 10.5%, 2.6% and 3.9% respectively. The mean increase in BMD from 18 to 24 months was 1.4%, 1.2%, and 1.6% at the lumbar spine, total hip and femoral neck, respectively.

Male osteoporosis:

437 patients (mean age 58.7 years) were enrolled in a clinical trial for men with hypogonadal (defined as low-morning free testosterone or an elevated FSH or LH) or idiopathic osteoporosis. Baseline spinal and femoral neck bone mineral density mean T-scores were -2.2 and -2.1, respectively. At baseline, 35% of patients had a vertebral fracture and 59% had a non-vertebral fracture.

All patients were offered 1,000mg calcium per day and at least 400IU vitamin D per day. Lumbar spine BMD significantly increased by 3 months. After 12 months, BMD had increased in the lumbar spine and total hip by 5% and 1%, respectively, compared with placebo. However, no significant effect on fracture rates was demonstrated.

Glucocorticoid-induced osteoporosis:

The efficacy of FORSTEO in men and women (N =428) receiving sustained systemic glucocorticoid therapy (equivalent to 5 mg or greater of prednisone for at least 3 months) was demonstrated in the 18-month primary phase of a 36-month, randomised, double-blind, comparator-controlled study (alendronate 10 mg/day). Twenty-eight percent of patients had one or more radiographic vertebral fractures at baseline. All patients were offered 1000 mg calcium per day and 800 IU vitamin D per day.

This study included postmenopausal women (N =277), premenopausal women (N =67), and men (N =83). At baseline, the postmenopausal women had a mean age of 61 years, mean lumbar spine BMD T-score of −2.7, median prednisone equivalent dose of 7.5 mg/day, and 34% had one or more radiographic vertebral fractures; premenopausal women had a mean age of 37 years, mean lumbar spine BMD T-score of −2.5, median prednisone equivalent dose of 10 mg/day, and 9% had one or more radiographic vertebral fractures; and men had a mean age of 57 years, mean lumbar spine BMD T-score of −2.2, median prednisone equivalent dose of 10 mg/day, and 24% had one or more radiographic vertebral fractures.

Sixty-nine percent of patients completed the 18-month primary phase. At the 18-month endpoint, FORSTEO significantly increased lumbar spine BMD (7.2%) compared with alendronate (3.4%) ($p < 0.001$). FORSTEO increased BMD at the total hip (3.6%) compared with alendronate (2.2%) ($p < 0.01$), as well as at the femoral neck (3.7%) compared with alendronate (2.1%) ($p < 0.05$). In patients treated with teriparatide, lumbar spine, total hip and femoral neck BMD increased between 18 and 24 months by an additional 1.7%, 0.9%, and 0.4%, respectively.

At 36 months, analysis of spinal X-rays from 169 alendronate patients and 173 FORSTEO patients showed that 13 patients in the alendronate group (7.7%) had experienced a new vertebral fracture compared with 3 patients in the FORSTEO group (1.7%) (p=0.01). In addition, 15 of 214 patients in the alendronate group (7.0%) had experienced a non-vertebral fracture compared with 16 of 214 patients in the FORSTEO group (7.5%) (p =0.84).

In premenopausal women, the increase in BMD from baseline to 18-month endpoint was significantly greater in the FORSTEO group compared with the alendronate group at the lumbar spine (4.2% versus −1.9%; (p <0.001) and total hip (3.8% versus 0.9%; p =0.005). However, no significant effect on fracture rates was demonstrated.

5.2 Pharmacokinetic properties

FORSTEO is eliminated through hepatic and extra-hepatic clearance (approximately 62 l/hr in women and 94 l/hr in men). The volume of distribution is approximately 1.7 l/kg. The half-life of FORSTEO is approximately 1 hour when administered subcutaneously, which reflects the time required for absorption from the injection site. No metabolism or excretion studies have been performed with FORSTEO, but the peripheral metabolism of parathyroid hormone is believed to occur predominantly in liver and kidney.

Patient characteristics

Geriatrics: No differences in FORSTEO pharmacokinetics were detected with regard to age (range 31 to 85 years). Dosage adjustment based on age is not required.

5.3 Preclinical safety data

Teriparatide was not genotoxic in a standard battery of tests. It produced no teratogenic effects in rats, mice or rabbits. There were no important effects observed in pregnant rats or mice administered teriparatide at daily doses of 30 to 1000 μg/kg. However, foetal resorption and reduced litter size occurred in pregnant rabbits administered daily doses of 3 to 100 μg/kg. The embryotoxicity observed in rabbits may be related to their much greater sensitivity to the effects of PTH on blood-ionised calcium compared with rodents.

Rats treated with near-lifetime daily injections had dose-dependent exaggerated bone formation and increased incidence of osteosarcoma most probably due to an epigenetic mechanism. Teriparatide did not increase the incidence of any other type of neoplasia in rats. Due to the differences in bone physiology in rats and humans, the clinical relevance of these findings is probably minor. No bone tumours were observed in ovariectomised monkeys treated for 18 months or during a 3-year follow-up period after treatment cessation. In addition, no osteosarcomas have been observed in clinical trials or during the post-treatment follow-up study.

Animal studies have shown that severely reduced hepatic blood flow decreases exposure of PTH to the principal cleavage system (Kupffer cells) and consequently clearance of PTH(1-84).

6. PHARMACEUTICAL PARTICULARS

6.1 List of excipients

Glacial acetic acid

Sodium acetate (anhydrous)

Mannitol

Metacresol

Hydrochloric acid

Sodium hydroxide

Water for injections

Hydrochloric acid and/or sodium hydroxide solution may be added to adjust pH.

6.2 Incompatibilities

In the absence of compatibility studies, this medicinal product must not be mixed with other medicinal products.

6.3 Shelf life

2 years.

Chemical, physical and microbiological in-use stability has been demonstrated for 28 days at 2°C-8°C. Once opened, the product may be stored for a maximum of 28 days at 2°C to 8°C. Other in-use storage times and conditions are the responsibility of the user.

6.4 Special precautions for storage

Store in a refrigerator (2°C-8°C) at all times. The pen should be returned to the refrigerator immediately after use. Do not freeze.

Do not store the injection device with the needle attached.

6.5 Nature and contents of container

3ml solution in cartridge (siliconised Type I glass) with a plunger (halobutyl rubber), disc seal (polyisoprene/bromobutyl rubber laminate) and crimp cap (aluminium) assembled into a disposable pen.

or

2.4 ml solution in cartridge (siliconised Type I glass) with a plunger (halobutyl rubber), disc seal (polyisoprene/bromobutyl rubber laminate)/aluminium assembled into a disposable pen.

FORSTEO is available in pack sizes of 1 or 3 pens. Each pen contains 28 doses of 20 micrograms (per 80 microlitres).

Not all pack sizes may be marketed.

6.6 Special precautions for disposal and other handling

FORSTEO is supplied in a pre-filled pen. Each pen should be used by only one patient. A new, sterile needle must be used for every injection. Each FORSTEO pack is provided with a User Manual that fully describes the use of the pen. No needles are supplied with the product. The device can be used with insulin pen injection needles. After each injection, the FORSTEO pen should be returned to the refrigerator.

FORSTEO should not be used if the solution is cloudy, coloured or contains particles.

Please also refer to the User Manual for instructions on how to use the pen.

Any unused product or waste material should be disposed of in accordance with local requirements.

7. MARKETING AUTHORISATION HOLDER

Eli Lilly Nederland BV, Grootslag 1-5, NL-3991 RA Houten, The Netherlands.

8. MARKETING AUTHORISATION NUMBER(S)

EU/1/03/247/001: 1 pre-filled pen

EU/1/03/247/002: 3 pre-filled pens

9. DATE OF FIRST AUTHORISATION/RENEWAL OF THE AUTHORISATION

Date of first authorisation: 10 June 2003

Date of last renewal: 10 June 2008

10. DATE OF REVISION OF THE TEXT

28 August 2009

LEGAL CATEGORY

POM

*FORSTEO (teriparatide) is a trademark of Eli Lilly and Company. FS9M

Fortum 1g Injection

(GlaxoSmithKline UK)

1. NAME OF THE MEDICINAL PRODUCT

Fortum® for Injection

Ceftazidime (as pentahydrate) (INN) Injection

2. QUALITATIVE AND QUANTITATIVE COMPOSITION

Fortum for Injection: Vials contain 1g ceftazidime (as pentahydrate) with sodium carbonate (118mg per gram of ceftazidime).

3. PHARMACEUTICAL FORM

Sterile Powder for constitution for Injection

4. CLINICAL PARTICULARS

4.1 Therapeutic indications

Single infections

Mixed infections caused by two or more susceptible organisms

Severe infections in general

Respiratory tract infections

Ear, nose and throat infections

Urinary tract infections

Skin and soft tissue infections

Gastrointestinal, biliary and abdominal infections

Bone and joint infections

Dialysis: infections associated with haemo - and peritoneal dialysis and with continuous ambulatory peritoneal dialysis (CAPD)

In meningitis it is recommended that the results of a sensitivity test are known before treatment with ceftazidime as a single agent. It may be used for infections caused by organisms resistant to other antibiotics including aminoglycosides and many cephalosporins. When appropriate, however, it may be used in combination with an aminoglycoside or other beta-lactam antibiotic for example, in the presence of severe neutropenia, or with an antibiotic active against anaerobes when the presence of bacteroides fragilis is suspected. In addition, ceftazidime is indicated in the perioperative prophylaxis of transurethral prostatectomy.

In vitro the activities of ceftazidime and aminoglycoside antibiotics in combination have been shown to be at least additive; there is evidence of synergy in some strains tested. This property may be important in the treatment of febrile neutropenic patients.

Consideration should be given to official guidance on the appropriate use of antibacterial agents.

4.2 Posology and method of administration

Ceftazidime is to be used by the parenteral route, the dosage depending upon the severity, sensitivity and type of infection and the age, weight and renal function of the patient.

Adults: The adult dosage range for ceftazidime is 1 to 6g per day 8 or 12 hourly (im or iv). In the majority of infections, 1g 8-hourly or 2g 12-hourly should be given. In urinary tract infections and in many less serious infections, 500mg or 1g 12-hourly is usually adequate. In very severe infections, especially immunocompromised patients, including those with neutropenia, 2g 8 or 12-hourly or 3g 12-hourly should be administered.

When used as a prophylactic agent in prostatic surgery 1g (from the 1g vial) should be given at the induction of anaesthesia. A second dose should be considered at the time of catheter removal.

Elderly: In view of the reduced clearance of ceftazidime in acutely ill elderly patients, the daily dosage should not normally exceed 3g, especially in those over 80 years of age.

Cystic fibrosis: In fibrocystic adults with normal renal function who have pseudomonal lung infections, high doses of 100 to 150mg/kg/day as three divided doses should be used. In adults with normal renal function 9g/day has been used.

Infants and children: The usual dosage range for children aged over two months is 30 to 100mg/kg/day, given as two or three divided doses.

Doses up to 150mg/kg/day (maximum 6g daily) in three divided doses may be given to infected immunocompromised or fibrocystic children or children with meningitis.

Neonates and children up to 2 months of age: Whilst clinical experience is limited, a dose of 25 to 60mg/kg/day given as two divided doses has proved to be effective. In the neonate the serum half-life of ceftazidime can be three to four times that in adults.

Dosage in impaired renal function: Ceftazidime is excreted by the kidneys almost exclusively by glomerular filtration. Therefore, in patients with impaired renal function it is recommended that the dosage of ceftazidime should be reduced to compensate for its slower excretion, except in mild impairment, i.e. glomerular filtration rate (GFR) greater than 50ml/min. In patients with suspected renal insufficiency, an initial loading dose of 1g of ceftazidime may be given. An estimate of GFR should be made to determine the appropriate maintenance dose.

Renal impairment: For patients in renal failure on continuous arteriovenous haemodialysis or high-flux haemofiltration in intensive therapy units, it is recommended that the dosage should be 1g daily in divided doses. For low-flux haemofiltration it is recommended that the dosage should be that suggested under impaired renal function.

Recommended maintenance doses are shown below:

RECOMMENDED MAINTENANCE DOSES OF CEFTAZIDIME IN RENAL INSUFFICIENCY

(see Table 1 below)

In patients with severe infections, especially in neutropenics, who would normally receive 6g of ceftazidime daily were it not for renal insufficiency, the unit dose given in the table above may be increased by 50% or the dosing frequency increased appropriately. In such patients it is recommended that ceftazidime serum levels should be monitored and trough levels should not exceed 40mg/litre.

When only serum creatinine is available, the following formula (Cockcroft's equation) may be used to estimate creatinine clearance. The serum creatinine should represent a steady state of renal function:

Males:

$$\text{Creatinine clearance (ml/min)} = \frac{\text{Weight (kg)} \times (140 - \text{age in years})}{72 \times \text{serum creatinine (mg/dl)}}$$

Females:

0.85 × above value.

To convert serum creatinine in µmol/litre into mg/dl divide by 88.4.

In children the creatinine clearance should be adjusted for body surface area or lean body mass and the dosing frequency reduced in cases of renal insufficiency as for adults.

The serum half-life of ceftazidime during haemodialysis ranges from 3 to 5 hours. The appropriate maintenance dose of ceftazidime should be repeated following each haemodialysis period.

Dosage in peritoneal dialysis: Ceftazidime may also be used in peritoneal dialysis and continuous ambulatory peritoneal dialysis (CAPD). As well as using ceftazidime intravenously, it can be incorporated into the dialysis fluid (usually 125 to 250mg for 2L of dialysis fluid).

Administration: Ceftazidime may be given intravenously or by deep intramuscular injection into a large muscle mass such as the upper outer quadrant of the gluteus maximus or lateral part of the thigh.

4.3 Contraindications

Ceftazidime is contraindicated in patients with known hypersensitivity to cephalosporin antibiotics.

4.4 Special warnings and precautions for use

Hypersensitivity reactions:

As with other beta-lactam antibiotics, before therapy with ceftazidime is instituted, careful inquiry should be made for a history of hypersensitivity reactions to ceftazidime, cephalosporins, penicillins or other drugs. Special care is indicated in patients who have experienced an allergic reaction to penicillins or beta-lactams. Ceftazidime should be given only with special caution to patients with type I or immediate hypersensitivity reactions to penicillin. If an allergic reaction to ceftazidime occurs, discontinue the drug. Serious hypersensitivity reactions may require adrenaline (epinephrine), hydrocortisone, antihistamine or other emergency measures.

Renal function:

Cephalosporin antibiotics at high dosage should be given with caution to patients receiving concurrent treatment with nephrotoxic drugs, e.g. aminoglycoside antibiotics, or potent diuretics such as furosemide, as these combinations are suspected of affecting renal function adversely. Clinical experience with ceftazidime has shown that this is not likely to be a problem at the recommended dose levels. There is no evidence that ceftazidime adversely affects renal function at normal therapeutic doses: however, as for all antibiotics eliminated via the kidneys, it is necessary to reduce the dosage according to the degree of reduction in renal function to avoid the clinical consequences of elevated antibiotic levels, e.g. neurological sequelae, which have occasionally been reported when the dose has not been reduced appropriately (see 4.2 Dosage in Impaired Renal Function and 4.8 Undesirable Effects).

Overgrowth of non-susceptible organisms:

As with other broad spectrum antibiotics, prolonged use of ceftazidime may result in the overgrowth of non-susceptible organisms (e.g. Candida, Enterococci and Serratia spp) which may require interruption of treatment or adoption of appropriate measures. Repeated evaluation of the patient's condition is essential.

4.5 Interaction with other medicinal products and other forms of interaction

Ceftazidime does not interfere with enzyme-based tests for glycosuria. Slight interference with copper reduction methods (Benedict's, Fehling's, Clinitest) may be observed. Ceftazidime does not interfere in the alkaline picrate assay for creatinine. The development of a positive Coombs' test associated with the use of ceftazidime in about 5% of patients may interfere with the cross-matching of blood.

Chloramphenicol is antagonistic in vitro with ceftazidime and other cephalosporins. The clinical relevance of this finding is unknown, but if concurrent administration of ceftazidime with chloramphenicol is proposed, the possibility of antagonism should be considered.

In common with other antibiotics, ceftazidime may affect the gut flora, leading to lower oestrogen reabsorption and reduced efficacy of combined oral contraceptives. Therefore, alternative non-hormonal methods of contraception are recommended.

4.6 Pregnancy and lactation

There is no experimental evidence of embryopathic or teratogenic effects attributable to ceftazidime but, as with all drugs, it should be administered with caution during the early months of pregnancy and in early infancy. Use in pregnancy requires that the anticipated benefit be weighed against the possible risks.

Ceftazidime is excreted in human milk in low concentrations and consequently caution should be exercised when ceftazidime is administered to a nursing mother.

4.7 Effects on ability to drive and use machines

None reported.

4.8 Undesirable effects

Data from large clinical trials (internal and published) were used to determine the frequency of very common to uncommon undesirable effects. The frequencies assigned to all other undesirable effects were mainly determined using post-marketing data and refer to a reporting rate rather than a true frequency.

The following convention has been used for the classification of frequency:

very common ⩾1/10,

common ⩾1/100 and <1/10,

uncommon ⩾1/1000 and <1/100,

rare ⩾1/10,000 and <1/1000,

very rare <1/10,000.

Infections and infestations

Uncommon: Candidiasis (including vaginitis and oral thrush).

Blood and lymphatic system disorders

Common: Eosinophilia and thrombocytosis.

Uncommon: Leucopenia, neutropenia, and thrombocytopenia,

Very Rare: Lymphocytosis, haemolytic anaemia, and agranulocytosis.

Immune system disorders

Very Rare: Anaphylaxis (including bronchospasm and/or hypotension).

Nervous system disorders

Uncommon: Headache and dizziness

Very Rare: Paraesthesia

There have been reports of neurological sequelae including tremor, myoclonia, convulsions, encephalopathy, and coma in patients with renal impairment in whom the dose of ceftazidime has not been appropriately reduced.

Vascular disorders

Common: Phlebitis or thrombophlebitis with IV administration.

Gastrointestinal disorders

Common: Diarrhoea

Uncommon: Nausea, vomiting, abdominal pain, and colitis

Very Rare: Bad taste

As with other cephalosporins, colitis may be associated with *Clostridium difficile* and may present as pseudomembranous colitis.

Renal and urinary disorders

Very Rare: Interstitial nephritis, acute renal failure.

Hepatobiliary disorders

Common: Transient elevations in one or more of the hepatic enzymes, ALT (SGPT), AST (SOGT), LDH, GGT and alkaline phosphatase.

Very Rare: Jaundice.

Skin and subcutaneous tissue disorders

Common: Maculopapular or urticarial rash

Uncommon: Pruritus

Very Rare: Angioedema, erythema multiforme, Stevens-Johnson syndrome, and toxic epidermal necrolysis.

General disorders and administration site conditions

Common: Pain and/or inflammation after IM injection.

Uncommon: Fever

Investigations

Common: Positive Coombs test.

Uncommon: As with some other cephalosporins, transient elevations of blood urea, blood urea nitrogen and/or serum creatinine have been observed.

4.9 Overdose

Overdosage can lead to neurological sequelae including encephalopathy, convulsions and coma.

Serum levels of ceftazidime can be reduced by dialysis.

5. PHARMACOLOGICAL PROPERTIES

5.1 Pharmacodynamic properties

ATC classification

Pharmacotherapeutic group: cephalosporins ATC code: J01DD02

Mode of action

Ceftazidime inhibits bacterial cell wall synthesis following attachment to penicillin binding proteins (PBPs). This results in the interruption of cell wall (peptidoglycan) biosynthesis, which leads to bacterial cell lysis and death.

Mechanism of Resistance

Ceftazidime is effectively stable to hydrolysis by most classes of beta-lactamases, including penicillinases and cephalosporinases but not extended spectrum beta-lactamases.

Table 1 RECOMMENDED MAINTENANCE DOSES OF CEFTAZIDIME IN RENAL INSUFFICIENCY

Creatinine clearance Ml/min	Approx. serum creatinine* µmol/l(mg/dl)	Recommended unit dose of ceftazidime (g)	Frequency of dosing (hourly)
50-31	150-200 (1.7-2.3)	1	12
30-16	200-350 (2.3-4.0)	1	24
15-6	350-500 (4.0-5.6)	0.5	24
<5	>500 (>5.6)	0.5	48

* These values are guidelines and may not accurately predict renal function in all patients especially in the elderly in whom the serum creatinine concentration may over estimate renal function.

Bacterial resistance to ceftazidime may be due to one or more of the following mechanisms:

- hydrolysis by beta-lactamases. Ceftazidime may be efficiently hydrolysed by certain of the extended-spectrum beta-lactamases (ESBLs) including the SHV plasmid mediated ESBLs and by the chromosomally-encoded (AmpC) enzyme that may be induced or stably derepressed in certain aerobic gram-negative bacterial species

- reduced affinity of penicillin-binding proteins for ceftazidime

- outer membrane impermeability, which restricts access of ceftazidime to penicillin binding proteins in gram-negative organisms

- drug efflux pumps.

Breakpoints

Minimum inhibitory concentration (MIC) breakpoints established by the European Committee on Antimicrobial Susceptibility Testing (EUCAST) are as follows:

- Enterobacteriaceae: S =< 1 mg/l and R> 8 mg/l

- *Pseudomonas aeruginosa*: S =< 8 mg/l and R> 8 mg/l

Microbiological Susceptibility

The prevalence of acquired resistance may vary geographically and with time for selected species and local information on resistance is desirable, particularly when treating severe infections. As necessary, expert advice should be sought when the local prevalence of resistance is such that the utility of ceftazidime in at least some types of infections is questionable.

Commonly Susceptible Species
Gram-positive aerobes: Methicillin-susceptible-staphylococci (including *Staphylococcus aureus*) *Streptococcus pneumoniae* *Streptococcus pyogenes* *Streptococcus agalactiae*
Gram-negative aerobes: *Escherichia coli* *Proteus mirabilis* *Proteus spp* (other) *Providencia* spp. *Pseudomonas aeruginosa* *Pseudomonas* spp. (other) *Salmonella* spp. *Shigella* spp *Haemophilus influenzae* (including ampicillin-resistant strains)
Species for which acquired resistance may be a problem
Gram-negative aerobes: *Enterobacter aerogenes* *Enterobacter spp* (other) *Klebsiella pneumoniae* *Klebsiella spp* (other) *Serratia* spp *Morganella morganii*
Gram-positive anaerobes: *Peptococcus spp.* *Peptostreptococcus spp.* *Propionibacterium spp.* *Clostridium perfringens*
Gram-negative anaerobes *Fusobacterium* spp.
Inherently resistant organisms
Gram-positive aerobes: Enterococci including *Enterococcus faecalis* and *Enterococcus faecium* *Listeria spp* Methicillin-resistant-staphylococci
Gram-negative aerobes: *Acinetobacter spp* *Campylobacter spp*
Gram-positive anaerobes: *Clostridium difficile*
Gram-negative anaerobes *Bacteroides* spp. (many strains of *Bacteroides fragilis* resistant).
Others: *Chlamydia* species *Mycoplasma* species *Legionella* species

5.2 Pharmacokinetic properties

Ceftazidime administered by the parenteral route reaches high and prolonged serum levels in man. After intramuscular administration of 500mg and 1g serum mean peak levels of 18 and 37mg/litre respectively are rapidly achieved. Five minutes after an intravenous bolus injection of 500mg, 1g or 2g, serum mean levels are respectively 46, 87 and 170mg/litre.

Therapeutically effective concentrations are still found in the serum 8 to 12 hours after both intravenous and intramuscular administration. The serum half-life is about 1.8 hours in normal volunteers and about 2.2 hours in patients with apparently normal renal function. The serum protein binding of ceftazidime is low at about 10%.

Ceftazidime is not metabolised in the body and is excreted unchanged in the active form into the urine by glomerular filtration. Approximately 80 to 90% of the dose is recovered in the urine within 24 hours. Less than 1% is excreted via the bile, significantly limiting the amount entering the bowel.

Concentrations of ceftazidime in excess of the minimum inhibitory levels for common pathogens can be achieved in tissues such as bone, heart, bile, sputum, aqueous humour, synovial and pleural and peritoneal fluids. Transplacental transfer of the antibiotic readily occurs. Ceftazidime penetrates the intact blood brain barrier poorly and low levels are achieved in the csf in the absence of inflammation. Therapeutic levels of 4 to 20mg/litre or more are achieved in the csf when the meninges are inflamed.

5.3 Preclinical safety data

No additional data of relevance.

6. PHARMACEUTICAL PARTICULARS

6.1 List of excipients

Sodium carbonate (anhydrous sterile)

6.2 Incompatibilities

Ceftazidime is less stable in Sodium Bicarbonate Injection than other intravenous fluids. It is not recommended as a diluent.

Ceftazidime and aminoglycosides should not be mixed in the same giving set or syringe.

Precipitation has been reported when vancomycin has been added to ceftazidime in solution. It is recommended that giving sets and intravenous lines are flushed been administration of these two agents.

6.3 Shelf life

Three years when stored below 25°C and protected from light.

Two years for Fortum Monovials when stored below 30°C and protected from light.

6.4 Special precautions for storage

The unconstituted product should be stored below 25°C and protected from light. Constituted solutions may be stored in the refrigerator (2 - 8°C) for up to 24 hours.

6.5 Nature and contents of container

Individually cartoned vials containing 1g ceftazidime (as pentahydrate) for intramuscular or intravenous use in packs of 1 or 5.

Not all pack sizes may be marketed.

6.6 Special precautions for disposal and other handling

Instructions for constitution: See table for addition volumes and solution concentrations, which may be useful when fractional doses are required.

PREPARATION OF SOLUTION

(see Table 2 below)

All sizes of vials as supplied are under reduced pressure. As the product dissolves, carbon dioxide is released and a positive pressure develops. For ease of use, it is recommended that the following techniques of reconstitution are adopted.

250mg i.m./i.v., 500mg i.m./i.v., 1g i.m./i.v., and 2g and 3g i.v. bolus vials:

1. Insert the syringe needle through the vial closure and inject the recommended volume of diluent. The vacuum may assist entry of the diluent. Remove the syringe needle.

2. Shake to dissolve: carbon dioxide is released and a clear solution will be obtained in about 1 to 2 minutes.

3. Invert the vial. With the syringe plunger fully depressed, insert the needle through the vial closure and withdraw the total volume of solution into the syringe (the pressure in the vial may aid withdrawal). Ensure that the needle remains within the solution and does not enter the head space. The withdrawn solution may contain small bubbles of carbon dioxide; they may be disregarded.

These solutions may be given directly into the vein or introduced into the tubing of a giving set if the patient is receiving parenteral fluids. Ceftazidime is compatible with the most commonly used intravenous fluids.

Vials of Fortum for Injection as supplied are under reduced pressure; a positive pressure is produced on constitution due to the release of carbon dioxide.

Vials of Fortum for Injection should be stored at a temperature below 25°C.

Vials of Fortum for Injection do not contain any preservatives and should be used as single-dose preparations.

In keeping with good pharmaceutical practice, it is preferable to use freshly constituted solutions of Fortum for Injection. If this is not practicable, satisfactory potency is retained for 24 hours in the refrigerator (2 - 8°C) when prepared in Water for Injection BP or any of the injections listed below.

At ceftazidime concentrations between 1mg/ml and 40mg/ml in:

0.9% Sodium Chloride Injection BP

M/6 Sodium Lactate Injection BP

Compound Sodium Lactate Injection BP (Hartmann's Solution)

5% Dextrose Injection BP

0.225% Sodium Chloride and 5% Dextrose Injection BP

0.45% Sodium Chloride and 5% Dextrose Injection BP

0.9% Sodium Chloride and 5% Dextrose Injection BP

0.18% Sodium Chloride and 4% Dextrose Injection BP

10% Dextrose Injection BP

Dextran 40 Injection BP 10% in 0.9% Sodium Chloride Injection BP

Dextran 40 Injection BP 10% in 5% Dextrose Injection BP

Dextran 70 Injection BP 6% in 0.9% Sodium Chloride Injection BP

Dextran 70 Injection BP 6% in 5% Dextrose Injection BP

(Ceftazidime is less stable in Sodium Bicarbonate Injection than in other intravenous fluids. It is not recommended as a diluent)

At concentrations of between 0.05mg/ml and 0.25mg/ml in Intraperitoneal Dialysis Fluid (Lactate) BPC 1973.

When reconstituted for intramuscular use with: 0.5% or 1% Lidocaine Hydrochloride Injection BP

When admixed at 4mg/ml with (both components retain satisfactory potency):

Hydrocortisone (hydrocortisone sodium phosphate) 1mg/ml in 0.9% Sodium Chloride Injection BP or 5% Dextrose Injection BP

Cefuroxime (cefuroxime sodium) 3mg/ml in 0.9% Sodium Chloride Injection BP

Cloxacillin (cloxacillin sodium) 4mg/ml in 0.9% Sodium Chloride Injection BP

Heparin 10u/ml or 50u/ml in 0.9% Sodium Chloride Injection BP

Potassium Chloride 10mEq/L or 40 mEq/L in 0.9% Sodium Chloride Injection BP

Solutions range from light yellow to amber depending on concentration, diluent and storage conditions used. Within the stated recommendations, product potency is not adversely affected by such colour variations.

Administrative Data

7. MARKETING AUTHORISATION HOLDER

Glaxo Operations UK Ltd

Greenford

Middlesex

UB6 OHE

Trading as

GlaxoSmithKline UK

Stockley Park West

Uxbridge

Middlesex UB11 1BT

Table 2 PREPARATION OF SOLUTION

Vial size		Amount of Diluent to be added (ml)	Approximate Concentration (mg/ml)
250mg 250mg	Intramuscular Intravenous	1.0 2.5	210 90
500mg 500mg	Intramuscular Intravenous	1.5 5.0	260 90
1g 1g	Intramuscular Intravenous	3.0 10.0	260 90
2g 2g	Intravenous bolus Intravenous Infusion	10.0 50.0*	170 40‡
3g 3g	Intravenous bolus Intravenous Infusion	15.0 75.0*	170 40‡

* Note: Addition should be in two stages.

‡ Note: Use Sodium Chloride Injection 0.9%, Dextrose Injection 5% or other approved diluent (see pharmaceutical precautions) as Water for Injections produces hypotonic solutions at this concentration.

8. MARKETING AUTHORISATION NUMBER(S)
PL 00004/0293

9. DATE OF FIRST AUTHORISATION/RENEWAL OF THE AUTHORISATION
18 May 2001

10. DATE OF REVISION OF THE TEXT
31 July 2009

11. Legal Status
POM

Fortum 2g and 3g Injection

(GlaxoSmithKline UK)

1. NAME OF THE MEDICINAL PRODUCT
Fortum® for Injection

Ceftazidime (as pentahydrate) (INN) Injection

2. QUALITATIVE AND QUANTITATIVE COMPOSITION
Fortum for Injection: Vials contain 2g or 3g ceftazidime (as pentahydrate) with sodium carbonate (118mg per gram of ceftazidime).

Fortum Monovial in a vial containing 2g ceftazidime pentahydrate.

3. PHARMACEUTICAL FORM
Sterile Powder for constitution for Injection

4. CLINICAL PARTICULARS
4.1 Therapeutic indications
Single infections

Mixed infections caused by two or more susceptible organisms

Severe infections in general

Respiratory tract infections

Ear, nose and throat infections

Urinary tract infections

Skin and soft tissue infections

Gastrointestinal, biliary and abdominal infections

Bone and joint infections

Dialysis: infections associated with haemo - and peritoneal dialysis and with continuous ambulatory peritoneal dialysis (CAPD)

In meningitis it is recommended that the results of a sensitivity test are known before treatment with ceftazidime as a single agent. It may be used for infections caused by organisms resistant to other antibiotics including aminoglycosides and many cephalosporins. When appropriate, however, it may be used in combination with an aminoglycoside or other beta-lactam antibiotic for example, in the presence of severe neutropenia, or with an antibiotic active against anaerobes when the presence of bacteroides fragilis is suspected. In addition, ceftazidime is indicated in the perioperative prophylaxis of transurethral prostatectomy.

In vitro the activities of ceftazidime and aminoglycoside antibiotics in combination have been shown to be at least additive; there is evidence of synergy in some strains tested. This property may be important in the treatment of febrile neutropenic patients.

Consideration should be given to official guidance on the appropriate use of antibacterial agents.

4.2 Posology and method of administration
Ceftazidime is to be used by the parenteral route, the dosage depending upon the severity, sensitivity and type of infection and the age, weight and renal function of the patient.

Adults: The adult dosage range for ceftazidime is 1 to 6g per day 8 or 12 hourly (im or iv). In the majority of infections, 1g 8-hourly or 2g 12-hourly should be given. In urinary tract infections and in many less serious infections, 500mg or 1g 12-hourly is usually adequate. In very severe infections, especially immunocompromised patients, including those with neutropenia, 2g 8 or 12-hourly or 3g 12-hourly should be administered.

When used as a prophylactic agent in prostatic surgery 1g (from the 1g vial) should be given at the induction of anaesthesia. A second dose should be considered at the time of catheter removal.

Elderly: In view of the reduced clearance of ceftazidime in acutely ill elderly patients, the daily dosage should not normally exceed 3g, especially in those over 80 years of age.

Cystic fibrosis: In fibrocystic adults with normal renal function who have pseudomonal lung infections, high doses of 100 to 150mg/kg/day as three divided doses should be used. In adults with normal renal function 9g/day has been used.

Infants and children: The usual dosage range for children aged over two months is 30 to 100mg/kg/day, given as two or three divided doses.

Doses up to 150mg/kg/day (maximum 6g daily) in three divided doses may be given to infected immunocompromised or fibrocystic children or children with meningitis.

Table 1 RECOMMENDED MAINTENANCE DOSES OF CEFTAZIDIME IN RENAL INSUFFICIENCY

Creatinine clearance ml/min	Approx. serum creatinine* µmol/l(mg/dl)	Recommended unit dose of ceftazidime (g)	Frequency of dosing (hourly)
50-31	150-200 (1.7-2.3)	1	12
30-16	200-350 (2.3-4.0)	1	24
15-6	350-500 (4.0-5.6)	0.5	24
<5	>500 (>5.6)	0.5	48

* These values are guidelines and may not accurately predict renal function in all patients especially in the elderly in whom the serum creatinine concentration may overestimate renal function.

Neonates and children up to 2 months of age: Whilst clinical experience is limited, a dose of 25 to 60mg/kg/day given as two divided doses has proved to be effective. In the neonate the serum half-life of ceftazidime can be three to four times that in adults.

Dosage in impaired renal function: Ceftazidime is excreted by the kidneys almost exclusively by glomerular filtration. Therefore, in patients with impaired renal function it is recommended that the dosage of ceftazidime should be reduced to compensate for its slower excretion, except in mild impairment, i.e. glomerular filtration rate (GFR) greater than 50ml/min. In patients with suspected renal insufficiency, an initial loading dose of 1g of ceftazidime may be given. An estimate of GFR should be made to determine the appropriate maintenance dose.

Renal impairment: For patients in renal failure on continuous arteriovenous haemodialysis or high-flux haemofiltration in intensive therapy units, it is recommended that the dosage should be 1g daily in divided doses. For low-flux haemofiltration it is recommended that the dosage should be that suggested under impaired renal function.

Recommended maintenance doses are shown below:

RECOMMENDED MAINTENANCE DOSES OF CEFTAZIDIME IN RENAL INSUFFICIENCY

(see Table 1 above)

In patients with severe infections, especially in neutropenics, who would normally receive 6g of ceftazidime daily were it not for renal insufficiency, the unit dose given in the table above may be increased by 50% or the dosing frequency increased appropriately. In such patients it is recommended that ceftazidime serum levels should be monitored and trough levels should not exceed 40mg/litre.

When only serum creatinine is available, the following formula (Cockcroft's equation) may be used to estimate creatinine clearance. The serum creatinine should represent a steady state of renal function:

Males:

$$\text{Creatinine clearance (ml/min)} = \frac{\text{Weight (kg)} \times (140 - \text{age in years})}{72 \times \text{serum creatinine (mg/dl)}}$$

Females:

0.85 × above value.

To convert serum creatinine in µmol/litre into mg/dl divide by 88.4.

In children the creatinine clearance should be adjusted for body surface area or lean body mass and the dosing frequency reduced in cases of renal insufficiency as for adults.

The serum half-life of ceftazidime during haemodialysis ranges from 3 to 5 hours. The appropriate maintenance dose of ceftazidime should be repeated following each haemodialysis period.

Dosage in peritoneal dialysis: Ceftazidime may also be used in peritoneal dialysis and continuous ambulatory peritoneal dialysis (CAPD). As well as using ceftazidime intravenously, it can be incorporated into the dialysis fluid (usually 125 to 250mg for 2L of dialysis fluid).

Administration: Ceftazidime may be given intravenously or by deep intramuscular injection into a large muscle mass such as the upper outer quadrant of the gluteus maximus or lateral part of the thigh.

4.3 Contraindications
Ceftazidime is contraindicated in patients with known hypersensitivity to cephalosporin antibiotics.

4.4 Special warnings and precautions for use
Hypersensitivity reactions:

As with other beta-lactam antibiotics, before therapy with ceftazidime is instituted, careful inquiry should be made for a history of hypersensitivity reactions to ceftazidime, cephalosporins, penicillins or other drugs. Special care is indicated in patients who have experienced an allergic reaction to penicillins or beta-lactams. Ceftazidime should be given only with special caution to patients with type I or immediate hypersensitivity reactions to penicillin. If an allergic reaction to ceftazidime occurs, discontinue the drug. Serious hypersensitivity reactions may require adrenaline (epinephrine), hydrocortisone, antihistamine or other emergency measures.

Renal function:

Cephalosporin antibiotics at high dosage should be given with caution to patients receiving concurrent treatment with nephrotoxic drugs, e.g. aminoglycoside antibiotics, or potent diuretics such as furosemide, as these combinations are suspected of affecting renal function adversely. Clinical experience with ceftazidime has shown that this is not likely to be a problem at the recommended dose levels. There is no evidence that ceftazidime adversely affects renal function at normal therapeutic doses: however, as for all antibiotics eliminated via the kidneys, it is necessary to reduce the dosage according to the degree of reduction in renal function to avoid the clinical consequences of elevated antibiotic levels, e.g. neurological sequelae, which have occasionally been reported when the dose has not been reduced appropriately (see 4.2 Dosage in Impaired Renal Function and 4.8 Undesirable Effects).

Overgrowth of non-susceptible organisms:

As with other broad spectrum antibiotics, prolonged use of ceftazidime may result in the overgrowth of non-susceptible organisms (e.g. Candida, Enterococci and Serratia spp) which may require interruption of treatment or adoption of appropriate measures. Repeated evaluation of the patient's condition is essential.

4.5 Interaction with other medicinal products and other forms of interaction
Ceftazidime does not interfere with enzyme-based tests for glycosuria. Slight interference with copper reduction methods (Benedict's, Fehling's, Clinitest) may be observed. Ceftazidime does not interfere in the alkaline picrate assay for creatinine. The development of a positive Coombs' test associated with the use of ceftazidime in about 5% of patients may interfere with the cross-matching of blood.

Chloramphenicol is antagonistic in vitro with ceftazidime and other cephalosporins. The clinical relevance of this finding is unknown, but if concurrent administration of ceftazidime with chloramphenicol is proposed, the possibility of antagonism should be considered.

In common with other antibiotics, ceftazidime may affect the gut flora, leading to lower oestrogen reabsorption and reduced efficacy of combined oral contraceptives. Therefore, alternative non-hormonal methods of contraception are recommended.

4.6 Pregnancy and lactation
There is no experimental evidence of embryopathic or teratogenic effects attributable to ceftazidime but, as with all drugs, it should be administered with caution during the early months of pregnancy and in early infancy. Use in pregnancy requires that the anticipated benefit be weighed against the possible risks.

Ceftazidime is excreted in human milk in low concentrations and consequently caution should be exercised when ceftazidime is administered to a nursing mother.

4.7 Effects on ability to drive and use machines
None reported.

4.8 Undesirable effects
Data from large clinical trials (internal and published) were used to determine the frequency of very common to uncommon undesirable effects. The frequencies assigned to all other undesirable effects were mainly determined using post-marketing data and refer to a reporting rate rather than a true frequency.

The following convention has been used for the classification of frequency:

very common ≥1/10,

common ≥1/100 and <1/10,

uncommon ≥1/1000 and <1/100,

rare ≥1/10,000 and <1/1000,

very rare <1/10,000.

Infections and infestations

Uncommon: Candidiasis (including vaginitis and oral thrush).

Blood and lymphatic system disorders

Common: Eosinophilia and thrombocytosis.

Uncommon: Leucopenia, neutropenia, and thrombocytopenia,

Very Rare:	Lymphocytosis, haemolytic anaemia, and agranulocytosis.

Immune system disorders

Very Rare:	Anaphylaxis (including bronchospasm and/or hypotension).

Nervous system disorders

Uncommon:	Headache and dizziness
Very Rare:	Paraesthesia

There have been reports of neurological sequelae including tremor, myoclonia, convulsions, encephalopathy, and coma in patients with renal impairment in whom the dose of ceftazidime has not been appropriately reduced.

Vascular disorders

Common:	Phlebitis or thrombophlebitis with IV administration.

Gastrointestinal disorders

Common:	Diarrhoea
Uncommon:	Nausea, vomiting, abdominal pain, and colitis
Very Rare:	Bad taste

As with other cephalosporins, colitis may be associated with *Clostridium difficile* and may present as pseudomembranous colitis.

Renal and urinary disorders

Very Rare:	Interstitial nephritis, acute renal failure

Hepatobiliary disorders

Common:	Transient elevations in one or more of the hepatic enzymes, ALT (SGPT), AST (SOGT), LDH, GGT and alkaline phosphatase.
Very Rare:	Jaundice.

Skin and subcutaneous tissue disorders

Common:	Maculopapular or urticarial rash
Uncommon:	Pruritus
Very Rare:	Angioedema, erythema multiforme, Stevens Johnson syndrome, and toxic epidermal necrolysis.

General disorders and administration site conditions

Common:	Pain and/or inflammation after IM injection.
Uncommon:	Fever

Investigations

Common:	Positive Coombs test.
Uncommon:	As with some other cephalosporins, transient elevations of blood urea, blood urea nitrogen and/or serum creatinine have been observed.

4.9 Overdose

Overdosage can lead to neurological sequelae including encephalopathy, convulsions and coma.

Serum levels of ceftazidime can be reduced by dialysis.

5. PHARMACOLOGICAL PROPERTIES

5.1 Pharmacodynamic properties

ATC classification

Pharmacotherapeutic group: cephalosporins ATC code: J01DD02

Mode of action

Ceftazidime inhibits bacterial cell wall synthesis following attachment to penicillin binding proteins (PBPs). This results in the interruption of cell wall (peptidoglycan) biosynthesis, which leads to bacterial cell lysis and death.

Mechanism of Resistance

Ceftazidime is effectively stable to hydrolysis by most classes of beta-lactamases, including penicillinases and cephalosporinases but not extended spectrum beta-lactamases.

Bacterial resistance to ceftazidime may be due to one or more of the following mechanisms:

- hydrolysis by beta-lactamases. Ceftazidime may be efficiently hydrolysed by certain of the extended-spectrum beta-lactamases (ESBLs) including the SHV plasmid mediated ESBLs and by the chromosomally-encoded (AmpC) enzyme that may be induced or stably derepressed in certain aerobic gram-negative bacterial species
- reduced affinity of penicillin-binding proteins for ceftazidime
- outer membrane impermeability, which restricts access of ceftazidime to penicillin binding proteins in gram-negative organisms
- drug efflux pumps.

Breakpoints

Minimum inhibitory concentration (MIC) breakpoints established by the European Committee on Antimicrobial Susceptibility Testing (EUCAST) are as follows:

- Enterobacteriaceae: S =< 1 mg/l and R > 8 mg/l
- *Pseudomonas aeruginosa*: S =< 8 mg/l and R > 8 mg/l

Microbiological Susceptibility

The prevalence of acquired resistance may vary geographically and with time for selected species and local information on resistance is desirable, particularly when treating severe infections. As necessary, expert advice should be sought when the local prevalence of resistance is such that the utility of ceftazidime in at least some types of infections is questionable.

Commonly Susceptible Species
Gram-positive aerobes: Methicillin-susceptible-staphylococci (including *Staphylococcus aureus)* *Streptococcus pneumoniae* *Streptococcus pyogenes* *Streptococcus agalactiae*
Gram-negative aerobes: *Escherichia coli* *Proteus mirabilis* *Proteus spp* (other) *Providencia* spp. *Pseudomonas aeruginosa* *Pseudomonas* spp. (other) *Salmonella* spp. *Shigella* spp *Haemophilus influenzae* (including ampicillin-resistant strains)
Species for which acquired resistance may be a problem
Gram-negative aerobes: *Enterobacter aerogenes* *Enterobacter spp* (other) *Klebsiella pneumoniae* *Klebsiella spp* (other) *Serratia spp* *Morganella morganii*
Gram-positive anaerobes: *Peptococcus spp.* *Peptostreptococcus spp.* *Propionibacterium spp.* *Clostridium perfringens*
Gram-negative anaerobes *Fusobacterium* spp.
Inherently resistant organisms
Gram-positive aerobes: Enterococci including *Enterococcus faecalis* and *Enterococcus faecium* *Listeria spp* Methicillin-resistant-staphylococci
Gram-negative aerobes: *Acinetobacter spp* *Campylobacter spp*
Gram-positive anaerobes: *Clostridium difficile*
Gram-negative anaerobes *Bacteroides* spp. (many strains of *Bacteroides fragilis* resistant).
Others: *Chlamydia* species *Mycoplasma* species *Legionella* species

5.2 Pharmacokinetic properties

Ceftazidime administered by the parenteral route reaches high and prolonged serum levels in man. After intramuscular administration of 500mg and 1g serum mean peak levels of 18 and 37mg/litre respectively are rapidly achieved. Five minutes after an intravenous bolus injection of 500mg, 1g or 2g, serum mean levels are respectively 46, 87 and 170mg/litre.

Therapeutically effective concentrations are still found in the serum 8 to 12 hours after both intravenous and intramuscular administration. The serum half-life is about 1.8 hours in normal volunteers and about 2.2 hours in patients with apparently normal renal function. The serum protein binding of ceftazidime is low at about 10%.

Ceftazidime is not metabolised in the body and is excreted unchanged in the active form into the urine by glomerular filtration. Approximately 80 to 90% of the dose is recovered in the urine within 24 hours. Less than 1% is excreted via the bile, significantly limiting the amount entering the bowel.

Concentrations of ceftazidime in excess of the minimum inhibitory levels for common pathogens can be achieved in tissues such as bone, heart, bile, sputum, aqueous humour, synovial and pleural and peritoneal fluids. Transplacental transfer of the antibiotic readily occurs. Ceftazidime penetrates the intact blood brain barrier poorly and low levels are achieved in the csf in the absence of inflammation. Therapeutic levels of 4 to 20mg/litre or more are achieved in the csf when the meninges are inflamed.

5.3 Preclinical safety data

No additional data of relevance.

6. PHARMACEUTICAL PARTICULARS

6.1 List of excipients

Sodium carbonate (anhydrous sterile)

6.2 Incompatibilities

Ceftazidime is less stable in Sodium Bicarbonate Injection than other intravenous fluids. It is not recommended as a diluent.

Ceftazidime and aminoglycosides should not be mixed in the same giving set or syringe.

Precipitation has been reported when vancomycin has been added to ceftazidime in solution. It is recommended that giving sets and intravenous lines are flushed between administration of these two agents.

6.3 Shelf life

Fortum Monovial - Two years for the unconstituted product and 24 hours for the constituted product when stored below 30°C and protected from light.

Three years when stored below 25°C and protected from light.

6.4 Special precautions for storage

The unconstituted product should be stored below 30°C and protected from light. Constituted solutions may be stored in the refrigerator (2 - 8°C) for up to 24 hours.

6.5 Nature and contents of container

Individually cartoned vials containing 2g ceftazidime (as pentahydrate) for intravenous use in packs of 1 or 5.

Individually cartoned Monovials containing 2g (as pentahydrate) for intravenous infusion.

Individually cartoned vials containing 2g ceftazidime (as pentahydrate) for intravenous infusion in packs of 1 or 5.

Individually cartoned vials containing 3g ceftazidime (as pentahydrate) for intravenous and intravenous infusion use.

Not all pack sizes may be marketed.

6.6 Special precautions for disposal and other handling

Instructions for constitution: See table for addition volumes and solution concentrations, which may be useful when fractional doses are required.

PREPARATION OF SOLUTION

(see Table 2 on next page)

All sizes of vials as supplied are under reduced pressure. As the product dissolves, carbon dioxide is released and a positive pressure develops. For ease of use, it is recommended that the following techniques of reconstitution are adopted.

250mg i.m./i.v., 500mg i.m./i.v., 1g i.m./i.v., and 2g and 3g i.v. bolus vials:

1. Insert the syringe needle through the vial closure and inject the recommended volume of diluent. The vacuum may assist entry of the diluent. Remove the syringe needle.
2. Shake to dissolve: carbon dioxide is released and a clear solution will be obtained in about 1 to 2 minutes.
3. Invert the vial. With the syringe plunger fully depressed, insert the needle through the vial closure and withdraw the total volume of solution into the syringe (the pressure in the vial may aid withdrawal). Ensure that the needle remains within the solution and does not enter the head space. The withdrawn solution may contain small bubbles of carbon dioxide; they may be disregarded.

2g and 3g i.v. infusion vials:

This vial may be constituted for short intravenous infusion (e.g. up to 30 minutes) as follows (mini-bag or burette-type set):

Prepare using a total of 50ml (for 2g vials) and 75ml (for 3g vials) of compatible diluent, added in TWO stages as below:-

1. Insert the syringe needle through the vial closure and inject 10ml of diluent for 2g vial and 15ml for 3g vial. The vacuum may assist entry of the diluent. Remove the syringe needle.
2. Shake to dissolve: carbon dioxide is released and a clear solution obtained in about 1 to 2 minutes.
3. Do not insert a gas relief needle until the product has dissolved. Insert a gas relief needle through the vial closure to relieve the internal pressure.
4. Transfer the reconstituted solution to final delivery vehicle (e.g. mini-bag or burette-type set) making up a total volume of a least 50ml (75ml for the 3g vial), and administer by intravenous infusion over 15-30 minutes.

NOTE: To preserve product sterility, it is important that a gas relief needle is not inserted through the vial closure before the product has dissolved.

Fortum Monovial:

The contents of the Monovial are added to small volume infusion bags containing 0.9% Sodium Chloride Injection or 5% Dextrose Injection, or another compatible fluid.

The 2g presentation must be constituted in not less than 100mL infusion bag.

1) Peel off the removable top part of the label and remove the cap.

2) Insert the needle of the Monovial into the additive port of the infusion bag.

3) To activate, push the plastic needle holder of the Monovial down onto the vial shoulder until a "click" is heard.

4) Holding it upright, fill the vial to approximately two-thirds capacity by squeezing the bag several times.

5) Shake the vial to reconstitute the Fortum.

6) On constitution, the Fortum will effervesce slightly.

Table 2 PREPARATION OF SOLUTION

Vial size		Amount of Diluent to be added (ml)	Approximate Concentration (mg/ml)
250mg 250mg	Intramuscular Intravenous	1.0 2.5	210 90
500mg 500mg	Intramuscular Intravenous	1.5 5.0	260 90
1g 1g	Intramuscular Intravenous	3.0 10.0	260 90
2g 2g	Intravenous bolus Intravenous Infusion	10.0 50.0*	170 40‡
3g 3g	Intravenous bolus Intravenous Infusion	15.0 75.0*	170 40‡

* Note: Addition should be in two stages.

‡ Note: Use Sodium Chloride Injection 0.9%, Dextrose Injection 5% or other approved diluent (see pharmaceutical precautions) as Water for Injections produces hypotonic solutions at this concentration.

7) With the vial uppermost, transfer the reconstituted Fortum into the infusion bag by squeezing and releasing the bag.

8) Repeat the steps 4 to 7 to rinse the inside of the vial. Dispose of the empty Monovial safely. Check that the powder is completely dissolved and that the bag has no leaks.

Fortum Monovial is for i.v. infusion only.

These solutions may be given directly into the vein or introduced into the tubing of a giving set if the patient is receiving parenteral fluids. Ceftazidime is compatible with the most commonly used intravenous fluids.

Vials of Fortum for Injection and Fortum Monovials as supplied are under reduced pressure; a positive pressure is produced on constitution due to the release of carbon dioxide.

Vials of Fortum for Injection should be stored at a temperature below 25°C.

Vials of Fortum for Injection do not contain any preservatives and should be used as single-dose preparations.

In keeping with good pharmaceutical practice, it is preferable to use freshly constituted solutions of Fortum for Injection. If this is not practicable, satisfactory potency is retained for 24 hours in the refrigerator (2 - 8°C) when prepared in Water for Injection BP or any of the injections listed below.

At ceftazidime concentrations between 1mg/ml and 40mg/ml in:

0.9% Sodium Chloride Injection BP

M/6 Sodium Lactate Injection BP

Compound Sodium Lactate Injection BP (Hartmann's Solution)

5% Dextrose Injection BP

0.225% Sodium Chloride and 5% Dextrose Injection BP

0.45% Sodium Chloride and 5% Dextrose Injection BP

0.9% Sodium Chloride and 5% Dextrose Injection BP

0.18% Sodium Chloride and 4% Dextrose Injection BP

10% Dextrose Injection BP

Dextran 40 Injection BP 10% in 0.9% Sodium Chloride Injection BP

Dextran 40 Injection BP 10% in 5% Dextrose Injection BP

Dextran 70 Injection BP 6% in 0.9% Sodium Chloride Injection BP

Dextran 70 Injection BP 6% in 5% Dextrose Injection BP

(Ceftazidime is less stable in Sodium Bicarbonate Injection than in other intravenous fluids. It is not recommended as a diluent)

At concentrations of between 0.05mg/ml and 0.25mg/ml in Intraperitoneal Dialysis Fluid (Lactate) BPC 1973.

When reconstituted for intramuscular use with: 0.5% or 1% Lidocaine Hydrochloride Injection BP

When admixed at 4mg/ml with (both components retain satisfactory potency):

Hydrocortisone (hydrocortisone sodium phosphate) 1mg/ml in 0.9% Sodium Chloride Injection BP or 5% Dextrose Injection BP

Cefuroxime (cefuroxime sodium) 3mg/ml in 0.9% Sodium Chloride Injection BP

Cloxacillin (cloxacillin sodium) 4mg/ml in 0.9% Sodium Chloride Injection BP

Heparin 10u/ml or 50u/ml in 0.9% Sodium Chloride Injection BP

Potassium Chloride 10mEq/L or 40 mEq/L in 0.9% Sodium Chloride Injection BP

Solutions range from light yellow to amber depending on concentration, diluent and storage conditions used. Within the stated recommendations, product potency is not adversely affected by such colour variations.

Administrative Data

7. MARKETING AUTHORISATION HOLDER

Glaxo Operations UK Ltd

Greenford

Middlesex

UB6 OHE

Trading as

GlaxoSmithKline UK

Stockley Park West

Uxbridge

Middlesex UB11 1BT

8. MARKETING AUTHORISATION NUMBER(S)

PL 00004/0294

9. DATE OF FIRST AUTHORISATION/RENEWAL OF THE AUTHORISATION

18 May 2001

10. DATE OF REVISION OF THE TEXT

31st July 2009

11. Legal Status

POM

Fortum 500 Injection

(GlaxoSmithKline UK)

1. NAME OF THE MEDICINAL PRODUCT

Fortum ® for Injection

Ceftazidime (as pentahydrate) (INN) Injection

2. QUALITATIVE AND QUANTITATIVE COMPOSITION

Fortum for Injection: Vials contain 500mg ceftazidime (as pentahydrate) with sodium carbonate (118mg per gram of ceftazidime).

3. PHARMACEUTICAL FORM

Sterile Powder for constitution for Injection

4. CLINICAL PARTICULARS

4.1 Therapeutic indications

Single infections

Mixed infections caused by two or more susceptible organisms

Severe infections in general

Respiratory tract infections

Ear, nose and throat infections

Urinary tract infections

Skin and soft tissue infections

Gastrointestinal, biliary and abdominal infections

Bone and joint infections

Dialysis: infections associated with haemo - and peritoneal dialysis and with continuous ambulatory peritoneal dialysis (CAPD)

In meningitis it is recommended that the results of a sensitivity test are known before treatment with ceftazidime as a single agent. It may be used for infections caused by organisms resistant to other antibiotics including aminoglycosides and many cephalosporins. When appropriate, however, it may be used in combination with an aminoglycoside or other beta-lactam antibiotic for example, in the presence of severe neutropenia, or with an antibiotic active against anaerobes when the presence of bacteroides fragilis is suspected. In addition, ceftazidime is indicated in the perioperative prophylaxis of transurethral prostatectomy.

In vitro the activities of ceftazidime and aminoglycoside antibiotics in combination have been shown to be at least additive; there is evidence of synergy in some strains tested. This property may be important in the treatment of febrile neutropenic patients.

Consideration should be given to official guidance on the appropriate use of antibacterial agents.

4.2 Posology and method of administration

Ceftazidime is to be used by the parenteral route, the dosage depending upon the severity, sensitivity and type of infection and the age, weight and renal function of the patient.

Adults: The adult dosage range for ceftazidime is 1 to 6g per day 8 or 12 hourly (im or iv). In the majority of infections, 1g 8-hourly or 2g 12-hourly should be given. In urinary tract infections and in many less serious infections, 500mg or 1g 12-hourly is usually adequate. In very severe infections, especially immunocompromised patients, including those with neutropenia, 2g 8 or 12-hourly or 3g 12-hourly should be administered.

When used as a prophylactic agent in prostatic surgery 1g (from the 1g vial) should be given at the induction of anaesthesia. A second dose should be considered at the time of catheter removal.

Elderly: In view of the reduced clearance of ceftazidime in acutely ill elderly patients, the daily dosage should not normally exceed 3g, especially in those over 80 years of age.

Cystic fibrosis: In fibrocystic adults with normal renal function who have pseudomonal lung infections, high doses of 100 to 150mg/kg/day as three divided doses should be used. In adults with normal renal function 9g/day has been used.

Infants and children: The usual dosage range for children aged over two months is 30 to 100mg/kg/day, given as two or three divided doses.

Doses up to 150mg/kg/day (maximum 6g daily) in three divided doses may be given to infected immunocompromised or fibrocystic children or children with meningitis.

Neonates and children up to 2 months of age: Whilst clinical experience is limited, a dose of 25 to 60mg/kg/day given as two divided doses has proved to be effective. In the neonate the serum half-life of ceftazidime can be three to four times that in adults.

Dosage in impaired renal function: Ceftazidime is excreted by the kidneys almost exclusively by glomerular filtration. Therefore, in patients with impaired renal function it is recommended that the dosage of ceftazidime should be reduced to compensate for its slower excretion, except in mild impairment, i.e. glomerular filtration rate (GFR) greater than 50ml/min. In patients with suspected renal insufficiency, an initial loading dose of 1g of ceftazidime may be given. An estimate of GFR should be made to determine the appropriate maintenance dose.

Renal impairment: For patients in renal failure on continuous arteriovenous haemodialysis or high-flux haemofiltration in intensive therapy units, it is recommended that the dosage should be 1g daily in divided doses. For low-flux haemofiltration it is recommended that the dosage should be that suggested under impaired renal function.

Recommended maintenance doses are shown overleaf:

RECOMMENDED MAINTENANCE DOSES OF CEFTAZIDIME IN RENAL INSUFFICIENCY

(see Table 1 on next page)

In patients with severe infections, especially in neutropenics, who would normally receive 6g of ceftazidime daily were it not for renal insufficiency, the unit dose given in the table above may be increased by 50% or the dosing frequency increased appropriately. In such patients it is recommended that ceftazidime serum levels should be monitored and trough levels should not exceed 40mg/litre.

When only serum creatinine is available, the following formula (Cockcroft's equation) may be used to estimate creatinine clearance. The serum creatinine should represent a steady state of renal function:

Males:

Creatinine clearance = (ml/min)	Weight (kg) × (140 - age in years) / 72 × serum creatinine (mg/dl)

Females:

0.85 × above value.

To convert serum creatinine in μmol/litre into mg/dl divide by 88.4.

In children the creatinine clearance should be adjusted for body surface area or lean body mass and the dosing frequency reduced in cases of renal insufficiency as for adults.

The serum half-life of ceftazidime during haemodialysis ranges from 3 to 5 hours. The appropriate maintenance dose of ceftazidime should be repeated following each haemodialysis period.

Dosage in peritoneal dialysis: Ceftazidime may also be used in peritoneal dialysis and continuous ambulatory peritoneal dialysis (CAPD). As well as using ceftazidime intravenously, it can be incorporated into the dialysis fluid (usually 125 to 250mg for 2L of dialysis fluid).

Administration: Ceftazidime may be given intravenously or by deep intramuscular injection into a large muscle mass such as the upper outer quadrant of the gluteus maximus or lateral part of the thigh.

4.3 Contraindications

Ceftazidime is contraindicated in patients with known hypersensitivity to cephalosporin antibiotics.

Table 1 RECOMMENDED MAINTENANCE DOSES OF CEFTAZIDIME IN RENAL INSUFFICIENCY

Creatinine clearance ml/min	Approx. serum creatinine* μmol/l(mg/dl)	Recommended unit dose of ceftazidime (g)	Frequency of dosing (hourly)
50-31	150-200 (1.7-2.3)	1	12
30-16	200-350 (2.3-4.0)	1	24
15-6	350-500 (4.0-5.6)	0.5	24
<5	>500 (>5.6)	0.5	48

* These values are guidelines and may not accurately predict renal function in all patients especially in the elderly in whom the serum creatinine concentration may overestimate renal function.

4.4 Special warnings and precautions for use

Hypersensitivity reactions:

As with other beta-lactam antibiotics, before therapy with ceftazidime is instituted, careful inquiry should be made for a history of hypersensitivity reactions to ceftazidime, cephalosporins, penicillins or other drugs. Special care is indicated in patients who have experienced an allergic reaction to penicillins or beta-lactams. Ceftazidime should be given only with special caution to patients with type I or immediate hypersensitivity reactions to penicillin. If an allergic reaction to ceftazidime occurs, discontinue the drug. Serious hypersensitivity reactions may require adrenaline (epinephrine), hydrocortisone, antihistamine or other emergency measures.

Renal function:

Cephalosporin antibiotics at high dosage should be given with caution to patients receiving concurrent treatment with nephrotoxic drugs, e.g. aminoglycoside antibiotics, or potent diuretics such as furosemide, as these combinations are suspected of affecting renal function adversely. Clinical experience with ceftazidime has shown that this is not likely to be a problem at the recommended dose levels. There is no evidence that ceftazidime adversely affects renal function at normal therapeutic doses: however, as for all antibiotics eliminated via the kidneys, it is necessary to reduce the dosage according to the degree of reduction in renal function to avoid the clinical consequences of elevated antibiotic levels, e.g. neurological sequelae, which have occasionally been reported when the dose has not been reduced appropriately (see 4.2 Dosage in Impaired Renal Function and 4.8 Undesirable Effects).

Overgrowth of non-susceptible organisms:

As with other broad spectrum antibiotics, prolonged use of ceftazidime may result in the overgrowth of non-susceptible organisms (e.g. Candida, Enterococci and Serratia spp) which may require interruption of treatment or adoption of appropriate measures. Repeated evaluation of the patient's condition is essential.

4.5 Interaction with other medicinal products and other forms of interaction

Ceftazidime does not interfere with enzyme-based tests for glycosuria. Slight interference with copper reduction methods (Benedict's, Fehling's, Clinitest) may be observed. Ceftazidime does not interfere in the alkaline picrate assay for creatinine. The development of a positive Coombs' test associated with the use of ceftazidime in about 5% of patients may interfere with the cross-matching of blood.

Chloramphenicol is antagonistic in vitro with ceftazidime and other cephalosporins. The clinical relevance of this finding is unknown, but if concurrent administration of ceftazidime with chloramphenicol is proposed, the possibility of antagonism should be considered.

In common with other antibiotics, ceftazidime may affect the gut flora, leading to lower oestrogen reabsorption and reduced efficacy of combined oral contraceptives. Therefore, alternative non-hormonal methods of contraception are not recommended.

4.6 Pregnancy and lactation

There is no experimental evidence of embryopathic or teratogenic effects attributable to ceftazidime but, as with all drugs, it should be administered with caution during the early months of pregnancy and in early infancy. Use in pregnancy requires that the anticipated benefit be weighed against the possible risks.

Ceftazidime is excreted in human milk in low concentrations and consequently caution should be exercised when ceftazidime is administered to a nursing mother.

4.7 Effects on ability to drive and use machines

None reported.

4.8 Undesirable effects

Data from large clinical trials (internal and published) were used to determine the frequency of very common to uncommon undesirable effects. The frequencies assigned to all other undesirable effects were mainly determined using post-marketing data and refer to a reporting rate rather than a true frequency.

The following convention has been used for the classification of frequency:

very common $\geqslant 1/10$,
common $\geqslant 1/100$ and $< 1/10$,
uncommon $\geqslant 1/1000$ and $< 1/100$,
rare $\geqslant 1/10{,}000$ and $< 1/1000$,
very rare $< 1/10{,}000$.

Infections and infestations

Uncommon:	Candidiasis (including vaginitis and oral thrush).

Blood and lymphatic system disorders

Common:	Eosinophilia and thrombocytosis.
Uncommon:	Leucopenia, neutropenia, and thrombocytopenia.
Very Rare:	Lymphocytosis, haemolytic anaemia, and agranulocytosis.

Immune system disorders

Very Rare:	Anaphylaxis (including bronchospasm and/or hypotension).

Nervous system disorders

Uncommon:	Headache and dizziness
Very Rare:	Paraesthesia

There have been reports of neurological sequelae including tremor, myoclonia, convulsions, encephalopathy, and coma in patients with renal impairment in whom the dose of ceftazidime has not been appropriately reduced.

Vascular disorders

Common:	Phlebitis or thrombophlebitis with IV administration.

Gastrointestinal disorders

Common:	Diarrhoea
Uncommon:	Nausea, vomiting, abdominal pain, and colitis
Very Rare:	Bad taste

As with other cephalosporins, colitis may be associated with *Clostridium difficile* and may present as pseudomembranous colitis.

Renal and urinary disorders

Very Rare:	Interstitial nephritis, acute renal failure.

Hepatobiliary disorders

Common:	Transient elevations in one or more of the hepatic enzymes, ALT (SGPT), AST (SOGT), LDH, GGT and alkaline phosphatase.
Very Rare:	Jaundice.

Skin and subcutaneous tissue disorders

Common:	Maculopapular or urticarial rash
Uncommon:	Pruritus
Very Rare:	Angioedema, erythema multiforme, Stevens-Johnson syndrome, and toxic epidermal necrolysis.

General disorders and administration site conditions

Common:	Pain and/or inflammation after IM injection.
Uncommon:	Fever

Investigations

Common:	Positive Coombs test.
Uncommon:	As with some other cephalosporins, transient elevations of blood urea, blood urea nitrogen and/or serum creatinine have been observed.

4.9 Overdose

Overdosage can lead to neurological sequelae including encephalopathy, convulsions and coma.

Serum levels of ceftazidime can be reduced by dialysis.

5. PHARMACOLOGICAL PROPERTIES

5.1 Pharmacodynamic properties

ATC classification

Pharmacotherapeutic group: cephalosporins ATC code: J01DD02

Mode of action

Ceftazidime inhibits bacterial cell wall synthesis following attachment to penicillin binding proteins (PBPs). This results in the interruption of cell wall (peptidoglycan) biosynthesis, which leads to bacterial cell lysis and death.

Mechanism of Resistance

Ceftazidime is effectively stable to hydrolysis by most classes of beta-lactamases, including penicillinases and cephalosporinases but not extended spectrum beta-lactamases.

Bacterial resistance to ceftazidime may be due to one or more of the following mechanisms:

- hydrolysis by beta-lactamases. Ceftazidime may be efficiently hydrolysed by certain of the extended-spectrum beta-lactamases (ESBLs) including the SHV plasmid mediated ESBLs and by the chromosomally-encoded (AmpC) enzyme that may be induced or stably derepressed in certain aerobic gram-negative bacterial species
- reduced affinity of penicillin-binding proteins for ceftazidime
- outer membrane impermeability, which restricts access of ceftazidime to penicillin binding proteins in gram-negative organisms
- drug efflux pumps.

Breakpoints

Minimum inhibitory concentration (MIC) breakpoints established by the European Committee on Antimicrobial Susceptibility Testing (EUCAST) are as follows:

- Enterobacteriaceae: S =< 1 mg/l and R > 8 mg/l
- *Pseudomonas aeruginosa*: S =< 8 mg/l and R > 8 mg/l

Microbiological Susceptibility

The prevalence of acquired resistance may vary geographically and with time for selected species and local information on resistance is desirable, particularly when treating severe infections. As necessary, expert advice should be sought when the local prevalence of resistance is such that the utility of ceftazidime in at least some types of infections is questionable.

Commonly Susceptible Species
Gram-positive aerobes: Methicillin-susceptible-staphylococci (including *Staphylococcus aureus*) *Streptococcus pneumoniae* *Streptococcus pyogenes* *Streptococcus agalactiae*
Gram-negative aerobes: *Escherichia coli* *Proteus mirabilis* *Proteus spp* (other) *Providencia* spp. *Pseudomonas aeruginosa* *Pseudomonas* spp. (other) *Salmonella* spp. *Shigella* spp *Haemophilus influenzae* (including ampicillin-resistant strains)
Species for which acquired resistance may be a problem
Gram-negative aerobes: *Enterobacter aerogenes* *Enterobacter spp* (other) *Klebsiella pneumoniae* *Klebsiella spp* (other) *Serratia* spp *Morganella morganii*
Gram-positive anaerobes: *Peptococcus spp.* *Peptostreptococcus spp.* *Propionibacterium spp.* *Clostridium perfringens*
Gram-negative anaerobes *Fusobacterium* spp.

Inherently resistant organisms
Gram-positive aerobes: Enterococci including *Enterococcus faecalis* and *Enterococcus faecium* *Listeria spp* Methicillin-resistant-staphylococci
Gram-negative aerobes: *Acinetobacter spp* *Campylobacter spp*
Gram-positive anaerobes: *Clostridium difficile*
Gram-negative anaerobes *Bacteroides* spp. (many strains of *Bacteroides fragilis* resistant).
Others: *Chlamydia* species *Mycoplasma* species *Legionella* species

5.2 Pharmacokinetic properties

Ceftazidime administered by the parenteral route reaches high and prolonged serum levels in man. After intramuscular administration of 500mg and 1g serum mean peak levels of 18 and 37mg/litre respectively are rapidly achieved. Five minutes after an intravenous bolus injection of 500mg, 1g or 2g, serum mean levels are respectively 46, 87 and 170mg/litre.

Therapeutically effective concentrations are still found in the serum 8 to 12 hours after both intravenous and intramuscular administration. The serum half-life is about 1.8 hours in normal volunteers and about 2.2 hours in patients with apparently normal renal function. The serum protein binding of ceftazidime is low at about 10%.

Ceftazidime is not metabolised in the body and is excreted unchanged in the active form into the urine by glomerular filtration. Approximately 80 to 90% of the dose is recovered in the urine within 24 hours. Less than 1% is excreted via the bile, significantly limiting the amount entering the bowel.

Concentrations of ceftazidime in excess of the minimum inhibitory levels for common pathogens can be achieved in tissues such as bone, heart, bile, sputum, aqueous humour, synovial and pleural and peritoneal fluids. Transplacental transfer of the antibiotic readily occurs. Ceftazidime penetrates the intact blood brain barrier poorly and low levels are achieved in the csf in the absence of inflammation. Therapeutic levels of 4 to 20mg/litre or more are achieved in the csf when the meninges are inflamed.

5.3 Preclinical safety data

No additional data of relevance.

6. PHARMACEUTICAL PARTICULARS

6.1 List of excipients

Sodium carbonate (anhydrous sterile)

6.2 Incompatibilities

Ceftazidime is less stable in Sodium Bicarbonate Injection than other intravenous fluids. It is not recommended as a diluent.

Ceftazidime and aminoglycosides should not be mixed in the same giving set or syringe.

Precipitation has been reported when vancomycin has been added to ceftazidime in solution. It is recommended that giving sets and intravenous lines are flushed been administration of these two agents.

6.3 Shelf life

Three years when stored below 25°C and protected from light.

6.4 Special precautions for storage

Fortum for Injection should be below 25°C. Protect from light.

6.5 Nature and contents of container

Individually cartoned vials containing 500mg ceftazidime (as pentahydrate) for intravenous use in packs of 1 or 5.

Not all pack sizes may be marketed.

6.6 Special precautions for disposal and other handling

Instructions for constitution: See table for addition volumes and solution concentrations, which may be useful when fractional doses are required.

PREPARATION OF SOLUTION

(see Table 2 below)

All sizes of vials as supplied are under reduced pressure. As the product dissolves, carbon dioxide is released and a positive pressure develops. For ease of use, it is recommended that the following techniques of reconstitution are adopted.

250mg i.m./i.v., 500mg i.m./i.v., 1g i.m./i.v., and 2g and 3g i.v. bolus vials:

1. Insert the syringe needle through the vial closure and inject the recommended volume of diluent. The vacuum may assist entry of the diluent. Remove the syringe needle.

2. Shake to dissolve: carbon dioxide is released and a clear solution will be obtained in about 1 to 2 minutes.

3. Invert the vial. With the syringe plunger fully depressed, insert the needle through the vial closure and withdraw the total volume of solution into the syringe (the pressure in the vial may aid withdrawal). Ensure that the needle remains within the solution and does not enter the head space. The withdrawn solution may contain small bubbles of carbon dioxide; they may be disregarded.

These solutions may be given directly into the vein or introduced into the tubing of a giving set if the patient is receiving parenteral fluids. Ceftazidime is compatible with the most commonly used intravenous fluids.

Vials of Fortum for Injection as supplied are under reduced pressure; a positive pressure is produced on constitution due to the release of carbon dioxide.

Vials of Fortum for Injection should be stored at a temperature below 25°C.

Vials of Fortum for Injection do not contain any preservatives and should be used as single-dose preparations.

In keeping with good pharmaceutical practice, it is preferable to use freshly constituted solutions of Fortum for Injection. If this is not practicable, satisfactory potency is retained for 24 hours in the refrigerator (2 - 8°C) when prepared in Water for Injection BP or any of the injections listed below.

At ceftazidime concentrations between 1mg/ml and 40mg/ml in:

0.9% Sodium Chloride Injection BP

M/6 Sodium Lactate Injection BP

Compound Sodium Lactate Injection BP (Hartmann's Solution)

5% Dextrose Injection BP

0.225% Sodium Chloride and 5% Dextrose Injection BP

0.45% Sodium Chloride and 5% Dextrose Injection BP

0.9% Sodium Chloride and 5% Dextrose Injection BP

0.18% Sodium Chloride and 4% Dextrose Injection BP

10% Dextrose Injection BP

Dextran 40 Injection BP 10% in 0.9% Sodium Chloride Injection BP

Dextran 40 Injection BP 10% in 5% Dextrose Injection BP

Dextran 70 Injection BP 6% in 0.9% Sodium Chloride Injection BP

Dextran 70 Injection BP 6% in 5% Dextrose Injection BP

(Ceftazidime is less stable in Sodium Bicarbonate Injection than in other intravenous fluids. It is not recommended as a diluent)

At concentrations of between 0.05mg/ml and 0.25mg/ml in Intraperitoneal Dialysis Fluid (Lactate) BPC 1973.

When reconstituted for intramuscular use with: 0.5% or 1% Lidocaine Hydrochloride Injection BP

When admixed at 4mg/ml with (both components retain satisfactory potency):

Hydrocortisone (hydrocortisone sodium phosphate) 1mg/ml in 0.9% Sodium Chloride Injection BP or 5% Dextrose Injection BP

Cefuroxime (cefuroxime sodium) 3mg/ml in 0.9% Sodium Chloride Injection BP

Cloxacillin (cloxacillin sodium) 4mg/ml in 0.9% Sodium Chloride Injection BP

Heparin 10u/ml or 50u/ml in 0.9% Sodium Chloride Injection BP

Potassium Chloride 10mEq/L or 40 mEq/L in 0.9% Sodium Chloride Injection BP

The contents of a 500mg vial of Fortum for Injection, constituted with 1.5ml water for injections, may be added to metronidazole injection (500mg in 100ml) and both retain their activity.

Solutions range from light yellow to amber depending on concentration, diluent and storage conditions used. Within the stated recommendations, product potency is not adversely affected by such colour variations.

Administrative Data

7. MARKETING AUTHORISATION HOLDER

Glaxo Operations UK Ltd
Greenford
Middlesex
UB6 OHE
Trading as
GlaxoSmithKline UK
Stockley Park West
Uxbridge
Middlesex UB11 1BT

8. MARKETING AUTHORISATION NUMBER(S)

PL 00004/0292

9. DATE OF FIRST AUTHORISATION/RENEWAL OF THE AUTHORISATION

18 May 2001

10. DATE OF REVISION OF THE TEXT

31st July 2009

11. Legal Status

POM

Table 2 PREPARATION OF SOLUTION

Vial size		Amount of Diluent to be added (ml)	Approximate Concentration (mg/ml)
250mg 250mg	Intramuscular Intravenous	1.0 2.5	210 90
500mg 500mg	Intramuscular Intravenous	1.5 5.0	260 90
1g 1g	Intramuscular Intravenous	3.0 10.0	260 90
2g 2g	Intravenous bolus Intravenous Infusion	10.0 50.0*	170 40‡
3g 3g	Intravenous bolus Intravenous Infusion	15.0 75.0*	170 40‡

* Note: Addition should be in two stages.

‡ Note: Use Sodium Chloride Injection 0.9%, Dextrose Injection 5% or other approved diluent (see pharmaceutical precautions) as Water for Injections produces hypotonic solutions at this concentration.

Fosamax

(Merck Sharp & Dohme Limited)

1. NAME OF THE MEDICINAL PRODUCT

FOSAMAX® 10 mg Tablets

2. QUALITATIVE AND QUANTITATIVE COMPOSITION

Each tablet contains 13.05 mg of alendronate sodium, which is the molar equivalent to 10 mg of alendronic acid.

Excipients:

Each tablet contains 103.95 mg lactose anhydrous.

For a full list of excipients see section 6.1

3. PHARMACEUTICAL FORM

Tablets

Oval white tablets marked with '936' on one side, and plain on the other.

4. CLINICAL PARTICULARS

4.1 Therapeutic indications

'Fosamax' is indicated for the treatment of osteoporosis in post-menopausal women to prevent fractures.

'Fosamax' is indicated for the treatment of osteoporosis in men to prevent fractures.

'Fosamax' is indicated for the treatment of glucocorticoid-induced osteoporosis and prevention of bone loss in post-menopausal women considered at risk of developing the disease.

Risk factors often associated with the development of osteoporosis include thin body build, family history of osteoporosis, early menopause, moderately low bone mass and long-term glucocorticoid therapy, especially with high doses (⩾15 mg/day).

4.2 Posology and method of administration

Treatment of osteoporosis in post-menopausal women: The recommended dosage is 10 mg once a day.

Treatment of osteoporosis in men: The recommended dosage is 10 mg once a day.

Treatment and prevention of glucocorticoid-induced osteoporosis: For post-menopausal women not receiving hormone replacement therapy (HRT) with an oestrogen, the recommended dosage is 10 mg once a day.

To permit adequate absorption of 'Fosamax':

'Fosamax' must be taken at least 30 minutes before the first food, beverage, or medication of the day with plain water only. Other beverages (including mineral water), food and some medications are likely to reduce the absorption of 'Fosamax' (see 4.5 'Interaction with other medicinal products and other forms of interaction').

To facilitate delivery to the stomach and thus reduce the potential for local and oesophageal irritation/adverse experiences (see 4.4 'Special warnings and precautions for use'):

- 'Fosamax' should only be swallowed upon arising for the day with a full glass of water (not less than 200 ml or 7 fl.oz.).
- Patients should not chew the tablet or allow the tablet to dissolve in their mouths because of a potential for oropharyngeal ulceration.
- Patients should not lie down until after their first food of the day which should be at least 30 minutes after taking the tablet.
- Patients should not lie down for at least 30 minutes after taking 'Fosamax'.
- 'Fosamax' should not be taken at bedtime or before arising for the day.

Patients should receive supplemental calcium and vitamin D if dietary intake is inadequate (see 4.4 'Special warnings and precautions for use').

Use in the elderly: In clinical studies there was no age-related difference in the efficacy or safety profiles of 'Fosamax'. Therefore no dosage adjustment is necessary for the elderly.

Use in renal impairment: No dosage adjustment is necessary for patients with GFR greater than 35 ml/min. 'Fosamax' is not recommended for patients with renal impairment where GFR is less than 35 ml/min, due to lack of experience.

Use in children (under 18 years): Alendronate has been studied in a small number of patients with osteogenesis imperfecta under 18 years of age. Results are insufficient to support its use in children.

4.3 Contraindications

- Abnormalities of the oesophagus and other factors which delay oesophageal emptying such as stricture or achalasia.
- Inability to stand or sit upright for at least 30 minutes.
- Hypersensitivity to any component of this product.
- Hypocalcaemia (see 4.4 'Special warnings and precautions for use').

4.4 Special warnings and precautions for use

'Fosamax' can cause local irritation of the upper gastro-intestinal mucosa. Because there is a potential for worsening of the underlying disease, caution should be used when 'Fosamax' is given to patients with active upper gastro-intestinal problems, such as dysphagia, oesophageal disease, gastritis, duodenitis, or ulcers (see 4.3 'Contraindications').

Oesophageal reactions (sometimes severe and requiring hospitalisation), such as oesophagitis, oesophageal ulcers and oesophageal erosions, rarely followed by oesophageal stricture or perforation, have been reported in patients receiving 'Fosamax'. Physicians should therefore be alert to any signs or symptoms signalling a possible oesophageal reaction and patients should be instructed to discontinue 'Fosamax' and seek medical attention if they develop symptoms of oesophageal irritation such as dysphagia, pain on swallowing or retrosternal pain, new or worsening heartburn.

The risk of severe oesophageal adverse experiences appears to be greater in patients who fail to take 'Fosamax' properly and/or who continue to take 'Fosamax' after developing symptoms suggestive of oesophageal irritation. It is very important that the full dosing instructions are provided to, and understood by the patient (see 4.2 'Posology and method of administration'). Patients should be informed that failure to follow these instructions may increase their risk of oesophageal problems.

While no increased risk was observed in extensive clinical trials, there have been rare (post-marketing) reports of gastric and duodenal ulcers, some severe and with complications.

Osteonecrosis of the jaw, generally associated with tooth extraction and/or local infection (including osteomyelitis) has been reported in patients with cancer receiving treatment regimens including primarily intravenously administered bisphosphonates. Many of these patients were also receiving chemotherapy and corticosteroids. Osteonecrosis of the jaw has also been reported in patients with osteoporosis receiving oral bisphosphonates.

A dental examination with appropriate preventive dentistry should be considered prior to treatment with bisphosphonates in patients with concomitant risk factors (e.g. cancer, chemotherapy, radiotherapy, corticosteroids, poor oral hygiene, periodontal disease).

While on treatment, these patients should avoid invasive dental procedures if possible. For patients who develop osteonecrosis of the jaw while on bisphosphonate therapy, dental surgery may exacerbate the condition. For patients requiring dental procedures, there are no data available to suggest whether discontinuation of bisphosphonate treatment reduces the risk of osteonecrosis of the jaw.

Clinical judgement of the treating physician should guide the management plan of each patient based on individual benefit/risk assessment.

Bone, joint, and/or muscle pain has been reported in patients taking bisphosphonates. In post-marketing experience, these symptoms have rarely been severe and/or incapacitating (see '4.8 Undesirable effects'). The time to onset of symptoms varied from one day to several months after starting treatment. Most patients had relief of symptoms after stopping. A subset had recurrence of symptoms when rechallenged with the same drug or another bisphosphonate.

'Fosamax' is not recommended for patients with renal impairment where GFR is less than 35 ml/min, (see 4.2 'Posology and method of administration').

Causes of osteoporosis other than oestrogen deficiency, ageing and glucocorticoid use should be considered.

Hypocalcaemia must be corrected before initiating therapy with alendronate (see 4.3 'Contra-indications'). Other disorders affecting mineral metabolism (such as vitamin D deficiency and hypoparathyroidism) should also be effectively treated. In patients with these conditions, serum calcium and symptoms of hypocalcaemia should be monitored during therapy with 'Fosamax'.

Due to the positive effects of alendronate in increasing bone mineral, decreases in serum calcium and phosphate may occur. These are usually small and asymptomatic. However, there have been rare reports of symptomatic hypocalcaemia, which have occasionally been severe and often occurred in patients with predisposing conditions (e.g. hypoparathyroidism, vitamin D deficiency and calcium malabsorption).

Ensuring adequate calcium and vitamin D intake is particularly important in patients receiving glucocorticoids.

Excipients

This medicinal product contains lactose. Patients with rare hereditary problems of galactose intolerance, the Lapp lactase deficiency or glucose-galactose malabsorption should not take this medicinal product.

4.5 Interaction with other medicinal products and other forms of interaction

If taken at the same time, it is likely that calcium supplements, antacids, and some oral medications will interfere with absorption of 'Fosamax'. Therefore, patients must wait at least 30 minutes after taking 'Fosamax' before taking any other oral medication.

No other drug interactions of clinical significance are anticipated. Concomitant use of HRT (oestrogen ± progestin) and 'Fosamax' was assessed in two clinical studies of one or two years duration in post-menopausal osteoporotic women (5.1 'Pharmacodynamic properties, *concomitant use with oestrogen/hormone replacement therapy (HRT)*'). Combined use of 'Fosamax' and HRT resulted in greater increases in bone mass, together with greater decreases in bone turnover, than seen with either treatment alone. In these studies, the safety and tolerability profile of the combination was consistent with those of the individual treatments.

Although specific interaction studies were not performed, in clinical studies 'Fosamax' was used concomitantly with a wide range of commonly prescribed drugs without evidence of clinical adverse interactions (see 5.1 'Pharmacodynamic properties' *'Concomitant use with oestrogen/hormone replacement therapy (HRT)'*).

4.6 Pregnancy and lactation

Use during pregnancy

'Fosamax' has not been studied in pregnant women and should not be given to them.

In developmental toxicity studies in animals, there were no adverse effects at doses up to 25 mg/kg/day in rats and 35 mg/kg/day in rabbits.

Use during lactation

'Fosamax' has not been studied in breast-feeding women and should not be given to them.

4.7 Effects on ability to drive and use machines

There are no data to suggest that 'Fosamax' affects the ability to drive or use machines.

4.8 Undesirable effects

'Fosamax' has been studied in nine major clinical studies (n=5,886). In the longest running trials in post-menopausal women up to five years experience has been collected. Two years safety data are available in both men with osteoporosis and men and women on glucocorticoids.

The following adverse experiences have been reported during clinical studies and/or post-marketing use:

[Common (≥1/100, < 1/10), Uncommon (≥1/1000, < 1/100), Rare (≥1/10,000, < 1/1000), Very rare (< 1/10,000 including isolated cases)]

Immune system disorders:

Rare: hypersensitivity reactions including urticaria and angioedema

Metabolism and nutrition disorders:

Rare: symptomatic hypocalcaemia, often in association with predisposing conditions. (see section 4.4)

Nervous system disorders:

Common: headache

Eye disorders:

Rare: uveitis, scleritis, episcleritis

Gastrointestinal disorders:

Common: abdominal pain, dyspepsia, constipation, diarrhoea, flatulence, oesophageal ulcer*, dysphagia*, abdominal distension, acid regurgitation

Uncommon: nausea, vomiting, gastritis, oesophagitis*, oesophageal erosions*, melena

Rare: oesophageal stricture*, oropharyngeal ulceration*, upper gastro-intestinal PUBs (perforation, ulcers, bleeding) (see section 4.4)

*See sections 4.2 and 4.4

Skin and subcutaneous tissue disorders:

Uncommon: rash, pruritus, erythema

Rare: rash with photosensitivity

Very rare and isolated cases: isolated cases of severe skin reactions including Stevens-Johnson syndrome and toxic epidermal necrolysis

Musculoskeletal, connective tissue and bone disorders:

Common: musculoskeletal (bone, muscle or joint) pain

Rare: osteonecrosis of the jaw has been reported in patients treated by bisphosphonates. The majority of the reports refer to cancer patients, but such cases have also been reported in patients treated for osteoporosis. Osteonecrosis of the jaw is generally associated with tooth extraction and / or local infection (including osteomyelitis). Diagnosis of cancer, chemotherapy, radiotherapy, corticosteroids and poor oral hygiene are also deemed as risk factors; severe musculoskeletal (bone, muscle or joint) pain (see 4.4 'Special warnings and precautions for use')

General disorders and administration site conditions:

Rare: transient symptoms as in an acute-phase response (myalgia, malaise and rarely, fever), typically in association with initiation of treatment.

During post-marketing experience the following reactions have been reported (frequency unknown):

Nervous system disorders: dizziness

Ear and labyrinth disorders: vertigo

Skin and subcutaneous tissue disorders: alopecia

Musculoskeletal, connective tissue and bone disorders: joint swelling

General disorders and administration site conditions: asthenia, peripheral oedema

Laboratory test findings

In clinical studies, asymptomatic, mild and transient decreases in serum calcium and phosphate were observed in approximately 18 and 10%, respectively, of patients taking 'Fosamax' versus approximately 12 and 3% of those taking placebo. However, the incidences of decreases in serum calcium to <8.0 mg/dl (2.0 mmol/l) and serum phosphate to ≤2.0 mg/dl (0.65 mmol/l) were similar in both treatment groups.

4.9 Overdose

No specific information is available on the treatment of overdosage with 'Fosamax'. Hypocalcaemia, hypophosphataemia and upper gastro-intestinal adverse events, such as upset stomach, heartburn, oesophagitis, gastritis, or ulcer, may result from oral overdosage. Milk or antacids should be given to bind alendronate. Owing to the risk of oesophageal irritation, vomiting should not be induced and the patient should remain fully upright.

5. PHARMACOLOGICAL PROPERTIES

5.1 Pharmacodynamic properties

'Fosamax' is a bisphosphonate that inhibits osteoclastic bone resorption with no direct effect on bone formation. The bone formed during treatment with 'Fosamax' is of normal quality.

Treatment of post-menopausal osteoporosis

The effects of 'Fosamax' on bone mass and fracture incidence in post-menopausal women were examined in two initial efficacy studies of identical design (n=994) as well as in the Fracture Intervention Trial (FIT: n=6,459).

In the initial efficacy studies, the mean bone mineral density (BMD) increases with 'Fosamax' 10 mg/day relative to placebo at three years were 8.8%, 5.9% and 7.8% at the spine, femoral neck and trochanter, respectively. Total body BMD also increased significantly. There was a 48% reduction in the proportion of patients treated with 'Fosamax' experiencing one or more vertebral fractures relative to those treated with placebo. In the two-year extension of these studies BMD at the spine and trochanter continued to increase and BMD at the femoral neck and total body were maintained.

FIT consisted of two placebo-controlled studies: a three-year study of 2,027 patients who had at least one baseline vertebral (compression) fracture and a four-year study of 4,432 patients with low bone mass but without a baseline vertebral fracture, 37% of whom had osteoporosis as defined by a baseline femoral neck BMD at least 2.5 standard deviations below the mean for young, adult women. In all FIT patients with osteoporosis from both studies, 'Fosamax' reduced the incidence of: ≥1 vertebral fracture by 48%, multiple vertebral fractures by 87%, ≥1 painful vertebral fracture by 45%, any painful fracture by 31% and hip fracture by 54%.

Overall these results demonstrate the consistent effect of 'Fosamax' to reduce the incidence of fractures, including those of the spine and hip, which are the sites of osteoporotic fracture associated with the greatest morbidity.

Prevention of post-menopausal osteoporosis

The effects of 'Fosamax' to prevent bone loss were examined in two studies of post-menopausal women aged ≤60 years. In the larger study of 1,609 women (≥6 months post-menopausal) those receiving 'Fosamax' 5 mg daily for two years had BMD increases of 3.5%, 1.3%, 3.0% and 0.7% at the spine, femoral neck, trochanter and total body, respectively. In the smaller study (n=447), similar results were observed in women (6 to 36 months post-menopausal) treated with 'Fosamax' 5 mg daily for three years. In contrast, in both studies, women receiving placebo lost bone mass at a rate of approximately 1% per year. The longer term effects of 'Fosamax' in an osteoporosis prevention population are not known but clinical trial extensions of up to 10 years of continuous treatment are currently in progress.

Concomitant use with oestrogen/hormone replacement therapy (HRT)

The effects on BMD of treatment with 'Fosamax' 10 mg once-daily and conjugated oestrogen (0.625 mg/day) either alone or in combination were assessed in a two-year study of hysterectomised, post-menopausal, osteoporotic women. At two years, the increases in lumbar spine BMD from baseline were significantly greater with the combination (8.3%) than with either oestrogen or 'Fosamax' alone (both 6.0%).

The effects on BMD when 'Fosamax' was added to stable doses (for at least one year) of HRT (oestrogen ± progestin) were assessed in a one-year study in post-menopausal, osteoporotic women. The addition of 'Fosamax' 10 mg once-daily to HRT produced, at one year, significantly greater increases in lumbar spine BMD (3.7%) vs. HRT alone (1.1%).

In these studies, significant increases or favourable trends in BMD for combined therapy compared with HRT alone were seen at the total hip, femoral neck and trochanter. No significant effect was seen for total body BMD.

Treatment of osteoporosis in men

The efficacy of 'Fosamax' 10 mg once daily in men (ages 31 to 87; mean, 63) with osteoporosis was demonstrated in a two-year study. At two years, the mean increases relative to placebo in BMD in men receiving 'Fosamax' 10 mg/day were: lumbar spine, 5.3%; femoral neck, 2.6%; trochanter, 3.1%; and total body, 1.6%. 'Fosamax' was effective regardless of age, race, gonadal function, baseline rate of bone turnover, or baseline BMD. Consistent with much larger studies in post-menopausal women, in these 127 men, 'Fosamax' 10 mg/day reduced the incidence of new vertebral fracture (assessed by quantitative radiography) relative to placebo (0.8% vs. 7.1%) and, correspondingly, also reduced height loss (-0.6 vs. -2.4 mm).

Glucocorticoid-induced osteoporosis

The efficacy of 'Fosamax' 5 and 10 mg once-daily in men and women receiving at least 7.5 mg/day of prednisone (or equivalent) was demonstrated in two studies. At two years of treatment, spine BMD increased by 3.7% and 5.0% (relative to placebo) with 'Fosamax' 5 and 10 mg/day respectively. Significant increases in BMD were also observed at the femoral neck, trochanter, and total body. In post-menopausal women not receiving oestrogen, greater increases in lumbar spine and trochanter BMD were seen in those receiving 10 mg 'Fosamax' than those receiving 5 mg. 'Fosamax' was effective regardless of dose or duration of glucocorticoid use. Data pooled from three dosage groups (5 or 10 mg for two years or 2.5 mg for one year followed by 10 mg for one year) showed a significant reduction in the incidence of patients with a new vertebral fracture at two years ('Fosamax' 0.7% vs. placebo 6.8%).

5.2 Pharmacokinetic properties

Absorption

Relative to an intravenous (IV) reference dose, the oral bioavailability of alendronate in women was 0.7% for doses ranging from 5 to 40 mg when administered after an overnight fast and two hours before a standardised breakfast. Oral bioavailability in men (0.6%) was similar to that in women. Bioavailability was decreased similarly to an estimated 0.46% and 0.39% when alendronate was administered one hour or half an hour before a standardised breakfast. In osteoporosis studies, 'Fosamax' was effective when administered at least 30 minutes before the first food or beverage of the day.

Bioavailability was negligible whether alendronate was administered with, or up to two hours after, a standardised breakfast. Concomitant administration of alendronate with coffee or orange juice reduced bioavailability by approximately 60%.

In healthy subjects, oral prednisone (20 mg three times daily for five days) did not produce a clinically meaningful change in oral bioavailability of alendronate (a mean increase ranging from 20% to 44%).

Distribution

Studies in rats show that alendronate transiently distributes to soft tissues following 1 mg/kg IV administration but is then rapidly redistributed to bone or excreted in the urine. The mean steady-state volume of distribution, exclusive of bone, is at least 28 litres in humans. Concentrations of drug in plasma following therapeutic oral doses are too low for analytical detection (<5 ng/ml). Protein binding in human plasma is approximately 78%.

Biotransformation

There is no evidence that alendronate is metabolised in animals or humans.

Elimination

Following a single IV dose of [^{14}C] alendronate, approximately 50% of the radioactivity was excreted in the urine within 72 hours and little or no radioactivity was recovered in the faeces. Following a single 10 mg IV dose, the renal clearance of alendronate was 71 ml/min, and systemic clearance did not exceed 200 ml/min. Plasma concentrations fell by more than 95% within six hours following IV administration. The terminal half-life in humans is estimated to exceed ten years, reflecting release of alendronate from the skeleton. Alendronate is not excreted through the acidic or basic transport systems of the kidney in rats, and thus it is not anticipated to interfere with the excretion of other drugs by those systems in humans.

Characteristics in patients

Preclinical studies show that the drug that is not deposited in bone is rapidly excreted in the urine. No evidence of saturation of bone uptake was found after chronic dosing with cumulative IV doses up to 35 mg/kg in animals. Although no clinical information is available, it is likely that, as in animals, elimination of alendronate via the kidney will be reduced in patients with impaired renal function. Therefore, somewhat greater accumulation of alendronate in bone might be expected in patients with impaired renal function (see 4.2 'Posology and method of administration').

5.3 Preclinical safety data

In test animal species the main target organs for toxicity were kidneys and gastro-intestinal tract. Renal toxicity was seen only at doses >2 mg/kg/day orally (ten times the recommended dose) and was evident only on histological examination as small widely scattered foci of nephritis, with no evidence of effect on renal function. The gastro-intestinal toxicity, seen in rodents only, occurred at doses >2.5 mg/kg/day and appears to be due to a direct effect on the mucosa. There is no additional relevant information.

Significant lethality after single oral doses was seen in female rats and mice at 552 mg/kg (3,256 mg/m^2) and 966 mg/kg (2,898 mg/m^2) (equivalent to human oral doses* of 27,600 and 48,300 mg), respectively. In males, these values were slightly higher, 626 and 1,280 mg/kg, respectively. There was no lethality in dogs at oral doses up to 200 mg/kg (4,000 mg/m^2) (equivalent to a human oral dose* of 10,000 mg).

* Based on a patient weight of 50 kg.

6. PHARMACEUTICAL PARTICULARS

6.1 List of excipients

10 mg tablets: microcrystalline cellulose, anhydrous lactose, croscarmellose sodium, magnesium stearate and carnauba wax.

6.2 Incompatibilities

None known.

6.3 Shelf life

3 years.

6.4 Special precautions for storage

Do not store above 30°C.

6.5 Nature and contents of container

Blisters of opaque white PVC lidded with aluminium foil.

Pack size: 28 tablets.

6.6 Special precautions for disposal and other handling

None.

7. MARKETING AUTHORISATION HOLDER

Merck Sharp & Dohme Limited

Hertford Road, Hoddesdon, Hertfordshire EN11 9BU, UK

8. MARKETING AUTHORISATION NUMBER(S)

10 mg tablets: PL 0025/0326

9. DATE OF FIRST AUTHORISATION/RENEWAL OF THE AUTHORISATION

10 mg tablets: 28 July 1995/ 3 June 2008

10. DATE OF REVISION OF THE TEXT

30 March 2009

LEGAL CATEGORY

P.O.M.

® denotes registered trademark of Merck & Co., Inc., Whitehouse Station, NJ, USA.

Merck Sharp & Dohme Limited

Hertford Road, Hoddesdon, Hertfordshire EN11 9BU, UK

SPC.FSM.10 mg.09.3018

Fosamax Once Weekly 70mg Tablets

(Merck Sharp & Dohme Limited)

1. NAME OF THE MEDICINAL PRODUCT

'Fosamax' Once Weekly 70 mg tablets

2. QUALITATIVE AND QUANTITATIVE COMPOSITION

Each tablet contains the equivalent of 70 mg alendronic acid as 91.37 mg of alendronate sodium trihydrate.

Excipients:

Each tablet contains 113.4 mg lactose anhydrous.

For a full list of excipients, see section 6.1.

3. PHARMACEUTICAL FORM

Tablet.

Oval white tablets, marked with an outline of a bone image on one side, and '31' on the other.

4. CLINICAL PARTICULARS

4.1 Therapeutic indications

Treatment of postmenopausal osteoporosis. 'Fosamax' reduces the risk of vertebral and hip fractures.

4.2 Posology and method of administration

The recommended dosage is one 70 mg tablet once weekly.

To permit adequate absorption of alendronate:

'Fosamax' must be taken at least 30 minutes before the first food, beverage, or medicinal product of the day with plain water only. Other beverages (including mineral water), food and some medicinal products are likely to reduce the absorption of alendronate (see section 4.5).

To facilitate delivery to the stomach and thus reduce the potential for local and oesophageal irritation/adverse experiences (see section 4.4):

• 'Fosamax' should only be swallowed upon arising for the day with a full glass of water (not less than 200 ml or 7 fl.oz.).

• Patients should not chew the tablet or allow the tablet to dissolve in their mouths because of a potential for oropharyngeal ulceration.

• Patients should not lie down until after their first food of the day which should be at least 30 minutes after taking the tablet.

• Patients should not lie down for at least 30 minutes after taking 'Fosamax'.

• 'Fosamax' should not be taken at bedtime or before arising for the day.

Patients should receive supplemental calcium and vitamin D if dietary intake is inadequate (see section 4.4).

Use in the elderly: In clinical studies there was no age-related difference in the efficacy or safety profiles of alendronate. Therefore no dosage adjustment is necessary for the elderly.

Use in renal impairment: No dosage adjustment is necessary for patients with GFR greater than 35 ml/min. Alendronate is not recommended for patients with renal impairment where GFR is less than 35 ml/min, due to lack of experience.

Use in children: (under 18 years): Alendronate has not been studied in a small number of patients with osteogenesis imperfecta under 18 years of age. Results are insufficient to support its use in children.

'Fosamax' Once Weekly 70 mg has not been investigated in the treatment of glucocorticoid-induced osteoporosis.

4.3 Contraindications

• Abnormalities of the oesophagus and other factors which delay oesophageal emptying such as stricture or achalasia.

• Inability to stand or sit upright for at least 30 minutes.

• Hypersensitivity to alendronate or to any of the excipients.

• Hypocalcaemia.

• See also section 4.4.

4.4 Special warnings and precautions for use

Alendronate can cause local irritation of the upper gastro-intestinal mucosa. Because there is a potential for worsening of the underlying disease, caution should be used when alendronate is given to patients with active upper gastro-intestinal problems, such as dysphagia, oesophageal disease, gastritis, duodenitis, ulcers, or with a recent history (within the previous year) of major gastro-intestinal disease such as peptic ulcer, or active gastro-intestinal bleeding, or surgery of the upper gastro-intestinal tract other than pyloroplasty (see section 4.3).

Oesophageal reactions (sometimes severe and requiring hospitalisation), such as oesophagitis, oesophageal ulcers and oesophageal erosions, rarely followed by oesophageal stricture, have been reported in patients receiving alendronate. Physicians should therefore be alert to any signs or symptoms signalling a possible oesophageal reaction and patients should be instructed to discontinue alendronate and seek medical attention if they develop symptoms of oesophageal irritation such as dysphagia, pain on swallowing or retrosternal pain, new or worsening heartburn.

The risk of severe oesophageal adverse experiences appears to be greater in patients who fail to take alendronate properly and/or who continue to take alendronate after developing symptoms suggestive of oesophageal irritation. It is very important that the full dosing instructions are provided to, and understood by the patient (see section 4.2). Patients should be informed that failure to follow these instructions may increase their risk of oesophageal problems.

While no increased risk was observed in extensive clinical trials, there have been rare (post-marketing) reports of gastric and duodenal ulcers, some severe and with complications.

Osteonecrosis of the jaw, generally associated with tooth extraction and/or local infection (including osteomyelitis), has been reported in patients with cancer receiving treatment regimens including primarily intravenously administered bisphosphonates. Many of these patients were also receiving chemotherapy and corticosteroids. Osteonecrosis of the jaw has also been reported in patients with osteoporosis receiving oral bisphosphonates.

A dental examination with appropriate preventive dentistry should be considered prior to treatment with bisphosphonates in patients with concomitant risk factors (e.g. cancer, chemotherapy, radiotherapy, corticosteroids, poor oral hygiene, periodontal disease).

While on treatment, these patients should avoid invasive dental procedures if possible. For patients who develop osteonecrosis of the jaw while on bisphosphonate therapy, dental surgery may exacerbate the condition. For patients requiring dental procedures, there are no data available to suggest whether discontinuation of bisphosphonate treatment reduces the risk of osteonecrosis of the jaw.

Clinical judgement of the treating physician should guide the management plan of each patient based on individual benefit/risk assessment.

Bone, joint, and/or muscle pain has been reported in patients taking bisphosphonates. In post-marketing experience, these symptoms have rarely been severe and/or incapacitating (see section 4.8). The time to onset of symptoms varied from one day to several months after starting treatment. Most patients had relief of symptoms after stopping. A subset had recurrence of symptoms when rechallenged with the same drug or another bisphosphonate.

Stress fractures (also known as insufficiency fractures) of the proximal femoral shaft have been reported in patients treated long-term with alendronic acid (time to onset in the majority of cases ranged from 18 months to 10 years). The fractures occurred after minimal or no trauma and some patients experienced thigh pain, often associated with imaging features of stress fractures, weeks to months before presenting with a completed femoral fracture. Fractures were often bilateral; therefore the contralateral femur should be examined in bisphosphonate-treated patients who have sustained a femoral shaft fracture. Poor healing of these fractures was also reported. Discontinuation of bisphosphonate therapy in patients with stress fracture is advisable pending evaluation of the patient, based on an individual benefit risk assessment.

Patients should be instructed that if they miss a dose of 'Fosamax' Once Weekly, they should take one tablet on the morning after they remember. They should not take two tablets on the same day but should return to taking one tablet once a week, as originally scheduled on their chosen day.

Alendronate is not recommended for patients with renal impairment where GFR is less than 35 ml/min, (see section 4.2).

Causes of osteoporosis other than oestrogen deficiency and ageing should be considered.

Hypocalcaemia must be corrected before initiating therapy with alendronate (see section 4.3). Other disorders affecting mineral metabolism (such as vitamin D deficiency and hypoparathyroidism) should also be effectively treated. In patients with these conditions, serum calcium and symptoms of hypocalcaemia should be monitored during therapy with 'Fosamax'.

Due to the positive effects of alendronate in increasing bone mineral, decreases in serum calcium and phosphate may occur. These are usually small and asymptomatic. However, there have been rare reports of symptomatic hypocalcaemia, which have occasionally been severe and often occurred in patients with predisposing conditions (e.g. hypoparathyroidism, vitamin D deficiency and calcium malabsorption). Ensuring adequate calcium and vitamin D intake is particularly important in patients receiving glucocorticoids.

Excipients

This medicinal product contains lactose. Patients with rare hereditary problems of galactose intolerance, the Lapp lactase deficiency or glucose-galactose malabsorption should not take this medicinal product

4.5 Interaction with other medicinal products and other forms of interaction

If taken at the same time, it is likely that food and beverages (including mineral water), calcium supplements, antacids, and some oral medicinal products will interfere with absorption of alendronate. Therefore, patients must wait at least 30 minutes after taking alendronate before taking any other oral medicinal product (see section 4.2 and 5.2).

No other interactions with medicinal products of clinical significance are anticipated. A number of patients in the clinical trials received oestrogen (intravaginal, transdermal, or oral) while taking alendronate. No adverse experiences attributable to their concomitant use were identified.

Although specific interaction studies were not performed, in clinical studies alendronate was used concomitantly with a wide range of commonly prescribed medicinal products without evidence of clinical adverse interactions.

4.6 Pregnancy and lactation

Use during pregnancy

There are no adequate data from the use of alendronate in pregnant women. Animal studies do not indicate direct harmful effects with respect to pregnancy, embryonal/foetal development, or postnatal development. Alendronate given during pregnancy in rats caused dystocia related to hypocalcemia (see section 5.3). Given the indication, alendronate should not be used during pregnancy.

Use during lactation

It is not known whether alendronate is excreted into human breast milk. Given the indication, alendronate should not be used by breast-feeding women.

4.7 Effects on ability to drive and use machines

No studies on the effects on the ability to drive and use machines have been performed.

4.8 Undesirable effects

In a one-year study in post-menopausal women with osteoporosis the overall safety profiles of 'Fosamax' Once Weekly 70 mg (n=519) and alendronate 10 mg/day (n=370) were similar.

In two three-year studies of virtually identical design, in post-menopausal women (alendronate 10 mg: n=196, placebo: n=397) the overall safety profiles of alendronate 10 mg/day and placebo were similar.

Adverse experiences reported by the investigators as possibly, probably or definitely drug-related are presented below if they occurred in ⩾1% in either treatment group in the one-year study, or in ⩾1% of patients treated with alendronate 10 mg/day and at a greater incidence than in patients given placebo in the three-year studies:

(see Table 1 below)

The following adverse experiences have also been reported during clinical studies and/or post-marketing use:

[Common (⩾1/100, < 1/10), Uncommon (⩾1/1000, < 1/100), Rare (⩾1/10,000, < 1/1000), Very rare (< 1/10,000 including isolated cases)]

Immune system disorders:

Rare: hypersensitivity reactions including urticaria and angioedema

Metabolism and nutrition disorders:

Rare: symptomatic hypocalcaemia, often in association with predisposing conditions. (see section 4.4)

Nervous system disorders:

Common: headache

Eye disorders:

Rare: uveitis, scleritis, episcleritis

Gastrointestinal disorders:

Common: abdominal pain, dyspepsia, constipation, diarrhoea, flatulence, oesophageal ulcer*, dysphagia*, abdominal distension, acid regurgitation

Uncommon: nausea, vomiting, gastritis, oesophagitis*, oesophageal erosions*, melena

Rare: oesophageal stricture*, oropharyngeal ulceration*, upper gastrointestinal PUBs (perforation, ulcers, bleeding)(see section 4.4)

*See sections 4.2 and 4.4

Skin and subcutaneous tissue disorders:

Uncommon: rash, pruritus, erythema

Rare: rash with photosensitivity

Very rare and isolated cases: isolated cases of severe skin reactions including Stevens-Johnson syndrome and toxic epidermal necrolysis

Musculoskeletal, connective tissue and bone disorders:

Common: musculoskeletal (bone, muscle or joint) pain

Rare: Osteonecrosis of the jaw has been reported in patients treated by bisphosphonates. The majority of the reports refer to cancer patients, but such cases have also been reported in patients treated for osteoporosis. Osteonecrosis of the jaw is generally associated with tooth extraction and / or local infection (including osteomyelitis). Diagnosis of cancer, chemotherapy, radiotherapy, corticosteroids and poor oral hygiene are also deemed as risk factors; severe musculoskeletal (bone, muscle or joint) pain (see section 4.4)

General disorders and administration site conditions:

Rare: transient symptoms as in an acute-phase response (myalgia, malaise and rarely, fever), typically in association with initiation of treatment.

During post-marketing experience the following reactions have been reported (frequency unknown):

Nervous system disorders: dizziness

Ear and labyrinth disorders: vertigo

Skin and subcutaneous tissue disorders: alopecia

Musculoskeletal, connective tissue and bone disorders: joint swelling, stress fractures of the proximal femoral shaft (see section 4.4)

General disorders and administration site conditions: asthenia, peripheral oedema

Laboratory test findings

In clinical studies, asymptomatic, mild and transient decreases in serum calcium and phosphate were observed in approximately 18 and 10%, respectively, of patients taking alendronate 10 mg/day versus approximately 12 and 3% of those taking placebo. However, the incidences of decreases in serum calcium to <8.0 mg/dl (2.0 mmol/l) and serum phosphate to ⩽2.0 mg/dl (0.65 mmol/l) were similar in both treatment groups.

4.9 Overdose

Hypocalcaemia, hypophosphataemia and upper gastrointestinal adverse events, such as upset stomach, heartburn, oesophagitis, gastritis, or ulcer, may result from oral overdosage.

No specific information is available on the treatment of overdosage with alendronate. Milk or antacids should be

Table 1

	One-Year Study		Three-Year Studies	
	'Fosamax' Once Weekly 70 mg (n = 519) %	alendronate 10 mg/day (n = 370) %	alendronate 10 mg/day (n = 196) %	Placebo (n = 397) %
Gastro-intestinal				
abdominal pain	3.7	3.0	6.6	4.8
dyspepsia	2.7	2.2	3.6	3.5
acid regurgitation	1.9	2.4	2.0	4.3
nausea	1.9	2.4	3.6	4.0
abdominal distention	1.0	1.4	1.0	0.8
constipation	0.8	1.6	3.1	1.8
diarrhoea	0.6	0.5	3.1	1.8
dysphagia	0.4	0.5	1.0	0.0
flatulence	0.4	1.6	2.6	0.5
gastritis	0.2	1.1	0.5	1.3
gastric ulcer	0.0	1.1	0.0	0.0
oesophageal ulcer	0.0	0.0	1.5	0.0
Musculoskeletal				
musculoskeletal (bone, muscle or joint) pain	2.9	3.2	4.1	2.5
muscle cramp	0.2	1.1	0.0	1.0
Neurological				
headache	0.4	0.3	2.6	1.5

given to bind alendronate. Owing to the risk of oesophageal irritation, vomiting should not be induced and the patient should remain fully upright.

5. PHARMACOLOGICAL PROPERTIES

5.1 Pharmacodynamic properties

Pharmacotherapeutic group: Bisphosphonate, for the treatment of bone diseases.

ATC Code: M05B A04

The active ingredient of 'Fosamax', alendronate sodium trihydrate, is a bisphosphonate that inhibits osteoclastic bone resorption with no direct effect on bone formation. Preclinical studies have shown preferential localisation of alendronate to sites of active resorption. Activity of osteoclasts is inhibited, but recruitment or attachment of osteoclasts is not affected. The bone formed during treatment with alendronate is of normal quality.

Treatment of post-menopausal osteoporosis

Osteoporosis is defined as BMD of the spine or hip 2.5 SD below the mean value of a normal young population or as a previous fragility fracture, irrespective of BMD.

The therapeutic equivalence of 'Fosamax' Once Weekly 70 mg (n=519) and alendronate 10 mg daily (n=370) was demonstrated in a one-year multicentre study of post-menopausal women with osteoporosis. The mean increases from baseline in lumbar spine BMD at one year were 5.1% (95% CI: 4.8, 5.4%) in the 70 mg once-weekly group and 5.4% (95% CI: 5.0, 5.8%) in the 10 mg daily group. The mean BMD increases were 2.3% and 2.9% at the femoral neck and 2.9% and 3.1% at the total hip in the 70 mg once weekly and 10 mg daily groups, respectively. The two treatment groups were also similar with regard to BMD increases at other skeletal sites.

The effects of alendronate on bone mass and fracture incidence in post-menopausal women were examined in two initial efficacy studies of identical design (n=994) as well as in the Fracture Intervention Trial (FIT: n=6,459).

In the initial efficacy studies, the mean bone mineral density (BMD) increases with alendronate 10 mg/day relative to placebo at three years were 8.8%, 5.9% and 7.8% at the spine, femoral neck and trochanter, respectively. Total body BMD also increased significantly. There was a 48% reduction (alendronate 3.2% vs placebo 6.2%) in the proportion of patients treated with alendronate experiencing one or more vertebral fractures relative to those treated with placebo. In the two-year extension of these studies BMD at the spine and trochanter continued to increase and BMD at the femoral neck and total body were maintained.

FIT consisted of two placebo-controlled studies using alendronate daily (5 mg daily for two years and 10 mg daily for either one or two additional years):

- FIT 1: A three-year study of 2,027 patients who had at least one baseline vertebral (compression) fracture. In this study alendronate daily reduced the incidence of $\geqslant$1 new vertebral fracture by 47% (alendronate 7.9% vs. placebo 15.0%). In addition, a statistically significant reduction was found in the incidence of hip fractures (1.1% vs. 2.2%, a reduction of 51%).
- FIT 2: A four-year study of 4,432 patients with low bone mass but without a baseline vertebral fracture. In this study, a significant difference was observed in the analysis of the subgroup of osteoporotic women (37% of the global population who correspond with the above definition of osteoporosis) in the incidence of hip fractures (alendronate 1.0% vs. placebo 2.2%, a reduction of 56%) and in the incidence of $\geqslant$1 vertebral fracture (2.9% vs. 5.8%, a reduction of 50%).

5.2 Pharmacokinetic properties

Absorption

Relative to an intravenous reference dose, the oral mean bioavailability of alendronate in women was 0.64% for doses ranging from 5 to 70 mg when administered after an overnight fast and two hours before a standardised breakfast. Bioavailability was decreased similarly to an estimated 0.46% and 0.39% when alendronate was administered one hour or half an hour before a standardised breakfast. In osteoporosis studies, alendronate was effective when administered at least 30 minutes before the first food or beverage of the day.

Bioavailability was negligible whether alendronate was administered with, or up to two hours after, a standardised breakfast. Concomitant administration of alendronate with coffee or orange juice reduced bioavailability by approximately 60%.

In healthy subjects, oral prednisone (20 mg three times daily for five days) did not produce a clinically meaningful change in oral bioavailability of alendronate (a mean increase ranging from 20% to 44%).

Distribution

Studies in rats show that alendronate transiently distributes to soft tissues following 1 mg/kg intravenous administration but is then rapidly redistributed to bone or excreted in the urine. The mean steady-state volume of distribution, exclusive of bone, is at least 28 litres in humans. Concentrations of drug in plasma following therapeutic oral doses are too low for analytical detection (<5 ng/ml). Protein binding in human plasma is approximately 78%.

Biotransformation

There is no evidence that alendronate is metabolised in animals or humans.

Elimination

Following a single intravenous dose of [^{14}C]alendronate, approximately 50% of the radioactivity was excreted in the urine within 72 hours and little or no radioactivity was recovered in the faeces. Following a single 10 mg intravenous dose, the renal clearance of alendronate was 71 ml/min, and systemic clearance did not exceed 200 ml/min. Plasma concentrations fell by more than 95% within six hours following intravenous administration. The terminal half-life in humans is estimated to exceed ten years, reflecting release of alendronate from the skeleton. Alendronate is not excreted through the acidic or basic transport systems of the kidney in rats, and thus it is not anticipated to interfere with the excretion of other medicinal products by those systems in humans.

Characteristics in patients

Preclinical studies show that the drug that is not deposited in bone is rapidly excreted in the urine. No evidence of saturation of bone uptake was found after chronic dosing with cumulative intravenous doses up to 35 mg/kg in animals. Although no clinical information is available, it is likely that, as in animals, elimination of alendronate via the kidney will be reduced in patients with impaired renal function. Therefore, somewhat greater accumulation of alendronate in bone might be expected in patients with impaired renal function (see section 4.2).

5.3 Preclinical safety data

Non-clinical data reveal no special hazard for humans based on conventional studies of safety pharmacology, repeated dose toxicity, genotoxicity and carcinogenic potential. Studies in rats have shown that treatment with alendronate during pregnancy was associated with dystocia in dams during parturition which was related to hypocalcaemia. In studies, rats given high doses showed an increased incidence of incomplete foetal ossification. The relevance to humans is unknown.

6. PHARMACEUTICAL PARTICULARS

6.1 List of excipients

Microcrystalline cellulose

Lactose anhydrous

Croscarmellose sodium

Magnesium stearate

6.2 Incompatibilities

Not applicable.

6.3 Shelf life

3 years.

6.4 Special precautions for storage

No special precautions for storage.

6.5 Nature and contents of container

Aluminum/aluminum blisters in packs containing 2, 4, 8 (2 × 4 packs), 12 (3 × 4 packs) or 40 (10 × 4 packs) tablets.

Not all pack sizes may be marketed.

6.6 Special precautions for disposal and other handling

No special requirements.

7. MARKETING AUTHORISATION HOLDER

Merck Sharp & Dohme Limited

Hertford Road, Hoddesdon, Hertfordshire EN11 9BU, UK

8. MARKETING AUTHORISATION NUMBER(S)

PL 0025/0399

9. DATE OF FIRST AUTHORISATION/RENEWAL OF THE AUTHORISATION

10 November 2000/ 9 November 2005

10. DATE OF REVISION OF THE TEXT

June 2009

LEGAL CATEGORY

POM

® denotes registered trademark of Merck & Co., Inc., Whitehouse Station, NJ, USA.

SPC.FSM70.09.UK.3052 -II-026

FOSAVANCE Tablets

(Merck Sharp & Dohme Limited)

1. NAME OF THE MEDICINAL PRODUCT

FOSAVANCE ▼ 70 mg/2800 IU tablets

2. QUALITATIVE AND QUANTITATIVE COMPOSITION

Each tablet contains 70 mg alendronic acid as alendronate sodium trihydrate, and 70 micrograms (2800 IU) colecalciferol (vitamin D_3).

Excipients:

Each tablet contains 62 mg lactose anhydrous and 8 mg sucrose.

For a full list of excipients, see section 6.1.

3. PHARMACEUTICAL FORM

Tablet.

Capsule-shaped, white to off-white tablets, marked with an outline of a bone image on one side, and '710' on the other.

4. CLINICAL PARTICULARS

4.1 Therapeutic indications

Treatment of postmenopausal osteoporosis in patients at risk of vitamin D insufficiency.

FOSAVANCE reduces the risk of vertebral and hip fractures.

4.2 Posology and method of administration

The recommended dosage is one FOSAVANCE tablet once weekly.

Due to the nature of the disease process in osteoporosis, FOSAVANCE is intended for long-term use.

To permit adequate absorption of alendronate:

FOSAVANCE must be taken with water only (**not** mineral water) at least 30 minutes before the first food, beverage, or medicinal product (including antacids, calcium supplements and vitamins) of the day. Other beverages (including mineral water), food and some medicinal products are likely to reduce the absorption of alendronate (see section 4.5).

The following instructions should be followed exactly in order to minimize the risk of oesophageal irritation and related adverse reactions (see section 4.4):

- FOSAVANCE should only be swallowed after getting up for the day with a full glass of water (not less than 200ml or 7fl.oz.).
- Patients should only swallow FOSAVANCE whole. Patients should not crush or chew the tablet or allow the tablet to dissolve in their mouths because of a potential for oropharyngeal ulceration.
- Patients should not lie down until after their first food of the day which should be at least 30 minutes after taking the tablet.
- Patients should not lie down for at least 30 minutes after taking FOSAVANCE.
- FOSAVANCE should not be taken at bedtime or before arising for the day.

Patients should receive supplemental calcium if intake from diet is inadequate (see section 4.4). Additional supplementation with vitamin D should be considered on an individual basis taking into account any vitamin D intake from vitamins and dietary supplements. The equivalence of intake of 2800 IU of vitamin D_3 weekly in FOSAVANCE to daily dosing of vitamin D 400 IU has not been studied.

Use in the elderly:

In clinical studies there was no age-related difference in the efficacy or safety profiles of alendronate. Therefore no dosage adjustment is necessary for the elderly.

Use in renal impairment:

No dosage adjustment is necessary for patients with a glomerular filtration rate (GFR) greater than 35ml/min. FOSAVANCE is not recommended for patients with renal impairment where GFR is less than 35ml/min, due to lack of experience.

Use in children and adolescents:

FOSAVANCE has not been studied in children and adolescents and therefore should not be given to them.

4.3 Contraindications

- Hypersensitivity to the active substances or to any of the excipients.
- Abnormalities of the oesophagus and other factors which delay oesophageal emptying such as stricture or achalasia.
- Inability to stand or sit upright for at least 30 minutes.
- Hypocalcaemia.

4.4 Special warnings and precautions for use

Alendronate

Alendronate can cause local irritation of the upper gastrointestinal mucosa. Because there is a potential for worsening of the underlying disease, caution should be used when alendronate is given to patients with active upper gastrointestinal problems, such as dysphagia, oesophageal disease, gastritis, duodenitis, ulcers, or with a recent history (within the previous year) of major gastrointestinal disease such as peptic ulcer, or active gastrointestinal bleeding, or surgery of the upper gastrointestinal tract other than pyloroplasty (see section 4.3).

Oesophageal reactions (sometimes severe and requiring hospitalisation), such as oesophagitis, oesophageal ulcers and oesophageal erosions, rarely followed by oesophageal stricture, have been reported in patients receiving alendronate. Physicians should therefore be alert to any signs or symptoms signalling a possible oesophageal reaction and patients should be instructed to discontinue alendronate and seek medical attention if they develop symptoms of oesophageal irritation such as dysphagia, pain on swallowing or retrosternal pain or new or worsening heartburn (see section 4.8).

The risk of severe oesophageal adverse reactions appears to be greater in patients who fail to take alendronate properly and/or who continue to take alendronate after developing symptoms suggestive of oesophageal irritation. It is very important that the full dosing instructions are provided to, and are understood by the patient (see section 4.2). Patients should be informed that failure to follow these instructions may increase their risk of oesophageal problems.

While no increased risk was observed in extensive clinical trials with alendronate, there have been rare (post-marketing) reports of gastric and duodenal ulcers, some of which were severe and with complications (see section 4.8).

Osteonecrosis of the jaw, generally associated with tooth extraction and/or local infection (including osteomyelitis), has been reported in patients with cancer who are receiving treatment regimens including primarily intravenously administered bisphosphonates. Many of these patients were also receiving chemotherapy and corticosteroids. Osteonecrosis of the jaw has also been reported in patients with osteoporosis receiving oral bisphosphonates.

A dental examination with appropriate preventive dentistry should be considered prior to treatment with bisphosphonates in patients with concomitant risk factors (e.g. cancer, chemotherapy, radiotherapy, corticosteroids, poor oral hygiene, periodontal disease).

While on treatment, these patients should avoid invasive dental procedures if possible. For patients who develop osteonecrosis of the jaw while on bisphosphonate therapy, dental surgery may exacerbate the condition. For patients requiring dental procedures, there are no data available to suggest whether discontinuation of bisphosphonate treatment reduces the risk of osteonecrosis of the jaw.

Clinical judgement of the treating physician should guide the management plan of each patient based on individual benefit/risk assessment.

Bone, joint, and/or muscle pain has been reported i n patients taking bisphosphonates. In post-marketing experience, these symptoms have rarely been severe and/or incapacitating (see section 4.8). The time to onset of symptoms varied from one day to several months after starting treatment. Most patients had relief of symptoms after stopping treatment. A subset had recurrence of symptoms when rechallenged with the same medicinal product or another bisphosphonate.

Stress fractures (also known as insufficiency fractures) of the proximal femoral shaft have been reported in patients treated long-term with alendronic acid (time to onset in the majority of cases ranged from 18 months to 10 years). The fractures occurred after minimal or no trauma and some patients experienced thigh pain, often associated with imaging features of stress fractures, weeks to months before presenting with a completed femoral fracture. Fractures were often bilateral; therefore the contralateral femur should be examined in bisphosphonate-treated patients who have sustained a femoral shaft fracture. Poor healing of these fractures was also reported. Discontinuation of bisphosphonate therapy in patients with stress fracture is advisable pending evaluation of the patient, based on an individual benefit risk assessment.

Patients should be instructed that if they miss a dose of FOSAVANCE they should take one tablet on the morning after they remember. They should not take two tablets on the same day but should return to taking one tablet once a week, as originally scheduled on their chosen day.

FOSAVANCE is not recommended for patients with renal impairment where GFR is less than 35ml/min (see section 4.2).

Causes of osteoporosis other than oestrogen deficiency and ageing should be considered.

Hypocalcaemia must be corrected before initiating therapy with FOSAVANCE (see section 4.3). Other disorders affecting mineral metabolism (such as vitamin D deficiency and hypoparathyroidism) should also be effectively treated before starting FOSAVANCE. The content of vitamin D in FOSAVANCE is not suitable for correction of vitamin D deficiency. In patients with these conditions, serum calcium and symptoms of hypocalcaemia should be monitored during therapy with FOSAVANCE.

Due to the positive effects of alendronate in increasing bone mineral, decreases in serum calcium and phosphate may occur especially in patients taking glucocrticoids in whom calcium absorption may be decreased. These are usually small and asymptomatic. However, there have been rare reports of symptomatic hypocalcaemia, which have occasionally been severe and often occurred in patients with predisposing conditions (e.g. hypoparathyroidism, vitamin D deficiency and calcium malabsorption) (see section 4.8).

Colecalciferol

Vitamin D_3 may increase the magnitude of hypercalcaemia and/or hypercalciuria when administered to patients with disease associated with unregulated overproduction of calcitriol (e.g. leukaemia, lymphoma, sarcoidosis). Urine and serum calcium should be monitored in these patients.

Patients with malabsorption may not adequately absorb vitamin D

Excipients

This medicinal product contains lactose and sucrose. Patients with rare hereditary problems of fructose intolerance, galactose intolerance, the Lapp lactase deficiency, glucose-galactose malabsorption or sucrase-isomaltase insufficiency should not take this medicinal product.

4.5 Interaction with other medicinal products and other forms of interaction

Alendronate

If taken at the same time, it is likely that food and beverages (including mineral water), calcium supplements, antacids, and some oral medicinal products will interfere with absorption of alendronate. Therefore, patients must wait at least 30 minutes after taking alendronate before taking any other oral medicinal product (see sections 4.2 and 5.2).

No other clinically significant interactions with medicinal products are anticipated. A number of patients in the clinical trials received oestrogen (intravaginal, transdermal, or oral) while taking alendronate. No adverse reactions attributable to their concomitant use were identified.

Since NSAID use is associated with gastrointestinal irritation, caution should be used during concomitant use with alendronate.

Although specific interaction studies were not performed, in clinical studies alendronate was used concomitantly with a wide range of commonly prescribed medicinal products without evidence of interactions of clinical relevance.

Colecalciferol

Olestra, mineral oils, orlistat, and bile acid sequestrants (e.g. cholestyramine, colestipol) may impair the absorption of vitamin D. Anticonvulsants, cimetidine and thiazides may increase the catabolism of vitamin D. Additional vitamin D supplements may be considered on an individual basis.

4.6 Pregnancy and lactation

FOSAVANCE is only intended for use in postmenopausal women and therefore it should not be used during pregnancy or in breast-feeding women.

There are no adequate data from the use of FOSAVANCE in pregnant women. Animal studies with alendronate do not indicate direct harmful effects with respect to pregnancy, embryonal/foetal development, or postnatal development. Alendronate given during pregnancy in rats caused dystocia related to hypocalcaemia (see section 5.3). Studies in animals have shown hypercalcaemia and reproductive toxicity with high doses of vitamin D (see section 5.3).

It is not known whether alendronate is excreted into human breast milk. Colecalciferol and some of its active metabolites pass into breast milk.

4.7 Effects on ability to drive and use machines

No studies on the effects on the ability to drive and use machines have been performed.

However, certain adverse reactions that have been reported with FOSAVANCE may affect some patients' ability to drive or operate machinery. Individual responses to FOSAVANCE may vary (see section 4.8).

4.8 Undesirable effects

The following adverse reactions have been reported during clinical studies and/or post-marketing use with alendronate.

No additional adverse reactions have been identified for FOSAVANCE.

[Common ($\geqslant$ 1/100, < 1/10), uncommon ($\geqslant$ 1/1000, < 1/100), rare ($\geqslant$ 1/10,000, < 1/1000), very rare (< 1/10,000)]

(see Table 1 below)

During post-marketing experience the following reactions have been reported (frequency not known):

Nervous system disorders:	Dizziness, dysgeusia
Ear and labyrinth disorders:	Vertigo
Skin and subcutaneous tissue disorders:	Alopecia
Musculoskeletal, connective tissue and bone disorders:	Osteonecrosis of the jaw has been reported in patients treated by bisphosphonates. The majority of the reports refer to cancer patients, but such cases have also been reported in patients treated for osteoporosis. Osteonecrosis of the jaw is generally associated with tooth extraction and / or local infection (including osteomyelitis). Diagnosis of cancer, chemotherapy, radiotherapy, corticosteroids and poor oral hygiene are also deemed as risk factors (see section 4.4); joint swelling; stress fractures of the proximal femoral shaft (see section 4.4).
General disorders and administration site conditions:	Asthenia, peripheral oedema

Laboratory test findings

In clinical studies, asymptomatic, mild and transient decreases in serum calcium and phosphate were observed in approximately 18 % and 10 %, respectively, of patients taking alendronate 10 mg/day versus approximately 12 % and 3 % of those taking placebo. However, the incidences of decreases in serum calcium to < 8.0 mg/dl (2.0 mmol/l) and serum phosphate to $\leqslant$ 2.0 mg/dl (0.65 mmol/l) were similar in both treatment groups.

4.9 Overdose

Alendronate

Hypocalcaemia, hypophosphataemia and upper gastrointestinal adverse reactions, such as upset stomach, heartburn, oesophagitis, gastritis, or ulcer, may result from oral overdose.

No specific information is available on the treatment of overdose with alendronate. In case of overdose with FOSAVANCE, milk or antacids should be given to bind alendronate. Owing to the risk of oesophageal irritation, vomiting should not be induced and the patient should remain fully upright.

Colecalciferol

Vitamin D toxicity has not been documented during chronic therapy in generally healthy adults at a dose less than 10,000 IU/day. In a clinical study of healthy adults a 4000 IU daily dose of vitamin D_3 for up to five months was not associated with hypercalciuria or hypercalcaemia.

5. PHARMACOLOGICAL PROPERTIES

5.1 Pharmacodynamic properties

Pharmacotherapeutic group: Bisphosphonates, combinations, ATC code: M05BB03.

FOSAVANCE is a combination tablet containing the two active substances alendronate sodium trihydrate and colecalciferol (vitamin D_3).

Alendronate

Alendronate sodium is a bisphosphonate that inhibits osteoclastic bone resorption with no direct effect on bone formation. Preclinical studies have shown preferential localisation of alendronate to sites of active resorption. Activity of osteoclasts is inhibited, but recruitment or attachment of osteoclasts is not affected. The bone formed during treatment with alendronate is of normal quality.

Table 1 *[Common ($\geqslant$ 1/100, < 1/10), uncommon ($\geqslant$ 1/1000, < 1/100), rare ($\geqslant$ 1/10,000, < 1/1000), very rare (< 1/10,000)]*

Nervous system disorders:	*Common:* headache
Eye disorders:	*Rare:* uveitis, scleritis, episcleritis
Gastrointestinal disorders:	*Common:* abdominal pain, dyspepsia, constipation, diarrhoea, flatulence, oesophageal ulcer*, dysphagia*, abdominal distension, acid regurgitation *Uncommon:* nausea, vomiting, gastritis, oesophagitis*, oesophageal erosions*, melena *Rare:* oesophageal stricture*, oropharyngeal ulceration*, upper gastrointestinal PUBs (perforation, ulcers, bleeding) (see section 4.4). *See sections 4.2 and 4.4
Skin and subcutaneous tissue disorders:	*Uncommon:* rash, pruritus, erythema *Rare:* rash with photosensitivity *Very rare:* severe skin reactions including Stevens-Johnson syndrome and toxic epidermal necrolysis
Musculoskeletal and connective tissue disorders:	*Common:* musculoskeletal (bone, muscle or joint) pain *Rare:* severe musculoskeletal (bone, muscle or joint) pain (see section 4.4)
Metabolism and nutrition disorders:	*Rare:* symptomatic hypocalcaemia, often in association with predisposing conditions. (see section 4.4)
General disorders and administration site conditions:	*Rare:* transient symptoms as in an acute-phase response (myalgia, malaise and rarely, fever), typically in association with initiation of treatment.
Immune system disorders:	*Rare:* hypersensitivity reactions including urticaria and angioedema

Colecalciferol (vitamin D_3)

Vitamin D_3 is produced in the skin by conversion of 7-dehydrocholesterol to vitamin D_3 by ultraviolet light. In the absence of adequate sunlight exposure, vitamin D_3 is an essential dietary nutrient. Vitamin D_3 is converted to 25-hydroxyvitamin D_3 in the liver, and stored until needed. Conversion to the active calcium-mobilizing hormone 1,25-dihydroxyvitamin D_3 (calcitriol) in the kidney is tightly regulated. The principal action of 1,25-dihydroxyvitamin D_3 is to increase intestinal absorption of both calcium and phosphate as well as regulate serum calcium, renal calcium and phosphate excretion, bone formation and bone resorption.

Vitamin D_3 is required for normal bone formation. Vitamin D insufficiency develops when both sunlight exposure and dietary intake are inadequate. Insufficiency is associated with negative calcium balance, bone loss, and increased risk of skeletal fracture. In severe cases, deficiency results in secondary hyperparathyroidism, hypophosphataemia, proximal muscle weakness and osteomalacia, further increasing the risk of falls and fractures in osteoporotic individuals. Supplemental vitamin D reduces these risks and their consequences.

Osteoporosis is defined as bone mineral density (BMD) of the spine or hip 2.5 standard deviations (SD) below the mean value of a normal young population or as a previous fragility fracture, irrespective of BMD.

FOSAVANCE studies

The effect of FOSAVANCE (alendronate 70 mg/vitamin D_3 2800 IU) on vitamin D status was demonstrated in a 15-week, multinational study that enrolled 682 osteoporotic post-menopausal women (serum 25-hydroxyvitamin D at baseline: mean, 56 nmol/l [22.3 ng/ml]; range, 22.5-225 nmol/l [9-90 ng/ml]). Patients received the lower strength (70 mg/2800 IU) of FOSAVANCE (n=350) or FOSAMAX (alendronate) 70 mg (n=332) once a week; additional vitamin D supplements were prohibited. After 15 weeks of treatment, the mean serum 25-hydroxyvitamin D levels were significantly higher (26 %) in the FOSAVANCE (70 mg/2800 IU) group (56 nmol/l [23 ng/ml]) than in the alendronate-only group (46 nmol/l [18.2 ng/ml]). The percentage of patients with vitamin D insufficiency (serum 25-hydroxyvitamin D < 37.5 nmol/l [< 15 ng/ml]) was significantly reduced by 62.5 % with FOSAVANCE (70 mg/2800 IU) vs. alendronate-only (12 % vs. 32 %, respectively), through week 15. The percentage of patients with vitamin D deficiency (serum 25-hydroxyvitamin D < 22.5 nmol/l [< 9 ng/ml]) was significantly reduced by 92 % with FOSAVANCE (70 mg/2800 IU) vs. alendronate-only (1 % vs 13 %, respectively). In this study, mean 25-hydroxyvitamin D levels in patients with vitamin D insufficiency at baseline (25- hydroxyvitamin D, 22.5 to 37.5 nmol/l [9 to < 15 ng/ml]) increased from 30 nmol/l (12.1 ng/ml) to 40 nmol/l (15.9 ng/ml) at week 15 in the FOSAVANCE (70 mg/2800 IU) group (n=75) and decreased from 30 nmol/l (12.0 ng/ml) at baseline to 26 nmol/l (10.4 ng/ml) at week 15 in the alendronate-only group (n=70). There were no differences in mean serum calcium, phosphate, or 24-hour urine calcium between treatment groups.

Alendronate studies

The therapeutic equivalence of alendronate once weekly 70 mg (n=519) and alendronate 10 mg daily (n=370) was demonstrated in a one-year multicentre study of post-menopausal women with osteoporosis. The mean increases from baseline in lumbar spine BMD at one year were 5.1 % (95 % CI: 4.8, 5.4 %) in the 70 mg once-weekly group and 5.4 % (95 % CI: 5.0, 5.8 %) in the 10 mg daily group. The mean BMD increases were 2.3 % and 2.9 % at the femoral neck and 2.9 % and 3.1 % at the total hip in the 70 mg once weekly and 10 mg daily groups, respectively. The two treatment groups were also similar with regard to BMD increases at other skeletal sites.

The effects of alendronate on bone mass and fracture incidence in post-menopausal women were examined in two initial efficacy studies of identical design (n=994) as well as in the Fracture Intervention Trial (FIT: n=6,459).

In the initial efficacy studies, the mean BMD increases with alendronate 10 mg/day relative to placebo at three years were 8.8 %, 5.9 % and 7.8 % at the spine, femoral neck and trochanter, respectively. Total body BMD also increased significantly. There was a 48 % reduction (alendronate 3.2 % vs placebo 6.2 %) in the proportion of patients treated with alendronate experiencing one or more vertebral fractures relative to those treated with placebo. In the two-year extension of these studies BMD at the spine and trochanter continued to increase and BMD at the femoral neck and total body were maintained.

FIT consisted of two placebo-controlled studies using alendronate daily (5 mg daily for two years and 10 mg daily for either one or two additional years):

- FIT 1: A three-year study of 2,027 patients who had at least one baseline vertebral (compression) fracture. In this study alendronate daily reduced the incidence of ≥1 new vertebral fracture by 47 % (alendronate 7.9 % vs. placebo 15.0 %). In addition, a statistically significant reduction was found in the incidence of hip fractures (1.1 % vs. 2.2 %, a reduction of 51 %).
- FIT 2: A four-year study of 4,432 patients with low bone mass but without a baseline vertebral fracture. In this study, a significant difference was observed in the analysis of the subgroup of osteoporotic women (37 % of the global population who correspond with the above definition of osteoporosis) in the incidence of hip fractures (alendronate 1.0 % vs. placebo 2.2 %, a reduction of 56 %) and in the incidence of ≥1 vertebral fracture (2.9 % vs. 5.8 %, a reduction of 50 %).

5.2 Pharmacokinetic properties

Alendronate

Absorption

Relative to an intravenous reference dose, the oral mean bioavailability of alendronate in women was 0.64 % for doses ranging from 5 to 70 mg when administered after an overnight fast and two hours before a standardised breakfast. Bioavailability was decreased similarly to an estimated 0.46 % and 0.39 % when alendronate was administered one hour or half an hour before a standardised breakfast. In osteoporosis studies, alendronate was effective when administered at least 30 minutes before the first food or beverage of the day.

The alendronate component in the FOSAVANCE (70 mg/2800 IU) combination tablet is bioequivalent to the alendronate 70 mg tablet.

Bioavailability was negligible whether alendronate was administered with, or up to two hours after, a standardised breakfast. Concomitant administration of alendronate with coffee or orange juice reduced bioavailability by approximately 60 %.

In healthy subjects, oral prednisone (20 mg three times daily for five days) did not produce a clinically meaningful change in oral bioavailability of alendronate (a mean increase ranging from 20 % to 44 %).

Distribution

Studies in rats show that alendronate transiently distributes to soft tissues following 1 mg/kg intravenous administration but is then rapidly redistributed to bone or excreted in the urine. The mean steady-state volume of distribution, exclusive of bone, is at least 28 litres in humans. Concentrations of alendronate in plasma following therapeutic oral doses are too low for analytical detection (< 5 ng/ml). Protein binding in human plasma is approximately 78 %.

Biotransformation

There is no evidence that alendronate is metabolised in animals or humans.

Elimination

Following a single intravenous dose of [^{14}C]alendronate, approximately 50 % of the radioactivity was excreted in the urine within 72 hours and little or no radioactivity was recovered in the faeces. Following a single 10 mg intravenous dose, the renal clearance of alendronate was 71 ml/min, and systemic clearance did not exceed 200 ml/min. Plasma concentrations fell by more than 95 % within six hours following intravenous administration. The terminal half-life in humans is estimated to exceed ten years, reflecting release of alendronate from the skeleton. Alendronate is not excreted through the acidic or basic transport systems of the kidney in rats, and thus it is not anticipated to interfere with the excretion of other medicinal products by those systems in humans.

Colecalciferol

Absorption

In healthy adult subjects (males and females), following administration of FOSAVANCE after an overnight fast and two hours before a meal, the mean area under the serum-concentration-time curve ($AUC_{0\text{-}120\ hrs}$) for vitamin D_3 (unadjusted for endogenous vitamin D_3 levels) was 296.4 ng•hr/ml. The mean maximal serum concentration (C_{max}) of vitamin D_3 was 5.9 ng/ml, and the median time to maximal serum concentration (T_{max}) was 12 hours. The bioavailability of the 2800 IU vitamin D_3 in FOSAVANCE is similar to 2800 IU vitamin D_3 administered alone.

Distribution

Following absorption, vitamin D_3 enters the blood as part of chylomicrons. Vitamin D_3 is rapidly distributed mostly to the liver where it undergoes metabolism to 25-hydroxyvitamin D_3, the major storage form. Lesser amounts are distributed to adipose and muscle tissue and stored as vitamin D_3 at these sites for later release into the circulation. Circulating vitamin D_3 is bound to vitamin D-binding protein.

Biotransformation

Vitamin D_3 is rapidly metabolized by hydroxylation in the liver to 25-hydroxyvitamin D_3, and subsequently metabolized in the kidney to 1,25-dihydroxyvitamin D_3, which represents the biologically active form. Further hydroxylation occurs prior to elimination. A small percentage of vitamin D_3 undergoes glucuronidation prior to elimination.

Elimination

When radioactive vitamin D_3 was administered to healthy subjects, the mean urinary excretion of radioactivity after 48 hours was 2.4 %, and the mean faecal excretion of radioactivity after 4 days was 4.9 %. In both cases, the excreted radioactivity was almost exclusively as metabolites of the parent. The mean half-life of vitamin D_3 in the serum following an oral dose of FOSAVANCE (70 mg/2800 IU) is approximately 24 hours.

Characteristics in patients

Preclinical studies show that alendronate that is not deposited in bone is rapidly excreted in the urine. No evidence of saturation of bone uptake was found after chronic dosing with cumulative intravenous doses up to 35 mg/kg in animals. Although no clinical information is available, it is likely that, as in animals, elimination of alendronate via the kidney will be reduced in patients with impaired renal function. Therefore, somewhat greater accumulation of alendronate in bone might be expected in patients with impaired renal function (see section 4.2).

5.3 Preclinical safety data

Non-clinical studies with the combination of alendronate and colecalciferol have not been conducted.

Alendronate

Non-clinical data reveal no special hazard for humans based on conventional studies of safety pharmacology, repeated dose toxicity, genotoxicity and carcinogenic potential. Studies in rats have shown that treatment with alendronate during pregnancy was associated with dystocia in dams during parturition which was related to hypocalcaemia. In studies, rats given high doses showed an increased incidence of incomplete foetal ossification. The relevance to humans is unknown.

Colecalciferol

At doses far higher than the human therapeutic range, reproductive toxicity has been observed in animal studies.

6. PHARMACEUTICAL PARTICULARS

6.1 List of excipients

Microcrystalline cellulose (E460)

Lactose anhydrous

Medium chain triglycerides

Gelatin

Croscarmellose sodium

Sucrose

Colloidal silicon dioxide

Magnesium stearate (E572)

Butyl hydroxytoluene (E321)

Modified starch (maize)

Sodium aluminium silicate (E554)

6.2 Incompatibilities

Not applicable.

6.3 Shelf life

18 months.

6.4 Special precautions for storage

Store in the original blister in order to protect from moisture and light.

6.5 Nature and contents of container

Wallet with sealed aluminium/aluminium blisters, in cartons containing 2 (1 wallet × 2 tablets), 4 (1 wallet × 4 tablets), 6 (3 wallets × 2 tablets), 12 (3 wallets × 4 tablets) or 40 (10 wallets × 4 tablets) tablets.

Not all pack sizes may be marketed.

6.6 Special precautions for disposal and other handling

No special requirements.

7. MARKETING AUTHORISATION HOLDER

Merck Sharp & Dohme Ltd.

Hertford Road, Hoddesdon

Hertfordshire EN11 9BU

United Kingdom

8. MARKETING AUTHORISATION NUMBER(S)

EU/1/05/310/001 – 2 tablets

EU/1/05/310/002 – 4 tablets

EU/1/05/310/003 – 6 tablets

EU/1/05/310/004 – 12 tablets

EU/1/05/310/005 – 40 tablets

9. DATE OF FIRST AUTHORISATION/RENEWAL OF THE AUTHORISATION

24 August 2005

10. DATE OF REVISION OF THE TEXT

07 July 2009

SPC.FSP.09.UK.3109 II-011

Foscavir

(AstraZeneca UK Limited)

1. NAME OF THE MEDICINAL PRODUCT

Brand name: Foscavir

Non-proprietary name: Foscarnet trisodium hexahydrate

2. QUALITATIVE AND QUANTITATIVE COMPOSITION

Foscarnet trisodium hexahydrate 24 mg/ml.

3. PHARMACEUTICAL FORM

Intravenous infusion.

4. CLINICAL PARTICULARS

4.1 Therapeutic indications

Foscavir is indicated for induction and maintenance therapy of cytomegalovirus (CMV) retinitis in patients with AIDS. Induction therapy of mucocutaneous Herpes Simplex Virus (HSV) infections, unresponsive to acyclovir in immunocompromised patients.

Following induction therapy over 2–3 weeks Foscavir produced stabilisation of retinal lesions in approximately 80% of cases treated. However, since CMV causes latent infections and since Foscavir exerts a virustatic activity, relapses are likely in the majority of patients with persistent immunodeficiency once treatment is discontinued. Following completion of induction therapy, maintenance therapy should be instituted with a once daily regimen at an initial dose of 60 mg/kg increasing to 90–120 mg/kg if tolerated. A number of patients have received 90 mg/kg over a two hour period as a maintenance therapy starting dose. Maintenance therapy has produced a delay in time to retinitis progression. In patients experiencing progression of retinitis while receiving maintenance therapy or off-therapy, reinstitution of induction therapy has shown equal efficacy equivalent to that of the initial course.

Foscavir is also indicated for the treatment of mucocutaneous HSV infections, clinically unresponsive to acyclovir in immunocompromised patients. The safety and efficacy of Foscavir for the treatment of other HSV infections (e.g. retinitis, encephalitis); congenital or neonatal disease; or HSV in immunocompetent individuals has not been established.

The diagnosis of acyclovir unresponsiveness can be made either clinically by treatment with intravenous acyclovir (5–10 mg/kg t.i.d) for 10 days without response or by *in vitro* testing.

For treatment of acyclovir unresponsive mucocutaneous infections Foscavir was administered at 40 mg/kg every 8 hours over 2–3 weeks or until healing. In a prospective randomised study in patients with AIDS, Foscavir-treated patients healed within 11–25 days, had a complete relief of pain within 9 days and stopped shedding HSV virus within 7 days.

Foscavir is not recommended for treatment of CMV infections other than retinitis or HSV or for use in non-AIDS or non-immunocompromised patients.

4.2 Posology and method of administration

Method of administration: Foscarnet should be administered by the intravenous route only, either by a central venous line or in a peripheral vein.

When peripheral veins are used, the solution of foscarnet 24 mg/ml must be diluted. Individually dispensed doses of foscarnet should be aseptically transferred and diluted with equal parts of 0.9% sodium chloride (9 mg/ml) or 5% dextrose (50 mg/ml) by the hospital pharmacy. The diluted solutions should be used as soon as possible after preparation but can be stored for up to 24 hours if kept refrigerated.

The solution of foscarnet 24 mg/ml may be given without dilution via a central vein.

Adults: Induction therapy for CMV retinitis: Foscavir is administered over 2–3 weeks depending on the clinical response, as intermittent infusions every 8 hours at a dose of 60 mg/kg in patients with normal renal function. Dosage must be individualised for patient's renal function (see dosing chart below). The infusion time should not be shorter than 1 hour.

Maintenance therapy: For maintenance therapy, following induction therapy of CMV retinitis, Foscavir is administered seven days a week as long as therapy is considered appropriate. In patients with normal renal function, it is recommended to initiate therapy at 60 mg/kg. Increase to a dose of 90–120 mg/kg may then be considered in patients tolerating the initial dose level and/or those with progressive retinitis. A number of patients have received 90 mg/kg over a 2 hour period as a starting dose for maintenance therapy. Dosage must be reduced in patients with renal insufficiency (see dosage chart at end of dosage section).

Patients who experience progression of retinitis while receiving maintenance therapy may be re-treated with the induction regimen.

Induction therapy of mucocutaneous HSV infections unresponsive to acyclovir: Foscavir is administered for 2–3 weeks or until healing of lesions, as intermittent infusions at a dose of 40 mg/kg over one hour every 8 hours in patients with normal renal function. Dosage must be individualised for patients renal function (see dosing chart below). The infusion time should not be shorter than 1 hour.

Efficacy of Foscavir maintenance therapy following induction therapy of acyclovir unresponsive HSV infections has not been established.

Caution: Do not administer Foscavir by rapid intravenous injection.

Foscavir Dosing Chart

Induction Therapy

Creatinine Clearance (ml/kg/min)	CMV Every 8 Hours (mg/kg)	HSV Every 8 Hours (mg/kg)
> 1.6	60	40
1.6–1.4	55	37
1.4–1.2	49	33
1.2–1.0	42	28
1.0–0.8	35	24
0.8–0.6	28	19
0.6–0.4	21	14
< 0.4	Treatment not recommended	

CMV Maintenance Therapy

Creatinine Clearance (ml/kg/min)	One Infusion Dose (mg/kg/day in not less than one hour)
> 1.6	60*
1.6–1.4	55
1.4–1.2	49
1.2–1.0	42
1.0–0.8	35
0.8–0.6	28
0.6–0.4	21
< 0.4	Treatment not recommended

*A number of patients have received 90 mg/kg as a starting dose for maintenance therapy.

Foscavir is not recommended in patients undergoing haemodialysis since dosage guidelines have not been established.

Hydration: Renal toxicity of Foscavir can be reduced by adequate hydration of the patient. It is recommended to establish diuresis by hydration with 0.5-1.0 L of normal saline at each infusion.

Elderly: As for adults.

Children: There is very limited experience in treating children.

Renal or hepatic insufficiency: The dose must be reduced in patients with renal insufficiency according to the creatinine clearance level as described in the table above. Dose adjustment is not required in patients with hepatic insufficiency.

4.3 Contraindications

Hypersensitivity to Foscavir, pregnancy and lactation.

4.4 Special warnings and precautions for use

Foscavir should be used with caution in patients with reduced renal function. Since renal functional impairment may occur at any time during Foscavir administration, serum creatinine should be monitored every second day during induction therapy and once weekly during maintenance therapy, and appropriate dose adjustments should be performed according to renal function. Adequate hydration should be maintained in all patients. (See Posology and method of administration).

Due to Foscavir's propensity to chelate bivalent metal ions, such as calcium, Foscavir administration may be associated with an acute decrease of ionised serum calcium, which may not be reflected in total serum calcium levels. The electrolytes, especially calcium and magnesium, should be assessed prior to and during Foscavir therapy and deficiencies corrected.

Foscavir has local irritating properties and when excreted in high concentrations in the urine it may induce genital irritation or even ulcerations. Close attention to personal hygiene is recommended after micturition to lessen the potential of local irritation.

When diuretics are indicated, thiazides are recommended.

Following treatment with foscarnet, clinical unresponsiveness can appear which may be due to appearance of virus strains with decreased sensitivity towards foscarnet. Termination of treatment with foscarnet should then be considered.

Mutagenicity studies showed that foscarnet has a genotoxic potential. The possible explanation for the observed effect in the mutagenicity studies is an inhibition of the DNA polymerase in the cell line used. Foscarnet therapeutically acts by inhibition of the herpes virus specific DNA polymerase. The human cellular polymerase α is about 100 times less sensitive to foscarnet. The carcinogenicity studies performed did not disclose any oncogenic potential.

4.5 Interaction with other medicinal products and other forms of interaction

Since Foscavir can impair renal function, additive toxicity may occur when used in combination with other nephrotoxic drugs such as aminoglycoside antibiotics, amphotericin B and ciclosporin A. Moreover, since Foscavir can reduce serum levels of ionised calcium, extreme caution is advised when used concurrently with other drugs known to influence serum calcium levels, like i.v. pentamidine. Renal impairment and symptomatic hypocalcaemia (Trousseau's and Chvostek's signs) have been observed during concurrent treatment with Foscavir and i.v. pentamidine. Abnormal renal function has been reported in connection with the use of foscarnet in combination with protease inhibitors associated with impaired renal function e.g. ritonavir and saquinavir.

The elimination of Foscavir may be impaired by drugs which inhibit renal tubular secretion.

There is no evidence of an increased myelotoxicity when foscarnet is used in combination with zidovudine (AZT). Neither is there any pharmacokinetic interaction between the two drugs.

4.6 Pregnancy and lactation

Foscavir is contraindicated in pregnancy. Breast-feeding should be discontinued before starting Foscavir treatment.

4.7 Effects on ability to drive and use machines

Adverse effects such as dizziness and convulsions may occur during Foscavir therapy. The physician is advised to discuss this issue with the patient, and based upon the condition of the disease and the tolerance of medication, give his recommendation in the individual case.

4.8 Undesirable effects

In different patient populations Foscavir has been administered to more than 11,500 patients the majority severely immunocompromised and suffering from serious viral infections. The patient's physical status, the severity of the underlying disease, other infections and concurrent therapy also contribute to the observed adverse event profile of Foscavir.

Consistent findings associated with Foscavir administration are renal function impairment, impact on serum electrolytes and haemoglobin concentration, convulsions and local genital irritation/ulceration.

The adverse events discussed and tabulated below refer to results for 188 AIDS patients in prospective clinical trials and include those events related, unrelated and of unknown relationship to Foscavir. The adverse event profile from the market is similar to that reported in clinical studies.

Renal function impairment: Twenty-seven percent of the above 188 study patients experienced renal functional impairment recorded as a rise in serum creatinine (19%), decreases in creatinine clearance (6%), abnormal renal function (9%), acute renal failure (2%), uraemia (1%) and polyuria in 2%. Metabolic acidosis was seen in 1%. The overall pattern of these symptoms is consistent with previous experiences although the incidence may vary. Most patients with increased serum creatinine have shown normalisation or return to pre-treatment levels within 1–10 weeks of treatment discontinuation.

Electrolytes: Among the above 188 patients, hypocalcaemia was recorded in 14%. Also, hypomagnesaemia was recorded in 15%. Frequently recorded were also hypokalaemia in 16% and hypophosphataemia and hyperphosphataemia in 8 and 6% respectively. Foscarnet chelates with metal ions (Ca^{2+}, Mg^{2+}, Fe^{2+}, Zn^{2+}) and acute hypocalcaemia, sometimes symptomatic, has been a common observation in some 30% of AIDS patients receiving foscarnet. Experimental and clinical data have shown that foscarnet acutely decreases ionised calcium in a dose-related manner. The drop in serum calcium is reversible. It is reasonable to assume that the infusion rate significantly affects the decrease rate of ionised calcium.

Convulsions: Among the AIDS patients referred to above, convulsions including grand mal were recorded in 10%. Based on the occurrence of convulsions among immunocompromised patients receiving foscarnet, an association between foscarnet-induced hypocalcaemia or a direct action of foscarnet *per se* and convulsions has been discussed. Although many of the patients experiencing convulsions had pre-existing CNS abnormalities such as cryptococcal meningitis, space occupying lesions or other CNS tumours, an association with foscarnet can not be excluded.

Haemoglobin concentration: Decreases of the haemoglobin concentration have been observed in 25–33% of patients. Generally, there has been no consistent pattern of simultaneous decreases in white blood cell and platelet counts. Some 30% of the above study patients were also on concurrent AZT treatment. Many AIDS patients were anaemic already before foscarnet administration.

Local irritation in terms of thrombophlebitis in peripheral veins following infusion of undiluted foscarnet solution and genital irritation/ulcerations have been observed. Since foscarnet is excreted in high concentrations in the urine local irritation/ulceration may ensue especially during induction therapy when high doses of foscarnet are being administered.

Other adverse events: Other adverse events that were recorded in the 188 study patients include a variety of symptoms varying in frequency from 1% to approximately 60%, the latter being the incidence for fever. Subgrouped by body system the following adverse events, related, unrelated or of unknown relationship to foscarnet therapy were recorded.

Body as a whole: Asthenia, fatigue, malaise and chills were observed in 12, 20, 7 and 13% respectively and sepsis in 7%.

Gastrointestinal system disorders: Nausea and vomiting were observed in 45 and 25% respectively and diarrhoea in 32%. Abdominal pain and occasionally dyspepsia and constipation were observed in 10, 3 and 6% respectively. Isolated cases of pancreatitis have been reported from marketed use.

Metabolic and nutritional disorders: Hyponatraemia and oedema in legs were seen in 4 and 1% respectively and increase in LDH and alkaline phosphatases in 2 and 3% respectively. Increased levels of amylase have been reported from marketed use.

Central/Peripheral nervous system disorders: Paraesthesia was observed in 18%, headache in 25% and dizziness in 12%. Involuntary muscle contractions and tremor were seen in 9 and 5% respectively. Hypoaesthesia, ataxia and neuropathy were observed in 7, 4 and 6% respectively.

Psychiatric disorders: Anorexia, anxiety and nervousness were observed in 15 and 5% respectively and depression in 10%, confusion in 7%, psychosis in 1%, agitation in 3% and aggressive reaction in 2%.

White blood cells: Adverse events related to white blood cells included leukopenia 9%, granulocytopenia 17%. In these patients over 90% had some degree of leukopenia already before foscarnet administration, in 8% severe or even life-threatening. Moreover in some patients, it is noteworthy that mean WBC counts increased during treatment with foscarnet. Although a few patients worsened in this respect, there is no clear evidence to indicate that foscarnet is myelosuppressive.

Platelet, bleeding, clotting disorders: Thrombocytopenia was observed in 4%.

Skin and appendages: Rash was observed in 16%.

Liver and biliary system disorders: Abnormal liver function was observed in 4% and increase in serum ALAT and ASAT in 3 and 2% respectively and gamma GT in 2%.

Cardiovascular disorders: Abnormal ECG, hypertension and hypotension were observed in 1, 4 and 2% respectively.

Heart rate and rhythm disorders: Ventricular arrhythmia has been reported in 2 patients from marketed use.

Urinary system disorders: A few cases of diabetes insipidus, usually of the nephrogenic type, have been reported from marketed use.

Musculoskeletal disorders: Muscle weakness has been reported from marketed use.

4.9 Overdose

Overdose has been reported during the use of Foscavir, the highest dose being some 20 times the recommended dose. Some of the cases were relative overdoses, in that the dose of drug used had not been promptly adjusted for a patient experiencing reduced renal function. There are cases where it has been reported that no clinical sequelae were consequent on the overdose.

The pattern of adverse events reported in association with an overdose of Foscavir is in accordance with the known adverse event profile of the drug.

Haemodialysis increases Foscavir elimination and may be of benefit in relevant cases.

5. PHARMACOLOGICAL PROPERTIES

5.1 Pharmacodynamic properties

Foscarnet is an antiviral agent with a broad spectrum inhibiting all known human viruses of the herpes group: herpes simplex virus type 1 and 2; human herpes virus 6; varicella zoster virus; Epstein-Barr virus and cytomegalovirus (CMV) and some retroviruses, including human immunodeficiency virus (HIV) at concentrations not affecting normal cell growth. Foscarnet also inhibits the viral DNA polymerase from hepatitis B virus.

Foscarnet exerts its antiviral activity by a direct inhibition of viral specific DNA polymerase a reverse transcriptase at concentrations that do not affect cellular DNA polymerases. Foscarnet does not require activation (phosphorylation) by thymidine kinase or other kinases and therefore is active *in vitro* against HSV mutants deficient in thymidine kinase. CMV strains resistant to ganciclovir may be sensitive to foscarnet. Sensitivity test results expressed as concentration of the drug required to inhibit growth of virus by 50% in cell culture (IC_{50}) vary greatly depending on the assay method used and cell type employed. A number of sensitive viruses and their IC_{50} are listed below.

Foscarnet inhibition of virus multiplication cell culture

Virus	IC_{50}(μm)
CMV	50–800 *
HSV-1, HSV-2	10–130
VZV	48–90
EBV	<500**
HHV-6	49
Ganciclovir resistant CMV	190
HSV - TK Minus Mutant	67
HSV - DNA Polymerase Mutant	5–443
HIV-1	11–32
Zidovudine resistant HIV-1	10–32

* Mean = 269 micrograms

** 97% of viral antigen synthesis inhibited at 500 micrograms

If no clinical response to foscarnet is observed, viral isolates should be tested for sensitivity to foscarnet since naturally resistant mutants may exist or emerge under selective pressure both *in vitro* and *in vivo*.

The mean foscarnet 50% inhibition value for more than one hundred clinical CMV isolates was approximately 270 micrograms/L, while a reversible inhibition of normal cell growth was observed at about 1000 micrograms/L.

5.2 Pharmacokinetic properties

Foscarnet is eliminated by the kidneys mainly through glomerular filtration. The plasma clearance after intravenous administration to man varies between 130–160 ml/min and the renal clearance is about 130 ml/min. The half-life is in the order of 2–4 hours in patients with normal renal function.

The mean volume of distribution of foscarnet at steady state varies between 0.4–0.6 L/kg. There is no metabolic conversion of foscarnet and the binding to human plasma proteins is low (<20%). Foscarnet is distributed to the cerebrospinal fluid and concentrations ranging from 10 to 70% of the concurrent plasma concentrations have been observed in HIV-infected patients.

5.3 Preclinical safety data

The most pronounced effects noted during general toxicity studies performed with foscarnet are perturbation of some serum electrolytes, and kidney and bone changes.

An observed reduction of serum electrolytes such as calcium and magnesium can be explained by the property of foscarnet to form chelate with divalent metal ions. The reduction of ionised calcium and magnesium is, most probably the explanation to seizures/convulsions seen during and shortly after the infusion of high doses of foscarnet. This reduction may also have a bearing on heart function (e.g. ECG) although the toxicological studies performed did not disclose any such effects. The rate of infusion of foscarnet is critical to disturbances in the homeostasis of some serum divalent cations.

The mechanism behind the kidney changes e.g. tubular atrophy, mainly confined to juxtamedullary nephrons, is less clear. The changes were noted in all species investigated. It is known that other complex binders of divalent cations (EDTA and biphosphonates) can cause changes of the kidney similar to those of foscarnet. It has been shown that hydration, to induce diuresis, significantly reduces kidney changes during foscarnet treatment.

The bone changes were characterised as increased osteoclast activity and bone resorption. This effect has only been seen in the dog. The reason to these changes may be that foscarnet, due to the structural similarity to phosphate is incorporated into the hydroxyapatite. Autoradiographic studies showed that foscarnet has a pronounced affinity to bone tissue. Recovery studies revealed that the bone changes were reversible.

Mutagenicity studies showed that foscarnet has a genotoxic potential. The possible explanation for the observed effect in the mutagenicity studies is an inhibition of the DNA polymerase in the cell line used. Foscarnet therapeutically acts by inhibition of the herpes virus specific DNA polymerase. The human cellular polymerase is about 100 times less sensitive to foscarnet. The carcinogenicity studies performed did not disclose any oncogenic potential. The information gained from teratogenicity and fertility studies did not reveal any adverse events upon the reproductive process. However, the results are of limited value since the dose levels used in these studies are below or at most similar (75–150 mg/kg sc) to those used in man for treatment of CMV retinitis.

6. PHARMACEUTICAL PARTICULARS

6.1 List of excipients

Water for injection, hydrochloric acid.

6.2 Incompatibilities

Foscarnet is not compatible with dextrose 30% solution, amphotericin B, acyclovir sodium, ganciclovir, pentamidine isethionate, trimethoprimsulfamtoxazole and vancomycin hydrochloride. Neither is foscarnet compatible with solutions containing calcium. It is recommended that other drugs should not be infused concomitantly in the same line until further experience is gained.

6.3 Shelf life

3 years.

6.4 Special precautions for storage

Do not store above 30°C. Do not refrigerate. If refrigerated or exposed to temperatures below freezing point precipitation may occur. By keeping the bottle at room temperature with repeated shaking, the precipitate can be brought into solution again.

6.5 Nature and contents of container

Infusion glass bottles of 250 ml and 500 ml.

6.6 Special precautions for disposal and other handling

Foscarnet contains no preservatives and once the sterility seal of a bottle has been broken the solution should be used within 24 hours.

Individually dispensed doses of foscarnet can be aseptically transferred to plastic infusion bags by the hospital pharmacy. The physico-chemical stability of foscarnet and dilutions thereof in equal parts with 0.9% sodium chloride (9 mg/ml) or 5% dextrose (50 mg/ml) in PVC bags is 7 days. However, diluted solutions should be refrigerated and storage restricted to 24 hours.

Each bottle of Foscavir should only be used to treat one patient with a single infusion. Unused solution should be discarded.

Accidental skin and eye contact with the foscarnet sodium solution may cause local irritation and burning sensation. If accidental contact occurs, the exposed area should be rinsed with water.

7. MARKETING AUTHORISATION HOLDER

AstraZeneca UK Ltd.,
600 Capability Green,
Luton, LU1 3LU, UK.

8. MARKETING AUTHORISATION NUMBER(S)

PL 17901/0124

9. DATE OF FIRST AUTHORISATION/RENEWAL OF THE AUTHORISATION

16th October 2002

10. DATE OF REVISION OF THE TEXT

30th May 2007

Fosrenol 250mg, 500mg, 750mg & 1000mg chewable tablets

(Shire Pharmaceuticals Limited)

1. NAME OF THE MEDICINAL PRODUCT

Fosrenol▼ 250 mg chewable tablets

Fosrenol▼ 500 mg chewable tablets

Fosrenol▼ 750 mg chewable tablets

Fosrenol▼ 1000 mg chewable tablets

2. QUALITATIVE AND QUANTITATIVE COMPOSITION

Each chewable tablet contains lanthanum carbonate hydrate corresponding to 250 mg lanthanum.

Each chewable tablet contains lanthanum carbonate hydrate corresponding to 500 mg lanthanum.

Each chewable tablet contains lanthanum carbonate hydrate corresponding to 750 mg lanthanum.

Each chewable tablet contains lanthanum carbonate hydrate corresponding to 1000 mg lanthanum.

For excipients, see section 6.1.

3. PHARMACEUTICAL FORM

Chewable tablet.

250 mg: White, round, beveled-edge flat tablets embossed with 'S405/250' on one side.

500 mg: White, round, beveled-edge flat tablets embossed with 'S405/500' on one side.

750 mg: White, round, beveled-edge flat tablets embossed with 'S405/750' on one side.

1000 mg: White, round, beveled-edge flat tablets embossed with 'S405/1000' on one side.

4. CLINICAL PARTICULARS

4.1 Therapeutic indications

Fosrenol is indicated as a phosphate binding agent for use in the control of hyperphosphataemia in chronic renal failure patients on haemodialysis or continuous ambulatory peritoneal dialysis (CAPD).

4.2 Posology and method of administration

Fosrenol is for oral administration.

Tablets must be chewed and not swallowed whole.

The experience with therapy beyond two years is limited (see section 4.4). The risk /benefit from longer-term administration over two years should be carefully considered.

Adults, including elderly (> 65 years)

Fosrenol should be taken with or immediately after food, with the daily dose divided between meals. Patients should adhere to recommended diets in order to control phosphate and fluid intake. Fosrenol is presented as a chewable tablet therefore avoiding the need to take additional fluid. Serum phosphate levels should be monitored and the dose of Fosrenol titrated every 2-3 weeks until an acceptable serum phosphate level is reached, with regular monitoring thereafter.

Control of serum phosphate level has been demonstrated at doses starting from 750 mg per day. The maximum dose studied in clinical trials, in a limited number of patients, is 3750mg. Patients who respond to lanthanum therapy, usually achieve acceptable serum phosphate levels at doses of 1500 – 3000 mg lanthanum per day.

Children and Adolescents

The safety and efficacy of Fosrenol has not been established in patients below the age of 18 years (see section 4.4).

Hepatic impairment

The effect of hepatic impairment on Fosrenol pharmacokinetics has not been assessed. Due to its mechanism of action and the lack of liver metabolism doses in hepatic impairment should not be modified, but patients should be monitored carefully (see sections 4.4 and 5.2).

4.3 Contraindications

Hypersensitivity to lanthanum carbonate hydrate or to any of the excipients.

Hypophosphataemia.

4.4 Special warnings and precautions for use

Tissue deposition of lanthanum has been shown with Fosrenol in animal studies. In 105 bone biopsies from patients treated with Fosrenol, some for up to 4.5 years, rising levels of lanthanum were noted over time (see section 5.1). No clinical data are available on deposition of lanthanum in other human tissues. Safety data exceeding 24 months are currently limited. The risk /benefit from longer-term administration should be carefully considered.

Patients with acute peptic ulcer, ulcerative colitis, Crohn's disease or bowel obstruction were not included in clinical studies with Fosrenol. Fosrenol should be used in these patients following careful assessment of benefit and risk.

Patients with renal insufficiency may develop hypocalcaemia. Fosrenol does not contain calcium. Serum calcium levels should therefore be monitored at regular time intervals for this patient population and appropriate supplements given.

No pharmacokinetic data are available in patients with hepatic impairment. Lanthanum is not metabolised by liver enzymes but it is most likely excreted in the bile. Conditions resulting in a marked reduction of bile flow may be associated with incrementally slower elimination of lanthanum, which may result in higher plasma levels and increased tissue deposition of lanthanum (see sections 5.2 and 5.3). Caution should, therefore, be exercised in these patients, and monitoring of liver function may be required.

Safety and efficacy of Fosrenol have not been established in paediatric patients; use in children is not recommended (see section 4.2).

Fosrenol should be discontinued if hypophosphataemia develops.

Abdominal x-rays of patients taking lanthanum carbonate may have a radio-opaque appearance typical of an imaging agent.

4.5 Interaction with other medicinal products and other forms of interaction

Lanthanum carbonate hydrate may increase gastric pH. It is recommended that compounds, which are known to interact with antacids, should not be taken within 2 hours of dosing with Fosrenol (e.g. chloroquine, hydroxychloroquine and ketoconazole).

In healthy subjects, the absorption and pharmacokinetics of lanthanum were not affected by co-administration of citrate.

Serum levels of fat-soluble vitamins A, D, E and K, were not affected by Fosrenol administration in clinical studies.

Human volunteer studies have shown that co-administration of Fosrenol with digoxin, warfarin or metoprolol does not produce clinically-relevant changes in the pharmacokinetic profiles of these drugs.

In simulated gastric juice, lanthanum carbonate hydrate did not form insoluble complexes with warfarin, digoxin, frusemide, phenytoin, metoprolol or enalapril, suggesting a low potential to affect the absorption of these drugs.

However, interactions with drugs such as tetracycline, doxycycline and the floxacins are theoretically possible and if these compounds are to be co-administered, it is recommended that they not be taken within 2 hours of dosing with Fosrenol.

Lanthanum carbonate hydrate is not a substrate for cytochrome P450 and does not significantly inhibit the activities of the major human cytochrome P450 isoenzymes, CYP1A2, CYP2D6, CYP3A4, CYP2C9 or CYP2C19 in vitro.

4.6 Pregnancy and lactation

There are no adequate data from the use of Fosrenol in pregnant women.

One study in rats showed reproductive foetotoxicity (delayed eye opening and sexual maturation) and reduced pup weights at high doses (see section 5.3). The potential risk for humans is unknown. Fosrenol is not recommended for use during pregnancy.

It is unknown whether lanthanum is excreted in human breast milk. The excretion of lanthanum in milk has not been studied in animals. Caution should be used in taking a decision whether to continue/discontinue breast feeding or to continue/discontinue therapy with Fosrenol, taking into account the potential benefit of breast feeding to the child and the potential benefit of Fosrenol therapy to the nursing mother.

4.7 Effects on ability to drive and use machines

Fosrenol may induce dizziness and vertigo, which may impair the ability to drive and use machinery.

4.8 Undesirable effects

The safety of Fosrenol for use in patients with end-stage renal failure (ESRF) on maintenance haemodialysis and peritoneal dialysis has been examined in three short-term, placebo-controlled, double-blind studies, three long-term, comparator-controlled studies, and three long-term open-label studies. These studies have provided a total safety database of 1754 patients treated with lanthanum carbonate hydrate with 495 patients with more than 1 year of treatment and 130 patients with more than 2 years of treatment and represents a mean exposure of 272.1 days (median 184.0 days, range 1-1123 days).

Approximately 24% of all ESRF patients who participated in these clinical studies, reported a drug related adverse reaction, as determined by the investigator. No individual ADR was reported at a frequency greater than 10%. The most commonly reported adverse drug reactions, with the exception of hypocalcaemia, are gastrointestinal in nature; these are minimized by taking Fosrenol with food and generally abated with time with continued dosing (see section 4.2).

(see Table 1 below)

Although there have been a number of additional isolated reactions reported, none of these reactions are considered unexpected in this patient population.

Transient QT changes have been observed but these were not associated with an increase of cardiac adverse events.

4.9 Overdose

No case of overdose has been reported. The highest daily dose of lanthanum administered to healthy volunteers during Phase I studies was 4718mg given for 3 days. The adverse events seen were mild to moderate and included nausea and headache.

5. PHARMACOLOGICAL PROPERTIES

5.1 Pharmacodynamic properties

Pharmacotherapeutic group: Drugs for treatment of hyperkalaemia and hyperphosphataemia.

ATC code: V03A E03

Fosrenol contains lanthanum carbonate hydrate. The activity of lanthanum carbonate hydrate as a phosphate binder is dependent on the high affinity of lanthanum ions, which are released from the carbonate salt in the acid environment of the stomach, for dietary phosphate. Insoluble lanthanum phosphate is formed which reduces the absorption of phosphate from the gastro-intestinal tract.

A total of 1130 patients with chronic renal failure treated with maintenance haemodialysis or CAPD were studied in two phase II and two phase III studies. Three studies were placebo controlled (1 fixed dose and 2 titrated dose designs) and one included calcium carbonate as an active comparator. During these studies, 1016 patients received lanthanum carbonate, 267 received calcium carbonate and 176 received placebo.

Two placebo-controlled, randomised studies enrolled patients on dialysis after a washout from previous phosphate binders. After titration of lanthanum carbonate to achieve a serum phosphate level between 1.3 and 1.8mmol/L in one study (doses up to 2250mg/day), or ≤1.8mmol/L in a second study (doses up to 3000mg/day), patients were randomised to lanthanum carbonate or placebo as maintenance treatment. After the 4-week randomised placebo-controlled phase, the serum phosphate concentration rose between 0.5 and 0.6mmol/L in the placebo group, in both studies, relative to patients who remained on lanthanum carbonate therapy. There were 61% patients on lanthanum carbonate who maintained their response, compared to 23% on placebo.

The active comparator study demonstrated that serum phosphate levels were reduced to target levels of 1.8mmol/l at the end of the 5 week titration period, in 51% of the lanthanum group compared with 57% of the calcium carbonate group. At week 25 the percentage of randomised patients showing controlled serum phosphate levels was similar in the two treatment groups, 29% on lanthanum and 30% on calcium carbonate (using a missing=failure approach). Mean serum phosphate levels were reduced by a similar amount in both treatment groups.

Further long-term extension studies have demonstrated maintenance of phosphate reduction for some patients following continued administration of at least 2 years of lanthanum carbonate.

Hypercalcaemia was reported in 0.4% of patients with Fosrenol compared with 20.2% on calcium-based binders in comparative studies. Serum PTH concentrations may fluctuate depending on a patient's serum calcium, phosphate and vitamin D status. Fosrenol has not been shown to have any direct effects on serum PTH concentrations.

In the long-term bone studies a trend towards increasing bone lanthanum concentrations with time in the control population was observed from the averaged data, the median rising 3-fold from a baseline of 53 μg/kg at 24 months. In patients treated with lanthanum carbonate, the bone lanthanum concentration increased during the first 12 months of lanthanum carbonate treatment up to a median of 1328μg/kg (range 122-5513μg/kg). Median and range concentrations at 18 and 24 months were similar to 12 months. The median at 54 months was 4246μg/kg (range 1673-9792μg/kg).

Paired bone biopsies (at baseline and at one or two years) in patients randomised to either Fosrenol or calcium carbonate in one study and patients randomised to either Fosrenol or alternative therapy in a second study, showed no differences in the development of mineralization defects between the groups.

5.2 Pharmacokinetic properties

As binding between lanthanum and dietary phosphorus occurs in the lumen of the stomach and upper small intestine, the therapeutic effectiveness of Fosrenol is not dependent on levels of lanthanum in the plasma.

Lanthanum is present in the environment. Measurement of background levels in non-lanthanum carbonate hydrate-treated chronic renal failure patients during Phase III clinical trials revealed concentrations of <0.05 to 0.90 ng/mL in plasma, and <0.006 to 1.0 μg/g in bone biopsy samples.

Absorption

Lanthanum carbonate hydrate has low aqueous solubility (<0.01 mg/mL at pH 7.5) and is minimally absorbed following oral administration. Absolute oral bioavailability is estimated to be <0.002% in humans.

In healthy subjects, plasma AUC and C_{max} increased as a function of dose, but in a less than proportional manner, after single oral doses of 250 to 1000 mg lanthanum, consistent with dissolution-limited absorption. The apparent plasma elimination half-life in healthy subjects was 36 hours.

In renal dialysis patients dosed for 10 days with 1000 mg lanthanum 3 times daily, the mean (± sd) peak plasma concentration was 1.06 (± 1.04) ng/mL, and mean AUC_{last} was 31.1 (± 40.5) ng.h/mL. Regular blood level monitoring in 1707 renal dialysis patients taking lanthanum carbonate hydrate for up to 2 years showed no increase in plasma lanthanum concentrations over this time period.

Distribution

Lanthanum does not accumulate in plasma in patients or in animals after repeated oral administration of lanthanum carbonate hydrate. The small fraction of orally administered lanthanum absorbed is extensively bound to plasma proteins (>99.7%) and in animal studies, was widely distributed to systemic tissues, predominantly bone, liver and

Table 1

Organ System	Common Reactions (>1/100, <1/10)	Uncommon Reactions (>1/1,000 to <1/100)
Infections and Infestations		Gastroenteritis, laryngitis
Blood and lymphatic system disorders		Eosinophilia
Endocrine disorders		Hyperparathyroidism
Metabolism and nutrition disorders	Hypocalcaemia	Hypercalcaemia, hyperglycaemia, hyperphosphataemia, hypophosphataemia, anorexia, appetite increased
Nervous system disorders		Dizziness, headache, taste alteration
Ear and Labyrinth disorders		Vertigo
Gastrointestinal disorders	Abdominal pain, constipation, diarrhoea, dyspepsia, flatulence, nausea, vomiting	Eructation, indigestion, irritable bowel syndrome, dry mouth, oesophagitis, stomatitis, loose stools, tooth disorder, gastro-intestinal disorder NOS*
Skin and subcutaneous tissue disorders		Alopecia, itching, pruritus, erythematous rash, sweating increased
Musculoskeletal and connective tissue disorders		Arthralgia, myalgia, osteoporosis
General disorders		Asthenia, chest pain, fatigue, malaise, peripheral oedema, pain, thirst.
Investigations		Blood aluminium increased, increase in GGT, increases in hepatic transaminases, alkaline phosphatase increased, weight decrease.

* Not otherwise specified

the gastrointestinal tract, including the mesenteric lymph nodes. In long-term animal studies, lanthanum concentrations in several tissues, including the gastrointestinal tract, bone and liver increased over time to levels several orders of magnitude above those in plasma. An apparent steady-state level of lanthanum was attained in some tissues, e.g. the liver whereas levels in gastrointestinal tract increased with duration of treatment. Changes in tissue lanthanum levels after withdrawal of treatment varied between tissues. A relatively high proportion of lanthanum was retained in tissues for longer than 6 months after cessation of dosing (median % retained in bone ⩽100% (rat) and ⩽87% (dog), and in the liver ⩽6% (rat) and ⩽82 % (dog). No adverse effects were associated with the tissue deposition of lanthanum seen in long-term animal studies with high oral doses of lanthanum carbonate (see 5.3) (See section 5.1 for information regarding changes in lanthanum concentrations in bone biopsies taken from renal dialysis patients after one year of treatment with lanthanum containing versus calcium containing phosphate binders).

Metabolism

Lanthanum is not metabolised.

Studies in chronic renal failure patients with hepatic impairment have not been conducted. In patients with co-existing hepatic disorders at the time of entry into Phase III clinical studies, there was no evidence of increased plasma exposure to lanthanum or worsening hepatic function after treatment with Fosrenol for periods up to 2 years.

Elimination

Lanthanum is excreted mainly in the faeces with only around 0.000031% of an oral dose excreted via the urine in healthy subjects (renal clearance approximately 1mL/min, representing <2% of total plasma clearance).

After intravenous administration to animals, lanthanum is excreted mainly in the faeces (74% of the dose), both via the bile and direct transfer across the gut wall. Renal excretion was a minor route.

5.3 Preclinical safety data

Preclinical data reveal no special hazards for humans based on conventional studies of safety pharmacology, repeated dose toxicity or genotoxicity.

Lanthanum carbonate hydrate reduced gastric acidity in the rat in a safety pharmacology study.

In rats administered high doses of lanthanum carbonate hydrate from day 6 of gestation to day 20 post partum there were no maternal effects, but reduced pup weight and delays in some developmental markers (eye and vaginal opening) were seen. In rabbits given high daily doses of lanthanum carbonate hydrate during gestation, maternal toxicity with reduced maternal food intake and body weight gain, increased pre- and post-implantation losses and decreased pup weight were seen.

Lanthanum carbonate hydrate was not carcinogenic in mice or rats. In mice, an increase in gastric glandular adenomas was seen in the high-dose group (1500 mg/kg/day). The neoplastic response in the mouse is considered to be related to an exacerbation of spontaneous pathological stomach changes and to be of little clinical significance.

Studies in animals have shown deposition of lanthanum in tissues, mainly the gastrointestinal tract, mesenteric lymph nodes, liver and bone (see section 5.2). However, life-time studies in healthy animals do not indicate a hazard for man from the use of Fosrenol. Specific immunotoxicity studies have not been performed.

6. PHARMACEUTICAL PARTICULARS

6.1 List of excipients

Dextrates (hydrated)

Colloidal anhydrous silica

Magnesium stearate.

6.2 Incompatibilities

Not applicable.

6.3 Shelf life

3 years.

6.4 Special precautions for storage

This medicinal product does not require any special storage conditions.

6.5 Nature and contents of container

White cylindrical HDPE bottles containing a rayon coil fitted with a tamper evident, child resistant polypropylene screw cap.

Pack sizes

250 mg: 90 tablets.

500 mg: 90 tablets

750 mg: 90 tablets

1000 mg: 90 tablets

6.6 Special precautions for disposal and other handling

No special requirements.

7. MARKETING AUTHORISATION HOLDER

Shire Pharmaceutical Contracts Ltd

Hampshire International Business Park

Chineham

Basingstoke

Hampshire, RG24 8EP

United Kingdom

8. MARKETING AUTHORISATION NUMBER(S)

PL 08081/0041

PL 08081/0042

PL 08081/0043

PL 08081/0044

9. DATE OF FIRST AUTHORISATION/RENEWAL OF THE AUTHORISATION

12 September 2006

10. DATE OF REVISION OF THE TEXT

17 July 2008

Fragmin - Extended Treatment in Oncology (5000, 7500, 10000, 12500, 15000, 18000 I.U Syringes)

(Pharmacia Limited)

1. NAME OF THE MEDICINAL PRODUCT

Single Dose Syringes

1. Fragmin ▼® 5,000 IU/0.2ml Solution for injection
2. Fragmin ▼® 7,500 IU/0.3ml Solution for Injection
3. Fragmin ▼® 10,000 IU/0.4ml Solution for Injection
4. Fragmin ▼® 12,500 IU/0.5ml Solution for Injection
5. Fragmin ▼® 15,000 IU/0.6ml Solution for Injection
6. Fragmin ▼® 18,000 IU/0.72ml Solution for Injection

2. QUALITATIVE AND QUANTITATIVE COMPOSITION

Active ingredient

Dalteparin sodium (INN)

Quality according to Ph Eur and in-house specification

1. Fragmin 5,000 IU: Single dose syringe containing dalteparin sodium 5,000IU (anti-Factor Xa*) in 0.2ml solution for injection equivalent to 25,000IU/ml.
2. Fragmin 7,500 IU: Single dose syringe containing dalteparin sodium 7,500IU (anti-Factor Xa*) in 0.3ml solution for injection equivalent to 25,000 IU/ml.
3. Fragmin 10,000 IU: Single dose syringe containing dalteparin sodium 10,000IU (anti-Factor Xa*) in 0.4ml solution for injection equivalent to 25,000 IU/ml.
4. Fragmin 12,500 IU: Single dose syringe containing dalteparin sodium 12,500IU (anti-Factor Xa*) in 0.5ml solution for injection equivalent to 25,000 IU/ml.
5. Fragmin 15,000 IU: Single dose syringe containing dalteparin sodium 15,000IU (anti-Factor Xa*) in 0.6ml solution for injection equivalent to 25,000 IU/ml.
6. Fragmin 18,000 IU: Single dose syringe containing dalteparin sodium 18,000IU (anti-Factor Xa*) in 0.72ml solution for injection equivalent to 25,000 IU/ml.

For excipients see section 6.1.

1 – 6: Fragmin does not contain preservatives

*Potency is described in International anti-Factor Xa units (IU) of the 1st International Standard for Low Molecular Weight Heparin.

3. PHARMACEUTICAL FORM

Solution for injection for subcutaneous administration.

4. CLINICAL PARTICULARS

4.1 Therapeutic indications

Patients with solid tumours: Extended treatment of symptomatic venous thromboembolism (VTE) and prevention of its recurrence.

4.2 Posology and method of administration

Recommended dosage for adults: Single Dose Syringes

Patients with solid tumours: Extended treatment of symptomatic venous thromboembolism (VTE) and prevention of its recurrence.

Month 1

Administer Fragmin 200 IU/kg total body weight subcutaneously (SC) once daily for the first 30 days of treatment. The total daily dose should not exceed 18,000 IU daily.

Body Weight (kg)	Dose (IU)
<46	7 500
46-56	10 000
57-68	12 500
69-82	15 000
83 and over	18 000*

Maximum dose of 18, 000 IU was used in patient weighing up to 132 kg in the CLOT study.

In the case of chemotherapy-induced thrombocytopenia, Fragmin dose should be adopted as follows:

- In patients receiving Fragmin who experience platelet counts between 50,000 and 100,000/mm³, the daily dose of Fragmin should be reduced by 2,500 IU until the platelet count recovers to ⩾100,000/mm³.

- In patients receiving Fragmin who experience platelet counts <50,000/mm³, Fragmin should be discontinued until the platelet count recovers above 50,000/mm³.

Months 2-6

Fragmin should be administered at a dose of approximately 150 IU/kg, subcutaneously, once daily using fixed dose syringes and the table shown below.

Body Weight (kg)	Dose (IU)
⩽56	7 500
57 to 68	10 000
69 to 82	12 500
83 to 98	15 000
⩾99	18 000

Recommended duration of treatment is 6 months (first month of Fragmin treatment is included). Relevance of continuing treatment beyond this period will be evaluated according to individual risk/benefit ratio, taking into account particularly the progression of cancer. No data is available with dalteparin beyond 6 months of treatment in the CLOT study.

In the case of chemotherapy-induced thrombocytopenia, Fragmin dose should be adopted as follows:

- With platelet counts <50,000/mm³, Fragmin dosing should be interrupted until the platelet count recovers above 50,000/mm³

- For platelet counts between 50,000 and 100,000/mm³, Fragmin should be reduced as illustrated in the table below depending on the patient's weight. Once the platelet count has recovered to ⩾100,000/mm³, Fragmin should be re-instituted at full dose.

Body Weight (kg)	Scheduled Fragmin Dose (IU)	Reduced Fragmin Dose (IU)
⩽56	7 500	5 000
57 to 68	10 000	7 500
69 to 82	12 500	10 000
83 to 98	15 000	12 500
⩾99	18 000	15 000

Renal failure:

In the case of significant renal failure, defined as a creatinine clearance <30 ml/min, the dose of Fragmin should be adjusted based on anti-Factor Xa activity. If the anti-Factor Xa level is below or above the desired range, the dose of Fragmin should be increased or reduced respectively, and the anti-Factor Xa measurement should be repeated after 3-4 new doses. This dose adjustment should be repeated until the desired anti-Factor Xa level is achieved.

As an indication, on the basis of the data available in CLOT, the observed mean levels (min, max) between 4 and 6 hours after administration in patients without severe renal insufficiency were 1.11 IU anti-Factor Xa/ml (0.6; 1.88) and 1.03 IU anti-Factor Xa/ml (0.54; 1.70), respectively, on week 1 and 4 of dalteparin 200 IU/kg OD. Anti-Factor Xa activity determinations were conducted by the chromogenic method.

Children

Not recommended for children.

Elderly

Fragmin has been used safely in elderly patients without the need for dosage adjustment.

Method of Administration

By subcutaneous injection, preferably into the abdominal subcutaneous tissue anterolaterally or posterolaterally, or into the lateral part of the thigh. Patients should be supine and the total length of the needle should be introduced vertically, not at an angle, into the thick part of a skin fold, produced by squeezing the skin between thumb and forefinger; the skin fold should be held throughout the injection.

4.3 Contraindications

Known hypersensitivity to Fragmin or other low molecular weight heparins and/or heparins e.g. history of confirmed or suspected immunologically mediated heparin induced thrombocytopenia, acute gastroduodenal ulcer; cerebral haemorrhage; known haemorrhagic diathesis; subacute endocarditis; haemorrhagic pericardial effusion and haemorrhagic pleural effusion; injuries to and operations on the central nervous system, eyes and ears.

In patients receiving Fragmin for treatment rather than prophylaxis, local and/or regional anaesthesia in elective surgical procedures is contra-indicated.

In cancer patients with body weight < 40kg at time of venous thromboembolic event, Fragmin should not be used for extended treatment of symptomatic VTE and prevention of its recurrences due to lack of data.

Dalteparin should not be used in patients who have suffered a recent (within 3months) stroke unless due to systemic emboli.

4.4 Special warnings and precautions for use

Do not administer by the intramuscular route.

Caution should be exercised in patients in whom there is an increased risk of bleeding complications, e.g. following surgery or trauma, haemorrhagic stroke, severe liver or renal failure, thrombocytopenia or defective platelet function, uncontrolled hypertension, hypertensive or diabetic retinopathy, patients receiving concurrent anticoagulant/antiplatelet agents (see interactions section).

Limited data are available regarding the safety and efficacy of antithrombotic therapy in patients with primary or metastatic tumours of the brain who develop concurrent thromboembolic events. There is a risk of fatal intracranial bleeding with use of anticoagulation in this category of patients. Therefore, if the treatment with Fragmin was considered, it should be monitored closely with regular re-assessment of the status of tumour involvement of the brain and other individual risks.

Thrombocytopenia, should it occur, usually appears within three weeks following the beginning of therapy. Therefore, it is recommended that the platelet counts are measured before starting treatment with Fragmin and monitored closely in first three weeks and regularly thereafter during treatment. Special caution is necessary in rapidly developing thrombocytopenia and severe thrombocytopenia (<100,000/µl) associated with positive or unknown results of in-vitro tests for anti-platelet antibody in the presence of Fragmin or other low molecular weight (mass) heparins and/or heparin.

Fragmin induces only a moderate prolongation of the APTT and thrombin time. Accordingly, dosage increments based upon prolongation of the APTT may cause overdosage and bleeding. Therefore, prolongation of the APTT should only be used as a test of overdosage.

Fragmin induces only a moderate prolongation of the APTT and thrombin time. Accordingly, dosage increments based upon prolongation of the APTT may cause overdosage and bleeding. Therefore, prolongation of the APTT should only be used as a test of overdosage.

Monitoring Anti-Xa Levels

Monitoring of Anti-Xa Levels in patients using Fragmin is not usually required but should be considered for specific patient populations such as those with renal failure, those who are very thin or morbidly obese, pregnant or at increased risk for bleeding or rethrombosis

Where monitoring is necessary, laboratory assays using a chromogenic substrate are considered the method of choice for measuring anti-Xa levels. Activated partial thromboplastin time (APTT) or thrombin time should not be used because these tests are relatively insensitive to the activity of dalteparin. Increasing the dose of dalteparin in an attempt to prolong APTT may result in bleeding (see section 4.9 Overdosage).

Patients with severely disturbed hepatic function, significant renal failure or chemotherapy induced thrombocytopenia may need a reduction in dosage and should be monitored accordingly.

If a transmural myocardial infarction occurs in patients where thrombolytic treatment might be appropriate, this does not necessitate discontinuation of treatment with Fragmin but might increase the risk of bleeding.

As individual low molecular weight (mass) heparins have differing characteristics, switching to an alternative low molecular weight heparin should be avoided. The directions for use relating to each specific product must be observed as different dosages may be required.

Interchangeability with other anticoagulants

Dalteparin cannot be used interchangeably (unit for unit) with unfractionated heparin, other low molecular weight heparins, or synthetic polysaccharides. Each of these medicines differ in their starting raw materials, manufacturing process, physico-chemical, biological, and clinical properties, leading to differences in biochemical identity, dosing and possibly clinical efficacy and safety. Each of these medicines is unique and has its own instructions for use.

Heparin can suppress adrenal secretion of aldosterone leading to hyperkalaemia, particularly in patients such as those with diabetes mellitus, chronic renal failure, pre-existing metabolic acidosis, a raised plasma potassium or taking potassium sparing drugs. The risk of hyperkalaemia appears to increase with duration of therapy but is usually reversible. Plasma potassium should be measured in patients at risk before starting heparin therapy and monitored regularly thereafter particularly if treatment is prolonged beyond about 7 days.

In patients undergoing spinal or epidural anaesthesia, the prophylactic use of heparin may be very rarely associated with spinal haematomas resulting in prolonged or permanent paralysis. The risk is increased by use of an epidural or spinal catheter for anaesthesia, by the concomitant use of drugs (NSAIDs), platelet inhibitors or anti-coagulants and by traumatic or repeated puncture.

In decision-making on the interval between the last administration of Fragmin at prophylactic doses and the placement or removal of a peridural or spinal catheter for anaesthesia, the product characteristics and the patient profile should be taken into account. Readministration should be delayed until at least four hours after the surgical procedure is completed.

Table 1

MedDRA System Organ Class	Frequency	Undesirable Effects
Blood and lymphatic system disorders	Common Rare	Reversible non-immunologically-mediated thrombocytopenia (type I) Immunologically-mediated heparin-induced thrombocytopenia (type II, with or without associated thrombotic complications – arterial and/or thrombosis or thromboembolism)
Immune system disorders	Uncommon	Allergic reactions
Endocrine disorders	Uncommon	Hyperkalaemia
Vascular disorders	Common	Haemorrhage (bleeding at any site)
Hepato-biliary disorders	Common	Transient elevation of liver transaminases (ASAT, ALAT)
Skin and subcutaneous tissue disorders	Uncommon Rare	Urticaria, pruritus Skin necrosis
Musculoskeletal and connective tissue disorders	Uncommon	Osteoporosis
General disorders and administration site conditions	Uncommon Common	Pain at injection site, Haematoma at injection site

Should a physician, as a clinical judgement, decide to administer anticoagulation in the context of peridual spinal anaesthesia, extreme vigilance and frequent monitoring must be exercised to detect any signs and symptoms of neurologic impairment such as back pain, sensory or motor deficits (numbness and weakness in lower limbs) and bowel or bladder dysfunction. Nurses should be trained to detect such signs and symptoms. Patients should be instructed to inform immediately a nurse or a clinician if they experience any of these.

If signs or symptoms of epidural or spinal haematoma are suspected, urgent diagnosis and treatment may include spinal cord decompression.

There have been no adequate studies to assess the safe and effective use of Fragmin in preventing valve thrombosis in patients with prosthetic heart valves. Prophylactic doses of Fragmin are not sufficient to prevent valve thrombosis in patients with prosthetic heart valves. The use of Fragmin cannot be recommended for this purpose.

4.5 Interaction with other medicinal products and other forms of interaction

The possibility of the following interactions with Fragmin should be considered:

(i) An enhancement of the anticoagulant effect by anticoagulant/antiplatelet agents e.g. aspirin/ dipyridamole, vitamin K antagonists, NSAIDs e.g. indometacin, cytostatics, dextran, sulfinpyrazone, probenecid, and etacrynic acid.

(ii) A reduction of the anticoagulant effect may occur with concomitant administration of antihistamines, cardiac glycosides, tetracycline and ascorbic acid.

4.6 Pregnancy and lactation

Pregnancy

Animal studies do not indicate direct or indirect harmful effects with respect to pregnancy, embryonal/foetal developments, parturition or postnatal development (see Section 5.3 Preclinical Safety Data).

If dalteparin is used during pregnancy, the possibility of foetal harm appears remote. However, because the possibility of harm cannot be completely ruled out, dalteparin should be used during pregnancy only if clearly needed (see Section 5.3 Preclinical Safety Data).

Therefore, caution should be exercised when prescribing to pregnant women.

Therapeutic failures have been reported in pregnant women with prosthetic heart valves on full anti-coagulant doses of low molecular weight heparin. In the absence of clear dosing, efficacy and safety information in this circumstance, Fragmin is not recommended for use in pregnant women with prosthetic heart valves.

<u>Lactation</u>

Limited data are available for excretion of dalteparin in human milk. One study in 15 lactating women receiving prophylactic doses of dalteparin detected small amounts of anti-Xa activity in breast milk, equivalent to a milk/plasma ratio of <0.025-0.224. As oral absorption of low molecular weight heparin is extremely low the clinical implications, if any, of this small amount of anticoagulant activity on the nursing infant are unknown.

A risk to the suckling child cannot be excluded. A decision on whether to continue/discontinue breast-feeding or to continue/discontinue therapy with Fragmin should be made taking into account the benefit of breast-feeding to the child and the benefit of Fragmin therapy to the woman.

4.7 Effects on ability to drive and use machines

Fragmin does not affect the ability to drive or operate machinery.

4.8 Undesirable effects

In the table below, the adverse reactions are listed by system organ class and frequency (very common (≥1/10), common (≥1/100 to <1/10), uncommon (≥1/1,000 to <1/100), rare (≥1/10,000 to <1/1,000), very rare (<1/10,000) and not known (cannot be estimated from the available data)).

Within each frequency grouping, undesirable effects are presented in order of decreasing seriousness.

Adverse events associated with dalteparin therapy, in patients participating in controlled clinical studies were:

(see Table 1 above)

In post-marketing experience, the following additional undesirable effects have been reported:

MedDRA System Organ Class	Undesirable Effects
Immune system disorders	Anaphylactic reactions
Endocrine Disorders	Hypoaldosteronism
Nervous system disorders	Intracranial bleeds
Cardiac Disorders	Prosthetic cardiac valve thrombosis
Gastrointestinal disorders	Retroperitoneal bleeds
Skin and subcutaneous tissue disorders	Alopecia
Injury, poisoning and procedural complications	Spinal or epidural haematoma

4.9 Overdose

The anticoagulant effect (i.e. prolongation of the APTT) induced by Fragmin is inhibited by protamine. Since protamine itself has an inhibiting effect on primary haemostasis it should be used only in an emergency.

The prolongation of the clotting time induced by Fragmin may be fully neutralised by protamine, but the anti-Factor Xa activity is only neutralised to about 25-50%. 1 mg of protamine inhibits the effect of 100 IU (anti-Factor Xa) of Fragmin.

Protamine should be given by intravenous injection over approximately 10 minutes.

5. PHARMACOLOGICAL PROPERTIES

5.1 Pharmacodynamic properties

ATC Code BO1 AB 04: Antithrombotics

Dalteparin sodium is a low molecular weight heparin fraction (average molecular weight 4000-6000 Daltons) produced from porcine-derived sodium heparin.

Dalteparin sodium is an antithrombotic agent, which acts mainly through its ability to potentiate the inhibition of Factor Xa and thrombin by antithrombin. It has a relatively higher ability to potentiate Factor Xa inhibition than to prolong plasma clotting time (APTT).

Compared with standard, unfractionated heparin, dalteparin sodium has a reduced adverse effect on platelet function and platelet adhesion, and thus has only a minimal effect on primary haemostasis. Some of the antithrombotic properties of dalteparin sodium are thought to be mediated through the effects on vessel walls or the fibrinolytic system.

The randomized, open-label, controlled, multicenter CLOT study (Randomized Comparison of Low-Molecular Weight Heparin Versus Oral Anticoagulant Therapy for Long Term Anticoagulation in Cancer patients with Venous Thomboembolism) compared dalteparin to standard oral anticoagulant (OAC) therapy in the long term treatment of venous thromboembolism (VTE) in 676 patients with active malignancy who had experienced an acute symptomatic VTE (deep venous thrombosis (DVT) and/or a pulmonary embolism (PE)).

Patients were randomized to one of two groups:

- dalteparin arm prescribed at 200 IU/kg/day administered by subcutaneous (SC) injections (maximum 18,000 IU/day) during 1 month, then approximately 150 IU/kg/day from 2nd– 6th month

or

- VKA arm prescribed during 6 months (target INR 2-3), preceded by SC dalteparin 200 IU/kg/day OD (maximum 18,000 IU/day) during 5 to 7 days.

The most frequent diagnoses were: tumors of the gastro-intestinal tract and pancreas (23.7%), genitourinary tumors (prostate, testicle, cervix, uterus, ovary and bladder) (21.5%), breast (16.0%), lung (13.3%). 10.4% of patients had haematological malignancies; 75.1% of patients had metastatic disease.

The index VTE event was DVT alone in nearly 70% and PE with or without DVT in 30% of patients.

The primary endpoint was the time to first recurrence of symptomatic VTE (DVT and/or PE) during 6 months.

A total of 27 patients of 338 (8.0%) in the dalteparin arm and 53 patients of 338 (15.7%) in the VKA arm experienced at least one of the events of the composite primary end-point. A significant 52% risk reduction in VTE recurrence at 6 months was seen with dalteparin (RR= 0.48, 95% CI [0.30-0.77], p=0.0016).

In the dalteparin arm, 19 patients (5.6%) experienced at least one episode of major bleeding compared to 12 patients (3.6%) in the VKA arm. The cumulative probability of experiencing a major bleeding at 6 months was respectively 6.5% and 4.9%, respectively. Any bleeding occurred with a higher frequency in the VKA arm (18.5% VKA vs 13.6% dalteparin). The comparison of the cumulative probability of first bleeding episode for the 2 treatments was of statistical significance in favour of dalteparin treatment (p=0.0487).

There was no significant difference in mortality between the two groups in deaths at 6 and 12 months (131 vs. 137 and 190 vs. 194 in the dalteparin and VKA arms, respectively).

There was no significant difference in the assessment of Quality of Life between the two groups of treatment.

5.2 Pharmacokinetic properties

The half life following iv and sc. administration is 2 hours and 3.5-4 hours respectively, twice that of unfractionated heparin.

The bioavailability following sc. injection is approximately 87 per cent and the pharmacokinetics are not dose dependent. The half life is prolonged in uraemic patients as dalteparin sodium is eliminated primarily through the kidneys.

Special Populations

Haemodialysis:

In patients with chronic renal insufficiency requiring haemodialysis, the mean terminal half-life of anti-Factor Xa activity following a single intravenous dose of 5000 IU dalteparin was 5.7 ± 2.0 hours, i.e. considerably longer than values observed in healthy volunteers; therefore, greater accumulation can be expected in these patients.

5.3 Preclinical safety data

The acute toxicity of dalteparin sodium is considerably lower than that of heparin. The only significant finding, which occurred consistently throughout the toxicity studies after subcutaneous administration of the higher dose levels was local haemorrhage at the injection site, dose-related in incidence and severity. There was no cumulative effect on injection site haemorrhages.

The haemorrhagic reaction was reflected in dose related changes in the anticoagulant effects as measured by APTT and anti-Factor Xa activities.

It was concluded that dalteparin sodium may have an osteopenic effect at very high concentrations, and that this effect is less than that of unfractionated heparin at equivalent doses.

The results revealed no organ toxicity irrespective of the route of administration, doses or the duration of treatment. No mutagenic effect was found. No embryotoxic or teratogenic effects and no effect on fertility reproductive capacity or peri- and postnatal development was shown.

6. PHARMACEUTICAL PARTICULARS

6.1 List of excipients

1	Fragmin 5,000 IU/0.2ml (1) Water for injections (Ph. Eur)
2	Fragmin 7,500 IU/0.3ml (2) Water for injections (Ph. Eur) Sodium hydroxide or hydrochloric acid for pH adjustment
3 – 6	Fragmin 10,000 IU/0.4ml (3) Fragmin 12,500 IU/0.5ml (4) Fragmin 15,000 IU/0.6ml (5) Framgin 18,000 IU/0.72ml (6) Water for Injections (Ph. Eur) Sodium Chloride (Ph. Eur) Sodium hydroxide or hydrochloric acid for pH adjustment

6.2 Incompatibilities

Not applicable.

6.3 Shelf life

1	Fragmin 5,000 IU/0.2ml	36 months
2	Fragmin 7,500 IU/0.3ml	36 months
3	Fragmin 10,000 IU/0.4ml	24 months
4	Fragmin 12,500 IU/0.5ml	24 months
5	Fragmin 15,000 IU/0.6ml	24 months
6	Fragmin 18,000 IU/0.72ml	24 months

6.4 Special precautions for storage

1 – 6: Do not store above 25°C

6.5 Nature and contents of container

1	Fragmin 5,000 IU/0.2ml Solution for Injection is supplied in 0.5ml glass Ph.Eur type I single dose syringes with chlorobutyl (Type I) rubber and polypropylene rod. Each pack contains 10 syringes.
2	Fragmin 7,500 IU/0.3ml Solution for Injection is supplied in 0.5ml glass Ph.Eur type I single dose syringes with chlorobutyl (Type I) rubber and polypropylene rod. Each pack contains 10 syringes.
3	Fragmin 10,000 IU/0.4 ml Solution for Injection is supplied in 1 ml glass Ph. Eur. Type I single dose syringes with chlorobutyl (Type I) rubber stopper and polypropylene rod. Each pack contains 5 syringes.
4	Fragmin 12,500 IU/0.5 ml solution for injection is supplied in 1 ml glass Ph. Eur. Type I single dose syringes with chlorobutyl (Type I) rubber stopper and polypropylene rod. Each pack contains 5 syringes.
5	Fragmin 15 000 IU/0.6 ml solution for injection is supplied in 1 ml glass Ph. Eur. Type I single dose syringes with chlorobutyl (Type I) rubber stopper and polypropylene rod. Each pack contains 5 syringes.
6	1 ml single dose syringe (glass Ph. Eur. Type I) with chlorobutyl rubber stopper containing dalteparin sodium 18,000 IU (anti-Factor Xa) in 0.72 ml. Each pack contains 5 syringes.

6.6 Special precautions for disposal and other handling

Not applicable

7. MARKETING AUTHORISATION HOLDER

Pharmacia Limited

Ramsgate Road

Sandwich KENT

CT13 9NJ

United Kingdom

8. MARKETING AUTHORISATION NUMBER(S)

1	PL 0032/0383
2	PL 0032/0483
3	PL 0032/0375
4	PL 0032/0379
5	PL 0032/0380
6	PL 0032/0381

9. DATE OF FIRST AUTHORISATION/RENEWAL OF THE AUTHORISATION

1: 18 March 2002

2: 26 June 2002

3 – 6: 18 March 2002

10. DATE OF REVISION OF THE TEXT

May 2009

Legal Category

POM

Ref: FR 2_0

Fragmin - Haemodialysis/Haemofiltration (1ml and 4ml Ampoules)

(Pharmacia Limited)

1. NAME OF THE MEDICINAL PRODUCT

1. Fragmin 10,000 IU/1 ml

2. Fragmin 10,000 IU/4ml

2. QUALITATIVE AND QUANTITATIVE COMPOSITION

Active ingredient

Dalteparin sodium (INN)

Quality according to Ph Eur and in-house specification.

Potency is described in International anti-Factor Xa units (IU) of the 1st International Standard for Low Molecular Weight Heparin.

Content of active ingredient

1. Ampoules containing dalteparin sodium, 10,000 IU (anti-Factor Xa) in 1 ml.

2. Fragmin 10,000 IU/4ml: Ampoules containing dalteparin sodium corresponding to 2,500 IU (anti-Factor Xa)/ml.

3. PHARMACEUTICAL FORM

Solution for injection for intravenous or subcutaneous administration

4. CLINICAL PARTICULARS

4.1 Therapeutic indications

Prevention of clotting in the extracorporeal circulation during haemodialysis or haemofiltration, in patients with chronic renal insufficiency or acute renal failure.

4.2 Posology and method of administration

Recommended dosage for adults

(i) Prevention of clotting during haemodialysis and haemofiltration

In chronic renal insufficiency for patients with no known additional bleeding risk, the dosage is:

(a) Long-term haemodialysis or haemofiltration - duration of haemodialysis/haemofiltration more than 4 hours;

An I.V. bolus injection of Fragmin 30-40 IU (anti-Factor Xa)/kg bodyweight, followed by an infusion of 10-15 IU (anti-Factor Xa)/kg bodyweight/hour.

(b) Short-term haemodialysis or haemofiltration - duration of haemodialysis/haemofiltration less than 4 hours:

Either as above, or, a single IV bolus injection of Fragmin 5000 IU (anti-Factor Xa).

Both for long and short-term haemodialysis and haemofiltration, the plasma anti-Factor Xa levels should be within the range 0.5-1.0 IU (anti-Factor Xa)/ml.

In acute renal failure, or chronic renal failure in patients with a high risk of bleeding, the dosage is:

An I.V. bolus injection of Fragmin 5-10 IU (anti-Factor Xa)/kg bodyweight, followed by an infusion of 4-5 IU (anti-Factor Xa)/kg bodyweight/hour.

The plasma anti-Factor Xa levels should be within the range 0.2-0.4 IU (anti-Factor Xa)/ml.

When considered necessary, it is recommended that the antithrombotic effect of Fragmin be monitored by analysing anti-Factor Xa activity using a suitable chromogenic substrate assay. This is because Fragmin has only a moderate prolonging effect on clotting time assays such as APTT or thrombin time.

Children

Not recommended for children.

Elderly

Fragmin has been used safely in elderly patients without the need for dosage adjustment.

4.3 Contraindications

Known hypersensitivity to Fragmin or other low molecular weight heparins and/or heparins e.g. history of confirmed or suspected immunologically mediated heparin induced thrombocytopenia, acute gastroduodenal ulcer; cerebral haemorrhage; known haemorrhagic diathesis; subacute endocarditis; injuries to and operations on the central nervous system, eyes and ears.

In patients receiving Fragmin for treatment rather than prophylaxis, local and/or regional anaesthesia in elective surgical procedures is contra-indicated.

4.4 Special warnings and precautions for use

Do not administer by the intramuscular route.

Caution should be exercised in patients in whom there is an increased risk of bleeding complications, e.g. following surgery or trauma, haemorrhagic stroke, severe liver or renal failure, thrombocytopenia or defective platelet function, uncontrolled hypertension, hypertensive or diabetic retinopathy, patients receiving concurrent anticoagulant/antiplatelet agents (see interactions section).

It is recommended that platelets be counted before starting treatment with Fragmin and monitored regularly. Special caution is necessary in rapidly developing thrombocytopenia and severe thrombocytopenia ($<100{,}000/\mu l$) associated with positive or unknown results of in-vitro tests for anti-platelet antibody in the presence of Fragmin or other low molecular weight (mass) heparins and/or heparin

Fragmin induces only a moderate prolongation of the APTT and thrombin time. Accordingly, dosage increments based upon prolongation of the APTT may cause overdosage and bleeding. Therefore, prolongation of the APTT should only be used as a test of overdosage.

Monitoring Anti-Xa Levels

Monitoring of Anti-Xa Levels in patients using Fragmin is not usually required but should be considered for specific patient populations such as those with renal failure, those who are very thin or morbidly obese, pregnant or at increased risk for bleeding or rethrombosis

Anti-Factor Xa levels should be regularly monitored in new patients on chronic haemodialysis during the first weeks, later less frequent monitoring is generally required. Patients undergoing acute haemodialysis have a narrower therapeutic dose range and should be monitored frequently in accordance with the individual course of the disease (See Section 5.2 Pharmacokinetic properties).

Where monitoring is necessary, laboratory assays using a chromogenic substrate are considered the method of choice for measuring anti-Xa levels. Activated partial thromboplastin time (APTT) or thrombin time should not be used because these tests are relatively insensitive to the activity of dalteparin. Increasing the dose of dalteparin in an attempt to prolong APTT may result in bleeding (see section 4.9 Overdosage).

Patients with severely disturbed hepatic function may need a reduction in dosage and should be monitored accordingly.

If a transmural myocardial infarction occurs in patients where thrombolytic treatment might be appropriate, this does not necessitate discontinuation of treatment with Fragmin, but might increase the risk of bleeding.

As individual low molecular weight (mass) heparins have differing characteristics, switching to an alternative low molecular weight heparin should be avoided. The directions for use relating to each specific product must be observed as different dosages may be required.

Interchangeability with other anticoagulants

Dalteparin cannot be used interchangeably (unit for unit) with unfractionated heparin, other low molecular weight heparins, or synthetic polysaccharides. Each of these medicines differ in their starting raw materials, manufacturing process, physico-chemical, biological, and clinical properties, leading to differences in biochemical identity, dosing, and possibly clinical efficacy and safety. Each of these medicines is unique and has its own instructions for use.

Heparin can suppress adrenal secretion of aldosterone leading to hyperkalaemia, particularly in patients such as those with diabetes mellitus, chronic renal failure, pre-existing metabolic acidosis, a raised plasma potassium or taking potassium sparing drugs. The risk of hyperkalaemia appears to increase with duration of therapy but is usually reversible. Plasma potassium should be measured in patients at risk before starting heparin therapy and monitored regularly thereafter particularly if treatment is prolonged beyond about 7 days.

In patients undergoing spinal or epidural anaesthesia, the prophylactic use of heparin may be very rarely associated with spinal haematomas resulting in prolonged or permanent paralysis. The risk is increased by use of an epidural or spinal catheter for anaesthesia, by the concomitant use of drugs (NSAIDs), platelet inhibitors or anti-coagulants and by traumatic or repeated puncture.

In decision-making on the interval between the last administration of Fragmin at prophylactic doses and the placement or removal of a peridural or spinal catheter for anaesthesia, the product characteristics and the patient profile should be taken into account. Readministration should be delayed until at least four hours after the surgical procedure is completed.

Should a physician, as a clinical judgement, decide to administer anticoagulation in the context of peridural or spinal anaesthesia, extreme vigilance and frequent monitoring must be exercised to detect any signs and symptoms of neurologic impairment such as back pain, sensory or motor deficits (numbness and weakness in lower limbs) and bowel or bladder dysfunction. Nurses should be trained to detect such signs and symptoms. Patients should be instructed to inform immediately a nurse or a clinician if they experience any of these.

If signs or symptoms of epidural or spinal haematoma are suspected, urgent diagnosis and treatment may include spinal cord decompression.

There have been no adequate studies to assess the safe and effective use of Fragmin in preventing valve thrombosis in patients with prosthetic heart valves. Prophylactic doses of Fragmin are not sufficient to prevent valve thrombosis in patients with prosthetic heart valves. The use of Fragmin cannot be recommended for this purpose

4.5 Interaction with other medicinal products and other forms of interaction

The possibility of the following interactions with Fragmin should be considered:

(i) An enhancement of the anticoagulant effect by anticoagulant/antiplatelet agents e.g. aspirin/ dipyridamole, vitamin K antagonists, NSAIDs e.g. indometacin, cytostatics, dextran, sulfinpyrazone, probenecid, and etacrynic acid.

(ii) A reduction of the anticoagulant effect may occur with concomitant administration of antihistamines, cardiac glycosides, tetracycline and ascorbic acid.

4.6 Pregnancy and lactation

Pregnancy

Animal studies do not indicate direct or indirect harmful effects with respect to pregnancy, embryonal/foetal developments, parturition or postnatal development (see Section 5.3 Preclinical Safety Data).

If dalteparin is used during pregnancy, the possibility of foetal harm appears remote. However, because the possibility of harm cannot be completely ruled out, dalteparin should be used during pregnancy only if clearly needed (see Section 5.3 Preclinical Safety Data).

Therefore, caution should be exercised when prescribing to pregnant women.

Therapeutic failures have been reported in pregnant women with prosthetic heart valves on full anti-coagulant doses of low molecular weight heparin. In the absence of clear dosing, efficacy and safety information in this circumstance, Fragmin is not recommended for use in pregnant women with prosthetic heart valves.

Lactation

Limited data are available for excretion of dalteparin in human milk. One study in 15 lactating women receiving prophylactic doses of dalteparin detected small amounts of anti-Xa activity in breast milk, equivalent to a milk/plasma ratio of <0.025-0.224. As oral absorption of low molecular weight heparin is extremely low the clinical implications, if any, of this small amount of anticoagulant activity on the nursing infant are unknown.

A risk to the suckling child cannot be excluded. A decision on whether to continue/discontinue breast-feeding or to continue/discontinue therapy with Fragmin should be made taking into account the benefit of breast-feeding to the child and the benefit of Fragmin therapy to the woman.

4.7 Effects on ability to drive and use machines

Fragmin does not affect the ability to drive or operate machinery.

4.8 Undesirable effects

In the table below, the adverse reactions are listed by system organ class and frequency (very common (≥1/10), common (≥1/100 to <1/10), uncommon (≥1/1,000 to <1/100), rare (≥1/10,000 to <1/1,000), very rare (<1/10,000) and not known (cannot be estimated from the available data).

Within each frequency grouping, undesirable effects are presented in order of decreasing seriousness.

Adverse events associated with dalteparin therapy, in patients participating in controlled clinical studies were:

(see Table 1 above)

Table 1

MedDRA System Organ Class	Frequency	Undesirable Effects
Blood and lymphatic system disorders	Common Rare	Reversible non-immunologically-mediated thrombocytopenia (type I) Immunologically-mediated heparin-induced thrombocytopenia (type II, with or without associated thrombotic complications – arterial and/or thrombosis or thromboembolism)
Immune system disorders	Uncommon	Allergic reactions
Endocrine disorders	Uncommon	Hyperkalaemia
Vascular disorders	Common	Haemorrhage (bleeding at any site)
Hepato-biliary disorders	Common	Transient elevation of liver transaminases (ASAT, ALAT)
Skin and subcutaneous tissue disorders	Uncommon Rare	Urticaria, pruritus Skin necrosis
Musculoskeletal and connective tissue disorders	Uncommon	Osteoporosis
General disorders and administration site conditions	Uncommon Common	Pain at injection site, Haematoma at injection site

In post-marketing experience, the following additional undesirable effects have been reported:

MedDRA System Organ Class	Undesirable Effects
Immune system disorders	Anaphylactic reactions
Endocrine Disorders	Hypoaldosteronism
Nervous system disorders	Intracranial bleeds
Cardiac Disorders	Prosthetic cardiac valve thrombosis
Gastrointestinal disorders	Retroperitoneal bleeds
Skin and subcutaneous tissue disorders	Alopecia
Injury, poisoning and procedural complications	Spinal or epidural haematoma

4.9 Overdose

The anticoagulant effect (i.e. prolongation of the APTT) induced by Fragmin is inhibited by protamine. Since protamine itself has an inhibiting effect on primary haemostasis it should be used only in an emergency.

The prolongation of the clotting time induced by Fragmin may be fully neutralised by protamine, but the anti-Factor Xa activity is only neutralised to about 25-50%. 1 mg of protamine inhibits the effect of 100 IU (anti-Factor Xa) of Fragmin.

5. PHARMACOLOGICAL PROPERTIES

5.1 Pharmacodynamic properties

Dalteparin sodium is a low molecular weight heparin fraction (average molecular weight 4000-6000 Daltons) produced from porcine-derived sodium heparin.

Dalteparin sodium is an antithrombotic agent, which acts mainly through its ability to potentiate the inhibition of Factor Xa and thrombin by antithrombin. It has a relatively higher ability to potentiate Factor Xa inhibition than to prolong plasma clotting time (APTT).

Compared with standard, unfractionated heparin, dalteparin sodium has a reduced adverse effect on platelet function and platelet adhesion, and thus has only a minimal effect on primary haemostasis. Some of the antithrombotic properties of dalteparin sodium are thought to be mediated through the effects on vessel walls or the fibrinolytic system.

5.2 Pharmacokinetic properties

The half life following iv and sc. administration is 2 hours and 3.5-4 hours respectively, twice that of unfractionated heparin.

The bioavailability following sc. injection is approximately 87 per cent and the pharmacokinetics are not dose dependent. The half life is prolonged in uraemic patients as dalteparin sodium is eliminated primarily through the kidneys.

Special Populations

Haemodialysis:

In patients with chronic renal insufficiency requiring haemodialysis, the mean terminal half-life of anti-Factor Xa activity following a single intravenous dose of 5000 IU dalteparin was 5.7 ± 2.0 hours, i.e. considerably longer than values observed in healthy volunteers; therefore, greater accumulation can be expected in these patients.

5.3 Preclinical safety data

The acute toxicity of dalteparin sodium is considerably lower than that of heparin. The only significant finding, which occurred consistently throughout the toxicity studies after subcutaneous administration of the higher dose levels was local haemorrhage at the injection site, dose-related in incidence and severity. There was no cumulative effect on injection site haemorrhages.

The haemorrhagic reaction was reflected in dose related changes in the anticoagulant effects as measured by APTT and anti-Factor Xa activities.

It was concluded that dalteparin sodium did not have a greater osteopenic effect than heparin since at equivalent doses the osteopenic effect was comparable.

The results revealed no organ toxicity irrespective of the route of administration, doses or the duration of treatment. No mutagenic effect was found. No embryotoxic or teratogenic effects and no effect on fertility reproductive capacity or peri- and postnatal development were shown.

6. PHARMACEUTICAL PARTICULARS

6.1 List of excipients

10,000 IU/ml and 10,000 IU/4ml

Sodium chloride (Ph Eur)
Water for injections (Ph Eur)

6.2 Incompatibilities

The compatibility of Fragmin with products other than those mentioned under 6.6 has not been investigated.

6.3 Shelf life

10,000 IU/ml and 10,000 IU/4ml

36 months.

6.4 Special precautions for storage
10,000 IU/ml and 10,000 IU/4ml

Store at room temperature (below 30°C).

6.5 Nature and contents of container
1. Clear glass ampoules (Ph Eur Type 1) containing dalteparin sodium, 10,000 IU (anti-factor Xa) in 1 ml.

2. Clear glass ampoules (Ph Eur Type 1) containing dalteparin sodium, 10,000 IU (anti-factor Xa) in 4 ml.

6.6 Special precautions for disposal and other handling
10,000 IU/ml and 10,000 IU/4ml

Fragmin solution for injection is compatible with isotonic sodium chloride (9 mg/ml) or isotonic glucose (50 mg/ml) infusion solutions in glass bottles and plastic containers for up to 24 hours. Compatibility between Fragmin and other products has not been studied.

7. MARKETING AUTHORISATION HOLDER
Pharmacia Limited

Ramsgate Road

Sandwich KENT

CT13 9NJ

United Kingdom

8. MARKETING AUTHORISATION NUMBER(S)
PL 0032/0376: 10,000 IU/ml

PL 0032/0377: 10,000 IU/4ml

9. DATE OF FIRST AUTHORISATION/RENEWAL OF THE AUTHORISATION
5 April 2002: 10,000 IU/ml

27 March 2002: 10,000 IU/4ml

10. DATE OF REVISION OF THE TEXT
May 2009

Legal Category: POM: 10,000 IU/ml

10,000 IU/4ml

Ref: FR 5_0

Fragmin - Surgical & Medical Thromboprophylaxis (2500IU/5000IU Syringes)

(Pharmacia Limited)

1. NAME OF THE MEDICINAL PRODUCT
Fragmin® 2500IU/5000 IU

2. QUALITATIVE AND QUANTITATIVE COMPOSITION
Active ingredient

Dalteparin sodium (INN)

Quality according to Ph.Eur. and in-house specification.

Potency is described in International anti-Factor Xa units (IU) of the 1st International Standard for Low Molecular Weight Heparin.

Content of active ingredient

Fragmin 2500 IU: single dose syringe containing dalteparin sodium 2,500 IU (anti-Factor Xa) in 0.2 ml solution.

Fragmin 5000 IU: single dose syringe containing dalteparin sodium 5000 IU (anti-Factor Xa) in 0.2 ml solution.

Fragmin syringes do not contain preservatives.

3. PHARMACEUTICAL FORM
Solution for injection for subcutaneous administration.

4. CLINICAL PARTICULARS
4.1 Therapeutic indications
Peri- and post-operative surgical thromboprophylaxis.

For the 5000 IU Presentation Only:

The prophylaxis of proximal deep venous thrombosis in patients bedridden due to a medical condition, including, but not limited to; congestive cardiac failure (NYHA class III or IV), acute respiratory failure or acute infection, who also have a predisposing risk factor for venous thromboembolism such as age over 75 years, obesity, cancer or previous history of VTE.

4.2 Posology and method of administration
Adults

a) Surgical thromboprophylaxis in patients at moderate risk of thrombosis

2,500IU is administered subcutaneously 1-2 hours before the surgical procedure and thereafter 2,500 IU subcutaneously each morning until the patient is mobilised, in general 5-7 days or longer.

b) Surgical thromboprophylaxis in patients at high risk of thrombosis

2,500 IU is administered subcutaneously 1-2 hours before the surgical procedure and 2,500 IU subcutaneously 8-12 hours later. On the following days, 5,000 IU subcutaneously each morning.

As an alternative, 5,000 IU is administered subcutaneously the evening before the surgical procedure and 5,000 IU subcutaneously the following evenings.

Treatment is continued until the patient is mobilised, in general 5-7 days or longer.

c) Prolonged thromboprophylaxis in hip replacement surgery

5,000IU is given subcutaneously the evening before the operation and 5,000IU subcutaneously the following evenings. Treatment is continued for five post-operative weeks.

If pre-operative administration of Fragmin is not considered appropriate because the patient is at high risk of haemorrhage during the procedure, post-operative Fragmin may be administered (see Section 5.1).

d) Prophylaxis of venous thromboembolism in medical patients: The recommended dose of dalteparin sodium is 5,000 IU once daily. Treatment with dalteparin sodium is prescribed for up to 14 days.

Children

Not recommended for children.

Elderly

Fragmin has been used safely in elderly patients without the need for dosage adjustment.

Method of Administration

By subcutaneous injection, preferably into the abdominal subcutaneous tissue anterolaterally or posterolaterally, or into the lateral part of the thigh. Patients should be supine and the total length of the needle should be introduced vertically, not at an angle, into the thick part of a skin fold, produced by squeezing the skin between the thumb and forefinger; the skin fold should be held throughout the injection.

4.3 Contraindications
Known hypersensitivity to Fragmin or other low molecular weight heparins and/or heparins e.g. history of confirmed or suspected immunologically mediated heparin induced thrombocytopenia; acute gastroduodenal ulcer; cerebral haemorrhage; known haemorrhagic diathesis; subacute endocarditis; injuries to and operations on the central nervous system, eyes and ears.

In patients receiving Fragmin for treatment rather than prophylaxis, local and/or regional anaesthesia in elective surgical procedures is contra-indicated.

For the 5000 IU Presentation Only:

Dalteparin should not be used in patients who have suffered a recent (within 3 months) stroke unless due to systemic emboli.

4.4 Special warnings and precautions for use
Caution should be exercised in patients in whom there is an increased risk of bleeding complications, e.g. following trauma, haemorrhagic stroke, severe liver or renal failure, thrombocytopenia or defective platelet function, uncontrolled hypertension, hypertensive or diabetic retinopathy, patients receiving concurrent anticoagulant/antiplatelet agents (see Interactions Section).

It is recommended that platelets be counted before starting treatment with Fragmin and monitored regularly. Special caution is necessary in rapidly developing thrombocytopenia and severe thrombocytopenia (<100,000/µl) associated with positive or unknown results of in-vitro tests for anti-platelet antibody in the presence of Fragmin or other low molecular weight (mass) heparins and/or heparin.

Fragmin induces only a moderate prolongation of the APTT and thrombin time. Accordingly, dosage increments based upon prolongation of the APTT may cause overdosage and bleeding. Therefore, prolongation of the APTT should only be used as a test of overdosage.

Monitoring Anti-Xa Levels

Monitoring of Anti-Xa Levels in patients using Fragmin is not usually required but should be considered for specific patient populations such as those with renal failure, those who are very thin or morbidly obese, pregnant or at increased risk for bleeding or rethrombosis

Where monitoring is necessary, laboratory assays using a chromogenic substrate are considered the method of choice for measuring anti-Xa levels. Activated partial thromboplastin time (APTT) or thrombin time should not be used because these tests are relatively insensitive to the activity of dalteparin. Increasing the dose of dalteparin in an attempt to prolong APTT may result in bleeding (see section 4.9 Overdosage).

Patients with severely disturbed hepatic function may need a reduction in dosage and should be monitored accordingly.

If a transmural myocardial infarction occurs in patients where thrombolytic treatment might be appropriate, this does not necessitate discontinuation of treatment with Fragmin but might increase the risk of bleeding.

As individual low molecular weight (mass) heparins have differing characteristics, switching to an alternative low molecular weight heparin should be avoided. The directions for use relating to each specific product must be observed as different dosages may be required.

Interchangeability with other anticoagulants

Dalteparin cannot be used interchangeably (unit for unit) with unfractionated heparin, other low molecular weight heparins, or synthetic polysaccharides. Each of these medicines differ in their starting raw materials, manufacturing process, physico-chemical, biological, and clinical properties, leading to differences in biochemical identity, dosing, and possibly clinical efficacy and safety. Each of these medicines is unique and has its own instructions for use.

Do not administer by the intramuscular route.

Heparin can suppress adrenal secretion of aldosterone leading to hyperkalaemia, particularly in patients such as those with diabetes mellitus, chronic renal failure, pre-existing metabolic acidosis, a raised plasma potassium or taking potassium sparing drugs. The risk of hyperkalaemia appears to increase with duration of therapy but is usually reversible. Plasma potassium should be measured in patients at risk before starting heparin therapy and monitored regularly thereafter particularly if treatment is prolonged beyond about 7 days.

In patients undergoing spinal or epidural anaesthesia, the prophylactic use of heparin maybe very rarely associated with spinal haematomas resulting in prolonged or permanent paralysis. The risk is increased by use of an epidural or spinal catheter for anaesthesia, by the concomitant use of drugs (NSAIDs), platelet inhibitors or anti-coagulants and by traumatic or repeated puncture.

In decision-making on the interval between the last administration of Fragmin at prophylactic doses and the placement or removal of a peridural or spinal catheter for anaesthesia, the product characteristics and the patient profile should be taken into account. Re-administration should be delayed until at least four hours after the surgical procedure is completed.

Should a physician, as a clinical judgement, decide to administer anticoagulation in the context of peridural or spinal anaesthesia, extreme vigilance and frequent monitoring must be exercised to detect any signs and symptoms of neurologic impairment such as back pain, sensory or motor deficits (numbness and weakness in lower limbs) and bowel or bladder dysfunction. Nurses should be trained to detect such signs and symptoms. Patients should be instructed to inform immediately a nurse or a clinician if they experience any of these.

If signs or symptoms of epidural or spinal haematoma are suspected, urgent diagnosis and treatment may include spinal cord decompression.

There have been no adequate studies to assess the safe and effective use of Fragmin in preventing valve thrombosis in patients with prosthetic heart valves. Prophylactic doses of Fragmin are not sufficient to prevent valve thrombosis in patients with prosthetic heart valves. The use of Fragmin cannot be recommended for this purpose

4.5 Interaction with other medicinal products and other forms of interaction
The possibility of the following interactions with Fragmin should be considered:

i) An enhancement of the anticoagulant effect by anticoagulant/antiplatelet agents e.g. aspirin/dipyridamole, Vitamin K antagonists, NSAIDs e.g. indometacin, cytostatics, dextran, sulfinpyrazone, probenecid, and etacrynic acid.

ii) A reduction of the anticoagulant effect may occur with concomitant administration of antihistamines, cardiac glycosides, tetracycline and ascorbic acid.

4.6 Pregnancy and lactation
Pregnancy

Animal studies do not indicate direct or indirect harmful effects with respect to pregnancy, embryonal/foetal developments, parturition or postnatal development (see Section 5.3 Preclinical Safety Data).

If dalteparin is used during pregnancy, the possibility of foetal harm appears remote. However, because the possibility of harm cannot be completely ruled out, dalteparin should be used during pregnancy only if clearly needed (see Section 5.3 Preclinical Safety Data).

Therefore, caution should be exercised when prescribing to pregnant women.

Therapeutic failures have been reported in pregnant women with prosthetic heart valves on full anti-coagulant doses of low molecular weight heparin. In the absence of clear dosing, efficacy and safety information in this circumstance, Fragmin is not recommended for use in pregnant women with prosthetic heart valves.

Lactation

Limited data are available for excretion of dalteparin in human milk. One study in 15 lactating women receiving prophylactic doses of dalteparin detected small amounts of anti-Xa activity in breast milk, equivalent to a milk/plasma ratio of <0.025-0.224. As oral absorption of low molecular weight heparin is extremely low the clinical implications, if any, of this small amount of anticoagulant activity on the nursing infant are unknown.

A risk to the suckling child cannot be excluded. A decision on whether to continue/discontinue breast-feeding or to continue/discontinue therapy with Fragmin should be made taking into account the benefit of breast-feeding to the child and the benefit of Fragmin therapy to the woman.

4.7 Effects on ability to drive and use machines
Fragmin does not affect the ability to drive or operate machinery.

4.8 Undesirable effects
In the table below, the adverse reactions are listed by system organ class and frequency (very common

Table 1

MedDRA System Organ Class	Frequency	Undesirable Effects
Blood and lymphatic system disorders	Common Rare	Reversible non-immunologically-mediated thrombocytopenia (type I) Immunologically-mediated heparin-induced thrombocytopenia (type II, with or without associated thrombotic complications – arterial and/or thrombosis or thromboembolism)
Immune system disorders	Uncommon	Allergic reactions
Endocrine disorders	Uncommon	Hyperkalaemia
Vascular disorders	Common	Haemorrhage (bleeding at any site)
Hepato-biliary disorders	Common	Transient elevation of liver transaminases (ASAT, ALAT)
Skin and subcutaneous tissue disorders	Uncommon Rare	Urticaria, pruritus Skin necrosis
Musculoskeletal and connective tissue disorders	Uncommon	Osteoporosis
General disorders and administration site conditions	Uncommon Common	Pain at injection site, Haematoma at injection site

Table 2

Phase 1	Pre-op Dalteparin		Post-op Dalteparin		Warfarin	
	n/N	%	n/N	%	n/N	%
DVT and or PE	37/338*	10.9	44/336*	13.1	81/338	24.0
Proximal DVT	3/354	0.8	3/358	0.8	11/363	3.0

*p 0.001 vs warfarin (Cocharan-Mantel-Haenszel test, two-sided)

Abbreviations: n/N = number of patients affected/number of efficacy-evaluable patients; post-op = treatment at earliest 4 hours after surgery;

Pre-op, = treatment within 2 hours before surgery

(≥1/10), common (≥1/100 to <1/10), uncommon (≥1/1,000 to <1/100), rare (≥1/10,000 to <1/1,000), very rare (<1/10,000) and not known (cannot be estimated from the available data)).

Within each frequency grouping, undesirable effects are presented in order of decreasing seriousness.

Adverse events associated with dalteparin therapy, in patients participating in controlled clinical studies were:

(see Table 1 above)

In post-marketing experience, the following additional undesirable effects have been reported:

MedDRA System Organ Class	Undesirable Effects
Immune system disorders	Anaphylactic reactions
Endocrine Disorders	Hypoaldosteronism
Nervous system disorders	Intracranial bleeds
Cardiac Disorders	Prosthetic cardiac valve thrombosis
Gastrointestinal disorders	Retroperitoneal bleeds
Skin and subcutaneous tissue disorders	Alopecia
Injury, poisoning and procedural complications	Spinal or epidural haematoma

4.9 Overdose

The anticoagulant effect (i.e. prolongation of the APTT) induced by Fragmin is inhibited by protamine. Since protamine itself has an inhibiting effect on primary haemostasis it should be used only in an emergency. The prolongation of the clotting time induced by Fragmin may be fully neutralised by protamine, but the anti-Factor Xa activity is only neutralised to about 25-50%. 1 mg of protamine inhibits the effect of 100 IU (anti-Factor Xa) of Fragmin.

5. PHARMACOLOGICAL PROPERTIES

5.1 Pharmacodynamic properties

Dalteparin sodium is a low molecular weight heparin fraction (average molecular weight 4000-6000 daltons) produced from porcine-derived sodium heparin.

Dalteparin sodium is an antithrombotic agent, which acts mainly through its ability to potentiate the inhibition of Factor Xa and thrombin by antithrombin.

It has a relatively higher ability to potentiate Factor Xa inhibition than to prolong plasma clotting time (APTT)

Compared with standard, unfractionated heparin, dalteparin sodium has a reduced adverse effect on platelet function and platelet adhesion, and thus has only a minimal effect on primary haemostasis. Still some of the antithrombotic properties of dalteparin sodium are thought to be mediated through the effects on vessel walls or the fibrinolytic system.

In a randomised, actively controlled, double – blind trial in 1500 patients undergoing hip replacement surgery (North American Fragmin Trial), both pre-operative and post operative Fragmin were found to be superior to warfarin (see table below). There was a numerical superiority for pre-operative Fragmin over post-operative Fragmin. Thus in patients where the risk of bleeding is perceived to be too great for pre-operative Fragmin administration other means of reducing thromboembolic risk such as post-oeperative Fragmin administration may be considered.

Incidence of verified thromboembolic events in ITT efficacy population within 6 ± 2 post operative days

(see Table 2 above)

In a randomised; placebo-controlled double-blind trial (PREVENT) in 3700 patients with acute medical conditions requiring a projected stay in hospital of >4 days and with recent (<3 days) immobilisation (defined as patients mainly confined to bed during waking hours), the incidence of clinically relevant thromboembolic events was reduced by 45% in patients randomised to receive Fragmin compared with those who received placebo. The incidence of the events comprising the primary endpoint was 2.77% compared with 4.96% in placebo treated patients (difference: - 2.19; 95% CI: - 3.57 to - 0.81; p=0.0015. Therefore, a clinically meaningful reduction in the risk of venous thromboembolism was seen in this study.

5.2 Pharmacokinetic properties

The half-life following i.v. and s.c. administration is 2 hours and 3.5-4 hours respectively, twice that of unfractionated heparin.

The bioavailability following s.c. injection is approximately 87 per cent and the pharmacokinetics are not dose dependent. The half life is prolonged in uraemic patients as dalteparin sodium is eliminated primarily through the kidneys.

Special Populations

Haemodialysis:

In patients with chronic renal insufficiency requiring haemodialysis, the mean terminal half-life of anti-Factor Xa activity following a single intravenous dose of 5000 IU dalteparin was 5.7 ± 2.0 hours, i.e. considerably longer than values observed in healthy volunteers; therefore, greater accumulation can be expected in these patients.

5.3 Preclinical safety data

The acute toxicity of dalteparin sodium is considerably lower than that of heparin. The only significant finding, which occurred consistently throughout the toxicity studies after subcutaneous administration of the higher dose levels was local haemorrhage at the injection sites, dose-related in incidence and severity. There was no cumulative effect on injection site haemorrhages.

The haemorrhagic reaction was reflected in dose related changes in the anticoagulant effects as measured by APTT and anti-Factor Xa activities.

It was concluded that dalteparin sodium did not have a greater osteopenic effect than heparin since at equivalent doses the osteopenic effect was comparable.

The results revealed no organ toxicity irrespective of the route of administration, doses or duration of treatment. No mutagenic effect was found. No embryotoxic or teratogenic effects and no effect on fertility, reproductive capacity or peri- and post natal development was shown.

6. PHARMACEUTICAL PARTICULARS

6.1 List of excipients

Sodium Chloride (Ph.Eur)

(2,500 IU presentation only)

Water for Injections (Ph. Eur.)

(2,500IU and 5,000IU presentations)

6.2 Incompatibilities

Not applicable.

6.3 Shelf life

36 months

6.4 Special precautions for storage

Do not store above 25°C

6.5 Nature and contents of container

Single dose syringe (glass Ph. Eur. Type I) with chlorobutyl rubber stopper containing dalteparin sodium 2500 IU (anti-Factor Xa) in 0.2 ml

Single dose syringe (glass Ph. Eur. Type I) with chlorobutyl rubber stopper containing dalteparin sodium 5000 IU (anti-Factor Xa) in 0.2 ml.

6.6 Special precautions for disposal and other handling

Not applicable

7. MARKETING AUTHORISATION HOLDER

Pharmacia Limited

Ramsgate Road

Sandwich KENT

CT13 9NJ

United Kingdom

8. MARKETING AUTHORISATION NUMBER(S)

Fragmin 2500 IU: PL 00032/0382

Fragmin 5000 IU: PL 00032/0383

9. DATE OF FIRST AUTHORISATION/RENEWAL OF THE AUTHORISATION

18 March 2002

10. DATE OF REVISION OF THE TEXT

May 2009

LEGAL CATEGORY

POM

Ref: FR 6_0

Fragmin - Treatment of VTE

(Pharmacia Limited)

1. NAME OF THE MEDICINAL PRODUCT

Single Dose Syringes

1. Fragmin 7,500 IU/0.3ml Solution for Injection
2. Fragmin 10,000 IU/0.4ml Solution for Injection
3. Fragmin 12,500 IU/0.5ml Solution for Injection
4. Fragmin 15,000 IU/0.6ml Solution for Injection
5. Fragmin 18,000 IU/0.72ml Solution for Injection

Ampoules/Vials

6. Fragmin 10,000 IU/1 ml Ampoule
7. Fragmin 100,000 IU/4ml Multidose-Vial

2. QUALITATIVE AND QUANTITATIVE COMPOSITION

Active ingredient

Dalteparin sodium (INN)

Quality according to Ph Eur and in-house specification

1. Fragmin 7,500 IU: Single dose syringe containing dalteparin sodium 7,500IU (anti-Factor Xa*) in 0.3ml solution for injection equivalent to 25,000 IU/ml.
2. Fragmin 10,000 IU: Single dose syringe containing dalteparin sodium 10,000IU (anti-Factor Xa*) in 0.4ml solution for injection equivalent to 25,000 IU/ml.
3. Fragmin 12,500 IU: Single dose syringe containing dalteparin sodium 12,500IU (anti-Factor Xa*) in 0.5ml solution for injection equivalent to 25,000 IU/ml.

4. Fragmin 15,000 IU: Single dose syringe containing dalteparin sodium 15,000IU (anti-Factor Xa*) in 0.3ml solution for injection equivalent to 25,000 IU/ml.

5. Fragmin 18,000 IU: Single dose syringe containing dalteparin sodium 18,000IU (anti-Factor Xa*) in 0.72ml solution for injection equivalent to 25,000 IU/ml.

6. Ampoules containing dalteparin sodium 10,000 IU (anti-Factor Xa*) in 1ml

7. Fragmin 100,000 IU/4ml: Multidose vial containing dalteparin sodium corresponding to 25,000 IU (anti-Factor Xa*)/ml.

For excipients see section 6.1.

1 – 6: Fragmin does not contain preservatives

7: Contains a preservative (Benzyl alcohol (Ph. Eur))

*Potency is described in International anti-Factor Xa units (IU) of the 1st International Standard for Low Molecular Weight Heparin.

3. PHARMACEUTICAL FORM

Solution for injection for subcutaneous administration.

4. CLINICAL PARTICULARS

4.1 Therapeutic indications

Treatment of venous thromboembolism (VTE) presenting clinically as deep vein thrombosis (DVT), pulmonary embolism (PE) or both.

4.2 Posology and method of administration

Recommended dosage for adults: Single Dose Syringes

1 – 5: A single daily dose of Fragmin is administered subcutaneously, once daily according to the following weight ranges. Monitoring of the anticoagulant effect is not usually necessary:

Weight (kg)	Dose
<46	7,500 IU (1)
46-56	10,000 IU (2)
57-68	12,500 IU (3)
69-82	15,000 IU (4)
83 and over	18,000 IU (5)

The single daily dose should not exceed 18,000 IU.

For patients with an increased risk of bleeding, it is recommended that Fragmin be administered according to the twice daily regimen detailed for Fragmin 10,000 IU/ml ampoules or Fragmin Multidose Vial.

Recommended dosage for adults: Ampoule and Multidose Vial:

Fragmin can be administered subcutaneously either as a single daily injection or as twice daily injections:

(a) Once daily administration

200 IU/kg body weight is administered sc. once daily. Monitoring of the anticoagulant effect is not necessary. The single daily dose should not exceed 18,000 IU.

(b) Twice daily administration

A dose of 100 IU/kg body weight administered sc. twice daily can be used for patients with increased risk of bleeding. Monitoring of the treatment is generally not necessary but can be performed with a functional anti-Factor Xa assay. Maximum plasma levels are obtained 3-4 hours after sc. injection, when samples should be taken. Recommended plasma levels are between 0.5-1.0 IU (anti-Factor Xa)/ml.

Simultaneous anticoagulation with oral vitamin K antagonists can be started immediately. Treatment with Fragmin is continued until the prothrombin complex levels (factor II, VII, IX and X) have decreased to a therapeutic level. At least five days of combined treatment is normally required.

Children

Not recommended for children.

Elderly

Fragmin has been used safely in elderly patients without the need for dosage adjustment.

Method of Administration

By subcutaneous injection, preferably into the abdominal subcutaneous tissue anterolaterally or posterolaterally, or into the lateral part of the thigh. Patients should be supine and the total length of the needle should be introduced vertically, not at an angle, into the thick part of a skin fold, produced by squeezing the skin between thumb and forefinger; the skin fold should be held throughout the injection.

4.3 Contraindications

Known hypersensitivity to Fragmin or other low molecular weight heparins and/or heparins e.g. history of confirmed or suspected immunologically mediated heparin induced thrombocytopenia, acute gastroduodenal ulcer; cerebral haemorrhage; known haemorrhagic diathesis; subacute endocarditis; injuries to and operations on the central nervous system, eyes and ears.

In patients receiving Fragmin for treatment rather than prophylaxis, local and/or regional anaesthesia in elective surgical procedures is contra-indicated.

Table 1

MedDRA System Organ Class	Frequency	Undesirable Effects
Blood and lymphatic system disorders	Common	Reversible non-immunologically-mediated thrombocytopenia (type I)
	Rare	Immunologically-mediated heparin-induced thrombocytopenia (type II, with or without associated thrombotic complications – arterial and/or thrombosis or thromboembolism)
Immune system disorders	Uncommon	Allergic reactions
Endocrine disorders	Uncommon	Hyperkalaemia
Vascular disorders	Common	Haemorrhage (bleeding at any site)
Hepato-biliary disorders	Common	Transient elevation of liver transaminases (ASAT, ALAT)
Skin and subcutaneous tissue disorders	Uncommon	Urticaria, pruritus
	Rare	Skin necrosis
Musculoskeletal and connective tissue disorders	Uncommon	Osteoporosis
General disorders and administration site conditions	Uncommon	Pain at injection site,
	Common	Haematoma at injection site

4.4 Special warnings and precautions for use

Do not administer by the intramuscular route.

Caution should be exercised in patients in whom there is an increased risk of bleeding complications, e.g. following surgery or trauma, haemorrhagic stroke, severe liver or renal failure, thrombocytopenia or defective platelet function, uncontrolled hypertension, hypertensive or diabetic retinopathy, patients receiving concurrent anticoagulant/antiplatelet agents (see interactions section).

It is recommended that platelets be counted before starting treatment with Fragmin and monitored regularly. Special caution is necessary in rapidly developing thrombocytopenia and severe thrombocytopenia (<100,000/μl) associated with positive or unknown results of in-vitro tests for anti-platelet antibody in the presence of Fragmin or other low molecular weight (mass) heparins and/or heparin

Fragmin induces only a moderate prolongation of the APTT and thrombin time. Accordingly, dosage increments based upon prolongation of the APTT may cause overdosage and bleeding. Therefore, prolongation of the APTT should only be used as a test of overdosage.

Monitoring Anti-Xa Levels

Monitoring ofAnti-Xa Levels in patients using Fragmin is not usually required but should be considered for specific patient populations such as those with renal failure, those who are very thin or morbidly obese, pregnant or at increased risk for bleeding or rethrombosis

Where monitoring is necessary, laboratory assays using a chromogenic substrate are considered the method of choice for measuring anti-Xa levels. Activated partial thromboplastin time (APTT) or thrombin time should not be used because these tests are relatively insensitive to the activity of dalteparin. Increasing the dose of dalteparin in an attempt to prolong APTT may result in bleeding (see section 4.9 Overdosage).

Patients with severely disturbed hepatic function may need a reduction in dosage and should be monitored accordingly.

If a transmural myocardial infarction occurs in patients where thrombolytic treatment might be appropriate, this does not necessitate discontinuation of treatment with Fragmin but might increase the risk of bleeding.

As individual low molecular weight (mass) heparins have differing characteristics, switching to an alternative low molecular weight heparin should be avoided. The directions for use relating to each specific product must be observed as different dosages may be required.

Interchangeability with other anticoagulants

Dalteparin cannot be used interchangeably (unit for unit) with unfractionated heparin, other low molecular weight heparins, or synthetic polysaccharides. Each of these medicines differ in their starting raw materials, manufacturing process, physico-chemical, biological, and clinical properties, leading to differences in biochemical identity, dosing and possibly clinical efficacy and safety. Each of these medicines is unique and has its own instructions for use.

Pregnancy

The administration of medications containing benzyl alcohol as a preservative to premature neonates has been associated with a fatal "Gasping Syndrome". Because benzyl alcohol may cross the placenta, (dalteparin) multiple-dose vials, preserved with benzyl alcohol, should be used with caution in pregnant women and only if clearly needed

Heparin can suppress adrenal secretion of aldosterone leading to hyperkalaemia, particularly in patients such as those with diabetes mellitus, chronic renal failure, pre-existing metabolic acidosis, a raised plasma potassium or taking potassium sparing drugs. The risk of hyperkalaemia appears to increase with duration of therapy but is usually reversible. Plasma potassium should be measured in patients at risk before starting heparin therapy and monitored regularly thereafter particularly if treatment is prolonged beyond about 7 days.

In patients undergoing spinal or epidural anaesthesia, the prophylactic use of heparin may be very rarely associated with spinal haematomas resulting in prolonged or permanent paralysis. The risk is increased by use of an epidural or spinal catheter for anaesthesia, by the concomitant use of drugs (NSAIDs), platelet inhibitors or anti-coagulants and by traumatic or repeated puncture.

In decision-making on the interval between the last administration of Fragmin at prophylactic doses and the placement or removal of a peridural or spinal catheter for anaesthesia, the product characteristics and the patient profile should be taken into account. Readministration should be delayed until at least four hours after the surgical procedure is completed.

Should a physician, as a clinical judgement, decide to administer anticoagulation in the context of peridural spinal anaesthesia, extreme vigilance and frequent monitoring must be exercised to detect any signs and symptoms of neurologic impairment such as back pain, sensory or motor deficits (numbness and weakness in lower limbs) and bowel or bladder dysfunction. Nurses should be trained to detect such signs and symptoms. Patients should be instructed to inform immediately a nurse or a clinician if they experience any of these.

If signs or symptoms of epidural or spinal haematoma are suspected, urgent diagnosis and treatment may include spinal cord decompression.

There have been no adequate studies to assess the safe and effective use of Fragmin in preventing valve thrombosis in patients with prosthetic heart valves. Prophylactic doses of Fragmin are not sufficient to prevent valve thrombosis in patients with prosthetic heart valves. The use of Fragmin cannot be recommended for this purpose

4.5 Interaction with other medicinal products and other forms of interaction

The possibility of the following interactions with Fragmin should be considered:

(i) An enhancement of the anticoagulant effect by anticoagulant/antiplatelet agents e.g. aspirin/ dipyridamole, vitamin K antagonists, NSAIDs e.g. indometacin, cytostatics, dextran, sulfinpyrazone, probenecid, and etacrynic acid.

(ii) A reduction of the anticoagulant effect may occur with concomitant administration of antihistamines, cardiac glycosides, tetracycline and ascorbic acid.

4.6 Pregnancy and lactation

Pregnancy

Animal studies do not indicate direct or indirect harmful effects with respect to pregnancy, embryonal/foetal developments, parturition or postnatal development (see Section 5.3 Preclinical Safety Data).

If dalteparin is used during pregnancy, the possibility of foetal harm appears remote. However, because the possibility of harm cannot be completely ruled out, dalteparin should be used during pregnancy only if clearly needed (see Section 5.3 Preclinical Safety Data).

Therefore, caution should be exercised when prescribing to pregnant women.

Therapeutic failures have been reported in pregnant women with prosthetic heart valves on full anti-coagulant doses of low molecular weight heparin. In the absence of clear dosing, efficacy and safety information in this circumstance, Fragmin is not recommended for use in pregnant women with prosthetic heart valves.

7 Only

Fragmin multidose vial contains benzyl alcohol as a preservative and is not recommended for use during pregnancy. Benzyl alcohol may cross the placenta. One should bear in mind the potential toxicity for premature infants **Medications containing benzyl alcohol - (**see Section 4.4 Special Warnings and Precaution for use – Pregnancy).

Lactation

Limited data are available for excretion of dalteparin in human milk. One study in 15 lactating women receiving prophylactic doses of dalteparin detected small amounts of anti-Xa activity in breast milk, equivalent to a milk/plasma ratio of <0.025-0.224. As oral absorption of low molecular weight heparin is extremely low the clinical implications, if any, of this small amount of anticoagulant activity on the nursing infant are unknown.

A risk to the suckling child cannot be excluded. A decision on whether to continue/discontinue breast-feeding or to continue/discontinue therapy with Fragmin should be made taking into account the benefit of breast-feeding to the child and the benefit of Fragmin therapy to the woman.

4.7 Effects on ability to drive and use machines

Fragmin does not affect the ability to drive or operate machinery.

4.8 Undesirable effects

In the table below, the adverse reactions are listed by system organ class and frequency (very common (≥1/10), common (≥1/100 to <1/10), uncommon (≥1/1,000 to <1/100), rare (≥1/10,000 to <1/1,000), very rare (<1/10,000) and not known (cannot be estimated from the available data)).

Within each frequency grouping, undesirable effects are presented in order of decreasing seriousness.

Adverse events associated with dalteparin therapy, in patients participating in controlled clinical studies were:

(see Table 1 on previous page)

In post-marketing experience, the following additional undesirable effects have been reported:

MedDRA System Organ Class	Undesirable Effects
Immune system disorders	Anaphylactic reactions
Endocrine Disorders	Hypoaldosteronism
Nervous system disorders	Intracranial bleeds
Cardiac Disorders	Prosthetic cardiac valve thrombosis
Gastrointestinal disorders	Retroperitoneal bleeds
Skin and subcutaneous tissue disorders	Alopecia
Injury, poisoning and procedural complications	Spinal or epidural haematoma

4.9 Overdose

The anticoagulant effect (i.e. prolongation of the APTT) induced by Fragmin is inhibited by protamine. Since protamine itself has an inhibiting effect on primary haemostasis it should be used only in an emergency.

The prolongation of the clotting time induced by Fragmin may be fully neutralised by protamine, but the anti-Factor Xa activity is only neutralised to about 25-50%. 1 mg of protamine inhibits the effect of 100 IU (anti-Factor Xa) of Fragmin.

Protamine should be given by intravenous injection over approximately 10 minutes.

5. PHARMACOLOGICAL PROPERTIES

5.1 Pharmacodynamic properties

ATC Code BO1A B

Dalteparin sodium is a low molecular weight heparin fraction (average molecular weight 4000-6000 Daltons) produced from porcine-derived sodium heparin.

Dalteparin sodium is an antithrombotic agent, which acts mainly through its ability to potentiate the inhibition of Factor Xa and thrombin by antithrombin. It has a relatively higher ability to potentiate Factor Xa inhibition than to prolong plasma clotting time (APTT).

Compared with standard, unfractionated heparin, dalteparin sodium has a reduced adverse effect on platelet function and platelet adhesion, and thus has only a minimal effect on primary haemostasis. Some of the antithrombotic properties of dalteparin sodium are thought to be mediated through the effects on vessel walls or the fibrinolytic system.

5.2 Pharmacokinetic properties

The half life following iv and sc. administration is 2 hours and 3.5-4 hours respectively, twice that of unfractionated heparin.

The bioavailability following sc. injection is approximately 87 per cent and the pharmacokinetics are not dose dependent. The half life is prolonged in uraemic patients as dalteparin sodium is eliminated primarily through the kidneys.

Special Populations

Haemodialysis:

In patients with chronic renal insufficiency requiring haemodialysis, the mean terminal hal-life of anti-Factor Xa activity following a single intravenous dose of 5000 IU dalteparin was 5.7 ± 2.0 hours, i.e. considerably longer than values observed in healthy volunteers, therefore, greater accumulation can be expected in these patients.

5.3 Preclinical safety data

The acute toxicity of dalteparin sodium is considerably lower than that of heparin. The only significant finding, which occurred consistently throughout the toxicity studies after subcutaneous administration of the higher dose levels was local haemorrhage at the injection site, dose-related in incidence and severity. There was no cumulative effect on injection site haemorrhages.

The haemorrhagic reaction was reflected in dose related changes in the anticoagulant effects as measured by APTT and anti-Factor Xa activities.

It was concluded that dalteparin sodium did not have a greater osteopenic effect than heparin since at equivalent doses the osteopenic effect was comparable.

The results revealed no organ toxicity irrespective of the route of administration, doses or the duration of treatment. No mutagenic effect was found. No embryotoxic or teratogenic effects and no effect on fertility reproductive capacity or peri- and postnatal development was shown.

6. PHARMACEUTICAL PARTICULARS

6.1 List of excipients

1	Fragmin 7,500 IU/0.3ml (1) Water for injections (Ph. Eur) Sodium hydroxide or hydrochloric acid for pH adjustment
2 – 5	Fragmin 10,000 IU/0.4ml (2) Fragmin 12,500 IU/0.5ml (3) Fragmin 15,000 IU/0.6ml (4) Framgin 18,000 IU/0.72ml (5) Water for Injections (Ph. Eur) Sodium Chloride (Ph. Eur) Sodium hydroxide or hydrochloric acid for pH adjustment
6	Fragmin 10,000 IU/ml Ampoule (6) Sodium chloride (Ph. Eur) Water for Injections (Ph. Eur)
7	Fragmin 100,000 IU/4ml Multidose Vial (7) Benzyl Alcohol (Ph. Eur) Water for Injections (Ph. Eur)

6.2 Incompatibilities

Not applicable.

6.3 Shelf life

1	Fragmin 7,500 IU/0.3ml	36 months
2	Fragmin 10,000 IU/0.4ml	24 months
3	Fragmin 12,500 IU/0.5ml	24 months
4	Fragmin 15,000 IU/0.6ml	24 months
5	Fragmin 18,000 IU/0.72ml	24 months
6	Fragmin 10,000 IU/ml Ampoule	36 months
7	Fragmin 100,000 IU/4ml Multidose Vial	24 months Once opened the solution should be used within 14 days

6.4 Special precautions for storage

1 – 5: Do no store above 25°C

6 – 7: Store at room temperature (below 30°C)

6.5 Nature and contents of container

1	Fragmin 7,500 IU/0.3ml Solution for Injection is supplied in 0.5ml glass Ph.Eur type I single dose syringes with chlorobutyl (Type I) rubber and polypropylene rod. Each pack contains 10 syringes.
2	Fragmin 10,000 IU/0.4 ml Solution for Injection is supplied in 1 ml glass Ph. Eur. Type I single dose syringes with chlorobutyl (Type I) rubber stopper and polypropylene rod. Each pack contains 5 syringes.
3	Fragmin 12,500 IU/0.5 ml solution for injection is supplied in 1 ml glass Ph. Eur. Type I single dose syringes with chlorobutyl (Type I) rubber stopper and polypropylene rod. Each pack contains 5 syringes.
4	Fragmin 15 000 IU/0.6 ml solution for injection is supplied in 1 ml glass Ph. Eur. Type I single dose syringes with chlorobutyl (Type I) rubber stopper and polypropylene rod. Each pack contains 5 syringes.
5	1 ml single dose syringe (glass Ph. Eur. Type I) with chlorobutyl rubber stopper containing dalteparin sodium 18,000 IU (anti-Factor Xa) in 0.72 ml. Each pack contains 5 syringes.
6	Clear glass ampoules (Ph Eur Type 1) containing dalteparin sodium, 10,000 IU (anti-factor Xa) in 1 ml
7	Multidose vial (Ph Eur Type 1) with bromobutyl rubber stopper, secured with aluminium overseal with flip off cap, containing dalteparin sodium 100,000 IU (anti-Factor Xa) in 4 ml.

6.6 Special precautions for disposal and other handling

1 – 6: Not applicable

7: As with other multidose preparations, care should be taken to avoid any risk of cross-contamination during use.

7. MARKETING AUTHORISATION HOLDER

Pharmacia Limited

Ramsgate Road

Sandwich KENT

CT13 9NJ

United Kingdom

8. MARKETING AUTHORISATION NUMBER(S)

1	PL 0032/0483
2	PL 0032/0375
3	PL 0032/0379
4	PL 0032/0380
5	PL 0032/0381
6	PL 0032/0376
7	PL 0032/0378

9. DATE OF FIRST AUTHORISATION/RENEWAL OF THE AUTHORISATION

1: 24 April 2001

2 – 5: 18 March 2002

6: 5 April 2002

7: 27 March 2002

10. DATE OF REVISION OF THE TEXT

May 2009

Legal Category

POM (1-7)

Ref: FR 5_0

Fragmin - Unstable Angina

(Pharmacia Limited)

1. NAME OF THE MEDICINAL PRODUCT

1. Fragmin Graduated Syringe 10,000 IU/1 ml solution for Injection

2. Fragmin 7,500 IU/0.3 ml solution for injection

3. Fragmin 10,000 IU/1 ml Ampoule

2. QUALITATIVE AND QUANTITATIVE COMPOSITION

Pre-filled, single dose syringes containing dalteparin sodium 10,000 IU (anti-Factor Xa*) in 1.0ml solution for injection

Fragmin 7,500 IU: single dose syringe containing dalteparin sodium 7,500 IU (anti-Factor Xa*) in 0.3 ml solution for injection equivalent to 25,000 IU/ml

Fragmin Syringes do not contain preservatives

Ampoules containing dalteparin sodium, 10,000 IU (anti-Factor Xa*) in 1 ml.

*Potency is described in International anti-Factor Xa units (IU) of the 1st International Standard for Low Molecular Weight Heparin.

3. PHARMACEUTICAL FORM

Solution for injection for intravenous or subcutaneous administration.

4. CLINICAL PARTICULARS

4.1 Therapeutic indications

Unstable angina and non-Q wave myocardial infarction (unstable coronary artery disease-UCAD), administered concurrently with aspirin.

Extended Use
Fragmin may be used beyond 8 days in patients awaiting angiography/revascularisation procedures (see Section 5.1)

4.2 Posology and method of administration

Recommended dosage for adults

120 IU/kg body weight are administered subcutaneously 12 hourly for up to 8 days if considered of benefit by the physician. Maximum dose is 10,000 IU/12 hours.

Patients needing treatment beyond 8 days, while awaiting angiography/ revascularisation, should receive a fixed dose of either 5,000 IU (women < 80 kg and men <70 kg) or 7,500 IU (women ≥80 kg and men ≥70 kg) 12 hourly. Treatment is recommended to be given until the day of the revascularisation procedure (PTCA or CA BG) but not for more than 45 days.

Children

Not recommended for children.

Elderly

Fragmin has been used safely in elderly patients without the need for dosage adjustment.

Method of Administration

Following the determination of the required dose, excess solution should be ejected from the syringe.

Administration is by subcutaneous injection, preferably into the abdominal subcutaneous tissue anterolaterally or poterolaterally, or into the lateral part of the thigh. Patients should be supine and the total length of the needle should be introduced vertically, not at an angle, into the thick part of a skin fold, produced by squeezing the skin between thumb and forefinger; the skin fold should be held throughout the injection.

Syringes should be discarded after use.

4.3 Contraindications

Known hypersensitivity to Fragmin or other low molecular weight heparins and/or heparins e.g. history of confirmed or suspected immunologically mediated heparin induced thrombocytopenia, acute gastroduodenal ulcer; cerebral haemorrhage; known haemorrhagic diathesis; subacute endocarditis; injuries to and operations on the central nervous system, eyes and ears.

In patients receiving Fragmin for treatment rather than prophylaxis, local and/or regional anaesthesia in elective surgical procedures is contra-indicated.

4.4 Special warnings and precautions for use

Do not administer by the intramuscular route.

Caution should be exercised in patients in whom there is an increased risk of bleeding complications, e.g. following surgery or trauma, haemorrhagic stroke, severe liver or renal failure, thrombocytopenia or defective platelet function, uncontrolled hypertension, hypertensive or diabetic retinopathy, patients receiving concurrent anticoagulant/ antiplatelet agents (see interactions section).

It is recommended that platelets be counted before starting treatment with Fragmin and monitored regularly. Special caution is necessary in rapidly developing thrombocytopenia and severe thrombocytopenia (<100,000/μl) associated with positive or unknown results of in-vitro tests for anti-platelet antibody in the presence of Fragmin or other low molecular weight (mass) heparins and/or heparin.

Fragmin induces only a moderate prolongation of the APTT and thrombin time. Accordingly, dosage increments based upon prolongation of the APTT may cause overdosage and bleeding. Therefore, prolongation of the APTT should only be used as a test of overdosage.

Monitoring Anti-Xa Levels

Monitoring of Anti-Xa Levels in patients using Fragmin is not usually required but should be considered for specific patient populations such as those with renal failure, those who are very thin or morbidly obese, pregnant or at increased risk for bleeding or rethrombosis

Where monitoring is necessary, laboratory assays using a chromogenic substrate are considered the method of choice for measuring anti-Xa levels. Activated partial thromboplastin time (APTT) or thrombin time should not be used because these tests are relatively insensitive to the activity of dalteparin. Increasing the dose of dalteparin in an attempt to prolong APTT may result in bleeding (see section 4.9 Overdosage).

Patients with severely disturbed hepatic function may need a reduction in dosage and should be monitored accordingly.

If a transmural myocardial infarction occurs in patients with unstable coronary artery disease, thrombolytic treatment might be appropriate. This does not necessitate discontinuation of treatment with Fragmin, but might increase the risk of bleeding.

As individual low molecular weight (mass) heparins have differing characteristics, switching to an alternative low molecular weight heparin should be avoided. The directions for use relating to each specific product must be observed as different dosages may be required.

Interchangeability with other anticoagulants

Dalteparin cannot be used interchangeably (unit for unit) with unfractionated heparin, other low molecular weight heparins, or synthetic polysaccharides. Each of these medicines differ in their starting raw materials, manufacturing process, physico-chemical, biological, and clinical properties, leading to differences in biochemical identity, dosing, and possibly clinical efficacy and safety. Each of these medicines is unique and has its own instructions for use.

Heparin can suppress adrenal secretion of aldosterone leading to hyperkalaemia, particularly in patients such as those with diabetes mellitus, chronic renal failure, pre-existing metabolic acidosis, a raised plasma potassium or taking potassium sparing drugs. The risk of hyperkalaemia appears to increase with duration of therapy but is usually reversible. Plasma potassium should be measured in patients at risk before starting heparin therapy and monitored regularly thereafter particularly if treatment is prolonged beyond about 7 days.

In patients undergoing spinal or epidural anaesthesia, the prophylactic use of heparin may be very rarely associated with spinal haematomas resulting in prolonged or permanent paralysis. The risk is increased by use of an epidural or spinal catheter for anaesthesia, by the concomitant use of drugs (NSAIDs), platelet inhibitors or anti-coagulants and by traumatic or repeated puncture.

In decision-making on the interval between the last administration of Fragmin at prophylactic doses and the placement or removal of a peridural or spinal catheter for anaesthesia, the product characteristics and the patient profile should be taken into account. Readministration should be delayed until at least four hours after the surgical procedure is completed.

Should a physician, as a clinical judgement, decide to administer anticoagulation in the context of peridural or spinal anaesthesia, extreme vigilance and frequent monitoring must be exercised to detect any signs and symptoms of neurologic impairment such as back pain, sensory or motor deficits (numbness and weakness in lower limbs) and bowel or bladder dysfunction. Nurses should be trained to detect such signs and symptoms. Patients should be instructed to inform immediately a nurse or a clinician if they experience any of these.

If signs or symptoms of epidural or spinal haematoma are suspected, urgent diagnosis and treatment may include spinal cord decompression.

There have been no adequate studies to assess the safe and effective use of Fragmin in preventing valve thrombosis in patients with prosthetic heart valves. Prophylactic doses of Fragmin are not sufficient to prevent valve thrombosis in patients with prosthetic heart valves. The use of Fragmin cannot be recommended for this purpose

4.5 Interaction with other medicinal products and other forms of interaction

The possibility of the following interactions with Fragmin should be considered:

(i) An enhancement of the anticoagulant effect by anticoagulant/antiplatelet agents e.g. aspirin/ dipyridamole, vitamin K antagonists, NSAIDs e.g. indometacin, cytostatics, dextran, sulfinpyrazone, probenecid, and etacrynic acid.

However, unless specifically contraindicated, patients with unstable coronary artery disease should receive oral low dose aspirin.

(ii) A reduction of the anticoagulant effect may occur with concomitant administration of antihistamines, cardiac glycosides, tetracycline and ascorbic acid.

4.6 Pregnancy and lactation

Pregnancy

Animal studies do not indicate direct or indirect harmful effects with respect to pregnancy, embryonal/foetal developments, parturition or postnatal development (see Section 5.3 Preclinical Safety Data).

If dalteparin is used during pregnancy, the possibility of foetal harm appears remote. However, because the possibility of harm cannot be completely ruled out, dalteparin should be used during pregnancy only if clearly needed (see Section 5.3 Preclinical Safety Data).

Therefore, caution should be exercised when prescribing to pregnant women.

Therapeutic failures have been reported in pregnant women with prosthetic heart valves on full anti-coagulant doses of low molecular weight heparin. In the absence of clear dosing, efficacy and safety information in this circumstance, Fragmin is not recommended for use in pregnant women with prosthetic heart valves.

Lactation

Limited data are available for excretion of dalteparin in human milk. One study in 15 lactating women receiving prophylactic doses of dalteparin detected small amounts of anti-Xa activity in breast milk, equivalent to a milk/ plasma ratio of <0.025-0.224. As oral absorption of low molecular weight heparin is extremely low the clinical implications, if any, of this small amount of anticoagulant activity on the nursing infant are unknown.

A risk to the suckling child cannot be excluded. A decision on whether to continue/discontinue breast-feeding or to continue/discontinue therapy with Fragmin should be made taking into account the benefit of breast-feeding to the child and the benefit of Fragmin therapy to the woman.

4.7 Effects on ability to drive and use machines

Fragmin does not affect the ability to drive or operate machinery.

4.8 Undesirable effects

In the table below, the adverse reactions are listed by system organ class and frequency (very common (≥1/10), common (≥1/100 to <1/10), uncommon (≥1/1,000 to <1/100), rare (≥1/10,000 to <1/1,000), very rare (<1/10,000) and not known (cannot be estimated from the available data)).

Within each frequency grouping, undesirable effects are presented in order of decreasing seriousness.

Adverse events associated with dalteparin therapy, in patients participating in controlled clinical studies were:

(see Table 1 above)

Table 1

MedDRA System Organ Class	Frequency	Undesirable Effects
Blood and lymphatic system disorders	Common	Reversible non-immunologically-mediated thrombocytopenia (type I)
	Rare	Immunologically-mediated heparin-induced thrombocytopenia (type II, with or without associated thrombotic complications arterial and/or thrombosis or thromboembolism)
Immune system disorders	Uncommon	Allergic reactions
Endocrine disorders	Uncommon	Hyperkalaemia
Vascular disorders	Common	Haemorrhage (bleeding at any site)
Hepato-biliary disorders	Common	Transient elevation of liver transaminases (ASAT, ALAT)
Skin and subcutaneous tissue disorders	Uncommon	Urticaria, pruritus
	Rare	Skin necrosis
Musculoskeletal and connective tissue disorders	Uncommon	Osteoporosis
General disorders and administration site conditions	Uncommon	Pain at injection site,
	Common	Haematoma at injection site

In post-marketing experience, the following additional undesirable effects have been reported:

MedDRA System Organ Class	Undesirable Effects
Immune system disorders	Anaphylactic reactions
Endocrine Disorders	Hypoaldosteronism
Nervous system disorders	Intracranial bleeds
Cardiac Disorders	Prosthetic cardiac valve thrombosis
Gastrointestinal disorders	Retroperitoneal bleeds
Skin and subcutaneous tissue disorders	Alopecia
Injury, poisoning and procedural complications	Spinal or epidural haematoma

4.9 Overdose

The anticoagulant effect (i.e. prolongation of the APTT) induced by Fragmin is inhibited by protamine. Since protamine itself has an inhibiting effect on primary haemostasis it should be used only in an emergency.

The prolongation of the clotting time induced by Fragmin may be fully neutralised by protamine, but the anti-Factor Xa activity is only neutralised to about 25-50%. 1 mg of protamine inhibits the effect of 100 IU (anti-Factor Xa) of Fragmin. Protamine should be given by intravenous injection over approximately 10 minutes.

5. PHARMACOLOGICAL PROPERTIES

5.1 Pharmacodynamic properties

ATC Code BO1A B

Dalteparin sodium is a low molecular weight heparin fraction (average molecular weight 4000-6000 Daltons) produced from porcine-derived sodium heparin.

Dalteparin sodium is an antithrombotic agent, which acts mainly through its ability to potentiate the inhibition of Factor Xa and thrombin by antithrombin. It has a relatively higher ability to potentiate Factor Xa inhibition than to prolong plasma clotting time (APTT).

Compared with standard, unfractionated heparin, dalteparin sodium has a reduced adverse effect on platelet function and platelet adhesion, and thus has only a minimal effect on primary haemostasis. Some of the antithrombotic properties of dalteparin sodium are thought to be mediated through the effects on vessel walls or the fibrinolytic system.

In a prospectively randomised study in 3489 patients (FRISC II) with acute coronary syndromes, early invasive strategy was clearly superior to non –invasive strategy.

In a post-hoc analysis, the extended use of Fragmin, up to Day 45 reduced the incidence of death and/or MI compared with placebo in the non-invasive group (revascularisation only if necessary).

The use of Fragmin beyond 8 days did not significantly reduce the incidence of death and/or MI, compared to placebo, in patients who were contraindicated to early angiography and revascularisation.

5.2 Pharmacokinetic properties

The half life following iv and sc. administration is 2 hours and 3.5-4 hours respectively, twice that of unfractionated heparin.

The bioavailability following sc. injection is approximately 87 per cent and the pharmacokinetics are not dose dependent. The half life is prolonged in uraemic patients as dalteparin sodium is eliminated primarily through the kidneys.

Special Populations

Haemodialysis:

In patients with chronic renal insufficiency requiring haemodialysis, the mean terminal hal-life of anti-Factor Xa activity following a single intravenous dose of 5000 IU dalteparin was 5.7 ± 2.0 hours, i.e. considerably longer than values observed in healthy volunteers; therefore, greater accumulation can be expected in these patients.

5.3 Preclinical safety data

The acute toxicity of dalteparin sodium is considerably lower than that of heparin. The only significant finding, which occurred consistently throughout the toxicity studies after subcutaneous administration of the higher dose levels was local haemorrhage at the injection site, dose-related in incidence and severity. There was no cumulative effect on injection site haemorrhages.

The haemorrhagic reaction was reflected in dose related changes in the anticoagulant effects as measured by APTT and anti-Factor Xa activities.

It was concluded that dalteparin sodium did not have a greater osteopenic effect than heparin since at equivalent doses the osteopenic effect was comparable.

The results revealed no organ toxicity irrespective of the route of administration, doses or the duration of treatment. No mutagenic effect was found. No embryotoxic or teratogenic effects and no effect on fertility reproductive capacity or peri- and postnatal development was shown.

6. PHARMACEUTICAL PARTICULARS

6.1 List of excipients

Graduated Syringe 10,000 IU/ml

Sodium chloride (Ph Eur)

Water for injections (Ph Eur)

Sodium Hydroxide or hydrochloric acid for pH adjustment

7,500 IU/0.3 ml solution for injection

Water for injections (Ph Eur)

Sodium Hydroxide or hydrochloric acid for pH adjustment

Fragmin 10,000 IU/ml Ampoule

Sodium chloride (Ph Eur)

Water for injections (Ph Eur)

6.2 Incompatibilities

Not applicable.

6.3 Shelf life

36 months.

6.4 Special precautions for storage

1 – 2: Do not store above 25°C

3: Store at room temperature (below 30°C).

6.5 Nature and contents of container

1 ml single dose syringe (glass Ph. Eur. Type I) with chlorobutyl rubber stopper containing dalteparin sodium 10,000 IU (anti-Factor Xa) in 1ml solution for injection, Each box contains 5 × 1 ml syringes.

Fragmin 7,500 IU/0.3 ml Solution for Injection is supplied in 0.5 ml glass Ph. Eur. Type I single dose syringes with chlorobutyl (Type I) rubber and polypropylene rod. Each pack contains 10 syringes.

Clear glass ampoules (Ph Eur Type 1) containing dalteparin sodium, 10,000 IU (anti-factor Xa) in 1 ml

6.6 Special precautions for disposal and other handling

Not applicable

7. MARKETING AUTHORISATION HOLDER

Pharmacia Limited
Ramsgate Road
Sandwich KENT
CT13 9NJ
United Kingdom

8. MARKETING AUTHORISATION NUMBER(S)

Graduated Syringe 10,000 IU/ml

PL 0032/0384

7,500 IU/0.3 ml solution for injection

PL 0032/0483

Fragmin 10,000 IU/ml Ampoule

PL 0032/0376

9. DATE OF FIRST AUTHORISATION/RENEWAL OF THE AUTHORISATION

Graduated Syringe 10,000 IU/ml

29 April 2002

7,500 IU/0.3 ml solution for injection

26 June 2002

Fragmin 10,000 IU/ml Ampoule

5 April 2002

10. DATE OF REVISION OF THE TEXT

May 2009

Legal Category: POM

Ref: FR 5_0

Frisium Tablets 10 mg

(sanofi-aventis)

1. NAME OF THE MEDICINAL PRODUCT

Frisium™

2. QUALITATIVE AND QUANTITATIVE COMPOSITION

Clobazam 10 mg.

3. PHARMACEUTICAL FORM

Tablet

4. CLINICAL PARTICULARS

4.1 Therapeutic indications

Frisium is a 1,5-benzodiazepine indicated for the short-term relief (2-4 weeks) only of anxiety that is severe, disabling or subjecting the individual to unacceptable distress, occurring alone or in association with insomnia or short term psychosomatic, organic or psychotic illness. The use of Frisium to treat short-term "mild" anxiety is inappropriate and unsuitable.

Before treatment of anxiety states associated with emotional instability, it must first be determined whether the patient suffers from a depressive disorder requiring adjunctive or different treatment. Indeed, in patients with anxiety associated with depression, Frisium must be used only in conjunction with adequate concomitant treatment. Use of benzodiazepine (such as Frisium) alone, can precipitate suicide in such patients.

In patients with schizophrenic or other psychotic illnesses, use of benzodiazepines is recommended only for adjunctive, i.e. not for primary treatment.

Frisium may be used as adjunctive therapy in epilepsy.

4.2 Posology and method of administration

Treatment of anxiety

The usual anxiolytic dose for adults and adolescents over 15 years of age is 20-30 mg daily in divided doses or as a single dose given at night. Doses up to 60mg daily have been used in the treatment of adult in-patients with severe anxiety.

The lowest dose that can control symptoms should be used. After improvement of the symptoms, the dose may be reduced.

It should not be used for longer than 4 weeks. Long term chronic use as an anxiolytic is not recommended. In certain cases, extension beyond the maximum treatment period may be necessary; treatment must not be extended without re-evaluation of the patient's status using special expertise. It is strongly recommended that prolonged periods of uninterrupted treatment be avoided, since they may lead to dependence. Treatment should always be withdrawn gradually. Patients who have taken Frisium for a long time may require a longer period during which doses are reduced.

Treatment of epilepsy in association with one or more other anticonvulsants

In epilepsy a starting dose of 20-30 mg/day is recommended, increasing as necessary up to a maximum of 60 mg daily. The patient must be re-assessed after a period not exceeding 4 weeks and regularly thereafter in order to evaluate the need for continued treatment. A break in therapy may be beneficial if drug exhaustion develops, recommencing therapy at a low dose. At the end of treatment (including in poor-responding patients), since the risk of withdrawal phenomena/rebound phenomena is greater after abrupt discontinuation of treatment, it is recommended to gradually decrease the dosage.

Elderly: Doses of 10-20 mg daily in anxiety may be used in the elderly, who are more sensitive to the effects of psychoactive agents. Treatment requires low initial doses and gradual dose increments under careful observation.

Children: When prescribed for children over three years of age, dosage should not exceed half the recommended adult dose. Treatment requires low initial doses and gradual dose increments under careful observation. There is insufficient experience of the use of Frisium in children under three years of age to enable any dosage recommendation to be made.

Tablets should to be swallowed without chewing with sufficient amount of liquid (1/2 glass).

4.3 Contraindications

Frisium must not be used:

– In patients with hypersensitivity to benzodiazepines or any of the excipients of Frisium.

– In patients with any history of drug or alcohol dependence (increased risk of development of dependence).

– In patients with myasthenia gravis (risk of aggravation of muscle weakness).

– In patients with severe respiratory insufficiency (risk of deterioration).

– In patients with sleep apnoea syndrome (risk of deterioration).

– In patients with severe hepatic insufficiencies (risk of precipitating encephalopathy).

– During the first trimester of pregnancy (for use during second and third trimester, see section 4.6 Pregnancy and Lactation).

– In breast-feeding women.

Benzodiazepines must not be given to children without careful assessment of the need for their use. Frisium must not be used in children between the ages of 6 months and 3 years, other than in exceptional cases for anticonvulsant treatment where there is a compelling indication.

4.4 Special warnings and precautions for use

Amnesia may occur with benzodiazepines. In case of loss or bereavement psychological adjustment may be inhibited by benzodiazepines.

Special caution is necessary if clobazam is used in patients with myasthenia gravis, spinal or cerebellar ataxia or sleep apnoea. A dose reduction may be necessary.

Disinhibiting effects may be manifested in various ways. Suicide may be precipitated in patients who are depressed and aggressive behaviour towards self and others may be precipitated. Extreme caution should therefore be used in prescribing benzodiazepines in patients with personality disorders.

Use of benzodiazepines - including clobazam - may lead to the development of physical and psychic dependence upon these products. The risk of dependence increases with dose and duration of treatment; it is also greater in patients with a history of alcohol or drug abuse. Therefore the duration of treatment should be as short as possible (see Posology).

Once physical dependence has developed, abrupt termination of treatment will be accompanied by withdrawal symptoms (or rebound phenomena). Rebound phenomena are characterised by a recurrence in enhanced form of the symptoms which originally led to clobazam treatment. This may be accompanied by other reactions including mood changes, anxiety or sleep disturbances and restlessness.

A withdrawal syndrome may also occur when abruptly changing over from a benzodiazepine with a long duration of action (for example, Frisium) to one with a short duration of action.

Respiratory function should be monitored in patients with chronic or acute severe respiratory insufficiency and a dose reduction of clobazam may be necessary.

In patients with impairment of renal or hepatic function, responsiveness to clobazam and susceptibility to adverse effects are increased, and a dose reduction may be necessary. In long-term treatment renal and hepatic function must be checked regularly.

In the treatment of epilepsy with benzodiazepines - including clobazam - consideration must be given to the possibility of a decrease in anticonvulsant efficacy (development of tolerance) in the course of treatment.

4.5 Interaction with other medicinal products and other forms of interaction

Especially when clobazam is administered at higher doses, an enhancement of the central depressive effect may occur in cases of concomitant use with antipsychotics (neuroleptics), hypnotics, anxiolytics/sedatives, antidepressant agents, narcotic analgesics, anticonvulsant drugs, anaesthetics and sedative antihistamines. Special caution is also necessary when clobazam is administered in cases of intoxication with such substances or with lithium.

Concomitant consumption of alcohol can increase the bioavailability of clobazam by 50% and therefore increase the effects of clobazam (e.g.; sedation). This affects the ability to drive or use machines.

Addition of clobazam to established anticonvulsant medication (eg, phenytoin, valproic acid) may cause a change in plasma levels of these drugs. If used as an adjuvant in epilepsy the dosage of Frisium should be determined by monitoring the EEG and the plasma levels of the other drugs checked.

Phenytoin and carbamazepine may cause an increase in the metabolic conversion of clobazam to the active metabolite N-desmethyl clobazam.

The effects of muscle relaxants, analgesics and nitrous oxide may be enhanced. If clobazam is used concomitantly with narcotic analgesics, possible euphoria may be enhanced; this may lead to increased psychological dependence.

Concurrent treatment with drugs that inhibit the cytochrome P-450 enzyme (mono-oxygenase) system (eg cimetidine) may enhance and prolong the effect of clobazam.

4.6 Pregnancy and lactation

If the product is prescribed to a woman of childbearing potential, she should be warned to contact her physician regarding discontinuation of the product if she intends to become pregnant or suspects that she is pregnant.

If, for compelling medical reasons, the product is administered during the late phase of pregnancy, or during labour at high doses, effects on the neonate such as hypothermia, hypotonia, moderate respiratory depression and difficulties in drinking (signs and symptoms of so-called "floppy infant syndrome"), can be expected due to the pharmacological action of the compound.

Moreover, infants born to mothers who took benzodiazepines during the latter stage of pregnancy may have developed physical dependence and may be at some risk for developing withdrawal symptoms in the postnatal period.

Since benzodiazepines are found in the breast milk, benzodiazepines should not be given to breast feeding mothers.

4.7 Effects on ability to drive and use machines

Sedation, amnesia, impaired concentration and impaired muscular function may adversely affect the ability to drive or to use machines. If insufficient sleep duration occurs, the likelihood of impaired alertness may be increased (see also Interactions).

4.8 Undesirable effects

Clobazam may cause sedation, leading to fatigue and sleepiness, especially at the beginning of treatment and when higher doses are used. Side-effects such as drowsiness, dizziness or dryness of the mouth, constipation, loss of appetite, nausea, or a fine tremor of the fingers have been reported. These are more likely to occur at the beginning of treatment and often disappear with continued treatment or a reduction in dose.

Paradoxical reactions, such as restlessness, irritability, difficulty in sleeping, anxiety, delusion, nightmare, hallucinations or suicidal tendencies may occur, especially in elderly and in children. In the event of such reactions, treatment with clobazam must be discontinued.

Anterograde amnesia may occur, especially at higher dose levels. Amnesia effects may be associated with inappropriate behaviour.

Clobazam may cause respiratory depression, especially if administered in high doses. Therefore, particularly in patients with pre-existing compromised respiratory function (i.e., in patients with bronchial asthma) or brain damage, respiratory insufficiency may occur or deteriorate.

Isolated cases of skin reactions, such as rashes or urticaria, have been observed.

Slowing of reaction time, ataxia, confusion and headaches may occasionally occur.

Disorders of articulation, unsteadiness of gait and other motor functions, visual disorders (e.g., double vision), weight gain, or loss of libido may occur, particularly with high doses or in long-term treatment. These reactions are reversible.

Pre-existing depression may be unmasked during benzodiazepine use.

After prolonged use of benzodiazepines, impairment of consciousness, sometimes combined with respiratory disorders, has been reported in very rare cases, particularly in elderly patients: it sometimes persists for some length of time. These disorders have not been seen so far under clobazam treatment.

Tolerance and physical and/or psychic dependence may develop, especially during prolonged use. Discontinuation of the therapy may result in withdrawal or rebound phenomena (see Warnings and Precautions). Abuse of benzodiazepines has been reported.

When used as an adjuvant in the treatment of epilepsy, this preparation may in rare cases cause restlessness and muscle weakness.

As with other benzodiazepines, the therapeutic benefit must be balanced against the risk of habituation and dependence during prolonged use.

4.9 Overdose

Overdose of benzodiazepines is usually manifested by degrees of central nervous system depression ranging from drowsiness to coma. In mild cases, symptoms include drowsiness, mental confusion and lethargy, in more serious cases, symptoms may include ataxia, hypotonia, hypotension, respiratory depression, rarely coma and very rarely death. As with other benzodiazepines, overdose should not present a threat to life unless combined with other CNS depressants (including alcohol).

In the management of overdose, it is recommended that the possible involvement of multiple agents be taken into consideration.

Following overdose with oral benzodiazepines, vomiting should be induced (within one hour) if the patient is conscious, or gastric lavage undertaken with the airway protected if the patient is unconscious. If there is no advantage in emptying the stomach, activated charcoal should be given to reduce absorption. Special attention should be paid to respiratory and cardiovascular functions in intensive care.

Secondary elimination of clobazam (by forced diuresis or haemodialysis) is ineffective.

Consideration should be given to the use of flumazenil as a benzodiazepine antagonist.

5. PHARMACOLOGICAL PROPERTIES

5.1 Pharmacodynamic properties

Clobazam is a 1,5-benzodiazepine. In single doses up to 20mg or in divided doses up to 30mg, clobazam does not affect psychomotor function, skilled performance, memory or higher mental functions.

5.2 Pharmacokinetic properties

Absorption of clobazam is virtually complete after oral administration. Approximately 85% is protein bound in man. It is metabolised by demethylation and hydroxylation. It is excreted unchanged and as metabolites in the urine (87%) and faeces.

5.3 Preclinical safety data

None applicable

6. PHARMACEUTICAL PARTICULARS

6.1 List of excipients

Lactose monohydrate, maize starch, colloidal silicon dioxide, talc, magnesium stearate.

6.2 Incompatibilities

None.

6.3 Shelf life

Five years.

6.4 Special precautions for storage

Store below 25°C.

6.5 Nature and contents of container

Blister pack (Alufoil/PVC) containing 30 tablets.

6.6 Special precautions for disposal and other handling

None.

Administrative Data

7. MARKETING AUTHORISATION HOLDER

Sanofi-aventis

One Onslow Street

Guildford

Surrey

GU1 4YS

8. MARKETING AUTHORISATION NUMBER(S)

PL 04425/0214

9. DATE OF FIRST AUTHORISATION/RENEWAL OF THE AUTHORISATION

15 January 2002

10. DATE OF REVISION OF THE TEXT

November 2006

11. LEGAL CLASSIFICATION

POM

Froben 100mg Tablets

(Abbott Laboratories Limited)

1. NAME OF THE MEDICINAL PRODUCT

Froben Tablets 100 mg

2. QUALITATIVE AND QUANTITATIVE COMPOSITION

Froben Tablets 100 mg contain 100 mg Flurbiprofen BP.

3. PHARMACEUTICAL FORM

The tablets are sugar-coated and yellow in colour. They may be either unprinted or printed in black with an identifying motif.

4. CLINICAL PARTICULARS

4.1 Therapeutic indications

For the treatment of rheumatoid disease, osteoarthritis, ankylosing spondylitis, musculoskeletal disorders and trauma such as periarthritis, frozen shoulder, bursitis, tendinitis, tenosynovitis, low back pain, sprains and strains.

Froben is also indicated for its analgesic effect in the relief of mild to moderate pain in conditions such as dental pain, post-operative pain, dysmenorrhoea and migraine.

4.2 Posology and method of administration

For oral administration. To be taken preferably with or after food.

Undesirable effects may be minimised by using the lowest effective dose for the shortest duration necessary to control symptoms (see Section 4.4).

Adults:

150 to 200 mg daily in two, three or four divided doses. In patients with severe symptoms or disease of recent origin, or during acute exacerbations, the total daily dosage may be increased to 300 mg in divided doses.

For dysmenorrhoea, a dosage of 100 mg may be administered at the start of symptoms followed by 50 or 100 mg given at four- to six-hour intervals. The maximum total daily dosage should not exceed 300 mg.

Children:

Not recommended for use in children under 12 years.

Elderly:

The elderly are at increased risk of the serious consequences of adverse reactions. Although flurbiprofen is generally well tolerated in the elderly, some patients, especially those with impaired renal function, may eliminate NSAIDs more slowly than normal. In these cases, flurbiprofen should be used with caution and dosage should be assessed individually.

If an NSAID is considered necessary, the lowest effective dose should be used and for the shortest possible duration. The patient should be monitored regularly for GI bleeding during NSAID therapy.

4.3 Contraindications

Froben is contraindicated in patients with hypersensitivity (asthma, urticaria or allergic type) to flurbiprofen or to any of the inactive ingredients.

Froben is contraindicated in patients who have previously shown hypersensitivity reactions (*e.g.* asthma, rhinitis, angioedema or urticaria) in response to flurbiprofen, aspirin or other NSAIDs.

Froben is also contraindicated in patients with a history of gastrointestinal bleeding or perforation, related to previous NSAID therapy. Froben should not be used in patients with active, or history of, ulcerative colitis, Crohn's disease, recurrent peptic ulceration or gastrointestinal haemorrhage (defined as two or more distinct episodes of proven ulceration or bleeding).

Froben is contraindicated in patients with severe heart failure, hepatic failure and renal failure (see section 4.4).

Froben is contraindicated during the last trimester of pregnancy (see section 4.6).

4.4 Special warnings and precautions for use

Undesirable effects may be minimised by using the lowest effective dose for the shortest duration necessary to control symptoms (see Section 4.2 and GI and cardiovascular risks below).

Patients with rare hereditary problems of galactose intolerance, fructose intolerance, the Lapp lactose deficiency, sucrase-isomaltase insufficiency or glucose-galactose malabsorption should not take this medication.

The use of Froben with concomitant NSAIDs, including cyclooxygenase-2 selective inhibitors, should be avoided due to the potential for additive effects (see section 4.5).

Elderly

The elderly have an increased frequency of adverse reactions to NSAIDs, especially gastrointestinal bleeding and perforation, which may be fatal (see section 4.2).

Gastrointestinal bleeding, ulceration and perforation

GI bleeding, ulceration or perforation has been reported with all NSAIDs at any time during treatment. These adverse events can be fatal and may occur with or without warning symptoms or a previous history of serious GI events.

The risk of GI bleeding, ulceration or perforation is higher with increasing NSAID doses, in patients with a history of ulcer, particularly if complicated with haemorrhage or perforation (see section 4.3), and in the elderly. These patients should commence treatment on the lowest dose available. Combination therapy with protective agents (e.g. misoprostol or proton pump inhibitors) should be considered for these patients, and also for patients requiring concomitant low dose aspirin, or other drugs likely to increase gastrointestinal risk (see below and section 4.5).

Patients with a history of gastrointestinal disease, particularly when elderly, should report any unusual abdominal symptoms (especially gastrointestinal bleeding) particularly in the initial stages of treatment.

Caution should be advised in patients receiving concomitant medications which could increase the risk of ulceration or bleeding, such as oral corticosteroids, anticoagulants such as warfarin, selective serotonin-reuptake inhibitors or anti-platelet agents such as aspirin (see section 4.5).

When GI bleeding or ulceration occurs in patients receiving Froben, the treatment should be withdrawn.

Respiratory disorders

Caution is required if Froben is administered to patients suffering from, or with a previous history of, bronchial asthma since NSAIDs have been reported to precipitate bronchospasm in such patients.

Cardiovascular, renal and hepatic impairment

The administration of an NSAID may cause a dose dependent reduction in prostaglandin formation and precipitate renal failure. Patients at greatest risk of this reaction are those with impaired renal function, cardiac impairment, liver dysfunction, those taking diuretics and the elderly. Renal function should be monitored in these patients (see also section 4.3).

Froben should be given with care to patients with a history of heart failure or hypertension since oedema has been reported in association with flurbiprofen administration.

Cardiovascular and cerebrovascular effects

Appropriate monitoring and advice are required for patients with a history of hypertension and/or mild to moderate congestive heart failure as fluid retention and oedema have been reported in association with flurbiprofen administration and NSAID therapy.

Clinical trial and epidemiological data suggest that use of some NSAIDs (particularly at high doses and in long term treatment) may be associated with a small increased risk of arterial thrombotic events such as myocardial infarction or stroke. There are insufficient data to exclude such a risk for flurbiprofen.

Patients with uncontrolled hypertension, congestive heart failure, established ischaemic heart disease, peripheral arterial disease, and/or cerebrovascular disease should only be treated with flurbiprofen after careful consideration. Similar consideration should be made before initating longer-term treatment of patients with risk factors for cardiovascular disease (eg hypertension, hyperlipidaemia, diabetes mellitus, smoking).

Renal effects

Caution should be used when initiating treatment with NSAIDs such as flurbiprofen in patients with considerable dehydration.

SLE and mixed connective tissue disease

In patients with systemic lupus erythematosus (SLE) and mixed connective tissue disorders there may be an increased risk of aseptic meningitis (see section 4.8).

Dermatological effects

Serious skin reactions, some of them fatal, including exfoliative dermatitis, Stevens-Johnson syndrome and toxic epidermal necrolysis, have been reported very rarely in association with the use of NSAIDs (see section 4.8). Patients appear to be at highest risk of these reactions early in the course of therapy, the onset of the reaction occurring within the first month of treatment in the majority of cases. Froben should be discontinued at the first appearance of skin rash, mucosal lesions or any other sign of hypersensitivity.

Haematological effects

Flurbiprofen, like other NSAIDs, may inhibit platelet aggregation and prolong bleeding time. Froben should be used with caution in patients with a potential for abnormal bleeding.

Impaired female fertility

The use of Froben may impair female fertility and is not recommended in women attempting to conceive. In women who have difficulties conceiving or who are undergoing investigation of infertility, withdrawal of Froben should be considered.

4.5 Interaction with other medicinal products and other forms of interaction

Care should be taken in patients treated with any of the following drugs as interactions have been reported in some patients.

Diuretics, ACE inhibitors and Angiotensin II Antagonists: NSAIDs may reduce the effect of diuretics and other antihypertensive drugs. In some patients with compromised renal function (e.g. dehydrated patients or elderly patients with compromised renal function) the co-administration of an ACE inhibitor or Angiotensin II antagonist and agents that inhibit cyclo-oxygenase may result in further deterioration of renal function, including possible acute renal failure, which is usually reversible. These interactions should be considered in patients taking flurbiprofen concomitantly with ACE inhibitors or angiotensin II antagonists. Therefore, the combination should be administered with caution, especially in the elderly. Patients should be adequately hydrated and consideration should be given to monitoring of renal function after initiation of concomitant therapy, and periodically thereafter.

Cardiac glycosides: NSAIDs may exacerbate cardiac failure, reduce GFR and increase plasma cardiac glycoside levels.

Anticoagulants: NSAIDs may enhance the effects of anticoagulants such as warfarin (see section 4.4).

Aspirin: As with other products containing NSAIDs, concomitant administration of flurbiprofen and aspirin is not generally recommended because of the potential of increased adverse effects.

Anti-platelet agents: Increased risk of gastrointestinal bleeding with NSAIDs (see section 4.4).

Selective serotonin reuptake inhibitors (SSRIs): Increased risk of gastrointestinal bleeding with NSAIDs (see section 4.4).

Lithium salts: Decreased elimination of lithium.

Methotrexate: Caution is advised in the concomitant administration of flurbiprofen and methotrexate since NSAIDs may increase methotrexate levels.

Ciclosporin: Increased risk of nephrotoxicity.

Corticosteroids: Increased risk of gastrointestinal ulceration or bleeding with NSAIDs (see section 4.4).

Other analgesics and cyclooxygenase-2 selective inhibitors: Avoid concomitant use of two or more NSAIDs, including Cox-2 inhibitors, as this may increase the risk of adverse effects (see section 4.4).

Quinolone antibiotics: Animal data indicate that NSAIDs can increase the risk of convulsions associated with quinolone antibiotics. Patients taking NSAIDs and quinolones may have an increased risk of developing convulsions.

Mifepristone: NSAIDs should not be used for 8-12 days after mifepristone administration as NSAIDs can reduce the effects of mifepristone.

Tacrolimus: Possible increased risk of nephrotoxicity when NSAIDs are given with tacrolimus.

Zidovudine: Increased risk of haematological toxicity when NSAIDs are given with zidovudine. There is evidence of an increased risk of haemarthroses and haematoma in HIV(+) haemophiliacs receiving concurrent treatment with zidovudine and other NSAIDs.

Studies have failed to show any interaction between flurbiprofen and tolbutamide or antacids. There is no evidence so far that flurbiprofen interferes with standard laboratory tests.

4.6 Pregnancy and lactation

Pregnancy

Inhibition of prostaglandin synthesis may adversely affect the pregnancy and/or the embryo/foetal development. Data from epidemiological studies suggest an increased risk of miscarriage and of cardiac malformation and gastroschisis after use of a prostaglandin synthesis inhibitor in early pregnancy. The absolute risk for cardiovascular malformation was increased from less than 1%, up to approximately 1.5 %. The risk is believed to increase with dose and duration of therapy. In animals, administration of a prostaglandin synthesis inhibitor has been shown to result in increased pre- and post-implantation loss and embryo-foetal lethality. In addition, increased incidences of various malformations, including cardiovascular, have been reported in animals given a prostaglandin synthesis inhibitor during the organogenetic period. During the first and second trimester of pregnancy, flurbiprofen should not be given unless clearly necessary. If flurbiprofen is used by a woman attempting to conceive, or during the first and second trimester of pregnancy, the dose should be kept as low and duration of treatment as short as possible.

During the third trimester of pregnancy, all prostaglandin synthesis inhibitors may expose the foetus to:

- cardiopulmonary toxicity (with premature closure of the ductus arteriosus and pulmonary hypertension);
- renal dysfunction, which may progress to renal failure with oligo-hydroamniosis;

the mother and the neonate, at the end of pregnancy, to:

- possible prolongation of bleeding time, an anti-aggregating effect which may occur even at very low doses.
- inhibition of uterine contractions resulting in delayed or prolonged labour.

Consequently, flurbiprofen is contraindicated during the third trimester of pregnancy.

Lactation

In the limited studies so far available, NSAIDs can appear in the breast milk in very low concentrations. NSAIDs should, if possible, be avoided when breastfeeding.

See section 4.4 Special warnings and precautions for use, regarding female fertility.

4.7 Effects on ability to drive and use machines

Undesirable effects such as dizziness, drowsiness, fatigue and visual disturbances are possible after taking NSAIDs. If affected, patients should not drive or operate machinery.

4.8 Undesirable effects

Gastrointestinal disorders: The most commonly observed adverse events are gastrointestinal in nature. Peptic ulcers, perforation or GI bleeding, sometimes fatal, particularly in the elderly, may occur (see section 4.4). Nausea, vomiting, diarrhoea, dyspepsia, flatulence, constipation, abdominal pain, melaena, haematemesis, ulcerative stomatitis, exacerbation of colitis and Crohn's disease (see section 4.3 and 4.4) have been reported following flurbiprofen administration. Less frequently, gastritis, has been observed. Pancreatitis has been reported very rarely.

Immune system disorders: Hypersensitivity reactions have been reported following treatment with NSAIDs. These may consist of (a) non-specific allergic reactions and anaphylaxis, (b) respiratory tract reactivity comprising asthma, aggravated asthma, bronchospasm or dyspnoea, or (c) assorted skin disorders, including rashes of various types, pruritus, urticaria, purpura, angioedema and, more rarely exfoliative and bullous dermatoses (including toxic epidermal necrolysis and erythema multiforme).

Cardiac disorders and Vascular disorders: Oedema, hypertension and cardiac failure have been reported in association with NSAID treatment.

Clinical trial and epidemiological data suggest that use of some NSAIDs (particularly at high doses and in long term treatment) may be associated with an increased risk of arterial thrombotic events (for example myocardial infarction or stroke) (see section 4.4).

Respiratory, thoracic and mediastinal disorders: Respiratory tract reactivity (asthma, bronchospasm, dyspnoea).

Other adverse events reported less commonly and for which causality has not necessarily been established include:

Blood and lymphatic system disorders: Thrombocytopenia, neutropenia, agranulocytosis, aplastic anaemia and haemolytic anaemia.

Psychiatric disorders: Depression, confusional state, hallucination

Nervous system disorders: Cerebrovascular accident, optic neuritis, headache, paraesthesia, dizziness, and somnolence.

Aseptic meningitis (especially in patients with existing autoimmune disorders, such as systemic lupus erythematosus and mixed connective tissue disease) with symptoms of stiff neck, headache, nausea, vomiting, fever or disorientation) (see section 4.4).

Eye disorders: Visual disturbance

Ear and labyrinth disorders: Tinnitus, vertigo

Hepatobiliary disorders: Abnormal liver function, hepatitis and jaundice.

Skin and subcutaneous tissue disorders: Skin disorders including rash, pruritis, urticaria, purpura and very rarely, bullous dermatoses (including Stevens-Johnson syndrome, toxic epidermal necrolysis and erythema multiforme) and photosensitivity reaction.

Renal and urinary disorders: Toxic nephropathy in various forms, including interstitial nephritis, nephrotic syndrome and renal failure.

General disorders and administration site conditions: Malaise, fatigue

4.9 Overdose

Symptoms

Symptoms of overdosage may include headache, nausea, vomiting, epigastric pain, gastrointestinal bleeding, rarely diarrhoea, disorientation, excitation, coma, drowsiness, dizziness, tinnitus, fainting and occasionally convulsions. In cases of significant poisoning, acute renal failure and liver damage are possible.

Therapeutic measures

Patients should be treated symptomatically as required. Within one hour of ingestion of a potentially toxic amount, activated charcoal should be considered. Alternatively, in adults, gastric lavage should be considered within one hour of ingestion of a potentially life-threatening overdose.

Good urine output should be ensured.

Renal and liver function should be closely monitored.

Patients should be observed for at least four hours after ingestion of potentially toxic amounts.

Frequent or prolonged convulsions should be treated with intravenous diazepam. Other measures may be indicated by the patient's clinical condition.

5. PHARMACOLOGICAL PROPERTIES

5.1 Pharmacodynamic properties

Flurbiprofen has analgesic, anti-inflammatory and antipyretic properties. These are thought to result from the drug's ability to inhibit prostaglandin synthesis.

5.2 Pharmacokinetic properties

Flurbiprofen is readily absorbed from the gastrointestinal tract, with peak plasma concentrations occurring about 90 minutes after ingestion. It is about 99% protein-bound and has an elimination half-life of about three to four hours.

The rate of urinary excretion of flurbiprofen and its two major metabolites ([2-(2-fluoro-4′-hydroxy-4-biphenylyl) propionic acid] and [2-(2-fluoro-3′-hydroxy-4′-methoxy-4-biphenylyl) propionic acid]) in both free and conjugated states is similar for both the oral and rectal routes of administration. Metabolic patterns are quantitatively similar for both routes of administration.

5.3 Preclinical safety data

Not applicable.

6. PHARMACEUTICAL PARTICULARS

6.1 List of excipients

Maize starch powder EP, lactose NF anhydrous, povidone BPC, industrial alcohol FRP, magnesium stearate EP, stearic acid PDR BPC, *sandarac BPC 49 tablet varnish WMR, isopropyl alcohol, sucrose, purified water

Coat

Liquid glucose BPC 63, French chalk for tablets HSE, titanium dioxide BP, colloidal silicon dioxide NF, opalux yellow ASF 2230 HSE, carnauba wax PDR BP, **opacode S-1-8152HV black HSE

* Alternatively sandarac tablet varnish BPC 49

** Alternatively fine black ink markem

6.2 Incompatibilities

None known.

6.3 Shelf life

Blister pack: 36 months (unopened)

Bulk pack: 12 months (unopened)

6.4 Special precautions for storage

None for the blister pack.

Store in a cool, dry place for the bulk pack.

6.5 Nature and contents of container

A blister pack consisting of a PVC blister heat sealed to hard temper aluminium foil packed in a cardboard carton. Each blister contains 10 tablets.

Pack sizes: 10, 20, 30, 100 and 500 tablets. Also a sample pack of 5 tablets in a blister.

A bulk pack of a low density polyethylene bag in a rectangular white plastic tub having a snap-on lid.

Pack sizes: Approx. 25,000 or 50,000 tablets.

6.6 Special precautions for disposal and other handling

None stated.

7. MARKETING AUTHORISATION HOLDER

Abbott Laboratories Limited

Queenborough

Kent

ME11 5EL

United Kingdom

8. MARKETING AUTHORISATION NUMBER(S)

Froben Tablets 100 mg: PL 00037/0347

9. DATE OF FIRST AUTHORISATION/RENEWAL OF THE AUTHORISATION

31 December 2001

10. DATE OF REVISION OF THE TEXT

17 March 2009

Froben 50mg Tablets

(Abbott Laboratories Limited)

1. NAME OF THE MEDICINAL PRODUCT

Froben Tablets 50 mg

2. QUALITATIVE AND QUANTITATIVE COMPOSITION

Froben Tablets 50mg contain 50 mg Flurbiprofen BP.

3. PHARMACEUTICAL FORM

The tablets are sugar-coated and yellow in colour. They may be either unprinted or printed in black with an identifying motif.

4. CLINICAL PARTICULARS

4.1 Therapeutic indications

For the treatment of rheumatoid disease, osteoarthritis, ankylosing spondylitis, musculoskeletal disorders and trauma such as periarthritis, frozen shoulder, bursitis, tendinitis, tenosynovitis, low back pain, sprains and strains.

Froben is also indicated for its analgesic effect in the relief of mild to moderate pain in conditions such as dental pain, post-operative pain, dysmenorrhoea and migraine.

4.2 Posology and method of administration

For oral administration. To be taken preferably with or after food.

Undesirable effects may be minimised by using the lowest effective dose for the shortest duration necessary to control symptoms (see Section 4.4).

Adults:

150 to 200 mg daily in two, three or four divided doses. In patients with severe symptoms or disease of recent origin, or during acute exacerbations, the total daily dosage may be increased to 300 mg in divided doses.

For dysmenorrhoea, a dosage of 100 mg may be administered at the start of symptoms followed by 50 or 100 mg given at four- to six-hour intervals. The maximum total daily dosage should not exceed 300 mg.

Children:

Not recommended for use in children under 12 years.

Elderly:

The elderly are at increased risk of the serious consequences of adverse reactions. Although flurbiprofen is generally well tolerated in the elderly, some patients, especially those with impaired renal function, may eliminate NSAIDs more slowly than normal. In these cases, flurbiprofen should be used with caution and dosage should be assessed individually.

If an NSAID is considered necessary, the lowest effective dose should be used and for the shortest possible duration. The patient should be monitored regularly for GI bleeding during NSAID therapy.

4.3 Contraindications

Froben is contraindicated in patients with hypersensitivity (asthma, urticaria or allergic type) to flurbiprofen or to any of the inactive ingredients.

Froben is contraindicated in patients who have previously shown hypersensitivity reactions (*e.g.* asthma, rhinitis, angioedema or urticaria) in response to flurbiprofen, aspirin or other NSAIDs.

Froben is also contraindicated in patients with a history of gastrointestinal bleeding or perforation, related to previous NSAID therapy. Froben should not be used in patients with active, or history of, ulcerative colitis, Crohn's disease, recurrent peptic ulceration or gastrointestinal haemorrhage (defined as two or more distinct episodes of proven ulceration or bleeding).

Froben is contraindicated in patients with severe heart failure, hepatic failure and renal failure (see section 4.4).

Froben is contraindicated during the last trimester of pregnancy (see section 4.6).

4.4 Special warnings and precautions for use

Undesirable effects may be minimised by using the lowest effective dose for the shortest duration necessary to control symptoms (see Section 4.2 and GI and cardiovascular risks below).

Patients with rare hereditary problems of galactose intolerance, fructose intolerance, the Lapp lactose deficiency, sucrase-isomaltase insufficiency or glucose-galactose malabsorption should not take this medication.

The use of Froben with concomitant NSAIDs, including cyclooxygenase-2 selective inhibitors, should be avoided due to the potential for additive effects (see section 4.5).

Elderly

The elderly have an increased frequency of adverse reactions to NSAIDs, especially gastrointestinal bleeding and perforation, which may be fatal (see section 4.2).

Gastrointestinal bleeding, ulceration and perforation

GI bleeding, ulceration or perforation has been reported with all NSAIDs at any time during treatment. These adverse events can be fatal and may occur with or without warning symptoms or a previous history of serious GI events.

The risk of GI bleeding, ulceration or perforation is higher with increasing NSAID doses, in patients with a history of ulcers, particularly if complicated with haemorrhage or perforation (see section 4.3), and in the elderly. These patients should commence treatment on the lowest dose available. Combination therapy with protective agents (e.g. misoprostol or proton pump inhibitors) should be considered for these patients, and also for patients requiring concomitant low dose aspirin, or other drugs likely to increase gastrointestinal risk (see below and section 4.5).

Patients with a history of gastrointestinal disease, particularly when elderly, should report any unusual abdominal symptoms (especially gastrointestinal bleeding) particularly in the initial stages of treatment.

Caution should be advised in patients receiving concomitant medications which could increase the risk of ulceration or bleeding, such as oral corticosteroids, anticoagulants such as warfarin, selective serotonin-reuptake inhibitors or anti-platelet agents such as aspirin (see section 4.5).

When GI bleeding or ulceration occurs in patients receiving Froben, the treatment should be withdrawn.

Respiratory disorders

Caution is required if Froben is administered to patients suffering from, or with a previous history of, bronchial asthma since NSAIDs have been reported to precipitate bronchospasm in such patients.

Cardiovascular, renal and hepatic impairment

The administration of an NSAID may cause a dose dependent reduction in prostaglandin formation and precipitate renal failure. Patients at greatest risk of this reaction are those with impaired renal function, cardiac impairment, liver dysfunction, those taking diuretics and the elderly. Renal function should be monitored in these patients (see also section 4.3).

Froben should be given with care to patients with a history of heart failure or hypertension since oedema has been reported in association with flurbiprofen administration.

Cardiovascular and cerebrovascular effects

Appropriate monitoring and advice are required for patients with a history of hypertension and/or mild to moderate congestive heart failure as fluid retention and oedema have been reported in association with flurbiprofen administration and NSAID therapy.

Clinical trial and epidemiological data suggest that use of some NSAIDs (particularly at high doses and in long term treatment) may be associated with a small increased risk of arterial thrombotic events such as myocardial infarction or stroke. There are insufficient data to exclude such a risk for flurbiprofen.

Patients with uncontrolled hypertension, congestive heart failure, established ischaemic heart disease, peripheral arterial disease, and/or cerebrovascular disease should only be treated with flurbiprofen after careful consideration. Similar consideration should be made before initating longer-term treatment of patients with risk factors for cardiovascular disease (eg hypertension, hyperlipidaemia, diabetes mellitus, smoking).

Renal effects

Caution should be used when initiating treatment with NSAIDs such as flurbiprofen in patients with considerable dehydration.

SLE and mixed connective tissue disease

In patients with systemic lupus erythematosus (SLE) and mixed connective tissue disorders there may be an increased risk of aseptic meningitis (see section 4.8).

Dermatological effects

Serious skin reactions, some of them fatal, including exfoliative dermatitis, Stevens-Johnson syndrome and toxic epidermal necrolysis, have been reported very rarely in association with the use of NSAIDs (see section 4.8). Patients appear to be at highest risk of these reactions early in the course of therapy. In the majority of cases, the onset of the reaction occurs within the first month of treatment. Froben should be discontinued at the first appearance of skin rash, mucosal lesions or any other signs of hypersensitivity.

Haematological effects

Flurbiprofen, like other NSAIDs, may inhibit platelet aggregation and prolong bleeding time. Froben should be used with caution in patients with a potential for abnormal bleeding.

Impaired female fertility

The use of Froben may impair female fertility and is not recommended in women attempting to conceive. In women who have difficulties conceiving or who are undergoing investigation of infertility, withdrawal of Froben should be considered.

4.5 Interaction with other medicinal products and other forms of interaction

Care should be taken in patients treated with any of the following drugs as interactions have been reported in some patients.

Diuretics, ACE inhibitors and Angiotensin II Antagonists: NSAIDs may reduce the effect of diuretics and other antihypertensive drugs. In some patients with compromised renal function (e.g. dehydrated patients or elderly patients with compromised renal function) the co-administration of an ACE inhibitor or Angiotensin II antagonist and agents that inhibit cyclo-oxygenase may result in further deterioration of renal function, including possible acute renal failure, which is usually reversible. These interactions should be considered in patients taking flurbiprofen concomitantly with ACE inhibitors or angiotensin II antagonists. Therefore, the combination should be administered with caution, especially in the elderly. Patients should be adequately hydrated and consideration should be given to monitoring of renal function after initiation of concomitant therapy, and periodically thereafter.

Cardiac glycosides: NSAIDs may exacerbate cardiac failure, reduce GFR and increase plasma cardiac glycoside levels.

Anticoagulants: NSAIDs may enhance the effects of anticoagulants such as warfarin (see section 4.4).

Aspirin: As with other products containing NSAIDs, concomitant administration of flurbiprofen and aspirin is not generally recommended because of the potential of increased adverse effects.

Anti-platelet agents: Increased risk of gastrointestinal bleeding (see section 4.4).

Selective serotonin reuptake inhibitors (SSRIs): Increased risk of gastrointestinal bleeding with NSAIDs (see section 4.4).

Lithium salts: Decreased elimination of lithium.

Methotrexate: Caution is advised in the concomitant administration of flurbiprofen and methotrexate since NSAIDs may increase methotrexate levels.

Ciclosporin: Increased risk of nephrotoxicity.

Corticosteroids: Increased risk of gastrointestinal ulceration or bleeding with NSAIDs (see section 4.4).

Other analgesics and cyclooxygenase-2 selective inhibitors: Avoid concomitant use of two or more NSAIDs, including Cox-2 inhibitors, as this may increase the risk of adverse effects (see section 4.4).

Quinolone antibiotics: Animal data indicate that NSAIDs can increase the risk of convulsions associated with quinolone antibiotics. Patients taking NSAIDs and quinolones may have an increased risk of developing convulsions.

Mifepristone: NSAIDs should not be used for 8-12 days after mifepristone administration as NSAIDs can reduce the effects of mifepristone.

Tacrolimus: Possible increased risk of nephrotoxicity when NSAIDs are given with tacrolimus.

Zidovudine: Increased risk of haematological toxicity when NSAIDs are given with zidovudine. There is evidence of an increased risk of haemarthroses and haematoma in HIV(+) haemophiliacs receiving concurrent treatment with zidovudine and other NSAIDs.

Studies have failed to show any interaction between flurbiprofen and tolbutamide or antacids. There is no evidence so far that flurbiprofen interferes with standard laboratory tests.

4.6 Pregnancy and lactation

Pregnancy

Inhibition of prostaglandin synthesis may adversely affect the pregnancy and/or the embryo/foetal development. Data from epidemiological studies suggest an increased risk of miscarriage and of cardiac malformation and gastroschisis after use of a prostaglandin synthesis inhibitor in early pregnancy. The absolute risk for cardiovascular malformation was increased from less than 1%, up to approximately 1.5 %. The risk is believed to increase with dose and duration of therapy. In animals, administration of a prostaglandin synthesis inhibitor has been shown to result in increased pre- and post-implantation loss and embryo-foetal lethality. In addition, increased incidences of various malformations, including cardiovascular, have been reported in animals given a prostaglandin synthesis inhibitor during the organogenetic period. During the first and second trimester of pregnancy, flurbiprofen should not be given unless clearly necessary. If flurbiprofen is used by a woman attempting to conceive, or during the first and second trimester of pregnancy, the dose should be kept as low and duration of treatment as short as possible.

During the third trimester of pregnancy, all prostaglandin synthesis inhibitors may expose the foetus to:

• cardiopulmonary toxicity (with premature closure of the ductus arteriosus and pulmonary hypertension);

• renal dysfunction, which may progress to renal failure with oligo-hydroamniosis;

the mother and the neonate, at the end of pregnancy, to:

• possible prolongation of bleeding time, an anti-aggregating effect which may occur even at very low doses.

• inhibition of uterine contractions resulting in delayed or prolonged labour.

Consequently, flurbiprofen is contraindicated during the third trimester of pregnancy.

Lactation

In the limited studies so far available, NSAIDs can appear in the breast milk in very low concentrations. NSAIDs should, if possible, be avoided when breastfeeding.

See section 4.4 Special warnings and precautions for use, regarding female fertility.

4.7 Effects on ability to drive and use machines

Undesirable effects such as dizziness, drowsiness, fatigue and visual disturbances are possible after taking NSAIDs. If affected, patients should not drive or operate machinery.

4.8 Undesirable effects

Gastrointestinal disorders: The most commonly observed adverse events are gastrointestinal in nature. Peptic ulcers, perforation or GI bleeding, sometimes fatal, particularly in the elderly, may occur (see section 4.4). Nausea, vomiting, diarrhoea, dyspepsia, flatulence, constipation, abdominal pain, melaena, haematemesis, ulcerative stomatitis, exacerbation of colitis and Crohn's disease (see section 4.3 and 4.4) have been reported following flurbiprofen administration. Less frequently, gastritis, has been observed. Pancreatitis has been reported very rarely.

Immune system disorders: Hypersensitivity reactions have been reported following treatment with NSAIDs. These may consist of (a) non-specific allergic reactions and anaphylaxis, (b) respiratory tract reactivity comprising asthma, aggravated asthma, bronchospasm or dyspnoea, or (c) assorted skin disorders, including rashes of various types, pruritus, urticaria, purpura, angioedema and, more rarely exfoliative and bullous dermatoses (including toxic epidermal necrolysis and erythema multiforme).

Cardiac disorders and Vascular disorders: Oedema, hypertension and cardiac failure have been reported in association with NSAID treatment.

Clinical trial and epidemiological data suggest that use of some NSAIDs (particularly at high doses and in long term treatment) may be associated with an increased risk of arterial thrombotic events (for example myocardial infarction or stroke) (see section 4.4).

Respiratory, thoracic and mediastinal disorders: Respiratory tract reactivity (asthma, bronchospasm, dyspnoea).

Other adverse events reported less commonly and for which causality has not necessarily been established include:

Blood and lymphatic system disorders: Thrombocytopenia, neutropenia, agranulocytosis, aplastic anaemia and haemolytic anaemia.

Psychiatric disorders: Depression, confusional state, hallucination

Nervous system disorders: Cerebrovascular accident, optic neuritis, headache, paraesthesia, dizziness, and somnolence.

Aseptic meningitis (especially in patients with existing autoimmune disorders, such as systemic lupus erythematosus and mixed connective tissue disease) with symptoms of stiff neck, headache, nausea, vomiting, fever or disorientation) (see section 4.4).

Eye disorders: Visual disturbance

Ear and labyrinth disorders: Tinnitus, vertigo

Hepatobiliary disorders: Abnormal liver function, hepatitis and jaundice.

Skin and subcutaneous tissue disorders: Skin disorders including rash, pruritis, urticaria, purpura and very rarely, bullous dermatoses (including Stevens-Johnson syndrome, toxic epidermal necrolysis and erythema multiforme) and photosensitivity reaction.

Renal and urinary disorders: Toxic nephropathy in various forms, including interstitial nephritis, nephrotic syndrome and renal failure.

General disorders and administration site conditions: Malaise, fatigue

4.9 Overdose

Symptoms

Symptoms of overdosage may include headache, nausea, vomiting, epigastric pain, gastrointestinal bleeding, rarely diarrhoea, disorientation, excitation, coma, drowsiness, dizziness, tinnitus, fainting and occasionally convulsions. In cases of significant poisoning, acute renal failure and liver damage are possible.

Therapeutic measures

Patients should be treated symptomatically as required. Within one hour of ingestion of a potentially toxic amount, activated charcoal should be considered. Alternatively, in adults, gastric lavage should be considered within one hour of ingestion of a potentially life-threatening overdose.

Good urine output should be ensured.

Renal and liver function should be closely monitored.

Patients should be observed for at least four hours after ingestion of potentially toxic amounts.

Frequent or prolonged convulsions should be treated with intravenous diazepam. Other measures may be indicated by the patient's clinical condition.

5. PHARMACOLOGICAL PROPERTIES

5.1 Pharmacodynamic properties

Flurbiprofen has analgesic, anti-inflammatory and antipyretic properties. These are thought to result from the drug's ability to inhibit prostaglandin synthesis.

5.2 Pharmacokinetic properties

Flurbiprofen is readily absorbed from the gastrointestinal tract, with peak plasma concentrations occurring about 90 minutes after ingestion. It is about 99% protein-bound and has an elimination half-life of about three to four hours.

The rate of urinary excretion of flurbiprofen and its two major metabolites ([2-(2-fluoro-4′-hydroxy-4-biphenylyl) propionic acid] and [2-(2-fluoro-3′-hydroxy-4′-methoxy-4-biphenylyl) propionic acid]) in both free and conjugated states is similar for both the oral and rectal routes of administration. Metabolic patterns are quantitatively similar for both routes of administration.

5.3 Preclinical safety data

Not applicable.

6. PHARMACEUTICAL PARTICULARS

6.1 List of excipients

Maize starch powder EP, lactose NF anhydrous, povidone BPC, industrial alcohol FRP, magnesium stearate EP, stearic acid PDR BPC, *sandarac BPC 49 tablet varnish WMR, isopropyl alcohol, sucrose, purified water

Coat

Liquid glucose BPC 63, French chalk for tablets HSE, titanium dioxide BP, colloidal silicon dioxide NF, opalux yellow ASF 2230 HSE, carnauba wax PDR BP, **opacode S-1-8152HV black HSE

* Alternatively sandarac tablet varnish BPC 49

** Alternatively fine black ink markem

6.2 Incompatibilities

None known.

6.3 Shelf life

Blister pack: 36 months (unopened)

Bulk pack: 12 months (unopened)

6.4 Special precautions for storage

None for the blister pack.

Store in a cool, dry place for the bulk pack.

6.5 Nature and contents of container

A blister pack consisting of a PVC blister heat sealed to hard temper aluminium foil packed in a cardboard carton. Each blister contains 10 tablets.

Pack sizes: 10, 20, 30, 100 and 500 tablets. Also a sample pack of 5 tablets in a blister.

A bulk pack of a low density polyethylene bag in a rectangular white plastic tub having a snap-on lid.

Pack sizes: Approx. 25,000 or 50,000 tablets.

6.6 Special precautions for disposal and other handling

None stated.

7. MARKETING AUTHORISATION HOLDER

Abbott Laboratories Limited

Queenborough

Kent

ME11 5EL

United Kingdom

8. MARKETING AUTHORISATION NUMBER(S)

Froben Tablets 50 mg: PL 00037/0349

9. DATE OF FIRST AUTHORISATION/RENEWAL OF THE AUTHORISATION

31 December 2001

10. DATE OF REVISION OF THE TEXT

17 March 2009

Froben SR

(Abbott Laboratories Limited)

1. NAME OF THE MEDICINAL PRODUCT

Froben SR Slow-Release Capsule 200mg

2. QUALITATIVE AND QUANTITATIVE COMPOSITION

Flurbiprofen (milled) HSE 200.0mg.

3. PHARMACEUTICAL FORM

A hard geletine capsule with a yellow opaque cap and a transparent yellow body.

4. CLINICAL PARTICULARS

4.1 Therapeutic indications

Froben is indicated for the treatment of rheumatoid disease, osteoarthritis, ankylosing spondylitis, musculoskeletal disorders and trauma such as periarthritis; frozen shoulder, bursitis, tendinitis, tenosynovitis, low back pain, sprains and strains.

4.2 Posology and method of administration

For oral administration. To be taken preferably with or after food.

Undesirable effects may be minimised by using the lowest effective dose for the shortest duration necessary to control symptoms (see section 4.4).

Adult: The recommended daily dose is one 200 mg capsule taken preferably in the evening with or after food.

Children: Paediatric dosage not established. For this reason, Froben SR is not recommended for use in children under 12 years.

Elderly: The elderly are at increased risk of the serious consequences of adverse reactions. Although flurbiprofen is generally well tolerated in the elderly, some patients, especially those with impaired renal function, may eliminate NSAIDs more slowly than normal. In these cases, flurbiprofen should be used with caution and dosage should be assessed individually.

If an NSAID is considered necessary, the lowest effective dose should be used and for the shortest possible duration. The patient should be monitored regularly for GI bleeding during NSAID therapy.

4.3 Contraindications

Froben is contraindicated in patients with hypersensitivity (asthma, urticaria or allergic type) to flurbiprofen or to any of the inactive ingredients.

Froben is contraindicated in patients who have previously shown hypersensitivity reactions (*e.g.* asthma, rhinitis, angioedema or urticaria) in response to flurbiprofen, aspirin or other NSAIDs.

Froben is also contraindicated in patients with a history of gastrointestinal bleeding or perforation, related to previous NSAID therapy. Froben should not be used in patients with active, or history of, ulcerative colitis, Crohn's disease, recurrent peptic ulceration or gastrointestinal haemorrhage (defined as two or more distinct episodes of proven ulceration or bleeding).

Froben is contraindicated in patients with severe heart failure, hepatic failure and renal failure (see section 4.4).

Froben is contraindicated during the last trimester of pregnancy (see section 4.6).

4.4 Special warnings and precautions for use

Undesirable effects may be minimised by using the lowest effective dose for the shortest duration necessary to control symptoms (see Section 4.2 and GI and cardiovascular risks below).

The use of Froben with concomitant NSAIDs, including cyclooxygenase-2 selective inhibitors, should be avoided due to the potential for additive effects (see section 4.5).

Elderly

The elderly have an increased frequency of adverse reactions to NSAIDs, especially gastrointestinal bleeding and perforation, which may be fatal (see section 4.2).

Gastrointestinal bleeding, ulceration and perforation

GI bleeding, ulceration or perforation has been reported with all NSAIDs at any time during treatment. These adverse events can be fatal and may occur with or without warning symptoms or a previous history of serious GI events.

The risk of GI bleeding, ulceration or perforation is higher with increasing NSAID doses, in patients with a history of ulcers, particularly if complicated with haemorrhage or perforation (see section 4.3), and in the elderly. These patients should commence treatment on the lowest dose available. Combination therapy with protective agents (e.g. misoprostol or proton pump inhibitors) should be considered for these patients, and also for patients requiring concomitant low dose aspirin, or other drugs likely to increase gastrointestinal risk (see below and section 4.5).

Patients with a history of gastrointestinal disease, particularly when elderly, should report any unusual abdominal symptoms (especially gastrointestinal bleeding) particularly in the initial stages of treatment.

Caution should be advised in patients receiving concomitant medications which could increase the risk of ulceration or bleeding, such as oral corticosteroids, anticoagulants such as warfarin, selective serotonin-reuptake inhibitors or anti-platelet agents such as aspirin (see section 4.5).

When GI bleeding or ulceration occurs in patients receiving Froben, the treatment should be withdrawn.

Respiratory disorders

Caution is required if Froben is administered to patients suffering from, or with a previous history of, bronchial asthma since NSAIDs have been reported to precipitate bronchospasm in such patients.

Cardiovascular, renal and hepatic impairment

The administration of an NSAID may cause a dose dependent reduction in prostaglandin formation and precipitate renal failure. Patients at greatest risk of this reaction are those with impaired renal function, cardiac impairment, liver dysfunction, those taking diuretics and the elderly. Renal function should be monitored in these patients (see also section 4.3).

Froben should be given with care to patients with a history of heart failure or hypertension since oedema has been reported in association with flurbiprofen administration.

Cardiovascular and cerebrovascular effects

Appropriate monitoring and advice are required for patients with a history of hypertension and/or mild to moderate congestive heart failure as fluid retention and oedema have been reported in association with flurbiprofen administration and NSAID therapy.

Clinical trial and epidemiological data suggest that use of some NSAIDs (particularly at high doses and in long term treatment) may be associated with a small increased risk of arterial thrombotic events such as myocardial infarction or stroke. There are insufficient data to exclude such a risk for flurbiprofen.

Patients with uncontrolled hypertension, congestive heart failure, established ischaemic heart disease, peripheral arterial disease, and/or cerebrovascular disease should only be treated with flurbiprofen after careful consideration. Similar consideration should be made before initating longer-term treatment of patients with risk factors for cardiovascular disease (eg hypertension, hyperlipidaemia, diabetes mellitus, smoking).

Renal effects

Caution should be used when initiating treatment with NSAIDs such as flurbiprofen in patients with considerable dehydration.

SLE and mixed connective tissue disease

In patients with systemic lupus erythematosus (SLE) and mixed connective tissue disorders there may be an increased risk of aseptic meningitis (see section 4.8).

Dermatological effects

Serious skin reactions, some of them fatal, including exfoliative dermatitis, Stevens-Johnson syndrome and toxic epidermal necrolysis, have been reported very rarely in association with the use of NSAIDs (see section 4.8). Patients appear to be at highest risk of these reactions early in the course of therapy, the onset of the reaction occurring within the first month of treatment in the majority of cases. Froben should be discontinued at the first appearance of skin rash, mucosal lesions or any other sign of hypersensitivity.

Haematological effects

Flurbiprofen, like other NSAIDs, may inhibit platelet aggregation and prolong bleeding time. Froben should be used with caution in patients with a potential for abnormal bleeding.

Impaired female fertility

The use of Froben may impair female fertility and is not recommended in women attempting to conceive. In women who have difficulties conceiving or who are undergoing investigation of infertility, withdrawal of Froben should be considered.

4.5 Interaction with other medicinal products and other forms of interaction

Care should be taken in patients treated with any of the following drugs as interactions have been reported in some patients.

Diuretics, ACE inhibitors and Angiotensin II Antagonists: NSAIDs may reduce the effect of diuretics and other antihypertensive drugs. In some patients with compromised renal function (e.g. dehydrated patients or elderly patients with compromised renal function) the co-administration of an ACE inhibitor or Angiotensin II antagonist and agents that inhibit cyclo-oxygenase may result in further deterioration of renal function, including possible acute renal failure, which is usually reversible. These interactions should be considered in patients taking flurbiprofen concomitantly with ACE inhibitors or angiotensin II antagonists. Therefore, the combination should be administered with caution, especially in the elderly. Patients should be adequately hydrated and consideration should be given to monitoring of renal function after initiation of concomitant therapy, and periodically thereafter.

Cardiac glycosides: NSAIDs may exacerbate cardiac failure, reduce GFR and increase plasma cardiac glycoside levels.

Anticoagulants: NSAIDs may enhance the effects of anticoagulants such as warfarin (see section 4.4).

Aspirin: As with other products containing NSAIDs, concomitant administration of flurbiprofen and aspirin is not generally recommended because of the potential of increased adverse effects.

Anti-platelet agents: Increased risk of gastrointestinal bleeding (see section 4.4).

Selective serotonin reuptake inhibitors (SSRIs): Increased risk of gastrointestinal bleeding with NSAIDs (see section 4.4).

Lithium salts: Decreased elimination of lithium.

Methotrexate: Caution is advised in the concomitant administration of flurbiprofen and methotrexate since NSAIDs may increase methotrexate levels.

Ciclosporin: Increased risk of nephrotoxicity.

Corticosteroids: Increased risk of gastrointestinal ulceration or bleeding with NSAIDs (see section 4.4).

Other analgesics and cyclooxygenase-2 selective inhibitors: Avoid concomitant use of two or more NSAIDs, including Cox-2 inhibitors, as this may increase the risk of adverse effects (see section 4.4).

Quinolone antibiotics: Animal data indicate that NSAIDs can increase the risk of convulsions associated with quinolone antibiotics. Patients taking NSAIDs and quinolones may have an increased risk of developing convulsions.

Mifepristone: NSAIDs should not be used for 8-12 days after mifepristone administration as NSAIDs can reduce the effects of mifepristone.

Tacrolimus: Possible increased risk of nephrotoxicity when NSAIDs are given with tacrolimus.

Zidovudine: Increased risk of haematological toxicity when NSAIDs are given with zidovudine. There is evidence of an increased risk of haemarthroses and haematoma in HIV(+) haemophiliacs receiving concurrent treatment with zidovudine and other NSAIDs.

Studies have failed to show any interaction between flurbiprofen and tolbutamide or antacids. There is no evidence so far that flurbiprofen interferes with standard laboratory tests.

4.6 Pregnancy and lactation

Pregnancy

Inhibition of prostaglandin synthesis may adversely affect the pregnancy and/or the embryo/foetal development. Data from epidemiological studies suggest an increased risk of miscarriage and of cardiac malformation and gastroschisis after use of a prostaglandin synthesis inhibitor in early pregnancy. The absolute risk for cardiovascular malformation was increased from less than 1%, up to approximately 1.5 %. The risk is believed to increase with dose and duration of therapy. In animals, administration of a prostaglandin synthesis inhibitor has been shown to result in increased pre- and post-implantation loss and embryo-foetal lethality. In addition, increased incidences of various malformations, including cardiovascular, have been reported in animals given a prostaglandin synthesis inhibitor during the organogenetic period. During the first and second trimester of pregnancy, flurbiprofen should not be given unless clearly necessary. If flurbiprofen is used by a woman attempting to conceive, or during the first and second trimester of pregnancy, the dose should be kept as low and duration of treatment as short as possible.

During the third trimester of pregnancy, all prostaglandin synthesis inhibitors may expose the foetus to:

- cardiopulmonary toxicity (with premature closure of the ductus arteriosus and pulmonary hypertension);
- renal dysfunction, which may progress to renal failure with oligo-hydroamniosis;

the mother and the neonate, at the end of pregnancy, to:

- possible prolongation of bleeding time, an anti-aggregating effect which may occur even at very low doses.
- inhibition of uterine contractions resulting in delayed or prolonged labour.

Consequently, flurbiprofen is contraindicated during the third trimester of pregnancy.

Lactation

In the limited studies so far available, NSAIDs can appear in the breast milk in very low concentrations. NSAIDs should, if possible, be avoided when breastfeeding.

See section 4.4 Special warnings and precautions for use, regarding female fertility.

4.7 Effects on ability to drive and use machines

Undesirable effects such as dizziness, drowsiness, fatigue and visual disturbances are possible after taking NSAIDs. If affected, patients should not drive or operate machinery.

4.8 Undesirable effects

Gastrointestinal disorders: The most commonly observed adverse events are gastrointestinal in nature. Peptic ulcers, perforation or GI bleeding, sometimes fatal, particularly in the elderly, may occur (see section 4.4). Nausea, vomiting, diarrhoea, dyspepsia, flatulence, constipation, abdominal pain, melaena, haematemesis, ulcerative stomatitis, exacerbation of colitis and Crohn's disease (see section 4.3 and 4.4) have been reported following flurbiprofen administration. Less frequently, gastritis, has been observed. Pancreatitis has been reported very rarely.

Immune system disorders: Hypersensitivity reactions have been reported following treatment with NSAIDs. These may consist of (a) non-specific allergic reactions and anaphylaxis, (b) respiratory tract reactivity comprising asthma, aggravated asthma, bronchospasm or dyspnoea, or (c) assorted skin disorders, including rashes of various types, pruritus, urticaria, purpura, angioedema and, more rarely exfoliative and bullous dermatoses (including toxic epidermal necrolysis and erythema multiforme).

Cardiac disorders and Vascular disorders: Oedema, hypertension and cardiac failure have been reported in association with NSAID treatment.

Clinical trial and epidemiological data suggest that use of some NSAIDs (particularly at high doses and in long term treatment) may be associated with an increased risk of arterial thrombotic events (for example myocardial infarction or stroke) (see section 4.4).

Respiratory, thoracic and mediastinal disorders: Respiratory tract reactivity (asthma, bronchospasm, dyspnoea).

Other adverse events reported less commonly and for which causality has not necessarily been established include:

Blood and lymphatic system disorders: Thrombocytopenia, neutropenia, agranulocytosis, aplastic anaemia and haemolytic anaemia.

Psychiatric disorders: Depression, confusional state, hallucination

Nervous system disorders: Cerebrovascular accident, optic neuritis, headache, paraesthesia, dizziness, and somnolence.

Aseptic meningitis (especially in patients with existing autoimmune disorders, such as systemic lupus erythematosus and mixed connective tissue disease) with symptoms of stiff neck, headache, nausea, vomiting, fever or disorientation) (see section 4.4).

Eye disorders: Visual disturbance

Ear and labyrinth disorders: Tinnitus, vertigo

Hepatobiliary disorders: Abnormal liver function, hepatitis and jaundice.

Skin and subcutaneous tissue disorders: Skin disorders including rash, pruritis, urticaria, purpura and very rarely, bullous dermatoses (including Stevens-Johnson syndrome, toxic epidermal necrolysis and erythema multiforme) and photosensitivity reaction.

Renal and urinary disorders: Toxic nephropathy in various forms, including interstitial nephritis, nephrotic syndrome and renal failure.

General disorders and administration site conditions: Malaise, fatigue

4.9 Overdose

Symptoms

Symptoms of overdosage may include headache, nausea, vomiting, epigastric pain, gastrointestinal bleeding, rarely diarrhoea, disorientation, excitation, coma, drowsiness, dizziness, tinnitus, fainting and occasionally convulsions. In cases of significant poisoning, acute renal failure and liver damage are possible.

Therapeutic measures

Patients should be treated symptomatically as required. Within one hour of ingestion of a potentially toxic amount, activated charcoal should be considered. Alternatively, in adults, gastric lavage should be considered within one hour of ingestion of a potentially life-threatening overdose.

Good urine output should be ensured.

Renal and liver function should be closely monitored.

Patients should be observed for at least four hours after ingestion of potentially toxic amounts.

Frequent or prolonged convulsions should be treated with intravenous diazepam. Other measures may be indicated by the patient's clinical condition.

5. PHARMACOLOGICAL PROPERTIES

5.1 Pharmacodynamic properties

Flurbiprofen has analgesic, anti-inflammatory and antipyretic properties. These are thought to result from the drug's ability to inhibit prostaglandin synthesis.

5.2 Pharmacokinetic properties

Following oral administration, flurbiprofen in sustained-release formulation is readily absorbed from the gastrointestinal tract, with peak plasma concentrations occurring 4 to 6 hours after ingestion. It is approximately 99%

protein-bound and has an elimination half-life of about three to four hours.

The rate of urinary excretion of flurbiprofen and its two major metabolites ([2-(2-fluoro-4'hydroxy-4-biphenylyl) propionic acid] and [2-(2-fluoro-3'hydroxy-4'methoxy-4-biphenylyl) propionic acid]) in both free and conjugated states is the same for Froben SR as for the other oral forms of flurbiprofen. Metabolic patterns are the same for Froben SR as for the other oral forms of flurbiprofen.

5.3 Preclinical safety data
Not applicable.

6. PHARMACEUTICAL PARTICULARS

6.1 List of excipients
Microcrystalline Cellulose
Eudragit RS 100
Magnesium Stearate
Polyethylene Glycol 6000 (PDR)
Purified Water
Industrial Methylated Spirit
Colloidal Silicon Dioxide
Erythrosine
Quinoline Yellow
Red Iron Oxide Glycerin
Titanium Dioxide
Gelatin
Shellac
Soya Lecithin
Dimethylpolysiloxane
Black Iron Oxide
Purified Water
Industrial Methylated Spirit or Industrial Alcohol
2-Ethoxyethanol

6.2 Incompatibilities
None known.

6.3 Shelf life
36 months.

6.4 Special precautions for storage
None.

6.5 Nature and contents of container
White high density polyethylene bottle with a plastic screw-cap containing 4, 30 or 210 capsules

6.6 Special precautions for disposal and other handling
None stated.

7. MARKETING AUTHORISATION HOLDER
Abbott Laboratories Limited
Queenborough
Kent
ME11 5EL
United Kingdom

8. MARKETING AUTHORISATION NUMBER(S)
PL 00037/0353

9. DATE OF FIRST AUTHORISATION/RENEWAL OF THE AUTHORISATION
31 December 2001

10. DATE OF REVISION OF THE TEXT
17 March 2009

Frumil, Frumil LS

(sanofi-aventis)

1. NAME OF THE MEDICINAL PRODUCT
Frumil
Frumil LS

2. QUALITATIVE AND QUANTITATIVE COMPOSITION
The active ingredient is Furosemide 40.0mg and amiloride hydrochloride equivalent to 5.0mg anhydrous amiloride hydrochloride.

The active ingredient is Furosemide 20.0mg and amiloride hydrochloride equivalent to 2.5mg anhydrous amiloride hydrochloride.

For excipients, see section 6.1

3. PHARMACEUTICAL FORM
Tablets for oral administration.

4. CLINICAL PARTICULARS

4.1 Therapeutic indications
Frumil/Frumil LS is a potassium sparing diuretic which is indicated where a prompt diuresis is required. It is of particular value in conditions where potassium conservation is important: congestive cardiac failure, nephrosis, corticosteroid therapy, oestrogen therapy and for ascites associated with cirrhosis.

4.2 Posology and method of administration
Adults: One or two tablets to be taken in the morning.

Children: Not recommended for children under 18 years of age as safety and efficacy have not been established.

Elderly: The dosage should be adjusted according to the diuretic response; serum electrolytes and urea should be carefully monitored.

4.3 Contraindications
Patients with hypovolaemia or dehydration (with or without accompanying hypotension). Patients with an impaired renal function and a creatinine clearance below 30ml/min per 1.73 m^2 body surface area, anuria or renal failure with anuria not responding to furosemide, renal failure as a result of poisoning by nephrotoxic or hepatotoxic agents or renal failure associated with hepatic coma, hyperkalaemia, severe hypokalaemia, severe hyponatraemia, concomitant potassium supplements or potassium sparing diuretics, precomatose states associated with cirrhosis, Addison's disease, and breast feeding women.

Frumil/Frumil LS is contraindicated in children and adolescents under 18 years of age as safety in this age group has not yet been established.

Hypersensitivity to furosemide, amiloride, sulphonamides or sulphonamide derivatives, or any of the excipients of the product.

4.4 Special warnings and precautions for use
Frumil/Frumil LS should be discontinued before a glucose tolerance test.

Frumil/Frumil LS should be used with particular caution in elderly patients or those with potential obstruction of the urinary tract or disorders rendering electrolyte balance precarious.

Urinary output must be secured. Patients with partial obstruction of urinary outflow, for example patients with prostatic hypertrophy or impairment of micturition have an increased risk of developing acute retention and require careful monitoring.

Where indicated, steps should be taken to correct hypotension or hypovolaemia before commencing therapy.

Particularly careful monitoring is necessary in:

- patients with hypotension.
- patients who are at risk from a pronounced fall in blood pressure.
- patients where latent diabetes may become manifest or the insulin requirements of diabetic patients may increase.
- patients with gout.
- patients with hepatic cirrhosis together with impaired renal function.
- patients with hypoproteinaemia, e.g. associated with nephrotic syndrome (the effect of furosemide may be weakened and its ototoxicity potentiated). Cautious dose titration is required.

Caution should be observed in patients liable to electrolyte deficiency. Regular monitoring of serum sodium, potassium, creatinine and glucose is generally recommended during therapy; particularly close monitoring is required in patients at high risk of developing electrolyte imbalances or in case of significant additional fluid loss. Hypovolaemia or dehydration as well as any significant electrolyte and acid-base disturbances must be corrected. This may require temporary discontinuation of Frumil/Frumil LS.

Frequent checks of the serum potassium level are necessary in patients with impaired renal function and a creatinine clearance below 60ml/min per 1.73m^2 body surface area as well as in cases where Frumil/Frumil LS is taken in combination with certain other drugs which may lead to an increase in potassium levels.

In patients who are at high risk for radiocontrast nephropathy, furosemide is not recommended to be used for diuresis as part of the preventative measures against radiocontrast-induced nephropathy.

Patients with rare hereditary problems of galactose intolerance, the Lapp lactase deficiency or glucose-galactose malabsorption should not take this medicine.

4.5 Interaction with other medicinal products and other forms of interaction
The dosage of concurrently administered cardiac glycosides, diuretics, anti-hypertensive agents, or other drugs with blood-pressure-lowering potential may require adjustment as a more pronounced fall in blood pressure must be anticipated if given concomitantly with Frumil/Frumil LS. A marked fall in blood pressure and deterioration in renal function may be seen when ACE inhibitors or angiotensin II receptor antagonists are added to furosemide therapy, or their dose level increased. The dose of Frumil/Frumil LS should be reduced for at least three days, or the drug stopped, before initiating the ACE inhibitor or angiotensin II receptor antagonist or increasing their dose.

When amiloride is taken in combination with potassium salts, with drugs which reduce potassium excretion, with nonsteroidal anti-inflammatory drugs or with ACE inhibitors, an increase in serum potassium concentration and hyperkalaemia may occur.

The toxic effects of nephrotoxic drugs may be increased by concomitant administration of potent diuretics such as furosemide.

Oral Frumil/Frumil LS and sucralfate must not be taken within 2 hours of each other because sucralfate decreases the absorption of furosemide from the intestine and so reduces its effect.

In common with other diuretics, serum lithium levels may be increased when lithium is given concomitantly with Frumil/Frumil LS, resulting in increased lithium toxicity, including increased risk of cardiotoxic and neurotoxic effects of lithium. Therefore, it is recommended that lithium levels are carefully monitored and where necessary the lithium dosage is adjusted in patients receiving this combination.

Certain non-steroidal anti-inflammatory agents (e.g. indometacin, acetylsalicylic acid) may attenuate the action of Frumil/Frumil LS and may cause acute renal failure in cases of pre-existing hypovolaemia or dehydration. Salicylic toxicity may be increased by furosemide. Frumil/Frumil LS may sometimes attenuate the effects of other drugs (e.g. the effects of anti-diabetics and of pressor amines) and sometimes potentiate them (e.g. the effects of salicylates, theophylline and curare-type muscle relaxants).

Furosemide may potentiate the ototoxicity of aminoglycosides and other ototoxic drugs. Since this may lead to irreversible damage, these drugs must only be used with Frumil/Frumil LS if there are compelling medical reasons.

There is a risk of ototoxic effects if cisplatin and furosemide are given concomitantly. In addition, nephrotoxicity of cisplatin may be enhanced if furosemide is not given in low doses (e.g. 40 mg in patients with normal renal function) and with positive fluid balance when used to achieve forced diuresis during cisplatin treatment.

Amiloride may cause raised blood digoxin levels. Some electrolyte disturbances (e.g. hypokalaemia, hypomagnesaemia) may increase the toxicity of certain other drugs (e.g. digitalis preparations and drugs inducing QT interval prolongation syndrome).

Attenuation of the effect of Frumil/Frumil LS may occur following concurrent administration of phenytoin.

Concomitant administration of carbamazepine or aminoglutethimide may increase the risk of hyponatraemia.

Corticosteroids administered concurrently may cause sodium retention.

Corticosteroids, carbenoxolone, liquorice, B_2 sympathomimetics in large amounts, and prolonged use of laxatives, reboxetine and amphotericin may increase the risk of developing hypokalaemia.

Probenecid, methotrexate and other drugs which, like furosemide, undergo significant renal tubular secretion may reduce the effect of Frumil/Frumil LS. Conversely, furosemide may decrease renal elimination of these drugs. In case of high-dose treatment (in particular, of both furosemide and the other drugs), this may lead to increased serum levels and an increased risk of adverse effects due to furosemide or the concomitant medication.

Impairment of renal function may develop in patients receiving concurrent treatment with furosemide and high doses of certain cephalosporins

Concomitant use of ciclosporin and furosemide is associated with increased risk of gouty arthritis.

4.6 Pregnancy and lactation
Pregnancy:

Results of animal work, in general, show no hazardous effect of furosemide in pregnancy. There is clinical evidence of safety of the drug in the third trimester of human pregnancy; however, furosemide crosses the placental barrier. It must not be given during pregnancy unless there are compelling medical reasons. Treatment during pregnancy requires monitoring of foetal growth.

The safety of Amiloride Hydrochloride has not been established and is therefore not recommended for use during pregnancy.

Lactation:

Furosemide passes into breast milk and may inhibit lactation. It is not known whether Amiloride Hydrochloride is excreted in breast milk. Breastfeeding must be avoided during treatment with Frumil/Frumil LS.

4.7 Effects on ability to drive and use machines
None stated.

4.8 Undesirable effects
Frumil/Frumil LS Tablets are generally well tolerated.

Eosinophilia is rare.

Occasionally, thrombocytopenia may occur. In rare cases, leucopenia and, in isolated cases, agranulocytosis, aplastic anaemia or haemolytic anaemia may develop.

Bone marrow depression has been reported as a rare complication and necessitates withdrawal of treatment.

Rarely, paraesthesiae or hepatic encephalopathy in patients with hepatocellular insufficiency may occur.

Serum calcium levels may be reduced; in very rare cases tetany has been observed. Nephrocalcinosis / Nephrolithiasis has been reported in premature infants.

Serum cholesterol and triglyceride levels may rise during furosemide treatment. During long term therapy they will usually return to normal within six months.

Glucose tolerance may decrease with furosemide. In patients with diabetes mellitus this may lead to a deterioration of metabolic control; latent diabetes mellitus may become manifest.

Hearing disorders and tinnitus, although usually transitory, may occur in rare cases, particularly in patients with renal failure, hypoproteinaemia (e.g. in nephritic syndrome) and/or when intravenous furosemide has been given too rapidly.

Furosemide may cause a reduction in blood pressure which, if pronounced may cause signs and symptoms such as impairment of concentration and reactions, light-headedness, sensations of pressure in the head, headache, dizziness, drowsiness, weakness, disorders of vision, dry mouth, orthostatic intolerance.

In isolated cases, intrahepatic cholestasis, an increase in liver transaminases or acute pancreatitis may develop.

The incidence of allergic reactions, such as skin rashes, photosensitivity, vasculitis, fever, interstitial nephritis, or shock is very low, but when these occur treatment should be withdrawn. Skin and mucous membrane reactions may occasionally occur, e.g. itching, urticaria, other rashes or bullous lesions, erythema multiforme, bullous pemphigoid, exfoliative dermatitis, purpura.

As with other diuretics, electrolytes and water balance may be disturbed as a result of diuresis after prolonged therapy. Furosemide leads to increased excretion of sodium and chloride and consequently water. In addition excretion of other electrolytes (in particular potassium, calcium and magnesium) is increased. However, as treatment is continued, the serum potassium concentration may increase due to the later onset of action of amiloride, especially in patients with impaired renal function. Symptomatic electrolyte disturbances and metabolic alkalosis may develop in the form of a gradually increasing electrolyte deficit or, e.g. where higher furosemide doses are administered to patients with normal renal function, acute severe electrolyte losses, although amiloride may contribute to the development or aggravation of metabolic acidosis. Warning signs of electrolyte disturbances include increased thirst, headache, hypotension, confusion, muscle cramps, tetany, muscle weakness, disorders of cardiac rhythm and gastrointestinal symptoms. Disturbances of electrolyte balance, particularly if pronounced, must be corrected. Pre-existing metabolic alkalosis (e.g. in decompensated cirrhosis of the liver) may be aggravated by furosemide treatment.

Rare complications may include minor psychiatric disturbances.

The diuretic action of furosemide may lead to or contribute to hypovolaemia and dehydration, especially in elderly patients. Severe fluid depletion may lead to haemoconcentration with a tendency for thromboses to develop.

Increased production of urine may provoke or aggravate complaints in patients with an obstruction of urinary outflow. Thus, acute retention of urine with possible secondary complications may occur. for example, in patients with bladder-emptying disorders, prostatic hyperplasia or narrowing of the urethra.

If furosemide is administered to premature infants during the first weeks of life, it may increase the risk of persistence of patent ductus arteriosus.

Severe anaphylactic or anaphylactoid reactions (e.g. with shock) occur rarely.

Side-effects of a minor nature such as nausea, malaise or gastric upset (vomiting or diarrhoea) and constipation may occur but are not usually severe enough to necessitate withdrawal of treatment.

As with other diuretics, treatment with furosemide may lead to transitory increases in blood creatinine and urea levels. Serum levels of uric acid may increase and attacks of gout may occur.

4.9 Overdose

Treatment of overdosage should be aimed at reversing dehydration and correcting electrolyte imbalance, particularly hyperkalaemia. Emesis should be induced or gastric lavage performed. Treatment should be symptomatic and supportive.

If hyperkalaemia is seen, appropriate measures to reduce serum potassium must be instituted.

5. PHARMACOLOGICAL PROPERTIES

5.1 Pharmacodynamic properties

ATC code: CO3C A01

FUROSEMIDE:

Furosemide is a loop diuretic which acts primarily to inhibit electrolyte re-absorption in the thick ascending Loop of Henle. Excretion of sodium, potassium and chloride ions is increased and water excretion enhanced.

AMILORIDE:

Amiloride is a mild diuretic which moderately increases the excretion of sodium and chloride and reduces potassium excretion, and appears to act mainly on the distal renal tubules. It does not appear to act by inhibition of aldosterone and does not inhibit carbonic anhydrase. Amiloride adds to the natiuretic but diminishes the kaliuretic effect of other diuretics.

A combination of Furosemide and Amiloride is a diuretic which reduces the potassium loss of furosemide alone while avoiding the possible gastro-intestinal disturbances of potassium supplements.

5.2 Pharmacokinetic properties

FUROSEMIDE:

Approximately 65% of the dose is absorbed after oral administration. The plasma half-life is biphasic with a terminal elimination phase of about 1 ½ hours. Furosemide is up to 99% bound to plasma proteins and is mainly excreted in the urine, largely unchanged, but also excreted in the bile, non-renal elimination being considerably increased in renal failure. Furosemide crosses the placental barrier and is excreted in the milk.

AMILORIDE:

Approximately 50% of the dose is absorbed after oral administration and peak serum concentrations are achieved by about 3 - 4 hours. The serum half-life is estimated to be about 6 hours. Amiloride is not bound to plasma proteins. Amiloride is not metabolised and is excreted unchanged in the urine.

Pharmacokinetic studies have been completed on Frumil, a combination tablet of furosemide and amiloride which is of a higher strength than Frumil LS.

FUROSEMIDE

Cp MAX = 1/14 μg/ml SD = 0.67

Tmax = 3.0 hours

AUC = 3.17μg/ml hr SD = + 1.25

AMILORIDE

Cp MAX = 13.42 ng/ml SD = 5.74

Tmax = 4.0 hours

AUC = 154 ng/ml hr SD = + 65.2

5.3 Preclinical safety data

No further information available

6. PHARMACEUTICAL PARTICULARS

6.1 List of excipients

Frumil tablets contain the following excipients:

Lactose

Starch Maize

Microcrystalline Cellulose

Sodium Starch Glycollate

Sunset Yellow Dye (E110)

French Chalk Powdered

Colloidal Anhydrous Silica

Magnesium Stearate

Frumil LS tablets contain the following excipients:

Lactose

Starch Maize

Microcrystalline Cellulose

Sodium Starch Glycollate

Sunset Yellow Dye (E110)

French Chalk Powdered

Colloidal Anhydrous Silica

Magnesium Stearate

6.2 Incompatibilities

None stated

6.3 Shelf life

The shelf-life of Frumil and Frumil LS is 3 years.

6.4 Special precautions for storage

Store below 25°C in a dry place. Protect from light.

6.5 Nature and contents of container

PVC/Aluminium foil blisters (14's) in cartons with 28 or 56 tablets

6.6 Special precautions for disposal and other handling

None

7. MARKETING AUTHORISATION HOLDER

Sanofi-aventis
One Onslow Street
Guildford
Surrey
GU1 4YS
UK

8. MARKETING AUTHORISATION NUMBER(S)

Frumil PL 04425/0573

Frumil LS PL 04425/0574

9. DATE OF FIRST AUTHORISATION/RENEWAL OF THE AUTHORISATION

20th June 2006

10. DATE OF REVISION OF THE TEXT

18 June 2008

11. LEGAL CLASSIFICATION

POM

Frusene Tablets

(Orion Pharma (UK) Limited)

1. NAME OF THE MEDICINAL PRODUCT

Frusene Tablets

2. QUALITATIVE AND QUANTITATIVE COMPOSITION

Furosemide 40.0 mg

Triamterene 50.0 mg

For excipients, refer to 6.1.

3. PHARMACEUTICAL FORM

Tablet.

Pale-yellowish, convex, scored, uncoated tablet, diameter 9 mm.

4. CLINICAL PARTICULARS

4.1 Therapeutic indications

For the treatment of oedematous conditions, where a prompt diuresis is required and where potassium conservation is important: congestive heart failure, pulmonary oedema, cardiac oedema, hepatic oedema, and ascites.

A fixed ratio combination should only be used if titration with component drugs separately indicates that this product is appropriate.

4.2 Posology and method of administration

The dosage depends on individual requirements.

Tablets should be taken with a sufficient quantity of liquid, preferably one hour before food because concomitant intake of food can reduce the absorption of furosemide by 30%.

Adults:

The usual adult dose is ½ to 2 tablets, taken in the morning. Maximum daily dose is 6 tablets.

Children:

Not recommended for use in children.

Hepatic insufficiency:

Treatment must be initiated using a small dose with careful monitoring of the serum electrolyte concentrations (refer to section 4.4. Special warnings and precautions for use). The natriuretic potency of Furosemide may be weakened in patients with hepatic insufficiency but the kaliuretic potency usually remains. Elimination of triamterene is slowed down and its efficacy is increased in severe hepatic insufficiency.

4.3 Contraindications

Moderate or severe renal impairment (Creatinine Clearance < 25 ml/min). Hepatic coma and severe hepatic insufficiency. Anuria. Hyperkalaemia. Sodium depletion and accompanying hypovolemia. Hypersensitivity to Furosemide, triamterene or to the excipients of the preparation. Hypersensitivity to sulphonamides (because of cross-sensitivity between sulphonamides and furosemide.

4.4 Special warnings and precautions for use

Electrolyte balance of the patients receiving furosemide and triamterene must be monitored. More frequent and careful monitoring are required for the following patient groups: diabetics, patients with cardiac, renal or hepatic impairment and elderly patients. Of note, the risk of electrolyte disturbances can be increased even in mild renal failure. Hepatic failure and alcoholic cirrhosis particularly predispose to hypokalaemia and hypomagnesaemia. Refer to section 4.8 for details of electrolyte and metabolic abnormalities.

In elderly patients there is no requirement for dosage adjustments unless a clinically significant impairment of renal or hepatic function also exists. Creatinine and serum electrolytes should be monitored.

Diuretics must be administered carefully to avoid hypotension and circulatory collapse in patients with pulmonary oedema caused by acute myocardial infarction.

Daily weight loss should not exceed 1 kg daily to avoid relative intravascular dehydration; particular care is required in hepatic failure and ascites. Caution should also be exercised in the presence of liver disease as hepatic coma may be precipitated in susceptible cases.

Development of megaloblastic anaemia is possible in patients having folic acid deficiency (e.g. in hepatic cirrhosis). Triamterene may worsen this condition as it is a weak folic acid antagonist. In patients considered at risk, red cell folate levels should be measured and replacement given as appropriate.

Furosemide and, to a lesser extent, triamterene may predispose the patient to the development of hyperuricaemia and precipitate gout attacks (refer to section 4.8).

Acute diuresis may cause urinary retention in patients with urinary outflow obstruction (such as prostatic hyperplasia). Urinary output must be monitored in these patients.

Co-administration with nonsteriodal anti-inflammatory analgesics (NSAIDs) should be avoided wherever possible. Where this is not possible particularly careful monitoring is required to ensure that the diuretic effect is not attenuated (Refer to section 4.5)

Triamterene may cause blue discolouration of the urine.

4.5 Interaction with other medicinal products and other forms of interaction

Triamterene reduces the risk of hypokalaemia induced by use of furosemide. This is the rationale for using the two medications in a combination product.

Effect of drugs and other substances on Frusene

Drugs likely to increase the hypotensive effect:

ACE inhibitors, angiotensin receptor antagonists, beta-blockers, calcium-channel blockers, diuretics, nitrates, other antihypertensive drugs and other drugs such as dipyridamole, moxisylate, tizanidine, alprostadil.

Drugs likely to exacerbate hyponatraemia:

Diuretics, carbamazepine, aminoglutethamide, trimethoprim.

Table 1 Furosemide

Blood and lymphatic system disorders	Rare or very rare (<1/1000, including case reports)	bone marrow depression, aplastic anaemia, agranulocytosis, thrombocytopenia, haemolytic anaemia
Metabolism and nutrition disorders	Very common or common (>1/100)	dehydration*, hyponatraemia*, hypochloremic metabolic alkalosis*, hypokalaemia*, hypocalcaemia*, hypomagnesemia* (incidences of the last three are reduced by triamterene)
	Uncommon (>1/1,000, <1/100)	impaired glucose tolerance (by hypokalaemia)*, hyperuricaemia, gout, reduction of serum HDL-cholesterol, elevation of serum LDL-cholesterol, elevation of serum triglycerides
Nervous system disorders	Uncommon (>1/1,000, <1/100)	tiredness*, dizziness*, headache*, paresthesias*, restlessness*
Eye disorders	Uncommon (>1/1,000, <1/100)	visual disturbance*
Ear and labyrinth disorders	Rare or very rare (<1/1000, including case reports)	Tinnitus, reversible or irreversible loss of hearing (after large doses or prolonged use of Furosemide)
Cardiac disorders	Uncommon (>1/1,000, <1/100)	Cardiac arrhythmias*
Vascular disorders	Very common or common (>1/100)	decreased blood pressure*
	Uncommon (>1/1,000, <1/100)	hypotension*, hypovolaemia
	Rare or very rare (<1/1000, including case reports)	Vasculitis
Gastrointestinal disorders	Uncommon (>1/1,000, <1/100)	dry mouth*, thirst*, nausea*, bowel motility disturbances*
	Rare or very rare (<1/1000, including case reports)	Pancreatitis
Hepato-biliary disorders	Rare or very rare (<1/1000, including case reports)	Cholestasis
Skin and subcutaneous tissue disorders	Rare or very rare (<1/1000, including case reports)	Urticaria, purpura, *erythema multiforme*, exfoliative dermatitis, photosensitivity reactions
Musculoskeletal, connective tissue and bone disorders	Uncommon (>1/1,000, <1/100)	muscle cramps*
Renal and urinary disorders	Uncommon (>1/1,000, <1/100)	Reduced diuresis*, urinary incontinence, urinary obstruction (in patients with hyperplasia of the prostate)
	Rare or very rare (<1/1000, including case reports)	nephrocalcinosis (in pre-term infants treated with Furosemide), interstitial nephritis, acute renal failure
General disorders and administration site conditions	Uncommon (>1/1,000, <1/100)	fatigue*
	Rare or very rare (<1/1000, including case reports)	Fever

Table 2 Triamterene

Blood and lymphatic system disorders	Rare or very rare (<1/1000, including case reports)	megaloblastic anaemia, pancytopenia
Metabolism and nutrition disorders	Very common or common (>1/100)	hyperkalaemia (incidence is reduced by Furosemide)
	Uncommon (>1/1,000, <1/100)	hyperuricaemia
Nervous system disorders	Uncommon (>1/1,000, <1/100)	Headache
Vascular disorders	Uncommon (>1/1,000, <1/100)	hypovolaemia
Gastrointestinal disorders	Very common or common (>1/100)	nausea, vomiting, diarrhoea
	Uncommon (>1/1,000, <1/100)	dry mouth
Skin and subcutaneous tissue disorders	Uncommon (>1/1,000, <1/100)	Rashes
	Rare or very rare (<1/1000, including case reports)	photosensitivity reactions, pseudoporphyria
Renal and urinary disorders	Uncommon (>1/1,000, <1/100)	elevation of s-creatinine, transient renal insufficiency
	Rare or very rare (<1/1000, including case reports)	Interstitial nephritis, urinary stones
General disorders and administration site conditions	Rare or very rare (<1/1000, including case reports)	serum sickness

Drugs and other substances likely to exacerbate hypokalaemia:

Thiazide and loop diuretics, corticosteroids, glychyrrizin (contained in liquorice), amphotericin B.

Drugs and other substances likely to exacerbate hyperkalaemia:

Potassium salts or supplements, potassium-sparing diuretics (such as amiloride and spironolactone), ACE inhibitors, angiotensin receptor antagonists, ciclosporin, tacrolimus, trilostane and drosperinone.

Drugs and other substances likely to decrease the hypotensive and natriuretic effect:

Nonsteroidal anti-inflammatory analgesics (NSAIDs), probenecid, phenytoin, tobacco smoking. Cholestyramine and cholestipol prevent the absorption of Frusene, so they should be taken at different times, preferably 4 to 6 hours after Frusene administration.

Drugs likely to exacerbate nephrotoxicity:

Aminoglycoside and cephalosporin antibiotics, amphotericin B. Concomitant use of NSAIDs and Frusene increases the risk of acute renal failure (refer to section 4.4).

Drugs likely to exacerbate ototoxicity:

Aminoglycoside antibiotics, cisplatin.

Concomitant intake of food may reduce the absorption of furosemide by approximately 30%.

Effect of Frusene on other drugs

Frusene induced electrolyte disturbances (such as hypokalaemia) may predispose the patient to arrhythmogenic effect of other drugs (such as digoxin and drugs that prolong the QT interval). Effect of competitive muscle relaxants may also be reduced in hypokalaemia.

Frusene may reduce the elimination of lithium, phenobarbital, and amantadine causing toxic drug concentrations. Drug concentrations and/or signs of toxicity should be monitored in concomitant use and if Frusene is discontinued.

Frusene may reduce the efficacy of antihyperglycaemic medications. Adjustment of the dose of antihyperglycaemic medications may be needed in concomitant use.

Warfarin and clofibrate compete with Furosemide in the binding to serum albumin. This may have clinical significance in patients with low serum albumin levels (e.g. in nephrotic syndrome). Furosemide does not change the pharmacokinetics of warfarin to a significant extent, but the strong diuresis with associated dehydration may weaken the antithrombotic effect of warfarin.

4.6 Pregnancy and lactation

Furosemide crosses the placenta and has been shown to reduce placental circulation. It may predispose the foetus to hypercalciuria, nephrocalcinosis, and secondary hyperparathyroidism. Closure of the patent arterial duct can also be hindered after birth. Use of Furosemide in premature infants has led to development of sensorineural hearing loss. Triamterene crosses the placenta, but has not been associated with causing birth defects.

Furosemide and triamterene are excreted in the breast milk in small quantities and Furosemide may impair lactation.

Frusene Tablets should be used during pregnancy or lactation only if clearly needed.

4.7 Effects on ability to drive and use machines

Occasionally Frusene may cause hypotension, especially at the start of therapy. This may manifest itself as dizziness or faintness. If affected, avoid driving or the use of machinery.

4.8 Undesirable effects

Of the adverse events caused by Furosemide and triamterene, most are linked to the pharmacological effects of the compounds, and they are more common in patients with multiple illnesses or compromised physical condition.

Furosemide:

(see Table 1 opposite)

Triamterene:

(see Table 2 below)

4.9 Overdose

Symptoms of overdose include increased diuresis, natriuresis, hypovolaemia, and decrease of blood pressure (refer to section 4.8. Undesirable effects). After an overdose, activated charcoal should be administered as soon as possible to decrease absorption of the drug. Fluid and electrolyte balance must be monitored. Sodium chloride -infusion can be used to sustain blood pressure. Otherwise, the treatment is symptomatic.

5. PHARMACOLOGICAL PROPERTIES

5.1 Pharmacodynamic properties

Furosemide:

Furosemide is a potent diuretic with a rapid action. Its effects are evident within 1 hour after a dose by mouth and lasts for about 4 to 6 hours. It has been reported to exert inhibiting effects on electrolyte reabsorption in the proximal and distal renal tubules and in the ascending Loop of Henle.

Excretion of sodium, potassium and chloride ions is increased and water excretion enhanced.

Unlike thiazide diuretics where, owing to their flat dose-response curve, very little is gained by increasing the dose, furosemide has a steep dose-response curve, which gives it a wide therapeutic range.

Triamterene:

Triamterene is a mild diuretic which appears to mainly act on the distal renal tubules. It produces a diuresis in about 2 to 4 hours, reaching a maximum effect in about 6 hours. Triamterene adds to the natriuretic but diminishes the kaliuretic affects of other diuretics and is used as an adjunct to frusemide to conserve potassium, in the treatment of refractory oedema associated with hepatic cirrhosis, congestive heart failure and the nephrotic syndrome.

5.2 Pharmacokinetic properties

Furosemide:

Furosemide is incompletely but fairly rapidly absorbed from the gastrointestinal tract. It has a biphasic half-life in the plasma with a terminal elimination phase that has been estimated to range up to about 1½ hours. It is up to 99% bound to plasma proteins and is mainly excreted in the urine, largely unchanged, but also in the form of the glucuronide and free amine metabolites. Variable amounts are also excreted in the bile, non renal elimination being considerably increased in renal failure. Furosemide crosses the placental barrier and is excreted in the breast milk.

Triamterene:

Triamterene is incompletely but fairly rapidly absorbed from the gastrointestinal tract. It has been estimated to have a plasma half-life of about 2 hours. It is extensively metabolised and is excreted in the urine in the form of metabolites with some unchanged triamterene. Variable amounts are also excreted in the bile. Animal studies have indicated that triamterene crosses the placental barrier and is excreted in the breast milk.

5.3 Preclinical safety data
None stated

6. PHARMACEUTICAL PARTICULARS
6.1 List of excipients
Lactose monohydrate
Corn starch
Starch, pregelatinised
Polysorbate 80
Gelatin
Sodium starch glycolate
Magnesium stearate

6.2 Incompatibilities
Not applicable.

6.3 Shelf life
5 years.

6.4 Special precautions for storage
Do not store above 30 °C. Store in the original container.

6.5 Nature and contents of container
PVC-Al-foil blister strip, 14 or 56 tablets.
PE-bottle with LDPE snap cap, 28, 100, or 1000 tablets.
PE-bottle with HDPE screw cap, 100 tablets.

6.6 Special precautions for disposal and other handling
No special instructions.

7. MARKETING AUTHORISATION HOLDER
Orion Corporation
P.O. Box 65
FIN-02200, Espoo
Finland

8. MARKETING AUTHORISATION NUMBER(S)
PL 27925/0007

9. DATE OF FIRST AUTHORISATION/RENEWAL OF THE AUTHORISATION
20 December 1996 /

10. DATE OF REVISION OF THE TEXT
July 2006

Frusol 20mg/5ml Oral Solution

(Rosemont Pharmaceuticals Limited)

1. NAME OF THE MEDICINAL PRODUCT
Frusol 20mg/5ml Oral Solution

2. QUALITATIVE AND QUANTITATIVE COMPOSITION
Furosemide Ph.Eur 20mg/5ml

3. PHARMACEUTICAL FORM
Oral Solution

4. CLINICAL PARTICULARS
4.1 Therapeutic indications
Furosemide is indicated in all conditions requiring prompt diuresis, including cardiac, pulmonary, hepatic and renal oedema, peripheral oedema due to mechanical obstruction or venous insufficiency and hypertension.

It is also indicated for the maintenance therapy of mild oedema of any origin.

4.2 Posology and method of administration
This liquid should only be taken orally.

The medication should be administered in the morning to avoid nocturnal diuresis.

Adults: The usual initial daily dose is 40mg. This may be adjusted until an effective dose is achieved.

Children: 1 to 3mg/Kg body weight daily up to a maximum total dose of 40mg/day.

Elderly: In the elderly, Furosemide is generally eliminated more slowly. Dosage should be titrated until the required response is achieved.

4.3 Contraindications
Hypovolaemia or dehydration. Anuria. Renal failure with anuria not responding to furosemide, or as a result of poisoning by nephrotoxic or hepatotoxic agents, or associated with hepatic coma. Severe hyperkalaemia, severe hyponatraemia. Pre-comatose and comatose states associated with hepatic encephalopathy. Breast feeding.

Contra-indicated in hypersensitivity to Furosemide, sulphonamides or any of the excipients listed.

4.4 Special warnings and precautions for use
Caution is required in patients liable to electrolyte deficiency. Regular monitoring of serum sodium, potassium and creatinine is generally recommended during furosemide therapy; particularly close monitoring is required in patients at high risk of developing electrolyte imbalances or in case of significant additional fluid loss. Hypovolaemia or dehydration as well as any significant electrolyte and acid-base disturbances must be corrected. This may require temporary discontinuation of furosemide. Where indicated, steps should be taken to correct hypotension or hypovolaemia before commencing therapy.

Urinary output must be secured. Patients with partial obstructions of urinary outflow for example patients with prostatic hypertrophy or impairment of micturition have an increased risk of developing acute urinary retention.

Particularly careful monitoring is necessary in:

- Patients with hypotension
- Patients who are at risk from a pronounced fall in blood pressure
- Patients with gout
- Patients with hepatorenal syndrome
- Patients with hypoproteinaemia, e.g. associated with nephrotic syndrome (the effect of furosemide may be weakened and its ototoxicity potentiated). Cautious dose titration is required
- Premature infants (possible development nephrocalcinosus/nephrolithiasis; renal function must be monitored and renal ultrasonography performed).

The use of some diuretics is considered to be unsafe in acute porphyria therefore caution should be exercised.

Latent diabetes may become manifest or the insulin requirements of diabetic patients may increase.

Excipient Warnings
This product contains:

Ethanol 10%v/v (alcohol) – each dose contains up to 0.4g of alcohol.

It is harmful to those suffering from alcoholism. It should be taken into account in pregnant and lactating women, children and other high-risk groups (those suffering from liver disease, epilepsy, brain injury or disease). It may modify or increase the effect of other medicines.

Liquid maltitol – patients with a rare hereditary problem of fructose intolerance should not take this medicine.

Quinoline Yellow (E104) – can cause allergic-type reactions including asthma. The allergy is more common in people who are allergic to aspirin.

4.5 Interaction with other medicinal products and other forms of interaction
ACE Inhibitors: Enhanced hypotensive effect when given with diuretics

Alpha-blockers: Enhanced hypotensive effect when diuretics are given with alpha-blockers, also increased risk of first dose hypotension with post-synaptic alpha-blockers such as prazosin.

Analgesics: Diuretics can increase the risk of nephrotoxicity of NSAIDs, also antagonism of diuretic effect. Antagonism of diuretic effect (especially with indomethacin and ketorolac). Salicylic toxicity may be increased by furosemide.

Angiotensin –II Receptor Antagonists: Enhanced hypotensive effect when diuretics given with angiotensin-II receptor antagonists.

Anti-arrhythmics: Hypokalaemia caused by loop diuretics increases cardiac toxicity with amiodarone, disopyramide, flecainide, and antagonises the action of lidocaine and mexiletine.

Antibacterials: Avoid the use of diuretics in lymecycline treatment. There is an increased risk of ototoxicity when loop diuretics are given with aminoglycosides, polymyxins or vancomycin. Impairment of renal function may develop in patients receiving concurrent treatment with furosemide and high doses of certain cephalosporins.

Antidepressants: Possible increase of hypokalaemia when loop diuretics are given with reboxetine. There is an enhanced hypotensive effect when diuretics are given with MAOIs. There is an increased risk of postural hypotension when diuretics are given with tricyclic antidepressants.

Antiepileptics: There is an increased risk of hyponatraemia when diuretics are given with carbemazepine. The effects of furosemide are antagonised by phenytoin.

Antifungals: There is an increased risk of hypokalaemia when loop diuretics are given with amphotericin.

Antipsychotics: Hypokalaemia caused by diuretics increase the risk of ventricular arrhythmias with amisulpiride or sertindole. An enhanced hypotensive effect may be seen when diuretics are given with phenothiazines. Hypokalaemia caused by diuretics increases risk of ventricular arrhythmias with pimozide (avoid concomitant use).

Antivirals: Plasma concentration of diuretics may be increased by nelfinavir, ritonavir or saquinavir.

Atomoxetine: Hypokalaemia caused by diuretics increases the risk of ventricular arrhythmias with atomoxetine.

Barbiturates: Plasma concentrations of diuretics may be decreased. There may be an increased risk of osteomalacia when diuretics are taken in combination with Phenobarbital.

Beta-blockers: There is an enhanced hypotensive effect when diuretics are given with beta-blockers. Hypokalaemia caused by loop diuretics increases the risk of ventricular arrhythmias with sotalol.

Cardiac glycosides: Hypokalaemia caused by loop diuretics increases cardiac toxicity with cardiac glycosides.

Ciclosporin: there is an increased risk of nephrotoxicity and possibly hypermagnesaemia when diuretics are given with ciclosporin.

Cisplatin: There is a risk of increased ototoxic effects if cisplatin and furosemide are given concomitantly.

Corticosteroids: The diuretic effect of diuretics is antagonised by corticosteroids. There is an increased risk of hypokalaemia when loop diuretics are given with corticosteroids.

Other Diuretics: There is an increased risk of hypokalaemia when loop diuretics are given with acetazolamide. Profound diuresis is possible when metolazone is given with furosemide. There is an increased risk of hypokalaemia when loop diuretics are given with thiazides and related diuretics.

Lithium: Loop diuretics reduce the excretion of lithium, which may lead to increased plasma concentrations and a risk of toxicity. However loop diuretics are safer than thiazides.

Potassium salts: There is an increased risk of hypokalaemia when given with potassium salts.

Sucralfate: Frusol and sucralfate must not be taken within 2 hours of each other as sucralfate decreases the absorption of furosemide from the intestine and so reduces its effect.

Sympathomimetics, Beta $_2$: There is an increased risk of hypokalameia when loop diuretics are given with high doses of beta$_2$ synpathomimetics.

Tacrolimus: There is an increased risk of hypokalaemia when given with tacrolimus.

Theophylline: There is an increased risk of hypokalaemia when loop diuretics are given with theophylline.

Carbenoxolone, prolonged use of laxatives, liquorice: May increase the risk of developing hypokalaemia.

Warfarin and clofibrate: Warfarin and clofibrate compete with furosemide in the binding to serum albumin. This may have clinical significance in patients with low serum albumin levels (e.g. in nephrotic syndrome). Furosemide does not change the pharmacokinetics of warfarin to a significant extent, but a strong diuresis with associated dehydration may weaken the antithrombotic effect of warfarin.

4.6 Pregnancy and lactation
Frusol must not be given during pregnancy unless there are compelling medical reasons

Furosemide may inhibit lactation and may pass into breast milk. Women must not breastfeed if they are treated with furosemide.

4.7 Effects on ability to drive and use machines
Mental alertness may be reduced and the ability to drive or operate machinery may be impaired.

4.8 Undesirable effects
The side effects are generally minor and Furosemide is well tolerated.

General
Side effects of a minor nature such as nausea, malaise, gastric upset (vomiting or diarrhoea) may occur but are not usually severe enough to necessitate withdrawal of treatment.

Disturbance of electrolytes and water balance (see also section 4.4).

Furosemide leads to increased excretion of sodium, chloride, water and other electrolytes (in particular potassium, calcium and magnesium). Symptomatic electrolyte disturbances and metabolic acidosis may develop either gradually or acutely (with higher furosemide doses). Pre-existing metabolic alkalosis (e.g. in decompensated cirrhosis of the liver) may be aggravated by furosemide treatment.

Signs of electrolyte disturbances include increased thirst, headache, hypotension, confusion, muscle cramps, tetany, muscle weakness, disorders of cardiac rhythm and gastrointestinal symptoms.

The diuretic action of furosemide may lead to or contribute to hypovolaemia and dehydration, especially in dehydrated patients. Severe fluid depletion may lead to haemoconcentration with a tendency for thrombosis to develop.

Furosemide may cause a reduction in blood pressure which if pronounced may cause signs and symptoms such as impairment of concentration and reactions, light-headedness, sensations of pressure in the head, headache, dizziness, drowsiness, weakness, disorders of vision, dry mouth, orthostatic intolerance.

Other blood biochemistry
Treatment with furosemide may lead to transitory increases in blood creatinine and urea levels and to an increase in cholesterol and triglyceride levels. Serum levels of uric acid may increase and attacks of gout may occur (see section 4.4).

Bladder outlet obstruction
Increased production of urine may provoke or aggravate any obstruction of urinary outflow (including prostatic hyperplasia or narrowing of the urethra) and acute retention of urine with possible secondary complications may occur.

Haematological
Aplastic anaemia and bone marrow depression has been reported as a rare complication and necessitate withdrawal of treatment.

Occasionally, thrombocytopenia may occur with rare cases of leucopenia and eoisinophilia, and isolated cases of agranulocytosis and haemolytic anaemia.

Tetany and reduced serum calcium

Serum calcium levels may be reduced; in very rare cases tetany has been observed. Nephrocalcinosis/nephrolithiasis has been reported in premature infants.

Control of glucose

Glucose tolerance may decrease with furosemide. In patients with diabetes mellitus this may lead to deterioration of metabolic control; latent diabetes mellitus may become manifest.

Hearing disorders

Hearing disorders and tinnitus, although usually transitory, may occur in rare cases, particularly in patients with renal failure with hypoproteinaemia (e.g. in nephrotic syndrome.) See also section 4.4.

Anaphylaxis and allergic reactions

Severe anaphylactic or anaphylactoid reactions (e.g. with shock) occur rarely. The incidence of allergic reactions such as skin rash, photosensitivity, vasculitis, fever, interstitial nephritis, or shock is very low but treatment should be withdrawn when these occur.

Pancreatitis/jaundice

Isolated cases of acute pancreatitis and jaundice have been reported after long term diuretic therapy.

Skin and mucous membrane

Skin and mucous membrane reactions may occasionally occur, e.g. itching, urticaria, other rashes or bullous lesions, erythema multiforme, exfoliative dermatitis, purpura.

Nervous system

Rarely, paraethesiae may occur.

Premature infants

If furosemide is administered to premature infants during the first weeks of life, it may increase the risk of persistence of patent ductus arteriosus. Risk of nephrocalcinosis/nephroliathisis (see *Tetany and reduced serum calcium* and section 4.4 re monitoring)

4.9 Overdose

Overdosing may lead to dehydration and electrolyte depletion through excessive diuresis. Severe potassium loss may lead to serious cardiac arrhythmias.

Treatment of overdose consists of fluid replacement and electrolyte imbalance correction.

5. PHARMACOLOGICAL PROPERTIES

5.1 Pharmacodynamic properties

Pharmacotherapeutic group:

High-Ceiling Diuretic Sulfonamide - CO3C A 01

Furosemide is a potent loop diuretic which inhibits sodium and chloride reabsorption at the Loop of Henlé. The drug eliminates both positive and negative free water production. Furosemide acts at the luminal face of the epithelial cells by inhibiting co-transport mechanisms for the entry of sodium and chloride. Furosemide gains access to its site of action by being transported through the secretory pathway for organic acids in the proximal tubule. It reduces the renal excretion of uric acid. Furosemide causes an increased loss of potassium in the urine and also increases the excretion of ammonia by the kidney.

5.2 Pharmacokinetic properties

When oral doses of Furosemide are given to normal subjects the mean bioavailability of the drug is approximately 52% but the range is wide. In plasma, Furosemide is extensively bound to proteins mainly to albumin. The unbound fraction in plasma averages 2 - 4% at therapeutic concentrations. The volume of distribution ranges between 170 - 270ml/Kg. The half life of the β phase ranges from 45 - 60 min. The total plasma clearance is about 200ml/min. Renal excretion of unchanged drug and elimination by metabolism plus faecal excretion contribute almost equally to the total plasma clearance. Furosemide is in part cleared by the kidneys in the form of the glucuronide conjugate.

5.3 Preclinical safety data

Furosemide is a widely used diuretic which has been available for over thirty years and its safety profile in man is well established.

6. PHARMACEUTICAL PARTICULARS

6.1 List of excipients

Ethanol, sodium hydroxide, quinoline yellow (E104), cherry flavour (containing ethanol and propylene glycol), liquid maltitol (E965), disodium hydrogen phosphate (E339), citric acid monohydrate (E330) and purified water.

6.2 Incompatibilities

None known

6.3 Shelf life

24 months

3 months once open

6.4 Special precautions for storage

Store at or below 25°C.

6.5 Nature and contents of container

Bottles: Amber (Type III) glass

Closures: a) Aluminium, EPE wadded, Roll-On Pilfer Proof Closures (ROPP)

b) HDPE, EPE wadded, tamper evident

c) HDPE, EPE wadded, tamper evident, child resistant

Capacity: 150ml, 200ml or 300ml.

6.6 Special precautions for disposal and other handling

Keep out of the reach of children.

Administrative Data

7. MARKETING AUTHORISATION HOLDER

Rosemont Pharmaceuticals Ltd

Yorkdale Industrial Park

Braithwaite Street

Leeds

LS11 9XE

UK

8. MARKETING AUTHORISATION NUMBER(S)

00427/0109

9. DATE OF FIRST AUTHORISATION/RENEWAL OF THE AUTHORISATION

6 April 1998

10. DATE OF REVISION OF THE TEXT

17 April 2009

Frusol 40mg/5ml Oral Solution

(Rosemont Pharmaceuticals Limited)

1. NAME OF THE MEDICINAL PRODUCT

Frusol 40mg/5ml Oral Solution

2. QUALITATIVE AND QUANTITATIVE COMPOSITION

Furosemide Ph.Eur 40mg/5ml

3. PHARMACEUTICAL FORM

Oral Solution

4. CLINICAL PARTICULARS

4.1 Therapeutic indications

Furosemide is indicated in all conditions requiring prompt diuresis, including cardiac, pulmonary, hepatic and renal oedema, peripheral oedema due to mechanical obstruction or venous insufficiency and hypertension.

It is also indicated for the maintenance therapy of mild oedema of any origin.

4.2 Posology and method of administration

This liquid should only be taken orally.

The medication should be administered in the morning to avoid nocturnal diuresis.

Adults: The usual initial daily dose is 40mg. This may be adjusted until an effective dose is achieved.

Children: 1 to 3mg/Kg body weight daily up to a maximum total dose of 40mg/day.

Elderly: In the elderly, Furosemide is generally eliminated more slowly. Dosage should be titrated until the required response is achieved.

4.3 Contraindications

Hypovolaemia or dehydration. Anuria. Renal failure with anuria not responding to furosemide, or as a result of poisoning by nephrotoxic or hepatotoxic agents, or associated with hepatic coma. Severe hyperkalaemia, severe hyponatraemia. Pre-comatose and comatose states associated with hepatic encephalopathy. Breast feeding.

Contra-indicated in hypersensitivity to Furosemide, sulphonamides or any of the excipients listed.

4.4 Special warnings and precautions for use

Caution is required in patients liable to electrolyte deficiency. Regular monitoring of serum sodium, potassium and creatinine is generally recommended during furosemide therapy; particularly close monitoring is required in patients at high risk of developing electrolyte imbalances or in case of significant additional fluid loss. Hypovolaemia or dehydration as well as any significant electrolyte and acid-base disturbances must be corrected. This may require temporary discontinuation of furosemide. Where indicated, steps should be taken to correct hypotension or hypovolaemia before commencing therapy.

Urinary output must be secured. Patients with partial obstructions of urinary outflow for example patients with prostatic hypertrophy or impairment of micturition have an increased risk of developing acute urinary retention.

Particularly careful monitoring is necessary in:

- Patients with hypotension
- Patients who are at risk from a pronounced fall in blood pressure
- Patients with gout
- Patients with hepatorenal syndrome
- Patients with hypoproteinaemia, e.g. associated with nephrotic syndrome (the effect of furosemide may be weakened and its ototoxicity potentiated). Cautious dose titration is required
- Premature infants (possible development nephrocalcinosus/nephrolithiasis; renal function must be monitored and renal ultrasonography performed).

The use of some diuretics is considered to be unsafe in acute porphyria therefore caution should be exercised.

Latent diabetes may become manifest or the insulin requirements of diabetic patients may increase.

Excipient Warnings

This product contains:

Ethanol 10%v/v (alcohol) – each dose contains up to 0.4g of alcohol.

It is harmful to those suffering from alcoholism. It should be taken into account in pregnant and lactating women, children and other high-risk groups (those suffering from liver disease, epilepsy, brain injury or disease). It may modify or increase the effect of other medicines.

Liquid maltitol – patients with a rare hereditary problem of fructose intolerance should not take this medicine.

4.5 Interaction with other medicinal products and other forms of interaction

ACE Inhibitors: Enhanced hypotensive effect when given with diuretics

Alpha-blockers: Enhanced hypotensive effect when diuretics are given with alpha-blockers, also increased risk of first dose hypotension with post-synaptic alpha-blockers such as prazosin.

Analgesics: Diuretics can increase the risk of nephrotoxicity of NSAIDs, also antagonism of diuretic effect. Antagonism of diuretic effect (especially with indomethacin and ketorolac). Salicylic toxicity may be increased by furosemide.

Angiotensin –II Receptor Antagonists: Enhanced hypotensive effect when diuretics given with angiotensin-II receptor antagonists.

Anti-arrhythmics: Hypokalaemia caused by loop diuretics increases cardiac toxicity with amiodarone, disopyramide, flecainide, and antagonises the action of lidocaine and mexiletine.

Antibacterials: Avoid the use of diuretics in lymecycline treatment. There is an increased risk of ototoxicity when loop diuretics are given with aminoglycosides, polymyxins or vancomycin. Impairment of renal function may develop in patients receiving concurrent treatment with furosemide and high doses of certain cephalosporins.

Antidepressants: Possible increase of hypokalaemia when loop diuretics are given with reboxetine. There is an enhanced hypotensive effect when diuretics are given with MAOIs. There is an increased risk of postural hypotension when diuretics are given with tricyclic antidepressants.

Antiepileptics: There is an increased risk of hyponatraemia when diuretics are given with carbemazepine. The effects of furosemide are antagonised by phenytoin.

Antifungals: There is an increased risk of hypokalaemia when loop diuretics are given with amphotericin.

Antipsychotics: Hypokalaemia caused by diuretics increase the risk of ventricular arrhythmias with amisulpiride or sertindole. An enhanced hypotensive effect may be seen when diuretics are given with phenothiazines. Hypokalaemia caused by diuretics increases risk of ventricular arrhythmias with pimozide (avoid concomitant use).

Antivirals: Plasma concentration of diuretics may be increased by nelfinavir, ritonavir or saquinavir.

Atomoxetine: Hypokalaemia caused by diuretics increases the risk of ventricular arrhythmias with atomoxetine.

Barbiturates: Plasma concentrations of diuretics may be decreased. There may be an increased risk of osteomalacia when diuretics are taken in combination with Phenobarbital.

Beta-blockers: There is an enhanced hypotensive effect when diuretics are given with beta-blockers. Hypokalaemia caused by loop diuretics increases the risk of ventricular arrhythmias with sotalol.

Cardiac glycosides: Hypokalaemia caused by loop diuretics increases cardiac toxicity with cardiac glycosides.

Ciclosporin: there is an increased risk of nephrotoxicity and possibly hypermagnesaemia when diuretics are given with ciclosporin.

Cisplatin: There is a risk of increased ototoxic effects if cisplatin and furosemide are given concomitantly.

Corticosteroids: The diuretic effect of diuretics is antagonised by corticosteroids. There is an increased risk of hypokalaemia when loop diuretics are given with corticosteroids.

Other Diuretics: There is an increased risk of hypokalaemia when loop diuretics are given with acetazolamide. Profound diuresis is possible when metolazone is given with furosemide. There is an increased risk of hypokalaemia when loop diuretics are given with thiazides and related diuretics.

Lithium: Loop diuretics reduce the excretion of lithium, which may lead to increased plasma concentrations and a risk of toxicity. However loop diuretics are safer than thiazides.

Potassium salts: There is an increased risk of hypokalaemia when given with potassium salts.

Sucralfate: Frusol and sucralfate must not be taken within 2 hours of each other as sucralfate decreases the absorption of furosemide from the intestine and so reduces its effect.

Sympathomimetics, Beta$_2$: There is an increased risk of hypokalameia when loop diuretics are given with high doses of beta$_2$ synpathomimetics.

Tacrolimus: There is an increased risk of hypokalaemia when given with tacrolimus.

Theophylline: There is an increased risk of hypokalaemia when loop diuretics are given with theophylline.

Carbenoxolone, prolonged use of laxatives, liquorice: May increase the risk of developing hypokalaemia.

Warfarin and clofibrate: Warfarin and clofibrate compete with furosemide in the binding to serum albumin. This may have clinical significance in patients with low serum albumin levels (e.g. in nephrotic syndrome). Furosemide does not change the pharmacokinetics of warfarin to a significant extent, but a strong diuresis with associated dehydration may weaken the antithrombotic effect of warfarin.

4.6 Pregnancy and lactation

Frusol must not be given during pregnancy unless there are compelling medical reasons

Furosemide may inhibit lactation and may pass into breast milk. Women must not breastfeed if they are treated with furosemide.

4.7 Effects on ability to drive and use machines

Mental alertness may be reduced and the ability to drive or operate machinery may be impaired.

4.8 Undesirable effects

The side effects are generally minor and Furosemide is well tolerated.

General

Side effects of a minor nature such as nausea, malaise, gastric upset (vomiting or diarrhoea) may occur but are not usually severe enough to necessitate withdrawal of treatment.

Disturbance of electrolytes and water balance (see also section 4.4).

Furosemide leads to increased excretion of sodium, chloride, water and other electrolytes (in particular potassium, calcium and magnesium). Symptomatic electrolyte disturbances and metabolic acidosis may develop either gradually or acutely (with higher furosemide doses). Pre-existing metabolic alkalosis (e.g. in decompensated cirrhosis of the liver) may be aggravated by furosemide treatment.

Signs of electrolyte disturbances include increased thirst, headache, hypotension, confusion, muscle cramps, tetany, muscle weakness, disorders of cardiac rhythm and gastrointestinal symptoms.

The diuretic action of furosemide may lead to or contribute to hypovolaemia and dehydration, especially in dehydrated patients. Severe fluid depletion may lead to haemoconcentration with a tendency for thrombosis to develop.

Furosemide may cause a reduction in blood pressure which if pronounced may cause signs and symptoms such as impairment of concentration and reactions, light-headedness, sensations of pressure in the head, headache, dizziness, drowsiness, weakness, disorders of vision, dry mouth, orthostatic intolerance.

Other blood biochemistry

Treatment with furosemide may lead to transitory increases in blood creatinine and urea levels and to an increase in cholesterol and triglyceride levels. Serum levels of uric acid may increase and attacks of gout may occur (see section 4.4).

Bladder outlet obstruction

Increased production of urine may provoke or aggravate any obstruction of urinary outflow (including prostatic hyperplasia or narrowing of the urethra) and acute retention of urine with possible secondary complications may occur.

Haematological

Aplastic anaemia and bone marrow depression has been reported as a rare complication and necessitate withdrawal of treatment.

Occasionally, thrombocytopenia may occur with rare cases of leucopenia and eoisinophilia, and isolated cases of agranulocytosis and haemolytic anaemia.

Tetany and reduced serum calcium

Serum calcium levels may be reduced; in very rare cases tetany has been observed. Nephrocalcinosis/nephrolithiasis has been reported in premature infants.

Control of glucose

Glucose tolerance may decrease with furosemide. In patients with diabetes mellitus this may lead to deterioration of metabolic control; latent diabetes mellitus may become manifest.

Hearing disorders

Hearing disorders and tinnitus, although usually transitory, may occur in rare cases, particularly in patients with renal failure with hypoproteinaemia (e.g. in nephrotic syndrome.) See also section 4.4.

Anaphylaxis and allergic reactions

Severe anaphylactic or anaphylactoid reactions (e.g. with shock) occur rarely. The incidence of allergic reactions such as skin rash, photosensitivity, vasculitis, fever, interstitial nephritis, or shock is very low but treatment should be withdrawn when these occur.

Pancreatitis/jaundice

Isolated cases of acute pancreatitis and jaundice have been reported after long term diuretic therapy.

Skin and mucous membrane

Skin and mucous membrane reactions may occasionally occur, e.g. itching, urticaria, other rashes or bullous lesions, erythema multiforme, exfoliative dermatitis, purpura.

Nervous system

Rarely, paraethesiae may occur.

Premature infants

If furosemide is administered to premature infants during the first weeks of life, it may increase the risk of persistence of patent ductus arteriosus. Risk of nephrocalcinosis/nephroliathiasis (see *Tetany and reduced serum calcium* and section 4.4 re monitoring).

4.9 Overdose

Overdosing may lead to dehydration and electrolyte depletion through excessive diuresis. Severe potassium loss may lead to serious cardiac arrhythmias.

Treatment of overdose consists of fluid replacement and electrolyte imbalance correction.

5. PHARMACOLOGICAL PROPERTIES

5.1 Pharmacodynamic properties

Pharmacotherapeutic group:

High-Ceiling Diuretic Sulfonamide - CO3C A 01

Furosemide is a potent loop diuretic which inhibits sodium and chloride reabsorption at the Loop of Henlé. The drug eliminates both positive and negative free water production. Furosemide acts at the luminal face of the epithelial cells by inhibiting co-transport mechanisms for the entry of sodium and chloride. Furosemide gains access to its site of action by being transported through the secretory pathway for organic acids in the proximal tubule. It reduces the renal excretion of uric acid. Furosemide causes an increased loss of potassium in the urine and also increases the excretion of ammonia by the kidney.

5.2 Pharmacokinetic properties

When oral doses of Furosemide are given to normal subjects the mean bioavailability of the drug is approximately 52% but the range is wide. In plasma, Furosemide is extensively bound to proteins mainly to albumin. The unbound fraction in plasma averages 2 - 4% at therapeutic concentrations. The volume of distribution ranges between 170 - 270ml/Kg. The half life of the β phase ranges from 45 - 60 min. The total plasma clearance is about 200ml/min. Renal excretion of unchanged drug and elimination by metabolism plus faecal excretion contribute almost equally to the total plasma clearance. Furosemide is in part cleared by the kidneys in the form of the glucuronide conjugate.

5.3 Preclinical safety data

Furosemide is a widely used diuretic which has been available for over thirty years and its safety profile in man is well established.

6. PHARMACEUTICAL PARTICULARS

6.1 List of excipients

Ethanol, sodium hydroxide, cherry flavour (containing ethanol and propylene glycol), liquid maltitol (E965), disodium hydrogen phosphate (E339), citric acid monohydrate (E330) and purified water.

6.2 Incompatibilities

None known

6.3 Shelf life

24 months

3 months after opening

6.4 Special precautions for storage

Store at or below 25°C.

6.5 Nature and contents of container

Bottles: Amber (Type III) glass

Closures: a) Aluminium, EPE wadded, Roll-On Pilfer Proof Closures (ROPP)

b) HDPE, EPE wadded, tamper evident

c) HDPE, EPE wadded, tamper evident, child resistant

Capacity: 150ml, 200ml or 300ml.

6.6 Special precautions for disposal and other handling

Keep out of the reach of children.

Administrative Data

7. MARKETING AUTHORISATION HOLDER

Rosemont Pharmaceuticals Ltd

Yorkdale Industrial Park

Braithwaite Street

Leeds

LS11 9XE

UK

8. MARKETING AUTHORISATION NUMBER(S)

00427/0110

9. DATE OF FIRST AUTHORISATION/RENEWAL OF THE AUTHORISATION

6 April 1998

10. DATE OF REVISION OF THE TEXT

17 April 2009

Frusol 50mg/5ml Oral Solution

(Rosemont Pharmaceuticals Limited)

1. NAME OF THE MEDICINAL PRODUCT

Frusol 50mg/5ml Oral Solution

2. QUALITATIVE AND QUANTITATIVE COMPOSITION

Furosemide Ph.Eur 50mg/5ml

3. PHARMACEUTICAL FORM

Oral Solution

4. CLINICAL PARTICULARS

4.1 Therapeutic indications

Furosemide is indicated in all conditions requiring prompt diuresis, including cardiac, pulmonary, hepatic and renal oedema, peripheral oedema due to mechanical obstruction or venous insufficiency and hypertension.

It is also indicated for the maintenance therapy of mild oedema of any origin.

4.2 Posology and method of administration

This liquid should only be taken orally.

The medication should be administered in the morning to avoid nocturnal diuresis.

Adults: The usual initial daily dose is 40mg. This may be adjusted until an effective dose is achieved.

Children: 1 to 3mg/Kg body weight daily up to a maximum total dose of 40mg/day.

Elderly: In the elderly, Furosemide is generally eliminated more slowly. Dosage should be titrated until the required response is achieved.

4.3 Contraindications

Hypovolaemia or dehydration. Anuria. Renal failure with anuria not responding to furosemide, or as a result of poisoning by nephrotoxic or hepatotoxic agents, or associated with hepatic coma. Severe hyperkalaemia, severe hyponatraemia. Pre-comatose and comatose states associated with hepatic encephalopathy. Breast feeding.

Contra-indicated in hypersensitivity to Furosemide, sulphonamides or any of the excipients listed.

4.4 Special warnings and precautions for use

Caution is required in patients liable to electrolyte deficiency. Regular monitoring of serum sodium, potassium and creatinine is generally recommended during furosemide therapy; particularly close monitoring is required in patients at high risk of developing electrolyte imbalances or in case of significant additional fluid loss. Hypovolaemia or dehydration as well as any significant electrolyte and acid-base disturbances must be corrected. This may require temporary discontinuation of furosemide. Where indicated, steps should be taken to correct hypotension or hypovolaemia before commencing therapy.

Urinary output must be secured. Patients with partial obstructions of urinary outflow for example patients with prostatic hypertrophy or impairment of micturition have an increased risk of developing acute urinary retention.

Particularly careful monitoring is necessary in:

- Patients with hypotension
- Patients who are at risk from a pronounced fall in blood pressure
- Patients with gout
- Patients with hepatorenal syndrome
- Patients with hypoproteinaemia, e.g. associated with nephrotic syndrome (the effect of furosemide may be weakened and its ototoxicity potentiated). Cautious dose titration is required
- Premature infants (possible development nephrocalcinosus/nephrolithiasis; renal function must be monitored and renal ultrasonography performed).

The use of some diuretics is considered to be unsafe in acute porphyria therefore caution should be exercised.

Latent diabetes may become manifest or the insulin requirements of diabetic patients may increase.

Excipient Warnings

This product contains:

Ethanol 10%v/v (alcohol) – each dose contains up to 0.4g of alcohol.

It is harmful to those suffering from alcoholism. It should be taken into account in pregnant and lactating women, children and other high-risk groups (those suffering from liver disease, epilepsy, brain injury or disease). It may modify or increase the effect of other medicines.

Liquid maltitol – patients with a rare hereditary problem of fructose intolerance should not take this medicine.

4.5 Interaction with other medicinal products and other forms of interaction

ACE Inhibitors: Enhanced hypotensive effect when given with diuretics

Alpha-blockers: Enhanced hypotensive effect when diuretics are given with alpha-blockers, also increased risk of first dose hypotension with post-synaptic alpha-blockers such as prazosin.

Analgesics: Diuretics can increase the risk of nephrotoxicity of NSAIDs, also antagonism of diuretic effect. Antagonism of diuretic effect (especially with indomethacin and ketorolac). Salicylic toxicity may be increased by furosemide.

Angiotensin –II Receptor Antagonists: Enhanced hypotensive effect when diuretics given with angiotensin-II receptor antagonists.

Anti-arrhythmics: Hypokalaemia caused by loop diuretics increases cardiac toxicity with amiodarone, disopyramide, flecainide, and antagonises the action of lidocaine and mexiletine.

Antibacterials: Avoid the use of diuretics in lymecycline treatment. There is an increased risk of ototoxicity when loop diuretics are given with aminoglycosides, polymyxins or vancomycin. Impairment of renal function may develop in patients receiving concurrent treatment with furosemide and high doses of certain cephalosporins.

Antidepressants: Possible increase of hypokalaemia when loop diuretics are given with reboxetine. There is an enhanced hypotensive effect when diuretics are given with MAOIs. There is an increased risk of postural hypotension when diuretics are given with tricyclic antidepressants.

Antiepileptics: There is an increased risk of hyponatraemia when diuretics are given with carbemazepine. The effects of furosemide are antagonised by phenytoin.

Antifungals: There is an increased risk of hypokalaemia when loop diuretics are given with amphotericin.

Antipsychotics: Hypokalaemia caused by diuretics increase the risk of ventricular arrhythmias with amisulpiride or sertindole. An enhanced hypotensive effect may be seen when diuretics are given with phenothiazines. Hypokalaemia caused by diuretics increases risk of ventricular arrhythmias with pimozide (avoid concomitant use).

Antivirals: Plasma concentration of diuretics may be increased by nelfinavir, ritonavir or saquinavir.

Atomoxetine: Hypokalaemia caused by diuretics increases the risk of ventricular arrhythmias with atomoxetine.

Barbiturates: Plasma concentrations of diuretics may be decreased. There may be an increased risk of osteomalacia when diuretics are taken in combination with Phenobarbital.

Beta-blockers: There is an enhanced hypotensive effect when diuretics are given with beta-blockers. Hypokalaemia caused by loop diuretics increases the risk of ventricular arrhythmias with sotalol.

Cardiac glycosides: Hypokalaemia caused by loop diuretics increases cardiac toxicity with cardiac glycosides.

Ciclosporin: there is an increased risk of nephrotoxicity and possibly hypermagnesaemia when diuretics are given with ciclosporin.

Cisplatin: There is a risk of increased ototoxic effects if cisplatin and furosemide are given concomitantly.

Corticosteroids: The diuretic effect of diuretics is antagonised by corticosteroids. There is an increased risk of hypokalaemia when loop diuretics are given with corticosteroids.

Other Diuretics: There is an increased risk of hypokalaemia when loop diuretics are given with acetazolamide. Profound diuresis is possible when metolazone is given with furosemide. There is an increased risk of hypokalaemia when loop diuretics are given with thiazides and related diuretics.

Lithium: Loop diuretics reduce the excretion of lithium, which may lead to increased plasma concentrations and a risk of toxicity. However loop diuretics are safer than thiazides.

Potassium salts: There is an increased risk of hypokalaemia when given with potassium salts.

Sucralfate: Frusol and sucralfate must not be taken within 2 hours of each other as sucralfate decreases the absorption of furosemide from the intestine and so reduces its effect.

Sympathomimetics, Beta $_2$: There is an increased risk of hypokalameia when loop diuretics are given with high doses of beta$_2$ synpathomimetics.

Tacrolimus: There is an increased risk of hypokalaemia when given with tacrolimus.

Theophylline: There is an increased risk of hypokalaemia when loop diuretics are given with theophylline.

Carbenoxolone, prolonged use of laxatives, liquorice: May increase the risk of developing hypokalaemia.

Warfarin and clofibrate: Warfarin and clofibrate compete with furosemide in the binding to serum albumin. This may have clinical significance in patients with low serum albumin levels (e.g. in nephrotic syndrome). Furosemide does not change the pharmacokinetics of warfarin to a significant extent, but a strong diuresis with associated dehydration may weaken the antithrombotic effect of warfarin.

4.6 Pregnancy and lactation

Frusol must not be given during pregnancy unless there are compelling medical reasons

Furosemide may inhibit lactation and may pass into breast milk. Women must not breastfeed if they are treated with furosemide.

4.7 Effects on ability to drive and use machines

Mental alertness may be reduced and the ability to drive or operate machinery may be impaired.

4.8 Undesirable effects

The side effects are generally minor and Furosemide is well tolerated.

General

Side effects of a minor nature such as nausea, malaise, gastric upset (vomiting or diarrhoea) may occur but are not usually severe enough to necessitate withdrawal of treatment.

Disturbance of electrolytes and water balance (see also section 4.4).

Furosemide leads to increased excretion of sodium, chloride, water and other electrolytes (in particular potassium, calcium and magnesium). Symptomatic electrolyte disturbances and metabolic acidosis may develop either gradually or acutely (with higher furosemide doses). Pre-existing metabolic alkalosis (e.g. in decompensated cirrhosis of the liver) may be aggravated by furosemide treatment.

Signs of electrolyte disturbances include increased thirst, headache, hypotension, confusion, muscle cramps, tetany, muscle weakness, disorders of cardiac rhythm and gastrointestinal symptoms.

The diuretic action of furosemide may lead to or contribute to hypovolaemia and dehydration, especially in dehydrated patients. Severe fluid depletion may lead to haemoconcentration with a tendency for thrombosis to develop.

Furosemide may cause a reduction in blood pressure which if pronounced may cause signs and symptoms such as impairment of concentration and reactions, light-headedness, sensations of pressure in the head, headache, dizziness, drowsiness, weakness, disorders of vision, dry mouth, orthostatic intolerance.

Other blood biochemistry

Treatment with furosemide may lead to transitory increases in blood creatinine and urea levels and to an increase in cholesterol and triglyceride levels. Serum levels of uric acid may increase and attacks of gout may occur (see section 4.4).

Bladder outlet obstruction

Increased production of urine may provoke or aggravate any obstruction of urinary outflow (including prostatic hyperplasia or narrowing of the urethra) and acute retention of urine with possible secondary complications may occur.

Haematological

Aplastic anaemia and bone marrow depression has been reported as a rare complication and necessitate withdrawal of treatment.

Occasionally, thrombocytopenia may occur with rare cases of leucopenia and eoisinophilia, and isolated cases of agranulocytosis and haemolytic anaemia.

Tetany and reduced serum calcium

Serum calcium levels may be reduced; in very rare cases tetany has been observed. Nephrocalcinosis/nephrolithiasis has been reported in premature infants.

Control of glucose

Glucose tolerance may decrease with furosemide. In patients with diabetes mellitus this may lead to deterioration of metabolic control; latent diabetes mellitus may become manifest.

Hearing disorders

Hearing disorders and tinnitus, although usually transitory, may occur in rare cases, particularly in patients with renal failure with hypoproteniaemia (e.g. in nephrotic syndrome.) See also section 4.4.

Anaphylaxis and allergic reactions

Severe anaphylactic or anaphylactoid reactions (e.g. with shock) occur rarely. The incidence of allergic reactions such as skin rash, photosensitivity, vasculitis, fever, interstitial nephritis, or shock is very low but treatment should be withdrawn when these occur.

Pancreatitis/jaundice

Isolated cases of acute pancreatitis and jaundice have been reported after long term diuretic therapy.

Skin and mucous membrane

Skin and mucous membrane reactions may occasionally occur, e.g. itching, urticaria, other rashes or bullous lesions, erythema multiforme, exfoliative dermatitis, purpura.

Nervous system

Rarely, paraesthesiae may occur.

Premature infants

If furosemide is administered to premature infants during the first weeks of life, it may increase the risk of persistence of patent ductus arteriosus. Risk of nephrocalcinosis/nephroliathiasis (see *Tetany and reduced serum calcium* and section 4.4 re monitoring).

4.9 Overdose

Overdosing may lead to dehydration and electrolyte depletion through excessive diuresis. Severe potassium loss may lead to serious cardiac arrhythmias.

Treatment of overdose consists of fluid replacement and electrolyte imbalance correction.

5. PHARMACOLOGICAL PROPERTIES

5.1 Pharmacodynamic properties

Pharmacotherapeutic group:

High-Ceiling Diuretic Sulfonamide - CO3C A 01

Furosemide is a potent loop diuretic which inhibits sodium and chloride reabsorption at the Loop of Henlé. The drug eliminates both positive and negative free water production. Furosemide acts at the luminal face of the epithelial cells by inhibiting co-transport mechanisms for the entry of sodium and chloride. Furosemide gains access to its site of action by being transported through the secretory pathway for organic acids in the proximal tubule. It reduces the renal excretion of uric acid. Furosemide causes an increased loss of potassium in the urine and also increases the excretion of ammonia by the kidney.

5.2 Pharmacokinetic properties

When oral doses of Furosemide are given to normal subjects the mean bioavailability of the drug is approximately 52% but the range is wide. In plasma, Furosemide is extensively bound to proteins mainly to albumin. The unbound fraction in plasma averages 2 - 4% at therapeutic concentrations. The volume of distribution ranges between 170 - 270ml/Kg. The half life of the β phase ranges from 45 - 60 min. The total plasma clearance is about 200ml/min. Renal excretion of unchanged drug and elimination by metabolism plus faecal excretion contribute almost equally to the total plasma clearance. Furosemide is in part cleared by the kidneys in the form of the glucuronide conjugate.

5.3 Preclinical safety data

Furosemide is a widely used diuretic which has been available for over thirty years and its safety profile in man is well established.

6. PHARMACEUTICAL PARTICULARS

6.1 List of excipients

Ethanol, sodium hydroxide, cherry flavour (containing ethanol and propylene glycol), liquid maltitol (E965), disodium hydrogen phosphate (E339), citric acid monohydrate (E330) and purified water.

6.2 Incompatibilities

None known

6.3 Shelf life

24 months

3 months after opening

6.4 Special precautions for storage

Store at or below 25°C.

6.5 Nature and contents of container

Bottles: Amber (Type III) glass

Closures: a) Aluminium, EPE wadded, Roll-On Pilfer Proof Closures (ROPP)

b) HDPE, EPE wadded, tamper evident

c) HDPE, EPE wadded, tamper evident, child resistant

Capacity: 150ml, 200ml or 300ml.

6.6 Special precautions for disposal and other handling

Keep out of the reach of children.

Administrative Data

7. MARKETING AUTHORISATION HOLDER

Rosemont Pharmaceuticals Ltd

Yorkdale Industrial Park

Braithwaite Street

Leeds

LS11 9XE

UK

8. MARKETING AUTHORISATION NUMBER(S)

00427/0111

9. DATE OF FIRST AUTHORISATION/RENEWAL OF THE AUTHORISATION

6 April 1998

10. DATE OF REVISION OF THE TEXT

17 April 2009

FuciBET Cream

(Leo Laboratories Limited)

1. NAME OF THE MEDICINAL PRODUCT

Fucibet® cream

2. QUALITATIVE AND QUANTITATIVE COMPOSITION

Fucibet® cream contains Fusidic acid Ph.Eur. 2% and Betamethasone 0.1% (as the valerate ester Ph.Eur)

3. PHARMACEUTICAL FORM

Cream for topical administration

4. CLINICAL PARTICULARS

4.1 Therapeutic indications

Fucibet® cream is indicated for the treatment of eczematous dermatoses including atopic eczema, infantile eczema, discoid eczema, stasis eczema, contact eczema and seborrhoeic eczema when secondary bacterial infection is confirmed or suspected.

4.2 Posology and method of administration

A small quantity should be applied to the affected area twice daily until a satisfactory response is obtained. A single treatment course should not normally exceed 2 weeks. In the more resistant lesions the effect of Fucibet®-cream can be enhanced by occlusion with polythene film. Overnight occlusion is usually adequate.

4.3 Contraindications
Acne rosacea and perioral dermatitis. Skin lesions of viral, fungal or bacterial origin. Hypersensitivity to the preparation.

4.4 Special warnings and precautions for use
Long-term continuous topical therapy should be avoided, particularly in infants and children. Adrenal suppression can occur even without occlusion. Atrophic changes may occur on the face and to a lesser degree in other parts of the body, after prolonged treatment with potent topical steroids. Caution should be exercised if Fucibet® cream is used near the eye. Glaucoma might result if the preparation enters the eye. Systemic chemotherapy is required if bacterial infection persists.

Bacterial resistance has been reported to occur with the use of fusidic acid applied topically. As with all topical antibiotics, extended or recurrent application may increase the risk of contact sensitisation and the development of antibiotic resistance.

Steroid-antibiotic combinations should not be continued for more than 7 days in the absence of any clinical improvement since in this situation occult extension of the infection may occur due to the masking of the steroid. Similarly, steroids may also mask hypersensitivity reactions.

4.5 Interaction with other medicinal products and other forms of interaction
None known

4.6 Pregnancy and lactation
Topical administration of any corticosteroid to pregnant animals can cause abnormalities of foetal development. The relevance of this finding to human beings has not been established; however, topical steroids should not be used extensively in pregnancy, i.e. in large amounts or for prolonged periods.

4.7 Effects on ability to drive and use machines
Not applicable

4.8 Undesirable effects
Prolonged and intensive treatment with potent corticosteroids may cause local atrophic changes in the skin, including striae, thinning and dilation of superficial blood vessels, particularly when applied to the flexures or when occlusion is employed. As with other topical corticosteroids sufficient systemic absorption to produce hypercorticism can occur with prolonged or extensive use. Infants and children are at particular risk, more so if occlusive dressings are used. A napkin may act as an occlusive dressing in infants. Hypersensitivity reactions to fusidic acid are rare and Fucibet® cream does not contain lanolin. However, if signs of hypersensitivity occur, treatment should be withdrawn.

4.9 Overdose
Not applicable

5. PHARMACOLOGICAL PROPERTIES

5.1 Pharmacodynamic properties
Fucibet® cream combines the well-known anti-inflammatory and antipruritic effects of betamethasone with the potent topical antibacterial action of fusidic acid. Betamethasone valerate is a topical steroid rapidly effective in those inflammatory dermatoses which normally respond to this form of therapy. More refractory conditions can often be treated successfully. When applied topically, fusidic acid is effective against *Staphyloccus aureus*, Streptococci, Corynebacteria, Neisseria and certain Clostridia and Bacteroides. Concentrations of 0.03 to 0.12 microgram per ml inhibit nearly all strains of *S. aureus*. The antibacterial activity of fusidic acid is not diminished in the presence of betamethasone.

5.2 Pharmacokinetic properties
There are no data which define the pharmacokinetics of Fucibet® cream, following topical administration in man.

However, *in vitro* studies show that fusidic acid can penetrate intact human skin. The degree of penetration depends on factors such as the duration of exposure to fusidic acid and the condition of the skin. Fusidic acid is excreted mainly in the bile with little excreted in the urine.

Betamethasone is absorbed following topical administration. The degree of absorption is dependent on various factors including skin condition and site of application. Betamethasone is metabolised largely in the liver but also to a limited extent in the kidneys, and the inactive metabolites are excreted with the urine.

5.3 Preclinical safety data
There are no pre-clinical data of relevance to the prescriber which are additional to that already included in other sections of the SPC.

6. PHARMACEUTICAL PARTICULARS

6.1 List of excipients
Macrogol cetostearyl ether, cetostearyl alcohol, chlorocresol, liquid paraffin, sodium dihydrogen phosphate, white soft paraffin, purified water, sodium hydroxide.

6.2 Incompatibilities
Not applicable

6.3 Shelf life
3 years

6.4 Special precautions for storage
Nil

6.5 Nature and contents of container
Aluminium tube of 30 gram and 60 gram.

6.6 Special precautions for disposal and other handling
None

7. MARKETING AUTHORISATION HOLDER
LEO Laboratories Limited

Princes Risborough

Bucks

HP27 9RR

8. MARKETING AUTHORISATION NUMBER(S)
PL 0043/0091

9. DATE OF FIRST AUTHORISATION/RENEWAL OF THE AUTHORISATION
17/01/2006

10. DATE OF REVISION OF THE TEXT
17/01/2006

11. Legal Category
POM

Fucibet Lipid cream

(Leo Laboratories Limited)

1. NAME OF THE MEDICINAL PRODUCT
Fucibet® Lipid cream

2. QUALITATIVE AND QUANTITATIVE COMPOSITION
Fucibet® Lipid cream contains Fusidic acid 2% and Betamethasone 0.1% (as the valerate ester).

Fucibet® Lipid cream also contains methyl parahydroxybenzoate 0.1% and propyl parahydroxybenzoate 0.02%. For full list of excipients, see Section 6.1.

3. PHARMACEUTICAL FORM
White Cream.

4. CLINICAL PARTICULARS

4.1 Therapeutic indications
Fucibet® Lipid cream is indicated for the treatment of eczematous dermatoses including atopic eczema, discoid eczema, stasis eczema and seborrhoeic eczema when secondary bacterial infection is confirmed or suspected.

4.2 Posology and method of administration
Adults and children aged 6 years and over:

A small quantity should be applied to the affected area twice daily until a satisfactory response is obtained. A single treatment course should not normally exceed 2 weeks. In the more resistant lesions the effect of Fucibet® lipid cream can be enhanced by occlusion with polyethylene film. Overnight occlusion is usually adequate.

4.3 Contraindications
Known hypersensitivity to the drug substances or to any of the ingredients.

Acne rosacea and perioral dermatitis. Skin lesions of viral, fungal or bacterial origin.

4.4 Special warnings and precautions for use
Long-term continuous topical therapy should be avoided, particularly in children. Adrenal suppression can occur even without occlusion. Atrophic changes may occur on the face and to a lesser degree in other parts of the body, after prolonged treatment with potent topical steroids. Caution should be exercised if Fucibet® Lipid cream is used near the eye. Glaucoma might result if the preparation enters the eye. Systemic chemotherapy is required if bacterial infection persists.

Bacterial resistance has been reported to occur with the use of fusidic acid applied topically. As with all topical antibiotics, extended or recurrent application may increase the risk of contact sensitisation and the development of antibiotic resistance.

Steroid-antibiotic combinations should not be continued for more than 7 days in the absence of any clinical improvement since in this situation occult extension of the infection may occur due to the masking of the steroid. Similarly, steroids may also mask hypersensitivity reactions.

4.5 Interaction with other medicinal products and other forms of interaction
None known.

4.6 Pregnancy and lactation
Topical administration of any corticosteroid to pregnant animals can cause abnormalities of foetal development. The relevance of this finding to human beings has not been established; however, topical steroids should not be used extensively in pregnancy, i.e. in large amounts or for prolonged periods.

4.7 Effects on ability to drive and use machines
Not applicable.

4.8 Undesirable effects
Prolonged and intensive treatment with potent corticosteroids may cause local atrophic changes in the skin, including striae, thinning and dilation of superficial blood vessels, particularly when applied to the flexures or when occlusion is employed. As with other topical corticosteroids sufficient systemic absorption to produce hypercorticism can occur with prolonged or extensive use. Children are at particular risk. Hypersensitivity reactions to fusidic acid are rare and Fucibet® Lipid cream does not contain lanolin. However, if signs of hypersensitivity occur, treatment should be withdrawn.

4.9 Overdose
Not applicable.

5. PHARMACOLOGICAL PROPERTIES

5.1 Pharmacodynamic properties
Fucibet® Lipid cream combines the well-known anti-inflammatory and antipruritic effects of betamethasone with the potent topical antibacterial action of fusidic acid. Betamethasone valerate is a topical steroid rapidly effective in those inflammatory dermatoses which normally respond to this form of therapy. More refractory conditions can often be treated successfully. When applied topically, fusidic acid is effective against *Staphyloccus aureus*, Streptococci, Corynebacteria, Neisseria and certain Clostridia and Bacteroides. Concentrations of 0.03 to 0.12 microgram per ml inhibit nearly all strains of *S. aureus*. The antibacterial activity of fusidic acid is not diminished in the presence of betamethasone.

5.2 Pharmacokinetic properties
There are no data which define the pharmacokinetics of Fucibet® Lipid cream, following topical administration in man.

However, *in vitro* studies show that fusidic acid can penetrate intact human skin. The degree of penetration depends on factors such as the duration of exposure to fusidic acid and the condition of the skin. Fusidic acid is excreted mainly in the bile with little excreted in the urine.

Betamethasone is absorbed following topical administration. The degree of absorption is dependent on various factors including skin condition and site of application. Betamethasone is metabolised largely in the liver but also to a limited extent in the kidneys, and the inactive metabolites are excreted with the urine.

5.3 Preclinical safety data
There are no pre-clinical data of relevance to the prescriber which are additional to that already included in other sections of the SPC.

6. PHARMACEUTICAL PARTICULARS

6.1 List of excipients
Steareth-21

Cetostearyl alcohol

White soft paraffin

Liquid paraffin

Hypromellose

Citric acid monohydrate

Methyl parahydroxybenzoate (E218)

Propyl parahydroxybenzoate (E216)

Potassium sorbate

Purified water

6.2 Incompatibilities
Not applicable.

6.3 Shelf life
Unopened container: 2 years.

After first opening of container: 3 months.

6.4 Special precautions for storage
Do not store above 25°C. Store in original container.

6.5 Nature and contents of container
Aluminium tubes of 5 gram, 15 gram, 30 gram, and 60 grams.

Not all pack sizes are marketed.

6.6 Special precautions for disposal and other handling
None.

7. MARKETING AUTHORISATION HOLDER
LEO Laboratories Limited

Princes Risborough

Bucks

HP27 9RR

8. MARKETING AUTHORISATION NUMBER(S)
PL 00043/0218

9. DATE OF FIRST AUTHORISATION/RENEWAL OF THE AUTHORISATION
06/02/2007

10. DATE OF REVISION OF THE TEXT
06/02/2007

LEGAL CATEGORY
POM

Fucidin Cream

(Leo Laboratories Limited)

1. NAME OF THE MEDICINAL PRODUCT
Fucidin® Cream

2. QUALITATIVE AND QUANTITATIVE COMPOSITION
Fucidin Cream contains fusidic acid Ph.Eur. 2%.

3. PHARMACEUTICAL FORM
Cream for topical administration

4. CLINICAL PARTICULARS
4.1 Therapeutic indications
Indicated either alone or in combination with systemic therapy, in the treatment of primary and secondary skin infections caused by sensitive strains of *Staphylococcus aureus,* Streptococcus spp and *Corynebacterium minutissimum*. Primary skin infections that may be expected to respond to treatment with fusidic acid applied topically include: impetigo contagiosa, superficial folliculitis, sycosis barbae, paronychia and erythrasma; also such secondary skin infections as infected eczematoid dermatitis, infected contact dermatitis and infected cuts / abrasions.

4.2 Posology and method of administration
Adults and Children:

Uncovered lesions - apply gently three or four times daily.

Covered lesions - less frequent applications may be adequate.

4.3 Contraindications
Infection caused by non-susceptible organisms, in particular, Pseudomonas aeruginosa.

Fucidin Cream is contraindicated in patients with hypersensitivity to fusidic acid and its salts.

4.4 Special warnings and precautions for use
Bacterial resistance has been reported to occur with the use of fusidic acid applied topically. As with all topical antibiotics, extended or recurrent application may increase the risk of contact sensitisation and the development of antibiotic resistance.

Fusidic acid does not appear to cause conjunctival irritation in experimental animals. Caution should still be exercised, however, when Fucidin Cream is used near the eyes.

4.5 Interaction with other medicinal products and other forms of interaction
Not applicable.

4.6 Pregnancy and lactation
There is inadequate evidence of safety in human pregnancy. Animal studies and many years of clinical experience have suggested that fusidic acid is devoid of teratogenic effect. There is evidence to suggest that when given systemically, fusidic acid can penetrate the placental barrier. The use of topical Fucidin in pregnancy requires that the potential benefits be weighed against the possible hazards to the foetus.

Safety in nursing mothers has not been established. When fusidic acid (as the sodium salt) has been given systemically, levels have been detected in breast milk, but with topical use the possible amount of drug present is unlikely to affect the infant.

4.7 Effects on ability to drive and use machines
Not applicable

4.8 Undesirable effects
Hypersensitivity reactions to the active ingredient in the form of skin rashes; mild stinging and irritation on application have been reported rarely.

4.9 Overdose
Not applicable

5. PHARMACOLOGICAL PROPERTIES
5.1 Pharmacodynamic properties
Fusidic acid is a potent antibacterial agent. Fusidic acid and its salts show fat and water solubility and strong surface activity and exhibit unusual ability to penetrate intact skin. Concentrations of 0.03 - 0.12 mcg fusidic acid per ml inhibit nearly all strains of *Staphylococcus aureus.* Topical application of fusidic acid is also effective against streptococci, corynebacteria, neisseria and certain clostridia.

5.2 Pharmacokinetic properties
In Vitro studies show that fusidic acid can penetrate intact human skin. The degree of penetration depends on factors such as the duration of exposure to fusidic acid and the condition of the skin. Fusidic acid is excreted mainly in the bile with little excreted in the urine.

5.3 Preclinical safety data
There are no pre-clinical data of relevance to the prescribe which are additional to that already included in other sections of the SPC.

6. PHARMACEUTICAL PARTICULARS
6.1 List of excipients
Butylated hydroxyanisole, cetanol, glycerol, liquid paraffin, potassium sorbate, Tween 60, white soft paraffin, purified water.

6.2 Incompatibilities
Not applicable

6.3 Shelf life
3 years

6.4 Special precautions for storage
Nil

6.5 Nature and contents of container
Aluminium tubes of 15 gram and 30 gram.

6.6 Special precautions for disposal and other handling
None

7. MARKETING AUTHORISATION HOLDER
Leo Laboratories Limited

Princes Risborough

Bucks

HP27 9RR

8. MARKETING AUTHORISATION NUMBER(S)
PL 0043/0065

9. DATE OF FIRST AUTHORISATION/RENEWAL OF THE AUTHORISATION
14 August 1979.

10. DATE OF REVISION OF THE TEXT
June 1999

11. Legal Category
POM

Fucidin H Cream

(Leo Laboratories Limited)

1. NAME OF THE MEDICINAL PRODUCT
Fucidin® H Cream

2. QUALITATIVE AND QUANTITATIVE COMPOSITION
Fucidin H Cream contains Fusidic acid Ph.Eur.2% and Hydrocortisone acetate Ph.Eur.1%.

3. PHARMACEUTICAL FORM
Cream for topical administration

4. CLINICAL PARTICULARS
4.1 Therapeutic indications
Fucidin H Cream is indicated in eczema and dermatitis with secondary bacterial infections, including atopic eczema, primary irritant dermatitis and allergic and seborrhoeic dermatitis where the organisms responsible are known to be or believed to be sensitive to fusidic acid.

4.2 Posology and method of administration
Adults and Children:

Uncovered lesions – a small quantity should be applied to the affected area twice daily until a satisfactory response is obtained. A single treatment course should not normally exceed 2 weeks.

Covered lesions - less frequent applications may be adequate.

4.3 Contraindications
Hypersensitivity to fusidic acid and its salts. As with other topical corticosteroid preparations, Fucidin H Cream is contraindicated in primary bacterial, viral and fungal skin infections, skin manifestations in relation to tuberculosis or syphilis, perioral dermatitis and rosacea.

4.4 Special warnings and precautions for use
Fusidic acid does not appear to cause conjunctival irritation in experimental animals. Caution should still be exercised, however, when Fucidin H Cream is used near the eyes.

Bacterial resistance has been reported to occur with the use of fusidic acid applied topically. As with all topical antibiotics, extended or recurrent application may increase the risk of contact sensitisation and the development of antibiotic resistance.

Steroid-antibiotic combinations should not be continued for more than 7 days in the absence of any clinical improvement since in this situation occult extension of the infection may occur due to the masking of the steroid. Similarly, steroids may also mask hypersensitivity reactions.

As Fucidin® H cream contains a corticosteroid it is not recommended in the following conditions: atrophic skin, cutaneous ulcer, acne vulgaris, fragile skin veins and perianal and genital pruritus. Contact with open wounds and mucous membranes should be avoided. As with all corticosteroids, prolonged use on the face should be avoided.

In infants and children, long-term continuous topical therapy with corticosteroids should be avoided. Adrenal suppression can occur even without occlusion.

4.5 Interaction with other medicinal products and other forms of interaction
None known.

4.6 Pregnancy and lactation
There is inadequate evidence of safety in human pregnancy. Topical administration of corticosteroids to pregnant animals can cause abnormalities of foetal development including cleft palate and intra-uterine growth retardation. There may, therefore, be a very small risk of such effects in the human foetus.

Animal studies and many years of clinical experience have suggested that fusidic acid is devoid of teratogenic effect. There is evidence to suggest that when given systemically, fusidic acid can penetrate the placental barrier. The use of topical Fucidin in pregnancy requires that the potential benefits be weighed against the possible hazards to the foetus.

Safety in nursing mothers has not been established.

When fusidic acid (as the sodium salt) has been given systemically, levels have been detected in breast milk, but with topical use the possible amount of drug present is unlikely to affect the infant.

4.7 Effects on ability to drive and use machines
Not known.

4.8 Undesirable effects
Very common > 1/10

Common > 1/100 and < 1/10

Uncommon > 1/1,000 and < 1/100

Rare > 1/10,000 and < 1/1,000

Very rare < 1/10,000

Based on clinical data for Fucidin® H approximately 5% of patients can be expected to experience an undesirable effect. The most frequently reported undesirable effects for Fucidin® H are various symptoms of application site irritation. Pruritus, skin irritation, skin rash, worsening of eczema, transient stinging and burning sensation were uncommon. Allergic reactions have been reported.

Undesirable effects, starting with the most frequently reported, are:

Skin and subcutaneous tissue disorders

Pruritus

Skin irritation

Skin burning sensation

Skin stinging sensation

Rash

Eczema aggravated

Immune system disorders

Allergic reaction

Although it has not been observed in the clinical studies for Fucidin® H, topical use of steroids may result in skin atrophy, telangiectasia or skin striae, especially during prolonged application.

As with all other corticosteroids, folliculitis, hypertrichosis, perioral dermatitis, contact dermatitis, depigmentation and systemic activity, although rare, may occur.

4.9 Overdose
Acute overdosage is very unlikely to occur. However, chronic overdosage or misuse may result in increased risk of topical or systemic side effects.

5. PHARMACOLOGICAL PROPERTIES
5.1 Pharmacodynamic properties
Fucidin H Cream combines the potent topical antibacterial action of fusidic acid with the anti-inflammatory and anti-pruritic effects of hydrocortisone. Concentrations of 0.03 - 0.12 micrograms fusidic acid per ml inhibit nearly all strains of *Staphylococcus aureus.* Topical application of fusidic acid is also effective against streptococci, corynebacteria, neisseria and certain clostridia.

5.2 Pharmacokinetic properties
There are no data which define the pharmacokinetics of Fucidin H Cream, following topical administration in man.

However, *in vitro* studies show that fusidic acid can penetrate intact human skin. The degree of penetration depends on factors such as the duration of exposure to fusidic acid and the condition of the skin. Fusidic acid is excreted mainly in the bile with little excreted in the urine.

Hydrocortisone is absorbed following topical administration. The degree of absorption is dependent on various factors including skin condition and site of application. Absorbed hydrocortisone is extensively metabolised and rapidly eliminated in the urine.

5.3 Preclinical safety data
There are no pre-clinical data of relevance to the prescriber which are additional to that already included in other sections of the SPC.

6. PHARMACEUTICAL PARTICULARS
6.1 List of excipients
Butylhydroxyanisole (E320), cetyl alcohol, glycerol, liquid paraffin, potassium sorbate, polysorbate 60, white soft paraffin, de-ionised water.

6.2 Incompatibilities
Not applicable

6.3 Shelf life
3 years

6.4 Special precautions for storage
Do not store above 30°C

6.5 Nature and contents of container
Aluminium tube of 30 gram and 60 gram.

6.6 Special precautions for disposal and other handling
None

7. MARKETING AUTHORISATION HOLDER
LEO Laboratories Limited

Princes Risborough

Bucks

HP27 9RR

8. MARKETING AUTHORISATION NUMBER(S)
PL 0043/0093

9. DATE OF FIRST AUTHORISATION/RENEWAL OF THE AUTHORISATION
16/10/2006

10. DATE OF REVISION OF THE TEXT
03/01/2007

LEGAL CATEGORY
POM

Fucidin Ointment

(Leo Laboratories Limited)

1. NAME OF THE MEDICINAL PRODUCT
Fucidin®Ointment.

2. QUALITATIVE AND QUANTITATIVE COMPOSITION
Fucidin Ointment contains Sodium Fusidate Ph. Eur. 2%.

3. PHARMACEUTICAL FORM
Ointment for topical administration.

4. CLINICAL PARTICULARS

4.1 Therapeutic indications
Indicated either alone or in combination with systemic therapy, in the treatment of primary and secondary skin infections caused by sensitive strains of *Staphylococcus aureus, streptococcus spp* and *Corynebacterium minutissimum.* Primary skin infections that may be expected to respond to treatment with fusidic acid applied topically include: impetigo contagiosa, superficial folliculitis, sycosis barbae, paronychia and erythrasma; also such secondary skin infections as infected eczematoid dermatitis, infected contact dermatitis and infected cuts /abrasions.

4.2 Posology and method of administration
Adults and Children: Uncovered lesions - apply gently, three or four times daily. Covered lesions - less frequent applications may be adequate.

4.3 Contraindications
Infection caused by non-susceptible organisms, in particular, Pseudomonas aeruginosa.

Fucidin ointment is contra-indicated in patients with hypersensitivity to fusidic acid and its salts.

4.4 Special warnings and precautions for use
The sodium salt of fusidic acid has been shown to cause conjunctival irritation. The ointment should not be used in or near the eye. Bacterial resistance has been reported to occur with the use of fusidic acid applied topically. As with all topical antibiotics, extended or recurrent application may increase the risk of contact sensitisation and the development of antibiotic resistance.

4.5 Interaction with other medicinal products and other forms of interaction
Not applicable.

4.6 Pregnancy and lactation
There is inadequate evidence of safety in human pregnancy. Animal studies and many years of clinical experience have suggested that fusidic acid is devoid of teratogenic effects.

There is evidence to suggest that when given systemically, fusidic acid can penetrate the placental barrier. The use of topical fucidin in pregnancy requires that the potential benefits be weighed against the possible hazards to the foetus.

Safety in nursing mothers has not been established. When fusidic acid (as the sodium salt) has been given systemically, levels have been detected in breast milk but with topical use the possible amount of drug present is unlikely to affect the infant.

4.7 Effects on ability to drive and use machines
Not applicable.

4.8 Undesirable effects
Hypersensitivity reactions to the active ingredient in the form of skin rashes, mild stinging and irritation on application have been reported rarely.

4.9 Overdose
Not applicable.

5. PHARMACOLOGICAL PROPERTIES

5.1 Pharmacodynamic properties
Fusidic acid is a potent topical antibacterial agent. Fusidic acid and its salts show fat and water solubility and strong surface activity and exhibit unusual ability to penetrate intact skin. Concentrations of 0.03-0.12 microgram/ml inhibit nearly all strains of *Staphylococcus aureus.* Topical application of fusidic acid is also effective against streptococci, corynebacteria, neisseria and certain clostridia.

5.2 Pharmacokinetic properties
In vitro studies show that fusidic acid can penetrate intact human skin. The degree of penetration depends on factors such as the duration of exposure to fusidic acid and the condition of the skin. Fusidic acid is excreted mainly in the bile with little excreted in the urine.

5.3 Preclinical safety data
There are no pre-clinical data of relevance to the prescriber which are additional to that already included in other sections of the SPC.

6. PHARMACEUTICAL PARTICULARS

6.1 List of excipients
Cetyl alcohol, lanolin, white soft paraffin, liquid paraffin.

6.2 Incompatibilities
Not applicable.

6.3 Shelf life
3 years.

6.4 Special precautions for storage
None.

6.5 Nature and contents of container
Aluminium tubes of 15 gram and 30 gram.

6.6 Special precautions for disposal and other handling
None.

7. MARKETING AUTHORISATION HOLDER
LEO Laboratories Limited
Longwick Road
Princes Risborough
Bucks
HP27 9RR

8. MARKETING AUTHORISATION NUMBER(S)
PL 0043/5005R

9. DATE OF FIRST AUTHORISATION/RENEWAL OF THE AUTHORISATION
24.10.1986.

10. DATE OF REVISION OF THE TEXT
May 1998

LEGAL CATEGORY
POM

Fucidin Suspension

(Leo Laboratories Limited)

1. NAME OF THE MEDICINAL PRODUCT
FUCIDIN® SUSPENSION

2. QUALITATIVE AND QUANTITATIVE COMPOSITION
Each 5ml of Suspension contains 250mg Fusidic Acid Ph.Eur. (therapeutically equivalent to 175mg Sodium Fusidate Ph.Eur.).

3. PHARMACEUTICAL FORM
Suspension for oral administration.

4. CLINICAL PARTICULARS

4.1 Therapeutic indications
Fucidin® is indicated in the treatment of all staphylococcal infections due to susceptible organisms such as: osteomyelitis, pneumonia, septicaemia, wound infections, endocarditis, superinfected cystic fibrosis, cutaneous infections.

Fucidin® should be administered intravenously whenever oral therapy is inappropriate, which includes cases where absorption from the gastro-intestinal tract is unpredictable.

4.2 Posology and method of administration
Each 5ml of Fucidin® Suspension is therapeutically equivalent to 175mg of sodium fusidate owing to its lower oral bioavailability. Therefore the following dosages are recommended:

Adults: 15ml three times daily

Children:

- 0-1 year: 1ml/kg bodyweight daily, divided into 3 equal doses
- 1-5 years: 5ml three times daily
- 5-12 years: 10ml three times daily

Elderly: No dosage alterations are necessary in the elderly.

Since Fucidin® is excreted in the bile, no dosage modifications are needed in renal impairment.

The dosage in patients undergoing haemodialysis needs no adjustment as Fucidin® is not significantly dialysed.

The Suspension should be shaken before use and dilution is not recommended.

4.3 Contraindications
Contra-indicated in patients with known hypersensitivity to fusidic acid and its salts.

4.4 Special warnings and precautions for use
Caution should be exercised with other antibiotics which have similar biliary excretion pathways, e.g. lincomycin and rifampicin. Periodic liver function tests should be carried out when high oral doses are used, when the drug is given for prolonged periods and in patients with liver dysfunction.

Fucidin® displaces bilirubin from its albumin binding site in vitro. The clinical significance of this finding is uncertain and kernicterus has not been observed in neonates receiving Fucidin®. However, this observation should be borne in mind when the drug is given to pre-term, jaundiced, acidotic or seriously ill neonates.

The use of Fucidin® in combination with drugs that are CYP-3A4 biotransformed should be avoided. See Section 4.5

Patients given Fucidin®systemically in combination with HMG-CoA reductase inhibitors should be closely clinically monitored. See Section 4.5

4.5 Interaction with other medicinal products and other forms of interaction
Specific pathways of Fucidin® metabolism in the liver are not known, however, an interaction between Fucidin® and drugs being CYP-3A4 biotransformed can be suspected. The mechanism of this interaction is presumed to be a mutual inhibition of metabolism. There is insufficient data to characterise the effect of fusidic acid on CYPs *in-vitro*. The use of Fucidin® systemically should be avoided in patients treated with CYP-3A4 biotransformed drugs.

Fucidin® administered systemically and concomitantly with oral anticoagulants such as coumarin derivatives or anticoagulants with similar actions may increase the plasma concentration of these agents enhancing the anticoagulant effect. Anticoagulation should be closely monitored and a decrease of the oral anticoagulant dose may be necessary in order to maintain the desired level of anticoagulation. Similarly, discontinuation of Fucidin®may require the maintenance dose of anticoagulant to be reassessed. The mechanism of this suspected interaction remains unknown.

Co-administration of Fucidin® systemically and HMG-CoA reductase inhibitors such as statins may cause increased plasma concentrations of both agents and rare cases of rhabdomyolysis have been reported for this combination. Patients on this combination should be closely clinically monitored.

Co-administration of Fucidin®systemically and ciclosporin has been reported to cause increased plasma concentration of ciclosporin.

4.6 Pregnancy and lactation
There is inadequate evidence of safety in human pregnancy. Animal studies and many years of clinical experience suggest that fusidic acid is devoid of teratogenic effects. There is evidence to suggest that when given systemically, fusidic acid can cross the placental barrier. If the administration of Fucidin®to pregnant patients is considered essential, its use requires that the potential benefits be weighed against the possible hazards to the foetus.

Safety in nursing mothers has not been established. When fusidic acid (as the sodium salt) has been given systemically, levels have been detected in the breast milk. Caution is therefore required when Fucidin®is used in mothers who wish to breast feed.

4.7 Effects on ability to drive and use machines
None known.

4.8 Undesirable effects
In some patients, given Fucidin®, particularly in the young and elderly, a reversible jaundice has been reported. Jaundice has been seen most frequently in patients receiving intravenous Fucidin®in high dosage, or where the drug has been infused too rapidly or at too high a concentration in the infusion fluid. In some instances instituting oral therapy may be beneficial. If the jaundice persists Fucidin®should be withdrawn, following which the serum bilirubin will invariably return to normal. Reported reactions are gastro-intestinal upsets and, rarely, skin rashes and other allergic reactions including anaphylaxis. Isolated cases of haematological abnormalities which can affect the 3 blood cell lines but mainly white blood cells e.g. bone marrow depression, neutropenia, granulocytopenia, agranulocytosis and pancytopenia have been reported. Reported less often is a depressive effect on the platelets and red blood cells with reports of thrombocytopenia and various anaemias. These abnormalities have been observed especially with treatment of more than 15 days. Acute renal failure has been described in patients with jaundice, particularly in the presence of other factors predisposing to renal failure.

4.9 Overdose
There has been no experience of overdosage with Fucidin®. Treatment should be restricted to symptomatic and supportive measures. Dialysis is of no benefit since the drug is not significantly dialysed.

5. PHARMACOLOGICAL PROPERTIES

5.1 Pharmacodynamic properties
Fusidic acid and its salts are potent anti-staphylococcal agents with unusual ability to penetrate tissue. Bactericidal levels have been assayed in bone and necrotic tissue. Concentrations of 0.03-0.12 mcg/ml inhibit nearly all strains of *staphylococcus aureus*. Fusidic acid is active against *staphylococcus epidermidis* and methicillin resistant staphylococci.

5.2 Pharmacokinetic properties
Blood levels are cumulative, reaching concentrations of 50-100 mcg/ml after oral administration of 1.5g daily for three to four days.

Fucidin® is excreted mainly in the bile, little or none being excreted in the urine.

In severe or deep-seated infections and when prolonged therapy may be required, systemic Fucidin®should generally be given concurrently with other anti-staphylococcal antibiotic therapy.

5.3 Preclinical safety data
There are no pre-clinical data of relevance to the prescriber which are additional to that already included in other sections of the SPC.

6. PHARMACEUTICAL PARTICULARS

6.1 List of excipients
Acesulfame potassium, banana flavour, citric acid, disodium phosphate dihydrate, hydroxyethylcellulose, glucose liquid, methylcellulose, orange dry flavour, sodium benzoate, sorbitol, purified water.

6.2 Incompatibilities
Not applicable.

6.3 Shelf life
3 years.

6.4 Special precautions for storage
Protect from direct sunlight and heat.

6.5 Nature and contents of container
Bottles of 50ml.

6.6 Special precautions for disposal and other handling
None.

7. MARKETING AUTHORISATION HOLDER
LEO Laboratories Limited
Longwick Road
Princes Risborough
Bucks
HP27 9RR

8. MARKETING AUTHORISATION NUMBER(S)
PL 0043/5014R

9. DATE OF FIRST AUTHORISATION/RENEWAL OF THE AUTHORISATION
United Kingdom 11.11.1986.

10. DATE OF REVISION OF THE TEXT
January 2004

Fucidin Tablets

(Leo Laboratories Limited)

1. NAME OF THE MEDICINAL PRODUCT
Fucidin® Tablets

2. QUALITATIVE AND QUANTITATIVE COMPOSITION
Each tablet contains Sodium Fusidate Ph.Eur.250mg

3. PHARMACEUTICAL FORM
Tablet.

4. CLINICAL PARTICULARS

4.1 Therapeutic indications
Fucidin® is indicated in the treatment of all staphylococcal infections due to susceptible organisms such as: cutaneous infections, osteomyelitis, pneumonia, septicaemia, wound infections, endocarditis, superinfected cystic fibrosis.

Fucidin® should be administered intravenously whenever oral therapy is inappropriate, which includes cases where absorption from the gastro-intestinal tract is unpredictable.

4.2 Posology and method of administration
For staphylococcal cutaneous infections:

Adults: Standard Dose: 250mg (one tablet) sodium fusidate (equivalent to 240mg fusidic acid) twice daily for 5-10 days.

For staphylococcal infections such as osteomyelitis, pneumonia, septicaemia, wound infections, endocarditis, superinfected cystic fibrosis.

Adults: Standard dose: 500mg (two tablets) sodium fusidate (equivalent to 480mg fusidic acid) three times daily.

In severe cases of fulminating infections, the dosage may be doubled or appropriate combined therapy may be used.

Elderly: No dosage alterations are necessary in the elderly.

Since Fucidin® is excreted in the bile, no dosage modifications are needed in renal impairment.

The dosage in patients undergoing haemodialysis needs no adjustment as Fucidin® is not significantly dialysed.

4.3 Contraindications
Contra-indicated in patients with known hypersensitivity to fusidic acid and its salts.

Patients with rare hereditary problems of galactose intolerance, the Lapp lactose deficiency or glucose-galactose malabsorption should not take this medicine.

4.4 Special warnings and precautions for use
Caution should be exercised with other antibiotics which have similar biliary excretion pathways e.g. lincomycin and rifampicin. Periodic liver function tests should be carried out when high oral doses are used, when the drug is given for prolonged periods and in patients with liver dysfunction.

Fucidin® displaces bilirubin from its albumin binding site *in vitro*. The clinical significance of this finding is uncertain and kernicterus has not been observed in neonates receiving Fucidin®. However, this observation should be borne in mind when the drug is given to pre-term, jaundiced, acidotic or seriously ill neonates.

The use of Fucidin® in combination with drugs that are CYP-3A4 biotransformed should be avoided. See Section 4.5

Patients given Fucidin® systemically in combination with HMG-CoA reductase inhibitors should be closely clinically monitored. See Section 4.5

4.5 Interaction with other medicinal products and other forms of interaction
Specific pathways of Fucidin® metabolism in the liver are not known, however, an interaction between Fucidin® and drugs being CYP-3A4 biotransformed can be suspected. The mechanism of this interaction is presumed to be a mutual inhibition of metabolism. There is insufficient data to characterise the effect of fusidic acid on CYPs *in-vitro*. The use of Fucidin® systemically should be avoided in patients treated with CYP-3A4 biotransformed drugs.

Fucidin® administered systemically and concomitantly with oral anticoagulants such as coumarin derivatives or anticoagulants with similar actions may increase the plasma concentration of these agents enhancing the anticoagulant effect. Anticoagulation should be closely monitored and a decrease of the oral anticoagulant dose may be necessary in order to maintain the desired level of anticoagulation. Similarly, discontinuation of Fucidin® may require the maintenance dose of anticoagulant to be reassessed. The mechanism of this suspected interaction remains unknown.

Co-administration of Fucidin® systemically and HMG-CoA reductase inhibitors such as statins may cause increased plasma concentrations of both agents and rare cases of rhabdomyolysis have been reported for this combination. Patients on this combination should be closely clinically monitored.

Co-administration of Fucidin® systemically and ciclosporin has been reported to cause increased plasma concentration of ciclosporin.

4.6 Pregnancy and lactation
There is inadequate evidence of safety in human pregnancy. Animal studies and many years of clinical experience suggest that fusidic acid is devoid of teratogenic effects. There is evidence to suggest that when given systemically, fusidic acid can cross the placental barrier. If the administration of Fucidin® to pregnant patients is considered essential, its use requires that the potential benefits be weighed against the possible hazards to the foetus.

Safety in nursing mothers has not been established. When fusidic acid (as the sodium salt) has been given systemically, levels have been detected in the breastmilk. Caution is therefore required when Fucidin® is used in mothers who wish to breast feed.

4.7 Effects on ability to drive and use machines
None known.

4.8 Undesirable effects
In some patients, given Fucidin®, particularly in the young and elderly, a reversible jaundice has been reported. Jaundice has been seen most frequently in patients receiving intravenous Fucidin® in high dosage, or where the drug has been infused too rapidly or at too high a concentration in the infusion fluid. In some instances instituting oral therapy may be beneficial. If the jaundice persists Fucidin® should be withdrawn, following which the serum bilirubin will invariably return to normal. Reported reactions are gastro-intestinal upsets and, rarely, skin rashes and other allergic reactions including anaphylaxis. Isolated cases of haematological abnormalities which can affect the 3 blood cell lines but mainly white blood cells e.g. bone marrow depression, neutropenia, granulocytopenia, agranulocytosis and pancytopenia have been reported. Reported less often is a depressive effect on the platelets and red blood cells with reports of thrombocytopenia and various anaemias. These abnormalities have been observed especially with treatment of more than 15 days. Acute renal failure has been described in patients with jaundice, particularly in the presence of other factors predisposing to renal failure.

4.9 Overdose
There has been no experience of overdosage with Fucidin®. Treatment should be restricted to symptomatic and supportive measures. Dialysis is of no benefit, since the drug is not significantly dialysed.

5. PHARMACOLOGICAL PROPERTIES

5.1 Pharmacodynamic properties
Fusidic acid and its salts are potent anti-staphylococcal agents with unusual ability to penetrate tissue. Bactericidal levels have been assayed in bone and necrotic tissue. Concentrations of 0.03 - 0.12 micrograms/ml inhibit nearly all strains of *Staphylococcus aureus*. Fusidic acid is active against *Staphylococcus epidermidis* and methicillin resistant staphylococci.

5.2 Pharmacokinetic properties
Blood levels are cumulative, reaching concentrations of 20-35 micrograms/ml after oral administration of 250mg twice daily for seven days and 50-100 micrograms/ml after oral administration of 500mg three times daily for three to four days.

Fucidin® is excreted mainly in the bile, little or none being excreted in the urine.

In severe or deep-seated infections and when prolonged therapy may be required, Fucidin® should generally be given concurrently with other anti-staphylococcal antibiotic therapy.

5.3 Preclinical safety data
There are no pre-clinical data of relevance to the prescriber which are additional to that already included in other sections of the SPC.

6. PHARMACEUTICAL PARTICULARS

6.1 List of excipients
Cellulose microcrystalline, crospovidone, hypromellose, lactose monohydrate, magnesium stearate, silica, *all-rac*-α-tocopherol, talc, titanium dioxide.

6.2 Incompatibilities
None.

6.3 Shelf life
3 years.

6.4 Special precautions for storage
This medicinal product does not require any special storage conditions.

6.5 Nature and contents of container
Blister packs of 10 and 10 × 10 tablets.

6.6 Special precautions for disposal and other handling
None.

7. MARKETING AUTHORISATION HOLDER
LEO Laboratories Limited, Longwick Road, Princes Risborough, Bucks. HP27 9RR.

8. MARKETING AUTHORISATION NUMBER(S)
0043/5000R

9. DATE OF FIRST AUTHORISATION/RENEWAL OF THE AUTHORISATION
4.6.87 (after review).

10. DATE OF REVISION OF THE TEXT
April 2006.

LEGAL CATEGORY
POM

Fucithalmic

(Leo Laboratories Limited)

1. NAME OF THE MEDICINAL PRODUCT
Fucithalmic®

2. QUALITATIVE AND QUANTITATIVE COMPOSITION
Each gram contains fusidic acid, hemihydrate Ph.Eur. 10mg.

3. PHARMACEUTICAL FORM
Sterile viscous eye drops.

4. CLINICAL PARTICULARS

4.1 Therapeutic indications
Fucithalmic is indicated for the topical treatment of bacterial conjunctivitis where the organism is known to be sensitive to the antibiotic.

4.2 Posology and method of administration
For all ages: One Fucithalmic drop to be instilled into the eye twice daily. Treatment should be continued for at least 48 hours after the eye returns to normal.

4.3 Contraindications
Hypersensitivity to any of its components.

4.4 Special warnings and precautions for use
Should not be used when contact lenses are being worn.

4.5 Interaction with other medicinal products and other forms of interaction
Not applicable.

4.6 Pregnancy and lactation
Not applicable.

4.7 Effects on ability to drive and use machines
Not applicable.

4.8 Undesirable effects
Transient stinging after application has been encountered. Hypersensitivity may occur.

4.9 Overdose
Not applicable.

5. PHARMACOLOGICAL PROPERTIES

5.1 Pharmacodynamic properties
Fucithalmic is active against a wide range of gram-positive organisms, particularly *Staphylococcus aureus*. Other species against which Fucithalmic has been shown to have *in*

vitro activity include *Streptococcus*, *Neisseria*, *Haemophilus*, *Moraxella* and *Corynebacteria*.

5.2 Pharmacokinetic properties
The sustained release formulation of Fucithalmic ensures a prolonged contact with the conjunctival sac. Twice daily application provides sufficient fusidic acid concentrations in all relevant tissues of the eye. Fusidic acid penetrates well into the aqueous humour.

5.3 Preclinical safety data
There are no pre-clinical data of relevance to the prescriber which are additional to that already included in other sections of the SPC.

6. PHARMACEUTICAL PARTICULARS
6.1 List of excipients
Benzalkonium chloride, disodium edetate, mannitol, carbomer, sodium hydroxide, water for injections.

6.2 Incompatibilities
None known.

6.3 Shelf life
3 years.

6.4 Special precautions for storage
Store below 25°C. Keep the tube tightly closed. The tube should be discarded one month after opening.

6.5 Nature and contents of container
Available in 5g tubes.

6.6 Special precautions for disposal and other handling
None.

7. MARKETING AUTHORISATION HOLDER
Leo Laboratories Limited, Longwick Road, Princes Risborough, Bucks. HP27 9RR.

8. MARKETING AUTHORISATION NUMBER(S)
0043/0137

9. DATE OF FIRST AUTHORISATION/RENEWAL OF THE AUTHORISATION
10.8.1987

10. DATE OF REVISION OF THE TEXT
June 1997.

LEGAL CATEGORY
POM

Furosemide Injection BP Minijet 10mg/ml Solution for Injection

(International Medication Systems (UK) Ltd)

1. NAME OF THE MEDICINAL PRODUCT
Furosemide Injection BP Minijet 10mg/ml. Solution for Injection.

2. QUALITATIVE AND QUANTITATIVE COMPOSITION
Furosemide 10mg per ml. 80mg per vial.

For excipients see section 6.1.

3. PHARMACEUTICAL FORM
Solution for Injection.

Sterile aqueous solution for intravenous or intramuscular administration.

4. CLINICAL PARTICULARS
4.1 Therapeutic indications
Conditions requiring prompt diuresis, where oral therapy is precluded.

Indications include oedema of cardiac, pulmonary, hepatic or renal origin, forced diuresis and severe hypercalcaemia.

4.2 Posology and method of administration
Parenteral administration should be replaced with oral therapy as soon as possible.

The intravenous injection should be given slowly (maximum 4mg/minute). Usually a prompt diuresis ensues.

Adults:

Acute pulmonary oedema: 40mg should be given immediately by slow intravenous injection, followed by further doses depending upon the patient's response. If there is no satisfactory response within 1 hour, 80mg may be given slowly intravenously.

Oedema: The usual initial dose of furosemide is 20 to 40mg given as a single dose, injected intravenously or intramuscularly.

If the diuretic response with a single dose of 20 to 40mg is not satisfactory, the dose may be increased in 20mg increments at 2 hourly intervals until the desired diuretic effect is obtained.

Very high doses may be required in patients with renal failure (see below).

Hypercalcaemia: Doses ranging from 20-240mg daily have been used. The aim is to increase diuresis to about 6 litres daily.

Forced diuresis: intravenous isotonic fluid at the rate of 500ml/hour is administered together with repeated doses of 20-80mg furosemide to produce a diuresis of 11-12 litres daily.

Acute or chronic renal failure: To avoid ototoxicity furosemide should be administered by intravenous infusion at a rate not exceeding 4mg/minute. The recommended initial dose in patients with acute or chronic renal failure is 25ml (250mg), diluted in approximately 225ml Sodium Chloride Injection BP or Ringer's Solution for Injection, administered over one hour. This gives an approximate drip rate of 80 drops/minute ensuring that the infusion is at the rate of 4mg/minute.

If a satisfactory increase in urine output, such as 40-50ml/hour, is not attained within the next hour, a second infusion of 50ml (500mg) in an appropriate infusion fluid should be given over 2 hours, the total volume of the infusion being governed by the patient's state of hydration. If a satisfactory output is still not achieved within one hour of the end of the second infusion, a third infusion of 100ml (1000mg) can be given over 4 hours. If the third infusion is not effective, then dialysis will probably be required.

In oliguric or anuric patients with significant fluid overload it may not be practicable to administer high dose furosemide by the above method. Under these circumstances the use of a constant rate infusion pump with micrometer screw-gauge adjustment may be considered for direct administration of the injection into the vein.

If the furosemide infusion produces a satisfactory response of 40-50ml/hour, the effective dose (up to 1000mg) can be repeated every 24 hours. Alternatively maintenance therapy can be continued with oral furosemide. Approximate dosage adjustments may then be made according to the observed clinical response.

Elderly: As for adults; the dose should be kept as low as possible.

Children: The usual initial dose is 0.5-1.5mg/kg up to 20mg/day. If the diuretic response after the initial dose is not satisfactory, the dose may be increased by 1mg/kg at 2 hourly intervals until the desired effect has been obtained. Doses greater than 6mg/kg are not recommended. For maintenance therapy, the dosage should be adjusted to the minimum effective level.

4.3 Contraindications
Furosemide is contra-indicated in women of child-bearing potential because animal reproductive studies have shown that it may cause foetal abnormalities. Exceptions to the above are life-threatening situations where the use of a diuretic such as furosemide is especially indicated as opposed to the use of alternative drugs. The physician of course should balance this efficacy potential against teratogenic and embryotoxic potential demonstrated to occur in animal studies.

Furosemide is contraindicated in patients with known hypersensitivity to the drug or to sulphonamides, renal failure associated with anuria or hepatic coma and in the presence of severe sodium and fluid depletion.

4.4 Special warnings and precautions for use
Fluid balance should be carefully monitored. Furosemide may cause profound diuresis, resulting in fluid and electrolyte depletion. Serum electrolytes (especially sodium, potassium, chloride and bicarbonate) should be determined, and abnormalities corrected or the drug withdrawn. If increasing azotemia and oliguria occur during the treatment of progressive renal disease, the drug should be discontinued.

Initiation of furosemide therapy in patients with hepatic cirrhosis and ascites is best carried out in hospital. Sudden alteration of fluid and electrolyte balance in patients with cirrhosis may precipitate hepatic coma, therefore strict observation is necessary during the period of diuresis.

Patients should be regularly observed for the possible occurrence of blood dyscrasias, liver damage or other idiosyncratic reactions.

Periodic checks on urine and blood glucose should be made in diabetics and those suspected of latent diabetes when receiving furosemide. Increases in blood glucose and alterations in glucose tolerance test, with abnormalities of the fasting and 2-hour post-prandial sugar have been observed and rare cases of precipitation of diabetes mellitus have been reported.

Furosemide may lower serum calcium levels and rare cases of tetany have been reported. Accordingly, calcium should be determined periodically.

Patients with prostatic hypertrophy or impaired micturition have an increased risk of developing acute retention.

Care is advised when prescribing Furosemide to patients with either gout or porphyria.

4.5 Interaction with other medicinal products and other forms of interaction
Furosemide -induced hypokalaemia may induce potentially fatal cardiac arrhythmias during treatment with cardiac glycosides. Furosemide may increase the ototoxicity of aminoglycoside antibiotics. Furosemide may enhance the nephrotoxicity of cephalosporins. Due to diuretic-induced sodium depletion, renal clearance of lithium is reduced, which may result in increased lithium concentrations leading to lithium toxicity. Fluid retention caused by steroids may potentially antagonise the diuretic effect but potentiate the potassium loss. In oedematous hypertensive patients being treated with antihypertensive agents, care should be taken to reduce the dose of these drugs since furosemide potentiates the hypotensive effect.

Severe hypotension and/or renal failure may occur if treatment with angiotensin-coverting enzyme-inhibitors is initiated while patients are receiving high doses of loop diuretics. The dose of furosemide should be reduced and severe salt and water depletion corrected before starting the ACE-inhibitor.

Sulphonamide diuretics have been reported to decrease arterial responsiveness to pressor amines and to enhance the effect of tubocurarine. Great caution should be exercised in administering curare or its derivatives to patients undergoing therapy with furosemide and it is advisable to discontinue furosemide two days before elective surgery.

Non-steroidal anti-inflammatory drugs may partially antagonise the action of furosemide. Because of competition for renal excretion, patients receiving high doses of salicylates together with furosemide may experience salicylate toxicity.

The following drugs have been reported to result in a disturbance in the electrolyte balance if given concurrently with furosemide: hormone antagonists, sympathetomimetics, carbamazepine, ulcer healing drugs e.g. carbenoxolone and metalozone.

Estrogens, antiepileptics, probenicid and lipid lowering resins may result in reduction in the diuretic effects of furosemide if administered concurrently.

Flushing, tachycardia, elevated blood pressure and severe diaphoresis have been seen in patients receiving intravenous furosemide having taken oral chloral hydrate in the preceding 24 hours.

Concurrent administration of furosemide and clofibrate may result in marked diuresis and muscle symptoms in patients with marked nephrotic syndrome.

The muscle relaxants baclofen and tizanidine may increase the hypotensive effect of furosemide.

Furosemide may enhance the hyperglycaemic action of diazoxide.

4.6 Pregnancy and lactation
Animal teratology studies indicate that furosemide may cause foetal abnormalities. Therefore, furosemide should only be used in women of child-bearing age when appropriate contraceptive measures are taken or if the potential benefits justify the potential risks to the foetus.

Furosemide is excreted in breast milk and breast-feeding should be discontinued if treatment is essential.

4.7 Effects on ability to drive and use machines
Furosemide may reduce mental alertness. Patients should be warned not to drive or operate machinery if affected.

4.8 Undesirable effects
Excessive diuresis may result in dehydration and reduction in blood volume, with circulatory collapse and with the possibility of vascular thrombosis and embolism, particularly in elderly patients. Serious depletion of potassium and magnesium may lead to cardiac arrhythmias.

Electrolyte depletion may manifest itself by weakness, fatigue, light-headedness or dizziness, muscle cramps, thirst, increased perspiration, urinary bladder spasm and symptoms of urinary frequency.

Transient pain after intramuscular injection has been reported at the injection site. Thrombophlebitis has occurred with intravenous administration.

Various forms of dermatitis, including urticaria and rare cases of exfoliative dermatitis, erythema multiforme, pruritus, paraesthesia, blurring of vision, postural hypotension, nausea, vomiting or diarrhoea, photosensitivity, or hypersensitivity reactions, including vasculitis/arteritis, fever, bullous pemphigoid or vesiculobullous eruptions may occur. Anaemia, leucopenia, aplastic anaemia and thrombocytopenia (with purpura) may occur. Very rarely, agranulocytosis has occurred which has responded to treatment. If a rash or thrombocytopenia occur, furosemide should be stopped immediately.

Cases of tinnitus and reversible hearing impairment have been reported. There have also been some reports of cases in which hearing impairment was irreversible. Usually ototoxicity is associated with rapid injection in patients with severe renal impairment at doses several times more than the usual recommended dose and in whom other drugs of known ototoxicity were given.

Acute diuresis in male patients with prostatic obstruction may cause acute retention of urine.

In addition, the following rare adverse events have been reported although the relationship to the drug has not been confirmed: sweet taste, oral and gastric burning, paradoxical swelling, headache, jaundice and acute pancreatitis.

In children, complaints of mild to moderate abdominal pain and cramping have been reported after intravenous furosemide. Nephrocalcaemia has been reported in premature infants.

Asymptomatic hyperuricaemia can occur and rarely gout may be precipitated. These are associated with dehydration which should be avoided particularly in patients with renal insufficiency.

4.9 Overdose
Symptoms: Overdose with furosemide may lead to excessive loss of water and electrolytes. Severe potassium loss may cause serious cardiac arrhythmias.

Treatment: Restoration of fluid and electrolytes balance by administration of sodium chloride and water, intravenously if necessary.

5. PHARMACOLOGICAL PROPERTIES

5.1 Pharmacodynamic properties

Furosemide is a short-acting sulphonamide diuretic, chemically similar to the thiazides. With parenteral administration, the diuretic effect is immediate and lasts approximately two hours. Furosemide primarily inhibits the reabsorption of sodium in the proximal and distal tubules as well as in the Loop of Henle, thus increasing the urinary excretion of sodium, chloride and water. Urinary excretion of potassium, calcium and magnesium are also increased, together with bicarbonate; urinary pH rises.

5.2 Pharmacokinetic properties

Furosemide is 91% to 99% bound to serum albumin but protein binding is reduced in patients with uraemia and nephrosis. The plasma half life ranges from 45 to 60 minutes. Furosemide crosses the placenta and enters breast milk. It is eliminated by renal excretion of unchanged drug, metabolism to a glucuronide conjugate and faecal excretion.

5.3 Preclinical safety data

Toxicity studies in animals have not demonstrated toxic effects relevant to clinical use. There is no evidence of mutagenic or carcinogenic potential.

6. PHARMACEUTICAL PARTICULARS

6.1 List of excipients

Sodium Hydroxide

Sodium Chloride

Water for Injections

6.2 Incompatibilities

Furosemide is soluble in alkaline solutions. The injection is a mildly buffered alkaline solution which should not be mixed with highly acidic solutions.

6.3 Shelf life

36 months.

6.4 Special precautions for storage

Do not store above 25°C.

6.5 Nature and contents of container

The solution is contained in a USP type I glass vial with an elastomeric closure which meets all the relevant USP specifications. The product is available as 8ml.

6.6 Special precautions for disposal and other handling

The container is specially designed for use with the IMS Minijet injector.

7. MARKETING AUTHORISATION HOLDER

International Medication Systems (UK) Limited

208 Bath Road

Slough

Berkshire

SL1 3WE

UK

8. MARKETING AUTHORISATION NUMBER(S)

PL 03265/0025

9. DATE OF FIRST AUTHORISATION/RENEWAL OF THE AUTHORISATION

28 June 2003

10. DATE OF REVISION OF THE TEXT

Approved: February 2009

POM

Fuzeon

(Roche Products Limited)

1. NAME OF THE MEDICINAL PRODUCT

Fuzeon 90 mg/ml powder and solvent for solution for injection

2. QUALITATIVE AND QUANTITATIVE COMPOSITION

Each vial contains 108 mg enfuvirtide.

Each ml of reconstituted solution contains 90 mg enfuvirtide.

For a full list of excipients, see section 6.1.

3. PHARMACEUTICAL FORM

Powder and solvent for solution for injection.

White to off-white lyophilised powder.

4. CLINICAL PARTICULARS

4.1 Therapeutic indications

Fuzeon is indicated in combination with other antiretroviral medicinal products for the treatment of HIV-1 infected patients who have received treatment with and failed on regimens containing at least one medicinal product from each of the following antiretroviral classes: protease inhibitors, non-nucleoside reverse transcriptase inhibitors and nucleoside reverse transcriptase inhibitors, or who have intolerance to previous antiretroviral regimens. (see section 5.1)

In deciding on a new regimen for patients who have failed an antiretroviral regimen, careful consideration should be given to the treatment history of the individual patient and the patterns of mutations associated with different medicinal products. Where available, resistance testing may be appropriate. (See sections 4.4 and 5.1)

4.2 Posology and method of administration

Fuzeon should be prescribed by physicians who are experienced in the treatment of HIV infection.

Fuzeon is only to be administered by subcutaneous injection.

Adults and adolescents ⩾ 16 years: The recommended dose of Fuzeon is 90 mg twice daily injected subcutaneously into the upper arm, anterior thigh or abdomen.

Elderly: There is no experience in patients > 65 years old.

Children ⩾ 6 years and adolescents: The experience in children is limited (See section 5.2). In clinical trials the dosage regimen in table 1 below was used:

Table 1: Paediatric Dosing

Weight (kg)	Dose per bid injection (mg/dose)	Injection volume (90 mg enfuvirtide per ml)
11.0 to 15.5	27	0.3 ml
15.6 to 20.0	36	0.4 ml
20.1 to 24.5	45	0.5 ml
24.6 to 29.0	54	0.6 ml
29.1 to 33.5	63	0.7 ml
33.6 to 38.0	72	0.8 ml
38.1 to 42.5	81	0.9 ml
⩾42.6	90	1.0 ml

Fuzeon is not recommended for use in children below age 6 due to insufficient data on safety and efficacy (see section 5.2).

Renal impairment: No dose adjustment is required for patients with renal impairment including those receiving dialysis. (See sections 4.4 and 5.2).

Hepatic impairment: No data are available to establish a dose recommendation for patients with hepatic impairment. (See sections 4.4 and 5.2).

4.3 Contraindications

Hypersensitivity to the active substance or to any of the excipients.

4.4 Special warnings and precautions for use

Fuzeon must be taken as part of a combination regimen. Please also refer to the respective summary of product characteristics of the other antiretroviral medicinal products used in the combination. As with other antiretrovirals, enfuvirtide should optimally be combined with other antiretrovirals to which the patient's virus is sensitive. (See section 5.1)

Patients must be advised that antiretroviral therapies including enfuvirtide have not been proved to prevent the risk of transmission to HIV to others through sexual contact or blood contamination. They must continue to use appropriate precautions. Patients should also be informed that Fuzeon is not a cure for HIV-1 infection.

Animal studies have shown that enfuvirtide may impair some immune functions (see section 5.3). An increased rate of some bacterial infections, most notably a higher rate of pneumonia, has been seen in patients treated with Fuzeon. Patients should be monitored closely for signs and symptoms of pneumonia. (See section 4.8)

Hypersensitivity reactions have occasionally been associated with therapy with enfuvirtide and in rare cases hypersensitivity reactions have recurred on rechallenge. Events included rash, fever, nausea and vomiting, chills, rigors, low blood pressure and elevated serum liver transaminases in various combinations, and possibly primary immune complex reaction, respiratory distress and glomerulonephritis. Patients developing signs/symptoms of a systemic hypersensitivity reaction should discontinue enfuvirtide treatment and should seek medical evaluation immediately. Therapy with enfuvirtide should not be restarted following systemic signs and symptoms consistent with a hypersensitivity reaction considered related to enfuvirtide. Risk factors that may predict the occurrence or severity of hypersensitivity to enfuvirtide have not been identified.

Liver disease: The safety and efficacy of enfuvirtide has not been specifically studied in patients with significant underlying liver disorders. Patients with chronic hepatitis B and C and treated with antiretroviral therapy are at an increased risk for severe and potentially fatal hepatic adverse events. Few patients included in the phase III trials were co-infected with hepatitis B/C. In these the addition of Fuzeon did not increase the incidence of hepatic events. In case of concomitant antiviral therapy for hepatitis B or C, please refer also to the relevant product information for these medicinal products.

Administration of Fuzeon to non-HIV-1 infected individuals may induce anti-enfuvirtide antibodies that cross-react with HIV gp41. This may result in a false positive HIV test with the anti-HIV ELISA test.

There is no experience in patients with reduced hepatic function. Data is limited in patients with moderate to severe renal impairment, and in patients maintained on dialysis. Fuzeon should be used with caution in these populations. (See sections 4.2 and 5.2)

Immune Reactivation Syndrome: In HIV-infected patients with severe immune deficiency at the time of institution of combination antiretroviral therapy (CART), an inflammatory reaction to asymptomatic or residual opportunistic pathogens may arise and cause serious clinical conditions, or aggravation of symptoms. Typically, such reactions have been observed within the first few weeks or months of initiation of CART. Relevant examples are cytomegalovirus retinitis, generalised and/or focal mycobacterial infections, and Pneumocystis carinii pneumonia. Any inflammatory symptoms should be evaluated and treatment instituted when necessary.

Osteonecrosis:

Although the aetiology is considered to be multifactorial (including corticosteroid use, alcohol consumption, severe immunosuppression, higher body mass index), cases of osteonecrosis have been reported particularly in patients with advanced HIV-disease and/or long-term exposure to CART. Patients should be advised to seek medical advice if they experience joint aches and pain, joint stiffness or difficulty in movement.

4.5 Interaction with other medicinal products and other forms of interaction

Interactions studies have only been performed in adults.

No clinically significant pharmacokinetic interactions are expected between enfuvirtide and concomitantly given medicinal products metabolised by CYP450 enzymes.

Influence of enfuvirtide on metabolism of concomitant medicinal products: In an in-vivo human metabolism study enfuvirtide, at the recommended dose of 90 mg twice daily, did not inhibit the metabolism of substrates by CYP3A4 (dapsone), CYP2D6 (debrisoquine), CYP1A2 (caffeine), CYP2C19 (mephenytoin), and CYP2E1 (chlorzoxazone).

Influence of concomitant medicinal products on enfuvirtide metabolism: In separate pharmacokinetic interaction studies, co-administration of ritonavir (potent CYP3A4 inhibitor) or saquinavir in combination with a booster dose of ritonavir or rifampicin (potent CYP34A inducer) did not result in clinically significant changes of the pharmacokinetics of enfuvirtide.

4.6 Pregnancy and lactation

There are no adequate and well-controlled studies in pregnant women. Animal studies do not indicate harmful effects with respect to foetal development. Enfuvirtide should be used during pregnancy only if the potential benefit justifies the potential risk to the foetus.

It is not known whether enfuvirtide is secreted in human milk. Mothers should be instructed not to breast-feed if they are receiving enfuvirtide because of the potential for HIV transmission and any possible undesirable effects in breast-fed infants.

4.7 Effects on ability to drive and use machines

No studies on the effects on the ability to drive and use machines have been performed. There is no evidence that enfuvirtide may alter the patient's ability to drive and use machines, however, the adverse event profile of enfuvirtide should be taken into account. (See section 4.8)

4.8 Undesirable effects

Safety data mainly refer to 48-week data from studies TORO 1 and TORO 2 combined (see section 5.1). Safety results are expressed as the number of patients with an adverse reaction per 100 patient-years of exposure (except for injection site reactions).

Injection site reactions

Injection site reactions (ISRs) were the most frequently reported adverse reaction and occurred in 98% of the patients (Table 2). The vast majority of ISRs occurred within the first week of Fuzeon administration and were associated with mild to moderate pain or discomfort at the injection site without limitation of usual activities. The severity of the pain and discomfort did not increase with treatment duration. The signs and symptoms generally lasted equal to or less than 7 days. Infections at the injection site (including abscess and cellulitis) occurred in 1.5% of patients.

Table 2: Summary of individual signs/symptoms characterising local injection site reactions in studies TORO 1 and TORO 2 combined (% of patients)

(see Table 2 on next page)

Other adverse reactions

The addition of Fuzeon to background antiretroviral therapy generally did not increase the frequency or severity of most adverse reactions. The most frequently reported events occurring in the TORO 1 and TORO 2 studies were diarrhoea (38 versus 73 patients with event per 100 patient years for Fuzeon + OB versus OB) and nausea (27 versus 50 patients with event per 100 patient years for Fuzeon + OB versus OB).

Table 2: Summary of individual signs/symptoms characterising local injection site reactions in studies TORO 1 and TORO 2 combined (% of patients)

	n=663		
Withdrawal Rate due to ISRs	4%		
Event Category	**Fuzeon +Optimised background[a]**	**% of Event comprising Grade 3 reactions**	**% of Event comprising Grade 4 reactions**
Pain / discomfort	96.1%	11.0%[b]	0%[b]
Erythema	90.8%	23.8%[c]	10.5%[c]
Induration	90.2%	43.5%[d]	19.4%[d]
Nodules and cysts	80.4%	29.1%[e]	0.2%[e]
Pruritus	65.2%	3.9%[f]	NA
Ecchymosis	51.9%	8.7%[g]	4.7%[g]

[a]Any severity grade.
[b]Grade 3= severe pain requiring analgesics (or narcotic analgesics for ≤ 72 hours) and/or limiting usual activities; Grade 4= severe pain requiring hospitalisation or prolongation of hospitalisation, resulting in death, or persistent or significant disability/incapacity, or life-threatening, or medically significant.
[c]Grade 3= ≥ 50 mm but < 85 mm average diameter; Grade 4= ≥ 85 mm average diameter.
[d]Grade 3= ≥ 25 mm but < 50 mm average diameter; Grade 4= ≥ 50 mm average diameter.
[e]Grade 3= ≥ 3 cm; Grade 4= If draining.
[f]Grade 3= refractory to topical treatment or requiring oral or parenteral treatment; Grade 4= not defined.
[g]Grade 3=> 3 cm but ≤ 5 cm; Grade 4=> 5 cm.

The following list presents events seen at a higher rate among patients receiving Fuzeon+OB regimen than among patients on the OB alone regimen with an exposure adjusted increase of at least 2 patients with event per 100 patient-years. These events are then designated frequency estimation ("very common" (≥1/10), or "common" (≥1/100, <1/10)). A statistically significant increase was seen for pneumonia and lymphadenopathy. Most adverse reactions were of mild or moderate intensity.

Infections and Infestations

Common: - sinusitis, skin papilloma, influenza, pneumonia, ear infection.

Blood and Lymphatic System Disorders

Common: - lymphadenopathy.

Metabolism and Nutrition Disorders

Common: - appetite decreased, anorexia, hypertriglyceridaemia, diabetes mellitus.

Psychiatric Disorders

Common: - anxiety, nightmare, irritability.

Nervous System Disorders

Very Common: - peripheral neuropathy.

Common: -hypoaesthesia, disturbance in attention, tremor.

Eye Disorders

Common: - conjunctivitis.

Ear and Labyrinth disorders

Common: - vertigo.

Respiratory, Thoracic and Mediastinal Disorders

Common: - nasal congestion.

Gastrointestinal Disorders

Common: - pancreatitis, gastro-oesophageal reflux disease.

Skin and Subcutaneous Tissue Disorders

Common: - dry skin, eczema seborrhoeic, erythema, acne.

Musculoskeletal, Connective Tissue and Bone Disorders

Common: - myalgia.

Renal and Urinary Disorders

Common: - Calculus renal.

General Disorders and Administration Site Conditions

Common: - influenza like illness, weakness.

Investigations

Very Common: - weight decreased

Common: - blood triglycerides increased, haematuria present.

In addition there have been a small number of hypersensitivity reactions attributed to enfuvirtide and in some cases recurrence has occurred upon re-challenge. (See section 4.4)

In HIV-infected patients with severe immune deficiency at the time of initiation of combination antiretroviral therapy (CART), an inflammatory reaction to asymptomatic or residual opportunistic infections may arise (see section 4.4).

Cases of osteonecrosis have been reported, particularly in patients with generally acknowledged risk factors, advanced HIV disease or long-term exposure to CART. The frequency of this is unknown (see section 4.4).

Laboratory abnormalities

The majority of patients had no change in the toxicity grade of any laboratory parameter during the study except for those listed in Table 3. Through week 48, eosinophilia [greater than the Upper Limit of Normal of > 0.7 × 10^9/l] occurred at a higher rate amongst patients in the Fuzeon containing group (12.4 patients with event per 100 patient-years) compared with OB alone regimen (5.6 patients with event per 100 patient-years). When using a higher threshold for eosinophilia (>1.4 × 10^9/l), the patient exposure adjusted rate of eosinophilia is equal in both groups (1.8 patients with event per 100 patient-years).

Table 3: Exposure adjusted Grade 3 & 4 laboratory abnormalities among patients on Fuzeon+OB and OB alone regimens, reported at more than 2 patients with event per 100 patient years

(see Table 3 below)

4.9 Overdose

No case of overdose has been reported. The highest dose administered to 12 patients in a clinical trial was 180 mg as a single dose subcutaneously. These patients did not experience any adverse reactions that were not seen with the recommended dose. In an Early Access Program study, one patient administered 180 mg of Fuzeon as a single dose on one occasion. He did not experience an adverse reaction as a result.

There is no specific antidote for overdose with enfuvirtide. Treatment of overdose should consist of general supportive measures.

5. PHARMACOLOGICAL PROPERTIES

5.1 Pharmacodynamic properties

Pharmacotherapeutic group: Other antivirals, ATC code: J05AX07

Mechanism of Action: Enfuvirtide is a member of the therapeutic class called fusion inhibitors. It is an inhibitor of the structural rearrangement of HIV-1 gp41 and functions by specifically binding to this virus protein extracellularly thereby blocking fusion between the viral cell membrane and the target cell membrane, preventing the viral RNA from entering into the target cell.

Antiviral activity *in vitro*: The susceptibility to enfuvirtide of 612 HIV recombinants containing the env genes from HIV RNA samples taken at baseline from patients in Phase III studies gave a geometric mean EC_{50} of 0.259 µg/ml (geometric mean + 2SD = 1.96 µg/ml) in a recombinant phenotype HIV entry assay. Enfuvirtide also inhibited HIV-1 envelope mediated cell-cell fusion. Combination studies of enfuvirtide with representative members of the various antiretroviral classes exhibited additive to synergistic antiviral activities and an absence of antagonism. The relationship between the *in vitro* susceptibility of HIV-1 to enfuvirtide and inhibition of HIV-1 replication in humans has not been established.

Antiretroviral drug resistance: Incomplete viral suppression may lead to the development of drug resistance to one or more components of the regimen.

In Vitro resistance to enfuvirtide: HIV-1 isolates with reduced susceptibility to enfuvirtide have been selected *in vitro* which harbour substitutions in amino acids (aa) 36-38 of the gp41 ectodomain. These substitutions were correlated with varying levels of reduced enfuvirtide susceptibility in HIV site-directed mutants.

In Vivo resistance to enfuvirtide: In phase III clinical studies HIV recombinants containing the env genes from HIV RNA samples taken up to week 24 from 187 patients showed > 4 fold reduced susceptibility to enfuvirtide compared with the corresponding pre-treatment samples. Of these, 185 (98.9%) env genes carried specific substitutions in region of aa 36 - 45 of gp41. The substitutions observed in decreasing frequency were at aa positions 38, 43, 36, 40, 42 and 45. Specific single substitutions at these residues in gp41 each resulted in a range of decreases from baseline in recombinant viral susceptibility to enfuvirtide. The geometric mean changes ranged from 15.2 fold for V38M to 41.6 fold for V38A. There were insufficient examples of multiple substitutions to determine any consistent patterns of substitutions or their effect on viral susceptibility to enfuvirtide. The relationship of these substitutions to *in vivo* effectiveness of enfuvirtide has not been established. Decrease in viral sensitivity was correlated to the degree of pre-treatment resistance to background therapy. (See Table 5)

Cross-resistance: Due to its novel viral target enfuvirtide is equally active *in vitro* against both wild-type laboratory and clinical isolates and those with resistance to 1, 2 or 3 other classes of antiretrovirals (nucleoside reverse transcriptase inhibitors, non-nucleoside reverse transcriptase inhibitors and protease inhibitors). Conversely, mutations in aa 36-45 of gp41 which give resistance to enfuvirtide would not be expected to give cross resistance to other classes of antiretrovirals.

Clinical Pharmacodynamic data

Studies in Antiretroviral Experienced Patients: The clinical activity of Fuzeon (in combination with other antiretroviral agents) on plasma HIV RNA levels and CD4 counts have been investigated in two randomised, multicentre, controlled studies (TORO 1 and TORO 2) of Fuzeon of 48 weeks duration. 995 patients comprised the intent-to-treat population. Patient demographics include a median baseline HIV-1 RNA of 5.2 $\log_{10}$ copies/ml and 5.1 $\log_{10}$ copies/ml and median baseline CD4 cell count of 88 cells/mm^3 and 97 cells/mm^3 for Fuzeon + OB and OB, respectively. Patients had prior exposure to a median of 12 antiretrovirals for a median of 7 years. All patients received an optimised background (OB) regimen consisting of 3 to 5 antiretroviral agents selected on the basis of the patient's prior treatment history, as well as baseline genotypic and phenotypic viral resistance measurements.

The proportion of patients achieving viral load of <400 copies/ml at week 48 was 30.4% among patients on the Fuzeon+OB regimen compared to 12% among patients receiving OB regimen only. The mean CD4 cell count increase was greater in patients on the Fuzeon + OB regimen than in patients on OB regimen only. (see Table 4)

Table 4 Outcomes of Randomised Treatment at Week 48 (Pooled Studies TORO 1 and TORO 2, ITT)

(see Table 4 on next page)

Fuzeon+OB therapy was associated with a higher proportion of patients reaching <400 copies/ml (or <50 copies/ml) across all subgroups based on baseline CD4, baseline

Table 3: Exposure adjusted Grade 3 & 4 laboratory abnormalities among patients on Fuzeon+OB and OB alone regimens, reported at more than 2 patients with event per 100 patient years

Laboratory Parameters Grading	Fuzeon+OB regimen Per 100 patient years	OB alone regimen Per 100 patient years
n (Total Exposure patient years)	663 (557.0)	334 (162.1)
ALAT		
Gr. 3 (>5-10 × ULN)	4.8	4.3
Gr. 4 (>10 × ULN)	1.4	1.2
Haemoglobin		
Gr. 3 (6.5-7.9 g/dL)	2.0	1.9
Gr. 4 (<6.5 g/dL)	0.7	1.2
Creatinine phosphokinase		
Gr. 3 (>5-10 × ULN)	8.3	8.0
Gr. 4 (>10 × ULN)	3.1	8.6

Table 4 Outcomes of Randomised Treatment at Week 48 (Pooled Studies TORO 1 and TORO 2, ITT)

Outcomes	Fuzeon +OB 90 mg bid (N=661)	OB (N=334)	Treatment Difference	95% Confidence Interval	p-value
HIV-1 RNA Log Change from baseline (log_{10} copies/ml)*	-1.48	-0.63	LSM -0.85	-1.073, -0.628	<.0001
CD4+ cell count Change from baseline (cells/mm^3)#	+91	+45	LSM 46.4	25.1, 67.8	<.0001
HIV RNA ≥1 log below Baseline**	247 (37.4%)	57 (17.1%)	Odds Ratio 3.02	2.16, 4.20	<.0001
HIV RNA <400 copies/ml**	201 (30.4%)	40 (12.0%)	Odds Ratio 3.45	2.36, 5.06	<.0001
HIV RNA <50 copies/ml**	121 (18.3%)	26 (7.8%)	Odds Ratio 2.77	1.76, 4.37	<.0001
Discontinued due to adverse reactions/ intercurrent illness/labs†	9%	11%			
Discontinued due to injection site reactions†	4%	N/A			
Discontinued due to other reasons†Φ§	13%	25%			

* Based on results from pooled data of TORO 1 and TORO 2 on ITT population, week 48 viral load for subjects who were lost to follow-up, discontinued therapy, or had virological failure replaced by their last observation (LOCF).

Last value carried forward.

** M-H test: Discontinuations or virological failure considered as failures.

† Percentages based on safety population Fuzeon+background (N=663) and background (N=334). Denominator for non-switch patients: N=112.

Φ As per the judgment of the investigator.

§ Includes discontinuations from loss to follow-up, treatment refusal, and other reasons.

Table 5 Proportion of Patients achieving <400 copies/ml and <50 copies/ml at Week 48 by subgroup (pooled TORO 1 and TORO 2, ITT)

Subgroups	HIV-1 RNA < 400 copies/ml		HIV-1 RNA < 50 copies/ml	
	Fuzeon + OB 90 mg bid (N=661)	OB (N=334)	Fuzeon + OB 90 mg bid (N=661)	OB (N=334)
BL HIV-1 RNA < 5.0 log_{10}[1] copies/ml	118/269 (43.9%)	26/144 (18.1%)	77/269 (28.6%)	18/144 (12.5%)
BL HIV-1 RNA ⩾ 5.0 log_{10}[1] copies/ml	83/392 (21.2%)	14/190 (7.4%)	44/392 (11.2%)	8/190 (4.2%)
Total prior ARVs ⩽ 10[1]	100/215 (46.5%)	29/120 (24.2%)	64/215 (29.8%)	19/120 (15.8%)
Total prior ARVs > 10[1]	101/446 (22.6%)	11/214 (5.1%)	57/446 (12.8%)	7/214 (3.3%)
0 Active ARVs in background[1,2]	9/112 (8.0%)	0/53 (0%)	4/112 (3.5%)	0/53 (0%)
1 Active ARV in background[1,2]	56/194 (28.9%)	7/95 (7.4%)	34/194 (17.5%)	3/95 (3.2%)
⩾ 2 Active ARVs in background[1,2]	130/344 (37.8%)	32/183 (17.5%)	77/334 (22.4%)	22/183 (12.0%)

[1]Discontinuations or virological failures considered as failures.

[2]Based on GSS score.

HIV-1 RNA, number of prior antiretrovirals (ARVs) or number of active ARVs in the OB regimen. However, subjects with baseline CD4 >100 cells/mm^3, baseline HIV-1 RNA <5.0 log_{10} copies/ml, ⩽ 10 prior ARVs, and/or other active ARVs in their OB regimen were more likely to achieve a HIV-1 RNA of <400 copies/ml (or <50 copies/ml) on either treatment. (see Table 5)

Table 5 Proportion of Patients achieving <400 copies/ ml and <50 copies/ml at Week 48 by subgroup (pooled TORO 1 and TORO 2, ITT)

(see Table 5 above)

5.2 Pharmacokinetic properties

The pharmacokinetic properties of enfuvirtide have been evaluated in HIV-1-infected adult and paediatric patients.

Absorption: The absolute bioavailability after subcutaneous administration of enfuvirtide 90 mg in the abdomen was 84.3 ± 15.5%. Mean (± SD) C_{max} was 4.59 ± 1.5 μg/ml, AUC was 55.8 ± 12.1 μg*hr/ml The subcutaneous absorption of enfuvirtide is proportional to the administered dose over the 45 to 180 mg dose range. Subcutaneous absorption at the 90 mg dose is comparable when injected into abdomen, thigh or arm. In four separate studies (N = 9 to 12) the mean steady state trough plasma concentration ranged from 2.6 to 3.4 μg/ml.

Distribution: The steady state volume of distribution with intravenous administration of a 90 mg dose of enfuvirtide was 5.5 ± 1.1 l. Enfuvirtide is 92% bound to plasma proteins in HIV infected plasma over a plasma concentration range of 2 to 10 μg/ml. It is bound predominantly to albumin and to a lower extent to α-1 acid glycoprotein. In *in vitro* studies, enfuvirtide was not displaced from its binding sites by other medicinal products, nor did enfuvirtide displace other medicinal products from their binding sites. In HIV patients, enfuvirtide levels in the cerebrospinal fluid have been reported to be negligible.

Metabolism: As a peptide, enfuvirtide is expected to undergo catabolism to its constituent amino acids, with subsequent recycling of the amino acids in the body pool. *In vitro* human microsomal studies and in *in vivo* studies indicate that enfuvirtide is not an inhibitor of CYP450 enzymes. In *in vitro* human microsomal and hepatocyte studies, hydrolysis of the amide group of the C-terminus amino acid, phenylalanine results in a deamidated metabolite and the formation of this metabolite is not NADPH dependent. This metabolite is detected in human plasma following administration of enfuvirtide, with an AUC ranging from 2.4 to 15% of the enfuvirtide AUC.

Elimination: Clearance of enfuvirtide after intravenous administration 90 mg was 1.4 ± 0.28 l/h and the elimination half-life was 3.2 ± 0.42 h. Following a 90 mg subcutaneous dose of enfuvirtide the half-life of enfuvirtide is 3.8 ± 0.6 h. Mass balance studies to determine elimination pathway(s) of enfuvirtide have not been performed in humans.

Hepatic Insufficiency: The pharmacokinetics of enfuvirtide have not been studied in patients with hepatic impairment.

Renal Insufficiency: Analysis of plasma concentration data from patients in clinical trials indicated that the clearance of enfuvirtide is not affected to any clinically relevant extent in patients with mild to moderate renal impairment. In a renal impairment study AUC of enfuvirtide was increased on average by 43-62% in patients with severe or end stage renal disease compared to patients with normal renal function. Haemodialysis did not significantly alter enfuvirtide clearance. Less than 13% of the dose was removed during haemodialysis. No dose adjustment is required for patients with impaired renal function.

Elderly: The pharmacokinetics of enfuvirtide have not been formally studied in elderly patients over 65 years of age.

Gender and Weight: Analysis of plasma concentration data from patients in clinical trials indicated that the clearance of enfuvirtide is 20% lower in females than males irrespective of weight and is increased with increased body weight irrespective of gender (20% higher in a 100 kg and 20% lower in a 40 kg body weight patient relative to a 70 kg reference patient). However, these changes are not clinically significant and no dose adjustment is required.

Race: Analysis of plasma concentration data from patients in clinical trials indicated that the clearance of enfuvirtide was not different in Afro-Americans compared to Caucasians. Other PK studies suggest no difference between Asians and Caucasians after adjusting exposure for body weight.

Paediatric Patients: The pharmacokinetics of enfuvirtide have been studied in 37 paediatric patients. A dose of 2 mg/kg bid (maximum 90 mg bid) provided enfuvirtide plasma concentrations similar to those obtained in adult patients receiving 90 mg bid dosage. In 25 paediatric patients ranging in age from 5 to 16 years and receiving the 2 mg/kg bid dose into the upper arm, anterior thigh or abdomen, the mean steady-state AUC was 54.3 ± 23.5 μg*h/ml, C_{max} was 6.14 ± 2.48 μg/ml, and C_{trough} was 2.93 ± 1.55 μg/ml.

5.3 Preclinical safety data

Non-clinical data reveal no special hazard for humans based on conventional studies of safety pharmacology, repeated dose toxicity, genotoxicity and late embryonal development. Long-term animal carcinogenicity studies have not been performed.

Studies in guinea pigs indicated a potential for enfuvirtide to produce delayed contact hypersensitivity. In a rat model on the resistance to influenza infection, an impairment of IFN-γ production was observed. The resistance to influenza and streptococcal infection in rats was only weakly compromised. The clinical relevance of these findings is unknown.

6. PHARMACEUTICAL PARTICULARS

6.1 List of excipients

Powder

Sodium carbonate

Mannitol

Sodium hydroxide

Hydrochloric Acid

Solvent

Water for Injections

6.2 Incompatibilities

This medicinal product must not be mixed with other medicinal products except those mentioned in section 6.6.

6.3 Shelf life

Powder

3 years

Solvent

3 years

Shelf life after reconstitution

After reconstitution: Store in a refrigerator (2°C – 8°C).

Chemical and physical in-use stability has been demonstrated for 48 hours at 5°C when protected from light.

From a microbiological point of view, the product should be used immediately. If not used immediately, in-use storage times and conditions prior to use are the responsibility of the user and would normally not be longer than 24 hours at 2°C to 8°C, unless reconstitution has taken place in controlled and validated aseptic conditions.

6.4 Special precautions for storage

Powder

Keep the vial in the outer carton in order to protect from light. For storage conditions of the reconstituted medicinal product, see section 6.3.

Solvent

This medicinal product does not require any special storage conditions.

6.5 Nature and contents of container

Powder

Vial: 3 ml vial, colourless glass type 1

Closure: lyophilisate stopper, rubber (latex free)

Seal: aluminum seal with flip-off cap

Solvent

Vial: 2 ml vial, colourless glass type 1

Closure: rubber stopper (latex free)

Seal: aluminum seal with flip-off cap

Pack sizes

Pack 1

60 vials powder for solution for injection

60 vials solvent

60 3 ml syringes

60 1 ml syringes

180 alcohol swabs

Pack 2

60 vials powder for solution for injection

60 vials solvent

6.6 Special precautions for disposal and other handling

Any unused product should be disposed of in accordance with local requirements.

Patients should be instructed on the use and administration of Fuzeon by a healthcare professional before using for the first time.

Fuzeon must only be reconstituted with 1.1 ml of Water for Injections. Patients must be instructed to add the water for injections and then gently tap the vial with their fingertip until the powder begins to dissolve. **They must never shake the vial or turn it upside down to mix—this will cause excessive foaming**. After the powder begins to dissolve they can set the vial aside to allow it to completely dissolve. The powder may take up to 45 minutes to dissolve into solution. The patient can gently roll the vial between their hands after adding the water for injections until it is fully dissolved and this may reduce the time it takes for the powder to dissolve. Before the solution is withdrawn for administration, the patient should inspect the vial visually to ensure that the contents are fully in solution, and that the solution is clear and without bubbles or particulate matter. If there is evidence of particulate matter, the vial must not be used and should be discarded or returned to the pharmacy.

The solvent vials contain 2 ml Water for Injections, of which 1.1 ml must be withdrawn for the reconstitution of the powder. Patients should be instructed to discard the remaining volume in the solvent vials.

Fuzeon contains no preservative. Once reconstituted, the solution should be injected immediately. If the reconstituted solution cannot be injected immediately, it must be kept refrigerated until use and used within 24 hours. Refrigerated reconstituted solution should be brought to room temperature before injection.

1 ml of the reconstituted solution should be injected subcutaneously in the upper arm, abdomen or anterior thigh. The injection should be given at a site different from the preceding injection site and where there is no current injection site reaction. A vial is suitable for single use only; unused portions must be discarded.

7. MARKETING AUTHORISATION HOLDER

Roche Registration Limited
6 Falcon Way
Shire Park
Welwyn Garden City
AL7 1TW
United Kingdom

8. MARKETING AUTHORISATION NUMBER(S)

EU/1/03/252/001-002

9. DATE OF FIRST AUTHORISATION/RENEWAL OF THE AUTHORISATION

Date of first authorisation: 27 May 2003

Date of last renewal: 27 May 2008

10. DATE OF REVISION OF THE TEXT

8 July 2008

Detailed information on this medicinal product is available on the web site of the European Medicines Agency (EMEA) http://www.emea.europa.eu

Gabitril 5mg, Gabitril 10mg, Gabitril 15mg

(Cephalon (UK) Limited)

1. NAME OF THE MEDICINAL PRODUCT

Gabitril® 5 mg film-coated tablets

Gabitril® 10 mg film-coated tablets

Gabitril® 15 mg film-coated tablets

2. QUALITATIVE AND QUANTITATIVE COMPOSITION

Each Gabitril 5 mg tablet contains:

Tiagabine anhydrous, INN 5 mg (as hydrochloride monohydrate)

Each Gabitril 10 mg tablet contains:

Tiagabine anhydrous, INN 10 mg (as hydrochloride monohydrate)

Each Gabitril 15 mg tablet contains:

Tiagabine anhydrous, INN 15 mg (as hydrochloride monohydrate)

3. PHARMACEUTICAL FORM

5 mg: Tablet. White, round biconvex film-coated tablet embossed on one side with '251'.

10 mg: Tablet. White, oval biconvex film-coated tablet embossed on one side with '252'.

15 mg: Tablet. White, oval biconvex film-coated tablet embossed on one side with '253'.

4. CLINICAL PARTICULARS

4.1 Therapeutic indications

Gabitril is an anti-epileptic drug indicated as add-on therapy for partial seizures with or without secondary generalisation where control is not achieved by optimal doses of at least one other anti-epileptic drug.

4.2 Posology and method of administration

Gabitril should be taken orally with meals.

Dosing schemes may need to be individualised based upon a patient's particular characteristics such as age and concomitant medications.

Concomitant use with drugs involving CYP 3A4/5 metabolism: As CYP3A4/5 is involved in the metabolism of tiagabine, it is recommended that the dose of tiagabine is adjusted when it is taken in combination with CYP3A4/5 inducers (see section 4.5 Interactions with other medicinal products and other forms of interactions).

Following a given dose of tiagabine, the estimated plasma concentration in non-induced patients is more than twice that in patients receiving enzyme-inducing agents. To achieve similar systemic exposures of tiagabine, non-induced patients require lower and less frequent doses of tiagabine than induced patients. These patients may also require a slower titration of tiagabine compared to that of induced patients.

Adults and children over 12 years: The initial daily dose is 5-10 mg tiagabine, followed by weekly increments of 5-10 mg/day. The usual maintenance dose in patients taking enzyme-inducing drugs is 30-45 mg/day. In patients not taking enzyme-inducing drugs, the maintenance dose should initially be reduced to 15-30 mg/day. The initial daily dose should be taken as a single dose or divided into two doses. The daily maintenance dose should be divided into two or three single doses.

Children under 12 years: There is no experience with Gabitril in children under 12 years of age and as such Gabitril should not be used in this age group.

Use in the elderly: There is limited information available on the use of Gabitril in elderly patients, but pharmacokinetics of tiagabine are unchanged, hence there should be no need for dose modification.

Patients with renal insufficiency: Renal insufficiency does not affect the pharmacokinetics of tiagabine, therefore the dosage does not need to be modified in this type of patient.

Use in patients with impaired liver function: In patients with mild to moderate hepatic dysfunction (Child Pugh Score 5 – 9) the initial daily maintenance dosage should be 5-10 mg given once or twice daily. Gabitril should not be used in patients with severely impaired hepatic function.

4.3 Contraindications

Gabitril should not be given to patients with a history of hypersensitivity to tiagabine or one of the excipients.

4.4 Special warnings and precautions for use

Suicidal ideation and behaviour have been reported in patients treated with anti-epileptic agents in several indications. A meta-analysis of randomised placebo controlled trials of anti-epileptic drugs has also shown a small increased risk of suicidal ideation and behaviour. The mechanism of this risk is not known and the available data do not exclude the possibility of an increased risk for Gabitril.

Therefore patients should be monitored for signs of suicidal ideation and behaviours and appropriate treatment should be considered. Patients (and caregivers of patients) should be advised to seek medical advice should signs of suicidal ideation or behaviour emerge.

Post-marketing reports have shown that Gabitril use has been associated with new onset seizures and status epilepticus in patients without epilepsy. Confounding factors that may have contributed to development of seizures include underlying medical conditions or concomitant medications that can reduce seizure threshold, reported overdose and manner of dose administration (e.g. high dosage, fast titration rate).

Safety and effectiveness of Gabitril have not been established for any indication other than as adjunctive therapy for partial seizures in adults and adolescents over 12 years.

Gabitril is eliminated by hepatic metabolism and therefore caution should be exercised when administering the product to patients with impaired hepatic function. Reduced doses and/or dose intervals should be used and patients should be monitored closely for adverse events such as dizziness and tiredness.

Gabitril should not be used in patients with severely impaired hepatic function.

Although Gabitril may slightly prolong the CNS depressant effect of triazolam, this interaction is unlikely to be relevant to clinical practice.

Anti-epileptic agents that induce hepatic enzymes (such as phenytoin, carbamazepine, phenobarbital and primidone) enhance the metabolism of tiagabine. Consequently, patients taking enzyme-inducing drugs may require doses of tiagabine above the usual dose range.

Although there is no evidence of withdrawal seizures following Gabitril, it is recommended to taper off treatment over a period of 2-3 weeks.

Spontaneous bruising has been reported. Therefore, if bruising is observed full blood count, including platelet count is to be performed.

Rare cases of visual field defects have been reported with tiagabine. If visual symptoms develop, the patient should be referred to an ophthalmologist for further evaluation including perimetry.

Gabitril tablets contain lactose and therefore should not be used in patients with rare hereditary problems of galactose intolerance, the Lapp lactase deficiency, or glucose-galactose malabsorption.

4.5 Interaction with other medicinal products and other forms of interaction

Anti-epileptic agents that induce hepatic enzymes (such as phenytoin, carbamazepine, phenobarbital and primidone) enhance the metabolism of tiagabine. The plasma concentration of tiagabine may be reduced by a factor 1.5-3 by concomitant use of these drugs.

Gabitril does not have any clinically significant effect on the plasma concentrations of phenytoin, carbamazepine, phenobarbital, warfarin, digoxin, theophylline and hormones from oral contraceptive pills. Gabitril reduces the plasma concentration of valproate by about 10%, and cimetidine increases the bioavailability of tiagabine by about 5%. Neither of these findings are considered clinically important and do not warrant a dose modification.

4.6 Pregnancy and lactation

Animal experiments have not shown a teratogenic effect of tiagabine. Studies in animals have however, revealed peri- and post-natal toxicity of tiagabine at very high doses.

Clinical experience of the use of Gabitril in pregnant women is limited.

No information on Gabitril during breast-feeding is available.

Consequently, as a precautionary measure, it is preferable not to use Gabitril during pregnancy or breast-feeding unless in the opinion of the physician, the potential benefits of treatment outweigh the potential risks.

4.7 Effects on ability to drive and use machines

Gabitril may cause dizziness or other CNS related symptoms, especially during initial treatment. Therefore caution should be shown by patients driving vehicles or operating machinery.

4.8 Undesirable effects

Adverse events are mainly CNS related.

In placebo controlled parallel group add-on epilepsy trials of Gabitril in combination with other anti-epileptic drugs, the adverse events that occurred statistically more frequently with Gabitril than with placebo are tabulated below.

	Gabitril	Placebo
	N=493	N=276
	%	%
Dizziness	29	16
Tiredness	22	15
Nervousness (non-specific)	11	4
Tremor	10	4
Diarrhoea	8	3
Concentration difficulties	6	3
Depressed mood	4	1
Emotional lability	4	1
Slowness in speech	2	0

In clinical trials, about 15% of patients receiving Gabitril reported serious adverse events; the causal relationship of these events with Gabitril treatment has not been established and some may be associated with the underlying condition or concomitant treatment. Accidental injury (2.8%) was the only adverse event which occurred with a frequency of more than 1%; others included confusion (1.0%), depression (0.8%), somnolence (0.8%) and psychosis (0.7%). However, none of these adverse events led to the withdrawal of more than 0.2% of patients.

In patients with a history of serious behavioural problems there is a risk of recurrence of these symptoms during treatment with Gabitril, as occurs with certain other anti-epileptic drugs.

Although not statistically significant, routine laboratory screening during placebo controlled trials showed a low white blood cell count ($<2.5 \times 10^9$ per litre) more frequently during Gabitril treatment (4.1%) than placebo (1.5%).

Rarely, cases of non-convulsive status epilepticus, hallucinations and delusion have been reported.

Infrequent cases of bruising can occur.

Rare cases of visual field defects have been reported (see section 4.4 Special Warnings and Precautions for use).

Post-marketing:

Post-marketing reports have shown that Gabitril use has been associated with new onset seizures and status epilepticus in patients without epilepsy (see section 4.4 Special warnings and special precautions for use).

Cases of encephalopathy have been reported (frequency unknown).

4.9 Overdose

Symptoms most often accompanying Gabitril overdose, alone or in combination with other drugs, have included seizures, including status epilepticus, in patients with and without underlying seizure disorders, coma, ataxia or incoordination, somnolence, dizziness, impaired speech, agitation, myoclonus, spike wave stupor, tremors, vomiting and hostility. In more severe instances, mute and withdrawn appearance of the patient, risk of convulsion have been reported.

From post-marketing experience, there have been no reports of fatal overdoses involving Gabitril alone (doses up to 720 mg), although a number of patients required intubation and ventilatory support as part of the management of their status epilepticus.

Standard medical observation and supportive care should be given.

5. PHARMACOLOGICAL PROPERTIES

5.1 Pharmacodynamic properties

Gabitril is an anti-epileptic drug.

Tiagabine is a potent and selective inhibitor of both neuronal and glial GABA uptake, which results in an increase in GABAergic medicated inhibition in the brain.

Tiagabine lacks significant affinity for other neurotransmitter receptor binding sites and/or uptake sites.

5.2 Pharmacokinetic properties

Tiagabine is rapidly and virtually completely absorbed from Gabitril tablets, with an absolute bioavailability of 89%. Administration with food results in a decreased rate and not extent of absorption.

The volume of distribution is approximately 1 L/kg.

Plasma protein binding of tiagabine is about 96%.

Renal clearance is negligible. Hepatic metabolism is the principle route for elimination of tiagabine. Less than 2% of the dose is excreted unchanged in urine and faeces. No active metabolites have been identified. Other anti-epileptic drugs such as phenytoin, carbamazepine, phenobarbital and primidone induce hepatic drug metabolism and the hepatic clearance of tiagabine is increased when given concomitantly with these drugs.

There is no evidence that tiagabine causes clinically significant induction or inhibition of hepatic drug metabolising enzymes at clinical doses.

The plasma elimination half-life of tiagabine is 7–9 hours, except in induced patients where it is 2-3 hours.

Absorption and elimination of tiagabine are linear within the therapeutic dose range.

5.3 Preclinical safety data

Animal safety data carried out in the rat, mouse and dog gave no clear evidence of specific organ toxicity nor any findings of concern for the therapeutic use of tiagabine. The dog appears to be particularly sensitive to the pharmacological actions of tiagabine and clinical signs such as sedation, insensibility, ataxia and visual impairment reflecting CNS effects were seen at daily doses of 0.5 mg/kg and above in a dose related manner. The results of a wide range of mutagenicity tests showed that tiagabine is unlikely to be genotoxic to humans. Clastogenic activity was seen only at cytotoxic concentrations (>>200-fold human plasma levels) using the *in-vitro* human lymphocyte test in the absence of a metabolising system. In long-term carcinogenicity studies conducted in the rat and mouse, only the rat study revealed slightly increased incidences of hepatocellular adenomas in females and benign Leydig cell tumours in the high dose (200 mg/kg/day) group only. These changes are considered to be rat-specific and macrophages and inflammation were seen at a higher incidence than normal. The significance of this latter finding is unknown.

6. PHARMACEUTICAL PARTICULARS

6.1 List of excipients

Tablet Core:

Cellulose, microcrystalline (E460)

Ascorbic acid (E300)

Lactose, anhydrous

Starch, pregelatinised (maize)

Crospovidone

Silica, colloidal anhydrous (E551)

Hydrogenated vegetable oil (Type 1)

Stearic acid

Magnesium stearate

Film-coating:

Hypromellose

Hydroxypropylcellulose (E463)

Titanium Dioxide (E171)

6.2 Incompatibilities

None.

6.3 Shelf life

3 years

6.4 Special precautions for storage

Do not refrigerate or freeze. Store in the original package.

6.5 Nature and contents of container

Child resistant, white polyethylene bottles with white polypropylene screw closures. Each bottle contains a high density polyethylene canister of activated clay desiccant.

Packs containing 50 and 100 tablets. Not all pack sizes may be marketed.

6.6 Special precautions for disposal and other handling

No special instructions

7. MARKETING AUTHORISATION HOLDER

Cephalon UK Limited

1 Albany Place

Hyde Way

Welwyn Garden City

Hertfordshire

AL7 3BT

United Kingdom

8. MARKETING AUTHORISATION NUMBER(S)

Gabitril 5 mg PL 16260/0009

Gabitril 10 mg PL 16260/0010

Gabitril 15 mg PL 16260/0011

9. DATE OF FIRST AUTHORISATION/RENEWAL OF THE AUTHORISATION

30th September 2002

10. DATE OF REVISION OF THE TEXT

June 2009

Legal Category

POM

GANFORT

(Allergan Ltd)

1. NAME OF THE MEDICINAL PRODUCT

GANFORT®▼300 micrograms/ml + 5 mg/ml eye drops, solution

2. QUALITATIVE AND QUANTITATIVE COMPOSITION

One ml of solution contains 0.3 mg of bimatoprost and 5 mg of timolol (as 6.8 mg of timolol maleate).

Contains benzalkonium chloride 0.05 mg/ml. For a full list of excipients, see section 6.1.

3. PHARMACEUTICAL FORM

Eye drops, solution.

Colourless to slightly yellow solution.

4. CLINICAL PARTICULARS

4.1 Therapeutic indications

Reduction of intraocular pressure (IOP) in patients with open-angle glaucoma or ocular hypertension who are insufficiently responsive to topical beta-blockers or prostaglandin analogues.

4.2 Posology and method of administration

Recommended dosage in adults (including the elderly)

The recommended dose is one drop of GANFORT in the affected eye(s) once daily, administered in the morning.

If one dose is missed, treatment should continue with the next dose as planned. The dose should not exceed one drop in the affected eye(s) daily.

If more than one topical ophthalmic product is to be used, the different products should be instilled at least 5 minutes apart.

Use in renal and hepatic impairment

GANFORT has not been studied in patients with hepatic or renal impairment. Therefore caution should be used in treating such patients.

Use in children and adolescents

GANFORT has only been studied in adults and therefore its use is not recommended in children or adolescents.

4.3 Contraindications

• Hypersensitivity to the active substances or to any of the excipients.

• Reactive airway disease including bronchial asthma or a history of bronchial asthma, severe chronic obstructive pulmonary disease.

• Sinus bradycardia, second or third degree atrioventricular block, overt cardiac failure, cardiogenic shock.

4.4 Special warnings and precautions for use

Like other topically applied ophthalmic agents, GANFORT may be absorbed systemically. No enhancement of the systemic absorption of the individual active substances has been observed.

Due to the beta-adrenergic component, timolol, the same types of cardiovascular and pulmonary adverse reactions as seen with systemic beta-blockers may occur.

Cardiac failure should be adequately controlled before beginning GANFORT therapy. Patients with a history of severe cardiac disease should be watched for signs of cardiac failure and have their pulse rates checked. Cardiac and respiratory reactions, including death due to bronchospasm in patients with asthma, and, rarely, death in association with cardiac failures have been reported following administration of timolol maleate.

Beta-blockers may also mask the signs of hyperthyroidism and cause worsening of Prinzmetal angina, severe peripheral and central circulatory disorders and hypotension.

Beta-adrenergic blocking agents should be administered with caution in patients subject to spontaneous hypoglycemia or to diabetic patients (especially those with labile diabetes) as beta-blockers may mask the signs and symptoms of acute hypoglycemia.

While taking beta-blockers, patients with a history of atopy or a history of severe anaphylactic reaction to a variety of allergens may be unresponsive to the usual dose of adrenaline used to treat anaphylactic reactions.

In patients with a history of mild liver disease or abnormal alanine aminotransferase (ALT), aspartate aminotransferase (AST) and/or bilirubin at baseline, bimatoprost had no adverse reactions on liver function over 24 months. There are no known adverse reactions of ocular timolol on liver function.

Before treatment is initiated, patients should be informed of the possibility of eyelash growth, darkening of the eyelid skin and increased iris pigmentation since these have been observed during treatment with bimatoprost and GANFORT. Some of these changes may be permanent, and may lead to differences in appearance between the eyes if only one eye is treated. After discontinuation of GANFORT, pigmentation of iris may be permanent. After 12 months treatment with GANFORT, the incidence of iris pigmentation was 0.2%. After 12 months treatment with bimatoprost eye drops alone, the incidence was 1.5% and did not increase following 3 years treatment.

Cystoid macular oedema has been reported with GANFORT. Therefore, GANFORT should be used with caution in patients with known risk factors for macular oedema (e.g. aphakic patients, pseudophakic patients with a torn posterior lens capsule).

The preservative in GANFORT, benzalkonium chloride, may cause eye irritation. Contact lenses must be removed prior to application, with at least a 15-minute wait before reinsertion. Benzalkonium chloride is known to discolour soft contact lenses. Contact with soft contact lenses must be avoided.

Benzalkonium chloride has been reported to cause punctate keratopathy and/or toxic ulcerative keratopathy. Therefore monitoring is required with frequent or prolonged use of GANFORT in dry eye patients or where the cornea is compromised.

GANFORT has not been studied in patients with inflammatory ocular conditions, neovascular, inflammatory, angle-closure glaucoma, congenital glaucoma or narrow-angle glaucoma.

4.5 Interaction with other medicinal products and other forms of interaction

No interaction studies have been performed.

There is a potential for additive effects resulting in hypotension, and/or marked bradycardia when eye drops containing timolol are administered concomitantly with oral calcium channel blockers, guanethidine, or beta-blocking agents, anti-arrhythmics, digitalis glycosides or parasympathomimetics.

Beta-blockers may increase the hypoglycaemic effect of antidiabetic agents. Beta-blockers can mask the signs and symptoms of hypoglycaemia (see section 4.4).

The hypertensive reaction to sudden withdrawal of clonidine can be potentiated when taking beta-blockers.

4.6 Pregnancy and lactation

Pregnancy

There are no adequate data from the use of GANFORT in pregnant women.

Bimatoprost

No adequate clinical data in exposed pregnancies are available. Animal studies have shown reproductive toxicity at high maternotoxic doses (see section 5.3).

Timolol

Epidemiological studies have not revealed malformative effects but shown a risk for intra uterine growth retardation when beta-blockers are administered by the oral route. In addition, signs and symptoms of beta-blockade (e.g. bradycardia, hypotension, respiratory distress and hypoglycaemia) have been observed in the neonate when beta-blockers have been administered until delivery. If GANFORT is administered until delivery, the neonate should be carefully monitored during the first days of life. Animal studies with timolol have shown reproductive toxicity at doses significantly higher than would be used in clinical practice (see section 5.3).

Consequently, GANFORT should not be used during pregnancy unless clearly necessary.

Lactation

Timolol is excreted in breast milk. It is not known if bimatoprost is excreted in human breast milk but it is excreted in the milk of the lactating rat. GANFORT should not be used by breast-feeding women.

4.7 Effects on ability to drive and use machines

GANFORT has negligible influence on the ability to drive and use machines. As with any ocular treatment, if transient blurred vision occurs at instillation, the patient should wait until the vision clears before driving or using machinery.

4.8 Undesirable effects

No adverse drug reactions (ADRs) specific for GANFORT have been observed in clinical studies. The ADRs have been limited to those earlier reported for bimatoprost and timolol.

The majority of ADRs were ocular, mild in severity and none were serious. Based on 12-month clinical data, the most commonly reported ADR was conjunctival hyperaemia (mostly trace to mild and thought to be of a non-inflammatory nature) in approximately 26% of patients and led to discontinuation in 1.5% of patients.

The following ADRs were reported during clinical trials with GANFORT (within each frequency grouping, undesirable effects are presented in order of decreasing seriousness):

Nervous system disorders

Uncommon (≥1/1000 to <1/100): headache

Eye disorders

Very common (≥1/10): conjunctival hyperaemia, growth of eyelashes.

Common (≥1/100 to <1/10): superficial punctuate keratitis, corneal erosion, burning sensation, eye pruritus, stinging sensation in the eye, foreign body sensation, eye dryness, eyelid erythema, eye pain, photophobia, eye discharge, visual disturbance, eyelid pruritus.

Uncommon (≥1/1000 to <1/100): iritis, eye irritation, conjunctival oedema, blepharitis, epiphora, eyelid oedema, eyelid pain, visual acuity worsened, asthenopia, trichiasis.

Not known: cystoid macular oedema.

Respiratory, thoracic and mediastinal disorders

Uncommon (≥1/1000 to <1/100): rhinitis

Skin and subcutaneous tissue disorders

Common (≥1/100 to <1/10): blepharal pigmentation

Uncommon (≥1/1000 to <1/100): hirsutism

Additional adverse events that have been seen with one of the components and may potentially occur also with GANFORT:

Bimatoprost

Infections and infestations: infection (primarily colds and upper respiratory symptoms).

Nervous system disorders: dizziness

Eye disorders: allergic conjunctivitis, cataract, eyelash darkening, increased iris pigmentation, blepharospasm, eyelid retraction, retinal haemorrhage, uveitis.

Vascular disorders: hypertension.

General disorders and administration site condition: asthenia, peripheral oedema.

Investigations: liver function tests (LFT) abnormal.

Timolol

Psychiatric disorders: insomnia, nightmares, decreased libido

Nervous system disorders: dizziness, memory loss, increase in signs and symptoms of myasthenia gravis, paresthaesia, cerebral ischaemia

Eye disorders: decreased corneal sensitivity, diplopia, ptosis, choroidal detachment (following filtration surgery), refractive changes (due to withdrawal of miotic therapy in some cases), keratitis.

Ear and labyrinth disorders: tinnitus.

Cardiac disorders: heart block, cardiac arrest, arrhythmia, syncope, bradycardia, cardiac failure, congestive heart failure.

Vascular disorders: hypotension, cerebrovascular accident, claudication, Raynaud's phenomenon, cold hands and feet, palpitation.

Respiratory, thoracic and mediastinal disorders: bronchospasm (predominantly in patients with pre-existing bronchospastic disease) dyspnoea, cough.

Gastrointestinal disorders: nausea, diarrhoea, dyspepsia, dry mouth.

Skin and subcutaneous tissue disorders: alopecia, psoriasiform rash or exacerbation of psoriasis.

Musculoskeletal and connective tissue disorders: systemic lupus erythematosus.

Renal and urinary disorders: Peyronie's disease.

General disorders and administration site conditions: oedema, chest pain, fatigue.

4.9 Overdose

No case of overdose has been reported, and is unlikely to occur after ocular administration.

Bimatoprost

If GANFORT is accidentally ingested, the following information may be useful: in two-week oral rat and mouse studies, doses of bimatoprost up to 100 mg/kg/day did not produce any toxicity. This dose expressed as mg/m^2 is at least 70-times higher than the accidental dose of one bottle of GANFORT in a 10 kg child.

Timolol

Symptoms of systemic timolol overdose are: bradycardia, hypotension, bronchospasm, headache, dizziness, shortness of breath, and cardiac arrest. A study of patients showed that timolol did not dialyse readily.

If overdose occurs treatment should be symptomatic and supportive.

5. PHARMACOLOGICAL PROPERTIES

5.1 Pharmacodynamic properties

Pharmacotherapeutic group: Ophthalmological – beta-blocking agents – timolol, combinations, ATC code: S01ED 51

Mechanism of action:

GANFORT consists of two active substances: bimatoprost and timolol maleate. These two components decrease elevated intraocular pressure (IOP) by complementary mechanisms of action and the combined effect results in additional IOP reduction compared to either compound administered alone. GANFORT has a rapid onset of action.

Bimatoprost is a potent ocular hypotensive agent. It is a synthetic prostamide, structurally related to prostaglandin $F_{2\alpha}$ ($PGF_{2\alpha}$) that does not act through any known prostaglandin receptors. Bimatoprost selectively mimics the effects of newly discovered biosynthesised substances called prostamides. The prostamide receptor, however, has not yet been structurally identified. The mechanism of action by which bimatoprost reduces intraocular pressure in man is by increasing aqueous humour outflow through the trabecular meshwork and enhancing uveoscleral outflow.

Timolol is a $beta_1$ and $beta_2$ non-selective adrenergic receptor blocking agent that does not have significant intrinsic sympathomimetic, direct myocardial depressant, or local anaesthetic (membrane-stabilising) activity. Timolol lowers IOP by reducing aqueous humour formation. The precise mechanism of action is not clearly established, but inhibition of the increased cyclic AMP synthesis caused by endogenous beta-adrenergic stimulation is probable.

Clinical effects:

The IOP-lowering effect of GANFORT is non-inferior to that achieved by adjunctive therapy of bimatoprost (once daily) and timolol (twice daily).

There are no studies with evening dosing of GANFORT. Morning dosing of GANFORT is therefore recommended to ensure maximal IOP-lowering effect at the time of the physiological IOP rise. However, if necessary for patient compliance, an evening dosing may be considered. Once-daily dosing of timolol 0.5% has a rapid onset of maximal effect, corresponding with the time of this rise, and maintains clinically meaningful IOP-lowering over the 24-hour period. Bimatoprost studies show comparable IOP control regardless of morning or evening dosing.

5.2 Pharmacokinetic properties

GANFORT:

Plasma bimatoprost and timolol concentrations were determined in a crossover study comparing the monotherapy treatments to GANFORT treatment in healthy subjects. Systemic absorption of the individual components was minimal and not affected by co-administration in a single formulation.

In two 12-month studies where systemic absorption was measured, no accumulation was observed with either of the individual components.

Bimatoprost:

Bimatoprost penetrates the human cornea and sclera well *in vitro*. After ocular administration, the systemic exposure of bimatoprost is very low with no accumulation over time. After once daily ocular administration of one drop of 0.03% bimatoprost to both eyes for two weeks, blood concentrations peaked within 10 minutes after dosing and declined to below the lower limit of detection (0.025 ng/ml) within 1.5 hours after dosing. Mean C_{max} and AUC $_{0\text{-}24hrs}$ values were similar on days 7 and 14 at approximately 0.08 ng/ml and 0.09 ng•hr/ml respectively, indicating that a steady drug concentration was reached during the first week of ocular dosing.

Bimatoprost is moderately distributed into body tissues and the systemic volume of distribution in humans at steady-state was 0.67 1/kg. In human blood, bimatoprost resides mainly in the plasma. The plasma protein binding of bimatoprost is approximately 88%.

Bimatoprost is the major circulating species in the blood once it reaches the systemic circulation following ocular dosing. Bimatoprost then undergoes oxidation, N-deethylation and glucuronidation to form a diverse variety of metabolites.

Bimatoprost is eliminated primarily by renal excretion, up to 67% of an intravenous dose administered to healthy volunteers was excreted in the urine, 25% of the dose was excreted via the faeces. The elimination half-life, determined after intravenous administration, was approximately 45 minutes; the total blood clearance was 1.5 1/hr/kg.

Characteristics in elderly patients:

After twice daily dosing, the mean AUC $_{0\text{-}24hrs}$ value of 0.0634 ng•hr/ml bimatoprost in the elderly (subjects 65 years or older) were significantly higher than 0.0218 ng•hr/ml in young healthy adults. However, this finding is not clinically relevant as systemic exposure for both elderly and young subjects remained very low from ocular dosing. There was no accumulation of bimatoprost in the blood over time and the safety profile was similar in elderly and young patients.

Timolol:

After ocular administration of a 0.5% eye drops solution in humans undergoing cataract surgery, peak timolol concentration was 898 ng/ml in the aqueous humour at one hour post-dose. Part of the dose is absorbed systemically where it is extensively metabolised in the liver. The half-life of timolol in plasma is about 4 to 6 hours. Timolol is partially metabolised by the liver with timolol and its metabolites excreted by the kidney. Timolol is not extensively bound to plasma.

5.3 Preclinical safety data

GANFORT:

Repeated dose ocular toxicity studies on GANFORT showed no special hazard for humans. The ocular and systemic safety profile of the individual components is well established.

Bimatoprost:

Non-clinical data reveal no special hazard for humans based on conventional studies of safety pharmacology, genotoxicity, carcinogenic potential. Studies in rodents produced species-specific abortion at systemic exposure levels 33- to 97-times that achieved in humans after ocular administration.

Monkeys administered ocular bimatoprost concentrations of ⩾0.03% daily for 1 year had an increase in iris pigmentation and reversible dose-related periocular effects characterised by a prominent upper and/or lower sulcus and widening of the palpebral fissure. The increased iris pigmentation appears to be caused by increased stimulation of melanin production in melanocytes and not by an increase in melanocyte number. No functional or microscopic changes related to the periocular effects have been observed, and the mechanism of action for the periocular changes is unknown.

Timolol:

Non-clinical data reveal no special hazard for humans based on conventional studies of safety pharmacology, repeated dose toxicity, genotoxicity, carcinogenic potential, toxicity to reproduction.

6. PHARMACEUTICAL PARTICULARS

6.1 List of excipients

Benzalkonium chloride

Sodium chloride

Sodium phosphate dibasic heptahydrate

Citric acid monohydrate

Hydrochloric acid or sodium hydroxide (to adjust pH)

Purified water

6.2 Incompatibilities

Not applicable.

6.3 Shelf life

2 years.

Chemical and physical in-use stability has been demonstrated for 28 days at 25°C.

From a microbiological point of view, the in-use storage times and conditions are the responsibility of the user and would normally not be longer than 28 days at 25°C.

6.4 Special precautions for storage

This medicinal product does not require any special storage conditions.

6.5 Nature and contents of container

White opaque low-density polyethylene bottles with polystyrene screw cap. Each bottle has a fill volume of 3 ml.

The following pack sizes are available: cartons containing 1 or 3 bottles of 3 ml. Not all pack sizes may be marketed.

6.6 Special precautions for disposal and other handling

No special requirements.

7. MARKETING AUTHORISATION HOLDER

Allergan Pharmaceuticals Ireland

Castlebar Road

Westport

Co. Mayo

Ireland

8. MARKETING AUTHORISATION NUMBER(S)

EU/1/06/340/001-002

9. DATE OF FIRST AUTHORISATION/RENEWAL OF THE AUTHORISATION

19 May 2006

10. DATE OF REVISION OF THE TEXT

02 March 2009

Gastrocote Liquid

(Actavis UK Ltd)

1. NAME OF THE MEDICINAL PRODUCT

Gastrocote Liquid

2. QUALITATIVE AND QUANTITATIVE COMPOSITION

Sodium Alginate 220mg

Dried aluminium hydroxide gel 80mg

Magnesium trisilicate 40mg

Sodium bicarbonate 70mg

Also contains:

Sodium Methylhydroxybenzoate (E219)

Sodium Propylhydroxybenzoate (E217)

3. PHARMACEUTICAL FORM

Oral suspension

4. CLINICAL PARTICULARS

4.1 Therapeutic indications

Gastrocote Liquid is indicated in heartburn, including heartburn of pregnancy, reflux oesophagitis, particularly where associated with hiatus hernia and in all cases of epigastric distress with gastric reflux or regurgitations. It is also indicated in acid indigestion.

4.2 Posology and method of administration

Oral

Adults and children over 12: One - three 5ml spoonfuls to be taken four times daily, that is, after main meals and at bedtime.

Children 6 to 12 years: One – two 5ml spoonfuls to be taken four times daily, that is, after main meals and at bedtime.

Not recommended for children under 6 years of age.

4.3 Contraindications

Hypersensitivity to any of the ingredients.

4.4 Special warnings and precautions for use

This medicinal product contains 2.13mmol (or 49mg) sodium per 5ml dose. To be taken into account by patients on a controlled sodium diet.

Use with caution in patients with renal impairment or on a low phosphate diet.

If symptoms persist consult your doctor.

May cause allergic reactions (possibly delayed).

4.5 Interaction with other medicinal products and other forms of interaction
Although conventional doses of antacids interfere with the absorption of some drugs, the lower doses of antacids present in Gastrocote Liquid are less likely to cause interactions.

4.6 Pregnancy and lactation
Gastrocote Liquid can be used in pregnancy. (General literature indicates no adverse effects for the active ingredients of Gastrocote Liquid on pregnancy or on the health of the foetus/newborn child).

4.7 Effects on ability to drive and use machines
No known effects.

4.8 Undesirable effects
Adverse effects are unlikely.

Flatulence may occur.

4.9 Overdose
In the event of overdose symptomatic treatment should be given. Abdominal distension may occur.

5. PHARMACOLOGICAL PROPERTIES

5.1 Pharmacodynamic properties
Alginate antacid products form an alginate foam raft on top of the gastric contents. The antacid components remain entrained in the alginate raft and exert little of no effect on gastric pH.

The presence of the foam raft helps to impede gastro-oesophageal reflux. If reflux is forced the alginate antacid foam enters the oesophagus first coating it with a protective demulcent and antacid layer. This coating process is repeated as the reflux subsides. Any refluxed gastric acid is thus rapidly neutralised, the oesophageal mucosa is protected and any pre-existing oesophagitis or ulceration can heal normally.

5.2 Pharmacokinetic properties
There is very little absorption of aluminium hydroxide from the gastrointestinal tract. Only 5% of magnesium is absorbed. However, there is a theoretical possibility of accumulation of aluminium or magnesium in cases of severe renal failure. There is negligible absorption of alginate.

5.3 Preclinical safety data
Not applicable.

6. PHARMACEUTICAL PARTICULARS

6.1 List of excipients
Aluminium magnesium silicate

Sunset yellow FCF (E110)

Butterscotch liquid flavour

Peppermint liquid

Saccharin sodium

Sodium methyl hydroxybenzoate (E219)

Sodium propyl hydroxybenzoate (E217)

Purified water.

6.2 Incompatibilities
None known.

6.3 Shelf life
18 months unopened.

1 month after opening.

6.4 Special precautions for storage
Store below 25°C.

6.5 Nature and contents of container
100ml, 150ml, 200ml, 250ml, 500ml: HDPE bottle with a tamper evident screw cap with EPE/Saranex liner.

6.6 Special precautions for disposal and other handling
Not applicable.

7. MARKETING AUTHORISATION HOLDER
Actavis Group PTC ehf

Reykjavíkurvegi 76-78

220 Hafnarfjordur

Iceland.

8. MARKETING AUTHORISATION NUMBER(S)
PL 30306/0076

9. DATE OF FIRST AUTHORISATION/RENEWAL OF THE AUTHORISATION
16 May 2003

10. DATE OF REVISION OF THE TEXT
08/05/2009

11. DOSIMETRY (IF APPLICABLE)

12 INSTRUCTIONS FOR PREPARATION OF RADIOPHARMACEUTICALS (IF APPLICABLE)

Gastrocote Tablets

(Actavis UK Ltd)

1. NAME OF THE MEDICINAL PRODUCT
Gastrocote Tablets

2. QUALITATIVE AND QUANTITATIVE COMPOSITION

Alginic acid BP	200mg/tablet
Dried aluminium hydroxide gel BP	80mg/tablet
Magnesium trisilicate BP	40mg/tablet
Sodium bicarbonate BP	70mg/tablet

3. PHARMACEUTICAL FORM
Tablet uncoated

4. CLINICAL PARTICULARS

4.1 Therapeutic indications
Gastrocote is indicated in heartburn, including heartburn of pregnancy, reflux oesophagitis, particularly where associated with hiatus hernia and in all cases of epigastric distress with gastric reflux or regurgitations. It is also indicated in acid indigestion.

4.2 Posology and method of administration
Oral

Adults and older children

One to two tablets to be chewed four times a day, that is, after main meals and at bedtime.

Not to be given to children under six years of age.

IMPORTANT: Tablets must be chewed before swallowing.

4.3 Contraindications
There are no specific contraindications in the use of gastrocote.

4.4 Special warnings and precautions for use
Care should be exercised in treating diabetic patients as the tablets contain approximately 1 g of sugar. Each tablet also contains 21mg (0.91Meq) of sodium, which may be important for patients on a low sodium diet. As gastrocote contains aluminium hydroxide, use with caution in patients with renal dysfunction or on a low phosphate diet.

4.5 Interaction with other medicinal products and other forms of interaction
None stated.

4.6 Pregnancy and lactation
Gastrocote Tablets can be used in pregnancy. (General literature indicates no adverse effects for the active ingredients of Gastrocote Tablets on pregnancy or the health of the foetus/newborn child).

4.7 Effects on ability to drive and use machines
None stated.

4.8 Undesirable effects
None stated.

4.9 Overdose
Overdose is virtually free of hazard although gastric bloating may occur.

5. PHARMACOLOGICAL PROPERTIES

5.1 Pharmacodynamic properties
Alginate antacid products form an alginate foam raft on top of the gastric contents. The antacid components remain entrained in the alginate raft and exert little or no effect on gastric pH.

The presence of the foam raft helps to impede gastro-oesophageal reflux. If reflux is forced the alginate antacid foam enters the oesophagus first coating it with a protective demulcent and antacid layer. This coating process is repeated as the reflux subsides. Any refluxed gastric acid is thus rapidly neutralised, the oesophageal mucosa is protected and any pre-existing oesophagitis or ulceration can heal normally.

5.2 Pharmacokinetic properties
There is very little absorption of aluminium hydroxide from the gastrointestinal tract. Only 5% of magnesium is absorbed. However, there is a theoretical possibility of accumulation of aluminium or magnesium in cases of severe renal failure. There is negligible absorption of alginate.

5.3 Preclinical safety data
Not applicable.

6. PHARMACEUTICAL PARTICULARS

6.1 List of excipients
Microcrystalline cellulose or powdered cellulose, carmellose sodium, butterscotch flavour, magnesium stearate, directly compressible sugar.

6.2 Incompatibilities
None stated.

6.3 Shelf life
60 months unopened.

6.4 Special precautions for storage
Store in a cool dry place below 25°C

6.5 Nature and contents of container
10, 12, 20, 40 or 100 tablets: securitainers or high-density polyethylene container with tamper evident low density polyethylene lid or blister pack of plastic/aluminium foil.

6.6 Special precautions for disposal and other handling
Not applicable.

7. MARKETING AUTHORISATION HOLDER
Actavis Group PTC ehf

Reykjavíkurvegi 76-78

220 Hafnarfjordur

Iceland.

8. MARKETING AUTHORISATION NUMBER(S)
PL 30306/0077

9. DATE OF FIRST AUTHORISATION/RENEWAL OF THE AUTHORISATION
1 March 2003

10. DATE OF REVISION OF THE TEXT

11. DOSIMETRY
Not Applicable

12. INSTRUCTIONS FOR PREPARATION OF RADIOPHARMACEUTICALS
Not Applicable

Gastromiro

(Bracco UK Limited)

1. NAME OF THE MEDICINAL PRODUCT
Gastromiro

2. QUALITATIVE AND QUANTITATIVE COMPOSITION

Active component	Quantity per ml
iopamidol (I.N.N.)	612.4 mg

Iopamidol 61.24 % w/v

3. PHARMACEUTICAL FORM
Gastromiro is an aqueous solution for oral or rectal administration (enema)

4. CLINICAL PARTICULARS

4.1 Therapeutic indications
All forms of radiological investigations of gastrointestinal tract, in particular:-

1. Paediatric radiology of the gastro-intestinal tract (GIT) where there is the possibility of:

i) Spill into the respiratory tract, for example in:

a) swallowing disorders

b) oesophageal obstruction with a foreign body, atresia or stricture

c) tracheo-oesophageal fistula.

ii. Spill into the mediastinum, pleura, peritoneum or retroperitoneal tissues, for example due to perforation of the GIT.

iii. Inspissation of fluid, for example in:

a) Meconium ileus equivalent.

b) Intussusception.

c) Colonic obstruction.

d) Hirschsprung's disease.

2. Adult radiology of the gastro-intestinal tract, such as:

i. Suspected upper gastro-intestinal perforation for example in:

Oesophagogastrectomy, endoscopy, partial gastrectomy, pneumonectomy, ingestion of foreign body, duodenal ulceration, small bowel resection, Whipples procedure and blunt abdominal trauma.

ii. Computer Tomography (CT) of the abdominal and pelvic regions, for example:

a) Suspicion of expanding lesions of pancreas, liver and gall bladder.

b) Space occupying metastatic lesions originating from prostate or recto-sigmoidal region in post-surgical staging of cancer.

4.2 Posology and method of administration
Adults:

Radiology of gastro-intestinal tract

Oral: 40-100ml undiluted

Rectal: 200ml of a 50% dilution, up to 1000ml of a 2% dilution

Computer Tomography

Oral:

Abdominal CT: 100ml of a 17% dilution, up to 600ml of a 3% dilution.

Rectal - Pelvic CT: 500-700ml of a 3% dilution

Infants and Children:

Radiology of gastro-intestinal tract

Oral: 10-100ml undiluted or, for use in infants 20-200ml of up to a 50% dilution to provide isotonic contrast medium

Rectal: 200ml of 50-60% dilution

Elderly:

Dosage as for adults.

Dilution of Gastromiro should be carried out using sterile water. Any unused solution should be discarded after 6 hours.

4.3 Contraindications
Proven or suspected hypersensitivity to iodine containing preparations of this type. It must not be used for parenteral administration.

4.4 Special warnings and precautions for use
Disturbances in water or electrolyte balance must first be corrected. This product is formulated for gastro-intestinal use only and should not be used parenterally.

Care should also be exercised in patients with severe functional impairment of the liver, kidney or myocardium, severe systemic disease and in myelomatosis. In such patients adequate hydration should be maintained and parameters of hepatic and renal function, especially urinary output should be monitored after the procedure.

Patients with hepato-renal insufficiency should not be examined unless benefits clearly outweigh risks and re-examination should be delayed for 5-7 days.

In patients with a history of adverse reactions during similar investigations additional caution should be exercised and the procedure should only be carried out if benefits clearly outweigh any risks.

X-ray examination of women should be conducted as far as possible during the pre-ovulation phase of the menstrual cycle. This product may interfere with tests of thyroid function.

4.5 Interaction with other medicinal products and other forms of interaction
None known

4.6 Pregnancy and lactation
The safety of iopamidol during pregnancy and lactation has not been demonstrated clinically. Due, however, to the extremely low absorption of iopamidol from the gastro-intestinal tract it is unlikely that a foetus could be exposed to significant levels. In animal experiments iopamidol is neither teratogenic nor foetotoxic. Similarly, during lactation breast fed infants are unlikely to be exposed to significant levels of iopamidol. However, the product should not be used during pregnancy or when breast feeding unless considered essential.

4.7 Effects on ability to drive and use machines
None known.

4.8 Undesirable effects
Systemic effects are rare since Gastromiro is only poorly absorbed from the alimentary tract. Owing to slight hypertonicity Gastromiro may occasionally cause diarrhoea in infants and children.

4.9 Overdose
The contrast agent is not absorbed from the gastrointestinal tract, therefore any systemic accumulation of the contrast medium following overdosage will not occur. Any treatment should be symptomatic.

5. PHARMACOLOGICAL PROPERTIES

5.1 Pharmacodynamic properties
Iopamidol is a contrast medium belonging to the new generation of non-ionic compounds whose solubility is due to the presence of hydrophilic substituents in the molecule. This results in a solution of low osmolality when compared with ionic media.

Iopamidol has been shown to be effective as an X-ray contrast medium in neuroradiology, angiography, venography, arthrography, urography, cerebral angiography, and left ventriculography, coronary arteriography, and investigations of the gastrointestinal tract. Its toxicity, particularly cardiac and CNS toxicity, is less than those of ionic contrast media.

5.2 Pharmacokinetic properties
Serum iopamidol concentration curves conform to an open two compartment pharmacokinetic model with first order elimination. Iopamidol is very poorly absorbed (about 1-2%) after oral or rectal administration.

Distribution volume is equivalent to extracellular fluid.

Following parenteral administration elimination is almost completely through the kidneys. Less than 1% of the administered dose has been recovered in the faeces up to seventy two hours after dosing. Renal elimination is rapid and up to half the administered dose may be recovered in the urine within the first two hours of dosing.

There is no evidence of biotransformation.

Serum protein binding is negligible.

5.3 Preclinical safety data
In animals, Gastromiro was well tolerated after repeated oral administration. After 4 weeks adminstration of Gastromiro equivalent to 9 gl/kg day, i.e. about 20 times higher than the recommended clinical dose, no severe symptoms of sub-acute intoxication were observed in rats. Following intraperitoneal injection of Gastromiro in rats, iopamidol was rapidly cleared and almost totally eliminated by the renal route within the first 24 hours.

The intraperitoneal acute toxicity was relatively low. Necroscopic examination revealed no irritant effects on the peritoneal membrane. Gastromiro also showed good local tolerability after both local intratracheal installation and systemic administration. It therefore offers a good margin of safety for examination in which there is the risk of an accidental inspiration of the diagnostic medium.

6. PHARMACEUTICAL PARTICULARS

6.1 List of excipients
Quantity per ml
Orange flavour 2.2 mg
Sodium cyclamate 1.5 mg
Red Curaçao flavour 1.1 mg
Disodium edetate dihydrate 0.3 mg
Sodium saccharinate 0.176 mg
Citric acid monohydrate 0.055 mg
Water for injections

6.2 Incompatibilities
No incompatibility studies have been performed: other drugs should not be mixed with Gastromiro.

6.3 Shelf life
Three years.

6.4 Special precautions for storage
Protect from light.

6.5 Nature and contents of container
The containers are amber glass bottles (Type III) with aluminium screw caps, guarantee seals, and elastomer inserts.

Boxes of 1 bottle 20ml
Boxes of 1 bottle 50ml
Boxes of 1 bottle 100ml

6.6 Special precautions for disposal and other handling
Gastromiro is formulated for gastro-intestinal use only and should not be administered parenterally.

The dosage of Gastromiro should be adjusted according to age, total weight, the segment of the digestive tract to be examined and the X-ray procedure.

The bottle once opened has to be used immediately. Solutions not used in one examination session must be discarded.

Gastromiro formulation is a colourless to pale yellow solution containing undissolved solids. Discard in case of discolouration.

7. MARKETING AUTHORISATION HOLDER
Bracco U.K. Ltd,
Bracco House, Mercury Park,
Wycombe Lane, Wooburn Green,
Buckinghamshire HP10 OHH

8. MARKETING AUTHORISATION NUMBER(S)
PL 18920/0012

9. DATE OF FIRST AUTHORISATION/RENEWAL OF THE AUTHORISATION
9 January 1991/ 9 January 1996

10. DATE OF REVISION OF THE TEXT
7 March 2002

LEGAL STATUS
POM

Gemcitabine medac 38 mg/ml powder for solution for infusion

(medac GmbH)

1. NAME OF THE MEDICINAL PRODUCT
Gemcitabine medac 38 mg/ml powder for solution for infusion

2. QUALITATIVE AND QUANTITATIVE COMPOSITION
One vial contains gemcitabine hydrochloride equivalent to 200 mg gemcitabine.

One vial contains gemcitabine hydrochloride equivalent to 1,000 mg gemcitabine.

One vial contains gemcitabine hydrochloride equivalent to 1,500 mg gemcitabine.

After reconstitution, the solution contains 38 mg/ml of gemcitabine.

Excipients
Each 200 mg vial contains 3.5 mg (< 1 mmol) sodium.
Each 1,000 mg vial contains 17.5 mg (< 1 mmol) sodium.
Each 1,500 mg vial contains 26.3 mg (< 1 mmol) sodium.
For a full list of excipients see section 6.1.

3. PHARMACEUTICAL FORM
Powder for solution for infusion
White to off-white powder.

4. CLINICAL PARTICULARS

4.1 Therapeutic indications
Gemcitabine is indicated for the treatment of locally advanced or metastatic bladder cancer in combination with cisplatin.

Gemcitabine is indicated for treatment of patients with locally advanced or metastatic adenocarcinoma of the pancreas.

Gemcitabine, in combination with cisplatin is indicated as first line treatment of patients with locally advanced or metastatic non-small cell lung cancer (NSCLC). Gemcitabine monotherapy can be considered in elderly patients or those with performance status 2.

Gemcitabine is indicated for the treatment of patients with locally advanced or metastatic epithelial ovarian carcinoma, in combination with carboplatin, in patients with relapsed disease following a recurrence-free interval of at least 6 months after platinum-based, first-line therapy.

Gemcitabine, in combination with paclitaxel, is indicated for the treatment of patients with unresectable, locally recurrent or metastatic breast cancer who have relapsed following adjuvant/neoadjuvant chemotherapy. Prior chemotherapy should have included an anthracycline unless clinically contraindicated.

4.2 Posology and method of administration
Gemcitabine should only be prescribed by a physician qualified in the use of anti-cancer chemotherapy.

Recommended posology

Bladder cancer

Combination use

The recommended dose for gemcitabine is 1000 mg/m^2, given by 30-minute intravenous infusion. The dose should be given on Days 1, 8 and 15 of each 28-day cycle in combination with cisplatin. Cisplatin is given at a recommended dose of 70 mg/m^2 on Day 1 following gemcitabine or day 2 of each 28-day cycle. This 4-week cycle is then repeated. Dosage reduction with each cycle or within a cycle may be applied based upon the grade of toxicity experienced by the patient.

Pancreatic cancer

The recommended dose of gemcitabine is 1000 mg/m^2, given by 30-minute intravenous infusion. This should be repeated once weekly for up to 7 weeks followed by a week of rest. Subsequent cycles should consist of injections once weekly for 3 consecutive weeks out of every 4 weeks. Dosage reduction with each cycle or within a cycle may be applied based upon the grade of toxicity experienced by the patient.

Non small Cell lung cancer

Monotherapy

The recommended dose of gemcitabine is 1000 mg/m^2, given by 30-minute intravenous infusion. This should be repeated once weekly for 3 weeks, followed by a 1-week rest period. This 4-week cycle is then repeated. Dosage reduction with each cycle or within a cycle may be applied based upon the grade of toxicity experienced by the patient.

Combination use

The recommended dose for gemcitabine is 1250 mg/m^2 body surface area given as a 30-minute intravenous infusion on Day 1 and 8 of the treatment cycle (21 days). Dosage reduction with each cycle or within a cycle may be applied based upon the grade of toxicity experienced by the patient.

Cisplatin has been used at doses between 75-100 mg/m^2 once every 3 weeks.

Breast cancer

Combination use

Gemcitabine in combination with paclitaxel is recommended using paclitaxel (175 mg/m^2) administered on Day 1 over approximately 3-hours as an intravenous infusion, followed by gemcitabine (1250 mg/m^2) as a 30-minute intravenous infusion on Days 1 and 8 of each 21-day cycle. Dose reduction with each cycle or within a cycle may be applied based upon the grade of toxicity experienced by the patient. Patients should have an absolute granulocyte count of at least 1,500 (x 10^6/l) prior to initiation of gemcitabine + paclitaxel combination.

Ovarian cancer

Combination use

Gemcitabine in combination with carboplatin is recommended using gemcitabine 1000 mg/m^2 administered on Days 1 and 8 of each 21-day cycle as a 30-minute intravenous infusion. After gemcitabine, carboplatin will be given on Day 1 consistent with a target Area under curve (AUC) of 4.0 mg/ml•min. Dosage reduction with each cycle or within a cycle may be applied based upon the grade of toxicity experienced by the patient.

Monitoring for toxicity and dose modification due to toxicity

Dose modification due to non haematological toxicity

Periodic physical examination and checks of renal and hepatic function should be made to detect non-haematological toxicity. Dosage reduction with each cycle or within a cycle may be applied based upon the grade of toxicity experienced by the patient. In general, for severe (Grade 3 or 4) non-haematological toxicity, except nausea/vomiting, therapy with gemcitabine should be withheld or decreased depending on the judgement of the treating physician. Doses should be withheld until toxicity has resolved in the opinion of the physician.

For cisplatin, carboplatin, and paclitaxel dosage adjustment in combination therapy, please refer to the corresponding Summary of Product Characteristics.

Dose modification due to haematological toxicity

Initiation of a cycle

For all indications, the patient must be monitored before each dose for platelet and granulocyte counts. Patients should have an absolute granulocyte count of at least 1,500 (x 10^6/l) and platelet account of 100,000 (x 10^6/l) prior to the initiation of a cycle.

Within a cycle

Dose modifications of gemcitabine within a cycle should be performed according to the following tables:

Dose modification of gemcitabine within a cycle for bladder cancer, NSCLC and pancreatic cancer, given in monotherapy or in combination with cisplatin		
Absolute granulocyte count (x 10^6/l)	**Platelet count (x 10^6/l)**	**Percentage of standard dose of gemcitabine (%)**
> 1,000 and	> 100,000	100
500-1,000 or	50,000-100,000	75
<500 or	< 50,000	Omit dose *

*Treatment omitted will not be re-instated within a cycle before the absolute granulocyte count reaches at least 500 (x10^6/l) and the platelet count reaches 50,000 (x10^6/l).

Dose modification of gemcitabine within a cycle for breast cancer, given in combination with paclitaxel		
Absolute granulocyte count (x 10^6/l)	**Platelet count (x 10^6/l)**	**Percentage of standard dose of gemcitabine (%)**
⩾ 1,200 and	>75,000	100
1,000- <1,200 or	50,000-75,000	75
700- <1,000 and	⩾ 50,000	50
<700 or	<50,000	Omit dose*

*Treatment omitted will not be re-instated within a cycle. Treatment will start on day 1 of the next cycle once the absolute granulocyte count reaches at least 1,500 (x10^6/l) and the platelet count reaches 100,000 (x10^6/l).

Dose modification of gemcitabine within a cycle for ovarian cancer, given in combination with carboplatin		
Absolute granulocyte count (x 10^6/l)	**Platelet count (x 10^6/l)**	**Percentage of standard dose of gemcitabine (%)**
> 1,500 and	⩾ 100,000	100
1000-1,500 or	75,000-100,000	50
<1000 or	< 75,000	Omit dose*

*Treatment omitted will not be re-instated within a cycle. Treatment will start on day 1 of the next cycle once the absolute granulocyte count reaches at least 1,500 (x10^6/l) and the platelet count reaches 100,000 (x10^6/l).

Dose modifications due to haematological toxicity in subsequent cycles, for all indications

The gemcitabine dose should be reduced to 75% of the original cycle initiation dose, in the case of the following haematological toxicities:

- Absolute granulocyte count < 500 × 10^6/l for more than 5 days
- Absolute granulocyte count < 100 × 10^6/l for more than 3 days
- Febrile neutropenia
- Platelets < 25,000 × 10^6/l
- Cycle delay of more than 1 week due to toxicity

Method of administration

Gemcitabine is tolerated well during infusion and may be administered ambulant. If extravasation occurs, generally the infusion must be stopped immediately and started again in another blood vessel. The patient should be monitored carefully after the administration.

For instructions on reconstitution, see section 6.6

Special populations

Patients with renal or hepatic impairment

Gemcitabine should be used with caution in patients with hepatic or renal insufficiency as there is insufficient information from clinical studies to allow for clear dose recommendations for these patient populations (see sections 4.4 and 5.2).

Elderly population (> 65 years)

Gemcitabine has been well tolerated in patients over the age of 65. There is no evidence to suggest that dose adjustments, other than those already recommended for all patients, are necessary in the elderly (see section 5.2).

Children

Gemcitabine has been studied in limited Phase I and II trials in children in a variety of tumour types. These studies did not provide sufficient data to establish the efficacy and safety of gemcitabine in children.

4.3 Contraindications

Hypersensitivity to the active substance gemcitabine or to any of the excipients.

Breast-feeding during treatment with gemcitabine.

4.4 Special warnings and precautions for use

Prolongation of the infusion time and increased dosing frequency have been shown to increase toxicity.

Haematological toxicity

Gemcitabine can suppress bone marrow function as manifested by leucopenia, thrombocytopenia and anaemia.

Patients receiving gemcitabine should be monitored prior to each dose for platelet, leucocyte and granulocyte counts. Suspension or modification of therapy should be considered when drug-induced bone marrow depression is detected (see section 4.2). However, myelosuppression is short lived and usually does not result in dose reduction and rarely in discontinuation.

Peripheral blood counts may continue to deteriorate after gemcitabine administration has been stopped. In patients with impaired bone marrow function, the treatment should be started with caution. As with other cytotoxic treatments, the risk of cumulative bone-marrow suppression must be considered when gemcitabine treatment is given together with other chemotherapy.

Hepatic insufficiency

Administration of gemcitabine in patients with concurrent liver metastases or a pre-existing medical history of hepatitis, alcoholism or liver cirrhosis may lead to exacerbation of the underlying hepatic insufficiency.

Laboratory evaluation of renal and hepatic function (including virological tests) should be performed periodically.

Gemcitabine should be used with caution in patients with hepatic insufficiency or with impaired renal function as there is insufficient information from clinical studies to allow clear dose recommendations for this patient population (see section 4.2).

Concomitant radiotherapy

Concomitant radiotherapy (given together or ⩽ 7 days apart): Toxicity has been reported (see section 4.5 for details and recommendations for use).

Live vaccinations

Yellow fever vaccine and other live attenuated vaccines are not recommended in patients treated with gemcitabine (see section 4.5).

Cardiovascular

Due to the risk of cardiac and/or vascular disorders with gemcitabine, particular caution must be exercised with patients presenting a history of cardiovascular events.

Pulmonary

Pulmonary effects, sometimes severe (such as pulmonary oedema, interstitial pneumonitis or adult respiratory distress syndrome (ARDS)) have been reported in association with gemcitabine therapy. The aetiology of these effects is unknown. If such effects develop, consideration should be made to discontinuing gemcitabine therapy. Early use of supportive care measures may help ameliorate the condition.

Renal

Clinical findings consistent with the haemolytic uraemic syndrome (HUS) were rarely reported in patients receiving gemcitabine (see section 4.8). Gemcitabine should be discontinued at the first signs of any evidence of microangiopathic haemolytic anaemia, such as rapidly falling haemoglobin with concomitant thrombocytopenia, elevation of serum bilirubin, serum creatinine, blood urea nitrogen, or LDH. Renal failure may not be reversible with discontinuation of therapy and dialysis may be required.

Fertility

In fertility studies gemcitabine caused hypospermatogenesis in male mice (see section 5.3). Therefore, men being treated with gemcitabine are advised not to father a child during and up to 6 months after treatment and to seek further advice regarding cryoconservation of sperm prior to treatment because of the possibility of infertility due to therapy with gemcitabine (see section 4.6).

Sodium

The 200 mg vial of Gemcitabine medac contains 3.5 mg (< 1 mmol) sodium per vial.

The 1,000 mg vial of Gemcitabine medac contains 17.5 mg (< 1 mmol) sodium per vial.

The 1,500 mg vial of Gemcitabine medac contains 26.3 mg (< 1 mmol) sodium per vial.

This should be taken into consideration by patients on a controlled sodium diet.

4.5 Interaction with other medicinal products and other forms of interaction

No specific interaction studies have been performed (see section 5.2)

Radiotherapy

Concurrent (given together or ⩽ 7 days apart) - Toxicity associated with this multimodality therapy is dependent on many different factors, including dose of gemcitabine, frequency of gemcitabine administration, dose of radiation, radiotherapy planning technique, the target tissue, and target volume. Pre-clinical and clinical studies have shown that gemcitabine has radiosensitising activity. In a single trial, where gemcitabine at a dose of 1,000 mg/m^2 was administered concurrently for up to 6 consecutive weeks with therapeutic thoracic radiation to patients with non-small cell lung cancer, significant toxicity in the form of severe, and potentially life threatening mucositis, especially oesophagitis, and pneumonitis was observed, particularly in patients receiving large volumes of radiotherapy [median treatment volumes 4,795 cm^3]. Studies done subsequently have suggested that it is feasible to administer gemcitabine at lower doses with concurrent radiotherapy with predictable toxicity, such as a phase II study in non-small cell lung cancer, where thoracic radiation doses of 66 Gy were applied concomitantly with an administration with gemcitabine (600 mg/m^2, four times) and cisplatin (80 mg/m^2 twice) during 6 weeks. The optimum regimen for safe administration of gemcitabine with therapeutic doses of radiation has not yet been determined in all tumour types.

Non-concurrent (given > 7 days apart)- Analysis of the data does not indicate any enhanced toxicity when gemcitabine is administered more than 7 days before or after radiation, other than radiation recall. Data suggest that gemcitabine can be started after the acute effects of radiation have resolved or at least one week after radiation.

Radiation injury has been reported on targeted tissues (e.g. oesophagitis, colitis, and pneumonitis) in association with both concurrent and non-concurrent use of gemcitabine.

Others

Yellow fever and other live attenuated vaccines are not recommended due to the risk of systemic, possibly fatal, disease, particularly in immunosuppressed patients.

4.6 Pregnancy and lactation

Pregnancy

There are no adequate data from the use of gemcitabine in pregnant women. Studies in animals have shown reproductive toxicity (see section 5.3). Based on results from animal studies and the mechanism of action of gemcitabine, this substance should not be used during pregnancy unless clearly necessary. Women should be advised not to become pregnant during treatment with gemcitabine and to warn their attending physician immediately, should this occur after all.

Breast-feeding

It is not known whether gemcitabine is excreted in human milk and adverse effects on the suckling child cannot be excluded. Breast-feeding must be discontinued during gemcitabine therapy.

Fertility

In fertility studies gemcitabine caused hypospermatogenesis in male mice (see section 5.3). Therefore, men being treated with gemcitabine are advised not to father a child during and up to 6 months after treatment and to seek further advice regarding cryoconservation of sperm prior to treatment because of the possibility of infertility due to therapy with gemcitabine.

4.7 Effects on ability to drive and use machines

No studies on the effects on the ability to drive and use machines have been performed. However, gemcitabine has been reported to cause mild to moderate somnolence, especially in combination with alcohol consumption. Patients should be cautioned against driving or operating machinery until it is established that they do not become somnolent.

4.8 Undesirable effects

The most commonly reported adverse drug reactions associated with gemcitabine treatment include: nausea with or without vomiting, raised liver transaminases (AST/ALT) and alkaline phosphatase, reported in approximately 60% of patients; proteinuria and haematuria reported in approximately 50% of patients; dyspnoea reported in 10-40% of patients (highest incidence in lung cancer patients); allergic skin rashes occur in approximately 25% of patients and are associated with itching in 10% of patients.

The frequency and severity of the adverse reactions are affected by the dose, infusion rate and intervals between doses (see section 4.4). Dose-limiting adverse reactions are reductions in thrombocyte, leucocyte and granulocyte counts (see section 4.2).

Clinical trial data

Frequencies are defined as: Very common (⩾1/10), Common (⩾1/100 to <1/10), Uncommon (⩾1/1000 to <1/100), Rare (⩾1/10,000 to <1/1000), Very Rare (<1/10,000).

The following table of undesirable effects and frequencies is based on data from clinical trials. Within each frequency grouping, undesirable effects are presented in order of decreasing seriousness.

System Organ Class	Frequency grouping
Blood and lymphatic system disorders	Very common • Leucopenia (Neutropenia Grade 3 = 19.3 %; Grade 4 = 6 %). Bone-marrow suppression is usually mild to moderate and mostly affects the granulocyte count (see section 4.2). • Thrombocytopenia • Anaemia Common • Febrile neutropenia Very rare •Thrombocytosis
Immune system disorders	Very Rare • Anaphylactoid reaction
Metabolism and nutrition disorders	Common • Anorexia
Nervous system disorders	Common • Headache • Insomnia • Somnolence
Cardiac disorders	Rare • Myocardial infarct
Vascular disorders	Rare • Hypotension
Respiratory, thoracic and mediastinal disorders	Very Common • Dyspnoea – usually mild and passes rapidly without treatment Common • Cough • Rhinitis Uncommon • Interstitial pneumonitis (see section 4.4) • Bronchospasm – usually mild and transient but may require parenteral treatment
Gastrointestinal disorders	Very common • Vomiting • Nausea Common • Diarrhoea • Stomatitis and ulceration of the mouth • Constipation
Hepatobiliary disorders	Very common • Elevation of liver transaminases (AST and ALT) and alkaline phosphatase Common • Increased bilirubin Rare • Increased gamma-glutamyl transferase (GGT)
Skin and subcutaneous tissue disorders	Very common • Allergic skin rash frequently associated with pruritus • Alopecia Common • Itching • Sweating Rare • Ulceration • Vesicle and sore formation • Scaling Very rare • Severe skin reactions, including desquamation and bullous skin eruptions
Musculoskeletal and connective tissue disorders	Common • Back pain • Myalgia
Renal and urinary disorders	Very Common • Haematuria • Mild proteinuria
General disorders and administration site conditions	Very common • Influenza-like symptoms - the most common symptoms are fever, headache, chills, myalgia, asthenia and anorexia. Cough, rhinitis, malaise, perspiration and sleeping difficulties have also been reported. • Oedema/peripheral oedema-including facial oedema. Oedema is usually reversible after stopping treatment Common • Fever • Asthenia • Chills Rare • Injection site reactions-mainly mild in nature
Injury, poisoning, and procedural complications	Radiation toxicity (see section 4.5).

Postmarketing experience (spontaneous reports) frequency not known (can't be estimated from the available data)

Nervous system disorders

Cerebrovascular accident

Cardiac disorders

Arrythmias, predominantly supraventricular in nature

Heart failure

Vascular disorders

Clinical signs of peripheral vasculitis and gangrene

Respiratory, thoracic and mediastinal disorder s

Pulmonary oedema

Adult respiratory distress syndrome (see section 4.4)

Gastrointestinal disorders

Ischaemic colitis

Hepatobiliary disorders

Serious hepatotoxicity, including liver failure and death

Skin and subcutaneous tissue disorders

Severe skin reactions, including desquamation and bullous skin eruptions, Lyell's Syndrome, Steven-Johnson Syndrome

Renal and urinary disorders

Renal failure (see section 4.4)

Haemolytic uraemic syndrome (see section 4.4)

Injury, poisoning and procedural complications

Radiation recall

Combination use in breast cancer

The frequency of grade 3 and 4 haematological toxicities, particularly neutropenia, increases when gemcitabine is used in combination with paclitaxel. However, the increase in these adverse reactions is not associated with an increased incidence of infections or haemorrhagic events. Fatigue and febrile neutropenia occur more frequently when gemcitabine is used in combination with paclitaxel. Fatigue, which is not associated with anaemia, usually resolves after the first cycle.

(see Table 1 below)

Combination use in bladder cancer

(see Table 2 on next page)

Combination use in ovarian cancer

(see Table 3 on next page)

Sensory neuropathy was also more frequent in the combination arm than with single agent carboplatin.

4.9 Overdose

There is no known antidote for overdose of gemcitabine. Doses as high as 5700 mg/m^2 have been administered by intravenous infusion over 30-minutes every 2 weeks with clinically acceptable toxicity. In the event of suspected overdose, the patient should be monitored with appropriate blood counts and receive supportive therapy, as necessary.

5. PHARMACOLOGICAL PROPERTIES

5.1 Pharmacodynamic properties

Pharmacotherapeutic group: pyrimidine analogues ATC code: L01BC05

Cytotoxic activity in cell cultures

Gemcitabine shows significant cytotoxic effects against a variety of cultured murine and human tumour cells. Its action is phase-specific such that gemcitabine primarily kills cells that are undergoing DNA synthesis (S-phase) and, under certain circumstances, blocks the progression of cells at the junction of the G_1/S phase boundary. *In vitro*, the cytotoxic effect of gemcitabine is dependent on both concentration and time.

Antitumoral activity in preclinical models

In animal tumour models, antitumoural activity of gemcitabine is schedule-dependent. When gemcitabine is administered daily, high mortality among the animals but minimal antitumoural activity is observed. If, however, gemcitabine is given every third or fourth day, it can be administered in non-lethal doses with substantial antitumoural activity against a broad spectrum of mouse tumours.

Mechanism of action

Cellular metabolism and mechanism of action: Gemcitabine (dFdC), which is a pyrimidine antimetabolite, is metabolised intracellularly by nucleoside kinase to the active diphosphate (dFdCDP) and triphosphate (dFdCTP) nucleosides. The cytotoxic effect of gemcitabine is due to inhibition of DNA synthesis by two mechanisms of action by dFdCDP and dFdCTP. First, dFdCDP inhibits ribonucleotide reductase, which is uniquely responsible for catalysing the reactions that produce deoxynucleoside triphosphates (dCTP) for DNA synthesis. Inhibition of this enzyme by dFdCDP reduces the concentration of deoxynucleosides in general and, in particular, dCTP. Second, dFdCTP competes with dCTP for incorporation into DNA (self-potentiation).

Likewise, a small amount of gemcitabine may also be incorporated into RNA. Thus, the reduced intracellular concentration of dCTP potentiates the incorporation of dFdCTP into DNA. DNA polymerase epsilon lacks the ability to eliminate gemcitabine and to repair the growing DNA strands. After gemcitabine is incorporated into DNA, one additional nucleotide is added to the growing DNA strands. After this addition there is essentially a complete inhibition in further DNA synthesis (masked chain termination). After incorporation into DNA, gemcitabine appears to induce the programmed cell death process known as apoptosis.

Clinical data

Bladder cancer

A randomised phase III study of 405 patients with advanced or metastatic urothelial transitional cell carcinoma showed no difference between the two treatment arms, gemcitabine/cisplatin versus methotrexate/vinblastine/adriamycin/cisplatin (MVAC), in terms of median survival (12.8 and 14.8 months respectively, p=0.547), time to disease progression (7.4 and 7.6 months respectively, p=0.842) and response rate (49.4% and 45.7% respectively, p=0.512). However, the combination of gemcitabine and cisplatin had a better toxicity profile than MVAC.

Pancreatic cancer

In a randomised phase III study of 126 patients with advanced or metastatic pancreatic cancer, gemcitabine showed a statistically significant higher clinical benefit response rate than 5-fluorouracil (23.8% and 4.8% respectively, p=0.0022). Also, a statistically significant prolongation of the time to progression from 0.9 to 2.3 months (log-rank $p < 0.0002$) and a statistically significant prolongation of median survival from 4.4 to 5.7 months (log-rank $p < 0.0024$) was observed in patients treated with gemcitabine compared to patients treated with 5-fluorouracil.

Table 1

Grade 3 and 4 Adverse Events Paclitaxel versus gemcitabine plus paclitaxel	Number (%) of Patients			
	Paclitaxel arm (N=259)		Gemcitabine plus paclitaxel arm (N=262)	
	Grade 3	Grade 4	Grade 3	Grade 4
Laboratory				
Anaemia	5 (1.9)	1 (0.4)	15 (5.7)	3 (1.1)
Thrombocytopenia	0	0	14 (5.3)	1 (0.4)
Neutropenia	11 (4.2)	17 (6.6)*	82 (31.3)	45 (17.2)*
Non-laboratory				
Febrile neutropenia	3 (1.2)	0	12 (4.6)	1(0.4)
Fatigue	3 (1.2)	1 (0.4)	15 (5.7)	2 (0.8)
Diarrhoea	5 (1.9)	0	8 (3.1)	0
Motor neuropathy	2(0.8)	0	6(2.3)	1(0.4)
Sensory neuropathy	9(3.5)	0	14(5.3)	1(0.4)

* Grade 4 neutropenia lasting for more than 7 days occurred in 12.6% of patients in the combination arm and 5.0% of patients in the paclitaxel arm.

Table 2 Combination use in bladder cancer

Grade 3 and 4 Adverse Events MVAC versus gemcitabine plus cisplatin				
	Number (%) of Patients			
	MVAC (methotrexate, vinblastine, doxorubicin and cisplatin) arm (N=196)		Gemcitabine plus cisplatin arm (N=200)	
Laboratory	Grade 3	Grade 4	Grade 3	Grade 4
Anaemia	30(16)	4(2)	47(24)	7(4)
Thrombocytopenia	15(8)	25(13)	57(29)	57(29)
Non-laboratory				
Nausea and vomiting	37(19)	3(2)	44(22)	0(0)
Diarrhoea	15(8)	1(1)	6(3)	0(0)
Infection	19(10)	10(5)	4(2)	1(1)
Stomatitis	34(18)	8(4)	2(1)	0(0)

Table 3 Combination use in ovarian cancer

Grade 3 and 4 Adverse Events Carboplatin versus gemcitabine plus carboplatin				
	Number (%) of Patients			
	Carboplatin arm (N=174)		Gemcitabine plus carboplatin arm (N=175)	
	Grade 3	Grade 4	Grade 3	Grade 4
Laboratory				
Anaemia	10(5.7)	4(2.3)	39(22.3)	9(5.1)
Neutropenia	19(10.9)	2(1.1)	73(41.7)	50(28.6)
Thrombocytopenia	18(10.3)	2(1.1)	53(30.3)	8(4.6)
Leucopenia	11(6.3)	1(0.6)	84(48.0)	9(5.1)
Non-laboratory				
Haemorrhage	0(0.0)	0(0.0)	3(1.8)	(0.0)
Febrile neutropenia	0(0.0)	0(0.0)	2(1.1)	(0.0)
Infection without neutropenia	0(0)	0(0.0)	(0.0)	1(0.6)

Non small cell lung cancer

In a randomised phase III study of 522 patients with inoperable, locally advanced or metastatic NSCLC, gemcitabine in combination with cisplatin showed a statistically significant higher response rate than cisplatin alone (31.0% and 12.0%, respectively, p<0.0001). A statistically significant prolongation of the time to progression, from 3.7 to 5.6 months (log-rank p<0.0012) and a statistically significant prolongation of median survival from 7.6 months to 9.1 months (log-rank p<0.004) was observed in patients treated with gemcitabine/cisplatin compared to patients treated with cisplatin.

In another randomised phase III study of 135 patients with stage IIIB or IV NSCLC, a combination of gemcitabine and cisplatin showed a statistically significant higher response rate than a combination of cisplatin and etoposide (40.6% and 21.2%, respectively, p=0.025). A statistically significant prolongation of the time to progression, from 4.3 to 6.9 months (p=0.014) was observed in patients treated with gemcitabine/cisplatin compared to patients treated with etoposide/cisplatin.

In both studies it was found that tolerability was similar in the two treatment arms.

Ovarian carcinoma

In a randomised phase III study, 356 patients with advanced epithelial ovarian carcinoma who had relapsed at least 6 months after completing platinum based therapy were randomised to therapy with gemcitabine and carboplatin (GCb), or carboplatin (Cb). A statistically significant prolongation of the time to progression of disease, from 5.8 to 8.6 months (log-rank p=0.0038) was observed in the patients treated with GCb compared to patients treated with Cb. Differences in response rate of 47.2% in the GCb arm versus 30.9% in the Cb arm (p=0.0016) and median survival 18 months (GCb) versus 17.3 (Cb) (p=0.73) favoured the GCb arm.

Breast cancer

In a randomised phase III study of 529 patients with inoperable, locally recurrent or metastatic breast cancer with relapse after adjuvant/neoadjuvant chemotherapy, gemcitabine in combination with paclitaxel showed a statistically significant prolongation of time to documented disease progression from 3.98 to 6.14 months (log-rank p=0.0002) in patients treated with gemcitabine/paclitaxel compared to patients treated with paclitaxel. After 377 deaths, the overall survival was 18.6 months versus 15.8 months (log rank p=0.0489, HR 0.82) in patients treated with gemcitabine/paclitaxel compared to patients treated with paclitaxel and the overall response rate was 41.4% and 26.2% respectively (p= 0.0002).

5.2 Pharmacokinetic properties

The pharmacokinetics of gemcitabine have been examined in 353 patients in seven studies. The 121 women and 232 men ranged in age from 29 to 79 years. Of these patients, approximately 45% had non-small cell lung cancer and 35% were diagnosed with pancreatic cancer. The following pharmacokinetic parameters were obtained for doses ranging from 500 to 2,592 mg/m^2 that were infused from 0.4 to 1.2 hours.

Peak plasma concentrations (obtained within 5 minutes of the end of the infusion) were 3.2 to 45.5 μg/ml. Plasma concentrations of the parent compound following a dose of 1,000 mg/m^2/30-minutes are greater than 5 μg/ml for approximately 30-minutes after the end of the infusion, and greater than 0.4 μg/ml for an additional hour.

Distribution

The volume of distribution of the central compartment was 12.4 l/m^2 for women and 17.5 l/m^2 for men (inter-individual variability was 91.9%). The volume of distribution of the peripheral compartment was 47.4 l/m^2. The volume of the peripheral compartment was not sensitive to gender.

The plasma protein binding was considered to be negligible.

Half-life: This ranged from 42 to 94 minutes depending on age and gender. For the recommended dosing schedule, gemcitabine elimination should be virtually complete within 5 to 11 hours of the start of the infusion. Gemcitabine does not accumulate when administered once weekly.

Metabolism

Gemcitabine is rapidly metabolised by cytidine deaminase in the liver, kidney, blood and other tissues. Intracellular metabolism of gemcitabine produces the gemcitabine mono, di and triphosphates (dFdCMP, dFdCDP and dFdCTP) of which dFdCDP and dFdCTP are considered active. These intracellular metabolites have not been detected in plasma or urine. The primary metabolite, 2'-deoxy-2', 2'-difluorouridine (dFdU), is not active and is found in plasma and urine.

Excretion

Systemic clearance ranged from 29.2 l/hr/m^2 to 92.2 /hr/m^2 depending on gender and age (inter-individual variability was 52.2%). Clearance for women is approximately 25% lower than the values for men. Although rapid, clearance for both men and women appears to decrease with age. For the recommended gemcitabine dose of 1000 mg/m^2 given as a 30-minute infusion, lower clearance values for women and men should not necessitate a decrease in the gemcitabine dose.

Urinary excretion: Less than 10% is excreted as unchanged drug.

Renal clearance was 2 to 7 l/hr/m^2.

During the week following administration, 92 to 98% of the dose of gemcitabine administered is recovered, 99% in the urine, mainly in the form of dFdU and 1% of the dose is excreted in faeces.

dFdCTP kinetics

This metabolite can be found in peripheral blood mononuclear cells and the information below refers to these cells. Intracellular concentrations increase in proportion to gemcitabine doses of 35-350 mg/m^2/30-minutes, which give steady state concentrations of 0.4-5 μg/ml. At gemcitabine plasma concentrations above 5 μg/ml, dFdCTP levels do not increase, suggesting that the formation is saturable in these cells.

Half-life of terminal elimination: 0.7-12 hours.

dFdU kinetics

Peak plasma concentrations (3-15 minutes after end of 30-minute infusion, 1000 mg/m^2): 28-52 μg/ml. Trough concentration following once weekly dosing: 0.07-1.12 μg/ml, with no apparent accumulation. Triphasic plasma concentration versus time curve, mean half-life of terminal phase - 65 hours (range 33-84 hr).

Formation of dFdU from parent compound: 91%-98%.

Mean volume of distribution of central compartment: 18 l/m^2 (range 11-22 l/m^2).

Mean steady state volume of distribution (V_{ss}): 150 l/m^2 (range 96-228 l/m^2).

Tissue distribution: Extensive.

Mean apparent clearance: 2.5 l/hr/m^2 (range 1-4 l/hr/m^2).

Urinary excretion: All.

Gemcitabine and paclitaxel combination therapy

Combination therapy did not alter the pharmacokinetics of either gemcitabine or paclitaxel.

Gemcitabine and carboplatin combination therapy

When given in combination with carboplatin the pharmacokinetics of gemcitabine were not altered

Renal impairment

Mild to moderate renal insufficiency (GFR from 30 ml/min to 80 ml/min) has no consistent, significant effect on gemcitabine pharmacokinetics.

5.3 Preclinical safety data

In repeat-dose studies of up to 6 months in duration in mice and dogs, the principal finding was schedule and dose-dependent haematopoietic suppression which was reversible.

Gemcitabine is mutagenic in an *in vitro* mutation test and an *in vivo* bone marrow micronucleus test. Long term animal studies evaluating the carcinogenic potential have not been performed.

In fertility studies, gemcitabine caused reversible hypospermatogenesis in male mice. No effect on the fertility of females has been detected.

Evaluation of experimental animal studies has shown reproductive toxicity e.g. birth defects and other effects on the development of the embryo or foetus, the course of gestation or peri- and postnatal development.

6. PHARMACEUTICAL PARTICULARS

6.1 List of excipients

Gemcitabine medac 38 mg/ml contains:

Mannitol (E421)

Sodium acetate trihydrate (E262)

Hydrochloric acid (E507) (for pH-adjustment)

Sodium hydroxide (E524) (for pH-adjustment)

6.2 Incompatibilities

This medicinal product must not be mixed with other medicinal product except those mentioned in section 6.6.

Table 4

Presentation	Presentation volume of sodium chloride 9 mg/ml (0.9 %) solution for injection to be added	Reconstituted volume	Final concentration
200 mg	5 ml	5.26 ml	38 mg/ml
1,000 mg	25 ml	26.3 ml	38 mg/ml
1,500 mg	37.5 ml	39.5 ml	38 mg/ml

6.3 Shelf life
2 years

After reconstitution:

Chemical and physical in-use stability has been demonstrated for 35 days at 25 °C. From a microbiological point of view, the product should be used immediately.

If not used immediately, in-use storage times and conditions prior to use are the responsibility of the user and would normally not be longer than 24 hours at 25 °C, unless reconstitution / dilution has taken place in controlled and validated aseptic conditions.

6.4 Special precautions for storage
This medicinal product does not require any special storage conditions.

Reconstituted solution:

Do not refrigerate (crystallisation may occur).

For storage condition of the reconstituted medicinal product, see section 6.3.

6.5 Nature and contents of container
Type I clear glass vials of 10 ml, 50 ml or 100 ml, closed with chlorobutyl rubber stoppers.

Pack sizes: carton containing a single vial containing 200 mg, 1,000 mg or 1,500 mg gemcitabine.

6.6 Special precautions for disposal and other handling
Reconstitution:

For single use only.

This medicinal product has only been shown to be compatible with sodium chloride 9 mg/ml (0.9 %) solution for injection. Accordingly, only this diluent should be used for reconstitution. Compatibility with other active substances has not been studied. Therefore, it is not recommended to mix this medicinal product with other active substances when reconstituted.

Reconstitution at concentrations greater than 38 mg/ml may result in incomplete dissolution, and should be avoided.

To reconstitute, slowly add the appropriate volume of sodium chloride 9 mg/ml (0.9 %) solution for injection (as stated in the table below) and shake to dissolve.

(see Table 4 above)

The appropriate amount of medicinal product may be further diluted with sodium chloride 9 mg/ml (0.9 %) solution for injection.

Parenteral medicinal products should be inspected visually for particulate matter and discolouration, prior to administration, whenever solution and container permit.

Any unused solution should be discarded as described below.

Guidelines for the Safe Handling of Cytotoxic Medicinal Products:

Local guidelines on safe preparation and handling of cytotoxic medicinal products must be adhered to. Cytotoxic preparations should not be handled by pregnant staff. The preparation of injectable solutions of cytotoxic agents must be carried out by trained specialist personnel with knowledge of the medicines used. This should be performed in a designated area. The work surface should be covered with disposable plastic-backed absorbent paper.

Suitable eye protection, disposable gloves, face mask and disposable apron should be worn. Precautions should be taken to avoid the medicinal product accidentally coming into contact with the eyes. If accidental contamination occurs, the eye should be washed with water thoroughly and immediately.

Syringes and infusion sets should be assembled carefully to avoid leakage (use of Luer lock fittings is recommended). Large bore needles are recommended to minimise pressure and the possible formation of aerosols. The latter may also be reduced by the use of a venting needle.

Actual spillage or leakage should be mopped up wearing protective gloves. Excreta and vomit must be handled with care.

Disposal:

Adequate care and precaution should be taken in the disposal of items used to reconstitute this medicinal product. Any unused dry product or contaminated materials should be placed in a high-risk waste bag. Sharp objects (needles, syringes, vials, etc) should be placed in a suitable rigid container. Personnel concerned with the collection and disposal of this waste should be aware of the hazard involved. Waste material should be destroyed by incineration. Any unused product or waste material should be disposed of in accordance with local requirements.

7. MARKETING AUTHORISATION HOLDER
medac
Gesellschaft für klinische
Spezialpräparate mbH
Fehlandtstr. 3
20354 Hamburg
Germany
Phone: +49 4103 8006-0
Fax: +49 4103 8006-100

8. MARKETING AUTHORISATION NUMBER(S)
PL 11587/0045

9. DATE OF FIRST AUTHORISATION/RENEWAL OF THE AUTHORISATION
30/03/2009

10. DATE OF REVISION OF THE TEXT
30/03/2009

Gemeprost

(sanofi-aventis)

1. NAME OF THE MEDICINAL PRODUCT
Gemeprost Pessary 1.0mg

2. QUALITATIVE AND QUANTITATIVE COMPOSITION
Each pessary contains gemeprost 1.0mg.

3. PHARMACEUTICAL FORM
White to yellowish-white spindle shaped vaginal pessary.

4. CLINICAL PARTICULARS
4.1 Therapeutic indications
1. Softening and dilatation of the cervix uteri to transcervical intra-uterine operative procedures in pregnant patients in the first trimester of gestation.

2. Therapeutic termination of pregnancy conducted in licensed premises during the second trimester of pregnancy.

3. Induction of abortion of second trimester pregnancy complicated by intra-uterine foetal death.

Gemeprost is not indicated in the induction of labour or for cervical dilatation at term as foetal effects have not yet been sufficiently studied.

4.2 Posology and method of administration
Adults:

1. Softening & dilatation of cervix
   One pessary to be inserted into the posterior vaginal fornix 3 hours before surgery.
2. Therapeutic termination of pregnancy
   One pessary to be inserted into the posterior vaginal fornix at 3 hourly intervals to a maximum of 5 administrations. A second course of treatment may be instituted starting 24 hours after the initial commencement of treatment. If abortion is not well established after 10 pessaries, a further course of Gemeprost treatment is not recommended and alternative means should be employed to effect uterine emptying.
3. Intra-uterine foetal death
   One pessary to be inserted into the posterior vaginal fornix at 3 hourly intervals up to a maximum of 5 administrations.

Elderly: Not applicable

Children: Not applicable.

4.3 Contraindications
Known hypersensitivity to prostaglandins, renal function disturbances. Gemeprost is also contraindicated in women experiencing uterine fragility related to uterine scarring, and in placenta previa.

Gemeprost pessaries should be not be used for the induction of labour or cervical softening at term as foetal effects have not been ascertained.

4.4 Special warnings and precautions for use
Gemeprost should be used with caution in patients with obstructive airways disease, those with cardiovascular insufficiency, elevated intraocular pressure, cervicitis or vaginitis. Serious, potentially fatal, cardiovascular accidents (myocardial infarction and/or spasm of the coronary arteries and severe hypotension) have been reported with prostaglandins including gemeprost. Cardiac and vascular parameters should be monitored by taking regular measurements of the patients pulse and blood pressure.

Coagulopathy may occur following intra-uterine foetal death and should be monitored and managed actively according to current clinical standard practice.

Adequate follow up of a patient having a pregnancy terminated is essential to ensure that the process has been completed, as the embryopathic hazards of gemeprost have not been determined.

Patients with the following diseases have not been studied: ulcerative colitis; diabetes mellitus; sickle-cell anaemia; epilepsy; disorders of blood coagulation; cardiovascular or pulmonary disease.

When used for cervical dilatation, if it is necessary to postpone surgery much beyond the recommended 3 hour interval patients should be kept under observation, as there is a possibility that spontaneous abortion may occur.

4.5 Interaction with other medicinal products and other forms of interaction
Oxytocin and other labour inducers or accelerators can potentiate the action of Gemeprost.

4.6 Pregnancy and lactation
Not applicable.

4.7 Effects on ability to drive and use machines
Not applicable.

4.8 Undesirable effects
Vaginal bleeding and mild uterine pain, similar to menstrual pain, may occur in the interval between the administration of the pessary and surgery, especially if this interval is prolonged beyond the recommended 3 hours. Nausea, vomiting, loose stools or diarrhoea may occur but are rarely severe enough to require treatment. However, standard anti-emetic or anti-diarrhoeal agents may be administered if required. Other reported side effects include: headache, muscle weakness; dizziness; flushing; chills; backache; dyspnoea; chest pain; palpitations and mild pyrexia. Uterine rupture has been reported on rare occasions, most commonly in multiparous women and in those women with a history of uterine surgery. Anaphylactic reactions have not occurred with gemeprost but such reactions have very rarely been noted with other prostaglandins. In very rare cases, severe hypotension and coronary spasms with subsequent myocardial infarctions have been reported.

4.9 Overdose
The toxic dose of gemeprost in women has not been established. Cumulative dosage of 10mg in 24 hours was accompanied by a significant increase in incidence and severity of side-effects. In animals the acute toxic effects are similar to those of prostaglandin E1 and include relaxation of smooth muscle, leading to hypotension and depression of the CNS. Clinically valuable signs of impending toxicity are likely to be sedation; tremor; convulsion; dyspnoea; abdominal pain and diarrhoea, which may be bloody; palpitations or bradycardia. Treatment should be symptomatic. A vaginal douche may be of value depending on elapsed time since insertion of the pessary.

5. PHARMACOLOGICAL PROPERTIES
5.1 Pharmacodynamic properties
Gemeprost (16, 16-dimethyl-trans-delta^2 PGE1 methyl ester) is a prostaglandin E1 analogue. Both in pregnant and non-pregnant animals, it causes contraction of the uterus and causes softening and decreases resistance of cervical tissue. Gemeprost depresses placental and uterine blood flow but those actions are secondary to the main uterine stimulation. In women, Gemeprost is an effective cervical dilator in the first trimester in pregnancy, Gemeprost is also effective at terminating pregnancy in the second trimester of gestation.

5.2 Pharmacokinetic properties
In pregnant women, although plasma levels of both the active drug and the main metabolite (de-esterified gemeprost) are very low, Gemeprost induces cervical softening within three hours of insertion. Between 12 and 28% of the vaginal dose is eventually absorbed into the circulation, and 50% of this is excreted in the urine. The unabsorbed dose is largely recovered from the genital area, either washed out in the urine or from pads used to absorb post-operative blood loss.

5.3 Preclinical safety data
No drug related toxicity has been observed in rodents given 6 times the therapeutic dose (3.2mmol Kg^{-1} daily) for up to 26 weeks.

In cynomolgus monkeys subcutaneous administration of doses up to 40 times the human therapeutic dose for 1 month caused effects such as muscular tremor, excessive salivation, poorly formed faeces and mild local reactions at injection sites.

No teratogenic effects observed in either rats or rabbits receiving intra vaginal doses 10 to 40 times the human therapeutic dose.

No mutagenic effects have been observed.

6. PHARMACEUTICAL PARTICULARS

6.1 List of excipients

Witepsol S 52

Dehydrated Ethanol

6.2 Incompatibilities

None known.

6.3 Shelf life

The shelf-life of Gemeprost pessaries is 3 years. Once the foil sachet has been opened, any pessary not used within 12 hours should be destroyed.

6.4 Special precautions for storage

Store below minus 10 °C in the original pack. Temperature cycling should be avoided.

6.5 Nature and contents of container

Container of 5 unit dose foil pessaries.

6.6 Special precautions for disposal and other handling

Before administration, the pessary should be allowed to warm to room temperature for 30 minutes away from direct heat and sunlight in the unopened foil sachet.

Administrative Data

7. MARKETING AUTHORISATION HOLDER

Sanofi-aventis

One Onslow Street

Guildford

Surrey, GU1 4YS, UK

8. MARKETING AUTHORISATION NUMBER(S)

PL 04425/0373

9. DATE OF FIRST AUTHORISATION/RENEWAL OF THE AUTHORISATION

16 September 2005

10. DATE OF REVISION OF THE TEXT

October 2006

LEGAL CATEGORY:

POM

Gemzar 200mg powder for solution for infusion, Gemzar 1g powder for solution for infusion

(Eli Lilly and Company Limited)

1. NAME OF THE MEDICINAL PRODUCT

GEMZAR* 200 mg powder for solution for infusion.

GEMZAR 1000 mg powder for solution for infusion.

2. QUALITATIVE AND QUANTITATIVE COMPOSITION

One vial contains gemcitabine hydrochloride equivalent to 200 mg gemcitabine.

One vial contains gemcitabine hydrochloride equivalent to 1,000 mg gemcitabine.

After reconstitution, the solution contains 38 mg/ml of gemcitabine.

Excipients:

Each 200 mg vial contains 3.5 mg (<1 mmol) sodium.

Each 1,000 mg vial contains 17.5 mg (<1 mmol) sodium.

For a full list of excipients see section 6.1.

3. PHARMACEUTICAL FORM

Powder for solution for infusion.

White to off-white plug or powder.

4. CLINICAL PARTICULARS

4.1 Therapeutic indications

Gemcitabine is indicated for the treatment of locally advanced or metastatic bladder cancer in combination with cisplatin.

Gemcitabine is indicated for treatment of patients with locally advanced or metastatic adenocarcinoma of the pancreas.

Gemcitabine, in combination with cisplatin, is indicated as first-line treatment of patients with locally advanced or metastatic non-small cell lung cancer (NSCLC). Gemcitabine monotherapy can be considered in elderly patients or those with performance status 2.

Gemcitabine is indicated for the treatment of patients with locally advanced or metastatic epithelial ovarian carcinoma, in combination with carboplatin, in patients with relapsed disease following a recurrence-free interval of at least 6 months after platinum-based, first-line therapy.

Gemcitabine, in combination with paclitaxel, is indicated for the treatment of patients with unresectable, locally recurrent or metastatic breast cancer who have relapsed following adjuvant/neoadjuvant chemotherapy. Prior chemotherapy should have included an anthracycline unless clinically contraindicated.

4.2 Posology and method of administration

Gemcitabine should only be prescribed by a physician qualified in the use of anti-cancer chemotherapy.

Recommended posology:

Bladder cancer

Combination use

The recommended dose for gemcitabine is 1,000 mg/m^2, given by 30-minute infusion. The dose should be given on Days 1, 8 and 15 of each 28-day cycle in combination with cisplatin. Cisplatin is given at a recommended dose of 70 mg/m^2 on Day 1 following gemcitabine or Day 2 of each 28-day cycle. This 4-week cycle is then repeated. Dosage reduction with each cycle or within a cycle may be applied based upon the grade of toxicity experienced by the patient.

Pancreatic cancer

The recommended dose of gemcitabine is 1,000 mg/m^2, given by 30-minute intravenous infusion. This should be repeated once weekly for up to 7 weeks followed by a week of rest. Subsequent cycles should consist of injections once weekly for 3 consecutive weeks out of every 4 weeks. Dosage reduction with each cycle or within a cycle may be applied based upon the grade of toxicity experienced by the patient.

Non-small cell lung cancer

Monotherapy

The recommended dose of gemcitabine is 1,000 mg/m^2, given by 30-minute intravenous infusion. This should be repeated once weekly for 3 weeks, followed by a 1-week rest period. This 4-week cycle is then repeated. Dosage reduction with each cycle or within a cycle may be applied based upon the grade of toxicity experienced by the patient.

Combination use

The recommended dose for gemcitabine is 1,250 mg/m^2 body surface area given as a 30-minute intravenous infusion on Days 1 and 8 of the treatment cycle (21 days). Dosage reduction with each cycle or within a cycle may be applied based upon the grade of toxicity experienced by the patient.

Cisplatin has been used at doses between 75-100 mg/m^2 once every 3 weeks.

Breast cancer

Combination use

Gemcitabine, in combination with paclitaxel, is recommended using paclitaxel (175 mg/m^2) administered on Day 1 over approximately 3-hours as an intravenous infusion, followed by gemcitabine (1,250 mg/m^2) as a 30-minute intravenous infusion on Days 1 and 8 of each 21-day cycle. Dose reduction with each cycle or within a cycle may be applied based upon the grade of toxicity experienced by the patient. Patients should have an absolute granulocyte count of at least 1,500 (x 10^6/l) prior to initiation of gemcitabine + paclitaxel combination.

Ovarian cancer

Combination use

Gemcitabine, in combination with carboplatin, is recommended using gemcitabine 1,000 mg/m^2 administered on Days 1 and 8 of each 21-day cycle as a 30-minute intravenous infusion. After gemcitabine, carboplatin will be given on Day 1 consistent with a target area under curve (AUC) of 4.0 mg/ml•min. Dosage reduction with each cycle or within a cycle may be applied based upon the grade of toxicity experienced by the patient.

Monitoring for toxicity and dose modification due to toxicity

Dose modification due to non-haematological toxicity

Periodic physical examination and checks of renal and hepatic function should be made to detect non-haematological toxicity. Dosage reduction with each cycle or within a cycle may be applied based upon the grade of toxicity experienced by the patient. In general, for severe (Grade 3 or 4) non-haematological toxicity, except nausea/vomiting, therapy with gemcitabine should be withheld or decreased depending on the judgement of the treating physician. Doses should be withheld until toxicity has resolved, in the opinion of the physician.

For cisplatin, carboplatin, and paclitaxel dosage adjustment in combination therapy, please refer to the corresponding Summary of Product Characteristics.

Dose modification due to haematological toxicity

Initiation of a cycle

For all indications, the patient must be monitored before each dose for platelet and granulocyte counts. Patients should have an absolute granulocyte count of at least 1,500 (x 10^6/l) and platelet count of 100,000 (x 10^6/l) prior to the initiation of a cycle.

Within a cycle

Dose modifications of gemcitabine within a cycle should be performed according to the following tables:

Dose modification of gemcitabine within a cycle for bladder cancer, NSCLC and pancreatic cancer, given in monotherapy or in combination with cisplatin

Absolute granulocyte count (x 10^6/l)	Platelet count (x 10^6/l)	Percentage of standard dose of GEMZAR (%)
> 1,000 and	> 100,000	100
500-1,000 or	50,000-100,000	75
< 500 or	< 50,000	Omit dose *

*Treatment omitted will not be reinstated within a cycle before the absolute granulocyte count reaches at least 500 (x10^6/l) and the platelet count reaches 50,000 (x10^6/l).

Dose modification of gemcitabine within a cycle for breast cancer, given in combination with paclitaxel

Absolute granulocyte count (x 10^6/l)	Platelet count (x 10^6/l)	Percentage of standard dose of GEMZAR (%)
⩾ 1,200 and	> 75,000	100
1,000- < 1,200 or	50,000-75,000	75
700- < 1,000 and	⩾ 50,000	50
< 700 or	< 50,000	Omit dose*

*Treatment omitted will not be reinstated within a cycle. Treatment will start on Day 1 of the next cycle once the absolute granulocyte count reaches at least 1,500 (x10^6/l) and the platelet count reaches 100,000 (x10^6/l).

Dose modification of gemcitabine within a cycle for ovarian cancer, given in combination with carboplatin

Absolute granulocyte count (x 10^6/l)	Platelet count (x 10^6/l)	Percentage of standard dose of GEMZAR (%)
> 1,500 and	⩾ 100,000	100
1,000-1,500 or	75,000-100,000	50
< 1,000 or	< 75,000	Omit dose*

*Treatment omitted will not be reinstated within a cycle. Treatment will start on Day 1 of the next cycle once the absolute granulocyte count reaches at least 1,500 (x10^6/l) and the platelet count reaches 100,000 (x10^6/l).

Dose modifications due to haematological toxicity in subsequent cycles, for all indications

The gemcitabine dose should be reduced to 75% of the original cycle initiation dose, in the case of the following haematological toxicities:

- Absolute granulocyte count < 500 × 10^6/l for more than 5 days
- Absolute granulocyte count < 100 × 10^6/l for more than 3 days
- Febrile neutropenia
- Platelets < 25,000 × 10^6/l
- Cycle delay of more than 1 week due to toxicity

Method of administration

GEMZAR is tolerated well during infusion and may be administered ambulant. If extravasation occurs, generally the infusion must be stopped immediately and started again in another blood vessel. The patient should be monitored carefully after the administration.

For instructions on reconstitution, see section 6.6.

Special populations

Patients with renal or hepatic impairment

Gemcitabine should be used with caution in patients with hepatic or renal insufficiency as there is insufficient information from clinical studies to allow for clear dose recommendations for these patient populations (see sections 4.4 and 5.2).

Elderly population (> 65 years)

Gemcitabine has been well tolerated in patients over the age of 65. There is no evidence to suggest that dose adjustments, other than those already recommended for all patients, are necessary in the elderly (see section 5.2).

Paediatric population (< 18 years)

Gemcitabine is not recommended for use in children under 18 years of age due to insufficient data on safety and efficacy.

4.3 Contraindications

Hypersensitivity to the active substance or to any of the excipients.

Breast-feeding (see section 4.6).

4.4 Special warnings and precautions for use

Prolongation of the infusion time and increased dosing frequency have been shown to increase toxicity.

Haematological toxicity

Gemcitabine can suppress bone marrow function as manifested by leucopenia, thrombocytopenia and anaemia.

Patients receiving gemcitabine should be monitored prior to each dose for platelet, leucocyte and granulocyte counts. Suspension or modification of therapy should be considered when drug-induced bone marrow depression is detected (see section 4.2). However, myelosuppression is short-lived and usually does not result in dose reduction and rarely in discontinuation.

Peripheral blood counts may continue to deteriorate after gemcitabine administration has been stopped. In patients with impaired bone marrow function, the treatment should be started with caution. As with other cytotoxic treatments, the risk of cumulative bone-marrow suppression must be considered when gemcitabine treatment is given together with other chemotherapy.

Hepatic insufficiency

Administration of gemcitabine in patients with concurrent liver metastases or a pre-existing medical history of hepatitis, alcoholism or liver cirrhosis may lead to exacerbation of the underlying hepatic insufficiency.

Laboratory evaluation of renal and hepatic function (including virological tests) should be performed periodically.

Gemcitabine should be used with caution in patients with hepatic insufficiency or with impaired renal function as there is insufficient information from clinical studies to allow clear dose recommendation for this patient population (see section 4.2).

Concomitant radiotherapy

Concomitant radiotherapy (given together or ⩽7 days apart): Toxicity has been reported (see section 4.5 for details and recommendations for use).

Live vaccinations

Yellow fever vaccine and other live attenuated vaccines are not recommended in patients treated with gemcitabine (see section 4.5).

Cardiovascular

Due to the risk of cardiac and/or vascular disorders with gemcitabine, particular caution must be exercised with patients presenting a history of cardiovascular events.

Pulmonary

Pulmonary effects, sometimes severe (such as pulmonary oedema, interstitial pneumonitis or adult respiratory distress syndrome (ARDS)) have been reported in association with gemcitabine therapy. The aetiology of these effects is unknown. If such effects develop, consideration should be made to discontinuing gemcitabine therapy. Early use of supportive care measure may help ameliorate the condition.

Renal

Clinical findings consistent with the haemolytic uraemic syndrome (HUS) were rarely reported in patients receiving gemcitabine (see section 4.8). Gemcitabine should be discontinued at the first signs of any evidence of microangiopathic haemolytic anaemia, such as rapidly falling haemoglobin with concomitant thrombocytopenia, elevation of serum bilirubin, serum creatinine, blood urea nitrogen, or LDH. Renal failure may not be reversible with discontinuation of therapy and dialysis may be required.

Fertility

In fertility studies, gemcitabine caused hypospermatogenesis in male mice (see section 5.3). Therefore, men being treated with gemcitabine are advised not to father a child during and up to 6 months after treatment and to seek further advice regarding cryoconservation of sperm prior to treatment because of the possibility of infertility due to therapy with gemcitabine (see section 4.6).

Sodium

GEMZAR 200 mg contains 3.5 mg (<1 mmol) sodium per vial. This should be taken into consideration by patients on a controlled sodium diet.

GEMZAR 1000 mg contains 17.5 mg (<1 mmol) sodium per vial. This should be taken into consideration by patients on a controlled sodium diet.

4.5 Interaction with other medicinal products and other forms of interaction

No specific interaction studies have been performed (see section 5.2).

Radiotherapy

Concurrent (given together or ⩽ 7 days apart) - Toxicity associated with this multimodality therapy is dependent on many different factors, including dose of gemcitabine, frequency of gemcitabine administration, dose of radiation, radiotherapy planning technique, the target tissue, and target volume. Pre-clinical and clinical studies have shown that gemcitabine has radiosensitising activity. In a single trial, where gemcitabine at a dose of 1,000 mg/m^2 was administered concurrently for up to 6 consecutive weeks with therapeutic thoracic radiation to patients with non-small cell lung cancer, significant toxicity in the form of severe, and potentially life-threatening mucositis, especially oesophagitis, and pneumonitis was observed, particularly in patients receiving large volumes of radiotherapy [median treatment volumes 4,795 cm^3]. Studies done subsequently have suggested that it is feasible to administer gemcitabine at lower doses with concurrent radiotherapy with predictable toxicity, such as a phase II study in non-small cell lung cancer, where thoracic radiation doses of 66 Gy were applied concomitantly with an administration with gemcitabine (600 mg/m^2, four times) and cisplatin (80 mg/m^2, twice) during 6 weeks. The optimum regimen for safe administration of gemcitabine with therapeutic doses of radiation has not yet been determined in all tumour types.

Non-concurrent (given >7 days apart) - Analysis of the data does not indicate any enhanced toxicity when gemcitabine is administered more than 7 days before or after radiation, other than radiation recall. Data suggest that gemcitabine can be started after the acute effects of radiation have resolved or at least one week after radiation.

Radiation injury has been reported on targeted tissues (e.g., oesophagitis, colitis, and pneumonitis) in association with both concurrent and non-concurrent use of gemcitabine.

Others

Yellow fever and other live attenuated vaccines are not recommended due to the risk of systemic, possibly fatal, disease, particularly in immunosuppressed patients.

4.6 Pregnancy and lactation

Pregnancy

There are no adequate data from the use of gemcitabine in pregnant women. Studies in animals have shown reproductive toxicity (see section 5.3). Based on results from animal studies and the mechanism of action of gemcitabine, this substance should not be used during pregnancy unless clearly necessary. Women should be advised not to become pregnant during treatment with gemcitabine and to warn their attending physician immediately, should this occur after all.

Breast-feeding

It is not known whether gemcitabine is excreted in human milk, and adverse effects on the suckling child cannot be excluded. Breast-feeding must be discontinued during gemcitabine therapy.

Fertility

In fertility studies, gemcitabine caused hypospermatogenesis in male mice (see section 5.3). Therefore, men being treated with gemcitabine are advised not to father a child during and up to 6 months after treatment, and to seek further advice regarding cryoconservation of sperm prior to treatment because of the possibility of infertility due to therapy with gemcitabine.

4.7 Effects on ability to drive and use machines

No studies on the effects on the ability to drive and use machines have been performed. However, gemcitabine has been reported to cause mild to moderate somnolence, especially in combination with alcohol consumption. Patients should be cautioned against driving or operating machinery until it is established that they do not become somnolent.

4.8 Undesirable effects

The most commonly reported adverse drug reactions associated with GEMZAR treatment include: nausea with or without vomiting, raised liver transaminases (AST/ALT) and alkaline phosphatase, reported in approximately 60% of patients; proteinuria and haematuria reported in approximately 50% of patients; dyspnoea reported in 10-40% of patients (highest incidence in lung cancer patients); allergic skin rashes occur in approximately 25% of patients and are associated with itching in 10% of patients.

The frequency and severity of the adverse reactions are affected by the dose, infusion rate and intervals between doses (see section 4.4). Dose-limiting adverse reactions are reductions in thrombocyte, leucocyte and granulocyte counts (see section 4.2).

Clinical trial data

Frequencies are defined as: Very common (⩾1/10), Common (⩾1/100 to <1/10), Uncommon (⩾1/1,000 to <1/100), Rare (⩾1/10,000 to <1/1,000), Very Rare (<1/10,000).

The following table of undesirable effects and frequencies is based on data from clinical trials. Within each frequency grouping, undesirable effects are presented in order of decreasing seriousness.

System Organ Class	Frequency grouping
Blood and lymphatic system disorders	*Very Common* • Leucopenia (Neutropenia Grade 3 = 19.3 %; Grade 4 = 6 %). Bone-marrow suppression is usually mild to moderate and mostly affects the granulocyte count (see section 4.2). • Thrombocytopenia • Anaemia *Common* • Febrile neutropenia *Very Rare* • Thrombocytosis
Immune system disorders	*Very Rare* • Anaphylactoid reaction
Metabolism and nutrition disorders	*Common* • Anorexia
Nervous system disorders	*Common* • Headache • Insomnia • Somnolence
Cardiac disorders	*Rare* • Myocardial infarct
Vascular disorders	*Rare* • Hypotension
Respiratory, thoracic and mediastinal disorders	*Very Common* • Dyspnoea – usually mild and passes rapidly without treatment *Common* • Cough • Rhinitis *Uncommon* • Interstitial pneumonitis (see section 4.4) • Bronchospasm – usually mild and transient but may require parenteral treatment
Gastro-intestinal disorders	*Very Common* • Vomiting • Nausea *Common* • Diarrhoea • Stomatitis and ulceration of the mouth • Constipation
Hepato-biliary disorders	*Very Common* • Elevation of liver transaminases (AST and ALT) and alkaline phosphatase *Common* • Increased bilirubin *Rare* • Increased gamma-glutamyl transferase (GGT)
Skin and subcutaneous tissue disorders	*Very Common* • Allergic skin rash frequently associated with pruritus • Alopecia *Common* • Itching • Sweating *Rare* • Ulceration • Vesicle and sore formation • Scaling *Very Rare* • Severe skin reactions, including desquamation and bullous skin eruptions
Musculoskeletal and connective tissue disorders	*Common* • Back pain • Myalgia
Renal and urinary disorders	*Very Common* • Haematuria • Mild proteinuria
General disorders and administration site conditions	*Very Common* • Influenza-like symptoms - the most common symptoms are fever, headache, chills, myalgia, asthenia and anorexia. Cough, rhinitis, malaise, perspiration and sleeping difficulties have also been reported. • Oedema/peripheral oedema - including facial oedema. Oedema is usually reversible after stopping treatment. *Common* • Fever • Asthenia • Chills *Rare* • Injection site reactions - mainly mild in nature
Injury, poisoning, and procedural complications	Radiation toxicity (see section 4.5).

Post-marketing experience (spontaneous reports): frequency not known (cannot be estimated from the available data)

Nervous system disorders

Cerebrovascular accident

Cardiac disorders

Arrythmias, predominantly supraventricular in nature

Heart failure

Vascular disorders

Clinical signs of peripheral vasculitis and gangrene

Respiratory, thoracic and mediastinal disorders

Pulmonary oedema

Adult respiratory distress syndrome (see section 4.4)

Gastro-intestinal disorders

Ischaemic colitis

Hepato-biliary disorders

Serious hepatotoxicity, including liver failure and death

Skin and subcutaneous tissue disorders

Severe skin reactions, including desquamation and bullous skin eruptions, Lyell's syndrome, Stevens-Johnson syndrome

Renal and urinary disorders

Renal failure (see section 4.4)

Haemolytic uraemic syndrome (see section 4.4)

Injury, poisoning and procedural complications

Radiation recall

Combination use in breast cancer

The frequency of Grade 3 and 4 haematological toxicities, particularly neutropenia, increases when gemcitabine is used in combination with paclitaxel. However, the increase in these adverse reactions is not associated with an increased incidence of infections or haemorrhagic events. Fatigue and febrile neutropenia occur more frequently when gemcitabine is used in combination with paclitaxel. Fatigue, which is not associated with anaemia, usually resolves after the first cycle.

(see Table 1 opposite)

Combination use in bladder cancer

(see Table 2 below)

Combination use in ovarian cancer

(see Table 3 below)

Sensory neuropathy was also more frequent in the combination arm than with single-agent carboplatin.

4.9 Overdose

There is no known antidote for overdose of gemcitabine. Doses as high as 5,700 mg/m^2 have been administered by intravenous infusion over 30 minutes every 2 weeks with clinically acceptable toxicity. In the event of suspected overdose, the patient should be monitored with appropriate blood counts and receive supportive therapy, as necessary.

5. PHARMACOLOGICAL PROPERTIES

5.1 Pharmacodynamic properties

Pharmacotherapeutic group: Pyrimidine analogues. *ATC code:* L01BC05

Cytotoxic activity in cell cultures

Gemcitabine shows significant cytotoxic effects against a variety of cultured murine and human tumour cells. Its action is phase-specific such that gemcitabine primarily kills cells that are undergoing DNA synthesis (S-phase) and, under certain circumstances, blocks the progression of cells at the junction of the G_1/S phase boundary. *In vitro*, the cytotoxic effect of gemcitabine is dependent on both concentration and time.

Anti-tumoural activity in preclinical models

In animal tumour models, anti-tumoural activity of gemcitabine is schedule-dependent. When gemcitabine is administered daily, high mortality among the animals, but minimal anti-tumoural activity, is observed. If, however, gemcitabine is given every third or fourth day, it can be administered in non-lethal doses with substantial anti-tumoural activity against a broad spectrum of mouse tumours.

Mechanism of action

Cellular metabolism and mechanism of action: Gemcitabine (dFdC), which is a pyrimidine antimetabolite, is metabolised intracellularly by nucleoside kinase to the active diphosphate (dFdCDP) and triphosphate (dFdCTP) nucleosides. The cytotoxic effect of gemcitabine is due to inhibition of DNA synthesis by two mechanisms of action by dFdCDP and dFdCTP. First, dFdCDP inhibits ribonucleotide reductase, which is uniquely responsible for catalysing the reactions that produce deoxynucleoside triphosphates (dCTP) for DNA synthesis. Inhibition of this enzyme by dFdCDP reduces the concentration of deoxynucleosides in general and, in particular, dCTP. Second, dFdCTP competes with dCTP for incorporation into DNA (self-potentiation).

Likewise, a small amount of gemcitabine may also be incorporated into RNA. Thus, the reduced intracellular concentration of dCTP potentiates the incorporation of dFdCTP into DNA. DNA polymerase epsilon lacks the ability to eliminate gemcitabine and to repair the growing DNA strands. After gemcitabine is incorporated into DNA, one additional nucleotide is added to the growing DNA strands. After this addition there is essentially a complete inhibition in further DNA synthesis (masked chain termination). After incorporation into DNA, gemcitabine appears to induce the programmed cell death process known as apoptosis.

Clinical data

Bladder cancer

A randomised phase III study of 405 patients with advanced or metastatic urothelial transitional cell carcinoma showed no difference between the two treatment arms, gemcitabine/cisplatin versus methotrexate/vinblastine/adriamycin/cisplatin (MVAC), in terms of median survival (12.8 and 14.8 months respectively, p=0.547), time to disease progression (7.4 and 7.6 months respectively, p=0.842) and response rate (49.4% and 45.7% respectively, p=0.512). However, the combination of gemcitabine and cisplatin had a better toxicity profile than MVAC.

Table 1

Grade 3 and 4 Adverse Events Paclitaxel versus Gemcitabine plus paclitaxel				
	Number (%) of Patients			
	Paclitaxel arm (N=259)		Gemcitabine plus paclitaxel arm (N=262)	
	Grade 3	Grade 4	Grade 3	Grade 4
Laboratory				
Anaemia	5 (1.9)	1 (0.4)	15 (5.7)	3 (1.1)
Thrombocytopenia	0	0	14 (5.3)	1 (0.4)
Neutropenia	11 (4.2)	17 (6.6)*	82 (31.3)	45 (17.2)*
Non-laboratory				
Febrile neutropenia	3 (1.2)	0	12 (4.6)	1(0.4)
Fatigue	3 (1.2)	1 (0.4)	15 (5.7)	2 (0.8)
Diarrhoea	5 (1.9)	0	8 (3.1)	0
Motor neuropathy	2(0.8)	0	6(2.3)	1(0.4)
Sensory neuropathy	9(3.5)	0	14(5.3)	1(0.4)

*Grade 4 neutropenia lasting for more than 7 days occurred in 12.6% of patients in the combination arm and 5.0% of patients in the paclitaxel arm.

Table 2 Combination use in bladder cancer

Grade 3 and 4 Adverse Events MVAC versus Gemcitabine plus cisplatin				
	Number (%) of Patients			
	MVAC (methotrexate, vinblastine, doxorubicin and cisplatin) arm (N=196)		Gemcitabine plus cisplatin arm (N=200)	
	Grade 3	Grade 4	Grade 3	Grade 4
Laboratory				
Anaemia	30(16)	4(2)	47(24)	7(4)
Thrombocytopenia	15(8)	25(13)	57(29)	57(29)
Non-laboratory				
Nausea and vomiting	37(19)	3(2)	44(22)	0(0)
Diarrhoea	15(8)	1(1)	6(3)	0(0)
Infection	19(10)	10(5)	4(2)	1(1)
Stomatitis	34(18)	8(4)	2(1)	0(0)

Table 3 Combination use in ovarian cancer

Grade 3 and 4 Adverse Events Carboplatin versus Gemcitabine plus carboplatin				
	Number (%) of Patients			
	Carboplatin arm (N=174)		Gemcitabine plus carboplatin arm (N=175)	
	Grade 3	Grade 4	Grade 3	Grade 4
Laboratory				
Anaemia	10(5.7)	4(2.3)	39(22.3)	9(5.1)
Neutropenia	19(10.9)	2(1.1)	73(41.7)	50(28.6)
Thrombocytopenia	18(10.3)	2(1.1)	53(30.3)	8(4.6)
Leucopenia	11(6.3)	1(0.6)	84(48.0)	9(5.1)
Non-laboratory				
Haemorrhage	0(0.0)	0(0.0)	3(1.8)	(0.0)
Febrile neutropenia	0(0.0)	0(0.0)	2(1.1)	(0.0)
Infection without neutropenia	0(0)	0(0.0)	(0.0)	1(0.6)

Pancreatic cancer

In a randomised phase III study of 126 patients with advanced or metastatic pancreatic cancer, gemcitabine showed a statistically significant higher clinical benefit response rate than 5-fluorouracil (23.8% and 4.8% respectively, p=0.0022). Also, a statistically significant prolongation of the time to progression from 0.9 to 2.3 months (log-rank $p<0.0002$) and a statistically significant prolongation of median survival from 4.4 to 5.7 months (log-rank $p<0.0024$) was observed in patients treated with gemcitabine compared to patients treated with 5-fluorouracil.

Non-small cell lung cancer

In a randomised phase III study of 522 patients with inoperable, locally advanced or metastatic NSCLC, gemcitabine in combination with cisplatin showed a statistically significant higher response rate than cisplatin alone (31.0% and 12.0%, respectively, $p<0.0001$). A statistically significant prolongation of the time to progression, from 3.7 to 5.6 months (log-rank $p<0.0012$) and a statistically significant prolongation of median survival from 7.6 months to 9.1 months (log-rank $p<0.004$) was observed in patients treated with gemcitabine/cisplatin compared to patients treated with cisplatin.

In another randomised phase III study of 135 patients with stage IIIB or IV NSCLC, a combination of gemcitabine and cisplatin showed a statistically significant higher response rate than a combination of cisplatin and etoposide (40.6% and 21.2%, respectively, p=0.025). A statistically significant prolongation of the time to progression, from 4.3 to 6.9 months (p=0.014) was observed in patients treated with gemcitabine/cisplatin compared to patients treated with etoposide/cisplatin. In both studies it was found that tolerability was similar in the two treatment arms.

Ovarian carcinoma

In a randomised phase III study, 356 patients with advanced epithelial ovarian carcinoma who had relapsed at least 6 months after completing platinum-based therapy were randomised to therapy with gemcitabine and carboplatin (GCb), or carboplatin (Cb). A statistically significant prolongation of the time to progression of disease, from 5.8 to 8.6 months (log-rank p=0.0038) was observed in the patients treated with GCb compared to patients treated with Cb. Differences in response rate of 47.2% in the GCb arm versus 30.9% in the Cb arm (p=0.0016) and median survival 18 months (GCb) versus 17.3 (Cb) (p=0.73) favoured the GCb arm.

Breast cancer

In a randomised phase III study of 529 patients with inoperable, locally recurrent or metastatic breast cancer with relapse after adjuvant/neoadjuvant chemotherapy, gemcitabine in combination with paclitaxel showed a statistically significant prolongation of time to documented disease progression from 3.98 to 6.14 months (log-rank p=0.0002) in patients treated with gemcitabine/paclitaxel compared to patients treated with paclitaxel. After 377 deaths, the overall survival was 18.6 months versus 15.8 months (log-rank p=0.0489, HR 0.82) in patients treated with gemcitabine/paclitaxel compared to patients treated with paclitaxel, and the overall response rate was 41.4% and 26.2% respectively (p= 0.0002).

5.2 Pharmacokinetic properties

The pharmacokinetics of gemcitabine have been examined in 353 patients in seven studies. The 121 women and 232 men ranged in age from 29 to 79 years. Of these patients, approximately 45% had non-small cell lung cancer and 35% were diagnosed with pancreatic cancer. The following pharmacokinetic parameters were obtained for doses ranging from 500 to 2,592 mg/m^2 that were infused from 0.4 to 1.2 hours.

Peak plasma concentrations (obtained within 5 minutes of the end of the infusion) were 3.2 to 45.5 µg/ml. Plasma concentrations of the parent compound following a dose of 1,000 mg/m^2/30 minutes are greater than 5 µg/ml for approximately 30 minutes after the end of the infusion, and greater than 0.4 µg/ml for an additional hour.

Distribution

The volume of distribution of the central compartment was 12.4 l/m^2 for women and 17.5 l/m^2 for men (inter-individual variability was 91.9%). The volume of distribution of the peripheral compartment was 47.4 l/m^2. The volume of the peripheral compartment was not sensitive to gender.

The plasma protein binding was considered to be negligible.

Half-life: This ranged from 42 to 94 minutes depending on age and gender. For the recommended dosing schedule, gemcitabine elimination should be virtually complete within 5 to 11 hours of the start of the infusion. Gemcitabine does not accumulate when administered once weekly.

Metabolism

Gemcitabine is rapidly metabolised by cytidine deaminase in the liver, kidney, blood and other tissues. Intracellular metabolism of gemcitabine produces the gemcitabine mono, di and triphosphates (dFdCMP, dFdCDP and dFdCTP) of which dFdCDP and dFdCTP are considered active. These intracellular metabolites have not been detected in plasma or urine. The primary metabolite, 2'-deoxy-2', 2'-difluorouridine (dFdU), is not active and is found in plasma and urine.

Excretion

Systemic clearance ranged from 29.2 l/hr/m^2 to 92.2 l/hr/m^2 depending on gender and age (inter-individual variability was 52.2%). Clearance for women is approximately 25% lower than the values for men. Although rapid, clearance for both men and women appears to decrease with age. For the recommended gemcitabine dose of 1,000 mg/m^2 given as a 30-minute infusion, lower clearance values for women and men should not necessitate a decrease in the gemcitabine dose.

Urinary excretion: Less than 10% is excreted as unchanged drug.

Renal clearance was 2 to 7 l/hr/m^2.

During the week following administration, 92 to 98% of the dose of gemcitabine administered is recovered, 99% in the urine, mainly in the form of dFdU and 1% of the dose is excreted in faeces.

dFdCTP kinetics

This metabolite can be found in peripheral blood mononuclear cells and the information below refers to these cells. Intracellular concentrations increase in proportion to gemcitabine doses of 35-350 mg/m^2/ 30 minutes, which give steady-state concentrations of 0.4-5 µg/ml. At gemcitabine plasma concentrations above 5 µg/ml, dFdCTP levels do not increase, suggesting that the formation is saturable in these cells.

Half-life of terminal elimination: 0.7-12 hours.

dFdU kinetics

Peak plasma concentrations (3-15 minutes after end of 30-minute infusion, 1,000 mg/m^2): 28-52 µg/ml. Trough concentration following once weekly dosing: 0.07-1.12 µg/ml, with no apparent accumulation. Triphasic plasma concentration versus time curve, mean half-life of terminal phase - 65 hours (range 33-84 hr).

Formation of dFdU from parent compound: 91%-98%.

Mean volume of distribution of central compartment: 18 l/m^2 (range 11-22 l/m^2).

Mean steady-state volume of distribution (Vss): 150 l/m^2 (range 96-228 l/m^2).

Tissue distribution: Extensive.

Mean apparent clearance: 2.5 l/hr/m^2 (range 1-4 l/hr/m^2).

Urinary excretion: All.

Gemcitabine and paclitaxel combination therapy

Combination therapy did not alter the pharmacokinetics of either gemcitabine or paclitaxel.

Gemcitabine and carboplatin combination therapy

When given in combination with carboplatin the pharmacokinetics of gemcitabine were not altered.

Renal impairment

Mild to moderate renal insufficiency (GFR from 30 ml/min to 80 ml/min) has no consistent, significant effect on gemcitabine pharmacokinetics.

5.3 Preclinical safety data

In repeat-dose studies of up to 6 months in duration in mice and dogs, the principal finding was schedule and dose-dependent haematopoietic suppression which was reversible.

Gemcitabine is mutagenic in an *in vitro* mutation test and an *in vivo* bone marrow micronucleus test. Long-term animal studies evaluating the carcinogenic potential have not been performed.

In fertility studies, gemcitabine caused reversible hypospermatogenesis in male mice. No effect on the fertility of females has been detected.

Evaluation of experimental animal studies has shown reproductive toxicity, e.g., birth defects and other effects on the development of the embryo or foetus, the course of gestation or perinatal and postnatal development.

6. PHARMACEUTICAL PARTICULARS

6.1 List of excipients

GEMZAR 200 mg contains:

Mannitol (E421)

Sodium acetate (E262)

Hydrochloric acid (E507) (for pH adjustment)

Sodium hydroxide (E524) (for pH adjustment)

GEMZAR 1000 mg contains:

Mannitol (E421)

Sodium acetate (E262)

Hydrochloric acid (E507) (for pH adjustment)

Sodium hydroxide (E524) (for pH adjustment)

6.2 Incompatibilities

This medicinal product must not be mixed with other medicinal products except those mentioned in section 6.6.

6.3 Shelf life

Unopened vials: 3 years.

Reconstituted solution:

Chemical and physical in-use stability has been demonstrated for 24 hours at 30°C. From a microbiological point of view, the product should be used immediately. If not used immediately, in-use storage times and conditions prior to use are the responsibility of the user and would normally not be longer than 24 hours at room temperature, unless reconstitution (and further dilution, if applicable) has taken place in controlled and validated aseptic conditions.

Solutions of reconstituted gemcitabine should not be refrigerated, as crystallisation may occur.

6.4 Special precautions for storage

Unopened vial: Store below 30°C.

For storage conditions of the reconstituted medicinal product, see section 6.3.

6.5 Nature and contents of container

Type I flint glass vials, stoppered with a grey bromobutyl rubber stopper and sealed with an aluminium seal, combined with a polypropylene cap.

Each pack contains 1 vial.

6.6 Special precautions for disposal and other handling

Handling

The normal safety precautions for cytostatic agents must be observed when preparing and disposing of the infusion solution. Handling of the solution for infusion should be done in a safety box and protective coats and gloves should be used. If no safety box is available, the equipment should be supplemented with a mask and protective glasses.

If the preparation comes into contact with the eyes, this may cause serious irritation. The eyes should be rinsed immediately and thoroughly with water. If there is lasting irritation, a doctor should be consulted. If the solution is spilled on the skin, rinse thoroughly with water.

Instructions for reconstitution (and further dilution, if performed)

The only approved diluent for reconstitution of gemcitabine sterile powder is sodium chloride 9 mg/ml (0.9%) solution for injection (without preservative). Due to solubility considerations, the maximum concentration for gemcitabine upon reconstitution is 40 mg/ml. Reconstitution at concentrations greater than 40 mg/ml may result in incomplete dissolution and should be avoided.

1. Use aseptic technique during the reconstitution and any further dilution of gemcitabine for intravenous infusion administration.

2. To reconstitute, add 5 ml of sterile sodium chloride 9 mg/ml (0.9 %) solution for injection, without preservative, to the 200 mg vial or 25 ml sterile sodium chloride 9 mg/ml (0.9 %) solution for injection, without preservative, to the 1,000 mg vial. The total volume after reconstitution is 5.26 ml (200 mg vial) or 26.3 ml (1,000 mg vial) respectively. This yields a gemcitabine concentration of 38 mg/ml, which includes accounting for the displacement volume of the lyophilised powder. Shake to dissolve. Further dilution with sterile sodium chloride 9 mg/ml (0.9 %) solution for injection, without preservative, can be done. Reconstituted solution is a clear, colourless to light straw-coloured solution.

3. Parenteral medicinal products should be inspected visually for particulate matter and discolouration prior to administration. If particulate matter is observed, do not administer.

Any unused product or waste material should be disposed of in accordance with local requirements.

7. MARKETING AUTHORISATION HOLDER

Eli Lilly and Company Limited

Lilly House

Priestley Road

Basingstoke

Hampshire

RG24 9NL

United Kingdom

8. MARKETING AUTHORISATION NUMBER(S)

GEMZAR 200 mg vial: PL 00006/0301

GEMZAR 1000mg vial: PL 00006/0302

9. DATE OF FIRST AUTHORISATION/RENEWAL OF THE AUTHORISATION

Date of first authorisation: 26 October 1995

Date of last renewal of the authorisation: 16 February 2006

10. DATE OF REVISION OF THE TEXT

18 February 2009

LEGAL CATEGORY

POM

*GEMZAR (gemcitabine hydrochloride) is a trademark of Eli Lilly and Company.

GE27M

Genotropin 5.3mg, 12mg

(Pharmacia Limited)

1. NAME OF THE MEDICINAL PRODUCT

Genotropin 5.3 mg powder and solvent for solution for injection.

Genotropin 12 mg powder and solvent for solution for injection.

2. QUALITATIVE AND QUANTITATIVE COMPOSITION

Somatropin (INN) recombinant DNA-derived human growth hormone produced in E.coli.

Presentations
Genotropin 5.3 mg powder and solvent for solution for injection, with preservative. One cartridge contains 5.3 mg somatropin. After reconstitution one cartridge contains 5.3 mg somatropin in 1ml.
Genotropin 12 mg powder and solvent for solution for injection, with preservative. One cartridge contains 12 mg somatropin. After reconstitution one cartridge contains 12 mg somatropin in 1ml.

For a full list of excipients, see section 6.1

3. PHARMACEUTICAL FORM

Powder and solvent for solution for injection. In the two-chamber cartridge there is a white powder in the front compartment and a clear solution in the rear compartment.

4. CLINICAL PARTICULARS

4.1 Therapeutic indications

Children

Growth disturbance due to insufficient secretion of growth hormone (growth hormone deficiency, GHD) and growth disturbance associated with Turner syndrome or chronic renal insufficiency.

Growth disturbance (current height SDS < -2.5 and parental adjusted height SDS < -1) in short children born small for gestational age (SGA), with a birth weight and/or length below –2SD, who failed to show catch-up growth (HV SDS < 0 during the last year) by 4 years of age or later.

Prader-Willi syndrome (PWS), for improvement of growth and body composition. The diagnosis of PWS should be confirmed by appropriate genetic testing.

Adults

Replacement therapy in adults with pronounced growth hormone deficiency.

Adult Onset: Patients who have severe growth hormone deficiency associated with multiple hormone deficiencies as a result of known hypothalamic or pituitary pathology and who have at least one known deficiency of a pituitary hormone not being prolactin. These patients should undergo an appropriate dynamic test in order to diagnose or exclude a growth hormone deficiency.

Childhood Onset: Patients who were growth hormone deficient during childhood as a result of congenital, genetic, acquired, or idiopathic causes. Patients with childhood onset GHD should be re-evaluated for growth hormone secretory capacity after completion of longitudinal growth. In patients with a high likelihood for persistent GHD, i.e. a congenital cause or GHD secondary to a pituitary/hypothalamic disease or insult, an IGF-I SDS < -2 off growth hormone treatment for at least 4 weeks should be considered sufficient evidence of profound GHD.

All other patients will require IGF-I assay and one growth hormone stimulation test

4.2 Posology and method of administration

The dosage and administration schedule should be individualised.

The injection should be given subcutaneously and the site varied to prevent lipoatrophy.

Growth disturbance due to insufficient secretion of growth hormone in children: Generally a dose of 0.025 - 0.035 mg/kg body weight per day or 0.7 - 1.0 mg/m^2 body surface area per day is recommended. Even higher doses have been used.

Where childhood onset GHD persists into adolescence, treatment should be continued to achieve full somatic development (e.g. body composition, bone mass). For monitoring, the attainment of a normal peak bone mass defined as a T score > −1 (i.e. standardized to average adult peak bone mass measured by dual energy X-ray absorptiometry taking into account sex and ethnicity) is one of the therapeutic objectives during the transition period. For guidance on dosing see adult section below.

Prader-Willi syndrome, for improvement of growth and body composition in children: Generally a dose of 0.035 mg/kg body weight per day or 1.0 mg/m^2 body surface area per day is recommended. Daily doses of 2.7 mg should not be exceeded. Treatment should not be used in children with a growth velocity less than 1 cm per year and near closure of epiphyses.

Growth disturbance due to Turner syndrome: A dose of 0.045 - 0.050 mg/kg body weight per day or 1.4 mg/m^2 body surface area per day is recommended.

Growth disturbance in chronic renal insufficiency: A dose of 1.4 mg/m^2 body surface area per day (approximately 0.045 - 0.050 mg/kg body weight per day) is recommended. Higher doses can be needed if growth velocity is too low. A dose correction can be needed after six months of treatment.

Growth disturbance in short children born small for gestational age (SGA): A dose of 0.035 mg/kg body weight per day (1 mg/m^2 body surface area per day) is usually recommended until final height is reached (see section 5.1). Treatment should be discontinued after the first year of treatment if the height velocity SDS is below +1. Treatment should be discontinued if the height velocity is < 2 cm/year and, if confirmation is required, bone age is > 14 years (girls) or > 16 years (boys), corresponding to closure of the epiphyseal growth plates.

Dosage Recommendations for Paediatric Patients

Indication	mg/kg body weight	mg/m^2 body surface area
	dose per day	dose per day
Growth hormone deficiency in children	0.025 - 0.035	0.7 - 1.0
Prader-Willi Syndrome in children	0.035	1.0
Turner syndrome	0.045 - 0.050	1.4
Chronic renal insufficiency	0.045 - 0.050	1.4
Children born small for gestational age (SGA)	0.035	1.0

Growth hormone deficient adult patients: In patients who continue growth hormone therapy after childhood GHD, the recommended dose to restart is 0.2 – 0.5 mg/day. The dose should be gradually increased or decreased according to individual patient requirements as determined by the IGF-I concentration.

In patients with adult-onset GHD, therapy should start with a low dose, 0.15 - 0.3 mg per day. The dose should be gradually increased according to individual patient requirements as determined by the IGF-I concentration.

In both cases treatment goal should be insulin-like growth factor-I (IGF-I) concentrations within 2 SDS from the age corrected mean. Patients with normal IGF-I concentrations at the start of the treatment should be administered growth hormone up to an IGF-I level into upper range of normal, not exceeding the 2 SDS. Clinical response and side effects may also be used as guidance for dose titration. It is recognised that there are patients with GHD who do not normalize IGF-I levels despite a good clinical response, and thus do not require dose escalation. The daily maintenance dose seldom exceeds 1.0 mg per day. Women may require higher doses than men, with men showing an increasing IGF-I sensitivity over time.

This means that there is a risk that women, especially those on oral oestrogen replacement are under-treated while men are over-treated. The accuracy of the growth hormone dose should therefore be controlled every 6 months. As normal physiological growth hormone production decreases with age, dose requirements are reduced. In patients above 60 years, therapy should start with a dose of 0.1 - 0.2 mg per day and should be slowly increased according to individual patient requirements. The minimum effective dose should be used. Daily maintenance dose in these patients seldom exceeds 0.5 mg per day.

4.3 Contraindications

Genotropin should not be used when there is any evidence of tumour activity and anti-tumour therapy must be completed prior to starting therapy.

Genotropin should not be used for growth promotion in children with closed epiphyses.

Patients with acute critical illness suffering complications following open heart surgery, abdominal surgery, multiple accidental trauma, acute respiratory failure or similar conditions should not be treated with Genotropin. (Regarding patients undergoing substitution therapy, see 4.4 "Special Warnings and Precautions for Use".)

Hypersensitivity to the active substance or to any of the excipients.

4.4 Special warnings and precautions for use

Diagnosis and therapy with Genotropin should be initiated and monitored by physicians who are appropriately qualified and experienced in the diagnosis and management of patients with the therapeutic indication of use.

Myositis is a very rare adverse event that may be related to the preservative metacresol. In the case of myalgia or disproportionate pain at the injection site, myositis should be considered and, if confirmed, a Genotropin presentation without metacresol should be used.

Somatropin may induce a state of insulin resistance and in some patients hyperglycaemia. Therefore patients should be observed for evidence of glucose intolerance. In rare cases the diagnostic criteria for diabetes mellitus type II may be fulfilled as a result of the somatropin therapy, but risk factors such as obesity (including obese PWS patients), family history, steroid treatment, or pre-existing impaired glucose tolerance have been present in most cases where this has occurred. In patients with an already manifest diabetes mellitus, the anti-diabetic therapy might require adjustment when somatropin is instituted.

During treatment with somatropin, an enhanced T4 to T3 conversion has been found which may result in a reduction in serum T4 and an increase in serum T3 concentrations. In general, the peripheral thyroid hormone levels have remained within the reference ranges for healthy subjects. The effects of somatropin on thyroid hormone levels may be of clinical relevance in patients with central subclinical hypothyroidism in whom hypothyroidism theoretically may develop. Conversely, in patients receiving replacement therapy with thyroxin, mild hyperthyroidism may occur. It is therefore particularly advisable to test thyroid function after starting treatment with somatropin and after dose adjustments.

In growth hormone deficiency secondary to treatment of malignant disease, it is recommended to pay attention to signs of relapse of the malignancy.

In patients with endocrine disorders, including growth hormone deficiency, slipped epiphyses of the hip may occur more frequently than in the general population. Children limping during treatment with somatropin should be examined clinically.

In case of severe or recurrent headache, visual problems, nausea and/or vomiting, a funduscopy for papilloedema is recommended. If papilloedema is confirmed, a diagnosis of benign intracranial hypertension should be considered and, if appropriate, the growth hormone treatment should be discontinued. At present there is insufficient evidence to give specific advice on the continuation of growth hormone treatment in patients with resolved intracranial hypertension. However, clinical experience has shown that reinstitution of the therapy is often possible without recurrence of the intracranial hypertension. If growth hormone treatment is restarted, careful monitoring for symptoms of intracranial hypertension is necessary.

Experience in patients above 80 years is limited. Elderly patients may be more sensitive to the action of Genotropin, and therefore may be more prone to develop adverse reactions.

In patients with PWS, treatment should always be in combination with a calorie-restricted diet.

There have been reports of fatalities associated with the use of growth hormone in paediatric patients with Prader-Willi syndrome who had one or more of the following risk factors: severe obesity (those patients exceeding a weight/height of 200%), history of respiratory impairment or sleep apnoea, or unidentified respiratory infection. Patients with one or more of these factors may be at increased risk.

Before initiation of treatment with somatropin in patients with Prader-Willi syndrome, signs for upper airway obstruction, sleep apnoea, or respiratory infections should be assessed.

If during the evaluation of upper airway obstruction, pathological findings are observed, the child should be referred to an ENT specialist for treatment and resolution of the respiratory disorder prior to initiating growth hormone treatment.

Sleep apnoea should be assessed before onset of growth hormone treatment by recognised methods such as polysomnography or overnight oxymetry, and monitored if sleep apnoea is suspected.

If during treatment with somatropin patients show signs of upper airway obstruction (including onset of or increased snoring), treatment should be interrupted, and a new ENT assessment performed.

All patients with Prader-Willi syndrome should be monitored if sleep apnoea is suspected.

Patients should be monitored for signs of respiratory infections, which should be diagnosed as early as possible and treated aggressively.

All patients with Prader-Willi syndrome should also have effective weight control before and during growth hormone treatment.

Scoliosis is common in patients with PWS. Scoliosis may progress in any child during rapid growth. Signs of scoliosis should be monitored during treatment. However, growth hormone treatment has not been shown to increase the incidence or severity of scoliosis.

Experience with prolonged treatment in adults and in patients with PWS is limited.

In short children born SGA other medical reasons or treatments that could explain growth disturbance should be ruled out before starting treatment.

In SGA children it is recommended to measure fasting insulin and blood glucose before start of treatment and annually thereafter. In patients with increased risk of diabetes mellitus (e.g. familial history of diabetes, obesity, severe insulin resistance, acanthosis nigricans) oral glucose tolerance testing (OGTT) should be performed. If overt diabetes occurs, growth hormone should not be administered.

In SGA children it is recommended to measure the IGF-I level before start of treatment and twice a year thereafter. If on repeated measurements IGF-I levels exceed +2 SD compared to references for age and pubertal status, the IGF-I / IGFBP-3 ratio could be taken into account to consider dose adjustment.

Experience in initiating treatment in SGA patients near onset of puberty is limited. It is therefore not recommended to initiate treatment near onset of puberty. Experience in patients with Silver-Russell syndrome is limited.

Some of the height gain obtained with treating short children born SGA with growth hormone may be lost if treatment is stopped before final height is reached.

In chronic renal insufficiency, renal function should be below 50 percent of normal before institution of therapy. To verify growth disturbance, growth should be followed for a year preceding institution of therapy. During this period, conservative treatment for renal insufficiency (which includes control of acidosis, hyperparathyroidism and nutritional status) should have been established and should be maintained during treatment. The treatment should be discontinued at renal transplantation.

To date, no data on final height in patients with chronic renal insufficiency treated with Genotropin are available.

The effects of Genotropin on recovery were studied in two placebo controlled trials involving 522 critically ill adult patients suffering complications following open heart surgery, abdominal surgery, multiple accidental trauma or acute respiratory failure. Mortality was higher in patients treated with 5.3 or 8 mg Genotropin daily compared to patients receiving placebo, 42% vs. 19%. Based on this information, these types of patients should not be treated with Genotropin. As there is no information available on the safety of growth hormone substitution therapy in acutely critically ill patients, the benefits of continued treatment in this situation should be weighed against the potential risks involved.

In all patients developing other or similar acute critical illness, the possible benefit of treatment with Genotropin must be weighed against the potential risk involved.

4.5 Interaction with other medicinal products and other forms of interaction

Data from an interaction study performed in growth hormone deficient adults suggests that somatropin administration may increase the clearance of compounds known to be metabolised by cytochrome P450 isoenzymes. The clearance of compounds metabolised by cytochrome P450 3A4 (e.g. sex steroids, corticosteroids, anticonvulsants and ciclosporin) may be especially increased resulting in lower plasma levels of these compounds. The clinical significance of this is unknown.

Also see Section 4.4 for statements regarding diabetes mellitus and thyroid disorder and Section 4.2 for statement on oral oestrogen replacement therapy.

4.6 Pregnancy and lactation

No clinical experience of use in pregnant women is available. Animal experimental data are incomplete. Treatment with Genotropin should be interrupted if pregnancy occurs.

During normal pregnancy, levels of pituitary growth hormone fall markedly after 20 gestation weeks, being replaced almost entirely by placental growth hormone by 30 weeks. In view of this, it is unlikely that continued replacement therapy with somatropin would be necessary in growth hormone deficient women in the third trimester of pregnancy.

It is not known if somatropin is excreted into breast milk, but absorption of intact protein from the gastrointestinal tract of the infant is extremely unlikely.

4.7 Effects on ability to drive and use machines

No effects on the ability to drive and use machines have been observed.

4.8 Undesirable effects

Within each frequency grouping, undesirable effects are presented in order of decreasing seriousness.

Patients with growth hormone deficiency are characterised by extracellular volume deficit. When treatment with somatropin is started, this deficit is rapidly corrected. In adult patients, adverse effects related to fluid retention such as peripheral oedema, stiffness in the extremities, arthralgia, myalgia and paraesthesia are common. In general, these adverse effects are mild to moderate, arise within the first months of treatment and subside spontaneously or with dose reduction.

The incidence of these adverse effects is related to the administered dose, the age of patients and possibly inversely related to the age of patients at the onset of growth hormone deficiency. In children, such adverse effects are uncommon.

Transient local skin reactions at the injection site in children are common.

Rare cases of diabetes mellitus type II have been reported.

Rare cases of benign intracranial hypertension have been reported.

Carpal tunnel syndrome is an uncommon event among adults.

Somatropin has given rise to the formation of antibodies in approximately 1% of patients. The binding capacity of these antibodies has been low and no clinical changes have been associated with their formation.

(see Table 1 below)

Somatropin has been reported to reduce serum cortisol levels, possibly by affecting carrier proteins or by increased hepatic clearance. The clinical relevance of these findings may be limited. Nevertheless, corticosteroid replacement therapy should be optimised before initiation of Genotropin therapy.

Very rare cases of leukaemia have been reported in growth hormone deficient children treated with somatropin, but the incidence appears to be similar to that in children without growth hormone deficiency.

In the post-marketing experience rare cases of sudden death have been reported in patients affected by Prader-Willi syndrome treated with somatropin, although no causal relationship has been demonstrated.

4.9 Overdose

No case of overdose or intoxication has been reported.

Acute overdosage could lead initially to hypoglycaemia and subsequently to hyperglycaemia.

Long term overdosage could result in signs and symptoms consistent with the known effects of human growth hormone excess.

5. PHARMACOLOGICAL PROPERTIES

5.1 Pharmacodynamic properties

Pharmacotherapeutic group: Anterior pituitary lobe hormones and analogues

ATC code: H01A C01

Somatropin is a potent metabolic hormone of importance for the metabolism of lipids, carbohydrates and proteins. In children with inadequate endogenous growth hormone, somatropin stimulates linear growth and increases growth rate. In adults, as well as in children, somatropin maintains a normal body composition by increasing nitrogen retention and stimulation of skeletal muscle growth, and by mobilisation of body fat. Visceral adipose tissue is particularly responsive to somatropin. In addition to enhanced lipolysis, somatropin decreases the uptake of triglycerides into body fat stores. Serum concentrations of IGF-I (Insulin-like Growth Factor-I) and IGFBP3 (Insulin-like Growth Factor Binding Protein 3) are increased by somatropin. In addition, the following actions have been demonstrated:

- Lipid metabolism: Somatropin induces hepatic LDL cholesterol receptors, and affects the profile of serum lipids and lipoproteins. In general, administration of somatropin to growth hormone deficient patients results in reductions in serum LDL and apolipoprotein B. A reduction in serum total cholesterol may also be observed.

- Carbohydrate metabolism: Somatropin increases insulin but fasting blood glucose is commonly unchanged. Children with hypopituitarism may experience fasting hypoglycaemia. This condition is reversed by somatropin.

- Water and mineral metabolism: Growth hormone deficiency is associated with decreased plasma and extracellular volumes. Both are rapidly increased after treatment with somatropin. Somatropin induces the retention of sodium, potassium and phosphorus.

- Bone metabolism: Somatropin stimulates the turnover of skeletal bone. Long-term administration of somatropin to growth hormone deficient patients with osteopenia results in an increase in bone mineral content and density at weight bearing sites.

- Physical capacity: Muscle strength and physical exercise capacity are improved after long-term treatment with somatropin. Somatropin also increases cardiac output, but the mechanism has yet to be clarified. A decrease in peripheral vascular resistance may contribute to this effect.

In clinical trials in short children born SGA doses of 0.033 and 0.067 mg/kg body weight per day have been used for treatment until final height. In 56 patients who were continuously treated and have reached (near) final height, the mean change from height at start of treatment was +1.90 SDS (0.033 mg/kg body weight per day) and +2.19 SDS (0.067 mg/kg body weight per day). Literature data from untreated SGA children without early spontaneous catch-up suggest a late growth of 0.5 SDS. Long-term safety data are still limited.

5.2 Pharmacokinetic properties

Absorption: The bioavailability of subcutaneously administered somatropin is approximately 80% in both healthy subjects and growth hormone deficient patients. A subcutaneous dose of 0.035 mg/kg of somatropin results in plasma C_{max} and t_{max} values in the range of 13-35 ng/ml and 3-6 hours, respectively.

Elimination: The mean terminal half-life of somatropin after intravenous administration in growth hormone deficient adults is about 0.4 hours. However, after subcutaneous administration, half-lives of 2-3 hours are achieved. The observed difference is likely due to slow absorption from the injection site following subcutaneous administration.

Sub-populations: The absolute bioavailability of somatropin seems to be similar in males and females following s.c. administration.

Information about the pharmacokinetics of somatropin in geriatric and paediatric populations, in different races and in patients with renal, hepatic or cardiac insufficiency is either lacking or incomplete.

5.3 Preclinical safety data

In studies regarding general toxicity, local tolerance and reproduction toxicity no clinically relevant effects have been observed.

In vitro and in vivo genotoxicity studies on gene mutations and induction of chromosome aberrations have been negative.

An increased chromosome fragility has been observed in one in-vitro study on lymphocytes taken from patients after long term treatment with somatropin and following the addition of the radiomimetic drug bleomycin. The clinical significance of this finding is unclear.

In another study, no increase in chromosomal abnormalities was found in the lymphocytes of patients who had received long term somatropin therapy.

6. PHARMACEUTICAL PARTICULARS

6.1 List of excipients

Powder: Front compartment	Solvent: Rear compartment
Glycine (E640), Sodium dihydrogen phosphate anhydrous (E339), Disodium phosphate anhydrous (E339), Mannitol (E421)	Water for injections, Metacresol, Mannitol (E421)

6.2 Incompatibilities

This medicinal product must not be mixed with other medicinal products except those mentioned in 6.6.

6.3 Shelf life

3 years

Chemical and physical in-use stability has been demonstrated for 4 weeks at 2°C – 8°C

From a microbiological point of view, once reconstituted, the product may be stored at 2°C - 8°C for 4 weeks.

Other in-use storage times and conditions are the responsibility of the user.

6.4 Special precautions for storage

Before reconstitution:

Store in a refrigerator (2°C – 8°C), with up to 1 month at or below 25°C allowed. Keep container in the outer carton in order to protect from light.

Table 1

	Common >1/100, <1/10	Uncommon >1/1000, <1/100	Rare >1/10,000, <1/1000	Very rare <1/10,000
Neoplasms, benign and malignant				**Leukaemia**
Immune system disorders	**Formation of antibodies**			
Endocrine disorders			**Diabetes mellitus type II**	
Nervous system disorders	**In adults paraesthesia**	**In adults carpal tunnel syndrome. In children paraesthesia**	**Benign intracranial hypertension**	
Skin and subcutaneous tissue disorders	**In children transient local skin reactions**			
Musculoskeletal, connective tissue and bone disorders	**In adults stiffness in the extremities, arthralgia, myalgia**	**In children stiffness in the extremities, arthralgia, myalgia**		
General disorders and administration site disorders	**In adults peripheral oedema**	**In children peripheral oedema**		

After reconstitution:

Store in a refrigerator (2°C – 8°C). Do not freeze. Keep container in the outer carton in order to protect from light. For storage conditions of the reconstituted medicinal product see section 6.3

6.5 Nature and contents of container
Powder and 1.15 ml solvent in a two-chamber glass cartridge (type I glass) separated by a rubber plunger (bromobutyl). The cartridge is sealed at one end with a rubber disc (bromobutyl) and an aluminium cap and at the other end by a rubber stopper (bromobutyl).

The two-chamber cartridge is supplied in a reconstitution device, KabiVial, or for use in an injection device, Genotropin Pen, or reconstitution device, Genotropin Mixer.

Pack size:

Presentation	Package Size
1. Genotropin 5.3 mg	1 × 5.3 mg 5 × 5.3 mg
2. Genotropin 12 mg	1 × 12 mg 5 × 12 mg

6.6 Special precautions for disposal and other handling
Only reconstitute the powder with the solvent supplied.

Two-chamber cartridge: The solution is prepared by screwing the reconstitution device or injection device together so that the solvent will be mixed with the powder in the two chamber cartridge. Gently dissolve the drug with a slow, swirling motion. Do not shake vigorously; this might cause denaturation of the active ingredient. The reconstituted solution is almost colourless or slightly opalescent. The reconstituted solution for injection is to be inspected prior to use and only clear solutions without particles should be used.

When using an injection device, the injection needle should be screwed on before reconstitution.

Any unused product or waste material should be disposed of in accordance with local requirements.

7. MARKETING AUTHORISATION HOLDER
Pharmacia Laboratories Ltd
Ramsgate Road
Sandwich
Kent CT13 9NJ
United Kingdom

8. MARKETING AUTHORISATION NUMBER(S)
Genotropin 5.3 mg PL 00022/0085
Genotropin 12 mg PL 00022/0098

9. DATE OF FIRST AUTHORISATION/RENEWAL OF THE AUTHORISATION
1 February 1995/ 1 February 2005

10. DATE OF REVISION OF THE TEXT
March 2009

11. LEGAL CATEGORY
POM
Ref: GN18_1 UK

Genotropin Miniquick

(Pharmacia Limited)

1. NAME OF THE MEDICINAL PRODUCT
1. Genotropin MiniQuick 0.2 mg powder and solvent for solution for injection
2. Genotropin MiniQuick 0.4 mg powder and solvent for solution for injection
3. Genotropin MiniQuick 0.6 mg powder and solvent for solution for injection
4. Genotropin MiniQuick 0.8 mg powder and solvent for solution for injection
5. Genotropin MiniQuick 1.0 mg powder and solvent for solution for injection
6. Genotropin MiniQuick 1.2 mg powder and solvent for solution for injection
7. Genotropin MiniQuick 1.4 mg powder and solvent for solution for injection
8. Genotropin MiniQuick 1.6 mg powder and solvent for solution for injection
9. Genotropin MiniQuick 1.8 mg powder and solvent for solution for injection
10. Genotropin MiniQuick 2.0 mg powder and solvent for solution for injection

2. QUALITATIVE AND QUANTITATIVE COMPOSITION
Somatropin (INN) recombinant DNA-derived human growth hormone produced in E.coli. Powder and solvent for solution for injection.

Presentation
Genotropin MiniQuick 0.2 mg powder and solvent for solution for injection. One cartridge contains 0.2 mg somatropin. After reconstition one cartridge contains 0.2 mg somatropin in 0.25 ml.
Genotropin MiniQuick 0.4 mg powder and solvent for solution for injection. One cartridge contains 0.4 mg somatropin. After reconstition one cartridge contains 0.4 mg somatropin in 0.25 ml.
Genotropin MiniQuick 0.6 mg powder and solvent for solution for injection. One cartridge contains 0.6 mg somatropin. After reconstition one cartridge contains 0.6 mg somatropin in 0.25 ml.
Genotropin MiniQuick 0.8 mg powder and solvent for solution for injection. One cartridge contains 0.8 mg somatropin. After reconstition one cartridge contains 0.8 mg somatropin in 0.25 ml.
Genotropin MiniQuick 1 mg. One cartridge contains 1.0 mg somatropin powder and solvent for solution for injection. After reconstitution one cartridge contains 1.0 mg somatropin in 0.25 ml.
Genotropin MiniQuick 1.2 mg. One cartridge contains 1.2 mg somatropin powder and solvent for solution for injection. After reconstitution one cartridge contains 1.2 mg somatropin in 0.25 ml.
Genotropin MiniQuick 1.4 mg. One cartridge contains 1.4 mg somatropin powder and solvent for solution for injection. After reconstitution one cartridge contains 1.4 mg somatropin in 0.25 ml.
Genotropin MiniQuick 1.6 mg. One cartridge contains 1.6 mg somatropin powder and solvent for solution for injection. After reconstitution one cartridge contains 1.6 mg somatropin in 0.25 ml.
Genotropin MiniQuick 1.8 mg. One cartridge contains 1.8 mg somatropin powder and solvent for solution for injection. After reconstitution one cartridge contains 1.8 mg somatropin in 0.25 ml.
Genotropin MiniQuick 2 mg. One cartridge contains 2.0 mg somatropin powder and solvent for solution for injection. After reconstitution one cartridge contains 2.0 mg somatropin in 0.25 ml.

For a full list of excipients, see section 6.1

3. PHARMACEUTICAL FORM
Powder and solvent for solution for injection. A two chamber cartridge with a white powder in the front compartment and a clear solution in the rear compartment.

4. CLINICAL PARTICULARS
4.1 Therapeutic indications
<u>Children</u>
Growth disturbance due to insufficient secretion of growth hormone (growth hormone deficiency, GHD) and growth disturbance associated with Turner syndrome or chronic renal insufficiency.

Growth disturbance (current height SDS < -2.5 and parental adjusted height SDS <-1) in short children born small for gestational age (SGA), with a birth weight and/or length below –2SD, who failed to show catch-up growth (HV SDS < 0 during the last year) by 4 years of age or later.

Prader-Willi syndrome (PWS), for improvement of growth and body composition. The diagnosis of PWS should be confirmed by appropriate genetic testing.

<u>Adults</u>
Replacement therapy in adults with pronounced growth hormone deficiency.

Adult Onset: Patients who have severe growth hormone deficiency associated with multiple hormone deficiencies as a result of known hypothalamic or pituitary pathology and who have at least one known deficiency of a pituitary hormone not being prolactin. These patients should undergo an appropriate dynamic test in order to diagnose or exclude a growth hormone deficiency.

Childhood Onset: Patients who were growth hormone deficient during childhood as a result of congenital, genetic, acquired, or idiopathic causes. Patients with childhood onset GHD should be re-evaluated for growth hormone secretory capacity after completion of longitudinal growth. In patients with a high likelihood for persistent GHD, i.e. a congenital cause or GHD secondary to a pituitary/hypothalamic disease or an insult IGF-I SDS <-2 off growth hormone treatment for at least 4 weeks should be considered sufficient evidence of profound GHD.

All other patients will require IGF-I assay and one growth hormone stimulation test.

4.2 Posology and method of administration
The dosage and administration schedule should be individualised.

The injection should be given subcutaneously and the site varied to prevent lipoatrophy.

Growth disturbance due to insufficient secretion of growth hormone in children: Generally a dose of 0.025 - 0.035 mg/kg body weight per day or 0.7 - 1.0 mg/m2 body surface area per day is recommended. Even higher doses have been used.

Where childhood onset GHD persists into adolescence, treatment should be continued to achieve full somatic development (e.g. body composition, bone mass). For monitoring, the attainment of a normal peak bone mass defined as a T score > −1 (i.e. standardized to average adult peak bone mass measured by dual energy X-ray absorptiometry taking into account sex and ethnicity) is one of the therapeutic objectives during the transition period. For guidance on dosing see adult section below

Prader-Willi syndrome, for improvement of growth and body composition in children: Generally a dose of 0.035 mg/kg body weight per day or 1.0 mg/m2 body surface area per day is recommended. Daily doses of 2.7 mg should not be exceeded. Treatment should not be used in children with a growth velocity less than 1 cm per year and near closure of epiphyses.

Growth disturbance due to Turner syndrome: A dose of 0.045 - 0.050 mg/kg body weight per day or 1.4 mg/m2 body surface area per day is recommended.

Growth disturbance in chronic renal insufficiency: A dose of 1.4 mg/m2 body surface area per day (approximately 0.045 - 0.050 mg/kg body weight per day) is recommended. Higher doses can be needed if growth velocity is too low. A dose correction can be needed after six months of treatment.

Growth disturbance in short children born small for gestational age (SGA): A dose of 0.035 mg/kg body weight per day (1 mg/m2 body surface area per day) is usually recommended until final height is reached (see section 5.1). Treatment should be discontinued after the first year of treatment if the height velocity SDS is below +1. Treatment should be discontinued if the height velocity is < 2 cm/year and, if confirmation is required, bone age is > 14 years (girls) or > 16 years (boys), corresponding to closure of the epiphyseal growth plates.

Dosage Recommendations In Paediatric Patients

Indication	mg/kg body weight	mg/m2 body surface area
	dose per day	dose per day
Growth hormone deficiency in children	0.025 - 0.035	0.7 - 1.0
Prader-Willi Syndrome in children	0.035	1.0
Turner syndrome	0.045 - 0.050	1.4
Chronic renal insufficiency	0.045 - 0.050	1.4
Children born small for gestational age (SGA)	0.035	1.0

Growth hormone deficient adult patients: In patients who continue growth hormone therapy after childhood GHD, the recommended dose to restart is 0.2 – 0.5 mg/day. The dose should be gradually increased or decreased according to individual patient requirements as determined by the IGF-I concentration.

In patients with adult-onset GHD, therapy should start with a low dose, 0.15 - 0.3 mg per day. The dose should be gradually increased according to individual patient requirements as determined by the IGF-I concentration.

In both cases treatment goal should be insulin-like growth factor-I (IGF-I) concentrations within 2 SDS from the age corrected mean. Patients with normal IGF-I concentrations at the start of the treatment should be administered growth hormone up to an IGF-I level into upper range of normal, not exceeding the 2 SDS. Clinical response and side effects may also be used as guidance for dose titration. It is recognised that there are patients with GHD who do not normalize IGF-I levels despite a good clinical response, and thus do not require dose escalation. The daily maintenance dose seldom exceeds 1.0 mg per day. Women may require higher doses than men, with men showing an increasing IGF-I sensitivity over time. This means that there is a risk that women, especially those on oral oestrogen replacement are under-treated while men are over-treated. The accuracy of the growth hormone dose should therefore be controlled every 6 months. As normal physiological growth hormone production decreases with age, dose requirements are reduced. In patients above 60 years, therapy should start with a dose of 0.1 - 0.2 mg per day and should be slowly increased according to individual patient requirements. The minimum effective dose should be used. Daily maintenance dose in these patients seldom exceeds 0.5 mg per day.

4.3 Contraindications

Genotropin MiniQuick should not be used when there is any evidence of tumour activity and anti-tumour therapy must be completed prior to starting therapy.

Genotropin MiniQuick should not be used for growth promotion in children with closed epiphyses.

Patients with acute critical illness suffering complications following open heart surgery, abdominal surgery, multiple accidental trauma, acute respiratory failure or similar conditions should not be treated with Genotropin MiniQuick. (Regarding patients undergoing substitution therapy, see 4.4 "Special Warnings and Precautions for Use".)

Hypersensitivity to the active substance or to any of the excipients.

4.4 Special warnings and precautions for use

Diagnosis and therapy with Genotropin MiniQuick should be initiated and monitored by physicians who are appropriately qualified and experienced in the diagnosis and management of patients with the therapeutic indication of use.

Somatropin may induce a state of insulin resistance and in some patients hyperglycaemia. Therefore patients should be observed for evidence of glucose intolerance. In rare cases the diagnostic criteria for diabetes mellitus type II may be fulfilled as a result of the somatropin therapy, but risk factors such as obesity (including obese PWS patients), family history, steroid treatment, or pre-existing impaired glucose tolerance have been present in most cases where this has occurred. In patients with an already manifest diabetes mellitus, the anti-diabetic therapy might require adjustment when somatropin is instituted.

During treatment with somatropin, an enhanced T4 to T3 conversion has been found which may result in a reduction in serum T4 and an increase in serum T3 concentrations. In general, the peripheral thyroid hormone levels have remained within the reference ranges for healthy subjects. The effects of somatropin on thyroid hormone levels may be of clinical relevance in patients with central subclinical hypothyroidism in whom hypothyroidism theoretically may develop. Conversely, in patients receiving replacement therapy with thyroxin, mild hyperthyroidism may occur. It is therefore particularly advisable to test thyroid function after starting treatment with somatropin and after dose adjustments.

In growth hormone deficiency secondary to treatment of malignant disease, it is recommended to pay attention to signs of relapse of the malignancy.

In patients with endocrine disorders, including growth hormone deficiency, slipped epiphyses of the hip may occur more frequently than in the general population. Children limping during treatment with somatropin should be examined clinically.

In case of severe or recurrent headache, visual problems, nausea and/or vomiting, a funduscopy for papilloedema is recommended. If papilloedema is confirmed, a diagnosis of benign intracranial hypertension should be considered and, if appropriate, the growth hormone treatment should be discontinued. At present there is insufficient evidence to give specific advice on the continuation of growth hormone treatment in patients with resolved intracranial hypertension. However, clinical experience has shown that reinstitution of the therapy is often possible without recurrence of the intracranial hypertension. If growth hormone treatment is restarted, careful monitoring for symptoms of intracranial hypertension is necessary.

Experience in patients above 80 years is limited. Elderly patients may be more sensitive to the action of Genotropin, and therefore may be more prone to develop adverse reactions.

In patients with PWS, treatment should always be in combination with a calorie-restricted diet.

There have been reports of fatalities associated with the use of growth hormone in paediatric patients with Prader-Willi syndrome who had one or more of the following risk factors: severe obesity (those patients exceeding a weight/height of 200%), history of respiratory impairment or sleep apnoea, or unidentified respiratory infection. Patients with one or more of these factors may be at increased risk.

Before initiation of treatment with somatropin in patients with Prader-Willi syndrome, signs for upper airway obstruction, sleep apnoea, or respiratory infections should be assessed.

If during the evaluation of upper airway obstruction, pathological findings are observed, the child should be referred to an ENT specialist for treatment and resolution of the respiratory disorder prior to initiating growth hormone treatment.

Sleep apnoea should be assessed before onset of growth hormone treatment by recognised methods such as polysomnography or overnight oxymetry, and monitored if sleep apnoea is suspected.

If during treatment with somatropin patients show signs of upper airway obstruction (including onset of or increased snoring), treatment should be interrupted, and a new ENT assessment performed.

All patients with Prader-Willi syndrome should be monitored if sleep apnoea is suspected.

Patients should be monitored for signs of respiratory infections, which should be diagnosed as early as possible and treated aggressively.

All patients with Prader-Willi syndrome should also have effective weight control before and during growth hormone treatment.

Scoliosis is common in patients with PWS. Scoliosis may progress in any child during rapid growth. Signs of scoliosis should be monitored during treatment. However, growth hormone treatment has not been shown to increase the incidence or severity of scoliosis.

Experience with prolonged treatment in adults and in patients with PWS is limited.

In short children born SGA other medical reasons or treatments that could explain growth disturbance should be ruled out before starting treatment.

In SGA children it is recommended to measure fasting insulin and blood glucose before start of treatment and annually thereafter. In patients with increased risk of diabetes mellitus (e.g. familial history of diabetes, obesity, severe insulin resistance, acanthosis nigricans) oral glucose tolerance testing (OGTT) should be performed. If overt diabetes occurs, growth hormone should not be administered.

In SGA children it is recommended to measure the IGF-I level before start of treatment and twice a year thereafter. If on repeated measurements IGF-I levels exceed +2 SD compared to references for age and pubertal status, the IGF-I / IGFBP-3 ratio could be taken into account to consider dose adjustment.

Experience in initiating treatment in SGA patients near onset of puberty is limited. It is therefore not recommended to initiate treatment near onset of puberty. Experience in patients with Silver-Russell syndrome is limited.

Some of the height gain obtained with treating short children born SGA with growth hormone may be lost if treatment is stopped before final height is reached.

In chronic renal insufficiency, renal function should be below 50 percent of normal before institution of therapy. To verify growth disturbance, growth should be followed for a year preceding institution of therapy. During this period, conservative treatment for renal insufficiency (which includes control of acidosis, hyperparathyroidism and nutritional status) should have been established and should be maintained during treatment. The treatment should be discontinued at renal transplantation. To date, no data on final height in patients with chronic renal insufficiency treated with Genotropin are available.

The effects of Genotropin on recovery were studied in two placebo controlled trials involving 522 critically ill adult patients suffering complications following open heart surgery, abdominal surgery, multiple accidental trauma or acute respiratory failure. Mortality was higher in patients treated with 5.3 or 8 mg Genotropin daily compared to patients receiving placebo, 42% vs. 19%. Based on this information, these types of patients should not be treated with Genotropin. As there is no information available on the safety of growth hormone substitution therapy in acutely critically ill patients, the benefits of continued treatment in this situation should be weighed against the potential risks involved. In all patients developing other or similar acute critical illness, the possible benefit of treatment with Genotropin must be weighed against the potential risk involved.

4.5 Interaction with other medicinal products and other forms of interaction

Data from an interaction study performed in growth hormone deficient adults suggests that somatropin administration may increase the clearance of compounds known to be metabolised by cytochrome P450 isoenzymes. The clearance of compounds metabolised by cytochrome P450 3A4 (e.g. sex steroids, corticosteroids, anticonvulsants and ciclosporin) may be especially increased resulting in lower plasma levels of these compounds. The clinical significance of this is unknown.

Also see Section 4.4 for statements regarding diabetes mellitus and thyroid disorder and Section 4.2 for statement on oral oestrogen replacement therapy.

4.6 Pregnancy and lactation

No clinical experience of use in pregnant women is available. Animal experimental data are incomplete. Treatment with Genotropin should be interrupted if pregnancy occurs.

During normal pregnancy, levels of pituitary growth hormone fall markedly after 20 gestation weeks, being replaced almost entirely by placental growth hormone by 30 weeks. In view of this, it is unlikely that continued replacement therapy with somatropin would be necessary in growth hormone deficient women in the third trimester of pregnancy.

It is not known if somatropin is excreted into breast milk, but absorption of intact protein from the gastrointestinal tract of the infant is extremely unlikely.

4.7 Effects on ability to drive and use machines

No effects on the ability to drive and use machines have been observed.

4.8 Undesirable effects

Within each frequency grouping, undesirable effects are presented in order of decreasing seriousness.

Patients with growth hormone deficiency are characterised by extracellular volume deficit. When treatment with somatropin is started, this deficit is rapidly corrected. In adult patients, adverse effects related to fluid retention such as peripheral oedema, stiffness in the extremities, arthralgia, myalgia and paraesthesia are common. In general, these adverse effects are mild to moderate, arise within the first months of treatment and subside spontaneously or with dose reduction.

The incidence of these adverse effects is related to the administered dose, the age of patients and possibly inversely related to the age of patients at the onset of growth hormone deficiency. In children, such adverse effects are uncommon.

Transient local skin reactions at the injection site in children are common.

Rare cases of diabetes mellitus type II have been reported.

Rare cases of benign intracranial hypertension have been reported.

Carpal tunnel syndrome is an uncommon event among adults.

Somatropin has given rise to the formation of antibodies in approximately 1% of patients. The binding capacity of these antibodies has been low and no clinical changes have been associated with their formation.

(see Table 1 below)

Somatropin has been reported to reduce serum cortisol levels, possibly by affecting carrier proteins or by increased hepatic clearance. The clinical relevance of these findings may be limited. Nevertheless, corticosteroid replacement therapy should be optimised before initiation of Genotropin therapy.

Very rare cases of leukaemia have been reported in growth hormone deficient children treated with somatropin, but

Table 1

	Common >1/100, <1/10	Uncommon >1/1000, <1/100	Rare >1/10,000, < 1/1000	Very rare <1/10,000
Neoplasms, benign and malignant				Leukaemia
Immune system disorders	Formation of antibodies			
Endocrine disorders			Diabetes mellitus type II	
Nervous system disorders	In adults paraesthesia	In adults carpal tunnel syndrome In children paraesthesia	Benign intracranial hypertension	
Skin and subcutaneous tissue disorders	In children transient local skin reactions			
Musculoskeletal, connective tissue and bone disorders	In adults stiffness in the extremities, arthralgia, myalgia	In children stiffness in the extremities, arthralgia, myalgia		
General disorders and administration site disorders	In adults peripheral oedema	In children peripheral oedema		

the incidence appears to be similar to that in children without growth hormone deficiency.

In the post-marketing experience rare cases of sudden death have been reported in patients affected by Prader-Willi syndrome treated with somatropin, although no causal relationship has been demonstrated.

4.9 Overdose
No case of overdose or intoxication has been reported.
Acute overdosage could lead initially to hypoglycaemia and subsequently to hyperglycaemia.

Long term overdosage could result in signs and symptoms consistent with the known effects of human growth hormone excess.

5. PHARMACOLOGICAL PROPERTIES
5.1 Pharmacodynamic properties
Pharmacotherapeutic group: Anterior pituitary lobe hormones and analogues

ATC code: H01A C01

Somatropin is a potent metabolic hormone of importance for the metabolism of lipids, carbohydrates and proteins. In children with inadequate endogenous growth hormone, somatropin stimulates linear growth and increases growth rate. In adults, as well as in children, somatropin maintains a normal body composition by increasing nitrogen retention and stimulation of skeletal muscle growth, and by mobilisation of body fat. Visceral adipose tissue is particularly responsive to somatropin. In addition to enhanced lipolysis, somatropin decreases the uptake of triglycerides into body fat stores. Serum concentrations of IGF-I (Insulin-like Growth Factor-I) and IGFBP3 (Insulin-like Growth Factor Binding Protein 3) are increased by somatropin. In addition, the following actions have been demonstrated:

– Lipid metabolism: Somatropin induces hepatic LDL cholesterol receptors, and affects the profile of serum lipids and lipoproteins. In general, administration of somatropin to growth hormone deficient patients results in reductions in serum LDL and apolipoprotein B. A reduction in serum total cholesterol may also be observed.

– Carbohydrate metabolism: Somatropin increases insulin but fasting blood glucose is commonly unchanged. Children with hypopituitarism may experience fasting hypoglycaemia. This condition is reversed by somatropin.

– Water and mineral metabolism: Growth hormone deficiency is associated with decreased plasma and extracellular volumes. Both are rapidly increased after treatment with somatropin. Somatropin induces the retention of sodium, potassium and phosphorus.

– Bone metabolism: Somatropin stimulates the turnover of skeletal bone. Long-term administration of somatropin to growth hormone deficient patients with osteopenia results in an increase in bone mineral content and density at weight bearing sites.

– Physical capacity: Muscle strength and physical exercise capacity are improved after long-term treatment with somatropin. Somatropin also increases cardiac output, but the mechanism has yet to be clarified. A decrease in peripheral vascular resistance may contribute to this effect.

In clinical trials in short children born SGA doses of 0.033 and 0.067 mg/kg body weight per day have been used for treatment until final height. In 56 patients who were continuously treated and have reached (near) final height, the mean change from height at start of treatment was +1.90 SDS (0.033 mg/kg body weight per day) and +2.19 SDS (0.067 mg/kg body weight per day). Literature data from untreated SGA children without early spontaneous catch-up suggest a late growth of 0.5 SDS. Long-term safety data are still limited.

5.2 Pharmacokinetic properties
Absorption: The bioavailability of subcutaneously administered somatropin is approximately 80% in both healthy subjects and growth hormone deficient patients. A subcutaneous dose of 0.035 mg/kg of somatropin results in plasma Cmax and tmax values in the range of 13-35 ng/ml and 3-6 hours, respectively.

Elimination: The mean terminal half-life of somatropin after intravenous administration in growth hormone deficient adults is about 0.4 hours. However, after subcutaneous administration, half-lives of 2-3 hours are achieved. The observed difference is likely due to slow absorption from the injection site following subcutaneous administration.

Sub-populations: The absolute bioavailability of somatropin seems to be similar in males and females following s.c. administration.

Information about the pharmacokinetics of somatropin in geriatric and paediatric populations, in different races and in patients with renal, hepatic or cardiac insufficiency is either lacking or incomplete.

5.3 Preclinical safety data
In studies regarding general toxicity, local tolerance and reproduction toxicity no clinically relevant effects have been observed.

In vitro and in vivo genotoxicity studies on gene mutations and induction of chromosome aberrations have been negative.

An increased chromosome fragility has been observed in one in-vitro study on lymphocytes taken from patients after long term treatment with somatropin and following the addition of the radiomimetic drug bleomycin. The clinical significance of this finding is unclear.

In another study, no increase in chromosomal abnormalities was found in the lymphocytes of patients who had received long term somatropin therapy.

6. PHARMACEUTICAL PARTICULARS
6.1 List of excipients

Powder: front compartment	Solvent: rear compartment
Glycine (E640) Sodium dihydrogen phosphate anhydrous (E339) Disodium phosphate anhydrous (E339) Mannitol (E421)	Water for Injections Mannitol (E421)

6.2 Incompatibilities
This medicinal product must not be mixed with other medicinal products except those mentioned in section 6.6.

6.3 Shelf life
3 years

Chemical and physical in-use stability has been demonstrated for 24 hours for the reconstituted solution at 2°C - 8°C.

From a microbiological point of view, once reconstituted, the product may be stored for 24 hours at 2°C - 8°C.

6.4 Special precautions for storage
Before reconstitution:

Store in a refrigerator (2°C – 8°C). Keep the container in the outer carton in order to protect from light.

For the only purpose of ambulatory use, the product may be stored at or below 25°C by the end user for a single period of not more than 6 months. During and/or at the end of this 6 months period, the product should not be put back in the refrigerator.

After reconstitution:

The reconstituted solution should be stored in a refrigerator (2°C – 8°C). Do not freeze. Keep the container in the outer carton in order to protect from light.

6.5 Nature and contents of container
Powder and 0.275 ml solvent in a two chamber glass cartridge (type I glass) separated by a rubber plunger (bromobutyl), supplied as a single dose syringe. The cartridge is sealed at both ends with rubber stoppers (bromobutyl) and is enclosed in a plastic sleeve with a plunger rod and a finger grip.

Pack size: 7 × 0.2 mg, 28 (4 × 7 × 0.2 mg)

Not all pack sizes may be marketed.

6.6 Special precautions for disposal and other handling
The solution is prepared by screwing the plunger rod inwards so that the solvent will be mixed with the powder in the two chamber cartridge. Do not shake vigorously; this might cause denaturation of the active ingredient. The injection needle should be screwed on before reconstitution. The reconstituted solution is colourless or slightly opalescent. The reconstituted solution for injection is to be inspected prior to use and only clear solutions without particles should be used.

Genotropin MiniQuick is for single use only. Any unused product should be disposed of in accordance with local requirements.

7. MARKETING AUTHORISATION HOLDER
Pharmacia Laboratories Limited

Ramsgate Road

Sandwich

Kent CT13 9NJ

United Kingdom

8. MARKETING AUTHORISATION NUMBER(S)

Presentation	PL number
1. Genotropin MiniQuick 0.2 mg	PL 00022/0186
2. Genotropin MiniQuick 0.4 mg	PL 00022/0187
3. Genotropin MiniQuick 0.6 mg	PL 00022/0188
4. Genotropin MiniQuick 0.8 mg	PL 00022/0189
5. Genotropin MiniQuick 1 mg	PL 00022/0190
6. Genotropin MiniQuick 1.2 mg	PL 00022/0191
7. Genotropin MiniQuick 1.4 mg	PL 00022/0192
8. Genotropin MiniQuick 1.6 mg	PL 00022/0193
9. Genotropin MiniQuick 1.8 mg	PL 00022/0194
10. Genotropin MiniQuick 2 mg	PL 00022/0195

9. DATE OF FIRST AUTHORISATION/RENEWAL OF THE AUTHORISATION
14 September 1998/1 February 2005

10. DATE OF REVISION OF THE TEXT
March 2009

11. LEGAL CATEGORY
CD (Sch 4, Part 1), POM
Ref: GN 13_0 UK

GHRH Ferring

(Ferring Pharmaceuticals Ltd)

1. NAME OF THE MEDICINAL PRODUCT
GHRH Ferring

2. QUALITATIVE AND QUANTITATIVE COMPOSITION
Active Ingredient

Somatorelin as acetate, 50 micrograms per ampoule.

3. PHARMACEUTICAL FORM
Lyophilised powder for injection.

Sterile solution for reconstitution of an injectable preparation.

4. CLINICAL PARTICULARS
4.1 Therapeutic indications
The product is applied to determine the somatotropic function of the anterior pituitary gland in cases of suspected growth hormone deficiency. The test distinguishes between hypophysic and hypothalamic disorders but is not suitable as a screening test for growth hormone deficiencies.

The diluent is supplied for the reconstitution of an injectable preparation.

4.2 Posology and method of administration
The recommended dosage for adult patients of standard weight is the content of one ampoule of GHRH Ferring (50 micrograms somatorelin) dissolved in 1ml of the supplied solvent. The solution is administered intravenously as a bolus injection.

In cases of highly overweight adult patients and in children, a dosage of 1 microgram per kg body weight is indicated.

GHRH Test: After withdrawal of approximately 2ml of venous blood from the fasted patient, the increase of basal growth hormone levels in plasma or serum after a single intravenous injection of the product is measured. For this procedure, the content of one ampoule is dissolved in 1ml of solvent (0.9% NaCl), or a volume corresponding to 1 microgram per kg body weight if appropriate, is administered intravenously to the fasted patient as a bolus injection (within 30 seconds).

To evaluate the growth hormone increment in plasma or serum, a second blood sample is taken 30 minutes after the injection. Peak growth hormone values may occasionally occur sooner or later. Therefore, additional blood samples may be taken 15, 45, 60 and 90 minutes after GHRH injection for better assessment of growth hormone release.

4.3 Contraindications
Hypersensitivity to growth hormone releasing hormone.

4.4 Special warnings and precautions for use
Because of possible inhibitory influence of human growth hormone on the somatotropic function of the pituitary gland, the GHRH Ferring test should not be carried out earlier than one week after discontinuation of treatment with human growth hormone.

The test results may be affected in conditions such as:

– untreated hyperthyroidism

– obesity, hyperglycaemia, elevated plasma fatty acids

– high levels of somatostatin

Although no hypersensitivity reactions have yet been reported, the possibility of this kind of adverse event cannot be completely ruled out because of the peptide nature of this product and the intravenous route of administration. It is recommended that emergency facilities should be available to treat such a reaction if it occurs.

4.5 Interaction with other medicinal products and other forms of interaction
The concomitant administration of substances which influence the release of growth hormone, such as growth hormone itself, somatostatin or its analogues, atropine, levodopa, dopamine, clonidine, arginine, ornithine, glycine, glucagon, insulin, oral glucose, anti thyroid drugs and propranolol should be avoided. High levels of glucocorticoids as well as somatostatin may inhibit the growth hormone response.

4.6 Pregnancy and lactation
GHRH Ferring is not indicated during pregnancy and lactation.

4.7 Effects on ability to drive and use machines
None.

4.8 Undesirable effects
Occasionally, a mild sensation of warmth may appear in the head, neck and upper part of the body, and there may

be disturbances of smell and taste. These side effects are short lasting and will fade rapidly. In combination with "hot flush", a slight increase or decrease in blood pressure may occur occasionally in conjunction with the corresponding alterations in heart rate. The described side effects are insignificant when the suggested dose is applied and they do not need any special treatment.

4.9 Overdose
In cases of higher dosage, the known side effects may occur. The undesirable effects fade rapidly and do not need any special treatment.

5. PHARMACOLOGICAL PROPERTIES

5.1 Pharmacodynamic properties
Somatorelin is normally synthesised in the hypothalamus and stimulates the secretion of growth hormone from the pituitary gland.

GHRH Ferring is the synthetic form of somatorelin and is identical in structure and function to the somatorelin released by the hypothalamus.

Somatorelin physiologically increases plasma growth hormone levels.

5.2 Pharmacokinetic properties
After intravenous application of different doses of somatorelin in man, the concentrations of somatorelin in plasma increase within 5 minutes to the maximum value, followed by a rapid decrease. The basal values are reached again after 30-40 minutes.

5.3 Preclinical safety data
Not applicable.

6. PHARMACEUTICAL PARTICULARS

6.1 List of excipients
GHRH Ferring

None.

Diluent for GHRH Ferring

Each diluent ampoule contains:

Sodium chloride Ph. Eur. 9mg

Water for injection Ph. Eur. to 1.0ml

6.2 Incompatibilities
GHRH Ferring should not be administered together with other preparations for parenteral use (e.g. mixed injections or infusion solutions).

6.3 Shelf life
Shelf life of the unopened powder and diluent ampoule is 33 months.

6.4 Special precautions for storage
Do not store above 25°C.

6.5 Nature and contents of container
GHRH Ferring is supplied in clear glass ampoules of high hydrolytic resistance (hydrolytic Class 1 according to Ph. Eur.).

The diluent is supplied in clear glass ampoules of high hydrolytic resistance (hydrolytic Class 1 according to Ph. Eur.).

6.6 Special precautions for disposal and other handling
Reconstitute GHRH Ferring with the solvent supplied, immediately prior to use.

7. MARKETING AUTHORISATION HOLDER
Ferring Pharmaceuticals Limited

The Courtyard

Waterside Drive

Langley

Berkshire SL3 6EZ.

8. MARKETING AUTHORISATION NUMBER(S)
GHRH Ferring PL 03194/0050

Diluent for GHRH Ferring PL 03194/0051

9. DATE OF FIRST AUTHORISATION/RENEWAL OF THE AUTHORISATION
28th June 2002

10. DATE OF REVISION OF THE TEXT
May 2005

11. LEGAL CATEGORY
POM

Glibenese

(Pfizer Limited)

1. NAME OF THE MEDICINAL PRODUCT
GLIBENESE™ TABLETS 5mg.

2. QUALITATIVE AND QUANTITATIVE COMPOSITION
Each tablet contains 5mg glipizide as the active ingredient.

3. PHARMACEUTICAL FORM
Tablets.

4. CLINICAL PARTICULARS

4.1 Therapeutic indications
Glipizide is indicated as an adjunct to diet and exercise to improve glycaemic control in adults with type 2 diabetes mellitus.

4.2 Posology and method of administration
Route of administration: Oral.

There is no fixed dosage regimen for the management of diabetes mellitus with Glibenese or any other hypoglycaemic agent. In addition to the usual monitoring of urinary glucose, the patient's blood glucose must also be monitored periodically to determine the minimum effective dose for the patient, to detect primary failure: i.e. inadequate lowering of blood glucose at the maximum recommended dose of medication, and to detect secondary failure, i.e. loss of adequate blood-glucose-lowering response after an initial period of effectiveness. Glycosylated haemoglobin levels may also be of value in monitoring the patient's response to therapy.

Short term administration of Glibenese may be sufficient during periods of transient loss of control in patients usually controlled well on diet.

In general, Glibenese should be given approximately 30 minutes before a meal to achieve the greatest reduction in post-prandial hyperglycaemia.

Initial dose: The recommended starting dose is 5mg, given before breakfast or the midday meal. Elderly patients and other patients at risk for hypoglycaemia may be started on 2.5mg (see Use in Elderly and in High Risk Patients).

Titration: Dosage adjustments should ordinarily be in increments of 2.5 or 5mg, as determined by blood glucose response. At least several days should elapse between titration steps. The maximum recommended single dose is 15mg. Doses above 15mg should ordinarily be divided.

Maintenance: Some patients may be effectively controlled on a once-a-day regimen. Total daily dosage above 15mg should ordinarily be divided. Patients can usually be stabilized on a dosage ranging from 2.5 to 20mg daily. The maximum recommended daily dosage is 20mg.

Use in elderly and in high risk patients: Elderly diabetics are more sensitive to the hypoglycaemic effects of sulphonylurea drugs and should therefore be prescribed a low starting dose of 2.5mg daily. The elderly are also particularly susceptible to the effects of hypoglycaemia. Hypoglycaemia may be difficult to recognise in the elderly.

To decrease the risk of hypoglycaemia in patients at risk including elderly, debilitated or malnourished patients, patients with irregular calorie intake and patients with an impaired renal or hepatic function, the initial maintenance dosing should be conservative to avoid hypoglycaemic reactions (see 'Initial Dose' and Section 4.4 'Special warnings and special precautions for use').

Use in children: Safety and effectiveness in children have not been established.

Patients receiving insulin: As with other sulphonylurea-class hypoglycaemics, many stable non-insulin-dependent diabetic patients receiving insulin may be safely placed on Glibenese. When transferring patients from insulin to Glibenese, the following general guidelines should be considered:

For patients whose daily insulin requirement is 20 units or less, insulin may be discontinued and Glibenese therapy begun at usual dosages. Several days should elapse between Glibenese titration steps.

For patients whose daily insulin requirement is greater than 20 units, the insulin dose should be reduced by 50% and Glibenese therapy initiated at usual dosages. Subsequent reductions in insulin dosage should depend on individual patient response. Several days should elapse between Glibenese titration steps.

During the insulin withdrawal period, the patient should self-monitor glucose levels. Patients should be instructed to contact the prescriber immediately if these tests are abnormal. In some cases, especially when the patient has been receiving greater than 40 units of insulin daily, it may be advisable to consider hospitalisation during the transition period.

Patients receiving other oral hypoglycaemic agents: As with other sulphonylurea class hypoglycaemics, no transition period is necessary when transferring patients to Glibenese. Patients should be observed carefully (1-2 weeks) for hypoglycaemia when being transferred from longer half-life sulphonylureas (e.g. chlorpropamide) to Glibenese due to potential overlapping of drug effect.

Combination Use: When adding other blood-glucose-lowering agents to glipizide for combination therapy, the agent should be initiated at the lowest recommended dose and patients should be observed carefully for hypoglycaemia. Refer to the product information supplied with the oral agent for additional information.

When adding glipizide to other blood-glucose-lowering agents, glipizide can be initiated at 5mg. Those patients who may be more sensitive to hypoglycaemic drugs may be started at a lower dose. Titration should be based on clinical judgement.

4.3 Contraindications
Glipizide is contra-indicated in patients with:

1. Hypersensitivity to glipizide or any excipients in the tablets.

2. Type 1 diabetes, diabetic ketoacidosis, diabetic coma.

3. Severe renal, hepatic or thyroid impairment; co-existent renal and hepatic disease.

4. Pregnancy and lactation.

5. Patients treated with miconazole (see 4.5 Interactions)

4.4 Special warnings and precautions for use
G6PD-deficiency: Since glipizide belongs to the class of sulfonylurea agents, caution should be used in patients with G6PD-deficiency. Treatment of patients with G6PD-deficiency with sulfonylurea agents can lead to haemolytic anaemia and a non-sulfonylurea alternative should be considered

Hypoglycaemia: All sulphonylurea drugs including glipizide are capable of producing severe hypoglycaemia which may result in coma, and may require hospitalization. Patients experiencing severe hypoglycaemia should be managed with appropriate glucose therapy and be monitored for a minimum of 24 to 48 hours. Proper patient selection, dosage and instructions are important to avoid hypoglycaemic episodes. Regular, timely carbohydrate intake is important to avoid hypoglycaemic events occurring when a meal is delayed or insufficient food is eaten or carbohydrate intake is unbalanced. Renal or hepatic insufficiency may affect the disposition of glipizide and the latter may also diminish gluconeogenic capacity, both of which increase the risk of serious hypoglycaemic reactions. Elderly, debilitated or malnourished patients and those with adrenal or pituitary insufficiency are particularly susceptible to the hypoglycaemic action of glucose-lowering drugs. Hypoglycaemia may be difficult to recognise in the elderly and in people who are taking beta-adrenergic blocking drugs. Hypoglycaemia is more likely to occur when calorific intake is deficient, after severe or prolonged exercise, when alcohol is ingested or when more than one glucose-lowering drug is used.

Loss of control of blood glucose: When a patient stabilised on any diabetic regimen is exposed to stress such as fever, trauma, infection or surgery, a loss of control may occur. At such times, it may be necessary to discontinue glipizide and administer insulin.

The effectiveness of any oral hypoglycaemic drug, including glipizide, in lowering blood glucose to a desired level decreases in many patients over a period of time. This may be due to progression of the severity of the diabetes or to diminished responsiveness to the drug. This phenomenon is known as secondary failure, to distinguish it from primary failure in which the drug is ineffective in an individual patient when first given. Adequate adjustment of dose and adherence to diet should be assessed before classifying a patient as a secondary failure.

Renal and hepatic disease: The pharmacokinetics and/or pharmacodynamics of glipizide may be affected in patients with impaired renal or hepatic function. If hypoglycaemia should occur in such patients, it may be prolonged and appropriate management should be instituted.

Information for patients: Patients should be informed of the potential risks and advantages of glipizide and of alternative modes of therapy. They should also be informed about the importance of adherence to dietary instructions, of a regular exercise programme and of regular testing of blood glucose.

The risk of hypoglycaemia, its symptoms and treatment and conditions that predispose to its development should be explained to patients and responsible family members. Primary and secondary failure should also be explained.

Laboratory tests: Blood glucose should be monitored periodically. Measurement of glycosylated haemoglobin should be performed and goals assessed by the current standard of care.

4.5 Interaction with other medicinal products and other forms of interaction
The following products are likely to increase the hypoglycaemic effect:

Miconazole: Increase in hypoglycaemic effect, possibly leading to symptoms of hypoglycaemia or even coma.

Fluconazole: There have been reports of hypoglycaemia following the co-administration of glipizide and fluconazole, possibly the result of an increased half-life of glipizide.

Voriconazole – Although not studied, voriconazole may increase the plasma levels of sulfonylureas, (e.g. tolbutamide, glipizide and glyburide) and therefore cause hypoglycemia. Careful monitoring of blood glucose is recommended during co-administration.

Nonsteroidal anti-inflammatory agents (NSAIDS) (e.g. phenylbutazone): increase in hypoglycaemic effect of sulphonylureas (displacement of sulphonylurea binding to plasma proteins and /or decrease in sulphonylurea elimination).

Salicylates (acetylsalicylic acid): Increase in hypoglycaemic effect by high doses of acetylsalicylic acid (hypoglycaemic action of the acetylsalicylic acid).

Alcohol: Increase in hypoglycaemic reaction which can lead to hypoglyaemic coma.

Beta-blockers: All beta-blockers mask some of the symptoms of hypoglycaemia, e.g., palpitations and tachycardia. Most noncardioselective beta-blockers increase the incidence and severity of hypoglycaemia.

Angiotensin converting enzyme inhibitors: The use of angiotensin converting enzyme inhibitors may lead to an increased hypoglycaemic effect in diabetic patients treated with sulphonylureas, including glipizide. Therefore, a reduction in glipizide dosage may be required.

H_2Receptor Antagonists: The use of H_2 receptor antagonists may potentiate the hypoglycaemic effects of sulphonylureas, including glipizide.

The hypoglycaemic action of sulphonylureas in general may also be potentiated by monoamine oxidase inhibitors and drugs that are highly protein bound, such as sulphonamides, chloramphenicol, probenecid and coumarins.

When such drugs are administered to (or withdrawn from) a patient receiving glipizide, the patient should be observed closely for hypoglycaemia (or loss of control).

In vitro binding studies with human serum proteins indicate that glipizide binds to different sites on albumin than does tolbutamide and does not interact with salicylate or dicoumarol. However, caution must be exercised in extrapolating these findings to the clinical situation in the use of glipizide with these drugs.

The following products could lead to hyperglycaemia:

Danazol: diabetogenic effect of danazol.

If it cannot be avoided, warn the patient and step up self-monitoring of blood glucose and urine Possibly adjust the dosage of antidiabetic agent during treatment with danazol and after its discontinuation

Phenothiazines (e.g. chlorpromazine) at high doses (> 100mg per day of chlorpromazine): elevation in blood glucose (reduction in insulin release).

Corticosteroids elevation in blood glucose.

Sympathomimetics (e.g., ritodrine, salbutamol, terbutaline): elevation in blood glucose due to beta-2-adrenoceptor stimulation.

Other drugs that may produce hyperglycaemia and lead to a loss of control include the thiazides and other diuretics, thyroid products, oestrogens, progestogens, oral contraceptives, phenytoin, nicotinic acid, calcium channel blocking drugs and isoniazid.

When such drugs are withdrawn from (or administered to) a patient receiving glipizide, the patient should be observed closely for hypoglycaemia (or loss of control).

4.6 Pregnancy and lactation

Use in pregnancy: Glipizide is contra-indicated during pregnancy. Diabetes in pregnancy should be treated with insulin and not sulphonylureas. Recent evidence suggests that hyperglycaemia in pregnancy is associated with a higher incidence of congenital abnormalities.

Lactation: Although it is not known whether glipizide is excreted in human milk, some sulphonylurea drugs are known to be excreted in human milk. Therefore glipizide is contra-indicated during lactation.

4.7 Effects on ability to drive and use machines

The effect of glipizide on the ability to drive or operate machinery has not been studied, however, there is no evidence to suggest that glipizide may affect these abilities. Patients should be aware of the symptoms of hypoglycaemia and be careful about driving and the use of machinery.

4.8 Undesirable effects

The majority of side-effects have been dose related, transient, and have responded to dose reduction or withdrawal of the medication. However, clinical experience thus far has shown that, as with other sulphonylureas some side-effects associated with hypersensitivity may be severe and deaths have been reported in some instances.

Side effects listed in this section marked with * are usually transient and do not require discontinuance of therapy; however, they may also be symptoms of hypoglycaemia.

Blood and Lymphatic System Disorders: leucopenia, thrombocytopenia, haemolytic anaemia and pancytopenia have been reported. Aplastic anaemia and agranulocytosis have been reported with other sulphonylureas.

Metabolism and Nutritional Disorders: Hypoglycaemia (see 'Special warnings and precautions for use' section 4.4 and 'Overdose' section 4.9). Hyponatraemia has been reported. Disulfiram-like reactions have been reported with other sulphonylureas.

Psychiatric Disorders: Confusion*

Nervous System Disorders: Dizziness*, drowsiness, headache* and tremor*

Eye Disorders: Visual disturbances such as blurred vision*, diplopia* and abnormal vision* including visual impairment* and decreased vision* have each been reported in patients treated with glipizide.

Gastrointestinal Disorders: Nausea, diarrhoea, constipation and gastralgia. They appear to be dose related and usually disappear on division or reduction of dosage. Abdominal pain and vomiting.

Hepatobiliary disorders: Cholestatic jaundice, impaired hepatic function and hepatitis have been reported. Discontinue treatment if jaundice occurs. Hepatic porphyria and porphyria cutanea tarda have been reported.

Skin and Subcutaneous Tissue Disorders: Allergic skin reactions including erythema, morbilliform or maculopapular reactions, urticaria, pruritus and eczema have been reported. They frequently disappear with continued therapy. However, if they persist, the drug should be discontinued. As with other sulphonylureas, photosensitivity reactions have been reported.

General Disorders and Administration Site Conditions: Malaise*.

Laboratory Investigations: Occasional mild to moderate elevations of AST (SGOT), LDH, alkaline phosphatase, BUN and creatinine were noted. The relationship of these abnormalities to glipizide is uncertain and they have rarely been associated with clinical symptoms.

4.9 Overdose

There is no well documented experience with glipizide overdosage.

Overdosage of sulphonylureas including glipizide can produce hypoglycaemia. Mild hypoglycaemic symptoms without loss of consciousness or neurological findings should be treated aggressively with oral glucose and adjustments in drug dosage and/or meal patterns. Close monitoring should continue until the physician is assured that the patient is out of danger. Severe hypoglycaemic reactions with coma, seizure or other neurological impairment occur infrequently but constitute medical emergencies requiring immediate hospitalisation. If hypoglycaemic coma is diagnosed or suspected, the patient should be given a rapid intravenous injection of concentrated (50%) glucose solution. This should be followed by continuous infusion of a more dilute (10%) glucose solution at a rate that will maintain the blood glucose at a level above 5.6mmol/1 (100mg/dl).

Patients should be closely monitored for a minimum of 48 hours and depending on the status of the patient at this time the physician should decide whether further monitoring is required. Clearance of glipizide from plasma would be prolonged in persons with liver disease. Because of the extensive protein binding of glipizide, dialysis is unlikely to be of benefit.

5. PHARMACOLOGICAL PROPERTIES

5.1 Pharmacodynamic properties

Glipizide is an oral blood glucose lowering drug of the sulphonylurea class.

The primary mode of action of glipizide is the stimulation of insulin secretion from the beta-cells of pancreatic islet tissue. Stimulation of insulin secretion by glipizide in response to a meal is of major importance. Fasting insulin levels are not elevated even on long-term glipizide administration but the post-prandial insulin response continues to be enhanced after at least 6 months of treatment. The insulinotropic response to a meal occurs within 30 minutes after an oral dose of glipizide in diabetic patients but elevated insulin levels do not persist beyond the time of the meal challenge. There is also increasing evidence that extrapancreatic effects involving potentiation of insulin action form a significant component of the activity of glipizide.

Blood sugar control persists for up to 24 hours after a single dose of glipizide, even though plasma levels have declined to a small fraction of peak levels by that time. See 'Pharmacokinetic properties' (section 5.2).

Some patients fail to respond initially, or gradually lose their responsiveness to sulphonylurea drugs, including glipizide. Alternatively, glipizide may be effective in some patients who have not responded or have ceased to respond to other sulphonylureas.

5.2 Pharmacokinetic properties

Gastrointestinal absorption of glipizide in man is uniform, rapid and essentially complete. Peak plasma concentrations occur 1-3 hours after a single oral dose. The half-life of elimination ranges from 2-4 hours in normal subjects, whether given intravenously or orally. The metabolic and excretory patterns are similar with the two routes of administration, indicating that first-pass metabolism is not significant. glipizide does not accumulate in plasma on repeated oral administration. Total absorption and disposition of an oral dose was unaffected by food in normal volunteers but absorption was delayed by about 40 minutes. Thus, glipizide was more effective when administered about 30 minutes before, rather than with a test meal in diabetic patients. Protein binding was studied in serum from volunteers who received either oral or intravenous glipizide and found to be 98%-99% one hour after either route of administration. The apparent volume of distribution of glipizide after intravenous administration was 11 litres, indicative of localisation within the extracellular fluid compartment.

The metabolism of glipizide is extensive and occurs mainly in the liver. The primary metabolites are inactive hydroxylation products and polar conjugates and are excreted mainly in the urine. Less than 10% unchanged glipizide is found in the urine.

5.3 Preclinical safety data

Acute toxicity studies showed no specific susceptibility. The acute oral toxicity of glipizide was extremely low in all species tested (LD_{50} greater than 4 g/kg). Chronic toxicity tests in rats and dogs at doses up to 8.0 mg/kg did not show any evidence of toxic effects.

A 20-month study in rats and an 18-month study in mice at doses up to 75 times the maximum human dose revealed no evidence of drug related carcinogenicity. Bacterial and *in vivo* mutagenicity tests were uniformly negative. Studies in rats of both sexes at doses up to 75 times the human dose showed no effects on fertility.

6. PHARMACEUTICAL PARTICULARS

6.1 List of excipients

The tablets contain the following ingredients: lactose, maize starch, microcrystalline cellulose and stearic acid.

6.2 Incompatibilities

None known.

6.3 Shelf life

2 years.

6.4 Special precautions for storage

Store below 25°C.

6.5 Nature and contents of container

Original packs of 56 tablets per carton. Blister pack formed from 250 μm white opaque PVC, coated 40g/m^2 PVdC and backed with 20μm hard tempered aluminium foil, coated with 5-6g/m^2 sealing lacquer.

6.6 Special precautions for disposal and other handling

None.

7. MARKETING AUTHORISATION HOLDER

Pfizer Limited

Ramsgate Road

Sandwich

CT13 9NJ

United Kingdom.

8. MARKETING AUTHORISATION NUMBER(S)

PL 00057/0113R.

9. DATE OF FIRST AUTHORISATION/RENEWAL OF THE AUTHORISATION

2 September 1997.

10. DATE OF REVISION OF THE TEXT

June 2008

11. Legal Category

POM

Ref: GL_8_0

GlucaGen Hypokit 1 mg

(Novo Nordisk Limited)

1. NAME OF THE MEDICINAL PRODUCT

GlucaGen 1 mg powder and solvent for solution for injection.

GlucaGen HypoKit 1 mg powder and solvent for solution for injection.

2. QUALITATIVE AND QUANTITATIVE COMPOSITION

Active substance: Glucagon, rDNA (produced by recombinant DNA technology in *Saccharomyces Cerevisiae*).

Glucagon, rDNA is structurally identical to human glucagon.

- Glucagon 1 mg (1 IU) as hydrochloride.

One vial contains 1 mg glucagon corresponding to 1 mg glucagon/ml after reconstitution.

For excipients, see section 6.1.

3. PHARMACEUTICAL FORM

Powder and solvent for solution for injection.

Before reconstitution the powder should be a white or nearly white powder. The solvent should be clear and colourless without particles.

4. CLINICAL PARTICULARS

4.1 Therapeutic indications

Therapeutic indication

Treatment of severe hypoglycaemic reactions, which may occur in the management of insulin treated persons with diabetes mellitus.

Diagnostic indication

Motility inhibition in examinations of the gastrointestinal tract.

4.2 Posology and method of administration

Dissolve the freeze-dried product in the accompanying solvent, as described under item 6.6.

Therapeutic indication (Severe hypoglycaemia)

Dosage for adult patients:

Administer 1 mg.

Dosage for paediatric patients:

Administer 1 mg (children above 25 kg or older than 6-8 years) or 0.5 mg (children below 25 kg or younger than 6-8 years).

Administer by subcutaneous or intramuscular injection. The patient will normally respond within 10 minutes. When the patient has responded to the treatment, give oral carbohydrate to restore the liver glycogen and prevent relapse of hypoglycaemia. If the patient does not respond within 10 minutes, intravenous glucose should be given.

Medical consultation is required for all patients with severe hypoglycaemia.

Diagnostic indication (Inhibition of motility)

GlucaGen must be administered by medical personnel. Onset of action after an intravenous injection of 0.2-0.5 mg occurs within one minute and the duration of effect is between 5 and 20 minutes depending on the organ under examination. The onset of action after an intramuscular injection of 1-2 mg occurs after 5-15 minutes and lasts approximately 10-40 minutes depending on the organ.

After end of the diagnostic procedure oral carbohydrate should be given, if this is compatible with the diagnostic procedure applied.

Dose range from 0.2-2 mg depending on the diagnostic technique used and the route of administration. The usual diagnostic dose for relaxation of the stomach, duodenal bulb, duodenum and small bowel is 0.2-0.5 mg given intravenously or 1 mg given intramuscularly; the usual dose to relax the colon is 0.5-0.75 mg intravenously or 1-2 mg intramuscularly.

4.3 Contraindications

Hypersensitivity to glucagon or lactose.

Phaeochromocytoma.

4.4 Special warnings and precautions for use

Therapeutic indication

To prevent relapse of the hypoglycaemia oral carbohydrates should be given to restore the liver glycogen, when the patient has responded to the treatment.

Diagnostic indication

Persons who have been given glucagon in connection with diagnostic procedures may experience discomfort, in particular if they have been fasting. Nausea, hypoglycaemia and blood pressure changes have been reported in these situations. After the end of a diagnostic procedure oral carbohydrates should be given to patients, who have been fasting, if this is compatible with the diagnostic procedure applied. If fasting is needed post-examination or in case of severe hypoglycaemia, intravenously given glucose may be required.

Glucagon reacts antagonistically towards insulin and caution should be observed if GlucaGen is used in patients with insulinoma. Caution should also be observed in patients with glucagonoma.

Caution should also be observed when GlucaGen is used as an adjunct in endoscopic or radiographic procedures in diabetic patients or in elderly patients with known cardiac disease.

GlucaGen should not be given via intravenous infusion.

4.5 Interaction with other medicinal products and other forms of interaction

Insulin: Reacts antagonistically towards glucagon.

Indomethacin: Glucagon may lose its ability to raise blood glucose or paradoxically may even produce hypoglycaemia.

Warfarin: Glucagon may increase the anticoagulant effect of warfarin.

Interactions between GlucaGen and other drugs are not known when GlucaGen is used in the approved indications.

4.6 Pregnancy and lactation

Glucagon does not cross the human placenta barrier. The use of glucagon has been reported in pregnant women with diabetes and no harmful effects are known with respect to the course of pregnancy and the health of the unborn and the neonate.

Glucagon is cleared from the bloodstream very fast (mainly by the liver) ($t_{1/2}$= 3-6 min.); thus the amount excreted in the milk of nursing mothers following treatment of severe hypoglycaemic reactions will be extremely small. As glucagon is degraded in the digestive tract and cannot be absorbed in its intact form, it will not exert any metabolic effect in the child.

4.7 Effects on ability to drive and use machines

No studies on the effects on the ability to drive and use machines have been performed.

After diagnostic procedures hypoglycaemia has been reported infrequently. Therefore driving a car should be avoided until the patient has had a meal with oral carbohydrates.

4.8 Undesirable effects

Frequencies of undesirable effects considered related to GlucaGen treatment during clinical trials and/or post marketing surveillance is presented below. Undesirable effects which have not been observed in clinical trials, but have been reported spontaneously are presented as "very rare". During marketed use reporting of adverse drug reactions is very rare (< 1/10,000). However, post-marketing experience is subject to under-reporting and this reporting rate should be interpreted in that light. The estimated number of treatment episodes is 46.9 millions over a 16 year period.

Therapeutic indication

System Organ Class	Subject incidence	Adverse drug reaction
Immune system disorders	Very rare ⩽ 1/10,000	Hypersensitivity reactions including anaphylactic reaction/shock
Gastrointestinal disorders	Common > 1/100 and < 1/10	Nausea
	Uncommon > 1/1,000 and ⩽ 1/100	Vomiting
	Rare > 1/10,000 and ⩽ 1/1,000	Abdominal pain

Diagnostic indication

System Organ Class	Subject incidence	Adverse drug reaction
Immune system disorders	Very rare ⩽ 1/10,000	Hypersensitivity reactions including anaphylactic reaction/shock
Metabolism and nutrition disorders	Uncommon > 1/1,000 and ⩽ 1/100	Hypoglycaemia*1
	Very rare ⩽ 1/10,000	Hypoglycaemic coma
Cardiac disorders	Very rare ⩽ 1/10,000	Bradycardia*2
	Very rare ⩽ 1/10,000	Tachycardia*2
Vascular disorders	Very rare ⩽ 1/10,000	Hypotension*2
	Very rare ⩽ 1/10,000	Hypertension*2
Gastrointestinal disorders	Common > 1/100 and < 1/10	Nausea
	Uncommon >1/1,000 and ⩽ 1/100	Vomiting
	Rare > 1/10,000 and ⩽ 1/1,000	Abdominal pain

*1 After a diagnostic procedure it can be more pronounced in patients having fasted, (see section 4.4 Special warnings and precautions for use).

*2 Cardio-vascular adverse events have only been reported, when GlucaGen is used as an adjunct in endoscopic or radiographic procedures.

4.9 Overdose

Adverse effects of overdose have not been reported. See section 4.8

In case of dosages substantially above the approved range, the serum potassium may decrease and should be monitored and corrected if needed.

5. PHARMACOLOGICAL PROPERTIES

5.1 Pharmacodynamic properties

Pharmacotherapeutic group: H 04 AA 01.

Glucagon is a hyperglycaemic agent that mobilizes hepatic glycogen, which is released into the blood as glucose. Glucagon will not be effective in patients whose liver glycogen is depleted. For that reason, glucagon has little or no effect when the patient has been fasting for a prolonged period, or is suffering from adrenal insufficiency, chronic hypoglycaemia or alcohol induced hypoglycaemia.

Glucagon, unlike adrenaline, has no effect upon muscle phosphorylase and therefore cannot assist in the transference of carbohydrate from the much larger stores of glycogen that are present in the skeletal muscle.

Glucagon stimulates the release of catecholamines. In the presence of phaeochromocytoma, glucagon can cause the tumour to release large amounts of catecholamines, which will cause an acute hypertensive reaction.

Glucagon inhibits the tone and motility of the smooth muscle in the gastrointestinal tract.

5.2 Pharmacokinetic properties

Metabolic clearance rate of glucagon in humans is approximately 10 ml/kg/min. It is degraded enzymatically in the blood plasma and in the organs to which it is distributed. The liver and kidney are major sites of glucagon clearance, each organ contributing about 30% to the overall metabolic clearance rate.

Glucagon has a short half-life in the blood of about 3-6 minutes.

Onset of effect occurs within 1 minute after an intravenous injection. Duration of action is in the range 5-20 minutes depending on dose and on the organ under examination. The onset of effect occurs within 5-15 minutes after an intramuscular injection, with a duration of 10-40 minutes depending on dose and organ.

When used in treatment of severe hypoglycaemia, an effect on blood glucose is usually seen within 10 minutes.

5.3 Preclinical safety data

No relevant pre-clinical data exist that provide information useful to the prescriber.

6. PHARMACEUTICAL PARTICULARS

6.1 List of excipients

Lactose monohydrate

Hydrochloric acid for pH adjustment

Sodium hydroxide for pH adjustment

Water for injections

The reconstituted solution contains glucagon 1 mg/ml and lactose monohydrate 107 mg/ml.

6.2 Incompatibilities

There are no known incompatibilities with GlucaGen.

6.3 Shelf life

Prior to reconstitution, the shelf life of the product is 3 years.

The reconstituted GlucaGen should be used immediately after preparation.

6.4 Special precautions for storage

The sealed container should be protected from light and stored in a refrigerator (+2°C to 8°C).

The user can store GlucaGen HypoKit at room temperature (25°C) for up to 18 months within the shelf life period.

Freezing should be avoided.

If in rare cases, the reconstituted product shows any signs of fibril formation (viscous appearance) or insoluble matter it should be discarded.

6.5 Nature and contents of container

Container for GlucaGen:

Vial made of glass type I, Ph. Eur., closed with a bromobutyl stopper and covered with an aluminium cap.

Containers for solvent:

Vial made of glass type I, Ph. Eur., closed with a bromobutyl disc with teflon and covered with an aluminium cap

or

pre-filled syringe of glass type I, Ph. Eur., with plunger (bromobutyl rubber) and needle.

The vials are provided with a tamperproof plastic cap which must be removed before use.

Not all presentations of GlucaGen are necessarily marketed.

6.6 Special precautions for disposal and other handling

Reconstitution

GlucaGen 1 mg:

Draw up the water for injections (1.1 ml) in a disposable syringe. Inject the water for injections into the vial containing the freeze-dried glucagon.

Shake the vial gently until the glucagon is completely dissolved and the solution is clear. Withdraw the solution back into the syringe.

GlucaGen HypoKit 1 mg:

Inject the water for injections (1.1 ml) into the vial containing the freeze-dried glucagon. Shake the vial gently until the glucagon is completely dissolved and the solution is clear. Withdraw the solution back into the syringe.

Note that a syringe with a thinner needle and a finer graduation may be more suitable for use in diagnostic procedures.

The reconstituted solution appears clear and colourless and forms an injection of 1 mg (1 IU) per ml to be administered subcutaneously, intramuscularly or intravenously.

Any unused product or waste material should be disposed of in accordance with local requirements.

7. MARKETING AUTHORISATION HOLDER

Novo Nordisk A/S

Novo Allé

DK-2880 Bagsvaerd

Denmark

8. MARKETING AUTHORISATION NUMBER(S)

PL 04668/0027

9. DATE OF FIRST AUTHORISATION/RENEWAL OF THE AUTHORISATION

Date of first authorisation: 30 September 1991

Date of last renewal: 15 October 2006

10. DATE OF REVISION OF THE TEXT

June 2008

Legal Category

POM.

GLUCOPHAGE 500 mg and 1000mg powder for oral solution in sachets

(Merck Serono)

1. NAME OF THE MEDICINAL PRODUCT

GLUCOPHAGE 500 mg powder for oral solution in sachets

GLUCOPHAGE 1000 mg powder for oral solution in sachets

2. QUALITATIVE AND QUANTITATIVE COMPOSITION

Each 500mg sachet contains 500 mg metformin hydrochloride corresponding to 390 mg metformin base.

Each 1000mg sachet contains 1000 mg metformin hydrochloride corresponding to 780 mg metformin base.

Excipients: contains aspartame.

For a full list of excipients, see section 6.1.

3. PHARMACEUTICAL FORM

Powder for oral solution.

White, odourless powder

4. CLINICAL PARTICULARS

4.1 Therapeutic indications

Treatment of type 2 diabetes mellitus, particularly in overweight patients, when dietary management and exercise alone does not result in adequate glycaemic control.

• In adults, Glucophage may be used as monotherapy or in combination with other oral anti-diabetic agents or with insulin.

• In children from 10 years of age and adolescents, Glucophage may be used as monotherapy or in combination with insulin.

A reduction of diabetic complications has been shown in overweight type 2 diabetic adult patients treated with metformin as first-line therapy after diet failure (see section 5.1).

4.2 Posology and method of administration

Adults:

Monotherapy and combination with other oral antidiabetic agents:

The usual starting dose is 500 mg or 850mg metformin hydrochloride 2 or 3 times daily given during or after meals.

After 10 to 15 days the dose should be adjusted on the basis of blood glucose measurements. A slow increase of dose may improve gastrointestinal tolerability. In patients receiving a high metformin hydrochloride dose (2 to 3 grams per day), it is possible to replace two Glucophage 500 mg doses with one Glucophage 1000 mg dose. The maximum recommended dose of metformin hydrochloride is 3 g daily, taken as 3 divided doses.

If transfer from another oral antidiabetic agent is intended: discontinue the other agent and initiate metformin at the dose indicated above.

Combination with insulin:

Metformin and insulin may be used in combination therapy to achieve better blood glucose control. Metformin hydrochloride is given at the usual starting dose of 500 mg or 850mg 2 or 3 times daily, while insulin dosage is adjusted on the basis of blood glucose measurements.

Elderly:

Due to the potential for decreased renal function in elderly subjects, the metformin dosage should be adjusted based on renal function. Regular assessment of renal function is necessary (see section 4.4).

Children and adolescents:

Monotherapy and combination with insulin

• Glucophage can be used in children from 10 years of age and adolescents.

• The usual starting dose is 500 mg or 850 mg metformin hydrochloride once daily, given during or after meals.

After 10 to 15 days the dose should be adjusted on the basis of blood glucose measurements. A slow increase of dose may improve gastrointestinal tolerability. The maximum recommended dose of metformin hydrochloride is 2 g daily, taken as 2 or 3 divided doses.

Preparation:

The powder should be poured into a glass and 150 ml water should be added to obtain a clear to slightly opalescent solution. The solution should be taken immediately after being prepared. If necessary, the solution may be stirred.

4.3 Contraindications

• Hypersensitivity to metformin or to any of the excipients.

• Diabetic ketoacidosis, diabetic pre-coma.

• Renal failure or renal dysfunction (creatinine clearance < 60 ml/min).

• Acute conditions with the potential to alter renal function such as: dehydration, severe infection, shock, intravascular administration of iodinated contrast agents (see section 4.4).

• Acute or chronic disease which may cause tissue hypoxia such as: cardiac or respiratory failure, recent myocardial infarction, shock.

• Hepatic insufficiency, acute alcohol intoxication, alcoholism.

• Lactation.

4.4 Special warnings and precautions for use

Lactic acidosis:

Lactic acidosis is a rare, but serious (high mortality in the absence of prompt treatment), metabolic complication that can occur due to metformin accumulation. Reported cases of lactic acidosis in patients on metformin have occurred primarily in diabetic patients with significant renal failure. The incidence of lactic acidosis can and should be reduced by assessing also other associated risk factors such as poorly controlled diabetes, ketosis, prolonged fasting, excessive alcohol intake, hepatic insufficiency and any condition associated with hypoxia.

Diagnosis:

The risk of lactic acidosis must be considered in the event of non-specific signs such as muscle cramps with digestive disorders as abdominal pain and severe asthenia. Lactic acidosis is characterised by acidotic dyspnea, abdominal pain and hypothermia followed by coma. Diagnostic laboratory findings are decreased blood pH, plasma lactate levels above 5 mmol/l, and an increased anion gap and lactate/pyruvate ratio. If metabolic acidosis is suspected, metformin should be discontinued and the patient should be hospitalised immediately (see section 4.9).

Renal function:

As metformin is excreted by the kidney, serum creatinine levels should be determined before initiating treatment and regularly thereafter:

• at least annually in patients with normal renal function,

• at least two to four times a year in patients with serum creatinine levels at the upper limit of normal and in elderly subjects.

Decreased renal function in elderly subjects is frequent and asymptomatic. Special caution should be exercised in situations where renal function may become impaired, for example when initiating antihypertensive therapy or diuretic therapy and when starting therapy with a non-steroidal anti-inflammatory drug.

Administration of iodinated contrast agent:

As the intravascular administration of iodinated contrast materials in radiologic studies can lead to renal failure, metformin must be discontinued prior to, or at the time of the test and not be reinstituted until 48 hours afterwards, and only after renal function has been re-evaluated and found to be normal (see sections 4.3 and 4.5).

Surgery:

Metformin must be discontinued 48 hours before elective surgery under general, spinal or peridural anaesthesia. Therapy may be restarted no earlier than 48 hours following surgery or resumption of oral nutrition and only if normal renal function has been established.

Children and adolescents:

The diagnosis of type 2 diabetes mellitus should be confirmed before treatment with metformin is initiated.

No effect of metformin on growth and puberty has been detected during controlled clinical studies of one-year duration but no long-term data on these specific points are available. Therefore, a careful follow-up of the effect of metformin on these parameters in metformin-treated children, especially pre-pubescent children, is recommended.

Children aged between 10 and 12 years:

Only 15 subjects aged between 10 and 12 years were included in the controlled clinical studies conducted in children and adolescents. Although efficacy and safety of metformin in these children did not differ from efficacy and safety in older children and adolescents, particular caution is recommended when prescribing to children aged between 10 and 12 years.

Other precautions:

All patients should continue their diet with a regular distribution of carbohydrate intake during the day. Overweight patients should continue their energy-restricted diet.

The usual laboratory tests for diabetes monitoring should be performed regularly.

Metformin alone does not cause hypoglycaemia, but caution is advised when it is used in combination with insulin or sulfonylureas.

Glucophage powder for oral solution contains aspartame, a source of phenylalanine. It is recommended to consider this fact before treatment is initiated in patients with phenylketonuria.

4.5 Interaction with other medicinal products and other forms of interaction

Concomitant use not recommended:

Alcohol:

Acute alcohol intoxication is associated with an increased risk of lactic acidosis, particularly in case of:

fasting or malnutrition, hepatic insufficiency.

Avoid consumption of alcohol and alcohol-containing medicinal product.

Iodinated contrast agents:

Intravascular administration of iodinated contrast agents may lead to renal failure, resulting in metformin accumulation and an increased risk of lactic acidosis.

Metformin must be discontinued prior to, or at the time of the test and not be reinstituted until 48 hours afterwards, and only after renal function has been re-evaluated and found to be normal (see sections 4.3 and 4.4).

Combinations requiring precautions for use:

Glucocorticoids (systemic and local routes), beta-2-agonists, and diuretics

have intrinsic hyperglycaemic activity. Inform the patient and perform more frequent blood glucose monitoring, especially at the beginning of treatment. If necessary, adjust the dosage of the antidiabetic medicinal product during therapy with the other medicinal product and upon its discontinuation.

ACE-inhibitors

may decrease the blood glucose levels. Therefore, dose adjustment of metformin may be necessary during and after addition or discontinuation of such medicinal products.

4.6 Pregnancy and lactation

Pregnancy

To date, no relevant epidemiological data are available. Animal studies do not indicate harmful effects with respect to pregnancy, embryonal or fetal development, parturition or postnatal development (see section 5.3).

When the patient plans to become pregnant and during pregnancy, diabetes should not be treated with metformin but insulin should be used to maintain blood glucose levels as close to normal as possible in order to lower the risk of fetal malformations associated with abnormal blood glucose levels.

Lactation

Metformin is excreted into milk in lactating rats. Similar data are not available in humans and a decision should be made whether to discontinue breast-feeding or to discontinue metformin, taking into account the importance of the medicinal product to the mother.

4.7 Effects on ability to drive and use machines

Metformin monotherapy does not cause hypoglycaemia and therefore has no effect on the ability to drive or to use machines.

However, patients should be alerted to the risk of hypoglycaemia when metformin is used in combination with other antidiabetic agents (sulfonylureas, insulin, repaglinide).

4.8 Undesirable effects

The following undesirable effects may occur under treatment with metformin. Frequencies are defined as follows: very common: $\geqslant$1/10; common $\geq$1/100, <1/10; uncommon $\geq$1/1,000, <1/100; rare $\geq$1/10,000, <1/1,000; very rare <1/10,000, not known (cannot be estimated from the available data).

Within each frequency grouping, undesirable effects are presented in order of decreasing seriousness.

Nervous system disorders:

Common: Taste disturbance

Gastrointestinal disorders:

very common: Gastrointestinal disorders such as nausea, vomiting, diarrhoea, abdominal pain and loss of appetite. These undesirable effects occur most frequently during initiation of therapy and resolve spontaneously in most cases. To prevent them, it is recommended that metformin be taken in 2 or 3 daily doses during or after meals. A slow increase of the dose may also improve gastrointestinal tolerability.

Skin and subcutaneous tissue disorders:

very rare: Skin reactions such as erythema, pruritus, urticaria

Metabolism and nutrition disorders:

very rare:

Lactic acidosis (see section 4.4).

Decrease of vitamin B12 absorption with decrease of serum levels during long-term use of metformin. Consideration of such aetiology is recommended if a patient presents with megaloblastic anaemia.

Hepatobiliary disorders:

very rare: Isolated reports of liver function tests abnormalities or hepatitis resolving upon metformin discontinuation.

Children and adolescents

In published and post marketing data and in controlled clinical studies in a limited paediatric population aged 10-16 years treated during 1 year, adverse event reporting was similar in nature and severity to that reported in adults.

4.9 Overdose

Hypoglycaemia has not been seen with metformin hydrochloride doses of up to 85 g, although lactic acidosis has occurred in such circumstances. High overdose of metformin or concomitant risks may lead to lactic acidosis. Lactic acidosis is a medical emergency and must be treated in hospital. The most effective method to remove lactate and metformin is haemodialysis.

5. PHARMACOLOGICAL PROPERTIES

5.1 Pharmacodynamic properties

Pharmacotherapeutic group: Blood glucose lowering drugs. Biguanides; ATC code: A10BA02

Metformin is a biguanide with antihyperglycaemic effects, lowering both basal and postprandial plasma glucose. It does not stimulate insulin secretion and therefore does not produce hypoglycaemia.

Metformin may act via 3 mechanisms:

(1) reduction of hepatic glucose production by inhibiting gluconeogenesis and glycogenolysis.

(2) in muscle, by increasing insulin sensitivity, improving peripheral glucose uptake and utilization.

(3) and delay of intestinal glucose absorption.

Metformin stimulates intracellular glycogen synthesis by acting on glycogen synthase.

Metformin increases the transport capacity of all types of membrane glucose transporters (GLUTs) known to date.

In humans, independently of its action on glycaemia, metformin has favourable effects on lipid metabolism. This has been shown at therapeutic doses in controlled, medium-term or long-term clinical studies: metformin reduces total cholesterol, LDL cholesterol and triglyceride levels.

Clinical efficacy:

The prospective randomised study (UKPDS) has established the long-term benefit of intensive blood glucose control in adult patients with type 2 diabetes.

Analysis of the results for overweight patients treated with metformin after failure of diet alone showed:

- a significant reduction of the absolute risk of any diabetes-related complication in the metformin group (29.8 events/1000 patient-years) versus diet alone (43.3 events/1000 patient-years), p=0.0023, and versus the combined sulfonylurea and insulin monotherapy groups (40.1 events/1000 patient-years), p=0.0034;
- a significant reduction of the absolute risk of diabetes-related mortality: metformin 7.5 events/1000 patient-years, diet alone 12.7 events/1000 patient-years, p=0.017;
- a significant reduction of the absolute risk of overall mortality: metformin 13.5 events/1000 patient-years versus diet alone 20.6 events/1000 patient-years (p=0.011), and versus the combined sulfonylurea and insulin monotherapy groups 18.9 events/1000 patient-years (p=0.021);
- a significant reduction in the absolute risk of myocardial infarction: metformin 11 events/1000 patient-years, diet alone 18 events/1000 patient-years (p=0.01).

Benefit regarding clinical outcome has not been shown for metformin used as second-line therapy, in combination with a sulfonylurea.

In type 1 diabetes, the combination of metformin and insulin has been used in selected patients, but the clinical benefit of this combination has not been formally established.

Controlled clinical studies in a limited paediatric population aged 10-16 years treated during 1 year demonstrated a similar response in glycaemic control to that seen in adults.

5.2 Pharmacokinetic properties

Absorption:

After an oral dose of metformin hydrochloride tablet, maximum plasma concentration (C_{max}) is reached in 2.5 hours (t_{max}). Absolute bioavailability of a 500 mg or 850 mg metformin hydrochloride tablet is approximately 50-60% in healthy subjects. After an oral dose, the non-absorbed fraction recovered in faeces was 20-30%.

After oral administration, metformin absorption is saturable and incomplete. It is assumed that the pharmacokinetics of metformin absorption is non-linear.

At the recommended metformin doses and dosing schedules, steady state plasma concentrations are reached within 24 to 48 hours and are generally less than 1 microgram/ml. In controlled clinical trials, maximum metformin plasma levels (C_{max}) did not exceed 4 microgram/ml, even at maximum doses.

Food decreases the extent and slightly delays the absorption of metformin tablets. Following oral administration of a 850 mg tablet, a 40% lower plasma peak concentration, a 25% decrease in AUC (area under the curve) and a 35-minute prolongation of the time to peak plasma concentration were observed. The clinical relevance of these findings is unknown.

Metformin hydrochloride powder for oral solution was shown to be bioequivalent to metformin hydrochloride tablet at a 500 mg dose with respect to C_{max} and AUC in healthy fed subjects.

Distribution:

Plasma protein binding is negligible. Metformin partitions into erythrocytes. The blood peak is lower than the plasma peak and appears at approximately the same time. The red blood cells most likely represent a secondary compartment of distribution. The mean volume of distribution (Vd) ranged between 63-276 l.

Metabolism:

Metformin is excreted unchanged in the urine. No metabolites have been identified in humans.

Elimination:

Renal clearance of metformin is > 400 ml/min, indicating that metformin is eliminated by glomerular filtration and tubular secretion. Following an oral dose, the apparent terminal elimination half-life is approximately 6.5 hours.

When renal function is impaired, renal clearance is decreased in proportion to that of creatinine and thus the elimination half-life is prolonged, leading to increased levels of metformin in plasma.

Children and adolescents:

Single dose study: After single doses of metformin hydrochloride 500 mg paediatric patients have shown similar pharmacokinetic profile to that observed in healthy adults.

Multiple dose study: Data are restricted to one study. After repeated doses of 500 mg twice daily for 7 days in paediatric patients the peak plasma concentration (C_{max}) and systemic exposure (AUC0-t) were reduced by approximately 33% and 40%, respectively compared to diabetic adults who received repeated doses of 500 mg twice daily for 14 days. As the dose is individually titrated based on glycaemic control, this is of limited clinical relevance.

5.3 Preclinical safety data

Preclinical data reveal no special hazard for humans based on conventional studies on safety, pharmacology, repeated dose toxicity, genotoxicity, carcinogenic potential and reproductive toxicity.

6. PHARMACEUTICAL PARTICULARS

6.1 List of excipients

Acesulfame potassium

Aspartame (E951)

Citric acid, anhydrous

Erythritol

Maize starch

Pullulan PI-20

6.2 Incompatibilities

Not applicable.

6.3 Shelf life

2 years

6.4 Special precautions for storage

This medicinal product does not require any special storage conditions

6.5 Nature and contents of container

Powder in paper/aluminium/polyethylene sachets

Pack of 20, 30 or 60 single-dose sachets

Not all pack sizes may be marketed.

6.6 Special precautions for disposal and other handling

Any unused product or waste material should be disposed of in accordance with local requirements.

7. MARKETING AUTHORISATION HOLDER

Lipha Pharmaceuticals Limited

Bedfont Cross, Stanwell Road

Feltham, Middlesex

TW14 8NX

United Kingdom

8. MARKETING AUTHORISATION NUMBER(S)

GLUCOPHAGE 500 mg powder for oral solution in sachets: PL 03759/0252

GLUCOPHAGE 1000 mg powder for oral solution in sachets: PL 03759/0254

9. DATE OF FIRST AUTHORISATION/RENEWAL OF THE AUTHORISATION

19th November 2008

10. DATE OF REVISION OF THE TEXT

GLUCOPHAGE 500 mg powder for oral solution in sachets: 4th December 2008

GLUCOPHAGE 1000 mg powder for oral solution in sachets: 12th March 2009

Glucophage 500 mg and 850 mg film coated tablets

(Merck Serono)

1. NAME OF THE MEDICINAL PRODUCT

Glucophage 500 mg film-coated tablet

Glucophage 850 mg film-coated tablet

2. QUALITATIVE AND QUANTITATIVE COMPOSITION

Glucophage 500 mg: One film-coated tablet contains 500mg metformin hydrochloride corresponding to 390 mg metformin base.

Glucophage 850 mg: One film-coated tablet contains 850mg metformin hydrochloride corresponding to 662.9 mg metformin base.

For a full list of excipients, see section 6.1.

3. PHARMACEUTICAL FORM

Film-coated tablet.

White, circular, convex film-coated tablet.

4. CLINICAL PARTICULARS

4.1 Therapeutic indications

Treatment of type 2 diabetes mellitus, particularly in overweight patients, when dietary management and exercise alone does not result in adequate glycaemic control.

- In adults, Glucophage film-coated tablets may be used as monotherapy or in combination with other oral anti-diabetic agents or with insulin.
- In children from 10 years of age and adolescents, Glucophage film-coated tablets may be used as monotherapy or in combination with insulin.

A reduction of diabetic complications has been shown in overweight type 2 diabetic adult patients treated with metformin hydrochloride as first-line therapy after diet failure (see section 5.1).

4.2 Posology and method of administration

Adults:

Monotherapy and combination with other oral antidiabetic agents:

The usual starting dose is one tablet 2 or 3 times daily given during or after meals.

After 10 to 15 days the dose should be adjusted on the basis of blood glucose measurements. A slow increase of dose may improve gastrointestinal tolerability. The maximum recommended dose of metformin hydrochloride is 3 g daily taken as 3 divided doses.

If transfer from another oral antidiabetic agent is intended: discontinue the other agent and initiate metformin hydrochloride at the dose indicated above.

Combination with insulin:

Metformin hydrochloride and insulin may be used in combination therapy to achieve better blood glucose control. Metformin hydrochloride is given at the usual starting dose of one tablet 2 or 3 times daily, while insulin dosage is adjusted on the basis of blood glucose measurements.

Elderly: Due to the potential for decreased renal function in elderly subjects, the metformin hydrochloride dosage should be adjusted based on renal function. Regular assessment of renal function is necessary (see section 4.4).

Children and adolescents:

Monotherapy and combination with insulin

- Glucophage film-coated tablets can be used in children from 10 years of age and adolescents.
- The usual starting dose is 500 mg or 850 mg metformin hydrochloride once daily, given during meals or after meals.

After 10 to 15 days the dose should be adjusted on the basis of blood glucose measurements. A slow increase of dose may improve gastrointestinal tolerability. The maximum recommended dose of metformin hydrochloride is 2 g daily, taken as 2 or 3 divided doses.

4.3 Contraindications

- Hypersensitivity to metformin hydrochloride or to any of the excipients.
- Diabetic ketoacidosis, diabetic pre-coma.
- Renal failure or renal dysfunction (creatinine clearance < 60 mL/min).
- Acute conditions with the potential to alter renal function such as: dehydration, severe infection, shock, intravascular administration of iodinated contrast agents (see section 4.4).
- Acute or chronic disease which may cause tissue hypoxia such as: cardiac or respiratory failure, recent myocardial infarction, shock
- Hepatic insufficiency, acute alcohol intoxication, alcoholism
- Lactation

4.4 Special warnings and precautions for use

Lactic acidosis.

Lactic acidosis is a rare, but serious (high mortality in the absence of prompt treatment), metabolic complication that can occur due to metformin hydrochloride accumulation. Reported cases of lactic acidosis in patients on metformin hydrochloride have occurred primarily in diabetic patients with significant renal failure. The incidence of lactic acidosis can and should be reduced by assessing also other associated risk factors such as poorly controlled diabetes, ketosis, prolonged fasting, excessive alcohol intake, hepatic insufficiency and any condition associated with hypoxia.

Diagnosis:

The risk of lactic acidosis must be considered in the event of non-specific signs such as muscle cramps with digestive disorders as abdominal pain and severe asthenia.

Lactic acidosis is characterised by acidotic dyspnea, abdominal pain and hypothermia followed by coma.

Diagnostic laboratory findings are decreased blood pH, plasma lactate levels above 5 mmol/L, and an increased anion gap and lactate/pyruvate ratio. If metabolic acidosis is suspected, metformin hydrochloride should be discontinued and the patient should be hospitalised immediately (see section 4.9).

Renal function:

As metformin hydrochloride is excreted by the kidney, serum creatinine levels should be determined before initiating treatment and regularly thereafter:

* at least annually in patients with normal renal function,

* at least two to four times a year in patients with serum creatinine levels at the upper limit of normal and in elderly subjects.

Decreased renal function in elderly subjects is frequent and asymptomatic. Special caution should be exercised in situations where renal function may become impaired, for example when initiating antihypertensive therapy or diuretic therapy and when starting therapy with a non-steroidal anti-inflammatory drug.

Administration of iodinated contrast agent

As the intravascular administration of iodinated contrast materials in radiologic studies can lead to renal failure, metformin hydrochloride should be discontinued prior to, or at the time of the test and not be reinstituted until 48 hours afterwards, and only after renal function has been re-evaluated and found to be normal (see section 4.5).

Surgery

Metformin hydrochloride must be discontinued 48 hours before elective surgery with general spinal or peridural anaesthesia. Therapy may be restarted no earlier than 48 hours following surgery or resumption of oral nutrition and only if normal renal function has been established.

Children and adolescents:

The diagnosis of type 2 diabetes mellitus should be confirmed before treatment with metformin hydrochloride is initiated.

No effect of metformin hydrochloride on growth and puberty has been detected during controlled clinical studies of one-year duration but no long-term data on these specific points are available. Therefore, a careful follow-up of the effect of metformin hydrochloride on these parameters in metformin hydrochloride-treated children, especially prepubescent children, is recommended.

Children aged between 10 and 12 years:

Only 15 subjects aged between 10 and 12 years were included in the controlled clinical studies conducted in children and adolescents. Although efficacy and safety of metformin hydrochloride in these children did not differ from efficacy and safety in older children and adolescents, particular caution is recommended when prescribing to children aged between 10 and 12 years.

Other precautions:

All patients should continue their diet with a regular distribution of carbohydrate intake during the day. Overweight patients should continue their energy-restricted diet.

The usual laboratory tests for diabetes monitoring should be performed regularly.

Metformin hydrochloride alone does not cause hypoglycaemia, but caution is advised when it is used in combination with insulin or sulfonylureas.

4.5 Interaction with other medicinal products and other forms of interaction

Concomitant use not recommended

Alcohol

Increased risk of lactic acidosis in acute alcohol intoxication, particularly in case of: fasting or malnutrition, hepatic insufficiency

Avoid consumption of alcohol and alcohol-containing medicinal product

Iodinated contrast agents (see section 4.4)

Intravascular administration of iodinated contrast agents may lead to renal failure, resulting in metformin hydrochloride accumulation and an increased risk of lactic acidosis.

Metformin hydrochloride must be discontinued prior to, or at the time of the test and not reinstituted until 48 hours afterwards, and only after renal function has been re-evaluated and found to be normal.

Combinations requiring precautions for use

Glucocorticoids (systemic and local routes), beta-2-agonists, and diuretics have intrinsic hyperglycaemic activity. Inform the patient and perform more frequent blood glucose monitoring, especially at the beginning of treatment. If necessary, adjust the dosage of the antidiabetic medicinal product during therapy with the other medicinal product and upon its discontinuation.

ACE-inhibitors may decrease the blood glucose levels. Therefore, dose adjustment of metformin hydrochloride may be necessary during and after addition or discontinuation of such medicinal products.

4.6 Pregnancy and lactation

To date, no relevant epidemiological data are available. Animal studies do not indicate harmful effects with respect to pregnancy, embryonal or foetal development, parturition or postnatal development (see section 5.3).

When the patient plans to become pregnant and during pregnancy, diabetes should not be treated with metformin hydrochloride but insulin should be used to maintain blood glucose levels as close to normal as possible in order to lower the risk of foetal malformations associated with abnormal blood glucose levels.

Metformin hydrochloride is excreted into milk in lactating rats. Similar data are not available in humans and a decision should be made whether to discontinue breast-feeding or to discontinue metformin hydrochloride, taking into account the importance of the medicinal product to the mother.

4.7 Effects on ability to drive and use machines

Metformin hydrochloride monotherapy does not cause hypoglycaemia and therefore has no effect on the ability to drive or to use machines.

However, patients should be alerted to the risk of hypoglycaemia when metformin hydrochloride is used in combination with other antidiabetic agents (sulphonylureas, insulin, repaglinide).

4.8 Undesirable effects

The following undesirable effects may occur under treatment with metformin hydrochloride. Frequencies are defined as follows: very common: ≥1/10; common ≥1/100, <1/10; uncommon ≥1/1,000, <1/100; rare ≥1/10,000, <1/1,000; very rare <1/10,000, not known (cannot be estimated from the available data).

Within each frequency grouping, undesirable effects are presented in order of decreasing seriousness.

Nervous system disorders:

Common: Taste disturbance

Gastrointestinal disorders:

Very common: Gastrointestinal disorders such as nausea, vomiting, diarrhoea, abdominal pain and loss of appetite. These undesirable effects occur most frequently during initiation of therapy and resolve spontaneously in most cases. To prevent them, it is recommended that metformin hydrochloride be taken in 2 or 3 daily doses during or after meals. A slow increase of the dose may also improve gastrointestinal tolerability.

Skin and subcutaneous tissue disorders:

Very rare: Skin reactions such as erythema, pruritus, urticaria

Metabolism and nutrition disorders:

Very rare: Lactic acidosis (see section 4.4)

Decrease of vitamin B12 absorption with decrease of serum levels during long-term use of metformin hydrochloride. Consideration of such aetiology is recommended if a patient presents with megaloblastic anaemia.

Hepatobiliary disorders:

Not known: Isolated reports of liver function tests abnormalities or hepatitis resolving upon metformin hydrochloride discontinuation.

In published and post marketing data and in controlled clinical studies in a limited paediatric population aged 10-16 years treated during 1 year, adverse event reporting was similar in nature and severity to that reported in adults.

4.9 Overdose

Hypoglycaemia has not been seen with metformin hydrochloride doses of up to 85g, although lactic acidosis has occurred in such circumstances. High overdose of metformin hydrochloride or concomitant risks may lead to lactic acidosis. Lactic acidosis is a medical emergency and must be treated in hospital. The most effective method to remove lactate and metformin hydrochloride is haemodialysis.

5. PHARMACOLOGICAL PROPERTIES

5.1 Pharmacodynamic properties

Pharmacotherapeutic group: Blood glucose lowering drugs. Biguanides; ATC code: A10BA02

Metformin hydrochloride is a biguanide with antihyperglycaemic effects, lowering both basal and postprandial plasma glucose. It does not stimulate insulin secretion and therefore does not produce hypoglycaemia.

Metformin hydrochloride may act via 3 mechanisms:

(1) reduction of hepatic glucose production by inhibiting gluconeogenesis and glycogenolysis

(2) in muscle, by increasing insulin sensitivity, improving peripheral glucose uptake and utilisation

(3) and delay of intestinal glucose absorption.

Metformin hydrochloride stimulates intracellular glycogen synthesis by acting on glycogen synthase.

Metformin hydrochloride increases the transport capacity of all types of membrane glucose transporters (GLUTs) known to date.

In humans, independently of its action on glycaemia, metformin hydrochloride has favourable effects on lipid metabolism. This has been shown at therapeutic doses in controlled, medium-term or long-term clinical studies: metformin hydrochloride reduces total cholesterol, LDL cholesterol and triglyceride levels.

Clinical efficacy:

The prospective randomised (UKPDS) study has established the long-term benefit of intensive blood glucose control in adult patients with type 2 diabetes.

Analysis of the results for overweight patients treated with metformin hydrochloride after failure of diet alone showed:

- a significant reduction of the absolute risk of any diabetes-related complication in the metformin hydrochloride group (29.8 events/1000 patient-years) versus diet alone (43.3 events/1000 patient-years), p=0.0023, and versus the combined sulphonylurea and insulin monotherapy groups (40.1 events/1000 patient-years), p=0.0034.
- a significant reduction of the absolute risk of diabetes-related mortality: metformin hydrochloride 7.5 events/1000 patient-years, diet alone 12.7 events/1000 patient-years, p=0.017;
- a significant reduction of the absolute risk of overall mortality: metformin hydrochloride 13.5 events/1000 patient-years versus diet alone 20.6 events/1000 patient-years (p=0.011), and versus the combined sulphonylurea and insulin monotherapy groups 18.9 events/1000 patient-years (p=0.021);
- a significant reduction in the absolute risk of myocardial infarction: metformin hydrochloride 11 events/1000 patient-years, diet alone 18 events/1000 patient-years (p=0.01)

Benefit regarding clinical outcome has not been shown for metformin hydrochloride used as second-line therapy, in combination with a sulfonylurea.

In type 1 diabetes, the combination of metformin hydrochloride and insulin has been used in selected patients, but the clinical benefit of this combination has not been formally established.

Controlled clinical studies in a limited paediatric population aged 10-16 years treated during 1 year demonstrated a similar response in glycaemic control to that seen in adults.

5.2 Pharmacokinetic properties

Absorption:

After an oral dose of metformin, Tmax is reached in 2.5 hours. Absolute bioavailability of a 500mg or 850mg metformin hydrochloride tablet is approximately 50-60% in healthy subjects. After an oral dose, the non-absorbed fraction recovered in faeces was 20-30%.

After oral administration, metformin hydrochloride absorption is saturable and incomplete. It is assumed that the pharmacokinetics of metformin hydrochloride absorption are non-linear.

At the recommended metformin hydrochloride doses and dosing schedules, steady state plasma concentrations are reached within 24 to 48 hours and are generally less than 1 microgram/ml. In controlled clinical trials, maximum metformin hydrochloride plasma levels (Cmax) did not exceed 4 microgram/ml, even at maximum doses.

Food decreases the extent and slightly delays the absorption of metformin hydrochloride. Following administration of a dose of 850 mg, a 40% lower plasma peak concentration, a 25% decrease in AUC (area under the curve) and a 35 minute prolongation of the time to peak plasma concentration were observed. The clinical relevance of these decreases is unknown.

Distribution:

Plasma protein binding is negligible. Metformin hydrochloride partitions into erythrocytes. The blood peak is lower than the plasma peak and appears at approximately the same time. The red blood cells most likely represent a secondary compartment of distribution. The mean volume of distribution (Vd) ranged between 63-276 L.

Metabolism:

Metformin hydrochloride is excreted unchanged in the urine. No metabolites have been identified in humans.

Elimination:

Renal clearance of metformin hydrochloride is > 400 ml/min, indicating that metformin hydrochloride is eliminated by glomerular filtration and tubular secretion. Following an oral dose, the apparent terminal elimination half-life is approximately 6.5 hours.

When renal function is impaired, renal clearance is decreased in proportion to that of creatinine and thus the elimination half-life is prolonged, leading to increased levels of metformin hydrochloride in plasma.

Children and adolescents:

Single dose study: After single doses of metformin 500 mg, paediatric patients have shown a similar pharmacokinetic profile to that observed in healthy adults.

Multiple dose study: Data are restricted to one study. After repeated doses of 500 mg twice daily for 7 days in paediatric patients the peak plasma concentration (Cmax) and systemic exposure (AUC0-t) were reduced by approximately 33% and 40%, respectively compared to diabetic adults who received repeated doses of 500 mg twice daily for 14 days. As the dose is individually titrated based on glycaemic control, this is of limited clinical relevance.

5.3 Preclinical safety data

Preclinical data reveal no special hazard for humans based on conventional studies on safety pharmacology, repeated dose toxicity, genotoxicity, carcinogenic potential and reproductive toxicity.

6. PHARMACEUTICAL PARTICULARS

6.1 List of excipients

Tablet core:

Povidone K 30

Magnesium stearate

Film-coating:

Hypromellose

6.2 Incompatibilities

Not applicable

6.3 Shelf life

5 years

6.4 Special precautions for storage

This medicinal product does not require any special storage conditions.

6.5 Nature and contents of container

500 mg tablets

1 (x 100), 9, 20, 21, 30, 40, 50, 56, 60, 84, 90, 100, 120, 200, 500, 600 or 1000 tablets in blister packs (PVC-aluminium)

21, 30, 40, 50, 60, 100, 120, 300, 400, 500, 600 or 1000 tablets in plastic bottles (high-density polyethylene) with caps (polypropylene),

Not all pack sizes may be marketed.

850 mg tablets:

1 (x 100), 8, 9, 10,14, 20, 21, 30, 40, 50, 56, 60, 84, 90, 100, 120, 300, 600 or 1000 tablets in blister packs (PVC-aluminium)

30, 60, 200, 300 or 600 tablets in plastic bottles (high-density polyethylene) with caps (polypropylene),

Not all pack sizes may be marketed.

6.6 Special precautions for disposal and other handling

No special requirements.

7. MARKETING AUTHORISATION HOLDER

Lipha Pharmaceuticals Limited

Trading from Bedfont Cross, Stanwell Road, Feltham, Middlesex, TW14 8NX, UK

8. MARKETING AUTHORISATION NUMBER(S)

PL 03759/0012-0013

9. DATE OF FIRST AUTHORISATION/RENEWAL OF THE AUTHORISATION

01/10/2007

10. DATE OF REVISION OF THE TEXT

01/10/2007

Glucophage SR 500mg, 750mg and 1000mg prolonged release tablets

(Merck Serono)

1. NAME OF THE MEDICINAL PRODUCT

Glucophage SR 500 mg prolonged release tablets

Glucophage SR 750 mg prolonged release tablets

Glucophage SR 1000 mg prolonged release tablets

2. QUALITATIVE AND QUANTITATIVE COMPOSITION

500 mg: One prolonged release tablet contains 500mg metformin hydrochloride corresponding to 390 mg metformin base.

750 mg: One prolonged release tablet contains 750 mg metformin hydrochloride corresponding to 585 mg metformin base.

1000 mg: One prolonged release tablet contains 1000 mg metformin hydrochloride corresponding to 780 mg metformin base.

For excipients, see section 6.1.

3. PHARMACEUTICAL FORM

Prolonged release tablet.

500 mg: White to off-white, capsule-shaped, biconvex tablet, debossed on one side with '500'.

750 mg: White capsule-shaped, biconvex tablet, debossed on one side with '750' and on the other side with 'Merck'.

1000 mg: White to off-white capsule-shaped, biconvex tablet, debossed on one side with '1000' and on the other side with 'MERCK'.

4. CLINICAL PARTICULARS

4.1 Therapeutic indications

Treatment of type 2 diabetes mellitus in adults, particularly in overweight patients, when dietary management and exercise alone does not result in adequate glycaemic control. Glucophage SR may be used as monotherapy or in combination with other oral antidiabetic agents, or with insulin.

4.2 Posology and method of administration

Monotherapy and combination with other oral antidiabetic agents:

- The usual starting dose is one tablet of Glucophage SR 500 mg once daily.
- After 10 to 15 days the dose should be adjusted on the basis of blood glucose measurements. A slow increase of dose may improve gastro-intestinal tolerability. The maximum recommended dose is 4 tablets of Glucophage SR 500 mg daily.
- Dosage increases should be made in increments of 500 mg every 10-15 days, up to a maximum of 2000 mg once daily with the evening meal. If glycaemic control is not achieved on Glucophage SR 2000 mg once daily, Glucophage SR 1000 mg twice daily should be considered, with both doses being given with food. If glycaemic control is still not achieved, patients may be switched to standard metformin tablets to a maximum dose of 3000 mg daily.
- In patients already treated with metformin tablets, the starting dose of Glucophage SR should be equivalent to the daily dose of metformin immediate release tablets. In patients treated with metformin at a dose above 2000 mg daily, switching to Glucophage SR is not recommended.
- If transfer from another oral antidiabetic agent is intended: discontinue the other agent and initiate Glucophage SR at the dose indicated above.
- Glucophage SR 750 mg and Glucophage SR 1000 mg are intended for patients who are already treated with metformin tablets (prolonged or immediate release).
- The dose of Glucophage SR 750 mg or Glucophage SR 1000 mg should be equivalent to the daily dose of metformin tablets (prolonged or immediate release), up to a maximum dose of 1500 mg or 2000 mg respectively, given with the evening meal.

Combination with insulin:

Metformin and insulin may be used in combination therapy to achieve better blood glucose control. The usual starting dose of Glucophage SR is one 500 mg tablet once daily, while insulin dosage is adjusted on the basis of blood glucose measurements.

For patients already treated with metformin and insulin in combination therapy, the dose of Glucophage SR 750 mg or Glucophage SR 1000 mg should be equivalent to the daily dose of metformin tablets up to a maximum of 1500 mg or 2000 mg respectively, given with the evening meal, while insulin dosage is adjusted on the basis of blood glucose measurements.

Elderly: due to the potential for decreased renal function in elderly subjects, the metformin dosage should be adjusted based on renal function. Regular assessment of renal function is necessary (see section 4.4).

Children: In the absence of available data, Glucophage SR should not be used in children.

4.3 Contraindications

- Hypersensitivity to metformin hydrochloride or to any of the excipients.
- Diabetic ketoacidosis, diabetic pre-coma.
- Renal failure or renal dysfunction (creatinine clearance < 60 ml/min).
- Acute conditions with the potential to alter renal function such as:

- dehydration,
- severe infection,
- shock,
- intravascular administration of iodinated contrast agents (see 4.4 Special warnings and precautions for use).

- Acute or chronic disease which may cause tissue hypoxia such as:

- cardiac or respiratory failure,
- recent myocardial infarction,
- shock

- Hepatic insufficiency, acute alcohol intoxication, alcoholism
- Lactation (see section 4.6).

4.4 Special warnings and precautions for use

Lactic acidosis:

Lactic acidosis is a rare, but serious (high mortality in the absence of prompt treatment), metabolic complication that can occur due to metformin accumulation. Reported cases of lactic acidosis in patients on metformin have occurred primarily in diabetic patients with significant renal failure. The incidence of lactic acidosis can and should be reduced by assessing also other associated risk factors such as poorly controlled diabetes, ketosis, prolonged fasting, excessive alcohol intake, hepatic insufficiency and any condition associated with hypoxia.

Diagnosis:

Lactic acidosis is characterised by acidotic dyspnoea, abdominal pain and hypothermia followed by coma. Diagnostic laboratory findings are decreased blood pH, plasma lactate levels above 5 mmol/L, and an increased anion gap and lactate/pyruvate ratio. If metabolic acidosis is suspected, metformin should be discontinued and the patient should be hospitalised immediately (see section 4.9).

Renal function:

As metformin is excreted by the kidney, creatinine clearance (this can be estimated using the Cockcroft-Gault formula) and/or serum creatinine levels should be determined before initiating treatment and regularly thereafter:

- at least annually in patients with normal renal function,
- at least two to four times a year in patients with creatinine clearance levels at the limit of normal and in elderly subjects.

Decreased renal function in elderly subjects is frequent and asymptomatic. Special caution should be exercised in situations where renal function may become impaired, for example when initiating antihypertensive therapy or diuretic therapy and when starting therapy with an NSAID.

Administration of iodinated contrast agent:

As the intravascular administration of iodinated contrast materials in radiologic studies can lead to renal failure, metformin should be discontinued prior to, or at the time of the test and not reinstituted until 48 hours afterwards, and only after renal function has been re-evaluated and found to be normal.

Surgery:

Metformin hydrochloride should be discontinued 48 hours before elective surgery with general anaesthesia and should not be usually resumed earlier than 48 hours afterwards.

Other precautions:

- All patients should continue their diet with a regular distribution of carbohydrate intake during the day. Overweight patients should continue their energy-restricted diet.
- The usual laboratory tests for diabetes monitoring should be performed regularly.
- Metformin alone never causes hypoglycaemia, although caution is advised when it is used in combination with insulin or sulphonylureas.
- The tablet shells may be present in the faeces. Patients should be advised that this is normal.

4.5 Interaction with other medicinal products and other forms of interaction

Inadvisable combinations

Alcohol

Increased risk of lactic acidosis in acute alcohol intoxication, particularly in case of:

- fasting or malnutrition,
- hepatic insufficiency.

Avoid consumption of alcohol and alcohol-containing medications.

Iodinated contrast agents

Intravascular administration of iodinated contrast agents may lead to renal failure, resulting in metformin accumulation and a risk of lactic acidosis.

Metformin should be discontinued prior to, or at the time of the test and not reinstituted until 48 hours afterwards, and only after renal function has been re-evaluated and found to be normal (see 4.4 special warnings and precautions for use).

Associations requiring precautions for use

Glucocorticoids (systemic and local routes), beta-2-agonists, and diuretics have intrinsic hyperglycaemic activity. Inform the patient and perform more frequent blood glucose monitoring, especially at the beginning of treatment. If necessary, adjust the dosage of the antidiabetic drug during therapy with the other drug and upon its discontinuation.

ACE-inhibitors may decrease the blood glucose levels. If necessary, adjust the dosage of the antidiabetic drug during therapy with the other drug and upon its discontinuation.

4.6 Pregnancy and lactation

Pregnancy:

To date, no relevant epidemiological data are available. Animal studies do not indicate harmful effects with respect to pregnancy, embryonal or fœtal development, parturition or postnatal development (see also section 5.3)

When the patient plans to become pregnant and during pregnancy, diabetes should not be treated with metformin but insulin should be used to maintain blood glucose levels as close to normal as possible in order to lower the risk of foetal malformations associated with abnormal blood glucose levels.

Lactation:

Metformin is excreted into milk in lactating rats. Similar data is not available in humans and a decision should be made whether to discontinue nursing or to discontinue metformin, taking into account the importance of the compound to the mother.

4.7 Effects on ability to drive and use machines

Glucophage SR monotherapy does not cause hypoglycaemia and therefore has no effect on the ability to drive or to use machines.

However, patients should be alerted to the risk of hypoglycaemia when metformin is used in combination with other antidiabetic agents (sulphonylureas, insulin, repaglinide).

4.8 Undesirable effects

In post marketing data and in controlled clinical studies, adverse event reporting in patients treated with Glucophage SR was similar in nature and severity to that reported in patients treated with Glucophage immediate release.

The following undesirable effects may occur with metformin:

Frequencies are defined as follows: very common: >1/10; common ≥1/100, <1/10; uncommon ≥1/1,000, <1/100; rare ≥1/10,000, <1/1,000; very rare <1/10,000 and isolated reports.

Nervous system disorders

Common: Taste disturbance

Gastrointestinal disorders

Very common: Gastrointestinal disorders such as nausea, vomiting, diarrhoea, abdominal pain and loss of appetite. These undesirable effects occur most frequently during initiation of therapy and resolve spontaneously in most cases. A slow increase of the dose may also improve gastrointestinal tolerability.

Skin and subcutaneous tissue disorders

Very rare: Skin reactions such as erythema, pruritus, urticaria

Metabolism and nutrition disorders

Very rare: Lactic acidosis (see section 4.4). Decrease of vitamin B12 absorption with decrease of serum levels during long-term use of metformin. Consideration of such aetiology is recommended if a patient presents with megaloblastic anaemia.

Hepatobiliary disorders

Not known: Isolated reports of liver function tests abnormalities or hepatitis resolving upon metformin discontinuation.

4.9 Overdose

Hypoglycaemia has not been seen with metformin doses of up to 85 g, although lactic acidosis has occurred in such circumstances. High overdose or concomitant risks of metformin may lead to lactic acidosis. Lactic acidosis is a medical emergency and must be treated in hospital. The most effective method to remove lactate and metformin is haemodialysis.

5. PHARMACOLOGICAL PROPERTIES

5.1 Pharmacodynamic properties

ORAL ANTI-DIABETICS

(A10BA02: Gastrointestinal tract and metabolism)

Metformin is a biguanide with antihyperglycaemic effects, lowering both basal and postprandial plasma glucose. It does not stimulate insulin secretion and therefore does not produce hypoglycaemia.

Metformin may act via 3 mechanisms:

(1) reduction of hepatic glucose production by inhibiting gluconeogenesis and glycogenolysis

(2) in muscle, by increasing insulin sensitivity, improving peripheral glucose uptake and utilisation

(3) and delay of intestinal glucose absorption.

Metformin stimulates intracellular glycogen synthesis by acting on glycogen synthase.

Metformin increases the transport capacity of all types of membrane glucose transporters (GLUT).

In humans, independently of its action on glycaemia, immediate release metformin has favourable effects on lipid metabolism. This has been shown at therapeutic doses in controlled, medium-term or long-term clinical studies: immediate release metformin reduces total cholesterol, LDL cholesterol and triglyceride levels. A similar action has not been demonstrated with the prolonged release formulation, possibly due to the evening administration, and an increase in triglycerides may occur.

Clinical efficacy:

The prospective randomised (UKPDS) study has established the long-term benefit of intensive blood glucose control in overweight type 2 diabetic patients treated with immediate release metformin as first-line therapy after diet failure. Analysis of the results for overweight patients treated with metformin after failure of diet alone showed:

• a significant reduction of the absolute risk of any diabetes-related complication in the metformin group (29.8 events/ 1000 patient-years) versus diet alone (43.3 events/ 1000 patient-years), p=0.0023, and versus the combined sulphonylurea and insulin monotherapy groups (40.1 events/ 1000 patient-years), p=0.0034.

• a significant reduction of the absolute risk of diabetes-related mortality: metformin 7.5 events/1000 patient-years, diet alone 12.7 events/ 1000 patient-years, p=0.017;

• a significant reduction of the absolute risk of overall mortality: metformin 13.5 events/ 1000 patient-years versus diet alone 20.6 events/ 1000 patient-years (p=0.011), and versus the combined sulphonylurea and insulin monotherapy groups 18.9 events/ 1000 patient-years (p=0.021);

• a significant reduction in the absolute risk of myocardial infarction: metformin 11 events/ 1000 patient-years, diet alone 18 events/ 1000 patient-years (p=0.01)

For metformin used as second-line therapy, in combination with a sulphonylurea, benefit regarding clinical outcome has not been shown.

In type 1 diabetes, the combination of metformin and insulin has been used in selected patients, but the clinical benefit of this combination has not been formally established.

5.2 Pharmacokinetic properties

Absorption

After an oral dose of the prolonged release tablet, metformin absorption is significantly delayed compared to the immediate release tablet with a Tmax at 7 hours (Tmax for the immediate release tablet is 2.5 hours).

At steady state, similar to the immediate release formulation, Cmax and AUC are not proportionally increased to the administered dose. The AUC after a single oral administration of 2000mg of metformin prolonged release tablets is similar to that observed after administration of 1000mg of metformin immediate release tablets b.i.d.

Intrasubject variability of Cmax and AUC of metformin prolonged release is comparable to that observed with metformin immediate release tablets.

When the prolonged release tablet is administered in fasting conditions the AUC is decreased by 30% (both Cmax and Tmax are unaffected).

Mean metformin absorption from the prolonged release formulation is almost not altered by meal composition.

No accumulation is observed after repeated administration of up to 2000mg of metformin as prolonged release tablets.

Following a single oral administration of 1500 mg of Glucophage SR 750 mg, a mean peak plasma concentration of 1193 ng/ml is achieved with a median value of 5 hours and a range of 4 to 12 hours.

Glucophage SR 750 mg was shown to be bioequivalent to Glucophage SR 500 mg at a 1500 mg dose with respect to Cmax and AUC in healthy fed and fasted subjects.

Following a single oral administration in the fed state of one tablet of Glucophage SR 1000 mg, a mean peak plasma concentration of 1214 ng/ml is achieved with a median time of 5 hours (range of 4 to 10 hours).

Glucophage SR 1000 mg was shown to be bioequivalent to Glucophage SR 500 mg at a 1000 mg dose with respect to Cmax and AUC in healthy fed and fasted subjects.

When the 1000 mg prolonged release tablet is administered in fed conditions the AUC is increased by 77% (Cmax is increased by 26% and Tmax is slightly prolonged by about 1 hour).

Distribution

Plasma protein binding is negligible. Metformin partitions into erythrocytes. The blood peak is lower than the plasma peak and appears at approximately the same time. The red blood cells most likely represent a secondary compartment of distribution. The mean Vd ranged between 63-276 L.

Metabolism

Metformin is excreted unchanged in the urine. No metabolites have been identified in humans.

Elimination

Renal clearance of metformin is > 400 ml/min, indicating that metformin is eliminated by glomerular filtration and tubular secretion. Following an oral dose, the apparent terminal elimination half-life is approximately 6.5 hours.

When renal function is impaired, renal clearance is decreased in proportion to that of creatinine and thus the elimination half-life is prolonged, leading to increased levels of metformin in plasma.

5.3 Preclinical safety data

Preclinical data reveal no special hazard for humans based on conventional studies on safety pharmacology, repeated dose toxicity, genotoxicity, carcinogenic potential, toxicity reproduction.

6. PHARMACEUTICAL PARTICULARS

6.1 List of excipients

500 mg: Magnesium stearate, carmellose sodium, hypromellose, microcrystalline cellulose.

750 mg: Magnesium stearate, carmellose sodium, hypromellose.

1000 mg: Carmellose sodium, hypromellose, magnesium stearate.

6.2 Incompatibilities

None

6.3 Shelf life

3 years

6.4 Special precautions for storage

This medicinal product does not require any special storage conditions.

6.5 Nature and contents of container

500mg:

20, 28, 30, 50, 56, 60, 84, 90, 100, 112, 120, 180, 600 tablets in blister strips composed of PVC/PVDC 90g.

20, 28, 30, 50, 56, 60, 84, 90, 100, 112, 120, 180, 600 tablets in blister strips composed of PVC-Aclar aluminium.

20, 28, 30, 50, 56, 60, 84, 90, 100, 112, 120, 180, 600 tablets in HDPE (High Density Polyethylene) bottles. HDPE bottles are composed of a two-piece plastic child-resistant closure or plastic continuous thread closure with aluminium-foil induction seal (innerseal).

750 mg:

14, 20, 28, 30, 50, 56, 60, 84, 90, 100, 112, 120, 180 or 600 tablets in blister strips composed of aluminium foil + PVC or PVC/PVDC (60 g/m^2 or 90g/m^2).

1000 mg:

14, 20, 28, 30, 50, 56, 60, 84, 90, 100, 112, 120, 180 or 600 tablets in blister strips composed of aluminium foil + PVC/ PVDC (60 g/m^2 or 90g/m^2).

Not all pack sizes may be marketed.

6.6 Special precautions for disposal and other handling

No special requirements. Any unused product or waste material should be disposed of in accordance with local requirements.

7. MARKETING AUTHORISATION HOLDER

Merck Serono Ltd
Bedfont Cross
Stanwell Road
Feltham
Middlesex
TW14 8NX
United Kingdom

8. MARKETING AUTHORISATION NUMBER(S)

500 mg: PL 11648/0054

750 mg: PL 11648/0066

1000 mg: PL 11648/0067

9. DATE OF FIRST AUTHORISATION/RENEWAL OF THE AUTHORISATION

500 mg: 26th November 2004

750 mg: 21st February 2008

1000 mg: 16th September 2008

10. DATE OF REVISION OF THE TEXT

5 March 2009

Glucose Injection BP Minijet (International Medication Systems)

(International Medication Systems (UK) Ltd)

1. NAME OF THE MEDICINAL PRODUCT

Glucose Injection BP Minijet 50%w/v

2. QUALITATIVE AND QUANTITATIVE COMPOSITION

Glucose anhydrous 500 mg in 1ml.

For excipients see 6.1

3. PHARMACEUTICAL FORM

Solution for injection.

The clear, colourless solution is contained in a USP Type I glass vial with an elastomeric closure. The container is specially designed for use with the IMS Minijet injector supplied.

4. CLINICAL PARTICULARS

4.1 Therapeutic indications

a) As a source of energy in parenteral nutrition.

b) In severe hypoglycaemia due to insulin excess or other causes.

c) For reduction of cerebrospinal pressure and/or cerebral oedema due to *delirium tremens* or acute alcohol intoxication.

Glucose injection 50% w/v is strongly hypertonic and is used partly because of its dehydrating effects.

4.2 Posology and method of administration

Hypertonic solutions of glucose should be administered via a central vein. The dose is variable and depends upon the indication, clinical condition and size of the individual.

The rate of utilisation of glucose varies considerably from patient to patient. In general, the maximal rate has been estimated at 500-800mg/kg body weight/hour. If the patient's capacity to utilise glucose is exceeded, glycosuria and diuresis will occur.

Adults, elderly, children over 6 years:

Hypoglycaemia: 20-50ml of a 50% w/v solution, repeated as necessary according to the patient's response, by slow intravenous injection, e.g. 3ml/minute. After 25g of glucose has been given, it is advisable to interrupt the injection and evaluate the effect. The exact dose required to relieve hypoglycaemia will vary. After the patient responds, supplemental oral feeding is indicated to avoid relapse, especially after insulin shock therapy.

Acute alcoholism: 50ml of glucose 50% w/v solution should be administered intravenously. Unmodified insulin (20 units) and thiamine hydrochloride (100mg) should be added to the infusion.

4.3 Contraindications

The intravenous use of strongly hypertonic solutions of glucose is contraindicated in patients with anuria, intracranial or intraspinal haemorrhage, or delirium tremens *if the patient is already dehydrated.*

Known sensitivity to corn or corn products, hyperglycaemic coma, or ischaemic stroke.

4.4 Special warnings and precautions for use

Hypertonic solutions of glucose should be administered via a large central vein to minimise the damage at the site of injection.

Use with caution in patients with diabetes mellitus, severe undernutrition, carbohydrate intolerance, thiamine deficiency, hypophosphataemia, haemodilution, sepsis and trauma. Rapid infusion of hypertonic glucose solution may lead to hyperglycaemia. Patients should be observed for signs of mental confusion or loss of consciousness.

Prolonged use in parenteral nutrition may affect insulin production; blood and urine glucose should be monitored. Fluid and acid-base balance and electrolyte status should also be determined during therapy with dextrose.

4.5 Interaction with other medicinal products and other forms of interaction
None known.

4.6 Pregnancy and lactation
Intravenous glucose may result in considerable foetal insulin production, with an associated risk of rebound hypoglycaemia in the new-born. Infusion should not exceed 5-10g/hour during labour or Caesarean section.

4.7 Effects on ability to drive and use machines
This preparation is intended for use only in emergencies.

4.8 Undesirable effects
Anaphylactoid reactions have been reported in patients with asthma and diabetes mellitus.

Local pain, inflammation, irritation, thrombophlebitis and fever may occur.

Hypokalaemia, hypomagnesaemia or hypophosphataemia may result from the use of hypertonic solutions via the intravenous route.

Prolonged or rapid administration of hyperosmotic (>5%) solutions may lead to dehydration.

The administration of glucose without adequate levels of thiamine (which form the coenzyme systems in its metabolism), may precipitate overt deficiency states, e.g. Wernicke's encephalopathy.

Excess glucose infusion produces increased CO_2, which may be important in respiratory failure, and stimulates catecholamine secretion.

4.9 Overdose
The patient becomes hyperglycaemic and glycosuria may occur. This can lead to dehydration, hyperosmolar coma and death.

Treatment: The infusion should be discontinued and the patient evaluated. Insulin may be administered and appropriate supportive measures taken.

5. PHARMACOLOGICAL PROPERTIES

5.1 Pharmacodynamic properties
Glucose, the natural sugar occurring in the blood, is the principle source of energy for the body. It is readily converted to fat and is also stored in the liver and muscles as glycogen. When a rapid rise in blood sugar is demanded by the body, glycogen is quickly liberated as d-glucose. When the supply of glucose is insufficient, the body mobilises fat stores which are converted to acetate with production of energy by the same oxidative pathways employed in the combustion of glucose.

It may decrease body protein and nitrogen losses. Glucose is also the probable source of glucuronic acid with which many foreign substances and their metabolites combine to form excretion products. It probably provides the basic substances required for the formation of hyalluronates and chondroitin sulphates, the supporting structures of the organism. It can be converted to a pentose essential for the formation of nucleic acids by the cells.

5.2 Pharmacokinetic properties
Glucose is metabolised to carbon dioxide and water with the release of energy.

5.3 Preclinical safety data
Not applicable since glucose has been used in clinical practice for many years and its effects in man are well known.

6. PHARMACEUTICAL PARTICULARS

6.1 List of excipients
Water for Injection

6.2 Incompatibilities
Glucose solutions which do not contain electrolytes should not be administered concomitantly with blood through the same infusion set as haemolysis and clumping may occur.

6.3 Shelf life
3 years.

6.4 Special precautions for storage
Store below 25°C.

6.5 Nature and contents of container
The solution is contained in a USP type I glass vial with an elastomeric closure which meets all the relevant USP specifications. The product is available as 10ml and 50ml.

6.6 Special precautions for disposal and other handling
The container is specially designed for use with the IMS Minijet injector. Do not use the injection if crystals have separated.

Administrative Data

7. MARKETING AUTHORISATION HOLDER
International Medication Systems (UK) Ltd
208 Bath Road
Slough
Berkshire
SL1 3WE
UK

8. MARKETING AUTHORISATION NUMBER(S)
PL 03265/0008R

9. DATE OF FIRST AUTHORISATION/RENEWAL OF THE AUTHORISATION
Date first granted: 28 February 1991
Date renewed: 28 February 1996

10. DATE OF REVISION OF THE TEXT
April 2001

POM

Glutarol 10% w/v Cutaneous Solution

(Dermal Laboratories Limited)

1. NAME OF THE MEDICINAL PRODUCT
GLUTAROL™ 10% w/v CUTANEOUS SOLUTION

2. QUALITATIVE AND QUANTITATIVE COMPOSITION
Glutaraldehyde 10.0% w/v.

3. PHARMACEUTICAL FORM
Cutaneous solution.

Colourless, evaporative wart paint.

4. CLINICAL PARTICULARS

4.1 Therapeutic indications
For the topical treatment of warts, especially plantar warts.

4.2 Posology and method of administration
For adults, children and the elderly:

1. Gently rub the surface of the wart with a piece of pumice stone or manicure emery board, or pare down any hard skin.

2. Using the applicator provided, carefully apply a few drops of the paint to the wart, taking care to localise the application to the affected area. Allow each drop to dry before the next is applied.

3. Repeat twice daily.

4. On subsequent days, repeat steps 1 to 3.

It is not necessary to cover the treated wart(s) with an adhesive plaster.

4.3 Contraindications
Not to be used in cases of sensitivity to any of the ingredients. Not to be used on the face, anal or perineal region. Not to be used on moles or on any other skin lesion for which it is not indicated.

4.4 Special warnings and precautions for use
Keep away from the eyes and mucous membranes. Avoid spreading onto surrounding uninvolved skin. Avoid spillage. Avoid inhaling vapour. Replace cap tightly after use. For external use only.

4.5 Interaction with other medicinal products and other forms of interaction
None known.

4.6 Pregnancy and lactation
No special precautions.

4.7 Effects on ability to drive and use machines
None known.

4.8 Undesirable effects
Undesirable effects occur very occasionally and mostly involve mild local skin rashes and irritation. Very rarely, a severe reaction may occur particularly on the hands or when the product is used excessively and allowed to spread onto surrounding normal skin. If mild irritation should occur, apply a reduced amount (taking special care to avoid spreading beyond the wart or verruca) and apply less often. If the irritation is severe, patients should stop treatment immediately and seek medical advice.

4.9 Overdose
Accidental oral ingestion should be treated immediately by gastric lavage with 2 to 5% aqueous sodium bicarbonate solution. Fluid and electrolyte balance should be monitored and appropriate supportive measures should be provided. Symptoms include headache, nausea, vomiting, diarrhoea and respiratory depression.

5. PHARMACOLOGICAL PROPERTIES

5.1 Pharmacodynamic properties
Glutaraldehyde is virucidal and thus inactivates the wart virus. On the skin, it also acts as an anhidrotic, drying the warts and surrounding skin, thus reducing the spread of lesions and simplifying the removal of persistent warts by curettage.

As glutaraldehyde stains the outer layer of the skin brown, treatment can be seen to be carried out. This stain soon disappears after cessation of treatment.

5.2 Pharmacokinetic properties
Addition of ethanol to the formulation stabilises the glutaraldehyde against irreversible polymerisation during storage but at the same time diminishes its activity. However, when the aqueous ethanolic solution is applied to the skin, the alcohol rapidly evaporates leaving a concentrated aqueous solution of glutaraldehyde which is highly reactive and attacks the wart before it has time to polymerise. Thus, the ethanolic formulation is stable in storage, as confirmed by stability tests, but is immediately activated when applied to the skin and the alcohol is allowed to evaporate.

5.3 Preclinical safety data
No relevant information additional to that contained elsewhere in the SPC.

6. PHARMACEUTICAL PARTICULARS

6.1 List of excipients
IMS; Purified Water.

6.2 Incompatibilities
None known.

6.3 Shelf life
36 months.

6.4 Special precautions for storage
Flammable. Keep away from flames. Keep upright. Do not store above 25°C.

6.5 Nature and contents of container
10 ml amber glass bottle incorporating a specially designed spatula for ease of application.

6.6 Special precautions for disposal and other handling
Not applicable.

7. MARKETING AUTHORISATION HOLDER
Dermal Laboratories
Tatmore Place, Gosmore
Hitchin, Herts SG4 7QR, UK.

8. MARKETING AUTHORISATION NUMBER(S)
00173/0022.

9. DATE OF FIRST AUTHORISATION/RENEWAL OF THE AUTHORISATION
15 September 2005.

10. DATE OF REVISION OF THE TEXT
July 2006.

Glypressin 0.12mg/ml Solution for Injection

(Ferring Pharmaceuticals Ltd)

1. NAME OF THE MEDICINAL PRODUCT
Glypressin 0.12 mg/ml solution for injection

2. QUALITATIVE AND QUANTITATIVE COMPOSITION
One ampoule contains 1mg terlipressin acetate in 8.5ml solution for injection.

For excipients, see section 6.1

3. PHARMACEUTICAL FORM
Solution for injection.

Clear, colourless liquid.

4. CLINICAL PARTICULARS

4.1 Therapeutic indications
Glypressin is indicated in the treatment of bleeding oesophageal varices.

4.2 Posology and method of administration
In acute variceal bleeding, 2mg Glypressin should be administered by intravenous bolus, followed by 1 – 2 mg every 4 – 6 hours until bleeding is controlled, up to a maximum of 72 hours.

Administration is by intravenous injection.

4.3 Contraindications
Contraindicated in pregnancy.

Hypersensitivity to terlipressin or any other excipients of the product.

4.4 Special warnings and precautions for use
Since Glypressin has antidiuretic and pressor activity it should be used with great caution in patients with hypertension, atherosclerosis, cardiac dysrhythmias or coronary insufficiency. Constant monitoring of blood pressure, serum sodium and potassium and fluid balance is essential.

4.5 Interaction with other medicinal products and other forms of interaction
None known

4.6 Pregnancy and lactation
Glypressin® may stimulate contraction of smooth muscle and is therefore contraindicated in pregnancy. There is no data concerning its use in lactation.

4.7 Effects on ability to drive and use machines
Not applicable

4.8 Undesirable effects
Glypressin® is only recommended for the short-term treatment of bleeding oesophageal varices, so few side effects have been reported. Those noted have included abdominal cramps, headache, transient blanching and increased arterial blood pressure.

4.9 Overdose
The recommended dose (2mg/4 hours) should not be exceeded as the risk of severe circulatory adverse effects is dose-dependent.

5. PHARMACOLOGICAL PROPERTIES

5.1 Pharmacodynamic properties
Pharmacotherapeutic group: Posterior pituitary lobe hormones (vasopressin and analogues) (H 01 BA 04)

Glypressin® may be regarded as a circulating depot of lysine vasopressin. Following intravenous injection, three glycyl moieties are enzymatically cleaved from the N-terminus to release lysine vasopressin.

The slowly released vasopressin reduces blood flow in the splanchnic circulation in a prolonged manner, thereby helping to control bleeding from ruptured oesophageal varices.

5.2 Pharmacokinetic properties

Glypressin® is administered by bolus intravenous injection. It shows a biphasic plasma level curve which indicates that a two compartment model can be applied.

The half-life of distribution ($T_{1/2\alpha}$) is about 8 -10 minutes.

The half-life of elimination ($T_{1/2\beta}$) is about 50 -70 minutes.

Lysine vasopressin reaches maximum plasma levels about 1 - 2 hours following intravenous administration and has a duration of activity of 4 - 6 hours.

5.3 Preclinical safety data

There are no pre-clinical data of relevance to the prescriber which are additional to that already included in other sections of the SPC.

6. PHARMACEUTICAL PARTICULARS

6.1 List of excipients

Sodium chloride

Acetic acid

Sodium acetate

Water for injections

6.2 Incompatibilities

In the absence of compatibility studies, this medicinal product must not be mixed with other medicinal products.

6.3 Shelf life

2 years

6.4 Special precautions for storage

Store in a refrigerator (2-8 °C). Keep the ampoules in the ourter carton in order to protect from light.

6.5 Nature and contents of container

Type I clear glass ampoules.

Pack size: 5 × 8.5ml

6.6 Special precautions for disposal and other handling

Unused drug and waste should be destroyed in accordance with local requirements.

7. MARKETING AUTHORISATION HOLDER

Ferring Pharmaceuticals Ltd.,

The Courtyard

Waterside Drive

Langley, Berkshire

SL3 6EZ

UK

8. MARKETING AUTHORISATION NUMBER(S)

PL 03194/0101

9. DATE OF FIRST AUTHORISATION/RENEWAL OF THE AUTHORISATION

11/05/2009

10. DATE OF REVISION OF THE TEXT

11/05/2009

Glypressin Injection

(Ferring Pharmaceuticals Ltd)

1. NAME OF THE MEDICINAL PRODUCT

Glypressin® Injection

2. QUALITATIVE AND QUANTITATIVE COMPOSITION

Each vial contains 1mg Terlipressin Acetate

For excipients, see 6.1

3. PHARMACEUTICAL FORM

Powder and solvent for solution for injection

Vial contains white, freeze-dried powder.

Ampoule contains solvent.

4. CLINICAL PARTICULARS

4.1 Therapeutic indications

Glypressin® is indicated in the treatment of bleeding oesophageal varices.

4.2 Posology and method of administration

In acute variceal bleeding, 2mg Glypressin® should be administered by intravenous bolus, followed by 1 - 2mg every 4 - 6 hours until bleeding is controlled, up to a maximum of 72 hours.

Administration is by intravenous injection.

4.3 Contraindications

Pregnancy

4.4 Special warnings and precautions for use

Since Glypressin® has antidiuretic and pressor activity it should be used with great caution in patients with hypertension, atherosclerosis, cardiac dysrhythmias or coronary insufficiency. Constant monitoring of blood pressure, serum sodium and potassium and fluid balance is essential.

4.5 Interaction with other medicinal products and other forms of interaction

None known

4.6 Pregnancy and lactation

Glypressin® may stimulate contraction of smooth muscle and is therefore contraindicated in pregnancy. There is no data concerning its use in lactation.

4.7 Effects on ability to drive and use machines

Not applicable

4.8 Undesirable effects

Glypressin® is only recommended for the short-term treatment of bleeding oesophageal varices, so few side effects have been reported. Those noted have included abdominal cramps, headache, transient blanching and increased arterial blood pressure.

4.9 Overdose

Increase in blood pressure in patients with known hypertension has been controlled with clonidine, 150mcg iv.

5. PHARMACOLOGICAL PROPERTIES

5.1 Pharmacodynamic properties

Glypressin® may be regarded as a circulating depot of lysine vasopressin. Following intravenous injection, three glycyl moieties are enzymatically cleaved from the N-terminus to release lysine vasopressin.

The slowly released vasopressin reduces blood flow in the splanchnic circulation in a prolonged manner, thereby helping to control bleeding from ruptured oesophageal varices.

5.2 Pharmacokinetic properties

Glypressin® is administered by bolus iv injection. It shows a biphasic plasma level curve which indicates that a two compartment model can be applied.

The half-life of distribution is about 8 -10 minutes.

The half-life of elimination is about 50 -70 minutes.

Lysine vasopressin reaches maximum plasma levels about 1 - 2 hours following iv administration and has a duration of activity of 4 - 6 hours.

5.3 Preclinical safety data

There are no pre-clinical data of relevance to the prescriber which are additional to that already included in other sections of the SPC.

6. PHARMACEUTICAL PARTICULARS

6.1 List of excipients

Vial:

Mannitol

Hydrochloric Acid 1M

Solvent Ampoule:

Sodium Chloride

Hydrochloric Acid 1M

Water for Injection

6.2 Incompatibilities

None known

6.3 Shelf life

36 months

6.4 Special precautions for storage

Do not store above 25°C. Keep container in the outer carton.

6.5 Nature and contents of container

Powder: Type I glass vial

Solvent: Type I glass ampoule

Pack size: Cartons containing 5 packs, each with one vial of powder and one ampoule of 5ml solvent.

6.6 Special precautions for disposal and other handling

Prior to injection, the powder should be reconstituted with the solvent provided. Use immediately after reconstitution.

7. MARKETING AUTHORISATION HOLDER

Ferring Pharmaceuticals Limited, The Courtyard, Waterside Drive, Langley, Berkshire SL3 6EZ (UK)

8. MARKETING AUTHORISATION NUMBER(S)

PL 3194/0018

9. DATE OF FIRST AUTHORISATION/RENEWAL OF THE AUTHORISATION

18th July 2001

10. DATE OF REVISION OF THE TEXT

June 2002

11. Legal Category

POM

Glytrin, 400 micrograms per metered dose, sublingual spray

(sanofi-aventis)

1. NAME OF THE MEDICINAL PRODUCT

Glytrin, 400 micrograms per metered dose, Sublingual Spray

2. QUALITATIVE AND QUANTITATIVE COMPOSITION

Active Ingredient:

Glyceryl Trinitrate: 400 micrograms per metered dose

This product contains small amounts of ethanol (alcohol) less than 100mg per spray.

For full list of excipients, see Section 6.1

3. PHARMACEUTICAL FORM

Metered dose oromucosal (sublingual) spray solution.

Small aerosol canister

4. CLINICAL PARTICULARS

4.1 Therapeutic indications

Treatment of acute angina pectoris

Prevention of inducible angina (e.g. physical effort, emotional stress, exposure to cold)

Route of Administration

Oromucosal (Sublingual)

4.2 Posology and method of administration

Oromucosal Dosage

Adults including the elderly

At the onset of an attack, one or two metered doses (400 to 800 micrograms glyceryl trinitrate) to be sprayed under the tongue for the relief of anginal pain while breath is held. No more than three doses are recommended at any one time.

For the prevention of inducible angina (e.g. physical effort, emotional stress, exposure to cold), one or two 400 microgram metered doses sprayed under the tongue within 2 – 3 minutes of the event starting.

Children

Glytrin is not recommended for children

Administration

During application the patient should rest, ideally in the sitting position. The canister should be held vertically with the valve head uppermost and the spray orifice as close to the mouth as possible. The dose should be sprayed under the tongue and the mouth should be closed immediately after each dose. The spray should not be inhaled. Patients should be instructed to familiarize themselves with the position of the spray orifice, which can be identified by the finger rest on top of the valve, in order to facilitate orientation, for administration at night.

4.3 Contraindications

Hypersensitivity to nitrates or to any of the excipients. Severe hypotension (systolic blood pressure lower than 90mm Hg). Hypotensive shock, severe anaemia, constrictive pericarditis, extreme bradycardia, Glucose-6-phosphatedehydrogenase-deficiency, cerebral haemorrhage and brain trauma, aortic and / or mitral stenosis and angina caused by hypertrophic obstructive cardiomyopathy. Circulatory collapse, cardiogenic shock and toxic pulmonary oedema.

Concomitant use with phosphodiesterase inhibitors, such as sildenafil, tadalafil, or vardenafil.

4.4 Special warnings and precautions for use

Tolerance to this drug and cross-tolerance to other nitrates may occur.

Glytrin should be administered with particular caution in:

- Pericardial tamponade
- Low filling pressures (e.g. acute myocardial infarction, left ventricular failure)
- Tendancy to dysregulation of orthostatic blood pressure
- Diseases accompanied by an increase in intracranial pressure (so far further pressure has been observed solely in high doses of glyceryl trinitrate).

Alcohol should be avoided because of the hypotensive effect and medical controls of the intraocular pressure of glaucoma patients are advisable.

Particular caution should also be exercised when using Glytrin in patients with volume depletion from diuretic therapy, severe hepatic or renal impairment and hypothyroidism.

4.5 Interaction with other medicinal products and other forms of interaction

Alcohol may potentiate the hypotensive effect. Vasodilators, antihypertensives, β-blockers, calcium antagonists, neuroleptics, tricyclic antidepressants and diuretics can increase nitrate-induced hypotension.

The hypotensive effects of nitrates are potentiated by the concurrent administration of phosphodiesterase inhibitors, such as sildenafil, tadalafil, or vardenafil.

The bioavailability of dihydroergotamine may be increased by concomitant use of Glytrin, which can result in vasoconstriction since dihydroergotamine can antagonise the effects of glyceryl trinitrate. The concomitant administration of Glytrin and heparin can reduce the antithrombotic effect of heparin. Regular monitoring of coagulation parameters and adjustment of the heparin dose may be necessary.

In patients pre-treated with organic nitrates a higher dose of glyceryl trinitrate may be necessary to achieve the desired haemodynamic effect.

4.6 Pregnancy and lactation

The safety of glyceryl trinitrate in human pregnancy, especially during the first trimester has not been established. It

Table 1

System Organ Class	Very Common (≥ 10%)	Common (≥ 1% < 10%)	Uncommon (≥0.1% <1%)	Rare (≥0.01% <0.1%)	Rare (≥0.01% <0.1%)
Nervous system disorders	Headache	Vertigo			
Skin and subcutaneous tissue disorders		Facial Flushing			
Vascular disorders		Dizziness		Postural Hypotension	
General disorders and administration site conditions		Weakness	Burning sensation Stinging sensation Tongue blistering		
Gastrointestinal disorders		Nausea			
Cardiac disorders				Tachycardia Bradycardia	
Skin and subcutaneous tissue disorders				Allergic skin reactions	Exfoliative dermatitis

is not known whether glyceryl trinitrate is excreted into human breast milk. Glytrin should be used only after weighing the benefit for the mother against possible risks for the child.

Nursing should be discontinued during treatment with this product.

4.7 Effects on ability to drive and use machines

The ability to react may be diminished because of the side effects or interactions due to the nitrates. This effect is potentiated by alcohol consumption. Therefore, driving and / or using machines should be avoided during treatment with Glytrin.

4.8 Undesirable effects

The following adverse reactions have been reported:

(see Table 1 above)

Rarely collapse states with bradycardia and syncope, a severe fall in blood pressure accompanied by an enhancement of the anginal symptoms may occur.

Use of Glytrin may give rise to transient hypoxaemia and, in patients with coronary heart disease, ischaemia as a result of a relative redistribution of the bloodstream, which is to hypoventilated alveolar areas.

Tolerance development and the occurrence of crossed tolerance of other nitro compounds have been found in chronic, continuous treatment using high doses. To avoid a decrease in efficacy or a loss of efficacy, high continuous doses should be avoided.

4.9 Overdose

Signs and symptoms

Flushing, severe headache, vertigo, tachycardia, a feeling of suffocation, hypotension, fainting and rarely cyanosis and methaemoglobinaemia may occur. In a few patients, there may be a reaction comparable to shock with nausea, vomiting, weakness, sweating and syncope.

Treatment

Recovery often occurs without special treatment. Hypotension may be corrected by elevation of the legs to promote venous return. Methaemoglobinaemia should be treated by intravenous methylthioninium chloride and / or toluidine blue. Symptomatic treatment should be given for respiratory and circulatory defects in more serious cases.

5. PHARMACOLOGICAL PROPERTIES

5.1 Pharmacodynamic properties

ATC-Code: COIDAO2

Glyceryl trinitrate acts on vascular smooth muscles to produce arterial and venous vasodilatation. The vasodilatation results in a reduction of venous return and an improvement in myocardial perfusion with the result of a reduction in the work performed by the heart and hence reduced oxygen demand.

5.2 Pharmacokinetic properties

Glyceryl trinitrate is rapidly absorbed through the buccal and sublingual mucosa, and in man, peak concentrations in plasma are observed within four minutes of sublingual administration.

The absolute bioavailability after sublingual administration is approximately 39%. After sublingual administration the plasma levels have shown a wide range of intra and inter individual variability.

The compound is extensively metabolised by liver enzymes and has a plasma half-life of 1 – 3 minutes. The principle mechanism of metabolism involves denitration.

5.3 Preclinical safety data

Preclinical data reveal no special hazard for humans based on conventional studies of safety pharmacology, repeated dose toxicity, genotoxicity, carcinogenic potential, or toxicity to reproduction.

6. PHARMACEUTICAL PARTICULARS

6.1 List of excipients

Peppermint Oil EP

Propellant 1,1,1,2-tetrafluoroethane (HFC 134A)

Ethanol BP

6.2 Incompatibilities

None

6.3 Shelf life

Two years

6.4 Special precautions for storage

Do not store above 25°C. Do not refrigerate or freeze.

6.5 Nature and contents of container

Internally lacquered monobloc aluminium pressurised container, sealed with a metered spray valve.

The product is presented in packs with one metered dose spray.

One metered dose spray (= one aluminium container) contains 1760.0mg of solution (according to 11400.0mg of solution and propellant) providing 200 single metered doses.

6.6 Special precautions for disposal and other handling

Glytrin is an aerosol spray and contains a pressurized liquid. Do not expose to temperature higher than 50°C, and do not pierce the canister, even when empty. It should not be sprayed at a naked flame or any incandescent material.

Patients, especially those who smoke, should be warned not to use Glytrin near a naked flame.

7. MARKETING AUTHORISATION HOLDER

Ayrton Saunders Ltd.

Peninsular Business Park

Reeds Lane

Wirral

CH46 1DW

United Kingdom

8. MARKETING AUTHORISATION NUMBER(S)

PL 16431/0017

9. DATE OF FIRST AUTHORISATION/RENEWAL OF THE AUTHORISATION

25 February 2003

10. DATE OF REVISION OF THE TEXT

August 2007

Legal Category: P

Goddard's Muscle Lotion

(Actavis UK Ltd)

1. NAME OF THE MEDICINAL PRODUCT

Goddard's Muscle Lotion

2. QUALITATIVE AND QUANTITATIVE COMPOSITION

Turpentine Oil	BP	22.0% v/v
Dilute Acetic Acid	BP	30.0% v/v
Dilute Ammonia	BP	14.0% v/v

3. PHARMACEUTICAL FORM

Topical Emulsion

4. CLINICAL PARTICULARS

4.1 Therapeutic indications

For the symptomatic relief of muscular pain and stiffness, including backache, sciatica, lumbago, fibrositis, rheumatic pain and pain caused by bruises, sprains, strains, stiff muscles and unbroken chilblains.

4.2 Posology and method of administration

Once or twice daily. Shake the bottle thoroughly. Pour into palm of hand and rub well until dry.

4.3 Contraindications

None known.

4.4 Special warnings and precautions for use

If symptoms persist, consult your doctor.

Do not use if skin is broken.

For external use only.

Keep all medicines out of the reach of children.

4.5 Interaction with other medicinal products and other forms of interaction

None known.

4.6 Pregnancy and lactation

As with all medicines, medical advice should be sought prior to use.

4.7 Effects on ability to drive and use machines

None known.

4.8 Undesirable effects

None known.

4.9 Overdose

Treatment is generally supportive.

Emesis should not be induced.

Lavage should not be performed.

5. PHARMACOLOGICAL PROPERTIES

5.1 Pharmacodynamic properties

Goddards Muscle Lotion is a traditional rub for the symptomatic relief of muscular pain and stiffness.

5.2 Pharmacokinetic properties

Not applicable.

5.3 Preclinical safety data

Not applicable.

6. PHARMACEUTICAL PARTICULARS

6.1 List of excipients

Arlacel 83V

PEG-8-Oleate

Purified Water

6.2 Incompatibilities

None known.

6.3 Shelf life

22 months unopened.

6.4 Special precautions for storage

None.

6.5 Nature and contents of container

Ribbed or non-ribbed, amber or white glass bottle with a plastic cap containing a PVDC/steran faced wad (100 ml or 200 ml).

6.6 Special precautions for disposal and other handling

Not applicable.

7. MARKETING AUTHORISATION HOLDER

Actavis Group PTC ehf

Reykjavíkurvegi 76-78

220 Hafnarfjordur

Iceland.

8. MARKETING AUTHORISATION NUMBER(S)

PL 30306/0078

9. DATE OF FIRST AUTHORISATION/RENEWAL OF THE AUTHORISATION

10 March 2003

10. DATE OF REVISION OF THE TEXT

07/0409

GONAL-f 1050 IU/1.75 ml (77mcg/1.75 ml)

(Merck Serono)

1. NAME OF THE MEDICINAL PRODUCT

GONAL-f 1050 IU/1.75 ml (77 micrograms/1.75 ml) powder and solvent for solution for injection.

2. QUALITATIVE AND QUANTITATIVE COMPOSITION

One multidose vial contains 87 micrograms follitropin alfa, recombinant human follicle stimulating hormone (FSH) in order to deliver 77 micrograms, equivalent to 1050 IU. Follitropin alfa is produced in genetically engineered Chinese Hamster Ovary (CHO) cells.

Excipients: 30 mg sucrose, 1.11 mg disodium phosphate dihydrate, 0.45 mg sodium dihydrogen phosphate monohydrate

For full list of excipients, see section 6.1.

3. PHARMACEUTICAL FORM

Powder and solvent for solution for injection in a pre-filled syringe.

Appearance of the powder: white lyophilised pellet.

Appearance of the solvent: clear colourless solution.

The pH of the reconstituted solution is 6.5 – 7.5.

4. CLINICAL PARTICULARS

4.1 Therapeutic indications

• Anovulation (including polycystic ovarian disease, PCOD) in women who have been unresponsive to treatment with clomiphene citrate.

• Stimulation of multifollicular development in patients undergoing superovulation for assisted reproductive technologies (ART) such as *in vitro* fertilisation (IVF), gamete intra-fallopian transfer (GIFT) and zygote intra-fallopian transfer (ZIFT).

• GONAL-f in association with a luteinising hormone (LH) preparation is recommended for the stimulation of follicular development in women with severe LH and FSH deficiency. In clinical trials these patients were defined by an endogenous serum LH level <1.2 IU/l.

• GONAL-f is indicated for the stimulation of spermatogenesis in men who have congenital or acquired hypogonadotrophic hypogonadism with concomitant human Chorionic Gonadotrophin (hCG) therapy.

4.2 Posology and method of administration

Treatment with GONAL-f should be initiated under the supervision of a physician experienced in the treatment of fertility problems.

GONAL-f is intended for subcutaneous administration. The powder should be reconstituted prior to the first use with the solvent provided. GONAL-f 1050 IU/1.75 ml (77 micrograms/1.75 ml) preparation must not be reconstituted with any other GONAL-f container.

The dosage recommendations given for GONAL-f are those in use for urinary FSH. Clinical assessment of GONAL-f indicates that its daily doses, regimens of administration, and treatment monitoring procedures should not be different from those currently used for urinary FSH-containing preparations.

It is advised to adhere to the recommended starting doses indicated below.

Comparative clinical studies have shown that on average patients require a lower cumulative dosage and shorter treatment duration with GONAL-f compared with urinary FSH. Therefore, it is considered appropriate to give a lower total dosage of GONAL-f than generally used for urinary FSH, not only in order to optimise follicular development but also to minimise the risk of unwanted ovarian hyperstimulation. See section 5.1.

Bioequivalence has been demonstrated between equivalent doses of the monodose presentation and the multidose presentation of GONAL-f.

Women with anovulation (including PCOD):

The object of GONAL-f therapy is to develop a single mature Graafian follicle from which the ovum will be liberated after the administration of hCG.

GONAL-f may be given as a course of daily injections. In menstruating patients treatment should commence within the first 7 days of the menstrual cycle.

Treatment should be tailored to the individual patient's response as assessed by measuring follicle size by ultrasound and/or oestrogen secretion. A commonly used regimen commences at 75-150 IU FSH daily and is increased preferably by 37.5 or 75 IU at 7 or preferably 14 day intervals if necessary, to obtain an adequate, but not excessive, response. The maximal daily dose is usually not higher than 225 IU FSH. If a patient fails to respond adequately after 4 weeks of treatment, that cycle should be abandoned and the patient should recommence treatment at a higher starting dose than in the abandoned cycle.

When an optimal response is obtained, a single injection of 5 000 IU, up to 10 000 IU hCG should be administered 24-48 hours after the last GONAL-f injection. The patient is recommended to have coitus on the day of, and the day following, hCG administration. Alternatively intrauterine insemination (IUI) may be performed.

If an excessive response is obtained, treatment should be stopped and hCG withheld (see section 4.4). Treatment should recommence in the next cycle at a dosage lower than that of the previous cycle.

Women undergoing ovarian stimulation for multiple follicular development prior to *in vitro* fertilisation or other assisted reproductive technologies:

A commonly used regimen for superovulation involves the administration of 150-225 IU of GONAL-f daily, commencing on days 2 or 3 of the cycle. Treatment is continued until adequate follicular development has been achieved (as assessed by monitoring of serum oestrogen concentrations and/or ultrasound examination), with the dose adjusted according to the patient's response, to usually not higher than 450 IU daily. In general adequate follicular development is achieved on average by the tenth day of treatment (range 5 to 20 days).

A single injection of up to 10 000 IU hCG is administered 24-48 hours after the last GONAL-f injection to induce final follicular maturation.

Down-regulation with a gonadotrophin-releasing hormone (GnRH) agonist is now commonly used in order to suppress the endogenous LH surge and to control tonic levels of LH. In a commonly used protocol, GONAL-f is started approximately 2 weeks after the start of agonist treatment, both being continued until adequate follicular development is achieved. For example, following two weeks of treatment with an agonist, 150-225 IU GONAL-f are administered for the first 7 days. The dose is then adjusted according to the ovarian response.

Overall experience with IVF indicates that in general the treatment success rate remains stable during the first four attempts and gradually declines thereafter.

Women with anovulation resulting from severe LH and FSH deficiency:

In LH and FSH deficient women (hypogonadotrophic hypogonadism), the objective of GONAL-f therapy in association with lutropin alfa is to develop a single mature Graafian follicle from which the oocyte will be liberated after the administration of human chorionic gonadotrophin (hCG). GONAL-f should be given as a course of daily injections simultaneously with lutropin alfa. Since these patients are amenorrhoeic and have low endogenous oestrogen secretion, treatment can commence at any time.

Treatment should be tailored to the individual patient's response as assessed by measuring follicle size by ultrasound and oestrogen response. A recommended regimen commences at 75 IU of lutropin alfa daily with 75-150 IU FSH.

If an FSH dose increase is deemed appropriate, dose adaptation should preferably be after 7-14 day intervals and preferably by 37.5-75 IU increments. It may be acceptable to extend the duration of stimulation in any one cycle to up to 5 weeks.

When an optimal response is obtained, a single injection of 5,000 IU to 10,000 IU hCG should be administered 24-48 hours after the last GONAL-f and lutropin alfa injections. The patient is recommended to have coitus on the day of, and on the day following, hCG administration. Alternatively, intrauterine insemination (IUI) may be performed.

Luteal phase support may be considered since lack of substances with luteotrophic activity (LH/hCG) after ovulation may lead to premature failure of the corpus luteum.

If an excessive response is obtained, treatment should be stopped and hCG withheld. Treatment should recommence in the next cycle at a dose of FSH lower than that of the previous cycle.

Men with hypogonadotrophic hypogonadism:

GONAL-f should be given at a dosage of 150 IU three times a week, concomitantly with hCG, for a minimum of 4 months. If after this period, the patient has not responded, the combination treatment may be continued; current clinical experience indicates that treatment for at least 18 months may be necessary to achieve spermatogenesis.

4.3 Contraindications

GONAL-f must not be used in:

• hypersensitivity to the active substance follitropin alfa, FSH or to any of the excipients

• case of tumours of the hypothalamus and pituitary gland

and in women:

• ovarian enlargement or cyst not due to polycystic ovarian disease

• gynaecological haemorrhages of unknown aetiology

• ovarian, uterine or mammary carcinoma

GONAL-f should not be used when an effective response cannot be obtained, such as:

In women:

• primary ovarian failure

• malformations of sexual organs incompatible with pregnancy

• fibroid tumours of the uterus incompatible with pregnancy

In men:

• primary testicular insufficiency

4.4 Special warnings and precautions for use

GONAL-f is a potent gonadotrophic substance capable of causing mild to severe adverse reactions, and should only be used by physicians who are thoroughly familiar with infertility problems and their management.

Gonadotrophin therapy requires a certain time commitment by physicians and supportive health professionals, as well as the availability of appropriate monitoring facilities. In women, safe and effective use of GONAL-f calls for monitoring of ovarian response with ultrasound, alone or preferably in combination with measurement of serum oestradiol levels, on a regular basis. There may be a degree of interpatient variability in response to FSH administration, with a poor response to FSH in some patients. The lowest effective dose in relation to the treatment objective should be used in both men and women.

Self-administration of GONAL-f should only be performed by patients who are well motivated, adequately trained and with access to expert advice. During training of the patient for self-administration, special attention should be given to specific instructions for the use of the multidose presentation.

As GONAL-f multidose is intended for several injections, clear instructions should be provided to the patients to avoid misuse of the multidose presentation.

Due to a local reactivity to benzyl alcohol, the same site of injection should not be used on consecutive days.

The first injection of GONAL-f should be performed under direct medical supervision.

Patients with porphyria or a family history of porphyria should be closely monitored during treatment with GONAL-f. Deterioration or a first appearance of this condition may require cessation of treatment.

GONAL-f contains less than 1 mmol sodium (23 mg) per dose, i.e. essentially "sodium-free".

Treatment in women

Before starting treatment, the couple's infertility should be assessed as appropriate and putative contraindications for pregnancy evaluated. In particular, patients should be evaluated for hypothyroidism, adrenocortical deficiency, hyperprolactinemia and pituitary or hypothalamic tumours, and appropriate specific treatment given.

Patients undergoing stimulation of follicular growth, whether in the frame of a treatment for anovulatory infertility or ART procedures, may experience ovarian enlargement or develop hyperstimulation. Adherence to recommended GONAL-f dosage and regimen of administration, and careful monitoring of therapy will minimise the incidence of such events. Acute interpretation of the indices of follicle development and maturation require a physician whom is experienced in the interpretation of the relevant tests.

In clinical trials, an increase of the ovarian sensitivity to GONAL-f was shown when administered with lutropin alfa. If an FSH dose increase is deemed appropriate, dose adaptation should preferably be at 7-14 day intervals and preferably with 37.5-75 IU increments.

No direct comparison of GONAL-f/LH versus human menopausal gonadotrophin (hMG) has been performed. Comparison with historical data suggests that the ovulation rate obtained with GONAL-f/LH is similar to what can be obtained with hMG.

Ovarian Hyperstimulation Syndrome (OHSS)

OHSS is a medical event distinct from uncomplicated ovarian enlargement. OHSS is a syndrome that can manifest itself with increasing degrees of severity. It comprises marked ovarian enlargement, high serum sex steroids, and an increase in vascular permeability which can result in an accumulation of fluid in the peritoneal, pleural and, rarely, in the pericardial cavities.

The following symptomatology may be observed in severe cases of OHSS: abdominal pain, abdominal distension, severe ovarian enlargement, weight gain, dyspnoea, oliguria and gastrointestinal symptoms including nausea, vomiting and diarrhoea. Clinical evaluation may reveal hypovolaemia, haemoconcentration, electrolyte imbalances, ascites, haemoperitoneum, pleural effusions, hydrothorax, acute pulmonary distress, and thromboembolic events. Very rarely, severe OHSS may be complicated by pulmonary embolism, ischemic stroke and myocardial infarction.

Excessive ovarian response to gonadotrophin treatment seldom gives rise to OHSS unless hCG is administered to trigger ovulation. Therefore in cases of ovarian hyperstimulation it is prudent to withhold hCG and advise the patient to refrain from coitus or to use barrier methods for at least 4 days. OHSS may progress rapidly (within 24 hours to several days) to become a serious medical event, therefore patients should be followed for at least two weeks after hCG administration.

To minimise the risk of OHSS or of multiple pregnancy, ultrasound scans as well as oestradiol measurements are recommended. In anovulation the risk of OHSS and multiple pregnancy is increased by a serum oestradiol > 900 pg/ml (3300 pmol/l) and more than 3 follicles of 14 mm or more in diameter. In ART there is an increased risk of OHSS with a serum oestradiol > 3000 pg/ml (11000 pmol/l) and 20 or more follicles of 12 mm or more in diameter. When the oestradiol level is > 5500 pg/ml (20200 pmol/l) and where there are 40 or more follicles in total, it may be necessary to withhold hCG administration.

Adherence to recommended GONAL-f dosage, regimen of administration and careful monitoring of therapy will minimise the incidence of ovarian hyperstimulation and multiple pregnancy (see Sections 4.2 and 4.8). In ART, aspiration of all follicles prior to ovulation may reduce the occurrence of hyperstimulation.

OHSS may be more severe and more protracted if pregnancy occurs. Most often, OHSS occurs after hormonal treatment has been discontinued and reaches its maximum at about seven to ten days following treatment. Usually, OHSS resolves spontaneously with the onset of menses.

If severe OHSS occurs, gonadotrophin treatment should be stopped if still ongoing, the patient hospitalised and specific therapy for OHSS started.

This syndrome occurs with higher incidence in patients with polycystic ovarian disease.

Multiple pregnancy

Multiple pregnancy, specially high order, carries an increase risk in adverse maternal and perinatal outcomes.

In patients undergoing ovulation induction with GONAL-f, the incidence of multiple pregnancies is increased as compared with natural conception. The majority of multiple conceptions are twins. To minimise the risk of multiple

Table 1

Treatment in women		
Immune system disorders	Very rare (<1/10,000)	Mild systemic allergic reactions (e.g. mild forms of erythema, rash, facial swelling, urticaria, oedema, difficulty breathing). Serious cases of allergic reactions, including anaphylactic reactions, have also been reported.
Nervous system disorders	Very Common (>1/10)	Headache
Vascular disorders	Very rare (<1/10,000)	Thromboembolism, usually associated with severe OHSS
Respiratory, thoracic and mediastinal disorders	Very rare (<1/10,000)	Exacerbation or worsening of asthma
Gastrointestinal disorders	Common (>1/100, <1/10)	Abdominal pain and gastrointestinal symptoms such as nausea, vomiting, diarrhoea, abdominal cramps and bloating
Reproductive system and breast disorders	Very Common (>1/10)	Ovarian cysts
	Common (>1/100, <1/10)	Mild to moderate OHSS (see section 4.4)
	Uncommon (>1/1,000, <1/100)	Severe OHSS (see section 4.4)
	Rare (>1/10,000, <1/1,000)	Ovarian torsion, a complication of OHSS
General disorders and administration site conditions	Very Common (>1/10)	Mild to severe injection site reaction (pain, redness, bruising, swelling and/or irritation at the site of injection)
Treatment in men		
Skin and subcutaneous tissue disorders	Common (>1/100, <1/10)	Acne
Reproductive system and breast disorders	Common (>1/100, <1/10)	Gynaecomastia Varicocele
General disorders and administration site conditions	Very Common (>1/10)	Mild to severe injection site reaction (pain, redness, bruising, swelling and/or irritation at the site of injection)
Investigations	Common (>1/100, <1/10)	Weight gain

pregnancy, careful monitoring of ovarian response is recommended.

In patients undergoing ART procedures the risk of multiple pregnancy is related mainly to the number of embryos replaced, their quality and the patient age.

The patients should be advised of the potential risk of multiple births before starting treatment.

Pregnancy wastage

The incidence of pregnancy wastage by miscarriage or abortion is higher in patients undergoing stimulation of follicular growth for ovulation induction or ART than in the normal population.

Ectopic pregnancy

Women with a history of tubal disease are at risk of ectopic pregnancy, whether the pregnancy is obtained by spontaneous conception or with fertility treatments. The prevalence of ectopic pregnancy after IVF was reported to be 2 to 5%, as compared to 1 to 1.5% in the general population.

Reproductive system neoplasms

There have been reports of ovarian and other reproductive system neoplasms, both benign and malignant, in women who have undergone multiple drug regimens for infertility treatment. It is not yet established whether or not treatment with gonadotrophins increases the baseline risk of these tumors in infertile women.

Congenital malformation

The prevalence of congenital malformations after ART may be slightly higher than after spontaneous conceptions. This is thought to be due to differences in parental characteristics (e.g. maternal age, sperm characteristics) and multiple pregnancies.

Thromboembolic events

In women with generally recognised risk factors for thrombo-embolic events, such as personal or family history, treatment with gonadotrophins may further increase the risk. In these women, the benefits of gonadotrophin administration need to be weighed against the risks. It should be noted however, that pregnancy itself also carries an increased risk of thrombo-embolic events.

Treatment in men

Elevated endogenous FSH levels are indicative of primary testicular failure. Such patients are unresponsive to GONAL-f/hCG therapy.

Semen analysis is recommended 4 to 6 months after the beginning of treatment in assessing the response.

4.5 Interaction with other medicinal products and other forms of interaction

Concomitant use of GONAL-f with other agents used to stimulate ovulation (e.g. hCG, clomiphene citrate) may potentiate the follicular response, whereas concurrent use of a GnRH agonist to induce pituitary desensitisation may increase the dosage of GONAL-f needed to elicit an adequate ovarian response. No other clinically significant drug interaction has been reported during GONAL-f therapy.

GONAL-f should not be administered as mixture with other medicinal products in the same injection.

4.6 Pregnancy and lactation

Use during pregnancy

There is no indication for use of GONAL-f during pregnancy. No teratogenic risk has been reported, following controlled ovarian hyperstimulation, in clinical use with gonadotrophins. In case of exposure during pregnancy, clinical data are not sufficient to exclude a teratogenic effect of recombinant hFSH. However, to date, no particular malformative effect has been reported. No teratogenic effect has been observed in animal studies.

Use during lactation

GONAL-f is not indicated during lactation. During lactation, the secretion of prolactin can entail a poor prognosis to ovarian stimulation.

4.7 Effects on ability to drive and use machines

No studies on the effects on the ability to drive and use machines have been performed.

4.8 Undesirable effects

Within each frequency grouping, undesirable effects are presented in order of decreasing seriousness.

(see Table 1 above)

4.9 Overdose

The effects of an overdose of GONAL-f are unknown, nevertheless one could expect ovarian hyperstimulation syndrome to occur, which is further described in section 4.4.

5. PHARMACOLOGICAL PROPERTIES

5.1 Pharmacodynamic properties

Pharmacotherapeutic group: gonadotrophins, ATC code: G03GA05.

GONAL-f is a preparation of follicle stimulating hormone produced by genetically engineered Chinese Hamster Ovary (CHO) cells.

In women, the most important effect resulting from parenteral administration of FSH is the development of mature Graafian follicles.

In clinical trials, patients with severe FSH and LH deficiency were defined by an endogenous serum LH level <1.2 IU/l as measured in a central laboratory. However, it should be taken into account that there are variations between LH measurements performed in different laboratories.

In clinical studies comparing r-hFSH (follitropin alfa) and urinary FSH in assisted reproduction technologies (see table below) and in ovulation induction, GONAL-f was more potent than urinary FSH in terms of a lower total dose and a shorter treatment period needed to trigger follicular maturation.

In assisted reproduction technologies, GONAL-f at a lower total dose and shorter treatment period than urinary FSH, resulted in a higher number of oocytes retrieved when compared to urinary FSH.

Table: Results of study GF 8407 (randomised parallel group study comparing efficacy and safety of Gonal-f with u-FSH in assisted reproduction technologies)

	GONAL-f (n = 130)	u-FSH (n = 116)
No. of oocytes retrieved	11.0 ± 5.9	8.8 ± 4.8
Days of FSH stimulation required	11.7 ± 1.9	14.5 ± 3.3
Total dose of FSH required (no. of FSH 75 IU ampoules)	27.6 ± 10.2	40.7 ± 13.6
Need to increase the dosage (%)	56.2	85.3

Differences between the 2 groups were statistically significant ($p<0.05$) for all criteria listed.

In men deficient in FSH, GONAL-f administered concomitantly with hCG for at least 4 months induces spermatogenesis.

5.2 Pharmacokinetic properties

Following intravenous administration, GONAL-f is distributed to the extracellular fluid space with an initial half-life of around 2 hours and eliminated from the body with a terminal half-life of about one day. The steady state volume of distribution and total clearance are 10 l and 0.6 l/h, respectively. One-eighth of the GONAL-fdose is excreted in the urine.

Following subcutaneous administration, the absolute bioavailability is about 70%. Following repeated administration, GONAL-f accumulates 3-fold achieving a steady-state within 3-4 days. In women whose endogenous gonadotrophin secretion is suppressed, GONAL-f has nevertheless been shown to effectively stimulate follicular development and steroidogenesis, despite unmeasurable LH levels.

5.3 Preclinical safety data

Non-clinical data reveal no special hazard for humans based on conventional studies of single and repeated dose toxicity and genotoxicity additional to that already stated in other sections of this SPC.

In rabbits, the formulation reconstituted with 0.9% benzyl alcohol and 0.9% benzyl alcohol alone, both resulted in a slight haemorrhage and subacute inflammation after single subcutaneous injection or mild inflammatory and degenerative changes after single intramuscular injection respectively.

Impaired fertility has been reported in rats exposed to pharmacological doses of follitropin alfa (≥ 40 IU/kg/day) for extended periods, through reduced fecundity.

Given in high doses (≥ 5 IU/kg/day) follitropin alfa caused a decrease in the number of viable foetuses without being a teratogen, and dystocia similar to that observed with urinary hMG. However, since GONAL-f is not indicated in pregnancy, these data are of limited clinical relevance.

6. PHARMACEUTICAL PARTICULARS

6.1 List of excipients

Powder:

Sucrose

Sodium dihydrogen phosphate monohydrate

Disodium phosphate dihydrate

Phosphoric acid, concentrated

Sodium hydroxide

Solvent:

Water for Injections

Benzyl alcohol

6.2 Incompatibilities

In the absence of compatibility studies, this medicinal product must not be mixed with other medicinal products.

6.3 Shelf life

2 years.

The reconstituted solution is stable for 28 days.

6.4 Special precautions for storage

Prior to reconstitution, do not store above 25°C. Store in the original package.

After reconstitution, do not store above 25°C. Do not freeze. Store in the original container.

6.5 Nature and contents of container

GONAL-f is presented as a powder and solvent for injection. The powder is presented in 3 ml vials (Type I glass), with rubber stopper (bromobutyl rubber) and aluminium flip-off cap. The solvent for reconstitution is presented in 2 ml pre-filled syringes (Type I glass) with a rubber stopper. The administration syringes made of polypropylene with a stainless steel pre-fixed needle are also provided.

The product is supplied as a pack of 1 vial of powder with 1 pre-filled syringe of solvent for reconstitution and 15 disposable syringes for administration graduated in FSH units.

6.6 Special precautions for disposal and other handling

GONAL-f 1050 IU/1.75 ml (77 micrograms/1.75 ml) must be reconstituted with the 2 ml solvent provided before use.

GONAL-f 1050 IU/1.75 ml (77 micrograms/1.75 ml) preparation must not be reconstituted with any other GONAL-f containers.

The solvent pre-filled syringe provided should be used for reconstitution only and then disposed of in accordance with local requirements. A set of administration syringes graduated in FSH units is supplied in the GONAL-f Multi-dose box. Alternatively, a 1 ml syringe, graduated in ml, with pre-fixed needle for subcutaneous administration could be used. Each ml of reconstituted solution contains 600 IU r-hFSH.

The following table states the volume to be administered to deliver the prescribed dose:

Dose (IU)	Volume to be injected (ml)
75	0.13
150	0.25
225	0.38
300	0.50
375	0.63
450	0.75

Individual reconstituted vials should be for single patient use only. The next injection should be done at the same time the next day.

The reconstituted solution should not be administered if it contains particles or is not clear.

Any unused product or waste material should be disposed of in accordance with local requirements.

7. MARKETING AUTHORISATION HOLDER

Serono Europe Ltd.

56 Marsh Wall

London E14 9TP

United Kingdom

8. MARKETING AUTHORISATION NUMBER(S)

EU/1/95/001/021

9. DATE OF FIRST AUTHORISATION/RENEWAL OF THE AUTHORISATION

Date of first authorisation: 20 October 1995.

Date of last renewal: 19 October 2005.

10. DATE OF REVISION OF THE TEXT

24th July 2009

GONAL-f 300IU (22 mcg) pen

(Merck Serono)

1. NAME OF THE MEDICINAL PRODUCT

GONAL-f 300 IU/0.5 ml (22 micrograms/0.5 ml) solution for injection in a pre-filled pen.

2. QUALITATIVE AND QUANTITATIVE COMPOSITION

Follitropin alfa*, 600 IU/ml (equivalent to 44 micrograms/ml).

Each cartridge delivers 300 IU (equivalent 22 micrograms) in 0.5 ml.

* Follitropin alfa is recombinant human follicle stimulating hormone (FSH) produced by recombinant DNA technology in Chinese Hamster Ovary (CHO) cell line.

Excipients: 30 mg sucrose, 0.555 mg disodium phosphate dihydrate, 0.225 mg sodium dihydrogen phosphate monohydrate, 0.05 mg methionine, 1.5 mg m-cresol, 0.05 mg poloxamer 188.

For a full list of excipients, see section 6.1.

3. PHARMACEUTICAL FORM

Solution for injection in a pre-filled pen.

Clear colourless solution.

The pH of the solution is 6.7 - 7.3.

4. CLINICAL PARTICULARS

4.1 Therapeutic indications

• Anovulation (including polycystic ovarian disease, PCOD) in women who have been unresponsive to treatment with clomiphene citrate.

• Stimulation of multifollicular development in patients undergoing superovulation for assisted reproductive technologies (ART) such as *in vitro* fertilisation (IVF), gamete intra-fallopian transfer (GIFT) and zygote intra-fallopian transfer (ZIFT).

• GONAL-f in association with a luteinising hormone (LH) preparation is recommended for the stimulation of follicular development in women with severe LH and FSH deficiency. In clinical trials these patients were defined by an endogenous serum LH level < 1.2 IU/l.

• GONAL-f is indicated for the stimulation of spermatogenesis in men who have congenital or acquired hypogonadotrophic hypogonadism with concomitant human Chorionic Gonadotrophin (hCG) therapy.

4.2 Posology and method of administration

Treatment with GONAL-f should be initiated under the supervision of a physician experienced in the treatment of fertility problems.

GONAL-f is intended for subcutaneous administration.

The dosage recommendations given for GONAL-f are those in use for urinary FSH. Clinical assessment of GONAL-f indicates that its daily doses, regimens of administration and treatment monitoring procedures should not be different from those currently used for urinary FSH-containing preparations.

It is advised to adhere to the recommended starting doses indicated below.

Comparative clinical studies have shown that on average patients require a lower cumulative dosage and shorter treatment duration with GONAL-f compared with urinary FSH. Therefore, it is considered appropriate to give a lower total dosage of GONAL-f than generally used for urinary FSH, not only in order to optimise follicular development but also to minimise the risk of unwanted ovarian hyperstimulation. See section 5.1.

Bioequivalence has been demonstrated between equivalent doses of the monodose presentation and the multidose presentation of GONAL-f.

Women with anovulation (including PCOD):

The object of GONAL-f therapy is to develop a single mature Graafian follicle from which the ovum will be liberated after the administration of hCG.

GONAL-f may be given as a course of daily injections. In menstruating patients treatment should commence within the first 7 days of the menstrual cycle.

Treatment should be tailored to the individual patient's response as assessed by measuring follicle size by ultrasound and/or oestrogen secretion. A commonly used regimen commences at 75-150 IU FSH daily and is increased preferably by 37.5 or 75 IU at 7 or preferably 14 day intervals if necessary, to obtain an adequate, but not excessive, response. The maximal daily dose is usually not higher than 225 IU FSH. If a patient fails to respond adequately after 4 weeks of treatment, that cycle should be abandoned and the patient should recommence treatment at a higher starting dose than in the abandoned cycle.

When an optimal response is obtained, a single injection of 250 micrograms r-hCG or 5 000 IU up to 10 000 IU hCG should be administered 24-48 hours after the last GONAL-f injection. The patient is recommended to have coitus on the day of, and the day following, hCG administration. Alternatively intrauterine insemination (IUI) may be performed.

If an excessive response is obtained, treatment should be stopped and hCG withheld (see section 4.4). Treatment should recommence in the next cycle at a dosage lower than that of the previous cycle.

Women undergoing ovarian stimulation for multiple follicular development prior to *in vitro* fertilisation or other assisted reproductive technologies:

A commonly used regimen for superovulation involves the administration of 150-225 IU of GONAL-f daily, commencing on days 2 or 3 of the cycle. Treatment is continued until adequate follicular development has been achieved (as assessed by monitoring of serum oestrogen concentrations and/or ultrasound examination), with the dose adjusted according to the patient's response, to usually not higher than 450 IU daily. In general adequate follicular development is achieved on average by the tenth day of treatment (range 5 to 20 days).

A single injection of 250 micrograms r-hCG or 5 000 IU up to 10 000 IU hCG is administered 24-48 hours after the last GONAL-f injection to induce final follicular maturation.

Down-regulation with a gonadotrophin-releasing hormone (GnRH) agonist or antagonist is now commonly used in order to suppress the endogenous LH surge and to control tonic levels of LH. In a commonly used protocol, GONAL-f is started approximately 2 weeks after the start of agonist treatment, both being continued until adequate follicular development is achieved. For example, following two weeks of treatment with an agonist, 150-225 IU GONAL-f are administered for the first 7 days. The dose is then adjusted according to the ovarian response.

Overall experience with IVF indicates that in general the treatment success rate remains stable during the first four attempts and gradually declines thereafter.

Women with anovulation resulting from severe LH and FSH deficiency:

In LH and FSH deficient women (hypogonadotropic hypogonadism), the objective of GONAL-f therapy in association with lutropin alfa is to develop a single mature Graafian follicle from which the oocyte will be liberated after the administration of human chorionic gonadotrophin (hCG). GONAL-f should be given as a course of daily injections simultaneously with lutropin alfa. Since these patients are amenorrhoeic and have low endogenous oestrogen secretion, treatment can commence at any time.

Treatment should be tailored to the individual patient's response as assessed by measuring follicle size by ultrasound and oestrogen response. A recommended regimen commences at 75 IU of lutropin alfa daily with 75-150 IU FSH.

If an FSH dose increase is deemed appropriate, dose adaptation should preferably be after 7-14 day intervals and preferably by 37.5-75 IU increments. It may be acceptable to extend the duration of stimulation in any one cycle to up to 5 weeks.

When an optimal response is obtained, a single injection of 250 micrograms r-hCG or 5 000 IU up to 10 000 IU hCG should be administered 24-48 hours after the last GONAL-f and lutropin alfa injections. The patient is recommended to have coitus on the day of, and on the day following, hCG administration.

Alternatively, intrauterine insemination (IUI) may be performed.

Luteal phase support may be considered since lack of substances with luteotrophic activity (LH/hCG) after ovulation may lead to premature failure of the corpus luteum.

If an excessive response is obtained, treatment should be stopped and hCG withheld. Treatment should recommence in the next cycle at a dose of FSH lower than that of the previous cycle.

Men with hypogonadotrophic hypogonadism:

GONAL-f should be given at a dosage of 150 IU three times a week, concomitantly with hCG, for a minimum of 4 months. If after this period, the patient has not responded, the combination treatment may be continued; current clinical experience indicates that treatment for at least 18 months may be necessary to achieve spermatogenesis.

4.3 Contraindications

• Hypersensitivity to the active substance follitropin alfa, FSH or to any of the excipients

• Tumours of the hypothalamus and pituitary gland

In women:

• ovarian enlargement or cyst not due to polycystic ovarian disease

• gynaecological haemorrhages of unknown aetiology

• ovarian, uterine or mammary carcinoma

Must not be used when an effective response cannot be obtained, such as:

In women:

• primary ovarian failure

• malformations of sexual organs incompatible with pregnancy

• fibroid tumours of the uterus incompatible with pregnancy

In men:

• primary testicular insufficiency

4.4 Special warnings and precautions for use

GONAL-f is a potent gonadotrophic substance capable of causing mild to severe adverse reactions, and should only be used by physicians who are thoroughly familiar with infertility problems and their management.

Gonadotrophin therapy requires a certain time commitment by physicians and supportive health professionals, as well as the availability of appropriate monitoring facilities. In women, safe and effective use of GONAL-f calls for monitoring of ovarian response with ultrasound, alone or preferably in combination with measurement of serum oestradiol levels, on a regular basis. There may be a degree of interpatient variability in response to FSH administration, with a poor response to FSH in some patients. The lowest effective dose in relation to the treatment objective should be used in both men and women.

Self-administration of GONAL-f should only be performed by patients who are well motivated, adequately trained and have access to expert advice. During training of the patient for self-administration, special attention should be given to specific instructions for the use of the prefilled pen.

The first injection of GONAL-f should be performed under direct medical supervision.

Patients with porphyria or a family history of porphyria should be closely monitored during treatment with GONAL-f. Deterioration or a first appearance of this condition may require cessation of treatment.

GONAL-f contains less than 1 mmol sodium (23 mg) per dose, i.e. essentially "sodium-free".

Treatment in women

Before starting treatment, the couple's infertility should be assessed as appropriate and putative contraindications for pregnancy evaluated. In particular, patients should be evaluated for hypothyroidism, adrenocortical deficiency, hyperprolactinemia and pituitary or hypothalamic tumours, and appropriate specific treatment given.

Patients undergoing stimulation of follicular growth, whether as treatment for anovulatory infertility or for ART procedures, may experience ovarian enlargement or develop hyperstimulation. Adherence to the recommended GONAL-f dosage and regimen of administration, and careful monitoring of therapy will minimise the incidence of such events. For accurate interpretation of the indices of follicle development and maturation, the physician should be experienced in the interpretation of the relevant tests.

In clinical trials, an increase of the ovarian sensitivity to GONAL-f was shown when administered with lutropin alfa. If an FSH dose increase is deemed appropriate, dose adaptation should preferably be at 7-14 day intervals and preferably with 37.5-75 IU increments.

No direct comparison of GONAL-f/LH versus human menopausal gonadotrophin (hMG) has been performed. Comparison with historical data suggests that the ovulation rate obtained with GONAL-f/LH is similar to that obtained with hMG.

Ovarian Hyperstimulation Syndrome (OHSS)

OHSS is a medical event distinct from uncomplicated ovarian enlargement. OHSS is a syndrome that can manifest itself with increasing degrees of severity. It comprises marked ovarian enlargement, high serum sex steroids, and an increase in vascular permeability which can result in an accumulation of fluid in the peritoneal, pleural and, rarely, in the pericardial cavities.

The following symptomatology may be observed in severe cases of OHSS: abdominal pain, abdominal distension, severe ovarian enlargement, weight gain, dyspnoea, oliguria and gastrointestinal symptoms including nausea, vomiting and diarrhoea. Clinical evaluation may reveal hypovolaemia, haemoconcentration, electrolyte imbalances, ascites, haemoperitoneum, pleural effusions, hydrothorax, acute pulmonary distress, and thromboembolic events. Very rarely, severe OHSS may be complicated by pulmonary embolism, ischemic stroke and myocardial infarction.

Excessive ovarian response to gonadotrophin treatment seldom gives rise to OHSS unless hCG is administered to trigger ovulation. Therefore in cases of ovarian hyperstimulation it is prudent to withhold hCG and advise the patient to refrain from coitus or to use barrier methods for at least 4 days. OHSS may progress rapidly (within 24 hours to several days) to become a serious medical event, therefore patients should be followed for at least two weeks after hCG administration.

To minimise the risk of OHSS or of multiple pregnancy, ultrasound scans as well as oestradiol measurements are recommended. In anovulation the risk of OHSS and multiple pregnancy is increased by a serum oestradiol > 900 pg/ml (3300 pmol/l) and more than 3 follicles of 14 mm or more in diameter. In ART there is an increased risk of OHSS with a serum oestradiol > 3000 pg/ml (11000 pmol/l) and 20 or more follicles of 12 mm or more in diameter. When the oestradiol level is > 5500 pg/ml (20200 pmol/l) and where there are 40 or more follicles in total, it may be necessary to withhold hCG administration.

Adherence to recommended GONAL-f dosage, regimen of administration and careful monitoring of therapy will minimise the incidence of ovarian hyperstimulation and multiple pregnancy (see sections 4.2 and 4.8).

In ART, aspiration of all follicles prior to ovulation may reduce the occurrence of hyperstimulation.

OHSS may be more severe and more protracted if pregnancy occurs. Most often, OHSS occurs after hormonal treatment has been discontinued and reaches its maximum at about seven to ten days following treatment. Usually, OHSS resolves spontaneously with the onset of menses.

If severe OHSS occurs, gonadotrophin treatment should be stopped if still ongoing, the patient hospitalised and specific therapy for OHSS started.

This syndrome occurs with higher incidence in patients with polycystic ovarian disease.

Multiple pregnancy

Multiple pregnancy, specially high order, carries an increase risk in adverse maternal and perinatal outcomes.

In patients undergoing ovulation induction with GONAL-f, the incidence of multiple pregnancies is increased as compared with natural conception. The majority of multiple conceptions are twins. To minimise the risk of multiple pregnancy, careful monitoring of ovarian response is recommended.

In patients undergoing ART procedures the risk of multiple pregnancy is related mainly to the number of embryos replaced, their quality and the patient age.

The patients should be advised of the potential risk of multiple births before starting treatment.

Pregnancy wastage

The incidence of pregnancy wastage by miscarriage or abortion is higher in patients undergoing stimulation of follicular growth for ovulation induction or ART than in the normal population.

Ectopic pregnancy

Women with a history of tubal disease are at risk of ectopic pregnancy, whether the pregnancy is obtained by spontaneous conception or with fertility treatments. The prevalence of ectopic pregnancy after IVF was reported to be 2 to 5%, as compared to 1 to 1.5% in the general population.

Reproductive system neoplasms

There have been reports of ovarian and other reproductive system neoplasms, both benign and malignant, in women who have undergone multiple drug regimens for infertility treatment. It is not yet established whether or not treatment with gonadotrophins increases the baseline risk of these tumours in infertile women.

Congenital malformation

The prevalence of congenital malformations after ART may be slightly higher than after spontaneous conceptions. This is thought to be due to differences in parental characteristics (e.g. maternal age, sperm characteristics) and multiple pregnancies.

Thromboembolic events

In women with generally recognised risk factors for thrombo-embolic events, such as personal or family history, treatment with gonadotrophins may further increase the risk. In these women, the benefits of gonadotrophin administration need to be weighed against the risks. It should be noted however, that pregnancy itself also carries an increased risk of thrombo-embolic events.

Treatment in men

Elevated endogenous FSH levels are indicative of primary testicular failure. Such patients are unresponsive to GONAL-f/hCG therapy.

Semen analysis is recommended 4 to 6 months after the beginning of treatment as part of the assessment of the response.

4.5 Interaction with other medicinal products and other forms of interaction

Concomitant use of GONAL-f with other agents used to stimulate ovulation (e.g. hCG, clomiphene citrate) may potentiate the follicular response, whereas concurrent use of a GnRH agonist or antagonist to induce pituitary desensitisation may increase the dosage of GONAL-f needed to elicit an adequate ovarian response. No other clinically significant drug interaction has been reported during GONAL-f therapy.

4.6 Pregnancy and lactation

There is no indication for use of GONAL-f during pregnancy. No teratogenic risk has been reported, following controlled ovarian hyperstimulation, in clinical use with gonadotrophins. In case of exposure during pregnancy, clinical data are not sufficient to exclude a teratogenic effect of recombinant hFSH. However, to date, no particular malformative effect has been reported. No teratogenic effect has been observed in animal studies.

GONAL-f is not indicated during lactation. During lactation, the secretion of prolactin can entail a poor prognosis to ovarian stimulation.

4.7 Effects on ability to drive and use machines

No studies on the effects on the ability to drive and use machines have been performed.

4.8 Undesirable effects

Within each frequency grouping, undesirable effects are presented in order of decreasing seriousness.

(see Table 1 below)

4.9 Overdose

The effects of an overdose of GONAL-f are unknown, nevertheless one could expect ovarian hyperstimulation syndrome to occur (see section 4.4).

5. PHARMACOLOGICAL PROPERTIES

5.1 Pharmacodynamic properties

Pharmacotherapeutic group: gonadotrophins, ATC code: G03GA05.

GONAL-f is a preparation of follicle stimulating hormone produced by genetically engineered Chinese Hamster Ovary (CHO) cells.

In women, the most important effect resulting from parenteral administration of FSH is the development of mature Graafian follicles.

In clinical trials, patients with severe FSH and LH deficiency were defined by an endogenous serum LH level <1.2 IU/l as measured in a central laboratory. However, it should be taken into account that there are variations between LH measurements performed in different laboratories.

Table 1

Treatment in women		
Immune system disorders	Very rare (<1/10,000)	Mild systemic allergic reactions (e.g. mild forms of erythema, rash, facial swelling, urticaria, oedema, difficulty breathing). Serious cases of allergic reactions, including anaphylactic reactions, have also been reported.
Nervous system disorders	Very Common (>1/10)	Headache
Vascular disorders	Very rare (<1/10,000)	Thromboembolism, usually associated with severe OHSS
Respiratory, thoracic and mediastinal disorders	Very rare (<1/10,000)	Exacerbation or worsening of asthma
Gastrointestinal disorders	Common (>1/100, <1/10)	Abdominal pain and gastrointestinal symptoms such as nausea, vomiting, diarrhoea, abdominal cramps and bloating
Reproductive system and breast disorders	Very Common (>1/10)	Ovarian cysts
	Common (>1/100, <1/10)	Mild to moderate OHSS (see section 4.4)
	Uncommon (>1/1,000, <1/100)	Severe OHSS (see section 4.4)
	Rare (>1/10,000, <1/1,000)	Ovarian torsion, a complication of OHSS
General disorders and administration site conditions	Very Common (>1/10)	Mild to severe injection site reaction (pain, redness, bruising, swelling and/or irritation at the site of injection)
Treatment in men		
Skin and subcutaneous tissue disorders	Common (>1/100, <1/10)	Acne
Reproductive system and breast disorders	Common (>1/100, <1/10)	Gynaecomastia Varicocele
General disorders and administration site conditions	Very Common (>1/10)	Mild to severe injection site reaction (pain, redness, bruising, swelling and/or irritation at the site of injection)
Investigations	Common (>1/100, <1/10)	Weight gain

In clinical studies comparing r-hFSH (follitropin alfa) and urinary FSH in assisted reproduction technologies (see table below) and in ovulation induction, GONAL-f was more potent than urinary FSH in terms of a lower total dose and a shorter treatment period needed to trigger follicular maturation.

In assisted reproduction technologies, GONAL-f at a lower total dose and shorter treatment period than urinary FSH, resulted in a higher number of oocytes retrieved when compared to urinary FSH.

Table: Results of study GF 8407 (randomised parallel group study comparing efficacy and safety of Gonal-f with u-FSH in assisted reproduction technologies)

	GONAL-f (n = 130)	u-FSH (n = 116)
No. of oocytes retrieved	11.0 ± 5.9	8.8 ± 4.8
Days of FSH stimulation required	11.7 ± 1.9	14.5 ± 3.3
Total dose of FSH required (no. of FSH 75 IU ampoules)	27.6 ± 10.2	40.7 ± 13.6
Need to increase the dosage (%)	56.2	85.3

Differences between the 2 groups were statistically significant ($p < 0.05$) for all criteria listed.

In men deficient in FSH, GONAL-f administered concomitantly with hCG for at least 4 months induces spermatogenesis.

5.2 Pharmacokinetic properties

Following intravenous administration, follitropin alfa is distributed to the extracellular fluid space with an initial half-life of around 2 hours and eliminated from the body with a terminal half-life of about one day. The steady state volume of distribution and total clearance are 10 l and 0.6 l/h, respectively. One-eighth of the follitropin alfadose is excreted in the urine.

Following subcutaneous administration, the absolute bioavailability is about 70%. Following repeated administration, follitropin alfa accumulates 3-fold achieving a steady-state within 3-4 days. In women whose endogenous gonadotrophin secretion is suppressed, follitropin alfa has nevertheless been shown to effectively stimulate follicular development and steroidogenesis, despite unmeasurable LH levels.

5.3 Preclinical safety data

Non-clinical data reveal no special hazard for humans based on conventional studies of single and repeated dose toxicity and genotoxicity additional to that already stated in other sections of this SPC.

Impaired fertility has been reported in rats exposed to pharmacological doses of follitropin alfa (⩾ 40 IU/kg/day) for extended periods, through reduced fecundity.

Given in high doses (⩾5 IU/kg/day) follitropin alfa caused a decrease in the number of viable foetuses without being a teratogen, and dystocia similar to that observed with urinary hMG. However, since GONAL-f is not indicated in pregnancy, these data are of limited clinical relevance.

6. PHARMACEUTICAL PARTICULARS

6.1 List of excipients

Poloxamer 188

Sucrose

Methionine

Sodium dihydrogen phosphate monohydrate

Disodium phosphate dihydrate

m-Cresol

Phosphoric acid, concentrated

Sodium hydroxide

Water for Injections

6.2 Incompatibilities

Not applicable.

6.3 Shelf life

2 years

Once opened, the product may be stored for a maximum of 28 days at or below 25°C.

6.4 Special precautions for storage

Store in a refrigerator (2°C - 8°C). Do not freeze.

Within its shelf life, the product may be stored at or below 25°C for up to 3 months without being refrigerated again and must be discarded if it has not been used after 3 months. Store in the original package in order to protect from light.

For in-use storage conditions, see section 6.3.

6.5 Nature and contents of container

0.5 ml of solution for injection in 3 ml cartridge (Type I glass), with a plunger stopper (halobutyl rubber) and an aluminium crimp cap with a black rubber inlay.

Pack of one pre-filled pen and 5 needles to be used with the pen for administration.

6.6 Special precautions for disposal and other handling

The solution should not be administered if it contains particles or is not clear.

Any unused solution must be discarded not later than 28 days after first opening.

GONAL-f 300 IU/0.5 ml (22 micrograms/0.5 ml) is not designed to allow the cartridge to be removed.

Discard used needles immediately after injection.

Any unused product or waste material should be disposed of in accordance with local requirements.

7. MARKETING AUTHORISATION HOLDER

Serono Europe Ltd.
56 Marsh Wall
London E14 9TP
United Kingdom

8. MARKETING AUTHORISATION NUMBER(S)

EU/1/95/001/033

9. DATE OF FIRST AUTHORISATION/RENEWAL OF THE AUTHORISATION

Date of first authorisation: 20 October 1995

Date of last renewal: 19 October 2005.

10. DATE OF REVISION OF THE TEXT

24th July 2009

GONAL-f 450 IU (33 mcg) pen

(Merck Serono)

1. NAME OF THE MEDICINAL PRODUCT

GONAL-f 450 IU/0.75 ml (33 micrograms/0.75 ml) solution for injection in a pre-filled pen.

2. QUALITATIVE AND QUANTITATIVE COMPOSITION

Follitropin alfa*, 600 IU/ml (equivalent to 44 micrograms/ml).

Each cartridge delivers 450 IU (equivalent 33 micrograms) in 0.75 ml.

* Follitropin alfa is recombinant human follicle stimulating hormone (FSH) produced by recombinant DNA technology in Chinese Hamster Ovary (CHO) cell line.

Excipients: 45 mg sucrose, 0.8325 mg disodium phosphate dihydrate, 0.3375 mg sodium dihydrogen phosphate monohydrate, 0.075 mg methionine, 2.25 mg m-cresol, 0.075 mg poloxamer 188.

For a full list of excipients, see section 6.1.

3. PHARMACEUTICAL FORM

Solution for injection in a pre-filled pen.

Clear colourless solution.

The pH of the solution is 6.7 - 7.3.

4. CLINICAL PARTICULARS

4.1 Therapeutic indications

• Anovulation (including polycystic ovarian disease, PCOD) in women who have been unresponsive to treatment with clomiphene citrate.

• Stimulation of multifollicular development in patients undergoing superovulation for assisted reproductive technologies (ART) such as in vitro fertilisation (IVF), gamete intra-fallopian transfer (GIFT) and zygote intra-fallopian transfer (ZIFT).

• GONAL-f in association with a luteinising hormone (LH) preparation is recommended for the stimulation of follicular development in women with severe LH and FSH deficiency. In clinical trials these patients were defined by an endogenous serum LH level <1.2 IU/l.

• GONAL-f is indicated for the stimulation of spermatogenesis in men who have congenital or acquired hypogonadotrophic hypogonadism with concomitant human Chorionic Gonadotrophin (hCG) therapy.

4.2 Posology and method of administration

Treatment with GONAL-f should be initiated under the supervision of a physician experienced in the treatment of fertility problems.

GONAL-f is intended for subcutaneous administration.

The dosage recommendations given for GONAL-f are those in use for urinary FSH. Clinical assessment of GONAL-f indicates that its daily doses, regimens of administration and treatment monitoring procedures should not be different from those currently used for urinary FSH-containing preparations.

It is advised to adhere to the recommended starting doses indicated below.

Comparative clinical studies have shown that on average patients require a lower cumulative dosage and shorter treatment duration with GONAL-f compared with urinary FSH. Therefore, it is considered appropriate to give a lower total dosage of GONAL-f than generally used for urinary FSH, not only in order to optimise follicular development but also to minimise the risk of unwanted ovarian hyperstimulation. See section 5.1.

Bioequivalence has been demonstrated between equivalent doses of the monodose presentation and the multidose presentation of GONAL-f.

Women with anovulation (including PCOD):

The object of GONAL-f therapy is to develop a single mature Graafian follicle from which the ovum will be liberated after the administration of hCG.

GONAL-f may be given as a course of daily injections. In menstruating patients treatment should commence within the first 7 days of the menstrual cycle.

Treatment should be tailored to the individual patient's response as assessed by measuring follicle size by ultrasound and/or oestrogen secretion. A commonly used regimen commences at 75-150 IU FSH daily and is increased preferably by 37.5 or 75 IU at 7 or preferably 14 day intervals if necessary, to obtain an adequate, but not excessive, response. The maximal daily dose is usually not higher than 225 IU FSH. If a patient fails to respond adequately after 4 weeks of treatment, that cycle should be abandoned and the patient should recommence treatment at a higher starting dose than in the abandoned cycle.

When an optimal response is obtained, a single injection of 250 micrograms r-hCG or 5 000 IU up to 10 000 IU hCG should be administered 24-48 hours after the last GONAL-f injection. The patient is recommended to have coitus on the day of, and the day following, hCG administration. Alternatively intrauterine insemination (IUI) may be performed.

If an excessive response is obtained, treatment should be stopped and hCG withheld (see section 4.4). Treatment should recommence in the next cycle at a dosage lower than that of the previous cycle.

Women undergoing ovarian stimulation for multiple follicular development prior to in vitro fertilisation or other assisted reproductive technologies:

A commonly used regimen for superovulation involves the administration of 150-225 IU of GONAL-f daily, commencing on days 2 or 3 of the cycle. Treatment is continued until adequate follicular development has been achieved (as assessed by monitoring of serum oestrogen concentrations and/or ultrasound examination), with the dose adjusted according to the patient's response, to usually not higher than 450 IU daily. In general adequate follicular development is achieved on average by the tenth day of treatment (range 5 to 20 days).

A single injection of 250 micrograms r-hCG or 5 000 IU up to 10 000 IU hCG is administered 24-48 hours after the last GONAL-f injection to induce final follicular maturation.

Down-regulation with a gonadotrophin-releasing hormone (GnRH) agonist or antagonist is now commonly used in order to suppress the endogenous LH surge and to control tonic levels of LH. In a commonly used protocol, GONAL-f is started approximately 2 weeks after the start of agonist treatment, both being continued until adequate follicular development is achieved. For example, following two weeks of treatment with an agonist, 150-225 IU GONAL-f are administered for the first 7 days. The dose is then adjusted according to the ovarian response.

Overall experience with IVF indicates that in general the treatment success rate remains stable during the first four attempts and gradually declines thereafter.

Women with anovulation resulting from severe LH and FSH deficiency:

In LH and FSH deficient women (hypogonadotrophic hypogonadism), the objective of GONAL-f therapy in association with lutropin alfa is to develop a single mature Graafian follicle from which the oocyte will be liberated after the administration of human chorionic gonadotrophin (hCG). GONAL-f should be given as a course of daily injections simultaneously with lutropin alfa. Since these patients are amenorrhoeic and have low endogenous oestrogen secretion, treatment can commence at any time.

Treatment should be tailored to the individual patient's response as assessed by measuring follicle size by ultrasound and oestrogen response. A recommended regimen commences at 75 IU of lutropin alfa daily with 75-150 IU FSH.

If an FSH dose increase is deemed appropriate, dose adaptation should preferably be after 7-14 day intervals and preferably by 37.5-75 IU increments. It may be acceptable to extend the duration of stimulation in any one cycle to up to 5 weeks.

When an optimal response is obtained, a single injection of 250 micrograms r-hCG or 5 000 IU up to 10 000 IU hCG should be administered 24-48 hours after the last GONAL-f and lutropin alfa injections. The patient is recommended to have coitus on the day of, and on the day following, hCG administration.

Alternatively, intrauterine insemination (IUI) may be performed.

Luteal phase support may be considered since lack of substances with luteotrophic activity (LH/hCG) after ovulation may lead to premature failure of the corpus luteum.

If an excessive response is obtained, treatment should be stopped and hCG withheld. Treatment should recommence in the next cycle at a dose of FSH lower than that of the previous cycle.

Men with hypogonadotrophic hypogonadism:

GONAL-f should be given at a dosage of 150 IU three times a week, concomitantly with hCG, for a minimum of 4 months. If after this period, the patient has not responded, the combination treatment may be continued; current clinical experience indicates that treatment for at least 18 months may be necessary to achieve spermatogenesis.

4.3 Contraindications

• Hypersensitivity to the active substance follitropin alfa, FSH or to any of the excipients

• Tumours of the hypothalamus and pituitary gland

In women:

• ovarian enlargement or cyst not due to polycystic ovarian disease

• gynaecological haemorrhages of unknown aetiology

• ovarian, uterine or mammary carcinoma

Must not be used when an effective response cannot be obtained, such as:

In women:

• primary ovarian failure

• malformations of sexual organs incompatible with pregnancy

• fibroid tumours of the uterus incompatible with pregnancy

In men:

• primary testicular insufficiency

4.4 Special warnings and precautions for use

GONAL-f is a potent gonadotrophic substance capable of causing mild to severe adverse reactions, and should only be used by physicians who are thoroughly familiar with infertility problems and their management.

Gonadotrophin therapy requires a certain time commitment by physicians and supportive health professionals, as well as the availability of appropriate monitoring facilities. In women, safe and effective use of Gonal-f calls for monitoring of ovarian response with ultrasound, alone or preferably in combination with measurement of serum oestradiol levels, on a regular basis. There may be a degree of interpatient variability in response to FSH administration, with a poor response to FSH in some patients. The lowest effective dose in relation to the treatment objective should be used in both men and women.

Self-administration of Gonal-f should only be performed by patients who are well motivated, adequately trained and have access to expert advice. During training of the patient for self-administration, special attention should be given to specific instructions for the use of the prefilled pen.

The first injection of GONAL-f should be performed under direct medical supervision.

Patients with porphyria or a family history of porphyria should be closely monitored during treatment with GONAL-f. Deterioration or a first appearance of this condition may require cessation of treatment.

GONAL-f contains less than 1 mmol sodium (23 mg) per dose, i.e. essentially "sodium-free".

Treatment in women

Before starting treatment, the couple's infertility should be assessed as appropriate and putative contraindications for pregnancy evaluated. In particular, patients should be evaluated for hypothyroidism, adrenocortical deficiency, hyperprolactinemia and pituitary or hypothalamic tumours, and appropriate specific treatment given.

Patients undergoing stimulation of follicular growth, whether as treatment for anovulatory infertility or for ART procedures, may experience ovarian enlargement or develop hyperstimulation. Adherence to the recommended Gonal-f dosage and regimen of administration, and careful monitoring of therapy will minimise the incidence of such events. For accurate interpretation of the indices of follicle development and maturation, the physician should be experienced in the interpretation of the relevant tests.

In clinical trials, an increase of the ovarian sensitivity to GONAL-f was shown when administered with lutropin alfa. If an FSH dose increase is deemed appropriate, dose adaptation should preferably be at 7-14 day intervals and preferably with 37.5-75 IU increments.

No direct comparison of GONAL-f/LH versus human menopausal gonadotrophin (hMG) has been performed. Comparison with historical data suggests that the ovulation rate obtained with GONAL-f/LH is similar to that obtained with hMG.

Ovarian Hyperstimulation Syndrome (OHSS)

OHSS is a medical event distinct from uncomplicated ovarian enlargement. OHSS is a syndrome that can manifest itself with increasing degrees of severity. It comprises marked ovarian enlargement, high serum sex steroids, and an increase in vascular permeability which can result in an accumulation of fluid in the peritoneal, pleural and, rarely, in the pericardial cavities.

The following symptomatology may be observed in severe cases of OHSS: abdominal pain, abdominal distension, severe ovarian enlargement, weight gain, dyspnoea, oliguria and gastrointestinal symptoms including nausea, vomiting and diarrhoea. Clinical evaluation may reveal hypovolaemia, haemoconcentration, electrolyte imbalances, ascites, haemoperitoneum, pleural effusions, hydrothorax, acute pulmonary distress, and thromboembolic events. Very rarely, severe OHSS may be complicated by pulmonary embolism, ischemic stroke and myocardial infarction.

Excessive ovarian response to gonadotrophin treatment seldom gives rise to OHSS unless hCG is administered to trigger ovulation. Therefore in cases of ovarian hyperstimulation it is prudent to withhold hCG and advise the patient to refrain from coitus or to use barrier methods for at least 4 days. OHSS may progress rapidly (within 24 hours to several days) to become a serious medical event, therefore patients should be followed for at least two weeks after hCG administration.

To minimise the risk of OHSS or of multiple pregnancy, ultrasound scans as well as oestradiol measurements are recommended. In anovulation the risk of OHSS and multiple pregnancy is increased by a serum oestradiol > 900 pg/ml (3300 pmol/l) and more than 3 follicles of 14 mm or more in diameter. In ART there is an increased risk of OHSS with a serum oestradiol > 3000 pg/ml (11000 pmol/l) and 20 or more follicles of 12 mm or more in diameter. When the oestradiol level is > 5500 pg/ml (20200 pmol/l) and where there are 40 or more follicles in total, it may be necessary to withhold hCG administration.

Adherence to recommended GONAL-f dosage, regimen of administration and careful monitoring of therapy will minimise the incidence of ovarian hyperstimulation and multiple pregnancy (see sections 4.2 and 4.8).

In ART, aspiration of all follicles prior to ovulation may reduce the occurrence of hyperstimulation.

OHSS may be more severe and more protracted if pregnancy occurs. Most often, OHSS occurs after hormonal treatment has been discontinued and reaches its maximum at about seven to ten days following treatment. Usually, OHSS resolves spontaneously with the onset of menses.

If severe OHSS occurs, gonadotrophin treatment should be stopped if still ongoing, the patient hospitalised and specific therapy for OHSS started.

This syndrome occurs with higher incidence in patients with polycystic ovarian disease.

Multiple pregnancy

Multiple pregnancy, specially high order, carries an increase risk in adverse maternal and perinatal outcomes.

In patients undergoing ovulation induction with GONAL-f, the incidence of multiple pregnancies is increased as compared with natural conception. The majority of multiple conceptions are twins. To minimise the risk of multiple pregnancy, careful monitoring of ovarian response is recommended.

In patients undergoing ART procedures the risk of multiple pregnancy is related mainly to the number of embryos replaced, their quality and the patient age.

The patients should be advised of the potential risk of multiple births before starting treatment.

Pregnancy wastage

The incidence of pregnancy wastage by miscarriage or abortion is higher in patients undergoing stimulation of follicular growth for ovulation induction or ART than in the normal population.

Ectopic pregnancy

Women with a history of tubal disease are at risk of ectopic pregnancy, whether the pregnancy is obtained by spontaneous conception or with fertility treatments. The prevalence of ectopic pregnancy after IVF was reported to be 2 to 5%, as compared to 1 to 1.5% in the general population.

Reproductive system neoplasms

There have been reports of ovarian and other reproductive system neoplasms, both benign and malignant, in women who have undergone multiple drug regimens for infertility treatment. It is not yet established whether or not treatment with gonadotrophins increases the baseline risk of these tumours in infertile women.

Congenital malformation

The prevalence of congenital malformations after ART may be slightly higher than after spontaneous conceptions. This is thought to be due to differences in parental characteristics (e.g. maternal age, sperm characteristics) and multiple pregnancies.

Thromboembolic events

In women with generally recognised risk factors for thrombo-embolic events, such as personal or family history, treatment with gonadotrophins may further increase the risk. In these women, the benefits of gonadotrophin administration need to be weighed against the risks. It should be noted however, that pregnancy itself also carries an increased risk of thrombo-embolic events.

Treatment in men

Elevated endogenous FSH levels are indicative of primary testicular failure. Such patients are unresponsive to GONAL-f/hCG therapy.

Semen analysis is recommended 4 to 6 months after the beginning of treatment as part of the assessment of the response.

Table 1

Treatment in women		
Immune system disorders	Very rare (< 1/10,000)	Mild systemic allergic reactions (e.g. mild forms of erythema, rash, facial swelling, urticaria, oedema, difficulty breathing). Serious cases of allergic reactions, including anaphylactic reactions, have also been reported.
Nervous system disorders	Very Common (> 1/10)	Headache
Vascular disorders	Very rare (< 1/10,000)	Thromboembolism, usually associated with severe OHSS
Respiratory, thoracic and mediastinal disorders	Very rare (< 1/10,000)	Exacerbation or worsening of asthma
Gastrointestinal disorders	Common (> 1/100, < 1/10)	Abdominal pain and gastrointestinal symptoms such as nausea, vomiting, diarrhoea, abdominal cramps and bloating
Reproductive system and breast disorders	Very Common (> 1/10)	Ovarian cysts
	Common (> 1/100, < 1/10)	Mild to moderate OHSS (see section 4.4)
	Uncommon (> 1/1,000, < 1/100)	Severe OHSS (see section 4.4)
	Rare (> 1/10,000, < 1/1,000)	Ovarian torsion, a complication of OHSS
General disorders and administration site conditions	Very Common (> 1/10)	Mild to severe injection site reaction (pain, redness, bruising, swelling and/ or irritation at the site of injection)
Treatment in men		
Skin and subcutaneous tissue disorders	Common (> 1/100, < 1/10)	Acne
Reproductive system and breast disorders	Common (> 1/100, < 1/10)	Gynaecomastia Varicocele
General disorders and administration site conditions	Very Common (> 1/10)	Mild to severe injection site reaction (pain, redness, bruising, swelling and/ or irritation at the site of injection)
Investigations	Common (> 1/100, < 1/10)	Weight gain

4.5 Interaction with other medicinal products and other forms of interaction

Concomitant use of GONAL-f with other agents used to stimulate ovulation (e.g. hCG, clomiphene citrate) may potentiate the follicular response, whereas concurrent use of a GnRH agonist or antagonist to induce pituitary desensitisation may increase the dosage of GONAL-f needed to elicit an adequate ovarian response. No other clinically significant drug interaction has been reported during GONAL-f therapy.

4.6 Pregnancy and lactation

There is no indication for use of GONAL-f during pregnancy. No teratogenic risk has been reported, following controlled ovarian hyperstimulation, in clinical use with gonadotrophins. In case of exposure during pregnancy, clinical data are not sufficient to exclude a teratogenic effect of recombinant hFSH. However, to date, no particular malformative effect has been reported. No teratogenic effect has been observed in animal studies.

GONAL-f is not indicated during lactation. During lactation, the secretion of prolactin can entail a poor prognosis to ovarian stimulation.

4.7 Effects on ability to drive and use machines

No studies on the effects on the ability to drive and use machines have been performed.

4.8 Undesirable effects

Within each frequency grouping, undesirable effects are presented in order of decreasing seriousness.

(see Table 1 on previous page)

4.9 Overdose

The effects of an overdose of GONAL-f are unknown, nevertheless one could expect ovarian hyperstimulation syndrome to occur (see section 4.4).

5. PHARMACOLOGICAL PROPERTIES

5.1 Pharmacodynamic properties

Pharmacotherapeutic group: gonadotrophins, ATC code: G03GA05.

GONAL-f is a preparation of follicle stimulating hormone produced by genetically engineered Chinese Hamster Ovary (CHO) cells.

In women, the most important effect resulting from parenteral administration of FSH is the development of mature Graafian follicles.

In clinical trials, patients with severe FSH and LH deficiency were defined by an endogenous serum LH level <1.2 IU/l as measured in a central laboratory. However, it should be taken into account that there are variations between LH measurements performed in different laboratories.

In clinical studies comparing r-hFSH (follitropin alfa) and urinary FSH in assisted reproduction technologies (see table below) and in ovulation induction, GONAL-f was more potent than urinary FSH in terms of a lower total dose and a shorter treatment period needed to trigger follicular maturation.

In assisted reproduction technologies, GONAL-f at a lower total dose and shorter treatment period than urinary FSH, resulted in a higher number of oocytes retrieved when compared to urinary FSH.

Table: Results of study GF 8407 (randomised parallel group study comparing efficacy and safety of Gonal-f with u-FSH in assisted reproduction technologies)

	GONAL-f (n = 130)	u-FSH (n = 116)
No. of oocytes retrieved	11.0 ± 5.9	8.8 ± 4.8
Days of FSH stimulation required	11.7 ± 1.9	14.5 ± 3.3
Total dose of FSH required (no. of FSH 75 IU ampoules)	27.6 ± 10.2	40.7 ± 13.6
Need to increase the dosage (%)	56.2	85.3

Differences between the 2 groups were statistically significant ($p < 0.05$) for all criteria listed.

In men deficient in FSH, GONAL-f administered concomitantly with hCG for at least 4 months induces spermatogenesis.

5.2 Pharmacokinetic properties

Following intravenous administration, follitropin alfa is distributed to the extracellular fluid space with an initial half-life of around 2 hours and eliminated from the body with a terminal half-life of about one day. The steady state volume of distribution and total clearance are 10 l and 0.6 l/h, respectively. One-eighth of the follitropin alfa dose is excreted in the urine.

Following subcutaneous administration, the absolute bioavailability is about 70%. Following repeated administration, follitropin alfa accumulates 3-fold achieving a steady-state within 3-4 days. In women whose endogenous gonadotrophin secretion is suppressed, follitropin alfa has nevertheless been shown to effectively stimulate follicular development and steroidogenesis, despite unmeasurable LH levels.

5.3 Preclinical safety data

Non-clinical data reveal no special hazard for humans based on conventional studies of single and repeated dose toxicity and genotoxicity additional to that already stated in other sections of this SPC.

Impaired fertility has been reported in rats exposed to pharmacological doses of follitropin alfa (≥ 40 IU/kg/day) for extended periods, through reduced fecundity.

Given in high doses (5 IU/kg/day) follitropin alfa caused a decrease in the number of viable foetuses without being a teratogen, and dystocia similar to that observed with urinary hMG. However, since GONAL-f is not indicated in pregnancy, these data are of limited clinical relevance.

6. PHARMACEUTICAL PARTICULARS

6.1 List of excipients

Poloxamer 188

Sucrose

Methionine

Sodium dihydrogen phosphate monohydrate

Disodium phosphate dihydrate

m-Cresol

Phosphoric acid, concentrated

Sodium hydroxide

Water for Injections

6.2 Incompatibilities

Not applicable.

6.3 Shelf life

2 years.

Once opened, the product may be stored for a maximum of 28 days at or below 25°C.

6.4 Special precautions for storage

Store in a refrigerator (2°C - 8°C). Do not freeze.

Within its shelf life, the product may be stored at or below 25°C for up to 3 months without being refrigerated again and must be discarded if it has not been used after 3 months.

Store in the original package in order to protect from light.

For in-use storage conditions, see section 6.3.

6.5 Nature and contents of container

0.75 ml of solution for injection in 3 ml cartridge (Type I glass), with a plunger stopper (halobutyl rubber) and an aluminium crimp cap with a black rubber inlay.

Pack of one pre-filled pen and 7 needles to be used with the pen for administration.

6.6 Special precautions for disposal and other handling

The solution should not be administered if it contains particles or is not clear.

Any unused solution must be discarded not later than 28 days after first opening.

GONAL-f 450 IU/0.75 ml (33 micrograms/0.75 ml) is not designed to allow the cartridge to be removed.

Discard used needles immediately after injection.

Any unused product or waste material should be disposed of in accordance with local requirements.

7. MARKETING AUTHORISATION HOLDER

Serono Europe Ltd.
56 Marsh Wall
London E14 9TP
United Kingdom

8. MARKETING AUTHORISATION NUMBER(S)

EU/1/95/001/034

9. DATE OF FIRST AUTHORISATION/RENEWAL OF THE AUTHORISATION

Date of first authorisation: 20 October 1995.

Date of last renewal: 19 October 2005.

10. DATE OF REVISION OF THE TEXT

24th July 2009

GONAL-f 450 IU/0.75 ml (33 mcg/0.75ml)

(Merck Serono)

1. NAME OF THE MEDICINAL PRODUCT

GONAL-f 450 IU/0.75 ml (33 micrograms/0.75 ml) powder and solvent for solution for injection.

2. QUALITATIVE AND QUANTITATIVE COMPOSITION

One multidose vial contains 44 micrograms follitropin alfa, recombinant human follicle stimulating hormone (FSH) in order to deliver 33 micrograms, equivalent to 450 IU. Follitropin alfa is produced in genetically engineered Chinese Hamster Ovary (CHO) cells.

Excipients: 30 mg sucrose, 1.11 mg disodium phosphate dihydrate, 0.45 mg sodium dihydrogen phosphate monohydrate.

For a full list of excipients, see section 6.1.

3. PHARMACEUTICAL FORM

Powder and solvent for solution for injection in a pre-filled syringe.

Appearance of the powder: white lyophilised pellet.

Appearance of the solvent: clear colourless solution.

The pH of the reconstituted solution is 6.5 - 7.5.

4. CLINICAL PARTICULARS

4.1 Therapeutic indications

- Anovulation (including polycystic ovarian disease, PCOD) in women who have been unresponsive to treatment with clomiphene citrate.
- Stimulation of multifollicular development in patients undergoing superovulation for assisted reproductive technologies (ART) such as *in vitro* fertilisation (IVF), gamete intra-fallopian transfer (GIFT) and zygote intra-fallopian transfer (ZIFT).
- GONAL-f in association with a luteinising hormone (LH) preparation is recommended for the stimulation of follicular development in women with severe LH and FSH deficiency. In clinical trials these patients were defined by an endogenous serum LH level <1.2 IU/l.
- GONAL-f is indicated for the stimulation of spermatogenesis in men who have congenital or acquired hypogonadotrophic hypogonadism with concomitant human Chorionic Gonadotrophin (hCG) therapy.

4.2 Posology and method of administration

Treatment with GONAL-f should be initiated under the supervision of a physician experienced in the treatment of fertility problems.

GONAL-f is intended for subcutaneous administration. The powder should be reconstituted prior to the first use with the solvent provided. GONAL-f 450 IU/0.75 ml (33 micrograms/0.75 ml) preparation must not be reconstituted with any other GONAL-f containers.

The dosage recommendations given for GONAL-f are those in use for urinary FSH. Clinical assessment of GONAL-f indicates that its daily doses, regimens of administration, and treatment monitoring procedures should not be different from those currently used for urinary FSH-containing preparations.

It is advised to adhere to the recommended starting doses indicated below.

Comparative clinical studies have shown that on average patients require a lower cumulative dosage and shorter treatment duration with GONAL-f compared with urinary FSH. Therefore, it is considered appropriate to give a lower total dosage of GONAL-f than generally used for urinary FSH, not only in order to optimise follicular development but also to minimise the risk of unwanted ovarian hyperstimulation. See section 5.1.

Bioequivalence has been demonstrated between equivalent doses of the monodose presentation and the multi-dose presentation of GONAL-f.

Women with anovulation (including PCOD):

The object of GONAL-f therapy is to develop a single mature Graafian follicle from which the ovum will be liberated after the administration of hCG.

GONAL-f may be given as a course of daily injections. In menstruating patients treatment should commence within the first 7 days of the menstrual cycle.

Treatment should be tailored to the individual patient's response as assessed by measuring follicle size by ultrasound and/or oestrogen secretion. A commonly used regimen commences at 75-150 IU FSH daily and is increased preferably by 37.5 or 75 IU at 7 or preferably 14 day intervals if necessary, to obtain an adequate, but not excessive, response. The maximal daily dose is usually not higher than 225 IU FSH. If a patient fails to respond adequately after 4 weeks of treatment, that cycle should be abandoned and the patient should recommence treatment at a higher starting dose than in the abandoned cycle.

When an optimal response is obtained, a single injection of 5 000 IU, up to 10 000 IU hCG should be administered 24-48 hours after the last GONAL-f injection. The patient is recommended to have coitus on the day of, and the day following, hCG administration. Alternatively intrauterine insemination (IUI) may be performed.

If an excessive response is obtained, treatment should be stopped and hCG withheld (see section 4.4). Treatment should recommence in the next cycle at a dosage lower than that of the previous cycle.

Women undergoing ovarian stimulation for multiple follicular development prior to *in vitro* fertilisation or other assisted reproductive technologies:

A commonly used regimen for superovulation involves the administration of 150-225 IU of GONAL-f daily, commencing on days 2 or 3 of the cycle. Treatment is continued until adequate follicular development has been achieved (as assessed by monitoring of serum oestrogen concentrations and/or ultrasound examination), with the dose adjusted according to the patient's response, to usually not higher than 450 IU daily. In general adequate follicular development is achieved on average by the tenth day of treatment (range 5 to 20 days).

A single injection of up to 10 000 IU hCG is administered 24-48 hours after the last GONAL-f injection to induce final follicular maturation.

Down-regulation with a gonadotrophin-releasing hormone (GnRH) agonist is now commonly used in order to suppress the endogenous LH surge and to control tonic levels of LH. In a commonly used protocol, GONAL-f is started approximately 2 weeks after the start of agonist treatment, both being continued until adequate follicular development is achieved. For example, following two weeks of treatment with an agonist, 150-225 IU GONAL-f are administered for the first 7 days. The dose is then adjusted according to the ovarian response.

Overall experience with IVF indicates that in general the treatment success rate remains stable during the first four attempts and gradually declines thereafter.

Women with anovulation resulting from severe LH and FSH deficiency:

In LH and FSH deficient women (hypogonadotrophic hypogonadism), the objective of GONAL-f therapy in association with lutropin alfa is to develop a single mature Graafian follicle from which the oocyte will be liberated after the administration of human chorionic gonadotrophin (hCG). GONAL-f should be given as a course of daily injections simultaneously with lutropin alfa. Since these patients are amenorrhoeic and have low endogenous oestrogen secretion, treatment can commence at any time.

Treatment should be tailored to the individual patient's response as assessed by measuring follicle size by ultrasound and oestrogen response. A recommended regimen commences at 75 IU of lutropin alfa daily with 75-150 IU FSH.

If an FSH dose increase is deemed appropriate, dose adaptation should preferably be after 7-14 day intervals and preferably by 37.5-75 IU increments. It may be acceptable to extend the duration of stimulation in any one cycle to up to 5 weeks.

When an optimal response is obtained, a single injection of 5,000 IU to 10,000 IU hCG should be administered 24-48 hours after the last GONAL-f and lutropin alfa injections. The patient is recommended to have coitus on the day of, and on the day following, hCG administration. Alternatively, intrauterine insemination (IUI) may be performed.

Luteal phase support may be considered since lack of substances with luteotrophic activity (LH/hCG) after ovulation may lead to premature failure of the corpus luteum.

If an excessive response is obtained, treatment should be stopped and hCG withheld. Treatment should recommence in the next cycle at a dose of FSH lower than that of the previous cycle.

Men with hypogonadotrophic hypogonadism:

GONAL-f should be given at a dosage of 150 IU three times a week, concomitantly with hCG, for a minimum of 4 months. If after this period, the patient has not responded, the combination treatment may be continued; current clinical experience indicates that treatment for at least 18 months may be necessary to achieve spermatogenesis.

4.3 Contraindications

GONAL-f must not be used in:

- hypersensitivity to the active substance follitropin alfa, FSH or to any of the excipients
- case of tumours of the hypothalamus and pituitary gland

and in women:

- ovarian enlargement or cyst not due to polycystic ovarian disease
- gynaecological haemorrhages of unknown aetiology
- ovarian, uterine or mammary carcinoma

GONAL-f should not be used when an effective response cannot be obtained, such as:

In women:

- primary ovarian failure
- malformations of sexual organs incompatible with pregnancy
- fibroid tumours of the uterus incompatible with pregnancy

In men:

- primary testicular insufficiency

4.4 Special warnings and precautions for use

GONAL-f is a potent gonadotrophic substance capable of causing mild to severe adverse reactions, and should only be used by physicians who are thoroughly familiar with infertility problems and their management.

Gonadotrophin therapy requires a certain time commitment by physicians and supportive health professionals, as well as the availability of appropriate monitoring facilities. In women, safe and effective use of GONAL-f calls for monitoring of ovarian response with ultrasound, alone or preferably in combination with measurement of serum oestradiol levels, on a regular basis. There may be a degree of interpatient variability in response to FSH administration, with a poor response to FSH in some patients. The lowest effective dose in relation to the treatment objective should be used in both men and women.

Self-administration of GONAL-f should only be performed by patients who are well motivated, adequately trained and with access to expert advice. During training of the patient for self-administration, special attention should be given to specific instructions for the use of the multidose presentation.

As GONAL-f multidose is intended for several injections, clear instructions should be provided to the patients to avoid misuse of the multidose presentation.

Due to a local reactivity to benzyl alcohol, the same site of injection should not be used on consecutive days.

The first injection of GONAL-f should be performed under direct medical supervision.

Patients with porphyria or a family history of porphyria should be closely monitored during treatment with GONAL-f. Deterioration or a first appearance of this condition may require cessation of treatment.

GONAL-f contains less than 1 mmol sodium (23 mg) per dose, i.e. essentially "sodium-free".

Treatment in women

Before starting treatment, the couple's infertility should be assessed as appropriate and putative contraindications for pregnancy evaluated. In particular, patients should be evaluated for hypothyroidism, adrenocortical deficiency, hyperprolactinemia and pituitary or hypothalamic tumours, and appropriate specific treatment given.

Patients undergoing stimulation of follicular growth, whether in the frame of a treatment for anovulatory infertility or ART procedures, may experience ovarian enlargement or develop hyperstimulation. Adherence to recommended GONAL-f dosage and regimen of administration, and careful monitoring of therapy will minimise the incidence of such events. Acute interpretation of the indices of follicle development and maturation require a physician whom is experienced in the interpretation of the relevant tests.

In clinical trials, an increase of the ovarian sensitivity to GONAL-f was shown when administered with lutropin alfa. If an FSH dose increase is deemed appropriate, dose adaptation should preferably be at 7-14 day intervals and preferably with 37.5-75 IU increments.

No direct comparison of GONAL-f/LH versus human menopausal gonadotrophin (hMG) has been performed. Comparison with historical data suggests that the ovulation rate obtained with GONAL-f/LH is similar to what can be obtained with hMG.

Ovarian Hyperstimulation Syndrome (OHSS)

OHSS is a medical event distinct from uncomplicated ovarian enlargement. OHSS is a syndrome that can manifest itself with increasing degrees of severity. It comprises marked ovarian enlargement, high serum sex steroids, and an increase in vascular permeability which can result in an accumulation of fluid in the peritoneal, pleural and, rarely, in the pericardial cavities.

The following symptomatology may be observed in severe cases of OHSS: abdominal pain, abdominal distension, severe ovarian enlargement, weight gain, dyspnoea, oliguria and gastrointestinal symptoms including nausea, vomiting and diarrhoea. Clinical evaluation may reveal hypovolaemia, haemoconcentration, electrolyte imbalances, ascites, haemoperitoneum, pleural effusions, hydrothorax, acute pulmonary distress, and thromboembolic events. Very rarely, severe OHSS may be complicated by pulmonary embolism, ischemic stroke and myocardial infarction.

Excessive ovarian response to gonadotrophin treatment seldom gives rise to OHSS unless hCG is administered to trigger ovulation. Therefore in cases of ovarian hyperstimulation it is prudent to withhold hCG and advise the patient to refrain from coitus or to use barrier methods for at least 4 days. OHSS may progress rapidly (within 24 hours to several days) to become a serious medical event, therefore patients should be followed for at least two weeks after hCG administration.

To minimise the risk of OHSS or of multiple pregnancy, ultrasound scans as well as oestradiol measurements are recommended. In anovulation the risk of OHSS and multiple pregnancy is increased by a serum oestradiol $>$ 900 pg/ml (3300 pmol/l) and more than 3 follicles of 14 mm or more in diameter. In ART there is an increased risk of OHSS with a serum oestradiol $>$ 3000 pg/ml (11000 pmol/l) and 20 or more follicles of 12 mm or more in diameter. When the oestradiol level is $>$ 5500 pg/ml (20200 pmol/l) and where there are 40 or more follicles in total, it may be necessary to withhold hCG administration.

Adherence to recommended GONAL-f dosage, regimen of administration and careful monitoring of therapy will minimise the incidence of ovarian hyperstimulation and multiple pregnancy (see Sections 4.2 and 4.8).

In ART, aspiration of all follicles prior to ovulation may reduce the occurrence of hyperstimulation.

OHSS may be more severe and more protracted if pregnancy occurs. Most often, OHSS occurs after hormonal treatment has been discontinued and reaches its maximum at about seven to ten days following treatment. Usually, OHSS resolves spontaneously with the onset of menses.

If severe OHSS occurs, gonadotrophin treatment should be stopped if still ongoing, the patient hospitalised and specific therapy for OHSS started.

This syndrome occurs with higher incidence in patients with polycystic ovarian disease.

Multiple pregnancy

Multiple pregnancy, specially high order, carries an increase risk in adverse maternal and perinatal outcomes.

In patients undergoing ovulation induction with GONAL-f, the incidence of multiple pregnancies is increased as compared with natural conception. The majority of multiple conceptions are twins. To minimise the risk of multiple pregnancy, careful monitoring of ovarian response is recommended.

In patients undergoing ART procedures the risk of multiple pregnancy is related mainly to the number of embryos replaced, their quality and the patient age.

The patients should be advised of the potential risk of multiple births before starting treatment.

Pregnancy wastage

The incidence of pregnancy wastage by miscarriage or abortion is higher in patients undergoing stimulation of follicular growth for ovulation induction or ART than in the normal population.

Ectopic pregnancy

Women with a history of tubal disease are at risk of ectopic pregnancy, whether the pregnancy is obtained by spontaneous conception or with fertility treatments. The prevalence of ectopic pregnancy after IVF was reported to be 2 to 5%, as compared to 1 to 1.5% in the general population.

Reproductive system neoplasms

There have been reports of ovarian and other reproductive system neoplasms, both benign and malignant, in women who have undergone multiple drug regimens for infertility treatment. It is not yet established whether or not treatment with gonadotrophins increases the baseline risk of these tumors in infertile women.

Congenital malformation

The prevalence of congenital malformations after ART may be slightly higher than after spontaneous conceptions. This is thought to be due to differences in parental characteristics (e.g. maternal age, sperm characteristics) and multiple pregnancies.

Thromboembolic events

In women with generally recognised risk factors for thrombo-embolic events, such as personal or family history, treatment with gonadotrophins may further increase the risk. In these women, the benefits of gonadotrophin administration need to be weighed against the risks. It should be noted however, that pregnancy itself also carries an increased risk of thrombo-embolic events.

Treatment in men

Elevated endogenous FSH levels are indicative of primary testicular failure. Such patients are unresponsive to GONAL-f/hCG therapy.

Semen analysis is recommended 4 to 6 months after the beginning of treatment in assessing the response.

4.5 Interaction with other medicinal products and other forms of interaction

Concomitant use of GONAL-f with other agents used to stimulate ovulation (e.g. hCG, clomiphene citrate) may potentiate the follicular response, whereas concurrent use of a GnRH agonist to induce pituitary desensitisation may increase the dosage of GONAL-f needed to elicit an adequate ovarian response. No other clinically significant drug interaction has been reported during GONAL-f therapy.

GONAL-f should not be administered as mixture with other medicinal products in the same injection.

4.6 Pregnancy and lactation

Use during pregnancy

There is no indication for use of GONAL-f during pregnancy. No teratogenic risk has been reported, following controlled ovarian hyperstimulation, in clinical use with gonadotrophins. In case of exposure during pregnancy, clinical data are not sufficient to exclude a teratogenic effect of recombinant hFSH. However, to date, no particular malformative effect has been reported. No teratogenic effect has been observed in animal studies.

Use during lactation

GONAL-f is not indicated during lactation. During lactation, the secretion of prolactin can entail a poor prognosis to ovarian stimulation.

4.7 Effects on ability to drive and use machines

No studies on the effects on ability to drive and use machines have been performed.

4.8 Undesirable effects

Within each frequency grouping, undesirable effects are presented in order of decreasing seriousness.

(see Table 1 on next page)

4.9 Overdose

The effects of an overdose of GONAL-f are unknown, nevertheless one could expect ovarian hyperstimulation syndrome to occur, which is further described in section 4.4.

5. PHARMACOLOGICAL PROPERTIES

5.1 Pharmacodynamic properties

Pharmacotherapeutic group: gonadotrophins, ATC code: G03GA05.

Table 1

Treatment in women		
Immune system disorders	Very rare (<1/10,000)	Mild systemic allergic reactions (e.g. mild forms of erythema, rash, facial swelling, urticaria, oedema, difficulty breathing). Serious cases of allergic reactions, including anaphylactic reactions, have also been reported.
Nervous system disorders	Very Common (>1/10)	Headache
Vascular disorders	Very rare (<1/10,000)	Thromboembolism, usually associated with severe OHSS
Respiratory, thoracic and mediastinal disorders	Very rare (<1/10,000)	Exacerbation or worsening of asthma
Gastrointestinal disorders	Common (>1/100, <1/10)	Abdominal pain and gastrointestinal symptoms such as nausea, vomiting, diarrhoea, abdominal cramps and bloating
Reproductive system and breast disorders	Very Common (>1/10)	Ovarian cysts
	Common (>1/100, <1/10)	Mild to moderate OHSS (see section 4.4)
	Uncommon (>1/1,000, <1/100)	Severe OHSS (see section 4.4)
	Rare (>1/10,000, <1/1,000)	Ovarian torsion, a complication of OHSS
General disorders and administration site conditions	Very Common (>1/10)	Mild to severe injection site reaction (pain, redness, bruising, swelling and/or irritation at the site of injection)
Treatment in men		
Skin and subcutaneous tissue disorders	Common (>1/100, <1/10)	Acne
Reproductive system and breast disorders	Common (>1/100, <1/10)	Gynaecomastia Varicocele
General disorders and administration site conditions	Very Common (>1/10)	Mild to severe injection site reaction (pain, redness, bruising, swelling and/or irritation at the site of injection)
Investigations	Common (>1/100, <1/10)	Weight gain

GONAL-f is a preparation of follicle stimulating hormone produced by genetically engineered Chinese Hamster Ovary (CHO) cells.

In women, the most important effect resulting from parenteral administration of FSH is the development of mature Graafian follicles.

In clinical trials, patients with severe FSH and LH deficiency were defined by an endogenous serum LH level <1.2 IU/l as measured in a central laboratory. However, it should be taken into account that there are variations between LH measurements performed in different laboratories.

In clinical studies comparing r-hFSH (follitropin alfa) and urinary FSH in assisted reproduction technologies (see table below) and in ovulation induction, GONAL-f was more potent than urinary FSH in terms of a lower total dose and a shorter treatment period needed to trigger follicular maturation.

In assisted reproduction technologies, GONAL-f at a lower total dose and shorter treatment period than urinary FSH, resulted in a higher number of oocytes retrieved when compared to urinary FSH.

Table: Results of study GF 8407 (randomised parallel group study comparing efficacy and safety of Gonal-f with u-FSH in assisted reproduction technologies)

	GONAL-f (n = 130)	u-FSH (n = 116)
No. of oocytes retrieved	11.0 ± 5.9	8.8 ± 4.8
Days of FSH stimulation required	11.7 ± 1.9	14.5 ± 3.3
Total dose of FSH required (no. of FSH 75 IU ampoules)	27.6 ± 10.2	40.7 ± 13.6
Need to increase the dosage (%)	56.2	85.3

Differences between the 2 groups were statistically significant ($p<0.05$) for all criteria listed.

In men deficient in FSH, GONAL-f administered concomitantly with hCG for at least 4 months induces spermatogenesis.

5.2 Pharmacokinetic properties

Following intravenous administration, GONAL-f is distributed to the extracellular fluid space with an initial half-life of around 2 hours and eliminated from the body with a terminal half-life of about one day. The steady state volume of distribution and total clearance are 10 l and 0.6 l/h, respectively. One-eighth of the GONAL-f dose is excreted in the urine.

Following subcutaneous administration, the absolute bioavailability is about 70%. Following repeated administration, GONAL-f accumulates 3-fold achieving a steady-state within 3-4 days. In women whose endogenous gonadotrophin secretion is suppressed, GONAL-f has nevertheless been shown to effectively stimulate follicular development and steroidogenesis, despite unmeasurable LH levels.

5.3 Preclinical safety data

Non-clinical data reveal no special hazard for humans based on conventional studies of single and repeated dose toxicity and genotoxicity additional to that already stated in other sections of this SPC.

In rabbits, the formulation reconstituted with 0.9% benzyl alcohol and 0.9% benzyl alcohol alone, both resulted in a slight haemorrhage and subacute inflammation after single subcutaneous injection or mild inflammatory and degenerative changes after single intramuscular injection respectively.

Impaired fertility has been reported in rats exposed to pharmacological doses of follitropin alfa (≥ 40 IU/kg/day) for extended periods, through reduced fecundity.

Given in high doses (≥5 IU/kg/day) follitropin alfa caused a decrease in the number of viable foetuses without being a teratogen, and dystocia similar to that observed with urinary hMG. However, since GONAL-f is not indicated in pregnancy, these data are of limited clinical relevance.

6. PHARMACEUTICAL PARTICULARS

6.1 List of excipients

Powder:

Sucrose

Sodium dihydrogen phosphate monohydrate

Disodium phosphate dihydrate

Phosphoric acid, concentrated

Sodium hydroxide

Solvent:

Water for Injections

Benzyl alcohol

6.2 Incompatibilities

In the absence of compatibility studies, this medicinal product must not be mixed with other medicinal products.

6.3 Shelf life

2 years.

The reconstituted solution is stable for 28 days.

6.4 Special precautions for storage

Prior to reconstitution, do not store above 25°C. Store in the original package.

After reconstitution, do not store above 25°C. Do not freeze. Store in the original container.

6.5 Nature and contents of container

GONAL-f is presented as a powder and solvent for injection. The powder is presented in 3 ml vials (Type I glass), with rubber stopper (bromobutyl rubber) and aluminium flip-off cap. The solvent for reconstitution is presented in 1 ml pre-filled syringes (Type I glass) with a rubber stopper. The Administration syringes made of polypropylene with a stainless steel pre-fixed needle are also provided.

The product is supplied as a pack of 1 vial of powder with 1 pre-filled syringe of solvent for reconstitution and 6 disposable syringes for administration graduated in FSH units.

6.6 Special precautions for disposal and other handling

GONAL-f 450 IU/0.75 ml (33 micrograms/0.75 ml) must be reconstituted with the 1 ml solvent provided before use.

GONAL-f 450 IU/0.75 ml (33 micrograms/0.75 ml) preparation must not be reconstituted with any other GONAL-f containers.

The solvent pre-filled syringe provided should be used for reconstitution only and then disposed of in accordance with local requirements. A set of administration syringes graduated in FSH units is supplied in the GONAL-f Multi-dose box. Alternatively, a 1 ml syringe, graduated in ml, with pre-fixed needle for subcutaneous administration could be used. Each ml of reconstituted solution contains 600 IU r-hFSH.

The following table states the volume to be administered to deliver the prescribed dose:

Dose (IU)	Volume to be injected (ml)
75	0.13
150	0.25
225	0.38
300	0.50
375	0.63
450	0.75

Individual reconstituted vials should be for single patient use only. The next injection should be done at the same time the next day.

The reconstituted solution should not be administered if it contains particles or is not clear.

Any unused product or waste material should be disposed of in accordance with local requirements.

7. MARKETING AUTHORISATION HOLDER

Serono Europe Ltd.

56 Marsh Wall

London E14 9TP

United Kingdom

8. MARKETING AUTHORISATION NUMBER(S)

EU/1/95/001/031

9. DATE OF FIRST AUTHORISATION/RENEWAL OF THE AUTHORISATION

Date of first authorisation: 20 October 1995.

Date of last renewal: 19 October 2005.

10. DATE OF REVISION OF THE TEXT

24th July 2009

GONAL-f 75 IU (5.5 micrograms)

(Merck Serono)

1. NAME OF THE MEDICINAL PRODUCT

GONAL-f 75 IU (5.5 micrograms) powder and solvent for solution for injection.

2. QUALITATIVE AND QUANTITATIVE COMPOSITION

One vial contains 6 micrograms follitropin alfa, recombinant human follicle stimulating hormone (FSH) in order to deliver 5.5 micrograms, equivalent to 75 IU. The reconstituted solution contains 75 IU/ml. Follitropin alfa is produced in genetically engineered Chinese Hamster Ovary (CHO) cells.

Excipients: 30 mg sucrose, 1.11 mg disodium phosphate dihydrate, 0.45 mg sodium dihydrogen phosphate monohydrate, 0.1 mg methionine, 0.05 mg polysorbate 20.

For a full list of excipients, see section 6.1.

3. PHARMACEUTICAL FORM

Powder and solvent for solution for injection.

Appearance of the powder: white lyophilised pellet.

Appearance of the solvent: clear colourless solution.

The pH of the reconstituted solution is 6.5 - 7.5.

4. CLINICAL PARTICULARS

4.1 Therapeutic indications

• Anovulation (including polycystic ovarian disease, PCOD) in women who have been unresponsive to treatment with clomiphene citrate.

- Stimulation of multifollicular development in patients undergoing superovulation for assisted reproductive technologies (ART) such as *in vitro* fertilisation (IVF), gamete intra-fallopian transfer (GIFT) and zygote intra-fallopian transfer (ZIFT).
- GONAL-f in association with a luteinising hormone (LH) preparation is recommended for the stimulation of follicular development in women with severe LH and FSH deficiency. In clinical trials these patients were defined by an endogenous serum LH level <1.2 IU/l.
- GONAL-f is indicated for the stimulation of spermatogenesis in men who have congenital or acquired hypogonadotrophic hypogonadism with concomitant human Chorionic Gonadotrophin (hCG) therapy.

4.2 Posology and method of administration

Treatment with GONAL-f should be initiated under the supervision of a physician experienced in the treatment of fertility problems.

GONAL-f is intended for subcutaneous administration. The powder should be reconstituted immediately prior to use with the solvent provided. In order to avoid the injection of large volumes, up to 3 vials of product may be dissolved in 1 ml of solvent.

The dosage recommendations given for GONAL-f are those in use for urinary FSH. Clinical assessment of GONAL-f indicates that its daily doses, regimens of administration, and treatment monitoring procedures should not be different from those currently used for urinary FSH-containing preparations. It is advised to adhere to the recommended starting doses indicated below.

Comparative clinical studies have shown that on average patients require a lower cumulative dosage and shorter treatment duration with GONAL-f compared with urinary FSH. Therefore, it is considered appropriate to give a lower total dosage of GONAL-f than generally used for urinary FSH, not only in order to optimise follicular development but also to minimise the risk of unwanted ovarian hyperstimulation. See section 5.1.

Women with anovulation (including PCOD):

The object of GONAL-f therapy is to develop a single mature Graafian follicle from which the ovum will be liberated after the administration of hCG.

GONAL-f may be given as a course of daily injections. In menstruating patients treatment should commence within the first 7 days of the menstrual cycle.

Treatment should be tailored to the individual patient's response as assessed by measuring follicle size by ultrasound and/or oestrogen secretion. A commonly used regimen commences at 75-150 IU FSH daily and is increased preferably by 37.5 or 75 IU at 7 or preferably 14 day intervals if necessary, to obtain an adequate, but not excessive, response. The maximal daily dose is usually not higher than 225 IU FSH. If a patient fails to respond adequately after 4 weeks of treatment, that cycle should be abandoned and the patient should recommence treatment at a higher starting dose than in the abandoned cycle.

When an optimal response is obtained, a single injection of 5 000 IU, up to 10 000 IU hCG should be administered 24-48 hours after the last GONAL-f injection. The patient is recommended to have coitus on the day of, and the day following, hCG administration. Alternatively intrauterine insemination (IUI) may be performed.

If an excessive response is obtained, treatment should be stopped and hCG withheld (see section 4.4). Treatment should recommence in the next cycle at a dosage lower than that of the previous cycle.

Women undergoing ovarian stimulation for multiple follicular development prior to *in vitro* fertilisation or other assisted reproductive technologies:

A commonly used regimen for superovulation involves the administration of 150-225 IU of GONAL-f daily, commencing on days 2 or 3 of the cycle. Treatment is continued until adequate follicular development has been achieved (as assessed by monitoring of serum oestrogen concentrations and/or ultrasound examination), with the dose adjusted according to the patient's response, to usually not higher than 450 IU daily. In general adequate follicular development is achieved on average by the tenth day of treatment (range 5 to 20 days).

A single injection of up to 10 000 IU hCG is administered 24-48 hours after the last GONAL-f injection to induce final follicular maturation.

Down-regulation with a gonadotrophin-releasing hormone (GnRH) agonist is now commonly used in order to suppress the endogenous LH surge and to control tonic levels of LH. In a commonly used protocol, GONAL-f is started approximately 2 weeks after the start of agonist treatment, both being continued until adequate follicular development is achieved. For example, following two weeks of treatment with an agonist, 150-225 IU GONAL-f are administered for the first 7 days. The dose is then adjusted according to the ovarian response.

Overall experience with IVF indicates that in general the treatment success rate remains stable during the first four attempts and gradually declines thereafter.

Women with anovulation resulting from severe LH and FSH deficiency:

In LH and FSH deficient women (hypogonadotrophic hypogonadism), the objective of GONAL-f therapy in association with lutropin alfa is to develop a single mature Graafian follicle from which the oocyte will be liberated after the administration of human chorionic gonadotrophin (hCG). GONAL-f should be given as a course of daily injections simultaneously with lutropin alfa. Since these patients are amenorrhoeic and have low endogenous oestrogen secretion, treatment can commence at any time.

Treatment should be tailored to the individual patient's response as assessed by measuring follicle size by ultrasound and oestrogen response. A recommended regimen commences at 75 IU of lutropin alfa daily with 75-150 IU FSH.

If an FSH dose increase is deemed appropriate, dose adaptation should preferably be after 7-14 day intervals and preferably by 37.5-75 IU increments. It may be acceptable to extend the duration of stimulation in any one cycle to up to 5 weeks.

When an optimal response is obtained, a single injection of 5,000 IU to 10,000 IU hCG should be administered 24-48 hours after the last GONAL-f and lutropin alfa injections. The patient is recommended to have coitus on the day of, and on the day following, hCG administration.

Alternatively, intrauterine insemination (IUI) may be performed.

Luteal phase support may be considered since lack of substances with luteotrophic activity (LH/hCG) after ovulation may lead to premature failure of the corpus luteum.

If an excessive response is obtained, treatment should be stopped and hCG withheld. Treatment should recommence in the next cycle at a dose of FSH lower than that of the previous cycle.

Men with hypogonadotrophic hypogonadism:

GONAL-f should be given at a dosage of 150 IU three times a week, concomitantly with hCG, for a minimum of 4 months. If after this period, the patient has not responded, the combination treatment may be continued; current clinical experience indicates that treatment for at least 18 months may be necessary to achieve spermatogenesis.

4.3 Contraindications

GONAL-f must not be used in:

- hypersensitivity to the active substance follitropin alfa, FSH or to any of the excipients
- case of tumours of the hypothalamus and pituitary gland

and in women:

- ovarian enlargement or cyst not due to polycystic ovarian disease
- gynaecological haemorrhages of unknown aetiology
- ovarian, uterine or mammary carcinoma

GONAL-f should not be used when an effective response cannot be obtained, such as:

In women:

- primary ovarian failure
- malformations of sexual organs incompatible with pregnancy
- fibroid tumours of the uterus incompatible with pregnancy

In men:

- primary testicular insufficiency

4.4 Special warnings and precautions for use

GONAL-f is a potent gonadotrophic substance capable of causing mild to severe adverse reactions, and should only be used by physicians who are thoroughly familiar with infertility problems and their management.

Gonadotrophin therapy requires a certain time commitment by physicians and supportive health professionals, as well as the availability of appropriate monitoring facilities. In women, safe and effective use of GONAL-f calls for monitoring of ovarian response with ultrasound, alone or preferably in combination with measurement of serum oestradiol levels, on a regular basis. There may be a degree of interpatient variability in response to FSH administration, with a poor response to FSH in some patients. The lowest effective dose in relation to the treatment objective should be used in both men and women.

Self-administration of GONAL-f should only be performed by patients who are well motivated, adequately trained and with access to expert advice.

The first injection of GONAL-f should be performed under direct medical supervision.

Patients with porphyria or a family history of porphyria should be closely monitored during treatment with GONAL-f. Deterioration or a first appearance of this condition may require cessation of treatment.

GONAL-f contains less than 1 mmol sodium (23 mg) per dose, i.e. essentially "sodium-free".

Treatment in women

Before starting treatment, the couple's infertility should be assessed as appropriate and putative contraindications for pregnancy evaluated. In particular, patients should be evaluated for hypothyroidism, adrenocortical deficiency, hyperprolactinemia and pituitary or hypothalamic tumours, and appropriate specific treatment given.

Patients undergoing stimulation of follicular growth, whether in the frame of a treatment for anovulatory infertility or ART procedures, may experience ovarian enlargement or develop hyperstimulation. Adherence to recommended GONAL-f dosage and regimen of administration, and careful monitoring of therapy will minimise the incidence of such events. Acute interpretation of the indices of follicle development and maturation require a physician whom is experienced in the interpretation of the relevant tests.

In clinical trials, an increase of the ovarian sensitivity to GONAL-f was shown when administered with lutropin alfa. If an FSH dose increase is deemed appropriate, dose adaptation should preferably be at 7-14 day intervals and preferably with 37.5-75 IU increments.

No direct comparison of GONAL-f/LH versus human menopausal gonadotrophin (hMG) has been performed. Comparison with historical data suggests that the ovulation rate obtained with GONAL-f/LH is similar to what can be obtained with hMG.

Ovarian Hyperstimulation Syndrome (OHSS)

OHSS is a medical event distinct from uncomplicated ovarian enlargement. OHSS is a syndrome that can manifest itself with increasing degrees of severity. It comprises marked ovarian enlargement, high serum sex steroids, and an increase in vascular permeability which can result in an accumulation of fluid in the peritoneal, pleural and, rarely, in the pericardial cavities.

The following symptomatology may be observed in severe cases of OHSS: abdominal pain, abdominal distension, severe ovarian enlargement, weight gain, dyspnoea, oliguria and gastrointestinal symptoms including nausea, vomiting and diarrhoea. Clinical evaluation may reveal hypovolaemia, haemoconcentration, electrolyte imbalances, ascites, haemoperitoneum, pleural effusions, hydrothorax, acute pulmonary distress, and thromboembolic events. Very rarely, severe OHSS may be complicated by pulmonary embolism, ischemic stroke and myocardial infarction.

Excessive ovarian response to gonadotrophin treatment seldom gives rise to OHSS unless hCG is administered to trigger ovulation. Therefore in cases of ovarian hyperstimulation it is prudent to withhold hCG and advise the patient to refrain from coitus or to use barrier methods for at least 4 days. OHSS may progress rapidly (within 24 hours to several days) to become a serious medical event, therefore patients should be followed for at least two weeks after hCG administration.

To minimise the risk of OHSS or of multiple pregnancy, ultrasound scans as well as oestradiol measurements are recommended. In anovulation the risk of OHSS and multiple pregnancy is increased by a serum oestradiol > 900 pg/ml (3300 pmol/l) and more than 3 follicles of 14 mm or more in diameter. In ART there is an increased risk of OHSS with a serum oestradiol > 3000 pg/ml (11000 pmol/l) and 20 or more follicles of 12 mm or more in diameter. When the oestradiol level is > 5500 pg/ml (20200 pmol/l) and where there are 40 or more follicles in total, it may be necessary to withhold hCG administration.

Adherence to recommended GONAL-f dosage, regimen of administration and careful monitoring of therapy will minimise the incidence of ovarian hyperstimulation and multiple pregnancy (see Sections 4.2 and 4.8).

In ART, aspiration of all follicles prior to ovulation may reduce the occurrence of hyperstimulation.

OHSS may be more severe and more protracted if pregnancy occurs. Most often, OHSS occurs after hormonal treatment has been discontinued and reaches its maximum at about seven to ten days following treatment. Usually, OHSS resolves spontaneously with the onset of menses.

If severe OHSS occurs, gonadotrophin treatment should be stopped if still ongoing, the patient hospitalised and specific therapy for OHSS started.

This syndrome occurs with higher incidence in patients with polycystic ovarian disease.

Multiple pregnancy

Multiple pregnancy, specially high order, carries an increase risk in adverse maternal and perinatal outcomes.

In patients undergoing ovulation induction with GONAL-f, the incidence of multiple pregnancies is increased as compared with natural conception. The majority of multiple conceptions are twins. To minimise the risk of multiple pregnancy, careful monitoring of ovarian response is recommended.

In patients undergoing ART procedures the risk of multiple pregnancy is related mainly to the number of embryos replaced, their quality and the patient age.

The patients should be advised of the potential risk of multiple births before starting treatment.

Pregnancy wastage

The incidence of pregnancy wastage by miscarriage or abortion is higher in patients undergoing stimulation of follicular growth for ovulation induction or ART than in the normal population.

Ectopic pregnancy

Women with a history of tubal disease are at risk of ectopic pregnancy, whether the pregnancy is obtained by spontaneous conception or with fertility treatments. The prevalence of ectopic pregnancy after IVF was reported to be 2 to 5%, as compared to 1 to 1.5% in the general population.

Table 1

Treatment in women		
Immune system disorders	Very rare (<1/10,000)	Mild systemic allergic reactions (e.g. mild forms of erythema, rash, facial swelling, urticaria, oedema, difficulty breathing). Serious cases of allergic reactions, including anaphylactic reactions, have also been reported.
Nervous system disorders	Very Common (>1/10)	Headache
Vascular disorders	Very rare (<1/10,000)	Thromboembolism, usually associated with severe OHSS
Respiratory, thoracic and mediastinal disorders	Very rare (<1/10,000)	Exacerbation or worsening of asthma
Gastrointestinal disorders	Common (>1/100, <1/10)	Abdominal pain and gastrointestinal symptoms such as nausea, vomiting, diarrhoea, abdominal cramps and bloating
Reproductive system and breast disorders	Very Common (>1/10)	Ovarian cysts
	Common (>1/100, <1/10)	Mild to moderate OHSS (see section 4.4)
	Uncommon (>1/1,000, <1/100)	Severe OHSS (see section 4.4)
	Rare (>1/10,000, <1/1,000)	Ovarian torsion, a complication of OHSS
General disorders and administration site conditions	Very Common (>1/10)	Mild to severe injection site reaction (pain, redness, bruising, swelling and/ or irritation at the site of injection)
Treatment in men		
Skin and subcutaneous tissue disorders	Common (>1/100, <1/10)	Acne
Reproductive system and breast disorders	Common (>1/100, <1/10)	Gynaecomastia Varicocele
General disorders and administration site conditions	Very Common (>1/10)	Mild to severe injection site reaction (pain, redness, bruising, swelling and/ or irritation at the site of injection)
Investigations	Common (>1/100, <1/10)	Weight gain

Reproductive system neoplasms

There have been reports of ovarian and other reproductive system neoplasms, both benign and malignant, in women who have undergone multiple drug regimens for infertility treatment. It is not yet established whether or not treatment with gonadotrophins increases the baseline risk of these tumors in infertile women.

Congenital malformation

The prevalence of congenital malformations after ART may be slightly higher than after spontaneous conceptions. This is thought to be due to differences in parental characteristics (e.g. maternal age, sperm characteristics) and multiple pregnancies.

Thromboembolic events

In women with generally recognised risk factors for thrombo-embolic events, such as personal or family history, treatment with gonadotrophins may further increase the risk. In these women, the benefits of gonadotrophin administration need to be weighed against the risks. It should be noted however, that pregnancy itself also carries an increased risk of thrombo-embolic events.

<u>Treatment in men</u>

Elevated endogenous FSH levels are indicative of primary testicular failure. Such patients are unresponsive to GONAL-f/hCG therapy.

Semen analysis is recommended 4 to 6 months after the beginning of treatment in assessing the response.

4.5 Interaction with other medicinal products and other forms of interaction

Concomitant use of GONAL-f with other agents used to stimulate ovulation (e.g. hCG, clomiphene citrate) may potentiate the follicular response, whereas concurrent use of a GnRH agonist to induce pituitary desensitisation may increase the dosage of GONAL-f needed to elicit an adequate ovarian response. No other clinically significant drug interaction has been reported during GONAL-f therapy.

4.6 Pregnancy and lactation

Use during pregnancy

There is no indication for use of GONAL-f during pregnancy. No teratogenic risk has been reported, following controlled ovarian hyperstimulation, in clinical use with gonadotrophins. In case of exposure during pregnancy, clinical data are not sufficient to exclude a teratogenic effect of recombinant hFSH. However, to date, no particular malformative effect has been reported. No teratogenic effect has been observed in animal studies.

Use during lactation

GONAL-f is not indicated during lactation. During lactation, the secretion of prolactin can entail a poor prognosis to ovarian stimulation.

4.7 Effects on ability to drive and use machines

No studies on the effects on ability to drive and use machines have been performed.

4.8 Undesirable effects

Within each frequency grouping, undesirable effects are presented in order of decreasing seriousness.

(see Table 1 above)

4.9 Overdose

The effects of an overdose of GONAL-f are unknown, nevertheless one could expect ovarian hyperstimulation syndrome to occur, which is further described in section 4.4.

5. PHARMACOLOGICAL PROPERTIES

5.1 Pharmacodynamic properties

Pharmacotherapeutic group: gonadotrophins, ATC code: G03GA05.

GONAL-f is a preparation of follicle stimulating hormone produced by genetically engineered Chinese Hamster Ovary (CHO) cells.

In women, the most important effect resulting from parenteral administration of FSH is the development of mature Graafian follicles.

In clinical trials, patients with severe FSH and LH deficiency were defined by an endogenous serum LH level <1.2 IU/l as measured in a central laboratory. However, it should be taken into account that there are variations between LH measurements performed in different laboratories.

In clinical studies comparing r-hFSH (follitropin alfa) and urinary FSH in assisted reproduction technologies (see table below) and in ovulation induction, GONAL-f was more potent than urinary FSH in terms of a lower total dose and a shorter treatment period needed to trigger follicular maturation.

In assisted reproduction technologies, GONAL-f at a lower total dose and shorter treatment period than urinary FSH, resulted in a higher number of oocytes retrieved when compared to urinary FSH.

Table: Results of study GF 8407 (randomised parallel group study comparing efficacy and safety of Gonal-f with u-FSH in assisted reproduction technologies)

	GONAL-f (n = 130)	u-FSH (n = 116)
No. of oocytes retrieved	11.0 ± 5.9	8.8 ± 4.8
Days of FSH stimulation required	11.7 ± 1.9	14.5 ± 3.3
Total dose of FSH required (no. of FSH 75 IU ampoules)	27.6 ± 10.2	40.7 ± 13.6
Need to increase the dosage (%)	56.2	85.3

Differences between the 2 groups were statistically significant ($p<0.05$) for all criteria listed.

In men deficient in FSH, GONAL-f administered concomitantly with hCG for at least 4 months induces spermatogenesis.

5.2 Pharmacokinetic properties

Following intravenous administration, GONAL-f is distributed to the extracellular fluid space with an initial half-life of around 2 hours and eliminated from the body with a terminal half-life of about one day. The steady state volume of distribution and total clearance are 10 l and 0.6 l/h, respectively. One-eighth of the GONAL-f dose is excreted in the urine.

Following subcutaneous administration, the absolute bioavailability is about 70%. Following repeated administration, GONAL-f accumulates 3-fold achieving a steady-state within 3-4 days. In women whose endogenous gonadotrophin secretion is suppressed, GONAL-f has nevertheless been shown to effectively stimulate follicular development and steroidogenesis, despite unmeasurable LH levels.

5.3 Preclinical safety data

Non-clinical data reveal no special hazard for humans based on conventional studies of single and repeated dose toxicity and genotoxicity additional to that already stated in other sections of this SPC.

Impaired fertility has been reported in rats exposed to pharmacological doses of follitropin alfa (⩾ 40 IU/kg/ day) for extended periods, through reduced fecundity.

Given in high doses (≥5 IU/kg/day) follitropin alfa caused a decrease in the number of viable foetuses without being a teratogen, and dystocia similar to that observed with urinary hMG. However, since GONAL-f is not indicated in pregnancy, these data are of limited clinical relevance.

6. PHARMACEUTICAL PARTICULARS

6.1 List of excipients

<u>Powder:</u>

Sucrose

Sodium dihydrogen phosphate monohydrate

Disodium phosphate dihydrate

Methionine

Polysorbate 20

Phosphoric acid, concentrated

Sodium hydroxide

<u>Solvent:</u>

Water for Injections

6.2 Incompatibilities

This medicinal product must not be mixed with other medicinal products except those mentioned in section 6.6.

6.3 Shelf life

2 years.

For immediate and single use following first opening and reconstitution.

6.4 Special precautions for storage

Do not store above 25°C.

Store in the original package.

6.5 Nature and contents of container

GONAL-f is presented as a powder and solvent for injection. The powder is presented in 3 ml vials (Type I glass), with stopper (bromobutyl rubber) and aluminium flip-off cap. The solvent for reconstitution is presented in either 2 or 3 ml vials (Type I glass) with stopper (teflon-coated rubber) or in 1 ml pre-filled syringes (Type I glass) with a rubber stopper.

The product is supplied in packs of 1 vials with the corresponding number of solvent vials or packs of 1, 5 or 10 vials with the corresponding number of solvent pre-filled syringes. Not all pack sizes may be marketed.

6.6 Special precautions for disposal and other handling

For single use only.

GONAL-f must be reconstituted with the solvent before use.

GONAL-f may be co-reconstituted with lutropin alfa and co-administered as a single injection. In this case lutropin alfa should be reconstituted first and then used to reconstitute GONAL-f powder.

The reconstituted solution should not be administered if it contains particles or is not clear.

Any unused product or waste material should be disposed of in accordance with local requirements.

7. MARKETING AUTHORISATION HOLDER

Serono Europe Ltd.

56 Marsh Wall

London E14 9TP

United Kingdom

8. MARKETING AUTHORISATION NUMBER(S)

EU/1/95/001/005

EU/1/95/001/025

EU/1/95/001/026

EU/1/95/001/027

9. DATE OF FIRST AUTHORISATION/RENEWAL OF THE AUTHORISATION

Date of first authorisation: 20 October 1995.

Date of last renewal: 19 October 2005.

10. DATE OF REVISION OF THE TEXT

24th July 2009

GONAL-f 900 IU (66mcg) pen

(Merck Serono)

1. NAME OF THE MEDICINAL PRODUCT

GONAL-f 900 IU/1.5 ml (66 micrograms/1.5 ml) solution for injection in a pre-filled pen.

2. QUALITATIVE AND QUANTITATIVE COMPOSITION

Follitropin alfa*, 600 IU/ml (equivalent to 44 micrograms/ml).

Each cartridge delivers 900 IU (equivalent 66 micrograms) in 1.5 ml.

* Follitropin alfa is recombinant human follicle stimulating hormone (FSH) produced by recombinant DNA technology in Chinese Hamster Ovary (CHO) cell line.

Excipients: 90 mg sucrose, 1.665 mg disodium phosphate dihydrate, 0.675 mg sodium dihydrogen phosphate monohydrate, 0.15 mg methionine, 4.5 mg m-cresol, 0.15 mg poloxamer 188.

For a full list of excipients, see section 6.1.

3. PHARMACEUTICAL FORM

Solution for injection in a pre-filled pen.

Clear colourless solution.

The pH of the solution is 6.7 - 7.3.

4. CLINICAL PARTICULARS

4.1 Therapeutic indications

• Anovulation (including polycystic ovarian disease, PCOD) in women who have been unresponsive to treatment with clomiphene citrate.

• Stimulation of multifollicular development in patients undergoing superovulation for assisted reproductive technologies (ART) such as in vitro fertilisation (IVF), gamete intra-fallopian transfer (GIFT) and zygote intra-fallopian transfer (ZIFT).

• GONAL-f in association with a luteinising hormone (LH) preparation is recommended for the stimulation of follicular development in women with severe LH and FSH deficiency. In clinical trials these patients were defined by an endogenous serum LH level <1.2 IU/l.

• GONAL-f is indicated for the stimulation of spermatogenesis in men who have congenital or acquired hypogonadotrophic hypogonadism with concomitant human Chorionic Gonadotrophin (hCG) therapy.

4.2 Posology and method of administration

Treatment with GONAL-f should be initiated under the supervision of a physician experienced in the treatment of fertility problems.

GONAL-f is intended for subcutaneous administration.

The dosage recommendations given for GONAL-f are those in use for urinary FSH. Clinical assessment of GONAL-f indicates that its daily doses, regimens of administration and treatment monitoring procedures should not be different from those currently used for urinary FSH-containing preparations.

It is advised to adhere to the recommended starting doses indicated below.

Comparative clinical studies have shown that on average patients require a lower cumulative dosage and shorter treatment duration with GONAL-f compared with urinary FSH. Therefore, it is considered appropriate to give a lower total dosage of GONAL-f than generally used for urinary FSH, not only in order to optimise follicular development but also to minimise the risk of unwanted ovarian hyperstimulation. See section 5.1

Bioequivalence has been demonstrated between equivalent doses of the monodose presentation and the multidose presentation of GONAL-f.

Women with anovulation (including PCOD):

The object of GONAL-f therapy is to develop a single mature Graafian follicle from which the ovum will be liberated after the administration of hCG.

GONAL-f may be given as a course of daily injections. In menstruating patients treatment should commence within the first 7 days of the menstrual cycle.

Treatment should be tailored to the individual patient's response as assessed by measuring follicle size by ultrasound and/or oestrogen secretion. A commonly used regimen commences at 75-150 IU FSH daily and is increased preferably by 37.5 or 75 IU at 7 or preferably 14 day intervals if necessary, to obtain an adequate, but not excessive, response. The maximal daily dose is usually not higher than 225 IU FSH. If a patient fails to respond adequately after 4 weeks of treatment, that cycle should be abandoned and the patient should recommence treatment at a higher starting dose than in the abandoned cycle.

When an optimal response is obtained, a single injection of 250 micrograms r-hCG or 5 000 IU up to 10 000 IU hCG should be administered 24-48 hours after the last GONAL-f injection. The patient is recommended to have coitus on the day of, and the day following, hCG administration. Alternatively intrauterine insemination (IUI) may be performed.

If an excessive response is obtained, treatment should be stopped and hCG withheld (see section 4.4). Treatment should recommence in the next cycle at a dosage lower than that of the previous cycle.

Women undergoing ovarian stimulation for multiple follicular development prior to in vitro fertilisation or other assisted reproductive technologies:

A commonly used regimen for superovulation involves the administration of 150-225 IU of GONAL-f daily, commencing on days 2 or 3 of the cycle. Treatment is continued until adequate follicular development has been achieved (as assessed by monitoring of serum oestrogen concentrations and/or ultrasound examination), with the dose adjusted according to the patient's response, to usually not higher than 450 IU daily. In general adequate follicular development is achieved on average by the tenth day of treatment (range 5 to 20 days).

A single injection of 250 micrograms r-hCG or 5 000 IU up to 10 000 IU hCG is administered 24-48 hours after the last GONAL-f injection to induce final follicular maturation.

Down-regulation with a gonadotrophin-releasing hormone (GnRH) agonist or antagonist is now commonly used in order to suppress the endogenous LH surge and to control tonic levels of LH. In a commonly used protocol, GONAL-f is started approximately 2 weeks after the start of agonist treatment, both being continued until adequate follicular development is achieved. For example, following two weeks of treatment with an agonist, 150-225 IU GONAL-f are administered for the first 7 days. The dose is then adjusted according to the ovarian response.

Overall experience with IVF indicates that in general the treatment success rate remains stable during the first four attempts and gradually declines thereafter.

Women with anovulation resulting from severe LH and FSH deficiency:

In LH and FSH deficient women (hypogonadotrophic hypogonadism), the objective of GONAL-f therapy in association with lutropin alfa is to develop a single mature Graafian follicle from which the oocyte will be liberated after the administration of human chorionic gonadotrophin (hCG). GONAL-f should be given as a course of daily injections simultaneously with lutropin alfa. Since these patients are amenorrhoeic and have low endogenous oestrogen secretion, treatment can commence at any time.

Treatment should be tailored to the individual patient's response as assessed by measuring follicle size by ultrasound and oestrogen response. A recommended regimen commences at 75 IU of lutropin alfa daily with 75-150 IU FSH.

If an FSH dose increase is deemed appropriate, dose adaptation should preferably be after 7-14 day intervals and preferably by 37.5-75 IU increments. It may be acceptable to extend the duration of stimulation in any one cycle to up to 5 weeks.

When an optimal response is obtained, a single injection of 250 micrograms r-hCG or 5 000 IU up to 10 000 IU hCG should be administered 24-48 hours after the last GONAL-f and lutropin alfa injections. The patient is recommended to have coitus on the day of, and on the day following, hCG administration.

Alternatively, intrauterine insemination (IUI) may be performed.

Luteal phase support may be considered since lack of substances with luteotrophic activity (LH/hCG) after ovulation may lead to premature failure of the corpus luteum.

If an excessive response is obtained, treatment should be stopped and hCG withheld. Treatment should recommence in the next cycle at a dose of FSH lower than that of the previous cycle.

Men with hypogonadotrophic hypogonadism:

GONAL-f should be given at a dosage of 150 IU three times a week, concomitantly with hCG, for a minimum of 4 months. If after this period, the patient has not responded, the combination treatment may be continued; current clinical experience indicates that treatment for at least 18 months may be necessary to achieve spermatogenesis.

4.3 Contraindications

• Hypersensitivity to the active substance follitropin alfa, FSH or to any of the excipients

• Tumours of the hypothalamus and pituitary gland

In women:

• ovarian enlargement or cyst not due to polycystic ovarian disease

• gynaecological haemorrhages of unknown aetiology

• ovarian, uterine or mammary carcinoma

Must not be used when an effective response cannot be obtained, such as:

In women:

• primary ovarian failure

• malformations of sexual organs incompatible with pregnancy

• fibroid tumours of the uterus incompatible with pregnancy

In men:

• primary testicular insufficiency

4.4 Special warnings and precautions for use

GONAL-f is a potent gonadotrophic substance capable of causing mild to severe adverse reactions, and should only be used by physicians who are thoroughly familiar with infertility problems and their management.

Gonadotrophin therapy requires a certain time commitment by physicians and supportive health professionals, as well as the availability of appropriate monitoring facilities. In women, safe and effective use of Gonal-f calls for monitoring of ovarian response with ultrasound, alone or preferably in combination with measurement of serum oestradiol levels, on a regular basis. There may be a degree of interpatient variability in response to FSH administration, with a poor response to FSH in some patients. The lowest effective dose in relation to the treatment objective should be used in both men and women.

Self-administration of Gonal-f should only be performed by patients who are well motivated, adequately trained and have access to expert advice. During training of the patient for self-administration, special attention should be given to specific instructions for the use of the prefilled pen.

The first injection of GONAL-f should be performed under direct medical supervision.

Patients with porphyria or a family history of porphyria should be closely monitored during treatment with GONAL-f. Deterioration or a first appearance of this condition may require cessation of treatment.

GONAL-f contains less than 1 mmol sodium (23 mg) per dose, i.e. essentially "sodium-free".

Treatment in women

Before starting treatment, the couple's infertility should be assessed as appropriate and putative contraindications for pregnancy evaluated. In particular, patients should be evaluated for hypothyroidism, adrenocortical deficiency, hyperprolactinemia and pituitary or hypothalamic tumours, and appropriate specific treatment given.

Patients undergoing stimulation of follicular growth, whether as treatment for anovulatory infertility or for ART procedures, may experience ovarian enlargement or develop hyperstimulation. Adherence to the recommended Gonal-f dosage and regimen of administration, and careful monitoring of therapy will minimise the incidence of such events. For accurate interpretation of the indices of follicle development and maturation, the physician should be experienced in the interpretation of the relevant tests.

In clinical trials, an increase of the ovarian sensitivity to GONAL-f was shown when administered with lutropin alfa. If an FSH dose increase is deemed appropriate, dose adaptation should preferably be at 7-14 day intervals and preferably with 37.5-75 IU increments.

No direct comparison of GONAL-f/LH versus human menopausal gonadotrophin (hMG) has been performed. Comparison with historical data suggests that the ovulation rate obtained with GONAL-f/LH is similar to that obtained with hMG.

Ovarian Hyperstimulation Syndrome (OHSS)

OHSS is a medical event distinct from uncomplicated ovarian enlargement. OHSS is a syndrome that can manifest itself with increasing degrees of severity. It comprises marked ovarian enlargement, high serum sex steroids, and an increase in vascular permeability which can result in an accumulation of fluid in the peritoneal, pleural and, rarely, in the pericardial cavities.

The following symptomatology may be observed in severe cases of OHSS: abdominal pain, abdominal distension, severe ovarian enlargement, weight gain, dyspnoea, oliguria and gastrointestinal symptoms including nausea, vomiting and diarrhoea. Clinical evaluation may reveal hypovolaemia, haemoconcentration, electrolyte imbalances, ascites, haemoperitoneum, pleural effusions, hydrothorax, acute pulmonary distress, and thromboembolic events. Very rarely, severe OHSS may be complicated by pulmonary embolism, ischemic stroke and myocardial infarction.

Excessive ovarian response to gonadotrophin treatment seldom gives rise to OHSS unless hCG is administered to trigger ovulation. Therefore in cases of ovarian hyperstimulation it is prudent to withhold hCG and advise the patient to refrain from coitus or to use barrier methods for at least 4 days. OHSS may progress rapidly (within 24 hours to several days) to become a serious medical event, therefore patients should be followed for at least two weeks after hCG administration.

To minimise the risk of OHSS or of multiple pregnancy, ultrasound scans as well as oestradiol measurements are recommended. In anovulation the risk of OHSS and multiple pregnancy is increased by a serum oestradiol > 900 pg/ml (3300 pmol/l) and more than 3 follicles of 14 mm or more in diameter. In ART there is an increased risk of OHSS with a serum oestradiol > 3000 pg/ml (11000 pmol/l) and 20 or more follicles of 12 mm or more in diameter. When the oestradiol level is > 5500 pg/ml (20200 pmol/l) and where there are 40 or more follicles in total, it may be necessary to withhold hCG administration.

Adherence to recommended GONAL-f dosage, regimen of administration and careful monitoring of therapy will minimise the incidence of ovarian hyperstimulation and multiple pregnancy (see sections 4.2 and 4.8).

In ART, aspiration of all follicles prior to ovulation may reduce the occurrence of hyperstimulation.

OHSS may be more severe and more protracted if pregnancy occurs. Most often, OHSS occurs after hormonal treatment has been discontinued and reaches its maximum at about seven to ten days following treatment. Usually, OHSS resolves spontaneously with the onset of menses.

If severe OHSS occurs, gonadotrophin treatment should be stopped if still ongoing, the patient hospitalised and specific therapy for OHSS started.

This syndrome occurs with higher incidence in patients with polycystic ovarian disease.

Multiple pregnancy

Multiple pregnancy, specially high order, carries an increase risk in adverse maternal and perinatal outcomes.

In patients undergoing ovulation induction with GONAL-f, the incidence of multiple pregnancies is increased as compared with natural conception. The majority of multiple conceptions are twins. To minimise the risk of multiple pregnancy, careful monitoring of ovarian response is recommended.

In patients undergoing ART procedures the risk of multiple pregnancy is related mainly to the number of embryos replaced, their quality and the patient age.

The patients should be advised of the potential risk of multiple births before starting treatment.

Pregnancy wastage

The incidence of pregnancy wastage by miscarriage or abortion is higher in patients undergoing stimulation of follicular growth for ovulation induction or ART than in the normal population.

Ectopic pregnancy

Women with a history of tubal disease are at risk of ectopic pregnancy, whether the pregnancy is obtained by spontaneous conception or with fertility treatments. The prevalence of ectopic pregnancy after IVF was reported to be 2 to 5%, as compared to 1 to 1.5% in the general population.

Reproductive system neoplasms

There have been reports of ovarian and other reproductive system neoplasms, both benign and malignant, in women who have undergone multiple drug regimens for infertility treatment. It is not yet established whether or not treatment with gonadotrophins increases the baseline risk of these tumours in infertile women.

Congenital malformation

The prevalence of congenital malformations after ART may be slightly higher than after spontaneous conceptions. This is thought to be due to differences in parental characteristics (e.g. maternal age, sperm characteristics) and multiple pregnancies.

Thromboembolic events

In women with generally recognised risk factors for thrombo-embolic events, such as personal or family history, treatment with gonadotrophins may further increase the risk. In these women, the benefits of gonadotrophin administration need to be weighed against the risks. It should be noted however, that pregnancy itself also carries an increased risk of thrombo-embolic events.

Treatment in men

Elevated endogenous FSH levels are indicative of primary testicular failure. Such patients are unresponsive to GONAL-f/hCG therapy.

Semen analysis is recommended 4 to 6 months after the beginning of treatment as part of the assessment of the response.

Table 1

Treatment in women		
Immune system disorders	Very rare (<1/10,000)	Mild systemic allergic reactions (e.g. mild forms of erythema, rash, facial swelling, urticaria, oedema, difficulty breathing). Serious cases of allergic reactions, including anaphylactic reactions, have also been reported.
Nervous system disorders	Very Common (>1/10)	Headache
Vascular disorders	Very rare (<1/10,000)	Thromboembolism, usually associated with severe OHSS
Respiratory, thoracic and mediastinal disorders	Very rare (<1/10,000)	Exacerbation or worsening of asthma
Gastrointestinal disorders	Common (>1/100, <1/10)	Abdominal pain and gastrointestinal symptoms such as nausea, vomiting, diarrhoea, abdominal cramps and bloating
Reproductive system and breast disorders	Very Common (>1/10)	Ovarian cysts
	Common (>1/100, <1/10)	Mild to moderate OHSS (see section 4.4)
	Uncommon (>1/1,000, <1/100)	Severe OHSS (see section 4.4)
	Rare (>1/10,000, <1/1,000)	Ovarian torsion, a complication of OHSS
General disorders and administration site conditions	Very Common (>1/10)	Mild to severe injection site reaction (pain, redness, bruising, swelling and/ or irritation at the site of injection)
Treatment in men		
Skin and subcutaneous tissue disorders	Common (>1/100, <1/10)	Acne
Reproductive system and breast disorders	Common (>1/100, <1/10)	Gynaecomastia Varicocele
General disorders and administration site conditions	Very Common (>1/10)	Mild to severe injection site reaction (pain, redness, bruising, swelling and/ or irritation at the site of injection)
Investigations	Common (>1/100, <1/10)	Weight gain

4.5 Interaction with other medicinal products and other forms of interaction

Concomitant use of GONAL-f with other agents used to stimulate ovulation (e.g. hCG, clomiphene citrate) may potentiate the follicular response, whereas concurrent use of a GnRH agonist or antagonist to induce pituitary desensitisation may increase the dosage of Gonal-f needed to elicit an adequate ovarian response. No other clinically significant drug interaction has been reported during Gonal-f therapy.

4.6 Pregnancy and lactation

There is no indication for use of GONAL-f during pregnancy. No teratogenic risk has been reported, following controlled ovarian hyperstimulation, in clinical use with gonadotrophins. In case of exposure during pregnancy, clinical data are not sufficient to exclude a teratogenic effect of recombinant hFSH. However, to date, no particular malformative effect has been reported. No teratogenic effect has been observed in animal studies.

GONAL-f is not indicated during lactation. During lactation, the secretion of prolactin can entail a poor prognosis to ovarian stimulation.

4.7 Effects on ability to drive and use machines

No studies on the effects on the ability to drive and use machines have been performed.

4.8 Undesirable effects

Within each frequency grouping, undesirable effects are presented in order of decreasing seriousness.

(see Table 1 above)

4.9 Overdose

The effects of an overdose of GONAL-f are unknown, nevertheless one could expect ovarian hyperstimulation syndrome to occur (see section 4.4).

5. PHARMACOLOGICAL PROPERTIES

5.1 Pharmacodynamic properties

Pharmacotherapeutic group: gonadotrophins, ATC code: G03GA05.

GONAL-f is a preparation of follicle stimulating hormone produced by genetically engineered Chinese Hamster Ovary (CHO) cells.

In women, the most important effect resulting from parenteral administration of FSH is the development of mature Graafian follicles.

In clinical trials, patients with severe FSH and LH deficiency were defined by an endogenous serum LH level <1.2 IU/l as measured in a central laboratory. However, it should be taken into account that there are variations between LH measurements performed in different laboratories.

In clinical studies comparing r-hFSH (follitropin alfa) and urinary FSH in assisted reproduction technologies (see table below) and in ovulation induction, GONAL-f was more potent than urinary FSH in terms of a lower total dose and a shorter treatment period needed to trigger follicular maturation.

In assisted reproduction technologies, GONAL-f at a lower total dose and shorter treatment period than urinary FSH, resulted in a higher number of oocytes retrieved when compared to urinary FSH.

Table: Results of study GF 8407 (randomised parallel group study comparing efficacy and safety of Gonal-f with u-FSH in assisted reproduction technologies)

	GONAL-f (n = 130)	**u-FSH (n = 116)**
No. of oocytes retrieved	11.0 ± 5.9	8.8 ± 4.8
Days of FSH stimulation required	11.7 ± 1.9	14.5 ± 3.3
Total dose of FSH required (no. of FSH 75 IU ampoules)	27.6 ± 10.2	40.7 ± 13.6
Need to increase the dosage (%)	56.2	85.3

Differences between the 2 groups were statistically significant ($p<0.05$) for all criteria listed.

In men deficient in FSH, GONAL-f administered concomitantly with hCG for at least 4 months induces spermatogenesis.

5.2 Pharmacokinetic properties

Following intravenous administration, follitropin alfa is distributed to the extracellular fluid space with an initial half-life of around 2 hours and eliminated from the body with a terminal half-life of about one day. The steady state volume of distribution and total clearance are 10 l and 0.6 l/h, respectively. One-eighth of the follitropin alfa dose is excreted in the urine.

Following subcutaneous administration, the absolute bioavailability is about 70%. Following repeated administration, follitropin alfa accumulates 3-fold achieving a steady-state within 3-4 days. In women whose endogenous gonadotrophin secretion is suppressed, follitropin alfa has nevertheless been shown to effectively stimulate follicular development and steroidogenesis, despite unmeasurable LH levels.

5.3 Preclinical safety data

Non-clinical data reveal no special hazard for humans based on conventional studies of single and repeated dose toxicity and genotoxicity additional to that already stated in other sections of this SPC.

Impaired fertility has been reported in rats exposed to pharmacological doses of follitropin alfa (≥ 40 IU/kg/day) for extended periods, through reduced fecundity.

Given in high doses (≥ 5 IU/kg/day) follitropin alfa caused a decrease in the number of viable foetuses without being a teratogen, and dystocia similar to that observed with urinary hMG. However, since GONAL-f is not indicated in pregnancy, these data are of limited clinical relevance.

6. PHARMACEUTICAL PARTICULARS

6.1 List of excipients

Poloxamer 188

Sucrose

Methionine

Sodium dihydrogen phosphate monohydrate

Disodium phosphate dihydrate

m-Cresol

Phosphoric acid, concentrated

Sodium hydroxide

Water for Injections

6.2 Incompatibilities

Not applicable.

6.3 Shelf life

2 years.

Once opened, the product may be stored for a maximum of 28 days at or below 25°C.

6.4 Special precautions for storage

Store in a refrigerator (2°C - 8°C). Do not freeze.

Within its shelf life, the product may be stored at or below 25°C for up to 3 months without being refrigerated again and must be discarded if it has not been used after 3 months.

Store in the original package in order to protect from light.

For in-use storage conditions, see section 6.3.

6.5 Nature and contents of container

1.5 ml of solution for injection in 3 ml cartridge (Type I glass), with a plunger stopper (halobutyl rubber) and an aluminium crimp cap with a black rubber inlay.

Pack of one pre-filled pen and 14 needles to be used with the pen for administration.

6.6 Special precautions for disposal and other handling

The solution should not be administered if it contains particles or is not clear.

Any unused solution must be discarded not later than 28 days after first opening.

GONAL-f 900 IU/1.5 ml (66 micrograms/1.5 ml) is not designed to allow the cartridge to be removed.

Discard used needles immediately after injection.

Any unused product or waste material should be disposed of in accordance with local requirements.

7. MARKETING AUTHORISATION HOLDER

Serono Europe Ltd.

56 Marsh Wall

London E14 9TP

United Kingdom

8. MARKETING AUTHORISATION NUMBER(S)

EU/1/95/001/035

9. DATE OF FIRST AUTHORISATION/RENEWAL OF THE AUTHORISATION

Date of first authorisation: 20 October 1995.

Date of last renewal: 19 October 2005.

10. DATE OF REVISION OF THE TEXT

24th July 2009

Gonapeptyl Depot 3.75 mg

(Ferring Pharmaceuticals Ltd)

1. NAME OF THE MEDICINAL PRODUCT

GONAPEPTYL DEPOT

3.75 mg

Powder and solvent for suspension for injection.

2. QUALITATIVE AND QUANTITATIVE COMPOSITION

One pre-filled syringe contains 3.75 mg triptorelin (as acetate) to be suspended in one ml suspension agent.

For excipients, see 6.1.

3. PHARMACEUTICAL FORM

Powder and solvent for suspension for injection prolonged release in pre-filled syringes.

4. CLINICAL PARTICULARS

4.1 Therapeutic indications

Men:

Treatment of advanced, hormone-dependent prostate carcinoma.

Women:

Preoperative reduction of myoma size to reduce the symptoms of bleeding and pain in women with symptomatic uterine myomas.

Symptomatic endometriosis confirmed by laparoscopy when suppression of the ovarian hormonogenesis is indicated to the extent that surgical therapy is not primarily indicated.

Children:

Treatment of confirmed central precocious puberty (girls under 9 years, boys under 10 years).

4.2 Posology and method of administration

The product should only be used under the supervision of an appropriate specialist having requisite facilities for regular monitoring of response.

It is important that the injection of the sustained release form be performed strictly in accordance with the instructions given in section 6.6.

Following reconstitution, the suspension has to be injected immediately.

Dosage and method of administration

The dosage of one syringe, equivalent to 3.75 mg triptorelin, is injected every 28 days either subcutaneously (e.g. into the skin of the abdomen, the buttock or thigh) or deep intramuscularly. The injection site should be changed each time.

Men:

Once every four weeks an injection with one syringe, equivalent to 3.75 mg triptorelin. In order to continually suppress testosterone levels, it is important to comply with a 4-weekly administration.

Women:

– Uterine myomas and endometriosis:

Once every four weeks an injection with one syringe, equivalent to 3.75 mg triptorelin. The treatment must be initiated in the first 5 days of the cycle.

Children:

At the beginning of treatment one injection with one syringe, equivalent to 3.75 mg triptorelin, on days 0, 14, and 28. Thereafter one injection every 4 weeks. Should the effect be insufficient, the injections may be given every 3 weeks. Dosing should be based on body weight. Children weighing less than 20 kg are injected with 1.875 mg (half dose), children between 20 and 30 kg receive 2.5 mg (2/3 dose), and children with more than 30 kg body weight are injected with 3.75 mg triptorelin (full dose).

Note for specific patient groups:

– There is no need to adjust the dose for the elderly.

– According to current data, dose reduction or prolongation of the dosage interval in patients with impaired renal function is not necessary.

Duration of administration

– Prostate carcinoma:

Treatment with *Gonapeptyl Depot* is usually a long-term therapy.

- Uterine myomas and endometriosis:

The duration of treatment depends on the initial degree of severity of endometriosis and on the evolution of its clinical manifestations (functional and anatomical) and on the evolution of the volume of the uterine myomas, determined by ultrasonography during treatment. Normally, the maximum attainable result is achieved after 3 to 4 injections.

In view of the possible effect on bone density, therapy should not exceed a duration of 6 months (see 4.4).

- Central precocious puberty (CPP):

Treatment should be stopped if a bone maturation of older than 12 years in girls and older than 13 years in boys has been achieved.

4.3 Contraindications

General:

Known hypersensitivity to triptorelin, poly-(d,l lactide coglycolide), dextran, or to any of the excipients.

In men:

– Hormone independent prostate carcinoma

– As sole treatment in prostate cancer patients with spinal cord compression or evidence of spinal metastases (see also section 4.4)

– After orchiectomy (in case of surgical castration *Gonapeptyl Depot* does not cause further decrease of serum testosterone)

In women:

– Pregnancy

– Clinically manifest osteoporosis

– Lactation period

In children:

– Progressive brain tumours

4.4 Special warnings and precautions for use

Men:

The initial transient increase of serum testosterone has, in few patients, been associated with a temporary aggravation of symptoms of the disease (see 4.8). The patient should be advised to consult the physician, if any of these symptoms aggravates. For that reason, the use of *Gonapeptyl Depot* has to be carefully evaluated in patients with premonitory signs of medullary compression and the medical surveillance has to be closer in the first weeks of treatment, particularly in patients with urinary tract obstructions due to metastases and/or in patients with spinal metastases.

In order to prevent accentuation of the clinical symptoms, supplementary administration of an appropriate antiandrogen agent should be considered in the initial phase of the treatment.

In order to control the therapeutic effect, the prostate-specific antigen (PSA) and the testosterone plasma levels should be regularly monitored during treatment. Testosterone levels should not exceed 1 ng/ml.

Women:

Gonapeptyl Depot should only be prescribed after careful diagnosis (e.g. laparoscopy). Pregnancy should be precluded prior to treatment.

- Uterine myomas and endometriosis:

Menstruation does not occur during treatment. A supervening metrorrhagia in the course of treatment is abnormal (apart from the first month), and should lead to verification of plasma oestrogen level. Should this level be less than 50 pg/ml, possible associated organic lesions should be sought. After withdrawal of treatment, ovarian function resumes, e.g. menstrual bleeding will resume after 7-12 weeks after the final injection.

Non-hormonal contraception should be used during the initial month of treatment as ovulation may be triggered by the initial release of gonadotrophins. It should also be used from 4 weeks after the last injection until resumption of menstruation or until another contraceptive method has been established.

During treatment of uterine myomas the size of uterus and myoma should be determined regularly, e.g. by means of ultrasonography. Disproportionally fast reduction of uterus size in comparison with the reduction of myoma tissue has in isolated cases led to bleeding and sepsis.

Treatment with *Gonapeptyl Depot* over several months can lead to a decrease of bone density (see 4.8). For this reason, therapy should not exceed a duration of 6 months. After withdrawal of treatment, the bone loss is generally reversible within 6 - 9 months.

Particular caution is therefore advised in patients with additional risk factors in view of osteoporosis.

Children:

The chronological age at the beginning of therapy should be under 9 years in girls and under 10 years in boys.

After finalising the therapy, development of puberty characteristics will occur. Information with regards to future fertility is still limited. In most girls menses will start on average one year after ending the therapy, which in most cases is regular.

Pseudo-precocious puberty (gonadal or adrenal tumour or hyperplasia) and gonadotropin-independent precocious puberty (testicular toxicosis, familial Leydig cell hyperplasia) should be precluded.

Allergic and anaphylactic reactions have been reported in adults and children. These include both local site reactions and systemic symptoms. The pathogenesis could not be elucidated. A higher reporting rate was seen in children.

General:

When triptorelin is co-administered with drugs affecting pituitary secretion of gonadotrophins caution should be given and the patient's hormonal status should be supervised.

4.5 Interaction with other medicinal products and other forms of interaction

Oestrogen containing medicinal products should not be used during treatment with Gonapeptyl Depot.

4.6 Pregnancy and lactation

Very limited data on the use of triptorelin during pregnancy do not indicate an increased risk of congenital malformations. However, long-term follow-up studies on development are far too limited. Animal data do not indicate direct or indirect harmful effects with respect to pregnancies or postnatal developments, but there are indications for foetotoxicity and delayed parturition. Based on the pharmacological effects disadvantageous influence on the pregnancy and the offspring cannot be excluded and *Gonapeptyl Depot* should not be used during pregnancy. Women of childbearing potential should use effective non-hormonal contraception. It is not known whether triptorelin is excreted in human milk. Because of the potential for adverse reactions from triptorelin in nursing infants, breast-feeding should be discontinued prior to and throughout administration.

4.7 Effects on ability to drive and use machines

Gonapeptyl Depot has no or negligible influence on the ability to drive and use machines.

4.8 Undesirable effects

Adverse experiences reported among patients treated with triptorelin during clinical trials and from post-marketing surveillance are shown below. As a consequence of decreased testosterone or oestrogen levels, most patients are expected to experience adverse reactions, with hot flushes being the most frequently reported (30% in men and 75-100% in women). Additionally, impotence and decreased libido should be expected in 30-40% of male patients, while bleeding/spotting, sweating, vaginal dryness and/or dyspareunia, decrease in libido and mood changes are expected in more than 10% of women.

Due to the fact that the testosterone levels normally increase during the first week of treatment, worsening of symptoms and complaints may occur (e.g. urinary obstruction, skeletal pain due to metastases, compression of the spinal cord, muscular fatigue and lymphatic oedema of the legs). In some cases urinary tract obstruction decreases the kidney function. Neurological compression with asthenia and paraesthesia in the legs has been observed.

Organ class	Common Adverse Reactions (> 1/100, < 1/10)	Uncommon Adverse Reactions (> 1/1000, < 1/100)
Men and women		
Endocrine	Depressive mood; irritation	
Metabolic and nutritional		Elevated enzyme levels (LDH, γGT, SGOT, SGPT)
Gastrointestinal	Nausea	
Musculo-skeletal system	Myalgia; arthralgia	
Body as a whole – general:	Tiredness; sleep disturbances; hypersensitivity reactions (itching; skin rash; fever)	Anaphylaxis
Application site disorders	Temporary pain at injection site	Foreign body reaction at injection site
Men		
Platelet, bleeding and clotting disorders		Thrombo-embolic disorder
Endocrine	Gynecomastia; headache; perspiration	Testicular atrophy; reduced growth of beard; hair loss on chest, arms and legs
Cardiovascular		Hypertension
Gastro-intestinal		Loss of appetite; gastralgia; dry mouth
Respiratory system disorders		Recurrence of asthma
General		Weight changes
Women		
Metabolic and nutritional		Slight rise in serum cholesterol
Central and peripheral nervous system		Visual disturbances; paraesthesia
General		Aching of back
Children		
Endocrine		Vaginal bleeding and discharge
Gastrointestinal		Vomiting; nausea
Body as a whole – general		Anaphylaxis

Slight trabecular bone loss may occur. This is generally reversible within 6-9 months after treatment discontinuation (see section 4.4).

Two cases of epiphysiolysis capitis femoris have been reported during use with triptorelin. Whether or not a causal relationship exists is unknown.

4.9 Overdose

There is insufficient experience of overdosing with triptorelin to draw conclusions on possible adverse effects. Considering the package form and the pharmaceutical form, overdosing is not expected.

5. PHARMACOLOGICAL PROPERTIES

5.1 Pharmacodynamic properties

Pharmacotherapeutic group: Gonadorelinanaloga

ATC code: L02AE04

Triptorelin is a synthetic decapeptide analogue of the natural gonadotrophin-releasing hormone (GnRH). GnRH is a decapeptide, which is synthesised in the hypothalamus and regulates the biosynthesis and release of the gonadotrophins LH (luteinising hormone) and FSH (follicle stimulating hormone) by the pituitary. Triptorelin stimulates the pituitary more strongly to secretion of LH and FSH than a comparable dose of gonadorelin, whereas the duration of action is longer. The increase of LH and FSH levels will initially lead to an increase of serum testosterone concentrations in men or serum oestrogen concentrations in women. Chronic administration of a GnRH agonist results in an inhibition of pituitary LH- and FSH-secretion. This inhibition leads to a reduction in steroidogenesis, by which the serum estradiol concentration in women and the serum testosterone concentration in men fall to within the post-menopausal or castrate range, respectively, i.e. a hypogonadotrophic hypogonadal state. In children with precocious puberty, the concentration of estradiol or testosterone will decrease to within the prepubertal range. Plasma DHEAS (dihydroepiandrostenedion sulphate) levels are not influenced. Therapeutically, this leads to a decrease in growth of testosterone-sensitive prostate tumours in men, and to reduction of endometriosis foci and oestrogen-dependent uterus myomas in women. Regarding uterine myoma, maximal benefit of treatment is observed in women with anaemia (haemoglobin inferior or equal to 8 g/dl). In children suffering from CPP triptorelin treatment leads to a suppression of the secretion of gonadotropins, estradiol, and testosterone to prepubertal levels. This results in arrest or even regression of pubertal signs and an increase in adult height prediction in CPP patients.

5.2 Pharmacokinetic properties

After intramuscular administration of *Gonapeptyl Depot*, the plasma concentrations of triptorelin are determined by the (slow) degradation of the poly-(d,l lactide coglycolide) polymer. The mechanism inherent to this administration form enables this slow release of triptorelin from the polymer.

After I.M. or S.C. application of a triptorelin depot-formulation (sustained-release microcapsules), a rapid increase in the concentration of triptorelin in plasma is recorded, with a maximum in the first hours. Then the triptorelin concentration declines notably within 24 hours. On day 4 the value reaches a second maximum, falling below the detection limit in a biexponential course after 44 days. After S.C. injections the triptorelin increase is more gradual and in a somewhat lower concentration than after I.M. injections. After S.C. injection, the decline in the triptorelin concentration takes longer, with values falling below the detection limit after 65 days.

During treatment over a period of 6 months and an administration every 28 days, there was no evidence of triptorelin accumulation in both modes of administration. Plasma triptorelin values decreased to approx. 100 pg/ml before the next application after I.M. or S.C. application (median values). It is to be assumed that the non-systemically available proportion of triptorelin is metabolized at the injection site, e.g. by macrophages.

In the pituitary, the systemically available triptorelin is inactivated by N-terminal cleavage via pyroglutamyl-peptidase and a neutral endopeptidase. In the liver and the kidneys, triptorelin is degraded to biologically inactive peptides and amino acids.

40 minutes after the end of an infusion of 100 µg triptorelin (over 1 hour) 3-14% of the administered dose has already been eliminated by the kidney.

For patients with an impaired renal function, adaptation and individualization of therapy with the triptorelin depot-formulation seems to be unnecessary, on account of the subordinate significance of the renal elimination route and the broad therapeutic range of triptorelin as an active component.

Bioavailability:

Men:

The systemic bioavailability of the active component triptorelin from the intramuscular depot is 38.3% in the first 13 days. Further release is linear at 0.92% of the dose per day on average. Bioavailability after S.C. application is 69% of I.M. availability.

Women:

After 27 test days, 35.7% of the applied dose can be detected on average, with 25.5% being released in the first 13 days and further release being linear at 0.73% of the dose per day on average.

General:

Calculation of the model-depending kinetic parameters ($t_{½}$, K_{el}, etc.) is inapplicable in presentations with a strongly protracted release of the active component.

5.3 Preclinical safety data

In rats, but not in mice treated over a long period of time with triptorelin, an increase in pituitary tumors has been detected. The influence of triptorelin on pituitary abnormalities in humans is unknown. The observation is considered not to be relevant to humans. Pituitary tumors in rodents in connection with other LHRH analogues have also been known to occur. Triptorelin has been shown to be embryo-/foetotoxic and to cause a delay in embryo-/foetal development as well as delay in parturition in rats. Preclinical data reveal no special hazard to humans based on repeat dose toxicity and genotoxicity studies. Single I.M. or S.C. injection of *Gonapeptyl Depot* or its suspension agent produced delayed foreign body reactions at the injection site. Within 8 weeks, these late reactions were nearly reversed after I.M. injection but only slightly reversed after S.C. injection. Local tolerance of *Gonapeptyl Depot* after I.V. injection was limited

6. PHARMACEUTICAL PARTICULARS

6.1 List of excipients

One pre-filledsyringe with powder contains:

Poly-(d,l lactide coglycolide)

Propyleneglycol octanoate decanoate

One pre-filledsyringe with one ml suspension agent contains:

Dextran 70

Polysorbate 80

Sodium chloride

Sodium hydrogen phosphate dihydrate

Sodium hydroxide

Water for injection

6.2 Incompatibilities

In the absence of compatibility studies this medicinal product should not be mixed with other medicinal products.

6.3 Shelf life

3 years

Reconstituted suspension: 3 minutes

6.4 Special precautions for storage

Store at 2°C - 8°C (in a refrigerator). Keep the container in the outer carton.

6.5 Nature and contents of container

Powder: Pre-filled syringe

Solvent: Pre-filled syringe

Pre-filled syringes (borosilicate glass type I, clear) with a connector (polypropylene), black chlorobutyl rubber stopper (plunger stopper, type I) and injection needle.

Pack sizes:

1 pre-filled syringe (powder) plus

1 pre-filled syringe (solvent)

3 pre-filled syringes (powder) plus

3 pre-filled syringes (solvent)

6.6 Special precautions for disposal and other handling

GonapeptylDepot is for single use only and any unused suspension should be discarded.

1. Preparation

Instructions for the physician how to prepare the suspension.

Since successful treatment depends upon correct preparation of the suspension, the following instructions must be strictly followed.

- Take the package of *Gonapeptyl Depot* from the refrigerator.

- Remove the cap from the disposable syringe containing the powder. Keep upright to prevent spilling.

- Open the package with the connector without removing the connector.

- Screw the syringe containing the sustained release microparticles on the connector in the package, then remove it.

Screw the syringe containing the suspension agent tightly on the free end of the connector and ensure that it fits tightly.

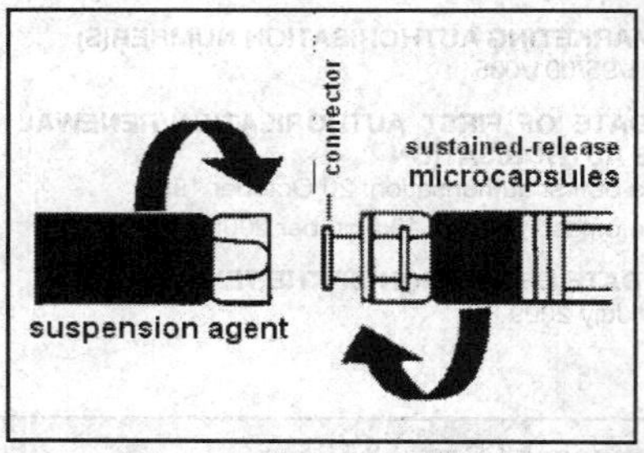

2. Reconstitution of a suspension

Empty the liquid into the syringe with the powder, then shoot it back and forth into the first syringe – the first two or three times without pushing the injection rod all the way in. Repeat this about 10 times or until you have a homogeneous milky-like suspension. While preparing the suspension, you might possibly create some foam. It is important that the foam be dissolved or removed from the syringe before giving the injection.

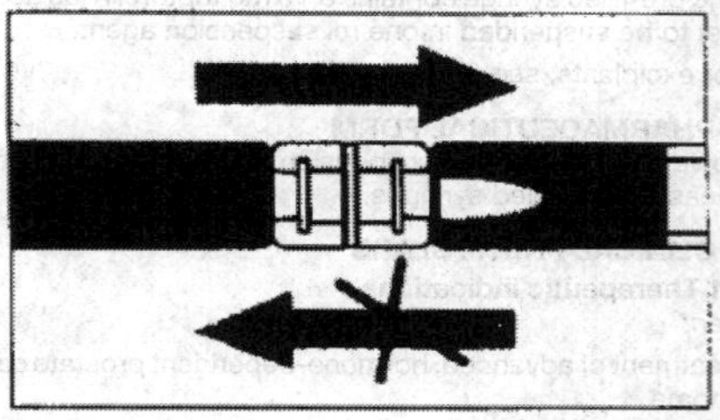

Mixing

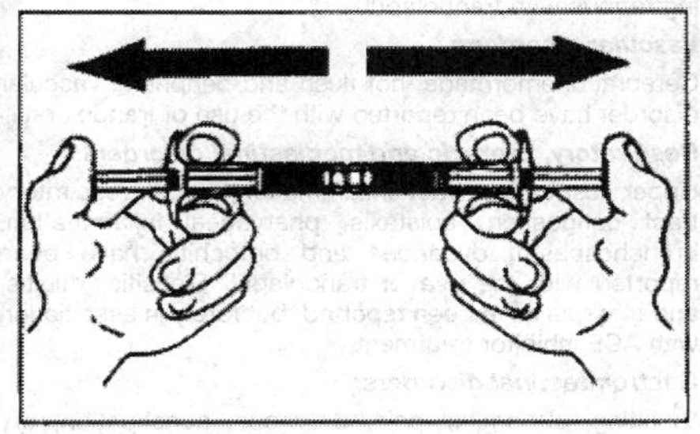

Mix approximately 10 times

3. Injection

- Remove the connector together with the empty syringe.

- Mount the injection needle on the syringe with the ready-to-use suspension.

- Inject subcutaneously or deep into the muscle immediately.

7. MARKETING AUTHORISATION HOLDER

Ferring Pharmaceuticals Ltd.

The Courtyard

Waterside Drive

Langley

Berkshire SL3 6EZ

United Kingdom

8. MARKETING AUTHORISATION NUMBER(S)

PL 03194/0085

9. DATE OF FIRST AUTHORISATION/RENEWAL OF THE AUTHORISATION

14th May 2003

10. DATE OF REVISION OF THE TEXT

Gopten

(Abbott Laboratories Limited)

1. NAME OF THE MEDICINAL PRODUCT

Gopten®

2. QUALITATIVE AND QUANTITATIVE COMPOSITION

Trandolapril, 0.5mg

Trandolapril, 1.0mg

Trandolapril, 2.0mg

Trandolapril, 4.0mg

For excipients see section 6.1

3. PHARMACEUTICAL FORM

Capsules, Hard

0.5mg: opaque red/yellow capsules

1.0mg: opaque red/orange capsules

2.0mg: opaque red/red capsules

4.0mg: opaque red/maroon capsules

4. CLINICAL PARTICULARS

4.1 Therapeutic indications

Mild or moderate hypertension.

Left ventricular dysfunction after myocardial infarction.

It has been demonstrated that Gopten improves survival following myocardial infarction in patients with left ventricular dysfunction (ejection fraction ≤35 percent), with or without symptoms of heart failure, and/or with or without residual ischaemia.

Long-term treatment with Gopten significantly reduces the overall cardiovascular mortality. It significantly decreases the risk of sudden death and the occurrence of severe or resistant heart failure.

4.2 Posology and method of administration

Adults

Hypertension

For adults not taking diuretics, without congestive heart failure and without renal or hepatic insufficiency, the recommended initial dosage is 0.5mg as a single daily dose. A 0.5mg dose will only achieve a therapeutic response in a minority of patients. Dosage should be doubled incrementally at intervals of 2 to 4 weeks, based on patient response, up to a maximum of 4mg as a single daily dose.

The usual maintenance dose range is 1 to 2mg as a single daily dose. If the patient response is still unsatisfactory at a dose of 4mg Gopten, combination therapy should be considered.

Left ventricular dysfunction after myocardial infarction

Following a myocardial infarction, therapy may be initiated as early as the third day. Treatment should be initiated at a daily dose of 0.5mg. The dose should be progressively increased to a maximum of 4mg as a single daily dose. Depending upon the tolerability such as symptomatic hypotension, this forced titration can be temporarily suspended.

In the event of hypotension, all concomitant hypotensive therapies such as vasodilators, including nitrates and diuretics must be carefully checked and if possible, their dose reduced.

The dose of Gopten should be lowered only if the previous measures are not effective or not feasible.

Elderly

The dose in elderly patients is the same as in adults. There is no need to reduce the dose in elderly patients with normal renal and hepatic function. Caution is required in elderly patients with concomitant use of diuretics, congestive heart failure or renal or hepatic insufficiency. The dose should be titrated according to the need to control blood pressure.

Prior diuretic treatment

In patients who are at risk from a stimulated renin-angiotensin system (e.g. patients with water and sodium depletion), the diuretic should be discontinued 2-3 days before beginning therapy with 0.5mg trandolapril to reduce the likelihood of symptomatic hypotension. The diuretic may be resumed later if required.

Cardiac failure

In hypertensive patients who also have congestive heart failure, with or without associated renal insufficiency, symptomatic hypotension has been observed after treatment with ACE inhibitors. In these patients, therapy should be started at a dose of 0.5mg Gopten once daily under close medical supervision in hospital.

Dosage adjustment in renal impairment

For patients with mild or moderate renal impairment (creatinine clearance of 10-70ml/min), the usual adult and elderly doses are recommended.

For patients with severe renal impairment (creatinine clearance of <10ml/min), the usual adult and elderly starting doses are also recommended but the maximum daily dose should not exceed 2mg. In these patients, therapy should be under close medical supervision.

Dialysis: It is not known for certain if trandolapril or trandolaprilat are removed by dialysis. However, it would be expected that dialysis could remove the active moiety, trandolaprilat, from the circulation, resulting in a possible loss of control of blood pressure. Therefore careful monitoring of the patient's blood pressure during dialysis is required, and the dosage of trandolapril adjusted if needed.

Dosage adjustment in hepatic impairment

In patients with severely impaired liver function, a decrease in the metabolic clearance of the parent compound, trandolapril and the active metabolite, trandolaprilat results in a large increase in plasma trandolapril levels and to a lesser extent, an increase in trandolaprilat levels. Treatment with Gopten should therefore be initiated at a dose of 0.5mg once daily under close medical supervision.

Children

Gopten has not been studied in children and therefore use in this age group is not recommended.

4.3 Contraindications

Known hypersensitivity to trandolapril.

History of angioedema associated with administration of an ACE inhibitor.

Hereditary/idiopathic angioneurotic oedema.

Second and third trimester of pregnancy (see sections 4.4 and 4.6).

Lactation.

Use in children.

4.4 Special warnings and precautions for use

Gopten should not be used in patients with aortic stenosis or outflow obstruction.

Assessment of renal function

Evaluation of the patient should include assessment of renal function prior to initiation of therapy and during treatment. Proteinuria may occur if renal impairment is present prior to therapy or relatively high doses are used.

Impaired renal function

Patients with severe renal insufficiency may require reduced doses of Gopten; their renal function should be closely monitored. In the majority, renal function will not alter. In patients with renal insufficiency, congestive heart failure or unilateral or bilateral renal artery stenosis, in the single kidney as well as after renal transplantation, there is a risk of impairment of renal function.

If recognised early, such impairment of renal function is reversible upon discontinuation of therapy.

Some hypertensive patients with no apparent pre-existing renal disease may develop minor and usually transient increases in blood urea nitrogen and serum creatinine when Gopten is given concomitantly with a diuretic. Dosage reduction of Gopten and/or discontinuation of the diuretic may be required. Additionally, in patients with renal insufficiency, the risk of hyperkalaemia should be considered and the patient's electrolyte status checked regularly.

Impaired liver function

As trandolapril is a prodrug metabolised to its active moiety in the liver, particular caution and close monitoring should be applied to patients with impaired liver function.

Symptomatic hypotension

In patients with uncomplicated hypertension, symptomatic hypotension has been observed rarely after the initial dose of Gopten, as well as after increasing the dose of Gopten. It is more likely to occur in patients who have been volume- and salt-depleted by prolonged diuretic therapy, dietary salt restriction, dialysis, diarrhoea or vomiting. Therefore, in these patients, diuretic therapy should be discontinued and volume and/or salt depletion should be corrected before initiating therapy with Gopten.

If symptomatic hypotension occurs, the patient should be placed in a supine position and, if necessary, receive an intravenous infusion of physiological saline. Intravenous atropine may be necessary if there is associated bradycardia. Treatment with Gopten may usually be continued following restoration of effective blood volume and blood pressure.

Surgery/anaesthesia

In patients undergoing surgery or during anaesthesia with agents producing hypotension, Gopten may block angiotensin II formation secondary to compensatory renin release. If hypotension occurs and is considered to be due to this mechanism, it can be corrected by appropriate treatment.

Agranulocytosis and bone marrow depression

In patients on ACE inhibitors, agranulocytosis and bone marrow depression have been seen rarely. They are more frequent in patients with renal impairment, especially if they have a collagen vascular disease. However, regular monitoring of white blood cell counts and protein levels in urine should be considered in patients with collagen vascular disease (e.g. lupus erythematosus and scleroderma), especially associated with impaired renal function and concomitant therapy, particularly with corticosteroids and antimetabolites.

Hyperkalaemia

Elevated serum potassium has been observed very rarely in hypertensive patients. Risk factors for the development of hyperkalaemia include renal insufficiency, potassium-sparing diuretics, the concomitant use of agents to treat hypokalaemia, diabetes mellitus and/or left ventricular dysfunction after myocardial infarction.

Angioedema:

Rarely, ACE inhibitors (such as trandolapril) may cause angioedema that includes swelling of the face, extremities, tongue, glottis, and/or larynx. Patients experiencing angioneurotic oedema must immediately discontinue Gopten therapy and be monitored until oedema resolution.

Angioedema of the face will usually resolve spontaneously. Oedema involving not only the face but also the glottis may be life-threatening because of the risk of airway obstruction.

Angioedema involving the tongue, glottis or larynx requires immediate subcutaneous administration of 0.3-0.5ml of adrenaline solution (1:1000) along with other therapeutic measures as appropriate.

Caution must be exercised in patients with a history of idiopathic angioneurotic oedema, and Gopten is contraindicated if angioneurotic oedema was an adverse reaction to an ACE inhibitor (section 4.3).

ACE inhibitors have been shown to cause a higher rate of angioedema in black patients than in non-black patients.

Intestinal angioedema has also been reported in patients treated with ACE inhibitors. This should be considered in patients on trandolapril presenting with abdominal pain (with or without nausea or vomiting).

Cough:

During treatment with an ACE inhibitor, a dry and non-productive cough may occur which disappears after discontinuation.

Hereditary disorders:

Patients with rare hereditary problems of galactose intolerance, the Lapp lactase deficiency or glucose-galactose malabsorption should not take this medicine.

Pregnancy

ACE inhibitors should not be initiated during pregnancy. Unless continued ACE inhibitor use is considered essential, patients planning pregnancy should be changed to alternative anti-hypertensive treatments which have an established safety profile for use in pregnancy. When pregnancy is diagnosed, treatment with ACE inhibitors should be stopped immediately, and, if appropriate, alternative therapy should be started (see sections 4.3 and 4.6).

4.5 Interaction with other medicinal products and other forms of interaction

Drug interactions

Combination with diuretics or other antihypertensive agents may potentiate the antihypertensive response to Gopten. Adrenergic-blocking drugs should only be combined with trandolapril under careful supervision.

Potassium-sparing diuretics (spironolactone, amiloride, triamterene) or potassium supplements may increase the risk of hyperkalaemia, particularly in renal failure. Gopten may attenuate the potassium loss caused by thiazide-type diuretics. If concomitant use of these agents is indicated, they should be given with caution and serum potassium should be monitored regularly.

Antidiabetic agents

As with all ACE inhibitors, concomitant use of antidiabetic medicines (insulin or oral hypoglycaemic agents) may cause an increased blood glucose lowering effect with greater risk of hypoglycaemia. Therefore, blood glucose should be closely monitored in diabetics treated with a hypoglycaemic agent and Gopten, particularly when starting or increasing the dose of ACE inhibitor, or in patients with impaired renal function.

Combinations necessitating a warning

In some patients already receiving diuretic treatment, particularly if this treatment has been recently instituted, the fall in blood pressure on initiation of treatment with Gopten may be excessive. The risk of symptomatic hypotension may be reduced by stopping the diuretic a few days before starting treatment with Gopten. If it is necessary to continue the diuretic treatment, the patient should be monitored, at least after the initial administration of Gopten. As with all antihypertensives, combination with a neuroleptic or tricyclic antidepressant increases the risk of orthostatic hypotension. Gopten may reduce the elimination of lithium and serum levels of lithium should be monitored.

Anaphylactoid reactions to high-flux polyacrylonitrile membranes used in haemodialysis have been reported in patients treated with ACE inhibitors. As with other antihypertensives of this chemical class, this combination should be avoided when prescribing ACE inhibitors to renal dialysis patients.

The hypotensive effects of certain inhalation anaesthetics may be enhanced by ACE inhibitors.

Allopurinol, cytostatic or immunosuppressive agents, systemic corticosteroids or procainamide may increase the risk of leucopoenia, if used concomitantly with ACE inhibitors.

As with all antihypertensives, NSAIDs may reduce the antihypertensive effects of trandolapril. Blood pressure monitoring should be increased when any NSAID is added or discontinued in a patient treated with trandolapril. An additive effect on serum potassium increase has been described when NSAIDs and ACE inhibitors have been used concomitantly, while renal function may be reduced.

Antacids may cause reduced bioavailability of ACE inhibitors.

The antihypertensive effects of ACE inhibitors may be reduced by sympathomimetics; patients should be carefully monitored.

No clinical interaction has been observed in patients with left ventricular dysfunction after myocardial infarction when Gopten has been concomitantly administered with thrombolytics, aspirin, beta-blockers, calcium channel blockers, nitrates, anticoagulants, diuretics or digoxin.

4.6 Pregnancy and lactation

The use of ACE inhibitors is not recommended during the first trimester of pregnancy (see section 4.4). The use of ACE inhibitors is contra-indicated during the second and third trimester of pregnancy (see sections 4.3 and 4.4).

Epidemiological evidence regarding the risk of teratogenicity following exposure to ACE inhibitors during the first trimester of pregnancy has not been conclusive; however, a small increase in the risk cannot be excluded. Unless continued ACE inhibitor therapy is considered essential, patients planning pregnancy should be changed to alternative anti-hypertensive treatments, which have an established safety profile for use in pregnancy. When pregnancy is diagnosed, treatment with ACE inhibitors should be stopped immediately and, if appropriate, alternative therapy should be started.

ACE inhibitor therapy exposure during the second and third trimesters is known to induce human fetotoxicity (decreased, renal function, oligohydramnios, skull ossification retardation) and neonatal toxicity (renal failure, hypotension, hyperkalemia). Should exposure to trandolapril have occurred from the second trimester of pregnancy, an ultrasound check of renal function and skull is recommended. Infants whose mothers have taken ACE inhibitors should be closely observed for hypotension.

Lactation:

Because no information is available regarding the use of Gopten during breastfeeding, Gopten is not recommended and alternative treatments with better established safety profiles during breast-feeding are preferable, especially while nursing a newborn or preterm infant.

4.7 Effects on ability to drive and use machines

Given the pharmacological properties of Gopten, no particular effect is expected. However, in some individuals, ACE inhibitors may affect the ability to drive or operate machinery, particularly at the start of treatment, when changing over from other medication or during concomitant use of alcohol. Therefore, after the first dose or subsequent increases in dose, it is not advisable to drive or operate machinery for several hours.

4.8 Undesirable effects

The following adverse reactions have been reported in long-term hypertension clinical trials with trandolapril. Within each system organ class, the reactions are ranked under headings of frequency, using the following convention: common (>1/100 to ≤1/10), uncommon (>1/1000 to ≤1/100).

Adverse Reactions Reported In Long Term Hypertension Trials With Trandolapril (n = 1049) That Occurred At A Frequency Greater Than Or Equal To 0.5%

Body System	Preferred Term	Frequency
Nervous system disorders	Headache Dizziness	Common (2.3%) Common (1.7%)
Cardiac disorders	Palpitations	Uncommon (0.7%)
Vascular disorders	Hypotension	Uncommon (0.5%)
Respiratory, thoracic and mediastinal disorders	Cough	Common (3.9%)
Gastrointestinal disorders	Nausea	Uncommon (0.5%)
Skin and subcutaneous tissue disorders	Pruritus	Uncommon (0.5%)
General disorders and administration site conditions	Asthenia Malaise	Common (2.1%) Uncommon (0.5%)

The following adverse reactions have been reported in the post myocardial infarction clinical trial with trandolapril. Within each system organ class, the reactions are ranked under headings of frequency, using the following convention: common (>1/100, ≤ 1/10), uncommon (>1/1000, ≤ 1/100).

Adverse Reactions Reported With Trandolapril In Post Myocardial Infarction Patients In The TRACE Study (n = 876) That Occurred At A Frequency Greater Than Or Equal To 0.5%

Body System	Preferred Term	Frequency
Nervous system disorders	Dizziness	Common (1.9%)
Cardiac disorders	Heart failure	Uncommon (0.8%)
Vascular disorders	Hypotension	Common (2.1%)
Respiratory, thoracic and mediastinal disorders	Cough	Common (3.9%)
Investigations	Creatinine Increased	Uncommon (0.6%)

In addition, other significant adverse events seen in clinical trials and postmarketing surveillance seen with trandolapril and those reported with other ACE inhibitors are listed below:

Infections and infestations:

Upper respiratory tract infection has been reported with the use of trandolapril.

Blood and lymphatic system disorders:

Anaemia has been reported with the use of trandolapril.

Metabolism and nutrition disorders:

Hyperuricaemia has been reported with the use of trandolapril.

Psychiatric disorders:

Insomnia, libido decreased, depression and sleep disorder have been reported with the use of trandolapril.

Nervous system disorders:

Transient ischaemic attacks, somnolence, syncope, myoclonus, migraine and dysgeusia have been reported with the use of trandolapril. Confusion has also been reported with the use of ACE inhibitors.

Eye disorders:

Visual disturbance has been reported with the use of trandolapril. Vision blurred has also been reported with the use ACE inhibitors.

Ear and labyrinth disorders:

Vertigo and tinnitus have been reported with the use of trandolapril.

Cardiac disorders:

Tachycardia, arrhythmias, angina pectoris, and myocardial infarction have been reported in association with hypotension during the use of trandolapril. Atrioventricular block and cardiac arrest have also been observed in postmarketing reports with trandolapril.

Vascular disorders:

Cerebral haemorrhage, hot flush and peripheral vascular disorder have been reported with the use of trandolapril.

Respiratory, thoracic and mediastinal disorders:

Upper respiratory tract inflammation, upper respiratory tract congestion, epistaxis, pharyngeal inflammation, bronchospasm, dyspnoea and bronchitis have been reported with the use of trandolapril. Sinusitis, rhinitis, and glossitis have been reported, but rarely in association with ACE inhibitor treatment.

Gastrointestinal disorders:

Vomiting, abdominal pain, diarrhoea, constipation, dry mouth, dyspepsia, ileus and gastrointestinal pain have been reported with the use of trandolapril. Pancreatitis has also been observed in postmarketing reports with trandolapril.

Hepatobiliary disorders:

There have been reports of individual incidents of cholestatic jaundice and hepatitis connected with the use of trandolapril.

Skin and subcutaneous tissue disorders:

Allergic hypersensitivity reactions such as pruritus and rash have been reported. Urticaria, erythema multiforme, Stevens-Johnson syndrome, toxic epidermal necrolysis, psoriasis-like efflorescences, and alopecia, which may be accompanied by fever, myalgia, arthralgia, eosinophilia and/or increased ANA (anti-nuclear antibody) -titres have been occasionally reported with ACE inhibitor treatment. Alopecia and hyperhidrosis have also been observed in postmarketing reports with trandolapril.

In very rare cases, angioedema has occurred. If laryngeal stridor or angioedema of the face, tongue or glottis occurs, treatment with Gopten must be discontinued and appropriate therapy instituted immediately.

Musculoskeletal and connective tissue disorders:

Back pain, muscle spasms and pain in extremity have been reported with the use of trandolapril.

Renal and urinary disorders:

Pollakiuria, deterioration of renal function and acute renal failure have been reported with the use of trandolapril.

Reproductive system and breast disorders:

Erectile dysfunction has been reported with the use of trandolapril.

General disorders and administration site conditions:

Chest pain, oedema peripheral, feeling abnormal and fatigue have been reported with the use of trandolapril.

Investigations:

Reversible (on stopping treatment) increases in blood urea and plasma creatinine may result, particularly if renal insufficiency, severe heart failure or renovascular hypertension are present. Decreased haemoglobin, haematocrit, platelets and white cell count, and increased blood alkaline phosphatase and blood lactate dehydrogenase, have been reported with the use of trandolapril. Individual cases of agranulocytosis or pancytopenia and increased serum bilirubin have also been reported with trandolapril use.

Haemolytic anaemia has been reported in some patients with a congenital deficiency concerning G-6 PDH (glucose-6-phosphate dehydrogenase) during treatment with ACE inhibitors. Leucopoenia and elevated liver enzymes (including SGOT and SGPT) have also been observed in postmarketing reports with trandolapril.

4.9 Overdose

Symptoms expected with ACE inhibitors are severe hypotension, shock, stupor, bradycardia, electrolyte disturbance and renal failure. In the event of overdosage following recent ingestion, consideration should be given to emptying the stomach contents. Blood pressure should be monitored and if hypotension develops, volume expansion should be considered.

5. PHARMACOLOGICAL PROPERTIES

5.1 Pharmacodynamic properties

ATC Code: C 09A A10

Gopten capsules contain the prodrug, trandolapril, a non-peptide ACE inhibitor with a carboxyl group but without a sulphydryl group. Trandolapril is rapidly absorbed and then non-specifically hydrolysed to its potent, long-acting active metabolite, trandolaprilat.

Trandolaprilat binds tightly and in a saturable manner to ACE.

The administration of trandolapril causes decreases in the concentrations of angiotensin II, aldosterone and atrial natriuretic factor and increases in plasma renin activity and concentrations of angiotensin I. Gopten thus modulates the renin-angiotensin-aldosterone system which plays a major part in regulating blood volume and blood pressure and consequently has a beneficial antihypertensive effect.

The administration of usual therapeutic doses of Gopten to hypertensive patients produces a marked reduction in both supine and erect blood pressure. The antihypertensive effect is evident after 1 hour, with a peak effect between 8 and 12 hours, persisting for at least 24 hours.

The properties of trandolapril might explain the results obtained in the regression of cardiac hypertrophy with improvement of diastolic function, and improvement of arterial compliance in humans. In addition, a decrease in vascular hypertrophy has been shown in animals.

5.2 Pharmacokinetic properties

Trandolapril is very rapidly absorbed after oral administration. The amount absorbed is equivalent to 40 to 60% of the administered dose and is not affected by food consumption.

The peak plasma concentration of trandolapril is observed 30 minutes after administration. Trandolapril disappears rapidly from the plasma with a half-life of less than one hour.

Trandolapril is hydrolysed to trandolaprilat, a specific ACE inhibitor. The amount of trandolaprilat formed is not modified by food consumption. The median peak plasma concentration values of trandolaprilat are reached after 3 to 8 hours. The absolute bioavailability of trandolaprilat following trandolapril dose is about 13%.

In the plasma, trandolaprilat is more than 80% protein-bound. It binds saturably, with a high affinity, to ACE. The major proportion of circulating trandolaprilat is also non-saturably bound to albumin.

After repeated administration of Gopten in a single daily dose, steady state of trandolaprilat is reached on average in four days, both in healthy volunteers and in young or elderly hypertensives. The effective half-life of trandolaprilat is between 15 and 23 hours. The terminal half-life of elimination is between 47 hours and 98 hours depending on dose. This terminal phase probably represents binding/dissociation kinetics of the trandolaprilat/ACE complex.

About 9-14% of an administered trandolapril dose is excreted as trandolaprilat in urine. A negligible amount of trandolapril is excreted unchanged in the urine (<0.5%). After oral administration of the labelled product in man, 33% of the radioactivity is found in the urine and 66% in the faeces.

Special Patient Populations

Pediatric: Trandolapril pharmacokinetics have not been evaluated in patients less than 18 years of age.

Geriatric and Gender: Trandolapril pharmacokinetics have been investigated in the elderly (over 65 years) and in both genders. The plasma concentration of trandolapril is increased in elderly hypertensive patients, but the plasma concentration of trandolaprilat and inhibition of ACE activity are similar in elderly and young hypertensive patients. The pharmacokinetics of trandolapril and trandolaprilat and inhibition of ACE activity are similar in male and female elderly hypertensive patients.

Race: Pharmacokinetic differences have not been evaluated in different races.

Renal Insufficiency: Compared to normal subjects, the plasma concentrations of trandolapril and trandolaprilat are approximately two-fold greater and renal clearance is reduced by about 85% in patients with creatinine clearance below 30 mL/min and in patients on hemodialysis. Dosage adjustment is recommended in renally impaired patients.

Hepatic Insufficiency: Following oral administration in patients with mild to moderate alcoholic cirrhosis, plasma concentrations of trandolapril and trandolaprilat were, respectively, nine-fold and twofold greater than in normal subjects, but inhibition of ACE activity was not affected. Lower doses should be considered in patients with hepatic insufficiency.

5.3 Preclinical safety data

There are no relevant pre-clinical findings which are additional to those already included in other section of the SPC.

6. PHARMACEUTICAL PARTICULARS

6.1 List of excipients

Excipients

Maize starch

Lactose monohydrate

Povidone

Sodium stearyl fumarate

Capsule Shell

Gelatin

Titanium dioxide (E171)

Erythrosine (E127)

Black iron oxide (E172) (Gopten 4mg)

Yellow iron oxide (E172)

Sodium laurylsulphate

6.2 Incompatibilities

None

6.3 Shelf life

Gopten 0.5mg: 24 Months

Gopten 1.0mg: 24 Months

Gopten 2.0mg: 48 months

Gopten 4.0mg: 36 months

6.4 Special precautions for storage

Do not store above 25 °C.

6.5 Nature and contents of container

Gopten 0.5mg: PVC/PVDC/AL calendar pack containing 14 capsules or 56 capsules.

Gopten 1.0mg, 2.0mg and 4.0mg: PVC/PVDC/AL calendar pack containing 28 capsules or 56 capsules.

6.6 Special precautions for disposal and other handling

None

7. MARKETING AUTHORISATION HOLDER

Abbott Laboratories Limited

Queenborough

Kent

ME11 5EL

United Kingdom

8. MARKETING AUTHORISATION NUMBER(S)

PL 00037/0356

PL 00037/0357

PL 00037/0358

PL 00037/0406

9. DATE OF FIRST AUTHORISATION/RENEWAL OF THE AUTHORISATION

Gopten 0.5mg, 1.0mg and 2.0mg: 31 December 2001

Gopten 4.0mg: 12 January 2004

10. DATE OF REVISION OF THE TEXT

7 July 2009 (24 July 2009 for 1mg)

Granocyte 13 million IU, and 34 million IU

(Chugai Pharma UK Limited)

1. NAME OF THE MEDICINAL PRODUCT

GRANOCYTE 13 million IU/mL, powder and solvent for solution for injection/infusion.

GRANOCYTE 13 million IU/mL, powder and solvent for solution for injection/infusion in a pre-filled syringe.

GRANOCYTE 34 million IU/mL, powder and solvent for solution for injection/infusion.

GRANOCYTE 34 million IU/mL, powder and solvent for solution for injection/infusion in a pre-filled syringe.

2. QUALITATIVE AND QUANTITATIVE COMPOSITION

Lenograstim* (rHuG-CSF) 13.4 million International Units (equivalent to 105 micrograms) per mL after reconstitution

Lenograstim* (rHuG-CSF) 33.6 million International Units (equivalent to 263 micrograms) per mL after reconstitution

*Produced by recombinant DNA technology in Chinese Hamster Ovary (CHO) cells.

Excipients known to have a recognised action or effect: phenylalanine

For a full list of excipients, see section 6.1.

3. PHARMACEUTICAL FORM

Powder and solvent for solution for injection/infusion.

Powder and solvent for solution for injection/infusion in a pre-filled syringe.

– White powder

– Solvent: clear, colourless solution

4. CLINICAL PARTICULARS

4.1 Therapeutic indications

• Reduction in the duration of neutropenia in patients (with non myeloid malignancy) undergoing myeloablative therapy followed by bone marrow transplantation (BMT) in patients considered to be at increased risk of prolonged severe neutropenia.

• Reduction of duration of severe neutropenia and its associated complications in patients undergoing established cytotoxic chemotherapy associated with a significant incidence of febrile neutropenia.

• Mobilisation of peripheral blood progenitor cells (PBPCs).

4.2 Posology and method of administration

Therapy should only be given in collaboration with an experienced oncology and/or haematology centre.

GRANOCYTE can be administered by sub-cutaneous injection or by intravenous infusion. Particular handling of the product or instructions for preparation are given in sections 6.6.

• The recommended dose of GRANOCYTE is 150 µg (19.2 MIU) per m^2 per day, therapeutically equivalent to 5 µg (0.64 MIU) per kg per day for:

• Peripheral Stem Cells or bone marrow transplantation,

• established cytotoxic chemotherapy

• PBPC mobilisation after chemotherapy.

GRANOCYTE 13 million IU/mL can be used in patients with body surface area up to 0.7 m^2.

GRANOCYTE 34 million IU/mL can be used in patients with body surface area up to 1.8 m^2.

For PBPC mobilisation with GRANOCYTE alone, the recommended dose is 10 µg (1.28 MIU) per kg per day.

4.2.1 Adults

• In Peripheral Stem Cells or Bone Marrow Transplantation

GRANOCYTE should be administered daily at the recommended dose of 150 µg (19.2 MIU) per m^2 per day as a 30-minute intravenous infusion diluted in isotonic saline solution or as a subcutaneous injection. The first dose should not be administered within 24 hours of the bone marrow infusion. Dosing should continue until the expected nadir has passed and the neutrophil count returns to a stable level compatible with treatment discontinuation, with, if necessary, a maximum of 28 consecutive days of treatment.

It is anticipated that by day 14 following bone marrow transplantation, 50% of patients will achieve neutrophil recovery.

• In Established Cytotoxic Chemotherapy

GRANOCYTE should be administered daily at the recommended dose of 150 µg (19.2 MIU) per m^2 per day as a subcutaneous injection. The first dose should not be administered less than 24 hours following cytotoxic chemotherapy (see 4.4 and 4.5). Daily administration of GRANOCYTE should continue until the expected nadir has passed and the neutrophil count returns to a stable level compatible with treatment discontinuation, with, if necessary, a maximum of 28 consecutive days of treatment.

A transient increase in neutrophil count may occur within the first 2 days of treatment, however GRANOCYTE treatment should not be stopped, since the subsequent nadir usually occurs earlier and recovers more quickly if treatment continues.

• In Peripheral Blood Progenitor Cells (PBPCs) Mobilisation

After chemotherapy, GRANOCYTE should be administered daily, at the recommended dose of 150 µg (19.2 MIU) per m^2 per day as a subcutaneous injection starting within 1 to 5 days after completion of chemotherapy, according to the chemotherapy regimen administered for mobilisation.

Granocyte should be maintained until the last leukapheresis.

Leukapheresis should be performed when the post nadir leukocyte count is rising or after assessment of $CD34^+$ cells in blood with a validated method. For patients who have not had extensive chemotherapy, one leukapheresis is often sufficient to obtain the acceptable minimum yield ($\geqslant 2.0 \times 10^6$ $CD34^+$ cells per kg).

In PBPC mobilisation with GRANOCYTE alone, GRANOCYTE should be administered daily at the recommended dose of 10 µg (1.28 MIU) per kg per day as a subcutaneous injection for 4 to 6 days. Leukapheresis should be performed between day 5 and 7.

In patients who have not had extensive chemotherapy one leukapheresis is often sufficient to obtain the acceptable minimum yield ($\geqslant 2.0 \times 10^6$ $CD34^+$ cells per kg).

In healthy donors, a 10µg/kg daily dose administered subcutaneously for 5-6 days allows a $CD34^+$ cells collection $\geqslant 3 \times 10^6$ /kg body weight with a single leukapheresis in 83% of subjects and with 2 leukapheresis in 97%.

Therapy should only be given in collaboration with an experienced oncology and/ or haematology centre.

4.2.2 Elderly

Clinical trials with GRANOCYTE have included a small number of patients up to the age of 70 years but special studies have not been performed in the elderly and therefore specific dosage recommendations cannot be made.

4.2.3 Children

The safety and efficacy of GRANOCYTE have been established in patients older than 2 years in BMT.

4.3 Contraindications

GRANOCYTE should not be administered to patients with known hypersensitivity to lenograstim or to any of the excipients.

GRANOCYTE should not be used to increase the dose intensity of cytotoxic chemotherapy beyond established doses and dosage regimens since the drug could reduce myelo-toxicity but not overall toxicity of cytotoxic drugs.

It should not be administered concurrently with cytotoxic chemotherapy.

It should not be administered to patients

• with myeloid malignancy other than *de novo* acute myeloid leukaemia,

• with *de novo* acute myeloid leukaemia aged below 55 years, and/or

• with *de novo* acute myeloid leukaemia with good cytogenetics, i.e. t(8;21), t(15;17) and inv (16).

4.4 Special warnings and precautions for use

• Malignant Cell Growth

Granulocyte colony stimulating factor can promote growth of myeloid cells *in vitro* and similar effects may be seen on some non-myeloid cells *in vitro*.

The safety and efficacy of GRANOCYTE administration in patients with myelodysplasia or secondary AML or chronic myelogenous leukaemia have not been established. Therefore, it should not be used in these indications. Particular care should be taken to distinguish the diagnosis of blast transformation of chronic myeloid leukaemia from acute myeloid leukaemia.

Clinical trials have not established whether GRANOCYTE influences the progression of myelodysplastic syndrome to acute myeloid leukaemia. Caution should be exercised in using it in any pre-malignant myeloid condition. As some tumours with non-specific characteristics can exceptionally express a G-CSF receptor, caution should be exerted in the event of unexpected tumour regrowth concomitantly observed with rHuG-CSF therapy

• Leukocytosis

A leukocyte count greater than 50 × 10^9/L has not been observed in any of the 174 clinical trials patients treated with 5 μg/kg/day (0.64 million units/kg/day) following bone marrow transplantation. White blood cell counts of 70 × 10^9/L or greater have been observed in less than 5% of patients who received cytotoxic chemotherapy and were treated by GRANOCYTE at 5 μg/kg/day (0.64 million units/kg/day). No adverse events directly attributable to this degree of leukocytosis have been reported. In view of the potential risks associated with severe leukocytosis, a white blood cell count should, however, be performed at regular intervals during GRANOCYTE therapy.

If leukocyte counts exceed 50 × 10^9/L after the expected nadir, GRANOCYTE should be discontinued immediately.

During PBPC mobilisation, GRANOCYTE should be discontinued if the leukocyte counts rise to > 70 × 109/L.

• Pulmonary adverse effects

Rare (>0.01% and <0.1%) pulmonary adverse effects, in particular interstitial pneumonia, have been reported after G-CSFs administration.

Patients with a recent history of pulmonary infiltrates or pneumonia may be at higher risk.

The onset of pulmonary symptoms or signs, such as cough, fever and dyspnoea, in association with radiological signs of pulmonary infiltrates and deterioration in pulmonary function may be preliminary signs of acute respiratory distress syndrome (ARDS).

GRANOCYTE should be immediately discontinued and appropriate treatment given.

• In Peripheral Stem Cells or Bone Marrow Transplantation

Special attention should be paid to platelet recovery since in double-blind placebo-controlled trials the mean platelet count was lower in patients treated with GRANOCYTE as compared with placebo.

The effect of GRANOCYTE on the incidence and severity of acute and chronic graft-versus-host disease has not been accurately determined.

• In Established Cytotoxic Chemotherapy

The use of GRANOCYTE is not recommended from 24 hours before, until 24 hours after chemotherapy ends (see section 4.5).

The safety of the use of GRANOCYTE with antineoplastic agents characterized by cumulative or predominant platelet lineage myelotoxicity (nitrosurea, mitomycin) has not been established. Administration of GRANOCYTE might enhance the toxicity of these agents, particularly to the platelets.

• Risks Associated with Increased Doses of Chemotherapy

The safety and efficacy of GRANOCYTE have yet to be established in the context of intensified chemotherapy. It should not be used to decrease, beyond the established limits, intervals between chemotherapy courses and/or to increase the doses of chemotherapy. Non-myeloid toxicities were limiting factors in a phase II chemotherapy intensification trial with GRANOCYTE.

• Special precautions in Peripheral Blood Progenitor Cells mobilisation.

Choice of the mobilisation method

Clinical trials carried out among the same patient population have shown that PBPC mobilisation, as assessed within the same laboratory, was higher when GRANOCYTE was used after chemotherapy than when used alone. Nevertheless the choice between the two mobilisation methods should be considered in relation to the overall objectives of treatment for an individual patient.

Prior exposure to radiotherapy and/or cytotoxic agents

Patients, who have undergone extensive prior myelosuppressive therapy and/or radiotherapy, may not show sufficient PBPC mobilisation to achieve the acceptable minimum yield (⩾ 2 x10^6 $CD34^+$ /kg) and therefore adequate haematological reconstitution.

A PBPC transplantation program should be defined early in the treatment course of the patient and particular attention should be paid to the number of PBPC mobilised before the administration of high-dose chemotherapy. If yields are low, other forms of treatment should replace the PBPC transplantation program.

Assessment of progenitor cell yields

Particular attention should be paid to the method of quantification of progenitor cell yields as the results of flow cytometric analysis of $CD34^+$ cell number vary among laboratories.

The minimum yield of $CD34^+$ cells is not well defined. The recommendation of a minimum yield of ⩾ 2.0 × 10^6 CD34+ cells/kg is based on published experience in order to achieve adequate haematological reconstitution. Yields higher than ⩾ 2.0 × 10^6 $CD34^+$ cells/kg are associated with more rapid recovery, including platelets, while lower yields result in slower recovery.

• In healthy donors

The PBPC mobilisation, which is a procedure without direct benefit for healthy people, should only be considered through a clear regular delimitation in accordance with local regulations as for bone marrow donation when applicable.

The efficacy and safety of GRANOCYTE has not been assessed in donors aged over 60 years, therefore the procedure cannot be recommended. Based on some local regulations and lack of studies, minor donors should not be considered.

PBPC mobilisation procedure should be considered for donors who fit usual clinical and laboratory eligibility criteria for bone marrow donation especially normal haematological values.

Marked leukocytosis (WBC ⩾ 50 × 10^9/L) was observed in 24% of subjects studied.

Apheresis-related thrombocytopenia (platelets < 100 × 10^9/L) was observed in 42% of subjects studied and values < 50 × 10^9/L were occasionally noted following leukapheresis without related clinical adverse events, all recovered. Therefore leukapheresis should not be performed in donors who are anticoagulated or who have known defects in haemostasis. If more than one leukapheresis is required particular attention should be paid to donors with platelets < 100 × 10^9/L prior to apheresis; in general apheresis should not be performed if platelets < 75 × 10^9/L.

Insertion of a central venous catheter should be avoided if possible with consideration given to venous access in selection of donors.

Transient cytogenetic modifications have been observed in normal donors following G-CSF use. The significance of these changes is unknown.

Long-term safety follow up of donors is ongoing. Nevertheless, a risk of promotion of a malignant myeloid clone cannot be excluded. It is recommended that the apheresis centre perform a systematic record and tracking of the stem cell donors for at least 10 years to ensure monitoring of long-term safety.

• In recipients of allogeneic peripheral stem-cells mobilised with GRANOCYTE

Allogeneic stem-cell grafting may be associated with an increased risk for chronic GVH (Graft Versus Host Disease), and long-term data of graft functioning are sparse.

• Other Special Precautions

In patients with severe impairment of hepatic or renal function, the safety and efficacy of GRANOCYTE have not been established.

In patients with substantially reduced myeloid progenitor cells (e.g. due to prior intensive radiotherapy/chemotherapy), neutrophil response is sometimes diminished and the safety of GRANOCYTE has not been established.

Common but generally asymptomatic cases of splenomegaly and very rare cases of splenic rupture have been reported in either healthy donors or patients following administration of Granulocyte-colony stimulating factors (G-CSFs). Therefore, spleen size should be carefully monitored (e.g. clinical examination, ultrasound). A diagnosis of splenic rupture should be considered when left upper abdominal pain or shoulder tip pain is reported.

GRANOCYTE contains phenylalanine, which may be harmful for people with phenylketonuria.

4.5 Interaction with other medicinal products and other forms of interaction

In view of the sensitivity of rapidly dividing myeloid cells to cytotoxic chemotherapy, the use of GRANOCYTE is not recommended from 24 hours before until 24 hours after chemotherapy ends (see section 4.4).

Possible interactions with other haematopoietic growth factors and cytokines have yet to be investigated in clinical trials.

4.6 Pregnancy and lactation

• Pregnancy

There are no adequate data from the use of lenograstim in pregnant women.

Studies in animals have shown reproductive toxicity (see section 5.3). The potential risk for humans is unknown.

GRANOCYTE should not be used during pregnancy unless clearly necessary.

• Lactation

It is unknown whether lenograstim is excreted in human milk. The excretion of lenograstim in milk has not been studied in animals. Breast-feeding should be discontinued during therapy with GRANOCYTE.

4.7 Effects on ability to drive and use machines

No studies on the effects on the ability to drive and use machines have been performed.

4.8 Undesirable effects

• In Peripheral Stem Cells or Bone Marrow Transplantation

In double-blind placebo-controlled trials the mean platelet count was lower in patients treated with GRANOCYTE as compared with placebo without an increase in incidence of adverse events related to blood loss and the median number of days following BMT to last platelet infusion was similar in both groups (see section 4.4).

• In Peripheral Stem Cells or Bone Marrow Transplantation and Chemotherapy-Induced Neutropenia

In clinical trials, the most frequently reported adverse events (15%) were the same in patients treated with either GRANOCYTE or placebo. These adverse events were those usually encountered with conditioning regimens and those observed in cancer patients treated with chemotherapy. The most commonly reported adverse events were infection/inflammatory disorder of the buccal cavity, sepsis and infection, fever, diarrhoea, abdominal pain, vomiting, nausea, rash, alopecia, and headache.

Frequency of adverse reactions issued from clinical trials and post-marketing surveillance data. Very common (⩾ 10%); common (⩾ 1/100 to < 1/10); uncommon (⩾ 1/1000 to ⩽ 1/100); rare (⩾ 1/10000 to ⩽ 1/1000); very rare (⩽ 1/10000); not known (cannot be estimated from the available data).

(see Table 1 on next page)

4.9 Overdose

The effects of GRANOCYTE overdose have not been established (see section 5.3). Discontinuation of GRANOCYTE therapy usually results in a 50% decrease in circulating, neutrophils within 1 to 2 days, with a return to normal levels in 1 to 7 days. A white blood cell count of approximately 50 × 10^9/L was observed in one patient out of three receiving the highest GRANOCYTE dose of 40 μg/kg/day (5.12 MIU/kg/day) on the 5th day of treatment. In humans, doses up to 40 μg/kg/day were not associated with toxic side effects except musculoskeletal pain.

5. PHARMACOLOGICAL PROPERTIES

5.1 Pharmacodynamic properties

Pharmacotherapeutic group: Cytokines, ATC code: L03AA10

Lenograstim(rHuG-CSF) belongs to the cytokine group of biologically active proteins which regulate cell differentiation and cell growth.

rHuG-CSF is a factor that stimulates neutrophil precursor cells as demonstrated by the CFU-S and CFU-GM cell count which increases in peripheral blood.

GRANOCYTE induces a marked increase in peripheral blood neutrophil counts within 24 hours of administration.

Elevations of neutrophil count are dose-dependent over the 1-10 μg/kg/day range. At the recommended dose, repeated doses induce an enhancement of the neutrophil response. Neutrophils produced in response to GRANOCYTE show normal chemotactic and phagocytic functions.

As with other hematopoietic growth factors, G-CSF has shown in vitro stimulating properties on human endothelial cells.

Use of GRANOCYTE in patients who underwent Bone Marrow Transplantation or who are treated with cytotoxic chemotherapy leads to significant reductions in duration of neutropenia and its associated complications.

Use of GRANOCYTE either alone or after chemotherapy mobilises haematopoietic progenitor cells into the peripheral blood. These autologous Peripheral Blood Progenitor Cells (PBPCs) can be harvested and infused after high dose cytotoxic chemotherapy, either in place of, or in addition to bone marrow transplantation.

Reinfused PBPCs, as obtained following mobilisation with GRANOCYTE have been shown to reconstitute haemopoiesis and reduce the time to engraftment, leading to a marked decrease of the days to platelets independence when compared to autologous bone marrow transplantation.

A pooled analysis of data from 3 double-blind placebo-controlled studies conducted in 861 patients (n=411 ⩾ 55 years) demonstrated a favourable benefit/risk ratio of lenograstim administration in patients over 55 years of age undergoing conventional chemotherapy for *de novo* acute myeloid leukaemia, in the exception of AML with good cytogenetics, i.e. t(8;21), t(15;17) and inv (16).

The benefit in the sub-group of patients over 55 years appeared in terms of lenograstim-induced acceleration of neutrophil recovery, increase in the percentage of patients without infectious episode, reduction in infection duration, reduction in the duration of hospitalisation, reduction in the duration of IV antibiotherapy. However, these beneficial results were not associated with decreased severe or life-threatening infections incidence, nor with decreased infection-related mortality.

Data from a double-blind placebo-controlled study conducted in 446 patients with *de novo* AML showed that, in the 99 patients subgroup with good cytogenetics, the event-free survival was significantly lower in the lenograstim arm than in the placebo arm, and there was a trend towards a lower overall survival in the lenograstim arm when compared to data from the not good cytogenetics subgroup.

5.2 Pharmacokinetic properties

The pharmacokinetics of GRANOCYTE are dose and time dependent.

During repeated dosing (IV and SC routes), peak serum concentration (immediately after IV infusion or after SC injection) is proportional to the injected dose. Repeated

Table 1

Medra System Organ Class	Very common	Common	Uncommon	Rare	Very rare
Investigations	Elevated LDH				
Blood and lymphatic system disorders	Leucocytosis Thrombocytopenia	Enlarged spleen size			Splenic rupture (5)
Nervous system disorders	Headache Asthenia				
Respiratory, thoracic and madiastinal disorders				Pulmonary edema Interstitial pneumonia (3) Pulmonary infiltrates Pulmonary fibrosis	
Gastrointestinal disorders		Abdominal pain			
Skin and subcutaneous tissue disorders					Cutaneous vasculitis Sweet's syndrome (4) Erythema nodosum Pyoderma gangrenosum Lyell's syndrome
Musculoskeletal and connective tissue disorders	Bone pain Back pain	Pain (1)			
General disorders and administration site condition		Injection site reaction			
Immune system disorders					Allergic reaction Anaphylactic shock
Hepatobiliary disorders	Elevated ASAT/ALAT (2) Elevated Alkaline-phosphatase				

1 / The risk of occurrence of pain is increased in subjects with high peak WBC values, especially when WBC $\geqslant 50 \times 10^9/L$

2 / Transient increase of ASAT and/or ALAT was observed. In most cases, liver function abnormalities improved after lenograstim discontinuation.

3 / Some of the respiratory reported cases have resulted in respiratory failure or acute respiratory distress syndrome (ADRS) which may be fatal.

4 / Sweet's syndrome, erythema nodosum and pyoderma gangrenosum were mainly described in patients with hematological malignancies, a condition known to be associated with neutrophilic dermatosis, but also in non-malignant related neutropenia.

5 / Splenic ruptures have been reported in either healthy donors or patients receiving G-CSFs (see section 4.4)

dosing with GRANOCYTE by the two administration routes showed no evidence of drug accumulation.

At the recommended dose, the absolute bioavailability of GRANOCYTE is 30%. The apparent volume of distribution (Vd) is approximately 1 L/kg body weight and the mean residence time close to 7 h following subcutaneous dosing.

The apparent serum elimination half-life of GRANOCYTE (S.C. route) is about 3-4 h, at steady state (repeated dosing) and is shorter (1-1.5 h) following repeated IV infusion.

Plasma clearance of rHuG-CSF increased 3-fold (from 50 up to 150 mL/min) during repeated S.C. dosing. Less than 1% of lenograstim is excreted in urine unchanged and it is considered to be metabolised to peptides. During multiple S.C. dosing, peak serum concentrations of lenograstim are close to 100 pg/mL/kg body weight at the recommended dosage. There is a positive correlation between the dose and the serum concentration of GRANOCYTE and between the neutrophil response and the total amount of lenograstim recovered in serum.

5.3 Preclinical safety data

In animals, acute toxicity studies (up to 1000 µg/kg/day in mice) and sub-acute toxicity studies (up to 100 µg/kg/day in monkey) showed the effects of overdose were restricted to an exaggerated and reversible pharmacological effect.

There is no evidence from studies in rats and rabbits that GRANOCYTE is teratogenic. An increased incidence of embryo-loss has been observed in rabbits, but no malformation has been seen.

6. PHARMACEUTICAL PARTICULARS

6.1 List of excipients

Powder

Arginine

Phenylalanine

Methionine

Mannitol (E421)

Polysorbate 20

Diluted hydrochloric acid (for pH adjustment)

Solvent

Water for injections

6.2 Incompatibilities

This medicinal product must not be mixed with other medicinal products, except those mentioned in section 6.6.

6.3 Shelf life

2 years.

After reconstitution or dilution, an immediate use is recommended. However, in-use stability of the reconstituted/diluted medicinal product has been demonstrated for 24 hours at 2°C - 8°C (in a refrigerator)

6.4 Special precautions for storage

Do not store above + 30°C.

Do not freeze.

For storage conditions of the reconstituted/diluted medicinal product, see section 6.3.

6.5 Nature and contents of container

105 micrograms of powder in vial (type I glass) with a rubber stopper (type I butyl rubber) + 1 mL of solvent in pre-filled syringe (type I glass) + 2 needles (19G and 26G); pack size of 1 or 5.

263 micrograms of powder in vial (type I glass) with a rubber stopper (type I butyl rubber) + 1 mL of solvent in pre-filled syringe (type I glass) + 2 needles (19G and 26 G); pack size of 1 or 5.

or

105 micrograms of powder in vial (type I glass) with a rubber stopper (type I butyl rubber) + 1 mL of solvent in ampoule (type I glass); pack size of 1 or 5.

263 micrograms of powder in vial (type I glass) with a rubber stopper (type I butyl rubber) + 1 mL of solvent in ampoule (type I glass); pack size of 1 or 5.

Not all pack sizes may be marketed.

6.6 Special precautions for disposal and other handling

Any unused product/solution or waste material should be disposed of in accordance with local requirements.

In view of the possible risk of microbial contamination, pre-filled syringe with solvent is for single use only.

Instructions for preparation

GRANOCYTE vials are for single-dose use only.

GRANOCYTE must be reconstituted before sub-cutaneous or intravenous administration.

Preparation of the reconstituted GRANOCYTE solution

Using a graduated syringe fitted with a needle, aseptically withdraw the entire extractable contents of one ampoule of solvent for GRANOCYTE. Inject the entire contents of the syringe into the corresponding GRANOCYTE vial.

Using the 19G needle provided in the pack, and the pre-filled disposable syringe with the solvent for GRANOCYTE ready for immediate use aseptically add the extractable contents of one pre-filled syringe of solvent for GRANOCYTE to the GRANOCYTE vial.

Agitate gently until completely dissolved. Do not shake vigorously.

The reconstituted parenteral solution appears transparent and free of particles.

The reconstituted solution should preferably be used immediately after preparation. For storage conditions of the reconstituted/diluted medicinal product, see section 6.3.

Preparation for the subcutaneous administration

Prepare a reconstituted GRANOCYTE solution as described above.

Keeping the needle and the syringe attached to the vial, withdraw the required volume of reconstituted solution from the vial. Replace the needle used for reconstitution and fit the syringe with an appropriate needle for subcutaneous injection.

Keeping the needle 19G and the syringe attached to the vial, withdraw the required volume of reconstituted solution from the vial. Replace the needle used for reconstitution and fit the syringe with the 26G needle provided for subcutaneous injection.

Administer immediately by sub-cutaneous injection (refer to section 4.2 for administration requirements).

Preparation of the infusion solution for the intravenous administration:

When intravenous use GRANOCYTE has to be diluted after reconstitution.

Prepare a reconstituted GRANOCYTE solution as described above.

Keeping the needle and the syringe attached to the vial, withdraw the required volume of reconstituted solution from the vial.

Dilute the reconstituted GRANOCYTE solution to the required concentration by injecting the required volume into either 0.9% sodium chloride or 5% dextrose solution.

Administer by IV route (refer to section 4.2 for administration requirements)

GRANOCYTE is compatible with the commonly used administration sets for injection when diluted either in a 0.9% saline solution (polyvinyl chloride bags and glass bottles) or in a 5% dextrose solution (glass bottles)

Dilution of GRANOCYTE 13 million IU/mL to a final concentration of less than 0.26 million IU/mL (2 µg/mL) is not recommended. 1 vial of reconstituted GRANOCYTE 13 million IU/mL should not be diluted in more than 50 mL.

Dilution of GRANOCYTE 34 million IU/mL to a final concentration of less than 0.32 million IU/mL (2.5 µg/mL) is not recommended. 1 vial of reconstituted GRANOCYTE 34 million IU/mL should not be diluted in more than 100 mL.

7. MARKETING AUTHORISATION HOLDER

Chugai Pharma UK Ltd

Mulliner House

Flanders Road

Turnham Green

London.

W4 1NN

8. MARKETING AUTHORISATION NUMBER(S)

PL 12185/0002

PL 12185/0005 (Water for Injections in pre-filled syringe)

9. DATE OF FIRST AUTHORISATION/RENEWAL OF THE AUTHORISATION

November 1993

10. DATE OF REVISION OF THE TEXT

May 2009

GRAZAX 75,000 SQ-T oral lyophilisate

(ALK-Abello Ltd)

1. NAME OF THE MEDICINAL PRODUCT

GRAZAX▼ 75,000 SQ-T oral lyophilisate.

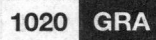

2. QUALITATIVE AND QUANTITATIVE COMPOSITION

Standardised allergen extract of grass pollen from Timothy (*Phleum pratense*) 75,000 SQ-T* per oral lyophilisate.

* [Standardised Quality units Tablet (SQ-T)]

For a full list of excipients, see section 6.1.

3. PHARMACEUTICAL FORM

Oral lyophilisate

White to off-white circular oral lyophilisate marked with a debossed image on one side.

4. CLINICAL PARTICULARS

4.1 Therapeutic indications

Treatment of grass pollen induced rhinitis and conjunctivitis in adults and children (5 years or older) with clinically relevant symptoms and diagnosed with a positive skin prick test and/or specific IgE test to grass pollen.

Children should be carefully selected for treatment (see section 4.2).

4.2 Posology and method of administration

The recommended dose for adults and children (5 years or older) is one oral lyophilisate (75,000 SQ-T) daily. Clinical experience on immunotherapy with Grazax in children (younger than 5 years) and the elderly (65 years or older) is lacking.

Grazax treatment should only be initiated by physicians with experience in treatment of allergic diseases and the capability to treat allergic reactions.

For treatment of children physicians should be experienced in treating allergic diseases in children and the patients should be carefully selected considering the expected level of efficacy in this age group (see section 5.1).

In order to enable patient and physician to discuss any side effects and possible actions it is recommended that the first oral lyophilisate is taken under medical supervision (20-30 minutes).

Efficacy data on treatment with Grazax for two years of continuous treatment is available in adult patients. If no relevant improvement of symptoms is observed during the first pollen season, there is no indication for continuing the treatment.

No data on treatment with Grazax in children beyond one grass pollen season is available.

Clinical effect in the first grass pollen season is expected when treatment is initiated at least 4 months prior to the expected start of the grass pollen season. If treatment is initiated 2-3 months before the season some efficacy may also be obtained. Continuous daily treatment with Grazax in adult patients for, at least 2 years resulted in a progressive immunomodulatory effect. It is recommended to continue treatment with Grazax for a period of 3 years.

Grazax is an oral lyophilisate. The oral lyophilisate should be taken from the blister unit with dry fingers, and placed under the tongue, where it will disperse.

Swallowing should be avoided for about 1 minute. Food and beverage should not be taken for the following 5 minutes.

The oral lyophilisate should be taken immediately after opening the blister.

4.3 Contraindications

Hypersensitivity to any of the excipients (for a full list of excipients, see section 6.1).

Malignancy or systemic diseases affecting the immune system e.g. autoimmune diseases, immune complex diseases or immune deficiency diseases.

Inflammatory conditions in the oral cavity with severe symptoms such as oral lichen planus with ulcerations or severe oral mycosis.

Patients with uncontrolled or severe asthma (in adults: $FEV_1 < 70\%$ of predicted value after adequate pharmacologic treatment; in children: $FEV_1 < 80\%$ of predicted value after adequate pharmacologic treatment) should not be treated with Grazax immunotherapy.

4.4 Special warnings and precautions for use

In case of oral surgery, including dental extraction and shedding of a deciduous tooth in children, treatment with Grazax should be stopped for 7 days to allow healing of the oral cavity.

In children with concomitant asthma and experiencing an acute upper respiratory tract infection, Grazax treatment should be temporarily discontinued until the infection has resolved.

When treated with Grazax the patient is exposed to the allergen that causes the allergic symptoms. Therefore, primarily mild or moderate local allergic reactions are to be expected during the treatment period. If the patient experiences significant local adverse reactions from the treatment, anti-allergic medication (e.g. antihistamines) should be considered.

In post marketing experience, rare cases of severe systemic allergic reactions have been reported and therefore the medical supervision at start of treatment is an important precaution.

The onset of systemic symptoms may include flushing, intensive itching in palms of hand and soles of the feet, and other areas of the body (like a nettle rash). Sense of

Table 1

System Organ Class	Frequency	Adverse Drug Reaction
Cardiac disorders	*Rare*	Palpitations
Infections and infestations	*Uncommon*	Upper respiratory tract infection
Blood and lymphatic system disorders	*Uncommon*	Lymphadenopathy
Nervous system disorders	*Common*	Headache, oral paraesthesia
	Uncommon	Dizziness
Eye disorders	*Common*	Eye pruritus, conjunctivitis
	Uncommon	Eye swelling
Ear and labyrinth disorders	*Very common*	Ear pruritus
Respiratory, thoracic and mediastinal disorders	*Very common*	Throat irritation, sneezing
	Common	Cough, asthma, pharyngitis, rhinorrhoea, nasal congestion, nasal passage irritation, rhinitis, throat tightness
	Uncommon	Nasopharyngitis, bronchospasm, dyspnoea, wheezing, hoarseness, laryngeal discomfort, pharyngeal oedema
Gastrointestinal disorders	*Very common*	Oedema mouth, oral pruritus
	Common	Oropharyngeal swelling, dyspepsia and nausea, oral hypoaesthesia or oral discomfort, oral mucosal blistering, swollen tongue or glossodynia
	Uncommon	Lip blister, mouth ulceration, odynophagia, oral pain, stomatitis, dry mouth and dry throat, tongue disorders, salivary gland disorders, abdominal pain, dysphagia, epigastric discomfort, vomiting, diarrhoea
Skin and subcutaneous tissue disorders	*Common*	Pruritus
	Uncommon	Angioneurotic oedema such as swollen face, oral cavity and pharynx, urticaria
General disorders and administration site conditions	*Common*	Fatigue
	Uncommon	Chest discomfort, chest pain, chest tightness, feeling hot, malaise, pyrexia, sensation of foreign body

Table 2 Efficacy in adults

	Grazax Mean (Median)	Placebo Mean (Median)	Absolute Diff. mean [CI $_{95\%}$]	Relative Diff.* (%) [CI $_{95\%}$]	p-value ANOVA
Number of subjects included in the full analysis set	282	286			
Primary endpoints					
Rhinoconjunctivitis symptom score [A]	2.85 (2.6)	4.14 (3.8)	1.29 [0.90; 1.68]	31% [22%; 41%]	<0.0001
Rhinoconjunctivitis symptom score adjusted for the use of rescue medication			0.91 [0.54; 1.27]		<0.0001
Rhinoconjunctivitis medication score [B]	1.65 (1.0)	2.68 (2.2)	1.03 [0.63; 1.44]	39% [24%; 54%]	<0.0001
Secondary endpoints					
Quality of life score [C]	1.03 (0.9)	1.40 (1.4)	0.37 [0.23; 0.50]	26% [16%; 36%]	<0.0001
Global evaluation [D]	82%	55%	27% [20%; 34%]	49% [36%; 63%]	<0.0001
Well days [E]	45% (40%)	33% (22%)	12% [8%; 17%]	38% [23%; 53%]	<0.0001
Excellent rhinoconjunctivitis control [F]	40%	24%	16% [8%; 24%]	66% [34%; 98%]	<0.0001

[A] Symptom score: Mean daily rhinoconjunctivitis symptom score for each subject for the grass pollen season. Rhinoconjunctivitis symptoms included runny nose, blocked nose, sneezing, itchy nose, gritty feeling/red/itchy eyes and watery eyes.

[B] Medication score: Mean daily rhinoconjunctivitis medication score for each subject for the grass pollen season. Medications used were loratadine (6 points per tablet), budesonide nasal spray (1 point per puff) and prednisone 5 mg (1.6 point per tablet).

[C] Quality of life was assessed by the Rhinoconjunctivitis Quality of Life Questionnaire. A higher score is reflecting a worse quality of life.

[D] Global evaluation: percentage of subjects with improvement in rhinoconjunctivitis symptoms in the treatment season as compared to previous seasons

[E] Well days: percentage of days where the subjects did not use any rescue medication and had a symptom score not larger than 2

[F] Excellent rhinoconjunctivitis control: percentage of subjects with more than 50% well days during the grass pollen season

*Relative difference = Absolute difference / Placebo

Table 3

	Grazax Mean (Median)	Placebo Mean (Median)	Absolute Diff. mean [CI $_{95\%}$]	Relative Diff.* (%) [CI $_{95\%}$]	p-value ANOVA
Number of subjects included in the full analysis set[A]	172	144			
Primary endpoints					
Rhinoconjunctivitis symptom score [B]	2.40 (1.94)	3.76 (3.45)	1.36 [0.86; 1.86]	36% [23%; 49%]	<0.0001
Rhinoconjunctivitis medication score [C]	1.74 (0.46)	3.19 (1.71)	1.45 [0.75; 2.16]	46% [24%; 68%]	<0.0001
Secondary endpoints					
Quality of life score [D]	0.85 (0.63)	1.26 (1.05)	0.41 [0.23; 0.59]	33% [18%; 49%]	<0.0001
Well days [E]	49.6% (47.5%)	33.4% (26.5%)	16.2% [9.4% -22.9%]	48% [28%; 69%]	<0.0001
Excellent rhinoconjunctivitis control [F]	47.1%	28.5%	18.6% [7.5; 29.7]	65% [26%; 104%]	0.0008
Symptom and medication free days [G]	45.8% (42.6%)	31.7% (24.1%)	14.2% [6.0%; 20.5%]	45% [19%; 65%]	<0.0001

[A] The trial was initially planned as a 1-year trial. 546 of the original 634 subjects completed the first year. The trial was extended with 2 more years of treatment and 2 years of follow-up. At inclusion into the extension, 351 subjects chose to enrol (74 were not offered enrolment due to closure of sites), and these were a representative subgroup of the original 634 subjects.

[B] Symptom score: Mean daily rhinoconjunctivitis symptom score for each subject for the grass pollen season. Rhinoconjunctivitis symptoms included runny nose, blocked nose, sneezing, itchy nose, gritty feeling/red/itchy eyes and watery eyes.

[C] Medication score: Mean daily rhinoconjunctivitis medication score for each subject for the grass pollen season. Medications used were loratadine (6 points per tablet), olopatadine eye drops (1.5 point per drop), budesonide nasal spray (1 point per puff) and prednisone 5 mg (1.6 point per tablet).

[D] Quality of life was assessed by the Rhinoconjunctivitis Quality of Life Questionnaire. A higher score is reflecting a worse quality of life.

[E] Well days: percentage of days where the subjects did not use any rescue medication and had a symptom score not larger than 2

[F] Excellent rhinoconjunctivitis control: percentage of subjects with more than 50% well days during the grass pollen season

[G] Symptom and medication free days: percentage of days where the subjects did not use any rescue medication and had no symptoms

*Relative difference = Absolute difference / Placebo

heat, general discomfort and agitation/anxiety may also occur. In case of severe systemic reactions, angioedema, difficulty in swallowing, difficulty in breathing, changes in voice, hypotension or feeling of fullness in the throat a physician should be contacted immediately. In such cases treatment should be discontinued permanently or until otherwise advised by the physician. If patients with concomitant asthma experience symptoms and signs indicating asthma deterioration, treatment should be discontinued and a physician consulted immediately in order to evaluate the continuation of treatment.

In patients who have previously had a systemic reaction to grass pollen subcutaneous immunotherapy, the risk of experiencing a severe reaction with Grazax may be increased. Initiation of Grazax should be carefully considered and measures to treat reactions should be available.

Severe allergic reactions may be treated with adrenaline. The effects of adrenaline may be potentiated in patients treated with tricyclic antidepressants and monoamine oxidase inhibitors (MAOIs) with possible fatal consequences; this should be taken into consideration prior to initiating specific immunotherapy.

Clinical experience in relation to simultaneous vaccination and treatment with Grazax is missing. Vaccination may be given without interrupting treatment with Grazax after medical evaluation of the general condition of the patient.

Grazax contains fish-derived gelatine. The available data have not indicated an increased risk of allergic reactions in severe fish allergic patients. However, awareness is suggested when initiating treatment with Grazax in these patients.

4.5 Interaction with other medicinal products and other forms of interaction

Concomitant therapy with symptomatic anti-allergic agents (e.g. antihistamines, corticosteroids and mast cell stabilisers) may increase the tolerance level of the patient to immunotherapy.

There are no data available on possible risks of simultaneous immunotherapy with other allergens during treatment with Grazax.

4.6 Pregnancy and lactation

Pregnancy

There is no data on the clinical experience for the use of Grazax in pregnant women. Animal studies do not indicate increased risk to the foetus. Treatment with Grazax should not be initiated during pregnancy. If pregnancy occurs during treatment, the treatment may continue after evaluation of the general condition (including lung function) of the patient and reactions to previous administration of Grazax.

In patients with pre-existing asthma close supervision during pregnancy is recommended.

Lactation

No clinical data are available for the use of Grazax during lactation. No effects on the breastfed infants are anticipated.

4.7 Effects on ability to drive and use machines

Treatment with Grazax has no or negligible influence on the ability to drive or use machines.

4.8 Undesirable effects

In studies investigating treatment with Grazax 75,000 SQ-T daily in adult patients, 70% of the patients receiving Grazax reported side effects during the first treatment year. This number decreased markedly in the second year of continuous treatment.

Very commonly reported adverse reactions in adult patients, with seasonal grass pollen induced allergic rhinoconjunctivitis, treated with Grazax were local allergic reactions in the mouth which mostly were mild to moderate. In the majority of patients these reactions started early in therapy, lasted from minutes to hours after each intake of Grazax and tended to subside spontaneously within 1 to 7 days.

The following Table of undesirable effects is based on data from controlled clinical trials investigating Grazax in adult patients with seasonal grass-pollen induced rhinoconjunctivitis including patients with mild to moderate co-existing grass-pollen induced asthma, during the first treatment year.

Adverse reactions are divided into groups according to the MedDRA- Convention frequencies: **Very common (>1/10), Common (>1/100, <1/10), Uncommon (>1/1,000, <1/100), and Rare (>1/10,000, <1/1,000).**

(see Table 1 on previous page)

If the patient experiences significant adverse events from the treatment, anti-allergic medication should be considered.

In post marketing experience, rare cases of severe systemic allergic reactions have been reported and therefore the medical supervision at start of treatment is an important precaution, please refer to section 4.2 and 4.4.

In case of severe systemic reactions, angioedema, difficulty in swallowing, difficulty in breathing, changes in voice, hypotension or feeling of fullness in the throat a physician should be contacted immediately. In such cases treatment should be discontinued permanently or until otherwise advised by the physician.

Experience in children

Overall, the adverse events profile in children and adolescents treated with Grazax was similar to that observed in adults. Upper respiratory tract infections, abdominal pain, vomiting and swollen lips were reported more frequently in the paediatric population than in the adult population (all common).

4.9 Overdose

In phase I studies adult patients with grass pollen allergy were exposed to doses up to 1,000,000 SQ-T. No data is available in children regarding exposure to doses above the recommended daily dose of 75,000 SQ-T.

If doses higher than the recommended daily dose are taken, the risk of side effects may increase, including the risk of systemic reactions or severe local reactions. In case of severe reactions such as angioedema, difficulty in swallowing, difficulty in breathing, changes in voice, or feeling of fullness in the throat, immediate medical evaluation is needed. These reactions should be treated with relevant symptomatic medication.

In such cases treatment should be discontinued permanently or until otherwise advised by the physician.

5. PHARMACOLOGICAL PROPERTIES

5.1 Pharmacodynamic properties

Pharmacotherapeutic group: Allergen extracts, Grass pollen.

ATC code: V01AA02.

Mode of action

Grazax is used for treatment of patients with specific IgE-mediated allergy with symptoms such as rhinitis and rhinoconjunctivitis caused by grass pollen.

The immune system is the target for the pharmacodynamic effect. The aim is to induce an immune response against the allergen with which the patient is treated. The complete and exact mechanism of action regarding clinical effect of specific immunotherapy is not fully understood and documented. Treatment with Grazax has shown to induce a systemic competitive antibody response towards grass pollen, and it induces a continuous increase in specific IgG over at least 2 years of treatment. The clinical significance of these findings has not been established.

Clinical efficacy in adults

In a placebo controlled, double-blind, randomised multinational study, the efficacy of Grazax once daily was evaluated in 634 adult patients with grass pollen induced rhinoconjunctivitis. 72% of the patients had positive skin prick tests to one or more allergens other than grass pollen. The efficacy was based on the average daily rhinoconjunctivitis symptom and medication score during one grass pollen season. Treatment was initiated at least 16 weeks before the anticipated start of the first grass pollen season and was continued all year round.

The efficacy and safety of Grazax has not been established in patients with significant allergic symptoms in the grass pollen season caused by other allergens than grass pollen.

Results after the first grass pollen season with Grazax treatment initiated at least 16 weeks prior to the anticipated start of the grass pollen season and continued throughout the year:

Efficacy in adults

(see Table 2 on previous page)

Results after two years of continuous Grazax treatment:

(see Table 3 above)

Statistically significant effect was demonstrated for each of the scored rhinoconjunctivitis symptoms (runny nose, blocked nose, sneezing, itchy nose, gritty feeling/red/itchy eyes and watery eyes).

In a trial with shorter pre-treatment, less reductions in symptom and medication scores were found; Grazax treatment approximately 2 months prior to and during the grass pollen season resulted in a symptom score reduction of 16% (p=0.071) and a medication score reduction of 28% (p=0.047) (full analysis set).

Clinical efficacy in children

The efficacy of Grazax has been investigated in children (5–16 years) with grass pollen induced rhinoconjunctivitis with/without asthma in a randomised, double-blind, placebo controlled study. Patients received treatment prior to the grass pollen season and continued throughout the entire season. Data on the clinical efficacy of Grazax on rhinoconjunctivitis in children are found below.

Efficacy in children

(see Table 4 on next page)

5.2 Pharmacokinetic properties

The main part of the allergens in Grazax is polypeptides and proteins, which are expected to be broken down to amino acids and small polypeptides in the lumen of the gastrointestinal tract and in tissues. It is expected that allergens from Grazax are not absorbed into the vascular system to any significant extent. Thus, no pharmacokinetic studies in animals or clinical studies investigating the pharmacokinetic profile and metabolism of Grazax have been conducted.

5.3 Preclinical safety data

Conventional studies in general toxicity and of toxicity to reproduction in mice revealed no special hazard for

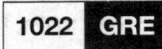

Table 4 Efficacy in children

	Grazax	Placebo	Absolute Diff. [CI $_{95\%}$]	Relative Diff.* (%) [CI $_{95\%}$]	p-value
Number of subjects included in the full analysis set	117	121			
Primary endpoints					
Rhinoconjunctivitis symptom score [A]	2.18	2.80	0.62 [0.10; 1.15]	22% [4%; 38%]	0.0215
Rhinoconjunctivitis medication score [B]	0.78	1.19	0.41	34%	0.0156
Key Secondary endpoints					
Rhinoconjunctivitis symptom score [A], peak grass pollen season	2.84	3.91	1.07 [0.32; 1.81]	27% [9%;43%]	0.0059
Rhinoconjunctivitis medication score [B], peak grass pollen season	0.87	2.40	1.53	64%	0.0013
Well days [C]	52%	42%	9% [1%; 17%]	22% [3%; 45%]	0.0225

[A] Symptom score: Mean daily rhinoconjunctivitis symptom score for each subject for the grass pollen season. Rhinoconjunctivitis symptoms included runny nose, blocked nose, sneezing, itchy nose, gritty feeling/red/itchy eyes and watery eyes. Parametric analysis (square-root-transformed data), relative difference of back-transformed, adjusted means.

[B] Medication score: Mean daily rhinoconjunctivitis medication score for each subject for the grass pollen season. Medications used were loratadine tablets, levocabastine eye drops, budesonide nasal spray, prednisolone tablets. Non-parametric analysis, relative difference of medians.

[C] Well days: percentage of days where the subjects did not use any rescue medication and had a symptom score not larger than 2. Parametric analysis (untransformed data), relative difference of adjusted means.

*Relative difference = Absolute difference / Placebo

humans. In toxicological studies in dogs, daily dosing for 52 weeks was associated with vasculitis / perivasculitis in males, but not in females. It is not expected that there is a risk of developing vasculitis/perivasculitis in humans.

6. PHARMACEUTICAL PARTICULARS

6.1 List of excipients

Gelatin (fish source)

Mannitol

Sodium hydroxide

6.2 Incompatibilities

Not applicable.

6.3 Shelf life

4 years.

6.4 Special precautions for storage

This medical product does not require any special storage conditions.

6.5 Nature and contents of container

Aluminium blister cards with removable aluminium foil in an outer carton box.

Pack sizes: 30 oral lyophilisates, 90 oral lyophilisates and 100 oral lyophilisates.

Not all pack sizes may be marketed.

6.6 Special precautions for disposal and other handling

Any unused product or waste material should be disposed of in accordance with local requirements.

7. MARKETING AUTHORISATION HOLDER

ALK-Abelló A/S

Bøge Allé 6-8

DK- 2970 Hørsholm

Denmark

8. MARKETING AUTHORISATION NUMBER(S)

PL 10085/0039

9. DATE OF FIRST AUTHORISATION/RENEWAL OF THE AUTHORISATION

14 March 2006

10. DATE OF REVISION OF THE TEXT

19 January 2009

Grepid (clopidogrel) 75mg tablets × 30

(Beacon Pharmaceuticals)

1. NAME OF THE MEDICINAL PRODUCT

Grepid 75 mg film-coated tablets

2. QUALITATIVE AND QUANTITATIVE COMPOSITION

Each film-coated tablet contains 75 mg of clopidogrel (as besilate). Excipients: Each film-coated tablet contains 2.6 mg lactose monohydrate. For a full list of excipients, see section 6.1.

3. PHARMACEUTICAL FORM

Film-coated tablet. Pink, round, biconvex, film-coated tablets.

4. CLINICAL PARTICULARS

4.1 Therapeutic indications

Clopidogrel is indicated in adults for the prevention of atherothrombotic events in: Patients suffering from myocardial infarction (from a few days until less than 35 days), ischaemic stroke (from 7 days until less than 6 months) or established peripheral arterial disease. For further information please refer to section 5.1.

4.2 Posology and method of administration

Adults and elderly: Clopidogrel should be given as a single daily dose of 75 mg with or without food. Paediatric patients: The safety and efficacy of clopidogrel in children and adolescents have not yet been established. Renal impairment: Therapeutic experience is limited in patients with renal impairment (see section 4.4). Hepatic impairment: Therapeutic experience is limited in patients with moderate hepatic disease who may have bleeding diatheses (see section 4.4).

4.3 Contraindications

Hypersensitivity to the active substance or to any of the excipients. Severe liver impairment. Active pathological bleeding such as peptic ulcer or intracranial haemorrhage.

4.4 Special warnings and precautions for use

Due to the risk of bleeding and haematological undesirable effects, blood cell count determination and/or other appropriate testing should be promptly considered whenever clinical symptoms suggestive of bleeding arise during the course of treatment (see section 4.8). As with other antiplatelet agents, clopidogrel should be used with caution in patients who may be at risk of increased bleeding from trauma, surgery or other pathological conditions and in patients receiving treatment with ASA, heparin, glycoprotein IIb/IIIa inhibitors or non-steroidal anti-inflammatory drugs including Cox-2 inhibitors. Patients should be followed carefully for any signs of bleeding including occult bleeding, especially during the first weeks of treatment and/or after invasive cardiac procedures or surgery. The concomitant administration of clopidogrel with oral anticoagulants is not recommended since it may increase the intensity of bleedings (see section 4.5).

If a patient is to undergo elective surgery and antiplatelet effect is temporarily not desirable, clopidogrel should be discontinued 7 days prior to surgery. Patients should inform physicians and dentists that they are taking clopidogrel before any surgery is scheduled and before any new medicinal product is taken. Clopidogrel prolongs bleeding time and should be used with caution in patients who have lesions with a propensity to bleed (particularly gastrointestinal and intraocular).

Patients should be told that it might take longer than usual to stop bleeding when they take clopidogrel (alone or in combination with ASA), and that they should report any unusual bleeding (site or duration) to their physician.

Thrombotic Thrombocytopenic Purpura (TTP) has been reported very rarely following the use of clopidogrel, sometimes after a short exposure. It is characterised by thrombocytopenia and microangiopathic haemolytic anaemia associated with either neurological findings, renal dysfunction or fever. TTP is a potentially fatal condition requiring prompt treatment including plasmapheresis.

In view of the lack of data, clopidogrel cannot be recommended during the first 7 days after acute ischaemic stroke.

Therapeutic experience with clopidogrel is limited in patients with renal impairment. Therefore clopidogrel should be used with caution in these patients (see section 4.2).

Experience is limited in patients with moderate hepatic disease who may have bleeding diatheses. Clopidogrel should therefore be used with caution in this population (see section 4.2).

Grepid contains lactose. Patients with rare hereditary problems of galactose intolerance, the Lapp lactase deficiency or glucose galactose malabsorption should not take this medicinal product.

4.5 Interaction with other medicinal products and other forms of interaction

Oral anticoagulants: the concomitant administration of clopidogrel with oral anticoagulants is not recommended since it may increase the intensity of bleedings (see section 4.4).

Glycoprotein IIb/IIIa inhibitors: clopidogrel should be used with caution in patients who may be at risk of increased bleeding from trauma, surgery or other pathological conditions that receive concomitant glycoprotein IIb/IIIa inhibitors (see section 4.4).

Acetylsalicylic acid (ASA): ASA did not modify the clopidogrel-mediated inhibition of ADP-induced platelet aggregation, but clopidogrel potentiated the effect of ASA on collagen-induced platelet aggregation. However, concomitant administration of 500 mg of ASA twice a day for one day did not significantly increase the prolongation of bleeding time induced by clopidogrel intake. A pharmacodynamic interaction between clopidogrel and acetylsalicylic acid is possible, leading to increased risk of bleeding. Therefore, concomitant use should be undertaken with caution (see section 4.4). However, clopidogrel and ASA have been administered together for up to one year (see section 5.1).

Heparin: in a clinical study conducted in healthy subjects, clopidogrel did not necessitate modification of the heparin dose or alter the effect of heparin on coagulation. Coadministration of heparin had no effect on the inhibition of platelet aggregation induced by clopidogrel. A pharmacodynamic interaction between clopidogrel and heparin is possible, leading to increased risk of bleeding. Therefore, concomitant use should be undertaken with caution (see section 4.4).

Thrombolytics: the safety of the concomitant administration of clopidogrel, fibrin or non-fibrin specific thrombolytic agents and heparins was assessed in patients with acute myocardial infarction. The incidence of clinically significant bleeding was similar to that observed when thrombolytic agents and heparin are co-administered with ASA (see section 4.8)

Non-Steroidal Anti-Inflammatory Drugs (NSAIDs): in a clinical study conducted in healthy volunteers, the concomitant administration of clopidogrel and naproxen increased occult gastrointestinal blood loss. However, due to the lack of interaction studies with other NSAIDs it is presently unclear whether there is an increased risk of gastrointestinal bleeding with all NSAIDs. Consequently, NSAIDs including Cox-2 inhibitors and clopidogrel should be coadministered with caution (see section 4.4).

Other concomitant therapy: a number of other clinical studies have been conducted with clopidogrel and other concomitant medicinal products to investigate the potential for pharmacodynamic and pharmacokinetic interactions. No clinically significant pharmacodynamic interactions were observed when clopidogrel was coadministered with atenolol, nifedipine, or both atenolol and nifedipine.

Furthermore, the pharmacodynamic activity of clopidogrel was not significantly influenced by the coadministration of phenobarbital, cimetidine, or oestrogen.

The pharmacokinetics of digoxin or theophylline were not modified by the co-administration of clopidogrel. Antacids did not modify the extent of clopidogrel absorption.

Data from studies with human liver microsomes indicated that the carboxylic acid metabolite of clopidogrel could inhibit the activity of Cytochrome P450 2C9. This could potentially lead to increased plasma levels of medicinal products such as phenytoin and tolbutamide and the NSAIDs, which are metabolised by Cytochrome P450 2C9. Data from the CAPRIE study indicate that phenytoin and tolbutamide can be safely co-administered with clopidogrel.

Apart from the specific medicinal product interaction information described above, interaction studies with clopidogrel and some medicinal products commonly administered in patients with atherothrombotic disease have not been performed. However, patients entered into clinical trials with clopidogrel received a variety of concomitant medicinal products including diuretics, beta blockers, ACEI, calcium antagonists, cholesterol lowering agents, coronary vasodilators, antidiabetic agents (including insulin), antiepileptic agents and GPIIb/IIIa antagonists without evidence of clinically significant adverse interactions.

4.6 Pregnancy and lactation

As no clinical data on exposure to clopidogrel during pregnancy are available, it is preferable not to use clopidogrel during pregnancy as a precautionary measure.

Animal studies do not indicate direct or indirect harmful effects with respect to pregnancy, embryonal/foetal development, parturition or postnatal development (see section 5.3).

It is unknown whether clopidogrel is excreted in human breast milk. Animal studies have shown excretion of clopidogrel in breast milk. As a precautionary measure, breast feeding should not be continued during treatment with Grepid.

4.7 Effects on ability to drive and use machines

Clopidogrel has no or negligible influence on the ability to drive and use machines.

4.8 Undesirable effects

Clopidogrel has been evaluated for safety in more than 42,000 patients who have participated in clinical studies, including over 9,000 patients treated for 1 year or more. The clinically relevant adverse reactions observed in the CAPRIE, CURE, CLARITY and COMMIT studies are discussed below. Overall, clopidogrel 75 mg/day was comparable to ASA 325 mg/day in CAPRIE regardless of age, gender and race. In addition to clinical studies experience, adverse reactions have been spontaneously reported.

Bleeding is the most common reaction reported both in clinical studies as well as in post-marketing experience where it was mostly reported during the first month of treatment.

In CAPRIE, in patients treated with either clopidogrel or ASA, the overall incidence of any bleeding was 9.3%. The incidence of severe cases was 1.4% for clopidogrel and 1.6% for ASA.

In CURE, the major bleeding event rate for clopidogrel+ASA was dose-dependent on ASA (<100mg: 2.6%; 100-200mg: 3.5%; >200mg: 4.9%) as was the major bleeding event rate for placebo+ASA (<100mg: 2.0%; 100-200mg: 2.3%; >200mg: 4.0%). The risk of bleeding (life-threatening, major, minor, other) decreased during the course of the trial: 0-1 months (clopidogrel: 9.6%; placebo: 6.6%), 1-3 months (clopidogrel: 4.5%; placebo: 2.3%), 3-6 months (clopidogrel: 3.8%; placebo: 1.6%), 6-9 months (clopidogrel: 3.2%; placebo: 1.5%), 9-12 months (clopidogrel: 1.9%; placebo: 1.0%). There was no excess in major bleeds with clopidogrel + ASA within 7 days after coronary bypass graft surgery in patients who stopped therapy more than five days prior to surgery (4.4% clopidogrel+ASA vs. 5.3% placebo+ASA). In patients who remained on therapy within five days of bypass graft surgery, the event rate was 9.6% for clopidogrel+ASA, and 6.3% for placebo+ASA.

In CLARITY, there was an overall increase in bleeding in the clopidogrel + ASA group (17.4%) vs. the placebo + ASA group (12.9%). The incidence of major bleeding was similar between groups (1.3% versus 1.1% for the clopidogrel + ASA and the placebo + ASA groups, respectively). This was consistent across subgroups of patients defined by baseline characteristics, and type of fibrinolytic or heparin therapy.

In COMMIT, the overall rate of noncerebral major bleeding or cerebral bleeding was low and similar in both groups (0.6% versus 0.5% in the clopidogrel + ASA and the placebo + ASA groups, respectively).

Adverse reactions that occurred either during clinical studies or that were spontaneously reported are presented in the table below. Their frequency is defined using the following conventions: common (≥1/100 to <1/10); uncommon (≥1/1,000 to <1/100); rare (≥1/10,000 to <1/1,000); very rare (<1/10,000). Within each system organ class, adverse drug reactions are presented in order of decreasing seriousness.

(see Table 1 opposite)

Table 1

System Organ Class	Common	Uncommon	Rare	Very rare
Blood and the lymphatic system disorders		Thrombocytopenia, leucopenia, eosinophilia	Neutropenia, including severe neutropenia	Thrombotic thrombocytopenic purpura (TTP) (see section 4.4), aplastic anaemia, pancytopenia, agranulocytosis, severe thrombocytopenia, granulocytopenia, anaemia
Immune system disorders				Serum sickness, anaphylactoid reactions
Psychiatric disorders				Hallucinations, confusion
Nervous system disorders		Intracranial bleeding (some cases were reported with fatal outcome), headache, paraesthesia, dizziness		Taste disturbances
Eye disorders		Eye bleeding (conjunctival, ocular, retinal)		
Ear and labyrinth disorders			Vertigo	
Vascular disorders	Haematoma			Serious haemorrhage, haemorrhage of operative wound, vasculitis, hypotension
Respiratory, thoracic and mediastinal disorders	Epistaxis			Respiratory tract bleeding (haemoptysis, pulmonary haemorrhage), bronchospasm, interstitial pneumonitis
Gastrointestinal disorders	Gastrointestinal haemorrhage, diarrhoea, abdominal pain, dyspepsia	Gastric ulcer and duodenal ulcer, gastritis, vomiting, nausea, constipation, flatulence	Retroperitoneal haemorrhage	Gastrointestinal and retroperitoneal haemorrhage with fatal outcome, pancreatitis, colitis (including ulcerative or lymphocytic colitis), stomatitis
Hepato-biliary disorders				Acute liver failure, hepatitis, abnormal liver function test
Skin and subcutaneous tissue disorders	Bruising	Rash, pruritus, skin bleeding (purpura)		Bullous dermatitis (toxic epidermal necrolysis, Stevens Johnson Syndrome, erythema multiforme), angioedema, rash erythematous, urticaria, eczema, lichen planus
Musculoskeletal, connective tissue and bone disorders				Musculo-skeletal bleeding (haemarthrosis), arthritis, arthralgia, myalgia
Renal and urinary disorders		Haematuria		Glomerulonephritis, blood creatinine increased
General disorders and administration site conditions	Bleeding at puncture site			Fever
Investigations		Bleeding time prolonged, neutrophil count decreased, platelet count decreased		

4.9 Overdose

Overdose following clopidogrel administration may lead to prolonged bleeding time and subsequent bleeding complications. Appropriate therapy should be considered if bleedings are observed.

No antidote to the pharmacological activity of clopidogrel has been found. If prompt correction of prolonged bleeding time is required, platelet transfusion may reverse the effects of clopidogrel.

5. PHARMACOLOGICAL PROPERTIES

5.1 Pharmacodynamic properties

Pharmacotherapeutic group: Platelet aggregation inhibitors excl. heparin, ATC code: B01AC04.

Clopidogrel selectively inhibits the binding of adenosine diphosphate (ADP) to its platelet receptor, and the subsequent ADP-mediated activation of the GPIIb/IIIa complex, thereby inhibiting platelet aggregation. Biotransformation of clopidogrel is necessary to produce inhibition of platelet aggregation. Clopidogrel also inhibits platelet aggregation induced by other agonists by blocking the amplification of platelet activation by released ADP. Clopidogrel acts by irreversibly modifying the platelet ADP receptor. Consequently, platelets exposed to clopidogrel are affected for the remainder of their lifespan and recovery of normal platelet function occurs at a rate consistent with platelet turnover.

Repeated doses of 75 mg per day produced substantial inhibition of ADP-induced platelet aggregation from the first day; this increased progressively and reached steady state between Day 3 and Day 7. At steady state, the average inhibition level observed with a dose of 75 mg per day was between 40% and 60%. Platelet aggregation and bleeding time gradually returned to baseline values, generally within 5 days after treatment was discontinued.

The safety and efficacy of clopidogrel have been evaluated in 4 double-blind studies involving over 80,000 patients: the CAPRIE study, a comparison of clopidogrel to ASA, and the CURE, CLARITY and COMMIT studies comparing clopidogrel to placebo, both medicinal products given in combination with ASA and other standard therapy.

Recent myocardial infarction (MI), recent stroke or established peripheral arterial disease

The CAPRIE study included 19,185 patients with atherothrombosis as manifested by recent myocardial infarction (<35 days), recent ischaemic stroke (between 7 days and 6 months) or established peripheral arterial disease (PAD). Patients were randomised to clopidogrel 75 mg/day or ASA 325 mg/day, and were followed for 1 to 3 years.

In the myocardial infarction subgroup, most of the patients received ASA for the first few days following the acute myocardial infarction.

Clopidogrel significantly reduced the incidence of new ischaemic events (combined end point of myocardial infarction, ischaemic stroke and vascular death) when compared to ASA. In the intention to treat analysis, 939 events were observed in the clopidogrel group and 1,020 events with ASA (relative risk reduction (RRR) 8.7%, [95% CI: 0.2 to 16.4]; p = 0.045), which corresponds, for every 1000 patients treated for 2 years, to 10 [CI: 0 to 20] additional patients being prevented from experiencing a new ischaemic event. Analysis of total mortality as a secondary endpoint did not show any significant difference between clopidogrel (5.8%) and ASA (6.0%).

In a subgroup analysis by qualifying condition (myocardial infarction, ischaemic stroke, and PAD) the benefit appeared to be strongest (achieving statistical significance at p = 0.003) in patients enrolled due to PAD (especially those who also had a history of myocardial infarction) (RRR = 23.7%; CI: 8.9 to 36.2) and weaker (not significantly different from ASA) in stroke patients (RRR = 7.3%; CI: -5.7 to 18.7 [p=0.258]). In patients who were enrolled in the trial on the sole basis of a recent myocardial infarction, clopidogrel was numerically inferior, but not statistically different from ASA (RRR = -4.0%; CI: -22.5 to 11.7 [p=0.639]). In addition, a subgroup analysis by age suggested that the benefit of clopidogrel in patients over 75 years was less than that observed in patients ≤75 years.

Since the CAPRIE trial was not powered to evaluate efficacy of individual subgroups, it is not clear whether the differences in relative risk reduction across qualifying conditions are real, or a result of chance.

5.2 Pharmacokinetic properties

After repeated oral doses of 75 mg per day, clopidogrel is rapidly absorbed. However, plasma concentrations of the parent compound are very low and below the quantification limit (0.00025 mg/l) beyond 2 hours. Absorption is at least 50%, based on urinary excretion of clopidogrel metabolites.

Clopidogrel is extensively metabolised by the liver and the main metabolite, which is inactive, is the carboxylic acid derivative, which represents about 85% of the circulating compound in plasma. Peak plasma levels of this metabolite (approx. 3mg/l after repeated 75 mg oral doses) occurred approximately 1 hour after dosing.

Clopidogrel is a prodrug. The active metabolite, a thiol derivative, is formed by oxidation of clopidogrel to 2-oxo-clopidogrel and subsequent hydrolysis. The oxidative step is regulated primarily by Cytochrome P450 isoenzymes 2B6 and 3A4 and to a lesser extent by 1A1, 1A2 and 2C19. The active thiol metabolite, which has been isolated *in vitro*, binds rapidly and irreversibly to platelet receptors, thus inhibiting platelet aggregation. This metabolite has not been detected in plasma.

The kinetics of the main circulating metabolite were linear (plasma concentrations increased in proportion to dose) in the dose range of 50 to 150 mg of clopidogrel.

Clopidogrel and the main circulating metabolite bind reversibly *in vitro* to human plasma proteins (98% and 94% respectively). The binding is non-saturable *in vitro* over a wide concentration range.

Following an oral dose of ^{14}C-labelled clopidogrel in man, approximately 50% was excreted in theurine and approximately 46% in the faeces in the 120-hour interval after dosing. The elimination half-life of the main circulating metabolite was 8 hours after single and repeated administration.

After repeated doses of 75 mg clopidogrel per day, plasma levels of the main circulating metabolite were lower in subjects with severe renal disease (creatinine clearance from 5 to 15 ml/min) compared to subjects with moderate renal disease (creatinine clearance from 30 to 60 ml/min) and to levels observed in other studies with healthy subjects. Although inhibition of ADP-induced platelet aggregation was lower (25%) than that observed in healthy subjects, the prolongation of bleeding was similar to that seen in healthy subjects receiving 75 mg of clopidogrel per day. In addition, clinical tolerance was good in all patients.

The pharmacokinetics and pharmacodynamics of clopidogrel were assessed in a single and multiple dose study in both healthy subjects and those with cirrhosis (Child-Pugh class A or B). Daily dosing for 10 days with clopidogrel 75 mg/day was safe and well tolerated. Clopidogrel Cmax for both single dose and steady state for cirrhotics was many fold higher than in normal subjects. However, plasma levels of the main circulating metabolite together with the effect of clopidogrel on ADP-induced platelet aggregation and bleeding time were comparable between these groups.

5.3 Preclinical safety data

During non clinical studies in rat and baboon, the most frequently observed effects were liver changes. These occurred at doses representing at least 25 times the exposure seen in humans receiving the clinical dose of 75 mg/day and were a consequence of an effect on hepatic metabolising enzymes. No effect on hepatic metabolising enzymes was observed in humans receiving clopidogrel at the therapeutic dose.

At very high doses, a poor gastric tolerability (gastritis, gastric erosions and/or vomiting) of clopidogrel was also reported in rat and baboon.

There was no evidence of carcinogenic effect when clopidogrel was administered for 78 weeks to mice and 104 weeks to rats when given at doses up to 77 mg/kg per day (representing at least 25 times the exposure seen in humans receiving the clinical dose of 75 mg/day).

Clopidogrel has been tested in a range of *in vitro* and *in vivo* genotoxicity studies, and showed no genotoxic activity.

Clopidogrel was found to have no effect on the fertility of male and female rats and was not teratogenic in either rats or rabbits. When given to lactating rats, clopidogrel caused a slight delay in the development of the offspring. Specific pharmacokinetic studies performed with radiolabelled clopidogrel have shown that the parent compound or its metabolites are excreted in the milk. Consequently, a direct effect (slight toxicity), or an indirect effect (low palatability) cannot be excluded.

6. PHARMACEUTICAL PARTICULARS

6.1 List of excipients

Tablet core: Cellulose, microcrystalline; Hydroxypropylcellulose (E463); Mannitol (E421); Crospovidone (type A); Citric acid, monohydrate; Macrogol 6000; Stearic acid; Talc

Film-coating: Hypromellose (E464); Iron oxide red (E172); Lactose monohydrate; Triacetin (E1518); Titanium dioxide (E171)

6.2 Incompatibilities

Not applicable

6.3 Shelf life

2 years

6.4 Special precautions for storage

This medicinal product does not require any special storage conditions.

6.5 Nature and contents of container

Blisters of white PVC/PE/PVDC-aluminium foil or PA/ALL/PVC-aluminium foil. Packs of 14, 28, 30, 50, 84, 90 or 100 film-coated tablets. Not all pack sizes may be marketed.

6.6 Special precautions for disposal and other handling

No special requirements.

7. MARKETING AUTHORISATION HOLDER

Pharmathen S.A., 6 Dervenakion, 15351 Pallini Attiki, Greece

8. MARKETING AUTHORISATION NUMBER(S)

EU/1/09/535/003

9. DATE OF FIRST AUTHORISATION/RENEWAL OF THE AUTHORISATION

July 2009.

10. DATE OF REVISION OF THE TEXT

Detailed information on this product is available on the website of the European Medicines Agency (EMEA): http://www.emea.europa.eu/

Gyno-Daktarin 20mg/g Cream

(Janssen-Cilag Ltd)

1. NAME OF THE MEDICINAL PRODUCT

Gyno-Daktarin 20mg/g cream

2. QUALITATIVE AND QUANTITATIVE COMPOSITION

Miconazole nitrate 2% w/w.

(Each gram of cream contains 20mg miconazole nitrate)

For a full list of excipients, see section 6.1.

3. PHARMACEUTICAL FORM

Vaginal cream.

The cream is white and homogeneous.

4. CLINICAL PARTICULARS

4.1 Therapeutic indications

For the treatment of mycotic vulvovaginitis and superinfections due to gram-positive bacteria.

4.2 Posology and method of administration

Gyno-Daktarin cream is for vaginal administration.

Recommended dosage

Administer the contents of one applicator (about 5g of cream) once daily deeply into vagina for 10 – 14 days or twice daily for 7 days. For vulvitis the cream should be applied topically twice daily. Continue the course of treatment even after pruritus and leukorrhoea have disappeared or menstruation begins.

4.3 Contraindications

Gyno-Daktarin cream is contraindicated in individuals with a known hypersensitivity to miconazole or another ingredient of the cream.

4.4 Special warnings and precautions for use

Should local sensitisation or an allergic reaction occur, treatment should be discontinued.

Appropriate therapy is indicated when the sexual partner is also infected.

Gyno-Daktarin cream does not stain skin or clothes.

The concurrent use of latex condoms or diaphragms with vaginal anti-infective preparations may decrease the effectiveness of latex contraceptive agents. Therefore Gyno-Daktarin cream should not be used concurrently with a latex condom or latex diaphragm.

4.5 Interaction with other medicinal products and other forms of interaction

Miconazole administered systemically is known to inhibit CYP3A4/2C9. Due to the limited systemic availability after vaginal application, clinically relevant interactions occur very rarely. In patients on oral anticoagulants, such as warfarin, caution should be exercised and anticoagulant effect should be monitored. The effects and side effects of other drugs metabolized by CYP2C9 (e.g., oral hypoglycemics and phenytoin) and also CYP3A4 (e.g., HMG-CoA reductase inhibitors such as simvastatin and lovastatin and calcium channel blockers such as dihydropyridines and verapamil), when co-administered with miconazole, can be increased and caution should be exercised.

Contact should be avoided between certain latex products such as contraceptive diaphragms or condoms and Gyno-Daktarin cream since the constituents of the cream may damage the latex. (see section 4.4).

4.6 Pregnancy and lactation

Pregnancy

Although intravaginal absorption is limited, Gyno-Daktarin cream should only be used in the first trimester of pregnancy only if, in the judgement of the physician, the potential benefits outweigh the possible risks.

Lactation

It is not known whether miconazole nitrate is excreted in human milk. Caution should be exercised when using Gyno-Daktarin cream during lactation.

4.7 Effects on ability to drive and use machines

None known.

4.8 Undesirable effects

The safety of GYNO-DAKTARIN was evaluated in a total of 537 women with microbiologically confirmed candidiasis and symptoms (e.g., vulvovaginal itching, burning/irritation), or signs of vulvar erythema, edema, excoriation, or vaginal erythema or edema who participated in 2 single-blind clinical trials. Subjects were treated with miconazole intravaginally, randomly assigned to either a single 1,200 mg capsule, or a 7-day application of 2% vaginal cream. Adverse Drug Reactions (ADRs) reported by ≥1% of GYNO-DAKTARIN-treated subjects in these trials are shown in Table 1.

In the table, the frequencies are provided according to the following convention:

Very common ≥1/10

Common ≥1/100 and <1/10

Uncommon ≥1/1,000 and <1/100

Rare ≥1/10,000, <1/1,000

Very rare <1/10,000, including isolated reports

Table 1. Adverse Drug Reactions Reported by Gyno-Daktarin-treated Subjects in 2 Single Blind Clinical Trials

Body System/ Organ Class *Frequency Category*	**Undesirable effects**
Skin and subcutaneous tissue disorders	
Common	Rash
Uncommon	Rash pruritic, urticaria
Reproductive System and Breast Disorders	
Very common	Genital pruritus female, vaginal burning sensation, vulvovaginal discomfort
Common	Dysmenorrhoea

A range of additional reactions were reported during the clinical trials, such as: vaginal discharge, vaginal haemorrhage, vaginal pain, headache, dysuria, urinary tract infection, abdominal pain, rosacea, swelling face and nausea. However due to the design of these studies, a definitive causal relationship could not be established.

Table 2. Adverse Drug Reactions Identified During Postmarketing Experience with Gyno-Daktarin by Frequency Category Estimated from Spontaneous Reporting Rates

Immune System Disorders	
Not known	Hypersensitivity including Anaphylactic and Anaphylactoid reactions, Angioedema

Skin and Subcutaneous Tissue Disorders	
Not known	Pruritis
Reproductive System and Breast Disorders	
Not known	Vaginal irritation, pelvic cramps

4.9 Overdose

Symptoms

In case of accidental ingestion, no problems are expected.

Treatment

In the event of accidental ingestion of large quantities, an appropriate method of gastric emptying may be used if considered appropriate.

5. PHARMACOLOGICAL PROPERTIES

5.1 Pharmacodynamic properties

Pharmacotherapeutic classification:

(Anti-infectives and antiseptics, excl. combinations with corticosteroids, imidazole derivatives)

ATC code: G01A F04

Miconazole combines a potent antifungal activity against common dermatophytes and yeasts with an antibacterial activity against certain gram-positive bacilli and cocci.

Miconazole inhibits the biosynthesis of ergosterol in fungi and changes the composition of other lipid components in the membrane, resulting in fungal cell necrosis.

In general, miconazole exerts a very rapid effect on pruritus, a symptom that frequently accompanies dermatophyte and yeast infections.

5.2 Pharmacokinetic properties

Absorption: Miconazole persists in the vagina for up to 72 hours after a single dose. Systemic absorption of miconazole after intravaginal administration is limited, with a bioavailability of 1 to 2% following intravaginal administration of a 1200 mg dose. Plasma concentrations of miconazole are measurable within 2 hours of administration in some subjects, with maximal levels seen 12 to 24 hours after administration. Plasma concentrations decline slowly thereafter and were still measurable in most subjects 96 hours post-dose. A second dose administered 48 hours later resulted in a plasma profile similar to that of the first dose.

Distribution: Absorbed miconazole is bound to plasma proteins (88.2%) and red blood cells (10.6%).

Metabolism and Excretion: The small amount of miconazole that is absorbed is eliminated predominantly in faeces as both unchanged drug and metabolites over a four-day post-administration period. Smaller amounts of unchanged drug and metabolites also appear in urine. The mean apparent elimination half-life is 57 hours.

5.3 Preclinical safety data

No relevant information additional to that contained elsewhere in the Summary of Product Characteristics.

6. PHARMACEUTICAL PARTICULARS

6.1 List of excipients

PEG-6, PEG-32 and glycol stearate

Oleoyl macroglycerides

Liquid paraffin

Benzoic acid (E210)

Butylated hydroxyanisole (E320)

Purified water

6.2 Incompatibilities

None known.

6.3 Shelf life

24 months.

6.4 Special precautions for storage

Do not store above 25°C.

6.5 Nature and contents of container

Tube containing 15 g, 40 g or 78 g of cream.

The aluminium tube inner is lined with heat polymerised epoxy-phenol resin with a white polypropylene cap.

The cream is supplied with disposable cardboard vaginal applicators.

*Not all pack sizes are marketed.

6.6 Special precautions for disposal and other handling

No special requirements.

7. MARKETING AUTHORISATION HOLDER

Janssen-Cilag Ltd

50-100 Holmers Farm Way

High Wycombe

Buckinghamshire

HP12 4EG

UK

8. MARKETING AUTHORISATION NUMBER(S)

PL 0242/0015

9. DATE OF FIRST AUTHORISATION/RENEWAL OF THE AUTHORISATION

12 December 2008

10. DATE OF REVISION OF THE TEXT

23rd July 09

Gyno-Pevaryl 1 Vaginal Pessary

(Janssen-Cilag Ltd)

1. NAME OF THE MEDICINAL PRODUCT

Gyno-Pevaryl 1 Vaginal Pessary.

2. QUALITATIVE AND QUANTITATIVE COMPOSITION

Each pessary contains econazole nitrate PhEur 150 mg.

3. PHARMACEUTICAL FORM

Light beige torpedo shaped pessary,

4. CLINICAL PARTICULARS

4.1 Therapeutic indications

Vaginitis due to Candida Albicans and other yeasts.

4.2 Posology and method of administration

For vaginal administration.

Adults:

Insert one pessary high into the vagina at night prior to retiring.

Children:

Gyno-Pevaryl 1 pessary is not indicated for use in children under the age of 16 years.

Elderly:

No specific dosage recommendations or precautions apply.

4.3 Contraindications

Hypersensitivity to any imidazole preparation (or other vaginal antifungal products).

4.4 Special warnings and precautions for use

Hypersensitivity has rarely been recorded; if it should occur administration should be discontinued.

4.5 Interaction with other medicinal products and other forms of interaction

Contact between contraceptive diaphragms or condoms and this product must be avoided since the rubber may be damaged by the preparation.

Although not studied, based on the chemical similarity of econazole with other imidazole compounds, a theoretical potential for competitive interaction with compounds metabolized by CYP3A4/2C9 exists. Due to the limited systemic availability after vaginal application (see 5.2. Pharmacokinetic Properties), clinically relevant interactions are unlikely to occur. In patients on oral anticoagulants, such as warfarin and acenocoumarol, caution should be exercised and monitoring of the anticoagulant effect should be considered.

4.6 Pregnancy and lactation

In animals, econazole nitrate has shown no teratogenic effects but is foetotoxic at high doses. The significance of this to man is unknown as there is no evidence of an increased risk when taken in human pregnancy. However, as with other imidazoles, econazole should be used in pregnancy only if the practitioner considers it to be necessary.

4.7 Effects on ability to drive and use machines

None known.

4.8 Undesirable effects

The most frequently reported adverse events in clinical trials were application site reactions, such as burning and stinging sensations, pruritus, and erythema.

Based on post-marketing experience, the following adverse reactions have also been reported:

Skin and subcutaneous tissue disorders; general disorders and administration site conditions

Very rare (< 1/10,000): Localized application site (mucocutaneous) reactions, such as erythema, rash, burning and pruritus.

Isolated reports of localized allergic reactions. Isolated reports of generalized allergic reactions, including angioedema and urticaria.

4.9 Overdose

This product is intended for vaginal use. If accidental ingestion of large quantities of the product occurs, an appropriate method of gastric emptying may be used if considered desirable.

5. PHARMACOLOGICAL PROPERTIES

5.1 Pharmacodynamic properties

Pharmacotherapeutic classification: (Antiinfectives and antiseptics, excl. combinations with corticosteroids, imidazole derivatives)

ATC code: G01A F05

Econazole is an imidazole derivative. The compound acts by damaging the membranes of bacterial and fungal cells; both the cellular and subcellular membranes are affected. Econazole apparently disturbs the permeability characteristics of the membrane which allow leakage of potassium and sodium ions and other intra cellular components. Macro-molecular synthesis may also be inhibited. Econazole is active against dermatophytes, yeast, moulds and Gram positive bacteria. Gram negative bacteria are generally resistant to econazole.

5.2 Pharmacokinetic properties

Econazole nitrate is poorly absorbed after vaginal application. Using radiolabelled techniques, it has been determined that between 2.5% and 7% of vaginally applied econazole nitrate is absorbed. However, no antimycotic activity could be detected in the serum after vaginal application of 5 g or 1% econazole nitrate cream or a suppository containing 50 mg econazole nitrate.

5.3 Preclinical safety data

No relevant information other than that contained elsewhere in the Summary of Product Characteristics.

6. PHARMACEUTICAL PARTICULARS

6.1 List of excipients

Polygel

Colloidal silicon dioxide

Witepsol H19

Wecobee FS

Stearyl heptanoate

6.2 Incompatibilities

None stated.

6.3 Shelf life

3 years.

6.4 Special precautions for storage

Do not store above 30°C.

6.5 Nature and contents of container

Multi-plast strip or PVC/PE moulds, containing one pessary.

1 applicator

Gyno-Pevaryl 1 Vaginal Pessary (PL 0242/0226) is also contained in:

Gyno-Pevaryl 1 C.P. PACK Vaginal Pessary and Cream (PL 0242/0226 & PL 0242/0229)

6.6 Special precautions for disposal and other handling

Not applicable.

7. MARKETING AUTHORISATION HOLDER

Janssen-Cilag Limited

50-100 Holmers Farm Way

High Wycombe

Buckinghamshire

HP12 4EG

UK

8. MARKETING AUTHORISATION NUMBER(S)

PL 00242/0226

9. DATE OF FIRST AUTHORISATION/RENEWAL OF THE AUTHORISATION

1 October 1995/June 2003

10. DATE OF REVISION OF THE TEXT

28th April 2009

Legal category POM

Gyno-Pevaryl 150 mg Vaginal Pessaries

(Janssen-Cilag Ltd)

1. NAME OF THE MEDICINAL PRODUCT

GYNO-PEVARYL® 150 mg Vaginal Pessaries

2. QUALITATIVE AND QUANTITATIVE COMPOSITION

Vaginal pessaries each containing 150 mg econazole nitrate.

3. PHARMACEUTICAL FORM

White to off-white torpedo-shaped pessaries.

4. CLINICAL PARTICULARS

4.1 Therapeutic indications

Vaginitis due to *Candida albicans* and other yeasts.

4.2 Posology and method of administration

For vaginal administration.

Adults:

One pessary should be inserted high into the vagina each evening for three consecutive days.

Children:

Gyno-Pevaryl 150 mg pessary is not indicated for use in children under the age of 16 years.

Elderly:

No specific dosage recommendations or precautions apply.

4.3 Contraindications

Hypersensitivity to any imidazole preparation or other vaginal antifungal products.

4.4 Special warnings and precautions for use

Hypersensitivity has rarely been recorded; if it should occur administration should be discontinued.

4.5 Interaction with other medicinal products and other forms of interaction

Contact between contraceptive diaphragms or condoms and this product must be avoided since the rubber may be damaged by this preparation.

Although not studied, based on the chemical similarity of econazole with other imidazole compounds, a theoretical potential for competitive interaction with compounds metabolized by CYP3A4/2C9 exists. Due to the limited systemic availability after vaginal application (see 5.2. Pharmacokinetic Properties), clinically relevant interactions are unlikely to occur. In patients on oral anticoagulants, such as warfarin and acenocoumarol, caution should be exercised and monitoring of the anticoagulant effect should be considered.

4.6 Pregnancy and lactation

In animals, econazole nitrate has shown no teratogenic effects but is foetotoxic at high doses. The significance of this to man is unknown as there is no evidence of an increased risk when taken in human pregnancy. However, as with other imidazoles, econazole should be used in pregnancy only if the practitioner considers it to be necessary.

4.7 Effects on ability to drive and use machines

None known.

4.8 Undesirable effects

The most frequently reported adverse events in clinical trials were application site reactions, such as burning and stinging sensations, pruritus, and erythema.

Based on post-marketing experience, the following adverse reactions have also been reported:

Skin and subcutaneous tissue disorders; general disorders and administration site conditions

Very rare (< 1/10,000): Localized application site (mucocutaneous) reactions, such as erythema, rash, burning and pruritus.

Isolated reports of localized allergic reactions. Isolated reports of generalized allergic reactions, including angioedema and urticaria.

4.9 Overdose

Gyno-Pevaryl 150 mg Vaginal Pessaries are intended for intra-vaginal use and by that route overdose is extremely unlikely. If accidental ingestion of large quantities of the product occurs an appropriate method of gastric emptying may be used if considered desirable.

5. PHARMACOLOGICAL PROPERTIES

5.1 Pharmacodynamic properties

Pharmacotherapeutic classification: (Antiinfectives and antiseptics, excl. combinations with corticosteroids, imidazole derivatives)

ATC code: G01A F05

Econazole nitrate has no anti-inflammatory action, no effects on the circulation, no central or autonomic nervous effects, no effects on respiration, no effect on α or β receptors, no anticholinergic or antiserotonic reactions.

A broad spectrum of antimycotic activity has been demonstrated against dermatophytes, yeasts and moulds. A clinically relevant action against Gram positive bacteria has also been found.

Econazole acts by damaging cell membranes. The permeability of the fungal cell is increased. Sub-cellular membranes in the cytoplasm are damaged. The site of action is most probably the unsaturated fatty acid acyl moiety of membrane phospholipids.

5.2 Pharmacokinetic properties

Econazole nitrate is poorly absorbed from the vagina and skin. If given orally, peak plasma levels occur six hours after dosing. About 90% of the absorbed dose is bound to plasma proteins. Metabolism is limited, but primarily occurs in the liver. Metabolites are excreted in the urine. Five major and two minor metabolites have been identified.

5.3 Preclinical safety data

No relevant information other than that contained elsewhere in the Summary of Product Characteristics.

6. PHARMACEUTICAL PARTICULARS

6.1 List of excipients

Wecobee M

Wecobee FS

6.2 Incompatibilities

None stated.

6.3 Shelf life

Three years.

6.4 Special precautions for storage

Do not store above 30°C.

Keep out of reach and sight of children.

6.5 Nature and contents of container

Available in PVC/PE strips containing three pessaries.

6.6 Special precautions for disposal and other handling

Not applicable.

7. MARKETING AUTHORISATION HOLDER

Janssen-Cilag Ltd

50-100 Holmers Farm Way

High Wycombe

Buckinghamshire

HP12 4EG

UK

8. MARKETING AUTHORISATION NUMBER(S)

PL 00242/0227

9. DATE OF FIRST AUTHORISATION/RENEWAL OF THE AUTHORISATION

1st October 1995/June 2003

10. DATE OF REVISION OF THE TEXT

26th March 2009

Legal Category: POM

Haemate P 500 and 1000 IU

(CSL Behring UK Limited)

1. NAME OF THE MEDICINAL PRODUCT

Haemate P 500 and 1000 Powder and solvent for solution for injection or infusion

2. QUALITATIVE AND QUANTITATIVE COMPOSITION

Haemate P 500

Haemate P 500 is presented as a powder and solvent for solution for injection or infusion containing nominally 1200 International Units (IU) human plasma-derived von Willebrand Factor-ristocetin co-factor activity (VWF:RCo) and 500 IU human coagulation factor VIII activity (FVIII:C) per vial.

Haemate P 500 contains approximately 120 IU/ml (1200 IU/10ml) human plasma-derived VWF:RCo when reconstituted with 10 ml water for injections.

Haemate P 500 contains approximately 50 IU/ml (500 IU/10ml) human plasma-derived coagulation Factor VIII:C when reconstituted with 10 ml water for injections.

Haemate P 1000

Haemate P 1000 is presented as a powder and solvent for solution for injection or infusion containing nominally 2400 International Units (IU) human plasma-derived von Willebrand Factor-ristocetin co-factor activity (VWF:RCo) and 1000 IU human coagulation factor VIII activity (FVIII:C) per vial.

Haemate P 1000 contains approximately 160 IU/ml (2400 IU/10ml15ml) human plasma-derived VWF:RCo when reconstituted with 15 ml water for injections.

Haemate P 1000 contains approximately 66.6 IU/ml (1000 IU/10ml15ml) human plasma-derived coagulation Factor VIII:C when reconstituted with 15 ml water for injections.

The specific activity of Haemate P is approximately 3-17 IU VWF:RCo/mg protein.

The factor VIII (FVIII) potency (IU) is determined using the European Pharmacopoeia chromogenic assay. The specific activity of Haemate P is approximately 2-6 IU FVIII:C/mg protein.

For a full list of excipients, see 6.1

3. PHARMACEUTICAL FORM

Powder and solvent for solution for injection or infusion

4. CLINICAL PARTICULARS

4.1 Therapeutic indications

von Willebrand Disease (VWD):

Prophylaxis and treatment of haemorrhage or surgical bleeding, when desmopressin (DDAVP) treatment alone is ineffective or contra-indicated

Haemophilia A (congenital factor VIII deficiency):

Prophylaxis and treatment of bleeding

This product may be used in the management of acquired factor VIII deficiency and for the treatment of patients with antibodies against factor VIII (see section 4.4).

4.2 Posology and method of administration

Treatment of VWD and Haemophilia A should be supervised by a physician experienced in the treatment of haemostatic disorders.

Posology

von Willebrand Disease:

Generally, 1 IU/kg VWF:RCo raises the circulating level of VWF:RCo by 0.02 IU/ml (2%).

Levels of VWF:RCo greater than 0.6 IU/ml (60%) and of FVIII:C greater than 0.4 IU/ml (40%) should be achieved.

Usually, 40-80 IU/kg bodyweight VWF:RCo and 20-40 IU/kg bodyweight FVIII:C are recommended to achieve haemostasis.

An initial dose of 80 IU/kg VWF:RCo may be required, especially in patients with type 3 von Willebrand disease where maintenance of adequate levels may require higher doses than in other types of von Willebrand disease.

Prevention of haemorrhage in case of surgery or severe trauma

For prevention of excessive bleeding during or after surgery, the injection should be started 1 to 2 hours before the surgical procedure.

An appropriate dose should be re-administered every 12 - 24 hours. The dose and duration of treatment will depend on the clinical status of the patient, the type and severity of bleeding and both the VWF:RCo and FVIII:C levels.

When using a factor VIII-containing von Willebrand factor product, the treating physician should be aware that continued treatment may cause an excessive rise in FVIII:C. After 24 - 48 hours of treatment, in order to avoid an uncontrolled rise in FVIII:C, reduced doses and/or prolongation of the dose interval should be considered.

Dosing in children is based on bodyweight and is therefore generally based on the same guidelines as for adults. The frequency of administration should always be tailored to clinical effectiveness in the individual case.

Haemophilia A:

The dosage and duration of the substitution therapy depend on the severity of the factor VIII deficiency, on the location and extent of the bleeding and on the patient's clinical condition.

The number of units of factor VIII administered is expressed in International Units, which are related to the current World Health Organisation (WHO) standard for factor VIII products. Factor VIII activity in plasma is expressed either as a percentage (relative to normal human plasma) or in International Units (relative to an International Standard for factor VIII in plasma).

One IU of factor VIII activity is equivalent to that quantity of factor VIII in one ml of normal human plasma.

The calculation of the required dosage of FVIII:C is based on the empirical finding that 1 IU factor VIII:C per kg bodyweight raises the plasma factor VIII activity by about 2% of normal activity (2 IU/dl). The required dosage is determined using the following formula:

Required units = body weight (kg) × desired factor VIII:C rise (% or IU/dl) × 0.5.

The amount to be administered and the frequency of administration should always be tailored to clinical effectiveness in the individual case.

In the case of the following haemorrhagic events, the factor VIII activity should not fall below the indicated plasma activity level (in % of normal or IU/dl) within the corresponding period.

The following table can be used to guide dosing in bleeding episodes and surgery:

Degree of haemorrhage / Type of surgical procedure	FVIII:C level required (% or IU/dl)	Frequency of Doses (hours) / Duration of therapy (days)
Haemorrhage		
Early haemarthrosis, muscle bleeding or oral bleeding	20 - 40	Repeat every 12 - 24 hours (at least 1 day) until the bleeding episode, as indicated by pain, is resolved or healing is achieved.
More extensive haemarthrosis, muscle bleeding or haematoma	30 - 60	Repeat infusion every 12 - 24 hours for 3 - 4 days or more until pain and disability are resolved.
Life-threatening haemorrhages	60 - 100	Repeat infusion every 8 - 24 hours until threat is resolved.
Surgery		
Minor including tooth extraction	30 - 60	Every 24 hours (at least 1 day) until healing is achieved.
Major	80 - 100 (pre- and postoperative)	Repeat infusion every 8 - 24 hours until adequate wound healing, then treat for at least another 7 days to maintain a FVIII:C activity of 30 to 60% or IU/dl.

During the course of treatment, appropriate determination of FVIII:C levels is advised, to guide the dose to be administered and the frequency of repeated infusions. In the case of major surgical interventions in particular, precise monitoring of the substitution therapy by means of coagulation analysis (plasma FVIII:C activity) is indispensable. Individual patients may vary in their response to factor VIII, achieving different levels of *in vivo* recovery and demonstrating different half-lives.

For long term prophylaxis against bleeding in patients with severe haemophilia A, the usual doses are 20 - 40 IU factor VIII:C per kg bodyweight at intervals of 2 to 3 days. In some cases, especially in younger patients, shorter dosage intervals or higher doses may be necessary.

Patients should be monitored for the development of factor VIII inhibitors. If the expected FVIII:C activity levels are not attained, or if bleeding is not controlled with an appropriate dose, an assay should be performed to determine if a factor VIII inhibitor is present. In patients with high levels of inhibitor, factor VIII therapy may not be effective and other therapeutic options should be considered. Management of such patients should be directed by physicians with experience in the care of patients with haemophilia. See section 4.4.

There are no data from clinical studies regarding the dosage of Haemate P in children with haemophilia A.

Method of administration

The preparation should be warmed to room or body temperature, then reconstituted as described in section 6.6. Then the product should be administered slowly via the intravenous route, at a rate comfortable for the patient.

Where a large volume is required, infusion is an alternative option. The reconstituted preparation should be transferred to an approved infusion system.

The injection or infusion rate should not exceed 4 ml per minute. The patient should be observed for any immediate reaction. Should any reaction occur which might be related to administration of Haemate P, the rate of infusion should be decreased or administration stopped, as appropriate. See section 4.4.

4.3 Contraindications

Hypersensitivity to any of the constituents of Haemate P.

4.4 Special warnings and precautions for use

As with any intravenous infusion of a plasma-derived protein, allergic type hypersensitivity reactions are possible. Patients must be closely monitored and carefully observed for any symptoms throughout the infusion period. Patients should be informed of the early signs of hypersensitivity reactions including hives, generalised urticaria, tightness of the chest, wheezing, hypotension and anaphylaxis. If these symptoms occur, the patient should be advised to discontinue use of the product immediately and contact their physician.

In case of shock, the current medical standards for shock treatment should be implemented.

Haemate P contains up to 140 mg sodium per 1000 IU. This should be taken into consideration for patients on a sodium-controlled diet.

Standard measures to prevent infections resulting from the use of medicinal products prepared from human blood or plasma include selection of donors, screening of individual donations and plasma pools for specific markers of infection and the inclusion of effective manufacturing steps for the inactivation/removal of viruses. Despite this, when medicinal products prepared from human blood or plasma are administered, the possibility of transmitting infective agents cannot be totally excluded. This also applies to unknown or emerging viruses and other pathogens.

The measures taken are considered effective for enveloped viruses such as HIV, HBV and HCV and for the non-enveloped virus HAV. The measures taken may be of limited value against other non-enveloped viruses such as parvovirus B19. Parvovirus B19 infection may be serious for pregnant women (foetal infection) and for individuals with immunodeficiency or increased erythropoiesis (e.g. haemolytic anaemia).

Appropriate vaccination (hepatitis A and B) should be considered for patients in regular/repeated receipt of human plasma-derived products.

It is strongly recommended that every time that Haemate P is administered to a patient, the name and batch number of the product are recorded in order to maintain a link between the patient and the batch of the product.

von Willebrand Disease:

There is a risk of occurrence of thrombotic events, particularly in patients with known clinical or laboratory risk factors. Therefore, patients at risk must be monitored for early signs of thrombosis. Prophylaxis against venous thromboembolism should be instituted, according to the current recommendations.

When using a factor VIII-containing VWF product, the treating physician should be aware that continued treatment may cause an excessive rise in FVIII:C. In patients receiving FVIII-containing VWF products, plasma levels of FVIII:C should be monitored to avoid sustained excessive FVIII:C plasma levels which may increase the risk of thrombotic events, and anti-thrombotic measures should be considered.

Patients with von Willebrand disease, especially type 3 patients, may develop neutralising antibodies (inhibitors) to VWF. If the expected VWF:RCo activity plasma levels are not attained, or if bleeding is not controlled with an appropriate dose, an appropriate assay should be performed to determine if a VWF inhibitor is present. In patients with high levels of inhibitor, VWF therapy may not be effective and other therapeutic options should be considered.

Haemophilia A:

The formation of neutralising antibodies (inhibitors) to factor VIII is a known complication in the management of individuals with haemophilia A. These inhibitors are usually IgG immunoglobulins directed against the factor VIII procoagulant activity, which are quantified in Bethesda Units per ml of plasma using the modified assay. The risk of developing inhibitors is correlated to the exposure to anti-haemophilic factor VIII, this risk being highest within the first 20 exposure days. Rarely, inhibitors may develop after the first 100 exposure days. Patients treated with human coagulation factor VIII should be carefully monitored for the development of inhibitory antibodies by appropriate clinical observations and laboratory tests. In patients with high levels of inhibitor, therapy may not be effective and other therapeutic options should be considered. See section 4.8.

4.5 Interaction with other medicinal products and other forms of interaction

No interactions of human coagulation factor VIII or von Willebrand factor products with other medicinal products are known.

4.6 Pregnancy and lactation

Animal reproduction studies have not been conducted with Haemate P.

Based on the rare occurrence of haemophilia A in women, experience regarding the use of factor VIII during pregnancy and breast-feeding is not available.

The situation is different in von Willebrand disease because of its autosomal heredity. Women are affected more than men because of additional bleeding risks such as menstruation, pregnancy, labour, childbirth and gynaecological complications. Based on post-marketing experience, substitution of VWF in the prevention and treatment of acute bleeding is not contra-indicated. There are no clinical studies available on substitution therapy in pregnant or lactating women.

Therefore, Haemate P should be administered to pregnant and lactating women only if clearly indicated and the benefit outweighs the risk.

4.7 Effects on ability to drive and use machines

No effects on ability to drive and use machines have been observed.

4.8 Undesirable effects

The following adverse reactions are based on experience from clinical trials and on post-marketing experience. The following standard categories of frequency are used:

Very common $\geqslant$1/10, Common $\geqslant$1/100 and $\leqslant$1/10, Uncommon $\geqslant$1/1000 and $\leqslant$1/100, Rare $\geqslant$1/10,000 and $\leqslant$1/1000, Very rare $\leqslant$1/10,000

Hypersensitivity or allergic reactions (which may include angioedema, burning and stinging at the infusion site, chills, flushing, generalised urticaria, headache, hives, hypotension, lethargy, nausea, restlessness, tachycardia, tightness of the chest, tingling, vomiting, wheezing) have been observed in very rare cases, and may in some cases progress to severe anaphylaxis (allergic shock).

On rare occasions, fever has been observed.

When very large or frequently repeated doses are needed, or when inhibitors are present or when pre-or post-surgical care is involved, all patients should be monitored for signs of hypervolaemia. In addition, those patients with blood groups A, B and AB should be monitored for signs of intravascular haemolysis and/or decreasing haematocrit values.

Patients with von Willebrand disease, especially type 3 patients, may very rarely develop neutralising antibodies (inhibitors) to VWF. If such inhibitors occur, the condition will manifest itself as an inadequate clinical response. Such antibodies are precipitation and occur in close association with anaphylactic reactions. Therefore, patients experiencing anaphylactic reaction should be evaluated for the presence of an inhibitor.

There is a risk of occurrence of thrombotic events, particularly in patients with known clinical or laboratory risk factors.

In patients receiving factor VIII-containing von Willebrand factor products sustained excessive FVIII:C plasma levels may increase the risk of thrombotic events. See section 4.4.

Patients with haemophilia A may develop neutralising antibodies (inhibitors) to factor VIII. If such inhibitors occur, the condition will manifest itself as an insufficient clinical response. The experience from clinical trials with Haemate P in previously untreated patients (PUPs) is very limited. Therefore, no valid figures on incidence of clinically relevant specific inhibitors can be provided. See section 4.2.

In all such cases, it is recommended that a specialised haemophilia centre be contacted.

For safety with respect to transmissible agents, see section 4.4.

4.9 Overdose

No symptoms of overdose with human von Willebrand factor and/or coagulation factor VIII have been reported. Thromboembolic events may occur in case of major overdose.

5. PHARMACOLOGICAL PROPERTIES

5.1 Pharmacodynamic properties

Pharmacotherapeutic Group: Antihaemorrhagics: blood coagulation factors, von Willebrand factor and coagulation factor VIII in combination. ATC code: B02BD06.

<u>von Willebrand factor:</u>

Haemate P behaves in the same way as endogenous von Willebrand factor.

Administration of von Willebrand factor allows correction of the haemostatic abnormalities exhibited by patients who suffer from VWF deficiency (VWD) at two levels:

- VWF re-establishes platelet adhesion to the vascular sub-endothelium at the site of vascular damage (as it binds both to the vascular sub-endothelium and to the platelet membrane), providing primary haemostasis as shown by the shortening of the bleeding time. This effect occurs immediately and is known to depend to a large extent on the level of polymerisation of the protein, i.e. content of high molecular weight VWF-multimers.

- VWF produces delayed correction of the associated factor VIII deficiency. Administered intravenously, VWF binds to endogenous factor VIII (which is produced normally by the patient), and by stabilising this factor, avoids its rapid degradation.

Because of this, administration of pure VWF (VWF product with a low FVIII level) restores the FVIII:C level to normal as a secondary effect after the first infusion.

Administration of a FVIII:C-containing VWF preparation restores the FVIII:C level to normal immediately after the first infusion.

<u>Factor VIII:</u>

Haemate P behaves in the same way as endogenous factor VIII.

The factor VIII/von Willebrand factor complex consists of two molecules (FVIII and VWF) with different physiological functions. When infused into a haemophiliac patient, factor VIII binds to VWF in the patient's circulation.

- Activated factor VIII acts as a cofactor for activated factor IX, accelerating the conversion of factor X to activated factor X. Activated factor X converts prothrombin into thrombin. Thrombin then converts fibrinogen into fibrin and a clot can be formed. Haemophilia A is a sex-linked hereditary disorder of blood coagulation due to decreased levels of factor VIII:C and results in profuse bleeding into joints, muscles or internal organs, either spontaneously or as a result of accidental or surgical trauma. By replacement therapy the plasma levels of factor VIII are increased, thereby enabling a temporary correction of the factor deficiency and correction of the bleeding tendency.

5.2 Pharmacokinetic properties

<u>von Willebrand factor:</u>

The pharmacokinetics of Haemate P has been evaluated in 28 VWD patients (type 1, n=10; type 2A, n=10; type 2M, n=1; type3, n=7) in the non-bleeding state.

The median half-life of VWF:RCo (one compartment model) was 7.1 hours (range: 2.9 to 22.0 hours). The median *in vivo* recovery for VWF:RCo activity was 1.9 IU/dldL per IU/kg (range: 0.8 to 3.6 IU/dl per IU/kg. The median area under the curve (AUC) was 1729 IU/dl × h (range: 423 to 8319 IU/dl × h, the median residence time (MRT) was 10.3 hours (range: 4.2 to 31.8 hours) and the median clearance was 4.24 ml/kg/h (range: 0.97 to 17.75 ml/kg/h).

Peak plasma levels of VWF usually occur at around 50 minutes after injection.

<u>Factor VIII:</u>

After intravenous injection, there is a rapid increase in plasma factor VIII (FVIII:C) activity, followed by a rapid decrease in activity and a subsequent slower rate of decrease in activity. Studies in patients with Haemophilia A have demonstrated a median half-life of 12.6 hours (range: 5.0 to 27.7 hours). An overall median FVIII *in vivo* recovery of 1.73 IU/dl per IU/kg (range: 0.5 to 4.13 IU/dl per IU/kg) was obtained. The MRT was found to be 19.0 hours (range: 14.8 to 40.0 hours), the median AUC was 36.1 % × hours/IU/kg (range: 14.8 to 72.4 % × hours/IU/kg) and the median clearance was 2.8 ml/kg/h (range: 1.4 to 6.7 ml/kg/h).

5.3 Preclinical safety data

Haemate P contains the active ingredients, factor VIII and von Willebrand factor, both of which are derived from human plasma and act like the endogenous constituents of plasma.

Single dose toxicity testing revealed no adverse findings in different species even at dose levels several times higher than the recommended human dose. Repeated dose toxicity testing is impracticable due to the development of antibodies to heterologous protein. To date Haemate P has not been reported to be associated with embryo-foetal toxicity, oncogenic or mutagenic potential.

6. PHARMACEUTICAL PARTICULARS

6.1 List of excipients

Human albumin

Glycine

Sodium chloride

Sodium citrate

Sodium hydroxide or hydrochloric acid (in small amounts for pH adjustment)

Supplied diluent: Water for injections 10ml (for Haemate P 500 IU) or15ml (for Haemate P 1000IU)

6.2 Incompatibilities

This medicinal product must not be mixed with other medicinal products, diluents and solvents, except those mentioned in section 6.1.

Only the provided injection/infusion sets should be used because treatment failure can occur as a consequence of human factor VIII adsorption to the internal surfaces of some infusion equipment.

6.3 Shelf life

3 years.

Following reconstitution, physico-chemical stability has been demonstrated for 48 hours at room temperature (max +25°C). Since Haemate P contains no preservatives, the reconstituted product should be used immediately, and should be used up within 8 hours.

6.4 Special precautions for storage

Do not store above 25 °C. Do not freeze. Keep the container in the outer carton.

6.5 Nature and contents of container

6.5.1 <u>Immediate containers:</u>

Substance vial:

Injection vial of colourless, moulded glass type II (Ph. Eur.), sealed with rubber infusion stopper (latex-free), plastic disc and aluminium cap.

1 vial (hermetically sealed under vacuum) with dried substance

Solvent (diluent) vial (Water for Injections):

Injection vial of tubular glass with inner surface treatment, colourless glass type I (Ph. Eur.), sealed with rubber infusion stopper (latex-free), plastic disc and aluminium cap.

1 vial with 10 or 15 ml water for injections.

6.5.2 <u>Administration set: (in separate box)</u>

1 filter transfer device 20/20

1 disposable 10 or 15 ml syringe

1 venipuncture set

2 alcohol swabs

1 plaster

6.6 Special precautions for disposal and other handling

General instructions

- The solution should be clear or slightly opalescent. After filtering/withdrawal (see below), the reconstituted product should be inspected visually for particulate matter prior to administration. Even if the directions for use for the reconstitution procedure are precisely followed, it is not uncommon for a few flakes or particles to remain.

Note: the filter included in the Mix2Vial transfer device will remove any particles.

Filtration does not influence dosage calculations. Do not use visibly cloudy solutions or solutions containing flakes or particles after filtration.

- Reconstitution and withdrawal must be carried out under aseptic conditions.

- Any unused product or waste material should be disposed of in accordance with local requirements.

Reconstitution

Bring the solvent to room or body temperature. Remove the product and diluent vial flip caps, wipe both stoppers with an alcohol swab and allow to dry before opening the Mix2Vial package.

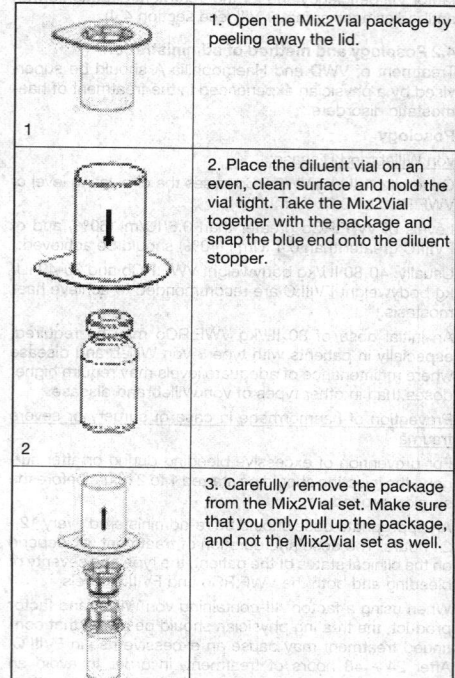

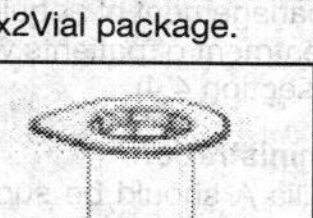 1	1. Open the Mix2Vial package by peeling away the lid.
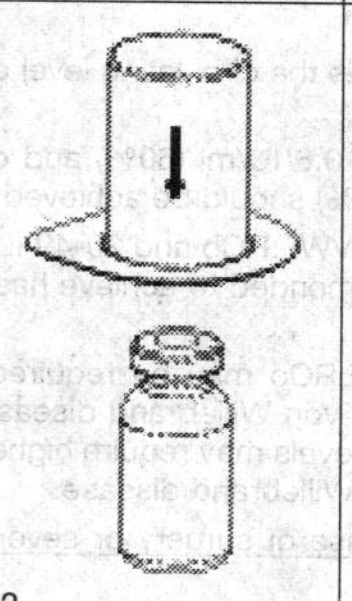 2	2. Place the diluent vial on an even, clean surface and hold the vial tight. Take the Mix2Vial together with the package and snap the blue end onto the diluent stopper.
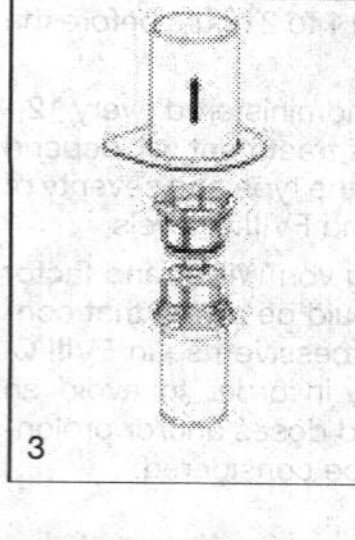 3	3. Carefully remove the package from the Mix2Vial set. Make sure that you only pull up the package, and not the Mix2Vial set as well.

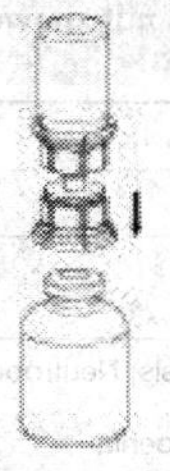

4

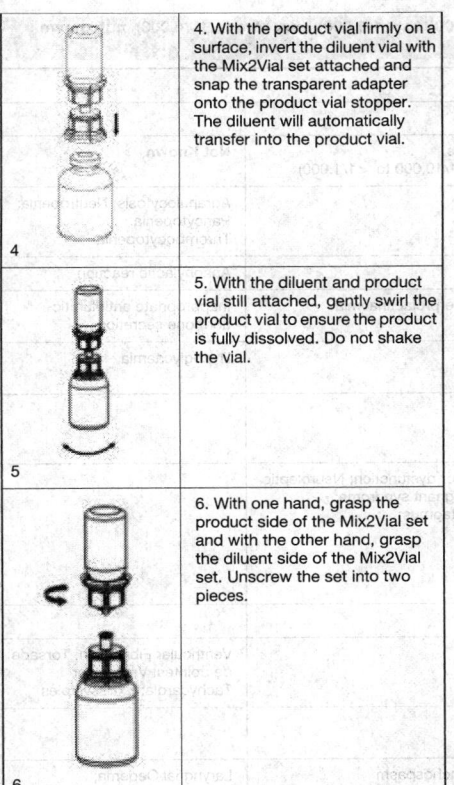

4. With the product vial firmly on a surface, invert the diluent vial with the Mix2Vial set attached and snap the transparent adapter onto the product vial stopper. The diluent will automatically transfer into the product vial.

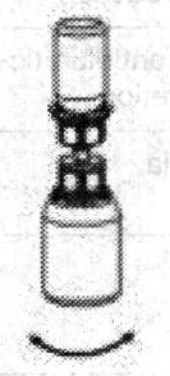

5

5. With the diluent and product vial still attached, gently swirl the product vial to ensure the product is fully dissolved. Do not shake the vial.

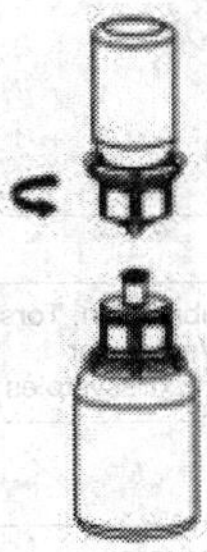

6

6. With one hand, grasp the product side of the Mix2Vial set and with the other hand, grasp the diluent side of the Mix2Vial set. Unscrew the set into two pieces.

Withdrawal and application

Draw air into an empty, sterile syringe. With the product vial upright, connect the syringe to the Mix2Vial set. Inject air into the product vial.

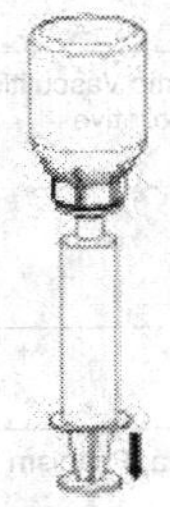

7

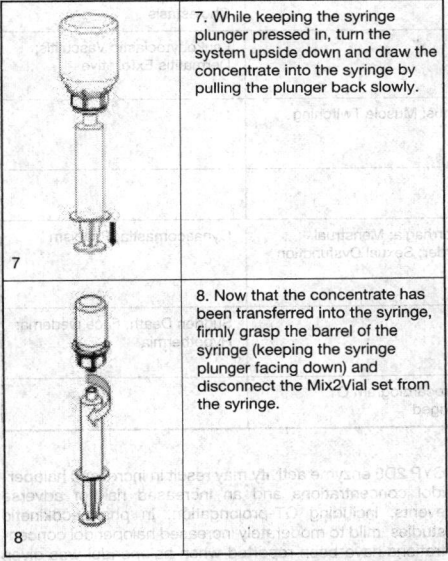

7. While keeping the syringe plunger pressed in, turn the system upside down and draw the concentrate into the syringe by pulling the plunger back slowly.

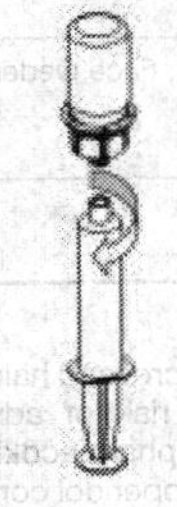

8

8. Now that the concentrate has been transferred into the syringe, firmly grasp the barrel of the syringe (keeping the syringe plunger facing down) and disconnect the Mix2Vial set from the syringe.

Administer the solution slowly via the intravenous route, taking care that no blood enters the syringe. See section 4.2.

7. MARKETING AUTHORISATION HOLDER

CSL Behring GmbH

Emil-von-Behring-Strasse 76

35041 Marburg

Germany

8. MARKETING AUTHORISATION NUMBER(S)

PL 15036/0009

PL 15036/0010

9. DATE OF FIRST AUTHORISATION/RENEWAL OF THE AUTHORISATION

12 April 2005

10. DATE OF REVISION OF THE TEXT

25 February 2008

Haldol 10mg Tablets

(Janssen-Cilag Ltd)

1. NAME OF THE MEDICINAL PRODUCT

HALDOL Tablets 10 mg

2. QUALITATIVE AND QUANTITATIVE COMPOSITION

Haloperidol 10 mg.

3. PHARMACEUTICAL FORM

Tablets.

4. CLINICAL PARTICULARS

4.1 Therapeutic indications

Adults:

- Schizophrenia: treatment of symptoms and prevention of relapse
- Other psychoses: especially paranoid
- Mania and hypomania
- Mental or behavioural problems such as aggression, hyperactivity and self mutilation in the mentally retarded and in patients with organic brain damage
- As an adjunct to short term management of moderate to severe psychomotor agitation, excitement, violent or dangerously impulsive behaviour
- Intractable hiccup
- Restlessness and agitation in the elderly
- Gilles de la Tourette syndrome and severe tics.

Children:

- Childhood behavioural disorders, especially when associated with hyperactivity and aggression
- Gilles de la Tourette syndrome
- Childhood schizophrenia.

4.2 Posology and method of administration

For oral administration.

Dosage for all indications should be individually determined and is best initiated and titrated under close clinical supervision. To determine initial dose, consideration should be given to the patient's age, severity of symptoms and previous response to neuroleptic drugs.

Patients who are elderly or debilitated or those with previously reported adverse reactions to neuroleptic drugs may require less Haldol. The normal starting dose should be halved, followed by a gradual titration to achieve optimal response.

Haldol should be used at the minimum dose that is clinically effective.

Adults

Schizophrenia, psychoses, mania and hypomania, mental or behavioural problems, psychomotor agitation, excitement, violent or dangerously impulsive behaviour, organic brain damage

Initial dose:

Moderate symptomatology: 1.5-3.0 mg bd or tds.

Severe symptomatology/resistant patients: 3.0-5.0 mg bd or tds.

The same starting dose may be employed in adolescents and resistant schizophrenics, who may require up to 30 mg/day.

Maintenance dosage:

Once satisfactory control of symptoms has been achieved dosage should be gradually reduced to the lowest effective maintenance dose, often as low as 5 or 10 mg/day. Too rapid a dosage reduction should be avoided.

Restlessness or agitation in the elderly

Initial dose: 1.5-3.0 mg bd or tds titrated as required, to attain an effective maintenance dose (1.5-30 mg daily).

Gilles de la Tourette syndrome, severe tics, intractable hiccup

Starting dose 1.5 mg tds adjusted according to response. A daily maintenance dose of 10 mg may be required in Gilles de la Tourette syndrome.

Children

Childhood behavioural disorders and schizophrenia

Total daily maintenance dose of 0.025-0.05 mg/kg/day. Half the total dose should be given in the morning and the other half in the evening, up to a maximum of 10 mg daily.

Gilles de la Tourette syndrome

Oral maintenance doses up to 10 mg/day in most patients.

4.3 Contraindications

Comatose states, CNS depression, Parkinson's disease, known hypersensitivity to haloperidol, lesions of basal ganglia.

In common with other neuroleptics, haloperidol has the potential to cause rare prolongation of the QT interval. Use of haloperidol is therefore contra-indicated in patients with clinically significant cardiac disorders e.g. recent acute myocardial infarction, uncompensated heart failure, arrhythmias treated with class IA and III antiarrhythmic medicinal products, QTc interval prolongation, history of ventricular arrhythmia or torsades de pointes clinically significant bradycardia, second or third degree heart block and uncorrected hypokalaemia. Haloperidol should not be used concomitantly with other QT prolonging drugs (see section 4.5, Interactions)

4.4 Special warnings and precautions for use

Cases of sudden death have been reported in psychiatric patients receiving antipsychotic drugs, including haloperidol.

Elderly patients with dementia-related psychosis treated with antipsychotic drugs are at an increased risk of death. Analyses of seventeen placebo-controlled trials (modal duration of 10 weeks), largely in patients taking atypical antipsychotic drugs, revealed a risk of death in drug-treated patients of between 1.6 to 1.7 times the risk of death in placebo-treated patients. Over the course of a typical 10 week controlled trial, the rate of death in drug-treated patients was about 4.5%, compared to a rate of about 2.6% in the placebo group. Although the causes of death were varied, most of the deaths appeared to be either cardiovascular (e.g., heart failure, sudden death) or infectious (e.g., pneumonia) in nature. Observational studies suggest that, similar to atypical antipsychotic drugs, treatment with conventional antipsychotic drugs may increase mortality. The extent to which the findings of increased mortality in observational studies may be attributed to the antipsychotic drug as opposed to some characteristic(s) of the patients is not clear.

Cardiovascular effects

Very rare reports of QT prolongation and/or ventricular arrhythmias, in addition to rare reports of sudden death, have been reported with haloperidol. They may occur more frequently with high doses and in predisposed patients.

The risk-benefit of haloperidol treatment should be fully assessed before treatment is commenced and patients with risk factors for ventricular arrhythmias such as cardiac disease, family history of sudden death and/or QT prolongation; uncorrected electrolyte disturbances, subarachnoid haemorrhage, starvation or alcohol abuse, should be monitored carefully (ECGs and potassium levels), particularly during the initial phase of treatment, to obtain steady plasma levels. The risk of QT prolongation and/or ventricular arrhythmias may be increased with higher doses (see Sections 4.8 and 4.9) or with parenteral use, particularly intravenous administration. ECG monitoring should be performed for QT interval prolongation and for serious cardiac dysrhythmias if Haldol is administered intravenously.

Haloperidol should be used with caution in patients known to be slow metabolisers of CYP2D6, and during use of cytochrome P450 inhibitors. Concomitant use of antipsychotics should be avoided. (See Section 4.5)

Baseline ECG is recommended prior to treatment in all patients, especially in the elderly and patients with a positive personal or family history of cardiac disease or abnormal findings on cardiac clinical examination. During therapy, the need for ECG monitoring (e.g. at dose escalation) should be assessed on an individual basis. Whilst on therapy, the dose should be reduced if QT is prolonged, and haloperidol should be discontinued if the QTc exceeds 500 ms.

Periodic electrolyte monitoring is recommended, especially for patients taking diuretics, or during intercurrent illness.

An approximately 3-fold increase risk of cerebrovascular adverse events have been seen in randomised placebo controlled clinical trials in the dementia population with some atypical antipsychotics. The mechanism for this increased risk is not known. An increased risk cannot be excluded for other antipsychotics or other patient populations. Haloperidol should be used in caution in patients with risk factors for stroke.

Neuroleptic malignant syndrome

In common with other antipsychotic drugs, Haldol has been associated with neuroleptic malignant syndrome: a rare idiosyncratic response characterised by hyperthermia, generalised muscle rigidity, autonomic instability, altered consciousness. Hyperthermia is often an early sign of this syndrome. Antipsychotic treatment should be withdrawn immediately and appropriate supportive therapy and careful monitoring instituted.

Tardive dyskinesia

As with all antipsychotic agents, tardive dyskinesia may appear in some patients on long-term therapy or after drug discontinuation. The syndrome is mainly characterised by rhythmic involuntary movements of the tongue, face, mouth or jaw.

The manifestations may be permanent in some patients. The syndrome may be masked when treatment is reinstituted, when the dosage is increased or when a switch is made to a different antipsychotic drug. Treatment should be discontinued as soon as possible.

Extrapyramidal symptoms

In common with all neuroleptics, extrapyramidal symptoms may occur, e.g. tremor, rigidity, hypersalivation, bradykinesia, akathisia, acute dystonia.

Antiparkinson drugs of the anticholinergic type may be prescribed as required, but should not be prescribed routinely as a preventive measure. If concomitant antiparkinson medication is required, it may have to be continued after stopping Haldol if its excretion is faster than that of Haldol in order to avoid the development or aggravation of extrapyramidal symptoms. The physician should keep in mind the possible increase in intraocular pressure when anticholinergic drugs, including antiparkinson agents, are administered concomitantly with Haldol.

Table 1 Very common (≥ 1/10); common (≥ 1/100 to < 1/10); uncommon (≥ 1/1,000 to < 1/100); rare (≥ 1/10,000 to < 1/1,000); very rare (< 1/10,000), not known (cannot be estimated form the available data)

System Organ Class	Adverse Drug Reactions				
	Frequency Category				
	Very Common (≥ 1/10)	Common (≥ 1/100 to < 1/10)	Uncommon (≥ 1/1,000 to < 1/100)	Rare (≥ 1/10,000 to < 1/1,000)	Not Known
Blood and lymphatic System Disorders			Leukopenia		Agranulocytosis; Neutropenia; Pancytopenia; Thrombocytopenia
Immune System Disorders			Hypersensitivity		Anaphylactic reaction
Endocrine Disorders				Hyperprolactinaemia	Inappropriate antidiuretic hormone secretion
Metabolic and Nutritional Disorders					Hypoglycaemia
Psychiatric Disorders	Agitation; Insomnia	Depression; Psychotic disorder	Confusional state; Libido Decreased; Loss of libido; Restlessness		
Nervous System Disorders	Extrapyramidal disorder; Hyperkinesia; Headache	Tardive dyskinesia; Oculogyric Crisis; Dystonia; Dyskinesia; Akathisia; Bradykinesia; Hypokinesia; Hypertonia; Somnolence; Masked Facies, Tremor; Dizziness	Convulsion; Parkinsonism; Akinesia; Cogwheel rigidity; Sedation; Muscle Contractions Involuntary	Motor dysfunction; Neuroleptic malignant syndrome; Nystagmus;	
Eye Disorders		Visual disturbance;	Vision blurred		
Cardiac Disorders			Tachycardia		Ventricular Fibrillation; Torsade de pointes; Ventricular Tachycardia; Extrasystoles
Vascular Disorders		Orthostatic Hypotension; Hypotension			
Respiratory, thoracic and mediastinal Disorders			Dyspnoea	Bronchospasm	Laryngeal Oedema; Laryngospasm
Gastrointestinal Disorders		Constipation; Dry mouth; Salivary hypersecretion; Nausea; Vomiting			
Hepatobiliary Disorders		Liver function test abnormal	Hepatitis; Jaundice		Acute Hepatic Failure; Cholestasis
Skin and subcutaneous tissue disorders		Rash	Photosensitivity Reaction; Urticaria; Pruritis; Hyperhidrosis		Leukocytoclastic Vasculitis; Dermatitis Exfoliative
Musculoskeletal and Connective Tissue Disorders			Torticollis; Muscle rigidity; Muscle Spasms; Musculoskeletal stiffness	Trismus; Muscle Twitching	
Renal and Urinary Disorders		Urinary retention			
Reproductive System and Breast Disorders		Erectile dysfunction	Amenorrhoea; Dysmenorrhoea; Galactorrhoea; Breast Discomfort; Breast Pain;	Menorrhagia; Menstrual Disorder; Sexual Dysfunction	Gynaecomastia, Priapism
General Disorders and Administration Site Conditions			Gait disturbance; Hyperthermia; Oedema		Sudden Death; Face Oedema; Hypothermia
Investigations		Weight increased; Weight decreased		Electrocardiogram QT prolonged	

Seizures/Convulsions

It has been reported that seizures can be triggered by Haldol. Caution is advised in patients suffering from epilepsy and in conditions predisposing to convulsions (e.g., alcohol withdrawal and brain damage).

Hepatobiliary concerns

As Haldol is metabolised by the liver, caution is advised in patients with liver disease. Isolated cases of liver function abnormalities or hepatitis, most often cholestatic, have been reported.

Endocrine system concerns

Thyroxin may facilitate Haldol toxicity. Antipsychotic therapy in patients with hyperthyroidism should be used only with great caution and must always be accompanied by therapy to achieve a euthyroid state.

Hormonal effects of antipsychotic neuroleptic drugs include hyperprolactinaemia, which may cause galactorrhoea, gynaecomastia and oligo- or amenorrhoea. Very rare cases of hypoglycaemia and of Syndrome of Inappropriate ADH Secretion have been reported.

Additional considerations

In schizophrenia, the response to antipsychotic drug treatment may be delayed. Also, if drugs are withdrawn, recurrence of symptoms may not become apparent for several weeks or months. Acute withdrawal symptoms including nausea, vomiting and insomnia have very rarely been described after abrupt cessation of high doses of antipsychotic drugs. Relapse may also occur and gradual withdrawal is advisable.

As with all antipsychotic agents, Haldol should not be used alone where depression is predominant. It may be combined with antidepressants to treat those conditions in which depression and psychosis coexist.

Caution is advised in patients with renal failure and phaeochromocytoma.

4.5 Interaction with other medicinal products and other forms of interaction

Concomitant use of haloperidol with drugs known to prolong the QT interval may increase the risk of ventricular arrhythmias, including torsade de pointes. Therefore concomitant use of these products is not recommended (see section 4.3-Contraindications).

Examples include certain antiarrhythmics, such as those of Class 1A (such as quinidine, disopyramide and procainamide) and class III (such as amiodarone, sotalol and dofetilide), certain antimicrobials (sparfloxacin, moxifloxacin, erythromycin IV), tricyclic antidepressants (such as amitriptyline), certain tetracyclic antidepressants (such as maprotiline), other neuroleptics (e.g. phenothiazines, pimozide and sertindole), certain antihistamines (such as terfenadine), cisapride, bretylium and certain antimalarials such as quinine and mefloquine. This list is not comprehensive.

Concurrent use of drugs causing electrolyte imbalance may increase the risk of ventricular arrhythmias and is not recommended (see section 4.4-Special Warnings and Precautions for Use). Diuretics, in particular those causing hypokalaemia, should be avoided but, if necessary, potassium-sparing diuretics are preferred.

Haloperidol is metabolised by several routes, including glucuronidation and the cytochrome P450 enzyme system (particularly CYP 3A4 or CYP 2D6). Inhibition of these routes of metabolism by another drug or a decrease in CYP 2D6 enzyme activity may result in increased haloperidol concentrations and an increased risk of adverse events, including QT-prolongation. In pharmacokinetic studies, mild to moderately increased haloperidol concentrations have been reported when haloperidol was given concomitantly with drugs characterised as substrates or inhibitors of CYP 3A4 or CYP 2D6 isozymes, such as, itraconazole, buspirone, venlafaxine, alprazolam, fluvoxamine, quinidine, fluoxetine, sertraline, chlorpromazine, and promethazine. A decrease in CYP2D6 enzyme activity may result in increased haloperidol concentrations. Increases in QTc and extrapyramidal symptoms have been observed when haloperidol was given with a combination of the metabolic inhibitors ketoconazole (400 mg/day) and paroxetine (20 mg/day). It may be necessary to reduce the haloperidol dosage.

Effect of Other Drugs on Haloperidol

When prolonged treatment with enzyme-inducing drugs such as carbamazepine, phenobarbital, rifampicin is added to Haldol therapy, this results in a significant reduction of haloperidol plasma levels. Therefore, during combination treatment, the Haldol dose should be adjusted, when necessary. After stopping such drugs, it may be necessary to reduce the dosage of Haldol.

Sodium valproate, a drug known to inhibit glucuronidation, does not affect haloperidol plasma concentrations.

Effect of Haloperidol on Other Drugs

In common with all neuroleptics, Haldol can increase the central nervous system depression produced by other CNS-depressant drugs, including alcohol, hypnotics, sedatives or strong analgesics. An enhanced CNS effect, when combined with methyldopa, has also been reported.

Haldol may antagonise the action of adrenaline and other sympathomimetic agents and reverse the blood-pressure-lowering effects of adrenergic-blocking agents such as guanethidine.

Haldol may impair the antiparkinson effects of levodopa.

Haloperidol is an inhibitor of CYP 2D6. Haldol inhibits the metabolism of tricyclic antidepressants, thereby increasing plasma levels of these drugs.

Other Forms of Interaction

In rare cases, an encephalopathy-like syndrome has been reported in combination with lithium and haloperidol. It remains controversial whether these cases represent a distinct clinical entity or whether they are in fact cases of NMS and/or lithium toxicity. Signs of encephalopathy-like syndrome include confusion, disorientation, headache, disturbances of balance and drowsiness. One report showing symptomless EEG abnormalities on the combination has suggested that EEG monitoring might be advisable. When lithium and haloperidol therapy are used concomitantly, haloperidol should be given in the lowest effective dose and lithium levels should be monitored and kept below 1 mmol/l. If symptoms of encephalopathy-like syndrome occur, therapy should be stopped immediately.

Antagonism of the effect of the anticoagulant phenindione has been reported.

The dosage of anticonvulsants may need to be increased to take account of the lowered seizure threshold.

4.6 Pregnancy and lactation

The safety of haloperidol in pregnancy has not been established. There is some evidence of harmful effects in some, but not all animal studies. There have been a number of reports of birth defects following foetal exposure to haloperidol for which a causal role for haloperidol cannot be excluded. Reversible extrapyrimidal symptoms have been observed in neonates exposed to haloperidol in utero during the last trimester of pregnancy. Haldol should be used during pregnancy only if the anticipated benefit outweighs the risk and the administered dose and duration of treatment should be as low and as short as possible.

Haloperidol is excreted in breast milk. There have been isolated cases of extrapyramidal symptoms in breast-fed children. If the use of Haldol is essential, the benefits of breast feeding should be balanced against its potential risks.

4.7 Effects on ability to drive and use machines

Some degree of sedation or impairment of alertness may occur, particularly with higher doses and at the start of treatment, and may be potentiated by alcohol or other CNS depressants. Patients should be advised not to undertake activities requiring alertness such as driving or operating machinery during treatment, until their susceptibility is known.

4.8 Undesirable effects

The data provided below covers all haloperidol formulations including the Haldol Decanoate formulations.

The safety of Haldol was evaluated in 284 haloperidol-treated subjects who participated in 3 placebo-controlled, and in 1295 haloperidol-treated subjects who participated in sixteen double-blind active comparator-controlled clinical trials. The safety of Haldol decanoate was evaluated in 410 subjects who participated in 3 comparator trials (one comparing haloperidol vs. fluphenazine and two comparing the decanoate formulation to the oral formulation), 9 open label trials and 1 dose responsive trial. Based on pooled safety data from these clinical trials, the most commonly reported (% incidence) Adverse Drug Reactions (ADRs) were: Extrapyramidal disorder (34), Insomnia (19), Agitation (15), Hyperkinesia (13), Headache (12), Psychotic disorder (9), Depression (8), Weight increased (8), Orthostatic hypotension (7) and Somnolence (5).

Including the above mentioned ADRs, the following ADRs have been observed from clinical trials and post-marketing experiences reported with the use of Haldol and Haldol Decanoate. Frequencies displayed use the following convention:

Very common (≥ 1/10); common (≥ 1/100 to < 1/10); uncommon (≥ 1/1,000 to < 1/100); rare (≥ 1/10,000 to <1/1,000); very rare (<1/10,000), not known (cannot be estimated form the available data).

(see Table 1 on previous page)

Additional Information

Cardiac effects such as QT-interval prolongation, torsade de pointes, ventricular arrhythmias, including ventricular fibrillation and ventricular tachycardia), and cardiac arrest have been reported. These effects may occur more frequently with high doses, and in predisposed patients

Toxic epidermal necrolysis and Stevens-Johnson syndrome have been reported in patients taking haloperidol. The true incidence of these reports in not known.

4.9 Overdose

Symptoms

In general, the manifestations of haloperidol overdosage are an extension of its pharmacological actions, the most prominent of which would be severe extrapyramidal symptoms, hypotension and psychic indifference with a transition to sleep. The risk of ventricular arrhythmias possibly associated with QT-prolongation should be considered.

The patient may appear comatose with respiratory depression and hypotension which could be severe enough to produce a shock-like state. Paradoxically hypertension rather than hypotension may occur. Convulsions may also occur.

Treatment

There is no specific antidote to haloperidol. A patent airway should be established and maintained with mechanically assisted ventilation if necessary. In view of isolated reports of arrhythmia ECG monitoring is strongly advised. Hypotension and circulatory collapse should be treated by plasma volume expansion and other appropriate measures. Adrenaline should not be used. The patient should be monitored carefully for 24 hours or longer, body temperature and adequate fluid intake should be maintained.

In cases of severe extrapyramidal symptoms, appropriate anti-Parkinsonian medication should be administered.

5. PHARMACOLOGICAL PROPERTIES

5.1 Pharmacodynamic properties

Haloperidol acts as a central and peripheral dopamine receptor antagonist. It also has some anticholinergic activity and binds to opiate receptors.

5.2 Pharmacokinetic properties

Pharmacotherapeutic group: Butyrophenone Derivatives: ATC code: NP5A DO1

Haloperidol is rapidly absorbed after oral administration with a bioavailability of 44-74% (mean 60%) after tablets. Variable bioavailability is likely due to inter-individual differences in gastro-intestinal absorption and extent of first-pass hepatic metabolism.

Distribution is rapid to extravascular tissue, haloperidol crosses the blood-brain barrier and is excreted in human breast milk.

Metabolism is by oxidative dealkylation. The elimination half-life is approximately 20 hours, with considerable diurnal variation.

5.3 Preclinical safety data

No relevant information additional to that contained elsewhere in the Summary of Product Characteristics.

6. PHARMACEUTICAL PARTICULARS

6.1 List of excipients

Calcium hydrogen phosphate dihydrate

Maize starch

Calcium stearate

Quinoline yellow (E104)

Purified water*

* not present in final product.

6.2 Incompatibilities

Not applicable.

6.3 Shelf life

60 months

6.4 Special precautions for storage

Do not store above 25°C.

Keep out of reach and sight of children.

6.5 Nature and contents of container

Blister packs of aluminium foil and polyvinylchloride genotherm glass clear.

or

* Bottles of polystyrene and stopper of low density polyethylene.

The strips are packed in cardboard cartons containing 84* or 100 tablets per pack.

* Not marketed.

6.6 Special precautions for disposal and other handling

None.

7. MARKETING AUTHORISATION HOLDER

Janssen-Cilag Ltd

50-100 Holmers Farm Way

High Wycombe

Buckinghamshire

HP12 4EG

UK

8. MARKETING AUTHORISATION NUMBER(S)

PL 0242/0039R

9. DATE OF FIRST AUTHORISATION/RENEWAL OF THE AUTHORISATION

17 June 1986/04 February 2002

10. DATE OF REVISION OF THE TEXT

06 August 2009

Legal category POM.

Haldol 2mg/ml oral liquid

(Janssen-Cilag Ltd)

1. NAME OF THE MEDICINAL PRODUCT

HALDOL 2 mg/ml oral liquid

2. QUALITATIVE AND QUANTITATIVE COMPOSITION

Each ml of liquid contains haloperidol 2mg

3. PHARMACEUTICAL FORM

Oral solution

For excipients, see 6.1.

4. CLINICAL PARTICULARS

4.1 Therapeutic indications

Adults:

- Schizophrenia: treatment of symptoms and prevention of relapse
- Other psychoses: especially paranoid
- Mania and hypomania
- Mental or behavioural problems such as aggression, hyperactivity and self mutilation in the mentally retarded and in patients with organic brain damage
- As an adjunct to short term management of moderate to severe psychomotor agitation, excitement, violent or dangerously impulsive behaviour
- Intractable hiccup
- Gilles de la Tourette syndrome and severe tics

Children:

- Childhood behavioural disorders, especially when associated with hyperactivity and aggression
- Gilles de la Tourette syndrome
- Childhood schizophrenia.

4.2 Posology and method of administration

For oral administration.

Since this product is not intended for administration in multiples of 5 ml, the quantities given are expressed per ml.

Dosage for all indications should be individually determined and is best initiated and titrated under close clinical supervision. To determine the initial dose, consideration should be given to the patient's age, severity of symptoms and previous response to other neuroleptic drugs.

Patients who are elderly or debilitated or those with previously reported adverse reactions to neuroleptic drugs may require less Haldol. The normal starting dose should be halved, followed by a gradual titration to achieve optimal response.

Haldol liquid should be used at the minimum dose that is clinically effective.

Adults:

Schizophrenia, psychoses, mania and hypomania, mental or behavioural problems, psychomotor agitation, excitement, violent or dangerously impulsive behaviour, organic brain damage

Initial dose:

Moderate symptomatology 1.5-3.0 mg bd or tds

Severe symptomatology/resistant patients 3.0-5.0mg bd or tds

The same starting doses may be employed in adolescents and resitant schizophrenics who may require up to 30 mg/day.

Maintenance dosage:

Once satisfactory control of symptoms has been achieved, dosage should be gradually reduced to the lowest effective maintenance dose, often as low as 5 or 10 mg/day. Too rapid a dosage reduction should be avoided.

Restlessness or agitation in the elderly

Initial dose 1.5-3.0 mg bd or tds. Titrated as required, to attain an effective maintenance dose(1.5 – 30mg daily).

Gilles de la Tourette syndrome, severe tics, intractable hiccup

Starting dose 1.5 mg tds adjusted according to response. A daily maintenance dose of 10 mg may be required in Gilles de la Tourette syndrome.

Children:

Childhood behavioural disorders/schizophrenia

Total daily maintenance dose of 0.025-0.05 mg/kg/day. Half the dose should be given in the morning and the other half in the evening, up to a maximum of 10 mg daily.

Gilles de la Tourette syndrome

Oral maintenance doses of up to 10 mg/day in most patients.

4.3 Contraindications

Comatose states, CNS depression, Parkinson's disease, known hypersensitivity to haloperidol, lesions of basal ganglia.

In common with other neuroleptics, haloperidol has the potential to cause rare prolongation of the QT interval. Use of haloperidol is therefore contra-indicated in patients with clinically significant cardiac disorders e.g. recent acute myocardial infarction, uncompensated heart failure, arrhythmias treated with class IA and III antiarrhythmic medicinal products, QTc interval prolongation, history of ventricular arrhythmia or torsades de pointes clinically significant bradycardia, second or third degree heart block and uncorrected hypokalaemia. Haloperidol should not be used concomitantly with other QT prolonging drugs (see section 4.5, Interactions)

4.4 Special warnings and precautions for use

Cases of sudden death have been reported in psychiatric patients receiving antipsychotic drugs, including haloperidol.

Elderly patients with dementia-related psychosis treated with antipsychotic drugs are at an increased risk of death. Analyses of seventeen placebo-controlled trials (modal duration of 10 weeks), largely in patients taking atypical antipsychotic drugs, revealed a risk of death in drug-treated patients of between 1.6 to 1.7 times the risk of death in placebo-treated patients. Over the course of a typical 10 week controlled trial, the rate of death in drug-treated patients was about 4.5%, compared to a rate of about 2.6% in the placebo group. Although the causes of death were varied, most of the deaths appeared to be either cardiovascular (e.g., heart failure, sudden death) or infectious (e.g., pneumonia) in nature. Observational studies suggest that, similar to atypical antipsychotic drugs, treatment with conventional antipsychotic drugs may increase mortality. The extent to which the findings of increased mortality in observational studies may be attributed to the antipsychotic drug as opposed to some characteristic(s) of the patients is not clear.

Cardiovascular effects

Very rare reports of QT prolongation and/or ventricular arrhythmias, in addition to rare reports of sudden death, have been reported with haloperidol. They may occur more frequently with high doses and in predisposed patients.

The risk-benefit of haloperidol treatment should be fully assessed before treatment is commenced and patients with risk factors for ventricular arrhythmias such as cardiac disease, family history of sudden death and/or QT prolongation; uncorrected electrolyte disturbances; subarachnoid haemorrhage, starvation or alcohol abuse should be monitored carefully (ECGs and potassium levels), particularly during the initial phase of treatment to obtain steady plasma levels. The risk of QT prolongation and/or ventricular arrhythmias may be increased with higher doses (see Sections 4.8 and 4.9) or with parenteral use, particularly intravenous administration. ECG monitoring should be performed for QT interval prolongation and for serious cardiac dysrhythmias if Haldol is administered intravenously.

Haloperidol should be used with caution in patients known to be slow metabolisers of CYP2D6, and during use of cytochrome P450 inhibitors. Concomitant use of antipsychotics should be avoided. (See Section 4.5)

Baseline ECG is recommended prior to treatment in all patients, especially in the elderly and patients with a positive personal or family history of cardiac disease or abnormal findings on cardiac clinical examination. During therapy, the need for ECG monitoring (e.g. at dose escalation) should be assessed on an individual basis. Whilst on therapy, the dose should be reduced if QT is prolonged, and haloperidol should be discontinued if the QTc exceeds 500 ms.

Periodic electrolyte monitoring is recommended, especially for patients taking diuretics, or during intercurrent illness.

An approximately 3-fold increase risk of cerebrovascular adverse events have been seen in randomised placebo controlled clinical trials in the dementia population with some atypical antipsychotics. The mechanism for this increased risk is not known. An increased risk cannot be excluded for other antipsychotics or other patient populations. Haloperidol should be used in caution in patients with risk factors for stroke.

Neuroleptic malignant syndrome

In common with other antipsychotic drugs, Haldol has been associated with neuroleptic malignant syndrome: a rare idiosyncratic response characterised by hyperthermia, generalised muscle rigidity, autonomic instability, altered consciousness. Hyperthermia is often an early sign of this syndrome. Antipsychotic treatment should be withdrawn immediately and appropriate supportive therapy and careful monitoring instituted.

Tardive dyskinesia

As with all antipsychotic agents, tardive dyskinesia may appear in some patients on long-term therapy or after drug discontinuation. The syndrome is mainly characterised by rhythmic involuntary movements of the tongue, face, mouth or jaw. The manifestations may be permanent in some patients. The syndrome may be masked when treatment is reinstituted, when the dosage is increased or when a switch is made to a different antipsychotic drug. Treatment should be discontinued as soon as possible.

Extrapyramidal symptoms

In common with all neuroleptics, extrapyramidal symptoms may occur, e.g. tremor, rigidity, hypersalivation, bradykinesia, akathisia, acute dystonia.

Antiparkinson drugs of the anticholinergic type may be prescribed as required, but should not be prescribed routinely as a preventive measure. If concomitant antiparkinson medication is required, it may have to be continued after stopping Haldol if its excretion is faster than that of Haldol in order to avoid the development or aggravation of extrapyramidal symptoms. The physician should keep in mind the possible increase in intraocular pressure when anticholinergic drugs, including antiparkinson agents, are administered concomitantly with Haldol.

Seizures/Convulsions

It has been reported that seizures can be triggered by Haldol. Caution is advised in patients suffering from epilepsy and in conditions predisposing to convulsions (e.g., alcohol withdrawal and brain damage).

Hepatobiliary concerns

As Haldol is metabolised by the liver, caution is advised in patients with liver disease. Isolated cases of liver function abnormalities or hepatitis, most often cholestatic, have been reported.

Endocrine system concerns

Thyroxin may facilitate Haldol toxicity. Antipsychotic therapy in patients with hyperthyroidism should be used only with great caution and must always be accompanied by therapy to achieve a euthyroid state.

Hormonal effects of antipsychotic neuroleptic drugs include hyperprolactinaemia, which may cause galactorrhoea, gynaecomastia and oligo- or amenorrhoea. Very rare cases of hypoglycaemia and of Syndrome of Inappropriate ADH Secretion have been reported.

Additional considerations

In schizophrenia, the response to antipsychotic drug treatment may be delayed. Also, if drugs are withdrawn, recurrence of symptoms may not become apparent for several weeks or months. Acute withdrawal symptoms including nausea, vomiting and insomnia have very rarely been described after abrupt cessation of high doses of antipsychotic drugs. Relapse may also occur and gradual withdrawal is advisable.

As with all antipsychotic agents, Haldol should not be used alone where depression is predominant. It may be combined with antidepressants to treat those conditions in which depression and psychosis coexist.

Caution is advised in patients with renal failure and phaeochromocytoma.

4.5 Interaction with other medicinal products and other forms of interaction

Concomitant use of haloperidol with drugs known to prolong the QT interval may increase the risk of ventricular arrhythmias, including torsade de pointes. Therefore concomitant use of these products is not recommended (see section 4.3-Contraindications).

Examples include certain antiarrhythmics, such as those of Class 1A (such as quinidine, disopyramide and procainamide) and class III (such as amiodarone, sotalol and dofetilide), certain antimicrobials (sparfloxacin, moxifloxacin, erythromycin IV), tricyclic antidepressants (such as amitriptyline), certain tetracyclic antidepressants (such as maprotiline), other neuroleptics (e.g. phenothiazines, pimozide and sertindole), certain antihistamines (such as terfenadine), cisapride, bretylium and certain antimalarials such as quinine and mefloquine. This list is not comprehensive.

Concurrent use of drugs causing electrolyte imbalance may increase the risk of ventricular arrhythmias and is not recommended (see section 4.4-Special Warnings and Precautions for Use). Diuretics, in particular those causing hypokalaemia, should be avoided but, if necessary, potassium-sparing diuretics are preferred.

Haloperidol is metabolised by several routes, including glucuronidation and the cytochrome P450 enzyme system (particularly CYP 3A4 or CYP 2D6). Inhibition of these routes of metabolism by another drug or a decrease in CYP 2D6 enzyme activity may result in increased haloperidol concentrations and an increased risk of adverse events, including QT-prolongation. In pharmacokinetic studies, mild to moderately increased haloperidol concentrations have been reported when haloperidol was given concomitantly with drugs characterised as substrates or inhibitors of CYP 3A4 or CYP 2D6 isozymes, such as, itraconazole, buspirone, venlafaxine, alprazolam, fluvoxamine, quinidine, fluoxetine, sertraline, chlorpromazine, and promethazine. A decrease in CYP2D6 enzyme activity may result in increased haloperidol concentrations. Increases in QTc and extrapyramidal symptoms have been observed when haloperidol was given with a combination of the metabolic inhibitors ketoconazole (400 mg/day) and paroxetine (20 mg/day). It may be necessary to reduce the haloperidol dosage.

Effect of Other Drugs on Haloperidol

When prolonged treatment with enzyme-inducing drugs such as carbamazepine, phenobarbital, rifampicin is added to Haldol therapy, this results in a significant reduction of haloperidol plasma levels. Therefore, during combination treatment, the Haldol dose should be adjusted, when necessary. After stopping such drugs, it may be necessary to reduce the dosage of Haldol.

Sodium valproate, a drug known to inhibit glucuronidation, does not affect haloperidol plasma concentrations.

Effect of Haloperidol on Other Drugs

In common with all neuroleptics, Haldol can increase the central nervous system depression produced by other CNS-depressant drugs, including alcohol, hypnotics, sedatives or strong analgesics. An enhanced CNS effect, when combined with methyldopa, has also been reported.

Haldol may antagonise the action of adrenaline and other sympathomimetic agents and reverse the blood-pressure-lowering effects of adrenergic-blocking agents such as guanethidine.

Haldol may impair the antiparkinson effects of levodopa.

Haloperidol is an inhibitor of CYP 2D6. Haldol inhibits the metabolism of tricyclic antidepressants, thereby increasing plasma levels of these drugs.

Other Forms of Interaction

In rare cases, an encephalopathy-like syndrome has been reported in combination with lithium and haloperidol. It remains controversial whether these cases represent a distinct clinical entity or whether they are in fact cases of NMS and/or lithium toxicity. Signs of encephalopathy-like syndrome include confusion, disorientation, headache, disturbances of balance and drowsiness. One report showing symptomless EEG abnormalities on the combination has suggested that EEG monitoring might be advisable. When lithium and haloperidol therapy are used concomitantly, haloperidol should be given in the lowest effective dose and lithium levels should be monitored and kept below 1 mmol/l. If symptoms of encephalopathy-like syndrome occur, therapy should be stopped immediately.

Antagonism of the effect of the anticoagulant phenindione has been reported.

The dosage of anticonvulsants may need to be increased to take account of the lowered seizure threshold.

4.6 Pregnancy and lactation

The safety of haloperidol in pregnancy has not been established. There is some evidence of harmful effects in some but not all animal studies. There have been a number of reports of birth defects following foetal exposure to haloperidol for which a causal role for haloperidol cannot be excluded. Reversible extrapyramidal symptoms have been observed in neonates exposed to haloperidol in utero during the last trimester of pregnancy. Haldol should be used during pregnancy only if the anticipated benefit outweighs the risk and the administered dose and duration of treatment should be as low and as short as possible.

Haloperidol is excreted in breast milk. There have been isolated cases of extrapyramidal symptoms in breast-fed children. If the use of Haldol is essential, the benefits of breast feeding should be balanced against its potential risks.

4.7 Effects on ability to drive and use machines

Some degree of sedation or impairment of alertness may occur, particularly with higher doses and at the start of treatment, and may be potentiated by alcohol or other CNS depressants. Patients should be advised not to undertake activities requiring alertness such as driving or operating machinery during treatment, until their susceptibility is known.

4.8 Undesirable effects

The data provided below covers all haloperidol formulations including the Haldol Decanoate formulations.

The safety of Haldol was evaluated in 284 haloperidol-treated subjects who participated in 3 placebo-controlled, and in 1295 haloperidol-treated subjects who participated in sixteen double-blind active comparator-controlled clinical trials. The safety of Haldol decanoate was evaluated in 410 subjects who participated in 3 comparator trials (one comparing haloperidol vs. fluphenazine and two comparing the decanoate formulation to the oral formulation), 9 open label trials and 1 dose responsive trial. Based on pooled safety data from these clinical trials, the most commonly reported (% incidence) Adverse Drug Reactions (ADRs) were: Extrapyramidal disorder (34), Insomnia (19), Agitation (15), Hyperkinesia (13), Headache (12), Psychotic disorder (9), Depression (8), Weight increased (8), Orthostatic hypotension (7) and Somnolence (5).

Including the above mentioned ADRs, the following ADRs have been observed from clinical trials and post-marketing experiences reported with the use of Haldol and Haldol decanoate. Frequencies displayed use the following convention:

Very common ($\geqslant$ 1/10); common ($\geqslant$ 1/100 to < 1/10); uncommon ($\geqslant$ 1/1,000 to < 1/100); rare ($\geqslant$ 1/10,000 to <1/1,000); very rare (<1/10,000), not known (cannot be estimated from the available data).

(see Table 1 on next page)

Additional Information

Cardiac effects such as QT-interval prolongation, torsade de pointes, ventricular arrhythmias, including ventricular fibrillation and ventricular tachycardia), and cardiac arrest have been reported. These effects may occur more frequently with high doses, and in predisposed patients.

Toxic epidermal necrolysis and Stevens-Johnson syndrome have been reported in patients taking haloperidol. The true incidence of these reports is not known.

4.9 Overdose

Symptoms:

In general, the manifestations of haloperidol overdosage are an extension of its pharmacological actions. The most prominent of which would be severe extrapyramidal symptoms, hypotension and psychic indifference with a transition to sleep. The risk of ventricular arrhythmias possibly associated with QT-prolongation should be considered. The patient may appear comatose with respiratory depression and hypotension which could be severe enough to

Table 1 Very common (≥ 1/10); common (≥ 1/100 to < 1/10); uncommon (≥ 1/1,000 to < 1/100); rare (≥ 1/10,000 to < 1/1,000); very rare (< 1/10,000), not known (cannot be estimated from the available data)

System Organ Class	Adverse Drug Reactions				
	Frequency Category				
	Very Common (≥ 1/10)	Common (≥ 1/100 to < 1/10)	Uncommon (≥ 1/1,000 to < 1/100)	Rare (≥ 1/10,000 to < 1/1,000)	Not Known
Blood and lymphatic System Disorders			Leukopenia		Agranulocytosis; Neutropenia; Pancytopenia; Thrombocytopenia
Immune System Disorders			Hypersensitivity		Anaphylactic reaction
Endocrine Disorders				Hyperprolactinaemia	Inappropriate antidiuretic hormone secretion
Metabolic and Nutritional Disorders					Hypoglycaemia
Psychiatric Disorders	Agitation; Insomnia	Depression; Psychotic disorder	Confusional state; Libido Decreased; Loss of libido; Restlessness		
Nervous System Disorders	Extrapyramidal disorder; Hyperkinesia; Headache	Tardive dyskinesia; Oculogyric Crisis; Dystonia; Dyskinesia; Akathisia; Bradykinesia; Hypokinesia; Hypertonia; Somnolence; Masked Facies, Tremor; Dizziness	Convulsion; Parkinsonism; Akinesia; Cogwheel rigidity; Sedation; Muscle Contractions Involuntary	Motor dysfunction; Neuroleptic malignant syndrome; Nystagmus;	
Eye Disorders		Visual disturbance;	Vision blurred		
Cardiac Disorders			Tachycardia		Ventricular Fibrillation; Torsade de pointes; Ventricular Tachycardia; Extrasystoles
Vascular Disorders		Orthostatic Hypotension; Hypotension			
Respiratory, thoracic and mediastinal Disorders			Dyspnoea	Bronchospasm	Laryngeal Oedema; Laryngospasm
Gastrointestinal Disorders		Constipation; Dry mouth; Salivary hypersecretion; Nausea; Vomiting			
Hepatobiliary Disorders		Liver function test abnormal	Hepatitis; Jaundice		Acute Hepatic Failure; Cholestasis
Skin and subcutaneous tissue disorders		Rash	Photosensitivity Reaction; Urticaria; Pruritis; Hyperhidrosis		Leukocytoclastic Vasculitis; Dermatitis Exfoliative
Musculoskeletal and Connective Tissue Disorders			Torticollis; Muscle rigidity; Muscle Spasms; Musculoskeletal stiffness	Trismus; Muscle Twitching	
Renal and Urinary Disorders		Urinary retention			
Reproductive System and Breast Disorders		Erectile dysfunction	Amenorrhoea; Dysmenorrhoea; Galactorrhoea; Breast Discomfort; Breast Pain;	Menorrhagia; Menstrual Disorder; Sexual Dysfunction	Gynaecomastia, Priapism
General Disorders and Administration Site Conditions			Gait disturbance; Hyperthermia; Oedema		Sudden Death; Face Oedema; Hypothermia
Investigations		Weight increased; Weight decreased		Electrocardiogram QT prolonged	

produce a shock-like state. Paradoxically hypertension rather than hypotension may occur. Convulsions may also occur.

Treatment:

There is no specific antidote to haloperidol. A patent airway should be established and maintained with mechanically assisted ventilation if necessary. In view of isolated reports of arrhythmia ECG monitoring is strongly advised. Hypotension and circulatory collapse should be treated by plasma volume expansion and other appropriate measures. Adrenaline should not be used. The patient should be monitored carefully for 24 hours or longer, body temperature and adequate fluid intake should be maintained.

In cases of severe extrapyramidal symptoms, appropriate anti-Parkinson medication should be administered.

5. PHARMACOLOGICAL PROPERTIES

5.1 Pharmacodynamic properties

Haloperidol acts as a central dopamine receptor antagonist. It also has some anticholinergic activity and binds to opiate receptors. It also acts at peripheral dopamine receptors.

5.2 Pharmacokinetic properties

Haloperidol is absorbed rapidly with a bioavailability of 38-86% (mean 58%) after oral solution. Variable bioavailability is likely to be due to interindividual differences in gastro-intestinal absorption and extent of first-pass metabolism.

Haloperidol is rapidly distributed to extravascular tissues especially liver and adipose tissue. It is approximately 92% bound to plasma proteins.

Haloperidol is extensively metabolised by oxidative dealkylation and ultimately conjugated with glycine. Half-life is approximately 20 hours.

5.3 Preclinical safety data

No relevant information other than that contained elsewhere in the Summary of Product Characteristics.

6. PHARMACEUTICAL PARTICULARS

6.1 List of excipients

Lactic acid

Methyl parahydroxybenzoate

Purified water

6.2 Incompatibilities

None known.

6.3 Shelf life

5 years.

6.4 Special precautions for storage

Do not store above 25°C.

Do not refrigerate or freeze

6.5 Nature and contents of container

Bottle:

Amber glass (Type III, Ph.Eur); 100 ml

Closure:

Aluminium screw-cap, tamper resistant, coated on the inner side with polyvinylchloride.

OR

Child resistant, polypropylene screw-cap with low density polyethylene insert.

Dosing Device:

A blunt ended 2.5ml plastic dosing pipette with minor graduations of 0.25ml

6.6 Special precautions for disposal and other handling

Fig. 1: The 100 ml amber glass bottle comes with a child-resistant cap, and should be opened as follows:

- Push the plastic screw cap down while turning it counter clockwise.
- Remove the unscrewed cap.

Fig. 2: Insert the pipette into the bottle.

While holding the bottom ring, pull the top ring up to the mark that corresponds to the number of millilitres or milligrams you need to give.

Fig. 3: Holding the bottom ring, remove the entire pipette from the bottle.

Empty the pipette into a cup by sliding the upper ring down and drink it immediately.

Close the bottle.

Rinse the pipette with some water for future use.

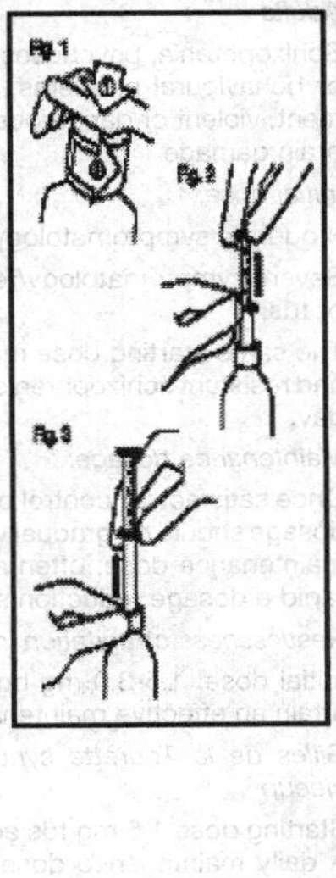

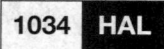

7. MARKETING AUTHORISATION HOLDER

Janssen-Cilag Limited
50-100 Holmers Farm Way
High Wycombe
Buckinghamshire
HP12 4EG
UK

8. MARKETING AUTHORISATION NUMBER(S)

PL 00242/0035R

9. DATE OF FIRST AUTHORISATION/RENEWAL OF THE AUTHORISATION

7 June 1989/30 March 2005

10. DATE OF REVISION OF THE TEXT

06 August 2009

Legal category POM

Haldol 5mg Tablets

(Janssen-Cilag Ltd)

1. NAME OF THE MEDICINAL PRODUCT

HALDOL Tablets 5 mg

2. QUALITATIVE AND QUANTITATIVE COMPOSITION

Haloperidol 5 mg.

3. PHARMACEUTICAL FORM

Tablets.

4. CLINICAL PARTICULARS

4.1 Therapeutic indications

Adults:

- Schizophrenia: treatment of symptoms and prevention of relapse
- Other psychoses: especially paranoid
- Mania and hypomania
- Mental or behavioural problems such as aggression, hyperactivity and self mutilation in the mentally retarded and in patients with organic brain damage
- As an adjunct to short term management of moderate to severe psychomotor agitation, excitement, violent or dangerously impulsive behaviour
- Intractable hiccup
- Restlessness and agitation in the elderly
- Gilles de la Tourette syndrome and severe tics.

Children:

- Childhood behavioural disorders, especially when associated with hyperactivity and aggression
- Gilles de la Tourette syndrome
- Childhood schizophrenia

4.2 Posology and method of administration

For oral administration.

Dosage for all indications should be individually determined and is best initiated and titrated under close clinical supervision. To determine initial dose, consideration should be given to the patient's age, severity of symptoms and previous response to neuroleptic drugs.

Patients who are elderly or debilitated or those with previously reported adverse reactions to neuroleptic drugs may require less Haldol. The normal starting dose should be halved, followed by a gradual titration to achieve optimal response.

Haldol should be used at the minimum dose that is clinically effective.

Adults

Schizophrenia, psychoses, mania and hypomania, mental or behavioural problems, psychomotor agitation, excitement, violent or dangerously impulsive behaviour, organic brain damage

Initial dose:

Moderate symptomatology: 1.5-3.0 mg bd or tds.

Severe symptomatology/resistant patients: 3.0-5.0 mg bd or tds.

The same starting dose may be employed in adolescents and resistant schizophrenics who may require up to 30 mg/day.

Maintenance dosage:

Once satisfactory control of symptoms has been achieved dosage should be gradually reduced to the lowest effective maintenance dose, often as low as 5 or 10 mg/day. Too rapid a dosage reduction should be avoided.

Restlessness or agitation in the elderly

Initial dose: 1.5-3.0 mg bd or tds titrated as required, to attain an effective maintenance dose (1.5-30 mg daily).

Gilles de la Tourette syndrome, severe tics, intractable hiccup

Starting dose 1.5 mg tds adjusted according to response. A daily maintenance dose of 10 mg may be required in Gilles de la Tourette syndrome.

Children

Childhood Behavioural Disorders and Schizophrenia

Total daily maintenance dose of 0.025-0.05 mg/kg/day. Half the total dose should be given in the morning and the other half in the evening, up to a maximum of 10 mg daily.

Gilles de la Tourette syndrome

Oral maintenance doses up to 10 mg/day in most patients.

4.3 Contraindications

Comatose states, CNS depression, Parkinson's disease, known hypersensitivity to haloperidol, lesions of basal ganglia.

In common with other neuroleptics, haloperidol has the potential to cause rare prolongation of the QT interval. Use of haloperidol is therefore contra-indicated in patients with clinically significant cardiac disorders e.g. recent acute myocardial infarction, uncompensated heart failure, arrhythmias treated with class IA and III antiarrhythmic medicinal products, QTc interval prolongation, history of ventricular arrhythmia or torsades de pointes clinically significant bradycardia, second or third degree heart block and uncorrected hypokalaemia. Haloperidol should not be used concomitantly with other QT prolonging drugs (see section 4.5, Interactions)

4.4 Special warnings and precautions for use

Cases of sudden death have been reported in psychiatric patients receiving antipsychotic drugs, including haloperidol.

Elderly patients with dementia-related psychosis treated with antipsychotic drugs are at an increased risk of death. Analyses of seventeen placebo-controlled trials (modal duration of 10 weeks), largely in patients taking atypical antipsychotic drugs, revealed a risk of death in drug-treated patients of between 1.6 to 1.7 times the risk of death in placebo-treated patients. Over the course of a typical 10 week controlled trial, the rate of death in drug-treated patients was about 4.5%, compared to a rate of about 2.6% in the placebo group. Although the causes of death were varied, most of the deaths appeared to be either cardiovascular (e.g., heart failure, sudden death) or infectious (e.g., pneumonia) in nature. Observational studies suggest that, similar to atypical antipsychotic drugs, treatment with conventional antipsychotic drugs may increase mortality. The extent to which the findings of increased mortality in observational studies may be attributed to the antipsychotic drug as opposed to some characteristic(s) of the patients is not clear.

Cardiovascular effects

Very rare reports of QT prolongation and/or ventricular arrhythmias, in addition to rare reports of sudden death, have been reported with haloperidol. They may occur more frequently with high doses and in predisposed patients.

The risk-benefit of haloperidol treatment should be fully assessed before treatment is commenced and patients with risk factors for ventricular arrhythmias such as cardiac disease, family history of sudden death and/or QT prolongation; uncorrected electrolyte disturbances, subarachnoid haemorrhage, starvation or alcohol abuse, should be monitored carefully (ECGs and potassium levels), particularly during the initial phase of treatment, to obtain steady plasma levels. The risk of QT prolongation and/or ventricular arrhythmias may be increased with higher doses (see Sections 4.8 and 4.9) or with parenteral use, particularly intravenous administration. ECG monitoring should be performed for QT interval prolongation and for serious cardiac dysrhythmias if Haldol is administered intravenously.

Haloperidol should be used with caution in patients known to be slow metabolisers of CYP2D6, and during use of cytochrome P450 inhibitors. Concomitant use of antipsychotics should be avoided. (See Section 4.5)

Baseline ECG is recommended prior to treatment in all patients, especially in the elderly and patients with a positive personal or family history of cardiac disease or abnormal findings on cardiac clinical examination. During therapy, the need for ECG monitoring (e.g. at dose escalation) should be assessed on an individual basis. Whilst on therapy, the dose should be reduced if QT is prolonged, and haloperidol should be discontinued if the QTc exceeds 500 ms.

Periodic electrolyte monitoring is recommended, especially for patients taking diuretics, or during intercurrent illness.

An approximately 3-fold increase risk of cerebrovascular adverse events have been seen in randomised placebo controlled clinical trials in the dementia population with some atypical antipsychotics. The mechanism for this increased risk is not known. An increased risk cannot be excluded for other antipsychotics or other patient populations. Haloperidol should be used in caution in patients with risk factors for stroke.

Neuroleptic malignant syndrome

In common with other antipsychotic drugs, Haldol has been associated with neuroleptic malignant syndrome: a rare idiosyncratic response characterised by hyperthermia, generalised muscle rigidity, autonomic instability, altered consciousness. Hyperthermia is often an early sign of this syndrome. Antipsychotic treatment should be withdrawn immediately and appropriate supportive therapy and careful monitoring instituted.

Tardive dyskinesia

As with all antipsychotic agents, tardive dyskinesia may appear in some patients on long-term therapy or after drug discontinuation. The syndrome is mainly characterised by rhythmic involuntary movements of the tongue, face, mouth or jaw. The manifestations may be permanent in some patients. The syndrome may be masked when treatment is reinstituted, when the dosage is increased or when a switch is made to a different antipsychotic drug. Treatment should be discontinued as soon as possible.

Extrapyramidal symptoms

In common with all neuroleptics, extrapyramidal symptoms may occur, e.g. tremor, rigidity, hypersalivation, bradykinesia, akathisia, acute dystonia.

Antiparkinson drugs of the anticholinergic type may be prescribed as required, but should not be prescribed routinely as a preventive measure. If concomitant antiparkinson medication is required, it may have to be continued after stopping Haldol if its excretion is faster than that of Haldol in order to avoid the development or aggravation of extrapyramidal symptoms. The physician should keep in mind the possible increase in intraocular pressure when anticholinergic drugs, including antiparkinson agents, are administered concomitantly with Haldol.

Seizures/Convulsions

It has been reported that seizures can be triggered by Haldol. Caution is advised in patients suffering from epilepsy and in conditions predisposing to convulsions (e.g., alcohol withdrawal and brain damage).

Hepatobiliary concerns

As Haldol is metabolised by the liver, caution is advised in patients with liver disease. Isolated cases of liver function abnormalities or hepatitis, most often cholestatic, have been reported.

Endocrine system concerns

Thyroxin may facilitate Haldol toxicity. Antipsychotic therapy in patients with hyperthyroidism should be used only with great caution and must always be accompanied by therapy to achieve a euthyroid state.

Hormonal effects of antipsychotic neuroleptic drugs include hyperprolactinaemia, which may cause galactorrhoea, gynaecomastia and oligo- or amenorrhoea. Very rare cases of hypoglycaemia and of Syndrome of Inappropriate ADH Secretion have been reported.

Additional considerations

In schizophrenia, the response to antipsychotic drug treatment may be delayed. Also, if drugs are withdrawn, recurrence of symptoms may not become apparent for several weeks or months.

Acute withdrawal symptoms including nausea, vomiting and insomnia have very rarely been described after abrupt cessation of high doses of anti-psychotic drugs. Relapse may also occur and gradual withdrawal is advisable.

As with all antipsychotic agents, Haldol should not be used alone where depression is predominant. It may be combined with antidepressants to treat those conditions in which depression and psychosis coexist.

Caution is advised in patients with renal failure and phaeochromocytoma.

4.5 Interaction with other medicinal products and other forms of interaction

Concomitant use of haloperidol with drugs known to prolong the QT interval may increase the risk of ventricular arrhythmias, including torsade de pointes. Therefore concomitant use of these products is not recommended (see section 4.3-Contraindications).

Examples include certain antiarrhythmics, such as those of Class 1A (such as quinidine, disopyramide and procainamide) and class III (such as amiodarone, sotalol and dofetilide), certain antimicrobials (sparfloxacin, moxifloxacin, erythromycin IV), tricyclic antidepressants (such as amitriptyline), certain tetracyclic antidepressants (such as maprotiline), other neuroleptics (e.g. phenothiazines, pimozide and sertindole), certain antihistamines (such as terfenadine), cisapride, bretylium and certain antimalarials such as quinine and mefloquine. This list is not comprehensive.

Concurrent use of drugs causing electrolyte imbalance may increase the risk of ventricular arrhythmias and is not recommended (see section 4.4-Special Warnings and Precautions for Use). Diuretics, in particular those causing hypokalaemia, should be avoided but, if necessary, potassium-sparing diuretics are preferred.

Haloperidol is metabolised by several routes, including glucuronidation and the cytochrome P450 enzyme system (particularly CYP 3A4 or CYP 2D6). Inhibition of these routes of metabolism by another drug or a decrease in CYP 2D6 enzyme activity may result in increased haloperidol concentrations and an increased risk of adverse events, including QT-prolongation. In pharmacokinetic studies, mild to moderately increased haloperidol concentrations have been reported when haloperidol was given concomitantly with drugs characterised as substrates or inhibitors of CYP 3A4 or CYP 2D6 isozymes, such as, itraconazole, buspirone, venlafaxine, alprazolam, fluvoxamine, quinidine, fluoxetine, sertraline, chlorpromazine, and promethazine. A decrease in CYP2D6 enzyme activity may result in increased haloperidol concentrations. Increases in

Table 1 Very common (⩾ 1/10); common (⩾ 1/100 to < 1/10); uncommon (⩾ 1/1,000 to < 1/100); rare (⩾ 1/10,000 to < 1/1,000); very rare (< 1/10,000), not known (cannot be estimated form the available data)

System Organ Class	Adverse Drug Reactions				
	Frequency Category				
	Very Common (⩾ 1/10)	Common (⩾ 1/100 to < 1/10)	Uncommon (⩾ 1/1,000 to < 1/100)	Rare (⩾ 1/10,000 to < 1/1,000)	Not Known
Blood and lymphatic System Disorders			Leukopenia		Agranulocytosis; Neutropenia; Pancytopenia; Thrombocytopenia
Immune System Disorders			Hypersensitivity		Anaphylactic reaction
Endocrine Disorders				Hyperprolactinaemia	Inappropriate antidiuretic hormone secretion
Metabolic and Nutritional Disorders					Hypoglycaemia
Psychiatric Disorders	Agitation; Insomnia	Depression; Psychotic disorder	Confusional state; Libido Decreased; Loss of libido; Restlessness		
Nervous System Disorders	Extrapyramidal disorder; Hyperkinesia; Headache	Tardive dyskinesia; Oculogyric Crisis; Dystonia; Dyskinesia; Akathisia; Bradykinesia; Hypokinesia; Hypertonia; Somnolence; Masked Facies, Tremor; Dizziness	Convulsion; Parkinsonism; Akinesia; Cogwheel rigidity; Sedation; Muscle Contractions Involuntary	Motor dysfunction; Neuroleptic malignant syndrome; Nystagmus	
Eye Disorders		Visual disturbance;	Vision blurred		
Cardiac Disorders			Tachycardia		Ventricular Fibrillation; Torsade de pointes; Ventricular Tachycardia; Extrasystoles
Vascular Disorders		Orthostatic Hypotension; Hypotension			
Respiratory, thoracic and mediastinal Disorders			Dyspnoea	Bronchospasm	Laryngeal Oedema; Laryngospasm
Gastrointestinal Disorders		Constipation; Dry mouth; Salivary hypersecretion; Nausea; Vomiting			
Hepatobiliary Disorders		Liver function test abnormal	Hepatitis; Jaundice		Acute Hepatic Failure; Cholestasis
Skin and subcutaneous tissue disorders		Rash	Photosensitivity Reaction; Urticaria; Pruritis; Hyperhidrosis		Leukocytoclastic Vasculitis; Dermatitis Exfoliative
Musculoskeletal and Connective Tissue Disorders			Torticollis; Muscle rigidity; Muscle Spasms; Musculoskeletal stiffness	Trismus; Muscle Twitching	
Renal and Urinary Disorders		Urinary retention			
Reproductive System and Breast Disorders		Erectile dysfunction	Amenorrhoea; Dysmenorrhoea; Galactorrhoea; Breast Discomfort; Breast Pain;	Menorrhagia; Menstrual Disorder; Sexual Dysfunction	Gynaecomastia, Priapism
General Disorders and Administration Site Conditions			Gait disturbance; Hyperthermia; Oedema		Sudden Death; Face Oedema; Hypothermia
Investigations		Weight increased; Weight decreased		Electrocardiogram QT prolonged	

QTc and extrapyramidal symptoms have been observed when haloperidol was given with a combination of the metabolic inhibitors ketoconazole (400 mg/day) and paroxetine (20 mg/day). It may be necessary to reduce the haloperidol dosage.

Effect of Other Drugs on Haloperidol

When prolonged treatment with enzyme-inducing drugs such as carbamazepine, phenobarbital, rifampicin is added to Haldol therapy, this results in a significant reduction of haloperidol plasma levels. Therefore, during combination treatment, the Haldol dose should be adjusted, when necessary. After stopping such drugs, it may be necessary to reduce the dosage of Haldol.

Sodium valproate, a drug known to inhibit glucuronidation, does not affect haloperidol plasma concentrations.

Effect of Haloperidol on Other Drugs

In common with all neuroleptics, Haldol can increase the central nervous system depression produced by other CNS-depressant drugs, including alcohol, hypnotics, sedatives or strong analgesics. An enhanced CNS effect, when combined with methyldopa, has also been reported.

Haldol may antagonise the action of adrenaline and other sympathomimetic agents and reverse the blood-pressure-lowering effects of adrenergic-blocking agents such as guanethidine.

Haldol may impair the antiparkinson effects of levodopa.

Haloperidol is an inhibitor of CYP 2D6. Haldol inhibits the metabolism of tricyclic antidepressants, thereby increasing plasma levels of these drugs.

Other Forms of Interaction

In rare cases, an encephalopathy-like syndrome has been reported in combination with lithium and haloperidol. It remains controversial whether these cases represent a distinct clinical entity or whether they are in fact cases of NMS and/or lithium toxicity. Signs of encephalopathy-like syndrome include confusion, disorientation, headache, disturbances of balance and drowsiness. One report showing symptomless EEG abnormalities on the combination has suggested that EEG monitoring might be advisable. When lithium and haloperidol therapy are used concomitantly, haloperidol should be given in the lowest effective dose and lithium levels should be monitored and kept below 1 mmol/l. If symptoms of encephalopathy-like syndrome occur, therapy should be stopped immediately.

Antagonism of the effect of the anticoagulant phenindione has been reported.

The dosage of anticonvulsants may need to be increased to take account of the lowered seizure threshold.

4.6 Pregnancy and lactation

The safety of haloperidol in pregnancy has not been established. There is some evidence of harmful effects in some, but not all animal studies. There have been a number of reports of birth defects following foetal exposure to haloperidol for which a causal role for haloperidol cannot be excluded. Reversible extrapyramidal symptoms have been observed in neonates exposed to haloperidol in utero during the last trimester of pregnancy. Haldol should be used during pregnancy only if the anticipated benefit outweighs the risk and the administered dose and duration of treatment should be as low and as short as possible.

Haloperidol is excreted in breast milk. There have been isolated cases of extrapyramidal symptoms in breast-fed children. If the use of Haldol is essential, the benefits of breast feeding should be balanced against its potential risks.

4.7 Effects on ability to drive and use machines

Some degree of sedation or impairment of alertness may occur, particularly with higher doses and at the start of treatment, and may be potentiated by alcohol or other CNS depressants. Patients should be advised not to undertake activities requiring alertness such as driving or operating machinery during treatment, until their susceptibility is known.

4.8 Undesirable effects

The data provided below covers all haloperidol formulations including the Haldol Decanoate formulations.

The safety of Haldol was evaluated in 284 haloperidol-treated subjects who participated in 3 placebo-controlled, and in 1295 haloperidol-treated subjects who participated in sixteen double-blind active comparator-controlled clinical trials. The safety of Haldol decanoate was evaluated in 410 subjects who participated in 3 comparator trials (one comparing haloperidol vs. fluphenazine and two comparing the decanoate formulation to the oral formulation), 9 open label trials and 1 dose responsive trial. Based on pooled safety data from these clinical trials, the most commonly reported (% incidence) Adverse Drug Reactions (ADRs) were: Extrapyramidal disorder (34), Insomnia (19), Agitation (15), Hyperkinesia (13), Headache (12), Psychotic disorder (9), Depression (8), Weight increased (8), Orthostatic hypotension (7) and Somnolence (5).

Including the above mentioned ADRs, the following ADRs have been observed from clinical trials and post-marketing experiences reported with the use of Haldol and Haldol Decanoate. Frequencies displayed use the following convention:

Very common (⩾ 1/10); common (⩾ 1/100 to < 1/10); uncommon (⩾ 1/1,000 to < 1/100); rare (⩾ 1/10,000 to

<1/1,000); very rare (<1/10,000), not known (cannot be estimated form the available data).

(see Table 1 on previous page)

Additional Information

Cardiac effects such as QT-interval prolongation, torsade de pointes, ventricular arrhythmias, including ventricular fibrillation and ventricular tachycardia), and cardiac arrest have been reported. These effects may occur more frequently with high doses, and in predisposed patients.

Toxic epidermal necrolysis and Stevens-Johnson syndrome have been reported in patients taking haloperidol. The true incidence of these reports is not known.

4.9 Overdose
Symptoms

In general, the manifestations of haloperidol overdosage are an extension of its pharmacological actions, the most prominent of which would be severe extrapyramidal symptoms, hypotension and psychic indifference with a transition to sleep. The risk of ventricular arrhythmias possibly associated with QT-prolongation should be considered. The patient may appear comatose with respiratory depression and hypotension which could be severe enough to produce a shock-like state. Paradoxically hypertension rather than hypotension may occur. Convulsions may also occur.

Treatment

There is no specific antidote to haloperidol. A patent airway should be established and maintained with mechanically assisted ventilation if necessary. In view of isolated reports of arrhythmia ECG monitoring is strongly advised. Hypotension and circulatory collapse should be treated by plasma volume expansion and other appropriate measures. Adrenaline should not be used. The patient should be monitored carefully for 24 hours or longer, body temperature and adequate fluid intake should be maintained.

In cases of severe extrapyramidal symptoms, appropriate anti-Parkinsonian medication should be administered.

5. PHARMACOLOGICAL PROPERTIES

5.1 Pharmacodynamic properties

Haloperidol acts as a central and peripheral dopamine receptor antagonist. It also has some anticholinergic activity and binds to opiate receptors.

5.2 Pharmacokinetic properties

Pharmacotherapeutic group: Butyrophenone Derivatives: ATC code: NO5A DO1

Haloperidol is rapidly absorbed after oral administration with a bioavailability of 44-74% (mean 60%) after tablets. Variable bioavailability is likely due to inter-individual differences in gastro-intestinal absorption and extent of first-pass hepatic metabolism.

Distribution is rapid to extravascular tissue, haloperidol crosses the blood-brain barrier and is excreted in human breast milk.

Metabolism is by oxidative dealkylation. The elimination half-life is approximately 20 hours, with considerable diurnal variation.

5.3 Preclinical safety data

No relevant information additional to that contained elsewhere in the Summary of Product Characteristics.

6. PHARMACEUTICAL PARTICULARS

6.1 List of excipients

Lactose monohydrate

Maize starch

Talc

Cottonseed oil - hydrogenated

Indigotindisulphonate sodium (E132)

Purified water*

* not present in final product.

6.2 Incompatibilities

None.

6.3 Shelf life

60 months.

6.4 Special precautions for storage

Do not store above 25°C.

Keep out of reach and sight of children.

6.5 Nature and contents of container

Blister packs of aluminium foil and polyvinylchloride genotherm glass clear.

or

*Bottles of polystyrene (white) and stoppers of low density polyethylene.

or

*Bottles of white polypropylene and stoppers of low density polyethylene.

The strips are packed in cardboard cartons containing 100 tablets per pack.

* Not marketed

6.6 Special precautions for disposal and other handling

None.

7. MARKETING AUTHORISATION HOLDER

Janssen-Cilag Ltd

50-100 Holmers Farm Way

High Wycombe

Buckinghamshire

HP12 4EG

UK

8. MARKETING AUTHORISATION NUMBER(S)

00242/0031R

9. DATE OF FIRST AUTHORISATION/RENEWAL OF THE AUTHORISATION

Date of First Authorisation: 20 June 1986

Date of Renewal of Authorisation: 11 January 2003

10. DATE OF REVISION OF THE TEXT

06 August 2009

Legal category POM

Haldol Decanoate

(Janssen-Cilag Ltd)

1. NAME OF THE MEDICINAL PRODUCT

HALDOL® decanoate 50 mg/ml

HALDOL® decanoate 100 mg/ml

2. QUALITATIVE AND QUANTITATIVE COMPOSITION

HALDOL® decanoate 50 mg/ml

Haloperidol decanoate 70.52 mg, equivalent to 50 mg haloperidol base, per millilitre.

HALDOL® decanoate 100 mg/ml

Haloperidol decanoate 141.04 mg, equivalent to 100 mg haloperidol base, per millilitre.

3. PHARMACEUTICAL FORM

Straw-coloured viscous solution for intramuscular injection.

4. CLINICAL PARTICULARS

4.1 Therapeutic indications

Haldol decanoate is indicated for long term maintenance treatment where a neuroleptic is required; for example in schizophrenia, other psychoses (especially paranoid), and other mental or behavioural problems where maintenance treatment is clearly indicated.

4.2 Posology and method of administration

By intramuscular administration.

Haldol decanoate is for use in adults only and has been formulated to provide one month's therapy for most patients following a single deep intramuscular injection in the gluteal region. Haldol decanoate should not be administered intravenously.

Since individual response to neuroleptic drugs is variable, dosage should be individually determined and is best initiated and titrated under close clinical supervision.

The size of the initial dose will depend on both the severity of the symptomatology and the amount of oral medication required to maintain the patient before starting depot treatment. Haldol decanoate injection should be used at the minimum dose that is clinically effective.

An initial dose of 50 mg every four weeks is recommended, increasing if necessary by 50 mg increments to 300 mg every four weeks. If, for clinical reasons, two-weekly administration is preferred, these doses should be halved.

In patients with severe symptomatology, or in those who require large oral doses as maintenance therapy, higher doses of Haldol decanoate will be required. However, clinical experience with Haldol decanoate at doses greater than 300 mg per month is limited.

Routine administration of volumes greater than 3 mls at any one injection site is not recommended as larger volumes of injection are uncomfortable for the patient.

Haldol decanoate should be administered by deep intramuscular injection using an appropriate needle, preferably 2-2.5 inches long, of at least 21 gauge. Local reactions and medication oozing from the injection site may be reduced by the use of a good injection technique, eg the 'Z-track' method. As with all oily injections, it is important to ensure, by aspiration before injection, that intravenous entry has not occurred.

For patients previously maintained on oral neuroleptics, an approximate guide to the starting dose of Haldol decanoate is as follows: 500 mg of chlorpromazine a day is equivalent to 100 mg of Haldol decanoate monthly.

The approximate equivalence for transferring patients previously maintained on fluphenazine decanoate or flupenthixol decanoate is as follows: 25 mg of fluphenazine decanoate 2-weekly or 40 mg of flupenthixol decanoate 2-weekly is equivalent to 100 mg of Haldol decanoate monthly. This dose should be adjusted to suit the individual patient's response.

Use in elderly:

It is recommended to start with low doses, for example 12.5 mg - 25 mg every four weeks, only increasing the dose according to the individual patient's response.

4.3 Contraindications

Comatose states, CNS depression, Parkinson's disease, known hypersensitivity to haloperidol, lesions of basal ganglia.

In common with other neuroleptics, haloperidol has the potential to cause rare prolongation of the QT interval. Use of haloperidol is therefore contra-indicated in patients with clinically significant cardiac disorders e.g. recent acute myocardial infarction, uncompensated heart failure, arrhythmias treated with class IA and III antiarrhythmic medicinal products, QTc interval prolongation, history of ventricular arrhythmia or Torsades de pointes clinically significant bradycardia, second or third degree heart block and uncorrected hypokalaemia. Haloperidol should not be used concomitantly with other QT prolonging drugs (see section 4.5, Interactions).

4.4 Special warnings and precautions for use

Cases of sudden death have been reported in psychiatric patients receiving antipsychotic drugs, including haloperidol.

Elderly patients with dementia-related psychosis treated with antipsychotic drugs are at an increased risk of death. Analyses of seventeen placebo-controlled trials (modal duration of 10 weeks), largely in patients taking atypical antipsychotic drugs, revealed a risk of death in drug-treated patients of between 1.6 to 1.7 times the risk of death in placebo-treated patients. Over the course of a typical 10 week controlled trial, the rate of death in drug-treated patients was about 4.5%, compared to a rate of about 2.6% in the placebo group. Although the causes of death were varied, most of the deaths appeared to be either cardiovascular (e.g., heart failure, sudden death) or infectious (e.g., pneumonia) in nature. Observational studies suggest that, similar to atypical antipsychotic drugs, treatment with conventional antipsychotic drugs may increase mortality. The extent to which the findings of increased mortality in observational studies may be attributed to the antipsychotic drug as opposed to some characteristic(s) of the patients is not clear.

Cardiovascular effects

Very rare reports of QT prolongation and/or ventricular arrhythmias, in addition to rare reports of sudden death, have been reported with haloperidol. They may occur more frequently with high doses and in predisposed patients.

The risk-benefit of haloperidol treatment should be fully assessed before treatment is commenced and patients with risk factors for ventricular arrhythmias such as cardiac disease, family history of sudden death and/or QT prolongation, uncorrected electrolyte disturbances, subarachnoid haemorrhage, starvation or alcohol abuse, should be monitored carefully (ECGs and potassium levels), particularly during the initial phase of treatment, to obtain steady plasma levels.

The risk of QT prolongation and/or ventricular arrhythmias may be increased with higher doses (see Sections 4.8, and 4.9) or with parenteral use, particularly intravenous administration. Haldol Decanoate should not be administered intravenously.

Haloperidol should be used with caution in patients known to be slow metabolisers of CYP2D6, and during use of cytochrome P450 inhibitors. Concomitant use of antipsychotics should be avoided. (See Section 4.5)

Baseline ECG is recommended prior to treatment in all patients, especially in the elderly and patients with a positive personal or family history of cardiac disease or abnormal findings on cardiac clinical examination. During therapy, the need for ECG monitoring (e.g. at dose escalation) should be assessed on an individual basis. Whilst on therapy, the dose should be reduced if QT is prolonged, and haloperidol should be discontinued if the QTc exceeds 500 ms.

Periodic electrolyte monitoring is recommended, especially for patients taking diuretics, or during intercurrent illness.

An approximately 3-fold increase risk of cerebrovascular adverse events have been seen in randomised placebo controlled clinical trials in the dementia population with some atypical antipsychotics. The mechanism for this increased risk is not known. An increased risk cannot be excluded for other antipsychotics or other patient populations. Haloperidol should be used in caution in patients with risk factors for stroke.

Neuroleptic malignant syndrome

In common with other antipsychotic drugs, Haldol Decanoate has been associated with neuroleptic malignant syndrome: a rare idiosyncratic response characterised by hyperthermia, generalised muscle rigidity, autonomic instability, altered consciousness. Hyperthermia is often an early sign of this syndrome. Antipsychotic treatment should be withdrawn immediately and appropriate supportive therapy and careful monitoring instituted.

Tardive dyskinesia

As with all antipsychotic agents, tardive dyskinesia may appear in some patients on long-term therapy or after drug discontinuation. The syndrome is mainly characterised by rhythmic involuntary movements of the tongue, face, mouth or jaw. The manifestations may be permanent in some patients. The syndrome may be masked when treatment is reinstituted, when the dosage is increased or when

Table 1 Very common (≥ 1/10); common (≥ 1/100 to < 1/10); uncommon (≥ 1/1,000 to < 1/100); rare (≥ 1/10,000 to <1/1,000); very rare (<1/10,000), not known (cannot be estimated form the available data)

System Organ Class	Adverse Drug Reactions				
	Frequency Category				
	Very Common (≥ 1/10)	Common (≥ 1/100 to < 1/10)	Uncommon (≥ 1/1,000 to < 1/100)	Rare (≥ 1/10,000 to <1/1,000)	Not Known
Blood and lymphatic System Disorders			Leukopenia		Agranulocytosis; Neutropenia; Pancytopenia; Thrombocytopenia
Immune System Disorders			Hypersensitivity		Anaphylactic reaction
Endocrine Disorders				Hyperprolactinaemia	Inappropriate Antidiuretic Hormone Secretion
Metabolic and Nutritional Disorders					Hypoglycaemia
Psychiatric Disorders	Agitation; Insomnia	Depression; Psychotic Disorder	Confusional State; Libido Decreased; Loss of Libido; Restlessness		
Nervous System Disorders	Extrapyramidal Disorder; Hyperkinesia; Headache	Tardive dyskinesia; Oculogyric Crisis; Dystonia; Dyskinesia; Akathisia; Bradykinesia; Hypokinesia; Hypertonia; Masked Facies; Somnolence; Tremor; Dizziness;	Convulsion; Parkinsonism; Akinesia; Cogwheel Rigidity; Muscle Contractions Involuntary; Sedation	Neuroleptic Malignant Syndrome; Motor Dysfunction; Nystagmus;	
Eye Disorders		Visual Disturbance;	Vision Blurred		
Cardiac Disorders			Tachycardia		Ventricular fibrillation; Torsade de pointes; Ventricular tachycardia; Extrasystoles
Vascular Disorders		Orthostatic Hypotension; Hypotension			
Respiratory, thoracic and mediastinal Disorders			Dyspnoea	Bronchospasm	Laryngeal Oedema; Laryngospasm
Gastro-intestinal Disorders		Constipation; Dry Mouth; Salivary Hypersecretion; Nausea; Vomiting			
Hepatobiliary Disorders		Liver function test abnormal	Hepatitis; Jaundice		Acute Hepatic Failure; Cholestasis
Skin and subcutaneous tissue disorders		Rash	Photosensitivity reaction; Urticaria; Pruritis; Hyperhidrosis		Leukocytoclastic Vasculitis; Dermatitis exfoliative
Musculoskeletal and Connective Tissue Disorders			Torticollis; Muscle rigidity; Muscle Spasms; Musculoskeletal stiffness	Trismus; Muscle Twitching	
Renal and Urinary Disorders		Urinary Retention			
Reproductive System and Breast Disorders		Erectile Dysfunction	Amenorrhoea; Dysmenorrhoea; Galactorrhoea; Breast pain; Breast discomfort	Menorrhagia; Menstrual Disorder; Sexual Dysfunction	Gynaecomastia, Priapism
General Disorders and Administration Site Conditions		Injection Site Reaction	Gait Disturbance; Hyperthermia; Oedema		Sudden Death; Face Oedema; Hypothermia
Investigations		Weight Increased; Weight Decreased		Electrocardiogram QT Prolonged	

a switch is made to a different antipsychotic drug. Treatment should be discontinued as soon as possible.

Extrapyramidal symptoms

In common with all neuroleptics, extrapyramidal symptoms may occur, e.g. tremor, rigidity, hypersalivation, bradykinesia, akathisia, acute dystonia.

Antiparkinson drugs of the anticholinergic type may be prescribed as required, but should not be prescribed routinely as a preventive measure. If concomitant antiparkinson medication is required, it may have to be continued after stopping Haldol Decanoate if its excretion is faster than that of Haldol in order to avoid the development or aggravation of extrapyramidal symptoms. The physician should keep in mind the possible increase in intraocular pressure when anticholinergic drugs, including antiparkinson agents, are administered concomitantly with Haldol Decanoate.

Seizures/Convulsions

It has been reported that seizures can be triggered by Haldol Decanoate. Caution is advised in patients suffering from epilepsy and in conditions predisposing to convulsions (e.g., alcohol withdrawal and brain damage).

Hepatobiliary concerns

As Haldol Decanoate is metabolised by the liver, caution is advised in patients with liver disease. Isolated cases of liver function abnormalities or hepatitis, most often cholestatic, have been reported.

Endocrine system concerns

Thyroxine may facilitate Haldol Decanoate toxicity. Therefore, it should only be used with great caution in patients with hyperthyroidism. Antipsychotic therapy in those patients with hyperthyroidism should be used only with great caution and must always be accompanied by therapy to achieve a euthyroid state.

Hormonal effects of antipsychotic neuroleptic drugs include hyperprolactinaemia, which may cause galactorrhoea, gynaecomastia and oligo- or amenorrhoea. Very rare cases of hypoglycaemia and of Syndrome of Inappropriate ADH Secretion have been reported.

Additional considerations

It is recommended that patients being considered for Haldol Decanoate therapy be initially put on oral haloperidol to exclude the possibility of an unexpected adverse sensitivity to haloperidol.

As with all antipsychotic agents, Haldol Decanoate should not be used alone where depression is predominant. It may be combined with antidepressants to treat those conditions in which depression and psychosis coexist. Haloperidol may impair the metabolism of tricyclic antidepressants (clinical significance unknown).

In schizophrenia, the response to antipsychotic drug treatment may be delayed. If drugs are withdrawn, recurrence of symptoms may not become apparent for several weeks or months.

Caution is advised in patients with renal failure and phaeochromocytoma.

4.5 Interaction with other medicinal products and other forms of interaction

Concomitant use of haloperidol with drugs known to prolong the QT interval may increase the risk of ventricular arrhythmias, including torsade de pointes. Therefore concomitant use of these products is not recommended (see section 4.3-Contraindications).

Examples include certain antiarrhythmics, such as those of Class 1A (such as quinidine, disopyramide and procainamide) and class III (such as amiodarone, sotalol and dofetilide), certain antimicrobials (sparfloxacin, moxifloxacin, erythromycin IV), tricyclic antidepressants (such as amitriptyline), certain tetracyclic antidepressants (such as maprotiline), other neuroleptics (e.g. phenothiazines, pimozide and sertindole), certain antihistamines (such as terfenadine), cisapride, bretylium and certain antimalarials such as quinine and mefloquine. This list is not comprehensive.

Concurrent use of drugs causing electrolyte imbalance may increase the risk of ventricular arrhythmias and is not recommended (see section 4.4-Special Warnings and Precautions for Use). Diuretics, in particular those causing hypokalaemia, should be avoided but, if necessary, potassium-sparing diuretics are preferred.

Haloperidol is metabolised by several routes, including glucuronidation and the cytochrome P450 enzyme system (particularly CYP 3A4 or CYP 2D6). Inhibition of these routes of metabolism by another drug or a decrease in CYP 2D6 enzyme activity may result in increased haloperidol concentrations and an increased risk of adverse events, including QT-prolongation. In pharmacokinetic studies, mild to moderately increased haloperidol concentrations have been reported when haloperidol was given concomitantly with drugs characterised as substrates or inhibitors of CYP 3A4 or CYP 2D6 isozymes, such as, itraconazole, buspirone, venlafaxine, alprazolam, fluvoxamine, quinidine, fluoxetine, sertraline, chlorpromazine, and promethazine. A decrease in CYP2D6 enzyme activity may result in increased haloperidol concentrations. Increases in QTc and extrapyramidal symptoms have been observed when haloperidol was given with a combination of the metabolic inhibitors ketoconazole (400 mg/day) and paroxetine (20 mg/day). It may be necessary to reduce the haloperidol dosage.

Effect of Other Drugs on Haloperidol

When prolonged treatment with enzyme-inducing drugs such as carbamazepine, phenobarbital, rifampicin is added to Haldol Decanoate therapy, this results in a significant reduction of haloperidol plasma levels. Therefore, during combination treatment, the Haldol Decanoate dose or the dosage interval should be adjusted, when necessary. After stopping such drugs, it may be necessary to reduce the dosage of Haldol Decanoate.

Sodium valproate, a drug known to inhibit glucuronidation, does not affect haloperidol plasma concentrations.

Effect of Haloperidol on Other Drugs

In common with all neuroleptics, Haldol Decanoate can increase the central nervous system depression produced by other CNS-depressant drugs, including alcohol, hypnotics, sedatives or strong analgesics. An enhanced CNS effect, when combined with methyldopa, has been reported.

Haldol Decanoate may antagonise the action of adrenaline and other sympathomimetic agents and reverse the blood-pressure lowering effects of adrenergic blocking agents such as guanethidine.

Haldol Decanoate may impair the antiparkinsonian effects of levodopa.

Haloperidol is an inhibitor of CYP 2D6. Haldol Decanoate inhibits the metabolism of tricyclic antidepressants, thereby increasing plasma levels of these drugs.

Other Forms of Interaction

In rare cases, an encephalopathy-like syndrome has been reported in combination with lithium and Haldol decanoate. It remains controversial whether these cases represent a distinct clinical entity or whether they are in fact cases of NMS and/or lithium toxicity. Signs of encephalopathy-like syndrome include confusion, disorientation, headache, disturbances of balance and drowsiness. One report showing symptomless EEG abnormalities on the combination has suggested that EEG monitoring might be advisable. When lithium and haloperidol therapy are used concomitantly, haloperidol should be given in the lowest effective dosage and lithium levels should be monitored and kept below 1 mmol/l. If symptoms of encephalopathy-like syndrome occur, therapy should be stopped immediately

Antagonism of the effect of the anticoagulant phenindione has been reported.

The dosage of anticonvulsants may need to be increased to take account of the lowered seizure threshold.

4.6 Pregnancy and lactation

The safety of haloperidol in pregnancy has not been established. There is some evidence of harmful effects in some, but not all, animal studies. There have been a number of reports of birth defects following foetal exposure to haloperidol for which a causal role for haloperidol cannot be excluded. Reversible extrapyramidal symptoms have been observed in neonates exposed to haloperidol in utero during the last trimester of pregnancy. Haldol decanoate should be used during pregnancy only if the anticipated benefit outweighs the risk and the administered dose and duration of treatment should be as low and as short as possible.

Haloperidol is excreted in breast milk. There have been isolated cases of extrapyramidal symptoms in breast-fed children. If the use of Haldol decanoate is essential, the benefits of breast feeding should be balanced against its potential risks.

4.7 Effects on ability to drive and use machines

Some degree of sedation or impairment of alertness may occur, particularly with higher doses and at the start of treatment, and may be potentiated by alcohol or other CNS depressants. Patients should be advised not to undertake activities requiring alertness such as driving or operating machinery during treatment, until their susceptibility is known.

4.8 Undesirable effects

The safety of Haldol Decanoate was evaluated in 410 subjects who participated in 3 comparator trials (one comparing haloperidol vs. fluphenazine and two comparing the decanoate formulation to the oral formulation), 9 open label trials and 1 dose responsive trial. The safety of Haldol was evaluated in 284 haloperidol-treated subjects who participated in 3 placebo-controlled, and in 1295 haloperidol-treated subjects who participated in sixteen double-blind active comparator-controlled clinical trials. Based on pooled safety data from these clinical trials, the most commonly reported (% incidence) Adverse Drug Reactions (ADRs) were: Extrapyramidal disorder (34), Insomnia (19), Agitation (15), Hyperkinesia (13), Headache (12), Psychotic disorder (9), Depression (8), Weight increased (8), Orthostatic hypotension (7) and Somnolence (5).

Including the above mentioned ADRs, the following ADRs have been observed from clinical trials and post-marketing experiences reported with the use of Haldol and Haldol Decanoate. Frequencies displayed use the following convention: Very common (≥ 1/10); common (≥ 1/100 to < 1/10); uncommon (≥ 1/1,000 to < 1/100); rare (≥ 1/10,000 to <1/1,000); very rare (<1/10,000), not known (cannot be estimated form the available data).

(see Table 1 on previous page)

Additional Information

Cardiac effects such as QT-interval prolongation, torsade de pointes, ventricular arrhythmias, including ventricular fibrillation and ventricular tachycardia, and cardiac arrest, have been reported. These effects may occur more frequently with high doses, and in predisposed patients

Toxic epidermal necrolysis and Stevens-Johnson syndrome have been reported in patients taking haloperidol. The true incidence of these reports is not known

4.9 Overdose

Symptoms

In general, the manifestations of haloperidol overdosage are an extension of its pharmacological actions, the most prominent of which would be severe extrapyramidal symptoms, hypotension and psychic indifference with a transition to sleep. The risk of ventricular arrhythmias possibly associated with QT-prolongation should be considered. The patient may appear comatose with respiratory depression and hypotension which could be severe enough to produce a shock-like state. Paradoxically, hypertension rather than hypotension may occur. Convulsions may also occur.

Treatment

There is no specific antidote to haloperidol. A patent airway should be established and maintained with mechanically assisted ventilation if necessary. In view of isolated reports of arrhythmia, ECG monitoring is strongly advised. Hypotension and circulatory collapse should be treated by plasma volume expansion and other appropriate measures. Adrenaline should not be used. The patient should be monitored, body temperature and adequate fluid intake should be maintained.

In cases of severe extrapyramidal symptoms, appropriate anti-Parkinson medication should be administered.

5. PHARMACOLOGICAL PROPERTIES

5.1 Pharmacodynamic properties

Pharmacotherapeutic group: Butyrophenone Derivatives:

ATC Code: NO5A DO1

The antipsychotic activity of haloperidol is principally due to its central dopamine blocking activity.

It has some activity against noradrenaline and less against serotonin. There is only very minimal activity against histamine and acetylcholine receptors.

5.2 Pharmacokinetic properties

Haloperidol decanoate in solution is slowly released from the injection site and enters the systemic circulation, where it is hydrolysed by esterases to haloperidol. After an initial dose of 30-300 mg of haloperidol decanoate, plasma concentrations ranged from 0.8-3.2 ng/ml. After the second dose they were raised to 2.8 ng/ml which was steady state. A monthly dose of approximately 20 times the previous oral maintenance dose has been shown to be approximately clinically equivalent. Blood levels will vary considerably between patients.

5.3 Preclinical safety data

Only limited data are available, however these show no specific hazards apart from decreased fertility, limited teratogenicity as well as embryo-toxic effects in rodents.

Haloperidol has been shown to block the cardiac hERG channel in several published studies *in vitro*. In a number of *in vivo* studies intravenous administration of haloperidol in some animal models has caused significant QTc prolongation, at doses around 0.3 mg/kg i.v., giving C_{max} plasma levels 3 to 7 times higher than the effective human plasma concentrations of 4 to 20ng/ml These intravenous doses which prolonged QTc did not cause arrhythmias. In some studies higher intravenous doses of 1 to 5 mg/kg haloperidol i.v. caused QTc prolongation and/or ventricular arrhythmias at C_{max} plasma levels 19 to 68 times higher than the effective human plasma concentrations.

6. PHARMACEUTICAL PARTICULARS

6.1 List of excipients

Benzyl alcohol

Sesame oil

6.2 Incompatibilities

None known.

6.3 Shelf life

36 months.

6.4 Special precautions for storage

Do not store above 25°C.

Do not refrigerate or freeze.

Keep ampoule in the outer carton to protect from light.

Lengthy storage in the cold may produce precipitation; if this does not clear after further storage at room temperature, the contents of the ampoule should be discarded.

6.5 Nature and contents of container

1 ml amber glass ampoule, in packs containing 5 ampoules.

6.6 Special precautions for disposal and other handling

Before use warm the ampoule in the hands to aid withdrawal of the contents.

1. Hold the body of the ampoule between the thumb and the index finger with the spot facing you.

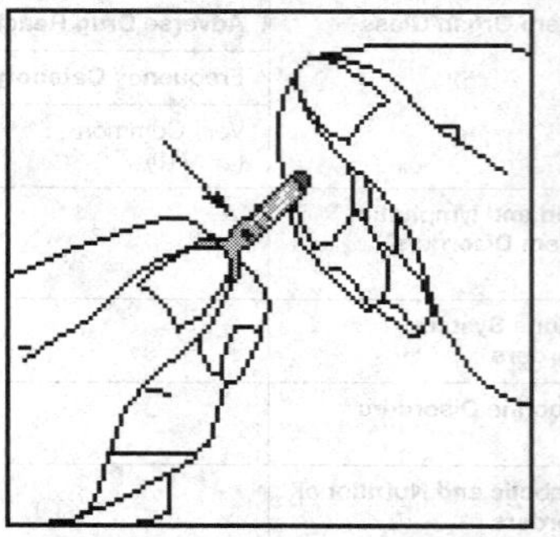

2. Position the index finger of the other hand so that it is supporting the neck of the ampoule. Position the thumb so that it covers the spot as shown below.

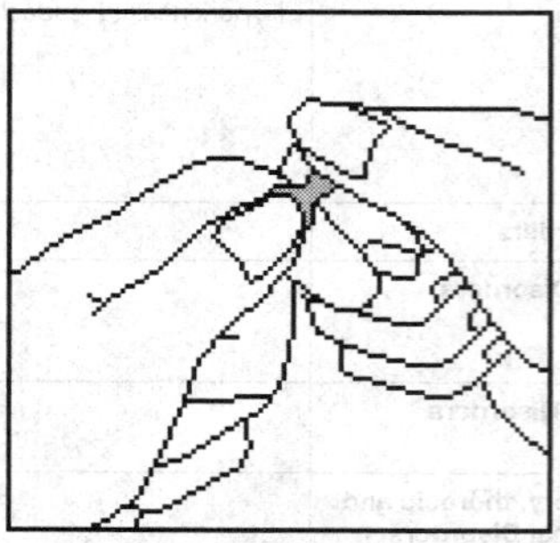

3. With the index fingers close together, apply firm downward pressure on the spot to snap the ampoule open.

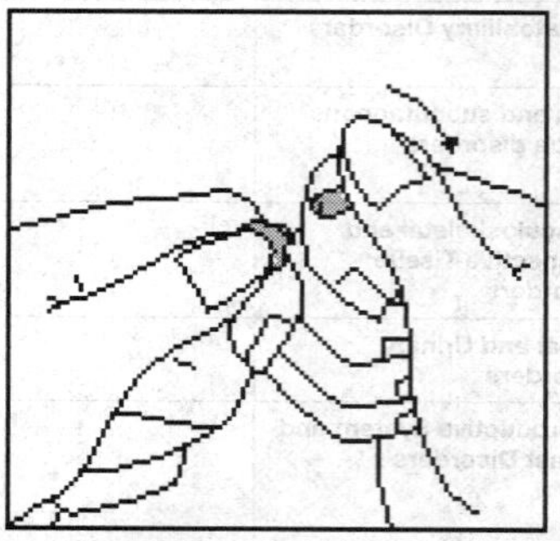

7. MARKETING AUTHORISATION HOLDER

Janssen-Cilag Ltd

50-100 Holmers Farm Way

High Wycombe

Bucks

HP12 4EG

UK

8. MARKETING AUTHORISATION NUMBER(S)

HALDOL DECANOATE 50 mg/ml: PL 0242/0094

HALDOL DECANOATE 100 mg/ml: PL 0242/0095

9. DATE OF FIRST AUTHORISATION/RENEWAL OF THE AUTHORISATION

Date of First Authorisation: 23 July 1982

Date of Renewal of Authorisation: 07 January 2003

10. DATE OF REVISION OF THE TEXT

06 August 2009

Legal category POM.

Haldol Injection

(Janssen-Cilag Ltd)

1. NAME OF THE MEDICINAL PRODUCT

HALDOL Injection

2. QUALITATIVE AND QUANTITATIVE COMPOSITION

Haloperidol 5 mg/ml

3. PHARMACEUTICAL FORM

Solution for injection

4. CLINICAL PARTICULARS

4.1 Therapeutic indications

Adults:

• Schizophrenia: treatment of symptoms and prevention of relapse.

- Other psychoses; especially paranoid.
- Mania and hypomania.
- Mental or behavioural problems such as aggression, hyperactivity and self-mutilation in the mentally retarded and in patients with organic brain damage.
- As an adjunct to short term management of moderate to severe psychomotor agitation, excitement, violent or dangerously impulsive behaviour.
- Nausea and vomiting.

4.2 Posology and method of administration

For intramuscular administration

Dosage for all indications should be individually determined and is best initiated and titrated under close clinical supervision. To determine the initial dose, consideration should be given to the patient's age, severity of symptoms and previous response to other neuroleptics.

Patients who are elderly or debilitated or those with previously reported adverse reactions to neuroleptic drugs may require less haloperidol. The normal starting dose should be halved, followed by a gradual titration to achieve optimal response.

Haldol injection should be used at the minimum dose that is clinically effective.

Adults:

Schizophrenia, psychoses, mania and hypomania, mental or behavioural problems, psychomotor agitation, excitement, violent or dangerously impulsive behaviour, organic brain damage:

For control of acutely agitated patients with moderate symptoms: 2-10 mg IM. Depending on the response of the patient, subsequent doses may be given every 4-8 hours, up to a maximum of 18 mg/day.

Infrequently, severely disturbed patients may require an initial dose of up to 18 mg.

Oral treatment should succeed intramuscular administration as soon as practicable. Bioavailability from the oral route is about 60% of that from the IM route, and readjustment of dose may be required.

Haldol can also be administered by the IV route.

Nausea and vomiting

1-2 mg IM

Children:

Not recommended for parenteral use in children.

4.3 Contraindications

Comatose states, CNS depression, Parkinson's disease, known hypersensitivity to haloperidol, lesions of basal ganglia.

In common with other neuroleptics, haloperidol has the potential to cause rare prolongation of the QT interval. Use of haloperidol is therefore contra-indicated in patients with clinically significant cardiac disorders e.g. recent acute myocardial infarction, uncompensated heart failure, arrhythmias treated with class IA and III antiarrhythmic medicinal products, QTc interval prolongation, history of ventricular arrhythmia or torsades de pointes clinically significant bradycardia, second or third degree heart block and uncorrected hypokalaemia. Haloperidol should not be used concomitantly with other QT prolonging drugs (see section 4.5, Interactions)

4.4 Special warnings and precautions for use

Cases of sudden death have been reported in psychiatric patients receiving antipsychotic drugs, including haloperidol.

Elderly patients with dementia-related psychosis treated with antipsychotic drugs are at an increased risk of death. Analyses of seventeen placebo-controlled trials (modal duration of 10 weeks), largely in patients taking atypical antipsychotic drugs, revealed a risk of death in drug-treated patients of between 1.6 to 1.7 times the risk of death in placebo-treated patients. Over the course of a typical 10 week controlled trial, the rate of death in drug-treated patients was about 4.5%, compared to a rate of about 2.6% in the placebo group. Although the causes of death were varied, most of the deaths appeared to be either cardiovascular (e.g., heart failure, sudden death) or infectious (e.g., pneumonia) in nature. Observational studies suggest that, similar to atypical antipsychotic drugs, treatment with conventional antipsychotic drugs may increase mortality. The extent to which the findings of increased mortality in observational studies may be attributed to the antipsychotic drug as opposed to some characteristic(s) of the patients is not clear.

Cardiovascular effects

Very rare reports of QT prolongation and/or ventricular arrhythmias, in addition to rare reports of sudden death, have been reported with haloperidol. They may occur more frequently with high doses and in predisposed patients.

The risk-benefit of haloperidol treatment should be fully assessed before treatment is commenced and patients with risk factors for ventricular arrhythmias such as cardiac disease; family history of sudden death and/or QT prolongation; uncorrected electrolyte disturbances; subarachnoid haemorrhage; starvation; or alcohol abuse should be monitored carefully (ECGs and potassium levels), particularly during the initial phase of treatment, to obtain steady plasma levels. The risk of QT prolongation and/or ventricular arrhythmias may be increased with higher doses (see Sections 4.8 and 4.9) or with parenteral use, particularly intravenous administration. ECG monitoring should be performed for QT interval prolongation and for serious cardiac dysrhythmias if Haldol is administered intravenously.

Haloperidol should be used with caution in patients known to be slow metabolisers of CYP2D6, and during use of cytochrome P450 inhibitors. Concomitant use of antipsychotics should be avoided. (See Section 4.5)

Baseline ECG is recommended prior to treatment in all patients, especially in the elderly and patients with a positive personal or family history of cardiac disease or abnormal findings on cardiac clinical examination. During therapy, the need for ECG monitoring (e.g. at dose escalation) should be assessed on an individual basis. Whilst on therapy, the dose should be reduced if QT is prolonged, and haloperidol should be discontinued if the QTc exceeds 500 ms.

Periodic electrolyte monitoring is recommended, especially for patients taking diuretics, or during intercurrent illness.

An approximately 3-fold increase risk of cerebrovascular adverse events have been seen in randomised placebo controlled clinical trials in the dementia population with some atypical antipsychotics. The mechanism for this increased risk is not known. An increased risk cannot be excluded for other antipsychotics or other patient populations. Haloperidol should be used in caution in patients with risk factors for stroke.

Neuroleptic malignant syndrome

In common with other antipsychotic drugs, Haldol has been associated with neuroleptic malignant syndrome: a rare idiosyncratic response characterised by hyperthermia, generalised muscle rigidity, autonomic instability, altered consciousness. Hyperthermia is often an early sign of this syndrome. Antipsychotic treatment should be withdrawn immediately and appropriate supportive therapy and careful monitoring instituted.

Tardive dyskinesia

As with all antipsychotic agents, tardive dyskinesia may appear in some patients on long-term therapy or after drug discontinuation. The syndrome is mainly characterised by rhythmic involuntary movements of the tongue, face, mouth or jaw. The manifestations may be permanent in some patients. The syndrome may be masked when treatment is reinstituted, when the dosage is increased or when a switch is made to a different antipsychotic drug. Treatment should be discontinued as soon as possible.

Extrapyramidal symptoms

In common with all neuroleptics, extrapyramidal symptoms may occur, e.g. tremor, rigidity, hypersalivation, bradykinesia, akathisia, acute dystonia.

Antiparkinson drugs of the anticholinergic type may be prescribed as required, but should not be prescribed routinely as a preventive measure. If concomitant antiparkinson medication is required, it may have to be continued after stopping Haldol if its excretion is faster than that of Haldol in order to avoid the development or aggravation of extrapyramidal symptoms. The physician should keep in mind the possible increase in intraocular pressure when anticholinergic drugs, including antiparkinson agents, are administered concomitantly with Haldol.

Seizures/Convulsions

It has been reported that seizures can be triggered by Haldol. Caution is advised in patients suffering from epilepsy and in conditions predisposing to convulsions (e.g., alcohol withdrawal and brain damage).

Hepatobiliary concerns

As Haldol is metabolised by the liver, caution is advised in patients with liver disease. Isolated cases of liver function abnormalities or hepatitis, most often cholestatic, have been reported.

Endocrine system concerns

Thyroxin may facilitate Haldol toxicity. Antipsychotic therapy in patients with hyperthyroidism should be used only with great caution and must always be accompanied by therapy to achieve a euthyroid state.

Hormonal effects of antipsychotic neuroleptic drugs include hyperprolactinaemia, which may cause galactorrhoea, gynaecomastia and oligo- or amenorrhoea. Very rare cases of hypoglycaemia and of Syndrome of Inappropriate ADH Secretion have been reported.

Additional considerations

In schizophrenia, the response to antipsychotic drug treatment may be delayed. Also, if drugs are withdrawn, recurrence of symptoms may not become apparent for several weeks or months. Acute withdrawal symptoms including nausea, vomiting and insomnia have very rarely been described after abrupt cessation of high doses of antipsychotic drugs. Relapse may also occur and gradual withdrawal is advisable.

As with all antipsychotic agents, Haldol should not be used alone where depression is predominant. It may be combined with antidepressants to treat those conditions in which depression and psychosis coexist.

Caution is advised in patients with renal failure and phaeochromocytoma.

4.5 Interaction with other medicinal products and other forms of interaction

Concomitant use of haloperidol with drugs known to prolong the QT interval may increase the risk of ventricular arrhythmias, including torsade de pointes. Therefore concomitant use of these products is not recommended (see section 4.3-Contraindications).

Examples include certain antiarrhythmics, such as those of Class 1A (such as quinidine, disopyramide and procainamide) and class III (such as amiodarone, sotalol and dofetilide), certain antimicrobials (sparfloxacin, moxifloxacin, erythromycin IV), tricyclic antidepressants (such as amitriptyline), certain tetracyclic antidepressants (such as maprotiline), other neuroleptics (e.g. phenothiazines, pimozide and sertindole), certain antihistamines (such as terfenadine), cisapride, bretylium and certain antimalarials such as quinine and mefloquine. This list is not comprehensive.

Concurrent use of drugs causing electrolyte imbalance may increase the risk of ventricular arrhythmias and is not recommended (see section 4.4-Special Warnings and Precautions for Use). Diuretics, in particular those causing hypokalaemia, should be avoided but, if necessary, potassium-sparing diuretics are preferred.

Haloperidol is metabolised by several routes, including glucuronidation and the cytochrome P450 enzyme system (particularly CYP 3A4 or CYP 2D6). Inhibition of these routes of metabolism by another drug or a decrease in CYP 2D6 enzyme activity may result in increased haloperidol concentrations and an increased risk of adverse events, including QT-prolongation. In pharmacokinetic studies, mild to moderately increased haloperidol concentrations have been reported when haloperidol was given concomitantly with drugs characterised as substrates or inhibitors of CYP 3A4 or CYP 2D6 isozymes, such as, itraconazole, buspirone, venlafaxine, alprazolam, fluvoxamine, quinidine, fluoxetine, sertraline, chlorpromazine, and promethazine. A decrease in CYP2D6 enzyme activity may result in increased haloperidol concentrations. Increases in QTc and extrapyramidal symptoms have been observed when haloperidol was given with a combination of the metabolic inhibitors ketoconazole (400 mg/day) and paroxetine (20 mg/day). It may be necessary to reduce the haloperidol dosage.

Effect of Other Drugs on Haloperidol

When prolonged treatment with enzyme-inducing drugs such as carbamazepine, phenobarbital, rifampicin is added to Haldol therapy, this results in a significant reduction of haloperidol plasma levels. Therefore, during combination treatment, the Haldol dose should be adjusted, when necessary. After stopping such drugs, it may be necessary to reduce the dosage of Haldol.

Sodium valproate, a drug known to inhibit glucuronidation, does not affect haloperidol plasma concentrations.

Effect of Haloperidol on Other Drugs

In common with all neuroleptics, Haldol can increase the central nervous system depression produced by other CNS-depressant drugs, including alcohol, hypnotics, sedatives or strong analgesics. An enhanced CNS effect, when combined with methyldopa, has also been reported.

Haldol may antagonise the action of adrenaline and other sympathomimetic agents and reverse the blood-pressure-lowering effects of adrenergic-blocking agents such as guanethidine.

Haldol may impair the antiparkinson effects of levodopa.

Haloperidol is an inhibitor of CYP 2D6. Haldol inhibits the metabolism of tricyclic antidepressants, thereby increasing plasma levels of these drugs.

Other Forms of Interaction

In rare cases, an encephalopathy-like syndrome has been reported in combination with lithium and haloperidol. It remains controversial whether these cases represent a distinct clinical entity or whether they are in fact cases of NMS and/or lithium toxicity. Signs of encephalopathy-like syndrome include confusion, disorientation, headache, disturbances of balance and drowsiness. One report showing symptomless EEG abnormalities on the combination has suggested that EEG monitoring might be advisable. When lithium and haloperidol therapy are used concomitantly, haloperidol should be given in the lowest effective dose and lithium levels should be monitored and kept below 1 mmol/l. If symptoms of encephalopathy-like syndrome occur, therapy should be stopped immediately.

Antagonism of the effect of the anticoagulant phenindione has been reported.

The dosage of anticonvulsants may need to be increased to take account of the lowered seizure threshold.

4.6 Pregnancy and lactation

The safety of haloperidol in pregnancy has not been established. There is some evidence of harmful effects in some but not all animal studies. There have been a number of reports of birth defects following foetal exposure to haloperidol for which a causal role for haloperidol cannot be excluded. Reversible extrapyramidal symptoms have been observed in neonates exposed to haloperidol in utero during the last trimester of pregnancy. Haldol should be used during pregnancy only if the anticipated benefit outweighs the risk and the administered dose and duration of treatment should be as low and as short as possible.

Table 1 Very common (⩾ 1/10); common (⩾ 1/100 to < 1/10); uncommon (⩾ 1/1,000 to < 1/100); rare (⩾ 1/10,000 to < 1/1,000); very rare (< 1/10,000), not known (cannot be estimated form the available data)

System Organ Class	Adverse Drug Reactions Frequency Category				
	Very Common (⩾ 1/10)	Common (⩾ 1/100 to < 1/10)	Uncommon (⩾ 1/1,000 to < 1/100)	Rare (⩾ 1/10,000 to < 1/1,000)	Not Known
Blood and lymphatic System Disorders			Leukopenia		Agranulocytosis; Neutropenia; Pancytopenia; Thrombocytopenia
Immune System Disorders			Hypersensitivity		Anaphylactic reaction
Endocrine Disorders				Hyperprolactinaemia	Inappropriate antidiuretic hormone secretion
Metabolic and Nutritional Disorders					Hypoglycaemia
Psychiatric Disorders	Agitation; Insomnia	Depression; Psychotic disorder	Confusional state; Libido Decreased; Loss of libido; Restlessness		
Nervous System Disorders	Extrapyramidal disorder; Hyperkinesia; Headache	Tardive dyskinesia; Oculogyric Crisis; Dystonia; Dyskinesia; Akathisia; Bradykinesia; Hypokinesia; Hypertonia; Somnolence; Masked Facies, Tremor; Dizziness	Convulsion; Parkinsonism; Akinesia; Cogwheel rigidity; Sedation; Muscle Contractions Involuntary	Motor dysfunction; Neuroleptic malignant syndrome; Nystagmus;	
Eye Disorders		Visual disturbance;	Vision blurred		
Cardiac Disorders			Tachycardia		Ventricular Fibrillation; Torsade de pointes; Ventricular Tachycardia; Extrasystoles
Vascular Disorders		Orthostatic Hypotension; Hypotension			
Respiratory, thoracic and mediastinal Disorders			Dyspnoea	Bronchospasm	Laryngeal Oedema; Laryngospasm
Gastrointestinal Disorders		Constipation; Dry mouth; Salivary hypersecretion; Nausea; Vomiting			
Hepatobiliary Disorders		Liver function test abnormal	Hepatitis; Jaundice		Acute Hepatic Failure; Cholestasis
Skin and subcutaneous tissue disorders		Rash	Photosensitivity Reaction; Urticaria; Pruritis; Hyperhidrosis		Leukocytoclastic Vasculitis; Dermatitis Exfoliative
Musculoskeletal and Connective Tissue Disorders			Torticollis; Muscle rigidity; Muscle Spasms; Musculoskeletal stiffness	Trismus; Muscle Twitching	
Renal and Urinary Disorders		Urinary retention			
Reproductive System and Breast Disorders		Erectile dysfunction	Amenorrhoea; Dysmenorrhoea; Galactorrhoea; Breast Discomfort; Breast Pain;	Menorrhagia; Menstrual Disorder; Sexual Dysfunction	Gynaecomastia, Priapism
General Disorders and Administration Site Conditions		Injection Site Reaction	Gait disturbance; Hyperthermia; Oedema		Sudden Death; Face Oedema; Hypothermia
Investigations		Weight increased; Weight decreased		Electrocardiogram QT prolonged	

Haloperidol is excreted in breast milk. There have been isolated cases of extrapyramidal symptoms in breast-fed children. If the use of Haldol is essential, the benefits of breast feeding should be balanced against its potential risks.

4.7 Effects on ability to drive and use machines

Some degree of sedation or impairment of alertness may occur, particularly with higher doses and at the start of treatment, and may be potentiated by alcohol or other CNS depressants. Patients should be advised not to undertake activities requiring alertness such as driving or operating machinery during treatment, until their susceptibility is known.

4.8 Undesirable effects

The data provided below covers all haloperidol formulations including the Haldol Decanoate formulations.

The safety of Haldol was evaluated in 284 haloperidol-treated subjects who participated in 3 placebo-controlled, and in 1295 haloperidol-treated subjects who participated in sixteen double-blind active comparator- controlled clinical trials. The safety of Haldol decanoate was evaluated in 410 subjects who participated in 3 comparator trials (one comparing haloperidol vs. fluphenazine and two comparing the decanoate formulation to the oral formulation), 9 open label trials and 1 dose responsive trial. Based on pooled safety data from these clinical trials, the most commonly reported (% incidence) Adverse Drug Reactions (ADRs) were: Extrapyramidal disorder (34), Insomnia (19), Agitation (15), Hyperkinesia (13), Headache (12), Psychotic disorder (9), Depression (8), Weight increased (8), Orthostatic hypotension (7) and Somnolence (5).

Including the above mentioned ADRs, the following ADRs have been observed from clinical trials and post-marketing experiences reported with the use of Haldol and Haldol decanoate. Frequencies displayed use the following convention:

Very common (⩾ 1/10); common (⩾ 1/100 to < 1/10); uncommon (⩾ 1/1,000 to < 1/100); rare (⩾ 1/10,000 to < 1/1,000); very rare (< 1/10,000), not known (cannot be estimated form the available data).

(see Table 1 above)

Additional Information

Cardiac effects such as QT-interval prolongation, torsade de pointes, ventricular arrhythmias, including ventricular fibrillation and ventricular tachycardia), and cardiac arrest have been reported. These effects may occur more frequently with high doses, and in predisposed patients.

Toxic epidermal necrolysis and Stevens-Johnson syndrome have been reported in patients taking haloperidol. The true incidence of these reports is not known.

4.9 Overdose

Symptoms: In general, the manifestations of haloperidol overdosage are an extension of its pharmacological actions, the most prominent of which would be severe extrapyramidal symptoms, hypotension and psychic indifference with a transition to sleep. The risk of ventricular arrhythmias possibly associated with QT-prolongation should be considered. The patient may appear comatose with respiratory depression and hypotension which could be severe enough to produce a shock-like state. Paradoxically hypertension rather than hypotension may occur. Convulsions may also occur.

Treatment: There is no specific antidote to haloperidol. A patent airway should be established and maintained with mechanically assisted ventilation if necessary. In view of isolated reports of arrhythmia, ECG monitoring is strongly advised. Hypotension and circulatory collapse should be treated by plasma volume expansion and other appropriate measures. Adrenaline should not be used. The patient should be monitored carefully for 24 hours or longer, body temperature and adequate fluid intake should be maintained.

In cases of severe extrapyramidal symptoms, appropriate anti-Parkinson medication should be administered.

5. PHARMACOLOGICAL PROPERTIES

5.1 Pharmacodynamic properties

Haloperidol is a central dopamine antagonist. It also has some anticholinergic properties and is an opiate receptor antagonist, and acts at peripheral dopamine receptors.

5.2 Pharmacokinetic properties

A 10 mg IV dose of haloperidol given over 2 mins produced a peak serum concentration of 34μg/ml at the end of infusion, declining to 1μg/ml by 40 hours. Following IM administration of 2 mg, peak plasma concentrations were similar to after oral ie. 10μg/ml but are reached within 20 minutes.

Haloperidol is rapidly distributed throughout the body.

Haloperidol is excreted in human breast milk, milk concentrations being 59-69% of maternal plasma.

Haloperidol is extensively metabolised by oxidative dealkylation. Metabolites are ultimately conjugated with glycine.

5.3 Preclinical safety data

No relevant information additional to that contained elsewhere in the Summary of Product Characteristics.

6. PHARMACEUTICAL PARTICULARS

6.1 List of excipients

Lactic Acid

Water for Injections

6.2 Incompatibilities
None known.

6.3 Shelf life
5 years

6.4 Special precautions for storage
Keep the ampoule in the outer carton.

6.5 Nature and contents of container
Amber glass ampoules containing 1 or 2ml of solution for injection. Boxes of 5 ampoules.

6.6 Special precautions for disposal and other handling
None stated.

7. MARKETING AUTHORISATION HOLDER
Janssen-Cilag Limited
50-100 Holmers Farm Way
High Wycombe
Bucks
HP12 4EG
UK

8. MARKETING AUTHORISATION NUMBER(S)
PL 00242/0036R

9. DATE OF FIRST AUTHORISATION/RENEWAL OF THE AUTHORISATION
23 November 1988/25 May 2004

10. DATE OF REVISION OF THE TEXT
06 August 2009

Legal category POM

Half Inderal LA 80mg

(AstraZeneca UK Limited)

1. NAME OF THE MEDICINAL PRODUCT
Half Inderal LA 80mg

2. QUALITATIVE AND QUANTITATIVE COMPOSITION
Propranolol hydrochloride Ph Eur 80 mg

3. PHARMACEUTICAL FORM
Pink/lavender or white opaque capsules containing propranolol hydrochloride in a prolonged release formulation.

4. CLINICAL PARTICULARS
4.1 Therapeutic indications
a) Management of angina
b) Prophylaxis of migraine
c) Management of essential tremor
d) Relief of situational anxiety and generalised anxiety, particularly those of somatic type
e) Adjunctive management of thyrotoxicosis
f) Prophylaxis of upper gastro-intestinal bleeding in patients with portal hypertension and oesophageal varices
g) Control of hypertension

4.2 Posology and method of administration
For oral administration.

Adults

Hypertension: The usual starting dose is one 160 mg Inderal LA capsule daily, taken either morning or evening. An adequate response is seen in most patients at this dosage. If necessary, it can be increased in 80 mg Half-Inderal LA increments until an adequate response is achieved. A further reduction in blood pressure can be obtained if a diuretic or other antihypertensive agent is given in addition to Inderal LA and Half-Inderal LA.

Angina, essential tremor, thyrotoxicosis and the prophylaxis of migraine: One Half-Inderal LA capsule daily, taken either morning or evening, may be sufficient to provide adequate control in many patients. If necessary the dose may be increased to one Inderal LA capsule per day and an additional Half-Inderal LA increment may be given.

Situational and generalised anxiety: One Half-Inderal LA capsule taken daily should be sufficient to provide short-term relief of acute situational anxiety. Generalised anxiety, requiring longer term therapy, usually responds adequately at the same dosage. In individual cases, the dosage may be increased to one Inderal LA capsule per day. Treatment should be continued according to response. Patients should be reviewed after 6 to 12 months' treatment.

Portal hypertension: Dosage should be titrated to achieve approximately 25% reduction in resting heart rate. Dosing should begin with one 80 mg Half-Inderal LA capsule daily, increasing to one 160 mg Inderal LA capsule daily depending on heart rate response. Further 80 mg Half-Inderal LA increments may be added up to a maximum dose of 320 mg once daily.

Patients who are already established on equivalent daily doses of Inderal tablets should be transferred to the equivalent doses of Half-Inderal LA or Inderal LA daily, taken either morning or evening.

Children
Inderal LA and Half-Inderal LA are not intended for use in children.

Elderly Patients
Evidence concerning the relation between blood level and age is conflicting. It is suggested that treatment should start with one Half-Inderal LA capsule once daily. The dose may be increased to one Inderal LA capsule daily or higher as appropriate.

4.3 Contraindications
Inderal LA and Half-Inderal LA must not be used if there is a history of bronchial asthma or bronchospasm. The product label states the following warning: "Do not take Inderal LA if you have a history of asthma or wheezing". A similar warning appears in the Patient Information Leaflet.

Bronchospasm can usually be reversed by $beta_2$ agonist bronchodilators such as salbutamol. Large doses of the $beta_2$ agonist bronchodilator may be required to overcome the beta blockade produced by propranolol and the dose should be titrated according to the clinical response; both intravenous and inhalational administration should be considered. The use of intravenous aminophylline and/or the use of ipratropium (given by nebuliser) may also be considered. Glucagon (1 to 2 mg given intravenously) has also been reported to produce a bronchodilator effect in asthmatic patients. Oxygen or artificial ventilation may be required in severe cases.

Inderal LA and Half-Inderal LA, as with other beta-blockers, must not be used in patients with any of the following conditions: known hypersensitivity to the substance, bradycardia, cardiogenic shock, hypotension, metabolic acidosis, after prolonged fasting, severe peripheral arterial circulatory disturbances, second or third degree heart block, sick sinus syndrome, untreated phaeochromocytoma, uncontrolled heart failure or Prinzmetal's angina.

Inderal LA and Half-Inderal LA must not be used in patients prone to hypoglycaemia, i.e. patients after prolonged fasting or patients with restricted counter-regulatory reserves.

4.4 Special warnings and precautions for use
Inderal LA and Half-Inderal LA as with other beta-blockers:

- although contra-indicated in uncontrolled heart failure (see Section 4.3) may be used in patients whose signs of heart failure have been controlled. Caution must be exercised in patients whose cardiac reserve is poor.
- should not be used in combination with calcium channel blockers with negative inotropic effects (e.g. verapamil, diltiazem), as it can lead to an exaggeration of these effects particularly in patients with impaired ventricular function and/or SA or AV conduction abnormalities. This may result in severe hypotension, bradycardia and cardiac failure. Neither the beta blocker nor the calcium channel blocker should be administered intravenously within 48 hours of discontinuing the other.
- should not be used in patients with Prinzmetal's angina and beta-1 selective agents should be used with care (see section 4.3).
- although contra-indicated in severe peripheral arterial circulatory disturbances (see section 4.3) may also aggravate less severe peripheral arterial circulatory disturbances.
- due to its negative effect on conduction time, caution must be exercised if it is given to patients with first degree heart block.
- may block/modify the signs and symptoms of the hypoglycaemia (especially tachycardia). Inderal LA and Half-Inderal LA occasionally causes hypoglycaemia, even in non-diabetic patients, e.g., elderly patients, patients on haemodialysis or patients suffering from chronic liver disease and patients suffering from overdose. Severe hypoglycaemia associated with Inderal LA and Half-Inderal LA has rarely presented with seizures and/or coma in isolated patients. Caution must be exercised in the concurrent use of Inderal LA and Half-Inderal LA and hypoglycaemic therapy in diabetic patients. Inderal LA and Half-Inderal LA may prolong the hypoglycaemic response to insulin (see section 4.3).
- may mask the signs of thyrotoxicosis.
- should not be used in untreated phaeochromocytoma. However, in patients with phaeochromocytoma, an alpha-blocker may be given concomitantly.
- should be used to treat the elderly with caution starting with a lower dose (see section 4.2).
- will reduce heart rate as a result of its pharmacological action. In the rare instances when a treated patient develops symptoms that may be attributable to a slow heart rate, the dose may be reduced.
- may cause a more severe reaction to a variety of allergens, when given to patients with a history of anaphylactic reaction to such allergens. Such patients may be unresponsive to the usual doses of adrenaline used to treat the allergic reactions.

Abrupt withdrawal of beta-blockers is to be avoided. The dosage should be withdrawn gradually over a period of 7 to 14 days. An equivalent dosage of another beta-blocker may be substituted during the withdrawal period to facilitate a reduction in dosage below Inderal LA 80mg. Patients should be followed during withdrawal especially those with ischaemic heart disease.

When a patient is scheduled for surgery and a decision is made to discontinue beta-blocker therapy, this should be done at least 24 hours prior to the procedure. The risk/benefit of stopping beta blockade should be made for each patient.

Since the half-life may be increased in patients with significant hepatic or renal impairment, caution must be exercised when starting treatment and selecting the initial dose.

Inderal LA and Half-Inderal LA must be used with caution in patients with decompensated cirrhosis (see section 4.2).

In patients with portal hypertension, liver function may deteriorate and hepatic encephalopathy may develop. There have been reports suggesting that treatment with propranolol may increase the risk of developing hepatic encephalopathy (see section 4.2).

Interference with laboratory tests: Inderal LA and Half-Inderal LA have been reported to interfere with the estimation of serum bilirubin by the diazo method and with the determination of catecholamines by methods using fluorescence.

4.5 Interaction with other medicinal products and other forms of interaction
Inderal LA and Half-Inderal LA modify the tachycardia of hypoglycaemia. Caution must be exercised in the concurrent use of Inderal LA or Half-Inderal LA and hypoglycaemic therapy in diabetic patients. Propranolol may prolong the hypoglycaemic response to insulin (see section 4.3 and 4.4).

Class I anti-arrhythmic drugs (e.g. disopyramide) and amiodarone may have potentiating effect on atrial-conduction time and induce negative inotropic effect.

Digitalis glycosides, in association with beta-blockers, may increase atrio-ventricular conduction time.

Combined use of beta-blockers and calcium channel blockers with negative inotropic effects eg, verapamil, diltiazem, can lead to an exaggeration of these effects, particularly in patients with impaired ventricular function and/or sino-atrial or atrio-ventricular conduction abnormalities. This may result in severe hypotension, bradycardia and cardiac failure. Neither the beta-blocker nor the calcium channel blocker should be administered intravenously within 48 hours of discontinuing the other.

Concomitant therapy with dihydropyridine calcium channel blockers eg, nifedipine, may increase the risk of hypotension, and cardiac failure may occur in patients with latent cardiac insufficiency.

Concomitant use of sympathomimetic agents, eg, adrenaline, may counteract the effect of beta-blockers. Caution must be exercised in the parenteral administration of preparations containing adrenaline to patients taking beta-blockers as, in rare cases, vasoconstriction, hypertension and bradycardia may result.

Administration of propranolol during infusion of lidocaine may increase the plasma concentration of lidocaine by approximately 30%. Patients already receiving propranolol tend to have higher lidocaine levels than controls. The combination should be avoided.

Concomitant use of cimetidine will increase the plasma levels of propranolol, and concomitant use of alcohol may increase the plasma levels of propranolol.

Beta-blockers may exacerbate the rebound hypertension which can follow the withdrawal of clonidine. If the two drugs are co-administered, the beta-blocker should be withdrawn several days before discontinuing clonidine. If replacing clonidine by beta-blocker therapy, the introduction of beta-blockers should be delayed for several days after clonidine administration has stopped.

Caution must be exercised if ergotamine, dihydroergotamine or related compounds are given in combination with propranolol since vasospastic reactions have been reported in a few patients.

Concomitant use of prostaglandin synthetase inhibiting drugs, e.g. ibuprofen or indometacin, may decrease the hypotensive effects of propranolol.

Concomitant administration of propranolol and chlorpromazine may result in an increase in plasma levels of both drugs. This may lead to an enhanced antipsychotic effect for chlorpromazine and an increased antihypertensive effect for propranolol.

Caution must be exercised when using anaesthetic agents with Inderal LA and Half-Inderal LA. The anaesthetist should be informed and the choice of anaesthetic should be the agent with as little negative inotropic activity as possible. Use of beta-blockers with anaesthetic drugs may result in attenuation of the reflex tachycardia and increase the risk of hypotension. Anaesthetic agents causing myocardial depression are best avoided.

Pharmacokinetic studies have shown that the following agents may interact with propranolol due to effects on enzyme systems in the liver which metabolise propranolol and these agents: quinidine, propafenone, rifampicin, theophylline, warfarin, thioridazine and dihydropyridine calcium channel blockers such as nifedipine, nisoldipine, nicardipine, isradipine and lacidipine. Owing to the fact that blood concentrations of either agent may be affected, dosage adjustments may be needed according to clinical judgement, (see also the interaction above concerning concomitant therapy with dihydropyridine calcium channel blockers).

4.6 Pregnancy and lactation

Pregnancy: As with all drugs, Inderal LA and Half-Inderal LA should not be given during pregnancy unless their use is essential. There is no evidence of teratogenicity with Inderal.

However beta-blockers reduce placental perfusion, which may result in intra-uterine foetal death, immature and premature deliveries. In addition, adverse effects (especially hypoglycaemia and bradycardia in the neonate and bradycardia in the foetus) may occur. There is an increased risk of cardiac and pulmonary complications in the neonate in the post-natal period.

Lactation: Most beta-blockers, particularly lipophilic compounds, will pass into breast milk although to a variable extent. Breast feeding is therefore not recommended following administration of these compounds.

4.7 Effects on ability to drive and use machines

The use of Inderal LA or Half-Inderal LA is unlikely to result in any impairment of the ability of patients to drive or operate machinery. However, it should be taken into account that occasionally dizziness or fatigue may occur.

4.8 Undesirable effects

Inderal LA and Half-Inderal LA are usually well tolerated. In clinical studies, the undesired events reported are usually attributable to the pharmacological actions of propranolol.

The following undesired events, listed by body system, have been reported.

Common (1-9.9%)

General: Fatigue and/or lassitude (often transient)

Cardiovascular: Bradycardia, cold extremities, Raynaud's phenomenon.

CNS: Sleep disturbances, nightmares.

Uncommon (0.1-0.9%)

GI: Gastrointestinal disturbance, such as nausea, vomiting, diarrhoea.

Rare (0.01-0.09%)

General: Dizziness.

Blood: Thrombocytopaenia.

Cardiovascular: Heart failure deterioration, precipitation of heart block, postural hypotension, which may be associated with syncope, exacerbation of intermittent claudication.

CNS: Hallucinations, psychoses, mood changes, confusion, memory loss.

Skin: Purpura, alopecia, psoriasiform skin reactions, exacerbation of psoriasis, skin rashes.

Neurological: Paraesthesia.

Eyes: Dry eyes, visual disturbances.

Respiratory: Bronchospasm may occur in patients with bronchial asthma or a history of asthmatic complaints, sometimes with fatal outcome.

Very rare (<0.01%)

Endocrine system: Hypoglycaemia in neonates, infants, children, elderly patients, patients on haemodialysis, patients on concomitant antidiabetic therapy, patients with prolonged fasting and patients with chronic liver disease has been reported.

Investigations: an increase in ANA (Antinuclear Antibodies) has been observed, however the clinical relevance of this is not clear.

Nervous system: Isolated reports of myasthenia gravis like syndrome or exacerbation of myasthenia gravis have been reported.

Discontinuance of the drug should be considered if, according to clinical judgement, the well being of the patient is adversely affected by any of the above reactions. Cessation of therapy with a beta-blocker should be gradual. In the rare event of intolerance manifested as bradycardia and hypotension, the drug should be withdrawn and, if necessary, treatment for overdosage instituted.

4.9 Overdose

The symptoms of overdosage may include bradycardia, hypotension, acute cardiac insufficiency and bronchospasm.

General treatment should include: close supervision, treatment in an intensive care ward, the use of gastric lavage, activated charcoal and a laxative to prevent absorption of any drug still present in the gastrointestinal tract, the use of plasma or plasma substitutes to treat hypotension and shock.

Excessive bradycardia can be countered with atropine 1 to 2 mg intravenously and/or a cardiac pacemaker. If necessary, this may be followed by a bolus dose of glucagon 10 mg intravenously. If required, this may be repeated or followed by an intravenous infusion of glucagon 1 to 10 mg/hour depending on response. If no response to glucagon occurs or if glucagon is unavailable, a beta-adrenoceptor stimulant such as dobutamine 2.5 to 10 microgram/kg/minute by intravenous infusion may be given. Dobutamine, because of its positive inotropic effect, could also be used to treat hypotension and acute cardiac insufficiency. It is likely that these doses would be inadequate to reverse the cardiac effects of beta blockade if a large overdose has been taken. The dose of dobutamine should therefore be increased if necessary to achieve the required response according to the clinical condition of the patient.

5. PHARMACOLOGICAL PROPERTIES

5.1 Pharmacodynamic properties

Propranolol is a competitive antagonist at both $beta_1$ and $beta_2$-adrenoceptors. It has no agonist activity at the beta adrenoceptor, but has membrane stabilising activity at concentrations exceeding 1 to 3 mg/litre, though such concentrations are rarely achieved during oral therapy. Competitive beta blockade has been demonstrated in man by a parallel shift to the right in the dose-heart rate response curve to beta agonists such as isoprenaline.

Propranolol, as with other beta-blockers, has negative inotropic effects, and is therefore contra-indicated in uncontrolled heart failure.

Propranolol is a racemic mixture and the active form is the S (-) isomer. With the exception of inhibition of the conversion of thyroxine to triiodothyronine it is unlikely that any additional ancillary properties possessed by R (+) propranolol, in comparison with the racemic mixture will give rise to different therapeutic effects.

Propranolol is effective and well tolerated in most ethnic populations, although the response may be less in black patients.

The sustained release preparation of propranolol maintains a higher degree of $beta_1$-blockade 24 hours after dosing compared with conventional propranolol.

5.2 Pharmacokinetic properties

Propranolol is completely absorbed after oral administration and peak plasma concentrations occur 1-2 hours after dosing in fasting patients. Following oral dosing with the sustained release preparation of propranolol, the blood profile is flatter than after conventional Inderal but the half-life is increased to between 10 and 20 hours. The liver removes up to 90% of an oral dose with an elimination half-life of 3 to 6 hours. Propranolol is widely and rapidly distributed throughout the body with highest levels occurring in the lungs, liver, kidney, brain and heart. Propranolol is highly protein bound (80 to 95%).

5.3 Preclinical safety data

Propranolol is a drug on which extensive clinical experience has been obtained. Relevant information for the prescriber is provided elsewhere in this Summary of Product Characteristics.

6. PHARMACEUTICAL PARTICULARS

6.1 List of excipients

Erythrosine (E127)

Ethyl cellulose Ph Eur. (E462)

Gelatin Ph Eur. (E441)

Iron oxide, red (E172)

Iron oxide, black (E172)

Methylhydroxypropylcellulose Ph Eur. (E464)

Microcrystalline cellulose Ph Eur. (E460)

Titanium dioxide Ph Eur. (E171)

Sodium lauryl sulphate Ph Eur.

Shellac (E904)

6.2 Incompatibilities

None known.

6.3 Shelf life

3 years.

6.4 Special precautions for storage

Store below 25°C, protected from light and moisture.

6.5 Nature and contents of container

Patient calendar pack of 28 capsules.

6.6 Special precautions for disposal and other handling

Use as directed by the prescriber.

7. MARKETING AUTHORISATION HOLDER

AstraZeneca UK Limited

600 Capability Green

Luton

LU1 3LU

UK

8. MARKETING AUTHORISATION NUMBER(S)

PL 17901/0020

9. DATE OF FIRST AUTHORISATION/RENEWAL OF THE AUTHORISATION

11th June 2000

10. DATE OF REVISION OF THE TEXT

19th May 2009

Half Securon SR

(Abbott Laboratories Limited)

1. NAME OF THE MEDICINAL PRODUCT

Half Securon SR

2. QUALITATIVE AND QUANTITATIVE COMPOSITION

Verapamil Hydrochloride Ph Eur – 120 mg

3. PHARMACEUTICAL FORM

Modified-release tablets.

The tablets are round, white, biconvex and embossed with the word 'Knoll' on one side and '120 SR' on the reverse.

4. CLINICAL PARTICULARS

4.1 Therapeutic indications

Half Securon SR is indicated for:

The treatment of mild to moderate hypertension.

The treatment and prophylaxis of angina pectoris.

Secondary prevention of reinfarction after an acute myocardial infarction in patients without heart failure, and not receiving diuretics (apart from low-dose diuretics when used for indications other than heart failure), and where beta-blockers are not appropriate. Treatment is to be started at least one week after an acute myocardial infarction.

4.2 Posology and method of administration

Half Securon SR tablets should not be chewed.

Adults

Hypertension: One tablet of Securon SR daily. For patients new to verapamil therapy, the physician should consider halving the initial dose to 120 mg (one tablet Half Securon SR). Most patients respond to 240 mg daily (one tablet Securon SR) given as a single dose. If control is not achieved after a period of at least one week, the dosage may be increased to a maximum of two Securon SR tablets daily (one in the morning and one in the evening at an interval of about twelve hours). A further reduction in blood pressure may be achieved by combining Securon SR with other antihypertensive agents, in particular diuretics. Half Securon SR may be used for dose titration purposes.

Angina pectoris: One tablet of Securon SR twice daily. A small number of patients respond to a lower dose and where indicated, adjustment down to one tablet of Securon SR daily could be made. Half Securon SR may be used for dose titration purposes.

Secondary prevention of reinfarction after an acute myocardial infarction in patients without heart failure, and not receiving diuretics (apart from low-dose diuretics when used for indications other than heart failure), and where beta-blockers are not appropriate: Treatment is to be started at least one week after an acute myocardial infarction. 360 mg/day in divided doses, to be taken either as one Half Securon SR (120 mg) tablet three times daily, or as one Securon SR (240 mg) tablet in the morning and one Half Securon SR (120 mg) tablet in the evening, on a daily basis.

Elderly patients

The adult dose is recommended unless renal or hepatic function is impaired (see Section 4.4, 'Special Warnings and Precautions for Use').

Children

Securon SR and Half Securon SR are not recommended for children.

4.3 Contraindications

Hypersensitivity to the active substance or to any of the excipients.

Cardiogenic shock; acute myocardial infarction complicated by bradycardia, marked hypotension or left ventricular failure; second or third degree atrioventricular (AV) block (except in patients with a functioning artificial pacemaker); sino-atrial block; sick sinus syndrome (except in patients with a functioning artificial pacemaker); uncompensated heart failure; bradycardia of less than 50 beats/minute; hypotension of less than 90 mmHg systolic.

Patients with atrial flutter/fibrillation in the presence of an accessory pathway (*e.g.* WPW syndrome) may develop increased conduction across the anomalous pathway and ventricular tachycardia may be precipitated.

4.4 Special warnings and precautions for use

Since verapamil is extensively metabolised in the liver, careful dose titration is required in patients with liver disease. The disposition of verapamil in patients with renal impairment has not been fully established and therefore careful patient monitoring is recommended. Verapamil is not removed during dialysis.

Verapamil may affect impulse conduction and should therefore be used with caution in patients with bradycardia or first degree AV block. Verapamil may affect left ventricular contractility; this effect is small and normally not important but cardiac failure may be precipitated or aggravated. In patients with incipient cardiac failure, therefore, verapamil should be given only after such cardiac failure has been controlled with appropriate therapy, e.g. digitalis.

When treating hypertension with verapamil, monitoring of the patient's blood pressure at regular intervals is required.

Caution should be exercised in treatment with HMG CoA reductase inhibitors (e.g., simvastatin, atorvastatin or lovastatin) for patients taking verapamil. These patients should be started at the lowest possible dose of verapamil and titrated upwards. If verapamil treatment is to be added to patients already taking an HMG CoA reductase inhibitor (e.g., simvastatin, atorvastatin or lovastatin), refer to advice in the respective statin product information.

4.5 Interaction with other medicinal products and other forms of interaction

In vitro metabolic studies indicate that verapamil hydrochloride is metabolized by cytochrome P450 CYP3A4, CYP1A2, CYP2C8, CYP2C9 and CYP2C18. Verapamil has been shown to be an inhibitor of CYP3A4 enzymes and P-glycoprotein (P-gp). Clinically significant interactions have been reported with inhibitors of CYP3A4 causing elevation of plasma levels of verapamil hydrochloride while inducers of CYP3A4 have caused a lowering of plasma levels of verapamil hydrochloride, therefore, patients should be monitored for drug interactions.

The following are potential drug interactions associated with verapamil:

Acetylsalicylic acid

Concomitant use of verapamil with aspirin may increase the risk of bleeding.

Alcohol

Increase in blood *alcohol* has been reported.

Alpha blockers

Verapamil may increase the plasma concentrations of *prazosin* and *terazosin* which may have an additive hypotensive effect.

Antiarrhythmics

Verapamil may slightly decrease the plasma clearance of *flecainide* whereas *flecainide* has no effect on the verapamil plasma clearance.

Verapamil may increase the plasma concentrations of *quinidine*. Pulmonary oedema may occur in patients with hypertrophic cardiomyopathy

The combination of verapamil and *antiarrhythmic agents* may lead to additive cardiovascular effects (e.g. AV block, bradycardia, hypotension, heart failure).

Anticonvulsants

Verapamil may increase the plasma concentrations of *carbamazepine*. This may produce side effects such as diplopia, headache, ataxia or dizziness. Verapamil may also increase the plasma concentrations of *phenytoin*.

Antidepressants

Verapamil may increase the plasma concentrations of *imipramine*.

Antidiabetics

Verapamil may increase the plasma concentrations of *glibenclamide (glyburide)*.

Antihypertensives, diuretics, vasodilators

Potentiation of the hypotensive effect.

Anti-infectives

Rifampicin may reduce the plasma concentrations of verapamil which may produce a reduced blood pressure lowering effect. *Erythromycin* and *telithromycin* may increase the plasma concentrations of verapamil.

Antineoplastics

Verapamil may increase the plasma concentrations of *doxorubicin*.

Barbiturates

Phenobarbital may reduce the plasma concentrations of verapamil.

Benzodiazepines and other anxiolytics

Verapamil may increase the plasma concentrations of *buspirone* and *midazolam*.

Beta blockers

Verapamil may increase the plasma concentrations of *metoprolol* and *propranolol* which may lead to additive cardiovascular effects (e.g. AV block, bradycardia, hypotension, heart failure).

Intravenous *beta-blockers* should not be given to patients under treatment with verapamil.

Cardiac glycosides

Verapamil may increase the plasma concentrations of *digitoxin* and *digoxin*. Verapamil has been shown to increase the serum concentration of *digoxin* and caution should be exercised with regard to digitalis toxicity. The digitalis level should be determined and the glycoside dose reduced, if required.

Colchicine

Colchicine is a substrate for both CYP3A and the efflux transporter, P-glycoprotein (P-gp). Verapamil is known to inhibit CYP3A and P-gp. When verapamil and *colchicine* are administered together, inhibition of P-gp and/or CYP3A by verapamil may lead to increased exposure to *colchicine*. Combined use is not recommended.

H_2 Receptor antagonists

Cimetidine may increase the plasma concentrations of verapamil.

HIV antiviral agents

Due to the metabolic inhibitory potential of some of the *HIV antiviral agents*, such as *ritonavir*, plasma concentrations of verapamil may increase. Caution should be used or dose of verapamil may be decreased.

Immunosuppressants

Verapamil may increase the plasma concentrations of *ciclosporin, everolimus, sirolimus* and *tacrolimus*.

Inhaled anaesthetics

When used concomitantly, *inhalation anaesthetics* and calcium antagonists, such as verapamil hydrochloride, should each be titrated carefully to avoid additive cardiovascular effects (e.g. AV block, bradycardia, hypotension, heart failure).

Lipid lowering agents

Verapamil may increase the plasma concentrations *atorvastatin, lovastatin* and *simvastatin.*

Treatment with HMG *CoA reductase inhibitors* (e.g., *simvastatin, atorvastatin* or *lovastatin*) in a patient taking verapamil should be started at the lowest possible dose and titrated upwards. If verapamil treatment is to be added to patients already taking an *HMG CoA reductase inhibitor* (e.g., *simvastatin, atorvastatin* or *lovastatin*), consider a reduction in the statin dose and retitrate against serum cholesterol concentrations.

Atorvastatin may increase verapamil levels. Although there is no direct in vivo clinical evidence, there is strong potential for verapamil to significantly affect *atorvastatin* pharmacokinetics in a similar manner to *simvastatin* or *lovastatin*. Consider using caution when *atorvastatin* and verapamil are concomitantly administered.

Fluvastatin, pravastatin and *rosuvastatin* are not metabolized by CYP3A4 and are less likely to interact with verapamil.

Lithium

Serum levels of *lithium* may be reduced. However there may be increased sensitivity to *lithium* causing enhanced neurotoxicity.

Neuromuscular blocking agents employed in anaesthesia

The effects may be potentiated.

Serotonin receptor agonists

Verapamil may increase the plasma concentrations of *almotriptan*.

Theophylline

Verapamil may increase the plasma concentrations of *theophylline*.

Uricosurics

Sulfinpyrazone may reduce the plasma concentrations of verapamil which may produce a reduced blood pressure lowering effect.

Other

St. John's Wort may reduce the plasma concentrations of verapamil, whereas *grapefruit juice* may increase the plasma concentrations of verapamil.

4.6 Pregnancy and lactation

Although animal studies have not shown any teratogenic effects, verapamil should not be given during the first trimester of pregnancy unless, in the clinician's judgement, it is essential for the welfare of the patient.

Verapamil is excreted into the breast milk in small amounts and is unlikely to be harmful. However, rare hypersensitivity reactions have been reported with verapamil and therefore it should only be used during lactation if, in the clinician's judgement, it is essential for the welfare of the patient.

4.7 Effects on ability to drive and use machines

Depending on individual susceptibility, the patient's ability to drive a vehicle, operate machinery or work under hazardous conditions may be impaired. This is particularly true in the initial stages of treatment, when changing over from another drug or when the dose is raised. Like many other common medicines, verapamil has been shown to increase the blood levels of alcohol and slow its elimination. Therefore, the effects of alcohol may be exaggerated.

4.8 Undesirable effects

Reactions from Postmarketing Surveillance or Phase IV Clinical Trials

The following adverse events reported with verapamil are listed below by system organ class:

Immune system disorders: allergic reactions (e.g. erythema, pruritus, urticaria) are very rarely seen.

Nervous system disorders: headache, dizziness, paresthesia, tremor and extrapyramidal syndrome.

Ear and labyrinth disorders: vertigo and tinnitus.

Cardiac disorders/vascular disorders: bradycardic arrhythmias such as sinus bradycardia, sinus arrest with asystole, 2nd and 3rd degree AV block, bradyarrhythmia in atrial fibrillation, peripheral oedema, palpitations, tachycardia, development or aggravation of heart failure and hypotension. There have been rare reports of flushing.

Gastrointestinal disorders: nausea, vomiting, constipation, ileus and abdominal pain/discomfort. Gingival hyperplasia may occur very rarely when the drug is administered over prolonged periods, and is fully reversible when the drug is discontinued.

Skin and subcutaneous tissue disorders: ankle oedema, Quincke's oedema, Steven-Johnson syndrome, erythema multiforme, erythromelalgia, alopecia and purpura.

Musculoskeletal and connective tissue disorders: muscular weakness, myalgia and arthralgia.

Reproductive system and breast disorders: impotence (erectile dysfunction) has been rarely reported and isolated cases of galactorrhoea. On very rare occasions, gynaecomastia has been observed in elderly male patients under long-term verapamil treatment, and is fully reversible in all cases when the drug was discontinued.

General disorders and administration site conditions: fatigue.

Investigations: A reversible impairment of liver function characterized by an increase of transaminase and/or alkaline phosphatase may occur on very rare occasions during verapamil treatment and is most probably a hypersensitivity reaction. Rises in blood prolactin levels have been reported.

4.9 Overdose

The course of symptoms in verapamil intoxication depends on the amount taken, the point in time at which detoxification measures are taken and myocardial contractility (age-related). The main symptoms are as follows: blood pressure fall (at times to values not detectable), shock symptoms, loss of consciousness, 1st and 2nd degree AV block (frequently as Wenckebach's phenomenon with or without escape rhythms), total AV block with total AV dissociation, escape rhythm, asystole, bradycardia up to high degree AV block and sinus arrest, hyperglycaemia, stupor and metabolic acidosis. Fatalities have occurred as a result of overdose.

The therapeutic measures to be taken depend on the point in time at which verapamil was taken and the type and severity of intoxication symptoms. In intoxications with large amounts of slow-release preparations (Securon SR and Half Securon SR), it should be noted that the release of the active drug and the absorption in the intestine may take more than 48 hours. Verapamil hydrochloride cannot be removed by haemodialysis. Depending on the time of ingestion, it should be taken into account that there may be some lumps of incompletely dissolved tablets along the entire length of the gastrointestinal tract, which function as active drug depots.

General measures to be taken: Gastric lavage with the usual precautions, even later than 12 hours after ingestion, if no gastrointestinal motility (peristaltic sounds) is detectable. Where intoxication by Securon SR or Half Securon SR is suspected, extensive elimination measures are indicated, such as induced vomiting, removal of the contents of the stomach and the small intestine under endoscopy, intestinal lavage, laxative, high enemas. The usual intensive resuscitation measures apply, such as extrathoracic heart massage, respiration, defibrillation and/or pacemaker therapy.

Specific measures to be taken: Elimination of cardiodepressive effects, hypotension or bradycardia. The specific antidote is calcium, e.g. 10 -20 ml of a 10% calcium gluconate solution administered intravenously (2.25 - 4.5 mmol), repeated if necessary or given as a continuous drip infusion (e.g. 5 mmol/hour).

The following measures may also be necessary: In case of 2nd or 3rd degree AV block, sinus bradycardia, asystole - atropine, isoprenaline, orciprenaline or pacemaker therapy. In case of hypotension - dopamine, dobutamine, noradrenaline. If there are signs of continuing myocardial failure - dopamine, dobutamine, if necessary repeated calcium injections.

5. PHARMACOLOGICAL PROPERTIES

5.1 Pharmacodynamic properties

Verapamil, a phenylalkylamine calcium antagonist, has a balanced profile of cardiac and peripheral effects. It lowers heart rate, increases myocardial perfusion and reduces coronary spasm. In a clinical study in patients after myocardial infarction, verapamil reduced total mortality, sudden cardiac death and reinfarction rate.

Verapamil reduces total peripheral resistance and lowers high blood pressure by vasodilation, without reflex tachycardia. Because of its use-dependent action on the voltage-operated calcium channel, the effects of verapamil are more pronounced on high than on normal blood pressure.

As early as day one of treatment, blood pressure falls; the effect is found to persist also in long-term therapy. Verapamil is suitable for the treatment of all types of hypertension: for monotherapy in mild to moderate hypertension; combined with other antihypertensives (in particular with diuretics and, according to more recent findings, with ACE inhibitors) in more severe types of hypertension. In hypertensive diabetic patients with nephropathy, verapamil in combination with ACE inhibitors led to a marked reduction of albuminuria and to an improvement of creatinine clearance.

5.2 Pharmacokinetic properties

Absorption: More than 90% of an orally-administered dose of verapamil is absorbed. Due to an intensive hepatic first-pass metabolism, the absolute bioavailability is about 22% with a variability of about 10 - 35%. Under multiple dosing, bioavailability increases by about 30%. Bioavailability is not affected by food consumption.

Distribution, biotransformation and elimination: Plasma concentrations reach their peak 4 - 8 hours after drug intake. Plasma protein binding of verapamil is about 90%. The elimination half-life is about 5 - 8 hours. The mean residence time of modified-release verapamil is 13 hours. After repeated single daily doses, steady-state conditions are reached between 3 - 4 days.

Within 5 days, approximately 70% of an orally-administered dose is excreted in the urine and about 16% with the faeces. Only 3 - 4 % is eliminated renally as unchanged drug. The drug is extensively metabolized. A number of metabolites are generated in humans (twelve have been identified). Of these metabolites only norverapamil has any appreciable pharmacological effect (approximately 20% that of the parent compound, which was observed in a study with dogs). Norverapamil represents about 6% of the dose eliminated in urine. Norverapamil can reach steady-state plasma concentrations approximately equal to those of verapamil itself. Renal insufficiency does not affect the kinetics of verapamil.

At-risk patients: In patients with liver cirrhosis, bioavailability is increased and elimination half-life is prolonged. In patients with compensated hepatic insufficiency, no influence on the kinetics of verapamil was observed.

5.3 Preclinical safety data
None stated.

6. PHARMACEUTICAL PARTICULARS

6.1 List of excipients
Microcrystalline cellulose, sodium alginate, povidone, magnesium stearate, purified water, hydroxypropyl methylcellulose, polyethylene glycol 400, polyethylene glycol 6000, talc, titanium dioxide (E171), montan glycol wax.

6.2 Incompatibilities
None stated.

6.3 Shelf life
5 years.

6.4 Special precautions for storage
Do not store above 25°C and store in the original package – blister pack.

Do not store above 25°C and keep the container tightly closed – bottle pack.

6.5 Nature and contents of container
Calendar pack consisting of a PVC/PVDC blister in a cardboard outer container. Pack size: 28 tablets.

Polypropylene bottle with polyethylene stopper. Pack size: 100 tablets.

6.6 Special precautions for disposal and other handling
There are no specific instructions for use/handling. The tablets should not be chewed.

7. MARKETING AUTHORISATION HOLDER
Abbott Laboratories Limited
Queenborough
Kent
ME11 5EL
United Kingdom

8. MARKETING AUTHORISATION NUMBER(S)
PL 00037/0370

9. DATE OF FIRST AUTHORISATION/RENEWAL OF THE AUTHORISATION
14 March 2002

10. DATE OF REVISION OF THE TEXT
02nd April 2009

Harmogen 1.5mg Tablets

(Pharmacia Limited)

1. NAME OF THE MEDICINAL PRODUCT
Harmogen 1.5 mg

2. QUALITATIVE AND QUANTITATIVE COMPOSITION
Each tablet contains Estropipate USP (piperazine estrone sulphate) equivalent to 0.93 mg estrone.

For excipients, see 6.1

3. PHARMACEUTICAL FORM
Tablets for oral administration

4. CLINICAL PARTICULARS

4.1 Therapeutic indications
Hormone Replacement Therapy (HRT) for estrogen deficiency symptoms in post- and peri-menopausal women.

Prevention of osteoporosis in postmenopausal women at high risk of future fractures who are intolerant of, or contra-indicated for, other medicinal products approved for the prevention of osteoporosis, (See also Section 4.4).

4.2 Posology and method of administration
Harmogen is an estrogen-only product for oral use.

Adults and the Elderly:

Post-menopausal osteoporosis: 1.5 mg daily.

Estrogen-deficiency symptoms: 1.5 mg - 3.0 mg daily taken as a single or divided dose.

For initiation and continuation of treatment of peri- and postmenopausal symptoms, the lowest effective dose for the shortest duration (see also Section 4.4) should be used.

Dosage Schedule (for both indications):

Therapy may start at any time in women with established amenorrhoea or who are experiencing long intervals between spontaneous menses. In women who are menstruating, it is advised that therapy starts within five days of the start of bleeding. Patients changing from a cyclical or continuous sequential preparation should complete the cycle, and after a withdrawal bleed, may then change to Harmogen 1.5mg. Patients changing from a continuous combined preparation may start therapy at any time if amenorrhoea is established, or otherwise start within five days of the start of bleeding.

Harmogen should be given continuously and, in women with an intact uterus, a progestogen is recommended and should be added for at least 12-14 days each cycle. The benefits of the lower risk of endometrial hyperplasia and endometrial cancer, due to adding progestogen, should be weighed against the increased risk of Breast cancer, (See Sections 4.4 and 4.8). Unless there is a previous diagnosis of endometriosis, it is not recommended to add a progestogen in hysterectomised women.

If a tablet is missed it should be taken within a few hours of when normally taken, otherwise the forgotten tablet should be discarded, and the usual tablet should be taken at the next scheduled time. If one extra tablet is taken inadvertently, the usual tablet should be taken at the next scheduled time. There is an increased likelihood of break-through bleeding and spotting when a dose is missed.

4.3 Contraindications
Known, past or suspected breast cancer;

Known or suspected estrogen-dependent malignant tumours, (e.g. endometrial cancer);

Undiagnosed genital bleeding;

Untreated endometrial hyperplasia;

Previous idiopathic or current venous thromboembolism (deep vein thrombosis, pulmonary embolism);

Active or recent arterial thromboembolic disease (e.g. angina, myocardial infarction);

Acute liver disease, or a history of liver disease as long as liver function tests have failed to return to normal;

Known hypersensitivity to the active substances or to any of the excipients;

Porphyria.

4.4 Special warnings and precautions for use
For the treatment of menopausal symptoms, HRT should only be initiated for symptoms that adversely affect quality of life. In all cases, a careful appraisal of the risks and benefits should be undertaken at least annually and HRT should only be continued as long as the benefit outweighs the risk

Medical Examination/Follow Up

Assessment of each woman prior to taking hormone replacement therapy (and at regular intervals thereafter) should include a personal and family medical history. Physical examination should be guided by this and by the contra-indications (see Section 4.3) and warnings (see Section 4.4) for this product. During assessment of each individual woman, clinical examination of the breasts and pelvic examination should be performed where clinically indicated rather than as a routine procedure. Women should be encouraged to participate in the national breast screening programme (mammography) and the national cervical screening programme (cervical cytology) as appropriate for their age. Breast awareness should also be encouraged and women advised to report any changes in their breasts to their doctor or nurse, (see "Breast Cancer" below).

Conditions which need supervision:

If any of the following conditions are present, have occurred previously, and/or have been aggravated during pregnancy or previous hormone treatment, the patient should be closely supervised. It should be taken into account that these conditions may recur or be aggravated during treatment with Harmogen, in particular:

Risk factors for estrogen dependent tumours, e.g. 1st degree heredity for breast cancer (see below);

Diabetes mellitus with or without vascular involvement;

Migraine or (severe) headache;

Epilepsy;

A history of, or risk of factors for, thromboembolic disorders (see below);

Systemic lupus erythematosus, SLE;

Liver disorders (e.g. liver adenoma);

Leiomyoma (uterine fibroids) or endometriosis;

Otosclerosis;

Cholelithiasis;

A history of endometrial hyperplasia (see below);

Hypertension;

Asthma.

Reasons for immediate withdrawal of therapy:

Therapy should be discontinued in case a contra-indication is discovered and in the following situations:

- Jaundice or deterioration in liver function
- Significant increase in blood pressure
- New onset of migraine-type headache
- Pregnancy

Endometrial Hyperplasia

The risk of endometrial hyperplasia and carcinoma is increased when estrogens are administered alone for prolonged periods, (see Section 4.8). The addition of progestogen for at least 12 days per cycle in non-hysterectomised women greatly reduces this risk (See Section 4.8).

The endometrial safety of added progestogen has not been studied for Harmogen 1.5mg.

The reduction in risk to the endometrium should be weighed against the increase in the risk of breast cancer of added progestogen (See 'Breast cancer' below, and in Section 4.8)

Breakthrough bleeding and spotting may occur during the first months of treatment. If breakthrough bleeding or spotting appears after some time on therapy or continues after treatment has been discontinued, the reason should be investigated which may include endometrial biopsy to exclude endometrial malignancy.

Unopposed estrogen stimulation may lead to premalignant transformation in the residual foci of endometriosis. Therefore, the addition of progestogens to estrogen replacement therapy should be considered in women who have undergone hysterectomy because of endometriosis, if they are known to have residual endometriosis (but see above).

Breast Cancer

A randomised placebo-controlled trial, the Women's Health Initiative study (WHI), and epidemiological studies, including the Million Women Study (MWS), have reported an increased risk of breast cancer in women taking estrogens, estrogen-progestogen combinations or tibolone for HRT for several years (see Section 4.8). For all HRT, an excess risk becomes apparent within a few years of use and increases with duration of intake but returns to baseline within a few (at most five) years after stopping treatment.

In the MWS, the relative risk of breast cancer with conjugated equine estrogens (CEE) or estradiol (E2) was greater when a progestogen was added, either sequentially or continuously, and regardless of type of progestogen. There was no evidence of a difference in risk between the different routes of administration.

In the WHI study, the continuous combined conjugated equine estrogen and medroxyprogesterone acetate (CEE + MPA) product used was associated with breast cancers that were slightly larger in size and more frequently had local lymph node metastases compared to placebo.

HRT, especially estrogen-progestogen combined treatment, increases the density of mammographic images which may adversely affect the radiological detection of breast cancer.

Venous Thromboembolism

HRT is associated with a higher relative risk of developing venous thromboembolism (VTE), i.e. deep vein thrombosis or pulmonary embolism. One randomised controlled trial and epidemiological studies found a two to threefold higher risk for users compared with non-users. For non-users, it is estimated that the number of cases of VTE that will occur over a 5 year period is about 3 per 1000 women aged 50-59 years and 8 per 1000 women aged between 60-69 years. It is estimated that in healthy women who use HRT for 5 years, the number of additional cases of VTE over a 5 year period will be between 2 and 6 (best estimate = 4) per 1000 women aged 50-59 years and between 5 and 15 (best estimate = 9) per 1000 women aged 60-69 years. The occurrence of such an event is more likely in the first year of HRT than later.

Generally recognised risk factors for VTE include a personal history or family history, severe obesity (BMI >30 kg/m²) and systemic lupus erythematosus (SLE). There is no consensus about the possible role of varicose veins in VTE.

Patients with a history of VTE or known thrombophilic states have an increased risk of VTE. HRT may add to this risk. Personal or strong family history of thromboembolism or recurrent spontaneous abortion should be investigated in order to exclude a thrombophilic predisposition. Until a thorough evaluation of thrombophilic factors has been made or anticoagulant treatment initiated, use of HRT in such patients should be viewed as contraindicated. Those women already on anticoagulant treatment require careful consideration of the benefit-risk of use of HRT.

The risk of VTE may be temporarily increased with prolonged immobilisation, major trauma or major surgery. As in all postoperative patients, scrupulous attention should be given to prophylactic measures to prevent VTE following surgery. Where prolonged immobilisation is liable to follow elective surgery, particularly abdominal or orthopaedic surgery to the lower limbs, consideration should be given to temporarily stopping HRT 4 to 6 weeks earlier, if possible. Treatment should not be restarted until the woman is completely mobilised.

If VTE develops after initiating therapy, the drug should be discontinued. Patients should be told to contact their doctor immediately when they are aware of a potential thromboembolic symptom (e.g. painful swelling of a leg, sudden pain in the chest, dyspnoea).

Coronary Artery Disease

There is no evidence from randomised controlled trials of cardiovascular benefit with continuous combined conjugated estrogens and medroxyprogesterone acetate (MPA). Two large clinical trials (WHI and HERS, i.e. Heart and Estrogen/progestin Replacement Study) showed a possible increased risk of cardiovascular morbidity in the first year of use and no overall benefit. For other HRT products there are only limited data from randomised controlled trials examining effects in cardiovascular morbidity or mortality. Therefore, it is uncertain whether these findings also extend to other HRT products.

Stroke

One large randomised clinical trial (WHI-trial) found, as a secondary outcome, an increased risk of ischaemic stroke in healthy women during treatment with continuous combined conjugated estrogens and medroxyprogesterone acetate. For women who do not use HRT, it is estimated that the number of cases of stroke that will occur over a 5 year period is about 3 per 1000 women aged 50-59 years and 11 per 1000 women aged 60-69 years. It is estimated that for women who use conjugated estrogens and medroxyprogesterone acetate for 5 years, the number of additional cases will be between 0 and 3 (best estimate = 1) per 1000 users aged 50-59 years and between 1 and 9 (best estimate = 4) per 1000 users aged 60-69 years. It is unknown whether the increased risk also extends to other HRT products.

Ovarian Cancer

Long-term (at least 5 to 10 years) use of estrogen-only HRT products in hysterectomised women has been associated with an increased risk of ovarian cancer in some epidemiological studies. It is uncertain whether long-term use of combined HRT confers a different risk than estrogen-only products.

Other Conditions

Estrogens may cause fluid retention and therefore patients with cardiac or renal dysfunction should be carefully observed. Patients with terminal renal insufficiency should be closely observed, since it is expected that the level of circulating active ingredients in Harmogen 1.5 mg tablets is increased.

Women with pre-existing hypertriglyceridaemia should be followed closely during estrogen replacement or hormone replacement therapy, since rare cases of large increases of plasma triglycerides leading to pancreatitis have been reported with estrogen therapy in this condition.

Estrogens increase thyroid binding globulin (TBG), leading to increased circulating total thyroid hormone, as measured by protein-bound iodine (PBI), T4 levels (by column or by radio-immunoassay) or T3 levels (by radio-immunoassay). T3 resin uptake is decreased, reflecting the elevated TBG. Free T4 and free T3 concentrations are unaltered. Other binding proteins may be elevated in serum, i.e. corticoid binding globulin (CBG), sex-hormone-binding globulin (SHBG) leading to increased circulating corticosteroids and sex steroids, respectively. Free or biologically active hormone concentrations are unchanged. Other plasma proteins may be increased (angiotensinogen/renin substrate, alpha-1-antitrypsin, ceruloplasmin).

There is no conclusive evidence for improvement of cognitive function. There is some evidence from the WHI trial of increased risk of probable dementia in women who start using continuous combined CEE and MPA after the age of 65. It is unknown whether the findings apply to younger post-menopausal women or other HRT products.

In rare cases benign, and in even rarer cases malignant liver tumours leading in isolated cases to life-threatening intra-abdominal haemorrhage have been observed after the use of hormonal substances such as those contained in Harmogen 1.5mg. If severe upper abdominal complaints, enlarged liver or signs of intra-abdominal haemorrhage occur, a liver tumour should be considered in the differential diagnosis.

Women who may be at risk of pregnancy should be advised to adhere to non-hormonal contraceptive methods.

The requirement for oral anti-diabetics or insulin can change as a result of the effect on glucose tolerance.

4.5 Interaction with other medicinal products and other forms of interaction

The metabolism of estrogen may be increased by concomitant use of substances known to induce drug-metabolising enzymes, specifically cytochrome P450 enzymes, such as anticonvulsants (e.g. phenobarbital, phenytoin, carbamazepine) and anti-infectives (e.g. rifampicin, rifabutin, nevirapine, efavirenz).

Ritonavir and nelfinavir, although known as strong inhibitors by contrast exhibit inducing properties when used concomitantly with steroid hormones. Herbal preparations containing St John's Wort (Hypericum Perforatum) may induce the metabolism of estrogens.

Clinically, an increased metabolism of estrogens and progestogens may lead to decreased effect and changes in the uterine bleeding profile.

Some laboratory tests can be influenced by estrogens such as tests for thyroid function (see Section 4.4).

4.6 Pregnancy and lactation

Pregnancy

Harmogen 1.5 mg is not indicated during pregnancy. If pregnancy occurs during medication with Harmogen 1.5 mg treatment should be withdrawn immediately.

The results of most epidemiological studies to date relevant to inadvertent foetal exposure to estrogens indicate no teratogenic or foetoxic effects.

Lactation

Harmogen 1.5mg is not indicated during lactation.

4.7 Effects on ability to drive and use machines

None known

4.8 Undesirable effects

The following adverse reactions have been reported with Harmogen 1.5 mg estrogen therapy:

1. *Genito-urinary tract:* Endometrial neoplasia*, intermenstrual bleeding, increase in the size of uterine fibromyomata, endometrial proliferation or aggravation of endometriosis, changes in cervical eversion and excessive production of cervical mucus, candidal infections, thrush;
2. *Breast:* Tenderness, pain, enlargement or secretion, breast cancer*
3. *Gastro-intestinal tract*: Nausea, vomiting, abdominal cramp, bloating;
4. *Cardiovascular system*: Hypertension, thrombosis, thrombophlebitis, venous thromboembolism*, myocardial infarction* and stroke*;
5. *Liver/biliary system*: In rare cases benign, and in even rarer cases malignant liver tumours, cholelithiasis, cholestatic jaundice, gall bladder disease;
6. *Skin*: Chloasma which may persist when the drug is discontinued, erythema multiforme, erythema nodosum, vascular purpura, rash, loss of scalp hair, hirsutism;
7. *Eyes*: Steepening of corneal curvature, intolerance to contact lenses;
8. *CNS*: Headache, migraine, dizziness, mood changes (elation or depression), chorea, probable dementia (see Section 4.4);
9. Miscellaneous: Sodium and water retention, reduced glucose tolerance, change in body weight, muscle cramps, aggravation of porphyria, changes in libido.

* See sections 4.3, Contraindications and Section 4.4 Special Warnings and Special Precautions for Use.

Breast cancer

According to evidence from a large number of epidemiological studies and one randomised placebo-controlled trial, the Women's Health Initiative (WHI), the overall risk of breast cancer increases with increasing duration of HRT use in current or recent HRT users.

For *estrogen-only* HRT, estimates of relative risk (RR) from a reanalysis of original data from 51 epidemiological studies (in which >80% of HRT use was estrogen-only HRT) and from the epidemiological Million Women Study (MWS) are similar at 1.35 (95% CI 1.21 – 1.49) and 1.30 (95% CI 1.21 – 1.40), respectively.

For *estrogen plus progestogen* combined HRT, several epidemiological studies have reported an overall higher risk for breast cancer than with estrogens alone.

The MWS reported that, compared to never users, the use of various types of estrogen-progestogen combined HRT was associated with a higher risk of breast cancer (RR = 2.00, 95% CI: 1.88 – 2.12) than use of estrogens alone (RR = 1.30, 95% CI: 1.21 – 1.40) or use of tibolone (RR=1.45; 95%CI 1.25-1.68).

The WHI trial reported a risk estimate of 1.24 (95% CI 1.01 – 1.54) after 5.6 years of use of estrogen-progestogen combined HRT (CEE + MPA) in all users compared with placebo.

The absolute risks calculated from the MWS and the WHI trial are presented below:

The MWS has estimated, from the known average incidence of breast cancer in developed countries, that:

- *For women not using HRT, about 32 in every 1000 are expected to have breast cancer diagnosed between the ages of 50 and 64 years.*
- For 1000 current or recent users of HRT, the number of *additional* cases during the corresponding period will be
  - For users of *estrogen-only* replacement therapy
    - o between 0 and 3 (best estimate = 1.5) for 5 years' use
    - o between 3 and 7 (best estimate = 5) for 10 years' use.
  - For users of *estrogen plus progestogen* combined HRT
    - o between 5 and 7 (best estimate = 6) for 5 years' use
    - o between 18 and 20 (best estimate = 19) for 10 years' use

The WHI trial estimated that after 5.6 years of follow-up of women between the ages of 50 and 79 years, an *additional* 8 cases of invasive breast cancer would be due to *estrogen-progestogen combined* HRT (CEE + MPA) per 10,000 women years.

According to calculations from the trial data, it is estimated that:

- For 1000 women in the placebo group,
  - o about 16 cases of invasive breast cancer would be diagnosed in 5 years.
- For 1000 women who used estrogen + progestogen combined HRT (CEE + MPA), the number of *additional* cases would be
  - o between 0 and 9 (best estimate = 4) for 5 years' use.

The number of additional cases of breast cancer in women who use HRT is broadly similar for women who start HRT irrespective of age at start of use (between the ages of 45-65) (see Section 4.4).

Endometrial cancer

In women with an intact uterus, the risk of endometrial hyperplasia and endometrial cancer increases with increasing duration of use of unopposed estrogens. According to data from epidemiological studies, the best estimate of the risk is that for women not using HRT, about 5 in every 1000 are expected to have endometrial cancer diagnosed between the ages of 50 and 65. Depending on the duration of treatment and estrogen dose, the reported increase in endometrial cancer risk among unopposed estrogen users varies from 2-to 12-fold greater compared with non-users. Adding a progestogen to estrogen-only therapy greatly reduces this increased risk.

4.9 Overdose

Overdosage is unlikely to cause serious problems, although the following symptoms may be present, i.e. nausea and withdrawal bleeding in women. However gastric lavage or emesis may be used when considered appropriate.

5. PHARMACOLOGICAL PROPERTIES

5.1 Pharmacodynamic properties

Pharmacotherapeutic group: Natural and semisynthetic estrogens, plain.

ATC Code G03C A

Estropipate is a semi-synthetic estrogen conjugate, sulphate ester of estrone. This substitutes for the loss of estrogen production in menopausal women, and alleviates menopausal symptoms. Estrogens prevent bone loss following menopause or ovariectemy.

Estrogen deficiency at menopause is associated with an increasing bone turnover and decline in bone mass. The effect of estrogens on the bone mineral density is dose-dependent. Protection appears to be effective for as long as treatment is continued. After discontinuation of HRT, bone mass is lost at a rate similar to that in untreated women.

Evidence from the WHI trial and meta-analysed trials shows that current use of HRT, alone or in combination with a progestagen – given to predominantly healthy women – reduces the risk of hip, vertebral, and other osteoporotic fractures. HRT may also prevent fractures in women with low bone density and/or established osteoporosis, but the evidence for that is limited.

Women with an increased risk of osteoporosis include those suffering from an early menopause, receiving recent prolonged corticosteroid therapy, having a family history of osteoporosis, of small frame, who are thin, smokers and those with an excess alcohol intake.

5.2 Pharmacokinetic properties

Estropipate is metabolised in the liver, so any form of liver impairment will result in reduced metabolism.

Gastro-intestinal absorption of orally administered (tablets) estrogens is usually prompt and complete, inactivation of estrogens in the body occurs mainly in the liver. During cyclic passage through the liver, estrogens in the body are degraded to less active estrogenic compounds and conjugated with sulphuric and glucuronic acids. Estrone is 50-80% bound as it circulates in the blood, primarily as a conjugate with sulphate.

5.3 Preclinical safety data

No additional information is available.

6. PHARMACEUTICAL PARTICULARS

6.1 List of excipients

Lactose (monohydrate) NF

Lactose (anhydrous) NF

Dibasic potassium phosphate USP

Tromethamine USP

Hydroxypropyl cellulose NF

Sodium starch glycollate NF

Microcrystalline cellulose NF

Colloidal silicon dioxide NF

Magnesium stearate NF

Hydrogenated vegetable oil wax

Dye E110

Purified water USP

Alcohol 200 proof

6.2 Incompatibilities

None known

6.3 Shelf life

Three years

6.4 Special precautions for storage

None

6.5 Nature and contents of container

The containers comprise an HDPE container with tamper-evident cap or securitainer holding 100 estropipate tablets or a PVC/Aluminium foil blister pack, holding 28 tablets, which, together with a Patient Information Leaflet are packed in a carton.

6.6 Special precautions for disposal and other handling

No special instructions

Administrative Data

7. MARKETING AUTHORISATION HOLDER
Pharmacia Limited

Ramsgate Road

Sandwich

Kent CT13 9NJ

UK

8. MARKETING AUTHORISATION NUMBER(S)
PL 0032/0252

9. DATE OF FIRST AUTHORISATION/RENEWAL OF THE AUTHORISATION
7th June 2001/7th June 2003

10. DATE OF REVISION OF THE TEXT
April 2008

Legal category
POM
Ref: HA 5_0

Havrix Junior Monodose Vaccine

(GlaxoSmithKline UK)

1. NAME OF THE MEDICINAL PRODUCT
Havrix® Junior Monodose® vaccine

2. QUALITATIVE AND QUANTITATIVE COMPOSITION
Hepatitis A virus antigen, 720 ELISA units/0.5 ml dose.

For excipients, see Section 6.1.

3. PHARMACEUTICAL FORM
Vaccine for injection

4. CLINICAL PARTICULARS

4.1 Therapeutic indications
Havrix Junior Monodose vaccine is indicated for active immunisation against HAV infection. The vaccine is particularly indicated for those at increased risk of infection or transmission. It is also indicated for use during outbreaks of hepatitis A infection.

4.2 Posology and method of administration
Havrix Junior Monodose vaccine should be injected intramuscularly in the deltoid region. The vaccine should never be administered intravenously.

Dosage

Children/adolescents (1-15 years)

Primary immunisation consists of a single dose of Havrix Junior Monodose vaccine (720 ELISA units/0.5 ml) given intramuscularly. This provides anti-HAV antibodies for at least one year.

Havrix Junior Monodose confers protection against hepatitis A within two to four weeks.

In order to obtain more persistent immunity, for at least 10 years, a booster dose is recommended between 6 and 12 months after primary immunisation.

Booster vaccination with Havrix Junior Monodose delayed up to 3 years after the primary dose induces similar antibody levels as a booster dose administered within the recommended time interval.

Current recommendations do not support the need for further booster vaccination among immunocompetent subjects after a 2 dose vaccination course.

Havrix Junior Monodose can be used as a booster in subjects previously immunised with any inactivated hepatitis A vaccine.

In the event of a subject being exposed to a high risk of contracting hepatitis A within two weeks of the primary immunisation dose, human normal immunoglobulin may be given simultaneously with Havrix Junior Monodose at different injection sites.

4.3 Contraindications
Hypersensitivity to any component of the vaccine.

Severe febrile illness.

4.4 Special warnings and precautions for use
As with all vaccinations, appropriate medication e.g.epinephrine (adrenaline) should be readily available for immediate use in case of anaphylaxis. Havrix Junior Monodose may contain traces of the antibiotic neomycin B sulphate.

It is possible that subjects may be in the incubation period of a hepatitis A infection at the time of immunisation. It is not known whether Havrix Junior Monodose will prevent hepatitis A in such cases.

In haemodialysis patients and in subjects with an impaired immune system, adequate anti-HAV antibody titres may not be obtained after the primary immunisation and such patients may therefore require administration of additional doses of vaccine.

4.5 Interaction with other medicinal products and other forms of interaction
Simultaneous administration of Havrix with normal immunoglobulin does not influence the seroconversion rate to Havrix, however, it may result in a lower antibody titre. A similar effect could be observed with Havrix Junior Monodose.

Preliminary data on the concomitant administration of Havrix, at a dose of 720 ELISA units/ml, with recombinant hepatitis B virus vaccine suggests that there is no interference in the immune response to either antigen. On this basis and since it is an inactivated vaccine interference with immune response is unlikely to occur when Havrix Junior Monodose is administered with other inactivated or live vaccines. When concomitant administration is considered necessary the vaccines must be given at different injection sites.

Havrix Junior Monodose must not be mixed with other vaccines in the same syringe.

4.6 Pregnancy and lactation
The effect of Havrix Junior Monodose on foetal development has not been assessed. However, as with all inactivated viral vaccines the risks to the foetus are considered to be negligible. Havrix Junior Monodose should be used during pregnancy only when clearly needed.

The effect on breast-fed infants of the administration of Havrix Junior Monodose to their mothers has not been evaluated in clinical studies. Havrix Junior Monodose should therefore be used with caution in breast-feeding women.

4.7 Effects on ability to drive and use machines
Not applicable.

4.8 Undesirable effects
These are usually mild and confined to the first few days after vaccination. The most common reactions are mild transient soreness, erythema and induration at the injection site. Less common general complaints, not necessarily related to the vaccination, include headache, fever, malaise, fatigue, nausea, vomiting, diarrhoea and loss of appetite and rash. Arthralgia, myalgia, convulsions and allergic reactions including anaphylactoid reactions have been reported very rarely. Elevations of serum liver enzymes (usually transient) have been reported occasionally. However, a causal relationship with the vaccine has not been established.

Neurological manifestations occurring in temporal association have been reported extremely rarely with the vaccine and include transverse myelitis, Guillain-Barré syndrome and neuralgic amyotrophy. No causal relationship has been established.

4.9 Overdose
Not applicable.

5. PHARMACOLOGICAL PROPERTIES

5.1 Pharmacodynamic properties
Havrix confers immunisation against HAV by stimulating specific immune responses evidenced by the induction of antibodies against HAV.

In clinical studies involving subjects of 1 – 18 years of age, specific humoral antibodies against HAV were detected in 93% of vaccines at day 15 and 99% of vaccines one month following administration of Havrix Junior Monodose.

The efficacy of Havrix was evaluated in different community outbreaks. These studies indicated that administration of a single dose of Havrix contributed to termination of the outbreaks. In one study, vaccine coverage in excess of 80% was followed by termination of the outbreak within 4 to 8 weeks.

Long term persistence of hepatitis A antibody titres following 2 doses of Havrix given 6 to 12 months apart has been evaluated in adults. Data available after 10 years allows prediction that at least 97% of subjects will remain seropositive (>20 mIU/ml) 25 years after vaccination.

5.2 Pharmacokinetic properties
Not applicable.

5.3 Preclinical safety data
Not applicable to vaccine products.

6. PHARMACEUTICAL PARTICULARS

6.1 List of excipients
Aluminium hydroxide gel (3% w/w)

2 Phenoxyethanol

Polysorbate 20

Amino acids for injection

Disodium phosphate

Monopotassium phosphate

Sodium chloride

Potassium Chloride

Water for injections

6.2 Incompatibilities
Not applicable.

6.3 Shelf life
Havrix Junior Monodose vaccine has a shelf-life of three years from the date of manufacture when stored at 2-8°C.

6.4 Special precautions for storage
Store at 2 - 8°C in a refrigerator. Keep in outer container. Do not freeze.

6.5 Nature and contents of container
Neutral glass vials (type 1, PhEur) with grey butyl rubber stoppers and aluminium overcaps fitted with flip-off tops. 0.5 ml of suspension in prefilled syringe (type I glass) with a plunger stopper (rubber butyl) with or without needles - pack size of 1 or 10.

Not all pack sizes may be marketed.

6.6 Special precautions for disposal and other handling
The vaccine should be inspected visually for any foreign particulate matter and/or variation of physical aspect prior to administration. Before use, the vaccine should be well shaken to obtain a slightly opaque white suspension. Discard the vaccine if the content appears otherwise.

Administrative Data

7. MARKETING AUTHORISATION HOLDER
SmithKline Beecham plc

980 Great West Road, Brentford, Middlesex TW8 9GS

Trading as:

GlaxoSmithKline UK

Stockley Park West

Uxbridge

Middlesex UB11 1BT

8. MARKETING AUTHORISATION NUMBER(S)
PL 10592/0080.

9. DATE OF FIRST AUTHORISATION/RENEWAL OF THE AUTHORISATION
14 March 2003

10. DATE OF REVISION OF THE TEXT
15 March 2006

11. Legal Status
POM

Havrix Monodose Vaccine

(GlaxoSmithKline UK)

1. NAME OF THE MEDICINAL PRODUCT
Havrix® Monodose® Vaccine

2. QUALITATIVE AND QUANTITATIVE COMPOSITION
Each vial or syringe contains 1440 ELISA units/1 ml dose of hepatitis A virus antigen.

3. PHARMACEUTICAL FORM
Vaccine suspension for injection.

4. CLINICAL PARTICULARS

4.1 Therapeutic indications
Active immunisation against infections caused by hepatitis A virus. The vaccine is particularly indicated for those at increased risk of infection or transmission. For example immunisation should be considered for the following risk groups:

travellers visiting areas of medium or high endemicity, i.e. anywhere outside northern or western Europe, Australia, North America and New Zealand.

military and diplomatic personnel, haemophiliacs and patients, intravenous drug abusers, homosexual men, laboratory workers working directly with the hepatitis A virus, sanitation workers in contact with untreated sewage.

patients with chronic liver disease (including alcoholic cirrhosis, chronic hepatitis B, chronic hepatitis C, autoimmune hepatitis, primary biliary cirrhosis).

close contacts of hepatitis A cases.

Since virus shedding from infected persons may occur for a prolonged period, active immunisation of close contacts may be considered.

Under certain circumstances additional groups could be at increased risk of infection or transmission. Immunisation of such groups should be considered in the light of local circumstances. Such groups might include:

staff and inmates of residential institutions for the mentally handicapped and other institutions where standards of personal hygiene are poor.

staff working in day care centres and other settings with children who are not yet toilet trained.

food packagers or handlers.

In addition there may be other groups at risk or specific circumstances such as an outbreak of hepatitis A infection when immunisation should be given.

4.2 Posology and method of administration
Posology

Adults (16 years and over)

Primary immunisation consists of a single dose of Havrix Monodose vaccine (1440 ELISA units/ml) given intramuscularly. This provides anti-HAV antibodies for at least one year.

Havrix Monodose confers protection against hepatitis A within 2-4 weeks.

In order to obtain more persistent immunity, a booster dose is recommended between 6 and 12 months after primary immunisation.

Although a booster should be given within 6 – 12 months of the initial vaccination with Havrix Monodose, it has been shown that immunocompetent subjects given a booster up to 3 years after the initial vaccination can develop similar antibody levels to subjects given a booster within the recommended time period. Subjects given a booster up to 5 years after initial vaccination can also show a satisfactory antibody response but approximately 30% of individuals receiving a delayed booster have no detectable anti-HAV antibodies prior to booster dosing.

It is unnecessary to restart the primary vaccination schedule of Havrix Monodose if the booster is administered within 5 years of the primary vaccination.

Current recommendations do not support the need for further booster vaccination among immunocompetent subjects after a 2 dose vaccination course.

The results described above should be considered to apply only to immunocompetent adults.

Havrix Monodose can be used as a booster in subjects previously immunised with any inactivated hepatitis A vaccine.

In the event of a subject being exposed to a high risk of contracting hepatitis A within 2 weeks of the primary immunisation dose human normal immunoglobulin may be given simultaneously with Havrix Monodose at different injection sites.

Children/adolescents (1-15 years)

Havrix Monodose is not recommended (Havrix Junior Monodose should be used).

Method of administration

Havrix Monodose vaccine should be injected intramuscularly in the deltoid region.

The vaccine should never be administered intravenously.

4.3 Contraindications

Hypersensitivity to any component of the vaccine. Severe febrile illness.

4.4 Special warnings and precautions for use

As for all vaccinations, appropriate medication e.g.epinephrine (adrenaline) should be readily available for immediate use in case of anaphylaxis. Havrix Monodose may contain traces of the antibiotic neomycin B sulphate.

It is possible that subjects may be in the incubation period of a hepatitis A infection at the time of immunisation. It is not known whether Havrix Monodose will prevent hepatitis A in such cases.

In haemodialysis patients and in subjects with an impaired immune system, adequate anti-HAV antibody titres may not be obtained after the primary immunisation and such patients may therefore require administration of additional doses of vaccine.

4.5 Interaction with other medicinal products and other forms of interaction

Simultaneous administration of Havrix at a dose of 720 ELISA units/ml with ISG does not influence the seroconversion rate to Havrix, however, it may result in a lower antibody titre. A similar effect could be observed with Havrix Monodose.

Preliminary data on the concomitant administration of Havrix at a dose of 720 ELISA units/ml, with recombinant hepatitis B virus vaccine suggest that there is no interference in the immune response to either antigen. On this basis and since it is an inactivated vaccine interference with immune response is unlikely to occur when Havrix Monodose is administered with other inactivated or live vaccines. When concomitant administration is considered necessary the vaccines must be given at different injection sites.

Havrix Monodose must not be mixed with other vaccines in the same syringe.

4.6 Pregnancy and lactation

The effect of Havrix Monodose on foetal development has not been assessed.

However, as with all inactivated viral vaccines the risks to the foetus are considered negligible. Havrix Monodose should be used during pregnancy only when clearly needed.

The effect on breast fed infants of the administration of Havrix Monodose to their mothers has not been evaluated in clinical studies. Havrix Monodose should therefore be used with caution in breast feeding women.

4.7 Effects on ability to drive and use machines

Not applicable.

4.8 Undesirable effects

These are usually mild and confined to the first few days after vaccination. The most common reactions are mild transient soreness, erythema and induration at the injection site. Less common general complaints, not necessarily related to the vaccination, include headache, fever, malaise, fatigue, nausea, diarrhoea and loss of appetite and rash. Arthralgia, myalgia, convulsions and allergic reactions including anaphylactoid reactions have been reported very rarely. Elevations of serum liver enzymes (usually transient) have been reported occasionally. However, a causal relationship with the vaccine has not been established.

Neurological manifestations occurring in temporal association have been reported extremely rarely with the vaccine and included transverse myelitis, Guillain-Barre syndrome and neuralgic amyotrophy. No causal relationship has been established.

4.9 Overdose

Not applicable.

5. PHARMACOLOGICAL PROPERTIES

5.1 Pharmacodynamic properties

Havrix confers immunisation against HAV by stimulating specific immune responses evidenced by the induction of antibodies against HAV.

In clinical studies, 99% of vaccinees seroconverted 30 days after the first dose. In a subset of clinical studies where the kinetics of the immune response was studied, early and rapid seroconversion was demonstrated following administration of a single dose of Havrix in 79% of vaccinees at day 13, 86.3% at day 15, 95.2% at day 17 and 100% at day 19, which is shorter than the average incubation period of hepatitis A (4 weeks).

The efficacy of Havrix was evaluated in different community outbreaks. These studies indicated that administration of a single dose of Havrix contributed to termination of the outbreaks. In one study, vaccine coverage in excess of 80% was followed by termination of the outbreak within 4 to 8 weeks.

In order to ensure long term protection, a booster dose should be given between 6 and 12 months after the primary dose of Havrix Monodose. In clinical trials, virtually all vaccinees were seropositive one month after the booster dose.

Long term persistence of hepatitis A antibody titres following 2 doses of Havrix given 6 to 12 months apart has been evaluated. Data available after 10 years allows prediction that at least 97% of subjects will remain seropositive (>20 mIU/ml) 25 years after vaccination.

5.2 Pharmacokinetic properties

Not applicable to vaccine products.

5.3 Preclinical safety data

Not applicable to vaccine products.

6. PHARMACEUTICAL PARTICULARS

6.1 List of excipients

Aluminium hydroxide, polysorbate 20, amino acids for injection, disodium phosphate, monopotassium phosphate, sodium chloride, potassium chloride and water for injections.

6.2 Incompatibilities

Not applicable.

6.3 Shelf life

36 months.

6.4 Special precautions for storage

Store at 2°C - 8°C in a refrigerator. Keep in outer container. Do not freeze.

6.5 Nature and contents of container

Colourless glass vials (Type I, Ph Eur) with grey butyl rubber stoppers and aluminium overcaps fitted with avocado coloured flip-off tops containing 1 ml of suspension in packs of one and 10.

1 ml of suspension in prefilled syringe (type I glass) with a plunger stopper (rubber butyl) with or without needles - pack size of 1 or 10.

Not all pack sizes may be marketed.

6.6 Special precautions for disposal and other handling

The vaccine should be inspected visually for any foreign particulate matter and/or variation of physical aspect prior to administration. Before use, the vaccine should be well shaken to obtain a slightly opaque white suspension. Discard the vaccine if the content appears otherwise.

Administrative Data

7. MARKETING AUTHORISATION HOLDER

SmithKline Beecham plc

Great West Road, Brentford, Middlesex TW8 9GS

Trading as:

GlaxoSmithKline UK

Stockley Park West

Uxbridge

Middlesex

UB11 1BT

8. MARKETING AUTHORISATION NUMBER(S)

PL 10592/0037

9. DATE OF FIRST AUTHORISATION/RENEWAL OF THE AUTHORISATION

18 May 1999

10. DATE OF REVISION OF THE TEXT

1 April 2009

11. Legal category

POM

Helixate NexGen

(CSL Behring UK Limited)

1. NAME OF THE MEDICINAL PRODUCT

Helixate NexGen 250/500/1000/2000 IU Powder and solvent for solution for injection.

2. QUALITATIVE AND QUANTITATIVE COMPOSITION

Recombinant Coagulation factor VIII, 250/500/1000/2000 IU/vial.

INN: octocog alfa.

Recombinant Coagulation factor VIII is produced from genetically engineered baby hamster kidney cells containing the human factor VIII gene.

Solvent: water for injections.

Helixate NexGen 250/500/1000 IU:

The product reconstituted with the accompanying 2.5 ml of water for injections contains approximately 100/200/400 IU octocog alfa/ml.

Helixate NexGen 2000 IU:

The product reconstituted with the accompanying 5.0 ml of water for injections contains approximately 400 IU octocog alfa/ml.

The potency (IU) is determined using the one-stage clotting assay against the FDA Mega standard which was calibrated against WHO standard in IU.

The specific activity is approximately 4000 IU/mg protein.

For a full list of excipients, see section 6.1.

3. PHARMACEUTICAL FORM

Powder and solvent for solution for injection.

The powder is provided in a vial as a dry white to slightly yellow powder or cake.

The solvent is water for injections provided in a vial.

4. CLINICAL PARTICULARS

4.1 Therapeutic indications

Treatment and prophylaxis of bleeding in patients with haemophilia A (congenital factor VIII deficiency).

This preparation does not contain von Willebrand factor and is therefore not indicated in von Willebrand's disease.

4.2 Posology and method of administration

Treatment should be initiated under the supervision of a physician experienced in the treatment of haemophilia.

Posology

The number of units of factor VIII administered is expressed in International Units (IU), which are related to the current WHO standard for factor VIII products. Factor VIII activity in plasma is expressed either as a percentage (relative to normal human plasma) or in International Units (relative to the International Standard for factor VIII in plasma). One International Unit (IU) of factor VIII activity is equivalent to that quantity of factor VIII in one ml of normal human plasma. The calculation of the required dosage of factor VIII is based on the empirical finding that 1 International Unit (IU) factor VIII per kg body weight raises the plasma factor VIII activity by 1.5% to 2.5% of normal activity. The required dosage is determined using the following formulae:

I. Required IU = body weight (kg) × desired factor VIII rise (% of normal) × 0.5

II. Expected factor VIII rise (% of normal) = $\frac{2 \times \text{administered IU}}{\text{body weight (kg)}}$

The dosage and duration of the substitution therapy must be individualised according to the patient's needs (weight, severity of disorder of the haemostatic function, the site and extent of the bleeding, the titre of inhibitors, and the factor VIII level desired).

The following table provides a guide for factor VIII minimum blood levels. In the case of the haemorrhagic events listed, the factor VIII activity should not fall below the given level (in % of normal) in the corresponding period:

Degree of haemorrhage/ Type of surgical procedure	Factor VIII level required (%) (IU/dl)	Frequency of doses (hours)/ Duration of therapy (days)
Haemorrhage		
Early haemarthrosis, muscle bleed or oral bleed	20 - 40	Repeat every 12 to 24 hours. At least 1 day, until the bleeding episode as indicated by pain is resolved or healing is achieved.
More extensive haemarthrosis, muscle bleed or haematoma	30 - 60	Repeat infusion every 12 - 24 hours for 3 - 4 days or more until pain and disability are resolved.
Life threatening bleeds such as intracranial bleed, throat bleed, severe abdominal bleed	60 - 100	Repeat infusion every 8 to 24 hours until threat is resolved
Surgery		
Minor including tooth extraction	30 - 60	Every 24 hours, at least 1 day, until healing is achieved.

Major	80 - 100 (pre- and postoperative)	a) By bolus infusions Repeat infusion every 8 - 24 hours until adequate wound healing occurs, then continue with therapy for at least another 7 days to maintain a factor VIII activity of 30% to 60% b) By continuous infusion Raise factor VIII activity pre-surgery with an initial bolus infusion and immediately follow with continuous infusion (in IU/Kg/h) adjusting according to patient's daily clearance and desired factor VIII levels for at least 7 days.

The amount to be administered and the frequency of administration should always be adapted according to the clinical effectiveness in the individual case. Under certain circumstances larger amounts than those calculated may be required, especially in the case of the initial dose.

During the course of treatment, appropriate determination of factor VIII levels is advised in order to guide the dose to be administered and the frequency at which to repeat the infusions. In the case of major surgical interventions in particular, precise monitoring of the substitution therapy by means of coagulation analysis (plasma factor VIII activity) is indispensable. Individual patients may vary in their response to factor VIII, achieving different levels of *in vivo* recovery and demonstrating different half-lives.

It has been shown in a clinical study performed with adult haemophilia A patients who undergo a major surgery that Helixate NexGen can be used for continuous infusion in surgeries (pre-, during and postoperative). In this study heparin was used to prevent thrombophlebitis at the infusion site as with any other long term intravenous infusions. For the calculation of the initial infusion rate, clearance can be obtained by performing a pre-surgery decay curve, or by starting from an average population value (3.0-3.5 ml/h/Kg) and then adjust accordingly.

Infusion rate (in IU/Kg/h) = Clearance (in ml/h/Kg) × desired factor VIII level (in IU/ml)

For continuous infusion, clinical and *in vitro* stability has been demonstrated using ambulatory pumps with a PVC reservoir. Helixate NexGen contains low level of polysorbate-80 as an excipient, which is known to increase the rate of di-(2-ethylhexyl)phthalate (DEHP) extraction from polyvinyl chloride (PVC) materials. This should be considered for a continuous infusion administration.

For scheduled prophylaxis against bleeds in patients with severe haemophilia A, doses of 20 to 60 IU of Helixate NexGen per kg body weight should be given at intervals of 2 to 3 days. In some cases, especially in younger patients, shorter dosage intervals or higher doses may be necessary. Data have been obtained in 61 children under 6 years of age.

Patients with inhibitors

Patients should be monitored for the development of factor VIII inhibitors. If the expected plasma factor VIII activity levels are not attained, or if bleeding is not controlled with an appropriate dose, an assay should be performed to determine if a factor VIII inhibitor is present. If the inhibitor is present at levels less than 10 Bethesda Units (BU) per ml, administration of additional recombinant coagulation factor VIII may neutralise the inhibitor and permit continued clinically effective therapy with Helixate NexGen. However, in the presence of an inhibitor the doses required are variable and must be adjusted according to clinical response and monitoring of plasma factor VIII activity. In patients with inhibitor titres above 10 BU or with high anamnestic response, the use of (activated) prothrombin complex concentrate (PCC) or recombinant activated factor VII (rFVIIa) preparations has to be considered. These therapies should be directed by physicians with experience in the care of patients with haemophilia.

Administration

Dissolve the preparation as described in section 6.6.

Table 2

Medical Entity (PTs)			
System Organ Class	***Common**	***Uncommon**	***Rare**
Blood and the Lymphatic System Disorders	*Inhibitor Formation to FVIII (*Reported in PUP/MTP clinical trials)	**Inhibitor Formation to FVIII (**Reported in PTP and PMS)	
General Disorders and Administration Site Conditions	Infusion site reaction		Infusion related febrile reaction (pyrexia)
Immune System Disorders	Skin associated hypersensitivity reactions, (pruritus, urticaria and rash)		Systemic Hypersensitivity reactions (including one anaphylactic reaction, nausea, blood pressure abnormal and, dizziness)

Helixate NexGen should be injected intravenously over several minutes. The rate of administration should be determined by the patient's comfort level (maximal rate of infusion: 2 ml/min).

Helixate NexGen can be infused by continuous infusion. The infusion rate should be calculated based on the clearance and the desired FVIII level.

Example: for a 75 kg patient with a clearance of 3 ml/h/kg, the initial infusion rate would be 3 IU/h/kg to achieve a FVIII level of 100%. For calculation of ml/hour, multiply infusion rate in IU/h/kg by kg bw/concentration of solution (IU/ml).

(see Table 1 below)

Higher infusion rates may be required in conditions with accelerated clearance during major bleedings or extensive tissue damage during surgical interventions.

Subsequent infusion rates should be calculated based on the actual FVIII levels and recalculated clearance for each day post surgery based on the equation: clearance = infusion rate/actual FVIII level.

4.3 Contraindications

Known hypersensitivity to the active substance, to mouse or hamster protein or to any of the excipients.

4.4 Special warnings and precautions for use

As with any intravenous protein product, allergic type hypersensitivity reactions are possible.

Patients should be made aware that the potential occurrence of chest tightness, dizziness, mild hypotension and nausea during infusion can constitute an early warning for hypersensitivity and anaphylactic reactions. Symptomatic treatment and therapy for hypersensitivity should be instituted as appropriate. If allergic or anaphylactic reactions occur, the injection/infusion should be stopped immediately and patients should contact their physician. In case of shock, the current medical standards for shock treatment should be observed.

The formation of neutralising antibodies (inhibitors) to factor VIII is a known complication in the management of individuals with haemophilia A. These inhibitors are invariably IgG immunoglobulins directed against the factor VIII procoagulant activity, which are quantified in Modified Bethesda Units (BU) per ml of plasma. The risk of developing inhibitors is correlated to the exposure to anti-haemophilic factor VIII and to genetic factors among others, this risk being highest within the first 20 exposure days. Rarely, inhibitors may develop after the first 100 exposure days.

Cases of recurrence of inhibitors (low titre) have been observed after switching from one recombinant factor VIII product to another in previously treated patients with more than 100 exposure days who have a history of inhibitor development.

Patients treated with recombinant coagulation factor VIII should be carefully monitored for the development of inhibitors by appropriate clinical observations and laboratory tests. See also section 4.8 Undesirable effects.

In a clinical study about the use of continuous infusion in surgeries, heparin was used to prevent thrombophlebitis at the infusion site as with any other long term intravenous infusions.

In the interest of the patients, it is recommended that, whenever possible, every time that Helixate NexGen is administered to them, the name and the batch number of the product is registered.

This medicinal product contains less than 1 mmol sodium (23 mg) per vial, i.e. essentially "sodium free".

4.5 Interaction with other medicinal products and other forms of interaction

No interactions of Helixate NexGen with other medicinal products are known.

4.6 Pregnancy and lactation

Animal reproduction studies have not been conducted with Helixate NexGen.

Based on the rare occurrence of haemophilia A in women, experience regarding the use of Helixate NexGen during pregnancy and breast-feeding is not available. Therefore, Helixate NexGen should be used during pregnancy and lactation only if clearly indicated.

4.7 Effects on ability to drive and use machines4.7 Effects on ability to drive or use machines

Helixate NexGen has no influence on the ability to drive or to use machines.

4.8 Undesirable effects

The frequencies of adverse drug reactions reported with Helixate NexGen are summarized in the table below. Within each frequency group, undesirable effects are presented in order of decreasing seriousness. Frequencies are defined as common (≥ 1/100 to < 1/10), uncommon (≥ 1/1,000 to < 1/100), and rare (≥ 1/10,000 to < 1/1,000).

(see Table 2 above)

The formation of neutralising antibodies to factor VIII (inhibitors) is a known complication in the management of individuals with haemophilia A. In studies with recombinant factor VIII preparations, development of inhibitors is predominantly observed in previously untreated haemophiliacs. Patients should be carefully monitored for the development of inhibitors by appropriate clinical observations and laboratory tests.

In clinical studies, Helixate NexGen has been used in the treatment of bleeding episodes in 37 previously untreated patients (PUPs) and 23 minimally treated pediatric patients (MTPs, defined as having equal to or less than 4 exposure days). Five out of 37 (14%) PUP and 4 out of 23 (17%) MTP patients treated with Helixate NexGen developed inhibitors: Overall 6 out of 60 (10%) with a titre above 10 BU and 3 out of 60 (5%) with a titre below 10 BU. The median number of exposure days at the time of inhibitor detection in these patients was 9 days (range 3 - 18 days).

The median number of exposure days in the clinical studies was 114 (range: 4-478). Four of the five patients, who had not achieved 20 exposure days at the end of the study, ultimately achieved more than 20 exposure days in post-study follow-up and one of them developed a low titre inhibitor. The fifth patient was lost to follow-up.

In clinical studies with 73 previously treated patients (PTP, defined as having more than 100 exposure days), followed over four years, no de-novo inhibitors were observed.

In extensive post-registration studies with Helixate NexGen, involving more than 1000 patients the following was observed: Less than 0.2% PTP developed de-novo inhibitors. In a subset defined as having less than 20 exposure days at study entry, less than 11% developed de-novo inhibitors.

During studies, no patient developed clinically relevant antibody titres against the trace amounts of mouse protein and hamster protein present in the preparation. However, the possibility of allergic reactions to constituents, e.g. trace amounts of mouse and hamster protein in the preparation exists in certain predisposed patients (see sections 4.3 and 4.4).

4.9 Overdose

No symptoms of overdose with recombinant coagulation factor VIII have been reported.

5. PHARMACOLOGICAL PROPERTIES

5.1 Pharmacodynamic properties

Pharmacotherapeutic group: blood coagulation factor VIII, ATC-Code B02B D02.

Table 1

	Desired plasma FVIII level	Infusion rate IU/h/kg	Infusion rate for 75 kg patient ml/h
Clearance: 3 ml/h/kg			Concentrations of rFVIII solution 100 IU/ml 200 IU/ml 400 IU/ml
	100 % (1 IU/ml)	3.0	2.25 1.125 0.56
	60% (0.6 IU/ml)	1.8	1.35 0.68 0.34
	40% (0.4 IU/ml)	1.2	0.9 0.45 0.225

The factor VIII/von Willebrand factor (vWF) complex consists of two molecules (factor VIII and vWF) with different physiological functions. When infused into a haemophiliac patient, factor VIII binds to vWF in the patient's circulation. Activated factor VIII acts as a cofactor for activated factor IX, accelerating the conversion of factor X to activated factor X. Activated factor X converts prothrombin into thrombin. Thrombin then converts fibrinogen into fibrin and a clot can be formed. Haemophilia A is a sex-linked hereditary disorder of blood coagulation due to decreased levels of factor VIII:C and results in profuse bleeding into joints, muscles or internal organs, either spontaneously or as a results of accidental or surgical trauma. By replacement therapy the plasma levels of factor VIII are increased, thereby enabling a temporary correction of the factor deficiency and correction of the bleeding tendencies.

Determination of activated partial thromboplastin time (aPTT) is a conventional *in vitro* assay method for biological activity of factor VIII. The aPTT is prolonged in all haemophiliacs. The degree and duration of aPTT normalisation observed after administration of Helixate NexGen is similar to that achieved with plasma-derived factor VIII.

5.2 Pharmacokinetic properties

The analysis of all recorded *in vivo* recoveries in previously treated patients demonstrated a mean rise of 2 % per IU/kg body weight for Helixate NexGen. This result is similar to the reported values for factor VIII derived from human plasma.

After administration of Helixate NexGen, peak factor VIII activity decreased by a two-phase exponential decay with a mean terminal half-life of about 15 hours. This is similar to that of plasma-derived factor VIII which has a mean terminal half-life of approx. 13 hours. Additional pharmacokinetic parameters for Helixate NexGen for bolus injectionare: mean residence time [MRT (0-48)] of about 22 hours and clearance of about 160 ml/h. Mean baseline clearance for 14 adult patients undergoing major surgeries with continuous infusion are 188 ml/h corresponding to 3.0 ml/h/kg (range 1.6-4.6 ml/h/kg).

5.3 Preclinical safety data

Even doses several fold higher than the recommended clinical dose (related to body weight) failed to demonstrate any acute or subacute toxic effects for Helixate NexGen in laboratory animals (mouse, rat, rabbit, and dog).

Specific studies with repeated administration such as reproduction toxicity, chronic toxicity, and carcinogenicity were not performed with octocog alfa due to the immune response to heterologous proteins in all non-human mammalian species.

No studies were performed on the mutagenic potential of Helixate NexGen, since no mutagenic potential could be detected *in vitro* or *in vivo* for the predecessor product of Helixate NexGen.

6. PHARMACEUTICAL PARTICULARS

6.1 List of excipients

Powder

Glycine

Sodium chloride

Calcium chloride

Histidine

Polysorbate 80

Sucrose

Solvent

Water for injections

6.2 Incompatibilities

This medicinal product must not be mixed with other medicinal products or solvents.

Only the provided administration sets can be used because treatment failure can occur as a consequence of human coagulation factor VIII adsorption to the internal surfaces of some infusion equipment.

6.3 Shelf life

30 months.

After reconstitution, the product should be used immediately. However, chemical and physical in-use stability has been demonstrated for 48 hours at 30°C.

6.4 Special precautions for storage

Store in a refrigerator (2°C – 8°C). Do not freeze.

Keep the vials in the outer carton in order to protect from light.

The product when kept in its outer carton may be stored at ambient room temperature (up to 25°C) for a limited period of 3 months. In this case, the product expires at the end of this 3-month period; the new expiry date must be noted on the top of the outer carton.

Do not refrigerate after reconstitution.

For single use only.

Any unused solution must be discarded.

For storage conditions of the reconstituted medicinal product, see section 6.3.

6.5 Nature and contents of container

Each package of Helixate NexGen contains:

- one vial with powder (10 ml clear glass type 1 vial with latex-free grey halogenobutyl rubber blend stopper and aluminium seal)
- one vial with solvent (6 ml clear glass type 1 vial with latex-free grey chlorobutyl rubber blend stopper and aluminium seal)
- an additional package with:

- 1 filter transfer device 20/20
- 1 venipuncture set
- 1 disposable 5 ml syringe
- 2 sterile alcohol swabs for single use

6.6 Special precautions for disposal and other handling

Detailed instructions for preparation and administration are contained in the package leaflet provided with Helixate NexGen.

Helixate NexGen powder should only be reconstituted with the supplied solvent (2.5 or 5.0 ml water for injections) using the supplied sterile Mix2Vial filter transfer device. Reconstitution should be performed in accordance with good practices rules, particularly with attention to asepsis. Gently rotate the vial until all powder is dissolved. After reconstitution the solution is clear. Do not use Helixate NexGen if you notice visible particulate matter or turbidity.

After reconstitution, the solution is drawn through the Mix2Vial filter transfer device into the sterile disposable syringe (both supplied).

Use the provided venipuncture set for intravenous injection.

Any unused product or waste material should be disposed of in accordance with local requirements.

7. MARKETING AUTHORISATION HOLDER

Bayer Schering Pharma AG
13342 Berlin
Germany

8. MARKETING AUTHORISATION NUMBER(S)

Helixate NexGen 250 IU: EU/1/00/144/001

Helixate NexGen 500 IU: EU/1/00/144/002

Helixate NexGen 1000 IU: EU/1/00/144/003

Helixate NexGen 2000 IU: EU/1/00/144/004

9. DATE OF FIRST AUTHORISATION/RENEWAL OF THE AUTHORISATION

Date of first authorisation: 04 August 2000

Date of last renewal: 04 August 2005

10. DATE OF REVISION OF THE TEXT

01 October 2009

Hemabate Sterile Solution

(Pharmacia Limited)

1. NAME OF THE MEDICINAL PRODUCT

Hemabate Sterile Solution

2. QUALITATIVE AND QUANTITATIVE COMPOSITION

Each 1 ml contains carboprost tromethamine equivalent to carboprost 250 micrograms.

3. PHARMACEUTICAL FORM

Colourless, sterile, aqueous solution for intramuscular injection.

4. CLINICAL PARTICULARS

4.1 Therapeutic indications

Treatment of post-partum haemorrhage due to uterine atony and refractory to conventional methods of treatment with oxytocic agents and ergometrine used either alone or in combination.

Conventional therapy should usually consist of 0.5 - 1 mg ergometrine with up to 50 units of oxytocin infused intravenously over periods of time from 20 minutes to 12 hours. The dosage and duration of administration should reflect the seriousness of the clinical situation.

4.2 Posology and method of administration

Parenteral drug products should be inspected visually for particulate matter and discoloration prior to administration whenever solution and container permit.

An initial dose of 250 micrograms (1.0 ml) of Hemabate should be administered as a deep intramuscular injection.

If necessary, further doses of 250 micrograms may be administered at intervals of approximately 1.5 hours. In severe cases the interval between doses may be reduced at the discretion of the attending physician, but it should not be less than 15 minutes. The total dose of Hemabate should not exceed 2 mg (8 doses).

Elderly: Not applicable

Children: Not applicable

4.3 Contraindications

Hemabate should not be used where the patient is sensitive to carboprost tromethamine or any of the excipients.

Hemabate is not recommended in the following circumstances:

1. Acute pelvic inflammatory disease.
2. Patients with known cardiac, pulmonary, renal or hepatic disease.

4.4 Special warnings and precautions for use

Warnings

This preparation should not be used for induction of labour.

Hemabate, as with other potent oxytocic agents, should be used only with strict adherence to recommended dosages. Hemabate should be used by medically trained personnel and is available only to hospitals and clinics with specialised obstetric units where 24 hour resident medical cover is provided.

Hemabate must not be given intravenously.

Very rare cases of cardiovascular collapse have been reported following the use of prostaglandins. This should always be considered when using Hemabate.

Precautions

Hemabate should be used with caution in patients with a history of glaucoma or raised intra-ocular pressure, asthma, hypertension or hypotension, cardiovascular disease, renal disease, hepatic disease, anaemia, jaundice, diabetes or epilepsy.

Animal studies lasting several weeks at high doses have shown that prostaglandins of the E and F series can induce proliferation of bone. Such effects have also been noted in newborn infants who have received prostaglandin E_1 during prolonged treatment. There is no evidence that short-term administration of Hemabate can cause similar bone effects.

Decreases in maternal arterial oxygen content have been observed in patients treated with carboprost tromethamine. A causal relationship to carboprost tromethamine has not been established, however, it is recommended that patients with pre-existing cardio-pulmonary problems receiving Hemabate are monitored during treatment and given additional oxygen if necessary.

4.5 Interaction with other medicinal products and other forms of interaction

Prostaglandins may potentiate the effect of oxytocin

4.6 Pregnancy and lactation

Hemabate is contra-indicated in pregnancy.

In the unlikely event of a mother breastfeeding her baby whilst receiving Hemabate, no adverse effects to the nursing infant would be anticipated.

4.7 Effects on ability to drive and use machines

Not applicable

4.8 Undesirable effects

The adverse effects of Hemabate are generally transient and reversible when therapy ends.

The most frequent side-effects observed with the use of Hemabate are related to its contractile effect on smooth muscle. Thus nausea, vomiting and diarrhoea have been reported as commonly encountered. The incidence of vomiting and diarrhoea may be decreased by pre-treatment and concomitant use during treatment of anti-emetic and antidiarrhoeal agents.

Hyperthermia and flushing have been observed after intramuscular Hemabate, but if not complicated by endometritis, the temperature will usually return to normal within several hours of the last injection.

Asthma and wheezing have been noted with Hemabate treatment.

Less frequent, but potentially more serious adverse effects are elevated blood pressure, dyspnoea and pulmonary oedema. Other less serious adverse effects noted include chills, headache, diaphoresis, dizziness and injection site erythema and pain.

4.9 Overdose

Treatment of overdosage must be symptomatic at this time, as clinical studies with prostaglandin antagonists have not progressed to the point where recommendations may be made.

If evidence of excessive side-effects appears, the frequency of administration should be decreased or administration discontinued.

5. PHARMACOLOGICAL PROPERTIES

5.1 Pharmacodynamic properties

Carboprost is a synthetic 15-methyl analogue of dinoprost (prostaglandin F2 alpha). It is a uterine stimulant with a more prolonged action than dinoprost and when used in post-partum haemorrhage, it stimulates the uterus to contract in a manner similar to that normally observed in the uterus following delivery. The resulting myometrial contractions provide haemostasis at the site of placentation and hence prevent further blood loss. Whether or not this action results from a direct effect on the myometrium has not been determined with certainty at this time. The fundamental actions of the prostaglandins include inhibition or stimulation of smooth muscle contraction and inhibition of the release of noradrenaline or modulation of its effects at neuroeffector sites. They affect the uterus, the cardiovascular system, the gastro-intestinal system, the nervous system, the urinary system and metabolic processes.

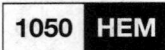

5.2 Pharmacokinetic properties
The presence of the methyl group delays inactivation by enzymic dehydrogenation.

Peak plasma levels vary depending on the route of administration. In the Rhesus monkey after a single i.m. injection of 20 - 30 micrograms of 15-methyl PGF2 alpha peak levels of 0.4 - 5 nanograms/ml resulted at 30 - 60 minutes, declining to baseline levels 6 - 8 hours after injection. In pregnant women, an i.m. injection of 100 - 400 micrograms resulted in peak plasma levels of 1 - 1.6 nanograms/ml 20 - 30 minutes after injection. Levels declined to 0.2 - 0.4 nanograms/ml after 3 hours. When i.m. doses of 250 micrograms were given every two hours, pre-injection plasma levels stabilised after four injections at 1.2 nanograms/ml.

After administration of 2.5 mg 15-methyl PGF2 alpha intra-amniotically to 5 subjects, plasma levels were from 100 - 580 picograms/ml during the first 15 hours after administration. In three subjects the levels were low and fairly constant, while the two other had higher, but more variable levels.

6. PHARMACEUTICAL PARTICULARS
6.1 List of excipients
Benzyl alcohol
Sodium chloride
Tromethamine
Sodium hydroxide
Hydrochloric acid
Water for injections

6.2 Incompatibilities
None known

6.3 Shelf life
Ampoules: 48 months
Vial: 24 months

6.4 Special precautions for storage
The ampoules must be stored in a refrigerator at 2 - 8°C.
The vial must be stored in a refrigerator at 0 - 6°C

6.5 Nature and contents of container
Ampoule: Type 1 glass ampoule containing 1 ml solution, packed in cartons of two or ten ampoules.

Vial: Type 1 glass with butyl rubber closure, containing 10 ml solution, packed individually in a carton.

6.6 Special precautions for disposal and other handling
Parenteral drug products should be inspected visually for particulate matter and discoloration prior to administration whenever solution and container permit.

Administrative Data
7. MARKETING AUTHORISATION HOLDER
Pharmacia Limited
Ramsgate Road
Sandwich
Kent CT13 9NJ
UK

8. MARKETING AUTHORISATION NUMBER(S)
PL 0032/0152

9. DATE OF FIRST AUTHORISATION/RENEWAL OF THE AUTHORISATION
16 August 1990/23 February 1996

10. DATE OF REVISION OF THE TEXT
May 2007

Legal category:
POM
Company Ref: HM 2_0

Heminevrin Capsules
(AstraZeneca UK Limited)

1. NAME OF THE MEDICINAL PRODUCT
Heminevrin 192 mg Capsules.

2. QUALITATIVE AND QUANTITATIVE COMPOSITION
Clomethiazole 192 mg (base) per capsule.
10 mg Sorbitol (E420) per capsule.
For a full list of excipients, see 6.1.

3. PHARMACEUTICAL FORM
Soft Capsules
Greyish-brown, soft gelatin capsules

4. CLINICAL PARTICULARS
4.1 Therapeutic indications
Heminevrin is a short acting hypnotic and sedative with anticonvulsant effect. It is used for the: management of restlessness and agitation in the elderly, short term treatment of severe insomnia in the elderly and treatment of alcohol withdrawal symptoms where close hospital supervision is also provided.

4.2 Posology and method of administration
For oral use.
The capsules should be swallowed whole.

Management of restlessness and agitation in the elderly: one capsule three times daily.

Severe insomnia in the elderly: 1 - 2 capsules before going to bed. The lower dose should be tried first. As with all psychotropic drugs, treatment should be kept to a minimum, reviewed regularly and discontinued as soon as possible.

Alcohol withdrawal states: Heminevrin is not a specific 'cure' for alcoholism. Alcohol withdrawal should be treated in hospital or, in exceptional circumstances, on an out-patient basis by specialist units when the daily dosage of Heminevrin must be monitored closely by community health staff. The dosage should be adjusted to patient response. The patient should be sedated but rousable. A suggested regimen is:

Initial dose:	2 to 4 capsules, if necessary repeated after some hours.
Day 1, first 24 hours:	9 to 12 capsules, divided into 3 or 4 doses.
Day 2:	6 to 8 capsules, divided into 3 or 4 doses.
Day 3:	4 to 6 capsules, divided into 3 or 4 doses.
Days 4 to 6:	A gradual reduction in dosage until the final dose.

Administration for more than nine (9) days is not recommended.

4.3 Contraindications
Known sensitivity to clomethiazole. Acute pulmonary insufficiency.

4.4 Special warnings and precautions for use
Heminevrin should be used cautiously in patients with sleep apnoea syndrome and chronic pulmonary insufficiency. Heminevrin may potentiate or be potentiated by centrally acting depressant drugs including alcohol and benzodiazepines. Fatal cardiorespiratory collapse has been reported when clomethiazole was combined with other CNS depressant drugs. When used concomitantly dosage should be appropriately reduced.

Hypoxia, resulting from, for example, cardiac and/or respiratory insufficiency, can manifest itself as an acute confusional state. Recognition and specific treatment of the cause is essential in such patients and in such cases sedatives/hypnotics should be avoided.

Moderate liver disorders associated with alcoholism do not preclude the use of clomethiazole, though an associated increase in systemic availability of oral doses and delayed elimination of the drug may require reduced dosage. Great caution should be observed in patients with gross liver damage and decreased liver function, particularly as sedation can mask the onset of liver coma.

Caution should be observed in patients with chronic renal disease.

Caution must be exercised in prescribing for individuals known to be addiction prone or for those whose histories suggest they may increase the dose on their own initiative since clomethiazole is not free from the risk of producing psychological and/or physical dependence. After prolonged administration of high doses, physical dependence has been reported with withdrawal symptoms such as convulsions, tremors, and organic psychosis. These reports have mainly been associated with indiscriminate prescribing to outpatient alcoholics and Heminevrin should not be prescribed to patients who continue to drink or abuse alcohol.

Alcoholism: Alcohol combined with clomethiazole particularly in alcoholics with cirrhosis can lead to fatal respiratory depression even with short term use. It should not therefore be prescribed for alcoholics who continue to drink alcoholic beverages.

Elderly: Caution is advised as there may be increased bioavailability and delayed elimination of clomethiazole.

Children: Oral Heminevrin is not recommended for use in children.

One capsule of Heminevrin contains 10 mg of sorbitol. When taken according to the dosage recommendations each dose supplies up to 40 mg of sorbitol. Unsuitable in hereditary fructose intolerance.

4.5 Interaction with other medicinal products and other forms of interaction
A combination of clomethiazole and diazoxide should be avoided as an adverse neonatal reaction suspected to be due to the maternal administration of this combination has been reported.

The combination of propranolol and clomethiazole has produced profound bradycardia in one patient possibly due to increased bioavailability of propranolol.

There is evidence to indicate that the metabolism of clomethiazole is inhibited by cimetidine, thus the co-administration of these drugs may lead to increased blood/plasma levels of clomethiazole.

When clomethiazole was administered by intravenous infusion in combination with carbamazepine, the clearance of clomethiazole increased by 30%, resulting in decreased plasma concentrations to the same extent. This interaction has not been studied after oral administration of clomethiazole. However, co-administration of carbamazepine and oral clomethiazole could result in both decreased bioavailability and increased clearance. Higher doses of clomethiazole could therefore be needed to obtain an effect when co-administered with carbamazepine or another potent inducer of the CYP3A4 enzyme.

4.6 Pregnancy and lactation
Do not use in pregnancy especially during the first and last trimesters, unless there are compelling reasons. There is no evidence of safety in human pregnancy, nor is there evidence from animal studies that it is entirely free from hazard.

Clomethiazole is excreted into the breast milk. The effect of even small quantities of sedative/hypnotic and anticonvulsant drugs on the infant brain is not established.

Clomethiazole should only be used in nursing mothers where the physician considers that the benefit outweighs the possible hazard to the infant.

4.7 Effects on ability to drive and use machines
As with all centrally acting depressant drugs, the driving of vehicles and the operating of machinery are to be avoided when under treatment.

4.8 Undesirable effects
The most common side-effect is nasal congestion and irritation, which may occur 15 to 20 minutes after drug ingestion. Conjunctival irritation has also been noted in some cases. Occasionally, these symptoms may be severe and may be associated with severe headache. This is commonest with the initial dose following which it decreases in severity with subsequent doses. Increased nasopharyngeal/bronchial secretions can occur.

Rash and urticaria have been reported. In rare cases, bullous skin eruptions have been reported.

Gastrointestinal disturbances have been reported.

Reversible increases of transaminases or bilirubin have been reported.

In rare cases anaphylactic reactions have occurred.

When Heminevrin has been given at higher than recommended doses for other than recommended indications over prolonged periods of time, physical dependence, tolerance and withdrawal reactions have been reported.

Great caution is required in prescribing Heminevrin for patients with a history of chronic alcoholism, drug abuse or marked personality disorder.

When used as a night-time hypnotic, hangover effects in the elderly may occur but are uncommon due to the short half-life.

Excessive sedation may occur, especially with higher doses or when given to the elderly for daytime sedation. Paradoxical excitement or confusion may occur rarely.

4.9 Overdose
The main effects to be expected with overdose of Heminevrin are: coma, respiratory depression, hypotension and hypothermia.

Hypothermia is thought to be due to a direct central effect as well as a result of lying unconscious for several hours. In addition, patients have increased secretion in the upper airways, which in one series was associated with a high incidence of pneumonia. The effects of overdosage are not usually severe in patients with no evidence of alcoholic liver disease, but they may be exacerbated when clomethiazole is taken in combination with alcohol and/or CNS depressant drugs, particularly those that are metabolised by the liver. There is no specific antidote to clomethiazole. Treatment of overdosage should therefore be carried out on a symptomatic basis, applying similar principles to those used in the treatment of barbiturate overdosage.

Charcoal column haemoperfusion is not and cannot be expected to be effective in treating clomethiazole poisoning.

5. PHARMACOLOGICAL PROPERTIES
5.1 Pharmacodynamic properties
Clomethiazole is pharmacologically distinct from both the benzodiazepines and the barbiturates

Clomethiazole has sedative, muscle relaxant and anticonvulsant properties. It is used for hypnosis in elderly and institutionalised patients, for preanaesthetic sedation and especially in the management of withdrawal from ethanol. Given alone its effects on respiration are slight and the therapeutic index high.

5.2 Pharmacokinetic properties
Clomethiazole has a short half-life, low oral bioavailability, high plasma clearance and shows no evidence of accumulation or altered pharmacokinetics after repeated dosage. It is excreted in urine after extensive metabolism in the liver. The rate of elimination is decreased by about 30% in liver cirrhosis.

5.3 Preclinical safety data
Extensive clinical use and experience with clomethiazole has provided a well established safety profile for this drug.

6. PHARMACEUTICAL PARTICULARS
6.1 List of excipients
Medium-chain triglycerides, Gelatin, Glycerol (85%), Sorbitol (E420), Mannitol, Oligosaccharides, Titanium Dioxide (E171), Brown Iron Oxide (E172).

6.2 Incompatibilities
Not applicable.

6.3 Shelf life
Amber glass bottles: 24 months.

Aluminium foil blister packs: 24 months.

6.4 Special precautions for storage
Do not store above 25°C.

Store in the original container.

6.5 Nature and contents of container
Amber glass bottle with either a screw cap or clic-loc cap containing 60 or 100 capsules.

Transparent plastic bag in a cardboard outer for bulk packaging of 20,000 capsules.

Aluminium foil blister packs each containing 10 capsules.
Not all pack sizes may be marketed.

6.6 Special precautions for disposal and other handling
The capsules should remain in the container in which they are supplied.

The capsules should be swallowed whole.

7. MARKETING AUTHORISATION HOLDER
AstraZeneca UK Ltd.,

600 Capability Green,

Luton,

LU1 3LU,

UK.

8. MARKETING AUTHORISATION NUMBER(S)
PL 17901/0126

9. DATE OF FIRST AUTHORISATION/RENEWAL OF THE AUTHORISATION
18th March 2002 / 7th March 2003

10. DATE OF REVISION OF THE TEXT
12th August 2009

Heminevrin Syrup

(AstraZeneca UK Limited)

1. NAME OF THE MEDICINAL PRODUCT
Heminevrin 31.5 mg/ml Syrup.

2. QUALITATIVE AND QUANTITATIVE COMPOSITION
Clomethiazole edisilate 50 mg/ml (equivalent to 31.5 mg/ml of clomethiazole).

Heminevrin syrup contains 0.13 vol % of ethanol.

1 ml of syrup contains 350 mg of Sorbitol (E420).

For a full list of excipients, see 6.1

3. PHARMACEUTICAL FORM
Syrup.

4. CLINICAL PARTICULARS

4.1 Therapeutic indications
Heminevrin is a short acting hypnotic and sedative with anticonvulsant effect. It is used for the: management of restlessness and agitation in the elderly, short term treatment of severe insomnia in the elderly and treatment of alcohol withdrawal symptoms where close hospital supervision is also provided.

4.2 Posology and method of administration
For oral use

Management of restlessness and agitation in the elderly: 5ml of syrup three times daily.

Severe insomnia in the elderly: 5 - 10ml of the syrup before going to bed. The lower dose should be tried first. As with all psychotropic drugs, treatment should be kept to a minimum, reviewed regularly and discontinued as soon as possible.

Alcohol withdrawal states: Heminevrin is not a specific 'cure' for alcoholism. Alcohol withdrawal should be treated in hospital or, in exceptional circumstances, on an out-patient basis by specialist units when the daily dosage of Heminevrin must be monitored closely by community health staff. The dosage should be adjusted to patient response. The patient should be sedated but rousable. A suggested regimen is:

Initial dose:	10 to 20ml, if necessary repeated after some hours.
Day 1, first 24 hours:	45 to 60ml, divided into 3 or 4 doses.
Day 2:	30 to 40ml, divided into 3 or 4 doses.
Day 3:	20 to 30ml, divided into 3 or 4 doses.
Days 4 to 6:	A gradual reduction in dosage until the final dose.

Administration for more than nine (9) days is not recommended.

4.3 Contraindications
Known sensitivity to clomethiazole. Acute pulmonary insufficiency.

4.4 Special warnings and precautions for use
Heminevrin should be used cautiously in patients with sleep apnoea syndrome and chronic pulmonary insufficiency. Heminevrin may potentiate or be potentiated by centrally acting depressant drugs including alcohol and benzodiazepines. Fatal cardiorespiratory collapse has been reported when clomethiazole was combined with other CNS depressant drugs. When used concomitantly dosage should be appropriately reduced.

Hypoxia, resulting from, for example, cardiac and/or respiratory insufficiency, can manifest itself as an acute confusional state. Recognition and specific treatment of the cause is essential in such patients and in such cases sedatives/hypnotics should be avoided.

Moderate liver disorders associated with alcoholism do not preclude the use of clomethiazole, though an associated increase in systemic availability of oral doses and delayed elimination of the drug may require reduced dosage. Great caution should be observed in patients with gross liver damage and decreased liver function, particularly as sedation can mask the onset of liver coma.

Caution should be observed in patients with chronic renal disease.

Caution must be exercised in prescribing for individuals known to be addiction prone or for those whose histories suggest they may increase the dose on their own initiative since clomethiazole is not free from the risk of producing psychological and/or physical dependence. After prolonged administration of high doses, physical dependence has been reported with withdrawal symptoms such as convulsions, tremors, and organic psychosis. These reports have mainly been associated with indiscriminate prescribing to outpatient alcoholics and Heminevrin should not be prescribed to patients who continue to drink or abuse alcohol.

Alcoholism: Alcohol combined with clomethiazole particularly in alcoholics with cirrhosis can lead to fatal respiratory depression even with short term use. It should not therefore be prescribed for alcoholics who continue to drink alcoholic beverages.

Elderly: Caution is advised as there may be increased bioavailability and delayed elimination of clomethiazole.

Children: Oral Heminevrin is not recommended for use in children.

Heminevrin syrup contains 0.13 vol % of ethanol. Each dose contains up to 20 mg of alcohol. Harmful for those suffering from liver disease, alcoholism, epilepsy, brain injury or disease, as well as for pregnant women and children. May modify or increase the effect of other medicines.

One ml of Heminevrin syrup contains 350 mg of sorbitol. When taken according to the dosage recommendations each dose supplies up to 7 g of sorbitol. Unsuitable in hereditary fructose intolerance. Can cause stomach upset and diarrhoea.

4.5 Interaction with other medicinal products and other forms of interaction
A combination of clomethiazole and diazoxide should be avoided as an adverse neonatal reaction suspected to be due to the maternal administration of this combination has been reported.

The combination of propranolol and clomethiazole has produced profound bradycardia in one patient possibly due to increased bioavailability of propranolol.

There is evidence to indicate that the metabolism of clomethiazole is inhibited by cimetidine, thus the co-administration of these drugs may lead to increased blood/plasma levels of clomethiazole.

When clomethiazole was administered by intravenous infusion in combination with carbamazepine, the clearance of clomethiazole increased by 30%, resulting in decreased plasma concentrations to the same extent. This interaction has not been studied after oral administration of clomethiazole. However, co-administration of carbamazepine and oral clomethiazole could result in both decreased bioavailability and increased clearance. Higher doses of clomethiazole could therefore be needed to obtain an effect when co-administered with carbamazepine or another potent inducer of the CYP3A4 enzyme.

4.6 Pregnancy and lactation
Do not use in pregnancy especially during the first and last trimesters, unless there are compelling reasons. There is no evidence of safety in human pregnancy, nor is there evidence from animal studies that it is entirely free from hazard.

Clomethiazole is excreted into the breast milk. The effect of even small quantities of sedative/hypnotic and anticonvulsant drugs on the infant brain is not established.

Clomethiazole should only be used in nursing mothers where the physician considers that the benefit outweighs the possible hazard to the infant.

4.7 Effects on ability to drive and use machines
As with all centrally acting depressant drugs, the driving of vehicles and the operating of machinery are to be avoided when under treatment.

4.8 Undesirable effects
The most common side-effect is nasal congestion and irritation, which may occur 15 to 20 minutes after drug ingestion. Conjunctival irritation has also been noted in some cases. Occasionally, these symptoms may be severe and may be associated with severe headache. This is commonest with the initial dose following which it decreases in severity with subsequent doses. Increased nasopharyngeal/bronchial secretions can occur.

Rash and urticaria have been reported. In rare cases, bullous skin eruptions have been reported.

Gastrointestinal disturbances have been reported.

Reversible increases of transaminases or bilirubin have been reported.

In rare cases anaphylactic reactions have occurred.

When Heminevrin has been given at higher than recommended doses for other than recommended indications over prolonged periods of time, physical dependence, tolerance and withdrawal reactions have been reported.

Great caution is required in prescribing Heminevrin for patients with a history of chronic alcoholism, drug abuse or marked personality disorder.

When used as a night-time hypnotic, hangover effects in the elderly may occur but are uncommon due to the short half-life.

Excessive sedation may occur, especially with higher doses or when given to the elderly for daytime sedation. Paradoxical excitement or confusion may occur rarely.

4.9 Overdose
The main effects to be expected with overdose of Heminevrin are: coma, respiratory depression, hypotension and hypothermia.

Hypothermia is thought to be due to a direct central effect as well as a result of lying unconscious for several hours. In addition, patients have increased secretion in the upper airways, which in one series was associated with a high incidence of pneumonia. The effects of overdosage are not usually severe in patients with no evidence of alcoholic liver disease, but they may be exacerbated when clomethiazole is taken in combination with alcohol and/or CNS depressant drugs, particularly those that are metabolised by the liver. There is no specific antidote to clomethiazole. Treatment of overdosage should therefore be carried out on a symptomatic basis, applying similar principles to those used in the treatment of barbiturate overdosage.

Charcoal column haemoperfusion is not and cannot be expected to be effective in treating clomethiazole poisoning.

5. PHARMACOLOGICAL PROPERTIES

5.1 Pharmacodynamic properties
Clomethiazole is pharmacologically distinct from both the benzodiazepines and the barbiturates

Clomethiazole has sedative, muscle relaxant and anticonvulsant properties. It is used for hypnosis in elderly and institutionalised patients, for preanaesthetic sedation and especially in the management of withdrawal from ethanol. Given alone its effects on respiration are slight and the therapeutic index high.

5.2 Pharmacokinetic properties
Clomethiazole has a short half-life, low oral bioavailability, high plasma clearance and shows no evidence of accumulation or altered pharmacokinetics after repeated dosage. It is excreted in urine after extensive metabolism in the liver. The rate of elimination is decreased by about 30% in liver cirrhosis.

5.3 Preclinical safety data
Extensive clinical use and experience with clomethiazole has provided a well established safety profile for this drug.

6. PHARMACEUTICAL PARTICULARS

6.1 List of excipients
Liquid Sorbitol (non-crystallising), Cineole, Levomenthol, Ethanol 99.5% vol, Sodium hydroxide, Purified water.

6.2 Incompatibilities
Not applicable.

6.3 Shelf life
2 years.

6.4 Special precautions for storage
Store in a refrigerator (2° to 8°C). Do not freeze.

6.5 Nature and contents of container
300ml amber glass type III bottle with a white polypropylene cap.

6.6 Special precautions for disposal and other handling
No special requirements.

7. MARKETING AUTHORISATION HOLDER
AstraZeneca UK Ltd.,

600 Capability Green,

Luton, LU1 3LU, UK.

8. MARKETING AUTHORISATION NUMBER(S)
PL 17901/0127

9. DATE OF FIRST AUTHORISATION/RENEWAL OF THE AUTHORISATION
18th March 2002 / 7th March 2003

10. DATE OF REVISION OF THE TEXT
13th December 2007

Hepatyrix

(GlaxoSmithKline UK)

1. NAME OF THE MEDICINAL PRODUCT
Hepatyrix, suspension for injection

Hepatitis A (inactivated) and Typhoid Polysaccharide vaccine (adsorbed).

2. QUALITATIVE AND QUANTITATIVE COMPOSITION
1 dose (1 ml) contains:

Hepatitis A virus (HM175 strain) (inactivated)[1] 1440 ELISA Units

Vi polysaccharide of *Salmonella typhi* (Ty2 strain) 25 micrograms

[1] Produced in human diploid (MRC-5) cells

Adsorbed on aluminium hydroxide, hydrated 0.5 milligrams Al^{3+}

For a full list of excipients, see section 6.1.

3. PHARMACEUTICAL FORM
Suspension for injection.

Slightly opaque white suspension.

4. CLINICAL PARTICULARS
4.1 Therapeutic indications
Active immunisation against hepatitis A virus infection and typhoid fever for adults and adolescents 15 years of age and older.

Hepatyrix should be given in accordance with official recommendations.

4.2 Posology and method of administration
Posology

Primary vaccination

A single dose of 1.0 ml is recommended for both adults and adolescents aged 15 years and older.

The vaccine should be given at least two weeks prior to risk of exposure to typhoid and hepatitis A (see section 5.1 for immunogenicity data).

Booster vaccination

In order to provide long term protection against infection caused by hepatitis A virus, a booster dose of an inactivated hepatitis A vaccine is recommended at any time between 6 and 12 months after a single dose of Hepatyrix.

Hepatyrix may also be given as a single dose of 1.0 ml for booster vaccination between 6 and 12 months following primary immunisation with an inactivated hepatitis A vaccine to subjects who also require protection against typhoid fever.

Subjects who remain at risk of typhoid fever should be revaccinated using a single dose of Vi polysaccharide vaccine every 3 years (see section 5.1). Hepatyrix may be used to revaccinate against typhoid fever in subjects that also need to have a dose of hepatitis A vaccine.

As Hepatyrix has not been studied in subjects under 15 years of age, it is not recommended for use in this age group.

Method of administration

Hepatyrix is for intramuscular administration in the deltoid region.

The vaccine should not be administered in the gluteal region.

Hepatyrix should under no circumstances be administered intravascularly.

Hepatyrix should not be administered subcutaneously/intradermally since administration by these routes may result in a suboptimal response to the vaccine.

In exceptional circumstances, Hepatyrix may be administered subcutaneously to subjects with thrombocytopenia or bleeding disorders since bleeding may occur following an intramuscular administration to these subjects. Firm pressure should be applied to the injection site (without rubbing) for at least two minutes after the injection.

4.3 Contraindications
Hepatyrix should not be administered to subjects who have had a hypersensitivity reaction to a previous dose of Hepatyrix or a dose of either of the monovalent vaccines Havrix and Typherix.

Hepatyrix should not be administered to subjects who are known to be hypersensitive to any component of the vaccine.

Hepatyrix contains traces of neomycin. The vaccine should not be used in subjects with known hypersensitivity to neomycin.

As with other vaccines, the administration of Hepatyrix should be postponed in subjects suffering from acute severe febrile illness. The presence of a minor infection, however, is not a contra-indication for vaccination.

4.4 Special warnings and precautions for use
As with all injectable vaccines, appropriate medical treatment and supervision should always be readily available in case of a rare anaphylactic event following the administration of the vaccine.

In subjects with an impaired immune system, adequate anti-HAV and anti-Vi antibody titres may not be obtained after a single dose of Hepatyrix and such patients may therefore require administration of additional doses of vaccine. If possible, vaccination should be delayed until the completion of any immunosuppressive treatment. Subjects with chronic immunodeficiency such as HIV infection may be vaccinated if the underlying immunodeficiency allows the induction of an antibody response, even if limited.

It is possible that subjects may be in the incubation period of a hepatitis A infection at the time of vaccination. It is not known whether Hepatyrix will prevent clinically apparent hepatitis A infections in such cases.

Hepatyrix will not prevent infection caused by other hepatitis-causing agents such as hepatitis B virus, hepatitis C virus, hepatitis E virus or other pathogens known to infect the liver.

Hepatyrix protects only against typhoid fever caused by *Salmonella enterica serotype Typhi*. Protection is not conferred against paratyphoid fever or infections with any other serotypes of *S. enterica*.

As with any vaccine, a protective immune response may not be elicited in all vaccinees.

4.5 Interaction with other medicinal products and other forms of interaction
Hepatyrix must not be mixed with any other vaccine in the same syringe.

If Hepatyrix is to be given at the same time as (an)other injectable vaccine(s), the vaccines should always be administered at different injection sites.

Hepatyrix contains purified inactivated hepatitis A antigen and purified Vi capsular polysaccharide. Although concomitant use with other inactivated vaccines has not specifically been studied, it is anticipated that no interaction will be observed.

Concomitant administration of yellow fever vaccine with Hepatyrix has not been specifically assessed. However, based on data obtained from the concomitant administration of various monovalent vaccines (purified Vi polysaccharide typhoid vaccine or inactivated hepatitis A vaccine) with yellow fever vaccine, no interference with the immune responses to any of these antigens would be expected.

The effect of concomitant administration of immunoglobulins on the immunogenicity of Hepatyrix has not been assessed. Therefore, interference with the immune response cannot be ruled out.

4.6 Pregnancy and lactation
Pregnancy

Adequate human data on use during pregnancy and adequate animal reproduction studies are not available. Hepatyrix should only be used after careful consideration of the risk-benefit relationship.

Lactation

Adequate data on the administration of Hepatyrix to women who are breast-feeding their infants are not available. Hepatyrix should be used during breast-feeding only when clearly needed.

4.7 Effects on ability to drive and use machines
Some of the effects mentioned under section 4.8 "Undesirable effects" may affect the ability to drive or operate machinery.

4.8 Undesirable effects
• Clinical trials

In controlled clinical studies, the most commonly reported reactions after administration of Hepatyrix were those at the site of injection. All local and general symptoms resolved without any sequelae.

Frequencies are reported as:

Very common: (≥ 1/10)

Common: (≥1/100 to <1/10)

Uncommon: (≥1/1,000 to <1/100)

Rare: (≥1/10,000 to <1/1,000)

Very rare: (<1/10,000)

Within each frequency grouping, undesirable effects are presented in order of decreasing seriousness

Nervous system disorders:

Common: headache

Gastrointestinal disorders:

Common: nausea

Skin and subcutaneous tissue disorders:

Very common: erythema

Common: itching

General disorders and administration site conditions:

Very common: pain

Common: fever, general aches, malaise, swelling

• Post-marketing surveillance

The following undesirable events have been reported in temporal association with Hepatyrix vaccination:

Immune system disorders:

Very rare: allergic reactions, including anaphylaxis and anaphylactoid reactions

Nervous system disorders:

Very rare: syncope

Skin and subcutaneous tissue disorders:

Very rare: skin rashes

Experience with the GlaxoSmithKline monovalent hepatitis A vaccine:

• Clinical trials:

The following undesirable effects have been reported during clinical trials conducted with the GlaxoSmithKline monovalent hepatitis A vaccine:

Metabolism and nutrition disorders:

Common: loss of appetite

Gastrointestinal disorders:

Common: vomiting

• Post-marketing surveillance:

During post-marketing surveillance, the following undesirable effects have been reported with the GlaxoSmithKline monovalent hepatitis A vaccine:

Nervous system disorders:

Very rare: neurological manifestations including transverse myelitis, Guillain-Barre syndrome and neuralgic amyotrophy, convulsions

Musculoskeletal and connective tissue disorders:

Very rare: arthralgia, myalgia

4.9 Overdose
No case of overdose has been reported.

5. PHARMACOLOGICAL PROPERTIES
5.1 Pharmacodynamic properties
Pharmacotherapeutic group: Bacterial and viral vaccines combined, ATC code J07CA10

Hepatyrix confers immunity against typhoid fever and HAV infection by inducing specific anti-Vi and anti-HAV antibodies.

In clinical studies involving 462 subjects of 15-50 years of age, seropositivity rates for anti-HAV and anti-Vi antibodies were 89.8% and 97.5% respectively two weeks after primary immunisation. At month 1, seropositivity rates for anti-HAV and anti-Vi antibodies were 99.0% and 95.7% respectively.

In a clinical study where a group of 99 subjects received a booster dose of hepatitis A vaccine 12 months following the initial dose of Hepatyrix, all subjects were seropositive for anti-HAV antibodies one month later (i.e. at month 13).

When Hepatyrix was given 12 months following primary vaccination with the hepatitis A vaccine in a cohort of 97 subjects, the seropositivity rates for anti-Vi and anti-HAV antibodies were 88.2% and 100% respectively one month later (i.e. at month 13).

In two long-term clinical studies (TypHA-002 and TypHA-009), the persistence of anti-Vi and anti-HAV antibodies has been evaluated up to 36 months after vaccination with Hepatyrix and a booster dose of Havrix 1440 (GlaxoSmithKline Biologicals monovalent inactivated hepatitis A vaccine) administered six months later. In one of these two studies TypHA-009) the seropositivity rates obtained with Hepatyrix were compared to those obtained with co-administration of Typherix (GlaxoSmithKline Biologicals monovalent purified Vi polysaccharide vaccine) and Havrix 1440, followed by a booster dose of Havrix 1440 administered six months later.

The anti-Vi seropositivity rates observed in these two studies are presented below:

(see Table 1 on next page)

In another clinical study (TypHA-010/011), subjects who had received a dose of Hepatyrix six years previously were given a dose of Typherix. Before Typherix was administered 15 of 39 subjects (38%) were seropositive for anti-Vi antibody. At one month after vaccination with Typherix the seropositivity rate was 92%. At one year after the dose of Typherix the anti-Vi seropositivity rate was 84%. The anti-Vi seropositivity rates and the geometric means concentrations of anti-Vi antibody at Months 1 and 12 after the dose of Typherix were comparable with the corresponding values observed previously in these subjects after a dose of Hepatyrix.

In studies TypHA-002 and TypHA-009, one month after the booster dose of Havrix 1440 (i.e. at month 7) the anti-HAV seropositivity rate observed was 100%. At month 36 at least 99% of the vaccinees were still seropositive with respect to anti-HAV antibodies.

Based on data generated after administration of a booster dose of a monovalent hepatitis A vaccine between six and twelve months following the initial dose of the monovalent hepatitis A vaccine, it is predicted that anti-HAV antibodies persist for many years (at least 10 years).

5.2 Pharmacokinetic properties
Evaluation of pharmacokinetic properties is not required for vaccines.

5.3 Preclinical safety data
Preclinical data reveal no special hazard for humans based on general safety studies.

6. PHARMACEUTICAL PARTICULARS
6.1 List of excipients
Sodium chloride

Water for injections

For adjuvants, see section 2.

Table 1

	TypHA-002		TypHA-009			
	Hepatyrix		Hepatyrix		Typherix +Havrix 1440	
	N	Anti-Vi seropositivity rate (%)	N	Anti-Vi seropositivity rate (%)	N	Anti-Vi seropositivity rate (%)
Day 14	128	97.7	217	96.3	230	97.4
Month 1	138	97.8	223	96.4	232	97.4
Month 12	120	73.3	211	80.6	210	85.7
Month 24	97	46.4	209	68.4	207	72.0
Month 36	113	53.1	195	55.9	192	65.1

N: number of vaccinees

Anti-Vi seropositivity rate (%): percentage of vaccinees with antibody titres ⩾ assay cut-off (⩾ 150 EL.U/ml)

6.2 Incompatibilities

In the absence of compatibility studies, this medicinal product must not be mixed with other medicinal products.

6.3 Shelf life

2 years.

6.4 Special precautions for storage

Store in a refrigerator (2°C - 8°C).

Store in the original package in order to protect from light.

Do not freeze. Discard if vaccine has been frozen.

6.5 Nature and contents of container

1 ml of suspension in a pre-filled syringe (type I glass) with a plunger stopper (butyl rubber).

Pack sizes of 1 and 10 with needles.

Packs of 1, 10, 20 and 50 without needles.

Not all pack sizes may be marketed.

6.6 Special precautions for disposal and other handling

The vaccine's normal appearance is a cloudy white suspension, which may sediment during storage. Shake the container well to distribute the suspension uniformly before administering the vaccine.

The vaccine should be inspected visually for extraneous particulate matter and/or discolouration prior to administration. Any unused vaccine or waste material should be disposed of safely in accordance with local regulations.

7. MARKETING AUTHORISATION HOLDER

SmithKline Beecham plc

Trading as:

GlaxoSmithKline UK,

Stockley Park West,

Uxbridge,

Middlesex, UB11 1BT

8. MARKETING AUTHORISATION NUMBER(S)

PL10592/0136

9. DATE OF FIRST AUTHORISATION/RENEWAL OF THE AUTHORISATION

19/06/2009

10. DATE OF REVISION OF THE TEXT

19/06/2009

Hepsera 10 mg tablets

(Gilead Sciences Ltd)

1. NAME OF THE MEDICINAL PRODUCT

Hepsera 10 mg tablets

2. QUALITATIVE AND QUANTITATIVE COMPOSITION

Each tablet contains 10 mg adefovir dipivoxil.

Excipient(s):

Each tablet contains 113 mg lactose monohydrate.

For a full list of excipients, see section 6.1.

3. PHARMACEUTICAL FORM

Tablet.

White to off-white, round, flat-faced, bevelled-edge tablets, debossed with "GILEAD" and "10" on one side and a stylised shape of a liver on the other side.

4. CLINICAL PARTICULARS

4.1 Therapeutic indications

Hepsera is indicated for the treatment of chronic hepatitis B in adults with:

- compensated liver disease with evidence of active viral replication, persistently elevated serum alanine aminotransferase (ALT) levels and histological evidence of active liver inflammation and fibrosis
- decompensated liver disease.

4.2 Posology and method of administration

Therapy should be initiated by a physician experienced in the management of chronic hepatitis B.

Adults: The recommended dose of Hepsera is 10 mg (one tablet) once daily taken orally with or without food.

Higher doses must not be administered.

The optimum duration of treatment is unknown. The relationship between treatment response and long-term outcomes such as hepatocellular carcinoma or decompensated cirrhosis is not known.

Patients should be monitored every six months for hepatitis B biochemical, virological and serological markers.

Treatment discontinuation may be considered as follows:

- In HBeAg positive patients without cirrhosis, treatment should be administered for at least 6-12 months after HBe seroconversion (HBeAg loss and HBV DNA loss with anti-HBe detection) is confirmed or until HBs seroconversion or there is loss of efficacy (see section 4.4). Serum ALT and HBV DNA levels should be followed regularly after treatment discontinuation to detect any late virological relapse.

- In HBeAg negative patients without cirrhosis, treatment should be administered at least until HBs seroconversion or there is evidence of loss of efficacy. With prolonged treatment for more than 2 years, regular reassessment is recommended to confirm that continuing the selected therapy remains appropriate for the patient.

In patients with decompensated liver disease or cirrhosis, treatment cessation is not recommended (see section 4.4).

Children and adolescents: Hepsera is not recommended for use in children below the age of 18 years due to insufficient data on safety and efficacy (see section 5.1).

Elderly: No data are available to support a dose recommendation for patients over the age of 65 years (see section 4.4).

Renal insufficiency: Adefovir is eliminated by renal excretion and adjustments of the dosing interval are required in patients with a creatinine clearance < 50 ml/min or on dialysis. The recommended dosing frequency according to renal function must not be exceeded (see sections 4.4 and 5.2). The proposed dose interval modification is based on extrapolation of limited data in patients with end stage renal disease (ESRD) and may not be optimal.

Patients with creatinine clearance between 30 and 49 ml/min:

It is recommended to administer adefovir dipivoxil (one 10 mg tablet) every 48 hours in these patients. There are only limited data on the safety and efficacy of this dosing interval adjustment guideline. Therefore, clinical response to treatment and renal function should be closely monitored in these patients (see section 4.4).

Patients with creatinine clearance < 30 ml/min and dialysis patients:

There are no safety and efficacy data to support the use of adefovir dipivoxil in patients with a creatinine clearance < 30 ml/min or on dialysis. Therefore, use of adefovir dipivoxil is not recommended in these patients and should only be considered if the potential benefits outweigh the potential risks. In that case, the limited data available suggest that for patients with creatinine clearance between 10 and 29 ml/min, adefovir dipivoxil (one 10 mg tablet) may be administered every 72 hours; for haemodialysis patients, adefovir dipivoxil (one 10 mg tablet) may be administered every 7 days following 12 hours continuous dialysis (or 3 dialysis sessions, each of 4 hours duration). These patients should be closely monitored for possible adverse reactions and to ensure efficacy is maintained (see sections 4.4 and 4.8). No dosing interval recommendations are available for other dialysis patients (e.g. ambulatory peritoneal dialysis patients) or non-haemodialysed patients with creatinine clearance less than 10 ml/min.

Hepatic impairment: No dose adjustment is required in patients with hepatic impairment (see section 5.2).

Clinical resistance: Lamivudine-refractory patients and patients harbouring HBV with evidence of resistance to lamivudine (mutations at rtL180M, rtA181T and/or rtM204I/V) should not be treated with adefovir dipivoxil monotherapy in order to reduce the risk of resistance to adefovir. Adefovir may be used in combination with lamivudine in lamivudine-refractory patients and in patients harbouring HBV with mutations at rtL180M and/or rtM204I/V. However, for patients harbouring HBV that contains the rtA181T mutation, consideration should be given to alternative treatment regimens due to the risk of reduced susceptibility to adefovir (see section 5.1).

In order to reduce the risk of resistance in patients receiving adefovir dipivoxil monotherapy, a modification of treatment should be considered if serum HBV DNA remains above 1,000 copies/ml at or beyond 1 year of treatment.

4.3 Contraindications

- Hypersensitivity to the active substance or to any of the excipients.

4.4 Special warnings and precautions for use

Renal function: Adefovir is excreted renally, by a combination of glomerular filtration and active tubular secretion. Treatment with adefovir dipivoxil may result in renal impairment. While the overall risk of renal impairment in patients with adequate renal function is low, this is of special importance in patients at risk of, or having underlying renal dysfunction and in patients receiving medicinal products that may affect renal function.

It is recommended that creatinine clearance is calculated in all patients prior to initiating therapy with adefovir dipivoxil.

In patients who develop renal insufficiency and have advanced liver disease or cirrhosis, dosing interval adjustment of adefovir or switch to an alternative therapy for hepatitis B infection should be considered. Treatment cessation for chronic hepatitis B in these patients is not recommended.

Patients with normal renal function:

Patients with normal renal function should be monitored for changes in serum creatinine every 3 months and creatinine clearance calculated. In patients at risk of renal impairment (see section 4.8), consideration should be given to more frequent monitoring of renal function.

Patients with creatinine clearance between 30 and 49 ml/min:

The dosing interval of adefovir dipivoxil should be adjusted in these patients (see section 4.2). In addition, renal function should be closely monitored with a frequency tailored to the individual patient's medical condition.

Patients with creatinine clearance < 30 ml/min and dialysis patients:

Adefovir dipivoxil is not recommended in patients with a creatinine clearance of < 30 ml/min or on dialysis. Administration of adefovir dipivoxil in these patients should only be considered if the potential benefits outweigh the potential risks. If treatment with adefovir dipivoxil is considered essential, then the dosing interval should be adjusted (see section 4.2). These patients should be closely monitored for possible adverse reactions and to ensure efficacy is maintained.

Patients receiving medicinal products that may affect renal function:

Adefovir dipivoxil should not be administered concurrently with tenofovir disoproxil fumarate (Viread).

Caution is advised in patients receiving other medicinal products that may affect renal function or are excreted renally (e.g. cyclosporin and tacrolimus, intravenous aminoglycosides, amphotericin B, foscarnet, pentamidine, vancomycin, or medicinal products which are secreted by the same renal transporter, human Organic Anion Transporter 1 (hOAT1), such as cidofovir). Co-administration of 10 mg adefovir dipivoxil with medicinal products in these patients may lead to an increase in serum concentrations of either adefovir or a co-administered medicinal product. The renal function of these patients should be closely monitored with a frequency tailored to the individual patient's medical condition.

For renal safety in patients pre- and post-transplantation with lamivudine-resistant HBV, see section 4.8.

Hepatic function: Spontaneous exacerbations in chronic hepatitis B are relatively common and are characterised by transient increases in serum ALT. After initiating antiviral therapy, serum ALT may increase in some patients as serum HBV DNA levels decline. In patients with compensated liver disease, these increases in serum ALT are generally not accompanied by an increase in serum bilirubin concentrations or hepatic decompensation (see section 4.8). Patients with advanced liver disease or cirrhosis may be at a higher risk for hepatic decompensation following hepatitis exacerbation which may be fatal. In these patients, including patients with decompensated liver disease, treatment cessation is not recommended and these patients should be monitored closely during therapy.

In the event of these patients developing renal insufficiency, see above *Renal function*.

If treatment cessation is necessary, patients should be closely monitored for several months after stopping treatment as exacerbations of hepatitis have occurred after discontinuation of 10 mg adefovir dipivoxil. These exacerbations occurred in the absence of HBeAg seroconversion and presented as serum ALT elevations and increases in serum HBV DNA. Elevations in serum ALT that occurred in patients with compensated liver function treated with 10 mg adefovir dipivoxil were not accompanied by clinical and laboratory changes associated with liver decompensation. Patients should be closely monitored after stopping treatment. Most post-treatment exacerbations of hepatitis were seen within 12 weeks of discontinuation of 10 mg adefovir dipivoxil.

Lactic acidosis and severe hepatomegaly with steatosis: Occurrences of lactic acidosis (in the absence of hypoxaemia), sometimes fatal, usually associated with severe hepatomegaly and hepatic steatosis, have been reported with the use of nucleoside analogues. As adefovir is structurally related to nucleoside analogues, this risk cannot be excluded. Treatment with nucleoside analogues should be discontinued when rapidly elevating aminotransferase levels, progressive hepatomegaly or metabolic/lactic acidosis of unknown aetiology occur. Benign digestive symptoms, such as nausea, vomiting and abdominal pain, might be indicative of lactic acidosis development. Severe cases, sometimes with fatal outcome, were associated with pancreatitis, liver failure/hepatic steatosis, renal failure and higher levels of serum lactate. Caution should be exercised when prescribing nucleoside analogues to any patient (particularly obese women) with hepatomegaly, hepatitis or other known risk factors for liver disease. These patients should be followed closely.

To differentiate between elevations in transaminases due to response to treatment and increases potentially related to lactic acidosis, physicians should ensure that changes in ALT are associated with improvements in other laboratory markers of chronic hepatitis B.

Co-infection with hepatitis C or D: There are no data on the efficacy of adefovir dipivoxil in patients co-infected with hepatitis C or hepatitis D.

Co-infection with HIV: Limited data are available on the safety and efficacy of 10 mg adefovir dipivoxil in patients with chronic hepatitis B, co-infected with HIV. To date there is no evidence that daily dosing with 10 mg adefovir dipivoxil results in emergence of adefovir-associated resistance mutations in the HIV reverse transcriptase. Nonetheless, there is a potential risk of selection of HIV strains resistant to adefovir with possible cross-resistance to other antiviral medicinal products.

As far as possible, treatment of hepatitis B by adefovir dipivoxil in an HIV co-infected patient should be reserved for patients whose HIV RNA is controlled. Treatment with 10 mg adefovir dipivoxil has not been shown to be effective against HIV replication and therefore should not be used to control HIV infection.

Elderly: The clinical experience in patients $>$ 65 years of age is very limited. Caution should be exercised when prescribing adefovir dipivoxil to the elderly, keeping in mind the greater frequency of decreased renal or cardiac function in these patients, and the increase in concomitant diseases or concomitant use of other medicinal products in the elderly.

Resistance: Resistance to adefovir dipivoxil (see section 5.1) can result in viral load rebound which may result in exacerbation of hepatitis B and, in the setting of diminished hepatic function, lead to liver decompensation and possible fatal outcome. Virological response should be closely monitored in patients treated with adefovir dipivoxil, with HBV DNA measured every 3 months. If viral rebound occurs, resistance testing should be performed. In case of emergence of resistance, treatment should be modified.

General: Patients should be advised that therapy with adefovir dipivoxil has not been proven to reduce the risk of transmission of hepatitis B virus to others and therefore appropriate precautions should still be taken.

Hepsera contains lactose monohydrate. Consequently, patients with rare hereditary problems of galactose intolerance, the Lapp lactase deficiency, or glucose-galactose malabsorption should not take this medicinal product.

4.5 Interaction with other medicinal products and other forms of interaction

Interaction studies have only been performed in adults.

The potential for CYP450 mediated interactions involving adefovir with other medicinal products is low, based on the results of *in vitro* experiments in which adefovir did not influence any of the common CYP isoforms known to be involved in human drug metabolism and based on the known elimination pathway of adefovir. A clinical study in liver-transplant patients has shown that no pharmacokinetic interaction occurs when adefovir dipivoxil 10 mg once daily is administered concomitantly with tacrolimus, an immunosuppressant which is predominantly metabolised via the CYP450 system. A pharmacokinetic interaction between adefovir and the immunosuppressant, cyclosporin, is also considered unlikely as cyclosporin shares the same metabolic pathway as tacrolimus. Nevertheless, given that tacrolimus and cyclosporin can affect renal function, close monitoring is recommended when either of these agents is coadministered with adefovir dipivoxil (see section 4.4).

Concomitant administration of 10 mg adefovir dipivoxil and 100 mg lamivudine did not alter the pharmacokinetic profile of either medicinal product.

Adefovir is excreted renally, by a combination of glomerular filtration and active tubular secretion. Co-administration of 10 mg adefovir dipivoxil with other medicinal products that are eliminated by tubular secretion or alter tubular function may increase serum concentrations of either adefovir or the co-administered medicinal product (see section 4.4).

Due to the high pharmacokinetic variability of pegylated interferon, no definitive conclusion can be drawn regarding the effect of adefovir and pegylated interferon co-administration on the pharmacokinetic profile of either medicinal product. Even though a pharmacokinetic interaction is unlikely given the two products are eliminated via different pathways, caution is recommended if both products are co-administered.

4.6 Pregnancy and lactation

Pregnancy: There are no adequate data on the use of adefovir dipivoxil in pregnant women.

Studies in animals administered adefovir intravenously have shown reproductive toxicity (see section 5.3). Studies in orally dosed animals do not indicate teratogenic or foetotoxic effects.

Adefovir dipivoxil should be used during pregnancy only if the potential benefit justifies the potential risk to the foetus.

There are no data on the effect of adefovir dipivoxil on transmission of HBV from mother to infant. Therefore, the standard recommended procedures for immunisation of infants should be followed to prevent neonatal acquisition of HBV.

Given that the potential risks to developing human foetuses are unknown, it is recommended that women of child-bearing potential treated with adefovir dipivoxil use effective contraception.

Lactation: It is not known whether adefovir is excreted in human milk. Mothers should be instructed not to breast-feed if they are taking adefovir dipivoxil tablets.

4.7 Effects on ability to drive and use machines

No studies on the effects on the ability to drive and use machines have been performed. However, based on the safety profile and mechanism of action, adefovir dipivoxil is expected to have no or negligible influence on these abilities.

4.8 Undesirable effects

In patients with compensated liver disease, the most frequently reported adverse reactions during 48 weeks of adefovir dipivoxil therapy were asthenia (13 %), headache (9 %), abdominal pain (9 %) and nausea (5 %).

Assessment of adverse reactions is based on experience from post-marketing surveillance and from three pivotal clinical studies in patients with chronic hepatitis B:

- two placebo-controlled studies in which 522 patients with chronic hepatitis B and compensated liver disease received double-blind treatment with 10 mg adefovir dipivoxil (n=294) or placebo (n=228) for 48 weeks.
- an open-label study in which pre- (n=226) and post-liver transplantation patients (n=241) with lamivudine-resistant HBV were treated with 10 mg adefovir dipivoxil once daily, for up to 203 weeks (median 51 and 99 weeks, respectively).

The adverse reactions considered at least possibly related to treatment are listed below, by body system organ class, and frequency. Within each frequency grouping, undesirable effects are presented in order of decreasing seriousness. Frequencies are defined as very common ($\geq$ 1/10), common ($\geq$ 1/100, $<$ 1/10) or not known (identified through post-marketing safety surveillance and the frequency cannot be estimated from the available data).

Nervous system disorders:

Common ($\geq$ 1/100, $<$ 1/10): headache.

Gastrointestinal disorders:

Common ($\geq$ 1/100, $<$ 1/10): diarrhoea, vomiting, abdominal pain, dyspepsia, nausea, flatulence.

Frequency not known: pancreatitis.

Skin and subcutaneous tissue disorders:

Common ($\geq$ 1/100, $<$ 1/10): rash, pruritus.

Musculoskeletal and connective tissue disorders:

Frequency not known: myopathy, osteomalacia (both associated with proximal renal tubulopathy).

Renal and urinary disorders:

Very common ($\geq$ 1/10): increases in creatinine.

Common ($\geq$ 1/100, $<$ 1/10): renal failure, abnormal renal function, hypophosphatemia.

Frequency not known: Fanconi syndrome, proximal renal tubulopathy.

General disorders and administration site conditions:

Very common ($\geq$ 1/10): asthenia.

Exacerbation of hepatitis:

Clinical and laboratory evidence of exacerbations of hepatitis have occurred after discontinuation of treatment with 10 mg adefovir dipivoxil (see section 4.4).

Long-term safety data in patients with compensated disease:

In a long-term safety study of 125 HBeAg negative patients with compensated liver disease, the adverse event profile was overall unchanged after a median exposure of 226 weeks. No clinically significant changes in renal function were observed. However, mild to moderate increases in serum creatinine concentrations, hypophosphatemia and a decrease in carnitine concentrations were reported in 3 %, 4 % and 6 % of patients, respectively, on extended treatment.

In a long-term safety study of 65 HBeAg positive patients with compensated liver disease (after a median exposure of 234 weeks), 6 patients (9 %) had confirmed increases in serum creatinine of at least 0.5 mg/dl from baseline with 2 patients discontinuing from the study due to the elevated serum creatinine concentration. Patients with a confirmed increase in creatinine of $\geq$ 0.3 mg/dl by week 48 were at a statistically significant higher risk of a subsequent confirmed increase in creatinine of $\geq$ 0.5 mg/dl. Hypophosphatemia and a decrease in carnitine concentrations were reported each in 3 % of patients on extended treatment.

Safety in patients with decompensated disease:

In patients with decompensated liver disease, the most frequently reported adverse reactions during up to 203 weeks of adefovir dipivoxil therapy were increased creatinine (7 %) and asthenia (5 %). Renal toxicity is an important feature of the safety profile of adefovir dipivoxil in patients with decompensated liver disease. In clinical studies of wait-listed and post-liver transplantation patients, four percent (19/467) of patients discontinued treatment with adefovir dipivoxil due to renal adverse events.

4.9 Overdose

Administration of 500 mg adefovir dipivoxil daily for 2 weeks and 250 mg daily for 12 weeks has been associated with the gastrointestinal disorders listed above and anorexia.

If overdose occurs, the patient must be monitored for evidence of toxicity, and standard supportive treatment applied as necessary.

Adefovir can be removed by haemodialysis; the median haemodialysis clearance of adefovir is 104 ml/min. The elimination of adefovir by peritoneal dialysis has not been studied.

5. PHARMACOLOGICAL PROPERTIES

5.1 Pharmacodynamic properties

Pharmacotherapeutic group: Nucleoside and nucleotide reverse transcriptase inhibitors, ATC code: J05AF08.

Adefovir dipivoxil is an oral prodrug of adefovir, an acyclic nucleotide phosphonate analogue of adenosine monophosphate, which is actively transported into mammalian cells where it is converted by host enzymes to adefovir diphosphate. Adefovir diphosphate inhibits viral polymerases by competing for direct binding with the natural substrate (deoxyadenosine triphosphate) and, after incorporation into viral DNA, causes DNA chain termination. Adefovir diphosphate selectively inhibits HBV DNA polymerases at concentrations 12-, 700-, and 10-fold lower than those needed to inhibit human DNA polymerases α, β, and γ, respectively. Adefovir diphosphate has an intracellular half-life of 12 to 36 hours in activated and resting lymphocytes.

Adefovir is active against hepadnaviruses *in vitro*, including all common forms of lamivudine-resistant HBV (rtL180M, rtM204I, rtM204V, rtL180M/rtM204V), famciclovir-associated mutations (rtV173L, rtP177L, rtL180M, rtT184S or rtV207I) and hepatitis B immunoglobulin escape mutations (rtT128N and rtW153Q), and in *in vivo* animal models of hepadnavirus replication.

Clinical experience: The demonstration of the benefit of adefovir dipivoxil is based on histological, virological, biochemical, and serological responses in adults with:

- HBeAg positive and HBeAg negative chronic hepatitis B with compensated liver disease.
- lamivudine-resistant HBV with either compensated or decompensated liver disease, including patients pre- and post-liver transplantation or co-infected with HIV. In the majority of these studies adefovir dipivoxil 10 mg was added to ongoing lamivudine treatment in patients failing lamivudine therapy.

In these clinical studies patients had active viral replication (HBV DNA $\geq$ 100,000 copies/ml) and elevated ALT levels ($\geq$ 1.2 $\times$ Upper Limit of Normal (ULN)).

Experience in patients with compensated liver disease: In two placebo-controlled studies (total n=522) in HBeAg positive or in HBeAg negative chronic hepatitis B patients with compensated liver disease, significantly more patients ($p < 0.001$) in the 10 mg adefovir dipivoxil groups (53 and 64 %, respectively) had histological improvement from baseline at week 48 than in the placebo groups (25 and 33 %). Improvement was defined as a reduction from baseline of two points or more in the Knodell necro-inflammatory score with no concurrent worsening in the Knodell fibrosis score. Histological improvement was seen regardless of baseline demographic and hepatitis B characteristics, including prior interferon-alpha therapy. High baseline ALT levels ($\geq$ 2 $\times$ ULN) and Knodell Histology Activity Index (HAI) scores ($\geq$ 10) and low HBV DNA ($<$ 7.6 $\log_{10}$ copies/ml) were associated with greater histological improvement. Blinded, ranked assessments of both necro-inflammatory activity and fibrosis at baseline and week 48, demonstrated that patients treated with 10 mg adefovir dipivoxil had improved necro-inflammatory and fibrosis scores relative to placebo-treated patients.

Assessment of the change in fibrosis after 48 weeks treatment using the Knodell scores confirms that patients treated with adefovir dipivoxil 10 mg had more regression and less progression of fibrosis than patients treated with placebo.

In the two studies mentioned above, treatment with 10 mg adefovir dipivoxil was associated with significant reductions in serum HBV DNA (3.52 and 3.91 $\log_{10}$ copies/ml, respectively, *versus* 0.55 and 1.35 $\log_{10}$ copies/ml), increased proportion of patients with normalisation of ALT (48 and 72 % *versus* 16 and 29 %) or increased proportion of patients with serum HBV DNA below the limits of quantification (< 400 copies/ml Roche Amplicor Monitor PCR assay) (21 and 51 % *versus* 0 %) when compared with placebo. In the study in HBeAg positive patients, HBeAg seroconversion (12 %) and HBeAg loss (24 %) was observed significantly more frequently in patients receiving 10 mg adefovir dipivoxil than in patients receiving placebo (6 % and 11 %, respectively) after 48 weeks of treatment.

In the HBeAg positive study, treatment beyond 48 weeks resulted in further reductions in serum HBV DNA levels and increases in the proportion of patients with ALT normalisation, HBeAg loss and seroconversion.

In the HBeAg negative study patients on adefovir dipivoxil (0-48 weeks) were re-randomised in a blinded-manner to continue on adefovir dipivoxil or receive placebo for an additional 48 weeks. At week 96, patients continuing on adefovir dipivoxil 10 mg had sustained suppression of serum HBV with maintenance of the reduction seen at week 48. In over two thirds of patients suppression of serum HBV DNA was associated with normalisation of ALT levels. In most patients who stopped treatment with adefovir dipivoxil, serum HBV DNA and ALT levels returned towards baseline.

Treatment with adefovir dipivoxil resulted in improvement in the liver fibrosis from baseline to 96 weeks therapy when analysed using the Ishak score (median change: Δ= -1). No differences in the median fibrosis score were seen between groups using the Knodell fibrosis score.

Patients who completed the first 96 weeks of the HBeAg negative study and received adefovir dipivoxil treatment during weeks 49 to 96, were offered the opportunity to receive open-label treatment with adefovir dipivoxil from study week 97 through to week 240. Serum HBV DNA levels remained undetectable and ALT levels normalised in approximately two thirds of patients following treatment with adefovir dipivoxil for up to 240 weeks. Clinically and statistically significant improvement in fibrosis was seen in the changes in Ishak scores from the start of adefovir dipivoxil treatment to the end of the study (week 240) (median change: Δ= -1). By the end of the study, 7 of 12 patients (58 %) with bridging fibrosis or cirrhosis at baseline, had an improved Ishak fibrosis score of ⩾ 2 points. Five patients achieved and maintained HBsAg seroconversion (HBsAg negative/HBsAb positive).

Experience in patients pre- and post-liver transplantation with lamivudine-resistant HBV: In a clinical study in 394 chronic hepatitis B patients with lamivudine-resistant HBV (pre-liver transplantation (n=186) and post-liver transplantation (n=208)), treatment with 10 mg adefovir dipivoxil resulted in a median reduction in serum HBV DNA of 4.1 and 4.2 $\log_{10}$ copies/ml, respectively, at week 48. In the pre-liver transplantation and post-liver transplantation cohorts 77 of 109 (71 %) patients and 64 of 159 (40 %) patients, respectively, achieved undetectable HBV DNA levels at week 48 (< 1,000 copies/ml Roche Amplicor Monitor PCR assay). Treatment with 10 mg adefovir dipivoxil showed similar efficacy regardless of the patterns of lamivudine-resistant HBV DNA polymerase mutations at baseline. Improvements or stabilisation were seen in Child-Pugh-Turcotte score. Normalisation of ALT, albumin, bilirubin and prothrombin time was seen at week 48 in 51-85 % of the patients.

In the pre-liver transplantation cohort, 25 of 33 (76 %) patients achieved undetectable HBV DNA levels and 84 % of patients had ALT normalisation at 96 weeks. In the post-liver transplantation cohort, 61 of 94 (65 %) and 35 of 45 (78 %) of patients achieved undetectable HBV DNA levels at 96 and 144 weeks, respectively, and 70 % and 58 % of patients had ALT normalisation at these study visits. The clinical significance of these findings as they relate to histological improvement is not known.

Experience in patients with compensated liver disease and lamivudine-resistant HBV: In a double-blind comparative study in chronic hepatitis B patients with lamivudine-resistant HBV (n=58), there was no median reduction in HBV DNA from baseline after 48 weeks of treatment with lamivudine. Forty-eight weeks of treatment with adefovir dipivoxil 10 mg alone or in combination with lamivudine resulted in a similar significant decrease in median serum HBV DNA levels from baseline (4.04 $\log_{10}$ copies/ml and 3.59 $\log_{10}$ copies/ml, respectively). The clinical significance of these observed changes in HBV DNA has not been established.

Experience in patients with decompensated liver disease and lamivudine-resistant HBV: In 40 HBeAg positive or HBeAg negative patients with lamivudine-resistant HBV and decompensated liver disease receiving treatment with 100 mg lamivudine, addition of 10 mg adefovir dipivoxil treatment for 52 weeks resulted in a median reduction in HBV DNA of 4.6 $\log_{10}$ copies/ml. Improvement in liver function was also seen after one year of therapy.

Experience in patients with HIV co-infection and lamivudine-resistant HBV: In an open-label investigator study in 35 chronic hepatitis B patients with lamivudine-resistant HBV and co-infected with HIV, continued treatment with 10 mg adefovir dipivoxil resulted in progressive reductions in serum HBV DNA levels and ALT levels throughout the course of treatment up to 144 weeks.

In a second open-label, one-arm study, 10 mg adefovir dipivoxil and pegylated interferon alpha-2a were added to ongoing lamivudine therapy in 18 HIV/HBV co-infected patients with lamivudine-resistant HBV. Patients were all HBeAg positive and had median CD4 cell count of 441 cells/mm^3 (no patient had CD4 count < 200 cells/mm^3). During therapy, serum HBV DNA levels were significantly lower compared to baseline for up to 48 weeks of treatment while ALT levels declined progressively from week 12. However, on-treatment HBV DNA response was not maintained off-therapy since all the patients had a rebound in HBV DNA after adefovir dipivoxil and pegylated interferon alpha-2a discontinuation. No patients became HBsAg- or HBeAg-negative during the study. Due to the small sample size and the study design, in particular the lack of treatment arms with pegylated interferon alpha-2a monotherapy and with adefovir monotherapy, it is not possible to draw formal conclusions on the best therapeutic management of HIV co-infected patients with lamivudine-resistant HBV.

Paediatric population: The efficacy and safety of a daily dose of 0.25 mg/kg to 10 mg adefovir dipivoxil in children (aged from 2 to < 18 years) was examined in a double-blind, randomised, placebo-controlled study in 173 paediatric patients (115 on adefovir dipivoxil, 58 on placebo) who had HBeAg positive chronic hepatitis B, serum ALT levels ⩾ 1.5 × upper limit of normal (ULN) and compensated liver disease. At week 48, in children aged 2 to 11 years old, no statistically significant difference was observed in the proportions of patients that achieved the primary endpoint of serum HBV DNA < 1,000 copies/ml and normal ALT levels between the placebo arm and the adefovir dipivoxil arm. In the adolescent population (n=83) (aged from 12 to < 18 years), significantly more patients treated with adefovir dipivoxil achieved the primary efficacy endpoint and obtained significant reductions in serum HBV DNA (23 %) compared to placebo-treated patients (0 %). However, the proportions of subjects who achieved HBeAg seroconversion at week 48 were similar (11 %) between the placebo arm and the adefovir dipivoxil 10 mg arm in adolescent patients.

Overall, the safety profile of adefovir dipivoxil in children was consistent with the known safety profile in adult patients. However, a signal towards a higher rate of decreased appetite and/or food intake was observed in the adefovir arm as compared to the placebo arm. At week 48 and 96, mean changes from baseline in weight and BMI Z scores tended to decrease in adefovir dipivoxil-treated patients. No long-term safety data or long-term resistance data are available with adefovir dipivoxil in children.

The clinical data available are insufficient to draw definitive conclusions on the benefit/risk ratio of the adefovir treatment in children with chronic hepatitis B (see section 4.2).

Clinical resistance in patients receiving adefovir dipivoxil as monotherapy and in combination with lamivudine: In several clinical studies (HBeAg positive, HBeAg negative, pre- and post-liver transplantation with lamivudine-resistant HBV and lamivudine-resistant HBV co-infected with HIV patients), genotypic analyses were conducted on HBV isolates from 379 of a total of 629 patients, treated with adefovir dipivoxil for 48 weeks. No HBV DNA polymerase mutations associated with resistance to adefovir were identified when patients were genotyped at baseline and at week 48. After 96, 144, 192 and 240 weeks of treatment with adefovir dipivoxil, resistance surveillance was performed for 293, 221, 116 and 64 patients, respectively. Two novel conserved site mutations were identified in the HBV polymerase gene (rtN236T and rtA181V), which conferred clinical resistance to adefovir dipivoxil. The cumulative probabilities of developing these adefovir-associated resistance mutations in all patients treated with adefovir dipivoxil were 0 % at 48 weeks and approximately 2 %, 7 %, 14 % and 25 % after 96, 144, 192 and 240 weeks, respectively.

Clinical resistance in monotherapy studies in nucleoside naïve patients: In patients receiving adefovir dipivoxil monotherapy (HBeAg negative study) the cumulative probability of developing adefovir-associated resistance mutations was 0 %, 3 %, 11 %, 18 % and 29 % at 48, 96, 144, 192 and 240 weeks respectively. In addition, the long-term (4 to 5 years) development of resistance to adefovir dipivoxil was significantly lower in patients who had serum HBV DNA below the limit of quantification (< 1,000 copies/ml) at week 48 as compared to patients with serum HBV DNA above 1,000 copies/ml at week 48. In HBeAg positive patients, the incidence of adefovir-associated resistance mutations was 3 % (2/65), 17 % (11/65) and 20 % (13/65) after a median duration exposure of 135, 189 and 235 weeks respectively.

Clinical resistance in studies where adefovir dipivoxil was added to ongoing lamivudine in patients with lamivudine-resistance: In an open-label study of pre- and post-liver transplantation patients with clinical evidence of lamivudine-resistant HBV, no adefovir-associated resistance mutations were observed at week 48. With up to 3 years of exposure, no patients receiving both adefovir dipivoxil and lamivudine developed resistance to adefovir dipivoxil. However, 4 patients who discontinued lamivudine treatment developed the rtN236T mutation while receiving adefovir dipivoxil monotherapy and all experienced serum HBV rebound.

The currently available data both *in vitro* and in patients suggest that HBV expressing the adefovir-associated resistance mutation rtN236T is susceptible to lamivudine. Preliminary clinical data suggest the adefovir-associated resistance mutation rtA181V may confer a reduced susceptibility to lamivudine, and the lamivudine-associated mutation rtA181T may confer a reduced susceptibility to adefovir dipivoxil.

5.2 Pharmacokinetic properties

Absorption: Adefovir dipivoxil is a dipivaloyloxymethyl ester prodrug of the active substance adefovir. The oral bioavailability of adefovir from 10 mg adefovir dipivoxil is 59 %. Following oral administration of a single dose of 10 mg adefovir dipivoxil to chronic hepatitis B patients, the median (range) peak serum concentration (C_{max}) was achieved after 1.75 h (0.58-4.0 h). Median C_{max} and $AUC_{0-\infty}$ values were 16.70 (9.66-30.56) ng/ml and 204.40 (109.75-356.05) ng·h/ml, respectively. Systemic exposure to adefovir was not affected when 10 mg adefovir dipivoxil was taken with a high fat meal. The t_{max} was delayed by two hours.

Distribution: Preclinical studies show that after oral administration of adefovir dipivoxil, adefovir is distributed to most tissues with the highest concentrations occurring in kidney, liver and intestinal tissues. *In vitro* binding of adefovir to human plasma or human serum proteins is ⩽ 4 %, over the adefovir concentration range of 0.1 to 25 µg/ml. The volume of distribution at steady-state following intravenous administration of 1.0 or 3.0 mg/kg/day is 392±75 and 352±9 ml/kg, respectively.

Biotransformation: Following oral administration, adefovir dipivoxil is rapidly converted to adefovir. At concentrations substantially higher (> 4,000-fold) than those observed *in vivo*, adefovir did not inhibit any of the following human CYP450 isoforms, CYP1A2, CYP2D6, CYP2C9, CYP2C19, CYP3A4. Based on the results of these *in vitro* experiments and the known elimination pathway of adefovir, the potential for CYP450 mediated interactions involving adefovir with other medicinal products is low.

Elimination: Adefovir is excreted renally by a combination of glomerular filtration and active tubular secretion. The median (min-max) renal clearance of adefovir in subjects with normal renal function (Cl_{cr} > 80 ml/min) is 211 ml/min (172-316 ml/min), approximately twice calculated creatinine clearance (Cockroft-Gault method). After repeated administration of 10 mg adefovir dipivoxil, 45 % of the dose is recovered as adefovir in the urine over 24 hours. Plasma adefovir concentrations declined in a biexponential manner with a median terminal elimination half-life of 7.22 h (4.72-10.70 h).

Linearity/non-linearity: The pharmacokinetics of adefovir are proportional to dose when given as adefovir dipivoxil over the dose range of 10 to 60 mg. Repeated dosing of adefovir dipivoxil 10 mg daily did not influence the pharmacokinetics of adefovir.

Gender, age and ethnicity: The pharmacokinetics of adefovir were similar in male and female patients. Pharmacokinetic studies have not been conducted in children or in the elderly. Pharmacokinetic studies were principally conducted in Caucasian patients. The available data do not appear to indicate any difference in pharmacokinetics with regard to race.

The pharmacokinetics of adefovir dipivoxil were studied in an efficacy and safety study of a daily dose of 0.25 mg/kg to 10 mg adefovir dipivoxil in children (aged 2 to < 18 years). Pharmacokinetic analysis revealed that adefovir exposure was comparable among 3 age groups, 2 to 6 years (0.3 mg/kg), 7 to 11 years (0.25 mg/kg) and 12 to 17 years (10 mg) and all age groups achieved adefovir exposure in the target range (for efficacy results see section 5.1), which was based on adefovir plasma concentrations in adult patients with chronic hepatitis B with established safety and efficacy profiles.

Renal impairment: The mean (± SD) pharmacokinetic parameters of adefovir following administration of a single dose of 10 mg adefovir dipivoxil to patients with varying degrees of renal impairment are described in the table below:

(see Table 1 on next page)

A four-hour period of haemodialysis removed approximately 35 % of the adefovir dose. The effect of peritoneal dialysis on adefovir removal has not been evaluated.

It is recommended that the dosing interval of 10 mg adefovir dipivoxil is modified in patients with creatinine clearance between 30 and 49 ml/min. Adefovir dipivoxil is not recommended in patients with creatinine clearance of < 30 ml/min or in patients on dialysis (see section 4.2 and 4.4).

Hepatic impairment: Pharmacokinetic properties were similar in patients with moderate and severe hepatic impairment compared to healthy volunteers (see section 4.2).

Table 1

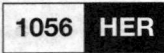

Renal Function Group	Unimpaired	Mild	Moderate	Severe
Baseline Creatinine Clearance (ml/min)	> 80 (n=7)	50-80 (n=8)	30-49 (n=7)	10-29 (n=10)
C_{max} (ng/ml)	17.8±3.2	22.4±4.0	28.5±8.6	51.6±10.3
$AUC_{0-\infty}$ (ng·h/ml)	201±40.8	266±55.7	455±176	1240±629
CL/F (ml/min)	469±99.0	356±85.6	237±118	91.7±51.3
CL_{renal} (ml/min)	231±48.9	148±39.3	83.9±27.5	37.0±18.4

5.3 Preclinical safety data

The primary dose-limiting toxic effect associated with administration of adefovir dipivoxil in animals (mice, rats and monkeys) was renal tubular nephropathy characterised by histological alterations and/or increases in blood urea nitrogen and serum creatinine. Nephrotoxicity was observed in animals at systemic exposures at least 3-10 times higher than those achieved in humans at the recommended therapeutic dose of 10 mg/day.

No effects on male or female fertility, or reproductive performance, occurred in rats and there was no embryotoxicity or teratogenicity in rats or rabbits administered adefovir dipivoxil orally.

When adefovir was administered intravenously to pregnant rats at doses associated with notable maternal toxicity (systemic exposure 38 times that achieved in humans at the therapeutic dose) embryotoxicity and an increased incidence of foetal malformations (anasarca, depressed eye bulge, umbilical hernia and kinked tail) were observed. No adverse effects on development were seen at systemic exposures approximately 12 times that achieved in humans at the therapeutic dose.

Adefovir dipivoxil was mutagenic in the *in vitro* mouse lymphoma cell assay (with or without metabolic activation), but was not clastogenic in the *in vivo* mouse micronucleus assay.

Adefovir was not mutagenic in microbial mutagenicity assays involving *Salmonella typhimurium* (Ames) and *Escherichia coli* in the presence and absence of metabolic activation. Adefovir induced chromosomal aberrations in the *in vitro* human peripheral blood lymphocyte assay without metabolic activation.

In long-term carcinogenicity studies in rats and mice with adefovir dipivoxil, no treatment-related increase in tumour incidence was found in mice or rats (systemic exposures approximately 10 and 4 times those achieved in humans at the therapeutic dose of 10 mg/day, respectively).

6. PHARMACEUTICAL PARTICULARS

6.1 List of excipients

Pregelatinised starch

Croscarmellose sodium

Lactose monohydrate

Talc

Magnesium stearate

6.2 Incompatibilities

Not applicable.

6.3 Shelf life

2 years.

6.4 Special precautions for storage

Do not store above 30°C. Store in the original package in order to protect from moisture. Keep the bottle tightly closed.

6.5 Nature and contents of container

Hepsera is supplied in high-density polyethylene (HDPE) bottles with a child-resistant closure. Each bottle contains 30 tablets, silica gel desiccant and fibre packing material.

The following pack sizes are available: outer cartons containing 1 × 30 tablet and 3 × 30 tablet bottles. Not all pack sizes may be marketed.

6.6 Special precautions for disposal and other handling

Any unused product or waste material should be disposed of in accordance with local requirements.

7. MARKETING AUTHORISATION HOLDER

Gilead Sciences International Limited

Cambridge

CB21 6GT

United Kingdom

8. MARKETING AUTHORISATION NUMBER(S)

EU/1/03/251/001

EU/1/03/251/002

9. DATE OF FIRST AUTHORISATION/RENEWAL OF THE AUTHORISATION

Date of first authorisation: 06 March 2003

Date of last renewal: 06 March 2008

10. DATE OF REVISION OF THE TEXT

06/2009

Detailed information on this medicinal product is available on the website of the European Medicines Agency (EMEA) http://www.emea.europa.eu/.

Herceptin

(Roche Products Limited)

1. NAME OF THE MEDICINAL PRODUCT

Herceptin ▼ 150 mg Powder for concentrate for solution for infusion

2. QUALITATIVE AND QUANTITATIVE COMPOSITION

1 vial contains 150 mg of trastuzumab, a humanised IgG1 monoclonal antibody manufactured from a mammalian cell line (Chinese hamster ovary, CHO) by continuous perfusion. Reconstituted Herceptin solution contains 21 mg/ml of trastuzumab.

For a full list of excipients, see section 6.1.

3. PHARMACEUTICAL FORM

Powder for concentrate for solution for infusion.

Herceptin is a white to pale yellow lyophilised powder.

4. CLINICAL PARTICULARS

4.1 Therapeutic indications

Metastatic Breast Cancer (MBC)

Herceptin is indicated for the treatment of patients with metastatic breast cancer whose tumours overexpress HER2:

a) as monotherapy for the treatment of those patients who have received at least two chemotherapy regimens for their metastatic disease. Prior chemotherapy must have included at least an anthracycline and a taxane unless patients are unsuitable for these treatments. Hormone receptor positive patients must also have failed hormonal therapy, unless patients are unsuitable for these treatments.

b) in combination with paclitaxel for the treatment of those patients who have not received chemotherapy for their metastatic disease and for whom an anthracycline is not suitable.

c) in combination with docetaxel for the treatment of those patients who have not received chemotherapy for their metastatic disease.

d) in combination with an aromatase inhibitor for the treatment of postmenopausal patients with hormone-receptor positive metastatic breast cancer, not previously treated with trastuzumab.

Early Breast Cancer (EBC)

Herceptin is indicated for the treatment of patients with HER2 positive early breast cancer following surgery, chemotherapy (neoadjuvant or adjuvant) and radiotherapy (if applicable) (see 5.1).

Herceptin should only be used in patients whose tumours have either HER2 overexpression or HER2 gene amplification as determined by an accurate and validated assay (see 4.4 and 5.1).

4.2 Posology and method of administration

HER2 testing is mandatory prior to initiation of Herceptin therapy (see 4.4 and 5.1). Herceptin treatment should only be initiated by a physician experienced in the administration of cytotoxic chemotherapy (see 4.4).

MBC Weekly schedule:

The following loading and subsequent doses are recommended for monotherapy and in combination with paclitaxel, docetaxel or an aromatase inhibitor.

Loading dose

The recommended initial loading dose of Herceptin is 4 mg/kg body weight.

Subsequent doses

The recommended weekly dose of Herceptin is 2 mg/kg body weight, beginning one week after the loading dose.

Method of administration

Herceptin is administered as a 90-minute intravenous infusion. Patients should be observed for at least six hours after the start of the first infusion and for two hours after the start of the subsequent infusions for symptoms like fever and chills or other infusion-related symptoms (see 4.4 and 4.8). Interruption of the infusion may help control such symptoms. The infusion may be resumed when symptoms abate.

If the initial loading dose was well tolerated, the subsequent doses can be administered as a 30-minute infusion. Emergency equipment must be available.

Administration in combination with paclitaxel or docetaxel

In the pivotal trials, paclitaxel or docetaxel was administered the day following the first dose of Herceptin (for dose, see the Summary of Product Characteristics for paclitaxel or docetaxel) and immediately after the subsequent doses of Herceptin if the preceding dose of Herceptin was well tolerated.

Administration in combination with an aromatase inhibitor

In the pivotal trial Herceptin and anastrozole were administered from day 1. There were no restrictions on the relative timing of Herceptin and anastrozole at administration (for dose, see the Summary of Product Characteristics for anastrozole or other aromatase inhibitors).

Duration of treatment

Herceptin should be administered until progression of disease.

MBC 3-weekly schedule:

Alternatively the following loading and subsequent doses are recommended for monotherapy and in combination with paclitaxel, docetaxel or an aromatase inhibitor.

Initial loading dose of 8 mg/kg body weight, followed by 6 mg/kg body weight 3 weeks later and then 6 mg/kg repeated at 3-weekly intervals administered as infusions over approximately 90 minutes.

Duration of treatment

Herceptin should be administered until progression of disease.

EBC 3-weekly schedule:

In the HERA trial, Herceptin was initiated after completions of standard chemotherapy (most commonly, anthracycline-containing regimens or anthracyclines plus a taxane).

Initial loading dose of 8 mg/kg body weight, followed by 6 mg/kg body weight 3 weeks later and then 6 mg/kg repeated at 3-weekly intervals administered as infusions over approximately 90 minutes.

Patients with early breast cancer should be treated for 1 year or until disease recurrence.

EBC weekly schedule:

In the adjuvant setting, Herceptin has also been investigated as a weekly regimen (an initial loading dose of 4 mg/kg followed by 2 mg/kg every week for one year) concomitantly with paclitaxel (administered weekly (80 mg/m^2) or every 3 weeks (175 mg/m^2) for a total of 12 weeks) following 4 cycles of AC (doxorubicin 60 mg/m^2 IV push concurrently with cyclophosphamide 600 mg/m^2 over 20–30 minutes).

MBC and EBC:

Do not administer as an intravenous push or bolus.

For instructions for use and handling refer to 6.6.

Dose reduction

No reductions in the dose of Herceptin were made during clinical trials. Patients may continue Herceptin therapy during periods of reversible, chemotherapy-induced myelosuppression but they should be monitored carefully for complications of neutropenia during this time. Refer to the Summary of Product Characteristics for paclitaxel, docetaxel or aromatase inhibitor for information on dose reduction or delays.

Missed doses during 3-weekly schedule

If the patient misses a dose of Herceptin by one week or less, then the usual dose of Herceptin (6 mg/kg) should be given as soon as possible (do not wait until the next planned cycle). Subsequent maintenance Herceptin doses of 6 mg/kg should then be given every 3 weeks, according to the previous schedule.

If the patient misses a dose of Herceptin by more than one week, a re-loading dose of Herceptin should be given (8 mg/kg over approximately 90 minutes). Subsequent maintenance Herceptin doses of 6 mg/kg should then be given every 3 weeks from that point.

Special patient populations

Clinical data show that the disposition of Herceptin is not altered based on age or serum creatinine (see 5.2). In clinical trials, elderly patients did not receive reduced doses of Herceptin. Dedicated pharmacokinetic studies in the elderly and those with renal or hepatic impairment have not been carried out. However in a population pharmacokinetic analysis, age and renal impairment were not shown to affect trastuzumab disposition.

Paediatric use

Herceptin is not recommended for use in children below 18 due to insufficient data on safety and efficacy.

4.3 Contraindications

Patients with known hypersensitivity to trastuzumab, murine proteins, or to any of the excipients.

Patients with severe dyspnoea at rest due to complications of advanced malignancy or requiring supplementary oxygen therapy.

4.4 Special warnings and precautions for use

HER2 testing must be performed in a specialised laboratory which can ensure adequate validation of the testing procedures (see 5.1).

Currently no data from clinical trials are available on Herceptin re-treatment of patients with previous exposure to Herceptin in the adjuvant setting.

The use of Herceptin is associated with cardiotoxicity. All candidates for treatment should undergo careful cardiac monitoring (see "*cardiotoxicity*"section below). The risk of cardiotoxicity is greatest when Herceptin is used in combination with anthracyclines. Therefore Herceptin and anthracyclines should not be used currently in combination except in a well-controlled clinical trial setting with cardiac monitoring. Patients who have previously received anthracyclines are also at risk of cardiotoxicity with Herceptin treatment, although the risk is lower than with concurrent use of Herceptin and anthracyclines. Because the half-life of Herceptin is approximately 28.5 days (95 % confidence interval, 25.5 – 32.8 days), Herceptin may persist in the circulation for up to 24 weeks after stopping Herceptin treatment. Patients who receive anthracyclines after stopping Herceptin may possibly be at increased risk of cardiotoxicity. If possible, physicians should avoid anthracycline-based therapy for up to 24 weeks after stopping Herceptin. If anthracyclines are used, the patient's cardiac function should be monitored carefully (see "*cardiotoxicity*" section below). Serious adverse reactions including infusion reactions, hypersensitivity, allergic-like reactions and pulmonary events have been observed in patients receiving Herceptin therapy. Patients who are experiencing dyspnoea at rest due to complications of advanced malignancy and comorbidities may be at increased risk of a fatal infusion reaction. These severe reactions were usually associated with the first infusion of Herceptin and generally occurred during or immediately following the infusion. For some patients, symptoms progressively worsened and led to further pulmonary complications. Initial improvement followed by clinical deterioration and delayed reactions with rapid clinical deterioration have also been reported. Fatalities have occurred within hours and up to one week following infusion. On very rare occasions, patients have experienced the onset of infusion symptoms or pulmonary symptoms more than six hours after the start of the Herceptin infusion. Patients should be warned of the possibility of such a late onset and should be instructed to contact their physician if these symptoms occur.

Infusion reactions, allergic-like reactions and hypersensitivity

Serious adverse reactions to Herceptin infusion that have been reported infrequently include dyspnoea, hypotension, wheezing, hypertension, bronchospasm, supraventricular tachyarrythmia, reduced oxygen saturation, anaphylaxis, respiratory distress, urticaria and angioedema (see 4.8). The majority of these events occur during or within 2.5 hours of the start of the first infusion. Should an infusion reaction occur the Herceptin infusion should be discontinued and the patient monitored until resolution of any observed symptoms (see 4.2). The majority of patients experienced resolution of symptoms and subsequently received further infusions of Herceptin. Serious reactions have been treated successfully with supportive therapy such as oxygen, beta-agonists, and corticosteroids. In rare cases, these reactions are associated with a clinical course culminating in a fatal outcome. Patients who are experiencing dyspnoea at rest due to complications of advanced malignancy and comorbidities may be at increased risk of a fatal infusion reaction. Therefore, these patients should not be treated with Herceptin (see 4.3).

Pulmonary events

Severe pulmonary events have been reported rarely with the use of Herceptin in the post-marketing setting (see 4.8). These rare events have occasionally been fatal. In addition, rare cases of pulmonary infiltrates, acute respiratory distress syndrome, pneumonia, pneumonitis, pleural effusion, respiratory distress, acute pulmonary oedema and respiratory insufficiency have been reported. These events may occur as part of an infusion-related reaction or with a delayed onset. Patients who are experiencing dyspnoea at rest due to complications of advanced malignancy and comorbidities may be at increased risk of pulmonary events. Therefore, these patients should not be treated with Herceptin (see 4.3). Caution should be exercised for pneumonitis, especially in patients being treated concomitantly with taxanes.

Cardiotoxicity

Heart failure (New York Heart Association [NYHA] class II-IV) has been observed in patients receiving Herceptin therapy alone or in combination with paclitaxel or docetaxel, particularly following anthracycline (doxorubicin or epirubicin)–containing chemotherapy. This may be moderate to severe and has been associated with death (see 4.8).

All candidates for treatment with Herceptin, but especially those with prior anthracycline and cyclophosphamide (AC) exposure, should undergo baseline cardiac assessment including history and physical examination, ECG, echocardiogram, or MUGA scan or magnetic resonance imaging. A careful risk-benefit assessment should be made before deciding to treat with Herceptin.

In EBC, the following patients were excluded from the HERA trial, there are no data about the benefit:risk balance, and therefore treatment can not be recommended in such patients:

- History of documented CHF
- High-risk uncontrolled arrhythmias
- Angina pectoris requiring medication
- Clinically significant valvular disease
- Evidence of transmural infarction on ECG
- Poorly controlled hypertension

Formal cardiological assessment should be considered in patients in whom there are cardiovascular concerns following baseline screening. Cardiac function should be further monitored during treatment (e.g. every three months). Monitoring may help to identify patients who develop cardiac dysfunction. For early breast cancer patients, cardiac assessment, as performed at baseline, should be repeated every 3 months during treatment and at 6, 12 and 24 months following cessation of treatment. Patients who develop asymptomatic cardiac dysfunction may benefit from more frequent monitoring (e.g. every 6-8 weeks). If patients have a continued decrease in left ventricular function, but remain asymptomatic, the physician should consider discontinuing therapy if no clinical benefit of Herceptin therapy has been seen. Caution should be exercised in treating patients with symptomatic heart failure, a history of hypertension or documented coronary artery disease, and in early breast cancer, in those patients with an LVEF of 55 % or less.

If LVEF drops 10 ejection points from baseline AND to below 50 %, Herceptin should be suspended and a repeat LVEF assessment performed within approximately 3 weeks. If LVEF has not improved, or declined further, discontinuation of Herceptin should be strongly considered, unless the benefits for the individual patient are deemed to outweigh the risks. All such patients should be referred for assessment by a cardiologist and followed up.

If symptomatic cardiac failure develops during Herceptin therapy, it should be treated with the standard medications for this purpose. Discontinuation of Herceptin therapy should be strongly considered in patients who develop clinically significant heart failure unless the benefits for an individual patient are deemed to outweigh the risks.

The safety of continuation or resumption of Herceptin in patients who experience cardiotoxicity has not been prospectively studied. However, most patients who developed heart failure in the pivotal trials improved with standard medical treatment. This included diuretics, cardiac glycosides, beta-blockers and/or angiotensin-converting enzyme inhibitors. The majority of patients with cardiac symptoms and evidence of a clinical benefit of Herceptin treatment continued on weekly therapy with Herceptin without additional clinical cardiac events.

4.5 Interaction with other medicinal products and other forms of interaction

No interaction studies have been performed. A risk for interactions with concomitant medication cannot be excluded.

4.6 Pregnancy and lactation

Pregnancy

Reproduction studies have been conducted in cynomolgus monkeys at doses up to 25 times that of the weekly human maintenance dose of 2 mg/kg Herceptin and have revealed no evidence of impaired fertility or harm to the foetus. Placental transfer of trastuzumab during the early (Days 20–50 of gestation) and late (Days 120–150 of gestation) foetal development period was observed. It is not known whether Herceptin can cause foetal harm when administered to a pregnant woman or whether it can affect reproductive capacity. As animal reproduction studies are not always predictive of human response, Herceptin should be avoided during pregnancy unless the potential benefit for the mother outweighs the potential risk to the foetus.

In the postmarketing setting, cases of oligohydramnios have been reported in pregnant women receiving Herceptin.

Lactation

A study conducted in lactating cynomolgus monkeys at doses 25 times that of the weekly human maintenance dose of 2 mg/kg Herceptin demonstrated that trastuzumab is secreted in the milk. The presence of trastuzumab in the serum of infant monkeys was not associated with any adverse effects on their growth or development from birth to 1 month of age. It is not known whether trastuzumab is secreted in human milk. As human IgG1 is secreted into human milk, and the potential for harm to the infant is unknown, women should not breast-feed during Herceptin therapy and for 6 months after the last dose of Herceptin.

4.7 Effects on ability to drive and use machines

No studies on the effects on the ability to drive and to use machines have been performed. Patients experiencing infusion-related symptoms should be advised not to drive and use machines until symptoms abate.

4.8 Undesirable effects

MBC

The adverse event data reflect the clinical trial and post marketing experience of using Herceptin at the recommended dose regimen, either alone or in combination with paclitaxel.

Patients received Herceptin as monotherapy or in combination with paclitaxel in the two pivotal clinical trials. The most common adverse reactions are infusion-related symptoms, such as fever and chills, usually following the first infusion of Herceptin.

Adverse reactions attributed to Herceptin in ⩾ 10 % of patients in the two pivotal clinical trials were the following:

Body as a Whole:	abdominal pain, asthenia, chest pain, chills, fever, headache, pain
Digestive:	diarrhoea, nausea, vomiting
Musculoskeletal:	arthralgia, myalgia
Skin and appendages:	Rash

Adverse reactions attributed to Herceptin in > 1 % and < 10 % of patients in the two pivotal clinical trials were the following:

Body as a Whole:	influenza-like illness, back pain, infection, neck pain, malaise, hypersensitivity reaction, mastitis, weight loss
Cardiovascular:	vasodilation, supraventricular tachyarrythmia, hypotension, heart failure, cardiomyopathy, palpitation
Digestive:	anorexia, constipation, dyspepsia, liver tenderness, dry mouth, rectal disorder (haemorrhoids)
Blood and lymphatic:	leucopenia, ecchymosis
Metabolic:	peripheral oedema, oedema
Musculoskeletal:	bone pain, leg cramps, arthritis
Nervous:	dizziness, paraesthesia, somnolence, hypertonia, peripheral neuropathy, tremor
Psychiatric disorders	anxiety, depression, insomnia,
Respiratory:	asthma, cough increased, dyspnoea, epistaxis, lung disorders, pharyngitis, rhinitis, sinusitis
Urogenital:	urinary tract infection
Skin and appendages:	pruritus, sweating, nail disorder, dry skin, alopecia, acne, maculopapular rash
Special senses:	taste perversion

In a further randomised clinical trial (M77001), patients with metastatic breast cancer received docetaxel, with or without Herceptin. The following table displays adverse events which were reported in ⩾ 10% of patients, by study treatment:

Table 1 Common Non-haematological Adverse Events Reported in ⩾ 10% of Patients, by Study Treatment

(see Table 1 on next page)

There was an increased incidence of SAEs (40 % vs. 31%) and Grade 4 AEs (34 % vs. 23 %) in the combination arm compared to docetaxel monotherapy.

In a further randomised clinical trial (BO16216), patients with HER2 positive and hormone receptor positive metastatic breast cancer received anastrozole with or without Herceptin. In this trial, there was no change in the safety profile compared with previous trials in the metastatic population. The following table displays adverse events which were reported in ⩾ 10% of patients, by study treatment:

Table 2 Summary of Adverse Events with an Incidence Rate of at Least 10 % by Trial Treatment

Adverse Event	Arimidex Plus Herceptin N=103 No. (%)	Arimidex Alone N=104 No. (%)
Fatigue	22 (21)	10 (10)
Diarrhoea	21 (20)	8 (8)
Vomiting	22 (21)	5 (5)
Arthralgia	15 (15)	10 (10)
Pyrexia	18 (17)	7 (7)
Back pain	15 (15)	7 (7)
Dyspnoea	13 (13)	9 (9)
Nausea	17 (17)	5 (5)
Cough	14 (14)	6 (6)

Headache	14 (14)	6 (6)
Nasopharyngitis	17 (17)	2 (2)
Bone pain	11 (11)	6 (6)
Constipation	12 (12)	5 (5)
Chills	15 (15)	-

Percentages are based on N.
Multiple occurrences of the same adverse event in one individual counted only once.
Note: For patients from the Arimidex Alone arm who switched to Herceptin, only AEs before the 1st Herceptin administration are displayed

There was an increased incidence of SAEs (23% vs. 6%) and Grade 3/4 AEs (25% vs. 15%) in the combination arm compared to anastrozole monotherapy.

EBC

The HERA trial is a randomised, open label study in patients with HER2-positive early breast cancer (see section 5.1 Pharmacodynamic properties). Table 3 displays adverse events which were reported at 1 year in ≥ 1% of patients, by study treatment.

Table 3 Adverse Events Reported at 1 year in ≥ 1% of Patients, by Study Treatment

(see Table 3 on next page)

The following information is relevant to all indications:

Serious Adverse Reactions

At least one case of the following serious adverse reactions has occurred in at least one patient treated with Herceptin alone or in combination with chemotherapy in clinical trials or has been reported during post marketing experience:

Body System	Adverse Event
Body as a Whole	hypersensitivity reaction, anaphylaxis and anaphylactic shock, angioedema, ataxia, sepsis, chills and fever, asthenia, fever, rigor, headache, paresis, chest pain, fatigue, infusion-related symptoms, peripheral oedema, bone pain, coma, meningitis, cerebral oedema, thinking abnormal, progression of neoplasia
Cardiovascular	cardiomyopathy, congestive heart failure, increased congestive heart failure, decreased ejection fraction, hypotension, pericardial effusion, bradycardia, cerebrovascular disorder, cardiac failure, cardiogenic shock, pericarditis
Digestive	hepatocellular damage, liver tenderness, diarrhoea, nausea and vomiting, pancreatitis, hepatic failure, jaundice
Blood and Lymphatic	leukaemia, febrile neutropenia, neutropenia, thrombocytopenia, anaemia, hypoprothrombinemia
Infections	cellulitis, erysipelas
Metabolic	hyperkalaemia
Musculoskeletal	myalgia
Nervous	paraneoplastic cerebellar degeneration
Renal	membranous glomerulonephritis, glomerulonephropathy, renal failure
Respiratory	bronchospasm, respiratory distress, acute pulmonary oedema, respiratory insufficiency, dyspnoea, hypoxia, laryngeal oedema, acute respiratory distress, acute respiratory distress syndrome, Cheyne-Stokes breathing, pulmonary infiltrates, pneumonia, pneumonitis, pulmonary fibrosis
Skin and appendages	rash, dermatitis, urticaria, Stevens-Johnson syndrome
Special Senses	papilloedema, abnormal lacrimation, retinal haemorrhage, deafness

Infusion-Related Symptoms

During the first infusion of Herceptin chills and/or fever are observed commonly in patients. Other signs and/or symptoms may include nausea, hypertension, vomiting, pain, rigors, headache, cough, dizziness, rash, and asthenia. These symptoms are usually mild to moderate in severity, and occur infrequently with subsequent Herceptin infusions. These symptoms can be treated with an analgesic/antipyretic such as meperidine or paracetamol, or an antihistamine such as diphenhydramine (see 4.2). Some adverse reactions to Herceptin infusion including dys-

Table 1 Common Non-haematological Adverse Events Reported in ≥ 10% of Patients, by Study Treatment

Body System	Adverse Event	Herceptin plus docetaxel N = 92 (%)	docetaxel N = 94 (%)
General disorders and administration site conditions	asthenia	45	41
	oedema peripheral	40	35
	fatigue	24	21
	mucosal inflammation	23	22
	pyrexia	29	15
	pain	12	9
	lethargy	7	11
	chest pain	11	5
	influenza like illness	12	2
	rigors	11	1
Skin and subcutaneous tissue disorders	alopecia	67	54
	nail disorder	17	21
	rash	24	12
	erythema	23	11
Gastrointestinal disorders	nausea	43	41
	diarrhoea	43	36
	vomiting	29	22
	constipation	27	23
	stomatitis	20	14
	abdominal pain	12	12
	dyspepsia	14	5
Nervous system disorders	paraesthesia	32	21
	headache	21	18
	dysgeusia	14	12
	hypoaesthesia	11	5
Blood and lymphatic system disorders	febrile neutropenia[1] / neutropenic sepsis	23	17
Musculoskeletal and connective tissue disorders	myalgia	27	26
	arthralgia	27	20
	pain in extremity	16	16
	back pain	10	14
	bone pain	14	6
Respiratory, thoracic and mediastinal disorders	cough	13	16
	dyspnoea	14	15
	pharyngolaryngeal pain	16	9
	epistaxis	18	5
	rhinorrhoea	12	1
Infections and infestations	nasopharyngitis	15	6
Eye disorders	lacrimation increased	21	10
	conjunctivitis	12	7
Vascular disorders	lymphoedema	11	6
Metabolism and nutrition disorders	anorexia	22	13
Investigations	weight increased	15	6
Psychiatric disorders	insomnia	11	4
Injury, poisoning and procedural complications	nail toxicity	11	7

[1] These numbers include patients with preferred terms of 'febrile neutropenia', 'neutropenic sepsis' or 'neutropenia' that was associated with fever (and antibiotic use). See also section 4.8

Table 3 Adverse Events Reported at 1 year in ⩾ 1% of Patients, by Study Treatment

Body System	Adverse Event	Observation Only N = 1708 No. (%)	Herceptin 1 year N = 1678 No. (%)
	Total Pts with at least one AE **Total number of AEs**	**792 (46)** **2251**	**1179 (70)** **5248**
Musculoskeletal and connective tissue disorders	arthralgia*	98 (6)	137 (8)
	back pain*	59 (3)	91 (5)
	pain in extremity	45 (3)	60 (4)
	myalgia*	17 (<1)	63 (4)
	bone pain	26 (2)	49 (3)
	shoulder pain	29 (2)	30 (2)
	chest wall pain	24 (1)	26 (2)
	muscle spasms*	3 (<1)	45 (3)
	musculoskeletal pain	11 (<1)	17 (1)
Infections and infestations	nasopharyngitis*	43 (3)	135 (8)
	influenza*	9 (<1)	69 (4)
	upper respiratory tract infection*	20 (1)	46 (3)
	urinary tract infection	13 (<1)	39 (2)
	rhinitis	6 (<1)	36 (2)
	sinusitis	5 (<1)	26 (2)
	cystitis	11 (<1)	19 (1)
	pharyngitis	9 (<1)	20 (1)
	bronchitis	9 (<1)	18 (1)
	herpes zoster	9 (<1)	17 (1)
General disorders and administration site conditions	fatigue*	44 (3)	128 (8)
	oedema peripheral	38 (2)	79 (5)
	pyrexia*	6 (<1)	100 (6)
	asthenia*	30 (2)	75 (4)
	chills*	-	85 (5)
	chest pain*	22 (1)	45 (3)
	influenza illness	3 (<1)	40 (2)
	oedema	7 (<1)	18 (1)
	chest discomfort	2 (<1)	20 (1)
Gastrointestinal disorders	diarrhoea*	16 (<1)	123 (7)
	nausea*	19 (1)	108 (6)
	vomiting*	10 (<1)	58 (3)
	abdominal pain	16 (<1)	40 (2)
	constipation	17 (<1)	33 (2)
	abdominal pain upper	15 (<1)	29 (2)
	dyspepsia	9 (<1)	30 (2)
	gastritis	11 (<1)	20 (1)
	stomatitis	1 (<1)	26 (2)
Nervous system disorders	headache*	49 (3)	161 (10)
	dizziness*	29 (2)	60 (4)
	paraesthesia	11 (<1)	29 (2)
	vertigo	7 (<1)	25 (1)
Vascular disorders	hot flush	84 (5)	98 (6)
	hypertension*	35 (2)	64 (4)
	lymphoedema	40 (2)	42 (3)
Skin and subcutaneous tissue	rash*	10 (<1)	70 (4)
	pruritus	10 (<1)	40 (2)
	nail disorder*	-	43 (3)
	onychorrhexis	1 (<1)	36 (2)
	erythema	7 (<1)	24 (1)
Respiratory, thoracic and mediastinal disorders	cough*	34 (2)	81 (5)
	dyspnoea	26 (2)	56 (3)
	pharyngolaryngeal pain	8 (<1)	32 (2)
	dyspnoea exertional	15 (<1)	21 (1)
	rhinorrhoea	5 (<1)	24 (1)
	epistaxis	1 (<1)	24 (1)
Reproductive system and breast disorders	breast pain	19 (1)	24 (1)
Psychiatric	insomnia	31 (2)	58 (3)
	depression	34 (2)	51 (3)
	anxiety	19 (1)	39 (2)
Cardiac disorders	palpitations*	12 (<1)	48 (3)
	cardiac failure congestive	5 (<1)	30 (2)
	tachycardia	5 (<1)	20 (1)
Investigations	ejection fraction decreased*	11 (<1)	58 (3)
	weight increased	17 (<1)	29 (2)
Renal and urinary disorders	dysuria	2 (<1)	17 (1)

** Adverse Events that were reported at higher incidence (≥ 2 % difference) in the Herceptin group compared with the observation group and therefore may be attributable to Herceptin.*

pnoea, hypotension, wheezing, bronchospasm, supraventricular tachyarrythmia, reduced oxygen saturation and respiratory distress can be serious and potentially fatal (see 4.4).

Allergic-like and hypersensitivity reactions

Allergic reactions, anaphylaxis and anaphylactic shock, urticaria and angioedema occurring during the first infusion of Herceptin, have been reported rarely. Over a third of these patients had a negative re-challenge and continued to receive Herceptin. Some of these reactions can be serious and potentially fatal (see 4.4).

Serious pulmonary events

Single cases of pulmonary infiltrates, pneumonia, pulmonary fibrosis, pleural effusion, respiratory distress, acute pulmonary oedema, acute respiratory distress syndrome (ARDS) and respiratory insufficiency have been reported rarely. These events have been reported rarely with fatal outcome (see 4.4).

Cardiac toxicity

Reduced ejection fraction and signs and symptoms of heart failure, such as dyspnoea, orthopnoea, increased cough, pulmonary oedema, and S_3 gallop, have been observed in patients treated with Herceptin. (see 4.4).

The incidence of cardiac adverse events from retrospective analysis of data from the combination therapy study (Herceptin plus paclitaxel versus paclitaxel alone and the Herceptin monotherapy study is shown in the following table:

Cardiac Adverse Event Incidence; n,% [95 %-confidence limits]

(see Table 4 on next page)

The incidence of symptomatic congestive heart failure in the study of Herceptin plus docetaxel versus docetaxel alone (M77001), is shown in the following table:

	Herceptin plus docetaxel N = 92	docetaxel N = 94
Symptomatic heart failure	2 (2.2 %)	0 %

In this study, all patients had a baseline cardiac ejection fraction of greater than 50 %. In the Herceptin plus docetaxel arm, 64 % had received a prior anthracycline compared with 55 % in the docetaxel alone arm.

Summary of Patients with an LVEF Decrease by at least an Absolute 15% from Baseline and the Absolute LVEF Value below 50%, Safety Population (Before Cross-over)

	Anastrozole plus Herceptin n=103	Anastrozole alone n=104
Symptomatic CHF	1 (<1%)	0[a]
Confirmed LVEF drops of ⩾ 15% from Baseline and below 50%	1 (<1%)	0[b]
At least one LVEF drop of ⩾ 15% from baseline and below 50%	6 (5.8%)	0[c]

[a] One patient experienced symptomatic CHF after cross over to Herceptin-containing regimen following progression

[b] Two patients experienced confirmed LVEF drops after cross over to Herceptin-containing regimen following progression

[c] Four patients experienced one LVEF drops after cross over to Herceptin-containing regimen following progression

In the HERA trial, NYHA class III-IV heart failure was observed in 0.6 % of patients in the one-year arm. Asymptomatic or mildly symptomatic NYHA class I – II events were observed in 3.0% of patients in the Herceptin arm compared to 0.5% of patients in the observation arm. The percentage of patients with at least one significant LVEF drop (decrease of ⩾ 10 EF points and to < 50%) during the study was 7.4% in the 1 year Herceptin arm versus 2.3% in the observation arm.

Haematological toxicity

Haematological toxicity was infrequent following the administration of Herceptin as a single agent in the metastatic setting, WHO Grade 3 leucopenia, thrombocytopenia and anaemia occurring in < 1 % of patients. No WHO Grade 4 toxicities were observed.

There was an increase in WHO Grade 3 or 4 haematological toxicity in patients treated with the combination of Herceptin and paclitaxel compared with patients receiving paclitaxel alone (34 % versus 21 %). Haematological toxicity was also increased in patients receiving Herceptin and docetaxel, compared with docetaxel alone (32 % grade 3/4 neutropenia versus 22 %, using NCI-CTC criteria). Note that this is likely to be an underestimate since docetaxel alone at a dose of 100mg/m^2 is known to result in

Table 4 Cardiac Adverse Event Incidence; n,% [95 %-confidence limits]

	Herceptin plus paclitaxel N=91	paclitaxel N=95	Herceptin N=213
Symptomatic heart failure	8, 8.8 % [3.9-16.6]	4, 4.2 % [1.2-10.4]	18, 8.5 % [5.1-13.0]
Cardiac diagnosis other than heart failure	4, 4.4 % [1.2-10.9]	7, 7.4 % [3.0-14.6]	7, 3.3 % [1.3-6.7]

neutropenia in 97 % of patients, 76% grade 4, based on nadir blood counts. The incidence of febrile neutropenia/ neutropenic sepsis was also increased in patients treated with Herceptin plus docetaxel (23 % versus 17 % for patients treated with docetaxel alone).

Using NCI-CTC criteria, in the HERA trial, 0.4% of Herceptin-treated patients experienced a shift of 3 or 4 grades from baseline, compared with 0.6% in the observation arm.

Hepatic and renal toxicity

WHO Grade 3 or 4 hepatic toxicity was observed in 12 % of patients following administration of Herceptin as single agent, in the metastatic setting. This toxicity was associated with progression of disease in the liver in 60 % of these patients. WHO Grade 3 or 4 hepatic toxicity was less frequently observed among patients receiving Herceptin and paclitaxel than among patients receiving paclitaxel (7 % compared with 15 %). No WHO Grade 3 or 4 renal toxicity was observed in patients treated with Herceptin.

Diarrhoea

Of patients treated with Herceptin as a single agent in the metastatic setting, 27 % experienced diarrhoea. An increase in the incidence of diarrhoea, primarily mild to moderate in severity, has also been observed in patients receiving Herceptin in combination with paclitaxel or docetaxel compared with patients receiving paclitaxel or docetaxel alone.

In the HERA trial, 7 % of Herceptin-treated patients had diarrhoea.

Infection

An increased incidence of infections, primarily mild upper respiratory infections of minor clinical significance or catheter infections, has been observed primarily in patients treated with Herceptin plus paclitaxel or docetaxel compared with patients receiving paclitaxel or docetaxel alone.

4.9 Overdose

There is no experience with overdosage in human clinical trials. Single doses of Herceptin alone greater than 10 mg/kg have not been administered in the clinical trials. Doses up to this level were well tolerated.

5. PHARMACOLOGICAL PROPERTIES

5.1 Pharmacodynamic properties

Pharmacotherapeutic group: Antineoplastic agents, ATC code: L01XC03

Trastuzumab is a recombinant humanised IgG1 monoclonal antibody against the human epidermal growth factor receptor 2 (HER2). Overexpression of HER2 is observed in 20 %-30 % of primary breast cancers. Studies indicate that patients whose tumours overexpress HER2 have a shortened disease-free survival compared to patients whose tumours do not overexpress HER2. The extracellular domain of the receptor (ECD, p105) can be shed into the blood stream and measured in serum samples.

Trastuzumab has been shown, in both *in vitro* assays and in animals, to inhibit the proliferation of human tumour cells that overexpress HER2. Additionally, trastuzumab is a potent mediator of antibody-dependent cell-mediated cytotoxicity (ADCC). In vitro, trastuzumab-mediated ADCC has been shown to be preferentially exerted on HER2 overexpressing cancer cells compared with cancer cells that do not overexpress HER2.

Detection of HER2 overexpression or HER2 gene amplification

Herceptin should only be used in patients whose tumours have HER2 overexpression or HER2 gene amplification as determined by an accurate and validated assay. HER2 overexpression should be detected using an immunohistochemistry (IHC)-based assessment of fixed tumour blocks (see 4.4). HER2 gene amplification should be detected using fluorescence in situ hybridisation (FISH) or chromogenic in situ hybridisation (CISH) of fixed tumour blocks. Patients are eligible for Herceptin treatment if they show strong HER2 overexpression as described by a 3+ score by IHC or a positive FISH or CISH result.

To ensure accurate and reproducible results, the testing must be performed in a specialised laboratory, which can ensure validation of the testing procedures.

The recommended scoring system to evaluate the IHC staining patterns is as follows:

(see Table 5 below)

In general, FISH is considered positive if the ratio of the HER2 gene copy number per tumour cell to the chromosome 17 copy number is greater than or equal to 2, or if there are more than 4 copies of the HER2 gene per tumour cell if no chromosome 17 control is used.

In general, CISH is considered positive if there are more than 5 copies of the HER2 gene per nucleus in greater than 50 % of tumour cells.

For full instructions on assay performance and interpretation please refer to the package inserts of validated FISH and CISH assays. Official recommendations on HER2 testing may also apply.

For any other method that may be used for the assessment of HER2 protein or gene expression, the analyses should only be performed by laboratories that provide adequate state-of-the-art performance of validated methods. Such methods must clearly be precise and accurate enough to demonstrate overexpression of HER2 and must be able to distinguish between moderate (congruent with 2+) and strong (congruent with 3+) overexpression of HER2.

Clinical Data

Herceptin has been used in clinical trials as monotherapy for patients with metastatic breast cancer who have tumours that overexpress HER2 and who have failed one or more chemotherapy regimens for their metastatic disease (Herceptin alone).

Herceptin has also been used in combination with paclitaxel or docetaxel for the treatment of patients who have not received chemotherapy for their metastatic disease. Patients who had previously received anthracycline-based adjuvant chemotherapy were treated with paclitaxel (175 mg/m^2 infused over 3 hours) with or without Herceptin. In the pivotal trial of docetaxel (100 mg/m^2 infused over 1 hour) with or without Herceptin, 60 % of the patients had received prior anthracycline-based adjuvant chemotherapy. Patients were treated with Herceptin until progression of disease.

The efficacy of Herceptin in combination with paclitaxel in patients who did not receive prior adjuvant anthracyclines has not been studied. However, Herceptin plus docetaxel was efficacious in patients whether or not they had received prior adjuvant anthracyclines.

The test method for HER2 overexpression used to determine eligibility of patients in the pivotal Herceptin monotherapy and Herceptin plus paclitaxel clinical trials employed immunohistochemical staining for HER2 of fixed material from breast tumours using the murine monoclonal antibodies CB11 and 4D5. These tissues were fixed in formalin or Bouin's fixative. This investigative clinical trial assay performed in a central laboratory utilised a 0 to 3+ scale. Patients classified as staining 2+ or 3+ were included, while those staining 0 or 1+ were excluded.

Table 5

Staining Intensity Score	Staining pattern	HER2 Overexpression Assessment
0	No staining is observed or membrane staining is observed in < 10 % of the tumour cells	Negative
1+	A faint/barely perceptible membrane staining is detected in > 10 % of the tumour cells. The cells are only stained in part of their membrane.	Negative
2+	A weak to moderate complete membrane staining is detected in > 10 % of the tumour cells.	Weak to moderate overexpression
3+	A moderate to strong complete membrane staining is detected in > 10 % of the tumour cells.	Moderate to strong overexpression

Greater than 70 % of patients enrolled exhibited 3+ overexpression. The data suggest that beneficial effects were greater among those patients with higher levels of overexpression of HER2 (3+).

The main test method used to determine HER2 positivity in the pivotal trial of docetaxel, with or without Herceptin, was immunohistochemistry. A minority of patients were tested using fluorescence *in-situ* hybridisation (FISH). In this trial, 87 % of patients entered had disease that was IHC3+, and 95 % of patients entered had disease that was IHC3+ and/ or FISH-positive.

Efficacy

Weekly dosing in MBC

The efficacy results from the monotherapy and combination therapy studies are summarised in the following table:

(see Table 6 on next page)

Combination treatment with Herceptin and anastrozole

Herceptin has been studied in combination with anastrozole for first line treatment of metastatic breast cancer in HER2 overexpressing, hormone-receptor (i.e. estrogen-receptor (ER) and/or progesterone-receptor (PR)) positive postmenopausal patients. Progression free survival was doubled in the Herceptin plus anastrozole arm compared to anastrozole (4.8 months versus 2.4 months). For the other parameters the improvements seen for the combination were for overall response (16.5% versus 6.7%); clinical benefit rate (42.7% versus 27.9%); time to progression (4.8 months versus 2.4 months). For time to response and duration of response no difference could be recorded between the arms. The median overall survival was extended by 4.6 months for patients in the combination arm. The difference was not statistically significant, however more than half of the patients in the anastrozole alone arm crossed over to a Herceptin containing regimen after progression of disease.

3 -weekly dosing in MBC

The efficacy results from the non-comparative monotherapy and combination therapy studies are summarised in the following table:

(see Table 7 on next page)

EBC

Early breast cancer is defined as non-metastatic primary invasive carcinoma of the breast. Early breast cancer in the HERA trial was limited to operable, primary, invasive adenocarcinoma of the breast, with axillary nodes positive or axillary nodes negative if tumours at least 1 cm in diameter.

In the adjuvant setting, Herceptin was investigated in a multicentre, randomised, trial (HERA) designed to compare one year of three-weekly Herceptin treatment versus observation in patients with HER2 positive early breast cancer following surgery, established chemotherapy and radiotherapy (if applicable). Patients assigned to receive Herceptin were given an initial loading dose of 8 mg/kg, followed by 6 mg/kg every three weeks for one year.

The efficacy results from the Hera trial are summarized in the following table:

(see Table 8 on next page)

For the primary endpoint, DFS, the hazard ratio translates into an absolute benefit, in terms of a 2-year disease-free survival rate, of 7.6 percentage points (85.8 % vs 78.2 %) in favour of the Herceptin arm.

Immunogenicity

Nine hundred and three patients treated with Herceptin, alone or in combination with chemotherapy, have been evaluated for antibody production. Human anti-trastuzumab antibodies were detected in one patient, who had no allergic manifestations.

Sites of progression

After Herceptin and paclitaxel therapy for metastatic breast cancer in patients in the pivotal trial the following sites of disease progression were found:

(see Table 9 on next page)

The frequency of progression in the liver was significantly reduced in patients treated with the combination of Herceptin and paclitaxel. More patients treated with Herceptin and paclitaxel progressed in the central nervous system than those treated with paclitaxel alone.

5.2 Pharmacokinetic properties

The pharmacokinetics of trastuzumab have been studied in patients with metastatic breast cancer and early breast cancer. Short duration intravenous infusions of 10, 50, 100, 250, and 500 mg trastuzumab once weekly in patients demonstrated dose-dependent pharmacokinetics. Drug interaction studies have not been performed with Herceptin.

Half-life

The half-life is approximately 28.5 days (95 % confidence interval, 25.5 –32.8 days). The washout period is up to 24 weeks (95 % confidence interval, 18-24 weeks)

Steady State Concentration

Steady state pharmacokinetics should be reached by approximately 20 weeks (95 % confidence interval, 18 – 24 weeks). In a population pharmacokinetic assessment of Phase I, II and III clinical trials in metastatic breast cancer, the estimated mean AUC was 578 mg day/L and the estimated mean peak and trough concentrations were

Table 6

Parameter	Monotherapy	Combination Therapy			
	Herceptin[1] N=172	Herceptin plus paclitaxel[2] N=68	Paclitaxel[2] N=77	Herceptin plus docetaxel[3] N=92	Docetaxel[3] N=94
Response rate(95%CI)	18% (13 - 25)	49% (36 - 61)	17% (9 - 27)	61% (50-71)	34% (25-45)
Median duration of response (months) (95%CI)	9.1 (5.6-10.3)	8.3 (7.3-8.8)	4.6 (3.7-7.4)	11.7 (9.3 – 15.0)	5.7 (4.6-7.6)
Median TTP (months) (95%CI)	3.2 (2.6-3.5)	7.1 (6.2-12.0)	3.0 (2.0-4.4)	11.7 (9.2-13.5)	6.1 (5.4-7.2)
Median Survival (months) (95%CI)	16.4 (12.3-ne)	24.8 (18.6-33.7)	17.9 (11.2-23.8)	31.2 (27.3-40.8)	22.74 (19.1-30.8)

TTP = time to progression; "ne" indicates that it could not be estimated or it was not yet reached.

1. Study H0649g: IHC3+ patient subset
2. Study H0648g: IHC3+ patient subset
3. Study M77001: Full analysis set (intent-to-treat)

Table 7

Parameter	Monotherapy		Combination Therapy	
	Herceptin[1] N=105	Herceptin[2] N=72	Herceptin plus paclitaxel [3] N=32	Herceptin plus docetaxel[4] N=110
Response rate(95%CI)	24% (15 - 35)	27% (14 - 43)	59% (41-76)	73% (63-81)
Median duration of response (months) (range)	10.1 (2.8-35.6)	7.9 (2.1-18.8)	10.5 (1.8-21)	13.4 (2.1-55.1)
Median TTP (months) (95%CI)	3.4 (2.8-4.1)	7.7 (4.2-8.3)	12.2 (6.2-ne)	13.6 (11-16)
Median Survival (months) (95%CI)	ne	ne	ne	47.3 (32-ne)

TTP = time to progression; "ne" indicates that it could not be estimated or it was not yet reached.

1. Study WO16229: loading dose 8 mg/kg, followed by 6 mg/kg 3 weekly schedule
2. Study MO16982: loading dose 6mg/kg weekly × 3; followed by 6mg/kg 3-weekly schedule
3. BO15935
4. MO16419

Table 8

Parameter	Observation N=1693	Herceptin 1 Year N = 1693	P-value vs Observation	Hazard Ratio vs Observation
Disease-free survival				
- No. patients with event	219 (12.9 %)	127 (7.5 %)	< 0.0001	0.54
- No. patients without event	1474 (87.1 %)	1566 (92.5 %)		
Recurrence-free survival				
- No. patients with event	208 (12.3 %)	113 (6.7 %)	< 0.0001	0.51
- No. patients without event	1485 (87.7 %)	1580 (93.3 %)		
Distant disease-free survival				
- No. patients with event	184 (10.9 %)	99 (5.8 %)	< 0.0001	0.50
- No. patients without event	1508 (89.1 %)	1594 (94.6 %)		

Table 9

Site*	Herceptin plus paclitaxel (N=87) %	paclitaxel (N=92) %	p-value
Any site	**70.1**	**95.7**	
Abdomen	0	0	-
Bone	17.2	16.3	0.986
Chest	5.7	13.0	0.250
Liver	21.8	45.7	**0.004**
Lung	16.1	18.5	0.915
Dist. Node	3.4	6.5	0.643
Mediastinum	4.6	2.2	0.667
CNS	12.6	6.5	0.377
Other	4.6	9.8	0.410

*Patients may have had multiple sites of disease progression

110 mg/L and 66 mg/L, respectively. In patients with early breast cancer administered Herceptin at a loading dose of 8 mg/kg followed every three weeks by 6 mg/kg, steady state trough concentrations of 63 mg/L were achieved by cycle 13 (week 37). The concentrations were comparable to those reported previously in patients with metastatic breast cancer.

Clearance

Clearance decreased with increased dose level. In clinical trials where a loading dose of 4 mg/kg trastuzumab followed by a subsequent weekly dose of 2 mg/kg was used, the mean clearance was 0.225L/day.

The effects of patient characteristics (such as age or serum creatinine) on the disposition of trastuzumab have been evaluated. The data suggest that the disposition of trastuzumab is not altered in any of these groups of patients (see 4.2), however, studies were not specifically designed to investigate the impact of renal impairment upon pharmacokinetics.

Volume of Distribution

In all clinical studies, volume of distribution approximated serum volume, 2.95 L.

Circulating Shed Antigen

Detectable concentrations of the circulating extracellular domain of the HER2 receptor (shed antigen) are found in the serum of some patients with HER2 overexpressing breast cancers. Determination of shed antigen in baseline serum samples revealed that 64 % (286/447) of patients had detectable shed antigen, which ranged as high as 1880 ng/ml (median = 11 ng/ml). Patients with higher baseline shed antigen levels were more likely to have lower serum trough concentrations of trastuzumab. However, with weekly dosing, most patients with elevated shed antigen levels achieved target serum concentrations of trastuzumab by week 6 and no significant relationship has been observed between baseline shed antigen and clinical response.

5.3 Preclinical safety data

There was no evidence of acute or multiple dose-related toxicity in studies of up to 6 months, or reproductive toxicity in teratology, female fertility or late gestational toxicity/placental transfer studies. Herceptin is not genotoxic. A study of trehalose, a major formulation excipient did not reveal any toxicities.

No long-term animal studies have been performed to establish the carcinogenic potential of Herceptin, or to determine its effects on fertility in males.

6. PHARMACEUTICAL PARTICULARS

6.1 List of excipients

L-histidine hydrochloride

L-histidine

α,α-trehalose dihydrate

polysorbate 20

6.2 Incompatibilities

Do not dilute with glucose solutions since these cause aggregation of the protein.

Herceptin should not be mixed or diluted with other products except those mentioned under section 6.6.

6.3 Shelf life

4 years

After reconstitution with sterile water for injections the reconstituted solution is physically and chemically stable for 48 hours at 2°C – 8°C. Any remaining reconstituted solution should be discarded.

Solutions of Herceptin for infusion are physically and chemically stable in polyvinylchloride, polyethylene or polypropylene bags containing 0.9 % sodium chloride for 24 hours at temperatures not exceeding 30°C.

From a microbiological point of view, the reconstituted solution and Herceptin infusion solution should be used immediately. The product is not intended to be stored after reconstitution and dilution unless this has taken place under controlled and validated aseptic conditions. If not used immediately, in-use storage times and conditions are the responsibility of the user.

6.4 Special precautions for storage

Store in a refrigerator (2°C – 8°C)

Do not freeze the reconstituted solution.

6.5 Nature and contents of container

Herceptin vial:

One 15 ml clear glass type I vial with butyl rubber stopper laminated with a fluoro-resin film.

Each carton contains one vial.

6.6 Special precautions for disposal and other handling

Preparation for Administration

Appropriate aseptic technique should be used. Each vial of Herceptin is reconstituted with 7.2 ml of sterile water for injections (not supplied). Use of other reconstitution solvents should be avoided.

This yields a 7.4 ml solution for single-dose use, containing approximately 21 mg/ml trastuzumab, at a pH of approximately 6.0. A volume overage of 4 % ensures that the labelled dose of 150 mg can be withdrawn from each vial.

Formula 1

$$\text{Volume (ml)} = \frac{\text{Body weight (kg)} \times \text{dose (4 mg/kg for loading or 2 mg/kg for maintenance)}}{\text{21 (mg/ml, concentration of reconstituted solution)}}$$

Formula

$$\text{Volume (ml)} = \frac{\text{Body weight (kg)} \times \text{dose (8 mg/kg for loading or 6 mg/kg for maintenance)}}{\text{21 (mg/ml, concentration of reconstituted solution)}}$$

Herceptin should be carefully handled during reconstitution. Causing excessive foaming during reconstitution or shaking the reconstituted Herceptin may result in problems with the amount of Herceptin that can be withdrawn from the vial.

Instructions for Reconstitution:

1) Using a sterile syringe, slowly inject 7.2 ml of sterile water for injections in the vial containing the lyophilised Herceptin, directing the stream into the lyophilised cake.

2) Swirl vial gently to aid reconstitution. DO NOT SHAKE!

Slight foaming of the product upon reconstitution is not unusual. Allow the vial to stand undisturbed for approximately 5 minutes. The reconstituted Herceptin results in a colourless to pale yellow transparent solution and should be essentially free of visible particulates.

Determine the volume of the solution required:

• based on a loading dose of 4 mg trastuzumab/kg body weight, or a subsequent weekly dose of 2 mg trastuzumab/kg body weight:

(see Formula 1 above)

• based on a loading dose of 8 mg trastuzumab/kg body weight, or a subsequent 3-weekly dose of 6 mg trastuzumab/kg body weight:

(see Formula 2 above)

The appropriate amount of solution should be withdrawn from the vial and added to an infusion bag containing 250 ml of 0.9 % sodium chloride solution. Do not use with glucose-containing solutions (see 6.2). The bag should be gently inverted to mix the solution in order to avoid foaming. Parenteral solutions should be inspected visually for particulates and discoloration prior to administration. Once the infusion is prepared it should be administered immediately. If diluted aseptically, it may be stored for 24 hours (do not store above 30°C).

No incompatibilities between Herceptin and polyvinylchloride, polyethylene or polypropylene bags have been observed.

7. MARKETING AUTHORISATION HOLDER

Roche Registration Limited
6 Falcon Way
Shire Park
Welwyn Garden City
AL7 1TW
United Kingdom

8. MARKETING AUTHORISATION NUMBER(S)

EU/1/00/145/001

9. DATE OF FIRST AUTHORISATION/RENEWAL OF THE AUTHORISATION

28 August 2000/ 28 August 2005

10. DATE OF REVISION OF THE TEXT

2nd December 2008

Herpid

(Astellas Pharma Ltd)

1. NAME OF THE MEDICINAL PRODUCT

Herpid.

2. QUALITATIVE AND QUANTITATIVE COMPOSITION

A clear, colourless solution containing idoxuridine BP 5% in dimethyl sulfoxide.

3. PHARMACEUTICAL FORM

Topical Solution.

4. CLINICAL PARTICULARS

4.1 Therapeutic indications

Cutaneous herpes simplex and herpes zoster (shingles).

4.2 Posology and method of administration

Administration: Herpid should be painted on the lesions and their erythematous bases four times daily for four days.

Adults and children over 12 years:

Treatment should start as soon as the condition has been diagnosed, ideally within two or three days after the rash appears. Good results are less likely if treatment is not started within seven days.

Children under 12 years:

The use of Herpid in children with malignant disease might be justified but, although not a contra-indication, its use in children under the age of 12 years is not recommended.

No specific information on the use of this product in the elderly is available. Clinical trials have included patients over 65 years and no adverse reactions specific to this age group have been reported.

4.3 Contraindications

Known hypersensitivity to either idoxuridine or dimethyl sulfoxide.

Dermographia.

4.4 Special warnings and precautions for use

Herpid in the eye causes stinging: treat by washing out with water. The dimethyl sulfoxide in Herpid may be irritant to the skin.

4.5 Interaction with other medicinal products and other forms of interaction

Since the solvent in Herpid can increase the absorption of many substances it is important that no other topical medication be used on the same areas of skin treated with Herpid.

4.6 Pregnancy and lactation

Animal studies have shown idoxuridine to be teratogenic. Consequently, Herpid should not be prescribed for women who are pregnant or at risk of becoming pregnant. In a small number of cases of women who used Herpid inadvertently in early pregnancy and who were followed to term, the infant was normal in each case.

4.7 Effects on ability to drive and use machines

None.

4.8 Undesirable effects

Patients often experience stinging when applying Herpid and a distinctive taste during a course of treatment; both effects are transient.

Skin reactions have occasionally been reported.

Over-usage of the solution may lead to maceration of the skin.

4.9 Overdose

There is no clinical evidence of overdosage. Standard supportive measures should be adopted.

5. PHARMACOLOGICAL PROPERTIES

5.1 Pharmacodynamic properties

Idoxuridine is an antiviral agent which acts by blocking the uptake of thymidine into the deoxyribonucleic acid (DNA) of the virus and inhibits replication of viruses such as adenovirus, cytomegalovirus, herpes simplex (herpes virus hominus), varicella zoster or herpes zoster (herpes virus varicella) and vaccinia. It has no action against latent forms of the virus. It does not inhibit RNA viruses such as influenza virus or poliovirus.

5.2 Pharmacokinetic properties

The idoxuridine is dissolved in dimethyl sulfoxide which penetrates the skin and carries the antiviral agent to the deeper levels of the epidermis where the virus is replicating.

Idoxuridine is rapidly metabolised in the body to iodouracil, uracil and iodine which are rapidly excreted in the urine.

5.3 Preclinical safety data

6. PHARMACEUTICAL PARTICULARS

6.1 List of excipients

Dimethyl sulfoxide.

6.2 Incompatibilities

None stated.

6.3 Shelf life

2 years.

6.4 Special precautions for storage

Herpid should be stored in its box below 25°C. Do not refrigerate as the contents of the bottle may solidify. If crystals do form, allow to re-dissolve before use by warming the bottle gently (in the palm of the hand) until the solution is clear. Because the solution is hygroscopic, any remaining after completion of treatment should be discarded.

6.5 Nature and contents of container

5 ml bottle with brush (OP):

Bottle: Type III amber glass

Cap liner: high density natural polyethylene

Brush stem: low density natural polyethylene

6.6 Special precautions for disposal and other handling

Instructions for use:

1) Carefully unscrew the white cap and discard. Replace it with the black cap and brush.

2) Apply the liquid sparingly with the brush 4 times a day to the affected area of skin.

It is important to treat only the affected areas.

3) Wash your hands thoroughly after using Herpid.

4) Do not continue a course of treatment on one area of the skin for more than four days.

5) Discard any solution remaining in the bottle as soon as the treatment period is complete.

Herpid can damage some synthetic materials (e.g. artificial silk and Terylene) and printed cotton fabrics. Contact between Herpid and these materials should therefore be avoided.

7. MARKETING AUTHORISATION HOLDER

Astellas Pharma Ltd
Lovett House
Lovett Road
Staines
TW18 3AZ
United Kingdom

8. MARKETING AUTHORISATION NUMBER(S)

PL 00166/0177

9. DATE OF FIRST AUTHORISATION/RENEWAL OF THE AUTHORISATION

Date of first authorisation 13.03.74

Date of latest renewal 15th March 2007

10. DATE OF REVISION OF THE TEXT

30 January 2008

11. LEGAL CATEGORY

POM

Hexopal 500mg Tablets

(Genus Pharmaceuticals)

1. NAME OF THE MEDICINAL PRODUCT

Hexopal Tablets 500mg / Inositol Nicotinate Tablets BP 500mg.

2. QUALITATIVE AND QUANTITATIVE COMPOSITION

Inositol Nicotinate BP 500mg.

3. PHARMACEUTICAL FORM

Tablet.

4. CLINICAL PARTICULARS

4.1 Therapeutic indications

Hexopal is indicated for the symptomatic relief of severe intermittent claudication and Raynaud's phenomenon.

4.2 Posology and method of administration

For oral administration.

Adults (including the elderly): The usual dose is 3g daily (i.e. 2 tablets three times a day). The dose may be increased to 4g daily if necessary.

Children: Not recommended.

4.3 Contraindications

Use in patients who have suffered a recent myocardial infarction or are in the acute phase of a cerebrovascular accident.

Use in patients hypersensitive to the active ingredient.

4.4 Special warnings and precautions for use

This product should be used with caution in the presence of cerebrovascular insufficiency or unstable angina.

4.5 Interaction with other medicinal products and other forms of interaction

None.

4.6 Pregnancy and lactation

There is no evidence of the safety of Hexopal in human pregnancy nor is there adequate evidence from animal work that it is free from hazard. The use of Hexopal in pregnancy should therefore be avoided unless there is no safer alternative.

4.7 Effects on ability to drive and use machines

None.

4.8 Undesirable effects

Side effects are uncommon, but may include flushing, dizziness, headache, nausea, vomiting, syncope, paraesthesia, rash, oedema, and postural hypotension.

4.9 Overdose

Despite extensive clinical experience in Britain since 1959, no case of poisoning or overdosage with Hexopal has been reported. In an emergency, it is suggested that the stomach be emptied by gastric lavage and the patient be treated symptomatically.

5. PHARMACOLOGICAL PROPERTIES

5.1 Pharmacodynamic properties

The mode of action of inositol nicotinate in Raynaud's phenomenon and in intermittent claudication remains to be determined. Inositol nicotinate does not appear to produce general peripheral vasodilation.

5.2 Pharmacokinetic properties
Radiolabelled tracer studies indicate that with orally administered inositol nicotinate very low concentrations of nicotinic acid are found in the plasma. These levels appear to be maintained for approximately 24 hours.

5.3 Preclinical safety data
There are no preclinical safety data of relevance to the prescriber which are additional to that already included in other sections of the SPC.

6. PHARMACEUTICAL PARTICULARS

6.1 List of excipients
Pregelatinised starch, Maize starch, Purified talc, Magnesium stearate, Stearic acid, Sodium lauryl sulphate.

6.2 Incompatibilities
None.

6.3 Shelf life
60 months.

6.4 Special precautions for storage
Store below 25°C.

6.5 Nature and contents of container
Amber glass bottle with wadless polypropylene screws caps.

Pack size: 100 and 500 tablets.

200μm white opaque PVC/20μm aluminium blister pack.

Pack size: 100 tablets.

6.6 Special precautions for disposal and other handling
None.

7. MARKETING AUTHORISATION HOLDER
Genus Pharmaceuticals Limited (*trading as Genus Pharmaceuticals*)

Park View House

65 London Road

Newbury

Berkshire

RG14 1JN UK

8. MARKETING AUTHORISATION NUMBER(S)
PL 06831/0147

9. DATE OF FIRST AUTHORISATION/RENEWAL OF THE AUTHORISATION
10th May 2005

10. DATE OF REVISION OF THE TEXT
15 January 2008

Hexopal Forte 750mg Tablets / Inositol Nicotinate750mg Tablets

(Genus Pharmaceuticals)

1. NAME OF THE MEDICINAL PRODUCT
Hexopal Forte Tablets / Inositol Nicotinate Tablets

2. QUALITATIVE AND QUANTITATIVE COMPOSITION
Each tablet contains Inositol Nicotinate BP 750 mg.

3. PHARMACEUTICAL FORM
Tablets

4. CLINICAL PARTICULARS

4.1 Therapeutic indications
Hexopal is indicated for the symptomatic relief of severe intermittent claudication and Raynauds phenomenon.

4.2 Posology and method of administration
Adults: The usual dose is 3g daily (two Hexopal Forte Tablets twice daily). The dose of Hexopal may be increased up to 4g daily if necessary.

Oral administration.

4.3 Contraindications
Use in patients who have suffered a recent myocardial infarction or are in the acute phase of a cerebrovascular accident.

Use in patients hypersensitive to the active ingredient.

4.4 Special warnings and precautions for use
This product should be used with caution in the presence of cerebrovascular insufficiency or unstable angina.

4.5 Interaction with other medicinal products and other forms of interaction
None.

4.6 Pregnancy and lactation
There is no evidence of the safety of Hexopal in human pregnancy nor is there any evidence from animal work that it is free from hazard. The use of Hexopal in pregnancy should therefore be avoided unless there is no safer alternative.

4.7 Effects on ability to drive and use machines
None.

4.8 Undesirable effects
Side effects are uncommon, but may include flushing, dizziness, headache, nausea, vomiting, syncope, paraesthesia, rash, oedema, and postural hypotension.

4.9 Overdose
Despite extensive clinical experience in Britain since 1959, no case of poisoning or overdosage with Hexopal has been reported. In an emergency, it is suggested that the stomach be emptied by gastric lavage and the patient be treated symptomatically.

5. PHARMACOLOGICAL PROPERTIES

5.1 Pharmacodynamic properties
In addition to a vasodilator effect, thought to be due to the slow release of nicotinic acid, Hexopal has been reported to reduce fibrinogen and blood viscosity and to have a beneficial effect on the fibrinolytic system and on blood lipids.

5.2 Pharmacokinetic properties
Radiolabelled tracer studies indicate that with orally administered inositol nicotinate very low concentrations of nicotinic acid are found in the plasma. These levels appear to be maintained for approximately 24 hours.

5.3 Preclinical safety data
None.

6. PHARMACEUTICAL PARTICULARS

6.1 List of excipients
Pregelatinised starch, Talc, Magnesium stearate, Maize starch, Stearic acid, Sodium lauryl sulphate.

6.2 Incompatibilities
None.

6.3 Shelf life
60 months.

6.4 Special precautions for storage
The product should be stored below 25°C.

6.5 Nature and contents of container
Amber glass bottles containing 100, 250 and 500 tablets.

250μm clear PVC/20μm aluminium blister pack containing 112 tablets.

Not all pack sizes may be marketed.

6.6 Special precautions for disposal and other handling
No special requirements.

7. MARKETING AUTHORISATION HOLDER
Genus Pharmaceuticals Limited (*trading as Genus Pharmaceuticals*)

Park View House

65 London Road

Newbury

Berkshire

RG14 1JN UK

8. MARKETING AUTHORISATION NUMBER(S)
PL 06831/0148

9. DATE OF FIRST AUTHORISATION/RENEWAL OF THE AUTHORISATION
10th May 2005

10. DATE OF REVISION OF THE TEXT
15 January 2008

Hirudoid Cream

(Genus Pharmaceuticals)

1. NAME OF THE MEDICINAL PRODUCT
Hirudoid Cream

2. QUALITATIVE AND QUANTITATIVE COMPOSITION
Heparinoid 0.3% w/w (Equivalent to 25 000 Units per 100 g cream).

3. PHARMACEUTICAL FORM
Topical cream.

4. CLINICAL PARTICULARS

4.1 Therapeutic indications
Hirudoid is indicated for the treatment of superficial thrombophlebitis and the soothing relief of superficial bruising and haematoma.

4.2 Posology and method of administration
Adults, the elderly and children over 5 years of age:

Two to six inches (5-15 cm) to be applied up to four times daily to the affected area and gently massaged into the skin.

4.3 Contraindications
Not to be used on large areas of skin, broken skin, sensitive areas of skin or mucous membranes. Not to be used in individuals with a known sensitivity to any active or inactive component of the formulation. Not to be used in children under 5 years of age.

4.4 Special warnings and precautions for use
For external use only. If symptoms persist or worsen, seek medical advice. Do not exceed the stated dose.

4.5 Interaction with other medicinal products and other forms of interaction
None known.

4.6 Pregnancy and lactation
There is no evidence to suggest that Hirudoid should not be used during pregnancy and lactation.

4.7 Effects on ability to drive and use machines
None.

4.8 Undesirable effects
None known.

4.9 Overdose
In the absence of any reports of the accidental ingestion of Hirudoid, no specific advice is available. General supportive measures may be appropriate.

5. PHARMACOLOGICAL PROPERTIES

5.1 Pharmacodynamic properties
Heparinoid is recognised as having: a weak inhibitory effect on PGE_2 synthesis and an indirect effect on LTB_4 production (based on in vitro studies), anti-coagulant activity (as a heparinoid), thrombolytic activity (through potentiation of urokinase activity), anti-exudatory activity (through inhibition of hyaluronidase).

5.2 Pharmacokinetic properties
Radiochemical studies of absorption following cutaneous application of heparinoid (mucopolysaccharide polysulphate) have shown that between 0.3 and 4% of the mucopolysaccharide administered is absorbed by various tissues (other than the treated area) within the first 8 hours. Typically between 1.7% and 4.6% will be absorbed within 2 to 4 days. Animal studies have also shown that mucopolysaccharide is bound intracellularly within the subcutis. Peak serum concentrations following cutaneous application are below the threshold of physiological relevance for coagulation. Mucopolysaccharide is excreted in the urine partly unchanged and partly as depolymerized, shorter chain length molecules.

5.3 Preclinical safety data
None stated.

6. PHARMACEUTICAL PARTICULARS

6.1 List of excipients
Anhydrous eucerine

Emulsifying cetostearyl alcohol type A

Glycerol

Isopropyl alcohol

Methyl parahydroxybenzoate (E218)

Myristyl alcohol, potassium hydroxide

Propyl parahydroxybenzoate (E216)

Purified water

Stearic acid

Thymol

6.2 Incompatibilities
None.

6.3 Shelf life
5 years.

6.4 Special precautions for storage
Store below 25°C.

6.5 Nature and contents of container
Lacquered aluminium tubes 14, 40, 50 g.

6.6 Special precautions for disposal and other handling
Not applicable.

7. MARKETING AUTHORISATION HOLDER
Genus Pharmaceuticals Limited

T/A Genus Pharmaceuticals

Park View House

65 London Road

Newbury

Berkshire RG14 1JN

United Kingdom

8. MARKETING AUTHORISATION NUMBER(S)
PL 06831/0175

9. DATE OF FIRST AUTHORISATION/RENEWAL OF THE AUTHORISATION
02 February 2006

10. DATE OF REVISION OF THE TEXT
23 July 2008

Hirudoid Gel

(Genus Pharmaceuticals)

1. NAME OF THE MEDICINAL PRODUCT
Hirudoid Gel

2. QUALITATIVE AND QUANTITATIVE COMPOSITION
Heparinoid 0.3% w/w (Equivalent to 25 000 Units per 100 g gel).

3. PHARMACEUTICAL FORM
Topical gel.

4. CLINICAL PARTICULARS

4.1 Therapeutic indications

Hirudoid is indicated for the treatment of superficial thrombophlebitis and the soothing relief of superficial bruising and haematoma.

4.2 Posology and method of administration

Adults, the elderly and children over 5 years of age:

Two to six inches (5-15 cm) to be applied, as a thin layer, up to four times a day to the affected area. Recommended when its cooling effect and rapid action are required.

4.3 Contraindications

Not to be used on large areas of skin, broken skin, sensitive areas of skin or mucous membranes. Not to be used in individuals with a known sensitivity to any active or inactive component of the formulation. Not to be used in children under 5 years of age.

4.4 Special warnings and precautions for use

For external use only. If symptoms persist or worsen, seek medical advice. Do not exceed the stated dose.

4.5 Interaction with other medicinal products and other forms of interaction

None known.

4.6 Pregnancy and lactation

There is no evidence to suggest that Hirudoid should not be used during pregnancy and lactation.

4.7 Effects on ability to drive and use machines

None.

4.8 Undesirable effects

None known.

4.9 Overdose

In the absence of any reports of the accidental ingestion of Hirudoid, no specific advice is available. General supportive measures may be appropriate.

5. PHARMACOLOGICAL PROPERTIES

5.1 Pharmacodynamic properties

Heparinoid is recognised as having: a weak inhibitory effect on PGE_2 synthesis and an indirect effect on LTB_4 production (based on in vitro studies), anti-coagulant activity (as a heparinoid), thrombolytic activity (through potentiation of urokinase activity), anti-exudatory activity (through inhibition of hyaluronidase).

5.2 Pharmacokinetic properties

Radiochemical studies of absorption following cutaneous application of heparinoid (mucopolysaccharide polysulphate) have shown that between 0.3 and 4% of the mucopolysaccharide administered is absorbed by various tissues (other than the treated area) within the first 8 hours. Typically between 1.7% and 4.6% will be absorbed within 2 to 4 days. Animal studies have also shown that mucopolysaccharide is bound intracellularly within the subcutis. Peak serum concentrations following cutaneous application are below the threshold of physiological relevance for coagulation. Mucopolysaccharide is excreted in the urine partly unchanged and partly as depolymerized, shorter chain length molecules.

5.3 Preclinical safety data

None stated.

6. PHARMACEUTICAL PARTICULARS

6.1 List of excipients

Isopropyl alcohol

Perfume oil No 8185

Polyacrylic acid

Propylene glycol

Purified water

Sodium hydroxide

6.2 Incompatibilities

None.

6.3 Shelf life

5 years.

6.4 Special precautions for storage

Store below 25°C.

6.5 Nature and contents of container

Lacquered aluminium tubes 14, 50, 50 g.

6.6 Special precautions for disposal and other handling

Not applicable.

7. MARKETING AUTHORISATION HOLDER

Genus Pharmaceuticals Limited

T/A Genus Pharmaceuticals

Park View House

65 London Road

Newbury

Berkshire RG14 1JN

United Kingdom

8. MARKETING AUTHORISATION NUMBER(S)

PL 06831/0174

9. DATE OF FIRST AUTHORISATION/RENEWAL OF THE AUTHORISATION

02 February 2006

10. DATE OF REVISION OF THE TEXT

27 July 2008

HRF 100 Microgram

(Intrapharm Laboratories Ltd)

1. NAME OF THE MEDICINAL PRODUCT

HRF 100 microgram.

2. QUALITATIVE AND QUANTITATIVE COMPOSITION

Each vial contains 100 micrograms of Gonadorelin as Gonadorelin Hydrochloride.

3. PHARMACEUTICAL FORM

Powder and solvent for solution for injection.

4. CLINICAL PARTICULARS

4.1 Therapeutic indications

HRF as a single injection is indicated for evaluating the functional capacity and response of the gonadotropes of the anterior pituitary. The LH/FSH-RH response is used in testing patients with suspected gonadotropin deficiency, whether due to the hypothalamus alone or in combination with anterior pituitary failure. HRF is also indicated for evaluating residual gonadolropic function of the pituitary following removal of a pituitary tumour or surgery and/or irradiation.

The HRF test complements the clinical assessment of patients with a variety of endocrine disorders involving the hypothalamic-pituitary axis. In cases where there is a normal response, it indicates the presence of functional pituitary gonadotropes. The single injection test does not determine the patho-physiological cause for the subnormal response and does not measure pituitary gonadotropic reserve.

4.2 Posology and method of administration

Route of administration

For subcutaneous and intravenous administration.

Adults and elderly

100 micrograms, subcutaneously or intravenously. In females for whom the phase of the menstrual cycle can be established, the test should be performed in early follicular phase (days 1—7).

Children

Do not use in children under one year of age as diluent contains 2 % benzyl alcohol.

Test Methodology:

To determine the status of the gonadotropin secretory capacity of the anterior pituitary, a test procedure requiring seven venous blood samples for LH/FSH-RH is recommended.

Procedure:

1. Venous blood samples should be drawn at *- 15* minutes and immediately prior to HRF administration. The LH/FSH-RH baseline is obtained by averaging the LH/FSH-RH values of the two samples.

2. Administer a bolus of HRF subcutaneously or intravenously.

3. Draw venous blood samples at *15*, 30, *45*, 60 and 120 minutes after administration.

4. Blood samples should be handled as recommended by the laboratory that will determine the LH/FSH-RH content. It must be emphasised that the reliability of the test is directly related to the inter-assay and intra-assay reliability of the laboratory performing the assay.

Interpretation of Test Results: Interpretation of the LH/FSH-RH response to HRF requires an understanding of the hypothalamic-pituitary physiology, knowledge of the clinical status of the individual patient, and familiarity with the normal ranges and the standards used in the laboratory performing the LH/FSH-RH assays.

Curves provided represent the LH/FSH-RH response curves after administration in normal subjects. The normal LH/FSH-RH response curves were established between the 10th percentile (B line) and 90th percentile (A line) of all LH/FSH-RH responses in normal subjects analysed from the results of clinical studies.

Individual patient responses should be plotted on the appropriate curve. A subnormal response in patients is defined as three or more LH/FSH-RH values which fall below the B line of the normal LH/FSH-RH response curve.

In cases where there is a blunted or borderline response, the HRF test should be repeated.

The HRF test complements the clinical assessment of patients with a variety of endocrine disorders involving the hypothalamic-pituitary axis. In cases where there is a normal response, it indicates the presence of functional pituitary gonadotropes. The single injection test does not determine the patho-physiological cause for the subnormal response and does not measure pituitary gonadotropic reserve.

4.3 Contraindications

Hypersensitivity to HRF or any of the components. Known or suspected pregnancy. Do not use in children under one year of age as diluent contains 2% benzyl alcohol.

4.4 Special warnings and precautions for use

Although allergic and hypersensitivity reactions have been observed with other polypeptide hormones, to date no such reactions have been encountered following the administration of a single 100 micrograms dose of HRF used for diagnostic purposes. Rare instances of hypersensitivity reactions have been reported. Therefore, patients treated by intermittent pulsatile therapy in whom re-administration is considered, particularly by the intravenous route, should be carefully observed. Administration during the follicular phase of a normal cycle may result in premature ovulation and appropriate measures are advised to prevent an unwanted pregnancy in these circumstances.

4.5 Interaction with other medicinal products and other forms of interaction

The HRF test should be conducted in the absence of other drugs which directly affect the pituitary secretion of the gonadotropins. These would include a variety of preparations which contain androgens, oestrogens, progestins, or glucocorticoids. The gonadotropin levels may be transiently elevated by spironolactone, minimally elevated by levodopa, and suppressed by oral contraceptives and digoxin. The response to HRF may be blunted by phenothiazines and dopamine antagonists which cause a rise in prolactin.

4.6 Pregnancy and lactation

HRF should not be administered to pregnant or nursing mothers.

4.7 Effects on ability to drive and use machines

None known.

4.8 Undesirable effects

Systemic complaints such as headaches, nausea, lightheadedness, abdominal discomfort and flushing have been reported rarely following administration of FIRE. Local swelling, occasionally with pain and pruritus at the injection site may occur if I-IRE is administered subcutaneously. Local and generalised skin rash have been noted after chronic subcutaneous administration.

Thrombophlebitis with septicaemia, mild and severe, has been reported in isolated cases at the site of intravenous injection. Rare instances of hypersensitivity reaction (bronchospasm, tachycardia, flushing, urticaria, swelling, itching and redness of face, eyelids and lips, induration at injection site) have been reported following multiple-dose administration of large doses. Antibody formation has also been reported rarely after chronic administration of large doses.

4.9 Overdose

HRF has been administered parenterally in doses up to 3 mg bd for 28 days without any signs of symptoms of overdosage. In cases of overdosage or idiosyncrasy, symptomatic treatment should be administered as required.

5. PHARMACOLOGICAL PROPERTIES

5.1 Pharmacodynamic properties

Gonadorelin stimulates the synthesis of follicle stimulating hormone and luteinising hormone in the anterior lobe of the pituitary as well as their release.

5.2 Pharmacokinetic properties

Gonadorelin is rapidly hydrolysed in plasma and excreted in urine with a half life of about 4 minutes

5.3 Preclinical safety data

Not applicable.

6. PHARMACEUTICAL PARTICULARS

6.1 List of excipients

Lactose monohydrate USP

Solvent:

Benzyl alcohol BP

Water for injections BP

6.2 Incompatibilities

HRF should not be mixed with any other substance.

6.3 Shelf life

Unopened:48 months

After reconstitution: 24 hours

6.4 Special precautions for storage

Store below 25C.

6.5 Nature and contents of container

HRF is supplied in a USP Type 1 clear glass vial with grey butyl rubber stopper and aluminium collar. The sterile solvent is *5* ml water for injections with 2% benzyl alcohol supplied in a Pb. Eur Type I clear glass ampoule.

6.6 Special precautions for disposal and other handling

Preparation for single injection administration: Reconstitute 100 micrograms vial with 1.0 ml of the accompanying sterile solvent of 2% benzyl alcohol. Prepare solution immediately before use. After reconstitution, refrigerate and use within 1 day. Discard unused reconstituted solution and solvent.

Administrative Data

7. MARKETING AUTHORISATION HOLDER

Intrapharm Laboratories Limited

60 Boughton Lane

Maidstone

Kent

ME15 9QS

United Kingdom

8. MARKETING AUTHORISATION NUMBER(S)
PL 17509/0005

9. DATE OF FIRST AUTHORISATION/RENEWAL OF THE AUTHORISATION
25 May 2001

10. DATE OF REVISION OF THE TEXT
February 2005

Humalog 100U/ml, solution for injection in vial, Humalog 100U/ml, solution for injection in Cartridge, Humalog Pen 100U/ml, solution for injection

(Eli Lilly and Company Limited)

1. NAME OF THE MEDICINAL PRODUCT
HUMALOG* 100U/ml, solution for injection in vial.

HUMALOG 100U/ml, solution for injection in cartridge.

HUMALOG Pen 100U/ml, solution for injection.

HUMALOG 100U/ml KwikPen, solution for injection.

2. QUALITATIVE AND QUANTITATIVE COMPOSITION
One ml contains 100U (equivalent to 3.5mg) insulin lispro (recombinant DNA origin produced in *E. coli*).

Vial: Each container includes 10ml equivalent to 1000U insulin lispro.

3 ml cartridge: Each container includes 3ml equivalent to 300U insulin lispro.

HUMALOG Pen 3ml/KwikPen: Each container includes 3ml equivalent to 300U insulin lispro.

For a full list of excipients, see section 6.1.

3. PHARMACEUTICAL FORM
Solution for injection.

HUMALOG, HUMALOG Pen and HUMALOG KwikPen are sterile, clear, colourless, aqueous solutions.

4. CLINICAL PARTICULARS

4.1 Therapeutic indications
For the treatment of adults and children with diabetes mellitus who require insulin for the maintenance of normal glucose homeostasis. HUMALOG, HUMALOG Pen or HUMALOG KwikPen is also indicated for the initial stabilisation of diabetes mellitus.

4.2 Posology and method of administration
The dosage should be determined by the physician, according to the requirement of the patient.

HUMALOG may be given shortly before meals. When necessary, HUMALOG can be given soon after meals.

HUMALOG preparations should be given by subcutaneous injection or by continuous subcutaneous infusion pump (see section 4.2) and may, although not recommended, also be given by intramuscular injection. If necessary, HUMALOG may also be administered intravenously, for example, for the control of blood glucose levels during ketoacidosis, acute illnesses, or during intraoperative and postoperative periods.

Subcutaneous administration should be in the upper arms, thighs, buttocks, or abdomen. Use of injection sites should be rotated so that the same site is not used more than approximately once a month.

When administered subcutaneously, care should be taken when injecting HUMALOG, HUMALOG Pen or HUMALOG KwikPen to ensure that a blood vessel has not been entered. After injection, the site of injection should not be massaged. Patients must be educated to use the proper injection techniques.

HUMALOG, HUMALOG Pen or HUMALOG KwikPen takes effect rapidly and has a shorter duration of activity (2 to 5 hours) given subcutaneously as compared with soluble insulin. This rapid onset of activity allows a HUMALOG injection (or, in the case of administration by continuous subcutaneous infusion, a HUMALOG bolus) to be given very close to mealtime. The time course of action of any insulin may vary considerably in different individuals or at different times in the same individual. The faster onset of action compared to soluble human insulin is maintained regardless of injection site. As with all insulin preparations, the duration of action of HUMALOG, HUMALOG Pen or HUMALOG KwikPen is dependent on dose, site of injection, blood supply, temperature, and physical activity.

HUMALOG can be used in conjunction with a longer-acting human insulin or oral sulphonylurea agents, on the advice of a physician.

Use of HUMALOG in an insulin infusion pump:

Only certain CE-marked insulin infusion pumps may be used to infuse insulin lispro. Before infusing insulin lispro, the manufacturer's instructions should be studied to ascertain the suitability or otherwise for the particular pump. Read and follow the instructions that accompany the infusion pump. Use the correct reservoir and catheter for the pump. Change the infusion set every 48 hours. Use aseptic technique when inserting the infusion set. In the event of a hypoglycaemic episode, the infusion should be stopped until the episode is resolved. If repeated or severe low blood glucose levels occur, notify your health care professional and consider the need to reduce or stop your insulin infusion. A pump malfunction or obstruction of the infusion set can result in a rapid rise in glucose levels. If an interruption to insulin flow is suspected, follow the instructions in the product literature and if appropriate, notify your health care professional. When used with an insulin infusion pump, HUMALOG should not be mixed with any other insulin.

Intravenous administration of insulin:

Intravenous injection of insulin lispro should be carried out following normal clinical practise for intravenous injections, for example by an intravenous bolus or by an infusion system. Frequent monitoring of the blood glucose levels is required.

Infusion systems at concentrations from 0.1U/ml to 1.0U/ml insulin lispro in 0.9% sodium chloride or 5% dextrose are stable at room temperature for 48 hours. It is recommended that the system is primed before starting the infusion to the patient.

4.3 Contraindications
Hypersensitivity to insulin lispro or to any of the excipients.

Hypoglycaemia.

4.4 Special warnings and precautions for use
Transferring a patient to another type or brand of insulin should be done under strict medical supervision. Changes in strength, brand (manufacturer), type (soluble, isophane, lente, etc), species (animal, human, human insulin analogue), and/or method of manufacture (recombinant DNA versus animal-source insulin) may result in the need for a change in dosage. For fast-acting insulins, any patient also on basal insulin must optimise dosage of both insulins to obtain glucose control across the whole day, particularly nocturnal/fasting glucose control.

Vials: The shorter-acting HUMALOG should be drawn into the syringe first, to prevent contamination of the vial by the longer-acting insulin. Mixing of the insulins ahead of time or just before the injection should be on advice of the physician. However, a consistent routine must be followed.

Conditions which may make the early warning symptoms of hypoglycaemia different or less pronounced include long duration of diabetes, intensified insulin therapy, diabetic nerve disease, or medications such as beta-blockers.

A few patients who have experienced hypoglycaemic reactions after transfer from animal-source insulin to human insulin have reported that the early warning symptoms of hypoglycaemia were less pronounced or different from those experienced with their previous insulin. Uncorrected hypoglycaemic or hyperglycaemic reactions can cause loss of consciousness, coma, or death.

The use of dosages which are inadequate or discontinuation of treatment, especially in insulin-dependent diabetics, may lead to hyperglycaemia and diabetic ketoacidosis; conditions which are potentially lethal.

Insulin requirements may be reduced in the presence of renal impairment. Insulin requirements may be reduced in patients with hepatic impairment due to reduced capacity for gluconeogenesis and reduced insulin breakdown; however, in patients with chronic hepatic impairment, an increase in insulin resistance may lead to increased insulin requirements.

Insulin requirements may be increased during illness or emotional disturbances.

Adjustment of dosage may also be necessary if patients undertake increased physical activity or change their usual diet. Exercise taken immediately after a meal may increase the risk of hypoglycaemia. A consequence of the pharmacodynamics of rapid-acting insulin analogues is that if hypoglycaemia occurs, it may occur earlier after an injection when compared with soluble human insulin.

If the 40U/ml vial is the product normally prescribed, do not take insulin from a 100U/ml cartridge using a 40U/ml syringe.

HUMALOG should only be used in children in preference to soluble insulin when a fast action of insulin might be beneficial. For example, in the timing of the injection in relation to meals.

4.5 Interaction with other medicinal products and other forms of interaction
Insulin requirements may be increased by medicinal products with hyperglycaemic activity, such as oral contraceptives, corticosteroids, or thyroid replacement therapy, danazol, beta$_2$ stimulants (such as ritodrine, salbutamol, terbutaline).

Insulin requirements may be reduced in the presence of medicinal products with hypoglycaemic activity, such as oral hypoglycaemics, salicylates (for example, acetylsalicylic acid), sulpha antibiotics, certain antidepressants (monoamine oxidase inhibitors, selective serotonin reuptake inhibitors), certain angiotensin converting enzyme inhibitors (captopril, enalapril), angiotensin II receptor blockers, beta-blockers, octreotide, or alcohol.

The physician should be consulted when using other medications in addition to HUMALOG, HUMALOG Pen or HUMALOG KwikPen.

4.6 Pregnancy and lactation
Data on a large number of exposed pregnancies do not indicate any adverse effect of insulin lispro on pregnancy or on the health of the foetus/newborn.

It is essential to maintain good control of the insulin-treated (insulin-dependent or gestational diabetes) patient throughout pregnancy. Insulin requirements usually fall during the first trimester and increase during the second and third trimesters. Patients with diabetes should be advised to inform their doctor if they are pregnant or are contemplating pregnancy. Careful monitoring of glucose control, as well as general health, is essential in pregnant patients with diabetes.

Patients with diabetes who are breast-feeding may require adjustments in insulin dose, diet or both.

4.7 Effects on ability to drive and use machines
The patient's ability to concentrate and react may be impaired as a result of hypoglycaemia. This may constitute a risk in situations where these abilities are of special importance (e.g., driving a car or operating machinery).

Patients should be advised to take precautions to avoid hypoglycaemia whilst driving, this is particularly important in those who have reduced or absent awareness of the warning signs of hypoglycaemia or have frequent episodes of hypoglycaemia. The advisability of driving should be considered in these circumstances.

4.8 Undesirable effects
Hypoglycaemia is the most frequent undesirable effect of insulin therapy that a patient with diabetes may suffer. Severe hypoglycaemia may lead to loss of consciousness and in extreme cases, death. No specific frequency for hypoglycaemia is presented, since hypoglycaemia is a result of both the insulin dose and other factors, e.g., a patient's level of diet and exercise.

Local allergy in patients is common (1/100 to $<1/10$). Redness, swelling, and itching can occur at the site of insulin injection. This condition usually resolves in a few days to a few weeks. In some instances, this condition may be related to factors other than insulin, such as irritants in the skin cleansing agent or poor injection technique. Systemic allergy, which is rare (1/10,000 to $<1/1,000$) but potentially more serious, is a generalised allergy to insulin. It may cause a rash over the whole body, shortness of breath, wheezing, reduction in blood pressure, fast pulse, or sweating. Severe cases of generalised allergy may be life-threatening.

Lipodystrophy at the injection site is uncommon (1/1,000 to $<1/100$).

4.9 Overdose
Insulins have no specific overdose definitions because serum glucose concentrations are a result of complex interactions between insulin levels, glucose availability and other metabolic processes. Hypoglycaemia may occur as a result of an excess of insulin activity relative to food intake and energy expenditure.

Hypoglycaemia may be associated with listlessness, confusion, palpitations, headache, sweating and vomiting.

Mild hypoglycaemic episodes will respond to oral administration of glucose or other sugar or saccharated products.

Correction of moderately severe hypoglycaemia can be accomplished by intramuscular or subcutaneous administration of glucagon, followed by oral carbohydrate when the patient recovers sufficiently. Patients who fail to respond to glucagon must be given glucose solution intravenously.

If the patient is comatose, glucagon should be administered intramuscularly or subcutaneously. However, glucose solution must be given intravenously if glucagon is not available or if the patient fails to respond to glucagon. The patient should be given a meal as soon as consciousness is recovered.

Sustained carbohydrate intake and observation may be necessary because hypoglycaemia may recur after apparent clinical recovery.

5. PHARMACOLOGICAL PROPERTIES

5.1 Pharmacodynamic properties
Pharmacotherapeutic group: Fast-acting human insulin analogue. *ATC code:* A10A B04.

The primary activity of insulin lispro is the regulation of glucose metabolism.

In addition, insulins have several anabolic and anti-catabolic actions on a variety of different tissues. Within muscle tissue this includes increasing glycogen, fatty acid, glycerol and protein synthesis and amino acid uptake, while decreasing glycogenolysis, gluconeogenesis, ketogenesis, lipolysis, protein catabolism and amino acid output.

Insulin lispro has a rapid onset of action (approximately 15 minutes), thus allowing it to be given closer to a meal (within zero to 15 minutes of the meal) when compared to soluble insulin (30 to 45 minutes before). Insulin lispro takes effect rapidly and has a shorter duration of activity (2 to 5 hours) when compared to soluble insulin.

Clinical trials in patients with Type 1 and Type 2 diabetes have demonstrated reduced postprandial hyperglycaemia with insulin lispro compared to soluble human insulin.

As with all insulin preparations, the time course of insulin lispro action may vary in different individuals or at different times in the same individual and is dependent on dose, site of injection, blood supply, temperature, and physical activity. The typical activity profile following subcutaneous injection is illustrated below.

Figure 1

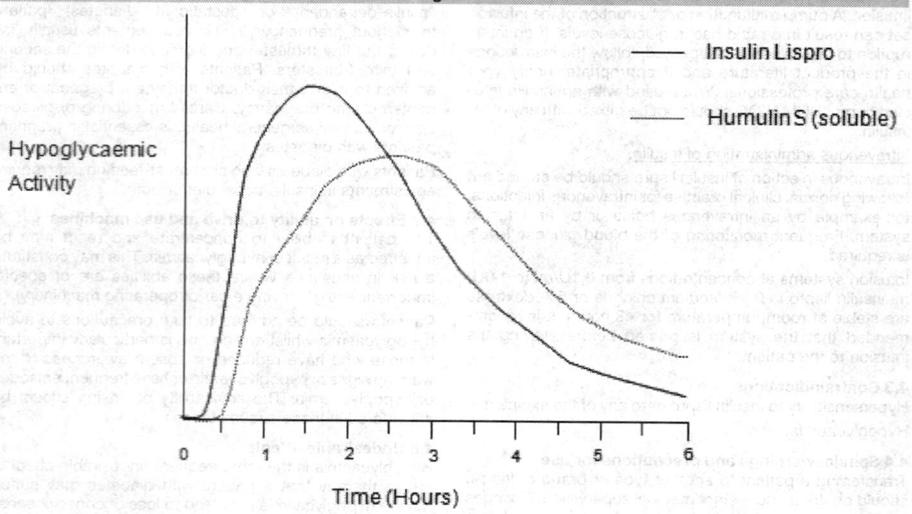

(see Figure 1 above)

The above representation reflects the relative amount of glucose over time required to maintain the subject's whole blood glucose concentrations near fasting levels and is an indicator of the effect of these insulins on glucose metabolism over time.

Clinical trials have been performed in children (61 patients aged 2 to 11) and children and adolescents (481 patients aged 9 to 19 years), comparing insulin lispro to human soluble insulin. The pharmacodynamic profile of insulin lispro in children is similar to that seen in adults.

When used in subcutaneous infusion pumps, treatment with insulin lispro has been shown to result in lower glycosylated haemoglobin levels compared to soluble insulin. In a double-blind, crossover study, the reduction in glycosylated haemoglobin levels after 12 weeks dosing was 0.37 percentage points with insulin lispro compared to 0.03 percentage points for soluble insulin ($P = 0.004$).

In patients with Type 2 diabetes on maximum doses of sulphonylurea agents, studies have shown that the addition of insulin lispro significantly reduces HbA_{1c} compared to sulphonylurea alone. The reduction of HbA_{1c} would also be expected with other insulin products, e.g., soluble or isophane insulins.

Clinical trials in patients with Type 1 and Type 2 diabetes have demonstrated a reduced number of episodes of nocturnal hypoglycaemia with insulin lispro compared to soluble human insulin. In some studies, reduction of nocturnal hypoglycaemia was associated with increased episodes of daytime hypoglycaemia.

The glucodynamic response to insulin lispro is not affected by renal or hepatic function impairment. Glucodynamic differences between insulin lispro and soluble human insulin, as measured during a glucose clamp procedure, were maintained over a wide range of renal function.

Insulin lispro has been shown to be equipotent to human insulin on a molar basis but its effect is more rapid and of a shorter duration.

5.2 Pharmacokinetic properties

The pharmacokinetics of insulin lispro reflect a compound that is rapidly absorbed and achieves peak blood levels 30 to 70 minutes following subcutaneous injection. When considering the clinical relevance of these kinetics, it is more appropriate to examine the glucose utilisation curves (as discussed in section 5.1).

Insulin lispro maintains more rapid absorption when compared to soluble human insulin in patients with renal impairment. In patients with Type 2 diabetes, over a wide range of renal function, the pharmacokinetic differences between insulin lispro and soluble human insulin were generally maintained and shown to be independent of renal function. Insulin lispro maintains more rapid absorption and elimination when compared to soluble human insulin in patients with hepatic impairment.

5.3 Preclinical safety data

In *in vitro* tests, including binding to insulin receptor sites and effects on growing cells, insulin lispro behaved in a manner that closely resembled human insulin. Studies also demonstrate that the dissociation of binding to the insulin receptor of insulin lispro is equivalent to human insulin. Acute, one-month and twelve-month toxicology studies produced no significant toxicity findings.

Insulin lispro did not induce fertility impairment, embryotoxicity, or teratogenicity in animal studies.

6. PHARMACEUTICAL PARTICULARS

6.1 List of excipients

m-cresol (3.15mg/ml), glycerol, dibasic sodium phosphate.$7H_2O$, zinc oxide, water for injections. Hydrochloric acid and sodium hydroxide may be used to adjust pH to 7.0-7.8.

6.2 Incompatibilities

HUMALOG, HUMALOG Pen or HUMALOG KwikPen preparations should not be mixed with insulin produced by other manufacturers or with animal insulin preparations. This medicinal product must not be mixed with other medicinal products except those mentioned in section 6.6.

6.3 Shelf life

Unopened vials,

2 years

Unused cartridges and unused pre-filled pens

3 years

After cartridge insertion, or after first use (vial and prefilled pen)

28 days

6.4 Special precautions for storage

Unused cartridge and unused pre-filled pens

Store in a refrigerator (2°C-8°C). Do not freeze. Do not expose to excessive heat or direct sunlight.

After cartridge insertion or first use (pre-filled pen)

Store below 30°C. Do not refrigerate. The pen with the inserted cartridge and the pre-filled pen should not be stored with the needle attached.

Vials

Do not freeze. Do not expose to excessive heat or direct sunlight.

Unopened vials

Store in a refrigerator (2°C - 8°C).

After first use (vials only)

Store in a refrigerator (2°C - 8°C) or below 30°C.

6.5 Nature and contents of container

Vials: The solution is contained in Type I flint glass vials, sealed with butyl or halobutyl stoppers, and secured with aluminium seals. Dimeticone or silicone emulsion may be used to treat the vial stoppers.

Cartridges/HUMALOG Pens: The solution is contained in Type I flint glass cartridges, sealed with butyl or halobutyl disc seals and plunger heads, and are secured with aluminium seals. Dimeticone or silicone emulsion may be used to treat the cartridge plunger and/or the glass cartridge.

HUMALOG Pens: The 3ml cartridges are sealed in a disposable pen injector. Needles are not included.

HUMALOG KwikPen: The 3ml cartridges are sealed in a disposable pen injector, called the 'KwikPen'. Needles are not included.

Not all packs may be marketed.

1 × 10ml HUMALOG vial.

2 × 10ml HUMALOG vials.

5 × (1 × 10ml) HUMALOG vials.

5 × 3ml HUMALOG cartridges for a 3ml pen.

2 × (5 × 3ml) HUMALOG cartridges for a 3ml pen.

5 × 3ml HUMALOG Pens.

2 × (5 × 3ml) HUMALOG Pens.

5 × 3ml HUMALOG 100 U/ml KwikPens.

2 × (5 × 3ml) HUMALOG 100 U/ml KwikPens.

6.6 Special precautions for disposal and other handling

Instructions for use and handling

Any unused product or waste material should be disposed of in accordance with local requirements.

HUMALOG Vials

The vial is to be used in conjunction with an appropriate syringe (100 U markings).

a) Preparing a dose

Inspect the HUMALOG solution. It should be clear and colourless. Do not use HUMALOG if it appears cloudy, thickened, or slightly coloured or if solid particles are visible.

i) HUMALOG

1. Wash your hands.

2. If using a new vial, flip off the plastic protective cap, but **do not** remove the stopper.

3. If the therapeutic regimen requires the injection of basal insulin and HUMALOG at the same time, the two can be mixed in the syringe. If mixing insulins, refer to the instructions for mixing that follow in section (ii) and section 6.2.

4. Draw air into the syringe equal to the prescribed HUMALOG dose. Wipe the top of the vial with an alcohol swab. Put the needle through the rubber top of the HUMALOG vial and inject the air into the vial.

5. Turn the vial and syringe upside down. Hold the vial and syringe firmly in one hand.

6. Making sure the tip of the needle is in the HUMALOG, withdraw the correct dose into the syringe.

7. Before removing the needle from the vial, check the syringe for air bubbles that reduce the amount of HUMALOG in it. If bubbles are present, hold the syringe straight up and tap its side until the bubbles float to the top. Push them out with the plunger and withdraw the correct dose.

8. Remove the needle from the vial and lay the syringe down so that the needle does not touch anything.

ii) Mixing HUMALOG with longer-acting Human Insulins (see section 6.2)

1. HUMALOG should be mixed with longer-acting human insulins only on the advice of a doctor.

2. Draw air into the syringe equal to the amount of longer-acting insulin being taken. Insert the needle into the longer-acting insulin vial and inject the air. Withdraw the needle.

3. Now inject air into the HUMALOG vial in the same manner, but **do not** withdraw the needle.

4. Turn the vial and syringe upside down.

5. Making sure the tip of the needle is in the HUMALOG, withdraw the correct dose of HUMALOG into the syringe.

6. Before removing the needle from the vial, check the syringe for air bubbles that reduce the amount of HUMALOG in it. If bubbles are present, hold the syringe straight up and tap its side until the bubbles float to the top. Push them out with the plunger and withdraw the correct dose.

7. Remove the needle from the vial of HUMALOG and insert it into the vial of the longer-acting insulin. Turn the vial and syringe upside down. Hold the vial and syringe firmly in one hand and shake gently. Making sure the tip of the needle is in the insulin, withdraw the dose of longer-acting insulin.

8. Withdraw the needle and lay the syringe down so that the needle does not touch anything.

b) Injecting a dose

1. Choose a site for injection.

2. Clean the skin as instructed.

3. Stabilise the skin by spreading it or pinching up a large area. Insert the needle and inject as instructed.

4. Pull the needle out and apply gentle pressure over the injection site for several seconds. Do not rub the area.

5. Dispose of the syringe and needle safely.

6. Use of the injection sites should be rotated so that the same is not used more than approximately once a month.

c) Mixing insulins

Do not mix insulin in vials with insulin in cartridges. See section 6.2.

HUMALOG cartridges

HUMALOG cartridges are to be used with a CE marked pen as recommended in the information provided by the device manufacturer.

a) Preparing a dose

Inspect the HUMALOG solution. It should be clear and colourless. Do not use HUMALOG if it appears cloudy, thickened, or slightly coloured, or if solid particles are visible.

The following is a general description. The manufacturer's instructions with each individual pen must be followed for loading the cartridge, attaching the needle, and administering the insulin injection.

b) Injecting a dose

1. Wash your hands.

2. Choose a site for injection.

3. Clean the skin as instructed.

4. Remove outer needle cap.

5. Stabilise the skin by spreading it or pinching up a large area. Insert the needle as instructed.

6. Press the knob.

7. Pull the needle out and apply gentle pressure over the injection site for several seconds. Do not rub the area.

8. Using the outer needle cap, unscrew the needle and dispose of it safely.

9. Use of injection sites should be rotated so that the same site is not used more than approximately once a month.

c) Mixing insulins

Do not mix insulin in vials with insulin in cartridges. See section 6.2.

HUMALOG Pens (excluding Kwikpen)

a) Preparing a dose

1. Inspect the HUMALOG Pen solution.

It should be clear and colourless. Do not use HUMALOG Pen if it appears cloudy, thickened, or slightly coloured, or if solid particles are visible.

2. Put on the needle.

Wipe the rubber seal with alcohol. Remove the paper tab from the capped needle. Screw the capped needle clockwise onto the pen until it is tight. Hold the pen with needle pointing up and remove the outer needle cap and inner needle cover.

3. Priming the pen (check insulin flow).

(a) The arrow should be visible in the dose window. If the arrow is not present, turn the dose knob clockwise until the arrow appears and notch is felt or visually aligned.

(b) Pull dose knob out (in direction of the arrow) until a '0' appears in the dose window. A dose cannot be dialled until the dose knob is pulled out.

(c) Turn dose knob clockwise until a '2' appears in the dose window.

(d) Hold the pen with needle pointing up and tap the clear cartridge holder gently with your finger so any air bubbles collect near the top. Depress the injection button fully until you feel or hear a click. You should see a drop of insulin at the tip of the needle. If insulin does not appear, repeat the procedure until insulin appears.

(e) Always prime the pen (check the insulin flow) before each injection. Failure to prime the pen may result in an inaccurate dose.

4. Setting the dose.

(a) Turn the dose knob clockwise until the arrow appears in the dose window and a notch is felt or visually aligned.

(b) Pull the dose knob out (in the direction of the arrow) until a '0' appears in the dose window. A dose cannot be dialled until the dose knob is pulled out.

(c) Turn the dose knob clockwise until the dose appears in the dose window. If too high a dose is dialled, turn the dose knob backward (anti-clockwise) until the correct dose appears in the window. A dose greater than the number of units remaining in the cartridge cannot be dialled.

b) Injecting a dose

1. Wash your hands.
2. Choose a site for injection.
3. Clean the skin as instructed.
4. Remove outer needle cap.
5. Stabilise the skin by spreading it or pinching up a large area. Insert the needle as instructed.
6. Press the injection button down with the thumb (until you hear or feel a click); wait 5 seconds.
7. Pull the needle out and apply gentle pressure over the injection site for several seconds. Do not rub the area.
8. Immediately after an injection, use the outer needle cap to unscrew the needle. Remove the needle from the pen. This will ensure sterility, and prevent leakage, re-entry of air, and potential needle clogs. Do not reuse the needle. Dispose of the needle in a responsible manner. Needles and pens must not be shared.

The prefilled pen can be used until it is empty. Please properly discard or recycle.

9. Replace the cap on the pen.
10. Use of injection sites should be rotated so that the same site is not used more than approximately once a month.
11. The injection button should be fully depressed before using the pen again.

c) Mixing insulins

Do not mix insulin in vials with insulin in cartridges. See section 6.2.

HUMALOG KwikPen

Inspect the HUMALOG solution. It should be clear and colourless. Do not use HUMALOG if it appears cloudy, thickened, or slightly coloured or if solid particles are visible.

a) Handling of the pre-filled pen

Before using the KwikPen the user manual included in the package leaflet must be read carefully. The KwikPen has to be used as recommended in the user manual.

b) Mixing insulins

Do not mix insulin in vials with insulin in cartridges. See section 6.2.

7. MARKETING AUTHORISATION HOLDER

Eli Lilly Nederland B.V., Grootslag 1-5, 3991 RA Houten, The Netherlands.

8. MARKETING AUTHORISATION NUMBER(S)

HUMALOG vials

1 × 10ml HUMALOG vial: EU/1/96/007/002

2 × 10ml HUMALOG vials: EU/1/96/007/020

5 × (1 × 10ml) HUMALOG vials: EU/1/96/007/021

HUMALOG cartridges

5 × 3ml HUMALOG cartridges for a 3ml pen: EU/1/96/007/004

2 × (5 × 3ml) HUMALOG cartridges for a 3ml pen: EU/1/96/007/023

HUMALOG Pens

5 × 3ml HUMALOG Pens: EU/1/96/007/015

2 × (5 × 3ml) HUMALOG Pens: EU/1/96/007/026

HUMALOG KwikPen

5 × 3ml HUMALOG 100 U/ml KwikPen: EU/1/96/007/031

2 × (5 × 3ml) HUMALOG 100 U/ml KwikPen: EU/1/96/007/032

9. DATE OF FIRST AUTHORISATION/RENEWAL OF THE AUTHORISATION

Date of first authorisation: 30 April 1996

Date of last renewal: 30 April 2006

10. DATE OF REVISION OF THE TEXT

01 July 2009

LEGAL CATEGORY

POM (United Kingdom)

For further information in the United Kingdom contact:

Eli Lilly and Company Limited

Lilly House, Priestley Road

Basingstoke, Hampshire, RG24 9NL

Telephone: Basingstoke (01256) 315 999

For further information in the Republic of Ireland contact:

Eli Lilly and Company (Ireland) Limited

Hyde House, 65 Adelaide Road

Dublin 2, Republic of Ireland

Telephone: Dublin (01) 661 4377

*HUMALOG (insulin lispro) and KWIKPEN are trademarks of Eli Lilly and Company. HLG33M

Humalog Mix25 100U/ml suspension for injection in cartridge, 100U/ml Pen suspension for injection. Mix50 100U/ml suspension for injection in cartridge, 100U/ml Pen suspension for injection

(Eli Lilly and Company Limited)

1. NAME OF THE MEDICINAL PRODUCT

HUMALOG* Mix25 100U/ml suspension for injection in cartridge.

HUMALOG Mix25 100U/ml Pen, suspension for injection.

HUMALOG Mix25 100U/ml KwikPen, suspension for injection.

HUMALOG Mix50 100U/ml suspension for injection in cartridge.

HUMALOG Mix50 100U/ml Pen, suspension for injection.

HUMALOG Mix50 100U/ml KwikPen, suspension for injection.

2. QUALITATIVE AND QUANTITATIVE COMPOSITION

One ml contains 100U (equivalent to 3.5mg) insulin lispro (recombinant DNA origin produced in *E. coli*).

Each container includes 3ml equivalent to 300U insulin lispro.

HUMALOG Mix25 consists of 25% insulin lispro solution and 75% insulin lispro protamine suspension.

HUMALOG Mix50 consists of 50% insulin lispro solution and 50% insulin lispro protamine suspension.

For a full list of excipients, see section 6.1.

3. PHARMACEUTICAL FORM

Suspension for injection.

HUMALOG Mix25 and HUMALOG Mix50 are white, sterile suspensions.

4. CLINICAL PARTICULARS

4.1 Therapeutic indications

HUMALOG Mix25 or HUMALOG Mix50 is indicated for the treatment of patients with diabetes mellitus who require insulin for the maintenance of normal glucose homeostasis.

4.2 Posology and method of administration

The dosage should be determined by the physician, according to the requirement of the patient.

HUMALOG Mix25 or HUMALOG Mix50 may be given shortly before meals. When necessary, HUMALOG Mix25 or HUMALOG Mix50 can be given soon after meals. HUMALOG Mix25 or HUMALOG Mix50 should only be given by subcutaneous injection. Under no circumstances should HUMALOG Mix25 or HUMALOG Mix50 be given intravenously.

Subcutaneous administration should be in the upper arms, thighs, buttocks, or abdomen. Use of injection sites should be rotated so that the same site is not used more than approximately once a month.

When administered subcutaneously, care should be taken when injecting HUMALOG Mix25 or HUMALOG Mix50 to ensure that a blood vessel has not been entered. After injection, the site of injection should not be massaged. Patients must be educated to use the proper injection techniques.

The rapid onset and early peak of activity of HUMALOG itself is observed following the subcutaneous administration of HUMALOG Mix25 or HUMALOG Mix50. This allows HUMALOG Mix25 or HUMALOG Mix50 to be given very close to mealtime. The duration of action of the insulin lispro protamine suspension (BASAL) component of HUMALOG Mix25 or HUMALOG Mix50 is similar to that of a basal insulin (NPH [isophane]).

The time course of action of any insulin may vary considerably in different individuals or at different times in the same individual. As with all insulin preparations, the duration of action of HUMALOG Mix25 or HUMALOG Mix50 is dependent on dose, site of injection, blood supply, temperature and physical activity.

4.3 Contraindications

Hypoglycaemia.

Hypersensitivity to insulin lispro or to any of the excipients.

4.4 Special warnings and precautions for use

Under no circumstances should HUMALOG Mix25 or HUMALOG Mix50 be given intravenously.

Transferring a patient to another type or brand of insulin should be done under strict medical supervision. Changes in strength, brand (manufacturer), type (soluble, NPH, lente, etc), species (animal, human, human insulin analogue), and/or method of manufacture (recombinant DNA versus animal-source insulin) may result in the need for a change in dosage.

Conditions which may make the early warning symptoms of hypoglycaemia different or less pronounced include long duration of diabetes, intensified insulin therapy, diabetic nerve disease, or medications such as beta-blockers.

A few patients who have experienced hypoglycaemic reactions after transfer from animal-source insulin to human insulin have reported that the early warning symptoms of hypoglycaemia were less pronounced or different from those experienced with their previous insulin. Uncorrected hypoglycaemic or hyperglycaemic reactions can cause loss of consciousness, coma, or death.

The use of dosages which are inadequate or discontinuation of treatment, especially in insulin-dependent diabetics, may lead to hyperglycaemia and diabetic ketoacidosis; conditions which are potentially lethal.

Insulin requirements may be reduced in the presence of renal impairment. Insulin requirements may be reduced in patients with hepatic impairment due to reduced capacity for gluconeogenesis and reduced insulin breakdown; however, in patients with chronic hepatic impairment, an increase in insulin resistance may lead to increased insulin requirements.

Insulin requirements may be increased during illness or emotional disturbances.

Adjustment of dosage may also be necessary if patients undertake increased physical activity or change their usual diet. Exercise taken immediately after a meal may increase the risk of hypoglycaemia.

Administration of insulin lispro to children below 12 years of age should be considered only in case of an expected benefit when compared to soluble insulin.

4.5 Interaction with other medicinal products and other forms of interaction

Insulin requirements may be increased by substances with hyperglycaemic activity, such as oral contraceptives, corticosteroids, or thyroid replacement therapy, danazol, $beta_2$ stimulants (such as ritodrine, salbutamol, terbutaline).

Insulin requirements may be reduced in the presence of substances with hypoglycaemic activity, such as oral hypoglycaemics, salicylates (for example, acetylsalicylic acid), sulpha antibiotics, certain antidepressants (monoamine oxidase inhibitors, selective serotonin reuptake inhibitors), certain angiotensin converting enzyme inhibitors (captopril, enalapril), angiotensin II receptor blockers, beta-blockers, octreotide or alcohol.

Mixing HUMALOG Mix25 or HUMALOG Mix50 with other insulins has not been studied.

The physician should be consulted when using other medications in addition to HUMALOG Mix25 or HUMALOG Mix50.

4.6 Pregnancy and lactation

Data on a large number of exposed pregnancies do not indicate any adverse effect of insulin lispro on pregnancy or on the health of the foetus/newborn.

It is essential to maintain good control of the insulin-treated (insulin-dependent or gestational diabetes) patient throughout pregnancy. Insulin requirements usually fall during the first trimester and increase during the second and third trimesters. Patients with diabetes should be advised to inform their doctor if they are pregnant or are contemplating pregnancy. Careful monitoring of glucose control, as well as general health, is essential in pregnant patients with diabetes.

Patients with diabetes who are breast-feeding may require adjustments in insulin dose, diet or both.

Figure 1

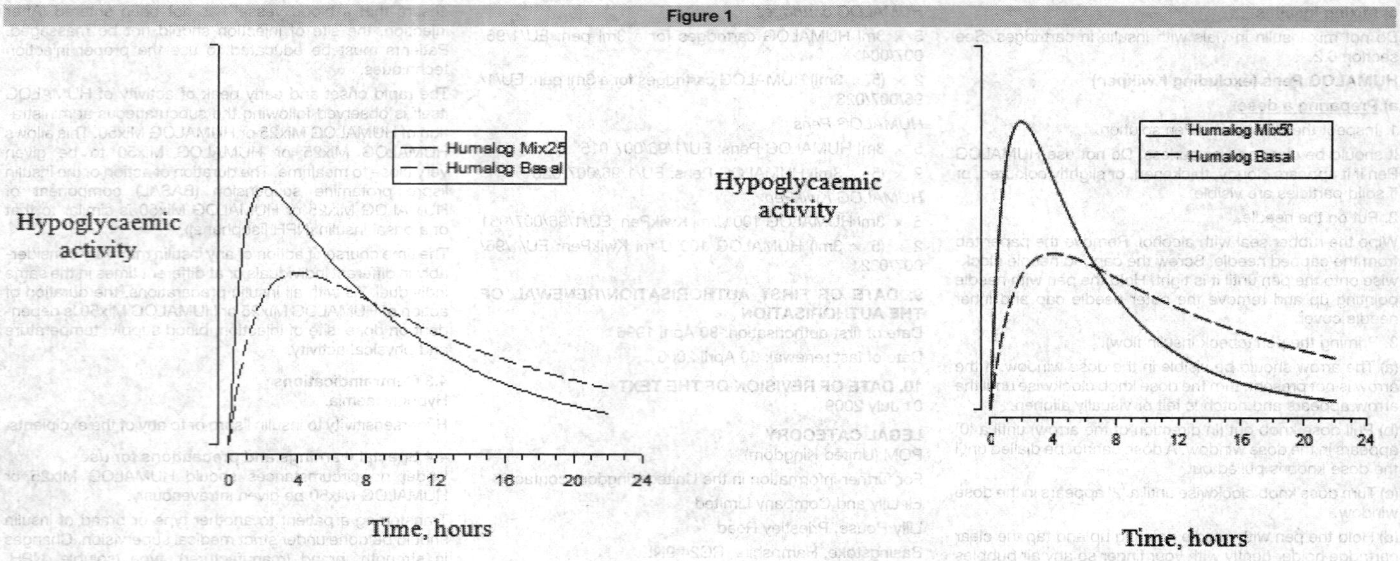

4.7 Effects on ability to drive and use machines

The patient's ability to concentrate and react may be impaired as a result of hypoglycaemia. This may constitute a risk in situations where these abilities are of special importance (e.g., driving a car or operating machinery).

Patients should be advised to take precautions to avoid hypoglycaemia whilst driving; this is particularly important in those who have reduced or absent awareness of the warning signs of hypoglycaemia or have frequent episodes of hypoglycaemia. The advisability of driving should be considered in these circumstances.

4.8 Undesirable effects

Hypoglycaemia is the most frequent undesirable effect of insulin therapy that a patient with diabetes may suffer. Severe hypoglycaemia may lead to loss of consciousness and in extreme cases, death. No specific frequency for hypoglycaemia is presented, since hypoglycaemia is a result of both the insulin dose and other factors, e.g., a patient's level of diet and exercise.

Local allergy in patients is common (1/100 to <1/10). Redness, swelling, and itching can occur at the site of insulin injection. This condition usually resolves in a few days to a few weeks. In some instances, this condition may be related to factors other than insulin, such as irritants in the skin cleansing agent or poor injection technique. Systemic allergy, which is rare (1/10,000 to <1/1,000) but potentially more serious, is a generalised allergy to insulin. It may cause a rash over the whole body, shortness of breath, wheezing, reduction in blood pressure, fast pulse, or sweating. Severe cases of generalised allergy may be life-threatening.

Lipodystrophy at the injection site is uncommon (1/1,000 to <1/100).

4.9 Overdose

Insulins have no specific overdose definitions because serum glucose concentrations are a result of complex interactions between insulin levels, glucose availability and other metabolic processes. Hypoglycaemia may occur as a result of an excess of insulin activity relative to food intake and energy expenditure.

Hypoglycaemia may be associated with listlessness, confusion, palpitations, headache, sweating and vomiting.

Mild hypoglycaemic episodes will respond to oral administration of glucose or other sugar or saccharated products.

Correction of moderately severe hypoglycaemia can be accomplished by intramuscular or subcutaneous administration of glucagon, followed by oral carbohydrate when the patient recovers sufficiently. Patients who fail to respond to glucagon must be given glucose solution intravenously.

If the patient is comatose, glucagon should be administered intramuscularly or subcutaneously. However, glucose solution must be given intravenously if glucagon is not available or if the patient fails to respond to glucagon. The patient should be given a meal as soon as consciousness is recovered.

Sustained carbohydrate intake and observation may be necessary because hypoglycaemia may recur after apparent clinical recovery.

5. PHARMACOLOGICAL PROPERTIES

5.1 Pharmacodynamic properties

Pharmacotherapeutic group: HUMALOG Mix25 and HUMALOG Mix50 are premixed suspensions consisting of insulin lispro (fast-acting human insulin analogue) and insulin lispro protamine suspension (intermediate-acting human insulin analogue). *ATC code:* A10A D04.

The primary activity of insulin lispro is the regulation of glucose metabolism.

In addition, insulins have several anabolic and anti-catabolic actions on a variety of different tissues. Within muscle tissue this includes increasing glycogen, fatty acid, glycerol and protein synthesis and amino acid uptake, while decreasing glycogenolysis, gluconeogenesis, ketogenesis, lipolysis, protein catabolism and amino acid output.

Insulin lispro has a rapid onset of action (approximately 15 minutes), thus allowing it to be given closer to a meal (within zero to 15 minutes of the meal) when compared to soluble insulin (30 to 45 minutes before). The rapid onset and early peak of activity of insulin lispro is observed following the subcutaneous administration of HUMALOG Mix25 or HUMALOG Mix50. BASAL has an activity profile that is very similar to that of a basal insulin (NPH) over a period of approximately 15 hours.

Clinical trials in patients with Type 1 and Type 2 diabetes have demonstrated reduced postprandial hyperglycaemia with HUMALOG Mix25 compared to human insulin mixture 30/70. In one clinical study there was a small (0.38mmol/l) increase in blood glucose levels at night (3 a.m.).

In the figures below the pharmacodynamics of HUMALOG Mix25, HUMALOG Mix50 and BASAL are illustrated.

(see Figure 1 above)

The above representations reflect the relative amount of glucose over time required to maintain the subject's whole blood glucose concentrations near fasting levels and is an indicator of the effect of these insulins on glucose metabolism over time.

The glucodynamic response to insulin lispro is not affected by renal or hepatic function impairment. Glucodynamic differences between insulin lispro and soluble human insulin, as measured during a glucose clamp procedure, were maintained over a wide range of renal function.

Insulin lispro has been shown to be equipotent to human insulin on a molar basis but its effect is more rapid and of a shorter duration.

In two 8-month open label crossover studies, Type 2 diabetes patients who were either new to insulin therapy or already using one or two injections of insulin received 4 months of treatment with HUMALOG Mix25 (used twice daily with metformin) and insulin glargine (used once daily with metformin) in a randomised sequence. Detailed information can be found in the following table.

(see Table 1 below)

5.2 Pharmacokinetic properties

The pharmacokinetics of insulin lispro reflect a compound that is rapidly absorbed and achieves peak blood levels 30 to 70 minutes following subcutaneous injection. The pharmacokinetics of insulin lispro protamine suspension are consistent with those of an intermediate-acting insulin, such as NPH. The pharmacokinetics of HUMALOG Mix25 or HUMALOG Mix50 are representative of the individual pharmacokinetic properties of the two components. When considering the clinical relevance of these kinetics, it is more appropriate to examine the glucose utilisation curves (as discussed in section 5.1).

Insulin lispro maintains more rapid absorption when compared to soluble human insulin in patients with renal impairment. In patients with Type 2 diabetes, over a wide range of renal function, the pharmacokinetic differences between insulin lispro and soluble human insulin were generally maintained and shown to be independent of renal function. Insulin lispro maintains more rapid absorption and elimination when compared to soluble human insulin in patients with hepatic impairment.

5.3 Preclinical safety data

In *in vitro* tests, including binding to insulin receptor sites and effects on growing cells, insulin lispro behaved in a manner that closely resembled human insulin. Studies also demonstrate that the dissociation of binding to the insulin receptor of insulin lispro is equivalent to human insulin. Acute, one-month and twelve-month toxicology studies produced no significant toxicity findings.

Insulin lispro did not induce fertility impairment, embryo-toxicity or teratogenicity in animal studies.

6. PHARMACEUTICAL PARTICULARS

6.1 List of excipients

HUMALOG Mix25: Protamine sulphate, *m*-cresol (1.76mg/ml), phenol (0.80mg/ml), glycerol, dibasic sodium phosphate.7H_2O, zinc oxide, water for injections. Hydrochloric acid and sodium hydroxide may be used to adjust pH to 7.0-7.8.

HUMALOG Mix50: Protamine sulphate, *m*-cresol (2.20mg/ml), phenol (1.00mg/ml), glycerol, dibasic sodium phosphate.7H_2O, zinc oxide, water for injections. Hydrochloric acid and sodium hydroxide may be used to adjust pH to 7.0-7.8.

6.2 Incompatibilities

Mixing HUMALOG Mix25 or HUMALOG Mix50 with other insulins has not been studied. In the absence of compatibility studies, this medicinal product must not be mixed with other medicinal products.

6.3 Shelf life

Unused cartridges & pre-filled pens

3 years

After cartridge insertion, or after first use (prefilled pen)

28 days

Table 1

	Insulin-Naive Patients n = 78	**Not Insulin-Naive Patients n = 97**
Mean total daily insulin dose at endpoint	0.63U/kg	0.42U/kg
Haemoglobin A_{1c} - reduction[1]	1.30% (mean at baseline = 8.7%)	1.00% (mean at baseline = 8.5%)
Reduction of the mean of combined morning/evening two-hour postprandial blood glucose[1]	3.46mM	2.48mM
Reduction of the mean fasting blood glucose[1]	0.55mM	0.65mM
Incidence of hypoglycaemia at endpoint	25%	25%
Bodyweight gain[2]	2.33 kg	0.96 kg

[1]From baseline to end of HUMALOG Mix25 treatment.

[2]In patients randomised to HUMALOG Mix25 during the first crossover period.

6.4 Special precautions for storage

Unused cartridge and unused pre-filled pens

Store in a refrigerator (2°C-8°C). Do not freeze. Do not expose to excessive heat or direct sunlight.

After cartridge insertion or first use (pre-filled pen)

Store below 30°C. Do not refrigerate. The pen with the inserted cartridge and the pre-filled pen should not be stored with the needle attached.

6.5 Nature and contents of container

HUMALOG Mix25 or HUMALOG Mix50 100U/ml suspension for injection in cartridge

The suspension is contained in Type I flint glass cartridges, sealed with butyl or halobutyl disc seals and plunger heads, and secured with aluminium seals. Dimeticone or silicone emulsion may have been used to treat the cartridge plunger and/or the glass cartridge.

5 × 3ml HUMALOG Mix25 cartridges for a 3ml pen.

2 × (5 × 3ml) HUMALOG Mix25 cartridges for a 3ml pen.

5 × 3ml HUMALOG Mix50 cartridges for a 3ml pen.

2 × (5 × 3ml) HUMALOG Mix50 cartridges for a 3ml pen.

HUMALOG Mix25 or HUMALOG Mix50 100U/ml Pen, suspension for injection

The suspension is contained in Type I flint glass cartridges, sealed with halobutyl disc seals and plunger heads and secured with aluminium seals. Dimeticone or silicone emulsion may have been used to treat the cartridge plunger and/or the glass cartridge. The 3ml cartridges are sealed in a disposable pen injector, called the 'Pen' or 'KwikPen'. Needles are not included.

5 × 3ml HUMALOG Mix25 100U/ml Pens.

2 × (5 × 3ml) HUMALOG Mix25 100U/ml Pens.

5 × 3ml HUMALOG Mix25 100U/ml KwikPens.

2 × (5 × 3ml) HUMALOG Mix25 100U/ml KwikPens.

5 × 3ml HUMALOG Mix50 100U/ml Pens.

2 × (5 × 3ml) HUMALOG Mix50 100U/ml Pens.

5 × 3ml HUMALOG Mix50 100U/ml KwikPens.

2 × (5 × 3ml) HUMALOG Mix50 100U/ml KwikPens.

Not all packs may be marketed.

6.6 Special precautions for disposal and other handling

Any unused product or waste material should be disposed of in accordance with local requirements.

HUMALOG Mix25 or HUMALOG Mix50 100U/ml suspension for injection in cartridges

Instructions for Use and Handling

HUMALOG Mix25 or HUMALOG Mix50 cartridges are to be used with a CE marked pen as recommended in the information provided by the device manufacturer.

a) Cartridge - Preparing a dose

Cartridges containing HUMALOG Mix25 or HUMALOG Mix50 should be rotated in the palms of the hands ten times and inverted 180° ten times immediately before use to resuspend the insulin until it appears uniformly cloudy or milky. If not, repeat the above procedure until contents are mixed. Cartridges contain a small glass bead to assist mixing. Do not shake vigorously as this may cause frothing, which may interfere with the correct measurement of the dose.

The cartridges should be examined frequently and should not be used if clumps of material are present or if solid white particles stick to the bottom or wall of the cartridge, giving a frosted appearance.

HUMALOG Mix25 or HUMALOG Mix50 cartridges are not designed to allow any other insulin to be mixed in the cartridge. Cartridges are not designed to be refilled.

The following is a general description. The manufacturer's instructions with each individual pen must be followed for loading the cartridge, attaching the needle and administering the insulin injection.

b) Cartridge - Injecting a dose

1. Wash your hands.
2. Choose a site for injection.
3. Clean the skin as instructed.
4. Remove outer needle cap.
5. Stabilise the skin by spreading it or pinching up a large area. Insert the needle as instructed.
6. Press the knob.
7. Pull the needle out and apply gentle pressure over the injection site for several seconds. Do not rub the area.
8. Using the outer needle cap, unscrew the needle and dispose of it safely.
9. Use of injection sites should be rotated so that the same site is not used more than approximately once a month.

HUMALOG Mix25 or HUMALOG Mix50 100U/ml Pen, suspension for injection (excluding Kwikpen)

Instructions for Use and Handling

a) Pen - Preparing a dose

1. Inspect the HUMALOG Mix25 or HUMALOG Mix50 100U/ml Pen

The Pen should be rotated in the palms of the hands ten times and inverted 180° ten times immediately before use to resuspend the insulin until it appears uniformly cloudy or milky. If not, repeat the above procedure until contents are mixed. Cartridges contain a small glass bead to assist mixing. Do not shake vigorously as this may cause frothing, which may interfere with the correct measurement of the dose.

The cartridges should be examined frequently and should not be used if clumps of material are present or if solid white particles stick to the bottom or wall of the cartridge, giving a frosted appearance.

2. Put on the needle.

Wipe the rubber seal with alcohol. Remove the paper tab from the capped needle. Screw the capped needle clockwise onto the pen until it is tight. Hold the pen with needle pointing up and remove the outer needle cap and inner needle cover.

3. Priming Pen (check insulin flow).

(a) The arrow should be visible in the dose window. If the arrow is not present, turn the dose knob clockwise until the arrow appears and notch is felt or visually aligned.

(b) Pull dose knob out (in direction of the arrow) until a '0' appears in the dose window. A dose cannot be dialled until the dose knob is pulled out.

(c) Turn dose knob clockwise until a '2' appears in the dose window.

(d) Hold the pen with needle pointing up and tap the clear cartridge holder gently with your finger so any air bubbles collect near the top. Depress the injection button fully until you feel or hear a click. You should see a drop of insulin at the tip of the needle. If insulin does not appear, repeat the procedure until insulin appears.

(e) Always prime the pen (check the insulin flow) before each injection. Failure to prime the pen may result in an inaccurate dose.

4. Setting the dose.

(a) Turn the dose knob clockwise until the arrow appears in the dose window and a notch is felt or visually aligned.

(b) Pull the dose knob out (in the direction of the arrow) until a '0' appears in the dose window. A dose cannot be dialled until the dose knob is pulled out.

(c) Turn the dose knob clockwise until the dose appears in the dose window. If too high a dose is dialled, turn the dose knob backward (anti-clockwise) until the correct dose appears in the window. A dose greater than the number of units remaining in the cartridge cannot be dialled.

b) Pen - Injecting a dose

1. Wash your hands.
2. Choose a site for injection.
3. Clean the skin as instructed.
4. Remove outer needle cap.
5. Stabilise the skin by spreading it or pinching up a large area. Insert the needle as instructed.
6. Press the injection button down with the thumb (until you hear or feel a click); wait 5 seconds.
7. Pull the needle out and apply gentle pressure over the injection site for several seconds. Do not rub the area.
8. Immediately after an injection, use the outer needle cap to unscrew the needle. Remove the needle from the pen. This will ensure sterility, and prevent leakage, re-entry of air, and potential needle clogs. Do not reuse the needle. Dispose of the needle in a responsible manner. Needles and pens must not be shared. The pre-filled pen can be used until it is empty. Please properly discard or recycle.
9. Replace the cap on the pen.
10. Use of injection sites should be rotated so that the same site is not used more than approximately once a month.
11. The injection button should be fully depressed before using the pen again.

HUMALOG Mix25 or HUMALOG Mix50 100U/ml Kwik-Pen, suspension for injection

a) Instructions for use and handling

The KwikPen should be rotated in the palms of the hands ten times and inverted 180° ten times immediately before use to resuspend the insulin until it appears uniformly cloudy or milky. If not, repeat the above procedure until contents are mixed. Cartridges contain a small glass bead to assist mixing. Do not shake vigorously as this may cause frothing which may interfere with the correct measurement of the dose.

The cartridges should be examined frequently and should not be used if clumps of material are present or if solid white particles stick to the bottom or wall of the cartridge, giving a frosted appearance.

b) Handling of the pre-filled pen

Before using the KwikPen the user manual included in the package leaflet must be read carefully. The KwikPen has to be used as recommended in the user manual.

7. MARKETING AUTHORISATION HOLDER

Eli Lilly Nederland B.V., Grootslag 1-5, 3991 RA Houten, The Netherlands.

8. MARKETING AUTHORISATION NUMBER(S)

5 × 3ml HUMALOG Mix25 cartridges for a 3ml pen: EU/1/96/007/008

2 × (5 × 3ml) HUMALOG Mix25 cartridges for a 3ml pen: EU/1/96/007/024

5 × 3ml HUMALOG Mix50 cartridges for a 3ml pen: EU/1/96/007/006

2 × (5 × 3ml) HUMALOG Mix50 cartridges for a 3ml pen: EU/1/96/007/025

5 × 3ml HUMALOG Mix25 100U/ml Pens: EU/1/96/007/016

2 × (5 × 3ml) HUMALOG Mix25 100U/ml Pens: EU/1/96/007/027

5 × 3ml HUMALOG Mix50 100U/ml Pens: EU/1/96/007/017

2 × (5 × 3ml) HUMALOG Mix50 100U/ml Pens: EU/1/96/007/028

5 × 3 ml Humalog Mix25 100 U/ml KwikPens EU/1/96/007/033

2 × (5 × 3 ml) Humalog Mix25 100 U/ml KwikPens EU/1/96/007/034

5 × 3 ml Humalog Mix50 100 U/ml KwikPens EU/1/96/007/035

2 × (5 × 3 ml) Humalog Mix50 100 U/ml KwikPens EU/1/96/007/036

9. DATE OF FIRST AUTHORISATION/RENEWAL OF THE AUTHORISATION

Date of first authorisation: 30 April 1996

Date of last renewal: 30 April 2006

10. DATE OF REVISION OF THE TEXT

01 July 2009

LEGAL CATEGORY

POM

For further information in the United Kingdom contact:

Eli Lilly and Company Limited
Lilly House, Priestley Road
Basingstoke, Hampshire, RG24 9NL
Telephone: Basingstoke (01256) 315 999

For further information in the Republic of Ireland contact:

Eli Lilly and Company (Ireland) Limited
Hyde House, 65 Adelaide Road
Dublin 2, Republic of Ireland
Telephone: Dublin (01) 661 4377

*HUMALOG, HUMALOG MIX25, HUMALOG MIX50 (insulin lispro) and KWIKPEN are trademarks of Eli Lilly and Company.

HLG34M

Humatrope 6mg, 12mg, or 24mg powder and solvent for solution for injection

(Eli Lilly and Company Limited)

1. NAME OF THE MEDICINAL PRODUCT

HUMATROPE* 6mg, 12mg, or 24mg powder and solvent for solution for injection.

2. QUALITATIVE AND QUANTITATIVE COMPOSITION

HUMATROPE 6 mg: The cartridge contains 6 mg of somatropin. When reconstituted contains 1.9 mg/ml.

HUMATROPE 12 mg: The cartridge contains 12 mg of somatropin. When reconstituted contains 3.8 mg/ml.

HUMATROPE 24 mg: The cartridge contains 24 mg of somatropin. When reconstituted contains 7.6 mg/ml.

The above mentioned concentrations after reconstitution are theoretical values.

Somatropin is produced in *Escherichia coli cells* by recombinant DNA technology.

HUMATROPE contains less than 1mmol sodium per dose, i.e. essentially sodium free.

For a full list of excipients, see section 6.1.

3. PHARMACEUTICAL FORM

Powder and solvent for solution for injection.

The powder is a white or almost white powder. The solvent is a clear solution.

4. CLINICAL PARTICULARS

4.1 Therapeutic indications

Paediatric Patients

HUMATROPE is indicated for the long-term treatment of children who have growth failure due to an inadequate secretion of normal endogenous growth hormone.

HUMATROPE is also indicated for the treatment of short stature in children with Turner syndrome, confirmed by chromosome analysis.

HUMATROPE is also indicated for the treatment of growth retardation in prepubertal children with chronic renal insufficiency.

HUMATROPE is also indicated for the treatment of patients who have growth failure associated with SHOX deficiency, as confirmed by DNA analysis.

HUMATROPE is also indicated for growth disturbance (current height SDS < -2.5 and parental adjusted height SDS < -1) in short children born small for gestational age (SGA), with a birth weight and/or length below -2 SD, who failed to show catch-up growth (height velocity SDS < 0 during the last year) by 4 years of age or later.

Adult Patients

HUMATROPE is indicated for replacement therapy in adults with pronounced growth hormone deficiency.

Patients with severe growth hormone deficiency in adulthood are defined as patients with known hypothalamic-pituitary pathology and at least one known deficiency of a pituitary hormone not being prolactin. These patients should undergo a single dynamic test in order to diagnose or exclude a growth deficiency. In patients with childhood onset isolated GH deficiency (no evidence of hypothalamic-pituitary disease or cranial irradiation), two dynamic tests should be recommended, except for those having low IGF-I concentrations (<-2 SDS), who may be considered for one test. The cut-off point of the dynamic test should be strict.

4.2 Posology and method of administration

HUMATROPE is administered by subcutaneous injection after reconstitution.

The dosage and administration schedule should be personalised for each individual; however, for:

Growth Hormone Deficient Paediatric Patients

The recommended dosage is 0.025-0.035mg/kg of body weight per day by subcutaneous injection. This is the equivalent to approximately 0.7-1.0mg/m^2 body surface area per day.

Growth Hormone Deficient Adult Patients

The recommended starting dose is 0.15-0.30mg/day. A lower starting dose may be necessary in older and obese patients.

This dose should be gradually increased according to individual patient requirements based on the clinical response and serum IGF-I concentrations. Total daily dose usually does not exceed 1mg.

IGF-I concentrations should be maintained below the upper limit of the age-specific normal range.

The minimum effective dose should be used and dose requirements may decline with increasing age.

The dosage of somatropin should be decreased in cases of persistent oedema or severe paraesthesia, in order to avoid the development of carpal tunnel syndrome (see section 4.8).

Patients With Turner Syndrome

The recommended dosage is 0.045-0.050mg/kg of body weight per day, given as a subcutaneous injection, to be administered preferably in the evening. This is equivalent to approximately 1.4mg/m^2 per day.

Prepubertal Paediatric Patients With Chronic Renal Insufficiency

The recommended dosage is 0.045-0.050mg/kg of body weight per day, given as a subcutaneous injection.

Paediatric Patients With SHOX Deficiency

The recommended dosage is 0.045-0.050mg/kg of body weight per day given as a subcutaneous injection.

Small For Gestational Age

The recommended dose is 0.035mg/kg of body weight per day (equivalent to 1mg/m^2 body surface area per day) given as a subcutaneous injection, until final height is reached (see section 5.1). Treatment should be discontinued after the first year of treatment, if the height velocity SDS is below +1.0 SDS. Treatment should be discontinued if height velocity is < 2cm/year and, if confirmation is required, bone age is > 14 years (girls) or > 16 years (boys), corresponding to closure of epiphyseal growth plates.

The subcutaneous injection sites should be varied in order to avoid lipo-atrophy.

4.3 Contraindications

HUMATROPE should not be used when there is any evidence of activity of a tumour. Intracranial lesions must be inactive and antitumour therapy complete prior to the institution of growth hormone therapy. HUMATROPE should be discontinued if there is evidence of tumour growth.

HUMATROPE should not be reconstituted with the supplied solvent for patients with a known sensitivity to either metacresol or glycerol.

HUMATROPE should not be used for growth promotion in children with closed epiphyses.

Growth hormone should not be initiated to treat patients with acute critical illness due to complications following open heart or abdominal surgery, multiple accidental trauma, or to patients having acute respiratory failure (see section 4.4).

4.4 Special warnings and precautions for use

Previous paediatric subjects who had been treated with growth hormone during childhood, until final height was attained, should be re-evaluated for growth hormone deficiency after epiphyseal closure before replacement therapy is commenced at the doses recommended for adults.

Diagnosis and therapy with HUMATROPE should be initiated and monitored by physicians who are appropriately qualified and experienced in the diagnosis and management of patients with growth hormone deficiency.

There is so far no evidence to suspect that growth hormone replacement influences the recurrence rate or regrowth of intracranial neoplasms, but standard clinical practice requires regular pituitary imaging in patients with a history of pituitary pathology. A baseline scan is recommended in these patients before instituting growth hormone replacement therapy.

In cases of severe or recurrent headache, visual problems, nausea and/or vomiting, a fundoscopy for papilloedema is recommended. If papilloedema is confirmed, a diagnosis of benign intracranial hypertension should be considered and, if appropriate, the growth hormone treatment should be discontinued.

At present there is insufficient evidence to guide clinical decision making in patients with resolved intracranial hypertension. If growth hormone treatment is restarted, careful monitoring for symptoms of intracranial hypertension is necessary.

Patients with endocrine disorders, including growth hormone deficiency, may develop slipped capital epiphyses more frequently. Any child with the onset of a limp during growth hormone therapy should be evaluated.

Growth hormone increases the extrathyroidal conversion of T4 to T3 and may, as such, unmask incipient hypothyroidism. Monitoring of thyroid function should therefore be conducted in all patients. In patients with hypopituitarism, standard replacement therapy must be closely monitored when somatropin therapy is administered.

For paediatric patients, the treatment should be continued until the end of the growth has been reached. It is advisable not to exceed the recommended dosage in view of the potential risks of acromegaly, hyperglycaemia and glucosuria.

Before instituting treatment with somatropin for growth retardation secondary to chronic renal insufficiency, patients should have been followed for one year to verify growth disturbance. Conservative treatment for renal insufficiency (which include control of acidosis, hyperparathyroidism and nutritional status for one year prior to the treatment) should have been established and should be maintained during treatment. Treatment with somatropin should be discontinued at the time of renal transplantation.

The effects of growth hormone on recovery were studied in two placebo-controlled clinical trials involving 522 adult patients who were critically ill due to complications following open heart or abdominal surgery, multiple accidental trauma, or who were having acute respiratory failure. Mortality was higher (41.9% versus 19.3%) among growth hormone-treated patients (doses 5.3-8mg/day) compared to those receiving placebo. The safety of continuing growth hormone in patients receiving replacement doses for approved indications who concurrently develop these illnesses has not been established. Therefore, the potential benefit of treatment continuation in patients having acute critical illnesses should be weighed against the potential risks.

Depending on dose and route of administration, oestrogen therapy may affect the response to growth hormone treatment. Higher doses of growth hormone may be required to achieve an equivalent increase in serum IGF-I in women, as compared to men, especially in women receiving oral oestrogen replacement. If a change of the route of oestrogen administration (oral to transdermal or vice versa) is made, growth hormone should be newly titrated (see section 4.5). An increasing sensitivity to growth hormone (expressed as change in serum IGF-I per growth hormone dose) over time may be observed, particularly in men.

Unless patients with Prader-Willi syndrome also have a diagnosis of growth hormone deficiency, HUMATROPE is not indicated for the treatment of patients who have growth failure due to genetically confirmed Prader-Willi syndrome. There have been reports of sleep apnoea and sudden death after initiating therapy with growth hormone in patients with Prader-Willi syndrome, who had one or more of the following risk factors: severe obesity, history of upper airway obstruction or sleep apnoea, or unidentified respiratory infection.

Subjects with diabetes mellitus should be carefully monitored during treatment with HUMATROPE. An adjustment of the insulin dose may be required.

Elderly patients (age ⩾ 65 years) are more sensitive to the action of HUMATROPE, they may be more prone to develop (severe) adverse events.

Experience in patients above 80 years is limited.

Experience with prolonged treatment in adults is lacking.

In short children born SGA other medical reasons or treatments that could explain growth disturbance should be ruled out before starting treatment.

In children born SGA it is recommended to measure fasting plasma insulin and blood glucose before start of treatment and annually thereafter. In patients with increased risk for diabetes mellitus (e.g. familial history of diabetes, obesity, severe insulin resistance, acanthosis nigricans) oral glucose tolerance testing (OGTT) should be performed. If overt diabetes occurs, growth hormone should not be administered until the patient has been stabilized for diabetes care. Then growth hormone may be introduced with careful monitoring of the diabetic metabolic control. An increase in insulin dosage may be required.

In children born SGA it is recommended to measure the plasma IGF-I concentration before the start of treatment and twice a year thereafter. If on repeated measurements IGF-I levels exceed +2 SD compared to references for sex, age and pubertal status, the IGF-I / IGFBP-3 ratio should be taken into account to consider dose adjustment.

Initiating HUMATROPE treatment in children born SGA and in children with SHOX deficiency, near onset of puberty, is not recommended because of limited experience.

Some of the height gain obtained with treating short children born SGA with growth hormone may be lost if treatment is stopped before reaching final height.

4.5 Interaction with other medicinal products and other forms of interaction

Because human growth hormone may induce a state of insulin resistance, patients should be monitored for evidence of glucose intolerance.

If glucocorticoid replacement therapy is required, glucocorticoid dosage and compliance should be monitored carefully to avoid either adrenal insufficiency or inhibition of growth promoting effects. In patients treated with somatropin, previously undiagnosed secondary hypoadrenalism may be unmasked, requiring glucocorticoid replacement therapy.

In women on oral oestrogen replacement, a higher dose of growth hormone may be required to achieve the treatment goal (see section 4.4).

4.6 Pregnancy and lactation

Animal reproduction studies have not been conducted with HUMATROPE. It is not known whether HUMATROPE can cause foetal harm when administered to a pregnant woman or can affect reproduction capacity. HUMATROPE should be given to a pregnant woman only if clearly needed.

There have been no studies conducted with HUMATROPE in nursing mothers. It is not known whether this drug is excreted in human milk. Because many drugs are excreted in human milk, caution should be exercised when HUMATROPE is administered to a nursing woman.

4.7 Effects on ability to drive and use machines

HUMATROPE has no known effect on ability to drive or use machines.

4.8 Undesirable effects

The following table of undesirable effects and frequencies is based on clinical trial and post-marketing spontaneous reports.

Immune System Disorders Hypersensitivity to solvent (metacresol/glycerol): 1%-10%.
Endocrine Disorders Hypothyroidism: 1%-10%.
Reproductive System and Breast Disorders Gynaecomastia: <0.01% paediatrics; 0.1%-1% adults.
Metabolism and Nutrition Disorders Mild hyperglycaemia: 1% paediatrics; 1%-10% adults. Insulin resistance.
Nervous System Disorders Benign intracranial hypertension: 0.01%-0.1%. Headache: >10% adults. Insomnia: <0.01% paediatrics; 1%-10% adults. Paraesthesia: 0.01%-0.1% paediatrics; 1%-10% adults. Carpal tunnel syndrome: 1%-10% adults.
Vascular Disorders Hypertension: <0.01% paediatrics; 1%-10% adults.
Musculoskeletal, Connective Tissue and Bone Disorders Localised muscle pain (myalgia): 1%-10% adults; 0.01%-0.1% paediatrics. Joint pain and disorder (arthralgia): >10% adults.
General Disorders and Administration Site Conditions Weakness: 0.1%-1%. Injection site pain (reaction): 1%-10%. Oedema (local and generalised): 1%-10% paediatrics; 10% adults.
Investigations Glucosuria: <0.01% paediatrics; 0.01%-0.1% adults.

Paediatric Patients

In clinical trials with growth hormone deficient patients, approximately 2% of the patients developed antibodies to growth hormone. In trials in Turner syndrome, where higher doses were used, up to 8% of patients developed antibodies to growth hormone. The binding capacity of these antibodies was low and growth rate was not affected adversely. Testing for antibodies to growth hormone should be carried out in any patient who fails to respond to therapy.

A mild and transient oedema was observed early during the course of treatment.

Leukaemia has been reported in a small number of children who have been treated with growth hormone. However, there is no evidence that leukaemia incidence is increased in growth hormone recipients without predisposing factors.

Adult Patients

In patients with adult onset growth hormone deficiency, oedema, muscle pain and joint pain and disorder, were reported early in therapy and tended to be transient.

Adult patients treated with growth hormone, following diagnosis of growth hormone deficiency in childhood, reported side-effects less frequently than those with adult onset growth hormone deficiency.

4.9 Overdose

Acute overdose could lead initially to hypoglycaemia and subsequently to hyperglycaemia. Long-term overdosage could result in signs and symptoms of acromegaly consistent with the known effects of excess human growth hormone.

5. PHARMACOLOGICAL PROPERTIES

5.1 Pharmacodynamic properties

Pharmacotherapeutic group: H01A C01.

Somatropin is a polypeptide hormone of recombinant DNA origin. It has 191 amino acid residues and a molecular weight of 22,125 daltons. The amino acid sequence of the product is identical to that of human growth hormone of pituitary origin. It is synthesised in a strain of *Escherichia coli* that has been modified by the addition of the gene for human growth hormone.

The biological effects of HUMATROPE are equivalent to human growth hormone of pituitary origin.

The most prominent effect of HUMATROPE is that it stimulates the growth plates of long bones. Additionally, it promotes cellular protein synthesis and nitrogen retention.

HUMATROPE stimulates lipid metabolism; it increases plasma fatty acids and HDL-cholesterols and decreases total plasma cholesterol.

HUMATROPE therapy has a beneficial effect on body composition in growth hormone deficient patients, in that body fat stores are reduced and lean body mass is increased. Long-term therapy in growth hormone deficient patients increases bone mineral density.

HUMATROPE may induce insulin resistance. Large doses of human growth hormone may impair glucose tolerance.

The data available from clinical trials so far in patients with Turner syndrome indicate that, while some patients may not respond to this therapy, an increase over predicted height has been observed, the average being 3.3 ± 3.9cm.

In a clinical trial, patients (mean age 9.5 ± 0.9 yr) who were treated with a HUMATROPE dose of 0.067mg/kg/day for two years showed a mean gain in height SDS of + 1.2 during treatment. The results obtained in this trial with HUMATROPE are comparable with those described for other recombinant growth hormone preparations. Long-term safety data are still limited.

5.2 Pharmacokinetic properties

A dose of 100μg/kg to adult male volunteers will give a peak serum level (C_{max}) of about 55ng/ml, a half-life ($t_{½}$) of nearly four hours and maximal absorption (AUC [0 to ∞]) of about 475ng/hr/ml.

5.3 Preclinical safety data

HUMATROPE is human growth hormone produced by recombinant technology. No serious events have been reported in subchronic toxicology studies. Long-term animal studies for carcinogenicity and impairment of fertility with this human growth hormone (HUMATROPE) have not been performed. There has been no evidence to date of HUMATROPE-induced mutagenicity.

6. PHARMACEUTICAL PARTICULARS

6.1 List of excipients

Cartridges of powder: Mannitol, glycine, dibasic sodium phosphate, phosphoric acid and sodium hydroxide.

Solvent syringes: Glycerol, metacresol, water for injections, hydrochloric acid, and sodium hydroxide.

6.2 Incompatibilities

In the absence of compatibility studies, this medicinal product must not be mixed with other medicinal products.

6.3 Shelf life

Before reconstitution: 3 years.

After reconstitution: The product may be stored for a maximum of 28 days at 2°C-8°C. Daily room temperature exposure should not exceed 30 minutes.

6.4 Special precautions for storage

Store in a refrigerator (2°C-8°C). Do not freeze.

6.5 Nature and contents of container

HUMATROPE is available in the following pack sizes:

HUMATROPE 6 mg: 1 cartridge (glass type I) with 6 mg of powder for solution for injection, and 3.17 ml of solvent solution in a pre-filled syringe (glass type I) with a plunger (rubber). Pack size of 1, 5 and 10.

HUMATROPE 12 mg: 1 cartridge (glass type I) with 12 mg of powder for solution for injection, and 3.15 ml of solvent solution in a pre-filled syringe (glass type I) with a plunger (rubber). Pack size of 1, 5 and 10.

HUMATROPE 24 mg: 1 cartridge (glass type I) with 24 mg of powder for solution for injection, and 3.15 ml of solvent solution in a pre-filled syringe (glass type I) with a plunger (rubber). Pack size of 1, 5 and 10.

Not all pack sizes may be marketed.

6.6 Special precautions for disposal and other handling

Instructions for preparation and handling:

Reconstitution: Each cartridge of HUMATROPE should be reconstituted using the accompanying solvent syringe. To reconstitute, attach the cartridge to the pre-filled solvent syringe and then inject the entire contents of the pre-filled solvent syringe into the cartridge. The solvent needle aims the stream of liquid against the glass wall of the cartridge. Following reconstitution, gently invert the cartridge up and down 10-times until the contents are completely dissolved. DO NOT SHAKE. The resulting solution should be clear, without particulate matter. If the solution is cloudy or contains particulate matter, the contents MUST NOT be injected.

HUMATROPE cartridges can be used in conjunction with compatible CE marked pen injection systems. The manufacturer's instructions with each individual pen must be followed for loading the cartridge, attaching the needle and administering the HUMATROPE injection.

The solvent syringe is for single use only. Discard it after use. A sterile needle should be used for each administration of HUMATROPE.

Any unused product or waste material should be disposed of in accordance with local requirements.

7. MARKETING AUTHORISATION HOLDER

Eli Lilly and Company Limited
Lilly House
Priestley Road
Basingstoke
Hampshire
RG24 9NL
UK

8. MARKETING AUTHORISATION NUMBER(S)

Cartridges 6mg:	PL 00006/0297
Cartridges 12mg:	PL 00006/0298
Cartridges 24mg:	PL 00006/0299
Solvent (6mg):	PL 00006/0254
Solvent(12 and 24mg):	PL 00006/0300

9. DATE OF FIRST AUTHORISATION/RENEWAL OF THE AUTHORISATION

Date of last renewal: 22 November 2006

10. DATE OF REVISION OF THE TEXT

25 March 2009

LEGAL CATEGORY

POM

*HUMATROPE (somatropin) is a trademark of Eli Lilly and Company.

HT20M

Humira Pen and Syringe

(Abbott Laboratories Limited)

1. NAME OF THE MEDICINAL PRODUCT

Humira▼ 40 mg solution for injection in pre-filled syringe

Humira▼ 40 mg solution for injection in pre-filled pen

2. QUALITATIVE AND QUANTITATIVE COMPOSITION

Each 0.8 ml single dose pre-filled syringe contains 40 mg of adalimumab.

Adalimumab is a recombinant human monoclonal antibody expressed in Chinese Hamster Ovary cells.

For a full list of excipients, see section 6.1.

3. PHARMACEUTICAL FORM

Clear solution for injection in pre-filled syringe.

Clear solution for injection in pre-filled pen

4. CLINICAL PARTICULARS

4.1 Therapeutic indications

Rheumatoid arthritis

Humira in combination with methotrexate, is indicated for:

- the treatment of moderate to severe, active rheumatoid arthritis in adult patients when the response to disease-modifying anti-rheumatic drugs including methotrexate has been inadequate.
- the treatment of severe, active and progressive rheumatoid arthritis in adults not previously treated with methotrexate.

Humira can be given as monotherapy in case of intolerance to methotrexate or when continued treatment with methotrexate is inappropriate.

Humira has been shown to reduce the rate of progression of joint damage as measured by X-ray and to improve physical function, when given in combination with methotrexate.

Polyarticular juvenile idiopathic arthritis

Humira in combination with methotrexate is indicated for the treatment of active polyarticular juvenile idiopathic arthritis, in adolescents aged 13 to 17 years who have had an inadequate response to one or more disease-modifying anti-rheumatic drugs (DMARDs). Humira can be given as monotherapy in case of intolerance to methotrexate or when continued treatment with methotrexate is inappropriate. (see section 5.1).

Psoriatic arthritis

Humira is indicated for the treatment of active and progressive psoriatic arthritis in adults when the response to previous disease-modifying anti-rheumatic drug therapy has been inadequate. Humira has been shown to reduce the rate of progression of peripheral joint damage as measured by X-ray in patients with polyarticular symmetrical subtypes of the disease (see Section 5.1) and to improve physical function.

Ankylosing spondylitis

Humira is indicated for the treatment of adults with severe active ankylosing spondylitis who have had an inadequate response to conventional therapy.

Crohn's disease

Humira is indicated for treatment of severe, active Crohn's disease, in patients who have not responded despite a full and adequate course of therapy with a corticosteroid and/or an immunosuppressant; or who are intolerant to or have medical contraindications for such therapies.

For induction treatment, Humira should be given in combination with corticosteroids. Humira can be given as monotherapy in case of intolerance to corticosteroids or when continued treatment with corticosteroids is inappropriate (see section 4.2).

Psoriasis

Humira is indicated for the treatment of moderate to severe chronic plaque psoriasis in adult patients who failed to respond to or who have a contraindication to, or are intolerant to other systemic therapy including cyclosporine, methotrexate or PUVA.

4.2 Posology and method of administration

Humira treatment should be initiated and supervised by specialist physicians experienced in the diagnosis and treatment of rheumatoid arthritis, polyarticular juvenile idiopathic arthritis, psoriatic arthritis, ankylosing spondylitis, Crohn's disease or psoriasis. Patients treated with Humira should be given the special alert card.

After proper training in injection technique, patients may self-inject with Humira if their physician determines that it is appropriate and with medical follow-up as necessary.

During treatment with Humira, other concomitant therapies (e.g., corticosteroids and/or immunomodulatory agents) should be optimised.

Adults

Rheumatoid arthritis

The recommended dose of Humira for adult patients with rheumatoid arthritis is 40 mg adalimumab administered every other week as a single dose via subcutaneous injection. Methotrexate should be continued during treatment with Humira.

Glucocorticoids, salicylates, nonsteroidal anti-inflammatory drugs, or analgesics can be continued during treatment with Humira. Regarding combination with disease modifying anti-rheumatic drugs other than methotrexate see sections 4.4 and 5.1.

In monotherapy, some patients who experience a decrease in their response may benefit from an increase in dose intensity to 40 mg adalimumab every week.

Dose Interruption

There may be a need for dose interruption, for instance before surgery or if a serious infection occurs. Available data suggest that re-introduction of Humira after discontinuation for 70 days or longer resulted in the same magnitudes of clinical response and similar safety profile as before dose interruption.

Psoriatic arthritis and ankylosing spondylitis

The recommended dose of Humira for patients with psoriatic arthritis or ankylosing spondylitis is 40 mg adalimumab administered every other week as a single dose via subcutaneous injection.

For all of the above indications, available data suggest that the clinical response is usually achieved within 12 weeks of treatment. Continued therapy should be carefully reconsidered in a patient not responding within this time period.

Crohn's disease

The recommended Humira induction dose regimen for adult patients with severe Crohn's disease is 80 mg at Week 0 followed by 40 mg at Week 2. In case there is a need for a more rapid response to therapy, the regimen 160 mg at Week 0 (dose can be administered as four injections in one day or as two injections per day for two consecutive days), 80 mg at Week 2, can be used with the awareness that the risk for adverse events is higher during induction.

After induction treatment, the recommended dose is 40 mg every other week via subcutaneous injection. Alternatively, if a patient has stopped Humira and signs and symptoms of disease recur, Humira may be re-administered. There is little experience from re-administration after more than 8 weeks since the previous dose.

During maintenance treatment, corticosteroids may be tapered in accordance with clinical practice guidelines.

Some patients who experience decrease in their response may benefit from an increase in dose intensity to 40 mg Humira every week.

Some patients who have not responded by Week 4 may benefit from continued maintenance therapy through Week 12. Continued therapy should be carefully reconsidered in a patient not responding within this time period.

Psoriasis

The recommended dose of Humira for adult patients is an initial dose of 80 mg administered subcutaneously, followed by 40 mg subcutaneously given every other week starting one week after the initial dose.

Continued therapy beyond 16 weeks should be carefully reconsidered in a patient not responding within this time period.

Elderly patients

No dose adjustment is required.

Children and adolescents (aged 13 to 17 years) Polyarticular Juvenile Idiopathic Arthritis

The recommended dose of Humira for patients with polyarticular juvenile idiopathic arthritis, aged 13 years and above is 40 mg adalimumab administered every other week as a single dose via subcutaneous injection.

Available data suggest that clinical response is usually achieved within 12 weeks of treatment. Continued therapy should be carefully reconsidered in a patient not responding within this time period.

Impaired renal and/or hepatic function

Humira has not been studied in these patient populations. No dose recommendations can be made.

4.3 Contraindications

Hypersensitivity to the active substance or to any of the excipients.

Active tuberculosis or other severe infections such as sepsis, and opportunistic infections (see section 4.4).

Moderate to severe heart failure (NYHA class III/IV) (see section 4.4).

4.4 Special warnings and precautions for use

Infections

Patients taking TNF-blockers are more susceptible to serious infections.

Patients must therefore be monitored closely for infections, including tuberculosis, before, during and after treatment with Humira. Because the elimination of adalimumab may take up to five months, monitoring should be continued throughout this period.

Treatment with Humira should not be initiated in patients with active infections including chronic or localized infections until infections are controlled. In patients who have been exposed to tuberculosis and patients who have travelled in areas of high risk of tuberculosis or endemic mycoses, such as histoplasmosis, coccidioidomycosis, or blastomycosis, the risk and benefits of treatment with Humira should be considered prior to initiating therapy (see *Opportunistic infections*).

Patients who develop a new infection while undergoing treatment with Humira should be monitored closely and undergo a complete diagnostic evaluation. Administration of Humira should be discontinued if a patient develops a new serious infection or sepsis, and appropriate antimicrobial or antifungal therapy should be initiated until the infectionis controlled. Physicians should exercise caution when considering the use of Humira in patients with a history of recurring infection or with underlying conditions which may predispose patients to infections, including the use of concomitant immunosuppressive medications.

Serious infections:

Serious infections, including sepsis, due to bacterial, mycobacterial, invasive fungal, parasitic, viral, or other opportunistic infections such as listeriosis, and pneumocystis have been reported in patients receiving Humira.

Other serious infections seen in clinical trials include pneumonia, pyelonephritis, septic arthritis and septicaemia. Hospitalisation or fatal outcomes associated with infections have been reported.

Tuberculosis:

There have been reports of tuberculosis in patients receiving Humira. It should be noted that in the majority of those reports, tuberculosis was extra-pulmonary, i.e. disseminated.

Before initiation of therapy with Humira, all patients must be evaluated for both, active or inactive (latent) tuberculosis infection. This evaluation should include a detailed medical history of patients with a personal history of tuberculosis or possible previous exposure to patients with active tuberculosis and previous and/or current immunosuppressive therapy. Appropriate screening tests, i.e. tuberculin skin test and chest X-ray, should be performed in all patients (local recommendations may apply). It is recommended that the conduct of these tests should be recorded in the patient alert card. Prescribers are reminded of the risk of false negative tuberculin skin test results, especially in patients who are severely ill or immunocompromised.

If active tuberculosis is diagnosed, Humira therapy must not be initiated (see section 4.3).

If latent tuberculosis is suspected, a physician with expertise in the treatment of tuberculosis should be consulted. In all situations described below, the benefit/risk balance of therapy should be very carefully considered.

If inactive ('latent') tuberculosis is diagnosed, appropriate treatment for latent tuberculosis must be started with anti-tuberculosis prophylaxis therapy before the initiation of Humira, and in accordance with local recommendations.

In patients who have several or significant risk factors for tuberculosis and have a negative test for latent tuberculosis, anti-tuberculosis therapy should also be considered before the initiation of Humira.

Use of anti-tuberculosis therapy should also be considered before the initiation of Humira in patients with a past history of latent or active tuberculosis in whom an adequate course of treatment cannot be confirmed. Some patients who have previously received treatment for latent or active tuberculosis have developed active tuberculosis while being treated with Humira.

Patients should be instructed to seek medical advice if signs/symptoms (e.g., persistent cough, wasting/weight loss, low grade fever) suggestive of a tuberculosis infection occur during or after therapy with Humira.

Other opportunistic infections:

Opportunistic infections, including invasive fungal infections have been observed in patients receiving Humira. These infections have not consistently been recognised in patients taking TNF-blockers and this resulted in delays in appropriate treatment, sometimes resulting in fatal outcomes.

For patients who develop the signs and symptoms such as fever, malaise, weight loss, sweats, cough, dyspnea, and/or pulmonary infiltrates or other serious systemic illness with or without concomitant shock an invasive fungal infection should be suspected and administration of Humira should be promptly discontinued and appropriate antifungal therapy should be initiated.

Hepatitis B Reactivation

Reactivation of hepatitis B has occurred in patients who are chronic carriers of this virus when receiving a TNF-antagonist including Humira. Some cases have had a fatal outcome. Patients at risk for HBV infection should be evaluated for prior evidence of HBV infection before initiating Humira therapy. Carriers of HBV who require treatment with Humira should be closely monitored for signs and symptoms of active HBV infection throughout therapy and for several months following termination of therapy. Adequate data from the treatment of patients who are carriers of HBV with anti-viral therapy in conjunction with TNF-antagonist therapy to prevent HBV reactivation are not available. In patients who develop HBV reactivation, Humira should be stopped and effective anti-viral therapy with appropriate supportive treatment should be initiated.

Neurological events

TNF-antagonists including Humira have been associated in rare instances with new onset or exacerbation of clinical symptoms and/or radiographic evidence of demyelinating disease including multiple sclerosis. Prescribers should exercise caution in considering the use of Humira in patients with pre-existing or recent-onset central nervous system demyelinating disorders.

Allergic reactions

Serious allergic adverse reactions have not been reported with subcutaneous administration of Humira during clinical trials. Non-serious allergic reactions associated with Humira were uncommon during clinical trials. In postmarketing, serious allergic reactions including anaphylaxis have been reported very rarely following Humira administration. If an anaphylactic reaction or other serious allergic reaction occurs, administration of Humira should be discontinued immediately and appropriate therapy initiated.

The needle cover of the syringe contains natural rubber (latex). This may cause severe allergic reactions in patients sensitive to latex.

Immunosuppression

In a study of 64 patients with rheumatoid arthritis that were treated with Humira, there was no evidence of depression of delayed-type hypersensitivity, depression of immunoglobulin levels, or change in enumeration of effector T-, B-, NK-cells, monocyte/macrophages, and neutrophils.

Malignancies and lymphoproliferative disorders

In the controlled portions of clinical trials of TNF-antagonists, more cases of malignancies including lymphoma have been observed among patients receiving a TNF-antagonist compared with control patients. However, the occurrence was rare. Furthermore, there is an increased background lymphoma risk in rheumatoid arthritis patients with long-standing, highly active, inflammatory disease, which complicates the risk estimation. With the current knowledge, a possible risk for the development of lymphomas or other malignancies in patients treated with a TNF-antagonist cannot be excluded.

Rare postmarketing cases of hepatosplenic T-cell lymphoma have been identified in patients treated with adalimumab. This rare type of T-cell lymphoma has a very aggressive disease course and is usually fatal. Some of these hepatosplenic T-cell lymphomas with Humira have occurred in young adult patients on concomitant treatment with azathioprine or 6-mercaptopurine used for Crohn's disease. A risk for the development of hepatosplenic T-cell lymphoma in patients treated with Humira cannot be excluded (see section 4.8).

No studies have been conducted that include patients with a history of malignancy or in whom treatment with Humira is continued following development of malignancy. Thus additional caution should be exercised in considering Humira treatment of these patients (see section 4.8).

All patients, and in particular patients with a medical history of extensive immunosuppressant therapy or psoriasis patients with a history of PUVA treatment should be examined for the presence of non-melanoma skin cancer prior to and during treatment with Humira.

In an exploratory clinical trial evaluating the use of another anti-TNF agent, infliximab, in patients with moderate to severe chronic obstructive pulmonary disease (COPD), more malignancies, mostly in the lung or head and neck, were reported in infliximab-treated patients compared with control patients. All patients had a history of heavy smoking. Therefore, caution should be exercised when using any TNF-antagonist in COPD patients, as well as in patients with increased risk for malignancy due to heavy smoking.

Haematologic reactions

Rare reports of pancytopenia including aplastic anaemia have been reported with TNF antagonists. Adverse events of the haematologic system, including medically significant cytopoenia (e.g. thrombocytopaenia, leucopaenia) have been infrequently reported with Humira. All patients should be advised to seek immediate medical attention if they develop signs and symptoms suggestive of blood dyscrasias (e.g. persistent fever, bruising, bleeding, pallor) while on Humira. Discontinuation of Humira therapy should be considered in patients with confirmed significant haematologic abnormalities.

Vaccinations

Similar antibody responses to the standard 23-valent pneumococcal vaccine and the influenza trivalent virus vaccination were observed in a study in 226 adult subjects with rheumatoid arthritis who were treated with adalimumab or placebo. No data are available on the secondary transmission of infection by live vaccines in patients receiving Humira.

It is recommended that polyarticular juvenile idiopathic arthritis patients, if possible, be brought up to date with all immunisations in agreement with current immunisation guidelines prior to initiating Humira therapy.

Patients on Humira may receive concurrent vaccinations, except for live vaccines.

Congestive heart failure

In a clinical trial with another TNF-antagonist worsening congestive heart failure and increased mortality due to congestive heart failure have been observed. Cases of worsening congestive heart failure have also been reported in patients receiving Humira. Humira should be used with caution in patients with mild heart failure (NYHA class I/II). Humira is contraindicated in moderate to severe heart failure (see section 4.3). Treatment with Humira must be discontinued in patients who develop new or worsening symptoms of congestive heart failure.

Autoimmune processes

Treatment with Humira may result in the formation of autoimmune antibodies. The impact of long-term treatment with Humira on the development of autoimmune diseases is unknown. If a patient develops symptoms suggestive of a lupus-like syndrome following treatment with Humira and is positive for antibodies against double-stranded DNA, further treatment with Humira should not be given (see section 4.8).

Concurrent administration of TNF-antagonists and anakinra

Serious infections were seen in clinical studies with concurrent use of anakinra and another TNF-antagonist, etanercept, with no added clinical benefit compared to etanercept alone. Because of the nature of the adverse events seen with the combination of etanercept and anakinra therapy, similar toxicities may also result from the combination of anakinra and other TNF-antagonists. Therefore, the combination of adalimumab and anakinra is not recommended. (See section 4.5).

Concurrent administration of TNF-antagonists and abatacept

Concurrent administration of TNF-antagonists and abatacept has been associated with an increased risk of infections including serious infections compared to TNF-antagonists alone, without increased clinical benefit. The combination of Humira and abatacept is not recommended. (See section 4.5).

Surgery

There is limited safety experience of surgical procedures in patients treated with Humira. The long half-life of adalimumab should be taken into consideration if a surgical procedure is planned. A patient who requires surgery while on Humira should be closely monitored for infections, and appropriate actions should be taken. There is limited safety experience in patients undergoing arthroplasty while receiving Humira.

Small bowel obstruction

Failure to respond to treatment for Crohn's disease may indicate the presence of fixed fibrotic stricture that may require surgical treatment. Available data suggest that Humira does not worsen or cause strictures.

4.5 Interaction with other medicinal products and other forms of interaction

Humira has been studied in rheumatoid arthritis, polyarticular juvenile idiopathic arthritis and psoriatic arthritis patients taking Humira as monotherapy and those taking concomitant methotrexate. Antibody formation was lower when Humira was given together with methotrexate in comparison with use as monotherapy. Administration of Humira without methotrexate resulted in increased formation of antibodies, increased clearance and reduced efficacy of adalimumab (see section 5.1).

The combination of Humira and anakinra is not recommended (see section 4.4 "Concurrent administration of TNF-antagonists and anakinra").

The combination of Humira and abatacept is not recommended (see section 4.4 "Concurrent administration of TNF-antagonists and abatacept").

4.6 Pregnancy and lactation

For Humira, no clinical data on exposed pregnancies are available

In a developmental toxicity study conducted in monkeys, there was no indication of maternal toxicity, embryotoxicity or teratogenicity. Preclinical data on postnatal toxicity and fertility effects of adalimumab are not available (see section 5.3).

Due to its inhibition of TNFα, adalimumab administered during pregnancy could affect normal immune responses in the newborn. Administration of adalimumab is not recommended during pregnancy. Women of childbearing potential are strongly recommended to use adequate contraception to prevent pregnancy and continue its use for at least five months after the last Humira treatment.

It is not known whether adalimumab is excreted in human milk or absorbed systemically after ingestion.

However, because human immunoglobulins are excreted in milk, women must not breast-feed for at least five months after the last Humira treatment.

4.7 Effects on ability to drive and use machines

Humira may have a minor influence on the ability to drive and use machines. Dizziness (including vertigo, vision disorder and fatigue) may occur following administration of Humira (see Section 4.8).

4.8 Undesirable effects

Clinical Trials

Humira was studied in 6,593 patients in controlled and open label trials for up to 60 months. These trials included rheumatoid arthritis patients with short term and long standing disease, polyarticular juvenile idiopathic arthritis as well as psoriatic arthritis, ankylosing spondylitis, Crohn's disease and psoriasis patients. The data in Table 1 is based on the pivotal controlled Studies involving 4,355 patients receiving Humira and 2,487 patients receiving placebo or active comparator during the controlled period.

The proportion of patients who discontinued treatment due to adverse events during the double-blind, controlled portion of pivotal studies was 4.5% for patients taking Humira and 4.5% for control treated patients.

Undesirable effects in paediatric patients with polyarticular juvenile idiopathic arthritis

In general, the adverse events in paediatric patients were similar in frequency and type to those seen in adult patients.

Adverse events at least possibly causally-related to adalimumab, for clinical studies both clinical and laboratory, are displayed by system organ class and frequency (very common $\geqslant$ 1/10; common $\geqslant$ 1/100 to < 1/10; uncommon $\geqslant$ 1/1,000 to < 1/100, rare $\geqslant$ 1/10,000 to < 1/1,000 and very rare < 1/10,000) in Table 1 below. Within each frequency grouping, undesirable effects are presented in order of decreasing seriousness. The highest frequency seen among the various indications has been included. An asterisk (*) appears in the SOC column if further information is found elsewhere in sections 4.3, 4.4 and 4.8.

Approximately 15% of patients can be expected to experience injection site reactions, based on the most common adverse event with adalimumab in controlled clinical studies.

Table 1

Undesirable Effects in Clinical Studies

(see Table 1 on next page)

Injection site reactions

In the pivotal controlled trials, 15% of patients treated with Humira developed injection site reactions (erythema and/or itching, haemorrhage, pain or swelling), compared to 9% of patients receiving placebo or active control. Injection site reactions generally did not necessitate discontinuation of the medicinal product.

Infections

In the pivotal controlled trials, the rate of infection was 1.58 per patient year in the Humira treated patients and 1.42 per patient year in the placebo and active control-treated patients. The infections consisted primarily nasopharyngitis, upper respiratory tract infection, and sinusitis. Most patients continued on Humira after the infection resolved.

The incidence of serious infections was 0.04 per patient year in Humira treated patients and 0.03 per patient year in placebo and active control – treated patients.

In controlled and open label studies with Humira, serious infections (including fatal infections, which occurred rarely) have been reported, which include reports of tuberculosis (including miliary and extra-pulmonary locations) and invasive opportunistic infections (e.g. disseminated or extrapulmonary histoplasmosis, blastomycosis, coccidioidomycosis, pneumocystis candidiasis, aspergillosis and listeriosis). Most of the cases of tuberculosis occurred within the first eight months after initiation of therapy and may reflect recrudescence of latent disease.

Malignancies and lymphoproliferative disorders

No malignancies were observed in 171 patients with an exposure of 192.5 patient years during a Humira trial in juvenile idiopathic arthritis patients.

During the controlled portions of pivotal Humira trials at least 12 weeks in duration in patients with moderately to severely active rheumatoid arthritis, psoriatic arthritis, ankylosing spondylitis, Crohn's disease or psoriasis, malignancies, other than lymphoma and non-melanoma skin cancer, were observed at a rate (95% confidence interval) of 5.9 (3.5, 9.9) per 1,000 patient-years among 3,853 Humira treated patients *versus* a rate of 4.3 (1.8, 10.4) per 1,000 patient-years among 2,183 control patients (median duration of treatment was 5.5 months for Humira and 3.9 months for control-treated patients). The rate (95% confidence interval) of non-melanoma skin cancers was 8.8 (5.7, 13.5) per 1,000 patient-years among Humira-treated patients and 2.6 (0.8, 8.0) per 1,000 patient-years among control patients. Of these skin cancers, squamous cell carcinomas occurred at rates (95% confidence interval) of 2.5 (1.1, 5.6) per 1,000 patient-years among Humira-treated patients and 0.9 (0.1, 6.1) per 1,000 patient-years among control patients. The rate (95% confidence interval) of lymphomas was 0.8 (0.2, 3.3) per 1,000 patient-years among Humira-treated patients and 0.9 (0.1, 6.1) per 1,000 patient-years among control patients.

When combining controlled portions of these trials and ongoing open label extension studies with a median duration of approximately 2.7 years including 4,767 patients and over 15,332 patient-years of therapy, the observed rate of malignancies, other than lymphoma and non-melanoma skin cancers is approximately 8.3 per 1,000 patient years. The observed rate of non-melanoma skin cancers is approximately 9.3 per 1,000 patient years, and the observed rate of lymphomas is approximately 1.2 per 1,000 patient years.

In post-marketing experience from January 2003, predominately in patients with rheumatoid arthritis, the reported rate of malignancies other than lymphomas and non-melanoma skin cancers is approximately 1.7 per 1,000 patient years. The reported rates for non-melanoma skin cancers and lymphomas are approximately 0.2 and 0.4 per 1,000 patient years, respectively (see section 4.4).

Rare post-marketing cases of hepatosplenic T-cell lymphoma have been reported in patients treated with adalimumab (see section 4.4).

Autoantibodies

Patients had serum samples tested for autoantibodies at multiple time points in rheumatoid arthritis Studies I – V. In these trials, 11.9% of patients treated with Humira and 8.1% of placebo and active control – treated patients that had negative baseline anti-nuclear antibody titres reported positive titres at Week 24. Two patients out of 3,441 treated with Humira in all rheumatoid arthritis and psoriatic arthritis studies developed clinical signs suggestive of new-onset lupus-like syndrome. The patients improved following discontinuation of therapy. No patients developed lupus nephritis or central nervous system symptoms.

Liver Enzyme Elevations

Rheumatoid arthritis clinical trials: in controlled rheumatoid arthritis clinical trials (RAstudies I – IV), elevations of ALT were similar in patients receiving adalimumab or placebo. In patients with early rheumatoid arthritis (disease duration of less than 3 years) (RAstudy V), elevations of ALT were more common in the combination arm (Humira /methotrexate) compared to the methotrexate monotherapy arm or the Humira monotherapy arm. In the JIA trial the few transaminase elevations were small and similar in the placebo and adalimumab exposed patients, and mostly occurred in combination with methotrexate.

Psoriatic arthritis clinical trials: elevations in ALT were more common in psoriatic arthritis patients (PsA studies I - II) compared with patients in rheumatoid arthritis clinical studies.

In all rheumatoid arthritis, polyarticular juvenile idiopathic arthritis and psoriatic arthritis studies, patients with raised ALT were asymptomatic and in most cases elevations were transient and resolved on continued treatment.

Crohn's disease clinical trials: in controlled clinical trials, elevations of ALT were similar in patients receiving adalimumab or placebo.

Psoriasis clinical trials: in controlled psoriasis clinical trials, elevations of ALT were similar in patients receiving adalimumab or placebo.

Additional Adverse Reactions from Postmarketing Surveillance or Phase IV Clinical Trials

The additional adverse reactions in Table 2 have been reported from postmarketing surveillance or Phase IV clinical trials:

Table 2

Undesirable Effects in Postmarketing Surveillance and Phase IV Clinical Studies

System Organ Class	Adverse Reaction
Neoplasm benign, malignant and unspecified (including cysts and polyps)*	hepatosplenic T-cell lymphoma
Immune system disorders*	anaphylaxis
Nervous system disorders*	demyelinating disorders (e.g. optic neuritis, Guillain-Barré syndrome); cerebrovascular accident
Gastrointestinal disorders*	intestinal perforation
Hepatobiliary disorders*	reactivation of hepatitis B
Skin and subcutaneous tissue disorders	cutaneous vasculitis, Stevens-Johnson syndrome, angioedema, new onset or worsening of psoriasis (including palmoplantar pustular psoriasis)
Musculoskeletal and connective tissue disorders	lupus-like syndrome
Cardiac disorders	myocardial infarction

* further information is found elsewhere in sections 4.3, 4.4 and 4.8

4.9 Overdose

No dose-limiting toxicity was observed during clinical trials. The highest dose level evaluated has been multiple intravenous doses of 10 mg/kg, which is approximately 15 times the recommended dose.

5. PHARMACOLOGICAL PROPERTIES

5.1 Pharmacodynamic properties

Pharmacotherapeutic group: Selective immunosuppressive agents. ATC code: L04AB04

Mechanism of action

Adalimumab binds specifically to TNF and neutralizes the biological function of TNF by blocking its interaction with the p55 and p75 cell surface TNF receptors.

Adalimumab also modulates biological responses that are induced or regulated by TNF, including changes in the levels of adhesion molecules responsible for leukocyte migration (ELAM-1, VCAM-1, and ICAM-1 with an IC_{50} of0.1-0.2 nM).

Pharmacodynamic effects

After treatment with Humira, a rapid decrease in levels of acute phase reactants of inflammation (C-reactive protein (CRP) and erythrocyte sedimentation rate (ESR)) and serum cytokines (IL-6) was observed compared to baseline in patients with rheumatoid arthritis. Serum levels of matrix metalloproteinases (MMP-1 and MMP-3) that produce tissue remodelling responsible for cartilage destruction were also decreased after Humira administration. Patients treated with Humira usually experienced improvement in haematological signs of chronic inflammation.

A rapid decrease in CRP levels was also observed in patients with Crohn's disease.

A rapid decrease in CRP levels was also observed in patients with polyarticular juvenile idiopathic arthritis.

Clinical trials

Rheumatoid arthritis

Humira was evaluated in over 3000 patients in all rheumatoid arthritis clinical trials. Some patients were treated for up to 60 months duration. The efficacy and safety of Humira for the treatment of rheumatoid arthritis were assessed in five randomised, double-blind and well-controlled studies.

RA study I evaluated 271 patients with moderately to severely active rheumatoid arthritis who were $\geqslant$ 18 years old, had failed therapy with at least one disease-modifying, anti rheumatic drug and had insufficient efficacy with methotrexate at doses of 12.5 to 25 mg (10 mg if methotrexate-intolerant) every week and whose methotrexate dose remained constant at 10 to 25 mg every week. Doses of 20, 40 or 80 mg of Humira or placebo were given every other week for 24 weeks.

Table 1 Undesirable Effects in Clinical Studies

System Organ Class	Frequency	Adverse Reaction
Infections and infestations*	Very common	respiratory tract infections (including lower and upper respiratory tract infection, pneumonia, sinusitis, pharyngitis, nasopharyngitis and pneumonia herpes viral)
	Common	systemic infections (including sepsis, candidiasis and influenza), intestinal infections (including gastroenteritis viral), skin and soft tissue infections (including paronychia, cellulitis, impetigo, necrotising fasciitis and herpes zoster), ear infections, oral infections (including herpes simplex, oral herpes and tooth infections), reproductive tract infections (including vulvovaginal mycotic infection), urinary tract infections (including pyelonephritis), fungal infections
	Uncommon	opportunistic infections and tuberculosis (including coccidioidomycosis, histoplasmosis and mycobacterium avum complex infection), neurological infections (including viral meningitis), eye infections, bacterial infections, joint infections
Neoplasms benign, malignant and unspecified (including cysts and polyps)*	Common	benign neoplasm, skin cancer excluding melanoma (including basal cell carcinoma and squamous cell carcinoma)
	Uncommon	lymphoma**, solid organ neoplasm (including breast cancer, lung neoplasm and thyroid neoplasm), melanoma**
Blood and the lymphatic system disorders*	Very common	leucopaenia (including neutropaenia and agranulocytosis), anaemia
	Common	thrombocytopaenia, leucocytosis
	Uncommon	idiopathic thrombocytopaenic purpura
	Rare	pancytopaenia
Immune system disorders*	Common	hypersensitivity, allergies (including seasonal allergy)
Metabolism and nutrition disorders	Very common	lipids increased
	Common	hypokalaemia, uric acid increased, blood sodium abnormal, hypocalcaemia, hyperglycemia, hypophosphotemia, blood potassium increased
	Uncommon	dehydration
Psychiatric disorders	Common	mood alterations (including depression), anxiety, insomnia
Nervous system disorders*	Very common	headache
	Common	paraesthesias (including hypoasthesia), migraine, sciatica
	Uncommon	tremor
	Rare	multiple sclerosis
Eye disorders	Common	visual impairment, conjunctivitis
	Uncommon	blepharitis, eye swelling, diplopia
Ear and labyrinth disorders	Common	vertigo
	Uncommon	deafness, tinnitus
Cardiac disorders*	Common	tachycardia
	Uncommon	arrhythmia, congestive heart failure
	Rare	cardiac arrest
Vascular disorders	Common	hypertension, flushing, haematoma
	Rare	vascular arterial occlusion, thrombophlebitis, aortic aneurysm
Respiratory, thoracic and mediastinal disorders*	Common	cough, asthma, dyspnoea
	Uncommon	chronic obstructive pulmonary disease, interstitial lung disease, pneumonitis
Gastrointestinal disorders	Very common	abdominal pain, nausea and vomiting
	Common	GI haemorrhage, dyspepsia, gastroesophageal reflux disease, sicca syndrome
	Uncommon	pancreatitis, dysphagia, face oedema
Hepato-biliary disorders*	Very Common	Elevated liver enzymes
	Uncommon	cholecystitis and cholelithiasis, bilirubin increased, hepatic steatosis
Skin and subcutaneous tissue disorders	Very Common	rash (including exfoliative rash),
	Common	pruritus, urticaria, bruising (including purpura), dermatitis (including eczema), onychoclasis, hyperhydrosis
	Uncommon	night sweats, scar
Musculoskeletal, connective tissue and bone disorders	Very common	musculoskeletal pain
	Common	muscle spasms (including blood creatine phosphokinase increased)
	Uncommon	rhabdomyolysis
	Rare	systemic lupus erythematosus
Renal and urinary disorders	Common	haematuria, renal impairment
	Uncommon	nocturia
Reproductive system and breast disorders	Uncommon	erectile dysfunction
General disorders and administration site conditions*	Very Common	injection site reaction (including injection site erythema)
	Common	chest pain, oedema
	Uncommon	inflammation
Investigations	Common	coagulation and bleeding disorders (including activated partial thromboplastin time prolonged), autoantibody test positive (including double stranded DNA antibody), blood lactate dehydrogenase increased
Injury and poisoning*	Common	impaired healing

* further information is found elsewhere in sections 4.3, 4.4 and 4.8

** including open label extension studies

Table 3 ACR Responses in Placebo-Controlled Trials (Percent of Patients)

Response	RA Study I[a**]		RA Study II[a**]		RA Study III[a**]	
	Placebo/ MTX[c] n=60	Humira[b]/ MTX[c] n=63	Placebo n=110	Humira[b] n=113	Placebo/ MTX[c] n=200	Humira[b]/ MTX[c] n=207
ACR 20						
6 months	13.3%	65.1%	19.1%	46.0%	29.5%	63.3%
12 months	NA	NA	NA	NA	24.0%	58.9%
ACR 50						
6 months	6.7%	52.4%	8.2%	22.1%	9.5%	39.1%
12 months	NA	NA	NA	NA	9.5%	41.5%
ACR 70						
6 months	3.3%	23.8%	1.8%	12.4%	2.5%	20.8%
12 months	NA	NA	NA	NA	4.5%	23.2%

[a] RA study I at 24 weeks, RA study II at 26 weeks, and RA study III at 24 and 52 weeks

[b] 40 mg Humira administered every other week

[c] MTX = methotrexate

**p < 0.01, Humira *versus* placebo

RA study II evaluated 544 patients with moderately to severely active rheumatoid arthritis who were ≥ 18 years old and had failed therapy with at least one disease-modifying, anti-rheumatic drugs. Doses of 20 or 40 mg of Humira were given by subcutaneous injection every other week with placebo on alternative weeks or every week for 26 weeks; placebo was given every week for the same duration. No other disease-modifying anti-rheumatic drugs were allowed.

RA study III evaluated 619 patients with moderately to severely active rheumatoid arthritis who were ≥ 18 years old, and who had an ineffective response to methotrexate at doses of 12.5 to 25 mg or have been intolerant to 10 mg of methotrexate every week. There were three groups in this study. The first received placebo injections every week for 52 weeks. The second received 20 mg of Humira every week for 52 weeks. The third group received 40 mg of Humira every other week with placebo injections on alternate weeks. Thereafter, patients enrolled in an open-label extension phase in which 40 mg of Humira was administered every other week up to 60 months.

RA study IV primarily assessed safety in 636 patients with moderately to severely active rheumatoid arthritis who were ≥ 18 years old. Patients were permitted to be either disease-modifying, anti-rheumatic drug-naïve or to remain on their pre-existing rheumatologic therapy provided that therapy was stable for a minimum of 28 days. These therapies include methotrexate, leflunomide, hydroxychloroquine, sulfasalazine and/or gold salts. Patients were randomised to 40 mg of Humira or placebo every other week for 24 weeks.

RA study V evaluated 799 methotrexate-naïve, adult patients with moderate to severely active early rheumatoid arthritis (mean disease duration less than 9 months). This study evaluated the efficacy of Humira 40 mg every other week/methotrexate combination therapy, Humira 40 mg every other week monotherapy and methotrexate monotherapy in reducing the signs and symptoms and rate of progression of joint damage in rheumatoid arthritis for 104 weeks.

The primary end point in RA studies I, II and III and the secondary endpoint in RA study IV was the percent of patients who achieved an ACR 20 response at Week 24 or 26. The primary endpoint in RA study V was the percent of patients who achieved an ACR 50 response at Week 52. RA studies III and V had an additional primary endpoint at 52 weeks of retardation of disease progression (as detected by X-ray results). RA study III also had a primary endpoint of changes in quality of life.

ACR response

The percent of Humira-treated patients achieving ACR 20, 50 and 70 responses was consistent across RA studies I, II and III. The results for the 40 mg every other week dose are summarised in Table 3.

(see Table 3 above)

In RA studies I-IV, all individual components of the ACR response criteria (number of tender and swollen joints, physician and patient assessment of disease activity and pain, disability index (HAQ) scores and CRP (mg/dl) values) improved at 24 or 26 weeks compared to placebo. In RA study III, these improvements were maintained throughout 52 weeks. In addition, ACR response rates were maintained in the majority of patients followed in the open-label extension phase to Week 104. There were 114 out of 207 patients who continued on Humira 40 mg every other week for 60 months. Among those, 86, 72, and 41 patients had ACR 20/50/70 response, respectively at Month 60.

In RA study IV, the ACR 20 response of patients treated with Humira plus standard of care was statistically significantly better than patients treated with placebo plus standard of care ($p < 0.001$).

In RA studies I-IV, Humira-treated patients achieved statistically significant ACR 20 and 50 responses compared to placebo as early as one to two weeks after initiation of treatment.

In RA study V with early rheumatoid arthritis patients who were methotrexate naïve, combination therapy with Humira and methotrexate led to faster and significantly greater ACR responses than methotrexate monotherapy and Humira monotherapy at Week 52 and responses were sustained at Week 104 (see Table 4).

(see Table 4 below)

At Week 52, 42.9% of patients who received Humira/methotrexate combination therapy achieved clinical remission (DAS28 < 2.6) compared to 20.6% of patients receiving methotrexate monotherapy and 23.4% of patients receiving Humira monotherapy. Humira/methotrexate combination therapy was clinically and statistically superior to methotrexate ($p < 0.001$) and Humira monotherapy ($p < 0.001$) in achieving a low disease state in patients with recently diagnosed moderate to severe rheumatoid arthritis. The response for the two monotherapy arms was similar (p = 0.447).

Radiographic response

In RA study III, where Humira treated patients had a mean duration of rheumatoid arthritis of approximately 11 years, structural joint damage was assessed radiographically and expressed as change in modified Total Sharp Score (TSS) and its components, the erosion score and joint space narrowing score. Humira/methotrexate patients demonstrated significantly less radiographic progression than patients receiving methotrexate alone at 6 and 12 months (see Table 5). Data from the open-label extension phase indicate that the reduction in rate of progression of structural damage is maintained for 60 months in a subset of patients. 113/207 of patients originally treated with 40 mg Humira every other week were evaluated radiographically at 5 years. Among those, 66 patients showed no progression of structural damage defined by a change in the TSS of zero or less.

(see Table 5 below)

In RA study V, structural joint damage was assessed radiographically and expressed as change in modified Total Sharp Score (see Table 6).

(see Table 6 on next page)

Following 52 weeks and 104 weeks of treatment, the percentage of patients without progression (change from baseline in modified Total Sharp Score ≤ 0.5) was significantly higher with Humira/methotrexate combination therapy (63.8% and 61.2% respectively) compared to methotrexate monotherapy (37.4% and 33.5% respectively, $p < 0.001$) and Humira monotherapy (50.7%, $p < 0.002$ and 44.5%, $p < 0.001$ respectively).

Quality of life and physical function

Health-related quality of life and physical function was assessed using the disability index of the Health Assessment Questionnaire (HAQ) in the four original adequate and well-controlled trials, which was a pre-specified primary endpoint at Week 52 in RA study III. All doses/schedules of Humira in all four studies showed statistically significantly greater improvement in the disability index of the HAQ from baseline to Month 6 compared to placebo and in RA study III the same was seen at Week 52. Results from the Short Form Health Survey (SF 36) for all doses/schedules of Humira in all four studies support these findings, with statistically significant physical component summary (PCS) scores, as well as statistically significant pain and vitality domain scores for the 40 mg every other week dose. A statistically significant decrease in fatigue as measured by functional assessment of chronic illness therapy (FACIT) scores was seen in all three studies in which it was assessed (RA studies I, III, IV).

In RA study III, improvement in physical function was maintained through Week 260 (60 months) of open-label

Table 4 ACR Responses in RA Study V (percent of patients)

Response	MTX n=257	Humira n=274	Humira/MTX n=268	p-value[a]	p-value[b]	p-value[c]
ACR 20						
Week 52	62.6%	54.4%	72.8%	0.013	< 0.001	0.043
Week 104	56.0%	49.3%	69.4%	0.002	< 0.001	0.140
ACR 50						
Week 52	45.9%	41.2%	61.6%	< 0.001	< 0.001	0.317
Week 104	42.8%	36.9%	59.0%	< 0.001	< 0.001	0.162
ACR 70						
Week 52	27.2%	25.9%	45.5%	< 0.001	< 0.001	0.656
Week 104	28.4%	28.1%	46.6%	< 0.001	< 0.001	0.864

a. p-value is from the pairwise comparison of methotrexate monotherapy and Humira/methotrexate combination therapy using the Mann-Whitney U test.

b. p-value is from the pairwise comparison of Humira monotherapy and Humira/methotrexate combination therapy using the Mann-Whitney U test

c. p-value is from the pairwise comparison of Humira monotherapy and methotrexate monotherapy using the Mann-Whitney U test

Table 5 Radiographic Mean Changes Over 12 Months in RA Study III

	Placebo/MTX[a]	HUMIRA/MTX 40 mg every other week	Placebo/MTX-HUMIRA/MTX (95% Confidence Interval[b])	p-value
Total Sharp Score	2.7	0.1	2.6 (1.4, 3.8)	< 0.001[c]
Erosion score	1.6	0.0	1.6 (0.9, 2.2)	< 0.001
JSN[d] score	1.0	0.1	0.9 (0.3, 1.4)	0.002

[a]methotrexate

[b]95% confidence intervals for the differences in change scores between methotrexate and Humira.

[c]Based on rank analysis

[d]Joint Space Narrowing

Table 6 Radiographic Mean Changes at Week 52 in RA Study V

	MTX n=257 (95% confidence interval)	Humira n=274 (95% confidence interval)	Humira/MTX n=268 (95% confidence interval)	p-value[a]	p-value[b]	p-value[c]
Total Sharp Score	5.7 (4.2-7.3)	3.0 (1.7-4.3)	1.3 (0.5-2.1)	< 0.001	0.0020	< 0.001
Erosion score	3.7 (2.7-4.7)	1.7 (1.0-2.4)	0.8 (0.4-1.2)	< 0.001	0.0082	< 0.001
JSN score	2.0 (1.2-2.8)	1.3 (0.5-2.1)	0.5 (0-1.0)	< 0.001	0.0037	0.151

[a] p-value is from the pairwise comparison of methotrexate monotherapy and Humira/methotrexate combination therapy using the Mann-Whitney U test.

[b] p-value is from the pairwise comparison of Humira monotherapy and Humira/methotrexate combination therapy using the Mann-Whitney U test

[c] p-value is from the pairwise comparison of Humira monotherapy and methotrexate monotherapy using the Mann-Whitney U test

Table 8 Ped ACR Responses in the JIA study

Stratum	MTX		Without MTX	
Phase				
OL-LI 16 weeks				
Ped ACR 30 response (n/N)	94.1% (80/85)		74.4% (64/86)	
Double Blind	Humira (n = 38)	Placebo (n = 37)	Humira (n = 30)	Placebo (n = 28)
Disease flares at the end of 32 weeks[a] (n/N)	36.8% (14/38)	64.9% (24/37)[b]	43.3% (13/30)	71.4% (20/28)[c]
Median time to disease flare	>32 weeks	20 weeks	>32 weeks	14 weeks

[a] Ped ACR 30/50/70 responses week 48 significantly greater than those of placebo treated patients

[b] p = 0.015

[c] p = 0.031

Table 9 ACR Response in Placebo-Controlled Psoriatic Arthritis Studies (Percent of Patients)

	PsA Study I		PsA Study II	
Response	Placebo N=162	Humira N=151	Placebo N=49	Humira N=51
ACR 20				
Week 12	14%	58%***	16%	39%*
Week 24	15%	57%***	N/A	N/A
ACR 50				
Week 12	4%	36%***	2%	25%***
Week 24	6%	39%***	N/A	N/A
ACR 70				
Week 12	1%	20%***	0%	14% *
Week 24	1%	23%***	N/A	N/A

*** p < 0.001 for all comparisons between Humira and placebo

* p < 0.05 for all comparisons between Humira and placebo

N/A not applicable

treatment. Improvement in quality of life was measured up to Week 156 (36 months) and improvement was maintained through that time.

In RA study V, the improvement in the HAQ disability index and the physical component of the SF 36 showed greater improvement ($p < 0.001$) for Humira/methotrexate combination therapy *versus* methotrexate monotherapy and Humira monotherapy at Week 52, which was maintained through Week 104.

Polyarticular juvenile idiopathic arthritis (JIA)

The safety and efficacy of Humira were assessed in a multicentre, randomised, double-blind, parallel – group study in 171 children (4-17 years old) with polyarticular JIA. In the open-label lead in phase (OL LI) patients were stratified into two groups, MTX (methotrexate)-treated or non-MTX-treated. Patients who were in the non-MTX stratum were either naïve to or had been withdrawn from MTX at least two weeks prior to study drug administration. Patients remained on stable doses of NSAIDs and or prednisone (⩽ 0.2 mg /kg/day or 10 mg/day maximum). In the OL LI phase all patients received 24 mg/m^2 up to a maximum of 40 mg Humira every other week for 16 weeks. The distribution of patients by age and minimum, median and maximum dose received during the OL LI phase is presented in Table 7.

Table 7

Distribution of patients by age and adalimumab dose received during the OL LI phase

Age Group	Number of patients at Baseline n (%)	Minimum, median and maximum dose
4 to 7 years	31 (18.1)	10, 20 and 25 mg
8 to 12 years	71 (41.5)	20, 25 and 40 mg
13 to 17 years	69 (40.4)	25, 40 and 40 mg

Patients demonstrating a Pediatric ACR 30 response at Week 16 were eligible to be randomised into the double blind (DB) phase and received either Humira 24 mg/m^2 up to a maximum of 40 mg, or placebo every other week for an additional 32 weeks or until disease flare. Disease flare criteria were defined as a worsening of ⩾ 30% from baseline in ⩾ 3 of 6 Pediatric ACR core criteria, ⩾ 2 active joints, and improvement of > 30% in no more than 1 of the 6 criteria. After 32 weeks or at disease flare, patients were eligible to enroll into the open label extension phase

Table 8

Ped ACR Responses in the JIA study

(see Table 8 below)

Amongst those who responded at Week 16 (n=144), the Pediatric ACR 30/50/70/90 responses were maintained for up to two years in the OLE phase in patients who received Humira throughout the study.

Overall responses were generally better and, fewer patients developed antibodies when treated with the combination of Humira and MTX compared to Humira alone. Taking these results into consideration, Humira is recommended for use in combination with MTX and for use as monotherapy in patients for whom MTX use is not appropriate (see section 4.2).

Psoriatic arthritis

Humira, 40 mg every other week, was studied in patients with moderately to severely active psoriatic arthritis in two placebo-controlled studies, PsA studies I and II. PsA study I with 24 week duration, treated 313 adult patients who had an inadequate response to non-steroidal anti-inflammatory drug therapy and of these, approximately 50% were taking methotrexate. PsA study II with 12-week duration, treated 100 patients who had an inadequate response to DMARD therapy. Upon completion of both studies, 383 patients enrolled in an open-label extension study, in which 40 mg Humira was administered eow.

There is insufficient evidence of the efficacy of Humira in patients with ankylosing spondylitis-like psoriatic arthropathy due to the small number of patients studied.

Table 9

ACR Response in Placebo-Controlled Psoriatic Arthritis Studies (Percent of Patients)

(see Table 9)

ACR responses in PsA study I were similar with and without concomitant methotrexate therapy.

ACR responses were maintained in the open-label extension study for up to 136 weeks.

Radiographic changes were assessed in the psoriatic arthritis studies. Radiographs of hands, wrists, and feet were obtained at baseline and Week 24 during the double-blind period when patients were on Humira or placebo and at Week 48 when all patients were on open-label Humira. A modified Total Sharp Score (mTSS), which included distal interphalangeal joints (i.e., not identical to the TSS used for rheumatoid arthritis), was used.

Humira treatment reduced the rate of progression of peripheral joint damage compared with placebo treatment as measured by change from baseline in mTSS (mean ± SD) 0.8 ± 2.5 in the placebo group (at Week 24) compared with 0.0 ± 1.9; ($p < 0.001$) in the Humira group (at Week 48).

In subjects treated with Humira with no radiographic progression from baseline to Week 48 (n=102), 84% continued to show no radiographic progression through 144 weeks of treatment.

Humira treated patients demonstrated statistically significant improvement in physical function as assessed by HAQ and Short Form Health Survey (SF 36) compared to placebo at Week 24. Improved physical function continued during the open label extension up to Week 136.

Ankylosing spondylitis

Humira 40 mg every other week was assessed in 393 patients in two randomised, 24 week double – blind, placebo – controlled studies in patients with active ankylosing spondylitis (mean baseline score of disease activity [Bath Ankylosing Spondylitis Disease Activity Index (BASDAI)] was 6.3 in all groups) who have had an inadequate response to conventional therapy. Seventy-nine (20.1%) patients were treated concomitantly with disease modifying anti – rheumatic drugs, and 37 (9.4%) patients with glucocorticoids. The blinded period was followed by an open – label period during which patients received Humira 40 mg every other week subcutaneously for up to an additional 28 weeks. Subjects (n=215, 54.7%) who failed to achieve ASAS 20 at Weeks 12, or 16 or 20 received early escape open-label adalimumab 40 mg every other week subcutaneously and were subsequently treated as non-responders in the double-blind statistical analyses.

In the larger AS study I with 315 patients, results showed statistically significant improvement of the signs and symptoms of ankylosing spondylitis in patients treated with Humira compared to placebo. Significant response was first observed at Week 2 and maintained through 24 weeks (Table 10).

Table 10 – Efficacy Responses in Placebo-Controlled AS Study – Study I

Reduction of Signs and Symptoms

Response	Placebo N=107	Humira N=208
ASAS[a] 20		
Week 2	16%	42%***
Week 12	21%	58%***
Week 24	19%	51%***

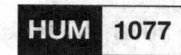

ASAS 50		
Week 2	3%	16%***
Week 12	10%	38%***
Week 24	11%	35%***
ASAS 70		
Week 2	0%	7%**
Week 12	5%	23%***
Week 24	8%	24%***
BASDAI[b] 50		
Week 2	4%	20%***
Week 12	16%	45%***
Week 24	15%	42%***

***,** Statistically significant at $p < 0.001$, < 0.01 for all comparisons between Humira and placebo at Weeks 2, 12 and 24

[a] ASsessments in Ankylosing Spondylitis

[b]Bath Ankylosing Spondylitis Disease Activity Index

Humira treated patients had significantly greater improvement at Week 12 which was maintained through Week 24 in both the SF36 and Ankylosing Spondylitis Quality of Life Questionnaire (ASQoL).

Similar trends (not all statistically significant) were seen in the smaller randomised, double – blind, placebo controlled AS study II of 82 adult patients with active ankylosing spondylitis.

Crohn's disease

The safety and efficacy of Humira were assessed in over 1400 patients with moderately to severely active Crohn's disease (Crohn's Disease Activity Index (CDAI) ⩾ 220 and ⩽ 450) in randomised, double-blind, placebo-controlled studies. 478 of the enrolled patients (32%) were defined as having a severe disease (CDAI score > 300 and concomitant corticosteroid and/or immunosuppressants) corresponding to the population defined in the indication (see section 4.1). Concomitant stable doses of aminosalicylates, corticosteroids, and/or immunomodulatory agents were permitted and 79% of patients continued to receive at least one of these medications.

Induction of clinical remission (defined as CDAI < 150) was evaluated in two studies, CD Study I (CLASSIC I) and CD Study II (GAIN). In CD Study I, 299 TNF-antagonist naive patients were randomised to one of four treatment groups; placebo at Weeks 0 and 2, 160 mg Humira at Week 0 and 80 mg at Week 2, 80 mg at Week 0 and 40 mg at Week 2, and 40 mg at Week 0 and 20 mg at Week 2. In CD Study II, 325 patients who had lost response or were intolerant to infliximab were randomised to receive either 160 mg Humira at Week 0 and 80 mg at Week 2 or placebo at Weeks 0 and 2. The primary non-responders were excluded from the studies and therefore these patients were not further evaluated.

Maintenance of clinical remission was evaluated in CD study III (CHARM). In CD Study III, 854 patients received open-label 80 mg at Week 0 and 40 mg at Week 2. At Week 4 patients were randomised to 40 mg every other Week, 40 mg every Week, or placebo with a total study duration of 56 Weeks. Patients in clinical response (decrease in CDAI ⩾ 70) at Week 4 were stratified and analysed separately from those not in clinical response at Week 4. Corticosteroid taper was permitted after Week 8.

CD study I and CD study II induction of remission and response rates are presented in Table 11.

(see Table 11 below)

Similar remission rates were observed for the 160/80 mg and 80/40 mg induction regimens by Week 8 and adverse events were more frequently noted in the 160/80 mg group.

InCD Study III, at Week 4, 58% (499/854) of patients were in clinical response and were assessed in the primary analysis. Of those in clinical response at Week 4, 48% had been previously exposed to other anti-TNF therapy. Maintenance of remission and response rates are presented in Table 12. Clinical remission results remained relatively constant irrespective of previous TNF-antagonist exposure.

(see Table 12 below)

Among patients who were not in response at Week 4, 43% of Humira maintenance patients responded by Week 12 compared to 30% of placebo maintenance patients. These results suggest that some patients who have not responded by Week 4 benefit from continued maintenance therapy through Week 12. Therapy continued beyond 12 Weeks did not result in significantly more responses (see section 4.2).

Quality of Life

In CD Study I and CD Study II, statistically significant improvement in the disease-specific inflammatory bowel disease questionnaire (IBDQ) total score was achieved at Week 4 in patients randomised to Humira 80/40 mg and 160/80 mg compared to placebo and was seen at Weeks 26 and 56 in CD Study III as well among the adalimumab treatment groups compared to the placebo group.

Psoriasis

The safety and efficacy of Humira were studied in adult patients with chronic plaque psoriasis (⩾ 10% BSA involvement and Psoriasis Area and Severity Index (PASI) ⩾ 12 or ⩾ 10) who were candidates for systemic therapy or phototherapy in randomised, double-blind studies. 73% of patients enrolled in Psoriasis Studies I and II had received prior systemic therapy or phototherapy.

Psoriasis Study I (REVEAL) evaluated 1,212 patients within three treatment periods. In period A, patients received placebo or Humira at an initial dose of 80 mg followed by 40 mg every other week starting one week after the initial dose. After 16 weeks of therapy, patients who achieved at least a PASI 75 response (PASI score improvement of at least 75% relative to baseline), entered period B and received open-label 40 mg Humira every other week. Patients who maintained ⩾PASI 75 response at Week 33 and were originally randomised to active therapy in Period A, were re-randomised in period C to receive 40 mg Humira every other week or placebo for an additional 19 weeks. Across all treatment groups, the mean baseline PASI score was 18.9 and the baseline Physician's Global Assessment (PGA) score ranged from "moderate" (53% of subjects included) to "severe" (41%) to "very severe" (6%).

Psoriasis Study II (CHAMPION) compared the efficacy and safety of Humira *versus* methotrexate and placebo in 271 patients. Patients received placebo, an initial dose of MTX 7.5 mg and thereafter dose increases up to Week 12, with a maximum dose of 25 mg or an initial dose of 80 mg Humira followed by 40 mg every other week (starting one week after the initial dose) for 16 weeks. There are no data available comparing Humira and MTX beyond 16 weeks of therapy. Patients receiving MTX who achieved a ⩾PASI 50 response at Week 8 and/or 12 did not receive further dose increases. Across all treatment groups, the mean baseline PASI score was 19.7 and the baseline PGA score ranged from "mild" (<1%) to "moderate" (48%) to "severe" (46%) to "very severe" (6%).

In Psoriasis Studies I and II, a primary endpoint was the proportion of patients who achieved a PASI 75 response from baseline at Week 16 (see Tables 13 and 14).

Table 13
Ps Study I (REVEAL) - Efficacy Results at 16 Weeks

	Placebo N=398 n (%)	Humira 40 mg eow N=814 n (%)
⩾ PASI 75[a]	26 (6.5)	578 (70.9)[b]
PASI 100	3 (0.8)	163 (20.0)[b]
PGA: Clear/minimal	17 (4.3)	506 (62.2)[b]

[a] Percent of patients achieving PASI75 response was calculated as center-adjusted rate

[b] p<0.001, Humira vs. placebo

(see Table 14 on next page)

In Psoriasis Study I, 28% of patients who were PASI 75 responders and were re-randomised to placebo at Week 33 compared to 5% continuing on Humira, p<0.001, experienced "loss of adequate response" (PASI score after Week 33 and on or before Week 52 that resulted in a <PASI 50 response relative to baseline with a minimum of a 6-point increase in PASI score relative to Week 33). Of the patients who lost adequate response after re-randomization to placebo who then enrolled into the open-label extension trial, 38% (25/66) and 55% (36/66) regained PASI 75 response after 12 and 24 weeks of re-treatment, respectively.

Significant improvements at Week 16 from baseline compared to placebo (Studies I and II) and MTX (Study II) were demonstrated in the DLQI (Dermatology Life Quality Index). In Study I, improvements in the physical and mental component summary scores of the SF-36 were also significant compared to placebo.

In an open-label extension study, for patients who dose escalated from 40 mg every other week to 40 mg weekly due to a PASI response below 50 and were evaluated at 12 weeks after dose escalation, 59/243 (24.3%) of patients regained PASI 75 response.

Immunogenicity

Formation of anti-adalimumab antibodies is associated with increased clearance and reduced efficacy of adalimumab. There is no apparent correlation between the presence of anti-adalimumab antibodies and the occurrence of adverse events.

Patients in RA Studies I, II and III were tested at multiple timepoints for anti-adalimumab antibodies during the 6 to 12 month period. In the pivotal trials, anti-adalimumab antibodies were identified in 58/1053 (5.5%) patients treated with adalimumab, compared to 2/370 (0.5%) on placebo. In patients not given concomitant methotrexate, the incidence was 12.4%, compared to 0.6% when adalimumab was used as add-on to methotrexate.

In patients with polyarticular juvenile idiopathic arthritis, adalimumab antibodies were identified in 27/171 subjects (15.8%) treated with adalimumab. In patients not given concomitant methotrexate, the incidence was 22/86 (25.6%), compared to 5/85 (5.9%) when adalimumab was used as add-on to methotrexate.

Table 11 Induction of Clinical Remission and Response (Percent of Patients)

	CDStudy I: Infliximab Naive Patients			CD Study II: Infliximab Experienced Patients	
	Placebo N=74	Humira 80/40 mg N = 75	Humira 160/80 mg N=76	Placebo N=166	Humira 160/80 mg N=159
Week 4					
Clinical remission	12%	24%	36%*	7%	21%*
Clinical response (CR-100)	24%	37%	49%**	25%	38%**

All p-values are pairwise comparisons of proportions for Humira *versus* placebo
* $p < 0.001$
** $p < 0.01$

Table 12 Maintenance of Clinical Remission and Response (Percent of Patients)

	Placebo	40 mg Humira every other week	40 mg Humira every week
Week 26	N=170	N=172	N=157
Clinical remission	17%	40%*	47%*
Clinical response (CR-100)	27%	52%*	52%*
Patients in steroid-free remission for >=90 days[a]	3% (2/66)	19% (11/58)**	15% (11/74)**
Week 56	N=170	N=172	N=157
Clinical remission	12%	36%*	41%*
Clinical response (CR-100)	17%	41%*	48%*
Patients in steroid-free remission for >=90 days[a]	5% (3/66)	29% (17/58)*	20% (15/74)**

* $p < 0.001$ for Humira *versus* placebo pairwise comparisons of proportions
** $p < 0.02$ for Humira *versus* placebo pairwise comparisons of proportions
[a] Of those receiving corticosteroids at baseline

Table 14 Ps Study II (CHAMPION) Efficacy Results at 16 Weeks

	Placebo N=53 n (%)	MTX N=110 n (%)	Humira 40 mg eow N=108 n (%)
≥ PASI 75	10 (18.9)	39 (35.5)	86 (79.6) [a, b]
PASI 100	1 (1.9)	8 (7.3)	18 (16.7) [c, d]
PGA: Clear/minimal	6 (11.3)	33 (30.0)	79 (73.1) [a, b]

[a] $p < 0.001$ Humira vs. placebo
[b] $p < 0.001$ Humira vs. methotrexate
[c] $p < 0.01$ Humira vs. placebo
[d] $p < 0.05$ Humira vs. methotrexate

In patients with psoriatic arthritis, anti-adalimumab antibodies were identified in 38/376 subjects (10%) treated with adalimumab. In patients not given concomitant methotrexate, the incidence was 13.5% (24/178 subjects), compared to 7% (14 of 198 subjects) when adalimumab was used as add-on to methotrexate.

In patients with ankylosing spondylitis anti-adalimumab antibodies were identified in 17/204 subjects (8.3%) treated with adalimumab. In patients not given concomitant methotrexate, the incidence was 16/185 (8.6%), compared to 1/19 (5.3%) when adalimumab was used as add-on to methotrexate.

In patients with Crohn's disease, anti-adalimumab antibodies were identified in 7/269 subjects (2.6%) treated with adalimumab.

In patients with psoriasis, anti-adalimumab antibodies were identified in 77/920 subjects (8.4%) treated with adalimumab monotherapy.

Because immunogenicity analyses are product-specific, comparison of antibody rates with those from other products is not appropriate.

5.2 Pharmacokinetic properties

After subcutaneous administration of a single 40 mg dose, absorption and distribution of adalimumab was slow, with peak serum concentrations being reached about 5 days after administration. The average absolute bioavailability of adalimumab estimated from three studies following a single 40 mg subcutaneous dose was 64%. After single intravenous doses ranging from 0.25 to 10 mg/kg, concentrations were dose proportional. After doses of 0.5 mg/kg (~40 mg), clearances ranged from 11 to 15 ml/hour, the distribution volume (V_{ss}) ranged from 5 to 6 litres and the mean terminal phase half-life was approximately two weeks. Adalimumab concentrations in the synovial fluid from several rheumatoid arthritis patients ranged from 31-96% of those in serum.

Following subcutaneous administration of 40 mg of Humira every other week in adult rheumatoid arthritis (RA) patients the mean steady-state trough concentrations were approximately 5 μg/ml (without concomitant methotrexate) and 8 to 9 μg/ml (with concomitant methotrexate), respectively. The serum adalimumab trough levels at steady-state increased roughly proportionally with dose following 20, 40 and 80 mg subcutaneous dosing every other week and every week.

Following the administration of 24 mg/m^2 (up to a maximum of 40 mg) subcutaneously every other week to patients with polyarticular juvenile idiopathic arthritis (JIA) the mean trough steady-state (values measured from Week 20 to 48) serum adalimumab concentration was 5.6 ± 5.6 μg/mL (102 %CV) Humira monotherapy and 10.9 ± 5.2 μg/mL (47.7% CV) with concomitant methotrexate.

In patients with Crohn's disease, the loading dose of 80 mg Humira on Week 0 followed by 40 mg Humira on Week 2 achieves serum adalimumab trough concentrations of approximately 5.5 μg/ml during the induction period. A loading dose of 160 mg Humira on Week 0 followed by 80 mg Humira on Week 2 achieves serum adalimumab trough concentrations of approximately 12 μg/ml during the induction period. Mean steady-state trough levels of approximately 7 μg/ml were observed in Crohn's disease patients who received a maintenance dose of 40 mg Humira every other week.

In patients with psoriasis, the mean steady-state trough concentration was 5 μg/mL during adalimumab 40 mg every other week monotherapy treatment.

Population pharmacokinetic analyses with data from over 1,300 RA patients revealed a trend toward higher apparent clearance of adalimumab with increasing body weight. After adjustment for weight differences, gender and age appeared to have a minimal effect on adalimumab clearance. The serum levels of free adalimumab (not bound to anti-adalimumab antibodies, AAA) were observed to be lower in patients with measurable AAA. Humira has not been studied in patients with hepatic or renal impairment.

5.3 Preclinical safety data

Non-clinical data reveal no special hazard for humans based on studies of single dose toxicity, repeated dose toxicity, and genotoxicity.

An embryo-foetal developmental toxicity/perinatal developmental study has been performed in cynomologous monkeys at 0, 30 and 100 mg/kg (9-17 monkeys/group) and has revealed no evidence of harm to the foetuses due to adalimumab. Neither carcinogenicity studies, nor a standard assessment of fertility and postnatal toxicity, were performed with adalimumab due to the lack of appropriate models for an antibody with limited cross-reactivity to rodent TNF and to the development of neutralizing antibodies in rodents.

6. PHARMACEUTICAL PARTICULARS

6.1 List of excipients

Mannitol
Citric acid monohydrate
Sodium citrate
Sodium dihydrogen phosphate dihydrate
Disodium phosphate dihydrate
Sodium chloride
Polysorbate 80
Sodium hydroxide
Water for injections

6.2 Incompatibilities

In the absence of compatibility studies, this medicinal product must not be mixed with other medicinal products.

6.3 Shelf life

24 months

6.4 Special precautions for storage

Store in a refrigerator (2°C – 8°C). Do not freeze. Keep the syringe in the outer carton.

Store in a refrigerator (2°C – 8°C). Do not freeze. Keep the pre-filled pen in the outer carton.

6.5 Nature and contents of container

Humira 40 mg solution for injection in single-use pre-filled syringe (type I glass) for patient use:

Packs of:

- 1 pre-filled syringe (0.8 ml sterile solution) with 1 alcohol pad in a blister.
- 2 pre-filled syringes (0.8 ml sterile solution), each with 1 alcohol pad, in a blister.
- 4 pre-filled syringes (0.8 ml sterile solution), each with 1 alcohol pad, in a blister.
- 6 pre-filled syringes (0.8 ml sterile solution), each with 1 alcohol pad, in a blister.

Humira 40 mg solution for injection in single-use pre-filled pen for patient use.

Packs of:

- 1 pre-filled pen with 1 alcohol pad in a blister.
- 2 pre-filled pen, each with 1 alcohol pad, in a blister.
- 4 pre-filled pen, each with 1 alcohol pad, in a blister.
- 6 pre-filled pen, each with 1 alcohol pad, in a blister.

Not all pack sizes may be marketed.

6.6 Special precautions for disposal and other handling

HUMIRA 40 mg solution for injection does not contain preservatives; therefore, any unused product or waste material should be disposed of in accordance with local requirements.

7. MARKETING AUTHORISATION HOLDER

Abbott Laboratories Ltd.
Queenborough
Kent ME11 5EL
United Kingdom

8. MARKETING AUTHORISATION NUMBER(S)

EU/1/03/256/002
EU/1/03/256/003
EU/1/03/256/004
EU/1/03/256/005
EU/1/03/256/007
EU/1/03/256/008
EU/1/03/256/009
EU/1/03/256/010

9. DATE OF FIRST AUTHORISATION/RENEWAL OF THE AUTHORISATION

8 September 2003

10. DATE OF REVISION OF THE TEXT

August 2009

Hycamtin 0.25mg and 1 mg hard capsule

(GlaxoSmithKline UK)

1. NAME OF THE MEDICINAL PRODUCT

HYCAMTIN ▼ 0.25 mg and 1 mg hard capsules

2. QUALITATIVE AND QUANTITATIVE COMPOSITION

Each capsule contains topotecan hydrochloride equivalent to 0.25 mg or 1 mg of topotecan.

For a full list of excipients, see section 6.1.

3. PHARMACEUTICAL FORM

Hard capsule.

0.25 mg: the capsules are opaque white to yellowish white and imprinted with 'HYCAMTIN' and '0.25 mg'.

1 mg: the capsules are opaque pink and imprinted with 'HYCAMTIN' and '1 mg'.

4. CLINICAL PARTICULARS

4.1 Therapeutic indications

HYCAMTIN capsules are indicated as monotherapy for the treatment of adult patients with relapsed small cell lung cancer (SCLC) for whom re-treatment with the first-line regimen is not considered appropriate (see section 5.1).

4.2 Posology and method of administration

HYCAMTIN capsules should only be prescribed and therapy supervised by a physician experienced in the use of chemotherapeutic agents.

Initial dose

The recommended dose of HYCAMTIN capsules is 2.3 mg/m^2 body surface area/day administered for 5 consecutive days with a 3 week interval between the start of each course. If well tolerated, treatment may continue until disease progression (see sections 4.8 and 5.1).

The capsule(s) must be swallowed whole, and must not be chewed crushed or divided.

Hycamtin capsules may be taken with or without food (see section 5.2).

Prior to administration of the first course of topotecan, patients must have a baseline neutrophil count of $\geq 1.5 \times 10^9$/l, a platelet count of $\geq 100 \times 10^9$/l and a haemoglobin level of ≥ 9 g/dl (after transfusion if necessary).

Subsequent doses

Topotecan should not be re-administered unless the neutrophil count is $\geq 1 \times 10^9$/l, the platelet count is $\geq 100 \times 10^9$/l, and the haemoglobin level is ≥ 9 g/dl (after transfusion if necessary).

Standard oncology practice for the management of neutropenia is either to administer topotecan with other medications (e.g. G-CSF) or to dose reduce to maintain neutrophil counts.

If dose reduction is chosen for patients who experience severe neutropenia (neutrophil count $< 0.5 \times 10^9$/l) for 7 days or more, or severe neutropenia associated with fever or infection, or who have had treatment delayed due to neutropenia, the dose should be reduced by 0.4 mg/m^2/day to 1.9 mg/m^2/day (or subsequently down to 1.5 mg/m^2/day if necessary).

Doses should be similarly reduced if the platelet count falls below 25×10^9/l. In clinical trials, topotecan was discontinued if the dose needed to be reduced below 1.5 mg/m^2.

For patients who experience Grade 3 or 4 diarrhoea, the dose should be reduced by 0.4 mg/m2/day for subsequent courses (see section 4.4). Patients with Grade 2 diarrhoea may need to follow the same dose modification guidelines.

Dosage in renally impaired patients

Patients with small cell lung carcinoma who participated in oral topotecan clinical trials had a serum creatinine less than or equal to 1.5 mg/dl (133 μmol/l) or a creatinine clearance of greater than or equal to 60 ml/min. Dosing recommendations for patients receiving oral topotecan with Cl_{cr} less than 60 ml/min have not been established (see section 4.4).

Dosage in hepatically impaired patients

Pharmacokinetics of HYCAMTIN capsules have not been specifically studied in patients with impaired hepatic function. There are insufficient data available with HYCAMTIN capsules to make a dose recommendation for this patient group (see section 4.4).

Paediatrics

The experience in children is limited, therefore no recommendation for treatment of paediatric patients with HYCAMTIN can be given (see section 5.1).

Elderly

No overall differences in effectiveness were observed between patients over 65 years and younger adult patients. However in the two studies administering both oral and intravenous topotecan, patients older than 65 years old receiving oral topotecan experienced an increase in drug related diarrhoea compared to those younger than 65 years of age (see section 4.4 and 4.8).

4.3 Contraindications

HYCAMTIN is contraindicated in patients who

– have a history of hypersensitivity to the active substance or to any of the excipients

– are breast feeding (see section 4.6)

– already have severe bone marrow depression prior to starting first course, as evidenced by baseline neutrophils $< 1.5 \times 10^9$/l and/or a platelet count of $< 100 \times 10^9$/l.

4.4 Special warnings and precautions for use

Haematological toxicity is dose-related and full blood count including platelets should be monitored regularly (see section 4.2).

As with other cytotoxic medicinal products, topotecan can cause severe myelosuppression. Myelosuppression leading to sepsis and fatalities due to sepsis have been reported in patients treated with topotecan (see section 4.8).

Topotecan-induced neutropenia can cause neutropenic colitis. Fatalities due to neutropenic colitis have been reported in clinical trials with topotecan. In patients presenting with fever, neutropenia, and a compatible pattern of abdominal pain, the possibility of neutropenic colitis should be considered.

Topotecan has been associated with reports of interstitial lung disease, some of which have been fatal (see section 4.8). Underlying risk factors include history of ILD, pulmonary fibrosis, lung cancer, thoracic exposure to radiation and use of pneumotoxic drugs and/or colony stimulating factors. Patients should be monitored for pulmonary symptoms indicative of interstitial lung disease (e.g. cough, fever, dyspnoea and/or hypoxia), and topotecan should be discontinued if a new diagnosis of ILD is confirmed.

Topotecan and topotecan in combination with cisplatin are commonly associated with clinically relevant thrombocytopenia. This should be taken into account, e.g. in case patients at increased risk of tumour bleeds are considered for therapy.

As expected, patients with poor performance status (PS>1) have a lower response rate and an increased incidence of complications such as fever, infection and sepsis (see section 4.8). Accurate assessment of performance status at the time therapy is given is important, to ensure that patients have not deteriorated to performance status 3.

Topotecan is partly eliminated via renal excretion and renal impairment might lead to increased exposure to topotecan. Dosing recommendations for patients receiving oral topotecan with Cl_{cr} less than 60 ml/min have not been established. There is insufficient experience of the use of oral or intravenous topotecan in patients with severely impaired renal function (creatinine clearance < 20 ml/min). Topotecan is not recommended to be used in these patients.

A small number of hepatically impaired patients (serum bilirubin between 1.5 and 10 mg/dl) were given intravenous topotecan at 1.5 mg/m^2 for five days every three weeks. A reduction in topotecan clearance was observed however there are insufficient data available to make a dose recommendation for this patient group. There is insufficient experience of the use of topotecan in patients with severely impaired hepatic function (serum bilirubin ⩾ 10 mg/dl). Topotecan is not recommended to be used in these patients.

Diarrhoea, including severe diarrhoea requiring hospitalization, has been reported during treatment with oral topotecan. Diarrhoea related to oral topotecan can occur at the same time as drug-related neutropenia and its sequelae. Communication with patients prior to drug administration regarding these side effects and proactive management of early and all signs and symptoms of diarrhoea is important. Cancer treatment-induced diarrhoea (CTID) is associated with significant morbidity and may be life-threatening. Should diarrhoea occur during treatment with oral topotecan, physicians are advised to aggressively manage diarrhoea. Clinical guidelines describing the aggressive management of CTID includes specific recommendations on patient communication and awareness, recognition of early warning signs, use of anti-diarrhoeals and antibiotics, changes in fluid intake and diet, and need for hospitalization.

Intravenous topotecan should be considered in the following clinical situations: uncontrolled emesis, swallowing disorders, uncontrolled diarrhoea, clinical conditions and medication that may alter gastrointestinal motility and drug absorption.

4.5 Interaction with other medicinal products and other forms of interaction

Topotecan does not inhibit human P450 enzymes (see section 5.2). In an intravenous population study, the co-administration of granisetron, ondansetron, morphine or corticosteroids did not appear to have a significant effect on the pharmacokinetics of total topotecan (active and inactive form).

Topotecan is a substrate for both ABCB1 (P-glycoprotein) and ABCG2 (BCRP). Inhibitors of ABCB1 and ABCG2 administered with oral topotecan have been shown to increase topotecan exposure.

Cyclosporin A (an inhibitor of ABCB1, ABCC1 [MRP-1], and CYP3A4) administered with oral topotecan increased topotecan AUC to approximately 2 - 2.5-fold of control.

Patients should be carefully monitored for adverse reactions when oral topotecan is administered with a drug known to inhibit ABCB1 or ABCG2 (see section 5.2).

In combining topotecan with other chemotherapy agents, reduction of the doses of each medicinal product may be required to improve tolerability. However, in combining with platinum agents, there is a distinct sequence-dependent interaction depending on whether the platinum agent is given on day 1 or 5 of the topotecan dosing. If either cisplatin or carboplatin is given on day 1 of the topotecan dosing, a lower dose of each agent must be given to improve tolerability compared to the dose of each agent which can be given if the platinum agent is given on day 5 of the topotecan dosing. Currently there is only limited experience in combining oral topotecan with other chemotherapy agents.

The pharmacokinetics of topotecan was generally unchanged when coadministered with ranitidine.

4.6 Pregnancy and lactation

As with all cytotoxic chemotherapy, effective contraceptive methods must be advised when either partner is treated with topotecan.

Topotecan has been shown to cause embryo-foetal lethality and malformations in preclinical studies (see section 5.3). As with other cytotoxic medicinal products, topotecan may cause foetal harm and therefore women of child bearing potential should be advised to avoid becoming pregnant during therapy with topotecan. If topotecan is used during pregnancy, or if the patient becomes pregnant during therapy with topotecan, the patient must be warned of the potential hazards to the foetus.

Topotecan is contra-indicated during breast-feeding (see section 4.3). Although it is not known whether topotecan is excreted in human breast milk, breast-feeding should be discontinued at the start of therapy.

No effects on male or female fertility have been observed in reproductive toxicity studies in rats (see section 5.3). However, as with other cytotoxic medicinal products topotecan is genotoxic and effects on fertility, including male fertility, cannot be excluded.

4.7 Effects on ability to drive and use machines

No studies on the effects on the ability to drive and use machines have been performed. However, caution should be observed when driving or operating machines if fatigue and asthenia persist.

4.8 Undesirable effects

In clinical trials involving patients with relapsed small cell lung cancer, the dose limiting toxicity of oral topotecan monotherapy was found to be haematological. Toxicity was predictable and reversible. There were no signs of cumulative haematological or non-haematological toxicity.

The frequencies associated with the haematological and non-haematological adverse events presented are for adverse events considered to be related/possibly related to oral topotecan therapy.

Adverse reactions are listed below, by system organ class and absolute frequency. Frequencies are defined as: very common (⩾ 1/10), common (⩾ 1/100 to < 1/10); uncommon (⩾ 1/1,000 to < 1/100); rare (⩾ 1/10,000 to < 1/1,000); very rare (< 1/10,000), including isolated reports and not known (cannot be estimated from the available data).

Within each frequency grouping, undesirable effects are presented in order of decreasing seriousness.

Blood and lymphatic system disorders
Very common: febrile neutropenia, neutropenia (see Gastrointestinal disorders), thrombocytopenia, anaemia, leucopenia.
Common: pancytopenia
Respiratory, thoracic and mediastinal disorders
Rare: interstitial lung disease
Gastrointestinal disorders
Very common: Nausea, vomiting and diarrhoea (all of which may be severe),
Common: abdominal pain*, constipation, stomatitis, dyspepsia
*Neutropenic colitis, including fatal neutropenic colitis, has been reported to occur as a complication of topotecan-induced neutropenia (see section 4.4).
Skin and subcutaneous tissue disorders
Very common: alopecia.
Common: pruritis
Metabolism and nutrition disorders
Very common: anorexia (which may be severe).
Infections and infestations
Very common: infection
Common: sepsis
General disorders and administration site conditions
Very common: fatigue.
Common: asthenia, pyrexia, malaise.
Immune system disorders
Common: hypersensitivity reaction including rash
Not known: anaphylactic reaction, angioedema, urticaria.
Hepato-biliary disorders
Uncommon: hyperbilirubinaemia.

The incidence of adverse events listed above have the potential to occur with a higher frequency in patients who have a poor performance status (see section 4.4).

Safety data are presented based on an integrated data set of 682 patients with relapsed lung cancer administered 2536 courses of oral topotecan monotherapy (275 patients with relapsed SCLC and 407 with relapsed non-SCLC).

Haematological

Neutropenia: Severe neutropenia (Grade 4 - neutrophil count $<0.5 \times 10^9$/l) occurred in 32% of patients in 13% of courses. Median time to onset of severe neutropenia was Day 12 with a median duration of 7 days. In 34% of courses with severe neutropenia, the duration was >7 days. In course 1 the incidence was 20%, by courses 4 the incidence was 8%. Infection, sepsis and febrile neutropenia occurred in 17%, 2%, and 4% of patients, respectively. Death due to sepsis occurred in 1% of patients. Pancytopenia has been reported. Growth factors were administered to 19% of patients in 8% of courses.

Thrombocytopenia: Severe thrombocytopenia (Grade 4 - platelets less than 10×10^9/l) occurred in 6 % of patients in 2 % of courses. Median time to onset of severe thrombocytopenia was Day 15 with a median duration of 2.5 days. In 18% of courses with severe thrombocytopenia the duration was >7 days. Moderate thrombocytopenia (Grade 3 - platelets between 10.0 and 50.0×10^9/l) occurred in 29% of patients in 14% of courses. Platelet transfusions were given to 10% of patients in 4 % of courses. Reports of significant sequelae associated with thrombocytopenia including fatalities due to tumour bleeds have been infrequent.

Anaemia: Moderate to severe anaemia (Grade 3 and 4 – Hb ⩽ 8.0 g/dl) occurred in 25 % of patients (12 % of courses). Median time to onset of moderate to severe anaemia was Day 12 with a median duration of 7 days. In 46% of courses with moderate to severe anaemia, the duration was >7 days. Red blood cell transfusions were given in 30 % of patients (13 % of courses). Erythropoietin was administered to 10% of patients in 8% of courses.

Non-haematological

The most frequently reported non-haematological effects were nausea (37 %), diarrhoea (29 %), fatigue (26 %), vomiting (24 %), alopecia (21 %) and anorexia (18 %). All cases were irrespective of associated causality. For severe cases (CTC grade 3/4) reported as related / possibly related to topotecan administration the incidence was diarrhoea 5% (see section 4.4), fatigue 4%, vomiting 3%, nausea 3% and anorexia 2%.

The overall incidence of drug-related diarrhoea was 22%, including 4% with Grade 3 and 0.4% with Grade 4. Drug-related diarrhoea was more frequent in patients ⩾65 years of age (28%) compared to those less than 65 years of age (19%).

Complete alopecia related/possibly related to topotecan administration was observed in 9 % of patients and partial alopecia related/possibly related to topotecan administration in 11 % of patients.

Therapeutic interventions associated with non-haematological effects included anti-emetic agents, given to 47% of patients in 38% of courses and anti-diarrhoeal agents, given to 15% of patients in 6% of courses. A 5-HT3 antagonist was administered to 30% of patients in 24% of courses. Loperamide was administered to 13% of patients in 5% of courses. The median time to onset of grade 2 or worse diarrhoea was 9 days.

4.9 Overdose

There is no known antidote for topotecan overdose. The primary complications of overdose are anticipated to be bone marrow suppression and mucositis.

5. PHARMACOLOGICAL PROPERTIES

5.1 Pharmacodynamic properties

Pharmacotherapeutic group: Other antineoplastic agents: ATC code: L01XX17.

The anti-tumour activity of topotecan involves the inhibition of topoisomerase-I, an enzyme intimately involved in DNA replication as it relieves the torsional strain introduced ahead of the moving replication fork. Topotecan inhibits topoisomerase-I by stabilising the covalent complex of enzyme and strand-cleaved DNA which is an intermediate of the catalytic mechanism. The cellular sequela of inhibition of topoisomerase-I by topotecan is the induction of protein-associated DNA single-strand breaks.

Table 1 Summary of survival, response rate, and time to progression in SCLC patients treated with oral HYCAMTIN or intravenous HYCAMTIN

	Study 065		Study 396	
	Oral topotecan	Intravenous topotecan	Oral topotecan	Intravenous topotecan
	(N = 52)	(N = 54)	(N = 153)	(N = 151)
Median survival (weeks)	32.3	25.1	33.0	35.0
(95% CI)	(26.3, 40.9)	(21.1, 33.0)	(29.1, 42.4)	(31.0, 37.1)
Hazard ratio (95% CI)	0.88 (0.59, 1.31)		0.88 (0.7, 1.11)	
Response rate (%)	23.1	14.8	18.3	21.9
(95% CI)	(11.6, 34.5)	(5.3, 24.3)	(12.2, 24.4)	(15.3, 28.5)
Difference in response rate (95% CI)	8.3 (-6.6, 23.1)		-3.6 (-12.6, 5.5)	
Median time to progression (weeks)	14.9	13.1	11.9	14.6
(95% CI)	(8.3, 21.3)	(11.6, 18.3)	(9.7, 14.1)	(13.3, 18.9)
Hazard ratio (95% CI)	0.90 (0.60, 1.35)		1.21 (0.96, 1.53)	

N = total number of patients treated.

CI = Confidence interval.

Relapsed SCLC

A phase III trial (study 478) compared oral topotecan plus Best Supportive Care [BSC] [n=71] with BSC alone [n=70] in patients who had relapsed following first line therapy [median time to progression [TTP] from first-line therapy: 84 days for oral topotecan + BSC, 90 days for BSC] and for whom retreatment with intravenous chemotherapy was not considered appropriate. Oral topotecan plus BSC group had a statistically significant improvement in overall survival compared with the BSC alone group (Log-rank p=0.0104). The unadjusted hazard ratio for oral topotecan plus BSC group relative to BSC alone group was 0.64 (95% CI: 0.45, 0.90). The median survival for patients treated with topotecan + BSC was 25.9 weeks [95 % C.I. 18.3, 31.6] compared to 13.9 weeks [95 % C.I. 11.1, 18.6] for patients receiving BSC alone.

Patient self-reports of symptoms using an unblinded assessment showed a consistent trend for symptom benefit for oral topotecan + BSC.

One Phase 2 study (Study 065) and one Phase 3 study (Study 396) were conducted to evaluate the efficacy of oral topotecan versus intravenous topotecan in patients who had relapsed ⩾ 90 days after completion of one prior regimen of chemotherapy.(see Table 1) Oral and intravenous topotecan were associated with similar symptom palliation in patients with relapsed sensitive SCLC in patient self-reports on an unblinded symptom scale assessment in each of these two studies.

Table 1. Summary of survival, response rate, and time to progression in SCLC patients treated with oral HYCAMTIN or intravenous HYCAMTIN

(see Table 1 above)

Paediatrics

Safety and effectiveness of oral topotecan in paediatric patients have not been established.

5.2 Pharmacokinetic properties

The pharmacokinetics of topotecan after oral administration have been evaluated in cancer patients following doses of 1.2 to 3.1 mg/m^2/day and 4 mg/m^2/day administered daily for 5 days. The bioavailability of oral topotecan (total and lactone) in humans is approximately 40%. Plasma concentrations of total topotecan (i.e. lactone and carboxylate forms) and topotecan lactone (active moiety) peak at approximately 2.0 hours and 1.5 hours, respectively, and decline bi-exponentially with mean terminal half-life of approximately 3.0 to 6.0 hour. Total exposure (AUC) increases approximately proportionally with dose. There is little or no accumulation of topotecan with repeated daily dosing and there is no evidence of a change in the PK after multiple doses. Preclinical studies indicate plasma protein binding of topotecan is low (35%) and distribution between blood cells and plasma was fairly homogeneous.

A major route of clearance of topotecan is by hydrolysis of the lactone ring to form the ring-opened carboxylate. Other than hydrolysis, topotecan is cleared predominantly renally, with a minor component metabolized to the N-desmethyl metabolite (SB-209780) identified in plasma, urine and faeces. Overall recovery of topotecan-related material following five daily doses of topotecan was 41 to 76 % (mean 57%) of the administered oral dose. Approximately 20% was excreted as total topotecan and 2 % was excreted as N-desmethyl topotecan in the urine. Faecal elimination of total topotecan accounted for 33 % while faecal elimination of N-desmethyl topotecan was 1.5%. Overall, the N-desmethyl metabolite contributed a mean of less than 6 % (range 4-8 %) of the total topotecan related material accounted for in the urine and faeces. O-glucuronides of both topotecan and N-desmethyl topotecan have been identified in the urine. The mean metabolite: parent plasma AUC ratio was less than 10% for both total topotecan and topotecan lactone.

In vitro, topotecan did not inhibit human P450 enzymes CYP1A2, CYP2A6, CYP2C8/9, CYP2C19, CYP2D6, CYP2E, CYP3A, or CYP4A nor did it inhibit the human cytosolic enzymes dihydropyrimidine or xanthine oxidase.

Following coadministration of the ABCB1 (P-gp) and ABCG2 (BCRP) inhibitor, elacridar (GF120918) at 100 to 1,000 mg with oral topotecan, the AUC0-∞ of topotecan lactone and total topotecan increased approximately 2.5-fold (see section 4.5 for guidance).

Administration of oral cyclosporine A (15 mg/kg), an inhibitor of transporters ABCB1 (P-gp) and ABCC1 (MRP-1) as well as the metabolising enzyme CYP3A4, within 4 hours of oral topotecan increased the dose normalised AUC0-24h of topotecan lactone and total topotecan approximately 2.0- and 2.5-fold, respectively (see section 4.5).

The extent of exposure was similar following a high fat meal and fasted state while tmax was delayed from 1.5 to 3 hours (topotecan lactone) and from 3 to 4 hours (total topotecan).

The pharmacokinetics of oral topotecan has not been studied in patients with renal or hepatic impairment (see section 4.2 and 4.4).

A cross-study analysis in 217 patients with advanced solid tumours indicated that gender did not affect the pharmacokinetics of HYCAMTIN capsules_to a clinically relevant extent. There are insufficient data to determine an effect of race on pharmacokinetics of oral topotecan.

5.3 Preclinical safety data

Resulting from its mechanism of action, topotecan is genotoxic to mammalian cells (mouse lymphoma cells and human lymphocytes) *in vitro* and mouse bone marrow cells *in vivo*. Topotecan was also shown to cause embryo-foetal lethality when given to rats and rabbits.

In reproductive toxicity studies with topotecan in rats there was no effect on male or female fertility; however, in females super-ovulation and slightly increased pre-implantation loss were observed.

The carcinogenic potential of topotecan has not been studied.

6. PHARMACEUTICAL PARTICULARS

6.1 List of excipients

Capsule contents (0.25 mg and 1 mg):

Hydrogenated vegetable oil

Glyceryl monostearate

Capsule shell (0.25 mg):

Gelatin

Titanium dioxide (E171)

Capsule shell (1 mg):

Gelatin,

Titanium dioxide (E171),

red iron oxide (E172)

Sealing band (0.25 mg and 1 mg):

Gelatin

Black ink comprising:

black iron oxide (E172)

shellac

anhydrous ethanol – see leaflet for further information

propylene glycol

isopropyl alcohol

butanol

concentrated ammonia solution

potassium hydroxide

6.2 Incompatibilities

Not applicable

6.3 Shelf life

3 years.

6.4 Special precautions for storage

Store in a refrigerator (2°C - 8°C).

Keep the blister card in the outer carton in order to protect from light.

Do not freeze.

6.5 Nature and contents of container

White polyvinyl chloride / polychlorotrifluoroethylene blister sealed with aluminium / Polyethyleneterephtalate (PET) / paper foil lidding.

The blisters are sealed with a peel-push child resistant opening feature.

Each blister card contains 10 capsules.

6.6 Special precautions for disposal and other handling

HYCAMTIN capsules should not be opened or crushed.

Any unused product or waste material should be disposed of in accordance with local requirements.

7. MARKETING AUTHORISATION HOLDER

SmithKline Beecham plc, 980 Great West Road, Brentford, Middlesex, TW8 9GS, United Kingdom.

8. MARKETING AUTHORISATION NUMBER(S)

0.25 mg: EU/1/96/027/006

1 mg: EU/1/96/027/007

9. DATE OF FIRST AUTHORISATION/RENEWAL OF THE AUTHORISATION

Date of first authorisation: 12/11/1996

Date of latest renewal: 12/11/2006

10. DATE OF REVISION OF THE TEXT

12 December 2008

POM

Detailed information on this medicinal product is available on the website of the European Medicines Agency (EMEA) http://www.emea.europa.eu/.

Hycamtin 1mg and 4mg powder for concentrate for solution for infusion

(GlaxoSmithKline UK)

1. NAME OF THE MEDICINAL PRODUCT

HYCAMTIN 1 mg and 4 mg powder for concentrate for solution for infusion

2. QUALITATIVE AND QUANTITATIVE COMPOSITION

Each 1 mg vial contains 1 mg topotecan (as hydrochloride), with a 10 % overage of fill.

Each 4 mg vial contains 4 mg topotecan (as hydrochloride).

For a full list of excipients, see section 6.1.

3. PHARMACEUTICAL FORM

Powder for concentrate for solution for infusion.

Light yellow to greenish powder.

4. CLINICAL PARTICULARS

4.1 Therapeutic indications

Topotecan monotherapy is indicated for the treatment of:

- patients with metastatic carcinoma of the ovary after failure of first-line or subsequent therapy.
- patients with relapsed small cell lung cancer [SCLC] for whom re-treatment with the first-line regimen is not considered appropriate (see section 5.1).

Topotecan in combination with cisplatin is indicated for patients with carcinoma of the cervix recurrent after radiotherapy and for patients with Stage IVB disease. Patients with prior exposure to cisplatin require a sustained treatment free interval to justify treatment with the combination (see section 5.1).

4.2 Posology and method of administration

The use of topotecan should be confined to units specialised in the administration of cytotoxic chemotherapy and should only be administered under the supervision of a physician experienced in the use of chemotherapy (see section 6.6).

When used in combination with cisplatin, the full prescribing information for cisplatin should be consulted.

Prior to administration of the first course of topotecan, patients must have a baseline neutrophil count of ⩾ 1.5 × 10^9/l, a platelet count of ⩾ 100 × 10^9/l and a haemoglobin level of ⩾ 9 g/dl (after transfusion if necessary).

Topotecan must be reconstituted and further diluted before use (see section 6.6).

Ovarian and Small Cell Lung Carcinoma

Initial dose

The recommended dose of topotecan is 1.5 mg/m^2 body surface area/day administered by intravenous infusion over 30 minutes daily for 5 consecutive days with a 3 week interval between the start of each course. If well tolerated, treatment may continue until disease progression (see sections 4.8 and 5.1).

Subsequent doses

Topotecan should not be re-administered unless the neutrophil count is $\geqslant 1 \times 10^9$/l, the platelet count is $\geqslant 100 \times 10^9$/l, and the haemoglobin level is $\geqslant$ 9 g/dl (after transfusion if necessary).

Standard oncology practice for the management of neutropenia is either to administer topotecan with other medications (e.g. G-CSF) or to dose reduce to maintain neutrophil counts.

If dose reduction is chosen for patients who experience severe neutropenia (neutrophil count $< 0.5 \times 10^9$/l) for 7 days or more, or severe neutropenia associated with fever or infection, or who have had treatment delayed due to neutropenia the dose should be reduced by 0.25 mg/m^2/day to 1.25 mg/m^2/day (or subsequently down to 1.0 mg/m^2/day if necessary).

Doses should be similarly reduced if the platelet count falls below 25×10^9/l. In clinical trials, topotecan was discontinued if the dose had been reduced to 1.0 mg/m^2 and a further dose reduction was required to manage adverse effects.

Cervical Carcinoma

Initial dose

The recommended dose of topotecan is 0.75 mg/m^2/day administered as 30 minute intravenous infusion daily on days 1, 2 and 3. Cisplatin is administered as an intravenous infusion on day 1 at a dose of 50 mg/m^2/day and following the topotecan dose. This treatment schedule is repeated every 21 days for 6 courses or until progressive disease.

Subsequent doses

Topotecan should not be re-administered unless the neutrophil count is more than or equal to 1.5×10^9/l, the platelet count is more than or equal to 100×10^9/l, and the haemoglobin level is more than or equal to 9g/dl (after transfusion if necessary).

Standard oncology practice for the management of neutropenia is either to administer topotecan with other medications (e.g. G-CSF) or to dose reduce to maintain neutrophil counts.

If dose reduction is chosen for patients who experience severe neutropenia (neutrophil count less than 0.5×10^9/l) for 7 days or more, or severe neutropenia associated with fever or infection or who have had treatment delayed due to neutropenia the dose should be reduced by 20% to 0.60 mg/m^2/day for subsequent courses (or subsequently down to 0.45 mg/m^2/day if necessary).

Doses should be similarly reduced if the platelet count falls below 25×10^9/l.

Dosage in renally impaired patients

Monotherapy (Ovarian and Small cell lung carcinoma)

Insufficient data are available to make a recommendation for patients with a creatinine clearance < 20 ml/min. Limited data indicate that the dose should be reduced in patients with moderate renal impairment. The recommended monotherapy dose of topotecan in patients with ovarian or small cell lung carcinoma and a creatinine clearance between 20 and 39 ml/min is 0.75 mg/m^2 /day for 5 consecutive days.

Combination therapy (Cervical carcinoma)

In clinical studies with topotecan in combination with cisplatin for the treatment of cervical cancer, therapy was only initiated in patients with serum creatinine less than or equal to 1.5 mg/dL. If, during topotecan/cisplatin combination therapy serum creatinine exceeds 1.5 mg/dL, it is recommended that the full prescribing information be consulted for any advice on cisplatin dose reduction/continuation. If cisplatin is discontinued, there are insufficient data regarding continuing monotherapy with topotecan in patients with cervical cancer.

Paediatrics

The experience in children is limited, therefore no recommendation for treatment of paediatric patients with HYCAMTIN can be given (see sections 5.1 and 5.2).

4.3 Contraindications

HYCAMTIN is contra-indicated in patients who

– have a history of severe hypersensitivity to the active substance or to any of the excipients

– are breast feeding (see section 4.6)

– already have severe bone marrow depression prior to starting first course, as evidenced by baseline neutrophils $< 1.5 \times 10^9$/l and/or a platelet count of $< 100 \times 10^9$/l.

4.4 Special warnings and precautions for use

Haematological toxicity is dose-related and full blood count including platelets should be monitored regularly (see section 4.2).

As with other cytotoxic medicinal products, topotecan can cause severe myelosuppression. Myelosuppression leading to sepsis and fatalities due to sepsis have been reported in patients treated with topotecan (see section 4.8).

Topotecan-induced neutropenia can cause neutropenic colitis. Fatalities due to neutropenic colitis have been reported in clinical trials with topotecan. In patients presenting with fever, neutropenia, and a compatible pattern of abdominal pain, the possibility of neutropenic colitis should be considered.

Topotecan has been associated with reports of interstitial lung disease, some of which have been fatal (see section 4.8). Underlying risk factors include history of ILD, pulmonary fibrosis, lung cancer, thoracic exposure to radiation and use of pneumotoxic drugs and/or colony stimulating factors. Patients should be monitored for pulmonary symptoms indicative of interstitial lung disease (e.g. cough, fever, dyspnoea and/or hypoxia), and topotecan should be discontinued if a new diagnosis of ILD is confirmed.

Topotecan and topotecan in combination with cisplatin are commonly associated with clinically relevant thrombocytopenia. This should be taken into account, e.g. in case patients at increased risk of tumour bleeds are considered for therapy.

As expected, patients with poor performance status (PS > 1) have a lower response rate and an increased incidence of complications such as fever, infection and sepsis (see section 4.8). Accurate assessment of performance status at the time therapy is given is important, to ensure that patients have not deteriorated to performance status 3.

There is insufficient experience of the use of topotecan in patients with severely impaired renal function (creatinine clearance < 20 ml/min) or severely impaired hepatic function (serum bilirubin $\geqslant$ 10 mg/dl) due to cirrhosis. Topotecan is not recommended to be used in these patient groups.

A small number of hepatically impaired patients (serum bilirubin between 1.5 and 10 mg/dl) were given 1.5 mg/m^2 for five days every three weeks. A reduction in topotecan clearance was observed however there are insufficient data available to make a dose recommendation for this patient group.

4.5 Interaction with other medicinal products and other forms of interaction

No *in vivo* human pharmacokinetic interaction studies have been performed.

Topotecan does not inhibit human P450 enzymes (see section 5.2). In a population study, the co-administration of granisetron, ondansetron, morphine or corticosteroids did not appear to have a significant effect on the pharmacokinetics of total topotecan (active and inactive form).

In combining topotecan with other chemotherapy agents, reduction of the doses of each medicinal product may be required to improve tolerability. However, in combining with platinum agents, there is a distinct sequence-dependent interaction depending on whether the platinum agent is given on day 1 or 5 of the topotecan dosing. If either cisplatin or carboplatin is given on day 1 of the topotecan dosing, a lower dose of each agent must be given to improve tolerability compared to the dose of each agent which can be given if the platinum agent is given on day 5 of the topotecan dosing.

When topotecan (0.75 mg/m^2/day for 5 consecutive days) and cisplatin (60 mg/m^2/day on Day 1) were administered in 13 patients with ovarian cancer, a slight increase in AUC (12%, n=9) and C_{max} (23%, n=11) was noted on day 5. This increase is considered unlikely to be of clinical relevance.

4.6 Pregnancy and lactation

As with all cytotoxic chemotherapy, effective contraceptive methods must be advised when either partner is treated with topotecan.

Topotecan has been shown to cause embryo-foetal lethality and malformations in preclinical studies (see section 5.3). As with other cytotoxic medicinal products, topotecan may cause foetal harm and therefore women of child bearing potential should be advised to avoid becoming pregnant during therapy with topotecan. If topotecan is used during pregnancy, or if the patient becomes pregnant during therapy with topotecan, the patient must be warned of the potential hazards to the foetus.

Topotecan is contra-indicated during breast-feeding (see section 4.3). Although it is not known whether topotecan is excreted in human breast milk, breast-feeding should be discontinued at the start of therapy.

No effects on male or female fertility have been observed in reproductive toxicity studies in rats (see section 5.3). However, as with other cytotoxic medicinal products topotecan is genotoxic and effects on fertility, including male fertility, cannot be excluded.

4.7 Effects on ability to drive and use machines

No studies on the effects on the ability to drive and use machines have been performed. However, caution should be observed when driving or operating machines if fatigue and asthenia persist.

4.8 Undesirable effects

In dose-finding trials involving 523 patients with relapsed ovarian cancer and 631 patients with relapsed small cell lung cancer, the dose limiting toxicity of topotecan monotherapy was found to be haematological. Toxicity was predictable and reversible. There were no signs of cumulative haematological or non-haematological toxicity.

The adverse event profile for topotecan when given in combination with cisplatin in the cervical cancer clinical trials is consistent with that seen with topotecan monotherapy. The overall haematological toxicity is lower in patients treated with topotecan in combination with cisplatin compared to topotecan monotherapy, but higher than with cisplatin alone.

Additional adverse events were seen when topotecan was given in combination with cisplatin, however, these events were seen with cisplatin monotherapy and not attributable to topotecan. The prescribing information for cisplatin should be consulted for a full list of adverse events associated cisplatin use.

The integrated safety data for topotecan monotherapy are presented below.

Adverse reactions are listed below, by system organ class and absolute frequency (all reported events). Frequencies are defined as: very common ($\geqslant$ 1/10), common ($\geqslant$ 1/100, < 1/10); uncommon ($\geqslant$ 1/1,000, < 1/100); rare ($\geqslant$ 1/10,000, < 1/1,000); very rare (< 1/10,000), including isolated reports and not known (cannot be estimated from the available data).

Within each frequency grouping, undesirable effects are presented in order of decreasing seriousness.

Blood and lymphatic system disorders
Very common: febrile neutropenia, neutropenia (see Gastrointestinal disorders), thrombocytopenia, anaemia, leucopenia.
Respiratory, thoracic and mediastinal disorders
Rare: interstitial lung disease
Gastrointestinal disorders
Very common: Nausea, vomiting and diarrhoea (all of which may be severe), constipation, abdominal pain* and mucositis. *Neutropenic colitis, including fatal neutropenic colitis, has been reported to occur as a complication of topotecan-induced neutropenia (see section 4.4).
Skin and subcutaneous tissue disorders
Very common: alopecia.
Common: pruritus.
Metabolism and nutrition disorders
Very common: anorexia (which may be severe).
Infections and infestations
Very common: infection
Common: sepsis
General disorders and administration site conditions
Very common: pyrexia, asthenia, fatigue.
Common: malaise.
Very rare: extravasation*. *Extravasation has been reported very rarely. Reactions have been mild and have not generally required specific therapy.
Immune system disorders
Common: hypersensitivity reaction including rash
Rare: anaphylactic reaction, angioedema, urticaria.
Hepato-biliary disorders
Common: hyperbilirubinaemia.

The incidence of adverse events listed above have the potential to occur with a higher frequency in patients who have a poor performance status (see section 4.4).

The frequencies associated with the haematological and non-haematological adverse events listed below represent the adverse event reports considered to be related/possibly related to topotecan therapy.

Haematological

Neutropenia: Severe (neutrophil count $< 0.5 \times 10^9$/l) during course 1 was seen in 55 % of the patients and with duration $\geqslant$ 7 days in 20 % and overall in 77 % of patients (39 % of courses). In association with severe neutropenia, fever or infection occurred in 16 % of patients during course 1 and overall in 23 % of patients (6 % of courses). Median time to onset of severe neutropenia was 9 days and the median duration was 7 days. Severe neutropenia lasted beyond 7 days in 11 % of courses overall. Among all patients treated in clinical trials (including both those with severe neutropenia and those who did not develop severe neutropenia), 11 % (4 % of courses) developed fever and 26 % (9 % of courses) developed infection. In addition, 5 % of all patients treated (1 % of courses) developed sepsis (see section 4.4).

Thrombocytopenia: Severe (platelets less than 25×10^9/l) in 25 % of patients (8 % of courses); moderate (platelets between 25.0 and 50.0 × 10^9/l) in 25 % of patients (15 % of courses). Median time to onset of severe thrombocytopenia was Day 15 and the median duration was 5 days. Platelet transfusions were given in 4 % of courses. Reports of significant sequelae associated with thrombocytopenia including fatalities due to tumour bleeds have been infrequent.

Anaemia: Moderate to severe (Hb ⩽ 8.0 g/dl) in 37 % of patients (14 % of courses). Red cell transfusions were given in 52 % of patients (21 % of courses).

Non-haematological

Frequently reported non-haematological effects were gastrointestinal such as nausea (52 %), vomiting (32 %), and diarrhoea (18 %), constipation (9 %) and mucositis (15 %). Severe (grade 3 or 4) nausea, vomiting, diarrhoea and mucositis incidence was 4, 3, 2 and 1 % respectively.

Mild abdominal pain was also reported amongst 4 % of patients.

Fatigue was observed in approximately 25 % and asthenia in 16 % of patients whilst receiving topotecan. Severe (grade 3 or 4) fatigue and asthenia incidence was 3 and 3 % respectively.

Total or pronounced alopecia was observed in 30 % of patients and partial alopecia in 15 % of patients.

Other severe events occurring in patients that were recorded as related or possibly related to topotecan treatment were anorexia (12 %), malaise (3 %) and hyperbilirubinaemia (1 %).

Hypersensitivity reactions including rash, urticaria, angioedema and anaphylactic reactions have been reported rarely. In clinical trials, rash was reported in 4 % of patients and pruritus in 1.5 % of patients.

4.9 Overdose

There is no known antidote for topotecan overdose. The primary complications of overdose are anticipated to be bone marrow suppression and mucositis.

5. PHARMACOLOGICAL PROPERTIES

5.1 Pharmacodynamic properties

Pharmacotherapeutic group: Other antineoplastic agents. ATC-code: L01XX17.

The anti-tumour activity of topotecan involves the inhibition of topoisomerase-I, an enzyme intimately involved in DNA replication as it relieves the torsional strain introduced ahead of the moving replication fork. Topotecan inhibits topoisomerase-I by stabilising the covalent complex of enzyme and strand-cleaved DNA which is an intermediate of the catalytic mechanism. The cellular sequela of inhibition of topoisomerase-I by topotecan is the induction of protein-associated DNA single-strand breaks.

Relapsed Ovarian Cancer

In a comparative study of topotecan and paclitaxel in patients previously treated for ovarian carcinoma with platinum based chemotherapy (n = 112 and 114, respectively), the response rate (95 % CI) was 20.5 % (13 %, 28 %) versus 14 % (8 %, 20 %) and median time to progression 19 weeks versus 15 weeks (hazard ratio 0.7 [0.6, 1.0]), for topotecan and paclitaxel, respectively. Median overall survival was 62 weeks for topotecan versus 53 weeks for paclitaxel (hazard ratio 0.9 [0.6, 1.3]).

The response rate in the whole ovarian carcinoma programme (n = 392, all previously treated with cisplatin or cisplatin and paclitaxel) was 16 %. The median time to response in clinical trials was 7.6-11.6 weeks. In patients refractory to, or relapsing within 3 months after cisplatin therapy (n = 186), the response rate was 10 %.

These data should be evaluated in the context of the overall safety profile of the medicinal product, in particular to the important haematological toxicity (see section 4.8).

A supplementary retrospective analysis was conducted on data from 523 patients with relapsed ovarian cancer. Altogether, 87 complete and partial responses were observed, with 13 of these occurring during cycles 5 and 6 and 3 occurring thereafter. For patients administered more than 6 cycles of therapy, 91 % completed the study as planned or were treated until disease progression with only 3 % withdrawn for adverse events.

Relapsed SCLC

A phase III trial compared oral topotecan plus Best Supportive Care [BSC] [n=71] with BSC alone [n=70] in patients who had relapsed following first line therapy [median time to progression [TTP] from first-line therapy: 84 days for oral topotecan + BSC, 90 days for BSC] and for whom retreatment with i.v chemotherapy was not considered appropriate. Oral topotecan plus BSC group had a statistically significant improvement in overall survival compared with the BSC alone group (Log-rank p=0.0104). The unadjusted hazard ratio for oral topotecan plus BSC group relative to BSC alone group was 0.64 (95% CI: 0.45, 0.90). The median survival for patients treated with topotecan + BSC was 25.9 weeks [95 % C.I. 18.3, 31.6] compared to 13.9 weeks [95 % C.I. 11.1, 18.6] for patients receiving BSC alone [p=0.0104].

Patient self-reports of symptoms using an unblinded assessment showed a consistent trend for symptom benefit for oral topotecan + BSC.

One Phase 2 study (Study 065) and one Phase 3 study (Study 396) were conducted to evaluate the efficacy of oral topotecan versus intravenous topotecan in patients who had relapsed ⩾ 90 days after completion of one prior regimen of chemotherapy.(see Table 1). Oral and intravenous topotecan were associated with similar symptom palliation in patients with relapsed sensitive SCLC in patient self-reports on an unblinded symptom scale assessment in each of these two studies.

Table 1 Summary of survival, response rate, and time to progression in SCLC patients treated with oral HYCAMTIN or intravenous HYCAMTIN

	Study 065		Study 396	
	Oral topotecan	Intravenous topotecan	Oral topotecan	Intravenous topotecan
	(N = 52)	(N = 54)	(N = 153)	(N = 151)
Median survival (weeks)	32.3	25.1	33.0	35.0
(95% CI)	(26.3, 40.9)	(21.1, 33.0)	(29.1, 42.4)	(31.0, 37.1)
Hazard ratio (95% CI)	0.88 (0.59, 1.31)		0.88 (0.7, 1.11)	
Response rate (%)	23.1	14.8	18.3	21.9
(95% CI)	(11.6, 34.5)	(5.3, 24.3)	(12.2, 24.4)	(15.3, 28.5)
Difference in response rate (95% CI)	8.3 (-6.6, 23.1)		-3.6 (-12.6, 5.5)	
Median time to progression (weeks)	14.9	13.1	11.9	14.6
(95% CI)	(8.3, 21.3)	(11.6, 18.3)	(9.7, 14.1)	(13.3, 18.9)
Hazard ratio (95% CI)	0.90 (0.60, 1.35)		1.21 (0.96, 1.53)	

N = total number of patients treated.

CI = Confidence interval.

Table 1. Summary of survival, response rate, and time to progression in SCLC patients treated with oral HYCAMTIN or intravenous HYCAMTIN

(see Table 1 above)

In another randomised phase III trial which compared IV topotecan to cyclophosphamide, Adriamycin (doxorubicin) and vincristine (CAV) in patients with relapsed, sensitive SCLC, the overall response rate was 24.3% for topotecan compared to 18.3% for the CAV group. Median time to progression was similar in the two groups (13.3 weeks and 12.3 weeks respectively). Median survivals for the two groups were 25.0 and 24.7 weeks respectively. The hazard ratio for survival of IV topotecan relative to CAV was 1.04 (95% CI 0.78 – 1.40).

The response rate to topotecan in the combined small cell lung cancer programme [n = 480] for patients with relapsed disease sensitive to first-line therapy, was 20.2 %. The median survival was 30.3 weeks (95 % CI: 27.6, 33.4).

In a population of patients with refractory SCLC (those not responding to first line therapy), the response rate to topotecan was 4.0%.

Cervical Carcinoma

In a randomised, comparative phase III trial conducted by the Gynaecological Oncology Group (GOG 0179), topotecan plus cisplatin (n=147) was compared with cisplatin alone (n=146) for the treatment of histologically confirmed persistent, recurrent or Stage IVB carcinoma of the cervix where curative treatment with surgery and/or radiation was not considered appropriate. Topotecan plus cisplatin had a statistically significant benefit in overall survival relative to cisplatin monotherapy after adjusting for interim analyses (Log-rank p =0.033).

Study results Study GOG-0179

ITT population		
	Cisplatin 50mg/m^2 d. 1 q21 d.	**Cisplatin 50mg/m^2 d. 1 + Topotecan 0.75mg/m^2 dx3 q21**
Survival (months)	**(n= 146)**	**(n = 147)**
Median (95% C.I.)	6.5 (5.8, 8.8)	9.4 (7.9, 11.9)
Hazard ratio (95% C.I.)	0.76 (0.59-0.98)	
Log rank p-value	0.033	
Patients without Prior Cisplatin Chemoradiotherapy		
	Cisplatin	**Topotecan/ Cisplatin**
Survival (months)	**(n= 46)**	**(n = 44)**
Median (95% C.I.)	8.8 (6.4, 11.5)	15.7 (11.9, 17.7)
Hazard ratio (95% C.I.)	0.51 (0.31, 0.82)	
Patients with Prior Cisplatin Chemoradiotherapy		
	Cisplatin	**Topotecan/ Cisplatin**
Survival (months)	**(n= 72)**	**(n = 69)**
Median (95% C.I)	5.9 (4.7, 8.8)	7.9 (5.5, 10.9)
Hazard ratio (95% C.I.)	0.85 (0.59, 1.21)	

In patients (n=39) with recurrence within 180 days after chemoradiotherapy with cisplatin, the median survival in the topotecan plus cisplatin arm was 4.6 months (95% C.I.: 2.6, 6.1) versus 4.5 months (95%C.I.: 2.9, 9.6) for the cisplatin arm with an hazard ratio of 1.15 (0.59, 2.23). In those (n=102) with recurrence after 180 days, the median survival in the topotecan plus cisplatin arm was 9.9 months (95% C.I.: 7, 12.6) versus 6.3 months (95%C.I.: 4.9, 9.5) for the cisplatin arm with an hazard ratio of 0.75 (0.49, 1.16).

Paediatrics

Topotecan was also evaluated in the paediatric population; however, only limited data on efficacy and safety are available.

In an open-label trial involving children (n = 108, age range: infant to 16 years) with recurrent or progressive solid tumours, topotecan was administered at a starting dose of 2.0 mg/m^2 given as a 30-minute infusion for 5 days repeated every 3 weeks for up to one year depending on response to therapy. Tumour types included were Ewing's Sarcoma/primitive neuroectodermal tumour, neuroblastoma, osteoblastoma, and rhabdomyosarcoma. Antitumour activity was demonstrated primarily in patients with neuroblastoma. Toxicities of topotecan in paediatric patients with recurrent and refractory solid tumours were similar to those historically seen in adult patients. In this study, forty-six (43%) patients received G-CSF over 192 (42.1%) courses; sixty-five (60%) received transfusions of Packed Red Blood Cells and fifty (46%) of platelets over 139 and 159 courses (30.5% and 34.9%) respectively. Based on the dose-limiting toxicity of myelosuppression, the maximum tolerated dose (MTD) was established at 2.0 mg/m^2/day with G-CSF and 1.4 mg/m^2/day without G-CSF in a pharmacokinetic study in paediatric patients with refractory solid tumours (see section 5.2).

5.2 Pharmacokinetic properties

Following intravenous administration of topotecan at doses of 0.5 to 1.5 mg/m^2 as a 30 minute infusion daily for five days, topotecan demonstrated a high plasma clearance of 62 l/h (SD 22), corresponding to approximately 2/3 of liver blood flow. Topotecan also had a high volume of distribution, about 132 l, (SD 57) and a relatively short half-life of 2-3 hours. Comparison of pharmacokinetic parameters did not suggest any change in pharmacokinetics over the 5 days of dosing. Area under the curve increased approximately in proportion to the increase in dose. There is little or no accumulation of topotecan with repeated daily dosing and there is no evidence of a change in the PK after multiple doses. Preclinical studies indicate plasma protein binding of topotecan is low (35%) and distribution between blood cells and plasma was fairly homogeneous.

The elimination of topotecan has only been partly investigated in man. A major route of clearance of topotecan was by hydrolysis of the lactone ring to form the ring-opened carboxylate.

Metabolism accounts for <10% of the elimination of topotecan. An N-desmethyl metabolite, which was shown to have similar or less activity than the parent in a cell-based assay, was found in urine, plasma, and faeces. The mean metabolite:parent AUC ratio was less than 10 % for both total topotecan and topotecan lactone. An O-glucuronidation metabolite of topotecan and N-desmethyl topotecan has been identified in the urine.

Overall recovery of medicinal product-related material following five daily doses of topotecan was 71 to 76 % of the administered IV dose. Approximately 51% was excreted as total topotecan and 3 % was excreted as N-desmethyl topotecan in the urine. Faecal elimination of total topotecan accounted for 18 % while faecal elimination of N-desmethyl topotecan was 1.7 %. Overall, the N-desmethyl metabolite contributed a mean of less than 7% (range 4-9 %) of the total medicinal product related material accounted for in the urine and faeces. The topotecan-O-glucuronide and N-desmethyl topotecan-O-glucuronide in the urine were less than 2.0 %.

In vitro data using human liver microsomes indicate the formation of small amounts of N-demethylated topotecan. In vitro, topotecan did not inhibit human P450 enzymes CYP1A2, CYP2A6, CYP2C8/9, CYP2C19, CYP2D6, CYP2E, CYP3A, or CYP4A nor did it inhibit the human cytosolic enzymes dihydropyrimidine or xanthine oxidase.

When given in combination with cisplatin (cisplatin day 1, topotecan days 1 to 5), the clearance of topotecan was reduced on day 5 compared to day 1 (19.1 L/h/m^2 compared to 21.3 L/h/m^2 [n=9]) (see section 4.5).

Plasma clearance in patients with hepatic impairment (serum bilirubin between 1.5 and 10 mg/dl) decreased to about 67 % when compared with a control group of patients. Topotecan half-life was increased by about 30 % but no clear change in volume of distribution was observed. Plasma clearance of total topotecan (active and inactive form) in patients with hepatic impairment only decreased by about 10 % compared with the control group of patients.

Plasma clearance in patients with renal impairment (creatinine clearance 41-60 ml/min.) decreased to about 67 % compared with control patients. Volume of distribution was slightly decreased and thus half-life only increased by 14 %. In patients with moderate renal impairment topotecan plasma clearance was reduced to 34 % of the value in control patients. Mean half-life increased from 1.9 hours to 4.9 hours.

In a population study, a number of factors including age, weight and ascites had no significant effect on clearance of total topotecan (active and inactive form).

Paediatrics

The pharmacokinetics of topotecan given as a 30-minute infusion for 5 days were evaluated in two studies. One study included a dose range of 1.4 mg/m^2 to 2.4 mg/m^2 in children (aged 2 up to 12 years, n = 18), adolescents (aged 12 up to 16 years, n = 9), and young adults (aged 16 to 21 years, n = 9) with refractory solid tumours. The second study included a dose range of 2.0 mg/m^2 to 5.2 mg/m^2 in children (n = 8), adolescents (n = 3), and young adults (n = 3) with leukaemia. In these studies, there were no apparent differences in the pharmacokinetics of topotecan among children, adolescents, and young adult patients with solid tumours or leukaemia, but data are too limited to draw definite conclusions.

5.3 Preclinical safety data

Resulting from its mechanism of action, topotecan is genotoxic to mammalian cells (mouse lymphoma cells and human lymphocytes) *in vitro* and mouse bone marrow cells *in vivo*. Topotecan was also shown to cause embryo-foetal lethality when given to rats and rabbits.

In reproductive toxicity studies with topotecan in rats there was no effect on male or female fertility; however, in females super-ovulation and slightly increased pre-implantation loss were observed.

The carcinogenic potential of topotecan has not been studied.

6. PHARMACEUTICAL PARTICULARS

6.1 List of excipients

Tartaric acid (E334)

Mannitol (E421)

Hydrochloric acid (E507)

Sodium hydroxide

6.2 Incompatibilities

None known.

6.3 Shelf life

Vials

3 years.

Reconstituted and diluted solutions

The product should be used immediately after reconstitution as it contains no antibacterial preservative. If reconstitution and dilution is performed under strict aseptic conditions (e.g. an LAF bench) the product should be used (infusion completed) within 12 hours at room temperature or 24 hours if stored at 2-8°C after the first puncture of the vial.

6.4 Special precautions for storage

Keep the vial in the outer carton in order to protect from light.

6.5 Nature and contents of container

HYCAMTIN 1 mg is supplied in 5 ml type I flint glass vials, together with 13 mm grey butyl rubber stoppers and 13 mm aluminium seals with plastic flip-off caps.

HYCAMTIN 1 mg is available in cartons containing 1 vial and 5 vials.

HYCAMTIN 4 mg is supplied in 17 ml type I flint glass vials, together with 20 mm grey butyl rubber stoppers and 20 mm aluminium seals with plastic flip-off caps.

HYCAMTIN 4 mg is available in cartons containing 1 vial and 5 vials.

Not all pack sizes may be marketed.

6.6 Special precautions for disposal and other handling

HYCAMTIN 1 mg vials must be reconstituted with 1.1 ml water for injections. Since HYCAMTIN contains a 10 % overage, the clear, reconstituted solution is yellow to yellow-green in colour and provides 1 mg per ml of topotecan.

HYCAMTIN 4 mg vials must be reconstituted with 4 ml water for injections. The reconstituted solution is yellow to yellow-green in colour and provides 1 mg per ml of topotecan.

Further dilution of the appropriate volume of the reconstituted solution with either 0.9 % w/v sodium chloride intravenous infusion or 5 % w/v glucose intravenous infusion is required to a final concentration of between 25 and 50 microgram/ml.

The normal procedures for proper handling and disposal of anticancer medicinal products should be adopted, namely:

– Personnel should be trained to reconstitute the medicinal product.

– Pregnant staff should be excluded from working with this medicinal product.

– Personnel handling this medicinal product during reconstitution should wear protective clothing including mask, goggles and gloves.

– All items for administration or cleaning, including gloves, should be placed in high-risk, waste disposal bags for high-temperature incineration. Liquid waste may be flushed with large amounts of water.

– Accidental contact with the skin or eyes should be treated immediately with copious amounts of water.

7. MARKETING AUTHORISATION HOLDER

SmithKline Beecham plc, 980 Great West Road, Brentford, Middlesex, TW8 9GS, United Kingdom.

8. MARKETING AUTHORISATION NUMBER(S)

1 mg vials:

5 vials EU/1/96/027/004

1 vial EU/1/96/027/005

4 mg vials:

5 vials EU/1/96/027/001

1 vial EU/1/96/027/003

9. DATE OF FIRST AUTHORISATION/RENEWAL OF THE AUTHORISATION

Date of first authorisation: 12/11/1996

Date of last renewal: 12/11/2006

10. DATE OF REVISION OF THE TEXT

12 December 2008

POM

Detailed information on this medicinal product is available on the website of the European Medicines Agency (EMEA) http://www.emea.europa.eu/.

Hydromol Bath & Shower Emollient

(Alliance Pharmaceuticals)

1. NAME OF THE MEDICINAL PRODUCT

Hydromol Bath & Shower Emollient

2. QUALITATIVE AND QUANTITATIVE COMPOSITION

Light Liquid Paraffin BP 37.80%

Isopropyl Myristate BP 13.00%

3. PHARMACEUTICAL FORM

Hydromol Bath & Shower Emollient is a clear, colourless bath additive.

4. CLINICAL PARTICULARS

4.1 Therapeutic indications

For the treatment of dry skin conditions such as eczema, ichthyosis and senile pruritus.

4.2 Posology and method of administration

Route of administration

Hydromol Bath & Shower Emollient should be used topically and is either added to water or applied to wet skin.

1. For use in the bath

a) Adults/Children and the Elderly:

Add 1—3 capfuls to an 8 inch bath of water. Soak for 10-15 minutes.

b) Infants:

Add ½ to 2 capfuls to a small bath of water.

2. For application to the skin as a sponge bath or in the shower.

Adults and Children and the Elderly:

Pour a small quantity on to a wet sponge or flannel and rub onto wet skin. Rinse and pat dry.

4.3 Contraindications

Known sensitivity to any of the ingredients.

4.4 Special warnings and precautions for use

Keep away from eyes. Take care to avoid slipping in the bath/shower. If there is aggravation of the condition consult the doctor.

4.5 Interaction with other medicinal products and other forms of interaction

None known.

4.6 Pregnancy and lactation

Hydromol Bath & Shower Emollient is not contra-indicated in pregnancy or lactation.

4.7 Effects on ability to drive and use machines

Not applicable.

4.8 Undesirable effects

Patients should be advised to take care to avoid slipping in the bath.

4.9 Overdose

Not applicable. Hydromol Bath & Shower Emollient is for topical use only.

5. PHARMACOLOGICAL PROPERTIES

5.1 Pharmacodynamic properties

The combination of oils used in Hydromol Bath & Shower Emollient are deposited on the skin surface during bathing and thus reduce moisture loss, provide anti-pruritic action, lubricate and soften the skin.

Hydromol Bath & Shower Emollient is particularly suitable for infant bathing. The preparation can also be used as a cleanser where soaps are best avoided.

5.2 Pharmacokinetic properties

Hydromol Bath & Shower Emollient is a water-dispersible bath additive resulting in an emulsion of dispersed oils together with a homogenised film on the surface.

5.3 Preclinical safety data

None stated.

6. PHARMACEUTICAL PARTICULARS

6.1 List of excipients

C12-C14 Alcohol with 3 molecules of Ethylene Oxide, Polyol Fatty Acid Ester, Iso-octyl Stearate.

6.2 Incompatibilities

Not applicable. Hydromol Bath & Shower Emollient is for topical use only.

6.3 Shelf life

3 years.

6.4 Special precautions for storage

Hydromol Bath & Shower Emollient should be stored in a dry place avoiding extremes of temperature ie above 30°C or below 5°C.

6.5 Nature and contents of container

Hydromol Bath & Shower Emollient is packed in printed polyethylene bottles of 25 ml, 150 ml, 200 ml, 350 ml, 500 ml and 1 litre capacity.

6.6 Special precautions for disposal and other handling

Hydromol Bath & Shower Emollient should be used topically and is either added to water or applied to wet skin.

1. For use in the bath

a) Adults/Children and the Elderly:

Add 1—3 capfuls to an 8 inch bath of water. Soak for 10-15 minutes.

b) Infants:

Add ½ to 2 capfuls to a small bath of water.

2. For application to the skin as a sponge bath or in the shower.

Adults and Children and the Elderly:

Pour a small quantity on to a wet sponge or flannel and rub onto wet skin. Rinse and pat dry.

7. MARKETING AUTHORISATION HOLDER

Alliance Pharmaceuticals Ltd., Avonbridge House, Bath Road, Chippenham, Wiltshire, SN15 2BB.

8. MARKETING AUTHORISATION NUMBER(S)

PL 16853/0090.

9. DATE OF FIRST AUTHORISATION/RENEWAL OF THE AUTHORISATION

29th June 2004

10. DATE OF REVISION OF THE TEXT

24th October 2008

Hydromol Cream

(Alliance Pharmaceuticals)

1. NAME OF THE MEDICINAL PRODUCT

Hydromol Cream.

2. QUALITATIVE AND QUANTITATIVE COMPOSITION

Sodium Pyrrolidone Carboxylate 2.5%.

Excipients: Cetomacrogol emulsifying wax contains cetostearyl alcohol.

For full list of excipients see Section 6.1.

3. PHARMACEUTICAL FORM

Hydromol Cream is a soft, white, oil-in-water cream which can be massaged easily into the skin.

4. CLINICAL PARTICULARS

4.1 Therapeutic indications

Any condition in which "dry skin" is a feature, including all forms of dermatitis/eczema and all degrees of ichthyosis and senile pruritus.

4.2 Posology and method of administration

Route of administration

For topical use only.

Adults, Children and the Elderly:

Apply liberally to the affected area and massage well into the skin. Hydromol Cream may be used as often as required.

Hydromol Cream is especially beneficial when used immediately after washing or bathing, when the resultant warmth of the skin enhances absorption.

4.3 Contraindications

There are no contra-indications except true hypersensitivity to any of the ingredients.

4.4 Special warnings and precautions for use

The formulation is not designed for use as a diluent.

4.5 Interaction with other medicinal products and other forms of interaction

None known.

4.6 Pregnancy and lactation

Hydromol Cream is not contra-indicated in pregnancy or lactation.

4.7 Effects on ability to drive and use machines

Not applicable.

4.8 Undesirable effects

Rarely a non serious allergic type reaction may be experienced, e.g. rash.

4.9 Overdose

Not applicable. Hydromol Cream is for topical use only.

5. PHARMACOLOGICAL PROPERTIES

5.1 Pharmacodynamic properties

The combination of oils used in Hydromol Cream helps to lubricate and hydrate the skin. Moisture loss from the stratum corneum is reduced by the formation of an occlusive film by liquid paraffin on the surface of the skin. Isopropyl myristate, a fatty acid ester, is easily absorbed into the skin and helps to improve skin softness.

5.2 Pharmacokinetic properties

Sodium pyrrolidone carboxylate positively aids the hydration of skin.

5.3 Preclinical safety data

None stated.

6. PHARMACEUTICAL PARTICULARS

6.1 List of excipients

Liquid Paraffin

Isopropyl Myristate

Sodium Lactate

Cetomacrogol Emulsifying Wax (contains cetostearyl alcohol)

Myristyl Myristate

Cetomacrogol 1000

Hydroxybenzoates (Parabens)

Phenoxyethanol

Purified Water.

6.2 Incompatibilities

Not applicable. Hydromol Cream is for topical use only.

6.3 Shelf life

2 years.

6.4 Special precautions for storage

Hydromol Cream should be stored in a dry place avoiding extremes of temperature ie not less than 5°C and not more than 30°C.

6.5 Nature and contents of container

Hydromol Cream is packed in low density polyethylene tubes of 10 g, 50 g and 100 g with a flush fitting cap. It is also available in polypropylene tubs containing 500 g with pump dispenser.

Not all pack sizes may be marketed.

6.6 Special precautions for disposal and other handling

No special instructions.

7. MARKETING AUTHORISATION HOLDER

Alliance Pharmaceuticals Ltd., Avonbridge House, Bath Road, Chippenham, Wiltshire, SN15 2BB.

8. MARKETING AUTHORISATION NUMBER(S)

PL 16853/0089.

9. DATE OF FIRST AUTHORISATION/RENEWAL OF THE AUTHORISATION

1st October 2004.

10. DATE OF REVISION OF THE TEXT

20th March 2009

Hydroxycarbamide medac 500 mg capsule, hard

(medac GmbH)

1. NAME OF THE MEDICINAL PRODUCT

Hydroxycarbamide medac 500 mg capsule, hard

2. QUALITATIVE AND QUANTITATIVE COMPOSITION

One capsule contains 500 mg hydroxycarbamide.

For excipients, see 6.1.

3. PHARMACEUTICAL FORM

Capsule, hard

White capsules.

4. CLINICAL PARTICULARS

4.1 Therapeutic indications

Treatment of patients with chronic myeloid leukaemia (CML) in the chronic or accelerated phase of the disease.

Treatment of patients with essential thrombocythemia or polycythemia vera with a high risk for thrombo-embolic complications.

4.2 Posology and method of administration

Therapy should only be conducted by a physician experienced in oncology or haematology. Doses are based on real or ideal bodyweight of the patient, whichever is the less.

In CML hydroxycarbamide is usually given at an initial dose of 40 mg/kg daily dependent on the white cell count. The dose is reduced by 50% (20 mg/kg daily) when the white cell count is dropped below 20×10^9/l. The dose is then adjusted individually to keep the white cell count at 5-10×10^9/l. Hydroxycarbamide dose should be reduced if white cell counts fall below 5×10^9/l and increased if white cell counts $>10 \times 10^9$/l are observed.

If white cell count falls below 2.5×10^9/l, or the platelet count below 100×10^9/l, therapy should be interrupted until the counts rise significantly towards normal.

An adequate trial period for determining the antineoplastic effect of Hydroxycarbamide medac is six weeks. Therapy should be interrupted indefinitely, if there is a significant progress of the disease. If there is a significant clinical response therapy may be continued indefinitely.

In essential thrombocythemia hydroxycarbamide is usually given at starting doses of 15 mg/kg/day with dose adjustment to maintain a platelet count below 600×10^9 /l without lowering the white blood cell count below 4×10^9/l.

In polycythemia vera hydroxycarbamide should be started at a dosage of 15-20 mg/kg/day. Hydroxycarbamide dose should be adjusted individually to maintain the hematocrit below 45% and platelet count below 400×10^9/l. In most patients this can be achieved with hydroxycarbamide given continuously at average daily doses of 500 to 1000 mg.

If hematocrit and platelet count can be sufficiently controlled therapy should be continued indefinitely.

Children:

Because of the rarity of these conditions in children, dosage regimens have not been established.

Elderly:

Elderly patients may be more sensitive to the effects of hydroxycarbamide, and may require a lower dosage regimen.

Dosage in conditions of impaired renal and/or liver function:

There are no data available. Dose recommendation cannot be given to patients with impaired renal and/or liver function (see 4.4 Special warnings and precautions for use).

The capsules should be swallowed whole and not allowed to disintegrate within the mouth.

4.3 Contraindications

Hydroxycarbamide medac is contraindicated in severe bone marrow depression, leucocytopenia ($<2{,}5 \times 10^9$ leukocytes/l), thrombocytopenia ($< 100 \times 10^9$ platelets/l) or severe anaemia.

Hydroxycarbamide medac is contraindicated in patients with hypersensitivity to hydroxycarbamide or to any of the excipients. Therapy should be discontinued if hypersensitivity to Hydroxycarbamide medac occurs.

4.4 Special warnings and precautions for use

Hydroxycarbamide can cause bone marrow depression with leucopenia as first and most often occurring sign of this depression. Thrombocytopenia and anaemia occur less frequently and are rare without preceding leucopenia. Complete blood counts including determination of haemoglobin level, total leukocyte differentiation counts, and platelet counts should be performed regularly also after the individual optimal dose has been established. The control interval should be individualised, but is normally once a week. If white cell count falls below 2.5×10^9/l, or the platelet count below 100×10^9/l, therapy should be interrupted until the counts rise significantly towards normal. (See 4.2 Posology and method of administration).

In case of anaemia before or during ongoing treatment red blood cells may be replaced when needed. Megaloblastic erythropoesis, which is self limiting, is often seen early in the course of hydroxycarbamide therapy. The morphologic change resembles pernicious anaemia, but is not related to vitamin B_{12} or folic acid deficiency.

During therapy with Hydroxycarbamide medac frequent monitoring of blood counts should be conducted as well as monitoring of hepatic and renal function. In patients with impaired renal and/or liver function the experience is limited. Therefore special care should be taken in the treatment of these patients, especially at the beginning of therapy.

Patients should be instructed to drink abundantly.

In patients receiving long-term treatment with hydroxycarbamide for myeloproliferative disorders, such as polycythemia vera and thrombocythemia, secondary leukemia may develop. To what extent this relates to the underlying disease or to treatment with hydroxycarbamide is presently unknown.

The monitoring of skin changes is advisable during hydroxycarbamide treatment as in single cases squamous cell carcinoma of the skin was reported.

Hydroxycarbamide can induce painful leg ulcers which are usually difficult to treat and require cessation of therapy. Discontinuation of hydroxycarbamide usually leads to slow resolution of the ulcers over some weeks.

Hydroxycarbamide should be administered with caution to patients who receive concomitant or have received previous therapy with other antineoplastic drugs or irradiation, since adverse reactions can occur more frequently and more severe than those reported with the use of hydroxycarbamide, other antineoplastic drugs or irradiation alone. These effects primarily include bone marrow depression, gastric irritation, and mucositis.

An exacerbation of erythema caused by previous or simultaneous irradiation may occur.

The combination of hydroxycarbamide and nucleoside reverse transcriptase inhibitors (NRTI) may enhance the risk of side effects of NRTI, see also section 4.5, Interaction with other medicinal products and other forms of interaction.

Hydroxycarbamide may be genotoxic. Therefore, men under therapy are advised to use safe contraceptive measures during and for at least 3 months after therapy. They should be informed about the possibility of sperm conservation before the start of therapy.

Hydroxycarbamide medac should not be administered to patients who are pregnant or to mothers who are breast feeding, unless the benefits outweigh the possible hazards (see 4.6 Pregnancy and lactation).

Hydroxycarbamide medac should not be administered to patients with rare hereditary problems of galactose intolerance, the Lapp lactase deficiency or glucose-galactose malabsorption.

4.5 Interaction with other medicinal products and other forms of interaction

Hydroxycarbamide should be administered with caution to patients who receive concomitant or have received previous therapy with other antineoplastic drugs or irradiation, since adverse reactions can occur more frequently and more severe than those reported with the use of hydroxycarbamide, other antineoplastic drugs or irradiation alone. These effects primarily include bone marrow depression, gastric irritation, and mucositis.

An exacerbation of erythema caused by previous or simultaneous irradiation may occur.

In-vitro studies have demonstrated hydroxycarbamide's ability to enhance the cytotoxicity of both ara-C and the fluoropyrimidines. Whether this interaction leads clinically to a co-operative toxicity or to the necessity of adjusting the doses is unclear.

Hydroxycarbamide may enhance the antiretroviral activity of nucleoside reverse transcriptase inhibitors like didanosine and stavudine. Hydroxycarbamide inhibits HIV DNA synthesis and HIV replication by decreasing the amount of intracellular deoxynucleotides. Hydroxycarbamide may also enhance the potential side effects of nucleoside reverse transcriptase inhibitors such as pancreatitis and peripheral neuropathy.

4.6 Pregnancy and lactation

Pregnancy

Hydroxycarbamide may be a potent mutagenic agent. Animal experiments with hydroxycarbamide indicated an increased incidence of congenital defects (see 5.3 Preclinical safety data). Hydroxycarbamide should not be administered to patients who are pregnant unless the benefits outweigh the possible hazards. Women of child-bearing potential have to take contraceptive precautions before the start of and during treatment with hydroxycarbamide.

If pregnancy still occurs during treatment the possibility of genetic consultation should be used. Hydroxycarbamide crosses the placenta.

Lactation:

As hydroxycarbamide passes into breast-milk, breast-feeding has to be interrupted before the start of treatment.

Fertility:

Hydroxycarbamide may be genotoxic, therefore, if a patient intends to become pregnant after a therapy with hydroxycarbamide a genetic consultation is recommended.

Men under therapy are advised to use safe contraceptive measures during and for at least 3 months after therapy. They should be informed about the possibility of sperm conservation before the start of therapy.

4.7 Effects on ability to drive and use machines
Ability to react may be impaired during treatment with Hydroxycarbamide medac. This should be borne in mind when heightened attention is required, e.g for driving and using machines.

4.8 Undesirable effects
Bone marrow depression is the dose limiting toxicity. Gastrointestinal side effects are common but require rarely dose reduction or cessation of treatment.

Common (> 1/100, < 1/10)

Blood: Bone marrow depression, leucopenia, megaloblastosis.

Gastrointestinal: Diarrhoea, constipation.

Uncommon (> 1/1,000, < 1/100)

Blood: Thrombocytopenia, anaemia

Body as a whole: Nausea, vomiting, anorexia, stomatitis. Drug fever, chills, malaise.

Skin: Maculopapular rash, facial erythema, acral erythema.

Liver: Elevation of liver enzymes, bilirubin.

Urogenital: Transient impairment of the renal tubular function accompanied by elevation in serum uric acid, urea and creatinine.

Rare: (> 1/10,000, < 1/1,000)

Body as a whole: Hypersensitive reactions

Skin: Alopecia.

Respiratory: Acute pulmonary reactions consisting of diffuse pulmonary infiltrates, fever and dyspnoe, allergic alveolitits.

Urogenital: Dysuria.

Neurological: Rare neurological disturbances including headache, dizziness, disorientation, hallucinations.

Very rare: (< 1/10,000)

Skin: Dermatomyositis-like skin changes, Hyperpigmentation or atrophy of skin and nails, cutaneous ulcers (especially leg ulcers), Pruritus, actinic keratosis, skin cancer (squamous cell cancer, basal cell carcinoma), violet papules, desquamation.

Urogenital: renal impairment.

In the therapy with hydroxycarbamide megaloblastosis may occur which does not respond to treatment with folic acid or B_{12}.

The bone-marrow suppression subsides, however, when therapy is discontinued.

Severe gastric distress (nausea, emesis, anorexia) resulting from combined hydroxycarbamide and irradiation therapy may usually be controlled by temporarily discontinuing hydroxycarbamide administration.

Hydroxycarbamide may aggravate the inflammation of mucous membranes secondary to irradiation. It can cause a recall of erythema and hyperpigmentation in previously irradiated tissues. Erythema, atrophy of skin and nails, desquamation, violet papules, alopecia, dermatomyositis-like skin changes, actinic keratosis, skin cancer (squamous cell cancer, basal cell carcinoma), cutaneous ulcers (especially leg ulcers), pruritus and hyperpigmentation of skin and nails have been observed in isolated cases partly after years of long-term daily maintenance therapy with hydroxycarbamide.

High doses may cause moderate drowsiness.

Rare neurological disturbances including headache, dizziness, disorientation, hallucinations, and convulsions have been reported.

In rare cases dysuria or renal impairment, hypersensitive reactions.

In individual cases allergic alveolitis.

In patients receiving long-term treatment with hydroxycarbamide for myeloproliferative disorders, such as polycythemia vera and thrombocythemia, secondary leukemia may develop. To what extent this relates to the underlying disease or to treatment with hydroxycarbamide is presently unknown.

Hydroxycarbamide can reduce plasma iron clearance and iron utilisation by erythrocytes. However, it does not appear to alter the red blood cell survival time.

4.9 Overdose
Acute mucocutaneous symptoms have been observed in patients receiving hydroxycarbamide dosages several times the recommended dose. Soreness, violet erythema, oedema on palms and soles followed by scaling of hands and feet, severe generalised hyperpigmentation of the skin, and stomatitis have also been observed.

Immediate treatment consists of gastric lavage, followed by supportive care and monitoring of the haematopoetic system.

5. PHARMACOLOGICAL PROPERTIES
5.1 Pharmacodynamic properties
Pharmacotherapeutic group: Other antineoplastic agents

ATC-code: L01XX05

The exact mechanism of action of hydroxycarbamide is unknown. The most important effect of hydroxycarbamide appears to be blocking of the ribonucleotide reductase system resulting in inhibition of DNA synthesis. Cellular resistance is usually caused by increased ribonucleotide reductase levels as a result of gene amplification.

5.2 Pharmacokinetic properties
The pharmacokinetic information is limited. Hydroxycarbamide is well absorbed and the oral bioavailability is complete. After oral administration maximum plasma concentrations are reached within 0.5 to 2 hours. Hydroxycarbamide is eliminated partly via renal excretion. The contribution of this route of elimination to the total elimination of hydroxycarbamide is unclear since the fractions of the given dose recovered in urine ranged from 9 to 95 %. Metabolism of hydroxycarbamide has not been thoroughly studied in humans.

Hydroxycarbamide crosses the blood-brain barrier.

5.3 Preclinical safety data
Repeated dose toxicity

Bone marrow damages, lymphoid atrophy in the spleen and degenerative changes in the epithelium of the small and large intestines are toxic effects which have been observed in animal studies. The potential risk for similar effects in humans must be considered.

Reproduction toxicity

Teratogenicity of hydroxycarbamide was demonstrated in many species, including rat, mouse and rabbit. The large variety of teratogenic effects were ranging from death of a large proportion of embryos to limb deformities, neural defects and even behavioural effects.

Additionally, hydroxycarbamide affected spermatogenesis and sperm motility of mice after repeated administration.

Genotoxicity

Hydroxycarbamide showed genotoxic properties in conventional testing systems.

Carcinogenicity

The preclinical information on the carcinogenic potential of hydroxycarbamide is meagre. A 12 months study on mice where the occurrence of lung tumours was studied did not show any carcinogenic potential in hydroxycarbamide.

6. PHARMACEUTICAL PARTICULARS
6.1 List of excipients
Capsule content:

calcium citrate, disodium citrate, magnesium stearate, lactose monohydrate

Capsule shell:

titanium dioxide (E 171), gelatin

6.2 Incompatibilities
Not applicable.

6.3 Shelf life
4 years

6.4 Special precautions for storage
No special precautions for storage.

6.5 Nature and contents of container
The capsules are packed in blisters made of Al/PVDC and PVC/PVDC opacified with titanium dioxide.
Available pack sizes: 50 and 100 capsules.

6.6 Special precautions for disposal and other handling
Procedures for proper handling and disposal of anticancer drugs should be considered.

7. MARKETING AUTHORISATION HOLDER
medac

Gesellschaft für klinische Spezialpräparate mbH

Fehlandtstraβe 3

20354 Hamburg

Germany

8. MARKETING AUTHORISATION NUMBER(S)
PL 11587/0019

9. DATE OF FIRST AUTHORISATION/RENEWAL OF THE AUTHORISATION
23 May 2001/9 January 2004

10. DATE OF REVISION OF THE TEXT
24 March 2005

Hygroton Tablets 50mg

(Alliance Pharmaceuticals)

1. NAME OF THE MEDICINAL PRODUCT
Hygroton® Tablets 50mg

2. QUALITATIVE AND QUANTITATIVE COMPOSITION
Chlortalidone PhEur 50mg.

3. PHARMACEUTICAL FORM
Pale yellow, round, flat tablets with bevelled edges, impressed Geigy on one side with a breakline, and the letters Z/A on the other side.

4. CLINICAL PARTICULARS
4.1 Therapeutic indications
Treatment of arterial hypertension, essential or nephrogenic or isolated systolic. Treatment of stable, chronic heart failure of mild to moderate degree (New York Heart Association, NYHA: functional class II or III).

Oedema of specific origin

- Ascites due to cirrhosis of the liver in stable patients under close control.
- Oedema due to nephrotic syndrome.

Diabetes Insipidus.

4.2 Posology and method of administration
The dosage of Hygroton should be individually titrated to give the lowest effective dose; this is particularly important in the elderly. Hygroton should be taken orally, preferably as a single daily dose at breakfast time.

Adults:

Hypertension

The recommended starting dose is 25mg/day. This is sufficient to produce the maximum hypotensive effect in most patients. If the decrease in blood pressure proves inadequate with 25mg/day, then the dose can be increased to 50mg/day. If a further reduction in blood pressure is required, additional hypertensive therapy may be added to the dosage regime.

Stable, chronic heart failure (NYHA: functional class II /III):

The recommended starting dose is 25 to 50mg/day, in severe cases it may be increased up to 100 to 200mg/day. The usual maintenance dose is the lowest effective dose, eg 25 to 50mg/day either daily or every other day. If the response proves inadequate, digitalis or an ACE inhibitor, or both, may be added. (See Section 4.4 "Special warnings and precautions for use").

Oedema of specific origin (see Section 4.1 "Therapeutic indications")

The lowest effective dose is to be identified by titration and administered over limited periods only. It is recommended that doses should not exceed 50mg/day.

Diabetes insipidus:

Initially 100mg twice daily but reducing where possible to a daily maintenance dose of 50mg.

Children:

The lowest effective dose should also be used in children. For example, an initial dose of 0.5 to 1mg/kg/48hours and a maximum dose of 1.7mg/kg/48hours have been used.

Elderly patients and patients with renal impairment:

The lowest effective dose of Hygroton is also recommended for patients with mild renal insufficiency and for elderly patients (see Section 5.2 "Pharmacokinetic properties").

In elderly patients, the elimination of chlortalidone is slower than in healthy young adults, although absorption is the same. Therefore, a reduction in the recommended adult dosage may be needed. Close medical observation is indicated when treating patients of advanced age with chlortalidone.

Hygroton and the thiazide diuretics lose their diuretic effect when the creatinine clearance is < 30ml/min.

4.3 Contraindications
Known hypersensitivity to chlortalidone or any of the excipients. Anuria, severe hepatic or renal failure (creatinine clearance < 30ml/min), hypersensitivity to chlortalidone and other sulphonamide derivatives, refractory hypokalaemia, hyponatraemia and hypercalcaemia, symptomatic hyperuricaemia (history of gout or uric acid calculi), hypertension during pregnancy, untreated Addison's disease and concomitant lithium therapy.

4.4 Special warnings and precautions for use
Warnings:

Hygroton should be used with caution in patients with impaired hepatic function or progressive liver disease since minor changes in the fluid and electrolyte balance due to thiazide diuretics may precipitate hepatic coma, especially in patients with liver cirrhosis (see Section 4.3 "Contra-indications").

Hygroton should also be used with caution in patients with severe renal disease. Thiazides may precipitate azotaemia in such patients, and the effects of repeated administration may be cumulative.

Precautions:

Electrolytes:

Treatment with thiazide diuretics has been associated with electrolyte disturbances such as hypokalaemia, hypomagnesaemia, hyperglycaemia and hyponatraemia. Since the excretion of electrolytes is increased, a very strict low-salt diet should be avoided.

Hypokalaemia can sensitise the heart or exaggerate its response to the toxic effects of digitalis.

Like all thiazide diuretics, kaluresis induced by Hygroton is dose dependent and varies in extent from one subject to another. With 25 to 50mg/day, the decrease in serum potassium concentrations averages 0.5mmol/l. Periodic serum electrolyte determinations should be carried out, particularly in digitalised patients.

If necessary, Hygroton may be combined with oral potassium supplements or a potassium-sparing diuretic (eg triamterene).

If hypokalaemia is accompanied by clinical signs (eg muscular weakness, paresis and ECG alteration), Hygroton should be discontinued.

Combined treatment consisting of Hygroton and a potassium salt or a potassium-sparing diuretic should be avoided in patients also receiving ACE inhibitors.

Monitoring of serum electrolytes is particularly indicated in the elderly, in patients with ascites due to liver cirrhosis, and in patients with oedema due to nephrotic syndrome. There have been isolated reports of hyponatraemia with neurological symptoms (eg nausea, debility, progressive disorientation and apathy) following thiazide treatment.

For nephrotic syndrome, Hygroton should be used only under close control in normokalaemic patients with no signs of volume depletion.

Metabolic effects:

Hygroton may raise the serum uric acid level, but attacks of gout are uncommon during chronic treatment.

As with the use of other thiazide diuretics, glucose intolerance may occur; this is manifest as hyperglycaemia and glycosuria. Hygroton may very seldom aggravate or precipitate diabetes mellitus; this is usually reversible on stopping therapy.

Small and partly reversible increases in plasma concentrations of total cholesterol, triglycerides, or low-density lipoprotein cholesterol were reported in patients during long-term treatment with thiazides and thiazide-like diuretics. The clinical relevance of these findings is a matter for debate.

Hygroton should not be used as a first-line drug for long-term treatment in patients with overt diabetes mellitus or in subjects receiving therapy for hypercholesterolaemia (diet or combined).

As with all antihypertensive agents, a cautious dosage schedule is indicated in patients with severe coronary or cerebral arteriosclerosis.

Other effects:

The antihypertensive effect of ACE inhibitors is potentiated by agents that increase plasma renin activity (diuretics). It is recommended that the diuretic be reduced in dosage or withdrawn for 2 to 3 days and/or that the ACE inhibitor therapy be started with a low initial dose of the ACE inhibitor. Patients should be monitored for several hours after the first dose.

4.5 Interaction with other medicinal products and other forms of interaction

Diuretics potentiate the action of curare derivatives and antihypertensive drugs (e.g. guanethidine, methyldopa, β-blockers, vasodilators, calcium antagonists and ACE inhibitors).

The hypokalaemic effect of diuretics may be potentiated by corticosteroids, ACTH, β_2– agonists, amphotericin and carbenoxolone.

It may prove necessary to adjust the dosage of insulin and oral anti-diabetic agents.

Thiazide-induced hypokalaemia or hypomagnesaemia may favour the occurrence of digitalis-induced cardiac arrhythmias (see Section 4.4 "Special warnings and precautions for use").

Concomitant administration of certain non-steroidal anti-inflammatory drugs (e.g. indometacin) may reduce the diuretic and antihypertensive activity of Hygroton; there have been isolated reports of a deterioration in renal function in predisposed patients.

The bioavailability of thiazide-type diuretics may be increased by anticholinergic agents (eg atropine, biperiden), apparently due to a decrease in gastrointestinal motility and stomach-emptying rate.

Absorption of thiazide diuretics is impaired in the presence of anionic exchange resins such as colestyramine. A decrease in the pharmacological effect may be expected.

Concurrent administration of thiazide diuretics may increase the incidence of hypersensitivity reactions to allopurinol, increase the risk of adverse effects caused by amantadine, enhance the hyperglycaemic effect of diazoxide, and reduce renal excretion of cytotoxic agents (eg cyclophosphamide, methotrexate) and potentiate their myelosuppressive effects.

The pharmacological effects of both calcium salts and vitamin D may be increased to clinically significant levels if given with thiazide diuretics. The resultant hypercalcaemia is usually transient but may be persistent and symptomatic (weakness, fatigue, anorexia) in patients with hyperparathyroidism.

Concomitant treatment with cyclosporin may increase the risk of hyperuricaemia and gout-type complications.

Thiazide and related diuretics can cause a rapid rise in serum lithium levels as the renal clearance of lithium is reduced by these compounds.

4.6 Pregnancy and lactation

Diuretics are best avoided for the management of oedema or hypertension in pregnancy as their use may be associated with hypovolaemia, increased blood viscosity and reduced placental perfusion. There have been reports of foetal bone marrow depression, thrombocytopenia, and foetal and neonatal jaundice associated with the use of thiazide diuretics.

Chlortalidone passes into the breast milk; mothers taking Hygroton should refrain from breast-feeding their infants.

4.7 Effects on ability to drive and use machines

Patients should be warned of the potential hazards of driving or operating machinery if they experience side effects such as dizziness.

4.8 Undesirable effects

Frequency estimate: very rare <0.01%, rare ⩽0.01% to ⩽0.1%;uncommon ⩽0.1% to <1%; common ⩽1% to <10%; very common ⩾10%.

Electrolytes and metabolic disorders:

Very common: mainly at higher doses, hypokalaemia, hyperuricaemia, and rise in blood lipids.

Common: hyponatraemia, hypomagnesaemia and hyperglycaemia.

Uncommon: gout.

Rare: hypercalcaemia, glycosuria, worsening of diabetic metabolic state.

Very rare: hypochloraemic alkalosis.

Skin:

Common: urticaria and other forms of skin rash.

Rare: photosensitisation.

Liver:

Rare: intrahepatic cholestasis or jaundice.

Cardiovascular system:

Common: postural hypotension.

Rare: cardiac arrhythmias.

Central nervous system:

Common: Dizziness.

Rare: paraesthesia, headache.

Gastro-intestinal tract:

Common: loss of appetite and minor gastrointestinal distress.

Rare: mild nausea and vomiting, gastric pain, constipation and diarrhoea.

Very rare: pancreatitis.

Blood:

Rare: Thrombocytopenia, leucopenia, agranulocytosis and eosinophilia.

Other effects:

Common: impotence

Rare: Idiosyncratic pulmonary oedema (respiratory disorders), allergic interstitial nephritis.

4.9 Overdose

Signs and symptoms: In poisoning due to an overdosage the following signs and symptoms may occur: dizziness, nausea, somnolence, hypovolaemia, hypotension and electrolyte disturbances associated with cardiac arrhythmias and muscle spasms.

Treatment: There is no specific antidote to Hygroton. Gastric lavage, emesis or activated charcoal should be employed to reduce absorption. Blood pressure and fluid and electrolyte balance should be monitored and appropriate corrective measures taken. Intravenous fluid and electrolyte replacement may be indicated.

5. PHARMACOLOGICAL PROPERTIES

5.1 Pharmacodynamic properties

Chlortalidone is a benzothiadiazine (thiazide)-related diuretic with a long duration of action.

Thiazide and thiazide-like diuretics act primarily on the distal renal tubule (early convoluted part), inhibiting NaCl reabsorption (by antagonising the Na^+Cl^- cotransporter) and promoting Ca^{++} reabsorption (by an unknown mechanism). The enhanced delivery of Na^+ and water to the cortical collection tubule and/or the increased flow rate leads to increased secretion and excretion of K^+ and H^+.

In persons with normal renal function, diuresis is induced after the administration of 12.5mg Hygroton. The resulting increase in urinary excretion of sodium and chloride and the less prominent increase in urinary potassium are dose dependent and occur both in normal and in oedematous patients. The diuretic effect sets in after 2 to 3 hours, reaches its maximum after 4 to 24 hours, and may persist for 2 to 3 days.

Thiazide-induced diuresis initially leads to decreases in plasma volume, cardiac output, and systemic blood pressure. The renin-angiotensin-aldosterone system may possibly become activated.

In hypertensive individuals, chlortalidone gently reduces blood pressure. On continued administration, the hypotensive effect is maintained, probably due to the fall in peripheral resistance; cardiac output returns to pretreatment values, plasma volume remains somewhat reduced and plasma renin activity may be elevated.

On chronic administration, the antihypertensive effect of Hygroton is dose dependent between 12.5 and 50mg/day. Raising the dose above 50mg increases metabolic complications and is rarely of therapeutic benefit.

As with other diuretics, when Hygroton is given as monotherapy, blood pressure control is achieved in about half of patients with mild to moderate hypertension. In general, elderly and black patients are found to respond well to diuretics given as primary therapy. Randomised clinical trials in the elderly have shown that treatment of hypertension or predominant systolic hypertension in older persons with low-dose thiazide diuretics, including chlortalidone, reduces cerebrovascular (stroke), coronary heart and total cardiovascular morbidity and mortality.

Combined treatment with other antihypertensives potentiates the blood-pressure lowering effects. In the large proportion of patients failing to respond adequately to monotherapy, a further decrease in blood pressure can thus be achieved.

In renal diabetes insipidus, Hygroton paradoxically reduces polyuria. The mechanism of action has not been elucidated.

5.2 Pharmacokinetic properties

Absorption and plasma concentration

The bioavailability of an oral dose of 50mg Hygroton is approximately 64%, peak blood concentrations being attained after 8 to 12 hours. For doses of 25 and 50mg, C_{max} values average 1.5μg/ml (4.4μmol/L) and 3.2μg/ml (9.4μmol/L) respectively. For doses up to 100mg there is a proportional increase in AUC. On repeated daily doses of 50mg, mean steady-state blood concentrations of 7.2μg/ml (21.2μmol/L), measured at the end of the 24 hour dosage interval, are reached after 1 to 2 weeks.

Distribution

In blood, only a small fraction of chlortalidone is free, due to extensive accumulation in erythrocytes and binding to plasma proteins. Owing to the large degree of high affinity binding to the carbonic anhydrase of erythrocytes, only some 1.4% of the total amount of chlortalidone in whole blood was found in plasma at steady state during treatment with 50mg doses. *In vitro*, plasma protein binding of chlortalidone is about 76% and the major binding protein is albumin.

Chlortalidone crosses the placental barrier and passes into the breast milk. In mothers treated with 50mg chlortalidone daily before and after delivery, chlortalidone levels in fetal whole blood are about 15% of those found in maternal blood. Chlortalidone concentrations in amniotic fluid and in the maternal milk are approximately 4% of the corresponding maternal blood level.

Metabolism

Metabolism and hepatic excretion into bile constitute a minor pathway of elimination. Within 120 hours, about 70% of the dose is excreted in the urine and the faeces, mainly in unchanged form.

Elimination

Chlortalidone is eliminated from whole blood and plasma with an elimination half-life averaging 50 hours. The elimination half-life is unaltered after chronic administration. The major part of an absorbed dose of chlortalidone is excreted by the kidneys, with a mean renal clearance of 60ml/min.

Special patient groups

Renal dysfunction does not alter the pharmacokinetics of chlortalidone, the rate-limiting factor in the elimination of the drug from blood or plasma being most probably the affinity of the drug to the carbonic anhydrase of erythrocytes.

No dosage adjustment is needed in patients with impaired renal function.

In elderly patients, the elimination of chlortalidone is slower than in healthy young adults, although absorption is the same. Therefore, close medical observation is indicated when treating patients of advanced age with chlortalidone.

5.3 Preclinical safety data

There are no pre-clinical data of relevance to the prescriber which are additional to those already included in other sections of the Summary of Product Characteristics.

6. PHARMACEUTICAL PARTICULARS

6.1 List of excipients

Microcrystalline cellulose, silicon dioxide, maize starch, magnesium stearate, sodium carboxymethyl cellulose, yellow iron oxide (E172).

6.2 Incompatibilities

None known.

6.3 Shelf life

Five years.

6.4 Special precautions for storage

None.

6.5 Nature and contents of container

Aluminium/PVC blister packs of 28 tablets.

6.6 Special precautions for disposal and other handling

None

Administrative Data

7. MARKETING AUTHORISATION HOLDER

Alliance Pharmaceuticals Ltd

Avonbridge House

Bath Road

Chippenham

Wiltshire

SN15 2BB

8. MARKETING AUTHORISATION NUMBER(S)
PL16853/0007

9. DATE OF FIRST AUTHORISATION/RENEWAL OF THE AUTHORISATION
25 June 1998

10. DATE OF REVISION OF THE TEXT
February 2004

11. Legal status
POM

Alliance, Alliance Pharmaceuticals and associated devices are registered Trademarks of Alliance Pharmaceuticals Ltd.

Hyoscine Injection BP 400mcg/ml (UCB Pharma Ltd)

(UCB Pharma Limited)

1. NAME OF THE MEDICINAL PRODUCT
Hyoscine Injection BP 400mcg/ml

2. QUALITATIVE AND QUANTITATIVE COMPOSITION
Hyoscine hydrobromide EP 0.04% w/v
For excipients, see 6.1

3. PHARMACEUTICAL FORM
Solution for Injection

4. CLINICAL PARTICULARS

4.1 Therapeutic indications
Due to its anticholinergic activity, hyoscine injection is used as a preoperative medication to control bronchial, nasal pharyngeal and salivary secretions, to prevent bronchospasms and laryngospasm and to block cardiac vagal inhibiting reflexes during induction of anaesthesia and intubation.

4.2 Posology and method of administration
Adults: For pre-medication a dose of 200 to 600 micrograms is given by the subcutaneous or intramuscular route 30 to 60 minutes before induction of anaesthesia.

The injection may if required also be given by the intravenous route for acute use.

Children: A dose of 15mcg/kg is recommended in children.

Elderly: Hyoscine is not recommended for use in the elderly.

4.3 Contraindications
Porphyria; hypersensitivity to hyoscine; narrow angle glaucoma.

4.4 Special warnings and precautions for use
Caution is necessary in treating patients with cardiovascular disease, gastrointestinal obstruction, paralytic ileus, prostatic enlargement, Down's Syndrome, myasthenia gravis, renal or hepatic impairment.

Because hyoscine may cause drowsiness, patients must not drive or operate machinery. Patients should avoid alcohol.

Heat prostration can occur, at high ambient temperatures due to decreased sweating.

There have been rare reports of an increase in frequency of seizures in epileptic patients.

4.5 Interaction with other medicinal products and other forms of interaction
Caution is necessary in treating patients with cardiovascular disease, gastrointestinal obstruction, paralytic ileus, prostatic enlargement, Down's Syndrome, myasthenia gravis, renal or hepatic impairment.

Because hyoscine may cause drowsiness, patients must not drive or operate machinery. Patients should avoid alcohol.

Heat prostration can occur, at high ambient temperatures due to decreased sweating.

There have been rare reports of an increase in frequency of seizures in epileptic patients.

4.6 Pregnancy and lactation
The antimuscarinic side-effect can be increased by concomitant administration of disopyramide, tricyclic and MAOI drugs, antihistamines, phenothiazines, amantadine and alcohol. Reduced effect of sub-lingual nitrates.

4.7 Effects on ability to drive and use machines
Because hyoscine may cause drowsiness, patients must not drive or operate machinery.

4.8 Undesirable effects
The most common side effects are drowsiness, dry mouth, dizziness, blurred vision and difficulty with micturition. Other reported effects include bradycardia, idiosyncratic reactions, mental confusion or excitement, dyspnoea, angioedema, anaphylaxis and anaphylactic shock.

4.9 Overdose
Symptoms of overdose may include dilated pupils, tachycardia, rapid respiration, hyperpyrexia, restlessness, excitement, delirium and hallucinations. In the unlikely event of overdosage, supportive therapy should be implemented. Physostigmine by slow intravenous injection in a dose of 1 to 4mg has been used to reverse the anticholinergic effects, but this drug is rapidly metabolised. Neostigmine by slow intravenous injection in a dose of 0.5 to 2 mg antagonises only the peripheral effects. Diazepam may be given to control excitement.

5. PHARMACOLOGICAL PROPERTIES

5.1 Pharmacodynamic properties
Hyoscine is an anticholinergic drug which inhibits the muscarinic actions of acetylcholine at post ganglionic parasympathetic neuroeffector sites including smooth muscle, secretary glands and CNS sites. Small doses effectively inhibit salivary and bronchial secretions and sweating and provide a degree of amnesia. Hyoscine is a more powerful suppressor of salivation than atropine and usually slows rather than increases heart rate.

5.2 Pharmacokinetic properties
Hyoscine is rapidly absorbed following IV or IM injection and is reversibly bound to plasma protein. Hyoscine is reported to cross the placenta and blood brain barrier. Hyoscine is almost completely metabolised by the liver and excreted in the urine. In one study in man, 3.4% of a single dose, administered by subcutaneous injection was excreted unchanged in urine within 72 hours.

5.3 Preclinical safety data
None stated.

6. PHARMACEUTICAL PARTICULARS

6.1 List of excipients
Hydrobromic acid

Sodium hydroxide

Water for Injections

6.2 Incompatibilities
None stated.

6.3 Shelf life
36 months.

6.4 Special precautions for storage
Store below 25°C and protect from light.

6.5 Nature and contents of container
1ml neutral glass (Type I) ampoules in packs of 5 or 10.

Not all pack sizes may be marketed.

6.6 Special precautions for disposal and other handling
None stated.

7. MARKETING AUTHORISATION HOLDER
UCB Pharma Limited

208 Bath Road

Slough

Berkshire

SL1 3WE

UK

8. MARKETING AUTHORISATION NUMBER(S)
PL 00039/5677R

9. DATE OF FIRST AUTHORISATION/RENEWAL OF THE AUTHORISATION
Granted: 5 June 1987

Renewed: 17 June 199310 November 1998

10. DATE OF REVISION OF THE TEXT
Approved: April 2009

Hypnomidate

(Janssen-Cilag Ltd)

1. NAME OF THE MEDICINAL PRODUCT
Hypnomidate® 2 mg/ml Injection

2. QUALITATIVE AND QUANTITATIVE COMPOSITION
Each ml of Hypnomidate contains etomidate 2 mg.

3. PHARMACEUTICAL FORM
Solution for injection.

4. CLINICAL PARTICULARS

4.1 Therapeutic indications
Hypnomidate is an intravenous induction agent of anaesthesia.

4.2 Posology and method of administration
For intravenous administration.

Adults and children:

A dose of 0.3 mg/kg given intravenously at induction of anaesthesia, gives sleep lasting from 6 to 10 minutes.

Elderly:

A dose of 0.15-0.2 mg/kg bodyweight should be given and the dose should be further adjusted according to effects. (see Section 4.4 Special Warnings and Precautions for Use).

Since Hypnomidate has no analgesic action, appropriate analgesics should be used in procedures involving painful stimuli.

Do not exceed a total dose of 30 ml (3 ampoules).

Hypnomidate should only be given by slow intravenous injection.

Hypnomidate may be diluted with sodium chloride infusion BP or dextrose infusion BP but it is not compatible with compound sodium lactate infusion BP (Hartmann's solution). Combinations with pancuronium bromide may show a very slight opalescence; for this reason the two should not be mixed together.

4.3 Contraindications
Hypnomidate is contraindicated in patients with known hypersensitivity to etomidate.

4.4 Special warnings and precautions for use
Warnings: In patients with liver cirrhosis, or in those who have already received neuroleptic, opiate or sedative agents, the dose of etomidate should be reduced.

When Hypnomidate is used, resuscitation equipment should be readily available to manage apnoea. In cases of adrenocortical gland dysfunction and during very long surgical procedures, a prophylactic cortisol supplement may be required (for example 50 to 100 mg hydrocortisone).

Reduced serum cortisol levels, unresponsive to ACTH injections, have been reported in some patients during induction of anaesthesia but particularly during maintenance of anaesthesia with etomidate; for this reason etomidate should not be used for maintenance. However, when etomidate is used for induction, the post-operative rise in serum cortisol which has been observed after thiopentone induction is delayed for approximately 3-6 hours.

Hypnomidate should not be administered to patients with evidence or suggestion of reduced adrenal cortical function.

Hypnomidate should be used with caution in elderly patients, since the potential exists for decreases in cardiac output, which have been reported with doses greater than recommended (see Section 4.2 Posology and Method of Administration for recommended dose in the elderly).

Convulsions may occur in unpremedicated patients.

Precautions: Hypnomidate by injection should be given slowly.

4.5 Interaction with other medicinal products and other forms of interaction
Sedative drugs potentiate the hypnotic effect of Hypnomidate.

Hypnomidate is pharmacologically compatible with the muscle relaxants, premedicant drugs and inhalation anaesthetics in current clinical use.

4.6 Pregnancy and lactation
Hypnomidate has no primary effect on fertility, nor primary embryotoxic or teratogenic effects. At maternally toxic doses in rats, decreased survival was noted. Safety in human pregnancy has not been established. As with other drugs, the possible risks should be weighed against the potential benefits before the drug is administered during pregnancy. Hypnomidate may cross the placental barrier during obstetric anaesthesia.

Lactation: It is not known whether etomidate is excreted in human milk. However, caution should be exercised when Hypnomidate is administered to a nursing mother.

4.7 Effects on ability to drive and use machines
Not applicable, but no effects likely. After very short surgical procedures (up to 15 minutes) the patient regains normal alertness 30 to 60 minutes after waking. After long operations, normal alertness is regained after 4 to 24 hours, depending on the duration of the operation.

4.8 Undesirable effects
The use of narcotic analgesics or diazepam as premedication and during surgery will reduce the uncontrolled spontaneous muscle movements shown by some patients after Hypnomidate administration.

Pain can occur after injection into the small veins of the dorsum of the hand. Use of larger veins or an intravenous application of a small dose of fentanyl 1-2 minutes before induction reduces pain on injection. In a small number of patients, thrombophlebitis has been reported.

Nausea and/or vomiting may occur although these are mainly as a result of concurrent use of opiates. Coughing, hiccough and/or shivering may also be experienced. Allergic reactions, including rare cases of bronchospasm and anaphylactoid reactions, have been reported. Rare cases of laryngospasm, cardiac arrhythmias and convulsions have also been reported.

A slight and transient drop in blood pressure may occur due to a reduction of the peripheral vascular resistance. In vulnerable patients, special care should be exercised to minimise this effect.

Respiratory depression and apnoea may occur.

4.9 Overdose
Overdosing is likely to result in prolonged anaesthesia with the possibility of respiratory depression and even arrest. Hypotension has also been observed. General supportive measures and close observation are recommended. In addition, administration of 50 -100 mg hydrocortisone (not ACTH) may be required for depression of cortisol secretion.

5. PHARMACOLOGICAL PROPERTIES

5.1 Pharmacodynamic properties
ATC code N01AX07

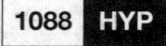

Etomidate is a short acting intravenous hypnotic which is rapidly inactivated by enzyme metabolism so that it does not give rise to a hangover effect. It does not release histamine, and has no effect on liver function. *In vitro* studies have shown etomidate to be an inhibitor of microsomal enzymes. Limited *in vivo* studies have demonstrated only minimal inhibition of hepatic metabolism.

5.2 Pharmacokinetic properties

Profile in Plasma

After intravenous administration, the time-course of the etomidate plasma levels can be described by a three-compartment model reflecting distribution, metabolism, and elimination processes. Plasma concentrations decrease rapidly for about 30 minutes and then more slowly; traces are still detectable after about 6 hours. Metabolites, chiefly of hydrolysis, are more slowly excreted.

Distribution

Etomidate is approximately 76.5% bound to plasma proteins. Etomidate is rapidly distributed to the brain and other tissues. Its volume of distribution is about 4.5 L/kg.

Metabolism and Elimination

Etomidate is metabolized in the liver. After 24 hours, 75% of the administered dose of etomidate has been eliminated in the urine primarily as metabolites. Only 2% of etomidate is excreted unchanged via the urine. The terminal half-life of about 3 to 5 hours reflects the slow distribution of etomidate from the deep peripheral compartment.

5.3 Preclinical safety data

No relevant information other than that contained elsewhere in the Summary of Product Characteristics.

6. PHARMACEUTICAL PARTICULARS

6.1 List of excipients

Propylene glycol

Water for injections

1N sodium hydroxide*

1N hydrochloric acid*

* for occasional pH adjustment only

6.2 Incompatibilities

Combinations with pancuronium bromide may show a very slight opalescence; for this reason the two should not be mixed together.

6.3 Shelf life

5 years.

6.4 Special precautions for storage

Store at room temperature.

6.5 Nature and contents of container

Colourless glass ampoule, PhEur Type I, containing 10 ml Hypnomidate, in packs of 5 and 10 ampoules.

Not all pack sizes may be marketed

6.6 Special precautions for disposal and other handling

None stated.

7. MARKETING AUTHORISATION HOLDER

Janssen-Cilag Limited

50-100 Holmers Farm Way

High Wycombe

Buckinghamshire

HP12 4EG

UK

8. MARKETING AUTHORISATION NUMBER(S)

PL 0242/0019

9. DATE OF FIRST AUTHORISATION/RENEWAL OF THE AUTHORISATION

27 October 1978/20 March 2004

10. DATE OF REVISION OF THE TEXT

17 March 2009

Hypnovel 10mg/2ml

(Roche Products Limited)

1. NAME OF THE MEDICINAL PRODUCT

Hypnovel Ampoules 10mg/2ml

2. QUALITATIVE AND QUANTITATIVE COMPOSITION

Active ingredient: midazolam as hydrochloride.

Ampoules 10mg/2ml; for i.v., i.m. and rectal administration.

For excipients, see 6.1.

3. PHARMACEUTICAL FORM

Solution for injection

4. CLINICAL PARTICULARS

4.1 Therapeutic indications

Hypnovel is a short-acting sleep-inducing drug that is indicated:

In adults

- CONSCIOUS SEDATION before and during diagnostic or therapeutic procedures with or without local anaesthesia
- ANAESTHESIA
  - Premedication before induction of anaesthesia
  - Induction of anaesthesia
  - As a sedative component in combined anaesthesia
- SEDATION IN INTENSIVE CARE UNITS

In children

- CONSCIOUS SEDATION before and during diagnostic or therapeutic procedures with or without local anaesthesia
- ANAESTHESIA
  - Premedication before induction of anaesthesia
- SEDATION IN INTENSIVE CARE UNITS

4.2 Posology and method of administration

STANDARD DOSAGE

Midazolam is a potent sedative agent that requires titration and slow administration. Titration is strongly recommended to safely obtain the desired level of sedation according to the clinical need, physical status, age and concomitant medication. In adults over 60 years, debilitated or chronically ill patients and paediatric patients, dose should be determined with caution and risk factors related to each patient should be taken into account. Standard dosages are provided in the table below. Additional details are provided in the text following the table.

(see Table 1 below)

CONSCIOUS SEDATION DOSAGE

For conscious sedation prior to diagnostic or surgical intervention, midazolam is administered i.v. The dose must be individualised and titrated, and should not be administered by rapid or single bolus injection. The onset of sedation may vary individually depending on the physical status of the patient and the detailed circumstances of dosing (e.g. speed of administration, amount of dose). If necessary, subsequent doses may be administered according to the individual need. The onset of action is about 2 minutes after the injection. Maximum effect is obtained in about 5 to 10 minutes.

Adults

The i.v. injection of midazolam should be given slowly at a rate of approximately 1 mg in 30 seconds.

In adults below the age of 60 the initial dose is 2 to 2.5 mg given 5 to 10 minutes before the beginning of the procedure. Further doses of 1mg may be given as necessary. Mean total doses have been found to range from 3.5 to 7.5 mg. A total dose greater than 5 mg is usually not necessary.

In *adults over 60 years of age*, debilitated or chronically ill patients, the initial dose must be reduced to 0.5-1.0 mg and given 5-10 minutes before the beginning of the procedure. Further doses of 0.5 to 1 mg may be given as necessary. Since in these patients the peak effect may be reached less rapidly, additional midazolam should be titrated very slowly and carefully. A total dose greater than 3.5 mg is usually not necessary.

Children

I.V. administration: midazolam should be titrated slowly to the desired clinical effect. The initial dose of midazolam should be administered over 2 to 3 minutes. One must wait an additional 2 to 5 minutes to fully evaluate the sedative effect before initiating a procedure or repeating a dose. If further sedation is necessary, continue to titrate with small increments until the appropriate level of sedation is achieved. Infants and young children less than 5 years of age may require substantially higher doses (mg/kg) than older children and adolescents.

- Paediatric patients less than 6 months of age: paediatric patients less than 6 months of age are particularly vulnerable to airway obstruction and hypoventilation. For this reason, the use in conscious sedation in children less than 6 months of age is not recommended.
- Paediatric patients 6 months to 5 years of age: initial dose 0.05 to 0.1 mg/kg. A total dose up to 0.6 mg/kg may be necessary to reach the desired endpoint, but the total dose should not exceed 6 mg. Prolonged sedation and risk of hypoventilation may be associated with the higher doses.
- Paediatric patients 6 to 12 years of age: initial dose 0.025 to 0.05 mg/kg. A total dose of up to 0.4 mg/kg to a maximum of 10mg may be necessary. Prolonged sedation and risk of hypoventilation may be associated with the higher doses.
- Paediatric patients 12 to 16 years of age: should be dosed as adults.

Rectal administration: the total dose of midazolam usually ranges from 0.3 to 0.5 mg/kg. Rectal administration of the ampoule solution is performed by means of a plastic applicator fixed on the end of the syringe. If the volume to be administered is too small, water may be added up to a total volume of 10 ml. Total dose should be administered at once and repeated rectal administration avoided.

The use in children less than 6 months of age is not recommended, as available data in this population are limited.

I.M. administration: the doses used range between 0.05 and 0.15 mg/kg. A total dose greater than 10.0 mg is usually not necessary. This route should only be used in exceptional cases. Rectal administration should be preferred as i.m. injection is painful.

In children less than 15 kg of body weight, midazolam solutions with concentrations higher than 1mg/ml are not recommended. Higher concentrations should be diluted to 1 mg/ml.

ANAESTHESIA DOSAGE

PREMEDICATION

Premedication with midazolam given shortly before a procedure produces sedation (induction of sleepiness or drowsiness and relief of apprehension) and preoperative impairment of memory. Midazolam can also be administered in combination with anticholinergics. For this indication midazolam should be administered i.v. or i.m., deep into a large muscle mass 20 to 60 minutes before induction of anaesthesia, or preferably via the rectal route in children (see below). Close and continuous monitoring of the patients after administration of premedication is mandatory as interindividual sensitivity varies and symptoms of overdose may occur.

Table 1

Indication	**Adults** < **60 y**	**Adults** ⩾ **60 y / debilitated or chronically ill**	**Children**
Conscious sedation	*i.v.* Initial dose: 2 - 2.5 mg Titration doses: 1 mg Total dose: 3.5 - 7.5 mg	*i.v* Initial dose: 0.5 - 1 mg Titration doses: 0.5 - 1 mg Total dose: < 3.5 mg	*i.v. in patients 6 months - 5 years* Initial dose: 0.05 - 0.1 mg/kg Total dose: < 6 mg *i.v. in patients 6-12 years* Initial dose: 0.025 - 0.05 mg/kg Total dose: < 10 mg *rectal > 6 months* 0.3 - 0.5 mg/kg *i.m. 1 - 15 years* 0.05 - 0.15 mg/kg
Anaesthesia premedication	*i.v.* 1-2 mg repeated *i.m.* 0.07 - 0.1 mg/kg	*i.v.* Initial dose: 0.5 mg Slow uptitration as needed *i.m.* 0.025 - 0.05 mg/kg	*rectal > 6 months* 0.3 - 0.5 mg/kg *i.m. 1 - 15 years* 0.08 - 0.2 mg/kg
Anaesthesia induction	*i.v.* 0.15 - 0.2 mg/kg (0.3 -0.35 without premedication)	*i.v.* 0.05-0.15 mg/kg (0.15 -0.3 without premedication)	
Sedative component in combined anaesthesia	*i.v.* intermittent doses of 0.03 - 0.1 mg/kg or continuous infusion of 0.03 -0.1 mg/kg/h	*i.v.* lower doses than recommended for adults <60 years	
Sedation in ICU	*i.v.* Loading dose: 0.03 - 0.3mg/kg in increments of 1 - 2.5 mg Maintenance dose: 0.03 - 0.2 mg/kg/h		*i.v. in neonates < 32 weeks gestational age* *0.03 mg/kg/h* *i.v in neonates > 32 weeks and children up to 6 months* *0.06 mg/kg/h* *i.v. in patients > 6 months of age* *Loading dose: 0.05 - 0.2 mg/kg* *Maintenance dose: 0.06 - 0.12 mg/kg/h*

Adults

For preoperative sedation and to impair memory of preoperative events, the recommended dose for adults of ASA Physical Status I & II and below 60 years is 1-2 mg i.v. repeated as needed, or 0.07 to 0.1 mg/kg administered i.m. The dose must be reduced and individualised when midazolam is administered to adults over 60 years of age, debilitated or chronically ill patients. The recommended initial i.v. dose is 0.5 mg and should be slowly uptitrated as needed. A dose of 0.025 to 0.05 mg/kg administered i.m. is recommended. In case of concomitant administration of narcotics the midazolam dose should be reduced. The usual dose is 2 to 3 mg.

Paediatric Patients

Neonates and children up to 6 months of age:

The use in children less than 6 months of age is not recommended as available data are limited.

Children over 6 months of age

Rectal administration: The total dose of midazolam, usually ranging from 0.3 to 0.5 mg/kg should be administered 15 to 30 minutes before induction of anaesthesia. Rectal administration of the ampoule solution is performed by means of a plastic applicator fixed on the end of the syringe. If the volume to be administered is too small, water may be added up to a total volume of 10 ml.

I.M. administration: As i.m. injection is painful, this route should only be used in exceptional cases. Rectal administration should be preferred. However, a dose range from 0.08 to 0.2 mg/kg of midazolam administered i.m. has been shown to be effective and safe. In children between ages 1 and 15 years, proportionally higher doses are required than in adults in relation to body-weight.

In children less than 15 kg of body weight, midazolam solutions with concentrations higher than 1 mg/ml are not recommended. Higher concentrations should be diluted to 1 mg/ml.

INDUCTION

Adults

If midazolam is used for induction of anaesthesia before other anaesthetic agents have been administered, the individual response is variable. The dose should be titrated to the desired effect according to the patient's age and clinical status. When midazolam is used before or in combination with other i.v. or inhalation agents for induction of anaesthesia, the initial dose of each agent should be significantly reduced, at times to as low as 25% of the usual initial dose of the individual agents.

The desired level of anaesthesia is reached by stepwise titration. The i.v. induction dose of midazolam should be given slowly in increments. Each increment of not more than 5 mg should be injected over 20 to 30 seconds allowing 2 minutes between successive increments.

- In *premedicated adults below the age of 60 years*, an i.v. dose of 0.15 to 0.2 mg/kg will usually suffice.
- In *non-premedicated adults below the age of 60* the dose may be higher (0.3 to 0.35 mg/kg i.v.). If needed to complete induction, increments of approximately 25% of the patient's initial dose may be used. Induction may instead be completed with inhalational anaesthetics. In resistant cases, a total dose of up to 0.6 mg/kg may be used for induction, but such larger doses may prolong recovery.
- In *premedicated adults over 60 years of age, debilitated or chronically ill patients,* the dose should significantly be reduced, eg., down to 0.05- 0.15 mg/kg administered i.v. over 20 -30 seconds and allowing 2 minutes for effect.
- *Non-premedicated adults over 60 years of age* usually require more midazolam for induction; an initial dose of 0.15 to 0.3 mg/kg is recommended. Non-premedicated patients with severe systemic disease or other debilitation usually require less midazolam for induction. An initial dose of 0.15 to 0.25 mg/kg will usually suffice.

SEDATIVE COMPONENT IN COMBINED ANAESTHESIA

Adults

Midazolam can be given as a sedative component in combined anaesthesia by either further intermittent small i.v. doses (range between 0.03 and 0.1 mg/kg) or continuous infusion of i.v. midazolam (range between 0.03 and 0.1 mg/kg/h) typically in combination with analgesics. The dose and the intervals between doses vary according to the patient's individual reaction.

In adults over 60 years of age, debilitated or chronically ill patients, lower maintenance doses will be required.

SEDATION IN INTENSIVE CARE UNITS

The desired level of sedation is reached by stepwise titration of midazolam followed by either continuous infusion or intermittent bolus, according to the clinical need, physical status, age and concomitant medication (see section 4.5).

Adults

I.V. loading dose: 0.03 to 0.3 mg/kg should be given slowly in increments. Each increment of 1 to 2.5 mg should be injected over 20 to 30 seconds allowing 2 minutes between successive increments. In hypovolaemic, vasoconstricted, or hypothermic patients the loading dose should be reduced or omitted. When midazolam is given with potent analgesics, the latter should be administered first so that the sedative effects of midazolam can be safely titrated on top of any sedation caused by the analgesic.

I.V. maintenance dose: doses can range from 0.03 to 0.2 mg/kg/h. In hypovolaemic, vasoconstricted, or hypothermic patients the maintenance dose should be reduced. The level of sedation should be assessed regularly. With long-term sedation, tolerance may develop and the dose may have to be increased.

Neonates and children up to 6 months of age

Midazolam should be given as a continuous i.v. infusion, starting at 0.03 mg/kg/h (0.5 µg/kg/min) in neonates with a gestational age <32 weeks, or 0.06 mg/kg/h (1 µg/kg/min) in neonates with a gestational age >32 weeks and children up to 6 months.

Intravenous loading doses is not recommended in premature infants, neonates and children up to 6 months, rather the infusion may be run more rapidly for the first several hours to establish therapeutic plasma levels. The rate of infusion should be carefully and frequently reassessed, particularly after the first 24 hours so as to administer the lowest possible effective dose and reduce the potential for drug accumulation.

Careful monitoring of respiratory rate and oxygen saturation is required.

Children over 6 months of age

In intubated and ventilated paediatric patients, a loading dose of 0.05 to 0.2 mg/kg i.v. should be administered slowly over at least 2 to 3 minutes to establish the desired clinical effect. Midazolam should not be administered as a rapid intravenous dose. The loading dose is followed by a continuous i.v. infusion at 0.06 to 0.12 mg/kg/h (1 to 2 µg/kg/min). The rate of infusion can be increased or decreased (generally by 25% of the initial or subsequent infusion rate) as required, or supplemental i.v. doses of midazolam can be administered to increase or maintain the desired effect.

When initiating an infusion with midazolam in haemodynamically compromised patients, the usual loading dose should be titrated in small increments and the patient monitored for haemodynamic instability, e.g., hypotension. These patients are also vulnerable to the respiratory depressant effects of midazolam and require careful monitoring of respiratory rate and oxygen saturation.

In premature infants, neonates and children less than 15 kg of body weight, midazolam solutions with concentrations higher than 1mg/ml are not recommended. Higher concentrations should be diluted to 1mg/ml.

Use in Special Populations

Renal Impairment

In patients with renal impairment (creatinine clearance < 10 ml/min) the pharmacokinetics of unbound midazolam following a single IV dose is similar to that reported in healthy volunteers. However, after prolonged infusion in intensive care unit (ICU) patients, the mean duration of the sedative effect in the renal failure population was considerably increased most likely due to accumulation of α-hydroxymidazolam glucuronide.

There is no specific data in patients with severe renal impairment (creatinine clearance below 30 ml/min) receiving midazolam for induction of anaesthesia.

Hepatic Impairment

Hepatic impairment reduces the clearance of i.v. midazolam with a subsequent increase in terminal half-life. Therefore the clinical effects may be stronger and prolonged. The required dose of midazolam may be reduced and proper monitoring of vital signs should be established. (See section 4.4).

Paediatric population

See above and section 4.4.

4.3 Contraindications

Use of this drug in patients with known hypersensitivity to benzodiazepines or to any excipient of the product.

Use of this drug for conscious sedation in patients with severe respiratory failure or acute respiratory depression.

4.4 Special warnings and precautions for use

Midazolam should be administered only by experienced physicians in a setting fully equipped for the monitoring and support of respiratory and cardiovascular function and by persons specifically trained in the recognition and management of expected adverse events including respiratory and cardiac resuscitation.

Severe cardiorespiratory adverse events have been reported. These have included respiratory depression, apnoea, respiratory arrest and/or cardiac arrest. Such life-threatening incidents are more likely to occur when the injection is given too rapidly or when a high dosage is administered (see section 4.8).

Special caution is required for the indication of conscious sedation in patients with impaired respiratory function.

Paediatric patients less than 6 months of age are particularly vulnerable to airway obstruction and hypoventilation, therefore titration with small increments to clinical effect and careful respiratory rate and oxygen saturation monitoring are essential.

When midazolam is used for premedication, adequate observation of the patient after administration is mandatory as interindividual sensitivity varies and symptoms of overdose may occur.

Special caution should be exercised when administering midazolam to high-risk patients:

- adults over 60 years of age
- chronically ill or debilitated patients, e.g.
- patients with chronic respiratory insufficiency
- patients with chronic renal failure, impaired hepatic function or with impaired cardiac function
- paediatric patients specially those with cardiovascular instability.

These high-risk patients require lower dosages (see section 4.2) and should be continuously monitored for early signs of alterations of vital functions.

As with any substance with CNS depressant and/or muscle-relaxant properties, particular care should be taken when administering midazolam to a patient with myasthenia gravis.

Tolerance

Some loss of efficacy has been reported when midazolam was used as long-term sedation in intensive care units (ICU).

Dependence

When midazolam is used in long-term sedation in ICU, it should be borne in mind that physical dependence on midazolam may develop. The risk of dependence increases with dose and duration of treatment it is also greater in patients with a medical history of alcohol and/or drug abuse (see section 4.8).

Withdrawal symptoms

During prolonged treatment with midazolam in ICU, physical dependence may develop. Therefore, abrupt termination of the treatment will be accompanied by withdrawal symptoms. The following symptoms may occur: headaches, muscle pain, anxiety, tension, restlessness, confusion, irritability, rebound insomnia, mood changes, hallucinations and convulsions. Since the risk of withdrawal symptoms is greater after abrupt discontinuation of treatment, it is recommended to decrease doses gradually.

Amnesia

Midazolam causes anterograde amnesia (frequently this effect is very desirable in situations such as before and during surgical and diagnostic procedures), the duration of which is directly related to the administered dose. Prolonged amnesia can present problems in outpatients, who are scheduled for discharge following intervention. After receiving midazolam parenterally, patients should be discharged from hospital or consulting room only if accompanied by an attendant.

Paradoxical reactions

Paradoxical reactions such as agitation, involuntary movements (including tonic/clonic convulsions and muscle tremor), hyperactivity, hostility, rage reaction, aggressiveness, paroxysmal excitement and assault, have been reported to occur with midazolam. These reactions may occur with high doses and/or when the injection is given rapidly. The highest incidence to such reactions has been reported among children and the elderly.

Altered elimination of midazolam

Midazolam elimination may be altered in patients receiving compounds that inhibit or induce CYP3A4 and the dose of midazolam may need to be adjusted accordingly (see section 4.5).

Midazolam elimination may also be delayed in patients with liver dysfunction, low cardiac output and in neonates (see section 5.2).

Preterm infants and neonates

Due to an increased risk of apnoea, extreme caution is advised when sedating preterm and former preterm non intubated patients. Careful monitoring of respiratory rate and oxygen saturation is required.

Rapid injection should be avoided in the neonatal population.

Neonates have reduced and/or immature organ function and are also vulnerable to profound and/or prolonged respiratory effects of midazolam.

Adverse haemodynamic events have been reported in paediatric patients with cardiovascular instability; rapid intravenous administration should be avoided in this population.

Paediatric patients less than 6 months

In this population, midazolam is indicated for sedation in ICU only. Paediatric patients less than 6 months of age are particularly vulnerable to airway obstruction and hypoventilation, therefore titration with small increments to clinical effect and careful respiratory rate and oxygen saturation monitoring are essential (see also section 'Preterm infants' above).

Concomitant use of alcohol / CNS depressants

The concomitant use of midazolam with alcohol or/and CNS depressants should be avoided. Such concomitant use has the potential to increase the clinical effects of midazolam possibly including severe sedation or clinically relevant respiratory depression (see section 4.5).

Medical history of alcohol or drug abuse

Midazolam as other benzodiazepines should be avoided in patients with a medical history of alcohol or drug abuse.

Discharging criteria

After receiving midazolam, patients should be discharged from hospital or consulting room only when recommended by treating physician and if accompanied by an attendant. It is recommended that the patient is accompanied when returning home after discharge.

4.5 Interaction with other medicinal products and other forms of interaction

Pharmacokinetic Interactions

Midazolam is metabolised by CYP3A4. Inhibitors and inducers of CYP3A4 have the potential to respectively increase and decrease the plasma concentrations and, subsequently, the effects of midazolam thus requiring dose adjustments accordingly. Pharmacokinetic interactions with CYP3A4 inhibitors or inducers are more pronounced for oral as compared to i.v. midazolam, in particular since CYP3A4 also exists in the upper gastro-intestinal tract. This is because for the oral route both systemic clearance and availability will be altered while for the parenteral route only the change in the systemic clearance becomes effective. After a single dose of IV midazolam, the consequence on the maximal clinical effect due to CYP3A4 inhibition will be minor while the duration of effect may be prolonged. However, after prolonged dosing of midazolam, both the magnitude and duration of effect will be increased in the presence of CYP3A4 inhibition.

There are no available studies on CYP3A4 modulation on the pharmacokinetics of midazolam after rectal and intramuscular administration. It is expected that these interactionswill be less pronouncedfor the rectal than for the oral route because the gastro-intestinal tract is by-passed whereas after i.m. administration the effects of CYP3A modulation should not substantially differ from those seen with i.v. midazolam.

It is therefore recommended to carefully monitor the clinical effects and vital signs during the use of midazolam, taking into account that they may be stronger and last longer after co-administration of a CYP3A4 inhibitor, be it given only once. Notably, administration of high doses or long-term infusions of midazolam to patients receiving strong CYP3A4 inhibitors, e.g. during intensive care, may result in long-lasting hypnotic effects, delayed recovery and respiratory depression, thus requiring dose adjustments.

With respect to induction, it should be considered that the inducing process needs several days to reach its maximum effect and also several days to dissipate. Contrary to a treatment of several days with an inducer, a short-term treatment is expected to result in less apparent DDI with midazolam. However, for strong inducers a relevant induction even after short-term treatment cannot be excluded.

Midazolam is not known to change the pharmacokinetics of other drugs.

Drugs that inhibit CYP3A4

Azole antifungals

- Ketoconazole increased the plasma concentrations of intravenous midazolam by 5-fold while the terminal half-life increased by about 3-fold. If parenteral midazolam is co-administered with the strong CYP3A4 inhibitor ketoconazole, it should be done in an intensive care unit (ICU) or similar setting which ensures close clinical monitoring and appropriate medical management in case of respiratory depression and/or prolonged sedation. Staggered dosing and dosage adjustment should be considered, especially if more than a single i.v. dose of midazolam is administered. The same recommendation may apply also for other azole antifungals (see further), since increased sedative effects of IV midazolam, although lesser, are reported.

- Voriconazole increased the exposure of intravenous midazolam by 3-fold whereas its elimination half-life increased by about 3-fold.

- Fluconazole and itraconazole both increased the plasma concentrations of intravenous midazolam by 2 – 3-fold associated with an increase in terminal half-life by 2.4-fold for itraconazole and 1.5-fold for fluconazole, respectively.

- Posaconazole increased the plasma concentrations of intravenous midazolam by about 2-fold.

- It should be kept in mind that if midazolam is given orally, its exposure will drastically be higher than the above-mentioned ones, notably with ketoconazole, itraconazole, voriconazole.

Midazolam ampoules are not indicated for oral administration.

Macrolide antibiotics

- Erythromycin resulted in an increase in the plasma concentrations of intravenous midazolam by about 1.6 – 2-fold associated with an increase of the terminal half-life of midazolam by 1.5 – 1.8-fold.

- Clarithromycin increased the plasma concentrations of midazolam by up to 2.5-fold associated with an increase in terminal half-life by 1.5 – 2-fold.

Additional information from oral midazolam

- Roxithromycin: While no information on roxithromycin with IV midazolam is available, the mild effect on the terminal half-life of oral midazolam tablet, increasing by 30%, indicates that the effects of roxithromycin on intravenous midazolam may be minor.

HIV Protease inhibitors

- Saquinavir and other HIV protease inhibitors: Co-administration with protease inhibitors may cause a large increase in the concentration of midazolam. Upon co-administration with ritonavir-boosted lopinavir, the plasma concentrations of intravenous midazolam increased by 5.4-fold, associated with a similar increase in terminal half-life. If parenteral midazolam is coadministered with HIV protease inhibitors, treatment setting should follow the description in the above section for azole antifungals, ketoconazole.

Additional information from oral midazolam

Based on data for other CYP3A4 inhibitors, plasma concentrations of midazolam are expected to be significantly higher when midazolam is given orally. Therefore protease inhibitors should not be co-administered with orally administered midazolam.

Calcium-channel blockers

- Diltiazem: A single dose of diltiazem increased the plasma concentrations of intravenous midazolam by about 25% and the terminal half-life was prolonged by 43%.

Additional information from oral midazolam

- Verapamil / diltiazem increased the plasma concentrations of oral midazolam by 3- and 4-fold, respectively. The terminal- half-life of midazolam was increased by 41% and 49% respectively.

Various drugs/Herbs

- Atorvastatin showed a 1.4-fold increase in plasma concentrations of IV midazolam compared to control group.

Additional information from oral midazolam

- Nefazodone increased the plasma concentrations of oral midazolam by 4.6-fold with an increase of its terminal half-life by 1.6-fold.

- Aprepitant dose dependently increased the plasma concentrations of oral midazolam by 3.3-fold after 80 mg/day associated with an increase in terminal half-life by ca. 2-fold.

Drugs that induce CYP3A4

- Rifampicin decreased the plasma concentrations of intravenous midazolam by about 60% after 7 days of rifampicin 600mg o.d. The terminal half-life decreased by about 50-60%.

Additional information from oral midazolam

- Rifampicin decreased the plasma concentrations of oral midazolam by 96% in healthy subjects and its psychomotor effects were almost totally lost.

- Carbamazepine / phenytoin: Repeat dosages of carbamezepine or phenytoin resulted in a decrease in plasma concentrations of oral midazolam by up to 90% and a shortening of the terminal half-life by 60%.

- Efavirenz: The 5-fold increase in the ratio of the CYP3A4 generated metabolite α-hydroxymidazolam to midazolam confirms its CYP3A4-inducing effect.

Herbs and food

- St John's Wort decreased plasma concentrations of midazolam by about 20 - 40 % associated with a decrease in terminal half-life of about 15 - 17%. Depending on the specific St John's Wort extract, the CYP3A4-inducing effect may vary.

Pharmacodynamic Drug-Drug Interactions (DDI)

The co-administration of midazolam with other sedative/hypnotic agents and CNS depressants, including alcohol, is likely to result in enhanced sedation and respiratory depression.

Examples include opiate derivatives (be they used as analgesics, antitussives or substitutive treatments), antipsychotics, other benzodiazepines used as anxiolytics or hypnotics, barbiturates, propofol, ketamine, etomidate; sedative antidepressants, non recent H1-antihistamines and centrally acting antihypertensive drugs.

Alcohol may markedly enhance the sedative effect of midazolam. Alcohol intake should be strongly avoided in case of midazolam administration (see section 4.4).

Midazolam decreases the minimum alveolar concentration (MAC) of inhalational anaesthetics.

4.6 Pregnancy and lactation

Insufficient data are available on midazolam to assess its safety during pregnancy. Animal studies do not indicate a teratogenic effect, but foetotoxicity was observed as with other benzodiazepines. No data on exposed pregnancies are available for the first two trimesters of pregnancy.

The administration of high doses of midazolam in the last trimester of pregnancy, during labour or when used as an induction agent of anaesthesia for caesarean section has been reported to produce maternal or foetal adverse effects (inhalation risk in mother, irregularities in the foetal heart rate, hypotonia, poor sucking, hypothermia and respiratory depression in the neonate).

Moreover, infants born from mothers who received benzodiazepines chronically during the latter stage of pregnancy may have developed physical dependence and may be at some risk of developing withdrawal symptoms in the postnatal period.

Consequently, midazolam may be used during pregnancy if clearly necessary but it is preferable to avoid using it for caesarean.

The risk for neonate should be taken into account in case of administration of midazolam for any surgery near the term.

Midazolam passes in low quantities into breast milk. Nursing mothers should be advised to discontinue breastfeeding for 24 hours following administration of midazolam.

4.7 Effects on ability to drive and use machines

Sedation, amnesia, impaired attention and impaired muscular function may adversely affect the ability to drive or use machines. Prior to receiving midazolam, the patient should be warned not to drive a vehicle or operate a machine until completely recovered. The physician should decide when these activities may be resumed. It is recommended that the patient is accompanied when returning home after discharge.

4.8 Undesirable effects

The following undesirable effects have been reported (very rarely) to occur when midazolam is injected:

Immune System Disorders: Generalised hypersensitivity reactions (skin reactions, cardiovascular reactions, bronchospasm), anaphylactic shock.

Psychiatric Disorders: Confusional state, euphoric mood, hallucinations.

Paradoxical reactions such as agitation, involuntary movements (including tonic/clonic movements and muscle tremor), hyperactivity, hostility, rage reaction, aggressiveness, paroxysmal excitement and assault, have been reported, particularly among children and the elderly.

Dependence: Use of midazolam - even in therapeutic doses - may lead to the development of physical dependence. After prolonged i.v. administration, discontinuation, especially abrupt discontinuation of the product, may be accompanied by withdrawal symptoms including withdrawal convulsions (see section 4.4).

Nervous System Disorders: Prolonged sedation, decreased alertness, somnolence, headache, dizziness, ataxia, postoperative sedation, anterograde amnesia, the duration of which is directly related to the administered dose. Anterograde amnesia may still be present at the end of the procedure and in isolated cases prolonged amnesia has been reported.

Convulsions have been reported in premature infants and neonates.

Cardiac Disorders: Severe cardiorespiratory adverse events have occurred. These have included cardiac arrest, hypotension, bradycardia, vasodilating effects. Life-threatening incidents are more likely to occur in adults over 60 years of age and those with pre-existing respiratory insufficiency or impaired cardiac function, particularly when the injection is given too rapidly or when a high dosage is administered (see section 4.4).

Respiratory Disorders: Severe cardiorespiratory adverse events including respiratory depression, apnoea, respiratory arrest, dyspnoea, laryngospasm have been reported. Life-threatening incidents are more likely to occur in adults over 60 years of age and those with pre-existing respiratory insufficiency or impaired cardiac function, particularly when the injection is given too rapidly or when a high dosage is administered (see section 4.4). Hiccup.

Gastrointestinal System Disorders: Nausea, vomiting, constipation, dry mouth.

Skin and Appendages Disorders: Skin rash urticaria, pruritus.

General and Application Site Disorders: Fatigue, erythema and pain on injection site, thrombophlebitis, thrombosis.

Injury, Poisoning and Procedural Complications: An increased risk for falls and fractures has been recorded in elderly benzodiazepine users.

4.9 Overdose

Symptoms

Like other benzodiazepines, midazolam commonly causes drowsiness, ataxia, dysarthria and nystagmus. Overdose of midazolam is seldom life-threatening if the drug is taken alone, but may lead to areflexia, apnoea, hypotension, cardiorespiratory depression and in rare cases to coma. Coma, if it occurs, usually lasts a few hours but it may be more protracted and cyclical, particularly in elderly patients. Benzodiazepine respiratory depressant effects are more serious in patients with respiratory disease.

Benzodiazepines increase the effects of other central nervous system depressants, including alcohol.

Treatment

Monitor the patient's vital signs and institute supportive measures as indicated by the patient's clinical state. In particular, patients may require symptomatic treatment for cardiorespiratory effects or central nervous system effects.

If taken orally further absorption should be prevented using an appropriate method e.g. treatment within 1-2 hours with activated charcoal. If activated charcoal is used airway protection is imperative for drowsy patients. In case of mixed ingestion gastric lavage may be considered, however not as a routine measure.

If CNS depression is severe consider the use of flumazenil, a benzodiazepine antagonist. This should only be administered under closely monitored conditions. It has a short half-life (about an hour), therefore patients administered flumazenil will require monitoring after its effects have worn off. Flumazenil is to be used with extreme caution in the presence of drugs that reduce seizure threshold (e.g. tricyclic antidepressants). Refer to the prescribing information for flumazenil, for further information on the correct use of this drug.

5. PHARMACOLOGICAL PROPERTIES

5.1 Pharmacodynamic properties

Pharmacotherapeutic group:

Hypnotics and sedatives (benzodiazepine derivatives), ATC code: N05CD08.

Midazolam is a derivative of the imidazobenzodiazepine group. The free base is a lipophilic substance with low solubility in water.

The basic nitrogen in position 2 of the imidazobenzodiazepine ring system enables the active ingredient of midazolam to form water-soluble salts with acids. These produce a stable and well tolerated injection solution.

The pharmacological action of midazolam is characterised by short duration because of rapid metabolic transformation. Midazolam has a sedative and sleep-inducing effect of pronounced intensity. It also exerts an anxiolytic, an anticonvulsant and a muscle-relaxant effect.

After i.m. or i.v. administration anterograde amnesia of short duration occurs (the patient does not remember events that occurred during the maximal activity of the compound).

5.2 Pharmacokinetic properties

Absorption after i.m. injection

Absorption of midazolam from the muscle tissue is rapid and complete. Maximum plasma concentrations are reached within 30 minutes. The absolute bioavailability after i.m. injection is over 90%.

Absorption after rectal administration

After rectal administration midazolam is absorbed quickly. Maximum plasma concentration is reached in about 30 minutes. The absolute bioavailability is about 50%.

Distribution

When midazolam is injected i.v., the plasma concentration-time curve shows one or two distinct phases of distribution. The volume of distribution at steady state is 0.7 - 1.2 l/kg. 96 - 98% of midazolam is bound to plasma proteins. The major fraction of plasma protein binding is due to albumin. There is a slow and insignificant passage of midazolam into the cerebrospinal fluid. In humans, midazolam has been shown to cross the placenta slowly and to enter foetal circulation. Small quantities of midazolam are found in human milk.

Metabolism

Midazolam is almost entirely eliminated by biotransformation. The fraction of the dose extracted by the liver has been estimated to be 30 - 60%. Midazolam is hydroxylated by the cytochrome P4503A4 isozyme and the major urinary and plasma metabolite is alpha-hydroxymidazolam. Plasma concentrations of alpha-hydroxymidazolam are 12% of those of the parent compound. Alpha-hydroxymidazolam is pharmacologically active, but contributes only minimally (about 10%) to the effects of intravenous midazolam.

Elimination

In healthy volunteers, the elimination half-life of midazolam is between 1.5 - 2.5 hours. Plasma clearance is in the range of 300 - 500ml/min. Midazolam is excreted mainly by renal route (60 - 80% of the injected dose) and recovered as glucuroconjugated alpha-hydroxymidazolam. Less than 1% of the dose is recovered in urine as unchanged drug. The elimination half-life of alpha-hydroxy-midazolam is shorter than 1 hour. When midazolam is given by i.v. infusion, its elimination kinetics do not differ from those following bolus injection.

Pharmacokinetics in special populations

Elderly

In adults over 60 years of age, the elimination half-life may be prolonged up to four times.

Children

The rate of rectal absorption in children is similar to that in adults but the bioavailability is lower (5 - 18%). The elimination half-life after i.v. and rectal administration is shorter in children 3 - 10 years old (1 - 1.5 hours) as compared with that in adults. The difference is consistent with an increased metabolic clearance in children.

Neonates

In neonates the elimination half-life is on average 6 - 12 hours, probably due to liver immaturity and the clearance is reduced (see section 4.4).

Obese

The mean half-life is greater in obese than in non-obese patients (5.9 vs 2.3 hours). This is due to an increase of approximately 50% in the volume of distribution corrected for total body weight. The clearance is not significantly different in obese and non-obese patients.

Patients with hepatic impairment

The elimination half-life in cirrhotic patients may be longer and the clearance smaller as compared to those in healthy volunteers (see section 4.4).

Patients with renal impairment

The elimination half-life in patients with chronic renal failure is similar to that in healthy volunteers.

Critically ill patients

The elimination half-life of midazolam is prolonged up to six times in the critically ill.

Patients with cardiac insufficiency

The elimination half-life is longer in patients with congestive heart failure compared with that in healthy subjects (see section 4.4).

5.3 Preclinical safety data

There are no preclinical data of relevance to the prescriber which are additional to that already included in other sections of the SPC.

6. PHARMACEUTICAL PARTICULARS

6.1 List of excipients

Sodium chloride, hydrochloric acid, sodium hydroxide, water for injection.

6.2 Incompatibilities

Admixture with Hartmann's solution is not recommended, as the potency of midazolam decreases.

6.3 Shelf life

60 months.

6.4 Special precautions for storage

Keep ampoules in the outer carton.

6.5 Nature and contents of container

Clear glass 2ml ampoules.

6.6 Special precautions for disposal and other handling

Hypnovel ampoule solution is stable, both physically and chemically, for up to 24 hours at room temperature when mixed with 500ml infusion fluids containing Dextrose 4% with Sodium Chloride 0.18%, Dextrose 5% or Sodium Chloride 0.9%.

There is no evidence of the adsorption of midazolam onto the plastic of infusion apparatus or syringes.

7. MARKETING AUTHORISATION HOLDER

Roche Products Limited, 6 Falcon Way, Shire Park, Welwyn Garden City, AL7 1TW, United Kingdom.

8. MARKETING AUTHORISATION NUMBER(S)

PL 0031/0126

9. DATE OF FIRST AUTHORISATION/RENEWAL OF THE AUTHORISATION

8 December 1982/22 April 1998

10. DATE OF REVISION OF THE TEXT

13 February 2008

Hypnovel Ampoules 10mg/5ml

(Roche Products Limited)

1. NAME OF THE MEDICINAL PRODUCT

Hypnovel Ampoules 10mg/5ml

2. QUALITATIVE AND QUANTITATIVE COMPOSITION

Active ingredient: midazolam as hydrochloride.

Ampoules 10mg/5ml for i.v., i.m. and rectal administration.

For excipients, see 6.1.

3. PHARMACEUTICAL FORM

Solution for injection.

4. CLINICAL PARTICULARS

4.1 Therapeutic indications

Hypnovel is a short-acting sleep-inducing drug that is indicated:

In adults

- CONSCIOUS SEDATION before and during diagnostic or therapeutic procedures with or without local anaesthesia
- ANAESTHESIA
  - o Premedication before induction of anaesthesia
  - o Induction of anaesthesia
  - o As a sedative component in combined anaesthesia
- SEDATION IN INTENSIVE CARE UNITS

In children

- CONSCIOUS SEDATION before and during diagnostic or therapeutic procedures with or without local anaesthesia
- ANAESTHESIA
  - o Premedication before induction of anaesthesia
- SEDATION IN INTENSIVE CARE UNITS

4.2 Posology and method of administration

STANDARD DOSAGE

Midazolam is a potent sedative agent that requires titration and slow administration. Titration is strongly recommended to safely obtain the desired level of sedation according to the clinical need, physical status, age and concomitant medication. In adults over 60 years, debilitated or chronically ill patients and paediatric patients, dose should be determined with caution and risk factors related to each patient should be taken into account. Standard dosages are provided in the table below. Additional details are provided in the text following the table.

(see Table 1 below)

CONSCIOUS SEDATION DOSAGE

For conscious sedation prior to diagnostic or surgical intervention, midazolam is administered i.v. The dose must be individualised and titrated, and should not be administered by rapid or single bolus injection. The onset of sedation may vary individually depending on the physical status of the patient and the detailed circumstances of dosing (e.g. speed of administration, amount of dose). If necessary, subsequent doses may be administered according to the individual need. The onset of action is about 2 minutes after the injection. Maximum effect is obtained in about 5 to 10 minutes.

Adults

The i.v. injection of midazolam should be given slowly at a rate of approximately 1 mg in 30 seconds.

Table 1

Indication	Adults < 60 y	Adults ≥ 60 y / debilitated or chronically ill	Children
Conscious sedation	*i.v.* Initial dose: 2 - 2.5mg Titration doses: 1mg Total dose: 3.5 - 7.5mg	*i.v.* Initial dose: 0.5 - 1mg Titration doses: 0.5 - 1mg Total dose: < 3.5mg	***i.v. in patients 6 months - 5 years Initial dose***: 0.05 - 0.1mg/kg Total dose: < 6mg ***i.v. in patients 6-12 years*** Initial dose: 0.025 - 0.05mg/kg Total dose: < 10mg ***rectal > 6 months*** 0.3 - 0.5mg/kg ***i.m. 1 - 15 years*** 0.05 - 0.15mg/kg
Anaesthesia premedication	*i.v.* 1-2 mg repeated *i.m.* 0.07 - 0.1mg/kg	*i.v.* Initial dose: 0.5mg Slow uptitration as needed *i.m.* 0.025 - 0.05mg/kg	***rectal > 6 months*** 0.3 - 0.5mg/kg ***i.m. 1 - 15 years*** 0.08 - 0.2mg/kg
Anaesthesia induction	*i.v.* 0.15 - 0.2mg/kg (0.3 -0.35 without premedication)	*i.v.* 0.05-0.15 mg/kg (0.15 -0.3 without premedication)	
Sedative component in combined anaesthesia	*i.v.* intermittent doses of 0.03 - 0.1mg/kg or continuous infusion of 0.03 -0.1mg/kg/h	*i.v.* lower doses than recommended for adults <60 years	
Sedation in ICU	*i.v.* Loading dose: 0.03 - 0.3mg/kg in increments of 1 - 2.5mg Maintenance dose: 0.03 - 0.2mg/kg/h		***i.v. in neonates < 32 weeks gestational age*** 0.03mg/kg/h ***i.v in neonates > 32 weeks and children up to 6 months*** 0.06mg/kg/h ***i.v. in patients > 6 months of age*** Loading dose: 0.05 - 0.2mg/kg Maintenance dose: 0.06 - 0.12mg/kg/h

In adults below the age of 60 the initial dose is 2 to 2.5 mg given 5 to10 minutes before the beginning of the procedure. Further doses of 1mg may be given as necessary. Mean total doses have been found to range from 3.5 to 7.5 mg. A total dose greater than 5 mg is usually not necessary.

In *adults over 60 years of age,* debilitated or chronically ill patients, the initial dose must be reduced to 0.5-1.0 mg and given 5-10 minutes before the beginning of the procedure. Further doses of 0.5 to 1 mg may be given as necessary. Since in these patients the peak effect may be reached less rapidly, additional midazolam should be titrated very slowly and carefully. A total dose greater than 3.5 mg is usually not necessary.

Children

I.V. administration: midazolam should be titrated slowly to the desired clinical effect. The initial dose of midazolam should be administered over 2 to 3 minutes. One must wait an additional 2 to 5 minutes to fully evaluate the sedative effect before initiating a procedure or repeating a dose. If further sedation is necessary, continue to titrate with small increments until the appropriate level of sedation is achieved. Infants and young children less than 5 years of age may require substantially higher doses (mg/kg) than older children and adolescents.

• Paediatric patients less than 6 months of age: paediatric patients less than 6 months of age are particularly vulnerable to airway obstruction and hypoventilation. For this reason, the use in conscious sedation in children less than 6 months of age is not recommended.

• Paediatric patients 6 months to 5 years of age: initial dose 0.05 to 0.1 mg/kg. A total dose up to 0.6 mg/kg may be necessary to reach the desired endpoint, but the total dose should not exceed 6 mg. Prolonged sedation and risk of hypoventilation may be associated with the higher doses.

• Paediatric patients 6 to 12 years of age: initial dose 0.025 to 0.05 mg/kg. A total dose of up to 0.4 mg/kg to a maximum of 10mg may be necessary. Prolonged sedation and risk of hypoventilation may be associated with the higher doses.

• Paediatric patients 12 to 16 years of age: should be dosed as adults.

Rectal administration: the total dose of midazolam usually ranges from 0.3 to 0.5 mg/kg. Rectal administration of the ampoule solution is performed by means of a plastic applicator fixed on the end of the syringe. If the volume to be administered is too small, water may be added up to a total volume of 10 ml. Total dose should be administered at once and repeated rectal administration avoided.

The use in children less than 6 months of age is not recommended, as available data in this population are limited.

I.M. administration: the doses used range between 0.05 and 0.15 mg/kg. A total dose greater than 10.0 mg is usually not necessary. This route should only be used in exceptional cases. Rectal administration should be preferred as i.m. injection is painful.

In children less than 15 kg of body weight, midazolam solutions with concentrations higher than 1mg/ml are not recommended. Higher concentrations should be diluted to 1 mg/ml.

ANAESTHESIA DOSAGE

PREMEDICATION

Premedication with midazolam given shortly before a procedure produces sedation (induction of sleepiness or drowsiness and relief of apprehension) and preoperative impairment of memory. Midazolam can also be administered in combination with anticholinergics. For this indication midazolam should be administered i.v. or i.m., deep into a large muscle mass 20 to 60 minutes before induction of anaesthesia, or preferably via the rectal route in children (see below). Close and continuous monitoring of the patients after administration of premedication is mandatory as interindividual sensitivity varies and symptoms of overdose may occur.

Adults

For preoperative sedation and to impair memory of preoperative events, the recommended dose for adults of ASA Physical Status I and II and below 60 years is 1-2 mg i.v. repeated as needed, or 0.07 to 0.1 mg/kg administered i.m. The dose must be reduced and individualised when midazolam is administered to adults over 60 years of age, debilitated or chronically ill patients. The recommended initial i.v. dose is 0.5 mg and should be slowly uptitrated as needed. A dose of 0.025 to 0.05 mg/kg administered i.m. is recommended. In case of concomitant administration of narcotics the midazolam dose should be reduced. The usual dose is 2 to 3 mg.

Paediatric Patients

Neonates and children up to 6 months of age:

The use in children less than 6 months of age is not recommended as available data are limited.

Children over 6 months of age

Rectal administration: The total dose of midazolam, usually ranging from 0.3 to 0.5 mg/kg should be administered 15 to 30 minutes before induction of anaesthesia. Rectal administration of the ampoule solution is performed by means of a plastic applicator fixed on the end of the syringe. If the volume to be administered is too small, water may be added up to a total volume of 10 ml.

I.M. administration: As i.m. injection is painful, this route should only be used in exceptional cases. Rectal administration should be preferred. However, a dose range from 0.08 to 0.2 mg/kg of midazolam administered i.m. has been shown to be effective and safe. In children between ages 1 and 15 years, proportionally higher doses are required than in adults in relation to body-weight.

In children less than 15 kg of body weight, midazolam solutions with concentrations higher than 1 mg/ml are not recommended. Higher concentrations should be diluted to 1 mg/ml.

INDUCTION

Adults

If midazolam is used for induction of anaesthesia before other anaesthetic agents have been administered, the individual response is variable. The dose should be titrated to the desired effect according to the patient's age and clinical status. When midazolam is used before or in combination with other i.v. or inhalation agents for induction of anaesthesia, the initial dose of each agent should be significantly reduced, at times to as low as 25% of the usual initial dose of the individual agents.

The desired level of anaesthesia is reached by stepwise titration. The i.v. induction dose of midazolam should be given slowly in increments. Each increment of not more than 5 mg should be injected over 20 to 30 seconds allowing 2 minutes between successive increments.

• In *premedicated adults below the age of 60 years,* an i.v. dose of 0.15 to 0.2 mg/kg will usually suffice.

• In *non-premedicated adults below the age of 60* the dose may be higher (0.3 to 0.35 mg/kg i.v.). If needed to complete induction, increments of approximately 25% of the patient's initial dose may be used. Induction may instead be completed with inhalational anaesthetics. In resistant cases, a total dose of up to 0.6 mg/kg may be used for induction, but such larger doses may prolong recovery.

• In *premedicated adults over 60 years of age, debilitated or chronically ill patients,* the dose should significantly be reduced, eg., down to 0.05- 0.15 mg/kg administered i.v. over 20 -30 seconds and allowing 2 minutes for effect.

•*Non-premedicated adults over 60 years* of age usually require more midazolam for induction; an initial dose of 0.15 to 0.3 mg/kg is recommended. Non-premedicated patients with severe systemic disease or other debilitation usually require less midazolam for induction. An initial dose of 0.15 to 0.25 mg/kg will usually suffice.

SEDATIVE COMPONENT IN COMBINED ANAESTHESIA

Adults

Midazolam can be given as a sedative component in combined anaesthesia by either further intermittent small i.v. doses (range between 0.03 and 0.1 mg/kg) or continuous infusion of i.v. midazolam (range between 0.03 and 0.1 mg/kg/h) typically in combination with analgesics. The dose and the intervals between doses vary according to the patient's individual reaction.

In adults over 60 years of age, debilitated or chronically ill patients, lower maintenance doses will be required.

SEDATION IN INTENSIVE CARE UNITS

The desired level of sedation is reached by stepwise titration of midazolam followed by either continuous infusion or intermittent bolus, according to the clinical need, physical status, age and concomitant medication (see section 4.5).

Adults

I.V. loading dose: 0.03 to 0.3 mg/kg should be given slowly in increments. Each increment of 1 to 2.5 mg should be injected over 20 to 30 seconds allowing 2 minutes between successive increments. In hypovolaemic, vasoconstricted, or hypothermic patients the loading dose should be reduced or omitted. When midazolam is given with potent analgesics, the latter should be administered first so that the sedative effects of midazolam can be safely titrated on top of any sedation caused by the analgesic.

I.V. maintenance dose: doses can range from 0.03 to 0.2 mg/kg/h. In hypovolaemic, vasoconstricted, or hypothermic patients the maintenance dose should be reduced. The level of sedation should be assessed regularly. With long-term sedation, tolerance may develop and the dose may have to be increased.

Neonates and children up to 6 months of age

Midazolam should be given as a continuous i.v. infusion, starting at 0.03 mg/kg/h (0.5 µg/kg/min) in neonates with a gestational age <32 weeks, or 0.06 mg/kg/h (1 µg/kg/min) in neonates with a gestational age >32 weeks and children up to 6 months.

Intravenous loading doses is not recommended in premature infants, neonates and children up to 6 months, rather the infusion may be run more rapidly for the first several hours to establish therapeutic plasma levels. The rate of infusion should be carefully and frequently reassessed, particularly after the first 24 hours so as to administer the lowest possible effective dose and reduce the potential for drug accumulation.

Careful monitoring of respiratory rate and oxygen saturation is required.

Children over 6 months of age

In intubated and ventilated paediatric patients, a loading dose of 0.05 to 0.2 mg/kg i.v. should be administered slowly over at least 2 to 3 minutes to establish the desired clinical effect. Midazolam should not be administered as a rapid intravenous dose. The loading dose is followed by a continuous i.v. infusion at 0.06 to 0.12 mg/kg/h (1 to 2 µg/kg/min). The rate of infusion can be increased or decreased (generally by 25% of the initial or subsequent infusion rate) as required, or supplemental i.v. doses of midazolam can be administered to increase or maintain the desired effect.

When initiating an infusion with midazolam in haemodynamically compromised patients, the usual loading dose should be titrated in small increments and the patient monitored for haemodynamic instability, e.g., hypotension. These patients are also vulnerable to the respiratory depressant effects of midazolam and require careful monitoring of respiratory rate and oxygen saturation.

In premature infants, neonates and children less than 15 kg of body weight, midazolam solutions with concentrations higher than 1mg/ml are not recommended. Higher concentrations should be diluted to 1mg/ml.

Use in Special Populations

Renal Impairment

In patients with renal impairment (creatinine clearance < 10 ml/min) the pharmacokinetics of unbound midazolam following a single IV dose is similar to that reported in healthy volunteers. However, after prolonged infusion in intensive care unit (ICU) patients, the mean duration of the sedative effect in the renal failure population was considerably increased most likely due to accumulation of α-hydroxymidazolam glucuronide.

There is no specific data in patients with severe renal impairment (creatinine clearance below 30 ml/min) receiving midazolam for induction of anaesthesia.

Hepatic Impairment

Hepatic impairment reduces the clearance of i.v. midazolam with a subsequent increase in terminal half-life. Therefore the clinical effects may be stronger and prolonged. The required dose of midazolam may be reduced and proper monitoring of vital signs should be established. (See section 4.4).

Paediatric population

See above and section 4.4.

4.3 Contraindications

Use of this drug in patients with known hypersensitivity to benzodiazepines or to any excipient of the product.

Use of this drug for conscious sedation in patients with severe respiratory failure or acute respiratory depression.

4.4 Special warnings and precautions for use

Midazolam should be administered only by experienced physicians in a setting fully equipped for the monitoring and support of respiratory and cardiovascular function and by persons specifically trained in the recognition and management of expected adverse events including respiratory and cardiac resuscitation.

Severe cardiorespiratory adverse events have been reported. These have included respiratory depression, apnoea, respiratory arrest and/or cardiac arrest. Such life-threatening incidents are more likely to occur when the injection is given too rapidly or when a high dosage is administered (see section 4.8).

Special caution is required for the indication of conscious sedation in patients with impaired respiratory function.

Paediatric patients less than 6 months of age are particularly vulnerable to airway obstruction and hypoventilation, therefore titration with small increments to clinical effect and careful respiratory rate and oxygen saturation monitoring are essential.

When midazolam is used for premedication, adequate observation of the patient after administration is mandatory as interindividual sensitivity varies and symptoms of overdose may occur.

Special caution should be exercised when administering midazolam to high-risk patients:

- adults over 60 years of age
- chronically ill or debilitated patients, e.g.
- patients with chronic respiratory insufficiency
- patients with chronic renal failure, impaired hepatic function or with impaired cardiac function
- paediatric patients specially those with cardiovascular instability.

These high-risk patients require lower dosages (see section 4.2) and should be continuously monitored for early signs of alterations of vital functions.

As with any substance with CNS depressant and/or muscle-relaxant properties, particular care should be taken when administering midazolam to a patient with myasthenia gravis.

Tolerance

Some loss of efficacy has been reported when midazolam was used as long-term sedation in intensive care units (ICU).

Dependence

When midazolam is used in long-term sedation in ICU, it should be borne in mind that physical dependence on midazolam may develop. The risk of dependence increases with dose and duration of treatment; it is also greater in patients with a medical history of alcohol and/or drug abuse (see section 4.8).

Withdrawal symptoms

During prolonged treatment with midazolam in ICU, physical dependence may develop. Therefore, abrupt termination of the treatment will be accompanied by withdrawal symptoms. The following symptoms may occur: headaches, muscle pain, anxiety, tension, restlessness, confusion, irritability, rebound insomnia, mood changes, hallucinations and convulsions. Since the risk of withdrawal symptoms is greater after abrupt discontinuation of treatment, it is recommended to decrease doses gradually.

Amnesia

Midazolam causes anterograde amnesia (frequently this effect is very desirable in situations such as before and during surgical and diagnostic procedures), the duration of which is directly related to the administered dose. Prolonged amnesia can present problems in outpatients, who are scheduled for discharge following intervention. After receiving midazolam parenterally, patients should be discharged from hospital or consulting room only if accompanied by an attendant.

Paradoxical reactions

Paradoxical reactions such as agitation, involuntary movements (including tonic/clonic convulsions and muscle tremor), hyperactivity, hostility, rage reaction, aggressiveness, paroxysmal excitement and assault, have been reported to occur with midazolam. These reactions may occur with high doses and/or when the injection is given rapidly. The highest incidence to such reactions has been reported among children and the elderly.

Altered elimination of midazolam

Midazolam elimination may be altered in patients receiving compounds that inhibit or induce CYP3A4 and the dose of midazolam may need to be adjusted accordingly (see section 4.5).

Midazolam elimination may also be delayed in patients with liver dysfunction, low cardiac output and in neonates (see section 5.2).

Preterm infants and neonates

Due to an increased risk of apnoea, extreme caution is advised when sedating preterm and former preterm non intubated patients. Careful monitoring of respiratory rate and oxygen saturation is required.

Rapid injection should be avoided in the neonatal population.

Neonates have reduced and/or immature organ function and are also vulnerable to profound and/or prolonged respiratory effects of midazolam.

Adverse haemodynamic events have been reported in paediatric patients with cardiovascular instability; rapid intravenous administration should be avoided in this population.

Paediatric patients less than 6 months

In this population, midazolam is indicated for sedation in ICU only. Paediatric patients less than 6 months of age are particularly vulnerable to airway obstruction and hypoventilation, therefore titration with small increments to clinical effect and careful respiratory rate and oxygen saturation monitoring are essential (see also section 'Preterm infants' above).

Concomitant use of alcohol / CNS depressants

The concomitant use of midazolam with alcohol or/and CNS depressants should be avoided. Such concomitant use has the potential to increase the clinical effects of midazolam possibly including severe sedation or clinically relevant respiratory depression (see section 4.5).

Medical history of alcohol or drug abuse

Midazolam as other benzodiazepines should be avoided in patients with a medical history of alcohol or drug abuse.

Discharging criteria

After receiving midazolam, patients should be discharged from hospital or consulting room only when recommended by treating physician and if accompanied by an attendant. It is recommended that the patient is accompanied when returning home after discharge.

4.5 Interaction with other medicinal products and other forms of interaction

Pharmacokinetic Interactions

Midazolam is metabolised by CYP3A4. Inhibitors and inducers of CYP3A4 have the potential to respectively increase and decrease the plasma concentrations and, subsequently, the effects of midazolam thus requiring dose adjustments accordingly. Pharmacokinetic interactions with CYP3A4 inhibitors or inducers are more pronounced for oral as compared to i.v. midazolam, in particular since CYP3A4 also exists in the upper gastro-intestinal tract. This is because for the oral route both systemic clearance and availability will be altered while for the parenteral route only the change in the systemic clearance becomes effective. After a single dose of IV midazolam, the consequence on the maximal clinical effect due to CYP3A4 inhibition will be minor while the duration of effect may be prolonged. However, after prolonged dosing of midazolam, both the magnitude and duration of effect will be increased in the presence of CYP3A4 inhibition.

There are no available studies on CYP3A4 modulation on the pharmacokinetics of midazolam after rectal and intramuscular administration. It is expected that these interactionswill be less pronouncedfor the rectal than for the oral route because the gastro-intestinal tract is by-passed whereas after i.m. administration the effects of CYP3A modulation should not substantially differ from those seen with i.v. midazolam.

It is therefore recommended to carefully monitor the clinical effects and vital signs during the use of midazolam, taking into account that they may be stronger and last longer after co-administration of a CYP3A4 inhibitor, be it given only once. Notably, administration of high doses or long-term infusions of midazolam to patients receiving strong CYP3A4 inhibitors, e.g. during intensive care, may result in long-lasting hypnotic effects, delayed recovery and respiratory depression, thus requiring dose adjustments.

With respect to induction, it should be considered that the inducing process needs several days to reach its maximum effect and also several days to dissipate. Contrary to a treatment of several days with an inducer, a short-term treatment is expected to result in less apparent DDI with midazolam. However, for strong inducers a relevant induction even after short-term treatment cannot be excluded.

Midazolam is not known to change the pharmacokinetics of other drugs.

Drugs that inhibit CYP3A4

Azole antifungals

- Ketoconazole increased the plasma concentrations of intravenous midazolam by 5-fold while the terminal half-life increased by about 3-fold. If parenteral midazolam is co-administered with the strong CYP3A4 inhibitor ketoconazole, it should be done in an intensive care unit (ICU) or similar setting which ensures close clinical monitoring and appropriate medical management in case of respiratory depression and/or prolonged sedation. Staggered dosing and dosage adjustment should be considered, especially if more than a single i.v. dose of midazolam is administered. The same recommendation may apply also for other azole antifungals (see further), since increased sedative effects of IV midazolam, although lesser, are reported.
- Voriconazole increased the exposure of intravenous midazolam by 3-fold whereas its elimination half-life increased by about 3-fold.
- Fluconazole and itraconazole both increased the plasma concentrations of intravenous midazolam by 2 – 3-fold associated with an increase in terminal half-life by 2.4-fold for itraconazole and 1.5-fold for fluconazole, respectively.
- Posaconazole increased the plasma concentrations of intravenous midazolam by about 2-fold.
- It should be kept in mind that if midazolam is given orally, its exposure will drastically be higher than the above-mentioned ones, notably with ketoconazole, itraconazole, voriconazole.

Midazolam ampoules are not indicated for oral administration.

Macrolide antibiotics

- Erythromycin resulted in an increase in the plasma concentrations of intravenous midazolam by about 1.6 – 2-fold associated with an increase of the terminal half-life of midazolam by 1.5 – 1.8-fold.
- Clarithromycin increased the plasma concentrations of midazolam by up to 2.5-fold associated with an increase in terminal half-life by 1.5 – 2-fold.

Additional information from oral midazolam

- Roxithromycin: While no information on roxithromycin with IV midazolam is available, the mild effect on the terminal half-life of oral midazolam tablet, increasing by 30%, indicates that the effects of roxithromycin on intravenous midazolam may be minor.

HIV Protease inhibitors

- Saquinavir and other HIV protease inhibitors: Co-administration with protease inhibitors may cause a large increase in the concentration of midazolam. Upon co-administration with ritonavir-boosted lopinavir, the plasma concentrations of intravenous midazolam increased by 5.4-fold, associated with a similar increase in terminal half-life. If parenteral midazolam is coadministered with HIV protease inhibitors, treatment setting should follow the description in the above section for azole antifungals, ketoconazole.

Additional information from oral midazolam

Based on data for other CYP3A4 inhibitors, plasma concentrations of midazolam are expected to be significantly higher when midazolam is given orally. Therefore protease inhibitors should not be co-administered with orally administered midazolam.

Calcium-channel blockers

- Diltiazem: A single dose of diltiazem increased the plasma concentrations of intravenous midazolam by about 25% and the terminal half-life was prolonged by 43%.

Additional information from oral midazolam

- Verapamil / diltiazem increased the plasma concentrations of oral midazolam by 3- and 4-fold, respectively. The terminal- half-life of midazolam was increased by 41% and 49% respectively.

Various drugs/Herbs

- Atorvastatin showed a 1.4-fold increase in plasma concentrations of IV midazolam compared to control group.

Additional information from oral midazolam

- Nefazodone increased the plasma concentrations of oral midazolam by 4.6-fold with an increase of its terminal half-life by 1.6-fold.
- Aprepitant dose dependently increased the plasma concentrations of oral midazolam by 3.3-fold after 80 mg/day associated with an increase in terminal half-life by ca. 2-fold.

Drugs that induce CYP3A4

- Rifampicin decreased the plasma concentrations of intravenous midazolam by about 60% after 7 days of rifampicin 600mg o.d. The terminal half-life decreased by about 50-60%.

Additional information from oral midazolam

- Rifampicin decreased the plasma concentrations of oral midazolam by 96% in healthy subjects and its psychomotor effects were almost totally lost.
- Carbamazepine / phenytoin: Repeat dosages of carbamezepine or phenytoin resulted in a decrease in plasma concentrations of oral midazolam by up to 90% and a shortening of the terminal half-life by 60%.
- Efavirenz: The 5-fold increase in the ratio of the CYP3A4 generated metabolite a-hydroxymidazolam to midazolam confirms its CYP3A4-inducing effect.

Herbs and food

- St John's Wort decreased plasma concentrations of midazolam by about 20 - 40 % associated with a decrease in terminal half-life of about 15 - 17%. Depending on the specific St John's Wort extract, the CYP3A4-inducing effect may vary.

Pharmacodynamic Drug-Drug Interactions (DDI)

The co-administration of midazolam with other sedative/hypnotic agents and CNS depressants, including alcohol, is likely to result in enhanced sedation and respiratory depression.

Examples include opiate derivatives (be they used as analgesics, antitussives or substitutive treatments), antipsychotics, other benzodiazepines used as anxiolytics or hypnotics, barbiturates, propofol, ketamine, etomidate; sedative antidepressants, non recent H1-antihistamines and centrally acting antihypertensive drugs.

Alcohol may markedly enhance the sedative effect of midazolam. Alcohol intake should be strongly avoided in case of midazolam administration (see section 4.4).

Midazolam decreases the minimum alveolar concentration (MAC) of inhalational anaesthetics.

4.6 Pregnancy and lactation

Insufficient data are available on midazolam to assess its safety during pregnancy. Animal studies do not indicate a teratogenic effect, but foetotoxicity was observed as with other benzodiazepines. No data on exposed pregnancies are available for the first two trimesters of pregnancy.

The administration of high doses of midazolam in the last trimester of pregnancy, during labour or when used as an induction agent of anaesthesia for caesarean section has been reported to produce maternal or foetal adverse effects (inhalation risk in mother, irregularities in the foetal heart rate, hypotonia, poor sucking, hypothermia and respiratory depression in the neonate).

Moreover, infants born from mothers who received benzodiazepines chronically during the latter stage of pregnancy may have developed physical dependence and may be at some risk of developing withdrawal symptoms in the postnatal period.

Consequently, midazolam may be used during pregnancy if clearly necessary but it is preferable to avoid using it for caesarean.

The risk for neonate should be taken into account in case of administration of midazolam for any surgery near the term.

Midazolam passes in low quantities into breast milk. Nursing mothers should be advised to discontinue breast-feeding for 24 hours following administration of midazolam.

4.7 Effects on ability to drive and use machines

Sedation, amnesia, impaired attention and impaired muscular function may adversely affect the ability to drive or use machines. Prior to receiving midazolam, the patient should be warned not to drive a vehicle or operate a machine until completely recovered. The physician should decide when these activities may be resumed. It is recommended that the patient is accompanied when returning home after discharge.

4.8 Undesirable effects

The following undesirable effects have been reported (very rarely) to occur when midazolam is injected:

Immune System Disorders: Generalised hypersensitivity reactions (skin reactions, cardiovascular reactions, bronchospasm), anaphylactic shock.

Psychiatric Disorders: Confusional state, euphoric mood, hallucinations.

Paradoxical reactions such as agitation, involuntary movements (including tonic/clonic movements and muscle tremor), hyperactivity, hostility, rage reaction, aggressiveness, paroxysmal excitement and assault, have been reported, particularly among children and the elderly.

Dependence: Use of midazolam - even in therapeutic doses - may lead to the development of physical dependence. After prolonged i.v. administration, discontinuation, especially abrupt discontinuation of the product, may be accompanied by withdrawal symptoms including withdrawal convulsions (see section 4.4).

Nervous System Disorders: Prolonged sedation, decreased alertness, somnolence, headache, dizziness, ataxia, postoperative sedation, anterograde amnesia, the duration of which is directly related to the administered dose. Anterograde amnesia may still be present at the end of the procedure and in isolated cases prolonged amnesia has been reported.

Convulsions have been reported in premature infants and neonates.

Cardiac Disorders: Severe cardiorespiratory adverse events have occurred. These have included cardiac arrest, hypotension, bradycardia, vasodilating effects. Life-threatening incidents are more likely to occur in adults over 60 years of age and those with pre-existing respiratory insufficiency or impaired cardiac function, particularly when the injection is given too rapidly or when a high dosage is administered (see section 4.4).

Respiratory Disorders: Severe cardiorespiratory adverse events including respiratory depression, apnoea, respiratory arrest, dyspnoea, laryngospasm have been reported. Life-threatening incidents are more likely to occur in adults over 60 years of age and those with pre-existing respiratory insufficiency or impaired cardiac function, particularly when the injection is given too rapidly or when a high dosage is administered (see section 4.4). Hiccup.

Gastrointestinal System Disorders: Nausea, vomiting, constipation, dry mouth.

Skin and Appendages Disorders: Skin rash urticaria, pruritus.

General and Application Site Disorders: Fatigue, erythema and pain on injection site, thrombophlebitis, thrombosis.

Injury, Poisoning and Procedural Complications: An increased risk for falls and fractures has been recorded in elderly benzodiazepine users.

4.9 Overdose

Symptoms

Like other benzodiazepines, midazolam commonly causes drowsiness, ataxia, dysarthria and nystagmus. Overdose of midazolam is seldom life-threatening if the drug is taken alone, but may lead to areflexia, apnoea, hypotension, cardiorespiratory depression and in rare cases to coma. Coma, if it occurs, usually lasts a few hours but it may be more protracted and cyclical, particularly in elderly patients. Benzodiazepine respiratory depressant effects are more serious in patients with respiratory disease.

Benzodiazepines increase the effects of other central nervous system depressants, including alcohol.

Treatment

Monitor the patient's vital signs and institute supportive measures as indicated by the patient's clinical state. In particular, patients may require symptomatic treatment for cardiorespiratory effects or central nervous system effects.

If taken orally further absorption should be prevented using an appropriate method e.g. treatment within 1-2 hours with activated charcoal. If activated charcoal is used airway protection is imperative for drowsy patients. In case of mixed ingestion gastric lavage may be considered, however not as a routine measure.

If CNS depression is severe consider the use of flumazenil, a benzodiazepine antagonist. This should only be administered under closely monitored conditions. It has a short half-life (about an hour), therefore patients administered flumazenil will require monitoring after its effects have worn off. Flumazenil is to be used with extreme caution in the presence of drugs that reduce seizure threshold (e.g. tricyclic antidepressants). Refer to the prescribing information for flumazenil, for further information on the correct use of this drug.

5. PHARMACOLOGICAL PROPERTIES

5.1 Pharmacodynamic properties

Pharmacotherapeutic group:

Hypnotics and sedatives (benzodiazepine derivatives), ATC code: N05CD08.

Midazolam is a derivative of the imidazobenzodiazepine group. The free base is a lipophilic substance with low solubility in water.

The basic nitrogen in position 2 of the imidazobenzodiazepine ring system enables the active ingredient of midazolam to form water-soluble salts with acids. These produce a stable and well tolerated injection solution.

The pharmacological action of midazolam is characterised by short duration because of rapid metabolic transformation. Midazolam has a sedative and sleep-inducing effect of pronounced intensity. It also exerts an anxiolytic, an anticonvulsant and a muscle-relaxant effect.

After i.m. or i.v. administration anterograde amnesia of short duration occurs (the patient does not remember events that occurred during the maximal activity of the compound).

5.2 Pharmacokinetic properties

Absorption after i.m. injection

Absorption of midazolam from the muscle tissue is rapid and complete. Maximum plasma concentrations are reached within 30 minutes. The absolute bioavailability after i.m. injection is over 90%.

Absorption after rectal administration

After rectal administration midazolam is absorbed quickly. Maximum plasma concentration is reached in about 30 minutes. The absolute bioavailability is about 50%.

Distribution

When midazolam is injected i.v., the plasma concentration-time curve shows one or two distinct phases of distribution. The volume of distribution at steady state is 0.7 - 1.2 l/kg. 96 - 98% of midazolam is bound to plasma proteins. The major fraction of plasma protein binding is due to albumin. There is a slow and insignificant passage of midazolam into the cerebrospinal fluid. In humans, midazolam has been shown to cross the placenta slowly and to enter foetal circulation. Small quantities of midazolam are found in human milk.

Metabolism

Midazolam is almost entirely eliminated by biotransformation. The fraction of the dose extracted by the liver has been estimated to be 30 - 60%. Midazolam is hydroxylated by the cytochrome P4503A4 isozyme and the major urinary and plasma metabolite is alpha-hydroxymidazolam. Plasma concentrations of alpha-hydroxymidazolam are 12% of those of the parent compound. Alpha-hydroxymidazolam is pharmacologically active, but contributes only minimally (about 10%) to the effects of intravenous midazolam.

Elimination

In healthy volunteers, the elimination half-life of midazolam is between 1.5 - 2.5 hours. Plasma clearance is in the range of 300 - 500ml/min. Midazolam is excreted mainly by renal route (60 - 80% of the injected dose) and recovered as glucuroconjugated alpha-hydroxymidazolam. Less than 1% of the dose is recovered in urine as unchanged drug. The elimination half-life of alpha-hydroxy-midazolam is shorter than 1 hour. When midazolam is given by i.v. infusion, its elimination kinetics do not differ from those following bolus injection.

Pharmacokinetics in special populations

Elderly

In adults over 60 years of age, the elimination half-life may be prolonged up to four times.

Children

The rate of rectal absorption in children is similar to that in adults but the bioavailability is lower (5 - 18%). The elimination half-life after i.v. and rectal administration is shorter in children 3 - 10 years old (1 - 1.5 hours) as compared with that in adults. The difference is consistent with an increased metabolic clearance in children.

Neonates

In neonates the elimination half-life is on average 6 - 12 hours, probably due to liver immaturity and the clearance is reduced (see section 4.4).

Obese

The mean half-life is greater in obese than in non-obese patients (5.9 vs 2.3 hours). This is due to an increase of approximately 50% in the volume of distribution corrected for total body weight. The clearance is not significantly different in obese and non-obese patients.

Patients with hepatic impairment

The elimination half-life in cirrhotic patients may be longer and the clearance smaller as compared to those in healthy volunteers (see section 4.4).

Patients with renal impairment

The elimination half-life in patients with chronic renal failure is similar to that in healthy volunteers.

Critically ill patients

The elimination half-life of midazolam is prolonged up to six times in the critically ill.

Patients with cardiac insufficiency

The elimination half-life is longer in patients with congestive heart failure compared with that in healthy subjects (see section 4.4).

5.3 Preclinical safety data

There are no preclinical data of relevance to the prescriber which are additional to that already included in other sections of the SPC.

6. PHARMACEUTICAL PARTICULARS

6.1 List of excipients

Sodium Chloride - Ph. Eur.

Hydrochloric Acid - Ph. Eur.

IM Sodium Hydroxide Solution - Ph. Eur.

Water for Injections - Ph. Eur

6.2 Incompatibilities

Admixture with Hartmann's solution is not recommended as the potency of midazolam decreases.

6.3 Shelf life

5 years.

6.4 Special precautions for storage

Keep ampoules in the outer carton.

6.5 Nature and contents of container

Type I Ph. Eur. 5ml colourless glass ampoules, in packs of 10.

6.6 Special precautions for disposal and other handling

Hypnovel ampoule solution is stable, both physically and chemically, for up to 24 hours at room temperature when mixed with 500ml infusion fluids containing Dextrose 4% with Sodium Chloride 0.18%, Dextrose 5% or Sodium Chloride 0.9%.

There is no evidence of the adsorption of midazolam on to the plastic of infusion apparatus or syringes.

7. MARKETING AUTHORISATION HOLDER

Roche Products Limited, 6 Falcon Way, Shire Park, Welwyn Garden City, AL7 1TW, United Kingdom.

8. MARKETING AUTHORISATION NUMBER(S)

PL 00031/0189

9. DATE OF FIRST AUTHORISATION/RENEWAL OF THE AUTHORISATION

15 November 1984/15 November 1994/24 March 2000/ 14 September 2005

10. DATE OF REVISION OF THE TEXT

13 February 2008

LEGAL STATUS

POM

Hypnovel is a registered trade mark.

Hypoloc 5 mg tablets

(A. Menarini Pharma U.K. S.R.L.)

1. NAME OF THE MEDICINAL PRODUCT

HYPOLOC® 5 mg tablets

2. QUALITATIVE AND QUANTITATIVE COMPOSITION

Each Hypoloc tablet contains 5 mg of nebivolol (as nebivolol hydrochloride): 2.5 mg of SRRR-nebivolol (or d-nebivolol) and 2.5 mg of RSSS-nebivolol (or l-nebivolol).

Excipients: amongst others lactose monohydrate (see section 4.4 and 6.1).

For a full list of excipients, see section 6.1.

3. PHARMACEUTICAL FORM

Tablets.

White, round, cross-scored tablets.

The tablets can be divided in equal quarters

4. CLINICAL PARTICULARS

4.1 Therapeutic indications

Hypertension

Treatment of essential hypertension.

Chronic heart failure (CHF)

Treatment of stable mild and moderate chronic heart failure in addition to standard therapies in elderly patients $\geq$ 70 years.

4.2 Posology and method of administration

Hypertension

Adults

The dose is one tablet (5 mg) daily, preferably at the same time of the day. Tablets may be taken with meals.

The blood pressure lowering effect becomes evident after 1-2 weeks of treatment. Occasionally, the optimal effect is reached only after 4 weeks.

Combination with other antihypertensive agents

Beta-blockers can be used alone or concomitantly with other antihypertensive agents. To date, an additional antihypertensive effect has been observed only when Hypoloc 5 mg is combined with hydrochlorothiazide 12.5-25 mg.

Patients with renal insufficiency

In patients with renal insufficiency, the recommended starting dose is 2.5 mg daily. If needed, the daily dose may be increased to 5 mg.

Patients with hepatic insufficiency

Data in patients with hepatic insufficiency or impaired liver function are limited. Therefore the use of Hypoloc in these patients is contra-indicated.

Elderly

In patients over 65 years, the recommended starting dose is 2.5 mg daily. If needed, the daily dose may be increased to 5 mg. However, in view of the limited experience in patients above 75 years, caution must be exercised and these patients monitored closely.

Children and adolescents

No studies have been conducted in children and adolescents. Therefore, use in children and adolescents is not recommended.

Chronic heart failure (CHF)

The treatment of stable chronic heart failure has to be initiated with a gradual uptitration of dosage until the optimal individual maintenance dose is reached.

Patients should have stable chronic heart failure without acute failure during the past six weeks. It is recommended that the treating physician should be experienced in the management of chronic heart failure.

For those patients receiving cardiovascular drug therapy including diuretics and/or digoxin and/or ACE inhibitors and/or angiotensin II antagonists, dosing of these drugs should be stabilised during the past two weeks prior to initiation of Hypoloc treatment.

The initial uptitration should be done according to the following steps at 1-2 weekly intervals based on patient tolerability:

1.25 mg nebivolol, to be increased to 2.5 mg nebivolol once daily, then to 5 mg once daily and then to 10 mg once daily.

The maximum recommended dose is 10 mg nebivolol once daily.

Initiation of therapy and every dose increase should be done under the supervision of an experienced physician over a period of at least 2 hours to ensure that the clinical status (especially as regards blood pressure, heart rate, conduction disturbances, signs of worsening of heart failure) remains stable.

Occurrence of adverse events may prevent all patients being treated with the maximum recommended dose. If necessary, the dose reached can also be decreased step by step and reintroduced as appropriate.

During the titration phase, in case of worsening of the heart failure or intolerance, it is recommended first to reduce the dose of nebivolol, or to stop it immediately if necessary (in case of severe hypotension, worsening of heart failure with acute pulmonary oedema, cardiogenic shock, symptomatic bradycardia or AV block).

Treatment of stable chronic heart failure with nebivolol is generally a long-term treatment.

The treatment with nebivolol is not recommended to be stopped abruptly since this might lead to a transitory worsening of heart failure. If discontinuation is necessary, the dose should be gradually decreased divided into halves weekly.

Tablets may be taken with meals.

Patients with renal insufficiency

No dose adjustment is required in mild to moderate renal insufficiency since uptitration to the maximum tolerated dose is individually adjusted. There is no experience in patients with severe renal insufficiency (serum creatinine ⩾ 250μmol/L). Therefore, the use of nebivolol in these patients is not recommended.

Patients with hepatic insufficiency

Data in patients with hepatic insufficiency are limited. Therefore the use of Hypoloc in these patients is contra-indicated.

Elderly

No dose adjustment is required since uptitration to the maximum tolerated dose is individually adjusted.

Children and adolescents

No studies have been conducted in children and adolescents. Therefore, use in children and adolescents is not recommended.

4.3 Contraindications

- Hypersensitivity to the active substance or to any of the excipients.
- Liver insufficiency or liver function impairment.
- Acute heart failure, cardiogenic shock or episodes of heart failure decompensation requiring i.v. inotropic therapy.

In addition, as with other beta-blocking agents, Hypoloc is contra-indicated in:

- sick sinus syndrome, including sino-atrial block.
- second and third degree heart block (without a pacemaker).
- history of bronchospasm and bronchial asthma.
- untreated phaeochromocytoma.
- metabolic acidosis.
- bradycardia (heart rate < 60 bpm prior to start therapy).
- hypotension (systolic blood pressure < 90 mmHg).
- severe peripheral circulatory disturbances.

4.4 Special warnings and precautions for use

See also 4.8 Undesirable effects.

The following warnings and precautions apply to beta-adrenergic antagonists in general.

Anaesthesia

Continuation of beta blockade reduces the risk of arrhythmias during induction and intubation. If beta blockade is interrupted in preparation for surgery, the beta-adrenergic antagonist should be discontinued at least 24 hours beforehand.

Caution should be observed with certain anaesthetics that cause myocardial depression. The patient can be protected against vagal reactions by intravenous administration of atropine.

Cardiovascular

In general, beta-adrenergic antagonists should not be used in patients with untreated congestive heart failure (CHF), unless their condition has been stabilised.

In patients with ischaemic heart disease, treatment with a beta-adrenergic antagonist should be discontinued gradually, i.e. over 1-2 weeks. If necessary replacement therapy should be initiated at the same time, to prevent exacerbation of angina pectoris.

Beta-adrenergic antagonists may induce bradycardia: if the pulse rate drops below 50-55 bpm at rest and/or the patient experiences symptoms that are suggestive of bradycardia, the dosage should be reduced.

Beta-adrenergic antagonists should be used with caution:

- in patients with peripheral circulatory disorders (Raynaud's disease or syndrome, intermittent claudication), as aggravation of these disorders may occur;
- in patients with first degree heart block, because of the negative effect of beta-blockers on conduction time;
- in patients with Prinzmetal's angina due to unopposed alphareceptor mediated coronary artery vasoconstriction: beta-adrenergic antagonists may increase the number and duration of anginal attacks.

Combination of nebivolol with calcium channel antagonists of the verapamil and diltiazem type, with Class I antiarrhythmic drugs, and with centrally acting antihypertensive drugs is generally not recommended, for details please refer to section 4.5.

Metabolic/Endocrinological

Hypoloc does not affect glucose levels in diabetic patients. Care should be taken in diabetic patients however, as nebivolol may mask certain symptoms of hypoglycaemia (tachycardia, palpitations).

Beta-adrenergic blocking agents may mask tachycardic symptoms in hyperthyroidism. Abrupt withdrawal may intensify symptoms.

Respiratory

In patients with chronic obstructive pulmonary disorders, beta-adrenergic antagonists should be used with caution as airway constriction may be aggravated.

Other

Patients with a history of psoriasis should take beta-adrenergic antagonists only after careful consideration.

Beta-adrenergic antagonists may increase the sensitivity to allergens and the severity of anaphylactic reactions.

The initiation of Chronic Heart Failure treatment with nebivolol necessitates regular monitoring. For the posology and method of administration please refer to section 4.2. Treatment discontinuation should not be done abruptly unless clearly indicated. For further information please refer to section 4.2.

This medicinal product contains lactose. Patients with rare hereditary problems of galactose intolerance, the Lapp-lactase deficiency or glucose-galactose malapsorption should not take this medicinal product.

4.5 Interaction with other medicinal products and other forms of interaction

Pharmacodynamic interactions:

The following interactions apply to beta-adrenergic antagonists in general.

Combinations not recommended:

Class I antiarrhythmics (quinidine, hydroquinidine, cibenzoline, flecainide, disopyramide, lidocaine, mexiletine, propafenone): effect on atrio-ventricular conduction time may be potentiated and negative inotropic effect increased (see section 4.4).

Calcium channel antagonists of verapamil/diltiazem type: negative influence on contractility and atrio-ventricular conduction. Intravenous administration of verapamil in patients with β-blocker treatment may lead to profound hypotension and atrio-ventricular block (see section 4.4).

Centrally-acting antihypertensives (clonidine, guanfacin, moxonidine, methyldopa, rilmenidine): concomitant use of centrally acting antihypertensive drugs may worsen heart failure by a decrease in the central sympathetic tonus (reduction of heart rate and cardiac output, vasodilation) (see section 4.4). Abrupt withdrawal, particularly if prior to beta-blocker discontinuation, may increase risk of "rebound hypertension".

Combinations to be used with caution

Class III antiarrhythmic drugs (Amiodarone): effect on atrio-ventricular conduction time may be potentiated.

Anaesthetics - volatile halogenated: concomitant use of beta-adrenergic antagonists and anaesthetics may attenuate reflex tachycardia and increase the risk of hypotension (see section 4.4). As a general rule, avoid sudden withdrawal of beta-blocker treatment. The anaesthesiologist should be informed when the patient is receiving Hypoloc.

Insulin and oral antidiabetic drugs: although nebivolol does not affect glucose level, concomitant use may mask certain symptoms of hypoglycaemia (palpitations, tachycardia).

Combinations to be considered

Digitalis glycosides: concomitant use may increase atrio-ventricular conduction time. Clinical trials with nebivolol have not shown any clinical evidence of an interaction. Nebivolol does not influence the kinetics of digoxin.

Calcium antagonists of the dihydropyridine type (amlodipine, felodipine, lacidipine, nifedipine, nicardipine, nimodipine, nitrendipine): concomitant use may increase the risk of hypotension, and an increase in the risk of a further deterioration of the ventricular pump function in patients with heart failure cannot be excluded.

Antipsychotics, antidepressants (tricyclics, barbiturates and phenothiazines): concomitant use may enhance the hypothensive effect of the beta-blockers (additive effect).

Non steroidal anti-inflammatory drugs (NSAID): no effect on the blood pressure lowering effect of nebivolol.

Sympathicomimetic agents: concomitant use may counteract the effect of beta-adrenergic antagonists. Beta-adrenergic agents may lead to unopposed alpha-adrenergic activity of sympathicomimetic agents with both alpha- and beta-adrenergic effects (risk of hypertension, severe bradycardia and heart block).

Pharmacokinetic interactions:

As nebivolol metabolism involves the CYP2D6 isoenzyme, co-administration with substances inhibiting this enzyme, especially paroxetine, fluoxetine, thioridazine and quinidine may lead to increased plasma levels of nebivolol associated with an increased risk of excessive bradycardia and adverse events.

Co-administration of cimetidine increased the plasma levels of nebivolol, without changing the clinical effect. Co-administration of ranitidine did not affect the pharmacokinetics of nebivolol. Provided Hypoloc is taken with the meal, and an antacid between meals, the two treatments can be co-prescribed.

Combining nebivolol with nicardipine slightly increased the plasma levels of both drugs, without changing the clinical effect. Co-administration of alcohol, furosemide or hydrochlorothiazide did not affect the pharmacokinetics of nebivolol. Nebivolol does not affect the pharmacokinetics and pharmacodynamics of warfarin.

4.6 Pregnancy and lactation

Use in pregnancy

Nebivolol has pharmacological effects that may cause harmful effects on pregnancy and/or the foetus/newborn. In general, beta-adrenoceptor blockers reduce placental perfusion, which has been associated with growth retardation, intrauterine death, abortion or early labour. Adverse effects (e.g. hypoglycaemia and bradycardia) may occur in the foetus and newborn infant. If treatment with beta-adrenoceptor blockers is necessary, $beta_1$-selective adrenoceptor blockers are preferable.

Nebivolol should not be used during pregnancy unless clearly necessary. If treatment with nebivolol is considered necessary, the uteroplacental blood flow and the foetal growth should be monitored. In case of harmful effects on pregnancy or the foetus alternative treatment should be considered. The newborn infant must be closely monitored. Symptoms of hypoglycaemia and bradycardia are generally to be expected within the first 3 days.

Use in lactation

Animal studies have shown that nebivolol is excreted in breast milk. It is not known whether this drug is excreted in human milk. Most beta-blockers, particularly lipophilic compounds like nebivolol and its active metabolites, pass into breast milk although to a variable extent. Therefore, breastfeeding is not recommended during administration of nebivolol.

4.7 Effects on ability to drive and use machines

No studies on the effects of Hypoloc on the ability to drive and use machines have been performed. Pharmacodynamic studies have shown that Hypoloc 5 mg does not affect psychomotor function. When driving vehicles or operating machines it should be taken into account that dizziness and fatigue may occasionally occur.

4.8 Undesirable effects

Adverse events are listed separately for hypertension and CHF because of differences in the background diseases.

Hypertension

The adverse reactions reported, which are in most of the cases of mild to moderate intensity, are tabulated below, classified by system organ class and ordered by frequency:

(see Table 1 on next page)

The following adverse reactions have also been reported with some beta adrenergic antagonists: hallucinations, psychoses, confusion, cold/cyanotic extremities, Raynaud phenomenon, dry eyes, and oculo-mucocutaneous toxicity of the practolol-type.

Chronic heart failure

Data on adverse reactions in CHF patients are available from one placebo-controlled clinical trial involving 1067 patients taking nebivolol and 1061 patients taking placebo. In this study, a total of 449 nebivolol patients (42.1%) reported at least possibly causally related adverse reactions compared to 334 placebo patients (31.5%). The most commonly reported adverse reactions in nebivolol patients were bradycardia and dizziness, both occurring in approximately 11% of patients. The corresponding frequencies among placebo patients were approximately 2% and 7%, respectively.

Table 1

SYSTEM ORGAN CLASS	Common (≥1/100 to <1/10)	Uncommon (≥1/1,000 to ≤1/100)	Very Rare (≤1/10,000)	Not Known
Immune system disorders				angioneurotic oedema, hypersensitivity
Psychiatric disorders		nightmares; depression		
Nervous system disorders	headache, dizziness, paraesthesia		syncope	
Eye disorders		impaired vision		
Cardiac disorders		bradycardia, heart failure, slowed AV conduction/AV-block		
Vascular disorders		hypotension, (increase of) intermittent claudication		
Respiratory, thoracic and mediastinal disorders	dyspnoea	bronchospasm		
Gastrointestinal disorders	constipation, nausea, diarrhoea	dyspepsia, flatulence, vomiting		
Skin and subcutaneous tissue disorders		pruritus, rash erythematous	psoriasis aggravated	
Reproductive system and breast disorders		impotence		
General disorders and administration site conditions	tiredness, oedema			

The following incidences were reported for adverse reactions (at least possibly drug-related) which are considered specifically relevant in the treatment of chronic heart failure:

- Aggravation of cardiac failure occurred in 5.8 % of nebivolol patients compared to 5.2% of placebo patients.

- Postural hypotension was reported in 2.1% of nebivolol patients compared to 1.0% of placebo patients.

- Drug intolerance occurred in 1.6% of nebivolol patients compared to 0.8% of placebo patients.

- First degree atrio-ventricular block occurred in 1.4% of nebivolol patients compared to 0.9% of placebo patients.

- Oedema of the lower limb were reported by 1.0% of nebivolol patients compared to 0.2% of placebo patients.

4.9 Overdose
No data are available on overdosage with Hypoloc.

Symptoms
Symptoms of overdosage with beta-blockers are: bradycardia, hypotension, bronchospasm and acute cardiac insufficiency.

Treatment
In case of overdosage or hypersensitivity, the patient should be kept under close supervision and be treated in an intensive care ward. Blood glucose levels should be checked. Absorption of any drug residues still present in the gastro-intestinal tract can be prevented by gastric lavage and the administration of activated charcoal and a laxative. Artificial respiration may be required. Bradycardia or extensive vagal reactions should be treated by administering atropine or methylatropine. Hypotension and shock should be treated with plasma/plasma substitutes and, if necessary, catecholamines. The beta-blocking effect can be counteracted by slow intravenous administration of isoprenaline hydrochloride, starting with a dose of approximately 5 μg/minute, or dobutamine, starting with a dose of 2.5 μg/minute, until the required effect has been obtained. In refractory cases isoprenaline can be combined with dopamine. If this does not produce the desired effect either, intravenous administration of glucagon 50-100 μg/kg i.v. may be considered. If required, the injection should be repeated within one hour, to be followed -if required- by an i.v. infusion of glucagon 70 μg/kg/h. In extreme cases of treatment-resistant bradycardia, a pacemaker may be inserted.

5. PHARMACOLOGICAL PROPERTIES

5.1 Pharmacodynamic properties
Pharmacotherapeutic group: Beta blocking agent, selective.

ATC code: C07AB12

Nebivolol is a racemate of two enantiomers, SRRR-nebivolol (or d-nebivolol) and RSSS-nebivolol (or l-nebivolol). It combines two pharmacological activities:

• It is a competitive and selective beta-receptor antagonist: this effect is attributed to the SRRR-enatiomer (d-enantiomer).

• It has mild vasodilating properties due to an interaction with the L-arginine/nitric oxide pathway.

Single and repeated doses of nebivolol reduce heart rate and blood pressure at rest and during exercise, both in normotensive subjects and in hypertensive patients. The antihypertensive effect is maintained during chronic treatment.

At therapeutic doses, nebivolol is devoid of alpha-adrenergic antagonism.

During acute and chronic treatment with nebivolol in hypertensive patients systemic vascular resistance is decreased. Despite heart rate reduction, reduction in cardiac output during rest and exercise may be limited due to an increase in stroke volume. The clinical relevance of these haemodynamic differences as compared to other beta1 receptor antagonists has not been fully established.

In hypertensive patients, nebivolol increases the NO-mediated vascular response to acetylcholine (ACh) which is reduced in patients with endothelial dysfunction.

In a mortality–morbidity, placebo-controlled trial performed in 2128 patients ≥ 70 years (median age 75.2 years) with stable chronic heart failure with or without impaired left ventricular ejection fraction (mean LVEF: 36 ± 12.3%, with the following distribution: LVEF less than 35% in 56% of patients, LVEF between 35% and 45% in 25% of patients and LVEF greater than 45% in 19% of patients) followed for a mean time of 20 months, nebivolol, on top of standard therapy, significantly prolonged the time to occurrence of deaths or hospitalisations for cardiovascular reasons (primary end-point for efficacy) with a relative risk reduction of 14% (absolute reduction: 4.2%). This risk reduction developed after 6 months of treatment and was maintained for all treatment duration (median duration: 18 months). The effect of nebivolol was independent from age, gender, or left ventricular ejection fraction of the population on study. The benefit on all cause mortality did not reach statistical significance in comparison to placebo (absolute reduction: 2.3%).

A decrease in sudden death was observed in nebivolol treated patients (4.1% vs 6.6%, relative reduction of 38%).

In vitro and in vivo experiments in animals showed that Nebivolol has no intrinsic sympathicomimetic activity.

In vitro and in vivo experiments in animals showed that at pharmacological doses nebivolol has no membrane stabilising action.

In healthy volunteers, nebivolol has no significant effect on maximal exercise capacity or endurance.

5.2 Pharmacokinetic properties
Both nebivolol enantiomers are rapidly absorbed after oral administration. The absorption of nebivolol is not affected by food; nebivolol can be given with or without meals.

Nebivolol is extensively metabolised, partly to active hydroxy-metabolites. Nebivol is metabolised via alicyclic and aromatic hydroxylation, N-dealkylation and glucuronidation; in addition, glucuronides of the hydroxy-metabolites are formed. The metabolism of nebivolol by aromatic hydroxylation is subject to the CYP2D6 dependent genetic oxidative polymorphism. The oral bioavailability of nebivolol averages 12% in fast metabolisers and is virtually complete in slow metabolisers. At steady state and at the same dose level, the peak plasma concentration of unchanged nebivolol is about 23 times higher in poor metabolisers than in extensive metabolisers. When unchanged drug plus active metabolites are considered, the difference in peak plasma concentrations is 1.3 to 1.4 fold. Because of the variation in rates of metabolism, the dose of Hypoloc should always be adjusted to the individual requirements of the patient: poor metabolisers therefore may require lower doses.

In fast metabolisers, elimination half-lives of the nebivolol enantiomers average 10 hours. In slow metabolisers, they are 3-5 times longer. In fast metabolisers, plasma levels of the RSSS-enantiomer are slightly higher than for the SRRR-enantiomer. In slow metabolisers, this difference is larger. In fast metabolisers, elimination half-lives of the hydroxymetabolites of both enantiomers average 24 hours, and are about twice as long in slow metabolisers.

Steady-state plasma levels in most subjects (fast metabolisers) are reached within 24 hours for nebivolol and within a few days for the hydroxy-metabolites.

Plasma concentrations are dose-proportional between 1 and 30 mg. The pharmacokinetics of nebivolol are not affected by age.

In plasma, both nebivolol enantiomers are predominantly bound to albumin.

Plasma protein binding is 98.1% for SRRR-nebivolol and 97.9% for RSSS-nebivolol.

One week after administration, 38% of the dose is excreted in the urine and 48% in the faeces. Urinary excretion of unchanged nebivolol is less than 0.5% of the dose.

5.3 Preclinical safety data
Preclinical data reveal no special hazard for humans based on conventional studies of genotoxicity and carcinogenic potential.

6. PHARMACEUTICAL PARTICULARS

6.1 List of excipients
Polysorbate 80

Hypromellose

Lactose monohydrate

Maize starch

Croscarmellose sodium

Microcrystalline cellulose

Colloidal anhydrous silica

Magnesium stearate

6.2 Incompatibilities
Not applicable

6.3 Shelf life
3 years.

6.4 Special precautions for storage
This medicinal product does not require any special storage precautions.

6.5 Nature and contents of container
Tablets are provided in blister packs (PVC/aluminium blister).

Pack sizes of 7, 14, 28, 30, 50, 56, 90, 100, 500 tablets (Not all pack sizes may be marketed)

6.6 Special precautions for disposal and other handling
No special requirements.

7. MARKETING AUTHORISATION HOLDER
Menarini International Operations Luxembourg S.A.

1, Avenue de la Gare,

L-1611 Luxembourg

8. MARKETING AUTHORISATION NUMBER(S)
PL 16239/0019

9. DATE OF FIRST AUTHORISATION/RENEWAL OF THE AUTHORISATION
Date of first authorisation: 11 December 2002

Date of last renewal: 18 October 2005

10. DATE OF REVISION OF THE TEXT
August 2007

Legal category
POM

Hypovase Tablets

(Pfizer Limited)

1. NAME OF THE MEDICINAL PRODUCT
HYPOVASE® TABLETS

2. QUALITATIVE AND QUANTITATIVE COMPOSITION
500 microgram tablets: prazosin hydrochloride Ph Eur equivalent to 500 micrograms prazosin base, based on potency of 93.1 % base activity.

1 mg tablets: prazosin hydrochloride Ph Eur equivalent to 1 mg prazosin based on a potency of 93.1 % base activity.

3. PHARMACEUTICAL FORM
500 microgram tablets: white and round marked "Pfizer" on one side.

1 mg tablets: white and oblong scored on both sides and engraved "M6" on one side.

4. CLINICAL PARTICULARS

4.1 Therapeutic indications
Hypertension: Hypovase is indicated in the treatment of all grades of essential (primary) hypertension and of all grades of secondary hypertension of varied aetiology. It can be used as the initial and sole agent or it may be employed in a treatment regimen in conjunction with a diuretic and/or other antihypertensive drug as needed for proper patient response.

Congestive heart failure: Hypovase may be used alone or added to the therapeutic regimen in those patients with congestive heart failure who are resistant or refractory to conventional therapy with diuretics and/or cardiac glycosides.

Raynaud's phenomenon and Raynaud's disease: Hypovase is indicated for the symptomatic treatment of patients with Raynaud's phenomenon and Raynaud's disease.

Benign prostatic hyperplasia: Hypovase is indicated as an adjunct in the symptomatic treatment of urinary obstruction caused by benign prostatic hyperplasia. It may therefore be of value in patients awaiting prostatic surgery.

4.2 Posology and method of administration

Hypovase tablets are for oral administration only.

Hypertension: The dosage range is from 500 micrograms – 20 mg daily. It is recommended that therapy be initiated at the lowest dose, 500 micrograms, twice or three times daily for three to seven days, with the starting dose administered in the evening. This dose should be increased to 1 mg twice or three times daily for a further three to seven days. Thereafter, the daily dose should be increased gradually as determined by the patient's response to the blood pressure lowering effect. Most patients are likely to be maintained on a dosage regimen of Hypovase alone of up to 15 mg daily in divided doses. Maximum recommended daily dosage: 20 mg in divided doses.

Patients receiving other antihypertensive therapy but with inadequate control: The dosage of the other drug should be reduced to a maintenance level and Hypovase initiated at 500 micrograms in the evening, then continuing with 500 micrograms twice or three times daily. Subsequent dosage increases should be made gradually depending upon the patient's response.

There is evidence that adding Hypovase to angiotensin converting enzyme inhibitor, beta-adrenergic antagonist or calcium antagonist therapy may bring about a substantial reduction in blood pressure. Therefore, the low initial dosage regimen is recommended.

Congestive cardiac failure: The recommended starting dose is 500 micrograms two, three or four times daily, increasing to 4 mg in divided doses. Dosage should be adjusted according to the patient's clinical response, based on careful monitoring of cardiopulmonary signs and symptoms, and when indicated, haemodynamic studies. Dosage may be adjusted as often as every two to three days in patients under close medical supervision. In severely ill, decompensated patients, rapid dosage adjustment over one to two days may be indicated and is best done when haemodynamic monitoring is available. In clinical studies the therapeutic dosages ranged from 4 mg to 20 mg daily in divided doses. Adjustment of dosage may be required in the course of Hypovase therapy in some patients to maintain optimal clinical improvement.

Usual daily maintenance dosage: 4 mg to 20 mg in divided doses.

Raynaud's phenomenon and Raynaud's disease: The recommended starting dosage is 500 micrograms twice daily given for a period of three to seven days and should be adjusted according to the patient's clinical response. Usual maintenance dosage is 1 mg or 2 mg twice daily.

Benign prostatic hyperplasia: The recommended dosage is 500 micrograms twice daily for a period of 3 to 7 days, with the initial dose administered in the evening. The dosage should then be adjusted according to clinical response. The usual maintenance dosage is 2 mg twice daily. This dose should not be exceeded unless the patient requires Hypovase as antihypertensive therapy. Patients with benign prostatic hyperplasia receiving hypertensive therapy, should be administered Hypovase only under the supervision of the practitioner responsible for treating the patient's hypertension.

Patients with moderate to severe grades of renal impairment

Evidence to date shows that Hypovase does not further compromise renal function when used in patients with renal impairment. As some patients in this category have responded to small doses of Hypovase, it is recommended that therapy be initiated at 500 micrograms daily and that dosage increases be instituted cautiously.

Patients with hepatic dysfunction: No information is available on the use of Hypovase in this patient group, however, since Hypovase normally undergoes substantial first pass metabolism and subsequent metabolism and excretion by the liver, it is recommended that therapy be initiated at 500 micrograms daily and that dosage increases be instituted cautiously.

Use in children: Hypovase is not recommended for the treatment of children under the age of 12 years since safe conditions for its use have not been established.

Use in the elderly: Since the elderly may be more susceptible to hypotension, therapy should be initiated with the lowest possible dose.

4.3 Contraindications

Hypovase is contraindicated in patients with known sensitivity to Hypovase, other quinazolines, prazosin or any of the excipients.

4.4 Special warnings and precautions for use

In patients with benign prostatic hyperplasia: Hypovase is not recommended for patients with a history of micturition syncope.

Hypovase decreases peripheral vascular resistance and since many patients with this disorder are elderly, careful monitoring of blood pressure during initial administration and during adjustment of dosage is recommended. The possibility of postural hypotension, or rarely, loss of consciousness, as reported in other patient groups should be borne in mind. Close observation is especially recommended. For patients taking medications that are known to lower blood pressure, Hypovase may augment the efficacy of antihypertensive therapy, consequently, close observation is especially recommended for patients taking medications that are known to lower blood pressure. Hypovase should not normally be administered to patients already receiving another alpha-1-antagonist.

In patients with congestive cardiac failure: Hypovase is not recommended in the treatment of congestive cardiac failure due to mechanical obstruction such as aortic valve stenosis, mitral valve stenosis, pulmonary embolism and restrictive pericardial disease. Adequate data are not yet available to establish efficacy in patients with heart failure due to recent myocardial infarction.

When Hypovase is initially administered to patients with congestive cardiac failure who have undergone vigorous diuretic or other vasodilator treatment, particularly in higher than the recommended starting dose, the resultant decrease in left ventricular filling pressure may be associated with a significant fall in cardiac output and systemic blood pressure. In such patients, observance of the recommended starting dose of Hypovase followed by gradual dosage increase is particularly important.

The clinical efficacy of Hypovase in congestive cardiac failure has been reported to diminish after several months of treatment, in a proportion of patients. In these patients there is usually evidence of weight gain or peripheral oedema indicating fluid retention. Since spontaneous deterioration may occur in such severely ill patients, a causal relationship to prazosin therapy has not been established. Thus, as with all patients with congestive cardiac failure, careful adjustment of diuretic dosage according to the patient's clinical condition is required to prevent excessive fluid retention and consequent relief of symptoms.

In those patients without evidence of fluid retention, when clinical improvement has diminished, an increase in the dosage of Hypovase will usually restore clinical efficacy.

In patients with hypertension: A very small percentage of patients may respond in an abrupt and exaggerated manner to the initial dose of Hypovase. Postural hypotension evidenced by dizziness and weakness, or rarely loss of consciousness, has been reported, particularly with the commencement of therapy, but this effect is readily avoided by initiating treatment with a low dose of Hypovase and with small increases in dosage during the first one to two weeks of therapy. The effect when observed is not related to the severity of hypertension, is self-limiting and in most patients does not recur after the initial period of therapy or during subsequent titration steps.

Raynaud's phenomenon and Raynaud's disease: Because Hypovase decreases peripheral vascular resistance, careful monitoring of blood pressure during initial administration and during subsequent dosage increments of Hypovase is suggested. Close observation is especially recommended for patients already taking medications that are known to lower blood pressure.

Use with phosphodiesterase-5 inhibitors (PDE-5 Inhibitors)

Concomitant use of PDE-5 inhibitors (e.g. sildenafil, tadalafil, vardenafil) and prazosin hydrochloride may lead to symptomatic hypotension in some patients. In order to minimise the risk for developing postural hypotension the patient should be stable on the alpha-blocker therapy before initiating use of PDE-5 inhibitors.

Cataract surgery

The 'Intraoperative Floppy Iris Syndrome' (IFIS, a variant of small pupil syndrome) has been observed during cataract surgery in some patients on or previously treated with tamsulosin.

Isolated reports have also been received with other alpha-1 blockers and the possibility of a class effect cannot be excluded. As IFIS may lead to increased procedural complications during the cataract operation current or past use of alpha-1 blockers should be made known to the ophthalmic surgeon in advance of surgery.

4.5 Interaction with other medicinal products and other forms of interaction

Hypovase has been administered without any adverse drug interaction in clinical experience to date with the following:

Cardiac glycosides: digitalis and digoxin.

Hypoglycaemic agents: insulin, chlorpropamide, phenformin, tolazamide and tolbutamide.

Tranquillizers and sedatives: chlordiazapoxide, diazepam and phenobarbital.

Agents for treatment of gout: allopurinol, colchicine and probenecid.

Anti-arrhythmic agents: procainamide and quinidine.

Analgesic, antipyretic and anti-inflammatory agents: dextropropoxyphene, aspirin, indomethacinand phenylbutazone.

There is evidence that adding Hypovase to beta-adrenergic antagonist or calcium antagonist therapy may produce a substantial reduction in blood pressure. Therefore the low initial dosage regimen is recommended.

PDE-5 Inhibitors: Concomitant use of PDE-5 inhibitors (e.g. sildenafil, tadalafil, vardenafil) and prazosin hydrochloride may lead to symptomatic hypotension in some patients (see section 4.4).

Drug/Laboratory Test Interactions: False positive results may occur in screening tests for phaeochromocytoma urinary vanillylmandelic acid (VMA) and methoxyhydroxyphenyl glycol (MHPG) metabolites of norepinephrine (noradrenaline) in patients who are being treated with Hypovase. Concomitant administration of prazosin hydrochloride with PDE-5 inhibitors may lead to symptomatic hypotension in some patients; **See section 4.4.**

4.6 Pregnancy and lactation

Although no teratogenic effects were seen in animal testing, the safety of Hypovase during pregnancy has not yet been established. The use of Hypovase and a beta-blocker for the control of severe hypertension in 44 pregnant women revealed no drug-related foetal abnormalities or adverse effects. Therapy with Hypovase was continued for as long as 14 weeks.

Hypovase has also been used alone or in combination with other hypotensive agents in severe hypertension of pregnancy. No foetal or neonatal abnormalities have been reported with the use of Hypovase.

Studies to date are inadequate to establish the safety of Hypovase in pregnancy, accordingly, it should be used only when, in the opinion of the physician, potential benefit outweighs potential risk. Hypovase has been shown to be excreted in small amounts in human milk. Caution should be exercised when Hypovase is administered to nursing mothers.

4.7 Effects on ability to drive and use machines

When instituting therapy with any effective antihypertensive agent, the patient should be advised on how to avoid symptoms resulting from postural hypotension and what measures to take should they develop. The patient should be cautioned to avoid situations where injury could result should dizziness or weakness occur during the initiation of Hypovase therapy (i.e. driving or operating machinery).

4.8 Undesirable effects

The following side-effects have been associated with Hypovase therapy:

MedDRA System Organ Class	Frequency	Undesirable effects
Immune System Disorders	Rare	Allergic reaction
Psychiatric Disorders	Common	Depression, nervousness
	Uncommon	Insomnia
	Rare	Hallucinations
Nervous System Disorders	Common	Dizziness, drowsiness, headache, faintness, syncope
	Uncommon	Paraesthesia
	Rare	Worsening of pre-existing narcolepsy
Eye Disorders	Common	Blurred vision
	Uncommon	Eye pain, reddened sclera
Ear and Labyrinth Disorders	Common	Vertigo
	Uncommon	Tinnitus
Cardiac Disorders	Common	Palpitations
	Uncommon	Angina pectoris, tachycardia,
	Rare	Bradycardia
Vascular Disorders	Rare	Flushing, hypotension, orthostatic hypotension, vasculitis
Respiratory, Thoracic and Mediastinal Disorders	Common	Dyspnoea, nasal congestion
	Uncommon	Epistaxis

Gastrointestinal Disorders	Common	Constipation, diarrhoea, dry mouth, nausea, vomiting
	Uncommon	Abdominal discomfort and/or pain
	Rare	Pancreatitis
Hepato-biliary Disorders	Rare	Liver function abnormalities
Skin and Subcutaneous Tissue Disorders	Common	Rash
	Uncommon	Diaphoresis, pruritis, urticaria
	Rare	Alopecia, lichen planus
Musculoskeletal and Connective Tissue Disorders	Uncommon	Arthralgia
Renal and Urinary Disorders	Common	Urinary frequency
	Rare	Incontinence
Reproductive System and Breast Disorders	Uncommon	Impotence
	Rare	Gynaecomastia, priapism
General Disorders and Administration Site Conditions	Common	Oedema, lack of energy, weakness
	Rare	Fever, pain
Investigations	Rare	Positive ANA titer

The frequency of side-effects observed in patients being managed for left ventricular failure with Hypovase when used in conjunction with cardiac glycosides and diuretics is shown below:

MedDRA System Organ Class	Frequency	Undesirable effects
Nervous System Disorders	Common	Dizziness
	Uncommon	Headache
	Rare	Drowsiness
Eye Disorders	Common	Blurred vision
Cardiac Disorders	Rare	Palpitations
Vascular Disorders	Common	Postural hypotension
Respiratory, Thoracic and Mediastinal Disorders	Rare	Nasal congestion
Gastrointestinal Disorders	Common	Dry mouth, nausea
	Uncommon	Diarrhoea
Reproductive System and Breast Disorders	Common	Impotence
General Disorders and Administration Site Conditions	Rare	Oedema

In most instances these occurrences have been mild to moderate in severity and have resolved with continued therapy or have been tolerated with no decrease in drug dosage.

4.9 Overdose

Should over-dosage lead to hypotension, support of the cardiovascular system is of first importance. Restoration of blood pressure and normalization of heart rate may be accomplished by keeping the patient in the supine position. If this measure is inadequate, shock should first be treated with volume expanders. If necessary, vasopressors including angiotensin should then be used. Renal function should be monitored and supported as needed. Laboratory data indicate Hypovase is not dialysable because it is protein bound.

5. PHARMACOLOGICAL PROPERTIES

5.1 Pharmacodynamic properties

Hypovase causes a decrease in total peripheral vascular resistance through selective inhibition of postsynaptic alpha-1-adrenoreceptors in vascular smooth muscle. The results of forearm plethysmographic studies in humans demonstrate that the resultant peripheral vasodilation is a balanced effect on both resistance vessels (arterioles) and capacitance vessels (veins).

In hypertensive patients, blood pressure is lowered in both the supine and standing positions; this effect is more pronounced on the diastolic blood pressure. Tolerance to the antihypertensive effect has not been observed in long-term clinical use; relatively little tachycardia or change in renin levels has been noted. Rebound elevation of blood pressure does not occur following abrupt cessation of Hypovase therapy.

The therapeutic efficacy of Hypovase in patients with congestive heart failure is ascribed to a reduction in left ventricular filling pressure, reduction in cardiac impedance and an augmentation of cardiac output. The use of Hypovase in congestive heart failure does not provoke a reflex tachycardia and blood pressure reduction is minimal in normotensive patients.

Hypovase has been found to successfully reduce the severity of the signs, symptoms, frequency and duration of attacks, in patients with Raynaud's disease.

In low dosage, antagonism of alpha-1-receptors on prostatic and urethral smooth muscle has been shown to improve the urinary pressure profile in men and to improve symptoms of benign prostatic hypertrophy.

Clinical studies have shown that Hypovase therapy is not associated with adverse changes in the serum lipid profile.

5.2 Pharmacokinetic properties

Following oral administration in normal volunteers and hypertensive patients plasma concentrations of prazosin reach a peak in one to two hours with a plasma half-life of two to three hours. Pharmacokinetic data in a limited number of patients with congestive heart failure, most of whom showed evidence of hepatic congestion, indicates that peak plasma concentrations are reached in 2.5 hours and plasma half life is approximately 7 hours. Hypovase is highly bound to plasma protein. Studies indicate that Hypovase is extensively metabolised, primarily by demethylation and conjugation, and excreted mainly via bile and faeces.

Renal blood flow and glomerular filtration rate are not impaired by long term oral administration and thus Hypovase can be used with safety in hypertensive patients with impaired renal function.

6. PHARMACEUTICAL PARTICULARS

6.1 List of excipients

Calcium phosphate dibasic anhydrous

Maize starch

Microcrystalline cellulose

Magnesium stearate

Sodium lauryl sulphate

6.2 Incompatibilities

None stated.

6.3 Shelf life

36 months

6.4 Special precautions for storage

Store below 30°C.

6.5 Nature and contents of container

PVC/PVdC/Aluminium blisters.

Hypovase 500 microgram: Original packs of 60 tablets, (in blister strips of 4 × 15 tablets).

PVC/Aluminium blisters.

Hypovase 1 mg: Original packs of 60 tablets, (in blister strips of 4 × 15 tablets).

6.6 Special precautions for disposal and other handling

No special requirements. Any unused product or waste should be disposed of in accordance with local requirements.

7. MARKETING AUTHORISATION HOLDER

Pfizer Limited

Ramsgate Road

Sandwich

Kent, CT13 9NJ

United Kingdom

8. MARKETING AUTHORISATION NUMBER(S)

PL 00057/0149R

PL 00057/0106R

9. DATE OF FIRST AUTHORISATION/RENEWAL OF THE AUTHORISATION

5 January 1994 / 22 November 2004

10. DATE OF REVISION OF THE TEXT

June 2009

11. LEGAL CATEGORY

POM

Ref: HY 9_1 UK

Ibugel

(Dermal Laboratories Limited)

1. NAME OF THE MEDICINAL PRODUCT
IBUGEL™

2. QUALITATIVE AND QUANTITATIVE COMPOSITION
Ibuprofen 5.0% w/w.

3. PHARMACEUTICAL FORM
Non-greasy, fragrance-free, clear, aqueous-alcoholic gel.

4. CLINICAL PARTICULARS

4.1 Therapeutic indications
For the topical treatment of backache, rheumatic and muscular pain, sprains, strains and neuralgia. Ibugel is also indicated for symptomatic relief of pain due to non-serious arthritic conditions.

4.2 Posology and method of administration
Apply the gel to the affected areas, up to three times daily, or as directed by the physician. On each occasion apply only enough gel to thinly cover the affected area, and gently massage well into the skin, until completely absorbed. Do not use excessively. Hands should be washed immediately after use (unless treating them). Treatment should not normally continue for more than a few weeks, unless recommended to do so by a doctor.

The same dosage and dosage schedule applies to all age groups, although Ibugel is not normally recommended for use on children under the age of 12 years, unless instructed by their doctor.

4.3 Contraindications
Not to be used in cases of sensitivity to any of the ingredients, particularly if asthmatic or suffer from allergic disease, and have previously shown hypersensitivity to aspirin, ibuprofen or related painkillers. Not to be used on broken skin.

4.4 Special warnings and precautions for use
Seek medical advice if symptoms worsen or persist. Oral NSAIDs, including ibuprofen, can sometimes be associated with renal impairment, aggravation of active peptic ulcers, and can induce allergic bronchial reactions in susceptible asthmatic patients. Although the systemic absorption of topically applied ibuprofen is less than for oral dosage forms, these complications can occur in rare cases. For these reasons, patients with an active peptic ulcer, a history of kidney problems, asthma or intolerance to aspirin or ibuprofen taken orally should seek medical advice before using Ibugel. Keep Ibugel away from the eyes and mucous membranes. For external use only.

The label will include statements to the following effect:

If symptoms persist, consult your doctor or pharmacist. Do not use if sensitive to any of the ingredients, particularly if asthmatic, suffer from rhinitis or urticaria and have previously shown hypersensitivity to aspirin, ibuprofen or related painkillers. Consult your doctor before use if you are taking aspirin or other pain-killers.

4.5 Interaction with other medicinal products and other forms of interaction
Non-steroidal anti-inflammatory drugs may interact with blood pressure lowering drugs, and may possibly enhance the effects of anticoagulants, although the chance of either of these occurring with a topically administered preparation is extremely remote. Concurrent aspirin or other NSAIDS may result in an increased incidence of adverse reactions.

4.6 Pregnancy and lactation
Do not use during pregnancy or lactation.

4.7 Effects on ability to drive and use machines
None known.

4.8 Undesirable effects
Very rarely, susceptible patients may experience the following side effects with ibuprofen, but these are extremely uncommon when ibuprofen is administered topically. If they occur, treatment should be discontinued:-

Hypersensitivity: hypersensitivity reactions have been reported following treatment with ibuprofen. These may consist of (a) non-specific allergic reactions and anaphylaxis, (b) respiratory tract reactivity comprising asthma, aggravated asthma, bronchospasm, or dyspnoea, or (c) assorted skin disorders, including rashes of various types, pruritus, urticaria, purpura, angioedema and, less commonly, bullous dermatoses (including epidermal necrolysis and erythema multiforme).

Renal: renal impairment can occur in patients with a history of kidney problems.

Gastrointestinal: side effects such as abdominal pain and dyspepsia have been reported.

4.9 Overdose
Not applicable. Any overdose with a topical presentation of ibuprofen is extremely unlikely.

5. PHARMACOLOGICAL PROPERTIES

5.1 Pharmacodynamic properties
Ibugel is a topical preparation which has anti-inflammatory and analgesic properties. It contains the active ingredient, ibuprofen, which exerts its effects directly in inflamed tissues underlying the site of application, mainly by inhibiting prostaglandin biosynthesis.

Because it is formulated in an aqueous/alcoholic gel, Ibugel also exerts a soothing and cooling effect when applied to the affected area.

5.2 Pharmacokinetic properties
Specially formulated for external application, the active ingredient penetrates through the skin rapidly and extensively, achieving high, therapeutically relevant local concentrations in underlying soft tissues, joints and synovial fluid, whilst producing plasma levels that are unlikely to be sufficient to cause any systemic side-effects, other than in rare individuals who are hypersensitive to ibuprofen.

Furthermore, there do not appear to be any appreciable differences between the oral and topical routes of administration regarding metabolism or excretion of ibuprofen.

5.3 Preclinical safety data
Published information on subchronic toxicity studies confirms that topically applied ibuprofen is well tolerated both locally and by the gastro-intestinal tract. Any local erythema is only mild and no signs of mucosal lesions or ulcerogenic effects have been determined in the gastro-intestinal tract.

In the course of assessing mucosal tolerance, topical ibuprofen has been found to cause acute, but reversible, irritant reactions in the eyes and mucous membranes.

6. PHARMACEUTICAL PARTICULARS

6.1 List of excipients
IMS; Carbomer; Propylene Glycol; Diethylamine; Purified Water.

6.2 Incompatibilities
None known.

6.3 Shelf life
36 months.

6.4 Special precautions for storage
Do not store above 25°C.

6.5 Nature and contents of container
100 g collapsible aluminium tube, fitted with a screw cap.

6.6 Special precautions for disposal and other handling
Not applicable.

7. MARKETING AUTHORISATION HOLDER
Dermal Laboratories
Tatmore Place, Gosmore
Hitchin, Herts SG4 7QR, UK.

8. MARKETING AUTHORISATION NUMBER(S)
00173/0050.

9. DATE OF FIRST AUTHORISATION/RENEWAL OF THE AUTHORISATION
2 September 2007.

10. DATE OF REVISION OF THE TEXT
October 2007.

Ibugel Forte 10%

(Dermal Laboratories Limited)

1. NAME OF THE MEDICINAL PRODUCT
IBUGEL™ FORTE 10%

2. QUALITATIVE AND QUANTITATIVE COMPOSITION
Ibuprofen 10.0% w/w.

3. PHARMACEUTICAL FORM
Aqueous-alcoholic, non-greasy, fragrance-free, clear or slightly hazy gel.

4. CLINICAL PARTICULARS

4.1 Therapeutic indications
For the topical treatment of rheumatic and muscular pain, sprains, strains, backache and neuralgia. Ibugel Forte 10% is also indicated for symptomatic relief of pain due to non-serious arthritic conditions.

4.2 Posology and method of administration
2 to 5 cm gel (50 to 125 mg ibuprofen) is to be applied to the affected area up to three times daily, or as directed by the physician. The gel should be massaged well into the skin until completely absorbed, and hands washed after use unless being treated.

Treatment should not normally continue for more than a few weeks, unless recommended to do so by a doctor.

The same dosage and dosage schedule applies to all age groups, although Ibugel Forte 10% is not normally recommended for use on children under the age of 12 years, unless instructed by the physician.

4.3 Contraindications
Not to be used if allergic to any of the ingredients, or in cases of hypersensitivity to aspirin, ibuprofen or related painkillers (including when taken by mouth), especially where associated with a history of asthma, rhinitis or urticaria. Not to be used on broken or damaged skin.

4.4 Special warnings and precautions for use
To be kept away from the eyes and mucous membranes. Oral NSAIDs, including ibuprofen, can sometimes be associated with renal impairment, aggravation of active peptic ulcers, and can induce allergic bronchial reactions in susceptible asthmatic patients. Although the systemic absorption of topically applied ibuprofen is less than for oral dosage forms, these complications can occur in rare cases. For these reasons, caution should be exercised before prescribing Ibugel Forte 10% for patients with an active peptic ulcer, a history of kidney problems, asthma or intolerance to aspirin or ibuprofen taken orally. Patients should seek medical advice if symptoms worsen or persist.

4.5 Interaction with other medicinal products and other forms of interaction
Non-steroidal anti-inflammatory drugs may interact with blood pressure lowering drugs, and may possibly enhance the effects of anticoagulants, although the chance of either of these occurring with a topically administered preparation is extremely remote. Where aspirin or other NSAID tablets are taken concurrently, it is important to bear in mind that these may increase the incidence of undesirable effects.

4.6 Pregnancy and lactation
Not to be used during pregnancy or lactation. Although no teratogenic effects have been demonstrated, ibuprofen should be avoided during pregnancy. The onset of labour may be delayed, and the duration of labour increased. Ibuprofen appears in breast milk in very low concentrations, but is unlikely to affect breast fed infants adversely.

4.7 Effects on ability to drive and use machines
None known.

4.8 Undesirable effects
Very rarely, susceptible patients may experience the following side effects with ibuprofen, but these are extremely uncommon when ibuprofen is administered topically. If they occur, treatment should be discontinued:-

Hypersensitivity: hypersensitivity reactions have been reported following treatment with ibuprofen. These may consist of (a) non-specific allergic reactions and anaphylaxis, (b) respiratory tract reactivity comprising asthma, aggravated asthma, bronchospasm, or dyspnoea, or (c) assorted skin disorders, including rashes of various types, pruritus, urticaria, purpura, angioedema and, less commonly, bullous dermatoses (including epidermal necrolysis and erythema multiforme).

Renal: renal impairment can occur in patients with a history of kidney problems.

Gastrointestinal: side effects such as abdominal pain and dyspepsia have been reported.

4.9 Overdose
Not applicable. Any overdose with a topical presentation of ibuprofen is extremely unlikely. Symptoms of severe ibuprofen overdosage (eg following accidental oral ingestion) include headache, vomiting, drowsiness and hypotension. Correction of severe electrolyte abnormalities should be considered.

5. PHARMACOLOGICAL PROPERTIES

5.1 Pharmacodynamic properties
Ibugel Forte 10% is a topical preparation which has anti-inflammatory and analgesic properties. It contains the active ingredient, ibuprofen, which exerts its effects directly in inflamed tissues underlying the site of application, mainly by inhibiting prostaglandin biosynthesis.

Because it is formulated in an aqueous/alcoholic gel, Ibugel Forte 10% also exerts a soothing and cooling effect when applied to the affected area.

5.2 Pharmacokinetic properties
Specially formulated for external application, the active ingredient penetrates through the skin rapidly and extensively, achieving high, therapeutically relevant local concentrations in underlying soft tissues, joints and synovial

fluid, whilst producing plasma levels that are unlikely to be sufficient to cause any systemic side effects, other than in rare individuals who are hypersensitive to ibuprofen. Furthermore, there do not appear to be any appreciable differences between the oral and topical routes of administration regarding metabolism or excretion of ibuprofen.

5.3 Preclinical safety data
Published information on subchronic toxicity studies confirms that topically applied ibuprofen is well tolerated both locally and by the gastro-intestinal tract. Any local erythema is only mild and no signs of mucosal lesions or ulcerogenic effects have been determined in the gastro-intestinal tract.

In the course of assessing mucosal tolerance, topical ibuprofen has been found to cause acute, but reversible, irritant reactions in the eyes and mucous membranes.

6. PHARMACEUTICAL PARTICULARS
6.1 List of excipients
IMS; Carbomers; Diethylamine; Purified Water.

6.2 Incompatibilities
None known.

6.3 Shelf life
36 months.

6.4 Special precautions for storage
Do not store above 25°C.

6.5 Nature and contents of container
100 g collapsible aluminium tube, fitted with a screw cap.

6.6 Special precautions for disposal and other handling
Not applicable.

7. MARKETING AUTHORISATION HOLDER
Dermal Laboratories

Tatmore Place, Gosmore

Hitchin, Herts SG4 7QR, UK.

8. MARKETING AUTHORISATION NUMBER(S)
00173/0175.

9. DATE OF FIRST AUTHORISATION/RENEWAL OF THE AUTHORISATION
22 May 2008.

10. DATE OF REVISION OF THE TEXT
October 2007.

Ibumousse
(Dermal Laboratories Limited)

1. NAME OF THE MEDICINAL PRODUCT
IBUMOUSSE™

2. QUALITATIVE AND QUANTITATIVE COMPOSITION
Ibuprofen 5.0% w/w.

3. PHARMACEUTICAL FORM
Non-greasy, fragrance-free, white aqueous cutaneous foam.

4. CLINICAL PARTICULARS
4.1 Therapeutic indications
For backache, rheumatic and muscular pain, and neuralgia. Ibumousse is also indicated for symptomatic relief of pain due to non-serious arthritic conditions.

4.2 Posology and method of administration
Shake container before use. Hold container upright, then press nozzle to dispense the mousse into the palm of your hand. Gently massage the mousse into and around the affected areas until absorbed. The exact amount to be applied will vary, depending on the extent and severity of the condition, but it should normally be sufficient to apply 1 to 2 g (1 to 2 golf-ball sized quantities of mousse dispensed into the palm of the hand). This amount may be repeated 3 to 4 times daily, unless otherwise directed by the doctor.

Treatment should not normally continue for more than a few weeks, unless recommended by a doctor.

The same dosage and dosage schedule applies to all age groups, although the mousse is not normally recommended for children under 12 years, unless instructed by their doctor.

4.3 Contraindications
Not to be used if allergic to any of the ingredients, or in cases of hypersensitivity to aspirin, ibuprofen or related painkillers (including when taken by mouth), especially where associated with a history of asthma, rhinitis or urticaria.

Not to be used on broken or damaged skin, or where there is infection or other skin disease.

4.4 Special warnings and precautions for use
This product is flammable. Do not spray near flames, burning cigarettes, electric heaters or similar objects.

Keep away from the eyes and mucous membranes.

Oral NSAIDs, including ibuprofen, can sometimes be associated with renal impairment or aggravation of active peptic ulcers, and they can induce allergic bronchial reactions in susceptible asthmatic patients. Although systemic absorption of topically applied ibuprofen is much less than for oral dosage forms, these complications can still occur in rare cases. For these reasons, patients with asthma, an active peptic ulcer or a history of kidney problems, should seek medical advice before using the mousse, as should patients already taking other painkillers.

Patients should seek medical advice if symptoms worsen or persist.

Keep out of the reach of children. For external use only. Wash hands after use unless treating them. Do not use excessively.

The label will include statements to the following effect:

Do not exceed the stated dose. Not recommended for children under 12 years without medical advice. For external use only. Not to be used during pregnancy or breastfeeding. Do not use if you are allergic to any of the ingredients or have experienced problems with aspirin, ibuprofen or related painkillers (including when taken by mouth). If symptoms persist consult your doctor or pharmacist. Keep out of the reach of children. Patients with asthma, an active peptic ulcer or a history of kidney problems should consult their doctor before use, as should patients already taking aspirin or other painkillers.

4.5 Interaction with other medicinal products and other forms of interaction
Non-steroidal anti-inflammatory drugs may interact with blood pressure lowering drugs, and may possibly enhance the effects of anticoagulants, although the chance of either of these occurring with a topically administered preparation is extremely remote. Concurrent aspirin or other NSAIDs may result in an increased incidence of undesirable effects.

4.6 Pregnancy and lactation
Not to be used during pregnancy or lactation. Although no teratogenic effects have been demonstrated, ibuprofen should be avoided during pregnancy. The onset of labour may be delayed, and the duration of labour increased. Ibuprofen appears in breast milk in very low concentrations, but is unlikely to affect breast-fed infants adversely.

4.7 Effects on ability to drive and use machines
None known.

4.8 Undesirable effects
The cooling effect of the mousse may result in a temporary paling of the skin. Very rarely, susceptible patients may experience the following side effects with ibuprofen, but these are extremely uncommon when ibuprofen is administered topically. If they occur, treatment should be discontinued:-

Hypersensitivity: hypersensitivity reactions have been reported following treatment with ibuprofen. These may consist of (a) non-specific allergic reactions and anaphylaxis, (b) respiratory tract reactivity comprising asthma, aggravated asthma, bronchospasm, or dyspnoea, or (c) assorted skin disorders, including rashes of various types, pruritus, urticaria, purpura, angioedema and, less commonly, bullous dermatoses (including epidermal necrolysis and erythema multiforme).

Renal: renal impairment can occur in patients with a history of kidney problems.

Gastrointestinal: side effects such as abdominal pain and dyspepsia have been reported.

4.9 Overdose
Any overdose with a topical presentation of ibuprofen is extremely unlikely.

Symptoms of severe ibuprofen overdosage (eg following accidental oral ingestion) include headache, vomiting, drowsiness and hypotension. Correction of severe electrolyte abnormalities should be considered.

5. PHARMACOLOGICAL PROPERTIES
5.1 Pharmacodynamic properties
The mousse is for topical application. Ibuprofen is a phenylpropionic acid derivative with analgesic and anti-inflammatory properties. It exerts its effects directly in inflamed tissues underlying the site of application, mainly by inhibiting prostaglandin biosynthesis.

Because it is formulated in an aqueous mousse, the preparation also exerts a soothing and cooling effect when applied to the affected area.

5.2 Pharmacokinetic properties
Ibumousse has been designed for external application. The formulation delivers the active ingredient through the skin rapidly and extensively, achieving high, therapeutically relevant local concentrations in underlying soft tissues, joints and the synovial fluid, whilst producing plasma levels that are unlikely to be sufficient to cause any systemic side-effects, other than in rare individuals who are hypersensitive to ibuprofen.

There do not appear to be any appreciable differences between the oral and topical routes of administration regarding metabolism or excretion of ibuprofen.

5.3 Preclinical safety data
No relevant information additional to that contained elsewhere in the SPC.

6. PHARMACEUTICAL PARTICULARS
6.1 List of excipients
Propylene Glycol; Carbomer; Phenoxyethanol; Diethylamine; Butane 40; Purified Water.

(The ozone-friendly aerosol propellent is a blend of C_2 - H_5 hydrocarbons consisting primarily of propane, iso-butane and n-butane).

6.2 Incompatibilities
None known.

6.3 Shelf life
48 months.

6.4 Special precautions for storage
Do not store above 25°C. Keep upright and away from direct heat or sunlight. Do not expose pressurised container to temperatures higher than 50°C. Do not pierce or burn container, even when empty.

6.5 Nature and contents of container
Aluminium pressurised container incorporating a spray valve and cap containing 125 g of product. This is supplied as an original pack (OP).

6.6 Special precautions for disposal and other handling
Not applicable.

7. MARKETING AUTHORISATION HOLDER
Dermal Laboratories

Tatmore Place, Gosmore

Hitchin, Herts SG4 7QR, UK.

8. MARKETING AUTHORISATION NUMBER(S)
00173/0169.

9. DATE OF FIRST AUTHORISATION/RENEWAL OF THE AUTHORISATION
22 May 2008.

10. DATE OF REVISION OF THE TEXT
October 2007.

Ibuspray
(Dermal Laboratories Limited)

1. NAME OF THE MEDICINAL PRODUCT
IBUSPRAY™

2. QUALITATIVE AND QUANTITATIVE COMPOSITION
Ibuprofen 5.0% w/w.

3. PHARMACEUTICAL FORM
Cutaneous spray solution.

Clear, colourless, fragrance-free, aqueous-alcoholic topical spray.

4. CLINICAL PARTICULARS
4.1 Therapeutic indications
For the topical treatment of backache, rheumatic and muscular pain, sprains, strains, and neuralgia. Ibuspray is also indicated for symptomatic relief of pain due to non-serious arthritic conditions.

4.2 Posology and method of administration
Hold the bottle upright or upside down and spray approximately 4 inches to 6 inches away from the skin. After every 2 to 3 sprays, gently massage the preparation into the skin, spreading the product over a wide area around the affected site. The exact amount to be applied will vary, depending on the extent and severity of the condition, but it should normally be sufficient to apply 5 to 10 sprays (1 to 2 ml). This amount may be repeated three to four times daily, or more often if required. Do not use excessively. Hands should be washed after use, unless treating them.

Treatment should not normally continue for more than a few weeks, unless recommended to do so by a doctor.

The same dosage and dosage schedule applies to all age groups, although Ibuspray is not normally recommended for use on children below the age of 12 years unless instructed by their doctor.

4.3 Contraindications
Not to be used in cases of sensitivity to any of the ingredients, particularly if asthmatic or suffer from rhinitis or urticaria, and have previously shown hypersensitivity to aspirin or ibuprofen or related painkillers. Not to be used on broken skin.

4.4 Special warnings and precautions for use
This product is flammable. Do not spray near flames, electric heaters or similar objects. Seek medical advice if symptoms worsen or persist. Oral NSAIDs, including ibuprofen, can sometimes be associated with renal impairment, aggravation of active peptic ulcers, and can induce allergic bronchial reactions in susceptible asthmatic patients. Although the systemic absorption of topically applied ibuprofen is much less than from oral dosage forms, these complications can occur in rare cases. For these reasons, patients with an active peptic ulcer, a history of kidney problems, asthma or intolerance to aspirin or ibuprofen should seek medical advice before using Ibuspray.

Keep away from the eyes and mucous membranes. For external use only.

The label will include statements to the following effect:

If symptoms persist, consult your doctor or pharmacist.

Do not use if sensitive to any of the ingredients, particularly if asthmatic, suffer from rhinitis or urticaria and have previously shown hypersensitivity to aspirin, ibuprofen or related painkillers.

Consult your doctor before use if you are taking aspirin or other painkillers.

4.5 Interaction with other medicinal products and other forms of interaction

Non-steroidal anti-inflammatory drugs may interact with blood pressure lowering drugs, and may possibly enhance the effects of anticoagulants, although the chance of either of these occurring with a topically administered preparation is extremely remote. Concurrent aspirin or other NSAIDs may result in an increased incidence of undesirable effects.

4.6 Pregnancy and lactation

Do not use during pregnancy or lactation.

4.7 Effects on ability to drive and use machines

None known.

4.8 Undesirable effects

Very rarely, susceptible patients may experience the following side effects with ibuprofen, but these are extremely uncommon when ibuprofen is administered topically. If they occur, treatment should be discontinued:-

Hypersensitivity: hypersensitivity reactions have been reported following treatment with ibuprofen. These may consist of (a) non-specific allergic reactions and anaphylaxis, (b) respiratory tract reactivity comprising asthma, aggravated asthma, bronchospasm, or dyspnoea, or (c) assorted skin disorders, including rashes of various types, pruritus, urticaria, purpura, angioedema and, less commonly, bullous dermatoses (including epidermal necrolysis and erythema multiforme).

Renal: renal impairment can occur in patients with a history of kidney problems.

Gastrointestinal: side effects such as abdominal pain and dyspepsia have been reported.

4.9 Overdose

Not applicable. Any overdose with a topical presentation of ibuprofen is unlikely.

5. PHARMACOLOGICAL PROPERTIES

5.1 Pharmacodynamic properties

Ibuspray is a topical preparation which has anti-inflammatory and analgesic properties. It contains the active ingredient, ibuprofen, which exerts its effects directly in inflamed tissues underlying the site of application, mainly by inhibiting prostaglandin biosynthesis. Because it is formulated in an evaporative aqueous/alcoholic solution, Ibuspray also exerts a soothing and cooling effect when applied to the affected area.

5.2 Pharmacokinetic properties

Specially formulated for external application, the active ingredient penetrates through the skin rapidly and extensively, achieving high, therapeutically relevant local concentrations in underlying soft tissues, joints and synovial fluid, whilst producing plasma levels that are unlikely to be sufficient to cause any systemic side effects, other than in rare individuals who are hypersensitive to ibuprofen. Furthermore, there do not appear to be any appreciable differences between the oral and topical routes of administration regarding metabolism or excretion of ibuprofen.

5.3 Preclinical safety data

No relevant information additional to that contained elsewhere in the SPC.

6. PHARMACEUTICAL PARTICULARS

6.1 List of excipients

IMS; Macrogol 300; Cetomacrogol 1000; Purified Water.

6.2 Incompatibilities

None known.

6.3 Shelf life

36 months.

6.4 Special precautions for storage

Do not store above 25°C.

6.5 Nature and contents of container

100 ml plastic bottle incorporating a controlled dose spray pump dispenser and overcap. This is supplied as an original pack (OP).

6.6 Special precautions for disposal and other handling

Not applicable.

7. MARKETING AUTHORISATION HOLDER

Dermal Laboratories

Tatmore Place, Gosmore

Hitchin, Herts SG4 7QR, UK.

8. MARKETING AUTHORISATION NUMBER(S)

00173/0150.

9. DATE OF FIRST AUTHORISATION/RENEWAL OF THE AUTHORISATION

11 August 2008.

10. DATE OF REVISION OF THE TEXT

October 2007.

Idrolax 10 g Powder for oral solution

(UCB Pharma Limited)

1. NAME OF THE MEDICINAL PRODUCT

Idrolax 10 g Powder for oral solution

2. QUALITATIVE AND QUANTITATIVE COMPOSITION

Each sachet contains 10 g of macrogol 4000.

For full list of excipients: see section 6:1

3. PHARMACEUTICAL FORM

Powder for oral solution in a sachet.

Almost white powder with an odour and taste of orange-grapefruit.

4. CLINICAL PARTICULARS

4.1 Therapeutic indications

Symptomatic treatment of constipation in adults and children aged 8 years and above.

An organic disorder should have been ruled out before initiation of treatment. Idrolax 10 g should remain a temporary adjuvant treatment to appropriate lifestyle and dietary management of constipation, with a maximum 3-month treatment course in children. If symptoms persist despite associated dietary measures, an underlying cause should be suspected and treated.

4.2 Posology and method of administration

Oral use

1 to 2 sachets per day, preferably taken as a single dose in the morning. Each sachet should be dissolved in a glass of water just before use.

The effect of Idrolax becomes apparent within 24 to 48 hours after its administration.

In children, treatment should not exceed 3 months due to a lack of clinical data for treatment lasting longer than 3 months. Treatment-induced restoration of bowel movements will be maintained by lifestyle and dietary measures.

The daily dose should be adapted according to the clinical effects and may range from one sachet every other day (especially in children) up to 2 sachets a day.

4.3 Contraindications

- severe inflammatory bowel disease (such as ulcerative colitis, Crohn's disease) or toxic megacolon, associated with symptomatic stenosis,
- digestive perforation or risk of digestive perforation,
- ileus or suspicion of intestinal obstruction,
- painful abdominal syndromes of indeterminate cause,
- hypersensitivity to macrogol (polyethylene glycol) or to any of the excipients.

4.4 Special warnings and precautions for use

<u>Warning</u>

The treatment of constipation with any medicinal product is only an adjuvant to a healthy lifestyle and diet, for example:

- increased intake of liquids and dietary fibre,
- appropriate physical activity and rehabilitation of the bowel reflex.

Patients with hereditary problems of fructose intolerance should not take this medicinal product.

In case of diarrhoea, caution should be exercised in patients who are prone to a disturbance of water electrolyte balance (e.g. patients with impaired hepatic or renal function or patients taking diuretics) and electrolyte control should be considered.

<u>Precautions for use</u>

Very rare cases of hypersensitivity reactions (rash, urticaria, oedema) have been reported with drugs containing macrogol (polyethylene glycol). Exceptional cases of anaphylactic shock have been reported.

Idrolax does not contain a significant quantity of sugar or polyol and can be prescribed to diabetic patients or patients on a galactose-free diet

4.5 Interaction with other medicinal products and other forms of interaction

Not applicable

4.6 Pregnancy and lactation

<u>Pregnancy</u>

Macrogol 4000 was not teratogenic in rats or rabbits

There are no adequate data from use of Idrolax in pregnant women

Therefore caution should be exercised when prescribing Idrolax to pregnant women.

<u>Lactation</u>

There are no data on the excretion of macrogol 4000 in breast milk. As macrogol 4000 is not significantly absorbed, Idrolax may be administered during lactation.

4.7 Effects on ability to drive and use machines

Not applicable

4.8 Undesirable effects

<u>Adults:</u>

Undesirable effects reported during clinical trial involving almost 600 patients with the following frequencies have always been minor and transitory and have mainly concerned the gastrointestinal system:

- common (⩾1/100, <1/10): abdominal distension and/or pain, nausea, diarrhoea,
- uncommon (⩾1/1000, <1/100): vomiting, and the more common consequence of diarrhoea: urgency to defecate and faecal incontinence.

Additional information from post-marketing surveillance included very rare (<1/10000) cases of hypersensitivity reactions: pruritus, urticaria, rash, face oedema, Quincke oedema and an isolated case of anaphylactic shock have been reported.

Excessive doses may cause diarrhoea, which generally disappears when the dosage is reduced or treatment temporarily interrupted

<u>Children:</u>

Undesirable effects reported during clinical trials involving 147 children aged from 6 months to 15 years with the following frequencies. These effects have always been minor and transitory and have concerned the gastrointestinal system.

Gastrointestinal disorders:

- common (⩾1/100, <1/10): diarrhoea and abdominal pain,
- uncommon (⩾1/1000, <1/100): bloating, vomiting and nausea.

There is no additional information from post-marketing surveillance: hypersensitivity reactions have not been reported in children so far. Nevertheless, such reactions may occur as reported in adults.

Excessive doses may cause diarrhoea which generally disappears when the dosage is reduced or treatment temporarily interrupted. Diarrhoea may cause perianal soreness.

4.9 Overdose

Overdose leads to diarrhoea which disappears when treatment is temporarily interrupted or the dosage is reduced.

Excessive fluid loss by diarrhoea or vomiting may require correction of electrolyte disturbances

Cases of aspiration have been reported when extensive volumes of polyethylene glycol and electrolytes were administered with nasogastric tube. Neurologically impaired children who have oromotor dysfunction are particularly at risk of aspiration.

5. PHARMACOLOGICAL PROPERTIES

5.1 Pharmacodynamic properties

Osmotically acting laxatives

ATC code: A06AD15

High molecular weight (4000) macrogols are long linear polymers which retain water molecules by means of hydrogen bonds. When administered by the oral route, they lead to an increase in volume of intestinal fluids.

The volume of unabsorbed intestinal fluid accounts for the laxative properties of the solution.

5.2 Pharmacokinetic properties

The pharmacokinetic data confirm that macrogol 4000 undergoes neither gastrointestinal resorption nor biotransformation following oral ingestion.

5.3 Preclinical safety data

Toxicological studies in different species of animals did not reveal any signs of systemic or local gastrointestinal toxicity of macrogol 4000. Macrogol 4000 had no teratogenic, mutagenic, nor carcinogenic effect. Potential drug interaction studies performed in rats on some NSAIDs, anticoagulants, gastric antisecretory agents, or on a hypoglycaemic sulfamide showed that Idrolax did not interfere with gastrointestinal absorption of these compounds.

6. PHARMACEUTICAL PARTICULARS

6.1 List of excipients

Saccharin sodium (E954), orange-grapefruit flavour**

** <u>Composition of the orange-grapefruit flavour</u>:

Orange and grapefruit oils, concentrated orange juice, citral, acetaldehyde, linalol, ethyl butyrate, alpha terpineol, octanal, beta gamma hexenol, maltodextrine, gum arabic, sorbitol.

6.2 Incompatibilities

Not applicable

6.3 Shelf life

5 years

6.4 Special precautions for storage

No special precaution for storage

6.5 Nature and contents of container

(Paper / Aluminium / PE) sachet.

Single dose sachets presented in pack sizes of 10, 20, 50 and 100 sachets

Not all pack sizes may be marketed

6.6 Special precautions for disposal and other handling

No special requirements

7. MARKETING AUTHORISATION HOLDER
SCHWARZ PHARMA Limited
5 Hercules Way
Leavesden Park
Watford
WD25 7GS
United Kingdom

8. MARKETING AUTHORISATION NUMBER(S)
04438/0062

9. DATE OF FIRST AUTHORISATION/RENEWAL OF THE AUTHORISATION
January 2002

10. DATE OF REVISION OF THE TEXT
July 2006

Ikorel Tablets

(sanofi-aventis)

1. NAME OF THE MEDICINAL PRODUCT
Ikorel™ Tablets 10mg and 20mg

2. QUALITATIVE AND QUANTITATIVE COMPOSITION
Nicorandil 10mg or 20mg

3. PHARMACEUTICAL FORM
Tablets, off-white, round, with faceted edges, scored on one side and bearing the inscription IK10 (10mg) or IK20 (20mg).

4. CLINICAL PARTICULARS

4.1 Therapeutic indications
Ikorel tablets are indicated for the following:

• The prevention and long term treatment of chronic stable angina pectoris

• A reduction in the risk of acute coronary syndromes in patients with chronic stable angina and at least one of the following risk factors:

Previous MI

Previous CABG

CHD on angiography **or** a positive exercise test together with one of the following: LVH on ECG, left ventricular dysfunction, Age ⩾ 65, diabetes mellitus (type I or II excluding those on sulphonylureas, see section 5.1), hypertension or documented vascular disease

4.2 Posology and method of administration
Route of administration: oral.

Adults: The recommended starting dose is 10mg nicorandil twice daily, although 5mg twice daily may be employed in patients particularly susceptible to headache. Subsequently the dosage should be titrated upward depending on the clinical response. The usual therapeutic dosage is in the range 10 to 20mg nicorandil twice daily, although up to 30mg twice daily may be employed if necessary.

Elderly: There is no special requirement for dosage reduction in elderly patients. As with all medicines, the lowest effective dosage should be used.

Children: A paediatric dosage has not been established and use of nicorandil is not recommended.

4.3 Contraindications
Ikorel is contraindicated in patients with cardiogenic shock, left ventricular failure with low filling pressures and in hypotension. It is also contraindicated in patients who have demonstrated an idiosyncratic response or hypersensitivity to nicorandil. Due to the risk of severe hypotension, the concomitant use of Ikorel and phosphodiesterase 5 inhibitors (e.g. sildenafil, tadalafil, vardenafil) is contraindicated.

4.4 Special warnings and precautions for use
The use of nicorandil should be avoided in patients with depleted blood volume, low systolic blood pressure, acute pulmonary oedema or acute myocardial infarction with acute left ventricular failure and low filling pressures.

Therapeutic doses of nicorandil may lower the blood pressure of hypertensive patients and therefore nicorandil, as with other antianginal agents, should be used with care when prescribed with antihypertensive drugs.

Gastrointestinal ulceration, skin ulceration, and ulcers of the mucosal membranes have been reported with nicorandil (see Section 4.8). These tend to be refractory to treatment and most only respond to withdrawal of nicorandil treatment.

4.5 Interaction with other medicinal products and other forms of interaction
No pharmacological or pharmacokinetic interactions have been observed in humans or animals with beta-blockers, digoxin, rifampicin, cimetidine, acenocoumarol, a calcium antagonist or a combination of digoxin and furosemide. Nevertheless, there is the possibility that nicorandil may potentiate the hypotensive effects of other vasodilators, tricyclic antidepressants or alcohol.

As the hypotensive effects of nitrates or nitric oxide donors are potentiated by phosphodiesterase 5 inhibitors, the concomitant use of Ikorel and phosphodiesterase 5 inhibitors is contraindicated.

Gastrointestinal perforations in the context of concomitant use of nicorandil and corticosteroids have been reported. Caution is advised when concomitant use is considered.

4.6 Pregnancy and lactation
Pregnancy: Animal studies have not revealed any harmful effect of nicorandil on the foetus although there is no experience in humans. It should not be used in pregnant patients unless there is no safer alternative.

Lactation: As it is not known whether nicorandil is excreted in human milk, breastfeeding should be avoided by lactating patients who require therapy.

4.7 Effects on ability to drive and use machines
Patients should be warned not to drive or operate machinery until it is established that their performance is unimpaired by nicorandil.

4.8 Undesirable effects
The following undesirable effects have been reported from the original clinical trials for the prevention and long-term treatment of chronic stable angina and post-marketing experience.

Very common (>1/10); common (>1/100, <1/10); uncommon (>1/1,000, <1/100); rare (>1/10,000, <1/1,000); very rare (<1/10,000), including isolated reports.

(see Table 1 below)

The following additional adverse reactions have been reported during postmarketing experience; they are derived from spontaneous reports, and therefore the frequency of these adverse reactions is not known:

Skin and subcutaneous tissue disorders
Skin and mucosal ulcerations (mainly peri-anal, genital, and para-stomal ulcerations).

Other Clinical Trials – IONA (Impact of Nicorandil in Angina)
In addition, the following undesirable effects occurred at a different frequency in the IONA trial which was a study of subjects at high risk of cardiovascular events.

Immune System disorders
Uncommon – angioedema

Gastrointestinal disorders
Common – rectal bleeding.

Uncommon -Cases of gastritis and oesophagitis were noted in the IONA study, but the difference in incidence between the nicorandil group and the placebo group was not statistically significant.

Uncommon – mouth ulcers

Very Rare – abdominal pain

The clinical expression of diverticular disease may possibly be increased with nicorandil[1]

Musculoskeletal & connective tissue disorders
Uncommon - myalgia

[1] A statistically significant difference (p=0.039) has been found between the nicorandil (20 cases = events) and the placebo group (5 cases = events) in the IONA study, with enrolement of 5126 patients.

4.9 Overdose
Acute overdosage is likely to be associated with peripheral vasodilation, decreased blood pressure and reflex tachycardia. Cardiac function should be monitored and general supportive measures employed. If necessary, circulating plasma volume should be increased by infusion of suitable fluid. In life-threatening situations, administration of vasopressors should be considered. There is no experience of massive overdosage in humans, although the LD_{50} in dogs is in the range 62.5 to 125 mg/kg and in rodents it is in the order of 1200 mg/kg.

5. PHARMACOLOGICAL PROPERTIES

5.1 Pharmacodynamic properties
Nicorandil provides a dual mode of action leading to relaxation of vascular smooth muscle. A potassium channel opening action provides arterial vasodilation, thus reducing afterload, while the nitrate component promotes venous relaxation and a reduction in preload. Nicorandil has a direct effect on coronary arteries without leading to a steal phenomenon. The overall action irnproves blood flow to post-stenotic regions and the oxygen balance in the myocardium.

A reduction of coronary heart disease complications has been shown in patients suffering from angina pectoris who were treated with nicorandil in the IONA study.

The study was a randomised, double blind, placebo controlled, cardiovascular endpoint study carried out in 5126 patients to determine if Nicorandil could reduce the frequency of coronary events in men and women with chronic stable angina and standard anti anginal treatment at high risk of cardiovascular events defined by either: 1) previous myocardial infarction, or 2) coronary artery bypass grafting, or 3) coronary artery disease confirmed by angiography, or a positive exercise test in the previous two years, together with one of the following: left ventricular hypertrophy on the ECG, left ventricular ejection fraction ⩽ 45%, or an end diastolic dimension of >55 mm, age ⩾ 65, diabetes (either type 1 or type 2), hypertension, peripheral vascular disease, or cerebrovascular disease. Patients were excluded from the study if they were receiving a sulphonylurea as it was felt these patients may not benefit; (sulphonylurea agents have the potential to close potassium channels and may thus antagonise some of the effects of nicorandil). Study follow up for endpoint analysis was between 12 and 36 months with a mean of 1.6 years.

The primary endpoint of coronary heart disease (CHD) death, non-fatal myocardial infarction, or unplanned hospital admission for cardiac chest pain, occurred in 13.1% of patients treated with nicorandil compared with 15.5% of patients receiving placebo (hazard ratio 0.83, p=0.014). The rate of acute coronary syndrome (CHD death, non fatal MI or unstable angina) was 6.1% in patients treated with nicorandil compared with 7.6% in patients receiving placebo (hazard ratio 0.79, p=0.028). All cardiovascular events were significantly less in the nicorandil than placebo group 14.7% vs 17.0% (hazard ratio 0.86 p=0.027). The validity of these findings was confirmed by re-analysing the primary endpoint using all cause rather than cardiovascular mortality (nicorandil 14.9% compared with placebo 17.3%, hazard ratio 0.85, p=0.021). The study was not expressly powered to, nor did it detect any statistically significant reduction in any individual component endpoints.

5.2 Pharmacokinetic properties
Nicorandil is well absorbed with no significant first-pass metabolism. Maximum plasma concentrations are achieved in 30 to 60 minutes and are directly related to the dosage. Metabolism is mainly by denitration of the

Table 1

SOC	FREQUENCY	ADR
Immune system disorders	Very rare	Angioedema
Nervous system disorders	Very common	Headache, usually of a transitory nature, especially when treatment is initiated
	Common	Dizziness
Cardiac disorders	Uncommon	An increase in heart rate at high doses
Vascular disorders	Common	Cutaneous vasodilation with flushing
	Uncommon	Hypotension at high therapeutic doses
Gastrointestinal disorders	Common	Nausea and vomiting
	Rare	Persistent aphtosis or mouth ulcers which were occasionally severe
	Very rare	Gastrointestinal ulcerations, such as small intestine ulcer, large intestine ulcer, and anal ulcerations and rectal bleeding. These ulcers may develop into perforation, fistulating disease, or abscess formation (see Sections 4.4 and 4.5)
Hepato-biliary disorders	Rare	Hepatic function abnormalities
Skin and subcutaneous tissue disorders	Rare	Various types of rash
Musculoskeletal & connective tissue disorders	Rare	Myalgia
General disorders and administration site conditions	Common	A feeling of weakness

molecule into the nicotinamide pathway with less than 20% of an administered dose being excreted in the urine. The main phase of elimination has a half-life of about 1 hour. Nicorandil is only slightly bound to plasma proteins.

No clinically relevant modifications in the pharmacokinetic profile have been seen in the elderly or in patients with liver disease or chronic renal failure.

5.3 Preclinical safety data
There are no preclinical data of relevance to the prescriber which are additional to that included in other sections of the SPC.

6. PHARMACEUTICAL PARTICULARS
6.1 List of excipients
Maize starch, croscarmellose sodium, stearic acid and mannitol.

6.2 Incompatibilities
None stated.

6.3 Shelf life
18 months.

Each blister strip should be used within 30 days of opening.

6.4 Special precautions for storage
Store in a dry place below 25°C.

6.5 Nature and contents of container
Ikorel tablets 10mg and 20mg are presented in hard tempered aluminium foil/ (Polyamide/aluminium/PVC) blister strips of 10 tablets, in which each tablet is linked to a silica gel capsule dessicant.

The blister strips are packaged in cartons of 60 tablets.

6.6 Special precautions for disposal and other handling
None stated.

7. MARKETING AUTHORISATION HOLDER
Sanofi-aventis

One Onslow Street

Guildford

Surrey, GU1 4YS, UK

8. MARKETING AUTHORISATION NUMBER(S)
Ikorel tablets 10mg: PL 04425/0327

Ikorel tablets 20mg: PL 04425/0328

9. DATE OF FIRST AUTHORISATION/RENEWAL OF THE AUTHORISATION
24 February 2009

10. DATE OF REVISION OF THE TEXT
February 2009

Legal category: POM

Imdur Tablets 60mg

(AstraZeneca UK Limited)

1. NAME OF THE MEDICINAL PRODUCT
Imdur® Tablets 60mg.

2. QUALITATIVE AND QUANTITATIVE COMPOSITION
Isosorbide mononitrate 60mg

For excipients, see Section 6.1.

3. PHARMACEUTICAL FORM
Extended release film coated tablet (Durules®)

4. CLINICAL PARTICULARS
4.1 Therapeutic indications
Prophylactic treatment of angina pectoris.

4.2 Posology and method of administration
Dosage

Adults:

Imdur 60mg (one tablet) once daily given in the morning. The dose may be increased to 120mg (two tablets) daily, both to be taken once daily in the morning. The dose can be titrated to minimise the possibility of headache, by initiating treatment with 30mg (half a tablet) for the first 2-4 days.

Administration:

Imdur Tablets must not be chewed or crushed. They should be swallowed whole with half a glass of water.

Children

The safety and efficacy of Imdur in children has not been established.

Elderly

No evidence of a need for routine dosage adjustment in the elderly has been found, but special care may be needed in those with increased susceptibility to hypotension or marked hepatic or renal insufficiency.

The core of the tablet is insoluble in the digestive juices but disintegrates into small particles when all active substance has been released. Very occasionally the matrix may pass through the gastrointestinal tract without disintegrating and be found visible in the stool, but all active substance has been released.

4.3 Contraindications
Hypersensitivity to any of the components. Constrictive cardiomyopathy and pericarditis, aortic stenosis, cardiac tamponade, mitral stenosis and severe anaemia.

Patients treated with Imdur must not be given Phosphodiesterase Type 5 Inhibitors (e.g. sildenafil).

Severe cerebrovascular insufficiency or hypotension are relative contraindications to the use of Imdur.

4.4 Special warnings and precautions for use
Imdur is not indicated for relief of acute angina attacks; in the event of an acute attack, sublingual or buccal glyceryl trinitrate tablets should be used.

4.5 Interaction with other medicinal products and other forms of interaction
Concomitant administration of Imdur and Phosphodiesterase Type 5 Inhibitors can potentiate the vasodilatory effect of Imdur with the potential result of serious side effects such as syncope or myocardial infarction. Therefore, Imdur and Phosphodiesterase Type 5 Inhibitors (e.g. sildenafil) must not be given concomitantly.

4.6 Pregnancy and lactation
The safety and efficacy of Imdur during pregnancy or lactation has not been established.

4.7 Effects on ability to drive and use machines
Patients may develop dizziness when first using Imdur. Patients should be advised to determine how they react to Imdur before they drive or operate machinery.

4.8 Undesirable effects
Most of the adverse reactions are pharmacodynamically mediated and dose dependent. Headache may occur when treatment is initiated, but usually disappears after 1-2 weeks of treatment. The dose can be titrated to minimise the possibility of headache, by initiating treatment with 30mg. Hypotension, with symptoms such as dizziness and nausea, has occasionally been reported. These symptoms generally disappear during continued treatment. Rash and pruritus have been reported rarely. Myalgia has been reported very rarely.

4.9 Overdose
Symptoms

Pulsing headache. More serious symptoms are excitation, flushing, cold perspiration, nausea, vomiting, vertigo, syncope, tachycardia and a fall in blood pressure.

Management

Induction of emesis, activated charcoal. In case of pronounced hypotension the patient should first be placed in the supine position with legs raised. If necessary fluids should be administered intravenously.

5. PHARMACOLOGICAL PROPERTIES
5.1 Pharmacodynamic properties
Pharmacotherapeutic group: Vasodilators used in cardiovascular disease (organic nitrates). ATC Code: C01D A.

The principal pharmacological action of isosorbide mononitrate, an active metabolite of isosorbide dinitrate, is relaxation of vascular smooth muscle, producing vasodilation of both arteries and veins with the latter effect predominating. The effect of the treatment is dependent on the dose. Low plasma concentrations lead to venous dilatation, resulting in peripheral pooling of blood, decreased venous return and reduction in left ventricular end-diastolic pressure (preload). High plasma concentrations also dilate the arteries reducing systemic vascular resistance and arterial pressure leading to a reduction in cardiac afterload. Isosorbide mononitrate may also have a direct dilatory effect on the coronary arteries. By reducing the end diastolic pressure and volume, the preparation lowers the intramural pressure, thereby leading to an improvement in the subendocardial blood flow.

The net effect when administering isosorbide mononitrate is therefore a reduced workload of the heart and an improved oxygen supply/demand balance in the myocardium.

5.2 Pharmacokinetic properties
Isosorbide mononitrate is completely absorbed and is not subject to first pass metabolism by the liver. This reduces the intra- and inter-individual variations in plasma levels and leads to predictable and reproducible clinical effects.

The elimination half-life of isosorbide mononitrate is around 5 hours. The plasma protein binding is less than 5%. The volume of distribution for isosorbide mononitrate is about 0.6 l/kg and total clearance around 115 ml/minute. Elimination is primarily by denitration and conjugation in the liver. The metabolites are excreted mainly via the kidneys. Only about 2% of the dose given is excreted intact via the kidneys.

Impaired liver or kidney function have no major influence on the pharmacokinetic properties.

Imdur is an extended release formulation (Durules). The active substance is released independently of pH, over a 10-hour period. Compared to ordinary tablets the absorption phase is prolonged and the duration of effect is extended.

The extent of bioavailability of Imdur is about 90% compared to immediate release tablets. Absorption is not significantly affected by food intake and there is no accumulation during steady state. Imdur exhibits dose proportional kinetics up to 120mg. After repeated peroral administration with 60mg once daily, maximal plasma concentration (around 3000 nmol/l) is achieved after around 4 hours. The plasma concentration then gradually falls to under 500 nmol/l at the end of the dosage interval (24 hours after dose intake). The tablets are divisible.

In placebo-controlled studies, Imdur once daily has been shown to effectively control angina pectoris both in terms of exercise capacity and symptoms, and also in reducing signs of myocardial ischaemia. The duration of the effect is at least 12 hours, at this point the plasma concentration is at the same level as at around 1 hour after dose intake (around 1300 nmol/l).

Imdur is effective as monotherapy as well as in combination with chronic -blocker therapy.

The clinical effects of nitrates may be attenuated during repeated administration owing to high and/or even plasma levels. This can be avoided by allowing low plasma levels for a certain period of the dosage interval. Imdur, when administered once daily in the morning, produces a plasma profile of high levels during the day and low levels during the night. With Imdur 60mg or 120mg once daily no development of tolerance with respect to antianginal effect has been observed. Rebound phenomenon between doses as described with intermittent nitrate patch therapy has not been seen with Imdur.

5.3 Preclinical safety data
The accessible data indicate that isosorbide mononitrate has expected pharmacodynamic properties of an organic nitrate ester, has simple pharmacokinetic properties, and is devoid of toxic, mutagenic or oncogenic effects.

6. PHARMACEUTICAL PARTICULARS
6.1 List of excipients
Aluminium silicate, paraffin special, hydroxypropylcellulose LF, magnesium stearate, colloidal anhydrous silica, hypromellose 6cps, macrogol 6000, titanium dioxide E171 and iron oxide yellow E172.

6.2 Incompatibilities
Not applicable for extended release products.

6.3 Shelf life
Glass bottle: 3 years

Blister pack: 3 years

6.4 Special precautions for storage
Store below 30°C.

6.5 Nature and contents of container
Amber glass bottles with a LD-polyethylene cap in a pack of 100 tablets.

Press-through package of thermoformed PVC, in packs of 7, 14, 28 and 98 tablets.

6.6 Special precautions for disposal and other handling
Do not crush or chew tablets. The tablets should be taken with half a glass of water.

7. MARKETING AUTHORISATION HOLDER
AstraZeneca UK Ltd.,

600 Capability Green,

Luton, LU1 3LU, UK.

8. MARKETING AUTHORISATION NUMBER(S)
PL 17901/0129

9. DATE OF FIRST AUTHORISATION/RENEWAL OF THE AUTHORISATION
18th May 2004

10. DATE OF REVISION OF THE TEXT
15th August 2007

Imigran 10mg and 20mg Nasal Spray

(GlaxoSmithKline UK)

1. NAME OF THE MEDICINAL PRODUCT
Imigran 10 mg Nasal Spray.

Imigran 20 mg Nasal Spray.

2. QUALITATIVE AND QUANTITATIVE COMPOSITION
Imigran 10 mg Nasal Spray: Unit dose spray device for intranasal administration. The device delivers 10 mg of sumatriptan in 0.1 mL of an aqueous buffered solution.

Imigran 20 mg Nasal Spray: Unit dose spray device for intranasal administration. The device delivers 20 mg of sumatriptan in 0.1 mL of an aqueous buffered solution.

For a full list of excipients, see section 6.1.

3. PHARMACEUTICAL FORM
Nasal Spray, solution.

Clear pale yellow to dark yellow liquid, in glass vials in a single dose nasal spray device.

4. CLINICAL PARTICULARS
4.1 Therapeutic indications
Imigran Nasal Spray is indicated for the acute treatment of migraine attacks with or without aura.

4.2 Posology and method of administration
Imigran Nasal Spray should not be used prophylactically.

Imigran is recommended as monotherapy for the acute treatment of a migraine attack and should not be given concomitantly with ergotamine or derivatives of ergotamine (including methysergide) (see Section 4.3 Contraindications).

It is advisable that Imigran be given as early as possible after the onset of a migraine headache. It is equally effective at whatever stage of the attack it is administered.

Adults (18 years of age and over)

The optimal dose of Imigran Nasal Spray is 20 mg for administration into one nostril. However, due to inter/intra patient variability of both the migraine attacks and the absorption of sumatriptan, 10 mg may be effective in some patients.

If a patient does not respond to the first dose of Imigran, a second dose should not be taken for the same attack. In these cases the attack can be treated with paracetamol, aspirin or non-steroidal anti-inflammatory drugs. Imigran may be taken for subsequent attacks.

If the patient has responded to the first dose but the symptoms recur, a second dose may be given in the following 24 hours, provided that there is a minimum interval of 2 hours between the two doses.

No more than two doses of Imigran 20 mg Nasal Spray should be taken in any 24-hour period.

Adolescents (12–17 years of age)

Use of sumatriptan in adolescents should be on the recommendation of a specialist or physician who has significant experience in treating migraine, taking into account local guidance.

The recommended dose of Imigran Nasal Spray is 10 mg for administration into one nostril.

If a patient does not respond to the first dose of Imigran, a second dose should not be taken for the same attack. In these cases the attack can be treated with paracetamol, aspirin or non-steroidal anti-inflammatory drugs.

Imigran may be taken for subsequent attacks.

If the patient has responded to the first dose but the symptoms recur, a second dose may be given in the following 24 hours, provided that there is a minimum interval of 2 hours between the two doses.

No more than two doses of Imigran 10 mg Nasal Spray should be taken in any 24-hour period.

Children (under 12 years of age)

Imigran Nasal Spray is not recommended for use in children under 12 years of age due to insufficient data on safety and efficacy.

Elderly (over 65)

There is no experience of the use of Imigran Nasal Spray in patients over 65. The pharmacokinetics in elderly patients have not been sufficiently studied. Therefore the use of sumatriptan is not recommended until further data are available.

4.3 Contraindications

Hypersensitivity to sumatriptan or to any of the excipients.

Sumatriptan should not be given to patients who have had myocardial infarction or have ischaemic heart disease, coronary vasospasm (Prinzmetal's angina), peripheral vascular disease or symptoms or signs consistent with ischaemic heart disease.

Sumatriptan should not be administered to patients with a history of cerebrovascular accident (CVA) or transient ischaemic attack (TIA).

Sumatriptan should not be administered to patients with severe hepatic impairment.

The use of sumatriptan in patients with moderate and severe hypertension and mild uncontrolled hypertension is contraindicated.

The concomitant administration of ergotamine, or derivatives of ergotamine (including methysergide) or any triptan/5-hydroxytryptamine$_1$ (5-HT$_1$) receptor agonist is contraindicated (see Section 4.5).

Concurrent administration of monoamine oxidase inhibitors (MAOIs) and sumatriptan is contraindicated.

Imigran must not be used within 2 weeks of discontinuation of therapy with monoamine oxidase inhibitors.

4.4 Special warnings and precautions for use

Imigran Nasal Spray should only be used where there is a clear diagnosis of migraine.

Sumatriptan is not indicated for use in the management of hemiplegic, basilar or ophthalmoplegic migraine.

As with other acute migraine therapies, before treating headaches in patients not previously diagnosed as migraineurs, and in migraineurs who present with atypical symptoms, care should be taken to exclude other potentially serious neurological conditions.

It should be noted that migraineurs may be at increased risk of certain cerebrovascular events (e.g. CVA, TIA).

Following administration, sumatriptan can be associated with transient symptoms including chest pain and tightness, which may be intense and involve the throat (see Section 4.8 Undesirable Effects). Where such symptoms are thought to indicate ischaemic heart disease, no further doses of sumatriptan should be given and an appropriate evaluation should be carried out.

Sumatriptan should not be given to patients with risk factors for ischaemic heart disease, including those patients who are heavy smokers or users of nicotine substitution therapies, without prior cardiovascular evaluation (see Section 4.3. Contraindications). Special consideration should be give to postmenopausal women and males over 40 with these risk factors. These evaluations however, may not identify every patient who has cardiac disease and, in very rare cases, serious cardiac events have occurred in patients without underlying cardiovascular disease and in adolescents *(see section 4.8).*

There have been rare post-marketing reports describing patients with serotonin syndrome (including altered mental status, autonomic instability and neuromuscular abnormalities) following the use of a selective serotonin reuptake inhibitor (SSRI) and sumatriptan. Serotonin syndrome has been reported following concomitant treatment with triptans and serotonin noradrenaline reuptake inhibitors (SNRIs).

If concomitant treatment with sumatriptan and an SSRI/SNRI is clinically warranted, appropriate observation of the patient is advised (see Section 4.5)

Sumatriptan should be administered with caution to patients with conditions that may affect significantly the absorption, metabolism, or excretion of the drug, e.g. impaired hepatic or renal function.

Sumatriptan should be used with caution in patients with a history of seizures or other risk factors which lower the seizure threshold, as seizures have been reported in association with sumatriptan (see Section 4.8).

Patients with known hypersensitivity to sulphonamides may exhibit an allergic reaction following administration of sumatriptan. Reactions may range from cutaneous hypersensitivity to anaphylaxis.

Undesirable effects may be more common during concomitant use of triptans and herbal preparations containing St John's Wort (*Hypericum perforatum*).

Prolonged use of any type of painkiller for headaches can make them worse. If this situation is experienced or suspected, medical advice should be obtained and treatment should be discontinued. The diagnosis of medication overuse headache (MOH) should be suspected in patients who have frequent or daily headaches despite (or because of) the regular use of headache medications.

The recommended dose of Imigran should not be exceeded

4.5 Interaction with other medicinal products and other forms of interaction

There is no evidence of interactions with propranolol, flunarizine, pizotifen or alcohol.

There are limited data on an interaction with preparations containing ergotamine or another triptan/5-HT$_1$ receptor agonist. The increased risk of coronary vasospasm is a theoretical possibility and concomitant administration is contraindicated (see section 4.3).

The period of time that should elapse between the use of sumatriptan and ergotamine-containing preparations or another triptan/5-HT$_1$ receptor agonist is not known. This will also depend on the doses and types of products used. The effects may be additive. It is advised to wait at least 24 hours following the use of ergotamine-containing preparations or another triptan/5-HT$_1$ receptor agonist before administering sumatriptan. Conversely, it is advised to wait at least 6 hours following use of sumatriptan before administering an ergotamine-containing product and at least 24 hours before administering another triptan/5-HT$_1$ receptor agonist.

An interaction may occur between sumatriptan and MAOIs and concomitant administration is contraindicated (see Section 4.3 Contraindications).

There have been rare post-marketing reports describing patients with serotonin syndrome (including altered mental status, autonomic instability and neuromuscular abnormalities) following the use of SSRIs and sumatriptan. Serotonin syndrome has also been reported following concomitant treatment with triptans and SNRIs (see Section 4.4).

4.6 Pregnancy and lactation

Post-marketing data on the use of sumatriptan during the first trimester of pregnancy in over 1,000 women are available. Although these data contain insufficient information to draw definitive conclusions, they do not point to an increased risk of congenital defects. Experience with the use of sumatriptan in the second and third trimester is limited.

Evaluation of experimental animal studies does not indicate direct teratogenic effects or harmful effects on peri- and postnatal development. However, embryo-foetal viability might be affected in the rabbit (see Section 5.3 Preclinical Safety Data). Administration of sumatriptan should only be considered if the expected benefit to the mother is greater than any possible risk to the foetus.

It has been demonstrated that following subcutaneous administration sumatriptan is secreted into breast milk. Infant exposure can be minimised by avoiding breast-feeding for 12 hours after treatment, during which time any breast milk expressed should be discarded.

4.7 Effects on ability to drive and use machines

No studies on the effects on the ability to drive and use machines have been performed. Drowsiness may occur as a result of migraine or its treatment with sumatriptan. This may influence the ability to drive and to operate machinery.

4.8 Undesirable effects

Adverse events are listed below by system organ class and frequency. Frequencies are defined as: very common (>1/10), common (>1/100, <1/10), uncommon (>1/1000, <1/100), rare (>1/10,000, <1/1000), very rare (<1/10,000), not known (cannot be estimated from the available data). Some of the symptoms reported as undesirable effects may be associated symptoms of migraine.

Adverse events reported in adults have also been observed in adolescents. These include very rare reports of coronary artery vasospasm and myocardial infarction (See section 4.4 Warnings and Precautions).

Immune system disorders

Very rare:

Hypersensitivity reactions ranging from cutaneous hypersensitivity (such as urticaria) to anaphylaxis.

Nervous system disorders

Very common:

Dysgeusia/unpleasant taste.

Common:

Dizziness, drowsiness, sensory disturbance including paraesthesia and hypoaesthesia.

Very rare:

Seizures, although some have occurred in patients with either a history of seizures or concurrent conditions predisposing to seizures. There are also reports in patients where no such predisposing factors are apparent; Tremor, dystonia, nystagmus, scotoma.

Eye disorders

Very rare:

Flickering, diplopia, reduced vision. Loss of vision including reports of permanent defects. However, visual disorders may also occur during a migraine attack itself.

Cardiac disorders

Very rare:

Bradycardia, tachycardia, palpitations, cardiac arrhythmias, transient ischaemic ECG changes, coronary artery vasospasm, angina, myocardial infarction (see Contraindications, Special Warnings and Precautions for Use).

Vascular disorders

Common:

Transient increases in blood pressure arising soon after treatment. Flushing.

Very rare:

Hypotension, Raynaud's phenomenon.

Respiratory, thoracic and mediastinal disorders

Common:

Following administration of sumatriptan nasal spray mild, transient irritation or burning sensation in the nose or throat or epistaxis have been reported. Dyspnoea.

Gastrointestinal disorders

Common:

Nausea and vomiting occurred in some patients but it is unclear if this is related to sumatriptan or the underlying condition.

Very rare:

Ischaemic colitis.

Not known:

Diarrhoea.

Musculoskeletal and connective tissue disorders

Common:

Sensations of heaviness (usually transient and may be intense and can affect any part of the body including the chest and throat). Myalgia.

Very rare:

Neck stiffness.

Not known:

Arthralgia.

General disorders and administration site conditions

Common:

Pain, sensations of heat or cold, pressure or tightness (these events are usually transient and may be intense and can affect any part of the body including the chest and throat); feelings of weakness, fatigue (both events are mostly mild to moderate in intensity and transient).

Investigations

Very rare:

Minor disturbances in liver function tests have occasionally been observed.

Psychiatric disorders

Not known:

Anxiety.

Skin and subcutaneous tissue disorders

Not known:

Hyperhidrosis.

4.9 Overdose

Single doses of sumatriptan up to 40 mg intranasally, in excess of 16 mg subcutaneously and 400 mg orally have not been associated with side effects other than those mentioned.

In clinical studies volunteers have received 20 mg of sumatriptan by the intranasal route three times a day for a period of 4 days without significant adverse effects.

If overdosage occurs, the patient should be monitored for at least 10 hours and standard supportive treatment applied as required. It is unknown what effect haemodialysis or peritoneal dialysis has on the plasma concentrations of sumatriptan.

5. PHARMACOLOGICAL PROPERTIES

5.1 Pharmacodynamic properties

Pharmacotherapeutic group: Selective 5-HT_1 receptor agonists.

ATC code: N02CC01.

Sumatriptan is a selective vascular 5-hydroxytryptamine-1-(5-HT_{1d}) receptor agonist with no effect on other 5-HT receptor (5-HT_2–5-HT_7) subtypes. The vascular 5-HT_{1d} receptor is found predominantly in cranial blood vessels and mediates vasoconstriction. In animals, sumatriptan selectively constricts the carotid arterial circulation, which supplies blood to the extracranial and intracranial tissues such as the meninges. Dilatation and/or oedema in these vessels is thought to be the underlying mechanism of migraine in man. In addition, evidence from animal studies suggests that sumatriptan inhibits trigeminal nerve activity. Both cranial vasoconstriction and inhibition of trigeminal nerve activity may contribute to the anti-migraine action of sumatriptan in humans.

Clinical response begins 15 minutes following a 20 mg dose given by intranasal administration.

Because of its route of administration, Imigran Nasal Spray may be particularly suitable for patients who suffer nausea and vomiting during a migraine attack.

The magnitude of treatment effect is smaller in adolescents compared with adults.

5.2 Pharmacokinetic properties

After intranasal administration, sumatriptan is rapidly absorbed, median times to maximum plasma concentrations being 1.5 (range: 0.25-3) hours in adults and 2 (range: 0.5-3) hours in adolescents. After a 20 mg dose, the mean maximum concentration is 13ng/mL. Mean intranasal bioavailability, relative to subcutaneous administration is about 16%, partly due to pre-systemic metabolism.

Following oral administration, presystemic clearance is reduced in patients with hepatic impairment resulting in increased plasma levels of sumatriptan. A similar increase is expected following intranasal administration.

Plasma protein binding is low (14–21%) and the mean volume of distribution is 170L. The elimination half-life is approximately 2 hours. The mean total plasma clearance is approximately 1160mL/min and the mean renal plasma clearance is approximately 260mL/min.

A pharmacokinetic study in adolescent subjects (12–17 years) indicated that the mean maximum plasma concentration was 13.9ng/mL and mean elimination half-life was approximately 2 hours following a 20 mg intranasal dose. Population pharmacokinetic modelling indicated that clearance and volume of distribution both increase with body size in the adolescent population resulting in higher exposure in lower bodyweight adolescents.

Non-renal clearance accounts for about 80% of the total clearance. Sumatriptan is eliminated primarily by oxidative metabolism mediated by monoamine oxidase A. The major metabolite, the indole acetic acid analogue of sumatriptan, is mainly excreted in urine, where it is present as a free acid and the glucuronide conjugate. It has no known 5-HT_1 or 5-HT_2 activity. Minor metabolites have not been identified. The pharmacokinetic profile of intranasal sumatriptan does not appear to be significantly affected by migraine attacks.

The kinetics in the elderly have been insufficiently studied to justify a statement on possible differences in kinetics between elderly and young volunteers.

5.3 Preclinical safety data

In non-clinical studies carried out to test for local and ocular irritancy, following administration of sumatriptan nasal spray, there was no nasal irritancy seen in laboratory animals and no ocular irritancy observed when the spray was applied directly to the eyes of rabbits.

Experimental studies of acute and chronic toxicity showed no evidence of toxic effects within the human therapeutic dose range. In a rat fertility study a reduction in success of insemination was seen at exposures sufficiently in excess of the maximum human exposure. In rabbits, embryolethality without marked teratogenic defects was seen.

Sumatriptan was devoid of genotoxic and carcinogenic activity in in-vitro systems and animal studies.

6. PHARMACEUTICAL PARTICULARS

6.1 List of excipients

Potassium Dihydrogen Phosphate

Dibasic Sodium Phosphate anhydrous

Sulphuric Acid

Sodium Hydroxide

Purified Water.

6.2 Incompatibilities

Not applicable.

6.3 Shelf life

3 years

6.4 Special precautions for storage

Do not store above 30°C. Do not freeze.

Imigran Nasal Spray should be kept in the sealed blister, preferably in the box, to protect from light.

6.5 Nature and contents of container

The container consists of a type I Ph.Eur. glass vial with rubber stopper and applicator.

Imigran 10 mg Nasal Spray: unit dose spray device containing 0.1mL solution.

Pack contains 1, 2, 4, 6, 12, or 18 sprays.

Imigran 20 mg Nasal Spray: unit dose spray device containing 0.1mL solution.

Pack contains 1, 2, 4, 6, 12, or 18 sprays.

Not all pack sizes may be marketed.

6.6 Special precautions for disposal and other handling

No special requirements.

7. MARKETING AUTHORISATION HOLDER

GlaxoSmithKline UK
Stockley Park West,
Uxbridge,
Middlesex,
UB11 1BT

8. MARKETING AUTHORISATION NUMBER(S)

PL 10949/0260; 0261

9. DATE OF FIRST AUTHORISATION/RENEWAL OF THE AUTHORISATION

Date of first authorisation: 29/05/1996

Date of last renewal: 29/03/2006

10. DATE OF REVISION OF THE TEXT

03/12/2007

Imigran Injection, Subject

(GlaxoSmithKline UK)

1. NAME OF THE MEDICINAL PRODUCT

Imigran Injection

Imigran Subject

2. QUALITATIVE AND QUANTITATIVE COMPOSITION

Each pre-filled syringe contains 6mg of sumatriptan base, as the succinate salt, in an isotonic solution of 0.5ml.

3. PHARMACEUTICAL FORM

Pre-filled syringes for use in conjunction with an auto injector for subcutaneous injection.

4. CLINICAL PARTICULARS

4.1 Therapeutic indications

Subcutaneous Injection is indicated for the acute relief of migraine attacks, with or without aura, and for the acute treatment of cluster headache. Imigran should only be used where there is a clear diagnosis of migraine or cluster headache.

4.2 Posology and method of administration

Imigran should not be used prophylactically.

It is recommended to start the treatment at the first sign of a migraine headache or associated symptoms such as nausea, vomiting or photophobia. It is equally effective at whatever stage of the attack it is administered. Imigran Injection should be injected subcutaneously using an auto-injector. Patients should be advised to observe strictly the instruction leaflet for the Imigran auto-injector especially regarding the safe disposal of syringes and needles.

Migraine:

Adult: The recommended adult dose of Imigran is a single 6mg subcutaneous injection. Patients who do not respond to this dose should not take a second dose of Imigran for the same attack. Imigran may be taken for subsequent attacks. Patients who respond initially but whose migraine returns may take a further dose at any time in the next 24 hours provided that one hour has elapsed since the first dose.

The maximum dose in 24 hours is two 6mg injections (12mg).

Imigran is recommended as monotherapy for the acute treatment of migraine and should not be given concomitantly with other acute migraine therapies. If a patient fails to respond to a single dose of Imigran there are no reasons, either on theoretical grounds or from limited clinical experience, to withhold products containing aspirin or non-steroidal anti-inflammatory drugs or paracetamol for further treatment of the attack.

Cluster headache:

Adult:

The recommended adult dose is a single 6mg subcutaneous injection for each cluster attack. The maximum dose in 24 hours is two 6mg injections (12mg) with a minimum interval of one hour between the two doses.

Children and Adolescents (under 18 years of age):

Sumatriptan Injection is not recommended for use in children and adolescents as sumatriptan injection has not been studied in these age categories.

Elderly (over 65):

Experience of the use of Imigran in patients aged over 65 years is limited. The pharmacokinetics do not differ significantly from a younger population but, until further clinical data are available, the use of Sumatriptan in patients aged over 65 years is not recommended.

4.3 Contraindications

Hypersensitivity to any component of the preparation.

Sumatriptan should not be given to patients who have had myocardial infarction or have ischaemic heart disease, coronary vasospasm (Prinzmetal's angina), peripheral vascular disease or patients who have symptoms or signs consistent with ischaemic heart disease.

Sumatriptan should not be administered to patients with a history of cerebrovascular accident (CVA) or transient ischaemic attack (TIA).

Sumatriptan should not be administered to patients with severe hepatic impairment.

The use of sumatriptan in patients with moderate and severe hypertension and mild uncontrolled hypertension is contraindicated.

The concomitant administration of ergotamine or derivatives of ergotamine (including methysergide) or any triptan/5-hydroxytryptamine$_1$ (5-HT_1) receptor agonist with sumatriptan is contraindicated. (see section 4.5)

Concurrent administration of monoamine oxidase inhibitors and sumatriptan is contraindicated.

Imigran Injection must not be used within two weeks of discontinuation of therapy with monoamine oxidase inhibitors.

4.4 Special warnings and precautions for use

Warnings: Imigran should only be used where there is a clear diagnosis of migraine or cluster headache.

Sumatriptan is not indicated for use in the management of hemiplegic, basilar or opthalmoplegic migraine.

The recommended doses of Sumatriptan should not be exceeded.

Imigran Injection should not be given intravenously because of its potential to cause vasospasm. The vasospasm may result in arrhythmias, ischaemic ECG changes or myocardial infarction.

Before treating headaches in patients not previously diagnosed as migraineurs, and in migraineurs who present with atypical symptoms, care should be taken to exclude other potentially serious neurological conditions. It should be noted that migraineurs may be at risk of certain cerebrovascular events (e.g. cerebrovascular accident, transient ischaemic attack).

Following administration, sumatriptan can be associated with transient symptoms including chest pain and tightness which may be intense and involve the throat. Where such symptoms are thought to indicate ischaemic heart disease, no further doses of sumatriptan should be given and appropriate evaluation should be carried out.

Sumatriptan should not be given to patients with risk factors for ischaemic heart disease without prior cardiovascular evaluation (See section 4.3). Special consideration should be given to postmenopausal women and males over 40 with these risk factors. These evaluations however, may not identify every patient who has cardiac disease and, in very rare cases, serious cardiac events have occurred in patients without underlying cardiovascular disease.

If the patient experiences symptoms which are severe or persistent or are consistent with angina, further doses should not be taken until appropriate investigations have been carried out to check for the possibility of ischaemic changes.

Precautions: Sumatriptan should be administered with caution to patients with controlled hypertension as transient increases in blood pressure and peripheral vascular resistance have been observed in a small proportion of patients.

There have been rare post-marketing reports describing patients with serotonin syndrome (including altered mental status, autonomic instability and neuromuscular abnormalities) following the use of a selective serotonin reuptake inhibitor (SSRI) and sumatriptan. Serotonin syndrome has been reported following concomitant treatment with triptans and serotonin noradrenaline reuptake inhibitors (SNRIs).

If concomitant treatment with sumatriptan and an SSRI/SNRI is clinically warranted, appropriate observation of the patient is advised.

Sumatriptan should be administered with caution to patients with conditions which may affect significantly the absorption, metabolism or excretion of the drug e.g. impaired hepatic or renal function.

Sumatriptan should be used with caution in patients with a history of seizures or other risk factors which lower the seizure threshold, as seizures have been reported in association with sumatriptan (see section 4.8).

Patients with known hypersensitivity to sulphonamides may exhibit an allergic reaction following administration of Sumatriptan. Reactions may range from cutaneous hypersensitivity to anaphylaxis.

Evidence of cross- sensitivity is limited, however, caution should be exercised before using sumatriptan in these patients.

Undesirable effects may be more common during concomitant use of triptans and herbal preparations containing St John's Wort (*Hypericum perforatum*).

Prolonged use of any type of painkiller for headaches can make them worse. If this situation is experienced or suspected, medical advice should be obtained and treatment should be discontinued. The diagnosis of medication overuse headache (MOH) should be suspected in patients who have frequent or daily headaches despite (or because of) the regular use of headache medications.

4.5 Interaction with other medicinal products and other forms of interaction

Studies in healthy subjects show that Imigran does not interact with propranolol, flunarizine, pizotifen or alcohol.

Sumatriptan has the potential to interact with monoamine oxidase inhibitors (MAOIs), ergotamine and derivatives of ergotamine (see also section 4.3).

There are limited data on an interaction with preparations containing ergotamine or another triptan/5-HT1 receptor agonist. The increased risk of coronary vasospasm is a theoretical possibility and concomitant administration is contraindicated (see section 4.3).

The period of time that should elapse between the use of sumatriptan and ergotamine-containing preparations or another triptan/5-HT1 receptor agonist is not known. This will also depend on the doses and types of products used. The effects may be additive. It is advised to wait at least 24 hours following the use of ergotamine-containing preparations or another triptan/5-HT1 receptor agonist before administering sumatriptan. Conversely, it is advised to wait at least 6 hours following use of sumatriptan before administering an ergotamine-containing product and at least 24 hours before administering another triptan/5-HT1 receptor agonist.

There have been rare post-marketing reports describing patients with serotonin syndrome (including altered mental status, autonomic instability and neuromuscular abnormalities) following the use of SSRIs and sumatriptan. Serotonin syndrome has also been reported following concomitant treatment with triptans and SNRIs (see section 4.4).

4.6 Pregnancy and lactation

Post-marketing data from the use of sumatriptan during the first trimester in over 1,000 women are available. Although these data contain insufficient information to draw definitive conclusions, they do not point to an increased risk of congenital defects. Experience with the use of sumatriptan in the second and third trimester is limited.

Evaluation of experimental animal studies does not indicate direct teratogenic effects or harmful effects on peri- and postnatal development. However, embryofoetal viability might be affected in the rabbit (see section 5.3). Administration of sumatriptan should only be considered if the expected benefit to the mother is greater than any possible risk to the foetus.

It has been demonstrated that following subcutaneous administration sumatriptan is excreted into breast milk. Infant exposure can be minimised by avoiding breast feeding for 12 hours after treatment, during which time any breast milk expressed should be discarded.

4.7 Effects on ability to drive and use machines

Drowsiness may occur as a result of migraine or its treatment with Sumatriptan. Caution is recommended in patients performing skilled tasks, e.g., driving or operating machinery.

4.8 Undesirable effects

Adverse events are listed below by system organ class and frequency [4]. Frequencies are defined as: very common (>1/10), common (>1/100, <1/10), uncommon (>1/1000, <1/100), rare (>1/10,000, <1/1000) and very rare (<1/10,000) including isolated reports.

Clinical Trial Data

Nervous System Disorders

Common: Dizziness, drowsiness, sensory disturbance including paraesthesia and hypoaesthesia.

Vascular Disorders

Common: Transient increases in blood pressure arising soon after treatment. Flushing.

Respiratory, Thoracic and Mediastinal Disorders

Common Dyspnoea.

Gastrointestinal Disorders

Common: Nausea and vomiting occurred in some patients but it is unclear if this is related to sumatriptan or the underlying condition.

Musculoskeletal and Connective Tissue Disorders

Common: Sensations of heaviness (usually transient and may be intense and can affect any part of the body including the chest and throat).

General Disorders and Administration Site Conditions

Very common: Transient injection site pain. Injection site stinging/burning, swelling, erythema, bruising and bleeding have also been reported.

Common: Pain, sensations of heat or cold, pressure or tightness (these events are usually transient and may be intense and can affect any part of the body including the chest and throat).

Feelings of weakness, fatigue (both events are mostly mild to moderate in intensity and transient).

Investigations

Very rare: Minor disturbances in liver function tests have occasionally been observed

Post-Marketing Data

Immune System Disorders

Very rare: Hypersensitivity reactions ranging from cutaneous hypersensitivity to anaphylaxis.

Nervous System Disorders

Very rare: Seizures, although some have occurred in patients with either a history of seizures or concurrent conditions predisposing to seizures there are also reports in patients where no such predisposing factors are apparent.

Tremor, dystonia, nystagmus, scotoma.

Eye Disorders

Very rare: Flickering, diplopia, reduced vision. Loss of vision including reports of permanent defects. However, visual disorders may also occur during a migraine attack itself.

Cardiac Disorders

Very rare: Bradycardia, tachycardia, palpitations, cardiac arrhythmias, transient ischaemic ECG changes, coronary artery vasospasm, angina, myocardial infarction (see Contraindications, Warnings and Precautions).

Vascular Disorders

Very rare: Hypotension, Raynaud's phenomenon.

Gastrointestinal Disorders

Very rare: Ischaemic colitis

Musculoskeletal, Connective Tissue and Bone Disorders

Very rare: Neck stiffness.

4.9 Overdose

There have been some reports of overdosage with Imigran Injection. Patients have received single injections of up to 12mg subcutaneously without significant adverse effects. Doses in excess of 16mg subcutaneously were not associated with side effects other than those mentioned.

If overdosage with Imigran occurs, the patient should be monitored for at least ten hours and standard supportive treatment applied as required.

It is unknown what effect haemodialysis or peritoneal dialysis has on the plasma concentrations of Imigran.

5. PHARMACOLOGICAL PROPERTIES

5.1 Pharmacodynamic properties

Pharmacotherapeutic group: Analgesics: Selective 5-HT_1 receptor agonists.

ATC Code: N02CC01

Sumatriptan has been demonstrated to be a specific and selective 5-hydroxytryptamine (5-HT_{1D}) receptor agonist with no effect on other 5-HT receptor (5-HT_2-5-HT_7) subtypes. The vascular 5-HT_{1D} receptor is found predominantly in cranial blood vessels and mediates vasoconstriction. In animals, sumatriptan selectively constricts the carotid arterial circulation but does not alter cerebral blood flow. The carotid arterial circulation supplies blood to the extracranial and intracranial tissues, such as the meninges and dilatation and/or oedema formation in these vessels is thought to be the underlying mechanism of migraine in man. In addition, experimental evidence from animal studies suggests that sumatriptan inhibits trigeminal nerve activity. Both these actions (cranial vasoconstriction and inhibition of trigeminal nerve activity) may contribute to the anti-migraine action of sumatriptan in humans.

Sumatriptan remains effective in treating menstrual migraine i.e. migraine without aura that occurs between 3 days prior and up to 5 days post onset of menstruation. Sumatriptan should be taken as soon as possible in an attack.

Clinical response begins 10 to 15 minutes following a 6mg subcutaneous injection.

Because of its route of administration Imigran Injection may be particularly suitable for patients who suffer with nausea and vomiting during an attack.

5.2 Pharmacokinetic properties

Following subcutaneous injection, sumatriptan has a high mean bioavailability (96%) with peak serum concentrations occurring in 25 minutes. Average peak serum concentration after a 6mg subcutaneous dose is 72ng/ml. The elimination phase half life is approximately two hours.

Plasma protein binding is low (14 to 21%), mean volume of distribution is 170 litres. Mean total plasma clearance is approximately 1160ml/min and the mean renal plasma clearance is approximately 260ml/min. Non-renal clearance accounts for about 80% of the total clearance. Sumatriptan is eliminated primarily by oxidative metabolism mediated by monoamine oxidase A.

The major metabolite, the indole acetic acid analogue of sumatriptan, is mainly excreted in the urine where it is present as a free acid and the glucuronide conjugate. It has no known 5-HT_1 or 5-HT_2 activity. Minor metabolites have not been identified.

In a pilot study no significant differences were found in the pharmacokinetic parameters between the elderly and young healthy volunteers.

5.3 Preclinical safety data

Sumatriptan was devoid of genotoxic and carcinogenic activity in *in-vitro* systems and animal studies.

In a rat fertility study oral doses of sumatriptan resulting in plasma levels approximately 150 times those seen in man after a 6 mg subcutaneous dose were associated with a reduction in the success of insemination.

This effect did not occur during a subcutaneous study where maximum plasma levels achieved approximately 100 times those in man by the subcutaneous route.

In rabbits embryolethality, without marked teratogenic defects, was seen. The relevance for humans of these findings is unknown.

6. PHARMACEUTICAL PARTICULARS

6.1 List of excipients

Sodium Chloride

Water for Injection

6.2 Incompatibilities

None Reported

6.3 Shelf life

Two years when stored below 30°C and protected from light

6.4 Special precautions for storage

Imigran Injection should be stored below 30°C and protected from light.

6.5 Nature and contents of container

Treatment pack: 2 pre-filled syringes (in cases) plus an auto-injector, in a plastic tray within a carton.

Refill pack: 2 pre-filled syringes (in cases) in a carton or 6 pre-filled syringes(ie three cases each containing 2 pre-filled syringes).

6.6 Special precautions for disposal and other handling

None stated.

Administrative Data

7. MARKETING AUTHORISATION HOLDER

Glaxo Wellcome UK Limited Trading as GlaxoSmithKline UK

Stockley Park West

Uxbridge

Middlesex, UB11 1BT

8. MARKETING AUTHORISATION NUMBER(S)

PL 10949/0113

9. DATE OF FIRST AUTHORISATION/RENEWAL OF THE AUTHORISATION

11/07/1997

10. DATE OF REVISION OF THE TEXT

30 December 2008

11. Legal Category

POM

Imigran Radis 50mg and 100mg Tablets

(GlaxoSmithKline UK)

1. NAME OF THE MEDICINAL PRODUCT

Imigran Radis 50mg Tablets

Imigran Radis 100mg Tablets

2. QUALITATIVE AND QUANTITATIVE COMPOSITION

50mg sumatriptan base as the succinate salt.

100mg sumatriptan base as the succinate salt.

3. PHARMACEUTICAL FORM

Film-coated dispersible tablet

Imigran Radis 50mg Tablets: Pink film-coated, triangular shaped, biconvex tablets debossed with 'GS 1YM' on one face and '50' on the other.

Imigran Radis 100mg Tablets: White film-coated, triangular shaped, biconvex tablets debossed with 'GS YE7' on one face and '100' on the other.

4. CLINICAL PARTICULARS

4.1 Therapeutic indications

Imigran Radis tablets are indicated for the acute relief of migraine attacks, with or without aura. Imigran should only be used where there is a clear diagnosis of migraine.

4.2 Posology and method of administration

Adults

Imigran Radis is indicated for the acute intermittent treatment of migraine. It should not be used prophylactically.

It is advisable that Imigran be given as early as possible after the onset of migraine attack but it is equally effective at whatever stage of the attack it is administered.

The recommended dose of oral Imigran is a single 50mg tablet. Some patients may require 100mg. If the patient has responded to the first dose but the symptoms recur a second dose may be given in the next 24 hours provided that there is a minimum interval of two hours between the two doses and no more than 300mg is taken in any 24 hour period.

Patients who do not respond to the prescribed dose of Imigran Radis should not take a second dose for the same attack. Imigran Radis may be taken for subsequent attacks.

Imigran Radis is recommended as monotherapy for the acute treatment of migraine and should not be given concomitantly with other acute migraine therapies. If a patient fails to respond to a single dose of Imigran Radis there are no reasons, either on theoretical grounds or from limited clinical experience, to withhold products containing aspirin or non-steroidal anti-inflammatory drugs for further treatment of the attack.

The tablets should be swallowed whole with water. Patients with swallowing difficulties may choose to disperse a tablet in a small amount of water before administration. Sumatriptan dispersed in water has a bitter taste.

Children(under 12 years of age)

Sumatriptan tablets are not recommended for use in children below 12 as sumatriptan tablets have not been studied in children.

Adolescents (12 to 17 years of age)

The efficacy of sumatriptan tablets in adolescents could not be demonstrated in the clinical studies performed in this age group. Therefore the use in adolescent is not recommended (see section 5.1 Pharmacodynamic Properties).

Elderly (Over 65)

Experience of the use of Imigran Radis in patients aged over 65 years is limited. The pharmacokinetics do not differ significantly from a younger population but until further clinical data are available, the use of Imigran Radis in patients aged over 65 years is not recommended

4.3 Contraindications

Hypersensitivity to any component of the preparation.

Sumatriptan should not be given to patients who have had myocardial infarction or have ischaemic heart disease, coronary vasospasm (Prinzmetal's angina), peripheral vascular disease or patients who have symptoms or sign consistent with ischaemic heart disease.

Sumatriptan should not be administered to patients with a history of cerebrovascular accident (CVA) or transient ischaemic attack (TIA).

Sumatriptan should not be administered to patients with severe hepatic impairment.

The use of sumatriptan in patients with moderate and severe hypertension and mild uncontrolled hypertension is contraindicated.

The concomitant administration of ergotamine or derivatives of ergotamine (including methysergide) or any triptan/ 5-hydroxytryptamine$_1$ (5-HT$_1$) receptor agonist with sumatriptan is contraindicated. (see section 4.5)

Concurrent administration of monoamine oxidase inhibitors and sumatriptan is contraindicated. Sumatriptan must not be used within two weeks of discontinuation of therapy with monoamine oxidase inhibitors.

4.4 Special warnings and precautions for use

Imigran Radis should only be used where there is a clear diagnosis of migraine.

Sumatriptan is not indicated for use in the management of hemiplegic, basilar or ophthalmoplegic migraine.

The recommended doses of sumatriptan should not be exceeded. As with other migraine therapies, before treating headaches in patients not previously diagnosed as migraineurs, and in migraineurs who present atypical symptoms, care should be taken to exclude other potentially serious neurological conditions.

It should be noted that migraineurs may be at risk of certain cerebrovascular events (e.g. cerebrovascular accident, transient ischaemic attack).

Following administration, sumatriptan can be associated with transient symptoms including chest pain and tightness which may be intense and involve the throat (see section 4.8). Where such symptoms are thought to indicate ischaemic heart disease, no further doses of sumatriptan should be given and appropriate evaluation should be carried out.

Sumatriptan should not be given to patients with risk factors for ischaemic heart disease without prior cardiovascular evaluation (see section 4.3). Special consideration should be given to postmenopausal women and males over 40 with these risk factors. These evaluations however, may not identify every patient who has cardiac disease and, in very rare cases, serious cardiac events have occurred in patients without underlying cardiovascular disease.

Sumatriptan should be administered with caution to patients with controlled hypertension as transient increases in blood pressure and peripheral vascular resistance have been observed in a small proportion of patients.

There have been rare post-marketing reports describing patients with serotonin syndrome (including altered mental status, autonomic instability and neuromuscular abnormalities) following the use of a selective serotonin reuptake inhibitor (SSRI) and sumatriptan. Serotonin syndrome has been reported following concomitant treatment with triptans and serotonin noradrenaline reuptake inhibitors (SNRIs).

If concomitant treatment with sumatriptan and an SSRI/ SNRI is clinically warranted, appropriate observation of the patient is advised.

Sumatriptan should be administered with caution to patients with conditions which may affect significantly the absorption, metabolism or excretion of drugs, e.g. impaired hepatic or renal function. A 50mg dose should be considered in patients with hepatic impairment.

Sumatriptan should be used with caution in patients with a history of seizures or other risk factors which lower the seizure threshold, as seizures have been reported in association with sumatriptan (see section 4.8).

Patients with known hypersensitivity to sulphonamides may exhibit an allergic reaction following administration of sumatriptan. Reactions may range from cutaneous hypersensitivity to anaphylaxis. Evidence of cross-sensitivity is limited, however, caution should be exercised before using sumatriptan in these patients.

Undesirable effects may be more common during concomitant use of triptans and herbal preparations containing St John's Wort (*Hypericum perforatum*).

Prolonged use of any type of painkiller for headaches can make them worse. If this situation is experienced or suspected, medical advice should be obtained and treatment should be discontinued. The diagnosis of medication overuse headache (MOH) should be suspected in patients who have frequent or daily headaches despite (or because of) the regular use of headache medications.

4.5 Interaction with other medicinal products and other forms of interaction

Studies in healthy subjects show that sumatriptan does not interact with propranolol, flunarizine, pizotifen or alcohol. Sumatriptan has the potential to interact with monoamine oxidase inhibitors (MAOIs), ergotamine and derivatives of ergotamine. The increased risk of coronary vasospasm is a theoretical possibility and concomitant administration is contra-indicated. (see also section 4.3).

There are limited data on an interaction with preparations containing ergotamine or another triptan/5-HT1 receptor agonist. The increased risk of coronary vasospasm is a theoretical possibility and concomitant administration is contraindicated (see section 4.3).

The period of time that should elapse between the use of sumatriptan and ergotamine-containing preparations or another triptan/5-HT1 receptor agonist is not known. This will also depend on the doses and types of products used. The effects may be additive. It is advised to wait at least 24 hours following the use of ergotamine-containing preparations or another triptan/5-HT1 receptor agonist before administering sumatriptan. Conversely, it is advised to wait at least 6 hours following use of sumatriptan before administering an ergotamine-containing product and at least 24 hours before administering another triptan/5-HT1 receptor agonist.

There have been rare post-marketing reports describing patients with serotonin syndrome (including altered mental status, autonomic instability and neuromuscular abnormalities) following the use of SSRIs and sumatriptan. Serotonin syndrome has also been reported following concomitant treatment with triptans and SNRIs (see section 4.4).

4.6 Pregnancy and lactation

Post-marketing data from the use of sumatriptan during the first trimester in over 1,000 women are available. Although these data contain insufficient information to draw definitive conclusions, they do not point to an increased risk of congenital defects. Experience with the use of sumatriptan in the second and third trimester is limited.

Evaluation of experimental animal studies does not indicate direct teratogenic effects or harmful effects on peri- and postnatal development. However, embryofoetal viability might be affected in the rabbit (see section 5.3). Administration of sumatriptan should only be considered if the expected benefit to the mother is greater than any possible risk to the foetus.

It has been demonstrated that following subcutaneous administration, sumatriptan is excreted into breast milk. Infant exposure can be minimised by avoiding breast feeding for 12 hours after treatment, during which time any breast milk expressed should be discarded.

4.7 Effects on ability to drive and use machines

Drowsiness may occur as a result of migraine or its treatment with sumatriptan. Caution is recommended in patients performing skilled tasks, e.g. driving or operating machinery

4.8 Undesirable effects

Adverse events are listed below by system organ class and frequency. Frequencies are defined as: very common (>1/10), common (>1/100, <1/10), uncommon (>1/1000, <1/100), rare (>1/10,000, <1/1000) and very rare (<1/10,000) including isolated reports.

Clinical Trial Data

Nervous System Disorders

Common: Dizziness, drowsiness, sensory disturbance including paraesthesia and hypoaesthesia.

Vascular Disorders

Common: Transient increases in blood pressure arising soon after treatment. Flushing.

Respiratory, Thoracic and Mediastinal Disorders

Common Dyspnoea.

Gastrointestinal Disorders

Common: Nausea and vomiting occurred in some patients but it is unclear if this is related to sumatriptan or the underlying condition.

Musculoskeletal and Connective Tissue Disorders

Common: Sensations of heaviness (usually transient and may be intense and can affect any part of the body including the chest and throat).

General Disorders and Administration Site Conditions

Common: Pain, sensations of heat or cold, pressure or tightness (these events are usually transient and may be intense and can affect any part of the body including the chest and throat).

Feelings of weakness, fatigue (both events are mostly mild to moderate in intensity and transient).

Investigations

Very rare: Minor disturbances in liver function tests have occasionally been observed.

Post-Marketing Data

Immune System Disorders

Very rare: Hypersensitivity reactions ranging from cutaneous hypersensitivity to anaphylaxis.

Nervous System Disorders

Very rare: Seizures, although some have occurred in patients with either a history of seizures or concurrent conditions predisposing to seizures there are also reports in patients where no such predisposing factors are apparent.

Tremor, dystonia, nystagmus, scotoma.

Eye Disorders

Very rare: Flickering, diplopia, reduced vision. Loss of vision including reports of permanent defects. However, visual disorders may also occur during a migraine attack itself.

Cardiac Disorders

Very rare: Bradycardia, tachycardia, palpitations, cardiac arrhythmias, transient ischaemic ECG changes, coronary artery vasospasm, angina, myocardial infarction (see Contraindications, Warnings and Precautions).

Vascular Disorders

Very rare: Hypotension, Raynaud's phenomenon.

Gastrointestinal Disorders

Very rare: Ischaemic colitis.

Musculoskeletal, Connective Tissue and Bone Disorders

Very rare: Neck stiffness.

4.9 Overdose

There have been some reports of overdosage with Imigran Tablets. Doses in excess of 400mg orally were not associated with side effects other than those mentioned.

If overdosage occurs, the patient should be monitored for at least ten hours and standard supportive treatment applied as required.

It is unknown what effect haemodialysis or peritoneal dialysis has on the plasma concentrations of Imigran

5. PHARMACOLOGICAL PROPERTIES

5.1 Pharmacodynamic properties

Pharmacotherapeutic group: Analgesics: Selective 5-HT$_1$ receptor agonists.

ATC code: N02CC01

Sumatriptan has been demonstrated to be a specific and selective 5-Hydroxytryptamine$_1$ (5HT$_{1D}$) receptor agonist with no effect on other 5HT receptor (5-HT$_2$-5-HT$_7$) subtypes. The vascular 5-HT$_{1D}$ receptor is found predominantly in cranial blood vessels and mediates vasoconstriction. In animals, sumatriptan selectively constricts the carotid arterial circulation but does not alter cerebral blood flow. The carotid arterial circulation supplies blood to the extracranial and intracranial tissues such as the meninges and dilatation of and/or oedema formation in these vessels is thought to be the underlying mechanism of migraine in man.

In addition, evidence from animal studies suggests that sumatriptan inhibits trigeminal nerve activity. Both these actions (cranial vasoconstriction and inhibition of trigeminal nerve activity) may contribute to the anti-migraine action of sumatriptan in humans.

Sumatriptan remains effective in treating menstrual migraine i.e. migraine without aura that occurs between 3 days prior and up to 5 days post onset of menstruation.

Sumatriptan should be taken as soon as possible in an attack.

Clinical response begins around 30 minutes following a 100mg oral dose.

Although the recommended dose of oral sumatriptan is 50mg, migraine attacks vary in severity both within and between patients. Doses of 25-100mg have shown greater efficacy than placebo in clinical trials, but 25mg is statistically significantly less effective than 50 and 100mg.

A number of placebo-controlled clinical studies assessed the safety and efficacy of oral sumatriptan in approximately 600 adolescent migraineurs aged 12 - 17 years. These studies failed to demonstrate relevant differences in headache relief at 2 hours between placebo and any sumatriptan dose. The undesirable effects profile of oral sumatriptan in adolescents aged 12 - 17 years was similar to that reported from studies in the adult population.

5.2 Pharmacokinetic properties

Following oral administration, sumatriptan is rapidly absorbed, 70% of maximum concentration occurring at 45 minutes. After 100mg dose, the maximum plasma concentration is 54ng/ml. Mean absolute oral bioavailability is 14% partly due to presystemic metabolism and partly due to incomplete absorption. The elimination phase half-life is approximately 2 hours, although there is an indication of a longer terminal phase. Plasma protein binding is low (14-21%), mean volume of distribution is 170 litres. Mean total plasma clearance is approximately 1160ml/min and the mean renal plasma clearance is approximately 260ml/min. Non-renal clearance accounts for about 80% of the total clearance. Sumatriptan is eliminated primarily by oxidative metabolism mediated by monoamine oxidase A. The major metabolite, the indole acetic acid analogue of Sumatriptan is mainly excreted in the urine, where it is present as a free acid and the glucuronide conjugate. It has no known $5HT_1$ or $5HT_2$ activity. Minor metabolites have not been identified. The pharmacokinetics of oral Sumatriptan do not appear to be significantly affected by migraine attacks.

In a pilot study, no significant differences were found in the pharmacokinetic parameters between the elderly and young healthy volunteers.

5.3 Preclinical safety data

Sumatriptan was devoid of genotoxic and carcinogenic activity in *in-vitro* systems and animal studies.

In a rat fertility study oral doses of sumatriptan resulting in plasma levels approximately 200 times those seen in man after a 100 mg oral dose were associated with a reduction in the success of insemination.

This effect did not occur during a subcutaneous study where maximum plasma levels achieved approximately 150 times those in man by the oral route.

In rabbits embryolethality, without marked teratogenic defects, was seen. The relevance for humans of these findings is unknown.

6. PHARMACEUTICAL PARTICULARS

6.1 List of excipients

Imigran Radis 50mg Tablets:

Calcium Hydrogen Phosphate, Anhydrous

Microcrystalline Cellulose

Sodium Hydrogen Carbonate

Croscarmellose Sodium

Magnesium Stearate

Hypromellose

Titanium Dioxide

Glycerol Triacetate

Iron Oxide Red

Imigran Radis 100mg Tablets:

Calcium Hydrogen Phosphate, Anhydrous

Microcrystalline Cellulose

Sodium Hydrogen Carbonate

Croscarmellose Sodium

Magnesium Stearate

Hypromellose

Titanium Dioxide

Glycerol Triacetate

6.2 Incompatibilities

None stated.

6.3 Shelf life

36 months

6.4 Special precautions for storage

Do not store above 30°C

6.5 Nature and contents of container

Aluminium double foil blister packs in a cardboard carton, containing either 2, 4, 6, 12 or 18 tablets.

Not all pack sizes may be marketed.

6.6 Special precautions for disposal and other handling

None stated

Administrative Data

7. MARKETING AUTHORISATION HOLDER

GlaxoSmithKline UK Ltd.

Stockley Park West

Uxbridge

Middlesex. UB11 1BT

8. MARKETING AUTHORISATION NUMBER(S)

Imigran Radis 50mg Tablets: PL 19494/0013

Imigran Radis 100mg Tablets: PL 19494/0014

9. DATE OF FIRST AUTHORISATION/RENEWAL OF THE AUTHORISATION

8th June 2004

10. DATE OF REVISION OF THE TEXT

30 December 2008

11. Legal Status

POM

Imigran Tablets 50mg Imigran Tablets 100mg

(GlaxoSmithKline UK)

1. NAME OF THE MEDICINAL PRODUCT

Imigran Tablets 50mg

Imigran Tablets 100mg

2. QUALITATIVE AND QUANTITATIVE COMPOSITION

50mg sumatriptan base as the succinate salt.

100mg sumatriptan base as the succinate salt.

3. PHARMACEUTICAL FORM

Tablet

50 mg tablet:

Pink, film-coated, capsule-shaped, biconvex tablet (nominal dimensions: 12 mm × 6.5 mm), engraved "GX ES3" on one face and plain on the other face

or "50" on one face and plain on the other face.

100 mg tablet:

White or off-white, film-coated, capsule-shaped, biconvex tablet engraved "GX ET2" on one face and plain on the other face

or "Glaxo" on one face and "Imigran" on the other face.

4. CLINICAL PARTICULARS

4.1 Therapeutic indications

Imigran tablets are indicated for the acute relief of migraine attacks, with or without aura. Imigran should only be used where there is a clear diagnosis of migraine.

4.2 Posology and method of administration

Adults

Imigran is indicated for the acute intermittent treatment of migraine. It should not be used prophylactically.

It is advisable that Imigran be given as early as possible after the onset of migraine attack but it is equally effective at whatever stage of the attack it is administered.

The recommended dose of oral Imigran is a single 50mg tablet. Some patients may require 100mg. If the patient has responded to the first dose but the symptoms recur a second dose may be given in the next 24 hours provided that there is a minimum interval of two hours between the two doses and no more than 300mg is taken in any 24 hour period.

Patients who do not respond to the prescribed dose of Imigran should not take a second dose for the same attack. Imigran may be taken for subsequent attacks.

Imigran is recommended as monotherapy for the acute treatment of migraine and should not be given concomitantly with other acute migraine therapies. If a patient fails to respond to a single dose of Imigran there are no reasons, either on theoretical grounds or from limited clinical experience, to withhold products containing aspirin or non-steroidal anti-inflammatory drugs for further treatment of the attack.

The tablets should be swallowed whole with water.

Children (under 12 years of age)

Sumatriptan tablets are not recommended for use in children below 12 as sumatriptan tablets have not been studied in children.

Adolescents (12 to 17 years of age)

The efficacy of sumatriptan tablets in adolescents could not be demonstrated in the clinical studies performed in this age group. Therefore the use in adolescent is not recommended (see section 5.1 Pharmacodynamic Properties).

Elderly (Over 65)

Experience of the use of Imigran in patients aged over 65 years is limited. The pharmacokinetics do not differ significantly from a younger population but until further clinical data are available, the use of Imigran in patients aged over 65 years is not recommended

4.3 Contraindications

Hypersensitivity to any component of the preparation.

Sumatriptan should not be given to patients who have had myocardial infarction or have ischaemic heart disease, coronary vasospasm (Prinzmetal's angina), peripheral vascular disease or patients who have symptoms or sign consistent with ischaemic heart disease.

Sumatriptan should not be administered to patients with a history of cerebovascular accident (CVA) or transient ischaemic attack (TIA).

Sumatriptan should not be administered to patients with severe hepatic impairment.

The use of sumatriptan in patients with moderate and severe hypertension and mild uncontrolled hypertension is contraindicated.

The concomitant administration of ergotamine or derivatives of ergotamine (including methysergide) or any triptan/5-hydroxytryptamine$_1$ (5-HT$_1$) receptor agonist with sumatriptan is contraindicated (see section 4.5).

Concurrent administration of monoamine oxidase inhibitors and sumatriptan is contraindicated.

Imigran Tablets must not be used within two weeks of discontinuation of therapy with monoamine oxidase inhibitors.

4.4 Special warnings and precautions for use

Imigran should only be used where there is a clear diagnosis of migraine.

Sumatriptan is not indicated for use in the management of hemiplegic, basilar or ophthalmoplegic migraine.

The recommended doses of sumatriptan should not be exceeded. As with other migraine therapies, before treating headaches in patients not previously diagnosed as migraineurs, and in migraineurs who present atypical symptoms, care should be taken to exclude other potentially serious neurological conditions.

It should be noted that migraineurs may be at risk of certain cerebrovascular events (e.g. cerebrovascular accident, transient ischaemic attack).

Following administration, sumatriptan can be associated with transient symptoms including chest pain and tightness which may be intense and involve the throat (see section 4.8). Where such symptoms are thought to indicate ischaemic heart disease, no further doses of sumatriptan should be given and appropriate evaluation should be carried out.

Sumatriptan should not be given to patients with risk factors for ischaemic heart disease without prior cardiovascular evaluation (see section 4.3). Special consideration should be given to postmenopausal women and males over 40 with these risk factors. These evaluations however, may not identify every patient who has cardiac disease and, in very rare cases, serious cardiac events have occurred in patients without underlying cardiovascular disease.

Sumatriptan should be administered with caution to patients with controlled hypertension as transient increases in blood pressure and peripheral vascular resistance have been observed in a small proportion of patients.

There have been rare post-marketing reports describing patients with serotonin syndrome (including altered mental status, autonomic instability and neuromuscular abnormalities) following the use of a selective serotonin reuptake inhibitor (SSRI) and sumatriptan. Serotonin syndrome has been reported following concomitant treatment with triptans and serotonin noradrenaline reuptake inhibitors (SNRIs).

If concomitant treatment with sumatriptan and an SSRI/SNRI is clinically warranted, appropriate observation of the patient is advised.

Sumatriptan should be administered with caution to patients with conditions which may affect significantly the absorption, metabolism or excretion of drugs, e.g. impaired hepatic or renal function. A 50mg dose should be considered in patients with hepatic impairment.

Sumatriptan should be used with caution in patients with a history of seizures or other risk factors which lower the seizure threshold, as seizures have been reported in association with sumatriptan (see section 4.8).

Patients with known hypersensitivity to sulphonamides may exhibit an allergic reaction following administration of sumatriptan. Reactions may range from cutaneous hypersensitivity to anaphylaxis. Evidence of cross-sensitivity is limited, however, caution should be exercised before using sumatriptan in these patients.

Undesirable effects may be more common during concomitant use of triptans and herbal preparations containing St John's Wort (*Hypericum perforatum*).

Prolonged use of any type of painkiller for headaches can make them worse. If this situation is experienced or suspected, medical advice should be obtained and treatment should be discontinued. The diagnosis of medication overuse headache (MOH) should be suspected in patients who have frequent or daily headaches despite (or because of) the regular use of headache medications.

Patients with rare hereditary problems of galactose intolerance, the Lapp lactase deficiency or glucose-galactose malabsorption should not take this medicine as it contains lactose.

4.5 Interaction with other medicinal products and other forms of interaction

Studies in healthy subjects show that sumatriptan does not interact with propranolol, flunarizine, pizotifen or alcohol.

Sumatriptan has the potential to interact with monoamine oxidase inhibitors (MAOIs), ergotamine and derivatives of ergotamine. The increased risk of coronary vasospasm is a theoretical possibility and concomitant administration is contra-indicated.(see also section 4.3).

There are limited data on an interaction with preparations containing ergotamine or another triptan/5-HT1 receptor agonist. The increased risk of coronary vasospasm is a theoretical possibility and concomitant administration is contraindicated (see section 4.3).

The period of time that should elapse between the use of sumatriptan and ergotamine-containing preparations or another triptan/5-HT1 receptor agonist is not known. This will also depend on the doses and types of products used. The effects may be additive. It is advised to wait at least 24 hours following the use of ergotamine-containing preparations or another triptan/5-HT1 receptor agonist before administering sumatriptan. Conversely, it is advised to wait at least 6 hours following use of sumatriptan before administering an ergotamine-containing product and at least 24 hours before administering another triptan/5-HT1 receptor agonist.

There have been rare post-marketing reports describing patients with serotonin syndrome (including altered mental status, autonomic instability and neuromuscular abnormalities) following the use of SSRIs and sumatriptan. Serotonin syndrome has also been reported following concomitant treatment with triptans and SNRIs (see section 4.4).

4.6 Pregnancy and lactation

Post-marketing data from the use of sumatriptan during the first trimester in over 1,000 women are available. Although these data contain insufficient information to draw definitive conclusions, they do not point to an increased risk of congenital defects. Experience with the use of sumatriptan in the second and third trimester is limited.

Evaluation of experimental animal studies does not indicate direct teratogenic effects or harmful effects on peri- and postnatal development. However, embryofoetal viability might be affected in the rabbit (see section 5.3). Administration of sumatriptan should only be considered if the expected benefit to the mother is greater than any possible risk to the foetus.

It has been demonstrated that following subcutaneous administration, sumatriptan is excreted into breast milk. Infant exposure can be minimised by avoiding breast feeding for 12 hours after treatment, during which time any breast milk expressed should be discarded.

4.7 Effects on ability to drive and use machines

Drowsiness may occur as a result of migraine or its treatment with sumatriptan. Caution is recommended in patients performing skilled tasks, e.g. driving or operating machinery

4.8 Undesirable effects

Adverse events are listed below by system organ class and frequency [4]. Frequencies are defined as: very common ($>1/10$), common ($>1/100$, $<1/10$), uncommon ($>1/1000$, $<1/100$), rare ($>1/10,000$, $<1/1000$) and very rare ($<1/10,000$) including isolated reports.

Clinical Trial Data

Nervous System Disorders

Common: Dizziness, drowsiness, sensory disturbance including paraesthesia and hypoaesthesia.

Vascular Disorders

Common: Transient increases in blood pressure arising soon after treatment. Flushing.

Respiratory, Thoracic and Mediastinal Disorders

Common Dyspnoea.

Gastrointestinal Disorders

Common: Nausea and vomiting occurred in some patients but it is unclear if this is related to sumatriptan or the underlying condition.

Musculoskeletal and Connective Tissue Disorders

Common: Sensations of heaviness (usually transient and may be intense and can affect any part of the body including the chest and throat).

General Disorders and Administration Site Conditions

Common: Pain, sensations of heat or cold, pressure or tightness (these events are usually transient and may be intense and can affect any part of the body including the chest and throat).

Feelings of weakness, fatigue (both events are mostly mild to moderate in intensity and transient).

Investigations

Very rare: Minor disturbances in liver function tests have occasionally been observed

Post-Marketing Data

Immune System Disorders

Very rare: Hypersensitivity reactions ranging from cutaneous hypersensitivity to anaphylaxis.

Nervous System Disorders

Very rare: Seizures, although some have occurred in patients with either a history of seizures or concurrent conditions predisposing to seizures there are also reports in patients where no such predisposing factors are apparent.

Tremor, dystonia, nystagmus, scotoma.

Eye Disorders

Very rare: Flickering, diplopia, reduced vision. Loss of vision including reports of permanent defects. However, visual disorders may also occur during a migraine attack itself.

Cardiac Disorders

Very rare: Bradycardia, tachycardia, palpitations, cardiac arrhythmias, transient ischaemic ECG changes, coronary artery vasospasm, angina, myocardial infarction (see Contraindications, Warnings and Precautions).

Vascular Disorders

Very rare: Hypotension, Raynaud's phenomenon.

Gastrointestinal Disorders

Very rare: Ischaemic colitis

Musculoskeletal, Connective Tissue and Bone Disorders

Very rare: Neck stiffness.

4.9 Overdose

There have been some reports of overdosage with Imigran Tablets. Doses in excess of 400mg orally were not associated with side effects other than those mentioned.

If overdosage occurs, the patient should be monitored for at least ten hours and standard supportive treatment applied as required.

It is unknown what effect haemodialysis or peritoneal dialysis has on the plasma concentrations of Imigran

5. PHARMACOLOGICAL PROPERTIES

5.1 Pharmacodynamic properties

Pharmacotherapeutic group: Analgesics: Selective 5-HT_1 receptor agonists.

ATC code: N02CC01

Sumatriptan has been demonstrated to be a specific and selective 5-Hydroxytryptamine$_1$ ($5HT_{1D}$) receptor agonist with no effect on other 5HT receptor ($5\text{-}HT_2\text{-}5\text{-}HT_7$) subtypes. The vascular 5-HT_{1D} receptor is found predominantly in cranial blood vessels and mediates vasoconstriction. In animals, sumatriptan selectively constricts the carotid arterial circulation but does not alter cerebral blood flow. The carotid arterial circulation supplies blood to the extracranial and intracranial tissues such as the meninges and dilatation of and/or oedema formation in these vessels is thought to be the underlying mechanism of migraine in man.

In addition, evidence from animal studies suggests that sumatriptan inhibits trigeminal nerve activity. Both these actions (cranial vasoconstriction and inhibition of trigeminal nerve activity) may contribute to the anti-migraine action of sumatriptan in humans.

Sumatriptan remains effective in treating menstrual migraine i.e. migraine without aura that occurs between 3 days prior and up to 5 days post onset of menstruation. Sumatriptan should be taken as soon as possible in an attack.

Clinical response begins around 30 minutes following a 100mg oral dose.

Although the recommended dose of oral sumatriptan is 50mg, migraine attacks vary in severity both within and between patients. Doses of 25-100mg have shown greater efficacy than placebo in clinical trials, but 25mg is statistically significantly less effective than 50 and 100mg.

A number of placebo-controlled clinical studies assessed the safety and efficacy of oral sumatriptan in approximately 600 adolescent migraineurs aged 12 - 17 years. These studies failed to demonstrate relevant differences in headache relief at 2 hours between placebo and any sumatriptan dose. The undesirable effects profile of oral sumatriptan in adolescents aged 12 - 17 years was similar to that reported from studies in the adult population.

5.2 Pharmacokinetic properties

Following oral administration, sumatriptan is rapidly absorbed, 70% of maximum concentration occurring at 45 minutes. After 100mg dose, the maximum plasma concentration is 54ng/ml. Mean absolute oral bioavailability is 14% partly due to presystemic metabolism and partly due to incomplete absorption. The elimination phase half-life is approximately 2 hours, although there is an indication of a longer terminal phase. Plasma protein binding is low (14-21%), mean volume of distribution is 170 litres. Mean total plasma clearance is approximately 1160ml/min and the mean renal plasma clearance is approximately 260ml/min. Non-renal clearance accounts for about 80% of the total clearance. Sumatriptan is eliminated primarily by oxidative metabolism mediated by monoamine oxidase A. The major metabolite, the indole acetic acid analogue of Sumatriptan is mainly excreted in the urine, where it is present as a free acid and the glucuronide conjugate. It has no known $5HT_1$ or $5HT_2$ activity. Minor metabolites have not been identified. The pharmacokinetics of oral Sumatriptan do not appear to be significantly affected by migraine attacks.

In a pilot study, no significant differences were found in the pharmacokinetic parameters between the elderly and young healthy volunteers.

5.3 Preclinical safety data

Sumatriptan was devoid of genotoxic and carcinogenic activity in *in-vitro* systems and animal studies.

In a rat fertility study oral doses of sumatriptan resulting in plasma levels approximately 200 times those seen in man after a 100 mg oral dose were associated with a reduction in the success of insemination.

This effect did not occur during a subcutaneous study where maximum plasma levels achieved approximately 150 times those in man by the oral route.

In rabbits embryolethality, without marked teratogenic defects, was seen. The relevance for humans of these findings is unknown.

6. PHARMACEUTICAL PARTICULARS

6.1 List of excipients

Imigran 50mg Tablets: Lactose, microcrystalline cellulose, croscarmellose sodium, magnesium stearate, methylhydroxypropylcellulose, titanium dioxide, triacetin and iron oxide.

Imigran 100mg Tablets: Lactose, microcrystalline cellulose, croscarmellose sodium, magnesium stearate, methylhydroxypropylcellulose and opaspray white.

6.2 Incompatibilities

None stated.

6.3 Shelf life

Imigran 50mg Tablets: 36 months

Imigran 100mg Tablets: 48 months

6.4 Special precautions for storage

Store below 30°C

6.5 Nature and contents of container

Imigran 50mg Tablets: Aluminium double foil blister packs in a cardboard carton, containing either 2, 3, 6, 12, 18 or 24 tablets.

Imigran 100mg Tablets: Aluminium double foil blister packs in a cardboard carton, containing either 2, 3, 6 or12 tablets.

6.6 Special precautions for disposal and other handling

None stated

Administrative Data

7. MARKETING AUTHORISATION HOLDER

Glaxo Wellcome UK Ltd. trading as GlaxoSmithKline UK.

Stockley Park West

Uxbridge

Middlesex. UB11 1BT

8. MARKETING AUTHORISATION NUMBER(S)

Imigran 50mg Tablets: PL 10949/0222

Imigran 100mg Tablets: PL 10949/0231

9. DATE OF FIRST AUTHORISATION/RENEWAL OF THE AUTHORISATION

Imigran 50mg Tablets: 29 December 2005

Imigran 100mg Tablets: 09 February 2003

10. DATE OF REVISION OF THE TEXT

24 August 2009

11. Legal Status

POM

ImmuCyst 81mg

(Cambridge Laboratories)

1. NAME OF THE MEDICINAL PRODUCT

Trade Name: ImmuCyst® 81 mg

Proper name: BCG Immunotherapy

2. QUALITATIVE AND QUANTITATIVE COMPOSITION

The product is presented as a lyophilisate, which is a white powder. This is reconstituted in sterile preservative-free normal saline.

ImmuCyst® 81 mg is freeze-dried preparation made from a culture of the Connaught strain of Bacillus of Calmette and Guérin (BCG), which is an attenuated strain of living bovine tubercle bacillus, *Mycobacterium bovis*. The bacilli are lyophilised (freeze-dried) and are viable upon reconstitution. The product contains no preservative.

Lyophilisate	Content per Vial
BCG (Bacillus of Calmette and Guérin)	81 mg (dry weight) 1.8 to 15.9 × 10^8 Colony Forming Units (CFU) throughout the shelf life
Monosodium glutamate	150 mg (5% w/v prior to lyophilisation)

3. PHARMACEUTICAL FORM

ImmuCyst® 81 mg is supplied as a lyophilisate for intravesicular use.

4. CLINICAL PARTICULARS

4.1 Therapeutic indications

ImmuCyst® 81 mg is indicated for intravesicular use in the treatment and prophylaxis of primary or recurrent carcinoma *in situ* (CIS) of the urinary bladder, and for the prophylaxis following transurethral resection (TUR) of primary or recurrent stage Ta and/or T1 papillary tumours, or any combination thereof, regardless of antecedent intravesicular treatment.

4.2 Posology and method of administration

Adults

One dose of ImmuCyst®81 mg consists of the intravesicular instillation of 81 mg (dry weight) BCG. This dose is prepared by reconstituting the vial containing freeze-dried BCG with preservative-free normal saline. The vial of reconstituted BCG is diluted in 50ml of sterile, preservative-free saline, to a total of 53 ml instillation volume (see instructions for use and handling).

A urethral catheter is inserted into the bladder under aseptic conditions. It is important to note that a sufficient quantity of lubricant is used to reduce the chance of traumatising the urinary mucosa and therefore the risk of severe complications including BCG infection and also to reduce the discomfort of the patient. From the limited evidence, bacteriostatic urethral lubricants have been shown to have an association with a reduction in the viability of BCG (see Section 4.5). As a precaution, to minimise the amount of lubricant in the bladder, it is recommended that catheterisation should be performed when the bladder is full. The bladder is drained, rinsing out with the urine any lubricant which may have reached the bladder. The 53ml suspension of ImmuCyst is instilled slowly by gravity, following which the catheter is withdrawn.

The patient retains the suspension for as long as possible for up to two hours. During the first 15 minutes following instillation, the patient should lie prone. Thereafter, the patient is allowed to be up. At the end of 2 hours, all patients should void in a seated position for environmental safety reasons. Patients should be instructed to maintain adequate hydration.

Clinical trials carried out with ImmuCyst® 81 mg included a percutaneous inoculation with each intravesicular dose. A 0.5 ml portion of the 53 ml intravesical dose of ImmuCyst® 81 mg was administered percutaneously (e.g., on inner, upper thigh). Some studies have suggested that there is no additional benefit of administering BCG systemically. If severe reactions occur, such as ulceration at the site of regional lymphadenitis, the percutaneous treatment should be discontinued.

Treatment Schedule

Intravesicular treatment of the urinary bladder should begin 10 to 14 days after biopsy of TUR, and consists of induction and maintenance treatments.

The induction treatment consists of one intravesicular instillation of ImmuCyst®81mg each week for 6 weeks. After a 6 week pause, one intravesical instillation should be given once each week for 1-3 weeks. Clinical studies have demonstrated that 3 weekly instillations significantly increase the complete response rate from 73% to 87% at 6 months, compared with no additional treatment given at 3 months. Three weekly instillations should definitely be given to patients who still have evidence of bladder cancer.

Based on clinical studies performed with ImmuCyst® 81 mg, maintenance therapy following induction is highly recommended. This consists of one dose given each week for 1 to 3 weeks at 6 months following the initial dose, and then every 6 months thereafter until 36 months.

Children

Safety and effectiveness in children have not been established.

4.3 Contraindications

ImmuCyst® 81 mg is contraindicated for patients:

- who have had a TUR or traumatic bladder catheterisation (associated with hematuria) in the previous 10 days,
- who are immunosuppressed as a result of malignancies or receiving immunosuppressive therapies, including irradiation, antimetabolites, alkylating agents, cytotoxic drugs, or who are otherwise immunocompromised (including HIV-infected individuals),
- with active tuberculosis, because of the danger of exacerbation or of concomitant systemic BCG infection,
- with current or previous evidence of a systemic BCG infection,
- with fever, unless the cause of the fever has been determined and evaluated, and
- with bacterial urinary tract infection, until all the infection has resolved.

4.4 Special warnings and precautions for use

Contains viable attenuated mycobacteria. Handle as infectious.

ImmuCyst® 81 mg should not be handled by persons with immune deficiency.

It is recommended that intravesicular ImmuCyst® 81 mg not be administered any sooner than 10 days following TUR. Given the specialised nature of BCG intravesical treatment, ImmuCyst® 81 mg should be administered under the supervision of a qualified physician, such as a urologist, experienced in the use of anti-cancer agents.

Care must be taken during administration of intravesicular ImmuCyst® 81 mg not to introduce contaminants into the urinary tract nor to traumatise unduly the urinary mucosa. If the physician believes that the bladder catheterisation has been traumatic (e.g. associated with bleeding), then ImmuCyst® 81 mg should not be administered and there must be a treatment delay of at least 10 days. Subsequent treatment should be resumed as if no interruption in the schedule had occurred.

Intravesicular treatment with ImmuCyst® 81 mg may induce a sensitivity to tuberculin purified protein derivative (PPD) which could complicate future interpretations of skin test reactions to tuberculin in the diagnosis of suspected mycobacterial infections. Determination of a patient's reactivity to tuberculin prior to administration of ImmuCyst® 81 mg may therefore be desirable.

For patients with small bladder capacity, increased risk of bladder contracture should be considered in decisions to treat with ImmuCyst® 81 mg.

If a bacterial urinary tract infection (UTI) occurs during the course of ImmuCyst® 81mg treatment, ImmuCyst® 81 mg instillation should be withheld until complete resolution of the bacterial UTI for two reasons: (1) the combination of a UTI and BCG- induced cystitis may lead to more severe adverse effects on the genitourinary tract, and (2) BCG bacilli are sensitive to a wide variety of antibiotics; antimicrobial administration may therefore diminish the efficacy of ImmuCyst® 81 mg.

Patients undergoing antimicrobial therapy for other infections should be evaluated to assess whether the therapy might diminish the efficacy of ImmuCyst® 81 mg.

BCG infection of aneurysms and prosthetic devices (including arterial grafts, cardiac devices, and artificial joints) have been reported following intravesicular administration of BCG. The risk of these ectopic BCG infections has not been determined, but is considered to be very small. The benefits of BCG therapy must carefully be weighed against the possibility of an ectopic BCG infection in patients with pre-existing arterial aneurysms or prosthetic devices of any kind.

4.5 Interaction with other medicinal products and other forms of interaction

Patients must be advised that drug combinations containing bone marrow depressants and/or immunosuppressants and/or radiation may impair the response to ImmuCyst® 81 mg and/or increase the risk of disseminated BCG infection. For patients with a condition that may in future require mandatory immunosuppression (e.g. awaiting an organ transplant, myasthenia gravis), the decision to treat with ImmuCyst® 81 mg should be considered carefully.

Limited in-vitro testing of bacteriostatic lubricants and BCG has shown a reduction in the number of BCG CFU. However, it has been shown in patients that when a bacteriostatic lubricant was used for catheterisation before instillation, the BCG CFU count remained above the required minimum microbial count and there was no significant reduction in the clinical efficacy of BCG therapy.

4.6 Pregnancy and lactation

Animal reproduction studies have not been conducted with ImmuCyst® 81 mg. It is also not known whether ImmuCyst® 81 mg can cause fetal harm when administered to a pregnant woman or can affect reproduction capacity. ImmuCyst® 81 mg should be given to a pregnant woman only if clearly needed.

A nursing woman with a systemic BCG infection could infect her infant.

It is not known whether this drug is excreted in human milk. Therefore, caution should be exercised when ImmuCyst® 81 mg is administered to a nursing woman.

4.7 Effects on ability to drive and use machines

There are no indications that ability to drive and use machines is impaired.

4.8 Undesirable effects

Administration of intravesicular ImmuCyst® 81 mg causes an inflammatory response in the bladder and has been frequently associated with transient fever, haematuria, urinary frequency and dysuria. Such reactions may to some degree be taken as evidence that BCG is evoking the desired response, but patients should be carefully monitored for serious adverse events. Serious adverse events have occurred in <1% of ImmuCyst® 81 mg recipients.

Local:

The most common local reactions are transient dysuria and urinary frequency. During the induction course, these reactions occurred on at least one occasion in 26% and 14% of patients, respectively. This rose to 46% and 34% respectively, among patients during maintenance therapy. Gross hematuria has occurred among 11-19% of ImmuCyst® 81 mg recipients, while more serious genitourinary adverse events have occurred in <0.5% of recipients. Infrequent associations include bacterial UTI, bladder contracture, symptomatic granulomatous prostatitis, epididymo-orchitis, urethral obstruction, and renal abscess.

Systemic:

Transient fever of <38.5° C of < 48 hours duration has occurred among 17% of ImmuCyst® 81 mg recipients during induction and among 31% during maintenance.

Skin rash, arthralgia, and migratory arthritis are rare, and are considered to be strictly allergic reactions.

Ocular symptoms (including uveitis, conjunctivitis, iritis, keratitis, and granulomatous choreoretinitis) alone, or in combination with joint symptoms (arthritis or arthralgia), urinary symptoms and/or skin rash, have been reported following administration of intravesicular BCG. The risk seems to be elevated among patients who are positive for HLA-B27.

BCG Infection

Systemic BCG infection is a serious side effect of ImmuCyst® 81 mg administration and fatalities have occurred.

BCG infection may be more common after traumatic bladder catheterisation or bladder perforation. BCG treatment should be delayed in such patients until mucosal damage has healed.

Treatment should be delayed for 10-14 days after TUR or biopsy of bladder lesions.

All patients receiving the product should be carefully monitored and advised to report all incidences of fever and other events outside the urinary tract. Fever lasting over 24 hours and any unusual event should be investigated to exclude another cause and to try and isolate organisms. Blood cultures and samples from affected sites should be cultured for BCG.

The infection may manifest as pneumonitis, hepatitis and/or cytopenia after a period of fever and malaise.

Fever lasting more than 48 hours for which there is no explanation and any other unexplained reactions should be treated with antituberculous therapy, following the regular treatment schedules for tuberculosis.

ImmuCyst® 81 mg is sensitive to Isoniazid, Rifampicin and Ethambutol.

No further treatment with BCG should be given.

Treatment of undesirable effects:

Table 1 summarises the recommended treatment of adverse events.

Irritative bladder side effects associated with ImmuCyst® 81 mg administration can be managed symptomatically with propantheline bromide. Paracetamol may be administered for symptomatic relief of transient fever or irritative bladder symptoms.

BCG organisms, including the Connaught strain, are susceptible to all currently used anti-tuberculosis drugs with the exception of pyrazinamide. Accordingly, for more serious reactions other than a systemic BCG infection (e.g., severe urinary tract adverse events or allergic reaction), Isoniazid with or without Rifampicin should be administered for 3-6 months.

If a systemic BCG infection occurs, an Infectious Diseases consultation should be sought. ImmuCyst® 81 mg should be permanently discontinued, and triple anti-tuberculosis therapy should be initiated promptly and continued for 6 months. Commonly, this will comprise Isoniazid (300 mg daily), Rifampicin (600 mg daily), and Ethambutol (1000 mg daily). In the presence of signs of septic shock as a manifestation of a systemic BCG infection, the addition of short-term corticosteroids (e.g. Prednisolone, 40 mg daily) has been shown to be beneficial, and should be considered.

If a systemic BCG infection has occurred, a report should be submitted to both the manufacturer and the appropriate health authorities. The report should include details of the treatment history with ImmuCyst® 81 mg, the symptoms and signs of the BCG infection, the treatment administered for the reaction, and the response to this treatment.

Patients must be advised to check with their doctor as soon as possible if there is an increase in their existing symptoms, or if their symptoms persist even after receiving a number of treatments, or if any of the following symptoms develop.

More common: Blood in the urine; painful or frequent urination lasting > 2 days; nausea and vomiting;fever and chill lasting > 24 hours.

Rare: Cough; skin rash; high or persistent fever; joint pains; jaundice; eye complaints.

Table 1

Recommended Treatment of Adverse Events Associated with ImmuCyst® 81mg

Symptom, Sign or Syndrome	Treatment
Irritative bladder symptoms < 48 hours duration	Symptomatic treatment.
Irritative bladder symptoms ≥48 hours duration	Symptomatic treatment; postpone next ImmuCyst® 81 mg treatment until complete resolution. If complete resolution has not occurred within one week, administer Isoniazid (INH), 300 mg daily until complete resolution.
Concomitant bacterial UTI	Postpone next ImmuCyst® 81 mg treatment until completion of antimicrobial therapy and negative urine culture.

Other genitourinary tract adverse events: symptomatic granulomatous prostatitis, epididymo-orchitis, urethral obstruction or renal abscess.	Discontinue ImmuCyst® 81 mg. Administer INH, 300 mg daily and Rifampicin, 600 mg daily for 3-6 months.
Fever <38.5° C of <48 hours duration.	Symptomatic treatment with Paracetamol
Skin rash, arthralgia, or migratory arthritis.	Anti-histamines or non-steroidal anti-inflammatories. If no response, discontinue ImmuCyst® 81 mg and administer INH 300 mg daily for 3 months. Consider administration of Prednisolone.
Systemic BCG infection without signs of septic shock.	Discontinue ImmuCyst® 81 mg. Seek an Infectious Disease consultation. Administer triple-drug anti-tuberculosis therapy for 6 months.
Systemic BCG infection with signs of septic shock.	As for immediately above. Consider addition of short-term high-dose systemic corticosteroids.
Ocular complaints	Consult Ophthalmologist for specific treatment

4.9 Overdose
In case of overdose, patients should be monitored closely, and any adverse events should be treated according to the recommendations in "Treatment of undesirable effects", above.

5. PHARMACOLOGICAL PROPERTIES
5.1 Pharmacodynamic properties
ATC Code: LO3AX

ImmuCyst® 81 mg promotes a local acute inflammatory and immunological reaction, and sub-acute granulomatous reaction with macrophage and lymphocyte infiltration in the urothelium and lamina propria of the urinary bladder.

5.2 Pharmacokinetic properties
ImmuCyst® 81 mg has been administered intravesically with concomitant percutaneous administration. Acid-fast bacteria have been observed in the urine. Cultures and strains for acid-fast bacilli at other sites have usually been negative even in the cases of suspected systemic BCG infection. However, traumatic catheterisation or treatment following extensive tumour resection or bladder perforation could result in systemic BCG infection.

5.3 Preclinical safety data
ImmuCyst® 81 mg administered intravesically induced no serious systemic toxicity in studies in guinea pigs and monkeys. Studies in animals suggest that there is a possibility of a potential for allergenicity to the product.

No animal reproduction studies have been performed. Studies on mutagenicity and carcinogenicity have also not been performed.

6. PHARMACEUTICAL PARTICULARS
6.1 List of excipients
Monosodium glutamate

6.2 Incompatibilities
BCG bacilli are sensitive to a wide variety of antibiotics. Antimicrobial administration may therefore diminish the efficacy of ImmuCyst® 81 mg. Patients undergoing antimicrobial therapy for infections should be evaluated to assess whether the therapy might diminish the efficacy of ImmuCyst® 81 mg.

ImmuCyst® 81 mg is contraindicated in persons receiving immunosuppressive therapies, including irradiation, antimetabolites, alkylating agents or cytotoxic drugs because of risk of disseminated BCG infection.

6.3 Shelf life
Twenty-four months from the date of initiation of the viability (potency:viable count) test when stored between 2° and 8° C.

6.4 Special precautions for storage
ImmuCyst® 81 mg should be kept in a refrigerator at a temperature between 2° and 8° C. it should not be used after the expiration date marked on the vial.

At no time should the freeze-dried or reconstituted ImmuCyst® 81 mg be exposed to sunlight, direct or indirect. Exposure to artificial light should be kept to a minimum.

6.5 Nature and contents of container
The lyophilisate is contained in a 5 ml type 1 amber glass vial sealed with a grey butyl silicone stopper and held closed with an aluminium seal with a blue flip-off plastic top.

6.6 Special precautions for disposal and other handling
Reconstitution of Freeze-Dried Product and Withdrawal from Rubber-Stoppered Vial

DO NOT REMOVE THE RUBBER STOPPERS FROM THE VIALS. HANDLE AS INFECTIOUS MATERIAL

Reconstitute and dilute immediately prior to use, using aseptic technique in a low traffic, high airflow area (e.g., in a biocontainment cabinet). Persons handling product should wear gloves. If and when the product is handled outside of a biocontainment cabinet, persons handling the product should also wear a mask and eye protection.

ImmuCyst® 81 mg should not be handled by persons with an immune deficiency.

ImmuCyst® 81 mg is to be reconstituted only with sterile preservative-free normal saline to ensure proper dispersion of the organisms.

Using a 5 ml sterile syringe and needle, draw up 3ml of saline from an ampoule.

Prepare the surface of the ImmuCyst® 81 mg vial using a suitable antiseptic and using a 5 ml syringe containing 3ml of saline, pierce the stopper of the vial. Holding the vial upright pull the plunger of the syringe back to the 5 ml marking on the barrel. This will create a mild vacuum in the vial. Release the plunger and allow the vacuum to pull the saline from the syringe into the vial. After all the saline has passed into the freeze-dried material, remove the needle and syringe.

Shake the vial gently.

Two options for intravesicular administration are possible:

Option 1:

Further dilute the reconstituted material from the vial (1 dose) in an additional 50 ml of sterile preservative-free normal saline to a final volume of 53 ml intravesicular instillation (and 0.5 ml of the 53 ml for percutaneous inoculation, if administered).

The reconstituted product is then transferred to a bladder syringe.

Option 2:

The entire contents from the reconstituted vial is added to a saline bladder irrigation bag.

The product should be used immediately after reconstitution. In the event of a delay between reconstitution and administration, the reconstituted and diluted suspension may be stored, protected from light, for up to 8 hours at room temperature (up to 25° C). Any reconstituted product, which exhibits flocculation or clumping that cannot be dispersed with gentle shaking should not be used.

At no time should the reconstituted product be exposed to sunlight, direct or indirect. Exposure to artificial light should be kept to a minimum.

Special Instructions

After use, unused product, packaging, and all equipment and materials used for instillation should be sterilised or disposed of properly as with any other biohazardous waste.

Urine voided over 6 hours following ImmuCyst® 81 mg instillation should be disinfected with an equal volume of 5% hypochlorite solution (undiluted household bleach) and allowed to stand for 15 minutes before flushing.

7. MARKETING AUTHORISATION HOLDER
Cambridge Laboratories Limited
Deltic House,
Kingfisher Way, Silverlink Business Park,
Wallsend, Tyne and Wear
NE28 9NX
United Kingdom

8. MARKETING AUTHORISATION NUMBER(S)
PL 12070/0024

9. DATE OF FIRST AUTHORISATION/RENEWAL OF THE AUTHORISATION
19 September 2001

10. DATE OF REVISION OF THE TEXT
April 2008

Immukin

(Boehringer Ingelheim Limited)

1. NAME OF THE MEDICINAL PRODUCT
Immukin 2 × 10^6 IU (0.1 mg) solution for injection

2. QUALITATIVE AND QUANTITATIVE COMPOSITION
Each vial (0.5 ml) contains 2 × 10^6 IU (0.1 mg) recombinant human interferon gamma-1b. Interferon gamma-1b is produced in an *E. coli* expression system.

For a full list of excipients, see section 6.1.

3. PHARMACEUTICAL FORM
Solution for injection

A clear, colourless solution

4. CLINICAL PARTICULARS
4.1 Therapeutic indications
Immukin is indicated for the reduction of the frequency of serious infections in patients with chronic granulomatous disease (CGD) (see also section 4.4).

Immukin is indicated for the reduction in frequency of serious infections in patients with severe, malignant osteopetrosis (see also section 4.4 and 5.1).

4.2 Posology and method of administration
Immukin is for subcutaneous use. The recommended dosage of Immukin for the treatment of patients with CGD or severe, malignant osteopetrosis is 50 mcg / m^2 for patients whose body surface area is greater than 0.5 m^2 and 1.5 mcg / kg / dose for patients whose body surface area is equal to or less than 0.5 m^2. The actually drawn volume has to be controlled before injection. Injections should be administered subcutaneously preferably in the evening three times weekly (for example, Monday, Wednesday, Friday). The optimum sites of injection are the right and the left deltoid and anterior thigh. Immukin can be administered by a physician, nurse, family member or patient when trained in the administration of subcutaneous injections.

Although the most beneficial dose of Immukin is not known yet higher doses are not recommended. Safety and efficacy has not been established for Immukin given in doses greater or less than the recommended dose of 50 mcg / m^2. If severe reactions occur, the dosage should be modified (50 % reduction) or therapy should be discontinued until the adverse reaction abates.

The experience in children is limited (see sections 4.4 and 5.1)

4.3 Contraindications
Hypersensitivity to the active substance (interferon gamma-1b) or known hypersensitivity to closely related interferons or to any of the excipients.

4.4 Special warnings and precautions for use
The use of Immukin does not exclude the need for any additional antimicrobial coverage that might be required for the management of CGD. In the pivotal clinical efficacy study the overwhelming majority of the patients were receiving prophylactic antimicrobial therapy (see section 5.1).

Patients with pre-existing cardiac disease may experience an acute, self-limiting exacerbation of their cardiac condition at doses of 250 mcg / m^2 / day or higher, as observed in early clinical trials, although no direct cardiotoxic effect has been demonstrated.

Caution should be exercised when treating patients with known seizure disorders and/or compromised central nervous system function.

Patients with serious hepatic insufficiency and patients with severe renal insufficiency should be treated with caution since the possibility of interferon gamma-1b accumulation exists in those patients.

Elevations of AST and /or ALT (up to 25-fold) have been observed during Immukin therapy. The incidence appeared to be higher in patients less than 1 year of age compared to older children with 6 out of 10 developing elevated enzyme levels. In one case this occurred as early as 7 days after starting therapy. Treatment with Immukin was interrupted in all 6 of these patients and restarted at a reduced dosage in 4. Liver transaminase values returned to baseline in all patients and did not recur with rechallenge except in one patient. Caution should be especially observed in patients with hepatic insufficiency.

Reversible neutropenia and thrombocytopenia that can be severe and may be dose related have been observed during Immukin therapy. Caution should be exercised when administering Immukin to patients with myelosuppression.

Simultaneous administration of interferon gamma-1b with other heterologous serum protein preparations or immunological preparations (e.g. vaccines) should be avoided because of the risk for unexpected amplified immune response.

In addition to tests normally required for monitoring patients with CGD or severe, malignant osteopetrosis, patients should have performed the following tests before beginning Immukin therapy and at appropriate periods during treatment: haematologic tests, including complete blood counts, differential and platelet counts; blood chemistries, including renal and liver function tests; urinalysis.

Interferon gamma-1b is an exogenous protein, which may lead to the occurrence of antibodies during the course of treatment. Up to now Immukin administered to CGD or severe, malignant osteopetrosis patients in the recommended dose does not seem to be associated with significant risk for the induction of neutralising antibodies to interferon gamma-1b.

Based on the information available it cannot be excluded that the presence of higher levels of interferon gamma-1b may impair male and female fertility.

4.5 Interaction with other medicinal products and other forms of interaction
Interaction studies have only been performed in adults. Immukin does not reduce the efficacy of antibiotics or glucocorticoids in CGD or severe, malignant osteopetrosis patients.

Drug interactions seen with Immukin are similar to those seen with other interferons in animal experiments.

It is theoretically possible that hepatotoxic and/or nephrotoxic drugs might have effects on the clearance of Immukin. Also the effects of anti-inflammatory drugs, NSAIDs, theophylline, immunosuppressive and cytostatic drugs on the acute cellular effects of Immukin and its therapeutic effects in CGD or severe, malignant osteopetrosis patients when such drugs are used concomitantly in chronic conditions are not known.

Immukin potentially can prolong the half-lives of simultaneously administered drugs, which are metabolised by the cytochrome P-450 system.

Concurrent use of drugs having neurotoxic (including effects on the central nervous system), haemotoxic, myelosuppressive or cardiotoxic effects may increase the toxicity of interferons in these systems.

4.6 Pregnancy and lactation

Pregnancy

There are no adequate data from the use of interferon gamma-1b in pregnant women. Higher levels of endogenous interferon gamma were found in women with recurrent first trimester miscarriage compared to women with normal pregnancy. There is no evidence of any clinical relevance for Immukin.

Studies in animals have shown reproductive toxicity (see 5.3). The potential risk for humans is unknown. Immukin should not be used during pregnancy unless vitally indicated.

Lactation

It is not known whether interferon gamma-1b is excreted in human milk. Because of the lack of data on neonatal effects, breastfeeding is not recommended.

4.7 Effects on ability to drive and use machines

Immukin may have minor or moderate influence on the ability to drive and use machines even when given at the recommended dosage of 50 mcg / m^2 by subcutaneous injection. This effect may be enhanced by alcohol.

4.8 Undesirable effects

a) General Description

The clinical and laboratory toxicity associated with multiple-dose Immukin therapy is dose- and schedule-dependent.

The most common adverse events are flu-like symptoms characterised by fever, headache, chills, myalgia or fatigue.

b) Table of Adverse Reactions

Adverse reactions have been ranked under headings of frequency using the following convention:

Very common (≥ 1/10); common (≥ 1/100 to < 1/10); uncommon (≥ 1/1,000 to < 1/100); rare (≥ 1/10,000 to < 1/1,000); very rare (< 1/10,000), not known (cannot be estimated from the available data)

Within each frequency grouping, undesirable effects are presented in order of decreasing seriousness.

System Organ Class	
MedDRA Term	Frequency
Blood and lymphatic disorders:	
Neutropenia (see section 4.4); Thrombocytopenia (see section 4.4)	Not known[2]
Psychiatric disorders	
Depression	Common
Confusion	Rare[1]
Nervous system disorders:	
Headache	Very common
Gastrointestinal disorders:	
Nausea; vomiting; abdominal pain; diarrhea	Common
Skin and subcutaneous tissue disorders:	
Rash	Very common
Musculoskeletal and connective tissue disorders	
Myalgia; arthralgia; back pain	Common
Systemic lupus erythematosus	Rare[1]
Renal and urinary disorders:	
Proteinuria	Not known[2]
General disorders and administration site conditions:	
Fever; chills; injection site pain	Very common
Fatigue	Common
Investigations:	
Autoantibody response	Rare[1]
AST increase (see section 4.4), ALT increase (see section 4.4)	Not known[2]

[1]It has been assumed that these events have a reporting frequency of less than 1/1,000 and, therefore, they have been systematically classified "rare".

[2]Because of the limitations of the applicable datasets available, no frequencies could be assigned.

In addition to the above mentioned undesirable effects reported in the registered indications CGD and osteopetrosis (see section 4.1) there were a number of undesirable effects seen in clinical trials of conditions other than in these indications. In these trials interferon gamma-1b was usually administered at higher doses than recommended for the registered indications (see also section 4.9: Overdose).

Since these events have not been seen in clinical trials involving CGD or osteopetrosis but are reported in trials of patients with very diverse indications and health statuses, it is not possible to provide meaningful frequencies.

System Organ Class:

MedDRA Term[1]

Metabolism and Nutritional disorders:

Hyponatremia, hyperglycemia and hypertriglyceridemia;

Nervous System disorders:

Confusional state, disorientation, gait disturbance, Parkinsonian gait and tremor, convulsion, hallucinations;

Cardiac disorders:

Tachyarrhythmia, atrioventricular block, cardiac failure, myocardial infarction;

Vascular disorders:

Hypotension, syncope, transient ischemic attack, deep venous thrombosis, pulmonary embolism;

Respiratory, Thoracic and Mediastinal disorders:

Tachypnea, bronchospasm, interstitial lung disease;

Gastrointestinal disorders:

Gastrointestinal haemorrhage, pancreatitis, including pancreatitis with fatal outcome;

Hepatobiliary disorders:

Hepatic failure;

Skin and Subcutaneous disorders:

Exacerbation of dermatomyositis;

Musculoskeletal and Connective Tissue disorders:

Systemic lupus erythematosus;

Renal and urinary disorders:

Reversible renal failure;

General disorders and Administration site conditions:

Chest discomfort;

Investigations:

Autoantibody positive.

c) Information Characterising Individual Serious and/or Frequently Occurring Adverse Reactions

The flu-like symptoms may decrease in severity as treatment continues. Some of these symptoms can be minimised by bedtime administration. Acetaminophen (paracetamol) may also be used to ameliorate these effects. Vomiting, nausea, arthralgia and injection site tenderness have been reported in some patients.

Transient cutaneous rashes, e.g. dermatitis, maculopapular rash, pustular and vesicular eruptions, and erythema at injection site have occurred in some patients following injection but have rarely necessitated treatment interruption.

The inclusion of autoantibody production and systemic lupus erythematosus is the result of case reports in the literature. The adverse reaction "confusion" is also in the literature as a case report.

4.9 Overdose

Immukin has been administered at higher doses (>100 mcg / m^2) to patients with advanced malignancies by the intravenous or intramuscular route.

Central nervous system adverse reactions including decreased mental status, gait disturbance and dizziness have been observed, particularly in cancer patients receiving doses greater than 100 mcg / m^2 / day. These abnormalities were reversible within a few days upon dose reduction or discontinuation of therapy.

Blood disorders including reversible neutropenia and thrombocytopenia as well as the onset of increased hepatic enzymes and of triglycerides have also been observed.

Patients with pre-existing cardiac disease may experience an acute, self-limited exacerbation of their cardiac condition at doses of 250 mcg / m^2 / day or higher, as observed in early clinical trials, although no direct cardiotoxic effect has been demonstrated.

Further undesirable effects which may occur as a consequence of overdosing as observed in respective clinical trials in other than the registered indications are outlined in section 4.8 above.

5. PHARMACOLOGICAL PROPERTIES

5.1 Pharmacodynamic properties

Pharmacotherapeutic group: Immunostimulants, Cytokines and immunomodulators

ATC code: L03A B03

Interferons are a family of functionally related proteins synthesised by eukaryotic cells in response to viruses and a variety of natural and synthetic stimuli. The real mechanism of action of interferon gamma-1b in CGD is still unknown. Findings related to superoxide anion production remain unequivocal. However, it is presumed that interferon gamma-1b increases macrophage cytotoxicity by enhancing the respiratory burst via generation of toxic oxygen metabolites capable of mediating the killing of intracellular micro-organisms. It increases HLA-DR expression on macrophages and augments Fc receptor expression, which results in increased antibody-dependent cell-mediated cytotoxicity.

In a placebo-controlled clinical trial in 128 patients with CGD, Immukin was shown to reduce the frequency of serious infections during the trial period of 12 months by 77 % in patients treated with Immukin compared to 30 % in the placebo group (p = 0.0006). The overwhelming majority of these patients were also receiving prophylactic antimicrobial therapy.

Data on the safety and efficacy of Immukin in 37 CGD patients under the age of 3 years was pooled from 4 uncontrolled post-marketing studies and 2 sequential post-marketing surveillance studies. The rate of serious infections per patient-year in this uncontrolled group was similar to the rate observed in the Immukin treatment groups in controlled trials.

In severe, malignant osteopetrosis (inherited disorder characterised by an osteoclast defect leading to bone overgrowth and deficient phagocyte oxidative metabolism), a treatment-related enhancement of superoxide production by phagocytes was observed *in situ*.

In a controlled randomised study in 16 patients with severe, malignant osteopetrosis, Immukin in combination with calcitriol was shown to reduce the frequency of serious infections versus calcitriol alone. In an analysis which combined data from two clinical studies, 19 of 24 patients treated with Immukin in combination with or without calcitriol for at least 6 months had reduced trabecular bone volume compared to baseline. The clinical relevance of this observed decrease in Immukin treated patients versus a control group could not be established.

5.2 Pharmacokinetic properties

Immukin is rapidly cleared after intravenous administration and slowly and well absorbed after intramuscular or subcutaneous administration.

With the recommended dosage regimen of subcutaneous administration of 0.05 mg / m^2 Immukin, the mean elimination half-lives were 4.9 hours and the mean residence time was 2.5 hours. Time to reach maximum plasma concentration ranged from 4 to 14 hours with a mean of 8 hours.

Interferon gamma-1b was not detected in the urine of healthy male subjects following administration of 100 mcg / m^2 by intramuscular or subcutaneous injection.

5.3 Preclinical safety data

Although difficult to interpret, due to species restrictions, non-clinical data reveal no hazard for humans based on conventional studies of safety pharmacology, repeated dose toxicity, genotoxicity, carcinogenic potential, toxicity to reproduction, local tolerance and skin sensitisation.

An increased incidence of abortion has been observed in pregnant non-human primates, which received the drug in doses manifold higher than that recommended for human use.

6. PHARMACEUTICAL PARTICULARS

6.1 List of excipients

D-Mannitol

Disodium succinate hexahydrate

Polysorbate 20

Succinic acid

Water for injections

6.2 Incompatibilities

In the absence of compatibility studies, this medicinal product must not be mixed with other medicinal products.

6.3 Shelf life

3 years

Immukin is for single use only.

The formulation does not contain a preservative. Once opened, the content of a vial should be used immediately. The unused portion of any vial should be discarded.

6.4 Special precautions for storage

Store in a refrigerator (2°C – 8°C). Do not freeze.

6.5 Nature and contents of container

3 ml glass vials (Type I borosilicate glass) which are stoppered with grey butyl rubber stoppers with aluminium/ polypropylene flip-off type caps.

Pack sizes: 1, 3, 5, 6 and 12 vial(s) in one folding box. Not all pack sizes may be marketed.

6.6 Special precautions for disposal and other handling

Vials of Immukin must not be shaken vigorously.

Parenteral drug products should be inspected visually for particulate matter and discolouration prior to administration.

Any unused product or waste material should be disposed of in accordance with local requirements.

7. MARKETING AUTHORISATION HOLDER

Boehringer Ingelheim Limited

Ellesfield Avenue

Bracknell

Berkshire

RG12 8YS

United Kingdom

8. MARKETING AUTHORISATION NUMBER(S)

PL 00015/0154

9. DATE OF FIRST AUTHORISATION/RENEWAL OF THE AUTHORISATION

29/09/2007

10. DATE OF REVISION OF THE TEXT
29/09/2007

Imodium Capsules

(Janssen-Cilag Ltd)

1. NAME OF THE MEDICINAL PRODUCT
Imodium^{TM} Capsules

2. QUALITATIVE AND QUANTITATIVE COMPOSITION
Loperamide hydrochloride 2 mg

Excipient: lactose

For a full list of excipients, see Section 6.1

3. PHARMACEUTICAL FORM
Capsule, hard.

Opaque green cap and grey body, hard gelatin capsule imprinted with 'Imodium' on cap and 'Janssen' on body containing white powder.

4. CLINICAL PARTICULARS

4.1 Therapeutic indications

POM

For the symptomatic treatment of acute diarrhoea of any aetiology including acute exacerbations of chronic diarrhoea for periods of up to 5 days in adults and children over 8 years. For the symptomatic treatment of chronic diarrhoea in adults.

P and GSL

For the symptomatic treatment of acute diarrhoea in adults and children aged 12 years and over.

For the symptomatic treatment of acute episodes of diarrhoea associated with Irritable Bowel Syndrome in adults aged 18 years and over following initial diagnosis by a doctor.

4.2 Posology and method of administration

ACUTE DIARRHOEA

P and POM

Adults and children over 12:

Two capsules initially, followed by one capsule after each loose stool. The usual dose is 3-4 capsules a day. The total daily dose should not exceed 8 capsules.

POM

Children 4-8 years:

Use Syrup.

Children 9 to12 years:

One capsule four times daily until diarrhoea is controlled (up to 5 days). This dose should not be exceeded.

Not recommended for children under 4 years of age.

Further investigation into the cause of the diarrhoea should be considered if there is no improvement within two days of starting treatment with Imodium.

GSL

Adults and children over 12:

2 capsules initially followed by 1 capsule after every loose stool.

The maximum daily dose should not exceed 6 capsules.

CHRONIC DIARRHOEA (POM)

Adults:

Studies have shown that patients may need widely differing amounts of Imodium. The starting dose should be between two and four capsules per day in divided doses, depending on severity. If required, this dose can be adjusted according to result up to a maximum of eight capsules daily.

Having established the patient's daily maintenance dose, the capsules may be administered on a twice daily regimen. Tolerance has not been observed and therefore subsequent dosage adjustment should be unnecessary.

SYMPTOMATIC TREATMENT OF ACUTE EPISODES OF DIARRHOEA ASSOCIATED WITH IRRITABLE BOWEL SYNDROME IN ADULTS AGED 18 YEARS AND OVER

P

Two capsules to be taken initially. The usual dose is between 2 and 4 capsules per day in divided doses, depending on severity. If required, this dose can be adjusted according to result, up to a maximum of 8 capsules daily.

GSL

Two capsules to be taken initially, followed by 1 capsule after every loose stool, or as previously advised by your doctor. The maximum daily dose should not exceed 6 capsules.

USE IN ELDERLY

No dose adjustment is required for the elderly.

RENAL IMPAIRMENT

No dose adjustment is required for patients with renal impairment.

HEPATIC IMPAIRMENT

Although no pharmacokinetic data are available in patients with hepatic impairment, Imodium should be used with caution in such patients because of reduced first pass metabolism (see 4.4 Special warnings and precautions for use).

Method of administration

Oral use.

4.3 Contraindications

Imodium is contraindicated in:

- patients with a known hypersensitivity to loperamide hydrochloride or to any of the excipients.
- children less than 4 years of age.
- when inhibition of peristalsis is to be avoided due to the possible risk of significant sequelae including ileus, megacolon and toxic megacolon, in particular:

- when ileus or constipation are present or when abdominal distension develops, particularly in severely dehydrated children,

- in patients with acute ulcerative colitis,

- in patients with bacterial enterocolitis caused by invasive organisms including Salmonella, Shigella, and Campylobacter,

- in patients with pseudomembranous colitis associated with the use of broad-spectrum antibiotics.

Imodium should not be used alone in acute dysentery, which is characterised by blood in stools and elevated body temperatures.

4.4 Special warnings and precautions for use

The priority in acute diarrhoea is the prevention or reversal of fluid and electrolyte depletion. This is particularly important in young children and in frail and elderly patients with acute diarrhoea. Use of Imodium does not preclude the administration of appropriate fluid and electrolyte replacement therapy.

Since persistent diarrhoea can be an indicator of potentially more serious conditions, Imodium should not be used for prolonged periods until the underlying cause of the diarrhoea has been investigated.

Imodium must be used with caution when the hepatic function necessary for the drug's metabolism is defective (eg in cases of severe hepatic disturbance), as this might result in a relative overdose leading to CNS toxicity.

Patients with AIDS treated with Imodium for diarrhoea should have therapy stopped at the earliest signs of abdominal distension. There have been isolated reports of toxic megacolon in AIDS patients with infectious colitis from both viral and bacterial pathogens treated with loperamide hydrochloride.

Patients with rare hereditary problems of galactose intolerance, the Lapp lactase deficiency or glucose-galactose malabsorption should not take this medicine because it contains lactose.

Also for P and GSL use

In cases of acute diarrhoea, if symptoms persist for more than 24 hours, consult your doctor.

If you are taking Imodium to control episodes of diarrhoea associated with Irritable Bowel Syndrome previously diagnosed by your doctor, you should return to him/her if the pattern of your symptoms changes. You should also return to your doctor if your episodes of diarrhoea continue for more than two weeks or there is a need for continued treatment of more than two weeks.

Special Warnings to be included on the GSL leaflet

Only take Imodium to treat acute episodes of diarrhoea associated with Irritable Bowel Syndrome if your doctor has previously diagnosed IBS.

If any of the following apply, do not use the product without first consulting your doctors, even if you know you have IBS:

- If you are 40 years or over and it is some time since your last attack of IBS or the symptoms are different this time
- If you have recently passed blood from the bowel
- If you suffer from severe constipation
- If you are sick or vomiting
- If you have lost your appetite or lost weight
- If you have difficulty or pain passing urine
- If you have a fever
- If you have recently traveled abroad

Consult your doctor if you develop new symptoms, or if your symptoms worsen, or your symptoms have not improved over two weeks.

4.5 Interaction with other medicinal products and other forms of interaction

Non-clinical data have shown that loperamide is a P-glycoprotein substrate. Concomitant administration of loperamide (16 mg single dose) with quinidine, or ritonavir, which are both P-glycoprotein inhibitors, resulted in a 2 to 3-fold increase in loperamide plasma levels. The clinical relevance of this pharmacokinetic interaction with P-glycoprotein inhibitors, when loperamide is given at recommended dosages (2 mg, up to 16 mg maximum daily dose), is unknown.

4.6 Pregnancy and lactation

Safety in human pregnancy has not been established although studies in animals have not demonstrated any teratogenic effects. As with other drugs, it is not advisable to administer Imodium in pregnancy.

Small amounts of loperamide may appear in human breast milk. Therefore, Imodium is not recommended during breast-feeding.

Women who are pregnant or breast feeding infants should therefore be advised to consult their doctor for appropriate treatment.

4.7 Effects on ability to drive and use machines

Tiredness, dizziness, or drowsiness may occur when diarrhoea is treated with Imodium. Therefore, it is advisable to use caution when driving a car or operating machinery. See section 4.8 Undesirable Effects.

4.8 Undesirable effects

In clinical trials, constipation and dizziness have been reported with greater frequency in loperamide hydrochloride treated patients than placebo treated patients.

The following adverse events have also been reported with use of loperamide hydrochloride:

Skin and appendages

Very rare: rash, urticaria and pruritus.

Isolated occurrences of angioedema, and bullous eruptions including Stevens-Johnson Syndrome, erythema multiforme, and toxic epidermal necrolysis.

Body as a whole, general

Very rare: isolated occurrences of allergic reactions and in some cases severe hypersensitivity reactions including anaphylactic shock and anaphylactoid reactions.

Gastrointestinal system disorders

Very rare: abdominal pain, ileus, abdominal distension, nausea, constipation, vomiting, megacolon including toxic megacolon, flatulence, and dyspepsia.

Genitourinary

Very rare: isolated reports of urinary retention.

Psychiatric

Very rare: drowsiness.

Central and peripheral nervous system

Very rare: dizziness.

A number of the adverse events reported during the clinical investigations and post-marketing experience with loperamide are frequent symptoms of the underlying diarrhoeal syndrome (abdominal pain/discomfort, nausea, vomiting, dry mouth, tiredness, drowsiness, dizziness, constipation, and flatulence). These symptoms are often difficult to distinguish from undesirable drug effects.

4.9 Overdose

In case of overdose the following effects may be observed: constipation, urinary retention, ileus and neurological symptoms (miosis, muscular hypertonia, somnolence and bradypnoea). If intoxication is suspected, naloxone may be given as an antidote. Since the duration of action of loperamide is longer than that of naloxone, the patient should be kept under constant observation for at least 48 hours in order to detect any possible depression of the central nervous system. Children, and patients with hepatic dysfunction, may be more sensitive to CNS effects. Gastric lavage, or induced emesis and or enema or laxatives may be recommended.

5. PHARMACOLOGICAL PROPERTIES

5.1 Pharmacodynamic properties

Pharmacotherapeutic Group: Antipropulsives; ATC code: A07DA03

Loperamide binds to the opiate receptor in the gut wall, reducing propulsive peristalsis and increasing intestinal transit time. Loperamide increases the tone of the anal sphincter.

In a double blind randomised clinical trial in 56 patients with acute diarrhoea receiving loperamide, onset of anti-diarrhoeal action was observed within one hour following a single 4 mg dose. Clinical comparisons with other antidiarrhoeal drugs confirmed this exceptionally rapid onset of action of loperamide.

5.2 Pharmacokinetic properties

The half-life of loperamide in man is 10.8 hours with a range of 9-14 hours. Studies on distribution in rats show high affinity for the gut wall with preference for binding to the receptors in the longitudinal muscle layer. Loperamide is well absorbed from the gut, but is almost completely extracted and metabolised by the liver where it is conjugated and excreted via the bile. Due to its high affinity for the gut wall and its high first pass metabolism, very little loperamide reaches the systemic circulation.

5.3 Preclinical safety data

No relevant information additional to that contained elsewhere in the Summary of Product Characteristics.

6. PHARMACEUTICAL PARTICULARS

6.1 List of excipients

Lactose

Maize starch

Talc

Magnesium stearate

Capsule cap:

Titanium dioxide

Yellow ferric oxide

Indigotindisulphonate sodium

Gelatin

Capsule body:

Titanium dioxide

Black ferrous oxide

Indigotindisulphonate sodium

Erythrosin

Gelatin

6.2 Incompatibilities
Not applicable.

6.3 Shelf life
60 months.

6.4 Special precautions for storage
None.

6.5 Nature and contents of container
Blister packs consisting of aluminium foil, hermetalu and polyvinyl chloride genotherm glass clear.

The blister strips are packed in cardboard cartons to contain 2, 6, 8, 12, 18 or 30 capsules (4, 28, 60 and 100 pack sizes not marketed).

OR

Tubs of capsules containing 250 capsules (500, 1000 and 10000 pack sizes not marketed).

6.6 Special precautions for disposal and other handling
Not applicable.

7. MARKETING AUTHORISATION HOLDER
Janssen-Cilag Ltd
50-100 Holmers Farm Way
High Wycombe
Buckinghamshire
HP12 4EG
UK

8. MARKETING AUTHORISATION NUMBER(S)
PL 00242/0028

9. DATE OF FIRST AUTHORISATION/RENEWAL OF THE AUTHORISATION
18 June 2001

10. DATE OF REVISION OF THE TEXT
10 September 2008

Legal category
POM/P/GSL

Imodium Syrup

(Janssen-Cilag Ltd)

1. NAME OF THE MEDICINAL PRODUCT
IMODIUM™ SYRUP

2. QUALITATIVE AND QUANTITATIVE COMPOSITION
Loperamide hydrochloride 0.2 mg/ml

Excipients: Methyl parahydroxybenzoate (E218)
Propyl parahydroxybenzoate (E216)
Ethanol

For a full list of excipients, see section 6.1

3. PHARMACEUTICAL FORM
Syrup for oral administration.

A clear, red, slightly viscous fruit-flavoured oral solution.

4. CLINICAL PARTICULARS

4.1 Therapeutic indications

P Classification: For the symptomatic treatment of acute diarrhoea in adults and children aged 12 years and over.

POM Classification: For the symptomatic treatment of acute diarrhoea of any aetiology including acute exacerbations of chronic diarrhoea for periods of up to 5 days in adults and children over 4 years. For the symptomatic treatment of chronic diarrhoea in adults.

4.2 Posology and method of administration

Acute diarrhoea

Adults:	Four 5 ml spoonfuls initially, followed by two 5 ml spoonfuls after each loose stool. The total daily dose should not exceed sixteen spoonfuls.
Children:	The following doses should not be exceeded.
Children over 8 years:	Two 5 ml spoonfuls four times daily with the duration limited to 5 days.
Children 4 - 8 years:	One 5 ml spoonful three or four times daily with the duration limited to 3 days.

Not recommended for children under 4 years of age.

Further investigation into the cause of the diarrhoea should be considered if there is no improvement within two days of starting treatment with Imodium.

Chronic Diarrhoea

Adults: Patients may need widely differing amounts of Imodium. The starting dose should be between four and eight 5 ml spoonfuls per day in divided doses, depending on severity. If required this dose can be adjusted up to a maximum of sixteen 5 ml spoonfuls daily.

Having established the patient's daily maintenance dose, Imodium may be administered on a twice daily regimen. Tolerance has not been observed and therefore subsequent dosage adjustment should be unnecessary.

Use in Elderly:

No dose adjustment is required for the elderly.

Renal impairment

No dose adjustment is required for patients with renal impairment.

Hepatic impairment

Although no pharmacokinetic data are available in patients with hepatic impairment, Imodium should be used with caution in such patients because of reduced first pass metabolism (see 4.4 Special warnings and special precautions for use).

Method of Administration: Oral Use.

4.3 Contraindications
Imodium is contraindicated in:

- patients with a known hypersensitivity to loperamide hydrochloride or to any of the excipients.
- children less than 4 years of age.
- when inhibition of peristalsis is to be avoided due to the possible risk of significant sequelae including ileus, megacolon and toxic megacolon, in particular:

- when ileus or constipation are present or when abdominal distension develops, particularly in severely dehydrated children,

- in patients with acute ulcerative colitis,

- in patients with bacterial enterocolitis caused by invasive organisms including Salmonella, Shigella, and Campylobacter,

- in patients with pseudomembranous colitis associated with the use of broad-spectrum antibiotics.

Imodium should not be used alone in acute dysentery, which is characterised by blood in stools and elevated body temperatures.

4.4 Special warnings and precautions for use
In patients with diarrhoea, especially young children, fluid and electrolyte depletion may occur. Use of Imodium does not preclude the administration of appropriate fluid and electrolyte replacement therapy.

Since persistent diarrhoea can be an indicator of potentially more serious conditions, Imodium should not be used for prolonged periods until the underlying cause of the diarrhoea has been investigated.

Imodium must be used with caution when the hepatic function necessary for the drug's metabolism is defective (eg in cases of severe hepatic disturbance), as this might result in a relative overdose leading to CNS toxicity.

Patients with AIDS treated with Imodium for diarrhoea should have therapy stopped at the earliest signs of abdominal distension. There have been isolated reports of toxic megacolon in AIDS patients with infectious colitis from both viral and bacterial pathogens treated with loperamide hydrochloride.

Also for P use only.

If symptoms persist for more than 24 hours, consult your doctor.

4.5 Interaction with other medicinal products and other forms of interaction
Non-clinical data have shown that loperamide is a P-glycoprotein substrate. Concomitant administration of loperamide (16 mg single dose) with quinidine, or ritonavir, which are both P-glycoprotein inhibitors, resulted in a 2 to 3-fold increase in loperamide plasma levels. The clinical relevance of this pharmacokinetic interaction with P-glycoprotein inhibitors, when loperamide is given at recommended dosages (2 mg, up to 16 mg maximum daily dose), is unknown.

4.6 Pregnancy and lactation
Safety in human pregnancy has not been established although studies in animals have not demonstrated any teratogenic effects. As with other drugs, it is not advisable to administer Imodium in pregnancy.

Small amounts of loperamide may appear in human breast milk. Therefore, Imodium is not recommended during breast feeding.

Women who are breast feeding infants should therefore be advised to consult their doctor for appropriate treatment.

4.7 Effects on ability to drive and use machines
Tiredness, dizziness, or drowsiness may occur when diarrhoea is treated with Imodium. Therefore, it is advisable to use caution when driving a car or operating machinery. See section 4.8 Undesirable effects.

4.8 Undesirable effects
In clinical trials, constipation and dizziness have been reported with greater frequency in loperamide hydrochloride treated patients than placebo treated patients.

The following adverse events have also been reported with use of loperamide hydrochloride:

Skin and appendages

Very rare: rash, urticaria and pruritus.

Isolated occurrences of angioedema, and bullous eruptions including Stevens-Johnson Syndrome, erythema multiforme, and toxic epidermal necrolysis.

Body as a whole, general

Very rare: isolated occurrences of allergic reactions and in some cases severe hypersensitivity reactions including anaphylactic shock and anaphylactoid reactions.

Gastrointestinal system disorders

Very rare: abdominal pain, ileus, abdominal distension, nausea, constipation, vomiting, megacolon including toxic megacolon, flatulence, and dyspepsia.

Genitourinary

Very rare: isolated reports of urinary retention.

Psychiatric

Very rare: drowsiness.

Central and peripheral nervous system

Very rare: dizziness.

A number of the adverse events reported during the clinical investigations and post-marketing experience with loperamide are frequent symptoms of the underlying diarrhoeal syndrome (abdominal pain/discomfort, nausea, vomiting, dry mouth, tiredness, drowsiness, dizziness, constipation, and flatulence). These symptoms are often difficult to distinguish from undesirable drug effects.

4.9 Overdose
In case of overdose the following effects may be observed: constipation, urinary retention, ileus and neurological symptoms (miosis, muscular hypertonia, somnolence and bradypnoea). If intoxication is suspected, naloxone may be given as an antidote. Since the duration of action of loperamide is longer than that of naloxone, the patient should be kept under constant observation for at least 48 hours in order to detect any possible depression of the central nervous system. Children, and patients with hepatic dysfunction, may be more sensitive to CNS effects. Gastric lavage, or induced emesis and /or enema or laxatives may be recommended.

5. PHARMACOLOGICAL PROPERTIES

5.1 Pharmacodynamic properties
Pharmacotherapeutic Group: Antipropulsives; ATC code: A07DA03

Loperamide binds to the opiate receptor in the gut wall, reducing propulsive peristalsis and increasing intestinal transit time. Loperamide increases the tone of the anal sphincter.

5.2 Pharmacokinetic properties
The half-life of loperamide in man is 10.8 hours with a range of 9-14 hours. Studies on distribution in rats show high affinity for the gut wall with preference for binding to the receptors in the longitudinal muscle layer. Loperamide is well absorbed from the gut, but is almost completely extracted and metabolised by the liver where it is conjugated and excreted via the bile. Due to its high affinity for the gut wall and its high first pass metabolism, very little loperamide reaches the systemic circulation.

5.3 Preclinical safety data
No relevant information additional to that contained elsewhere in the Summary of Product Characteristics.

6. PHARMACEUTICAL PARTICULARS

6.1 List of excipients
Glycerol

Sodium saccharin

Methyl parahydroxybenzoate (E218)

Propyl parahydroxybenzoate (E216)

Cochineal Red A

Raspberry Flavour

Red Currant Flavour

Ethanol (96%)

Citric acid monohydrate

Purified water

6.2 Incompatibilities
Not applicable.

6.3 Shelf life
60 months.

6.4 Special precautions for storage
None.

6.5 Nature and contents of container
Amber glass bottle with either a pilfer-proof aluminium screw cap coated on the inside with PVC or a child resistant polypropylene screw cap lined inside with an LDPE insert and a 5 ml or 10 ml polypropylene measuring cup.

Imodium syrup may be presented in bottle sizes of 30, 40, 50, 90 and 100 mls.

(Not all pack sizes may be marketed.)

6.6 Special precautions for disposal and other handling
Not applicable.

7. MARKETING AUTHORISATION HOLDER
Janssen-Cilag Ltd.
50-100 Holmers Farm Way
High Wycombe
Buckinghamshire
HP12 4EG
UK

8. MARKETING AUTHORISATION NUMBER(S)
PL 0242/0040

9. DATE OF FIRST AUTHORISATION/RENEWAL OF THE AUTHORISATION
Date of first authorisation: 03 December 1975
Date of renewal of authorisation: 20 December 1996

10. DATE OF REVISION OF THE TEXT
10 September 2008

Legal category POM/P

Imuran Injection

(GlaxoSmithKline UK)

1. NAME OF THE MEDICINAL PRODUCT
Imuran Injection.

2. QUALITATIVE AND QUANTITATIVE COMPOSITION
Azathioprine EP 50 mg/vial.

3. PHARMACEUTICAL FORM
Injection.

4. CLINICAL PARTICULARS

4.1 Therapeutic indications
Imuran is used as an immunosuppressant antimetabolite either alone or, more commonly, in combination with other agents (usually corticosteroids) and procedures which influence the immune response. Therapeutic effect may be evident only after weeks or months and can include a steroid-sparing effect, thereby reducing the toxicity associated with high dosage and prolonged usage of corticosteroids.

Imuran, in combination with corticosteroids and/or other immunosuppressive agents and procedures, is indicated to enhance the survival of organ transplants, such as renal transplants, cardiac transplants, and hepatic transplants, and to reduce the corticosteroid requirement of renal transplant recipients.

Imuran, either alone or more usually in combination with corticosteroids and/or other drugs and procedures, has been used with clinical benefit (which may include reduction of dosage or discontinuation of corticosteroids) in a proportion of patients suffering from the following:

severe rheumatoid arthritis;

systemic lupus erythematosus;

dermatomyositis and polymyositis;

auto-immune chronic active hepatitis;

pemphigus vulgaris;

polyarteritis nodosa;

auto-immune haemolytic anaemia;

chronic refractory idiopathic thrombocytopenic purpura.

4.2 Posology and method of administration
Imuran Injection should be used ONLY when the oral route is impractical, and should be discontinued as soon as oral therapy is tolerated. It must be administered only by the intravenous route.

Specialist medical literature should be consulted for guidance as to clinical experience in particular conditions.

<u>Dosage in transplantation - adults and children</u>

Depending on the immunosuppressive regimen employed, a dosage of up to 5 mg/kg bodyweight/day may be given on the first day of therapy, either orally or intravenously.

Maintenance dosage should range from 1 to 4 mg/kg bodyweight/day and must be adjusted according to clinical requirements and haematological tolerance.

Evidence indicates that Imuran therapy should be maintained indefinitely, even if only low doses are necessary, because of the risk of graft rejection.

<u>Dosage in other conditions - adults and children</u>

In general, starting dosage is from 1 to 3 mg/kg bodyweight/day, and should be adjusted, within these limits, depending on the clinical response (which may not be evident for weeks or months) and haematological tolerance.

When therapeutic response is evident, consideration should be given to reducing the maintenance dosage to the lowest level compatible with the maintenance of that response. If no improvement occurs in the patient's condition within 3 months, consideration should be given to withdrawing Imuran.

The maintenance dosage required may range from less than 1 mg/kg bodyweight/day to 3 mg/kg bodyweight/day, depending on the clinical condition being treated and the individual patient response, including haematological tolerance.

In patients with renal and/or hepatic insufficiency, dosages should be given at the lower end of the normal range (see Special Precautions for Use for further details).

<u>Use in the elderly</u> (see Renal and/or hepatic insufficiency)

There is a limited experience of the administration of Imuran to elderly patients. Although the available data do not provide evidence that the incidence of side effects among elderly patients is higher than that among other patients treated with Imuran, it is recommended that the dosages used should be at the lower end of the range.

Particular care should be taken to monitor haematological response and to reduce the maintenance dosage to the minimum required for clinical response.

<u>Reconstitution and dilution of Imuran Injection</u>

Precautions should always be taken when handling Imuran Injection (see section 6.6 Instructions for Use, Handling and Disposal).

No antimicrobial preservative is included. Therefore reconstitution and dilution must be carried out under full aseptic conditions, preferably immediately before use. Any unused solution should be discarded.

The contents of each vial should be reconstituted by the addition of 5 ml to 15 ml of Water for Injections BP. The reconstituted solution is stable for up to 5 days when stored between 5°C and 25°C.

When diluted on the basis of 5 ml of reconstituted solution to a volume of between 20 ml and 200 ml of one of the following infusion solutions, Imuran is stable for up to 24 hours at room temperature (15°C to 25°C):

Sodium Chloride Intravenous Infusion BP (0.45% w/v and 0.9% w/v)

Sodium Chloride (0.18% w/v) and Glucose (4.0% w/v) Intravenous Infusion BP.

Should any visible turbidity or crystallisation appear in the reconstituted or diluted solution the preparation must be discarded.

Imuran Injection should ONLY be reconstituted with the recommended volume of Water for Injections BP and should be diluted as specified above. Imuran Injection should not be mixed with other drugs or fluids, except those specified above, before administration.

<u>Administration of Imuran Injection</u>

Imuran Injection, when reconstituted as directed, is a very irritant solution with a pH of 10 to 12.

When the reconstituted solution is diluted as directed above, the pH of the resulting solution may be expected to be within the range pH 8.0 to 9.5 (the greater the dilution, the lower the pH).

Where dilution is not practicable, the reconstituted solution should be injected slowly over a period of not less than one minute and followed immediately by not less than 50 ml of one of the recommended infusion solutions.

Care must be taken to avoid perivenous injection, which may produce tissue damage.

4.3 Contraindications
Imuran is contra-indicated in patients known to be hypersensitive to azathioprine. Hypersensitivity to 6-mercaptopurine (6-MP) should alert the prescriber to probable hypersensitivity to Imuran.

Imuran therapy should not be initiated in patients who may be pregnant, or who are likely to become pregnant without careful assessment of risk versus benefit (see section 4.4 Special Warnings and Precautions for Use & section 4.6 Pregnancy and Lactation).

4.4 Special warnings and precautions for use
Monitoring

There are potential hazards in the use of Imuran. It should be prescribed only if the patient can be adequately monitored for toxic effects throughout the duration of therapy.

It is suggested that during the first 8 weeks of therapy, complete blood counts, including platelets, should be performed weekly or more frequently if high dosage is used or if severe renal and/or hepatic disorder is present. The blood count frequency may be reduced later in therapy, but it is suggested that complete blood counts are repeated monthly, or at least at intervals of not longer than 3 months.

Patients receiving Imuran should be instructed to report immediately any evidence of infection, unexpected bruising or bleeding or other manifestations of bone marrow depression.

There are individuals with an inherited deficiency of the enzyme thiopurine methyltransferase (TPMT) who may be unusually sensitive to the myelosuppressive effect of azathioprine and prone to developing rapid bone marrow depression following the initiation of treatment with Imuran. This problem could be exacerbated by co-administration with drugs that inhibit TPMT, such as olsalazine, mesalazine or sulfasalazine. Also it has been reported that decreased TPMT activity increases the risk of secondary leukaemias and myelodysplasia in individuals receiving 6-mercaptopurine (the active metabolite of azathioprine) in combination with other cytotoxics (see section 4.8 Undesirable effects).

Renal and/or hepatic insufficiency

It has been suggested that the toxicity of Imuran may be enhanced in the presence of renal insufficiency, but controlled studies have not supported this suggestion. Nevertheless, it is recommended that the dosages used should be at the lower end of the normal range and that haematological response should be carefully monitored. Dosage should be further reduced if haematological toxicity occurs.

Caution is necessary during the administration of Imuran to patients with hepatic dysfunction, and regular complete blood counts and liver function tests should be undertaken. In such patients the metabolism of Imuran may be impaired, and the dosage of Imuran should therefore be reduced if hepatic or haematological toxicity occurs.

Limited evidence suggests that Imuran is not beneficial to patients with hypoxanthine-guanine-phosphoribosyltransferase deficiency (Lesch-Nyhan syndrome). Therefore, given the abnormal metabolism in these patients, it is not prudent to recommend that these patients should receive Imuran.

Mutagenicity

Chromosomal abnormalities have been demonstrated in both male and female patients treated with Imuran. It is difficult to assess the role of Imuran in the development of these abnormalities.

Effects on fertility

Relief of chronic renal insufficiency by renal transplantation involving the administration of Imuran has been accompanied by increased fertility in both male and female transplant recipients.

Carcinogenicity (see also section 4.8 Undesirable Effects)

Patients receiving immunosuppressive therapy are at an increased risk of developing non-Hodgkin's lymphomas and other malignancies, notably skin cancers (melanoma and non-melanoma), sarcomas (Kaposi's and non-Kaposi's) and uterine cervical cancer in situ. The risk appears to be related to the intensity and duration of immunosuppression rather than to the use of any specific agent. It has been reported that reduction or discontinuation of immunosuppression may be associated with partial or complete regression of non-Hodgkin's lymphomas and Kaposi's sarcomas.

Patients receiving multiple immunosuppressive agents may be at risk of over-immunosuppression, therefore such therapy should be maintained at the lowest effective level.

Exposure to sunlight and UV light should be limited and patients should wear protective clothing and use a sunscreen with a high protection factor to minimize the risk of skin cancer and photosensitivity (see also section 4.8 Undesirable Effects).

Varicella Zoster Virus Infection (see also section 4.8 Undesirable Effects)

Infection with varicella zoster virus (VZV; chickenpox and herpes zoster) may become severe during the administration of immunosuppressants. Caution should be exercised especially with respect to the following:

Before starting the administration of immunosuppressants, the prescriber should check to see if the patient has a history of VZV. Serologic testing may be useful in determining previous exposure. Patients who have no history of exposure should avoid contact with individuals with chickenpox or herpes zoster. If the patient is exposed to VZV, special care must be taken to avoid patients developing chickenpox or herpes zoster, and passive immunisation with varicella-zoster immunoglobulin (VZIG) may be considered.

If the patient is infected with VZV, appropriate measures should be taken, which may include antiviral therapy and supportive care.

4.5 Interaction with other medicinal products and other forms of interaction
Allopurinol/ oxipurinol/ thiopurinol

Xanthine oxidase activity is inhibited by allopurinol, oxipurinol and thiopurinol which results in reduced conversion of biologically active 6-thioinosinic acid to biologically inactive 6-thiouric acid. When allopurinol, oxipurinol and/or thiopurinol are given concomitantly with 6-mercaptopurine or azathioprine, the dose of 6-mercaptopurine and azathioprine should be reduced to one-quarter of the original dose.

Neuromuscular blocking agents

Imuran can potentiate the neuromuscular blockade produced by depolarising agents such as succinylcholine and can reduce the blockade produced by non-depolarising agents such as tubocurarine. There is considerable variation in the potency of this interaction.

Warfarin

Inhibition of the anticoagulant effect of warfarin, when administered with azathioprine, has been reported.

Cytostatic/myelosuppressive agents

Where possible, concomitant administration of cytostatic drugs, or drugs which may have a myelosuppressive effect, such as penicillamine, should be avoided. There are conflicting clinical reports of interactions, resulting in serious haematological abnormalities, between Imuran and co-trimoxazole.

There has been a case report suggesting that haematological abnormalities may develop due to the concomitant administration of Imuran and captopril.

It has been suggested that cimetidine and indometacin may have myelosuppressive effects, which may be enhanced by concomitant administration of Imuran.

Other interactions

As there is *in vitro* evidence that aminosalicylate derivatives (eg. olsalazine, mesalazine or sulfasalazine) inhibit the TPMT enzyme, they should be administered with caution to patients receiving concurrent Imuran therapy (see section 4.4 Special Warnings and Special Precautions for Use).

Furosemide has been shown to impair the metabolism of azathioprine by human hepatic tissue *in vitro*. The clinical significance is unknown.

Vaccines

The immunosuppressive activity of Imuran could result in an atypical and potentially deleterious response to live vaccines and so the administration of live vaccines to patients receiving Imuran therapy is contra-indicated on theoretical grounds.

A diminished response to killed vaccines is likely and such a response to hepatitis B vaccine has been observed among patients treated with a combination of azathioprine and corticosteroids.

A small clinical study has indicated that standard therapeutic doses of Imuran do not deleteriously affect the response to polyvalent pneumococcal vaccine, as assessed on the basis of mean anti-capsular specific antibody concentration.

4.6 Pregnancy and lactation

Teratogenicity

Studies in pregnant rats, mice and rabbits using azathioprine in dosages from 5 to 15 mg/kg body weight/day over the period of organogenesis have shown varying degrees of foetal abnormalities. Teratogenicity was evident in rabbits at 10 mg/kg body weight/day.

Evidence of the teratogenicity of Imuran in man is equivocal. As with all cytotoxic chemotherapy, adequate contraceptive precautions should be advised when either partner is receiving Imuran.

Mutagenicity

Chromosomal abnormalities, which disappear with time, have been demonstrated in lymphocytes from the offspring of patients treated with Imuran. Except in extremely rare cases, no overt physical evidence of abnormality has been observed in the offspring of patients treated with Imuran. Azathioprine and long-wave ultraviolet light have been shown to have a synergistic clastogenic effect in patients treated with azathioprine for a range of disorders.

Use in Pregnancy and Lactation

Imuran should not be given to patients who are pregnant or likely to become pregnant without careful assessment of risk versus benefit.

There have been reports of premature birth and low birth weight following maternal exposure to azathioprine, particularly in combination with corticosteroids. There have also been reports of spontaneous abortion following either maternal or paternal exposure.

Azathioprine and/or its metabolites have been found in low concentrations in foetal blood and amniotic fluid after maternal administration of azathioprine.

Leucopenia and/or thrombocytopenia have been reported in a proportion of neonates whose mothers took azathioprine throughout their pregnancies. Extra care in haematological monitoring is advised during pregnancy.

Lactation

6-Mercaptopurine has been identified in the colostrum and breast-milk of women receiving azathioprine treatment.

4.7 Effects on ability to drive and use machines

None known.

4.8 Undesirable effects

For this product there is no modern clinical documentation that can be used as support for determining the frequency of undesirable effects. Undesirable effects may vary in their incidence depending on the indication. The following convention has been utilised for the classification of frequency: Very common, ⩾ 1/10; common, ⩾ 1/100 and < 1/10; uncommon, ⩾ 1/1000 and < 1/100; rare, ⩾ 1/10000 and < 1/1000; very rare, < 1/10000.

Infection and infestations

Transplant patients receiving Imuran in combination with other immunosuppressants.

Very common: Viral, fungal, and bacterial infections.

Other indications.

Uncommon: Viral, fungal and bacterial infections.

Patients receiving Imuran alone, or in combination with other immunosupressants, particularly corticosteroids, have shown increased susceptibility to viral, fungal and bacterial infections, including severe or atypical infection with varicella, herpes zoster and other infectious agents (see also section 4.4 Special Warnings and Precautions for Use).

Neoplasms benign and malignant (including cysts and polyps).

Rare: Neoplasms including non-Hodgkin's lymphomas, skin cancers (melanoma and non-melanoma), sarcomas (Kaposi's and non-Kaposi's) and uterine cervical cancer in situ, acute myeloid leukaemia and myelodysplasia (see also section 4.4 Special Warnings and Special Precautions for Use).

The risk of developing non-Hodgkin's lymphomas and other malignancies, notably skin cancers (melanoma and non-melanoma), sarcomas, (Kaposi's and non-Kaposi's) and uterine cervical cancer in situ, is increased in patients who receive immunosuppressive drugs, particularly in transplant recipients receiving aggressive treatment and such therapy should be maintained at the lowest effective levels. The increased risk of developing non-Hodgkin's lymphomas in immunosuppressed rheumatoid arthritis patients compared with the general population appears to be related at least in part to the disease itself.

There have been rare reports of acute myeloid leukaemia and myelodysplasia (some in association with chromosomal abnormalities).

Blood and lymphatic system disorders

Very common: Depression of bone marrow function; leucopenia.

Common: Thrombocytopenia.

Uncommon: Anaemia.

Rare: Agranulocytosis, pancytopenia, aplastic anaemia, megaloblastic anaemia, erythroid hypoplasia.

Imuran may be associated with a dose-related, generally reversible, depression of bone marrow function, most frequently expressed as leucopenia, but also sometimes as anaemia and thrombocytopenia, and rarely as agranulocytosis, pancytopenia and aplastic anaemia. These occur particularly in patients predisposed to myelotoxicity, such as those with TPMT deficiency and renal or hepatic insufficiency and in patients failing to reduce the dose of Imuran when receiving concurrent allopurinol therapy.

Reversible, dose-related increases in mean corpuscular volume and red cell haemoglobin content have occurred in association with Imuran therapy. Megaloblastic bone marrow changes have also been observed but severe megaloblastic anaemia and erythroid hypoplasia are rare.

Respiratory, thoracic and mediastinal disorders

Very rare: Reversible pneumonitis.

Reversible pneumonitis has been described very rarely.

Gastrointestinal disorders

Uncommon: Pancreatitis.

Rare: Colitis, diverticulitis and bowel perforation reported in transplant population, severe diarrhoea in inflammatory bowel disease population.

Serious complications, including colitis, diverticulitis and bowel perforation, have been described in transplant recipients receiving immunosuppressive therapy. However, the aetiology is not clearly established and high-dose corticosteroids may be implicated. Severe diarrhoea, recurring on re-challenge, has been reported in patients treated with Imuran for inflammatory bowel disease. The possibility that exacerbation of symptoms might be drug-related should be borne in mind when treating such patients.

Pancreatitis has been reported in a small percentage of patients on Imuran therapy, particularly in renal transplant patients and those diagnosed as having inflammatory bowel disease. There are difficulties in relating the pancreatitis to the administration of one particular drug, although re-challenge has confirmed an association with Imuran on occasions.

Hepato-biliary disorders

Uncommon: Cholestasis and degeneration of liver function tests.

Rare: Life-threatening hepatic damage.

Cholestasis and deterioration of liver function have occasionally been reported in association with Imuran therapy and are usually reversible on withdrawal of therapy. This may be associated with symptoms of a hypersensitivity reaction (see Hypersensitivity reactions).

Rare, but life-threatening hepatic damage associated with chronic administration of azathioprine has been described, primarily in transplant patients. Histological findings include sinusoidal dilatation, peliosis hepatis, veno-occlusive disease and nodular regenerative hyperplasia. In some cases withdrawal of azathioprine has resulted in either a temporary or permanent improvement in liver histology and symptoms.

Skin and subcutaneous tissue disorders

Rare: Alopecia, photosensitivity.

Hair loss has been described on a number of occasions in patients receiving azathioprine and other immunosuppressive agents. In many instances the condition resolved spontaneously despite continuing therapy. The relationship between alopecia and azathioprine treatment is uncertain.

Immune system disorders

Uncommon: Hypersensitivity reactions

Very rare: Stevens-Johnson syndrome and toxic epidermal necrolysis.

Several different clinical syndromes, which appear to be idiosyncratic manifestations of hypersensitivity, have been described occasionally following administration of Imuran. Clinical features include general malaise, dizziness, nausea, vomiting, diarrhoea, fever, rigors, exanthema, rash, vasculitis, myalgia, arthralgia, hypotension, renal dysfunction, hepatic dysfunction and cholestasis (see Hepato-biliary disorders).

In many cases, re-challenge has confirmed an association with Imuran.

Immediate withdrawal of azathioprine and institution of circulatory support where appropriate have led to recovery in the majority of cases.

Other marked underlying pathology has contributed to the very rare deaths reported.

Following a hypersensitivity reaction to Imuran, the necessity for continued administration of Imuran should be carefully considered on an individual basis.

4.9 Overdose

Symptoms and signs: Unexplained infection, ulceration of the throat, bruising and bleeding are the main signs of overdosage with Imuran and result from bone marrow depression which may be maximal after 9 to 14 days. These signs are more likely to be manifest following chronic overdosage, rather than after a single acute overdose. There has been a report of a patient who ingested a single overdose of 7.5 g of azathioprine. The immediate toxic effects of this overdose were nausea, vomiting and diarrhoea, followed by mild leucopenia and mild abnormalities in liver function. Recovery was uneventful.

Treatment: There is no specific antidote. Gastric lavage has been used. Subsequent monitoring, including haematological monitoring, is necessary to allow prompt treatment of any adverse effects which may develop. The value of dialysis in patients who have taken an overdose of Imuran is not known, though azathioprine is partially dialysable.

5. PHARMACOLOGICAL PROPERTIES

5.1 Pharmacodynamic properties

Azathioprine is an imidazole derivative of 6-mercaptopurine (6-MP). It is rapidly broken down *in vivo* into 6-MP and a methylnitroimidazole moiety. The 6-MP readily crosses cell membranes and is converted intracellularly into a number of purine thioanalogues, which include the main active nucleotide, thioinosinic acid. The rate of conversion varies from one person to another. Nucleotides do not traverse cell membranes and therefore do not circulate in body fluids. Irrespective of whether it is given directly or is derived *in vivo* from azathioprine, 6-MP is eliminated mainly as the inactive oxidised metabolite thiouric acid. This oxidation is brought about by xanthine oxidase, an enzyme that is inhibited by allopurinol. The activity of the methylnitroimidazole moiety has not been defined clearly. However, in several systems it appears to modify the activity of azathioprine as compared with that of 6-MP. Determination of plasma concentrations of azathioprine or 6-MP have no prognostic values as regards effectiveness or toxicity of these compounds.

Mode of action: While the precise modes of action remain to be elucidated, some suggested mechanisms include:

1. the release of 6-MP which acts as a purine antimetabolite.

2. the possible blockade of thiol (-SH) groups by alkylation.

3. the inhibition of many pathways in nucleic acid biosynthesis, hence preventing proliferation of cells involved in determination and amplification of the immune response.

4. damage to deoxyribonucleic acid (DNA) through incorporation of purine thio-analogues.

Because of these mechanisms, the therapeutic effect of Imuran may be evident only after several weeks or months of treatment.

Imuran appears to be well absorbed from the upper gastro-intestinal tract.

Studies in mice with [^{35}S]-azathioprine showed no unusually large concentration in any particular tissue, and there was very little [^{35}S]-label found in brain.

Plasma levels of azathioprine and 6-MP do not correlate well with the therapeutic efficacy or toxicity of Imuran.

5.2 Pharmacokinetic properties

Azathioprine is well absorbed following oral administration. After oral administration of [^{35}S]-azathioprine, the maximum plasma radioactivity occurs at 1-2 hours and decays with a half-life of 4-6 hours. This is not an estimate of the half-life of azathioprine itself, but reflects the elimination from plasma of azathioprine and the [^{35}S]-containing metabolites of the drug. As a consequence of the rapid and extensive metabolism of azathioprine, only a fraction of the radioactivity measured in plasma is comprised of unmetabolised drug. Studies in which the plasma concentration of azathioprine and 6-MP have been determined, following intravenous administration of azathioprine, have estimated the mean plasma $T_{1/2}$ for azathioprine to be in the range of 6-28 minutes and the mean plasma $T_{1/2}$ for 6-MP to be in the range 38-114 minutes.

Azathioprine is principally excreted as 6-thiouric uric acid in the urine. 1-methyl-4-nitro-5-thioimidazole has also been detected in urine as a minor excretory product. This would indicate that, rather than azathioprine being exclusive cleaved by nucleophilic attack at the 5-position of the nitroimidazole ring to generate 6-MP and 1-methyl-4-nitro-5-(S-glutathionyl)imidazole. A small proportion of the drug may be cleaved between the sulphur-atom and the purine ring. Only a small amount of the dose of azathioprine administered is excreted unmetabolised in the urine.

5.3 Preclinical safety data

No additional data of clinical relevance to the prescriber.

6. PHARMACEUTICAL PARTICULARS

6.1 List of excipients

Sodium hydroxide pellets* BP 7.2 mg

Sodium hydroxide pellets* to adjust pH

Water for Injections EP

*In the form of a 1M solution in water for injections.

6.2 Incompatibilities

Imuran Injection should ONLY be reconstituted with the recommended volume of Water for Injections BP and should be diluted as specified above. Imuran Injection should not be mixed with other drugs or fluids, except those specified above, before administration.

6.3 Shelf life

3 years unopened

5 days when reconstituted with 5 ml to 15 ml water for injections and stored at 5 to 25°C.

1 day for 5 ml of the reconstituted injection further diluted with between 20 ml and 200 ml of an appropriate infusion solution and stored at 15°C to 25°C.

6.4 Special precautions for storage

Store below 25°C

Keep dry

Protect from light

6.5 Nature and contents of container

Neutral glass vials with synthetic butyl rubber closures and aluminium collars. Each vial contains the equivalent of 50 mg azathioprine.

6.6 Special precautions for disposal and other handling

Health professionals who handle Imuran Injection should follow guidelines for the handling of cytotoxic drugs according to prevailing local recommendations and/or regulations (e.g., the Royal Pharmaceutical Society of Great Britain Working Party Report on the Handling of Cytotoxic Drugs, 1983).

Administrative Data

7. MARKETING AUTHORISATION HOLDER

The Wellcome Foundation Limited

Glaxo Wellcome House

Berkeley Avenue

Greenford

Middlesex

UB6 0NN

Trading as

GlaxoSmithKline UK

Stockley Park West

Uxbridge

Middlesex UB11 1BT

8. MARKETING AUTHORISATION NUMBER(S)

PL0003/5043R

9. DATE OF FIRST AUTHORISATION/RENEWAL OF THE AUTHORISATION

13 March 1988 / 06 March 2003

10. DATE OF REVISION OF THE TEXT

27-5-2009

11. Legal Status

POM

Imuran Tablets 25mg

(GlaxoSmithKline UK)

1. NAME OF THE MEDICINAL PRODUCT

Imuran tablets 25 mg

2. QUALITATIVE AND QUANTITATIVE COMPOSITION

Orange, round, biconvex, film-coated tablets, impressed 'GX EL5' and containing 25 mg Azathioprine BP in each tablet.

3. PHARMACEUTICAL FORM

Tablet.

4. CLINICAL PARTICULARS

4.1 Therapeutic indications

Imuran tablets are used as an immunosuppressant antimetabolite either alone or, more commonly, in combination with other agents (usually corticosteroids) and procedures which influence the immune response. Therapeutic effect may be evident only after weeks or months and can include a steroid-sparing effect, thereby reducing the toxicity associated with high dosage and prolonged usage of corticosteroids.

Imuran, in combination with corticosteroids and/or other immunosuppressive agents and procedures, is indicated to enhance the survival of organ transplants, such as renal transplants, cardiac transplants, and hepatic transplants; and to reduce the corticosteroid requirements of renal transplant recipients.

Imuran, either alone or more usually in combination with corticosteroids and/or other drugs and procedures, has been used with clinical benefit (which may include reduction of dosage or discontinuation of corticosteroids) in a proportion of patients suffering from the following:

severe rheumatoid arthritis;

systemic lupus erythematosus;

dermatomyositis and polymyositis;

auto-immune chronic active hepatitis;

pemphigus vulgaris;

polyarteritis nodosa;

auto-immune haemolytic anaemia;

chronic refractory idiopathic thrombocytopenic purpura.

4.2 Posology and method of administration

Transplantation - adults and children

Depending on the immunosuppressive regimen employed, a dosage of up to 5 mg/kg body weight/day may be given on the first day of therapy, either orally or intravenously.

Maintenance dosage should range from 1 to 4 mg/kg body weight/day and must be adjusted according to clinical requirements and haematological tolerance.

Evidence indicates that Imuran therapy should be maintained indefinitely, even if only low doses are necessary, because of the risk of graft rejection.

Dosage in other conditions - adults and children

In general, starting dosage is from 1 to 3 mg/kg body weight/day, and should be adjusted, within these limits, depending on the clinical response (which may not be evident for weeks or months) and haematological tolerance.

When therapeutic response is evident, consideration should be given to reducing the maintenance dosage to the lowest level compatible with the maintenance of that response. If no improvement occurs in the patient's condition within 3 months, consideration should be given to withdrawing Imuran.

The maintenance dosage required may range from less than 1 mg/kg body weight/day to 3 mg/kg body weight/day, depending on the clinical condition being treated and the individual patient response, including haematological tolerance.

In patients with renal and/or hepatic insufficiency, dosages should be given at the lower end of the normal range (see Special Warnings and Precautions for Use for further details).

Use in the elderly (see Renal and/or hepatic insufficiency)

There is limited experience of the administration of Imuran to elderly patients. Although the available data do not provide evidence that the incidence of side effects among elderly patients is higher than that among other patients treated with Imuran, it is recommended that the dosages used should be at the lower end of the range.

Particular care should be taken to monitor haematological response and to reduce the maintenance dosage to the minimum required for clinical response.

4.3 Contraindications

Imuran is contra-indicated in patients known to be hypersensitive to azathioprine. Hypersensitivity to 6-mercaptopurine (6-MP) should alert the prescriber to probable hypersensitivity to Imuran.

Imuran therapy should not be initiated in patients who may be pregnant, or who are likely to become pregnant without careful assessment of risk versus benefit (see Special Warnings and Precautions for Use and Pregnancy and Lactation).

4.4 Special warnings and precautions for use

Monitoring

There are potential hazards in the use of Imuran. It should be prescribed only if the patient can be adequately monitored for toxic effects throughout the duration of therapy.

It is suggested that during the first 8 weeks of therapy, complete blood counts, including platelets, should be performed weekly or more frequently if high dosage is used or if severe renal and/or hepatic disorder is present. The blood count frequency may be reduced later in therapy, but it is suggested that complete blood counts are repeated monthly, or at least at intervals of not longer than 3 months.

Patients receiving Imuran should be instructed to report immediately any evidence of infection, unexpected bruising or bleeding or other manifestations of bone marrow depression.

There are individuals with an inherited deficiency of the enzyme thiopurine methyltransferase (TPMT) who may be unusually sensitive to the myelosuppressive effect of azathioprine and prone to developing rapid bone marrow depression following the initiation of treatment with Imuran. This problem could be exacerbated by co-administration with drugs that inhibit TPMT, such as olsalazine, mesalazine or sulfasalazine. Also it has been reported that decreased TPMT activity increases the risk of secondary leukaemias and myelodysplasia in individuals receiving 6-mercaptopurine (the active metabolite of azathioprine) in combination with other cytotoxics (see section 4.8 Undesirable effects).

Renal and/or hepatic insufficiency

It has been suggested that the toxicity of Imuran may be enhanced in the presence of renal insufficiency, but controlled studies have not supported this suggestion. Nevertheless, it is recommended that the dosages used should be at the lower end of the normal range and that haematological response should be carefully monitored. Dosage should be further reduced if haematological toxicity occurs.

Caution is necessary during the administration of Imuran to patients with hepatic dysfunction, and regular complete blood counts and liver function tests should be undertaken. In such patients the metabolism of Imuran may be impaired, and the dosage of Imuran should therefore be reduced if hepatic or haematological toxicity occurs.

Limited evidence suggests that Imuran is not beneficial to patients with hypoxanthine-guanine-phosphoribosyltransferase deficiency (Lesch-Nyhan syndrome). Therefore, given the abnormal metabolism in these patients, it is not prudent to recommend that these patients should receive Imuran.

Mutagenicity

Chromosomal abnormalities have been demonstrated in both male and female patients treated with Imuran. It is difficult to assess the role of Imuran in the development of these abnormalities.

Effects on fertility

Relief of chronic renal insufficiency by renal transplantation involving the administration of Imuran has been accompanied by increased fertility in both male and female transplant recipients.

Carcinogenicity (see also section 4.8 Undesirable Effects)

Patients receiving immunosuppressive therapy are at an increased risk of developing non-Hodgkin's lymphomas and other malignancies, notably skin cancers (melanoma and non-melanoma), sarcomas (Kaposi's and non-Kaposi's) and uterine cervical cancer in situ. The risk appears to be related to the intensity and duration of immunosuppression rather than to the use of any specific agent. It has been reported that reduction or discontinuation of immunosuppression may be associated with partial or complete regression of non-Hodgkin's lymphomas and Kaposi's sarcomas.

Patients receiving multiple immunosuppressive agents may be at risk of over-immunosuppression, therefore such therapy should be maintained at the lowest effective level.

Exposure to sunlight and UV light should be limited and patients should wear protective clothing and use a sunscreen with a high protection factor to minimize the risk of skin cancer and photosensitivity (see also section 4.8 Undesirable Effects).

Varicella Zoster Virus Infection (see also section 4.8 Undesirable Effects)

Infection with varicella zoster virus (VZV; chickenpox and herpes zoster) may become severe during the administration of immunosuppressants. Caution should be exercised especially with respect to the following:

Before starting the administration of immunosuppressants, the prescriber should check to see if the patient has a history of VZV. Serologic testing may be useful in determining previous exposure. Patients who have no history of exposure should avoid contact with individuals with chickenpox or herpes zoster. If the patient is exposed to VZV, special care must be taken to avoid patients developing chickenpox or herpes zoster, and passive immunisation with varicella-zoster immunoglobulin (VZIG) may be considered.

If the patient is infected with VZV, appropriate measures should be taken, which may include antiviral therapy and supportive care.

4.5 Interaction with other medicinal products and other forms of interaction

Allopurinol/ oxipurinol/ thiopurinol

Xanthine oxidase activity is inhibited by allopurinol, oxipurinol and thiopurinol which results in reduced conversion of biologically active 6-thioinosinic acid to biologically inactive 6-thiouric acid. When allopurinol, oxipurinol and/or thiopurinol are given concomitantly with 6-mercaptopurine or azathioprine, the dose of 6-mercaptopurine and azathioprine should be reduced to one-quarter of the original dose.

Neuromuscular blocking agents

Imuran can potentiate the neuromuscular blockade produced by depolarising agents such as succinylcholine and can reduce the blockade produced by non-depolarising agents such as tubocurarine. There is considerable variation in the potency of this interaction.

Warfarin

Inhibition of the anticoagulant effect of warfarin, when administered with azathioprine, has been reported.

Cytostatic/myelosuppressive agents

Where possible, concomitant administration of cytostatic drugs, or drugs which may have a myelosuppressive effect, such as penicillamine, should be avoided. There are conflicting clinical reports of interactions, resulting in serious haematological abnormalities, between Imuran and co-trimoxazole.

There has been a case report suggesting that haematological abnormalities may develop due to the concomitant administration of Imuran and captopril.

It has been suggested that cimetidine and indometacin may have myelosuppressive effects, which may be enhanced by concomitant administration of Imuran.

Other interactions

As there is *in vitro* evidence that aminosalicylate derivatives (eg. olsalazine, mesalazine or sulfasalazine) inhibit the TPMT enzyme, they should be administered with caution to patients receiving concurrent Imuran therapy (see Special Warnings and Special Precautions for Use).

Furosemide has been shown to impair the metabolism of azathioprine by human hepatic tissue *in vitro*. The clinical significance is unknown.

Vaccines

The immunosuppressive activity of Imuran could result in an atypical and potentially deleterious response to live vaccines and so the administration of live vaccines to patients receiving Imuran therapy is contra-indicated on theoretical grounds.

A diminished response to killed vaccines is likely and such a response to hepatitis B vaccine has been observed among patients treated with a combination of azathioprine and corticosteroids.

A small clinical study has indicated that standard therapeutic doses of Imuran do not deleteriously affect the response to polyvalent pneumococcal vaccine, as assessed on the basis of mean anti-capsular specific antibody concentration.

4.6 Pregnancy and lactation

Teratogenicity

Studies in pregnant rats, mice and rabbits using azathioprine in dosages from 5 to 15 mg/kg body weight/day over the period of organogenesis have shown varying degrees of foetal abnormalities. Teratogenicity was evident in rabbits at 10 mg/kg body weight/day.

Evidence of the teratogenicity of Imuran in man is equivocal. As with all cytotoxic chemotherapy, adequate contraceptive precautions should be advised when either partner is receiving Imuran.

Mutagenicity

Chromosomal abnormalities, which disappear with time, have been demonstrated in lymphocytes from the offspring of patients treated with Imuran. Except in extremely rare cases, no overt physical evidence of abnormality has been observed in the offspring of patients treated with Imuran. Azathioprine and long-wave ultraviolet light have been shown to have a synergistic clastogenic effect in patients treated with azathioprine for a range of disorders.

Use in Pregnancy and Lactation

Imuran should not be given to patients who are pregnant or likely to become pregnant without careful assessment of risk versus benefit.

There have been reports of premature birth and low birth weight following maternal exposure to azathioprine, particularly in combination with corticosteroids. There have also been reports of spontaneous abortion following either maternal or paternal exposure.

Azathioprine and/or its metabolites have been found in low concentrations in foetal blood and amniotic fluid after maternal administration of azathioprine.

Leucopenia and/or thrombocytopenia have been reported in a proportion of neonates whose mothers took azathioprine throughout their pregnancies. Extra care in haematological monitoring is advised during pregnancy.

Lactation

6-Mercaptopurine has been identified in the colostrum and breast-milk of women receiving azathioprine treatment.

4.7 Effects on ability to drive and use machines

None known.

4.8 Undesirable effects

For this product there is no modern clinical documentation that can be used as support for determining the frequency of undesirable effects. Undesirable effects may vary in their incidence depending on the indication. The following convention has been utilised for the classification of frequency: Very common, ⩾ 1/10; common, ⩾ 1/100 and < 1/10; uncommon, ⩾ 1/1000 and < 1/100; rare, ⩾ 1/10000 and < 1/1000; very rare, < 1/10000.

Infection and infestations

Transplant patients receiving Imuran in combination with other immunosuppressants.

Very common: Viral, fungal and bacterial infections.

Other indications.

Uncommon: Viral, fungal and bacterial infections.

Patients receiving Imuran alone, or in combination with other immunosupressants, particularly corticosteroids, have shown increased susceptibility to viral, fungal and bacterial infections, including severe or atypical infection with varicella, herpes zoster and other infectious agents (see also section 4.4 Special Warnings and Precautions for Use).

Neoplasms benign and malignant (including cysts and polyps)

Rare: Neoplasms including non-Hodgkin's lymphomas, skin cancers melanoma and non-melanoma), sarcomas (Kaposi's and non-Kaposi's) and uterine cervical cancer in situ, acute myloid leukaemia and myelodysplasia (see also section 4.4 Special Warnings and Special Precautions for Use)

The risk of developing non-Hodgkin's lymphomas and other malignancies, notably skin cancers (melanoma and non-melanoma), sarcomas, (Kaposi's and non-Kaposi's) and uterine cervical cancer in situ, is increased in patients who receive immunosuppressive drugs, particularly in transplant recipients receiving aggressive treatment and such therapy should be maintained at the lowest effective levels. The increased risk of developing non-Hodgkin's lymphomas in immunosuppressed rheumatoid arthritis patients compared with the general population appears to be related at least in part to the disease itself.

There have been rare reports of acute myeloid leukaemia and myelodysplasia (some in association with chromasomal abnormalities)

Blood and lymphatic system disorders

Very common:	Depression of bone marrow function; leucopenia.
Common:	Thrombocytopenia.
Uncommon:	Anaemia.
Rare:	Agranulocytosis, pancytopenia, aplastic anaemia, megaloblastic anaemia, erythriod hypoplasia.

Imuran may be associated with a dose-related, generally reversible, depression of bone marrow function, most frequently expressed as leucopenia, but also sometimes as anaemia and thrombocytopenia, and rarely as agranulocytosis, pancytopenia and aplastic anaemia. These occur particularly in patients predisposed to myelotoxicity, such as those with TPMT deficiency and renal or hepatic insufficiency and in patients failing to reduce the dose of Imuran when receiving concurrent allopurinol therapy.

Reversible, dose-related increases in mean corpuscular volume and red cell haemoglobin content have occurred in association with Imuran therapy. Megaloblastic bone marrow changes have also been observed but severe megaloblastic anaemia and erythroid hypoplasia is rare.

Respiratory, thoracic and mediastinal disorders

Very rare: Reversible pneumonitis.

Reversible pneumonitis has been described very rarely.

Gastrointestinal disorders

Uncommon:	Pancreatitis.
Rare:	Colitis, diverticulitis and bowel perforation reported in transplant population, severe diarrhoea in inflammatory bowel disease population.

A minority of patients experience nausea when first given Imuran. This appears to be relieved by administering the tablets after meals.

Serious complications, including colitis, diverticulitis and bowel perforation, have been described in transplant recipients receiving immunosuppressive therapy. However, the aetiology is not clearly established and high-dose corticosteroids may be implicated. Severe diarrhoea, recurring on re-challenge, has been reported in patients treated with Imuran for inflammatory bowel disease. The possibility that exacerbation of symptoms might be drug-related should be borne in mind when treating such patients.

Pancreatitis has been reported in a small percentage of patients on Imuran therapy, particularly in renal transplant patients and those diagnosed as having inflammatory bowel disease. There are difficulties in relating the pancreatitis to the administration of one particular drug, although re-challenge has confirmed an association with Imuran on occasions.

Hepato-biliary disorders

Uncommon:	Cholestasis and degeneration of liver function tests.
Rare:	Life-threatening hepatic damage.

Cholestasis and deterioration of liver function have occasionally been reported in association with Imuran therapy and are usually reversible on withdrawal of therapy. This may be associated with symptoms of a hypersensitivity reaction (see Hypersensitivity reactions).

Rare, but life-threatening hepatic damage associated with chronic administration of azathioprine has been described primarily in transplant patients. Histological findings include sinusoidal dilatation, peliosis hepatis, veno-occlusive disease and nodular regenerative hyperplasia. In some cases withdrawal of azathioprine has resulted in either a temporary or permanent improvement in liver histology and symptoms.

Skin and subcutaneous tissue disorders

Rare: Alopecia, photosensitivity.

Hair loss has been described on a number of occasions in patients receiving azathioprine and other immunosuppressive agents. In many instances the condition resolved spontaneously despite continuing therapy. The relationship between alopecia and azathioprine treatment is uncertain.

Immune system disorders

Uncommon:	Hypersensitivity reactions
Very rare:	Stevens-Johnson syndrome and toxic epidermal necrolysis.

Several different clinical syndromes, which appear to be idiosyncratic manifestations of hypersensitivity, have been described occasionally following administration of Imuran. Clinical features include general malaise, dizziness, nausea, vomiting, diarrhoea, fever, rigors, exanthema, rash, vasculitis, myalgia, arthralgia, hypotension, renal dysfunction, hepatic dysfunction and cholestasis (see Hepato-biliary disorders).

In many cases, re-challenge has confirmed an association with Imuran.

Immediate withdrawal of azathioprine and institution of circulatory support where appropriate have led to recovery in the majority of cases.

Other marked underlying pathology has contributed to the very rare deaths reported.

Following a hypersensitivity reaction to Imuran, the necessity for continued administration of Imuran should be carefully considered on an individual basis.

4.9 Overdose

Symptoms and signs

Unexplained infection, ulceration of the throat, bruising and bleeding are the main signs of overdosage with Imuran and result from bone marrow depression which may be maximal after 9 to 14 days. These signs are more likely to be manifest following chronic overdosage, rather than after a single acute overdose. There has been a report of a patient who ingested a single overdose of 7.5 g of azathioprine. The immediate toxic effects of this overdose were nausea, vomiting and diarrhoea, followed by mild leucopenia and mild abnormalities in liver function. Recovery was uneventful.

Treatment

There is no specific antidote. Gastric lavage has been used. Subsequent monitoring, including haematological monitoring, is necessary to allow prompt treatment of any adverse effects which may develop. The value of dialysis in patients who have taken an overdose of Imuran is not known, though azathioprine is partially dialysable.

5. PHARMACOLOGICAL PROPERTIES

5.1 Pharmacodynamic properties

Azathioprine is an imidazole derivative of 6-mercaptopurine (6-MP). It is rapidly broken down *in vivo* into 6-MP and a methylnitroimidazole moiety. The 6-MP readily crosses cell membranes and is converted intracellularly into a number of purine thioanalogues, which include the main active nucleotide, thioinosinic acid. The rate of conversion varies from one person to another. Nucleotides do not traverse cell membranes and therefore do not circulate in body fluids. Irrespective of whether it is given directly or is derived *in vivo* from azathioprine, 6-MP is eliminated mainly as the inactive oxidised metabolite thiouric acid. This oxidation is brought about by xanthine oxidase, an enzyme that is inhibited by allopurinol. The activity of the methylnitroimidazole moiety has not been defined clearly. However, in several systems it appears to modify the activity of azathioprine as compared with that of 6-MP. Determination of plasma concentrations of azathioprine or 6-MP have no prognostic values as regards effectiveness or toxicity of these compounds.

While the precise modes of action remain to be elucidated, some suggested mechanisms include:

1. the release of 6-MP which acts as a purine antimetabolite.

2. the possible blockade of -SH groups by alkylation.

3. the inhibition of many pathways in nucleic acid biosynthesis, hence preventing proliferation of cells involved in determination and amplification of the immune response.

4. damage to deoxyribonucleic acid (DNA) through incorporation of purine thio-analogues.

Because of these mechanisms, the therapeutic effect of Imuran may be evident only after several weeks or months of treatment.

Imuran appears to be well absorbed from the upper gastrointestinal tract.

Studies in mice with [^{35}S]-azathioprine showed no unusually large concentration in any particular tissue, and there was very little [^{35}S]-label found in brain.

Plasma levels of azathioprine and 6-MP do not correlate well with the therapeutic efficacy or toxicity of Imuran.

5.2 Pharmacokinetic properties

Azathioprine is well absorbed following oral administration. After oral administration of [^{35}S]-azathioprine, the maximum plasma radioactivity occurs at 1-2 hours and decays with a half-life of 4-6 hours. This is not an estimate of the half-life of azathioprine itself, but reflects the elimination from plasma of azathioprine and the [^{35}S]-containing metabolites of the drug. As a consequence of the rapid and extensive metabolism of azathioprine, only a fraction of the radioactivity measured in plasma is comprised of unmetabolised drug. Studies in which the plasma concentration of azathioprine and 6-MP have been determined following intravenous administration of azathioprine have estimated the mean plasma $T^1/_2$ for azathioprine to be in the range of 6-28 minutes and the mean plasma $T^1/_2$ for 6-MP to be in the range 38-114 minutes after i.v. administration of the drug.

Azathioprine is principally excreted as 6-thiouric uric acid in the urine. 1-methyl-4-nitro-5-thioimidazole has also been detected in urine as a minor excretory product. This would indicate that, rather than azathioprine being exclusive cleaved by nucleophilic attack at the 5-position of the nitroimidazole ring to generate 6-MP and 1-methyl-4-nitro-5-(S-glutathionyl)imidazole. A small proportion of the drug may be cleaved between the S atom and the purine ring. Only a small amount of the dose of azathioprine administered is excreted unmetabolised in the urine.

5.3 Preclinical safety data

No additional data of clinical relevance to the prescriber.

6. PHARMACEUTICAL PARTICULARS

6.1 List of excipients

Lactose, pregelatinised starch, maize starch, stearic acid, magnesium sterate, methylhydroxylpropyl cellulose, polyethylene glycol 400, titanium dioxide (E171), iron oxide, yellow (E172), iron oxide, red (E172), industrial methylated spirit, purified water.

6.2 Incompatibilities

None known.

6.3 Shelf life

5 years.

6.4 Special precautions for storage

Store below 25°C. Protect from light.

6.5 Nature and contents of container

Blister strips in a pack.

Pack sizes: 28, 30, 56, 60 and 100 tablets.

6.6 Special precautions for disposal and other handling

Health professionals who handle Imuran Injection should follow guidelines for the handling of cytotoxic drugs (for example, the Royal Pharmaceutical Society of Great Britain Working Party Report on the Handling of Cytotoxic Drugs, 1983).

Provided that the film-coating is intact, there is no risk in handling film-coated Imuran Tablets. Imuran Tablets should not be divided and, provided the coating is intact, no additional precautions are required when handling them.

Administrative Data

7. MARKETING AUTHORISATION HOLDER

The Wellcome Foundation

Berkeley Avenue

Greenford

Middlesex

UB6 ONN

8. MARKETING AUTHORISATION NUMBER(S)

PL 00003/0225

9. DATE OF FIRST AUTHORISATION/RENEWAL OF THE AUTHORISATION

20 March 1992

10. DATE OF REVISION OF THE TEXT

27-5-2009

11. Legal Status

POM

Imuran Tablets 50mg

(GlaxoSmithKline UK)

1. NAME OF THE MEDICINAL PRODUCT

Imuran tablets 50 mg

2. QUALITATIVE AND QUANTITATIVE COMPOSITION

Yellow, round, biconvex, scored, film-coated tablets, impressed 'GX CH1' and containing 50 mg Azathioprine BP in each tablet.

3. PHARMACEUTICAL FORM

Tablet.

4. CLINICAL PARTICULARS

4.1 Therapeutic indications

Imuran tablets are used as an immunosuppressant antimetabolite either alone or, more commonly, in combination with other agents (usually corticosteroids) and procedures which influence the immune response. Therapeutic effect may be evident only after weeks or months and can include a steroid-sparing effect, thereby reducing the toxicity associated with high dosage and prolonged usage of corticosteroids.

Imuran, in combination with corticosteroids and/or other immunosuppressive agents and procedures, is indicated to enhance the survival of organ transplants, such as renal transplants, cardiac transplants, and hepatic transplants; and to reduce the corticosteroid requirements of renal transplant recipients.

Imuran, either alone or more usually in combination with corticosteroids and/or other drugs and procedures, has been used with clinical benefit (which may include reduction of dosage or discontinuation of corticosteroids) in a proportion of patients suffering from the following:

severe rheumatoid arthritis;

systemic lupus erythematosus;

dermatomyositis and polymyositis;

auto-immune chronic active hepatitis;

pemphigus vulgaris;

polyarteritis nodosa;

auto-immune haemolytic anaemia;

chronic refractory idiopathic thrombocytopenic purpura.

4.2 Posology and method of administration

Transplantation - adults and children

Depending on the immunosuppressive regimen employed, a dosage of up to 5 mg/kg body weight/day may be given on the first day of therapy, either orally or intravenously.

Maintenance dosage should range from 1 to 4 mg/kg body weight/day and must be adjusted according to clinical requirements and haematological tolerance.

Evidence indicates that Imuran therapy should be maintained indefinitely, even if only low doses are necessary, because of the risk of graft rejection.

Dosage in other conditions - adults and children

In general, starting dosage is from 1 to 3 mg/kg body weight/day, and should be adjusted, within these limits, depending on the clinical response (which may not be evident for weeks or months) and haematological tolerance.

When therapeutic response is evident, consideration should be given to reducing the maintenance dosage to the lowest level compatible with the maintenance of that response. If no improvement occurs in the patient's condition within 3 months, consideration should be given to withdrawing Imuran.

The maintenance dosage required may range from less than 1 mg/kg body weight/day to 3 mg/kg body weight/ day, depending on the clinical condition being treated and the individual patient response, including haematological tolerance.

In patients with renal and/or hepatic insufficiency, dosages should be given at the lower end of the normal range (see Special Warnings and Precautions for Use for further details).

Use in the elderly (see Renal and/or hepatic insufficiency)

There is limited experience of the administration of Imuran to elderly patients. Although the available data do not provide evidence that the incidence of side effects among elderly patients is higher than that among other patients treated with Imuran, it is recommended that the dosages used should be at the lower end of the range.

Particular care should be taken to monitor haematological response and to reduce the maintenance dosage to the minimum required for clinical response.

4.3 Contraindications

Imuran is contra-indicated in patients known to be hypersensitive to azathioprine. Hypersensitivity to 6-mercaptopurine (6-MP) should alert the prescriber to probable hypersensitivity to Imuran.

Imuran therapy should not be initiated in patients who may be pregnant, or who are likely to become pregnant without careful assessment of risk versus benefit (see Special Warnings and Precautions for Use and Pregnancy and Lactation).

4.4 Special warnings and precautions for use

Monitoring

There are potential hazards in the use of Imuran. It should be prescribed only if the patient can be adequately monitored for toxic effects throughout the duration of therapy.

It is suggested that during the first 8 weeks of therapy, complete blood counts, including platelets, should be performed weekly or more frequently if high dosage is used or if severe renal and/or hepatic disorder is present. The blood count frequency may be reduced later in therapy, but it is suggested that complete blood counts are repeated monthly, or at least at intervals of not longer than 3 months.

Patients receiving Imuran should be instructed to report immediately any evidence of infection, unexpected bruising or bleeding or other manifestations of bone marrow depression.

There are individuals with an inherited deficiency of the enzyme thiopurine methyltransferase (TPMT) who may be unusually sensitive to the myelosuppressive effect of azathioprine and prone to developing rapid bone marrow depression following the initiation of treatment with Imuran. This problem could be exacerbated by co-administration with drugs that inhibit TPMT, such as olsalazine, mesalazine or sulfasalazine. Also it has been reported that decreased TPMT activity increases the risk of secondary leukaemias and myelodysplasia in individuals receiving 6-mercaptopurine (the active metabolite of azathioprine) in combination with other cytotoxics (see section 4.8 Undesirable effects).

Renal and/or hepatic insufficiency

It has been suggested that the toxicity of Imuran may be enhanced in the presence of renal insufficiency, but controlled studies have not supported this suggestion. Nevertheless, it is recommended that the dosages used should be at the lower end of the normal range and that haematological response should be carefully monitored. Dosage should be further reduced if haematological toxicity occurs.

Caution is necessary during the administration of Imuran to patients with hepatic dysfunction, and regular complete blood counts and liver function tests should be undertaken. In such patients the metabolism of Imuran may be impaired, and the dosage of Imuran should therefore be reduced if hepatic or haematological toxicity occurs.

Limited evidence suggests that Imuran is not beneficial to patients with hypoxanthine-guanine-phosphoribosyltransferase deficiency (Lesch-Nyhan syndrome). Therefore, given the abnormal metabolism in these patients, it is not prudent to recommend that these patients should receive Imuran.

Mutagenicity

Chromosomal abnormalities have been demonstrated in both male and female patients treated with Imuran. It is difficult to assess the role of Imuran in the development of these abnormalities.

Effects on fertility

Relief of chronic renal insufficiency by renal transplantation involving the administration of Imuran has been accompanied by increased fertility in both male and female transplant recipients.

Carcinogenicity (see also section 4.8 Undesirable Effects)

Patients receiving immunosuppressive therapy are at an increased risk of developing non-Hodgkin's lymphomas and other malignancies, notably skin cancers (melanoma and non-melanoma), sarcomas (Kaposi's and non-Kaposi's) and uterine cervical cancer in situ. The risk appears to be related to the intensity and duration of immunosuppression rather than to the use of any specific agent. It has been reported that reduction or discontinuation of immunosuppression may be associated with partial or complete regression of non-Hodgkin's lymphomas and Kaposi's sarcomas.

Patients receiving multiple immunosuppressive agents may be at risk of over-immunosuppression, therefore such therapy should be maintained at the lowest effective level.

Exposure to sunlight and UV light should be limited and patients should wear protective clothing and use a sunscreen with a high protection factor to minimize the risk of skin cancer and photosensitivity (see also section 4.8 Undesirable Effects).

Varicella Zoster Virus Infection (see also section 4.8 Undesirable Effects)

Infection with varicella zoster virus (VZV; chickenpox and herpes zoster) may become severe during the administration of immunosuppressants. Caution should be exercised especially with respect to the following:

Before starting the administration of immunosuppressants, the prescriber should check to see if the patient has a history of VZV. Serologic testing may be useful in determining previous exposure. Patients who have no history of exposure should avoid contact with individuals with chickenpox or herpes zoster. If the patient is exposed to VZV, special care must be taken to avoid patients developing chickenpox or herpes zoster, and passive immunisation with varicella-zoster immunoglobulin (VZIG) may be considered.

If the patient is infected with VZV, appropriate measures should be taken, which may include antiviral therapy and supportive care.

4.5 Interaction with other medicinal products and other forms of interaction

Allopurinol/ oxipurinol/ thiopurinol

Xanthine oxidase activity is inhibited by allopurinol, oxipurinol and thiopurinol which results in reduced conversion of biologically active 6-thioinosinic acid to biologically inactive 6-thiouric acid. When allopurinol, oxipurinol and/or thiopurinol are given concomitantly with 6-mercaptopurine or azathioprine, the dose of 6-mercaptopurine and azathioprine should be reduced to one-quarter of the original dose.

Neuromuscular blocking agents

Imuran can potentiate the neuromuscular blockade produced by depolarising agents such as succinylcholine and can reduce the blockade produced by non-depolarising agents such as tubocurarine. There is considerable variation in the potency of this interaction.

Warfarin

Inhibition of the anticoagulant effect of warfarin, when administered with azathioprine, has been reported.

Cytostatic/myelosuppressive agents

Where possible, concomitant administration of cytostatic drugs, or drugs which may have a myelosuppressive effect, such as penicillamine, should be avoided. There are conflicting clinical reports of interactions, resulting in serious haematological abnormalities, between Imuran and co-trimoxazole.

There has been a case report suggesting that haematological abnormalities may develop due to the concomitant administration of Imuran and captopril.

It has been suggested that cimetidine and indometacin may have myelosuppressive effects, which may be enhanced by concomitant administration of Imuran.

Other interactions

As there is *in vitro* evidence that aminosalicylate derivatives (eg. olsalazine, mesalazine or sulfasalazine) inhibit the TPMT enzyme, they should be administered with caution to patients receiving concurrent Imuran therapy (see Special Warnings and Special Precautions for Use).

Furosemide has been shown to impair the metabolism of azathioprine by human hepatic tissue *in vitro*. The clinical significance is unknown.

Vaccines

The immunosuppressive activity of Imuran could result in an atypical and potentially deleterious response to live vaccines and so the administration of live vaccines to patients receiving Imuran therapy is contra-indicated on theoretical grounds.

A diminished response to killed vaccines is likely and such a response to hepatitis B vaccine has been observed among patients treated with a combination of azathioprine and corticosteroids.

A small clinical study has indicated that standard therapeutic doses of Imuran do not deleteriously affect the response to polyvalent pneumococcal vaccine, as assessed on the basis of mean anti-capsular specific antibody concentration.

4.6 Pregnancy and lactation

Teratogenicity

Studies in pregnant rats, mice and rabbits using azathioprine in dosages from 5 to 15 mg/kg body weight/day over the period of organogenesis have shown varying degrees of foetal abnormalities. Teratogenicity was evident in rabbits at 10 mg/kg body weight/day.

Evidence of the teratogenicity of Imuran in man is equivocal. As with all cytotoxic chemotherapy, adequate contraceptive precautions should be advised when either partner is receiving Imuran.

Mutagenicity

Chromosomal abnormalities, which disappear with time, have been demonstrated in lymphocytes from the offspring of patients treated with Imuran. Except in extremely rare cases, no overt physical evidence of abnormality has been observed in the offspring of patients treated with Imuran. Azathioprine and long-wave ultraviolet light have been shown to have a synergistic clastogenic effect in patients treated with azathioprine for a range of disorders.

Use in Pregnancy and Lactation

Imuran should not be given to patients who are pregnant or likely to become pregnant without careful assessment of risk versus benefit.

There have been reports of premature birth and low birth weight following maternal exposure to azathioprine, particularly in combination with corticosteroids. There have also been reports of spontaneous abortion following either maternal or paternal exposure.

Azathioprine and/or its metabolites have been found in low concentrations in foetal blood and amniotic fluid after maternal administration of azathioprine.

Leucopenia and/or thrombocytopenia have been reported in a proportion of neonates whose mothers took azathioprine throughout their pregnancies. Extra care in haematological monitoring is advised during pregnancy.

Lactation

6-Mercaptopurine has been identified in the colostrum and breast-milk of women receiving azathioprine treatment.

4.7 Effects on ability to drive and use machines

None known.

4.8 Undesirable effects

For this product there is no modern clinical documentation that can be used as support for determining the frequency of undesirable effects. Undesirable effects may vary in their incidence depending on the indication. The following convention has been utilised for the classification of frequency: Very common, $\geqslant 1/10$; common, $\geqslant 1/100$ and $< 1/10$; uncommon, $\geqslant 1/1000$ and $< 1/100$; rare, $\geqslant 1/10000$ and $< 1/1000$; very rare, $< 1/10000$.

Infection and infestations

Transplant patients receiving Imuran in combination with other immunosuppressants.

Very common: Viral, fungal, and bacterial infections.

Other indications.

Uncommon: Viral, fungal and bacterial infections.

Patients receiving Imuran alone, or in combination with other immunosupressants, particularly corticosteroids, have shown increased susceptibility to viral, fungal and bacterial infections, including severe or atypical infection with varicella, herpes zoster and other infectious agents (see also section 4.4 Special Warnings and Precautions for Use).

Neoplasms benign and malignant (including cysts and polyps)

Rare: Neoplasms including non-Hodgkin's lymphomas, skin cancers (melanoma and non-melanoma), sarcomas (Kaposi's and non-Kaposi's) and uterine cervical cancer in situ, acute myloid leukaemia and myelodysplasia (see also section 4.4 Special Warnings and Special Precautions for Use).

The risk of developing non-Hodgkin's lymphomas and other malignancies, notably skin cancers (melanoma and non-melanoma), sarcomas, (Kaposi's and non-Kaposi's) and uterine cervical cancer in situ, is increased in patients who receive immunosuppressive drugs, particularly in transplant recipients receiving aggressive treatment and such therapy should be maintained at the lowest effective levels. The increased risk of developing non-Hodgkin's lymphomas in immunosuppressed rheumatoid arthritis patients compared with the general population appears to be related at least in part to the disease itself.

There have been rare reports of acute myeloid leukaemia and myelodysplasia (some in association with chromasomal abnormalities).

Blood and lymphatic system disorders

Very common:	Depression of bone marrow function; leucopenia.
Common:	Thrombocytopenia.
Uncommon:	Anaemia.
Rare:	Agranulocytosis, pancytopenia, aplastic anaemia, megaloblastic anaemia, erythriod hypoplasia.

Imuran may be associated with a dose-related, generally reversible, depression of bone marrow function, most frequently expressed as leucopenia, but also sometimes as anaemia and thrombocytopenia, and rarely as agranulocytosis, pancytopenia and aplastic anaemia. These occur particularly in patients predisposed to myelotoxicity, such as those with TPMT deficiency and renal or hepatic insufficiency and in patients failing to reduce the dose of Imuran when receiving concurrent allopurinol therapy.

Reversible, dose-related increases in mean corpuscular volume and red cell haemoglobin content have occurred in association with Imuran therapy. Megaloblastic bone marrow changes have also been observed but severe megaloblastic anaemia and erythroid hypoplasia are rare.

Respiratory, thorasic and mediastinal disorders

Very rare: Reversible pneumonitis.

Reversible pneumonitis has been described very rarely.

Gastrointestinal disorders

Uncommon:	Pancreatitis.
Rare:	Colitis, diverticulitis and bowel perforation reported in transplant population, severe diarrhoea in inflammatory bowel disease population.

A minority of patients experience nausea when first given Imuran. This appears to be relieved by administering the tablets after meals.

Serious complications, including colitis, diverticulitis and bowel perforation, have been described in transplant recipients receiving immunosuppressive therapy. However, the aetiology is not clearly established and high-dose corticosteroids may be implicated. Severe diarrhoea, recurring on re-challenge, has been reported in patients treated with Imuran for inflammatory bowel disease. The possibility that exacerbation of symptoms might be drug-related should be borne in mind when treating such patients.

Pancreatitis has been reported in a small percentage of patients on Imuran therapy, particularly in renal transplant patients and those diagnosed as having inflammatory bowel disease. There are difficulties in relating the pancreatitis to the administration of one particular drug, although re-challenge has confirmed an association with Imuran on occasions.

Hepato-biliary disorders

Uncommon:	Cholestasis and degeneration of liver function tests.
Rare:	Life-threatening hepatic damage.

Cholestasis and deterioration of liver function have occasionally been reported in association with Imuran therapy and are usually reversible on withdrawal of therapy. This may be associated with symptoms of a hypersensitivity reaction (see Hypersensitivity reactions).

Rare, but life-threatening hepatic damage associated with chronic administration of azathioprine has been described primarily in transplant patients. Histological findings include sinusoidal dilatation, peliosis hepatis, veno-occlusive disease and nodular regenerative hyperplasia. In some cases withdrawal of azathioprine has resulted in either a temporary or permanent improvement in liver histology and symptoms.

Skin and subcutaneous tissue disorders

Rare: Alopecia, photosensitivity.

Hair loss has been described on a number of occasions in patients receiving azathioprine and other immunosuppressive agents. In many instances the condition resolved spontaneously despite continuing therapy. The relationship between alopecia and azathioprine treatment is uncertain.

Immune system disorders

Uncommon:	Hypersensitivity reactions
Very rare:	Stevens-Johnson syndrome and toxic epidermal necrolysis.

Several different clinical syndromes, which appear to be idiosyncratic manifestations of hypersensitivity, have been described occasionally following administration of Imuran. Clinical features include general malaise, dizziness, nausea, vomiting, diarrhoea, fever, rigors, exanthema, rash, vasculitis, myalgia, arthralgia, hypotension, renal dysfunction, hepatic dysfunction and cholestasis (see Hepatobiliary disorders).

In many cases, re-challenge has confirmed an association with Imuran.

Immediate withdrawal of azathioprine and institution of circulatory support where appropriate have led to recovery in the majority of cases.

Other marked underlying pathology has contributed to the very rare deaths reported.

Following a hypersensitivity reaction to Imuran, the necessity for continued administration of Imuran should be carefully considered on an individual basis.

4.9 Overdose

Symptoms and signs

Unexplained infection, ulceration of the throat, bruising and bleeding are the main signs of overdosage with Imuran and result from bone marrow depression which may be maximal after 9 to 14 days. These signs are more likely to be manifest following chronic overdosage, rather than after a single acute overdose. There has been a report of a patient who ingested a single overdose of 7.5 g of azathioprine. The immediate toxic effects of this overdose were nausea, vomiting and diarrhoea, followed by mild leucopenia and mild abnormalities in liver function. Recovery was uneventful.

Treatment

There is no specific antidote. Gastric lavage has been used. Subsequent monitoring, including haematological monitoring, is necessary to allow prompt treatment of any adverse effects which may develop. The value of dialysis in patients who have taken an overdose of Imuran is not known, though azathioprine is partially dialysable.

5. PHARMACOLOGICAL PROPERTIES

5.1 Pharmacodynamic properties

Azathioprine is an imidazole derivative of 6-mercaptopurine (6-MP). It is rapidly broken down *in vivo* into 6-MP and a methylnitroimidazole moiety. The 6-MP readily crosses cell membranes and is converted intracellularly into a number of purine thioanalogues, which include the main active nucleotide, thioinosinic acid. The rate of conversion varies from one person to another. Nucleotides do not traverse cell membranes and therefore do not circulate in body fluids. Irrespective of whether it is given directly or is derived *in vivo* from azathioprine, 6-MP is eliminated mainly as the inactive oxidised metabolite thiouric acid. This oxidation is brought about by xanthine oxidase, an enzyme that is inhibited by allopurinol. The activity of the methylnitroimidazole moiety has not been defined clearly. However, in several systems it appears to modify the activity of azathioprine as compared with that of 6-MP. Determination of plasma concentrations of azathioprine or 6-MP have no prognostic values as regards effectiveness or toxicity of these compounds.

While the precise modes of action remain to be elucidated, some suggested mechanisms include:

1. the release of 6-MP which acts as a purine antimetabolite.

2. the possible blockade of -SH groups by alkylation.

3. the inhibition of many pathways in nucleic acid biosynthesis, hence preventing proliferation of cells involved in determination and amplification of the immune response.

4. damage to deoxyribonucleic acid (DNA) through incorporation of purine thio-analogues.

Because of these mechanisms, the therapeutic effect of Imuran may be evident only after several weeks or months of treatment.

Imuran appears to be well absorbed from the upper gastrointestinal tract.

Studies in mice with [^{35}S]-azathioprine showed no unusually large concentration in any particular tissue, and there was very little [^{35}S]-label found in brain.

Plasma levels of azathioprine and 6-MP do not correlate well with the therapeutic efficacy or toxicity of Imuran.

5.2 Pharmacokinetic properties

Azathioprine is well absorbed following oral administration. After oral administration of [^{35}S]-azathioprine, the maximum plasma radioactivity occurs at 1-2 hours and decays with a half-life of 4-6 hours. This is not an estimate of the half-life of azathioprine itself, but reflects the elimination from plasma of azathioprine and the [^{35}S]-containing metabolites of the drug. As a consequence of the rapid and extensive metabolism of azathioprine, only a fraction of the radioactivity measured in plasma is comprised of unmetabolised drug. Studies in which the plasma concentration of azathioprine and 6-MP have been determined following intravenous administration of azathioprine have estimated the mean plasma $T^1/_2$ for azathioprine to be in the range of 6-28 minutes and the mean plasma $T^1/_2$ for 6-MP to be in the range 38-114 minutes after i.v. administration of the drug.

Azathioprine is principally excreted as 6-thiouric uric acid in the urine. 1-methyl-4-nitro-5-thioimidazole has also been detected in urine as a minor excretory product. This would indicate that, rather than azathioprine being exclusive cleaved by nucleophilic attack at the 5-position of the nitroimidazole ring to generate 6-MP and 1-methyl-4-nitro-5-(S-glutathionyl)imidazole. A small proportion of the drug may be cleaved between the sulphur-atom and the purine ring. Only a small amount of the dose of azathioprine administered is excreted unmetabolised in the urine.

5.3 Preclinical safety data

No additional data of clinical relevance to the prescriber.

6. PHARMACEUTICAL PARTICULARS

6.1 List of excipients

Lactose, pregelatinised starch, maize starch, stearic acid, magnesium sterate, purified water, methylhydroxylpropyl cellulose, polyethylene glycol 400.

6.2 Incompatibilities

None known.

6.3 Shelf life

5 years.

6.4 Special precautions for storage

Store below 25°C. Protect from light.

6.5 Nature and contents of container

Blister strips in a pack.

Pack sizes: 28, 30, 56, 60, 100 and 1000 tablets.

6.6 Special precautions for disposal and other handling

Health professionals who handle Imuran Injection should follow guidelines for the handling of cytotoxic drugs (for example, the Royal Pharmaceutical Society of Great Britain Working Party Report on the Handling of Cytotoxic Drugs, 1983).

Provided that the film-coating is intact, there is no risk in handling film-coated Imuran Tablets. Imuran Tablets should not be divided and, provided the coating is intact, no additional precautions are required when handling them.

Administrative Data

7. MARKETING AUTHORISATION HOLDER

The Wellcome Foundation

Berkeley Avenue

Greenford

Middlesex

UB6 ONN

8. MARKETING AUTHORISATION NUMBER(S)

PL00003/0226

9. DATE OF FIRST AUTHORISATION/RENEWAL OF THE AUTHORISATION

20 March 1992

10. DATE OF REVISION OF THE TEXT

27-5-2009

11. Legal Status

POM

Imuvac 2009/2010

(Solvay Healthcare Limited)

1. NAME OF THE MEDICINAL PRODUCT

Imuvac 2009/2010, suspension for injection (influenza vaccine, surface antigen, inactivated).

2. QUALITATIVE AND QUANTITATIVE COMPOSITION

Influenza virus surface antigens (haemagglutinin and neuraminidase) of the following strains*:

- A/Brisbane/59/2007 (H1N1)-like strain (A/Brisbane/59/2007 IVR-148 reass.) — 15 micrograms HA**
- A/Brisbane/10/2007 (H3N2)-like strain (A/Uruguay/716/2007 NYMC X-175C reass.) — 15 micrograms HA**
- B/ Brisbane/60/2008-like strain (B/Brisbane/60/2008) — 15 micrograms HA**

per 0.5 ml dose.

* propagated in fertilised hens' eggs from healthy chicken flocks.

** haemagglutinin.

This vaccine complies with the WHO recommendation (northern hemisphere), and EU decision for the 2009/2010 season.

For a full list of excipients see section 6.1.

3. PHARMACEUTICAL FORM

Suspension for injection in prefilled syringes; a colourless clear liquid, filled in single-dose syringes (glass, type I).

4. CLINICAL PARTICULARS

4.1 Therapeutic indications

Prophylaxis of influenza, especially in those who run an increased risk of associated complications.

The use of Imuvac 2009/2010 should be based on official recommendations.

4.2 Posology and method of administration

Adults and children from 36 months: 0.5 ml.

Children from 6 months to 35 months: Clinical data are limited. Dosages of 0.25 ml or 0.5 ml have been used.

For children who have not previously been vaccinated, a second dose should be given after an interval of at least 4 weeks.

Immunisation should be carried out by intramuscular or deep subcutaneous injection.

For instructions for preparation, see section 6.6.

4.3 Contraindications

Hypersensitivity to the active substances, to any of the excipients and to residues of eggs, chicken protein (Imuvac 2009/2010 does not contain more than 1 μg ovalbumin per dose), formaldehyde, cetyltrimethylammonium bromide, polysorbate 80, or gentamicin.

Immunisation shall be postponed in patients with febrile illness or acute infection.

4.4 Special warnings and precautions for use

As with all injectable vaccines, appropriate medical treatment and supervision should always be readily available in case of an anaphylactic event following the administration of the vaccine.

Imuvac 2009/2010 should under no circumstances be administered intravascularly.

Antibody response in patients with endogenous or iatrogenic immunosuppression may be insufficient.

4.5 Interaction with other medicinal products and other forms of interaction

Imuvac 2009/2010 may be given at the same time as other vaccines. Immunisation should be carried out on separate limbs. It should be noted that the adverse reactions may be intensified.

The immunological response may be diminished if the patient is undergoing immunosuppressant treatment.

Following influenza vaccination, false positive results in serology tests using the ELISA method to detect antibodies against HIV1, Hepatitis C and especially HTLV1 have been observed. The Western Blot technique disproves the false-positive ELISA test results. The transient false-positive reactions could be due to the IgM response by the vaccine.

4.6 Pregnancy and lactation

The limited data from vaccinations in pregnant women do not indicate that adverse fetal and maternal outcomes were attributable to the vaccine. The use of this vaccine may be considered from the second trimester of pregnancy. For pregnant women with medical conditions that increase their risk of complications from influenza, administration of the vaccine is recommended, irrespective of their stage of pregnancy.

Imuvac 2009/2010 may be used during lactation.

4.7 Effects on ability to drive and use machines

Imuvac 2009/2010 is unlikely to produce an effect on the ability to drive and use machines.

4.8 Undesirable effects

ADVERSE REACTIONS OBSERVED FROM CLINICAL TRIALS

The safety of trivalent inactivated influenza vaccines is assessed in open label, uncontrolled clinical trials performed as annual update requirement, including at least 50 adults aged 18 - 60 years of age and at least 50 elderly aged 61 years or older. Safety evaluation is performed during the first 3 days following vaccination.

The following undesirable effects have been observed during clinical trials with the following frequencies:

very common ($\geqslant 1/10$); common ($\geqslant 1/100$, $< 1/10$); uncommon ($\geqslant 1/1{,}000$, $< 1/100$); rare ($\geqslant 1/10{,}000$, $< 1/1{,}000$); very rare ($< 1/10{,}000$), including isolated reports.

(see Table 1 below)

ADVERSE REACTIONS REPORTED FROM POST-MARKETING SURVEILLANCE

Adverse reactions reported from post marketing surveillance are, next to the reactions which have also been observed during the clinical trials, the following:

Blood and lymphatic system disorders:

Transient thrombocytopenia, transient lymphadenopathy

Immune system disorders:

Allergic reactions, in rare cases leading to shock, angioedema

Nervous system disorders:

Neuralgia, paraesthesia, febril convulsions, neurological disorders, such as encephalomyelitis, neuritis and Guillain Barré syndrome

Vascular disorders:

Vasculitis associated in very rare cases with transient renal involvement

Skin and subcutaneous tissue disorders:

Generalised skin reactions including pruritus, urticaria or non-specific rash

4.9 Overdose

Overdosage is unlikely to have any untoward effect.

5. PHARMACOLOGICAL PROPERTIES

5.1 Pharmacodynamic properties

Pharmacotherapeutic group: Influenza vaccine, ATC Code: J07BB02.

Seroprotection is generally obtained within 2 to 3 weeks. The duration of post-vaccinal immunity to homologous strains or to strains closely related to the vaccine strains varies but is usually 6-12 months.

5.2 Pharmacokinetic properties

Not applicable.

5.3 Preclinical safety data

Not applicable.

6. PHARMACEUTICAL PARTICULARS

6.1 List of excipients

Potassium chloride, potassium dihydrogen phosphate, disodium phosphate dihydrate, sodium chloride, calcium chloride, magnesium chloride hexahydrate and water for injections.

6.2 Incompatibilities

In the absence of compatability studies, this medicinal product must not be mixed with other medicinal products.

6.3 Shelf life

1 year.

6.4 Special precautions for storage

Imuvac 2009/2010 should be stored in a refrigerator (+2°C to +8°C).

Do not freeze.

Protect from light.

6.5 Nature and contents of container

0.5 ml suspension for injection in prefilled syringe with/without needle (glass, type I), pack of 1 or 10.

Table 1

Organ class	Very common $\geqslant 1/10$	Common $\geqslant 1/100$, $< 1/10$	Uncommon $\geqslant 1/1{,}000$, $< 1/100$	Rare $\geqslant 1/10{,}000$, $< 1/1{,}000$	Very rare $< 1/10{,}000$
Nervous system disorders		Headache*			
Skin and subcutaneous tissue disorders		Sweating*			
Musculoskeletal and connective tissue disorders		Myalgia, arthralgia*			
General disorders and administration site conditions		fever, malaise, shivering, fatigue Local reactions: redness, swelling, pain, ecchymosis induration*			

* these reactions usually disappear within 1-2 days without treatment

6.6 Special precautions for disposal and other handling
Unused vaccine and other waste material should be disposed of in compliance with local rules for the disposal of products of this nature.

Imuvac 2009/2010 should be allowed to reach room temperature before use.

Shake before use.

For administration of a 0.25 ml dose from a syringe, push the front side of the plunger exactly to the edge of the hub (the knurled polypropylene ring); a reproducible volume of vaccine remains in the syringe, suitable for administration. See also section 4.2.

7. MARKETING AUTHORISATION HOLDER
Solvay Healthcare Limited

Mansbridge Road

West End

Southampton

SO18 3JD

8. MARKETING AUTHORISATION NUMBER(S)
PL 00512/0188

9. DATE OF FIRST AUTHORISATION/RENEWAL OF THE AUTHORISATION
31 March 2005

10. DATE OF REVISION OF THE TEXT
02/09/2009

Increlex 10mg/ml solution for injection

(Ipsen Ltd)

1. NAME OF THE MEDICINAL PRODUCT
INCRELEX®▼ 10 mg/mL solution for injection.

2. QUALITATIVE AND QUANTITATIVE COMPOSITION
Each mL contains 10 mg of mecasermin.

Each vial contains 40 mg of mecasermin.

Mecasermin is a recombinant DNA-derived human insulin-like growth factor-1 (IGF-1) produced in *Escherichia coli*.

Excipients:

One mL contains 9 mg of benzyl alcohol.

For a full list of excipients, see section 6.1.

3. PHARMACEUTICAL FORM
Solution for injection.

Aqueous, clear and colourless solution.

4. CLINICAL PARTICULARS
4.1 Therapeutic indications
For the long-term treatment of growth failure in children and adolescents with severe primary insulin-like growth factor-1 deficiency (primary IGFD).

Severe primary IGFD is defined by:

• height standard deviation score ⩽–3.0 and

• basal IGF-1 levels below the 2.5th percentile for age and gender and

• GH sufficiency.

• Exclusion of secondary forms of IGF-1 deficiency, such as malnutrition, hypothyroidism, or chronic treatment with pharmacologic doses of anti-inflammatory steroids.

Severe primary IGFD includes patients with mutations in the GH receptor (GHR), post-GHR signaling pathway, and IGF-1 gene defects; they are not GH deficient, and therefore, they cannot be expected to respond adequately to exogenous GH treatment. It is recommended to confirm the diagnosis by conducting an IGF-1 generation test.

4.2 Posology and method of administration
Treatment with INCRELEX should be directed by physicians who are experienced in the diagnosis and management of patients with growth disorders.

The dose should be individualised for each patient. The recommended starting dose of mecasermin is 0.04 mg/kg twice daily by subcutaneous injection. If no significant treatment-related adverse events occur for at least one week, the dose may be raised in increments of 0.04 mg/kg to the maximum dose of 0.12 mg/kg given twice daily. Doses greater than 0.12 mg/kg given twice daily have not been evaluated in children with severe primary IGFD.

If the recommended dose is not tolerated by the subject, treatment with a lower dose can be considered. Treatment success should be evaluated based on height velocities. The lowest dose that was associated with substantial growth increases on an individual basis was 0.04 mg/kg BID.

INCRELEX should be administered shortly before or after a meal or snack. If hypoglycaemia occurs with recommended doses, despite adequate food intake, the dose should be reduced. If the patient is unable to eat, for any reason, INCRELEX should be withheld. The dose of mecasermin should never be increased to make up for one or more omitted doses.

Injection sites should be rotated to a different site with each injection.

INCRELEX should be administered using sterile disposable syringes and injection needles. The syringes should be of small enough volume that the prescribed dose can be withdrawn from the vial with reasonable accuracy.

INCRELEX is not recommended for use in children below age 2 due to a lack of data on safety and efficacy (see section 5.1).

4.3 Contraindications
Hypersensitivity to the active substance or to any of the excipients.

Intravenous administration.

Active or suspected neoplasia. Therapy should be discontinued if evidence of neoplasia develops.

Benzyl alcohol must not be given to premature babies or neonates.

4.4 Special warnings and precautions for use
Thyroid and nutritional deficiencies should be corrected before initiating INCRELEX treatment.

INCRELEX is not a substitute for GH treatment.

INCRELEX should not be used for growth promotion in patients with closed epiphyses.

INCRELEX should be administered shortly before or after a meal or snack, because it may have insulin-like hypoglycaemic effects. Special attention should be paid to young children, children with a history of hypoglycaemia and children with inconsistent food intake. Patients should avoid engaging in any high-risk activities within 2-3 hours after dosing, particularly at the initiation of INCRELEX treatment, until a well tolerated dose of INCRELEX has been established. If a person with severe hypoglycemia is unconscious or otherwise unable to ingest food normally, an injection of glucagon may be required. Persons with a history of severe hypoglycemia should have glucagon available. At the time of initial prescription, physicians should educate parents on the signs, symptoms and treatment of hypoglycaemia, including injection of glucagon.

Doses of insulin and/or other hypoglycaemic agents may need to be reduced for diabetic subjects using INCRELEX.

Echocardiogram is recommended before initiation of INCRELEX treatment in all patients. Patients who terminate treatment should also have an echocardiogram. Patients with abnormal echocardiogram findings or cardiovascular symptoms should be followed regularly with echocardiogram procedures.

Lymphoid tissue (e.g., tonsillar) hypertrophy associated with complications, such as snoring, sleep apnoea, and chronic middle-ear effusions have been reported with the use of INCRELEX. Patients should have examinations periodically and at the occurrence of clinical symptoms to rule out such potential complications or to initiate appropriate treatment.

Intracranial hypertension (IH) with papilloedema, visual changes, headache, nausea and/or vomiting has been reported in patients treated with INCRELEX, as has been reported with therapeutic GH administration. IH-associated signs and symptoms resolved after interruption of dosing. Funduscopic examination is recommended at the initiation, periodically during the course of INCRELEX therapy and at the occurrence of clinical symptoms.

Slipped capital femoral epiphysis and progression of scoliosis can occur in patients who experience rapid growth. These conditions and other symptoms and signs known to be associated with GH treatment in general should be monitored during INCRELEX treatment. Any patient with the onset of a limp or complaint of hip or knee pain should be evaluated.

As with any exogenous protein administration, local or systemic allergic reactions may occur. Parents and patients should be informed that such reactions are possible and that if an allergic reaction occurs, treatment should be interrupted and prompt medical attention should be sought.

Treatment should be reconsidered if after a year patients remain non-responsive.

Persons who have allergic reactions to injected IGF-1, who have unexpectedly high blood values of IGF-1 after injection, or who fail to show a growth response may be having an antibody response to injected IGF-1. In such instances, follow the instructions for antibody testing.

INCRELEX contains 9 mg/mL benzyl alcohol as a preservative.

Benzyl alcohol may cause toxic reactions and anaphylactoid reactions in infants and children up to 3 years old.

4.5 Interaction with other medicinal products and other forms of interaction
No interaction studies have been performed.

4.6 Pregnancy and lactation
A negative pregnancy test and education about adequate contraception are recommended for all women of child bearing potential prior to treatment with INCRELEX.

There are no adequate data for the use of mecasermin in pregnant women.

Animal studies are insufficient with respect to pregnancy (see section 5.3). The potential risk for humans is unknown.

INCRELEX should not be used during pregnancy unless clearly necessary.

Breast-feeding while taking INCRELEX is not recommended.

4.7 Effects on ability to drive and use machines
No studies on the effects on the ability to drive and use machines have been performed. However, hypoglycaemia may impair the ability to drive or use machines.

4.8 Undesirable effects
An integrated safety database from clinical studies contains 76 subjects with severe primary IGFD treated for a mean duration of 4.4 years and representing 321 subject-years.

Hypoglycaemia is the most frequently reported adverse drug reaction. The thirty-six subjects (47%) who had one or more episodes of hypoglycaemia included 4 subjects who had hypoglycaemic seizure on one or more occasion. Of the 36 subjects, 12 (33%) had a history of hypoglycaemia prior to beginning treatment. The frequency of hypoglycaemia was highest in the first month of treatment, and episodes were more frequent in younger children. Symptomatic hypoglycaemia was generally avoided when a meal or snack was consumed either shortly before or after the administration of INCRELEX.

Injection site hypertrophy occurred in 24 subjects (32%). This reaction was generally associated with lack of proper rotation of injections. When injections were properly dispersed, the condition resolved.

Tonsillar hypertrophy was noted in 12 (16%) subjects, particularly in the first 1 to 2 years of therapy with lesser tonsillar growth in subsequent years.

Snoring, generally beginning in the first year of treatment, was reported in 17 subjects (22%).

Hypoacusis was reported in 15 subjects (20%).

Intracranial hypertension occurred in three subjects (4%). In two subjects the events resolved without interruption of INCRELEX treatment. INCRELEX treatment was discontinued in the third subject and resumed later at a lower dose without recurrence. Fourteen subjects (18%) had headache considered related to study drug.

As with all protein pharmaceuticals, some patients may develop antibodies to INCRELEX. Anti-IGF-1 antibodies were observed in 11 of 23 children with severe primary IGFD tested during the first year of therapy. However, no clinical consequences of these antibodies were observed (e.g., allergic reactions or attenuation of growth).

Table 1 contains very common (⩾ 1/10) and common (⩾ 1/100 to < 1/10) adverse reactions for which there is at least a reasonable suspicion of a causal relationship to INCRELEX treatment which occurred in clinical trials. Within each frequency grouping, undesirable effects are presented in order of decreasing seriousness.

Table 1: Adverse Drug Reactions in Clinical Trials

(see Table 1 on next page)

4.9 Overdose
No case of overdose has been reported.

Acute overdose could lead to hypoglycaemia. Long-term overdose may result in signs and symptoms of acromegaly or gigantism.

Treatment of acute overdose of mecasermin should be directed at alleviating any hypoglycaemic effects. Oral glucose or food should be consumed. If the overdose results in loss of consciousness, intravenous glucose or parenteral glucagon may be required to reverse the hypoglycaemic effects.

5. PHARMACOLOGICAL PROPERTIES
5.1 Pharmacodynamic properties
Pharmacotherapeutic group: Somatropin and agonists, ATC code: H01AC03

This medicinal product has been authorised under "Exceptional Circumstances".

This means that due to the rarity of the disease it has not been possible to obtain complete information on this medicinal product.

The European Medicines Agency (EMEA) will review any new information which may become available every year and this SPC will be updated as necessary.

Mecasermin is a human insulin-like growth factor-1 (rhIGF-1) produced by recombinant DNA technology. IGF-1 consists of 70 amino acids in a single chain with three intramolecular disulfide bridges and a molecular weight of 7649 daltons. The amino acid sequence of the product is identical to that of endogenous human IGF-1. The rhIGF-1 protein is synthesised in bacteria (*E. coli*) that have been modified by the addition of the gene for human IGF-1.

Insulin-like growth factor-1 (IGF-1) is the principal hormonal mediator of statural growth. Under normal circumstances, growth hormone (GH) binds to its receptor in the liver and other tissues, and stimulates the synthesis/secretion of IGF-1. In target tissues the Type 1 IGF-1 receptor, which is homologous to the insulin receptor, is activated by IGF-1, leading to intracellular signaling which stimulates multiple processes leading to statural growth. The metabolic actions of IGF-1 are in part directed at stimulating the uptake of glucose, fatty acids, and amino acids so that metabolism supports growing tissues.

Table 1: Adverse Drug Reactions in Clinical Trials

System Organ Class	Adverse Reaction	
	Very Common	Common
Investigations		Cardiac murmur, abnormal tympanometry, abnormal echocardiogram, increased alanine aminotransferase*, increased aspartate aminotransferase*, increased weight
Cardiac Disorders		Cardiomegaly, ventricular hypertrophy, atrial hypertrophy*, tachycardia, tachycardia paroxysmal*, mitral valve incompetence*, tricuspid valve incompetence*
Congenital, Familial and Genetic Disorders		Congenital jaw malformation, pigmented naevus*
Blood and Lymphatic System Disorders	Thymus hypertrophy	Lymphadenopathy*
Nervous System Disorders	Headache	Convulsions, febrile convulsion*, benign intracranial hypertension, loss of consciousness*, sleep apnoea syndrome, dizziness, tremor*, restless leg syndrome*
Eye Disorders		Papilloedema, reduced visual acuity*, myopia*
Ear and Labyrinth Disorders	Hypoacusis	Otorrhoea, ear disorder*, middle ear disorder*, tympanic membrane disorder*, ear pain, ear congestion*, fluid in middle ear
Respiratory, Thoracic and Mediastinal Disorders	Tonsillar hypertrophy, snoring	Adenoidal hypertrophy, nasal turbinate hypertrophy*, dyspnoea*, nasal mucosal disorder*, obstructive airway disorder*, abnormal respiration*, nasal congestion, mouth breathing
Gastrointestinal Disorders		Vomiting, retching*, abdominal pain*, upper abdominal pain*, abdominal distension*, dysphagia*
Renal and Urinary Disorders		Nephrolithiasis*, hydronephrosis*, renal colic*
Skin and Subcutaneous Tissue Disorders		Skin hypertrophy, acrochordons*, abnormal hair texture*
Musculoskeletal and Connective Tissue Disorders		Arthralgia, pain in extremity, myalgia, scoliosis*, spinal deformity*, soft tissue disorder*, muscle cramp*, flank pain*, musculoskeletal stiffness*
Metabolism and Nutrition Disorders	Hypoglycaemia	Hypoglycaemic seizure, hyperglycaemia, hyperlipidaemia*, obesity*
Infections and Infestations		Febrile infection*, upper respiratory tract infection*, otitis media, otitis media serous, chronic otitis media serous *, otitis externa*, pharyngitis*, tonsillitis, ear infection, oral candidiasis*
Surgical and Medical Procedures		Adenotonsillectomy*, adenoidectomy, ear tube insertion
General Disorders and Administration Site Conditions	Injection site hypertrophy	Mucosal membrane hyperplasia, hypertrophy, injection site pain, injection site bruising, injection site fibrosis*, injection site reaction*, injection site swelling*, injection site induration*, injection site pigmentation changes*, mucosal oedema*, asthenia*, lethargy*, chest discomfort*
Reproductive System and Breast Disorders		Gynaecomastia, ovarian cyst*
Psychiatric Disorders		Depression*, sleep terror, nervousness, abnormal behaviour*, disorientation*

* = occurred in only 1 subject (1%)

The following actions have been demonstrated for endogenous human IGF-1:

Tissue Growth

Skeletal growth is accomplished at the epiphyseal plates at the ends of a growing bone. Growth and metabolism of epiphyseal plate cells are directly stimulated by GH and IGF-1.

Organ growth: treatment of IGF-1 deficient rats with rhIGF-1 results in whole body and organ growth.

Cell growth: IGF-1 receptors are present on most types of cells and tissues. IGF-1 has mitogenic activity that leads to an increased number of cells in the body.

Carbohydrate Metabolism

IGF-1 suppresses hepatic glucose production, stimulates peripheral glucose utilization, and can reduce blood glucose and cause hypoglycaemia.

IGF-1 has inhibitory effects on insulin secretion.

Bone/Mineral Metabolism

Circulating IGF-1 plays an important role in the acquisition and maintenance of bone mass. IGF-1 increases bone density.

Clinical efficacy

Five clinical studies (4 open-label and 1 double-blind, placebo-controlled) were conducted with INCRELEX. Subcutaneous doses of mecasermin, generally ranging from 60 to 120 µg/kg given twice daily (BID), were administered to 76 paediatric subjects with severe primary IGFD. Patients were enrolled in the studies on the basis of extreme short stature, slow growth rates, low IGF-1 serum concentrations, and normal GH secretion. Baseline characteristics for the patients evaluated in the primary and secondary efficacy analyses from the combined studies were (mean ± SD): chronological age (years): 6.8 ± 3.8; height (cm): 85.0 ± 15.3; height standard deviation score (SDS): -6.7 ± 1.8; height velocity (cm/yr): 2.8 ± 1.8; height velocity SDS: -3.3 ± 1.7; IGF-1 (ng/mL): 21.9 ± 24.8; IGF-1 SDS: -4.4 ± 2.0; and bone age (years): 3.9 ± 2.8. Sixty-two subjects had at least one year of treatment. Of these, 53 (85%) had Laron syndrome-like phenotype; 7 (11%) had GH gene deletion, and 1 (2%) had neutralizing antibodies to GH. Thirty-eight (61%) of the subjects were male; 49 (79%) were Caucasian. Fifty-six (90%) of the subjects were prepubertal at baseline.

Annual results for height velocity, height velocity SDS, and height SDS are shown in Table 2. Pre-treatment height velocity data were available for 59 subjects. The height velocities at a given year of treatment were compared by paired t-tests to the pre-treatment height velocities of the same subjects completing that treatment year.

Table 2: Annual Height Results by Number of Years Treated with INCRELEX

(see Table 2 on next page)

Forty-seven subjects were included in an analysis of the effects of INCRELEX on bone age advancement. The mean ± SD change in chronological age was 5.1 ± 3.0 years and the mean ± SD change in bone age was 5.8 ± 2.9 years.

Efficacy is dose dependent. For subjects receiving doses between 100 and 120 µg/kg BID, the mean first year height velocity was approximately 8.7 cm/yr.

5.2 Pharmacokinetic properties

GENERAL CHARACTERISTICS

Absorption

The absolute subcutaneous bioavailability of mecasermin in severe primary IGFD subjects has not been determined. The bioavailability of mecasermin after subcutaneous administration in healthy subjects has been reported to be approximately 100%.

Distribution

In blood, IGF-1 is bound to six IGF binding proteins (IGFBPs), with ~80% bound as a complex with IGFBP-3 and an acid-labile subunit. IGFBP-3 is reduced in subjects with severe primary IGFD, resulting in increased clearance of IGF-1 in these subjects relative to healthy subjects. The total IGF-1 volume of distribution (mean ± SD) after subcutaneous administration of INCRELEX in 12 subjects with severe primary IGFD is estimated to be 0.257 (± 0.073) l/kg at a mecasermin dose of 0.045 mg/kg, and is estimated to increase as the dose of mecasermin increases. Limited information is available on the concentration of unbound IGF-1 after the administration of INCRELEX.

Metabolism

Both the liver and the kidney have been shown to metabolise IGF-1.

Excretion

The mean terminal $t_{1/2}$ of total IGF-1 after single subcutaneous administration of 0.12 mg/kg in three paediatric subjects with severe primary IGFD is estimated to be 5.8 hours. Clearance of total IGF-1 is inversely proportional to serum IGFBP-3 levels and total IGF-1 systemic clearance (CL/F) is estimated to be 0.04 l/hr/kg at 3 mg/l IGFBP-3 in 12 subjects.

CHARACTERISTICS IN SPECIAL POPULATIONS

Geriatric

The pharmacokinetics of INCRELEX have not been studied in subjects greater than 65 years of age.

Children

The pharmacokinetics of INCRELEX have not been studied in subjects younger than 12 years of age.

Gender

In children over 12 years old with primary IGFD and in healthy adults there were no apparent differences between males and females in the pharmacokinetics of INCRELEX.

Race

No information is available.

Renal insufficiency

No studies have been conducted in children with renal impairment.

Hepatic insufficiency

No studies have been conducted to determine the effect of hepatic impairment on the pharmacokinetics of mecasermin.

5.3 Preclinical safety data

Non-clinical data reveal no special hazard for humans based on conventional studies of safety pharmacology, repeated dose toxicity or genotoxicity.

Adverse reactions not observed in clinical studies, but seen in animals at exposure levels similar to clinical exposure levels and with possible relevance to clinical use were as follows:

Reproductive toxicity

In rats and rabbits reproductive toxicity was studied after intravenous but not after subcutaneous application (the normal clinical route). These studies did not indicate direct or indirect harmful effects with respect to fertility and pregnancy, but due to the different route of application the relevance of these findings is unclear. Placental transfer of mecasermin was not studied.

Carcinogenesis

Mecasermin was administered subcutaneously to Sprague Dawley rats at doses of 0, 0.25, 1, 4, and 10 mg/kg/day for up to 2 years. An increased incidence of adrenal medullary hyperplasia and pheochromocytoma was observed in male rats at doses of 1 mg/kg/day and above (⩾ 1 times the clinical exposure with the maximum recommended human dose [MRHD] based on AUC) and female rats at all dose levels (⩾ 0.3 times the clinical exposure with the MRHD based on AUC).

An increased incidence of keratoacanthoma in the skin was observed in male rats at doses of 4 and 10 mg/kg/day (⩾ 4 times the exposure with the MRHD based on AUC). An increased incidence of mammary gland carcinoma in both male and female rats was observed in animals treated with 10 mg/kg/day (7 times the exposure with the MRHD based on AUC). Excess mortality secondary to IGF-1 induced hypoglycaemia was observed in the carcinogenesis studies.

6. PHARMACEUTICAL PARTICULARS

6.1 List of excipients

Benzyl alcohol

Sodium chloride

Polysorbate 20

Glacial acetic acid

Sodium acetate

Water for injections

Table 2: Annual Height Results by Number of Years Treated with INCRELEX

	Pre-Tx	Year 1	Year 2	Year 3	Year 4	Year 5	Year 6	Year 7	Year 8
Height Velocity (cm/yr)									
N	59	59	54	48	39	21	20	16	14
Mean (SD)	2.8 (1.8)	8.0 (2.2)	5.8 (1.4)	5.5 (1.9)	4.7 (1.4)	4.7 (1.6)	4.8 (1.5)	4.6 (1.5)	4.5 (1.2)
Mean (SD) for change from pre-Tx		+5.2 (2.6)	+3.0 (2.3)	+2.6 (2.3)	+1.6 (2.1)	+1.5 (1.8)	+1.5 (1.7)	+1.0 (2.1)	+0.9 (2.4)
P-value for change from pre-Tx [1]		<0.0001	<0.0001	<0.0001	<0.0001	0.0015	0.0009	0.0897	0.2135
Height Velocity SDS									
N	59	59	53	47	38	19	18	15	12
Mean (SD)	-3.3 (1.7)	1.9 (2.9)	-0.2 (1.6)	-0.3 (2.0)	-0.7 (1.9)	-0.6 (2.1)	-0.4 (1.4)	-0.4 (1.9)	-0.3 (1.8)
Mean (SD) for change from pre-Tx P-value for change from pre-Tx [1]		+5.1 (3.1) <0.0001	+3.2 (2.2) <0.0001	+3.1 (2.4) <0.0001	+2.5 (2.1) <0.0001	+2.5 (2.2) 0.0001	+2.7 (1.7) <0.0001	+2.5 (2.1) 0.0003	+2.8 (2.7) 0.0041
Height SDS									
N	62	62	57	51	41	22	20	16	14
Mean (SD)	-6.7 (1.8)	-5.9 (1.7)	-5.6 (1.8)	-5.3 (1.8)	-5.3 (1.8)	-5.5 (1.8)	-5.4 (1.8)	-5.2 (2.0)	-5.2 (1.9)
Mean (SD) for change from pre-Tx P-value for change from pre-Tx [1]		+0.8 (0.5) <0.0001	+1.1 (0.8) <0.0001	+1.4 (1.0) <0.0001	+1.4 (1.1) <0.0001	+1.4 (1.3) <0.0001	+1.4 (1.2) <0.0001	+1.4 (1.1) 0.0001	+1.6 (1.1) <0.0001

Pre-Tx = Pre-treatment; SD = Standard Deviation; SDS = Standard Deviation Score

[1] P-values for comparison versus pre-Tx values were computed using paired t-tests.

6.2 Incompatibilities

In the absence of compatibility studies, this medicinal product must not be mixed with other medicinal products.

6.3 Shelf life

3 years

After opening:

Chemical and physical in-use stability has been demonstrated for 30 days at 2°C to 8°C.

From a microbiological point of view, once opened, the product may be stored for a maximum of 30 days at 2°C to 8°C. Other in-use storage times and conditions are the responsibility of the user.

6.4 Special precautions for storage

Store in a refrigerator (2°C - 8°C).

Do not freeze.

Keep the vial in the outer carton in order to protect from light.

6.5 Nature and contents of container

4 mL of solution in a 5 mL vial (type I glass) closed with a latex-free stopper (bromobutyl/isoprene polymer) and a seal (lacquered plastic).

Pack size of 1 vial.

6.6 Special precautions for disposal and other handling

INCRELEX is supplied as a sterile solution with preservative for multiple use.

The solution should be clear immediately after removal from the refrigerator. If the solution is cloudy, or contains particulate matter, it must not be injected.

Any unused product or waste material should be disposed of in accordance with local requirements.

7. MARKETING AUTHORISATION HOLDER

Tercica Europe Limited

Riverside One

Sir John Rogerson's Quay

Dublin 2

Republic of Ireland

8. MARKETING AUTHORISATION NUMBER(S)

EU/1/07/402/001

9. DATE OF FIRST AUTHORISATION/RENEWAL OF THE AUTHORISATION

3rd August 2007

10. DATE OF REVISION OF THE TEXT

17th March 2009

Inderal Injection

(AstraZeneca UK Limited)

1. NAME OF THE MEDICINAL PRODUCT

Inderal Injection.

2. QUALITATIVE AND QUANTITATIVE COMPOSITION

Propranolol Hydrochloride Ph. Eur. 0.1% w/v.

3. PHARMACEUTICAL FORM

Solution for intravenous injection.

4. CLINICAL PARTICULARS

4.1 Therapeutic indications

The emergency treatment of cardiac dysrhythmias and thyrotoxic crisis.

4.2 Posology and method of administration

For intravenous injection.

Adults

The initial dose of Inderal is 1 mg (1 ml) injected over 1 minute. This may be repeated at 2-minute intervals until a response is observed or to a maximum dose of 10 mg in conscious patients or 5 mg in patients under anaesthesia.

Elderly

Evidence concerning the relation between blood level and age is conflicting. Inderal should be used to treat the elderly with caution. It is suggested that treatment should start with the lowest dose. The optimum dose should be individually determined according to clinical response.

Children

Dysrhythmias, thyrotoxicosis

Dosage should be individually determined and the following is only a guide:

Intravenous: 0.025 to 0.05 mg/kg injected slowly under ECG control and repeated 3 or 4 times daily as required.

Fallot's tetralogy

The value of Inderal in this condition is confined mainly to the relief of right-ventricular outflow tract shut-down. It is also useful for treatment of associated dysrhythmias and angina. Dosage should be individually determined and the following is only a guide:

Intravenous: Up to 0.1 mg/kg injected slowly under ECG control, repeated 3 or 4 times daily as required.

4.3 Contraindications

Inderal must not be used if there is a history of bronchial asthma or bronchospasm. The product label and patient information leaflets state the following warnings:

Label: "Do not use Inderal if the patient has a history of asthma or wheezing".

Patient Information Leaflet: "If you have ever had asthma or wheezing, you should not be given Inderal injection. Talk to your doctor".

Bronchospasm can usually be reversed by beta$_2$ agonist bronchodilators such as salbutamol. Large doses of the beta$_2$ agonist bronchodilator may be required to overcome the beta blockade produced by propranolol and the dose should be titrated according to the clinical response; both intravenous and inhalational administration should be considered. The use of intravenous aminophylline and/or the use of ipratropium (given by nebuliser) may also be considered. Glucagon (1 to 2 mg given intravenously) has also been reported to produce a bronchodilator effect in asthmatic patients. Oxygen or artificial ventilation may be required in severe cases.

Inderal as with other beta-blockers must not be used in patients with any of the following conditions: known hypersensitivity to the substance; bradycardia; cardiogenic shock; hypotension; metabolic acidosis; after prolonged fasting; severe peripheral arterial circulatory disturbances; second or third degree heart block; sick sinus syndrome; untreated phaeochromocytoma; uncontrolled heart failure or Prinzmetal's angina.

Inderal must not be used in patients prone to hypoglycaemia, i.e., patients after prolonged fasting or patients with restricted counter-regulatory reserves. Patients with restricted counter regulatory reserves may have reduced autonomic and hormonal responses to hypoglycaemia which includes glycogenolysis, gluconeogenesis and /or impaired modulation of insulin secretion. Patients at risk for an inadequate response to hypoglycaemia includes individuals with malnutrition, prolonged fasting, starvation, chronic liver disease, diabetes and concomitant use of drugs which block the full response to catecholamines.

4.4 Special warnings and precautions for use

Inderal as with other beta-blockers:

- although contraindicated in uncontrolled heart failure (see Section 4.3), may be used in patients whose signs of heart failure have been controlled. Caution must be exercised in patients whose cardiac reserve is poor.

- Should not be used in combination with calcium channel blockers with negative inotropic effects (e.g. verapamil, diltiazem), as it can lead to an exaggeration of these effects particularly in patients with impaired ventricular function and/or SA or AV conduction abnormalities. This may result in severe hypotension, bradycardia and cardiac failure. Neither the beta-blocker nor the calcium channel blocker should be administered intravenously within 48 hours of discontinuing the other.

- although contraindicated in severe peripheral arterial circulatory disturbances (see Section 4.3), may also aggravate less severe peripheral arterial circulatory disturbances.

- due to its negative effect on conduction time, caution must be exercised if it is given to patients with first degree heart block.

- may block/modify the signs and symptoms of the hypoglycaemia (especially tachycardia). Inderal occasionally causes hypoglycaemia, even in non-diabetic patients, e.g., neonates, infants, children (Inderal is not recommended for use in children – see section 4.2), elderly patients, patients on haemodialysis or patients suffering from chronic liver disease and patients suffering from overdose. Severe hypoglycaemia associated with Inderal has rarely presented with seizures and/or coma in isolated patients. Caution must be exercised in the concurrent use of Inderal and hypoglycaemic therapy in diabetic patients. Inderal may prolong the hypoglycaemic response to insulin. (see section 4.3).

- may mask the signs of thyrotoxicosis.

- should not be used in untreated phaeochromocytoma. However, in patients with phaeochromocytoma, an alpha-blocker may be given concomitantly.

- will reduce heart rate as a result of its pharmacological action. In the rare instances when a treated patient develops symptoms which may be attributable to a slow heart rate, the dose may be reduced.

- may cause a more severe reaction to a variety of allergens when given to patients with a history of anaphylactic reaction to such allergens. Such patients may be unresponsive to the usual doses of adrenaline used to treat the allergic reactions.

Abrupt withdrawal of beta-blockers is to be avoided. The dosage should be withdrawn gradually over a period of 7 to 14 days. Patients should be followed during withdrawal especially those with ischaemic heart disease.

When a patient is scheduled for surgery and a decision is made to discontinue beta-blocker therapy, this should be done at least 24 hours prior to the procedure. The risk/benefit of stopping beta blockade should be made for each patient.

Since the half-life may be increased in patients with significant hepatic or renal impairment, caution must be exercised when starting treatment and selecting the initial dose.

Inderal must be used with caution in patients with decompensated cirrhosis (see section 4.2).

In patients with portal hypertension, liver function may deteriorate and hepatic encephalopathy may develop. There have been reports suggesting that treatment with propranolol may increase the risk of developing hepatic encephalopathy (see section 4.2).

Interference with laboratory tests. Inderal has been reported to interfere with the estimation of serum bilirubin by the diazo method and with the determination of catecholamines by methods using fluorescence.

4.5 Interaction with other medicinal products and other forms of interaction

Inderal modifies the tachycardia of hypoglycaemia. Caution must be exercised in the concurrent use of Inderal and hypoglycaemic therapy in diabetic patients. Inderal may prolong the hypoglycaemic response to insulin.

Class I anti-arrhythmic drugs (e.g. disopyramide) and amiodarone may have potentiating effect on atrial-conduction time and induce negative inotropic effect.

Digitalis glycosides in association with beta-blockers may increase atrioventricular conduction time.

Combined use of beta-blockers and calcium channel blockers with negative inotropic effects (eg, verapamil, diltiazem) can lead to an exaggeration of these effects particularly in patients with impaired ventricular function and/or SA or AV conduction abnormalities. This may result in severe hypotension, bradycardia and cardiac failure. Neither the beta-blocker nor the calcium channel blocker should be administered intravenously within 48 hours of discontinuing the other.

Concomitant therapy with dihydropyridines calcium channel blockers eg, nifedipine, may increase the risk of hypotension, and cardiac failure may occur in patients with latent cardiac insufficiency.

Concomitant use of sympathomimetic agents eg, adrenaline, may counteract the effect of beta-blockers. Caution must be exercised in the parenteral administration of preparations containing adrenaline to patients taking beta-blockers as, in rare cases, vasoconstriction, hypertension and bradycardia may result.

Administration of Inderal during infusion of lidocaine may increase the plasma concentration of lidocaine by approximately 30%. Patients already receiving Inderal tend to have higher lidocaine levels than controls. The combination should be avoided.

Concomitant use of cimetidine or hydralazine will increase the plasma levels of propranolol, and concomitant use of alcohol may increase the plasma levels of propranolol.

Beta-blockers may exacerbate the rebound hypertension which can follow the withdrawal of clonidine. If the two drugs are co-administered, the beta-blocker should be withdrawn several days before discontinuing clonidine. If replacing clonidine by beta-blocker therapy, the introduction of beta-blockers should be delayed for several days after clonidine administration has stopped.

Caution must be exercised if ergotamine, dihydroergotamine or related compounds are given in combination with Inderal since vasospastic reactions have been reported in a few patients.

Concomitant use of prostaglandin synthetase inhibiting drugs eg, ibuprofen and indometacin, may decrease the hypotensive effects of Inderal.

Concomitant administration of Inderal and chlorpromazine may result in an increase in plasma levels of both drugs. This may lead to an enhanced antipsychotic effect for chlorpromazine and an increased antihypertensive effect for Inderal.

Caution must be exercised when using anaesthetic agents with Inderal. The anaesthetist should be informed and the choice of anaesthetic should be an agent with as little negative inotropic activity as possible. Use of beta-blockers with anaesthetic drugs may result in attenuation of the reflex tachycardia and increase the risk of hypotension. Anaesthetic agents causing myocardial depression are best avoided.

Pharmacokinetic studies have shown that the following agents may interact with propranolol due to effects on enzyme systems in the liver which metabolise propranolol and these agents: quinidine, propafenone, rifampicin, theophylline, warfarin, thioridazine and dihydropyridine calcium channel blockers such as nifedipine, nisoldipine, nicardipine, isradipine and lacidipine. Owing to the fact that blood concentrations of either agent may be affected dosage adjustments may be needed according to clinical judgement. (See also the interaction above concerning the concomitant therapy with dihydropyridine calcium channel blockers).

4.6 Pregnancy and lactation

Pregnancy

As with all drugs Inderal should not be given during pregnancy unless its use is essential. There is no evidence of teratogenicity with Inderal. However beta-blockers reduce placental perfusion, which may result in intra-uterine foetal death, immature and premature deliveries. In addition, adverse effects (especially hypoglycaemia and bradycardia in the neonate and bradycardia in the foetus) may occur. There is an increased risk of cardiac and pulmonary complications in the neonate in the post-natal period.

Lactation

Most beta-blockers, particularly lipophilic compounds, will pass into breast milk although to a variable extent. Breast feeding is therefore not recommended following administration of these compounds.

4.7 Effects on ability to drive and use machines

Use is unlikely to result in any impairment of the ability of patients to drive or operate machinery. However it should be taken into account that occasionally dizziness or fatigue may occur.

4.8 Undesirable effects

Inderal is usually well tolerated. In clinical studies the undesired events reported are usually attributable to the pharmacological actions of propranolol.

The following undesired events, listed by body system, have been reported.

Common (1-9.9%)

General: Fatigue and/or lassitude (often transient)

Cardiovascular: Bradycardia, cold extremities, Raynaud's phenomenon.

CNS: Sleep disturbances, nightmares.

Uncommon (0.1-0.9%)

GI: Gastrointestinal disturbance, such as nausea, vomiting, diarrhoea.

Rare (0.01-0.09%)

General: Dizziness.

Blood: Thrombocytopaenia.

Cardiovascular: Heart failure deterioration, precipitation of heart block, postural hypotension, which may be associated with syncope, exacerbation of intermittent claudication.

CNS: Hallucinations, psychoses, mood changes, confusion, memory loss.

Skin: Purpura, alopecia, psoriasiform skin reactions, exacerbation of psoriasis, skin rashes.

Neurological: Paraesthesia.

Eyes: Dry eyes, visual disturbances.

Respiratory: Bronchospasm may occur in patients with bronchial asthma or a history of asthmatic complaints, sometimes with fatal outcome.

Very rare (<0.01%)

Endocrine system: Hypoglycaemia in neonates, infants, children, elderly patients, patients on haemodialysis, patients on concomitant antidiabetic therapy, patients with prolonged fasting and patients with chronic liver disease has been reported.

Investigations: an increase in ANA (Antinuclear Antibodies) has been observed, however the clinical relevance of this is not clear.

Nervous system: Isolated reports of myasthenia gravis like syndrome or exacerbation of myasthenia gravis have been reported.

Discontinuance of the drug should be considered if, according to clinical judgement, the well-being of the patient is adversely affected by any of the above reactions. Cessation of therapy with a beta-blocker should be gradual. In the rare event of intolerance, manifested as bradycardia and hypotension, the drug should be withdrawn and, if necessary, treatment for overdosage instituted.

4.9 Overdose

The symptoms of overdosage may include bradycardia, hypotension, acute cardiac insufficiency and bronchospasm.

General treatment should include: close supervision, treatment in an intensive care ward, the use of gastric lavage, activated charcoal and a laxative to prevent absorption of any drug still present in the gastrointestinal tract, the use of plasma or plasma substitutes to treat hypotension and shock.

Excessive bradycardia can be countered with atropine 1 to 2 mg intravenously and/or a cardiac pacemaker. If necessary, this may be followed by a bolus dose of glucagon 10 mg intravenously. If required, this may be repeated or followed by an intravenous infusion of glucagon 1 to 10 mg/hour depending on response. If no response to glucagon occurs or if glucagon is unavailable, a beta-adrenoceptor stimulant such as dobutamine 2.5 to 10 microgram/kg/minute by intravenous infusion may be given. Dobutamine, because of its positive inotropic effect, could also be used to treat hypotension and acute cardiac insufficiency. It is likely that these doses would be inadequate to reverse the cardiac effects of beta blockade if a large overdose has been taken. The dose of dobutamine should therefore be increased if necessary to achieve the required response according to the clinical condition of the patient.

5. PHARMACOLOGICAL PROPERTIES

5.1 Pharmacodynamic properties

Inderal is a competitive antagonist at both the $beta_1$- and $beta_2$ adrenoceptors. It has no agonist activity at the beta adrenoceptor, but has membrane stabilising activity at concentrations exceeding 1 to 3 mg/litre, though such concentrations are rarely achieved during oral therapy. Competitive beta blockade has been demonstrated in man by a parallel shift to the right in the dose-heart rate response curve to beta agonists such as isoprenaline.

Propranolol as with other beta-blockers, has negative inotropic effects, and is therefore contraindicated in uncontrolled heart failure.

Inderal is a racemic mixture and the active form is the S (-) isomer of propranolol. With the exception of inhibition of the conversion of thyroxine to triiodothyronine, it is unlikely that any additional ancillary properties possessed by R (+) propranolol, in comparison with the racemic mixture, will give rise to different therapeutic effects.

Inderal is effective and well tolerated in most ethnic populations, although the response may be less in black patients.

5.2 Pharmacokinetic properties

Following intravenous administration the plasma half-life of propranolol is about 2 hours and the ratio of metabolites to parent drug in the blood is lower than after oral administration. In particular 4-hydroxypropranolol is not present after intravenous administration. Propranolol is completely absorbed after oral administration and peak plasma concentrations occur 1 to 2 hours after dosing in fasting patients. The liver removes up to 90% of an oral dose with an elimination half-life of 3 to 6 hours. Propranolol is widely and rapidly distributed throughout the body with highest levels occurring in the lungs, liver, kidney, brain and heart. Propranolol is highly protein bound (80 to 95%).

5.3 Preclinical safety data

Propranolol is a drug on which extensive clinical experience has been obtained. Relevant information for the prescriber is provided elsewhere in this Summary of Product Characteristics.

6. PHARMACEUTICAL PARTICULARS

6.1 List of excipients

Citric acid (anhydrous) Ph. Eur.

Water for injections Ph. Eur.

6.2 Incompatibilities

None known.

6.3 Shelf life

5 years.

6.4 Special precautions for storage

Store below 30°C, protected from light

6.5 Nature and contents of container

Ampoule containing 1 ml.

6.6 Special precautions for disposal and other handling

None stated.

7. MARKETING AUTHORISATION HOLDER

AstraZeneca UK Limited,

600 Capability Green,

Luton, LU1 3LU, UK.

8. MARKETING AUTHORISATION NUMBER(S)

PL 17901/0018

9. DATE OF FIRST AUTHORISATION/RENEWAL OF THE AUTHORISATION

11th June 2000 / 4th June 2003

10. DATE OF REVISION OF THE TEXT

19th May 2009

Inderal LA 160mg

(AstraZeneca UK Limited)

1. NAME OF THE MEDICINAL PRODUCT

Inderal LA 160mg.

2. QUALITATIVE AND QUANTITATIVE COMPOSITION

Propranolol hydrochloride Ph Eur 160 mg

3. PHARMACEUTICAL FORM

Pink/lavender or white opaque capsules containing propranolol hydrochloride in a controlled release formulation.

4. CLINICAL PARTICULARS

4.1 Therapeutic indications

a) Control of hypertension

b) Management of angina

c) Prophylaxis of migraine

d) Management of essential tremor

e) Management of anxiety

f) Adjunctive management of thyrotoxicosis

g) Prophylaxis of upper gastro-intestinal bleeding in patients with portal hypertension and oesophageal varices

4.2 Posology and method of administration

For oral administration.

Adults

Hypertension: The usual starting dose is one 160 mg Inderal LA capsule daily, taken either morning or evening. An adequate response is seen in most patients at this dosage. If necessary, it can be increased in 80 mg Half-Inderal LA increments until an adequate response is achieved. A further reduction in blood pressure can be obtained if a diuretic or other antihypertensive agent is given in addition to Inderal LA and Half-Inderal LA.

Angina, anxiety, essential tremor, thyrotoxicosis and the prophylaxis of migraine: One Half-Inderal LA capsule daily, taken either morning or evening, may be sufficient to provide adequate control in many patients. If necessary the dose may be increased to one Inderal LA capsule per day and an additional Half-Inderal LA increment may be given.

Portal hypertension: Dosage should be titrated to achieve approximately 25% reduction in resting heart rate. Dosing should begin with one 80 mg Half-Inderal LA capsule daily, increasing to one 160 mg Inderal LA capsule daily depending on heart rate response. Further 80 mg Half-Inderal LA increments may be added up to a maximum dose of 320 mg once daily.

Patients who are already established on equivalent daily doses of Inderal tablets should be transferred to the equivalent doses of Half-Inderal LA or Inderal LA daily, taken either morning or evening.

Children

Inderal LA and Half-Inderal LA are not intended for use in children.

Elderly Patients

Evidence concerning the relation between blood level and age is conflicting. It is suggested that treatment should start with one Half-Inderal LA capsule once daily. The dose may be increased to one Inderal LA capsule daily or higher as appropriate.

4.3 Contraindications

Inderal LA and Half-Inderal LA must not be used if there is a history of bronchial asthma or bronchospasm. The product label states the following warning: "Do not take Inderal LA if you have a history of asthma or wheezing". A similar warning appears in the Patient Information Leaflet.

Bronchospasm can usually be reversed by $beta_2$ agonist bronchodilators such as salbutamol. Large doses of the $beta_2$ agonist bronchodilator may be required to overcome the beta blockade produced by propranolol and the dose should be titrated according to the clinical response; both intravenous and inhalational administration should be considered. The use of intravenous aminophylline and/or the use of ipratropium (given by nebuliser) may also be considered. Glucagon (1 to 2 mg given intravenously) has also been reported to produce a bronchodilator effect in asthmatic patients. Oxygen or artificial ventilation may be required in severe cases.

Inderal LA and Half-Inderal LA, as with other beta-blockers, must not be used in patients with any of the following conditions: known hypersensitivity to the substance, bradycardia, cardiogenic shock, hypotension, metabolic acidosis, after prolonged fasting, severe peripheral arterial circulatory disturbances, second or third degree heart block, sick sinus syndrome, untreated phaeochromocytoma, uncontrolled heart failure or Prinzmetal's angina.

Inderal LA and Half-Inderal LA must not be used in patients prone to hypoglycaemia, i.e., patients after prolonged fasting or patients with restricted counter-regulatory reserves.

4.4 Special warnings and precautions for use

Inderal LA and Half-Inderal LA as with other beta-blockers:

• although contra-indicated in uncontrolled heart failure (see Section 4.3) may be used in patients whose signs of heart failure have been controlled. Caution must be exercised in patients whose cardiac reserve is poor.

• should not be used in combination with calcium channel blockers with negative inotropic effects (e.g. verapamil, diltiazem), as it can lead to an exaggeration of these effects particularly in patients with impaired ventricular function and/or SA or AV conduction abnormalities. This may result in severe hypotension, bradycardia and cardiac failure. Neither the beta-blocker nor the calcium channel blocker should be administered intravenously within 48 hours of discontinuing the other.

• should not be used in patients with Prinzmetal's angina and beta-1 selective agents should be used with care. (see section 4.3).

• although contra-indicated in severe peripheral arterial circulatory disturbances (see Section 4.3) may also aggravate less severe peripheral arterial circulatory disturbances.

• due to its negative effect on conduction time, caution must be exercised if it is given to patients with first degree heart block.

• may block/modify the signs and symptoms of the hypoglycaemia (especially tachycardia). Inderal LA and Half-Inderal LA occasionally causes hypoglycaemia, even in non-diabetic patients, e.g., elderly patients, patients on haemodialysis or patients suffering from chronic liver disease and patients suffering from overdose. Severe hypoglycaemia associated with Inderal LA and Half-Inderal LA has rarely presented with seizures and/or coma in isolated patients. Caution must be exercised in the concurrent use of Inderal LA and Half-Inderal LA and hypoglycaemic therapy in diabetic patients. Inderal LA and Half-Inderal LA may prolong the hypoglycaemic response to insulin. (see section 4.3).

• may mask the signs of thyrotoxicosis.

• should not be used in untreated phaeochromocytoma. However, in patients with phaeochromocytoma, an alpha-blocker may be given concomitantly.

• should be used to treat the elderly with caution starting with a lower dose. (see section 4.2).

• will reduce heart rate as a result of its pharmacological action. In the rare instances when a treated patient develops symptoms that may be attributable to a slow heart rate, the dose may be reduced.

• may cause a more severe reaction to a variety of allergens, when given to patients with a history of anaphylactic reaction to such allergens. Such patients may be unresponsive to the usual doses of adrenaline used to treat the allergic reactions.

Abrupt withdrawal of beta-blockers is to be avoided. The dosage should be withdrawn gradually over a period of 7 to 14 days. An equivalent dosage of another beta-blocker may be substituted during the withdrawal period to facilitate a reduction in dosage below Inderal LA 80mg. Patients should be followed during withdrawal especially those with ischaemic heart disease.

When a patient is scheduled for surgery and a decision is made to discontinue beta-blocker therapy, this should be done at least 24 hours prior to the procedure.

The risk/benefit of stopping beta blockade should be made for each patient.

Since the half-life may be increased in patients with significant hepatic or renal impairment, caution must be exercised when starting treatment and selecting the initial dose.

Inderal LA and Half-Inderal LA must be used with caution in patients with decompensated cirrhosis. (see section 4.2)

In patients with portal hypertension, liver function may deteriorate and hepatic encephalopathy may develop. There have been reports suggesting that treatment with propranolol may increase the risk of developing hepatic encephalopathy (see section 4.2).

Interference with laboratory tests: Inderal LA and Half-Inderal LA have been reported to interfere with the estimation of serum bilirubin by the diazo method and with the determination of catecholamines by methods using fluorescence.

4.5 Interaction with other medicinal products and other forms of interaction

Inderal LA and Half-Inderal LA modify the tachycardia of hypoglycaemia. Caution must be exercised in the concurrent use of Inderal LA or Half-Inderal LA and hypoglycaemic therapy in diabetic patients. Propranolol may prolong the hypoglycaemic response to insulin.(see section 4.3 and 4.4).

Class I anti-arrhythmic drugs (e.g. disopyramide) and amiodarone may have potentiating effect on atrial-conduction time and induce negative inotropic effect.

Digitalis glycosides, in association with beta-blockers, may increase atrio-ventricular conduction time.

Combined use of beta-blockers and calcium channel blockers with negative inotropic effects eg, verapamil, diltiazem, can lead to an exaggeration of these effects, particularly in patients with impaired ventricular function and/or sino-atrial or atrio-ventricular conduction abnormalities. This may result in severe hypotension, bradycardia and cardiac failure. Neither the beta-blocker nor the calcium channel blocker should be administered intravenously within 48 hours of discontinuing the other.

Concomitant therapy with dihydropyridine calcium channel blockers eg, nifedipine, may increase the risk of hypotension, and cardiac failure may occur in patients with latent cardiac insufficiency.

Concomitant use of sympathomimetic agents, eg, adrenaline, may counteract the effect of beta-blockers. Caution must be exercised in the parenteral administration of preparations containing adrenaline to patients taking beta-blockers as, in rare cases, vasoconstriction, hypertension and bradycardia may result.

Administration of propranolol during infusion of lidocaine may increase the plasma concentration of lidocaine by approximately 30%. Patients already receiving propranolol tend to have higher lidocaine levels than controls. The combination should be avoided.

Concomitant use of cimetidine will increase plasma levels of propranolol, and concomitant use of alcohol may increase the plasma levels of propranolol.

Beta-blockers may exacerbate the rebound hypertension, which can follow the withdrawal of clonidine. If the two drugs are co-administered, the beta-blocker should be withdrawn several days before discontinuing clonidine. If replacing clonidine by beta-blocker therapy, the introduction of beta-blockers should be delayed for several days after clonidine administration has stopped.

Caution must be exercised if ergotamine, dihydroergotamine or related compounds are given in combination with propranolol since vasospastic reactions have been reported in a few patients.

Concomitant use of prostaglandin synthetase inhibiting drugs, eg, ibuprofen or indometacin, may decrease the hypotensive effects of propranolol.

Concomitant administration of propranolol and chlorpromazine may result in an increase in plasma levels of both drugs. This may lead to an enhanced antipsychotic effect for chlorpromazine and an increased antihypertensive effect for propranolol.

Caution must be exercised when using anaesthetic agents with Inderal LA and Half-Inderal LA. The anaesthetist should be informed and the choice of anaesthetic should be the agent with as little negative inotropic activity as possible. Use of beta-blockers with anaesthetic drugs may result in attenuation of the reflex tachycardia and increase the risk of hypotension. Anaesthetic agents causing myocardial depression are best avoided.

Pharmacokinetic studies have shown that the following agents may interact with propranolol due to effects on enzyme systems in the liver which metabolise propranolol and these agents: quinidine, propafenone, rifampicin, theophylline, warfarin, thioridazine and dihydropyridine calcium channel blockers such as nifedipine, nisoldipine, nicardipine, isradipine and lacidipine. Owing to the fact that blood concentrations of either agent may be affected, dosage adjustments may be needed according to clinical judgement. (See also the interaction above concerning concomitant therapy with dihydropyridine calcium channel blockers).

4.6 Pregnancy and lactation

Pregnancy: As with all drugs, Inderal LA and Half-Inderal LA should not be given during pregnancy unless their use is essential. There is no evidence of teratogenicity with Inderal. However beta-blockers reduce placental perfusion, which may result in intra-uterine foetal death, immature and premature deliveries. In addition, adverse effects (especially hypoglycaemia and bradycardia in the neonate and bradycardia in the foetus) may occur. There is an increased risk of cardiac and pulmonary complications in the neonate in the post-natal period.

Lactation: Most beta-blockers, particularly lipophilic compounds, will pass into breast milk although to a variable extent. Breast feeding is therefore not recommended following administration of these compounds.

4.7 Effects on ability to drive and use machines

The use of Inderal LA or Half-Inderal LA is unlikely to result in any impairment of the ability of patients to drive or operate machinery. However, it should be taken into account that occasionally dizziness or fatigue may occur.

4.8 Undesirable effects

Inderal LA and Half-Inderal LA are usually well tolerated. In clinical studies, the undesired events reported are usually attributable to the pharmacological actions of propranolol.

The following undesired events, listed by body system, have been reported.

Common (1-9.9%)

General: Fatigue and/or lassitude (often transient)

Cardiovascular: Bradycardia, cold extremities, Raynaud's phenomenon.

CNS: Sleep disturbances, nightmares.

Uncommon (0.1-0.9%)

GI: Gastrointestinal disturbance, such as nausea, vomiting, diarrhoea.

Rare (0.01-0.09%)

General: Dizziness.

Blood: Thrombocytopaenia.

Cardiovascular: Heart failure deterioration, precipitation of heart block, postural hypotension, which may be associated with syncope, exacerbation of intermittent claudication.

CNS: Hallucinations, psychoses, mood changes, confusion, memory loss.

Skin: Purpura, alopecia, psoriasiform skin reactions, exacerbation of psoriasis, skin rashes.

Neurological: Paraesthesia.

Eyes: Dry eyes, visual disturbances.

Respiratory: Bronchospasm may occur in patients with bronchial asthma or a history of asthmatic complaints, sometimes with fatal outcome.

Very rare (<0.01%)

Endocrine system: Hypoglycaemia in neonates, infants, children, elderly patients, patients on haemodialysis, patients on concomitant antidiabetic therapy, patients with prolonged fasting and patients with chronic liver disease has been reported.

Investigations: an increase in ANA (Antinuclear Antibodies) has been observed, however the clinical relevance of this is not clear.

Nervous system: Isolated reports of myasthenia gravis like syndrome or exacerbation of myasthenia gravis have been reported.

Discontinuance of the drug should be considered if, according to clinical judgement, the well-being of the patient is adversely affected by any of the above reactions. Cessation of therapy with a beta-blocker should be gradual. In the rare event of intolerance manifested as bradycardia and hypotension, the drug should be withdrawn and, if necessary, treatment for overdosage instituted.

4.9 Overdose

The symptoms of overdosage may include bradycardia, hypotension, acute cardiac insufficiency and bronchospasm.

General treatment should include: close supervision, treatment in an intensive care ward, the use of gastric lavage, activated charcoal and a laxative to prevent absorption of any drug still present in the gastrointestinal tract, the use of plasma or plasma substitutes to treat hypotension and shock.

Excessive bradycardia can be countered with atropine 1 to 2 mg intravenously and/or a cardiac pacemaker. If necessary, this may be followed by a bolus dose of glucagon 10 mg intravenously. If required, this may be repeated or followed by an intravenous infusion of glucagon 1 to 10 mg/hour depending on response. If no response to glucagon occurs or if glucagon is unavailable, a beta-adrenoceptor stimulant such as dobutamine 2.5 to 10 microgram/kg/minute by intravenous infusion may be given. Dobutamine, because of its positive inotropic effect, could also be used to treat hypotension and acute cardiac insufficiency. It is likely that these doses would be inadequate to reverse the cardiac effects of beta blockade if a large overdose has been taken. The dose of dobutamine should therefore be increased if necessary to achieve the required response according to the clinical condition of the patient.

5. PHARMACOLOGICAL PROPERTIES

5.1 Pharmacodynamic properties

Propranolol is a competitive antagonist at both $beta_1$ and $beta_2$-adrenoceptors. It has no agonist activity at the beta adrenoceptor, but has membrane stabilising activity at concentrations exceeding 1 to 3 mg/litre, though such concentrations are rarely achieved during oral therapy. Competitive beta blockade has been demonstrated in man by a parallel shift to the right in the dose-heart rate response curve to beta agonists such as isoprenaline.

Propranolol, as with other beta-blockers, has negative inotropic effects, and is therefore contra-indicated in uncontrolled heart failure.

Propranolol is a racemic mixture and the active form is the S (-) isomer. With the exception of inhibition of the conversion of thyroxine to triiodothyronine it is unlikely that any additional ancillary properties possessed by R (+) propranolol, in comparison with the racemic mixture will give rise to different therapeutic effects.

Propranolol is effective and well tolerated in most ethnic populations, although the response may be less in black patients.

The sustained release preparation of propranolol maintains a higher degree of $beta_1$-blockade 24 hours after dosing compared with conventional propranolol.

5.2 Pharmacokinetic properties

Propranolol is completely absorbed after oral administration and peak plasma concentrations occur 1-2 hours after dosing in fasting patients. Following oral dosing with the sustained release preparation of propranolol, the blood profile is flatter than after conventional Inderal but the half-life is increased to between 10 and 20 hours. The liver removes up to 90% of an oral dose with an elimination half-life of 3 to 6 hours. Propranolol is widely and rapidly distributed throughout the body with highest levels occurring in the lungs, liver, kidney, brain and heart. Propranolol is highly protein bound (80 to 95%).

5.3 Preclinical safety data

Propranolol is a drug on which extensive clinical experience has been obtained. Relevant information for the prescriber is provided elsewhere in this Summary of Product Characteristics.

6. PHARMACEUTICAL PARTICULARS

6.1 List of excipients

Erythrosine (E127)

Ethyl cellulose Ph Eur. (E462)

Gelatin Ph Eur. (E441)

Glycerol Ph Eur. (E422)

Iron oxide, red (E172)

Iron oxide, black (E172)

Methylhydroxypropylcellulose Ph Eur. (E464)

Microcrystalline cellulose Ph Eur. (E460)

Titanium dioxide Ph Eur. (E171)

6.2 Incompatibilities

None known.

6.3 Shelf life

3 years.

6.4 Special precautions for storage

Store below 25°C, protected from light and moisture.

6.5 Nature and contents of container

Patient calendar pack of 28 capsules.

6.6 Special precautions for disposal and other handling

Use as directed by the prescriber.

7. MARKETING AUTHORISATION HOLDER

AstraZeneca UK Limited

600 Capability Green

Luton

LU1 3LU

UK

8. MARKETING AUTHORISATION NUMBER(S)

PL 17901/0019

9. DATE OF FIRST AUTHORISATION/RENEWAL OF THE AUTHORISATION

11th June 2000

10. DATE OF REVISION OF THE TEXT

19th May 2009

Indivina

(Orion Pharma (UK) Limited)

1. NAME OF THE MEDICINAL PRODUCT

Indivina 1 mg/2.5 mg tablets

Indivina 1 mg/5 mg tablets

Indivina 2 mg/5 mg tablets

2. QUALITATIVE AND QUANTITATIVE COMPOSITION

One Indivina 1 mg/2.5 mg tablet contains:

Estradiol valerate 1 mg

Medroxyprogesterone acetate 2.5 mg

One Indivina 1 mg/5 mg tablet contains:

Estradiol valerate 1 mg

Medroxyprogesterone acetate 5 mg

One Indivina 2 mg/5 mg tablet contains:

Estradiol valerate 2 mg

Medroxyprogesterone acetate 5 mg

For excipients, see 6.1.

3. PHARMACEUTICAL FORM

Tablet. White, round, bevelled-edge, diameter 7 mm, flat tablets with a code on one side with 1+2,5, 1+5, and 2+5, respectively.

4. CLINICAL PARTICULARS

4.1 Therapeutic indications

Hormone replacement therapy (HRT) for estrogen deficiency symptoms in women with an intact uterus more than three years after menopause.

Prevention of osteoporosis in postmenopausal women at high risk of future fractures who are intolerant of, or contra-indicated for, other medicinal products approved for the prevention of osteoporosis.

The experience of treating women older than 65 years is limited.

4.2 Posology and method of administration

Indivina is a continuous combined HRT regimen in which estrogen and progestagen are given every day without interruption.

Dosage: One tablet each day orally without a tablet-free interval. Tablet should be taken approximately at the same time of the day.

Treatment is recommended to be initiated with Indivina 1 mg/2.5 mg tablet. Depending on the clinical response to treatment, the dosage can then be adjusted to individual needs.

Medroxyprogesterone acetate (MPA) 2.5 mg is usually sufficient to prevent breakthrough bleeding. If breakthrough bleeding occurs and persists, and endometrial abnormality has been ruled out, the dose can be increased to 5 mg (Indivina 1mg/5 mg tablet).

If 1 mg of estradiol valerate (E_2V) is not sufficient to alleviate estrogen deficiency symptoms, the dose can be increased to 2 mg (Indivina 2 mg/5 mg tablet).

In women with amenorrhea and not taking HRT or women who switch from another continuous combined HRT product, treatment with Indivina may be started on any day. Women who switch from cyclic HRT regimen should start Indivina treatment one week after completion of the cycle.

The effect of estrogen on bone mineral density is dose dependent and therefore the effect of 1 mg E_2V may be less than with 2 mg (see section 5.1).

If the patient has forgotten to take one tablet, the forgotten tablet is to be discarded. Forgetting a dose may increase the likelihood of breakthrough bleeding and spotting.

For initiation and continuation of treatment of postmenopausal symptoms, the lowest effective dose for the shortest duration (see also Section 4.4) should be used.

4.3 Contraindications

Known, past or suspected breast cancer

Known or suspected estrogen-dependent malignant tumours (e.g. endometrial cancer)

Undiagnosed genital bleeding

Untreated endometrial hyperplasia

Previous idiopathic or current venous thromboembolism [deep venous thrombosis (DVT), pulmonary embolism]

Active or recent arterial thromboembolic disease (e.g. angina, myocardial infarction)

Acute liver disease or a history of liver disease as long as liver function tests have failed to return to normal

Known hypersensitivity to the active substances or to any of the excipients

Porphyria.

4.4 Special warnings and precautions for use

For the treatment of postmenopausal symptoms, HRT should only be initiated for symptoms that adversely affect quality of life. In all cases, a careful appraisal of the risks and benefits should be undertaken at least annually and HRT should only be continued as long as the benefit outweighs the risk.

Medical examination/follow-up

Before initiating or reinstituting HRT, a complete personal and family medical history should be taken. Physical (including pelvic and breast) examination should be guided by this and by the contraindications and warnings for use.

During treatment, periodic check-ups are recommended of a frequency and nature adapted to the individual woman. Women should be advised what changes in their breasts should be reported to their doctor or nurse (see 'Breast cancer' below). Investigations, including mammography, should be carried out in accordance with currently accepted screening practices, modified to the clinical needs of the individual.

Conditions which need supervision

If any of the following conditions are present, have occurred previously and/or have been aggravated during pregnancy or previous hormone treatment, the patient should be closely supervised. It should be taken into account that these conditions may recur or be aggravated during treatment with Indivina, in particular:

Leiomyoma (uterine fibroids) or endometriosis

A history of or risk factors for thromboembolic disorders (see below)

Risk factors for estrogen dependent tumours, e.g. 1st degree heredity for breast cancer

Hypertension

Liver disorders (e.g. liver adenoma)

Diabetes mellitus with or without vascular involvement

Cholelithiasis

Migraine or (severe) headache

Systemic lupus erythematosus

A history of endometrial hyperplasia (see below)

Epilepsy

Asthma

Otosclerosis

Reasons for immediate withdrawal of therapy:

Therapy should be discontinued in case a contra-indication is discovered and in the following situations:

Jaundice or deterioration of liver function

Significant increase in blood pressure

New onset of migraine-type headache

Pregnancy

Endometrial hyperplasia

The risk of endometrial hyperplasia and carcinoma is increased when estrogens are administered alone for prolonged periods (see section 4.8). The addition of a progestagen for at least 12 days per cycle (for cyclic or sequential products) or every day (for combination products like Indivina) in non-hysterectomised women greatly reduces this risk.

Break-through bleeding and spotting may occur during the first months of treatment. If break-through bleeding or spotting appears after some time of therapy, or continues after treatment has been discontinued, the reason should be investigated, which may include endometrial biopsy to excluded endometrial malignancy.

Breast cancer

A randomised placebo-controlled trial, the Women's Health Initiative study (WHI), and epidemiological studies, including the Million Women Study (MWS), have reported an increased risk of breast cancer in women taking estrogens, estrogen-progestagen combinations or tibolone for HRT for several years (see section 4.8). For all HRT, an excess risk becomes apparent within a few years of use and increases with duration of intake but returns to baseline within a few (at most five) years after stopping treatment.

In the MWS, the relative risk of breast cancer with conjugated equine estrogens (CEE) or estradiol (E2) was greater when a progestagen was added, either sequentially or continuously, and regardless of type of progestagen. There was no evidence of a difference in risk between the different routes of administration.

In the WHI study, the continuous combined conjugated equine estrogen and medroxyprogesterone acetate (CEE + MPA) product used was associated with breast cancers that were slightly larger in size and more frequently had local lymph node metastases compared to placebo.

HRT, especially estrogen-progestagen combined treatment, increases the density of mammographic images which may adversely affect the radiological detection of breast cancer.

Venous thromboembolism

HRT is associated with a higher relative risk of developing venous thromboembolism (VTE), i.e. deep vein thrombosis or pulmonary embolism. One randomised controlled trial and epidemiological studies found a two- to threefold higher risk for users compared with non-users. For non-users it is estimated that the number of cases of VTE that will occur over a 5 year period is about 3 per 1000 women aged 50-59 years and 8 per 1000 women aged between 60-69 years. It is estimated that in healthy women who use HRT for 5 years, the number of additional cases of VTE over a 5 year period will be between 2 and 6 (best estimate = 4) per 1000 women aged 50-59 years and between 5 and 15 (best estimate = 9) per 1000 women aged 60-69 years. The occurrence of such an event is more likely in the first year of HRT than later.

Generally recognised risk factors for VTE include a personal history or family history, severe obesity (BMI > 30 kg/m^2) and systemic lupus erythematosus (SLE). There is no consensus about the possible role of varicose veins in VTE.

Patients with a history of VTE or known thrombophilic states have an increased risk of VTE. HRT may add to this risk. Personal or strong family history of thromboembolism or recurrent spontaneous abortion should be investigated in order to exclude a thrombophilic predisposition. Until a thorough evaluation of thrombophilic factors has been made or anticoagulant treatment initiated, use of HRT in such patients should be viewed as contraindicated. Those women already on anticoagulant treatment require careful consideration of the benefit-risk of use of HRT.

The risk of VTE may be temporarily increased with prolonged immobilisation, major trauma or major surgery. As in all postoperative patients, scrupulous attention should be given to prophylactic measures to prevent VTE following surgery. Where prolonged immobilisation is liable to follow elective surgery, particularly abdominal or orthopaedic surgery to the lower limbs, consideration should be given to temporarily stopping HRT 4 to 6 weeks earlier, if possible. Treatment should not be restarted until the woman is completely mobilised.

If VTE develops after initiating therapy, the drug should be discontinued. Patients should be told to contact their doctors immediately when they are aware of a potential thromboembolic symptom (e.g., painful swelling of a leg, sudden pain in the chest, dyspnea).

Coronary artery disease (CAD)

There is no evidence from randomised controlled trials of cardiovascular benefit with continuous combined conjugated estrogens and medroxyprogesterone acetate (MPA). Two large clinical trials (WHI and HERS i.e. Heart and Estrogen/progestin Replacement Study) showed a possible increased risk of cardiovascular morbidity in the first year of use and no overall benefit. For other HRT products there are only limited data from randomised controlled trials examining effects in cardiovascular morbidity and mortality. Therefore, it is uncertain whether these findings also extend to other HRT products.

Stroke

One large randomised clinical trial (WHI-trial) found, as a secondary outcome, an increased risk of ischaemic stroke in healthy women during treatment with continuous combined conjugated estrogens and MPA. For women who do not use HRT, it is estimated that the number of cases of stroke that will occur over a 5 year period is about 3 per 1000 women aged 50-59 years and 11 per 1000 women aged 60-69 years. It is estimated that for women who use conjugated estrogens and MPA for 5 years, the number of additional cases will be between 0 and 3 (best estimate = 1) per 1000 users aged 50-59 years and between 1 and 9 (best estimate = 4) per 1000 users aged 60-69 years. It is unknown whether the increased risk also extends to other HRT products.

Ovarian cancer

Long-term (at least 5-10 years) use of estrogen-only HRT products in hysterectomised women has been associated with an increased risk of ovarian cancer in some epidemiological studies. It is uncertain whether long-term use of combined HRT confers a different risk than estrogen-only products.

Other conditions

Estrogens may cause fluid retention and, therefore, patients with cardiac or renal dysfunction should be carefully observed. Patients with terminal renal insufficiency should be closely observed, since it is expected that the level of circulating active ingredients of Indivina is increased.

Women with pre-existing hypertriglyceridaemia should be followed closely during HRT, since rare cases of large increases of plasma triglycerides leading to pancreatitis have been reported with estrogen therapy in this condition.

Estrogens increase thyroid binding globulin (TBG), leading to increased circulating total thyroid hormone, as measured by protein-bound iodine (PBI), T4 levels (by column or by radio-immunoassay) or T3 levels (by radio-immunoassay). T3 resin uptake is decreased, reflecting the elevated TBG. Free T4 and free T3 concentrations are unaltered. Other binding proteins may be elevated in serum, i.e. corticoid binding globulin (CBG), sex-hormone-binding globulin (SHBG) leading to increased circulating corticosteroids and sex steroids, respectively. Free or biological active hormone concentrations are unchanged. Other plasma proteins may be increased (angiotensinogen/ennin substrate, alpha-1-antitrypsin, ceruloplasmin).

There is no conclusive evidence for improvement of cognitive function. There is some evidence from the WHI trial of increased risk of probable dementia in women who start using continuous combined CEE and MPA after the age of 65. It is unknown whether the findings apply to younger post-menopausal women or other HRT products.

Patients with rare hereditary problems of galactose intolerance, the Lapp lactase deficiency or glucose-galactose malabsorption should not take this medicine.

4.5 Interaction with other medicinal products and other forms of interaction

The metabolism of estrogens and progestagens may be increased by concomitant use of substances known to induce drug-metabolising enzymes, specifically cytochrome P450 enzymes, such as anticonvulsants (e.g. phenobarbital, phenytoin, carbamazepine) and anti-infectives (e.g. rifampicin, rifabutin, nevirapine, efavirenz).

Ritonavir and nelfinavir, although known as strong inhibitors, by contrast exhibit inducing properties when used concomitantly with steroid hormones. Herbal preparations containing St John's wort (*Hypericum perforatum*) may induce the metabolism of estrogens and progestagens.

Clinically, an increased metabolism of estrogens and progestagens may lead to decreased effect and changes in the uterine bleeding profile.

4.6 Pregnancy and lactation

Pregnancy

Indivina is not indicated during pregnancy. If pregnancy occurs during medication with Indivina, treatment should be withdrawn immediately. Data on limited number of exposed pregnancies indicate adverse effects of medroxyprogesterone acetate on sexual differentiation of the foetus. Studies in animals have shown reproductive toxicity (see section 5.3). The potential risk for humans is unknown.

The results of most epidemiological studies to date relevant to inadvertent foetal exposure to combinations of estrogens and progestagen indicate no teratogenic or foetotoxic effect.

Lactation

Indivina is not indicated during lactation.

4.7 Effects on ability to drive and use machines

No effects on ability to drive and use machines have been observed.

4.8 Undesirable effects

The most frequently reported undesirable effect during Indivina treatment in clinical trials was breast tenderness, which occurred in 10.6% of users.

Undesirable effects according to system organ class associated with Indivinatreatment are presented in the table below.

(see Table 1 below)

Breast cancer

According to evidence from a large number of epidemiological studies and one randomised placebo-controlled trial, the Women's Health Initiative (WHI), the overall risk of breast cancer increases with increasing duration of HRT use in current or recent HRT users.

For estrogen-only HRT, estimates of relative risk (RR) from a reanalysis of original data from 51 epidemiological studies (in which >80% of HRT use was estrogen-only HRT) and from the epidemiological Million Women Study (MWS) are similar at 1.35 (95% CI 1.21 – 1.49) and 1.30 (95% CI 1.21 – 1.40), respectively.

For oestrogen plus progestagen combined HRT, several epidemiological studies have reported an overall higher risk for breast cancer than with estrogens alone.

The MWS reported that, compared to never users, the use of various types of estrogen-progestagen combined HRT was associated with a higher risk of breast cancer (RR = 2.00, 95%CI: 1.88 – 2.12) than use of estrogens alone (RR = 1.30, 95%CI: 1.21 – 1.40) or use of tibolone (RR = 1.45; 95%CI 1.25-1.68).

The WHI trial reported a risk estimate of 1.24 (95%CI 1.01 – 1.54) after 5.6 years of use of estrogen-progestagen combined HRT (CEE + MPA) in all users compared with placebo.

The absolute risks calculated from the MWS and the WHI trial are presented below:

The MWS has estimated, from the known average incidence of breast cancer in developed countries, that:

For women not using HRT, about 32 in every 1000 are expected to have breast cancer diagnosed between the ages of 50 and 64 years.

For 1000 current or recent users of HRT, the number of additional cases during the corresponding period will be

For users of estrogen-only replacement therapy

- between 0 and 3 (best estimate = 1.5) for 5 years' use
- between 3 and 7 (best estimate = 5) for 10 years' use

For users of estrogen plus progestagen combined HRT,

- between 5 and 7 (best estimate = 6) for 5 years' use
- between 18 and 20 (best estimate = 19) for 10 years' use.

The WHI trial estimated that after 5.6 years of follow-up of women between the ages of 50 and 79 years, an additional 8 cases of invasive breast cancer would be due to estrogen- progestagen combined HRT (CEE + MPA) per 10,000 women years.

According to calculations from the trial data, it is estimated that:

For 1000 women in the placebo group,

- about 16 cases of invasive breast cancer would be diagnosed in 5 years.

For 1000 women who used estrogen + progestagen combined HRT (CEE + MPA), the number of additional cases would be

- between 0 and 9 (best estimate = 4) for 5 years' use.

The number of additional cases of breast cancer in women who use HRT is broadly similar for women who start HRT irrespective of age at start of use (between the ages of 45-65) (see section 4.4).'

Endometrial cancer

In women with an intact uterus, the risk of endometrial hyperplasia and endometrial cancer increases with increasing duration of use of unopposed estrogens. According to data from epidemiological studies, the best estimate of the risk is that for women not using HRT about 5 in every 1000 are expected to have endometrial cancer diagnosed between the ages of 50 and 65. Depending on the duration of treatment and estrogen dose, the reported increase in endometrial cancer risk among unopposed estrogen users varies from 2- to 12-fold greater compared with non-users. Adding a progestagen to estrogen-only therapy greatly reduces this increased risk.

Other adverse reactions have been reported in association with estrogen/progestagen treatment:

Estrogen-dependent neoplasms benign and malignant, e.g. endometrial cancer.

Venous thromboembolism, i.e. deep leg or pelvic venous thrombosis and pulmonary embolism, is more frequent among HRT users than among non-users. For further information see sections 4.3 and 4.4.

Myocardial infarction and stroke.

Gall bladder disease.

Skin and subcutaneous disorders: chloasma, erythema multiforme, erythema nodosum, vascular purpura.

Probable dementia (see section 4.4).

4.9 Overdose

Estrogen overdose may cause nausea, headache and uterine bleeding. Numerous reports on high doses of estrogen-containing oral contraceptives ingested by young children indicate that serious harmful effects do not occur. Treatment of estrogen overdose is symptomatic. High doses of medroxyprogesterone acetate (MPA) used for

Table 1

Organ group	Common (>1/100)	Uncommon (>1/1,000, <1/100)	Rare (>1/10,000; <1/1,000)
Gastrointestinal	Nausea, abdominal pain	Dyspepsia, vomiting, flatulence, gallbladder disease/ gall stones	
Skin			Alopecia, hirsutism, rash, itching
CNS	Headache	Dizziness, migraine	
Urogenital	Uterine bleeding, increase in size of uterine fibroids	Vaginal candidiasis	
Cardiovascular		Increase in blood pressure	Venous thromboembolism
Miscellaneous	Weight increase/ decrease, oedema, breast tenderness, breast enlargement, changes in mood including anxiety and depressive mood, changes in libido	Leg cramps	

cancer treatment have not resulted in serious undesirable effects.

5. PHARMACOLOGICAL PROPERTIES

5.1 Pharmacodynamic properties

Pharmacotherapeutic group: Progestagens and estrogens, fixed combinations; ATC code: G03FA12.

The active form of estradiol valerate, synthetic 17β-estradiol is chemically and biologically identical to endogenous human estradiol. It substitutes for the loss of estrogen production in menopausal women, and alleviates menopausal symptoms.

Estrogens prevent bone loss following menopause or ovariectomy.

Medroxyprogesterone acetate is a derivative of the natural progesterone, 17-alpha-hydroxy-6-methylprogesterone. Medroxyprogesterone acetate binds to progestin-specific receptors and acts on the endometrium to convert the status of the endometrium from proliferative to secretory.

As estrogens promote the growth of the endometrium, unopposed estrogens increase the risk of endometrial hyperplasia and cancer. The addition of medroxyprogesterone acetate greatly reduces the estrogen-induced risk of endometrial hyperplasia in non-hysterectomised women.

Clinical trial information

Relief of estrogen deficiency symptoms and bleeding patterns

Relief of menopausal symptoms was achieved during the first few weeks of treatment.

Bleeding and/or spotting appeared in 41% of the women receiving 1 mg estradiol valerate and 51% of women receiving 2 mg estradiol valerate during the first three months of treatment and in 9% of the women receiving 1 mg estradiol valerate and in 20% of women receiving 2 mg estradiol valerate during 10-12 months of treatment.

Amenorrhoea was seen in 91% of women receiving 1 mg estradiol valerate and in 80% of women receiving 2 mg estradiol valerate after 10-12 months of treatment.

Prevention of osteoporosis

Estrogen deficiency at menopause is associated with an increasing bone turnover and decline in bone mass. The effect of estrogens on bone mineral density (BMD) is dose dependent. Protection appears to be effective for as long as treatment is continued. After discontinuation of HRT, bone mass is lost at a rate similar to that in untreated women.

Evidence from the WHI trial and meta-analysed trials shows that current use of HRT, alone or in combination with a progestagen – given to predominantly healthy women – reduces the risk of hip, vertebral, and other osteoporotic fractures. HRT may also prevent fractures in women with low bone density and/or established osteoporosis, but the evidence for that is limited.

After 4 years of treatment with Indivina combinations containing the 1 mg dose, the increase in lumbar spine bone mineral density (BMD) was6.2 ± 0.5% (mean ± SE). The percentage of women who gained BMD in lumbar zone during treatment was 86.6%.

Indivina combinations containing the 1 mg dose also had an effect on hip BMD. The increase after 4 years was 2.9 ± 0.4% (mean ± SE) at femoral neck. The percentage of women who gained BMD in hip zone during treatment was 80.4%.

After 4 years of treatment with Indivina combinations containing the 2 mg dose, the increase in lumbar spine BMD was 7.4 ± 0.4% (mean ± SE). The percentage of women who gained BMD in lumbar zone during treatment was 95.8%.

Indivina combinations containing the 2 mg dose also had an effect on hip BMD. The increase after 4 years was 2.9 ± 0.4% (mean ± SE) at femoral neck. The percentage of women who gained BMD in hip zone during treatment was 72.3%.

5.2 Pharmacokinetic properties

Following oral administration estradiol valerate is absorbed from the gastrointestinal tract and rapidly hydrolysed to estradiol by esterases. In postmenopausal women aged 50-65 years the maximum concentration of estradiol in serum (C_{max}) was reached within 4 to 6 hours after multiple dosing of 1 mg or 2 mg estradiol valerate. After 1 mg dose C_{max} was about 166 pmol/l, trough concentration (C_{min}) about 101 pmol/l and average concentration ($C_{average}$) about 123 pmol/l. For 2 mg dose C_{max} was 308 pmol/l, C_{min} 171 pmol/l and $C_{average}$ 228 pmol/l. Comparable estradiol concentrations were observed in women over 65 years.

Circulating estradiol is bound to plasma proteins, mainly to sex hormone binding globulin (SHBG) and serum albumin. Estradiol undergoes extensive biotransformation. Its metabolites are excreted in the urine as glucuronide and sulphate conjugates together with a small proportion of unchanged estradiol. Besides urinary excretion, estrogen metabolites undergo an enterohepatic circulation. Only a small amount of a dose is excreted in the faeces.

The absorption of medroxyprogesterone acetate after oral administration is low due to low solubility and there is large individual variation. Medroxyprogesterone acetate undergoes virtually no first-pass metabolism. After multiple dosing of 2.5 mg or 5 mg medroxyprogesterone acetate to women aged 50-65 years, maximum concentration in serum was reached in less than 2 hours. After 2.5 mg dose C_{max} was about 0.37 ng/ml, C_{min} about 0.05 ng/ml and $C_{average}$ about 0.11 ng/ml. After 5 mg dose C_{max} was about 0.64 ng/ml, C_{min} about 0.12 ng/ml and $C_{average}$ about 0.21 ng/ml. Comparable medroxyprogesterone acetate concentrations were observed in women over 65 years.

Medroxyprogesterone acetate is over 90% bound to plasma proteins, mainly to albumin. The elimination half-life of oral medroxyprogesterone acetate is approximately 24 hours. Medroxyprogesterone acetate is extensively metabolised by hepatic hydroxylation and conjugation and excreted in the urine and the bile. Metabolism is poorly documented and the pharmacological activity of the metabolites is not known.

5.3 Preclinical safety data

Animal studies with estradiol and medroxyprogesterone acetate have shown expected estrogenic and gestagenic effect. Both compounds induced adverse effects in reproductive toxicity studies. Chiefly, estradiol showed embryotoxic effects and induced feminisation of male foetuses.

Medroxyprogesterone showed embryotoxic effects and induced anti-androgenic effects in male foetuses and masculinization in female foetuses. The relevance of these data for human exposure is unknown (see section 4.6). Concerning other preclinical effects, the toxicity profiles of estradiol valerate and medroxyprogesterone acetate are well known and reveal no particular human health risks beyond those discussed in other sections of the SPC and which generally apply to hormone replacement therapy.

6. PHARMACEUTICAL PARTICULARS

6.1 List of excipients

Lactose monohydrate, maize starch, elatine, magnesium stearate.

6.2 Incompatibilities

Not applicable.

6.3 Shelf life

3 years.

6.4 Special precautions for storage

Do not store above 30 °C. Store in the original package in order to protect from moisture.

6.5 Nature and contents of container

28 tablets in PVC/PVDC/Aluminium blister. Pack of 1x28 tablets and 3x28 tablets

6.6 Special precautions for disposal and other handling

No special requirements.

7. MARKETING AUTHORISATION HOLDER

Orion Corporation

Orionintie 1

FIN-02200 Espoo

Finland

8. MARKETING AUTHORISATION NUMBER(S)

Indivina 1 mg/2.5 mg: 27925/0011

Indivina 1 mg/5 mg: 27925/0012

Indivina 2 mg/5 mg: 27925/0013

9. DATE OF FIRST AUTHORISATION/RENEWAL OF THE AUTHORISATION

Date of first authorisation: 10 December 1999

Date of last renewal: 10 December 2004

10. DATE OF REVISION OF THE TEXT

July 2006

InductOs 12mg

(Wyeth Pharmaceuticals)

1. NAME OF THE MEDICINAL PRODUCT

InductOs 12 mg kit for implant

2. QUALITATIVE AND QUANTITATIVE COMPOSITION

One vial contains 12 mg dibotermin alfa*. After reconstitution, InductOs contains 1.5 mg/ml dibotermin alfa.

*dibotermin alfa (recombinant human Bone Morphogenetic Protein-2; rhBMP-2) is a human protein derived from a recombinant Chinese Hamster Ovary (CHO) cell line.

For a full list of excipients, see section 6.1.

3. PHARMACEUTICAL FORM

Kit for implant.

The kit consists of a white powder for solution, a clear colourless solvent and a white matrix.

4. CLINICAL PARTICULARS

4.1 Therapeutic indications

InductOs is indicated for single-level (L4– S1) anterior lumbar spine fusion as a substitute for autogenous bone graft in adults with degenerative disc disease who have had at least 6 months of non-operative treatment for this condition.

InductOs is indicated for the treatment of acute tibia fractures in adults, as an adjunct to standard care using open fracture reduction and intramedullary unreamed nail fixation.

See section 5.1.

4.2 Posology and method of administration

InductOs should be used by an appropriately qualified surgeon.

The directions for preparation for each kit should be followed exactly using the appropriate amount of InductOs for the intended indication.

InductOs is prepared immediately prior to use from a kit containing all necessary components. Once prepared, InductOs contains dibotermin alfa at a concentration of 1.5 mg/ml (12 mg per vial).

InductOs should not be used in concentrations higher than 1.5 mg/ml (see section 4.9).

There is very limited experience of the efficacy and safety of the medicinal product in the elderly (>65 years of age).

Paediatric use is not recommended until further data become available.

Product preparation

In the non-sterile field

1. Using sterile technique, place one syringe, one needle and the matrix inner package in the sterile field.

2. Disinfect the stoppers of the dibotermin alfa and solvent vials.

3. Using the remaining syringe and needle from the kit, reconstitute the dibotermin alfa vial with 8.4 ml of solvent. Slowly inject the solvent into the vial containing the lyophilised dibotermin alfa. Swirl the vial gently to aid reconstitution. Do not shake. Discard syringe and needle after use.

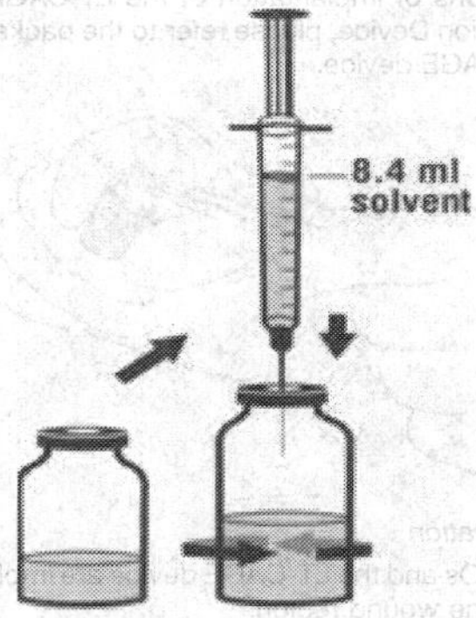

4. Disinfect the stopper of the reconstituted dibotermin alfa vial.

In the sterile field

5. Peel open the interior package of the matrix and leave the matrix in its tray.

6. Using aseptic transfer technique and the syringe and needle from step 1, withdraw 8 ml of the reconstituted dibotermin alfa solution from the vial in the non-sterile field holding up the inverted vial to facilitate withdrawal.

7. Leaving the matrix in its tray, UNIFORMLY distribute the dibotermin alfa solution on the matrix following the pattern in the figure below.

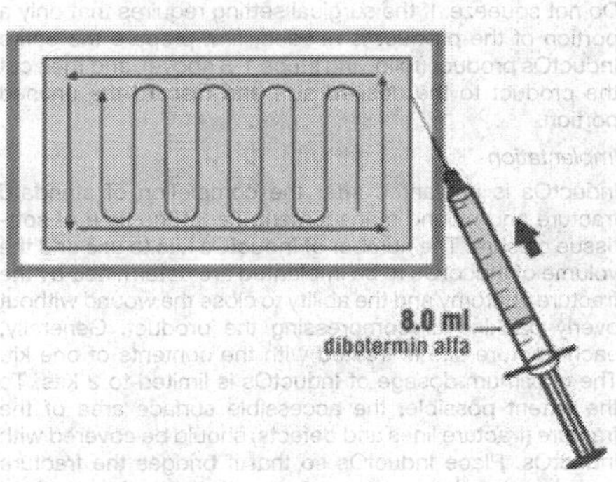

8. Wait a MINIMUM of 15 minutes before using the prepared InductOs product. The product must be used within 2 hours after preparation.

To prevent overloading the matrix, it is important to reconstitute the dibotermin alfa and to wet the entire sponge as described above.

9. Follow instructions relevant to the planned surgery – anterior lumbar spine fusion or acute tibia fracture repair.

Instructions for use in anterior lumbar spine fusion surgery

InductOs should not be used alone for this indication, but must be used with the LT-CAGE Lumbar Tapered Fusion Device.

Failure to follow the product preparation instructions for InductOs may compromise its safety and effectiveness. Care and caution should be used to prevent overfilling of the construct and/or intervertebral space. (see section 4.4)

Pre-Implantation

Cut the wetted matrix of InductOs into 6 equal (approximately 2.5 × 5 cm) pieces. During cutting and handling, avoid excessive fluid loss from InductOs. Do not squeeze.

The number of pieces of InductOs required is determined by the size of the LT-CAGE Lumbar Tapered Fusion Device being used. Using the table below, identify the number of 2.5 × 5 cm pieces of InductOs required for the size of LT-CAGE Lumbar Tapered Fusion Device.

LT-CAGE Lumbar Tapered Fusion Device size (lead diameter × length)	Number of 2.5 × 5 cm pieces of InductOs per LT-CAGE Lumbar Tapered Fusion Device
14 mm × 20 mm	1
14 mm × 23 mm	1
16 mm × 20 mm	1
16 mm × 23 mm	2
16 mm × 26 mm	2
18 mm × 23 mm	2
18 mm × 26 mm	2

Implantation

Using forceps to avoid excessive squeezing, carefully roll the required number of InductOs pieces for each LT-CAGE device and insert each roll into the matching LT-CAGE Lumbar Tapered Fusion Device, as shown in the figure below.

For instructions of implantation of the LT-CAGE Lumbar Tapered Fusion Device, please refer to the package leaflet for the LT-CAGE device.

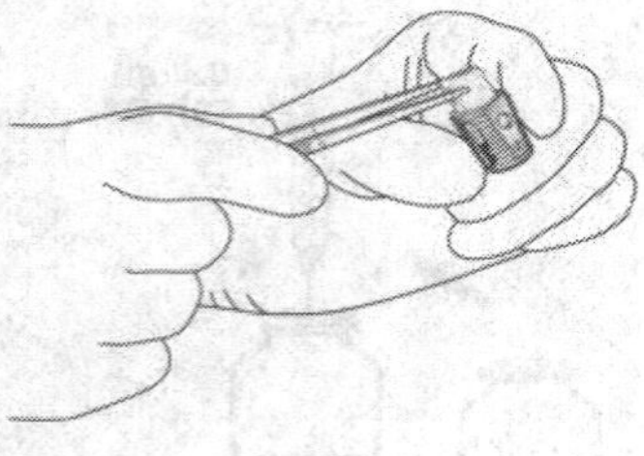

Post-Implantation

Once InductOs and the LT-CAGE device are implanted, do not irrigate the wound region.

If a surgical drain is required, place the drain remote from the implantation site or, preferably, one layer superficial to the implantation site.

Instructions for use in acute tibia fractures

Pre-Implantation

– Achieve definitive fracture reduction, fixation, and hemostasis prior to InductOs implantation.

– InductOs does not provide mechanical stability and should not be used to fill spaces in the presence of compressive forces.

– Fold or cut InductOs as needed prior to implantation. During handling, avoid excessive fluid loss from InductOs. Do not squeeze. If the surgical setting requires that only a portion of the product is needed, first prepare the entire InductOs product (following steps 1-8 above), and then cut the product to the desired size and discard the unused portion.

Implantation

InductOs is implanted after the completion of standard fracture and wound management, i.e. at the time of soft-tissue closure. The number of InductOs kits to use and the volume of InductOs to be implanted are determined by the fracture anatomy and the ability to close the wound without overly packing or compressing the product. Generally, each fracture site is treated with the contents of one kit. The maximum dosage of InductOs is limited to 2 kits. To the extent possible, the accessible surface area of the fracture (fracture lines and defects) should be covered with InductOs. Place InductOs so that it bridges the fracture region and makes good contact with the major proximal and distal fragments. It is not necessary to overlay the contents of multiple kits to achieve the desired effect.

During implantation, use forceps to handle InductOs to avoid excessive loss of fluid.

InductOs may be placed into a void (loosely packed), folded, rolled, or wrapped, as the geometry of the fracture requires. Do not squeeze.

Post-Implantation

Once InductOs is implanted, do not irrigate the wound.

If a surgical drain is required, place the drain remote from the implantation site or, preferably, one layer superficial to the implantation site.

In order to achieve maximum potential efficacy, it is important to achieve complete soft-tissue coverage of InductOs following its implantation.

4.3 Contraindications

InductOs is contraindicated for patients with:

- Hypersensitivity to the active substance or to any of the excipients
- Skeletal immaturity
- Any active malignancy or patient undergoing treatment for a malignancy
- An active infection at the operative site
- Persistent compartment syndrome or neurovascular residua of compartment syndrome
- Pathological fractures such as those observed in (but not limited to) Paget's disease or in metastatic bone

4.4 Special warnings and precautions for use

Failure to follow the product preparation instructions for InductOs may compromise its safety and effectiveness. Care and caution should be used to prevent overfilling of the construct and/or intervertebral space.

Localised oedema associated with the use of InductOs has been reported in patients undergoing cervical spine surgery. The oedema was delayed in onset and, in some cases, severe enough to result in airway compromise. The safety and efficacy of InductOs in cervical spine surgery have not been established and InductOs should not be used in this condition.

Formation of fluid collections (pseudocysts, localised oedema, implant site effusion), sometimes encapsulated, in some cases resulting in nerve compression and pain has been reported in patients undergoing spine surgery associated with the use of InductOs. Many of these reports have occurred when InductOs was used in unapproved approaches/devices or in a manner inconsistent with the instructions for use. Clinical intervention (aspiration and/or surgical removal) may be required if symptoms persist (see section 4.8).

There are no data on the efficacy and safety of the product in concomitant use with bone graft.

In the absence of any experience, the repeated use of the medicinal product is not recommended.

Nerve compression associated with ectopic bone formation and InductOs use has been reported. Additional surgical intervention may be required.

InductOs can cause initial resorption of surrounding trabecular bone. Therefore, in the absence of clinical data, the product should not be used for direct applications to trabecular bone when transient bone resorption may create a risk of bone fragility. When InductOs was used with the LT-CAGE device (section 4.2) in clinical trials for anterior lumbar spine fusion, the frequency and severity of resorption of bone as evidenced by radiolucencies and/or device migration was similar to that observed for patients treated with autogenous bone graft.

Use of InductOs may cause heterotopic ossification in the surrounding tissues, which can result in complications. Exuberant bone formation at the site of implantation and ectopic bone formation have been observed.

The safety and efficacy of the use of InductOs in patients with known autoimmune disease have not been established. These autoimmune diseases include rheumatoid arthritis, systemic lupus erythematosus, scleroderma, Sjögren's syndrome and dermatomyositis/polymyositis.

The safety and efficacy of InductOs have not been demonstrated in patients with metabolic bone diseases.

No studies have been performed in patients with hepatic or renal impairment.

Both dibotermin alfa and bovine Type I collagen have been found to elicit immune responses in patients.

Anti-dibotermin alfa antibodies: In anterior lumbar spine fusion studies, 0.7% of patients receiving InductOs developed antibodies vs 0.8% of patients receiving autogenous bone graft. In acute tibia fracture studies, 4.4% of patients receiving InductOs developed antibodies vs 0.6% in the control group.

Anti-bovine Type I collagen antibodies: In anterior lumbar spine fusion studies, 19% of patients receiving InductOs developed antibodies to bovine Type I collagen vs. 13% of patients receiving autogenous bone graft. In acute tibia fracture studies,15.7% of patients receiving InductOs developed antibodies to bovine Type I collagen vs. 11.8% of control patients. In either of the 2 indications, no patients who tested positive for anti-bovine Type I collagen antibodies developed antibodies to human Type I collagen.

Although no clear association with clinical outcome or undesirable effects could be observed in clinical studies, the possibility of developing neutralising antibodies or hypersensitivity-type reactions cannot be excluded. Special consideration of risks and benefits should be given for patients who have previously received injectable collagen (see section 4.3). The possibility of an immune response to the product should be evaluated in cases where an undesirable effect with immunological background is suspected.

Special warnings and precautions for use specific to anterior lumbar spine fusion

The safety and efficacy of InductOs have not been established in the following conditions:

- used with spinal implants other than the LT-CAGE device
- implanted at locations other than L4 –S1 in the lower lumbar spine
- used in surgical techniques other than anterior open or anterior laparoscopic approaches

When degenerative disc disease was treated by a posterior lumbar interbody fusion procedure with cylindrical threaded cages and dibotermin alfa, posterior bone formation was observed in some instances.

Special warnings and precautions for use specific to acute tibia fractures

InductOs is intended for use in patients with the following:

- adequate fracture reduction and stabilization to ensure mechanical stability
- adequate neurovascular status (e.g. absence of compartment syndrome, low risk of amputation)
- adequate hemostasis (providing a relatively dry implantation site)
- absence of large segmental defect repair of long bones, in which significant soft tissue compression can occur

The implant may only be administered to the fracture site under adequate vision and with utmost care (see section 4.2).

Efficacy information in tibia fracture is available only from controlled clinical trials in which open tibial fractures were treated using intramedullary nail fixation (see section 5.1). In a clinical study in which the intramedullary canal was reamed to cortical chatter, an increased rate of infection was observed in the InductOs-treated group versus the standard of care control group (see section 4.8). The use of InductOs with reamed nails in open tibial fracture repair is not recommended.

InductOs does not provide mechanical stability and should not be used to fill space in the presence of compressive forces. Long-bone fracture and soft-tissue management procedures should be based on standard practice, including control of infection.

4.5 Interaction with other medicinal products and other forms of interaction

No interaction studies have been performed. As dibotermin alfa is a protein and has not been identified in the general circulation, it is an unlikely candidate for pharmacokinetic drug-drug interactions.

Information from clinical studies in acute tibia fractures, indicated that the use of InductOs in patients receiving glucocorticoids was not associated with any apparent adverse effect. In preclinical studies, concurrent administration of glucocorticoids depressed bone repair (measured as a % change from control), but the effects of InductOs were not altered.

In acute tibia fracture clinical trials, more InductOs patients receiving concomitant NSAIDs for 14 consecutive days experienced mild or moderate adverse events related to wound healing (e.g. wound drainage) than InductOs patients not taking NSAIDs. Although patient outcome was not affected, an interaction between NSAIDs and InductOs cannot be excluded.

4.6 Pregnancy and lactation

Pregnancy

There are no adequate data from the use of dibotermin alfa in pregnant women.

Studies in animals have shown reproductive toxicity (see section 5.3). The potential risk for humans is unknown.

Animal studies have been conducted that cannot rule out effects of anti-dibotermin alfa antibodies on embryo-foetal development (see section 5.3). Due to the unknown risks to the fetus associated with the potential development of neutralising antibodies to dibotermin alfa, InductOs should not be used during pregnancy unless clearly necessary (see section 4.4). Women of childbearing potential should be advised to use effective contraception up to at least 12 months after treatment.

Lactation

It is unknown whether dibotermin alfa is excreted in human breast milk. The excretion of dibotermin alfa has not been studied in animals. Lactation is not recommended during treatment with InductOs.

4.7 Effects on ability to drive and use machines

No studies on the effects on the ability to drive and use machines have been performed, but since InductOs has no systemic effect, it is not likely to interfere with the ability to drive or use machinery.

4.8 Undesirable effects

Over 1490 patients have been evaluated in clinical studies, of which more than 955 received InductOs treatment. In the long bone fracture studies, over 418 patients received InductOs. In the anterior lumbar spine fusion studies, over 288 patients received InductOs.

There have been post-marketing reports of localised oedema in patients undergoing cervical spine surgery associated with the use of InductOs. The oedema was delayed in onset and, in some cases, severe enough to result in airway compromise (see section 4.4).

There have been post-marketing reports of formation of fluid collections (pseudocysts, localised oedema, implant site effusion), sometimes encapsulated, in some cases resulting in nerve compression and pain in patients undergoing spine surgery with Inductos (see section 4.4).

Nerve compression associated with ectopic bone formation has been reported in patients undergoing spine surgery with InductOs (see section 4.4).

Placement of InductOs can cause initial resorption of trabecular bone (see section 4.4 and section 5.1).

Undesirable effects specific to use in anterior lumbar spine fusion

The undesirable effects observed in anterior lumbar spine fusion patients were generally representative of the morbidity associated with spine fusion using autogenous bone graft taken from the iliac crest.

Very common (≥1/10) undesirable effects: accidental injury, neuralgia, back pain and bone disorder, were similar in both control and InductOs treatment groups.

Undesirable effects specific to use in acute tibia fractures

The undesirable effects observed in long bone fracture patients were generally representative of the morbidity associated with either orthopaedic trauma or the surgical procedure.

Localised infection specific to the fractured limb occurred in >1/10 patients in a clinical study in which the intramedullary canal was reamed to cortical chatter. An increased rate of infection was observed in the InductOs-treated group versus the standard of care control group (19% versus 9%, respectively; see section 4.4) For use with unreamed nails, estimated rates of infection were similar between treatment groups in a study (21% versus 23% respectively).

Common (≥1/100 to <1/10) undesirable effects were observed with equal incidence in control and InductOs treatment groups, with the following four exceptions which were observed significantly more frequently in the InductOs treatment group than in the control group:

- blood amylase increased (without overt signs of pancreatitis in InductOs treated patients),
- tachycardia,
- hypomagnesemia,
- headache.

4.9 Overdose

Use of InductOs in patients undergoing cervical spine surgery in concentrations or amounts greater than those recommended in section 4.2 for the approved indications has been associated with reports of localised oedema (see section 4.4).

In the case of patients receiving concentrations or amounts greater than those recommended, treatment should be supportive.

5. PHARMACOLOGICAL PROPERTIES

5.1 Pharmacodynamic properties

Pharmacotherapeutic group: Bone Morphogenetic Proteins, ATC code: M05BC01

Dibotermin alfa is an osteoinductive protein that results in the induction of new bone tissue at the site of implantation. Dibotermin alfa binds to receptors on the surface of mesenchymal cells and causes cells to differentiate into cartilage- and bone-forming cells. The differentiated cells form trabecular bone as the matrix is degraded, with vascular invasion evident at the same time. The bone formation process develops from the outside of the implant towards the center until the entire InductOs implant is replaced by trabecular bone.

Remodeling of the surrounding trabecular bone occurs in a manner that is consistent with the biomechanical forces placed on it. Placement of InductOs into trabecular bone resulted in transient resorption of the bone surrounding the implant, followed by replacement with new, more dense bone. The ability of InductOs to support bone remodeling may be responsible for the biological and biomechanical integration of the new bone induced by InductOs with that of the surrounding bone. Radiographic, biomechanical, and histologic evaluation of the induced bone indicates that it functions biologically and biomechanically as native bone. Furthermore, preclinical studies have indicated that the bone induced by InductOs, if fractured, can repair itself in a manner indistinguishable from native bone.

Preclinical studies have suggested that bone formation initiated by InductOs is a self-limiting process, forming a well-defined volume of bone. This self-limitation is likely due to the loss of dibotermin alfa from the implant site, as well as the presence of BMP inhibitors in the surrounding tissues. In addition, several preclinical studies indicate that there is a negative feedback mechanism at the molecular level that limits bone induction by BMPs.

Clinical pharmacology studies demonstrate that the matrix alone is not osteoinductive and is no longer present in biopsies taken as early as 16 weeks post-implantation.

Pharmacodynamic information specific to anterior lumbar spine fusion studies

The efficacy and safety of InductOs were demonstrated in a randomised, controlled, multicenter, non-inferiority study of 279 patients aged 19 – 78 years undergoing an open anterior lumbar interbody fusion procedure. Patients had received at least six months of non-operative treatment prior to treatment with InductOs for anterior lumbar spine fusion. Patients were randomised to receive the LT-CAGE Lumbar Tapered Fusion Device filled with either InductOs or autogenous bone graft taken from the iliac crest.

At 24 months post-operation, InductOs was demonstrated to be statistically non-inferior to autogenous bone graft. The success rate for radiologically determined fusion was 94.4% for InductOs versus 88.9% (95% two-sided CI of the difference: -1.53, 12.46) for autogenous bone graft. For pain and disability (Oswestry score), the success rate was 72.9% versus 72.5% (95% two-sided CI of the difference: -11.2, 12.0). A single, multi-component endpoint, known as overall success was the primary variable of the study. Overall success consists of the following primary efficacy and safety considerations:

1. Radiographically demonstrated fusion
2. Oswestry pain/disability improvement
3. Maintenance or improvement in neurological status
4. No Grade 3 or 4 adverse event classified as implant-associated or implant-/surgical procedure associated
5. No additional surgical procedure performed that was classified as a "failure"

At 24 months post-operation, the overall success rate was 57.5% for InductOs versus 55.8% (95% two-sided CI of the difference: -10.72, 14.01) for autogenous bone graft.

An additional, non-comparative study of 134 patients who received anterior lumbar interbody fusion procedures via a laparoscopic surgical technique yielded similar success rates of 92.9% for fusion, 85.6% for pain and disability and 90.3% for neurological status. The study confirmed the applicability of anterior lumbar spine fusion using InductOs via laparoscopic surgical implantation techniques.

Pharmacodynamic information specific to acute tibia fracture studies

The efficacy of InductOs was demonstrated in a multinational, randomized, controlled, single-blind study of 450 patients (age range 18 to 87 years; 81% male) with open tibial shaft fractures requiring surgical management. Patients received (in a 1:1:1 ratio) standard care (control group) consisting of intramedullary (IM) nail fixation and routine soft tissue management, standard care plus InductOs 0.75 mg/ml, or standard care plus InductOs 1.5 mg/ml. Patients were followed for 12 months after soft-tissue closure.

In the acute tibia fracture pivotal trial, InductOs increased the probability of fracture healing; patients treated with InductOs 1.5 mg/ml had a 44% reduced risk for treatment failure (secondary intervention to promote fracture healing) compared with patients in the standard-care group (RR = 0.56; 95% CI = 0.40 to 0.78). These results were independently corroborated by a radiology panel blinded to treatment. The number of secondary and subsequent interventions was significantly reduced for the InductOs patients, particularly with regard to more invasive interventions such as bone graft and exchange nailing (P=0.0326).

The proportion of patients healed after treatment with InductOs 1.5 mg/ml was significantly higher at all visits from 10 weeks to 12 months post-operative, suggesting accelerated fracture healing.

InductOs 1.5 mg/ml was significantly effective (compared to standard care) in patients both with or without a history of smoking.

Severity of fractures: Treatment with InductOs 1.5 mg/ml was significantly effective in all fracture classes, including severe Gustilo IIIB fractures (52% reduced risk of secondary interventions as compared to standard-care patients).

The proportion of patients with healed soft-tissue wounds was significantly higher at the 6-week post-treatment visit in the InductOs 1.5 mg/ml group compared with the standard-care group (83% vs. 65%; P=0.0010). The proportion of patients with hardware failure (locking screws bent or broken) was significantly lower in the InductOs 1.5 mg/ml group as compared to standard-care group (11% vs. 22%; P=0.0174).

5.2 Pharmacokinetic properties

InductOs is active at the site of implantation. In two exploratory studies, pre- and post-surgery serum samples were collected from a few long-bone fracture patients. Dibotermin alfa was not detectable in serum.

In animal studies (rats) using InductOs containing radiolabelled dibotermin alfa, the mean residence time at the site of implantation was 4-8 days. Peak levels of circulating dibotermin alfa (0.1% of the implanted dose) were observed within 6 hours following implantation. When injected intravenously, the terminal half-life of dibotermin alfa was 16 minutes in rats and 6.7 minutes in cynomolgus monkeys. It is concluded therefore that at the site of implantation dibotermin alfa is slowly released from the matrix and rapidly cleared when taken up into the systemic circulation.

5.3 Preclinical safety data

Non-clinical data reveal no special hazard for humans on conventional studies of pharmacology, acute and repeat exposure toxicity.

In reproductive toxicity studies in rats, where dibotermin alfa was administered intravenously to maximize systemic exposure, increased fetal weight and increased fetal ossification was observed and a treatment related effect could not be ruled out. The clinical relevance of these effects is unknown.

Anti-dibotermin antibodies have been investigated in pregnant rabbits following hyper-immunisation with dibotermin alfa to experimentally induce anti-BMP-2 antibodies. In some fetuses with decreased body weights there were decreases in ossification of frontal and parietal bones (4 out of 151 fetuses), which is generally considered to be reversible, and antibody related effects could not be ruled out. There were no other alterations in fetal external, visceral, or skeletal morphology. Other animal studies do not indicate direct or indirect harmful effects with respect to pregnancy, maternal toxicity, embryolethality, or fetotoxicity.

InductOs has not been tested for in vivo carcinogenicity. Dibotermin alfa has demonstrated variable effects on human tumour cell lines in vitro. Although the available in vitro data suggest a low potential for promotion of tumour growth, the use of InductOs is contraindicated in patients with an active malignancy or in patients undergoing treatment for a malignancy (see also section 4.3).

InductOs has been studied in a canine spinal implantation model. InductOs was implanted directly onto the exposed dura following a laminectomy. Although narrowing of the neuroforamen and stenosis was observed, no mineralization of the dura, no spinal cord stenosis, and no neurological deficits subsequent to the application of InductOs were observed. The significance of these data for humans is not known.

6. PHARMACEUTICAL PARTICULARS

6.1 List of excipients

Powder:

Sucrose

Glycine

Glutamic acid

Sodium chloride

Polysorbate 80

Sodium hydroxide

Solvent:

Water for injections

Matrix:

Bovine Type I collagen

6.2 Incompatibilities

This medicinal product must not be mixed with other medicinal products except those mentioned in section 6.6.

6.3 Shelf life

3 years

6.4 Special precautions for storage

Do not store above 30° C. Do not freeze.

Store in the original package.

6.5 Nature and contents of container

Each kit of InductOs is provided with:

- 12 mg of sterile dibotermin alfa powder in a 20 ml vial (Type I glass) stoppered with a bromobutyl rubber closure sealed with an aluminum flip-off seal and plastic cap.
- Solvent for reconstitution in a 10 ml vial (Type I glass) stoppered with a bromobutyl rubber closure sealed with an aluminum flip-off seal and plastic cap.
- One sterile matrix in a polyvinyl chloride (PVC) blister package sealed with a Tyvek lid.
- Two sterile 10 ml disposable polypropylene syringes.
- Two sterile needles (stainless steel).

6.6 Special precautions for disposal and other handling

Any unused product or waste material should be disposed of in accordance with local requirements.

Dibotermin alfa must be used only with the accompanying solvent and matrix provided in the InductOs kit. See section 4.2.

7. MARKETING AUTHORISATION HOLDER

Wyeth Europa Ltd.

Huntercombe Lane South

Taplow, Maidenhead

Berkshire, SL6 0PH

United Kingdom

8. MARKETING AUTHORISATION NUMBER(S)

EU/1/02/226/001

9. DATE OF FIRST AUTHORISATION/RENEWAL OF THE AUTHORISATION

Date of first authorisation: 9 September 2002

Date of latest renewal: 9 September 2007

10. DATE OF REVISION OF THE TEXT

19 June 2008

Detailed information on this product is available on the website of the European Medicines Agency (EMEA) http://www.emea.europa.eu

INEGY Tablets

(MSD-SP LTD)

1. NAME OF THE MEDICINAL PRODUCT

INEGY®▼ 10 mg/20 mg, 10 mg/40 mg, or 10 mg/80 mg Tablets

2. QUALITATIVE AND QUANTITATIVE COMPOSITION

Each tablet contains 10 mg ezetimibe and 20, 40 or 80 mg of simvastatin.

For a full list of excipients, see section 6.1.

3. PHARMACEUTICAL FORM

Tablet.

White to off-white capsule-shaped tablets with code "312", "313", or "315" on one side.

4. CLINICAL PARTICULARS

4.1 Therapeutic indications

Hypercholesterolaemia

INEGY is indicated as adjunctive therapy to diet for use in patients with primary (heterozygous familial and non-familial) hypercholesterolaemia or mixed hyperlipidaemia where use of a combination product is appropriate:

- patients not appropriately controlled with a statin alone
- patients already treated with a statin and ezetimibe

INEGY contains ezetimibe and simvastatin. Simvastatin (20-40 mg) has been shown to reduce the frequency of cardiovascular events (see section 5.1). Studies to demonstrate the efficacy of INEGY or ezetimibe in the prevention of complications of atherosclerosis have not been completed.

Homozygous Familial Hypercholesterolaemia (HoFH)

INEGY is indicated as adjunctive therapy to diet for use in patients with HoFH. Patients may also receive adjunctive treatments (e.g., low-density lipoprotein [LDL] apheresis).

4.2 Posology and method of administration

Hypercholesterolaemia

The patient should be on an appropriate lipid-lowering diet and should continue on this diet during treatment with INEGY.

Route of administration is oral. The dosage range of INEGY is 10/10 mg/day through 10/80 mg/day in the evening. All dosages may not be available in all member states. The typical dose is 10/20 mg/day or 10/40 mg/day given as a single dose in the evening. The 10/80 mg dose is only recommended in patients with severe hypercholesterolaemia and high risk for cardiovascular complications. The patient's low-density lipoprotein cholesterol (LDL-C) level, coronary heart disease risk status, and response to current cholesterol-lowering therapy should be considered when starting therapy or adjusting the dose.

The dose of INEGY should be individualised based on the known efficacy of the various dose strengths of INEGY (see section 5.1, Table 1) and the response to the current cholesterol-lowering therapy. Adjustments of dosage, if required, should be made at intervals of not less than 4 weeks. INEGY can be administered with or without food.

Homozygous Familial Hypercholesterolaemia

The recommended dosage for patients with homozygous familial hypercholesterolaemia is INEGY 10/40 mg/day or 10/80 mg/day in the evening. INEGY may be used as an adjunct to other lipid-lowering treatments (e.g., LDL apheresis) in these patients or if such treatments are unavailable.

Coadministration with other medicines

Dosing of INEGY should occur either ⩾2 hours before or ⩾4 hours after administration of a bile acid sequestrant.

In patients taking amiodarone or verapamil concomitantly with INEGY, the dose of INEGY should not exceed 10/20 mg/day (see sections 4.4 and 4.5).

In patients taking ciclosporin, danazol or lipid-lowering doses (⩾1 g/day) of niacin concomitantly with INEGY, the dose of INEGY should not exceed 10/10 mg/day (see sections 4.4 and 4.5).

Use in the Elderly

No dosage adjustment is required for elderly patients (see section 5.2).

Use in Children and adolescents

INEGY is not recommended for use in children due to a lack of data on safety and efficacy (see section 5.2).

Use in Hepatic Impairment

No dosage adjustment is required in patients with mild hepatic insufficiency (Child Pugh score 5 to 6). Treatment with INEGY is not recommended in patients with moderate (Child Pugh score 7 to 9) or severe (Child Pugh score >9) liver dysfunction. (See sections 4.4 and 5.2.)

Use in Renal Impairment

No modification of dosage should be necessary in patients with moderate renal insufficiency. If treatment in patients with severe renal insufficiency (creatinine clearance ⩽30 ml/min) is deemed necessary, dosages above 10/10 mg/day should be implemented cautiously (see section 5.2).

4.3 Contraindications

Hypersensitivity to ezetimibe, simvastatin, or to any of the excipients.

Pregnancy and lactation (see section 4.6).

Active liver disease or unexplained persistent elevations in serum transaminases.

Concomitant administration of potent CYP3A4 inhibitors (e.g., itraconazole, ketoconazole, erythromycin, clarithromycin, telithromycin, HIV protease inhibitors and nefazodone) (see sections 4.4 and 4.5).

4.4 Special warnings and precautions for use

Myopathy/Rhabdomyolysis

In post-marketing experience with ezetimibe, cases of myopathy and rhabdomyolysis have been reported. Most patients who developed rhabdomyolysis were taking a statin concomitantly with ezetimibe. However, rhabdomyolysis has been reported very rarely with ezetimibe monotherapy and very rarely with the addition of ezetimibe to other agents known to be associated with increased risk of rhabdomyolysis.

INEGY contains simvastatin. Simvastatin, like other inhibitors of HMG-CoA reductase, occasionally causes myopathy manifested as muscle pain, tenderness or weakness with creatine kinase (CK) above 10X the upper limit of normal (ULN). Myopathy sometimes takes the form of rhabdomyolysis with or without acute renal failure secondary to myoglobinuria, and very rare fatalities have occurred. The risk of myopathy is increased by high levels of HMG-CoA reductase inhibitory activity in plasma.

As with other HMG-CoA reductase inhibitors, the risk of myopathy/rhabdomyolysis is dose related for simvastatin. In a clinical trial database in which 41,050 patients were treated with simvastatin with 24,747 (approximately 60%) treated for at least 4 years, the incidence of myopathy was approximately 0.02%, 0.08% and 0.53% at 20, 40 and 80 mg/day, respectively. In these trials, patients were carefully monitored and some interacting medicinal products were excluded.

<u>Creatine Kinase measurement</u>

Creatine Kinase (CK) should not be measured following strenuous exercise or in the presence of any plausible alternative cause of CK increase as this makes value interpretation difficult. If CK levels are significantly elevated at baseline (>5 X ULN), levels should be re-measured within 5 to 7 days later to confirm the results.

<u>Before the treatment</u>

All patients starting therapy with INEGY, or whose dose of INEGY is being increased, should be advised of the risk of myopathy and told to report promptly any unexplained muscle pain, tenderness or weakness.

Caution should be exercised in patients with pre-disposing factors for rhabdomyolysis. In order to establish a reference baseline value, a CK level should be measured before starting treatment in the following situations:

- Elderly (age >70 years)
- Renal impairment
- Uncontrolled hypothyroidism
- Personal or familial history of hereditary muscular disorders
- Previous history of muscular toxicity with a statin or fibrate
- Alcohol abuse.

In such situations, the risk of treatment should be considered in relation to possible benefit, and clinical monitoring is recommended. If a patient has previously experienced a muscle disorder on a fibrate or a statin, treatment with any statin-containing product (such as INEGY) should only be initiated with caution. If CK levels are significantly elevated at baseline (>5 X ULN), treatment should not be started.

<u>Whilst on treatment</u>

If muscle pain, weakness or cramps occur whilst a patient is receiving treatment with INEGY, their CK levels should be measured. If these levels are found, in the absence of strenuous exercise, to be significantly elevated (>5 X ULN), treatment should be stopped. If muscular symptoms are severe and cause daily discomfort, even if CK levels are <5 X ULN, treatment discontinuation may be considered. If myopathy is suspected for any other reason, treatment should be discontinued.

If symptoms resolve and CK levels return to normal, then re-introduction of INEGY or introduction of another statin-containing product may be considered at the lowest dose and with close monitoring.

Therapy with INEGY should be temporarily stopped a few days prior to elective major surgery and when any major medical or surgical condition supervenes.

<u>Measures to reduce the risk of myopathy caused by medicinal product interactions (see also section 4.5)</u>

The risk of myopathy and rhabdomyolysis is significantly increased by concomitant use of INEGY with potent inhibitors of CYP3A4 (such as itraconazole, ketoconazole, erythromycin, clarithromycin, telithromycin, HIV protease inhibitors, nefazodone), as well as ciclosporin, danazol and gemfibrozil (see section 4.2).

Due to the simvastatin component of INEGY, the risk of myopathy and rhabdomyolysis is also increased by concomitant use of other fibrates, lipid-lowering doses (⩾1 g/day) of niacin or by concomitant use of amiodarone or verapamil with higher doses of INEGY (see sections 4.2 and 4.5). There is also a slight increase in risk when diltiazem is used with INEGY 10 mg/80 mg. The risk of myopathy including rhabdomyolysis may be increased by concomitant administration of fusidic acid with INEGY (see section 4.5).

Consequently, regarding CYP3A4 inhibitors, the use of INEGY concomitantly with itraconazole, ketoconazole, HIV protease inhibitors, erythromycin, clarithromycin, telithromycin, and nefazodone is contraindicated (see sections 4.3 and 4.5). If treatment with itraconazole, ketoconazole, erythromycin, clarithromycin or telithromycin is unavoidable, therapy with INEGY must be suspended during the course of treatment. Moreover, caution should be exercised when combining INEGY with certain other less potent CYP3A4 inhibitors: ciclosporin, verapamil, diltiazem (see sections 4.2 and 4.5). Concomitant intake of grapefruit juice and INEGY should be avoided.

The dose of INEGY should not exceed 10/10 mg daily in patients receiving concomitant medication with ciclosporin, danazol or lipid-lowering doses (⩾ 1 g/day) of niacin. The benefits of the combined use of INEGY 10 mg/10 mg daily with ciclosporin, danazol or niacin should be carefully weighed against the potential risks of these combinations. (See sections 4.2 and 4.5.)

The combined use of INEGY at doses higher than 10/20 mg daily with amiodarone or verapamil should be avoided unless the clinical benefit is likely to outweigh the increased risk of myopathy (see sections 4.2 and 4.5).

The safety and efficacy of INEGY administered with fibrates have not been studied. There is an increased risk of myopathy when simvastatin is used concomitantly with fibrates (especially gemfibrozil). Therefore, the concomitant use of INEGY with fibrates is not recommended. (See section 4.5.)

Patients on fusidic acid and INEGY should be closely monitored (see section 4.5). Temporary suspension of INEGY treatment may be considered.

Liver Enzymes

In controlled coadministration trials in patients receiving ezetimibe with simvastatin, consecutive transaminase elevations (⩾3 X ULN) have been observed (see section 4.8).

It is recommended that liver function tests be performed before treatment with INEGY begins and thereafter when clinically indicated. Patients titrated to the 10/80-mg dose should receive an additional test prior to titration, 3 months after titration to the 10/80-mg dose, and periodically thereafter (e.g., semiannually) for the first year of treatment. Special attention should be paid to patients who develop elevated serum transaminase levels, and in these patients, measurements should be repeated promptly and then performed more frequently. If the transaminase levels show evidence of progression, particularly if they rise to 3 X ULN and are persistent, the drug should be discontinued.

INEGY should be used with caution in patients who consume substantial quantities of alcohol.

Hepatic Insufficiency

Due to the unknown effects of the increased exposure to ezetimibe in patients with moderate or severe hepatic insufficiency, INEGY is not recommended (see section 5.2).

Fibrates

The safety and efficacy of ezetimibe administered with fibrates have not been established; therefore, coadministration of INEGY and fibrates is not recommended (see section 4.5).

Ciclosporin

Caution should be exercised when initiating INEGY in the setting of ciclosporin. Ciclosporin concentrations should be monitored in patients receiving INEGY and ciclosporin (see section 4.5).

Anticoagulants

If INEGY is added to warfarin, another coumarin anticoagulant, or fluindione, the International Normalised Ratio (INR) should be appropriately monitored (see section 4.5).

Excipient

Patients with rare hereditary problems of galactose intolerance, the Lapp lactase deficiency or glucose-galactose malabsorption should not take this medicine.

4.5 Interaction with other medicinal products and other forms of interaction

<u>Pharmacodynamic interactions</u>

Interactions with lipid-lowering medicinal products that can cause myopathy when given alone

The risk of myopathy, including rhabdomyolysis, is increased during concomitant administration of simvastatin with fibrates and niacin (nicotinic acid) (⩾1 g/day). Additionally, there is a pharmacokinetic interaction of simvastatin with gemfibrozil resulting in increased simvastatin plasma levels (see below *Pharmacokinetic interactions*).

Fibrates may increase cholesterol excretion into the bile, leading to cholelithiasis. In a preclinical study in dogs, ezetimibe increased cholesterol in the gallbladder bile (see section 5.3). Although the relevance of this preclinical finding to humans is unknown, coadministration of INEGY with fibrates is not recommended (see section 4.4).

<u>Pharmacokinetic interactions</u>

Prescribing recommendations for interacting agents are summarised in the table below (further details are provided in the text; see also sections 4.2, 4.3, and 4.4).

Drug Interactions Associated with Increased Risk of Myopathy/Rhabdomyolysis	
Interacting agents	**Prescribing recommendations**
Potent CYP3A4 inhibitors: Itraconazole Ketoconazole Erythromycin Clarithromycin Telithromycin HIV protease inhibitors Nefazodone	**Contraindicated with INEGY**
Fibrates	Not recommended with INEGY
Ciclosporin Danazol Niacin (≥1 g/day)	Do not exceed 10/10 mg INEGY daily
Amiodarone Verapamil	Do not exceed 10/20 mg INEGY daily
Diltiazem	Do not exceed 10/40 mg INEGY daily
Fusidic acid	Patients should be closely monitored. Temporary suspension of INEGY treatment may be considered.
Grapefruit juice	Avoid grapefruit juice when taking INEGY

Effects of other medicinal products on INEGY

Ezetimibe

Antacids: Concomitant antacid administration decreased the rate of absorption of ezetimibe but had no effect on the bioavailability of ezetimibe. This decreased rate of absorption is not considered clinically significant.

Colestyramine: Concomitant colestyramine administration decreased the mean area under the curve (AUC) of total ezetimibe (ezetimibe + ezetimibe glucuronide) approximately 55%. The incremental LDL-C reduction due to adding INEGY to colestyramine may be lessened by this interaction (see section 4.2).

Ciclosporin: In a study of eight post-renal transplant patients with creatinine clearance of >50 ml/min on a stable dose of ciclosporin, a single 10-mg dose of ezetimibe resulted in a 3.4-fold (range 2.3- to 7.9-fold) increase in the mean AUC for total ezetimibe compared to a healthy control population, receiving ezetimibe alone, from another study (n=17). In a different study, a renal transplant patient with severe renal insufficiency who was receiving ciclosporin and multiple other medications, demonstrated a 12-fold greater exposure to total ezetimibe compared to concurrent controls receiving ezetimibe alone. In a two-period crossover study in twelve healthy subjects, daily administration of 20 mg ezetimibe for 8 days with a single 100-mg dose of ciclosporin on Day 7 resulted in a mean 15% increase in ciclosporin AUC (range 10% decrease to 51% increase) compared to a single 100-mg dose of ciclosporin alone. A controlled study on the effect of coadministered ezetimibe on ciclosporin exposure in renal transplant patients has not been conducted. Caution should be exercised when initiating INEGY in the setting of ciclosporin. Ciclosporin concentrations should be monitored in patients receiving INEGY and ciclosporin (see section 4.4).

Fibrates: Concomitant fenofibrate or gemfibrozil administration increased total ezetimibe concentrations approximately 1.5- and 1.7-fold, respectively. Although these increases are not considered clinically significant, coadministration of INEGY with fibrates is not recommended (see section 4.4).

Simvastatin

Simvastatin is a substrate of cytochrome P450 3A4. Potent inhibitors of cytochrome P450 3A4 increase the risk of myopathy and rhabdomyolysis by increasing the concentration of HMG-CoA reductase inhibitory activity in plasma during simvastatin therapy. Such inhibitors include itraconazole, ketoconazole, erythromycin, clarithromycin, telithromycin, HIV protease inhibitors, and nefazodone. Concomitant administration of itraconazole resulted in a more than 10-fold increase in exposure to simvastatin acid (the active beta-hydroxyacid metabolite). Telithromycin caused an 11-fold increase in exposure to simvastatin acid.

Therefore, combination with itraconazole, ketoconazole, HIV protease inhibitors, erythromycin, clarithromycin, telithromycin, and nefazodone is contraindicated. If treatment with itraconazole, ketoconazole, erythromycin, clarithromycin or telithromycin is unavoidable, therapy with INEGY must be suspended during the course of treatment. Caution should be exercised when combining INEGY with certain other less potent CYP3A4 inhibitors: ciclosporin, verapamil, diltiazem (see sections 4.2 and 4.4).

Ciclosporin: The risk of myopathy/rhabdomyolysis is increased by concomitant administration of ciclosporin particularly with higher doses of INEGY (see sections 4.2 and 4.4). Therefore, the dose of INEGY should not exceed 10/10 mg daily in patients receiving concomitant medication with ciclosporin. Although the mechanism is not fully understood, ciclosporin has been shown to increase the AUC of HMG-CoA reductase inhibitors. The increase in AUC for simvastatin acid is presumably due, in part, to inhibition of CYP3A4.

Danazol: The risk of myopathy and rhabdomyolysis is increased by concomitant administration of danazol with higher doses of INEGY (see section 4.2 and section 4.4).

Gemfibrozil: Gemfibrozil increases the AUC of simvastatin acid by 1.9-fold, possibly due to inhibition of the glucuronidation pathway.

Amiodarone and verapamil: The risk of myopathy and rhabdomyolysis is increased by concomitant administration of amiodarone or verapamil with higher doses of simvastatin (see section 4.4). In an ongoing clinical trial, myopathy has been reported in 6% of patients receiving simvastatin 80 mg and amiodarone.

An analysis of the available clinical trials showed an approximately 1% incidence of myopathy in patients receiving simvastatin 40 mg or 80 mg and verapamil. In a pharmacokinetic study, concomitant administration of simvastatin with verapamil resulted in 2.3-fold increase in exposure of simvastatin acid, presumably due, in part, to inhibition of CYP3A4. Therefore, the dose of INEGY should not exceed 10/20 mg daily in patients receiving concomitant medication with amiodarone or verapamil, unless the clinical benefit is likely to outweigh the increased risk of myopathy and rhabdomyolysis.

Diltiazem: An analysis of the available clinical trials showed a 1% incidence of myopathy in patients receiving simvastatin 80 mg and diltiazem. The risk of myopathy in patients taking simvastatin 40 mg was not increased by concomitant diltiazem(see section 4.4). In a pharmacokinetic study, concomitant administration of diltiazem with simvastatin caused a 2.7-fold increase in exposure of simvastatin acid, presumably due to inhibition of CYP3A4. Therefore, the dose of INEGY should not exceed 10/40 mg daily in patients receiving concomitant medication with diltiazem, unless the clinical benefit is likely to outweigh the increased risk of myopathy and rhabdomyolysis.

Fusidic acid: The risk of myopathy including rhabdomyolysis may be increased by concomitant administration of fusidic acid with INEGY (see section 4.4). Specific pathways of fusidic acid metabolism in the liver are not known, however, an interaction between fusidic acid and HMG-CoA reductase inhibitors, which are metabolised by CYP-3A4, can be suspected.

Grapefruit juice: Grapefruit juice inhibits cytochrome P450 3A4. Concomitant intake of large quantities (over 1 litre daily) of grapefruit juice and simvastatin resulted in a 7-fold increase in exposure to simvastatin acid. Intake of 240 ml of grapefruit juice in the morning and administration of simvastatin in the evening also resulted in a 1.9-fold increase. Intake of grapefruit juice during treatment with INEGY should therefore be avoided.

Effects of INEGY on the pharmacokinetics of other medicinal products Ezetimibe

In preclinical studies, it has been shown that ezetimibe does not induce cytochrome P450 drug metabolising enzymes. No clinically significant pharmacokinetic interactions have been observed between ezetimibe and drugs known to be metabolised by cytochromes P450 1A2, 2D6, 2C8, 2C9, and 3A4, or N-acetyltransferase.

Anticoagulants: Concomitant administration of ezetimibe (10 mg once daily) had no significant effect on bioavailability of warfarin and prothrombin time in a study of twelve healthy adult males. However, there have been post-marketing reports of increased International Normalised Ratio (INR) in patients who had ezetimibe added to warfarin or fluindione. If INEGY is added to warfarin, another coumarin anticoagulant, or fluindione, INR should be appropriately monitored. (see section 4.4).

Simvastatin

Simvastatin does not have an inhibitory effect on cytochrome P450 3A4. Therefore, simvastatin is not expected to affect plasma concentrations of substances metabolised via cytochrome P450 3A4.

Oral anticoagulants: In two clinical studies, one in normal volunteers and the other in hypercholesterolaemic patients, simvastatin 20-40 mg/day modestly potentiated the effect of coumarin anticoagulants: the prothrombin time, reported as International Normalised Ratio (INR), increased from a baseline of 1.7 to 1.8 and from 2.6 to 3.4 in the volunteer and patient studies, respectively. Very rare cases of elevated INR have been reported. In patients taking coumarin anticoagulants, prothrombin time should be determined before starting INEGY and frequently enough during early therapy to ensure that no significant alteration of prothrombin time occurs. Once a stable prothrombin time has been documented, prothrombin times can be monitored at the intervals usually recommended for patients on coumarin anticoagulants. If the dose of INEGY is changed or discontinued, the same procedure should be repeated. Simvastatin therapy has not been associated with bleeding or with changes in prothrombin time in patients not taking anticoagulants.

4.6 Pregnancy and lactation

Pregnancy:

Atherosclerosis is a chronic process, and ordinarily discontinuation of lipid-lowering drugs during pregnancy should have little impact on the long-term risk associated with primary hypercholesterolaemia.

INEGY

INEGY is contraindicated during pregnancy. No clinical data are available on the use of INEGY during pregnancy. Animal studies on combination therapy have demonstrated reproduction toxicity. (See section 5.3.)

Simvastatin

The safety of simvastatin in pregnant women has not been established. No controlled clinical trials with simvastatin have been conducted in pregnant women. Rare reports of congenital anomalies following intrauterine exposure to HMG-CoA reductase inhibitors have been received. However, in an analysis of approximately 200 prospectively followed pregnancies exposed during the first trimester to simvastatin or another closely related HMG-CoA reductase inhibitor, the incidence of congenital anomalies was comparable to that seen in the general population. This number of pregnancies was statistically sufficient to exclude a 2.5-fold or greater increase in congenital anomalies over the background incidence.

Although there is no evidence that the incidence of congenital anomalies in offspring of patients taking simvastatin or another closely related HMG-CoA reductase inhibitor differs from that observed in the general population, maternal treatment with simvastatin may reduce the foetal levels of mevalonate which is a precursor of cholesterol biosynthesis. For this reason, INEGY should not be used in women who are pregnant, trying to become pregnant or suspect they are pregnant. Treatment with INEGY should be suspended for the duration of pregnancy or until it has been determined that the woman is not pregnant. (See section 4.3.)

Ezetimibe

No clinical data are available on the use of ezetimibe during pregnancy.

Lactation:

INEGY is contraindicated during lactation. Studies on rats have shown that ezetimibe is excreted into breast milk. It is not known if the active components of INEGY are secreted into human breast milk. (See section 4.3.)

4.7 Effects on ability to drive and use machines

No studies on the effects on the ability to drive and use machines have been performed. However, when driving vehicles or operating machines, it should be taken into account that dizziness has been reported.

4.8 Undesirable effects

INEGY (or coadministration of ezetimibe and simvastatin equivalent to INEGY) has been evaluated for safety in more than 3,800 patients in clinical trials.

The frequencies of adverse events are ranked according to the following: Very common (≥ 1/10), Common (≥ 1/100, < 1/10), Uncommon (≥ 1/1000), < 1/100), Rare (≥ 1/10,000, < 1/1000), Very rare (< 1/10,000) including isolated reports.

INEGY

Nervous system disorders:

Common: headache

Gastro-intestinal disorders:

Common: flatulence

Musculoskeletal and connective tissue disorders:

Common: myalgia

Laboratory Values

In coadministration trials, the incidence of clinically important elevations in serum transaminases (ALT and/or AST ≥3 X ULN, consecutive) was 1.7% for patients treated with INEGY. These elevations were generally asymptomatic, not associated with cholestasis, and returned to baseline after discontinuation of therapy or with continued treatment. (See section 4.4.)

Clinically important elevations of CK (≥10 X ULN) were seen in 0.2% of the patients treated with INEGY.

Post-marketing Experience

The following adverse reactions have been reported in post-marketing use with INEGY or during clinical studies or post-marketing use with one of the individual components.

Blood and lymphatic system disorders:

Thrombocytopaenia, anaemia

Nervous system disorders:

Dizziness, paraesthesia, peripheral neuropathy

Gastro-intestinal disorders:

Constipation, abdominal pain, dyspepsia, diarrhoea, nausea, vomiting, pancreatitis

Hepto-biliary disorders:

Hepatitis/jaundice, hepatic failure, cholelithiasis, cholecystitis

Skin and subcutaneous tissue disorders:

Pruritis, alopecia, hypersensitivity reactions, including rash, urticaria, anaphylaxis, angio-oedema

Musculoskeletal, connective tissue disorders:

arthralgia, muscle cramps, myopathy/rhabdomyolysis (see section 4.4)

General disorders and administration site conditions:

asthenia, fatigue

Psychiatric disorders: depression

An apparent hypersensitivity syndrome has been reported rarely which has included some of the following features: angio-oedema, lupus-like syndrome, polymyalgia rheumatica, dermatomyositis, vasculitis, thrombocytopaenia, eosinophilia, red blood cell sedimentation rate increased, arthritis and arthralgia, urticaria, photosensitivity reaction, pyrexia, flushing, dyspnoea and malaise.

Laboratory values

increased transaminases; increased CK, increases in γ-glutamyl transpeptidase, elevated alkaline phosphatase.

4.9 Overdose

INEGY

In the event of an overdose, symptomatic and supportive measures should be employed. Coadministration of ezetimibe (1000 mg/kg) and simvastatin (1000 mg/kg) was well-tolerated in acute, oral toxicity studies in mice and rats. No clinical signs of toxicity were observed in these animals. The estimated oral LD_{50} for both species was ezetimibe ≥1000 mg/kg/simvastatin ≥1000 mg/kg.

Ezetimibe

In clinical studies, administration of ezetimibe, 50 mg/day to 15 healthy subjects for up to 14 days, or 40 mg/day to 18 patients with primary hypercholesterolaemia for up to 56 days, was generally well tolerated. A few cases of overdosage have been reported; most have not been associated with adverse experiences. Reported adverse experiences have not been serious. In animals, no toxicity was observed after single oral doses of 5000 mg/kg of ezetimibe in rats and mice and 3000 mg/kg in dogs.

Simvastatin

A few cases of overdosage have been reported; the maximum dose taken was 3.6 g. All patients recovered without sequelae.

5. PHARMACOLOGICAL PROPERTIES

5.1 Pharmacodynamic properties

Pharmacotherapeutic group: HMG-CoA reductase inhibitors in combination with other lipid modifying agents, ATC code: C10BA02

INEGY (ezetimibe/simvastatin) is a lipid-lowering product that selectively inhibits the intestinal absorption of cholesterol and related plant sterols and inhibits the endogenous synthesis of cholesterol.

Mechanism of action:

INEGY

Plasma cholesterol is derived from intestinal absorption and endogenous synthesis. INEGY contains ezetimibe and simvastatin, two lipid-lowering compounds with complementary mechanisms of action. INEGY reduces elevated total cholesterol (total-C), LDL-C, apolipoprotein B (Apo B), triglycerides (TG), and non-high-density lipoprotein cholesterol (non-HDL-C), and increases high-density lipoprotein cholesterol (HDL-C) through dual inhibition of cholesterol absorption and synthesis.

Ezetimibe

Ezetimibe inhibits the intestinal absorption of cholesterol. Ezetimibe is orally active and has a mechanism of action that differs from other classes of cholesterol-reducing compounds (e.g., statins, bile acid sequestrants [resins], fibric acid derivatives, and plant stanols). The molecular target of ezetimibe is the sterol transporter, Niemann-Pick C1-Like 1 (NPC1L1), which is responsible for the intestinal uptake of cholesterol and phytosterols.

Ezetimibe localises at the brush border of the small intestine and inhibits the absorption of cholesterol, leading to a decrease in the delivery of intestinal cholesterol to the liver; statins reduce cholesterol synthesis in the liver and together these distinct mechanisms provide complementary cholesterol reduction. In a 2-week clinical study in 18 hypercholesterolaemic patients, ezetimibe inhibited intestinal cholesterol absorption by 54%, compared with placebo.

A series of preclinical studies was performed to determine the selectivity of ezetimibe for inhibiting cholesterol absorption. Ezetimibe inhibited the absorption of [^{14}C]-cholesterol with no effect on the absorption of triglycerides, fatty acids, bile acids, progesterone, ethinyl estradiol, or fat soluble vitamins A and D.

Simvastatin

After oral ingestion, simvastatin, which is an inactive lactone, is hydrolysed in the liver to the corresponding active β-hydroxyacid form which has a potent activity in inhibiting HMG-CoA reductase (3 hydroxy - 3 methylglutaryl CoA reductase). This enzyme catalyses the conversion of HMG-CoA to mevalonate, an early and rate-limiting step in the biosynthesis of cholesterol.

Simvastatin has been shown to reduce both normal and elevated LDL-C concentrations. LDL is formed from very-low-density protein (VLDL) and is catabolised predominantly by the high affinity LDL receptor. The mechanism of the LDL-lowering effect of simvastatin may involve both reduction of VLDL-cholesterol (VLDL-C) concentration and induction of the LDL receptor, leading to reduced production and increased catabolism of LDL-C. Apolipoprotein B also falls substantially during treatment with simvastatin. In addition, simvastatin moderately increases HDL-C and reduces plasma TG. As a result of these changes, the ratios of total- to HDL-C and LDL- to HDL-C are reduced.

CLINICAL TRIALS

In controlled clinical studies, INEGY significantly reduced total-C, LDL-C, Apo B, TG, and non-HDL-C, and increased HDL-C in patients with hypercholesterolaemia.

Primary Hypercholesterolaemia

In a double-blind, placebo-controlled, 8-week study, 240 patients with hypercholesterolaemia already receiving simvastatin monotherapy and not at National Cholesterol Education Program (NCEP) LDL-C goal (2.6 to 4.1 mmol/l [100 to 160 mg/dl], depending on baseline characteristics) were randomised to receive either ezetimibe 10 mg or placebo in addition to their on-going simvastatin therapy. Among simvastatin-treated patients not at LDL-C goal at baseline (~80%), significantly more patients randomised to ezetimibe coadministered with simvastatin achieved their LDL-C goal at study endpoint compared to patients randomised to placebo coadministered with simvastatin, 76% and 21.5%, respectively.

The corresponding LDL-C reductions for ezetimibe or placebo coadministered with simvastatin were also significantly different (27% or 3%, respectively). In addition, ezetimibe coadministered with simvastatin significantly decreased total-C, Apo B, and TG compared with placebo coadministered with simvastatin.

In a multicentre, double-blind, 24-week trial, 214 patients with type 2 diabetes mellitus treated with thiazolidinediones (rosiglitazone or pioglitazone) for a minimum of 3 months and simvastatin 20 mg for a minimum of 6 weeks with a mean LDL-C of 2.4 mmol/L (93 mg/dl), were randomised to receive either simvastatin 40 mg or the coadministered active ingredients equivalent to INEGY 10 mg/20 mg. INEGY 10 mg/20 mg was significantly more effective than doubling the dose of simvastatin to 40 mg in further reducing LDL-C (-21% and 0%, respectively), total-C (-14% and -1%, respectively), Apo B (-14% and -2%, respectively), and non-HDL-C (-20% and -2%, respectively) beyond the reductions observed with simvastatin 20 mg. Results for HDL-C and TG between the two treatment groups were not significantly different. Results were not affected by type of thiazolidinedione treatment.

The efficacy of the different dose-strengths of INEGY (10/10 to 10/80 mg/day) was demonstrated in a multicentre, double-blind, placebo-controlled 12-week trial that included all available doses of INEGY and all relevant doses of simvastatin. When patients receiving all doses of INEGY were compared to those receiving all doses of simvastatin, INEGY significantly lowered total-C, LDL-C, and TG (see Table 1) as well as Apo B (-42% and -29%, respectively), non-HDL-C (-49% and -34%, respectively) and C-reactive protein (-33% and -9%, respectively). The effects of INEGY on HDL-C were similar to the effects seen with simvastatin. Further analysis showed INEGY significantly increased HDL-C compared with placebo.

Table 1

Response to INEGY in Patients with Primary Hypercholesterolaemia

(Mean[a] % Change from Untreated Baseline[b])

(see Table 1 below)

In a similarly designed study, results for all lipid parameters were generally consistent. In a pooled analysis of these two studies, the lipid response to INEGY was similar in patients with TG levels greater than or less than 200 mg/dl.

INEGY contains simvastatin. In two large placebo-controlled clinical trials, the Scandinavian Simvastatin Survival Study (20-40 mg; N=4,444 patients) and the Heart Protection Study (40 mg; N=20,536 patients), the effects of treatment with simvastatin were assessed in patients at high risk of coronary events because of existing coronary heart disease, diabetes, peripheral vessel disease, history of stroke or other cerebrovascular disease. Simvastatin was proven to reduce: the risk of total mortality by reducing CHD deaths; the risk of non-fatal myocardial infarction and stroke; and the need for coronary and non-coronary revascularisation procedures.

Studies to demonstrate the efficacy of INEGY in the prevention of complications of atherosclerosis have not been completed.

Homozygous Familial Hypercholesterolaemia (HoFH)

A double-blind, randomised, 12-week study was performed in patients with a clinical and/or genotypic diagnosis of HoFH. Data were analysed from a subgroup of patients (n=14) receiving simvastatin 40 mg at baseline. Increasing the dose of simvastatin from 40 to 80 mg (n=5) produced a reduction of LDL-C of 13% from baseline on simvastatin 40 mg. Coadministered ezetimibe and simvastatin equivalent to INEGY (10 mg/40 mg and 10 mg/80 mg pooled, n=9), produced a reduction of LDL-C of 23% from baseline on simvastatin 40 mg. In those patients coadministered ezetimibe and simvastatin equivalent to INEGY (10 mg/80 mg, n=5), a reduction of LDL-C of 29% from baseline on simvastatin 40 mg was produced.

5.2 Pharmacokinetic properties

No clinically significant pharmacokinetic interaction was seen when ezetimibe was coadministered with simvastatin.

Absorption:

INEGY

INEGY is bioequivalent to coadministered ezetimibe and simvastatin.

Ezetimibe

After oral administration, ezetimibe is rapidly absorbed and extensively conjugated to a pharmacologically active phenolic glucuronide (ezetimibe-glucuronide). Mean maximum plasma concentrations (C_{max}) occur within 1 to 2 hours for ezetimibe-glucuronide and 4 to 12 hours for ezetimibe. The absolute bioavailability of ezetimibe cannot be determined as the compound is virtually insoluble in aqueous media suitable for injection.

Concomitant food administration (high fat or non-fat meals) had no effect on the oral bioavailability of ezetimibe when administered as 10-mg tablets.

Simvastatin

The availability of the active β-hydroxyacid to the systemic circulation following an oral dose of simvastatin was found to be less than 5% of the dose, consistent with extensive

Table 1 Response to INEGY in Patients with Primary Hypercholesterolaemia (Mean[a] % Change from Untreated Baseline[b])

Treatment (Daily Dose)	N	Total-C	LDL-C	HDL-C	TG[a]
Pooled data (All INEGY doses)[c]	353	-38	-53	+8	-28
Pooled data (All simvastatin doses)[c]	349	-26	-38	+8	-15
Ezetimibe10 mg	92	-14	-20	+7	-13
Placebo	93	+2	+3	+2	-2
INEGY by dose					
10/10	87	-32	-46	+9	-21
10/20	86	-37	-51	+8	-31
10/40	89	-39	-55	+9	-32
10/80	91	-43	-61	+6	-28
Simvastatin by dose					
10 mg	81	-21	-31	+5	-4
20 mg	90	-24	-35	+6	-14
40 mg	91	-29	-42	+8	-19
80 mg	87	-32	-46	+11	-26

[a] For triglycerides, median % change from baseline

[b] Baseline - on no lipid-lowering drug

[c] INEGY doses pooled (10/10-10/80) significantly reduced total-C, LDL-C, and TG, compared to simvastatin, and significantly increased HDL-C compared to placebo.

hepatic first-pass extraction. The major metabolites of simvastatin present in human plasma are the β-hydroxyacid and four additional active metabolites.

Relative to the fasting state, the plasma profiles of both active and total inhibitors were not affected when simvastatin was administered immediately before a test meal.

Distribution:

Ezetimibe

Ezetimibe and ezetimibe-glucuronide are bound 99.7% and 88 to 92% to human plasma proteins, respectively.

Simvastatin

Both simvastatin and the β-hydroxyacid are bound to human plasma proteins (95%).

The pharmacokinetics of single and multiple doses of simvastatin showed that no accumulation of drug occurred after multiple dosing. In all of the above pharmacokinetic studies, the maximum plasma concentration of inhibitors occurred 1.3 to 2.4 hours post-dose.

Biotransformation:

Ezetimibe

Ezetimibe is metabolised primarily in the small intestine and liver via glucuronide conjugation (a phase II reaction) with subsequent biliary excretion. Minimal oxidative metabolism (a phase I reaction) has been observed in all species evaluated. Ezetimibe and ezetimibe-glucuronide are the major drug-derived compounds detected in plasma, constituting approximately 10 to 20% and 80 to 90% of the total drug in plasma, respectively. Both ezetimibe and ezetimibe-glucuronide are slowly eliminated from plasma with evidence of significant enterohepatic recycling. The half-life for ezetimibe and ezetimibe-glucuronide is approximately 22 hours.

Simvastatin

Simvastatin is an inactive lactone which is readily hydrolyzed *in vivo* to the corresponding β-hydroxyacid, a potent inhibitor of HMG-CoA reductase. Hydrolysis takes place mainly in the liver; the rate of hydrolysis in human plasma is very slow.

In man simvastatin is well absorbed and undergoes extensive hepatic first-pass extraction. The extraction in the liver is dependent on the hepatic blood flow. The liver is its primary site of action, with subsequent excretion of drug equivalents in the bile. Consequently, availability of active drug to the systemic circulation is low.

Following an intravenous injection of the β-hydroxyacid metabolite, its half-life averaged 1.9 hours.

Elimination:

Ezetimibe

Following oral administration of ^{14}C-ezetimibe (20 mg) to human subjects, total ezetimibe accounted for approximately 93% of the total radioactivity in plasma. Approximately 78% and 11% of the administered radioactivity were recovered in the faeces and urine, respectively, over a 10-day collection period. After 48 hours, there were no detectable levels of radioactivity in the plasma.

Simvastatin

Following an oral dose of radioactive simvastatin to man, 13% of the radioactivity was excreted in the urine and 60% in the faeces within 96 hours. The amount recovered in the faeces represents absorbed drug equivalents excreted in bile as well as unabsorbed drug. Following an intravenous injection of the β-hydroxyacid metabolite, an average of only 0.3% of the IV dose was excreted in urine as inhibitors.

Special Populations:

Paediatric Patients

The absorption and metabolism of ezetimibe are similar between children and adolescents (10 to 18 years) and adults. Based on total ezetimibe, there are no pharmacokinetic differences between adolescents and adults. Pharmacokinetic data in the paediatric population < 10 years of age are not available. Clinical experience in paediatric and adolescent patients (ages 9 to 17) has been limited to patients with HoFH or sitosterolaemia. (See section 4.2.)

Geriatric Patients

Plasma concentrations for total ezetimibe are about 2-fold higher in the elderly (≥65 years) than in the young (18 to 45 years). LDL-C reduction and safety profile are comparable between elderly and younger subjects treated with ezetimibe. (See section 4.2.)

Hepatic Insufficiency

After a single 10-mg dose of ezetimibe, the mean AUC for total ezetimibe was increased approximately 1.7-fold in patients with mild hepatic insufficiency (Child Pugh score 5 or 6), compared to healthy subjects. In a 14-day, multiple-dose study (10 mg daily) in patients with moderate hepatic insufficiency (Child Pugh score 7 to 9), the mean AUC for total ezetimibe was increased approximately 4-fold on Day 1 and Day 14 compared to healthy subjects. No dosage adjustment is necessary for patients with mild hepatic insufficiency. Due to the unknown effects of the increased exposure to ezetimibe in patients with moderate or severe (Child Pugh score >9) hepatic insufficiency, ezetimibe is not recommended in these patients (see sections 4.2 and 4.4).

Renal Insufficiency

Ezetimibe

After a single 10-mg dose of ezetimibe in patients with severe renal disease (n=8; mean CrCl ≤30 ml/min), the mean AUC for total ezetimibe was increased approximately 1.5-fold, compared to healthy subjects (n=9). (See section 4.2.)

An additional patient in this study (post-renal transplant and receiving multiple medications, including ciclosporin) had a 12-fold greater exposure to total ezetimibe.

Simvastatin

In a study of patients with severe renal insufficiency (creatinine clearance <30 ml/min), the plasma concentrations of total inhibitors after a single dose of a related HMG-CoA reductase inhibitor were approximately two-fold higher than those in healthy volunteers.

Gender

Plasma concentrations for total ezetimibe are slightly higher (approximately 20%) in women than in men. LDL-C reduction and safety profile are comparable between men and women treated with ezetimibe.

5.3 Preclinical safety data

INEGY

In coadministration studies with ezetimibe and simvastatin, the toxic effects observed were essentially those typically associated with statins. Some of the toxic effects were more pronounced than observed during treatment with statins alone. This is attributed to pharmacokinetic and/or pharmacodynamic interactions following coadministration. No such interactions occurred in the clinical studies. Myopathies occurred in rats only after exposure to doses that were several times higher than the human therapeutic dose (approximately 20 times the AUC level for simvastatin and 1800 times the AUC level for the active metabolite). There was no evidence that coadministration of ezetimibe affected the myotoxic potential of simvastatin.

In dogs coadministered ezetimibe and statins, some liver effects were observed at low exposures (≤1 times human AUC). Marked increases in liver enzymes (ALT, AST) in the absence of tissue necrosis were seen. Histopathologic liver findings (bile duct hyperplasia, pigment accumulation, mononuclear cell infiltration and small hepatocytes) were observed in dogs coadministered ezetimibe and simvastatin. These changes did not progress with longer duration of dosing up to 14 months. General recovery of the liver findings was observed upon discontinuation of dosing. These findings were consistent with those described with HMG-CoA inhibitors or attributed to the very low cholesterol levels achieved in the affected dogs.

The coadministration of ezetimibe and simvastatin was not teratogenic in rats. In pregnant rabbits a small number of skeletal deformities (fused caudal vertebrae, reduced number of caudal vertebrae) were observed.

In a series of *in vivo* and *in vitro* assays, ezetimibe, given alone or coadministered with simvastatin, exhibited no genotoxic potential.

Ezetimibe

Animal studies on the chronic toxicity of ezetimibe identified no target organs for toxic effects. In dogs treated for four weeks with ezetimibe (≥0.03 mg/kg/day) the cholesterol concentration in the cystic bile was increased by a factor of 2.5 to 3.5. However, in a one-year study on dogs given doses of up to 300 mg/kg/day no increased incidence of cholelithiasis or other hepatobiliary effects were observed. The significance of these data for humans is not known. A lithogenic risk associated with the therapeutic use of ezetimibe cannot be ruled out.

Long-term carcinogenicity tests on ezetimibe were negative.

Ezetimibe had no effect on the fertility of male or female rats, nor was it found to be teratogenic in rats or rabbits, nor did it affect prenatal or postnatal development. Ezetimibe crossed the placental barrier in pregnant rats and rabbits given multiple doses of 1000 mg/kg/day.

Simvastatin

Based on conventional animal studies regarding pharmacodynamics, repeated dose toxicity, genotoxicity and carcinogenicity, there are no other risks for the patient than may be expected on account of the pharmacological mechanism. At maximally tolerated doses in both the rat and the rabbit, simvastatin produced no foetal malformations, and had no effects on fertility, reproductive function or neonatal development.

6. PHARMACEUTICAL PARTICULARS

6.1 List of excipients

Butylated hydroxyanisole

Citric acid monohydrate

Croscarmellose sodium

Hypromellose

Lactose monohydrate

Magnesium stearate

Microcrystalline cellulose

Propyl gallate

6.2 Incompatibilities

Not applicable.

6.3 Shelf life

2 years.

6.4 Special precautions for storage

Do not store above 30°C.

Blisters: Store in the original package.

Bottles: Keep bottles tightly closed.

6.5 Nature and contents of container

INEGY 10 mg/20 mg, and 10 mg/40 mg

White HDPE bottles with foil induction seals, white child-resistant polypropylene closure, and silica gel desiccant, containing 100 tablets.

INEGY 10/20 mg and 10/40 mg

Push-through blisters of opaque polychlorotrifluoroethylene/PVC sealed to vinyl coated aluminum in packs of 90 tablets.

INEGY 10 mg/20 mg, 10 mg/40 mg, and 10 mg/80 mg

Push-through blisters of opaque polychlorotrifluoroethylene/PVC sealed to vinyl coated aluminum in packs of 7, 10, 14, 28, 30, 50, 56, 84, 98, 100, or 300 tablets.

Unit dose push-through blisters of opaque polychlorotrifluoroethylene/PVC sealed to vinyl coated aluminum in packs of 30, 50, 100, or 300 tablets.

Not all pack sizes may be marketed.

6.6 Special precautions for disposal and other handling

No special requirements.

7. MARKETING AUTHORISATION HOLDER

MSD-SP Ltd
Hertford Road
Hoddesdon
Hertfordshire
EN11 9BU
United Kingdom

8. MARKETING AUTHORISATION NUMBER(S)

INEGY 10 mg/20 mg Tablets PL 19945/0008

INEGY 10 mg/40 mg Tablets PL 19945/0009

INEGY 10 mg/80 mg Tablets PL 19945/0010

9. DATE OF FIRST AUTHORISATION/RENEWAL OF THE AUTHORISATION

18 November 2004

10. DATE OF REVISION OF THE TEXT

09 September 2009

LEGAL CATEGORY

POM

® denotes registered trademark of MSP Singapore Company, LLC

INEGY SPC.VYT.08.UK.2872 II-026

Infacol

(Forest Laboratories UK Limited)

1. NAME OF THE MEDICINAL PRODUCT

INFACOL

2. QUALITATIVE AND QUANTITATIVE COMPOSITION

Simeticone 40mg/ml

3. PHARMACEUTICAL FORM

Oral suspension

4. CLINICAL PARTICULARS

4.1 Therapeutic indications

An antiflatulent for the relief of griping pain, colic or wind due to swallowed air.

4.2 Posology and method of administration

For adults and elderly:

Not applicable.

For infants:

20mg (0.5ml) administered before each feed. If necessary this may be increased to 40mg (1ml). Treatment with Infacol may provide a progressive improvement in symptoms over several days.

4.3 Contraindications

None stated

4.4 Special warnings and precautions for use

If symptoms persist, seek medical advice.

4.5 Interaction with other medicinal products and other forms of interaction

None stated

4.6 Pregnancy and lactation

Not applicable

4.7 Effects on ability to drive and use machines

Not applicable

4.8 Undesirable effects

None stated

4.9 Overdose

In the event of deliberate or accidental overdose, treat symptoms on appearance.

5. PHARMACOLOGICAL PROPERTIES

5.1 Pharmacodynamic properties

Physiologically the active ingredient is a chemically inert, non-systemic gastric defoaming agent that works by altering the elasticity of interfaces of mucus-embedded bubbles in the gastrointestinal tract.

The gas bubbles are thus broken down or coalesced and in this form gas is more easily eliminated through eructation or passing flatus.

5.2 Pharmacokinetic properties

Simeticone is not absorbed from the gastrointestinal tract.

5.3 Preclinical safety data

There are no preclinical data of relevance to the prescriber which are additional to that already included in other sections of the SPC.

6. PHARMACEUTICAL PARTICULARS

6.1 List of excipients

Saccharin Sodium

Hypromellose

Orange flavour

Methyl Hydroxybenzoate (E218)

Propyl Hydroxybenzoate (E216)

Purified Water

6.2 Incompatibilities

None stated.

6.3 Shelf life

As packaged for sale: 3 years

After first opening: 28 days.

6.4 Special precautions for storage

Do not store above 25°C.

6.5 Nature and contents of container

High-density polyethylene bottle fitted with a low-density polyethylene dropper and evoprene teat containing 50ml of liquid.

6.6 Special precautions for disposal and other handling

Not stated.

7. MARKETING AUTHORISATION HOLDER

Forest Laboratories UK Limited

Bourne Road

Bexley

Kent DA5 1NX

8. MARKETING AUTHORISATION NUMBER(S)

PL 0108/0100

9. DATE OF FIRST AUTHORISATION/RENEWAL OF THE AUTHORISATION

29th October 1986 / 26th November 2001

10. DATE OF REVISION OF THE TEXT

July 2009

11. Legal Category

GSL

Infanrix IPV

(GlaxoSmithKline UK)

1. NAME OF THE MEDICINAL PRODUCT

Infanrix-IPV, suspension for injection in pre-filled syringe.

Diphtheria, tetanus, pertussis (acellular, component) and poliomyelitis (inactivated) vaccine (adsorbed).

2. QUALITATIVE AND QUANTITATIVE COMPOSITION

One dose (0.5 ml) contains:

Diphtheria toxoid[1]	not less than 30 IU
Tetanus toxoid[1]	not less than 40 IU
Bordetella pertussis antigens	
Pertussis toxoid[1]	25 micrograms
Filamentous Haemagglutinin[1]	25 micrograms
Pertactin[1]	8 micrograms
Poliovirus (inactivated)[2]	
type 1 (Mahoney strain)	40 D-antigen unit
type 2 (MEF-1 strain)	8 D-antigen unit
type 3 (Saukett strain)	32 D-antigen unit
[1]adsorbed on aluminium hydroxide, hydrated	0.5 milligrams Al^{3+}

[2]propagated in VERO cells

For a full list of excipients, see section 6.1.

3. PHARMACEUTICAL FORM

Suspension for injection in pre-filled syringe.

Infanrix-IPV is a turbid white suspension.

4. CLINICAL PARTICULARS

4.1 Therapeutic indications

This vaccine is indicated for booster vaccination against diphtheria, tetanus, pertussis, and poliomyelitis diseases in individuals from 16 months to 13 years of age inclusive.

The administration of Infanrix-IPV should be based on official recommendations.

4.2 Posology and method of administration

Posology

A single dose of 0.5 ml should be administered.

Infanrix-IPV may be administered to subjects who have previously received whole cell or acellular pertussis-containing vaccines, and oral live attenuated or injected inactivated poliomyelitis vaccines. (See also sections 4.8 and 5.1).

Method of administration

The vaccine is for intramuscular injection, usually into the deltoid muscle. However, the anterolateral thigh may be used in very young subjects if preferred.

Do not administer intravascularly.

4.3 Contraindications

Hypersensitivity to the active substances or to any of the excipients or neomycin, polymyxin or formaldehyde.

Hypersensitivity after previous administration of diphtheria, tetanus, pertussis, or polio vaccines.

Infanrix-IPV should not be administered to subjects who experienced neurological complications (for convulsions or hypotonic-hyporesponsive episodes, see section 4.4) following previous immunisation with any of the antigens in the vaccine.

Infanrix-IPV should not be administered to subjects who have experienced an encephalopathy of unknown aetiology, occurring within 7 days following previous vaccination with a pertussis containing vaccine.

As with other vaccines, administration of Infanrix-IPV should be postponed in subjects suffering from an acute severe febrile illness. The presence of a minor infection is not a contra-indication.

4.4 Special warnings and precautions for use

As with all injectable vaccines, appropriate medical treatment and supervision should always be readily available in case of a rare anaphylactic event following the administration of the vaccine.

Vaccination should be preceded by a review of the medical history (especially with regard to previous vaccination and possible occurrence of undesirable events) and a clinical examination. A family history of convulsions or a family history of Sudden Infant Death Syndrome (SIDS) does not constitute a contra-indication.

If any of the following events are known to have occurred in temporal relation to receipt of pertussis-containing vaccine, the decision to give further doses of pertussis-containing vaccines should be carefully considered:

- temperature of ⩾ 40.0°C within 48 hours, not due to another identifiable cause,

- collapse or shock-like state (hypotonic-hyporesponsiveness episode) within 48 hours of vaccination,

- persistent, inconsolable crying lasting ⩾ 3 hours, occurring within 48 hours of vaccination,

- convulsions with or without fever, occurring within 3 days of vaccination.

There may be circumstances, such as a high incidence of pertussis, when the potential benefits outweigh possible risks.

Infanrix-IPV should be administered with caution to subjects with thrombocytopenia or a bleeding disorder since bleeding may occur following an intramuscular administration to these subjects.

HIV infection is not considered as a contra-indication. The expected immunological response may not be obtained after vaccination of immunosuppressed patients.

For children under immunosuppressive treatment (corticosteroid therapy, antimitotic chemotherapy, etc.), it is recommended to postpone vaccination until the end of treatment.

Infanrix-IPV should under no circumstances be administered intravascularly.

4.5 Interaction with other medicinal products and other forms of interaction

Infanrix-IPV has been administered concomitantly with measles-mumps-rubella vaccine or Hib vaccine in clinical trials. The data available do not suggest any clinically relevant interference in the antibody response to each of the individual antigens.

Interaction studies have not been carried out with other vaccines, biological products or therapeutic medications. However, in accordance with commonly accepted immunisation guidelines, since Infanrix-IPV is an inactivated product, there is no theoretical reason why it should not be administered concomitantly with other vaccines or immunoglobulins at separate sites.

As with other vaccines it may be expected that in patients receiving immunosuppressive therapy or patients with immunodeficiency, a protective immune response to one or more antigens in the vaccine may not be achieved.

4.6 Pregnancy and lactation

It is anticipated that Infanrix-IPV would only rarely be administered to subjects of child-bearing potential. Adequate human data on the use of Infanrix-IPV during pregnancy and lactation are not available and animal studies on reproductive toxicity have not been conducted. Consequently the use of this combined vaccine is not recommended during pregnancy. It is preferable to avoid the use of this vaccine during lactation.

4.7 Effects on ability to drive and use machines

It is anticipated that Infanrix-IPV would only rarely be administered to subjects who would be driving or using machines. However, somnolence, commonly reported after vaccination, may temporarily affect the ability to drive and use machines.

4.8 Undesirable effects

Clinical Trials: The safety of Infanrix-IPV has been evaluated in 2030 subjects in clinical studies. All vaccinees had previously received either 3 or 4 doses of a combined diphtheria, tetanus and pertussis vaccine. These vaccines contained either whole cell (Pw) or acellular (Pa) pertussis components as follows:

-736 children aged 15-26 months had previously been given 3 doses of DTP –37 had received DTPw, 699 had received DTPa,

– 593 children aged 4-7 years had previously been given either 3 or 4 doses of DTP – 128 had received 3 doses of DTPw, 211 had received 3 doses of DTPa, 73 had received 4 doses of DTPw, 181 had received 4 doses of DTPa

– 701 children aged 10-14 years had received 4 doses of DTPw

All had received a full primary course of either IPV or OPV. Vaccinees aged 10-14 years had also received an additional dose of diphtheria, tetanus and polio antigens at approximately 5-6 years.

Booster doses of DTPa-containing vaccines may be more reactogenic in children who have been previously primed with acellular pertussis-containing vaccines.

Adverse reactions reported during these studies were mostly reported within 48 hours following vaccination, were of mild to moderate severity and resolved spontaneously.

Frequencies are defined as follows:

Very common: ⩾ 10%

Common: ⩾ 1% and < 10%

Uncommon: ⩾ 0.1% and < 1%

Rare: ⩾ 0.01% and < 0.1%

Not known: cannot be estimated from the available data

<u>Infections and infestations</u>

Rare: pharyngitis

<u>Blood and lymphatic system disorders</u>

Uncommon: lymphadenopathy

<u>Metabolism and nutrition disorders</u>

Very common: loss of appetite

<u>Psychiatric disorders:</u>

Very common: irritability, restlessness, unusual crying

Uncommon: insomnia

<u>Nervous system disorders:</u>

Very common: headache, somnolence

<u>Eye disorders</u>

Rare: eye pain

<u>Ear and labyrinth disorders</u>

Rare: earache

<u>Respiratory, thoracic and mediastinal disorders</u>

Uncommon: rhinitis, coughing

<u>Gastrointestinal disorders:</u>

Common: nausea, vomiting, diarrhoea

Uncommon: abdominal pain

<u>Skin and subcutaneous tissue disorders</u>

Uncommon: rash

Rare: pruritis

<u>Musculoskeletal and connective tissue disorders</u>

Uncommon: back pain

<u>Renal and urinary disorders</u>

Uncommon: urinary incontinence

<u>General disorders and administration site conditions:</u>

Very common: pain, redness and swelling at the injection site*, fever, malaise

Common: asthenia

* Information on extensive swelling of the injected limb (defined as swelling with a diameter > 50 mm, noticeable diffuse swelling or noticeable increase of limb circumference) occurring after Infanrix-IPV was actively solicited in two clinical trials. When Infanrix-IPV was administered as either a fourth dose or a fifth dose of DTPa to children 4-6 years of age, extensive injection site swelling was reported with incidences of 13% and 25% respectively. The most frequent reactions were large, localised swelling (diameter > 50 mm) occurring around the injection site. A smaller percentage of children (3% and 6% respectively) experiences diffuse swelling of the injected limb, sometimes

Table 2

Antigen	Previous vaccination history/schedule (N subjects)	3 doses of DTPw + IPV 3, 5, 11 months (N = 128)	3 doses of DTPa + IPV or OPV 3, 5, 11-12 months (N = 208)	4 doses of DTPw + IPV 2, 3, 4 + 16-18 months (N = 73)	4 doses of DTPa + IPV or OPV 2, 4, 6 + 18 months (N = 166)
Diphtheria	% vaccinees with titres ⩾ 0.1 IU/ml by ELISA*	100	99.0	100	100
Tetanus	% vaccinees with titres ⩾ 0.1 IU/ml by ELISA*	100	100	100	100
Pertussis					
Pertussis toxoid	% vaccinees with titres ⩾ 5 EL.U/ml by ELISA	98.3	100	95.5	99.4
Filamentous haemagglutinin		100	100	100	100
Pertactin		100	100	100	100
Polio					
type 1	% vaccinees with titres ⩾ 8 by neutralisation*	100	100	100	100
type 2		100	100	100	100
type 3		100	99.5	100	100

* These levels are considered to be protective

involving adjacent joint. In general, these reactions began within 48 hours of vaccination and spontaneously resolved over an average of 4 days without sequelae.

Post marketing surveillance: Not known: For the following adverse events identified during post-marketing surveillance, an exact quantification of frequency cannot be established.

Immune system disorders

Allergic reactions, including anaphylactoid reactions

Nervous system disorders:

Convulsions, collapse or shock-like state (hypotonic-hyporesponsiveness episode)

Skin and subcutaneous tissue disorders

Urticaria

4.9 Overdose

No case of overdose has been reported.

5. PHARMACOLOGICAL PROPERTIES

Pharmaco-therapeutic group: Bacterial and viral vaccines combined, ATC code: J07CA02

5.1 Pharmacodynamic properties

The immune response after booster vaccination with Infanrix-IPV was evaluated in 917 vaccinees. The immune response observed was independent of the number of doses and type of vaccines administered previously (DTPw or DTPa, OPV or IPV) as shown in the tables below.

One month after vaccination of children aged 15 to 26 months, the immune responses were the following:

(see Table 1 below)

One month after vaccination of children aged 4-7 years, the immune responses were the following:

(see Table 2 above)

One month after vaccination of children/adolescents aged 10-13 years, the immune responses were the following:

(see Table 3 below)

After vaccination, ⩾ 99% of all subjects had protective antibody levels against diphtheria, tetanus and the three poliovirus types.

No serological correlate of protection has been defined for the pertussis antigens. The antibody titres to the three pertussis components were in all cases higher than those observed after primary vaccination with the paediatric acellular pertussis combination vaccine (DTPa, *Infanrix*™), for which efficacy has been demonstrated in a household contact efficacy study. Based on these comparisons, it can therefore be anticipated that Infanrix-IPV would provide protection against pertussis, although the degree and duration of protection afforded by the vaccine are undetermined.

5.2 Pharmacokinetic properties

Evaluation of pharmacokinetic properties is not required for vaccines.

5.3 Preclinical safety data

Non-clinical data reveal no special hazard for humans based on conventional studies of safety, specific toxicity and compatibility of ingredients.

Table 1

Antigen	Previous vaccination history/schedule (N subjects)	3 doses of DTPw + IPV 2, 3, 4 months (N = 37)	3 doses of DTPa + IPV 2, 3, 4 / 2, 4, 6 / 3, 4, 5 or 3, 4.5, 6 months (N = 252)
Diphtheria	% vaccinees with titres ⩾ 0.1 IU/ml by ELISA*	100	99.6
Tetanus	% vaccinees with titres ⩾ 0.1 IU/ml by ELISA*	100	100
Pertussis			
Pertussis toxoid	% vaccinees with titres ⩾ 5 EL.U/ml by ELISA	100	100
Filamentous haemagglutinin		100	100
Pertactin		100	100
Polio			
type 1	% vaccinees with titres ⩾ 8 by neutralisation*	100	100
type 2		100	100
type 3		100	100

* These levels are considered to be protective

Table 3

Antigen	Previous vaccination history/schedule (N subjects)	4 doses of DTPw+IPV at 2, 3, 4 + 16-18 months + 1 dose of DT-IPV at 5-6 years (N = 53)
Diphtheria	% vaccinees with titres ⩾ 0.1 IU/ml by ELISA*	100
Tetanus	% vaccinees with titres ⩾ 0.1 IU/ml by ELISA*	100
Pertussis		
Pertussis toxoid	% vaccinees with titres ⩾ 5 EL.U/ml by ELISA	100
Filamentous haemagglutinin		100
Pertactin		100
Polio		
type 1	% vaccinees with titres ⩾ 8 by neutralisation*	100
type 2		100
type 3		100

* These levels are considered to be protective

6. PHARMACEUTICAL PARTICULARS

6.1 List of excipients

Phenoxyethanol

Sodium chloride

Medium 199 (containing principally amino acids, mineral salts, vitamins)

Water for injections

For adjuvants, see section 2.

6.2 Incompatibilities

In the absence of compatibility studies, this medicinal product must not be mixed with other medicinal products.

6.3 Shelf life

3 years.

6.4 Special precautions for storage

Store in a refrigerator (2°C - 8°C).

Do not freeze.

Store in the original package, in order to protect from light.

6.5 Nature and contents of container

0.5 ml of suspension for injection in a pre-filled syringe (type I glass) with plunger stopper (butyl) - pack sizes of 1 or 20.

6.6 Special precautions for disposal and other handling

Upon storage, a white deposit and clear supernatant may be observed. This does not constitute a sign of deterioration.

The syringe should be well shaken in order to obtain a homogeneous turbid white suspension.

The suspension should be inspected visually for any foreign particulate matter and/or abnormal physical appearance. In the event of either being observed, discard the vaccine.

Any unused product or waste material should be disposed of in accordance with local requirements.

Administrative Data

7. MARKETING AUTHORISATION HOLDER

SmithKline Beecham plc

Trading as:

GlaxoSmithKline UK

Stockley Park West, Uxbridge

Middlesex UB11 1BT

8. MARKETING AUTHORISATION NUMBER(S)

PL10592/0209

9. DATE OF FIRST AUTHORISATION/RENEWAL OF THE AUTHORISATION

7 August 2006

10. DATE OF REVISION OF THE TEXT

29 October 2008

11. Legal Status

POM

Infanrix-IPV+Hib

(GlaxoSmithKline UK)

1. NAME OF THE MEDICINAL PRODUCT

INFANRIX-IPV+Hib powder and suspension for suspension for injection

Diphtheria, tetanus, pertussis (acellular component), poliomyelitis (inactivated) and Haemophilus type b conjugate vaccine (adsorbed)

2. QUALITATIVE AND QUANTITATIVE COMPOSITION

A 0.5 ml dose of vaccine contains

Diphtheria toxoid[1]	not less than 30 International Units (IU)
Tetanus toxoid[1]	not less than 40 International Units (IU)

Bordetella pertussis antigens	
Pertussis toxoid[1]	25 μg
Filamentous haemagglutinin[1]	25 μg
Pertactin[1]	8 μg
Poliovirus (inactivated)	
type 1 (Mahoney strain)[2]	40 D-antigen unit
type 2 (MEF-1 strain)[2]	8 D-antigen unit
type 3 (Saukett strain)[2]	32 D-antigen unit
Haemophilus type b polysaccharide	
(polyribosylribitol phosphate)	10 μg
conjugated to tetanus toxoid as carrier protein	approximately 30 μg
[1]Adsorbed on aluminium hydroxide, hydrated	0.5 milligrams Al
[2]Propagated in VERO cells	

For a full list of excipients, see section 6.1.

3. PHARMACEUTICAL FORM

Powder and suspension for suspension for injection.

The diphtheria, tetanus, acellular pertussis and inactivated poliomyelitis (DTPa-IPV) component is a turbid white suspension.

The lyophilised *Haemophilus influenzae* type b (Hib) component is a white powder.

4. CLINICAL PARTICULARS

4.1 Therapeutic indications

INFANRIX-IPV+Hib is indicated for active immunisation against diphtheria, tetanus, pertussis, poliomyelitis and *Haemophilus influenzae* type b disease from the age of 2 months.

INFANRIX-IPV+Hib is not suitable for use in children over 36 months of age.

4.2 Posology and method of administration

Posology

Primary vaccination:

The primary vaccination schedule consists of two or three doses given in accordance with official recommendations. The minimum age at the time of the first dose is 2 months. Subsequent doses of the primary course should be separated by a minimum interval of four weeks.

Booster vaccination:

After primary vaccination with two doses, a booster dose of INFANRIX-IPV+Hib must be given at least 6 months after the last priming dose, preferably between 11 and 13 months of age.

After primary vaccination with three doses, a booster dose of Hib conjugate vaccine (monovalent or combined) must be administered. The timing of this Hib conjugate vaccine booster dose should be in accordance with official recommendations. INFANRIX-IPV+Hib may be used for this booster dose if administration of the additional antigens at the same time is in accordance with official recommendations.

INFANRIX-IPV+Hib may be used as a booster dose for children who have previously been immunised with other vaccines that contain DTP, polio and Hib antigens.

Method of administration

INFANRIX-IPV+Hib is for deep intramuscular injection, in the anterolateral aspect of the thigh.

It is preferable that each subsequent dose is given into alternating limbs.

INFANRIX-IPV+Hib should be administered with caution to subjects with thrombocytopenia or a bleeding disorder since bleeding may occur following an intramuscular administration to these subjects. Firm pressure should be applied to the injection site (without rubbing) for at least two minutes.

INFANRIX-IPV+Hib should under no circumstances be administered intravascularly.

4.3 Contraindications

Hypersensitivity to the active substances or to any of the excipients or neomycin, polymyxin and polysorbate 80.

Hypersensitivity after previous administration of diphtheria, tetanus, pertussis, polio or Hib vaccines.

INFANRIX-IPV+Hib is contra-indicated if the child has experienced an encephalopathy of unknown aetiology, occurring within 7 days following previous vaccination with pertussis containing vaccine.

As with other vaccines, the administration of INFANRIX-IPV+Hib should be postponed in subjects suffering from an acute severe febrile illness. The presence of a minor infection, however, is not a contra-indication.

4.4 Special warnings and precautions for use

As with all injectable vaccines, appropriate medical treatment and supervision should always be readily available in case of a rare anaphylactic event following the administration of the vaccine.

If any of the following events have occurred in temporal relation to receipt of any DTP-containing vaccine, the decision to give subsequent doses of vaccine containing a pertussis component should be carefully considered.

- Temperature of ⩾ 40.0 °C (rectal) within 48 hours, not due to another identifiable cause.
- Collapse or shock-like state (hypotonic-hyporesponsive episode) within 48 hours of vaccination.
- Persistent, inconsolable crying lasting ⩾ 3 hours, occurring within 48 hours of vaccination.
- Convulsions with or without fever, occurring within 3 days of vaccination.

There may be circumstances, such as a high incidence of pertussis, when the potential benefits outweigh possible risks, particularly since the events are not associated with permanent sequelae. According to available clinical data, the risk of such reactions is lower with acellular pertussis vaccines than with whole cell pertussis vaccines.

As for any vaccination, the risk-benefit of immunising with INFANRIX-IPV+Hib or deferring this vaccination should be weighed carefully in an infant or in a child suffering from a new onset or progression of a severe neurological disorder.

The Hib component of the vaccine does not protect against diseases due to other types of *Haemophilus influenzae* nor against meningitis caused by other organisms.

A history of febrile convulsions, a family history of convulsions, a family history of Sudden Infant Death Syndrome (SIDS) and a family history of an adverse event following DTP, IPV and/or Hib vaccination do not constitute contra-indications to administration of INFANRIX-IPV+Hib.

Human Immunodeficiency Virus (HIV) infection is not considered to be a contra-indication to administration of INFANRIX-IPV+Hib.

The expected immunological response may not be obtained after vaccination of immunosuppressed patients, e.g. patients on immunosuppressive therapy.

Excretion of capsular polysaccharide antigen in the urine has been described following receipt of Hib vaccines. Therefore false positive antigen detection test results are possible within 1-2 weeks of vaccination.

Administration of INFANRIX-IPV+Hib should be recorded in the patient's International Vaccination Certificate.

The potential risk of apnoea and the need for respiratory monitoring for 48-72h should be considered when administering the primary immunisation series to very premature infants (born ⩽ 28 weeks of gestation) and particularly for those with a previous history of respiratory immaturity.

As the benefit of the vaccination is high in this group of infants, vaccination should not be withheld or delayed.

4.5 Interaction with other medicinal products and other forms of interaction

If INFANRIX-IPV+Hib is to be given at the same time as another injectable vaccine(s), the vaccines should always be administered at different injection sites.

As with other vaccines it may be expected that, in patients receiving immunosuppressive therapy or patients with immunodeficiency, an adequate response may not be achieved.

4.6 Pregnancy and lactation

As INFANRIX-IPV+Hib is not intended for use in adults, information on the safety of the vaccine when used during pregnancy or lactation is not available.

4.7 Effects on ability to drive and use machines

Not applicable.

4.8 Undesirable effects

- Clinical trials

The safety profile presented below is based on data from more than 3500 subjects.

As has been observed for DTPa and DTPa-containing combinations, an increase in local reactogenicity and fever was reported after booster vaccination with INFANRIX IPV+Hib with respect to the primary course.

Frequencies per dose are defined as follows:

Very common: (⩾1/10)

Common: (⩾ 1/100 to < 1/10)

Uncommon: (⩾ 1/1,000 to < 1/100)

Rare: (⩾ 1/10,000 to < 1/1,000)

Very rare: (< 1/10,000)

Within each frequency grouping, undesirable effects are presented in order of decreasing seriousness.

Blood and lymphatic system disorders

Uncommon: lymphadenopathy

Nervous system disorders:

Very common: somnolence

Respiratory, thoracic and mediastinal disorders:

Uncommon: bronchitis, cough, rhinorrhoea

Gastrointestinal disorders:

Common: diarrhoea, vomiting

Skin and subcutaneous tissue disorders

Uncommon: urticaria, rash

Rare: pruritus, dermatitis

Metabolism and nutrition disorders

Very common: appetite lost

Infections and infestations

Uncommon: upper respiratory tract infection

General disorders and administration site conditions:

Very common: fever (⩾38.0°C), injection site reactions such as pain and redness, local swelling at the injection site (⩽50 mm)

Common: injection site reactions including induration, local swelling at the injection site (>50 mm)[1]

Uncommon: diffuse swelling of the injected limb, sometimes involving the adjacent joint[1], fever[2] >39.5°C, fatigue

Psychiatric disorders:

Very common: crying abnormal, irritability, restlessness

- Post-marketing surveillance

Nervous system disorders:

Collapse or shock-like state (hypotonic-hyporesponsiveness episode), convulsions (with or without fever).

Respiratory, thoracic and mediastinal disorders:

Apnoea[3][see 4.4 for apnoea in very premature infants (⩽ 28 weeks of gestation)]

Skin and subcutaneous tissue disorders:

Angioneurotic oedema[3]

General disorders and administration site conditions:

Swelling of the entire injected limb[1], injection site vesicles[3]

Immune system disorders

Allergic reactions (including anaphylactic[3] and anaphylactoid reactions)

[1]Children primed with acellular pertussis vaccines are more likely to experience swelling reactions after booster administration in comparison with children primed with whole cell vaccines. These reactions resolve over an average of 4 days.

[2]common with booster vaccination

[3]reported with GSK's DTPa containing vaccines

4.9 Overdose

Not applicable.

5. PHARMACOLOGICAL PROPERTIES

5.1 Pharmacodynamic properties

Pharmaco-therapeutic group: Bacterial and viral vaccines combined, ATC code J07CA06

Results obtained in the clinical studies for each of the components are summarised in the tables below:

Percentage of subjects with antibody titres ⩾ assay cut-off after primary vaccination with INFANRIX-IPV+Hib:

(see Table 1 on next page)

Percentage of subjects with antibody titres ⩾ assay cut-off after booster vaccination with INFANRIX-IPV+Hib:

(see Table 2 on next page)

The effectiveness of the GlaxoSmithKline Biologicals' Hib component (when combined with DTPa, DTPa-IPV or DTPa-HBV-IPV) has been and continues to be investigated via an extensive post-marketing surveillance study conducted in Germany. Over a 4.5 year follow-up period, the effectiveness of DTPa/Hib or DTPa-IPV/Hib vaccines was 96.7% for a full primary series and 98.5% for a booster dose (irrespective of priming). Over a 3 year follow-up period, the effectiveness of hexavalent vaccines was 92.8% for a full primary series and 100% for a booster dose.

5.2 Pharmacokinetic properties

Evaluation of pharmacokinetic properties is not required for vaccines.

5.3 Preclinical safety data

Preclinical data reveal no special hazard for humans based on conventional studies of safety, specific toxicity and compatibility of ingredients.

6. PHARMACEUTICAL PARTICULARS

6.1 List of excipients

Lyophilised HIB component:

Lactose

Liquid DTPa-IPV component:

Sodium chloride

2-phenoxyethanol

Medium 199 (as stabilizer containing amino acids, mineral salts, vitamins and other substances)

Water for injections

For adjuvants, see section 2.

6.2 Incompatibilities

In the absence of compatibility studies, this medicinal product must not be mixed with other medicinal products.

6.3 Shelf life

The shelf life of the vaccine components before reconstitution is 36 months.

After reconstitution, the vaccine should be injected immediately. If not used immediately, in-use storage times and conditions prior to use are the responsibility of the user and should normally not be longer than 8 hours at +2°C to +8°C (in a refrigerator).

6.4 Special precautions for storage

Store in a refrigerator (2°C – 8°C)

Do not freeze.

Store in the original package, in order to protect from light.

Table 1 Percentage of subjects with antibody titres ≥ assay cut-off after primary vaccination with INFANRIX-IPV+Hib

Antibody (cut-off)	3-5 months N= 86 (1 trial) %	1.5-3.5-6 months N= 62 (1 trial)- %	2-3-4 months N= 337 (3 trials) %	2-4-6 months N= 624 (6 trials) %	3-4-5 months N= 127 (2 trials) %	3-4.5-6 months N=198 (1 trial) %
Anti-diphtheria (0.1 IU/ml)*	94.1	100	98.8	99.3	94.4	99.5
Anti-tetanus (0.1 IU/ml)*	100.0**	100	99.7	99.8	99.2	100
Anti-PT (5 EL.U/ml)	99.5**	100	99.4	100	98.4	100
Anti-FHA (5 EL.U/ml)	99.7**	100	100	100	100	100
Anti-PRN (5 EL.U/ml)	99.0**	100	100	100	100	100
Anti-Polio type 1 (1/8 dilution)*	93.0	ND	99.1	99.5	100	100
Anti-Polio type 2 (1/8 dilution)*	95.3	ND	95.7	99.0	99.2	100
Anti-Polio type 3 (1/8 dilution)*	98.8	ND	100	100	99.2	99.4
Anti-PRP (Hib) (0.15 µg/ml)*	83.7	100	98.5	98.5	100	98.4
Anti-PRP (Hib) (1.0 µg/ml)	51.2	87.1	68.5	76.0	97.6	81.2

* cut-off accepted as indicative of protection

** Post dose 2 results from studies where DTPa-HB-IPV/Hib was administered in a schedule 3, 5 and 11 Months of age.

Table 2 Percentage of subjects with antibody titres ≥ assay cut-off after booster vaccination with INFANRIX-IPV+Hib

Antibody (cut-off)	Booster vaccination at 11/12 months of age following a 3-5 month primary course N =184 (1 trial) %	Booster vaccination during the second year of life following a three dose primary course N = 1326 (9 trials) %
Anti-diphtheria (0.1 IU/ml)*	100	99.8
Anti-tetanus (0.1 IU/ml)*	99.9**	99.9
Anti-PT (5 EL.U/ml)	99.9**	99.7
Anti-FHA (5 EL.U/ml)	99.9**	100
Anti-PRN (5 EL.U/ml)	99.5**	99.9
Anti-Polio type 1 (1/8 dilution)*	99.4	99.9
Anti-Polio type 2 (1/8 dilution)*	100	100
Anti-Polio type 3 (1/8 dilution)*	99.4	100
Anti-PRP (Hib) (0.15 µg/ml)*	100	100
Anti-PRP (Hib) (1.0 µg/ml)	96.7	99.2

* cut-off accepted as indicative of protection

** Post dose 3 results from studies where DTPa-HB-IPV/Hib was administered in a schedule 3, 5 and 11 Months of age.

6.5 Nature and contents of container

Powder in vial (type I glass) with stopper (chlorobutyl).

0.5 ml of suspension in pre-filled syringe (type I glass) with a plunger stopper (chlorobutyl) with or without needles. Pack size of 1, 10, 20, 25, 40, 50 and 100.

Not all pack sizes may be marketed.

6.6 Special precautions for disposal and other handling

Upon storage of the DTPa-IPV suspension, a white deposit and clear supernatant can be observed in the syringe. This is not a sign of deterioration.

The syringe should be well shaken to obtain a homogeneous suspension. The DTPa-IPV suspension in the syringe, the Hib powder in the vial and the reconstituted vaccine should be inspected visually for any foreign particulate matter and/or abnormal physical appearance prior to administration. In the event either is observed, the vaccine should be discarded.

The vaccine is reconstituted by adding the entire contents of the pre-filled syringe of DTPa-IPV suspension to the vial containing the Hib powder. The mixture should then be injected immediately. The full reconstitution instructions are:

1. Shake the pre-filled syringe containing the DTPa-IPV suspension
2. Attach a needle to the pre-filled syringe of DTPa-IPV and inject the contents of the syringe into the Hib vial.
3. With the needle still inserted, shake the Hib vial vigorously and examine for complete dissolution.
4. Withdraw the entire mixture back into the syringe.
5. Replace the needle with an appropriate size needle for injection and administer the vaccine.
6. If the vaccine is not administered immediately, shake the solution vigorously again before injection.
7. Any unused reconstituted vaccine should be discarded safely in accordance with local regulations.

7. MARKETING AUTHORISATION HOLDER

SmithKline Beecham plc

Trading as:

GlaxoSmithKline UK

Stockley Park West, Uxbridge

Middlesex, UB11 1BT

8. MARKETING AUTHORISATION NUMBER(S)

PL10592/0216

9. DATE OF FIRST AUTHORISATION/RENEWAL OF THE AUTHORISATION

25 January 2005

10. DATE OF REVISION OF THE TEXT

4 February 2009

11. LEGAL CATEGORY

POM

Influenza vaccine (split virion, inactivated) Ph. Eur.

(Wyeth Pharmaceuticals)

1. NAME OF THE MEDICINAL PRODUCT

Influenza vaccine (split virion, inactivated) Ph. Eur., pre-filled syringe

2. QUALITATIVE AND QUANTITATIVE COMPOSITION

Split influenza virus*, inactivated with β-Propiolactone, containing antigens equivalent to:

A/Brisbane/59/2007 (H1N1)-like strain (A/Brisbane/59/2007 IVR-148)	15 micrograms HA**
A/Brisbane/10/2007 (H3N2)-like strain (A/Uruguay/716/2007NYMC X-175C)	15 micrograms HA**
B/Brisbane/60/2008-like strain (B/Brisbane/60/2008)	15 micrograms HA**

per 0.5 ml dose.

* propagated in fertilised hens' eggs from healthy chicken flocks

** haemagglutinin

This vaccine complies with the WHO recommendation (Northern Hemisphere) and EU decision for the 2009/2010 season.

For a full list of excipients, see section 6.1.

3. PHARMACEUTICAL FORM

Suspension for injection in a pre-filled syringe.

Clear to slightly opaque liquid with some sediment that resuspends upon shaking.

4. CLINICAL PARTICULARS

4.1 Therapeutic indications

Prophylaxis of influenza, especially in those who run an increased risk of associated complications.

The use of Influenza vaccine (split virion, inactivated) should be based on official recommendations.

4.2 Posology and method of administration

Posology

Adults and children from 36 months:	0.5 ml
Children from 6 months to 35 months:	Clinical data are limited. Dosages of 0.25 ml or 0.5 ml have been used.

For children who have not previously been vaccinated, a second dose should be given after an interval of at least 4 weeks.

Method of administration

Immunisation should be carried out by intramuscular or deep subcutaneous injection.

For instructions for preparation, see section 6.6.

4.3 Contraindications

Hypersensitivity to the active substances, to any of the excipients (see section 6.1), to eggs and/or chicken proteins.

Influenza vaccine (split virion, inactivated) does not contain more than 1 µg ovalbumin per dose.

The vaccine may contain residues of the following substances: neomycin, polymyxin.

Immunisation shall be postponed in patients with febrile illness or acute infection.

4.4 Special warnings and precautions for use

As with all injectable vaccines, appropriate medical treatment and supervision should always be readily available in case of an anaphylactic event following administration of the vaccine.

Influenza vaccine (split virion, inactivated) should under no circumstances be administered intravascularly.

Antibody response in patients with endogenous or iatrogenic immunosuppression may be insufficient.

4.5 Interaction with other medicinal products and other forms of interaction

Influenza vaccine (split virion, inactivated) may be given at the same time as other vaccines. Immunisation should be carried out on separate limbs. It should be noted that the adverse reactions may be intensified.

The immunological response may be diminished if the patient is undergoing immunosuppressant treatment.

Following influenza vaccination, false positive results in serological tests using the ELISA method to detect antibodies against HIV1, Hepatitis C and especially HTLV1 have been observed. The Western Blot technique disproves the false-positive ELISA test results. The transient false positive reactions could be due to the IgM response to the vaccine.

Table 1

Organ class	Very common >1/10	Common ⩾1/100, <1/10	Uncommon ⩾1/1,000, <1/100	Rare ⩾1/10,000, <1/1,000	Very rare <1/10,000
Nervous system disorders		Headache*			
Skin and subcutaneous tissue disorders		Sweating*			
Musculoskeletal and connective tissue disorders		Myalgia, arthralgia*			
General disorders and administration site conditions		Fever, malaise, shivering, fatigue. Local reactions: redness, swelling, pain, ecchymosis, induration*			

* These reactions usually disappear within 1-2 days without treatment

4.6 Pregnancy and lactation

Pregnancy

The limited data from vaccination in pregnant women do not indicate that adverse foetal and maternal outcomes were attributable to the vaccine. The use of this vaccine may be considered from the second trimester of pregnancy. For pregnant women with medical conditions that increase their risk of complications from influenza, administration of the vaccine is recommended, irrespective of their stage of pregnancy.

Lactation

Influenza vaccine (split virion, inactivated) may be used during lactation.

4.7 Effects on ability to drive and use machines

The vaccine is unlikely to produce an effect on the ability to drive and use machines.

4.8 Undesirable effects

Adverse reactions observed from clinical trials

The safety of trivalent inactivated influenza vaccines is assessed in open label, uncontrolled clinical trials performed as annual update requirements, including at least 50 adults aged 18 – 60 years of age and at least 50 elderly aged 61 years or older. Safety evaluation is performed during the first three days following vaccination.

The following undesirable effects have been observed during clinical trials with the following frequencies: Very common (>1/10), common (⩾1/100, <1/10), uncommon (⩾1/1,000, <1/100), rare (⩾1/10,000, <1/1,000), very rare (<1/10,000), including isolated reports.

(see Table 1 above)

Adverse reactions reported from post-marketing surveillance

Adverse reactions reported from post marketing surveillance for trivalent influenza vaccines are, next to the reactions which have also been observed during the clinical trials, the following:

Blood and lymphatic system disorders

Transient thrombocytopenia, transient lymphadenopathy

Immune system disorders

Allergic reactions, in rare cases leading to anaphylactic shock, angioedema

Nervous system disorders

Neuralgia, paraesthesia, convulsions

Neurological disorders, such as encephalomyelitis, neuritis and Guillain-Barré syndrome

Vascular disorders

Vasculitis associated in very rare cases with transient renal involvement

Skin and subcutaneous tissue disorders

Generalised skin reactions including pruritus, urticaria or non-specific rash

4.9 Overdose

Overdosage is unlikely to have any untoward effects.

5. PHARMACOLOGICAL PROPERTIES

5.1 Pharmacodynamic properties

Pharmacotherapeutic group: Influenza vaccine, ATC Code: J07B B02

Seroprotection is generally obtained within 2 to 3 weeks. The duration of postvaccinal immunity to homologous strains or to strains closely related to the vaccine strains varies but is usually 6 to 12 months.

5.2 Pharmacokinetic properties

Not applicable.

5.3 Preclinical safety data

Not applicable.

6. PHARMACEUTICAL PARTICULARS

6.1 List of excipients

Sodium chloride

Anhydrous disodium phosphate

Sodium dihydrogen phosphate dihydrate

Potassium chloride

Potassium dihydrogen phosphate

Calcium chloride

Water for injection

6.2 Incompatibilities

In the absence of compatibility studies, this medicinal product must not be mixed with other medicinal products.

6.3 Shelf life

1 year.

6.4 Special precautions for storage

Store in a refrigerator (2°C to 8°C). Do not freeze.

Keep the syringe in the outer carton in order to protect from light.

6.5 Nature and contents of container

0.5 ml suspension in pre-filled syringe (Type I glass) with plunger stopper (chlorobutyl rubber) with attached needle in pack sizes of 1 or 10.

Not all pack sizes may be marketed.

6.6 Special precautions for disposal and other handling

The vaccine should be allowed to reach room temperature before use. Shake before use. After shaking, the vaccine should appear as a homogenous suspension. The vaccine must be inspected visually prior to administration and should not be used if there is any variation of physical appearance (see section 3).

Influenza vaccine (split virion, inactivated) is presented as a single use syringe and any remaining contents should be disposed of in compliance with local rules for the disposal of products of this nature.

When a 0.25 ml dose is indicated, the pre-filled syringe should be held in an upright position and half the volume should be eliminated. To do so, depress the plunger to the half dose marking on the glass syringe barrel, the remaining volume should be injected.

7. MARKETING AUTHORISATION HOLDER

CSL Biotherapies GmbH

Emil-von-Behring-Strasse 76

35041 Marburg

Germany

8. MARKETING AUTHORISATION NUMBER(S)

PL 22236/0001

9. DATE OF FIRST AUTHORISATION/RENEWAL OF THE AUTHORISATION

19 April 2005 / 29 March 2009

10. DATE OF REVISION OF THE TEXT

11 August 2009

Influvac sub-unit 2009/2010

(Solvay Healthcare Limited)

1. NAME OF THE MEDICINAL PRODUCT

Influvac Sub-unit 2009/2010, suspension for injection (influenza vaccine, surface antigen, inactivated).

2. QUALITATIVE AND QUANTITATIVE COMPOSITION

Influenza virus surface antigens (haemagglutinin and neuraminidase) of the following strains*:

- A/Brisbane/59/2007 (H1N1)-like strain (A/Brisbane/59/2007 IVR-148 reass.) 15 micrograms HA**
- A/Brisbane/10/2007 (H3N2)-like strain (A/Uruguay/716/2007 NYMC X-175C reass.) 15 micrograms HA**
- B/ Brisbane/60/2008-like strain (B/Brisbane/60/2008) 15 micrograms HA**

per 0.5 ml dose.

* propagated in fertilised hens' eggs from healthy chicken flocks.

** haemagglutinin.

This vaccine complies with the WHO recommendation (northern hemisphere), and EU decision for the 2009/2010 season.

For a full list of excipients see section 6.1.

3. PHARMACEUTICAL FORM

Suspension for injection in prefilled syringes; a colourless clear liquid, filled in single-dose syringes (glass, type I).

4. CLINICAL PARTICULARS

4.1 Therapeutic indications

Prophylaxis of influenza, especially in those who run an increased risk of associated complications.

The use of Influvac Sub-unit 2009/2010 should be based on official recommendations.

4.2 Posology and method of administration

Adults and children from 36 months: 0.5 ml.

Children from 6 months to 35 months: Clinical data are limited. Dosages of 0.25 ml or 0.5 ml have been used.

For children who have not previously been vaccinated, a second dose should be given after an interval of at least 4 weeks.

Immunisation should be carried out by intramuscular or deep Subcutaneous injection.

For instructions for preparation, see section 6.6.

4.3 Contraindications

Hypersensitivity to the active substances, to any of the excipients and to residues of eggs, chicken protein (Influvac Sub-unit 2009/2010 does not contain more than 1 μg ovalbumin per dose), formaldehyde, cetyltrimethylammonium bromide, polysorbate 80, or gentamicin.

Immunisation shall be postponed in patients with febrile illness or acute infection.

4.4 Special warnings and precautions for use

As with all injectable vaccines, appropriate medical treatment and supervision should always be readily available in case of an anaphylactic event following the administration of the vaccine.

Influvac Sub-unit 2009/2010 should under no circumstances be administered intravascularly.

Antibody response in patients with endogenous or iatrogenic immunosuppression may be insufficient.

4.5 Interaction with other medicinal products and other forms of interaction

Influvac Sub-unit 2009/2010 may be given at the same time as other vaccines. Immunisation should be carried out on separate limbs. It should be noted that the adverse reactions may be intensified.

The immunological response may be diminished if the patient is undergoing immunosuppressant treatment.

Following influenza vaccination, false positive results in serology tests using the ELISA method to detect antibodies against HIV1, Hepatitis C and especially HTLV1 have been observed. The Western Blot technique disproves the false-positive ELISA test results. The transient false-positive reactions could be due to the IgM response by the vaccine.

4.6 Pregnancy and lactation

The limited data from vaccinations in pregnant women do not indicate that adverse fetal and maternal outcomes were attributable to the vaccine. The use of this vaccine may be considered from the second trimester of pregnancy. For pregnant women with medical conditions that increase their risk of complications from influenza, administration of the vaccine is recommended, irrespective of their stage of pregnancy.

Influvac Sub-unit 2009/2010 may be used during lactation.

4.7 Effects on ability to drive and use machines

Influvac Sub-unit 2009/2010 is unlikely to produce an effect on the ability to drive and use machines.

4.8 Undesirable effects

ADVERSE REACTIONS OBSERVED FROM CLINICAL TRIALS

The safety of trivalent inactivated influenza vaccines is assessed in open label, uncontrolled clinical trials performed as annual update requirement, including at least 50 adults aged 18 - 60 years of age and at least 50 elderly aged 61 years or older. Safety evaluation is performed during the first 3 days following vaccination.

The following undesirable effects have been observed during clinical trials with the following frequencies:

very common (⩾1/10); common (⩾1/100, <1/10); uncommon (⩾1/1,000, <1/100); rare (⩾1/10,000, <1/1,000); very rare (<1/10,000), including isolated reports.

(see Table 1 on next page)

ADVERSE REACTIONS REPORTED FROM POST-MARKETING SURVEILLANCE

Adverse reactions reported from post marketing surveillance are, next to the reactions which have also been observed during the clinical trials, the following:

Blood and lymphatic system disorders:

Transient thrombocytopenia, transient lymphadenopathy

Immune system disorders:

Allergic reactions, in rare cases leading to shock, angioedema

Nervous system disorders:

Neuralgia, paraesthesia, febril convulsions, neurological disorders, such as encephalomyelitis, neuritis and Guillain Barré syndrome

Vascular disorders:

Vasculitis associated in very rare cases with transient renal involvement

Table 1

Organ class	Very common ≥1/10	Common ≥1/100, <1/10	Uncommon ≥1/1,000, <1/100	Rare ≥1/10,000, <1/1,000	Very rare <1/10,000
Nervous system disorders		Headache*			
Skin and Subcutaneous tissue disorders		Sweating*			
Musculoskeletal and connective tissue disorders		Myalgia, arthralgia*			
General disorders and administration site conditions		fever, malaise, shivering, fatigue Local reactions: redness, swelling, pain, ecchymosis induration*			

* these reactions usually disappear within 1-2 days without treatment

Skin and Subcutaneous tissue disorders:
Generalised skin reactions including pruritus, urticaria or non-specific rash

4.9 Overdose
Overdosage is unlikely to have any untoward effect.

5. PHARMACOLOGICAL PROPERTIES

5.1 Pharmacodynamic properties
Pharmacotherapeutic group: Influenza vaccine, ATC Code: J07BB02.

Seroprotection is generally obtained within 2 to 3 weeks. The duration of post-vaccinal immunity to homologuous strains or to strains closely related to the vaccine strains varies but is usually 6-12 months.

5.2 Pharmacokinetic properties
Not applicable.

5.3 Preclinical safety data
Not applicable.

6. PHARMACEUTICAL PARTICULARS

6.1 List of excipients
Potassium chloride, potassium dihydrogen phosphate, disodium phosphate dihydrate, sodium chloride, calcium chloride, magnesium chloride hexahydrate and water for injections.

6.2 Incompatibilities
In the absence of compatability studies, this medicinal product must not be mixed with other medicinal products.

6.3 Shelf life
1 year.

6.4 Special precautions for storage
Influvac Sub-unit 2009/2010 should be stored in a refrigerator (+2°C to +8°C).

Do not freeze.

Protect from light.

6.5 Nature and contents of container
0.5 ml suspension for injection in prefilled syringe with/without needle (glass, type I), pack of 1 or 10.

6.6 Special precautions for disposal and other handling
Unused vaccine and other waste material should be disposed of in compliance with local rules for the disposal of products of this nature.

Influvac Sub-unit 2009/2010 should be allowed to reach room temperature before use.

Shake before use.

For administration of a 0.25 ml dose from a syringe, push the front side of the plunger exactly to the edge of the hub (the knurled polypropylene ring); a reproducible volume of vaccine remains in the syringe, suitable for administration. See also section 4.2.

7. MARKETING AUTHORISATION HOLDER
Solvay Healthcare Limited
Mansbridge Road
West End
Southampton
SO18 3JD

8. MARKETING AUTHORISATION NUMBER(S)
PL 00512/0156

9. DATE OF FIRST AUTHORISATION/RENEWAL OF THE AUTHORISATION
February 1998 / December 2007

10. DATE OF REVISION OF THE TEXT
02/09/2009

Innohep 10,000 IU/ml and Innohep Syringe 10,000 IU/ml

(Leo Laboratories Limited)

1. NAME OF THE MEDICINAL PRODUCT
INNOHEP® 10,000 IU/ML AND INNOHEP® SYRINGE 10,000 IU/ML.

2. QUALITATIVE AND QUANTITATIVE COMPOSITION
Tinzaparin sodium 10,000 anti-Factor Xa IU/ml.

3. PHARMACEUTICAL FORM
Solution for Injection.

4. CLINICAL PARTICULARS

4.1 Therapeutic indications
For the prevention of thromboembolic events, including deep vein thrombosis, in patients undergoing general and orthopaedic surgery.

For the prevention of clotting in the extracorporeal circuit during haemodialysis in patients with chronic renal insufficiency.

4.2 Posology and method of administration
For prevention of thromboembolic events:
Administration is by subcutaneous injection.

Adults at low to moderate risk, e.g. patients undergoing general surgery:

- 3,500 anti-Factor Xa IU two hours before surgery and then once daily for 7 to 10 days post-operatively.

Adults at high risk, e.g. patients undergoing orthopaedic surgery:

- In this high risk group the recommended dose is either a fixed dose of 4,500 anti-Factor Xa IU given 12 hours before surgery followed by a once daily dose, or 50 anti-Factor Xa IU/kilogram body weight 2 hours before surgery followed by a once daily dose for 7 to 10 days post-operatively.

For haemodialysis:
The dose of innohep® should be given into the arterial side of the dialyser or intravenously. The dialyser can be primed by flushing with 500-1000ml isotonic sodium chloride (9mg/ml) containing 5,000 anti-Factor Xa IU innohep® per litre.

Patients with chronic renal insufficiency:

a) Short-term haemodialysis (up to 4 hours)
A bolus dose of 2,000 - 2,500 anti-Factor Xa IU into the arterial side of the dialyser (or intravenously).

b) Long-term haemodialysis (more than 4 hours)
A bolus dose of 2,500 anti-Factor Xa IU into the arterial side of the dialyser (or intravenously) followed by 750 anti-Factor Xa IU/hour infused into the extracorporeal circuit.

Dosage adjustment
The bolus innohep® dose may be adjusted (increased or decreased) by 250 - 500 anti-Factor Xa IU until a satisfactory response is obtained.

Additional innohep® (500 - 1,000 anti-Factor Xa IU) may be given if concentrated red cells or blood transfusions (which may increase the likelihood of clotting in the dialyser) are given during dialysis or additional treatment beyond the normal dialysis duration is employed.

Dose monitoring
Determination of plasma anti-Factor Xa may be used to monitor the innohep® dose during haemodialysis. Plasma anti-Factor Xa, one hour after dosing should be within the range 0.4 - 0.5 IU/ml.

Use in the elderly
No dose modifications are necessary.

Use in children
There is no experience of use in children.

4.3 Contraindications

- Known hypersensitivity to constituents.
- Current or history of heparin-induced thrombocytopenia.
- Generalised or local haemorrhagic tendency, including uncontrolled severe hypertension, severe liver insufficiency, active peptic ulcer, acute or subacute septic endocarditis, intracranial haemorrhage, or injuries and operations on the central nervous system, eyes and ears, and in women with abortus imminens.
- The innohep® 10,000 IU/ml vial formulation contains 10 mg/ml of the preservative benzyl alcohol. This formulation must not be given to premature babies or neonates.

The innohep® 10,000 IU/ml syringe formulation does not contain the preservative benzyl alcohol.

- An epidural anaesthesia during birth in pregnant women treated with low molecular weight heparin is contraindicated (see section 4.6).
- In patients receiving heparin for treatment rather than prophylaxis, locoregional anaesthesia in elective surgical procedures is contra-indicated because the use of heparin may be very rarely associated with epidural or spinal haematoma resulting in prolonged or permanent paralysis.

4.4 Special warnings and precautions for use
Care should be taken when innohep® is administered to patients with increased risk of bleeding complications.

In patients undergoing peridural or spinal anaesthesia or spinal puncture, the prophylactic use of heparin may be very rarely associated with epidural or spinal haematoma resulting in prolonged or permanent paralysis. The risk is increased by the use of a peridural or spinal catheter for anaesthesia, by the concomitant use of drugs affecting haemostasis such as non-steroidal anti-inflammatory drugs (NSAIDs), platelet inhibitors or anticoagulants, and by traumatic or repeated puncture.

In decision making on the interval between the last administration of heparin at prophylactic doses and the placement or removal of a peridural or spinal catheter, the product characteristics and the patient profile should be taken into account. Subsequent dose should not take place before at least four hours have elapsed. Re-administration should be delayed until the surgical procedure is completed.

Should a physician decide to administer anti-coagulation in the context of peridural or spinal anaesthesia, extreme vigilance and frequent monitoring must be exercised to detect any signs and symptoms of neurologic impairment, such as back pain, sensory and motor deficits and bowel or bladder dysfunction. Patients should be instructed to inform immediately a nurse or a clinician if they experience any of these.

innohep® should not be administered by intramuscular injection due to the risk of haematoma.

Due to increased bleeding risk care should be taken when giving concomitant intramuscular injections, lumbar puncture and similar procedures.

innohep® should be used with caution in patients with hypersensitivity to heparin or to other low molecular weight heparins.

As there is a risk of antibody-mediated heparin-induced thrombocytopenia, platelet counts should be measured in patients receiving heparin treatment for longer than 5 days and the treatment should be stopped immediately in those who develop thrombocytopenia.

As with other low molecular weight heparins, in some patients undergoing surgical procedures (especially orthopaedic) or presenting with a concomitant inflammatory process, the administration of innohep® has coincided with an asymptomatic increase of platelet count, which in many cases subsided during continued administration. If an increase in platelet count occurs, evaluation of the benefit/risk of continuing therapy for that patient should be made.

Care should be taken when innohep® is administered to patients with kidney insufficiency who are undergoing general or orthopaedic surgery. In such cases a dose reduction should be considered.

Heparin can suppress adrenal secretion of aldosterone leading to hyperkalaemia, particularly in patients such as those with diabetes mellitus, chronic renal failure, pre-existing metabolic acidosis, a raised plasma potassium or taking potassium-sparing drugs. The risk of hyperkalaemia appears to increase with duration of therapy but is usually reversible. Plasma potassium should be measured in patients at risk before starting heparin therapy and monitored regularly thereafter particularly if treatment is prolonged beyond about 7 days.

The innohep® 10,000 IU/ml vial formulation contains the preservative benzyl alcohol 10 mg/ml. This should be administered with caution to infants and children up to 3 years old, as there is a risk that benzyl alcohol may cause toxic reactions and allergic reactions (anaphylactoid) in this age group (see section 4.3 for premature babies and neonates).

Drugs affecting platelet function or the coagulation system should in general not be given concomitantly with innohep® (see section 4.5).

Prosthetic Heart Valves:
There have been no adequate studies to assess the safe and effective use of tinzaparin sodium in preventing valve thrombosis in patients with prosthetic heart valves;

therefore no dosage recommendations can be given. High doses of tinzaparin sodium (175 IU/kg) may not be sufficient prophylaxis to prevent valve thrombosis in patients with prosthetic heart valves. The use of tinzaparin sodium cannot be recommended for this purpose.

4.5 Interaction with other medicinal products and other forms of interaction

The anticoagulant effect of innohep® may be enhanced by concomitant medication with other drugs affecting platelet function or the coagulation system, e.g. platelet aggregation inhibitors, thrombolytic agents, salicylates, non-steroidal anti-inflammatory drugs, vitamin K antagonists, dextrans, activated protein C.

innohep® does not appear to interact with other drugs used widely in chronic renal failure, including vitamin B supplements, aluminium hydroxide, calcium supplements, alfacalcidol, ranitidine, vitamin C supplements, ferrous sulphate, folic acid, nifedipine, erythropoietin and azatadine.

4.6 Pregnancy and lactation

Pregnancy

No transplacental passage of innohep® was found (assessed by anti-Factor Xa and anti-Factor IIa activity) in patients given a dose of 35 to 40 anti-Factor Xa IU/kg in the second trimester of pregnancy. In rabbits, no transplacental passage of anti-Factor Xa or anti-Factor IIa activity was observed after doses of 1750 anti-Factor Xa IU/kg. Toxicological studies in rats have shown no embryotoxic or teratogenic effects, although a lower birthweight was found.

Although these animal studies show no hazard, as a precaution innohep® should not be used in pregnancy unless no safer alternative is available.

As benzyl alcohol may cross the placenta, the use of innohep® formulations containing benzyl alcohol should be avoided during pregnancy.

The use of innohep® in women with abortus imminens is contraindicated (see section 4.3).

Prosthetic Heart Valves:

Therapeutic failures and maternal death have been reported in pregnant women with prosthetic heart valves on full anti-coagulant doses of low molecular weight heparins. In the absence of clear dosing, efficacy and safety information in this circumstance, tinzaparin sodium is not recommended for use in pregnant women with prosthetic heart valves.

Lactation

It is not known whether innohep® is excreted in breast milk. However, patients are advised to stop breast-feeding while receiving innohep®.

4.7 Effects on ability to drive and use machines

innohep® has no or negligible influence on the ability to drive or use machines.

4.8 Undesirable effects

Skin rashes and minor bruising at the site of injection have occurred occasionally. Systemic allergic reactions have been reported extremely rarely.

innohep®, like heparin, has been shown to increase the risk of haemorrhage. However, at the recommended dose this risk is low. As with heparin, thrombocytopenia may occur rarely.

As for heparin, a transient increase in aminotransferase levels is frequently seen. Cessation of treatment is not usually required.

Heparin products can cause hypoaldosteronism which may result in an increase in plasma potassium. Rarely, clinically significant hyperkalaemia may occur particularly in patients with chronic renal failure and diabetes mellitus (see Special Warnings and Precautions for Use).

Very rare cases of epidural and spinal haematoma have been reported in patients receiving heparin for prophylaxis undergoing spinal or epidural anaesthesia or spinal puncture. For further information, see Section 4.4, Special Warnings and Precautions for Use.

Skin necrosis has been reported. If this occurs treatment must be withdrawn immediately.

Priapism has been reported rarely.

Valve thrombosis in patients with prosthetic heart valves have been reported rarely in patients receiving low molecular weight heparins, usually associated with inadequate dosing (see Special warnings and precautions for use).

4.9 Overdose

Overdose of innohep® may be complicated by haemorrhage. With recommended dosages there should be no need for an antidote but in the event of accidental administration of an overdose, the effect of innohep® can be reversed by intravenous administration of 1% protamine sulphate solution.

The dose of protamine sulphate required for neutralisation should be accurately determined by titrating with the patient's plasma.

Studies in healthy volunteers indicate that 65-80% of the anti-Xa activity is neutralised by protamine sulphate 1 mg/100 anti-Xa IU of innohep®. A return of innohep® anti-Xa, anti-IIa and APTT activities are seen 3 hours after its reversal probably due to continuous absorption of innohep® from the s.c. depot. It may therefore be necessary to give protamine sulphate intermittently or as a continuous infusion to achieve and maintain neutralisation of s.c. innohep® for at least 24 hours. Potential side-effects of protamine sulphate must be considered and patients carefully observed.

Transfusion of fresh plasma may be used, if necessary. Plasma anti-Factor Xa and anti-Factor IIa activity should be measured during the management of overdose situations.

5. PHARMACOLOGICAL PROPERTIES

5.1 Pharmacodynamic properties

innohep® is an antithrombotic agent. It potentiates the inhibition of several activated coagulation factors, especially Factor Xa, its activity being mediated via antithrombin III.

5.2 Pharmacokinetic properties

The pharmacokinetics/pharmacodynamic activity of innohep® is monitored by anti-Factor Xa activity.

innohep® has a bioavailability of around 90% following a subcutaneous injection. The absorption half-life is 200 minutes, peak plasma activity being observed after 4 to 6 hours. The elimination half-life is about 90 minutes.

The half-life of innohep® in patients with renal insufficiency given a bolus intravenous dose of 2,500 anti-Factor Xa IU is about 2.5 hours.

There is a linear dose response relationship between plasma activity and the dose administered.

5.3 Preclinical safety data

There are no preclinical data of relevance to the prescriber which are additional to that already included in other sections of the SPC.

6. PHARMACEUTICAL PARTICULARS

6.1 List of excipients

innohep® 10,000 IU/ml: Benzyl alcohol, Sodium acetate, Sodium hydroxide, Water for Injections.

innohep® Syringe 10,000 IU/ml: Sodium acetate, Water for Injections. As pH adjuster: sodium hydroxide.

6.2 Incompatibilities

innohep® should not be mixed with any other injection.

6.3 Shelf life

2 years.

6.4 Special precautions for storage

Do not store above 25°C.

6.5 Nature and contents of container

- innohep® 10,000 IU/ml: 2ml glass vial containing 10,000 anti-Factor Xa IU/ml in packs of 10 vials.
- innohep® Syringe 10,000 IU/ml: A prefilled unit dose syringe containing:

o 2,500 anti-Factor Xa IU in 0.25ml

o 3,500 anti-Factor Xa IU in 0.35ml

o 4,500 anti-Factor Xa IU in 0.45ml

in packs of 10 syringes.

6.6 Special precautions for disposal and other handling

innohep® 10,000 IU/ml: The vial should be discarded 14 days after first use.

innohep® Syringe 10,000 IU/ml: Contains no preservative, any portion of the contents not used at once should be discarded with the syringe.

Administrative Data

7. MARKETING AUTHORISATION HOLDER

LEO Laboratories Limited

Longwick Road

Princes Risborough

Bucks HP27 9RR

8. MARKETING AUTHORISATION NUMBER(S)

innohep® 10,000 IU/ml: PL 00043/0205.

innohep® Syringe 10,000 IU/ml: PL 00043/0204.

9. DATE OF FIRST AUTHORISATION/RENEWAL OF THE AUTHORISATION

innohep® 10,000 IU/ml:

Date of First Authorisation: 30 September 1998

Date of last Renewal: 26 April 2004

innohep® Syringe 10,000 IU/ml:

Date of First Authorisation: 20 November 1997

Date of last Renewal: 23 January 2003

10. DATE OF REVISION OF THE TEXT

February 2008.

LEGAL CATEGORY

POM

Innohep 20,000 IU/ml and Innohep syringe 20,000 IU/ml

(Leo Laboratories Limited)

1. NAME OF THE MEDICINAL PRODUCT

INNOHEP® 20,000 IU/ML AND INNOHEP® SYRINGE 20,000 IU/ML

2. QUALITATIVE AND QUANTITATIVE COMPOSITION

Tinzaparin sodium 20,000 anti-Factor Xa IU/ml

3. PHARMACEUTICAL FORM

Solution for Injection

4. CLINICAL PARTICULARS

4.1 Therapeutic indications

Treatment of deep-vein thrombosis and of pulmonary embolus.

4.2 Posology and method of administration

Administration is by subcutaneous injection only.

Adults:	175 anti-Factor Xa IU/kg bodyweight once daily, for at least 6 days and until adequate oral anti-coagulation is established. There is no need to monitor the anticoagulant activity of innohep®.
Use in the elderly:	No dose modifications are necessary (see also section 4.3).
Use in children:	There is no experience of use in children.

4.3 Contraindications

- Known hypersensitivity to constituents.
- Current or history of heparin-induced thrombocytopenia.
- Generalised or local haemorrhagic tendency, including uncontrolled severe hypertension, severe liver insufficiency, active peptic ulcer, acute or subacute septic endocarditis, intracranial haemorrhage, or injuries and operations on the central nervous system, eyes and ears, and in women with abortus imminens.
- Patients aged 90 years or over who have renal insufficiency.
- The innohep® 20,000 IU/ml vial formulation contains 10 mg/ml of the preservative benzyl alcohol. This formulation must not be given to premature babies or neonates.

The innohep® 20,000 IU/ml syringe formulation does not contain the preservative benzyl alcohol.

- An epidural anaesthesia during birth in pregnant women treated with low molecular weight heparin is contraindicated (see section 4.6).
- In patients receiving heparin for treatment rather than prophylaxis, locoregional anaesthesia in elective surgical procedures is contra-indicated because the use of heparin may be very rarely associated with epidural or spinal haematoma resulting in prolonged or permanent paralysis.

4.4 Special warnings and precautions for use

Care should be taken when innohep® is administered to patients with increased risk of bleeding complications.

In patients undergoing peridural or spinal anaesthesia or spinal puncture, the prophylactic use of heparin may be very rarely associated with epidural or spinal haematoma resulting in prolonged or permanent paralysis. The risk is increased by the use of a peridural or spinal catheter for anaesthesia, by the concomitant use of drugs affecting haemostasis such as non-steroidal anti-inflammatory drugs (NSAIDs), platelet inhibitors or anticoagulants, and by traumatic or repeated puncture.

In decision making on the interval between the last administration of heparin at prophylactic doses and the placement or removal of a peridural or spinal catheter, the product characteristics and the patient profile should be taken into account. Subsequent dose should not take place before at least four hours have elapsed. Re-administration should be delayed until the surgical procedure is completed.

Should a physician decide to administer anti-coagulation in the context of peridural or spinal anaesthesia, extreme vigilance and frequent monitoring must be exercised to detect any signs and symptoms of neurologic impairment, such as back pain, sensory and motor deficits and bowel or bladder dysfunction. Patients should be instructed to inform immediately a nurse or a clinician if they experience any of these.

innohep® should not be administered by intramuscular injection due to the risk of haematoma.

Due to increased bleeding risk care should be taken when giving concomitant intramuscular injections, lumbar puncture and similar procedures.

innohep® should be used with caution in patients with hypersensitivity to heparin or to other low molecular weight heparins.

As there is a risk of antibody-mediated heparin-induced thrombocytopenia, platelet counts should be measured in patients receiving heparin treatment for longer than 5 days and the treatment should be stopped immediately in those who develop thrombocytopenia.

As with other low molecular weight heparins, in some patients undergoing surgical procedures (especially orthopaedic) or presenting with a concomitant inflammatory process, the administration of innohep® has coincided with an asymptomatic increase of platelet count, which in many cases subsided during continued administration. If an increase in platelet count occurs, evaluation of the benefit/risk of continuing therapy for that patient should be made.

Care should be taken when innohep® is administered to patients with kidney insufficiency. In such cases a dose reduction should be considered (see also section 4.3).

For some patients with pulmonary embolism (e.g. those with severe haemodynamic instability) alternative treatment, such as surgery or thrombolysis may be indicated.

Heparin can suppress adrenal secretion of aldosterone leading to hyperkalaemia, particularly in patients such as those with diabetes mellitus, chronic renal failure, pre-existing metabolic acidosis, a raised plasma potassium or taking potassium-sparing drugs. The risk of hyperkalaemia appears to increase with duration of therapy but is usually reversible. Plasma potassium should be measured in patients at risk before starting heparin therapy and monitored regularly thereafter particularly if treatment is prolonged beyond about 7 days.

The innohep® 20,000 IU/ml vial formulation contains sodium metabisulphite (E223). This may rarely cause severe hypersensitivity reactions and bronchospasm.

The innohep® 20,000 IU/ml vial formulation contains the preservative benzyl alcohol 10 mg/ml. This should be administered with caution to infants and children up to 3 years old, as there is a risk that benzyl alcohol may cause toxic reactions and allergic reactions (anaphylactoid) in this age group (see section 4.3 for premature babies and neonates).

Drugs affecting platelet function or the coagulation system should in general not be given concomitantly with innohep® (see section 4.5).

Prosthetic Heart Valves:

There have been no adequate studies to assess the safe and effective use of tinzaparin sodium in preventing valve thrombosis in patients with prosthetic heart valves; therefore no dosage recommendations can be given. High doses of tinzaparin sodium (175 IU/kg) may not be sufficient prophylaxis to prevent valve thrombosis in patients with prosthetic heart valves. The use of tinzaparin sodium cannot be recommended for this purpose.

4.5 Interaction with other medicinal products and other forms of interaction

The anticoagulant effect of innohep® may be enhanced by concomitant medication with other drugs affecting platelet function or the coagulation system, e.g. platelet aggregation inhibitors, thrombolytic agents, salicylates, non-steroidal anti-inflammatory drugs, vitamin K antagonists, dextrans, activated protein C.

4.6 Pregnancy and lactation

Pregnancy

No transplacental passage of innohep® was found (assessed by anti-Factor Xa and anti-Factor IIa activity) in patients given a dose of 35 to 40 anti-Factor Xa IU/kg in the second trimester of pregnancy. In rabbits, no transplacental passage of anti-Factor Xa or anti-Factor IIa activity was observed after doses of 1750 anti-Factor Xa IU/kg. Toxicological studies in rats have shown no embryotoxic or teratogenic effects, although a lower birthweight was found.

Although these animal studies show no hazard, as a precaution innohep® should not be used in pregnancy unless no safer alternative is available.

As benzyl alcohol may cross the placenta, the use of innohep® formulations containing benzyl alcohol should be avoided during pregnancy.

The use of innohep® in women with abortus imminens is contraindicated (see section 4.3).

Prosthetic Heart Valves:

Therapeutic failures and maternal death have been reported in pregnant women with prosthetic heart valves on full anti-coagulant doses of low molecular weight heparins. In the absence of clear dosing, efficacy and safety information in this circumstance, tinzaparin sodium is not recommended for use in pregnant women with prosthetic heart valves.

Lactation

It is not known whether innohep® is excreted in breast milk. However, patients are advised to stop breast-feeding while receiving innohep®.

4.7 Effects on ability to drive and use machines

innohep® has no or negligible influence on the ability to drive or use machines.

4.8 Undesirable effects

Skin rashes and minor bruising at the site of injection have occurred occasionally. Systemic allergic reactions have been reported extremely rarely.

innohep®, like heparin, has been shown to increase the risk of haemorrhage. However, at the recommended dose this risk is low. As with heparin, thrombocytopenia may occur rarely.

As for heparin, a transient increase in aminotransferase levels is frequently seen. Cessation of treatment is not usually required.

Heparin products can cause hypoaldosteronism which may result in an increase in plasma potassium. Rarely, clinically significant hyperkalaemia may occur particularly in patients with chronic renal failure and diabetes mellitus (see Special Warnings and Precautions for Use).

Very rare cases of epidural and spinal haematoma have been reported in patients receiving heparin for prophylaxis undergoing spinal or epidural anaesthesia or spinal puncture. For further information, see Section 4.4, Special Warnings and Precautions for Use.

Skin necrosis has been reported. If this occurs treatment must be withdrawn immediately.

Priapism has been reported rarely.

Valve thrombosis in patients with prosthetic heart valves have been reported rarely in patients receiving low molecular weight heparins, usually associated with inadequate dosing (see Special warnings and precautions for use).

4.9 Overdose

Overdose of innohep® may be complicated by haemorrhage. With recommended dosages there should be no need for an antidote but in the event of accidental administration of an overdose, the effect of innohep® can be reversed by intravenous administration of 1% protamine sulphate solution.

The dose of protamine sulphate required for neutralisation should be accurately determined by titrating with the patient's plasma.

Studies in healthy volunteers indicate that 65-80% of the anti-Xa activity is neutralised by protamine sulphate 1 mg/100 anti-Xa IU of innohep®. A return of innohep® anti-Xa, anti-IIa and APTT activities are seen 3 hours after its reversal probably due to continuous absorption of innohep® from the s.c. depot. It may therefore be necessary to give protamine sulphate intermittently or as a continuous infusion to achieve and maintain neutralisation of s.c. innohep® for at least 24 hours. Potential side-effects of protamine sulphate must be considered and patients carefully observed.

Transfusion of fresh plasma may be used, if necessary. Plasma anti-Factor Xa and anti-Factor IIa activity should be measured during the management of overdose situations.

5. PHARMACOLOGICAL PROPERTIES

5.1 Pharmacodynamic properties

innohep® is an antithrombotic agent. It potentiates the inhibition of several activated coagulation factors, especially Factor Xa, its activity being mediated via antithrombin III.

5.2 Pharmacokinetic properties

The pharmacokinetics/pharmacodynamic activity of innohep® is monitored by anti-Factor Xa activity. Following subcutaneous injection of innohep®, anti-Factor Xa activity reaches a maximum at 4-6 hours (peak anti-Factor Xa activity, after administration of 175 anti-Factor Xa IU/kg bodyweight once daily, is approximately 0.5-1.0 IU/ml). Detectable anti-Factor Xa activity persists for 24 hours.

5.3 Preclinical safety data

There are no preclinical data of relevance to the prescriber which are additional to that already included in other sections of the SPC.

6. PHARMACEUTICAL PARTICULARS

6.1 List of excipients

innohep® 20,000IU/ml - Sodium metabisulphite, Benzyl alcohol, Sodium hydroxide, Water for Injections.

innohep® Syringe 20,000IU/ml - Sodium metabisulphite, Sodium hydroxide, Water for Injections.

6.2 Incompatibilities

innohep® should be given by subcutaneous injection only. It should not be mixed with any other injection.

6.3 Shelf life

2 years.

6.4 Special precautions for storage

Do not store above 25°C.

6.5 Nature and contents of container

innohep® 20,000 IU/ml - A 2ml glass vial containing 20,000 anti-Factor Xa IU in packs of 1 vial.

innohep® Syringe 20,000 IU/ml - A prefilled variable dose graduated syringe containing: 0.5ml (10,000 anti-Factor Xa IU), 0.7ml (14,000 anti-Factor Xa IU), 0.9ml (18,000 anti-Factor Xa IU) in packs of 2 and 6 syringes.

6.6 Special precautions for disposal and other handling

innohep® 20,000 IU/ml - The vial should be discarded 14 days after first use.

innohep® Syringe 20,000 IU/ml - Contains no bactericide, any portion of the contents not used at once should be discarded together with the syringe.

7. MARKETING AUTHORISATION HOLDER

LEO Laboratories Limited

Longwick Road

Princes Risborough

Bucks HP27 9RR

8. MARKETING AUTHORISATION NUMBER(S)

innohep® 20,000 IU/ml - PL 0043/0192

innohep® Syringe 20,000 IU/ml - PL 0043/0197

9. DATE OF FIRST AUTHORISATION/RENEWAL OF THE AUTHORISATION

innohep® 20,000 IU/ml

Date of First Authorisation: 18 October 1994

Date of last Renewal: 26 March 2002

innohep® Syringe 20,000 IU/ml

Date of First Authorisation: 03 October 1996

Date of last Renewal: 21 December 2002

10. DATE OF REVISION OF THE TEXT

July 2008

LEGAL CATEGORY

POM

Innovace Tablets

(Merck Sharp & Dohme Limited)

1. NAME OF THE MEDICINAL PRODUCT

INNOVACE® 2.5 mg Tablets

INNOVACE® 5 mg Tablets

INNOVACE® 10 mg Tablets

INNOVACE® 20 mg Tablets

2. QUALITATIVE AND QUANTITATIVE COMPOSITION

Each tablet contains 2.5 mg, 5 mg, 10 mg or 20 mg of enalapril maleate.

For excipients, see 6.1.

3. PHARMACEUTICAL FORM

Tablets.

Strength	Appearance	Country
2.5 mg	White, oval shaped tablet, one side scored marked MSD 14, and the other side scored	Belgium, Denmark, Finland, France, Luxembourg, Germany, Norway, Sweden
	White, round shaped tablet, one side marked MSD 14, the other side plain	Ireland, United Kingdom
5 mg	White, rounded triangle shaped tablet, one side scored the other side marked MSD 712	Austria, Denmark, Finland, Iceland, Ireland, The Netherlands, Sweden, United Kingdom
	White, barrel shaped tablet, one side scored the other side marked RENITEC	Belgium, Luxemburg, France, Portugal, Spain
	White, round shaped tablet, one side scored, the other side marked 712	Italy
	White, round flat tablet, one side scored other side plain	Greece
	White, oval shaped tablet, one side scored, marked MSD 712 and the other side scored	Germany
10 mg	Rust Red, rounded triangle shaped tablet, one side scored, the other side marked MSD 713	Austria, Denmark, Finland, Iceland, Ireland, The Netherlands, Sweden, United Kingdom
	Rust Red, barrel shaped tablet, one side scored, the other side marked RENITEC	Belgium. Luxembourg
	Rust Red, oval shaped tablet, one side scored, and the other side scored, marked MSD 713	Germany
20 mg	Peach, triangle shaped tablet, one side scored, the other side marked MSD 714	Austria, Denmark, Finland, Iceland, Ireland, The Netherlands, Sweden, United Kingdom
	Peach, barrel shaped tablet, one side scored, the other side marked RENITEC	Belgium, France, Luxembourg, Portugal

Peach, round shaped tablet, one side scored quartersect, the other side marked 714	Italy
Peach, barrel shaped tablet, one side scored MSDE, the other side marked RENITEC	Spain
Peach, round flat tablet, one side scored other side plain	Greece
Peach, oval shaped tablet, one side scored, and the other side marked MSD 714, scored	Germany

4. CLINICAL PARTICULARS

4.1 Therapeutic indications

- Treatment of Hypertension
- Treatment of Symptomatic Heart Failure
- Prevention of Symptomatic Heart Failure in patients with Asymptomatic Left Ventricular Dysfunction (ejection fraction ⩽35%)

(See Section 5.1 'Pharmacodynamic properties'.)

4.2 Posology and method of administration

The absorption of Tablets 'Innovace' is not affected by food.

The dose should be individualised according to patient profile (see 4.4 'Special warnings and precautions for use') and blood pressure response.

Hypertension

The initial dose is 5 to maximally 20 mg, depending on the degree of hypertension and the condition of the patient (see below). 'Innovace' is given once daily. In mild hypertension, the recommended initial dose is 5 to 10 mg. Patients with a strongly activated renin-angiotensin-aldosterone system (e.g., renovascular hypertension, salt and/or volume depletion, cardiac decompensation, or severe hypertension) may experience an excessive blood pressure fall following the initial dose. A starting dose of 5 mg or lower is recommended in such patients and the initiation of treatment should take place under medical supervision.

Prior treatment with high dose diuretics may result in volume depletion and a risk of hypotension when initiating therapy with enalapril. A starting dose of 5 mg or lower is recommended in such patients. If possible, diuretic therapy should be discontinued for 2-3 days prior to initiation of therapy with 'Innovace'. Renal function and serum potassium should be monitored.

The usual maintenance dose is 20 mg daily. The maximum maintenance dose is 40 mg daily.

Heart Failure/Asymptomatic Left Ventricular Dysfunction

In the management of symptomatic heart failure, 'Innovace' is used in addition to diuretics and, where appropriate, digitalis or beta-blockers. The initial dose of 'Innovace' in patients with symptomatic heart failure or asymptomatic left ventricular dysfunction is 2.5 mg, and it should be administered under close medical supervision to determine the initial effect on the blood pressure. In the absence of, or after effective management of, symptomatic hypotension following initiation of therapy with 'Innovace' in heart failure, the dose should be increased gradually to the usual maintenance dose of 20 mg, given in a single dose or two divided doses, as tolerated by the patient. This dose titration is recommended to be performed over a 2 to 4 week period. The maximum dose is 40 mg daily given in two divided doses.

Suggested Dosage Titration of 'Innovace' in Patients with Heart Failure/Asymptomatic Left Ventricular Dysfunction

Week	Dose mg/day
Week 1	**Days 1 to 3:** 2.5 mg/day* in a single dose **Days 4 to 7:** 5 mg/day in two divided doses
Week 2	10 mg/day in a single dose or in two divided doses
Weeks 3 and 4	20 mg/day in a single dose or in two divided doses

*Special precautions should be followed in patients with impaired renal function or taking diuretics (See 4.4 'Special warnings and precautions for use').

Blood pressure and renal function should be monitored closely both before and after starting treatment with 'Innovace' (see 4.4 'Special warnings and precautions for use') because hypotension and (more rarely) consequent renal failure have been reported. In patients treated with diuretics, the dose should be reduced if possible before beginning treatment with 'Innovace'. The appearance of hypotension after the initial dose of 'Innovace' does not imply that hypotension will recur during chronic therapy with 'Innovace' and does not preclude continued use of the drug. Serum potassium and renal function also should be monitored.

Dosage in Renal Insufficiency

Generally, the intervals between the administration of enalapril should be prolonged and/or the dosage reduced.

Creatinine Clearance (CrCL) mL/min	Initial Dose mg/day
30 < CrCL < 80 ml/min.	5 - 10 mg
10 < CrCL ⩽ 30 ml/min.	2.5 mg
CrCL ⩽ 10 ml/min.	2.5 mg on dialysis days*

*See 4.4 'Special warnings and precautions for use' - Haemodialysis Patients.

Enalaprilat is dialysable. Dosage on nondialysis days should be adjusted depending on the blood pressure response.

Use in Elderly

The dose should be in line with the renal function of the elderly patient (see 4.4 'Special warnings and precautions for use', Renal Function Impairment).

Use in paediatrics

There is limited clinical trial experience of the use of 'Innovace' in hypertensive paediatric patients (see 4.4 'Special warnings and precautions for use', 5.1 'Pharmacodynamic properties' and 5.2 'Pharmacokinetic properties').

For patients who can swallow tablets, the dose should be individualised according to patient profile and blood pressure response. The recommended initial dose is 2.5 mg in patients 20 to <50 kg and 5 mg in patients ⩾ 50 kg. 'Innovace' is given once daily. The dosage should be adjusted according to the needs of the patient to a maximum of 20 mg daily in patients 20 to <50 kg and 40 mg in patients ⩾ 50 kg. (See 4.4 'Special warnings and precautions for use'.)

'Innovace' is not recommended in neonates and in pediatric patients with glomerular filtration rate <30 ml/min/1.73 m^2, as no data are available.

4.3 Contraindications

- Hypersensitivity to enalapril, to any of the excipients or any other ACE inhibitor
- History of angioedema associated with previous ACE inhibitor therapy
- Hereditary or idiopathic angioedema
- Second and third trimesters of pregnancy (see sections 4.4 and 4.6).

4.4 Special warnings and precautions for use

Symptomatic Hypotension

Symptomatic hypotension is rarely seen in uncomplicated hypertensive patients. In hypertensive patients receiving 'Innovace', symptomatic hypotension is more likely to occur if the patient has been volume - depleted, e.g., by diuretic therapy, dietary salt restriction, dialysis, diarrhoea or vomiting (see 4.5 'Interaction with other medicinal products and other forms of interaction' and 4.8 'Undesirable effects'). In patients with heart failure, with or without associated renal insufficiency, symptomatic hypotension has been observed. This is most likely to occur in those patients with more severe degrees of heart failure, as reflected by the use of high doses of loop diuretics, hyponatraemia or functional renal impairment. In these patients, therapy should be started under medical supervision and the patients should be followed closely whenever the dose of 'Innovace' and/or diuretic is adjusted. Similar considerations may apply to patients with ischemic heart or cerebrovascular disease in whom an excessive fall in blood pressure could result in a myocardial infarction or cerebrovascular accident.

If hypotension occurs, the patient should be placed in the supine position and, if necessary, should receive an intravenous infusion of normal saline. A transient hypotensive response is not a contraindication to further doses, which can be given usually without difficulty once the blood pressure has increased after volume expansion.

In some patients with heart failure who have normal or low blood pressure, additional lowering of systemic blood pressure may occur with 'Innovace'. This effect is anticipated, and usually is not a reason to discontinue treatment. If hypotension becomes symptomatic, a reduction of dose and/or discontinuation of the diuretic and/or 'Innovace' may be necessary.

Aortic or Mitral Valve Stenosis/Hypertrophic Cardiomyopathy

As with all vasodilators, ACE inhibitors should be given with caution in patients with left ventricular valvular and outflow tract obstruction and avoided in cases of cardiogenic shock and haemodynamically significant obstruction.

Renal Function Impairment

In cases of renal impairment (creatinine clearance <80 ml/min) the initial enalapril dosage should be adjusted according to the patient's creatinine clearance (see 4.2 'Posology and method of administration') and then as a function of the patient's response to treatment. Routine monitoring of potassium and creatinine are part of normal medical practice for these patients.

Renal failure has been reported in association with enalapril and has been mainly in patients with severe heart failure or underlying renal disease, including renal artery stenosis. If recognised promptly and treated appropriately, renal failure when associated with therapy with enalapril is usually reversible.

Some hypertensive patients, with no apparent pre-existing renal disease have developed increases in blood urea and creatinine when enalapril has been given concurrently with a diuretic. Dosage reduction of enalapril and/or discontinuation of the diuretic may be required. This situation should raise the possibility of underlying renal artery stenosis (see 4.4 'Special warnings and precautions for use', Renovascular hypertension).

Renovascular hypertension

There is an increased risk of hypotension and renal insufficiency when patients with bilateral renal artery stenosis or stenosis of the artery to a single functioning kidney are treated with ACE inhibitors. Loss of renal function may occur with only mild changes in serum creatinine. In these patients, therapy should be initiated under close medical supervision with low doses, careful titration, and monitoring of renal function.

Kidney Transplantation

There is no experience regarding the administration of 'Innovace' in patients with a recent kidney transplantation. Treatment with 'Innovace' is therefore not recommended.

Hepatic failure

Rarely, ACE inhibitors have been associated with a syndrome that starts with cholestatic jaundice or hepatitis and progresses to fulminant hepatic necrosis and (sometimes) death. The mechanism of this syndrome is not understood. Patients receiving ACE inhibitors who develop jaundice or marked elevations of hepatic enzymes should discontinue the ACE inhibitor and receive appropriate medical follow-up.

Neutropenia/Agranulocytosis

Neutropenia/agranulocytosis, thrombocytopenia and anaemia have been reported in patients receiving ACE inhibitors. In patients with normal renal function and no other complicating factors, neutropenia occurs rarely. Enalapril should be used with extreme caution in patients with collagen vascular disease, immunosuppressant therapy, treatment with allopurinol or procainamide, or a combination of these complicating factors, especially if there is pre-existing impaired renal function. Some of these patients developed serious infections which in a few instances did not respond to intensive antibiotic therapy. If enalapril is used in such patients, periodic monitoring of white blood cell counts is advised and patients should be instructed to report any sign of infection.

Hypersensitivity/Angioneurotic oedema

Angioneurotic oedema of the face, extremities, lips, tongue, glottis and/or larynx has been reported in patients treated with angiotensin converting enzyme inhibitors, including 'Innovace'. This may occur at any time during treatment. In such cases, 'Innovace' should be discontinued promptly and appropriate monitoring should be instituted to ensure complete resolution of symptoms prior to dismissing the patient. Even in those instances where swelling of only the tongue is involved, without respiratory distress, patients may require prolonged observation since treatment with antihistamines and corticosteroids may not be sufficient.

Very rarely, fatalities have been reported due to angioedema associated with laryngeal oedema or tongue oedema. Patients with involvement of the tongue, glottis or larynx are likely to experience airway obstruction, especially those with a history of airway surgery. Where there is involvement of the tongue, glottis or larynx, likely to cause airway obstruction, appropriate therapy, which may include subcutaneous epinephrine solution 1:1000 (0.3 ml to 0.5 ml) and/or measures to ensure a patent airway, should be administered promptly.

Black patients receiving ACE inhibitors have been reported to have a higher incidence of angioedema compared to non-blacks.

Patients with a history of angioedema unrelated to ACE inhibitor therapy may be at increased risk of angioedema while receiving an ACE inhibitor. (Also see 4.3 'Contraindications'.)

Anaphylactoid Reactions during Hymenoptera Desensitisation

Rarely, patients receiving ACE inhibitors during desensitisation with hymenoptera venom have experienced life-threatening anaphylactoid reactions. These reactions were avoided by temporarily withholding ACE-inhibitor therapy prior to each desensitisation.

Anaphylactoid Reactions during LDL Apheresis

Rarely, patients receiving ACE inhibitors during low density lipoprotein (LDL)-apheresis with dextran sulfate have experienced life-threatening anaphylactoid reactions. These reactions were avoided by temporarily withholding ACE-inhibitor therapy prior to each apheresis.

Haemodialysis Patients

Anaphylactoid reactions have been reported in patients dialysed with high-flux membranes (e.g., AN 69®) and treated concomitantly with an ACE inhibitor. In these patients consideration should be given to using a different type of dialysis membrane or a different class of antihypertensive agent.

Hypoglycaemia

Diabetic patients treated with oral antidiabetic agents or insulin starting an ACE inhibitor, should be told to closely monitor for hypoglycaemia, especially during the first month of combined use. (See 4.5 'Interaction with other medicinal products and other forms of interaction', Antidiabetics.)

Cough

Cough has been reported with the use of ACE inhibitors. Characteristically, the cough is nonproductive, persistent and resolves after discontinuation of therapy. ACE inhibitor-induced cough should be considered as part of the differential diagnosis of cough.

Surgery/Anaesthesia

In patients undergoing major surgery or during anaesthesia with agents that produce hypotension, enalapril blocks angiotensin II formation secondary to compensatory renin release. If hypotension occurs and is considered to be due to this mechanism, it can be corrected by volume expansion.

Hyperkalaemia

Elevations in serum potassium have been observed in some patients treated with ACE inhibitors, including enalapril. Risk factors for the development of hyperkalaemia include those with renal insufficiency, worsening of renal function, age (>70 years) diabetes mellitus, inter-current events in particular dehydration, acute cardiac decompensation, metabolic acidosis and concomitant use of potassium-sparing diuretics (e.g., spironolactone, eplerenone, triamterene, or amiloride), potassium supplements or potassium-containing salt substitutes; or those patients taking other drugs associated with increases in serum potassium (e.g. heparin). The use of potassium supplements, potassium-sparing diuretics, or potassium-containing salt substitutes particularly in patients with impaired renal function may lead to a significant increase in serum potassium. Hyperkalaemia can cause serious, sometimes fatal arrhythmias. If concomitant use of enalapril and any of the above-mentioned agents is deemed appropriate, they should be used with caution and with frequent monitoring of serum potassium. (See 4.5 'Interaction with other medicinal products and other forms of interaction'.)

Lithium

The combination of lithium and enalapril is generally not recommended (see 4.5 'Interaction with other medicinal products and other forms of interaction').

Lactose

'Innovace' contains lactose and therefore should not be used by patients with rare hereditary problems of galactose intolerance, the Lapp lactase deficiency or glucose-galactose malabsorption. 'Innovace' contains less than 200 mg of lactose per tablet.

Paediatric Use

There is limited efficacy and safety experience in hypertensive children >6 years old, but no experience in other indications. Limited pharmacokinetic data are available in children above 2 months of age. (Also see 4.2 'Posology and method of administration', 5.1 'Pharmacodynamic properties', and 5.2 'Pharmacokinetic properties'.) 'Innovace' is not recommended in children in other indications than hypertension.

'Innovace' is not recommended in neonates and in paediatric patients with glomerular filtration rate <30 ml/min/1.73 m^2, as no data are available. (See 4.2 'Posology and method of administration'.)

Pregnancy and lactation

ACE inhibitors should not be initiated during pregnancy. Unless continued ACE inhibitor therapy is considered essential, patients planning pregnancy should be changed to alternative antihypertensive treatments which have an established safety profile for use in pregnancy. When pregnancy is diagnosed, treatment with ACE inhibitors should be stopped immediately, and, if appropriate, alternative therapy should be started (see sections 4.3 and 4.6).

Use of enalapril is not recommended during breast feeding (see sections 4.6 and 5.2).

Ethnic differences

As with other angiotensin converting enzyme inhibitors, enalapril is apparently less effective in lowering blood pressure in black people than in non-blacks, possibly because of a higher prevalence of low-renin states in the black hypertensive population.

4.5 Interaction with other medicinal products and other forms of interaction

Potassium sparing diuretics or potassium supplements

ACE inhibitors attenuate diuretic induced potassium loss. Potassium sparing diuretics (e.g. spironolactone, eplerenone, triamterene or amiloride), potassium supplements, or potassium-containing salt substitutes may lead to significant increases in serum potassium. If concomitant use is indicated because of demonstrated hypokalaemia they should be used with caution and with frequent monitoring of serum potassium (see 4.4 'Special warnings and precautions for use').

Diuretics (thiazide or loop diuretics)

Prior treatment with high dose diuretics may result in volume depletion and a risk of hypotension when initiating therapy with enalapril (see 4.4 'Special warnings and precautions for use'). The hypotensive effects can be reduced by discontinuation of the diuretic, by increasing volume or salt intake or by initiating therapy with a low dose of enalapril.

Other antihypertensive agents

Concomitant use of these agents may increase the hypotensive effects of enalapril. Concomitant use with nitroglycerine and other nitrates, or other vasodilators, may further reduce blood pressure.

Lithium

Reversible increases in serum lithium concentrations and toxicity have been reported during concomitant administration of lithium with ACE inhibitors. Concomitant use of thiazide diuretics may further increase lithium levels and enhance the risk of lithium toxicity with ACE inhibitors. Use of enalapril with lithium is not recommended, but if the combination proves necessary, careful monitoring of serum lithium levels should be performed (see 4.4 'Special warnings and precautions for use').

Tricyclic antidepressants/Antipsychotics/Anesthetics/Narcotics

Concomitant use of certain anesthetic medicinal products, tricyclic antidepressants and antipsychotics with ACE inhibitors may result in further reduction of blood pressure (see 4.4 'Special warnings and precautions for use').

Non-Steroidal Anti-Inflammatory Drugs (NSAIDs)

Chronic administration of NSAIDs may reduce the antihypertensive effect of an ACE inhibitor.

NSAIDs (including COX-2 inhibitors) and ACE inhibitors exert an additive effect on the increase in serum potassium, and may result in a deterioration of renal function. These effects are usually reversible. Rarely, acute renal failure may occur, especially in patients with compromised renal function (such as the elderly or patients who are volume-depleted, including those on diuretic therapy).

Gold

Nitritoid reactions (symptoms include facial flushing, nausea, vomiting and hypotension) have been reported rarely in patients on therapy with injectable gold (sodium aurothiomalate) and concomitant ACE inhibitor therapy including enalapril.

Sympathomimetics

Sympathomimetics may reduce the antihypertensive effects of ACE inhibitors.

Antidiabetics

Epidemiological studies have suggested that concomitant administration of ACE inhibitors and antidiabetic medicines (insulins, oral hypoglycaemic agents) may cause an increased blood-glucose-lowering effect with risk of hypoglycaemia. This phenomenon appeared to be more likely to occur during the first weeks of combined treatment and in patients with renal impairment. (See 4.4 'Special warnings and precautions for use; Hypoglycaemia and 4.8 Undesirable effects; Metabolism and nutrition disorders').

Alcohol

Alcohol enhances the hypotensive effect of ACE inhibitors.

Acetyl salicylic acid, thrombolytics and β-blockers

Enalapril can be safely administered concomitantly with acetyl salicylic acid (at cardiologic doses), thrombolytics and β-blockers.

4.6 Pregnancy and lactation

Pregnancy

> The use of ACE inhibitors is not recommended during the first trimester of pregnancy (see section 4.4). The use of ACE inhibitors is contra-indicated during the second and third trimester of pregnancy (see sections 4.3 and 4.4).

Epidemiological evidence regarding the risk of teratogenicity following exposure to ACE inhibitors during the first trimester of pregnancy has not been conclusive; however a small increase in risk cannot be excluded. Unless continued ACE inhibitors therapy is considered essential, patients planning pregnancy should be changed to alternative anti-hypertensive treatments which have an established safety profile for use in pregnancy. When pregnancy is diagnosed, treatment with ACE inhibitors should be stopped immediately, and, if appropriate, alternative therapy should be started.

ACE inhibitors therapy exposure during the second and third trimesters is known to induce human foetotoxicity (decreased renal function, oligohydramnios, skull ossification retardation) and neonatal toxicity (renal failure, hypotension, hyperkalaemia). (See section 5.3).

Should exposure to ACE inhibitors have occurred from the second trimester of pregnancy, ultrasound check of renal function and skull is recommended.

Infants whose mothers have taken ACE inhibitors should be closely observed for hypotension (see sections 4.3 and 4.4).

Lactation

Limited pharmacokinetic data demonstrate very low concentrations in breast milk (see section 5.2). Although these concentrations seem to be clinically irrelevant the use of 'Innovace' in breast-feeding is not recommended for preterm infants and for the first few weeks after delivery, because of the hypothetical risk of cardiovascular and renal effects and because there is not enough clinical experience. In case of an older infant the use of 'Innovace' in breast-feeding mother may be considered if this treatment is necessary for the mother and the child is observed for any adverse effect.

4.7 Effects on ability to drive and use machines

When driving vehicles or operating machines it should be taken into account that occasionally dizziness or weariness may occur.

4.8 Undesirable effects

Undesirable effects reported for enalapril include:

[Very common (>1/10); common (>1/100, <1/10); uncommon (>1/1,000, <1/100); rare (>1/10,000, <1/1,000); very rare (<1/10,000), not known (cannot be estimated from the available data).]

Blood and the lymphatic system disorders:

uncommon: anaemia (including aplastic and hemolytic)

rare: neutropenia, decreases in hemoglobin, decreases in hematocrit, thrombocytopenia, agranulocytosis, bone marrow depression, pancytopenia, lymphadenopathy, autoimmune diseases

Endocrine disorders:

not known: syndrome of inappropriate antidiuretic hormone secretion (SIADH)

Metabolism and nutrition disorders:

uncommon: hypoglycaemia (see 4.4 'Special warnings and precautions for use', Hypoglycemia)

Nervous system and psychiatric disorders:

common: headache, depression

uncommon: confusion, somnolence, insomnia, nervousness, paresthaesia, vertigo

rare: dream abnormality, sleep disorders

Eye disorders:

very common: blurred vision

Cardiac and vascular disorders:

very common: dizziness

common: hypotension (including orthostatic hypotension), syncope, chest pain, rhythm disturbances, angina pectoris, tachycardia

uncommon: orthostatic hypotension, palpitations, myocardial infarction or cerebrovascular accident*, possibly secondary to excessive hypotension in high risk patients (see 4.4 'Special warnings and precautions for use')

rare: Raynaud's phenomenon

Respiratory, thoracic and mediastinal disorders:

very common: cough

common: dyspnea

uncommon: rhinorrhea, sore throat and hoarseness, bronchospasm/asthma

rare: pulmonary infiltrates, rhinitis, allergic alveolitis/eosinophilic pneumonia

Gastrointestinal disorders:

very common: nausea,

common: diarrhoea, abdominal pain, taste alteration

uncommon: ileus, pancreatitis, vomiting, dyspepsia, constipation, anorexia, gastric irritations, dry mouth, peptic ulcer

rare: stomatitis/aphthous ulcerations, glossitis

very rare: intestinal angioedema

Hepatobiliary disorders:

rare: hepatic failure, hepatitis – either hepatocellular or cholestatic, hepatitis including necrosis, cholestasis (including jaundice)

Skin and subcutaneous tissue disorders:

common: rash, hypersensitivity/angioneurotic oedema: angioneurotic oedema of the face, extremities, lips, tongue, glottis and/or larynx has been reported (see 4.4 'Special warnings and precautions for use')

uncommon: diaphoresis, pruritus, urticaria, alopecia

rare: erythema multiforme, Stevens-Johnson syndrome, exfoliative dermatitis, toxic epidermal necrolysis, pemphigus, erythroderma

A symptom complex has been reported which may include some or all of the following: fever, serositis, vasculitis, myalgia/myositis, arthralgia/arthritis, a positive ANA, elevated ESR, eosinophilia, and leukocytosis. Rash, photosensitivity or other dermatologic manifestations may occur.

Renal and urinary disorders:

uncommon: renal dysfunction, renal failure, proteinuria

rare: oliguria

Reproductive system and breast disorders:
uncommon: impotence
rare: gynecomastia
General disorders and administration site conditions:
very common: asthenia
common: fatigue
uncommon: muscle cramps, flushing, tinnitus, malaise, fever
Investigations:
common: hyperkalemia, increases in serum creatinine
uncommon: increases in blood urea, hyponatremia
rare: elevations of liver enzymes, elevations of serum bilirubin

* Incidence rates were comparable to those in the placebo and active control groups in the clinical trials

4.9 Overdose

Limited data are available for overdosage in humans. The most prominent features of overdosage reported to date are marked hypotension, beginning some six hours after ingestion of tablets, concomitant with blockade of the renin-angiotensin system, and stupor. Symptoms associated with overdosage of ACE inhibitors may include circulatory shock, electrolyte disturbances, renal failure, hyperventilation, tachycardia, palpitations, bradycardia, dizziness, anxiety, and cough. Serum enalaprilat levels 100- and 200-fold higher than usually seen after therapeutic doses have been reported after ingestion of 300 mg and 440 mg of enalapril, respectively.

The recommended treatment of overdosage is intravenous infusion of normal saline solution. If hypotension occurs, the patient should be placed in the shock position. If available, treatment with angiotensin II infusion and/or intravenous catecholamines may also be considered. If ingestion is recent, take measures aimed at eliminating enalapril maleate (e.g., emesis, gastric lavage, administration of absorbents, and sodium sulphate). Enalaprilat may be removed from the general circulation by haemodialysis. (See 4.4 'Special warnings and precautions for use', Haemodialysis Patients.) Pacemaker therapy is indicated for therapy-resistant bradycardia. Vital signs, serum electrolytes and creatinine concentrations should be monitored continuously.

5. PHARMACOLOGICAL PROPERTIES

5.1 Pharmacodynamic properties

Pharmacotherapeutic group: Angiotensin converting enzyme inhibitors, ATC Code: C09A A02

'Innovace' (enalapril maleate) is the maleate salt of enalapril, a derivative of two amino-acids, L-alanine and L-proline. Angiotensin converting enzyme (ACE) is a peptidyl dipeptidase which catalyzes the conversion of angiotensin I to the pressor substance angiotensin II. After absorption, enalapril is hydrolyzed to enalaprilat, which inhibits ACE. Inhibition of ACE results in decreased plasma angiotensin II, which leads to increased plasma renin activity (due to removal of negative feedback of renin release), and decreased aldosterone secretion.

ACE is identical to kininase II. Thus 'Innovace' may also block the degradation of bradykinin, a potent vasodepressor peptide. However, the role that this plays in the therapeutic effects of 'Innovace' remains to be elucidated.

While the mechanism through which 'Innovace' lowers blood pressure is believed to be primarily suppression of the renin-angiotensin-aldosterone system, 'Innovace' is antihypertensive even in patients with low-renin hypertension.

Administration of 'Innovace' to patients with hypertension results in a reduction of both supine and standing blood pressure without a significant increase in heart rate.

Symptomatic postural hypotension is infrequent. In some patients the development of optimal blood pressure reduction may require several weeks of therapy. Abrupt withdrawal of 'Innovace' has not been associated with rapid increase in blood pressure.

Effective inhibition of ACE activity usually occurs 2 to 4 hours after oral administration of an individual dose of enalapril. Onset of antihypertensive activity was usually seen at one hour, with peak reduction of blood pressure achieved by 4 to 6 hours after administration. The duration of effect is dose-related. However, at recommended doses, antihypertensive and haemodynamic effects have been shown to be maintained for at least 24 hours.

In haemodynamic studies in patients with essential hypertension, blood pressure reduction was accompanied by a reduction in peripheral arterial resistance with an increase in cardiac output and little or no change in heart rate. Following administration of 'Innovace' there was an increase in renal blood flow; glomerular filtration rate was unchanged. There was no evidence of sodium or water retention. However, in patients with low pretreatment glomerular filtration rates, the rates were usually increased.

In short term clinical studies in diabetic and nondiabetic patients with renal disease, decreases in albuminuria and urinary excretion of IgG and total urinary protein were seen after the administration of enalapril.

When given together with thiazide-type diuretics, the blood pressure-lowering effects of 'Innovace' are at least additive. 'Innovace' may reduce or prevent the development of thiazide-induced hypokalemia.

In patients with heart failure on therapy with digitalis and diuretics, treatment with oral or Injection 'Innovace' was associated with decreases in peripheral resistance and blood pressure. Cardiac output increased, while heart rate (usually elevated in patients with heart failure) decreased. Pulmonary capillary wedge pressure was also reduced. Exercise tolerance and severity of heart failure, as measured by New York Heart Association criteria, improved. These actions continued during chronic therapy.

In patients with mild to moderate heart failure, enalapril retarded progressive cardiac dilatation/enlargement and failure, as evidenced by reduced left ventricular end diastolic and systolic volumes and improved ejection fraction.

A multicentre, randomised, double-blind, placebo-controlled trial (SOLVD Prevention trial) examined a population with asymptomatic left ventricular dysfunction (LVEF < 35%). 4228 patients were randomised to receive either placebo (n=2117) or enalapril (n=2111). In the placebo group, 818 patients had heart failure or died (38.6%) as compared with 630 in the enalapril group (29.8%) (risk reduction: 29%; 95% CI; 21 - 36%; $p < 0.001$). 518 patients in the placebo group (24.5%) and 434 in the enalapril group (20.6%) died or were hospitalised for new or worsening heart failure (risk reduction 20%; 95% CI; 9 - 30%; $p < 0.001$).

A multicentre, randomised, double-blind, placebo-controlled trial (SOLVD Treatment trial) examined a population with symptomatic congestive heart failure due to systolic dysfunction (ejection fraction < 35%). 2569 patients receiving conventional treatment for heart failure were randomly assigned to receive either placebo (n=1284) or enalapril (n=1285). There were 510 deaths in the placebo group (39.7%) as compared with 452 in the enalapril group (35.2%) (reduction in risk, 16%; 95% CI, 5 - 26%; p=0.0036). There were 461 cardiovascular deaths in the placebo group as compared with 399 in the enalapril group (risk reduction 18%, 95% CI, 6 - 28%, $p < 0.002$), mainly due to a decrease of deaths due to progressive heart failure (251 in the placebo group vs 209 in the enalapril group, risk reduction 22%, 95% CI, 6 - 35%). Fewer patients died or were hospitalised for worsening heart failure (736 in the placebo group and 613 in the enalapril group; risk reduction, 26%; 95% CI, 18 - 34%; $p < 0.0001$). Overall in SOLVD study, in patients with left ventricular dysfunction, 'Innovace' reduced the risk of myocardial infarction by 23% (95% CI, 11 – 34%; $p < 0.001$) and reduced the risk of hospitalisation for unstable angina pectoris by 20% (95% CI, 9 – 29%; $p < 0.001$).

There is limited experience of the use in hypertensive paediatric patients > 6 years. In a clinical study involving 110 hypertensive paediatric patients 6 to 16 years of age with a body weight ⩾ 20 kg and a glomerular filtration rate > 30 ml/min/1.73 m^2, patients who weighed < 50 kg received either 0.625, 2.5 or 20 mg of enalapril daily and patients who weighed ⩾ 50 kg received either 1.25, 5 or 40 mg of enalapril daily. Enalapril administration once daily lowered trough blood pressure in a dose-dependent manner. The dose-dependent antihypertensive efficacy of enalapril was consistent across all subgroups (age, Tanner stage, gender, race). However, the lowest doses studied, 0.625 mg and 1.25 mg, corresponding to an average of 0.02 mg/kg once daily, did not appear to offer consistent antihypertensive efficacy. The maximum dose studied was 0.58 mg/kg (up to 40 mg) once daily. The adverse experience profile for paediatric patients is not different from that seen in adult patients.

5.2 Pharmacokinetic properties

Absorption

Oral enalapril is rapidly absorbed, with peak serum concentrations of enalapril occurring within one hour. Based on urinary recovery, the extent of absorption of enalapril from oral enalapril tablet is approximately 60%. The absorption of oral 'Innovace' is not influenced by the presence of food in the gastrointestinal tract.

Following absorption, oral enalapril is rapidly and extensively hydrolysed to enalaprilat, a potent angiotensin converting enzyme inhibitor. Peak serum concentrations of enalaprilat occur about 4 hours after an oral dose of enalapril tablet. The effective half-life for accumulation of enalaprilat following multiple doses of oral enalapril is 11 hours. In subjects with normal renal function, steady-state serum concentrations of enalaprilat were reached after 4 days of treatment.

Distribution

Over the range of concentrations which are therapeutically relevant, enalaprilat binding to human plasma proteins does not exceed 60%.

Biotransformation

Except for conversion to enalaprilat, there is no evidence for significant metabolism of enalapril.

Elimination

Excretion of enalaprilat is primarily renal. The principal components in urine are enalaprilat, accounting for about 40% of the dose, and intact enalapril (about 20%).

Renal impairment

The exposure of enalapril and enalaprilat is increased in patients with renal insufficiency. In patients with mild to moderate renal insufficiency (creatinine clearance 40-60 ml/min) steady state AUC of enalaprilat was approximately two-fold higher than in patients with normal renal function after administration of 5 mg once daily. In severe renal impairment (creatinine clearance ⩽ 30 ml/min), AUC was increased approximately 8-fold. The effective half-life of enalaprilat following multiple doses of enalapril maleate is prolonged at this level of renal insufficiency and time to steady state is delayed. (See 4.2 'Posology and method of administration'.) Enalaprilat may be removed from the general circulation by hemodialysis. The dialysis clearance is 62 ml/min.

Children and adolescents

A multiple dose pharmacokinetic study was conducted in 40 hypertensive male and female pediatric patients aged 2 months to ⩽ 16 years following daily oral administration of 0.07 to 0.14 mg/kg enalapril maleate. There were no major differences in the pharmacokinetics of enalaprilat in children compared with historic data in adults. The data indicate an increase in AUC (normalised to dose per body weight) with increased age; however, an increase in AUC is not observed when data are normalised by body surface area. At steady state, the mean effective half-life for accumulation of enalaprilat was 14 hours.

Lactation

After a single 20 mg oral dose in 5 postpartum women the average peak enalapril milk level was 1.7 μg/L (range 0.54 to 5.9 μg/L) at 4 to 6 hours after the dose. The average peak enalaprilat level was 1.7 μg/L (range 1.2 to 2.3 μg/L); peaks occurred at various times over the 24-hour period. Using the peak milk level data, the estimated maximum intake of an exclusively breastfed infant would be about 0.16% of the maternal weight-adjusted dosage.

A woman who had been taking oral enalapril 10 mg daily for 11 months had peak enalapril milk levels of 2 μg/L 4 hours after a dose and peak enalaprilat levels of 0.75 μg/L about 9 hours after the dose. The total amount of enalapril and enalaprilat measured in milk during the 24 hour period was 1.44 μg/L and 0.63 μg/L of milk respectively.

Enalaprilat milk levels were undetectable (< 0.2 μg/L) 4 hours after a single dose of enalapril 5 mg in 1 mother and 10 mg in 2 mothers; enalapril levels were not determined.

5.3 Preclinical safety data

Preclinical data reveal no special hazard for humans based on conventional studies of safety pharmacology, repeated dose toxicity, genotoxicity and carcinogenic potential. Reproductive toxicity studies suggest that enalapril has no effects on fertility and reproductive performance in rats, and is not teratogenic. In a study in which female rats were dosed prior to mating through gestation, an increased incidence of rat pup deaths occurred during lactation. The compound has been shown to cross the placenta and is secreted in milk. Angiotensin converting enzyme inhibitors, as a class, have been shown to be fetotoxic (causing injury and/or death to the fetus) when given in the second or third trimester.

6. PHARMACEUTICAL PARTICULARS

6.1 List of excipients

Sodium bicarbonate, corn starch, pregelatinized corn starch, magnesium stearate and lactose monohydrate (99 mg, 198 mg, 164 mg and 154 mg for the 2.5 mg, 5 mg, 10 mg and 20 mg tablet respectively).

The 10 mg and 20 mg tablets also contain iron oxide (E172).

6.2 Incompatibilities

Not applicable.

6.3 Shelf life

2 years for 'Innovace' 2.5 mg, 5 mg, 10 mg and 20 mg Tablets

6.4 Special precautions for storage

Do not store 'Innovace' above 25°C.

6.5 Nature and contents of container

'Innovace' tablets are available in aluminium foil blisters containing 28 tablets.

6.6 Special precautions for disposal and other handling

No special requirements

7. MARKETING AUTHORISATION HOLDER

Merck Sharp & Dohme Limited

Hertford Road, Hoddesdon, Hertfordshire, EN11 9BU, UK.

8. MARKETING AUTHORISATION NUMBER(S)

2.5 mg Tablet: PL 0025/0220

5 mg Tablet: PL 0025/0194

10 mg Tablet: PL 0025/0195

20 mg Tablet: PL 0025/0196

9. DATE OF FIRST AUTHORISATION/RENEWAL OF THE AUTHORISATION

2.5 mg tablets PL 0025/0220 first licensed 17 April 1986

2.5 mg tablets PL 0025/0220 last renewed 01 November 2004

5 mg tablets PL 0025/0194 first licensed 06 December 1984

5 mg tablets PL 0025/0194 last renewed 01 November 2004

10 mg tablets PL 0025/0195 first licensed 06 December 1984

10 mg tablets PL 0025/0195 last renewed 01 November 2004

20 mg tablets PL 0025/0196 first licensed 06 December 1984

20 mg tablets PL 0025/0196 last renewed 01 November 2004

10. DATE OF REVISION OF THE TEXT
August 2009

LEGAL CATEGORY
POM

SPC.RNT.08.UK.2979 (II-016)

Innozide Tablets

(Merck Sharp & Dohme Limited)

1. NAME OF THE MEDICINAL PRODUCT
INNOZIDE®

2. QUALITATIVE AND QUANTITATIVE COMPOSITION
Each tablet of 'Innozide' contains 20 mg enalapril maleate and 12.5 mg hydrochlorothiazide.

3. PHARMACEUTICAL FORM
'Innozide' is supplied as round, fluted, yellow tablets with 'MSD 718' on one side and scored on the other.

4. CLINICAL PARTICULARS

4.1 Therapeutic indications
'Innozide' is indicated for the treatment of mild to moderate hypertension in patients who have been stabilised on the individual components given in the same proportions.

4.2 Posology and method of administration
The dosage of 'Innozide' should be determined primarily by the experience with the enalapril maleate component.

Adults

Essential hypertension

The usual dosage is one tablet, taken once daily. If necessary, the dosage may be increased to two tablets, taken once daily.

Prior diuretic therapy: symptomatic hypotension may occur following the initial dose of 'Innozide'; this is more likely in patients who are volume and/or salt depleted as a result of prior diuretic therapy. The diuretic therapy should be discontinued for 2-3 days prior to initiation of therapy with 'Innozide'.

Dosage in renal insufficiency

Thiazides may not be appropriate diuretics for use in patients with renal impairment and are ineffective at creatinine clearance values of 30 ml/min or below (i.e. moderate or severe renal insufficiency).

In patients with creatinine clearance of >30 and <80 ml/min, 'Innozide' should be used only after titration of the individual components.

Use in the elderly

In clinical studies the efficacy and tolerability of enalapril maleate and hydrochlorothiazide, administered concomitantly, were similar in both elderly and younger hypertensive patients.

Paediatric use

Safety and effectiveness in children have not been established.

Route of administration: Oral.

4.3 Contraindications
'Innozide' is contra-indicated in patients with anuria.

'Innozide' is contra-indicated in patients who are hypersensitive to any component of this product and in patients with a history of angioneurotic oedema relating to previous treatment with an angiotensin-converting enzyme (ACE) inhibitor and in patients with hereditary or idiopathic angioedema.

'Innozide' is contra-indicated in patients who are hypersensitive to other sulphonamide-derived drugs.

'Innozide' is contra-indicated in patients with stenosis of the renal arteries.

'Innozide' is contra-indicated in the second and third trimester of pregnancy (see section 4.4 and 4.6).

4.4 Special warnings and precautions for use
Enalapril maleate - Hydrochorothiazide

Symptomatic Hypotension

Symptomatic hypotension is rarely seen in uncomplicated hypertensive patients. In hypertensive patients receiving 'Innozide', symptomatic hypotension is more likely to occur if the patient has been volume - depleted, e.g. by diuretic therapy, dietary salt restriction, dialysis, diarrhoea or vomiting (see 4.5 'Interaction with other medicinal products and other forms of interaction' and 4.8 'Undesirable effects'). Regular determination of serum electrolytes should be performed at appropriate intervals in such patients. In patients with heart failure, with or without associated renal insufficiency, symptomatic hypotension has been observed. This is most likely to occur in those patients with more severe degrees of heart failure, as reflected by the use of high doses of loop diuretics, hyponatraemia or functional renal impairment. In these patients, therapy should be started under medical supervision and the patients should be followed closely whenever the dose of 'Innozide' and/or diuretic is adjusted. Similar considerations may apply to patients with ischaemic heart or cerebrovascular disease in whom an excessive fall in blood pressure could result in a myocardial infarction or cerebrovascular accident.

If hypotension occurs, the patient should be placed in the supine position and, if necessary, should receive an intravenous infusion of normal saline. A transient hypotensive response is not a contra-indication to further doses, which can be given usually without difficulty once the blood pressure has increased after volume expansion.

In some patients with heart failure who have normal or low blood pressure, additional lowering of systemic blood pressure may occur with 'Innozide'. This effect is anticipated, and usually is not a reason to discontinue treatment. If hypotension becomes symptomatic, a reduction of dose and/or discontinuation of the diuretic and/or 'Innozide' may be necessary.

Renal function impairment

Renal failure has been reported in association with enalapril and has been mainly in patients with severe heart failure or underlying renal disease, including renal artery stenosis. If recognised promptly and treated appropriately, renal failure when associated with therapy with enalapril is usually reversible.

Some hypertensive patients, with no apparent pre-existing renal disease have developed increases in blood urea and creatinine when enalapril has been given concurrently with a diuretic. Dosage reduction of enalapril and/or discontinuation of the diuretic may be required. This situation should raise the possibility of underlying renal artery stenosis (see 4.4 'Special warnings and precautions for use', Renovascular hypertension).

Lithium

The combination of lithium and enalapril is generally not recommended (see 4.5 'Interaction with other medicinal products and other forms of interaction').

Lactose

'Innozide' contains lactose and therefore should not be used by patients with rare hereditary problems of galactose intolerance, the Lapp lactase deficiency or glucose-galactose malabsorption. 'Innozide' contains less than 200 mg of lactose per tablet.

Paediatric use

Safety and efficacy in children has not been established.

Enalapril maleate

Aortic or mitral valve stenosis/hypertrophic cardiomyopathy

As with all vasodilators, ACE inhibitors should be given with caution in patients with left ventricular valvular and outflow tract obstruction and avoided in cases of cardiogenic shock and haemodynamically significant obstruction.

Renovascular hypertension

There is an increased risk of hypotension and renal insufficiency when patients with bilateral renal artery stenosis or stenosis of the artery to a single functioning kidney are treated with ACE inhibitors. Loss of renal function may occur with only mild changes in serum creatinine. In these patients, therapy should be initiated under close medical supervision with low doses, careful titration, and monitoring of renal function.

Haemodialysis patients

Anaphylactoid reactions have been reported in patients dialysed with high-flux membranes (e.g. AN 69®) and treated concomitantly with an ACE inhibitor. In these patients consideration should be given to using a different type of dialysis membrane or a different class of antihypertensive agent.

Kidney transplantation

There is no experience regarding the administration of 'Innozide' in patients with a recent kidney transplantation. Treatment with 'Innozide' is therefore not recommended.

Hepatic failure

Rarely, ACE inhibitors have been associated with a syndrome that starts with cholestatic jaundice or hepatitis and progresses to fulminant hepatic necrosis and (sometimes) death. The mechanism of this syndrome is not understood. Patients receiving ACE inhibitors who develop jaundice or marked elevations of hepatic enzymes should discontinue the ACE inhibitor and receive appropriate medical follow-up.

Neutropenia/agranulocytosis

Neutropenia/agranulocytosis, thrombocytopenia and anaemia have been reported in patients receiving ACE inhibitors. In patients with normal renal function and no other complicating factors, neutropenia occurs rarely. Enalapril should be used with extreme caution in patients with collagen vascular disease, immunosuppressant therapy, treatment with allopurinol or procainamide, or a combination of these complicating factors, especially if there is pre-existing impaired renal function. Some of these patients developed serious infections which in a few instances did not respond to intensive antibiotic therapy. If enalapril is used in such patients, periodic monitoring of white blood cell counts is advised and patients should be instructed to report any sign of infection.

Hyperkalaemia

Elevations in serum potassium have been observed in some patients treated with ACE inhibitors, including enalapril. Risk factors for the development of hyperkalaemia include those with renal insufficiency, worsening of renal function, age (>70 years) diabetes mellitus, inter-current events in particular dehydration, acute decompensation, metabolic acidosis and concomitant use of potassium-sparing diuretics (e.g. spironolactone, eplerenone, triamterene, or amiloride), potassium supplements or potassium-containing salt substitutes; or those patients taking other drugs associated with increases in serum potassium (e.g. heparin). The use of potassium supplements, potassium-sparing diuretics, or potassium-containing salt substitutes particularly in patients with impaired renal function may lead to a significant increase in serum potassium. Hyperkalaemia can cause serious, sometimes fatal arrhythmias. If concomitant use of 'Innozide' and any of the above-mentioned agents is deemed appropriate, they should be used with caution and with frequent monitoring of serum potassium. (See 4.5 'Interaction with other medicinal products and other forms of interaction'.)

Hypoglycemia

Diabetic patients treated with oral antidiabetic agents or insulin starting an ACE inhibitor, should be told to closely monitor for hypoglycaemia, especially during the first month of combined use. (See 4.5 'Interaction with other medicinal products and other forms of interaction', Antidiabetics.)

Hypersensitivity/angioneurotic oedema

Angioneurotic oedema of the face, extremities, lips, tongue, glottis and/or larynx has been reported in patients treated with angiotensin converting enzyme inhibitors, including 'Innozide'. This may occur at any time during treatment. In such cases, 'Innozide' should be discontinued promptly and appropriate monitoring should be instituted to ensure complete resolution of symptoms prior to dismissing the patient. Even in those instances where swelling of only the tongue is involved, without respiratory distress, patients may require prolonged observation since treatment with antihistamines and corticosteroids may not be sufficient.

Very rarely, fatalities have been reported due to angioedema associated with laryngeal edema or tongue edema. Patients with involvement of the tongue, glottis or larynx are likely to experience airway obstruction, especially those with a history of airway surgery. Where there is involvement of the tongue, glottis or larynx, likely to cause airway obstruction, appropriate therapy, which may include subcutaneous epinephrine solution 1:1000 (0.3 ml to 0.5 ml) and/or measures to ensure a patent airway, should be administered promptly.

Black patients receiving ACE inhibitors have been reported to have a higher incidence of angioedema compared to non-blacks.

Patients with a history of angioedema unrelated to ACE inhibitor therapy may be at increased risk of angioedema while receiving an ACE inhibitor. (Also see 4.3 'Contra-indications'.)

Anaphylactoid reactions during hymenoptera desensitization

Rarely, patients receiving ACE inhibitors during desensitization with hymenoptera venom have experienced life-threatening anaphylactoid reactions. These reactions were avoided by temporarily withholding ACE-inhibitor therapy prior to each desensitisation.

Anaphylactoid reactions during LDL apheresis

Rarely, patients receiving ACE inhibitors during low density lipoprotein (LDL)-apheresis with dextran sulfate have experienced life-threatening anaphylactoid reactions. These reactions were avoided by temporarily withholding ACE-inhibitor therapy prior to each apheresis.

Cough

Cough has been reported with the use of ACE inhibitors. Characteristically, the cough is non-productive, persistent and resolves after discontinuation of therapy. ACE inhibitor-induced cough should be considered as part of the differential diagnosis of cough.

Surgery/anesthesia

In patients undergoing major surgery or during anaesthesia with agents that produce hypotension, enalapril blocks angiotensin II formation secondary to compensatory renin release. If hypotension occurs and is considered to be due to this mechanism, it can be corrected by volume expansion.

Pregnancy and lactation

Ace inhibitors should not be initiated during pregnancy. Unless continued ACE inhibitors is considered essential, patients planning pregnancy should be changed to alternative antihypertensive treatments which have an established safety profile for use in pregnancy. When pregnancy is diagnosed, treatment with ACE inhibitors should be stopped immediately, and, if appropriate, alternative therapy should be started (see sections 4.3 and 4.6).

Use of enalapril is not recommended during breast feeding.

Ethnic differences

As with other angiotensin converting enzyme inhibitors, enalapril is apparently less effective in lowering blood pressure in black people than in non-blacks, possibly because of a higher prevalence of low-renin states in the black hypertensive population.

Hydrochorothiazide

Renal function impairment

Thiazides may not be appropriate diuretics for use in patients with renal impairment and are ineffective at creatinine clearance values of 30 ml/min or below (i.e. moderate or severe renal insufficiency). (See section 4.2)

'Innozide' should not be administered to patients with renal insufficiency (creatinine clearance $\leq$80 ml/min) until titration of the individual components has shown the need for the doses present in the combination tablet.

Hepatic disease: thiazides should be used with caution in patients with impaired hepatic function or progressive liver disease, since minor alterations of fluid and electrolyte balance may precipitate hepatic coma.

Metabolic and endocrine effects:

Thiazide therapy may impair glucose tolerance. Dosage adjustment of antidiabetic agents, including insulin, may be required. Thaizides may decrease serum sodium, magnesium and potassium levels. Increases in cholesterol and triglyceride levels may be associated with thiazide diuretic therapy; however, at the 12.5 mg dose contained in 'Innozide', minimal or no effect was reported.

Thiazides may decrease urinary calcium excretion and may cause intermittent and slight elevation of serum calcium. Marked hypercalcaemia may be evidence of hidden hyperparathyroidism.

Thiazides should be discontinued before carrying out tests for parathyroid function.

Thiazide therapy may precipitate hyperuricaemia and/or gout in certain patients. However, enalapril may increase urinary uric acid and thus may attenuate the hyperuricaemic effect of hydrochlorothiazide.

Although no data exist for 'Innozide' from controlled clinical trials, as for any patient receiving diuretic therapy, periodic determination of serum electrolytes should be performed at appropriate intervals.

Thiazides (including hydrochlorothiazide) can cause fluid or electrolyte imbalance (hypokalaemia, hyponatraemia, and hypochloraemic alkalosis). Warning signs of fluid or electrolyte imbalance are xerostomia, thirst, weakness, lethargy, somnolence, restlessness, muscle pain or cramps, muscular fatigue, hypotension, oliguria, tachycardia, and gastro-intestinal disturbances such as nausea and vomiting.

Although hypokalaemia may develop during use of thiazide diuretics, concurrent therapy with enalapril may reduce diuretic-induced hypokalaemia. The risk of hypokalaemia is greatest in patients with cirrhosis of the liver, in patients experiencing brisk diuresis, in patients with inadequate oral intake of electrolytes and in patients receiving concomitant therapy with corticosteroids or ACTH.

Hyponatraemia may occur in oedematous patients in hot weather. Chloride deficit is generally mild and does not usually require treatment.

Thiazides may have been shown to increase the urinary excretion of magnesium, which may result in hypomagnesia.

Anti-doping test

Hydrochorothiazide contained in this product can produce a positive analytic result in an anti-doping test.

Hypersensitivity

In patients receiving thiazides, sensitivity reactions may occur with or without a history of allergy and bronchial asthma. Exacerbation or activation of systemic lupus erythematosus has been reported with the use of thiazides.

4.5 Interaction with other medicinal products and other forms of interaction

Enalapril maleate- hydrochlorothiazide

Other antihypertensive agents

Concomitant use of these agents may increase the hypotensive effects of enalapril. Concomitant use with nitroglycerine and other nitrates, or other vasodilators, may further reduce blood pressure.

Lithium

Reversible increases in serum lithium concentrations and toxicity have been reported during concomitant administration of lithium with ACE inhibitors. Concomitant use of thiazide diuretics may further increase lithium levels and enhance the risk of lithium toxicity with ACE inhibitors. Use of 'Innozide' with lithium is not recommended, but if the combination proves necessary, careful monitoring of serum lithium levels should be performed (see 4.4 'Special warnings and precautions for use').

Non-Steroidal Anti-Inflammatory Drugs (NSAIDs)

Chronic administration of NSAIDs may reduce the antihypertensive effect of an ACE inhibitor or may decrease the diuretic, natriuretic and antihypertensive effects of diuretics.

NSAIDs (including COX-2 inhibitors) and ACE inhibitors exert an additive effect on the increase in serum potassium, and may result in a deterioration of renal function. These effects are usually reversible. Rarely, acute renal failure may occur, especially in patients with compromised renal function (such as the elderly or patients who are volume-depleted including those on diuretic therapy).

Enalapril maleate

Potassium sparing diuretics or potassium supplements

ACE inhibitors attenuate diuretic induced potassium loss. Potassium sparing diuretics (e.g. spironolactone, eplerenone, triamterene or amiloride), potassium supplements, or potassium-containing salt substitutes may lead to significant increases in serum potassium. If concomitant use is indicated because of demonstrated hypokalaemia they should be used with caution and with frequent monitoring of serum potassium (see 4.4 'Special warnings and precautions for use').

Diuretics (thiazide or loop diuretics)

Prior treatment with high dose diuretics may result in volume depletion and a risk of hypotension when initiating therapy with enalapril (see 4.4 'Special warnings and precautions for use'). The hypotensive effects can be reduced by discontinuation of the diuretic, by increasing volume or salt intake or by initiating therapy with a low dose of enalapril.

Tricyclic antidepressants/antipsychotics/anesthetics/narcotics

Concomitant use of certain anaesthetic medicinal products, tricyclic antidepressants and antipsychotics with ACE inhibitors may result in further reduction of blood pressure (see 4.4 'Special warnings and precautions for use')

Gold

Nitritoid reactions (symptoms include facial flushing, nausea, vomiting and hypotension) have been reported rarely in patients on therapy with injectable gold (sodium aurothiomalate) and concomitant ACE inhibitor therapy including enalapril.

Sympathomimetics

Sympathomimetics may reduce the antihypertensive effects of ACE inhibitors.

Alcohol

Alcohol enhances the hypotensive effect of ACE inhibitors.

Antidiabetics

Epidemiological studies have suggested that concomitant administration of ACE inhibitors and antidiabetic medicines (insulins, oral hypoglycaemic agents) may cause an increased blood-glucose-lowering effect with risk of hypoglycaemia. This phenomenon appeared to be more likely to occur during the first weeks of combined treatment and in patients with renal impairment. (See 4.4 'Special warnings and precautions for use; Hypoglycaemia and 4.8 Undesirable effects; Metabolism and nutrition disorders').

Acetyl salicylic acid, thrombolytics and β-blockers

Enalapril can be safely administered concomitantly with acetyl salicylic acid (at cardiologic doses), thrombolytics and β-blockers.

Hydrochorothiazide

Non-depolarising muscle relaxants:

Thiazides may increase the responsiveness to tubocurarine.

Alcohol, barbiturates, or opioid analgesics

Potentiation of orthostatic hypotension may occur

Antidiabetic drugs (oral agents and insulin)

The use of antidiabetic drugs and thiazide diuretics may require dosage adjustment of the antidiabetic drug.

Cholestyramine and colestipol resins:

Absorption of hydrochlorothiazide is impaired in the presence of anionic exchange resins. Single doses of either cholestyramine or colestipol resins bind the hydrochlorothiazide and reduce its absorption from the gastro-intestinal tract by up to 85 and 43 percent respectively.

Increasing the QT Interval (e.g. procainamide, amiodarone, sotalol)

Increased risk of torsades de pointes

Digitalis glycosides

Hypokalaemia can sensitise or exaggerate the response of the heart to the toxic effects of digitalis (e.g. increased ventricular irritability)

Corticosteroids, ACTH: may result in intensified electrolyte depletion, particularly hypokalaemia with thiazide diuretics.

Pressor amines (e.g. adrenaline): possible decreased response to pressor amines but not sufficient to preclude their use.

Cytostatics (e.g. cyclophosphamide, methotrexate): Thiazides may reduce the renal excretion of cytotoxic drugs and potentiate their myelosuppressive effects.

4.6 Pregnancy and lactation

> The use of ACE inhibitors is not recommended during the first trimester of pregnancy (see section 4.4). The use of ACE inhibitors is contra-indicated during the second and third trimester of pregnancy (see sections 4.3 and 4.4).

Epidemiological evidence regarding the risk of teratogenicity following exposure to ACE inhibitors during the first trimester of pregnancy has not been conclusive; however a small increase in risk cannot be excluded. Unless continued ACE inhibitors therapy is considered essential, patients planning pregnancy should be changed to alternative anti-hypertensive treatments which have an established safety profile for use in pregnancy. When pregnancy is diagnosed, treatment with ACE inhibitors should be stopped immediately, and, if appropriate, alternative therapy should be started.

ACE inhibitors therapy exposure during the second and third trimesters is known to induce human foetotoxicity (decreased renal function, oligohydramnios, skull ossification retardation) and neonatal toxicity (renal failure, hypotension, hyperkalaemia). (See section 5.3).

Should exposure to ACE inhibitors have occurred from the second trimester of pregnancy, ultrasound check of renal function and skull is recommended.

Infants whose mothers have taken ACE inhibitors should be closely observed for hypotension (see sections 4.3 and 4.4).

Prolonged exposure to hydrochlorothiazide during the third trimester of pregnancy may cause a foetoplacental ischaemia and growth retardation. Moreover, rare cases of hypoglycaemia and thrombocytopenia in neonates have been reported following exposure near term. Neonatal jaundice may also occur.

Hydrochlorothiazide can reduce plasma volume as well as uteroplacental blood flow.

Lactation: Enalapril, enalaprilat and thiazides appear in human milk. If use of 'Innozide' is deemed essential, breast-feeding should stop.

4.7 Effects on ability to drive and use machines

When driving vehicles or operating machines it should be taken into account that occasionally dizziness or weariness may occur.

4.8 Undesirable effects

Undesirable effects reported for enalapril alone or hydrochlorothiazide alone either during clinical studies or after the drug was marketed include:

[Very common (>1/10); common (>1/100, <1/10); uncommon (>1/1,000, <1/100); rare (>1/10,000, <1/1,000); very rare (<1/10,000), not known (cannot be estimated from the available data).]

Blood and the lymphatic system disorders:

uncommon: anaemia (including aplastic and hemolytic)

rare: neutropenia, decreases in haemoglobin, decreases in haematocrit, thrombocytopenia, agranulocytosis, bone marrow depression, leukopenia, pancytopenia, lymphadenopathy, autoimmune diseases.

Endocrine disorders:

not known: syndrome of inappropriate antidiuretic hormone secretion (SIADH)

Metabolism and nutrition disorders:

common: hypokalaemia, increase of cholesterol, increase of triglycerides, hyperuricaemia

uncommon: hypoglycaemia (see 4.4 'Special warnings and precautions for use', Hypoglycaemia), gout

rare: increase in blood glucose

very rare: hypercalcaemia

Psychiatric disorders:

uncommon: decreased libido

Nervous system disorders:

common: headache, depression, syncope, taste alteration

uncommon: confusion, somnolence, insomnia, nervousness, paraesthesia, vertigo

rare: dream abnormality, sleep disorders

Eye disorders:

very common: blurred vision

Ear and labyrinth disorders:

uncommon: tinnitus

Cardiac and Vascular disorders:

very common: dizziness

common: hypotension (including orthostatic hypotension), rhythm disturbances, angina pectoris, tachycardia

uncommon: orthostatic hypotension, palpitations, myocardial infarction or cerebrovascular accident*, possibly secondary to excessive hypotension in high risk patients (see 4.4 'Special warnings and precautions for use')

rare: Raynaud's phenomenon

Respiratory, thoracic and mediastinal disorders:

very common: cough

common: dyspnoea

uncommon: rhinorrhoea, sore throat and hoarseness, bronchospasm/asthma

rare: pulmonary infiltrates, respiratory distress (including pneumonitis and pulmonary oedema), rhinitis, allergic alveolitis/eosinophilic pneumonia

Gastrointestinal disorders:

very common: nausea,

common: diarrhea, abdominal pain

uncommon: ileus, pancreatitis, vomiting, dyspepsia, constipation, anorexia, gastric irritations, dry mouth, peptic ulcer, flatulence

rare: stomatitis/aphthous ulcerations, glossitis

very rare: intestinal angioedema

Hepatobilliary disorders:

rare: hepatic failure, hepatitis – either hepatocellular or cholestatic, hepatitis including necrosis, cholestatsis (including jaundice)

Skin and subcutaneous tissue disorders:

common: rash, hypersensitivity/angioneurotic oedema: angioneurotic oedema of the face, extremities, lips, tongue, glottis and/or larynx has been reported (see 4.4 'Special warnings and precautions for use')

uncommon: diaphoresis, pruritus, urticaria, alopecia

rare: erythema multiforme, Stevens-Johnson syndrome, exfoliative dermatitis, toxic epidermal necrolysis, purpura, pemphigus, erythroderma

A symptom complex has been reported which may include some or all of the following: fever, serositis, vasculitis, myalgia/myositis, arthralgia/arthritis, a positive ANA, elevated ESR, eosinophilia, and leukocytosis. Rash, photosensitivity or other dermatologic manifestations may occur.

Renal and urinary disorders:

uncommon: renal dysfunction, renal failure, proteinuria

rare: oliguria, intestinal nephritis

Reproductive system and breast disorders:

uncommon: impotence

rare: gynecomastia

General disorders and administration site conditions:

very common: asthenia

common: chest pain, fatigue

uncommon: muscle cramps, flushing,, malaise, fever

Investigations:

common: increases in serum creatinine

uncommon: increases in blood urea, hyponatraemia

rare: elevations of liver enzymes, elevations of serum bilirubin

4.9 Overdose

No specific information is available on the treatment of overdosage with 'Innozide'. Treatment is symptomatic and supportive. Therapy with 'Innozide' should be discontinued and the patient observed closely. Suggested measures include induction of emesis and/or gastric lavage, and correction of dehydration, electrolyte imbalance and hypotension by established procedures.

Enalapril maleate

The most prominent feature of overdosage reported to date is marked hypotension, beginning some six hours after ingestion of tablets, concomitant with blockade of the renin-angiotensin-aldosterone system, and stupor. Serum enalaprilat levels 100 times and 200 times higher than usually seen after therapeutic doses have been reported after ingestion of 300 mg and 440 mg of enalapril maleate respectively.

The recommended treatment of overdosage is intravenous infusion of normal saline solution. If available angiotensin II infusion may be beneficial. Enalaprilat may be removed from the general circulation by haemodialysis (see section 4.4 'Special warnings and special precautions for use': haemodialysis patients).

Hydrochlorothiazide

The most common signs and symptoms observed are those caused by electrolyte depletion (hypokalaemia, hypochloraemia, hyponatraemia) and dehydration resulting from excessive diuresis. If digitalis has also been administered, hypokalaemia may accentuate cardiac arrhythmias.

5. PHARMACOLOGICAL PROPERTIES

5.1 Pharmacodynamic properties

Pharmacotherapeutic group: enalapril and diuretics, ATC code C09 BA02.

Enalapril maleate

Angiotensin-converting enzyme (ACE) is a peptidyl dipeptidase which catalyses the conversion of angiotensin I to the pressor substance angiotensin II. After absorption, enalapril is hydrolysed to enalaprilat, which inhibits ACE, which leads to increased plasma renin activity (due to removal of negative feedback on renin release), and decreased aldosterone secretion.

ACE is identical to kininase II. Thus enalapril may also block the degradation of bradykinin, a potential vasodepressor peptide. However, the role that this plays in the therapeutic effects of enalapril remains to be elucidated. While the mechanism through which enalapril lowers blood pressure is believed to be primarily suppression of the renin-angiotensin-aldosterone system, which plays a major role in the regulation of blood pressure, enalapril is antihypertensive even in patients with low-renin hypertension.

Enalapril maleate - hydrochlorothiazide

Hydrochlorothiazide is a diuretic and antihypertensive agent which increases plasma renin activity. Although enalapril alone is antihypertensive even in patients with low-renin hypertension, concomitant administration of hydrochlorothiazide in these patients leads to greater reduction of blood pressure.

5.2 Pharmacokinetic properties

Absorption

Oral enalapril maleate is rapidly absorbed, with peak serum concentrations of enalapril occurring within one hour. Based on urinary recovery, the extent of absorption of enalapril from oral enalapril maleate is approximately 60%. Following absorption, oral enalapril is rapidly and extensively hydrolysed to enalaprilat, a potent angiotensin-converting enzyme inhibitor. Peak serum concentrations of enalaprilat occur 3 to 4 hours after an oral dose of enalapril maleate. The principal components in urine are enalaprilat, accounting for about 40% of the dose, and intact enalapril. Except for conversion to enalaprilat, there is no evidence of significant metabolism of enalapril. The serum concentration profile of enalaprilat exhibits a prolonged terminal phase, apparently associated with binding to ACE. In subjects with normal renal function, steady state serum concentrations of enalaprilat were achieved by the fourth day of administration of enalapril maleate. The absorption of oral enalapril maleate is not influenced by the presence of food in the gastro-intestinal tract. The extent of absorption and hydrolysis of enalapril are similar for the various doses in the recommended therapeutic range.

Distribution

Studies in dogs indicate that enalapril crosses the blood-brain barrier poorly, if at all; enalaprilat does not enter the brain. Enalapril crosses the placental barrier. Hydrochlorothiazide crosses the placental but not the blood-brain barrier.

Biotransformation

Except for conversion to enalaprilat, there is no evidence for significant metabolism of enalapril. Hydrochlorothiazide is not metabolised but is eliminated rapidly by the kidney.

Elimination

Excretion of enalapril is primarily renal. The principal components in urine are enalaprilat, accounting for about 40% of the dose, and intact enalapril. The effective half-life for accumulation of enalaprilat following multiple doses of oral enalapril maleate is 11 hours. When plasma levels of hydrochlorothiazide have been followed for at least 24 hours, the plasma half-life has been observed to vary between 5.6 and 14.8 hours. Hydrochlorothiazide is not metabolised but is eliminated rapidly by the kidney. At least 61% of the oral dose is eliminated unchanged within 24 hours.

Characteristics in patients

Enalaprilat may be removed from the general circulation by haemodialysis.

5.3 Preclinical safety data

No relevant information.

6. PHARMACEUTICAL PARTICULARS

6.1 List of excipients

Sodium hydrogen carbonate E500, lactose, maize starch, yellow ferric oxide E172, pregelatinised starch, and magnesium stearate E572.

6.2 Incompatibilities

None

6.3 Shelf life

36 months.

6.4 Special precautions for storage

Do not store above 25°C. Store in the original container.

6.5 Nature and contents of container

PVC/nylon/aluminium blister calendar packs containing 28 tablets.

6.6 Special precautions for disposal and other handling

None.

7. MARKETING AUTHORISATION HOLDER

Merck Sharp & Dohme Limited

Hertford Road, Hoddesdon, Hertfordshire EN11 9BU, UK

8. MARKETING AUTHORISATION NUMBER(S)

PL 0025/0249

9. DATE OF FIRST AUTHORISATION/RENEWAL OF THE AUTHORISATION

First authorised: 8 May 1991.

Last renewed: 10 November 1999.

10. DATE OF REVISION OF THE TEXT

Revision approved: March 2009.

LEGAL CATEGORY

POM

® denotes registered trademark of Merck & Co., Inc., Whitehouse Station, NJ, USA.

MSD

Merck Sharp & Dohme Limited

Hertford Road, Hoddesdon, Hertfordshire EN11 9BU, UK

SPC.CRN.08.UK.2901

* Incidence rates were comparable to those in the placebo and active control groups in the clinical trials

Inovelon Tablets

(Eisai Ltd)

1. NAME OF THE MEDICINAL PRODUCT

100 mg: Inovelon ▼ 100 mg film-coated tablets.

200 mg: Inovelon ▼ 200 mg film-coated tablets.

400 mg: Inovelon ▼ 400 mg film-coated tablets.

2. QUALITATIVE AND QUANTITATIVE COMPOSITION

100 mg: Each film-coated tablet contains 100 mg rufinamide.

Excipient: 20 mg lactose monohydrate/film coated tablet.

200 mg: Each film-coated tablet contains 200 mg rufinamide.

Excipient: 40 mg lactose monohydrate/film coated tablet.

400 mg: Each film-coated tablet contains 400 mg rufinamide.

Excipient: 80 mg lactose monohydrate/film coated tablet.

For a full list of excipients, see section 6.1.

3. PHARMACEUTICAL FORM

Film-coated tablets.

100 mg: Pink, 'ovaloid', slightly convex, scored on both sides, embossed '€261' on one side and blank on the other side.

200 mg: Pink, 'ovaloid', slightly convex, scored on both sides, embossed '€262' on one side and blank on the other side.

400 mg: Pink, 'ovaloid', slightly convex, scored on both sides, embossed '€263' on one side and blank on the other side.

The tablets can be divided into equal halves.

4. CLINICAL PARTICULARS

4.1 Therapeutic indications

Inovelon is indicated as adjunctive therapy in the treatment of seizures associated with Lennox-Gastaut syndrome in patients 4 years and older.

4.2 Posology and method of administration

Treatment with Inovelon should be initiated by a physician specialised in paediatrics or neurology with experience in the treatment of epilepsy.

Inovelon is for oral use. It should be taken twice daily with water in the morning and in the evening, in two equally divided doses. As a food effect was observed, it will preferable to administer Inovelon with food (see Section 5.2). If the patient has difficulty with swallowing, tablets can be crushed and administered in half a glass of water.

Use in children four years of age or older and less than 30 kg

Patients <30 kg not receiving valproate:

Treatment should be initiated at a daily dose of 200 mg. According to clinical response and tolerability, the dose may be increased by 200 mg/day increments, as frequently as every two days, up to a maximum recommended dose of 1000 mg/day. Doses of up to 3600 mg/day have been studied in a limited number of patients.

Patients <30 kg also receiving valproate medication:

As valproate significantly decreases clearance of Inovelon, a lower maximum dose of Inovelon is recommended for patients <30 kg being co-administered valproate. Treatment should be initiated at a daily dose of 200 mg. According to clinical response and tolerability, after a minimum of 2 days the dose may be increased by 200 mg/day, to the maximum recommended dose of 600 mg/day.

Use in adults and children four years of age or older of 30 kg or over

Treatment should be initiated at a daily dose of 400 mg. According to clinical response and tolerability, the dose may be increased by 400 mg/day increments, as frequently as every two days, up to a maximum recommended dose as indicated in the table below.

Weight range	30.0 – 50.0 kg	50.1 – 70.0 kg	≥70.1 kg
Maximum recommended dose (mg/day)	1800	2400	3200

Doses of up to 4000 mg/day (in the 30-50 kg range) or 4800 mg/day (over 50 kg) have been studied in a limited number of patients.

Elderly

There is limited information on the use of Inovelon in the elderly. Since, the pharmacokinetics of rufinamide are not altered in the elderly (see Section 5.2), dosage adjustment is not required in patients over 65 years of age.

Patients with renal impairment

A study in patients with severe renal impairment indicated that no dose adjustments are required for these patients (see Section 5.2).

Patients with hepatic impairment

Use in patients with hepatic impairment has not been studied. Caution and careful dose titration is recommended when treating patients with mild to moderate hepatic impairment. Therefore, use in patients with severe hepatic impairment is not recommended.

Effect of food

Inovelon should preferably be taken with food (see Section 5.2).

Discontinuation of Inovelon

When Inovelon treatment is to be discontinued, it should be withdrawn gradually. In clinical trials Inovelon discontinuation was achieved by reducing the dose by approximately 25% every two days.

In the case of one or more missed doses, individualised clinical judgement is necessary.

Uncontrolled open-label studies suggest sustained long-term efficacy, although no controlled study has been conducted for longer than three months.

4.3 Contraindications

Hypersensitivity to the active substance, triazole derivatives or to any excipients.

4.4 Special warnings and precautions for use

Status epilepticus cases have been observed during clinical development studies, under rufinamide whereas no such cases have been observed under placebo. These events led to rufinamide discontinuation in 20 % of the cases. If patients develop new seizure types and/or experience an increased frequency of status epilepticus that is different from the patient's baseline condition, then the benefit risk ratio of the therapy should be reassessed.

Antiepileptic medicinal products, including Inovelon, should be withdrawn gradually to reduce the possibility of seizures on withdrawal. In clinical studies discontinuation was achieved by reducing the dose by approximately 25% every two days. There are insufficient data on the withdrawal of concomitant antiepileptic medicinal products once seizure control has been achieved with the addition of Inovelon.

Rufinamide treatment has been associated with dizziness, somnolence, ataxia and gait disturbances, which could increase the occurrence of accidental falls in this population (see Section 4.8). Patients and carers should exercise caution until they are familiar with the potential effects of this medicinal product.

Serious antiepileptic drug hypersensitivity syndrome has occurred in association with rufinamide therapy. Signs and symptoms of this disorder were diverse; however, patients typically, although not exclusively, presented with fever and rash associated with other organ system involvement. Other associated manifestations included lymphadenopathy, liver function tests abnormalities, and haematuria. Because the disorder is variable in its expression, other organ system signs and symptoms not noted here may occur. This syndrome occurred in close temporal association to the initiation of rufinamide therapy and in the paediatric population. If this reaction is suspected, rufinamide should be discontinued and alternative treatment started. All patients who develop a rash while taking rufinamide must be closely monitored.

In a thorough QT study, rufinamide produced a decrease in QTc interval proportional to concentration. Although the underlying mechanism and safety relevance of this finding is not known, clinicians should use clinical judgment when assessing whether to prescribe rufinamide to patients at risk from further shortening their QTc duration (eg. Congenital Short QT Syndrome or patients with a family history of such a syndrome).

Women of childbearing potential must use contraceptive measures during treatment with Inovelon. Physicians should try to ensure that appropriate contraception is used, and should use clinical judgement when assessing whether oral contraceptives, or the doses of the oral contraceptive components, are adequate based on the individual patients clinical situation (see Section 4.5).

Inovelon contains lactose, therefore patients with rare hereditary problems of galactose intolerance, the Lapp lactase deficiency or glucose-galactose malabsorption should not take this medicine.

4.5 Interaction with other medicinal products and other forms of interaction

Potential for other medicinal products to affect Inovelon

Other anti-epileptic medicinal products

Rufinamide concentrations may be decreased by co-administration with carbamazepine, phenobarbital, phenytoin, vigabatrin or primidone.

For patients on Inovelon treatment who have administration of valproate initiated, significant increases in rufinamide plasma concentrations may occur. The most pronounced increases were observed in patients of low body weight (<30 kg). Therefore, consideration should be given to a dose reduction of Inovelon in patients <30 kg who are initiated on valproate therapy (see Section 4.2).

The addition or withdrawal of these drugs or adjusting of the dose of these drugs during Inovelon therapy may require an adjustment in dosage of Inovelon.

No significant changes in rufinamide concentration are observed following co-administration with lamotrigine, topiramate or benzodiazepines.

Potential for Inovelon to affect other medicinal products

Other anti-epileptic medicinal products

The pharmacokinetic interactions between rufinamide and other anti-epileptic drugs have been evaluated in patients with epilepsy using population pharmacokinetic modelling. Rufinamide appears not to have clinically relevant effect on carbamazepine, lamotrigine, phenobarbital, topiramate or valproate steady state concentrations. Since rufinamide may decrease phenytoin clearance and increase average steady state plasma concentrations of co-administered phenytoin, consideration should be given to reducing the dose of phenytoin.

Oral contraceptives

Co-administration of rufinamide 800 mg b.i.d. and a combined oral contraceptive (ethinyloestradiol 35 μg and norethindrone 1 mg) for 14 days resulted in a mean decrease in the ethinyl estradiol AUC_{0-24} of 22% and in norethindrone AUC_{0-24} of 14%. Studies with other oral or implant contraceptives have not been conducted. Women of child-bearing potential using hormonal contraceptives are advised to use an additional safe and effective contraceptive method (see Section 4.4 and 4.6).

Cytochrome P450 enzymes

Rufinamide is metabolised by hydrolysis, and is not metabolised to any notable degree by cytochrome P450 enzymes. Furthermore, rufinamide does not inhibit the activity of cytochrome P450 enzymes (see Section 5.2). Thus, clinically significant interactions mediated through inhibition of cytochrome P450 system by rufinamide are unlikely to occur. Rufinamide has been shown to induce the cytochrome P450 enzyme CYP3A4 and may therefore reduce the plasma concentrations of drugs which are metabolised by this enzyme. The effect was modest to moderate. The mean CYP3A activity, assessed as clearance of triazolam, was increased by 55% after 11 days of treatment with rufinamide 400 mg b.i.d. The exposure of triazolam was reduced by 36%. Higher rufinamide doses may result in a more pronounced induction. It may not be excluded that rufinamide may decrease the exposure also of drugs metabolized by other enzymes, or transported by transport proteins such as P-glycoprotein.

It is recommended that patients treated with drugs that are metabolised by the CYP3A enzyme system are to be carefully monitored for two weeks at the start of, or after the end of treatment with Inovelon, or after any marked change in the dose. A dose adjustment of the concomitantly administered drug may need to be considered. These recommendations should also be considered when rufinamide is used concomitantly with drugs with a narrow therapeutic window such as warfarin and digoxin.

A specific interaction study in healthy subjects revealed no influence of rufinamide at a dose of 400 mg bid on the pharmacokinetics of olanzapine, a CYP1A2 substrate.

No data on the interaction of rufinamide with alcohol are available.

4.6 Pregnancy and lactation

Risk related to epilepsy and antiepileptic medicinal products in general:

It has been shown that in the offspring of women with epilepsy, the prevalence of malformations is two to three times greater than the rate of approximately 3% in the general population. In the treated population, an increase in malformations has been noted with polytherapy; however, the extent to which the treatment and/or the illness is responsible has not been elucidated.

Moreover, effective anti-epileptic therapy must not be interrupted, since the aggravation of the illness is detrimental to both the mother and the foetus.

Risk related to rufinamide:

Studies in animals revealed no teratogenic effect but foetotoxicity in presence of maternal toxicity (see Section 5.3). The potential risk for humans is unknown.

For rufinamide, no clinical data on exposed pregnancies are available

Taking these data into consideration, rufinamide should not be used during pregnancy unless clearly necessary and in women of childbearing age not using contraceptive measures.

Women of childbearing potential must use contraceptive measures during treatment with Inovelon. Physicians should try to ensure that appropriate contraception is used, and should use clinical judgement when assessing whether oral contraceptives, or the doses of the oral contraceptive components, are adequate based on the individual patients clinical situation (see Section 4.5).

If women treated with rufinamide plan to become pregnant, the indication of this product should be carefully weighed. During pregnancy, an effective antiepileptic rufinamide treatment must not be interrupted, since the aggravation of the illness is detrimental to both the mother and the foetus.

Is not known if rufinamide is excreted in human breast milk. Due to the potential harmful effects for the breast fed infant, the lactation should be avoided during maternal treatment with rufinamide.

4.7 Effects on ability to drive and use machines

Inovelon may cause dizziness, somnolence and blurred vision. Depending on the individual sensitivity, Inovelon may have a mild to severe influence on the ability to drive or use machines. Patients must be advised to exercise caution during activities requiring a high degree of alertness, e.g., driving or operating machinery.

4.8 Undesirable effects

The clinical development program has included over 1,900 patients, with different types of epilepsy, exposed to rufinamide. The most commonly reported adverse reactions overall were headache, dizziness, fatigue, and somnolence. The most common adverse reactions observed at a higher incidence than placebo in patients with Lennox-Gastaut syndrome were somnolence and vomiting. Adverse reactions were usually mild to moderate in severity. The discontinuation rate in Lennox-Gastaut syndrome due to adverse reactions was 8.2% for patients receiving Inovelon and 0% for patients receiving placebo. The most common adverse reactions resulting in discontinuation from the Inovelon treatment group were rash and vomiting.

Adverse reactions reported with an incidence greater than placebo, during the Lennox-Gastaut syndrome double-blind studies or in the overall rufinamide-exposed population, are listed in the table below by MedDRA preferred term, system organ class and by frequency.

Frequencies are defined as: very common (≥ 1/10), common (≥ 1/100 < 1/10), uncommon (≥ 1/1,000 < 1/100).

(see Table 1 on next page)

4.9 Overdose

After an acute overdose, the stomach may be emptied by gastric lavage or by induction of emesis. There is no specific antidote for Inovelon. Treatment should be supportive and may include haemodialysis (see Section 5.2).

Multiple dosing of 7,200 mg/day was associated with no major signs or symptoms.

5. PHARMACOLOGICAL PROPERTIES

5.1 Pharmacodynamic properties

Pharmacotherapeutic group: anti-epileptics, carboxamide derivatives; ATC-code: N03AF03.

Mechanism of action

Rufinamide modulates the activity of sodium channels, prolonging their inactive state. Rufinamide is active in a range of animal models of epilepsy.

Clinical experience

Inovelon was administered in a double blind, placebo-controlled study, at doses of up to 45 mg/kg/day for 84 days, to 139 patients with inadequately controlled seizures associated with Lennox-Gastaut Syndrome (including both atypical absence seizures and drop attacks). Male or female patients (between 4 and 30 years of age) were included if they were being treated with 1 to 3 concomitant fixed-dose antiepileptic drugs. Each patient had to have at least 90 seizures in the month prior to study entry. A significant improvement was observed for all three primary variables: the percentage change in total seizure frequency per 28 days during the maintenance phase relative to baseline (-35.8% on Inovelon vs. –1.6% on placebo, p= 0.0006), the number of tonic-atonic seizures (-42.9% on Inovelon vs. 2.2% on placebo, p = 0.0002), and the seizure severity rating from the Global Evaluation performed by the parent/guardian at the end of the double-blind phase (much or very much improved in 32.2% on Inovelon vs. 14.5% on the placebo arm, p=0.0041).

Population pharmacokinetic/pharmacodynamic modelling demonstrated that the reduction of total and tonic-atonic seizure frequencies, the improvement of the global evaluation of seizure severity and the increase in probability of reduction of seizure frequency were dependent on rufinamide concentrations.

5.2 Pharmacokinetic properties

Absorption

Maximum plasma levels are reached approximately 6 hours after administration. Peak concentration (C_{max}) and plasma AUC of rufinamide increase less than proportionally with doses in both fasted and fed healthy subjects and in patients, probably due to dose-limited absorption behaviour. After single doses food increases the bioavailability (AUC) of rufinamide by approximately 34% and the peak plasma concentration by 56%.

Distribution

In *in-vitro* studies, only a small fraction of rufinamide (34%) was bound to human serum proteins with albumin accounting for approximately 80% of this binding. This indicates minimal risk of drug-drug interactions by displacement from binding sites during concomitant administration of other drugs. Rufinamide was evenly distributed between erythrocytes and plasma.

Table 1 Frequencies are defined as: very common ($\geqslant 1/10$), common ($\geqslant 1/100 < 1/10$), uncommon ($\geqslant 1/1,000 < 1/100$)

System Organ Class	Very Common	Common	Uncommon	Rare
Infections and Infestations		Pneumonia		
		Influenza		
		Nasopharyngitis		
		Ear infection		
		Sinusitis		
		Rhinitis		
Immune system disorders			Hypersensitivity*	
Metabolism and Nutrition disorders		Anorexia		
		Eating disorder		
		Decreased appetite		
Psychiatric disorders		Anxiety		
		Insomnia		
Nervous system disorders	Somnolence*	Status epilepticus*		
	Headache	Convulsion		
	Dizziness*	Coordination Abnormal*		
		Nystagmus		
		Psychomotor hyperactivity		
		Tremor		
Eye Disorders		Diplopia		
		Vision blurred		
Ear and Labyrinth disorders		Vertigo		
Respiratory, thoracic and mediastinal disorders		Epistaxis		
Gastrointestinal disorders	Nausea	Abdominal pain upper		
	Vomiting	Constipation		
		Dyspepsia		
		Diarrhoea		
Hepato-biliary disorders			Hepatic enzyme increase	
Skin and subcutaneous tissue disorders		Rash*		
		Acne		
Musculoskeletal and connective tissue and bone disorders		Back pain		
Reproductive system and breast disorders		Oligomenorrhoea		
General disorders and administration site conditions	Fatigue	Gait disturbance*		
Investigations		Weight decrease		
Injury, poisoning		Head injury		
		Contusion		

*Cross refer to Section 4.4.

Biotransformation

Rufinamide is almost exclusively eliminated by metabolism. The main pathway of metabolism is hydrolysis of the carboxylamide group to the pharmacologically inactive acid derivative CGP 47292. Cytochrome P450-mediated metabolism is very minor. The formation of small amounts of glutathione conjugates cannot be completely excluded.

Rufinamide has demonstrated little or no significant capacity *in-vitro* to act as a competitive or mechanism-based inhibitor of the following human P450 enzymes: CYP1A2, CYP2A6, CYP2C9, CYP2C19, CYP2D6, CYP2E1, CYP3A4/5 or CYP4A9/11-2.

Elimination

The plasma elimination half-life is approximately 6-10 hours in healthy subjects and patients with epilepsy. When given twice daily at 12-hourly intervals, rufinamide accumulates to the extent predicted by its terminal half-life, indicating that the pharmacokinetics of rufinamide are time-independent (i.e. no autoinduction of metabolism).

In a radiotracer study in three healthy volunteers, the parent compound (rufinamide) was the main radioactive component in plasma, representing about 80% of the total radioactivity, and the metabolite CGP 47292 constituting only about 15%. Renal excretion was the predominant route of elimination for drug related material, accounting for 84.7% of the dose.

Linearity/non-linearity:

The bioavailability of rufinamide is dependent on dose. As dose increases the bioavailability decreases.

Pharmacokinetics in special patient groups

Sex

Population pharmacokinetic modelling has been used to evaluate the influence of sex on the pharmacokinetics of rufinamide. Such evaluations indicate that sex does not affect the pharmacokinetics of rufinamide to a clinically relevant extent.

Renal impairment

The pharmacokinetics of a single 400 mg dose of rufinamide were not altered in subjects with chronic and severe renal failure compared to healthy volunteers. However, plasma levels were reduced by approximately 30% when haemodialysis was applied after administration of rufinamide, suggesting that this may be a useful procedure in case of overdose (see Sections 4.2 and 4.9).

Hepatic impairment

No studies have been performed in patients with hepatic impairment and therefore Inovelon should not be administered to patients with severe hepatic impairment.

Children (2-12 years)

Children generally have lower clearance of rufinamide than adults, and this difference is related to body size. Studies in new-born infants or infants and toddlers under 2 years of age have not been conducted.

Elderly

A pharmacokinetic study in elderly healthy volunteers did not show a significant difference in pharmacokinetic parameters compared with younger adults.

5.3 Preclinical safety data

Conventional safety pharmacology studies revealed no special hazards at clinically relevant doses.

Toxicities observed in dogs at levels similar to human exposure at the maximum recommended dose were liver changes, including bile thrombi, cholestasis and liver enzyme elevations thought to be related to increased bile secretion in this species. No evidence of an associated risk was identified in the rat and monkey repeat dose toxicity studies.

In reproductive and developmental toxicity studies, there were reductions in foetal growth and survival, and some stillbirths secondary to maternal toxicity. However, no effects on morphology and function, including learning or memory, were observed in the offspring. Inovelon was not teratogenic in mice, rats or rabbits.

Rufinamide was not genotoxic and had no carcinogenic potential. Adverse effects not observed in clinical studies, but seen in animals at exposure levels similar to clinical exposure levels and with possible relevance to human use was myelofibrosis of the bone marrow in the mouse carcinogenicity study. Benign bone neoplasms (osteomas) and hyperostosis seen in mice were considered a result of the activation of a mouse specific virus by fluoride ions released during the oxidative metabolism of rufinamide.

Regarding the immunotoxic potential, small thymus and thymic involution were observed in dogs in a 13 week study with significant response at the high dose in male. In the 13 week study, female bone marrow and lymphoid changes are reported at the high dose with a weak incidence. In rats decreased cellularity of the bone marrow and thymic atrophy were observed only in the carcinogenicity study.

6. PHARMACEUTICAL PARTICULARS

6.1 List of excipients

Core:

Lactose monohydrate

Cellulose, microcrystalline

Maize starch

Croscarmellose sodium

Hypromellose

Magnesium stearate

Sodium laurilsulfate

Silica colloidal, anhydrous

Film coating:

Opadry 00F44042 [consists of hypromellose, macrogols (8000), titanium dioxide (E171), talc and ferric oxide red (E172)].

6.2 Incompatibilities

Not applicable.

6.3 Shelf life

3 years.

6.4 Special precautions for storage

Do not store above 30°C.

6.5 Nature and contents of container

100 mg: Aluminium/aluminium blisters, packs of 10, 30, 50, 60 and 100 film-coated tablets.

200mg: Aluminium/aluminium blisters, packs of 10, 30, 50, 60 and 100 film-coated tablets.

400 mg: Aluminium/aluminium blisters, packs of 10, 30, 50, 60, 100 and 200 film-coated tablets.

Not all pack sizes may be marketed.

6.6 Special precautions for disposal and other handling

No special requirements.

7. MARKETING AUTHORISATION HOLDER

Eisai Limited, European Knowledge Centre, Mosquito Way, Hatfield, Herts, AL10 9SN, UK

8. MARKETING AUTHORISATION NUMBER(S)

100 mg 10 film-coated tablets: EU/1/06/378/001

100 mg 30 film-coated tablets: EU/1/06/378/002

100 mg 50 film-coated tablets: EU/1/06/378/003

100 mg 60 film-coated tablets: EU/1/06/378/004

100 mg 100 film-coated tablets: EU/1/06/378/005

200 mg 10 film-coated tablets: EU/1/06/378/006

200 mg 30 film-coated tablets: EU/1/06/378/007

200 mg 50 film-coated tablets: EU/1/06/378/008

200 mg 60 film-coated tablets: EU/1/06/378/009

200 mg 100 film-coated tablets: EU/1/06/378/010

400 mg 10 film-coated tablets: EU/1/06/378/011

400 mg 30 film-coated tablets: EU/1/06/378/012

400 mg 50 film-coated tablets: EU/1/06/378/013

400 mg 60 film-coated tablets: EU/1/06/378/014

400 mg 100 film-coated tablets: EU/1/06/378/015

400 mg 200 film-coated tablets: EU/1/06/378/016

9. DATE OF FIRST AUTHORISATION/RENEWAL OF THE AUTHORISATION

16 January 2007

10. DATE OF REVISION OF THE TEXT

10th March 2009

11. LEGAL CATEGORY
POM - Medicinal product subject to medical prescription

Inspra 25mg & 50 mg film-coated tablets
(Pfizer Limited)

1. NAME OF THE MEDICINAL PRODUCT
INSPRA 25 mg film-coated tablets.

INSPRA 50 mg film-coated tablets.

2. QUALITATIVE AND QUANTITATIVE COMPOSITION
Each tablet contains 25 mg of eplerenone.

Each tablet contains 50 mg of eplerenone.

For excipients see section 6.1.

3. PHARMACEUTICAL FORM
Film-coated tablet.

25 mg tablet: yellow tablet with stylized "Pfizer" on one side of tablet, "NSR" over "25"on the other side of tablet.

50 mg tablet: yellow tablet with stylized "Pfizer" on one side of tablet, "NSR" over "50"on the other side of tablet.

4. CLINICAL PARTICULARS
4.1 Therapeutic indications
Eplerenone is indicated, in addition to standard therapy including beta-blockers, to reduce the risk of cardiovascular mortality and morbidity in stable patients with left ventricular dysfunction (LVEF ≤ 40 %) and clinical evidence of heart failure after recent myocardial infarction.

4.2 Posology and method of administration
For the individual adjustment of dose, the strengths of 25 mg and 50 mg are available.

The recommended maintenance dose of eplerenone is 50 mg once daily (OD). Treatment should be initiated at 25 mg once daily and titrated to the target dose of 50 mg once daily preferably within 4 weeks, taking into account the serum potassium level (see Table 1). Eplerenone therapy should usually be started within 3-14 days after an acute myocardial infarction.

Patients with a serum potassium of > 5.0 mmol/L should not be started on eplerenone (see section 4.3).

Serum potassium should be measured before initiating eplerenone therapy, within the first week and at one month after the start of treatment or dose adjustment. Serum potassium should be assessed as needed periodically thereafter.

After initiation, the dose should be adjusted based on the serum potassium level as shown in Table 1.

Table 1: Dose adjustment table after initiation

Serum potassium (mmol/L)	Action	Dose adjustment
< 5.0	Increase	25 mg EOD* to 25 mg OD 25 mg OD to 50 mg OD
5.0 – 5.4	Maintain	No dose adjustment
5.5 – 5.9	Decrease	50 mg OD to 25 mg OD 25 mg OD to 25 mg EOD* 25 mg EOD* to withhold
≥ 6.0	Withhold	N/A

* EOD: Every Other Day

Following withholding eplerenone due to serum potassium ≥ 6.0 mmol/L, eplerenone can be re-started at a dose of 25 mg every other day when potassium levels have fallen below 5.0 mmol/L.

Children and adolescents

There are no data to recommend the use of eplerenone in the paediatric population, and therefore, use in this age group is not recommended.

Elderly

No initial dose adjustment is required in the elderly. Due to an age-related decline in renal function, the risk of hyperkalaemia is increased in elderly patients. This risk may be further increased when co-morbidity associated with increased systemic exposure is also present, in particular mild-to-moderate hepatic impairment. Periodic monitoring of serum potassium is recommended (see section 4.4).

Renal impairment

No initial dose adjustment is required in patients with mild renal impairment. Periodic monitoring of serum potassium is recommended (see section 4.4).

Eplerenone is not dialysable.

Hepatic impairment

No initial dosage adjustment is necessary for patients with mild-to-moderate hepatic impairment. Due to an increased systemic exposure to eplerenone in patients with mild-to-moderate hepatic impairment, frequent and regular monitoring of serum potassium is recommended in these patients, especially when elderly (see section 4.4).

Concomitant treatment

In case of concomitant treatment with mild to moderate CYP3A4 inhibitors, e.g. amiodarone, diltiazem and verapamil, a starting dose of 25 mg OD may be initiated. Dosing should not exceed 25 mg OD (see section 4.5).

Eplerenone may be administered with or without food (see section 5.2).

4.3 Contraindications
• Hypersensitivity to eplerenone or any of the excipients (see section 6.1).

• Patients with serum potassium level > 5.0 mmol/L at initiation

• Patients with moderate to severe renal insufficiency (creatinine clearance < 50 mL/min)

• Patients with severe hepatic insufficiency (Child-Pugh Class C)

• Patients receiving potassium-sparing diuretics, potassium-supplements or strong inhibitors of CYP 3A4 (eg itraconazole, ketoconazole, ritonavir, nelfinavir, clarithromycin, telithromycin and nefazodone) (see section 4.5).

4.4 Special warnings and precautions for use
Hyperkalaemia: Consistent with its mechanism of action, hyperkalaemia may occur with eplerenone. Serum potassium levels should be monitored in all patients at initiation of treatment and with a change in dosage. Thereafter, periodic monitoring is recommended especially in patients at risk for the development of hyperkalaemia, such as (elderly) patients with renal insufficiency (see section 4.2) and patients with diabetes. The use of potassium supplements after initiation of eplerenone therapy is not recommended, due to an increased risk of hyperkalaemia. Dose reduction of eplerenone has been shown to decrease serum potassium levels. In one study, the addition of hydrochlorothiazide to eplerenone therapy has been shown to offset increases in serum potassium.

Impaired renal function: Potassium levels should be monitored regularly in patients with impaired renal function, including diabetic microalbuminuria. The risk of hyperkalaemia increases with decreasing renal function. While the data from EPHESUS in patients with type 2 diabetes and microalbuminuria is limited, an increased occurrence of hyperkalaemia was observed in this small number of patients. Therefore, these patients should be treated with caution. Eplerenone is not removed by haemodialysis.

Impaired hepatic function: No elevations of serum potassium above 5.5 mmol/L were observed in patients with mild to moderate hepatic impairment (Child Pugh class A and B). Electrolyte levels should be monitored in patients with mild to moderate hepatic impairment. The use of eplerenone in patients with severe hepatic impairment has not been evaluated and its use is therefore contraindicated (see section 4.3).

CYP3A4 inducers: Coadministration of eplerenone with strong CYP3A4 inducers is not recommended (see section 4.5).

Lithium, cyclosporin, tacromilus should be avoided during treatment with eplerenone (see section 4.5).

Lactose: The tablets contain lactose and should not be administered in patients with rare hereditary problems of galactose intolerance, the Lapp lactase deficiency or glucose-galactose malabsorption.

4.5 Interaction with other medicinal products and other forms of interaction
Pharmacodynamic interactions

Potassium-sparing diuretics and potassium supplements: Due to increased risk of hyperkalaemia, eplerenone should not be administered to patients receiving potassium-sparing diuretics and potassium supplements (see section 4.3). Potassium-sparing diuretics may potentiate the effect of anti-hypertensive agents and other diuretics.

Lithium: Drug interaction studies of eplerenone have not been conducted with lithium. However, lithium toxicity has been reported in patients receiving lithium concomitantly with diuretics and ACE inhibitors (see section 4.4). Coadministration of eplerenone and lithium should be avoided. If this combination appears necessary, lithium plasma concentrations should be monitored (see section 4.4).

Cyclosporin, tacrolimus: Cyclosporin and tacrolimus may lead to impaired renal function and increase the risk of hyperkalaemia. The concomitant use of eplerenone and cyclosporin or tacrolimus should be avoided. If needed, close monitoring of serum potassium and renal function are recommended when cyclosporine and tacrolimus are to be administered during treatment with eplerenone (see section 4.4).

Non-steroidal anti-inflammatory drugs (NSAIDs): Treatment with NSAIDs may lead to acute renal failure by acting directly on glomerular filtration, especially in at-risk patients (elderly and/or dehydrated patients). Patients receiving eplerenone and NSAIDs should be adequately hydrated and be monitored for renal function prior to initiating treatment.

Trimethroprim: The concomitant administration of trimethoprim with eplerenone increases the risk of hyperkalaemia. Monitoring of serum potassium and renal function should be made, particularly in patients with renal impairment and in the elderly.

ACE inhibitors, angiotensin-II receptors antagonists (AIIA): Eplerenone and ACE inhibitors or angiotensin-II receptors antagonists should be co-administered with caution. Combining eplerenone with these drugs may increase risk of hyperkalaemia in patients at risk for impaired renal function, e.g. the elderly. A close monitoring of serum potassium and renal function is recommended.

Alpha 1 blockers (e.g. prazosin, alfuzosine): When alpha-1-blockers are combined with eplerenone, there is the potential for increased hypotensive effect and/or postural hypotension. Clinical monitoring for postural hypotension is recommended during alpha-1-blocker co-administration.

Tricyclic anti-depressants, neuroleptics, amifostine, baclofene: Co-administration of these drugs with eplerenone may potentially increase antihypertensive effects and risk of postural hypotension.

Glucocorticoides, tetracosactide: Co-administration of these drugs with eplerenone may potentially decrease antihypertensive effects (sodium and fluid retention).

Pharmacokinetic interactions

In vitro studies indicate that eplerenone is not an inhibitor of CYP1A2, CYP2C19, CYP2C9, CYP2D6 or CYP3A4 isozymes. Eplerenone is not a substrate or an inhibitor of P-Glycoprotein.

Digoxin: Systemic exposure (AUC) to digoxin increases by 16% (90% CI: 4% - 30%) when co-administered with eplerenone. Caution is warranted when digoxin is dosed near the upper limit of therapeutic range.

Warfarin: No clinically significant pharmacokinetic interactions have been observed with warfarin. Caution is warranted when warfarin is dosed near the upper limit of therapeutic range.

CYP3A4 substrates: Results of pharmacokinetic studies with CYP3A4 probe-substrates, i.e. midazolam and cisapride, showed no significant pharmacokinetic interactions when these drugs were coadministered with eplerenone.

CYP3A4 inhibitors:

Strong CYP3A4 inhibitors: Significant pharmacokinetic interactions may occur when eplerenone is coadministered with drugs that inhibit the CYP3A4 enzyme. A strong inhibitor of CYP3A4 (ketoconazole 200 mg BID) led to a 441% increase in AUC of eplerenone (see section 4.3). The concomitant use of eplerenone with strong CYP3A4 inhibitors such as ketoconazole, itraconazole, ritonavir, nelfinavir, clarithromycin, telithromycin and nefazadone, is contra-indicated (see section 4.3).

Mild to moderate CYP3A4 inhibitors: Co-administration with erythromycin, saquinavir, amiodarone, diltiazem, verapamil, and fluconazole have led to significant pharmacokinetic interactions with rank order increases in AUC ranging from 98% to 187%. Eplerenone dosing should therefore not exceed 25 mg when mild to moderate inhibitors of CYP3A4 are coadministered with eplerenone (see sections 4.2).

CYP3A4 inducers: Co-administration of St John's Wort (a strong CYP3A4 inducer) with eplerenone caused a 30 % decrease in eplerenone AUC. A more pronounced decrease in eplerenone AUC may occur with stronger CYP3A4 inducers such as rifampicin. Due to the risk of decreased eplerenone efficacy, the concomitant use of strong CYP3A4 inducers (rifampicin, carbamazepine, phenytoin, phenobarbital, St John's Wort) with eplerenone is not recommended (see section 4.4).

Antacids: Based on the results of a pharmacokinetic clinical study, no significant interaction is expected when antacids are coadministered with eplerenone.

4.6 Pregnancy and lactation
Pregnancy: There are no adequate data on the use of eplerenone in pregnant women. Animal studies did not indicate direct or indirect adverse effects with respect to pregnancy, embryofoetal development, parturition and postnatal development (see section 5.3). Caution should be exercised prescribing eplerenone to pregnant women.

Lactation: It is unknown if eplerenone is excreted in human breast milk after oral administration. However, preclinical data show that eplerenone and/or metabolites are present in rat breast milk and that rat pups exposed by this route developed normally. Because of the unknown potential for adverse effects on the breast fed infant, a decision should be made whether to discontinue breast-feeding or discontinue the drug, taking into account the importance of the drug to the mother.

4.7 Effects on ability to drive and use machines
No studies on the effect of eplerenone on the ability to drive or use machines have been performed. Eplerenone does not cause drowsiness or impairment of cognitive function but when driving vehicles or operating machines it should be taken into account that dizziness may occur during treatment.

4.8 Undesirable effects
In the eplerenone post-acute myocardial infarction heart failure efficacy and survival study (EPHESUS), the overall incidence of adverse events reported with eplerenone (78.9%) was similar to placebo (79.5%). *The discontinuation rate due to adverse events in these studies was 4.4% for patients receiving eplerenone and for 4.3% patients receiving placebo.*

Adverse events reported below are either taken from EPHESUS and are those with suspected relationship to treatment and in excess of placebo or are serious and significantly in excess of placebo, or have been observed during post marketing surveillance. Adverse events are listed by body system and absolute frequency. Frequencies are defined as: common > 1/100, < 1/10; uncommon > 1/1000, < 1/100.

Infections and infestations

Uncommon: pyelonephritis

Blood and lymphatic system disorders

Uncommon: eosinophilia

Metabolism and nutrition disorders

Common: hyperkalaemia

Uncommon: hyponatraemia, dehydration, hypercholesterolaemia, hypertriglyceridaemia,

Psychiatric disorders

Uncommon: insomnia

Nervous system disorders

Common: dizziness

Uncommon: headache

Cardiac disorders

Uncommon: myocardial infarction, cardiac failure left, fibrillation atrial,

Vascular disorders

Common: hypotension

Uncommon: thrombosis arterial leg, hypotension postural,

Respiratory, thoracic and mediastinal disorders

Uncommon: pharyngitis

Gastrointestinal disorders

Common: diarrhoea, nausea

Uncommon: vomiting, flatulence,

Skin and subcutaneous tissue disorders

Common: rash

Uncommon: pruritus, sweating increased

Not known: angioneurotic oedema

Musculoskeletal and connective tissue disorders

Uncommon: back pain, cramp legs

Renal and urinary disorders

Common: renal function abnormal

Reproductive system and breast disorders

Uncommon: gynecomastia

General disorders and administration site conditions

Uncommon: asthenia, malaise

Investigations

Uncommon: BUN increased, creatinine increase

In EPHESUS, there were numerically more cases of stroke in the elderly group (≥ 75 years old). There was however no statistical significant difference between the occurrence of stroke in the eplerenone (30) vs placebo (22) groups.

4.9 Overdose

No cases of human overdosage with eplerenone have been reported. The most likely manifestation of human overdosage would be anticipated to be hypotension or hyperkalaemia. Eplerenone cannot be removed by haemodialysis. Eplerenone has been shown to bind extensively to charcoal. If symptomatic hypotension should occur, supportive treatment should be initiated. If hyperkalaemia develops, standard treatment should be initiated.

5. PHARMACOLOGICAL PROPERTIES

5.1 Pharmacodynamic properties

Pharmacotherapeutic group: aldosterone antagonists, ATC code: C03DA04

Eplerenone has relative selectivity in binding to recombinant human mineralocorticoid receptors compared to its binding to recombinant human glucocorticoid, progesterone and androgen receptors. Eplerenone prevents the binding of aldosterone, a key hormone in the renin-angiotensin-aldosterone-system (RAAS), which is involved in the regulation of blood pressure and the pathophysiology of cardiovascular disease.

Eplerenone has been shown to produce sustained increases in plasma renin and serum aldosterone, consistent with inhibition of the negative regulatory feedback of aldosterone on renin secretion. The resulting increased plasma renin activity and aldosterone circulating levels do not overcome the effects of eplerenone.

In dose-ranging studies of chronic heart failure (NYHA classification II-IV), the addition of eplerenone to standard therapy resulted in expected dose-dependent increases in aldosterone. Similarly, in a cardiorenal substudy of EPHESUS, therapy with eplerenone led to a significant increase in aldosterone. These results confirm the blockade of the mineralocorticoid receptor in these populations.

Eplerenone was studied in the eplerenone post-acute myocardial infarction heart failure efficacy and survival study (EPHESUS). EPHESUS was a double-blind, placebo-controlled study, of 3 year duration, in 6632 patients with acute myocardial infarction (MI), left ventricular dysfunction (as measured by left ventricular ejection fraction [LVEF] ⩽40%), and clinical signs of heart failure. Within 3-14 days (median 7 days) after an acute MI, patients received eplerenone or placebo in addition to standard therapies at an initial dose 25 mg once daily and titrated to the target dose of 50 mg once daily after 4 weeks if serum potassium was < 5.0 mmol/L. During the study patients received standard care including acetylsalicylic acid (92%), ACE inhibitors (90%), β-blockers (83%), nitrates (72%), loop diuretics (66%), or HMG CoA reductase inhibitors (60%).

In EPHESUS, the co-primary endpoints were all-cause mortality and the combined endpoint of CV death or CV hospitalisation; 14.4 % of patients assigned to eplerenone and 16.7 % of patients assigned to placebo died (all causes), while 26.7 % of patients assigned to eplerenone and 30.0 % assigned to placebo met the combined endpoint of CV death or hospitalisation. Thus, in EPHESUS, eplerenone reduced the risk of death from any cause by 15% (RR 0.85; 95% CI, 0.75-0.96; p= 0.008) compared to placebo, primarily by reducing cardiovascular (CV) mortality. The risk of CV death or CV hospitalisation was reduced by 13% with eplerenone (RR 0.87; 95% CI, 0.79-0.95; p=0.002). The absolute risk reductions for the endpoints all cause mortality and CV mortality/hospitalisation were 2.3 and 3.3%, respectively. Clinical efficacy was primarily demonstrated when eplerenone therapy was initiated in patients aged < 75 years old. The benefits of therapy in those patients over the age of 75 are unclear. NYHA functional classification improved or remained stable for a statistically significantly greater proportion of patients receiving eplerenone compared to placebo. The incidence of hyperkalaemia was 3.4 % in the eplerenone group vs 2.0 % in the placebo group (p < 0.001). The incidence of hypokalaemia was 0.5 % in the eplerenone group vs 1.5 % in the placebo group (p < 0.001).

No consistent effects of eplerenone on heart rate, QRS duration, or PR or QT interval were observed in 147 normal subjects evaluated for electrocardiographic changes during pharmacokinetic studies.

5.2 Pharmacokinetic properties

Absorption and Distribution:

The absolute bioavailability of eplerenone is unknown. Maximum plasma concentrations are reached after about 2 hours. Both peak plasma levels (Cmax) and area under the curve (AUC) are dose proportional for doses of 10 to 100 mg and less than proportional at doses above 100 mg. Steady state is reached within 2 days. Absorption is not affected by food.

The plasma protein binding of eplerenone is about 50% and is primarily bound to alpha 1-acid glycoproteins. The apparent volume of distribution at steady state is estimated at 50 (±7) L. Eplerenone does not preferentially bind to red blood cells.

Metabolism and Excretion:

Eplerenone metabolism is primarily mediated via CYP3A4. No active metabolites of eplerenone have been identified in human plasma.

Less than 5% of an eplerenone dose is recovered as unchanged drug in the urine and faeces. Following a single oral dose of radiolabeled drug, approximately 32% of the dose was excreted in the faeces and approximately 67% was excreted in the urine. The elimination half-life of eplerenone is approximately 3 to 5 hours. The apparent plasma clearance is approximately 10 L/hr.

Special Populations

Age, Gender, and Race: The pharmacokinetics of eplerenone at a dose of 100 mg once daily have been investigated in the elderly (⩾65 years), in males and females, and in blacks. The pharmacokinetics of eplerenone did not differ significantly between males and females. At steady state, elderly subjects had increases in C_{max} (22%) and AUC (45%) compared with younger subjects (18 to 45 years). At steady state, C_{max} was 19% lower and AUC was 26% lower in blacks. (see section 4.2.)

Renal Insufficiency: The pharmacokinetics of eplerenone were evaluated in patients with varying degrees of renal insufficiency and in patients undergoing haemodialysis. Compared with control subjects, steady-state AUC and Cmax were increased by 38% and 24%, respectively, in patients with severe renal impairment and were decreased by 26% and 3%, respectively, in patients undergoing haemodialysis. No correlation was observed between plasma clearance of eplerenone and creatinine clearance. Eplerenone is not removed by haemodialysis (see section 4.4.).

Hepatic Insufficiency: The pharmacokinetics of eplerenone 400 mg have been investigated in patients with moderate (Child-Pugh Class B) hepatic impairment and compared with normal subjects. Steady-state Cmax and AUC of eplerenone were increased by 3.6% and 42%, respectively (see section 4.2). Since the use of eplerenone has not been investigated in patients with severe hepatic impairment, eplerenone is contraindicated in this patients' group (see section 4.3).

Heart Failure: The pharmacokinetics of eplerenone 50 mg were evaluated in patients with heart failure (NYHA classification II-IV). Compared with healthy subjects matched according to age, weight and gender, steady state AUC and Cmax in heart failure patients were 38% and 30% higher, respectively. Consistent with these results, a population pharmacokinetic analysis of eplerenone based on a subset of patients from EPHESUS indicates that clearance of eplerenone in patients with heart failure was similar to that in healthy elderly subjects.

5.3 Preclinical safety data

Preclinical studies on safety pharmacology, genotoxicity, carcinogenic potential and toxicity to reproduction revealed no special hazard for humans.

In repeated dose toxicity studies, prostate atrophy was observed in rats and dogs at exposure levels slightly above clinical exposure levels. The prostatic changes were not associated with adverse functional consequences. The clinical relevance of these findings is unknown.

6. PHARMACEUTICAL PARTICULARS

6.1 List of excipients

Tablet core:

Lactose monohydrate

Microcrystalline cellulose (E460)

Croscarmellose sodium (E468)

Hypromellose (E464)

Sodium laurilsulfate

Talc (E553b)

Magnesium stearate (E470b)

Tablet coating:

Opadry yellow:

Hypromellose (E464)

Titanium dioxide (E171)

Macrogol 400

Polysorbate 80 (E433)

Iron oxide yellow (E172)

Iron oxide red (E172)

6.2 Incompatibilities

Not applicable.

6.3 Shelf life

3 years.

6.4 Special precautions for storage

No special precautions for storage.

6.5 Nature and contents of container

Opaque PVC/Al blisters containing 10, 20, 28, 30, 50, 90, 100 or 200 tablets

Opaque PVC/Al perforated unit dose blisters containing 20 × 1, 30 × 1, 50 × 1, 90 × 1, 100 × 1 or 200 × 1 (10 packs of 20 × 1) tablets

Not all pack sizes may be marketed.

6.6 Special precautions for disposal and other handling

No special requirements.

7. MARKETING AUTHORISATION HOLDER

Pfizer Limited

Ramsgate Road

Sandwich

Kent

CT13 9NJ

United Kingdom

8. MARKETING AUTHORISATION NUMBER(S)

PL 00057/0615-6

9. DATE OF FIRST AUTHORISATION/RENEWAL OF THE AUTHORISATION

21/09/2004

10. DATE OF REVISION OF THE TEXT

April 2007

Version IN 5_0

Instanyl 50, 100 and 200 mcg/dose nasal spray

(Nycomed UK Ltd)

1. NAME OF THE MEDICINAL PRODUCT

Instanyl®▼ 50, 100 and 200 micrograms/dose nasal spray, solution

2. QUALITATIVE AND QUANTITATIVE COMPOSITION

Each ml of solution contains fentanyl citrate equivalent to 500, 1,000 or 2,000 micrograms fentanyl.

1 dose (100 microliters) contains 50, 100 or 200 micrograms fentanyl.

For a full list of excipients, see section 6.1.

3. PHARMACEUTICAL FORM

Nasal spray, solution (nasal spray)

Clear, colourless solution.

4. CLINICAL PARTICULARS

4.1 Therapeutic indications

Instanyl is indicated for the management of breakthrough pain in adults already receiving maintenance opioid therapy for chronic cancer pain. Breakthrough pain is a transitory exacerbation of pain that occurs on a background of otherwise controlled persistent pain.

Patients receiving maintenance opioid therapy are those who are taking at least 60 mg of oral morphine daily, at least 25 micrograms of transdermal fentanyl per hour, at least 30 mg oxycodone daily, at least 8 mg of oral hydromorphone daily or an equianalgesic dose of another opioid for a week or longer.

4.2 Posology and method of administration

Treatment should be initiated by and remain under the supervision of a physician experienced in the management of opioid therapy in cancer patients. Physicians should keep in mind the potential of abuse of fentanyl.

Patients should be individually titrated to the dose that provides adequate analgesia with tolerable adverse drug reactions. Patients must be carefully monitored during the titration process.

Titration to a higher dose necessitates contact with the health care professional.

The dose of Instanyl for treatment of breakthrough pain was independent of the daily maintenance dose of opioid in the clinical studies (see section 5.1).

Maximum daily dose: Treatment of up to four breakthrough pain episodes, each with no more than two doses separated by at least 10 minutes.

Patient should wait at least 4 hours before treating another breakthrough pain episode with Instanyl during both titration and maintenance therapy.

Dose titration

Before patients are titrated with Instanyl, it is expected that their background persistent pain is controlled by use of chronic opioid therapy and that they are experiencing no more than four episodes of breakthrough pain per day.

Method of titration

The initial strength should be one dose of 50 micrograms in one nostril, titrating upwards as necessary through the range of available strengths (50, 100, and 200 micrograms). If adequate analgesia is not obtained redosing of the same strength may be administered at the earliest after 10 minutes. Each titration step (dose strength) should be evaluated in several episodes.

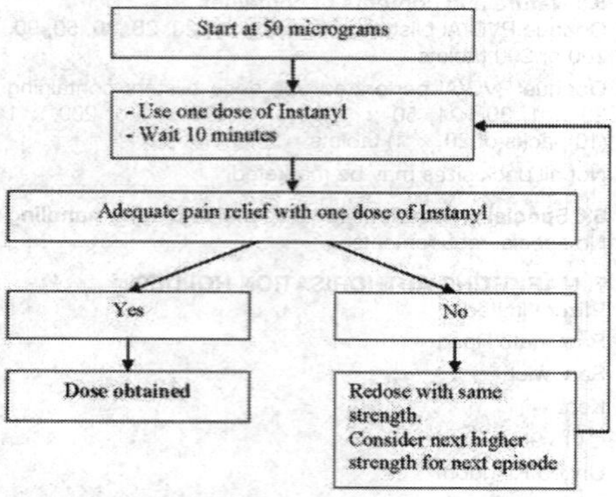

Maintenance therapy

Once the dose has been established according to the steps described above, the patient should be maintained on this strength of Instanyl. If the patient has insufficient pain relief, redosing with same strength can be done at the earliest after 10 minutes.

Dose adjustment

Generally, the maintenance strength of Instanyl should be increased when a patient requires more than one dose per breakthrough pain episode for several consecutive episodes.

Dose adjustment of the background opioid therapy may be required if the patient consistently present with more than four breakthrough pain episodes per 24 hours.

If adverse reactions are intolerable or persistent, the strength should be reduced or treatment with Instanyl replaced by other analgesics.

Discontinuation of therapy

Instanyl should be discontinued immediately if the patient no longer experience breakthrough pain episodes. The treatment for the persistent background pain should be kept as prescribed.

If discontinuation of all opioid therapy is required, the patient must be closely followed by the doctor as gradual downward opioid titration is necessary in order to avoid the possibility of abrupt withdrawal effects.

Method of administration

Instanyl is intended for nasal use.

It is recommended that the patient sit or stand in upright position when administrating Instanyl.

Cleaning of the nasal spray tip is required after each use.

Children and adolescents

Instanyl is not recommended for use in children and adolescent below 18 years of age, due to lack of data on safety and efficacy.

Elderly

Limited data on pharmacokinetics, efficacy and safety are available for the use of Instanyl in patients above >65 years of age. Elderly patients may have a reduced clearance, a prolonged half-life and higher sensitivity to fentanyl than younger patients. Caution should therefore be taken in treatment of elderly, cachectic or debilitated patients.

In clinical trials elderly patients tend to titrate to a lower effective strength than patients less than 65 years of age. Particular caution should be exercised when titrating Instanyl in elderly patients.

Hepatic impairment

Instanyl should be administered with caution to patients with moderate to severe hepatic impairment (see section 4.4).

Renal impairment

Instanyl should be administered with caution to patients with moderate to severe renal impairment (see section 4.4).

4.3 Contraindications

Hypersensitivity to the active substance or to any of the excipients.

Use in opioid-naïve patients.

Severe respiratory depression or severe obstructive lung conditions.

Previous facial radiotherapy.

Recurrent episodes of epistaxis (see section 4.4).

4.4 Special warnings and precautions for use

Respiratory depression

As with all potent opioids clinical significant respiratory depression may occur with fentanyl, and patients must be observed for these effects. Patients with pain who receives chronic opioid therapy develop tolerance to respiratory depression and hence the risk of respiratory depression in these patients is reduced. The use of concomitant central nervous system depressants may increase the risk of respiratory depression (see section 4.5).

Chronic pulmonary disease

In patients with chronic obstructive pulmonary diseases, fentanyl may have more severe adverse reactions. In these patients, opioids may decrease respiratory drive and increase airway resistance.

Impaired renal or hepatic function

Fentanyl should be administered with caution to patients with moderate to severe hepatic or renal impairment. The influence of hepatic and renal impairment on the pharmacokinetics of Instanyl have not been evaluated; however, when administered intravenously the clearance of fentanyl has shown to be altered due to hepatic and renal impairment caused by alterations in metabolic clearance and plasma proteins.

Increased intracranial pressure

Fentanyl should be used with caution in patients with evidence of increased intracranial pressure, impaired consciousness or coma.

Instanyl should be used with caution in patients with cerebral tumour or head injury.

Cardiac disease

Fentanyl may produce bradycardia. Fentanyl should therefore be administered with caution to patients with bradyarrhythmias. Opioids may cause hypotonia, especially in patients with hypovolaemia. Instanyl should therefore be used with caution in patients with hypotonia and/or hypovolaemia.

Nasal conditions

If the patient experience recurrent episodes of epistaxis or nasal discomfort while taking Instanyl, an alternative administration form for treatment of breakthrough pain should be considered.

Common cold

The overall extent of fentanyl exposure in subjects with common cold without prior treatment with nasal vasoconstrictor is comparable to that in healthy subjects. For concomitant use of nasal vasoconstrictor see section 4.5.

Abuse potential and dependence

Tolerance and physical and/or psychological dependence may develop upon repeated administration of opioids such as fentanyl. However, iatrogenic addiction following therapeutic use of opioids is rare in the treatment of cancer related pain.

Withdrawal symptoms

Withdrawal symptoms may be precipitated through the administration of substances with opioid antagonist activity, e.g. naloxone, or mixed agonist/antagonist analgesic (e.g. pentazocine, butorphanol, buprenorphine, nalbuphine).

Treatment with other nasally administered medicinal products

When initiating treatment with Instanyl, alternative administration forms should be considered for concurrent treatment of concomitant diseases that can be treated via nasal administration.

4.5 Interaction with other medicinal products and other forms of interaction

Instanyl is not recommended for use in patients who have received monoamine oxidase (MAO) inhibitors within 14 days because severe and unpredictable potentiation by MAO inhibitors has been reported with opioid analgesics.

Fentanyl is metabolised mainly via the human cytochrome P450 3A4 isoenzyme system (CYP3A4), therefore potential interactions may occur when Instanyl is given concurrently with agents that affect CYP3A4 activity. Co-administration with agents that induce 3A4 activity may reduce the efficacy of Instanyl. The concomitant use of Instanyl with strong CYP3A4 inhibitors (e.g. ritonavir, ketoconazole, itraconazole, troleandomycin, clarithromycin, and nelfinavir) or moderate CYP3A4 inhibitors (e.g., amprenavir, aprepitant, diltiazem, erythromycin, fluconazole, fosamprenavir, and verapamil) may result in increased fentanyl plasma concentrations, potentially causing serious adverse drug reactions including fatal respiratory depression.

Patients receiving Instanyl concomitantly with moderate or strong CYP3A4 inhibitors should be carefully monitored for an extended period of time. Dose increase should be done with caution.

In a pharmacokinetic interaction study it was found that the maximum plasma concentration of nasally applied fentanyl was reduced about 50% by the concomitant use of oxymetazoline, while the time to reach C_{max} (T_{max}) was doubled. This may reduce the efficacy of Instanyl. It is recommended that concomitant use of nasal decongestants is avoided (see section 5.2)

The concomitant use of other central nervous system depressants, including other opioids, sedatives or hypnotics, general anaesthetics, phenothiazines, tranquillisers, skeletal muscle relaxants, sedating antihistamines and alcohol may produce additive depressant effects.

The concomitant use of partial opioid agonists/antagonists (e.g. buprenorphine, nalbuphine, pentazocine) is not recommended. They have high affinity to opioid receptors with relatively low intrinsic activity and therefore partially antagonise the analgesic effect of fentanyl and may induce withdrawal symptoms in opioid dependent patients

Concomitant use of Instanyl and other medicinal products (other than oxymetazoline) administered via the nose has not been evaluated in the clinical trials. It is recommended that alternative administration forms should be considered for concomitant treatment of concurrent diseases that can be treated via nasal administration.

4.6 Pregnancy and lactation

There are no adequate data from the use of fentanyl in pregnant women. Studies in animals have shown reproductive toxicity (see section 5.3). The potential risk for humans is unknown. Instanyl should not be used in pregnancy unless clearly necessary.

Following long-term treatment, fentanyl may cause withdrawal in the new-born infant.

It is advised not to use fentanyl during labour and delivery (including caesarean section) because fentanyl passes through the placenta and may cause respiratory depression in the foetus. If Instanyl is administered, an antidote for the child should be readily available.

Fentanyl is excreted into human milk and may cause sedation and respiratory depression in the breast-fed infant. Fentanyl should only be used by breastfeeding women if the benefits outweigh the potential risks for both mother and child.

4.7 Effects on ability to drive and use machines

No studies of the effects on the ability to drive and use machines have been performed. However, opioid analgesics are known to impair the mental and/or physical ability required for driving or operating machinery. Patient should be advised not to drive or operate machinery if they experience somnolence, dizziness, visual disturbances or other adverse reaction which can impair their ability to drive and operate machinery.

4.8 Undesirable effects

Typical opioid adverse reactions are to be expected with Instanyl. Frequently, most of these will cease or decrease in intensity with continued use of the medicinal product. The most serious adverse reactions are respiratory depression (potentially leading to apnoea or respiratory arrest), circulatory depression, hypotension and shock and all patients should be closely monitored for these.

The clinical trials of Instanyl were designed to evaluate safety and efficacy in treating breakthrough pain. All patients were also taking concomitant opioids, such as sustained-release morphine or transdermal fentanyl, for their persistent pain. Thus, it is not possible to definitively separate the effects of Instanyl alone.

The adverse reactions considered to be at least possibly related to treatment in the clinical trials of Instanyl are included in the table below.

The following categories are used to rank the undesirable effects by frequency of occurrence: very common ($\geq 1/10$); common ($\geq 1/100$ to $< 1/10$); uncommon ($\geq 1/1000$ to $< 1/100$); rare ($\geq 1/10{,}000$ to $< 1/1000$); and very rare ($< 1/10{,}000$), not known (cannot be estimated from the available data).

Within each frequency grouping, adverse reactions are presented in order of decreasing seriousness.

System organ class	Common	Uncommon
Psychiatric disorders		Dependence, insomnia
Nervous system disorders	Somnolence, dizziness, headache	Sedation, myoclonus, paraesthesia, dysaesthesia, dysgeusia
Ear and Labyrinth disorders	Vertigo	Motion sickness
Cardiac disorders		Hypotension
Vascular disorders	Flushing, hot flush	
Respiratory, thoracic and mediastinal disorders	Throat irritation	Respiratory depression, epistaxis, nasal ulcer, rhinorrhea
Gastrointestinal disorders	Nausea, vomiting	Constipation, stomatitis, dry mouth
Skin and subcutaneous tissue disorders	Hyperhidrosis	Pain of skin, pruritus
General disorders and administration site conditions		Pyrexia

4.9 Overdose

Symptoms

The symptoms of fentanyl overdose are expected to be an extension of its pharmacological actions e.g. lethargy, coma and severe respiratory depression. Other symptoms may be hypothermia, decreased muscle tonus, bradycardia, hypotonia. Signs of toxicity are deep sedation, ataxia, miosis, convulsions and respiratory depression which is the main symptom.

Treatment

For management of respiratory depression immediate countermeasures should be started including physical or verbal stimulation of the patient. These actions can be followed by administration of a specific opioid antagonist such as naloxone. Respiratory depression following an overdose may outlast the duration of action of the opioid antagonist. The half-life of the antagonist may be short, therefore repeated administration or continuous infusion may be necessary. Reversal of the narcotic effect may result in acute onset of pain and release of catecholamines.

If the clinical situation warrants, a patent airway should be established and maintained, possibly with an oropharyngeal airway or endotracheal tube and oxygen should be administered and respiration assisted or controlled, as appropriate. Adequate body temperature and fluid intake should be maintained.

If severe or persistent hypotension occurs, hypovolemia should be considered and the condition should be managed with appropriate parenteral fluid therapy.

5. PHARMACOLOGICAL PROPERTIES

5.1 Pharmacodynamic properties

Pharmacotherapeutic group: Phenylpiperidine derivates. ATC code: N02AB03

Mechanism of action

Fentanyl is an opioid analgesic interacting primarily with the opioid μ-receptor as a pure agonist with low affinity for the δ- and κ-opioid receptors. The primary therapeutic action is analgesia. The secondary pharmacological effects are respiratory depression, bradycardia, hypothermia, constipation, miosis, physical dependence and euphoria.

Pharmacodynamic effects

The efficacy and safety of Instanyl (50, 100 and 200 micrograms) have been assessed in two randomised, double-blind, cross-over, placebo-controlled pivotal studies in 279 opioid-tolerant adult cancer patients (age 32-86 years) with breakthrough pain (BTP). The patients had an average of 1 to 4 episodes per day while taking maintenance opioid therapy. Patients in the second pivotal study had earlier participated in the Instanyl pharmacokinetic study or in the first pivotal study.

The clinical studies demonstrated the efficacy and safety of Instanyl. No distinct correlation between the maintenance opioid dose and Instanyl doses have been established, however in the second pivotal study patients with low maintenance opioid dose tended to achieve effective pain relief with a correspondingly lower strength of Instanyl compared to patients taking higher levels of maintenance opioid dose. This was most distinct for patients ending on Instanyl 50 micrograms.

In the clinical studies in cancer patients, the most frequent strength used were 100 and 200 micrograms

All three strengths of Instanyl showed statistically significant ($p < 0.001$) higher pain intensity difference at 10 minutes (PID_{10}) compared with placebo. Furthermore Instanyl was significantly superior to placebo in BTP relief at 10, 20, 40, and 60 minutes following administration. The results of summary of PID at 60 minutes ($SPID_{0-60}$) showed that all strengths of Instanyl had significantly higher mean $SPID_{0-60}$ scores compared with placebo ($p < 0.001$) demonstrating better pain relief of Instanyl compared to placebo during 60 minutes.

The safety and efficacy of Instanyl have been evaluated in patients taking the medicinal product at the onset of a breakthrough pain episode. Instanyl should not be used pre-emptively.

The clinical experience with Instanyl in patients with background opioid treatment equivalent to ≥ 500 mg/day morphine or ≥ 200 micrograms/hour transdermal fentanyl is limited.

Instanyl in doses above 400 micrograms have not been evaluated in clinical trials.

5.2 Pharmacokinetic properties

Absorption

Fentanyl is highly lipophilic. Fentanyl exhibits three compartment distribution kinetics. Animal data shows that following absorption, fentanyl is rapidly distributed to the brain, heart, lungs, kidneys and spleen followed by a slower redistribution to muscles and fat. The plasma protein binding of fentanyl is approximately 80%. The absolute bioavailability of Instanyl is about 89%.

Clinical data show that fentanyl is absorbed very rapidly through the nasal mucosa. Administration of Instanyl in single doses ranging from 50 to 200 micrograms fentanyl per dose in opioid tolerant cancer patients produces a rapid C_{max} level of 0.35 to 1.2 ng/ml. The corresponding median T_{max} are 12-15 minutes. However, higher values for T_{max} were observed in a dose-proportionality study in healthy volunteers.

Distribution

After intravenous administration of fentanyl the initial distribution half-life is approximately 6 minutes and a similar half-life is seen after the nasal administration of Instanyl. The elimination half-life is approximately 3-4 hours for Instanyl in cancer patients.

Biotransformation

Fentanyl is metabolised primarily in the liver via CYP3A4. The major metabolite, norfentanyl is inactive.

Elimination

About 75% of fentanyl is excreted into the urine, mostly as inactive metabolites, with less than 10% as unchanged active substance. About 9% of the dose is recovered in the faeces primarily as metabolites.

Dose linearity

Instanyl shows linear kinetics. Dose linearity from 50 micrograms to 400 micrograms of Instanyl has been demonstrated in healthy subjects.

A drug-drug-interaction study was performed with a nasal vasoconstrictor (oxymetazoline). Subjects with allergic rhinitis received oxymetazoline nasal spray one hour prior to Instanyl. Comparable bioavailability (AUC) of fentanyl was achieved with and without oxymetazoline, while fentanyl C_{max} decreased and T_{max} increased by a factor two when oxymetazoline was administered. The overall extent of fentanyl exposure in subjects with allergic rhinitis without prior treatment with nasal vasoconstrictor is comparable to that in healthy subjects. Concomitant use of nasal vasoconstrictor should be avoided (see section 4.5).

5.3 Preclinical safety data

Non-clinical data reveal no special hazard for humans based on conventional studies of safety pharmacology, repeated dose toxicity and genotoxicity.

Long-term carcinogenicity studies have not been performed.

Local tolerance studies with Instanyl in mini-pigs demonstrated that Instanyl administration was well tolerated.

Studies with female rats revealed reduced fertility and enhanced embryonal mortality. More recent studies showed that effects on the embryo were due to maternal toxicity and not to direct effects of the substances on the developing embryo. In a study on pre- and postnatal development the survival rate of offspring was significantly reduced at doses which slightly reduced maternal weight. This effect could either be due to altered maternal care or a direct effect of fentanyl on the pups. Effects on somatic development and behaviour of the offspring were not observed. Teratogenic effects have not been demonstrated.

6. PHARMACEUTICAL PARTICULARS

6.1 List of excipients

Sodium dihydrogen phosphate dihydrate

Disodium phosphate dihydrate

Purified water

6.2 Incompatibilities

Not applicable.

6.3 Shelf life

2 years

6.4 Special precautions for storage

Store below 30°C.

Do not freeze.

Keep the bottle stored upright.

6.5 Nature and contents of container

Bottle (brown Type 1 glass) with metering pump and dust cap packed in a child-resistant outer box.

Available in the following presentations:

1.8 ml containing 0.90, 1.80 or 3.60 mg fentanyl ensuring the delivery of 10 doses of 50, 100 or 200 micrograms

2.9 ml containing 1.45, 2.50 or 5.00 mg fentanyl ensuring the delivery of 20 doses of 50, 100 or 200 micrograms

5.0 ml containing 2.50, 5.00 or 10.00 mg fentanyl ensuring the delivery of 40 doses of 50, 100 or 200 micrograms

Not all pack sizes may be marketed.

6.6 Special precautions for disposal and other handling

Before using Instanyl for the first time, the nasal spray must be primed until a fine mist appears; 3 to 4 actuations of the nasal spray are usually required.

If the product has not been used during a period of more than seven days, the nasal spray must be actuated once to waste before the next dose is taken.

Because of the possible misuse of fentanyl and the possible amount of the solution left, the used and unused nasal spray solutions must be returned systematically and suitably in the child-resistant outer box according to local requirements or returned to the pharmacy.

7. MARKETING AUTHORISATION HOLDER

Nycomed Danmark ApS

Langebjerg 1

DK-4000 Roskilde

Denmark

Tel.: +45 4677 1111

info@nycomed.com

8. MARKETING AUTHORISATION NUMBER(S)

EU/1/09/531/001-009

9. DATE OF FIRST AUTHORISATION/RENEWAL OF THE AUTHORISATION

20 July 2009

10. DATE OF REVISION OF THE TEXT

11. LEGAL CATEGORY

CD (Sch 2), POM

Detailed information on this product is available on the website of the European Medicines Agency (EMEA) http://www.emea.europa.eu

Insulatard 100 IU/ml, Insulatard Penfill 100 IU/ml, Insulatard InnoLet 100 IU/ml

(Novo Nordisk Limited)

1. NAME OF THE MEDICINAL PRODUCT

Insulatard 100 IU/ml suspension for injection in a vial

Insulatard Penfill 100 IU/ml suspension for injection in a cartridge

Insulatard InnoLet 100 IU/ml suspension for injection in a pre-filled pen

2. QUALITATIVE AND QUANTITATIVE COMPOSITION

Insulin human, rDNA (produced by recombinant DNA technology in *Saccharomyces cerevisiae*).

1 ml contains 100 IU of insulin human

1 vial contains 10 ml equivalent to 1000 IU

1 cartridge contains 3 ml equivalent to 300 IU

1 pre-filled pen contains 3 ml equivalent to 300 IU

One IU (International Unit) corresponds to 0.035 mg of anhydrous human insulin.

Insulatard is a suspension of isophane (NPH) insulin.

For a full list of excipients, see section 6.1.

3. PHARMACEUTICAL FORM

Suspension for injection in a vial.

Suspension for injection in cartridge.

Suspension for injection in a pre-filled pen.

Cloudy, white, aqueous suspension.

4. CLINICAL PARTICULARS

4.1 Therapeutic indications

Treatment of diabetes mellitus.

4.2 Posology and method of administration

Insulatard is a long-acting insulin.

Dosage

Dosage is individual and determined in accordance with the needs of the patient. The individual insulin requirement is usually between 0.3 and 1.0 IU/kg/day. The daily insulin requirement may be higher in patients with insulin resistance (e.g. during puberty or due to obesity) and lower in patients with residual, endogenous insulin production.

The physician determines whether one or several daily injections are necessary. Insulatard may be used alone or mixed with fast-acting insulin. In intensive insulin therapy the suspension may be used as basal insulin (evening and/or morning injection) with fast-acting insulin given at meals.

In patients with diabetes mellitus optimised glycaemic control delays the onset of late diabetic complications. Close blood glucose monitoring is therefore recommended.

Dosage adjustment

Concomitant illness, especially infections and feverish conditions, usually increases the patient's insulin requirement.

Renal or hepatic impairment may reduce insulin requirement.

Adjustment of dosage may also be necessary if patients change physical activity or their usual diet.

Dosage adjustment may be necessary when transferring patients from one insulin preparation to another (see section 4.4).

Administration

For subcutaneous use. Insulin suspensions are never to be administered intravenously.

Insulatard is administered subcutaneously in the thigh. If convenient, the abdominal wall, the gluteal region or the deltoid region may also be used.

Subcutaneous injection into the thigh results in a slower and less variable absorption compared to the other injection sites.

Injection into a lifted skin fold minimises the risk of unintended intramuscular injection.

The needle should be kept under the skin for at least 6 seconds to make sure the entire dose is injected.

Injection sites should be rotated within an anatomic region in order to avoid lipodystrophy.

The vials are for use with insulin syringes with a corresponding unit scale. When two types of insulin are mixed, draw the amount of fast-acting insulin first, followed by the amount of long-acting insulin.

The cartridges are designed to be used with Novo Nordisk delivery systems (durable devices for repeated use) and NovoFine needles. Detailed instruction accompanying the delivery system must be followed.

Insulatard InnoLet is designed to be used with NovoFine short cap needles of 8 mm or shorter in length. The needle box is marked with an **S.**

InnoLet delivers 1-50 units in increments of 1 unit.

The pens should be primed before injection so that the dose selector returns to zero and a drop of insulin appears at the needle tip.

The dose is set by turning the selector, which returns to zero during the injection.

Insulatard is accompanied by a package leaflet with detailed instruction for use to be followed.

4.3 Contraindications

Hypersensitivity to the active ingredient or to any of the excipients (see section 6.1).

Hypoglycaemia.

4.4 Special warnings and precautions for use

Inadequate dosage or discontinuation of treatment, especially in type 1 diabetes, may lead to **hyperglycaemia**.

Usually the first symptoms of hyperglycaemia set in gradually, over a period of hours or days. They include thirst, increased frequency of urination, nausea, vomiting, drowsiness, flushed dry skin, dry mouth, loss of appetite as well as acetone odour of breath.

In type 1 diabetes, untreated hyperglycaemic events eventually lead to diabetic ketoacidosis, which is potentially lethal.

Hypoglycaemia may occur if the insulin dose is too high in relation to the insulin requirement (see sections 4.8 and 4.9).

Omission of a meal or unplanned, strenuous physical exercise may lead to hypoglycaemia.

Patients whose blood glucose control is greatly improved e.g. by intensified insulin therapy, may experience a change in their usual warning symptoms of hypoglycaemia and should be advised accordingly.

Usual warning symptoms may disappear in patients with long-standing diabetes.

Transferring a patient to another type or brand of insulin should be done under strict medical supervision. Changes in strength, brand (manufacturer), type (fast-, dual-, long-acting insulin etc.), origin (animal, human or analogue insulin) and/or method of manufacture (recombinant DNA versus animal source insulin) may result in a need for a change in dosage. If an adjustment is needed when switching the patients to Insulatard, it may occur with the first dose or during the first several weeks or months.

As with any insulin therapy, injection site reactions may occur and include pain, itching, hives, swelling and inflammation. Continuous rotation of the injection site within a given area may help to reduce or prevent these reactions. Reactions usually resolve in a few days to a few weeks. On rare occasions, injection site reactions may require discontinuation of Insulatard.

A few patients who have experienced hypoglycaemic reactions after transfer from animal source insulin have reported that early warning symptoms of hypoglycaemia were less pronounced or different from those experienced with their previous insulin.

Before travelling between different time zones, the patient should be advised to consult the physician, since this may mean that the patient has to take insulin and meals at different times.

Insulin suspensions are not to be used in insulin infusion pumps.

Insulatard contains metacresol, which may cause allergic reactions.

4.5 Interaction with other medicinal products and other forms of interaction

A number of medicinal products are known to interact with glucose metabolism. The physician must therefore take possible interactions into account and should always ask his patients about any medicinal products they take.

The following substances may reduce insulin requirement:

Oral hypoglycaemic agents (OHA), monoamine oxidase inhibitors (MAOI), non-selective beta-blocking agents, angiotensin converting enzyme (ACE) inhibitors, salicylates, alcohol, anabolic steroids and sulphonamides.

The following substances may increase insulin requirement:

Oral contraceptives, thiazides, glucocorticoids, thyroid hormones and beta-sympathomimetics, growth hormone and danazol.

Beta-blocking agents may mask the symptoms of hypoglycaemia and delay recovery from hypoglycaemia.

Octreotide/lanreotide may both decrease and increase insulin requirement.

Alcohol may intensify and prolong the hypoglycaemic effect of insulin.

4.6 Pregnancy and lactation

There are no restrictions on treatment of diabetes with insulin during pregnancy, as insulin does not pass the placental barrier.

Both hypoglycaemia and hyperglycaemia, which can occur in inadequately controlled diabetes therapy, increase the risk of malformations and death *in utero*. Intensified control in the treatment of pregnant women with diabetes is therefore recommended throughout pregnancy and when contemplating pregnancy.

Insulin requirements usually fall in the first trimester and subsequently increase during the second and third trimesters.

After delivery, insulin requirements return rapidly to pre-pregnancy values.

Insulin treatment of the nursing mother presents no risk to the baby. However, the Insulatard dosage may need to be adjusted.

4.7 Effects on ability to drive and use machines

The patient's ability to concentrate and react may be impaired as a result of hypoglycaemia. This may constitute a risk in situations where these abilities are of special importance (e.g. driving a car or operating machinery).

Patients should be advised to take precautions to avoid hypoglycaemia whilst driving. This is particularly important in those who have reduced or absent awareness of the warning signs of hypoglycaemia or have frequent episodes of hypoglycaemia. The advisability of driving should be considered in these circumstances.

4.8 Undesirable effects

As for other insulin products, in general, hypoglycaemia is the most frequently occurring undesirable effect. It may occur if the insulin dose is too high in relation to the insulin requirement. In clinical trials and during marketed use, the frequency varies with patient population and dose regimens. Therefore, no specific frequency can be presented. Severe hypoglycaemia may lead to unconsciousness and/or convulsions and may result in temporary or permanent impairment of brain function or even death.

Frequencies of adverse drug reactions from clinical trials, that are considered related to Insulatard are listed below. The frequencies are defined as: uncommon ($\geq$1/1000, $<$ 1/100). Isolated spontaneous cases are presented as very rare defined as $<$ 1/10,000 including isolated reports.

Within each frequency grouping, undesirable effects are presented in order of decreasing seriousness.

Nervous system disorders

Very rare – Peripheral neuropathy

Fast improvement in blood glucose control may be associated with a condition termed "acute painful neuropathy", which is usually reversible.

Eye disorders

Very rare – Refraction disorders

Refraction anomalies may occur upon initiation of insulin therapy. These symptoms are usually of transitory nature.

Uncommon – Diabetic retinopathy

Long-term improved glycaemic control decreases the risk of progression of diabetic retinopathy. However, intensification of insulin therapy with abrupt improvement in glycaemic control may be associated with temporary worsening of diabetic retinopathy.

Skin and subcutaneous tissue disorders

Uncommon – Lipodystrophy

Lipodystrophy may occur at the injection site as a consequence of failure to rotate injection sites within an area.

General disorders and administration site conditions

Uncommon – Injection site reactions

Injection site reactions (redness, swelling, itching, pain and haematoma at the injection site) may occur during treatment with insulin. Most reactions are transitory and disappear during continued treatment.

Uncommon – Oedema

Oedema may occur upon initiation of insulin therapy. These symptoms are usually of transitory nature.

Immune system disorders

Uncommon – Urticaria, rash

Very rare – Anaphylactic reactions

Symptoms of generalised hypersensitivity may include generalised skin rash, itching, sweating, gastrointestinal upset, angioneurotic oedema, difficulties in breathing, palpitation, reduction in blood pressure and fainting/loss of consciousness. Generalised hypersensitivity reactions are potentially life threatening.

4.9 Overdose

A specific overdose of insulin cannot be defined. However, hypoglycaemia may develop over sequential stages:

• Mild hypoglycaemic episodes can be treated by oral administration of glucose or sugary products. It is therefore recommended that the diabetic patients carry some sugar lumps, sweets, biscuits or sugary fruit juice.

• Severe hypoglycaemic episodes, where the patient has become unconscious, can be treated by glucagon (0.5 to 1 mg) given intramuscularly or subcutaneously by a person who has received appropriate instruction, or by glucose given intravenously by a medical professional. Glucose must also be given intravenously, if the patient does not respond to glucagon within 10 to 15 minutes.

Upon regaining consciousness, administration of oral carbohydrate is recommended for the patient in order to prevent relapse.

5. PHARMACOLOGICAL PROPERTIES

5.1 Pharmacodynamic properties

Pharmacotherapeutic group: Insulins and analogues for injection, intermediate-acting, insulin (human). ATC code: A10A C01.

The blood glucose lowering effect of insulin is due to the facilitated uptake of glucose following binding of insulin to receptors on muscle and fat cells and to the simultaneous inhibition of glucose output from the liver.

Insulatard is a long-acting insulin.

Onset of action is within 1½ hours, reaches a maximum effect within 4-12 hours and the entire time of duration is approximately 24 hours.

5.2 Pharmacokinetic properties

Insulin in the blood stream has a half-life of a few minutes. Consequently, the time-action profile of an insulin preparation is determined solely by its absorption characteristics.

This process is influenced by several factors (e.g. insulin dosage, injection route and site, thickness of subcutaneous fat, type of diabetes). The pharmacokinetics of insulin products are therefore affected by significant intra- and inter-individual variation.

Absorption

The maximum plasma concentration of the insulin is reached within 2-18 hours after subcutaneous administration.

Distribution

No profound binding to plasma proteins, except circulating insulin antibodies (if present) has been observed.

Metabolism

Human insulin is reported to be degraded by insulin protease or insulin-degrading enzymes and possibly protein disulfide isomerase. A number of cleavage (hydrolysis) sites on the human insulin molecule have been proposed; none of the metabolites formed following the cleavage are active.

Elimination

The terminal half-life is determined by the rate of absorption from the subcutaneous tissue. The terminal half-life ($t_{1/2}$) is therefore a measure of the absorption rather than of the elimination *per se* of insulin from plasma (insulin in the blood stream has a $t_{1/2}$ of a few minutes). Trials have indicated a $t_{1/2}$ of about 5-10 hours.

5.3 Preclinical safety data

Non-clinical data reveal no special hazard for humans based on conventional studies of safety pharmacology, repeated dose toxicity, genotoxicity, carcinogenic potential, toxicity to reproduction.

6. PHARMACEUTICAL PARTICULARS

6.1 List of excipients

Zinc chloride

Glycerol

Metacresol

Phenol

Disodium phosphate dihydrate

Sodium hydroxide (for pH adjustment)

Hydrochloric acid (for pH adjustment)

Protamine sulphate

Water for injections

6.2 Incompatibilities

Insulin products should only be added to compounds with which it is known to be compatible. Insulin suspensions should not be added to infusion fluids.

6.3 Shelf life

30 months when stored between 2°C-8°C.

Insulatard:

6 weeks when used or stored at room temperature (below 25°C).

Insulatard Penfill and Insulatard InnoLet:

6 weeks when used or carried as a spare (below 30°C).

6.4 Special precautions for storage

Before use; Store in a refrigerator (2°C - 8°C).

Do not store them in or too near the freezer section or cooling elements.

Do not freeze.

Insulatard:

During use: do not refrigerate. Do not store above 25°C.

Keep the vial in the outer carton in order to protect from light.

Protect from excessive heat and sunlight.

Insulatard Penfill:

During use: do not refrigerate. Do not store above 30°C.

Keep the cartridge in the outer carton in order to protect from light.

Protect from excessive heat and sunlight.

Insulatard InnoLet:

During use: do not refrigerate. Do not store above 30°C.

Keep the pen cap on in order to protect the insulin from light.

Protect from excessive heat and sunlight.

6.5 Nature and contents of container

10 ml glass vial (type 1) closed with a bromobutyl/polyisoprene rubber stopper and a protective tamper-proof plastic cap.

Pack size: 1 vial × 10 ml.

3 ml glass cartridge (type 1) with a bromobutyl rubber plunger and a bromobutyl/polyisoprene rubber stopper. The cartridge contains a glass ball to facilitate the re-suspension.

Pack size: 5 cartridges × 3 ml.

Pre-filled pen (multidose disposable pen) comprising a pen injector with a cartridge (3 ml). The cartridge is made of glass (type 1), containing a bromobutyl rubber plunger and a bromobutyl/polyisoprene rubber stopper. The cartridge contains a glass ball to facilitate the re-suspension. The pen injector is made of plastic.

Pack size: 5 pre-filled pens × 3 ml.

6.6 Special precautions for disposal and other handling

Cartridges and pens should only be used in combination with products that are compatible with them and allow the cartridge and pen to function safely and effectively.

Insulatard Penfill and Insulatard InnoLet are for single person use only. The container must not be refilled.

Insulin preparations which have been frozen, must not be used.

After removing Insulatard, Insulatard Penfill or Insulatard InnoLet from the refrigerator it is recommended to allow the vial, Penfill or InnoLet to reach room temperature (not above 25°C) before resuspending the insulin as instructed for first time use.

Insulin suspensions should not be used if they do not appear uniformly white and cloudy after re-suspension.

Any unused product or waste material should be disposed of in accordance with local requirements.

7. MARKETING AUTHORISATION HOLDER

Novo Nordisk A/S

Novo Allé

DK-2880 Bagsværd

Denmark

8. MARKETING AUTHORISATION NUMBER(S)

Insulatard 100 IU/ml	EU/1/02/233/003
Insulatard Penfill 100 IU/ml	EU/1/02/233/006
Insulatard InnoLet 100 IU/ml	EU/1/02/233/011

9. DATE OF FIRST AUTHORISATION/RENEWAL OF THE AUTHORISATION

Date of first authorisation: 07 October 2002

Date of last renewal: 18 October 2007

10. DATE OF REVISION OF THE TEXT

09/2007

Legal Status

POM

Insuman Basal Cartridges

(sanofi-aventis)

1. NAME OF THE MEDICINAL PRODUCT

Insuman Basal 100 IU/ml suspension for injection in a cartridge

2. QUALITATIVE AND QUANTITATIVE COMPOSITION

Each ml contains 100 IU insulin human (equivalent to 3.5 mg).

Each cartridge contains 3 ml of suspension for injection, equivalent to 300 IU insulin. One IU (International Unit) corresponds to 0.035 mg of anhydrous human insulin.

Insuman Basal is an isophane insulin suspension.

Human insulin is produced by recombinant DNA technology in *Escherichia coli*.

For a full list of excipients, see section 6.1.

3. PHARMACEUTICAL FORM

Suspension for injection in a cartridge.

After re-suspension, milky white suspension.

4. CLINICAL PARTICULARS

4.1 Therapeutic indications

Diabetes mellitus where treatment with insulin is required.

4.2 Posology and method of administration

The desired blood glucose levels, the insulin preparations to be used and the insulin dosage (doses and timings) must be determined individually and adjusted to suit the patient's diet, physical activity and life-style.

Daily doses and timing of administration

There are no fixed rules for insulin dosage. However, the average insulin requirement is often 0.5 to 1.0 IU per kg body weight per day. The basal metabolic requirement is 40% to 60% of the total daily requirement. Insuman Basal is injected subcutaneously 45 to 60 minutes before a meal.

Transfer to Insuman Basal

Dosage adjustment may be necessary when transferring patients from one insulin preparation to another. This applies, for example, when transferring from:

- an animal insulin (especially a bovine insulin) to human insulin,
- one human insulin preparation to another,
- a regimen with only regular insulin to one with a longer-acting insulin.

The need to adjust (e.g. reduce) the dose may become evident immediately after transfer. Alternatively, it may emerge gradually over a period of several weeks.

Following transfer from an animal insulin to human insulin, dosage reduction may be required in particular in patients who

- were previously already controlled on rather low blood glucose levels,
- have a tendency to hypoglycaemia,
- previously required high insulin doses due to the presence of insulin antibodies.

Close metabolic monitoring is recommended during the transition and in the initial weeks thereafter. In patients who require high insulin doses because of the presence of insulin antibodies, transfer under medical supervision in a hospital or similar setting must be considered.

Secondary dose adjustment

Improved metabolic control may result in increased insulin sensitivity, leading to a reduced insulin requirement. Dose adjustment may also be required, for example, if

- the patient's weight changes,
- the patient's life-style changes,
- other circumstances arise that may promote an increased susceptibility to hypo- or hyperglycaemia (see section 4.4).

Use in specific patient groups

In patients with hepatic or renal impairment as well as in the elderly, insulin requirements may be diminished (see section 4.4).

Administration

Insuman Basal in cartridges has been developed for use in the OptiPen series.

Insuman Basal is administered subcutaneously. Insuman Basal must never be injected intravenously.

Insulin absorption and hence the blood glucose lowering effect of a dose may vary from one injection area to another (e.g. the abdominal wall compared with the thigh). Injection sites within an injection area must be rotated from one injection to the next.

For further details on handling, see section 6.6.

4.3 Contraindications

Hypersensitivity to the active substance or to any of the excipients.

Insuman Basal must not be administered intravenously and must not be used in infusion pumps or external or implanted insulin pumps.

4.4 Special warnings and precautions for use

Patients hypersensitive to Insuman Basal for whom no better tolerated preparation is available must only continue treatment under close medical supervision and – where necessary – in conjunction with anti-allergic treatment.

In patients with an allergy to animal insulin intradermal skin testing is recommended prior to a transfer to Insuman Basal, since they may experience immunological cross-reactions.

In patients with renal impairment, insulin requirements may be diminished due to reduced insulin metabolism. In the elderly, progressive deterioration of renal function may lead to a steady decrease in insulin requirements.

In patients with severe hepatic impairment, insulin requirements may be diminished due to reduced capacity for gluconeogenesis and reduced insulin metabolism.

In case of insufficient glucose control or a tendency to hyper- or hypoglycaemic episodes, the patient's adherence to the prescribed treatment regimen, injection sites and proper injection technique and all other relevant factors must be reviewed before dose adjustment is considered.

Hypoglycaemia

Hypoglycaemia may occur if the insulin dose is too high in relation to the insulin requirement.

Particular caution should be exercised, and intensified blood glucose monitoring is advisable in patients in whom hypoglycaemic episodes might be of particular clinical relevance, such as in patients with significant stenoses of the coronary arteries or of the blood vessels supplying the brain (risk of cardiac or cerebral complications of hypoglycaemia) as well as in patients with proliferative retinopathy, particularly if not treated with photocoagulation (risk of transient amaurosis following hypoglycaemia).

Patients should be aware of circumstances where warning symptoms of hypoglycaemia are diminished. The warning symptoms of hypoglycaemia may be changed, be less pronounced or be absent in certain risk groups. These include patients:

- in whom glycaemic control is markedly improved,
- in whom hypoglycaemia develops gradually,
- who are elderly,
- after transfer from animal insulin to human insulin,
- in whom an autonomic neuropathy is present,
- with a long history of diabetes,
- suffering from a psychiatric illness,
- receiving concurrent treatment with certain other medicinal products (see section 4.5).

Such situations may result in severe hypoglycaemia (and possibly loss of consciousness) prior to the patient's awareness of hypoglycaemia.

If normal or decreased values for glycated haemoglobin are noted, the possibility of recurrent, unrecognised (especially nocturnal) episodes of hypoglycaemia must be considered.

Adherence of the patient to the dosage and dietary regimen, correct insulin administration and awareness of hypoglycaemia symptoms are essential to reduce the risk of hypoglycaemia. Factors increasing the susceptibility to hypoglycaemia require particularly close monitoring and may necessitate dose adjustment. These include:

- change in the injection area,
- improved insulin sensitivity (by, e.g., removal of stress factors),
- unaccustomed, increased or prolonged physical activity,
- intercurrent illness (e.g. vomiting, diarrhoea),
- inadequate food intake,
- missed meals,
- alcohol consumption,
- certain uncompensated endocrine disorders (e.g. in hypothyroidism and in anterior pituitary or adrenocortical insufficiency),
- concomitant treatment with certain other medicinal products.

Intercurrent illness

Intercurrent illness requires intensified metabolic monitoring. In many cases, urine tests for ketones are indicated, and often it is necessary to adjust the insulin dose. The insulin requirement is often increased. Patients with type 1 diabetes must continue to consume at least a small amount of carbohydrates on a regular basis, even if they are able to eat only little or no food, or are vomiting etc. and they must never omit insulin entirely.

4.5 Interaction with other medicinal products and other forms of interaction

A number of substances affect glucose metabolism and may require dose adjustment of human insulin.

Substances that may enhance the blood-glucose-lowering effect and increase susceptibility to hypoglycaemia include oral antidiabetic agents, angiotensin converting enzyme (ACE) inhibitors, disopyramide, fibrates, fluoxetine, monoamine oxidase (MAO) inhibitors, pentoxifylline, propoxyphene, salicylates and sulphonamide antibiotics.

Substances that may reduce the blood-glucose-lowering effect include corticosteroids, danazol, diazoxide, diuretics, glucagon, isoniazid, oestrogens and progestogens (e.g. in oral contraceptives), phenothiazine derivatives, somatropin, sympathomimetic agents (e.g. epinephrine [adrenaline], salbutamol, terbutaline), thyroid hormones, protease inhibitors and atypical antipsychotic medicinal products (e.g. olanzapine and clozapine).

Beta-blockers, clonidine, lithium salts or alcohol may either potentiate or weaken the blood-glucose-lowering effect of insulin. Pentamidine may cause hypoglycaemia which may sometimes be followed by hyperglycaemia.

In addition, under the influence of sympatholytic medicinal products such as beta-blockers, clonidine, guanethidine and reserpine, the signs of adrenergic counter-regulation may be reduced or absent.

4.6 Pregnancy and lactation

Pregnancy

For insulin human, no clinical data on exposed pregnancies are available. Insulin does not cross the placental barrier. Caution should be exercised when prescribing to pregnant women.

It is essential for patients with pre-existing or gestational diabetes to maintain good metabolic control throughout pregnancy. Insulin requirements may decrease during the first trimester and generally increase during the second and third trimesters. Immediately after delivery, insulin requirements decline rapidly (increased risk of hypoglycaemia). Careful monitoring of glucose control is essential.

Lactation

No effects on the suckling child are anticipated. Insuman Basal can be used during breastfeeding. Lactating women may require adjustments in insulin dose and diet.

4.7 Effects on ability to drive and use machines

The patient's ability to concentrate and react may be impaired as a result of hypoglycaemia or hyperglycaemia or, for example, as a result of visual impairment. This may constitute a risk in situations where these abilities are of special importance (e.g. driving a car or operating machinery).

Patients should be advised to take precautions to avoid hypoglycaemia whilst driving. This is particularly important in those who have reduced or absent awareness of the warning symptoms of hypoglycaemia or have frequent episodes of hypoglycaemia. It should be considered whether it is advisable to drive or operate machinery in these circumstances.

4.8 Undesirable effects

Hypoglycaemia, in general the most frequent undesirable effect of insulin therapy, may occur if the insulin dose is too high in relation to the insulin requirement. In clinical trials and during marketed use, the frequency varies with patient population and dose regimens. Therefore, no specific frequency can be presented.

Severe hypoglycaemic attacks, especially if recurrent, may lead to neurological damage. Prolonged or severe hypoglycaemic episodes may be life-threatening.

In many patients, the signs and symptoms of neuroglycopenia are preceded by signs of adrenergic counter-regulation. Generally, the greater and more rapid the decline in blood glucose, the more marked is the phenomenon of counter-regulation and its symptoms.

The following related adverse reactions from clinical investigations are listed below by system organ class and in order of decreasing incidence: very common (≥1/10); common (≥1/100, <1/10); uncommon (≥1/1,000, <1/100); rare (≥1/10,000, <1/1,000); very rare (<1/10,000), not known (cannot be estimated from the available data).

Within each frequency grouping, undesirable effects are presented in order of decreasing seriousness.

Immune system disorders

Uncommon: shock

Not known: immediate type allergic reactions (hypotension, angioneurotic oedema, bronchospasm, generalised skin reactions), anti-insulin antibodies

Immediate type allergic reactions to insulin or to the excipients may be life-threatening.

Insulin administration may cause anti-insulin antibodies to form. In rare cases, the presence of such anti-insulin antibodies may necessitate adjustment of the insulin dose in order to correct a tendency to hyper- or hypoglycaemia.

Metabolism and nutrition disorders

Common: oedema

Not known: sodium retention

Insulin may cause sodium retention and oedema, particularly if previously poor metabolic control is improved by intensified insulin therapy.

Eyes disorders

Not known: proliferative retinopathy, diabetic retinopathy, visual impairment

A marked change in glycaemic control may cause temporary visual impairment, due to temporary alteration in the turgidity and refractive index of the lens.

Long-term improved glycaemic control decreases the risk of progression of diabetic retinopathy. However, intensification of insulin therapy with abrupt improvement in glycaemic control may be associated with temporary worsening of diabetic retinopathy.

Skin and subcutaneous tissue disorders

Not known: lipodystrophy

As with any insulin therapy, lipodystrophy may occur at the injection site and delay local insulin absorption. Continuous rotation of the injection site within the given injection area may help to reduce or prevent these reactions.

General disorders and administration site conditions

Common: injection site reactions

Uncommon: injection site urticaria,

Not known: injection site inflammation, injection site swelling, injection site pain, injection site pruritus, injection site erythema.

Most minor reactions to insulins at the injection site usually resolve in a few days to a few weeks.

4.9 Overdose

Symptoms

Insulin overdose may lead to severe and sometimes long-term and life-threatening hypoglycaemia.

Management

Mild episodes of hypoglycaemia can usually be treated with oral carbohydrates. Adjustments in dosage of the medicinal product, meal patterns, or physical activity may be needed.

More severe episodes with coma, seizure, or neurologic impairment may be treated with intramuscular/subcutaneous glucagon or concentrated intravenous glucose. Sustained carbohydrate intake and observation may be necessary because hypoglycaemia may recur after apparent clinical recovery.

5. PHARMACOLOGICAL PROPERTIES

5.1 Pharmacodynamic properties

Pharmacotherapeutic group: Antidiabetic agent. Insulins and analogues, intermediate-acting, ATC Code: A10AC01.

Mode of action

Insulin

- lowers blood glucose and promotes anabolic effects as well as decreasing catabolic effects,

- increases the transport of glucose into cells as well as the formation of glycogen in the muscles and the liver, and improves pyruvate utilisation. It inhibits glycogenolysis and gluconeogenesis,

- increases lipogenesis in the liver and adipose tissue and inhibits lipolysis,

- promotes the uptake of amino acids into cells and promotes protein synthesis,

- enhances the uptake of potassium into cells.

Pharmacodynamic characteristics

Insuman Basal (an isophane insulin suspension) is an insulin with gradual onset and long duration of action. Following subcutaneous injection, onset of action is within 60 minutes, the phase of maximum action is between 3 and 4 hours after injection and the duration of action is 11 to 20 hours.

5.2 Pharmacokinetic properties

In healthy subjects, the serum half-life of insulin is approximately 4 to 6 minutes. It is longer in patients with severe renal insufficiency. However, it must be noted that the pharmacokinetics of insulin do not reflect its metabolic action.

5.3 Preclinical safety data

The acute toxicity was studied following subcutaneous administration in rats. No evidence of toxic effects was found. Studies of pharmacodynamic effects following subcutaneous administration in rabbits and dogs revealed the expected hypoglycaemic reactions.

6. PHARMACEUTICAL PARTICULARS

6.1 List of excipients

Protamine sulphate,

metacresol,

phenol,

zinc chloride,

sodium dihydrogen phosphate dihydrate,

glycerol,

sodium hydroxide,

hydrochloric acid (for pH adjustment),

water for injections.

6.2 Incompatibilities

This medicinal product must not be mixed with other medicinal products except those mentioned in section 6.6.

Concerning mixing or incompatibility with other insulins see section 6.6. Care must be taken to ensure that no alcohol or other disinfectants enter the insulin suspension.

6.3 Shelf life

2 years.

Shelf life after first use of the cartridge:

The cartridge in-use (in the insulin pen) or carried as a spare may be stored for a maximum of 4 weeks not above 25°C away from direct heat or direct light.

The pen containing a cartridge must not be stored in the refrigerator.

The pen cap must be put back on the pen after each injection in order to protect from light.

6.4 Special precautions for storage

Unopened cartridges:

Store in a refrigerator (2°C - 8°C).

Do not freeze.

Do not put Insuman Basal next to the freezer compartment or a freezer pack.

Keep the cartridge in the outer carton in order to protect from light.

In-use cartridges:

For storage precautions, see section 6.3.

6.5 Nature and contents of container

3 ml suspension in a cartridge (type 1 colourless glass) with a plunger (bromobutyl rubber (type 1)) and a flanged cap (aluminium) with a stopper (bromobutyl or laminate of polyisoprene and bromobutyl rubber (type 1)).

Each cartridge contains 3 balls (stainless steel).

Packs of 5 cartridges are available

6.6 Special precautions for disposal and other handling

Insulin pen

The cartridges are to be used in conjunction with an insulin pen such as OptiPen and other pens suitable for Insuman cartridges and as recommended in the information provided by the device manufacturer.

The manufacturer's instructions for using the pen must be followed carefully for loading the cartridge, attaching the injection needle, and administering the insulin injection.

If the insulin pen is damaged or not working properly (due to mechanical defects) it has to be discarded, and a new insulin pen has to be used.

If the pen malfunctions (see instructions for using the pen), the suspension may be drawn from the cartridge into an injection syringe (suitable for an insulin with 100 IU/ml) and injected.

Cartridges

Before insertion into the pen, Insuman Basal must be kept at room temperature for 1 to 2 hours and then resuspended to check the contents. This is best done by gently tilting the cartridge back and forth (at least ten times). Each cartridge contains three small metal balls to facilitate quick and thorough mixing of the contents.

Later on, when the cartridge has been inserted into the pen, the insulin must be resuspended again prior to each injection. This is best done by gently tilting the pen back and forth (at least ten times).

After resuspension, the fluid must have a uniformly milky appearance. Insuman Basal must not be used if this cannot be achieved, i.e. if the suspension remains clear, for example, or if clumps, particles or flocculation appear in the insulin or stick to the wall or bottom of the cartridge. These changes sometimes give the cartridge a frosted appearance. In such cases, a new cartridge yielding a uniform suspension must be used. It is also necessary to change to a new cartridge if the insulin requirement changes substantially.

Air bubbles must be removed from the cartridge before injection (see instructions for using the pen). Empty cartridges must not be refilled.

As with all insulin preparations, Insuman Basal must not be mixed with solutions containing reducing agents such as thioles and sulphites. It must also be remembered that insulin protamine crystals dissolve in an acid pH range.

Mixing of insulin

Insuman Basal may be mixed with all Sanofi-Aventis human insulins, but NOT with those designed specifically for use in insulin pumps. Insuman Basal must also NOT be mixed with insulins of animal origin or with insulin analogues.

Insuman Basal cartridges are not designed to allow any other insulin to be mixed in the cartridge.

Any unused product or waste material should be disposed of in accordance with local requirements.

7. MARKETING AUTHORISATION HOLDER

Sanofi-Aventis Deutschland GmbH, D-65926 Frankfurt am Main, Germany

8. MARKETING AUTHORISATION NUMBER(S)

EU/1/97/030/035

9. DATE OF FIRST AUTHORISATION/RENEWAL OF THE AUTHORISATION

Date of first authorisation: 21 February 1997

Date of latest renewal: 21 February 2007

10. DATE OF REVISION OF THE TEXT
June 2008

Legal Category: POM

Insuman Basal Optiset

(sanofi-aventis)

1. NAME OF THE MEDICINAL PRODUCT
Insuman Basal 100 IU/ml suspension for injection in a pre-filled pen.

2. QUALITATIVE AND QUANTITATIVE COMPOSITION
Each ml contains 100 IU insulin human (equivalent to 3.5 mg).

Each pen contains 3 ml of suspension for injection, equivalent to 300 IU insulin. One IU (International Unit) corresponds to 0.035 mg of anhydrous human insulin.

Insuman Basal is an isophane insulin suspension.

Human insulin is produced by recombinant DNA technology in *Escherichia coli*.

For a full list of excipients, see section 6.1.

3. PHARMACEUTICAL FORM
Suspension for injection in a pre-filled pen. OptiSet.

After re-suspension, milky white suspension.

4. CLINICAL PARTICULARS

4.1 Therapeutic indications
Diabetes mellitus where treatment with insulin is required.

4.2 Posology and method of administration
The desired blood glucose levels, the insulin preparations to be used and the insulin dosage (doses and timings) must be determined individually and adjusted to suit the patient's diet, physical activity and life-style.

Daily doses and timing of administration

There are no fixed rules for insulin dosage. However, the average insulin requirement is often 0.5 to 1.0 IU per kg body weight per day. The basal metabolic requirement is 40% to 60% of the total daily requirement. Insuman Basal is injected subcutaneously 45 to 60 minutes before a meal.

OptiSet delivers insulin in increments of 2 IU up to a maximum single dose of 40 IU.

Transfer to Insuman Basal

Dosage adjustment may be necessary when transferring patients from one insulin preparation to another. This applies, for example, when transferring from:

- an animal insulin (especially a bovine insulin) to human insulin,
- one human insulin preparation to another,
- a regimen with only regular insulin to one with a longer-acting insulin.

The need to adjust (e.g. reduce) the dose may become evident immediately after transfer. Alternatively, it may emerge gradually over a period of several weeks.

Following transfer from an animal insulin to human insulin, dosage reduction may be required in particular in patients who

- were previously already controlled on rather low blood glucose levels,
- have a tendency to hypoglycaemia,
- previously required high insulin doses due to the presence of insulin antibodies.

Close metabolic monitoring is recommended during the transition and in the initial weeks thereafter. In patients who require high insulin doses because of the presence of insulin antibodies, transfer under medical supervision in a hospital or similar setting must be considered.

Secondary dose adjustment

Improved metabolic control may result in increased insulin sensitivity, leading to a reduced insulin requirement. Dose adjustment may also be required, for example, if

- the patient's weight changes,
- the patient's life-style changes,
- other circumstances arise that may promote an increased susceptibility to hypo- or hyperglycaemia (see section 4.4).

Use in specific patient groups

In patients with hepatic or renal impairment as well as in the elderly, insulin requirements may be diminished (see section 4.4).

Administration

Insuman Basal is administered subcutaneously. Insuman Basal must never be injected intravenously.

Insulin absorption and hence the blood glucose lowering effect of a dose may vary from one injection area to another (e.g. the abdominal wall compared with the thigh). Injection sites within an injection area must be rotated from one injection to the next.

Before using OptiSet, the Instructions for Use included in the Package Leaflet must be read carefully.

For further details on handling, see section 6.6.

4.3 Contraindications
Hypersensitivity to the active substance or to any of the excipients.

4.4 Special warnings and precautions for use
Patients hypersensitive to Insuman Basal for whom no better tolerated preparation is available must only continue treatment under close medical supervision and – where necessary – in conjunction with anti-allergic treatment.

In patients with an allergy to animal insulin intradermal skin testing is recommended prior to a transfer to Insuman Basal, since they may experience immunological cross-reactions.

In patients with renal impairment, insulin requirements may be diminished due to reduced insulin metabolism. In the elderly, progressive deterioration of renal function may lead to a steady decrease in insulin requirements.

In patients with severe hepatic impairment, insulin requirements may be diminished due to reduced capacity for gluconeogenesis and reduced insulin metabolism.

In case of insufficient glucose control or a tendency to hyper- or hypoglycaemic episodes, the patient's adherence to the prescribed treatment regimen, injection sites and proper injection technique and all other relevant factors must be reviewed before dose adjustment is considered.

Hypoglycaemia

Hypoglycaemia may occur if the insulin dose is too high in relation to the insulin requirement.

Particular caution should be exercised, and intensified blood glucose monitoring is advisable in patients in whom hypoglycaemic episodes might be of particular clinical relevance, such as in patients with significant stenoses of the coronary arteries or of the blood vessels supplying the brain (risk of cardiac or cerebral complications of hypoglycaemia) as well as in patients with proliferative retinopathy, particularly if not treated with photocoagulation (risk of transient amaurosis following hypoglycaemia).

Patients should be aware of circumstances where warning symptoms of hypoglycaemia are diminished. The warning symptoms of hypoglycaemia may be changed, be less pronounced or be absent in certain risk groups. These include patients:

- in whom glycaemic control is markedly improved,
- in whom hypoglycaemia develops gradually,
- who are elderly,
- after transfer from animal insulin to human insulin,
- in whom an autonomic neuropathy is present,
- with a long history of diabetes,
- suffering from a psychiatric illness,
- receiving concurrent treatment with certain other medicinal products (see section 4.5).

Such situations may result in severe hypoglycaemia (and possibly loss of consciousness) prior to the patient's awareness of hypoglycaemia.

If normal or decreased values for glycated haemoglobin are noted, the possibility of recurrent, unrecognised (especially nocturnal) episodes of hypoglycaemia must be considered.

Adherence of the patient to the dosage and dietary regimen, correct insulin administration and awareness of hypoglycaemia symptoms are essential to reduce the risk of hypoglycaemia. Factors increasing the susceptibility to hypoglycaemia require particularly close monitoring and may necessitate dose adjustment. These include:

- change in the injection area,
- improved insulin sensitivity (by, e.g., removal of stress factors),
- unaccustomed, increased or prolonged physical activity,
- intercurrent illness (e.g. vomiting, diarrhoea),
- inadequate food intake,
- missed meals,
- alcohol consumption,
- certain uncompensated endocrine disorders (e.g. in hypothyroidism and in anterior pituitary or adrenocortical insufficiency),
- concomitant treatment with certain other medicinal products.

Intercurrent illness

Intercurrent illness requires intensified metabolic monitoring. In many cases, urine tests for ketones are indicated, and often it is necessary to adjust the insulin dose. The insulin requirement is often increased. Patients with type 1 diabetes must continue to consume at least a small amount of carbohydrates on a regular basis, even if they are able to eat only little or no food, or are vomiting etc. and they must never omit insulin entirely.

Handling of the pen

Before using OptiSet, the Instructions for Use included in the Package Leaflet must be read carefully. OptiSet has to be used as recommended in these Instructions for Use (see section 6.6).

4.5 Interaction with other medicinal products and other forms of interaction
A number of substances affect glucose metabolism and may require dose adjustment of human insulin.

Substances that may enhance the blood-glucose-lowering effect and increase susceptibility to hypoglycaemia include oral antidiabetic agents, angiotensin converting enzyme (ACE) inhibitors, disopyramide, fibrates, fluoxetine, monoamine oxidase (MAO) inhibitors, pentoxifylline, propoxyphene, salicylates and sulphonamide antibiotics.

Substances that may reduce the blood-glucose-lowering effect include corticosteroids, danazol, diazoxide, diuretics, glucagon, isoniazid, oestrogens and progestogens (e.g. in oral contraceptives), phenothiazine derivatives, somatropin, sympathomimetic agents (e.g. epinephrine [adrenaline], salbutamol, terbutaline), thyroid hormones, protease inhibitors and atypical antipsychotic medicinal products (e.g. olanzapine and clozapine).

Beta-blockers, clonidine, lithium salts or alcohol may either potentiate or weaken the blood-glucose-lowering effect of insulin. Pentamidine may cause hypoglycaemia which may sometimes be followed by hyperglycaemia.

In addition, under the influence of sympatholytic medicinal products such as beta-blockers, clonidine, guanethidine and reserpine, the signs of adrenergic counter-regulation may be reduced or absent.

4.6 Pregnancy and lactation
Pregnancy

For insulin human, no clinical data on exposed pregnancies are available. Insulin does not cross the placental barrier. Caution should be exercised when prescribing to pregnant women.

It is essential for patients with pre-existing or gestational diabetes to maintain good metabolic control throughout pregnancy. Insulin requirements may decrease during the first trimester and generally increase during the second and third trimesters. Immediately after delivery, insulin requirements decline rapidly (increased risk of hypoglycaemia). Careful monitoring of glucose control is essential.

Lactation

No effects on the suckling child are anticipated. Insuman Basal can be used during breastfeeding. Lactating women may require adjustments in insulin dose and diet.

4.7 Effects on ability to drive and use machines
The patient's ability to concentrate and react may be impaired as a result of hypoglycaemia or hyperglycaemia or, for example, as a result of visual impairment. This may constitute a risk in situations where these abilities are of special importance (e.g. driving a car or operating machinery).

Patients should be advised to take precautions to avoid hypoglycaemia whilst driving. This is particularly important in those who have reduced or absent awareness of the warning symptoms of hypoglycaemia or have frequent episodes of hypoglycaemia. It should be considered whether it is advisable to drive or operate machinery in these circumstances.

4.8 Undesirable effects
Hypoglycaemia, in general the most frequent undesirable effect of insulin therapy, may occur if the insulin dose is too high in relation to the insulin requirement. In clinical trials and during marketed use, the frequency varies with patient population and dose regimens. Therefore, no specific frequency can be presented.

Severe hypoglycaemic attacks, especially if recurrent, may lead to neurological damage. Prolonged or severe hypoglycaemic episodes may be life-threatening.

In many patients, the signs and symptoms of neuroglycopenia are preceded by signs of adrenergic counter-regulation. Generally, the greater and more rapid the decline in blood glucose, the more marked is the phenomenon of counter-regulation and its symptoms.

The following related adverse reactions from clinical investigations are listed below by system organ class and in order of decreasing incidence: very common ($\geqslant 1/10$); common ($\geqslant 1/100$, $< 1/10$); uncommon ($\geqslant 1/1{,}000$, $< 1/100$); rare ($\geqslant 1/10{,}000$, $< 1/1{,}000$); very rare ($< 1/10{,}000$), not known (cannot be estimated from the available data).

Within each frequency grouping, undesirable effects are presented in order of decreasing seriousness.

Immune system disorders

Uncommon: shock

Not known: immediate type allergic reactions (hypotension, angioneurotic oedema, bronchospasm, generalised skin reactions), anti-insulin antibodies

Immediate type allergic reactions to insulin or to the excipients may be life-threatening.

Insulin administration may cause anti-insulin antibodies to form. In rare cases, the presence of such anti-insulin antibodies may necessitate adjustment of the insulin dose in order to correct a tendency to hyper- or hypoglycaemia.

Metabolism and nutrition disorders

Common: oedema

Not known: sodium retention

Insulin may cause sodium retention and oedema, particularly if previously poor metabolic control is improved by intensified insulin therapy.

Eyes disorders

Not known: proliferative retinopathy, diabetic retinopathy, visual impairment

A marked change in glycaemic control may cause temporary visual impairment, due to temporary alteration in the turgidity and refractive index of the lens.

Long-term improved glycaemic control decreases the risk of progression of diabetic retinopathy. However, intensification of insulin therapy with abrupt improvement in glycaemic control may be associated with temporary worsening of diabetic retinopathy.

Skin and subcutaneous tissue disorders

Not known: lipodystrophy

As with any insulin therapy, lipodystrophy may occur at the injection site and delay local insulin absorption. Continuous rotation of the injection site within the given injection area may help to reduce or prevent these reactions.

General disorders and administration site conditions

Common: injection site reactions

Uncommon: injection site urticaria,

Not known: injection site inflammation, injection site swelling, injection site pain, injection site pruritus, injection site erythema.

Most minor reactions to insulins at the injection site usually resolve in a few days to a few weeks.

4.9 Overdose

Symptoms

Insulin overdose may lead to severe and sometimes long-term and life-threatening hypoglycaemia.

Management

Mild episodes of hypoglycaemia can usually be treated with oral carbohydrates. Adjustments in dosage of the medicinal product, meal patterns, or physical activity may be needed.

More severe episodes with coma, seizure, or neurologic impairment may be treated with intramuscular/subcutaneous glucagon or concentrated intravenous glucose. Sustained carbohydrate intake and observation may be necessary because hypoglycaemia may recur after apparent clinical recovery.

5. PHARMACOLOGICAL PROPERTIES

5.1 Pharmacodynamic properties

Pharmacotherapeutic group: Antidiabetic agent. Insulins and analogues, intermediate-acting, ATC Code: A10AC01.

Mode of action

Insulin

- lowers blood glucose and promotes anabolic effects as well as decreasing catabolic effects,

- increases the transport of glucose into cells as well as the formation of glycogen in the muscles and the liver, and improves pyruvate utilisation. It inhibits glycogenolysis and gluconeogenesis,

- increases lipogenesis in the liver and adipose tissue and inhibits lipolysis,

- promotes the uptake of amino acids into cells and promotes protein synthesis,

- enhances the uptake of potassium into cells.

Pharmacodynamic characteristics

Insuman Basal (an isophane insulin suspension) is an insulin with gradual onset and long duration of action. Following subcutaneous injection, onset of action is within 60 minutes, the phase of maximum action is between 3 and 4 hours after injection and the duration of action is 11 to 20 hours.

5.2 Pharmacokinetic properties

In healthy subjects, the serum half-life of insulin is approximately 4 to 6 minutes. It is longer in patients with severe renal insufficiency. However, it must be noted that the pharmacokinetics of insulin do not reflect its metabolic action.

5.3 Preclinical safety data

The acute toxicity was studied following subcutaneous administration in rats. No evidence of toxic effects was found. Studies of pharmacodynamic effects following subcutaneous administration in rabbits and dogs revealed the expected hypoglycaemic reactions.

6. PHARMACEUTICAL PARTICULARS

6.1 List of excipients

Protamine sulphate,

metacresol,

phenol,

zinc chloride,

sodium dihydrogen phosphate dihydrate,

glycerol,

sodium hydroxide,

hydrochloric acid (for pH adjustment),

water for injections.

6.2 Incompatibilities

This medicinal product must not be mixed with other medicinal products except those mentioned in section 6.6.

Concerning mixing or incompatibility with other insulins see section 6.6. Care must be taken to ensure that no alcohol or other disinfectants enter the insulin suspension.

6.3 Shelf life

2 years.

Handling of the pen

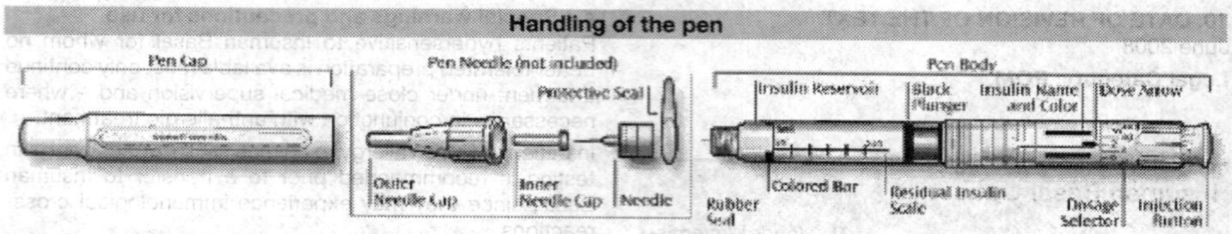

__Schematic diagram of the pen__

__Shelf life after first use of the pen:__

The pen in-use or carried as a spare may be stored for a maximum of 4 weeks not above 25°C away from direct heat or direct light.

Pens in-use must not be stored in the refrigerator.

The pen cap must be put back on the pen after each injection in order to protect from light.

6.4 Special precautions for storage

__Not in-use pens:__

Store in a refrigerator (2°C - 8°C).

Do not freeze.

Do not put Insuman Basal next to the freezer compartment or a freezer pack.

Keep the pre-filled pen in the outer carton in order to protect from light.

__In-use pens:__

For storage precautions, see section 6.3.

6.5 Nature and contents of container

3 ml suspension in a cartridge (type 1 colourless glass) with a plunger (bromobutyl rubber (type 1)) and a flanged cap (aluminium) with a stopper (bromobutyl or laminate of polyisoprene and bromobutyl rubber (type 1)).

The cartridges are sealed in a disposable pen injector. Injection needles are not included in the pack.

Each cartridge contains 3 balls (stainless steel).

Packs of 5 pens are available.

6.6 Special precautions for disposal and other handling

Before first use, Insuman Basal must be kept at room temperature for 1 to 2 hours and then resuspended to check the contents. This is best done by gently tilting the pen back and forth (at least ten times). Each cartridge contains three small metal balls to facilitate quick and thorough mixing of the contents. Later on, the insulin must be resuspended again prior to each injection.

After resuspension, the fluid must have a uniformly milky appearance. Insuman Basal must not be used if this cannot be achieved, i.e. if the suspension remains clear, for example, or if clumps, particles or flocculation appear in the insulin or stick to the wall or bottom of the cartridge. These changes sometimes give the cartridge a frosted appearance. In such cases, a new pen yielding a uniform suspension must be used. It is also necessary to change to a new pen if the insulin requirement changes substantially.

Empty pens must never be reused and must be properly discarded.

To prevent the possible transmission of disease, each pen must be used by one patient only.

As with all insulin preparations, Insuman Basal must not be mixed with solutions containing reducing agents such as thioles and sulphites. It must also be remembered that insulin protamine crystals dissolve in an acid pH range.

Mixing of insulins

Insuman Basal must not be mixed with any other insulin or with insulin analogues.

Any unused product or waste material should be disposed of in accordance with local requirements.

Handling of the pen

The Instructions for Use included in the Package Leaflet must be read carefully before using OptiSet.

(see Handling of the pen above)

Important information for use of OptiSet:

- Always attach a new needle before each use. Only use needles that are compatible for use with OptiSet.
- Always perform the safety test before each injection.
- If a new OptiSet is used the initial safety test must be done with the 8 units preset by the manufacturer.
- The dosage selector can only be turned in one direction.
- Never turn the dosage selector (change the dose) after injection button has been pulled out.
- This pen is only for the patients use. It must not be shared with anyone else.
- If the injection is given by another person, special caution must be taken by this person to avoid accidental needle injury and transmission of infection.
- Never use OptiSet if it is damaged or if you are not sure that it is working properly.
- Always have a spare OptiSet in case your OptiSet is lost or damaged.

Storage Instructions

Please check section 6.4 of this leaflet for instructions on how to store OptiSet.

If OptiSet is in cool storage, it should be taken out 1 to 2 hours before injection to allow it to warm up. Cold insulin is more painful to inject.

The used OptiSet must be discarded as required by your local authorities.

Maintenance

OptiSet has to be protected from dust and dirt.

You can clean the outside of your OptiSet by wiping it with a damp cloth.

Do not soak, wash or lubricate the pen as this may damage it.

OptiSet is designed to work accurately and safely. It should be handled with care. Avoid situations where OptiSet might be damaged. If you are concerned that your OptiSet may be damaged, use a new one.

Step 1. Check and mix the Insulin

After removing the pen cap, the label on the pen and the insulin reservoir should be checked to make sure it contains the correct insulin. The insulin should be mixed by turning OptiSet slowly up and down at least 10 times.

The appearance of the insulin should be checked: the insulin suspension must have an evenly milky white appearance.

Step 2. Attach the needle

The needle should be carefully attached straight onto the pen.

Step 3. Perform a safety test

Prior to each injection a safety test has to be performed.

For a new and unused OptiSet, a dose of 8 units is already preset by the manufacturer for the first safety test.

In-use OptiSet, select a dose of 2 units by turning the dosage selector forward till the dose arrow points to 2. The dosage selector will only turn in one direction.

Pull out the injection button completely in order to load the dose. Never turn the dosage selector after injection button has been pulled out.

The outer and inner needle caps should be removed. Keep the outer cap to remove the used needle.

While holding the pen with the needle pointing upwards, the insulin reservoir should be tapped with the finger so that any air bubbles rise up towards the needle

Then the injection button should be pressed all the way in.

If insulin has been expelled through the needle tip, then the pen and the needle are working properly.

If no insulin appears at the needle tip, step 3 should be repeated two more times until insulin appears at the needle tip. If still no insulin comes out, change the needle, as it might be blocked and try again. If no insulin comes out after changing the needle, the OptiSet may be damaged. Do not use this OptiSet.

Step 4. Select the dose

The dose can be set in steps of 2 units, from a minimum of 2 units to a maximum of 40 units. If a dose greater than 40 units is required, it should be given as two or more injections.

Check if you have enough insulin for the dose.

The residual insulin scale on the transparent insulin reservoir shows approximately how much insulin remains in the OptiSet. This scale must not be used to set the insulin dose.

If the black plunger is at the beginning of the coloured bar, then there are approximately 40 units of insulin available.

If the black plunger is at the end of the coloured bar, then there are approximately 20 units of insulin available.

The dosage selector should be turned forward until the dose arrow points to the required dose.

Step 5. Load the dose

The injection button should be pulled out as far as it will go in order to load the pen.

Check if the selected dose is fully loaded. Note that the injection button only goes out as far as the amount of insulin that is left in the reservoir.

The injection button allows checking the actual loaded dose. The injection button must be held out under tension during this check. The last thick line visible on the injection button shows the amount of insulin loaded. When the injection button is held out only the top part of this thick line can be seen.

Step 6. Inject the dose

The patient should be informed on the injection technique by his health care professional.

The needle should be inserted into the skin.

The injection button should be pressed all the way in. A clicking sound can be heard, which will stop when the injection button has been pressed in completely. Then the injection button should be held down 10 seconds before withdrawing the needle from the skin. This ensures that the full dose of insulin has been delivered.

Step 7. Remove and discard the needle

The needle should be removed after each injection and discarded. This helps prevent contamination and/or infection as well as entry of air into the insulin reservoir and leakage of insulin, which can cause inaccurate dosing. Needles must not be reused.

The pen cap should be replaced on the pen.

7. MARKETING AUTHORISATION HOLDER

Sanofi-Aventis Deutschland GmbH, D-65926 Frankfurt am Main, Germany

8. MARKETING AUTHORISATION NUMBER(S)

EU/1/97/030/071

9. DATE OF FIRST AUTHORISATION/RENEWAL OF THE AUTHORISATION

Date of first authorisation: 21 February 1997

Date of latest renewal: 21 February 2007

10. DATE OF REVISION OF THE TEXT

June 2008

Legal Category: POM

Insuman Basal Vials

(sanofi-aventis)

1. NAME OF THE MEDICINAL PRODUCT

Insuman Basal 100 IU/ml suspension for injection in a vial

2. QUALITATIVE AND QUANTITATIVE COMPOSITION

Each ml contains 100 IU insulin human (equivalent to 3.5 mg).

Each vial contains 5 ml of suspension for injection, equivalent to 500 IU insulin. One IU (International Unit) corresponds to 0.035 mg of anhydrous human insulin.

Insuman Basal is an isophane insulin suspension.

Human insulin is produced by recombinant DNA technology in *Escherichia coli*.

For a full list of excipients, see section 6.1.

3. PHARMACEUTICAL FORM

Suspension for injection in a vial.

After re-suspension, milky white suspension.

4. CLINICAL PARTICULARS

4.1 Therapeutic indications

Diabetes mellitus where treatment with insulin is required.

4.2 Posology and method of administration

The desired blood glucose levels, the insulin preparations to be used and the insulin dosage (doses and timings) must be determined individually and adjusted to suit the patient's diet, physical activity and life-style.

Daily doses and timing of administration

There are no fixed rules for insulin dosage. However, the average insulin requirement is often 0.5 to 1.0 IU per kg body weight per day. The basal metabolic requirement is 40% to 60% of the total daily requirement. Insuman Basal is injected subcutaneously 45 to 60 minutes before a meal.

Transfer to Insuman Basal

Dosage adjustment may be necessary when transferring patients from one insulin preparation to another. This applies, for example, when transferring from:

- an animal insulin (especially a bovine insulin) to human insulin,
- one human insulin preparation to another,
- a regimen with only regular insulin to one with a longer-acting insulin.

The need to adjust (e.g. reduce) the dose may become evident immediately after transfer. Alternatively, it may emerge gradually over a period of several weeks.

Following transfer from an animal insulin to human insulin, dosage reduction may be required in particular in patients who

- were previously already controlled on rather low blood glucose levels,
- have a tendency to hypoglycaemia,
- previously required high insulin doses due to the presence of insulin antibodies.

Close metabolic monitoring is recommended during the transition and in the initial weeks thereafter. In patients who require high insulin doses because of the presence of insulin antibodies, transfer under medical supervision in a hospital or similar setting must be considered.

Secondary dose adjustment

Improved metabolic control may result in increased insulin sensitivity, leading to a reduced insulin requirement. Dose adjustment may also be required, for example, if

- the patient's weight changes,
- the patient's life-style changes,
- other circumstances arise that may promote an increased susceptibility to hypo- or hyperglycaemia (see section 4.4).

Use in specific patient groups

In patients with hepatic or renal impairment as well as in the elderly, insulin requirements may be diminished (see section 4.4).

Administration

Insuman Basal contains 100 IU of insulin per ml suspension. Only injection syringes designed for this strength of insulin (100 IU per ml) are to be used. The injection syringes must not contain any other medicinal product or residue (e.g. traces of heparin).

Insuman Basal is administered subcutaneously. Insuman Basal must never be injected intravenously.

Insulin absorption and hence the blood glucose lowering effect of a dose may vary from one injection area to another (e.g. the abdominal wall compared with the thigh). Injection sites within an injection area must be rotated from one injection to the next.

For further details on handling, see section 6.6.

4.3 Contraindications

Hypersensitivity to the active substance or to any of the excipients.

Insuman Basal must not be administered intravenously and must not be used in infusion pumps or external or implanted insulin pumps.

4.4 Special warnings and precautions for use

Patients hypersensitive to Insuman Basal for whom no better tolerated preparation is available must only continue treatment under close medical supervision and – where necessary – in conjunction with anti-allergic treatment.

In patients with an allergy to animal insulin intradermal skin testing is recommended prior to a transfer to Insuman Basal, since they may experience immunological cross-reactions.

In patients with renal impairment, insulin requirements may be diminished due to reduced insulin metabolism. In the elderly, progressive deterioration of renal function may lead to a steady decrease in insulin requirements.

In patients with severe hepatic impairment, insulin requirements may be diminished due to reduced capacity for gluconeogenesis and reduced insulin metabolism.

In case of insufficient glucose control or a tendency to hyper- or hypoglycaemic episodes, the patient's adherence to the prescribed treatment regimen, injection sites and proper injection technique and all other relevant factors must be reviewed before dose adjustment is considered.

Hypoglycaemia

Hypoglycaemia may occur if the insulin dose is too high in relation to the insulin requirement.

Particular caution should be exercised, and intensified blood glucose monitoring is advisable in patients in whom hypoglycaemic episodes might be of particular clinical relevance, such as in patients with significant stenoses of the coronary arteries or of the blood vessels supplying the brain (risk of cardiac or cerebral complications of hypoglycaemia) as well as in patients with proliferative retinopathy, particularly if not treated with photocoagulation (risk of transient amaurosis following hypoglycaemia).

Patients should be aware of circumstances where warning symptoms of hypoglycaemia are diminished. The warning symptoms of hypoglycaemia may be changed, be less pronounced or be absent in certain risk groups. These include patients:

- in whom glycaemic control is markedly improved,
- in whom hypoglycaemia develops gradually,
- who are elderly,
- after transfer from animal insulin to human insulin,
- in whom an autonomic neuropathy is present,
- with a long history of diabetes,
- suffering from a psychiatric illness,
- receiving concurrent treatment with certain other medicinal products (see section 4.5).

Such situations may result in severe hypoglycaemia (and possibly loss of consciousness) prior to the patient's awareness of hypoglycaemia.

If normal or decreased values for glycated haemoglobin are noted, the possibility of recurrent, unrecognised (especially nocturnal) episodes of hypoglycaemia must be considered.

Adherence of the patient to the dosage and dietary regimen, correct insulin administration and awareness of hypoglycaemia symptoms are essential to reduce the risk of hypoglycaemia. Factors increasing the susceptibility to hypoglycaemia require particularly close monitoring and may necessitate dose adjustment. These include:

- change in the injection area,
- improved insulin sensitivity (by, e.g., removal of stress factors),
- unaccustomed, increased or prolonged physical activity,
- intercurrent illness (e.g. vomiting, diarrhoea),
- inadequate food intake,
- missed meals,
- alcohol consumption,
- certain uncompensated endocrine disorders (e.g. in hypothyroidism and in anterior pituitary or adrenocortical insufficiency),
- concomitant treatment with certain other medicinal products.

Intercurrent illness

Intercurrent illness requires intensified metabolic monitoring. In many cases, urine tests for ketones are indicated, and often it is necessary to adjust the insulin dose. The insulin requirement is often increased. Patients with type 1 diabetes must continue to consume at least a small amount of carbohydrates on a regular basis, even if they are able to eat only little or no food, or are vomiting etc. and they must never omit insulin entirely.

4.5 Interaction with other medicinal products and other forms of interaction

A number of substances affect glucose metabolism and may require dose adjustment of human insulin.

Substances that may enhance the blood-glucose-lowering effect and increase susceptibility to hypoglycaemia include oral antidiabetic agents, angiotensin converting enzyme (ACE) inhibitors, disopyramide, fibrates, fluoxetine, monoamine oxidase (MAO) inhibitors, pentoxifylline, propoxyphene, salicylates and sulphonamide antibiotics.

Substances that may reduce the blood-glucose-lowering effect include corticosteroids, danazol, diazoxide, diuretics, glucagon, isoniazid, oestrogens and progestogens (e.g. in oral contraceptives), phenothiazine derivatives, somatropin, sympathomimetic agents (e.g. epinephrine [adrenaline], salbutamol, terbutaline), thyroid hormones, protease inhibitors and atypical antipsychotic medicinal products (e.g. olanzapine and clozapine).

Beta-blockers, clonidine, lithium salts or alcohol may either potentiate or weaken the blood-glucose-lowering effect of insulin. Pentamidine may cause hypoglycaemia which may sometimes be followed by hyperglycaemia.

In addition, under the influence of sympatholytic medicinal products such as beta-blockers, clonidine, guanethidine and reserpine, the signs of adrenergic counter-regulation may be reduced or absent.

4.6 Pregnancy and lactation

Pregnancy

For insulin human, no clinical data on exposed pregnancies are available. Insulin does not cross the placental barrier. Caution should be exercised when prescribing to pregnant women.

It is essential for patients with pre-existing or gestational diabetes to maintain good metabolic control throughout pregnancy. Insulin requirements may decrease during the first trimester and generally increase during the second and third trimesters. Immediately after delivery, insulin requirements decline rapidly (increased risk of hypoglycaemia). Careful monitoring of glucose control is essential.

Lactation

No effects on the suckling child are anticipated. Insuman Basal can be used during breastfeeding. Lactating women may require adjustments in insulin dose and diet.

4.7 Effects on ability to drive and use machines

The patient's ability to concentrate and react may be impaired as a result of hypoglycaemia or hyperglycaemia or, for example, as a result of visual impairment. This may constitute a risk in situations where these abilities are of special importance (e.g. driving a car or operating machinery).

Patients should be advised to take precautions to avoid hypoglycaemia whilst driving. This is particularly important in those who have reduced or absent awareness of the warning symptoms of hypoglycaemia or have frequent episodes of hypoglycaemia. It should be considered whether it is advisable to drive or operate machinery in these circumstances.

4.8 Undesirable effects

Hypoglycaemia, in general the most frequent undesirable effect of insulin therapy, may occur if the insulin dose is too high in relation to the insulin requirement. In clinical trials and during marketed use, the frequency varies with patient population and dose regimens. Therefore, no specific frequency can be presented.

Severe hypoglycaemic attacks, especially if recurrent, may lead to neurological damage. Prolonged or severe hypoglycaemic episodes may be life-threatening.

In many patients, the signs and symptoms of neuroglycopenia are preceded by signs of adrenergic counter-regulation. Generally, the greater and more rapid the decline in blood glucose, the more marked is the phenomenon of counter-regulation and its symptoms.

The following related adverse reactions from clinical investigations are listed below by system organ class and in order of decreasing incidence: very common (≥1/10); common (≥1/100, <1/10); uncommon (≥1/1,000, <1/100); rare (≥1/10,000, <1/1,000); very rare (<1/10,000), not known (cannot be estimated from the available data).

Within each frequency grouping, undesirable effects are presented in order of decreasing seriousness.

Immune system disorders

Uncommon: shock

Not known: immediate type allergic reactions (hypotension, angioneurotic oedema, bronchospasm, generalised skin reactions), anti-insulin antibodies

Immediate type allergic reactions to insulin or to the excipients may be life-threatening.

Insulin administration may cause anti-insulin antibodies to form. In rare cases, the presence of such anti-insulin antibodies may necessitate adjustment of the insulin dose in order to correct a tendency to hyper- or hypoglycaemia.

Metabolism and nutrition disorders

Common: oedema

Not known: sodium retention

Insulin may cause sodium retention and oedema, particularly if previously poor metabolic control is improved by intensified insulin therapy.

Eyes disorders

Not known: proliferative retinopathy, diabetic retinopathy, visual impairment

A marked change in glycaemic control may cause temporary visual impairment, due to temporary alteration in the turgidity and refractive index of the lens.

Long-term improved glycaemic control decreases the risk of progression of diabetic retinopathy. However, intensification of insulin therapy with abrupt improvement in glycaemic control may be associated with temporary worsening of diabetic retinopathy.

Skin and subcutaneous tissue disorders

Not known: lipodystrophy

As with any insulin therapy, lipodystrophy may occur at the injection site and delay local insulin absorption. Continuous rotation of the injection site within the given injection area may help to reduce or prevent these reactions.

General disorders and administration site conditions

Common: injection site reactions

Uncommon: injection site urticaria,

Not known: injection site inflammation, injection site swelling, injection site pain, injection site pruritus, injection site erythema.

Most minor reactions to insulins at the injection site usually resolve in a few days to a few weeks.

4.9 Overdose

Symptoms

Insulin overdose may lead to severe and sometimes long-term and life-threatening hypoglycaemia.

Management

Mild episodes of hypoglycaemia can usually be treated with oral carbohydrates. Adjustments in dosage of the medicinal product, meal patterns, or physical activity may be needed.

More severe episodes with coma, seizure, or neurologic impairment may be treated with intramuscular/subcutaneous glucagon or concentrated intravenous glucose. Sustained carbohydrate intake and observation may be necessary because hypoglycaemia may recur after apparent clinical recovery.

5. PHARMACOLOGICAL PROPERTIES

5.1 Pharmacodynamic properties

Pharmacotherapeutic group: Antidiabetic agent. Insulins and analogues, intermediate-acting, ATC Code: A10AC01.

Mode of action

Insulin

- lowers blood glucose and promotes anabolic effects as well as decreasing catabolic effects,
- increases the transport of glucose into cells as well as the formation of glycogen in the muscles and the liver, and improves pyruvate utilisation. It inhibits glycogenolysis and gluconeogenesis,
- increases lipogenesis in the liver and adipose tissue and inhibits lipolysis,
- promotes the uptake of amino acids into cells and promotes protein synthesis,
- enhances the uptake of potassium into cells.

Pharmacodynamic characteristics

Insuman Basal (an isophane insulin suspension) is an insulin with gradual onset and long duration of action. Following subcutaneous injection, onset of action is within 60 minutes, the phase of maximum action is between 3 and 4 hours after injection and the duration of action is 11 to 20 hours.

5.2 Pharmacokinetic properties

In healthy subjects, the serum half-life of insulin is approximately 4 to 6 minutes. It is longer in patients with severe renal insufficiency. However, it must be noted that the pharmacokinetics of insulin do not reflect its metabolic action.

5.3 Preclinical safety data

The acute toxicity was studied following subcutaneous administration in rats. No evidence of toxic effects was found. Studies of pharmacodynamic effects following subcutaneous administration in rabbits and dogs revealed the expected hypoglycaemic reactions.

6. PHARMACEUTICAL PARTICULARS

6.1 List of excipients

Protamine sulphate,

metacresol,

phenol,

zinc chloride,

sodium dihydrogen phosphate dihydrate,

glycerol,

sodium hydroxide,

hydrochloric acid (for pH adjustment),

water for injections.

6.2 Incompatibilities

This medicinal product must not be mixed with other medicinal products except those mentioned in section 6.6.

Concerning mixing or incompatibility with other insulins see section 6.6. Care must be taken to ensure that no alcohol or other disinfectants enter the insulin suspension.

6.3 Shelf life

2 years.

Shelf life after first use of the vial:

The product may be stored for a maximum of 4 weeks not above 25°C away from direct heat or direct light.

Keep the vial in the outer carton in order to protect from light.

It is recommended that the date of the first use be noted on the label.

6.4 Special precautions for storage

Unopened vials:

Store in a refrigerator (2°C - 8°C).

Do not freeze.

Do not put Insuman Basal next to the freezer compartment or a freezer pack.

Keep the vial in the outer carton in order to protect from light.

Opened vials:

For storage precautions, see section 6.3.

6.5 Nature and contents of container

5 ml suspension in a vial (type 1 colourless glass) with a flanged cap (aluminium), a stopper (chlorobutyl rubber (type 1)) and a tear-off cap (polypropylene).

Packs of 1 vial are available.

6.6 Special precautions for disposal and other handling

Before withdrawing insulin from the vial for the first time, remove the plastic protective cap.

Immediately before withdrawal from the vial into the injection syringe, the insulin must be re-suspended. This is best done by rolling the vial at an oblique angle between the palms of the hands. Do not shake the vial vigorously as this may lead to changes in the suspension (giving the vial a frosted appearance; see below) and cause frothing. Froth may interfere with the correct measurement of the dose.

After resuspension, the fluid must have a uniformly milky appearance. Insuman Basal must not be used if this cannot be achieved, i.e. if the suspension remains clear, for example, or if clumps, particles or flocculation appear in the insulin or stick to the wall or bottom of the vial. These changes sometimes give the vial a frosted appearance. In such cases, a new vial yielding a uniform suspension must be used. It is also necessary to change to a new vial if the insulin requirement changes substantially.

As with all insulin preparations, Insuman Basal must not be mixed with solutions containing reducing agents such as thioles and sulphites. It must also be remembered that insulin protamine crystals dissolve in an acid pH range.

Mixing of insulins

Insuman Basal may be mixed with all Sanofi-Aventis human insulins, but NOT with those designed specifically for use in insulin pumps. Insuman Basal must also NOT be mixed with insulins of animal origin or with insulin analogues.

If two different insulins have to be drawn into one single injection syringe, it is recommended that the shorter-acting insulin be drawn first to prevent contamination of the vial by the longer-acting preparation. It is advisable to inject immediately after mixing. Insulins of different concentration (e.g. 100 IU per ml and 40 IU per ml) must not be mixed.

Any unused product or waste material should be disposed of in accordance with local requirements.

7. MARKETING AUTHORISATION HOLDER

Sanofi-Aventis Deutschland GmbH, D-65926 Frankfurt am Main, Germany

8. MARKETING AUTHORISATION NUMBER(S)

EU/1/97/030/033

9. DATE OF FIRST AUTHORISATION/RENEWAL OF THE AUTHORISATION

Date of first authorisation: 21 February 1997

Date of latest renewal: 21 February 2007

10. DATE OF REVISION OF THE TEXT

June 2008

Legal Category: POM

Insuman Comb 15 Optiset

(sanofi-aventis)

1. NAME OF THE MEDICINAL PRODUCT

Insuman Comb 15 100 IU/ml suspension for injection in a pre-filled pen.

2. QUALITATIVE AND QUANTITATIVE COMPOSITION

Each ml contains 100 IU insulin human (equivalent to 3.5 mg).

Each pen contains 3 ml of suspension for injection, equivalent to 300 IU insulin. One IU (International Unit) corresponds to 0.035 mg of anhydrous human insulin.

Insuman Comb 15 is a biphasic isophane insulin suspension consisting of 15% dissolved insulin and 85% crystalline protamine insulin.

Human insulin is produced by recombinant DNA technology in *Escherichia coli*.

For a full list of excipients, see section 6.1.

3. PHARMACEUTICAL FORM

Suspension for injection in a pre-filled pen. OptiSet.

After re-suspension, milky white suspension.

4. CLINICAL PARTICULARS

4.1 Therapeutic indications

Diabetes mellitus where treatment with insulin is required.

4.2 Posology and method of administration

The desired blood glucose levels, the insulin preparations to be used and the insulin dosage (doses and timings) must be determined individually and adjusted to suit the patient's diet, physical activity and life-style.

Daily doses and timing of administration

There are no fixed rules for insulin dosage. However, the average insulin requirement is often 0.5 to 1.0 IU per kg body weight per day. The basal metabolic requirement is 40% to 60% of the total daily requirement. Insuman Comb 15 is injected subcutaneously 30 to 45 minutes before a meal.

OptiSet delivers insulin in increments of 2 IU up to a maximum single dose of 40 IU.

Transfer to Insuman Comb 15

Dosage adjustment may be necessary when transferring patients from one insulin preparation to another. This applies, for example, when transferring from:

- an animal insulin (especially a bovine insulin) to human insulin,
- one human insulin preparation to another,
- a regimen with only regular insulin to one with a longer-acting insulin.

The need to adjust (e.g. reduce) the dose may become evident immediately after transfer. Alternatively, it may emerge gradually over a period of several weeks.

Following transfer from an animal insulin to human insulin, dosage reduction may be required in particular in patients who

- were previously already controlled on rather low blood glucose levels,
- have a tendency to hypoglycaemia,
- previously required high insulin doses due to the presence of insulin antibodies.

Close metabolic monitoring is recommended during the transition and in the initial weeks thereafter. In patients who require high insulin doses because of the presence of insulin antibodies, transfer under medical supervision in a hospital or similar setting must be considered.

Secondary dose adjustment

Improved metabolic control may result in increased insulin sensitivity, leading to a reduced insulin requirement. Dose adjustment may also be required, for example, if

- the patient's weight changes,
- the patient's life-style changes,
- other circumstances arise that may promote an increased susceptibility to hypo- or hyperglycaemia (see section 4.4).

Use in specific patient groups

In patients with hepatic or renal impairment as well as in the elderly, insulin requirements may be diminished (see section 4.4).

Administration

Insuman Comb 15 is administered subcutaneously. Insuman Comb 15 must never be injected intravenously.

Insulin absorption and hence the blood glucose lowering effect of a dose may vary from one injection area to another (e.g. the abdominal wall compared with the thigh). Injection sites within an injection area must be rotated from one injection to the next.

Before using OptiSet, the Instructions for Use included in the Package Leaflet must be read carefully.

For further details on handling, see section 6.6.

4.3 Contraindications

Hypersensitivity to the active substance or to any of the excipients.

4.4 Special warnings and precautions for use

Patients hypersensitive to Insuman Comb 15 for whom no better tolerated preparation is available must only continue treatment under close medical supervision and – where necessary – in conjunction with anti-allergic treatment.

In patients with an allergy to animal insulin intradermal skin testing is recommended prior to a transfer to Insuman Comb 15, since they may experience immunological cross-reactions.

In patients with renal impairment, insulin requirements may be diminished due to reduced insulin metabolism. In the elderly, progressive deterioration of renal function may lead to a steady decrease in insulin requirements.

In patients with severe hepatic impairment, insulin requirements may be diminished due to reduced capacity for gluconeogenesis and reduced insulin metabolism.

In case of insufficient glucose control or a tendency to hyper- or hypoglycaemic episodes, the patient's adherence to the prescribed treatment regimen, injection sites and proper injection technique and all other relevant factors must be reviewed before dose adjustment is considered.

Hypoglycaemia

Hypoglycaemia may occur if the insulin dose is too high in relation to the insulin requirement.

Particular caution should be exercised, and intensified blood glucose monitoring is advisable in patients in whom hypoglycaemic episodes might be of particular clinical relevance, such as in patients with significant stenoses of the coronary arteries or of the blood vessels supplying the brain (risk of cardiac or cerebral complications of hypoglycaemia) as well as in patients with proliferative retinopathy, particularly if not treated with photocoagulation (risk of transient amaurosis following hypoglycaemia).

Patients should be aware of circumstances where warning symptoms of hypoglycaemia are diminished. The warning symptoms of hypoglycaemia may be changed, be less pronounced or be absent in certain risk groups. These include patients:

- in whom glycaemic control is markedly improved,
- in whom hypoglycaemia develops gradually,
- who are elderly,
- after transfer from animal insulin to human insulin,
- in whom an autonomic neuropathy is present,
- with a long history of diabetes,
- suffering from a psychiatric illness,
- receiving concurrent treatment with certain other medicinal products (see section 4.5).

Such situations may result in severe hypoglycaemia (and possibly loss of consciousness) prior to the patient's awareness of hypoglycaemia.

If normal or decreased values for glycated haemoglobin are noted, the possibility of recurrent, unrecognised (especially nocturnal) episodes of hypoglycaemia must be considered.

Adherence of the patient to the dosage and dietary regimen, correct insulin administration and awareness of hypoglycaemia symptoms are essential to reduce the risk of hypoglycaemia. Factors increasing the susceptibility to hypoglycaemia require particularly close monitoring and may necessitate dose adjustment. These include:

- change in the injection area,
- improved insulin sensitivity (by, e.g., removal of stress factors),
- unaccustomed, increased or prolonged physical activity,
- intercurrent illness (e.g. vomiting, diarrhoea),
- inadequate food intake,
- missed meals,
- alcohol consumption,
- certain uncompensated endocrine disorders (e.g. in hypothyroidism and in anterior pituitary or adrenocortical insufficiency),
- concomitant treatment with certain other medicinal products.

Intercurrent illness

Intercurrent illness requires intensified metabolic monitoring. In many cases, urine tests for ketones are indicated, and often it is necessary to adjust the insulin dose. The insulin requirement is often increased. Patients with type 1 diabetes must continue to consume at least a small amount of carbohydrates on a regular basis, even if they are able to eat only little or no food, or are vomiting etc. and they must never omit insulin entirely.

Handling of the pen

Before using OptiSet, the Instructions for Use included in the Package Leaflet must be read carefully. OptiSet has to be used as recommended in these Instructions for Use (see section 6.6).

4.5 Interaction with other medicinal products and other forms of interaction

A number of substances affect glucose metabolism and may require dose adjustment of human insulin.

Substances that may enhance the blood-glucose-lowering effect and increase susceptibility to hypoglycaemia include oral antidiabetic agents, angiotensin converting enzyme (ACE) inhibitors, disopyramide, fibrates, fluoxetine, monoamine oxidase (MAO) inhibitors, pentoxifylline, propoxyphene, salicylates and sulphonamide antibiotics.

Substances that may reduce the blood-glucose-lowering effect include corticosteroids, danazol, diazoxide, diuretics, glucagon, isoniazid, oestrogens and progestogens (e.g. in oral contraceptives), phenothiazine derivatives, somatropin, sympathomimetic agents (e.g. epinephrine [adrenaline], salbutamol, terbutaline), thyroid hormones, protease inhibitors and atypical antipsychotic medicinal products (e.g. olanzapine and clozapine).

Beta-blockers, clonidine, lithium salts or alcohol may either potentiate or weaken the blood-glucose-lowering effect of insulin. Pentamidine may cause hypoglycaemia which may sometimes be followed by hyperglycaemia.

In addition, under the influence of sympatholytic medicinal products such as beta-blockers, clonidine, guanethidine and reserpine, the signs of adrenergic counter-regulation may be reduced or absent.

4.6 Pregnancy and lactation

Pregnancy

For insulin human, no clinical data on exposed pregnancies are available. Insulin does not cross the placental barrier. Caution should be exercised when prescribing to pregnant women.

It is essential for patients with pre-existing or gestational diabetes to maintain good metabolic control throughout pregnancy. Insulin requirements may decrease during the first trimester and generally increase during the second and third trimesters. Immediately after delivery, insulin requirements decline rapidly (increased risk of hypoglycaemia). Careful monitoring of glucose control is essential.

Lactation

No effects on the suckling child are anticipated. Insuman Comb 15 can be used during breastfeeding. Lactating women may require adjustments in insulin dose and diet.

4.7 Effects on ability to drive and use machines

The patient's ability to concentrate and react may be impaired as a result of hypoglycaemia or hyperglycaemia or, for example, as a result of visual impairment. This may constitute a risk in situations where these abilities are of special importance (e.g. driving a car or operating machinery).

Patients should be advised to take precautions to avoid hypoglycaemia whilst driving. This is particularly important in those who have reduced or absent awareness of the warning symptoms of hypoglycaemia or have frequent episodes of hypoglycaemia. It should be considered whether it is advisable to drive or operate machinery in these circumstances.

4.8 Undesirable effects

Hypoglycaemia, in general the most frequent undesirable effect of insulin therapy, may occur if the insulin dose is too high in relation to the insulin requirement. In clinical trials and during marketed use, the frequency varies with patient population and dose regimens. Therefore, no specific frequency can be presented.

Severe hypoglycaemic attacks, especially if recurrent, may lead to neurological damage. Prolonged or severe hypoglycaemic episodes may be life-threatening.

In many patients, the signs and symptoms of neuroglycopenia are preceded by signs of adrenergic counter-regulation. Generally, the greater and more rapid the decline in blood glucose, the more marked is the phenomenon of counter-regulation and its symptoms.

The following related adverse reactions from clinical investigations are listed below by system organ class and in order of decreasing incidence: very common ($\geqslant$1/10); common ($\geqslant$1/100, $<$1/10); uncommon ($\geqslant$1/1,000, $<$1/100); rare ($\geqslant$1/10,000, $<$1/1,000); very rare ($<$1/10,000), not known (cannot be estimated from the available data).

Within each frequency grouping, undesirable effects are presented in order of decreasing seriousness.

Immune system disorders

Uncommon: shock

Not known: immediate type allergic reactions (hypotension, angioneurotic oedema, bronchospasm, generalised skin reactions), anti-insulin antibodies

Immediate type allergic reactions to insulin or to the excipients may be life-threatening.

Insulin administration may cause anti-insulin antibodies to form. In rare cases, the presence of such anti-insulin antibodies may necessitate adjustment of the insulin dose in order to correct a tendency to hyper- or hypoglycaemia.

Metabolism and nutrition disorders

Common: oedema

Not known: sodium retention

Insulin may cause sodium retention and oedema, particularly if previously poor metabolic control is improved by intensified insulin therapy.

Eyes disorders

Not known: proliferative retinopathy, diabetic retinopathy, visual impairment

A marked change in glycaemic control may cause temporary visual impairment, due to temporary alteration in the turgidity and refractive index of the lens.

Long-term improved glycaemic control decreases the risk of progression of diabetic retinopathy. However, intensification of insulin therapy with abrupt improvement in glycaemic control may be associated with temporary worsening of diabetic retinopathy.

Skin and subcutaneous tissue disorders

Not known: lipodystrophy

As with any insulin therapy, lipodystrophy may occur at the injection site and delay local insulin absorption. Continuous rotation of the injection site within the given injection area may help to reduce or prevent these reactions.

General disorders and administration site conditions

Common: injection site reactions

Uncommon: injection site urticaria,

Not known: injection site inflammation, injection site swelling, injection site pain, injection site pruritus, injection site erythema.

Most minor reactions to insulins at the injection site usually resolve in a few days to a few weeks.

4.9 Overdose

Symptoms

Insulin overdose may lead to severe and sometimes long-term and life-threatening hypoglycaemia.

Management

Mild episodes of hypoglycaemia can usually be treated with oral carbohydrates. Adjustments in dosage of the medicinal product, meal patterns, or physical activity may be needed.

More severe episodes with coma, seizure, or neurologic impairment may be treated with intramuscular/subcutaneous glucagon or concentrated intravenous glucose. Sustained carbohydrate intake and observation may be necessary because hypoglycaemia may recur after apparent clinical recovery.

5. PHARMACOLOGICAL PROPERTIES

5.1 Pharmacodynamic properties

Pharmacotherapeutic group: Antidiabetic agent. Insulins and analogues, intermediate-acting combined with fast-acting, ATC Code: A10AD01.

Mode of action

Insulin

- lowers blood glucose and promotes anabolic effects as well as decreasing catabolic effects,
- increases the transport of glucose into cells as well as the formation of glycogen in the muscles and the liver, and improves pyruvate utilisation. It inhibits glycogenolysis and gluconeogenesis,
- increases lipogenesis in the liver and adipose tissue and inhibits lipolysis,
- promotes the uptake of amino acids into cells and promotes protein synthesis,
- enhances the uptake of potassium into cells.

Pharmacodynamic characteristics

Insuman Comb 15 (a biphasic isophane insulin suspension with 15% dissolved insulin) is an insulin with gradual onset and long duration of action. Following subcutaneous injection, onset of action is within 30 to 60 minutes, the phase of maximum action is between 2 and 4 hours after injection and the duration of action is 11 to 20 hours.

5.2 Pharmacokinetic properties

In healthy subjects, the serum half-life of insulin is approximately 4 to 6 minutes. It is longer in patients with severe renal insufficiency. However, it must be noted that the pharmacokinetics of insulin do not reflect its metabolic action.

5.3 Preclinical safety data

The acute toxicity was studied following subcutaneous administration in rats. No evidence of toxic effects was found. Studies of pharmacodynamic effects following subcutaneous administration in rabbits and dogs revealed the expected hypoglycaemic reactions.

6. PHARMACEUTICAL PARTICULARS

6.1 List of excipients

Protamine sulphate,

metacresol,

phenol,

zinc chloride,

sodium dihydrogen phosphate dihydrate,

glycerol,

sodium hydroxide,

hydrochloric acid (for pH adjustment),

water for injections.

6.2 Incompatibilities

This medicinal product must not be mixed with other medicinal products except those mentioned in section 6.6.

Concerning mixing or incompatibility with other insulins see section 6.6. Care must be taken to ensure that no alcohol or other disinfectants enter the insulin suspension.

Handling of the pen

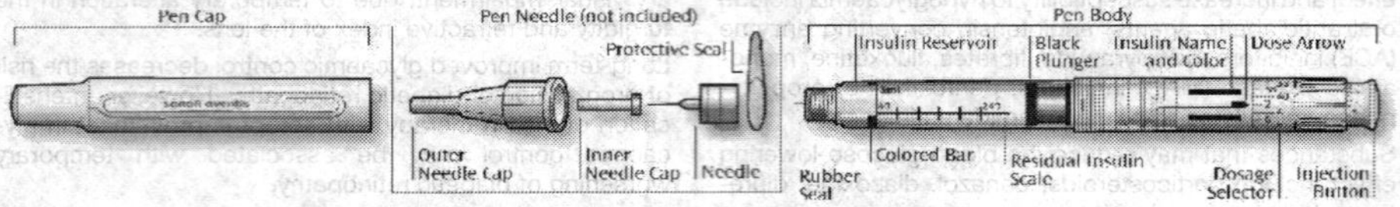

<u>Schematic diagram of the pen</u>

6.3 Shelf life
2 years.

<u>Shelf life after first use of the pen</u>:

The pen in-use or carried as a spare may be stored for a maximum of 4 weeks not above 25°C away from direct heat or direct light.

Pens in-use must not be stored in the refrigerator.

The pen cap must be put back on the pen after each injection in order to protect from light.

6.4 Special precautions for storage

<u>Not in-use pens</u>:

Store in a refrigerator (2°C - 8°C).

Do not freeze.

Do not put Insuman Comb 15 next to the freezer compartment or a freezer pack.

Keep the pre-filled pen in the outer carton in order to protect from light.

<u>In-use pens</u>:

For storage precautions, see section 6.3.

6.5 Nature and contents of container

3 ml suspension in a cartridge (type 1 colourless glass) with a plunger (bromobutyl rubber (type 1)) and a flanged cap (aluminium) with a stopper (bromobutyl or laminate of polyisoprene and bromobutyl rubber (type 1)).

The cartridges are sealed in a disposable pen injector. Injection needles are not included in the pack.

Each cartridge contains 3 balls (stainless steel).

Packs of 5 pens are available.

6.6 Special precautions for disposal and other handling

Before first use, Insuman Comb 15 must be kept at room temperature for 1 to 2 hours and then resuspended to check the contents. This is best done by gently tilting the pen back and forth (at least ten times). Each cartridge contains three small metal balls to facilitate quick and thorough mixing of the contents. Later on, the insulin must be resuspended again prior to each injection.

After resuspension, the fluid must have a uniformly milky appearance. Insuman Comb 15 must not be used if this cannot be achieved, i.e. if the suspension remains clear, for example, or if clumps, particles or flocculation appear in the insulin or stick to the wall or bottom of the cartridge. These changes sometimes give the cartridge a frosted appearance. In such cases, a new pen yielding a uniform suspension must be used. It is also necessary to change to a new pen if the insulin requirement changes substantially.

Empty pens must never be reused and must be properly discarded.

To prevent the possible transmission of disease, each pen must be used by one patient only.

As with all insulin preparations, Insuman Comb 15 must not be mixed with solutions containing reducing agents such as thioles and sulphites. It must also be remembered that

- insulin protamine crystals dissolve in an acid pH range,
- the soluble insulin part precipitates out at a pH of approximately 4.5 to 6.5.

Mixing of insulins

Insuman Comb 15 must not be mixed with any other insulin or with insulin analogues.

Any unused product or waste material should be disposed of in accordance with local requirements.

Handling of the pen

The Instructions for Use included in the Package Leaflet must be read carefully before using OptiSet.

(see Handling of the pen above)

Important information for use of OptiSet:

• Always attach a new needle before each use. Only use needles that are compatible for use with OptiSet.

• Always perform the safety test before each injection.

• If a new OptiSet is used the initial safety test must be done with the 8 units preset by the manufacturer.

• The dosage selector can only be turned in one direction.

• Never turn the dosage selector (change the dose) after injection button has been pulled out.

• This pen is only for the patients use. It must not be shared with anyone else.

• If the injection is given by another person, special caution must be taken by this person to avoid accidental needle injury and transmission of infection.

• Never use OptiSet if it is damaged or if you are not sure that it is working properly.

• Always have a spare OptiSet in case your OptiSet is lost or damaged.

Storage Instructions

Please check section 6.4 of this leaflet for instructions on how to store OptiSet.

If OptiSet is in cool storage, it should be taken out 1 to 2 hours before injection to allow it to warm up. Cold insulin is more painful to inject.

The used OptiSet must be discarded as required by your local authorities.

Maintenance

OptiSet has to be protected from dust and dirt.

You can clean the outside of your OptiSet by wiping it with a damp cloth.

Do not soak, wash or lubricate the pen as this may damage it.

OptiSet is designed to work accurately and safely. It should be handled with care. Avoid situations where OptiSet might be damaged. If you are concerned that your OptiSet may be damaged, use a new one.

Step 1. Check and mix the Insulin

After removing the pen cap, the label on the pen and the insulin reservoir should be checked to make sure it contains the correct insulin. The insulin should be mixed by turning OptiSet slowly up and down at least 10 times.

The appearance of the insulin should be checked: the insulin suspension must have an evenly milky white appearance.

Step 2. Attach the needle

The needle should be carefully attached straight onto the pen.

Step 3. Perform a safety test

Prior to each injection a safety test has to be performed.

For a new and unused OptiSet, a dose of 8 units is already preset by the manufacturer for the first safety test.

In-use OptiSet, select a dose of 2 units by turning the dosage selector forward till the dose arrow points to 2. The dosage selector will only turn in one direction.

Pull out the injection button completely in order to load the dose. Never turn the dosage selector after injection button has been pulled out.

The outer and inner needle caps should be removed. Keep the outer cap to remove the used needle.

While holding the pen with the needle pointing upwards, the insulin reservoir should be tapped with the finger so that any air bubbles rise up towards the needle

Then the injection button should be pressed all the way in.

If insulin has been expelled through the needle tip, then the pen and the needle are working properly.

If no insulin appears at the needle tip, step 3 should be repeated two more times until insulin appears at the needle tip. If still no insulin comes out, change the needle, as it might be blocked and try again. If no insulin comes out after changing the needle, the OptiSet may be damaged. Do not use this OptiSet.

Step 4. Select the dose

The dose can be set in steps of 2 units, from a minimum of 2 units to a maximum of 40 units. If a dose greater than 40 units is required, it should be given as two or more injections.

Check if you have enough insulin for the dose.

The residual insulin scale on the transparent insulin reservoir shows approximately how much insulin remains in the OptiSet. This scale must not be used to set the insulin dose.

If the black plunger is at the beginning of the coloured bar, then there are approximately 40 units of insulin available.

If the black plunger is at the end of the coloured bar, then there are approximately 20 units of insulin available.

The dosage selector should be turned forward until the dose arrow points to the required dose.

Step 5. Load the dose

The injection button should be pulled out as far as it will go in order to load the pen.

Check if the selected dose is fully loaded. Note that the injection button only goes out as far as the amount of insulin that is left in the reservoir.

The injection button allows checking the actual loaded dose. The injection button must be held out under tension during this check. The last thick line visible on the injection button shows the amount of insulin loaded. When the injection button is held out only the top part of this thick line can be seen.

Step 6. Inject the dose

The patient should be informed on the injection technique by his health care professional.

The needle should be inserted into the skin.

The injection button should be pressed all the way in. A clicking sound can be heard, which will stop when the injection button has been pressed in completely. Then the injection button should be held down 10 seconds before withdrawing the needle from the skin. This ensures that the full dose of insulin has been delivered.

Step 7. Remove and discard the needle

The needle should be removed after each injection and discarded. This helps prevent contamination and/or infection as well as entry of air into the insulin reservoir and leakage of insulin, which can cause inaccurate dosing. Needles must not be reused.

The pen cap should be replaced on the pen.

7. MARKETING AUTHORISATION HOLDER

Sanofi-Aventis Deutschland GmbH, D-65926 Frankfurt am Main, Germany

8. MARKETING AUTHORISATION NUMBER(S)

EU/1/97/030/075

9. DATE OF FIRST AUTHORISATION/RENEWAL OF THE AUTHORISATION

Date of first authorisation: 21 February 1997

Date of latest renewal: 21 February 2007

10. DATE OF REVISION OF THE TEXT

June 2008

Legal Category: POM

Insuman Comb 25 Cartridges

(sanofi-aventis)

1. NAME OF THE MEDICINAL PRODUCT

Insuman Comb 25 100 IU/ml suspension for injection in a cartridge

2. QUALITATIVE AND QUANTITATIVE COMPOSITION

Each ml contains 100 IU insulin human (equivalent to 3.5 mg).

Each cartridge contains 3 ml of suspension for injection, equivalent to 300 IU insulin. One IU (International Unit) corresponds to 0.035 mg of anhydrous human insulin.

Insuman Comb 25 is a biphasic isophane insulin suspension consisting of 25% dissolved insulin and 75% crystalline protamine insulin.

Human insulin is produced by recombinant DNA technology in *Escherichia coli*.

For a full list of excipients, see section 6.1.

3. PHARMACEUTICAL FORM

Suspension for injection in a cartridge.

After re-suspension, milky white suspension.

4. CLINICAL PARTICULARS

4.1 Therapeutic indications

Diabetes mellitus where treatment with insulin is required.

4.2 Posology and method of administration

The desired blood glucose levels, the insulin preparations to be used and the insulin dosage (doses and timings) must be determined individually and adjusted to suit the patient's diet, physical activity and life-style.

<u>Daily doses and timing of administration</u>

There are no fixed rules for insulin dosage. However, the average insulin requirement is often 0.5 to 1.0 IU per kg body weight per day. The basal metabolic requirement is 40% to 60% of the total daily requirement. Insuman Comb 25 is injected subcutaneously 30 to 45 minutes before a meal.

<u>Transfer to Insuman Comb 25</u>

Dosage adjustment may be necessary when transferring patients from one insulin preparation to another. This applies, for example, when transferring from:

- an animal insulin (especially a bovine insulin) to human insulin,
- one human insulin preparation to another,
- a regimen with only regular insulin to one with a longer-acting insulin.

The need to adjust (e.g. reduce) the dose may become evident immediately after transfer. Alternatively, it may emerge gradually over a period of several weeks.

Following transfer from an animal insulin to human insulin, dosage reduction may be required in particular in patients who

- were previously already controlled on rather low blood glucose levels,
- have a tendency to hypoglycaemia,
- previously required high insulin doses due to the presence of insulin antibodies.

Close metabolic monitoring is recommended during the transition and in the initial weeks thereafter. In patients who require high insulin doses because of the presence of insulin antibodies, transfer under medical supervision in a hospital or similar setting must be considered.

Secondary dose adjustment

Improved metabolic control may result in increased insulin sensitivity, leading to a reduced insulin requirement. Dose adjustment may also be required, for example, if

- the patient's weight changes,
- the patient's life-style changes,
- other circumstances arise that may promote an increased susceptibility to hypo- or hyperglycaemia (see section 4.4).

Use in specific patient groups

In patients with hepatic or renal impairment as well as in the elderly, insulin requirements may be diminished (see section 4.4).

Administration

Insuman Comb 25 in cartridges has been developed for use in the OptiPen series.

Insuman Comb 25 is administered subcutaneously. Insuman Comb 25 must never be injected intravenously.

Insulin absorption and hence the blood glucose lowering effect of a dose may vary from one injection area to another (e.g. the abdominal wall compared with the thigh). Injection sites within an injection area must be rotated from one injection to the next.

For further details on handling, see section 6.6.

4.3 Contraindications

Hypersensitivity to the active substance or to any of the excipients.

Insuman Comb 25 must not be administered intravenously and must not be used in infusion pumps or external or implanted insulin pumps.

4.4 Special warnings and precautions for use

Patients hypersensitive to Insuman Comb 25 for whom no better tolerated preparation is available must only continue treatment under close medical supervision and – where necessary – in conjunction with anti-allergic treatment.

In patients with an allergy to animal insulin intradermal skin testing is recommended prior to a transfer to Insuman Comb 25, since they may experience immunological cross-reactions.

In patients with renal impairment, insulin requirements may be diminished due to reduced insulin metabolism. In the elderly, progressive deterioration of renal function may lead to a steady decrease in insulin requirements.

In patients with severe hepatic impairment, insulin requirements may be diminished due to reduced capacity for gluconeogenesis and reduced insulin metabolism.

In case of insufficient glucose control or a tendency to hyper- or hypoglycaemic episodes, the patient's adherence to the prescribed treatment regimen, injection sites and proper injection technique and all other relevant factors must be reviewed before dose adjustment is considered.

Hypoglycaemia

Hypoglycaemia may occur if the insulin dose is too high in relation to the insulin requirement.

Particular caution should be exercised, and intensified blood glucose monitoring is advisable in patients in whom hypoglycaemic episodes might be of particular clinical relevance, such as in patients with significant stenoses of the coronary arteries or of the blood vessels supplying the brain (risk of cardiac or cerebral complications of hypoglycaemia) as well as in patients with proliferative retinopathy, particularly if not treated with photocoagulation (risk of transient amaurosis following hypoglycaemia).

Patients should be aware of circumstances where warning symptoms of hypoglycaemia are diminished. The warning symptoms of hypoglycaemia may be changed, be less pronounced or be absent in certain risk groups. These include patients:

- in whom glycaemic control is markedly improved,
- in whom hypoglycaemia develops gradually,
- who are elderly,
- after transfer from animal insulin to human insulin,
- in whom an autonomic neuropathy is present,
- with a long history of diabetes,
- suffering from a psychiatric illness,
- receiving concurrent treatment with certain other medicinal products (see section 4.5).

Such situations may result in severe hypoglycaemia (and possibly loss of consciousness) prior to the patient's awareness of hypoglycaemia.

If normal or decreased values for glycated haemoglobin are noted, the possibility of recurrent, unrecognised (especially nocturnal) episodes of hypoglycaemia must be considered.

Adherence of the patient to the dosage and dietary regimen, correct insulin administration and awareness of hypoglycaemia symptoms are essential to reduce the risk of hypoglycaemia. Factors increasing the susceptibility to hypoglycaemia require particularly close monitoring and may necessitate dose adjustment. These include:

- change in the injection area,
- improved insulin sensitivity (by, e.g., removal of stress factors),
- unaccustomed, increased or prolonged physical activity,
- intercurrent illness (e.g. vomiting, diarrhoea),
- inadequate food intake,
- missed meals,
- alcohol consumption,
- certain uncompensated endocrine disorders (e.g. in hypothyroidism and in anterior pituitary or adrenocortical insufficiency),
- concomitant treatment with certain other medicinal products.

Intercurrent illness

Intercurrent illness requires intensified metabolic monitoring. In many cases, urine tests for ketones are indicated, and often it is necessary to adjust the insulin dose. The insulin requirement is often increased. Patients with type 1 diabetes must continue to consume at least a small amount of carbohydrates on a regular basis, even if they are able to eat only little or no food, or are vomiting etc. and they must never omit insulin entirely.

4.5 Interaction with other medicinal products and other forms of interaction

A number of substances affect glucose metabolism and may require dose adjustment of human insulin.

Substances that may enhance the blood-glucose-lowering effect and increase susceptibility to hypoglycaemia include oral antidiabetic agents, angiotensin converting enzyme (ACE) inhibitors, disopyramide, fibrates, fluoxetine, monoamine oxidase (MAO) inhibitors, pentoxifylline, propoxyphene, salicylates and sulphonamide antibiotics.

Substances that may reduce the blood-glucose-lowering effect include corticosteroids, danazol, diazoxide, diuretics, glucagon, isoniazid, oestrogens and progestogens (e.g. in oral contraceptives), phenothiazine derivatives, somatropin, sympathomimetic agents (e.g. epinephrine [adrenaline], salbutamol, terbutaline), thyroid hormones, protease inhibitors and atypical antipsychotic medicinal products (e.g. olanzapine and clozapine).

Beta-blockers, clonidine, lithium salts or alcohol may either potentiate or weaken the blood-glucose-lowering effect of insulin. Pentamidine may cause hypoglycaemia which may sometimes be followed by hyperglycaemia.

In addition, under the influence of sympatholytic medicinal products such as beta-blockers, clonidine, guanethidine and reserpine, the signs of adrenergic counter-regulation may be reduced or absent.

4.6 Pregnancy and lactation

Pregnancy

For insulin human, no clinical data on exposed pregnancies are available. Insulin does not cross the placental barrier. Caution should be exercised when prescribing to pregnant women.

It is essential for patients with pre-existing or gestational diabetes to maintain good metabolic control throughout pregnancy. Insulin requirements may decrease during the first trimester and generally increase during the second and third trimesters. Immediately after delivery, insulin requirements decline rapidly (increased risk of hypoglycaemia). Careful monitoring of glucose control is essential.

Lactation

No effects on the suckling child are anticipated. Insuman Comb 25 can be used during breastfeeding. Lactating women may require adjustments in insulin dose and diet.

4.7 Effects on ability to drive and use machines

The patient's ability to concentrate and react may be impaired as a result of hypoglycaemia or hyperglycaemia or, for example, as a result of visual impairment. This may constitute a risk in situations where these abilities are of special importance (e.g. driving a car or operating machinery).

Patients should be advised to take precautions to avoid hypoglycaemia whilst driving. This is particularly important in those who have reduced or absent awareness of the warning symptoms of hypoglycaemia or have frequent episodes of hypoglycaemia. It should be considered whether it is advisable to drive or operate machinery in these circumstances.

4.8 Undesirable effects

Hypoglycaemia, in general the most frequent undesirable effect of insulin therapy, may occur if the insulin dose is too high in relation to the insulin requirement. In clinical trials and during marketed use, the frequency varies with patient population and dose regimens. Therefore, no specific frequency can be presented.

Severe hypoglycaemic attacks, especially if recurrent, may lead to neurological damage. Prolonged or severe hypoglycaemic episodes may be life-threatening.

In many patients, the signs and symptoms of neuroglycopenia are preceded by signs of adrenergic counter-regulation. Generally, the greater and more rapid the decline in blood glucose, the more marked is the phenomenon of counter-regulation and its symptoms.

The following related adverse reactions from clinical investigations are listed below by system organ class and in order of decreasing incidence: very common (≥1/10); common (≥1/100, <1/10); uncommon (≥1/1,000, <1/100); rare (≥1/10,000, <1/1,000); very rare (<1/10,000), not known (cannot be estimated from the available data).

Within each frequency grouping, undesirable effects are presented in order of decreasing seriousness.

Immune system disorders

Uncommon: shock

Not known: immediate type allergic reactions (hypotension, angioneurotic oedema, bronchospasm, generalised skin reactions), anti-insulin antibodies

Immediate type allergic reactions to insulin or to the excipients may be life-threatening.

Insulin administration may cause anti-insulin antibodies to form. In rare cases, the presence of such anti-insulin antibodies may necessitate adjustment of the insulin dose in order to correct a tendency to hyper- or hypoglycaemia.

Metabolism and nutrition disorders

Common: oedema

Not known: sodium retention

Insulin may cause sodium retention and oedema, particularly if previously poor metabolic control is improved by intensified insulin therapy.

Eyes disorders

Not known: proliferative retinopathy, diabetic retinopathy, visual impairment

A marked change in glycaemic control may cause temporary visual impairment, due to temporary alteration in the turgidity and refractive index of the lens.

Long-term improved glycaemic control decreases the risk of progression of diabetic retinopathy. However, intensification of insulin therapy with abrupt improvement in glycaemic control may be associated with temporary worsening of diabetic retinopathy.

Skin and subcutaneous tissue disorders

Not known: lipodystrophy

As with any insulin therapy, lipodystrophy may occur at the injection site and delay local insulin absorption. Continuous rotation of the injection site within the given injection area may help to reduce or prevent these reactions.

General disorders and administration site conditions

Common: injection site reactions

Uncommon: injection site urticaria,

Not known: injection site inflammation, injection site swelling, injection site pain, injection site pruritus, injection site erythema.

Most minor reactions to insulins at the injection site usually resolve in a few days to a few weeks.

4.9 Overdose

Symptoms

Insulin overdose may lead to severe and sometimes long-term and life-threatening hypoglycaemia.

Management

Mild episodes of hypoglycaemia can usually be treated with oral carbohydrates. Adjustments in dosage of the medicinal product, meal patterns, or physical activity may be needed.

More severe episodes with coma, seizure, or neurologic impairment may be treated with intramuscular/subcutaneous glucagon or concentrated intravenous glucose. Sustained carbohydrate intake and observation may be necessary because hypoglycaemia may recur after apparent clinical recovery.

5. PHARMACOLOGICAL PROPERTIES

5.1 Pharmacodynamic properties

Pharmacotherapeutic group: Antidiabetic agent. Insulins and analogues, intermediate-acting combined with fast-acting, ATC Code: A10AD01.

Mode of action

Insulin

- lowers blood glucose and promotes anabolic effects as well as decreasing catabolic effects,
- increases the transport of glucose into cells as well as the formation of glycogen in the muscles and the liver, and improves pyruvate utilisation. It inhibits glycogenolysis and gluconeogenesis,
- increases lipogenesis in the liver and adipose tissue and inhibits lipolysis,
- promotes the uptake of amino acids into cells and promotes protein synthesis,
- enhances the uptake of potassium into cells.

Pharmacodynamic characteristics

Insuman Comb 25 (a biphasic isophane insulin suspension with 25% dissolved insulin) is an insulin with gradual onset and long duration of action. Following subcutaneous injection, onset of action is within 30 to 60 minutes, the phase of maximum action is between 2 and 4 hours after injection and the duration of action is 12 to 19 hours.

5.2 Pharmacokinetic properties

In healthy subjects, the serum half-life of insulin is approximately 4 to 6 minutes. It is longer in patients with severe renal insufficiency. However, it must be noted that the pharmacokinetics of insulin do not reflect its metabolic action.

5.3 Preclinical safety data

The acute toxicity was studied following subcutaneous administration in rats. No evidence of toxic effects was found. Studies of pharmacodynamic effects following subcutaneous administration in rabbits and dogs revealed the expected hypoglycaemic reactions.

6. PHARMACEUTICAL PARTICULARS

6.1 List of excipients

Protamine sulphate,

metacresol,

phenol,

zinc chloride,

sodium dihydrogen phosphate dihydrate,

glycerol,

sodium hydroxide,

hydrochloric acid (for pH adjustment),

water for injections.

6.2 Incompatibilities

This medicinal product must not be mixed with other medicinal products except those mentioned in section 6.6.

Concerning mixing or incompatibility with other insulins see section 6.6. Care must be taken to ensure that no alcohol or other disinfectants enter the insulin suspension.

6.3 Shelf life

2 years.

Shelf life after first use of the cartridge:

The cartridge in-use (in the insulin pen) or carried as a spare may be stored for a maximum of 4 weeks not above 25°C away from direct heat or direct light.

The pen containing a cartridge must not be stored in the refrigerator.

The pen cap must be put back on the pen after each injection in order to protect from light.

6.4 Special precautions for storage

Unopened cartridges:

Store in a refrigerator (2°C - 8°C).

Do not freeze.

Do not put Insuman Comb 25 next to the freezer compartment or a freezer pack.

Keep the cartridge in the outer carton in order to protect from light.

In-use cartridges:

For storage precautions, see section 6.3.

6.5 Nature and contents of container

3 ml suspension in a cartridge (type 1 colourless glass) with a plunger (bromobutyl rubber (type 1)) and a flanged cap (aluminium) with a stopper (bromobutyl or laminate of polyisoprene and bromobutyl rubber (type 1)).

Each cartridge contains 3 balls (stainless steel).

Packs of 5 cartridges are available.

6.6 Special precautions for disposal and other handling

Insulin pen

The cartridges are to be used in conjunction with an insulin pen such as OptiPen and other pens suitable for Insuman cartridges and as recommended in the information provided by the device manufacturer.

The manufacturer's instructions for using the pen must be followed carefully for loading the cartridge, attaching the injection needle, and administering the insulin injection.

If the insulin pen is damaged or not working properly (due to mechanical defects) it has to be discarded, and a new insulin pen has to be used.

If the pen malfunctions (see instructions for using the pen), the suspension may be drawn from the cartridge into an injection syringe (suitable for an insulin with 100 IU/ml) and injected.

Cartridges

Before insertion into the pen, Insuman Comb 25 must be kept at room temperature for 1 to 2 hours and then resuspended to check the contents. This is best done by gently tilting the cartridge back and forth (at least ten times). Each cartridge contains three small metal balls to facilitate quick and thorough mixing of the contents.

Later on, when the cartridge has been inserted into the pen, the insulin must be resuspended again prior to each injection. This is best done by gently tilting the pen back and forth (at least ten times).

After resuspension, the fluid must have a uniformly milky appearance. Insuman Comb 25 must not be used if this cannot be achieved, i.e. if the suspension remains clear, for example, or if clumps, particles or flocculation appear in the insulin or stick to the wall or bottom of the cartridge. These changes sometimes give the cartridge a frosted appearance. In such cases, a new cartridge yielding a uniform suspension must be used. It is also necessary to change to a new cartridge if the insulin requirement changes substantially.

Air bubbles must be removed from the cartridge before injection (see instructions for using the pen). Empty cartridges must not be refilled.

As with all insulin preparations, Insuman Comb 25 must not be mixed with solutions containing reducing agents such as thioles and sulphites. It must also be remembered that

- insulin protamine crystals dissolve in an acid pH range,

- the soluble insulin part precipitates out at a pH of approximately 4.5 to 6.5.

Mixing of insulins

Insuman Comb 25 may be mixed with all Sanofi-Aventis human insulins, but NOT with those designed specifically for use in insulin pumps. Insuman Comb 25 must also NOT be mixed with insulins of animal origin or with insulin analogues.

Insuman Comb 25 cartridges are not designed to allow any other insulin to be mixed in the cartridge.

Any unused product or waste material should be disposed of in accordance with local requirements.

7. MARKETING AUTHORISATION HOLDER

Sanofi-Aventis Deutschland GmbH, D-65926 Frankfurt am Main, Germany

8. MARKETING AUTHORISATION NUMBER(S)

EU/1/97/030/045

9. DATE OF FIRST AUTHORISATION/RENEWAL OF THE AUTHORISATION

Date of first authorisation: 21 February 1997

Date of latest renewal: 21 February 2007

10. DATE OF REVISION OF THE TEXT

June 2008

Legal Category

POM

Insuman Comb 25 Optiset

(sanofi-aventis)

1. NAME OF THE MEDICINAL PRODUCT

Insuman Comb 25 100 IU/ml suspension for injection in a pre-filled pen.

2. QUALITATIVE AND QUANTITATIVE COMPOSITION

Each ml contains 100 IU insulin human (equivalent to 3.5 mg).

Each pen contains 3 ml of suspension for injection, equivalent to 300 IU insulin. One IU (International Unit) corresponds to 0.035 mg of anhydrous human insulin.

Insuman Comb 25 is a biphasic isophane insulin suspension consisting of 25% dissolved insulin and 75% crystalline protamine insulin.

Human insulin is produced by recombinant DNA technology in *Escherichia coli*.

For a full list of excipients, see section 6.1.

3. PHARMACEUTICAL FORM

Suspension for injection in a pre-filled pen. OptiSet.

After re-suspension, milky white suspension.

4. CLINICAL PARTICULARS

4.1 Therapeutic indications

Diabetes mellitus where treatment with insulin is required.

4.2 Posology and method of administration

The desired blood glucose levels, the insulin preparations to be used and the insulin dosage (doses and timings) must be determined individually and adjusted to suit the patient's diet, physical activity and life-style.

Daily doses and timing of administration

There are no fixed rules for insulin dosage. However, the average insulin requirement is often 0.5 to 1.0 IU per kg body weight per day. The basal metabolic requirement is 40% to 60% of the total daily requirement. Insuman Comb 25 is injected subcutaneously 30 to 45 minutes before a meal.

OptiSet delivers insulin in increments of 2 IU up to a maximum single dose of 40 IU.

Transfer to Insuman Comb 25

Dosage adjustment may be necessary when transferring patients from one insulin preparation to another. This applies, for example, when transferring from:

- an animal insulin (especially a bovine insulin) to human insulin,

- one human insulin preparation to another,

- a regimen with only regular insulin to one with a longer-acting insulin.

The need to adjust (e.g. reduce) the dose may become evident immediately after transfer. Alternatively, it may emerge gradually over a period of several weeks.

Following transfer from an animal insulin to human insulin, dosage reduction may be required in particular in patients who

- were previously already controlled on rather low blood glucose levels,

- have a tendency to hypoglycaemia,

- previously required high insulin doses due to the presence of insulin antibodies.

Close metabolic monitoring is recommended during the transition and in the initial weeks thereafter. In patients who require high insulin doses because of the presence of insulin antibodies, transfer under medical supervision in a hospital or similar setting must be considered.

Secondary dose adjustment

Improved metabolic control may result in increased insulin sensitivity, leading to a reduced insulin requirement. Dose adjustment may also be required, for example, if

- the patient's weight changes,

- the patient's life-style changes,

- other circumstances arise that may promote an increased susceptibility to hypo- or hyperglycaemia (see section 4.4).

Use in specific patient groups

In patients with hepatic or renal impairment as well as in the elderly, insulin requirements may be diminished (see section 4.4).

Administration

Insuman Comb 25 is administered subcutaneously. Insuman Comb 25 must never be injected intravenously.

Insulin absorption and hence the blood glucose lowering effect of a dose may vary from one injection area to another (e.g. the abdominal wall compared with the thigh). Injection sites within an injection area must be rotated from one injection to the next.

Before using OptiSet, the Instructions for Use included in the Package Leaflet must be read carefully.

For further details on handling, see section 6.6.

4.3 Contraindications

Hypersensitivity to the active substance or to any of the excipients.

4.4 Special warnings and precautions for use

Patients hypersensitive to Insuman Comb 25 for whom no better tolerated preparation is available must only continue treatment under close medical supervision and – where necessary – in conjunction with anti-allergic treatment.

In patients with an allergy to animal insulin intradermal skin testing is recommended prior to a transfer to Insuman Comb 25, since they may experience immunological cross-reactions.

In patients with renal impairment, insulin requirements may be diminished due to reduced insulin metabolism. In the elderly, progressive deterioration of renal function may lead to a steady decrease in insulin requirements.

In patients with severe hepatic impairment, insulin requirements may be diminished due to reduced capacity for gluconeogenesis and reduced insulin metabolism.

In case of insufficient glucose control or a tendency to hyper- or hypoglycaemic episodes, the patient's adherence to the prescribed treatment regimen, injection sites and proper injection technique and all other relevant factors must be reviewed before dose adjustment is considered.

Hypoglycaemia

Hypoglycaemia may occur if the insulin dose is too high in relation to the insulin requirement.

Particular caution should be exercised, and intensified blood glucose monitoring is advisable in patients in whom hypoglycaemic episodes might be of particular clinical relevance, such as in patients with significant stenoses of the coronary arteries or of the blood vessels supplying the brain (risk of cardiac or cerebral complications of hypoglycaemia) as well as in patients with proliferative retinopathy, particularly if not treated with photocoagulation (risk of transient amaurosis following hypoglycaemia).

Patients should be aware of circumstances where warning symptoms of hypoglycaemia are diminished. The warning symptoms of hypoglycaemia may be changed, be less pronounced or be absent in certain risk groups. These include patients:

- in whom glycaemic control is markedly improved,

- in whom hypoglycaemia develops gradually,

- who are elderly,

- after transfer from animal insulin to human insulin,

- in whom an autonomic neuropathy is present,

- with a long history of diabetes,

- suffering from a psychiatric illness,

- receiving concurrent treatment with certain other medicinal products (see section 4.5).

Such situations may result in severe hypoglycaemia (and possibly loss of consciousness) prior to the patient's awareness of hypoglycaemia.

If normal or decreased values for glycated haemoglobin are noted, the possibility of recurrent, unrecognised (especially nocturnal) episodes of hypoglycaemia must be considered.

Adherence of the patient to the dosage and dietary regimen, correct insulin administration and awareness of hypoglycaemia symptoms are essential to reduce the risk of hypoglycaemia. Factors increasing the susceptibility to hypoglycaemia require particularly close monitoring and may necessitate dose adjustment. These include:

- change in the injection area,

- improved insulin sensitivity (by, e.g., removal of stress factors),

- unaccustomed, increased or prolonged physical activity,

- intercurrent illness (e.g. vomiting, diarrhoea),

- inadequate food intake,
- missed meals,
- alcohol consumption,
- certain uncompensated endocrine disorders (e.g. in hypothyroidism and in anterior pituitary or adrenocortical insufficiency),
- concomitant treatment with certain other medicinal products.

Intercurrent illness

Intercurrent illness requires intensified metabolic monitoring. In many cases, urine tests for ketones are indicated, and often it is necessary to adjust the insulin dose. The insulin requirement is often increased. Patients with type 1 diabetes must continue to consume at least a small amount of carbohydrates on a regular basis, even if they are able to eat only little or no food, or are vomiting etc. and they must never omit insulin entirely.

Handling of the pen

Before using OptiSet, the Instructions for Use included in the Package Leaflet must be read carefully. OptiSet has to be used as recommended in these Instructions for Use (see section 6.6).

4.5 Interaction with other medicinal products and other forms of interaction

A number of substances affect glucose metabolism and may require dose adjustment of human insulin.

Substances that may enhance the blood-glucose-lowering effect and increase susceptibility to hypoglycaemia include oral antidiabetic agents, angiotensin converting enzyme (ACE) inhibitors, disopyramide, fibrates, fluoxetine, monoamine oxidase (MAO) inhibitors, pentoxifylline, propoxyphene, salicylates and sulphonamide antibiotics.

Substances that may reduce the blood-glucose-lowering effect include corticosteroids, danazol, diazoxide, diuretics, glucagon, isoniazid, oestrogens and progestogens (e.g. in oral contraceptives), phenothiazine derivatives, somatropin, sympathomimetic agents (e.g. epinephrine [adrenaline], salbutamol, terbutaline), thyroid hormones, protease inhibitors and atypical antipsychotic medicinal products (e.g. olanzapine and clozapine).

Beta-blockers, clonidine, lithium salts or alcohol may either potentiate or weaken the blood-glucose-lowering effect of insulin. Pentamidine may cause hypoglycaemia which may sometimes be followed by hyperglycaemia.

In addition, under the influence of sympatholytic medicinal products such as beta-blockers, clonidine, guanethidine and reserpine, the signs of adrenergic counter-regulation may be reduced or absent.

4.6 Pregnancy and lactation

Pregnancy

For insulin human, no clinical data on exposed pregnancies are available. Insulin does not cross the placental barrier. Caution should be exercised when prescribing to pregnant women.

It is essential for patients with pre-existing or gestational diabetes to maintain good metabolic control throughout pregnancy. Insulin requirements may decrease during the first trimester and generally increase during the second and third trimesters. Immediately after delivery, insulin requirements decline rapidly (increased risk of hypoglycaemia). Careful monitoring of glucose control is essential.

Lactation

No effects on the suckling child are anticipated. Insuman Comb 25 can be used during breastfeeding. Lactating women may require adjustments in insulin dose and diet.

4.7 Effects on ability to drive and use machines

The patient's ability to concentrate and react may be impaired as a result of hypoglycaemia or hyperglycaemia or, for example, as a result of visual impairment. This may constitute a risk in situations where these abilities are of special importance (e.g. driving a car or operating machinery).

Patients should be advised to take precautions to avoid hypoglycaemia whilst driving. This is particularly important in those who have reduced or absent awareness of the warning symptoms of hypoglycaemia or have frequent episodes of hypoglycaemia. It should be considered whether it is advisable to drive or operate machinery in these circumstances.

4.8 Undesirable effects

Hypoglycaemia, in general the most frequent undesirable effect of insulin therapy, may occur if the insulin dose is too high in relation to the insulin requirement. In clinical trials and during marketed use, the frequency varies with patient population and dose regimens. Therefore, no specific frequency can be presented.

Severe hypoglycaemic attacks, especially if recurrent, may lead to neurological damage. Prolonged or severe hypoglycaemic episodes may be life-threatening.

In many patients, the signs and symptoms of neuroglycopenia are preceded by signs of adrenergic counter-regulation. Generally, the greater and more rapid the decline in blood glucose, the more marked is the phenomenon of counter-regulation and its symptoms.

The following related adverse reactions from clinical investigations are listed below by system organ class and in order of decreasing incidence: very common (≥1/10); common (≥1/100, <1/10); uncommon (≥1/1,000, <1/100); rare (≥1/10,000, <1/1,000); very rare (<1/10,000), not known (cannot be estimated from the available data).

Within each frequency grouping, undesirable effects are presented in order of decreasing seriousness.

Immune system disorders

Uncommon: shock

Not known: immediate type allergic reactions (hypotension, angioneurotic oedema, bronchospasm, generalised skin reactions), anti-insulin antibodies

Immediate type allergic reactions to insulin or to the excipients may be life-threatening.

Insulin administration may cause anti-insulin antibodies to form. In rare cases, the presence of such anti-insulin antibodies may necessitate adjustment of the insulin dose in order to correct a tendency to hyper- or hypoglycaemia.

Metabolism and nutrition disorders

Common: oedema

Not known: sodium retention

Insulin may cause sodium retention and oedema, particularly if previously poor metabolic control is improved by intensified insulin therapy.

Eyes disorders

Not known: proliferative retinopathy, diabetic retinopathy, visual impairment

A marked change in glycaemic control may cause temporary visual impairment, due to temporary alteration in the turgidity and refractive index of the lens.

Long-term improved glycaemic control decreases the risk of progression of diabetic retinopathy. However, intensification of insulin therapy with abrupt improvement in glycaemic control may be associated with temporary worsening of diabetic retinopathy.

Skin and subcutaneous tissue disorders

Not known: lipodystrophy

As with any insulin therapy, lipodystrophy may occur at the injection site and delay local insulin absorption. Continuous rotation of the injection site within the given injection area may help to reduce or prevent these reactions.

General disorders and administration site conditions

Common: injection site reactions

Uncommon: injection site urticaria,

Not known: injection site inflammation, injection site swelling, injection site pain, injection site pruritus, injection site erythema.

Most minor reactions to insulins at the injection site usually resolve in a few days to a few weeks.

4.9 Overdose

Symptoms

Insulin overdose may lead to severe and sometimes long-term and life-threatening hypoglycaemia.

Management

Mild episodes of hypoglycaemia can usually be treated with oral carbohydrates. Adjustments in dosage of the medicinal product, meal patterns, or physical activity may be needed.

More severe episodes with coma, seizure, or neurologic impairment may be treated with intramuscular/subcutaneous glucagon or concentrated intravenous glucose. Sustained carbohydrate intake and observation may be necessary because hypoglycaemia may recur after apparent clinical recovery.

5. PHARMACOLOGICAL PROPERTIES

5.1 Pharmacodynamic properties

Pharmacotherapeutic group: Antidiabetic agent. Insulins and analogues, intermediate-acting combined with fast-acting, ATC Code: A10AD01.

Mode of action

Insulin

- lowers blood glucose and promotes anabolic effects as well as decreasing catabolic effects,
- increases the transport of glucose into cells as well as the formation of glycogen in the muscles and the liver, and improves pyruvate utilisation. It inhibits glycogenolysis and gluconeogenesis,
- increases lipogenesis in the liver and adipose tissue and inhibits lipolysis,
- promotes the uptake of amino acids into cells and promotes protein synthesis,
- enhances the uptake of potassium into cells.

Pharmacodynamic characteristics

Insuman Comb 25 (a biphasic isophane insulin suspension with 25% dissolved insulin) is an insulin with gradual onset and long duration of action. Following subcutaneous injection, onset of action is within 30 to 60 minutes, the phase of maximum action is between 2 and 4 hours after injection and the duration of action is 12 to 19 hours.

5.2 Pharmacokinetic properties

In healthy subjects, the serum half-life of insulin is approximately 4 to 6 minutes. It is longer in patients with severe renal insufficiency. However, it must be noted that the pharmacokinetics of insulin do not reflect its metabolic action.

5.3 Preclinical safety data

The acute toxicity was studied following subcutaneous administration in rats. No evidence of toxic effects was found. Studies of pharmacodynamic effects following subcutaneous administration in rabbits and dogs revealed the expected hypoglycaemic reactions.

6. PHARMACEUTICAL PARTICULARS

6.1 List of excipients

Protamine sulphate,

metacresol,

phenol,

zinc chloride,

sodium dihydrogen phosphate dihydrate,

glycerol,

sodium hydroxide,

hydrochloric acid (for pH adjustment),

water for injections.

6.2 Incompatibilities

This medicinal product must not be mixed with other medicinal products except those mentioned in section 6.6.

Concerning mixing or incompatibility with other insulins see section 6.6. Care must be taken to ensure that no alcohol or other disinfectants enter the insulin suspension.

6.3 Shelf life

2 years.

Shelf life after first use of the pen:

The pen in-use or carried as a spare may be stored for a maximum of 4 weeks not above 25°C away from direct heat or direct ligh.

Pens in-use must not be stored in the refrigerator.

The pen cap must be put back on the pen after each injection in order to protect from light.

6.4 Special precautions for storage

Not in-use pens:

Store in a refrigerator (2°C - 8°C).

Do not freeze.

Do not put Insuman Comb 25 next to the freezer compartment or a freezer pack.

Keep the pre-filled pen in the outer carton in order to protect from light.

In-use pens:

For storage precautions, see section 6.3.

6.5 Nature and contents of container

3 mlsuspension in a cartridge (type 1 colourless glass) with a plunger (bromobutyl rubber (type 1)) and a flanged cap (aluminium) with a stopper (bromobutyl or laminate of polyisoprene and bromobutyl rubber (type 1)).

Each cartridge contains 3 balls (stainless steel). The cartridges are sealed in a disposable pen injector. Injection needles are not included in the pack.

Packs of 5 pens are available.

6.6 Special precautions for disposal and other handling

Before first use, Insuman Comb 25 must be kept at room temperature for 1 to 2 hours and then resuspended to check the contents. This is best done by gently tilting the pen back and forth (at least ten times). Each cartridge contains three small metal balls to facilitate quick and thorough mixing of the contents. Later on, the insulin must be resuspended again prior to each injection.

After resuspension, the fluid must have a uniformly milky appearance. Insuman Comb 25 must not be used if this cannot be achieved, i.e. if the suspension remains clear, for example, or if clumps, particles or flocculation appear in the insulin or stick to the wall or bottom of the cartridge. These changes sometimes give the cartridge a frosted appearance. In such cases, a new pen yielding a uniform suspension must be used. It is also necessary to change to a new pen if the insulin requirement changes substantially.

Empty pens must never be reused and must be properly discarded.

To prevent the possible transmission of disease, each pen must be used by one patient only.

As with all insulin preparations, Insuman Comb 25 must not be mixed with solutions containing reducing agents such as thioles and sulphites. It must also be remembered that
- insulin protamine crystals dissolve in an acid pH range,
- the soluble insulin part precipitates out at a pH of approximately 4.5 to 6.5.

Mixing of insulins

Insuman Comb 25 must not be mixed with any other insulin or with insulin analogues.

Any unused product or waste material should be disposed of in accordance with local requirements.

Handling of the pen

The Instructions for Use included in the Package Leaflet must be read carefully before using OptiSet.

(see Handling of the pen on next page)

Handling of the pen

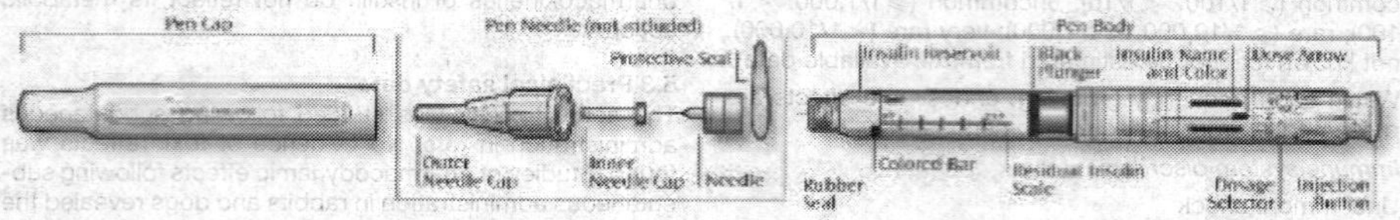

Schematic diagram of the pen

Important information for use of OptiSet:

• Always attach a new needle before each use. Only use needles that are compatible for use with OptiSet.

• Always perform the safety test before each injection.

• If a new OptiSet is used the initial safety test must be done with the 8 units preset by the manufacturer.

• The dosage selector can only be turned in one direction.

• Never turn the dosage selector (change the dose) after injection button has been pulled out.

• This pen is only for the patients use. It must not be shared with anyone else.

• If the injection is given by another person, special caution must be taken by this person to avoid accidental needle injury and transmission of infection.

• Never use OptiSet if it is damaged or if you are not sure that it is working properly.

• Always have a spare OptiSet in case your OptiSet is lost or damaged.

Storage Instructions

Please check section 6.4 of this leaflet for instructions on how to store OptiSet.

If OptiSet is in cool storage, it should be taken out 1 to 2 hours before injection to allow it to warm up. Cold insulin is more painful to inject.

The used OptiSet must be discarded as required by your local authorities.

Maintenance

OptiSet has to be protected from dust and dirt.

You can clean the outside of your OptiSet by wiping it with a damp cloth.

Do not soak, wash or lubricate the pen as this may damage it.

OptiSet is designed to work accurately and safely. It should be handled with care. Avoid situations where OptiSet might be damaged. If you are concerned that your OptiSet may be damaged, use a new one.

Step 1. Check and mix the Insulin

After removing the pen cap, the label on the pen and the insulin reservoir should be checked to make sure it contains the correct insulin. The insulin should be mixed by turning OptiSet slowly up and down at least 10 times.

The appearance of the insulin should be checked: the insulin suspension must have an evenly milky white appearance.

Step 2. Attach the needle

The needle should be carefully attached straight onto the pen.

Step 3. Perform a safety test

Prior to each injection a safety test has to be performed.

For a new and unused OptiSet, a dose of 8 units is already preset by the manufacturer for the first safety test.

In-use OptiSet, select a dose of 2 units by turning the dosage selector forward till the dose arrow points to 2. The dosage selector will only turn in one direction.

Pull out the injection button completely in order to load the dose. Never turn the dosage selector after injection button has been pulled out.

The outer and inner needle caps should be removed. Keep the outer cap to remove the used needle.

While holding the pen with the needle pointing upwards, the insulin reservoir should be tapped with the finger so that any air bubbles rise up towards the needle

Then the injection button should be pressed all the way in.

If insulin has been expelled through the needle tip, then the pen and the needle are working properly.

If no insulin appears at the needle tip, step 3 should be repeated until insulin appears at the needle tip. If still no insulin comes out, change the needle, as it might be blocked and try again. If no insulin comes out after changing the needle, the OptiSet may be damaged. Do not use this OptiSet.

Step 4. Select the dose

The dose can be set in steps of 2 units, from a minimum of 2 units to a maximum of 40 units. If a dose greater than 40 units is required, it should be given as two or more injections.

Check if you have enough insulin for the dose.

The residual insulin scale on the transparent insulin reservoir shows approximately how much insulin remains in the OptiSet. This scale must not be used to set the insulin dose.

If the black plunger is at the beginning of the coloured bar, then there are approximately 40 units of insulin available.

If the black plunger is at the end of the coloured bar, then there are approximately 20 units of insulin available.

The dosage selector should be turned forward until the dose arrow points to the required dose.

Step 5. Load the dose

The injection button should be pulled out as far as it will go in order to load the pen.

Check if the selected dose is fully loaded. Note that the injection button only goes out as far as the amount of insulin that is left in the reservoir.

The injection button allows checking the actual loaded dose. The injection button must be held out under tension during this check. The last thick line visible on the injection button shows the amount of insulin loaded. When the injection button is held out only the top part of this thick line can be seen.

Step 6. Inject the dose

The patient should be informed on the injection technique by his health care professional.

The needle should be inserted into the skin.

The injection button should be pressed all the way in. A clicking sound can be heard, which will stop when the injection button has been pressed in completely. Then the injection button should be held down 10 seconds before withdrawing the needle from the skin. This ensures that the full dose of insulin has been delivered.

Step 7. Remove and discard the needle

The needle should be removed after each injection and discarded. This helps prevent contamination and/or infection as well as entry of air into the insulin reservoir and leakage of insulin, which can cause inaccurate dosing. Needles must not be reused.

The pen cap should be replaced on the pen.

7. MARKETING AUTHORISATION HOLDER

Sanofi-Aventis Deutschland GmbH, D-65926 Frankfurt am Main, Germany

8. MARKETING AUTHORISATION NUMBER(S)

EU/1/97/030/079

9. DATE OF FIRST AUTHORISATION/RENEWAL OF THE AUTHORISATION

Date of first authorisation: 21 February 1997

Date of latest renewal: 21 February 2007

10. DATE OF REVISION OF THE TEXT

June 2008

Legal Category: POM

Insuman Comb 25 Vials

(sanofi-aventis)

1. NAME OF THE MEDICINAL PRODUCT

Insuman Comb 25 100 IU/ml suspension for injection in a vial

2. QUALITATIVE AND QUANTITATIVE COMPOSITION

Each ml contains 100 IU insulin human (equivalent to 3.5 mg).

Each vial contains 5 ml of suspension for injection, equivalent to 500 IU insulin. One IU (International Unit) corresponds to 0.035 mg of anhydrous human insulin.

Insuman Comb 25 is a biphasic isophane insulin suspension consisting of 25% dissolved insulin and 75% crystalline protamine insulin.

Human insulin is produced by recombinant DNA technology in *Escherichia coli*.

For a full list of excipients, see section 6.1.

3. PHARMACEUTICAL FORM

Suspension for injection in a vial.

After re-suspension, milky white suspension.

4. CLINICAL PARTICULARS

4.1 Therapeutic indications

Diabetes mellitus where treatment with insulin is required.

4.2 Posology and method of administration

The desired blood glucose levels, the insulin preparations to be used and the insulin dosage (doses and timings) must be determined individually and adjusted to suit the patient's diet, physical activity and life-style.

Daily doses and timing of administration

There are no fixed rules for insulin dosage. However, the average insulin requirement is often 0.5 to 1.0 IU per kg body weight per day. The basal metabolic requirement is 40% to 60% of the total daily requirement. Insuman Comb 25 is injected subcutaneously 30 to 45 minutes before a meal.

Transfer to Insuman Comb 25

Dosage adjustment may be necessary when transferring patients from one insulin preparation to another. This applies, for example, when transferring from:

- an animal insulin (especially a bovine insulin) to human insulin,

- one human insulin preparation to another,

- a regimen with only regular insulin to one with a longer-acting insulin.

The need to adjust (e.g. reduce) the dose may become evident immediately after transfer. Alternatively, it may emerge gradually over a period of several weeks.

Following transfer from an animal insulin to human insulin, dosage reduction may be required in particular in patients who

- were previously already controlled on rather low blood glucose levels,

- have a tendency to hypoglycaemia,

- previously required high insulin doses due to the presence of insulin antibodies.

Close metabolic monitoring is recommended during the transition and in the initial weeks thereafter. In patients who require high insulin doses because of the presence of insulin antibodies, transfer under medical supervision in a hospital or similar setting must be considered.

Secondary dose adjustment

Improved metabolic control may result in increased insulin sensitivity, leading to a reduced insulin requirement. Dose adjustment may also be required, for example, if

- the patient's weight changes,

- the patient's life-style changes,

- other circumstances arise that may promote an increased susceptibility to hypo- or hyperglycaemia (see section 4.4).

Use in specific patient groups

In patients with hepatic or renal impairment as well as in the elderly, insulin requirements may be diminished (see section 4.4).

Administration

Insuman Comb 25 contains 100 IU of insulin per ml suspension. Only injection syringes designed for this strength of insulin (100 IU per ml) are to be used. The injection syringes must not contain any other medicinal product or residue (e.g. traces of heparin).

Insuman Comb 25 is administered subcutaneously. Insuman Comb 25 must never be injected intravenously.

Insulin absorption and hence the blood glucose lowering effect of a dose may vary from one injection area to another (e.g. the abdominal wall compared with the thigh). Injection sites within an injection area must be rotated from one injection to the next.

For further details on handling, see section 6.6.

4.3 Contraindications

Hypersensitivity to the active substance or to any of the excipients.

Insuman Comb 25 must not be administered intravenously and must not be used in infusion pumps or external or implanted insulin pumps.

4.4 Special warnings and precautions for use

Patients hypersensitive to Insuman Comb 25 for whom no better tolerated preparation is available must only continue treatment under close medical supervision and – where necessary – in conjunction with anti-allergic treatment.

In patients with an allergy to animal insulin intradermal skin testing is recommended prior to a transfer to Insuman Comb 25, since they may experience immunological cross-reactions.

In patients with renal impairment, insulin requirements may be diminished due to reduced insulin metabolism. In the elderly, progressive deterioration of renal function may lead to a steady decrease in insulin requirements.

In patients with severe hepatic impairment, insulin requirements may be diminished due to reduced capacity for gluconeogenesis and reduced insulin metabolism.

In case of insufficient glucose control or a tendency to hyper- or hypoglycaemic episodes, the patient's adherence to the prescribed treatment regimen, injection sites and proper injection technique and all other relevant factors must be reviewed before dose adjustment is considered.

Hypoglycaemia

Hypoglycaemia may occur if the insulin dose is too high in relation to the insulin requirement.

Particular caution should be exercised, and intensified blood glucose monitoring is advisable in patients in whom hypoglycaemic episodes might be of particular clinical relevance, such as in patients with significant stenoses of the coronary arteries or of the blood vessels supplying the brain (risk of cardiac or cerebral complications of hypoglycaemia) as well as in patients with proliferative retinopathy, particularly if not treated with photocoagulation (risk of transient amaurosis following hypoglycaemia).

Patients should be aware of circumstances where warning symptoms of hypoglycaemia are diminished. The warning symptoms of hypoglycaemia may be changed, be less pronounced or be absent in certain risk groups. These include patients:

- in whom glycaemic control is markedly improved,
- in whom hypoglycaemia develops gradually,
- who are elderly,
- after transfer from animal insulin to human insulin,
- in whom an autonomic neuropathy is present,
- with a long history of diabetes,
- suffering from a psychiatric illness,
- receiving concurrent treatment with certain other medicinal products (see section 4.5).

Such situations may result in severe hypoglycaemia (and possibly loss of consciousness) prior to the patient's awareness of hypoglycaemia.

If normal or decreased values for glycated haemoglobin are noted, the possibility of recurrent, unrecognised (especially nocturnal) episodes of hypoglycaemia must be considered.

Adherence of the patient to the dosage and dietary regimen, correct insulin administration and awareness of hypoglycaemia symptoms are essential to reduce the risk of hypoglycaemia. Factors increasing the susceptibility to hypoglycaemia require particularly close monitoring and may necessitate dose adjustment. These include:

- change in the injection area,
- improved insulin sensitivity (by, e.g., removal of stress factors),
- unaccustomed, increased or prolonged physical activity,
- intercurrent illness (e.g. vomiting, diarrhoea),
- inadequate food intake,
- missed meals,
- alcohol consumption,
- certain uncompensated endocrine disorders (e.g. in hypothyroidism and in anterior pituitary or adrenocortical insufficiency),
- concomitant treatment with certain other medicinal products.

Intercurrent illness

Intercurrent illness requires intensified metabolic monitoring. In many cases, urine tests for ketones are indicated, and often it is necessary to adjust the insulin dose. The insulin requirement is often increased. Patients with type 1 diabetes must continue to consume at least a small amount of carbohydrates on a regular basis, even if they are able to eat only little or no food, or are vomiting etc. and they must never omit insulin entirely.

4.5 Interaction with other medicinal products and other forms of interaction

A number of substances affect glucose metabolism and may require dose adjustment of human insulin.

Substances that may enhance the blood-glucose-lowering effect and increase susceptibility to hypoglycaemia include oral antidiabetic agents, angiotensin converting enzyme (ACE) inhibitors, disopyramide, fibrates, fluoxetine, monoamine oxidase (MAO) inhibitors, pentoxifylline, propoxyphene, salicylates and sulphonamide antibiotics.

Substances that may reduce the blood-glucose-lowering effect include corticosteroids, danazol, diazoxide, diuretics, glucagon, isoniazid, oestrogens and progestogens (e.g. in oral contraceptives), phenothiazine derivatives, somatropin, sympathomimetic agents (e.g. epinephrine [adrenaline], salbutamol, terbutaline), thyroid hormones, protease inhibitors and atypical antipsychotic medicinal products (e.g. olanzapine and clozapine).

Beta-blockers, clonidine, lithium salts or alcohol may either potentiate or weaken the blood-glucose-lowering effect of insulin. Pentamidine may cause hypoglycaemia which may sometimes be followed by hyperglycaemia.

In addition, under the influence of sympatholytic medicinal products such as beta-blockers, clonidine, guanethidine and reserpine, the signs of adrenergic counter-regulation may be reduced or absent.

4.6 Pregnancy and lactation

Pregnancy

For insulin human, no clinical data on exposed pregnancies are available. Insulin does not cross the placental barrier. Caution should be exercised when prescribing to pregnant women.

It is essential for patients with pre-existing or gestational diabetes to maintain good metabolic control throughout pregnancy. Insulin requirements may decrease during the first trimester and generally increase during the second and third trimesters. Immediately after delivery, insulin requirements decline rapidly (increased risk of hypoglycaemia). Careful monitoring of glucose control is essential.

Lactation

No effects on the suckling child are anticipated. Insuman Comb 25 can be used during breastfeeding. Lactating women may require adjustments in insulin dose and diet.

4.7 Effects on ability to drive and use machines

The patient's ability to concentrate and react may be impaired as a result of hypoglycaemia or hyperglycaemia or, for example, as a result of visual impairment. This may constitute a risk in situations where these abilities are of special importance (e.g. driving a car or operating machinery).

Patients should be advised to take precautions to avoid hypoglycaemia whilst driving. This is particularly important in those who have reduced or absent awareness of the warning symptoms of hypoglycaemia or have frequent episodes of hypoglycaemia. It should be considered whether it is advisable to drive or operate machinery in these circumstances.

4.8 Undesirable effects

Hypoglycaemia, in general the most frequent undesirable effect of insulin therapy, may occur if the insulin dose is too high in relation to the insulin requirement. In clinical trials and during marketed use, the frequency varies with patient population and dose regimens. Therefore, no specific frequency can be presented.

Severe hypoglycaemic attacks, especially if recurrent, may lead to neurological damage. Prolonged or severe hypoglycaemic episodes may be life-threatening.

In many patients, the signs and symptoms of neuroglycopenia are preceded by signs of adrenergic counter-regulation. Generally, the greater and more rapid the decline in blood glucose, the more marked is the phenomenon of counter-regulation and its symptoms.

The following related adverse reactions from clinical investigations are listed below by system organ class and in order of decreasing incidence: very common ($\geqslant$1/10); common ($\geqslant$1/100, <1/10); uncommon ($\geqslant$1/1,000, <1/100); rare ($\geqslant$1/10,000, <1/1,000); very rare (<1/10,000), not known (cannot be estimated from the available data).

Within each frequency grouping, undesirable effects are presented in order of decreasing seriousness.

Immune system disorders

Uncommon: shock

Not known: immediate type allergic reactions (hypotension, angioneurotic oedema, bronchospasm, generalised skin reactions), anti-insulin antibodies

Immediate type allergic reactions to insulin or to the excipients may be life-threatening.

Insulin administration may cause anti-insulin antibodies to form. In rare cases, the presence of such anti-insulin antibodies may necessitate adjustment of the insulin dose in order to correct a tendency to hyper- or hypoglycaemia.

Metabolism and nutrition disorders

Common: oedema

Not known: sodium retention

Insulin may cause sodium retention and oedema, particularly if previously poor metabolic control is improved by intensified insulin therapy.

Eyes disorders

Not known: proliferative retinopathy, diabetic retinopathy, visual impairment

A marked change in glycaemic control may cause temporary visual impairment, due to temporary alteration in the turgidity and refractive index of the lens.

Long-term improved glycaemic control decreases the risk of progression of diabetic retinopathy. However, intensification of insulin therapy with abrupt improvement in glycaemic control may be associated with temporary worsening of diabetic retinopathy.

Skin and subcutaneous tissue disorders

Not known: lipodystrophy

As with any insulin therapy, lipodystrophy may occur at the injection site and delay local insulin absorption. Continuous rotation of the injection site within the given injection area may help to reduce or prevent these reactions.

General disorders and administration site conditions

Common: injection site reactions

Uncommon: injection site urticaria,

Not known: injection site inflammation, injection site swelling, injection site pain, injection site pruritus, injection site erythema.

Most minor reactions to insulins at the injection site usually resolve in a few days to a few weeks.

4.9 Overdose

Symptoms

Insulin overdose may lead to severe and sometimes long-term and life-threatening hypoglycaemia.

Management

Mild episodes of hypoglycaemia can usually be treated with oral carbohydrates. Adjustments in dosage of the medicinal product, meal patterns, or physical activity may be needed.

More severe episodes with coma, seizure, or neurologic impairment may be treated with intramuscular/subcutaneous glucagon or concentrated intravenous glucose. Sustained carbohydrate intake and observation may be necessary because hypoglycaemia may recur after apparent clinical recovery.

5. PHARMACOLOGICAL PROPERTIES

5.1 Pharmacodynamic properties

Pharmacotherapeutic group: Antidiabetic agent. Insulins and analogues, intermediate-acting combined with fast-acting, ATC Code: A10AD01.

Mode of action

Insulin

- lowers blood glucose and promotes anabolic effects as well as decreasing catabolic effects,
- increases the transport of glucose into cells as well as the formation of glycogen in the muscles and the liver, and improves pyruvate utilisation. It inhibits glycogenolysis and gluconeogenesis,
- increases lipogenesis in the liver and adipose tissue and inhibits lipolysis,
- promotes the uptake of amino acids into cells and promotes protein synthesis,
- enhances the uptake of potassium into cells.

Pharmacodynamic characteristics

Insuman Comb 25 (a biphasic isophane insulin suspension with 25% dissolved insulin) is an insulin with gradual onset and long duration of action. Following subcutaneous injection, onset of action is within 30 to 60 minutes, the phase of maximum action is between 2 and 4 hours after injection and the duration of action is 12 to 19 hours.

5.2 Pharmacokinetic properties

In healthy subjects, the serum half-life of insulin is approximately 4 to 6 minutes. It is longer in patients with severe renal insufficiency. However, it must be noted that the pharmacokinetics of insulin do not reflect its metabolic action.

5.3 Preclinical safety data

The acute toxicity was studied following subcutaneous administration in rats. No evidence of toxic effects was found. Studies of pharmacodynamic effects following subcutaneous administration in rabbits and dogs revealed the expected hypoglycaemic reactions.

6. PHARMACEUTICAL PARTICULARS

6.1 List of excipients

Protamine sulphate,

metacresol,

phenol,

zinc chloride,

sodium dihydrogen phosphate dihydrate,

glycerol,

sodium hydroxide,

hydrochloric acid (for pH adjustment),

water for injections.

6.2 Incompatibilities

This medicinal product must not be mixed with other medicinal products except those mentioned in section 6.6.

Concerning mixing or incompatibility with other insulins see section 6.6. Care must be taken to ensure that no alcohol or other disinfectants enter the insulin suspension.

6.3 Shelf life

2 years.

Shelf life after first use of the vial:

The product may be stored for a maximum of 4 weeks not above 25°C away from direct heat or direct light.

Keep the vial in the outer carton in order to protect from light.

It is recommended that the date of the first use be noted on the label.

6.4 Special precautions for storage

Unopened vials:

Store in a refrigerator (2°C - 8°C).

Do not freeze.

Do not put Insuman Comb 25 next to the freezer compartment or a freezer pack.

Keep the vial in the outer carton in order to protect from light.

Opened vials:

For storage precautions, see section 6.3.

6.5 Nature and contents of container

5 ml solution in a vial (type 1 colourless glass) with a flanged cap (aluminium), a stopper (chlorobutyl rubber (type 1)) and a tear-off cap (polypropylene).

Packs of 1 vials are available.

6.6 Special precautions for disposal and other handling

Before withdrawing insulin from the vial for the first time, remove the plastic protective cap.

Immediately before withdrawal from the vial into the injection syringe, the insulin must be re-suspended. This is best done by rolling the vial at an oblique angle between the palms of the hands. Do not shake the vial vigorously as this may lead to changes in the suspension (giving the vial a frosted appearance; see below) and cause frothing. Froth may interfere with the correct measurement of the dose.

After resuspension, the fluid must have a uniformly milky appearance. Insuman Comb 25 must not be used if this cannot be achieved, i.e. if the suspension remains clear, for example, or if clumps, particles or flocculation appear in the insulin or stick to the wall or bottom of the vial. These changes sometimes give the vial a frosted appearance. In such cases, a new vial yielding a uniform suspension must be used. It is also necessary to change to a new vial if the insulin requirement changes substantially.

As with all insulin preparations, Insuman Comb 25 must not be mixed with solutions containing reducing agents such as thioles and sulphites. It must also be remembered that
- insulin protamine crystals dissolve in an acid pH range,
- the soluble insulin part precipitates out at a pH of approximately 4.5 to 6.5.

Mixing of insulins

Insuman Comb 25 may be mixed with all Sanofi-Aventis human insulins, but NOT with those designed specifically for use in insulin pumps. Insuman Comb 25 must also NOT be mixed with insulins of animal origin or with insulin analogues.

If two different insulins have to be drawn into one single injection syringe, it is recommended that the shorter-acting insulin be drawn first to prevent contamination of the vial by the longer-acting preparation. It is advisable to inject immediately after mixing. Insulins of different concentration (e.g. 100 IU per ml and 40 IU per ml) must not be mixed.

Any unused product or waste material should be disposed of in accordance with local requirements.

7. MARKETING AUTHORISATION HOLDER

Sanofi-Aventis Deutschland GmbH, D-65926 Frankfurt am Main, Germany

8. MARKETING AUTHORISATION NUMBER(S)

EU/1/97/030/043

9. DATE OF FIRST AUTHORISATION/RENEWAL OF THE AUTHORISATION

Date of first authorisation: 21 February 1997

Date of latest renewal: 21 February 2007

10. DATE OF REVISION OF THE TEXT

June 2008

Legal Category
POM

Insuman Comb 50 Cartridges

(sanofi-aventis)

1. NAME OF THE MEDICINAL PRODUCT

Insuman Comb 50 100 IU/ml suspension for injection in a cartridge

2. QUALITATIVE AND QUANTITATIVE COMPOSITION

Each ml contains 100 IU insulin human (equivalent to 3,5 mg).

Each cartridge contains 3 ml of suspension for injection, equivalent to 300 IU insulin. One IU (International Unit) corresponds to 0.035 mg of anhydrous human insulin.

Insuman Comb 50 is a biphasic isophane insulin suspension consisting of 50% dissolved insulin and 50% crystalline protamine insulin.

Human insulin is produced by recombinant DNA technology in *Escherichia coli*.

For a full list of excipients, see section 6.1.

3. PHARMACEUTICAL FORM

Suspension for injection in a cartridge.

After re-suspension, milky white suspension.

4. CLINICAL PARTICULARS

4.1 Therapeutic indications

Diabetes mellitus where treatment with insulin is required.

4.2 Posology and method of administration

The desired blood glucose levels, the insulin preparations to be used and the insulin dosage (doses and timings) must be determined individually and adjusted to suit the patient's diet, physical activity and life-style.

Daily doses and timing of administration

There are no fixed rules for insulin dosage. However, the average insulin requirement is often 0.5 to 1.0 IU per kg body weight per day. The basal metabolic requirement is 40% to 60% of the total daily requirement. Insuman Comb 50 is injected subcutaneously 20 to 30 minutes before a meal.

Transfer to Insuman Comb 50

Dosage adjustment may be necessary when transferring patients from one insulin preparation to another. This applies, for example, when transferring from:
- an animal insulin (especially a bovine insulin) to human insulin,
- one human insulin preparation to another,
- a regimen with only regular insulin to one with a longer-acting insulin.

The need to adjust (e.g. reduce) the dose may become evident immediately after transfer. Alternatively, it may emerge gradually over a period of several weeks.

Following transfer from an animal insulin to human insulin, dosage reduction may be required in particular in patients who
- were previously already controlled on rather low blood glucose levels,
- have a tendency to hypoglycaemia,
- previously required high insulin doses due to the presence of insulin antibodies.

Close metabolic monitoring is recommended during the transition and in the initial weeks thereafter. In patients who require high insulin doses because of the presence of insulin antibodies, transfer under medical supervision in a hospital or similar setting must be considered.

Secondary dose adjustment

Improved metabolic control may result in increased insulin sensitivity, leading to a reduced insulin requirement. Dose adjustment may also be required, for example, if
- the patient's weight changes,
- the patient's life-style changes,
- other circumstances arise that may promote an increased susceptibility to hypo- or hyperglycaemia (see section 4.4).

Use in specific patient groups

In patients with hepatic or renal impairment as well as in the elderly, insulin requirements may be diminished (see section 4.4).

Administration

Insuman Comb 50 in cartridges has been developed for use in the OptiPen series.

Insuman Comb 50 is administered subcutaneously. Insuman Comb 50 must never be injected intravenously.

Insulin absorption and hence the blood glucose lowering effect of a dose may vary from one injection area to another (e.g. the abdominal wall compared with the thigh). Injection sites within an injection area must be rotated from one injection to the next.

For further details on handling, see section 6.6.

4.3 Contraindications

Hypersensitivity to the active substance or to any of the excipients.

Insuman Comb 50 must not be administered intravenously and must not be used in infusion pumps or external or implanted insulin pumps.

4.4 Special warnings and precautions for use

Patients hypersensitive to Insuman Comb 50 for whom no better tolerated preparation is available must only continue treatment under close medical supervision and – where necessary – in conjunction with anti-allergic treatment.

In patients with an allergy to animal insulin intradermal skin testing is recommended prior to a transfer to Insuman Comb 50, since they may experience immunological cross-reactions.

In patients with renal impairment, insulin requirements may be diminished due to reduced insulin metabolism. In the elderly, progressive deterioration of renal function may lead to a steady decrease in insulin requirements.

In patients with severe hepatic impairment, insulin requirements may be diminished due to reduced capacity for gluconeogenesis and reduced insulin metabolism.

In case of insufficient glucose control or a tendency to hyper- or hypoglycaemic episodes, the patient's adherence to the prescribed treatment regimen, injection sites and proper injection technique and all other relevant factors must be reviewed before dose adjustment is considered.

Hypoglycaemia

Hypoglycaemia may occur if the insulin dose is too high in relation to the insulin requirement.

Particular caution should be exercised, and intensified blood glucose monitoring is advisable in patients in whom hypoglycaemic episodes might be of particular clinical relevance, such as in patients with significant stenoses of the coronary arteries or of the blood vessels supplying the brain (risk of cardiac or cerebral complications of hypoglycaemia) as well as in patients with proliferative retinopathy, particularly if not treated with photocoagulation (risk of transient amaurosis following hypoglycaemia).

Patients should be aware of circumstances where warning symptoms of hypoglycaemia are diminished. The warning symptoms of hypoglycaemia may be changed, be less pronounced or be absent in certain risk groups. These include patients:
- in whom glycaemic control is markedly improved,
- in whom hypoglycaemia develops gradually,
- who are elderly,
- after transfer from animal insulin to human insulin,
- in whom an autonomic neuropathy is present,
- with a long history of diabetes,
- suffering from a psychiatric illness,
- receiving concurrent treatment with certain other medicinal products (see section 4.5).

Such situations may result in severe hypoglycaemia (and possibly loss of consciousness) prior to the patient's awareness of hypoglycaemia.

If normal or decreased values for glycated haemoglobin are noted, the possibility of recurrent, unrecognised (especially nocturnal) episodes of hypoglycaemia must be considered.

Adherence of the patient to the dosage and dietary regimen, correct insulin administration and awareness of hypoglycaemia symptoms are essential to reduce the risk of hypoglycaemia. Factors increasing the susceptibility to hypoglycaemia require particularly close monitoring and may necessitate dose adjustment. These include:
- change in the injection area,
- improved insulin sensitivity (by, e.g., removal of stress factors),
- unaccustomed, increased or prolonged physical activity,
- intercurrent illness (e.g. vomiting, diarrhoea),
- inadequate food intake,
- missed meals,
- alcohol consumption,
- certain uncompensated endocrine disorders (e.g. in hypothyroidism and in anterior pituitary or adrenocortical insufficiency),
- concomitant treatment with certain other medicinal products.

Intercurrent illness

Intercurrent illness requires intensified metabolic monitoring. In many cases, urine tests for ketones are indicated, and often it is necessary to adjust the insulin dose. The insulin requirement is often increased. Patients with type 1 diabetes must continue to consume at least a small amount of carbohydrates on a regular basis, even if they are able to eat only little or no food, or are vomiting etc. and they must never omit insulin entirely.

4.5 Interaction with other medicinal products and other forms of interaction

A number of substances affect glucose metabolism and may require dose adjustment of human insulin.

Substances that may enhance the blood-glucose-lowering effect and increase susceptibility to hypoglycaemia include oral antidiabetic agents, angiotensin converting enzyme (ACE) inhibitors, disopyramide, fibrates, fluoxetine, monoamine oxidase (MAO) inhibitors, pentoxifylline, propoxyphene, salicylates and sulphonamide antibiotics.

Substances that may reduce the blood-glucose-lowering effect include corticosteroids, danazol, diazoxide, diuretics, glucagon, isoniazid, oestrogens and progestogens (e.g. in oral contraceptives), phenothiazine derivatives, somatropin, sympathomimetic agents (e.g. epinephrine [adrenaline], salbutamol, terbutaline), thyroid hormones, protease inhibitors and atypical antipsychotic medicinal products (e.g. olanzapine and clozapine).

Beta-blockers, clonidine, lithium salts or alcohol may either potentiate or weaken the blood-glucose-lowering effect of insulin. Pentamidine may cause hypoglycaemia which may sometimes be followed by hyperglycaemia.

In addition, under the influence of sympatholytic medicinal products such as beta-blockers, clonidine, guanethidine and reserpine, the signs of adrenergic counter-regulation may be reduced or absent.

4.6 Pregnancy and lactation

Pregnancy

For insulin human, no clinical data on exposed pregnancies are available. Insulin does not cross the placental barrier. Caution should be exercised when prescribing to pregnant women.

It is essential for patients with pre-existing or gestational diabetes to maintain good metabolic control throughout pregnancy. Insulin requirements may decrease during the first trimester and generally increase during the second and third trimesters. Immediately after delivery, insulin requirements decline rapidly (increased risk of hypoglycaemia). Careful monitoring of glucose control is essential.

Lactation

No effects on the suckling child are anticipated. Insuman Comb 50 can be used during breastfeeding. Lactating women may require adjustments in insulin dose and diet.

4.7 Effects on ability to drive and use machines

The patient's ability to concentrate and react may be impaired as a result of hypoglycaemia or hyperglycaemia or, for example, as a result of visual impairment. This may constitute a risk in situations where these abilities are of special importance (e.g. driving a car or operating machinery).

Patients should be advised to take precautions to avoid hypoglycaemia whilst driving. This is particularly important in those who have reduced or absent awareness of the warning symptoms of hypoglycaemia or have frequent episodes of hypoglycaemia. It should be considered whether it is advisable to drive or operate machinery in these circumstances.

4.8 Undesirable effects

Hypoglycaemia, in general the most frequent undesirable effect of insulin therapy, may occur if the insulin dose is too high in relation to the insulin requirement. In clinical trials and during marketed use, the frequency varies with patient population and dose regimens. Therefore, no specific frequency can be presented.

Severe hypoglycaemic attacks, especially if recurrent, may lead to neurological damage. Prolonged or severe hypoglycaemic episodes may be life-threatening.

In many patients, the signs and symptoms of neuroglycopenia are preceded by signs of adrenergic counter-regulation. Generally, the greater and more rapid the decline in blood glucose, the more marked is the phenomenon of counter-regulation and its symptoms.

The following related adverse reactions from clinical investigations are listed below by system organ class and in order of decreasing incidence: very common (≥1/10); common (≥1/100, <1/10); uncommon (≥1/1,000, <1/100); rare (≥1/10,000, <1/1,000); very rare (<1/10,000), not known (cannot be estimated from the available data).

Within each frequency grouping, undesirable effects are presented in order of decreasing seriousness.

Immune system disorders

Uncommon: shock

Not known: immediate type allergic reactions (hypotension, angioneurotic oedema, bronchospasm, generalised skin reactions), anti-insulin antibodies

Immediate type allergic reactions to insulin or to the excipients may be life-threatening.

Insulin administration may cause anti-insulin antibodies to form. In rare cases, the presence of such anti-insulin antibodies may necessitate adjustment of the insulin dose in order to correct a tendency to hyper- or hypoglycaemia.

Metabolism and nutrition disorders

Common: oedema

Not known: sodium retention

Insulin may cause sodium retention and oedema, particularly if previously poor metabolic control is improved by intensified insulin therapy.

Eyes disorders

Not known: proliferative retinopathy, diabetic retinopathy, visual impairment

A marked change in glycaemic control may cause temporary visual impairment, due to temporary alteration in the turgidity and refractive index of the lens.

Long-term improved glycaemic control decreases the risk of progression of diabetic retinopathy. However, intensification of insulin therapy with abrupt improvement in glycaemic control may be associated with temporary worsening of diabetic retinopathy.

Skin and subcutaneous tissue disorders

Not known: lipodystrophy

As with any insulin therapy, lipodystrophy may occur at the injection site and delay local insulin absorption. Continuous rotation of the injection site within the given injection area may help to reduce or prevent these reactions.

General disorders and administration site conditions

Common: injection site reactions

Uncommon: injection site urticaria,

Not known: injection site inflammation, injection site swelling, injection site pain, injection site pruritus, injection site erythema.

Most minor reactions to insulins at the injection site usually resolve in a few days to a few weeks.

4.9 Overdose

Symptoms

Insulin overdose may lead to severe and sometimes long-term and life-threatening hypoglycaemia.

Management

Mild episodes of hypoglycaemia can usually be treated with oral carbohydrates. Adjustments in dosage of the medicinal product, meal patterns, or physical activity may be needed.

More severe episodes with coma, seizure, or neurologic impairment may be treated with intramuscular/subcutaneous glucagon or concentrated intravenous glucose. Sustained carbohydrate intake and observation may be necessary because hypoglycaemia may recur after apparent clinical recovery.

5. PHARMACOLOGICAL PROPERTIES

5.1 Pharmacodynamic properties

Pharmacotherapeutic group: Antidiabetic agent. Insulins and analogues, intermediate-acting combined with fast-acting, ATC Code: A10AD01.

Mode of action

Insulin

- lowers blood glucose and promotes anabolic effects as well as decreasing catabolic effects,

- increases the transport of glucose into cells as well as the formation of glycogen in the muscles and the liver, and improves pyruvate utilisation. It inhibits glycogenolysis and gluconeogenesis,

- increases lipogenesis in the liver and adipose tissue and inhibits lipolysis,

- promotes the uptake of amino acids into cells and promotes protein synthesis,

- enhances the uptake of potassium into cells.

Pharmacodynamic characteristics

Insuman Comb 50 (a biphasic isophane insulin suspension with 50% dissolved insulin) is an insulin with rapid onset and moderately long duration of action. Following subcutaneous injection, onset of action is within 30 minutes, the phase of maximum action is between 1.5 and 4 hours after injection and the duration of action is 12 to 16 hours.

5.2 Pharmacokinetic properties

In healthy subjects, the serum half-life of insulin is approximately 4 to 6 minutes. It is longer in patients with severe renal insufficiency. However, it must be noted that the pharmacokinetics of insulin do not reflect its metabolic action.

5.3 Preclinical safety data

The acute toxicity was studied following subcutaneous administration in rats. No evidence of toxic effects was found. Studies of pharmacodynamic effects following subcutaneous administration in rabbits and dogs revealed the expected hypoglycaemic reactions.

6. PHARMACEUTICAL PARTICULARS

6.1 List of excipients

Protamine sulphate,

metacresol,

phenol,

zinc chloride,

sodium dihydrogen phosphate dihydrate,

glycerol,

sodium hydroxide,

hydrochloric acid (for pH adjustment),

water for injections.

6.2 Incompatibilities

This medicinal product must not be mixed with other medicinal products except those mentioned in section 6.6.

Concerning mixing or incompatibility with other insulins see section 6.6. Care must be taken to ensure that no alcohol or other disinfectants enter the insulin suspension.

6.3 Shelf life

2 years.

<u>Shelf life after first use of the cartridge:</u>

The cartridge in-use (in the insulin pen) or carried as a spare may be stored for a maximum of 4 weeks not above 25°C away from direct heat or direct light.

The pen containing a cartridge must not be stored in the refrigerator.

The pen cap must be put back on the pen after each injection in order to protect from light.

6.4 Special precautions for storage

<u>Unopened cartridges:</u>

Store in a refrigerator (2°C - 8°C).

Do not freeze.

Do not put Insuman Comb 50 next to the freezer compartment or a freezer pack.

Keep the cartridge in the outer carton in order to protect from light.

<u>In-use cartridges:</u>

For storage precautions, see section 6.3.

6.5 Nature and contents of container

3 ml suspension in a cartridge (type 1 colourless glass) with a plunger (bromobutyl rubber (type 1)) and a flanged cap (aluminium) with a stopper (bromobutyl or laminate of polyisoprene and bromobutyl rubber (type 1)).

Each cartridge contains 3 balls (stainless steel).

Packs of 5 cartridges are available.

6.6 Special precautions for disposal and other handling

<u>Insulin pen</u>

The cartridges are to be used in conjunction with an insulin pen such as <u>OptiPen and other pens suitable for Insuman cartridges</u> and as recommended in the information provided by the device manufacturer.

The manufacturer's instructions for using the pen must be followed carefully for loading the cartridge, attaching the injection needle, and administering the insulin injection.

<u>If the insulin pen is damaged or not working properly (due to mechanical defects) it has to be discarded, and a new insulin pen has to be used.</u>

If the pen malfunctions (see instructions for using the pen), the suspension may be drawn from the cartridge into an injection syringe (suitable for an insulin with 100 IU/ml) and injected.

<u>Cartridges</u>

Before insertion into the pen, Insuman Comb 50 must be kept at room temperature for 1 to 2 hours and then resuspended to check the contents. This is best done by gently tilting the cartridge back and forth (at least ten times). Each cartridge contains three small metal balls to facilitate quick and thorough mixing of the contents.

Later on, when the cartridge has been inserted into the pen, the insulin must be resuspended again prior to each injection. This is best done by gently tilting the pen back and forth (at least ten times).

After resuspension, the fluid must have a uniformly milky appearance. Insuman Comb 50 must not be used if this cannot be achieved, i.e. if the suspension remains clear, for example, or if clumps, particles or flocculation appear in the insulin or stick to the wall or bottom of the cartridge. These changes sometimes give the cartridge a frosted appearance. In such cases, a new cartridge yielding a uniform suspension must be used. It is also necessary to change to a new cartridge if the insulin requirement changes substantially.

Air bubbles must be removed from the cartridge before injection (see instructions for using the pen). Empty cartridges must not be refilled.

As with all insulin preparations, Insuman Comb 50 must not be mixed with solutions containing reducing agents such as thioles and sulphites. It must also be remembered that

- insulin protamine crystals dissolve in an acid pH range,

- the soluble insulin part precipitates out at a pH of approximately 4.5 to 6.5.

Mixing of insulins

Insuman Comb 50 may be mixed with all Sanofi-Aventis human insulins, but NOT with those designed specifically for use in insulin pumps. Insuman Comb 50 must also NOT be mixed with insulins of animal origin or with insulin analogues.

Insuman Comb 50 cartridges are not designed to allow any other insulin to be mixed in the cartridge.

Any unused product or waste material should be disposed of in accordance with local requirements.

7. MARKETING AUTHORISATION HOLDER

Sanofi-Aventis Deutschland GmbH, D-65926 Frankfurt am Main, Germany

8. MARKETING AUTHORISATION NUMBER(S)

EU/1/97/030/050

9. DATE OF FIRST AUTHORISATION/RENEWAL OF THE AUTHORISATION

Date of first authorisation: 21 February 1997

Date of latest renewal: 21 February 2007

10. DATE OF REVISION OF THE TEXT

June 2008

Legal Category

POM

Insuman Comb 50 Optiset

(sanofi-aventis)

1. NAME OF THE MEDICINAL PRODUCT

Insuman Comb 50 100 IU/ml suspension for injection in a pre-filled pen.

2. QUALITATIVE AND QUANTITATIVE COMPOSITION

Each ml contains 100 IU insulin human (equivalent to 3.5 mg).

Each pen contains 3 ml of suspension for injection, equivalent to 300 IU insulin. One IU (International Unit) corresponds to 0.035 mg of anhydrous human insulin.

Insuman Comb 50 is a biphasic isophane insulin suspension consisting of 50% dissolved insulin and 50% crystalline protamine insulin.

Human insulin is produced by recombinant DNA technology in *Escherichia coli*.

For a full list of excipients, see section 6.1.

3. PHARMACEUTICAL FORM

Suspension for injection in a pre-filled pen. OptiSet.

After re-suspension, milky white suspension.

4. CLINICAL PARTICULARS

4.1 Therapeutic indications

Diabetes mellitus where treatment with insulin is required.

4.2 Posology and method of administration

The desired blood glucose levels, the insulin preparations to be used and the insulin dosage (doses and timings) must be determined individually and adjusted to suit the patient's diet, physical activity and life-style.

<u>Daily doses and timing of administration</u>

There are no fixed rules for insulin dosage. However, the average insulin requirement is often 0.5 to 1.0 IU per kg body weight per day. The basal metabolic requirement is 40% to 60% of the total daily requirement. Insuman Comb 50 is injected subcutaneously 20 to 30 minutes before a meal.

OptiSet delivers insulin in increments of 2 IU up to a maximum single dose of 40 IU.

<u>Transfer to Insuman Comb 50</u>

Dosage adjustment may be necessary when transferring patients from one insulin preparation to another. This applies, for example, when transferring from:

- an animal insulin (especially a bovine insulin) to human insulin,

- one human insulin preparation to another,

- a regimen with only regular insulin to one with a longer-acting insulin.

The need to adjust (e.g. reduce) the dose may become evident immediately after transfer. Alternatively, it may emerge gradually over a period of several weeks.

Following transfer from an animal insulin to human insulin, dosage reduction may be required in particular in patients who

- were previously already controlled on rather low blood glucose levels,
- have a tendency to hypoglycaemia,
- previously required high insulin doses due to the presence of insulin antibodies.

Close metabolic monitoring is recommended during the transition and in the initial weeks thereafter. In patients who require high insulin doses because of the presence of insulin antibodies, transfer under medical supervision in a hospital or similar setting must be considered.

Secondary dose adjustment

Improved metabolic control may result in increased insulin sensitivity, leading to a reduced insulin requirement. Dose adjustment may also be required, for example, if

- the patient's weight changes,
- the patient's life-style changes,
- other circumstances arise that may promote an increased susceptibility to hypo- or hyperglycaemia (see section 4.4).

Use in specific patient groups

In patients with hepatic or renal impairment as well as in the elderly, insulin requirements may be diminished (see section 4.4).

Administration

Insuman Comb 50 is administered subcutaneously. Insuman Comb 50 must never be injected intravenously.

Insulin absorption and hence the blood glucose lowering effect of a dose may vary from one injection area to another (e.g. the abdominal wall compared with the thigh). Injection sites within an injection area must be rotated from one injection to the next.

Before using OptiSet, the Instructions for Use included in the Package Leaflet must be read carefully.

For further details on handling, see section 6.6.

4.3 Contraindications

Hypersensitivity to the active substance or to any of the excipients.

4.4 Special warnings and precautions for use

Patients hypersensitive to Insuman Comb 50 for whom no better tolerated preparation is available must only continue treatment under close medical supervision and – where necessary – in conjunction with anti-allergic treatment.

In patients with an allergy to animal insulin intradermal skin testing is recommended prior to a transfer to Insuman Comb 50, since they may experience immunological cross-reactions.

In patients with renal impairment, insulin requirements may be diminished due to reduced insulin metabolism. In the elderly, progressive deterioration of renal function may lead to a steady decrease in insulin requirements.

In patients with severe hepatic impairment, insulin requirements may be diminished due to reduced capacity for gluconeogenesis and reduced insulin metabolism.

In case of insufficient glucose control or a tendency to hyper- or hypoglycaemic episodes, the patient's adherence to the prescribed treatment regimen, injection sites and proper injection technique and all other relevant factors must be reviewed before dose adjustment is considered.

Hypoglycaemia

Hypoglycaemia may occur if the insulin dose is too high in relation to the insulin requirement.

Particular caution should be exercised, and intensified blood glucose monitoring is advisable in patients in whom hypoglycaemic episodes might be of particular clinical relevance, such as in patients with significant stenoses of the coronary arteries or of the blood vessels supplying the brain (risk of cardiac or cerebral complications of hypoglycaemia) as well as in patients with proliferative retinopathy, particularly if not treated with photocoagulation (risk of transient amaurosis following hypoglycaemia).

Patients should be aware of circumstances where warning symptoms of hypoglycaemia are diminished. The warning symptoms of hypoglycaemia may be changed, be less pronounced or be absent in certain risk groups. These include patients:

- in whom glycaemic control is markedly improved,
- in whom hypoglycaemia develops gradually,
- who are elderly,
- after transfer from animal insulin to human insulin,
- in whom an autonomic neuropathy is present,
- with a long history of diabetes,
- suffering from a psychiatric illness,
- receiving concurrent treatment with certain other medicinal products (see section 4.5).

Such situations may result in severe hypoglycaemia (and possibly loss of consciousness) prior to the patient's awareness of hypoglycaemia.

If normal or decreased values for glycated haemoglobin are noted, the possibility of recurrent, unrecognised (especially nocturnal) episodes of hypoglycaemia must be considered.

Adherence of the patient to the dosage and dietary regimen, correct insulin administration and awareness of hypoglycaemia symptoms are essential to reduce the risk of hypoglycaemia. Factors increasing the susceptibility to hypoglycaemia require particularly close monitoring and may necessitate dose adjustment. These include:

- change in the injection area,
- improved insulin sensitivity (by, e.g., removal of stress factors),
- unaccustomed, increased or prolonged physical activity,
- intercurrent illness (e.g. vomiting, diarrhoea),
- inadequate food intake,
- missed meals,
- alcohol consumption,
- certain uncompensated endocrine disorders (e.g. in hypothyroidism and in anterior pituitary or adrenocortical insufficiency),
- concomitant treatment with certain other medicinal products.

Intercurrent illness

Intercurrent illness requires intensified metabolic monitoring. In many cases, urine tests for ketones are indicated, and often it is necessary to adjust the insulin dose. The insulin requirement is often increased. Patients with type 1 diabetes must continue to consume at least a small amount of carbohydrates on a regular basis, even if they are able to eat only little or no food, or are vomiting etc. and they must never omit insulin entirely.

Handling of the pen

Before using OptiSet, the Instructions for Use included in the Package Leaflet must be read carefully. OptiSet has to be used as recommended in these Instructions for Use (see section 6.6).

4.5 Interaction with other medicinal products and other forms of interaction

A number of substances affect glucose metabolism and may require dose adjustment of human insulin.

Substances that may enhance the blood-glucose-lowering effect and increase susceptibility to hypoglycaemia include oral antidiabetic agents, angiotensin converting enzyme (ACE) inhibitors, disopyramide, fibrates, fluoxetine, monoamine oxidase (MAO) inhibitors, pentoxifylline, propoxyphene, salicylates and sulphonamide antibiotics.

Substances that may reduce the blood-glucose-lowering effect include corticosteroids, danazol, diazoxide, diuretics, glucagon, isoniazid, oestrogens and progestogens (e.g. in oral contraceptives), phenothiazine derivatives, somatropin, sympathomimetic agents (e.g. epinephrine [adrenaline], salbutamol, terbutaline), thyroid hormones, protease inhibitors and atypical antipsychotic medicinal products (e.g. olanzapine and clozapine).

Beta-blockers, clonidine, lithium salts or alcohol may either potentiate or weaken the blood-glucose-lowering effect of insulin. Pentamidine may cause hypoglycaemia which may sometimes be followed by hyperglycaemia.

In addition, under the influence of sympatholytic medicinal products such as beta-blockers, clonidine, guanethidine and reserpine, the signs of adrenergic counter-regulation may be reduced or absent.

4.6 Pregnancy and lactation

Pregnancy

For insulin human, no clinical data on exposed pregnancies are available. Insulin does not cross the placental barrier. Caution should be exercised when prescribing to pregnant women.

It is essential for patients with pre-existing or gestational diabetes to maintain good metabolic control throughout pregnancy. Insulin requirements may decrease during the first trimester and generally increase during the second and third trimesters. Immediately after delivery, insulin requirements decline rapidly (increased risk of hypoglycaemia). Careful monitoring of glucose control is essential.

Lactation

No effects on the suckling child are anticipated. Insuman Comb 50 can be used during breastfeeding. Lactating women may require adjustments in insulin dose and diet.

4.7 Effects on ability to drive and use machines

The patient's ability to concentrate and react may be impaired as a result of hypoglycaemia or hyperglycaemia or, for example, as a result of visual impairment. This may constitute a risk in situations where these abilities are of special importance (e.g. driving a car or operating machinery).

Patients should be advised to take precautions to avoid hypoglycaemia whilst driving. This is particularly important in those who have reduced or absent awareness of the warning symptoms of hypoglycaemia or have frequent episodes of hypoglycaemia. It should be considered whether it is advisable to drive or operate machinery in these circumstances.

4.8 Undesirable effects

Hypoglycaemia, in general the most frequent undesirable effect of insulin therapy, may occur if the insulin dose is too high in relation to the insulin requirement. In clinical trials and during marketed use, the frequency varies with patient population and dose regimens. Therefore, no specific frequency can be presented.

Severe hypoglycaemic attacks, especially if recurrent, may lead to neurological damage. Prolonged or severe hypoglycaemic episodes may be life-threatening.

In many patients, the signs and symptoms of neuroglycopenia are preceded by signs of adrenergic counter-regulation. Generally, the greater and more rapid the decline in blood glucose, the more marked is the phenomenon of counter-regulation and its symptoms.

The following related adverse reactions from clinical investigations are listed below by system organ class and in order of decreasing incidence: very common ($\geq 1/10$); common ($\geq 1/100$, $< 1/10$); uncommon ($\geq 1/1,000$, $< 1/100$); rare ($\geq 1/10,000$, $< 1/1,000$); very rare ($< 1/10,000$), not known (cannot be estimated from the available data).

Within each frequency grouping, undesirable effects are presented in order of decreasing seriousness.

Immune system disorders

Uncommon: shock

Not known: immediate type allergic reactions (hypotension, angioneurotic oedema, bronchospasm, generalised skin reactions), anti-insulin antibodies

Immediate type allergic reactions to insulin or to the excipients may be life-threatening.

Insulin administration may cause anti-insulin antibodies to form. In rare cases, the presence of such anti-insulin antibodies may necessitate adjustment of the insulin dose in order to correct a tendency to hyper- or hypoglycaemia.

Metabolism and nutrition disorders

Common: oedema

Not known: sodium retention

Insulin may cause sodium retention and oedema, particularly if previously poor metabolic control is improved by intensified insulin therapy.

Eyes disorders

Not known: proliferative retinopathy, diabetic retinopathy, visual impairment

A marked change in glycaemic control may cause temporary visual impairment, due to temporary alteration in the turgidity and refractive index of the lens.

Long-term improved glycaemic control decreases the risk of progression of diabetic retinopathy. However, intensification of insulin therapy with abrupt improvement in glycaemic control may be associated with temporary worsening of diabetic retinopathy.

Skin and subcutaneous tissue disorders

Not known: lipodystrophy

As with any insulin therapy, lipodystrophy may occur at the injection site and delay local insulin absorption. Continuous rotation of the injection site within the given injection area may help to reduce or prevent these reactions.

General disorders and administration site conditions

Common: injection site reactions

Uncommon: injection site urticaria,

Not known: injection site inflammation, injection site swelling, injection site pain, injection site pruritus, injection site erythema.

Most minor reactions to insulins at the injection site usually resolve in a few days to a few weeks.

4.9 Overdose

Symptoms

Insulin overdose may lead to severe and sometimes long-term and life-threatening hypoglycaemia.

Management

Mild episodes of hypoglycaemia can usually be treated with oral carbohydrates. Adjustments in dosage of the medicinal product, meal patterns, or physical activity may be needed.

More severe episodes with coma, seizure, or neurologic impairment may be treated with intramuscular/subcutaneous glucagon or concentrated intravenous glucose. Sustained carbohydrate intake and observation may be necessary because hypoglycaemia may recur after apparent clinical recovery.

5. PHARMACOLOGICAL PROPERTIES

5.1 Pharmacodynamic properties

Pharmacotherapeutic group: Antidiabetic agent. Insulins and analogues, intermediate-acting combined with fast-acting, ATC Code: A10AD01.

Mode of action

Insulin

- lowers blood glucose and promotes anabolic effects as well as decreasing catabolic effects,
- increases the transport of glucose into cells as well as the formation of glycogen in the muscles and the liver, and

improves pyruvate utilisation. It inhibits glycogenolysis and gluconeogenesis,

- increases lipogenesis in the liver and adipose tissue and inhibits lipolysis,
- promotes the uptake of amino acids into cells and promotes protein synthesis,
- enhances the uptake of potassium into cells.

Pharmacodynamic characteristics

Insuman Comb 50 (a biphasic isophane insulin suspension with 50% dissolved insulin) is an insulin with rapid onset and moderately long duration of action. Following subcutaneous injection, onset of action is within 30 minutes, the phase of maximum action is between 1.5 and 4 hours after injection and the duration of action is 12 to 16 hours.

5.2 Pharmacokinetic properties

In healthy subjects, the serum half-life of insulin is approximately 4 to 6 minutes. It is longer in patients with severe renal insufficiency. However, it must be noted that the pharmacokinetics of insulin do not reflect its metabolic action.

5.3 Preclinical safety data

The acute toxicity was studied following subcutaneous administration in rats. No evidence of toxic effects was found. Studies of pharmacodynamic effects following subcutaneous administration in rabbits and dogs revealed the expected hypoglycaemic reactions.

6. PHARMACEUTICAL PARTICULARS

6.1 List of excipients

Protamine sulphate,

metacresol,

phenol,

zinc chloride,

sodium dihydrogen phosphate dihydrate,

glycerol,

sodium hydroxide,

hydrochloric acid (for pH adjustment),

water for injections.

6.2 Incompatibilities

This medicinal product must not be mixed with other medicinal products except those mentioned in section 6.6.

Concerning mixing or incompatibility with other insulins see section 6.6. Care must be taken to ensure that no alcohol or other disinfectants enter the insulin suspension.

6.3 Shelf life

2 years.

<u>Shelf life after first use of the pen</u>:

The pen in-use or carried as a spare may be stored for a maximum of 4 weeks not above 25°C away from direct heat or direct light.

Pens in-use must not be stored in the refrigerator.

The pen cap must be put back on the pen after each injection in order to protect from light.

6.4 Special precautions for storage

<u>Not in-use pens:</u>

Store in a refrigerator (2°C – 8°C).

Do not freeze.

Do not put Insuman Comb 50 next to the freezer compartment or a freezer pack.

Keep the pre-filled pen in the outer carton in order to protect from light.

<u>In-use pens</u>:

For storage precautions, see section 6.3.

6.5 Nature and contents of container

3 ml suspension in a cartridge (type 1 colourless glass) with a plunger (bromobutyl rubber (type 1)) and a flanged cap (aluminium) with a stopper (bromobutyl or laminate of polyisoprene and bromobutyl rubber (type 1)).

Each cartridge contains 3 balls (stainless steel). The cartridges are sealed in a disposable pen injector. Injection needles are not included in the pack.

Packs of 5 pens are available.

6.6 Special precautions for disposal and other handling

Before first use, Insuman Comb 50 must be kept at room temperature for 1 to 2 hours and then resuspended to check the contents. This is best done by gently tilting the pen back and forth (at least ten times). Each cartridge contains three small metal balls to facilitate quick and thorough mixing of the contents. Later on, the insulin must be resuspended again prior to each injection.

After resuspension, the fluid must have a uniformly milky appearance. Insuman Comb 50 must not be used if this cannot be achieved, i.e. if the suspension remains clear, for example, or if clumps, particles or flocculation appear in the insulin or stick to the wall or bottom of the cartridge. These changes sometimes give the cartridge a frosted appearance. In such cases, a new pen yielding a uniform suspension must be used. It is also necessary to change to a new pen if the insulin requirement changes substantially.

Empty pens must never be reused and must be properly discarded.

Handling of the pen

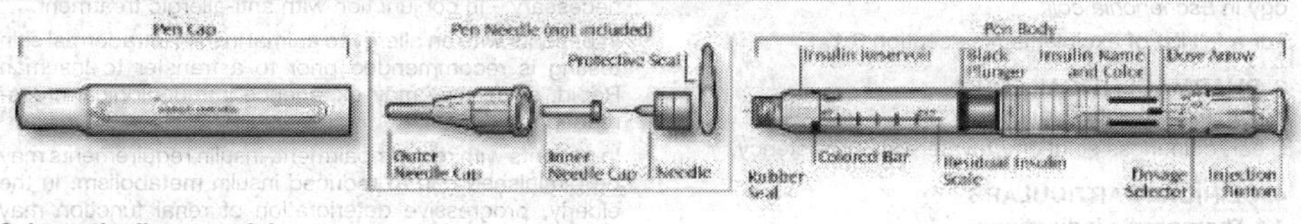

<u>**Schematic diagram of the pen**</u>

To prevent the possible transmission of disease, each pen must be used by one patient only.

As with all insulin preparations, Insuman Comb 50 must not be mixed with solutions containing reducing agents such as thioles and sulphites. It must also be remembered that

- insulin protamine crystals dissolve in an acid pH range,
- the soluble insulin part precipitates out at a pH of approximately 4.5 to 6.5.

Mixing of insulins

Insuman Comb 50 must not be mixed with any other insulin or with insulin analogues.

Any unused product or waste material should be disposed of in accordance with local requirements.

Handling of the pen

The Instructions for Use included in the Package Leaflet must be read carefully before using OptiSet.

<u>(see Handling of the pen above)</u>

Important information for use of OptiSet:

- Always attach a new needle before each use. Only use needles that are compatible for use with OptiSet.
- Always perform the safety test before each injection.
- If a new OptiSet is used the initial safety test must be done with the 8 units preset by the manufacturer.
- The dosage selector can only be turned in one direction.
- Never turn the dosage selector (change the dose) after injection button has been pulled out.
- This pen is only for the patients use. It must not be shared with anyone else.
- If the injection is given by another person, special caution must be taken by this person to avoid accidental needle injury and transmission of infection.
- Never use OptiSet if it is damaged or if you are not sure that it is working properly.
- Always have a spare OptiSet in case your OptiSet is lost or damaged.

Storage Instructions

Please check section 6.4 of this leaflet for instructions on how to store OptiSet.

If OptiSet is in cool storage, it should be taken out 1 to 2 hours before injection to allow it to warm up. Cold insulin is more painful to inject.

The used OptiSet must be discarded as required by your local authorities.

Maintenance

OptiSet has to be protected from dust and dirt.

You can clean the outside of your OptiSet by wiping it with a damp cloth.

Do not soak, wash or lubricate the pen as this may damage it.

OptiSet is designed to work accurately and safely. It should be handled with care. Avoid situations where OptiSet might be damaged. If you are concerned that your OptiSet may be damaged, use a new one.

Step 1. Check and mix the Insulin

After removing the pen cap, the label on the pen and the insulin reservoir should be checked to make sure it contains the correct insulin. The insulin should be mixed by turning OptiSet slowly up and down at least 10 times.

The appearance of the insulin should be checked: the insulin suspension must have an evenly milky white appearance.

Step 2. Attach the needle

The needle should be carefully attached straight onto the pen.

Step 3. Perform a safety test

Prior to each injection a safety test has to be performed.

For a new and unused OptiSet, a dose of 8 units is already preset by the manufacturer for the first safety test.

In-use OptiSet, select a dose of 2 units by turning the dosage selector forward till the dose arrow points to 2. The dosage selector will only turn in one direction.

Pull out the injection button completely in order to load the dose. Never turn the dosage selector after injection button has been pulled out

The outer and inner needle caps should be removed. Keep the outer cap to remove the used needle.

While holding the pen with the needle pointing upwards, the insulin reservoir should be tapped with the finger so that any air bubbles rise up towards the needle

Then the injection button should be pressed all the way in.

If insulin has been expelled through the needle tip, then the pen and the needle are working properly.

If no insulin appears at the needle tip, step 3 should be repeated two more times until insulin appears at the needle tip. If still no insulin comes out, change the needle, as it might be blocked and try again. If no insulin comes out after changing the needle, the OptiSet may be damaged. Do not use this OptiSet.

Step 4. Select the dose

The dose can be set in steps of 2 units, from a minimum of 2 units to a maximum of 40 units. If a dose greater than 40 units is required, it should be given as two or more injections.

Check if you have enough insulin for the dose.

The residual insulin scale on the transparent insulin reservoir shows approximately how much insulin remains in the OptiSet. This scale must not be used to set the insulin dose.

If the black plunger is at the beginning of the coloured bar, then there are approximately 40 units of insulin available.

If the black plunger is at the end of the coloured bar, then there are approximately 20 units of insulin available.

The dosage selector should be turned forward until the dose arrow points to the required dose.

Step 5. Load the dose

The injection button should be pulled out as far as it will go in order to load the pen.

Check if the selected dose is fully loaded. Note that the injection button only goes out as far as the amount of insulin that is left in the reservoir.

The injection button allows checking the actual loaded dose. The injection button must be held out under tension during this check. The last thick line visible on the injection button shows the amount of insulin loaded. When the injection button is held out only the top part of this thick line can be seen.

Step 6. Inject the dose

The patient should be informed on the injection technique by his health care professional.

The needle should be inserted into the skin.

The injection button should be pressed all the way in. A clicking sound can be heard, which will stop when the injection button has been pressed in completely. Then the injection button should be held down 10 seconds before withdrawing the needle from the skin. This ensures that the full dose of insulin has been delivered.

Step 7. Remove and discard the needle

The needle should be removed after each injection and discarded. This helps prevent contamination and/or infection as well as entry of air into the insulin reservoir and leakage of insulin, which can cause inaccurate dosing. Needles must not be reused.

The pen cap should be replaced on the pen.

7. MARKETING AUTHORISATION HOLDER

Sanofi-Aventis Deutschland GmbH, D-65926 Frankfurt am Main, Germany

8. MARKETING AUTHORISATION NUMBER(S)

EU/1/97/030/083

9. DATE OF FIRST AUTHORISATION/RENEWAL OF THE AUTHORISATION

Date of first authorisation: 21 February 1997

Date of latest renewal: 21 February 2007

10. DATE OF REVISION OF THE TEXT

June 2008

Legal Category: POM

Insuman Rapid Cartridges

(sanofi-aventis)

1. NAME OF THE MEDICINAL PRODUCT

Insuman Rapid 100 IU/ml solution for injection in a cartridge

2. QUALITATIVE AND QUANTITATIVE COMPOSITION

Each ml contains 100 IU insulin human (equivalent to 3.5 mg).

Each cartridge contains 3 ml of solution for injection, equivalent to 300 IU insulin. One IU (International Unit) corresponds to 0.035 mg of anhydrous human insulin.

Insuman Rapid is a neutral insulin solution (regular insulin).

Human insulin is produced by recombinant DNA technology in *Escherichia coli*.

For a full list of excipients, see section 6.1.

3. PHARMACEUTICAL FORM

Solution for injection in a cartridge.

Clear, colourless solution of water-like consistency.

4. CLINICAL PARTICULARS

4.1 Therapeutic indications

Diabetes mellitus where treatment with insulin is required. Insuman Rapid is also suitable for the treatment of hyperglycaemic coma and ketoacidosis, as well as for achieving pre-, intra- and post-operative stabilisation in patients with diabetes mellitus.

4.2 Posology and method of administration

The desired blood glucose levels, the insulin preparations to be used and the insulin dosage (doses and timings) must be determined individually and adjusted to suit the patient's diet, physical activity and life-style.

Daily doses and timing of administration

There are no fixed rules for insulin dosage. However, the average insulin requirement is often 0.5 to 1.0 IU per kg body weight per day. The basal metabolic requirement is 40% to 60% of the total daily requirement. Insuman Rapid is injected subcutaneously 15 to 20 minutes before a meal.

In the treatment of severe hyperglycaemia or ketoacidosis in particular, insulin administration is part of a complex therapeutic regimen which includes measures to protect patients from possible severe complications of a relatively rapid lowering of blood glucose. This regimen requires close monitoring (metabolic status, acid-base and electrolyte status, vital parameters etc.) in an intensive care unit or similar setting.

Transfer to Insuman Rapid

Dosage adjustment may be necessary when transferring patients from one insulin preparation to another. This applies, for example, when transferring from:

- an animal insulin (especially a bovine insulin) to human insulin,
- one human insulin preparation to another,
- a regimen with only regular insulin to one with a longer-acting insulin.

The need to adjust (e.g. reduce) the dose may become evident immediately after transfer. Alternatively, it may emerge gradually over a period of several weeks.

Following transfer from an animal insulin to human insulin, dosage reduction may be required in particular in patients who

- were previously already controlled on rather low blood glucose levels,
- have a tendency to hypoglycaemia,
- previously required high insulin doses due to the presence of insulin antibodies.

Close metabolic monitoring is recommended during the transition and in the initial weeks thereafter. In patients who require high insulin doses because of the presence of insulin antibodies, transfer under medical supervision in a hospital or similar setting must be considered.

Secondary dose adjustment

Improved metabolic control may result in increased insulin sensitivity, leading to a reduced insulin requirement. Dose adjustment may also be required, for example, if

- the patient's weight changes,
- the patient's life-style changes,
- other circumstances arise that may promote an increased susceptibility to hypo- or hyperglycaemia (see section 4.4).

Use in specific patient groups

In patients with hepatic or renal impairment as well as in the elderly, insulin requirements may be diminished (see section 4.4).

Administration

Insuman Rapid in cartridges has been developed for use in the OptiPen series.

Insuman Rapid is administered subcutaneously.

Insulin absorption and hence the blood glucose lowering effect of a dose may vary from one injection area to another (e.g. the abdominal wall compared with the thigh). Injection sites within an injection area must be rotated from one injection to the next.

Insuman Rapid may also be administered intravenously. Intravenous insulin therapy must generally take place in an intensive care unit or under comparable monitoring and treatment conditions (see "Daily doses and timing of administration").

For further details on handling, see section 6.6.

4.3 Contraindications

Hypersensitivity to the active substance or to any of the excipients.

Insuman Rapid must not be used in external or implanted insulin pumps or in peristaltic pumps with silicone tubing.

4.4 Special warnings and precautions for use

Patients hypersensitive to Insuman Rapid for whom no better tolerated preparation is available must only continue treatment under close medical supervision and – where necessary – in conjunction with anti-allergic treatment.

In patients with an allergy to animal insulin intradermal skin testing is recommended prior to a transfer to Insuman Rapid, since they may experience immunological cross-reactions.

In patients with renal impairment, insulin requirements may be diminished due to reduced insulin metabolism. In the elderly, progressive deterioration of renal function may lead to a steady decrease in insulin requirements.

In patients with severe hepatic impairment, insulin requirements may be diminished due to reduced capacity for gluconeogenesis and reduced insulin metabolism.

In case of insufficient glucose control or a tendency to hyper- or hypoglycaemic episodes, the patient's adherence to the prescribed treatment regimen, injection sites and proper injection technique and all other relevant factors must be reviewed before dose adjustment is considered.

Hypoglycaemia

Hypoglycaemia may occur if the insulin dose is too high in relation to the insulin requirement.

Particular caution should be exercised, and intensified blood glucose monitoring is advisable in patients in whom hypoglycaemic episodes might be of particular clinical relevance, such as in patients with significant stenoses of the coronary arteries or of the blood vessels supplying the brain (risk of cardiac or cerebral complications of hypoglycaemia) as well as in patients with proliferative retinopathy, particularly if not treated with photocoagulation (risk of transient amaurosis following hypoglycaemia).

Patients should be aware of circumstances where warning symptoms of hypoglycaemia are diminished. The warning symptoms of hypoglycaemia may be changed, be less pronounced or be absent in certain risk groups. These include patients:

- in whom glycaemic control is markedly improved,
- in whom hypoglycaemia develops gradually,
- who are elderly,
- after transfer from animal insulin to human insulin,
- in whom an autonomic neuropathy is present,
- with a long history of diabetes,
- suffering from a psychiatric illness,
- receiving concurrent treatment with certain other medicinal products (see section 4.5).

Such situations may result in severe hypoglycaemia (and possibly loss of consciousness) prior to the patient's awareness of hypoglycaemia.

If normal or decreased values for glycated haemoglobin are noted, the possibility of recurrent, unrecognised (especially nocturnal) episodes of hypoglycaemia must be considered.

Adherence of the patient to the dosage and dietary regimen, correct insulin administration and awareness of hypoglycaemia symptoms are essential to reduce the risk of hypoglycaemia. Factors increasing the susceptibility to hypoglycaemia require particularly close monitoring and may necessitate dose adjustment. These include:

- change in the injection area,
- improved insulin sensitivity (by, e.g., removal of stress factors),
- unaccustomed, increased or prolonged physical activity,
- intercurrent illness (e.g. vomiting, diarrhoea),
- inadequate food intake,
- missed meals,
- alcohol consumption,
- certain uncompensated endocrine disorders (e.g. in hypothyroidism and in anterior pituitary or adrenocortical insufficiency),
- concomitant treatment with certain other medicinal products.

Intercurrent illness

Intercurrent illness requires intensified metabolic monitoring. In many cases, urine tests for ketones are indicated, and often it is necessary to adjust the insulin dose. The insulin requirement is often increased. Patients with type 1 diabetes must continue to consume at least a small amount of carbohydrates on a regular basis, even if they are able to eat only little or no food, or are vomiting etc. and they must never omit insulin entirely.

4.5 Interaction with other medicinal products and other forms of interaction

A number of substances affect glucose metabolism and may require dose adjustment of human insulin.

Substances that may enhance the blood-glucose-lowering effect and increase susceptibility to hypoglycaemia include oral antidiabetic agents, angiotensin converting enzyme (ACE) inhibitors, disopyramide, fibrates, fluoxetine, monoamine oxidase (MAO) inhibitors, pentoxifylline, propoxyphene, salicylates and sulphonamide antibiotics.

Substances that may reduce the blood-glucose-lowering effect include corticosteroids, danazol, diazoxide, diuretics, glucagon, isoniazid, oestrogens and progestogens (e.g. in oral contraceptives), phenothiazine derivatives, somatropin, sympathomimetic agents (e.g. epinephrine [adrenaline], salbutamol, terbutaline), thyroid hormones, protease inhibitors and atypical antipsychotic medicinal products (e.g. olanzapine and clozapine).

Beta-blockers, clonidine, lithium salts or alcohol may either potentiate or weaken the blood-glucose-lowering effect of insulin. Pentamidine may cause hypoglycaemia which may sometimes be followed by hyperglycaemia.

In addition, under the influence of sympatholytic medicinal products such as beta-blockers, clonidine, guanethidine and reserpine, the signs of adrenergic counter-regulation may be reduced or absent.

4.6 Pregnancy and lactation

Pregnancy

For insulin human, no clinical data on exposed pregnancies are available. Insulin does not cross the placental barrier. Caution should be exercised when prescribing to pregnant women.

It is essential for patients with pre-existing or gestational diabetes to maintain good metabolic control throughout pregnancy. Insulin requirements may decrease during the first trimester and generally increase during the second and third trimesters. Immediately after delivery, insulin requirements decline rapidly (increased risk of hypoglycaemia). Careful monitoring of glucose control is essential.

Lactation

No effects on the suckling child are anticipated. Insuman Rapid can be used during breastfeeding. Lactating women may require adjustments in insulin dose and diet.

4.7 Effects on ability to drive and use machines

The patient's ability to concentrate and react may be impaired as a result of hypoglycaemia or hyperglycaemia or, for example, as a result of visual impairment. This may constitute a risk in situations where these abilities are of special importance (e.g. driving a car or operating machinery).

Patients should be advised to take precautions to avoid hypoglycaemia whilst driving. This is particularly important in those who have reduced or absent awareness of the warning symptoms of hypoglycaemia or have frequent episodes of hypoglycaemia. It should be considered whether it is advisable to drive or operate machinery in these circumstances.

4.8 Undesirable effects

Hypoglycaemia, in general the most frequent undesirable effect of insulin therapy, may occur if the insulin dose is too high in relation to the insulin requirement. In clinical trials and during marketed use, the frequency varies with patient population and dose regimens. Therefore, no specific frequency can be presented.

Severe hypoglycaemic attacks, especially if recurrent, may lead to neurological damage. Prolonged or severe hypoglycaemic episodes may be life-threatening.

In many patients, the signs and symptoms of neuroglycopenia are preceded by signs of adrenergic counter-regulation. Generally, the greater and more rapid the decline in blood glucose, the more marked is the phenomenon of counter-regulation and its symptoms.

The following related adverse reactions from clinical investigations are listed below by system organ class and in order of decreasing incidence: very common ($\geq$1/10); common ($\geq$1/100, $<$1/10); uncommon ($\geq$1/1,000, $<$1/100); rare ($\geq$1/10,000, $<$1/1,000); very rare ($<$1/10,000), not known (cannot be estimated from the available data).

Within each frequency grouping, undesirable effects are presented in order of decreasing seriousness.

Immune system disorders

Uncommon: shock

Not known: immediate type allergic reactions (hypotension, angioneurotic oedema, bronchospasm, generalised skin reactions), anti-insulin antibodies

Immediate type allergic reactions to insulin or to the excipients may be life-threatening.

Insulin administration may cause anti-insulin antibodies to form. In rare cases, the presence of such insulin antibodies may necessitate adjustment of the insulin dose in order to correct a tendency to hyper- or hypoglycaemia.

Metabolism and nutrition disorders

Common: oedema

Not known: sodium retention

Insulin may cause sodium retention and oedema, particularly if previously poor metabolic control is improved by intensified insulin therapy.

Eyes disorders

Not known: proliferative retinopathy, diabetic retinopathy, visual impairment

A marked change in glycaemic control may cause temporary visual impairment, due to temporary alteration in the turgidity and refractive index of the lens.

Long-term improved glycaemic control decreases the risk of progression of diabetic retinopathy. However, intensification of insulin therapy with abrupt improvement in glycaemic control may be associated with temporary worsening of diabetic retinopathy.

Skin and subcutaneous tissue disorders

Not known: lipodystrophy

As with any insulin therapy, lipodystrophy may occur at the injection site and delay local insulin absorption. Continuous rotation of the injection site within the given injection area may help to reduce or prevent these reactions.

General disorders and administration site conditions

Common: injection site reactions

Uncommon: injection site urticaria,

Not known: injection site inflammation, injection site swelling, injection site pain, injection site pruritus, injection site erythema.

Most minor reactions to insulins at the injection site usually resolve in a few days to a few weeks.

4.9 Overdose

Symptoms

Insulin overdose may lead to severe and sometimes long-term and life-threatening hypoglycaemia.

Management

Mild episodes of hypoglycaemia can usually be treated with oral carbohydrates. Adjustments in dosage of the medicinal product, meal patterns, or physical activity may be needed.

More severe episodes with coma, seizure, or neurologic impairment may be treated with intramuscular/subcutaneous glucagon or concentrated intravenous glucose. Sustained carbohydrate intake and observation may be necessary because hypoglycaemia may recur after apparent clinical recovery.

5. PHARMACOLOGICAL PROPERTIES

5.1 Pharmacodynamic properties

Pharmacotherapeutic group: Antidiabetic agent. Insulins and analogues, fast-acting, ATC Code: A10AB01.

Mode of action

Insulin

- lowers blood glucose and promotes anabolic effects as well as decreasing catabolic effects,
- increases the transport of glucose into cells as well as the formation of glycogen in the muscles and the liver, and improves pyruvate utilisation. It inhibits glycogenolysis and gluconeogenesis,
- increases lipogenesis in the liver and adipose tissue and inhibits lipolysis,
- promotes the uptake of amino acids into cells and promotes protein synthesis,
- enhances the uptake of potassium into cells.

Pharmacodynamic characteristics

Insuman Rapid is an insulin with rapid onset and short duration of action. Following subcutaneous injection, onset of action is within 30 minutes, the phase of maximum action is between 1 and 4 hours after injection and the duration of action is 7 to 9 hours.

5.2 Pharmacokinetic properties

In healthy subjects, the serum half-life of insulin is approximately 4 to 6 minutes. It is longer in patients with severe renal insufficiency. However, it must be noted that the pharmacokinetics of insulin do not reflect its metabolic action.

5.3 Preclinical safety data

The acute toxicity was studied following subcutaneous administration in rats. No evidence of toxic effects was found. Local tolerability studies following subcutaneous and intramuscular administration in rabbits gave no remarkable findings. Studies of pharmacodynamic effects following subcutaneous administration in rabbits and dogs revealed the expected hypoglycaemic reactions.

6. PHARMACEUTICAL PARTICULARS

6.1 List of excipients

Metacresol,

sodium dihydrogen phosphate dihydrate,

glycerol,

sodium hydroxide,

hydrochloric acid (for pH adjustment),

water for injections.

6.2 Incompatibilities

This medicinal product must not be mixed with other medicinal products except those mentioned in section 6.6.

Concerning mixing or incompatibility with other insulins see section 6.6. Care must be taken to ensure that no alcohol or other disinfectants enter the insulin solution.

6.3 Shelf life

2 years.

Shelf life after first use of the cartridge:

The cartridge in-use (in the insulin pen) or carried as a spare may be stored for a maximum of 4 weeks not above 25°C away from direct heat or direct light.

The pen containing a cartridge must not be stored in the refrigerator.

The pen cap must be put back on the pen after each injection in order to protect from light.

6.4 Special precautions for storage

Unopened cartridges:

Store in a refrigerator (2°C - 8°C).

Do not freeze.

Do not put Insuman Rapid next to the freezer compartment or a freezer pack.

Keep the cartridge in the outer carton in order to protect from light.

In-use cartridges:

For storage precautions, see section 6.3.

6.5 Nature and contents of container

3 ml solution in a cartridge (type 1 colourless glass) with a plunger (bromobutyl rubber (type 1)) and a flanged cap (aluminium) with a stopper (bromobutyl or laminate of polyisoprene and bromobutyl rubber (type 1)).

Packs of 5 cartridges are available.

6.6 Special precautions for disposal and other handling

Insulin pen

The cartridges are to be used in conjunction with an insulin pen such as OptiPen and other pens suitable for Insuman cartridges and as recommended in the information provided by the device manufacturer.

The manufacturer's instructions for using the pen must be followed carefully for loading the cartridge, attaching the injection needle, and administering the insulin injection.

If the insulin pen is damaged or not working properly (due to mechanical defects) it has to be discarded, and a new insulin pen has to be used.

If the pen malfunctions (see instructions for using the pen), the solution may be drawn from the cartridge into an injection syringe (suitable for an insulin with 100 IU/ml) and injected.

Cartridges

Before insertion into the pen, Insuman Rapid must be kept at room temperature for 1 to 2 hours.

Inspect the cartridge before use. Insuman Rapid must only be used if the solution is clear, colourless, with no solid particles visible, and if it is of a water-like consistency.

Air bubbles must be removed from the cartridge before injection (see instructions for using the pen). Empty cartridges must not be refilled.

As with all insulin preparations, Insuman Rapid must not be mixed with solutions containing reducing agents such as thioles and sulphites. It must also be remembered that neutral regular insulin precipitates out at a pH of approximately 4.5 to 6.5.

Mixing of insulins

Insuman Rapid may be mixed with all Sanofi-Aventis human insulins, but NOT with those designed specifically for use in insulin pumps. Insuman Rapid must also NOT be mixed with insulins of animal origin or with insulin analogues.

Insuman Rapid cartridges are not designed to allow any other insulin to be mixed in the cartridge.

Any unused product or waste material should be disposed of in accordance with local requirements.

7. MARKETING AUTHORISATION HOLDER

Sanofi-Aventis Deutschland GmbH, D-65926 Frankfurt am Main, Germany

8. MARKETING AUTHORISATION NUMBER(S)

EU/1/97/030/030

9. DATE OF FIRST AUTHORISATION/RENEWAL OF THE AUTHORISATION

Date of first authorisation: 21 February 1997

Date of latest renewal: 21 February 2007

10. DATE OF REVISION OF THE TEXT

June 2008

Legal Category

POM

Insuman Rapid Optiset

(sanofi-aventis)

1. NAME OF THE MEDICINAL PRODUCT

Insuman Rapid 100 IU/ml solution for injection in a pre-filled pen.

2. QUALITATIVE AND QUANTITATIVE COMPOSITION

Each ml contains 100 IU insulin human (equivalent to 3.5 mg).

Each pen contains 3 ml of solution for injection, equivalent to 300 IU insulin. One IU (International Unit) corresponds to 0.035 mg of anhydrous human insulin.

Insuman Rapid is a neutral insulin solution (regular insulin).

Human insulin is produced by recombinant DNA technology in *Escherichia coli*.

For a full list of excipients, see section 6.1.

3. PHARMACEUTICAL FORM

Solution for injection in a pre-filled pen. OptiSet.

Clear, colourless solution of water-like consistency.

4. CLINICAL PARTICULARS

4.1 Therapeutic indications

Diabetes mellitus where treatment with insulin is required.

4.2 Posology and method of administration

The desired blood glucose levels, the insulin preparations to be used and the insulin dosage (doses and timings) must be determined individually and adjusted to suit the patient's diet, physical activity and life-style.

Daily doses and timing of administration

There are no fixed rules for insulin dosage. However, the average insulin requirement is often 0.5 to 1.0 IU per kg body weight per day. The basal metabolic requirement is 40% to 60% of the total daily requirement. Insuman Rapid is injected subcutaneously 15 to 20 minutes before a meal.

OptiSet delivers insulin in increments of 2 IU up to a maximum single dose of 40 IU.

Transfer to Insuman Rapid

Dosage adjustment may be necessary when transferring patients from one insulin preparation to another. This applies, for example, when transferring from:

- an animal insulin (especially a bovine insulin) to human insulin,
- one human insulin preparation to another,
- a regimen with only regular insulin to one with a longer-acting insulin.

The need to adjust (e.g. reduce) the dose may become evident immediately after transfer. Alternatively, it may emerge gradually over a period of several weeks.

Following transfer from an animal insulin to human insulin, dosage reduction may be required in particular in patients who

- were previously already controlled on rather low blood glucose levels,
- have a tendency to hypoglycaemia,
- previously required high insulin doses due to the presence of insulin antibodies.

Close metabolic monitoring is recommended during the transition and in the initial weeks thereafter. In patients who require high insulin doses because of the presence of insulin antibodies, transfer under medical supervision in a hospital or similar setting must be considered.

Secondary dose adjustment

Improved metabolic control may result in increased insulin sensitivity, leading to a reduced insulin requirement. Dose adjustment may also be required, for example, if

- the patient's weight changes,
- the patient's life-style changes,
- other circumstances arise that may promote an increased susceptibility to hypo- or hyperglycaemia (see section 4.4).

Use in specific patient groups

In patients with hepatic or renal impairment as well as in the elderly, insulin requirements may be diminished (see section 4.4).

Administration

Insuman Rapid is administered subcutaneously.

Insulin absorption and hence the blood glucose lowering effect of a dose may vary from one injection area to another (e.g. the abdominal wall compared with the thigh). Injection sites within an injection area must be rotated from one injection to the next.

Before using OptiSet, the Instructions for Use included in the Package Leaflet must be read carefully

For further details on handling, see section 6.6.

4.3 Contraindications

Hypersensitivity to the active substance or to any of the excipients.

4.4 Special warnings and precautions for use

Patients hypersensitive to Insuman Rapid for whom no better tolerated preparation is available must only continue treatment under close medical supervision and – where necessary – in conjunction with anti-allergic treatment.

In patients with an allergy to animal insulin intradermal skin testing is recommended prior to a transfer to Insuman Rapid, since they may experience immunological cross-reactions.

In patients with renal impairment, insulin requirements may be diminished due to reduced insulin metabolism. In the elderly, progressive deterioration of renal function may lead to a steady decrease in insulin requirements.

In patients with severe hepatic impairment, insulin requirements may be diminished due to reduced capacity for gluconeogenesis and reduced insulin metabolism.

In case of insufficient glucose control or a tendency to hyper- or hypoglycaemic episodes, the patient's adherence to the prescribed treatment regimen, injection sites and proper injection technique and all other relevant factors must be reviewed before dose adjustment is considered.

Hypoglycaemia

Hypoglycaemia may occur if the insulin dose is too high in relation to the insulin requirement.

Particular caution should be exercised, and intensified blood glucose monitoring is advisable in patients in whom hypoglycaemic episodes might be of particular clinical relevance, such as in patients with significant stenoses of the coronary arteries or of the blood vessels supplying the brain (risk of cardiac or cerebral complications of hypoglycaemia) as well as in patients with proliferative retinopathy, particularly if not treated with photocoagulation (risk of transient amaurosis following hypoglycaemia).

Patients should be aware of circumstances where warning symptoms of hypoglycaemia are diminished. The warning symptoms of hypoglycaemia may be changed, be less pronounced or be absent in certain risk groups. These include patients:

- in whom glycaemic control is markedly improved,
- in whom hypoglycaemia develops gradually,
- who are elderly,
- after transfer from animal insulin to human insulin,
- in whom an autonomic neuropathy is present,
- with a long history of diabetes,
- suffering from a psychiatric illness,
- receiving concurrent treatment with certain other medicinal products (see section 4.5).

Such situations may result in severe hypoglycaemia (and possibly loss of consciousness) prior to the patient's awareness of hypoglycaemia.

If normal or decreased values for glycated haemoglobin are noted, the possibility of recurrent, unrecognised (especially nocturnal) episodes of hypoglycaemia must be considered.

Adherence of the patient to the dosage and dietary regimen, correct insulin administration and awareness of hypoglycaemia symptoms are essential to reduce the risk of hypoglycaemia. Factors increasing the susceptibility to hypoglycaemia require particularly close monitoring and may necessitate dose adjustment. These include:

- change in the injection area,
- improved insulin sensitivity (by, e.g., removal of stress factors),
- unaccustomed, increased or prolonged physical activity,
- intercurrent illness (e.g. vomiting, diarrhoea),
- inadequate food intake,
- missed meals,
- alcohol consumption,
- certain uncompensated endocrine disorders (e.g. in hypothyroidism and in anterior pituitary or adrenocortical insufficiency),
- concomitant treatment with certain other medicinal products.

Intercurrent illness

Intercurrent illness requires intensified metabolic monitoring. In many cases, urine tests for ketones are indicated, and often it is necessary to adjust the insulin dose. The insulin requirement is often increased. Patients with type 1 diabetes must continue to consume at least a small amount of carbohydrates on a regular basis, even if they are able to eat only little or no food, or are vomiting etc. and they must never omit insulin entirely.

Handling of the pen

Before using OptiSet, the Instructions for Use included in the Package Leaflet must be read carefully. OptiSet has to be used as recommended in these Instructions for Use (see section 6.6).

4.5 Interaction with other medicinal products and other forms of interaction

A number of substances affect glucose metabolism and may require dose adjustment of human insulin.

Substances that may enhance the blood-glucose-lowering effect and increase susceptibility to hypoglycaemia include oral antidiabetic agents, angiotensin converting enzyme (ACE) inhibitors, disopyramide, fibrates, fluoxetine, monoamine oxidase (MAO) inhibitors, pentoxifylline, propoxyphene, salicylates and sulphonamide antibiotics.

Substances that may reduce the blood-glucose-lowering effect include corticosteroids, danazol, diazoxide, diuretics, glucagon, isoniazid, oestrogens and progestogens (e.g.in oral contraceptives), phenothiazine derivatives, somatropin, sympathomimetic agents (e.g. epinephrine [adrenaline], salbutamol, terbutaline), thyroid hormones, protease inhibitors and atypical antipsychotic medicinal products (e.g. olanzapine and clozapine).

Beta-blockers, clonidine, lithium salts or alcohol may either potentiate or weaken the blood-glucose-lowering effect of insulin. Pentamidine may cause hypoglycaemia which may sometimes be followed by hyperglycaemia.

In addition, under the influence of sympatholytic medicinal products such as beta-blockers, clonidine, guanethidine and reserpine, the signs of adrenergic counter-regulation may be reduced or absent.

4.6 Pregnancy and lactation

Pregnancy

For insulin human, no clinical data on exposed pregnancies are available. Insulin does not cross the placental barrier. Caution should be exercised when prescribing to pregnant women.

It is essential for patients with pre-existing or gestational diabetes to maintain good metabolic control throughout pregnancy. Insulin requirements may decrease during the first trimester and generally increase during the second and third trimesters. Immediately after delivery, insulin requirements decline rapidly (increased risk of hypoglycaemia). Careful monitoring of glucose control is essential.

Lactation

No effects on the suckling child are anticipated. Insuman Rapid can be used during breastfeeding. Lactating women may require adjustments in insulin dose and diet.

4.7 Effects on ability to drive and use machines

The patient's ability to concentrate and react may be impaired as a result of hypoglycaemia or hyperglycaemia or, for example, as a result of visual impairment. This may constitute a risk in situations where these abilities are of special importance (e.g. driving a car or operating machinery).

Patients should be advised to take precautions to avoid hypoglycaemia whilst driving. This is particularly important in those who have reduced or absent awareness of the warning symptoms of hypoglycaemia or have frequent episodes of hypoglycaemia. It should be considered whether it is advisable to drive or operate machinery in these circumstances.

4.8 Undesirable effects

Hypoglycaemia, in general the most frequent undesirable effect of insulin therapy, may occur if the insulin dose is too high in relation to the insulin requirement. In clinical trials and during marketed use, the frequency varies with patient population and dose regimens. Therefore, no specific frequency can be presented.

Severe hypoglycaemic attacks, especially if recurrent, may lead to neurological damage. Prolonged or severe hypoglycaemic episodes may be life-threatening.

In many patients, the signs and symptoms of neuroglycopenia are preceded by signs of adrenergic counter-regulation. Generally, the greater and more rapid the decline in blood glucose, the more marked is the phenomenon of counter-regulation and its symptoms.

The following related adverse reactions from clinical investigations are listed below by system organ class and in order of decreasing incidence: very common (≥1/10); common (≥1/100, <1/10); uncommon (≥1/1,000, <1/100); rare (≥1/10,000, <1/1,000); very rare (<1/10,000), not known (cannot be estimated from the available data).

Within each frequency grouping, undesirable effects are presented in order of decreasing seriousness.

Immune system disorders

Uncommon: shock

Not known: immediate type allergic reactions (hypotension, angioneurotic oedema, bronchospasm, generalised skin reactions), anti-insulin antibodies

Immediate type allergic reactions to insulin or to the excipients may be life-threatening.

Insulin administration may cause anti-insulin antibodies to form. In rare cases, the presence of such anti-insulin antibodies may necessitate adjustment of the insulin dose in order to correct a tendency to hyper- or hypoglycaemia.

Metabolism and nutrition disorders

Common: oedema

Not known: sodium retention

Insulin may cause sodium retention and oedema, particularly if previously poor metabolic control is improved by intensified insulin therapy.

Eyes disorders

Not known: proliferative retinopathy, diabetic retinopathy, visual impairment

A marked change in glycaemic control may cause temporary visual impairment, due to temporary alteration in the turgidity and refractive index of the lens.

Long-term improved glycaemic control decreases the risk of progression of diabetic retinopathy. However, intensification of insulin therapy with abrupt improvement in glycaemic control may be associated with temporary worsening of diabetic retinopathy.

Skin and subcutaneous tissue disorders

Not known: lipodystrophy

As with any insulin therapy, lipodystrophy may occur at the injection site and delay local insulin absorption. Continuous rotation of the injection site within the given injection area may help to reduce or prevent these reactions.

General disorders and administration site conditions

Common: injection site reactions

Uncommon: injection site urticaria,

Not known: injection site inflammation, injection site swelling, injection site pain, injection site pruritus, injection site erythema.

Most minor reactions to insulins at the injection site usually resolve in a few days to a few weeks.

4.9 Overdose

Symptoms

Insulin overdose may lead to severe and sometimes long-term and life-threatening hypoglycaemia.

Management

Mild episodes of hypoglycaemia can usually be treated with oral carbohydrates. Adjustments in dosage of the medicinal product, meal patterns, or physical activity may be needed.

More severe episodes with coma, seizure, or neurologic impairment may be treated with intramuscular/subcutaneous glucagon or concentrated intravenous glucose. Sustained carbohydrate intake and observation may be necessary because hypoglycaemia may recur after apparent clinical recovery.

5. PHARMACOLOGICAL PROPERTIES

5.1 Pharmacodynamic properties

Pharmacotherapeutic group: Antidiabetic agent. Insulins and analogues, fast-acting, ATC Code: A10AB01.

Mode of action

Insulin

- lowers blood glucose and promotes anabolic effects as well as decreasing catabolic effects,
- increases the transport of glucose into cells as well as the formation of glycogen in the muscles and the liver, and improves pyruvate utilisation. It inhibits glycogenolysis and gluconeogenesis,
- increases lipogenesis in the liver and adipose tissue and inhibits lipolysis,
- promotes the uptake of amino acids into cells and promotes protein synthesis,
- enhances the uptake of potassium into cells.

Pharmacodynamic characteristics

Insuman Rapid is an insulin with rapid onset and short duration of action. Following subcutaneous injection, onset of action is within 30 minutes, the phase of maximum action is between 1 and 4 hours after injection and the duration of action is 7 to 9 hours.

5.2 Pharmacokinetic properties

In healthy subjects, the serum half-life of insulin is approximately 4 to 6 minutes. It is longer in patients with severe renal insufficiency. However, it must be noted that the pharmacokinetics of insulin do not reflect its metabolic action.

5.3 Preclinical safety data

The acute toxicity was studied following subcutaneous administration in rats. No evidence of toxic effects was found. Local tolerability studies following subcutaneous and intramuscular administration in rabbits gave no remarkable findings. Studies of pharmacodynamic effects following subcutaneous administration in rabbits and dogs revealed the expected hypoglycaemic reactions.

6. PHARMACEUTICAL PARTICULARS

6.1 List of excipients

Metacresol,

sodium dihydrogen phosphate dihydrate,

glycerol,

sodium hydroxide,

hydrochloric acid (for pH adjustment),

water for injections.

6.2 Incompatibilities

This medicinal product must not be mixed with other medicinal products except those mentioned in section 6.6.

Concerning mixing or incompatibility with other insulins see section 6.6. Care must be taken to ensure that no alcohol or other disinfectants enter the insulin solution.

6.3 Shelf life

2 years.

Shelf life after first use of the pen:

The pen in-use or carried as a spare may be stored for a maximum of 4 weeks not above 25°C away from direct heat or direct light.

Pens in-usemust not be stored in the refrigerator.

The pen cap must be put back on the pen after each injection in order to protect from light.

6.4 Special precautions for storage

Not in-use pens:

Store in a refrigerator (2°C - 8°C).

Do not freeze.

Do not put Insuman Rapid next to the freezer compartment or a freezer pack.

Keep the pre-filled pen in the outer carton in order to protect from light.

In-use pens:

For storage precautions, see section 6.3.

6.5 Nature and contents of container

3 ml solution in a cartridge (type 1 colourless glass) with a plunger (bromobutyl rubber (type 1)) and a flanged cap (aluminium) with a stopper (bromobutyl or laminate of polyisoprene and bromobutyl rubber (type 1)).

The cartridges are sealed in a disposable pen injector. Injection needles are not included in the pack.

Packs of 5 pens are available.

6.6 Special precautions for disposal and other handling

Insuman Rapid must only be used if the solution is clear, colourless, with no solid particles visible, and if it is of a water-like consistency.

Empty pens must never be reused and must be properly discarded.

Handling of the pen

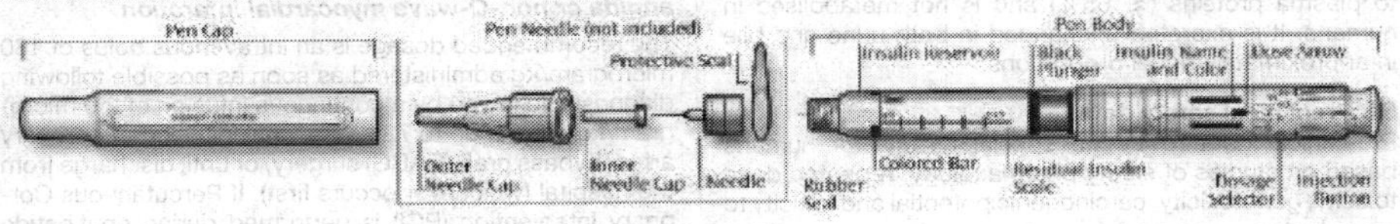

Schematic diagram of the pen

To prevent the possible transmission of disease, each pen must be used by one patient only.

As with all insulin preparations, Insuman Rapid must not be mixed with solutions containing reducing agents such as thioles and sulphites. It must also be remembered that neutral regular insulin precipitates out at a pH of approximately 4.5 to 6.5.

Mixing of insulins

Insuman Rapid must not be mixed with any other insulin or with insulin analogues.

Any unused product or waste material should be disposed of in accordance with local requirements.

Handling of the pen

The Instructions for Use included in the Package Leaflet must be read carefully before using OptiSet.

(see Handling of the pen above)

Important information for use of OptiSet:

- Always attach a new needle before each use. Only use needles that are compatible for use with OptiSet.
- Always perform the safety test before each injection.
- If a new OptiSet is used the initial safety test must be done with the 8 units preset by the manufacturer.
- The dosage selector can only be turned in one direction.
- Never turn the dosage selector (change the dose) after injection button has been pulled out.
- This pen is only for the patients use. It must not be shared with anyone else.
- If the injection is given by another person, special caution must be taken by this person to avoid accidental needle injury and transmission of infection.
- Never use OptiSet if it is damaged or if you are not sure that it is working properly.
- Always have a spare OptiSet in case your OptiSet is lost or damaged.

Storage Instructions

Please check section 6.4 of this leaflet for instructions on how to store OptiSet.

If OptiSet is in cool storage, it should be taken out 1 to 2 hours before injection to allow it to warm up. Cold insulin is more painful to inject.

The used OptiSet must be discarded as required by your local authorities.

Maintenance

OptiSet has to be protected from dust and dirt.

You can clean the outside of your OptiSet by wiping it with a damp cloth.

Do not soak, wash or lubricate the pen as this may damage it.

OptiSet is designed to work accurately and safely. It should be handled with care. Avoid situations where OptiSet might be damaged. If you are concerned that your OptiSet may be damaged, use a new one.

Step 1. Check the Insulin

After removing the pen cap, the label on the pen and the insulin reservoir should be checked to make sure it contains the correct insulin. The appearance of insulin should also be checked: the insulin solution must be clear, colourless, with no solid particles visible, and must have a water-like consistency. Do not use this OptiSet if insulin is cloudy, coloured or has particles.

Step 2. Attach the needle

The needle should be carefully attached straight onto the pen.

Step 3. Perform a safety test

Prior to each injection a safety test has to be performed.

For a new and unused OptiSet, a dose of 8 units is already preset by the manufacturer for the first safety test.

In-use OptiSet, select a dose of 2 units by turning the dosage selector forward till the dose arrow points to 2. The dosage selector will only turn in one direction.

Pull out the injection button completely in order to load the dose. Never turn the dosage selector after injection button has been pulled out.

The outer and inner needle caps should be removed. Keep the outer cap to remove the used needle.

While holding the pen with the needle pointing upwards, the insulin reservoir should be tapped with the finger so that any air bubbles rise up towards the needle

Then the injection button should be pressed all the way in.

If insulin has been expelled through the needle tip, then the pen and the needle are working properly.

If no insulin appears at the needle tip, step 3 should be repeated two more times until insulin appears at the needle tip. If still no insulin comes out, change the needle, as it might be blocked and try again. If no insulin comes out after changing the needle, the OptiSet may be damaged. Do not use this OptiSet.

Step 4. Select the dose

The dose can be set in steps of 2 units, from a minimum of 2 units to a maximum of 40 units. If a dose greater than 40 units is required, it should be given as two or more injections.

Check if you have enough insulin for the dose.

The residual insulin scale on the transparent insulin reservoir shows approximately how much insulin remains in the OptiSet. This scale must not be used to set the insulin dose.

If the black plunger is at the beginning of the coloured bar, then there are approximately 40 units of insulin available.

If the black plunger is at the end of the coloured bar, then there are approximately 20 units of insulin available.

The dosage selector should be turned forward until the dose arrow points to the required dose.

Step 5. Load the dose

The injection button should be pulled out as far as it will go in order to load the pen.

Check if the selected dose is fully loaded. Note that the injection button only goes out as far as the amount of insulin that is left in the reservoir.

The injection button allows checking the actual loaded dose. The injection button must be held out under tension during this check. The last thick line visible on the injection button shows the amount of insulin loaded. When the injection button is held out only the top part of this thick line can be seen.

Step 6. Inject the dose

The patient should be informed on the injection technique by his health care professional.

The needle should be inserted into the skin.

The injection button should be pressed all the way in completely. A clicking sound can be heard, which will stop when the injection button has been pressed in completely. Then the injection button should be held down 10 seconds before withdrawing the needle from the skin. This ensures that the full dose of insulin has been delivered.

Step 7. Remove and discard the needle

The needle should be removed after each injection and discarded. This will help prevent contamination and/or infection as well as entry of air into the insulin reservoir and leakage of insulin, which can cause inaccurate dosing. Needles must not be reused.

The pen cap should be replaced on the pen.

7. MARKETING AUTHORISATION HOLDER

Sanofi-Aventis Deutschland GmbH, D-65926 Frankfurt am Main, Germany

8. MARKETING AUTHORISATION NUMBER(S)

EU/1/97/030/067

9. DATE OF FIRST AUTHORISATION/RENEWAL OF THE AUTHORISATION

Date of first authorisation: 21 February 1997

Date of latest renewal: 21 February 2007

10. DATE OF REVISION OF THE TEXT

June 2008

Legal Category: POM

Intal CFC-free Inhaler

(sanofi-aventis)

1. NAME OF THE MEDICINAL PRODUCT

Intal CFC-free Inhaler

2. QUALITATIVE AND QUANTITATIVE COMPOSITION

The active component of Intal CFC-free is sodium cromoglicate 3.521% w/w. Each canister provides at least 112 actuations each containing 5 mg of sodium cromoglicate.

For excipients, see section 6.1.

3. PHARMACEUTICAL FORM

Intal CFC-free is presented as a metered dose inhaler, containing sodium cromoglicate as a suspension in a new non-CFC propellant, apaflurane (HFA-227), for inhalation. The product contains no chlorofluorocarbons (CFCs).

4. CLINICAL PARTICULARS

4.1 Therapeutic indications

Intal CFC-free is indicated for the preventative treatment of bronchial asthma, in adults and children.

4.2 Posology and method of administration

Intal CFC-free is for oral inhalation use only. It is essential to instruct the patient how to use the inhaler correctly.

Adults and Children

The initial dose is two inhalations of the aerosol four times daily. Once adequate control of symptoms has been achieved it may be possible to reduce to a maintenance dose of one inhalation four times daily. However, the dose may be increased to two inhalations six or eight times daily in more severe cases or during periods of severe antigen challenge. An additional dose before exercise may also be taken.

Elderly

No current evidence for alteration of the recommended adult dose

Concomitant Bronchodilator Therapy

Where a concomitant aerosol bronchodilator is prescribed it is recommended that this be administered prior to Intal CFC-free.

Concomitant Steroid Therapy

In patients currently treated with steroids, the addition of Intal CFC-free to the regimen may make it possible to reduce the maintenance dose of steroids, or discontinue steroid therapy completely. The patient must be carefully supervised while the steroid dose is reduced; a rate of 10% weekly is suggested.

If reduction of a steroid dosage has been possible, Intal CFC-free should not be withdrawn until steroid cover has been reinstituted.

Method of Administration

If the inhaler is new, it should be primed by actuating 4 times prior to inhalation. If not used for more than 3 days, additional priming with 1-2 actuations is advised.

The inhaler should be well shaken and the dustcap removed. The patient should be instructed to breathe in slowly and deeply and as inhalation begins the aerosol should be actuated by pressing the can down firmly with the first finger whilst continuing to breathe in. The breath should then be held for several seconds before exhaling into the air. To avoid condensation of moisture in the inhaler and blocking of the spray, exhalation through the inhaler should be avoided. The dustcap should be replaced following use. To prevent excessive accumulation of powder the plastic body and mouthpiece cover should be washed twice a week and then thoroughly dried. If the Fisonair holding chamber is used this should also should be washed twice a week and thoroughly dried.

Children and patients with difficulty in coordinating actuation of the inhaler with inhalation of the aerosol cloud, may benefit from using a holding chamber to assist inhalation of the medication. When using a holding chamber the procedure for inhalation is different from that with the standard mouthpiece. The medication is first released into the holding chamber from which it is subsequently inhaled (in one or more breaths) until the chamber is empty. Thus, there is no need to coordinate actuation of the inhaler with simultaneous breathing, but the medication must be inhaled slowly and deeply from the holding chamber. The standard mouthpiece, is suitable for use with a large volume holding chamber such as Fisonair.

Detailed instructions for the inhalation of Intal CFC-free from the devices are provided in the respective Patient Information Leaflet supplied with each pack.

4.3 Contraindications

Intal CFC-free is contraindicated in patients with known hypersensitivity to sodium cromoglicate or to any of the other constituents.

4.4 Special warnings and precautions for use

Intal CFC-free must not be used for relief of an acute attack of bronchospasm.

Since therapy is prophylactic, it is important that Intal CFC-free should be used regularly every day, in those patients who benefit, even if they become asymptomatic. The patient should also be advised that because several doses may be needed to establish benefit, relief may not be apparent immediately, but may take some weeks to develop.

Patients should have relief medication, such as an inhaled short-acting bronchodilator, available to relieve symptoms of acute asthma, and must be instructed to seek medical attention if their relief medication becomes less effective, or if more inhalations than usual are required to control symptoms.

In those cases where corticosteroid therapy has been reduced or discontinued, such therapy may need to be increased or reinstated if symptoms of asthma worsen - particularly during periods of stress, such as infection, illness, trauma, or severe antigen challenge. Alternative therapeutic management may also need to be considered.

Intal CFC-Free should be discontinued if eosinophilic pneumonia appears.

Withdrawal of INTAL CFC-free therapy

If it is necessary to withdraw this treatment, it should be done progressively over a period of one week. Symptoms of asthma may recur.

4.5 Interaction with other medicinal products and other forms of interaction

Sodium cromoglicate has been used for the treatment of a variety of indications in man for many years and no interactions with other drugs have been reported, nor are expected for sodium cromoglicate, due to its pharmacokinetic properties (no metabolism, moderate plasma protein binding, low plasma concentrations) and its high safety profile.

4.6 Pregnancy and lactation

As with all medication, caution should be exercised especially during the first trimester of pregnancy. Although there is no information with the new HFA-227 formulation in human pregnancy cumulative clinical experience with sodium cromoglicate formulated with CFC propellants, suggests that the active ingredient sodium cromoglicate has no adverse effects on foetal development. In addition, both the new HFA-227 propellant and sodium cromoglicate have been separately shown to be free of adverse effects on the foetus in laboratory animals. It should only be used in pregnancy where there is a clear need.

It is not known whether sodium cromoglicate is excreted in human breast milk but on the basis of its physico-chemical properties this is considered unlikely. There is no evidence to suggest that the use of sodium cromoglicate has any undesirable effects on the baby, however, there is no experience to date with either the new HFA-227 propellant alone or formulated with sodium cromoglicate, during lactation in asthmatic patients. It should only be used in lactation where there is a clear need.

4.7 Effects on ability to drive and use machines

Intal CFC-free has no known effect on ability to drive or operate machinery.

4.8 Undesirable effects

Mild throat irritation, coughing and transient bronchospasm may occur. Headache and rhinitis have also been reported in clinical trials of Intal CFC-free. Hypersensitivity reactions, including angioedema, bronchospasm, hypotension and collapse, have been reported extremely rarely, in patients using inhaled sodium cromoglicate.

As with other inhalation therapy, paradoxical bronchospasm may occur immediately after administration: in such cases immediate treatment with a fast-acting bronchodilator is required and immediate medical attention must be sought. Therapy with Intal CFC-free should be discontinued and alternative treatment instituted.

Very rare cases of eosinophilic pneumonia have been reported.

4.9 Overdose

Animal studies have shown that sodium cromoglicate has a very low local or systemic toxicity and extended human studies have not revealed any safety hazard with products containing sodium cromoglicate. Overdosage is therefore unlikely to cause problems, but, if suspected, treatment should be supportive and directed to the control of the relevant symptoms.

5. PHARMACOLOGICAL PROPERTIES

5.1 Pharmacodynamic properties

Sodium cromoglicate inhibits the activation of many of the cell types involved in the development and progression of asthma. Thus, sodium cromoglicate inhibits the release of inflammatory mediators including cytokines from mast cells and reduces the chemotactic activity of eosinophils and neutrophils. Activation of and mediator release from monocytes and macrophages in vitro is also reduced by sodium cromoglicate.

The diverse range of activities of the drug may be explained by the ability of sodium cromoglicate to block chloride channels in different cell types which are important in cell activation.

In acute bronchial provocation tests in humans, sodium cromoglicate has been shown to inhibit or diminish the asthmatic reaction to antigen, exercise and to a range of non-specific triggers including cold air, sulphur dioxide, hypertonic saline and bradykinin. Antigen-induced increased bronchial hyperactivity to histamine is prevented and a reduction in bronchial mucus eosinophils and antigen-specific IgE occurs after 4 weeks treatment of asthmatic subjects with sodium cromoglicate.

5.2 Pharmacokinetic properties

ACT code: Antiallergic agents, excl. corticosteroids RO3BC01.

After inhalation in man via a metered dose inhaler approximately 10% of a dose of sodium cromoglicate is absorbed from the respiratory tract. The remainder is either exhaled or deposited in the oropharynx, or swallowed and eliminated via the alimentary tract, as only a small amount (1%) of the dose is absorbed from the gastrointestinal tract. The rate of absorption of sodium cromoglicate from the respiratory tract is slower than the elimination rate ($t_{½}$ of 1.5-2h). Hence, the drug remains effectively in the lungs to produce its local therapeutic effect and is then cleared rapidly from the systemic circulation. No substantial increase in plasma concentration occurs during repeated dose therapy.

Sodium cromoglicate is moderately and reversibly bound to plasma proteins (≈ 65%) and is not metabolised in humans. It is excreted unchanged in both urine and bile in approximately equal proportions.

5.3 Preclinical safety data

Pre-clinical data reveal no special hazard for humans based on studies of safety pharmacology, repeated dose toxicity, genotoxicity, carcinogenic potential and toxicity to reproduction.

6. PHARMACEUTICAL PARTICULARS

6.1 List of excipients

Polyvidone K30

Polyethylene glycol (PEG) 600

Apaflurane (HFA 227 - a non ozone depleting propellant).

6.2 Incompatibilities

Not applicable.

6.3 Shelf life

30 months.

6.4 Special precautions for storage

Do not refrigerate or freeze.

As the aerosol inhaler canister is pressurised it should be protected from heat or direct sunlight and should not be punctured or incinerated even when empty.

6.5 Nature and contents of container

The aluminium can is fitted with a metering valve which delivers 112 actuations each containing 5 mg of sodium cromoglicate.

Intal CFC-free Inhaler: The cartoned pack consists of an aerosol canister and a plastic adaptor with a dustcap.

6.6 Special precautions for disposal and other handling

Not applicable.

7. MARKETING AUTHORISATION HOLDER

Sanofi-aventis

One Onslow Street

Guildford

Surrey

GU1 4YS, UK

8. MARKETING AUTHORISATION NUMBER(S)

PL 04425/0179

9. DATE OF FIRST AUTHORISATION/RENEWAL OF THE AUTHORISATION

23 May 2001

10. DATE OF REVISION OF THE TEXT

January 2009

Legal Classification

POM

Integrilin 2mg solution for injection, 0.75mg solution for infusion

(GlaxoSmithKline UK)

1. NAME OF THE MEDICINAL PRODUCT

INTEGRILIN 0.75 mg/ml, solution for infusion

INTEGRILIN 2 mg/ml, solution for injection

2. QUALITATIVE AND QUANTITATIVE COMPOSITION

INTEGRILIN solution for infusion contains 0.75 mg/ml of eptifibatide.

INTEGRILIN solution for injection contains 2 mg/ml of eptifibatide.

For a full list of excipients, see section 6.1.

3. PHARMACEUTICAL FORM

Solution for infusion and solution for injection

Clear, colourless solution

4. CLINICAL PARTICULARS

4.1 Therapeutic indications

INTEGRILIN is intended for use with acetylsalicylic acid and unfractionated heparin.

INTEGRILIN is indicated for the prevention of early myocardial infarction in patients presenting with unstable angina or non-Q-wave myocardial infarction with the last episode of chest pain occurring within 24 hours and with ECG changes and/or elevated cardiac enzymes.

Patients most likely to benefit from INTEGRILIN treatment are those at high risk of developing myocardial infarction within the first 3-4 days after onset of acute angina symptoms including for instance those that are likely to undergo an early PTCA (Percutaneous Transluminal Coronary Angioplasty) (see section 5.1).

4.2 Posology and method of administration

This product is for hospital use only, by specialist physicians experienced in the management of acute coronary syndromes.

INTEGRILIN solution for infusion must be used in conjunction with INTEGRILIN solution for injection.

Adults (⩾ 18 years of age) presenting with unstable angina or non-Q-wave myocardial infarction

The recommended dosage is an intravenous bolus of 180 microgram/kg administered as soon as possible following diagnosis, followed by a continuous infusion of 2.0 microgram/kg/min for up to 72 hours, until initiation of coronary artery bypass graft (CABG) surgery, or until discharge from the hospital (whichever occurs first). If Percutaneous Coronary Intervention (PCI) is performed during eptifibatide therapy, continue the infusion for 20-24 hours post-PCI for an overall maximum duration of therapy of 96 hours.

Emergency or semi-elective surgery

If the patient requires emergency or urgent cardiac surgery during the course of eptifibatide therapy, terminate the infusion immediately. If the patient requires semi-elective surgery, stop the eptifibatide infusion at an appropriate time to allow time for platelet function to return towards normal.

Hepatic impairment

Experience in patients with hepatic impairment is very limited. Administer with caution to patients with hepatic impairment in whom coagulation could be affected (see section 4.3, prothrombin time).

Renal impairment

In patients with moderate renal impairment (creatinine clearance ⩾ 30 - < 50 ml/min), an intravenous bolus of 180 microgram/kg should be administered followed by a continuous infusion dose of 1.0 microgram/kg/min for the duration of therapy. Experience in patients with more severe renal impairment is limited (see section 4.3).

Paediatric use

It is not recommended for use in children and adolescents below 18 years of age, due to a lack of data on safety and efficacy.

4.3 Contraindications

INTEGRILIN must not be used to treat patients with:

– hypersensitivity to the active substance or to any of the excipients

– evidence of gastrointestinal bleeding, gross genitourinary bleeding or other active abnormal bleeding within the previous 30 days of treatment

– history of stroke within 30 days or any history of haemorrhagic stroke

– known history of intracranial disease (neoplasm, arteriovenous malformation, aneurysm)

– major surgery or severe trauma within past 6 weeks

– a history of bleeding diathesis

– thrombocytopaenia (< 100,000 cells/mm^3)

– prothrombin time > 1.2 times control, or International Normalized Ratio (INR) ⩾ 2.0

– severe hypertension (systolic blood pressure > 200 mm Hg or diastolic blood pressure > 110 mm Hg on antihypertensive therapy)

– severe renal impairment (creatinine clearance < 30 ml/min) or dependency on renal dialysis;

– clinically significant hepatic impairment

– concomitant or planned administration of another parenteral GP IIb/IIIa inhibitor

4.4 Special warnings and precautions for use

Bleeding

INTEGRILIN is an antithrombotic agent that acts by inhibition of platelet aggregation; therefore the patient must be observed carefully for indications of bleeding during treatment (see section 4.8). Women, the elderly and patients with low body weight may have an increased risk of bleeding. Monitor these patients closely with regard to bleeding.

Bleeding is most common at the arterial access site in patients undergoing percutaneous arterial procedures. All potential bleeding sites, e.g., catheter insertion sites; arterial, venous, or needle puncture sites; cutdown sites; gastrointestinal and genitourinary tracts must be observed carefully. Other potential bleeding sites such as central and peripheral nervous system and retroperitoneal sites, must be carefully considered too.

Because INTEGRILIN inhibits platelet aggregation, caution must be employed when it is used with other medicinal products that affect haemostasis, including ticlopidine, clopidogrel, thrombolytics, oral anticoagulants, dextran solutions (see section 6.2), adenosine, sulfinpyrazone, prostacyclin, non-steroidal anti-inflammatory agents, or dypyridamole (see section 4.5).

There is no experience with INTEGRILIN and low molecular weight heparins.

There is limited therapeutic experience with INTEGRILIN in patients for whom thrombolytic therapy is generally indicated (e.g., acute transmural myocardial infarction with new pathological Q-waves or elevated ST-segments or left bundle branch block in the ECG). Consequently the use of INTEGRILIN is not recommended in these circumstances.

Stop the INTEGRILIN infusion immediately if circumstances arise that necessitate thrombolytic therapy or if the patient must undergo an emergency CABG surgery or requires an intraortic balloon pump.

If serious bleeding occurs that is not controllable with pressure, immediately stop the INTEGRILIN infusion and any unfractionated heparin that is given concomitantly.

Arterial procedures

During treatment with eptifibatide there is a significant increase in bleeding rates, especially in the femoral artery area, where the catheter sheath is introduced. Take care to ensure that only the anterior wall of the femoral artery is punctured. Arterial sheaths may be removed when coagulation has returned to normal (e.g., when activated clotting time [ACT] is less than 180 seconds (usually 2-6 hours after discontinuation of heparin). After removal of the introducer sheath, careful haemostasis must be ensured under close observation.

Thrombocytopaenia

INTEGRILIN inhibits platelet aggregation, but does not appear to affect the viability of platelets. As demonstrated in clinical trials, the incidence of thrombocytopaenia was low, and similar in patients treated with eptifibatide or placebo. Thrombocytopaenia, including acute profound thrombocytopaenia, has been observed with eptifibatide administration (see section 4.8). Platelet counts should be monitored prior to treatment, within 6 hours of administration, and at least once daily thereafter while on therapy and immediately at clinical signs of unexpected bleeding tendency. If the patient experiences a confirmed platelet decrease to < 100,000/mm^3, discontinue INTEGRILIN and unfractionated heparin and monitor and treat the patient appropriately. The decision to use platelet transfusions should be based upon clinical judgment on an individual basis. In patients with previous thrombocytopaenia from other parenteral GP IIb/IIIa inhibitors, there are no data with the use of INTEGRILIN, and thus these patients require close monitoring as noted above.

Heparin administration

Heparin administration is recommended unless a contra-indication (such as a history of thrombocytopaenia associated with use of heparin) is present.

UA/NQMI: For a patient who weighs ⩾ 70 kg, it is recommended that a bolus dose of 5,000 units is given, followed by a constant intravenous infusion of 1,000 units/hr. If the patient weighs < 70 kg, a bolus dose of 60 units/kg is recommended, followed by an infusion of 12 units/kg/hr. The activated partial thromboplastin time (aPTT) must be monitored in order to maintain a value between 50 and 70 seconds, above 70 seconds there may be an increased risk of bleeding.

If PCI is to be performed in the setting of UA/NQMI, monitor the activated clotting time (ACT) to maintain a value between 300-350 seconds. Stop heparin administration if the ACT exceeds 300 seconds; do not administer until the ACT falls below 300 seconds.

Monitoring of laboratory values

Before infusion of INTEGRILIN, the following laboratory tests are recommended before treatment to identify pre-existing haemostatic abnormalities: prothrombin time (PT) and aPTT, serum creatinine, platelet count, haemoglobin and haematocrit levels. Haemoglobin, haematocrit, and platelet count are to be monitored as well within 6 hours after start of therapy and at least once daily thereafter while on therapy (or more often if there is evidence of a marked decrease). If the platelet count falls below 100,000/mm^3, further platelet counts are required to rule out pseudo-thrombocytopaenia. Discontinue unfractionated heparin. In patients undergoing PCI, measure the ACT also.

Patients must be monitored for bleeding and treated if necessary (see section 4.9).

Immunogenicity

Immunogenic response or antibodies against eptifibatide have been observed in isolated cases in naïve patients or in rare cases of patients re-exposed to eptifibatide. Only limited experience exists for readministration of INTEGRILIN. If treatment with INTEGRILIN is repeated, no diminished therapeutic response is expected.

4.5 Interaction with other medicinal products and other forms of interaction

INTEGRILIN did not appear to increase the risk of major and minor bleeding associated with concomitant use of warfarin and dipyridamole. INTEGRILIN-treated patients who had a prothrombin time (PT) > 14.5 seconds and received warfarin concomitantly did not appear to be at an increased risk of bleeding.

Data are limited on the use of INTEGRILIN in patients receiving thrombolytic agents. There was no consistent evidence that eptifibatide increased the risk of major or minor bleeding associated with tissue plasminogen activator in either a PCI or an acute myocardial infarction study; however, eptifibatide appeared to increase the risk of bleeding when administered with streptokinase in an acute myocardial infarction study.

In an acute myocardial infarction study involving 181 patients, eptifibatide (in regimens up to a bolus injection of 180 microgram/kg, followed by an infusion up to 2 microgram/kg/min for up to 72 hours) was administered concomitantly with streptokinase (1.5 million units over 60 minutes). At the highest infusion rates (1.3 microgram/kg/min and 2.0 microgram/kg/min) studied, eptifibatide was associated with an increased incidence of bleeding and transfusions compared to the incidence seen when streptokinase was given alone.

4.6 Pregnancy and lactation

There are no adequate data from the use of eptifibatide in pregnant women.

Animal studies are insufficient with respect to effects on pregnancy, embryonal/foetal development, parturition or postnatal development (see section 5.3). The potential risk for humans is unknown.

INTEGRILIN should not be used during pregnancy unless clearly necessary.

It is not known whether eptifibatide is excreted in human milk. Interruption of breast-feeding during the treatment period is recommended.

4.7 Effects on ability to drive and use machines

Not relevant, as INTEGRILIN is intended for use in hospitalised patients.

4.8 Undesirable effects

The majority of undesirable effects experienced by patients treated with eptifibatide were generally related to bleeding, or to cardiovascular events that occur frequently in this patient population.

At the recommended therapeutic dose, as administered in the PURSUIT trial involving nearly 11,000 patients, bleeding was the most common complication encountered during eptifibatide therapy. Administration of eptifibatide is associated with an increase in major and minor bleeding, as classified by the criteria of the Thrombolysis in Myocardial Infarction (TIMI) study group.

Bleeding

Minor bleeding was a very common (> 1/10) complication of eptifibatide administration (13.1 % eptifibatide vs 7.6 % placebo). Minor bleeding was defined as spontaneous gross haematuria, spontaneous haematemesis, observed blood loss with a haemoglobin decrease of more than 3 g/dl, or more than 4 g/dl in the absence of an observed bleeding site. Bleeding events were more frequent in patients receiving concurrent heparin while undergoing PCI, when ACT exceeded 350 seconds (see section 4.4, heparin use).

Major bleeding was also very common (> 1/10) and reported more frequently in patients treated with eptifibatide than with placebo, i.e., 10.8 % vs 9.3 %, respectively. Major bleeding was defined as either an intracranial haemorrhage or a decrease in haemoglobin concentrations of more than 5 g/dl (see table 1).

The incidence of severe or life-threatening bleeding events with eptifibatide was common (> 1/100, < 1/10); 1.9 % vs 1.1 % with placebo. Eptifibatide treatment increased the need for blood transfusions modestly (11.8 % vs 9.3 %, placebo).

In the subgroup of patients undergoing PCI, major bleeding was observed commonly, in 9.7 % of eptifibatide-treated patients vs 4.6 % of placebo-treated patients.

Other undesirable effects

Overall, in the same trial, serious non-bleeding adverse events were reported at a similar rate in patients treated with eptifibatide and those treated with placebo.

Commonly (> 1/100, < 1/10) reported events (occurring in ⩾ 2 % across all groups) in PURSUIT were events related to the underlying disease, such as atrial fibrillation, hypotension, congestive heart failure, cardiac arrest and shock.

Adverse events reported within 30 days of initiation of eptifibatide treatment in PURSUIT are reported in Table 1 below. Patients with unstable angina/non-Q wave myocardial infarction (NQMI) [PURSUIT trial] received an IV bolus of 180 microgram/kg followed by continuous infusion of 2.0 microgram/kg/min for up to 72 hours (96 hours if PCI performed).

Within each frequency grouping in the tables below, undesirable effects are presented in decreasing order of seriousness.

Table 1. Reported Adverse Events in PURSUIT at 30 Days*

Very common (> 1/10), Common (> 1/100, < 1/10), Uncommon (> 1/1,000, < 1/100), Rare (> 1/10,000, < 1/1,000), Very rare (< 1/10,000)

Adverse Event	Placebo (N=4,696)	Eptifibatide (N=4,679)
Blood and lymphatic system disorders Very common Major Bleeding	9.3 %	10.8 %
Type or Location of Major Bleeding:		
Femoral Artery Access	1.3	2.7
CABG-related	6.7	6.5
Genitourinary	0.3	0.8
Gastrointestinal	0.4	1.5
Retroperitoneal	0.04	0.2
Oral/Oropharyngeal	0.2	1.6
Haemoglobin/Haematocrit decrease	1.5	1.4
Intracranial	0.06	0.1
Very common Minor Bleeding	7.6 %	13.1 %
Type or Location of Minor Bleeding:		
Femoral Artery Access	1.3	3.3
CABG-related	2.7	2.8
Genitourinary	1.6	3.9
Gastrointestinal	0.8	2.8
Oral/Oropharyngeal	0.3	3.0
Haemoglobin/Haematocrit decrease	1.4	1.4
Uncommon Thrombocytopaenia	< 0.1	0.2
Very common Any Non-Bleeding Adverse Event	18.7 %	19.0 %
Cardiac disorders Common		
Cardiac Arrest	2.7	2.3
Ventricular Fibrillation	1.4	1.3
Ventricular Tachycardia	1.1	1.1
Congestive Heart Failure	5.5	5.1
Atrioventricular Block	1.3	1.5
Atrial Fibrillation	6.4	6.3
Vascular disorder Common		
Shock	2.5	2.6
Hypotension	6.2	6.9
Phlebitis	1.5	1.4
Nervous system disorders Uncommon		
Cerebral ischaemia	0.5	0.4

* Causality has not been determined for all adverse events.

Table 2 (below) depicts the incidence of bleeding by TIMI criteria and by invasive cardiac procedures in the PURSUIT trial.

(see Table 2 on next page)

The most common bleeding complications were associated with cardiac invasive procedures (CABG-related or at femoral artery access site). Major bleeding was infrequent in the PURSUIT trial in the large majority of patients who did not undergo CABG within 30 days of enrollment.

Adverse events reported in the ESPRIT trial are listed in Table 3.

(see Table 3 on next page)

Post-marketing experience

Blood and lymphatic system disorders

Very rare: fatal bleeding (the majority involved central and peripheral nervous system disorders: cerebral or intracranial haemorrhages); pulmonary haemorrhage, acute profound thrombocytopaenia, haematoma, anaemia.

Immune system disorders

Very rare: anaphylactic reactions.

Skin and subcutaneous tissue disorders

Very rare: rash, application site disorders such as urticaria.

Laboratory values

Changes during eptifibatide treatment result from its known pharmacological action, i.e., inhibition of platelet aggregation. Thus, changes in laboratory parameters associated with bleeding (e.g., bleeding time) are common and expected. No apparent differences were observed between patients treated with eptifibatide or with placebo in values for liver function (SGOT/AST, SGPT/ALT, bilirubin, alkaline phosphatase) or renal function (serum creatinine, blood urea nitrogen).

4.9 Overdose

The experience in humans with overdosage of eptifibatide is extremely limited. There was no indication of severe adverse events associated with administration of accidental large bolus doses, rapid infusion reported as overdose or large cumulative doses. In the PURSUIT trial, there were 9 patients who received bolus and/or infusion doses more than double that specified in the protocol, or who were identified by the investigator as having received an overdose. There was no excessive bleeding in any of these patients, although one patient undergoing CABG surgery was reported as having had a moderate bleed. Specifically, no patients experienced an intracranial bleed.

Potentially, an overdose of eptifibatide could result in bleeding. Because of its short half-life and rapid clearance, the activity of eptifibatide may be halted readily by

Table 2. Bleeding (TIMI Criteria) by Procedures in the PURSUIT Trial

	Major		Minor	
	Placebon (%)	Eptifibatide n (%)	Placebo n (%)	Eptifibatide n (%)
Patients	**4,577**	**4,604**	**4,577**	**4,604**
Overall Incidence of Bleeding	425 (9.3 %)	498 (10.8 %)	347 (7.6 %)	604 (13.1 %)
Breakdown by Procedure: CABG	375 (8.2 %)	377 (8.2 %)	157 (3.4 %)	156 (3.4 %)
Angioplasty without CABG	27 (0.6 %)	64 (1.4 %)	102 (2.2 %)	197 (4.3 %)
Angiography without angioplasty or CABG	11 (0.2 %)	29 (0.6 %)	36 (0.8 %)	102 (2.2 %)
Medical Therapy Only	12 (0.3 %)	28 (0.6 %)	52 (1.1 %)	149 (3.2 %)

Denominators are based on the total number of patients whose TIMI classification was resolved.

Table 3. Reported Adverse Events in ESPRIT *
Very common (> 1/10), Common (> 1/100, < 1/10), Uncommon (> 1/1,000, < 1/100), Rare (> 1/10,000, <1/1,000), Very rare (< 1/10,000)

Adverse Event	Placebo (N=1,024)	Eptifibatide (N=1,040)
Blood and lymphatic system disorders		
Common		
Major Bleeding	(4) 0.4 %	(13) 1.3 %
Type or Location of Major Bleeding:		
Femoral Artery Access	0.1	0.8
Genitourinary	0.0	0.1
Retroperitoneal	0.0	0.3
Intracranial	0.1	0.2
Hematemesis	0.0	0.1
Hematuria	0.0	0.1
Other	0.2	0.4
Common		
Minor Bleeding	(18) 1.8 %	(29) 2.8 %
Type or Location of Minor Bleeding:		
Femoral Artery Access	0.9	1.0
Gastrointestinal	0.2	0.1
Hematemesis	0.4	0.6
Hematuria	0.9	1.4
Other	0.2	0.5
Uncommon		
Thrombocytopaenia	0.0	0.2
Common		
Any Non-Bleeding Adverse Event	(35) 3.4 %	(34) 3.3 %
Cardiac disorders		
Uncommon		
Cardiac Arrest	0.4	0.3
Ventricular Fibrillation	0.0	0.1
Ventricular Tachycardia	0.1	0.1
Heart Failure	0.5	0.0
Atrioventricular Block	0.1	0.0
Atrial Fibrillation	0.3	0.3
Vascular disorders		
Hypotension	0.2	0.0
Nervous system disorders		
Uncommon		
Cerebral ischaemia	0.1	0.2

* Causality has not been determined for all adverse events. Bleeding events were reported at 48 hours and non bleeding events are reported at 30 days.

discontinuing the infusion. Thus, although eptifibatide can be dialysed, the need for dialysis is unlikely.

5. PHARMACOLOGICAL PROPERTIES

5.1 Pharmacodynamic properties

Pharmacotherapeutic group: Antithrombotic agent (platelet aggregation inhibitor excl. heparin), ATC code: B01AC16

Eptifibatide, a synthetic cyclic heptapeptide containing six amino acids, including one cysteine amide and one mercaptopropionyl (desamino cysteinyl) residue, is an inhibitor of platelet aggregation and belongs to the class of RGD (arginine-glycine-aspartate)-mimetics.

Eptifibatide reversibly inhibits platelet aggregation by preventing the binding of fibrinogen, von Willebrand factor and other adhesive ligands to the glycoprotein (GP)IIb/IIIa receptors.

Eptifibatide inhibits platelet aggregation in a dose- and concentration-dependent manner as demonstrated by *ex vivo* platelet aggregation using adenosine diphosphate (ADP) and other agonists to induce platelet aggregation. The effect of eptifibatide is observed immediately after administration of a 180 microgram/kg intravenous bolus. When followed by a 2.0 microgram/kg/min continuous infusion, this regimen produces a > 80 % inhibition of ADP-induced *ex vivo* platelet aggregation, at physiologic calcium concentrations, in more than 80 % of patients.

Platelet inhibition was readily reversed, with a return of platelet function towards baseline (> 50 % platelet aggregation) 4 hours after stopping a continuous infusion of 2.0 microgram/kg/min. Measurements of ADP-induced *ex vivo* platelet aggregation at physiologic calcium concentrations (D-phenylalanyl-L-prolyl-L-arginine chloromethyl ketone [PPACK] anticoagulant) in patients presenting with unstable angina and Non Q-Wave Myocardial Infarction showed a concentration-dependent inhibition with an IC_{50} (50 % inhibitory concentration) of approximately 550 ng/ml and an IC_{80} (80 % inhibitory concentration) of approximately 1,100 ng/ml.

PURSUIT trial

The pivotal clinical trial for Unstable Angina (UA)/Non-Q Wave Myocardial Infarction (NQMI) was PURSUIT. This study was a 726-center, 27-country, double-blind, randomised, placebo-controlled study in 10,948 patients presenting with UA or NQMI. Patients could be enrolled only if they had experienced cardiac ischemia at rest (> 10 minutes) within the previous 24 hours and had:

- either ST-segment changes: ST depression > 0.5 mm of less than 30 minutes or persistent ST elevation > 0.5 mm not requiring reperfusion therapy or thrombolytic agents, T-wave inversion (> 1 mm),
- or increased CK-MB.

Patients were randomised to either placebo, eptifibatide 180 microgram/kg bolus followed by a 2.0 microgram/kg/min infusion (180/2.0), or eptifibatide 180 microgram/kg bolus followed by a 1.3 microgram/kg/min infusion (180/1.3).

The infusion was continued until hospital discharge, until the time of coronary artery bypass grafting (CABG) or for up to 72 hours, whichever occurred first. If PCI was performed, the eptifibatide infusion was continued for 24 hours after the procedure, allowing for a duration of infusion up to 96 hours.

The 180/1.3 arm was stopped after an interim analysis, as prespecified in the protocol, when the two active-treatment arms appeared to have a similar incidence of bleeding.

Patients were managed according to the usual standards of the investigational site; frequencies of angiography, PCI and CABG therefore differed widely from site to site and from country to country. Of the patients in PURSUIT, 13 % were managed with PCI during eptifibatide infusion, of whom approximately 50 % received intracoronary stents; 87 % were managed medically (without PCI during eptifibatide infusion).

The vast majority of patients received acetylsalicylic acid (75-325 mg once daily).

Unfractionated heparin was administered intravenously or subcutaneously at the physician's discretion, most commonly as an intravenous bolus of 5,000 U followed by a continuous infusion of 1,000 U/h. A target aPTT of 50-70 seconds was recommended. A total of 1,250 patients underwent PCI within 72 hours after randomisation, in which case they received intravenous unfractionated heparin to maintain an activated clotting time (ACT) of 300-350 seconds.

The primary endpoint of the study was the occurrence of death from any cause or new myocardial infarction (MI) (evaluated by a blinded Clinical Events Committee) within 30 days of randomisation. The component MI could be defined as asymptomatic with enzymatic elevation of CK-MB or new Q wave.

Compared to placebo, eptifibatide administered as 180/2.0 significantly reduced the incidence of the primary endpoint events (table 4): this represents around 15 events avoided for 1,000 patients treated:

Table 4
Incidence of Death/CEC-Assessed MI («Treated as Randomised» Population)

Time	Placebo	Eptifibatide	p-Value
30 days	743/4,697 (15.8 %)	667/4,680 (14.3 %)	0.034[a]

a: Pearson's chi-square test of difference between placebo and eptifibatide.

Results on the primary endpoint were principally attributed to the occurrence of myocardial infarction.

The reduction in the incidence of endpoint events in patients receiving eptifibatide appeared early during treatment (within the first 72-96 hours) and this reduction was maintained through 6 months, without any significant effect on mortality.

Patients most likely to benefit from eptifibatide treatment are those at high risk of developing myocardial infarction within the first 3-4 days after onset of acute angina.

According to epidemiological findings, a higher incidence of cardiovascular events has been associated with certain indicators, for instance:

– age
– elevated heart rate or blood pressure
– persistent or recurrent ischemic cardiac pain

– marked ECG changes (in particular ST-segment abnormalities)

– raised cardiac enzymes or markers (e.g. CK-MB, troponins) and

– heart failure

ESPRIT trial

ESPRIT (Enhanced Suppression of the Platelet IIb/IIIa Receptor with eptifibatide Therapy) was a double-blind, randomised, placebo-controlled trial (n= 2,064) for nonurgent PCI with intracoronary stenting.

All patients received routine standard of care and were randomised to either placebo or eptifibatide (2 bolus doses of 180 microgram/kg and a continuous infusion until discharge from hospital or a maximum of 18-24 hours).

The first bolus and the infusion were started simultaneously, immediately before the PCI procedure and were followed by a second bolus 10 minutes after the first. The rate of infusion was 2.0 microgram/kg/min for patients with serum creatinine ⩽ 175 micromols/l or 1.0 microgram/kg/min for serum creatinine > 175 up to 350 micromols/l.

In the eptifibatide arm of the trial, virtually all patients received aspirin (99.7 %), and 98.1 % received a thienopyridine, (clopidogrel in 95.4 % and ticlopidine in 2.7 %). On the day of PCI, prior to catheterization, 53.2 % received a thienopyridine (clopidogrel 52.7 %; ticlopidine 0.5 %) – mostly as a loading dose (300 mg or more). The placebo arm was comparable (aspirin 99.7 %, clopidogrel 95.9 %, ticlopidin 2.6 %).

The ESPRIT trial used a simplified regimen of heparin during PCI that consisted of an initial bolus of 60 units/kg, with a target ACT of 200 - 300 seconds. The primary endpoint of the trial was death (D), MI, urgent target vessel revascularisation (UTVR), and acute antithrombotic rescue with GP IIb/IIIa inhibitor therapy (RT) within 48 hours of randomisation.

MI was identified per the CK-MB core laboratory criteria. For this diagnosis, within 24 hours after the index PCI procedure, there had to be at least two CK-MB values ⩾ 3 × the upper limit of normal; thus, validation by the CEC was not required. MI could also be reported following CEC adjudication of an investigator report.

The primary endpoint analysis [quadruple composite of death, MI, urgent target vessel revascularisation (UTVR) and thrombolytic bail-out (TBO) at 48 hours] showed a 37 % relative and 3.9 % absolute reduction in the eptifibatide group (6.6 % events versus 10.5 %, p = 0.0015). Results on the primary endpoint were mainly attributed to the reduction of enzymatic MI occurrence, identified as the occurrence of early elevation of cardiac enzymes after PCI (80 out of 92 MIs in the placebo group vs. 47 out of 56 MIs in the eptifibitide group). The clinical relevance of such enzymatic MIs is still controversial.

Similar results were also obtained for the 2 secondary endpoints assessed at 30 days: a triple composite of death, MI and UTVR, and the more robust combination of death and MI.

The reduction in the incidence of endpoint events in patients receiving eptifibatide appeared early during treatment. There was no increased benefit thereafter, up to 1 year.

Prolongation of bleeding time

Administration of eptifibatide by intravenous bolus and infusion causes up to a 5-fold increase in bleeding time. This increase is readily reversible upon discontinuation of the infusion with bleeding times returning towards baseline inapproximately 6 (2-8) hours. When administered alone, eptifibatide has no measurable effect on prothrombin time (PT) or activated partial thromboplastin time (aPTT).

5.2 Pharmacokinetic properties

The pharmacokinetics of eptifibatide are linear and dose proportional for bolus doses ranging from 90 to 250 microgram/kg and infusion rates from 0.5 to 3.0 microgram/kg/min. For a 2.0 microgram/kg/min infusion, mean steady-state plasma eptifibatide concentrations range from 1.5 to 2.2 microgram/ml in patients with coronary artery disease. These plasma concentrations are achieved rapidly when the infusion is preceded by a 180 microgram/kg bolus. The extent of eptifibatide binding to human plasma protein is about 25 %. In the same population, plasma elimination half-life is approximately 2.5 hours, plasma clearance 55 to 80 ml/kg/hr and volume of distribution of approximately 185 to 260 ml/kg.

In healthy subjects, renal excretion accounted for approximately 50 % of total body clearance; approximately 50 % of the amount cleared is excreted unchanged. In patients with moderate to severe renal insufficiency (creatinine clearance < 50 ml/min), the clearance of eptifibatide is reduced by approximately 50% and steady-state plasma levels are approximately doubled.

No formal pharmacokinetic interaction studies have been conducted. However, in a population pharmacokinetic study there was no evidence of a pharmacokinetic interaction between eptifibatide and the following concomitant medicinal products: amlodipine, atenolol, atropine, captopril, cefazolin, diazepam, digoxin, diltiazem, diphenhydramine, enalapril, fentanyl, furosemide, heparin, lidocaine, lisinopril, metoprolol, midazolam, morphine, nitrates, nifedipine, and warfarin.

5.3 Preclinical safety data

Toxicology studies conducted with eptifibatide include single and repeated dose studies in the rat, rabbit and monkey, reproduction studies in the rat and rabbit, *in vitro* and *in vivo* genetic toxicity studies, and irritation, hypersensitivity and antigenicity studies. No unexpected toxic effects for an agent with this pharmacologic profile were observed and findings were predictive of clinical experience, with bleeding effects being the principal adverse event. No genotoxic effects were observed with eptifibatide.

Teratology studies have been performed by continuous intravenous infusion of eptifibatide in pregnant rats at total daily doses of up to 72 mg/kg/day (about 4 times the recommended maximum daily human dose on a body surface area basis) and in pregnant rabbits at total daily doses of up to 36 mg/kg/day (about 4 times the recommended maximum daily human dose on a body surface area basis). These studies revealed no evidence of impaired fertility or harm to the foetus due to eptifibatide. Reproduction studies in animal species where eptifibatide shows a similar pharmacologic activity as in humans are not available. Consequently these studies are not suitable to evaluate the toxicity of eptifibatide on reproductive function (see section 4.6).

The carcinogenic potential of eptifibatide has not been evaluated in long-term studies.

6. PHARMACEUTICAL PARTICULARS

6.1 List of excipients

Citric acid monohydrate

Sodium hydroxide

Water for injections

6.2 Incompatibilities

INTEGRILIN is not compatible with furosemide.

In the absence of compatibility studies, INTEGRILIN must not be mixed with other medicinal products except those mentioned in 6.6.

6.3 Shelf life

3 years

6.4 Special precautions for storage

Store in a refrigerator (2°C - 8°C). Store in the original carton in order to protect from light.

6.5 Nature and contents of container

INTEGRILIN 0.75 mg/ml, solution for infusion: One 100 ml Type I glass vial, closed with a butyl rubber stopper and sealed with a crimped aluminium seal.

INTEGRILIN 2 mg/ml, solution for injection: One 10 ml Type I glass vial, closed with a butyl rubber stopper and sealed with a crimped aluminium seal.

6.6 Special precautions for disposal and other handling

Physical and chemical compatibility testing indicate that INTEGRILIN may be administered through an intravenous line with atropine sulfate, dobutamine, heparin, lidocaine, meperidine, metoprolol, midazolam, morphine, nitroglycerin, tissue plasminogen activator, or verapamil. INTEGRILIN is compatible with 0.9 % sodium chloride solution for infusion and with Dextrose 5 % in Normosol R, in the presence or absence of potassium chloride.

Before using, inspect the vial contents. Do not use if particulate matter or discoloration is present. Protection of INTEGRILIN solution from light is not necessary during administration.

Discard any unused material after opening.

7. MARKETING AUTHORISATION HOLDER

Glaxo Group Ltd

Greenford

Middlesex

UB6 0NN

United Kingdom

8. MARKETING AUTHORISATION NUMBER(S)

INTEGRILIN 0.75 mg/ml, solution for infusion: EU/1/99/109/001

INTEGRILIN 2 mg/ml, solution for injection: EU/1/99/109/002

9. DATE OF FIRST AUTHORISATION/RENEWAL OF THE AUTHORISATION

Date of first authorisation: 1 July 1999

Date of latest renewal: 1 July 2004

10. DATE OF REVISION OF THE TEXT

1 March 2007

Intelence

(Janssen-Cilag Ltd)

1. NAME OF THE MEDICINAL PRODUCT

INTELENCE®▼ 100 mg tablets

2. QUALITATIVE AND QUANTITATIVE COMPOSITION

Each tablet contains 100 mg of etravirine.

Excipient: Each tablet contains 160 mg lactose.

For a full list of excipients, see section 6.1.

3. PHARMACEUTICAL FORM

White to off-white, oval tablet, debossed with "T125" on one side and "100" on the other side.

4. CLINICAL PARTICULARS

4.1 Therapeutic indications

INTELENCE, in combination with a boosted protease inhibitor and other antiretroviral medicinal products, is indicated for the treatment of human immunodeficiency virus type 1 (HIV-1) infection in antiretroviral treatment-experienced adult patients (see sections 4.4, 4.5 and 5.1).

This indication is based on week 48 analyses from 2 randomised, double-blind, placebo-controlled Phase III trials in highly pre-treated patients with viral strains harbouring mutations of resistance to non-nucleoside reverse transcriptase inhibitors and protease inhibitors, where INTELENCE was investigated in combination with an optimised background regimen (OBR) which included darunavir/ritonavir (see section 5.1).

4.2 Posology and method of administration

Therapy should be initiated by a physician experienced in the management of HIV infection.

INTELENCE must always be given in combination with other antiretroviral medicinal products.

Adults

The recommended dose of INTELENCE is 200 mg (two 100 mg tablets) taken orally twice daily (b.i.d.), following a meal (see section 5.2).

Patients who are unable to swallow INTELENCE tablets whole may disperse the tablets in a glass of water. Once dispersed, patients should stir the dispersion well and drink it immediately. The glass should be rinsed with water several times and each rinse completely swallowed to ensure the entire dose is consumed.

Paediatric population

INTELENCE is not recommended for use in children and adolescents due to insufficient data on safety and efficacy (see section 5.2).

Elderly

There is limited information regarding the use of INTELENCE in patients > 65 years of age (see section 5.2), therefore caution should be used in this population.

Hepatic impairment

No dose adjustment is suggested in patients with mild or moderate hepatic impairment (Child-Pugh Class A or B); INTELENCE should be used with caution in patients with moderate hepatic impairment. The pharmacokinetics of etravirine have not been studied in patients with severe hepatic impairment (Child-Pugh Class C). Therefore, INTELENCE is not recommended in patients with severe hepatic impairment (see sections 4.4 and 5.2).

Renal impairment

No dose adjustment is required in patients with renal impairment (see section 5.2).

If the patient misses a dose of INTELENCE within 6 hours of the time it is usually taken, the patient should be told to take it following a meal as soon as possible and then take the next dose at the regularly scheduled time. If a patient misses a dose by more than 6 hours of the time it is usually taken, the patient should be told not to take the missed dose and simply resume the usual dosing schedule.

4.3 Contraindications

Hypersensitivity to the active substance or to any of the excipients.

4.4 Special warnings and precautions for use

Patients should be advised that current antiretroviral therapy does not cure HIV and has not been proven to prevent the transmission of HIV to others through blood or sexual contact. Appropriate precautions should continue to be employed.

INTELENCE should optimally be combined with other antiretrovirals that exhibit activity against the patient's virus (see section 5.1).

A decreased virologic response to etravirine was observed in patients with viral strains harbouring 3 or more among the following mutations V90I, A98G, L100I, K101E/P, V106I, V179D/F, Y181C/I/V, and G190A/S (see section 5.1).

Conclusions regarding the relevance of particular mutations or mutational patterns are subject to change with additional data, and it is recommended to always consult current interpretation systems for analysing resistance test results.

No data other than drug-drug interaction data (see section 4.5) are available when etravirine is combined with raltegravir or maraviroc.

Cutaneous reactions

Severe cutaneous adverse drug reactions have been reported with INTELENCE; Stevens-Johnson Syndrome and erythema multiforme have been rarely (< 0.1%) reported. Treatment with INTELENCE should be discontinued if a severe cutaneous reaction develops. Cutaneous reactions were most frequently mild to moderate, mostly occurred in the second week of therapy, and were infrequent after week 4. Cutaneous reactions were mostly self-limiting and generally resolved within 1-2 weeks on continued therapy (see section 4.8).

The clinical data are limited and an increased risk of cutaneous reactions in patients with a history of NNRTI-associated cutaneous reactions cannot be excluded. Caution should be observed in such patients, especially in case of history of a severe cutaneous drug reaction.

When prescribing INTELENCE to women, prescribers should be aware that the incidence of cutaneous reactions was higher in women compared to men in the INTELENCE arm in the DUET trials.

Elderly

Experience in geriatric patients is limited: in the Phase III trials, 6 patients aged 65 years or older and 53 patients aged 56-64 years received INTELENCE. The type and incidence of adverse reactions in patients $>$ 55 years of age were similar to the ones in younger patients (see section 4.2 and 5.2).

Patients with coexisting conditions

Hepatic impairment

Etravirine is primarily metabolised and eliminated by the liver and highly bound to plasma proteins. Effects on unbound exposure could be expected (has not been studied) therefore caution is advised in patients with moderate hepatic impairment. INTELENCE has not been studied in patients with severe hepatic impairment (Child-Pugh Class C) and its use is therefore not recommended in this group of patients (see sections 4.2 and 5.2).

Co-infection with HBV or HCV

Caution should be exercised in patients co-infected with hepatitis B or C virus due to the current limited data available. A potential increased risk of liver enzymes increase cannot be excluded.

Fat redistribution

Combination antiretroviral therapy (CART) has been associated with redistribution of body fat (lipodystrophy) in HIV infected patients. The long-term consequences of these events are currently unknown. Knowledge about the mechanism is incomplete. A connection between visceral lipomatosis and protease inhibitors (PIs), and lipoatrophy and nucleoside reverse transcriptase inhibitors (NRTIs), has been hypothesised. A higher risk of lipodystrophy has been associated with individual factors such as older age, and with treatment related factors such as longer duration of antiretroviral treatment and associated metabolic disturbances. Clinical examination should include evaluation for physical signs of fat redistribution (see section 4.8).

Immune reconstitution syndrome

In HIV infected patients with severe immune deficiency at the time of institution of CART, an inflammatory reaction to asymptomatic or residual opportunistic pathogens may arise and cause serious clinical conditions, or aggravation of symptoms. Typically, such reactions have been observed within the first weeks or months of initiation of CART. Relevant examples are cytomegalovirus retinitis, generalised and/or focal mycobacterial infections and *Pneumocystis jiroveci* pneumonia. Any inflammatory symptoms should be evaluated and treatment instituted when necessary (see section 4.8).

Osteonecrosis

Although the etiology is considered to be multifactorial (including corticosteroid use, alcohol consumption, severe immunosuppression, higher body mass index), cases of osteonecrosis have been reported particularly in patients with advanced HIV disease and/or long-term exposure to CART. Patients should be advised to seek medical advice if they experience joint aches and pain, joint stiffness or difficulty in movement.

Interactions with medicinal products

It is not recommended to combine etravirine with tipranavir/ritonavir, due to a marked pharmacokinetic interaction (76% decrease of etravirine AUC) that could significantly impair the virologic response to etravirine.

For further information on interactions with medicinal products see section 4.5.

Lactose intolerance and lactase deficiency

Each tablet contains 160 mg of lactose. Patients with rare hereditary problems of galactose intolerance, the Lapp lactase deficiency or glucose-galactose malabsorption should not take this medicine.

4.5 Interaction with other medicinal products and other forms of interaction

Medicinal products that affect etravirine exposure

Etravirine is metabolised by CYP3A4, CYP2C9 and CYP2C19 followed by glucuronidation of the metabolites by uridine diphosphate glucuronosyl transferase (UDPGT). Medicinal products that induce CYP3A4, CYP2C9 or CYP2C19 may increase the clearance of etravirine, resulting in lowered plasma concentrations of etravirine.

Co-administration of INTELENCE and medicinal products that inhibit CYP3A4, CYP2C9 or CYP2C19 may decrease the clearance of etravirine and may result in increased plasma concentrations of etravirine.

Medicinal products that are affected by the use of etravirine

Etravirine is a weak inducer of CYP3A4. Co-administration of INTELENCE with medicinal products primarily metabolised by CYP3A4 may result in decreased plasma concentrations of such medicinal products, which could decrease or shorten their therapeutic effects.

Etravirine is a weak inhibitor of CYP2C9 and CYP2C19. Etravirine is also a weak inhibitor of P-glycoprotein. Co-administration with medicinal products primarily metabolised by CYP2C9 or CYP2C19 or transported by P-glycoprotein may result in increased plasma concentrations of such medicinal products, which could increase or prolong their therapeutic effect or alter their adverse events profile.

Known and theoretical interactions with selected antiretrovirals and non-antiretroviral medicinal products are listed in table1.

Interaction table

Interactions between etravirine and co-administered medicinal products are listed in table 1 (increase is indicated as "↑", decrease as "↓", no change as "↔", not done as "ND", once daily as "q.d.", twice daily as "b.i.d.", confidence interval as "CI").

(see Table 1 on next page)

4.6 Pregnancy and lactation

Pregnancy

There are no adequate and well-controlled studies with etravirine in pregnant women. Placental transfer has been seen in pregnant rats, but it is not known whether placental transfer of INTELENCE also occurs in pregnant women. Studies in animals do not indicate direct or indirect harmful effects with respect to pregnancy, embryonal/foetal development, parturition or postnatal development (see section 5.3).

INTELENCE should be used during pregnancy only if the potential benefit justifies the potential risk.

Breastfeeding

It is not known whether etravirine is excreted in human milk. Because of both the potential for HIV transmission and the potential for adverse reactions in breast-fed infants, mothers should be instructed not to breast-feed if they are receiving INTELENCE.

Fertility

No human data on the effect of etravirine on fertility are available. In rats, there was no effect on mating or fertility with etravirine treatment (see section 5.3).

4.7 Effects on ability to drive and use machines

No studies on the effects of INTELENCE on the ability to drive or operate machines have been performed. Adverse drug reactions such as somnolence and vertigo have been reported in INTELENCE treated subjects at incidences similar to placebo (see section 4.8). There is no evidence that INTELENCE may alter the patient's ability to drive and operate machines, however, the adverse drug reaction profile should be taken into account.

4.8 Undesirable effects

The safety assessment is based on all data from 1,203 patients in the Phase III placebo-controlled trials DUET-1 and DUET-2 in antiretroviral treatment-experienced HIV-1 infected adult patients, 599 of whom received INTELENCE (200 mg b.i.d.) (see section 5.1). In these pooled trials, the median exposure for patients in the INTELENCE arm was 52.3 weeks.

The most frequently reported adverse drug reactions (ADRs) (incidence $\geq$ 10% in the INTELENCE arm) of all intensities occurring in the Phase III studies were rash (19.2% in the INTELENCE arm versus 10.9% in the placebo arm), diarrhoea (18.0% in the INTELENCE arm versus 23.5% in the placebo arm), nausea (14.9% in the INTELENCE arm versus 12.7% in the placebo arm) and headache (10.9% in the INTELENCE arm versus 12.7% in the placebo arm). The rates of discontinuation due to any adverse reaction were 7.2% in patients receiving INTELENCE and 5.6% in patients receiving placebo. The most common ADR leading to discontinuation was rash (2.2% in the INTELENCE arm versus 0% in the placebo arm).

Rash was most frequently mild to moderate, generally macular to maculopapular or erythematous, mostly occurred in the second week of therapy, and was infrequent after week 4. Rash was mostly self-limiting, and generally resolved within 1-2 weeks on continued therapy (see section 4.4). The incidence of rash was higher in women compared to men in the INTELENCE arm in the DUET trials. There was no gender difference in severity or treatment discontinuation due to rash. The clinical data are limited and an increased risk of cutaneous reactions in patients with a history of NNRTI-associated cutaneous reaction cannot be excluded (see section 4.4).

ADRs of moderate intensity or greater ($\geq$ grade 2) reported in patients treated with INTELENCE are summarised in table 2 (background regimen is indicated as "BR"). Laboratory abnormalities considered ADRs are included in a paragraph below table 2. The ADRs are listed by system organ class (SOC) and frequency. Within each frequency grouping, ADRs are presented in order of decreasing seriousness. Frequencies are defined as very common ($\geq$ 1/10), common ($\geq$ 1/100 to $<$ 1/10) and uncommon ($\geq$ 1/1,000 to $<$ 1/100). Rare and very rare ADRs cannot be detected based on the number of patients included in the DUET trials.

(see Table 2 on page 4931186)

Additional ADRs of at least moderate intensity observed in other trials were acquired lipodystrophy, angioneurotic oedema, erythema multiforme and haemorrhagic stroke, each reported in no more than 0.5% of patients. Stevens-Johnson Syndrome has been reported rarely ($<$ 0.1%) during clinical development with INTELENCE.

Laboratory abnormalities

Treatment emergent clinical laboratory abnormalities (grade 3 or 4), considered ADRs, reported in $\geq$ 2% of patients in the INTELENCE arm versus the placebo arm, respectively, were increases in amylase (8.9% vs 9.4%), creatinine (2.0% vs 1.7%), lipase (3.4% vs 2.6%), total cholesterol (8.1% vs 5.3%), low density lipoprotein (LDL) (7.2% vs 6.6%), triglycerides (9.2% vs 5.8%), glucose (3.5% vs 2.4%), alanine aminotransferase (ALT) (3.7% vs 2.0%), aspartate amino transferase (AST) (3.2% vs 2.0%) and decreases in neutrophils (5.0% vs 7.4%) and white blood cell count (2.0% vs 4.3%).

Lipodystrophy

Combination antiretroviral therapy has been associated with redistribution of body fat (lipodystrophy) in HIV infected patients, including loss of peripheral and facial subcutaneous fat, increased intra-abdominal and visceral fat, breast hypertrophy and dorsocervical fat accumulation (buffalo hump) (see section 4.4).

Immune reconstitution syndrome

In HIV infected patients with severe immune deficiency at the time of initiation of combination antiretroviral therapy, an inflammatory reaction to asymptomatic or residual opportunistic infections may arise (immune reconstitution syndrome) (see section 4.4).

Osteonecrosis

Cases of osteonecrosis have been reported, particularly in patients with generally acknowledged risk factors, advanced HIV disease or long-term exposure to combination antiretroviral therapy. The frequency of this is unknown (see section 4.4).

Additional information on special populations

Patients co-infected with hepatitis B and/or hepatitis C virus

In the pooled analysis for DUET-1 and DUET-2, the incidence of hepatic events tended to be higher in co-infected subjects treated with INTELENCE compared to co-infected subjects in the placebo group. INTELENCE should be used with caution in these patients (see also sections 4.4 and 5.2).

4.9 Overdose

There is no specific antidote for overdose with INTELENCE. Treatment of overdose with INTELENCE consists of general supportive measures including monitoring of vital signs and observation of the clinical status of the patient. If indicated, elimination of unabsorbed active substance is to be achieved by emesis or gastric lavage. Administration of activated charcoal may also be used to aid in removal of unabsorbed active substance. Since etravirine is highly protein bound, dialysis is unlikely to result in significant removal of the active substance.

5. PHARMACOLOGICAL PROPERTIES

5.1 Pharmacodynamic properties

Pharmacotherapeutic group: NNRTI (non-nucleoside reverse transcriptase inhibitor), ATC code: J05AG04.

Mechanism of action

Etravirine is an NNRTI of human immunodeficiency virus type 1 (HIV-1). Etravirine binds directly to reverse transcriptase (RT) and blocks the RNA-dependent and DNA-dependent DNA polymerase activities by causing a disruption of the enzyme's catalytic site.

Antiviral activity *in vitro*

Etravirine exhibits activity against wild type HIV-1 in T-cell lines and primary cells with median EC_{50} values ranging from 0.9 to 5.5 nM. Etravirine demonstrates activity against HIV-1 group M (subtypes A, B, C, D, E, F, and G) and HIV-1 group O primary isolates with EC_{50} values ranging from 0.3 to 1.7 nM and from 11.5 to 21.7 nM, respectively. Although etravirine demonstrates in vitro activity against wild type HIV-2 with median EC_{50} values ranging from 5.7 to 7.2 μM, treatment of HIV-2 infection with etravirine is not recommended in the absence of clinical data. Etravirine retains activity against HIV-1 viral strains resistant to nucleoside reverse transcriptase and/or protease inhibitors. In addition, etravirine demonstrates a fold change (FC) in $EC_{50} \leq 3$ against 60% of 6,171 NNRTI-resistant clinical isolates.

Resistance

Etravirine efficacy in relation to NNRTI resistance at baseline has mainly been analysed with etravirine given in combination with darunavir/ritonavir (DUET-1 and -2). Boosted protease inhibitors, like darunavir/ritonavir, show a higher barrier to resistance compared to other classes of antiretrovirals. The breakpoints for reduced efficacy with etravirine ($>$ 2 etravirine-associated mutations at baseline, see clinical results section) applies when etravirine is given in combination with a boosted protease inhibitor. This breakpoint might be lower in antiretroviral combination therapy not including a boosted protease inhibitor.

In the Phase III trials DUET-1 and DUET-2, mutations that developed most commonly in patients with virologic failure to the INTELENCE containing regimen were V108I, V179F, V179I, Y181C and Y181I, which usually emerged in a background of multiple other NNRTI resistance-associated

Table 1: INTERACTIONS AND DOSE RECOMMENDATIONS WITH OTHER MEDICINAL PRODUCTS

Medicinal products by therapeutic areas	Effects on drug levels Least Squares Mean Ratio (90% CI; 1.00 = No effect)	Recommendations concerning co-administration
ANTI-INFECTIVES		
Antiretrovirals		
NRTIs		
Didanosine 400 mg q.d.	didanosine AUC ↔ 0.99 (0.79-1.25) didanosine C_{min} ND didanosine C_{max}↔ 0.91 (0.58-1.42) etravirine AUC ↔ 1.11 (0.99-1.25) etravirine C_{min}↔ 1.05 (0.93-1.18) etravirine C_{max}↔ 1.16 (1.02-1.32)	No significant effect on didanosine and etravirine PK parameters is seen. INTELENCE and didanosine can be used without dose adjustments.
Tenofovir 300 mg q.d.	tenofovir AUC ↔ 1.15 (1.09-1.21) tenofovir C_{min} ↑ 1.19 (1.13-1.26) tenofovir C_{max} ↑ 1.15 (1.04-1.27) etravirine AUC ↓ 0.81 (0.75-0.88) etravirine C_{min}↓ 0.82 (0.73-0.91) etravirine C_{max}↓ 0.81 (0.75-0.88)	No significant effect on tenofovir and etravirine PK parameters is seen. INTELENCE and tenofovir can be used without dose adjustments.
Other NRTIs	Not studied, but no interaction expected based on the primary renal elimination route for other NRTIs (e.g., abacavir, emtricitabine, lamivudine, stavudine and zidovudine).	Etravirine can be used with these NRTIs without dose adjustment.
NNRTIs		
Efavirenz Nevirapine	Combining two NNRTIs has not been shown to be beneficial. Concomitant use of INTELENCE with efavirenz or nevirapine may cause a significant decrease in the plasma concentration of etravirine and loss of therapeutic effect of INTELENCE.	It is not recommended to co-administer INTELENCE with other NNRTIs.
PIs - Unboosted (i.e. without co-administration of low-dose ritonavir)		
Nelfinavir	Not studied. INTELENCE is expected to increase nelfinavir plasma concentrations.	It is not recommended to co-administer INTELENCE with nelfinavir.
Indinavir	Concomitant use of INTELENCE with indinavir may cause a significant decrease in the plasma concentration of indinavir and loss of therapeutic effect of indinavir.	It is not recommended to co-administer INTELENCE with indinavir.
PIs - Boosted (with low-dose ritonavir)		
Tipranavir/ritonavir 500/200 mg b.i.d.	tipranavir AUC ↑ 1.18 (1.03-1.36) tipranavir C_{min} ↑ 1.24 (0.96-1.59) tipranavir C_{max} ↑ 1.14 (1.02-1.27) etravirine AUC ↓ 0.24 (0.18-0.33) etravirine C_{min}↓ 0.18 (0.13-0.25) etravirine C_{max}↓ 0.29 (0.22-0.40)	It is not recommended to co-administer tipranavir/ritonavir and INTELENCE (see section 4.4).
Fosamprenavir/ritonavir 700/100 mg b.i.d.	amprenavir AUC ↑ 1.69 (1.53-1.86) amprenavir C_{min} ↑ 1.77 (1.39-2.25) amprenavir C_{max} ↑ 1.62 (1.47-1.79) etravirine AUC ↔[a] etravirine C_{min}↔[a] etravirine C_{max}↔[a]	Amprenavir/ritonavir and fosamprenavir/ritonavir may require dose reduction when co-administered with INTELENCE. Using the oral solution may be considered for dose reduction.
Atazanavir/ritonavir 300/100 mg q.d.	atazanavir AUC ↓ 0.86 (0.79-0.93) atazanavir C_{min}↓ 0.62 (0.55-0.71) atazanavir C_{max}↔ 0.97 (0.89-1.05) etravirine AUC ↑ 1.30 (1.18-1.44) etravirine C_{min} ↑ 1.26 (1.12-1.42) etravirine C_{max} ↑ 1.30 (1.17-1.44)	INTELENCE and atazanavir/ritonavir can be used without dose adjustment.
Darunavir/ritonavir 600/100 mg b.i.d.	darunavir AUC ↔ 1.15 (1.05-1.26) darunavir C_{min}↔ 1.02 (0.90-1.17) darunavir C_{max}↔ 1.11 (1.01-1.22) etravirine AUC ↓ 0.63 (0.54-0.73) etravirine C_{min}↓ 0.51 (0.44-0.61) etravirine C_{max}↓ 0.68 (0.57-0.82)	INTELENCE and darunavir/ritonavir can be used without dose adjustments (see also section 5.1).
Lopinavir/ritonavir (soft capsule) 400/100 mg b.i.d.	lopinavir AUC ↓ 0.80 (0.49-1.07) lopinavir C_{min}↓ 0.92 (0.15-1.68) lopinavir C_{max}↓ 0.85 (0.62-1.05) etravirine AUC ↑ 1.17 (0.96-1.43) etravirine C_{min} ↑ 1.23 (0.98-1.53) etravirine C_{max} ↑ 1.15 (0.94-1.41)	INTELENCE and lopinavir/ritonavir can be used without dose adjustments.
Saquinavir/ritonavir 1,000/100 mg b.i.d.	saquinavir AUC ↔ 0.95 (0.64-1.42) saquinavir C_{min}↓ 0.80 (0.46-1.38) saquinavir C_{max}↔ 1.00 (0.70-1.42) etravirine AUC ↓ 0.67 (0.56-0.80) etravirine C_{min}↓ 0.71 (0.58-0.87) etravirine C_{max}↓ 0.63 (0.53-0.75)	INTELENCE and saquinavir/ritonavir can be used without dose adjustments.
CCR5 Antagonists		
Maraviroc 300 mg b.i.d. Maraviroc/darunavir/ ritonavir 150/600/100 mg b.i.d.	maraviroc AUC ↓ 0.47 (0.38-0.58) maraviroc C_{min}↓ 0.61 (0.53-0.71) maraviroc C_{max}↓ 0.40 (0.28-0.57) etravirine AUC ↔ 1.06 (0.99-1.14) etravirine C_{min}↔ 1.08 (0.98-1.19) etravirine C_{max}↔ 1.05 (0.95-1.17) maraviroc AUC ↑ 3.10* (2.57-3.74) maraviroc C_{min} ↑ 5.27* (4.51-6.15) maraviroc C_{max} ↑ 1.77* (1.20-2.60) * compared to maraviroc 150 mg b.i.d.	The recommended dose for maraviroc when combined with INTELENCE in the presence of potent CYP3A inhibitors (e.g. boosted PIs) is 150 mg b.i.d. except for fosamprenavir/ritonavir (maraviroc dose 300 mg b.i.d.). No dose adjustment for INTELENCE is necessary. See also section 4.4.
Fusion Inhibitors		
Enfuvirtide 90 mg b.i.d.	etravirine* AUC ↔[a] etravirine* C_{0h}↔[a] Enfuvirtide concentrations not studied, no effect is expected. * based on population pharmacokinetic analyses	No interaction is expected for either INTELENCE or enfuvirtide when co-administered.

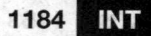

Medicinal products by therapeutic areas	Effects on drug levels Least Squares Mean Ratio (90% CI; 1.00 = No effect)	Recommendations concerning co-administration
Integrase Strand Transfer Inhibitors		
Raltegravir 400 mg b.i.d.	raltegravir AUC ↓ 0.90 (0.68-1.18) raltegravir C_{min}↓ 0.66 (0.34-1.26) raltegravir C_{max}↓ 0.89 (0.68-1.15) etravirine AUC ↔ 1.10 (1.03-1.16) etravirine C_{min}↔ 1.17 (1.10-1.26) etravirine C_{max}↔ 1.04 (0.97-1.12)	INTELENCE and raltegravir can be used without dose adjustments.
ANTIARRHYTHMICS		
Digoxin 0.5 mg single dose	digoxin AUC ↑ 1.18 (0.90-1.56) digoxin C_{min} ND digoxin C_{max} ↑ 1.19 (0.96-1.49)	INTELENCE and digoxin can be used without dose adjustments. It is recommended that digoxin levels be monitored when digoxin is combined with INTELENCE.
Amiodarone Bepridil Disopyramide Flecainide Lidocaine (systemic) Mexiletine Propafenone Quinidine	Not studied. INTELENCE is expected to decrease plasma concentrations of these antiarrhythmics.	Caution is warranted and therapeutic concentration monitoring, if available, is recommended for antiarrhythmics when co-administered with INTELENCE.
ANTIBIOTICS		
Azithromycin	Not studied. Based on the biliary elimination pathway of azithromycin, no drug interactions are expected between azithromycin and INTELENCE.	INTELENCE and azithromycin can be used without dose adjustments.
Clarithromycin 500 mg b.i.d.	clarithromycin AUC ↓ 0.61 (0.53-0.69) clarithromycin C_{min}↓ 0.47 (0.38-0.57) clarithromycin C_{max}↓ 0.66 (0.57-0.77) 14-OH-clarithromycin AUC ↑ 1.21 (1.05-1.39) 14-OH-clarithromycin C_{min}↔ 1.05 (0.90-1.22) 14-OH-clarithromycin C_{max} ↑ 1.33 (1.13-1.56) etravirine AUC ↑ 1.42 (1.34-1.50) etravirine C_{min} ↑ 1.46 (1.36-1.58) etravirine C_{max} ↑ 1.46 (1.38-1.56)	Clarithromycin exposure was decreased by etravirine; however, concentrations of the active metabolite, 14-OH-clarithromycin, were increased. Because 14-OH-clarithromycin has reduced activity against *Mycobacterium avium* complex (MAC), overall activity against this pathogen may be altered; therefore alternatives to clarithromycin should be considered for the treatment of MAC.
ANTICOAGULANTS		
Warfarin	Not studied. INTELENCE is expected to increase plasma concentrations of warfarin.	It is recommended that the international normalised ratio (INR) be monitored when warfarin is combined with INTELENCE.
ANTICONVULSANTS		
Carbamazepine Phenobarbital Phenytoin	Not studied. Carbazamepine, phenobarbital and phenytoin are expected to decrease plasma concentrations of etravirine.	Combination not recommended.
ANTIFUNGALS		
Fluconazole Itraconazole Ketoconazole Posaconazole Voriconazole	Not studied. Posaconazole is a potent inhibitor of CYP3A4 and fluconazole is a potent inhibitor of CYP2C9; both may increase plasma concentrations of etravirine. Itraconazole and ketoconazole are potent inhibitors as well as substrates of CYP3A4. Concomitant systemic use of itraconazole or ketoconazole and INTELENCE may increase plasma concentrations of etravirine. Simultaneously, plasma concentrations of itraconazole or ketoconazole may be decreased by INTELENCE. Voriconazole is a CYP2C19 substrate and CYP3A4 and CYP2C inhibitor. Concomitant use of voriconazole and INTELENCE may increase plasma concentrations of both drugs.	INTELENCE and antifungals can be used without dose adjustments.
ANTIMYCOBACTERIALS		
Rifampicin Rifapentine	Not studied. Rifampicin and rifapentine are expected to decrease plasma concentrations of etravirine. INTELENCE should be used in combination with a boosted protease inhibitor (PI). Rifampicin is contraindicated in combination with boosted PIs.	Combination not recommended.
Rifabutin 300 mg q.d.	rifabutin AUC ↓ 0.83 (0.75-0.94) rifabutin C_{min}↓ 0.76 (0.66-0.87) rifabutin C_{max}↓ 0.90 (0.78-1.03) 25-O-desacetyl-rifabutin AUC ↓ 0.83 (0.74-0.92) 25-O-desacetyl-rifabutin C_{min}↓ 0.78 (0.70-0.87) 25-O-desacetyl-rifabutin C_{max}↓ 0.85 (0.72-1.00) etravirine AUC ↓ 0.63 (0.54-0.74) etravirine C_{min}↓ 0.65 (0.56-0.74) etravirine C_{max}↓ 0.63 (0.53-0.74)	The combination of INTELENCE and rifabutin should be used with caution due to the risk of decrease in etravirine and rifabutin exposures.
ANTIVIRALS		
Ribavirin	Not studied, but no interaction expected based on the renal elimination pathway of ribavirin.	The combination of INTELENCE and ribavirin can be used without dose adjustments.
BENZODIAZEPINES		
Diazepam	Not studied, etravirine is expected to increase plasma concentrations of diazepam.	Alternatives to diazepam should be considered.
CORTICOSTEROIDS		
Dexamethasone (systemic)	Not studied. Dexamethasone is expected to decrease plasma concentrations of etravirine	Systemic dexamethasone should be used with caution or alternatives should be considered, particularly for chronic use.
ESTROGEN-BASED CONTRACEPTIVES		
Ethinylestradiol 0.035 mg q.d. Norethindrone 1 mg q.d.	ethinylestradiol AUC ↑ 1.22 (1.13-1.31) ethinylestradiol C_{min}↔ 1.09 (1.01-1.18) ethinylestradiol C_{max} ↑ 1.33 (1.21-1.46) norethindrone AUC ↔ 0.95 (0.90-0.99) norethindrone C_{min}↓ 0.78 (0.68-0.90) norethindrone C_{max}↔ 1.05 (0.98-1.12) etravirine AUC ↔[a] etravirine C_{min}↔[a] etravirine C_{max}↔[a]	The combination of estrogen- and/or progesterone-based contraceptives and INTELENCE can be used without dose adjustment.

Medicinal products by therapeutic areas	Effects on drug levels Least Squares Mean Ratio (90% CI; 1.00 = No effect)	Recommendations concerning co-administration
HERBAL PRODUCTS		
St John's wort *(Hypericum perforatum)*	Not studied. St John's wort is expected to decrease the plasma concentrations of etravirine.	Combination not recommended.
HMG CO-A REDUCTASE INHIBITORS		
Atorvastatin 40 mg q.d.	atorvastatin AUC ↓ 0.63 (0.58-0.68) atorvastatin C_{min} ND atorvastatin C_{max}↓ 1.04 (0.84-1.30) 2-OH-atorvastatin AUC ↑ 1.27 (1.19-1.36) 2-OH-atorvastatin C_{min} ND 2-OH-atorvastatin C_{max} ↑ 1.76 (1.60-1.94) etravirine AUC ↔ 1.02 (0.97-1.07) etravirine C_{min}↔ 1.10 (1.02-1.19) etravirine C_{max}↔ 0.97 (0.93-1.02)	The combination of INTELENCE and atorvastatin can be given without any dose adjustments, however, the dose of atorvastatin may need to be altered based on clinical response.
Fluvastatin Lovastatin Pravastatin Rosuvastatin Simvastatin	Not studied. No interaction between pravastatin and INTELENCE is expected. Lovastatin, rosuvastatin and simvastatin are CYP3A4 substrates and co-administration with INTELENCE may result in lower plasma concentrations of the HMG Co-A reductase inhibitor. Fluvastatin, and rosuvastatin are metabolised by CYP2C9 and co-administration with INTELENCE may result in higher plasma concentrations of the HMG Co-A reductase inhibitor.	Dose adjustments for these HMG Co-A reductase inhibitors may be necessary.
H_2-RECEPTOR ANTAGONISTS		
Ranitidine 150 mg b.i.d.	etravirine AUC ↓ 0.86 (0.76-0.97) etravirine C_{min} ND etravirine C_{max}↓ 0.94 (0.75-1.17)	INTELENCE can be co-administered with H_2-receptor antagonists without dose adjustments.
IMMUNOSUPPRESSANTS		
Cyclosporine Sirolimus Tacrolimus	Not studied. Etravirine is expected to decrease plasma concentrations of cyclosporine, sirolimus or tacrolimus.	Co-administration with systemic immunosuppressants should be done with caution because plasma concentrations of cyclosporine, sirolimus or tacrolimus may be affected when co-administered with INTELENCE.
NARCOTIC ANALGESICS		
Methadone individual dose ranging from 60 mg to 130 mg q.d.	R(-) methadone AUC ↔ 1.06 (0.99-1.13) R(-) methadone C_{min}↔ 1.10 (1.02-1.19) R(-) methadone C_{max}↔ 1.02 (0.96-1.09) S(+) methadone AUC ↔ 0.89 (0.82-0.96) S(+) methadone C_{min}↔ 0.89 (0.81-0.98) S(+) methadone C_{max}↔ 0.89 (0.83-0.97) etravirine AUC ↔[a] etravirine C_{min}↔[a] etravirine C_{max}↔[a]	No changes in methadone dosage were required based on clinical status during or after the period of INTELENCE co-administration.
PHOSPHODIESTERASE, TYPE 5 (PDE-5) INHIBITORS		
Sildenafil 50 mg single dose Vardenafil Tadalafil	sildenafil AUC ↓ 0.43 (0.36-0.51) sildenafil C_{min} ND sildenafil C_{max}↓ 0.55 (0.40-0.75) N-desmethyl-sildenafil AUC ↓ 0.59 (0.52-0.68) N-desmethyl-sildenafil C_{min} ND N-desmethyl-sildenafil C_{max}↓ 0.75 (0.59-0.96)	Concomitant use of PDE-5 inhibitors with INTELENCE may require dose adjustment of the PDE-5 inhibitor to attain the desired clinical effect.
PROTON PUMP INHIBITORS		
Omeprazole 40 mg q.d.	etravirine AUC ↑ 1.41 (1.22-1.62) etravirine C_{min} ND etravirine C_{max} ↑ 1.17 (0.96-1.43)	INTELENCE can be co-administered with proton pump inhibitors without dose adjustments.
SELECTIVE SEROTONIN REUPTAKE INHIBITORS (SSRIS)		
Paroxetine 20 mg q.d.	paroxetine AUC ↔ 1.03 (0.90-1.18) paroxetine C_{min}↓ 0.87 (0.75-1.02) paroxetine C_{max}↔ 1.06 (0.95-1.20) etravirine AUC ↔ 1.01 (0.93-1.10) etravirine C_{min}↔ 1.07 (0.98-1.17) etravirine C_{max}↔ 1.05 (0.96-1.15)	INTELENCE can be co-administered with paroxetine without dose adjustments.

[a] Comparison based on historic control.

Note: In drug-drug interaction studies, different formulations and/or doses of etravirine were used which led to similar exposures and, therefore, interactions relevant for one formulation are relevant for the other.

mutations (RAMs). In all the other trials conducted with INTELENCE in HIV-1 infected patients, the following mutations emerged most commonly: L100I, E138G, V179F, V179I, Y181C and H221Y.

Cross-resistance

Following virologic failure of an etravirine-containing regimen it is not recommended to treat patients with efavirenz and/or nevirapine.

Clinical experience

Treatment-experienced patients

Pivotal studies

The evidence of efficacy of INTELENCE is based on 48-week data from 2 ongoing Phase III trials DUET-1 and DUET-2. These trials were identical in design and similar efficacy for INTELENCE was seen in each trial. The results below are pooled data from the two trials.

Trial characteristics

(see Table 2a on next page)

Summary of efficacy results

(see Table 3 on page 4931187)

Since there was a significant interaction effect between treatment and ENF, the primary analysis was done for 2 ENF strata (patients reusing or not using ENF versus patients using ENF *de novo*). The week 48 results from the pooled analysis of DUET– 1 and DUET-2 demonstrated that the INTELENCE arm was superior to the placebo arm irrespective of whether ENF was used de novo (p = 0.0199) or not (p < 0.0001). Results of this analysis (week 48 data) by ENF stratum are shown in table 3.

Significantly fewer patients in the INTELENCE arm reached a clinical endpoint (AIDS-defining illness or death) as compared to the placebo arm (p = 0.0408)

A subgroup analysis of the virologic response (defined as a viral load < 50 HIV-1 RNA copies/ml) at week 48 by baseline viral load and baseline CD4 count (pooled DUET data) is presented in table 4.

(see Table 4 on next page)

Baseline genotype or phenotype and virologic outcome analyses

In DUET-1 and DUET-2, the presence at baseline of 3 or more of the following mutations: V90I, A98G, L100I, K101E, K101P, V106I, V179D, V179F, Y181C, Y181I, Y181V, G190A and G190S, (INTELENCE RAMs) was associated with a decreased virologic response to INTELENCE (see table 5). These individual mutations occurred in the presence of other NNRTI RAMs. V179F was never present without Y181C.

Conclusions regarding the relevance of particular mutations or mutational patterns are subject to change with additional data, and it is recommended to always consult current interpretation systems for analysing resistance test results.

(see Table 5493 on page 1187)

The presence of K103N alone, which was the most prevalent NNRTI mutation in DUET-1 and DUET-2 at baseline, was not identified as a mutation associated with resistance to INTELENCE. Furthermore, the presence of this mutation alone did not affect the response in the INTELENCE arm. Additional data is required to conclude on the influence of K103N when associated with other NNRTIs mutations.

Data from the DUET studies suggest that baseline fold change (FC) in EC_{50} to etravirine was a predictive factor of virologic outcome, with gradually decreasing responses observed above FC 3 and FC 13.

FC subgroups are based on the select patient populations in DUET-1 and DUET-2 and are not meant to represent definitive clinical susceptibility breakpoints for INTELENCE.

Table 2: DUET-1 and DUET-2 trials

System Organ Class (SOC)	Frequency Category	ADRs (INTELENCE + BR versus Placebo + BR)
Cardiac disorders	common	myocardial infarction (1.3% vs 0.3%)
	uncommon	atrial fibrillation (0.2% vs 0.2%), angina pectoris (0.5% vs 0.3%)
Blood and lymphatic system disorders	common	thrombocytopaenia (1.3% vs 1.5%), anaemia (4.0% vs 3.8%)
Nervous system disorders	common	peripheral neuropathy (3.8% vs 2.0%), headache (3.0% vs 4.5%)
	uncommon	convulsion (0.5% vs 0.7%), syncope (0.3% vs 0.3%), amnesia (0.3% vs 0.5%), tremor (0.2% vs 0.3%), somnolence (0.7% vs 0.5%), paraesthesia (0.7% vs 0.7%), hypoaesthesia (0.5% vs 0.2%), hypersomnia (0.2% vs 0%), disturbance in attention (0.2% vs 0.2%)
Eye disorders	uncommon	blurred vision (0.7% vs 0%)
Ear and labyrinth disorders	uncommon	vertigo (0.2% vs 0.5%)
Respiratory, thoracic and mediastinal disorders	uncommon	bronchospasm (0.2% vs 0%), exertional dyspnoea (0.5% vs 0.5%)
Gastrointestinal disorders	common	gastrooesophageal reflux disease (1.8% vs 1.0%), diarrhoea (7.0% vs 11.3%), vomiting (2.8% vs 2.8%), nausea (5.2% vs 4.8%), abdominal pain (3.5% vs 3.1%), flatulence (1.5% vs 1.0%), gastritis (1.5% vs 1.0%)
	uncommon	pancreatitis (0.7% vs 0.3%), haematemesis (0.2% vs 0%), stomatitis (0.2% vs 0.2%), constipation (0.3% vs 0.5%), abdominal distension (0.7% vs 1.0%), dry mouth (0.3% vs 0%), retching (0.2% vs 0%)
Renal and urinary disorders	common	renal failure (2.7% vs 2.0%)
Skin and subcutaneous tissue disorders	very common	rash (10.0% vs 3.5%)
	common	lipohypertrophy (1.0% vs 0.3%), night sweats (1.0% vs 1.0%)
	uncommon	swelling face (0.3% vs 0%), hyperhidrosis (0.5% vs 0.2%), prurigo (0.7% vs 0.5%), dry skin (0.3% vs 0.2%)
Metabolism and nutrition disorders	common	diabetes mellitus (1.3% vs 0.2%), hyperglycaemia (1.5% vs 0.7%), hypercholesterolaemia (4.3% vs 3.6%), hypertriglyceridaemia (6.3% vs 4.3%), hyperlipidaemia (2.5% vs 1.3%)
	uncommon	anorexia (0.8% vs 1.5%), dyslipidaemia (0.8% vs 0.3%)
Vascular disorders	common	hypertension (3.2% vs 2.5%)
General disorders and administration site conditions	common	fatigue (3.5% vs 4.6%)
	uncommon	sluggishness (0.2% vs 0%)
Immune system disorders	uncommon	immune reconstitution syndrome (0.2% vs 0.3%), drug hypersensitivity (0.8% vs 1.2%)
Hepatobiliary disorders	uncommon	hepatitis (0.2% vs 0.3%), hepatic steatosis (0.3% vs 0%), cytolytic hepatitis (0.3% vs 0%), hepatomegaly (0.5% vs 0.2%)
Reproductive system and breast disorders	uncommon	gynaecomastia (0.2% vs 0%)
Psychiatric disorders	common	anxiety (1.7% vs 2.6%), insomnia (2.7% vs 2.8%)
	uncommon	confusional state (0.2% vs 0.2%), disorientation (0.2% vs 0.3%), nightmares (0.2% vs 0.2%), sleep disorders (0.5% vs 0.5%), nervousness (0.2% vs 0.3%), abnormal dreams (0.2% vs 0.2%)

Table 2a Trial characteristics

- Design: randomized (1:1), double-blinded, placebo-controlled.
- Treatment: INTELENCE vs. placebo, in addition to a background regimen including darunavir/ritonavir (DRV/rtv), investigator-selected N(t)RTIs and optional enfuvirtide (ENF).
- Main inclusion criteria:
• HIV-1 plasma viral load > 5,000 HIV-1 RNA copies/ml at screening
• 1 or more NNRTI resistance-associated mutations (RAMs) at screening or from prior genotypic analysis (i.e., archived resistance)
• 3 or more primary PI mutations at screening
• on a stable antiretroviral regimen for at least 8 weeks.
- Stratification: Randomisation was stratified by the intended use of ENF in the BR, previous use of darunavir and screening viral load.
- Virologic response was defined as achieving a confirmed undetectable viral load (< 50 HIV-1 RNA copies/ml).

Table 4: DUET-1 and DUET-2 pooled data

Subgroups	Proportion of subjects with HIV-1 RNA < 50 copies/ml at week 48	
	INTELENCE + BR N=599	Placebo + BR N=604
Baseline HIV-1 RNA		
< 30,000 copies/ml	75.8%	55.7%
≥ 30,000 and < 100,000 copies/ml	61.2%	38.5%
≥ 100,000 copies/ml	49.1%	28.1%
Baseline CD4 count (x 10^6/l)		
< 50	45.1 %	21.5%
≥ 50 and < 200	65.4%	47.6%
≥ 200 and < 350	73.9%	52.0%
≥ 350	72.4%	50.8%

Note: Imputations according to the TLOVR algorithm (TLOVR = Time to Loss of Virologic Response)

Exploratory head to head comparison with protease inhibitor in protease inhibitor naïve patients (trial TMC125-C227)

TMC125-C227 was an exploratory, randomised, active-controlled open-label trial, which investigated the efficacy and safety of INTELENCE in a treatment regimen, which is not approved under the current indication. In the TMC125-C227 study, INTELENCE (N=59) was administered with 2 investigator-selected NRTIs (i.e. without a ritonavir-boosted PI) and compared to an investigator-selected combination of a PI with 2 NRTIs (N=57). The trial population included PI-naïve, NNRTI-experienced patients with evidence of NNRTI resistance.

At week 12, virologic response was greater in the control-PI arm (-2.2 $\log_{10}$ copies/ml from baseline; n=53) compared to the INTELENCE arm (-1.4 $\log_{10}$ copies/ml from baseline; n=40). This difference between treatment arms was statistically significant.

Based on these trial results, INTELENCE is not recommended for use in combination with N(t)RTIs only in patients who have experienced virological failure on an NNRTI- and N(t)RTI-containing regimen.

This medicinal product has been authorised under a so-called "conditional approval" scheme.

This means that further evidence on this medicinal product is awaited.

The European Medicines Agency (EMEA) will review new information on the product every year and this SPC will be updated as necessary.

5.2 Pharmacokinetic properties

The pharmacokinetic properties of etravirine have been evaluated in adult healthy subjects and in adult treatment-experienced HIV-1 infected patients. Exposure to etravirine was lower (35-50%) in HIV-1 infected patients than in healthy subjects.

Absorption

An intravenous formulation of etravirine is unavailable, thus, the absolute bioavailability of etravirine is unknown. After oral administration with food, the maximum plasma concentration of etravirine is generally achieved within 4 hours.

Table 3: DUET-1 and DUET-2 pooled 48-week data

	INTELENCE + BR N=599	Placebo + BR N=604	Treatment difference (95% CI)
Baseline characteristics			
Median plasma HIV-1 RNA	4.8 $\log_{10}$ copies/ml	4.8 $\log_{10}$ copies/ml	
Median CD4 cell count	99 $\times$ 10^6 cells/l	109 $\times$ 10^6 cells/l	
Outcomes			
Confirmed undetectable viral load (< 50 HIV-1 RNA copies/ml)[a] n (%)			
Overall	363 (60.6%)	240 (39.7%)	20.9% (15.3%; 26.4%)[d]
De novo ENF	109 (71.2%)	93 (58.5%)	12.8% (2.3%; 23.2%)[f]
Not *de novo* ENF	254 (57.0%)	147 (33.0%)	23.9% (17.6%; 30.3%)[f]
< 400 HIV-1 RNA copies/ml[a] n (%)	428 (71.5%)	286 (47.4%)	24.1% (18.7%; 29.5%)[d]
HIV-1 RNA $\log_{10}$ mean change from baseline ($\log_{10}$ copies/ml)[b]	-2.25	-1.49	-0.6 (-0.8; -0.5)[c]
CD4 cell count mean change from baseline (x 10^6/l)[b]	+98.2	+72.9	24.4 (10.4; 38.5)[c]
Any AIDS defining illness and/or death n (%)	35 (5.8%)	59 (9.8%)	-3.9% (-0.9%; -6.9%)[e]

[a] Imputations according to the TLOVR algorithm (TLOVR = Time to Loss of Virologic Response).

[b] Non-completer is failure (NC = F) imputation.

[c] Treatment differences are based on Least Square Means from an ANCOVA model including the stratification factors. P-value < 0.0001 for mean decrease in HIV-1 RNA; P-value = 0.0006 for mean change in CD4 cell count.

[d] Confidence interval around observed difference of response rates; P-value < 0.0001 from logistic regression model, including stratification factors.

[e] Confidence interval around observed difference of response rates; P-value = 0.0408

[f] Confidence interval around observed difference of response rates; P-value from CMH test controlling for stratification factors = 0.0199 for *de novo*, and < 0.0001 for not *de novo*

Table 5: Proportion of subjects with < 50 HIV-1 RNA copies/ml at week 48 by baseline number of INTELENCE RAMs in the non-viral failure excluded population of pooled DUET-1 and DUET-2 trials

Baseline number of INTELENCE RAMs*	Etravirine arms N=549	
	Reused/not used ENF	*De novo* ENF
All ranges	63.3% (254/401)	78.4% (109/139)
0	74.1% (117/158)	91.3% (42/46)
1	61.3% (73/119)	80.4% (41/51)
2	64.1% (41/64)	66.7% (18/27)
⩾ 3	38.3% (23/60)	53.3% (8/15)
	Placebo arms N=569	
All ranges	37.1% (147/396)	64.1% (93/145)

* INTELENCE RAMs = V90I, A98G, L100I, K101E/P, V106I, V179D/F, Y181C/I/V, G190A/S

Note: all patients in the DUET trials received a background regimen consisting of darunavir/rtv, investigator-selected NRTIs and optional enfuvirtide.

In healthy subjects, the absorption of etravirine is not affected by co-administration of oral ranitidine or omeprazole, medicinal products that are known to increase gastric pH.

Effect of food on absorption

The systemic exposure (AUC) to etravirine was decreased by about 50% when INTELENCE was administered under fasting conditions, as compared to administration following a meal. Therefore, INTELENCE should be taken following a meal.

Distribution

Etravirine is approximately 99.9% bound to plasma proteins, primarily to albumin (99.6%) and α1-acid glycoprotein (97.66%-99.02%) *in vitro*. The distribution of etravirine into compartments other than plasma (e.g., cerebrospinal fluid, genital tract secretions) has not been evaluated in humans.

Metabolism

In vitro experiments with human liver microsomes (HLMs) indicate that etravirine primarily undergoes oxidative metabolism by the hepatic cytochrome CYP450 (CYP3A) system and, to a lesser extent, by the CYP2C family, followed by glucuronidation.

Elimination

After administration of a radiolabeled ^{14}C-etravirine dose, 93.7% and 1.2% of the administered dose of ^{14}C-etravirine could be retrieved in faeces and urine, respectively. Unchanged etravirine accounted for 81.2% to 86.4% of the administered dose in faeces. Unchanged etravirine in faeces is likely to be unabsorbed drug. Unchanged etravirine was not detected in urine. The terminal elimination half-life of etravirine was approximately 30-40 hours.

Special populations

Paediatric population

The pharmacokinetics of etravirine in paediatric patients are under investigation. There are insufficient data at this time to recommend a dose (see section 4.2).

Elderly

Population pharmacokinetic analysis in HIV infected patients showed that etravirine pharmacokinetics are not considerably different in the age range (18 to 77 years) evaluated, with 6 subjects aged 65 years or older (see sections 4.2 and 4.4).

Gender

No significant pharmacokinetic differences have been observed between men and women. A limited number of women were included in the studies.

Race

Population pharmacokinetic analysis of etravirine in HIV infected patients indicated no apparent difference in the exposure to etravirine between Caucasian, Hispanic and Black subjects. The pharmacokinetics in other races have not been sufficiently evaluated.

Hepatic impairment

Etravirine is primarily metabolised and eliminated by the liver. In a study comparing 8 patients with mild (Child-Pugh Class A) hepatic impairment to 8 matched controls and 8 patients with moderate (Child-Pugh Class B) hepatic impairment to 8 matched controls, the multiple dose pharmacokinetic disposition of etravirine was not altered in patients with mild to moderate hepatic impairment. However, unbound concentrations have not been assessed. Increased unbound exposure could be expected. No dose adjustment is suggested but caution is adviced in patients with moderate hepatic impairment. INTELENCE has not been studied in patients with severe hepatic impairment (Child-Pugh Class C) and is therefore not recommended (see sections 4.2 and 4.4).

Hepatitis B and/or hepatitis C virus co-infection

Population pharmacokinetic analysis of the DUET-1 and DUET-2 trials showed reduced clearance (potentially leading to increased exposure and alteration of the safety profile) for INTELENCE in HIV-1 infected patients with hepatitis B and/or hepatitis C virus co-infection. In view of the limited data available in hepatitis B and/or C co-infected patients, particular caution should be paid when INTELENCE is used in these patients (see sections 4.4 and 4.8).

Renal impairment

The pharmacokinetics of etravirine have not been studied in patients with renal insufficiency. Results from a mass balance study with radioactive ^{14}C-etravirine showed that < 1.2% of the administered dose of etravirine is excreted in the urine. No unchanged drug was detected in urine so the impact of renal impairment on etravirine elimination is expected to be minimal. As etravirine is highly bound to plasma proteins, it is unlikely that it will be significantly removed by haemodialysis or peritoneal dialysis (see section 4.2).

5.3 Preclinical safety data

Animal toxicology studies have been conducted with etravirine in mice, rats, rabbits and dogs. In mice, the key target organs identified were the liver and the coagulation system. Haemorrhagic cardiomyopathy was only observed in male mice and was considered to be secondary to severe coagulopathy mediated via the vitamin K pathway. In the rat, the key target organs identified were the liver, the thyroid and the coagulation system. Exposure in mice was equivalent to human exposure while in rats it was below the clinical exposure at the recommended dose. In the dog, changes were observed in the liver and gall bladder at exposures approximately 8-fold higher than human exposure observed at the recommended dose (200 mg b.i.d.).

In a study conducted in rats, there were no effects on mating or fertility at exposure levels equivalent to those in humans at the clinically recommended dose. There was no teratogenicity with etravirine in rats and rabbits at exposures equivalent to those observed in humans at the recommended clinical dose. Etravirine had no effect on offspring development during lactation or post weaning at maternal exposures equivalent to those observed at the recommended clinical dose.

Etravirine was not carcinogenic in rats and in male mice. An increase in the incidences of hepatocellular adenomas and carcinomas were observed in female mice. The observed hepatocellular findings in female mice are generally considered to be rodent specific, associated with liver enzyme induction, and of limited relevance to humans. At the highest tested doses, the systemic exposures (based on AUC) to etravirine were 0.6-fold (mice) and between 0.2- and 0.7-fold (rats), relative to those observed in humans at the recommended therapeutic dose (200 mg b.i.d.).

In vitro and *in vivo* studies with etravirine revealed no evidence of a mutagenic potential.

6. PHARMACEUTICAL PARTICULARS

6.1 List of excipients

Hypromellose

Microcrystalline cellulose

Colloidal anhydrous silica

Croscarmellose sodium

Magnesium stearate

Lactose monohydrate

6.2 Incompatibilities

Not applicable.

6.3 Shelf life

2 years.

6.4 Special precautions for storage

Store in the original bottle. Keep the bottle tightly closed in order to protect from moisture. Do not remove the desiccant pouches.

6.5 Nature and contents of container

High-density polyethylene (HDPE) plastic bottles containing 120 tablets and 3 desiccant pouches, fitted with polypropylene (PP) child resistant closures.

Each carton contains one bottle.

6.6 Special precautions for disposal and other handling
No special requirements.

Any unused product or waste material should be disposed of in accordance with local requirements.

7. MARKETING AUTHORISATION HOLDER
Janssen-Cilag International NV
Turnhoutseweg 30
B-2340 Beerse
Belgium

8. MARKETING AUTHORISATION NUMBER(S)
EU/1/08/468/001

9. DATE OF FIRST AUTHORISATION/RENEWAL OF THE AUTHORISATION
28 August 2008

10. DATE OF REVISION OF THE TEXT
23 April 2009

Detailed information on this medicinal product is available on the website of the European Medicines Agency (EMEA) http://www.emea.europa.eu/

Intrinsa 300 micrograms/24 hours transdermal patch

(Procter & Gamble Pharmaceuticals UK Limited)

1. NAME OF THE MEDICINAL PRODUCT
Intrinsa 300 micrograms/24 hours transdermal patch ▼

2. QUALITATIVE AND QUANTITATIVE COMPOSITION
Each patch of 28 cm^2 contains 8.4 mg testosterone and provides 300 micrograms of testosterone per 24 hours.

For a full list of excipients, see section 6.1.

3. PHARMACEUTICAL FORM
Transdermal patch.

Thin, clear, oval matrix-type transdermal patch consisting of three layers: a translucent backing film, an adhesive matrix drug layer, and a protective release liner that is removed prior to application. Each patch surface is stamped with PG T001.

4. CLINICAL PARTICULARS

4.1 Therapeutic indications
Intrinsa is indicated for the treatment of hypoactive sexual desire disorder (HSDD) in bilaterally oophorectomised and hysterectomised (surgically induced menopause) women receiving concomitant estrogen therapy.

4.2 Posology and method of administration
The recommended daily dose of testosterone is 300 micrograms. This is achieved by applying the patch twice weekly on a continuous basis. The patch should be replaced with a fresh patch every 3 to 4 days. A particular application site should be rotated with an interval of at least 7 days between applications. Only one patch is to be worn at a time.

The adhesive side of the patch should be applied to a clean, dry area of skin on the lower abdomen below the waist. Patches should not be applied to the breasts or other body regions. A skin site with minimal wrinkling and not covered by tight clothing is recommended. The site should not be oily, damaged, or irritated. To prevent interference with the adhesive properties of Intrinsa, no creams, lotions or powder should be applied to the skin where the patch is to be applied.

The patch should be applied immediately after opening the sachet and removing both parts of the protective release liner. The patch should be pressed firmly in place for about 10 seconds, making sure there is good contact with the skin, especially around the edges. If an area of the patch lifts, pressure should be applied to that area. If the patch detaches prematurely, it may be reapplied. If the same patch cannot be reapplied, a new patch should be applied to another location. In either case, the original treatment regimen should be maintained. The patch is designed to remain in place during a shower, bath, swimming or exercising.

Concomitant estrogen treatment

The appropriate use and restrictions associated with estrogen therapy should be considered before Intrinsa therapy is initiated and during routine re-evaluation of treatment. Continued use of Intrinsa is only recommended while concomitant use of estrogen is considered appropriate (i.e. the lowest effective dose for the shortest possible duration).

Patients treated with conjugated equine estrogen (CEE) are not recommended to use Intrinsa, as efficacy has not been demonstrated (see sections 4.4 and 5.1).

Duration of treatment

Intrinsa treatment response should be evaluated within 3-6 months of initiation, to determine if continued therapy is appropriate. Patients who do not experience a meaningful benefit should be re-evaluated and discontinuation of therapy be considered.

As the efficacy and safety of Intrinsa have not been evaluated in studies of longer duration than 1 year, it is recommended that an appraisal of the treatment is undertaken every 6 months.

Children and adolescents:

There is no relevant indication for use of Intrinsa in children and adolescents.

4.3 Contraindications
Hypersensitivity to the active substance or to any of the excipients.

Known, suspected or past history of cancer of the breast or known or suspected estrogen-dependent neoplasia, or any other condition consistent with the contraindications for the use of estrogen.

4.4 Special warnings and precautions for use
At regular intervals during treatment, physicians should monitor patients for potential androgenic undesirable effects (e.g. acne, changes in hair growth or hair loss). Patients should be advised to self assess for androgenic undesirable effects. Signs of virilisation, such as voice deepening, hirsutism or clitoromegaly, may be irreversible and discontinuation of treatment should be considered. In clinical trials these reactions were reversible in the majority of patients (see section 4.8).

Severe skin erythema, local oedema and blistering may occur due to hypersensitivity to the patch at the site of application. Use of the patch should be discontinued if this occurs.

The safety of Intrinsa has not been evaluated in double blind placebo controlled studies of longer than 1 year duration. There is little information on long-term safety, including effects on breast tissue, the cardiovascular system and increase in insulin resistance.

Data in the literature regarding the influence of testosterone on the risk of breast cancer in women are limited, inconclusive and conflicting. The long-term effect of testosterone treatment on the breast is currently unknown, therefore patients should be carefully monitored with regard to breast cancer in accordance with currently accepted screening practises and individual patient needs.

Patients with known cardiovascular disease have not been studied. Patients with cardiovascular risk factors, in particular hypertension, and patients with known cardiovascular disease should be carefully monitored, specifically regarding changes in blood pressure and weight.

In diabetic patients the metabolic effects of testosterone may decrease blood glucose and therefore insulin requirements. Patients with diabetes mellitus have not been studied.

Little information is available on the effects of testosterone on the endometrium. The limited data evaluating the effect of testosterone on the endometrium neither allow conclusions nor reassurances on the incidence of endometrial cancer.

Oedema (with or without congestive heart failure) may be a serious complication from high doses of testosterone or other anabolic steroids in patients with pre-existing cardiac, renal, or hepatic disease. However, this is not expected from the low dose of testosterone delivered by the Intrinsa patch.

Intrinsa is recommended for use in surgically menopausal women up to the age of 60. Consistent with the prevalence of HSDD, there are limited data above the age of 60.

Efficacy and safety of Intrinsa 300 micrograms in naturally menopausal women with HSDD on concomitant estrogen, with or without progestogen, have not been evaluated. Intrinsa 300 micrograms is not recommended in naturally menopausal women.

Whereas Intrinsa is indicated with concomitant estrogen therapy, the subgroup of patients receiving oral conjugated equine estrogens (CEE) did not demonstrate a significant improvement in sexual function. Therefore, Intrinsa should not be used in women on concomitant CEE (see sections 4.2 and 5.1).

Androgens may decrease levels of thyroxin-binding globulin, resulting in decreased total T4 serum levels and increased resin uptake of T3 and T4. Free thyroid hormone levels remain unchanged, however, and there is no clinical evidence of thyroid dysfunction.

4.5 Interaction with other medicinal products and other forms of interaction
No interaction studies have been performed. When testosterone is given concomitantly with anticoagulants, the anticoagulant effect may increase. Patients receiving oral anticoagulants require close monitoring, especially when testosterone therapy is started or stopped.

4.6 Pregnancy and lactation
Intrinsa must not be used in women who are or may become pregnant or by breast-feeding women.

Testosterone may induce virilising effects on the female foetus when administered to a pregnant woman. Studies in animals have shown reproductive toxicity (see section 5.3).

Table 1

MedDRA System organ class	Very Common ⩾ 1/10	Common ⩾ 1/100, < 1/10	Uncommon ⩾ 1/1,000, < 1/100
Infections and infestations			Sinusitis
Blood and lymphatic system disorders			Abnormal clotting factor
Immune system disorders			Hypersensitivity
Metabolism and nutrition disorders			Increased appetite
Psychiatric disorders		Insomnia	Agitation, anxiety
Nervous system disorders		Migraine	Disturbance in attention, dysgeusia, impaired balance, hyperaesthesia, oral paraesthesia, transient ischemic attack
Eye disorders			Diplopia, eye redness
Cardiac disorders			Palpitations
Respiratory, thoracic and mediastinal disorders		Voice deepening	Nasal congestion, throat tightness
Gastrointestinal disorders		Abdominal pain	Diarrhoea, dry mouth, nausea
Skin and subcutaneous tissue disorders	Hirsutism	Acnes, alopecias	Eczema, increased sweating, rosacea
Musculoskeletal and connective tissue disorders			Arthritis
Reproductive system and breast disorders		Breast pain	Breast cyst, clitoral engorgement, enlarged clitoris, genital pruritus, vaginal burning sensation
General disorders and administration site conditions	Application site reaction (erythema, itching)		Anasarca, asthenia, chest tightness, chest discomfort
Investigations		Increased weight	Abnormal blood fibrinogen, increased heart rate, increased alanine aminotransferase, increased aspartate aminotransferase, increased blood bilirubin, abnormal liver function test, increased blood triglycerides

In case of inadvertent exposure during pregnancy, use of Intrinsa must be discontinued.

4.7 Effects on ability to drive and use machines

Intrinsa has no influence on the ability to drive and use machines.

4.8 Undesirable effects

The adverse reaction most often reported (30.4 %) was application site reactions. The majority of these adverse reactions consisted of mild erythema and itching and did not result in patient withdrawal.

Hirsutism was also very commonly reported. Most reports concerned the chin and upper lip, were mild (≥ 90 %), and less than 1 % of all patients withdrew from the studies due to hirsutism. Hirsutism was reversible in the majority of patients.

Other androgenic effects commonly reported were acne, voice deepening and alopecia. More than 90 % of these reports were considered mild. These reactions were reversible in the majority of patients. Less than 1 % of patients withdrew from the studies because of any of these reactions. All other common adverse events resolved in the majority of patients.

During 6-month double blind exposure the following adverse reactions occurred in the treatment group (n=549) at a greater incidence than placebo (n=545) and were assessed by the investigators as possibly or probably related to Intrinsa treatment. If an adverse reaction occurred at a higher frequency in the integrated phase III studies (Intrinsa patients n=1,498, placebo patients n=1,297), this frequency is reported in the table.

(see Table 1 on previous page)

No new or other adverse reactions have been identified from the post-marketing spontaneous reporting system.

4.9 Overdose

The mode of administration of Intrinsa makes overdose unlikely. Removal of the patch results in a rapid decrease in serum testosterone levels (see section 5.2).

5. PHARMACOLOGICAL PROPERTIES

5.1 Pharmacodynamic properties

Pharmacotherapeutic group: Androgens, testosterone, ATC code: G03BA03

Testosterone, the primary circulating androgen in women, is a naturally occurring steroid, secreted by the ovaries and adrenal glands. In premenopausal women, the rate of production of testosterone is 100 to 400 micrograms/24 hours, of which half is contributed by the ovary as either testosterone or a precursor. Serum levels of androgens fall as women age. In women, who have undergone bilateral oophorectomy, serum levels of testosterone decline by approximately 50 % within days after surgery.

Intrinsa is a transdermal therapy for HSDD, which improves sexual desire while achieving testosterone concentrations compatible with premenopausal levels.

Two multi-centre, double-blind, placebo-controlled six month studies in 562 (INTIMATE SM1) and 533 (INTIMATE SM2) oophorectomised and hysterectomised women (surgically induced menopause), aged 20 to 70 years, with HSDD on concomitant estrogen were used to evaluate the efficacy and safety of Intrinsa. Total satisfying sexual activity (primary endpoint), sexual desire, and distress associated with low sexual desire (secondary endpoints) were evaluated with validated instruments.

In the combined study analysis at 24 weeks, the difference in the mean frequency of total satisfying episodes between Intrinsa and placebo was 1.07 per 4 weeks.

A significantly higher percentage of women who received Intrinsa reported a benefit in the three endpoints, that they considered clinically meaningful compared to women who received placebo. In the combined phase III data, excluding patients taking oral CEE, in whom there was no significant improvement in sexual function, 50.7 % of women (n=274) treated with Intrinsa and 29.4 % of those treated with placebo (n=269) were responders with regard to total satisfying sexual activity (primary endpoint), when a responder was predefined as having an increase in the 4-week frequency of satisfying activities of > 1.

Effects of Intrinsa were observed at 4 weeks after initiation of therapy (the first measured time point) and at all monthly efficacy time points thereafter.

Efficacy versus placebo was significant across a range of subgroups which included patients separated by the following baseline characteristics: age (all subgroups up to age 65 years); body weight (up to 80 kg) and oophorectomy (up to 15 years ago).

Subgroup analyses suggested that the route and type of concomitant estrogen (transdermal oestradiol, oral conjugated equine estrogen (CEE), oral non-CEE) can influence patient response. A responder analysis of the pivotal phase II and III studies showed significant improvements in all three major clinical endpoints versus placebo in patients on concomitant transdermal and oral non-CEE estrogens. However, the subgroup of patients receiving oral CEE did not demonstrate a significant improvement in sexual activity compared to placebo (see sections 4.2 and 4.4).

5.2 Pharmacokinetic properties

Absorption:

Testosterone from Intrinsa is transported across intact skin by a passive diffusion process that is primarily controlled by permeation across the stratum corneum. Intrinsa is designed to systemically deliver 300 micrograms/day. Following application of the patch on abdominal skin, maximum serum concentrations of testosterone are reached within 24-36 hours, with a wide inter-individual variability. Serum concentrations of testosterone attain steady-state by the application of the second patch when applied in a twice-a-week regimen. Intrinsa did not influence serum concentrations of sex hormone binding globulin (SHBG), estrogens or adrenal hormones.

(see Table 2 below)

Distribution:

In women, circulating testosterone is primarily bound in the serum to SHBG (65-80 %) and to albumin (20-30 %) leaving only about 0.5-2 % as the free fraction. The affinity of binding to serum SHBG is relatively high and the SHBG bound fraction is regarded as not contributing to biological activity. Binding to albumin is of relatively low affinity and is reversible. The albumin-bound fraction and the unbound fraction are collectively termed 'bioavailable' testosterone. The amount of SHBG and albumin in serum and the total testosterone concentration determine the distribution of free and bioavailable testosterone. Serum concentration of SHBG is influenced by the route of administration of concomitant estrogen therapy.

Metabolism:

Testosterone is metabolised primarily in the liver. Testosterone is metabolised to various 17-ketosteroids and further metabolism results in inactive glucuronides and other conjugates. The active metabolites of testosterone are estradiol and dihydrotestosterone (DHT). DHT has a greater affinity to SHBG than does testosterone. DHT concentrations increased in parallel with testosterone concentrations during Intrinsa treatment. There were no significant differences in serum estradiol and estrone levels in patients treated with Intrinsa for up to 52 weeks compared to baseline.

On removal of an Intrinsa patch, testosterone serum concentrations return to near baseline values within 12 hours due to its short terminal exponential half-life (approximately 2 hours). There was no evidence of accumulation of testosterone over 52 weeks of treatment.

Elimination:

Testosterone is mainly excreted in the urine as glucuronic and sulphuric acid conjugates of testosterone and its metabolites.

5.3 Preclinical safety data

Toxicological studies of testosterone have only revealed effects which can be explained based on the hormone profile.

Testosterone has been found to be nongenotoxic. Nonclinical studies on a relationship between testosterone treatment and cancer suggest that high doses may promote tumour growth in sex organs, mammary glands and liver in laboratory animals. The significance of these data for the use of Intrinsa in patients is not known.

Testosterone has a masculinising effect on female rat foetuses when dosed subcutaneously at 0.5 or 1 mg/day (as the propionate ester) to pregnant rats during organogenesis.

Table 2

Serum Concentrations of Testosterone and SHBG in Patients Receiving Intrinsa in Clinical Safety and Efficacy Studies

Hormone	Baseline		Week 24		Week 52	
	N	Mean (SEM)	N	Mean (SEM)	N	Mean (SEM)
Free testosterone (pg/ml)	544	0.92 (0.03)	412	4.36 (0.16)	287	4.44 (0.31)
Total testosterone (ng/dl)	547	17.6 (0.4)	413	79.7 (2.7)	288	74.8 (3.6)
DHT (ng/dl)	271	7.65 (0.34)	143	20.98 (0.98)	169	21.04 (0.97)
SHBG (nmol/l)	547	91.7 (2.5)	415	93.9 (2.8)	290	90.0 (3.6)

DHT = dihydrotestosterone, SHBG = sex hormone binding globulin

SEM = Standard Error of the Mean

6. PHARMACEUTICAL PARTICULARS

6.1 List of excipients

Backing layer:

Translucent polyethylene backing film printed with proprietary ink containing sunset yellow FCF (E110), latolrubine BK (E180) and copper phthalocyanine blue pigment.

Self adhesive matrix drug layer:

Sorbitan oleate,

Acrylic co-polymer adhesive containing 2-Ethylhexylacrylate – 1-Vinyl-2-pyrrolidone co-polymer.

Protective release liner:

Siliconised polyester film.

6.2 Incompatibilities

Not applicable.

6.3 Shelf life

3 years

6.4 Special precautions for storage

Do not store above 30°C.

Do not refrigerate or freeze.

6.5 Nature and contents of container

Each patch is packed in a sealed laminated sachet. The sachet material comprises of food grade paper/polyethylene/aluminium foil/ethylene methacrylic acid copolymer (outer to inner layer). The ethylene methacrylic acid copolymer (Surlyn®) is the heat seal layer which allows the two laminate sachet stocks to be heat-sealed together to form the sachet.

Cartons of 2, 8 and 24 patches.

Not all pack sizes may be marketed.

6.6 Special precautions for disposal and other handling

Any unused product or waste material should be disposed of in accordance with local requirements.

7. MARKETING AUTHORISATION HOLDER

Procter & Gamble Pharmaceuticals UK Ltd.

Rusham Park Technical Centre

Whitehall Lane

Egham

Surrey

TW20 9NW

United Kingdom

8. MARKETING AUTHORISATION NUMBER(S)

EU/1/06/352/001-003

9. DATE OF FIRST AUTHORISATION/RENEWAL OF THE AUTHORISATION

28/07/2006

10. DATE OF REVISION OF THE TEXT

16/09/2008

INVANZ 1g powder for concentrate for solution for infusion

(Merck Sharp & Dohme Limited)

1. NAME OF THE MEDICINAL PRODUCT

INVANZ® 1 g powder for concentrate for solution for infusion.

2. QUALITATIVE AND QUANTITATIVE COMPOSITION

Each vial contains 1.0 g ertapenem equivalent to 1.046 g ertapenem sodium.

Excipients: each 1.0 g dose contains approximately 6.0 mEq of sodium (approximately 137 mg).

For a full list of excipients, see section 6.1.

3. PHARMACEUTICAL FORM

Powder for concentrate for solution for infusion. White to off-white powder.

4. CLINICAL PARTICULARS

4.1 Therapeutic indications

Treatment

Treatment of the following infections when caused by bacteria known or very likely to be susceptible to ertapenem and when parenteral therapy is required (see section 4.4 and section 5.1):

- Intra-abdominal infections
- Community acquired pneumonia
- Acute gynaecological infections
- Diabetic foot infections of the skin and soft tissue (see section 4.4)

Prevention

INVANZ is indicated in adults for the prophylaxis of surgical site infection following elective colorectal surgery.

Consideration should be given to official guidance on the appropriate use of antibacterial agents.

4.2 Posology and method of administration

Adults and adolescents (13 to 17 years of age): The dose of INVANZ is 1 gram (g) given once a day by the intravenous route (see section 6.6).

Prophylaxis of surgical site infection following elective colorectal surgery in adults: To prevent surgical site infections, the recommended dosage is 1 g administered as a single intravenous dose to be completed within 1 hour prior to the surgical incision.

For infants and children (3 months to 12 years of age): The dose of INVANZ is 15 mg/kg given twice daily (not to exceed 1 g/day) by the intravenous route (see section 6.6). INVANZ is not recommended for use in children below 3 months of age due to a lack of data on safety and efficacy (see sections 4.4; 5.1 and 5.2).

Intravenous administration: INVANZ should be infused over a period of 30 minutes.

The usual duration of therapy with INVANZ is 3 to 14 days but may vary depending on the type and severity of infection and causative pathogen(s). When clinically indicated, a switch to an appropriate oral antibacterial agent may be implemented if clinical improvement has been observed.

Renal insufficiency:

INVANZ may be used for the treatment of infections in adult patients with renal insufficiency. In patients whose creatinine clearance is > 30 ml/min/1.73 m^2, no dosage adjustment is necessary. There are inadequate data on the safety and efficacy of ertapenem in patients with advanced renal insufficiency to support a dose recommendation. Therefore, ertapenem should not be used in these patients. (See section 5.2.) There are no data in children and adolescents with renal insufficiency.

Patients on haemodialysis:

There are inadequate data on the safety and efficacy of ertapenem in patients on haemodialysis to support a dose recommendation. Therefore, ertapenem should not be used in these patients.

Hepatic insufficiency:

No dosage adjustment is recommended in patients with impaired hepatic function (see section 5.2).

Elderly:

The recommended dose of INVANZ should be administered, except in cases of advanced renal insufficiency (see *Renal insufficiency*).

4.3 Contraindications

- Hypersensitivity to the active substance or to any of the excipients
- Hypersensitivity to any other carbapenem antibacterial agent
- Severe hypersensitivity (e.g. anaphylactic reaction, severe skin reaction) to any other type of beta-lactam antibacterial agent (e.g. penicillins or cephalosporins).

4.4 Special warnings and precautions for use

Serious and occasionally fatal hypersensitivity (anaphylactic) reactions have been reported in patients receiving therapy with beta-lactams. These reactions are more likely to occur in individuals with a history of sensitivity to multiple allergens. Before initiating therapy with ertapenem, careful inquiry should be made concerning previous hypersensitivity reactions to penicillins, cephalosporins, other beta-lactams and other allergens (see section 4.3). If an allergic reaction to ertapenem occurs, discontinue the therapy immediately. **Serious anaphylactic reactions require immediate emergency treatment.**

As with other antibiotics, prolonged use of ertapenem may result in overgrowth of non-susceptible organisms. Repeated evaluation of the patient's condition is essential. If superinfection occurs during therapy, appropriate measures should be taken.

Antibiotic-associated colitis and pseudomembranous colitis have been reported with nearly all antibacterial agents, including ertapenem, and may range in severity from mild to life-threatening. Therefore, it is important to consider this diagnosis in patients who present with diarrhoea subsequent to the administration of antibacterial agents. Discontinuation of therapy with INVANZ and the administration of specific treatment for *Clostridium difficile* should be considered. Medicinal products that inhibit peristalsis should not be given.

Seizures have been reported during clinical investigation in adult patients treated with ertapenem sodium (1g once a day) during therapy or in the 14 -day follow-up period. Seizures occurred most commonly in elderly patients and those with pre-existing CNS disorders (e.g. brain lesions or history of seizures) and /or compromised renal function). Similar observations have been made in the post-marketing environment.

The efficacy of INVANZ in the treatment of community acquired pneumonia due to penicillin-resistant *Streptococcus pneumoniae* has not been established.

There is relatively little experience with ertapenem in children less than two years of age. In this age group, particular care should be taken to establish the susceptibility of the infecting organism(s) to ertapenem. No data are available in children under 3 months of age.

Experience in the use of ertapenem in the treatment of severe infections is limited. In clinical studies for the treatment of community-acquired pneumonia, in adults, 25 % of evaluable patients treated with ertapenem had severe disease (defined as pneumonia severity index > III). In a clinical study for the treatment of acute gynaecologic infections, in adults, 26 % of evaluable patients treated with ertapenem had severe disease (defined as temperature ⩾ 39°C and/or bacteraemia); ten patients had bacteraemia. Of evaluable patients treated with ertapenem in a clinical study for the treatment of intra-abdominal infections, in adults, 30 % had generalised peritonitis and 39 % had infections involving sites other than the appendix including the stomach, duodenum, small bowel, colon, and gallbladder; there were limited numbers of evaluable patients who were enrolled with APACHE II scores ⩾ 15 and efficacy in these patients has not been established.

Efficacy of ertapenem in the treatment of diabetic foot infections with concurrent osteomyelitis has not been established.

Based on the data available it cannot be excluded that in the few cases of surgical interventions exceeding 4 hours, patients could be exposed to sub-optimal ertapenem concentrations and consequently to a risk of potential treatment failure. Therefore, caution should be exercised in such unusual cases.

This medicinal product contains approximately 6.0 mEq (approximately 137 mg) of sodium per 1.0 g dose which should be taken into consideration by patients on a controlled sodium diet.

4.5 Interaction with other medicinal products and other forms of interaction

Interactions caused by inhibition of P-glycoprotein-mediated clearance or CYP-mediated clearance of medicinal products are unlikely (see section 5.2).

Penem and carbapenem antibacterial agents may decrease the serum levels of valproic acid. Monitoring of serum levels of valproic acid should be considered if ertapenem is to be co-administered with valproic acid.

4.6 Pregnancy and lactation

Adequate and well-controlled studies have not been performed in pregnant women. Animal studies do not indicate direct or indirect harmful effects with respect to pregnancy, embryo-foetal development, parturition or post-natal development. However, ertapenem should not be used during pregnancy unless the potential benefit outweighs the possible risk to the foetus.

Ertapenem is excreted in human milk. Because of the potential for adverse reactions on the infant, mothers should not breast-feed their infants while receiving ertapenem.

4.7 Effects on ability to drive and use machines

No studies on the effects on the ability to drive and use machines have been performed.

INVANZ may influence patient's ability to drive and use machines. Patients should be informed that dizziness and somnolence have been reported with INVANZ (see section 4.8).

4.8 Undesirable effects

Adults 18 years of age and older:

The total number of patients treated with ertapenem in clinical studies was over 2,200 of which over 2,150 received a 1 g dose of ertapenem. Adverse reactions (i.e. considered by the investigator to be possibly, probably, or definitely related to the medicinal product) were reported in approximately 20 % of patients treated with ertapenem. Treatment was discontinued due to adverse reactions in 1.3 % of patients. An additional 476 patients received ertapenem as a single 1 g dose prior to surgery in a clinical study for the prophylaxis of surgical site infections following colorectal surgery.

For patients who received only INVANZ, the most common adverse reactions reported during therapy plus follow-up for 14 days after treatment was stopped were: diarrhoea (4.8 %), infused vein complication (4.5 %) and nausea (2.8 %).

For patients who received only INVANZ, the most frequently reported laboratory abnormalities and their respective incidence rates during therapy plus follow-up for 14 days after treatment was stopped were: elevations in ALT (4.6 %), AST (4.6 %), alkaline phosphatase (3.8 %) and platelet count (3.0 %).

Children and adolescents (3 months to 17 years of age):

The total number of patients treated with ertapenem in clinical studies was 384. The overall safety profile is comparable to that in adult patients. Adverse reactions (i.e. considered by the investigator to be possibly, probably, or definitely related to the medicinal product) were reported in approximately 20.8 % of patients treated with ertapenem. Treatment was discontinued due to adverse reactions in 0.5 % of patients.

For patients who received only INVANZ, the most common adverse reactions reported during therapy plus follow-up for 14 days after treatment was stopped were: diarrhoea (5.2 %) and infusion site pain (6.1 %).

For patients who received only INVANZ, the most frequently reported laboratory abnormalities and their respective incidence rates during therapy plus follow-up for 14 days after treatment was stopped were: decreases in neutrophil count (3.0 %), and elevations in ALT (2.9 %) and AST (2.8 %).

For patients who received only INVANZ, the following adverse reactions were reported during therapy plus follow-up for 14 days after treatment was stopped:

Common (⩾ 1/100 to < 1/10); Uncommon (⩾ 1/ 1000 to < 1/100); Rare (⩾ 1/ 10,000 to < 1/1000); Very rare (< 1/ 10,000)

(see Table 1 on next page)

4.9 Overdose

No specific information is available on the treatment of overdose with ertapenem. Overdosing of ertapenem is unlikely. Intravenous administration of ertapenem at a 3 g daily dose for 8 days to healthy adult volunteers did not result in significant toxicity. In clinical studies in adults inadvertent administration of up to 3 g in a day did not result in clinically important adverse reactions. In paediatric clinical studies, a single IV dose of 40 mg/kg up to a maximum of 2 g did not result in toxicity.

However, in the event of an overdose, treatment with INVANZ should be discontinued and general supportive treatment given until renal elimination takes place.

Ertapenem can be removed to some extent by haemodialysis (see section 5.2); however, no information is available on the use of haemodialysis to treat overdose.

5. PHARMACOLOGICAL PROPERTIES

5.1 Pharmacodynamic properties

General properties

Pharmacotherapeutic group: carbapenems, ATC code: J01D H03

Mode of action

Ertapenem inhibits bacterial cell wall synthesis following attachment to penicillin binding proteins (PBPs). In *Escherichia coli*, affinity is strongest to PBPs 2 and 3.

Pharmacokinetic/Pharmacodynamic (PK/PD) relationship

Similar to other beta-lactam antimicrobial agents, the time that the plasma concentration of ertapenem exceeds the MIC of the infecting organism has been shown to best correlate with efficacy in pre-clinical PK/PD studies.

Mechanism of resistance

For species considered susceptible to ertapenem, resistance was uncommon in surveillance studies in Europe. In resistant isolates, resistance to other antibacterial agents of the carbapenem class was seen in some but not all isolates. Ertapenem is effectively stable to hydrolysis by most classes of beta-lactamases, including penicillinases, cephalosporinases and extended spectrum beta-lactamases, but not metallo-beta-lactamases.

Methicillin-resistant staphylococci and enterococci are resistant to ertapenem, owing to PBP target insensitivity; *P. aeruginosa* and other non-fermentative bacteria are generally resistant, probably owing to limited penetration and to active efflux.

Resistance is uncommon in Enterobacteriaceae and the drug is generally active against those with extended-spectrum beta-lactamases (ESBLs). Resistance can however be observed when ESBLs or other potent beta-lactamases (e.g. AmpC types) are present in conjunction with reduced permeability, arising by the loss of one or more outer membrane porins, or with up-regulated efflux. Resistance can also arise via the acquisition of betalactamases with significant carbapenem-hydrolysing activity (e.g. IMP and VIM metallo-beta-lactamases or KPC types), though these are rare.

The mechanism of action of ertapenem differs from that of other classes of antibiotics, such as quinolones, aminoglycosides, macrolides and tetracyclines. There is no target-based cross-resistance between ertapenem and these substances. However, micro-organisms may exhibit resistance to more than one class of antibacterial agents when the mechanism is, or includes, impermeability to some compounds and/or an efflux pump.

Breakpoints

The EUCAST MIC breakpoints are as follows:

- *Enterobacteriaceae: S ⩽ 0.5 mg/l and R > 1 mg/l*
- *Streptococcus A,B,C,G: S ⩽ 0.5 mg/l and R >0.5 mg/l*
- *Streptococcus pneumoniae: S ⩽ 0.5 mg/l and R > 0.5 mg/l*
- *Haemophilus influenzae: S ⩽ 0.5 mg/l and R > 0.5 mg/l*
- *M. catarrhalis: S ⩽ 0.5 mg/l and R > 0.5 mg/l*
- *Gram negative anaerobes: S ⩽ 1 mg/l and R>1 mg/l*
- *Non-species related breakpoints: S ⩽ 0.5 mg/l and R > 1 mg/l*

(NB: Susceptibilty of staphylococci to ertapenem is inferred from the methicillin susceptibility)

The prescribers are informed that local MIC breakpoints, if available, should be consulted.

Microbiological susceptibility

The prevalence of acquired resistance may vary geographically and with time for selected species and local information on resistance is desirable, particularly when treating severe infections. Localised clusters of infections due to carbapenem-resistant organisms have been reported in the European Union. The information below gives only approximate guidance on the probability as to

Table 1

	Adults 18 years of age and older	*Children and adolescents (3 months to 17 years of age)*
Infections and infestations:	*Uncommon*: Oral candidiasis	
Blood and lymphatic disorders:	*Rare*: Neutropenia, thrombocytopenia	
Metabolism and nutrition disorders:	*Uncommon*: Anorexia *Rare*: Hypoglycaemia	
Nervous system disorders:	*Common*: Headache *Uncommon*: Dizziness, somnolence, insomnia, confusion, seizure (see section 4.4) *Rare*: Agitation, anxiety, depression, tremor	*Uncommon*: Headache
Cardiac disorders:	*Uncommon*: Sinus bradycardia *Rare*: Arrhythmia, tachycardia	
Vascular disorders:	*Common*: Phlebitis/thrombophlebitis *Uncommon*: Hypotension *Rare*: Haemorrhage, increased blood pressure	*Uncommon*: Hot flush, hypertension, petechiae
Respiratory, thoracic and mediastinal disorders:	*Uncommon*: Dyspnoea, pharyngeal discomfort *Rare*: Nasal congestion, cough, epistaxis, pneumonia, rales/rhonchi, wheezing	
Gastro-intestinal disorders:	*Common*: Diarrhoea, nausea, vomiting *Uncommon*: Constipation, pseudomembranous enterocolitis, acid regurgitation, dry mouth, dyspepsia *Rare*: Dysphagia, faecal incontinence	*Common*: Diarrhoea *Uncommon*: Faeces discoloured, melaena
Hepato-biliary disorders:	*Rare*: Cholecystitis, jaundice, liver disorder	
Skin and subcutaneous tissue disorders:	*Common*: Rash, pruritus *Uncommon*: Erythema, urticaria *Rare*: Dermatitis, dermatomycosis, desquamation, post-operative wound infection	*Common*: Diaper dermatitis *Uncommon*: Erythema, rash
Musculoskeletal and connective tissue disorders:	*Rare*: Muscle cramp, shoulder pain	
Renal and urinary disorders:	*Rare*: Urinary tract infection, renal insufficiency, acute renal insufficiency	
Reproductive system and breast disorders:	*Uncommon*: Vaginitis *Rare*: Abortion, genital bleeding	
General disorders and administration site conditions:	*Common*: Infused vein complication *Uncommon*: Extravasation, abdominal pain, candidiasis, asthenia/fatigue, fungal infection, fever, oedema/swelling, chest pain, taste perversion *Rare*: Allergy, injection-site induration, malaise, pelvic peritonitis, scleral disorder, syncope	*Common*: Infusion site pain *Uncommon*: Infusion site burning, infusion site pruritus, infusion site erythema, injection site erythema, infusion site warmth
Laboratory test findings:		
Chemistry:	*Common*: Elevations in ALT, AST, alkaline phosphatase *Uncommon*: Increases in total serum bilirubin, direct serum bilirubin, indirect serum bilirubin, serum creatinine, serum urea, serum glucose *Rare*: Decreases in serum bicarbonate, serum creatinine, and serum potassium; increases in serum LDH, serum phosphorus, serum potassium	*Common*: Elevations in ALT and AST
Haematology:	*Common*: Elevation in platelet count *Uncommon*: Decreases in white blood cells, platelet count, segmented neutrophils, haemoglobin and haematocrit; increases in eosinophils, activated partial thromboplastin time, prothrombin time, segmented neutrophils, and white blood cells *Rare*: Decrease in lymphocytes; increases in band neutrophils, lymphocytes, metamyelocytes, monocytes, myelocytes; atypical lymphocytes	*Common*: Decreases in neutrophil count *Uncommon*: Increases in platelet count, activated partial thromboplastin time, prothrombin time, decreases in haemoglobin
Urinalysis:	*Uncommon*: Increases in urine bacteria, urine white blood cells, urine epithelial cells, and urine red blood cells; urine yeast present *Rare*: Increase in urobilinogen	
Miscellaneous:	*Uncommon*: Positive *Clostridium difficile* toxin	
Post-marketing experience		
Immune system disorder:	Anaphylaxis including anaphylactoid reactions	
Psychiatric disorders:	Altered mental status (including aggression, delirium, disorientation, mental status changes)	
Nervous system disorders:	Hallucinations, dyskinesia, myoclonus	

whether the micro-organism will be susceptible to ertapenem or not.

Commonly susceptible species:

Gram-positive aerobes:
Methicillin-susceptible-staphylococci (including *Staphylococcus aureus*)*
*Streptococcus agalactiae**
*Streptococcus pneumoniae**†
Streptococcus pyogenes

Gram-negative aerobes:
Citrobacter freundii
Enterobacter aerogenes
Enterobacter cloacae
*Escherichia coli**
*Haemophilus influenzae**
Haemophilus parainfluenzae
Klebsiella oxytoca
*Klebsiella pneumoniae**
*Moraxella catarrhalis**
Morganella morganii
*Proteus mirabilis**
Proteus vulgaris
Serratia marcescens

Anaerobes:
Bacteroides fragilis and species in the *B. fragilis* Group*
Clostridium species (excluding *C. difficile*)*
Eubacterium species*
Fusobacterium species*
Peptostreptococcus species*
*Porphyromonas asaccharolytica**
Prevotella species*

Species for which acquired resistance may be a problem:

Methicillin-resistant staphylococci +#

Inherently resistant organisms:

Gram-positive aerobes:
Corynebacterium jeikeium
Enterococci including *Enterococcus faecalis* and *Enterococcus faecium*

Gram-negative aerobes:
Aeromonas species
Acinetobacter species
Burkholderia cepacia
Pseudomonas aeruginosa
Stenotrophomonas maltophilia

Anaerobes:
Lactobacillus species

Others:
Chlamydia species
Mycoplasma species
Rickettsia species
Legionella species

* Activity has been satisfactorily demonstrated in clinical studies.

† The efficacy of INVANZ in the treatment of community acquired pneumonia due to penicillin-resistant *Streptococcus pneumoniae* has not been established.

+ Frequency of acquired resistance > 50 % in some Member States

Methicillin-resistant staphylococci (including MRSA) are always resistant to beta-lactams.

Information from clinical studies

Efficacy in paediatric studies

Ertapenem was evaluated primarily for paediatric safety and secondarily for efficacy in randomised comparative, multicentre studies in patients 3 months to 17 years of age.

The proportion of patients with a favourable clinical response assessment at post-treatment visit in the clinical MITT population is shown below:

(see Table 2 on next page)

5.2 Pharmacokinetic properties

Plasma concentrations

Average plasma concentrations of ertapenem following a single 30 minute intravenous infusion of a 1 g dose in healthy young adults (25 to 45 years of age) were 155 micrograms/ml (C_{max}) at 0.5 hour post-dose (end of infusion), 9 micrograms/ml at 12 hour post-dose, and 1 microgram/ml at 24 hour post-dose.

Area under the plasma concentration curve (AUC) of ertapenem in adults increases nearly dose-proportionally over the 0.5 to 2 g dose range.

There is no accumulation of ertapenem in adults following multiple intravenous doses ranging from 0.5 to 2 g daily.

Average plasma concentrations of ertapenem following a single 30 minute intravenous infusion of a 15 mg/kg (up to a maximum dose of 1 g) dose in patients 3 to 23 months of age were 103.8 micrograms/ml (C_{max}) at 0.5 hour post-dose (end of infusion), 13.5 micrograms/ml at 6 hour post-dose, and 2.5 micrograms/ml at 12 hour post-dose.

Average plasma concentrations of ertapenem following a single 30 minute intravenous infusion of a 15 mg/kg (up to a maximum dose of 1 g) dose in patients 2 to 12 years of age were 113.2 micrograms/ml (C_{max}) at 0.5 hour post-dose (end of infusion), 12.8 micrograms/ml at 6 hour post-dose, and 3.0 micrograms/ml at 12 hour post-dose.

Average plasma concentrations of ertapenem following a single 30 minute intravenous infusion of a 20 mg/kg (up to a

Table 2

Disease stratum†	Age stratum	Ertapenem		Ceftriaxone	
		n/m	%	n/m	%
Community Acquired Pneumonia (CAP)	3 to 23 months	31/35	88.6	13/13	100.0
	2 to 12 years	55/57	96.5	16/17	94.1
	13 to 17 years	3/3	100.0	3/3	100.0
Disease stratum	Age stratum	Ertapenem		Ticarcillin/clavulanate	
		n/m	%	n/m	%
Intra-abdominal Infections (IAI)	2 to 12 years	28/34	82.4	7/9	77.8
	13 to 17 years	15/16	93.8	4/6	66.7
Acute Pelvic Infections (API)	13 to 17 years	25/25	100.0	8/8	100.0

†. This includes 9 patients in the ertapenem group (7 CAP and 2 IAI), 2 patients in the ceftriaxone group (2 CAP), and 1 patient with IAI in the ticarcillin/clavulanate group with secondary bacteraemia at entry into the study.

maximum dose of 1 g) dose in patients 13 to 17 years of age were 170.4 micrograms/ml (C_{max}) at 0.5 hour post-dose (end of infusion), 7.0 micrograms/ml at 12 hour post-dose, and 1.1 microgram/ml at 24 hour post-dose.

Average plasma concentrations of ertapenem following a single 30 minute intravenous infusion of a 1 g dose in three patients 13 to 17 years of age were 155.9 micrograms/ml (C_{max}) at 0.5 hour post-dose (end of infusion), and 6.2 micrograms/ml at 12 hour post-dose.

Distribution

Ertapenem is highly bound to human plasma proteins. In healthy young adults (25 to 45 years of age), the protein binding of ertapenem decreases, as plasma concentrations increase, from approximately 95 % bound at an approximate plasma concentration of < 50 micrograms/ml to approximately 92 % bound at an approximate plasma concentration of 155 micrograms/ml (average concentration achieved at the end of infusion following 1 g intravenously).

The volume of distribution (V_{dss}) of ertapenem in adults is approximately 8 litres (0.11 litre/kg) and approximately 0.2 litre/kg in paediatric patients 3 months to 12 years of age and approximately 0.16 litre/kg in paediatric patients 13 to 17 years of age.

Concentrations of ertapenem achieved in adult skin blister fluid at each sampling point on the third day of 1 g once daily intravenous doses showed a ratio of AUC in skin blister fluid: AUC in plasma of 0.61.

In-vitro studies indicate that the effect of ertapenem on the plasma protein binding of highly protein bound medicinal products (warfarin, ethinyl estradiol, and norethindrone) was small. The change in binding was < 12 % at peak plasma ertapenem concentration following a 1 g dose. *In vivo*, probenecid (500 mg every 6 hours) decreased the bound fraction of ertapenem in plasma at the end of infusion in subjects administered a single 1 g intravenous dose from approximately 91 % to approximately 87 %. The effects of this change are anticipated to be transient. A clinically significant interaction due to ertapenem displacing another medicinal product or another medicinal product displacing ertapenem is unlikely.

In-vitro studies indicate that ertapenem does not inhibit P-glycoprotein-mediated transport of digoxin or vinblastine and that ertapenem is not a substrate for P-glycoprotein-mediated transport.

Metabolism

In healthy young adults (23 to 49 years of age), after intravenous infusion of radiolabelled 1 g ertapenem, the plasma radioactivity consists predominantly (94 %) of ertapenem. The major metabolite of ertapenem is the ring-opened derivative formed by dehydropeptidase-I-mediated hydrolysis of the beta-lactam ring.

In-vitro studies in human liver microsomes indicate that ertapenem does not inhibit metabolism mediated by any of the six major CYP isoforms: 1A2, 2C9, 2C19, 2D6, 2E1 and 3A4.

Elimination

Following administration of a 1 g radiolabelled intravenous dose of ertapenem to healthy young adults (23 to 49 years of age), approximately 80 % is recovered in urine and 10 % in faeces. Of the 80 % recovered in urine, approximately 38 % is excreted as unchanged ertapenem and approximately 37 % as the ring-opened metabolite.

In healthy young adults (18 to 49 years of age) and patients 13 to 17 years of age given a 1 g intravenous dose, the mean plasma half-life is approximately 4 hours. The mean plasma half-life in children 3 months to 12 years of age is approximately 2.5 hours. Average concentrations of ertapenem in urine exceed 984 micrograms/ml during the period 0 to 2 hours post-dose and exceed 52 micrograms/ml during the period 12 to 24 hours post-administration.

Special populations

Gender

The plasma concentrations of ertapenem are comparable in men and women.

Elderly

Plasma concentrations following a 1 g and 2 g intravenous dose of ertapenem are slightly higher (approximately 39 % and 22 %, respectively) in healthy elderly adults (≥ 65 years) relative to young adults (< 65 years). In the absence of advanced renal insufficiency, no dosage adjustment is necessary in elderly patients.

Paediatric patients

Plasma concentrations of ertapenem are comparable in paediatric patients 13 to 17 years of age and adults following a 1 g once daily intravenous dose.

Following the 20 mg/kg dose (up to a maximum dose of 1 g), the pharmacokinetic parameter values in patients 13 to 17 years of age were generally comparable to those in healthy young adults. To provide an estimate of the pharmacokinetic data if all patients in this age group were to receive a 1 g dose, the pharmacokinetic data were calculated adjusting for a 1 g dose, assuming linearity. A comparison of results show that a 1 g once daily dose of ertapenem achieves a pharmacokinetic profile in patients 13 to 17 years of age comparable to that of adults. The ratios (13 to 17 years/adults) for AUC, the end of infusion concentration and the concentration at the midpoint of the dosing interval were 0.99, 1.20, and 0.84, respectively.

Plasma concentrations at the midpoint of the dosing interval following a single 15 mg/kg intravenous dose of ertapenem in patients 3 months to 12 years of age are comparable to plasma concentrations at the midpoint of the dosing interval following a 1 g once daily intravenous dose in adults (see Plasma concentrations). The plasma clearance (ml/min/kg) of ertapenem in patients 3 months to 12 years of age is approximately 2-fold higher as compared to that in adults. At the 15 mg/kg dose, the AUC value and plasma concentrations at the midpoint of the dosing interval in patients 3 months to 12 years of age were comparable to those in young healthy adults receiving a 1 g intravenous dose of ertapenem.

Hepatic insufficiency

The pharmacokinetics of ertapenem in patients with hepatic insufficiency have not been established. Due to the limited extent of hepatic metabolism of ertapenem, its pharmacokinetics are not expected to be affected by hepatic impairment. Therefore, no dosage adjustment is recommended in patients with hepatic impairment.

Renal insufficiency

Following a single 1 g intravenous dose of ertapenem in adults, AUCs of total ertapenem (bound and unbound) and of unbound ertapenem are similar in patients with mild renal insufficiency (Cl_{cr} 60 to 90 ml/min/1.73 m^2) compared with healthy subjects (ages 25 to 82 years). AUCs of total ertapenem and of unbound ertapenem are increased in patients with moderate renal insufficiency (Cl_{cr} 31 to 59 ml/min/1.73 m^2) approximately 1.5-fold and 1.8-fold, respectively, compared with healthy subjects. AUCs of total ertapenem and of unbound ertapenem are increased in patients with advanced renal insufficiency (Cl_{cr} 5 to 30 ml/min/1.73 m^2) approximately 2.6-fold and 3.4-fold, respectively, compared with healthy subjects. AUCs of total ertapenem and of unbound ertapenem are increased in patients who require haemodialysis approximately 2.9-fold and 6.0-fold, respectively, between dialysis sessions, compared with healthy subjects. Following a single 1 g intravenous dose given immediately prior to a haemodialysis session, approximately 30 % of the dose is recovered in the dialysate. There are no data in paediatric patients with renal insufficiency.

There are inadequate data on the safety and efficacy of ertapenem in patients with advanced renal insufficiency and patients who require haemodialysis to support a dose recommendation. Therefore, ertapenem should not be used in these patients.

5.3 Preclinical safety data

Non-clinical data reveal no special hazard for humans based on conventional studies of safety, pharmacology, repeated-dose toxicity, genotoxicity and toxicity in reproduction. Decreased neutrophil counts, however, occurred in rats that received high doses of ertapenem, which was not considered a significant safety issue.

Long-term studies in animals to evaluate the carcinogenic potential of ertapenem have not been performed.

6. PHARMACEUTICAL PARTICULARS

6.1 List of excipients

Sodium bicarbonate (E500).

Sodium hydroxide (E524) to adjust pH to 7.5

6.2 Incompatibilities

Do not use solvents or infusion fluids containing dextrose for reconstitution or administration of ertapenem sodium.

In the absence of compatibility studies, this medicinal product must not be mixed with other medicinal products.

6.3 Shelf life

2 years.

After reconstitution:

Diluted solutions should be used immediately. If not used immediately, in use storage times are the responsibility of the user. Diluted solutions (approximately 20 mg/ml ertapenem) are physically and chemically stable for 6 hours at room temperature (25°C) or for 24 hours at 2 to 8°C (in a refrigerator). Solutions should be used within 4 hours of their removal from the refrigerator.

6.4 Special precautions for storage

Do not store above 25°C.

For storage instructions after reconstitution: see section 6.3.

Do not freeze solutions of INVANZ.

6.5 Nature and contents of container

20 ml Type I glass vials with a grey butyl stopper and a white plastic cap on a coloured aluminium band seal.

Supplied in packs of 1 vial or 10 vials.

Not all pack sizes may be marketed.

6.6 Special precautions for disposal and other handling

Instructions for use:

For single use only.

Reconstituted solutions should be diluted in sodium chloride 9 mg/ml (0.9 %) solution immediately after preparation.

Preparation for intravenous administration:

INVANZ must be reconstituted and then diluted prior to administration.

Adults and adolescents (13 to 17 years of age):

1. **Reconstitution**:

Reconstitute the contents of a 1 g vial of INVANZ with 10 ml of water for injection or sodium chloride 9 mg/ml (0.9 %) solution to yield a reconstituted solution of approximately 100 mg/ml. Shake well to dissolve. (See section 6.4)

2. **Dilution**:

For a 50 ml bag of diluent: For a 1 g dose, immediately transfer contents of the reconstituted vial to a 50 ml bag of sodium chloride 9 mg/ml (0.9 %) solution; or

For a 50 ml vial of diluent: For a 1 g dose, withdraw 10 ml from a 50 ml vial of sodium chloride 9 mg/ml (0.9 %) solution and discard. Transfer the contents of the reconstituted 1 g vial of INVANZ to the 50 ml vial of sodium chloride 9 mg/ml (0.9 %) solution.

3. **Infusion**:

Infuse over a period of 30 minutes.

Children (3 months to 12 years of age):

1. **Reconstitution**:

Reconstitute the contents of a 1 g vial of INVANZ with 10 ml of water for injection or sodium chloride 9 mg/ml (0.9 %) solution to yield a reconstituted solution of approximately 100 mg/ml. Shake well to dissolve. (See section 6.4.)

2. **Dilution**:

For a bag of diluent: Transfer a volume equal to 15 mg/kg of body weight (not to exceed 1 g/day) to a bag of sodium chloride 9 mg/ml (0.9 %) solution for a final concentration of 20 mg/ml or less; or

For a vial of diluent: Transfer a volume equal to 15 mg/kg of body weight (not to exceed 1 g/day) to a vial of sodium chloride 9 mg/ml (0.9 %) solution for a final concentration of 20 mg/ml or less.

3. **Infusion**:

Infuse over a period of 30 minutes.

Compatibility of INVANZ with intravenous solutions containing heparin sodium and potassium chloride has been demonstrated.

The reconstituted solutions should be inspected visually for particulate matter and discoloration prior to administration, whenever the container permits. Solutions of INVANZ range from colourless to pale yellow. Variations of colour within this range do not affect potency.

Any unused product or waste material should be disposed of in accordance with local requirements.

7. MARKETING AUTHORISATION HOLDER

Merck Sharp & Dohme Limited
Hertford Road, Hoddesdon
Hertfordshire EN11 9BU
United Kingdom

8. MARKETING AUTHORISATION NUMBER(S)

EU/1/02/216/001
EU/1/02/216/002

9. DATE OF FIRST AUTHORISATION/RENEWAL OF THE AUTHORISATION

Date of first authorisation: 18 April 2002
Date of latest renewal: 18 April 2007

10. DATE OF REVISION OF THE TEXT

August 2009

® denotes registered trademark of Merck & Co., Inc., Whitehouse Station, NJ, USA.

Detailed information on this medicine is available on the European Medicines Agency (EMEA) web site: http://www.emea.europa.eu/.

SPC.IVZ.09.UK.3125 (II-030)

INVEGA 1.5 mg, 3 mg, 6 mg, 9 mg, 12 mg prolonged-release tablets

(Janssen-Cilag Ltd)

1. NAME OF THE MEDICINAL PRODUCT

INVEGA®▼ 1.5 mg prolonged-release tablets
INVEGA®▼ 3 mg prolonged-release tablets
INVEGA®▼ 6 mg prolonged-release tablets
INVEGA®▼ 9 mg prolonged-release tablets
INVEGA®▼ 12 mg prolonged-release tablets

2. QUALITATIVE AND QUANTITATIVE COMPOSITION

Each prolonged-release tablet contains 1.5 mg of paliperidone.

Each prolonged-release tablet contains 3 mg of paliperidone.

Each prolonged-release tablet contains 6 mg of paliperidone.

Each prolonged-release tablet contains 9 mg of paliperidone.

Each prolonged-release tablet contains 12 mg of paliperidone.

FOR THE 3 mg TABLET:

Excipient: Each tablet contains 13.2 mg lactose.

For a full list of excipients, see section 6.1.

3. PHARMACEUTICAL FORM

Prolonged-release tablet

1.5 mg: Trilayer capsule-shaped orange brown tablets printed with "PAL 1.5"

3 mg: Trilayer capsule-shaped white tablets printed with "PAL 3"

6 mg: Trilayer capsule-shaped beige tablets printed with "PAL 6"

9 mg: Trilayer capsule-shaped pink tablets printed with "PAL 9"

12 mg: Trilayer capsule-shaped dark-yellow tablets printed with "PAL 12".

4. CLINICAL PARTICULARS

4.1 Therapeutic indications

INVEGA is indicated for the treatment of schizophrenia.

4.2 Posology and method of administration

Adults

INVEGA is for oral administration. The recommended dose of INVEGA is 6 mg once daily, administered in the morning. The administration of INVEGA should be standardised in relation to food intake (see section 5.2). The patient should be instructed to always take INVEGA in the fasting state or always take it together with breakfast and not to alternate between administration in the fasting state or in the fed state. Initial dose titration is not required. Some patients may benefit from lower or higher doses within the recommended range of 3 to 12 mg once daily. Dosage adjustment, if indicated, should occur only after clinical reassessment. When dose increases are indicated, increments of 3 mg/day are recommended and generally should occur at intervals of more than 5 days.

INVEGA must be swallowed whole with liquid, and must not be chewed, divided, or crushed. The active substance is contained within a non absorbable shell designed to release the active substance at a controlled rate. The tablet shell, along with insoluble core components, is eliminated from the body; patients should not be concerned if they occasionally notice in their stool something that looks like a tablet.

Patients with hepatic impairment

No dose adjustment is required in patients with mild or moderate hepatic impairment. As INVEGA has not been studied in patients with severe hepatic impairment, caution is recommended in such patients.

Patients with renal impairment

For patients with mild renal impairment (creatinine clearance ⩾ 50 to < 80 ml/min), the recommended initial dose is 3 mg once daily. The dose may be increased to 6 mg once daily based on clinical response and tolerability.

For patients with moderate to severe renal impairment (creatinine clearance ⩾ 10 to < 50 ml/min), the recommended dose of INVEGA is 1.5 mg every day, which may be increased to 3 mg once daily after clinical reassessment. As INVEGA has not been studied in patients with creatinine clearance below 10 ml/min, use is not recommended in such patients.

Elderly

Dosing recommendations for elderly patients with normal renal function (⩾ 80 ml/min) are the same as for adults with normal renal function. However, because elderly patients may have diminished renal function, dose adjustments may be required according to their renal function status (see Patients with Renal Impairment above). INVEGA should be used with caution in elderly patients with dementia with risk factors for stroke (see section 4.4).

Paediatric population

Safety and efficacy of INVEGA in patients < 18 years of age have not been studied. There is no experience in children.

Other special populations

No dose adjustment for INVEGA is recommended based on gender, race, or smoking status. (For pregnant women and breast-feeding mothers, see section 4.6)

Switching to other antipsychotic medicinal products

There are no systematically collected data to specifically address switching patients from INVEGA to other antipsychotic medicinal products. Due to different pharmacodynamic and pharmacokinetic profiles among antipsychotic medicinal products, supervision by a clinician is needed when switching to another antipsychotic product is considered medically appropriate.

4.3 Contraindications

Hypersensitivity to the active substance, risperidone, or to any of the excipients.

4.4 Special warnings and precautions for use

QT interval

As with other antipsychotics, caution should be exercised when INVEGA is prescribed in patients with known cardiovascular disease or family history of QT prolongation, and in concomitant use with other medicines thought to prolong the QT interval.

Neuroleptic malignant syndrome

Neuroleptic Malignant Syndrome (NMS), characterised by hyperthermia, muscle rigidity, autonomic instability, altered consciousness, and elevated serum creatine phosphokinase levels has been reported to occur with antipsychotics, including paliperidone. Additional clinical signs may include myoglobinuria (rhabdomyolysis) and acute renal failure. If a patient develops signs or symptoms indicative of NMS, all antipsychotics, including INVEGA, should be discontinued.

Tardive dyskinesia

Medicines with dopamine receptor antagonistic properties have been associated with the induction tardive dyskinesia characterised by rhythmical, involuntary movements, predominantly of the tongue and/or face. If signs and symptoms of tardive dyskinesia appear, the discontinuation of all antipsychotics, including INVEGA, should be considered.

Hyperglycemia

Rare cases of glucose related adverse reactions, e.g., increase in blood glucose, have been reported in clinical trials with INVEGA. As with other antipsychotics, appropriate clinical monitoring is advisable in diabetic patients and in patients with risk factors for the development of diabetes mellitus.

Orthostatic hypotension

Paliperidone may induce orthostatic hypotension in some patients based on its alpha-blocking activity.

Based on pooled data from the three, placebo-controlled, 6-week, fixed-dose trials with INVEGA (3, 6, 9, and 12 mg), orthostatic hypotension was reported by 2.5% of subjects treated with INVEGA compared with 0.8% of subjects treated with placebo. INVEGA should be used with caution in patients with known cardiovascular disease (e.g., heart failure, myocardial infarction or ischaemia, conduction abnormalities), cerebrovascular disease, or conditions that predispose the patient to hypotension (e.g., dehydration and hypovolemia).

Seizures

INVEGA should be used cautiously in patients with a history of seizures or other conditions that potentially lower the seizure threshold.

Potential for gastrointestinal obstruction

Because the INVEGA tablet is non-deformable and does not appreciably change shape in the gastrointestinal tract, INVEGA should not ordinarily be administered to patients with pre-existing severe gastrointestinal narrowing (pathologic or iatrogenic) or in patients with dysphagia or significant difficulty in swallowing tablets. There have been rare reports of obstructive symptoms in patients with known strictures in association with the ingestion of medicines in non-deformable controlled-release formulations. Due to the controlled-release design of the dosage form, INVEGA should only be used in patients who are able to swallow the tablet whole.

Conditions with decreased gastro-intestinal transit time

Conditions leading to shorter gastrointestinal transit time, e.g., diseases associated with chronic severe diarrhoea, may result in a reduced absorption of paliperidone.

Renal impairment

The plasma concentrations of paliperidone are increased in patients with renal impairment and, therefore, dosage adjustment may be required in some patients (see section 4.2 and 5.2). No data are available in patients with a creatinine clearance below 10 ml/min. Paliperidone should not be used in patients with creatinine clearance below 10 ml/min.

Hepatic impairment

No data are available in patients with severe hepatic impairment (Child-Pugh class C). Caution is recommended if paliperidone is used in such patients.

Elderly patients with dementia

INVEGA has not been studied in elderly patients with dementia. Hence, until data demonstrate otherwise the experience from risperidone is considered valid also for paliperidone.

Overall mortality

In a meta-analysis of 17 controlled clinical trials, elderly patients with dementia treated with other atypical antipsychotics, including risperidone, aripiprazole, olanzapine, and quetiapine had an increased risk of mortality compared to placebo. Among those treated with risperidone, the mortality was 4% compared with 3.1% for placebo.

Cerebrovascular adverse reactions

An approximately 3-fold increased risk of cerebrovascular adverse reactions have been seen in randomised placebo-controlled clinical trials in the dementia population with some atypical antipsychotics, including risperidone, aripiprazole, and olanzapine. The mechanism for this increased risk is not known. INVEGA should be used with caution in elderly patients with dementia who have risk factors for stroke.

Parkinson's disease and dementia with Lewy bodies

Physicians should weigh the risks versus the benefits when prescribing antipsychotic medicinal products, including INVEGA, to patients with Parkinson's Disease or Dementia with Lewy Bodies (DLB) since both groups may be at increased risk of Neuroleptic Malignant Syndrome as well as having an increased sensitivity to antipsychotics. Manifestation of this increased sensitivity can include confusion, obtundation, postural instability with frequent falls, in addition to extrapyramidal symptoms.

Priapism

Antipsychotic drugs (including risperidone) with α-adrenergic blocking effects have been reported to induce priapism. During post-marketing surveillance priapism has also been reported with paliperidone, which is the active metabolite of risperidone. Patients should be informed to seek urgent medical care in case that priapism has not been resolved within 3-4 hours.

Body temperature regulation

Disruption of the body's ability to reduce core body temperature has been attributed to antipsychotic medicines. Appropriate care is advised when prescribing INVEGA to patients who will be experiencing conditions which may contribute to an elevation in core body temperature, e.g., exercising strenuously, exposure to extreme heat, receiving concomitant medication with anticholinergic activity, or being subject to dehydration.

Antiemetic effect

An antiemetic effect was observed in preclinical studies with paliperidone. This effect, if it occurs in humans, may mask the signs and symptoms of overdosage with certain medicines or of conditions such as intestinal obstruction, Reye's syndrome, and brain tumour.

Lactose content (pertains only to the 3 mg tablets)

Patients with rare hereditary problems of galactose intolerance, the Lapp lactase deficiency or glucose-galactose malabsorption should not take this medicine.

4.5 Interaction with other medicinal products and other forms of interaction

Caution is advised when prescribing INVEGA with medicines known to prolong the QT interval, e.g., class IA antiarrhythmics (e.g., quinidine, disopyramide) and class III antiarrhythmics (e.g., amiodarone, sotalol), some antihistaminics, some other antipsychotics and some antimalarials (e.g., mefloquine).

Potential for INVEGA to affect other medicines

Paliperidone is not expected to cause clinically important pharmacokinetic interactions with medicines that are metabolised by cytochrome P-450 isozymes.

Table 1

System Organ Class	Adverse Drug Reaction Frequency			
	Very common	**Common**	**Uncommon**	**Not Known**
Immune system disorders			anaphylactic reaction	
Metabolism and nutrition disorders			increased appetite	
Psychiatric disorders			nightmare	
Nervous system disorders	headache	extrapyramidal disorder, parkinsonism, tremor, hypertonia, dystonia, akathisia, dizziness, sedation, somnolence,	grand mal convulsion, syncope, dyskinesia, dizziness postural,	
Eye disorders			oculogyration	
Cardiac disorders		tachycardia, sinus tachycardia, bundle branch block, atrioventricular block first degree, bradycardia	palpitations, sinus arrhythmia	
Vascular disorders		orthostatic hypotension	ischaemia, hypotension,	
Gastrointestinal disorders		vomiting, abdominal pain upper, salivary hypersecretion, dry mouth,		
Musculoskeletal, connective tissue and bone disorders			muscle rigidity	
Reproductive system and breast disorders			amenorrhoea, galactorrhoea, erectile dysfunction, gynaecomastia, breast discharge, menstruation irregular	priapism
General disorders		asthenia, fatigue	oedema	
Investigations		weight increased	electrocardiogram abnormal	

Given the primary CNS effects of paliperidone (see section 4.8), INVEGA should be used with caution in combination with other centrally acting medicines, e.g., anxiolytics, most antipsychotics, hypnotics, opiates, etc. or alcohol.

Paliperidone may antagonise the effect of levodopa and other dopamine agonists. If this combination is deemed necessary, particularly in end-stage Parkinson's disease, the lowest effective dose of each treatment should be prescribed.

Because of its potential for inducing orthostatic hypotension (see section 4.4), an additive effect may be observed when INVEGA is administered with other therapeutic agents that have this potential, e.g., other antipsychotics, tricyclics.

Caution is advised if paliperidone is combined with other medicines know to lower the seizure threshold (i.e., phenothiazines or butyrophenones, tricyclics or SSRIs, tramadol, mefloquine, etc.).

Potential for other medicines to affect INVEGA

In vitro studies indicate that CYP2D6 and CYP3A4 may be minimally involved in paliperidone metabolism, but there are no indications *in vitro* nor *in vivo* that these isozymes play a significant role in the metabolism of paliperidone. Concomitant administration of INVEGA with paroxetine, a potent CYP2D6 inhibitor, showed no clinically significant effect on the pharmacokinetics of paliperidone. *In vitro* studies have shown that paliperidone is a P-glycoprotein (P-gp) substrate.

Co-administration of INVEGA once daily with carbamazepine 200 mg twice daily caused a decrease of approximately 37% in the mean steady-state Cmax and AUC of paliperidone. This decrease is caused, to a substantial degree, by a 35% increase in renal clearance of paliperidone likely as a result of induction of renal P-gp by carbamazepine. A minor decrease in the amount of active substance excreted unchanged in the urine suggests that there was little effect on the CYP metabolism or bioavailability of paliperidone during carbamazepine co-administration. Larger decreases in plasma concentrations of paliperidone could occur with higher doses of carbamazepine. On initiation of carbamazepine, the dose of INVEGA should be re-evaluated and increased if necessary. Conversely, on discontinuation of carbamazepine, the dose of INVEGA should be re-evaluated and decreased if necessary. It takes 2-3 weeks for full induction to be achieved and upon discontinuation of the inducer the effect wears off over a similar time period. Other medicinal products or herbals which are inducers, e.g. rifampicin and St John's wort (*Hypericum perforatum*) may have similar effects on paliperidone.

Medicinal products affecting gastrointestinal transit time may affect the absorption of paliperidone, e.g. metoclopramide.

Concomitant use of INVEGA with risperidone

Concomitant use of INVEGA with oral risperidone is not recommended as paliperidone is the active metabolite of risperidone and the combination of the two may lead to additive paliperidone exposure.

4.6 Pregnancy and lactation

There are no adequate data from the use of paliperidone during pregnancy. Paliperidone was not teratogenic in animal studies, but other types of reproductive toxicity were observed(see section 5.3). The use of antipsychotics during the last trimester of pregnancy has resulted in long term but reversible neurological disturbances of extrapyramidal nature in the infant. INVEGA should not be used during pregnancy unless clearly necessary. If discontinuation during pregnancy is necessary, it should not be done abruptly.

Paliperidone is excreted in the breast milk to such an extent that effects on the breast-fed infant are likely if therapeutic doses are administered to breast-feeding women. INVEGA should not be used while breast feeding.

4.7 Effects on ability to drive and use machines

Paliperidone can have minor or moderate influence on the ability to drive and use machines due to potential nervous system and visual effects (see section 4.8). Therefore, patients should be advised not to drive or operate machines until their individual susceptibility to INVEGA is known.

4.8 Undesirable effects

The most frequently reported adverse drug reactions (ADRs) reported in clinical trials were headache, tachycardia, akathisia, sinus tachycardia, extrapyramidal disorder, somnolence, dizziness, sedation, tremor, hypertonia, dystonia, orthostatic hypotension, and dry mouth.

The ADRs that appeared to be dose-related included weight increased, headache, salivary hypersecretion, vomiting, dyskinesia, akathisia, dystonia, extrapyramidal disorder, hypertonia, and Parkinsonism.

The following are all ADRs that were reported in clinical trials and postmarketing. The following terms and frequencies are applied: *very common* (≥ 1/10), *common* (≥ 1/100 to < 1/10), *uncommon* (≥ 1/1000 to < 1/100), *rare* (≥ 1/10,000 to < 1/1000), *very rare* (< 1/10,000) and *not known* (cannot be estimated from the available clinical trial data). Within each frequency grouping, adverse reactions are presented in order of decreasing seriousness.

(see Table 1 above)

Paliperidone is an active metabolite of risperidone. The following is a list of additional ADRs that have been reported with risperidone.

System Organ Class	Adverse Drug Reaction
Infections and infestations	acarodermatitis, bronchitis, bronchopneumonia, cellulitis, cystitis, ear infection, eye infection, influenza, localised infection, nasopharyngitis, onychomycosis, otitis media, otitis media chronic, pharyngitis, pneumonia, respiratory tract infection, rhinitis, sinusitis, tonsillitis, tracheobronchitis, upper respiratory tract infection, urinary tract infection, viral infection
Blood and lymphatic system disorders	anaemia, granulocytopenia, neutropenia, thrombocytopenia
Immune system disorders	drug hypersensitivity, hypersensitivity
Endocrine disorders	hyperprolactaemia, inappropriate antidiuretic hormone secretion
Metabolism and nutrition disorders	anorexia, decreased appetite, diabetic ketoacidosis, polydipsia
Psychiatric disorders	agitation, anorgasmia, anxiety, blunted affect, confusional state, insomnia, libido decreased, listless, mania, middle insomnia, nervousness, restlessness, sleep disorder
Nervous system disorders	akinesia, balance disorder, bradykinesia, cerebral ischaemia, cerebrovascular accident, cerebrovascular disorder, cogwheel rigidity, convulsion, coordination abnormal, depressed level of consciousness, diabetic coma, disturbance in attention, drooling, dysarthria, hypersomnia, hypoaesthesia, hypokinesia, lethargy, loss of consciousness, masked facies, movement disorder, muscle contractions involuntary, neuroleptic malignant syndrome, parkinsonian rest tremor, speech disorder, tardive dyskinesia, transit ischaemic attack, unresponsive to stimuli
Eye disorders	conjunctivitis, dry eye, eye discharge, eye rolling, eye swelling, eyelid margin crusting, eyelid oedema, glaucoma, lacrimation increased, ocular hyperaemia, photophobia, vision blurred, visual acuity reduced
Ear and labyrinth disorders	ear pain, tinnitus
Cardiac disorders	atrial fibrillation, atrioventricular block
Vascular disorders	flushing
Respiratory, thoracic and mediastinal disorders	cough, dysphonia, dyspnoea, epistaxis, hyperventilation, nasal congestion, nasal oedema, pharyngolaryngeal pain, pneumonia aspiration, productive cough, pulmonary congestion, rales, respiratory disorder, respiratory tract congestion, rhinorrhoea, sinus congestion, sleep apnoea syndrome, wheezing
Gastrointestinal disorders	abdominal discomfort, abdominal pain, aptyalism, cheilitis, constipation, diarrhoea, dyspepsia, dysphagia, faecal incontinence, faecaloma, gastritis, intestinal obstruction, lip swelling, nausea, stomach discomfort
Hepatobiliary disorders	jaundice
Skin and subcutaneous tissue disorders	acne, angioneurotic oedema, dandruff, dry skin, erythema, hyperkeratosis, pruritus, rash, rash erythematous, rash generalised, rash maculo-papular, rash papular, seborrhoeic dermatitis, skin discolouration, skin disorder, skin lesion
Musculoskeletal and connective tissue disorders	arthralgia, back pain, joint stiffness, muscle spasms, muscle twitching, muscular weakness, musculoskeletal chest pain, musculoskeletal stiffness, myalgia, neck pain, pain in extremity, posture abnormal, rhabdomyolysis, torticollis
Renal and urinary disorders	dysuria, enuresis, pollakiuria, urinary incontinence
Reproductive system and breast disorders	breast enlargement, ejaculation disorder, ejaculation failure, menstrual disorder, priapism, retrograde ejaculation, sexual dysfunction, vaginal discharge
General disorders	adverse drug reaction, chest discomfort, chest pain, chills, discomfort, drug withdrawal syndrome, face oedema, feeling abnormal, gait disturbance, generalized oedema, influenza like illness, malaise, oedema peripheral, peripheral coldness, pitting oedema, pyrexia, sluggishness, thirst

Investigations	alanine aminotransferase increased, aspartate aminotransferase increased, blood creatine phosphokinase increased, blood glucose increased, blood pressure decreased, blood prolactin increased, body temperature decreased, body temperature increased, electrocardiogram QT prolonged, eosinophil count increased, haematocrit decreased, haemoglobin decreased, heart rate increased, transaminases increased, white blood cell count decreased

Elderly

In a study conducted in elderly subjects with schizophrenia, the safety profile was similar to that seen in non-elderly subjects. INVEGA has not been studied in elderly patients with dementia. In clinical trials with some other atypical antipsychotics, increased risks of death and cerebrovascular accidents have been reported (see section 4.4).

Events of Particular interest to the class

Extrapyramidal Symptoms (EPS). In clinical trials, there was no difference observed between placebo and the 3 and 6 mg doses of INVEGA. Dose dependence for EPS was seen with the two higher doses of INVEGA (9 and 12 mg). EPS included a pooled analysis of the following terms: dyskinesia, dystonia, hyperkinesia, Parkinsonism, and tremor.

Weight Gain. In clinical trials, the proportions of subjects meeting a weight gain criterion of ≥7% of body weight were compared, revealing a similar incidence of weight gain for INVEGA 3 mg and 6 mg compared with placebo, and a higher incidence of weight gain for INVEGA 9 mg and 12 mg compared with placebo.

Laboratory Tests: Serum Prolactin. In clinical trials, median increases in serum prolactin were observed with INVEGA in 67% of subjects. Adverse events that may suggest increase in prolactin levels (e.g., amenorrhoea, galactorrhoea, gynaecomastia) were reported overall in 2% of subjects. Maximum mean increases of serum prolactin concentrations were generally observed on Day 15 of treatment, but remained above baseline levels at study endpoint.

Class effects

QT prolongation, ventricular arrythmias (ventricular fibrillation, ventricular tachycardia), sudden unexplained death, cardiac arrest and Torsade de pointes may occur with antipsychotics.

4.9 Overdose

In general, expected signs and symptoms are those resulting from an exaggeration of paliperidone's known pharmacological effects, i.e., drowsiness and sedation, tachycardia and hypotension, QT prolongation, and extrapyramidal symptoms. In the case of acute overdosage, the possibility of multiple medicinal product involvement should be considered.

Consideration should be given to the prolonged-release nature of the product when assessing treatment needs and recovery. There is no specific antidote to paliperidone. General supportive measures should be employed. Establish and maintain a clear airway and ensure adequate oxygenation and ventilation.

Cardiovascular monitoring should commence immediately and should include continuous electrocardiographic monitoring for possible arrhythmias. Hypotension and circulatory collapse should be treated with appropriate measures such as intravenous fluid and/or sympathomimetic agents. Gastric lavage (after intubation if the patient is unconscious) and administration of activated charcoal together with a laxative should be considered. In case of severe extrapyramidal symptoms, anticholinergic agents should be administered. Close supervision and monitoring should continue until the patient recovers.

5. PHARMACOLOGICAL PROPERTIES

5.1 Pharmacodynamic properties

Pharmacologic group: other antipsychotics ATC code: N05AX13

INVEGA contains a racemic mixture of (+)- and (-)-paliperidone.

Mechanism of Action

Paliperidone is a selective blocking agent of monoamine effects, whose pharmacological properties are different from that of traditional neuroleptics. Paliperidone binds strongly to serotonergic 5-HT2- and dopaminergic D2-receptors. Paliperidone also blocks alfa1-adrenergic receptors and blocks, to a lesser extent, H1-histaminergic and alfa2-adrenergic receptors. The pharmacological activity of the (+)- and (-)-paliperidone enantiomers are qualitatively and quantitatively similar.

Paliperidone is not bound to cholinergic receptors. Even though paliperidone is a strong D2-antagonist, which is believed to relieve the positive symptoms of schizophrenia, it causes less catalepsy and decreases motor functions to a lesser extent than traditional neuroleptics. Dominating central serotonin antagonism may reduce the tendency of paliperidone to cause extrapyramidal side effects.

Table 2

	Placebo	3 mg	6 mg	9 mg	12 mg
R076477-SCH-303	(N=126)		(N=123)	(N=122)	(N=129)
Mean baseline (SD)	94.1 (10.74)		94.3 (10.48)	93.2 (11.90)	94.6 (10.98)
Mean change	4.1 (23.16)		-17.9 (22.23)	-17.2 (20.23)	-23.3 (20.12)
P-value (vs, Placebo)			<0.001	<0.001	<0.001
Diff. of LS Means (SE)			-13.7 (2.63)	-13.5 (2.63)	-18.9 (2.60)
R076477-SCH-304	(N=105)		(N=111)		(N=111)
Mean baseline (SD)	93.6 (11.71)		92.3 (11.96)		94.1 (11.42)
Mean change (SD)	-8.0 (21.48)		-15.7 (18.89)		-17.5 (19.83)
P-value (vs, Placebo)			0.006		<0.001
Diff. of LS Means (SE)			-7.0 (2.36)		-8.5 (2.35)
R076477-SCH-305	(N=120)	(N=123)		(N=123)	
Mean baseline (SD)	93.9 (12.66)	91.6 (12.19)		93.9 (13.20)	
Mean change (SD)	-2.8 (20.89)	15.0 (19.61)		-16.3 (21.81)	
P-value (vs, Placebo)		<0.001		<0.001	
Diff. of LS Means (SE)		-11.6 (2.35)		-12.9 (2.34)	

Note: Negative change in score indicates improvement. For all 3 studies, an active control (olanzapine at a dose of 10 mg) was included. LOCF = last observation carried forward. The 1-7 version of the PANSS was used. A 15 mg dose was also included in Study R076477-SCH-305, but results are not presented since this is above the maximum recommended daily dose of 12 mg.

Pharmacodynamic Effects

Clinical Efficacy

The efficacy of INVEGA was established in three multicentre, placebo-controlled, double-blind, 6-week trials in subjects who met DSM-IV criteria for schizophrenia. INVEGA doses, which varied across the three studies, ranged from 3 to 15 mg once daily. The primary efficacy endpoint was defined as a decrease in total Positive and Negative Syndrome Scale (PANSS) scores as shown in the following table. All tested doses of INVEGA separated from placebo on day 4 ($p<0.05$). Predefined secondary endpoints included the Personal and Social Performance (PSP) scale and the Clinical Global Impression – Severity (CGI-S) scale. In all three studies, INVEGA was superior to placebo on PSP and CGI-S.

Positive and Negative Syndrome Scale for Schizophrenia (PANSS) Total Score - Change From Baseline to End Point-LOCF for Studies R076477-SCH-303, R076477-SCH-304, and R076477-SCH-305: Intent-to-Treat Analysis Set

(see Table 2 above)

In a long-term trial designed to assess the maintenance of effect, INVEGA was significantly more effective than placebo in maintaining symptom control and delaying relapse of schizophrenia. After having been treated for an acute episode for 6 weeks and stabilized for an additional 8 weeks with INVEGA (doses ranging from 3 to 15 mg once daily) patients were then randomised in a double-blind manner to either continue on INVEGA or on placebo until they experienced a relapse in schizophrenia symptoms. The trial was stopped early for efficacy reasons by showing a significantly longer time to relapse in patients treated with INVEGA compared to placebo (p=0.0053).

5.2 Pharmacokinetic properties

The pharmacokinetics of paliperidone following INVEGA administration are dose proportional within the recommended clinical dose range (3 to 12 mg).

Absorption

Following a single dose, INVEGA exhibits a gradual ascending release rate, allowing the plasma concentrations of paliperidone to steadily rise to reach peak plasma concentration (Cmax) approximately 24 hours after dosing. With once-daily dosing of INVEGA, steady-state concentrations of paliperidone are attained within 4-5 days of dosing in most subjects.

Paliperidone is the active metabolite of risperidone. The release characteristics of INVEGA result in minimal peak-trough fluctuations as compared to those observed with immediate-release risperidone (fluctuation index 38% versus 125%).

The absolute oral bioavailability of paliperidone following INVEGA administration is 28% (90% CI of 23%-33%).

Administration of paliperidone prolonged-release tablets with a standard high-fat/high-caloric meal increases C_{max} and AUC of paliperidone by up to 50-60% compared with administration in the fasting state.

Distribution

Paliperidone is rapidly distributed. The apparent volume of distribution is 487 l. The plasma protein binding of paliperidone is 74%. It binds primarily to α1-acid glycoprotein and albumin.

Biotransformation and elimination

One week following administration of a single oral dose of 1 mg immediate-release ^{14}C-paliperidone, 59% of the dose was excreted unchanged into urine, indicating that paliperidone is not extensively metabolised by the liver. Approximately 80% of the administered radioactivity was recovered in urine and 11% in the faeces. Four metabolic pathways have been identified *in vivo*, none of which accounted for more than 6.5% of the dose: dealkylation, hydroxylation, dehydrogenation, and benzisoxazole scission. Although *in vitro* studies suggested a role for CYP2D6 and CYP3A4 in the metabolism of paliperidone, there is no evidence *in vivo* that these isozymes play a significant role in the metabolism of paliperidone. Population pharmacokinetics analyses indicated no discernable difference on the apparent clearance of paliperidone after administration of INVEGA between extensive metabolisers and poor metabolisers of CYP2D6 substrates. *In vitro* studies in human liver microsomes showed that paliperidone does not substantially inhibit the metabolism of medicines metabolised by cytochrome P450 isozymes, including CYP1A2, CYP2A6, CYP2C8/9/10, CYP2D6, CYP2E1, CYP3A4, and CYP3A5. The terminal elimination half-life of paliperidone is about 23 hours.

In vitro studies have shown that paliperidone is a P-gp substrate and a weak inhibitor of P-gp at high concentrations. No in vivo data are available and the clinical relevance is unknown.

Hepatic Impairment

Paliperidone is not extensively metabolized in the liver. In a study in subjects with moderate hepatic impairment (Child-Pugh class B), the plasma concentrations of free paliperidone were similar to those of healthy subjects. No data are available in patients with severe hepatic impairment (Child-Pugh class C).

Renal Impairment

Elimination of paliperidone decreased with decreasing renal function. Total clearance of paliperidone was reduced in subjects with impaired renal function by 32% in mild (Creatinine Clearance [CrCl] = 50 to < 80 ml/min), 64% in moderate (CrCl = 30 to < 50 ml/min), and 71% in severe (CrCl = < 30 ml/min) renal impairment. The mean terminal elimination half-life of paliperidone was 24, 40, and 51 hours in subjects with mild, moderate, and severe renal impairment, respectively, compared with 23 hours in subjects with normal renal function (CrCl ≥ 80 ml/min).

Elderly

Data from a pharmacokinetic study in elderly subjects (≥ 65 years of age, n = 26) indicated that the apparent steady-state clearance of paliperidone following INVEGA administration was 20% lower compared to that of adult subjects (18-45 years of age, n = 28). However, there was no discernable effect of age in the population pharmacokinetic analysis involving schizophrenia subjects after correction of age-related decreases in CrCl.

Race

Population pharmacokinetics analysis revealed no evidence of race-related differences in the pharmacokinetics of paliperidone following INVEGA administration.

Gender

The apparent clearance of paliperidone following INVEGA administration is approximately 19% lower in women than men. This difference is largely explained by differences in lean body mass and creatinine clearance between men and women.

Smoking Status

Based on *in vitro* studies utilising human liver enzymes, paliperidone is not a substrate for CYP1A2; smoking should, therefore, not have an effect on the pharmacokinetics of paliperidone. A population pharmacokinetic analysis showed a slightly lower exposure to paliperidone in smokers compared with non-smokers. The difference is unlikely to be of clinical relevance, though.

5.3 Preclinical safety data

Repeat-dose toxicity studies of paliperidone in rat and dog showed mainly pharmacological effects, such as sedation and prolactin-mediated effects on mammary glands and genitals. Paliperidone was not teratogenic in rat and rabbit. In rat reproduction studies using risperidone, which is extensively converted to paliperidone in rats and humans, a reduction was observed in the birth weight and survival of the offspring. Other dopamine antagonists, when administered to pregnant animals, have caused negative effects on learning and motor development in the offspring. Paliperidone was not genotoxic in a battery of tests. In oral carcinogenicity studies of risperidone in rats and mice, increases in pituitary gland adenomas (mouse), endocrine pancreas adenomas (rat), and mammary gland adenomas (both species) were seen. These tumours can be related to prolonged dopamine D2 antagonism and hyperprolactinemia. The relevance of these tumour findings in rodents in terms of human risk is unknown.

6. PHARMACEUTICAL PARTICULARS

6.1 List of excipients

Coated tablet core:

Polyethylene oxide 200K

Sodium chloride

Povidone (K29-32)

Stearic acid

Butyl hydroxytoluene (E321)

Ferric oxide (yellow) (E172) (3 mg and 12 mg only)

Polyethylene oxide 7000K

Ferric oxide (red) (E172)

Iron oxide (black) (E172) (1.5 mg and 9 mg only)

Hydroxyethyl cellulose

Polyethylene glycol 3350

Cellulose acetate

Colour overcoat:

Hypromellose

Titanium dioxide (E171)

Lactose monohydrate (3 mg only)

Triacetin (3 mg only)

Polyethylene glycol 400 (1.5 mg,6 mg,9 mg and 12 mg only)

Ferric oxide (yellow) (E172) (1.5 mg,6 mg and 12 mg only)

Ferric oxide (red) (E172) (1.5 mg,6 mg and 9 mg only)

Carnauba wax

Printing ink:

Iron oxide (black) (E172)

Propylene glycol

Hypromellose

6.2 Incompatibilities

Not applicable

6.3 Shelf life

2 years

6.4 Special precautions for storage

Bottles: Do not store above 30°C. Keep the bottle tightly closed in order to protect from moisture.

Blisters: Do not store above 30°C. Store in the original package in order to protect from moisture.

6.5 Nature and contents of container

Bottles:

White high-density polyethylene (HDPE) bottle with induction sealing and polypropylene child- resistant closure. Each bottle contains two 1g dessicant silica gel (silicone dioxide) pouches (pouch is food approved polyethylene).

Pack sizes of 30 and 350 prolonged-release tablets.

Blisters:

• Polyvinyl chloride (PVC) laminated with polychloro-trifluoroethylene (PCTFE)/aluminium push-through layer.

Pack sizes of 28, 30, 49, 56, and 98 prolonged-release tablets.

Or

• White polyvinyl chloride (PVC) laminated with polychlorotrifluoroethylene (PCTFE)/aluminium push-through layer.

Pack sizes of 28, 30, 49, 56, and 98 prolonged-release tablets.

Or

• Oriented polyamide (OPA)-aluminium-polyvinyl chloride (PVC)/aluminium push-through layer.

Pack sizes of 28, 49, 56, and 98 prolonged-release tablets.

Not all pack sizes may be marketed.

6.6 Special precautions for disposal and other handling

No special requirements.

7. MARKETING AUTHORISATION HOLDER

Janssen-Cilag International NV,

Turnhoutseweg 30,

B-2340 Beerse,

Belgium.

8. MARKETING AUTHORISATION NUMBER(S)

EU/1/07/395/078

EU/1/07/395/001

EU/1/07/395/006

EU/1/07/395/011

EU/1/07/395/016

9. DATE OF FIRST AUTHORISATION/RENEWAL OF THE AUTHORISATION

Date of first authorisation 25/06/ 2007

10. DATE OF REVISION OF THE TEXT

07/07/09

Detailed information on this product is available on the website of the European Medicines Agency (EMEA): http://www.emea.europa.eu/

Invirase 200 mg hard capsules

(Roche Products Limited)

1. NAME OF THE MEDICINAL PRODUCT

INVIRASE 200 mg hard capsules.

2. QUALITATIVE AND QUANTITATIVE COMPOSITION

One capsule contains 200 mg of saquinavir as saquinavir mesilate.

Excipient: Contains lactose anhydrous: 63.3 mg.

For a full list of excipients, see section 6.1.

3. PHARMACEUTICAL FORM

Hard capsule.

Light brown and green, opaque hard capsule with the marking "ROCHE" and the code "0245" on each half of the capsule shell.

4. CLINICAL PARTICULARS

4.1 Therapeutic indications

Invirase is indicated for the treatment of HIV-1 infected adult patients. Invirase should only be given in combination with ritonavir and other antiretroviral medicinal products (see section 4.2).

4.2 Posology and method of administration

Therapy with Invirase should be initiated by a physician experienced in the management of HIV infection.

Adults and adolescents over the age of 16 years:

In combination with ritonavir

The recommended dose of Invirase is 1000 mg (5 × 200 mg capsules) two times daily with ritonavir 100 mg two times daily in combination with other antiretroviral agents.

Invirase capsules should be swallowed whole and taken at the same time as ritonavir with or after food (see section 5.2).

Renal and hepatic impairment:

No dosage adjustment is necessary for patients with mild to moderate renal or mild hepatic impairment. Caution should be exercised in patients with severe renal or moderate hepatic impairment. Invirase/ritonavir is contraindicated in patients with decompensated hepatic impairment (see sections 4.3 and 4.4).

Children under the age of 16 and adults over 60 years:

The experience with Invirase in children below the age of 16 and adults over 60 years is limited. In children, as in adults, Invirase should only be given in combination with ritonavir.

4.3 Contraindications

Hypersensitivity to the active substance or to any of the excipients.

Invirase/ritonavir is contraindicated in decompensated liver disease (see section 4.4).

Invirase/ritonavir should not be given together with other medicinal products which may interact and result in potentially life threatening undesirable effects.

Medicinal products which should not be given with Invirase/ritonavir include:

• terfenadine, astemizole, pimozide, cisapride, amiodarone, propafenone and flecainide (potential for life threatening cardiac arrhythmia)

• midazolam administered orally (for caution on parenterally administered midazolam, see section 4.5), triazolam (potential for prolonged or increased sedation, respiratory depression)

• simvastatin, lovastatin (increased risk of myopathy including rhabdomyolysis)

• ergot alkaloids (e.g. ergotamine, dihydroergotamine, ergonovine, and methylergonovine) (potential for acute ergot toxicity)

• rifampicin (risk of severe hepatocellular toxicity) (see sections 4.4, 4.5, and 4.8).

4.4 Special warnings and precautions for use

Considerations when initiating Invirase therapy: Invirase should not be given as the sole protease inhibitor. Invirase should only be given in combination with ritonavir (see section 4.2).

Patients should be informed that saquinavir is not a cure for HIV infection and that they may continue to acquire illnesses associated with advanced HIV infection, including opportunistic infections. Patients should also be advised that they might experience undesirable effects associated with co-administered medications.

Liver disease: The safety and efficacy of saquinavir/ritonavir has not been established in patients with significant underlying liver disorders, therefore saquinavir/ritonavir should be used cautiously in this patient population. Invirase/ritonavir is contraindicated in patients with decompensated liver disease (see section 4.3). Patients with chronic hepatitis B or C and treated with combination antiretroviral therapy are at an increased risk for severe and potentially fatal hepatic adverse events. In case of concomitant antiviral therapy for hepatitis B or C, please refer also to the relevant product information for these medicinal products.

Patients with pre-existing liver dysfunction including chronic active hepatitis have an increased frequency of liver function abnormalities during combination antiretroviral therapy and should be monitored according to standard practice. If there is evidence of worsening liver disease in such patients, interruption or discontinuation of treatment must be considered.

In cases of mild hepatic impairment no initial dosage adjustment is necessary at the recommended dose. The use of Invirase in combination with ritonavir in patients with moderate hepatic impairment has not been studied. In the absence of such studies, caution should be exercised, as increases in saquinavir levels and/or increases in liver enzymes may occur.

There have been reports of exacerbation of chronic liver dysfunction, including portal hypertension, in patients with underlying hepatitis B or C, cirrhosis and other underlying liver abnormalities.

Renal impairment: Renal clearance is only a minor elimination pathway, the principal route of metabolism and excretion for saquinavir being via the liver. Therefore, no initial dose adjustment is necessary for patients with renal impairment. However, patients with severe renal impairment have not been studied and caution should be exercised when prescribing saquinavir/ritonavir in this population.

Patients with chronic diarrhoea or malabsorption: No information on boosted saquinavir and only limited information on the safety and efficacy of unboosted saquinavir is available for patients suffering from chronic diarrhoea or malabsorption. It is unknown whether patients with such conditions could receive subtherapeutic saquinavir levels.

Children under the age of 16 and adults over 60 years: The experience with Invirase in children below the age of 16 and adults over 60 years is limited. In children, as in adults, Invirase should only be given in combination with ritonavir.

Lactose intolerance: Invirase 200 mg capsules contain lactose. Patients with rare hereditary problems of galactose intolerance, the Lapp lactase deficiency or glucose-galactose malabsorption should not take this medicine.

Patients with haemophilia: There have been reports of increased bleeding, including spontaneous skin haematomas and haemarthroses, in haemophiliac patients type A and B treated with protease inhibitors. In some patients additional factor VIII was given. In more than half of the reported cases, treatment with protease inhibitors was continued or reintroduced if treatment had been discontinued. A causal relationship has been evoked, although the mechanism of action has not been elucidated. Haemophiliac patients should therefore be made aware of the possibility of increased bleeding.

Diabetes mellitus and hyperglycaemia: New onset diabetes mellitus, hyperglycaemia or exacerbation of existing diabetes mellitus has been reported in patients receiving protease inhibitors. In some of these patients, the hyperglycaemia was severe and in some cases was also associated with ketoacidosis. Many patients had confounding medical conditions, some of which required therapy with agents that have been associated with the development of diabetes mellitus or hyperglycaemia.

Lipodystrophy: Combination antiretroviral therapy has been associated with the redistribution of body fat (lipodystrophy) in HIV infected patients. The long-term consequences of these events are currently unknown. Knowledge about the mechanism is incomplete. A connection between visceral lipomatosis and PIs and lipoatrophy and Nucleoside Reverse Transcriptase Inhibitors (NRTIs) has been hypothesised. A higher risk of lipodystrophy has been associated with individual factors such as older age, and with drug related factors such as longer duration of antiretroviral treatment and associated metabolic disturbances. Clinical examination should include evaluation for physical signs of fat redistribution. Consideration should be given to the measurement of fasting serum lipids and blood glucose. Lipid disorders should be managed as clinically appropriate (see section 4.8).

Osteonecrosis: Although the aetiology is considered to be multifactorial (including corticosteroid use, alcohol consumption, severe immunosuppression, higher body mass index), cases of osteonecrosis have been reported particularly in patients with advanced HIV–disease and/or long-term exposure to combination antiretroviral therapy (CART). Patients should be advised to seek medical advice if they experience joint aches and pain, joint stiffness or difficulty in movement.

Immune Reactivation Syndrome: In HIV-infected patients with severe immune deficiency at the time of institution of combination antiretroviral therapy (CART), an inflammatory reaction to asymptomatic or residual opportunistic pathogens may arise and cause serious clinical conditions, or aggravation of symptoms. Typically, such reactions have been observed within the first few weeks or months of initiation of CART. Relevant examples are cytomegalovirus retinitis, generalised and/or focal mycobacterial infections, and Pneumocystis carinii pneumonia. Any inflammatory symptoms should be evaluated and treatment instituted when necessary.

Interaction with ritonavir: The recommended dose of Invirase and ritonavir is 1000 mg Invirase plus 100 mg ritonavir twice daily. Higher doses of ritonavir have been shown to be associated with an increased incidence of adverse events. Co-administration of saquinavir and ritonavir has led to severe adverse events, mainly diabetic ketoacidosis and liver disorders, especially in patients with pre-existing liver disease.

Interaction with tipranavir: Concomitant use of boosted saquinavir and tipranavir, co-administered with low dose ritonavir in a dual-boosted regimen, results in a significant decrease in saquinavir plasma concentrations (see section 4.5). Therefore, the co-administration of boosted saquinavir and tipranavir, co-administered with low dose ritonavir, is not recommended.

Interaction with HMG-CoA reductase inhibitors: Caution must be exercised if Invirase/ritonavir is used concurrently with atorvastatin, which is metabolised to a lesser extent by CYP3A4. In this situation a reduced dose of atorvastatin should be considered. If treatment with a HMG-CoA reductase inhibitor is indicated, pravastatin or fluvastatin is recommended (see section 4.5).

Oral contraceptives: Because concentration of ethinyl estradiol may be decreased when co-administered with Invirase/ritonavir, alternative or additional contraceptive measures should be used when oestrogen-based oral contraceptives are co-administered (see section 4.5).

Glucocorticoids: Concomitant use of boosted saquinavir and fluticasone or other glucocorticoids that are metabolised by CYP3A4 is not recommended unless the potential benefit of treatment outweighs the risk of systemic corticosteroid effects, including Cushing's syndrome and adrenal suppression (see section 4.5).

Interaction with efavirenz: The combination of saquinavir and ritonavir with efavirenz has been shown to be associated with an increased risk of liver toxicity; liver function should be monitored when saquinavir and ritonavir are co-administered with efavirenz. No clinically significant alterations of either saquinavir or efavirenz concentration were noted in studies in healthy volunteers or in HIV-infected patients (see section 4.5).

4.5 Interaction with other medicinal products and other forms of interaction

Most drug interaction studies with saquinavir have been completed with unboosted Invirase or unboosted saquinavir soft capsules (Fortovase). A limited number of studies have been completed with ritonavir boosted Invirase or ritonavir boosted saquinavir soft capsules.

Observations from drug interaction studies done with unboosted saquinavir might not be representative of the effects seen with saquinavir/ritonavir therapy. Furthermore, results seen with saquinavir soft capsules may not predict the magnitude of these interactions with Invirase/ritonavir.

The metabolism of saquinavir is mediated by cytochrome P450, with the specific isoenzyme CYP3A4 responsible for 90 % of the hepatic metabolism. Additionally, *in vitro* studies have shown that saquinavir is a substrate and an inhibitor for P-glycoprotein (P-gp). Therefore, medicinal products that either share this metabolic pathway or modify CYP3A4 and/or P-gp activity (see "*Other potential interactions*") may modify the pharmacokinetics of saquinavir. Similarly, saquinavir might also modify the pharmacokinetics of other medicinal products that are substrates for CYP3A4 or P-gp.

Ritonavir can affect the pharmacokinetics of other medicinal products because it is a potent inhibitor of CYP3A4 and P-gp. Therefore, when saquinavir is co-administered with ritonavir, consideration should be given to the potential effects of ritonavir on other medicinal products (see the Summary of Product Characteristics for Norvir).

Table 1: Interactions and dose recommendations with other medicinal products

(see Table 1 on next page)

4.6 Pregnancy and lactation

Pregnancy: Evaluation of experimental animal studies does not indicate direct or indirect harmful effects with respect to the development of the embryo or foetus, the course of gestation and peri- and post-natal development. Clinical experience in pregnant women is limited: Congenital malformations, birth defects and other disorders (without a congenital malformation) have been reported rarely in pregnant women who had received saquinavir in combination with other antiretroviral agents. However, so far the available data are insufficient and do not identify specific risks for the unborn child. Saquinavir should be used during pregnancy only if the potential benefit justifies the potential risk to the foetus (see section 5.3).

Lactation: There are no laboratory animal or human data available on secretion of saquinavir in breast milk. The potential for adverse reactions to saquinavir in nursing infants cannot be assessed, and therefore, breast-feeding should be discontinued prior to receiving saquinavir. It is recommended that HIV-infected women do not breast feed their infants under any circumstances in order to avoid transmission of HIV.

4.7 Effects on ability to drive and use machines

Invirase may have a minor influence on the ability to drive and use machines. Dizziness and fatigue have been reported during treatment with Invirase. No studies on the effects on the ability to drive and use machines have been performed.

4.8 Undesirable effects

The following adverse events with an at least possible relationship to ritonavir boosted saquinavir (i.e. adverse reactions) were reported most frequently: nausea, diarrhoea, fatigue, vomiting, flatulence, and abdominal pain.

For comprehensive dose adjustment recommendations and drug-associated adverse reactions for ritonavir and other medicinal products used in combination with saquinavir, physicians should refer to the Summary of Product Characteristics for each of these medicinal products.

Within each frequency grouping, undesirable effects are presented in order of decreasing seriousness.

Adverse reactions from clinical trials where saquinavir was boosted with ritonavir

Limited data is available from two studies where the safety of saquinavir soft capsule (1000 mg twice daily) used in combination with low dose ritonavir (100 mg twice daily) for at least 48 weeks was studied in 311 patients. Adverse reactions in these two pivotal studies are summarised in Table 2. The list also includes marked laboratory abnormalities that have been observed with the saquinavir soft capsule in combination with ritonavir (at 48 weeks).

Table 2: Incidences of Adverse Reactions and marked laboratory abnormalities from the MaxCmin1 and MaxCmin2 study. (Very common (≥ 10 %); common (≥ 1 % and < 10 %))

Body System Frequency of Reaction	Adverse Reactions	
	Grades 3&4	All Grades
Blood and the lymphatic system disorders		
Common	Anaemia	Anaemia
Immune system disorders		
Common		Hypersensitivity
Metabolism and nutrition disorders		
Common	Diabetes mellitus	Diabetes mellitus, anorexia, increased appetite
Psychiatric disorders		
Common		Decreased libido, sleep disorder
Nervous System Disorders		
Common		Paraesthesia, peripheral neuropathy, dizziness, dysgeusia, headache
Respiratory, thoracic and mediastinal disorders		
Common		Dyspnoea
Gastrointestinal disorders		
Very common		Diarrhoea, nausea
Common	Diarrhoea, nausea, vomiting	Vomiting, abdominal distension, abdominal pain, upper abdominal pain, constipation, dry mouth, dyspepsia, eructation, flatulence, lip dry, loose stools
Skin and subcutaneous tissue disorders		
Common	Acquired lipodystrophy	Acquired lipodystrophy, alopecia, dry skin, eczema, lipoatrophy, pruritus, rash
Musculoskeletal and connective tissue disorders		
Common		Muscle spasms
General disorders and administration site conditions		
Common	Fatigue	Asthenia, fatigue, increased fat tissue, malaise
Investigations		
Very common		Increased alanine aminotransferase, increased aspartate aminotransferase, increased blood cholesterol, increased blood triglycerides, increased low density lipoprotein, decreased platelet count
Common		Increased blood amylase, increased blood bilirubin, increased blood creatinine, decreased haemoglobin, decreased lymphocyte count, decreased white blood cell count

Post-marketing experience with saquinavir

Serious and non-serious adverse reactions from post-marketing spontaneous reports (where saquinavir was taken as the sole protease inhibitor or in combination with ritonavir), not mentioned previously in section 4.8, for which a causal relationship to saquinavir cannot be excluded, are summarised below. As these data come from the spontaneous reporting system, the frequency of the adverse reactions is unknown.

- Immune system disorders: Hypersensitivity.
- Metabolism and nutrition disorders:

- Diabetes mellitus or hyperglycaemia sometimes associated with ketoacidosis (see section 4.4).

- Lipodystrophy: Combination antiretroviral therapy has been associated with redistribution of body fat (lipodystrophy) in HIV infected patients including the loss of peripheral and facial subcutaneous fat, increased intra-abdominal and visceral fat, breast hypertrophy and dorsicervical fat accumulation (buffalo hump).

- Combination antiretroviral therapy has been associated with metabolic abnormalities such as hypertriglyceridaemia, hypercholesterolaemia, insulin resistance, hyperglycaemia and hyperlactataemia (see section 4.4).

- Nervous system disorders: Somnolence, convulsions.
- Vascular disorders: There have been reports of increased bleeding, including spontaneous skin haematomas and haemarthroses, in haemophilic patients type A and B treated with protease inhibitors (see section 4.4).
- Hepato-biliary disorders: Hepatitis.
- Musculoskeletal, connective tissue and bone disorders: Increased CPK, myalgia, myositis and rarely, rhabdomyolysis have been reported with protease inhibitors, particularly in combination with nucleoside analogues. Cases of osteonecrosis have been reported, particularly in patients with generally acknowledged risk factors, advanced HIV disease or long-term exposure to combination antiretroviral therapy (CART). The frequency of this is unknown (see section 4.4).
- Renal and urinary disorders: Renal impairment.
- In HIV-infected patients with severe immune deficiency at the time of initiation of combination antiretroviral therapy (CART), an inflammatory reaction to asymptomatic or residual opportunistic infections may arise (see section 4.4).

4.9 Overdose

There is limited experience of overdose with saquinavir. Whereas acute or chronic overdose of saquinavir alone did not result in major complications, in combination with other protease inhibitors, overdose symptoms and signs such as general weakness, fatigue, diarrhoea, nausea, vomiting, hair loss, dry mouth, hyponatraemia, weight loss and orthostatic hypotension have been observed. There is no specific antidote for overdose with saquinavir. Treatment of overdose with saquinavir should consist of general supportive measures, including monitoring of vital signs and ECG, and observations of the patient's clinical status. If indicated, prevention of further absorption can be considered. Since saquinavir is highly protein bound, dialysis is unlikely to be beneficial in significant removal of the active substance.

5. PHARMACOLOGICAL PROPERTIES

5.1 Pharmacodynamic properties

Pharmaco-therapeutic group: Antiviral agent, ATC code J05A E01

Mechanism of action: The HIV protease is an essential viral enzyme required for the specific cleavage of viral gag and gag-pol polyproteins. Saquinavir selectively inhibits the HIV protease, thereby preventing the creation of mature infectious virus particles.

Antiviral activity in vitro: Saquinavir demonstrates antiviral activity against a panel of laboratory strains and clinical isolates of HIV-1 with typical EC_{50} and EC_{90} values in the range 1-10 nM and 5-50 nM, respectively, with no

Table 1: Interactions and dose recommendations with other medicinal products

Medicinal product by therapeutic area (dose of Invirase used in study)	Interaction	Recommendations concerning co-administration
Antiretroviral agents ***Nucleoside reverse transcriptase inhibitors (NRTIs)***		
- Zalcitabine and/or Zidovudine (saquinavir/ritonavir)	- No pharmacokinetic interaction studies have been completed. Interaction with zalcitabine is unlikely due to different routes of metabolism and excretion. For zidovudine (200 mg every 8 hours) a 25 % decrease in AUC was reported when combined with ritonavir (300 mg every 6 hours). The pharmacokinetics of ritonavir remained unchanged.	- No dose adjustment required.
- Zalcitabine and/or Zidovudine (unboosted saquinavir)	- Saquinavir ↔ Zalcitabine ↔ Zidovudine ↔	
Didanosine 400 mg single dose (saquinavir/ritonavir 1600/100 mg qd)	Saquinavir AUC ↓ 30% Saquinavir C_{max}↓ 25% Saquinavir C_{min} ↔	No dose adjustment required.
Tenofovir disoproxil fumarate 300 mg qd (saquinavir/ritonavir 1000/100 mg bid)	Saquinavir AUC ↓ 1% Saquinavir C_{max}↓ 7% Saquinavir C_{min} ↔	No dose adjustment required.
Non-nucleoside reverse transcriptase inhibitors (NNRTIs)		
- Delavirdine (saquinavir/ritonavir)	- Interaction with Invirase/ritonavir not studied.	
- Delavirdine (unboosted saquinavir)	- Saquinavir AUC ↑ 348%. There are limited safety and no efficacy data available from the use of this combination. In a small, preliminary study, hepatocellular enzyme elevations occurred in 13 % of subjects during the first several weeks of the delavirdine and saquinavir combination (6 % Grade 3 or 4).	- Hepatocellular changes should be monitored frequently if this combination is prescribed.
Efavirenz 600 mg qd (saquinavir/ritonavir 1600/200 mg qd, *or* saquinavir/ritonavir 1000/100 mg bid, *or* saquinavir/ritonavir 1200/100 mg qd)	Saquinavir ↔ Efavirenz ↔	No dose adjustment required.
- Nevirapine (saquinavir/ritonavir)	- Interaction with Invirase/ritonavir not studied.	
- Nevirapine (unboosted saquinavir)	- Saquinavir AUC ↓ 24% Nevirapine AUC ↔	- No dose adjustment required.
HIV protease inhibitors (PIs)		
Atazanavir 300 mg qd (saquinavir/ritonavir 1600/100 mg qd)	Saquinavir AUC ↑ 60% Saquinavir C_{max} ↑ 42% Ritonavir AUC ↑ 41% Ritonavir C_{max} ↑ 34% Atazanavir ↔ No clinical data available for the combination of saquinavir/ritonavir 1000/100 mg bid and atazanavir.	
Fosamprenavir 700 mg bid (saquinavir/ritonavir 1000/100 mg bid)	Saquinavir AUC ↓ 15% Saquinavir C_{max}↓ 9% Saquinavir C_{min}↓ 24% (remained above the target threshold for effective therapy.)	No dose adjustment required for Invirase/ritonavir.
- Indinavir (saquinavir/ritonavir)	- Low dose ritonavir increases the concentration of indinavir.	Increased concentrations of indinavir may result in nephrolithiasis.
- Indinavir 800 mg tid (saquinavir 600-1200 mg single dose)	- Saquinavir AUC ↑ 4.6-7.2 fold Indinavir ↔ No safety and efficacy data available for this combination. Appropriate doses of combination not established.	
Lopinavir/ritonavir 400/100 mg bid (saquinavir/ritonavir 1000/100 mg bid in combination with 2 or 3 NRTIs)	Saquinavir ↔ Ritonavir ↓ (effectiveness as boosting agent not modified). Lopinavir ↔ (based on historical comparison with unboosted lopinavir)	No dose adjustment required.
-	-	
- Nelfinavir 1250 mg bid (saquinavir/ritonavir 1000/100 mg bid)	- Saquinavir AUC ↑ 13% (90% CI: 27 ↓ - 74 ↑) Saquinavir C_{max} ↑ 9% (90% CI: 27 ↓ - 61 ↑) Nelfinavir AUC ↓ 6% (90% CI: 28 ↓ - 22 ↑) Nelfinavir C_{max} ↓ 5% (90% CI: 23 ↓ - 16 ↑)	No dose adjustment required
- Nelfinavir 750 mg tid (unboosted saquinavir 1200 mg tid)	Saquinavir AUC ↑ 392% Saquinavir C_{max} ↑ 179% Nelfinavir AUC ↑ 18% Nelfinavir C_{max}↔	Quadruple therapy, including saquinavir soft capsules and nelfinavir in addition to two nucleoside reverse transcriptase inhibitors gave a more durable response (prolongation of time to virological relapse) than triple therapy with either single protease inhibitor. Concomitant administration of nelfinavir and saquinavir soft capsules resulted in a moderate increase in the incidence of diarrhoea.
Ritonavir 100 mg bid (saquinavir 1000 mg bid)	Saquinavir ↑ Ritonavir ↔ In HIV-infected patients, Invirase or saquinavir soft capsules in combination with ritonavir at doses of 1000/100 mg twice daily provide a systemic exposure of saquinavir over a 24 hour period similar to or greater than that achieved with saquinavir soft capsules 1200 mg three times daily (see section 5.2).	This is the approved combination regimen. No dose adjustment is recommended.
Tipranavir/ritonavir (saquinavir/ritonavir)	Saquinavir C_{min}↓ 78% Dual-boosted protease inhibitor combination therapy in multiple-treatment experienced HIV-positive adults.	Concomitant administration of tipranavir, co-administered with low dose ritonavir, with saquinavir/ ritonavir, is not recommended. If the combination is considered necessary, monitoring of the saquinavir plasma levels is strongly encouraged.

Medicinal product by therapeutic area (dose of Invirase used in study)	Interaction	Recommendations concerning co-administration
HIV fusion inhibitor		
Enfuvirtide (saquinavir/ritonavir 1000/100 mg bid)	Saquinavir ↔ Enfuvirtide ↔ No clinically significant interaction was noted.	No dose adjustment required.
Other medicinal products		
Antiarrhythmics		
Bepridil Lidocaine (systemic) Quinidine (saquinavir/ritonavir)	Concentrations of bepridil, systemic lidocaine or quinidine may be increased when co-administered with Invirase/ritonavir.	Caution is warranted. Therapeutic concentration monitoring is recommended, if available.
Amiodarone Flecainide Propafenone (saquinavir/ritonavir)	Concentrations of amiodarone, flecainide or propafenone may be increased when co-administered with Invirase/ritonavir.	Contraindicated in combination with saquinavir/ritonavir due to potentially life threatening cardiac arrhythmia (see section 4.3).
Anticoagulant		
Warfarin (saquinavir/ritonavir)	Concentrations of warfarin may be affected.	INR (international normalised ratio) monitoring recommended.
Anticonvulsants		
- Carbamazepine Phenobarbital Phenytoin (saquinavir/ritonavir)	- Interaction with Invirase/ritonavir not studied.	
- Carbamazepine Phenobarbital Phenytoin (unboosted saquinavir)	- These medicinal products will induce CYP3A4 and may therefore decrease saquinavir concentrations.	
Antidepressants		
Tricyclic antidepressants (e.g. amitriptyline, imipramine) (saquinavir/ritonavir)	Invirase/ritonavir may increase concentrations of tricyclic antidepressants.	Therapeutic concentration monitoring recommended.
- Nefazodone (saquinavir/ritonavir)	- Interaction with saquinavir/ritonavir not evaluated.	
- Nefazodone (unboosted saquinavir)	- Nefazodone inhibits CYP3A4. Saquinavir concentrations may be increased.	- Monitoring for saquinavir toxicity recommended.
Antihistamines		
Terfenadine Astemizole (saquinavir/ritonavir)	Terfenadine AUC ↑, associated with a prolongation of QTc intervals. A similar interaction with astemizole is likely.	Terfenadine and astemizole are contraindicated with boosted or unboosted saquinavir (see section 4.3).
Anti-infectives		
- Clarithromycin (saquinavir/ritonavir)	- Interaction with Invirase/ritonavir not studied.	
- Clarithromycin 500 mg bid (unboosted saquinavir 1200 mg tid)	- Saquinavir AUC ↑ 177 % Saquinavir C_{max} ↑ 187 % Clarithromycin AUC ↑ 40 % Clarithromycin C_{max} ↑ 40 %	- No dose adjustment is required when co-administered for a limited time at the doses studied.
- Erythromycin (saquinavir/ritonavir)	- Interaction with Invirase/ritonavir not studied.	
- Erythromycin 250 mg qid (unboosted saquinavir 1200 mg tid)	- Saquinavir AUC ↑ 99 % Saquinavir C_{max} ↑ 106 %	- No dose adjustment required.
- Streptogramin antibiotics (saquinavir/ritonavir)	- Interaction with Invirase/ritonavir not studied.	
- Streptogramin antibiotics (unboosted saquinavir)	- Streptogramin antibiotics such as quinupristin/dalfopristin inhibit CYP3A4. Saquinavir concentrations may be increased.	- Monitoring for saquinavir toxicity recommended.
Antifungals		
Ketoconazole 200 mg qd (saquinavir/ritonavir 1000/100 mg bid)	Saquinavir AUC ↔ Saquinavir C_{max} ↔ Ritonavir AUC ↔ Ritonavir C_{max} ↔ Ketoconazole AUC ↑ 168% (90% CI 146%-193%) Ketoconazole C_{max} ↑ 45% (90% CI 32%-59%)	No dose adjustment required when saquinavir/ritonavir combined with ≤ 200 mg/day ketoconazole. High doses of ketoconazole (> 200 mg/day) are not recommended.
- Itraconazole (saquinavir/ritonavir)	- Interaction with Invirase/ritonavir not studied.	
- Itraconazole (unboosted saquinavir)	- Itraconazole is a moderately potent inhibitor of CYP3A4. An interaction is possible.	Monitoring for saquinavir toxicity recommended.
Fluconazole/miconazole (saquinavir/ritonavir)	Interaction with Invirase/ritonavir not studied.	
Antimycobacterials		
Rifampicin 600 mg qd (saquinavir/ritonavir 1000/100 mg bid)	In a clinical study 11 of 17 (65 %) healthy volunteers developed severe hepatocellular toxicity with transaminase elevations up to > 20-fold the upper limit of normal after 1 to 5 days of co-administration.	Rifampicin is contraindicated in combination with Invirase/ritonavir (see section 4.3).
Rifabutin (saquinavir/ritonavir 1000/100 mg bid)	Interaction with saquinavir/ritonavir 1000/100 mg not studied.	A dosage reduction to rifabutin 150 mg every three days is recommended based on experience with low dose ritonavir boosted protease inhibitors. Patients receiving rifabutin with Invirase/ritonavir should be closely monitored for liver function test elevations and emergence of adverse events associated with rifabutin therapy. Further dosage reduction of rifabutin may be necessary. Therapeutic concentration monitoring for saquinavir is recommended.

Medicinal product by therapeutic area (dose of Invirase used in study)	Interaction	Recommendations concerning co-administration
Benzodiazepines		
Midazolam 7.5 mg single dose (oral) (saquinavir/ritonavir 1000/100 mg bid)	Midazolam AUC ↑ 12.4 fold Midazolam C_{max} ↑ 4.3 fold Midazolam $t_{1/2}$ ↑ from 4.7 h to 14.9 h No data are available on concomitant use of ritonavir boosted saquinavir with intravenous midazolam. Studies of other CYP3A modulators and i.v. midazolam suggest a possible 3-4 fold increase in midazolam plasma levels.	Co-administration of Invirase/ritonavir with orally administered midazolam is contraindicated (see section 4.3). Caution should be used with co-administration of Invirase and parenteral midazolam. If Invirase is co-administered with parenteral midazolam it should be done in an intensive care unit (ICU) or similar setting which ensures close clinical monitoring and appropriate medical management in case of respiratory depression and/or prolonged sedation. Dosage adjustment should be considered, especially if more than a single dose of midazolam is administered.
Alprazolam Clorazepate Diazepam Flurazepam (saquinavir/ritonavir)	Concentrations of these medicinal products may be increased when co-administered with Invirase/ritonavir.	Careful monitoring of patients with regard to sedative effects is warranted. A decrease in the dose of the benzodiazepine may be required.
Triazolam (saquinavir/ritonavir)	Concentrations of triazolam may be increased when co-administered with Invirase/ritonavir.	Contraindicated in combination with saquinavir/ritonavir, due to the risk of potentially prolonged or increased sedation and respiratory depression (see section 4.3).
Calcium channel blockers		
Felodipine, nifedipine, nicardipine, diltiazem, nimodipine, verapamil, amlodipine, nisoldipine, isradipine (saquinavir/ritonavir)	Concentrations of these medicinal products may be increased when co-administered with Invirase/ritonavir.	Caution is warranted and clinical monitoring of patients is recommended.
Corticosteroids		
- Dexamethasone (saquinavir/ritonavir)	- Interaction with Invirase/ritonavir not studied.	
- Dexamethasone (unboosted saquinavir)	- Dexamethasone induces CYP3A4 and may decrease saquinavir concentrations.	- Use with caution. Saquinavir may be less effective in patients taking dexamethasone.
Fluticasone propionate 50 mcg qid, intranasal (ritonavir 100 mg bid)	Fluticasone propionate ↑ Intrinsic cortisol ↓ 86% (90% CI 82%-89%) Greater effects may be expected when fluticasone propionate is inhaled. Systemic corticosteroid effects including Cushing's syndrome and adrenal suppression have been reported in patients receiving ritonavir and inhaled or intranasally administered fluticasone propionate; this could also occur with other corticosteroids metabolised via the P450 3A pathway e.g. budesonide. Effects of high fluticasone systemic exposure on ritonavir plasma levels yet unknown.	Concomitant administration of boosted saquinavir and fluticasone propionate and other corticosteroids metabolised via the P450 3A pathway (e.g. budesonide) is not recommended unless the potential benefit of treatment outweighs the risk of systemic corticosteroid effects (see section 4.4). Dose reduction of the glucocorticoid should be considered with close monitoring of local and systemic effects or a switch to a glucocorticoid, which is not a substrate for CYP3A4 (e.g. beclomethasone). In case of withdrawal of glucocorticoids progressive dose reduction may have to be performed over a longer period.
<u>Medicinal products that are substrates of P-glycoprotein</u>Digitalis glycosides		
Digoxin 0.5 mg single dose (saquinavir/ritonavir 1000/100 mg bid)	Digoxin AUC_{0-72} ↑ 49% Digoxin C_{max} ↑ 27% Digoxin levels may differ over time. Large increments of digoxin may be expected when saquinavir/ritonavir is introduced in patients already treated with digoxin.	Caution should be exercised when Invirase/ritonavir and digoxin are co-administered. The serum concentration of digoxin should be monitored and a dose reduction of digoxin should be considered if necessary.
Histamine H_2-receptor antagonist		
- Ranitidine (saquinavir/ritonavir)	- Interaction with Invirase/ritonavir not studied.	
- Ranitidine (unboosted saquinavir)	- Saquinavir AUC ↑ 67 %	- Increase not thought to be clinically relevant. No dose adjustment of saquinavir recommended.
HMG-CoA reductase inhibitors		
Pravastatin Fluvastatin (saquinavir/ritonavir)	Interaction not studied. Metabolism of pravastatin and fluvastatin is not dependent on CYP3A4. Interaction via effects on transport proteins cannot be excluded.	Interaction unknown. If no alternative treatment is available, use with careful monitoring.
Simvastatin Lovastatin (saquinavir/ritonavir)	Simvastatin ↑↑ Lovastatin ↑↑ Plasma concentrations highly dependent on CYP3A4 metabolism.	Increased concentrations of simvastatin and lovastatin have been associated with rhabdomyolysis. These medicinal products are contraindicated for use with Invirase/ritonavir (see section 4.3).
Atorvastatin (saquinavir/ritonavir)	Atorvastatin is less dependent on CYP3A4 for metabolism.	When used with Invirase/ritonavir, the lowest possible dose of atorvastatin should be administered and the patient should be carefully monitored for signs/symptoms of myopathy (muscle weakness, muscle pain, rising plasma creatinine kinase).
Immunosuppressants		
Ciclosporin Tacrolimus Rapamycin (saquinavir/ritonavir)	Concentrations of these medicinal products increase several fold when co-administered with Invirase/ritonavir.	Careful therapeutic drug monitoring is necessary for immunosuppressants when co-administered with Invirase/ritonavir.
Narcotic analgesics		
Methadone 60-120 mg qd (saquinavir/ritonavir 1000/100 mg bid)	Methadone AUC ↓ 19 % (90 % CI 9 % to 29 %) None of the 12 patients experienced withdrawal symptoms.	No dosage adjustment required.
Neuroleptics		
Pimozide (saquinavir/ritonavir)	Concentrations of pimozide may be increased when co-administered with Invirase/ritonavir.	Due to a potential for life threatening cardiac arrhythmias, Invirase/ritonavir is contra-indicated in combination with pimozide (see section 4.3).

Medicinal product by therapeutic area (dose of Invirase used in study)	Interaction	Recommendations concerning co-administration
Oral contraceptives		
Ethinyl estradiol (saquinavir/ritonavir)	Concentration of ethinyl estradiol may be decreased when co-administered with Invirase/ritonavir.	Alternative or additional contraceptive measures should be used when oestrogen-based oral contraceptives are co-administered.
Phosphodiesterase type 5 (PDE5) inhibitors		
- Sildenafil (saquinavir/ritonavir)	- Interaction with Invirase/ritonavir not studied.	
- Sildenafil 100 mg (single dose) (unboosted saquinavir 1200 mg tid)	- Saquinavir ↔ Sildenafil C_{max} ↑ 140 % Sildenafil AUC ↑ 210 % - Sildenafil is a substrate of CYP3A4.	- Use sildenafil with caution at reduced doses of no more than 25 mg every 48 hours with increased monitoring of adverse events when administered concomitantly with Invirase/ritonavir.
Vardenafil (saquinavir/ritonavir)	Concentrations of vardenafil may be increased when co-administered with Invirase/ritonavir.	Use vardenafil with caution at reduced doses of no more than 2.5 mg every 72 hours with increased monitoring of adverse events when administered concomitantly with Invirase/ritonavir.
Tadalafil (saquinavir/ritonavir)	Concentrations of tadalafil may be increased when co-administered with Invirase/ritonavir.	Use tadalafil with caution at reduced doses of no more than 10 mg every 72 hours with increased monitoring of adverse events when administered concomitantly with Invirase/ritonavir.
Proton pump inhibitors		
Omeprazole 40 mg qd (saquinavir/ritonavir 1000/100 mg bid)	Saquinavir AUC ↑ 82% (90 % CI 44-131 %) Saquinavir C_{max} ↑ 75% (90 % CI 38-123 %) Ritonavir ↔	Monitoring for potential saquinavir toxicities is recommended.
Other proton pump inhibitors (saquinavir/ritonavir 1000/100 mg bid)	No data are available on the concomitant administration of Invirase/ritonavir and other proton pump inhibitors.	If omeprazole or other proton pump inhibitors are taken concomitantly with Invirase/ritonavir, monitoring for potential saquinavir toxicities is recommended.
Others		
Ergot alkaloids (e.g. ergotamine, dihydroergotamine, ergonovine, and methylergonovine) (saquinavir/ritonavir)	Invirase/ritonavir may increase ergot alkaloids exposure, and consequently, increase the potential for acute ergot toxicity.	The concomitant use of Invirase/ritonavir and ergot alkaloids is contra-indicated (see section 4.3).
- Grapefruit juice (saquinavir/ritonavir)	- Interaction with Invirase/ritonavir not studied.	
- Grapefruit juice (single dose) (unboosted saquinavir)	- Saquinavir ↑ 50% (normal strength grapefruit juice) - Saquinavir ↑ 100% (double strength grapefruit juice)	- Increase not thought to be clinically relevant. No dose adjustment required.
- Garlic capsules (saquinavir/ritonavir)	- Interaction with Invirase/ritonavir not studied.	
- Garlic capsules (dose approx. equivalent to two 4 g cloves of garlic daily) (unboosted saquinavir 1200 mg tid)	- Saquinavir AUC ↓ 51 % Saquinavir C_{trough}↓ 49 % (8 hours post dose) Saquinavir C_{max}↓ 54 %.	- Patients on saquinavir treatment must not take garlic capsules due to the risk of decreased plasma concentrations and loss of virological response and possible resistance to one or more components of the antiretroviral regimen.
- St. John's wort (saquinavir/ritonavir)	- Interaction with Invirase/ritonavir not studied.	
- St. John's wort (unboosted saquinavir)	- Plasma levels of saquinavir can be reduced by concomitant use of the herbal preparation St. John's wort *(Hypericum perforatum)*. This is due to induction of drug metabolising enzymes and/or transport proteins by St. John's wort.	- Herbal preparations containing St. John's wort must not be used concomitantly with Invirase. If a patient is already taking St. John's wort, stop St. John's wort, check viral levels and if possible saquinavir levels. Saquinavir levels may increase on stopping St. John's wort, and the dose of saquinavir may need adjusting. The inducing effect of St. John's wort may persist for at least 2 weeks after cessation of treatment.
Other potential interactions ***Medicinal products that are substrates of CYP3A4***		
e.g. dapsone, disopyramide, quinine, fentanyl, and alfentanyl (unboosted saquinavir)	Although specific studies have not been performed, co-administration of Invirase/ritonavir with medicinal products that are mainly metabolised by CYP3A4 pathway may result in elevated plasma concentrations of these medicinal products.	These combinations should be given with caution.
Medicinal products reducing gastrointestinal transit time		
Metoclopramide	It is unknown whether medicinal products which reduce the gastrointestinal transit time could lead to lower saquinavir plasma concentrations.	

Key: ↓ reduced, ↑ increased, ↔ unchanged, ↑↑ markedly increased

apparent difference between subtype B and non-B clades. The corresponding serum (50% human serum) adjusted EC_{50} ranged from 25-250 nM. Clinical isolates of HIV-2 demonstrated EC_{50} values in the range of 0.3-2.4 nM.

Resistance

Antiviral activity according to baseline genotype and phenotype:

Genotypic and phenotypic clinical cut-offs predicting the clinical efficacy of ritonavir boosted saquinavir have been derived from retrospective analyses of the RESIST 1 and 2 clinical studies and analysis of a large hospital cohort (Marcelin et al 2007).

Baseline saquinavir phenotype (shift in susceptibility relative to reference, PhenoSense Assay) was shown to be a predictive factor of virological outcome. Virological response was first observed to decrease when the fold shift exceeded 2.3-fold; whereas virological benefit was not observed when the fold shift exceeded 12-fold.

Marcelin et al (2007) identified nine protease codons (L10F/I/M/R/V, I15A/V, K20I/M/R/T, L24I, I62V, G73S/T, V82A/F/S/T, I84V, L90M) that were associated with decreased virological response to saquinavir/ritonavir (1000/100 mg twice daily) in 138 saquinavir naive patients. The presence of 3 or more mutations was associated with reduced response to saquinavir/ritonavir.The association between the number of these saquinavir-associated resistance mutations and virological response was confirmed in an independent clinical study (RESIST 1 and 2) involving a more heavily treatment experienced patient population, including 54% who had received prior saquinavir (p=0.0133, see Table 3). The G48V mutation, previously identified in vitro as a saquinavir signature mutation, was present at baseline in virus from three patients, none of whom responded to therapy.

Table 3: Virological response to saquinavir/ritonavir stratified by the number of baseline saquinavir-associated resistance mutations

(see Table 3 on next page)

Clinical results from studies with treatment naïve and experienced patients

In the MaxCmin1 study, the safety and efficacy of saquinavir soft capsules/ritonavir 1000/100 mg twice daily plus 2 NRTIs/Non-Nucleoside Reverse Transcriptase Inhibitors (NNRTIs) was compared to indinavir/ritonavir 800/100 mg twice daily plus 2 NRTIs/NNRTIs in over 300 (both protease inhibitor treatment naïve and experienced) subjects. The

Table 3: Virological response to saquinavir/ritonavir stratified by the number of baseline saquinavir-associated resistance mutations

Number of Saquinavir Associated Resistance Mutations at Baseline*	Marcelin et al (2007)		RESIST 1 & 2	
	SQV Naive Population		SQV Naive/Experienced Population	
	N=138	Change in Baseline Plasma HIV-1 RNA at Weeks 12-20	N=114	Change in Baseline Plasma HIV-1 RNA at Week 4
0	35	-2.24	2	-2.04
1	29	-1.88	3	-1.69
2	24	-1.43	14	-1.57
3	30	-0.52	28	-1.41
4	9	-0.18	40	-0.75
5	6	-0.11	17	-0.44
6	5	-0.30	9	0.08
7	0	-	1	0.24

* Saquinavir Mutation Score Mutations: L10F/I/M/R/V, I15A/V, K20I/M/R/T, L24I, I62V, G73S/T, V82A/F/S/T, I84V, L90M

Table 4: Subject Demographics MaxCmin1 and MaxCmin2

	MaxCmin1		MaxCmin2	
	SQV/r	IDV/r	SQV/r	LPV/r
	N=148	N=158	N=161	N=163
Sex Male	82%	74%	81%	76%
Race (White/Black/Asian) %	86/9/1	82/12/4	75/19/1	74/19/2
Age, median, yrs	39	40	40	40
CDC Category C (%)	32%	28%	32%	31%
Antiretroviral naïve (%)	28%	22%	31%	34%
PI naïve (%)	41%	38%	48%	48%
Median Baseline HIV-1 RNA, log_{10} copies/ml (IQR)	4.0 (1.7-5.1)	3.9 (1.7-5.2)	4.4 (3.1-5.1)	4.6 (3.5-5.3)
Median Baseline $CD4^+$ Cell Count, cells/mm^3 (IQR)	272 (135-420)	280 (139-453)	241 (86-400)	239 (95-420)

†data from clinical study report

Table 5: Outcomes at Week 48 MaxCmin1 and MaxCmin2†

Outcomes	MaxCmin1		MaxCmin2	
	SQV/r	IDV/r	SQV/r	LPV/r
Initiated assigned treatment, n (%)	148 (94%)	158 (99%)	161 (94%)	163 (98%)
Discontinued assigned treatment, n (%)	40 (27%)	64 (41%)	48 (30%)	23 (14%)
	P=0.01		P=0.001	
Virological failure ITT/e*#	36/148 (24%)	41/158 (26%)	53/161 (33%)	29/163 (18%)
	P=0.76		P=0.002	
Proportion with VL < 50 copies/ml at week 48, ITT/e#	97/144 (67%)	106/154 (69%)	90/158 (57%)	106/162 (65%)
	P>0.05‡		P=0.12	
Proportion with VL < 50 copies/ml at week 48, On Treatment	82/104 (79%)	73/93 (78%)	84/113 (74%)	97/138 (70%)
	p>0.05‡		P=0.48	
Median increase in CD4 cell count at week 48 (cells/mm^3)	85	73	110	106

* For both studies: For patients entering study with VL < 200 copies/ml, VF defined as $\geq$ 200 copies/ml. MaxCmin1: For those entering with VL $\geq$ 200 copies/ml, VF defined as any increase $\geq$ 0.5 logs and/or VL $\geq$ 50,000 copies/ml at week 4, $\geq$ 5,000 copies/ml at week 12, or $\geq$ 200 copies/ml at week 24 or thereafter. MaxCmin2: any rise $\geq$ 0.5 log at a specific visit; $\leq$ 0.5 log reduction if VL $\geq$ 200 copies/ml at week 4; $\leq$ 1.0 log reduction from base line if VL $\geq$ 200 copies/ml at week 12; and a VL $\geq$ 200 copies/ml at week 24.

\# ITT/e = Intent-to-treat/exposed

†Data from clinical study report

‡Data fromMaxCmin1 publication

combination of saquinavir and ritonavir exhibited a superior virological activity compared with the indinavir and ritonavir arm when switch from the assigned treatment was counted as virological failure.

In the MaxCmin2 study, the safety and efficacy of saquinavir soft capsules/ritonavir 1000/100 mg twice daily plus 2 NRTIs/NNRTIs was compared with lopinavir/ritonavir 400/100 mg twice daily plus 2 NRTIs/NNRTIs in 324 (both protease inhibitor treatment naïve and experienced) subjects. None of the subjects in the lopinavir/ritonavir arm had been exposed to lopinavir prior to randomisation whereas 16 of the subjects in the saquinavir/ritonavir arm had previously been exposed to saquinavir.

Table 4: Subject Demographics MaxCmin1 and MaxCmin2†

(see Table 4 above)

Table 5: Outcomes at Week 48 MaxCmin1 and MaxCmin2†

(see Table 5 above)

5.2 Pharmacokinetic properties

Saquinavir is essentially completely metabolised by CYP3A4. Ritonavir inhibits the metabolism of saquinavir, thereby increasing ("boosting") the plasma levels of saquinavir.

Absorption and bioavailability in adults: In HIV-infected patients, Invirase in combination with ritonavir at doses of 1000/100 mg twice daily provides saquinavir systemic exposures over a 24-hour period similar to or greater than those achieved with saquinavir soft capsules 1200 mg tid (see Table 6). The pharmacokinetics of saquinavir is stable during long-term treatment.

Table 6: Mean (% CV) AUC, C_{max} and C_{min} of saquinavir in patients following multiple dosing of Invirase, saquinavir soft capsules, Invirase/ritonavir, and saquinavir soft capsules/ritonavir

(see Table 6 on next page)

Absolute bioavailability averaged 4 % (CV 73 %, range: 1 % to 9 %) in 8 healthy volunteers who received a single 600 mg dose (3 × 200 mg hard capsule) of Invirase following a heavy breakfast. The low bioavailability is thought to be due to a combination of incomplete absorption and extensive first-pass metabolism. Gastric pH has been shown to be only a minor component in the large increase in bioavailability seen when given with food. The absolute bioavailability of saquinavir co-administered with ritonavir has not been established in humans.

In combination with ritonavir, bioequivalence of Invirase hard capsules and film-coated tablets was demonstrated under fed conditions.

Effective therapy in treatment naïve patients is associated with a C_{min} of approximately 50 ng/ml and an AUC_{0-24} of about 20,000 ng·h/ml. Effective therapy in treatment experienced patients is associated with a C_{min} of approximately 100 ng/ml and an AUC_{0-24} of about 20,000 ng·h/ml.

In vitro studies have shown that saquinavir is a substrate for P-glycoprotein (P-gp).

Effect of food: In a cross-over study in 22 HIV-infected patients treated with Invirase/ritonavir 1000 mg/100 mg twice daily and receiving three consecutive doses under fasting conditions or after a high-fat, high-calorie meal (46 g fat, 1,091 Kcal), the AUC_{0-12}, C_{max} and C_{trough} values of saquinavir under fasting conditions were about 70 per cent lower than with a high-fat meal. All but one of the patients achieved C_{trough} values of saquinavir above the therapeutic threshold (100 ng/ml) in the fasted state. There were no clinically significant differences in the pharmacokinetic profile of ritonavir in fasting and fed conditions but the ritonavir C_{trough} (geometric mean 245 vs. 348 ng/ml) was lower in the fasting state compared to the administration with a meal. Invirase/ritonavir should be administered with or after food.

Distribution in adults: Saquinavir partitions extensively into the tissues. The mean steady-state volume of distribution following intravenous administration of a 12 mg dose of saquinavir was 700 l (CV 39 %). It has been shown that saquinavir is approximately 97 % bound to plasma proteins up to 30 µg/ml. In two patients receiving Invirase 600 mg three times daily, cerebrospinal fluid concentrations of saquinavir were negligible when compared to concentrations from matching plasma samples.

Metabolism and elimination in adults: *In vitro* studies using human liver microsomes have shown that the metabolism of saquinavir is cytochrome P450 mediated with the specific isoenzyme, CYP3A4, responsible for more than 90 % of the hepatic metabolism. Based on *in vitro* studies, saquinavir is rapidly metabolised to a range of mono- and di-hydroxylated inactive compounds. In a mass balance study using 600 mg ^{14}C-saquinavir (n = 8), 88 % and 1 % of the orally administered radioactivity, was recovered in faeces and urine, respectively, within 4 days of dosing. In an additional four subjects administered 10.5 mg ^{14}C-saquinavir intravenously, 81 % and 3 % of the intravenously administered radioactivity was recovered in faeces and urine, respectively, within 4 days of dosing. 13 % of circulating saquinavir in plasma was present as unchanged compound after oral administration and the remainder as metabolites. Following intravenous administration 66 % of circulating saquinavir was present as unchanged compound and the remainder as metabolites, suggesting that saquinavir undergoes extensive first pass metabolism. *In vitro* experiments have shown that the hepatic metabolism of saquinavir becomes saturable at concentrations above 2 µg/ml.

Systemic clearance of saquinavir was high, 1.14 l/h/kg (CV 12 %), slightly above the hepatic plasma flow, and constant after intravenous doses of 6, 36 and 72 mg. The mean residence time of saquinavir was 7 hours (n = 8).

__*Special populations*__

Effect of gender following treatment with Invirase/ritonavir: A gender difference was observed with females showing higher saquinavir exposure than males (AUC on average 56 % higher and C_{max} on average 26 % higher) in the bioequivalence study comparing Invirase 500 mg film coated tablets with Invirase 200 mg hard capsules both in combination with ritonavir. There was no evidence that age and body-weight explained the gender difference in this study. Limited data from controlled clinical studies with the approved dosage regimen do not indicate a major

Table 6: Mean (% CV) AUC, C_{max} and C_{min} of saquinavir in patients following multiple dosing of Invirase, saquinavir soft capsules, Invirase/ritonavir, and saquinavir soft capsules/ritonavir

Treatment	N	AUCτ (ng·h/ml)	AUC_{0-24} (ng·h/ml)†	C_{max} (ng/ml)	C_{min} (ng/ml)
Invirase (hard capsule) 600 mg tid	10	866 (62)	2,598	197 (75)	75 (82)
saquinavir soft capsule 1200 mg tid	31	7,249 (85)	21,747	2,181 (74)	216 (84)
Invirase (tablet) 1000 mg bid plus ritonavir 100 mg bid* (fasting condition)	22	10,320 (2,530-30,327)	20,640	1509 (355-4,101)	313 (70-1,725)††
Invirase (tablet) 1000 mg bid plus ritonavir 100 mg bid* (high fat meal)	22	34,926 (11,826-105,992)	69,852	5208 (1,536-14,369)	1,179 (334-5,176)††

τ = dosing interval, i.e. 8 hour for tid and 12 h for bid dosing

C_{min} = the observed plasma concentration at the end of the dose interval

bid = twice daily

tid = three times daily

* results are geometric mean (min - max)

†derived from tid or bid dosing schedule

††C_{trough} values

difference in the efficacy and safety profile between men and women.

5.3 Preclinical safety data

Acute and chronic toxicity: Saquinavir was well tolerated in oral acute and chronic toxicity studies in mice, rats, dogs and marmosets.

Mutagenesis: Mutagenicity and genotoxicity studies, with and without metabolic activation where appropriate, have shown that saquinavir has no mutagenic activity *in vitro* in either bacterial (Ames test) or mammalian cells (Chinese hamster lung V79/HPRT test). Saquinavir does not induce chromosomal damage *in vivo* in the mouse micronucleus assay or *in vitro* in human peripheral blood lymphocytes and does not induce primary DNA damage *in vitro* in the unscheduled DNA synthesis test.

Carcinogenesis: There was no evidence of carcinogenic activity after the administration of saquinavir mesilate for 96 to 104 weeks to rats and mice. The plasma exposures (AUC values) in rats (maximum dose 1000 mg/kg/day) and in mice (maximum dose 2500 mg/kg/day) were lower than the expected plasma exposures obtained in humans at the recommended clinical dose of ritonavir boosted Invirase.

Reproductive toxicity: Fertility, peri- and postnatal development were not affected, and embryotoxic / teratogenic effects were not observed in rats or rabbits at plasma exposures lower than those achieved in humans at the recommended clinical dose of ritonavir boosted Invirase. Distribution studies in these species showed that the placental transfer of saquinavir is low (less than 5% of maternal plasma concentrations).

6. PHARMACEUTICAL PARTICULARS

6.1 List of excipients

Capsule filling:

Lactose (anhydrous),

Microcrystalline cellulose,

Povidone,

Sodium starch glycollate,

Talc,

Magnesium stearate.

Capsule shell:

Gelatine,

Iron oxide black, red and yellow (E172),

Indigo carmine (E132),

Titanium dioxide (E171).

Printing ink:

Titanium dioxide (E 171),

Shellac,

Soya lecithin,

Polydimethylsiloxane.

6.2 Incompatibilities

Not applicable.

6.3 Shelf life

3 years.

6.4 Special precautions for storage

Store in the original container.

6.5 Nature and contents of container

Amber glass bottles with plastic screw cap containing 270 capsules of Invirase.

6.6 Special precautions for disposal and other handling

No special requirements.

7. MARKETING AUTHORISATION HOLDER

Roche Registration Limited

6 Falcon Way

Shire Park

WelwynGarden City

AL7 1TW

United Kingdom

8. MARKETING AUTHORISATION NUMBER(S)

EU/1/96/026/001

9. DATE OF FIRST AUTHORISATION/RENEWAL OF THE AUTHORISATION

Date of first authorisation: 04 October 1996

Date of last renewal: 04 October 2006

10. DATE OF REVISION OF THE TEXT

27 January 2009

Detailed information on this product is available on the website of the European Medicines Agency (EMEA) http://www.emea.europa.eu/.

Invirase 500mg Film-Coated Tablets

(Roche Products Limited)

1. NAME OF THE MEDICINAL PRODUCT

INVIRASE 500 mg film-coated tablets.

2. QUALITATIVE AND QUANTITATIVE COMPOSITION

One film-coated tablet contains 500 mg of saquinavir as saquinavir mesilate.

Excipient: Contains lactose monohydrate: 38.5 mg.

For a full list of excipients, see section 6.1.

3. PHARMACEUTICAL FORM

Film-coated tablet.

Light orange to greyish or brownish orange film-coated tablet of oval cylindrical biconvex shape with the marking "SQV 500" on the one side and "ROCHE" on the other side.

4. CLINICAL PARTICULARS

4.1 Therapeutic indications

Invirase is indicated for the treatment of HIV-1 infected adult patients. Invirase should only be given in combination with ritonavir and other antiretroviral medicinal products (see section 4.2).

4.2 Posology and method of administration

Therapy with Invirase should be initiated by a physician experienced in the management of HIV infection.

Adults and adolescents over the age of 16 years:

In combination with ritonavir

The recommended dose of Invirase is 1000 mg (2 × 500 mg film-coated tablets) two times daily with ritonavir 100 mg two times daily in combination with other antiretroviral agents.

Invirase film-coated tablets should be swallowed whole and taken at the same time as ritonavir with or after food (see section 5.2).

Renal and hepatic impairment:

No dosage adjustment is necessary for patients with mild to moderate renal or mild hepatic impairment. Caution should be exercised in patients with severe renal or moderate hepatic impairment. Invirase/ritonavir is contraindicated in patients with decompensated hepatic impairment (see sections 4.3 and 4.4).

Children under the age of 16 and adults over 60 years:

The experience with Invirase in children below the age of 16 and adults over 60 years is limited. In children, as in adults, Invirase should only be given in combination with ritonavir.

4.3 Contraindications

Hypersensitivity to the active substance or to any of the excipients.

Invirase/ritonavir is contraindicated in decompensated liver disease (see section 4.4).

Invirase/ritonavir should not be given together with other medicinal products which may interact and result in potentially life threatening undesirable effects.

Medicinal products which should not be given with Invirase/ritonavir include:

- terfenadine, astemizole, pimozide, cisapride, amiodarone, propafenone and flecainide (potential for life threatening cardiac arrhythmia)
- midazolam administered orally (for caution on parenterally administered midazolam, see section 4.5), triazolam (potential for prolonged or increased sedation, respiratory depression)
- simvastatin, lovastatin (increased risk of myopathy including rhabdomyolysis)
- ergot alkaloids (e.g. ergotamine, dihydroergotamine, ergonovine, and methylergonovine) (potential for acute ergot toxicity)
- rifampicin (risk of severe hepatocellular toxicity) (see sections 4.4, 4.5, and 4.8).

4.4 Special warnings and precautions for use

Considerations when initiating Invirase therapy: Invirase should not be given as the sole protease inhibitor. Invirase should only be given in combination with ritonavir (see section 4.2).

Patients should be informed that saquinavir is not a cure for HIV infection and that they may continue to acquire illnesses associated with advanced HIV infection, including opportunistic infections. Patients should also be advised that they might experience undesirable effects associated with co-administered medications.

Liver disease: The safety and efficacy of saquinavir/ritonavir has not been established in patients with significant underlying liver disorders, therefore saquinavir/ritonavir should be used cautiously in this patient population. Invirase/ritonavir is contraindicated in patients with decompensated liver disease (see section 4.3). Patients with chronic hepatitis B or C and treated with combination antiretroviral therapy are at an increased risk for severe and potentially fatal hepatic adverse events. In case of concomitant antiviral therapy for hepatitis B or C, please refer also to the relevant product information for these medicinal products.

Patients with pre-existing liver dysfunction including chronic active hepatitis have an increased frequency of liver function abnormalities during combination antiretroviral therapy and should be monitored according to standard practice. If there is evidence of worsening liver disease in such patients, interruption or discontinuation of treatment must be considered.

In cases of mild hepatic impairment no initial dosage adjustment is necessary at the recommended dose. The use of Invirase in combination with ritonavir in patients with moderate hepatic impairment has not been studied. In the absence of such studies, caution should be exercised, as increases in saquinavir levels and/or increases in liver enzymes may occur.

There have been reports of exacerbation of chronic liver dysfunction, including portal hypertension, in patients with underlying hepatitis B or C, cirrhosis and other underlying liver abnormalities.

Renal impairment: Renal clearance is only a minor elimination pathway, the principal route of metabolism and excretion for saquinavir being via the liver. Therefore, no initial dose adjustment is necessary for patients with renal impairment. However, patients with severe renal impairment have not been studied and caution should be exercised when prescribing saquinavir/ritonavir in this population.

Patients with chronic diarrhoea or malabsorption: No information on boosted saquinavir and only limited information on the safety and efficacy of unboosted saquinavir is available for patients suffering from chronic diarrhoea or malabsorption. It is unknown whether patients with such conditions could receive subtherapeutic saquinavir levels.

Children under the age of 16 and adults over 60 years: The experience with Invirase in children below the age of 16 and adults over 60 years is limited. In children, as in adults, Invirase should only be given in combination with ritonavir.

Lactose intolerance: Invirase 500 mg film-coated tablets contain lactose. Patients with rare hereditary problems of galactose intolerance, the Lapp lactase deficiency or glucose-galactose malabsorption should not take this medicine.

Patients with haemophilia: There have been reports of increased bleeding, including spontaneous skin haematomas and haemarthroses, in haemophiliac patients type A and B treated with protease inhibitors. In some patients additional factor VIII was given. In more than half of the reported cases, treatment with protease inhibitors was continued or reintroduced if treatment had been discontinued. A causal relationship has been evoked, although the mechanism of action has not been elucidated. Haemophiliac patients should therefore be made aware of the possibility of increased bleeding.

Diabetes mellitus and hyperglycaemia: New onset diabetes mellitus, hyperglycaemia or exacerbation of existing diabetes mellitus has been reported in patients receiving protease inhibitors. In some of these patients, the hyperglycaemia was severe and in some cases was also associated with ketoacidosis. Many patients had confounding medical conditions, some of which required therapy with agents that have been associated with the development of diabetes mellitus or hyperglycaemia.

Lipodystrophy: Combination antiretroviral therapy has been associated with the redistribution of body fat (lipodystrophy) in HIV infected patients. The long-term consequences of these events are currently unknown. Knowledge about the mechanism is incomplete. A connection between visceral lipomatosis and PIs and lipoatrophy and Nucleoside Reverse Transcriptase Inhibitors (NRTIs) has been hypothesised. A higher risk of lipodystrophy has been associated with individual factors such as older age, and with drug related factors such as longer duration of antiretroviral treatment and associated metabolic disturbances. Clinical examination should include evaluation for physical signs of fat redistribution. Consideration should be given to the measurement of fasting serum lipids and blood glucose. Lipid disorders should be managed as clinically appropriate (see section 4.8).

Osteonecrosis: Although the aetiology is considered to be multifactorial (including corticosteroid use, alcohol consumption, severe immunosuppression, higher body mass index), cases of osteonecrosis have been reported particularly in patients with advanced HIV–disease and/or long-term exposure to combination antiretroviral therapy (CART). Patients should be advised to seek medical advice if they experience joint aches and pain, joint stiffness or difficulty in movement.

Immune Reactivation Syndrome: In HIV-infected patients with severe immune deficiency at the time of institution of combination antiretroviral therapy (CART), an inflammatory reaction to asymptomatic or residual opportunistic pathogens may arise and cause serious clinical conditions, or aggravation of symptoms. Typically, such reactions have been observed within the first few weeks or months of initiation of CART. Relevant examples are cytomegalovirus retinitis, generalised and/or focal mycobacterial infections, and Pneumocystis carinii pneumonia. Any inflammatory symptoms should be evaluated and treatment instituted when necessary.

Interaction with ritonavir: The recommended dose of Invirase and ritonavir is 1000 mg Invirase plus 100 mg ritonavir twice daily. Higher doses of ritonavir have been shown to be associated with an increased incidence of adverse events. Co-administration of saquinavir and ritonavir has led to severe adverse events, mainly diabetic ketoacidosis and liver disorders, especially in patients with pre-existing liver disease.

Interaction with tipranavir: Concomitant use of boosted saquinavir and tipranavir, co-administered with low dose ritonavir in a dual-boosted regimen, results in a significant decrease in saquinavir plasma concentrations (see section 4.5). Therefore, the co-administration of boosted saquinavir and tipranavir, co-administered with low dose ritonavir, is not recommended.

Interaction with HMG-CoA reductase inhibitors: Caution must be exercised if Invirase/ritonavir is used concurrently with atorvastatin, which is metabolised to a lesser extent by CYP3A4. In this situation a reduced dose of atorvastatin should be considered. If treatment with a HMG-CoA reductase inhibitor is indicated, pravastatin or fluvastatin is recommended (see section 4.5).

Oral contraceptives: Because concentration of ethinyl estradiol may be decreased when co-administered with Invirase/ritonavir, alternative or additional contraceptive measures should be used when oestrogen-based oral contraceptives are co-administered (see section 4.5).

Glucocorticoids: Concomitant use of boosted saquinavir and fluticasone or other glucocorticoids that are metabolised by CYP3A4 is not recommended unless the potential benefit of treatment outweighs the risk of systemic corticosteroid effects, including Cushing's syndrome and adrenal suppression (see section 4.5).

Interaction with efavirenz: The combination of saquinavir and ritonavir with efavirenz has been shown to be associated with an increased risk of liver toxicity; liver function should be monitored when saquinavir and ritonavir are co-administered with efavirenz. No clinically significant alterations of either saquinavir or efavirenz concentration were noted in studies in healthy volunteers or in HIV-infected patients (see section 4.5).

4.5 Interaction with other medicinal products and other forms of interaction

Most drug interaction studies with saquinavir have been completed with unboosted Invirase or unboosted saquinavir soft capsules (Fortovase). A limited number of studies have been completed with ritonavir boosted Invirase or ritonavir boosted saquinavir soft capsules.

Observations from drug interaction studies done with unboosted saquinavir might not be representative of the effects seen with saquinavir/ritonavir therapy. Furthermore, results seen with saquinavir soft capsules may not predict the magnitude of these interactions with Invirase/ritonavir.

The metabolism of saquinavir is mediated by cytochrome P450, with the specific isoenzyme CYP3A4 responsible for 90 % of the hepatic metabolism. Additionally, *in vitro* studies have shown that saquinavir is a substrate and an inhibitor for P-glycoprotein (P-gp). Therefore, medicinal products that either share this metabolic pathway or modify CYP3A4 and/or P-gp activity (see "*Other potential interactions*") may modify the pharmacokinetics of saquinavir. Similarly, saquinavir might also modify the pharmacokinetics of other medicinal products that are substrates for CYP3A4 or P-gp.

Ritonavir can affect the pharmacokinetics of other medicinal products because it is a potent inhibitor of CYP3A4 and P-gp. Therefore, when saquinavir is co-administered with ritonavir, consideration should be given to the potential effects of ritonavir on other medicinal products (see the Summary of Product Characteristics for Norvir).

Table 1: Interactions and dose recommendations with other medicinal products

(see Table 1 on next page)

4.6 Pregnancy and lactation

Pregnancy: Evaluation of experimental animal studies does not indicate direct or indirect harmful effects with respect to the development of the embryo or foetus, the course of gestation and peri- and post-natal development. Clinical experience in pregnant women is limited: Congenital malformations, birth defects and other disorders (without a congenital malformation) have been reported rarely in pregnant women who had received saquinavir in combination with other antiretroviral agents. However, so far the available data are insufficient and do not identify specific risks for the unborn child. Saquinavir should be used during pregnancy only if the potential benefit justifies the potential risk to the foetus (see section 5.3).

Lactation: There are no laboratory animal or human data available on secretion of saquinavir in breast milk. The potential for adverse reactions to saquinavir in nursing infants cannot be assessed, and therefore, breast-feeding should be discontinued prior to receiving saquinavir. It is recommended that HIV-infected women do not breast feed their infants under any circumstances in order to avoid transmission of HIV.

4.7 Effects on ability to drive and use machines

Invirase may have a minor influence on the ability to drive and use machines. Dizziness and fatigue have been reported during treatment with Invirase. No studies on the effects on the ability to drive and use machines have been performed.

4.8 Undesirable effects

The following adverse events with an at least possible relationship to ritonavir boosted saquinavir (i.e. adverse reactions) were reported most frequently: nausea, diarrhoea, fatigue, vomiting, flatulence, and abdominal pain.

For comprehensive dose adjustment recommendations and drug-associated adverse reactions for ritonavir and other medicinal products used in combination with saquinavir, physicians should refer to the Summary of Product Characteristics for each of these medicinal products.

Within each frequency grouping, undesirable effects are presented in order of decreasing seriousness.

Adverse reactions from clinical trials where saquinavir was boosted with ritonavir

Limited data is available from two studies where the safety of saquinavir soft capsule (1000 mg twice daily) used in combination with low dose ritonavir (100 mg twice daily) for at least 48 weeks was studied in 311 patients. Adverse reactions in these two pivotal studies are summarised in Table 2. The list also includes marked laboratory abnormalities that have been observed with the saquinavir soft capsule in combination with ritonavir (at 48 weeks).

Table 2: Incidences of Adverse Reactions and marked laboratory abnormalities from the MaxCmin1 and MaxCmin2 study. (Very common (⩾ 10 %); common (⩾ 1 % and < 10 %))

Body System Frequency of Reaction	Adverse Reactions	
	Grades 3&4	All Grades
Blood and the lymphatic system disorders		
Common	Anaemia	Anaemia
Immune system disorders		
Common		Hypersensitivity
Metabolism and nutrition disorders		
Common	Diabetes mellitus	Diabetes mellitus, anorexia, increased appetite
Psychiatric disorders		
Common		Decreased libido, sleep disorder
Nervous System Disorders		
Common		Paraesthesia, peripheral neuropathy, dizziness, dysgeusia, headache
Respiratory, thoracic and mediastinal disorders		
Common		Dyspnoea
Gastrointestinal disorders		
Very common		Diarrhoea, nausea
Common	Diarrhoea, nausea, vomiting	Vomiting, abdominal distension, abdominal pain, upper abdominal pain, constipation, dry mouth, dyspepsia, eructation, flatulence, lip dry, loose stools
Skin and subcutaneous tissue disorders		
Common	Acquired lipodystrophy	Acquired lipodystrophy, alopecia, dry skin, eczema, lipoatrophy, pruritus, rash
Musculoskeletal and connective tissue disorders		
Common		Muscle spasms
General disorders and administration site conditions		
Common	Fatigue	Asthenia, fatigue, increased fat tissue, malaise
Investigations		
Very common		Increased alanine aminotransferase, increased aspartate aminotransferase, increased blood cholesterol, increased blood triglycerides, increased low density lipoprotein, decreased platelet count
Common		Increased blood amylase, increased blood bilirubin, increased blood creatinine, decreased haemoglobin, decreased lymphocyte count, decreased white blood cell count

Post-marketing experience with saquinavir

Serious and non-serious adverse reactions from post-marketing spontaneous reports (where saquinavir was taken as the sole protease inhibitor or in combination with ritonavir), not mentioned previously in section 4.8, for which a causal relationship to saquinavir cannot be excluded, are summarised below. As these data come from the spontaneous reporting system, the frequency of the adverse reactions is unknown.

• Immune system disorders: Hypersensitivity.

• Metabolism and nutrition disorders:

- Diabetes mellitus or hyperglycaemia sometimes associated with ketoacidosis (see section 4.4).

- Lipodystrophy: Combination antiretroviral therapy has been associated with redistribution of body fat (lipodystrophy) in HIV infected patients including the loss of peripheral and facial subcutaneous fat, increased intra-abdominal and visceral fat, breast hypertrophy and dorsicervical fat accumulation (buffalo hump).

- Combination antiretroviral therapy has been associated with metabolic abnormalities such as hypertriglyceridaemia, hypercholesterolaemia, insulin resistance, hyperglycaemia and hyperlactataemia (see section 4.4).

• Nervous system disorders: Somnolence, convulsions.

• Vascular disorders: There have been reports of increased bleeding, including spontaneous skin haematomas and haemarthroses, in haemophilic patients type A and B treated with protease inhibitors (see section 4.4).

• Hepato-biliary disorders: Hepatitis.

• Musculoskeletal, connective tissue and bone disorders: Increased CPK, myalgia, myositis and rarely, rhabdomyolysis have been reported with protease inhibitors, particularly in combination with nucleoside analogues. Cases of osteonecrosis have been reported, particularly in patients with generally acknowledged risk factors, advanced HIV disease or long-term exposure to combination antiretroviral therapy (CART). The frequency of this is unknown (see section 4.4).

Table 1: Interactions and dose recommendations with other medicinal products

Medicinal product by therapeutic area (dose of Invirase used in study)	Interaction	Recommendations concerning co-administration
Antiretroviral agents ***Nucleoside reverse transcriptase inhibitors (NRTIs)***		
- Zalcitabine and/or Zidovudine (saquinavir/ritonavir)	- No pharmacokinetic interaction studies have been completed. Interaction with zalcitabine is unlikely due to different routes of metabolism and excretion. For zidovudine (200 mg every 8 hours) a 25 % decrease in AUC was reported when combined with ritonavir (300 mg every 6 hours). The pharmacokinetics of ritonavir remained unchanged.	- No dose adjustment required.
- Zalcitabine and/or Zidovudine (unboosted saquinavir)	- Saquinavir ↔ Zalcitabine ↔ Zidovudine ↔	
Didanosine 400 mg single dose (saquinavir/ritonavir 1600/100 mg qd)	Saquinavir AUC ↓ 30% Saquinavir C_{max}↓ 25% Saquinavir C_{min} ↔	No dose adjustment required.
Tenofovir disoproxil fumarate 300 mg qd (saquinavir/ritonavir 1000/100 mg bid)	Saquinavir AUC ↓ 1% Saquinavir C_{max}↓ 7% Saquinavir C_{min} ↔	No dose adjustment required.
Non-nucleoside reverse transcriptase inhibitors (NNRTIs)		
- Delavirdine (saquinavir/ritonavir)	- Interaction with Invirase/ritonavir not studied.	
- Delavirdine (unboosted saquinavir)	- Saquinavir AUC ↑ 348%. There are limited safety and no efficacy data available from the use of this combination. In a small, preliminary study, hepatocellular enzyme elevations occurred in 13 % of subjects during the first several weeks of the delavirdine and saquinavir combination (6 % Grade 3 or 4).	- Hepatocellular changes should be monitored frequently if this combination is prescribed.
Efavirenz 600 mg qd (saquinavir/ritonavir 1600/200 mg qd, *or* saquinavir/ritonavir 1000/100 mg bid, *or* saquinavir/ritonavir 1200/100 mg qd)	Saquinavir ↔ Efavirenz ↔	No dose adjustment required.
- Nevirapine (saquinavir/ritonavir)	- Interaction with Invirase/ritonavir not studied.	
- Nevirapine (unboosted saquinavir)	- Saquinavir AUC ↓ 24% Nevirapine AUC ↔	- No dose adjustment required.
HIV protease inhibitors (PIs)		
Atazanavir 300 mg qd (saquinavir/ritonavir 1600/100 mg qd)	Saquinavir AUC ↑ 60% Saquinavir C_{max} ↑ 42% Ritonavir AUC ↑ 41% Ritonavir C_{max} ↑ 34% Atazanavir ↔ No clinical data available for the combination of saquinavir/ritonavir 1000/100 mg bid and atazanavir.	
Fosamprenavir 700 mg bid (saquinavir/ritonavir 1000/100 mg bid)	Saquinavir AUC ↓ 15% Saquinavir C_{max}↓ 9% Saquinavir C_{min}↓ 24% (remained above the target threshold for effective therapy.)	No dose adjustment required for Invirase/ritonavir.
- Indinavir (saquinavir/ritonavir)	- Low dose ritonavir increases the concentration of indinavir.	Increased concentrations of indinavir may result in nephrolithiasis.
- Indinavir 800 mg tid (saquinavir 600-1200 mg single dose)	- Saquinavir AUC ↑ 4.6-7.2 fold Indinavir ↔ No safety and efficacy data available for this combination. Appropriate doses of combination not established.	
Lopinavir/ritonavir 400/100 mg bid (saquinavir/ritonavir 1000/100 mg bid in combination with 2 or 3 NRTIs)	Saquinavir ↔ Ritonavir ↓ (effectiveness as boosting agent not modified). Lopinavir ↔ (based on historical comparison with unboosted lopinavir)	No dose adjustment required.
- Nelfinavir (saquinavir/ritonavir)	- Interaction with Invirase/ritonavir not studied.	
- Nelfinavir 1250 mg bid (saquinavir/ritonavir 1000/100 mg bid)	- Saquinavir AUC ↑ 13% (90% CI: 27 ↓ - 74 ↑) Saquinavir C_{max} ↑ 9% (90% CI: 27 ↓ - 61 ↑) Nelfinavir AUC ↓ 6% (90% CI: 28 ↓ - 22 ↑) Nelfinavir C_{max} ↓ 5% (90% CI: 23 ↓ - 16 ↑)	No dose adjustment required
- Nelfinavir 750 mg tid (unboosted saquinavir 1200 mg tid)	- Saquinavir AUC ↑ 392% Saquinavir C_{max} ↑ 179% Nelfinavir AUC ↑ 18% Nelfinavir C_{max}↔	- Quadruple therapy, including saquinavir soft capsules and nelfinavir in addition to two nucleoside reverse transcriptase inhibitors gave a more durable response (prolongation of time to virological relapse) than triple therapy with either single protease inhibitor. Concomitant administration of nelfinavir and saquinavir soft capsules resulted in a moderate increase in the incidence of diarrhoea.
Ritonavir 100 mg bid (saquinavir 1000 mg bid)	Saquinavir ↑ Ritonavir ↔ In HIV-infected patients, Invirase or saquinavir soft capsules in combination with ritonavir at doses of 1000/100 mg twice daily provide a systemic exposure of saquinavir over a 24 hour period similar to or greater than that achieved with saquinavir soft capsules 1200 mg three times daily (see section 5.2).	This is the approved combination regimen. No dose adjustment is recommended.
Tipranavir/ritonavir (saquinavir/ritonavir)	Saquinavir C_{min}↓ 78% Dual-boosted protease inhibitor combination therapy in multiple-treatment experienced HIV-positive adults.	Concomitant administration of tipranavir, co-administered with low dose ritonavir, with saquinavir/ritonavir, is not recommended. If the combination is considered necessary, monitoring of the saquinavir plasma levels is strongly encouraged.

Medicinal product by therapeutic area (dose of Invirase used in study)	Interaction	Recommendations concerning co-administration
HIV fusion inhibitor		
Enfuvirtide (saquinavir/ritonavir 1000/100 mg bid)	Saquinavir ↔ Enfuvirtide ↔ No clinically significant interaction was noted.	No dose adjustment required.
Other medicinal products ***Antiarrhythmics***		
Bepridil Lidocaine (systemic) Quinidine (saquinavir/ritonavir)	Concentrations of bepridil, systemic lidocaine or quinidine may be increased when co-administered with Invirase/ritonavir.	Caution is warranted. Therapeutic concentration monitoring is recommended, if available.
Amiodarone Flecainide Propafenone (saquinavir/ritonavir)	Concentrations of amiodarone, flecainide or propafenone may be increased when co-administered with Invirase/ritonavir.	Contraindicated in combination with saquinavir/ritonavir due to potentially life threatening cardiac arrhythmia (see section 4.3).
Anticoagulant		
Warfarin (saquinavir/ritonavir)	Concentrations of warfarin may be affected.	INR (international normalised ratio) monitoring recommended.
Anticonvulsants		
- Carbamazepine Phenobarbital Phenytoin (saquinavir/ritonavir)	- Interaction with Invirase/ritonavir not studied.	
- Carbamazepine Phenobarbital Phenytoin (unboosted saquinavir)	- These medicinal products will induce CYP3A4 and may therefore decrease saquinavir concentrations.	
Antidepressants		
Tricyclic antidepressants (e.g. amitriptyline, imipramine) (saquinavir/ritonavir)	Invirase/ritonavir may increase concentrations of tricyclic antidepressants.	Therapeutic concentration monitoring recommended.
- Nefazodone (saquinavir/ritonavir)	- Interaction with saquinavir/ritonavir not evaluated.	
- Nefazodone (unboosted saquinavir)	- Nefazodone inhibits CYP3A4. Saquinavir concentrations may be increased.	- Monitoring for saquinavir toxicity recommended.
Antihistamines		
Terfenadine Astemizole (saquinavir/ritonavir)	Terfenadine AUC ↑, associated with a prolongation of QTc intervals. A similar interaction with astemizole is likely.	Terfenadine and astemizole are contraindicated with boosted or unboosted saquinavir (see section 4.3).
Anti-infectives		
- Clarithromycin (saquinavir/ritonavir)	- Interaction with Invirase/ritonavir not studied.	
- Clarithromycin 500 mg bid (unboosted saquinavir 1200 mg tid)	- Saquinavir AUC ↑ 177 % Saquinavir C_{max} ↑ 187 % Clarithromycin AUC ↑ 40 % Clarithromycin C_{max} ↑ 40 %	- No dose adjustment is required when co-administered for a limited time at the doses studied.
- Erythromycin (saquinavir/ritonavir)	- Interaction with Invirase/ritonavir not studied.	
- Erythromycin 250 mg qid (unboosted saquinavir 1200 mg tid)	- Saquinavir AUC ↑ 99 % Saquinavir C_{max} ↑ 106 %	- No dose adjustment required.
- Streptogramin antibiotics (saquinavir/ritonavir)	- Interaction with Invirase/ritonavir not studied.	
- Streptogramin antibiotics (unboosted saquinavir)	- Streptogramin antibiotics such as quinupristin/dalfopristin inhibit CYP3A4. Saquinavir concentrations may be increased.	- Monitoring for saquinavir toxicity recommended.
Antifungals		
Ketoconazole 200 mg qd (saquinavir/ritonavir 1000/100 mg bid)	Saquinavir AUC ↔ Saquinavir C_{max} ↔ Ritonavir AUC ↔ Ritonavir C_{max} ↔ Ketoconazole AUC ↑ 168% (90% CI 146%-193%) Ketoconazole C_{max} ↑ 45% (90% CI 32%-59%)	No dose adjustment required when saquinavir/ritonavir combined with ≤ 200 mg/day ketoconazole. High doses of ketoconazole (> 200 mg/day) are not recommended.
- Itraconazole (saquinavir/ritonavir)	- Interaction with Invirase/ritonavir not studied.	
- Itraconazole (unboosted saquinavir)	- Itraconazole is a moderately potent inhibitor of CYP3A4. An interaction is possible.	Monitoring for saquinavir toxicity recommended.
Fluconazole/miconazole (saquinavir/ritonavir)	Interaction with Invirase/ritonavir not studied.	
Antimycobacterials		
Rifampicin 600 mg qd (saquinavir/ritonavir 1000/100 mg bid)	In a clinical study 11 of 17 (65 %) healthy volunteers developed severe hepatocellular toxicity with transaminase elevations up to > 20-fold the upper limit of normal after 1 to 5 days of co-administration.	Rifampicin is contraindicated in combination with Invirase/ritonavir (see section 4.3).
Rifabutin (saquinavir/ritonavir 1000/100 mg bid)	Interaction with saquinavir/ritonavir 1000/100 mg not studied.	A dosage reduction to rifabutin 150 mg every three days is recommended based on experience with low dose ritonavir boosted protease inhibitors. Patients receiving rifabutin with Invirase/ritonavir should be closely monitored for liver function test elevations and emergence of adverse events associated with rifabutin therapy. Further dosage reduction of rifabutin may be necessary. Therapeutic concentration monitoring for saquinavir is recommended.

Medicinal product by therapeutic area (dose of Invirase used in study)	Interaction	Recommendations concerning co-administration
Benzodiazepines		
Midazolam 7.5 mg single dose (oral) (saquinavir/ritonavir 1000/100 mg bid)	Midazolam AUC ↑ 12.4 fold Midazolam C_{max} ↑ 4.3 fold Midazolam $t_{1/2}$ ↑ from 4.7 h to 14.9 h No data are available on concomitant use of ritonavir boosted saquinavir with intravenous midazolam. Studies of other CYP3A modulators and i.v. midazolam suggest a possible 3-4 fold increase in midazolam plasma levels.	Co-administration of Invirase/ritonavir with orally administered midazolam is contraindicated (see section 4.3). Caution should be used with co-administration of Invirase and parenteral midazolam. If Invirase is co-administered with parenteral midazolam it should be done in an intensive care unit (ICU) or similar setting which ensures close clinical monitoring and appropriate medical management in case of respiratory depression and/or prolonged sedation. Dosage adjustment should be considered, especially if more than a single dose of midazolam is administered.
Alprazolam Clorazepate Diazepam Flurazepam (saquinavir/ritonavir)	Concentrations of these medicinal products may be increased when co-administered with Invirase/ritonavir.	Careful monitoring of patients with regard to sedative effects is warranted. A decrease in the dose of the benzodiazepine may be required.
Triazolam (saquinavir/ritonavir)	Concentrations of triazolam may be increased when co-administered with Invirase/ritonavir.	Contraindicated in combination with saquinavir/ritonavir, due to the risk of potentially prolonged or increased sedation and respiratory depression (see section 4.3).
Calcium channel blockers		
Felodipine, nifedipine, nicardipine, diltiazem, nimodipine, verapamil, amlodipine, nisoldipine, isradipine (saquinavir/ritonavir)	Concentrations of these medicinal products may be increased when co-administered with Invirase/ritonavir.	Caution is warranted and clinical monitoring of patients is recommended.
Corticosteroids		
- Dexamethasone (saquinavir/ritonavir)	- Interaction with Invirase/ritonavir not studied.	
- Dexamethasone (unboosted saquinavir)	- Dexamethasone induces CYP3A4 and may decrease saquinavir concentrations.	- Use with caution. Saquinavir may be less effective in patients taking dexamethasone.
Fluticasone propionate 50 mcg qid, intranasal (ritonavir 100 mg bid)	Fluticasone propionate ↑ Intrinsic cortisol ↓ 86% (90% CI 82%-89%) Greater effects may be expected when fluticasone propionate is inhaled. Systemic corticosteroid effects including Cushing's syndrome and adrenal suppression have been reported in patients receiving ritonavir and inhaled or intranasally administered fluticasone propionate; this could also occur with other corticosteroids metabolised via the P450 3A pathway e.g. budesonide. Effects of high fluticasone systemic exposure on ritonavir plasma levels yet unknown.	Concomitant administration of boosted saquinavir and fluticasone propionate and other corticosteroids metabolised via the P450 3A pathway (e.g. budesonide) is not recommended unless the potential benefit of treatment outweighs the risk of systemic corticosteroid effects (see section 4.4). Dose reduction of the glucocorticoid should be considered with close monitoring of local and systemic effects or a switch to a glucocorticoid, which is not a substrate for CYP3A4 (e.g. beclomethasone). In case of withdrawal of glucocorticoids progressive dose reduction may have to be performed over a longer period.
<u>Medicinal products that are substrates of P-glycoprotein</u> ***Digitalis glycosides***		
Digoxin 0.5 mg single dose (saquinavir/ritonavir 1000/100 mg bid)	Digoxin AUC_{0-72} ↑ 49% Digoxin C_{max} ↑ 27% Digoxin levels may differ over time. Large increments of digoxin may be expected when saquinavir/ritonavir is introduced in patients already treated with digoxin.	Caution should be exercised when Invirase/ritonavir and digoxin are co-administered. The serum concentration of digoxin should be monitored and a dose reduction of digoxin should be considered if necessary.
Histamine H_2-receptor antagonist		
- Ranitidine (saquinavir/ritonavir)	- Interaction with Invirase/ritonavir not studied.	
- Ranitidine (unboosted saquinavir)	- Saquinavir AUC ↑ 67 %	- Increase not thought to be clinically relevant. No dose adjustment of saquinavir recommended.
HMG-CoA reductase inhibitors		
Pravastatin Fluvastatin (saquinavir/ritonavir)	Interaction not studied. Metabolism of pravastatin and fluvastatin is not dependent on CYP3A4. Interaction via effects on transport proteins cannot be excluded.	Interaction unknown. If no alternative treatment is available, use with careful monitoring.
Simvastatin Lovastatin (saquinavir/ritonavir)	Simvastatin ↑↑ Lovastatin ↑↑ Plasma concentrations highly dependent on CYP3A4 metabolism.	Increased concentrations of simvastatin and lovastatin have been associated with rhabdomyolysis. These medicinal products are contraindicated for use with Invirase/ritonavir (see section 4.3).
Atorvastatin (saquinavir/ritonavir)	Atorvastatin is less dependent on CYP3A4 for metabolism.	When used with Invirase/ritonavir, the lowest possible dose of atorvastatin should be administered and the patient should be carefully monitored for signs/symptoms of myopathy (muscle weakness, muscle pain, rising plasma creatinine kinase).
Immunosuppressants		
Ciclosporin Tacrolimus Rapamycin (saquinavir/ritonavir)	Concentrations of these medicinal products increase several fold when co-administered with Invirase/ritonavir.	Careful therapeutic drug monitoring is necessary for immunosuppressants when co-administered with Invirase/ritonavir.
Narcotic analgesics		
Methadone 60-120 mg qd (saquinavir/ritonavir 1000/100 mg bid)	Methadone AUC ↓ 19 % (90 % CI 9 % to 29 %) None of the 12 patients experienced withdrawal symptoms.	No dosage adjustment required.
Neuroleptics		
Pimozide (saquinavir/ritonavir)	Concentrations of pimozide may be increased when co-administered with Invirase/ritonavir.	Due to a potential for life threatening cardiac arrhythmias, Invirase/ritonavir is contra-indicated in combination with pimozide (see section 4.3).

Medicinal product by therapeutic area (dose of Invirase used in study)	Interaction	Recommendations concerning co-administration
Oral contraceptives		
Ethinyl estradiol (saquinavir/ritonavir)	Concentration of ethinyl estradiol may be decreased when co-administered with Invirase/ritonavir.	Alternative or additional contraceptive measures should be used when oestrogen-based oral contraceptives are co-administered.
Phosphodiesterase type 5 (PDE5) inhibitors		
- Sildenafil (saquinavir/ritonavir)	- Interaction with Invirase/ritonavir not studied.	
- Sildenafil 100 mg (single dose) (unboosted saquinavir 1200 mg tid)	- Saquinavir ↔ Sildenafil C_{max} ↑ 140 % Sildenafil AUC ↑ 210 % - Sildenafil is a substrate of CYP3A4.	- Use sildenafil with caution at reduced doses of no more than 25 mg every 48 hours with increased monitoring of adverse events when administered concomitantly with Invirase/ritonavir.
Vardenafil (saquinavir/ritonavir)	Concentrations of vardenafil may be increased when co-administered with Invirase/ritonavir.	Use vardenafil with caution at reduced doses of no more than 2.5 mg every 72 hours with increased monitoring of adverse events when administered concomitantly with Invirase/ritonavir.
Tadalafil (saquinavir/ritonavir)	Concentrations of tadalafil may be increased when co-administered with Invirase/ritonavir.	Use tadalafil with caution at reduced doses of no more than 10 mg every 72 hours with increased monitoring of adverse events when administered concomitantly with Invirase/ritonavir.
Proton pump inhibitors		
Omeprazole 40 mg qd (saquinavir/ritonavir 1000/100 mg bid)	Saquinavir AUC ↑ 82% (90 % CI 44-131 %) Saquinavir C_{max} ↑ 75% (90 % CI 38-123 %) Ritonavir ↔	Monitoring for potential saquinavir toxicities is recommended.
Other proton pump inhibitors (saquinavir/ritonavir 1000/100 mg bid)	No data are available on the concomitant administration of Invirase/ritonavir and other proton pump inhibitors.	If omeprazole or other proton pump inhibitors are taken concomitantly with Invirase/ritonavir, monitoring for potential saquinavir toxicities is recommended.
Others		
Ergot alkaloids (e.g. ergotamine, dihydroergotamine, ergonovine, and methylergonovine) (saquinavir/ritonavir)	Invirase/ritonavir may increase ergot alkaloids exposure, and consequently, increase the potential for acute ergot toxicity.	The concomitant use of Invirase/ritonavir and ergot alkaloids is contra-indicated (see section 4.3).
- Grapefruit juice (saquinavir/ritonavir)	- Interaction with Invirase/ritonavir not studied.	
- Grapefruit juice (single dose) (unboosted saquinavir)	- Saquinavir ↑ 50% (normal strength grapefruit juice) - Saquinavir ↑ 100% (double strength grapefruit juice)	- Increase not thought to be clinically relevant. No dose adjustment required.
- Garlic capsules (saquinavir/ritonavir)	- Interaction with Invirase/ritonavir not studied.	
- Garlic capsules (dose approx. equivalent to two 4 g cloves of garlic daily) (unboosted saquinavir 1200 mg tid)	- Saquinavir AUC ↓ 51 % Saquinavir C_{trough}↓ 49 % (8 hours post dose) Saquinavir C_{max}↓ 54 %.	- Patients on saquinavir treatment must not take garlic capsules due to the risk of decreased plasma concentrations and loss of virological response and possible resistance to one or more components of the antiretroviral regimen.
- St. John's wort (saquinavir/ritonavir)	- Interaction with Invirase/ritonavir not studied.	
- St. John's wort (unboosted saquinavir)	- Plasma levels of saquinavir can be reduced by concomitant use of the herbal preparation St. John's wort *(Hypericum perforatum)*. This is due to induction of drug metabolising enzymes and/or transport proteins by St. John's wort.	- Herbal preparations containing St. John's wort must not be used concomitantly with Invirase. If a patient is already taking St. John's wort, stop St. John's wort, check viral levels and if possible saquinavir levels. Saquinavir levels may increase on stopping St. John's wort, and the dose of saquinavir may need adjusting. The inducing effect of St. John's wort may persist for at least 2 weeks after cessation of treatment.
Other potential interactions ***Medicinal products that are substrates of CYP3A4***		
e.g. dapsone, disopyramide, quinine, fentanyl, and alfentanyl (unboosted saquinavir)	Although specific studies have not been performed, co-administration of Invirase/ritonavir with medicinal products that are mainly metabolised by CYP3A4 pathway may result in elevated plasma concentrations of these medicinal products.	These combinations should be given with caution.
Medicinal products reducing gastrointestinal transit time		
Metoclopramide	It is unknown whether medicinal products which reduce the gastrointestinal transit time could lead to lower saquinavir plasma concentrations.	

Key: ↓ reduced, ↑ increased, ↔ unchanged, ↑ ↑ markedly increased

- Renal and urinary disorders: Renal impairment.
- In HIV-infected patients with severe immune deficiency at the time of initiation of combination antiretroviral therapy (CART), an inflammatory reaction to asymptomatic or residual opportunistic infections may arise (see section 4.4).

4.9 Overdose

There is limited experience of overdose with saquinavir. Whereas acute or chronic overdose of saquinavir alone did not result in major complications, in combination with other protease inhibitors, overdose symptoms and signs such as general weakness, fatigue, diarrhoea, nausea, vomiting, hair loss, dry mouth, hyponatraemia, weight loss and orthostatic hypotension have been observed. There is no specific antidote for overdose with saquinavir. Treatment of overdose with saquinavir should consist of general supportive measures, including monitoring of vital signs and ECG, and observations of the patient's clinical status. If indicated, prevention of further absorption can be considered. Since saquinavir is highly protein bound, dialysis is unlikely to be beneficial in significant removal of the active substance.

5. PHARMACOLOGICAL PROPERTIES

5.1 Pharmacodynamic properties

Pharmaco-therapeutic group: Antiviral agent, ATC code J05A E01

Mechanism of action: The HIV protease is an essential viral enzyme required for the specific cleavage of viral gag and gag-pol polyproteins. Saquinavir selectively inhibits the HIV protease, thereby preventing the creation of mature infectious virus particles.

Antiviral activity in vitro: Saquinavir demonstrates antiviral activity against a panel of laboratory strains and clinical isolates of HIV-1 with typical EC_{50} and EC_{90} values in the range 1-10 nM and 5-50 nM, respectively, with no apparent difference between subtype B and non-B clades. The corresponding serum (50% human serum) adjusted EC_{50} ranged from 25-250 nM. Clinical isolates of HIV-2 demonstrated EC_{50} values in the range of 0.3-2.4 nM.

Resistance

Antiviral activity according to baseline genotype and phenotype:

Genotypic and phenotypic clinical cut-offs predicting the clinical efficacy of ritonavir boosted saquinavir have been derived from retrospective analyses of the RESIST 1 and 2

Table 3: Virological response to saquinavir/ritonavir stratified by the number of baseline saquinavir-associated resistance mutations

Number of Saquinavir Associated Resistance Mutations at Baseline*	Marcelin et al (2007)		RESIST 1 & 2	
	SQV Naive Population		SQV Naive/Experienced Population	
	N=138	Change in Baseline Plasma HIV-1 RNA at Weeks 12-20	N=114	Change in Baseline Plasma HIV-1 RNA at Week 4
0	35	-2.24	2	-2.04
1	29	-1.88	3	-1.69
2	24	-1.43	14	-1.57
3	30	-0.52	28	-1.41
4	9	-0.18	40	-0.75
5	6	-0.11	17	-0.44
6	5	-0.30	9	0.08
7	0	-	1	0.24

* Saquinavir Mutation Score Mutations: L10F/I/M/R/V, I15A/V, K20I/M/R/T, L24I, I62V, G73S/T, V82A/F/S/T, I84V, L90M

Table 4: Subject Demographics MaxCmin1 and MaxCmin2[†]

	MaxCmin1		MaxCmin2	
	SQV/r	IDV/r	SQV/r	LPV/r
	N=148	N=158	N=161	N=163
Sex Male	82%	74%	81%	76%
Race (White/Black/Asian) %	86/9/1	82/12/4	75/19/1	74/19/2
Age, median, yrs	39	40	40	40
CDC Category C (%)	32%	28%	32%	31%
Antiretroviral naïve (%)	28%	22%	31%	34%
PI naïve (%)	41%	38%	48%	48%
Median Baseline HIV-1 RNA, log_{10} copies/ml (IQR)	4.0 (1.7-5.1)	3.9 (1.7-5.2)	4.4 (3.1-5.1)	4.6 (3.5-5.3)
Median Baseline CD4[+] Cell Count, cells/mm^3 (IQR)	272 (135-420)	280 (139-453)	241 (86-400)	239 (95-420)

[†]data from clinical study report

Table 5: Outcomes at Week 48 MaxCmin1 and MaxCmin2[†]

Outcomes	MaxCmin1		MaxCmin2	
	SQV/r	IDV/r	SQV/r	LPV/r
Initiated assigned treatment, n (%)	148 (94%)	158 (99%)	161 (94%)	163 (98%)
Discontinued assigned treatment, n (%)	40 (27%)	64 (41%)	48 (30%)	23 (14%)
	P=0.01		P=0.001	
Virological failure ITT/e*[#]	36/148 (24%)	41/158 (26%)	53/161 (33%)	29/163 (18%)
	P=0.76		P=0.002	
Proportion with VL < 50 copies/ml at week 48, ITT/e[#]	97/144 (67%)	106/154 (69%)	90/158 (57%)	106/162 (65%)
	P>0.05[‡]		P=0.12	
Proportion with VL < 50 copies/ml at week 48, On Treatment	82/104 (79%)	73/93 (78%)	84/113 (74%)	97/138 (70%)
	P >0.05[‡]		P=0.48	
Median increase in CD4 cell count at week 48 (cells/mm^3)	85	73	110	106

* For both studies: For patients entering study with VL < 200 copies/ml, VF defined as ≥ 200 copies/ml. MaxCmin1: For those entering with VL ≥ 200 copies/ml, VF defined as any increase ≥ 0.5 logs and/or VL ≥ 50,000 copies/ml at week 4, ≥ 5,000 copies/ml at week 12, or ≥ 200 copies/ml at week 24 or thereafter. MaxCmin2: any rise ≥ 0.5 log at a specific visit; ≤ 0.5 log reduction if VL ≥ 200 copies/ml at week 4; ≤ 1.0 log reduction from base line if VL ≥ 200 copies/ml at week 12; and a VL ≥ 200 copies/ml at week 24.

[#] ITT/e = Intent-to-treat/exposed

[†]Data from clinical study report

[‡]Data fromMaxCmin1 publication

clinical studies and analysis of a large hospital cohort (Marcelin et al 2007).

Baseline saquinavir phenotype (shift in susceptibility relative to reference, PhenoSense Assay) was shown to be a predictive factor of virological outcome. Virological response was first observed to decrease when the fold shift exceeded 2.3-fold; whereas virological benefit was not observed when the fold shift exceeded 12-fold.

Marcelin et al (2007) identified nine protease codons (L10F/I/M/R/V, I15A/V, K20I/M/R/T, L24I, I62V, G73S/T, V82A/F/S/T, I84V, L90M) that were associated with decreased virological response to saquinavir/ritonavir (1000/100 mg twice daily) in 138 saquinavir naive patients. The presence of 3 or more mutations was associated with reduced response to saquinavir/ritonavir.The association between the number of these saquinavir-associated resistance mutations and virological response was confirmed in an independent clinical study (RESIST 1 and 2) involving a more heavily treatment experienced patient population, including 54% who had received prior saquinavir (p=0.0133, see Table 3). The G48V mutation, previously identified in vitro as a saquinavir signature mutation, was present at baseline in virus from three patients, none of whom responded to therapy.

Table 3: Virological response to saquinavir/ritonavir stratified by the number of baseline saquinavir-associated resistance mutations

(see Table 3 opposite)

Clinical results from studies with treatment naïve and experienced patients

In the MaxCmin1 study, the safety and efficacy of saquinavir soft capsules/ritonavir 1000/100 mg twice daily plus 2 NRTIs/Non-Nucleoside Reverse Transcriptase Inhibitors (NNRTIs) was compared to indinavir/ritonavir 800/100 mg twice daily plus 2 NRTIs/NNRTIs in over 300 (both protease inhibitor treatment naïve and experienced) subjects. The combination of saquinavir and ritonavir exhibited a superior virological activity compared with the indinavir and ritonavir arm when switch from the assigned treatment was counted as virological failure.

In the MaxCmin2 study, the safety and efficacy of saquinavir soft capsules/ritonavir 1000/100 mg twice daily plus 2 NRTIs/NNRTIs was compared with lopinavir/ritonavir 400/100 mg twice daily plus 2 NRTIs/NNRTIs in 324 (both protease inhibitor treatment naïve and experienced) subjects. None of the subjects in the lopinavir/ritonavir arm had been exposed to lopinavir prior to randomisation whereas 16 of the subjects in the saquinavir/ritonavir arm had previously been exposed to saquinavir.

Table 4: Subject Demographics MaxCmin1 and MaxCmin2[†]

(see Table 4 opposite)

Table 5: Outcomes at Week 48 MaxCmin1 and MaxCmin2[†]

(see Table 5 below)

5.2 Pharmacokinetic properties

Saquinavir is essentially completely metabolised by CYP3A4. Ritonavir inhibits the metabolism of saquinavir, thereby increasing ("boosting") the plasma levels of saquinavir.

Absorption and bioavailability in adults: In HIV-infected patients, Invirase in combination with ritonavir at doses of 1000/100 mg twice daily provides saquinavir systemic exposures over a 24-hour period similar to or greater than those achieved with saquinavir soft capsules 1200 mg tid (see Table 6). The pharmacokinetics of saquinavir is stable during long-term treatment.

Table 6: Mean (% CV) AUC, C_{max} and C_{min} of saquinavir in patients following multiple dosing of Invirase, saquinavir soft capsules, Invirase/ritonavir, and saquinavir soft capsules/ritonavir

(see Table 6 on next page)

Absolute bioavailability averaged 4 % (CV 73 %, range: 1 % to 9 %) in 8 healthy volunteers who received a single 600 mg dose (3 × 200 mg hard capsule) of Invirase following a heavy breakfast. The low bioavailability is thought to be due to a combination of incomplete absorption and extensive first-pass metabolism. Gastric pH has been shown to be only a minor component in the large increase in bioavailability seen when given with food. The absolute bioavailability of saquinavir co-administered with ritonavir has not been established in humans.

In combination with ritonavir, bioequivalence of Invirase hard capsules and film-coated tablets was demonstrated under fed conditions.

Effective therapy in treatment naïve patients is associated with a C_{min} of approximately 50 ng/ml and an AUC_{0-24} of about 20,000 ng·h/ml. Effective therapy in treatment experienced patients is associated with a C_{min} of approximately 100 ng/ml and an AUC_{0-24} of about 20,000 ng·h/ml.

In vitro studies have shown that saquinavir is a substrate for P-glycoprotein (P-gp).

Effect of food: In a cross-over study in 22 HIV-infected patients treated with Invirase/ritonavir 1000 mg/100 mg twice daily and receiving three consecutive doses under fasting conditions or after a high-fat, high-calorie meal (46 g fat, 1,091 Kcal), the AUC_{0-12}, C_{max} and C_{trough} values of saquinavir under fasting conditions were about 70 per cent lower than with a high-fat meal. All but one of the patients achieved C_{trough} values of saquinavir above the therapeutic threshold (100 ng/ml) in the fasted state. There were no clinically significant differences in the pharmacokinetic profile of ritonavir in fasting and fed conditions but the ritonavir C_{trough} (geometric mean 245 vs. 348 ng/ml) was lower in the fasting state compared to the administration with a meal. Invirase/ritonavir should be administered with or after food.

Distribution in adults: Saquinavir partitions extensively into the tissues. The mean steady-state volume of distribution following intravenous administration of a 12 mg dose of saquinavir was 700 l (CV 39 %). It has been shown that saquinavir is approximately 97 % bound to plasma proteins up to 30 µg/ml. In two patients receiving Invirase 600 mg three times daily, cerebrospinal fluid concentrations of

Table 6: Mean (% CV) AUC, C_{max} and C_{min} of saquinavir in patients following multiple dosing of Invirase, saquinavir soft capsules, Invirase/ritonavir, and saquinavir soft capsules/ritonavir

Treatment	N	AUCτ (ng·h/ml)	AUC_{0-24} (ng·h/ml)†	C_{max} (ng/ml)	C_{min} (ng/ml)
Invirase (hard capsule) 600 mg tid	10	866 (62)	2,598	197 (75)	75 (82)
saquinavir soft capsule 1200 mg tid	31	7,249 (85)	21,747	2,181 (74)	216 (84)
Invirase (tablet) 1000 mg bid plus ritonavir 100 mg bid* (fasting condition)	22	10,320 (2,530-30,327)	20,640	1509 (355-4,101)	313 (70-1,725)††
Invirase (tablet) 1000 mg bid plus ritonavir 100 mg bid* (high fat meal)	22	34,926 (11,826-105,992)	69,852	5208 (1,536-14,369)	1,179 (334-5,176)††

τ = dosing interval, i.e. 8 hour for tid and 12 h for bid dosing.

C_{min} = the observed plasma concentration at the end of the dose interval.

bid = twice daily

tid = three times daily

* results are geometric mean (min - max)

†derived from tid or bid dosing schedule

††C_{trough} values

saquinavir were negligible when compared to concentrations from matching plasma samples.

Metabolism and elimination in adults: *In vitro* studies using human liver microsomes have shown that the metabolism of saquinavir is cytochrome P450 mediated with the specific isoenzyme, CYP3A4, responsible for more than 90 % of the hepatic metabolism. Based on *in vitro* studies, saquinavir is rapidly metabolised to a range of mono- and di-hydroxylated inactive compounds. In a mass balance study using 600 mg 14C-saquinavir (n = 8), 88 % and 1 % of the orally administered radioactivity, was recovered in faeces and urine, respectively, within 4 days of dosing. In an additional four subjects administered 10.5 mg 14C-saquinavir intravenously, 81 % and 3 % of the intravenously administered radioactivity was recovered in faeces and urine, respectively, within 4 days of dosing. 13 % of circulating saquinavir in plasma was present as unchanged compound after oral administration and the remainder as metabolites. Following intravenous administration 66 % of circulating saquinavir was present as unchanged compound and the remainder as metabolites, suggesting that saquinavir undergoes extensive first pass metabolism. *In vitro* experiments have shown that the hepatic metabolism of saquinavir becomes saturable at concentrations above 2 μg/ml.

Systemic clearance of saquinavir was high, 1.14 l/h/kg (CV 12 %), slightly above the hepatic plasma flow, and constant after intravenous doses of 6, 36 and 72 mg. The mean residence time of saquinavir was 7 hours (n = 8).

Special populations

Effect of gender following treatment with Invirase/ritonavir: A gender difference was observed with females showing higher saquinavir exposure than males (AUC on average 56 % higher and C_{max} on average 26 % higher) in the bioequivalence study comparing Invirase 500 mg film coated tablets with Invirase 200 mg hard capsules both in combination with ritonavir. There was no evidence that age and body-weight explained the gender difference in this study. Limited data from controlled clinical studies with the approved dosage regimen do not indicate a major difference in the efficacy and safety profile between men and women.

5.3 Preclinical safety data

Acute and chronic toxicity: Saquinavir was well tolerated in oral acute and chronic toxicity studies in mice, rats, dogs and marmosets.

Mutagenesis: Mutagenicity and genotoxicity studies, with and without metabolic activation where appropriate, have shown that saquinavir has no mutagenic activity *in vitro* in either bacterial (Ames test) or mammalian cells (Chinese hamster lung V79/HPRT test). Saquinavir does not induce chromosomal damage *in vivo* in the mouse micronucleus assay or *in vitro* in human peripheral blood lymphocytes and does not induce primary DNA damage *in vitro* in the unscheduled DNA synthesis test.

Carcinogenesis: There was no evidence of carcinogenic activity after the administration of saquinavir mesilate for 96 to 104 weeks to rats and mice. The plasma exposures (AUC values) in rats (maximum dose 1000 mg/kg/day) and in mice (maximum dose 2500 mg/kg/day) were lower than the expected plasma exposures obtained in humans at the recommended clinical dose of ritonavir boosted Invirase.

Reproductive toxicity: Fertility, peri- and postnatal development were not affected, and embryotoxic / teratogenic effects were not observed in rats or rabbits at plasma exposures lower than those achieved in humans at the recommended clinical dose of ritonavir boosted Invirase. Distribution studies in these species showed that the placental transfer of saquinavir is low (less than 5% of maternal plasma concentrations).

6. PHARMACEUTICAL PARTICULARS

6.1 List of excipients

Tablet core:

Microcrystalline cellulose,

Croscarmellose sodium,

Povidone,

Lactose (monohydrate),

Magnesium stearate.

Tablet coat:

Hypromellose,

Titanium dioxide (E 171),

Talc,

Glycerol triacetate,

Iron oxide yellow and red (E172).

6.2 Incompatibilities

Not applicable.

6.3 Shelf life

3 years.

6.4 Special precautions for storage

This medicinal product does not require any special storage conditions.

6.5 Nature and contents of container

Plastic bottles (HDPE) containing 120 tablets.

6.6 Special precautions for disposal and other handling

No special requirements.

7. MARKETING AUTHORISATION HOLDER

Roche Registration Limited

6 Falcon Way

Shire Park

Welwyn Garden City

AL7 1TW

United Kingdom

8. MARKETING AUTHORISATION NUMBER(S)

EU/1/96/026/002

9. DATE OF FIRST AUTHORISATION/RENEWAL OF THE AUTHORISATION

Date of first authorisation: 04 October 1996

Date of last renewal: 04 October 2006

10. DATE OF REVISION OF THE TEXT

27 January 2009

Detailed information on this product is available on the website of the European Medicines Agency (EMEA) http://www.emea.europa.eu/.

IOMERON 250

(Bracco UK Limited)

1. NAME OF THE MEDICINAL PRODUCT

Iomeron 250, solution for injection

2. QUALITATIVE AND QUANTITATIVE COMPOSITION

Contains 51.03% w/v of iomeprol equivalent to 25% iodine or 250mg iodine/ml.

For excipients, see 6.1.

3. PHARMACEUTICAL FORM

Solution for injection.

4. CLINICAL PARTICULARS

4.1 Therapeutic indications

X-ray contrast medium used for:

venography

cerebral arteriography

digital subtraction angiography

computed tomography enhancement

urography

cavernosography

myelography

4.2 Posology and method of administration

venography

adults	10 - 100ml* max 250ml 10 - 50ml upper extremity 50 - 100 lower extremity	

cerebral arteriography

adults	5 - 12ml*	
children	3 - 7ml or * *	

digital subtraction angiography

Intra arterial

visceral	adults	2 - 20ml per artery* aorta 25-50ml* both 250ml max
peripheral	adults	5 - 10ml per artery* max 250ml
intravenous	adults	30 - 60ml* max 250ml

computed tomography

brain	adults	50 - 150
	children	* *
body	adults	40 - 150ml max 250ml
	children	* *
urography intravenous	adults	50 - 150ml
	neonates	3 - 4.8ml/kg
	babies	2.5 - 4ml/kg
	children	1 - 2.5ml/kg or *
cavernosography	adults	40 - 250ml
myelography	adults	12 - 18ml by lumbar injection

* Repeat as necessary

* * According to body size and age

In elderly patients the lowest effective dose should be used.

In myelography, lower doses may be used for lumbar or thoracic studies and higher doses for cervical or total columnar studies. Regardless of the nature of the myelographic study, Iomeron should be injected slowly over 1-2 minutes.

The X ray can be taken up to 60 minutes following injection. Post myelographic CT of the spinal column should be delayed for approximately four hours to allow dilution and clearance of excessive contrast.

In patient with moderate to severe impairment of renal function, attention should be paid to renal function parameters before re-examining the patient with a contrast media.

4.3 Contraindications

Proven or suspected hypersensitivity to iodine containing preparations of this type.

Intrathecal concomitant administration of corticosteroids with contrast media is contraindicated.

4.4 Special warnings and precautions for use

A positive history of allergy, asthma or untoward reaction during previous similar investigations indicates a need for extra caution since, as with other contrast media, this product may provoke anaphylaxis or other manifestations of allergy with nausea, vomiting, dyspnoea, erythema, urticaria and hypotension. The benefits should clearly outweigh the risks in such patients and appropriate resuscitative measures should be immediately available. The primary treatments are as follows:

Effect	Major Symptoms	Primary Treatment
Vasomotor effect	warmth	reassurance
	nausea/vomiting	
Cutaneous	scattered hives	H_1-antihistamines
	severe urticaria	H_2 -antihistamines
Bronchospastic	wheezing	oxygen
		Beta-2-agonist inhalers
Anaphylactoid reaction	angioedema	oxygen
	urticaria	iv fluids

	bronchospasm	adrenergics (iv epinephrine)
	hypotension	Inhaled beta-2-adrenergics
		antihistamines (H_1-and H_2- blockers)
		corticosteroids
Hypotensive	hypotension	iv fluids
Vagal reaction	hypotension	iv fluids
	bradycardia	iv atropine

From: Bush WH; The Contrast Media Manual; Katzburg RW Ed.; Williams and Wilkins; Baltimore 1992; Chapter 2 p 23

In consideration of possible complications, the patient should be kept under observation for at least 60 minutes after the administration.

Extreme caution during injection of contrast media is necessary to avoid extravasation.

Special care is required when investigations are performed in patients with suspected thrombosis, phlebitis, severe ischemic disease, local infection or a totally obstructed artero-venous system.

Any severe disorders of water and electrolyte balance must be corrected prior to administration. Adequate hydration must be ensured particularly in patients with multiple myeloma, diabetes mellitus, polyuria, oliguria and hyperuricaemia; also in babies, small children and the elderly. Rehydration prior to use of iomeprol is recommended in patients with sickle cell disease.

Care should be taken in severe cardiac disease particularly heart failure and coronary artery disease. Reactions may include pulmonary oedema, haemodynamic changes, ischaemic ECG changes and arrhythmias. In severe, chronic hypertension the risk of renal damage following administration of a contrast medium is increased. In these cases the risks associated with the catheterization procedure are increased. Care should be taken in renal impairment and diabetes. In these patients it is important to maintain hydration in order to minimise deterioration in renal function.

A combination of severe hepatic and renal impairment delays excretion of the contrast medium therefore such patients should not be examined unless absolutely necessary.

The product should be used with caution in patients with hyperthyroidism or goitre. Use may interfere with thyroid function tests.

The administration of iodinated contrast media may aggravate myasthenia signs and symptoms.

Particular care is needed in patients with acute cerebral infarction, acute intracranial haemorrhage and any conditions involving damage to the blood brain barrier, brain oedema or acute demyelination. Convulsive seizures are more likely in patients with intracranial tumours or metastases or with a history of epilepsy.

Neurological symptoms related to cerebrovascular diseases, intracranial tumours/metastases or degenerative or inflammatory pathologies may be exacerbated.

There is an increased risk of transient neurological complications in patients with symptomatic cerebrovascular disease e.g. stroke, transient ischaemic attacks. Cerebral ischaemic phenomena may be caused by intravascular injection.

Treatment with drugs that lower the seizure threshold such as analgesics and anti-emetics of the phenotiazine class, and neuroleptics should be discontinued 48 hours before the examination. Treatment should not be resumed until 24 hours post-procedure.

In acute and chronic alcoholism the increase in blood brain barrier permeability facilitates the passage of the contrast medium into cerebral tissue possibly leading to CNS disorders. There is a possibility of a reduced seizure threshold in alcoholics.

In patients with a drug addiction there is also the possibility of a reduced seizure threshold.

Patients with phaeochromocytoma may develop severe, occasionally uncontrollable hypertensive crises during intravascular administration. Premedication with an alpha blocker is recommended in these patients. Pronounced excitement, anxiety and pain can cause side effects or intensify reaction to the contrast medium. A sedative may be given.

Since, on rare occasions, delayed reactions can occur, driving or operating machinery is not advisable for the first 24 hours after the procedure.

Anticonvulsant therapy should not be discontinued. A normal diet should be maintained until the patient refrains from eating 2 hours before the procedure.

Non ionic contrast media have less antiocoagulant activity in vitro than ionic media. Meticulous attention should therefore be paid to angiographic technique. Non ionic media should not be allowed to remain in contact with blood in a syringe, and intravascular catheters should be flushed frequently to minimise the risk of clotting which, rarely, has led to serious thromboembolic complications.

In patients with moderate to severe impairment of renal function, attention should be paid to renal function parameters before re-examining the patient with a contrast media.

In diabetic patients with diabetic nephropathy, metformin should be stopped at the time of, or prior to the procedure and withheld for 48 hours subsequent to the procedure and re-instituted only after renal function has been re-evaluated and found to be normal (see section 4.5 - Interaction with other medicaments and other forms of interaction).

Intravascular administration should be performed if possible with the patient lying down. The patient should be kept in this position and closely observed for at least 30 minutes after the procedure since the majority of severe incidents occur within this time.

Following intrathecal use, the patient should rest with the head and the chest elevated for 1 hour and be kept well hydrated. Thereafter, he/she may ambulate carefully, but bending down must be avoided. If remaining in bed, the head and chest should be kept elevated for 6 hours. Patients, suspected of having a lower seizure threshold should be observed during this period.

Children: Infants up to 1 year, especially the new-born, are particularly susceptible to electrolyte imbalance and haemodynamic alterations. Care should be taken regarding the dosage used.

Elderly: There is special risk of reactions involving the circulatory system such that myocardial ischaemia, major arrhythmias and extrasystoles are more likely to occur. A combination of neurological disturbances and vascular pathologies present a serious complication. The probability of acute renal insufficiencies is higher in these people.

4.5 Interaction with other medicinal products and other forms of interaction

Use of the product may interfere with tests for thyroid function. Vasopressor agents should not be administered prior to iomeprol.

The presence of renal damage in diabetic patients is one of the factors predisposing to renal impairment following contrast media administration. This may precipitate lactic acidosis in patients who are taking metformin (see section 4.4 - Special warnings and special precautions for use).

Epidural and intrathecal corticosteroids should never be concurrently administered when iodinated contrast media are used, because corticosteroids may promote and affect the signs and symptoms of arachnoiditis (see section 4.3 - Contraindications).

4.6 Pregnancy and lactation

Animal studies have not indicated any harmful effects with respect to the course of pregnancy or on the health of the unborn or neonate. The safety of iomeprol in human pregnancy however has not been established. Therefore avoid in pregnancy unless there is no safer alternative.

No human data exist concerning the excretion of iomeprol in breast milk. Animal studies have demonstrated that the excretion of iomeprol in breast milk is similar to that of other contrast agents and that these compounds are only minimally absorbed by the gastrointestinal tract of the young. Adverse effects on the nursing infant are therefore unlikely to occur.

As a precautionary measure, breast-feeding should be discontinued prior to the administration of iomeprol and should not be recommenced until at least 24 hours after the administration of the contrast medium.

4.7 Effects on ability to drive and use machines

There is no known effect on the ability to drive and operate machines. However, because of the risk of early reactions, driving or operating machinery is not advisable for one hour following the last injection.

4.8 Undesirable effects

General

The use of iodinated contrast media may cause untoward side effects. They are usually mild to moderate and transient in nature. However, severe and life-threatening reactions sometimes leading to death have been reported. In most cases, reactions occur within minutes of dosing but at times reactions may occur at later time.

After intra-thecal administration most side effects occur some hours (3 to 6 hours) after the procedure, due to the distribution of the contrast medium in the cerebro-spinal fluid (CSF) circulation from the site of administration to the intravascular space. Most reactions usually occur within 24 hours after injection.

After injection of an iodinated contrast media in body cavities, the majority of the reactions occur some hours after the contrast administration due to the slow absorption from the area of administration.

Anaphylaxis (anaphylactoid/hypersensitivity reactions) may manifest with various symptoms, and rarely does any one patient develop all the symptoms. Typically, in 1 to 15 min (but rarely after as long as 2 h), the patient complains of feeling abnormal, agitation, flushing, feeling hot, increased sweating, dizziness, increased lacrimation, rhinitis, palpitations, paresthesia, pruritus, sore throat and throat tightness, dysphagia, cough, sneezing, urticaria, erythema, mild localised oedema, angioneurotic oedema, dyspnoea due to glottic/laryngeal/pharyngeal oedema and/or spasm manifesting with wheezing and bronchospasm.

Nausea, vomiting, abdominal pain, and diarrhoea are also reported.

These reactions, which can occur independently of the dose administered or the route of administration, may represent the first signs of circulatory collapse.

Administration of the contrast medium must be discontinued immediately and, if needed, appropriate specific treatment urgently initiated via venous access.

Severe reactions involving the cardiovascular system, such as vasodilatation, with pronounced hypotension, tachycardia, dyspnoea, agitation, cyanosis and loss of consciousness progressing to respiratory and/or cardiac arrest may result in death. These events can occur rapidly and require full and aggressive cardio-pulmonary resuscitation.

Primary circulatory collapse, can occur as the only and/or initial presentation without respiratory symptoms or without other signs or symptoms outlined above.

From Clinical Studies

Adverse experiences reported among patients treated with iomeprol during clinical trials are shown below:

(see Table 1 on next page)

Some of these events may occur as a consequence of the procedure.

From Post Marketing Surveillance

The following undesirable effects have been reported during post-marketing:

Intravascular and intra-thecal administration.

- *Blood and lymphatic system disorders:* thrombocytopenia.
- *Psychiatric disorders:* anxiety, agitation
- *Nervous system disorders:* taste abnormality, headache, paralysis, dysarthria, parasthesia, dizziness, cerebral oedema, hypoxic encephalopathy, transient ischaemic attack, loss of consciousness, convulsions, tremor, syncope, meningitis, somnolence.
- *Eye disorders:* transient blindness, conjunctivitis, increased lacrimation, visual disturbance,, photopsia, photophobia.
- *Cardiac disorders:* cardiac arrest, myocardial infarction, cardiac failure, angina pectoris, pulmonary oedema, arrhythmias including extrasystoles, ventricular or atrial fibrillation, tachycardia, bradycardia, atrioventricular block, cyanosis.
- *Vascular disorders:* shock, flushing, circulatory collapse, hypotension, hypertension, thrombosis
- *Respiratory, thoracic and mediastinal disorders:* respiratory arrest, acute respiratory distress syndrome (ARDS), asthma, bronchospasm, stridor, dyspnoea, rhinitis, cough, sneezing, laryngospasm, pharyngeal/laryngeal oedema, hypoxia, dysphonia
- *Gastrointestinal disorders:* acute pancreatitis, nausea, vomiting, diarrhea, abdominal pain, salivary hypersecretion, dysphagia, ileus.
- *Skin and subcutaneous tissue disorders:* angioneurotic oedema, pruritis, urticaria, rash, erythema, dermatitis, eczema, sweat.
- *Musculoskeletal and connective tissue disorders:* muscle weakness.
- *Renal and urinary disorders:* renal failure.
- *General disorders and administration site conditions:* oedema, malaise, chest pain, feeling of warmth, chills, pain, fever, injection site reaction.
- *Investigations:* abnormal electrocardiogram, abnormal liver function tests.

Administration to body cavities.

Hypersensitivity reactions are rare, generally mild and in the form of dermatitis. However, the possibility of severe anaphylactoid reactions cannot be excluded.

After injection into body cavities, local pain may occur.

4.9 Overdose

The effects of overdose on the pulmonary and cardiovascular systems may become life-threatening. Treatment consists of support of the vital functions and prompt use of symptomatic therapy. Iomeprol does not bind to plasma or serum proteins and is therefore dialyzable.

5. PHARMACOLOGICAL PROPERTIES

5.1 Pharmacodynamic properties

ATC code: V08AB10

Iomeprol is a low osmolality, non-ionic organic molecule with radio-opacity conferred by an iodine content of 49% of the molecular weight. It is formulated for use as an intravascular/intracavitary/ intrathecal contrast medium in concentrations of up to 400mg iodine per ml. Even at this concentration the low viscosity allows delivery of high doses through thin catheters.

5.2 Pharmacokinetic properties

The pharmacokinetics of intravascularly administered iomeprol are similar to those of other iodinated contrast media and conform to a two-compartment model with a rapid distribution and a slower elimination phase. In healthy subjects, the mean distribution and elimination half-lives of iomeprol were 0.5 hours and 1.9 hours respectively.

Table 1

System Organ Class	Common (>1/100, <1/10)	Uncommon (>1/1,000, <1/100)	Rare (>1/10,000,<1/1,000)
Psychiatric Disorders		Agitation	
Nervous System Disorders	Headache	Dizziness, paralysis	Tremor, confusion, loss of consciousness, visual field defect, syncope, aphasia, convulsions, coma
Cardiac Disorders		Bradycardia, tachycardia	Cyanosis
Vascular Disorders (mainly after cardiovascular procedures/interventions)	Pallor	Hypertension, hypotension	Vasodilatation, circulatory collapse
Respiratory, Thoracic and Mediastinal Disorders		Dyspnoea, nasal congestion, laryngeal oedema	
Gastrointestinal Disorders	Nausea	Vomiting	
Skin and Subcutaneous Tissue Disorders		Rash, erythema, wheals, pruritus, sweating increased	
Musculoskeletal and Connective Tissue Disorders		Back pain	Muscle spasms
Renal and Urinary Disorders			Renal failure, oliguria, proteinuria
General Disorders and Administration Site Conditions	Injection site warmth and pain	Chest pain, rigors, injection site haemorrhage, pyrexia	Asthenia
Investigations			Blood creatinine increased
Injury, Poisoning and Procedural Complications			Anaphylactoid reaction (characterized by cardiovascular, respiratory and cutaneous symptoms)

Distribution volume is similar to that of extra cellular fluid. There is no significant serum protein binding and iomeprol is not metabolized.

Elimination is almost exclusively through the kidneys (90% of the dose recovered in the urine within 96 hours of its administration) and is rapid (50% of an intravascularly administered dose within 2 hours).

Following intrathecal administration to animals, iomeprol is completely cleared from the CSF and passes into the plasma compartment.

5.3 Preclinical safety data

Pre-clinical data reveal no special hazard for humans based on conventional studies of safety pharmacology, repeated dose toxicity, genotoxicity, toxicity to reproduction.

Results from studies in rats, mice and dogs demonstrate that iomeprol has an acute intravenous or intra-arterial toxicity similar to that of the other non-ionic contrast media, as well as a good systemic tolerability after repeated intravenous administrations in rats and dogs.

6. PHARMACEUTICAL PARTICULARS

6.1 List of excipients

trometamol

hydrochloric acid

water for injection

6.2 Incompatibilities

No other drug should be mixed with the contrast medium.

6.3 Shelf life

Five years

6.4 Special precautions for storage

Store below 30°C

Protect from light

6.5 Nature and contents of container

Colourless Type I glass ampoules and colourless Type I or Type II glass bottles with rubber/aluminium cap.

Quantities of 10, 20, 30, 50, 75, 100, 150, 200 or 250 ml of solution.

6.6 Special precautions for disposal and other handling

Bottles containing contrast media solution are not intended for the withdrawal of multiple doses. The rubber stopper should never be pierced more than once. The use of proper withdrawal cannulas for piercing the stopper and drawing up the contrast medium is recommended.

Before use, examine the product to assure that the container and closure have not been damaged. Do not use the solution if it is discolored or particulate matter is present.

The contrast medium should not be drawn into the syringe until immediately before use. Withdrawal of contrast agents from their containers should be accomplished under aseptic conditions with sterile syringes. Sterile techniques must be used with any spinal puncture or intravascular injection, and with catheters and guidewires. If non-disposable equipment is used, scrupulous care should be taken to prevent residual contamination with traces of cleansing agents.

It is desirable that solutions of contrast media for intravascular and intrathecal use should be at body temperature when injected.

Any residue of contrast medium in the syringe must be discarded. Solutions not used in one examination session or waste material, such as the connecting tubes, should be disposed in accordance with local requirements.

7. MARKETING AUTHORISATION HOLDER

Bracco U.K. Ltd,

Bracco House, Mercury Park,

Wycombe Lane, Wooburn Green,

Buckinghamshire HP10 OHH

8. MARKETING AUTHORISATION NUMBER(S)

18920/0003

9. DATE OF FIRST AUTHORISATION/RENEWAL OF THE AUTHORISATION

11 December 1992 / 29 December 1998

10. DATE OF REVISION OF THE TEXT

September 2008

IOMERON 300

(Bracco UK Limited)

1. NAME OF THE MEDICINAL PRODUCT

Iomeron 300, solution for injection

2. QUALITATIVE AND QUANTITATIVE COMPOSITION

Contains 61.24% w/v of iomeprol equivalent to 30% iodine or 300mg iodine/ml.

For excipients, see 6.1.

3. PHARMACEUTICAL FORM

Solution for injection.

4. CLINICAL PARTICULARS

4.1 Therapeutic indications

X-ray contrast medium used for:

peripheral arteriography

venography

angiogardiography and left ventriculography

cerebral arteriography

visceral arteriography

digital subtraction angiography

computed tomography enhancement

urography

ERCP

dacryocystography

sialography

fistulography

galactography

myelography

4.2 Posology and method of administration

(see Table 1 on next page)

In elderly patients the lowest effective dose should be used.

In myelography, lower doses may be used for lumbar or thoracic studies and higher doses for cervical or total columnar studies. Regardless of the nature of the myelographic study, Iomeron should be injected slowly over 1-2 minutes.

The X ray can be taken up to 60 minutes following injection. Post myelographic CT of the spinal column should be delayed for approximately four hours to allow dilution and clearance of excessive contrast.

4.3 Contraindications

Proven or suspected hypersensitivity to iodine containing preparations of this type.

Intrathecal concomitant administration of corticosteroids with contrast media is contraindicated.

4.4 Special warnings and precautions for use

A positive history of allergy, asthma or untoward reaction during previous similar investigations indicates a need for extra caution since, as with other contrast media, this product may provoke anaphylaxis or other manifestations of allergy with nausea, vomiting, dyspnoea, erythema, urticaria and hypotension. The benefits should clearly outweigh the risks in such patients and appropriate resuscitative measures should be immediately available. The primary treatments are as follows:

Effect	Major Symptoms	Primary Treatment
Vasomotor effect	warmth	reassurance
	nausea/vomiting	
Cutaneous	scattered hives	H_1 -antihistamines
	severe urticaria	H_2 -antihistamines
Bronchospastic	wheezing	oxygen
		Beta-2-agonist inhalers
Anaphylactoid reaction	angioedema	oxygen
	urticaria	iv fluids
	bronchospasm	adrenergics (iv epinephrine)
	hypotension	Inhaled beta-2-adrenergics
		antihistamines (H_1-and H_2- blockers)
		corticosteroids
Hypotensive	hypotension	iv fluids
Vagal reaction	hypotension	iv fluids
	bradycardia	iv atropine

From: Bush WH; The Contrast Media Manual; Katzburg RW Ed.; Williams and Wilkins; Baltimore 1992; Chapter 2 p 23

In consideration of possible complications, the patient should be kept under observation for at least 60 minutes after the administration.

Extreme caution during injection of contrast media is necessary to avoid extravasation.

Special care is required when investigations are performed in patients with thrombosis, phlebitis, severe ischaemic disease, local infection or a totally obstructed arterovenous system.

Any severe disorders of water and electrolyte balance must be corrected prior to administration. Adequate hydration must be ensured particularly in patients with multiple myeloma, diabetes mellitus, polyuria, oliguria and hyperuricaemia; also in babies, small children and the elderly. Rehydration prior to use of iomeprol is recommended in patients with sickle cell disease.

Care should be taken in severe cardiac disease particularly heart failure and coronary artery disease. Reactions may include pulmonary oedema, haemodynamic changes, ischaemic ECG changes and arrhythmias. In severe, chronic hypertension the risk of renal damage following administration of a contrast medium is increased. In these cases the risks associated with the catheterization procedure are increased. Care should be taken in renal impairment and diabetes. In these patients it is important to maintain hydration in order to minimise deterioration in renal function.

A combination of severe hepatic and renal impairment delays excretion of the contrast medium therefore such patients should not be examined unless absolutely necessary.

The product should be used with caution in patients with hyperthyroidism or goitre. Use may interfere with thyroid function tests.

The administration of iodinated contrast media may aggravate myasthenia signs and symptoms.

Particular care is needed in patients with acute cerebral infarction, acute intracranial haemorrhage and any conditions involving damage to the blood brain barrier, brain oedema or acute demyelination. Convulsive seizures are

Table 1

peripheral arteriography	adults	10 - 90ml *
	children	* *
venography	adults	10 - 100ml* max 250ml 10 - 50ml upper extremity 50 - 100ml lower extremity
angiocardiography and left ventriculography	adults	30 - 80ml max 250ml
	children	* *
cerebral arteriography	adults	5 - 12ml *
	children	3 - 7ml or * *
visceral arteriography	adults	5 - 50ml* or according to type of examination; max 250ml
	children	* *
digital subtraction angiography intra arterial		
visceral	adults	2 - 20ml per artery* aorta 25-50ml* both 250ml max
peripheral	adults	5 - 10ml per artery* max 250ml
intravenous	adults	30 - 60ml* max 250ml
computed tomography		
brain	adults	50 - 150ml
	children	* *
body	adults	40 - 150ml max 250ml
	children	* *
urography intravenous	adults	50 - 150ml
	neonates	3 - 4.8ml/kg
	babies	2.5 - 4ml
	children	1 - 2.5ml/kg or *
arthrography	adults	1 - 10ml
ERCP	adults	12 - 30ml
dacryocystography	adults	3 - 8ml
sialography	adults	1 - 3ml
fistulography	adults	1 - 50ml
galactography	adults	0.2 - 1.5ml
myelography	adults	10 - 15ml by lumbar injection

* Repeat as necessary

* * According to body size and age

more likely in patients with intracranial tumours or metastases or with a history of epilepsy.

Neurological symptoms related to cerebrovascular diseases, intracranial tumours/metastases or degenerative or inflammatory pathologies may be exacerbated.

There is an increased risk of transient neurological complications in patients with symptomatic cerebrovascular disease eg stroke, transient ischaemic attacks. Cerebral ischaemic phenomena may be caused by intravascular injection.

Treatment with drugs that lower the seizure threshold such as analgesics and anti-emetics of the phenotiazine class, and neuroleptics should be discontinued 48 hours before the examination. Treatment should not be resumed until 24 hours post-procedure.

In acute and chronic alcoholism the increase in blood brain barrier permeability facilitates the passage of the contrast medium into cerebral tissue possibly leading to CMS disorders. There is a possibility of a reduced seizure threshold facilitates the passage of contrast medium into cerebral tissue possibly leading to CNS disorders. There is a possibility of a reduced seizure threshold in alcoholics.

In patients with a drug addiction there is also the possibility of a reduced seizure threshold.

Patients with phaeochromocytoma may develop severe, occasionally uncontrollable hypertensive crises during intravascular administration. Premedication with an alpha blocker is recommended in these patients. Pronounced excitement, anxiety and pain can cause side effects or intensify reaction to the contrast medium. A sedative may be given.

Since, on rare occasions, delayed reactions can occur, driving or operating machinery is not advisable for the first 24 hours after the procedure.

Anticonvulsant therapy should not be discontinued. A normal diet should be maintained until the patient refrains from eating 2 hours before the procedure.

Non ionic contrast media have less antiocoagulant activity in vitro than ionic media. Meticulous attention should therefore be paid to angiographic technique. Non ionic media should not be allowed to remain in contact with blood in a syringe, and intravascular catheters should be flushed frequently to minimise the risk of clotting which, rarely, has led to serious thromboembolic complications.

In patients with moderate to severe impairment of renal function, attention should be paid to renal function parameters, in particular before re-examining the patient with contrast media.

In diabetic patients with diabetic nephropathy, metformin should be stopped at the time of, or prior to the procedure and withheld for 48 hours subsequent to the procedure and reinstituted only after renal function has been re-evaluated and found to be normal (see section 4.5 - Interaction with medicaments and other forms of interaction).

Intravascular administration should be performed if possible with the patient lying down. The patient should be kept in this position and closely observed for at least 30 minutes after the procedure since the majority of severe incidents occur with this time.

Following intrathecal use, the patient should rest with the head and the chest elevated for 1 hour and be kept well hydrated. Thereafter, he/she may ambulate carefully, but bending down must be avoided. If remaining in bed, the head and chest should be kept elevated for 6 hours. Patients, suspected of having a lower seizure threshold should be observed during this period.

Children: Infants up to 1 year, especially the new-born, are particularly susceptible to electrolyte imbalance and haemodynamic alterations. Care should be taken regarding the dosage used.

Elderly: There is special risk of reactions involving the circulatory system such that myocardial ischaemia, major arrhythmias and extrasystoles are more likely to occur. A combination of neurological disturbances and vascular pathologies present a serious complication. The probability of acute renal insufficiencies is higher in these people.

4.5 Interaction with other medicinal products and other forms of interaction

Use of the product may interfere with tests for thyroid function. Vasopressor agents should not be administered prior to iomeprol.

The presence of renal damage in diabetic patients is one of the factors predisposing to renal impairment following contrast media administration. This may precipitate lactic acidosis in patients who are taking metformin (see section 4.4 - Special warnings and special precautions for use).

Epidural and intrathecal corticosteroids should never be concurrently administered when iodinated contrast media are used, because corticosteroids may promote and affect the signs and symptoms of arachnoiditis. (see section 4.3 Contraindications)

4.6 Pregnancy and lactation

Animal studies have not indicated any harmful effects with respect to the course of pregnancy or on the health of the unborn or neonate. The safety of iomeprol in human pregnancy however has not been established. Therefore avoid in pregnancy unless there is no safer alternative.

No human data exist concerning the excretion of iomeprol in breast milk. Animal studies have demonstrated that the excretion of iomeprol in breast milk is similar to that of other contrast agents and that these compounds are only minimally absorbed by the gastrointestinal tract of the young. Adverse effects on the nursing infant are therefore unlikely to occur.

As a precautionary measure, breast-feeding should be discontinued prior to the administration of iomeprol and should not be recommenced until at least 24 hours after the administration of the contrast medium.

4.7 Effects on ability to drive and use machines

There is no known effect on the ability to drive and operate machines. However, because of the risk of early reactions, driving or operating machinery is not advisable for one hour following the last injection.

4.8 Undesirable effects

General

The use of iodinated contrast media may cause untoward side effects. They are usually mild to moderate and transient in nature. However, severe and life-threatening reactions sometimes leading to death have been reported. In most cases, reactions occur within minutes of dosing but at times reactions may occur at later time.

After intra-thecal administration most side effects occur some hours (3 to 6 hours) after the procedure, due to the distribution of the contrast medium in the cerebro-spinal fluid (CSF) circulation from the site of administration to the intravascular space. Most reactions usually occur within 24 hours after injection.

After injection of an iodinated contrast media in body cavities, the majority of the reactions occur some hours after the contrast administration due to the slow absorption from the area of administration.

Anaphylaxis (anaphylactoid/hypersensitivity reactions) may manifest with various symptoms, and rarely does any one patient develop all the symptoms. Typically, in 1 to 15 min (but rarely after as long as 2 h), the patient complains of feeling abnormal, agitation, flushing, feeling hot, sweating increased, dizziness, increased lacrimation, rhinitis, palpitations, paresthesia, pruritus, sore throat and throat tightness, dysphagia, cough, sneezing, urticaria, erythema, mild localised oedema, angioneurotic oedema and dyspnoea due to glottic/laryngeal/pharyngeal oedema and/or spasm manifesting with wheezing, and bronchospasm.

Nausea, vomiting, abdominal pain, and diarrhoea are also reported.

These reactions, which can occur independently of the dose administered or the route of administration, may represent the first signs of circulatory collapse.

Administration of the contrast medium must be discontinued immediately and, if needed, appropriate specific treatment urgently initiated via venous access.

Severe reactions involving the cardiovascular system, such as vasodilatation, with pronounced hypotension, tachycardia, dyspnoea, agitation, cyanosis and loss of consciousness progressing to respiratory and/or cardiac arrest may result in death. These events can occur rapidly and require full and aggressive cardio-pulmonary resuscitation.

Primary circulatory collapse can occur as the only and/or initial presentation without respiratory symptoms or without other signs or symptoms outlined above.

From Clinical Studies

Adverse experiences reported among patients treated with iomeprol during clinical trials are shown below:

(see Table 2 on next page)

Some of these events may occur as a consequence of the procedure.

From Post Marketing Surveillance

The following undesirable effects have been reported during post-marketing:

Intravascular and intra-thecal administration.

- *Blood and lymphatic system disorders:* thrombocytopenia.
- *Psychiatric disorders:* anxiety, agitation
- *Nervous system disorders:* taste abnormality, headache, paralysis, dysarthria, paraesthesia, dizziness, cerebral oedema, hypoxic encephalopathy, transient ischaemic attack, loss of consciousness, convulsions, tremor, syncope, meningitis, somnolence.
- *Eye disorders:* transient blindness, conjunctivitis, increased lacrimation, visual disturbance, photopsia, photophobia.
- *Cardiac disorders:* cardiac arrest, myocardial infarction, cardiac failure, angina pectoris, pulmonary oedema, arrhythmias including extrasystoles, and ventricular or atrial fibrillation, tachycardia, bradycardia, atrioventricular block, cyanosis.
- *Vascular disorders:* shock, flushing, circulatory collapse, hypotension, hypertension, thrombosis.
- *Respiratory, thoracic and mediastinal disorders:* respiratory arrest, acute respiratory distress syndrome (ARDS), asthma, bronchospasm, stridor, dyspnoea, rhinitis, cough, sneezing, laryngospasm, pharyngeal/ laryngeal oedema, hypoxia, dysphonia.

Table 2

System Organ Class	Common (>1/100, <1/10)	Uncommon (>1/1,000, <1/100)	Rare (>1/10,000, <1/1,000)
Psychiatric Disorders		Agitation	
Nervous System Disorders	Headache	Dizziness, paralysis	Tremor, confusion, loss of consciousness, visual field defect, syncope, aphasia, convulsions, coma
Cardiac Disorders		Bradycardia, tachycardia	Cyanosis
Vascular Disorders (mainly after cardiovascular procedures/interventions)	Pallor	Hypertension, hypotension	Vasodilatation, circulatory collapse
Respiratory, Thoracic and Mediastinal Disorders		Dyspnoea, nasal congestion, laryngeal oedema	
Gastrointestinal Disorders	Nausea	Vomiting	
Skin and Subcutaneous Tissue Disorders		Rash, erythema, wheals, pruritus, sweating increased	
Musculoskeletal and Connective Tissue Disorders		Back pain	Muscle spasms
Renal and Urinary Disorders			Renal failure, oliguria, proteinuria
General Disorders and Administration Site Conditions	Injection site warmth and pain	Chest pain, rigors, injection site haemorrhage, pyrexia	Asthenia
Investigations			Blood creatinine increased
Injury, Poisoning and Procedural Complications			Anaphylactoid reaction (characterized by cardiovascular, respiratory and cutaneous symptoms)

- *Gastrointestinal disorders:* acute pancreatitis, nausea, vomiting, diarrhea, abdominal pain, salivary hypersecretion, dysphagia, ileus.

- *Skin and subcutaneous tissue disorders:* angioneurotic oedema, pruritis, urticaria, rash, erythema, dermatitis, eczema, sweat.

- *Musculoskeletal and connective tissue disorders:* muscle weakness.

- *Renal and urinary disorders:* renal failure.

- *General disorders and administration site conditions:* oedema, malaise, chest pain, feeling of warmth, chills, pain, fever, injection site reaction.

- *Investigations:* electrocardiogram abnormal, abnormal liver function tests.

Administration to body cavities.

Hypersensitivity reactions are rare, generally mild and in the form of dermatitis. However, the possibility of severe anaphylactoid reactions cannot be excluded.

After injection into body cavities, local pain may occur.

4.9 Overdose

The effects of overdose on the pulmonary and cardiovascular systems may become life-threatening. Treatment consists of support of the vital functions and prompt use of symptomatic therapy. Iomeprol does not bind to plasma or serum proteins and is therefore dialyzable.

5. PHARMACOLOGICAL PROPERTIES

5.1 Pharmacodynamic properties

ATC code: V08AB10

Iomeprol is a low osmolality, non-ionic organic molecule with radio-opacity conferred by an iodine content of 49% of the molecular weight. It is formulated for use as an intravascular/intracavitary/intrathecal contrast medium in concentrations of up to 400mg iodine per ml. Even at this concentration the low viscosity allows delivery of high doses through thin catheters.

5.2 Pharmacokinetic properties

The pharmacokinetics of intravascularly administered iomeprol are similar to those of other iodinated contrast media and conform to a two-compartment model with a rapid distribution and a slower elimination phase. In healthy subjects, the mean distribution and elimination half-lives of iomeprol were 0.5 hours and 1.9 hours respectively.

Distribution volume is similar to that of extra cellular fluid. There is no significant serum protein binding and iomeprol is not metabolized.

Elimination is almost exclusively through the kidneys (90% of the dose recovered in the urine within 96 hours of its administration) and is rapid (50% of an intravascularly administered dose within 2 hours).

Following intrathecal administration to animals, iomeprol is completely cleared from the CSF and passes into the plasma compartment.

5.3 Preclinical safety data

Pre-clinical data reveal no special hazard for humans based on conventional studies of safety pharmacology, repeated dose toxicity, genotoxicity, toxicity to reproduction.

Results from studies in rats, mice and dogs demonstrate that iomeprol has an acute intravenous or intra-arterial toxicity similar to that of the other non-ionic contrast media, as well as a good systemic tolerability after repeated intravenous administrations in rats and dogs.

6. PHARMACEUTICAL PARTICULARS

6.1 List of excipients

trometamol

hydrochloric acid

water for injection

6.2 Incompatibilities

No other drug should be mixed with the contrast medium.

6.3 Shelf life

Five years

6.4 Special precautions for storage

Store below 30°C

Protect from light

6.5 Nature and contents of container

Colourless Type I glass ampoules and colourless Type I or Type II glass bottles with rubber/aluminium cap.

Quantities of 10, 20, 30, 50, 75, 100, 150, 200 or 250 ml of solution.

6.6 Special precautions for disposal and other handling

Bottles containing contrast media solution are not intended for the withdrawal of multiple doses. The rubber stopper should never be pierced more than once. The use of proper withdrawal cannulas for piercing the stopper and drawing up the contrast medium is recommended.

Before use, examine the product to assure that the container and closure have not been damaged. Do not use the solution if it is discolored or particulate matter is present.

The contrast medium should not be drawn into the syringe until immediately before use. Withdrawal of contrast agents from their containers should be accomplished under aseptic conditions with sterile syringes. Sterile techniques must be used with any spinal puncture or intravascular injection, and with catheters and guidewires. If non-disposable equipment is used, scrupulous care should be taken to prevent residual contamination with traces of cleansing agents.

It is desirable that solutions of contrast media for intravascular and intrathecal use should be at body temperature when injected.

Any residue of contrast medium in the syringe must be discarded. Solutions not used in one examination session or waste material, such as the connecting tubes, should be disposed in accordance with local requirements.

7. MARKETING AUTHORISATION HOLDER

Bracco U.K. Ltd,

Bracco House, Mercury Park,

Wycombe Lane, Wooburn Green,

Buckinghamshire HP10 OHH

8. MARKETING AUTHORISATION NUMBER(S)

18920/0004

9. DATE OF FIRST AUTHORISATION/RENEWAL OF THE AUTHORISATION

11 December 1992 / 29 December 1998

10. DATE OF REVISION OF THE TEXT

September 2008

IOMERON 350

(Bracco UK Limited)

1. NAME OF THE MEDICINAL PRODUCT

Iomeron 350, solution for injection

2. QUALITATIVE AND QUANTITATIVE COMPOSITION

Contains 71.44% w/v of iomeprol equivalent to 35% iodine or 350mg iodine/ml.

For excipients, see 6.1.

3. PHARMACEUTICAL FORM

Solution for injection.

4. CLINICAL PARTICULARS

4.1 Therapeutic indications

X-ray contrast medium used for:

peripheral arteriography

venography

aortography

angiocardiography and left ventriculography

coronary arteriography

visceral arteriography

digital subtraction angiography

computed tomography enhancement

urography

dacryocystography

sialography

fistulography

galactography

4.2 Posology and method of administration

peripheral arteriography	adults	10 - 90ml *
	children	* *
venography	adults	10 - 100ml* max 250ml 10 - 50ml upper extremity 50 - 100ml lower extremity
aortography	adults	50 - 80ml
	children	* *
angiocardiography and left ventriculography	adults	30 - 80ml max 250ml
	children	* *
coronary arteriography	adults	4 - 10ml per artery *
visceral arteriography	adults	5 - 50ml* or according to type of examination; max 250ml
	children	* *

digital subtraction angiography

intravenous	adults	30 - 60ml* max 250ml

computed tomography

brain	adults	50 - 150ml
	children	* *
body	adults	40 - 150ml max 250ml
	children	* *

Urography

intravenous	adults	50 - 150ml
	neonates	3 - 4.8ml/kg
	babies	2.5 - 4ml
	children	1 - 2.5ml/kg or *

arthrography	adults	up to 10ml
dacryocystography	adults	3 - 8ml
sialography	adults	1 - 3ml
fistulography	adults	1 - 50ml
galactography	adults	0.2 - 1.5ml

* Repeat as necessary

* * According to body size and age

In elderly patients the lowest effective dose should be used.

The X ray can be taken up to 60 minutes following injection.

4.3 Contraindications

Proven or suspected hypersensitivity to iodine containing preparations of this type.

4.4 Special warnings and precautions for use

A positive history of allergy, asthma or untoward reaction during previous similar investigations indicates a need for extra caution since, as with other contrast media, this product may provoke anaphylaxis or other manifestations of allergy with nausea, vomiting, dyspnoea, erythema, urticaria and hypotension. The benefits should clearly outweigh the risks in such patients and appropriate resuscitative measures should be immediately available. The primary treatments are as follows:

Effect	Major Symptoms	Primary Treatment
Vasomotor effect	warmth	reassurance
	nausea/vomiting	
Cutaneous	scattered hives	H_1 -antihistamines
	severe urticaria	H_2 -antihistamines
Bronchospastic	wheezing	oxygen
		Beta-2-agonist inhalers
Anaphylactoid	angioedema	oxygen
reaction	urticaria	iv fluids
	bronchospasm	adrenergics (iv epinephrine)
	hypotension	Inhaled beta-2-adrenergics
		antihistamines (H_1-and
		H_2- blockers)
		corticosteroids
Hypotensive	hypotension	iv fluids
Vagal reaction	hypotension	iv fluids
	bradycardia	iv atropine

From: Bush WH; The Contrast Media Manual; Katzburg RW Ed.; Williams and Wilkins; Baltimore 1992; Chapter 2 p 23

In consideration of possible complications, the patient should be kept under observation for at least 60 minutes after the administration.

Extreme caution during injection of contrast media is necessary to avoid extravasation.

Special care is required when investigations are performed in patients with suspected thrombosis, phlebitis, severe ischemic disease, local infection or a totally obstructed artero-venous system.

Any severe disorders of water and electrolyte balance must be corrected prior to administration. Adequate hydration must be ensured particularly in patients with multiple myeloma, diabetes mellitus, polyuria, oliguria and hyperuricaemia; also in babies, small children and the elderly. Rehydration prior to use of iomeprol is recommended in patients with sickle cell disease.

Care should be taken in severe cardiac disease particularly heart failure and coronary artery disease. Reactions may include pulmonary oedema, haemodynamic changes, ischaemic ECG changes and arrhythmias. In severe, chronic hypertension the risk of renal damage following administration of a contrast medium is increased. In these cases the risks associated with the catheterization procedure are increased. Care should be taken in renal impairment and diabetes. In these patients it is important to maintain hydration in order to minimise deterioration in renal function.

A combination of severe hepatic and renal impairment delays excretion of the contrast medium therefore such patients should not be examined unless absolutely necessary.

The product should be used with caution in patients with hyperthyroidism or goitre. Use may interfere with thyroid function tests.

The administration of iodinated contrast media may aggravate myasthenia signs and symptoms.

Particular care is needed in patients with acute cerebral infarction, acute intracranial haemorrhage and any conditions involving damage to the blood brain barrier, brain oedema or acute demyelination. Convulsive seizures are more likely in patients with intracranial tumours or metastases or with a history of epilepsy.

Neurological symptoms related to cerebrovascular diseases, intracranial tumours/metastases or degenerative or inflammatory pathologies may be exacerbated.

There is an increased risk of transient neurological complications in patients with symptomatic cerebrovascular disease eg stroke, transient ischaemic attacks. Cerebral ischaemic phenomena may be caused by intravascular injection.

Treatment with drugs that lower the seizure threshold such as analgesics and anti-emetics of the phenotiazine class should be discontinued 48 hours before the examination. Treatment should not be resumed until 24 hours post-procedure.

In acute and chronic alcoholism the increase in blood brain barrier permeability facilitates the passage of contrast medium into cerebral tissue possibly leading to CNS disorders. There is a possibility of a reduced seizure threshold in alcoholics.

In patients with a drug addiction there is also the possibility of a reduced seizure threshold.

Patients with phaeochromocytoma may develop severe, occasionally uncontrollable hypertensive crises during intravascular administration. Premedication with an alpha blocker is recommended in these patients. Pronounced excitement, anxiety and pain can cause side effects or intensify reaction to the contrast medium. A sedative may be given.

Since, on rare occasions, delayed reactions can occur, driving or operating machinery is not advisable for the first 24 hours after the procedure.

Anticonvulsant therapy should not be discontinued. A normal diet should be maintained until the patient refrains from eating 2 hours before the procedure.

Non ionic contrast media have less antiocoagulant activity in vitro than ionic media. Meticulous attention should therefore be paid to angiographic technique. Non ionic media should not be allowed to remain in contact with blood in a syringe, and intravascular catheters should be flushed frequently to minimise the risk of clotting which, rarely, has led to serious thromboembolic complications.

In patients with moderate to severe impairment of renal function, attention should be paid to renal function parameters before re-examining the patient with a contrast media.

In diabetic patients with diabetic nephropathy, metformin should be stopped at the time of, or prior to the procedure and withheld for 48 hours subsequent to the procedure and re-instituted only after renal function has been re-evaluated and found to be normal (see section 4.5 - Interaction with other medicaments and other forms of interaction).

Intravascular administration should be performed if possible with the patient lying down. The patient should be kept in this position and closely observed for at least 30 minutes after the procedure since the majority of severe incidents occur with this time.

Children: Infants up to 1 year, especially the new-born, are particularly susceptible to electrolyte imbalance and haemodynamic alterations. Care should be taken regarding the dosage used.

Elderly: There is special risk of reactions involving the circulatory system such that myocardial ischaemia, major arrhythmias and extrasystoles are more likely to occur. A combination of neurological disturbances and vascular pathologies present a serious complication. The probability of acute renal insufficiencies is higher in these people.

4.5 Interaction with other medicinal products and other forms of interaction

Use of the product may interfere with tests for thyroid function. Vasopressor agents should not be administered prior to iomeprol.

The presence of renal damage in diabetic patients is one of the factors predisposing to renal impairment following contrast media administration. This may precipitate lactic acidosis in patients who are taking metformin (see section 4.4 - Special warnings and special precautions for use).

4.6 Pregnancy and lactation

Animal studies have not indicated any harmful effects with respect to the course of pregnancy or on the health of the unborn or neonate. The safety of iomeprol in human pregnancy however has not been established. Therefore avoid in pregnancy unless there is no safer alternative.

No human data exist concerning the excretion of iomeprol in breast milk. Animal studies have demonstrated that the excretion of iomeprol in breast milk is similar to that of other contrast agents and that these compounds are only minimally absorbed by the gastrointestinal tract of the young. Adverse effects on the nursing infant are therefore unlikely to occur.

As a precautionary measure, breast-feeding should be discontinued prior to the administration of iomeprol and should not be recommenced until at least 24 hours after the administration of the contrast medium.

4.7 Effects on ability to drive and use machines

There is no known effect on the ability to drive and operate machines. However, because of the risk of early reactions, driving or operating machinery is not advisable for one hour following the last injection.

4.8 Undesirable effects

General

The use of iodinated contrast media may cause untoward side effects. They are usually mild to moderate and transient in nature. However, severe and life-threatening reactions sometimes leading to death have been reported. In most cases, reactions occur within minutes of dosing but at times reactions may occur at later time.

After injection of an iodinated contrast media in body cavities, the majority of the reactions occur some hours after the contrast administration due to the slow absorption from the area of administration.

Anaphylaxis (anaphylactoid/hypersensitivity reactions) may manifest with various symptoms, and rarely does any one patient develop all the symptoms. Typically, in 1 to 15 min (but rarely after as long as 2 h), the patient complains of feeling abnormal, agitation, flushing, feeling hot, increased weating, dizziness, increased lacrimation, rhinitis, palpitations, paresthesia, pruritus,, sore throat and throat tightness, dysphagia, cough, sneezing, urticaria, erythema, mild localised oedema, angioneurotic oedema, dyspnoea due to glottic/laryngeal/pharyngeal oedema and/or spasm manifesting with wheezing, and bronchospasm.

Nausea, vomiting, abdominal pain, and diarrhoea are also reported.

These reactions, which can occur independently of the dose administered or the route of administration, may represent the first signs of circulatory collapse.

Administration of the contrast medium must be discontinued immediately and, if needed, appropriate specific treatment urgently initiated via venous access.

Severe reactions involving the cardiovascular system, such as vasodilatation, with pronounced hypotension, tachycardia, dyspnoea, agitation, cyanosis and loss of consciousness progressing to respiratory and/or cardiac arrest may result in death. These events can occur rapidly and require full and aggressive cardio-pulmonary resuscitation.

Primary circulatory collapse, can occur as the only and/or initial presentation without respiratory symptoms or without other signs or symptoms outlined above.

From Clinical Studies

Adverse experiences reported among patients treated with iomeprol during clinical trials are shown below:

(see Table 1 on next page)

Some of these events may occur as a consequence of the procedure.

From Post Marketing Surveillance

The following undesirable effects have been reported during post-marketing:

Intravascular and intra-thecal administration.

- *Blood and lymphatic system disorders:* thrombocytopenia.
- *Psychiatric disorders:* anxiety, agitation
- *Nervous system disorders:* taste abnormality, headache, paralysis, dysarthria, parasthesia, dizziness, cerebral oedema, hypoxic encephalopathy, transient ischaemic attack, loss of consciousness, convulsions, tremor, syncope, meningitis, somnolence.
- *Eye disorders:* transient blindness, conjunctivitis, increased lacrimation, visual disturbance, photopsia, photophobia.
- *Cardiac disorders:* cardiac arrest, myocardial infarction, cardiac failure, angina pectoris, pulmonary oedema, arrhythmias including extrasystoles, ventricular or atrial fibrillation, tachycardia, bradycardia, atrioventricular block, cyanosis.
- *Vascular disorders:* shock, flushing, circulatory collapse, hypotension, hypertension, thrombosis
- *Respiratory, thoracic and mediastinal disorders:* respiratory arrest, acute respiratory distress syndrome (ARDS), asthma, bronchospasm, stridor, dyspnoea, rhinitis, cough, sneezing, laryngospasm, pharyngeal/laryngeal oedema, hypoxia, dysphonia
- *Gastrointestinal disorders:* acute pancreatitis, nausea, vomiting, diarrhea, abdominal pain, salivary hypersecretion, dysphagia, ileus.
- *Skin and subcutaneous tissue disorders:* angioneurotic oedema, pruritis, urticaria, rash, erythema, dermatitis, eczema, sweat.
- *Musculoskeletal and connective tissue disorders:* muscle weakness.
- *Renal and urinary disorders:* renal failure.
- *General disorders and administration site conditions:* oedema, malaise, chest pain, feeling of warmth, chills, pain, fever, injection site reaction.
- *Investigations:* abnormal electrocardiogram, abnormal liver function tests.

Administration to body cavities.

Hypersensitivity reactions are rare, generally mild and in the form of dermatitis. However, the possibility of severe anaphylactoid reactions cannot be excluded.

After injection into body cavities, local pain may occur.

Table 1

System Organ Class	Common (>1/100, <1/10)	Uncommon (>1/1,000, <1/100)	Rare (>1/10,000, <1/1,000)
Psychiatric Disorders		Agitation	
Nervous System Disorders	Headache	Dizziness, paralysis	Tremor, confusion, loss of consciousness, visual field defect, syncope, aphasia, convulsions, coma
Cardiac Disorders		Bradycardia, tachycardia	Cyanosis
Vascular Disorders (mainly after cardiovascular procedures/interventions)	Pallor	Hypertension, hypotension	Vasodilatation, circulatory collapse
Respiratory, Thoracic and Mediastinal Disorders		Dyspnoea, nasal congestion, laryngeal oedema	
Gastrointestinal Disorders	Nausea	Vomiting	
Skin and Subcutaneous Tissue Disorders		Rash, erythema, wheals, pruritus, sweating increased	
Musculoskeletal and Connective Tissue Disorders		Back pain	Muscle spasms
Renal and Urinary Disorders			Renal failure, oliguria, proteinuria
General Disorders and Administration Site Conditions	Injection site warmth and pain	Chest pain, rigors, injection site haemorrhage, pyrexia	Asthenia
Investigations			Blood creatinine increased
Injury, Poisoning and Procedural Complications			Anaphylactoid reaction (characterized by cardiovascular, respiratory and cutaneous symptoms)

4.9 Overdose
The effects of overdose on the pulmonary and cardiovascular systems may become life-threatening. Treatment consists of support of the vital functions and prompt use of symptomatic therapy. Iomeprol does not bind to plasma or serum proteins and is therefore dialyzable.

5. PHARMACOLOGICAL PROPERTIES

5.1 Pharmacodynamic properties
ATC code: V08AB10

Iomeprol is a low osmolality, non-ionic organic molecule with radio-opacity conferred by an iodine content of 49% of the molecular weight. It is formulated for use as an intravascular/intracavitary contrast medium in concentrations of up to 400mg iodine per ml. Even at this concentration the low viscosity allows delivery of high doses through thin catheters.

5.2 Pharmacokinetic properties
The pharmacokinetics of intravascularly administered iomeprol are similar to those of other iodinated contrast media and conform to a two-compartment model with a rapid distribution and a slower elimination phase. In healthy subjects, the mean distribution and elimination half-lives of iomeprol were 0.5 hours and 1.9 hours respectively.

Distribution volume is similar to that of extra cellular fluid. There is no significant serum protein binding and iomeprol is not metabolized.

Elimination is almost exclusively through the kidneys (90% of the dose recovered in the urine within 96 hours of its administration) and is rapid (50% of an intravascularly administered dose within 2 hours).

5.3 Preclinical safety data
Pre-clinical data reveal no special hazard for humans based on conventional studies of safety pharmacology, repeated dose toxicity, genotoxicity, toxicity to reproduction.

Results from studies in rats, mice and dogs demonstrate that iomeprol has an acute intravenous or intra-arterial toxicity similar to that of the other non-ionic contrast media, as well as a good systemic tolerability after repeated intravenous administrations in rats and dogs.

6. PHARMACEUTICAL PARTICULARS

6.1 List of excipients
trometamol

hydrochloric acid

water for injection

6.2 Incompatibilities
No other drug should be mixed with the contrast medium.

6.3 Shelf life
Five years

6.4 Special precautions for storage
Store below 30°C

Protect from light

6.5 Nature and contents of container
Colourless Type I glass ampoules and colourless Type I or Type II glass bottles with rubber/aluminium cap.

Quantities of 10, 20, 30, 50, 75, 100, 150, 200 or 250 ml of solution.

6.6 Special precautions for disposal and other handling
Bottles containing contrast media solution are not intended for the withdrawal of multiple doses. The rubber stopper should never be pierced more than once. The use of proper withdrawal cannulas for piercing the stopper and drawing up the contrast medium is recommended.

Before use, examine the product to assure that the container and closure have not been damaged. Do not use the solution if it is discolored or particulate matter is present.

The contrast medium should not be drawn into the syringe until immediately before use. Withdrawal of contrast agents from their containers should be accomplished under aseptic conditions with sterile syringes. Sterile techniques must be used with any spinal puncture or intravascular injection, and with catheters and guidewires. If non-disposable equipment is used, scrupulous care should be taken to prevent residual contamination with traces of cleansing agents.

It is desirable that solutions of contrast media for intravascular and intrathecal use should be at body temperature when injected.

Any residue of contrast medium in the syringe must be discarded. Solutions not used in one examination session or waste material, such as the connecting tubes, should be disposed in accordance with local requirements.

7. MARKETING AUTHORISATION HOLDER
Bracco U.K. Ltd,

Bracco House, MercuryPark,

Wycombe Lane, Wooburn Green,

Buckinghamshire HP10 0HH

8. MARKETING AUTHORISATION NUMBER(S)
18920/0005

9. DATE OF FIRST AUTHORISATION/RENEWAL OF THE AUTHORISATION
11 December 1992/ 29 December 1998

10. DATE OF REVISION OF THE TEXT
September 2008

IOMERON 400

(Bracco UK Limited)

1. NAME OF THE MEDICINAL PRODUCT
Iomeron 400, solution for injection

2. QUALITATIVE AND QUANTITATIVE COMPOSITION
Contains 81.65% w/v of iomeprol equivalent to 40% iodine or 400mg iodine/ml.

For excipients, see 6.1.

3. PHARMACEUTICAL FORM
Solution for injection.

4. CLINICAL PARTICULARS

4.1 Therapeutic indications
X-ray contrast medium used for:

peripheral arteriography

aortography

angiocardiography and left ventriculography

coronary arteriography

visceral arteriography

digital subtraction angiography

computed tomography enhancement

urography

dacryocystography

sialography

fistulography

galactography

4.2 Posology and method of administration

peripheral arteriography	adults	10 - 90ml *
	children	* *
aortography	adults	50 - 80ml
	children	* *
angiocardiography and left ventriculography	adults	30 - 80ml max 250ml
	children	* *
coronary arteriography	adults	4 - 10ml per artery *
visceral arteriography	adults	5 - 50ml* or according to type of examination;
	children	* *

digital subtraction angiography

intravenous	adults	30 - 60ml* max 250ml

computed tomography

body	adults	40 - 150ml max 250ml
	children	* *

urography

intravenous	adults	50 - 150ml
	neonates	3 - 4.8ml/kg
	babies	2.5 - 4ml
	children	1 - 2.5ml/kg or *
dacryocystography	adults	3 - 8ml
sialography	adults	1 - 3ml
fistulography	adults	1 - 50ml
galactography	adults	0.2 - 1.5ml

* Repeat as necessary

* * According to body size and age

In elderly patients the lowest effective dose should be used.

The X ray can be taken up to 60 minutes following injection.

4.3 Contraindications
Proven or suspected hypersensitivity to iodine containing preparations of this type.

4.4 Special warnings and precautions for use
A positive history of allergy, asthma or untoward reaction during previous similar investigations indicates a need for extra caution since, as with other contrast media, this product may provoke anaphylaxis or other manifestations of allergy with nausea, vomiting, dyspnoea, erythema, urticaria and hypotension. The benefits should clearly outweigh the risks in such patients and appropriate resuscitative measures should be immediately available. The primary treatments are as follows:

Effect	Major Symptoms	Primary Treatment
Vasomotor effect	warmth	reassurance
	nausea/ vomiting	
Cutaneous	scattered hives	H_1 - antihistamines
	severe urticaria	H_2 - antihistamines

Bronchospastic	wheezing	oxygen
		Beta-2-agonist inhalers
Anaphylactoid	angioedema	oxygen
reaction	urticaria	iv fluids
	bronchospasm	adrenergics (iv epinephrine)
	hypotension	Inhaled beta-2-adrenergics
		antihistamines (H_1-and
		H_2- blockers)
		corticosteroids
Hypotensive	hypotension	iv fluids
Vagal reaction	hypotension	iv fluids
	bradycardia	iv atropine

From: Bush WH; The Contrast Media Manual; Katzburg RW Ed.; Williams and Wilkins; Baltimore 1992; Chapter 2 p 23

In consideration of possible complications, the patient should be kept under observation for at least 60 minutes after the administration.

Extreme caution during injection of contrast media is necessary to avoid extravasation.

Special care is required when investigations are performed in patients with suspected thrombosis, phlebitis, severe ischemic disease, local infection or a totally obstructed artero-venous system.

Any severe disorders of water and electrolyte balance must be corrected prior to administration. Adequate hydration must be ensured particularly in patients with multiple myeloma, diabetes mellitus, polyuria, oliguria and hyperuricaemia; also in babies, small children and the elderly. Rehydration prior to use of iomeprol is recommended in patients with sickle cell disease.

Care should be taken in severe cardiac disease particularly heart failure and coronary artery disease. Reactions may include pulmonary oedema, haemodynamic changes, ischaemic ECG changes and arrhythmias. In severe, chronic hypertension the risk of renal damage following administration of a contrast medium is increased. In these cases the risks associated with the catheterization procedure are increased. Care should be taken in renal impairment and diabetes. In these patients it is important to maintain hydration in order to minimise deterioration in renal function.

A combination of severe hepatic and renal impairment delays excretion of the contrast medium therefore such patients should not be examined unless absolutely necessary.

The product should be used with caution in patients with hyperthyroidism or goitre. Use may interfere with thyroid function tests.

The administration of iodinated contrast media may aggravate myasthenia signs and symptoms.

Particular care is needed in patients with acute cerebral infarction, acute intracranial haemorrhage and any conditions involving damage to the blood brain barrier, brain oedema or acute demyelination. Convulsive seizures are more likely in patients with intracranial tumours or metastases or with a history of epilepsy.

Neurological symptoms related to cerebrovascular diseases, intracranial tumours/metastases or degenerative or inflammatory pathologies may be exacerbated.

There is an increased risk of transient neurological complications in patients with symptomatic cerebrovascular disease eg stroke, transient ischaemic attacks. Cerebral ischaemic phenomena may be caused by intravascular injection.

Treatment with drugs that lower the seizure threshold such as analgesics and anti-emetics of the phenotiazine class should be discontinued 48 hours before the examination. Treatment should not be resumed until 24 hours post-procedure.

In acute and chronic alcoholism the increase in blood brain barrier permeability facilitates the passage of the contrast medium into cerebral tissue possibly leading to CMS disorders. There is a possibility of a reduced seizure threshold facilitates the passage of contrast medium into cerebral tissue possibly leading to CNS disorders. There is a possibility of a reduced seizure threshold in alcoholics.

In patients with a drug addiction there is also the possibility of a reduced seizure threshold.

Patients with phaeochromocytoma may develop severe, occasionally uncontrollable hypertensive crises during intravascular administration. Premedication with an alpha blocker is recommended in these patients. Pronounced excitement, anxiety and pain can cause side effects or intensify reaction to the contrast medium. A sedative may be given.

Since, on rare occasions, delayed reactions can occur, driving or operating machinery is not advisable for the first 24 hours after the procedure.

Anticonvulsant therapy should not be discontinued. A normal diet should be maintained until the patient refrains from eating 2 hours before the procedure.

Non ionic contrast media have less antiocoagulant activity in vitro than ionic media. Meticulous attention should therefore be paid to angiographic technique. Non ionic media should not be allowed to remain in contact with blood in a syringe, and intravascular catheters should be flushed frequently to minimise the risk of clotting which, rarely, has led to serious thromboembolic complications.

In patients with moderate to severe impairment of renal function, attention should be paid to renal function parameters before re-examining the patient with a contrast media.

In diabetic patients with diabetic nephropathy, metformin should be stopped at the time of, or prior to the procedure and withheld for 48 hours subsequent to the procedure and re-instituted only after renal function has been re-evaluated and found to be normal (see section 4.5 - Interaction with other medicaments and other forms of interaction).

Intravascular administration should be performed if possible with the patient lying down. The patient should be kept in this position and closely observed for at least 30 minutes after the procedure since the majority of severe incidents occur with this time.

Children: Infants up to 1 year, especially the newborn, are particularly susceptible to electrolyte imbalance and haemodynamic alterations. Care should be taken regarding the dosage used.

Elderly: There is special risk of reactions involving the circulatory system such that myocardial ischaemia, major arrhythmias and extrasystoles are more likely to occur. A combination of neurological disturbances and vascular pathologies present a serious complication. The probability of acute renal insufficiencies is higher in these people.

4.5 Interaction with other medicinal products and other forms of interaction

Use of the product may interfere with tests for thyroid function. Vasopressor agents should not be administered prior to iomeprol.

The presence of renal damage in diabetic patients is one of the factors predisposing to renal impairment following contrast media administration. This may precipitate lactic acidosis in patients who are taking metformin (see section 4.4 - Special warnings and special precautions for use).

4.6 Pregnancy and lactation

Animal studies have not indicated any harmful effects with respect to the course of pregnancy or on the health of the unborn or neonate. The safety of iomeprol in human pregnancy however has not been established. Therefore avoid in pregnancy unless there is no safer alternative.

No human data exist concerning the excretion of iomeprol in breast milk. Animal studies have demonstrated that the excretion of iomeprol in breast milk is similar to that of other contrast agents and that these compounds are only minimally absorbed by the gastrointestinal tract of the young. Adverse effects on the nursing infant are therefore unlikely to occur.

As a precautionary measure, breast-feeding should be discontinued prior to the administration of iomeprol and should not be recommenced until at least 24 hours after the administration of the contrast medium.

4.7 Effects on ability to drive and use machines

There is no known effect on the ability to drive and operate machines. However, because of the risk of early reactions, driving or operating machinery is not advisable for one hour following the last injection.

4.8 Undesirable effects

General

The use of iodinated contrast media may cause untoward side effects. They are usually mild to moderate and transient in nature. However, severe and life-threatening reactions sometimes leading to death have been reported. In most cases, reactions occur within minutes of dosing but at times reactions may occur at later time.

After injection of an iodinated contrast media in body cavities, the majority of the reactions occur some hours after the contrast administration due to the slow absorption from the area of administration.

Anaphylaxis (anaphylactoid/hypersensitivity reactions) may manifest with various symptoms, and rarely does any one patient develop all the symptoms. Typically, in 1 to 15 min (but rarely after as long as 2 h), the patient complains of feeling abnormal, agitation, flushing, feeling hot, increased sweating increased, dizziness, increased lacrimation increased, rhinitis, palpitations, paresthesia, pruritus, head throbbing, sore throat sore and throat tightness, dysphagia, cough, sneezing, urticaria, erythema, and mild localised oedema, or angioneurotic oedema, and dyspnoea owing due to tongue and glottic/laryngeal/pharyngeal oedema and/or spasm manifesting with wheezing, and bronchospasm.

Nausea, vomiting, abdominal pain, and diarrhoea are also reported.

These reactions, which can occur independently of the dose administered or the route of administration, may represent the first signs of circulatory collapse.

Administration of the contrast medium must be discontinued immediately and, if needed, appropriate specific treatment urgently initiated via venous access.

Severe reactions involving the cardiovascular system, such as vasodilatation, with pronounced hypotension, tachycardia, dyspnoea, agitation, cyanosis and loss of consciousness progressing to respiratory and/or cardiac arrest may result in death. These events can occur rapidly and require full and aggressive cardio-pulmonary resuscitation.

Primary circulatory collapse can occur as the only and/or initial presentation without respiratory symptoms or without other signs or symptoms outlined above.

From Clinical Studies

Adverse experiences reported among patients treated with iomeprol during clinical trials are shown below:

(see Table 1 on next page)

Some of these events may occur as a consequence of the procedure.

From Post Marketing Surveillance

The following undesirable effects have been reported during post-marketing:

Intravascular and intra-thecal administration.

- *Blood and lymphatic system disorders:* thrombocytopenia.
- *Psychiatric disorders:* anxiety, agitation
- *Nervous system disorders:* taste abnormality, headache, paralysis, dysarthria, parasthesia, dizziness, cerebral oedema, hypoxic encephalopathy, transient ischaemic attack, loss of consciousness, convulsions, tremor, syncope, meningitis, somnolence.
- *Eye disorders:* transient blindness, conjunctivitis, increased lacrimation, visual disturbance, photopsia, photophobia.
- *Cardiac disorders:* cardiac arrest, myocardial infarction, cardiac failure, angina pectoris, pulmonary oedema, arrhythmias including extrasystoles, ventricular or atrial fibrillation, tachycardia, bradycardia, atrioventricular block, cyanosis.
- *Vascular disorders:* shock, flushing, circulatory collapse, hypotension, hypertension, thrombosis
- *Respiratory, thoracic and mediastinal disorders:* respiratory arrest, acute respiratory distress syndrome (ARDS), asthma, bronchospasm, stridor, dyspnoea, rhinitis, cough, sneezing, laryngospasm, pharyngeal/laryngeal oedema, hypoxia, dysphonia
- *Gastrointestinal disorders:* acute pancreatitis, nausea, vomiting, diarrhea, abdominal pain, salivary hypersecretion, dysphagia, ileus.
- *Skin and subcutaneous tissue disorders:* angioneurotic oedema, pruritis, urticaria, rash, erythema, dermatitis, eczema, sweat.
- *Musculoskeletal and connective tissue disorders:* muscle weakness.
- *Renal and urinary disorders:* renal failure.
- *General disorders and administration site conditions:* oedema, malaise, chest pain, feeling of warmth, chills, pain, fever, injection site reaction.
- *Investigations:* abnormal electrocardiogram, abnormal liver function tests.

Administration to body cavities.

Hypersensitivity reactions are rare, generally mild and in the form of dermatitis. However, the possibility of severe anaphylactoid reactions cannot be excluded.

After injection into body cavities, local pain may occur.

4.9 Overdose

The effects of overdose on the pulmonary and cardiovascular systems may become life-threatening. Treatment consists of support of the vital functions and prompt use of symptomatic therapy. Iomeprol does not bind to plasma or serum proteins and is therefore dialyzable.

5. PHARMACOLOGICAL PROPERTIES

5.1 Pharmacodynamic properties

ATC code: V08AB10

Iomeprol is a low osmolality, non-ionic organic molecule with radio-opacity conferred by an iodine content of 49% of the molecular weight. It is formulated for use as an intravascular/intracavitary contrast medium in concentrations of up to 400mg iodine per ml. Even at this concentration the low viscosity allows delivery of high doses through thin catheters.

5.2 Pharmacokinetic properties

The pharmacokinetics of intravascularly administered iomeprol are similar to those of other iodinated contrast media and conform to a two-compartment model with a rapid distribution and a slower elimination phase. In healthy subjects, the mean distribution and elimination half-lives of iomeprol were 0.5 hours and 1.9 hours respectively.

Table 1

System Organ Class	Common (>1/100, <1/10)	Uncommon (>1/1,000, <1/100)	Rare (>1/10,000, <1/1,000)
Psychiatric Disorders		Agitation	
Nervous System Disorders	Headache	Dizziness, paralysis	Tremor, confusion, loss of consciousness, visual field defect, syncope, aphasia, convulsions, coma
Cardiac Disorders		Bradycardia, tachycardia	Cyanosis
Vascular Disorders (mainly after cardiovascular procedures/interventions)	Pallor	Hypertension, hypotension	Vasodilatation, circulatory collapse
Respiratory, Thoracic and Mediastinal Disorders		Dyspnoea, nasal congestion, laryngeal oedema	
Gastrointestinal Disorders	Nausea	Vomiting	
Skin and Subcutaneous Tissue Disorders		Rash, erythema, wheals, pruritus, sweating increased	
Musculoskeletal and Connective Tissue Disorders		Back pain	Muscle spasms
Renal and Urinary Disorders			Renal failure, oliguria, proteinuria
General Disorders and Administration Site Conditions	Injection site warmth and pain	Chest pain, rigors, injection site haemorrhage, pyrexia	Asthenia
Investigations			Blood creatinine increased
Injury, Poisoning and Procedural Complications			Anaphylactoid reaction (characterized by cardiovascular, respiratory and cutaneous symptoms)

Distribution volume is similar to that of extra cellular fluid. There is no significant serum protein binding and iomeprol is not metabolized.

Elimination is almost exclusively through the kidneys (90% of the dose recovered in the urine within 96 hours of its administration) and is rapid (50% of an intravascularly administered dose within 2 hours).

5.3 Preclinical safety data
Pre-clinical data reveal no special hazard for humans based on conventional studies of safety pharmacology, repeated dose toxicity, genotoxicity, toxicity to reproduction.

Results from studies in rats, mice and dogs demonstrate that iomeprol has an acute intravenous or intra-arterial toxicity similar to that of the other non-ionic contrast media, as well as a good systemic tolerability after repeated intravenous administrations in rats and dogs.

6. PHARMACEUTICAL PARTICULARS

6.1 List of excipients
trometamol

hydrochloric acid

water for injection

6.2 Incompatibilities
No other drug should be mixed with the contrast medium.

6.3 Shelf life
Five years

6.4 Special precautions for storage
Store below 30°C

Protect from light

6.5 Nature and contents of container
Colourless Type I glass ampoules and colourless Type I or Type II glass bottles with rubber/aluminium cap.

Quantities of 10, 20, 30, 50, 75, 100, 150, 200 or 250 ml of solution.

6.6 Special precautions for disposal and other handling
Bottles containing contrast media solution are not intended for the withdrawal of multiple doses. The rubber stopper should never be pierced more than once. The use of proper withdrawal cannulas for piercing the stopper and drawing up the contrast medium is recommended.

Before use, examine the product to assure that the container and closure have not been damaged. Do not use the solution if it is discolored or particulate matter is present.

The contrast medium should not be drawn into the syringe until immediately before use. Withdrawal of contrast agents from their containers should be accomplished under aseptic conditions with sterile syringes. Sterile techniques must be used with any spinal puncture or intravascular injection, and with catheters and guidewires. If non-disposable equipment is used, scrupulous care should be taken to prevent residual contamination with traces of cleansing agents.

It is desirable that solutions of contrast media for intravascular and intrathecal use should be at body temperature when injected.

Any residue of contrast medium in the syringe must be discarded. Solutions not used in one examination session or waste material, such as the connecting tubes, should be disposed in accordance with local requirements.

7. MARKETING AUTHORISATION HOLDER
Bracco U.K. Ltd,

Bracco House, Mercury Park,

Wycombe Lane, Wooburn Green,

Buckinghamshire HP10 0HH

8. MARKETING AUTHORISATION NUMBER(S)
18920/0006

9. DATE OF FIRST AUTHORISATION/RENEWAL OF THE AUTHORISATION
11 December 1992/ 29 December 1998

10. DATE OF REVISION OF THE TEXT
September 2008

Iressa 250mg film-coated tablets

(AstraZeneca UK Limited)

1. NAME OF THE MEDICINAL PRODUCT
IRESSA▼ 250 mg film-coated tablets

2. QUALITATIVE AND QUANTITATIVE COMPOSITION
Each tablet contains 250 mg of gefitinib.

Excipient: Each tablet contains 163.5 mg of lactose (as monohydrate)

For a full list of excipients, see section 6.1.

3. PHARMACEUTICAL FORM
Film-coated tablet (tablet).

Tablets are brown, round, biconvex, impressed with "IRESSA 250" on one side and plain on the other.

4. CLINICAL PARTICULARS

4.1 Therapeutic indications
IRESSA is indicated for the treatment of adult patients with locally advanced or metastatic non-small cell lung cancer (NSCLC) with activating mutations of EGFR-TK (see section 5.1 Pharmacodynamic properties).

4.2 Posology and method of administration
Treatment with IRESSA should be initiated and supervised by a physician experienced in the use of anticancer therapies.

Posology
The recommended posology of IRESSA is one 250 mg tablet once a day. If a dose of IRESSA is missed, it should be taken as soon as the patient remembers. If it is less than 12 hours to the next dose, the patient should not take the missed dose. Patients should not take a double dose (two doses at the same time) to make up for a forgotten dose.

Paediatric population
There is no relevant indication for use of IRESSA in children and adolescents.

Hepatic impairment
Patients with moderate to severe hepatic impairment (Child Pugh B or C) due to cirrhosis have increased plasma concentrations of gefitinib. These patients should be closely monitored for adverse events. Plasma concentrations were not increased in patients with elevated aspartate transaminase (AST), alkaline phosphatase or bilirubin due to liver metastases (see section 5.2 Pharmacokinetic properties).

Renal impairment
No dose adjustment is required in patients with impaired renal function at creatinine clearance >20 ml/min. Only limited data are available in patients with creatinine clearance ≤ 20 ml/min and caution is advised in these patients (see section 5.2 Pharmacokinetic properties).

Elderly
No dose adjustment is required on the basis of patient age (see section 5.2 Pharmacokinetic properties).

CYP2D6 poor metabolisers
No specific dose adjustment is recommended in patients with known CYP2D6 poor metaboliser genotype, but these patients should be closely monitored for adverse events (see section 5.2 Pharmacokinetic properties).

Dose adjustment due to toxicity
Patients with poorly tolerated diarrhoea or skin adverse reactions may be successfully managed by providing a brief (up to 14 days) therapy interruption followed by reinstatement of the 250 mg dose (see section 4.8 Undesirable effects). For patients unable to tolerate treatment after a therapy interruption, IRESSA should be discontinued and an alternative treatment should be considered.

Method of administration
The tablet may be taken with or without food, at about the same time each day. The tablet can be swallowed whole with some water or if dosing of whole tablets is not possible, tablets may be administered as a dispersion in water (non-carbonated). No other liquids should be used. Without crushing it, the tablet should be dropped in half a glass of drinking water. The glass should be swirled occasionally, until the tablet is dispersed (this may take up to 20 minutes). The dispersion should be drunk immediately after dispersion is complete (i.e. within 60 minutes). The glass should be rinsed with half a glass of water, which should also be drunk. The dispersion can also be administered through a naso-gastric or gastrostomy tube.

4.3 Contraindications
Hypersensitivity to the active substance or to any of the excipients.

Breast-feeding (see section 4.6 Pregnancy and lactation).

4.4 Special warnings and precautions for use
Assessment of EGFR mutation status
When assessing the EGFR mutation status of a patient, it is important that a well-validated and robust methodology is chosen to avoid false negative or false positive determinations.

Interstitial lung disease (ILD)
ILD, which may be acute in onset, has been observed in 1.3 % of patients receiving IRESSA, and some cases have been fatal (see section 4.8 Undesirable effects). If patients experience worsening of respiratory symptoms such as dyspnoea, cough and fever, IRESSA should be interrupted and the patient should be promptly investigated. If ILD is confirmed, IRESSA should be discontinued and the patient treated appropriately.

In a Japanese pharmacoepidemiological case control study in 3159 patients with NSCLC receiving IRESSA or chemotherapy who were followed up for 12 weeks, the following risk factors for developing ILD (irrespective of whether the patient received IRESSA or chemotherapy) were identified: smoking, poor performance status (PS≥ 2), CT scan evidence of reduced normal lung (≤ 50 %), recent diagnosis of NSCLC (< 6 months), pre-existing ILD, older age (≥ 55 years old) and concurrent cardiac disease. An increased risk of ILD on gefitinib relative to chemotherapy was seen predominantly during the first 4 weeks of treatment (adjusted OR 3.8; 95 % CI 1.9 to 7.7); thereafter the relative risk was lower (adjusted OR 2.5; 95 % CI 1.1 to 5.8). Risk of mortality among patients who developed ILD on IRESSA or chemotherapy was higher in patients with the following risk factors: smoking, CT scan evidence of reduced normal lung (≤ 50 %), pre-existing ILD, older age (≥ 65 years old), and extensive areas adherent to pleura (≥ 50 %).

Hepatotoxicity and liver impairment
Although liver function test abnormalities (including increases in alanine aminotransferase, aspartate aminotransferase, bilirubin) were common, they were rarely observed as hepatitis (see section 4.8 Undesirable effects).

Table 1 Adverse reactions

Adverse reactions by system organ class and frequency		
Metabolism and nutrition disorders	Very Common	Anorexia mild or moderate (CTC grade 1 or 2).
Eye disorders	Common	Conjunctivitis, blepharitis, and dry eye*, mainly mild (CTC grade 1).
	Uncommon	Corneal erosion, reversible and sometimes in association with aberrant eyelash growth.
Vascular disorders	Common	Haemorrhage, such as epistaxis and haematuria.
Respiratory, thoracic and mediastinal disorders	Common	Interstitial lung disease (1.3 %), often severe (CTC grade 3-4). Cases with fatal outcomes have been reported.
Gastrointestinal disorders	Very Common	Diarrhoea, mainly mild or moderate (CTC grade 1 or 2).
		Vomiting, mainly mild or moderate (CTC grade 1 or 2).
		Nausea, mainly mild (CTC grade 1).
		Stomatitis, predominantly mild in nature (CTC grade 1).
	Common	Dehydration, secondary to diarrhoea, nausea, vomiting or anorexia.
		Dry mouth*, predominantly mild (CTC grade 1).
	Uncommon	Pancreatitis
Hepatobiliary disorders	Very Common	Elevations in alanine aminotransferase, mainly mild to moderate.
	Common	Elevations in aspartate aminotransferase, mainly mild to moderate.
		Elevations in total bilirubin, mainly mild to moderate.
	Rare	Hepatitis
Skin and subcutaneous tissue disorders	Very Common	Skin reactions, mainly a mild or moderate (CTC grade 1 or 2) pustular rash, sometimes itchy with dry skin, on an erythematous base.
	Common	Nail disorder
		Alopecia
	Uncommon	Allergic reactions**, including angioedema and urticaria
	Rare	Toxic epidermal necrolysis, Stevens Johnson syndrome and erythema multiforme
Renal and urinary disorders	Common	Asymptomatic laboratory elevations in blood creatinine
		Proteinuria
General disorders	Very Common	Asthenia, predominantly mild (CTC grade 1).
	Common	Pyrexia

Frequency of ADRs relating to abnormal laboratory values is based on patients with a change in baseline of 2 or more CTC grades in the relevant laboratory parameters.

*This event can occur in association with other dry conditions (mainly skin reactions) seen with IRESSA.

**The overall incidence of adverse events of allergic reaction reported in the pooled analysis of the ISEL, INTEREST and IPASS trials was 1.5 % (36 patients). Fourteen of the 36 patients were excluded from the reported frequency as their reports contained evidence of either a non allergic aetiology or that the allergic reaction was the result of treatment with another medicinal product.

Therefore, periodic liver function testing is recommended. IRESSA should be used cautiously in the presence of mild to moderate changes in liver function. Discontinuation should be considered if changes are severe.

Impaired liver function due to cirrhosis has been shown to lead to increased plasma concentrations of gefitinib (see section 5.2 Pharmacokinetic properties).

Interactions with other medicinal products

CYP3A4 inducers may increase metabolism of gefitinib and decrease gefitinib plasma concentrations. Therefore, concomitant administration of CYP3A4 inducers (e.g. phenytoin, carbamazepine, rifampicin, barbiturates or herbal preparations containing St John's wort/*Hypericum perforatum*) may reduce efficacy of the treatment and should be avoided (see section 4.5 Interaction with other medicinal products and other forms of interaction).

In individual patients with CYP2D6 poor metaboliser genotype, treatment with a potent CYP3A4 inhibitor might lead to increased plasma levels of gefitinib. At initiation of treatment with a CYP3A4 inhibitor, patients should be closely monitored for gefitinib adverse reactions (see section 4.5 Interaction with other medicinal products and other forms of interaction).

International normalised ratio (INR) elevations and/or bleeding events have been reported in some patients taking warfarin together with gefitinib (see section 4.5 Interaction with other medicinal products and other forms of interaction). Patients taking warfarin and gefitinib concomitantly should be monitored regularly for changes in prothrombin time (PT) or INR.

Medicinal products that cause significant sustained elevation in gastric pH, such as proton-pump inhibitors and h_2-antagonists may reduce bioavailability and plasma concentrations of gefitinib and, therefore, may reduce efficacy. Antacids if taken regularly close in time to administration of IRESSA may have a similar effect (see sections 4.5 Interaction with other medicinal products and other forms of interaction and 5.2 Pharmacokinetic properties).

Data from phase II clinical trials, where gefitinib and vinorelbine have been used concomitantly, indicate that gefitinib may exacerbate the neutropenic effect of vinorelbine.

Lactose

IRESSA contains lactose. Patients with rare hereditary problems of galactose intolerance, the Lapp lactose deficiency or glucose-galactose malabsorption should not take this medicinal product.

Further precautions for use

Patients should be advised to seek medical advice immediately if they experience:

- any eye symptoms.
- severe or persistent diarrhoea, nausea, vomiting or anorexia as these may indirectly lead to dehydration.

These symptoms should be managed as clinically indicated (see section 4.8 Undesirable effects).

In a phase I/II trial studying the use of gefitinib and radiation in paediatric patients, with newly diagnosed brain stem glioma or incompletely resected supratentorial malignant glioma, 4 cases (1 fatal) of Central Nervous System (CNS) haemorrhages were reported from 45 patients enrolled. A further case of CNS haemorrhage has been reported in a child with an ependymoma from a trial with gefitinib alone. An increased risk of cerebral haemorrhage in adult patients with NSCLC receiving gefitinib has not been established.

4.5 Interaction with other medicinal products and other forms of interaction

The metabolism of gefitinib is via the cytochrome P450 isoenzyme CYP3A4 (predominantly) and via CYP2D6.

Active substances that may increase gefitinib plasma concentrations

In vitro studies have shown that gefitinib is a substrate of p-glycoprotein (Pgp). Available data do not suggest any clinical consequences to this *in vitro* finding.

Substances that inhibit CYP3A4 may decrease the clearance of gefitinib. Concomitant administration with potent inhibitors of CYP3A4 activity (e.g. ketoconazole, posaconazole, voriconazole, protease inhibitors, clarithromycin, telithromycin) may increase gefitinib plasma concentrations. The increase may be clinically relevant since adverse reactions are related to dose and exposure. The increase might be higher in individual patients with CYP2D6 poor metaboliser genotype. Pre-treatment with itraconazole (a potent CYP3A4 inhibitor) resulted in an 80 % increase in the mean AUC of gefitinib in healthy volunteers. In situations of concomitant treatment with potent inhibitors of CYP3A4 the patient should be closely monitored for gefitinib adverse reactions.

There are no data on concomitant treatment with an inhibitor of CYP2D6 but potent inhibitors of this enzyme might cause increased plasma concentrations of gefitinib in CYP2D6 extensive metabolisers by about 2-fold (see section 5.2 Pharmacokinetic properties). If concomitant treatment with a potent CYP2D6 inhibitor is initiated, the patient should be closely monitored for adverse reactions.

Active substances that may reduce gefitinib plasma concentrations

Substances that are inducers of CYP3A4 activity may increase metabolism and decrease gefitinib plasma concentrations and thereby reduce the efficacy of IRESSA. Concomitant medicinal products that induce CYP3A4 (e.g. phenytoin, carbamazepine, rifampicin, barbiturates or St John's wort (*Hypericum perforatum*)), should be avoided. Pre-treatment with rifampicin (a potent CYP3A4 inducer) in healthy volunteers reduced mean gefitinib AUC by 83 % (see section 4.4 Special warnings and precautions for use).

Substances that cause significant sustained elevation in gastric pH may reduce gefitinib plasma concentrations and thereby reduce the efficacy of IRESSA. High doses of short-acting antacids may have a similar effect if taken regularly close in time to administration of gefitinib. Concomitant administration of gefitinib with ranitidine at a dose that caused sustained elevations in gastric pH $\geqslant 5$, resulted in a reduced mean gefitinib AUC by 47 % in healthy volunteers (see sections 4.4 Special warnings and precautions for use and 5.2 Pharmacokinetic properties).

Active substances that may have their plasma concentrations altered by gefitinib

In vitro studies have shown that gefitinib has limited potential to inhibit CYP2D6. In a clinical trial in patients, gefitinib was co-administered with metoprolol (a CYP2D6 substrate). This resulted in a 35 % increase in exposure to metoprolol. Such an increase might potentially be relevant for CYP2D6 substrates with narrow therapeutic index. When the use of CYP2D6 substrates are considered in combination with gefitinib, a dose modification of the CYP2D6 substrate should be considered especially for products with a narrow therapeutic window.

Gefitinib inhibits the transporter protein BCRP *in vitro*, but the clinical relevance of this finding is unknown.

Other potential interactions

INR elevations and/or bleeding events have been reported in some patients concomitantly taking warfarin (see section 4.4 Special warnings and precautions for use).

4.6 Pregnancy and lactation

There are no data from the use of gefitinib in pregnant women. Studies in animals have shown reproductive toxicity (see section 5.3 Preclinical safety data). The potential risk for humans is unknown. IRESSA should not be used during pregnancy unless clearly necessary, and women of childbearing potential must be advised not to get pregnant during therapy.

It is not known whether gefitinib is secreted in human milk. Gefitinib and metabolites of gefitinib accumulated in milk of lactating rats (see section 5.3 Preclinical safety data). IRESSA is contraindicated during breast-feeding and therefore breast-feeding must be discontinued while receiving IRESSA therapy (see section 4.3 Contraindications).

Table 2 Efficacy outcomes for gefitinib versus carboplatin/paclitaxel from the IPASS study

Population	N	Objective response rates and 95 % CI for difference between treatments[a]	Primary endpoint Progression free survival[ab]	Overall survival[abc]
Overall	1217	43.0 % vs 32.2 % [5.3 %, 16.1 %]	HR 0.74 [0.65, 0.85] 5.7 m vs 5.8 m p<0.0001	HR 0.91 [0.76, 1.10] 18.6 m vs 17. 3m
EGFR mutation-positive	261	71.2 % vs 47.3 % [12.0 %, 34.9 %]	HR 0.48 [0.36, 0.64] 9.5 m vs 6.3 m p<0.0001	HR 0.78 [0.50, 1.20] NR vs 19.5 m
EGFR mutation-negative	176	1.1 % vs 23.5 % [-32.5 %, -13.3 %]	HR 2.85 [2.05, 3.98] 1.5 m vs 5.5 m p<0.0001	HR 1.38 [0.92, 2.09] 12.1 m vs 12.6 m

a Values presented are for IRESSA versus carboplatin/paclitaxel.

b "m" is medians in months. Numbers in square brackets are 95 % confidence intervals for HR

c From early analysis, overall survival follow up is ongoing

NR Not reached

N Number of patients randomised.

HR Hazard ratio (hazard ratios <1 favour IRESSA)

Figures 1 and 2 Efficacy outcomes in subgroups of non-Asian patients in the INTEREST study

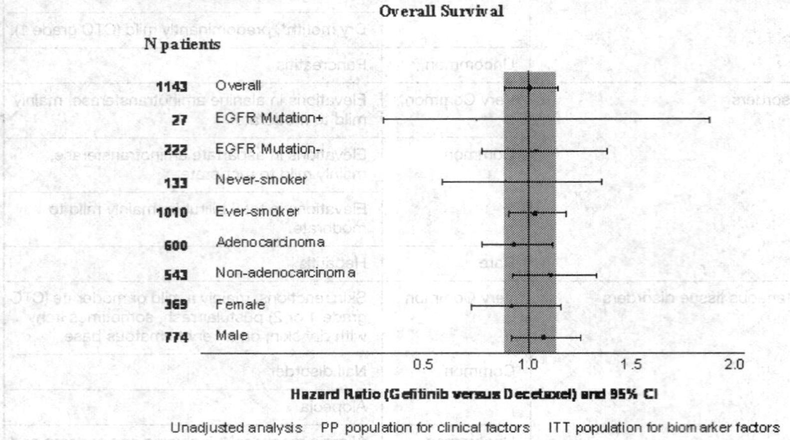

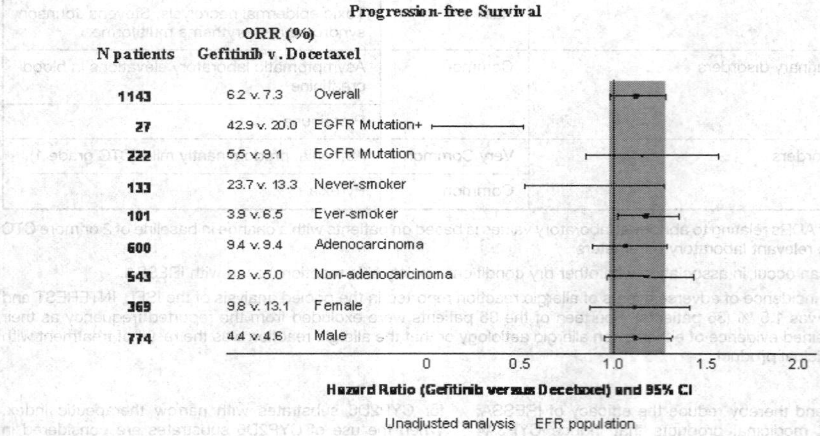

(N patients = Number of patients randomised)

4.7 Effects on ability to drive and use machines

IRESSA has no or negligible influence on the ability to drive and use machines.

However, during treatment with gefitinib, asthenia has been reported. Therefore, patients who experience this symptom should be cautious when driving or using machines.

4.8 Undesirable effects

In the pooled dataset from the ISEL, INTEREST and IPASS phase III clinical trials (2462 IRESSA-treated patients), the most frequently reported adverse drug reactions (ADRs), occurring in more than 20 % of the patients, are diarrhoea and skin reactions (including rash, acne, dry skin and pruritus). ADRs usually occur within the first month of therapy and are generally reversible. Approximately 8 % of patients had a severe ADR (common toxicity criteria, (CTC) grade 3 or 4). Approximately 3 % of patients stopped therapy due to an ADR.

Interstitial lung disease (ILD) has occurred in 1.3 % of patients, often severe (CTC grade 3-4). Cases with fatal outcomes have been reported.

The safety profile presented in Table 1 is based on the gefitinib clinical development programme and postmarketed experience. Adverse reactions have been assigned to the frequency categories in Table 1 based on the incidence of comparable adverse event reports in a pooled dataset from the ISEL, INTEREST and IPASS phase III clinical trials (2462 IRESSA-treated patients).

Frequencies of occurrence of undesirable effects are defined as: very common (⩾ 1/10); common (> 1/100 to < 1/10); uncommon (⩾ 1/1,000 to < 1/100); rare (⩾ 1/10,000 to < 1/1,000); very rare (< 1/10,000), not known (cannot be estimated from the available data).

Within each frequency grouping, undesirable effects are presented in order of decreasing seriousness.

Table 1 Adverse reactions

(see Table 1 on previous page)

Interstitial lung disease (ILD)

In the INTEREST trial, the incidence of ILD type events was 1.4 % (10) patients in the gefitinib group *vs.* 1.1 % (8) patients in the docetaxel group. One ILD-type event was fatal, and this occurred in a patient receiving gefitinib.

In the ISEL trial, the incidence of ILD-type events in the overall population was approximately 1 % in both treatment arms. The majority of ILD-type events reported was from patients of Asian ethnicity and the ILD incidence among patients of Asian ethnicity receiving gefitinib therapy and placebo was approximately 3 % and 4 % respectively. One ILD-type event was fatal, and this occurred in a patient receiving placebo.

In a post-marketing surveillance study in Japan (3350 patients) the reported rate of ILD-type events in patients receiving gefitinib was 5.8 %. The proportion of ILD-type events with a fatal outcome was 38.6 %.

In a phase III open-label clinical trial (IPASS) in 1217 patients comparing IRESSA to carboplatin/paclitaxel doublet chemotherapy as first-line treatment in selected patients with advanced NSCLC in Asia, the incidence of ILD-type events was 2.6 % on the IRESSA treatment arm versus 1.4 % on the carboplatin/paclitaxel treatment arm.

4.9 Overdose

There is no specific treatment in the event of overdose of gefitinib, and possible symptoms of overdose are not established. However, in phase I clinical trials, a limited number of patients were treated with daily doses of up to 1000 mg. An increase of frequency and severity of some adverse reactions was observed, mainly diarrhoea and skin rash. Adverse reactions associated with overdose should be treated symptomatically; in particular severe diarrhoea should be managed appropriately.

5. PHARMACOLOGICAL PROPERTIES

5.1 Pharmacodynamic properties

Pharmacotherapeutic group: Protein kinase inhibitors; ATC code: L01XE02

Mechanism of action

The epidermal growth factor (EGF) and its receptor (EGFR [HER1; ErbB1]) have been identified as key drivers in the process of cell growth and proliferation for normal and cancer cells. EGFR activating mutation within a cancer cell is an important factor in promotion of tumour cell growth, blocking of apoptosis, increasing the production of angiogenic factors and facilitating the processes of metastasis.

Gefitinib is a selective small molecule inhibitor of the epidermal growth factor receptor tyrosine kinase and is an effective treatment for patients with tumours with activating mutations of the EGFR tyrosine kinase domain regardless of line of therapy. No clinically relevant activity has been shown in patients with known EGFR mutation-negative tumours.

First line treatment

The randomised phase III first line IPASS study was conducted in patients in Asia[1] with advanced (stage IIIB or IV) NSCLC of adenocarcinoma histology who were ex-light smokers (ceased smoking ≥ 15 years ago and smoked ≤ 10 pack years) or never smokers (see Table 2).

[1]China, Hong Kong, Indonesia, Japan, Malaysia, Philippines, Singapore, Taiwan and Thailand.

Table 2 Efficacy outcomes for gefitinib versus carboplatin/paclitaxel from the IPASS study

(see Table 2 above)

Quality of life outcomes differed according to EGFR mutation status. In EGFR mutation-positive patients, significantly more IRESSA-treated patients experienced an improvement in quality of life and lung cancer symptoms vs carboplatin/paclitaxel (see Table 3).

Table 3 Quality of life outcomes for gefitinib versus carboplatin/paclitaxel from the IPASS study

Population	N	FACT-L QoL improvement rate [a] %	LCS symptom improvement rate [a] %
Overall	1151	(48.0 % vs 40.8 %) p=0.0148	(51.5 % vs 48.5 %) p=0.3037
EGFR mutation-positive	259	(70.2 % vs 44.5 %) p<0.0001	(75.6 % vs 53.9 %) p=0.0003
EGFR mutation-negative	169	(14.6 % vs 36.3 %) p=0.0021	(20.2 % vs 47.5 %) p=0.0002

Trial outcome index results were supportive of FACT-L and LCS results

[a] Values presented are for IRESSA versus carboplatin/paclitaxel.

N Number of patients evaluable for quality of life analyses

QoL Quality of life

FACT-L Functional assessment of cancer therapy-lung

LCS Lung cancer subscale

Pretreated Patients

The randomised phase III INTEREST study was conducted in patients with locally advanced or metastatic NSCLC who had previously received platinum-based chemotherapy. In the overall population, no statistically significant difference between gefitinib and docetaxel (75 mg/m2) was observed

Table 4 Efficacy outcomes for gefitinib versus docetaxel from the INTEREST study

Population	N	Objective response rates and 95 % CI for difference between treatments[a]	Progression free survival[ab]	Primary endpoint overall survival[ab]
Overall	1466	9.1 % vs 7.6 % [-1.5 %, 4.5 %]	HR 1.04 [0.93,1.18] 2.2 m vs 2.7 m p=0.4658	HR 1.020 [0.905, 1.150] [c] 7.6 m vs 8.0 m p=0.7332
EGFR mutation-positive	44	42.1 % vs 21.1 % [-8.2 %, 46.0 %]	HR 0.16 [0.05, 0.49] 7.0 m vs 4.1 m p=0.0012	HR 0.83 [0.41, 1.67] 14.2 m vs 16.6 m p=0.6043
EGFR mutation- negative	253	6.6 % vs 9.8 % [-10.5 %, 4.4 %]	HR 1.24 [0.94,1.64] 1.7 m vs 2.6 m p=0.1353	HR 1.02 [0.78, 1.33] 6.4 m vs 6.0 m p=0.9131
Asians[c]	323	19.7 % vs 8.7 % [3.1 %, 19.2 %]	HR 0.83 [0.64,1.08] 2.9 m vs 2.8 m p=0.1746	HR 1.04 [0.80, 1.35] 10.4 m vs 12.2 m p=0.7711
Non-Asians	1143	6.2 % vs 7.3 % [-4.3 %, 2.0 %]	HR 1.12 [0.98, 1.28] 2.0 m vs 2.7 m p=0.1041	HR 1.01 [0.89, 1.14] 6.9 m vs 6.9 m p=0.9259

a Values presented are for IRESSA versus docetaxel.

b "m" is medians in months. Numbers in square brackets are 96 % confidence interval for overall survival HR in the overall population, or otherwise 95 % confidence intervals for HR

c Confidence interval entirely below non-inferiority margin of 1.154

N Number of patients randomised.

HR Hazard ratio (hazard ratios <1 favour IRESSA)

Table 5 Efficacy outcomes for gefitinib versus placebo from the ISEL study

Population	N	Objective response rates and 95 % CI for difference between treatments[a]	Time to treatment failure[ab]	Primary endpoint overall survival[abc]
Overall	1692	8.0 % vs 1.3 % [4.7 %, 8.8 %]	HR 0.82 [0.73, 0.92] 3.0 m vs 2.6 m p=0.0006	HR 0.89 [0.77,1.02] 5.6 m vs 5.1 m p=0.0871
EGFR mutation- positive	26	37.5 % vs 0 % [-15.1 %, 61.4 %]	HR 0.79 [0.20, 3.12] 10.8 m vs 3.8m p=0.7382	HR NC NR vs 4.3 m
EGFR mutation- negative	189	2.6 % vs 0 % [-5.6 %, 7.3 %]	HR 1.10 [0.78, 1.56] 2.0 m vs 2.6 m p=0.5771	HR 1.16 [0.79, 1.72] 3.7 m vs 5.9 m p=0.4449
Never smoker	375	18.1 % vs 0 % [12.3 %, 24.0 %]	HR 0.55 [0.42, 0.72] 5.6 m vs 2.8 m p<0.0001	HR 0.67 [0.49, 0.92] 8.9 m vs 6.1 m p=0.0124
Ever smoker	1317	5.3 % vs 1.6 % [1.4 %, 5.7 %]	HR 0.89 [0.78, 1.01] 2.7 m vs 2.6 m p=0.0707	HR 0.92 [0.79, 1.06] 5.0 m vs 4.9 m p=0.2420
Asians[d]	342	12.4 % vs 2.1 % [4.0 %, 15.8 %]	HR 0.69 [0.52, 0.91] 4.4 m vs 2.2 m p=0.0084	HR 0.66 [0.48, 0.91] 9.5 m vs 5.5 m p=0.0100
Non-Asians	1350	6.8 % vs 1.0 % [3.5 %, 7.9 %]	HR 0.86 [0.76, 0.98] 2.9 m vs 2.7 m p=0.0197	HR 0.92 [0.80, 1.07] 5.2 m vs 5.1 m p=0.2942

a Values presented are for IRESSA versus placebo.

b "m" is medians in months. Numbers in square brackets are 95 % confidence intervals for HR

c Stratified log-rank test for overall; otherwise cox proportional hazards model

d Asian ethnicity excludes patients of Indian origin and refers to the racial origin of a patient group and not necessarily their place of birth

N Number of patients randomised

NC Not calculated for overall survival HR as the number of events is too few

NR Not reached

HR Hazard ratio (hazard ratios <1 favour IRESSA)

for overall survival, progression free survival and objective response rates (see table 4).

Table 4 Efficacy outcomes for gefitinib versus docetaxel from the INTEREST study

(see Table 4 above)

Figures 1 and 2 Efficacy outcomes in subgroups of non-Asian patients in the INTEREST study

(see Figures 1 and 2 on previous page)

The randomised phase III ISEL study, was conducted in patients with advanced NSCLC who had received 1 or 2 prior chemotherapy regimens and were refractory or intolerant to their most recent regimen. Gefitinib plus best supportive care was compared to placebo plus best supportive care. IRESSA did not prolong survival in the overall population. Survival outcomes differed by smoking status and ethnicity (see Table 5).

Table 5 Efficacy outcomes for gefitinib versus placebo from the ISEL study

(see Table 5 above)

EGFR mutation status and clinical characteristics

Clinical characteristics of never smoker, adenocarcinoma histology, and female gender have been shown to be independent predictors of positive EGFR mutation status in a multivariate analysis of 786 Caucasian patients from gefitinib studies* (see Table 6). Asian patients also have a higher incidence of EGFR mutation-positive tumours (see Tables 4 and 5).

*Table 6 Summary of multivariate logistic regression analysis to identify factors that independently predicted for the presence of EGFR mutations in 786 Caucasian patients**

(see Table 6 on next page)

5.2 Pharmacokinetic properties

Absorption

Following oral administration of gefitinib, absorption is moderately slow and peak plasma concentrations of gefitinib typically occur at 3 to 7 hours after administration. Mean absolute bioavailability is 59 % in cancer patients. Exposure to gefitinib is not significantly altered by food. In a trial in healthy volunteers where gastric pH was maintained above pH 5, gefitinib exposure was reduced by 47 %, likely due to impaired solubility of gefitinib in the stomach (see sections 4.4 Special warnings and precautions for use and 4.5 Interaction with other medicinal products and other forms of interaction).

Distribution

Gefitinib has a mean steady state volume of distribution of 1400 l indicating extensive distribution into tissue. Plasma protein binding is approximately 90 %. Gefitinib binds to serum albumin and alpha 1-acid glycoprotein.

In vitro data indicate that gefitinib is a substrate for the membrane transport protein Pgp.

Metabolism

In vitro data indicate that CYP3A4 and CYP2D6 are the major P450 isozyme involved in the oxidative metabolism of gefitinib.

In vitro studies have shown that gefitinib has limited potential to inhibit CYP2D6. Gefitinib shows no enzyme induction effects in animal studies and no significant inhibition (*in vitro*) of any other cytochrome P450 enzyme.

Gefitinib is extensively metabolised in humans. Five metabolites have been fully identified in excreta and 8 metabolites in plasma. The major metabolite identified was O-desmethyl gefitinib, which is 14-fold less potent than gefitinib at inhibiting EGFR stimulated cell growth and has no inhibitory effect on tumour cell growth in mice. It is therefore considered unlikely that it contributes to the clinical activity of gefitinib.

The formation of O-desmethyl gefitinib has been shown, *in vitro*, to be via CYP2D6. The role of CYP2D6 in the metabolic clearance of gefitinib has been evaluated in a clinical trial in healthy volunteers genotyped for CYP2D6 status. In poor metabolisers no measurable levels of O-desmethyl gefitinib were produced. The levels of exposure to gefitinib achieved in both the extensive and the poor metaboliser groups were wide and overlapping but the mean exposure to gefitinib was 2-fold higher in the poor metaboliser group. The higher average exposures that could be achieved by individuals with no active CYP2D6 may be clinically relevant since adverse effects are related to dose and exposure.

Elimination

Gefitinib is excreted mainly as metabolites via the faeces, with renal elimination of gefitinib and metabolites accounting for less than 4 % of the administered dose.

Gefitinib total plasma clearance is approximately 500 ml/min and the mean terminal half-life is 41 hours in cancer patients. Administration of gefitinib once daily results in 2 to 8-fold accumulation, with steady state exposures achieved after 7 to 10 doses. At steady state, circulating plasma concentrations are typically maintained within a 2- to 3-fold range over the 24-hour dosing interval.

Special populations

From analyses of population pharmacokinetic data in cancer patients, no relationships were identified between predicted steady state trough concentration and patient age, body weight, gender, ethnicity or creatinine clearance (above 20 ml/min).

Hepatic impairment

In a phase I open-label study of single dose gefitinib 250 mg in patients with mild, moderate or severe hepatic impairment due to cirrhosis (according to Child-Pugh classification), there was an increase in exposure in all groups compared with healthy controls. An average 3.1-fold increase in exposure to gefitinib in patients with moderate and severe hepatic impairment was observed. None of the patients had cancer, all had cirrhosis and some had hepatitis. This increase in exposure may be of clinical relevance since adverse experiences are related to dose and exposure to gefitinib.

Gefitinib has been evaluated in a clinical trial conducted in 41 patients with solid tumours and normal hepatic function, or moderate or severe hepatic impairment (classified according to baseline Common Toxicity Criteria grades for AST, alkaline phosphatase and bilirubin) due to liver metastases. It was shown that following daily administration of 250 mg gefitinib, time to steady state, total plasma clearance (C_{maxSS}) and steady-state exposure (AUC_{24SS}) were similar for the groups with normal and moderately impaired hepatic function. Data from 4 patients with severe hepatic impairment due to liver metastases suggested that steady-state exposures in these patients are also similar to those in patients with normal hepatic function.

5.3 Preclinical safety data

Adverse reactions not observed in clinical studies, but seen in animals at exposure levels similar to the clinical exposure levels and with possible relevance to clinical use were as follows:

- Corneal epithelia atrophy and corneal translucencies
- Renal papillary necrosis

Table 6 Summary of multivariate logistic regression analysis to identify factors that independently predicted for the presence of EGFR mutations in 786 Caucasian patients*

Factors that predicted for presence of EGFR mutation	p-value	Odds of EGFR mutation	Positive predictive value (9.5 % of the overall population are EGFR mutation-positive (M+))
Smoking status	<0.0001	6.5 times higher in never smokers than ever-smokers	28/70 (40 %) of never smokers are M+ 47/716 (7 %) of ever smokers are M+
Histology	<0.0001	4.4 times higher in adenocarcinoma than in non-adenocarcinoma	63/396 (16 %) of patients with adenocarcinoma histology are M+ 12/390 (3 %) of patients with non-adenocarcinoma histology are M+
Gender	0.0397	1.7 times higher in females than males	40/235 (17 %) of females are M+ 35/551 (6 %) of males are M+

* from the following studies: INTEREST, ISEL, INTACT 1&2, IDEAL 1&2, INVITE

– Hepatocellular necrosis and eosinophilic sinusoidal macrophage infiltration

Data from *in vitro* studies indicate that gefitinib has the potential to inhibit cardiac repolarization (e.g. QT interval). The clinical significance of these findings is unknown.

A reduction in female fertility was observed in the rat at a dose of 20 mg/kg/day.

Published studies have shown that genetically modified mice, lacking expression of EGFR, exhibit developmental defects, related to epithelial immaturity in a variety of organs including the skin, gastrointestinal tract and lung. When gefitinib was administered to rats during organogenesis, there were no effects on embryofoetal development at the highest dose (30 mg/kg/day). However, in the rabbit, there were reduced foetal weights at 20 mg/kg/day and above. There were no compound-induced malformations in either species. When administered to the rat throughout gestation and parturition, there was a reduction in pup survival at a dose of 20 mg/kg/day.

Following oral administration of C-14 labelled gefitinib to lactating rats 14 days post partum, concentrations of radioactivity in milk were 11-19 fold higher than in blood.

Gefitinib showed no genotoxic potential.

A 2-year carcinogenicity study in rats resulted in a small but statistically significant increased incidence of hepatocellular adenomas in both male and female rats and mesenteric lymph node haemangiosarcomas in female rats at the highest dose (10 mg/kg/day) only. The hepatocellular adenomas were also seen in a 2-year carcinogenicity study in mice, which demonstrated a small increased incidence of this finding in male mice at the mid dose, and in both male and female mice at the highest dose. The effects reached statistical significance for the female mice, but not for the males. At no-effect levels in both mice and rats there was no margin in clinical exposure. The clinical relevance of these findings is unknown.

The results of an *in vitro* phototoxicity study demonstrated that gefitinib may have phototoxicity potential.

6. PHARMACEUTICAL PARTICULARS

6.1 List of excipients

Tablet core:

Lactose monohydrate

Microcrystalline cellulose (E460)

Croscarmellose sodium

Povidone (K29-32) (E1201)

Sodium laurilsulfate

Magnesium stearate

Tablet coating:

Hypromellose (E464)

Macrogol 300

Titanium dioxide (E171)

Yellow iron oxide (E172)

Red iron oxide (E172)

6.2 Incompatibilities

Not applicable.

6.3 Shelf life

4 years.

6.4 Special precautions for storage

Store in the original package in order to protect from moisture.

6.5 Nature and contents of container

PVC/Aluminium blister containing 10 tablets.

3 blisters are combined with an aluminium foil laminate over-wrap in a carton.

Pack size of 30 film-coated tablets.

6.6 Special precautions for disposal and other handling

Any unused product or waste material should be disposed of in accordance with local requirements.

7. MARKETING AUTHORISATION HOLDER

AstraZeneca AB

S-151 85

Sodertalje

Sweden

8. MARKETING AUTHORISATION NUMBER(S)

EU/1/09/526/001

9. DATE OF FIRST AUTHORISATION/RENEWAL OF THE AUTHORISATION

24th June 2009

10. DATE OF REVISION OF THE TEXT

Detailed information on this medicinal product is available on the website of the European Medicines Agency (EMEA) http://www.emea.europa.eu/.

Isentress 400 mg Film-coated Tablets

(Merck Sharp & Dohme Limited)

1. NAME OF THE MEDICINAL PRODUCT

ISENTRESS® 400 mg film-coated tablets ▼

2. QUALITATIVE AND QUANTITATIVE COMPOSITION

Each film-coated tablet contains 400 mg of raltegravir (as potassium).

Excipient: Each tablet contains 26.06 mg lactose monohydrate.

For a full list of excipients, see section 6.1.

3. PHARMACEUTICAL FORM

Film-coated tablet.

Pink, oval tablet, marked with "227" on one side.

4. CLINICAL PARTICULARS

4.1 Therapeutic indications

ISENTRESS is indicated in combination with other anti-retroviral medicinal products for the treatment of human immunodeficiency virus (HIV-1) infection in adult patients.

This indication is based on safety and efficacy data from two double-blind, placebo-controlled trials of 48 weeks duration in treatment-experienced patients and one double-blind, active-controlled trial of 48 weeks duration in treatment-naïve patients (see sections 4.4 and 5.1).

4.2 Posology and method of administration

Therapy should be initiated by a physician experienced in the management of HIV infection. ISENTRESS should be used in combination with other active anti-retroviral therapies (ARTs) (see sections 4.4 and 5.1). The use of raltegravir in previously ART-naïve patients is based on a study in which it was co-administered with two NRTIs (see sections 4.4 and 5.1).

Posology

Adults

The recommended dosage of ISENTRESS is 400 mg administered twice daily with or without food. The effect of food on absorption of raltegravir is uncertain (see section 5.2). It is not recommended to chew, crush or split the tablets.

Elderly

There is limited information regarding the use of ISENTRESS in the elderly (see section 5.2). Therefore ISENTRESS should be used with caution in this population.

Children and adolescents

Safety and efficacy have not been established in patients below 16 years of age (see sections 5.1 and 5.2).

Renal impairment

No dosage adjustment is required for patients with renal impairment (see section 5.2).

Hepatic impairment

No dosage adjustment is required for patients with mild to moderate hepatic impairment. The safety and efficacy of ISENTRESS have not been established in patients with severe underlying liver disorders. Therefore ISENTRESS should be used with caution in patients with severe hepatic impairment (see sections 4.4 and 5.2).

Method of administration

Oral

4.3 Contraindications

Hypersensitivity to the active substance or to any of the excipients.

4.4 Special warnings and precautions for use

Patients should be advised that current anti-retroviral therapy does not cure HIV and has not been proven to prevent the transmission of HIV to others through blood or sexual contact. Appropriate precautions should continue to be employed.

Overall, considerable inter- and intra-subject variability was observed in the pharmacokinetics of raltegravir (see sections 4.5 and 5.2).

Raltegravir has a relatively low genetic barrier to resistance. Therefore, whenever possible, raltegravir should be administered with two other active ARTs to minimise the potential for virological failure and the development of resistance (see section 5.1).

In treatment naïve patients, the clinical study data on use of raltegravir are limited to use in combination with two nucleotide reverse transcriptase inhibitors (NRTIs) (emtricitabine and tenofovir disoproxil fumarate).

The safety and efficacy of ISENTRESS have not been established in patients with severe underlying liver disorders. Therefore ISENTRESS should be used with caution in patients with severe hepatic impairment (see sections 4.2 and 5.2).

Patients with pre-existing liver dysfunction including chronic hepatitis have an increased frequency of liver function abnormalities during combination anti-retroviral therapy and should be monitored according to standard practice. If there is evidence of worsening liver disease in such patients, interruption or discontinuation of treatment should be considered.

There are very limited data on the use of raltegravir in patients co-infected with HIV and hepatitis B virus (HBV) or hepatitis C virus (HCV). Patients with chronic hepatitis B or C and treated with combination anti-retroviral therapy are at an increased risk for severe and potentially fatal hepatic adverse events.

Osteonecrosis

Although the etiology is considered to be multifactorial (including corticosteroid use, alcohol consumption, severe immunosuppression, higher body mass index), cases of osteonecrosis have been reported particularly in patients with advanced HIV disease and/or long-term exposure to combination anti-retroviral therapy. Patients should be advised to seek medical advice if they experience joint aches and pain, joint stiffness or difficulty in movement.

Immune reactivation syndrome

In HIV-infected patients with severe immune deficiency at the time of institution of combination anti-retroviral therapy (CART), an inflammatory reaction to asymptomatic or residual opportunistic pathogens may arise and cause serious clinical conditions, or aggravation of symptoms. Typically, such reactions have been observed within the first weeks or months of initiation of CART. Relevant examples are cytomegalovirus retinitis, generalised and/or focal mycobacterial infections and pneumonia caused by *Pneumocystis jiroveci* (formerly known as *Pneumocystis carinii*). Any inflammatory symptoms should be evaluated and treatment instituted when necessary.

Caution should be used when co-administering ISENTRESS with strong inducers of uridine diphosphate glucuronosyltransferase (UGT) 1A1 (e.g., rifampicin). Rifampicin reduces plasma levels of raltegravir; the impact on the efficacy of raltegravir is unknown. However, if co-administration with rifampicin is unavoidable, a doubling of the dose of ISENTRESS can be considered (see section 4.5).

Myopathy and rhabdomyolysis have been reported; however, the relationship of ISENTRESS to these events is not known. Use with caution in patients who have had myopathy or rhabdomyolysis in the past or have any predisposing issues including other medicinal products associated with these conditions (see section 4.8).

ISENTRESS contains lactose. Patients with rare hereditary problems of galactose intolerance, the Lapp lactase deficiency or glucose-galactose malabsorption should not take this medicine.

4.5 Interaction with other medicinal products and other forms of interaction

In vitro studies indicated that raltegravir is not a substrate of cytochrome P450 (CYP) enzymes, does not inhibit CYP1A2, CYP2B6, CYP2C8, CYP2C9, CYP2C19, CYP2D6 or CYP3A, does not induce CYP3A4 and does not inhibit P-glycoprotein-mediated transport. Based on these data, ISENTRESS is not expected to affect the pharmacokinetics of medicinal products that are substrates of these enzymes or P-glycoprotein.

Based on *in vitro* and *in vivo* studies, raltegravir is eliminated mainly by metabolism via a UGT1A1-mediated glucuronidation pathway.

Although *in vitro* studies indicated that raltegravir is not an inhibitor of the UDP glucuronosyltransferases (UGTs) 1A1 and 2B7, one clinical study has suggested that some inhibition of UGT1A1 may occur *in vivo* based on effects observed on bilirubin glucuronidation. However, the magnitude of the effect seems unlikely to result in clinically important drug-drug interactions.

Considerable inter- and intra-individual variability was observed in the pharmacokinetics of raltegravir. The following drug interaction information is based on Geometric

Mean values; the effect for an individual patient cannot be predicted precisely.

Effect of raltegravir on the pharmacokinetics of other medicinal products

In interaction studies, raltegravir did not have a clinically meaningful effect on the pharmacokinetics of etravirine, maraviroc, tenofovir, hormonal contraceptives, methadone, or midazolam.

Effect of other agents on the pharmacokinetics of raltegravir

Given that raltegravir is metabolised primarily via UGT1A1, caution should be used when co-administering ISENTRESS with strong inducers of UGT1A1 (e.g., rifampicin). Rifampicin reduces plasma levels of raltegravir; the impact on the efficacy of raltegravir is unknown. However, if co-administration with rifampicin is unavoidable, a doubling of the dose of ISENTRESS can be considered (see section 4.4). The impact of other strong inducers of drug metabolising enzymes, such as phenytoin and phenobarbital, on UGT1A1 is unknown. Less potent inducers (e.g., efavirenz, nevirapine, etravirine, rifabutin, glucocorticoids, St. John's wort, pioglitazone) may be used with the recommended dose of ISENTRESS.

Co-administration of ISENTRESS with medicinal products that are known to be potent UGT1A1 inhibitors (e.g., atazanavir) may increase plasma levels of raltegravir. Less potent UGT1A1 inhibitors (e.g., indinavir, saquinavir) may also increase plasma levels of raltegravir, but to a lesser extent compared with atazanavir. In addition, tenofovir may increase plasma levels of raltegravir, however, the mechanism for this effect is unknown (see Table 1). From the clinical trials, a large proportion of patients used atazanavir and / or tenofovir, both agents that result in increases in raltegravir plasma levels, in the optimised background regimens. The safety profile observed in patients who used atazanavir and / or tenofovir was generally similar to the safety profile of patients who did not use these agents. Therefore no dose adjustment is required.

In healthy subjects, co-administration of ISENTRESS with omeprazole increases raltegravir plasma levels. As the effects of increasing gastric pH on the absorption of raltegravir in HIV-infected patients are uncertain, use ISENTRESS with medicinal products that increase gastric pH (e.g., proton pump inhibitors and H2 antagonists) only if unavoidable.

Table 1

Pharmacokinetic Interaction Data

(see Table 1 opposite)

4.6 Pregnancy and lactation

Pregnancy

There are no adequate data from the use of raltegravir in pregnant women. Studies in animals have shown reproductive toxicity (see section 5.3). The potential risk for humans is unknown. ISENTRESS should not be used during pregnancy.

Anti-retroviral Pregnancy Registry

To monitor maternal-foetal outcomes in patients inadvertently administered ISENTRESS while pregnant, an Antiretroviral Pregnancy Registry has been established. Physicians are encouraged to register patients in this registry.

Lactation

It is not known whether raltegravir is secreted in human milk. However, raltegravir is secreted in the milk of lactating rats. In rats, at a maternal dose of 600 mg/kg/day, mean active substance concentrations in milk were approximately 3-fold greater than in maternal plasma. Breastfeeding is not recommended while taking ISENTRESS. In addition, it is recommended that HIV-infected mothers should not breastfeed their infants to avoid risking postnatal transmission of HIV.

4.7 Effects on ability to drive and use machines

No studies have been performed on the effects of ISENTRESS on the ability to drive and use machines. However, dizziness has been reported in some patients during treatment with regimens containing ISENTRESS, which may influence some patients' ability to drive and use machines (see section 4.8).

4.8 Undesirable effects

The safety profile of ISENTRESS was based on the pooled safety data from two Phase III clinical studies in treatment-experienced patients and one Phase III clinical study in treatment-naïve patients; described below.

In treatment-experienced patients, the two randomised clinical studies used the recommended dose of 400 mg twice daily in combination with optimised background therapy (OBT) in 462 patients, in comparison to 237 patients taking placebo in combination with OBT. During double-blind treatment, the total follow-up was 470.5 patient-years in the group receiving ISENTRESS 400 mg twice daily, and 179.1 patient-years in the group receiving placebo.

In treatment-naïve patients, the multi-centre, randomised, double-blind, active-controlled clinical study used the recommended dose of 400 mg twice daily in combination with a fixed dose of emtricitabine 200 mg (+) tenofovir 245 mg in 281 patients, in comparison to 282 patients taking efavirenz (EFV) 600 mg (at bedtime) in combination with emtricitabine (+) tenofovir. During double-blind treatment,

Table 1 Pharmacokinetic Interaction Data

Medicinal products by therapeutic area	**Interaction** (mechanism, if known)	**Recommendations concerning co-administration**
ANTI-RETROVIRAL		
Protease inhibitors (PI)		
atazanavir /ritonavir (raltegravir 400 mg Twice Daily)	raltegravir AUC ↑ 41% raltegravir C_{12hr} ↑ 77% raltegravir C_{max} ↑ 24% (UGT1A1 inhibition)	No dose adjustment required for ISENTRESS.
tipranavir /ritonavir (raltegravir 400 mg Twice Daily)	raltegravir AUC ↓24% raltegravir C_{12hr}↓55% raltegravir C_{max}↓18% (UGT1A1 induction)	No dose adjustment required for ISENTRESS.
Non-nucleoside reverse transcriptase inhibitors (NNRTIs)		
efavirenz (raltegravir 400 mg Single Dose)	raltegravir AUC ↓36% raltegravir C_{12hr}↓21% raltegravir C_{max}↓36% (UGT1A1 induction)	No dose adjustment required for ISENTRESS.
etravirine (raltegravir 400 mg Twice Daily)	raltegravir AUC ↓ 10 % raltegravir C_{12hr}↓ 34 % raltegravir C_{max}↓ 11 % (UGT1A1 induction) etravirine AUC ↑ 10 % etravirine C_{12hr} ↑ 17 % etravirine C_{max} ↑ 4 %	No dose adjustment required for ISENTRESS or etravirine.
Nucleoside/tide reverse transcriptase inhibitors		
tenofovir (raltegravir 400 mg Twice Daily)	raltegravir AUC ↑ 49% raltegravir C_{12hr} ↑ 3% raltegravir C_{max} ↑ 64% (mechanism of interaction unknown) tenofovir AUC ↓10% tenofovir C_{12hr}↓13% tenofovir C_{max}↓23%	No dose adjustment required for ISENTRESS or tenofovir disoproxil fumarate.
CCR5 inhibitors		
maraviroc (raltegravir 400 mg Twice Daily)	raltegravir AUC ↓ 37 % raltegravir C_{12hr}↓ 28 % raltegravir C_{max}↓ 33% (mechanism of interaction unknown) maraviroc AUC ↓ 14 % maraviroc C_{12hr}↓ 10 % maraviroc C_{max}↓ 21 %	No dose adjustment required for ISENTRESS or maraviroc.
ANTIMICROBIALS		
Antimycobacterial		
rifampicin (raltegravir 400 mg Single Dose)	raltegravir AUC ↓40% raltegravir C_{12hr}↓61% raltegravir C_{max}↓38% (UGT1A1 induction)	Rifampicin reduces plasma levels of ISENTRESS. If co-administration with rifampicin is unavoidable, a doubling of the dose of ISENTRESS can be considered (see section 4.4).
SEDATIVE		
midazolam (raltegravir 400 mg Twice Daily)	midazolam AUC ↓8% midazolam C_{max} ↑ 3%	No dosage adjustment required for ISENTRESS or midazolam. These results indicate that raltegravir is not an inducer or inhibitor of CYP3A4, and raltegravir is thus not anticipated to affect the pharmacokinetics of medicinal products which are CYP3A4 substrates.
ANTI-ULCER		
omeprazole (raltegravir 400 mg Single Dose)	raltegravir AUC ↑ 212% raltegravir $C_{12\,hr}$ ↑ 46% raltegravir C_{max} ↑ 315%	Co-administration of proton pump inhibitors or other antiulcer medicinal products may increase plasma levels of raltegravir. Do not use ISENTRESS with medicinal products that increase gastric pH unless this is unavoidable.
HORMONAL CONTRACEPTIVES		
Ethinyl Estradiol Norelgestromin (raltegravir 400 mg Twice Daily)	Ethinyl Estradiol AUC ↓ 2 % Ethinyl Estradiol C_{max} ↑ 1 % Norelgestromin AUC ↑ 14 % Norelgestromin C_{max} ↑ 29 %	No dosage adjustment required for ISENTRESS or hormonal contraceptives (estrogen- and/or progesterone-based)
OPIOID ANALGESICS		
methadone (raltegravir 400 mg Twice Daily)	methadone AUC ↔ methadone C_{max}↔	No dose adjustment required for ISENTRESS or methadone.

the total follow-up was 333 patient-years in the group receiving ISENTRESS 400 mg twice daily, and 317 patient-years in the group receiving efavirenz 600 mg at bedtime.

In the pooled analysis of treatment-experienced patients, the rates of discontinuation of therapy due to adverse reactions were 2.4 % in patients receiving ISENTRESS + OBT and 3.0 % in patients receiving placebo + OBT. The rates of discontinuation of therapy in naïve patients due to adverse reactions were 3.2 % in patients receiving ISENTRESS + emtricitabine (+) tenofovir and 6.4 % in patients receiving efavirenz + emtricitabine (+) tenofovir.

Adverse reactions considered by investigators to be causally related to ISENTRESS (alone or in combination with other ART) are listed below by System Organ Class. Any term that includes at least one serious adverse reaction is identified with a dagger (†). Adverse reactions identified from post-marketing experience are included in italics.

Frequencies are defined as common (≥ 1/100 to < 1/10), uncommon (≥ 1/1,000 to < 1/100), and not known (cannot be estimated from the available data).

(see Table 1a opposite)

Table 1a

System Organ Class	Frequency	Adverse reactions ISENTRESS (alone or in combination with other ART)
Infections and infestations	uncommon	genital herpes†, folliculitis, gastro-enteritis, herpes simplex, herpes virus infection, herpes zoster, influenza, molluscum contagiosum, nasopharyngitis
Neoplasms benign, malignant and unspecified (including cysts and polyps)	uncommon	skin papilloma
Blood and lymphatic system disorders	uncommon	iron deficiency anaemia, lymph node pain, neutropenia
Immune system disorders	uncommon	immune reconstitution syndrome†, drug hypersensitivity, hypersensitivity
Metabolism and nutrition disorders	uncommon	anorexia, decreased appetite, diabetes mellitus, dyslipidaemia, hypercholesterolaemia, hyperglycaemia, hyperphagia, increased appetite, polydipsia
Psychiatric disorders	common	abnormal dreams, insomnia
	uncommon	mental disorder†, anxiety, confusional state, depressed mood, depression, middle insomnia, mood altered, nightmare, sleep disorder
	not known	*suicidal ideation, suicidal behaviour (particularly in patients with a pre-existing history of psychiatric illness)*
Nervous system disorders	common	dizziness, headache
	uncommon	amnesia, carpal tunnel syndrome, cognitive disorder, disturbance in attention, dizziness postural, dysgeusia, hypersomnia, hypoaesthesia, lethargy, memory impairment, migraine, neuropathy peripheral, paraesthesia, somnolence, tension headache, tremor
Eye disorders	uncommon	visual disturbance
Ear and labyrinth disorders	common	vertigo
	uncommon	tinnitus
Cardiac disorders	uncommon	palpitations, sinus bradycardia, ventricular extrasystoles
Vascular disorders	uncommon	hot flush, hypertension
Respiratory, thoracic and mediastinal disorders	uncommon	dysphonia, epistaxis, nasal congestion
Gastro-intestinal disorders	common	abdominal distention, abdominal pain, diarrhoea, flatulence, nausea, vomiting
	uncommon	gastritis†, abdominal discomfort, abdominal pain upper, abdominal tenderness, anorectal discomfort, dry mouth, constipation, dyspepsia, eructation, gastro-oesophageal reflux disease, odynophagia, pancreatitis acute, peptic ulcer, rectal haemorrhage, stomach discomfort
Hepato-biliary disorders	uncommon	hepatitis†
Skin and subcutaneous tissue disorders	common	rash
	uncommon	acne, alopecia, dermatitis acneiforme, dry skin, erythema, hyperhidrosis, lipodystrophy acquired, lipohypertrophy, night sweats, prurigo, pruritis, pruritis generalised, rash macular, rash maculo-papular, rash pruritic, skin lesion, urticaria, xeroderma
	not known	*Stevens Johnson syndrome*
Musculoskeletal and connective tissue disorders	uncommon	arthralgia, arthritis, back pain, lumbarisation, musculoskeletal pain, myalgia, neck pain, pain in extremity, tendonitis
Renal and urinary disorders	uncommon	renal failure†, nephritis interstitial, nephrolithiasis, nocturia, renal cyst
Reproductive system and breast disorders	uncommon	erectile dysfunction, gynaecomastia, menopausal symptoms
General disorders and administration site conditions	common	asthenia, fatigue
	uncommon	chest discomfort, chills, face oedema, fat tissue increased, feeling jittery, malaise, oedema peripheral, pain, pyrexia
Investigations	common	alanine aminotransferase increased, atypical lymphocytes, aspartate aminotransferase increased, blood triglycerides increased
	uncommon	absolute neutrophil count decreased, alkaline phosphatase increased, blood amylase increased, blood bilirubin increased, blood cholesterol increased, blood creatinine increased, blood glucose increased, blood urea nitrogen increased, creatine phosphokinase increased, fasting blood glucose increased, glucose urine present, high density lipoprotein increased, lipase increased, low density lipoprotein increased, platelet count decreased, red blood cells urine positive, waist circumference increased, weight increased, white blood cell count decreased
Injury, poisoning and procedural complications	uncommon	accidental overdose†

† includes at least one serious adverse reaction

Cancers were reported in treatment-experienced and treatment-naïve patients who initiated ISENTRESS in conjunction with other antiretroviral agents. The types and rates of specific cancers were those expected in a highly immunodeficient population. The risk of developing cancer in these studies was similar in the groups receiving ISENTRESS and in the groups receiving comparators.

Grade 2-4 creatine kinase laboratory abnormalities were observed in subjects treated with ISENTRESS. Myopathy and rhabdomyolysis have been reported; however, the relationship of ISENTRESS to these events is not known. Use with caution in patients who have had myopathy or rhabdomyolysis in the past or have any predisposing issues including other medicinal products associated with these conditions (see section 4.4).

Cases of osteonecrosis have been reported, particularly i n patients with generally acknowledged risk factors, advanced HIV disease or long-term exposure to combination antiretroviral therapy (CART). The frequency of this is unknown (see section 4.4).

Patients co-infected with hepatitis B and/or hepatitis C virus

In Phase III studies, treatment-experienced patients (N = 113/699 or 16.2%; HBV=6 %, HCV=9 %, HBV+HCV=1%) and treatment-naïve patients (N = 34/563 or 6 %; HBV=4.1 %, HCV=2.1 %, HBV+HCV=0.2 %) with chronic (but not acute) active hepatitis B and/or hepatitis C co-infection were permitted to enrol provided that baseline liver function tests did not exceed 5 times the upper limit of normal. In general the safety profile of ISENTRESS in patients with hepatitis B and/or hepatitis C virus co-infection was similar to that in patients without hepatitis B and/or hepatitis C virus co-infection, although the rates of AST and ALT abnormalities were somewhat higher in the subgroup with hepatitis B and/or hepatitis C virus co-infection for both treatment groups. In treatment-experienced patients, Grade 2 or higher laboratory abnormalities that represent a worsening from baseline of AST, ALT or total bilirubin occurred in 26%, 27% and 12%, respectively, of co-infected subjects treated with ISENTRESS as compared to 9%, 8% and 7% of all other subjects treated with ISENTRESS. In treatment-naïve patients, Grade 2 or higher laboratory abnormalities that represent a worsening from baseline of AST, ALT or total bilirubin occurred in 17 %, 22 % and 11 %, respectively, of co-infected subjects treated with ISENTRESS as compared to 4 %, 5 % and 3 % of all other subjects treated with ISENTRESS.

4.9 Overdose

No specific information is available on the treatment of overdosage with ISENTRESS.

In the event of an overdose, it is reasonable to employ the standard supportive measures, e.g., remove unabsorbed material from the gastro-intestinal tract, employ clinical monitoring (including obtaining an electrocardiogram), and institute supportive therapy if required. It should be taken into account that raltegravir is presented for clinical use as the potassium salt. The extent to which ISENTRESS may be dialysable is unknown.

5. PHARMACOLOGICAL PROPERTIES

5.1 Pharmacodynamic properties

Pharmacotherapeutic group: Antiviral for systemic use, Other Antivirals, ATC code: J05AX08.

Mechanism of action

Raltegravir is an integrase strand transfer inhibitor active against the Human Immunodeficiency Virus (HIV-1). Raltegravir inhibits the catalytic activity of integrase, an HIV-encoded enzyme that is required for viral replication. Inhibition of integrase prevents the covalent insertion, or integration, of the HIV genome into the host cell genome. HIV genomes that fail to integrate cannot direct the production of new infectious viral particles, so inhibiting integration prevents propagation of the viral infection.

Antiviral activity *in vitro*

Raltegravir at concentrations of 31 ± 20 nM resulted in 95% inhibition (IC_{95}) of HIV-1 replication (relative to an untreated virus-infected culture) in human T-lymphoid cell cultures infected with the cell-line adapted HIV-1 variant H9IIIB. In addition, raltegravir inhibited viral replication in cultures of mitogen-activated human peripheral blood mononuclear cells infected with diverse, primary clinical isolates of HIV-1, including isolates from 5 non–B subtypes, and isolates resistant to reverse transcriptase inhibitors and protease inhibitors. In a single-cycle infection assay, raltegravir inhibited infection of 23 HIV isolates representing 5 non-B subtypes and 5 circulating recombinant forms with IC50 values ranging from 5 to 12 nM.

Resistance

Most viruses isolated from patients failing raltegravir had high-level raltegravir resistance resulting from the appearance of two or more mutations. Most had a signature mutation at amino acid 155 (N155 changed to H), amino acid 148 (Q148 changed to H, K, or R), or amino acid 143 (Y143 changed to H, C, or R), along with one or more additional integrase mutations (e.g., L74M, E92Q, T97A, E138A/K, G140A/S, V151I, G163R, S230R). The signature mutations decrease viral susceptibility to raltegravir and addition of other mutations results in a further decrease in raltegravir susceptibility. Factors that reduced the likelihood of developing resistance included lower baseline viral load and use of other active anti-retroviral agents. Preliminary data indicate that there is potential for at least some degree of cross-resistance to occur between raltegravir and other integrase inhibitors.

Clinical experience

The evidence of efficacy of ISENTRESS is based on the analyses of 48-week data from two ongoing, randomised, double-blind, placebo-controlled trials, (BENCHMRK 1 and BENCHMRK 2, Protocols 018 and 019) in antiretroviral treatment-experienced HIV-1 infected adult patients and the analysis of 48-week data from an ongoing, randomised, double-blind, active-control trial, (STARTMRK, Protocol 021) in antiretroviral treatment-naïve HIV-1 infected adult patients. These efficacy results were supported by 96-week analysis of a randomised, double-blind, controlled, dose-ranging trial, Protocol 004, in antiretroviral treatment-naïve HIV-1 infected adult patients.

Efficacy

Treatment-experienced patients

BENCHMRK 1 and BENCHMRK 2 (ongoing multi-centre, randomised, double-blind, placebo-controlled trials) evaluate the safety and anti-retroviral activity of ISENTRESS 400 mg twice daily vs. placebo in a combination with optimised background therapy (OBT), in HIV-infected patients, 16 years or older, with documented resistance to at least 1 drug in each of 3 classes (NRTIs, NNRTIs, PIs) of anti-retroviral therapies. Prior to randomisation, OBT were selected by the investigator based on the patient's prior treatment history, as well as baseline genotypic and phenotypic viral resistance testing.

Patient demographics (gender, age and race) and baseline characteristics were comparable between the groups receiving ISENTRESS 400 mg twice daily and placebo. Patients had prior exposure to a median of 12 anti-retrovirals for a median of 10 years. A median of 4 ARTs was used in OBT.

Results 48-week analyses

Durable week 48 outcomes for patients on the recommended dose ISENTRESS 400 mg twice daily from the pooled studies BENCHMRK 1 and BENCHMRK 2 are shown in Table 2.

Table 2

Efficacy Outcome at Week 48

BENCHMRK 1 and 2 Pooled Parameter	ISENTRESS 400 mg twice daily + OBT (N = 462)	Placebo + OBT (N = 237)
Percent HIV-RNA < 400 copies/ml (95% CI)		
All patients†	72 (68, 76)	37 (31, 44)
Baseline Characteristic‡		
HIV-RNA > 100,000 copies/ml	62 (53, 69)	17 (9, 27)
≤ 100,000 copies/ml	82 (77, 86)	49 (41, 58)
CD4-count ≤ 50 cells/mm³	61 (53, 69)	21 (13, 32)
> 50 and ≤ 200 cells/mm³	80 (73, 85)	44 (33, 55)
> 200 cells/mm³	83 (76, 89)	51 (39, 63)
Sensitivity score (GSS) §		
0	52 (42, 61)	8 (3, 17)
1	81 (75, 87)	40 (30, 51)
2 and above	84 (77, 89)	65 (52, 76)
Percent HIV-RNA < 50 copies/ml (95% CI)		
All patients†	62 (57, 67)	33 (27, 39)
Baseline Characteristic‡		
HIV-RNA > 100,000 copies/ml	48 (40, 56)	16 (8, 26)
≤ 100,000 copies/ml	73 (68, 78)	43 (35, 52)
CD4-count ≤ 50 cells/mm³	50 (41, 58)	20 (12, 31)
> 50 and ≤ 200 cells/mm³	67 (59, 74)	39 (28, 50)
> 200 cells/mm³	76 (68, 83)	44 (32, 56)
Sensitivity score (GSS) §		
0	45 (35, 54)	3 (0, 11)
1	67 (59, 74)	37 (27, 48)
2 and above	75 (68, 82)	59 (46, 71)
Mean CD4 Cell Change (95% CI), cells/mm³		
All patients‡	109 (98, 121)	45 (32, 57)
Baseline Characteristic‡		
HIV-RNA > 100,000 copies/ml	126 (107, 144)	36 (17, 55)
≤ 100,000 copies/ml	100 (86, 115)	49 (33, 65)
CD4-count ≤ 50 cells/mm³	121 (100, 142)	33 (18, 48)
> 50 and ≤ 200 cells/mm³	104 (88, 119)	47 (28, 66)
> 200 cells/mm³	104 (80, 129)	54 (24, 84)
Sensitivity score (GSS) §		
0	81 (55, 106)	11 (4, 26)
1	113 (96, 130)	44 (24, 63)
2 and above	125 (105, 144)	76 (48, 103)

† Non-completer is failure imputation: patients who discontinued prematurely are imputed as failure thereafter. Percent of patients with response and associated 95% confidence interval (CI) are reported.

‡ For analysis by prognostic factors, virologic failures were carried forward for percent < 400 and 50 copies/ml. For mean CD4 changes, baseline-carry-forward was used for virologic failures.

§ The Genotypic Sensitivity Score (GSS) was defined as the total oral ARTs in the optimised background therapy (OBT) to which a patient's viral isolate showed genotypic sensitivity based upon genotypic resistance test. Enfuvirtide use in OBT in enfuvirtide-naïve patients was counted as one active drug in OBT. Similarly, darunavir use in OBT in darunavir-naïve patients was counted as one active drug in OBT.

Raltegravir achieved virologic responses (using Not Completer=Failure approach) of HIV RNA < 50 copies/ml in 61.7 % of patients at Week 16 and in 62.1 % at Week 48. Some patients experienced viral rebound between Week 16 and Week 48. Factors associated with failure include high baseline viral load and OBT that did not include at least one potent active agent.

Switch to raltegravir

The SWITCHMRK 1 & 2 studies evaluated HIV-infected patients receiving suppressive (screening HIV RNA <50 copies/ml; stable regimen >3 months) therapy with lopinavir 200 mg (+) ritonavir 50 mg 2 tablets twice daily plus at least 2 nucleoside reverse transcriptase inhibitors and randomized them 1:1 to continue lopinavir (+) ritonavir 2 tablets twice daily (n=174 and n=178, respectively) or replace lopinavir (+) ritonavir with raltegravir 400 mg twice daily (n=174 and n=176, respectively). Patients with a prior history of virological failure were not excluded and the number of previous antiretroviral therapies was not limited.

These studies were terminated after the primary efficacy analysis at Week 24 because they failed to demonstrate non-inferiority of raltegravir versus lopinavir (+) ritonavir. In both studies at Week 24, suppression of HIV RNA to less than 50 copies/ml was maintained in 84.4 % of the raltegravir group versus 90.6 % of the lopinavir (+) ritonavir group, (Non-completers = Failure). See section 4.4 regarding the need to administer raltegravir with two other active agents.

Treatment-naïve patients

STARTMRK (ongoing multi-centre, randomised, double-blind, active-control trial) evaluates the safety and anti-retroviral activity of ISENTRESS 400 mg twice daily vs. efavirenz 600 mg at bedtime, in a combination with emtricitabine (+) tenofovir, in treatment-naïve HIV-infected patients with HIV RNA > 5,000 copies/ml. Randomisation was stratified by screening HIV RNA level (≤50,000 copies/ml; and > 50,000 copies/ml) and by hepatitis B or C status (positive or negative).

Patient demographics (gender, age and race) and baseline characteristics were comparable between the group receiving ISENTRESS 400 mg twice daily and the group receiving efavirenz 600 mg at bedtime.

Results 48-week analyses

With respect to the primary efficacy endpoint, the proportion (%) of patients achieving HIV RNA < 50 copies/ml at Week 48 was 241/280 (86.1%) in the group receiving ISENTRESS and 230/281 (81.9%) in the group receiving efavirenz. The treatment difference (ISENTRESS – efavirenz) was 4.2% with an associated 95% CI of (-1.92, 10.32) establishing that ISENTRESS is non-inferior to efavirenz (p-value for non-inferiority < 0.001). Week 48 outcomes for patients on the recommended dose of ISENTRESS 400 mg twice daily from STARTMRK are shown in Table 3.

Table 3

Efficacy Outcome at Week 48

STARTMRK Study Parameter	ISENTRESS 400 mg twice daily (N = 281)	Efavirenz 600 mg at bedtime (N = 282)
Percent HIV-RNA < 50 copies/ml (95% CI)		
All patients†	86 (81, 90)	82 (77, 86)
Baseline Characteristic‡		
HIV-RNA > 100,000 copies/ml	91 (85, 95)	89 (83, 94)
≤ 100,000 copies/ml	93 (86, 97)	89 (82, 94)
CD4-count ≤ 50 cells/mm³	84 (64, 95)	86 (67, 96)
> 50 and ≤ 200 cells/mm³	89 (81, 95)	86 (77, 92)
> 200 cells/mm³	94 (89, 98)	92 (87, 96)
Viral Subtype Clade B	90 (85, 94)	89 (83, 93)
Non-Clade B	96 (87, 100)	91 (78, 97)
Mean CD4 Cell Change (95% CI), cells/mm³		
All patients‡	189 (174, 204)	163 (148, 178)
Baseline Characteristic‡		
HIV-RNA > 100,000 copies/ml	196 (174, 219)	192 (169, 214)
≤ 100,000 copies/ml	180 (160, 200)	134 (115, 153)
CD4-count ≤ 50 cells/mm³	170 (122, 218)	152 (123, 180)
> 50 and ≤ 200 cells/mm³	193 (169, 217)	175 (151, 198)
> 200 cells/mm³	190 (168, 212)	157 (134, 181)
Viral Subtype Clade B	187 (170, 204)	164 (147, 181)
Non-Clade B	189 (153, 225)	156 (121, 190)

† Non-completer is failure imputation: patients who discontinued prematurely are imputed as failure thereafter. Percent of patients with response and associated 95% confidence interval (CI) are reported.

‡ For analysis by prognostic factors, virologic failures were carried forward for percent < 50 and 400 copies/ml. For mean CD4 changes, baseline-carry-forward was used for virologic failures.

Notes: The analysis is based on all available data.

ISENTRESS and efavirenz were administered with emtricitabine (+) tenofovir.

Long-term results

Long-term efficacy data of ISENTRESS 400 mg twice daily + lamivudine and tenofovir in treatment-naïve patients up to 96 weeks is available from the Phase II dose-finding study (Protocol 004). Through 96 weeks of treatment, 84 % in the group receiving ISENTRESS 400 mg twice daily maintained HIV-1 RNA < 400 copies/ml and 83 % also maintained HIV-1 RNA < 50 copies/ml. The mean increase from baseline in CD4+ cell counts was +221 cells/mm³ in the group receiving ISENTRESS.

5.2 Pharmacokinetic properties

Absorption

As demonstrated in healthy volunteers administered single oral doses of raltegravir in the fasted state, raltegravir is rapidly absorbed with a t_{max} of approximately 3 hours postdose. Raltegravir AUC and C_{max} increase dose proportionally over the dose range 100 mg to 1600 mg. Raltegravir $C_{12\ hr}$ increases dose proportionally over the dose range of 100 to 800 mg and increases slightly less than dose proportionally over the dose range 100 mg to 1600 mg. Dose proportionality has not been established in patients.

With twice-daily dosing, pharmacokinetic steady state is achieved rapidly, within approximately the first 2 days of dosing. There is little to no accumulation in AUC and C_{max} and evidence of slight accumulation in $C_{12\ hr}$. The absolute bioavailability of raltegravir has not been established.

ISENTRESS may be administered with or without food. Raltegravir was administered without regard to food in the pivotal safety and efficacy studies in HIV-infected patients. Administration of multiple doses of raltegravir following a moderate-fat meal did not affect raltegravir AUC to a clinically meaningful degree with an increase of 13% relative to fasting. Raltegravir $C_{12\ hr}$ was 66% higher and C_{max} was 5% higher following a moderate-fat meal compared to fasting. Administration of raltegravir following a high-fat meal increased AUC and C_{max} by approximately 2-fold and increased $C_{12\ hr}$ by 4.1-fold. Administration of raltegravir following a low-fat meal decreased AUC and C_{max} by 46% and 52%, respectively; $C_{12\ hr}$ was essentially unchanged. Food appears to increase pharmacokinetic variability relative to fasting.

Overall, considerable variability was observed in the pharmacokinetics of raltegravir. For observed C_{12hr} in BENCHMRK 1 and 2 the coefficient of variation (CV) for inter-subject variability = 212% and the CV for intra-subject variability = 122%. Sources of variability may include differences in co-administration with food and concomitant medications.

Distribution

Raltegravir is approximately 83% bound to human plasma protein over the concentration range of 2 to 10 μM.

Raltegravir readily crossed the placenta in rats, but did not penetrate the brain to any appreciable extent.

Metabolism and excretion

The apparent terminal half-life of raltegravir is approximately 9 hours, with a shorter α-phase half-life (~1 hour) accounting for much of the AUC. Following administration of an oral dose of radiolabeled raltegravir, approximately 51 and 32 % of the dose was excreted in faeces and urine, respectively. In faeces, only raltegravir was present, most of which is likely to be derived from hydrolysis of raltegravir-glucuronide secreted in bile as observed in preclinical species. Two components, namely raltegravir and raltegravir-glucuronide, were detected in urine and accounted for approximately 9 and 23 % of the dose, respectively. The major circulating entity was raltegravir and represented approximately 70 % of the total radioactivity; the remaining radioactivity in plasma was accounted for by raltegravir-glucuronide. Studies using isoform-selective chemical inhibitors and cDNA-expressed UDP-glucuronosyltransferases (UGT) show that UGT1A1 is the main enzyme responsible for the formation of raltegravir-glucuronide. Thus the data indicate that the major mechanism of clearance of raltegravir in humans is UGT1A1-mediated glucuronidation.

UGT1A1 Polymorphism

In a comparison of 30 subjects with *28/*28 genotype to 27 subjects with wild-type genotype, the geometric mean ratio (90% CI) of AUC was 1.41 (0.96, 2.09) and the geometric mean ratio of $C_{12\ hr}$ was 1.91 (1.43, 2.55). Dose adjustment is not considered necessary in subjects with reduced UGT1A1 activity due to genetic polymorphism.

Special populations

Children

The pharmacokinetics of raltegravir in paediatric patients has not been established.

Elderly

There was no clinically meaningful effect of age on raltegravir pharmacokinetics over the age range studied (19 to 71 years, with few (8) subjects over the age of 65).

Gender, Race and BMI

There were no clinically important pharmacokinetic differences due to gender, race or body mass index (BMI).

Renal impairment

Renal clearance of unchanged medicinal product is a minor pathway of elimination. There were no clinically important pharmacokinetic differences between patients with severe renal insufficiency and healthy subjects (see section 4.2). Because the extent to which ISENTRESS may be dialysable is unknown, dosing before a dialysis session should be avoided.

Hepatic impairment

Raltegravir is eliminated primarily by glucuronidation in the liver. There were no clinically important pharmacokinetic differences between patients with moderate hepatic insufficiency and healthy subjects. The effect of severe hepatic insufficiency on the pharmacokinetics of raltegravir has not been studied (see sections 4.2 and 4.4).

5.3 Preclinical safety data

Non-clinical toxicology studies, including conventional studies of safety pharmacology, repeated-dose toxicity, genotoxicity, and developmental toxicity, have been conducted with raltegravir, in mice, rats, dogs and rabbits. Effects at exposure levels sufficiently in excess of clinical exposure levels indicate no special hazard for humans.

Mutagenicity

No evidence of mutagenicity or genotoxicity was observed in *in vitro* microbial mutagenesis (Ames) tests, *in vitro* alkaline elution assays for DNA breakage and *in vitro* and *in vivo* chromosomal aberration studies.

Carcinogenicity

A carcinogenicity study of raltegravir in mice did not show any carcinogenic potential. At the highest dose levels, 400 mg/kg/day in females and 250 mg/kg/day in males, systemic exposure was similar to that at the clinical dose of 400 mg twice daily In rats, tumours (squamous cell carcinoma) of the nose/nasopharynx were identified at 300 and 600 mg/kg/day in females and at 300 mg/kg/day in males. These neoplasia could result from local deposition and/or aspiration of drug on the mucosa of the nose/nasopharynx during oral gavage dosing and subsequent chronic irritation and inflammation; it is likely that they are of limited relevance for the intended clinical use. At the NOAEL, systemic exposure was similar to that at the clinical dose of 400 mg twice daily Standard genotoxicity studies to evaluate mutagenicity and clastogenicity were negative.

Developmental Toxicity

Raltegravir was not teratogenic in developmental toxicity studies in rats and rabbits. A slight increase in incidence of supernumerary ribs was observed in rat pups of dams exposed to raltegravir at approximately 4.4-fold human exposure at 400 mg twice daily based on $AUC_{0\text{-}24\ hr}$. No development effects were seen at 3.4-fold human exposure at 400 mg twice daily based on $AUC_{0\text{-}24\ hr}$ (see section 4.6). Similar findings were not observed in rabbits.

6. PHARMACEUTICAL PARTICULARS

6.1 List of excipients

Tablet core

- microcrystalline cellulose
- lactose monohydrate
- calcium phosphate dibasic anhydrous
- hypromellose 2208
- poloxamer 407
- sodium stearyl fumarate
- magnesium stearate

Film-coating

- polyvinyl alcohol
- titanium dioxide (E 171)
- polyethylene glycol 3350
- talc
- red iron oxide (E 172)
- black iron oxide (E 172)

6.2 Incompatibilities

Not applicable.

6.3 Shelf life

30 months

6.4 Special precautions for storage

This medicinal product does not require any special storage conditions.

6.5 Nature and contents of container

High density polyethylene (HDPE) bottle with a child-resistant polypropylene closure.

Two pack sizes are available: 1 bottle with 60 tablets, and a multi-pack containing 3 bottles of 60 tablets.

Not all pack sizes may be marketed.

6.6 Special precautions for disposal and other handling

No special requirements.

7. MARKETING AUTHORISATION HOLDER

Merck Sharp & Dohme Limited
Hertford Road, Hoddesdon
Hertfordshire EN11 9BU
United Kingdom

8. MARKETING AUTHORISATION NUMBER(S)

EU/1/07/436/001: 400 mg-Film-coated tablets-Oral use-Bottle (HDPE)-60 tablets

EU/1/07/436/002: 400 mg-Film-coated tablets-Oral use-Bottle (HDPE)-180 (3x60) tablets

9. DATE OF FIRST AUTHORISATION/RENEWAL OF THE AUTHORISATION

Date of first authorisation: 20 December 2007

Date of last renewal: 20 December 2008.

10. DATE OF REVISION OF THE TEXT

9 September 2009

Detailed information on this medicinal product is available on the website of the European Medicines Agency (EMEA) http://www.emea.europa.eu

® denotes registered trademark of Merck & Co., Inc., Whitehouse Station, NJ, USA.

SPC.IST.08.UK.2983 (II-010)

Isocarboxazid Tablets 10mg (Cambridge Laboratories)

(Cambridge Laboratories)

1. NAME OF THE MEDICINAL PRODUCT

Isocarboxazid Tablets 10mg

2. QUALITATIVE AND QUANTITATIVE COMPOSITION

Each tablet contains 10mg Isocarboxazid.

3. PHARMACEUTICAL FORM

Tablets

4. CLINICAL PARTICULARS

4.1 Therapeutic indications

For the treatment of the symptoms of depressive illness.

4.2 Posology and method of administration

Isocarboxazid Tablets are for oral administration.

Adults

A daily dose of 30mg, in single or divided doses, should be given until improvement is obtained. The maximal effect is only observed after a period varying from 1 - 4 weeks. If no improvement has been seen by 4 weeks, doses up to 60mg may be tried, according to the patient's tolerance, for no longer than 4 - 6 weeks, provided the patient is closely monitored because of the increased risk of adverse reactions occurring.

Once the optimal effect is achieved, the dose should be reduced to the lowest possible amount sufficient to maintain the improvement. Clinical experience has shown this to be usually 10 - 20mg daily but up to 40mg daily may be required in some cases.

The elderly

The elderly are more likely to experience adverse reactions such as agitation, confusion and postural hypotension. Half the normal maintenance dose may be sufficient to produce a satisfactory clinical response.

Children

Isocarboxazid Tablets are not indicated for paediatric use.

4.3 Contraindications

Isocarboxazid is contra-indicated in patients with any impairment of hepatic function, cerebrovascular disorders or severe cardiovascular disease, and in those with actual or suspected phaeochromocytoma.

4.4 Special warnings and precautions for use

Depression is associated with an increased risk of suicidal thoughts, self harm and suicide (suicide-related events). This risk persists until significant remission occurs. As improvement may not occur during the first few weeks or more of treatment, patients should be closely monitored until such improvement occurs. It is general clinical experience that the risk of suicide may increase in the early stages of recovery.

Patients with a history of suicide-related events, or those exhibiting a significant degree of suicidal ideation prior to commencement of treatment are known to be at greater risk of suicidal thoughts or suicide attempts, and should receive careful monitoring during treatment. A meta-analysis of placebo-controlled clinical trials of antidepressant drugs in adult patients with psychiatric disorders showed an increased risk of suicidal behaviour with antidepressants compared to placebo in patients less than 25 years old.

Close supervision of patients and in particular those at high risk should accompany drug therapy especially in early treatment and following dose changes. Patients (and caregivers of patients) should be alerted about the need to monitor for any clinical worsening, suicidal behaviour or thoughts and unusual changes in behaviour and to seek medical advice immediately if these symptoms present.

Some monoamine oxidase inhibitors have occasionally caused hepatic complications and jaundice in patients, therefore regular monitoring of liver function should be carried out during Isocarboxazid therapy. If there is any evidence of a hepatotoxic reaction, the drug should be withdrawn immediately.

The drug should be used cautiously in patients with impaired renal function, to prevent accumulation taking place, and also in the elderly or debilitated and those with cardiovascular disease, diabetes or blood dyscrasias.

In restless or agitated patients, Isocarboxazid may precipitate states of excessive excitement. Isocarboxazid appears to have varying effects in epileptic patients; while some have a decrease in frequency of seizures, others have more seizures.

4.5 Interaction with other medicinal products and other forms of interaction

Like other monoamine oxidase inhibitors, Isocarboxazid potentiates the action of a number of drugs and foods. Patients being treated with a monoamine oxidase inhibitor should not receive indirectly-acting sympathomimetic agents such as amphetamines, metaraminol, fenfluramine or similar anorectic agents, ephedrine or phenylpropanolamine (contained in many proprietary 'cold-cure' medications), dopamine or levodopa. Patients should also be warned to avoid foodstuffs and beverages with a high tyramine content: mature cheeses (including processed cheeses), hydrolysed yeast or meat extracts, alcoholic beverages, particularly heavy red wines such as Chianti, non-alcoholic beers, lagers and wines, and other foods which are not fresh and are fermented, pickled, 'hung', 'matured' or otherwise subject to protein degradation before consumption. Broad bean pods (which contain levodopa) and banana skins may also present a hazard. In extreme cases interactions may result in severe hypertensive episodes. Isocarboxazid should therefore be discontinued immediately upon the occurrence of palpitations or frequent headaches.

Pethidine should not be given to patients receiving monoamine oxidase inhibitors as serious, potentially fatal reactions, including central excitation, muscle rigidity, hyperpyrexia, circulatory collapse, respiratory depression and coma, can result. Such reactions are less likely with morphine, but experience of the interaction of Isocarboxazid with narcotic analgesics other than pethidine is limited and extreme caution is therefore necessary when administering morphine to patients undergoing therapy with Isocarboxazid.

Isocarboxazid should not be administered together with other monoamine oxidase inhibitors or most tricyclic antidepressants (clomipramine, desipramine, imipramine, butriptyline, nortriptyline or protriptyline). Although there is no proof that combined therapy will be effective, refractory cases of depression may be treated with Isocarboxazid in combination with amitriptyline or trimipramine, provided appropriate care is taken. Hypotensive and other adverse reactions are likely to be increased.

An interval of 1 - 2 weeks should be allowed after treatment with Isocarboxazid before the administration of antidepressants with a different mode of action or any other drug which may interact. A similar interval is recommended before administration of Isocarboxazid when another antidepressant has been used; in the case of drugs with a very long half-life (such as fluoxetine), it may be advisable to extend this interval.

Isocarboxazid should be discontinued for at least 2 weeks prior to elective surgery requiring general anaesthesia. The anaesthetist should be warned that a patient is being treated with Isocarboxazid, in the event of emergency surgery being necessary. Concurrent administration of Isocarboxazid with other central nervous system depressants (especially barbiturates and phenothiazines), stimulants, local anaesthetics, ganglion-blocking agents and other hypotensives (including methyl-dopa and reserpine), diuretics, vasopressors, anticholinergic drugs and hypoglycaemic agents may lead to potentiation of their effects. This should be borne in mind if dentistry, surgery or a change in treatment of a patient becomes necessary during treatment with Isocarboxazid.

All patients taking Isocarboxazid should be warned against self-medication with proprietary 'cold-cure' preparations and nasal decongestants and advised of the dietary restrictions listed under 'warnings'.

With Isocarboxazid, as with other drugs acting on the central nervous system, patients should be instructed to avoid alcohol while under treatment, since the individual response cannot be foreseen.

4.6 Pregnancy and lactation

Do not use in pregnancy, especially during the first and last trimesters, unless there are compelling reasons. There is no evidence as to drug safety in human pregnancy, nor is there evidence from animal work that it is free from hazard. In addition, the effect of psychotropic drugs on the fine brain structure of the foetus is unknown. Since there is no information on the secretion of the drug into breast milk, Isocarboxazid is contra-indicated during lactation.

4.7 Effects on ability to drive and use machines

Like all medicaments of this type, Isocarboxazid may modify patients' reactions (driving ability, operation of machinery etc.) to a varying extent, depending on dosage and individual susceptibility.

4.8 Undesirable effects

In general, Isocarboxazid is well tolerated by the majority of patients. Side-effects, if they occur, are those common to the group of monoamine oxidase inhibitors.

The most frequently reported have been orthostatic hypotension, associated in some patients with disturbances in cardiac rhythm, peripheral oedema, complaints of dizziness, dryness of the mouth, nausea and vomiting, constipation, blurred vision, insomnia, drowsiness, weakness and fatigue. These side-effects can usually be controlled by dosage reduction.

There have been infrequent reports of mild headaches, sweating, paraesthesiae, peripheral neuritis, hyperreflexia, agitation, overactivity, muscle tremor, confusion and other behavioural changes, difficulty in micturition, impairment of erection and ejaculation, and skin rashes. Although rare, blood dyscrasias (purpura, granulocytopenia) have been reported. Response to Isocarboxazid may be accompanied by increased appetite and weight gain.

Cases of suicidal ideation and suicidal behaviours have been reported during Isocarboxazid therapy or early after treatment discontinuation (see Section 4.4).

4.9 Overdose

The primary symptoms of overdosage include dizziness, ataxia and irritability. In acute cases, hypotension or hypertension, tachycardia, pyrexia, psychotic manifestations, convulsions, respiratory depression and coma may occur and continue for 8 - 14 days before recovery.

Gastric lavage should be performed soon after ingestion and intensive supportive therapy carried out. Sympathomimetic agents should not be given to treat hypotension but plasma expanders may be used in severe cases. Hypertensive crises may be treated by pentolinium or phentolamine, severe shock with hydrocortisone. Diazepam may be used to control convulsions or severe excitement. Dialysis is of value in eliminating the drug in severe cases.

5. PHARMACOLOGICAL PROPERTIES

5.1 Pharmacodynamic properties

Isocarboxazid is a monoamine oxidase inhibitor, effective in small doses. Its antidepressant action is thought to be related to its effect on physiological amines such as serotonin and noradrenaline, and this effect is cumulative and persistent.

5.2 Pharmacokinetic properties

Isocarboxazid is readily absorbed after oral administration. Most of the drug-related material is excreted as metabolites in the urine.

5.3 Preclinical safety data

There are no pre-clinical data of relevance to the prescriber which are additional to that already included in other sections of the SPC.

6. PHARMACEUTICAL PARTICULARS

6.1 List of excipients

Lactose

Starch

Talc

Magnesium stearate

Gelatin

Iron oxide yellow E172

Iron Oxide red E172

6.2 Incompatibilities

None known.

6.3 Shelf life

Three years.

6.4 Special precautions for storage

The recommended maximum storage temperature is 25°C.

Isocarboxazid Tablets should be stored in well-closed containers.

6.5 Nature and contents of container

HDPE bottles with snap closures, containing 56 tablets.

6.6 Special precautions for disposal and other handling

None.

Administrative Data

7. MARKETING AUTHORISATION HOLDER

Cambridge Laboratories Limited
Deltic House
Kingfisher Way
Silverlink Business Park
Wallsend
Tyne & Wear
NE28 9NX

8. MARKETING AUTHORISATION NUMBER(S)

PL 12070/0003

9. DATE OF FIRST AUTHORISATION/RENEWAL OF THE AUTHORISATION

21 April 1992

10. DATE OF REVISION OF THE TEXT

February 2008

Isoket 0.05%

(UCB Pharma Limited)

1. NAME OF THE MEDICINAL PRODUCT

Isoket 0.05 %

2. QUALITATIVE AND QUANTITATIVE COMPOSITION

Isosorbide dinitrate 500 micrograms (0.05% w/v) 5mg/10ml

For excipients, See 6.1

3. PHARMACEUTICAL FORM

Sterile colourless solution for intravenous infusion.

4. CLINICAL PARTICULARS

4.1 Therapeutic indications

1. Intravenous

Isoket is indicated in the treatment of unresponsive left ventricular failure secondary to acute myocardial infarction, unresponsive left ventricular failure of various aetiology and severe to unstable angina pectoris.

2. Intra-coronary

Isoket is indicated during percutaneous transluminal coronary angioplasty to facilitate prolongation of balloon inflation and to prevent or relieve coronary spasm.

4.2 Posology and method of administration

Adults, including the elderly

Intravenous route

Isoket 0.05% is intended for intravenous administration by slow infusion via a syringe pump.

A dose of between 2mg and 12mg per hour is usually satisfactory. However, dosages up to 20mg per hour may be required. In all cases the dose administered should be adjusted to the patient response.

Intra-coronary Route

Isoket 0.05% 10ml prefilled syringes may be used for direct administration (through a catheter by means of an adaptor, if necessary) during percutaneous transluminal coronary angioplasty.

The usual dose is 1mg given as a bolus injection prior to balloon inflation. Further doses may be given not exceeding 5mg within a 30 minute period.

Children

The safety and efficacy of Isoket has not yet been established in children.

4.3 Contraindications

These are common to all nitrates: known hypersensitivity to nitrates, marked anaemia, cerebral haemorrhage, head trauma, hypovolaemia, and severe hypotension. Use in circulatory collapse or low filling pressure is also contra-indicated. Isoket should not be used in the treatment of cardiogenic shock, unless some means of maintaining an adequate diastolic pressure is undertaken.

Sildenafil has been shown to potentiate the hypotensive effects of nitrates, and its co-administration with nitrates or nitric oxide donors is therefore contraindicated.

4.4 Special warnings and precautions for use

Isoket should be used with caution in patients who are suffering from hypothyroidism, malnutrition, severe liver or renal disease or hypothermia. Close attention to pulse and blood pressure is necessary during the administration of Isoket infusions.

4.5 Interaction with other medicinal products and other forms of interaction

Concurrent intake of drugs with blood pressure lowering properties e.g. beta-blockers, calcium antagonists, vasodilators etc. and/or alcohol may potentiate the hypotensive effect of Isoket.

The hypotensive effect of nitrates is potentiated by concurrent administration of sildenafil (Viagra®). This might also occur with neuroleptics and tricyclic antidepressants.

4.6 Pregnancy and lactation

No data have been reported which would indicate the possibility of adverse effects resulting from the use of isosorbide dinitrate in pregnancy. Safety in pregnancy, however, has not been established. Isosorbide dinitrate should only be used in pregnancy and during lactation if, in the opinion of the physician, the possible benefits of treatment outweigh the possible hazards.

4.7 Effects on ability to drive and use machines

None known.

4.8 Undesirable effects

In common with other nitrates, headaches, nausea and tachycardia may occur during administration. Whilst sharp falls in systemic arterial pressure can give rise to symptoms of cerebral flow deficiency and decreased coronary perfusion, clinical experience with Isoket has shown that this is not normally a problem.

4.9 Overdose

General supportive therapy is recommended.

5. PHARMACOLOGICAL PROPERTIES

ATC Code: C02D A 08 Vasodilators used in cardiac diseases.

5.1 Pharmacodynamic properties

Isosorbide dinitrate is an organic nitrate, which in common with other cardioactive nitrates, is a vasodilator. It produces decreased left and right ventricular end-diastolic pressures to a greater extent than the decrease in systemic arterial pressure, thereby reducing afterload and especially the preload of the heart.

Isosorbide dinitrate influences the oxygen supply to ischaemic myocardium by causing the redistribution of blood flow along collateral channels and from epicardial to endocardial regions by selective dilatation of large epicardial vessels.

It reduces the requirement of the myocardium for oxygen by increasing venous capacitance, causing a pooling of blood in peripheral veins, thereby reducing ventricular volume and heart wall distension.

5.2 Pharmacokinetic properties

Isosorbide dinitrate (ISDN) is eliminated from plasma with a short half-life (about 0.7h). The metabolic degradation of ISDN occurs via denitration and glucuronidation, like all organic nitrates. The rate of formation of the metabolites has been calculated for isosorbide-5-mononitrate (IS-5-MN) with $0.57h^{-1}$ followed by isosorbide-2-mononitrate (IS-2-MN) with $0.27h^{-1}$ and isosorbide (IS) with $0.16h^{-1}$. IS-5-MN and IS-2-MN are the primary metabolites, which are also pharmacologically active. IS-5-MN is metabolised to isosorbide 5-mononitrate-2-glucuronide (IS-5-MN-2-GLU). The half-life of this metabolite (about 2.5h) is shorter than that of IS-5-MN (about 5.1h). The half-life of ISDN is the shortest of all and that of IS-2-MN (about 3.2h) lies in between.

5.3 Preclinical safety data

None stated.

6. PHARMACEUTICAL PARTICULARS

6.1 List of excipients

Sodium chloride

Water for injection

Hydrochloric acid for pH adjustment

Sodium hydroxide for pH adjustment

6.2 Incompatibilities

Isoket contains isosorbide dinitrate in isotonic saline and is compatible with commonly employed infusion fluids, no incompatibilities have so far been demonstrated.

Isoket is compatible with glass infusion bottles and infusion packs made from polyethylene. Isoket may be infused slowly using a syringe pump with glass or plastic syringe. The use of PVC giving sets and containers should be avoided since significant losses of the active ingredient by adsorption can occur.

6.3 Shelf life

50ml glass bottles (glass type 1): 5 years as packaged for sale.

50ml glass bottles (glass type 2): 2 years as packaged for sale.

Admixtures are stable for approximately 24 hours at room temperature in the recommended containers.

Open ampoules or bottles should be used immediately and any unused drug discarded.

Prefilled glass syringes: 3 years

6.4 Special precautions for storage

There are no special precautions for storage of the product as packaged for sale.

6.5 Nature and contents of container

50ml glass bottles (glass type 1 or 2) with a laminated rubber stopper. The stopper consists of butyl rubber. The inner side of the stopper, coming into contact with the product is laminated with a film, consisting of a copolymer of tetrafluorethylene, ethylene and a fluorine containing vinyl monomer.

10ml prefilled glass syringes with rubber plunger, stopper and cap and polystyrene plunger rod.

6.6 Special precautions for disposal and other handling
None

7. MARKETING AUTHORISATION HOLDER
SCHWARZ PHARMA Limited

5 Hercules Way

Leavesden Park

Watford

WD25 7GS

United Kingdom

8. MARKETING AUTHORISATION NUMBER(S)
PL 04438/0017

9. DATE OF FIRST AUTHORISATION/RENEWAL OF THE AUTHORISATION
October 2003

10. DATE OF REVISION OF THE TEXT
July 2006

Isoket 0.1%
(UCB Pharma Limited)

1. NAME OF THE MEDICINAL PRODUCT
Isoket 0.1% w/v concentrate for solution for infusion and injection

2. QUALITATIVE AND QUANTITATIVE COMPOSITION
Isosorbide dinitrate 1 mg/ml.

For excipients, see 6.1.

3. PHARMACEUTICAL FORM
Concentrate for solution for infusion and injection.

4. CLINICAL PARTICULARS
4.1 Therapeutic indications
1. Intravenous

Isoket is indicated in the treatment of unresponsive left ventricular failure secondary to acute myocardial infarction, unresponsive left ventricular failure of various aetiology and severe or unstable angina pectoris.

2. Intra-coronary

Isoket is indicated during percutaneous transluminal coronary angioplasty to facilitate prolongation of balloon inflation and to prevent or relieve coronary spasm.

4.2 Posology and method of administration
Dosage: Adults, including the elderly

Intravenous route

A dose of between 2 mg and 12 mg per hour is usually satisfactory. However, dosages up to 20 mg per hour administered should be adjusted to the patient response.

Intra-coronary Route

The usual dose is 1 mg given as a bolus injection prior to balloon inflation. Further doses maybe given not exceeding 5 mg within a 30 minute period.

Children

The safety and efficacy of Isoket has not yet been established in children.

Administration:

Isoket is a concentrated solution and must be diluted prior use. The diluted solution should never be injected directly in the form of a bolus except via the intra-coronary route prior to balloon inflation. A dilution of 50% is advocated for intracoronary administration.

Isoket can be administered as an intravenous admixture with a suitable vehicle such as sodium chloride injection BP or dextrose injection BP.

Prepared Isoket admixtures should be given by intravenous infusion or with the aid of a syringe pump incorporating a glass or rigid plastic syringe. During administration the patient's blood pressure and pulse should be closely monitored.

4.3 Contraindications
These are common to all nitrates; known hypersensitivity to nitrates, marked anaemia, cerebral haemorrhage, head trauma, hypovolaemia, and severe hypotension. Use in circulatory collapse or low filling pressure is also contraindicated. Isoket should not be used in the treatment of cardiogenic shock, unless some means of maintaining an adequate diastolic pressure is undertaken.

Sildenafil has been shown to potentiate the hypotensive effects of nitrates, and its co-administration with nitrates or nitric oxide donors is therefore contraindicated.

4.4 Special warnings and precautions for use
Isoket should be used with caution in patients who are suffering from hypothyroidism, malnutrition, severe liver or renal disease or hypothermia. Close attention to pulse and blood pressure is necessary during the administration of Isoket infusions.

4.5 Interaction with other medicinal products and other forms of interaction
Concurrent intake of drugs with blood pressure lowering properties e.g. beta-blockers, calcium antagonists, vasodilators etc. and or/alcohol may potentiate the hypotensive effect of Isoket 0.1%.

The hypotensive effect of nitrates is potentiated by concurrent administration of sildenafil (Viagra®). This might also occur with neuroleptics and tricyclic antidepressants.

4.6 Pregnancy and lactation
No data have been reported which would indicate the possibility of adverse effects resulting from the use of isosorbide dinitrate in pregnancy. Safety in pregnancy, however, has not been established. Isosorbide dinitrate should only be used in pregnancy and during lactation if, in the opinion of the physician, the possible benefits of treatment outweigh the possible hazards.

4.7 Effects on ability to drive and use machines
Unknown.

4.8 Undesirable effects
In common with other nitrates, headaches, nausea and tachycardia may occur during administration. Whilst sharp falls in systemic arterial pressure can give rise to symptoms of cerebral flow deficiency and decreased coronary perfusion, clinical experience with Isoket has shown that this is not normally a problem.

4.9 Overdose
General supportive therapy.

5. PHARMACOLOGICAL PROPERTIES
5.1 Pharmacodynamic properties
ATC Code: CO1D A08 Vasodilators used in cardiac diseases – organic nitrates.

Isosorbide dinitrate is an organic nitrate, which in common with other cardioactive nitrates, is a vasodilator. It produces decreased left and right ventricular end-diastolic pressures to a greater extent than the decrease in systemic arterial pressure, thereby reducing afterload and especially the preload of the heart.

Isosorbide dinitrate influences the oxygen supply to ischaemic myocardium by causing the redistribution of blood flow along collateral channels and from epicardial to endocardial regions by selective dilatation of large epicardial vessels.

It reduces the requirement of the myocardium for oxygen by increasing venous capacitance, causing a pooling of blood in peripheral veins, thereby reducing ventricular volume and heart wall distension.

5.2 Pharmacokinetic properties
Isosorbide dinitrate (ISDN) is eliminated from plasma with a short half-life (about 0.7h). The metabolic degradation of ISDN occurs via denitration and glucuronidation, like all organic nitrates. The rate of formation of the metabolites has been calculated for isosorbide-5-mononitrate (IS-5-MN) with 0.27 h^{-1}, and isosorbide (IS) with 0.16 h^{-1}. IS-5-MN and IS-2-MN are the primary metabolites which are also pharmacologically active. IS-5-MN is metabolised to isosorbide 5-mononitrate-2-glucuronide (IS-5-MN-2-GLU). The half-life of this metabolite (about 2.5h) is shorter than that of IS-5-MN (about 5.1h). The half-life of ISDN is the shortest of all and that of IS-2-MN (about 3.2h) lies in between.

5.3 Preclinical safety data
None stated.

6. PHARMACEUTICAL PARTICULARS
6.1 List of excipients
Sodium chloride

Water for injection

Sodium hydroxide 1N

Hydrochloric acid solution 2N

6.2 Incompatibilities
Isoket contains isosorbide dinitrate in isotonic saline and is compatible with commonly employed infusion fluids, no incompatibilities have so far been demonstrated.

Isoket is compatible with glass infusion bottles and infusion packs made from polyethylene. Isoket may be infused slowly using a syringe pump with glass or plastic syringe. The use of PVC giving sets and containers should be avoided since significant losses of the active ingredient by adsorption can occur.

6.3 Shelf life
5 years, as packaged for sale.

Admixtures are stable for approximately 24 hours at room temperature in the recommended containers.

Open ampoules or bottles should be used immediately and any unused drug discarded.

6.4 Special precautions for storage
There are no special precautions for storage of the product as packaged for sale.

6.5 Nature and contents of container
Ten 10 ml clear glass ampoules.

Clear, Type I glass vials sealed with a grey stopper and a red flip-off aluminium cap, containing 50ml or 100ml of concentrate and packed in a cardboard carton.

Clear, Type I glass vials sealed with a grey stopper and a red flip-off aluminium cap, containing 50ml or 100ml of concentrate and packed in a cardboard carton containing a Sterifix Minispike to aid withdrawal of the product from the bottle.

6.6 Special precautions for disposal and other handling
Example of admixture preparation

To obtain a dose of 6 mg per hour, add 50 ml of Isoket 0.1% to 450 ml of a suitable vehicle, under aseptic conditions. The resultant admixture (500ml) contains 100 µg/ml (1mg/10ml) isosorbide dinitrate. An infusion rate of 60ml per hour (equivalent to 60 paediatric microdrops per minute or 20 standard drops per minute) will deliver the required dose of 6mg per hour.

Should it be necessary to reduce fluid intake, 100ml of Isoket 0.1% may be diluted to 500ml using a suitable vehicle. The resultant solution now contains 200 µg/ml (2mg/10ml) isosorbide dinitrate. An infusion rate of 30ml per hour (equivalent to 30 paediatric microdrops per minute or 10 standard drops per minute), will deliver the required dose of 6 mg per hour.

A dilution of 50% is advocated to produce a solution containing 0.5 mg/ml where fluid intake is strictly limited.

7. MARKETING AUTHORISATION HOLDER
SCHWARZ PHARMA Limited

5 Hercules Way

Leavesden Park

Watford

WD25 7GS

United Kingdom

8. MARKETING AUTHORISATION NUMBER(S)
PL 04438/0001

9. DATE OF FIRST AUTHORISATION/RENEWAL OF THE AUTHORISATION
10 February 2002

10. DATE OF REVISION OF THE TEXT
January 2007

Isoket Retard 20
(UCB Pharma Limited)

1. NAME OF THE MEDICINAL PRODUCT
Isoket Retard 20 Tablets

2. QUALITATIVE AND QUANTITATIVE COMPOSITION
Each tablet contains isosorbide dinitrate 20 mg in a prolonged release formulation.

For excipients see 6.1.

3. PHARMACEUTICAL FORM
Prolonged release tablets.

White with break score, marked IR 20 on the upper side and with SCHWARZ PHARMA on the reverse side.

4. CLINICAL PARTICULARS
4.1 Therapeutic indications
For the prophylaxis and treatment of angina pectoris.

4.2 Posology and method of administration
For oral administration.

Adults: One tablet to be taken twice daily without chewing and with a sufficient amount of fluid. The second dose should be given 6 to 8 hours after the first. For patients with higher nitrate requirements the dose may be increased to one tablet three times daily; the last dose should be taken around 6pm.

Elderly: Clinical experience has not necessitated alternative advice for use in elderly patients.

Children: The safety and efficacy of Isoket Retard has yet to be established.

4.3 Contraindications
This product should not be given to patients with a known sensitivity to nitrates (or any other ingredient in this product), very low blood pressure, acute myocardial infarction with low filling pressure, marked anaemia, head trauma, cerebral haemorrhage, acute circulatory failure, severe hypotension or hypovolaemia.

Phosphodiesterase inhibitors (e.g. Sildenafil) have been shown to potentiate the hypotensive effects of nitrates, and their co-administration with nitrates or nitric oxide donors is therefore contraindicated.

4.4 Special warnings and precautions for use
These tablets should be used with caution in patients who are suffering from hypothyroidism, hypothermia, malnutrition, severe liver disease or renal disease.

Symptoms of circulatory collapse may arise after the first dose, particularly in patients with labile circulation.

This product may give rise to symptoms of postural hypotension and sycope in some patients.

These tablets should be used with particular caution and under medical supervison in the following:

Hypertrophic obstructive cardiomyopathy (HOCM), constrictive pericarditis, cardiac tamponade, low cardiac filling pressures, aortic/mitral valve stenosis, and diseases associated with raised intracranial pressure.

Treatment with these tablets must not be interrupted or stopped to take phosphodiestearase inhibitor products due to the increased risk of inducing an attack of angina pectoris.

If these tablets are not taken as indicated with the appropriate dosing interval (see section 4.2) tolerance to the medication could develop.

4.5 Interaction with other medicinal products and other forms of interaction

Concurrent intake of drugs with blood pressure lowering properties e.g. beta-blockers, calcium antagonists, vasodilators etc. and/or alcohol may potentiate the hypotensive effect of the tablets. Symptoms of circulatory collapse can arise in patients already taking ACE inhibitors.

The hypotensive effect of nitrates is potentiated by concurrent administration of phosphodiesterase inhibitors (e.g. sildenafil). This might also occur with neuroleptics and tricyclic antidepressants.

Reports suggest that when administered concomitantly, nitrates may increase the blood level of dihydroergotamine and its hypertensive effect.

4.6 Pregnancy and lactation

This product should not be used during pregnancy or lactation unless considered essential by the physician.

4.7 Effects on ability to drive and use machines

Headaches, tiredness and dizziness may occur. These may affect the ability to drive and operate machinery. Patients should not drive or operate machinery if their ability is impaired.

4.8 Undesirable effects

A very common (> 10% of patients) adverse reaction to these tablets is headache. The incidence of headache diminishes gradually with time and continued use,

At start of therapy or when the dosage is increased, hypotension and/or light-headedness on standing are observed commonly (i.e. in 1-10% of patients.) These symptoms may be associated with dizziness, drowsiness, reflex tachycardia, and a feeling of weakness.

Infrequently (i.e. in less than 1% of patients), nausea, vomiting, flush and allergic skin reaction (e.g. rash), which may be sometimes severe may infrequently occur. In isolated cases exfoliative dermatitis may occur. Very rarely, Stevens-Johnson-Syndrome or angiodema may occur.

Severe hypotensive responses have been reported for organic nitrates and include nausea, vomiting, restlessness, pallor and excessive perspiration. Uncommonly collapse may occur (sometimes accompanied by bradyarrhythmia and syncope). Uncommonly severe hypotension may lead to enhanced angina symptoms.

A few reports on heartburn most likely due to a nitrate-induced sphincter relaxation have been recorded.

During treatment with these tablets, a temporary hypoxaemia may occur due to a relative redistribution of the blood flow in hypoventilated alveolar areas. Particularly in patients with coronary artery disease this may lead to a myocardial hypoxia.

4.9 Overdose

Clinical Features:

- Fall of blood pressure ⩽ 90mm Hg, paleness, sweating, weak pulse, tachycardia, light-headedness on standing, headache, weakness, dizziness, nausea and vomiting
- During isosorbide mononitrate biotransformation nitrite ions are released, which may include methaemoglobinaemia and cyanosis with subsequent tachypnoea, anxiety, loss of consciousness and cardiac arrest. It can not be excluded that an overdose of isosorbide dinitrate may cause this adverse reaction.
- In very high doses the intracranial pressure may be increased. This might lead to cerebral symptoms.

Supportive measures:

- Stop intake of the drug
- General procedures in the event of nitrate-related hypotension:

- Patient should be kept horizontal with the head lowered and legs raised
- Supply oxygen
- Expand plasma volume
- For specific shock treatment admit patient to intensive care unit

Specific Procedures:

- Raising the blood pressure if the blood pressure is very low
- Treatment of methaeglobinaemia

- Reduction therapy of choice with vitamin C, methylene-blue, or toluidine-blue
- Administer oxygen (if necessary)
- Initiate artificial ventilation
- Hemodialysis (if necessary)

- Resuscitation measures:

In case of signs of respiratory and circulatory arrest, initiate resuscitation measures immediately.

5. PHARMACODYNAMIC PROPERTIES

5.1 Pharmacodynamic properties

ATC Code: C01D A08 (Organic nitrates)

Isosorbide dinitrate causes a relaxation of vascular smooth muscle thereby inducing a vasodilation.

Both peripheral arteries and veins are relaxed by isosorbide dinitrate. The latter effect promotes venous pooling of blood and decreases venous return to the heart, thereby reducing ventricular end-diastolic pressure and volume (preload).

The action on arterial, and at higher dosages arteriolar vessels, reduce the systemic vascular resistance (afterload). This in turn reduces the cardiac work.

The effect on both preload and afterload lead subsequently to a reduced oxygen consumption of the heart.

Furthermore, isosorbide dinitrate causes redistribution of blood flow to the subendocardial regions of the heart when the coronary circulation is partially occluded by arteriosclerotic lesions. This last effect is likely to be due to a selective dilation of large coronary vessels. Nitrate-induced dilation of collateral arteries can improve the perfusion of poststenotic myocardium. Nitrates also dilate eccentric stenoses as they can counteract possible constricting factors acting on the residual arch of compliant smooth muscle at the site of the coronary narrowing. Furthermore, coronary spasms can be relaxed by nitrates.

Nitrates were shown to improve resting and exercise haemodynamics in patients suffering from congestive heart failure. In this beneficial effect several mechanisms including an improvement of valvular regurgitation (due to the lessening of ventricular dilation) and the reduction of myocardial oxygen demand are involved.

By decreasing the oxygen demand and increasing the oxygen supply, the area of myocardial damage is reduced. Therefore, isosorbide dinitrate may be useful in selected patients who suffered a myocardial infarction.

Effects on other organ systems include a relaxation of the bronchial muscle, the muscles of the gastrointestinal, the biliary and the urinary tract. Relaxation of the uterine smooth muscles is reported as well.

Mechanism of action:

Like all organic nitrates, isosorbide dinitrate acts as a donor of nitric oxide (NO). NO causes a relaxation of vascular smooth muscle via the stimulation of guanylyl cyclase and the subsequent increase of intracellular cyclic guanosine monophosphate (cGMP) concentration. A cGMP-dependent protein kinase is thus stimulated, with resultant alteration of the phosphorylation of various proteins in the smooth muscle cell. This eventually leads to the dephosphorylation of the light chain of myosin and the lowering of contractility

5.2 Pharmacokinetic properties

After administration of one tablet of Isoket Retard 20 at least two peak concentrations of ISDN occurred in the plasma. The initial peak (mean 1.9 ng/ml, range 1.0 to 3.4 ng/ml) occurred during 0.5 to 2 hours and then the mean plasma concentrations declined to 1.3 ng/ml at 3 hours. The concentration then increased again to reach a major peak level (mean 6.2 ng/ml range 1.6 to 12.3 ng/ml) during 4 to 6 hours after dosing. Plasma concentrations of ISDN have been measured after administration of increasing doses in the range 20 to 100 mg as Isoket Retard 20 tablets. Means of peak concentrations of 4.2 ng/ml, 13.1 ng/ml, 20.7 ng/ml, 36.8 ng/ml and 34.9 ng/ml were measured after doses of 20mg, 40mg, 60mg, 80mg and 100mg respectively.

Gastrointestinal absorption is slower than absorption through the oral mucosa. The first pass effect is higher when given orally. Isosorbide dinitrate is metabolised to isosorbide 2-mononitrate with a half life of 2.01 h (±0.4 h) to 2.5 h and isosorbide 5-mononitrate with a half-life of 4.6 h (±0.8 h). Both metabolites are pharmocologically active.

The relative bioavailability of Isoket Retard in comparison to the non-sustained-release tablet amounts to more than 80% after oral use.

5.3 Preclinical safety data

None stated.

6. PHARMACEUTICAL PARTICULARS

6.1 List of excipients

Lactose monohydrate

Talc

Polyvinyl acetate

Magnesium stearate

Potato starch

6.2 Incompatibilities

None known.

6.3 Shelf life

5 years.

6.4 Special precautions for storage

None

6.5 Nature and contents of container

Cartons of blister strips of polypropylene (PP) and aluminium or of PP/PP

Pack sizes 50, **56**, 60, 84 and 90 tablets.

Only the pack sizes marked in bold are currently marketed.

6.6 Special precautions for disposal and other handling

None

7. MARKETING AUTHORISATION HOLDER

UCB Pharma Limited

208 Bath Road

Slough

Berkshire

SL1 3WE

United Kingdom

8. MARKETING AUTHORISATION NUMBER(S)

PL 00039/0743

9. DATE OF FIRST AUTHORISATION/RENEWAL OF THE AUTHORISATION

30 June 2008

10. DATE OF REVISION OF THE TEXT

Isoket Retard 40

(UCB Pharma Limited)

1. NAME OF THE MEDICINAL PRODUCT

Isoket Retard 40 Tablets

2. QUALITATIVE AND QUANTITATIVE COMPOSITION

Each tablet contains isosorbide dinitrate 40 mg in a prolonged release formulation.

For excipients see 6.1

3. PHARMACEUTICAL FORM

Prolonged release tablets.

White with break score, marked IR 40 on the upper side and with SCHWARZ PHARMA on the reverse side.

4. CLINICAL PARTICULARS

4.1 Therapeutic indications

For the prophylaxis and treatment of angina pectoris.

4.2 Posology and method of administration

For oral administration.

Adults: One tablet to be taken once daily without chewing and with a sufficient amount of fluid. For patients with higher nitrate requirements the dose may be increased to one tablet twice daily; the second dose should be given 6 to 8 hours after the first.

Elderly: Clinical experience has not necessitated alternative advice for use in elderly patients.

Children: The safety and efficacy of Isoket Retard has yet to be established.

4.3 Contraindications

This product should not be given to patients with a known sensitivity to nitrates (or any other ingredient in this product), very low blood pressure, acute myocardial infarction with low filling pressure, marked anaemia, head trauma, cerebral haemorrhage, acute circulatory failure, severe hypotension or hypovolaemia.

Phosphodiesterase inhibitors (e.g. Sildenafil) have been shown to potentiate the hypotensive effects of nitrates, and their co-administration with nitrates or nitric oxide donors is therefore contraindicated.

4.4 Special warnings and precautions for use

These tablets should be used with caution in patients who are suffering from hypothyroidism, hypothermia, malnutrition, severe liver disease or renal disease.

Symptoms of circulatory collapse may arise after the first dose, particularly in patients with labile circulation.

This product may give rise to symptoms of postural hypotension and sycope in some patients.

These tablets should be used with particular caution and under medical supervison in the following:

Hypertrophic obstructive cardiomyopathy (HOCM), constrictive pericarditis, cardiac tamponade, low cardiac filling pressures, aortic/mitral valve stenosis, and diseases associated with raised intracranial pressure.

Treatment with these tablets must not be interrupted or stopped to take phosphodiestearase inhibitors due to the increased risk of inducing an attack of angina pectoris.

If these tablets are not taken as indicated with the appropriate dosing interval (see section 4.2) tolerance to the medication could develop.

4.5 Interaction with other medicinal products and other forms of interaction

Concurrent intake of drugs with blood pressure lowering properties e.g. beta blockers, calcium antagonists, vasodilators etc. and/or alcohol may potentiate the hypotensive effect of the tablets. Symptoms of circulatory collapse can arise in patients already taking ACE inhibitors.

The hypotensive effect of nitrates is potentiated by concurrent administration of phosphodiesterase inhibitors (e.g. sildenafil). This might also occur with neuroleptics and tricyclic antidepressants.

Reports suggest that when administered concomitantly, nitrates may increase the blood level of dihydroergotamine and its hypertensive effect.

4.6 Pregnancy and lactation
This product should not be used during pregnancy or lactation unless considered essential by the physician.

4.7 Effects on ability to drive and use machines
Headaches, tiredness and dizziness may occur. These may affect the ability to drive and operate machinery. Patients should not drive or operate machinery if their ability is impaired.

4.8 Undesirable effects
A very common (> 10% of patients) adverse reaction to these tablets is headache. The incidence of headache diminishes gradually with time and continued use.

At start of therapy or when the dosage is increased, hypotension and/or light-headedness on standing are observed commonly (i.e. in 1-10% of patients.) These symptoms may be associated with dizziness, drowsiness, reflex tachycardia, and a feeling of weakness.

Infrequently (i.e. in less than 1% of patients), nausea, vomiting, flush and allergic skin reaction (e.g. rash), which may be sometimes severe may infrequently occur. In isolated cases exfoliative dermatitis may occur. Very rarely, Stevens-Johnson-Syndrome or angiodema may occur.

Severe hypotensive responses have been reported for organic nitrates and include nausea, vomiting, restlessness, pallor and excessive perspiration. Uncommonly collapse may occur (sometimes accompanied by bradyarrhythmia and syncope). Uncommonly severe hypotension may lead to enhanced angina symptoms.

A few reports on heartburn most likely due to a nitrate-induced sphincter relaxation have been recorded.

During treatment with these tablets, a temporary hypoxaemia may occur due to a relative redistribution of the blood flow in hypoventilated alveolar areas. Particularly in patients with coronary artery disease this may lead to a myocardial hypoxia.

4.9 Overdose
Clinical Features:

• Fall of blood pressure ≤ 90mm Hg, paleness, sweating, weak pulse, tachycardia, light-headedness on standing, headache, weakness, dizziness, nausea and vomiting

• During isosorbide monintrate biotransformation nitrite ions are released, which may include methaemoglobinaemia and cyanosis with subsequent tachypnoea, anxiety, loss of consciousness and cardiac arrest. It can not be excluded that an overdose of isosorbide dinitrate may cause this adverse reaction.

• In very high doses the intracranial pressure may be increased. This might lead to cerebral symptoms.

Supportive measures

• Stop intake of the drug

• General procedures in the event of nitrate-related hypotension:

- Patient should be kept horizontal with the head lowered and legs raised
- Supply oxygen
- Expand plasma volume
- For specific shock treatment admit patient to intensive care unit

Specific Procedures

• Raising the blood pressure if the blood pressure is very low

• Treatment of methaeglobinaemia

- Reduction therapy of choice with vitamin C, methylene-blue, or toluidine-blue
- Administer oxygen (if necessary)
- Initiate artificial ventilation
- Hemodialysis (of necessary)

• Resuscitation measures:

In case of signs of respiratory and circulatory arrest, initiate resuscitation measures immediately.

5. PHARMACOLOGICAL PROPERTIES

5.1 Pharmacodynamic properties
ATC Code: C01D A08 (Organic nitrates)

Isosorbide dinitrate causes a relaxation of vascular smooth muscle thereby inducing a vasodilation.

Both peripheral arteries and veins are relaxed by isosorbide dinitrate. The latter effect promotes venous pooling of blood and decreases venous return to the heart, thereby reducing ventricular end-diastolic pressure and volume (preload).

The action on arterial, and at higher dosages arteriolar vessels, reduce the systemic vascular resistance (afterload). This in turn reduces the cardiac work.

The effects on both preload and afterload lead subsequently to a reduced oxygen consumption of the heart.

Furthermore, isosorbide dinitrate causes redistribution of blood flow to the subendocardial regions of the heart when the coronary circulation is partially occluded by arteriosclerotic lesions. This last effect is likely to be due to a selective dilation of large coronary vessels. Nitrate-induced dilation of collateral arteries can improve the perfusion of poststenotic myocardium. Nitrates also dilate eccentric stenoses as they can counteract possible constricting factors acting on the residual arch of compliant smooth muscle at the site of the coronary narrowing. Furthermore, coronary spasms can be relaxed by nitrates.

Nitrates were shown to improve resting and exercise haemodynamics in patients suffering from congestive heart failure. In this beneficial effect several mechansims including an improvement of valvular regurgitation (due to the lessening of ventricular dilation) and the reduction of myocardial oxygen demand are involved.

By decreasing the oxygen demand and increasing the oxygen supply, the area of myocardial damage is reduced. Therefore, isosorbide dinitrate may be useful in selected patients who suffered a myocardial infarction.

Effects on other organ systems include a relaxation of the bronchial muscle, the muscles of the gastrointestinal, the biliary and the urinary tract. Relaxation of the uterine smooth muscles is reported as well.

Mechanism of action:

Like all organic nitrates, isosorbide dinitrate acts as a donor of nitric oxide (NO). NO causes a relaxation of vascular smooth muscle via the stimulation of guanylyl cyclase and the subsequent increase of intracellular cyclic guanosine monophosphate (cGMP) concentration. A cGMP-dependent protein kinase is thus stimulated, with resultant alteration of the phosphorylation of various proteins in the smooth muscle cell. This eventually leads to the dephosphorylation of the light chain of myosin and the lowering of contractility

5.2 Pharmacokinetic properties
After administration of one tablet of Isoket Retard 40 mean peak plasma concentrations of ISDN (8.0 ± 12 ng/ml) at 7.7 ± 2.9 hours and IS-5N (190 ± 33 ng/ml) at 8.7 ± 2.1 hours. The terminal half life of IS-5N which was least affected by the absorption process was 5.4 hours ± 0.5 sd.

Gastrointestinal absorption is slower than absorption through the oral mucosa. The first pass effect is higher when given orally. Isosorbide dinitrate is metabolized to isosorbide 2-mononitrate with a half-life of 2.01 h (±0.4 h) to 2.5 h and isosorbide 5-mononitrate with a half-life of 4.6 h (± 8 h). Both metabolites are pharmacologically active.

The relative bioavailability of Isoket Retard in comparison to the non-sustained-release tablet amounts to more than 80% after oral use.

5.3 Preclinical safety data
None stated.

6. PHARMACEUTICAL PARTICULARS

6.1 List of excipients
Lactose monohydrate
Talc
Polyvinyl acetate
Magnesium stearate
Potato starch

6.2 Incompatibilities
None known.

6.3 Shelf life
5 years.

6.4 Special precautions for storage
None

6.5 Nature and contents of container
Cartons of blister strips of polypropylene (PP) and aluminium or of PP/PP

Pack sizes 50, **56**, 60, 84 and 90 tablets.

Only the pack sizes marked in bold are currently marketed.

6.6 Special precautions for disposal and other handling
None

7. MARKETING AUTHORISATION HOLDER
UCB Pharma Limited
208 Bath Road
Slough
Berkshire
SL1 3WE
United Kingdom

8. MARKETING AUTHORISATION NUMBER(S)
PL 00039/0744

9. DATE OF FIRST AUTHORISATION/RENEWAL OF THE AUTHORISATION
30 June 2008

10. DATE OF REVISION OF THE TEXT

Isoniazid Ampoules 50mg/2ml

(Cambridge Laboratories)

1. NAME OF THE MEDICINAL PRODUCT
Isoniazid Ampoules 50 mg/2 ml.

2. QUALITATIVE AND QUANTITATIVE COMPOSITION
Each ampoule contains 50 mg Isoniazid BP in 2 ml of solution.

3. PHARMACEUTICAL FORM
Ampoules

4. CLINICAL PARTICULARS

4.1 Therapeutic indications
For all forms of pulmonary and extra-pulmonary tuberculosis.

4.2 Posology and method of administration
Isoniazid ampoules are for intramuscular, intravenous, intrapleural, or intrathecal injection.

Adults and children

The usual intramuscular or intravenous dose for adults is 200 to 300 mg as a single daily dose, for children 100 to 300 mg daily (10 - 20 mg/kg), but doses much larger than these are sometimes given, especially in conditions such as tuberculous meningitis. It is recommended to give an intravenous dose slowly as an undiluted bolus injection, although other methods may be employed.

Neonates

The recommended intravenous or intramuscular dose for neonates is 3-5 mg/kg with a maximum of 10 mg/kg daily. Isoniazid may be present in the milk of lactating mothers.

The elderly

No dosage reduction is necessary in the elderly.

Intrapleural use

50 to 250 mg may be instilled intrapleurally after aspiration of pus, the dosage of oral isoniazid on that day being correspondingly reduced. The ampoule solution is also used for the local treatment of tuberculous ulcers, for irrigation of fistulae, etc.

Intrathecal use:

It should be noted that CSF concentrations of isoniazid are approximately 90% of plasma concentrations. Where intrathecal use is required, 25 - 50 mg daily has been given to adults and 10 - 20 mg daily for children, according to age.

It is usual to give Isoniazid together with other antituberculous therapy, as determined by current practice and/or sensitivity testing.

It is recommended that pyridoxine 10 - 50mg daily be given during Isoniazid therapy to minimise adverse reactions, especially in malnourished patients and those predisposed to neuropathy (eg. diabetics and alcoholics).

4.3 Contraindications
Isoniazid should not be given to patients with a history of sensitivity to isoniazid.

4.4 Special warnings and precautions for use
Use in renal and hepatic impairment: no dosage reduction of Isoniazid is necessary when given to patients with mild renal failure. Patients with severe renal failure (glomerular filtration rate of less than 10 ml/minute) and slow acetylator status might require a dose reduction of about 100mg to maintain trough plasma levels at less than 1 mcg/ml. The possible risks of administration of Isoniazid to patients with pre-existing non-tuberculous hepatic disease should be balanced against the benefits expected from treating tuberculosis.

Care is also required in chronic alcoholism and when prescribing isoniazid for patients with pre-existing hepatitis. Convulsions and psychotic reactions have occurred, especially in patients with a previous history of these conditions. These manifestations usually subside rapidly when the drug is withdrawn. Isoniazid should therefore be given with caution to patients with convulsive disorders and should be avoided in those with manic or hypomanic psychoses.

Isoniazid is metabolised by acetylation, which is subject to genetic variation. The 'slow acetylators' may be more susceptible to drug-induced peripheral neuropathy. However, dose adjustment is not normally required.

4.5 Interaction with other medicinal products and other forms of interaction
Isoniazid may inhibit the metabolism of phenytoin, primidone and carbamazepine. Plasma levels of these drugs should be monitored if concurrent therapy with Isoniazid is necessary. See also statement under 4.8 regarding Rifampicin.

4.6 Pregnancy and lactation
While Isoniazid is generally regarded to be safe in pregnancy, there is a possibility of an increased risk of foetal malformations occurring when Isoniazid is given in early pregnancy. If pregnancy cannot be excluded possible risks should be balanced against therapeutic benefits. Isoniazid is excreted in breast milk at concentrations equivalent to those found in maternal plasma, ie. 6-12 mcg/ml. this could result in an infant ingesting up to 2 mg/kg/day.

4.7 Effects on ability to drive and use machines
None known.

4.8 Undesirable effects
Isoniazid is generally well tolerated. Side-effects have been reported mainly in association with high doses or in slow acetylators who develop higher blood levels of the drug. Fever, peripheral neuropathy (preventable with pyridoxine), optic neuritis and atrophy, allergic skin conditions (including erythema multiforme), and rarely lupoid syndrome, pellagra, purpura and haematological reactions have occurred during isoniazid therapy. Hyperglycaemia and gynaeco-mastia have been reported with isoniazid treatment. Isoniazid, especially if given with rifampicin,

may induce abnormalities in liver function, particularly in patients with pre-existing liver disorders, in the elderly, the very young and the malnourished. Monthly review is suggested to detect and limit the severity of this side-effect by stopping treatment if plasma transaminases exceed three times the upper limit of normal. There is conflicting opinion as to the relationship of this side-effect to acetylator status.

4.9 Overdose

In severe poisoning the main risk is of epileptiform convulsions. In addition any of the side-effects listed above may occur together with metabolic acidosis and hyperglycaemia. Treatment should be directed to the control of convulsions and large doses of pyridoxine may limit the occurrence of other adverse effects. Metabolic acidosis may require sodium bicarbonate infusion. The drug is removed by dialysis.

5. PHARMACOLOGICAL PROPERTIES

5.1 Pharmacodynamic properties

Isoniazid is a highly active tuberculostatic drug, and at high concentrations it is bactericidal to mycobacterium tuberculosis, possibly acting by interference with the synthesis of mycolic acid (a constituent of the bacterial cell wall).

5.2 Pharmacokinetic properties

Isoniazid is not appreciably protein-bound and diffuses readily throughout the body. It affects intracellular as well as extracellular bacilli. The primary metabolic route involves acetylation the rate of which is determined genetically.

5.3 Preclinical safety data

There are no pre-clinical data of relevance to the prescriber which are additional to that already included in other sections of the SPC.

6. PHARMACEUTICAL PARTICULARS

6.1 List of excipients

Hydrochloric Acid

Water for Injections BP

6.2 Incompatibilities

None known.

6.3 Shelf life

Three years.

6.4 Special precautions for storage

The recommended maximum storage temperature is 25°C.

Protect from light.

6.5 Nature and contents of container

Colourless glass ampoules coded with dark red and orange colour rings, each containing 2 ml of solution, in packs of 10 ampoules.

6.6 Special precautions for disposal and other handling

None.

Administrative Data

7. MARKETING AUTHORISATION HOLDER

Cambridge Laboratories Limited

Deltic House

Kingfisher Way

Silverlink Business Park

Wallsend

Tyne & Wear

NE28 9NX

8. MARKETING AUTHORISATION NUMBER(S)

PL 12070/0005

9. DATE OF FIRST AUTHORISATION/RENEWAL OF THE AUTHORISATION

30 July 1997

10. DATE OF REVISION OF THE TEXT

April 2002

Isoniazid Tablets BP 100mg

(UCB Pharma Limited)

1. NAME OF THE MEDICINAL PRODUCT

Isoniazid Tablets BP 100mg

2. QUALITATIVE AND QUANTITATIVE COMPOSITION

Isoniazid BP 100mg

For excipients see 6.1

3. PHARMACEUTICAL FORM

White biconvex uncoated tablets embossed 100 152 on one face and EVANS on the obverse.

4. CLINICAL PARTICULARS

4.1 Therapeutic indications

Isoniazid is indicated in the treatment of all forms of pulmonary and extra-pulmonary tuberculosis.

4.2 Posology and method of administration

Official guidance should always be consulted when selecting the dose regimens to be used for adults and children (according to age and body weight), the duration of therapy and the total content of the combination treatment regimen.

Posology

Adults

The dose of isoniazid for the treatment of tuberculosis is commonly 4 to 5 mg per kilogram body-weight daily given by mouth in single or divided doses up to a maximum of 300 mg daily. Up to 10 mg per kilogram body-weight daily may be given particularly during the first 1 to 2 weeks of treatment of tuberculous meningitis. A dose of 15 mg per kilogram has been given two or three times weekly in intermittent treatment regimens.

Elderly

No dosage reduction is necessary in the elderly, but caution should be exercised due to the possible decrease in renal and hepatic function.

Children

The usual daily dose for children is from 5 up to 20 mg per kilogram body-weight daily in single or divided doses.

Method of Administration

Isoniazid tablets should be taken preferably on an empty stomach, i.e. at least 30 minutes before a meal or 2 hours after a meal.

4.3 Contraindications

Patients who are known to be hypersensitive to isoniazid or drug-induced liver disease.

4.4 Special warnings and precautions for use

All patients should have baseline liver function tests performed and repeated at regular intervals during treatment. If serum AST rises to more than three times normal, or there is any increase in bilirubin, treatment should be withdrawn. Special precautions are required in patients with impaired liver function. Any deterioration in liver function in these patients is an indication for stopping treatment.

Isoniazid should not be given to patients who have experience severe adverse reactions including drug-induced liver disease. Care should be taken in giving isoniazid to patients suffering from convulsive disorders, diabetes mellitus, chronic alcoholism, or impaired liver or kidney function or to patients taking other potentially hepatoxic agents. If symptoms of hepatitis such as malaise, fatigue, anorexia, and nausea develop isoniazid should be discontinued immediately.

Isoniazid should be used with caution in patients with a history of psychosis.

Advanced age, female gender, slow acetylators, malnutrition, HIV infection, preexisting liver disease, and extrapulmonary tuberculosis were identified as risk factors for isoniazid-induced hepatotoxicity.

Patients who are at risk of neuropathy or pyridoxine deficiency, including those who are diabetic, alcoholic, malnourished, uraemic, pregnant, or infected with HIV, should be given pyridoxine.

4.5 Interaction with other medicinal products and other forms of interaction

When isoniazid is given to patients who inactivate it slowly or to patients receiving paraminosalicyclic acid concurrently, tissue concentrations may be enhanced, and adverse effects are more likely to appear. There may be an increased risk of liver damage in patients receiving rifampicin and isoniazid but liver enzymes are raised only transiently.

Isoniazid can inhibit the hepatic metabolism of a number of drugs, in some cases leading to increased toxicity. These include the antiepileptics carbamazepine, primidone, and phenytoin, the benzodiazepines diazepam and triazolam, chlorzoxazone, and disulfiram.

Isoniazid has been reported to cause substantial elevations of serum concentrations of carbamazepine and symptoms of carbamazepine toxicity at isoniazid doses of 200 mg daily or more. The concurrent used is not recommended unless the effects can be closely monitored and suitable downward dosage adjustments made (a reduction between one-half or one-third was reported effective).

Concomitant benzodiazepine (diazepam) and isoniazid therapy has been reported to result in an increased risk of benzodiazepine toxicity (sedation, respiratory depression).

Isoniazid may reduce the therapeutic effects of levodopa.

Concomitant administration of isoniazid with itraconazole may result in significant decreases in itraconazole serum concentrations and therapeutic failure. Co administration is not recommended.

Isoniazid may decrease ketoconazole serum levels. Concurrent use should be well monitored and dosage increases made if necessary.

Because the clearance of isoniazid was found doubled when zalcitabine was given in HIV-positive patients, concurrent use of isoniazid and zalcitabine should be monitored to ensure isoniazid effectiveness.

There may be an increased risk of distal sensory neuropathy when isoniazid is used in patients taking stavudine (d4T).

There may be a potential interaction between isoniazid and foods containing histamine or tyramine.

4.6 Pregnancy and lactation

Isoniazid crosses the placenta. Therefore, isoniazid should only be used in pregnant women or in women of child-bearing potential if the potential benefit justifies the potential risk to the foetus. It is considered that untreated tuberculosis represents a far greater hazard to a pregnant woman and her fetus than does treatment of the disease. Pyridoxine supplementation is recommended.

Isoniazid passes into breast milk. When administered to nursing mother, breast-fed infants should be monitored for possible signs of isoniazid toxicity. Administration of pyridoxine to the breast-feeding mother and infant may be considered.

4.7 Effects on ability to drive and use machines

No specific statement, but unlikely to effect the ability to drive or use machinery.

4.8 Undesirable effects

Patients may experience fever, nausea, vomiting and other gastro-intestinal effects.

Many of the adverse effects of isoniazid are related to hypersensitivity or to the use of large doses; patients who are slow inactivators may experience a greater incidence of toxicity.

Interstitial pneumonitis.

Peripheral neuropathy, constipation, difficulty in starting urination, dryness of the mouth, and sometimes vertigo and hyperreflexia may be troublesome with doses of 10mg per kg body weight.

Convulsions, optic neuritis, systemic lupus erythematosus, lupus-like syndrome, gynaecomastia and psychotic reactions have been reported.

Liver damage, elevated liver enzymes, jaundice, hepatitis, and fulminant hepatic failure, has occurred especially over the age of 35; it may be serious and sometimes fatal with the development of necrosis.

Blood disorders include haemolytic and aplastic anaemia and agranulocytosis.

Acute pancreatitis.

Various skin reactions including erythema multiforme, Stevens-Johnson syndrome and toxic epidermal necrolysis have occurred.

Hyperglycaemia and acidosis.

Pellagra may be related to an isoniazid-induced pyridoxine deficiency which affects the conversion of tryptophan to nicotinic acid.

Although isoniazid usually has a mood elevating effect, mental disturbances, ranging from minor personality changes to major mental derangement have been reported; these are usually reversed on withdrawal of the drug.

Hearing loss and tinnitus have been reported in patients with end stage renal impairment.

Withdrawal symptoms, which may occur on the cessation of the treatment, include headache, insomnia, excessive dreaming, irritability and nervousness.

4.9 Overdose

The most commonly reported adverse events associated with isoniazid overdose are nausea, vomiting and central nervous system toxicity such as vertigo, seizures and coma.

Treatment of overdosage consists of gastric lavage following intubation and the control of convulsions by anticonvulsants given intravenously as well as the intravenous injection of large doses of pyridoxine. Any acidosis is corrected with sodium bicarbonate. Forced diuresis may be tried and haemodialysis or peritoneal dialysis has been used.

5. PHARMACOLOGICAL PROPERTIES

5.1 Pharmacodynamic properties

Isoniazid has no significant antibacterial action against any micro-organisms except the mycobacteria; against mycobacterium tuberculosis it is bacteriostatic in extremely low concentrations.

Isoniazid is used mainly in the treatment of pulmonary tuberculosis but it appears to be effective also in the treatment of extrapulmonary lesions, including meningitis and genito-urinary disease.

5.2 Pharmacokinetic properties

Absorption

Readily and completely absorbed after oral administration.

Distribution

Readily diffuses into all tissues and fluids including the cerebrospinal fluid. Isoniazid is retained in the skin and in infected tissue; it crosses the placenta and is secreted in the milk of lactating mothers.

Protein binding

Isoniazid does not appear to be bound in the blood.

Half-life

Plasma elimination half-life, in rapid acetylators about 1.2 hours and in slow acetylators about 3.5 hours.

Metabolic reactions

Acetylation, hydrolysis and glycine conjugation, hydrazone formation, and n-methylation; acetylation is polymorphic and two groups of acetylators have been identified, rapid and slow acetylators. The rate of hydrolysis is more rapid in the rapid acetylators than in the slow ones. The metabolites formed include acetyl isoniazid, isonicotinic acid, isonicotinuric acid, isonicotinoylhydrazones of pyruvic and glutaric acids, and n-methylisoniazid.

Excretion

Over 90% of a dose is excreted in the urine in 24 hours, most being excreted in the first 12 hours, 4-32% is unchanged, but no more than 10% of a dose is excreted in the faeces.

5.3 Preclinical safety data

Not applicable since isoniazid tablets have been used in clinical practice for many years and its effects in man are well known.

6. PHARMACEUTICAL PARTICULARS

6.1 List of excipients

Lactose 170 Mesh

Maize Starch

Microcrystalline Cellulose

Alginic Acid

Magnesium Stearate

Purified Water

6.2 Incompatibilities

None

6.3 Shelf life

36 months

6.4 Special precautions for storage

Store below 25°C

6.5 Nature and contents of container

Pigmented polypropylene container fitted with a tamper-evident closure containing 7, 14, 21, 28, 30, 50, 56, 60, 84, 90, 100, 112, 120 or 250 tablets.

Not all pack sizes may be marketed.

6.6 Special precautions for disposal and other handling

No special precautions are required.

7. MARKETING AUTHORISATION HOLDER

UCB Pharma Ltd

208 Bath Road

Slough

Berkshire

SL1 3WE

8. MARKETING AUTHORISATION NUMBER(S)

PL 00039/0552

9. DATE OF FIRST AUTHORISATION/RENEWAL OF THE AUTHORISATION

April 2007

10. DATE OF REVISION OF THE TEXT

Drafted July 2009

Isoniazid Tablets BP 50mg

(UCB Pharma Limited)

1. NAME OF THE MEDICINAL PRODUCT

Isoniazid Tablets BP 50mg

2. QUALITATIVE AND QUANTITATIVE COMPOSITION

Isoniazid BP 50mg

For excipients see 6.1

3. PHARMACEUTICAL FORM

White biconvex uncoated tablets embossed 50 151 on one face and EVANS on the obverse.

4. CLINICAL PARTICULARS

4.1 Therapeutic indications

Isoniazid is indicated in the treatment of all forms of pulmonary and extra-pulmonary tuberculosis.

4.2 Posology and method of administration

Official guidance should always be consulted when selecting the dose regimens to be used for adults and children (according to age and body weight), the duration of therapy and the total content of the combination treatment regimen.

Posology

Adults

The dose of isoniazid for the treatment of tuberculosis is commonly 4 to 5 mg per kilogram body-weight daily given by mouth in single or divided doses up to a maximum of 300 mg daily. Up to 10 mg per kilogram body-weight daily may be given particularly during the first 1 to 2 weeks of treatment of tuberculous meningitis. A dose of 15 mg per kilogram has been given two or three times weekly in intermittent treatment regimens.

Elderly

No dosage reduction is necessary in the elderly, but caution should be exercised due to the possible decrease in renal and hepatic function.

Children

The usual daily dose for children is from 5 to 20mg per kilogram body-weight daily in single or divided doses.

Method of Administration

Isoniazid Tablets should be taken preferably on an empty stomach, i.e. at least 30 minutes before a meal or 2 hours after a meal.

4.3 Contraindications

Patients who are known to be hypersensitive to isoniazid or drug-induced liver disease.

4.4 Special warnings and precautions for use

All patients should have baseline liver function tests performed and repeated at regular intervals during treatment. If serum AST rises to more than three times normal, or there is any increase in bilirubin, treatment should be withdrawn. Special precautions are required in patients with impaired liver function. Any deterioration in liver function in these patients is an indication for stopping treatment.

Isoniazid should not be given to patients who have experience severe adverse reactions including drug-induced liver disease. Care should be taken in giving isoniazid to patients suffering from convulsive disorders, diabetes mellitus, chronic alcoholism, or impaired liver or kidney function or to patients taking other potentially hepatoxic agents. If symptoms of hepatitis such as malaise, fatigue, anorexia, and nausea develop isoniazid should be discontinued immediately.

Isoniazid should be used with caution in patients with a history of psychosis.

Advanced age, female gender, slow acetylators, malnutrition, HIV infection, preexisting liver disease, and extra-pulmonary tuberculosis were identified as risk factors for isoniazid-induced hepatotoxicity.

Patients who are at risk of neuropathy or pyridoxine deficiency, including those who are diabetic, alcoholic, malnourished, uraemic, pregnant, or infected with HIV, should be given pyridoxine.

4.5 Interaction with other medicinal products and other forms of interaction

When isoniazid is given to patients who inactivate it slowly or to patients receiving paraminosalicyclic acid concurrently, tissue concentrations may be enhanced, and adverse effects are more likely to appear. There may be an increased risk of liver damage in patients receiving rifampicin and isoniazid but liver enzymes are raised only transiently.

Isoniazid can inhibit the hepatic metabolism of a number of drugs, in some cases leading to increased toxicity. These include the antiepileptics carbamazepine, primidone, and phenytoin, the benzodiazepines diazepam and triazolam, chlorzoxazone, and disulfiram.

Isoniazid has been reported to cause substantial elevations of serum concentrations of carbamazepine and symptoms of carbamazepine toxicity at isoniazid doses of 200 mg daily or more. The concurrent used is not recommended unless the effects can be closely monitored and suitable downward dosage adjustments made (a reduction between one-half or one-third was reported effective).

Concomitant benzodiazepine (diazepam) and isoniazid therapy has been reported to result in an increased risk of benzodiazepine toxicity (sedation, respiratory depression).

Isoniazid may reduce the therapeutic effects of levodopa.

Concomitant administration of isoniazid with itraconazole may result in significant decreases in itraconazole serum concentrations and therapeutic failure. Co administration is not recommended.

Isoniazid may decrease ketoconazole serum levels. Concurrent use should be well monitored and dosage increases made if necessary.

Because the clearance of isoniazid was found doubled when zalcitabine was given in HIV-positive patients, concurrent use of isoniazid and zalcitabine should be monitored to ensure isoniazid effectiveness.

There may be an increased risk of distal sensory neuropathy when isoniazid is used in patients taking stavudine (d4T).

There may be a potential interaction between isoniazid and foods containing histamine or tyramine.

4.6 Pregnancy and lactation

Isoniazid crosses the placenta. Therefore, isoniazid should only be used in pregnant women or in women of child-bearing potential if the potential benefit justifies the potential risk to the foetus. It is considered that untreated tuberculosis represents a far greater hazard to a pregnant woman and her fetus than does treatment of the disease. Pyridoxine supplementation is recommended.

Isoniazid passes into breast milk. When administered to nursing mother, breast-fed infants should be monitored for possible signs of isoniazid toxicity. Administration of pyridoxine to the breast-feeding mother and infant may be considered.

4.7 Effects on ability to drive and use machines

No specific statement, but unlikely to effect the ability to drive or use machinery.

4.8 Undesirable effects

Patients may experience fever, nausea, vomiting and other gastro-intestinal effects.

Many of the adverse effects of isoniazid are related to hypersensitivity or to the use of large doses; patients who are slow inactivators may experience a greater incidence of toxicity.

Interstitial pneumonitis.

Peripheral neuropathy, constipation, difficulty in starting urination, dryness of the mouth, and sometimes vertigo and hyperreflexia may be troublesome with doses of 10mg per kg body weight.

Convulsions, optic neuritis, systemic lupus erythematosus, lupus-like syndrome, gynaecomastia and psychotic reactions have been reported.

Liver damage, elevated liver enzymes, jaundice, hepatitis, and fulminant hepatic failure, has occurred especially over the age of 35; it may be serious and sometimes fatal with the development of necrosis.

Blood disorders include haemolytic and aplastic anaemia and agranulocytosis.

Acute pancreatitis.

Various skin reactions including erythema multiforme, Stevens-Johnson syndrome and toxic epidermal necrolysis have occurred.

Hyperglycaemia and acidosis.

Pellagra may be related to an isoniazid-induced pyridoxine deficiency which affects the conversion of tryptophan to nicotinic acid.

Although isoniazid usually has a mood elevating effect, mental disturbances, ranging from minor personality changes to major mental derangement have been reported; these are usually reversed on withdrawal of the drug.

Hearing loss and tinnitus have been reported in patients with end stage renal impairment.

Withdrawal symptoms, which may occur on the cessation of the treatment, include headache, insomnia, excessive dreaming, irritability and nervousness.

4.9 Overdose

The most commonly reported adverse events associated with isoniazid overdose are nausea, vomiting and central nervous system toxicity such as vertigo, seizures and coma.

Treatment of overdosage consists of gastric lavage following intubation and the control of convulsions by anti-convulsants given intravenously as well as the intravenous injection of large doses of pyridoxine. Any acidosis is corrected with sodium bicarbonate. Forced diuresis may be tried and haemodialysis or peritoneal dialysis has been used.

5. PHARMACOLOGICAL PROPERTIES

5.1 Pharmacodynamic properties

Isoniazid has no significant antibacterial action against any micro-organisms except the mycobacteria; against mycobacterium tuberculosis it is bacteriostatic in extremely low concentrations.

Isoniazid is used mainly in the treatment of pulmonary tuberculosis but it appears to be effective also in the treatment of extrapulmonary lesions, including meningitis and genito-urinary disease.

5.2 Pharmacokinetic properties

Absorption

Readily and completely absorbed after oral administration.

Distribution

Readily diffuses into all tissues and fluids including the cerebrospinal fluid. Isoniazid is retained in the skin and in infected tissue; it crosses the placenta and is secreted in the milk of lactating mothers.

Protein binding

Isoniazid does not appear to be bound in the blood.

Half-life

Plasma elimination half-life, in rapid acetylators about 1.2 hours and in slow acetylators about 3.5 hours.

Metabolic reactions

Acetylation, hydrolysis and glycine conjugation, hydrazone formation, and n-methylation; acetylation is polymorphic and two groups of acetylators have been identified, rapid and slow acetylators. The rate of hydrolysis is more rapid in the rapid acetylators than in the slow ones. The metabolites formed include acetyl isoniazid, isonicotinic acid, isonicotinuric acid, isonicotinoylhydrazones of pyruvic and glutaric acids, and n-methylisoniazid.

Excretion

Over 90% of a dose is excreted in the urine in 24 hours, most being excreted in the first 12 hours, 4-32% is unchanged, but no more than 10% of a dose is excreted in the faeces.

5.3 Preclinical safety data

Not applicable since isoniazid tablets have been used in clinical practice for many years and its effects in man are well known.

6. PHARMACEUTICAL PARTICULARS

6.1 List of excipients

Lactose 170 Mesh

Maize Starch

Microcrystalline Cellulose

Alginic Acid

Magnesium Stearate

Purified Water

6.2 Incompatibilities

None

6.3 Shelf life

36 months

6.4 Special precautions for storage

Store below 25°C.

6.5 Nature and contents of container

Pigmented polypropylene container fitted with a tamper-evident closure containing 7, 14, 21, 28, 30, 50, 56, 60, 84, 90, 100, 112, 120 or 250 tablets. Not all pack sizes may be marketed.

6.6 Special precautions for disposal and other handling

No special precautions are required.

7. MARKETING AUTHORISATION HOLDER

UCB Pharma Ltd

208 Bath Road

Slough

Berkshire

SL1 3WE

8. MARKETING AUTHORISATION NUMBER(S)

PL 00039/0551

9. DATE OF FIRST AUTHORISATION/RENEWAL OF THE AUTHORISATION

April 2007

10. DATE OF REVISION OF THE TEXT

Drafted July 2009

Isotard XL

(ProStrakan)

1. NAME OF THE MEDICINAL PRODUCT

Isotard 25XL, 40XL, 50XL and 60XL Tablets

2. QUALITATIVE AND QUANTITATIVE COMPOSITION

Isosorbide-5-mononitrate 25mg

Isosorbide-5-mononitrate 40mg

Isosorbide-5-mononitrate 50mg

Isosorbide-5-mononitrate 60mg

International non-proprietary name (INN): Isosorbide mononitrate.

Isosorbide mononitrate is also referred to as ISMN.

Chemical name: 1,4;3,6 dianhydro-D-glucitol-5-mononitrate.

3. PHARMACEUTICAL FORM

Tablets (modified release).

4. CLINICAL PARTICULARS

4.1 Therapeutic indications

Prophylactic treatment of angina pectoris.

4.2 Posology and method of administration

Adults

One tablet, once daily given in the morning. The dose may be increased to two tablets, the whole dose to be given together (dose range 25 to 120 mg).

For Isotard 60XL only, the dose can be titrated to minimise the possibility of headache by initiating treatment with half a tablet (30 mg) for the first two to four days.

The tablets should not be chewed or crushed and should be swallowed with half a glass of fluid.

Children

The safety and efficacy of Isotard XL ISMN modified release tablets has not been established.

Elderly

No need for routine dosage adjustment in the elderly has been found, but special care may be needed in those with increased susceptibility to hypotension or marked hepatic or renal insufficiency.

The lowest effective dose should be used.

Attenuation of effect has occurred in some patients being treated with prolonged release preparations. In such patients intermittent therapy may be more appropriate (see Section 4.4).

Therapy should not be discontinued suddenly. Both dosage and frequency should be tapered gradually (see Section 4.4).

4.3 Contraindications

Hypertrophic obstructive cardiomyopathy, constrictive pericarditis, cardiac tamponade, aortic/mitral valve stenosis, severe anaemia, closed-angle glaucoma, conditions associated with raised intracerebral pressure e.g. following head trauma, cerebral haemorrhage. Acute myocardial infarction with low filling pressures, acute circulatory failure (shock, vascular collapse) or very low blood pressure. Phosphodiesterase type-5 inhibitors e.g. sildenafil, tadalafil and vardenafil have been shown to potentiate the hypotensive effects of nitrates, and their co-administration with nitrates or nitric oxide donors is therefore contra-indicated (see section 4.5). Isotard XL should not be given to patients with a known sensitivity to nitrates.

4.4 Special warnings and precautions for use

Isotard XL ISMN modified release tablets are not indicated for relief of acute anginal attacks. In the event of an acute attack, sublingual or buccal glyceryl trinitrate tablets should be used.

Isotard XL ISMN should be used with caution in patients who have a recent history of myocardial infarction, or who are suffering from hypothyroidism, hypothermia, malnutrition and severe liver or renal disease.

The lowest effective dose should be used.

Attenuation of effect has occurred in some patients being treated with prolonged release preparations. In such patients intermittent therapy may be more appropriate (see Section 4.2).

Therapy should not be discontinued suddenly. Both dosage and frequency should be tapered gradually (see Section 4.2).

Hypotension induced by nitrates may be accompanied by paradoxical bradycardia and increased angina.

Severe postural hypotension with light-headedness and dizziness is frequently observed after the consumption of alcohol.

4.5 Interaction with other medicinal products and other forms of interaction

Alprostadil, aldesleukin, angiotensin II receptor antagonists.

This product may potentiate some of the effects of alcohol and the action of hypotensive agents. The hypotensive effects of nitrates are potentiated by concurrent administration of phosphodiesterase type-5 inhibitors e.g. sildenafil (see section 4.3).

4.6 Pregnancy and lactation

No data have been reported which would indicate the possibility of adverse effects resulting from the use of isosorbide mononitrate in pregnancy. Safety in pregnancy, however, has not been established. It is not known whether nitrates are excreted in human milk and therefore caution should be exercised when administered to nursing women.

Isosorbide mononitrate should only be used in pregnancy and during lactation if, in the opinion of the physician, the possible benefits of treatment outweigh the possible hazards.

4.7 Effects on ability to drive and use machines

The patient should be warned not to drive or operate machinery if hypotension, blurred vision or dizziness occurs.

4.8 Undesirable effects

Throbbing headache may occur when treatment is initiated, but usually disappears after 1–2 weeks of treatment. Hypotension with symptoms such as dizziness, nausea and fatigue has occasionally been reported. Infrequently, flushing and allergic rashes can occur. These symptoms generally disappear during long-term treatment.

Tachycardia and paroxysmal bradycardia have been reported.

4.9 Overdose

4.10

Symptoms: Nausea, vomiting, restlessness, warm flushed skin, blurred vision, headache, fainting, tachycardia, hypotension and palpitations. A rise in intracranial pressure with confusion and neurological deficits can sometimes occur.

Management: Consider oral activated charcoal if ingestion of a potentially toxic amount has occurred within 1 hour. Observe for at least 12 hours after the overdose. Monitor blood pressure and pulse. Correct hypotension by raising the foot of the bed and/or by expanding the intravascular volume. Other measures as indicated by the patient's clinical condition. If severe hypotension persists despite the above measures consider use of inotropes such as dopamine or dobutamine.

5. PHARMACOLOGICAL PROPERTIES

5.1 Pharmacodynamic properties

Organic nitrates (including GTN, ISDN, and ISMN) are potent relaxers of smooth muscle. They have a powerful effect on vascular smooth muscle with less effect on bronchiolar, gastrointestinal, ureteral and uterine smooth muscle. Low concentrations dilate both arteries and veins.

Venous dilatation pools blood in the periphery leading to a decrease in venous return, central blood volume, and ventricular filling volumes and pressures. Cardiac output may remain unchanged or it may decline as a result of the decrease in venous return. Arterial blood pressure usually declines secondary to a decrease in cardiac output or arteriolar vasodilatation, or both. A modest reflex increase in heart rate results from the decrease in arterial blood pressure. Nitrates can dilate epicardial coronary arteries including atherosclerotic stenoses.

The cellular mechanism of nitrate-induced smooth muscle relaxation has become apparent in recent years. Nitrates enter the smooth muscle cell and are cleaved to inorganic nitrate and eventually to nitric oxide. This cleavage requires the presence of sulphydryl groups, which apparently come from the amino acid cysteine. Nitric oxide undergoes further reduction to nitrosothiol by further interaction with sulphydryl groups. Nitrosothiol activates guanylate cyclase in the vascular smooth muscle cells, thereby generating cyclic guanosine monophosphate (cGMP). It is this latter compound, cGMP, that produces smooth muscle relaxation by accelerating the release of calcium from these cells.

5.2 Pharmacokinetic properties

Absorption

Isosorbide-5-mononitrate is readily absorbed from the gastro-intestinal tract.

Distribution

Following oral administration of conventional tablets, peak plasma levels are reached in about 1 hour. Unlike isosorbide dinitrate, ISMN does not undergo first-pass hepatic metabolism and bioavailability is 100%. ISMN has a volume of distribution of about 40 litres and is not significantly protein bound.

Elimination

ISMN is metabolised to inactive metabolites including isosorbide and isosorbide glucuronide. The pharmacokinetics are unaffected by the presence of heart failure, renal or hepatic insufficiency. Only 20% of ISMN is excreted unchanged in the urine. An elimination half life of about 4-5 hours has been reported.

5.3 Preclinical safety data

Not applicable.

6. PHARMACEUTICAL PARTICULARS

6.1 List of excipients

Stearic acid

Carnauba wax

Hydroxypropylmethylcellulose

Lactose

Magnesium stearate

Talc

Purified siliceous earth

Polyethylene glycol 4000

E171

E172.

6.2 Incompatibilities

None known.

6.3 Shelf life

36 months

6.4 Special precautions for storage

Do not store above 25°C. Store in the original package. Keep container in the outer carton

6.5 Nature and contents of container

The tablets are packed in blisters which consist of 250μm PVC with a 25μm PVdC coating which is sealed to 25μm thick aluminium foil with 20μm PVdC sealing lacquer. The tablets are packaged in boxes of 28 tablets.

Isotard 25XL, 40XL and 50XL tablets are round, biconvex, cream coloured tablets marked IM25, 40 or 50 on one side, as appropriate. The Isotard 60XL tablets, only, are oval, cream coloured tablets scored on both sides but with '6 (score) 0' on one side.

6.6 Special precautions for disposal and other handling

The tablets should be swallowed whole with half a glass of water. They must not be chewed or crushed.

Administrative Data

7. MARKETING AUTHORISATION HOLDER

ProStrakan Limited

Galabank Business Park

Galashiels

TD1 1QH

UK

8. MARKETING AUTHORISATION NUMBER(S)

Isotard 25XL: PL 16508/0018

Isotard 40XL: PL 16508/0020

Isotard 50XL: PL 16508/0021

Isotard 60XL: PL 16508/0022

9. DATE OF FIRST AUTHORISATION/RENEWAL OF THE AUTHORISATION

08 April 2002

10. DATE OF REVISION OF THE TEXT

February 2006

11. Legal Category

P

Isotretinoin 20mg capsules

(Beacon Pharmaceuticals)

1. NAME OF THE MEDICINAL PRODUCT

Isotretinoin 20mg Capsules

2. QUALITATIVE AND QUANTITATIVE COMPOSITION

Each capsule contains 20mg isotretinoin

For excipients, see section 6.1

3. PHARMACEUTICAL FORM

Soft capsules.

Red/orange soft gelatin capsules marked 'P20'.

4. CLINICAL PARTICULARS

4.1 Therapeutic indications

Isotretinoin capsules are indicated for the treatment of severe forms of acne (such as nodular or conglobate acne or acne at risk of permanent scarring), resistant to adequate courses of standard therapy with systemic antibacterials and topical therapy.

4.2 Posology and method of administration

Isotretinoin should only be prescribed by or under the supervision of physicians with expertise in the use of systemic retinoids for the treatment of severe acne and a full understanding of the risks of isotretinoin therapy and monitoring requirements.

The capsules should be taken with food once or twice daily.

Adults including adolescents and the elderly:

Isotretinoin therapy should be started at a dose of 0.5 mg/kg daily. The therapeutic response to isotretinoin and some of the adverse effects are dose-related and vary between patients. This necessitates individual dosage adjustment during therapy. For most patients, the dose ranges from 0.5-1.0 mg/kg per day.

Long-term remission and relapse rates are more closely related to the total dose administered than to either duration of treatment or daily dose. It has been shown that no substantial additional benefit is to be expected beyond a cumulative treatment dose of 120-150 mg/kg. The duration of treatment will depend on the individual daily dose. A treatment course of 16-24 weeks is normally sufficient to achieve remission.

In the majority of patients, complete clearing of the acne is obtained with a single treatment course. In the event of a definite relapse a further course of isotretinoin therapy may be considered using the same daily dose and cumulative treatment dose. As further improvement of the acne can be observed up to 8 weeks after discontinuation of treatment, a further course of treatment should not be considered until at least this period has elapsed.

Patients with severe renal insufficiency

In patients with severe renal insufficiency treatment should be started at a lower dose (e.g. 10 mg/day). The dose should then be increased up to 1 mg/kg/day or until the patient is receiving the maximum tolerated dose (see section 4.4 "Special warnings and special precautions for use").

Children

Isotretinoin is not indicated for the treatment of prepubertal acne and is not recommended in patients less than 12 years of age.

Patients with intolerance

In patients who show severe intolerance to the recommended dose, treatment may be continued at a lower dose with the consequences of a longer therapy duration and a higher risk of relapse. In order to achieve the maximum possible efficacy in these patients the dose should normally be continued at the highest tolerated dose.

4.3 Contraindications

Isotretinoin is contraindicated in women who are pregnant or breastfeeding. (see section 4.6 "Pregnancy and lactation").

Isotretinoin is contraindicated in women of childbearing potential unless all of the conditions of the Pregnancy Prevention Programme are met (see section 4.4 "Special warnings and special precautions for use").

Isotretinoin is also contraindicated in patients:

- With hepatic insufficiency
- With excessively elevated blood lipid values
- With hypervitaminosis A
- With hypersensitivity to isotretinoin or to any of the excipients (the medicine contains hydrogenated soya-bean oil and refined soya-bean oil). It is possible that some patients who are allergic to peanuts may suffer cross reactivity to products containing soya protein
- Receiving concomitant treatment with tetracyclines (see section 4.5 "Interaction with other medicinal products and other forms of interactions")

4.4 Special warnings and precautions for use

Pregnancy Prevention Programme

This medicinal product is TERATOGENIC

Isotretinoin is contraindicated in women of childbearing potential unless all of the following conditions of the Pregnancy Prevention Programme are met:

- She has severe acne (such as nodular or conglobate acne or acne at risk of permanent scarring) resistant to adequate courses of standard therapy with systemic antibacterials and topical therapy (see section 4.1 "Therapeutic indications").
- She understands the teratogenic risk.
- She understands the need for rigorous follow-up, on a monthly basis.
- She understands and accepts the need for effective contraception, without interruption, 1 month before starting treatment, throughout the duration of treatment and 1 month after the end of treatment. At least one and preferably two complementary forms of contraception including a barrier method should be used.
- Even if she has amenorrhea she must follow all of the advice on effective contraception.
- She should be capable of complying with effective contraceptive measures.
- She is informed and understands the potential consequences of pregnancy and the need to rapidly consult if there is a risk of pregnancy.
- She understands the need and accepts to undergo pregnancy testing before, during and 5 weeks after the end of treatment.
- She has acknowledged that she has understood the hazards and necessary precautions associated with the use of isotretinoin.

These conditions also concern women who are not currently sexually active unless the prescriber considers that there are compelling reasons to indicate that there is no risk of pregnancy.

The prescriber must ensure that:

- The patient complies with the conditions for pregnancy prevention as listed above, including confirmation that she has an adequate level of understanding.
- The patient has acknowledged the aforementioned conditions.
- The patient has used at least one and preferably two methods of effective contraception including a barrier method for at least 1 month prior to starting treatment and is continuing to use effective contraception throughout the treatment period and for at least 1 month after cessation of treatment.
- Negative pregnancy test results have been obtained before, during and 5 weeks after the end of treatment. The dates and results of pregnancy tests should be documented.

Contraception

Female patients must be provided with comprehensive information on pregnancy prevention and should be referred for contraceptive advice if they are not using effective contraception.

As a minimum requirement, female patients at potential risk of pregnancy must use at least one effective method of contraception. Preferably the patient should use two complementary forms of contraception including a barrier method. Contraception should be continued for at least 1 month after stopping treatment with isotretinoin, even in patients with amenorrhea.

Pregnancy testing

According to local practice, medically supervised pregnancy tests with a minimum sensitivity of 25mIU/mL are recommended to be performed in the first 3 days of the menstrual cycle, as follows.

Prior to starting therapy:

In order to exclude the possibility of pregnancy prior to starting contraception, it is recommended that an initial medically supervised pregnancy test should be performed and its date and result recorded. In patients without regular menses, the timing of this pregnancy test should reflect the sexual activity of the patient and should be undertaken approximately 3 weeks after the patient last had unprotected sexual intercourse. The prescriber should educate the patient about contraception.

A medically supervised pregnancy test should also be performed during the consultation when isotretinoin is prescribed or in the 3 days prior to the visit to the prescriber, and should have been delayed until the patient had been using effective contraception for at least 1 month. This test should ensure the patient is not pregnant when she starts treatment with isotretinoin.

Follow-up visits

Follow-up visits should be arranged at 28 day intervals. The need for repeated medically supervised pregnancy tests every month should be determined according to local practice including consideration of the patient's sexual activity and recent menstrual history (abnormal menses, missed periods or amenorrhea). Where indicated, follow-up pregnancy tests should be performed on the day of the prescribing visit or in the 3 days prior to the visit to the prescriber.

End of treatment

Five weeks after stopping treatment, women should undergo a final pregnancy test to exclude pregnancy.

Prescribing and dispensing restrictions

Prescriptions of isotretinoin for women of childbearing potential should be limited to 30 days of treatment and continuation of treatment requires a new prescription. Ideally, pregnancy testing, issuing a prescription and dispensing of isotretinoin should occur on the same day. Dispensing of isotretinoin should be completed within a maximum of 7 days of the prescription.

Male patients

The available data suggests that the level of maternal exposure from the semen of the patients receiving isotretinoin is not of sufficient magnitude to be associated with the teratogenic effects of isotretinoin.

Male patients should be reminded that they must not share their medication with anyone, particularly not females.

Additional precautions

Patients should be instructed never to give this medicinal product to another person and to return any unused capsules to their pharmacist at the end of treatment.

Patients should not donate blood during therapy and for 1 month following discontinuation of isotretinoin because of the potential risk to the foetus of a pregnant transfusion recipient.

Educational material

In order to assist prescribers, pharmacists and patients in avoiding foetal exposure to isotretinoin the Marketing Authorisation Holder will provide educational material to reinforce the warnings about the teratogenicity of isotretinoin, to provide advice on contraception before therapy is started and to provide guidance on the need for pregnancy testing.

Full patient information about the teratogenic risk and the strict pregnancy prevention measures as specified in the Pregnancy Prevention Programme should be given by the physician to all patients, both male and female.

Psychiatric disorders

Depression, depression aggravated, aggressive tendencies, mood alterations, psychotic symptoms and, very rarely, suicidal ideation, suicide attempts and suicide have been reported in patients treated with isotretinoin (see section 4.8 "Undesirable effects"). Particular care needs to be taken in patients with a history of depression and all patients should be monitored for signs of depression and referred for appropriate treatment if necessary. However, discontinuation of isotretinoin may be insufficient to alleviate symptoms and therefore further psychiatric or psychological evaluation may be necessary.

Skin and subcutaneous tissues disorders

Acute exacerbation of acne is occasionally seen during the initial period but this subsides with continued treatment, usually within 7-10 days, and usually does not require dose adjustment.

Exposure to intense sunlight or to UV rays should be avoided. Where necessary a sun-protection product with a high protection factor of at least SPF 15 should be used.

Aggressive chemical dermabrasion and cutaneous laser treatment should be avoided in patients on isotretinoin for a period of 5-6 months after the end of the treatment because of the risk of hypertrophic scarring in atypical areas and more rarely post inflammatory hyper or hypo-pigmentation in treated areas. Wax depilation should be avoided in patients on isotretinoin for at least a period of 6 months after treatment because of the risk of epidermal stripping.

Concurrent administration of isotretinoin with topical keratolytic or exfoliative anti-acne agents should be avoided as local irritation may increase (see section 4.5 Interaction with other medicinal products and other forms of interaction).

Patients should be advised to use a skin moisturising ointment or cream and a lip balm from the start of treatment as isotretinoin is likely to cause dryness of the skin and lips.

Eye disorders

Dry eyes, corneal opacities, decreased night vision and keratitis usually resolve after discontinuation of therapy. Dry eyes can be helped by the application of a lubricating eye ointment or by the application of tear replacement therapy. Intolerance to contact lenses may occur which may necessitate the patient to wear glasses during treatment.

Decreased night vision has also been reported and the onset in some patients was sudden (see section 4.7 "Effects on ability to drive and to use machines"). Patients experiencing visual difficulties should be referred for an expert ophthalmological opinion. Withdrawal of isotretinoin may be necessary.

Musculo-skeletal and connective tissue disorders

Myalgia, arthralgia and increased serum creatine phosphokinase values have been reported in patients receiving isotretinoin, particularly in those undertaking vigorous physical activity (see section 4.8 "Undesirable effects").

Bone changes including premature epiphyseal closure, hyperostosis, and calcification of tendons and ligaments have occurred after several years of administration at very high doses for treating disorders of keratinisation. The dose levels, duration of treatment and total cumulative dose in these patients generally far exceeded those recommended for the treatment of acne.

Benign intracranial hypertension

Cases of benign intracranial hypertension have been reported, some of which involved concomitant use of tetracyclines (see sections 4.3 "Contraindications" and

4.5 "Interactions with other medicinal products and other forms of interaction"). Signs and symptoms of benign intracranial hypertension include headache, nausea and vomiting, visual disturbances and papilloedema. Patients who develop benign intracranial hypertension should discontinue isotretinoin immediately.

Hepatobiliary disorders

Liver enzymes should be checked before treatment, 1 month after the start of treatment, and subsequently at 3 monthly intervals unless more frequent monitoring is clinically indicated. Transient and reversible increases in liver transaminases have been reported. In many cases these changes have been within the normal range and values have returned to baseline levels during treatment. However, in the event of persistent clinically relevant elevation of transaminase levels, reduction of the dose or discontinuation of treatment should be considered.

Renal insufficiency

Renal insufficiency and renal failure do not affect the pharmacokinetics of isotretinoin. Therefore, isotretinoin can be given to patients with renal insufficiency. However, it is recommended that patients are started on a low dose and titrated up to the maximum tolerated dose (see section 4.2 "Posology and Method of Administration").

Lipid Metabolism

Serum lipids (fasting values) should be checked before treatment, 1 month after the start of treatment, and subsequently at 3 monthly intervals unless more frequent monitoring is clinically indicated. Elevated serum lipid values usually return to normal on reduction of the dose or discontinuation of treatment and may also respond to dietary measures.

Isotretinoin has been associated with an increase in plasma triglyceride levels. Isotretinoin should be discontinued if hypertriglyceridaemia cannot be controlled at an acceptable level or if symptoms of pancreatitis occur (see section 4.8 "Undesirable effects"). Levels in excess of 800mg/dL or 9mmol/L are sometimes associated with acute pancreatitis, which may be fatal.

Gastrointestinal disorders

Isotretinoin has been associated with inflammatory bowel disease (inlcuding regional ileitis) in patients without a prior history of intestinal disorders. Patients experiencing severe (haemorrhagic) diarrhoea should discontinue isotretinoin immediately. Patients with rare hereditary problems of fructose intolerance should not take this medicine.

Allergic reactions

Anaphylactic reactions have been rarely reported, in some cases after previous topical exposure to retinoids. Allergic cutaneous reactions are reported infrequently. Serious cases of allergic vasculitis, often with purpura (bruises and red patches) of the extremities and extracutaneous involvement have been reported. Severe allergic reactions necessitate interruption of therapy and careful monitoring.

High Risk Patients

In patients with diabetes, obesity, alcoholism or a lipid metabolism disorder undergoing treatment with isotretinoin, more frequent checks of serum values for lipids and/or blood glucose may be necessary. Elevated fasting blood sugars have been reported, and new cases of diabetes have been diagnosed during isotretinoin therapy.

4.5 Interaction with other medicinal products and other forms of interaction

Patients should not take vitamin A as concurrent medication due to the risk of developing hypervitaminosis A.

Cases of benign intracranial hypertension (pseudotumor cerebri) have been reported with concomitant use of isotretinoin and tetracyclines. Therefore, concomitant treatment with tetracyclines must be avoided (see section 4.3 "Contraindications" and section 4.4 "Special warnings and special precautions for use").

Concurrent administration of isotretinoin with topical keratolytic or exfoliative anti-acne agents should be avoided as local irritation may increase (see section 4.4 Special warnings and special precautions for use).

4.6 Pregnancy and lactation

Pregnancy is an absolute contraindication to treatment with isotretinoin (see section 4.3 "Contraindications"). If pregnancy does occur in spite of these precautions during treatment with isotretinoin or in the month following, there is a great risk of very severe and serious malformation of the foetus.

The foetal malformations associated with exposure to isotretinoin include central nervous system abnormalities (hydrocephalus, cerebellar malformation/abnormalities, microcephaly), facial dysmorphia, cleft palate, external ear abnormalities (absence of external ear, small or absent external auditory canals), eye abnormalities (microphthalmia), cardiovascular abnormalities (conotruncal malformations such as tetralogy of Fallot, transposition of great vessels, septal defects), thymus gland abnormality and parathyroid gland abnormalities. There is also an increased incidence of spontaneous abortion.

If pregnancy occurs in a woman treated with isotretinoin, treatment must be stopped and the patient should be referred to a physician specialised or experienced in teratology for evaluation and advice.

Lactation:

Isotretinoin is highly lipophilic, therefore the passage of isotretinoin into human milk is very likely. Due to the potential for adverse effects in the mother and exposed child, the use of isotretinoin is contraindicated in nursing mothers.

4.7 Effects on ability to drive and use machines

A number of cases of decreased night vision have occurred during isotretinoin therapy and in rare instances have persisted after therapy (see section 4.4 "Special warnings and special precautions for use" and section 4.8 "Undesirable effects"). Because the onset in some patients was sudden, patients should be advised of this potential problem and warned to be cautious when driving or operating machines.

Drowsiness, dizziness and visual disturbances have been reported very rarely. Patients should be warned that if they experience these effects, they should not drive, operate machinery or take part in any other activities where the symptoms could put either themselves or others at risk.

4.8 Undesirable effects

The following symptoms are the most commonly reported undesirable effects with isotretinoin:

dryness of the mucosa e.g. of the lips, cheilitis, the nasal mucosa, epistaxis, and the eyes, conjunctivitis, dryness of the skin. Some of the side effects associated with the use of isotretinoin are dose-related. The side effects are generally reversible after altering the dose or discontinuation of treatment, however some may persist after treatment has stopped.

Infections:	
Very Rare (≤1/10 000)	Gram positive (mucocutaneous) bacterial infection
Blood and lymphatic system disorders:	
Very common (≥1/10)	Anaemia, Red blood cell sedimentation rate increased, Thrombocytopenia, Thrombocytosis
Common (≥1/100, <1/10)	Neutropenia
Very Rare (≤1/10000)	Lymphadenopathy
Immune system disorders:	
Rare (≥1/10 000, <1/1000)	Allergic skin reaction, Anaphylactic reactions, Hypersensitivity
Metabolism and nutrition disorders:	
Very Rare (≤1/10000)	Diabetes mellitus, Hyperuricaemia
Psychiatric disorders:	
Rare (≥1/10 000, <1/1000)	Depression, Depression aggravated, Aggressive tendencies, Anxiety, Mood alterations
Very Rare (≤1/10000)	Abnormal behaviour. Psychotic disorder. Suicidal ideation, Suicide attempt, Suicide
Nervous system disorders:	
Common (≥1/100, <1/10)	Headache
Very Rare (≤1/10 000)	Benign intracranial hypertension. Convulsions, Drowsiness, Dizziness
Eye disorders:	
Very common (≥1/10)	Blepharitis, Conjunctivitis, Dry eye. Eye irritation
Very Rare (≤1/10000)	Blurred vision, Cataract, Colour blindness (colour vision deficiencies). Contact lens intolerance, Corneal opacity, Decreased night vision, Keratitis, Papilloedema (as sign of benign intracranial hypertension). Photophobia, Visual disturbances
Ear and labyrinth disorders:	
Very Rare (≤1/10 000)	Hearing impaired
Vascular disorders:	
Very Rare (≤1/10000)	Vasculitis (for example Wegener's granulomatosis, allergic vasculitis)
Respiratory, thoracic and mediastinal disorders:	
Common (≥1/100, <1/10)	Epistaxis, Nasal dryness, Nasopharyngitis
Very Rare (≤1/10000)	Bronchospasm (particularly in patients with asthma), Hoarseness
Gastrointestinal disorders:	
Very Rare (≤1/10000)	Colitis, Ileitis, Dry throat, Gastrointestinal haemorrhage, haemorrhagic diarrhoea and inflammatory bowel disease, Nausea, Pancreatitis (see section 4.4 "Special warnings and special precautions for use")
Hepatobiliary disorders	
Very common (≥1/10)	Transaminase increased (see section 4.4 "Special warnings and special precautions for use")
Very Rare (≤1/10000)	Hepatitis
Skin and subcutaneous tissues disorders:	
Very common (≥1/10)	Cheilitis, Dermatitis, Dry skin. Localised exfoliation, Pruritus, Rash erythematous, Skin fragility (risk of frictional trauma)
Rare (≥l/10000, <l/1000)	Alopecia
Very Rare (≤1/10 000)	Acne fulminans. Acne aggravated (acne flare). Erythema (facial). Exanthema, Hair disorders, Hirsutism, Nail dystrophy, Paronychia, Photosensitivity reaction, Pyogenic granuloma. Skin hyperpigmentation, Sweating increased
Musculo-skeletal and connective tissue disorders:	
Very common (≥1/10)	Arthralgia, Myalgia, Back pain (particularly adolescent patients)
Very Rare (≤1/10 000)	Arthritis, Calcinosis (calcification of ligaments and tendons), Epiphyses premature fusion, Exostosis, (hyperostosis). Reduced bone density, Tendonitis
Renal and urinary disorders	
Very Rare (≤1/10 000)	Glomerulonephritis
General disorders and administration site conditions:	
Very Rare (≤1/10 000)	Granulation tissue (increased formation of). Malaise
Investigations:	
Very common (≥1/10)	Blood triglycerides increased, High density lipoprotein decreased
Common (≥1/100, <1/10)	Blood cholesterol increased. Blood glucose increased, Haematuria, Proteinuria
Very Rare (≤1/10000)	Blood creatine phosphokinase increased

The incidence of the adverse events was calculated from pooled clinical trial data involving 824 patients and from post-marketing data.

4.9 Overdose

Isotretinoin is a derivative of vitamin A. Although the acute toxicity of isotretinoin is low, signs of hypervitaminosis A could appear in cases of accidental overdose. Manifestations of acute vitamin A toxicity include severe headache, nausea or vomiting, drowsiness, irritability and pruritus. Signs and symptoms of accidental or deliberate overdosage with isotretinoin would probably be similar. These symptoms would be expected to be reversible and to subside without the need for treatment.

5. PHARMACOLOGICAL PROPERTIES

5.1 Pharmacodynamic properties

Pharmacotherapeutic group: anti-acne preparations for systemic use

ATC code: D10BA01

Mechanism of action

Isotretinoin is a stereoisomer of all-trans retinoic acid (tretinoin). The exact mechanism of action of isotretinoin has not yet been elucidated in detail, but it has been established that the improvement observed in the clinical picture of severe acne is associated with suppression of sebaceous gland activity and a histologically demonstrated reduction in the size of the sebaceous glands. Furthermore, a dermal anti-inflammatory effect of isotretinoin has been established.

Efficacy

Hypercornification of the epithelial lining of the pilosebaceous unit leads to shedding of corneocytes into the duct and blockage by keratin and excess sebum. This is followed by formation of a comedone and, eventually, inflammatory lesions. Isotretinoin inhibits proliferation of sebocytes and appears to act in acne by re-setting the orderly program of differentiation. Sebum is a major substrate for the growth of Propionibacterium acnes so that reduced sebum production inhibits bacterial colonisation of the duct.

5.2 Pharmacokinetic properties

Absorption

The absorption of isotretinoin from the gastro-intestinal tract is variable and dose-linear over the therapeutic range. The absolute bioavailability of isotretinoin has not been determined, since the compound is not available as an intravenous preparation for human use, but extrapolation from dog studies would suggest a fairly low and variable systemic bioavailability. When isotretinoin is taken with food, the bioavailability is doubled relative to fasting conditions.

Distribution

Isotretinoin is extensively bound to plasma proteins, mainly albumin (99.9%). The volume of distribution of isotretinoin in man has not been determined since isotretinoin is not available as an intravenous preparation for human use. In humans little information is available on the distribution of isotretinoin into tissue. Concentrations of isotretinoin in the epidermis are only half of those in serum. Plasma concentrations of isotretinoin are about 1.7 times those of whole blood due to poor penetration of isotretinoin into red blood cells.

Metabolism

After oral administration of isotretinoin, three major metabolites have been identified in plasma: 4-oxo-isotretinoin, tretinoin, (all-trans retinoic acid), and 4-oxo-tretinoin. These metabolites have shown biological activity in several in vitro tests. 4-oxo-isotretinoin has been shown in a clinical study to be a significant contributor to the activity of isotretinoin (reduction in sebum excretion rate despite no effect on plasma levels of isotretinoin and tretinoin). Other minor metabolites includes glucuronide conjugates. The major metabolite is 4-oxo-isotretinoin with plasma concentrations at steady state, that are 2.5 times higher than those of the parent compound.

Isotretinoin and tretinoin (all-trans retinoic acid) are reversibly metabolised (interconverted), and the metabolism of tretinoin is therefore linked with that of isotretinoin. It has been estimated that 20-30% of an isotretinoin dose is metabolised by isomerisation.

Enterohepatic circulation may play a significant role in the pharmacokinetics of isotretinoin in man. In vitro metabolism studies have demonstrated that several CYP enzymes are involved in the metabolism of isotretinoin to 4-oxo-isotretinoin and tretinoin. No single isoform appears to have a predominant role. Isotretinoin and its metabolites do not significantly affect CYP activity.

Elimination

After oral administration of radiolabelled isotretinoin approximately equal fractions of the dose were recovered in urine and faeces. Following oral administration of isotretinoin, the terminal elimination half-life of unchanged drug in patients with acne has a mean value of 19 hours. The terminal elimination half-life of 4-oxo-isotretinoin is longer, with a mean value of 29 hours.

Isotretinoin is a physiological retinoid and endogenous retinoid concentrations are reached within approximately two weeks following the end of isotretinoin therapy.

Pharmacokinetics in special populations

Since isotretinoin is contraindicated in patients with hepatic impairment, limited information on the kinetics of isotretinoin is available in this patient population. Renal failure does not significantly reduce the plasma clearance of isotretinoin or 4-oxo-isotretinoin.

5.3 Preclinical safety data

Acute toxicity

The acute oral toxicity of isotretinoin was determined in various animal species. LD50 is approximately 2000 mg/kg in rabbits, approximately 3000 mg/kg in mice, and over 4000 mg/kg in rats.

Chronic toxicity

A long-term study in rats over 2 years (isotretinoin dosage 2, 8 and 32 mg/kg/d) produced evidence of partial hair loss and elevated plasma triglycerides in the higher dose groups. The side effect spectrum of isotretinoin in the rodent thus closely resembles that of vitamin A, but does not include the massive tissue and organ calcifications observed with vitamin A in the rat. The liver cell changes observed with vitamin A did not occur with isotretinoin.

All observed side effects of hypervitaminosis A syndrome were spontaneously reversible after withdrawal of isotretinoin. Even experimental animals in a poor general state had largely recovered within 1-2 weeks.

Teratogenicity

Like other vitamin A derivatives, isotretinoin has been shown in animal experiments to be teratogenic and embryotoxic.

Due to the teratogenic potential of isotretinoin there are therapeutic consequences for the administration to women of a childbearing age (see section 4.3 "Contraindications", section 4.4 "Special warnings and special precautions for use" and section 4.6 "Pregnancy and lactation").

Fertility

Isotretinoin, in therapeutic dosages, does not affect the number, motility and morphology of sperm and does not jeopardise the formation and development of the embryo on the part of the men taking isotretinoin.

Mutagenicity

Isotretinoin has not been shown to be mutagenic nor carcinogenic in in vitro or in vivo animal tests respectively.

6. PHARMACEUTICAL PARTICULARS

6.1 List of excipients

Capsule contents:

refined soya-bean oil

yellow beeswax

hydrogenated soya-bean oil

partially hydrogenated vegetable oil.

Capsule shell:

Gelatin

Glycerol

titanium dioxide E171

ferrous oxide red E172

ferrous oxide yellow E172

Printing ink:

Brilliant Blue FCF Dye

sorbitol

maltitol

phosphatidylcholine

lysophosphatidylcholine.

6.2 Incompatibilities

Not applicable

6.3 Shelf life

Two years

6.4 Special precautions for storage

Do not store above 25°C. Store in the original container.

6.5 Nature and contents of container

PVC/PE/PVdC aluminium blisters in cardboard carton containing either 30 or 56 capsules

6.6 Special precautions for disposal and other handling

Not applicable

7. MARKETING AUTHORISATION HOLDER

Beacon Pharmaceuticals Ltd.

Tunbridge Wells

Kent TN1 1YG

8. MARKETING AUTHORISATION NUMBER(S)

PL 18157/0007

9. DATE OF FIRST AUTHORISATION/RENEWAL OF THE AUTHORISATION

18 October 2004

10. DATE OF REVISION OF THE TEXT

21 May 2009

Isotretinoin 5mg capsules

(Beacon Pharmaceuticals)

1. NAME OF THE MEDICINAL PRODUCT

Isotretinoin 5mg Capsules

2. QUALITATIVE AND QUANTITATIVE COMPOSITION

Each capsule contains 5mg isotretinoin

For excipients, see section 6.1

3. PHARMACEUTICAL FORM

Soft capsules.

Red/orange soft gelatin capsules marked 'P5'

4. CLINICAL PARTICULARS

4.1 Therapeutic indications

Isotretinoin capsules are indicated for the treatment of severe forms of acne (such as nodular or conglobate acne or acne at risk of permanent scarring), resistant to adequate courses of standard therapy with systemic antibacterials and topical therapy.

4.2 Posology and method of administration

Isotretinoin should only be prescribed by or under the supervision of physicians with expertise in the use of systemic retinoids for the treatment of severe acne and a full understanding of the risks of isotretinoin therapy and monitoring requirements.

The capsules should be taken with food once or twice daily.

Adults including adolescents and the elderly:

Isotretinoin therapy should be started at a dose of 0.5 mg/kg daily. The therapeutic response to isotretinoin and some of the adverse effects are dose-related and vary between patients. This necessitates individual dosage adjustment during therapy. For most patients, the dose ranges from 0.5-1.0 mg/kg per day.

Long-term remission and relapse rates are more closely related to the total dose administered than to either duration of treatment or daily dose. It has been shown that no substantial additional benefit is to be expected beyond a cumulative treatment dose of 120-150 mg/kg. The duration of treatment will depend on the individual daily dose. A treatment course of 16-24 weeks is normally sufficient to achieve remission.

In the majority of patients, complete clearing of the acne is obtained with a single treatment course. In the event of a definite relapse a further course of isotretinoin therapy may be considered using the same daily dose and cumulative treatment dose. As further improvement of the acne can be observed up to 8 weeks after discontinuation of treatment, a further course of treatment should not be considered until at least this period has elapsed.

Patients with severe renal insufficiency

In patients with severe renal insufficiency treatment should be started at a lower dose (e.g. 10 mg/day). The dose should then be increased up to 1 mg/kg/day or until the patient is receiving the maximum tolerated dose (see section 4.4 "Special warnings and special precautions for use").

Children

Isotretinoin is not indicated for the treatment of prepubertal acne and is not recommended in patients less than 12 years of age.

Patients with intolerance

In patients who show severe intolerance to the recommended dose, treatment may be continued at a lower dose with the consequences of a longer therapy duration and a higher risk of relapse. In order to achieve the maximum possible efficacy in these patients the dose should normally be continued at the highest tolerated dose.

4.3 Contraindications

Isotretinoin is contraindicated in women who are pregnant or breastfeeding. (see section 4.6 "Pregnancy and lactation").

Isotretinoin is contraindicated in women of childbearing potential unless all of the conditions of the Pregnancy Prevention Programme are met (see section 4.4 "Special warnings and special precautions for use").

Isotretinoin is also contraindicated in patients:

- With hepatic insufficiency
- With excessively elevated blood lipid values
- With hypervitaminosis A
- With hypersensitivity to isotretinoin or to any of the excipients (the medicine contains hydrogenated soya-bean oil and refined soya-bean oil). It is possible that some patients who are allergic to peanuts may suffer cross reactivity to products containing soya protein
- Receiving concomitant treatment with tetracyclines (see section 4.5 "Interaction with other medicinal products and other forms of interactions")

4.4 Special warnings and precautions for use

Pregnancy Prevention Programme

This medicinal product is TERATOGENIC

Isotretinoin is contraindicated in women of childbearing potential unless all of the following conditions of the Pregnancy Prevention Programme are met:

- She has severe acne (such as nodular or conglobate acne or acne at risk of permanent scarring) resistant to adequate courses of standard therapy with systemic antibacterials and topical therapy (see section 4.1 "Therapeutic indications").
- She understands the teratogenic risk.
- She understands the need for rigorous follow-up, on a monthly basis.
- She understands and accepts the need for effective contraception, without interruption, 1 month before starting treatment, throughout the duration of treatment and 1 month after the end of treatment. At least one and preferably two complementary forms of contraception including a barrier method should be used.
- Even if she has amenorrhea she must follow all of the advice on effective contraception.
- She should be capable of complying with effective contraceptive measures.
- She is informed and understands the potential consequences of pregnancy and the need to rapidly consult if there is a risk of pregnancy.
- She understands the need and accepts to undergo pregnancy testing before, during and 5 weeks after the end of treatment.
- She has acknowledged that she has understood the hazards and necessary precautions associated with the use of isotretinoin.

These conditions also concern women who are not currently sexually active unless the prescriber considers that there are compelling reasons to indicate that there is no risk of pregnancy.

The prescriber must ensure that:

- The patient complies with the conditions for pregnancy prevention as listed above, including confirmation that she has an adequate level of understanding.
- The patient has acknowledged the aforementioned conditions.
- The patient has used at least one and preferably two methods of effective contraception including a barrier

method for at least 1 month prior to starting treatment and is continuing to use effective contraception throughout the treatment period and for at least 1 month after cessation of treatment.

• Negative pregnancy test results have been obtained before, during and 5 weeks after the end of treatment. The dates and results of pregnancy tests should be documented.

Contraception

Female patients must be provided with comprehensive information on pregnancy prevention and should be referred for contraceptive advice if they are not using effective contraception.

As a minimum requirement, female patients at potential risk of pregnancy must use at least one effective method of contraception. Preferably the patient should use two complementary forms of contraception including a barrier method. Contraception should be continued for at least 1 month after stopping treatment with isotretinoin, even in patients with amenorrhea.

Pregnancy testing

According to local practice, medically supervised pregnancy tests with a minimum sensitivity of 25mIU/mL are recommended to be performed in the first 3 days of the menstrual cycle, as follows.

Prior to starting therapy:

In order to exclude the possibility of pregnancy prior to starting contraception, it is recommended that an initial medically supervised pregnancy test should be performed and its date and result recorded. In patients without regular menses, the timing of this pregnancy test should reflect the sexual activity of the patient and should be undertaken approximately 3 weeks after the patient last had unprotected sexual intercourse. The prescriber should educate the patient about contraception.

A medically supervised pregnancy test should also be performed during the consultation when isotretinoin is prescribed or in the 3 days prior to the visit to the prescriber, and should have been delayed until the patient had been using effective contraception for at least 1 month. This test should ensure the patient is not pregnant when she starts treatment with isotretinoin.

Follow-up visits

Follow-up visits should be arranged at 28 day intervals. The need for repeated medically supervised pregnancy tests every month should be determined according to local practice including consideration of the patient's sexual activity and recent menstrual history (abnormal menses, missed periods or amenorrhea). Where indicated, follow-up pregnancy tests should be performed on the day of the prescribing visit or in the 3 days prior to the visit to the prescriber.

End of treatment

Five weeks after stopping treatment, women should undergo a final pregnancy test to exclude pregnancy.

Prescribing and dispensing restrictions

Prescriptions of isotretinoin for women of childbearing potential should be limited to 30 days of treatment and continuation of treatment requires a new prescription. Ideally, pregnancy testing, issuing a prescription and dispensing of isotretinoin should occur on the same day. Dispensing of isotretinoin should be completed within a maximum of 7 days of the prescription.

Male patients

The available data suggests that the level of maternal exposure from the semen of the patients receiving isotretinoin is not of sufficient magnitude to be associated with the teratogenic effects of isotretinoin.

Male patients should be reminded that they must not share their medication with anyone, particularly not females.

Additional precautions

Patients should be instructed never to give this medicinal product to another person and to return any unused capsules to their pharmacist at the end of treatment.

Patients should not donate blood during therapy and for 1 month following discontinuation of isotretinoin because of the potential risk to the foetus of a pregnant transfusion recipient.

Educational material

In order to assist prescribers, pharmacists and patients in avoiding foetal exposure to isotretinoin the Marketing Authorisation Holder will provide educational material to reinforce the warnings about the teratogenicity of isotretinoin, to provide advice on contraception before therapy is started and to provide guidance on the need for pregnancy testing.

Full patient information about the teratogenic risk and the strict pregnancy prevention measures as specified in the Pregnancy Prevention Programme should be given by the physician to all patients, both male and female.

Psychiatric disorders

Depression, depression aggravated, aggressive tendencies, mood alterations, psychotic symptoms and, very rarely, suicidal ideation, suicide attempts and suicide have been reported in patients treated with isotretinoin (see section 4.8 "Undesirable effects"). Particular care needs to be taken in patients with a history of depression and all patients should be monitored for signs of depression and referred for appropriate treatment if necessary. However, discontinuation of isotretinoin may be insufficient to alleviate symptoms and therefore further psychiatric or psychological evaluation may be necessary.

Skin and subcutaneous tissues disorders

Acute exacerbation of acne is occasionally seen during the initial period but this subsides with continued treatment, usually within 7-10 days, and usually does not require dose adjustment.

Exposure to intense sunlight or to UV rays should be avoided. Where necessary a sun-protection product with a high protection factor of at least SPF 15 should be used.

Aggressive chemical dermabrasion and cutaneous laser treatment should be avoided in patients on isotretinoin for a period of 5-6 months after the end of the treatment because of the risk of hypertrophic scarring in atypical areas and more rarely post inflammatory hyper or hypopigmentation in treated areas. Wax depilation should be avoided in patients on isotretinoin for at least a period of 6 months after treatment because of the risk of epidermal stripping.

Concurrent administration of isotretinoin with topical keratolytic or exfoliative anti-acne agents should be avoided as local irritation may increase (see section 4.5 Interaction with other medicinal products and other forms of interaction).

Patients should be advised to use a skin moisturising ointment or cream and a lip balm from the start of treatment as isotretinoin is likely to cause dryness of the skin and lips.

Eye disorders

Dry eyes, corneal opacities, decreased night vision and keratitis usually resolve after discontinuation of therapy. Dry eyes can be helped by the application of a lubricating eye ointment or by the application of tear replacement therapy. Intolerance to contact lenses may occur which may necessitate the patient to wear glasses during treatment.

Decreased night vision has also been reported and the onset in some patients was sudden (see section 4.7 "Effects on ability to drive and to use machines"). Patients experiencing visual difficulties should be referred for an expert ophthalmological opinion. Withdrawal of isotretinoin may be necessary.

Musculo-skeletal and connective tissue disorders

Myalgia, arthralgia and increased serum creatine phosphokinase values have been reported in patients receiving isotretinoin, particularly in those undertaking vigorous physical activity (see section 4.8 "Undesirable effects").

Bone changes including premature epiphyseal closure, hyperostosis, and calcification of tendons and ligaments have occurred after several years of administration at very high doses for treating disorders of keratinisation. The dose levels, duration of treatment and total cumulative dose in these patients generally far exceeded those recommended for the treatment of acne.

Benign intracranial hypertension

Cases of benign intracranial hypertension have been reported, some of which involved concomitant use of tetracyclines (see sections 4.3 "Contraindications" and 4.5 "Interactions with other medicinal products and other forms of interaction"). Signs and symptoms of benign intracranial hypertension include headache, nausea and vomiting, visual disturbances and papilloedema. Patients who develop benign intracranial hypertension should discontinue isotretinoin immediately.

Hepatobiliary disorders

Liver enzymes should be checked before treatment, 1 month after the start of treatment, and subsequently at 3 monthly intervals unless more frequent monitoring is clinically indicated. Transient and reversible increases in liver transaminases have been reported. In many cases these changes have been within the normal range and values have returned to baseline levels during treatment. However, in the event of persistent clinically relevant elevation of transaminase levels, reduction of the dose or discontinuation of treatment should be considered.

Renal insufficiency

Renal insufficiency and renal failure do not affect the pharmacokinetics of isotretinoin. Therefore, isotretinoin can be given to patients with renal insufficiency. However, it is recommended that patients are started on a low dose and titrated up to the maximum tolerated dose (see section 4.2 "Posology and Method of Administration").

Lipid Metabolism

Serum lipids (fasting values) should be checked before treatment, 1 month after the start of treatment, and subsequently at 3 monthly intervals unless more frequent monitoring is clinically indicated. Elevated serum lipid values usually return to normal on reduction of the dose or discontinuation of treatment and may also respond to dietary measures.

Isotretinoin has been associated with an increase in plasma triglyceride levels. Isotretinoin should be discontinued if hypertriglyceridaemia cannot be controlled at an acceptable level or if symptoms of pancreatitis occur (see section 4.8 "Undesirable effects"). Levels in excess of 800mg/dL or 9mmol/L are sometimes associated with acute pancreatitis, which may be fatal.

Gastrointestinal disorders

Isotretinoin has been associated with inflammatory bowel disease (inlcuding regional ileitis) in patients without a prior history of intestinal disorders. Patients experiencing severe (haemorrhagic) diarrhoea should discontinue isotretinoin immediately. Patients with rare hereditary problems of fructose intolerance should not take this medicine.

Allergic reactions

Anaphylactic reactions have been rarely reported, in some cases after previous topical exposure to retinoids. Allergic cutaneous reactions are reported infrequently. Serious cases of allergic vasculitis, often with purpura (bruises and red patches) of the extremities and extracutaneous involvement have been reported. Severe allergic reactions necessitate interruption of therapy and careful monitoring.

High Risk Patients

In patients with diabetes, obesity, alcoholism or a lipid metabolism disorder undergoing treatment with isotretinoin, more frequent checks of serum values for lipids and/or blood glucose may be necessary. Elevated fasting blood sugars have been reported, and new cases of diabetes have been diagnosed during isotretinoin therapy.

4.5 Interaction with other medicinal products and other forms of interaction

Patients should not take vitamin A as concurrent medication due to the risk of developing hypervitaminosis A.

Cases of benign intracranial hypertension (pseudotumor cerebri) have been reported with concomitant use of isotretinoin and tetracyclines. Therefore, concomitant treatment with tetracyclines must be avoided (see section 4.3 "Contraindications" and section 4.4 "Special warnings and special precautions for use"). Concurrent administration of isotretinoin with topical keratolytic or exfoliative anti-acne agents should be avoided as local irritation may increase (see section 4.4 Special warnings and special precautions for use).

4.6 Pregnancy and lactation

Pregnancy is an absolute contraindication to treatment with isotretinoin (see section 4.3 "Contraindications"). If pregnancy does occur in spite of these precautions during treatment with isotretinoin or in the month following, there is a great risk of very severe and serious malformation of the foetus.

The foetal malformations associated with exposure to isotretinoin include central nervous system abnormalities (hydrocephalus, cerebellar malformation/abnormalities, microcephaly), facial dysmorphia, cleft palate, external ear abnormalities (absence of external ear, small or absent external auditory canals), eye abnormalities (microphthalmia), cardiovascular abnormalities (conotruncal malformations such as tetralogy of Fallot, transposition of great vessels, septal defects), thymus gland abnormality and parathyroid gland abnormalities. There is also an increased incidence of spontaneous abortion.

If pregnancy occurs in a woman treated with isotretinoin, treatment must be stopped and the patient should be referred to a physician specialised or experienced in teratology for evaluation and advice.

Lactation:

Isotretinoin is highly lipophilic, therefore the passage of isotretinoin into human milk is very likely. Due to the potential for adverse effects in the mother and exposed child, the use of isotretinoin is contraindicated in nursing mothers.

4.7 Effects on ability to drive and use machines

A number of cases of decreased night vision have occurred during isotretinoin therapy and in rare instances have persisted after therapy (see section 4.4 "Special warnings and special precautions for use" and section 4.8 "Undesirable effects"). Because the onset in some patients was sudden, patients should be advised of this potential problem and warned to be cautious when driving or operating machines.

Drowsiness, dizziness and visual disturbances have been reported very rarely. Patients should be warned that if they experience these effects, they should not drive, operate machinery or take part in any other activities where the symptoms could put either themselves or others at risk.

4.8 Undesirable effects

The following symptoms are the most commonly reported undesirable effects with isotretinoin:

dryness of the mucosa e.g. of the lips, cheilitis, the nasal mucosa, epistaxis, and the eyes, conjunctivitis, dryness of the skin. Some of the side effects associated with the use of isotretinoin are dose-related. The side effects are generally reversible after altering the dose or discontinuation of treatment, however some may persist after treatment has stopped.

Infections:	
Very Rare (≤1/10 000)	Gram positive (mucocutaneous) bacterial infection

Blood and lymphatic system disorders:	
Very common (≥1/10)	Anaemia, Red blood cell sedimentation rate increased, Thrombocytopenia, Thrombocytosis
Common (≥1/100, <1/10)	Neutropenia
Very Rare (≤1/10000)	Lymphadenopathy
Immune system disorders:	
Rare (≥1/10 000, <1/1000)	Allergic skin reaction, Anaphylactic reactions, Hypersensitivity
Metabolism and nutrition disorders:	
Very Rare (≤1/10000)	Diabetes mellitus, Hyperuricaemia
Psychiatric disorders:	
Rare (≥1/10 000, <1/1000)	Depression, Depression aggravated, Aggressive tendencies, Anxiety, Mood alterations
Very Rare (≤1/10000)	Abnormal behaviour. Psychotic disorder. Suicidal ideation, Suicide attempt, Suicide
Nervous system disorders:	
Common (≥1/100, <1/10)	Headache
Very Rare (≤1/10 000)	Benign intracranial hypertension. Convulsions, Drowsiness, Dizziness
Eye disorders:	
Very common (≥1/10)	Blepharitis, Conjunctivitis, Dry eye. Eye irritation
Very Rare (≤1/10000)	Blurred vision, Cataract, Colour blindness (colour vision deficiencies). Contact lens intolerance, Corneal opacity, Decreased night vision, Keratitis, Papilloedema (as sign of benign intracranial hypertension). Photophobia, Visual disturbances
Ear and labyrinth disorders:	
Very Rare (≤1/10 000)	Hearing impaired
Vascular disorders:	
Very Rare (≤1/10000)	Vasculitis (for example Wegener's granulomatosis, allergic vasculitis)
Respiratory, thoracic and mediastinal disorders:	
Common (≥1/100, <1/10)	Epistaxis, Nasal dryness, Nasopharyngitis
Very Rare (≤1/10000)	Bronchospasm (particularly in patients with asthma), Hoarseness
Gastrointestinal disorders:	
Very Rare (≤1/10000)	Colitis, Ileitis, Dry throat, Gastrointestinal haemorrhage, haemorrhagic diarrhoea and inflammatory bowel disease, Nausea, Pancreatitis (see section 4.4 "Special warnings and special precautions for use")
Hepatobiliary disorders	
Very common (≥1/10)	Transaminase increased (see section 4.4 "Special warnings and special precautions for use")
Very Rare (≤1/10000)	Hepatitis
Skin and subcutaneous tissues disorders:	
Very common (≥1/10)	Cheilitis, Dermatitis, Dry skin. Localised exfoliation, Pruritus, Rash erythematous, Skin fragility (risk of frictional trauma)
Rare (≥1/10000, <1/1000)	Alopecia
Very Rare (≤1/10 000)	Acne fulminans. Acne aggravated (acne flare). Erythema (facial). Exanthema, Hair disorders, Hirsutism, Nail dystrophy, Paronychia, Photosensitivity reaction, Pyogenic granuloma. Skin hyperpigmentation, Sweating increased
Musculo-skeletal and connective tissue disorders:	
Very common (≥1/10)	Arthralgia, Myalgia, Back pain (particularly adolescent patients)
Very Rare (≤1/10 000)	Arthritis, Calcinosis (calcification of ligaments and tendons), Epiphyses premature fusion, Exostosis, (hyperostosis). Reduced bone density, Tendonitis
Renal and urinary disorders	
Very Rare (≤1/10 000)	Glomerulonephritis
General disorders and administration site conditions:	
Very Rare (≤1/10 000)	Granulation tissue (increased formation of). Malaise
Investigations:	
Very common (≥1/10)	Blood triglycerides increased, High density lipoprotein decreased
Common (≥1/100, <1/10)	Blood cholesterol increased. Blood glucose increased, Haematuria, Proteinuria
Very Rare (≤1/10000)	Blood creatine phosphokinase increased

The incidence of the adverse events was calculated from pooled clinical trial data involving 824 patients and from post-marketing data.

4.9 Overdose

Isotretinoin is a derivative of vitamin A. Although the acute toxicity of isotretinoin is low, signs of hypervitaminosis A could appear in cases of accidental overdose. Manifestations of acute vitamin A toxicity include severe headache, nausea or vomiting, drowsiness, irritability and pruritus. Signs and symptoms of accidental or deliberate overdosage with isotretinoin would probably be similar. These symptoms would be expected to be reversible and to subside without the need for treatment.

5. PHARMACOLOGICAL PROPERTIES

5.1 Pharmacodynamic properties

Pharmacotherapeutic group: anti-acne preparations for systemic use

ATC code: D10BA01

Mechanism of action

Isotretinoin is a stereoisomer of all-trans retinoic acid (tretinoin). The exact mechanism of action of isotretinoin has not yet been elucidated in detail, but it has been established that the improvement observed in the clinical picture of severe acne is associated with suppression of sebaceous gland activity and a histologically demonstrated reduction in the size of the sebaceous glands. Furthermore, a dermal anti-inflammatory effect of isotretinoin has been established.

Efficacy

Hypercornification of the epithelial lining of the pilosebaceous unit leads to shedding of corneocytes into the duct and blockage by keratin and excess sebum. This is followed by formation of a comedone and, eventually, inflammatory lesions. Isotretinoin inhibits proliferation of sebocytes and appears to act in acne by re-setting the orderly program of differentiation. Sebum is a major substrate for the growth of Propionibacterium acnes so that reduced sebum production inhibits bacterial colonisation of the duct.

5.2 Pharmacokinetic properties

Absorption

The absorption of isotretinoin from the gastro-intestinal tract is variable and dose-linear over the therapeutic range. The absolute bioavailability of isotretinoin has not been determined, since the compound is not available as an intravenous preparation for human use, but extrapolation from dog studies would suggest a fairly low and variable systemic bioavailability. When isotretinoin is taken with food, the bioavailability is doubled relative to fasting conditions.

Distribution

Isotretinoin is extensively bound to plasma proteins, mainly albumin (99.9%). The volume of distribution of isotretinoin in man has not been determined since isotretinoin is not available as an intravenous preparation for human use. In humans little information is available on the distribution of isotretinoin into tissue. Concentrations of isotretinoin in the epidermis are only half of those in serum. Plasma concentrations of isotretinoin are about 1.7 times those of whole blood due to poor penetration of isotretinoin into red blood cells.

Metabolism

After oral administration of isotretinoin, three major metabolites have been identified in plasma: 4-oxo-isotretinoin, tretinoin, (all-trans retinoic acid), and 4-oxo-tretinoin. These metabolites have shown biological activity in several in vitro tests. 4-oxo-isotretinoin has been shown in a clinical study to be a significant contributor to the activity of isotretinoin (reduction in sebum excretion rate despite no effect on plasma levels of isotretinoin and tretinoin). Other minor metabolites includes glucuronide conjugates. The major metabolite is 4-oxo-isotretinoin with plasma concentrations at steady state, that are 2.5 times higher than those of the parent compound.

Isotretinoin and tretinoin (all-trans retinoic acid) are reversibly metabolised (interconverted), and the metabolism of tretinoin is therefore linked with that of isotretinoin. It has been estimated that 20-30% of an isotretinoin dose is metabolised by isomerisation.

Enterohepatic circulation may play a significant role in the pharmacokinetics of isotretinoin in man. In vitro metabolism studies have demonstrated that several CYP enzymes are involved in the metabolism of isotretinoin to 4-oxo-isotretinoin and tretinoin. No single isoform appears to have a predominant role. Isotretinoin and its metabolites do not significantly affect CYP activity.

Elimination

After oral administration of radiolabelled isotretinoin approximately equal fractions of the dose were recovered in urine and faeces. Following oral administration of isotretinoin, the terminal elimination half-life of unchanged drug in patients with acne has a mean value of 19 hours. The terminal elimination half-life of 4-oxo-isotretinoin is longer, with a mean value of 29 hours.

Isotretinoin is a physiological retinoid and endogenous retinoid concentrations are reached within approximately two weeks following the end of isotretinoin therapy.

Pharmacokinetics in special populations

Since isotretinoin is contraindicated in patients with hepatic impairment, limited information on the kinetics of isotretinoin is available in this patient population. Renal failure does not significantly reduce the plasma clearance of isotretinoin or 4-oxo-isotretinoin.

5.3 Preclinical safety data

Acute toxicity

The acute oral toxicity of isotretinoin was determined in various animal species. LD50 is approximately 2000 mg/kg in rabbits, approximately 3000 mg/kg in mice, and over 4000 mg/kg in rats.

Chronic toxicity

A long-term study in rats over 2 years (isotretinoin dosage 2, 8 and 32 mg/kg/d) produced evidence of partial hair loss and elevated plasma triglycerides in the higher dose groups. The side effect spectrum of isotretinoin in the rodent thus closely resembles that of vitamin A, but does not include the massive tissue and organ calcifications observed with vitamin A in the rat. The liver cell changes observed with vitamin A did not occur with isotretinoin.

All observed side effects of hypervitaminosis A syndrome were spontaneously reversible after withdrawal of isotretinoin. Even experimental animals in a poor general state had largely recovered within 1-2 weeks.

Teratogenicity

Like other vitamin A derivatives, isotretinoin has been shown in animal experiments to be teratogenic and embryotoxic.

Due to the teratogenic potential of isotretinoin there are therapeutic consequences for the administration to women of a childbearing age (see section 4.3 "Contraindications", section 4.4 "Special warnings and special precautions for use" and section 4.6 "Pregnancy and lactation").

Fertility

Isotretinoin, in therapeutic dosages, does not affect the number, motility and morphology of sperm and does not jeopardise the formation and development of the embryo on the part of the men taking isotretinoin.

Mutagenicity

Isotretinoin has not been shown to be mutagenic nor carcinogenic in in vitro or in vivo animal tests respectively.

6. PHARMACEUTICAL PARTICULARS

6.1 List of excipients

Capsule contents:

refined soya-bean oil

yellow beeswax

hydrogenated soya-bean oil

partially hydrogenated vegetable oil.

Capsule shell:

Gelatin

Glycerol

titanium dioxide E171

ferrous oxide red E172

ferrous oxide yellow E172

Printing ink:

Brilliant Blue FCF Dye

sorbitol

maltitol

phosphatidylcholine

lysophosphatidylcholine.

6.2 Incompatibilities
Not applicable

6.3 Shelf life
Two years

6.4 Special precautions for storage
Do not store above 25°C. Store in the original container.

6.5 Nature and contents of container
PVC/PE/PVdC aluminium blisters in cardboard carton containing either 30 or 56 capsules

6.6 Special precautions for disposal and other handling
Not applicable

7. MARKETING AUTHORISATION HOLDER
Beacon Pharmaceuticals Ltd.

Tunbridge Wells

Kent TN1 1YG

8. MARKETING AUTHORISATION NUMBER(S)
PL 18157/0005

9. DATE OF FIRST AUTHORISATION/RENEWAL OF THE AUTHORISATION
18 October 2004

10. DATE OF REVISION OF THE TEXT
21 May 2009

Isotrex Gel

(Stiefel Laboratories (UK) Limited)

1. NAME OF THE MEDICINAL PRODUCT
Isotrex Gel

2. QUALITATIVE AND QUANTITATIVE COMPOSITION
Isotretinoin 0.05% w/w

For excipients, see 6.1.

3. PHARMACEUTICAL FORM
Gel for topical application

4. CLINICAL PARTICULARS

4.1 Therapeutic indications
Isotrex Gel is intended for use in the treatment of mild to moderate inflammatory and non-flammatory acne vulgaris.

4.2 Posology and method of administration
Apply Isotrex Gel sparingly over the whole affected area once or twice daily.

Patients should be advised that 6-8 weeks of treatment may be required before a therapeutic effect is observed.

The safety and efficacy of Isotrex Gel has not been established in children since acne vulgaris rarely presents in this age group.

There are no specific recommendations for use in the elderly. Acne vulgaris does not present in the elderly.

4.3 Contraindications
Isotrex Gel should not be used in patients with known hypersensitivity to any of the ingredients.

4.4 Special warnings and precautions for use
Contact with the mouth, eyes and mucous membranes and with abraded or eczematous skin should be avoided. Care should be taken not to let the medication accumulate in skin fold areas and in the angles of the nose.

Application to sensitive areas of skin, such as the neck, should be made with caution.

Although tretinoin has not been shown to initiate or promote carcinogenesis in humans, tretinoin applied topically to albino hairless mice had resulted in a dose-related acceleration in ultraviolet-B radiation induced cutaneous tumours. The same author also observed the opposite effect in another study of low, non-irritating concentrations of tretinoin. The significance of these findings as related to man is unknown; however, caution should be observed in patients with a personal or family history of cutaneous epithelioma. Exposure to sunlight of areas treated with Isotrex Gel should be avoided or minimised. When exposure to strong sunlight cannot be avoided a sunscreen product and protective clothing should be used. Patients with sunburn should not use Isotrex Gel due to the possibility of increased sensitivity to sunlight. The use of sunlamps should be avoided during treatment.

4.5 Interaction with other medicinal products and other forms of interaction
Concomitant topical medication should be used with caution during therapy with Isotrex Gel. Particular caution should be exercised when using preparations containing a peeling agent (for example Benzoyl Peroxide) or abrasive cleansers.

4.6 Pregnancy and lactation
Category B1.

There is inadequate evidence of the safety of topically applied isotretinoin in human pregnancy.

Isotretinoin has been associated with teratogenicity in humans when administered systemically. Reproduction studies conducted in rabbits using Isotrex Gel applied topically at up to 60 times the human dose have, however, revealed no harm to the foetus. The use of Isotrex gel should be avoided during pregnancy.

Use during lactation

Percutaneous absorption of isotretinoin from Isotrex Gel is negligible. It is not known, however, whether isotretinoin is excreted in human milk. Isotrex Gel should not be used during lactation.

4.7 Effects on ability to drive and use machines
Not applicable; the product is a topical preparation which acts locally at the site of application.

4.8 Undesirable effects
In normal use, Isotrex Gel may cause stinging, burning or irritation; erythema and peeling at the site of application may occur.

If undue irritation occurs, treatment should be interrupted temporarily and resumed once the reaction subsides. If irritation persists, treatment should be discontinued. Reactions will normally resolve on discontinuation of therapy.

4.9 Overdose
Acute overdosage of Isotrex Gel has not been reported to date. Accidental ingestion of Isotrex Gel resulting in overdosage of isotretinoin could be expected to induce symptoms of hypervitaminosis A. These include severe headaches, nausea or vomiting, drowsiness, irritability and pruritus.

5. PHARMACOLOGICAL PROPERTIES

5.1 Pharmacodynamic properties
Isotretinoin is structurally and pharmacologically related to Vitamin A which regulates epithelial cell growth and differentiation.

The pharmacological action of isotretinoin remains to be fully elucidated. When used systemically it suppresses sebaceous gland activity and reduces sebum production; it also affects comedogenesis, suppresses *Propionibacterium acnes* and reduces inflammation.

When applied topically, the mode of action of isotretinoin may be comparable with its stereoisomer, tretinoin. Tretinoin stimulates mitosis in the epidermis and reduces intercellular cohesion in the stratum corneum; it contests the hyperkeratosis characteristic of acne vulgaris and aids desquamation, preventing the formation of lesions. Tretinoin also mediates an increased production of less cohesive epidermal sebaceous cells, this appears to promote the initial expulsion and subsequent prevention of comedones.

5.2 Pharmacokinetic properties
Percutaneous absorption of isotretinoin from the gel is negligible. After applying 30g per day of isotretinoin 0.05% gel to acne of the face, chest and back for 30 days, HPLC assays for isotretinoin and tretinoin demonstrated non-detectable levels in the plasma samples (0.02μg/ml). Applying ^{14}C isotretinoin in a cream base on the healthy skin of human volunteers resulted in only 0.03% of the topically applied dose being recovered through estimating the radioactivity of blood, urine and faecal samples

5.3 Preclinical safety data
Not applicable. The relevant information is given in Section 4.

6. PHARMACEUTICAL PARTICULARS

6.1 List of excipients
Butylated Hydroxytoluene

Hydroxypropylcellulose

Ethanol

6.2 Incompatibilities
Not applicable.

6.3 Shelf life

a) For the product as packaged for sale

3 years

b) After first opening the container

Two months

6.4 Special precautions for storage
Store below 25°C

6.5 Nature and contents of container
Aluminium tube of 5g, 15g, 25g, 30g, 50g, 60g fitted with a screw cap.

6.6 Special precautions for disposal and other handling
There are no special instructions for use or handling of Isotrex Gel.

7. MARKETING AUTHORISATION HOLDER
Stiefel Laboratories (UK) Ltd

Eurasia Headquarters

Concorde Road

Maidenhead

SL6 4BY

UK

8. MARKETING AUTHORISATION NUMBER(S)
PL 0174/0073

9. DATE OF FIRST AUTHORISATION/RENEWAL OF THE AUTHORISATION
20/12/2005

10. DATE OF REVISION OF THE TEXT
August 2009

Isotrexin Gel

(Stiefel Laboratories (UK) Limited)

1. NAME OF THE MEDICINAL PRODUCT
Isotrexin Gel

2. QUALITATIVE AND QUANTITATIVE COMPOSITION
Active Ingredients:

Isotretinoin 0.05% w/w

Erythromycin 2.00% w/w

1 g Gel contains:

Isotretinoin 0.5mg

Erythromycin 20.0mg

For excipients, see 6.1.

3. PHARMACEUTICAL FORM
Gel.

A pale yellow soft gel.

4. CLINICAL PARTICULARS

4.1 Therapeutic indications
Isotrexin is indicated for the topical treatment of moderate acne.

4.2 Posology and method of administration
Adults

Apply Isotrexin sparingly over the entire affected area once or twice daily, preferably after cleaning the skin.

Patients should be advised that, in some cases, six to eight weeks of treatment may be required before the full therapeutic effect is observed.

Patients should wash their hands after application of Isotrexin Gel.

The patient should be advised to avoid over-saturation with Isotrexin to the extent that excess medication could run into their eyes, and angles of the nose or other areas where treatment is not intended. Patients should be advised that if Isotrexin is applied excessively, no more rapid or better results would be obtained and marked redness, peeling or discomfort may occur. Should this occur accidentally or through over enthusiastic use application should be discontinued for a few days.

Use in children

Not established for prepubescent children, in whom acne vulgaris rarely presents.

Use in elderly

No specific recommendations as acne vulgaris does not present in the elderly.

4.3 Contraindications
Isotrexin should not be used in patients with known hypersensitivity to any of the ingredients.

Isotrexin should not be used in patients with acute eczema, rosacea and perioral dermatitis. Isotrexin is contraindicated in pregnancy, in women intending to conceive and in lactation (see section 4.6).

4.4 Special warnings and precautions for use
Contact with the mouth, eyes and mucous membranes and with abraded or eczematous skin should be avoided. The excipient butylated hydroxytoluene may cause local skin reactions (e.g. contact dermatitis), or irritation to the eyes and mucous membranes. Application to sensitive areas of skin, such as the neck, should be made with caution. As Isotrexin may cause increased sensitivity to sunlight, deliberate or prolonged exposure to sunlight or sunlamps should be avoided or minimised. In case of "sunburn" reaction the treatment should be temporarily interrupted.

When exposure to sunlight cannot be avoided use of sunscreen products providing adequate UVB and UVA protection and protective clothing over treated areas is recommended. Following prolonged use of a peeling agent it is advisable to "rest" a patient's skin until the effects of the peeling subside before starting to use Isotrexin. When Isotrexin and peeling agents are alternated, irritancy or dermatitis may result and the frequency of application may have to be reduced.

4.5 Interaction with other medicinal products and other forms of interaction
Concomitant topical antibiotics, medicated or abrasive soaps and cleaners, soaps and cosmetics that have a strong drying effect, and products with high concentrations of alcohol and/or astringents, should be used with caution as a cumulative irritant effect may occur. Particular caution should be exercised when using preparations containing a peeling agent (for example benzoyl peroxide.)

4.6 Pregnancy and lactation
The safety of Isotrexin for use in human pregnancy has not been established (see section 5.3).

Isotretinoin has been associated with teratogenicity in humans when administered systemically. Isotrexin is contraindicated in pregnant women and those intending to conceive. Treatment should be discontinued for one cycle prior to intended conception.

Use during lactation

Percutaneous absorption of isotretinoin from Isotrexin is negligible. However, as it is not known if isotretinoin is excreted into maternal milk, Isotrexin must not be used during lactation.

4.7 Effects on ability to drive and use machines

None

4.8 Undesirable effects

Isotrexin may cause stinging, burning or irritation; erythema and peeling at the site of application may occur. These local effects usually subside with continued treatment. If undue irritation occurs, treatment should be interrupted temporarily and resumed once the reaction subsides. If irritation persists, treatment should be discontinued. Reactions will usually resolve on discontinuation of therapy.

Heightened susceptibility to either sunlight or other sources of UVB light has been reported (See 4.4).

Long-term use of erythromycin-containing preparations may rarely trigger gram-negative folliculitis. In this case the product should be withdrawn and therapy continued with an antibiotic-free monopreparation.

4.9 Overdose

Acute overdose of Isotrexin has not been reported to date. The isotretinoin and erythromycin components are not expected to cause problems on ingestion of the topical gel.

Excessive application of Isotrexin does not improve the results of treatment and may induce marked irritation e.g. erythema, peeling, pruritis etc.

5. PHARMACOLOGICAL PROPERTIES

5.1 Pharmacodynamic properties

ATC Code: D10A X30

Isotretinoin is structurally and pharmacologically related to vitamin A, which regulates epithelial cell growth and differentiation. The pharmacological action of isotretinoin has not been fully determined. When used systemically, it suppresses sebaceous gland activity and reduces sebum production; it also affects comedogenesis, inhibits follicular keratinisation, suppresses *Propionibacterium acnes* and reduces inflammation. It is thought that topically applied isotretinoin stimulates mitosis in the epidermis and reduces intercellular cohesion in the stratum corneum; contests the hyperkeratosis characteristic of acne vulgaris and aids desquamation, preventing the formation of lesions. It is also thought that it mediates an increased production of less cohesive epidermal sebaceous cells. This appears to promote the initial expulsion and subsequent prevention of comedones.

Studies in animal models have shown similar activity when isotretinoin is applied topically. Inhibition of sebum production by topical isotretinoin has been demonstrated in the ears and flank organs of the Syrian hamster. Application of isotretinoin to the ear for 15 days led to a 50% reduction in sebaceous gland size, and application to the flank organ resulted in a 40% reduction. Topical application of isotretinoin has also been shown to have an effect on the epidermal differentiation of rhino mouse skin. Reduction in the size of the utriculi or superficial cysts leading to normal looking follicles was a predominant feature of isotretinoin treatment and has been used to quantify the antikeratinising effects of isotretinoin.

Isotretinoin has topical anti-inflammatory actions. Topically applied isotretinoin inhibits leukotriene-B4-induced migration of polymorphonuclear leukocytes, which accounts for topical isotretinoin's anti-inflammatory action. A significant inhibition was produced by topically applied isotretinoin but only a weak inhibition by topical tretinoin. This may account for the reduced rebound effect seen with topical isotretinoin when compared with topical tretinoin.

Erythromycin is a macrolide antibiotic which acts by interfering with bacterial protein synthesis by reversibly binding to ribosomal subunits, thereby inhibiting translocation of aminoacyl transfer-RNA and inhibiting polypeptide synthesis. In the treatment of acne, it is effective through reduction in the population of *Propionibacterium acnes* and through prevention of release of inflammatory mediators by the bacteria. Resistance of *P. acnes* to topical erythromycin can occur, but evidence exists that the combination of erythromycin and isotretinoin in Isotrexin is effective against erythromycin-resistant strains of *P. acnes*.

Isotrexin is effective in treating both inflammatory and non-inflammatory lesions. The isotretinoin component treats the comedonal phase of the disease. The erythromycin component is effective in the treatment of moderate inflammatory acne vulgaris.

5.2 Pharmacokinetic properties

Percutaneous absorption of isotretinoin and erythromycin from Isotrexin is negligible. In a maximised study of the topical absorption of the two components from Isotrexin in patients suffering from widespread acne, isotretinoin levels were shown to be only slightly raised from baseline levels (isotretinoin is normally present in plasma). Levels remained below 5 ng/ml, and were not increased in the presence of erythromycin when compared to topical isotretinoin alone. The levels of erythromycin were not detectable.

Under conditions of normal use in patients with acne, percutaneous absorption of the active components was negligible.

5.3 Preclinical safety data

Isotretinoin and erythromycin, the active ingredients in Isotrexin, are well-established pharmacopoeial substances which are regularly used in the topical and systemic treatment of acne vulgaris. Preclinical safety studies have not been conducted on Isotrexin, as an extensive range of toxicological studies has been conducted on isotretinoin and erythromycin as well as their respective topical formulations. A human patch test for irritation has shown the combination to be comparable to the application of either component alone, with an acceptably low potential for irritation.

Isotretinoin has been associated with teratogenicity in humans when administered systemically. However, reproduction studies conducted in rabbits using topical isotretinoin applied at up to 10 times the human therapeutic dose have revealed no harm to the foetus.

6. PHARMACEUTICAL PARTICULARS

6.1 List of excipients

Hydroxypropylcellulose,

Butylated Hydroxytoluene (BHT)

Anhydrous Ethanol

6.2 Incompatibilities

Not applicable

6.3 Shelf life

2 years

6.4 Special precautions for storage

Do not store above 25°C

6.5 Nature and contents of container

Internally lacquered membrane-sealed aluminium tubes fitted with a polypropylene screw-cap, packed into a carton. Pack sizes: 6g, 25g, 30g, 40g and 50g. Not all pack sizes may be marketed.

6.6 Special precautions for disposal and other handling

See section 4.2

7. MARKETING AUTHORISATION HOLDER

Stiefel Laboratories (UK) Ltd

Holtspur Lane

Wooburn Green

High Wycombe

Buckinghamshire

HP10 0AU

8. MARKETING AUTHORISATION NUMBER(S)

PL 0174/0200

9. DATE OF FIRST AUTHORISATION/RENEWAL OF THE AUTHORISATION

26th March 2007

10. DATE OF REVISION OF THE TEXT

26th March 2007

Isovorin

(Wyeth Pharmaceuticals)

1. NAME OF THE MEDICINAL PRODUCT

ISOVORIN* Solution for Injection 10mg/ml

2. QUALITATIVE AND QUANTITATIVE COMPOSITION

Calcium levofolinate (INN: calcium levofolinate) equivalent to 1.00% w/v (10mg/ml) of levoleucovorin (levofolinic acid).

The product is presented as vials containing 25mg, 50mg or 175mg of levofolinic acid (as calcium levofolinate) in 2.5ml, 5ml or 17.5ml of solution respectively.

3. PHARMACEUTICAL FORM

Solution for injection.

4. CLINICAL PARTICULARS

4.1 Therapeutic indications

4.1.1 Calcium Levofolinate Rescue

Calcium levofolinate is used to diminish the toxicity and counteract the action of folic acid antagonists such as methotrexate in cytotoxic therapy. This procedure is known as Calcium Levofolinate Rescue.

4.1.2 Advanced Colorectal Cancer - Enhancement of 5-Fluorouracil (5-FU) Cytotoxicity

Calcium levofolinate increases the thymine depleting effects of 5-FU resulting in enhanced cytotoxic activity. Combination regimens of 5-fluorouracil and levofolinate give greater efficacy compared to 5-FU given alone.

4.2 Posology and method of administration

For single use only.

4.2.1 Calcium Levofolinate Rescue

Adults, Children and the Elderly:

Calcium Levofolinate Rescue therapy should commence 24 hours after the beginning of methotrexate infusion. Dosage regimes vary depending upon the dose of methotrexate administered. In general, the calcium levofolinate should be administered at a dose of 7.5mg (approximately 5mg/m^2) every 6 hours for 10 doses by intramuscular injection, bolus intravenous injection or intravenous infusion, (refer to 4.2.2 for information concerning use of calcium levofolinate with infusion fluids). **Do not administer calcium levofolinate intrathecally.**

Where overdose of methotrexate is suspected, the dose of calcium levofolinate should be at least 50% of the offending dose of methotrexate and should be administered in the first hour. In the case of intravenous administration, no more than 160mg of calcium levofolinate should be injected per minute due to the calcium content of the solution.

In addition to calcium levofolinate administration, measures to ensure the prompt excretion of methotrexate are important as part of Calcium Levofolinate Rescue therapy. These measures include:

a. Alkalinisation of urine so that the urinary pH is greater than 7.0 before methotrexate infusion (to increase solubility of methotrexate and its metabolites).

b. Maintenance of urine output of 1800-2000 cc/m^2/24 hr by increased oral or intravenous fluids on days 2, 3 and 4 following methotrexate therapy.

c. Plasma methotrexate concentration, BUN and creatinine should be measured on days 2, 3 and 4.

These measures must be continued until the plasma methotrexate level is less than 10^{-7} molar (0.1μM).

Delayed methotrexate excretion may be seen in some patients. This may be caused by a third space accumulation (as seen in ascites or pleural effusion for example), renal insufficiency or inadequate hydration. Under such circumstances, higher doses of calcium levofolinate or prolonged administration may be indicated. Dosage and administration guidelines for these patients are given in Table 1. Patients who experience delayed early methotrexate elimination are likely to develop reversible renal failure.

TABLE 1:

Dosage and Administration Guidelines for Calcium Levofolinate Rescue

Clinical Situation	Laboratory Findings	Levofolinate Dosage and Duration
Normal Methotrexate Elimination	Serum methotrexate level approximately 10μM at 24 hours after administration, 1μM at 48 hours and less than 0.2μM at 72 hours.	7.5mg IM or IV every 6 hours for 60 hours (10 doses starting at 24 hours after start of methotrexate infusion).
Delayed Late Methotrexate Elimination	Serum methotrexate level remaining above 0.2μM at 72 hours, and more than 0.05μM at 96 hours after administration.	Continue 7.5mg IM or IV every 6 hours, until methotrexate level is less than 0.05μM.
Delayed Early Methotrexate Elimination and/or Evidence of Acute Renal Injury	Serum methotrexate level of 50μM or more at 24 hours or 5μM or more at 48 hours after administration, OR; a 100% or greater increase in serum creatinine level at 24 hours after methotrexate administration.	75mg IV every 3 hours, until methotrexate level is less than 1μM; then 7.5mg IV every 3 hours until methotrexate level is less than 0.05μM.

4.2.2 Colorectal Cancer: Enhancement of 5-FU Cytotoxicity

Adults and the Elderly:

Administration: The 175mg in 17.5ml vial of Calcium Levofolinate Solution for Injection should be used to administer the high doses of calcium levofolinate required in combination regimens.

When used in combination regimens with 5-FU, calcium levofolinate should only be given by the intravenous route. The agents should not be mixed together. Each vial of calcium levofolinate 175mg contains 0.7mEq (0.35mmol) of calcium per vial and it is recommended that the solution is administered over not less than 3 minutes.

For intravenous infusion, the 175mg in 17.5ml Solution for Injection may be diluted with any of the following infusion fluids before use: Sodium Chloride 0.9%; Glucose 5%; Glucose 10%; Glucose 10% and Sodium Chloride 0.9% Injection; Compound Sodium Lactate Injection.

Calcium levofolinate should not be mixed together with 5-FU in the same infusion and, because of the risk of degradation, the giving set should be protected from light.

Dosage: Based on the available clinical evidence, the following regimen is effective in advanced colorectal carcinoma:

Calcium levofolinate given at a dose of 100mg/m^2 by slow intravenous injection, followed immediately by 5-FU at an initial dose of 370mg/m^2 by intravenous injection. The injection of levofolinate should not be given more rapidly than over 3 minutes because of the calcium content of the solution. This treatment is repeated daily for 5 consecutive days. Subsequent courses may be given after a treatment-free interval of 21-28 days.

For the above regimen, modification of the 5-FU dosage and the treatment-free interval may be necessary depending on patient condition, clinical response and dose limiting toxicity. A reduction of calcium levofolinate dosage is not required. The number of repeat cycles used is at the discretion of the clinician.

On the basis of the available data, no specific dosage modifications are recommended in the use of the combination regimen with 5-FU in the elderly. However, particular care should be taken when treating elderly or debilitated patients as these patients are at increased risk of severe toxicity with this therapy (See 'Warnings and Precautions').

Children:

There are no data available on the use of this combination in children.

4.3 Contraindications

Known hypersensitivity to calcium levofolinate, or to any components of the excipients.

Calcium levofolinate should not be used for the treatment of pernicious anaemia or other megaloblastic anaemias due to vitamin B12 deficiency.

Regarding the use of calcium levofolinate with methotrexate or 5-FU during pregnancy and lactation, see section 4.6, and the Summaries of Product Characteristics for methotrexate and 5-FU-containing medicinal products.

4.4 Special warnings and precautions for use

Calcium levofolinate must not be administered intrathecally. When levofolinic acid has been administered intrathecally, following intrathecal overdose of methotrexate, a death has been reported.

General

Calcium levofolinate treatment may mask pernicious anaemia and other megaloblastic anaemias resulting from vitamin B12 deficiency.

Calcium levofolinate should only be used with 5-FU or methotrexate under the direct supervision of a clinician experienced in the use of cancer chemotherapeutic agents.

Many cytotoxic medicinal products – direct or indirect DNA synthesis inhibitors – lead to macrocytosis (hydroxycarbamide, cytarabine, mercaptopurine, thioguanine). Such macrocytosis should not be treated with folinic acid.

Calcium levofolinate / 5-FU

Calcium levofolinate may enhance the toxicity profile of 5-FU, particularly in elderly or debilitated patients. The most common manifestations are leucopenia, mucositis, stomatitis and / or diarrhoea, which may be dose limiting.

Combined 5-FU / calcium levofolinate treatment should neither be initiated nor maintained in patients with symptoms of GI toxicity, regardless of the severity, until all of these symptoms have completely disappeared.

Patients presenting with diarrhoea must be carefully monitored until the symptoms have disappeared completely, since a rapid clinical deterioration leading to death can occur. If diarrhoea and / or stomatitis occur, it is advisable to reduce the dose of 5-FU. The elderly and patients with a low physical performance due to their illness are especially prone to these toxicities. Therefore, particular care should be taken when treating these patients.

In elderly patients and patients who have undergone preliminary radiotherapy, it is recommended to begin with a reduced dosage of 5-FU.

Calcium levofolinate must not be mixed with 5-FU in the same IV injection or infusion.

Calcium levofolinate / methotrexate

An accidental overdose with a folate antagonist, such as methotrexate, should be treated quickly as a medical emergency. As the time interval between methotrexate administration and calcium levofolinate rescue increases, calcium levofolinate effectiveness in counteracting toxicity decreases.

Calcium levofolinate has no effect on non-haematological toxicities of methotrexate such as the nephrotoxicity resulting from methotrexate and / or metabolite precipitation in the kidney. Patients who experience delayed early methotrexate elimination are likely to develop reversible renal failure and all toxicities associated with methotrexate. The presence of pre-existing or methotrexate-induced renal insufficiency is potentially associated with delayed excretion of methotrexate and may increase the need for higher doses or more prolonged use of calcium levofolinate.

The possibility that the patient is taking other medications that interact with methotrexate (e.g. medications which may interfere with methotrexate elimination or binding to serum albumin) should always be considered when laboratory abnormalities or clinical toxicities are observed.

Excessive calcium levofolinate doses must be avoided since this might impair the anti-tumour activity of methotrexate, expecially in CNS tumours where calcium levofolinate accumulates after repeated courses.

Resistance to methotrexate as a result of decreased membrane transport implies also resistance to folinic acid rescue as both medicinal products share the same transport system.

4.5 Interaction with other medicinal products and other forms of interaction

When calcium levofolinate is given in conjunction with a folic acid antagonist (e.g. cotrimoxazole, pyrimethamine) the efficacy of the folic acid antagonist may either be reduced or completely neutralised.

Calcium levofolinate may diminish the antiepileptic effect of phenobarbital, phenytoin, primidone and succinimides, and may increase the frequency of seizures in susceptible patients. Clinical monitoring is therefore recommended.

4.6 Pregnancy and lactation

There are no adequate and well-controlled clinical studies conducted in pregnant or breast-feeding women.

Calcium levofolinate may be excreted in human milk and should only be administered where the benefits of the drug to the mother outweigh possible hazards to the infant. Calcium levofolinate can be used during breast-feeding when considered necessary according to the therapeutic indications.

4.7 Effects on ability to drive and use machines

There is no evidence that calcium levofolinate has an effect on the ability to drive or use machines.

4.8 Undesirable effects

Within the organ system classes, adverse reactions are listed under the headings of frequency (number of patients expected to experience the reaction), using the following categories: very common (>1/10); common (>1/100, <1/10); uncommon (>1/1000, <1/100); rare (>1/10,000, <1/1000); very rare (<1/10,000); not known (could not be accurately estimated through clinical studies).

Immune system disorders:

Very rare:	Anaphylactoid / anaphylactic reactions (including shock)
Not known:	Allergic reactions, urticaria

Nervous system disorders:

Rare: Seizures and syncope

General disorders and administration site conditions:

Not known: Fever

Cases of Stevens-Johnson Syndrome (SJS) and Toxic Epidermal Necrolysis (TEN), some fatal, have been reported in patients receiving calcium levofolinate in combination with other agents known to be associated with these disorders. A contributory role of calcium levofolinate in these cases cannot be excluded.

Calcium levofolinate may enhance 5-FU induced toxicities depending on the applied regimen. Additional undesirable effects when used in combination with 5-FU:

Gastrointestinal disorders:

Very common: Nausea, vomiting, diarrhoea

Hepatobiliary disorders:

Not known: Hyperammonemia

Skin and subcutaneous tissue disorders:

Not known: Palmer-Plantar Erythrodysaesthesia

General disorders and administration site conditions:

Not known:	Mucositis, including stomatitis and chelitis

Fatalities have occurred as a result of gastrointestinal toxicity (predominantly mucositis and diarrhoea) and myelosuppression.

4.9 Overdose

There have been no reported sequelae in patients who have received significantly more calcium levofolinate than the recommended dosage. However, excessive amounts of calcium levofolinate may nullify the chemotherapeutic effect of folic acid antagonists.

Should overdose of the combination of 5-FU with calcium levofolinate occur, the overdose instructions for 5-FU should be followed.

5. PHARMACOLOGICAL PROPERTIES

5.1 Pharmacodynamic properties

Levofolinate is the pharmacologically active isomer of 5-formyltetrahydrofolic acid. Levofolinate does not require reduction by the enzyme dihydrofolate reductase in order to participate in reactions utilising folates as a source of "one carbon" moieties. Levofolinate is actively and passively transported across cell membranes.

Administration of levofolinate can "rescue" normal cells and thereby prevent toxicity of folic acid antagonists such as methotrexate which act by inhibiting dihydrofolate reductase.

Levofolinate can enhance the therapeutic and toxic effects of fluoropyrimidines used in cancer therapy such as 5-fluorouracil. 5-fluorouracil is metabolised to 5-fluoro-2'-deoxyuridine-5'-monophosphate (FDUMP), which binds to and inhibits thymidylate synthase. Levofolinate is readily converted to another reduced folate, 5, 10-methylenetetrahydrofolate, which acts to stabilise the binding of FDUMP to thymidylate synthase and thereby enhances the inhibition of this enzyme.

Levofolinate is also effective in the treatment of megaloblastic anaemias due to folate deficiencies.

5.2 Pharmacokinetic properties

When levofolinate is injected intravenously it is 100% bioavailable.

The pharmacokinetics of levofolinate after intravenous administration of a 15mg dose were studied in healthy male volunteers. After rapid intravenous administration, serum total tetrahydrofolate (total-THF) concentrations reached a mean peak of 1722ng/ml. Serum levo-5-methyl-THF concentrations reached a mean peak of 275ng/ml and the mean time to peak concentration was 0.9 hours. The mean half-life for total-THF and levo-5-methyl-THF was 5.1 and 6.8 hours respectively.

The distribution and plasma levels of levofolinate following intramuscular administration have not been established.

The distribution in tissue and body fluids and protein binding have not been determined.

In vivo, levofolinate is converted to levo-5-methyltetrahydrofolic acid (levo-5-methyl-THF), the primary circulating form of active reduced folate. Levofolinate and levo-5-methyl-THF are polyglutamated intracellularly by the enzyme folylpolyglutamate synthetase. Folylpolyglutamates are active and participate in biochemical pathways that require reduced folate.

Levofolinate and levo-5-methyl-THF are excreted renally.

Due to the inherent lack of levofolinate toxicity, the influence of impaired renal or hepatic function on levofolinate disposition was not evaluated.

5.3 Preclinical safety data

The pre-clinical data raises no concerns for the clinical uses indicated.

6. PHARMACEUTICAL PARTICULARS

6.1 List of excipients

Sodium Chloride, Water for Injection, Hydrochloric Acid, Sodium Hydroxide

6.2 Incompatibilities

Calcium levofolinate should not be mixed together with 5-FU in the same intravenous injection or infusion.

6.3 Shelf life

2 years

6.4 Special precautions for storage

Store ISOVORIN Solution for Injection under refrigerated conditions (2 - 8°C) in original containers. Protect from light.

Discard any unused products.

When ISOVORIN Solution for Injection is diluted with the recommended infusion fluids, the resulting solutions are intended for immediate use but may be stored for up to 24 hours under refrigerated conditions (2 - 8°C). Because of the risk of degradation, reconstituted solutions should be protected from light prior to use if necessary.

6.5 Nature and contents of container

Type I amber glass vials each containing the equivalent of 25mg, 50mg or 175mg of calcium levofolinate in 2.5ml, 5ml or 17.5ml of solution respectively. Isovorin is packed in boxes of 1 vial.

6.6 Special precautions for disposal and other handling

See sections 4.2 and 6.4.

7. MARKETING AUTHORISATION HOLDER

John Wyeth and Brother Limited trading as Wyeth Pharmaceuticals

Huntercombe Lane South

Taplow, Maidenhead

Berkshire

SL6 OPH

8. MARKETING AUTHORISATION NUMBER(S)

PL 0011/0235

9. DATE OF FIRST AUTHORISATION/RENEWAL OF THE AUTHORISATION

12 June 1998

10. DATE OF REVISION OF THE TEXT

20 March 2009

* Registered Trademark

Istin

(Pfizer Limited)

1. NAME OF THE MEDICINAL PRODUCT

ISTIN™

2. QUALITATIVE AND QUANTITATIVE COMPOSITION

Active Ingredient: amlodipine

The tablets contain amlodipine besilate (equivalent to 5mg and 10mg amlodipine)

3. PHARMACEUTICAL FORM

Tablet for oral administration

5mg tablets: White emerald shaped tablets with imprint AML-5 on one side and Pfizer logo on the other.

10mg tablets: White emerald shaped tablets with imprint AML-10 on one side and Pfizer logo on the other.

4. CLINICAL PARTICULARS

4.1 Therapeutic indications

Hypertension

Prophylaxis of chronic stable angina pectoris

Prinzmetal's (variant) angina when diagnosed by a cardiologist

In hypertensive patients, Istin has been used in combination with a thiazide diuretic, alpha blocker, beta-adrenoceptor blocking agent, or an angiotensin converting enzyme inhibitor. For angina, Istin may be used as monotherapy or in combination with other antianginal drugs in patients with angina that is refractory to nitrates and/or adequate doses of beta blockers.

Istin is well tolerated in patients with heart failure and a history of hypertension or ischaemic heart disease.

4.2 Posology and method of administration

In adults: For both hypertension and angina the usual initial dose is 5mg Istin once daily which may be increased to a maximum dose of 10mg depending on the individual patient's response.

No dose adjustment of Istin is required upon concomitant administration of thiazide diuretics, beta blockers, and angiotensin-converting enzyme inhibitors.

Use in children: Not recommended.

Use in the elderly: Istin, used at similar doses in elderly or younger patients, is equally well tolerated. Therefore normal dosage regimens are recommended.

Patients with hepatic impairment: See section 4.4 Special warnings and precautions for use.

Patients with renal impairment: Changes in amlodipine plasma concentrations are not correlated with degree of renal impairment, therefore the normal dosage is recommended. Amlodipine is not dialysable.

4.3 Contraindications

Istin is contra-indicated in patients with a known sensitivity to dihydropyridines, amlodipine or any of the excipients.

Istin should not be used in cardiogenic shock, clinically significant aortic stenosis, unstable angina (excluding Prinzmetal's angina).

Pregnancy and lactation

4.4 Special warnings and precautions for use

Use in patients with Heart Failure: In a long-term, placebo controlled study (PRAISE-2) of Istin in patients with NYHA III and IV heart failure of nonischaemic aetiology, amlodipine was associated with increased reports of pulmonary oedema despite no significant difference in the incidence of worsening heart failure as compared to placebo. See section 5.1 "Pharmacodynamic Properties".

Use in patients with impaired hepatic function: As with all calcium antagonists, amlodipine's half-life is prolonged in patients with impaired liver function and dosage recommendations have not been established. The drug should therefore be administered with caution in these patients.

There are no data to support the use of Istin alone, during or within one month of a myocardial infarction.

The safety and efficacy of Istin in hypertensive crisis has not been established.

4.5 Interaction with other medicinal products and other forms of interaction

Istin has been safely administered with thiazide diuretics, alpha blockers, beta blockers, angiotensin-converting enzyme inhibitors, long-acting nitrates, sublingual glyceryl trinitrate, non-steroidal anti-inflammatory drugs, antibiotics, and oral hypoglycaemic drugs.

In vitro data from studies with human plasma, indicate that amlodipine has no effect on protein binding of digoxin, phenytoin, warfarin or indometacin.

Special Studies: Effect of other agents on amlodipine

Cimetidine: Co-administration of Istin with cimetidine did not alter the pharmacokinetics of Istin.

Grapefruit Juice: Co-administration of 240ml of grapefruit juice with a single oral dose of Istin 10mg in 20 healthy volunteers had no significant effect on the pharmacokinetics of Istin.

Sildenafil: When Istin and sildenafil were used in combination, each agent independently exerted its own blood pressure lowering effect.

Special Studies: Effect of amlodipine on other agents

Atorvastatin: Co-administration of multiple 10mg doses of Istin with 80mg of atorvastatin resulted in no significant change in the steady state pharmacokinetic parameters of atorvastatin.

Digoxin: Co-administration of Istin with digoxin did not change serum digoxin levels or digoxin renal clearance in normal volunteers.

Warfarin: In healthy male volunteers, the co-administration of Istin does not significantly alter the effect of warfarin on prothrombin response time. Co-administration of Istin with warfarin did not change the warfarin prothrombin response time.

Ciclosporin: Pharmacokinetic studies with ciclosporin have demonstrated that Istin does not significantly alter the pharmacokinetics of ciclosporin.

Drug/Laboratory test Interactions: None known.

4.6 Pregnancy and lactation

Although some dihydropyridine compounds have been found to be teratogenic in animals, data in the rat and rabbit for amlodipine provide no evidence for a teratogenic effect. There is, however, no clinical experience with the preparation in pregnancy or lactation. Accordingly, Istin should not be administered during pregnancy, or lactation, or to women of childbearing potential unless effective contraception is used.

4.7 Effects on ability to drive and use machines

Clinical experience with Istin indicates that therapy is unlikely to impair a patient's ability to drive or use machinery.

4.8 Undesirable effects

Adverse events that have been reported in amlodipine trials are categorised below, according to system organ class and frequency. Frequencies are defined as: very common (>10%); common (>1%, <10%); uncommon (>0.1%, <1%); rare (>0.01%, <0.1%) and very rare (<0.01%).

Blood and the Lymphatic System Disorders	thrombocytopenia	Very Rare
Immune System Disorders	allergic reaction	Very Rare
Metabolism and Nutrition Disorders	hyperglycaemia	Very Rare
Psychiatric Disorders	insomnia, mood changes	Uncommon
Nervous System Disorders	somnolence, dizziness, headache	Common
	tremor, taste perversion, syncope, hypoaesthesia, paraesthesia	Uncommon
	peripheral neuropathy	Very Rare
Eye Disorders	visual disturbances	Uncommon
Ear and Labyrinth Disorders	tinnitus	Uncommon
Cardiac Disorders	palpitations	Common
	myocardial infarction, arrhythmia, ventricular tachycardia and atrial fibrillation)	Very Rare
Vascular Disorders	flushing	Common
	hypotension	Uncommon
	vasculitis	Very Rare
Respiratory, Thoracic and Mediastinal Disorders	dyspnoea, rhinitis	Uncommon
	coughing	Very Rare
Gastrointestinal Disorders	abdominal pain, nausea	Common
	vomiting, dyspepsia, altered bowel habits, dry mouth	Uncommon
	pancreatitis, gastritis, gingival hyperplasia	Very Rare
Hepato-biliary Disorders	hepatitis, jaundice and hepatic enzyme elevations (mostly consistent with cholestasis)	Very Rare
Skin and Subcutaneous Tissue Disorders	alopecia, purpura, skin discolouration, increased sweating, pruritus, rash	Uncommon
	angioedema, erythema multiforme, urticaria	Very Rare
Musculoskeletal and Connective Tissue Disorders	arthralgia, myalgia, muscle cramps, back pain	Uncommon
Renal and Urinary Disorders	micturition disorder, nocturia, increased urinary frequency	Uncommon
Reproductive System and Breast Disorders	impotence, gynaecomastia	Uncommon
General Disorders and Administration Site Conditions	oedema, fatigue	Common
	chest pain, asthenia, pain, malaise	Uncommon
Investigations	weight increase, weight decrease	Uncommon

4.9 Overdose

Available data suggest that gross overdosage could result in excessive peripheral vasodilatation and possibly reflex tachycardia. Marked and probably prolonged systemic hypotension up to and including shock with fatal outcome have been reported.

Administration of activated charcoal to healthy volunteers immediately or up to two hours after ingestion of amlodipine 10mg has been shown to significantly decrease amlodipine absorption. Gastric lavage may be worthwhile in some cases. Clinically significant hypotension due to Istin overdosage calls for active cardiovascular support including frequent monitoring of cardiac and respiratory function, elevation of extremities, and attention to circulating fluid volume and urine output. A vasoconstrictor may be helpful in restoring vascular tone and blood pressure, provided that there is no contraindication to its use. Intravenous calcium gluconate may be beneficial in reversing the effects of calcium channel blockade. Since Istin is highly protein-bound, dialysis is not likely to be of benefit.

5. PHARMACOLOGICAL PROPERTIES

5.1 Pharmacodynamic properties

Istin is a calcium ion influx inhibitor of the dihydropyridine group (slow channel blocker or calcium ion antagonist) and inhibits the transmembrane influx of calcium ions into cardiac and vascular smooth muscle.

The mechanism of the antihypertensive action of Istin is due to a direct relaxant effect on vascular smooth muscle. The precise mechanism by which Istin relieves angina has not been fully determined but Istin reduces total ischaemic burden by the following two actions.

1) Istin dilates peripheral arterioles and thus, reduces the total peripheral resistance (afterload) against which the heart works. Since the heart rate remains stable, this unloading of the heart reduces myocardial energy consumption and oxygen requirements.

2) The mechanism of action of Istin also probably involves dilatation of the main coronary arteries and coronary arterioles, both in normal and ischaemic regions. This dilatation increases myocardial oxygen delivery in patients with coronary artery spasm (Prinzmetal's or variant angina).

In patients with hypertension, once daily dosing provides clinically significant reductions of blood pressure in both the supine and standing positions throughout the 24 hour interval. Due to the slow onset of action, acute hypotension is not a feature of Istin administration.

In patients with angina, once daily administration of Istin increases total exercise time, time to angina onset, and time to 1mm ST segment depression, and decreases both angina attack frequency and glyceryl trinitrate tablet consumption.

Istin has not been associated with any adverse metabolic effects or changes in plasma lipids and is suitable for use in patients with asthma, diabetes, and gout.

Use in Patients with Heart Failure: Haemodynamic studies and exercise based controlled clinical trials in NYHA Class II-IV heart failure patients have shown that Istin did not lead to clinical deterioration as measured by exercise tolerance, left ventricular ejection fraction and clinical symptomatology.

A placebo controlled study (PRAISE) designed to evaluate patients in NYHA Class III-IV heart failure receiving digoxin, diuretics and ACE inhibitors has shown that Istin did not lead to an increase in risk of mortality or combined mortality and morbidity with heart failure.

In a follow-up, long term, placebo controlled study (PRAISE-2) of Istin in patients with NYHA III and IV heart failure without clinical symptoms or objective findings suggestive or underlying ischaemic disease, on stable doses of ACE inhibitors, digitalis, and diuretics, Istin had no effect on total cardiovascular mortality. In this same population Istin was associated with increased reports of pulmonary oedema despite no significant difference in the incidence of worsening heart failure as compared to placebo.

A randomized double-blind morbidity-mortality study called the Antihypertensive and Lipid-Lowering Treatment to Prevent Heart Attack Trial (ALLHAT) was performed to compare newer drug therapies: amlodipine 2.5-10 mg/d (calcium channel blocker) or lisinopril 10-40 mg/d (ACE-inhibitor) as first-line therapies to that of the thiazide-diuretic, chlorthalidone 12.5-25 mg/d in mild to moderate hypertension."

A total of 33,357 hypertensive patients aged 55 or older were randomized and followed for a mean of 4.9 years. The patients had at least one additional CHD risk factor, including: previous myocardial infarction or stroke > 6 months prior to enrollment) or documentation of other atherosclerotic CVD (overall 51.5%), type 2 diabetes (36.1%), HDL-C < 35 mg/dL (11.6%), left ventricular hypertrophy diagnosed by electrocardiogram or echocardiography (20.9%), current cigarette smoking (21.9%).

The primary endpoint was a composite of fatal CHD or non-fatal myocardial infarction. There was no significant difference in the primary endpoint between amlodipine-based therapy and chlorthalidone-based therapy: RR 0.98 95% CI(0.90-1.07) p=0.65. Among Secondary Endpoints, the incidence of heart failure (component of a composite combined cardiovascular endpoint) was significantly higher in the amlodipine group as compared to the chlorthalidone group (10.2% % vs 7.7%, RR 1.38, 95% CI [1.25-1.52] p<0.001). However, there was no significant difference in all-cause mortality between amlodipine-based therapy and chlorthalidone-based therapy. RR 0.96 95% CI [0.89-1.02] p=0.20.

In a study involving 268 children aged 6-17 years with predominantly secondary hypertension, comparison of a 2.5mg dose, and 5.0mg dose of amlodipine with placebo, showed that both doses reduced Systolic Blood Pressure significantly more than placebo. The difference between the two doses was not statistically significant.

The long-term effects of amlodipine on growth, puberty and general development have not been studied. The long-term efficacy of amlodipine on therapy in childhood to reduce cardiovascular morbidity and mortality in adulthood have also not been established.

5.2 Pharmacokinetic properties

Absorption, distribution, plasma protein binding: After oral administration of therapeutic doses, amlodipine is well absorbed with peak blood levels between 6-12 hours post dose. Absolute bioavailability has been estimated to be between 64 and 80%. The volume of distribution is approximately 21 l/kg. *In vitro* studies have shown that approximately 97.5% of circulating amlodipine is bound to plasma proteins.

Biotransformation/elimination: The terminal plasma elimination half life is about 35-50 hours and is consistent with once daily dosing. Amlodipine is extensively metabolised by the liver to inactive metabolites with 10% of the parent compound and 60% of metabolites excreted in the urine.

Use in the elderly: The time to reach peak plasma concentrations of amlodipine is similar in elderly and younger subjects. Amlodipine clearance tends to be decreased with resulting increases in AUC and elimination half-life in elderly patients. Increases in AUC and elimination half-life in patients with congestive heart failure were as expected for the patient age group studied.

5.3 Preclinical safety data
None

6. PHARMACEUTICAL PARTICULARS

6.1 List of excipients
Microcrystalline cellulose, E460

Dibasic calcium phosphate anhydrous

Sodium starch glycollate

Magnesium stearate, E572

6.2 Incompatibilities
Not applicable

6.3 Shelf life
4 years

6.4 Special precautions for storage
Do not store above 25°C

6.5 Nature and contents of container
Istin is available as:

Calendar packs of 28 tablets. Aluminium/PVC blister strips, 14 tablets/strip, 2 strips in a carton box.

6.6 Special precautions for disposal and other handling
No special requirements

7. MARKETING AUTHORISATION HOLDER
Pfizer Limited
Ramsgate Road
Sandwich
Kent
CT13 9NJ
United Kingdom

8. MARKETING AUTHORISATION NUMBER(S)
Istin Tablets 5mg PL 00057/0297
Istin Tablets 10mg PL 00057/0298

9. DATE OF FIRST AUTHORISATION/RENEWAL OF THE AUTHORISATION
30 January 1995 / 25 April 2001

10. DATE OF REVISION OF THE TEXT
July 2007

11. LEGAL CATEGORY
POM

Ref: IS10_0

IVEMEND 115 mg powder for solution for infusion

(Merck Sharp & Dohme Limited)

1. NAME OF THE MEDICINAL PRODUCT
IVEMEND 115 mg powder for solution for infusion. ▼

2. QUALITATIVE AND QUANTITATIVE COMPOSITION
Each vial contains fosaprepitant dimeglumine equivalent to 115 mg fosaprepitant. After reconstitution and dilution 1 ml of solution contains 1 mg fosaprepitant (see section 6.6).

For a full list of excipients, see section 6.1.

3. PHARMACEUTICAL FORM
Powder for solution for infusion.

White to off-white amorphous powder.

4. CLINICAL PARTICULARS

4.1 Therapeutic indications
Prevention of acute and delayed nausea and vomiting associated with highly emetogenic cisplatin-based cancer chemotherapy in adults.

Prevention of nausea and vomiting associated with moderately emetogenic cancer chemotherapy in adults.

IVEMEND 115mg is given as part of a combination therapy (see section 4.2).

4.2 Posology and method of administration
IVEMEND is a lyophilized prodrug of aprepitant containing polysorbate 80 (PS80) for intravenous administration. Aprepitant is available as capsules for oral administration.

Posology

IVEMEND (115 mg) may be substituted for aprepitant (125 mg) prior to chemotherapy, on Day 1 only of the chemotherapy induced nausea and vomiting (CINV) regimen as an infusion administered over 15 minutes (see section 6.6).

The 3-day CINV regimen includes IVEMEND (115 mg) 30 minutes prior to chemotherapy treatment or aprepitant (125 mg) PO once daily one hour prior to chemotherapy treatment on Day 1; aprepitant (80 mg) PO on Days 2 and 3; in addition to a corticosteroid and a 5-HT_3 antagonist.

The following regimen is recommended, based on clinical studies with aprepitant, for the prevention of nausea and vomiting associated with emetogenic cancer chemotherapy.

Highly Emetogenic Chemotherapy Regimen

(see Table 1a below)

In clinical studies:

Aprepitant was administered orally 1 hour prior to chemotherapy treatment on Day 1 and in the morning on Days 2 and 3.

Dexamethasone was administered 30 minutes prior to chemotherapy treatment on Day 1 and in the morning on Days 2 to 4. The dose of dexamethasone was chosen to account for active substance interactions.

Ondansetron was administered intravenously 30 minutes prior to chemotherapy treatment on Day 1.

Moderately Emetogenic Chemotherapy Regimen

(see Table 1b on next page)

In clinical studies:

Aprepitant was administered orally 1 hour prior to chemotherapy treatment on Day 1 and in the morning on Days 2 and 3.

Dexamethasone was administered 30 minutes prior to chemotherapy treatment on Day 1. The dose of dexamethasone was chosen to account for active substance interactions.

One 8 mg capsule of ondansetron was administered 30 to 60 minutes prior to chemotherapy treatment and one 8 mg capsule was administered 8 hours after first dose on Day 1.

Efficacy data on combination with other corticosteroids and 5-HT_3 antagonists are limited. For additional information on the co-administration with corticosteroids, see section 4.5.

Refer to the Summary of Product Characteristics of co-administered antiemetic agents.

Elderly(≥65 years)

No dose adjustment is necessary for the elderly (see section 5.2)

Gender.

No dose adjustment is necessary based on gender (see section 5.2)

Renal Impairment

No dose adjustment is necessary for patients with renal impairment or for patients with end stage renal disease undergoing haemodialysis (see section 5.2).

Hepatic Impairment

No dose adjustment is necessary for patients with mild hepatic impairment. There are limited data in patients with moderate hepatic insufficiency and no data in patients with severe hepatic impairment (see sections 4.4 and 5.2).

Children and adolescents

IVEMEND is not recommended for use in children below the age of 18 years of age due to insufficient data on safety and efficacy.

Method of Administration

IVEMEND should be administered intravenously and should not be given by the intramuscular or subcutaneous route. Intravenous administration occurs preferably through a running intravenous infusion over 15 minutes (see section 6.6). Do not administer IVEMEND as a bolus injection or undiluted solution.

4.3 Contraindications
Hypersensitivity to the active substance, aprepitant, or to polysorbate 80 or any of the other excipients.

Co-administration with pimozide, terfenadine, astemizole or cisapride (see section 4.5).

4.4 Special warnings and precautions for use
There are limited data in patients with moderate hepatic insufficiency and no data in patients with severe hepatic impairment. IVEMEND should be used with caution in these patients (see section 5.2).

IVEMEND and oral aprepitant should be used with caution in patients receiving concomitant orally administered active substances that are metabolised primarily through CYP3A4 and with a narrow therapeutic range, such as ciclosporine, tacrolimus, sirolimus, everolimus, alfentanil, diergotamine, ergotamine, fentanyl, and quinidine (see section 4.5). Additionally, concomitant administration with irinotecan should be approached with particular caution as the combination might result in increased toxicity.

Co-administration of fosaprepitant with ergot alkaloid derivatives, which are CYP3A4 substrates, may result in elevated plasma concentrations of these active substances. Therefore, caution is advised due to the potential risk of ergot-related toxicity.

Co-administration of oral aprepitant with warfarin results in decreased prothrombin time, reported as International Normalised Ratio (INR). In patients on chronic warfarin therapy, the INR should be monitored closely during treatment with oral aprepitant and for 2 weeks following each 3-day regimen of fosaprepitant followed by oral aprepitant for chemotherapy induced nausea and vomiting (see section 4.5).

The efficacy of hormonal contraceptives may be reduced during and for 28 days after administration of aprepitant. Alternative or back-up methods of contraception should be used during treatment with fosaprepitant or aprepitant and for 2 months following the last dose of aprepitant (see section 4.5).

Table 1a Highly Emetogenic Chemotherapy Regimen

	Day 1	Day 2	Day 3	Day 4
IVEMEND	115 mg intravenously	none	none	none
Aprepitant	none	80 mg PO	80 mg PO	none
Dexamethasone	12 mg PO	8 mg PO	8 mg PO	8 mg PO
Ondansetron	32 mg intravenously	none	none	none

Table 1b Moderately Emetogenic Chemotherapy Regimen

	Day 1	Day 2	Day 3
IVEMEND	115 mg intravenously	none	none
Aprepitant	none	80 mg PO	80 mg PO
Dexamethasone	12 mg PO	none	none
Ondansetron	2 × 8 mg PO	none	none

Concomitant administration of fosaprepitant with active substances that strongly induce CYP3A4 activity (e.g. rifampicin, phenytoin, carbamazepine, phenobarbital) should be avoided as the combination results in reductions of the plasma concentrations of aprepitant (see section 4.5). Concomitant administration of fosaprepitant with herbal presentations containing St. John's Wort (*Hypericum perforatum*) is not recommended.

Concomitant administration of fosaprepitant with active substances that inhibit CYP3A4 activity (e.g. ketoconazole, itraconazole, voriconazole, posaconazole, clarithromycin, telithromycin, nefazodone, and protease inhibitors) should be approached cautiously as the combination is expected to result in increased plasma concentrations of aprepitant (see section 4.5).

IVEMEND should not be given as a bolus injection, but should always be diluted and given as a slow intravenous infusion (see section 4.2). IVEMEND should not be administered intramuscularly or subcutaneously. Mild injection site thrombosis has been observed at higher doses (see section 4.9). If signs or symptoms of local irritation occur, the injection or infusion should be terminated and restarted in another vein.

4.5 Interaction with other medicinal products and other forms of interaction

When administered intravenously fosaprepitant is rapidly converted to aprepitant.

Drug interactions following administration of fosaprepitant are likely to occur with active substances that interact with oral aprepitant. The following information was derived from data with oral aprepitant and studies conducted with fosaprepitant and midazolam or diltiazem.

Aprepitant (125mg/80mg) is a substrate, a moderate inhibitor, and an inducer of CYP3A4. Aprepitant is also an inducer of CYP2C9. During treatment with oral aprepitant, CYP3A4 is inhibited. After the end of treatment, oral aprepitant causes a transient mild induction of CYP2C9, CYP3A4 and glucuronidation. Fosaprepitant or aprepitant does not seem to interact with the P-glycoprotein transporter, as demonstrated by the lack of interaction of oral aprepitant with digoxin.

Effect of aprepitant on the pharmacokinetics of active substances.

CYP3A4 inhibition

As a moderate inhibitor of CYP3A4, aprepitant can increase plasma concentrations of orally co-administered active substances that are metabolised through CYP3A4. The total exposure of orally administered CYP3A4 substrates may increase up to approximately 3-fold during the 3-day treatment with fosaprepitant followed by oral aprepitant; the effect of aprepitant on the plasma concentrations of intravenously administered CYP3A4 substrates is expected to be smaller. Fosaprepitant must not be used concurrently with pimozide, terfenadine, astemizole, or cisapride. Inhibition of CYP3A4 by aprepitant could result in elevated plasma concentrations of these active substances, potentially causing serious or life-threatening reactions. (see section 4.3). Caution is advised during concomitant administration of fosaprepitant orally administered active substances that are metabolised primarily through CYP3A4 and with a narrow therapeutic range, such as ciclosporin, tacrolimus, sirolimus, everolimus, alfentanil, diergotamine, ergotamine, fentanyl, and quinidine (see section 4.4).

Corticosteroids:

Dexamethasone: The usual oral dexamethasone dose should be reduced by approximately 50 % when co-administered with a regimen of fosaprepitant followed by aprepitant. The dose of dexamethasone in clinical chemotherapy induced nausea and vomiting clinical trials was chosen to account for active substances interactions (see section 4.2). Oral aprepitant, when given as a regimen of 125 mg with dexamethasone co-administered orally as 20 mg on Day 1, and oral aprepitant when given as 80 mg/day with dexamethasone co-administered orally as 8 mg on Days 2 through 5, increased the AUC of dexamethasone, a CYP3A4 substrate, 2.2-fold on Days 1 and 5.

Methylprednisolone: The usual intravenously administered methylprednisolone dose should be reduced approximately 25 %, and the usual oral methylprednisolone dose should be reduced approximately 50 % when co-administered with a regimen of fosaprepitant followed by aprepitant. Oral aprepitant, when given as a regimen of 125 mg on Day 1 and 80 mg/day on Days 2 and 3, increased the AUC of methylprednisolone, a CYP3A4 substrate, by 1.3-fold on Day 1 and by 2.5-fold on Day 3, when methylprednisolone was co-administered intravenously as 125 mg on Day 1 and orally as 40 mg on Days 2 and 3.

During continuous treatment with methylprednisolone, the AUC of methylprednisolone may decrease at later time points within 2 weeks following initiation of dosing with oral aprepitant, due to the inducing effect of aprepitant on CYP3A4. This effect may be expected to be more pronounced for orally administered methylprednisolone.

Chemotherapeutic agents: In pharmacokinetic studies, oral aprepitant, when given as a regimen of 125 mg on Day 1 and 80 mg/day on Days 2 and 3, did not influence the pharmacokinetics of docetaxel administered intravenously on Day 1 or vinorelbine administered intravenously on Day 1 or Day 8. Because the effect of aprepitant on the pharmacokinetics of orally administered CYP3A4 substrates is greater than the effect of aprepitant on the pharmacokinetics of intravenously administered CYP3A4 substrates, an interaction with orally administered chemotherapeutic agents metabolised primarily or in part by CYP3A4 (e.g., etoposide, vinorelbine) cannot be excluded. Caution is advised and additional monitoring may be appropriate in patients receiving such agents (see section 4.4).

Immunosuppressants:

During the 3 day CINV regimen, a transient moderate increase followed by a mild decrease in exposure of immunosuppressants metabolised by CYP3A4 (e.g. ciclosporin, tacrolimus, everolimus and sirolimus) is expected. Given the short duration of the 3-day regimen and the time-dependent limited changes in exposure, dose reduction of the immunosuppressants is not recommended during the 3 days of co-administration with EMEND.

Midazolam: The potential effects of increased plasma concentrations of midazolam or other benzodiazepines metabolised via CYP3A4 (alprazolam, triazolam) should be considered when co-administering these agents with a 3-day regimen of fosaprepitant followed by aprepitant.

Fosaprepitant given at a dose of 100 mg over 15 minutes with a single dose of midazolam 2 mg increased the AUC of midazolam 1.6-fold. This effect was not considered clinically important.

Oral aprepitant increased the AUC of midazolam 2.3-fold on Day 1 and 3.3-fold on Day 5, when a single oral dose of midazolam 2 mg was co-administered on Days 1 and 5 of a regimen of oral aprepitant 125 mg on Day 1 and 80 mg/day on Days 2 to 5.

In another study with intravenous administration of midazolam, oral aprepitant was given as 125 mg on Day 1 and 80 mg/day on Days 2 and 3, and midazolam 2 mg was given intravenously prior to the administration of the 3-day regimen of oral aprepitant and on Days 4, 8, and 15. Oral aprepitant increased the AUC of midazolam 25 % on Day 4 and decreased the AUC of midazolam 19 % on Day 8 and 4 % on Day 15. These effects were not considered clinically important.

In a third study with intravenous and oral administration of midazolam, oral aprepitant was given as 125 mg on Day 1 and 80 mg/day on Days 2 and 3, together with ondansetron 32 mg Day 1, dexamethasone, 12 mg Day 1 and 8 mg Days 2-4. This combination (i.e. oral aprepitant, ondansetron and dexamethasone) decreased the AUC of oral midazolam 16 % on Day 6, 9 % on Day 8, 7 % on Day 15 and 17 % on Day 22. These effects were not considered clinically important.

A fourth study was completed with intravenous administration of midazolam and oral aprepitant. Intravenous midazolam 2 mg was given 1 hour after oral administration of a single dose of oral aprepitant 125 mg. The plasma AUC of midazolam was increased by 1.5-fold. This effect was not considered clinically important.

Diltiazem: In patients with mild to moderate hypertension, infusion of 100 mg fosaprepitant over 15 minutes with diltiazem 120 mg 3 times daily, resulted in a 1.4-fold increase in diltiazem AUC and a small but clinically meaningful decrease in blood pressure, but did not result in a clinically meaningful change in heart rate, or PR interval.

Induction

As a mild inducer of CYP2C9, CYP3A4 and glucuronidation, aprepitant can decrease plasma concentrations of substrates eliminated by these routes within two weeks following initiation of dosing regimen. This effect may become apparent only after the end of a 3 day regimen of fosaprepitant followed by aprepitant. For CYP2C9 and CYP3A4 substrates, the induction is transient with a maximum effect reached 3-5 days after end of the oral aprepitant 3-day treatment. The effect is maintained for a few days, thereafter slowly declines and is clinically insignificant by two weeks after end of oral aprepitant treatment. Mild induction of glucuronidation is also seen with 80 mg oral aprepitant given for 7 days. Data are lacking regarding effects on CYP2C8 and CYP2C19. Caution is advised when warfarin, acenocoumarol, tolbutamide, phenytoin or other active substances that are known to be metabolised by CYP2C9 are administered during this time period.

Warfarin: In patients on chronic warfarin therapy, the prothrombin time (INR) should be monitored closely during treatment with fosaprepitant or aprepitant and for 2 weeks following each 3-day regimen for chemotherapy induced nausea and vomiting (see section 4.4). When a single 125 mg dose of oral aprepitant was administered on Day 1 and 80 mg/day on Days 2 and 3 to healthy subjects who were stabilised on chronic warfarin therapy, there was no effect of oral aprepitant on the plasma AUC of R(+) or S(-) warfarin determined on Day 3; however, there was a 34 % decrease in S(-) warfarin (a CYP2C9 substrate) trough concentration accompanied by a 14 % decrease in INR 5 days after completion of dosing with oral aprepitant.

Tolbutamide: Oral aprepitant, when given as 125 mg on Day 1 and 80 mg/day on Days 2 and 3, decreased the AUC of tolbutamide (a CYP2C9 substrate) by 23 % on Day 4, 28 % on Day 8, and 15 % on Day 15, when a single dose of tolbutamide 500 mg was administered orally prior to the administration of the 3-day regimen of oral aprepitant and on Days 4, 8, and 15.

Hormonal contraceptives: The efficacy of hormonal contraceptives may be reduced during and for 28 days after administration of oral aprepitant. Alternative or back-up methods of contraception should be used during treatment with fosaprepitant or oral aprepitant and for 2 months following the last dose of aprepitant.

In a clinical study, single doses of an oral contraceptive containing ethinyl estradiol and norethindrone were administered on Days 1 through 21 with oral aprepitant, given as a regimen of 125 mg on Day 8 and 80 mg/day on Days 9 and 10 with ondansetron 32 mg intravenously on Day 8 and oral dexamethasone given as 12 mg on Day 8 and 8 mg/day on Days 9, 10, and 11. During days 9 through 21 in this study, there was as much as a 64 % decrease in ethinyl estradiol trough concentrations and as much as a 60 % decrease in norethindrone trough concentrations.

5 -HT_3 antagonists: In clinical interaction studies, aprepitant did not have clinically important effects on the pharmacokinetics of ondansetron, granisetron, or hydrodolasetron (the active metabolite of dolasetron).

Effect of other agents on the pharmacokinetics of aprepitant

Concomitant administration of fosaprepitant or aprepitant with active substances that inhibit CYP3A4 activity (e.g., ketoconazole, itraconazole, voriconazole, posaconazole, clarithromycin, telithromycin nefazodone, and protease inhibitors) should be approached cautiously, as the combination is expected to result in increased plasma concentrations of aprepitant (see section 4.4).

Concomitant administration of fosaprepitant or aprepitant with active substances that strongly induce CYP3A4 activity (e.g. rifampicin, phenytoin, carbamazepine, phenobarbital) should be avoided as the combination results in reductions of the plasma concentrations of aprepitant that may result in decreased efficacy. Concomitant administration of fosaprepitant with herbal preparations containing St. John's Wort *Hypericum perforatum*) is not recommended.

Ketoconazole: When a single 125 mg dose of oral aprepitant was administered on Day 5 of a 10-day regimen of 400 mg/day of ketoconazole, a strong CYP3A4 inhibitor, the AUC of aprepitant increased approximately 5-fold and the mean terminal half-life of aprepitant increased approximately 3-fold.

Diltiazem: Infusion of 100 mg fosaprepitant over 15 minutes with diltiazem 120 mg 3 times daily, resulted in a 1.5-fold increase of aprepitant AUC. This effect was not considered clinically important.

Rifampicin: When a single 375 mg dose of oral aprepitant was administered on Day 9 of a 14-day regimen of 600 mg/day of rifampicin, a strong CYP3A4 inducer, the AUC of aprepitant decreased 91 % and the mean terminal half-life decreased 68 %.

4.6 Pregnancy and lactation

For fosaprepitant and aprepitant no clinical data on exposed pregnancies are available.

The potential for reproductive toxicities of fosaprepitant and aprepitant have not been fully characterized, since exposure levels above the therapeutic exposure in humans were not attained in animal studies. These studies did not indicate direct or indirect harmful effects with respect to pregnancy, embryonal/foetal development, parturition or postnatal development (see section 5.3). The potential effects on reproduction of alterations in neurokinin regulation are unknown. IVEMEND should not be used during pregnancy unless clearly necessary.

Aprepitant is excreted in the milk of lactating rats after intravenous administration of fosaprepitant as well as after oral administration of aprepitant. It is not known whether aprepitant is excreted in human milk. Therefore, breastfeeding is not recommended during treatment with IVEMEND and oral aprepitant.

4.7 Effects on ability to drive and use machines

No studies on the effects of IVEMEND on the ability to drive and use machines have been performed. However, when driving vehicles or operating machines, it should be taken into account that dizziness and fatigue have been reported after using IVEMEND (see section 4.8).

4.8 Undesirable effects

Since fosaprepitant is converted to aprepitant, those adverse reactions associated with aprepitant areexpected to occur with fosaprepitant. The safety profile of aprepitant was evaluated in approximately 4900 individuals. Various formulations of fosaprepitant have been administered to a total of 729 individuals including 347 healthy subjects and 149 patients with CINV.

Adverse reactions considered as drug-related by the investigator were reported in approximately 17 % of patients treated with the aprepitant regimen compared with approximately 13 % of patients treated with standard therapy in patients receiving highly emetogenic chemotherapy. Aprepitant was discontinued due to adverse reactions in 0.6 % of patients treated with the aprepitant regimen compared with 0.4 % of patients treated with standard therapy. In a clinical study of patients receiving moderately emetogenic chemotherapy, clinical adverse reactions were reported in approximately 21 % of patients treated with the aprepitant regimen compared with approximately 20 % of patients treated with standard therapy. Aprepitant was discontinued due to adverse reactions in 1.1 % of patients treated with the aprepitant regimen compared with 0.5 % of patients treated with standard therapy.

The most common adverse reactions reported at a greater incidence in patients treated with the aprepitant regimen than with standard therapy in patients receiving highly emetogenic chemotherapy were: hiccups (4.6 % versus 2.9%), asthenia/fatigue (2.9 % versus 1.6%), alanine transferase (ALT) increased (2.8 % versus 1.5%), constipation (2.2 % versus 2.0%), headache (2.2 % versus 1.8%), and anorexia (2.0 % versus 0.5%). The most common adverse reaction reported at a greater incidence in patients treated with the aprepitant regimen than with standard therapy in patients receiving moderately emetogenic chemotherapy was fatigue (2.5 % versus 1.6%).

The following adverse reactions were observed in patients treated with the aprepitant regimen and at a greater incidence than with standard therapy:

Frequencies are defined as: very common (≥1/10); common (≥1/100 to <1/10); uncommon (≥1/1,000 to <1/100); rare (≥1/10,000 to <1/1,000) and very rare (<1/10,000), not known (cannot be estimated from the available data).

System Organ Class	Adverse reaction	Frequency
Investigations	ALT increased, AST increased	common
	alkaline phosphatase increased, hyperglycaemia, microscopic haematuria, hyponatraemia, weight decreased	uncommon
Cardiac disorders	Bradycardia	uncommon
Blood and lymphatic system disorders	febrile neutropenia, anaemia	uncommon
Nervous system disorders	headache, dizziness	common
	dream abnormality, cognitive disorder	uncommon
Eye disorders	Conjunctivitis	uncommon
Ear and labyrinth disorders	Tinnitus	uncommon
Respiratory, thoracic and mediastinal disorders	Hiccups	common
	pharyngitis, sneezing, cough, postnasal drip, throat irritation	uncommon
Gastrointestinal disorders	constipation, diarrhoea, dyspepsia, eructation	common
	perforating duodenal ulcer, nausea*, vomiting*, acid reflux, dysgeusia, epigastric discomfort, obstipation, gastroesophageal reflux disease, abdominal pain, dry mouth, enterocolitis, flatulence, stomatitis	uncommon
Renal and urinary disorders	polyuria, dysuria, pollakiuria	uncommon
Skin and subcutaneous tissue disorders	rash, acne, photosensitivity, hyperhidrosis, oily skin, pruritus, skin lesion	uncommon
Musculoskeletal and connective tissue disorders	muscle cramp, myalgia	uncommon
Metabolism and nutrition disorders	Anorexia	common
	weight gain, polydipsia	uncommon
Infection and infestations	candidiasis, staphylococcal infection	uncommon
Vascular disorders	flushing/hot flush	uncommon
General disorders and administration site conditions	asthaenia/fatigue	common
	oedema, chest discomfort, lethargy, thirst	uncommon
Psychiatric disorders	disorientation, euphoria, anxiety	uncommon

*Nausea and vomiting were efficacy parameters in the first 5 days of post-chemotherapy treatment and were reported as adverse reactions only thereafter.

The adverse reactions profiles in the Multiple-Cycle extension for up to 5 additional cycles of chemotherapy were generally similar to those observed in Cycle 1.

Additional adverse reactions were observed in patients treated with aprepitant (40 mg) for postoperative nausea and vomiting and a greater incidence than with ondansetron: abdominal pain upper, bowel sounds abnormal, dysarthria, dyspnoea, hypoaesthesia, insomnia, miosis, nausea, sensory disturbance, stomach discomfort, visual acuity reduced, wheezing.

In addition, two serious adverse reactions were reported in clinical studies in postoperative nausea and vomiting (PONV) in patients taking a higher dose of aprepitant: one case of constipation, and one case of sub-ileus.

One case of Stevens-Johnson syndrome was reported as a serious adverse event in a patient receiving aprepitant with cancer chemotherapy.

In addition, infusion site induration and infusion site pain were common adverse reactions in a bioequivalence study in which 66 subjects were dosed with 115 mg of fosaprepitant intravenously.

One case of angioedema and urticaria was reported as a serious adverse event in a patient receiving aprepitant in a non-CINV/non-PONV study.

<u>Post-marketing experience</u>

During post-marketing experience with aprepitant the following side effects have been reported (frequency not known):

Skin and subcutaneous tissue disorders: pruritus, rash, urticaria

Immune system disorders: hypersensitivity reactions including anaphylactic reactions

4.9 Overdose

No specific information is available on the treatment of overdose.

Drowsiness and headache were reported in one patient who ingested 1,440 mg of aprepitant.

Single doses up to 200 mg of fosaprepitant were generally well tolerated in healthy subjects.

Table 1 Percent of Patients Receiving Highly Emetogenic Chemotherapy Responding by Treatment Group and Phase — Cycle 1

COMPOSITE MEASURES	Aprepitant Regimen (N= 521)†	Standard Therapy (N= 524)†	Differences*	
	%	%	%	(95 % CI)
Complete Response (no emesis and no rescue therapy)				
Overall (0-120 hours) 0-24 hours 25-120 hours	67.7 86.0 71.5	47.8 73.2 51.2	19.9 12.7 20.3	(14.0, 25.8) (7.9, 17.6) (14.5, 26.1)
INDIVIDUAL MEASURES				
No Emesis (no emetic episodes regardless of use of rescue therapy)				
Overall (0-120 hours) 0-24 hours 25-120 hours	71.9 86.8 76.2	49.7 74.0 53.5	22.2 12.7 22.6	(16.4, 28.0) (8.0, 17.5) (17.0, 28.2)
No Significant Nausea (maximum VAS <25 mm on a scale of 0-100 mm)				
Overall (0-120 hours) 25-120 hours	72.1 74.0	64.9 66.9	7.2 7.1	(1.6, 12.8) (1.5, 12.6)

* The confidence intervals were calculated with no adjustment for gender and concomitant chemotherapy, which were included in the primary analysis of odds ratios and logistic models.

† One patient in the Aprepitant Regimen only had data in the acute phase and was excluded from the overall and delayed phase analyses; one patient in the Standard Regimen only had data in the delayed phase and was excluded from the overall and acute phase analyses.

Table 2 Percent of Patients Responding by Treatment Group and Phase — Cycle 1 Moderately Emetogenic Chemotherapy

COMPOSITE MEASURES	Aprepitant Regimen (N= 433)†	Standard Therapy (N= 424)	Differences*	
	%	%	%	(95 % CI)
Complete Response (no emesis and no rescue therapy)				
Overall (0-120 hours) 0-24 hours 25-120 hours	50.8 75.7 55.4	42.5 69.0 49.1	8.3 6.7 6.3	(1.6, 15.0) (0.7, 12.7) (-0.4, 13.0)
INDIVIDUAL MEASURES				
No Emesis (no emetic episodes regardless of use of rescue therapy)				
Overall (0-120 hours) 0-24 hours 25-120 hours	75.7 87.5 80.8	58.7 77.3 69.1	17.0 10.2 11.7	(10.8, 23.2) (5.1, 15.3) (5.9, 17.5)
No Significant Nausea (maximum VAS <25 mm on a scale of 0-100 mm)				
Overall (0-120 hours) 0-24 hours 25-120 hours	60.9 79.5 65.3	55.7 78.3 61.5	5.3 1.3 3.9	(-1.3, 11.9) (-4.2, 6.8) (-2.6, 10.3)

* The confidence intervals were calculated with no adjustment for age category (<55 years, ≥ 55 years) and investigator group, which were included in the primary analysis of odds ratios and logistic models.

† One patient in the Aprepitant Regimen only had data in the acute phase and was excluded from the overall and delayed phase analyses.

Figure 1 Percent of Patients Receiving Highly Emetogenic Chemotherapy Who Remain Emesis Free Over Time – Cycle 1

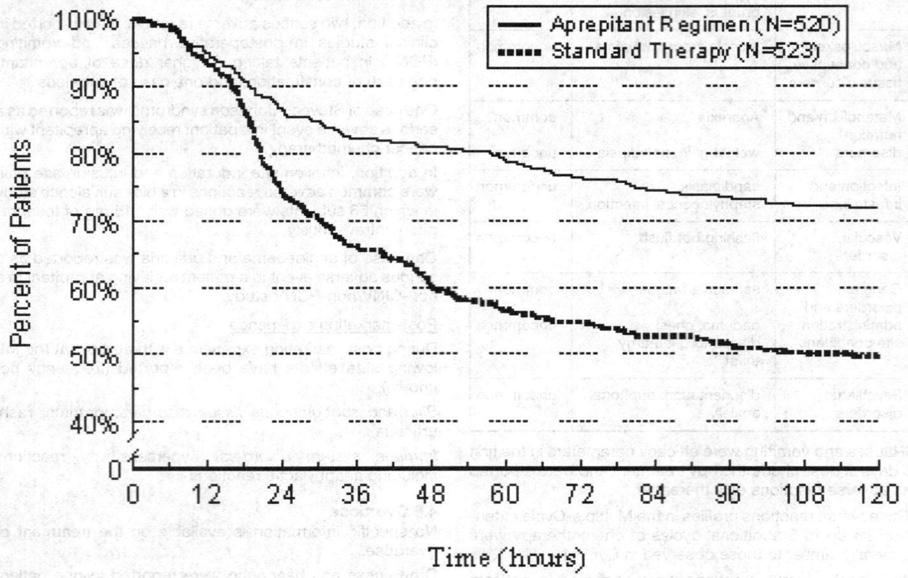

Figure 2 Percent of Patients Receiving Moderately Emetogenic Chemotherapy Who Remain Emesis Free Over Time – Cycle 1

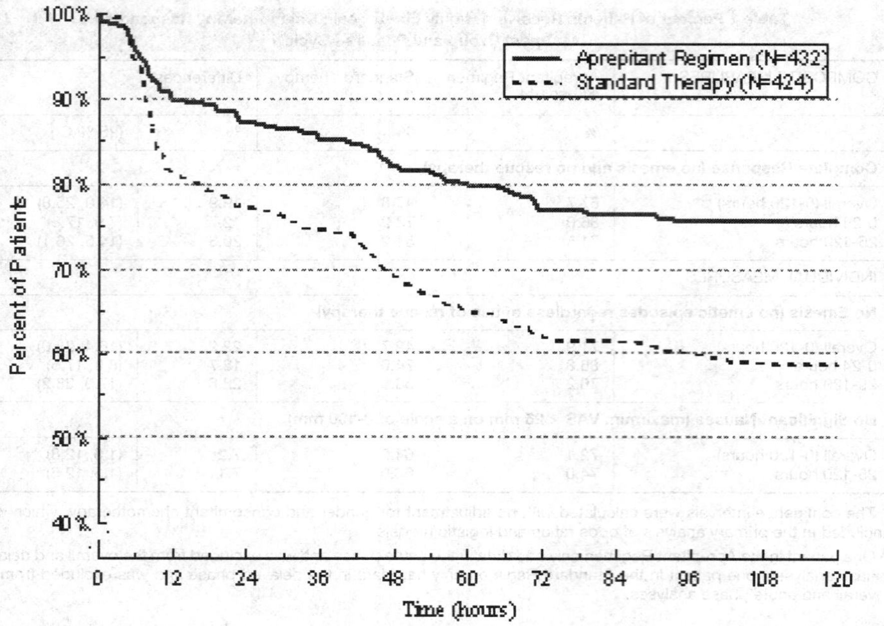

Three out of 33 subjects receiving 200 mg of fosaprepitant experienced mild injection site thrombosis.

In the event of overdose, fosaprepitant should be discontinued and general supportive treatment and monitoring should be provided. Because of the antiemetic activity of aprepitant, drug-induced emesis may not be effective.

Aprepitant cannot be removed by haemodialysis.

5. PHARMACOLOGICAL PROPERTIES

5.1 Pharmacodynamic properties

Pharmacotherapeutic group: Antiemetics and antinauseants, ATC code: A04A D12

Fosaprepitant is the prodrug of aprepitant and when administered intravenously is converted rapidly to aprepitant (see section 5.2). The contribution of fosaprepitant to the overall antiemetic effect has not fully been characterized, but a transient contribution during the initial phase cannot be ruled out. Aprepitant is a selective high-affinity antagonist at human substance P neurokinin 1 (NK_1) receptors. The pharmacological effect of fosaprepitant is attributed to aprepitant.

In 2 randomised, double-blind studies encompassing a total of 1,094 patients receiving chemotherapy that included cisplatin ⩾70 mg/m², aprepitant in combination with an ondansetron/dexamethasone regimen (see section 4.2) was compared with a standard regimen (placebo plus ondansetron 32 mg intravenously administered on Day 1 plus dexamethasone 20 mg orally on Day 1 and 8 mg orally twice daily on Days 2 to 4).

Efficacy was based on evaluation of the following composite measure: complete response (defined as no emetic episodes and no use of rescue therapy) primarily during Cycle 1. The results were evaluated for each individual study and for the 2 studies combined.

A summary of the key study results from the combined analysis is shown in Table 1.

Table 1

Percent of Patients Receiving Highly Emetogenic Chemotherapy Responding by Treatment Group and Phase — Cycle 1

(see Table 1 on previous page)

The estimated time to first emesis in the combined analysis is depicted by the Kaplan-Meier plot in Figure 1.

Figure 1

Percent of Patients Receiving Highly Emetogenic Chemotherapy Who Remain Emesis Free Over Time – Cycle 1

(see Figure 1 above)

Statistically significant differences in efficacy were also observed in each of the 2 individual studies.

In the same 2 clinical studies, 851 patients continued into the Multiple-Cycle extension for up to 5 additional cycles of chemotherapy. The efficacy of the aprepitant regimen was maintained during all cycles.

In a randomised, double-blind study in a total of 866 patients (864 females, 2 males) receiving chemotherapy that included cyclophosphamide 750-1500 mg/m²; or cyclophosphamide 500-1500 mg/m² and doxorubicin (⩽ 60 mg/m²) or epirubicin (⩽100 mg/m²), aprepitant in combination with an ondansetron/dexamethasone regimen (see section 4.2) was compared with standard therapy (placebo plus ondansetron 8 mg orally (twice on Day 1, and every 12 hours on Days 2 and 3) plus dexamethasone 20 mg orally on Day 1).

Efficacy was based on evaluation of the composite measure: complete response (defined as no emetic episodes and no use of rescue therapy) primarily during Cycle 1.

A summary of the key study results is shown in Table 2.

Table 2

(see Table 2 on previous page)

The estimated time to first emesis in the study is depicted by the Kaplan-Meier plot in Figure 2.

Figure 2

Percent of Patients Receiving Moderately Emetogenic Chemotherapy Who Remain Emesis Free Over Time – Cycle 1

(see Figure 2 below)

In the same clinical study, 744 patients continued into the Multiple-Cycle extension for up to 3 additional cycles of chemotherapy. The efficacy of the aprepitant regimen was maintained during all cycles.

5.2 Pharmacokinetic properties

Fosaprepitant, a prodrug of aprepitant, when administered intravenously is rapidly converted to aprepitant. Plasma concentrations of fosaprepitant are below quantifiable levels within 30 minutes of the completion of infusion.

Aprepitant after fosaprepitant administration

The AUC of aprepitant following 115 mg of fosaprepitant was equivalent to the AUC of 125 mg of oral aprepitant, while C_{max} was 2.5-fold higher.

Following a single intravenous dose of fosaprepitant administered as a 15-minute infusion to healthy volunteers the mean AUC_{0-24hr} of aprepitant was 19.8 μg•hr/ml and the mean maximal aprepitant concentration was 3.26 μg/ml. The mean aprepitant plasma concentrations from 4 hours after dosing (including the concentration at 24 hours post-dose) were similar between the 125 mg oral aprepitant dose and the 115 mg intravenous fosaprepitant dose.

Distribution

Aprepitant is highly protein bound, with a mean of 97 %. The geometric mean apparent volume of distribution at steady state (Vd_{ss}) is approximately 66 l in humans.

Metabolism

Fosaprepitant was rapidly converted to aprepitant in *in vitro* incubations with liver preparations from humans. Furthermore, fosaprepitant underwent rapid and nearly complete conversion to aprepitant in S9 preparations from other human tissues including kidney, lung and ileum. Thus, it appears that the conversion of fosaprepitant to aprepitant can occur in multiple tissues. In humans, fosaprepitant administered intravenously was rapidly converted to aprepitant within 30 minutes following the end of infusion.

Aprepitant undergoes extensive metabolism. In healthy young adults, aprepitant accounts for approximately 19 % of the radioactivity in plasma over 72 hours following a single intravenous administration 100 mg dose of [^{14}C]-fosaprepitant a prodrug, for aprepitant indicating a substantial presence of metabolites in the plasma. Twelve metabolites of aprepitant have been identified in human plasma. The metabolism of aprepitant occurs largely via oxidation at the morpholine ring and its side chains and the resultant metabolites were only weakly active. *In vitro* studies using human liver microsomes indicate that aprepitant is metabolised primarily by CYP3A4 and potentially with minor contribution by CYP1A2 and CYP2C19.

All metabolites observed in urine, faeces and plasma following an intravenous 100 mg [^{14}C]-fosaprepitant dose were also observed following an oral dose of [^{14}C]-aprepitant. Upon conversion of 115 mg of fosaprepitant to aprepitant, 18.3 mg of phosphate is liberated from fosaprepitant.

Elimination

Aprepitant is not excreted unchanged in urine. Metabolites are excreted in urine and via biliary excretion in faeces. Following a single intravenously administered 100 mg dose of [^{14}C]- fosaprepitant to healthy subjects, 57 % of the radioactivity was recovered in urine and 45 % in faeces.

The pharmacokinetics of aprepitant is non-linear across the clinical dose range. The terminal half-life of aprepitant after oral administration ranged from approximately 9 to 13 hours.

Pharmacokinetics in special populations

Fosaprepitant pharmacokinetics has not been evaluated in special populations. No clinically relevant differences in aprepitant pharmacokinetics is expected due to age and gender.

Hepatic impairment: Fosaprepitant is metabolized in various extrahepatic tissues; therefore hepatic impairment is not expected to alter the conversion of fosaprepitant to aprepitant. Mild hepatic impairment (Child-Pughclass A) does not affect the pharmacokinetics of aprepitant to a clinically relevant extent. No dose adjustment is necessary for patients with mild hepatic impairment. Conclusions regarding the influence of moderate hepatic impairment (Child-Pugh scoreClass B) on aprepitant pharmacokinetics cannot be drawn from available data. There are no clinical or pharmacokinetic data in patients with severe hepatic impairment (Child-PughClass C).

Renal impairment: A single 240 mg dose of oral aprepitant was administered to patients with severe renal impairment (CrCl< 30 ml/min) and to patients with end stage renal disease (ESRD) requiring haemodialysis.

In patients with severe renal impairment, the $AUC_{0-\infty}$ of total aprepitant (unbound and protein bound) decreased by 21 % and C_{max} decreased by 32 %, relative to healthy subjects. In patients with ESRD undergoing haemodialysis, the $AUC_{0-\infty}$ of total aprepitant decreased by 42 % and C_{max} decreased by 32 %. Due to modest decreases in protein binding of aprepitant in patients with renal disease, the AUC of pharmacologically active unbound aprepitant was not significantly affected in patients with renal impairment compared with healthy subjects. Haemodialysis conducted 4 or 48 hours after dosing had no significant effect on the pharmacokinetics of aprepitant; less than 0.2 % of the dose was recovered in the dialysate.

No dose adjustment is necessary for patients with renal impairment or for patients with ESRD undergoing haemodialysis.

Relationship between concentration and effect

Fosaprepitant is a prodrug of aprepitant. Positron emission tomography (PET) imaging studies, using a highly specific NK_1-receptor tracer, in healthy young men after administration of oral aprepitant have shown that aprepitant penetrates into the brain and occupies NK_1 receptors in a dose- and plasma-concentration-dependent manner. Aprepitant plasma concentrations achieved with the 3-day regimen of oral aprepitant are predicted to provide greater than 95 % occupancy of brain NK_1 receptors. The relationship between concentration and effect has not been evaluated after administration of fosaprepitant.

5.3 Preclinical safety data

Pre-clinical data obtained with intravenous administration of fosaprepitant and oral administration of aprepitant reveal no special hazard for humans based on conventional studies of single and repeated dose toxicity, genotoxicity (including *in vitro* tests), and toxicity to reproduction. In laboratory animals, fosaprepitant in non-commercial formulations caused vascular toxicity and hemolysis at concentrations below 1 mg/ml and higher, dependent on the formulation. In human washed blood cells also evidence of hemolysis was found with non-commercial formulations at fosaprepitant concentrations of 2.3 mg/ml and higher, although tests in human whole blood were negative. No hemolysis was found with the commercial formulation up to a fosaprepitant concentration of 1 mg/ml in human whole blood and washed human erythrocytes.

Carcinogenic potential in rodents was only investigated with orally administered aprepitant. However, it should be noted that the value of the toxicity studies carried out with rodents, rabbit and monkey, including the reproduction toxicity studies, are limited since systemic exposures to fosaprepitant and aprepitant were only similar or even lower than therapeutic exposure in humans. In the performed safety pharmacology and repeated dose toxicity studies with dogs, fosaprepitant Cmax and aprepitant AUC values were 4-7 times and 60-70 times, respectively, higher than clinical values.

6. PHARMACEUTICAL PARTICULARS

6.1 List of excipients

Disodium edetate (E386)

Polysorbate 80 (E433)

Lactose anhydrous

Sodium hydroxide (E524) (for pH adjustment) and/or

Hydrochloric acid diluted (E507) (for pH adjustment)

6.2 Incompatibilities

IVEMEND is incompatible with any solutions containing divalent cations (e.g., Ca^{2+}, Mg^{2+}), including Hartman's and Lactated Ringer's Solutions. This medicinal product must not be mixed with other medicinal products except those mentioned in section 6.6.

6.3 Shelf life

2 years.

After reconstitution and dilution, chemical and physical in-use stability has been demonstrated for 24 hours at 25°C.

From a microbiological point of view, the product should be used immediately. If not used immediately, in-use storage times and conditions prior to use are the responsibility of the user and would normally not be longer than 24 hours at 2 to 8°C.

6.4 Special precautions for storage

Store in a refrigerator (2°C - 8°C).

For storage conditions of the reconstituted and diluted medicinal product, see section 6.3.

6.5 Nature and contents of container

10 ml Type I clear glass vial with a chlorobutyl or bromobutyl rubberstopper and an aluminum seal with a blue plastic flip off cap.

IVEMEND will be available as a pack of 1 vial of 115 mg fosaprepitant or 10 vials of 115 mg fosaprepitant.

Not all pack sizes may be marketed.

6.6 Special precautions for disposal and other handling

No special requirements for disposal.

IVEMEND must be reconstituted and then diluted prior to administration.

Preparation for intravenous administration:

1. Inject 5 ml sodium chloride 9 mg/ml (0.9%) solution for injection into the vial. Assure that sodium chloride 9 mg/ml (0.9%) solution for injection is added to the vial along the vial wall in order to prevent foaming. Swirl the vial gently. Avoid shaking and jetting sodium chloride 9 mg/ml (0.9%) solution for injection into the vial.

2. Prepare an infusion bag filled with 110 ml of sodium chloride 9 mg/ml (0.9%) solution for injection (for example, by adding 10 ml of sodium chloride 9 mg/ml (0.9%) solution for injection to a 100 ml sodium chloride 9 mg/ml (0.9%) solution for injection infusion bag).

3. Withdraw the entire volume from the vial and transfer it into an infusion bag containing 110 ml of sodium chloride 9 mg/ml (0.9%) solution for injection to yield a total volume of 115 ml. Gently invert the bag 2-3 times.

The medicinal product must not be reconstituted or mixed with solutions for which physical and chemical compatibility has not been established (see section 6.2).

The appearance of the reconstituted solution is the same as the appearance of the diluent.

The reconstituted product should be inspected visually for particulate matter and discoloration before administration.

7. MARKETING AUTHORISATION HOLDER

Merck Sharp & Dohme Ltd.

Hertford Road, Hoddesdon

Hertfordshire EN 11 9BU

United Kingdom

8. MARKETING AUTHORISATION NUMBER(S)

10 ml × 1: EU/1/07/437/001

10 ml × 10: EU/1/07/437/002

9. DATE OF FIRST AUTHORISATION/RENEWAL OF THE AUTHORISATION

11 January 2008

10. DATE OF REVISION OF THE TEXT

6 August 2009

Detailed information on this medicinal product is available on the website of the European Medicines Agency (EMEA) website: http://www.emea.europa.eu/.

® denotes registered trademark of Merck & Co. Inc., Whitehouse Station, NJ, USA.

SPC.IVE.09.UK.3118

IXIARO suspension for injection - Japanese encephalitis vaccine (inactivated, adsorbed)

(Novartis Vaccines)

1. NAME OF THE MEDICINAL PRODUCT

IXIARO®▼suspension for injection

Japanese encephalitis vaccine (inactivated, adsorbed)

2. QUALITATIVE AND QUANTITATIVE COMPOSITION

1 dose (0.5 ml) of IXIARO®contains:

Japanese encephalitis virus strain SA_{14}-14-2 (inactivated)[1,2] 6 micrograms[3]

corresponding to a potency of ≤ 460 ng ED_{50}

[1] produced in Vero cells

[2] adsorbed on aluminium hydroxide, hydrated 0.25 milligrams Al^{3+}

[3] total protein content

For a full list of excipients, see section 6.1.

3. PHARMACEUTICAL FORM

Suspension for injection.

Clear liquid with a white precipitate.

4. CLINICAL PARTICULARS

4.1 Therapeutic indications

IXIARO®is indicated for active immunization against Japanese encephalitis for adults.

IXIARO®should be considered for use in individuals at risk of exposure through travel or in the course of their occupation.

4.2 Posology and method of administration

Posology

Adults

The primary vaccination series consists of two doses of 0.5 ml each according to the following schedule:

First dose at Day 0.

Second dose: 28 days after first dose.

Persistence of protective immunity is unknown. Timing and effect of booster immunisation is currently under investigation.

It is recommended that vaccinees who receive the first dose of IXIARO®complete the full vaccination course with IXIARO®.

Paediatric

IXIARO®is not recommended for use in children and adolescents due to lack of data on safety and efficacy.

Method of administration

The vaccine should be administered by intramuscular injection into the deltoid muscle. It should never be injected intravascularly.

Exceptionally, IXIARO®can also be administered subcutaneously to patients with thrombocytopenia or bleeding disorders since bleeding may occur following an intramuscular administration. Subcutaneous administration could lead to a suboptimal response to the vaccine (see section 4.4). However, it should be noted that there are no clinical efficacy data to support administration by the subcutaneous route.

4.3 Contraindications

Hypersensitivity to the active substance or to any of the excipients or to any residuals (e.g. protamine sulphate).

Individuals who show hypersensitivity reactions after receiving the first dose of the vaccine should not be given the second dose.

Administration must be postponed in persons with acute severe febrile conditions.

4.4 Special warnings and precautions for use

As with all injectable vaccines, appropriate medical treatment and supervision should always be available to treat rare cases of anaphylactic reactions following the administration of the vaccine.

Under no circumstances should IXIARO®be administered intravascularly.

As with any other vaccine, vaccination with IXIARO®may not result in protection in all cases.

IXIARO®will not protect against encephalitis caused by other micro-organisms.

Like other intramuscular injections, this vaccine should not be administered intramuscularly to persons with thrombocytopenia, haemophilia or other bleeding disorders (see section 4.2).

A seroconversion rate of 29.4 % has been observed 10 days after the first vaccination, and 97.3 % one week after the second vaccination. Hence, primary immunization should be completed at least one week prior to potential exposure to Japanese encephalitis virus (JEV).

4.5 Interaction with other medicinal products and other forms of interaction

Concomitant administration of IXIARO®with inactivated hepatitis A vaccine has been evaluated in one clinical study. There was no interference with the immune response to Japanese encephalitis virus (JEV) and hepatitis A virus (HAV) vaccines, respectively. Concomitant administration of IXIARO®and hepatitis A vaccine was shown to be non inferior to single vaccinations with regard to geometric mean titres (GMT) of anti JEV neutralizing antibody and HAV antibody, and for seroconversion rates (see section 5.1). There were no statistically significant higher rates in systemic or injection site adverse reactions among subjects who received concomitant vaccination with IXIARO®and hepatitis A vaccine compared with those who received IXIARO®or hepatitis A vaccine alone.

In patients receiving immunosuppressive therapy or patients with immunodeficiency an adequate immune response may not be obtained.

4.6 Pregnancy and lactation

Pregnancy

There are limited amount of data from the use of IXIARO®in pregnant or breast-feeding women.

In animal studies findings of unclear clinical relevance have been identified (see section 5.3).

As a precautionary measure, the use of IXIARO®during pregnancy or lactation should be avoided.

Lactation

It is unknown whether IXIARO®is excreted in human milk.

No effects on the breastfed newborn/infant are anticipated since the systemic exposure of the breast-feeding woman to IXIARO®is negligible.

4.7 Effects on ability to drive and use machines

No studies on the effects of IXIARO®on the ability to drive and use machines have been performed.

4.8 Undesirable effects

The safety of the vaccine was assessed in different controlled clinical studies in which more than 4,715 healthy adults were included of which 3,558 healthy adults received IXIARO®.

Approximately 40% of treated subjects can be expected to experience adverse reactions. They usually occur within the first three days after vaccination, are usually mild and disappear within a few days. No increase in the number of adverse reactions was noted between first and second doses.

Most commonly reported adverse reactions included headache and myalgia occurring in approximately 20% and 13% of subjects, respectively.

Table 2: Seroconversion rates (SCR) and geometric mean titers (GMT) at Month 2, 6 and 12 after vaccination with IXIARO® (ITT population)

SCR ITT population				GMT ITT population		
		N=181 % (n)	95% Confidence Interval		N=181	95% Confidence Interval
Month 2	Seroconverted Not seroconverted Missing	98.9 (179) 0.6 (1) 0.6 (1)	[96.1, 99.7]	**Month 2**	310.8	[268.8, 359.4]
Month 6	Seroconverted Not seroconverted	95.0 (172) 5.0 (9)	[90.8, 97.4]	**Month 6**	83.5	[70.9, 98.4]
Month 12	Seroconverted Not seroconverted	83.4 (151) 16.6 (30)	[77.3, 88.1]	**Month 12**	41.2	[34.4, 49.3]

Table 3: Seroconversion rates and geometric mean titer of anti JEV neutralizing antibody at Day 56 and seroconversion rates and geometric mean titer for HAV antibody at Day 28 in the Per Protocol Population

Seroconversion rates and geometric mean titer for anti-JEV neutralizing antibody at Day 56			
	% with SCR	GMT	95% CI
Group C: IXIARO®+ HAVRIX®1440	100.0	202.7	[153.7, 261.2]
Group A: IXIARO®+ Placebo	98.2	192.2	[147.9, 249.8]
Seroconversion rates and geometric mean titer for HAV antibody at Day 28			
	% with SCR	GMT	95% CI
Group C: IXIARO®+ HAVRIX®1440	100.0	150.0	[111.7, 202.3]
Group B: HAVRIX®+ Placebo	96.2	124.0	[91.4, 168.2]

Adverse reactions are listed according to the following frequencies:

Very common: ≥ 1/10

Common: ≥ 1/100 to < 1/10

Uncommon: ≥1/1,000 to < 1/100

Rare: ≥1/10,000 to < 1/1,000

Very rare: < 1/10,000, not known (cannot be estimated from the available data)

Infections and infestations

Uncommon: nasopharyngitis, rhinitis

Blood and lymphatic system disorders

Rare: lymphadenitis

Nervous system disorders

Very common: headache

Uncommon: migraine, dizziness

Ear and labyrinth disorders

Uncommon: vertigo

Respiratory, thoracic and mediastinal disorders

Uncommon: pharyngolaryngeal pain

Gastrointestinal disorders

Common: nausea

Uncommon: diarrhoea, vomiting

Skin and subcutaneous tissue disorders

Common: rash

Rare: pruritus

Musculoskeletal and connective tissue disorders

Very common: myalgia

General disorders and administration site conditions

Very common: injection site reactions (pain, tenderness)

Common: fatigue, influenza like illness, pyrexia, injection site reactions (erythema, hardening, swelling, itching)

Uncommon: chills, injection site reactions (haemorrhage, bruising)

Investigations

Uncommon: hepatic enzymes increased

4.9 Overdose

No case of overdose has been reported.

5. PHARMACOLOGICAL PROPERTIES

5.1 Pharmacodynamic properties

Pharmacotherapeutic group: Encephalitis vaccines. ATC code: J07BA02

Mechanism of action

The mechanism of action of Japanese encephalitis (JE) vaccines is not well understood. Studies in animals have shown that the vaccine triggers the immune system to produce antibodies against Japanese encephalitis virus that are most often protective. Challenge studies were performed in mice that were treated with human IXIARO®antisera. These studies showed that almost all mice that had a Plaque Reduction Neutralization Test titre of at least 1:10 were protected from a lethal Japanese encephalitis virus challenge.

Clinical studies

No prospective efficacy trials have been performed. Immunogenicity of IXIARO®was studied in approximately 2,060 healthy adult subjects included in five randomized, controlled clinical studies and one non controlled trial.

Immunogenicity of the vaccine was evaluated in a randomized, active controlled, observer blinded, multicenter Phase 3 clinical trial including 867 healthy male and female subjects given IXIARO®or the US licensed JEV vaccine JE VAX® (on a 0, 7 and 28 day schedule by subcutaneous injection). The co primary endpoint was seroconversion rate (anti JEV antibody titer ≥1:10) and geometric mean titers (GMT) at Day 56 as assessed by a Plaque Reduction Neutralization Test (PRNT) for the entire study population.

By Day 56, the proportion of subjects who had seroconverted was similar for both treatment groups (96.4% vs. 93.8% for IXIARO®and JE VAX®, respectively). GMT increased by Day 56 to 243.6 for IXIARO®and to 102.0 for JE VAX®, respectively. The immune responses elicited by IXIARO(r) were non inferior to those induced by JE VAX® (Table 1).

Table 1: Seroconversion rates and geometric mean titers of IXIARO(r) and JE VAX(r) in the Per Protocol Population. Neutralising antibody titers against JEV was measured against the JEV strain SA_{14}-14-2.

Seroconversion rate		
Timepoint	IXIARO® N=365 % (n)	JE-VAX® N=370 % (n)
Visit 0 (Screening)	0	0
Visit 3 (Day 28)	54 (197)	86.8 (321)
Visit 4 (Day 56)	96.4 (352)	93.8 (347)
Geometric mean titer (by plaque reduction neutralization test)		
Timepoint	IXIARO® N=365 GMT (n)	JE-VAX® N=370 GMT (n)
Visit 0 (Screening)	5.0 (365)	5.0 (370)
Visit 3 (Day 28)	17.4 (363)	76.9 (367)
Visit 4 (Day 56)	243.6 (361)	102.0 (364)

The effect of age on the immune response to IXIARO®and JE VAX®was assessed as a secondary endpoint in this active controlled study, comparing subjects over 50 years of age (N=262, mean age 59.8) with those below 50 years of age (N=605, mean age 33.9).

There was no significant difference between seroconversion rates of IXIARO®and JE VAX®in subjects aged <50 years compared to those aged ≥50 years at Day 28 or Day 56 following vaccination. Geometric mean titers were significantly higher at Day 28 in subjects aged <50 years than those aged ≥50 years in the JE VAX®group (80.9 vs. 45.9, p=0.0236) but there was no significant difference at Day 56 for this treatment group. There were no significant effects of age on geometric mean titer in the group receiving IXIARO®. There was no significant difference between seroconversion rates in subjects aged <50 years compared to those aged ≥50 years at Day 28 or Day 56 for either treatment group.

The 12 months immune response to IXIARO®was assessed in an uncontrolled Phase 3 follow up clinical trial, enrolling subjects who had completed two pivotal studies, and who received at least one dose of IXIARO®. The primary objective was the evaluation of the immune response to IXIARO®24 months after the first vaccination. Secondary objectives were the evaluation of the immune response to IXIARO®6 and 12 months after the first vaccination and to evaluate the safety of IXIARO®during the respective study period. A total of 3,258 healthy male and female subjects were enrolled of which 2,283 subjects had received IXIARO®, 338 subjects had received JE VAX®, and 637 subjects had received placebo in the respective previous study. Long term immunogenicity to IXIARO®was assessed in a subset of 181 subjects (Intent-to-treat (ITT) population). Immunogenicity data covering a period of 12 months after the first vaccination were as follows:

Seroconversion rates for anti JEV antibodies and GMT at Months 2, 6 and 12 are summarized in Table 2 for the ITT population. At Month 2, 98.9% of subjects had seroconverted (95% CI: 96.06, 99.70). By Month 12, the percentage of subjects who had seroconverted was 83.4% (95% CI: 77.33, 88.14). GMT at Months 2, 6, and 12 after vaccination with IXIARO®are summarized in Table 2. At Month 2, the GMT was 310.8 (95% CI: 268.76, 359.44) which decreased to 83.5 (95% CI: 70.89, 98.38) at Month 6 and to 41.2 (95% CI: 34.39, 49.33) at Month 12 after vaccination with IXIARO® (Table 2).

Table 2: Seroconversion rates (SCR) and geometric mean titers (GMT) at Month 2, 6 and 12 after vaccination with IXIARO® (ITT population)

(see Table 2 above)

The observed decline in GMT is as expected and compares well with data from other inactivated JE vaccines.

The concomitant use of IXIARO®with inactivated hepatitis A virus (HAV) vaccine (HAVRIX®1440) has been explored in one clinical trial. There was no interference with the immune response to the JE virus and HAV, respectively. Concomitant administration of IXIARO®and inactivated hepatitis A vaccine was shown to be non-inferior to single vaccinations with regard to GMT of anti-JE virus neutralizing antibody and HAV antibody, and for seroconversion rates of both antibody types (Table 3).

Table 3: Seroconversion rates and geometric mean titer of anti JEV neutralizing antibody at Day 56 and seroconversion rates and geometric mean titer for HAV antibody at Day 28 in the Per Protocol Population

(see Table 3 above)

5.2 Pharmacokinetic properties

Evaluation of pharmacokinetic properties is not required for vaccines.

5.3 Preclinical safety data

Non-clinical toxicity data are limited.

In a reproductive and pre-/post-natal toxicity study, no vaccine-related effects were detected on reproduction, foetal weight, survival and development of the off-spring. However, incomplete ossification of parts of the skeleton was observed in the group receiving 2 doses, but not in the group receiving 3 doses. It is currently difficult to explain if this phenomenon is treatment related or not.

6. PHARMACEUTICAL PARTICULARS

6.1 List of excipients

Phosphate buffered saline consisting of:

Sodium chloride

Potassium dihydrogen phosphate

Disodium hydrogen phosphate

Water for injections

For adjuvant, see section 2.

6.2 Incompatibilities

In the absence of compatibility studies, this vaccine must not be mixed with other medicinal products.

6.3 Shelf life

1 year

6.4 Special precautions for storage

Store in a refrigerator (2°C - 8°C). Do not freeze. Store in the original package in order to protect from light.

6.5 Nature and contents of container

0.5 ml of suspension in a pre-filled syringe (Type I glass) with a plunger stopper (chlorobutyl elastomer). Pack size of 1 syringe with or without a separate needle.

6.6 Special precautions for disposal and other handling

Do not use if the blister foil is not intact or packaging is damaged.

Upon storage, a fine white deposit with a clear colourless supernatant can be observed.

The pre-filled syringe is ready to use. If a needle is not provided, use a sterile needle. Shake before use. Thorough agitation immediately before administration is necessary to maintain suspension of the vaccine. The full recommended dose of the vaccine should be used.

Prior to agitation, IXIARO®may appear as a clear liquid with a white precipitate. After thorough agitation, it forms a white, cloudy liquid/suspension. The vaccine should be visually inspected for particulate matter and discoloration prior to administration. Discard the product if particulates are present or if it appears discoloured or if the syringe appears to be physically damaged.

Any unused product or waste material should be disposed of in accordance with local requirements.

7. MARKETING AUTHORISATION HOLDER

Intercell AG

Campus Vienna Biocenter 3

A-1030 Vienna

Austria

8. MARKETING AUTHORISATION NUMBER(S)

EU/1/08/501/001 and EU/1/08/501/002

9. DATE OF FIRST AUTHORISATION/RENEWAL OF THE AUTHORISATION

02 April 2009

10. DATE OF REVISION OF THE TEXT

April 2009

Detailed information on this medicinal product is available on the website of the European Medicines Agency (EMEA) http://www.emea.europa.eu/.

JE09ARR037 July 2009

JANUVIA 100mg film-coated tablets

(Merck Sharp & Dohme Limited)

1. NAME OF THE MEDICINAL PRODUCT

JANUVIA®▼ 100 mg film-coated tablets

2. QUALITATIVE AND QUANTITATIVE COMPOSITION

Each tablet contains sitagliptin phosphate monohydrate, equivalent to 100 mg sitagliptin.

For a full list of excipients, see section 6.1.

3. PHARMACEUTICAL FORM

Film-coated tablet (tablet)

Round, beige film-coated tablet with "277" on one side.

4. CLINICAL PARTICULARS

4.1 Therapeutic indications

For patients with type 2 diabetes mellitus, Januvia is indicated:

• to improve glycaemic control when diet and exercise alone do not provide adequate glycaemic control and when metformin is inappropriate due to contraindications or intolerance.

• to improve glycaemic control in combination with metformin when diet and exercise plus metformin alone do not provide adequate glycaemic control.

• to improve glycaemic control in combination with a sulphonylurea when diet and exercise plus maximal tolerated dose of a sulphonylurea alone do not provide adequate glycaemic control and when metformin is inappropriate due to contraindications or intolerance.

• to improve glycaemic control in combination with a sulphonylurea and metformin when diet and exercise plus dual therapy with these agents do not provide adequate glycaemic control.

For patients with type 2 diabetes mellitus in whom use of a PPARγ agonist (i.e. a thiazolidinedione) is appropriate, Januvia is indicated:

• in combination with the PPARγ agonist when diet and exercise plus the PPARγ agonist alone do not provide adequate glycaemic control.

• in combination with the PPARγ agonist and metformin when diet and exercise plus dual therapy with these agents do not provide adequate glycaemic control.

4.2 Posology and method of administration

The dose of Januvia is 100 mg once daily. When sitagliptin is used in combination with metformin and/or a PPARγ agonist, the dosage of metformin and/or PPARγ agonist should be maintained, and sitagliptin administered concomitantly.

When Januvia is used in combination with a sulphonylurea, a lower dose of the sulphonylurea may be considered to reduce the risk of hypoglycaemia. (See section 4.4.)

If a dose of Januvia is missed, it should be taken as soon as the patient remembers. A double dose should not be taken on the same day.

Januvia can be taken with or without food.

Patients with renal insufficiency

For patients with mild renal insufficiency (creatinine clearance [CrCl] ⩾50 ml/min), no dosage adjustment for Januvia is required.

Clinical study experience with Januvia in patients with moderate or severe renal insufficiency is limited. Therefore, use of Januvia is not recommended in this patient population (see section 5.2).

Patients with hepatic insufficiency

No dosage adjustment is necessary for patients with mild to moderate hepatic insufficiency. Januvia has not been studied in patients with severe hepatic insufficiency.

Elderly

No dosage adjustment is necessary based on age. Limited safety data is available in patients ⩾ 75 years of age and care should be exercised.

Paediatric population

Januvia is not recommended for use in children below 18 years of age due to a lack of data on its safety and efficacy.

4.3 Contraindications

Hypersensitivity to the active substance or to any of the excipients (see section 4.4 and 4.8).

4.4 Special warnings and precautions for use

General

Januvia should not be used in patients with type 1 diabetes or for the treatment of diabetic ketoacidosis.

Hypoglycaemia when used in combination with other anti-hyperglycaemic agents

In clinical trials of Januvia as monotherapy and as part of combination therapy with agents not known to cause hypoglycaemia (i.e. metformin and/or a PPARγ agonist), rates of hypoglycaemia reported with sitagliptin were similar to rates in patients taking placebo. When sitagliptin was added to a sulphonylurea, the incidence of hypoglycaemia was increased over that of placebo (see section 4.8). Therefore, to reduce the risk of hypoglycaemia, a lower dose of sulphonylurea may be considered (see section 4.2). The use of sitagliptin in combination with insulin has not been adequately studied.

Renal insufficiency

As the experience is limited, patients with moderate to severe renal insufficiency should not be treated with Januvia (see section 5.2).

Hypersensitivity Reactions

Postmarketing reports of serious hypersensitivity reactions in patients treated with Januvia have been reported. These reactions include anaphylaxis, angioedema, and exfoliative skin conditions including Stevens-Johnson syndrome. Onset of these reactions occurred within the first 3 months after initiation of treatment with Januvia, with some reports occurring after the first dose. If a hypersensitivity reaction is suspected, discontinue Januvia, assess for other potential causes for the event, and institute alternative treatment for diabetes. (See section 4.8).

4.5 Interaction with other medicinal products and other forms of interaction

Effects of other medicinal products on sitagliptin

Clinical data described below suggest that the risk for clinically meaningful interactions by co-administered medicinal products is low.

Metformin: Co-administration of multiple twice-daily doses of 1000 mg metformin with 50 mg sitagliptin did not meaningfully alter the pharmacokinetics of sitagliptin in patients with type 2 diabetes.

Ciclosporin: A study was conducted to assess the effect of ciclosporin, a potent inhibitor of p-glycoprotein, on the pharmacokinetics of sitagliptin. Coadministration of a single 100 mg oral dose of sitagliptin and a single 600 mg oral dose of ciclosporin increased the AUC and C_{max} of sitagliptin by approximately 29 % and 68 %, respectively. These changes in sitagliptin pharmacokinetics were not considered to be clinically meaningful. The renal clearance of sitagliptin was not meaningfully altered. Therefore, meaningful interactions would not be expected with other p-glycoprotein inhibitors.

In vitro studies indicated that the primary enzyme responsible for the limited metabolism of sitagliptin is CYP3A4, with contribution from CYP2C8. In patients with normal renal function, metabolism, including via CYP3A4, plays only a small role in the clearance of sitagliptin. Metabolism may play a more significant role in the elimination of sitagliptin in the setting of severe renal insufficiency or ESRD. For this reason, it is possible that potent CYP3A4 inhibitors (i.e. ketoconazole, itraconazole, ritonavir, clarithromycin) could alter the phamacokinetics of sitagliptin in patients with severe renal insufficiency or ESRD. The effects of potent CYP3A4 inhibitors in the setting of renal insufficiency has not been assessed in a clinical study.

In vitro transport studies showed that sitagliptin is a substrate for p-glycoprotein and OAT3. OAT3 mediated transport of sitagliptin was inhibited *in vitro* by probenecid, although the risk of clinically meaningful interactions is considered to be low. Concomitant administration of OAT3 inhibitors has not been evaluated *in vivo*.

Effects of sitagliptin on other medicinal products

In vitro data suggest that sitagliptin does not inhibit nor induce CYP450 isoenzymes. In clinical studies, sitagliptin did not meaningfully alter the pharmacokinetics of metformin, glyburide, simvastatin, rosiglitazone, warfarin, or oral contraceptives, providing *in vivo* evidence of a low propensity for causing interactions with substrates of CYP3A4, CYP2C8, CYP2C9, and organic cationic transporter (OCT).

Sitagliptin had a small effect on plasma digoxin concentrations, and may be a mild inhibitor of p-glycoprotein *in vivo*.

Digoxin: Sitagliptin had a small effect on plasma digoxin concentrations. Following administration of 0.25 mg digoxin concomitantly with 100 mg of Januvia daily for 10 days, the plasma AUC of digoxin was increased on average by 11 %, and the plasma C_{max} on average by 18 %. No dosage adjustment of digoxin is recommended. However, patients at risk of digoxin toxicity should be monitored for this when sitagliptin and digoxin are administered concomitantly.

4.6 Pregnancy and lactation

Pregnancy

There are no adequate data from the use of Januvia in pregnant women. Studies in animals have shown reproductive toxicity at high doses (see section 5.3). The potential risk for humans is unknown. Due to lack of human data, Januvia should not be used during pregnancy.

Lactation

It is unknown whether sitagliptin is excreted in human breast milk. Animal studies have shown excretion of sitagliptin in breast milk. Januvia should not be used during breast-feeding.

4.7 Effects on ability to drive and use machines

No studies on the effects on the ability to drive and use machines have been performed. However, when driving or operating machines, it should be taken into account that dizziness and somnolence have been reported.

4.8 Undesirable effects

In 10 large clinical trials of up to 2 years in duration, over 2,900 patients have received treatment with Januvia 100 mg per day alone or in combination with metformin, a sulphonylurea (with or without metformin) or a PPARγ agent (with or without metformin). In a pooled analysis of 9 of these trials, the rate of discontinuation due to adverse experiences considered drug-related was 0.8 % with 100 mg per day and 1.5 % with other treatments. No adverse reactions considered as drug-related were reported in patients treated with sitagliptin occurring in excess (> 0.2 % and difference > 1 patient) of that in patients treated with control. In an additional combination study with a PPARγ agent (rosiglitazone) and metformin, no patients were discontinued due to adverse experiences considered as drug-related.

Adverse reactions considered as drug-related reported in patients treated with sitagliptin occurring in excess (> 0.2 % and difference > 1 patient) of that in patients treated with placebo are listed below (Table 1) by system organ class and frequency. Frequencies are defined as: very common (⩾ 1/10); common (⩾ 1/100, < 1/10); uncommon (⩾ 1/1,000, < 1/100); rare (⩾ 1/10,000, < 1/1,000); and very rare (< 1/10,000).

Table 1. The frequency of adverse reactions identified from placebo-controlled clinical studies

(see Table 1 on next page)

In an additional 1-year study of sitagliptin 100 mg once daily in combination with metformin, the incidence of adverse reactions considered as drug-related in patients treated with sitagliptin/metformin compared to sulphonylurea/metformin was 14.5 % and 30.3 %, respectively.

In pooled studies of up to 1 year in duration comparing sitagliptin/metformin to a sulphonylurea agent/metformin, adverse reactions considered as drug-related reported in patients treated with sitagliptin 100 mg occurring in excess (> 0.2 % and difference > 1 patient) of that in patients receiving the sulphonylurea agent are as follows: anorexia (Metabolism and nutritional disorders; frequency uncommon) and weight decreased (Investigations; frequency uncommon).

[2] In this 24-week study of sitagliptin 100 mg once daily in combination with glimepiride, the incidence of adverse reactions considered as drug-related in patients treated with sitagliptin/glimepiride compared to treatment with placebo/glimepiride was 11.3 % and 6.6 %, respectively.

[3] In this 24-week study of sitagliptin 100 mg once daily in combination with glimepiride and metformin, the incidence of adverse reactions considered as drug-related in patients treated with sitagliptin in combination with glimepiride/metformin compared to treatment with placebo in combination with glimepiride/metformin was 18.1 % and 7.1 %, respectively.

[4] In this 24-week study of the combination of sitagliptin 100 mg once daily and pioglitazone, the incidence of adverse reactions considered as drug-related in patients treated with sitagliptin/pioglitazone compared to patients treated with placebo/pioglitazone was 9.1 % and 9.0 %, respectively.

[5] In this study of sitagliptin 100 mg once daily in combination with rosiglitazone and metformin, which continued through 54 weeks, the incidence of adverse reactions considered as drug-related in patients treated with sitagliptin combination compared to treatment with the placebo combination was 15.3 % and 10.9 %, respectively. Other drug-related adverse reactions reported in the 54-week analysis (frequency common) in patients treated with sitagliptin combination occurring in excess (> 0.2 % and difference > 1 patient) of that in patients treated with the placebo combination were: headache, cough, vomiting, hypoglycaemia, fungal skin infection, and upper respiratory tract infection.

In addition, in monotherapy studies of up to 24 weeks in duration of sitagliptin 100 mg once daily alone compared to placebo, adverse reactions considered as drug-related reported in patients treated with sitagliptin in excess (> 0.2 % and difference > 1 patient) of that in patients receiving placebo are headache, hypoglycaemia, constipation, and dizziness.

In addition to the drug-related adverse experiences described above, adverse experiences reported regardless

Table 1 The frequency of adverse reactions identified from placebo-controlled clinical studies

Adverse Reaction	Frequency of adverse reaction by treatment regimen				
	Sitagliptin with Metformin[1]	Sitagliptin with a Sulfonylurea[2]	Sitagliptin with a Sulfonylurea and Metformin [3]	Sitagliptin with a PPARγ Agent (pioglitazone)[4]	Sitagliptin with a PPARγ Agent (rosiglitazone) and Metformin[5]
Time-point	**24-week**	**24-week**	**24-week**	**24-week**	**18-week**
Investigations					
blood glucose decreased	Uncommon				
Nervous system disorders					
headache					Common
somnolence	Uncommon				
Gastrointestinal disorders					
diarrhoea	Uncommon				Common
nausea	Common				
flatulence				Common	
constipation			Common		
upper abdominal pain	Uncommon				
vomiting					Common
Metabolism and nutrition disorders					
Hypoglycaemia*		Very common	Very common	Common	Common
General disorders					
peripheral oedema				Common	Common†

* In clinical trials of Januvia as monotherapy and sitagliptin as part of combination therapy with metformin and/or a PPARγ agent, rates of hypoglycaemia reported with sitagliptin were similar to rates in patients taking placebo.

† Observed in the 54-week analysis.

[1] In this placebo-controlled 24-week study of sitagliptin 100 mg once daily in combination with metformin, the incidence of adverse reactions considered as drug-related in patients treated with sitagliptin/metformin compared to treatment with placebo/metformin was 9.3 % and 10.1 %, respectively.

of causal relationship to medication and occurring in at least 5 % and more commonly in patients treated with Januvia included upper respiratory tract infection and nasopharyngitis. Additional adverse experiences reported regardless of causal relationship to medication that occurred more frequently in patients treated with Januvia (not reaching the 5 % level, but occurring with an incidence of > 0.5 % higher with Januvia than that in the control group) included osteoarthritis and pain in extremity.

In an additional 24-week study of sitagliptin 100 mg once daily compared to metformin, the incidence of adverse reactions considered as drug-related in patients treated with sitagliptin compared to metformin was 5.9 % and 16.7 %, respectively, primarily due to a higher incidence of gastrointestinal adverse reactions in the metformin group. In this study 0.6 % of patients treated with sitagliptin and 2.3 % of patients treated with metformin were discontinued due to adverse experiences considered as drug-related.

In a 24-week study of initial combination therapy with sitagliptin and metformin administered twice daily (sitagliptin/metformin 50 mg/500 mg or 50 mg/1000 mg), the overall incidence of adverse reactions considered as drug-related in patients treated with the combination of sitagliptin and metformin compared to patients treated with placebo was 14.0 % and 9.7 %, respectively. The overall incidence of adverse reactions considered as drug-related in patients treated with the combination of sitagliptin and metformin was comparable to metformin alone (14.0 % each) and greater than sitagliptin alone (6.7 %), with the differences relative to sitagliptin alone primarily due to gastrointestinal adverse reactions.

Across clinical studies, a small increase in white blood cell count (approximately 200 cells/microl difference in WBC vs. placebo; mean baseline WBC approximately 6600 cells/microl) was observed due to an increase in neutrophils. This observation was seen in most but not all studies. This change in laboratory parameters is not considered to be clinically relevant.

No clinically meaningful changes in vital signs or in ECG (including in QTc interval) were observed with Januvia treatment.

Post-marketing Experience:

During post-marketing experience the following additional side effects have been reported (frequency not known): hypersensitivity reactions including anaphylaxis, angioedema, rash, urticaria, cutaneous vasculitis and exfoliative skin conditions including Stevens-Johnson syndrome (see section 4.4); pancreatitis.

4.9 Overdose

During controlled clinical trials in healthy subjects, single doses of up to 800 mg sitagliptin were generally well tolerated. Minimal increases in QTc, not considered to be clinically relevant, were observed in one study at a dose of 800 mg sitagliptin. There is no experience with doses above 800 mg in humans. In Phase I multiple-dose studies, there were no dose-related clinical adverse reactions observed with sitagliptin with doses of up to 600 mg per day for periods of up to 10 days and 400 mg per day for periods of up to 28 days.

In the event of an overdose, it is reasonable to employ the usual supportive measures, e.g., remove unabsorbed material from the gastrointestinal tract, employ clinical monitoring (including obtaining an electrocardiogram), and institute supportive therapy if required.

Sitagliptin is modestly dialyzable. In clinical studies, approximately 13.5 % of the dose was removed over a 3- to 4-hour haemodialysis session. Prolonged haemodialysis may be considered if clinically appropriate. It is not known if sitagliptin is dialyzable by peritoneal dialysis.

5. PHARMACOLOGICAL PROPERTIES

5.1 Pharmacodynamic properties

Pharmacotherapeutic group: DPP-4 Inhibitor, ATC code: A10BH01.

Januvia is a member of a class of oral anti-hyperglycaemic agents called dipeptidyl peptidase 4 (DPP-4) inhibitors. The improvement in glycaemic control observed with this agent may be mediated by enhancing the levels of active incretin hormones. Incretin hormones, including glucagon-like peptide-1 (GLP-1) and glucose-dependent insulinotropic polypeptide (GIP), are released by the intestine throughout the day, and levels are increased in response to a meal. The incretins are part of an endogenous system involved in the physiologic regulation of glucose homeostasis. When blood glucose concentrations are normal or elevated, GLP-1 and GIP increase insulin synthesis and release from pancreatic beta cells by intracellular signaling pathways involving cyclic AMP. Treatment with GLP-1 or with DPP-4 inhibitors in animal models of type 2 diabetes has been demonstrated to improve beta cell responsiveness to glucose and stimulate insulin biosynthesis and release. With higher insulin levels, tissue glucose uptake is enhanced. In addition, GLP-1 lowers glucagon secretion from pancreatic alpha cells. Decreased glucagon concentrations, along with higher insulin levels, lead to reduced hepatic glucose production, resulting in a decrease in blood glucose levels. The effects of GLP-1 and GIP are glucose-dependent such that when blood glucose concentrations are low, stimulation of insulin release and suppression of glucagon secretion by GLP-1 are not observed. For both GLP-1 and GIP, stimulation of insulin release is enhanced as glucose rises above normal concentrations. Further, GLP-1 does not impair the normal glucagon response to hypoglycaemia. The activity of GLP-1 and GIP is limited by the DPP-4 enzyme, which rapidly hydrolyzes the incretin hormones to produce inactive products. Sitagliptin prevents the hydrolysis of incretin hormones by DPP-4, thereby increasing plasma concentrations of the active forms of GLP-1 and GIP. By enhancing active incretin levels, sitagliptin increases insulin release and decreases glucagon levels in a glucose-dependent manner. In patients with type 2 diabetes with hyperglycaemia, these changes in insulin and glucagon levels lead to lower haemoglobin A_{1c} (HbA_{1c}) and lower fasting and postprandial glucose concentrations. The glucose-dependent mechanism of sitagliptin is distinct from the mechanism of sulphonylureas, which increase insulin secretion even when glucose levels are low and can lead to hypoglycaemia in patients with type 2 diabetes and in normal subjects. Sitagliptin is a potent and highly selective inhibitor of the enzyme DPP-4 and does not inhibit the closely-related enzymes DPP-8 or DPP-9 at therapeutic concentrations.

In a two-day study in healthy subjects, sitagliptin alone increased active GLP-1 concentrations, whereas metformin alone increased active and total GLP-1 concentrations to similar extents. Co-administration of sitagliptin and metformin had an additive effect on active GLP-1 concentrations. Sitagliptin, but not metformin, increased active GIP concentrations.

Overall, sitagliptin improved glycaemic control when given as monotherapy, when used in combination with metformin (initial or add-on therapy), in combination with a sulphonylurea (with or without metformin), in combination with a thiazolidinedione, and in combination with a thiazolidinedione and metformin, as measured by clinically relevant reductions in HbA_{1c} from baseline at study endpoint (see Table 2).

Two studies were conducted to evaluate the efficacy and safety of Januvia monotherapy. Treatment with sitagliptin at 100 mg once daily as monotherapy provided significant improvements in HbA_{1c}, fasting plasma glucose (FPG), and 2-hour post-prandial glucose (2-hour PPG), compared to placebo in two studies, one of 18- and one of 24-weeks duration. Improvement of surrogate markers of beta cell function, including HOMA-β (Homeostasis Model Assessment-β), proinsulin to insulin ratio, and measures of beta cell responsiveness from the frequently-sampled meal tolerance test were observed. The observed incidence of hypoglycaemia in patients treated with Januvia was similar to placebo. Body weight did not increase from baseline with sitagliptin therapy in either study, compared to a small reduction in patients given placebo.

In a study in patients with type 2 diabetes and chronic renal insufficiency (creatinine clearance < 50 ml/min), the safety and tolerability of reduced doses of sitagliptin were investigated and generally similar to placebo. In addition, the reductions in HbA_{1c} and FPG with sitagliptin compared to placebo were generally similar to those observed in other monotherapy studies in patients with normal renal function (see section 5.2). The number of patients with moderate to severe renal insufficiency was too low to confirm safe use of sitagliptin in this type of patients.

Sitagliptin 100 mg once daily provided significant improvements in glycaemic parameters compared with placebo in two 24-week studies of sitagliptin as add-on therapy, one in combination with metformin and one in combination with pioglitazone. Change from baseline in body weight was similar for patients treated with sitagliptin relative to placebo. In these studies there was a similar incidence of hypoglycaemia reported for patients treated with sitagliptin or placebo.

A 24-week placebo-controlled study was designed to evaluate the efficacy and safety of sitagliptin (100 mg once daily) added to glimepiride alone or glimepiride in combination with metformin. The addition of sitagliptin to either glimepiride alone or to glimepiride and metformin provided significant improvements in glycaemic parameters. Patients treated with sitagliptin had a modest increase in body weight compared to those given placebo.

A 54-week placebo-controlled study was designed to evaluate the efficacy and safety of sitagliptin (100 mg once daily) added to the combination of rosiglitazone and metformin. The addition of sitagliptin to rosiglitazone and metformin provided significant improvements in glycaemic parameters at the primary timepoint of Week 18, with improvements sustained through the end of the study.

Change from baseline in body weight was similar for patients treated with sitagliptin relative to placebo (1.9 vs. 1.3 kg).

In a 24-week placebo-controlled factorial study of initial therapy, sitagliptin 50 mg twice daily in combination with metformin (500 mg or 1000 mg twice daily) provided significant improvements in glycaemic parameters compared with either monotherapy. The decrease in body weight with the combination of sitagliptin and metformin was similar to that observed with metformin alone or placebo; there was no change from baseline for patients on sitagliptin alone. The incidence of hypoglycaemia was similar across treatment groups.

Table 2. HbA_{1c} results in placebo-controlled monotherapy and combination therapy studies*

(see Table 2 opposite)

A 24-week active (metformin)-controlled study was designed to evaluate the efficacy and safety of sitagliptin 100 mg once daily (N=528) compared to metformin (N=522) in patients with inadequate glycaemic control on diet and exercise and who were not on anti-hyperglycaemic therapy (off therapy for at least 4 months). The mean dose of metformin was approximately 1900 mg per day. The reduction in HbA_{1c} from mean baseline values of 7.2 % was -0.38 % for sitagliptin and -0.55 % for metformin. The overall incidence of gastrointestinal adverse reactions considered as drug-related in patients treated with sitagliptin was 2.7 % compared with 12.6 % in patients treated with metformin. The incidence of hypoglycaemia was not significantly different between the treatment groups (sitagliptin, 1.3 %; metformin, 1.9 %). Body weight decreased from baseline in both groups (sitagliptin, -0.6 kg; metformin -1.9 kg).

In a study comparing the efficacy and safety of the addition of Januvia 100 mg once daily or glipizide (a sulphonylurea agent) in patients with inadequate glycaemic control on metformin monotherapy, sitagliptin was similar to glipizide in reducing HbA_{1c}. The mean glipizide dose used in the comparator group was 10 mg per day with approximately 40 % of patients requiring a glipizide dose of ≤ 5 mg/day throughout the study. However, more patients in the sitagliptin group discontinued due to lack of efficacy than in the glipizide group. Patients treated with sitagliptin exhibited a significant mean decrease from baseline in body weight compared to a significant weight gain in patients administered glipizide (-1.5 vs. +1.1 kg). In this study, the proinsulin to insulin ratio, a marker of efficiency of insulin synthesis and release, improved with sitagliptin and deteriorated with glipizide treatment. The incidence of hypoglycaemia in the sitagliptin group (4.9 %) was significantly lower than that in the glipizide group (32.0 %).

Table 2 HbA_{1c} results in placebo-controlled monotherapy and combination therapy studies*

Study	Mean baseline HbA_{1c} (%)	Mean change from baseline HbA_{1c} (%)†	Placebo-corrected mean change in HbA_{1c} (%)† (95 % CI)
Monotherapy Studies			
Sitagliptin 100 mg once daily§ (N= 193)	8.0	-0.5	-0.6‡ (-0.8, -0.4)
Sitagliptin 100 mg once daily% (N= 229)	8.0	-0.6	-0.8‡ (-1.0, -0.6)
Combination Therapy Studies			
Sitagliptin 100 mg once daily added to ongoing metformin therapy% (N=453)	8.0	-0.7	-0.7‡ (-0.8, -0.5)
Sitagliptin 100 mg once daily added to ongoing pioglitazone therapy% (N=163)	8.1	-0.9	-0.7‡ (-0.9, -0.5)
Sitagliptin 100 mg once daily added to ongoing glimepiride therapy% (N=102)	8.4	-0.3	-0.6‡ (-0.8, -0.3)
Sitagliptin 100 mg once daily added to ongoing glimepiride + metformin therapy% (N=115)	8.3	-0.6	-0.9‡ (-1.1, -0.7)
Sitagliptin 100 mg once daily added to ongoing rosiglitazone + metformin therapy (N=170)			
Week 18	8.8	-1.0	-0.7‡ (-0.9, -0.5)
Week 54	8.8	-1.0	-0.8‡ (-1.0, -0.5)
Initial therapy (twice daily)%: Sitagliptin 50 mg + metformin 500 mg (N=183)	8.8	-1.4	-1.6‡ (-1.8, -1.3)
Initial therapy (twice daily)%: Sitagliptin 50 mg + metformin 1000 mg (N=178)	8.8	-1.9	-2.1‡ (-2.3, -1.8)

* All Patients Treated Population (an intention-to-treat analysis).

† Least squares means adjusted for prior antihyperglycaemic therapy status and baseline value.

‡ $p < 0.001$ compared to placebo or placebo + combination treatment.

§ HbA_{1c} (%) at week 18.

% HbA_{1c} (%) at week 24.

5.2 Pharmacokinetic properties

Absorption

Following oral administration of a 100-mg dose to healthy subjects, sitagliptin was rapidly absorbed, with peak plasma concentrations (median T_{max}) occurring 1 to 4 hours post-dose, mean plasma AUC of sitagliptin was 8.52 μM•hr, C_{max} was 950 nM. The absolute bioavailability of sitagliptin is approximately 87 %. Since coadministration of a high-fat meal with Januvia had no effect on the pharmacokinetics, Januvia may be administered with or without food.

Plasma AUC of sitagliptin increased in a dose-proportional manner. Dose-proportionality was not established for C_{max} and C_{24hr} (C_{max} increased in a greater than dose-proportional manner and C_{24hr} increased in a less than dose-proportional manner).

Distribution

The mean volume of distribution at steady state following a single 100-mg intravenous dose of sitagliptin to healthy subjects is approximately 198 litres. The fraction of sitagliptin reversibly bound to plasma proteins is low (38 %).

Metabolism

Sitagliptin is primarily eliminated unchanged in urine, and metabolism is a minor pathway. Approximately 79 % of sitagliptin is excreted unchanged in the urine.

Following a [^{14}C]sitagliptin oral dose, approximately 16 % of the radioactivity was excreted as metabolites of sitagliptin. Six metabolites were detected at trace levels and are not expected to contribute to the plasma DPP-4 inhibitory activity of sitagliptin. *In vitro* studies indicated that the primary enzyme responsible for the limited metabolism of sitagliptin was CYP3A4, with contribution from CYP2C8.

In vitro data showed that sitagliptin is not an inhibitor of CYP isozymes CYP3A4, 2C8, 2C9, 2D6, 1A2, 2C19 or 2B6, and is not an inducer of CYP3A4 and CYP1A2.

Elimination

Following administration of an oral [^{14}C]sitagliptin dose to healthy subjects, approximately 100 % of the administered radioactivity was eliminated in faeces (13 %) or urine (87 %) within one week of dosing. The apparent terminal $t_{1/2}$ following a 100-mg oral dose of sitagliptin was approximately 12.4 hours. Sitagliptin accumulates only minimally with multiple doses. The renal clearance was approximately 350 ml/min.

Elimination of sitagliptin occurs primarily via renal excretion and involves active tubular secretion. Sitagliptin is a substrate for human organic anion transporter-3 (hOAT-3), which may be involved in the renal elimination of sitagliptin. The clinical relevance of hOAT-3 in sitagliptin transport has not been established. Sitagliptin is also a substrate of p-glycoprotein, which may also be involved in mediating the renal elimination of sitagliptin. However, ciclosporin, a p-glycoprotein inhibitor, did not reduce the renal clearance of sitagliptin. Sitagliptin is not a substrate for OCT2 or OAT1 or PEPT1/2 transporters. *In vitro*, sitagliptin did not inhibit OAT3 (IC50=160 μM) or p-glycoprotein (up to 250 μM) mediated transport at therapeutically relevant plasma concentrations. In a clinical study sitagliptin had a small effect on plasma digoxin concentrations indicating that sitagliptin may be a mild inhibitor of p-glycoprotein.

Characteristics in patients

The pharmacokinetics of sitagliptin were generally similar in healthy subjects and in patients with type 2 diabetes.

Renal insufficiency

A single-dose, open-label study was conducted to evaluate the pharmacokinetics of a reduced dose of sitagliptin (50-mg) in patients with varying degrees of chronic renal insufficiency compared to normal healthy control subjects. The study included patients with renal insufficiency classified on the basis of creatinine clearance as mild (50 to < 80 ml/min), moderate (30 to < 50 ml/min), and severe (< 30 ml/min), as well as patients with end-stage renal disease (ESRD) on haemodialysis.

Patients with mild renal insufficiency did not have a clinically meaningful increase in the plasma concentration of sitagliptin as compared to normal healthy control subjects. An approximately 2-fold increase in the plasma AUC of sitagliptin was observed in patients with moderate renal insufficiency, and an approximately 4-fold increase was observed in patients with severe renal insufficiency and in patients with ESRD on haemodialysis, as compared to normal healthy control subjects. Sitagliptin was modestly removed by haemodialysis (13.5 % over a 3- to 4-hour haemodialysis session starting 4 hours postdose). Januvia is not recommended for use in patients with moderate or severe renal insufficiency including those with ESRD since experience in these patients is too limited. (See section 4.2.)

Hepatic insufficiency

No dosage adjustment for Januvia is necessary for patients with mild or moderate hepatic insufficiency (Child-Pugh score ≤ 9). There is no clinical experience in patients with severe hepatic insufficiency (Child-Pugh score > 9). However, because sitagliptin is primarily renally eliminated, severe hepatic insufficiency is not expected to affect the pharmacokinetics of sitagliptin.

Elderly

No dosage adjustment is required based on age. Age did not have a clinically meaningful impact on the pharmacokinetics of sitagliptin based on a population pharmacokinetic analysis of Phase I and Phase II data. Elderly subjects (65 to 80 years) had approximately 19 % higher plasma concentrations of sitagliptin compared to younger subjects.

Paediatric

No studies with Januvia have been performed in paediatric patients.

Other patient characteristics

No dosage adjustment is necessary based on gender, race, or body mass index (BMI). These characteristics had no clinically meaningful effect on the pharmacokinetics of sitagliptin based on a composite analysis of Phase I pharmacokinetic data and on a population pharmacokinetic analysis of Phase I and Phase II data.

5.3 Preclinical safety data

Renal and liver toxicity were observed in rodents at systemic exposure values 58 times the human exposure level, while the no-effect level was found at 19 times the human exposure level. Incisor teeth abnormalities were observed in rats at exposure levels 67 times the clinical exposure level; the no-effect level for this finding was 58-fold based on the 14-week rat study. The relevance of these findings for humans is unknown. Transient treatment-related physical signs, some of which suggest neural toxicity, such as open-mouth breathing, salivation, white foamy emesis, ataxia, trembling, decreased activity, and/or hunched posture were observed in dogs at exposure levels approximately 23 times the clinical exposure level. In addition, very slight to slight skeletal muscle degeneration was also observed histologically at doses resulting in systemic exposure levels of approximately 23 times the human exposure level. A no-effect level for these findings was found at an exposure 6-fold the clinical exposure level.

Sitagliptin has not been demonstrated to be genotoxic in preclinical studies. Sitagliptin was not carcinogenic in mice. In rats, there was an increased incidence of hepatic adenomas and carcinomas at systemic exposure levels 58 times the human exposure level. Since hepatotoxicity has been shown to correlate with induction of hepatic neoplasia in rats, this increased incidence of hepatic tumours in rats was likely secondary to chronic hepatic toxicity at this high dose. Because of the high safety margin (19-fold at this no-effect level), these neoplastic changes are not considered relevant for the situation in humans.

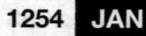

No adverse effects upon fertility were observed in male and female rats given sitagliptin prior to and throughout mating.

In a pre-/postnatal development study performed in rats sitagliptin showed no adverse effects.

Reproductive toxicity studies showed a slight treatment-related increased incidence of fetal rib malformations (absent, hypoplastic and wavy ribs) in the offspring of rats at systemic exposure levels more than 29 times the human exposure levels. Maternal toxicity was seen in rabbits at more than 29 times the human exposure levels. Because of the high safety margins, these findings do not suggest a relevant risk for human reproduction. Sitagliptin is secreted in considerable amounts into the milk of lactating rats (milk/plasma ratio: 4:1).

6. PHARMACEUTICAL PARTICULARS

6.1 List of excipients

Tablet core:

microcrystalline cellulose (E460)

calcium hydrogen phosphate, anhydrous (E341)

croscarmellose sodium (E468)

magnesium stearate (E470b)

sodium stearyl fumarate

Film coating:

polyvinyl alcohol

macrogol 3350

talc (E553b)

titanium dioxide (E171)

red iron oxide (E172)

yellow iron oxide (E172)

6.2 Incompatibilities

Not applicable.

6.3 Shelf life

3 years

6.4 Special precautions for storage

This medicinal product does not require any special storage conditions.

6.5 Nature and contents of container

Opaque blisters (PVC/PE/PVDC and aluminum). Packs of 14, 28, 56, 84 or 98 film-coated tablets and 50 × 1 film-coated tablets in perforated unit dose blisters.

Not all pack sizes may be marketed.

6.6 Special precautions for disposal and other handling

Any unused product or waste material should be disposed of in accordance with local requirements.

7. MARKETING AUTHORISATION HOLDER

Merck Sharp & Dohme Ltd.
Hertford Road, Hoddesdon
Hertfordshire EN11 9BU
United Kingdom

8. MARKETING AUTHORISATION NUMBER(S)

EU/1/07/383/014

9. DATE OF FIRST AUTHORISATION/RENEWAL OF THE AUTHORISATION

Date of first authorisation: 21 March 2007

10. DATE OF REVISION OF THE TEXT

21 August 2009

Detailed information on this medicinal product is available on the website of the European Medicines Agency (EMEA) web site: http://www.emea.europa.eu/.

® denotes registered trademark of Merck & Co. Inc., Whitehouse Station, NJ, USA.

JANUVIA.SPC.JAN.09.UK.3131-II-009

Kaletra 100mg/25mg film-coated tablets

(Abbott Laboratories Limited)

1. NAME OF THE MEDICINAL PRODUCT
Kaletra 100 mg/25 mg film-coated tablets

2. QUALITATIVE AND QUANTITATIVE COMPOSITION
Each film-coated tablet contains 100 mg of lopinavir co-formulated with 25 mg of ritonavir as a pharmacokinetic enhancer.

For a full list of excipients, see section 6.1.

3. PHARMACEUTICAL FORM
Film-coated tablet

Pale yellow debossed with [Abbott logo] and "KC".

4. CLINICAL PARTICULARS

4.1 Therapeutic indications
Kaletra is indicated for the treatment of HIV-1 infected children above the age of 2 years and adults, in combination with other antiretroviral agents.

Most experience with Kaletra is derived from the use of the product in antiretroviral therapy naïve patients. Data in heavily pretreated protease inhibitor experienced patients are limited. There are limited data on salvage therapy on patients who have failed therapy with Kaletra.

The choice of Kaletra to treat protease inhibitor experienced HIV-1 infected patients should be based on individual viral resistance testing and treatment history of patients (see sections 4.4 and 5.1).

4.2 Posology and method of administration
Kaletra should be prescribed by physicians who are experienced in the treatment of HIV infection.

Kaletra tablets should be swallowed whole and not chewed, broken or crushed.

Adult and adolescent use: the standard recommended dosage of Kaletra tablets is 400/100 mg (two 200/50 mg) tablets twice daily taken with or without food. In adult patients naive to antiretroviral therapy, in cases where once daily dosing is considered necessary for the management of the patient, Kaletra tablets may be administered as 800/200 mg (four 200/50 mg tablets) once daily with or without food. However, this once daily regimen might be associated with a lesser sustainability of the virologic suppression (see section 5.1) and the higher risk of diarrhoea (see section 4.8) compared to the recommended standard twice daily dosage. This once daily regimen is not validated in antiretroviral experienced patients. Oral solution is available to patients who have difficulty swallowing. Refer to the Summary of Product Characteristics for Kaletra oral solution for dosing instructions.

Paediatric use (2 years of age and above): the adult dose of Kaletra tablets (400/100 mg twice daily) may be used in children 40 kg or greater or with a Body Surface Area (BSA)* greater than 1.4 m^2. For children weighing less than 40 kg or with a BSA between 0.5 and 1.4 m^2 and able to swallow tablets, refer to the dosing guideline tables below. For children unable to swallow tablets, please refer to the Kaletra oral solution Summary of Product Characteristics. Kaletra dosed once daily has not been evaluated in paediatric patients.

Before prescribing Kaletra 100/25 mg tablets, infants and young children should be assessed for the ability to swallow intact tablets. If a child is unable to reliably swallow a Kaletra tablet, Kaletra oral solution formulation should be prescribed.

The following table contains dosing guidelines for Kaletra 100/25 mg tablets based on BSA.

Paediatric Dosing Guidelines

Body Surface Area (m^2)	Recommended number of 100/25 mg tablets twice-daily
≥ 0.5 to < 0.9	2 tablets (200/50 mg)
≥ 0.9 to < 1.4	3 tablets (300/75 mg)
≥ 1.4	4 tablets (400/100 mg)

If more convenient for patients, the Kaletra 200/50 mg tablets may also be considered alone or in combination with the Kaletra 100/25 mg tablet to achieve the recommended dose.

* Body surface area can be calculated with the following equation:

BSA (m^2) = $\sqrt{}$ (Height (cm) X Weight (kg) / 3600)

Children less than 2 years of age: Kaletra is not recommended for use in children below 2 years of age due to insufficient data on safety and efficacy (see section 5.1).

Concomitant Therapy: Efavirenz or nevirapine
The following table contains dosing guidelines for Kaletra 100/25 mg tablets based on BSA when used in combination with efavirenz or nevirapine in children.

Paediatric Dosing Guidelines with concomitant efavirenz or nevirapine

Body Surface Area (m^2)	Recommended number of 100/25 mg tablets twice-daily
≥ 0.5 to < 0.8	2 tablets (200/50 mg)
≥ 0.8 to < 1.2	3 tablets (300/75 mg)
≥ 1.2 to < 1.4	4 tablets (400/100 mg)
≥ 1.4	5 tablets (500/125 mg)

If more convenient for patients, the Kaletra 200/50 mg tablets may also be considered alone or in combination with the Kaletra 100/25 mg tablet to achieve the recommended dose.

Hepatic impairment: In HIV-infected patients with mild to moderate hepatic impairment, an increase of approximately 30% in lopinavir exposure has been observed but is not expected to be of clinical relevance (see section 5.2). No data are available in patients with severe hepatic impairment. Kaletra should not be given to these patients (see section 4.3).

Renal impairment: no dose adjustment is necessary in patients with renal impairment. Caution is warranted when Kaletra is used in patients with severe renal impairment (see section 4.4).

4.3 Contraindications
Hypersensitivity to the active substances or to any of the excipients.

Patients with severe hepatic insufficiency.

Kaletra contains lopinavir and ritonavir, both of which are inhibitors of the P450 isoform CYP3A. Kaletra should not be co-administered with medicinal products that are highly dependent on CYP3A for clearance and for which elevated plasma concentrations are associated with serious and/or life threatening events. These medicinal products include astemizole, terfenadine, oral midazolam (for caution on parenterally administered midazolam, see section 4.5), triazolam, cisapride, pimozide, amiodarone, ergot alkaloids (e.g. ergotamine, dihydroergotamine, ergonovine and methylergonovine) and vardenafil.

Herbal preparations containing St John's wort (*Hypericum perforatum*) must not be used while taking lopinavir and ritonavir due to the risk of decreased plasma concentrations and reduced clinical effects of lopinavir and ritonavir (see section 4.5).

4.4 Special warnings and precautions for use
Patients with coexisting conditions

Hepatic impairment: the safety and efficacy of Kaletra has not been established in patients with significant underlying liver disorders. Kaletra is contraindicated in patients with severe liver impairment (see section 4.3). Patients with chronic hepatitis B or C and treated with combination antiretroviral therapy are at an increased risk for severe and potentially fatal hepatic adverse reactions. In case of concomitant antiviral therapy for hepatitis B or C, please refer to the relevant product information for these medicinal products.

Patients with pre-existing liver dysfunction including chronic hepatitis have an increased frequency of liver function abnormalities during combination antiretroviral therapy and should be monitored according to standard practice. If there is evidence of worsening liver disease in such patients, interruption or discontinuation of treatment should be considered.

Renal impairment: since the renal clearance of lopinavir and ritonavir is negligible, increased plasma concentrations are not expected in patients with renal impairment. Because lopinavir and ritonavir are highly protein bound, it is unlikely that they will be significantly removed by haemodialysis or peritoneal dialysis.

Haemophilia: there have been reports of increased bleeding, including spontaneous skin haematomas and haemarthrosis in patients with haemophilia type A and B treated with protease inhibitors. In some patients additional factor VIII was given. In more than half of the reported cases, treatment with protease inhibitors was continued or reintroduced if treatment had been discontinued. A causal relationship had been evoked, although the mechanism of action had not been elucidated. Haemophiliac patients should therefore be made aware of the possibility of increased bleeding.

Lipid elevations

Treatment with Kaletra has resulted in increases, sometimes marked, in the concentration of total cholesterol and triglycerides. Triglyceride and cholesterol testing is to be performed prior to initiating Kaletra therapy and at periodic intervals during therapy. Particular caution should be paid to patients with high values at baseline and with history of lipid disorders. Lipid disorders are to be managed as clinically appropriate (see also section 4.5 for additional information on potential interactions with HMG-CoA reductase inhibitors).

Pancreatitis

Cases of pancreatitis have been reported in patients receiving Kaletra, including those who developed hypertriglyceridaemia. In most of these cases patients have had a prior history of pancreatitis and/or concurrent therapy with other medicinal products associated with pancreatitis. Marked triglyceride elevation is a risk factor for development of pancreatitis. Patients with advanced HIV disease may be at risk of elevated triglycerides and pancreatitis

Pancreatitis should be considered if clinical symptoms (nausea, vomiting, abdominal pain) or abnormalities in laboratory values (such as increased serum lipase or amylase values) suggestive of pancreatitis should occur. Patients who exhibit these signs or symptoms should be evaluated and Kaletra therapy should be suspended if a diagnosis of pancreatitis is made (see section 4.8).

Hyperglycaemia

New onset diabetes mellitus, hyperglycaemia or exacerbation of existing diabetes mellitus has been reported in patients receiving protease inhibitors. In some of these the hyperglycaemia was severe and in some cases also associated with ketoacidosis. Many patients had confounding medical conditions some of which required therapy with agents that have been associated with the development of diabetes mellitus or hyperglycaemia.

Fat redistribution and metabolic disorders

Combination antiretroviral therapy has been associated with redistribution of body fat (lipodystrophy) in HIV patients. The long-term consequences of these events are currently unknown. Knowledge about the mechanism is incomplete. A connection between visceral lipomatosis and protease inhibitors (PIs) and lipoatrophy and nucleoside reverse transcriptase inhibitors (NRTIs) has been hypothesised. A higher risk of lipodystrophy has been associated with individual factors such as older age, and with drug related factors such as longer duration of antiretroviral treatment and associated metabolic disturbances. Clinical examination should include evaluation for physical signs of fat redistribution. Consideration should be given to measurement of fasting serum lipids and blood glucose. Lipid disorders should be managed as clinically appropriate (see section 4.8).

Immune Reactivation Syndrome

In HIV-infected patients with severe immune deficiency at the time of institution of combination antiretroviral therapy (CART), an inflammatory reaction to asymptomatic or residual opportunistic pathogens may arise and cause serious clinical conditions, or aggravation of symptoms. Typically, such reactions have been observed within the first few weeks or months of initiation of CART. Relevant examples are cytomegalovirus retinitis, generalised and/or focal mycobacterial infections, and Pneumocystis carinii pneumonia. Any inflammatory symptoms should be evaluated and treatment instituted when necessary.

Osteonecrosis

Although the etiology is considered to be multifactorial (including corticosteroid use, alcohol consumption, severe immunosuppression, higher body mass index), cases of osteonecrosis have been reported particularly in patients with advanced HIV-disease and/or long-term exposure to combination antiretroviral therapy (CART). Patients should be advised to seek medical advice if they experience joint aches and pain, joint stiffness or difficulty in movement.

PR interval prolongation

Lopinavir/ritonavir has been shown to cause modest asymptomatic prolongation of the PR interval in some healthy adult subjects. Rare reports of 2nd or 3rd degree atroventricular block in patients with underlying structural heart disease and pre-existing conduction system abnormalities or in patients receiving drugs known to prolong the PR interval (such as verapamil or atazanavir) have been reported in patients receiving lopinavir/ritonavir. Kaletra should be used with caution in such patients (see section 5.1).

Interactions with medicinal products

Kaletra contains lopinavir and ritonavir, both of which are inhibitors of the P450 isoform CYP3A. Kaletra is likely to increase plasma concentrations of medicinal products that are primarily metabolised by CYP3A. These increases of plasma concentrations of co-administered medicinal products could increase or prolong their therapeutic effect and adverse events (see sections 4.3 and 4.5).

The HMG-CoA reductase inhibitors simvastatin and lovastatin are highly dependent on CYP3A for metabolism, thus concomitant use of Kaletra with simvastatin or lovastatin is not recommended due to an increased risk of myopathy including rhabdomyolysis. Caution must also be exercised and reduced doses should be considered if Kaletra is used concurrently with rosuvastatin or with atorvastatin, which is metabolised to a lesser extent by CYP3A4. If treatment with a HMG-CoA reductase inhibitor is indicated, pravastatin or fluvastatin is recommended (see section 4.5).

Particular caution must be used when prescribing Kaletra and medicinal products known to induce QT interval prolongation such as: chlorpheniramine, quinidine, erythromycin, clarithromycin. Indeed, Kaletra could increase concentrations of the co-administered medicinal products and this may result in an increase of their associated cardiac adverse events. Cardiac events have been reported with Kaletra in preclinical studies; therefore, the potential cardiac effects of Kaletra cannot be currently ruled out (see sections 4.8 and 5.3).

Co-administration of Kaletra with rifampicin is not recommended. Rifampicin in combination with Kaletra causes large decreases in lopinavir concentrations which may in turn significantly decrease the lopinavir therapeutic effect. Adequate exposure to lopinavir/ritonavir may be achieved when a higher dose of Kaletra is used but this is associated with a higher risk of liver and gastrointestinal toxicity. Therefore, this co-administration should be avoided unless judged strictly necessary (see section 4.5).

Other

Kaletra is not a cure for HIV infection or AIDS. It does not reduce the risk of passing HIV to others through sexual contact or blood contamination. Appropriate precautions should be taken. People taking Kaletra may still develop infections or other illnesses associated with HIV disease and AIDS.

Concomitant use of Kaletra and fluticasone or other glucocorticoids that are metabolised by CYP3A4 is not recommended unless the potential benefit of treatment outweighs the risk of systemic corticosteroid effects, including Cushing's syndrome and adrenal suppression (see section 4.5).

4.5 Interaction with other medicinal products and other forms of interaction

Kaletra contains lopinavir and ritonavir, both of which are inhibitors of the P450 isoform CYP3A *in vitro*. Co-administration of Kaletra and medicinal products primarily metabolised by CYP3A may result in increased plasma concentrations of the other medicinal product, which could increase or prolong its therapeutic and adverse reactions. Kaletra does not inhibit CYP2D6, CYP2C9, CYP2C19, CYP2E1, CYP2B6 or CYP1A2 at clinically relevant concentrations (see section 4.3).

Kaletra has been shown *in vivo* to induce its own metabolism and to increase the biotransformation of some medicinal products metabolised by cytochrome P450 enzymes and by glucuronidation. This may result in lowered plasma concentrations and potential decrease of efficacy of co-administered medicinal products.

Medicinal products that are contraindicated specifically due to the expected magnitude of interaction and potential for serious adverse events are listed in section 4.3.

All interaction studies, when otherwise not stated, were performed using Kaletra capsules, which gives an approximately 20% lower exposure of lopinavir than the 200/50 mg tablets.

Antiretroviral agents

Nucleoside/Nucleotide reverse transcriptase inhibitors (NRTIs):

Stavudine and Lamivudine: no change in the pharmacokinetics of lopinavir was observed when Kaletra was given alone or in combination with stavudine and lamivudine in clinical studies.

Didanosine: it is recommended that didanosine be administered on an empty stomach; therefore, didanosine may be co-administered with Kaletra tablets without food.

Zidovudine and Abacavir: Kaletra induces glucuronidation; therefore Kaletra has the potential to reduce zidovudine and abacavir plasma concentrations. The clinical significance of this potential interaction is unknown.

Tenofovir: when tenofovir disoproxil fumarate was co-administered with Kaletra, tenofovir concentrations were increased by approximately 30% with no changes noted in lopinavir or ritonavir concentrations. Higher tenofovir concentrations could potentiate tenofovir associated adverse events, including renal disorders.

Non-nucleoside reverse transcriptase inhibitors (NNRTIs):

In a study performed in healthy volunteers to explore the interaction between Kaletra tablets (400/100 mg twice daily) and efavirenz (600 mg once daily), efavirenz has been shown to decrease the lopinavir concentrations by 30 - 40%. When Kaletra tablet dosages were increased to 500/125 mg twice daily during co-administration of efavirenz 600 mg once daily in healthy volunteers, lopinavir pharmacokinetic parameters were similar to those obtained with Kaletra tablets 400/100 mg twice daily administered alone. Therefore, the Kaletra tablets dosage should be increased to 500/125 mg twice daily when co-administered with efavirenz 600 mg once daily. Kaletra must not be administered once daily in combination with efavirenz.

Similar pharmacokinetic interactions are expected for the co-administration of Kaletra tablets with the NNRTI nevirapine and with the protease inhibitors nelfinavir and amprenavir. The same recommendations for monitoring apply in these cases of co-administration. Kaletra must not be administered once daily in combination with nevirapine.

Co-administration with other HIV protease inhibitors (PIs):

Kaletra (400/100 mg twice daily) has been studied in combination with reduced doses of amprenavir, indinavir, nelfinavir and saquinavir in steady-state controlled healthy volunteer studies relative to clinical doses of each HIV protease inhibitor in the absence of ritonavir. Comparisons to published pharmacokinetic data with ritonavir-enhanced amprenavir and saquinavir regimens are also described. Additionally, the effect of additional ritonavir on the pharmacokinetics of lopinavir are discussed. Note that the historical comparisons to ritonavir-enhanced protease inhibitor regimens should be interpreted with caution (see details of combinations below). Appropriate doses of HIV-protease inhibitors in combination with Kaletra with respect to safety and efficacy have not been established. Therefore, the concomitant administration of Kaletra with PIs requires close monitoring.

Amprenavir: see recommendations described for Kaletra tablets co-administration with efavirenz. Kaletra must not be administered once daily in combination with amprenavir.

Fosamprenavir: co-administration of standard doses of lopinavir/ritonavir with fosamprenavir results in a significant reduction in amprenavir concentrations. Co-administration of increased doses of fosamprenavir 1400 mg twice daily with lopinavir/ritonavir 533/133 mg twice daily to protease inhibitor-experienced patients resulted in a higher incidence of gastrointestinal adverse events and elevations in triglycerides with the combination regimen without increases in virological efficacy, when compared with standard doses of fosamprenavir/ritonavir. Therefore, concomitant administration of these medicinal products is not recommended.

Indinavir: indinavir 600 mg twice daily in combination with Kaletra produces similar indinavir AUC, higher C_{min} (by 3.5-fold) and lower C_{max} relative to indinavir 800 mg three times daily alone. Furthermore, concentrations of lopinavir do not appear to be affected when both medicinal products, Kaletra and indinivir, are combined, based on historical comparison with Kaletra alone.

Nelfinavir: see recommendations described for Kaletra tablets co-administration with efavirenz. Kaletra must not be administered once daily in combination with nelfinavir.

Saquinavir: saquinavir 800 mg twice daily co-administered with Kaletra produces an increase of saquinavir AUC by 9.6-fold relative to saquinavir 1200 mg three times daily given alone.

Saquinavir 800 mg twice daily co-administered with Kaletra resulted in an increase of saquinavir AUC by approximately 30% relative to saquinavir/ritonavir 1000/100 mg twice daily, and produces similar exposure to those reported after saquinavir/ritonavir 400/400 mg twice daily.

When saquinavir 1200 mg twice daily was combined with Kaletra, no further increase of concentrations was noted. Furthermore, concentrations of lopinavir do not appear to be affected when both medicinal products, Kaletra and saquinavir, are combined, based on historical comparison with Kaletra alone.

Ritonavir: Kaletra co-administered with an additional 100 mg ritonavir twice daily resulted in an increase of lopinavir AUC and C_{min} of 33% and 64%, respectively, as compared to Kaletra alone.

Other medicinal products:

Acid reducing agents (omeprazole, ranitidine): in a study performed in healthy volunteers, no clinically relevant interaction has been observed when Kaletra tablets 400/100 mg twice daily or 800/200 mg once daily was co-administered with omeprazole or with ranitidine. Kaletra can be co-administered with acid reducing agents with no dose adjustment.

Antiarrhythmics: (bepridil, systemic lidocaine and quinidine): concentrations may be increased when co-administered with Kaletra. Caution is warranted and therapeutic concentration monitoring is recommended when available.

Anticancer agents (eg vincristine, vinblastine): these agents may have their serum concentrations increased when co-administered with lopinavir/ritonavir resulting in the potential for increased adverse events usually associated with these anticancer agents.

Anticoagulants: warfarin concentrations may be affected when co-administered with Kaletra. It is recommended that INR (international normalised ratio) be monitored.

Anticonvulsants (phenobarbital, phenytoin, carbamazepine): will induce CYP3A4 and may decrease lopinavir concentrations.

In addition, co-administration of phenytoin and lopinavir/ritonavir resulted in moderate decreases in steady-state phenytoin concentrations. Phenytoin levels should be monitored when co-administering with lopinavir/ritonavir. Kaletra must not be administered once daily in combination with carbamazepine, phenobarbital or phenytoin.

Bupropion: in healthy volunteers, the AUC and C_{max} of bupropion and of its active metabolite, hydroxybupropion, were decreased by about 50% when co-administered with lopinavir/ritonavir capsules 400/100 mg twice daily at steady-state. This effect may be due to induction of bupropion metabolism. Therefore, if the co-administration of lopinavir/ritonavir with bupropion is judged unavoidable, this should be done under close clinical monitoring for bupropion efficacy, without exceeding the recommended dosage, despite the observed induction.

Trazodone: in a pharmacokinetic study performed in healthy volunteers, concomitant use of low dose ritonavir (200 mg twice daily) with a single dose of trazodone led to an increase in plasma concentrations of trazodone (AUC increased by 2.4 fold). Adverse events of nausea, dizziness, hypotension and syncope were observed following co-administration of trazodone and ritonavir in this study. However, it is unknown whether the combination of lopinavir/ritonavir causes a similar increase in trazodone exposure. The combination should be used with caution and a lower dose of trazodone should be considered.

Digoxin: plasma concentrations of digoxin may be increased when co-administered with Kaletra. Caution is warranted and therapeutic drug monitoring of digoxin concentrations, if available, is recommended in case of co-administration of Kaletra and digoxin. Particular caution should be used when prescribing Kaletra in patients taking digoxin as the acute inhibitory effect of ritonavir on Pgp is expected to significantly increase digoxin levels. The increased digoxin level may lessen over time as Pgp induction develops. Initiation of digoxin in patients already taking Kaletra is expected to result in lower increase of digoxin concentrations.

Dihydropyridine calcium channel blockers: (e.g. felodipine, nifedipine, nicardipine): may have their serum concentrations increased by Kaletra.

Lipid lowering agents: HMG-CoA reductase inhibitors which are highly dependent on CYP3A4 metabolism, such as lovastatin and simvastatin, are expected to have markedly increased plasma concentrations when co-administered with Kaletra. Since increased concentrations of HMG-CoA reductase inhibitors may cause myopathy, including rhabdomyolysis, the combination of these medicinal products with Kaletra is not recommended. Atorvastatin is less dependent on CYP3A for metabolism. When atorvastatin was given concurrently with Kaletra, a mean 4.7-fold and 5.9-fold increase in atorvastatin C_{max} and AUC, respectively, was observed. When used with Kaletra, the lowest possible dose of atorvastatin should be administered. Rosuvastatin is not dependent on CYP3A. However, when given concurrently with Kaletra a mean 5-fold and 2-fold increase in rosuvastatin C_{max} and AUC, respectively, was observed. Caution should be exercised when Kaletra is co-administered with rosuvastatin. Results from an interaction study with Kaletra and pravastatin reveal no clinically significant interaction. The metabolism of pravastatin and fluvastatin is not dependent on CYP3A4, and interactions are not expected with Kaletra. If treatment with a HMG-CoA reductase inhibitor is indicated, pravastatin or fluvastatin is recommended.

Dexamethasone: may induce CYP3A4 and may decrease lopinavir concentrations.

Phosphodiesterase inhibitors: phosphodiesterase inhibitors which are dependent on CYP3A4 metabolism, such as tadalafil and sildenafil, are expected to result in an approximately 2-fold and 11-fold increase in AUC respectively, when co-administered with ritonavir containing regimens including Kaletra and may result in an increase in PDE5 inhibitor associated adverse reactions including hypotension, synope, visual changes and prolonged erection. Particular caution must be used when prescribing sildenafil or tadalafil in patients receiving Kaletra with increased monitoring for adverse events. Co-administration of vardenafil with ritonavir containing regimens including Kaletra is expected to result in 49-fold increase in vardenafil AUC. The use of vardenafil with Kaletra is contraindicated (see section 4.3).

Cyclosporin, sirolimus (rapamycin) and tacrolimus: concentrations may be increased when co-administered with Kaletra. More frequent therapeutic concentration monitoring is recommended until plasma levels of these products have been stabilised.

Ketoconazole and itraconazole: may have serum concentrations increased by Kaletra. High doses of ketoconazole and itraconazole (> 200 mg/day) are not recommended.

Voriconazole: due to the potential for reduced voriconazole concentrations, co-administration of voriconazole and low dose ritonavir (100 mg twice daily) as contained in Kaletra should be avoided unless an assessment of the benefit/risk to patient justifies the use of voriconazole.

Clarithromycin: moderate increases in clarithromycin AUC are expected when co-administered with Kaletra. For patients with renal or hepatic impairment dose reduction of clarithromycin should be considered (see section 4.4).

Buprenorphine: buprenorphine (dosed at 16 mg daily) co-administered with lopinavir/ritonavir (dosed at 400/100 mg twice daily) showed no clinically significant interaction. Kaletra can be co-administered with buprenorphine with no dose adjustment.

Methadone: Kaletra was demonstrated to lower plasma concentrations of methadone. Monitoring plasma concentrations of methadone is recommended.

Contraceptives: levels of ethinyl oestradiol were decreased when oestrogen-based oral contraceptives were co-administered with Kaletra. In case of co-administration of Kaletra with contraceptives containing ethinyl oestradiol (whatever the contraceptive formulation e.g. oral or patch), alternative methods of contraception are to be used.

Rifabutin: when rifabutin and Kaletra were co-administered for 10 days, rifabutin (parent substance and active 25-O-desacetyl metabolite) C_{max} and AUC were increased by 3.5- and 5.7-fold, respectively. On the basis of these data, a rifabutin dose reduction of 75% (i.e. 150 mg every other day or 3 times per week) is recommended when administered with Kaletra. Further reduction may be necessary.

Rifampicin: co-administration of Kaletra with rifampicin is not recommended. Rifampicin administered with Kaletra causes large decreases in lopinavir concentrations which may in turn significantly decrease the lopinavir therapeutic effect. A dose adjustment of Kaletra 400 mg/400 mg twice daily has allowed compensating for the CYP 3A4 inducer effect of rifampicin. However, such a dose adjustment might be associated with ALT/AST elevations and with increase in gastrointestinal disorders. Therefore, this co-administration should be avoided unless judged strictly necessary. If this co-administration is judged unavoidable, increased dose of Kaletra at 400 mg/400 mg twice daily may be administered with rifampicin under close safety and therapeutic drug monitoring. The Kaletra dose should be titrated upward only after rifampicin has been initiated (see section 4.4).

St John's wort: serum levels of lopinavir and ritonavir can be reduced by concomitant use of the herbal preparation St John's wort (*Hypericum perforatum*). This is due to the induction of drug metabolising enzymes by St John's wort. Herbal preparations containing St John's wort should therefore not be combined with lopinavir and ritonavir. If a patient is already taking St John's wort, stop St John's wort and if possible check viral levels. Lopinavir and ritonavir levels may increase on stopping St John's wort. The dose of Kaletra may need adjusting. The inducing effect may persist for at least 2 weeks after cessation of treatment with St John's wort (see section 4.3).

Midazolam: midazolam is extensively metabolised by CYP3A4. Co-administration with Kaletra may cause a large increase in the concentration of this benzodiazepine. A phenotyping cocktail study in 14 healthy volunteers showed an increase of AUC by about 13 fold with oral midazolam and an increase by about 4 fold with parenteral midazolam. Therefore, Kaletra should not be co-administered with orally administered midazolam (see section 4.3), whereas caution should be used with co-administration of Kaletra and parenteral midazolam. If Kaletra is co-administered with parenteral midazolam, it should be done in an intensive care unit (ICU) or similar setting which ensures close clinical monitoring and appropriate medical management in case of respiratory depression and/or prolonged sedation. Dosage adjustment for midazolam should be considered especially if more than a single dose of midazolam is administered.

Fluticasone propionate (interaction with ritonavir): in a clinical study where ritonavir 100 mg capsules twice daily were co – administered with 50 µg intranasal fluticasone propionate (4 times daily) for seven days in healthy subjects, the fluticasone propionate plasma levels increased significantly, whereas the intrinsic cortisol levels decreased by approximately 86% (90% confidence interval 82 – 89%). Greater effects may be expected when fluticasone propionate is inhaled. Systemic corticosteroid effects including Cushing's syndrome and adrenal suppression have been reported in patients receiving ritonavir and inhaled or intranasally administered fluticasone propionate; this could also occur with other corticosteroids metabolised via the P450 3A pathway eg budesonide. Consequently, concomitant administration of Kaletra and these glucocorticoids is not recommended unless the potential benefit of treatment outweighs the risk of systemic corticosteroid effects (see section 4.4). A dose reduction of the glucocorticoid should be considered with close monitoring of local and systemic effects or a switch to a glucocorticoid, which is not a substrate for CYP3A4 (eg beclomethasone). Moreover, in case of withdrawal of glucocorticoids progressive dose reduction may have to be performed over a longer period. The effects of high fluticasone systemic exposure on ritonavir plasma levels is yet unknown.

Based on known metabolic profiles, clinically significant interactions are not expected between Kaletra and fluvastatin, dapsone, trimethoprim/sulfamethoxazole, azithromycin or fluconazole.

4.6 Pregnancy and lactation

There are no data from the use of Kaletra in pregnant women. Studies in animals have shown reproductive toxicity (see section 5.3). The potential risk for humans is unknown. Kaletra should not be used during pregnancy unless clearly necessary.

Studies in rats revealed that lopinavir is excreted in the milk. It is not known whether this medicinal product is excreted in human milk. HIV infected women must not breast-feed their infants under any circumstances to avoid transmission of HIV.

4.7 Effects on ability to drive and use machines

No studies on the effects on the ability to drive and use machines have been performed. Patients should be

Table 1

Undesirable effects in clinical studies in adult patients

System organ class	Frequency	Adverse reaction
Investigations	Very common (Grade 3 or 4)	Blood triglycerides increased, blood cholesterol increased, glutamyltransferase increased
	Common (Grade 3 or 4)	Blood glucose increased, blood amylase increased, aspartate aminotransferase increased, alanine aminotransferase increased, liver function tests abnormal
	Uncommon	Glucose tolerance decreased, blood bilirubin increased, creatinine renal clearance decreased, lipase increased, weight increased, weight decreased, hormone level abnormal, laboratory test abnormal
	Rare	Blood alkaline phosphatase increased
Cardiac disorders	Uncommon	myocardial infarction[1], palpitations
	Rare	Atrioventricular block
Blood and lymphatic system disorders	Uncommon	Anaemia, leucopenia, lymphadenopathy
	Rare	Splenomegaly
Nervous system disorders	Common	Headache, paresthesia
	Uncommon	Extrapyramidal disorder, migraine, facial palsy, encephalopathy, dizziness, amnesia, coordination abnormal, hypertonia, neuropathy, neuropathy peripheral, somnolence, tremor, ageusia, dysgeusia, dyskinesia
Eye disorders	Uncommon	Visual disturbance
Ear and labyrinth disorders	Uncommon	Tinnitus
	Rare	Vertigo, hyperacusis
Respiratory, thoracic and mediastinal disorders	Uncommon	Pulmonary oedema, dyspnoea, cough
Gastrointestinal disorders	Very common	Diarrhoea
	Common	Nausea, vomiting, abdominal pain, abnormal faeces, dyspepsia, flatulence, gastrointestinal disorder
	Uncommon	Haemorrhagic colitis, pancreatitis[2], enterocolitis, oesophagitis, constipation, faecal incontinence, abdominal distension, gastroesophageal reflux disease, dry mouth, dysphagia, eructation, gastritis, mouth ulcerations, stomatitis, periodontitis
	Rare	Haemorrhoids
Renal and urinary disorders	Uncommon	Nephrolithiasis, nephritis, albuminuria, hypercalcinuria, urine abnormality,
Skin and subcutaneous tissue disorders	Common	Rash, lipodystrophy acquired, acne
	Uncommon	Alopecia, eczema, dermatitis exfoliative rash maculopapular, dermatitis allergic, dry skin, nail disorder, pruritis, seborrhoea, skin discoloration, skin ulcer, hyperhidrosis, skin striae
	Rare	Idiopathic capillaritis
Musculoskeletal and connective tissue disorders	Uncommon	Arthralgia, osteoarthritis, myalgia, back pain, arthropathy
Endocrine disorders	Uncommon	Cushing syndrome, hypothyroidism, hypogonadism male,
Metabolism and nutrition disorders	Uncommon	Diabetes mellitus, dehydration, lactic acidosis, oedema, increased appetite, obesity, anorexia, hyperglycaemia, hypocholesteremia, lipomatosis, hyperuricaemia, hypovitaminosis
	Rare	Hypophosphataemia, decreased appetite
Infections and infestations	Uncommon	Gastroenteritis, otitis media, bronchitis, sinusitis, sialadenitis, furunculosis, bacterial infection, viral infection, pharyngitis, influenza, rhinitis
	Rare	Cellulitis, folliculitis, perineal abscess
Neoplasms benign, malignant and unspecified (including cysts and polyps)	Uncommon	Benign neoplasm of skin
Vascular disorders	Uncommon	Hypertension, thrombophlebitis, deep vein thrombosis, vasculitis, varicose vein, angiopathy
General disorders and administration site conditions	Common	Asthenia, pain
	Uncommon	Chest pain, chest pain substernal, chills, pyrexia, malaise, oedema peripheral, face oedema, drug interaction, cyst
Immune system disorders	Uncommon	Drug hypersensitivity
	Rare	Immune reconstitution syndrome
Hepatobiliary disorders	Uncommon	Hepatitis, cholecystitis, hepatic steatosis, hepatomegaly, liver tenderness
Reproductive system and breast disorders	Uncommon	Amenorrhoea, menorrhagia, ejaculation disorder, erectile dysfunction, breast enlargement, gynecomastia
Psychiatric disorders	Common	Insomnia
	Uncommon	Agitation, anxiety, confusional state, affect lability, abnormal dreams, decreased libido, nervousness, abnormal thinking

[1] This event had a fatal outcome.

[2] See section 4.4: pancreatitis and lipids

informed that nausea has been reported during treatment with Kaletra (see section 4.8).

4.8 Undesirable effects

The safety of Kaletra has been investigated in over 1400 patients in Phase II/III clinical trials, of which 888 have received a dose of 400/100 mg (3 capsules or 2 tablets) twice daily and 408 received a dose of 800/200 mg (6 capsules or 4 tablets) once daily. In some studies, Kaletra was used in combination with efavirenz or nevirapine.

The most common adverse reaction associated with Kaletra therapy was diarrhoea and was generally of mild to moderate severity. The risk of diarrhoea may be greater with once daily dosing of Kaletra. Discontinuation due to adverse reactions was 4.5% (naïve patients) and 9% (experienced patients) over a 48 week period.

It is important to note that cases of pancreatitis have been reported in patients receiving Kaletra, including those who developed hypertriglyceridaemia. Furthermore, rare increases in PR interval have been reported during Kaletra therapy (see section 4.4: sections pancreatitis and lipid elevations).

Increased CPK, myalgia, myositis, and rarely, rhabdomyolysis have been reported with protease inhibitors, particularly in combination with nucleoside reverse transcriptase inhibitors.

Combination antiretroviral therapy has been associated with redistribution of body fat (lipodystrophy) in HIV patients including the loss of peripheral and facial subcutaneous fat, increased intra-abdominal and visceral fat, breast hypertrophy and dorsocervical fat accumulation (buffalo hump).

Combination antiretroviral therapy has been associated with metabolic abnormalities such as hypertriglyceridaemia, hypercholesterolaemia, insulin resistance, hyperglycaemia and hyperlactataemia (see section 4.4).

In HIV-infected patients with severe immune deficiency at the time of initiation of combination antiretroviral therapy (CART), an inflammatory reaction to asymptomatic or residual opportunistic infections may arise (see section 4.4).

Adult patients

Adverse reactions:

The following adverse reactions of moderate to severe intensity with possible or probable relationship to Kaletra have been reported. The adverse reactions are displayed by system organ class. Within each frequency grouping, undesirable effects are presented in order of decreasing seriousness: very common (≥ 1/10), common (≥ 1/100 to < 1/10), uncommon (≥ 1/1000 to < 1/100) and rare (≥ 1/10,000 to < 1/1,000).

(see Table 1 on previous page)

Paediatric patients

In children 2 years of age and older, the nature of the safety profile is similar to that seen in adults.

Undesirable effects in clinical studies in paediatric patients		
Infections and infestations	Common	Viral infection
Nervous system disorders	Common	Taste perversion
Gastrointestinal disorders	Common	Constipation, vomiting, pancreatitis*
Hepatobiliary disorders	Common	Hepatomegaly
Skin and subcutaneous tissue disorders	Common	Rash, dry skin
General disorders and administration site conditions	Common	Fever
Investigations	Common (Grade 3 or 4)	Increased activated partial thromboplastin time, decreased haemoglobin, decreased platelets, increased sodium, increased potassium, increased calcium, increased bilirubin, increased SGPT/ALT, increased SGOT/AST, increased total cholesterol, increased amylase, increased uric acid, decreased sodium, decreased potassium, decreased calcium, decreased neutrophils

*see section 4.4: pancreatitis and lipids

Post marketing experience

Hepatitis, and rarely jaundice, have been reported in patients on Kaletra therapy in the presence or absence of identifiable risk factors for hepatitis.

Stevens-Johnson syndrome and erythema multiforme have been reported.

Cases of osteonecrosis have been reported, particularly in patients with generally acknowledged risk factors, advanced HIV disease or long-term exposure to combination antiretroviral therapy (CART). The frequency of this is unknown (see section 4.4).

4.9 Overdose

To date, there is limited human experience of acute overdose with Kaletra.

The adverse clinical signs observed in dogs included salivation, emesis and diarrhoea/abnormal stool. The signs of toxicity observed in mice, rats or dogs included decreased activity, ataxia, emaciation, dehydration and tremors.

There is no specific antidote for overdose with Kaletra. Treatment of overdose with Kaletra is to consist of general supportive measures including monitoring of vital signs and observation of the clinical status of the patient. If indicated, elimination of unabsorbed active substance is to be achieved by emesis or gastric lavage. Administration of activated charcoal may also be used to aid in removal of unabsorbed active substance. Since Kaletra is highly protein bound, dialysis is unlikely to be beneficial in significant removal of the active substance.

5. PHARMACOLOGICAL PROPERTIES

5.1 Pharmacodynamic properties

Pharmaco-therapeutic group: protease inhibitor, ATC code: J05AE06

Mechanism of action: lopinavir provides the antiviral activity of Kaletra. Lopinavir is an inhibitor of the HIV-1 and HIV-2 proteases. Inhibition of HIV protease prevents cleavage of the *gag-pol* polyprotein resulting in the production of immature, non-infectious virus.

Effects on the electrocardiogram: QTcF interval was evaluated in a randomised, placebo and active (moxifloxacin 400 mg once daily) controlled crossover study in 39 healthy adults, with 10 measurements over 12 hours on Day 3. The maximum mean (95% upper confidence bound) differences in QTcF from placebo were 3.6 (6.3) and 13.1(15.8) for 400/100 mg twice daily and supratherapeutic 800/200 mg twice daily LPV/r, respectively. The induced QRS interval prolongation from 6 ms to 9.5 ms with high dose lopinavir/ritonavir (800/200 mg twice daily) contributes to QT prolongation. The two regimens resulted in exposures on Day 3 which were approximately 1.5 and 3-fold higher than those observed with recommended once daily or twice daily LPV/r doses at steady state. No subject experienced an increase in QTcF of ≥60 msec from baseline or a QTcF interval exceeding the potentially clinically relevant threshold of 500 msec.

Modest prolongation of the PR interval was also noted in subjects receiving lopinavir/ritonavir in the same study on Day 3. The mean changes from baseline in PR interval ranged from 11.6 ms to 24.4 ms in the 12 hour interval post dose. Maximum PR interval was 286 msec and no second or third degree heart block was observed (see section 4.4).

Antiviral activity in vitro: the *in vitro* antiviral activity of lopinavir against laboratory and clinical HIV strains was evaluated in acutely infected lymphoblastic cell lines and peripheral blood lymphocytes, respectively. In the absence of human serum, the mean IC_{50} of lopinavir against five different HIV-1 laboratory strains was 19 nM. In the absence and presence of 50% human serum, the mean IC_{50} of lopinavir against HIV-1_{IIIB} in MT4 cells was 17 nM and 102 nM, respectively. In the absence of human serum, the mean IC_{50}- of lopinavir was 6.5 nM against several HIV-1 clinical isolates.

Resistance

In vitro selection of resistance:

HIV-1 isolates with reduced susceptibility to lopinavir have been selected *in vitro*. HIV-1 has been passaged *in vitro* with lopinavir alone and with lopinavir plus ritonavir at concentration ratios representing the range of plasma concentration ratios observed during Kaletra therapy. Genotypic and phenotypic analysis of viruses selected in these passages suggest that the presence of ritonavir, at these concentration ratios, does not measurably influence the selection of lopinavir-resistant viruses. Overall, the *in vitro* characterisation of phenotypic cross-resistance between lopinavir and other protease inhibitors suggest that decreased susceptibility to lopinavir correlated closely with decreased susceptibility to ritonavir and indinavir, but did not correlate closely with decreased susceptibility to amprenavir, saquinavir, and nelfinavir.

Analysis of resistance in ARV-naïve patients:

In a Phase II study (M97-720) through 204 weeks of treatment, genotypic analysis of viral isolates was successfully conducted in 11 of 16 patients with confirmed HIV RNA above 400 copies/ml revealed no primary or active site mutations in protease (amino acids at positions 8, 30, 32, 46, 47, 48, 50, 82, 84 and 90) or protease inhibitor phenotypic resistance.

In a Phase III study (M98-863) of 653 patients randomised to receive stavudine plus lamivudine with either lopinavir/ritonavir or nelfinavir, 113 nelfinavir-treated subjects and 74 lopinavir/ritonavir-treated subjects had an HIV RNA above 400 copies/ml while on treatment from Week 24 through Week 96. Of these, isolates from 96 nelfinavir-treated subject and 51 lopinavir/ritonavir-treated subjects could be amplified for resistance testing. Resistance to nelfinavir, defined as the presence of the D30N or L90M mutation in protease, was observed in 41/96 (43%) subjects. Resistance to lopinavir, defined as the presence of any primary or active site mutations in protease (see above), was observed in 0/51 (0%) subjects. Lack of resistance to lopinavir was confirmed by phenotypic analysis.

Analysis of resistance in PI-experienced patients:

The selection of resistance to lopinavir in patients having failed prior protease inhibitor therapy was characterised by analysing the longitudinal isolates from 19 protease inhibitor-experienced subjects in 2 Phase II and one Phase III studies who either experienced incomplete virologic suppression or viral rebound subsequent to initial response to Kaletra and who demonstrated incremental in vitro resistance between baseline and rebound (defined as emergence of new mutations or 2-fold change in phenotypic susceptibility to lopinavir). Incremental resistance was most common in subjects whose baseline isolates had several protease inhibitor-associated mutations, but < 40-fold reduced susceptibility to lopinavir at baseline. Mutations V82A, I54V and M46I emerged most frequently. Mutations L33F, I50V and V32I combined with I47V/A were also observed. The 19 isolates demonstrated a 4.3-fold increase in IC_{50} compared to baseline isolates (from 6.2- to 43-fold, compared to wild-type virus).

Genotypic correlates of reduced phenotypic susceptibility to lopinavir in viruses selected by other protease inhibitors. The *in vitro* antiviral activity of lopinavir against 112 clinical isolates taken from patients failing therapy with one or more protease inhibitors was assessed. Within this panel, the following mutations in HIV protease were associated with reduced *in vitro* susceptibility to lopinavir: L10F/I/R/V, K20M/R, L24I, M46I/L, F53L, I54L/T/V, L63P, A71I/L/T/V, V82A/F/T, I84V and L90M. The median EC_{50} of lopinavir against isolates with 0 – 3, 4 – 5, 6 – 7 and 8 – 10 mutations at the above amino acid positions was 0.8, 2.7 13.5 and 44.0-fold higher than the EC_{50} against wild type HIV, respectively. The 16 viruses that displayed > 20-fold change in susceptibility all contained mutations at positions 10, 54, 63 plus 82 and/or 84. In addition, they contained a median of 3 mutations at amino acid positions 20, 24, 46, 53, 71 and 90. In addition to the mutations described above, mutations V32I and I47A have been observed in rebound isolates with reduced lopinavir susceptibility from protease inhibitor experienced patients receiving Kaletra therapy.

In addition to the mutations described above, mutations I47A and L76V have been observed in rebound isolates with reduced lopinavir susceptibility from patients receiving Kaletra therapy.

Conclusions regarding the relevance of particular mutations or mutational patterns are subject to change with additional data, and it is recommended to always consult current interpretation systems for analysing resistance test results.

Antiviral activity of Kaletra in patients failing protease inhibitor therapy: the clinical relevance of reduced *in vitro* susceptibility to lopinavir has been examined by assessing the virologic response to Kaletra therapy, with respect to baseline viral genotype and phenotype, in 56 patients previous failing therapy with multiple protease inhibitors. The EC_{50} of lopinavir against the 56 baseline viral isolates ranged from 0.6 to 96-fold higher than the EC_{50} against wild type HIV. After 48 weeks of treatment with Kaletra, efavirenz and nucleoside reverse transcriptase inhibitors, plasma HIV RNA ≤ 400 copies/ml was observed in 93% (25/27), 73% (11/15), and 25% (2/8) of patients with < 10-fold, 10 to 40-fold, and > 40-fold reduced susceptibility to lopinavir at baseline, respectively. In addition, virologic response was observed in 91% (21/23), 71% (15/21) and 33% (2/6) patients with 0 – 5, 6 – 7, and 8 – 10 mutations of the above mutations in HIV protease associated with reduced *in vitro* susceptibility to lopinavir. Since these patients had not previously been exposed to either Kaletra or efavirenz, part of the response may be attributed to the antiviral activity of efavirenz, particularly in patients harbouring highly lopinavir resistant virus. The study did not contain a control arm of patients not receiving Kaletra.

Cross-resistance: Activity of other protease inhibitors against isolates that developed incremental resistance to lopinavir after Kaletra therapy in protease inhibitor experienced patients: The presence of cross resistance to other protease inhibitors was analysed in 18 rebound isolates that had demonstrated evolution of resistance to lopinavir during 3 Phase II and one Phase III studies of Kaletra in protease inhibitor-experienced patients. The median fold IC_{50} of lopinavir for these 18 isolates at baseline and rebound was 6.9- and 63-fold, respectively, compared to wild type virus. In general, rebound isolates either retained (if cross-resistant at baseline) or developed significant cross-resistance to indinavir, saquinavir and atazanavir. Modest decreases in amprenavir activity were noted with a median increase of IC_{50} from 3.7- to 8-fold in the baseline and rebound isolates, respectively. Isolates retained susceptibility to tipranavir with a median increase of IC_{50} in baseline and rebound isolates of 1.9- and 1.8-fold, respectively, compared to wild type virus. Please refer to the Aptivus Summary of Product Characteristics for additional information on the use of tipranavir, including genotypic

Table 2

Virologic Response of Study Subjects at Week 48 and Week 96

	Week 48			Week 96		
	QD	BID	Difference [95% CI]	QD	BID	Difference [95% CI]
NC= Failure	257/333 (77.2%)	251/331 (75.8%)	1.3 % [-5.1, 7.8]	216/333 (64.9%)	229/331 (69.2%)	-4.3% [-11.5, 2.8]
Observed data	257/295 (87.1%)	250/280 (89.3%)	-2.2% [-7.4, 3.1]	216/247 (87.4%)	229/248 (92.3%)	-4.9% [-10.2, 0.4]

predictors of response, in treatment of lopinavir-resistant HIV-1 infection.

Clinical pharmacodynamic data

The effects of Kaletra (in combination with other antiretroviral agents) on biological markers (plasma HIV RNA levels and CD_4 counts) have been investigated in a controlled study of Kaletra of 48 weeks duration, and in additional studies of Kaletra of 360 weeks duration.

Adult Use

Patients without prior antiretroviral therapy

Study M98-863 is a randomised, double-blind trial of 653 antiretroviral treatment naïve patients investigating Kaletra (400/100 mg twice daily) compared to nelfinavir (750 mg three times daily) plus nucleoside reverse transcriptase inhibitors. By intent to treat analysis where patients with missing values are considered virologic failures, the proportion of patients at 48 weeks with HIV RNA < 400 copies/ml in the Kaletra arm was 75% and 63% in the nelfinavir arm. Mean baseline CD_4 cell count was 259 cells/ mm^3 (range: 2 to 949 cells/ mm^3) and mean baseline plasma HIV-1 RNA was 4.9 $\log_{10}$ copies/ml (range: 2.6 to 6.8 $\log_{10}$ copies/ml). Through 48 weeks of therapy, the proportion of patients in the Kaletra arm with plasma RNA < 50 copies/ml was 67% and 52% in the nelfinavir arm. The mean increase from baseline in CD_4 cell count was 207 cells/mm^3 in the Kaletra arm and 195 cells/mm^3 in the nelfinavir arm. Through 48 weeks of therapy, a statistically significantly higher proportion of patients in the Kaletra arm had HIV RNA < 50 copies/ml compared to the nelfinavir arm.

Study M05-730 was a randomised, open-label, multicentre trial comparing treatment with Kaletra 800/200 mg once daily plus tenofovir DF and emtricitabine versus Kaletra 400/100 mg twice daily plus tenofovir DF and emtricitabine in 664 antiretroviral treatment-naïve patients. Given the pharmacokinetic interaction between Kaletra and tenofovir (see section 4.5), the results of this study might not be strictly extrapolable when other backbone regimens are used with Kaletra. Patients were randomised in a 1:1 ratio to receive either Kaletra 800/200 mg once daily (n = 333) or Kaletra 400/100 mg twice daily (n = 331). Further stratification within each group was 1:1 (tablet versus. soft capsule). Patients were administered either the tablet or the soft capsule formulation for 8 weeks, after which all patients were administered the tablet formulation once daily or twice daily for the remainder of the study. Patients were administered emtricitabine 200 mg once daily and tenofovir DF 300 mg once daily. Protocol defined non-inferiority of once daily dosing compared with twice daily dosing was demonstrated if the lower bound of the 95% confidence interval for the difference in proportion of subjects responding (once dialy minus twice daily) excluded -12% at Week 48. Mean age of patients enrolled was 39 years (range: 19 to 71); 75% were Caucasian, and 78% were male. Mean baseline CD4+ cell count was 216 cells/mm3 (range: 20 to 775 cells/mm^3) and mean baseline plasma HIV-1 RNA was 5.0 $\log_{10}$ copies/ml (range: 1.7 to 7.0 $\log_{10}$ copies/ml).

(see Table 2 above)

Sustained virological response to Kaletra (in combination with nucleoside/nucleotide reverse transcriptase inhibitors) has been also observed in a small Phase II study (M97-720) through 360 weeks of treatment. One hundred patients were originally treated with Kaletra in the study (including 51 patients receiving 400/100 mg twice daily and 49 patients at either 200/100 mg twice daily or 400/200 mg twice daily). All patients converted to open-label Kaletra at the 400/100 mg twice daily dose between week 48 and week 72. Sixty-one patients completed the study (35 patients received the recommended 400/100 mg twice daily dose throughout the study). Through 360 weeks of treatment, the proportion of patients with HIV RNA < 400 (< 50) copies/ml was 61% (59%), and the corresponding mean increase in CD_4 cell count was 501 cells/mm^3. Thirty-nine patients (39%) discontinued the study, including 16 (16%) discontinuations due to adverse events, one of which was associated with a death.

Patients with prior antiretroviral therapy

Study M97-765 is a randomised, double-blind trial evaluating Kaletra at two dose levels (400/100 mg and 400/ 200 mg, both twice daily) plus nevirapine (200 mg twice daily) and two nucleoside reverse transcriptase inhibitors in 70 single protease inhibitor experienced, non-nucleoside reverse transcriptase inhibitor naïve patients. Median baseline CD_4 cell count was 349 cells/mm^3 (range 72 to 807 cells/mm^3) and median baseline plasma HIV-1 RNA was 4.0 $\log_{10}$ copies/ml (range 2.9 to 5.8 $\log_{10}$ copies/ml). By intent to treat analysis where patients with missing values are considered virologic failures, the proportion of patients with HIV RNA < 400 (< 50) copies/ml at 24 weeks was 75% (58%) and the mean increase from baseline in CD_4 cell count was 174 cells/mm^3 for the 36 patients receiving the 400/100 mg dose of Kaletra.

M98-957 is a randomised, open-label study evaluating Kaletra treatment at two dose levels (400/100 mg and 533/133 mg, both twice daily) plus efavirenz (600 mg once daily) and nucleoside reverse transcriptase inhibitors in 57 multiple protease inhibitor experienced, non-nucleoside reverse transcriptase inhibitor naïve patients. Between week 24 and 48, patients randomised to a dose of 400/ 100 mg were converted to a dose of 533/133 mg. Median baseline CD_4 cell count was 220 cells/mm^3 (range 13 to 1030 cells/mm^3). By intent-to-treat analysis of both dose groups combined (n=57), where patients with missing values are considered virologic failures, the proportion of patients with HIV RNA < 400 copies/ml at 48 weeks was 65% and the mean increase from baseline CD_4 cell count was 94 cells/mm^3.

Paediatric Use

M98-940 is an open-label study of a liquid formulation of Kaletra in 100 antiretroviral naïve (44%) and experienced (56%) paediatric patients. All patients were non-nucleoside reverse transcriptase inhibitor naïve. Patients were randomised to either 230 mg lopinavir/57.5 mg ritonavir per m^2 or 300 mg lopinavir/75 mg ritonavir per m^2. Naïve patients also received nucleoside reverse transcriptase inhibitors. Experienced patients received nevirapine plus up to two nucleoside reverse transcriptase inhibitors. Safety, efficacy and pharmacokinetic profiles of the two dose regimens were assessed after 3 weeks of therapy in each patient. Subsequently, all patients were continued on the 300/75 mg per m^2 dose. Patients had a mean age of 5 years (range 6 months to 12 years) with 14 patients less than 2 years old and 6 patients one year or less. Mean baseline CD_4 cell count was 838 cells/mm^3 and mean baseline plasma HIV-1 RNA was 4.7 $\log_{10}$ copies/ml. Through 48 weeks of therapy, the proportion of patients with HIV RNA < 400 copies/ml was 84% for antiretroviral naïve patients and 75% for antiretroviral experienced patients and the mean increases from baseline in CD_4 cell count were 404 cells/mm^3 and 284 cells/mm^3 respectively.

5.2 Pharmacokinetic properties

The pharmacokinetic properties of lopinavir co-administered with ritonavir have been evaluated in healthy adult volunteers and in HIV-infected patients; no substantial differences were observed between the two groups. Lopinavir is essentially completely metabolised by CYP3A. Ritonavir inhibits the metabolism of lopinavir, thereby increasing the plasma levels of lopinavir. Across studies, administration of Kaletra 400/100 mg twice daily yields mean steady-state lopinavir plasma concentrations 15 to 20-fold higher than those of ritonavir in HIV-infected patients. The plasma levels of ritonavir are less than 7% of those obtained after the ritonavir dose of 600 mg twice daily. The *in vitro* antiviral EC_{50} of lopinavir is approximately 10-fold lower than that of ritonavir. Therefore, the antiviral activity of Kaletra is due to lopinavir.

Absorption: multiple dosing with 400/100 mg Kaletra twice daily for 2 weeks and without meal restriction produced a mean ± SD lopinavir peak plasma concentration (C_{max}) of 12.3 ± 5.4 μg/ml, occurring approximately 4 hours after administration. The mean steady-state trough concentration prior to the morning dose was 8.1 ± 5.7 μg/ml. Lopinavir AUC over a 12 hour dosing interval averaged 113.2 ± 60.5 μg•h/ml. The absolute bioavailability of lopinavir co-formulated with ritonavir in humans has not been established.

Effects of food on oral absorption: Administration of a single 400/100 mg dose of Kaletra tablets under fed conditions (high fat, 872 kcal, 56% from fat) compared to fasted state was associated with no significant changes in C_{max} and AUC_{inf}. Therefore, Kaletra tablets may be taken with or without food. Kaletra tablets have also shown less pharmacokinetic variability under all meal conditions compared to Kaletra soft capsules.

Distribution: at steady state, lopinavir is approximately 98 – 99% bound to serum proteins. Lopinavir binds to both alpha-1-acid glycoprotein (AAG) and albumin, however, it has a higher affinity for AAG. At steady state, lopinavir protein binding remains constant over the range of observed concentrations after 400/100 mg Kaletra twice daily, and is similar between healthy volunteers and HIV-positive patients.

Metabolism: *in vitro* experiments with human hepatic microsomes indicate that lopinavir primarily undergoes oxidative metabolism. Lopinavir is extensively metabolised by the hepatic cytochrome P450 system, almost exclusively by isozyme CYP3A. Ritonavir is a potent CYP3A inhibitor which inhibits the metabolism of lopinavir and therefore, increases plasma levels of lopinavir. A ^{14}C-lopinavir study in humans showed that 89% of the plasma radioactivity after a single 400/100 mg Kaletra dose was due to parent active substance. At least 13 lopinavir oxidative metabolites have been identified in man. The 4-oxo and 4-hydroxymetabolite epimeric pair are the major metabolites with antiviral activity, but comprise only minute amounts of total plasma radioactivity. Ritonavir has been shown to induce metabolic enzymes, resulting in the induction of its own metabolism, and likely the induction of lopinavir metabolism. Pre-dose lopinavir concentrations decline with time during multiple dosing, stabilising after approximately 10 days to 2 weeks.

Elimination: after a 400/100 mg ^{14}C-lopinavir/ritonavir dose, approximately 10.4 ± 2.3% and 82.6 ± 2.5% of an administered dose of ^{14}C-lopinavir can be accounted for in urine and faeces, respectively. Unchanged lopinavir accounted for approximately 2.2% and 19.8% of the administered dose in urine and faeces, respectively. After multiple dosing, less than 3% of the lopinavir dose is excreted unchanged in the urine. The effective (peak to trough) half-life of lopinavir over a 12 hour dosing interval averaged 5 – 6 hours, and the apparent oral clearance (CL/F) of lopinavir is 6 to 7 l/h.

Once daily dosing: the pharmacokinetics of once daily Kaletra have been evaluated in HIV-infected subjects naïve to antiretroviral treatment. Kaletra 800/200 mg was administered in combination with emtricitabine 200 mg and tenofovir DF 300 mg as part of a once daily regimen. Multiple dosing of 800/200 mg Kaletra once daily for 2 weeks without meal restriction (n=16) produced a mean ± SD lopinavir peak plasma concentration (C_{max}) of 14.8 ± 3.5 μg/ml, occurring approximately 6 hours after administration. The mean steady-state trough concentration prior to the morning dose was 5.5 ± 5.4 μg/ml. Lopinavir AUC over a 24 hour dosing interval averaged 206.5 ± 89.7 μg·h/ml.

As compared to the BID regimen, the once daily dosing is associated with a reduction in the C_{min}/C_{trough} values of approximately 50%.

Special Populations

Paediatrics:

There are limited pharmacokinetic data in children below 2 years of age. The pharmacokinetics of Kaletra oral solution 300/75 mg/m^2 twice daily and 230/57.5 mg/m^2 twice daily have been studied in a total of 53 paediatric patients, ranging in age from 6 months to 12 years. The lopinavir mean steady-state AUC, C_{max}, and C_{min} were 72.6 ± 31.1 μg•h/ml, 8.2 ± 2.9 μg/ml and 3.4 ± 2.1 μg/ml, respectively after Kaletra oral solution 230/57.5 mg/m^2 twice daily without nevirapine (n=12), and were 85.8 ± 36.9 μg•h/ml, 10.0 ± 3.3 μg/ml and 3.6 ± 3.5 μg/ml, respectively after 300/ 75 mg/m^2 twice daily with nevirapine (n=12). The 230/ 57.5 mg/m^2 twice daily regimen without nevirapine and the 300/75 mg/m^2 twice daily regimen with nevirapine provided lopinavir plasma concentrations similar to those obtained in adult patients receiving the 400/100 mg twice daily regimen without nevirapine. Kaletra once daily has not been evaluated in paediatric patients.

Gender, Race and Age:

Kaletra pharmacokinetics have not been studied in the elderly. No age or gender related pharmacokinetic differences have been observed in adult patients. Pharmacokinetic differences due to race have not been identified.

Renal Insufficiency:

Kaletra pharmacokinetics have not been studied in patients with renal insufficiency; however, since the renal clearance of lopinavir is negligible, a decrease in total body clearance is not expected in patients with renal insufficiency.

Hepatic Insufficiency:

The steady state pharmacokinetic parameters of lopinavir in HIV-infected patients with mild to moderate hepatic impairment were compared with those of HIV-infected patients with normal hepatic function in a multiple dose study with lopinavir/ritonavir 400/100 mg twice daily. A limited increase in total lopinavir concentrations of approximately 30% has been observed which is not expected to be of clinical relevance (see section 4.2).

5.3 Preclinical safety data

Repeat-dose toxicity studies in rodents and dogs identified major target organs as the liver, kidney, thyroid, spleen and circulating red blood cells. Hepatic changes indicated cellular swelling with focal degeneration. While exposure eliciting these changes were comparable to or below human clinical exposure, dosages in animals were over 6-fold the recommended clinical dose. Mild renal tubular degeneration was confined to mice exposed with at least twice the recommended human exposure; the kidney was unaffected in rats and dogs. Reduced serum thyroxin led to an increased release of TSH with resultant follicular cell hypertrophy in the thyroid glands of rats. These changes were reversible with withdrawal of the active substance and were absent in mice and dogs. Coombs-negative anisocytosis and poikilocytosis were observed in rats, but not in mice or dogs. Enlarged spleens with histiocytosis were seen in rats but not other species. Serum cholesterol was elevated in rodents but not dogs, while triglycerides were elevated only in mice.

During *in vitro* studies, cloned human cardiac potassium channels (HERG) were inhibited by 30% at the highest concentrations of lopinavir/ritonavir tested, corresponding to a lopinavir exposure 7-fold total and 15-fold free peak plasma levels achieved in humans at the maximum recommended therapeutic dose. In contrast, similar concentrations of lopinavir/ritonavir demonstrated no repolarisation delay in the canine cardiac Purkinje fibres. Lower concentrations of lopinavir/ritonavir did not produce significant potassium (HERG) current blockade. Tissue distribution studies conducted in the rat did not suggest significant cardiac retention of the active substance; 72-hour AUC in heart was approximately 50% of measured plasma AUC. Therefore, it is reasonable to expect that cardiac lopinavir levels would not be significantly higher than plasma levels.

In dogs, prominent U waves on the electrocardiogram have been observed associated with prolonged PR interval and bradycardia. These effects have been assumed to be caused by electrolyte disturbance.

The clinical relevance of these preclinical data is unknown, however, the potential cardiac effects of this product in humans cannot be ruled out (see also sections 4.4 and 4.8).

In rats, embryofoetotoxicity (pregnancy loss, decreased foetal viability, decreased foetal body weights, increased frequency of skeletal variations) and postnatal developmental toxicity (decreased survival of pups) was observed at maternally toxic dosages. The systemic exposure to lopinavir/ritonavir at the maternal and developmental toxic dosages was lower than the intended therapeutic exposure in humans.

Long-term carcinogenicity studies of lopinavir/ritonavir in mice revealed a nongenotoxic, mitogenic induction of liver tumours, generally considered to have little relevance to human risk.

Carcinogenicity studies in rats revealed no tumourigenic findings. Lopinavir/ritonavir was not found to be mutagenic or clastogenic in a battery of *in vitro* and *in vivo* assays including the Ames bacterial reverse mutation assay, the mouse lymphoma assay, the mouse micronucleus test and chromosomal aberration assays in human lymphocytes.

6. PHARMACEUTICAL PARTICULARS

6.1 List of excipients

Tablet contents:

Copovidone

Sorbitan laurate

Colloidal anhydrous silica

Sodium stearyl fumarate

Film-coating:

Polyvinyl alcohol

Titanium dioxide

Talc

Macrogols type 3350 (Polyethylene glycol 3350)

Yellow ferric oxide E172

6.2 Incompatibilities

Not applicable.

6.3 Shelf life

2 years.

6.4 Special precautions for storage

This medicinal product does not require any special storage conditions.

6.5 Nature and contents of container

High density polyethylene (HDPE) bottles closed with propylene caps. Each bottle contains 60 tablets. Each pack contains 1 bottle (60 tablets).

6.6 Special precautions for disposal and other handling

No special requirements.

7. MARKETING AUTHORISATION HOLDER

Abbott Laboratories Limited

Queenborough

Kent ME11 5EL

United Kingdom

8. MARKETING AUTHORISATION NUMBER(S)

EU/1/01/172/00

9. DATE OF FIRST AUTHORISATION/RENEWAL OF THE AUTHORISATION

Date of first authorisation: 20 March 2001

Date of last renewal: 20 March 2006

10. DATE OF REVISION OF THE TEXT

21 August 2009

Kaletra 200 mg/50 mg film-coated tablets

(Abbott Laboratories Limited)

1. NAME OF THE MEDICINAL PRODUCT

Kaletra 200 mg/50 mg film-coated tablets

2. QUALITATIVE AND QUANTITATIVE COMPOSITION

Each film-coated tablet contains 200 mg of lopinavir co-formulated with 50 mg of ritonavir as a pharmacokinetic enhancer.

For a full list of excipients, see section 6.1.

3. PHARMACEUTICAL FORM

Film-coated tablet

Yellow embossed with [Abbott logo] and "KA".

4. CLINICAL PARTICULARS

4.1 Therapeutic indications

Kaletra is indicated for the treatment of HIV-1 infected adults and children above the age of 2 years, in combination with other antiretroviral agents.

Most experience with Kaletra is derived from the use of the product in antiretroviral therapy naïve patients. Data in heavily pretreated protease inhibitor experienced patients are limited. There are limited data on salvage therapy on patients who have failed therapy with Kaletra.

The choice of Kaletra to treat protease inhibitor experienced HIV-1 infected patients should be based on individual viral resistance testing and treatment history of patients (see sections 4.4 and 5.1).

4.2 Posology and method of administration

Kaletra should be prescribed by physicians who are experienced in the treatment of HIV infection.

Kaletra tablets should be swallowed whole and not chewed, broken or crushed

Adult and adolescent use: the standard recommended dosage of Kaletra tablets is 400/100 mg (two 200/50 mg) tablets twice daily taken with or without food. In adult patients naive to antiretroviral therapy, in cases where once daily dosing is considered necessary for the management of the patient, Kaletra tablets may be administered as 800/200 mg (four 200/50 mg tablets) once daily with or without food. However, this once daily regimen might be associated with a lesser sustainability of the virologic suppression (see section 5.1) and the higher risk of diarrhoea (see section 4.8) compared to the recommended standard twice daily dosage. This once daily regimen is not validated in antiretroviral experienced patients. Oral solution is available to patients who have difficulty swallowing. Refer to the Summary of Product Characteristics for Kaletra oral solution for dosing instructions.

Paediatric use (2 years of age and above): the adult dose of Kaletra tablets (400/100 mg twice daily) may be used in children 40 kg or greater or with a Body Surface Area (BSA)* greater than 1.4 m^2. For children weighing less than 40 kg or with a BSA between 0.5 and 1.4 m^2 and able to swallow tablets, please refer to the Kaletra 100 mg/25 mg tablets Summary of Product Characteristics. For children unable to swallow tablets, please refer to the Kaletra oral solution Summary of Product Characteristics. Kaletra dosed once daily has not been evaluated in paediatric patients.

* Body surface area can be calculated with the following equation:

BSA (m^2) = $\sqrt{}$ (Height (cm) X Weight (kg) / 3600)

Children less than 2 years of age: Kaletra is not recommended for use in children below 2 years of age due to insufficient data on safety and efficacy (see section 5.1).

Concomitant Therapy: Efavirenz or nevirapine

The following table contains dosing guidelines for Kaletra tablets based on BSA when used in combination with efavirenz or nevirapine in children.

Paediatric Dosing Guidelines with concomitant efavirenz or nevirapine

Body Surface Area (m^2)	Recommended lopinavir/ritonavir dosing (mg) twice daily. The adequate dosing may be achieved with the two available strengths of Kaletra tablets: 100/25 mg and 200/50 mg.*
≥ 0.5 to < 0.8	200/50 mg
≥ 0.8 to < 1.2	300/75 mg
≥ 1.2 to < 1.4	400/100 mg
≥ 1.4	500/125 mg

* Kaletra tablets must not be chewed, broken or crushed.

Hepatic impairment: In HIV-infected patients with mild to moderate hepatic impairment, an increase of approximately 30% in lopinavir exposure has been observed but is not expected to be of clinical relevance (see section 5.2). No data are available in patients with severe hepatic impairment. Kaletra should not be given to these patients (see section 4.3).

Renal impairment: no dose adjustment is necessary in patients with renal impairment. Caution is warranted when Kaletra is used in patients with severe renal impairment (see section 4.4).

4.3 Contraindications

Hypersensitivity to the active substances or to any of the excipients.

Patients with severe hepatic insufficiency.

Kaletra contains lopinavir and ritonavir, both of which are inhibitors of the P450 isoform CYP3A. Kaletra should not be co-administered with medicinal products that are highly dependent on CYP3A for clearance and for which elevated plasma concentrations are associated with serious and/or life threatening events. These medicinal products include astemizole, terfenadine, oral midazolam (for caution on parenterally administered midazolam, see section 4.5), triazolam, cisapride, pimozide, amiodarone, ergot alkaloids (e.g. ergotamine, dihydroergotamine, ergonovine and methylergonovine) and vardenafil.

Herbal preparations containing St John's wort (*Hypericum perforatum)* must not be used while taking lopinavir and ritonavir due to the risk of decreased plasma concentrations and reduced clinical effects of lopinavir and ritonavir (see section 4.5).

4.4 Special warnings and precautions for use

Patients with coexisting conditions

Hepatic impairment: the safety and efficacy of Kaletra has not been established in patients with significant underlying liver disorders. Kaletra is contraindicated in patients with severe liver impairment (see section 4.3). Patients with chronic hepatitis B or C and treated with combination antiretroviral therapy are at an increased risk for severe and potentially fatal hepatic adverse reactions. In case of concomitant antiviral therapy for hepatitis B or C, please refer to the relevant product information for these medicinal products.

Patients with pre-existing liver dysfunction including chronic hepatitis have an increased frequency of liver function abnormalities during combination antiretroviral therapy and should be monitored according to standard practice. If there is evidence of worsening liver disease in such patients, interruption or discontinuation of treatment should be considered.

Renal impairment: since the renal clearance of lopinavir and ritonavir is negligible, increased plasma concentrations are not expected in patients with renal impairment. Because lopinavir and ritonavir are highly protein bound, it is unlikely that they will be significantly removed by haemodialysis or peritoneal dialysis.

Haemophilia: there have been reports of increased bleeding, including spontaneous skin haematomas and haemarthrosis in patients with haemophilia type A and B treated with protease inhibitors. In some patients additional factor VIII was given. In more than half of the reported cases, treatment with protease inhibitors was continued or reintroduced if treatment had been discontinued. A causal relationship had been evoked, although the mechanism of action had not been elucidated. Haemophiliac patients should therefore be made aware of the possibility of increased bleeding.

Lipid elevations

Treatment with Kaletra has resulted in increases, sometimes marked, in the concentration of total cholesterol and triglycerides. Triglyceride and cholesterol testing is to be performed prior to initiating Kaletra therapy and at periodic intervals during therapy. Particular caution should be paid to patients with high values at baseline and with history of lipid disorders. Lipid disorders are to be managed as clinically appropriate (see also section 4.5 for additional information on potential interactions with HMG-CoA reductase inhibitors).

Pancreatitis

Cases of pancreatitis have been reported in patients receiving Kaletra, including those who developed hypertriglyceridaemia. In most of these cases patients have had a prior history of pancreatitis and/or concurrent therapy with other medicinal products associated with pancreatitis. Marked triglyceride elevation is a risk factor for development of pancreatitis. Patients with advanced HIV disease may be at risk of elevated triglycerides and pancreatitis

Pancreatitis should be considered if clinical symptoms (nausea, vomiting, abdominal pain) or abnormalities in laboratory values (such as increased serum lipase or amylase values) suggestive of pancreatitis should occur. Patients who exhibit these signs or symptoms should be evaluated and Kaletra therapy should be suspended if a diagnosis of pancreatitis is made (see section 4.8).

Hyperglycaemia

New onset diabetes mellitus, hyperglycaemia or exacerbation of existing diabetes mellitus has been reported in patients receiving protease inhibitors. In some of these the hyperglycaemia was severe and in some cases also associated with ketoacidosis. Many patients had confounding medical conditions some of which required therapy with agents that have been associated with the development of diabetes mellitus or hyperglycaemia.

Fat redistribution and metabolic disorders

Combination antiretroviral therapy has been associated with redistribution of body fat (lipodystrophy) in HIV patients. The long-term consequences of these events are currently unknown. Knowledge about the mechanism is incomplete. A connection between visceral lipomatosis and protease inhibitors (PIs) and lipoatrophy and nucleoside reverse transcriptase inhibitors (NRTIs) has been hypothesised. A higher risk of lipodystrophy has been associated with individual factors such as older age, and with drug related factors such as longer duration of antiretroviral treatment and associated metabolic disturbances. Clinical examination should include evaluation for physical signs of fat redistribution. Consideration should be given to measurement of fasting serum lipids and blood glucose. Lipid disorders should be managed as clinically appropriate (see section 4.8).

Immune Reactivation Syndrome

In HIV-infected patients with severe immune deficiency at the time of institution of combination antiretroviral therapy (CART), an inflammatory reaction to asymtomatic or residual opportunistic pathogens may arise and cause serious clinical conditions, or aggravation of symptoms. Typically, such reactions have been observed within the first few weeks or months of initiation of CART. Relevant examples are cytomegalovirus retinitis, generalised and/or focal mycobacterial infections, and Pneumocystis carinii pneumonia. Any inflammatory symptoms should be evaluated and treatment instituted when necessary.

Osteonecrosis

Although the etiology is considered to be multifactorial (including corticosteroid use, alcohol consumption, severe immunosuppression, higher body mass index), cases of osteonecrosis have been reported particularly in patients with advanced HIV-disease and/or long-term exposure to combination antiretroviral therapy (CART). Patients should be advised to seek medical advice if they experience joint aches and pain, joint stiffness or difficulty in movement.

PR interval prolongation

Lopinavir/ritonavir has been shown to cause modest asymptomatic prolongation of the PR interval in some healthy adult subjects. Rare reports of 2nd or 3rd degree atroventricular block in patients with underlying structural heart disease and pre-existing conduction system abnormalities or in patients receiving drugs known to prolong the PR interval (such as verapamil or atazanavir) have been reported in patients receiving lopinavir/ritonavir. Kaletra should be used with caution in such patients (see section 5.1).

Interactions with medicinal products

Kaletra contains lopinavir and ritonavir, both of which are inhibitors of the P450 isoform CYP3A. Kaletra is likely to increase plasma concentrations of medicinal products that are primarily metabolised by CYP3A. These increases of plasma concentrations of co-administered medicinal products could increase or prolong their therapeutic effect and adverse events (see sections 4.3 and 4.5).

The HMG-CoA reductase inhibitors simvastatin and lovastatin are highly dependent on CYP3A for metabolism, thus concomitant use of Kaletra with simvastatin or lovastatin is not recommended due to an increased risk of myopathy including rhabdomyolysis. Caution must also be exercised and reduced doses should be considered if Kaletra is used concurrently with rosuvastatin or with atorvastatin, which is metabolised to a lesser extent by CYP3A4. If treatment with a HMG-CoA reductase inhibitor is indicated, pravastatin or fluvastatin is recommended (see section 4.5).

Particular caution must be used when prescribing Kaletra and medicinal products known to induce QT interval prolongation such as: chlorpheniramine, quinidine, erythromycin, clarithromycin. Indeed, Kaletra could increase concentrations of the co-administered medicinal products and this may result in an increase of their associated cardiac adverse events. Cardiac events have been reported with Kaletra in preclinical studies; therefore, the potential cardiac effects of Kaletra cannot be currently ruled out (see sections 4.8 and 5.3).

Co-administration of Kaletra with rifampicin is not recommended. Rifampicin in combination with Kaletra causes large decreases in lopinavir concentrations which may in turn significantly decrease the lopinavir therapeutic effect. Adequate exposure to lopinavir/ritonavir may be achieved when a higher dose of Kaletra is used but this is associated with a higher risk of liver and gastrointestinal toxicity. Therefore, this co-administration should be avoided unless judged strictly necessary (see section 4.5).

Other

Kaletra is not a cure for HIV infection or AIDS. It does not reduce the risk of passing HIV to others through sexual contact or blood contamination. Appropriate precautions should be taken. People taking Kaletra may still develop infections or other illnesses associated with HIV disease and AIDS.

Concomitant use of Kaletra and fluticasone or other glucocorticoids that are metabolised by CYP3A4 is not recommended unless the potential benefit of treatment outweighs the risk of systemic corticosteroid effects, including Cushing's syndrome and adrenal suppression (see section 4.5).

4.5 Interaction with other medicinal products and other forms of interaction

Kaletra contains lopinavir and ritonavir, both of which are inhibitors of the P450 isoform CYP3A *in vitro*. Co-administration of Kaletra and medicinal products primarily metabolised by CYP3A may result in increased plasma concentrations of the other medicinal product, which could increase or prolong its therapeutic and adverse reactions. Kaletra does not inhibit CYP2D6, CYP2C9, CYP2C19, CYP2E1, CYP2B6 or CYP1A2 at clinically relevant concentrations (see section 4.3).

Kaletra has been shown *in vivo* to induce its own metabolism and to increase the biotransformation of some medicinal products metabolised by cytochrome P450 enzymes and by glucuronidation. This may result in lowered plasma concentrations and potential decrease of efficacy of co-administered medicinal products.

Medicinal products that are contraindicated specifically due to the expected magnitude of interaction and potential for serious adverse events are listed in section 4.3.

All interaction studies, when otherwise not stated, were performed using Kaletra capsules, which gives an approximately 20% lower exposure of lopinavir than the 200/50 mg tablets.

Antiretroviral agents

Nucleoside/Nucleotide reverse transcriptase inhibitors (NRTIs):

Stavudine and Lamivudine: no change in the pharmacokinetics of lopinavir was observed when Kaletra was given alone or in combination with stavudine and lamivudine in clinical studies.

Didanosine: it is recommended that didanosine be administered on an empty stomach; therefore, didanosine may be co-administered with Kaletra tablets without food.

Zidovudine and Abacavir: Kaletra induces glucuronidation; therefore Kaletra has the potential to reduce zidovudine and abacavir plasma concentrations. The clinical significance of this potential interaction is unknown.

Tenofovir: when tenofovir disoproxil fumarate was co-administered with Kaletra, tenofovir concentrations were increased by approximately 30% with no changes noted in lopinavir or ritonavir concentrations. Higher tenofovir concentrations could potentiate tenofovir associated adverse events, including renal disorders.

Non-nucleoside reverse transcriptase inhibitors (NNRTIs):

In a study performed in healthy volunteers to explore the interaction between Kaletra tablets (400/100 mg twice daily) and efavirenz (600 mg once daily), efavirenz has been shown to decrease the lopinavir concentrations by 30 - 40%. When Kaletra tablet dosages were increased to 500/125 mg twice daily during co-administration of efavirenz 600 mg once daily in healthy volunteers, lopinavir pharmacokinetic parameters were similar to those obtained with Kaletra tablets 400/100 mg twice daily administered alone. Therefore, the Kaletra tablets dosage should be increased to 500/125 mg twice daily when co-administered with efavirenz 600 mg once daily. Kaletra must not be administered once daily in combination with efavirenz.

Similar pharmacokinetic interactions are expected for the co-administration of Kaletra tablets with the NNRTI nevirapine and with the protease inhibitors nelfinavir and amprenavir. The same recommendations for monitoring apply in these cases of co-administration. Kaletra must not be administered once daily in combination with nevirapine.

Co-administration with other HIV protease inhibitors (PIs):

Kaletra (400/100 mg twice daily) has been studied in combination with reduced doses of amprenavir, indinavir, nelfinavir and saquinavir in steady-state controlled healthy volunteer studies relative to clinical doses of each HIV protease inhibitor in the absence of ritonavir. Comparisons to published pharmacokinetic data with ritonavir-enhanced amprenavir and saquinavir regimens are also described. Additionally, the effect of additional ritonavir on the pharmacokinetics of lopinavir are discussed. Note that the historical comparisons to ritonavir-enhanced protease inhibitor regimens should be interpreted with caution (see details of combinations below). Appropriate doses of HIV-protease inhibitors in combination with Kaletra with respect to safety and efficacy have not been established. Therefore, the concomitant administration of Kaletra with PIs requires close monitoring.

Amprenavir: see recommendations described for Kaletra tablets co-administration with efavirenz. Kaletra must not be administered once daily in combination with amprenavir.

Fosamprenavir: co-administration of standard doses of lopinavir/ritonavir with fosamprenavir results in a significant reduction in amprenavir concentrations. Co-administration of increased doses of fosamprenavir 1400 mg twice daily with lopinavir/ritonavir 533/133 mg twice daily to protease inhibitor-experienced patients resulted in a higher incidence of gastrointestinal adverse events and elevations in triglycerides with the combination regimen without increases in virological efficacy, when compared with standard doses of fosamprenavir/ritonavir. Therefore, concomitant administration of these medicinal products is not recommended.

Indinavir: indinavir 600 mg twice daily in combination with Kaletra produces similar indinavir AUC, higher C_{min} (by 3.5-fold) and lower C_{max} relative to indinavir 800 mg three times daily alone. Furthermore, concentrations of lopinavir do not appear to be affected when both medicinal products, Kaletra and indinivir, are combined, based on historical comparison with Kaletra alone.

Nelfinavir: see recommendations described for Kaletra tablets co-administration with efavirenz. Kaletra must not be administered once daily in combination with nelfinavir.

Saquinavir: saquinavir 800 mg twice daily co-administered with Kaletra produces an increase of saquinavir AUC by 9.6-fold relative to saquinavir 1200 mg three times daily given alone.

Saquinavir 800 mg twice daily co-administered with Kaletra resulted in an increase of saquinavir AUC by approximately 30% relative to saquinavir/ritonavir 1000/100 mg twice daily, and produces similar exposure to those reported after saquinavir/ritonavir 400/400 mg twice daily.

When saquinavir 1200 mg twice daily was combined with Kaletra, no further increase of concentrations was noted. Furthermore, concentrations of lopinavir do not appear to be affected when both medicinal products, Kaletra and saquinavir, are combined, based on historical comparison with Kaletra alone.

Ritonavir: Kaletra co-administered with an additional 100 mg ritonavir twice daily resulted in an increase of lopinavir AUC and C_{min} of 33% and 64%, respectively, as compared to Kaletra alone.

Other medicinal products:

Acid reducing agents (omeprazole, ranitidine): in a study performed in healthy volunteers, no clinically relevant interaction has been observed when Kaletra tablets 400/100 mg twice daily or 800/200 mg once daily was co-administered with omeprazole or with ranitidine. Kaletra can be co-administered with acid reducing agents with no dose adjustment.

Antiarrhythmics: (bepridil, systemic lidocaine and quinidine): concentrations may be increased when co-administered with Kaletra. Caution is warranted and therapeutic concentration monitoring is recommended when available.

Anticancer agents (eg vincristine, vinblastine): these agents may have their serum concentrations increased when co-administered with lopinavir/ritonavir resulting in the potential for increased adverse events usually associated with these anticancer agents.

Anticoagulants: warfarin concentrations may be affected when co-administered with Kaletra. It is recommended that INR (international normalised ratio) be monitored.

Anticonvulsants (phenobarbital, phenytoin, carbamazepine): will induce CYP3A4 and may decrease lopinavir concentrations.

In addition, co-administration of phenytoin and lopinavir/ritonavir resulted in moderate decreases in steady-state phenytoin concentrations. Phenytoin levels should be monitored when co-administering with lopinavir/ritonavir. Kaletra must not be administered once daily in combination with carbamazepine, phenobarbital or phenytoin.

Bupropion: in healthy volunteers, the AUC and C_{max} of bupropion and of its active metabolite, hydroxybupropion, were decreased by about 50% when co-administered with lopinavir/ritonavir capsules 400/100 mg twice daily at steady-state. This effect may be due to induction of bupropion metabolism. Therefore, if the co-administration of lopinavir/ritonavir with bupropion is judged unavoidable, this should be done under close clinical monitoring for bupropion efficacy, without exceeding the recommended dosage, despite the observed induction.

Trazodone: in a pharmacokinetic study performed in healthy volunteers, concomitant use of low dose ritonavir (200 mg twice daily) with a single dose of trazodone led to an increase in plasma concentrations of trazodone (AUC increased by 2.4 fold). Adverse events of nausea, dizziness, hypotension and syncope were observed following co-administration of trazodone and ritonavir in this study. However, it is unknown whether the combination of lopinavir/ritonavir causes a similar increase in trazodone exposure. The combination should be used with caution and a lower dose of trazodone should be considered.

Digoxin: plasma concentrations of digoxin may be increased when co-administered with Kaletra. Caution is warranted and therapeutic drug monitoring of digoxin concentrations, if available, is recommended in case of co-administration of Kaletra and digoxin. Particular caution should be used when prescribing Kaletra in patients taking digoxin as the acute inhibitory effect of ritonavir on Pgp is expected to significantly increase digoxin levels. The increased digoxin level may lessen over time as Pgp induction develops. Initiation of digoxin in patients already taking Kaletra is expected to result in lower increase of digoxin concentrations.

Dihydropyridine calcium channel blockers: (e.g. felodipine, nifedipine, nicardipine): may have their serum concentrations increased by Kaletra.

Lipid lowering agents: HMG-CoA reductase inhibitors which are highly dependent on CYP3A4 metabolism, such as lovastatin and simvastatin, are expected to have markedly increased plasma concentrations when co-administered with Kaletra. Since increased concentrations of HMG-CoA reductase inhibitors may cause myopathy, including rhabdomyolysis, the combination of these medicinal products with Kaletra is not recommended. Atorvastatin is less dependent on CYP3A for metabolism. When atorvastatin was given concurrently with Kaletra, a mean 4.7-fold and 5.9-fold increase in atorvastatin C_{max} and AUC, respectively, was observed. When used with Kaletra, the lowest possible dose of atorvastatin should be administered. Rosuvastatin is not dependent on CYP3A. However, when given concurrently with Kaletra a mean 5-fold and 2-fold increase in rosuvastatin C_{max} and AUC, respectively, was observed. Caution should be exercised when Kaletra is co-administered with rosuvastatin. Results from an interaction study with Kaletra and pravastatin reveal no clinically significant interaction. The metabolism of pravastatin and fluvastatin is not dependent on CYP3A4, and interactions are not expected with Kaletra. If treatment with a HMG-CoA reductase inhibitor is indicated, pravastatin or fluvastatin is recommended.

Dexamethasone: may induce CYP3A4 and may decrease lopinavir concentrations.

Phosphodiesterase inhibitors: phosphodiesterase inhibitors which are dependent on CYP3A4 metabolism, such as tadalafil and sildenafil, are expected to result in an approximately 2-fold and 11-fold increase in AUC respectively, when co-administered with ritonavir containing regimens including Kaletra and may result in an increase in PDE5 inhibitor associated adverse reactions including hypotension, synope, visual changes and prolonged erection. Particular caution must be used when prescribing sildenafil or tadalafil in patients receiving Kaletra with increased monitoring for adverse events. Co-administration of vardenafil with ritonavir containing regimens including Kaletra is expected to result in 49-fold increase in vardenafil AUC. The use of vardenafil with Kaletra is contraindicated (see section 4.3).

Cyclosporin, sirolimus (rapamycin) and tacrolimus: concentrations may be increased when co-administered with Kaletra. More frequent therapeutic concentration monitoring is recommended until plasma levels of these products have been stabilised.

Ketoconazole and itraconazole: may have serum concentrations increased by Kaletra. High doses of ketoconazole and itraconazole > 200 mg/day) are not recommended.

Voriconazole: due to the potential for reduced voriconazole concentrations, co-administration of voriconazole and low dose ritonavir (100 mg twice daily) as contained in Kaletra should be avoided unless an assessment of the benefit/risk to patient justifies the use of voriconazole.

Clarithromycin: moderate increases in clarithromycin AUC are expected when co-administered with Kaletra. For patients with renal or hepatic impairment dose reduction of clarithromycin should be considered (see section 4.4).

Buprenorphine: buprenorphine (dosed at 16 mg daily) co-administered with lopinavir/ritonavir (dosed at 400/100 mg twice daily) showed no clinically significant interaction. Kaletra can be co-administered with buprenorphine with no dose adjustment.

Methadone: Kaletra was demonstrated to lower plasma concentrations of methadone. Monitoring plasma concentrations of methadone is recommended.

Contraceptives: levels of ethinyl oestradiol were decreased when oestrogen-based oral contraceptives were co-administered with Kaletra. In case of co-administration of Kaletra with contraceptives containing ethinyl oestradiol (whatever the contraceptive formulation e.g. oral or patch), alternative methods of contraception are to be used.

Rifabutin: when rifabutin and Kaletra were co-administered for 10 days, rifabutin (parent substance and active 25-O-desacetyl metabolite) C_{max} and AUC were increased by 3.5- and 5.7-fold, respectively. On the basis of these data, a rifabutin dose reduction of 75% (i.e. 150 mg every other day or 3 times per week) is recommended when administered with Kaletra. Further reduction may be necessary.

Rifampicin: co-administration of Kaletra with rifampicin is not recommended. Rifampicin administered with Kaletra causes large decreases in lopinavir concentrations which may in turn significantly decrease the lopinavir therapeutic effect. A dose adjustment of Kaletra 400 mg/400 mg twice daily has allowed compensating for the CYP 3A4 inducer effect of rifampicin. However, such a dose adjustment might be associated with ALT/AST elevations and with increase in gastrointestinal disorders. Therefore, this co-administration should be avoided unless judged strictly necessary. If this co-administration is judged unavoidable, increased dose of Kaletra at 400 mg/400 mg twice daily may be administered with rifampicin under close safety and therapeutic drug monitoring. The Kaletra dose should be titrated upward only after rifampicin has been initiated (see section 4.4).

St John's wort: serum levels of lopinavir and ritonavir can be reduced by concomitant use of the herbal preparation St John's wort (*Hypericum perforatum)*. This is due to the induction of drug metabolising enzymes by St John's wort. Herbal preparations containing St John's wort should therefore not be combined with lopinavir and ritonavir. If a patient is already taking St John's wort, stop St John's wort and if possible check viral levels. Lopinavir and ritonavir levels may increase on stopping St John's wort. The dose of Kaletra may need adjusting. The inducing effect may persist for at least 2 weeks after cessation of treatment with St John's wort (see section 4.3).

Midazolam: midazolam is extensively metabolised by CYP3A4. Co-administration with Kaletra may cause a large increase in the concentration of this benzodiazepine. A phenotyping cocktail study in 14 healthy volunteers showed an increase of AUC by about 13 fold with oral midazolam and an increase by about 4 fold with parenteral midazolam. Therefore, Kaletra should not be co-administered with orally administered midazolam (see section 4.3), whereas caution should be used with co-administration of Kaletra and parenteral midazolam. If Kaletra is co-administered with parenteral midazolam, it should be done in an intensive care unit (ICU) or similar setting which ensures close clinical monitoring and appropriate medical management in case of respiratory depression and/or prolonged sedation. Dosage adjustment for midazolam should be considered especially if more than a single dose of midazolam is administered.

Fluticasone propionate (interaction with ritonavir): in a clinical study where ritonavir 100 mg capsules twice daily were co – administered with 50 µg intranasal fluticasone propionate (4 times daily) for seven days in healthy subjects, the fluticasone propionate plasma levels increased significantly, whereas the intrinsic cortisol levels decreased by approximately 86% (90% confidence interval 82 – 89%). Greater effects may be expected when fluticasone propionate is inhaled. Systemic corticosteroid effects including Cushing's syndrome and adrenal suppression have been reported in patients receiving ritonavir and inhaled or intranasally administered fluticasone propionate; this could also occur with other corticosteroids metabolised via the P450 3A pathway eg budesonide. Consequently, concomitant administration of Kaletra and these glucocorticoids is not recommended unless the potential benefit of treatment outweighs the risk of systemic corticosteroid effects (see section 4.4). A dose reduction of the glucocorticoid should be considered with close monitoring of local and systemic effects or a switch to a glucocorticoid, which is not a substrate for CYP3A4 (eg beclomethasone). Moreover, in case of withdrawal of glucocorticoids progressive dose reduction may have to be performed over a longer period. The effects of high fluticasone systemic exposure on ritonavir plasma levels is yet unknown.

Based on known metabolic profiles, clinically significant interactions are not expected between Kaletra and fluvastatin, dapsone, trimethoprim/sulfamethoxazole, azithromycin or fluconazole.

4.6 Pregnancy and lactation

There are no data from the use of Kaletra in pregnant women. Studies in animals have shown reproductive toxicity (see section 5.3). The potential risk for humans is unknown. Kaletra should not be used during pregnancy unless clearly necessary.

Studies in rats revealed that lopinavir is excreted in the milk. It is not known whether this medicinal product is excreted in human milk. HIV infected women must not breast-feed their infants under any circumstances to avoid transmission of HIV.

4.7 Effects on ability to drive and use machines

No studies on the effects on the ability to drive and use machines have been performed. Patients should be informed that nausea has been reported during treatment with Kaletra (see section 4.8).

4.8 Undesirable effects

The safety of Kaletra has been investigated in over 1400 patients in Phase II/III clinical trials, of which 888 have received a dose of 400/100 mg (3 capsules or 2 tablets) twice daily and 408 received a dose of 800/200 mg (6 capsules or 4 tablets) once daily. In some studies, Kaletra was used in combination with efavirenz or nevirapine.

The most common adverse reaction associated with Kaletra therapy was diarrhoea and was generally of mild to moderate severity. The risk of diarrhoea may be greater with once daily dosing of Kaletra. Discontinuation due to adverse reactions was 4.5% (naïve patients) and 9% (experienced patients) over a 48 week period.

It is important to note that cases of pancreatitis have been reported in patients receiving Kaletra, including those who developed hypertriglyceridaemia. Furthermore, rare increases in PR interval have been reported during Kaletra therapy (see section 4.4: sections pancreatitis and lipid elevations).

Increased CPK, myalgia, myositis, and rarely, rhabdomyolysis have been reported with protease inhibitors, particularly in combination with nucleoside reverse transcriptase inhibitors.

Combination antiretroviral therapy has been associated with redistribution of body fat (lipodystrophy) in HIV patients including the loss of peripheral and facial subcutaneous fat, increased intra-abdominal and visceral fat, breast hypertrophy and dorsocervical fat accumulation (buffalo hump).

Combination antiretroviral therapy has been associated with metabolic abnormalities such as hypertriglyceridaemia, hypercholesterolaemia, insulin resistance, hyperglycaemia and hyperlactataemia (see section 4.4).

In HIV-infected patients with severe immune deficiency at the time of initiation of combination antiretroviral therapy (CART), an inflammatory reaction to asymptomatic or residual opportunistic infections may arise (see section 4.4).

Adult patients

Adverse reactions:

The following adverse reactions of moderate to severe intensity with possible or probable relationship to Kaletra have been reported. The adverse reactions are displayed by system organ class. Within each frequency grouping, undesirable effects are presented in order of decreasing seriousness: very common (≥ 1/10), common (≥ 1/100 to < 1/10), uncommon (≥ 1/1000 to < 1/100) and rare (≥ 1/10,000 to < 1/1,000).

Undesirable effects in clinical studies in adult patients

System organ class	Frequency	Adverse reaction
Investigations	Very common (Grade 3 or 4)	Blood triglycerides increased, blood cholesterol increased, glutamyltransferase increased
	Common (Grade 3 or 4)	Blood glucose increased, blood amylase increased, aspartate aminotransferase increased, alanine aminotransferase increased, liver function tests abnormal
	Uncommon	Glucose tolerance decreased, blood bilirubin increased, creatinine renal clearance decreased, lipase increased, weight increased, weight decreased, hormone level abnormal, laboratory test abnormal
	Rare	Blood alkaline phosphatase increased
Cardiac disorders	Uncommon	Myocardial infarction[1], palpitations
	Rare	Atrioventricular block
Blood and lymphatic system disorders	Uncommon	Anaemia, leucopenia, lymphadenopathy
	Rare	Splenomegaly
Nervous system disorders	Common	Headache, paresthesia
	Uncommon	Extrapyramidal disorder, migraine, facial palsy, encephalopathy, dizziness, amnesia, coordination abnormal, hypertonia, neuropathy, neuropathy peripheral, somnolence, tremor, ageusia, dysgeusia, dyskinesia
Eye disorders	Uncommon	Visual disturbance
Ear and labyrinth disorders	Uncommon	Tinnitus
	Rare	Vertigo, hyperacusis
Respiratory, thoracic and mediastinal disorders	Uncommon	Pulmonary oedema, dyspnoea, cough
Gastrointestinal disorders	Very common	Diarrhoea
	Common	Nausea, vomiting, abdominal pain, abnormal faeces, dyspepsia, flatulence, gastrointestinal disorder
	Uncommon	Haemorrhagic colitis, pancreatitis[2], enterocolitis, oesophagitis, constipation, faecal incontinence, abdominal distension, gastrooesophageal reflux disease, dry mouth, dysphagia, eructation, gastritis, mouth ulcerations, stomatitis, periodontitis
	Rare	Haemorrhoids

Renal and urinary disorders	Uncommon	Nephrolithiasis, nephritis, albuminuria, hypercalcinuria, urine abnormality
Skin and subcutaneous tissue disorders	Common	Rash, lipodystrophy acquired, acne
	Uncommon	Alopecia, eczema, dermatitis exfoliative, rash maculopapular, dermatitis allergic, dry skin, nail disorder, pruritis, seborrhoea, skin discoloration, skin ulcer, hyperhidrosis, skin striae
	Rare	Idiopathic capillaritis
Musculoskeletal and connective tissue disorders	Uncommon	Arthralgia, osteoarthritis, myalgia, back pain, arthropathy
Endocrine disorders	Uncommon	Cushing syndrome, hypothyroidism, hypogonadism male,
Metabolism and nutrition disorders	Uncommon	Diabetes mellitus, dehydration, lactic acidosis, oedema, increased appetite, obesity, anorexia, hyperglycaemia, hypocholesteremia, lipomatosis, hyperuricaemia, hypovitaminosis
	Rare	Hypophosphataemia, decreased appetite
Infections and infestations	Uncommon	Gastroenteritis, otitis media, bronchitis, sinusitis, sialadenitis, furunculosis, bacterial infection, viral infection, pharyngitis, influenza, rhinitis
	Rare	Cellulitis, folliculitis, perineal abscess
Neoplasms benign, malignant and unspecified (including cysts and polyps)	Uncommon	Benign neoplasm of skin
Vascular disorders	Uncommon	Hypertension, thrombophlebitis, deep vein thrombosis, vasculitis, varicose vein, angiopathy
General disorders and administration site conditions	Common	Asthenia, pain
	Uncommon	Chest pain, chest pain substernal, chills, pyrexia, malaise, oedema peripheral, face oedema, drug interaction, cyst
Immune system disorders	Uncommon	Drug hypersensitivity
	Rare	Immune reconstitution syndrome
Hepatobiliary disorders	Uncommon	Hepatitis, cholecystitis, hepatic steatosis, hepatomegaly, liver tenderness
Reproductive system and breast disorders	Uncommon	Amenorrhoea, menorrhagia, ejaculation disorder, erectile dysfunction, breast enlargement, gynecomastia
Psychiatric disorders	Common	Insomnia
	Uncommon	Agitation, anxiety, confusional state, depression, affect lability, abnormal dreams, decreased libido, nervousness, abnormal thinking

[1] This event had a fatal outcome.

[2] See section 4.4: pancreatitis and lipids

Paediatric patients

In children 2 years of age and older, the nature of the safety profile is similar to that seen in adults.

Undesirable effects in clinical studies in paediatric patients		
Infections and infestations	Common	Viral infection
Nervous system disorders	Common	Taste perversion
Gastrointestinal disorders	Common	Constipation, vomiting, pancreatitis*
Hepatobiliary disorders	Common	Hepatomegaly
Skin and subcutaneous tissue disorders	Common	Rash, dry skin
General disorders and administration site conditions	Common	Fever
Investigations	Common (Grade 3 or 4)	Increased activated partial thromboplastin time, decreased haemoglobin, decreased platelets, increased sodium, increased potassium, increased calcium, increased bilirubin, increased SGPT/ALT, increased SGOT/AST, increased total cholesterol, increased amylase, increased uric acid, decreased sodium, decreased potassium, decreased calcium, decreased neutrophils

* see section 4.4: pancreatitis and lipids

Post marketing experience

Hepatitis, and rarely jaundice, have been reported in patients on Kaletra therapy in the presence or absence of identifiable risk factors for hepatitis.

Stevens-Johnson syndrome and erythema multiforme have been reported.

Cases of osteonecrosis have been reported, particularly in patients with generally acknowledged risk factors, advanced HIV disease or long-term exposure to combination antiretroviral therapy (CART). The frequency of this is unknown (see section 4.4).

4.9 Overdose

To date, there is limited human experience of acute overdose with Kaletra.

The adverse clinical signs observed in dogs included salivation, emesis and diarrhoea/abnormal stool. The signs of toxicity observed in mice, rats or dogs included decreased activity, ataxia, emaciation, dehydration and tremors.

There is no specific antidote for overdose with Kaletra. Treatment of overdose with Kaletra is to consist of general supportive measures including monitoring of vital signs and observation of the clinical status of the patient. If indicated, elimination of unabsorbed active substance is to be achieved by emesis or gastric lavage. Administration of activated charcoal may also be used to aid in removal of unabsorbed active substance. Since Kaletra is highly protein bound, dialysis is unlikely to be beneficial in significant removal of the active substance.

5. PHARMACOLOGICAL PROPERTIES

5.1 Pharmacodynamic properties

Pharmaco-therapeutic group: protease inhibitor, ATC code: J05AE06

Mechanism of action: Lopinavir provides the antiviral activity of Kaletra. Lopinavir is an inhibitor of the HIV-1 and HIV-2 proteases. Inhibition of HIV protease prevents cleavage of the *gag-pol* polyprotein resulting in the production of immature, non-infectious virus.

Effects on the electrocardiogram: QTcF interval was evaluated in a randomised, placebo and active (moxifloxacin 400 mg once daily) controlled crossover study in 39 healthy adults, with 10 measurements over 12 hours on Day 3. The maximum mean (95% upper confidence bound) differences in QTcF from placebo were 3.6 (6.3) and 13.1(15.8) for 400/100 mg twice daily and supratherapeutic 800/200 mg twice daily LPV/r, respectively. The induced QRS interval prolongation from 6 ms to 9.5 ms with high dose lopinavir/ritonavir (800/200 mg twice daily) contributes to QT prolongation. The two regimens resulted in exposures on Day 3 which were approximately 1.5 and 3-fold higher than those observed with recommended once daily or twice daily LPV/r doses at steady state. No subject experienced an increase in QTcF of $\geq$60 msec from baseline or a QTcF interval exceeding the potentially clinically relevant threshold of 500 msec.

Modest prolongation of the PR interval was also noted in subjects receiving lopinavir/ritonavir in the same study on Day 3. The mean changes from baseline in PR interval ranged from 11.6 ms to 24.4 ms in the 12 hour interval post dose. Maximum PR interval was 286 msec and no second or third degree heart block was observed (see section 4.4).

Antiviral activity *in vitro*: the *in vitro* antiviral activity of lopinavir against laboratory and clinical HIV strains was evaluated in acutely infected lymphoblastic cell lines and peripheral blood lymphocytes, respectively. In the absence of human serum, the mean IC_{50} of lopinavir against five different HIV-1 laboratory strains was 19 nM. In the absence and presence of 50% human serum, the mean IC_{50} of lopinavir against $HIV\text{-}1_{IIIB}$ in MT4 cells was 17 nM and 102 nM, respectively. In the absence of human serum, the mean IC_{50}- of lopinavir was 6.5 nM against several HIV-1 clinical isolates.

Resistance

In vitro selection of resistance:

HIV-1 isolates with reduced susceptibility to lopinavir have been selected *in vitro*. HIV-1 has been passaged *in vitro* with lopinavir alone and with lopinavir plus ritonavir at concentration ratios representing the range of plasma concentration ratios observed during Kaletra therapy. Genotypic and phenotypic analysis of viruses selected in these passages suggest that the presence of ritonavir, at these concentration ratios, does not measurably influence the selection of lopinavir-resistant viruses. Overall, the *in vitro* characterisation of phenotypic cross-resistance between lopinavir and other protease inhibitors suggest that decreased susceptibility to lopinavir correlated closely with decreased susceptibility to ritonavir and indinavir, but did not correlate closely with decreased susceptibility to amprenavir, saquinavir, and nelfinavir.

Analysis of resistance in ARV-naïve patients:

In a Phase II study (M97-720) through 204 weeks of treatment, genotypic analysis of viral isolates was successfully conducted in 11 of 16 patients with confirmed HIV RNA above 400 copies/ml revealed no primary or active site mutations in protease (amino acids at positions 8, 30, 32, 46, 47, 48, 50, 82, 84 and 90) or protease inhibitor phenotypic resistance.

In a Phase III study (M98-863) of 653 patients randomised to receive stavudine plus lamivudine with either lopinavir/ritonavir or nelfinavir, 113 nelfinavir-treated subjects and 74 lopinavir/ritonavir-treated subjects had an HIV RNA above 400 copies/ml while on treatment from Week 24 through Week 96. Of these, isolates from 96 nelfinavir-treated subject and 51 lopinavir/ritonavir-treated subjects could be amplified for resistance testing. Resistance to nelfinavir, defined as the presence of the D30N or L90M mutation in protease, was observed in 41/96 (43%) subjects. Resistance to lopinavir, defined as the presence of any primary or active site mutations in protease (see above), was observed in 0/51 (0%) subjects. Lack of resistance to lopinavir was confirmed by phenotypic analysis.

Analysis of resistance in PI-experienced patients:

The selection of resistance to lopinavir in patients having failed prior protease inhibitor therapy was characterised by analysing the longitudinal isolates from 19 protease inhibitor-experienced subjects in 2 Phase II and one Phase III studies who either experienced incomplete virologic suppression or viral rebound subsequent to initial response to Kaletra and who demonstrated incremental in vitro resistance between baseline and rebound (defined as emergence of new mutations or 2-fold change in phenotypic susceptibility to lopinavir). Incremental resistance was most common in subjects whose baseline isolates had several protease inhibitor-associated mutations, but $<$ 40-fold reduced susceptibility to lopinavir at baseline. Mutations V82A, I54V and M46I emerged most frequently. Mutations L33F, I50V and V32I combined with I47V/A were also observed. The 19 isolates demonstrated a 4.3-fold increase in IC_{50} compared to baseline isolates (from 6.2- to 43-fold, compared to wild-type virus).

Genotypic correlates of reduced phenotypic susceptibility to lopinavir in viruses selected by other protease inhibitors. The *in vitro* antiviral activity of lopinavir against 112 clinical isolates taken from patients failing therapy with one or more protease inhibitors was assessed. Within this panel, the following mutations in HIV protease were associated with reduced *in vitro* susceptibility to lopinavir: L10F/I/R/V, K20M/R, L24I, M46I/L, F53L, I54L/T/V, L63P, A71I/L/T/V, V82A/F/T, I84V and L90M. The median EC_{50} of lopinavir against isolates with 0 – 3, 4 – 5, 6 – 7 and 8 – 10 mutations at the above amino acid positions was 0.8, 2.7 13.5 and 44.0-fold higher than the EC_{50} against wild type HIV, respectively. The 16 viruses that displayed $>$ 20-fold change in susceptibility all contained mutations at positions 10, 54, 63 plus 82 and/or 84. In addition, they contained a median of 3 mutations at amino acid positions 20, 24, 46, 53, 71 and 90. In addition to the mutations described above, mutations V32I and I47A have been observed in rebound isolates with reduced lopinavir susceptibility from protease inhibitor experienced patients receiving Kaletra therapy.

In addition to the mutations described above, mutations I47A and L76V have been observed in rebound isolates with reduced lopinavir susceptibility from patients receiving Kaletra therapy.

Conclusions regarding the relevance of particular mutations or mutational patterns are subject to change with additional data, and it is recommended to always consult current interpretation systems for analysing resistance test results.

Antiviral activity of Kaletra in patients failing protease inhibitor therapy: the clinical relevance of reduced *in vitro* susceptibility to lopinavir has been examined by assessing the virologic response to Kaletra therapy, with respect to baseline viral genotype and phenotype, in 56 patients previous failing therapy with multiple protease inhibitors. The EC_{50} of lopinavir against the 56 baseline viral isolates ranged from 0.6 to 96-fold higher than the EC_{50} against wild type HIV. After 48 weeks of treatment with Kaletra, efavirenz and nucleoside reverse transcriptase inhibitors, plasma HIV RNA $\leqslant$ 400 copies/ml was observed in 93% (25/27), 73% (11/15), and 25% (2/8) of patients with < 10-fold, 10 to 40-fold, and > 40-fold reduced susceptibility to lopinavir at baseline, respectively. In addition, virologic response was observed in 91% (21/23), 71% (15/21) and 33% (2/6) patients with 0 – 5, 6 – 7, and 8 – 10 mutations of the above mutations in HIV protease associated with reduced *in vitro* susceptibility to lopinavir. Since these patients had not previously been exposed to either Kaletra or efavirenz, part of the response may be attributed to the antiviral activity of efavirenz, particularly in patients harbouring highly lopinavir resistant virus. The study did not contain a control arm of patients not receiving Kaletra.

Cross-resistance: Activity of other protease inhibitors against isolates that developed incremental resistance to lopinavir after Kaletra therapy in protease inhibitor experienced patients: The presence of cross resistance to other protease inhibitors was analysed in 18 rebound isolates that had demonstrated evolution of resistance to lopinavir during 3 Phase II and one Phase III studies of Kaletra in protease inhibitor-experienced patients. The median fold IC_{50} of lopinavir for these 18 isolates at baseline and rebound was 6.9- and 63-fold, respectively, compared to wild type virus. In general, rebound isolates either retained (if cross-resistant at baseline) or developed significant cross-resistance to indinavir, saquinavir and atazanavir. Modest decreases in amprenavir activity were noted with a median increase of IC_{50} from 3.7- to 8-fold in the baseline and rebound isolates, respectively. Isolates retained susceptibility to tipranavir with a median increase of IC_{50} in baseline and rebound isolates of 1.9- and 1.8–fold, respectively, compared to wild type virus. Please refer to the Aptivus Summary of Product Characteristics for additional information on the use of tipranavir, including genotypic predictors of response, in treatment of lopinavir-resistant HIV-1 infection.

Clinical pharmacodynamic data

The effects of Kaletra (in combination with other antiretroviral agents) on biological markers (plasma HIV RNA levels and CD_4 counts) have been investigated in a controlled study of Kaletra of 48 weeks duration, and in additional studies of Kaletra of 360 weeks duration.

Adult Use

Patients without prior antiretroviral therapy

Study M98-863 is a randomised, double-blind trial of 653 antiretroviral treatment naïve patients investigating Kaletra (400/100 mg twice daily) compared to nelfinavir (750 mg three times daily) plus nucleoside reverse transcriptase inhibitors. By intent to treat analysis where patients with missing values are considered virologic failures, the proportion of patients at 48 weeks with HIV RNA < 400 copies/ml in the Kaletra arm was 75% and 63% in the nelfinavir arm. Mean baseline CD_4 cell count was 259 cells/mm^3 (range: 2 to 949 cells/ mm^3) and mean baseline plasma HIV-1 RNA was 4.9 $\log_{10}$ copies/ml (range: 2.6 to 6.8 $\log_{10}$ copies/ml). Through 48 weeks of therapy, the proportion of patients in the Kaletra arm with plasma RNA < 50 copies/ml was 67% and 52% in the nelfinavir arm. The mean increase from baseline in CD_4 cell count was 207 cells/mm^3 in the Kaletra arm and 195 cells/mm^3 in the nelfinavir arm. Through 48 weeks of therapy, a statistically significantly higher proportion of patients in the Kaletra arm had HIV RNA < 50 copies/ml compared to the nelfinavir arm.

Study M05-730 was a randomised, open-label, multicentre trial comparing treatment with Kaletra 800/200 mg once daily plus tenofovir DF and emtricitabine versus Kaletra 400/100 mg twice daily plus tenofovir DF and emtricitabine in 664 antiretroviral treatment-naïve patients. Given the pharmacokinetic interaction between Kaletra and tenofovir (see section 4.5), the results of this study might not be strictly extrapolable when other backbone regimens are used with Kaletra. Patients were randomised in a 1:1 ratio to receive either Kaletra 800/200 mg once daily (n = 333) or Kaletra 400/100 mg twice daily (n = 331). Further stratification within each group was 1:1 (tablet versus. soft capsule). Patients were administered either the tablet or the soft capsule formulation for 8 weeks, after which all patients were administered the tablet formulation once daily or twice daily for the remainder of the study. Patients were administered emtricitabine 200 mg once daily and tenofovir DF 300 mg once daily. Protocol defined non-inferiority of once daily dosing compared with twice daily dosing was demonstrated if the lower bound of the 95% confidence interval for the difference in proportion of subjects responding (once dialy minus twice daily) excluded -12% at Week 48. Mean age of patients enrolled was 39 years (range: 19 to 71); 75% were Caucasian, and 78% were male. Mean baseline CD4+ cell count was 216 cells/mm3 (range: 20 to 775 cells/mm^3) and mean baseline plasma HIV-1 RNA was 5.0 $\log_{10}$ copies/ml (range: 1.7 to 7.0 $\log_{10}$ copies/ml).

(see Table 1 below)

Sustained virological response to Kaletra (in combination with nucleoside/nucleotide reverse transcriptase inhibitors) has been also observed in a small Phase II study (M97-720) through 360 weeks of treatment. One hundred patients were originally treated with Kaletra in the study (including 51 patients receiving 400/100 mg twice daily and 49 patients at either 200/100 mg twice daily or 400/200 mg twice daily). All patients converted to open-label Kaletra at the 400/100 mg twice daily dose between week 48 and week 72. Sixty-one patients completed the study (35 patients received the recommended 400/100 mg twice daily dose throughout the study). Through 360 weeks of treatment, the proportion of patients with HIV RNA < 400 (< 50) copies/ml was 61% (59%), and the corresponding mean increase in CD_4 cell count was 501 cells/mm^3. Thirty-nine patients (39%) discontinued the study, including 16 (16%) discontinuations due to adverse events, one of which was associated with a death.

Patients with prior antiretroviral therapy

Study M97-765 is a randomised, double-blind trial evaluating Kaletra at two dose levels (400/100 mg and 400/200 mg, both twice daily) plus nevirapine (200 mg twice daily) and two nucleoside reverse transcriptase inhibitors in 70 single protease inhibitor experienced, non-nucleoside reverse transcriptase inhibitor naïve patients. Median baseline CD_4 cell count was 349 cells/mm^3 (range 72 to 807 cells/mm^3) and median baseline plasma HIV-1 RNA was 4.0 $\log_{10}$ copies/ml (range 2.9 to 5.8 $\log_{10}$ copies/ml). By intent to treat analysis where patients with missing values are considered virologic failures, the proportion of patients with HIV RNA < 400 (< 50) copies/ml at 24 weeks was 75% (58%) and the mean increase from baseline in CD_4 cell count was 174 cells/mm^3 for the 36 patients receiving the 400/100 mg dose of Kaletra.

M98-957 is a randomised, open-label study evaluating Kaletra treatment at two dose levels (400/100 mg and 533/133 mg, both twice daily) plus efavirenz (600 mg once daily) and nucleoside reverse transcriptase inhibitors in 57 multiple protease inhibitor experienced, non-nucleoside reverse transcriptase inhibitor naïve patients. Between week 24 and 48, patients randomised to a dose of 400/100 mg were converted to a dose of 533/133 mg. Median baseline CD_4 cell count was 220 cells/mm^3 (range 13 to 1030 cells/mm^3). By intent-to-treat analysis of both dose groups combined (n=57), where patients with missing values are considered virologic failures, the proportion of patients with HIV RNA < 400 copies/ml at 48 weeks was 65% and the mean increase from baseline CD_4 cell count was 94 cells/mm^3.

Paediatric Use

M98-940 is an open-label study of a liquid formulation of Kaletra in 100 antiretroviral naïve (44%) and experienced (56%) paediatric patients. All patients were non-nucleoside reverse transcriptase inhibitor naïve. Patients were randomised to either 230 mg lopinavir/57.5 mg ritonavir per m^2 or 300 mg lopinavir/75 mg ritonavir per m^2. Naïve patients also received nucleoside reverse transcriptase inhibitors. Experienced patients received nevirapine plus up to two nucleoside reverse transcriptase inhibitors. Safety, efficacy and pharmacokinetic profiles of the two dose regimens were assessed after 3 weeks of therapy in each patient. Subsequently, all patients were continued on the 300/75 mg per m^2 dose. Patients had a mean age of 5 years (range 6 months to 12 years) with 14 patients less than 2 years old and 6 patients one year or less. Mean baseline CD_4 cell count was 838 cells/mm^3 and mean baseline plasma HIV-1 RNA was 4.7 $\log_{10}$ copies/ml. Through 48 weeks of therapy, the proportion of patients with HIV RNA < 400 copies/ml was 84% for antiretroviral naïve patients and 75% for antiretroviral experienced patients and the mean increases from baseline in CD_4 cell count were 404 cells/mm^3 and 284 cells/mm^3 respectively.

5.2 Pharmacokinetic properties

The pharmacokinetic properties of lopinavir co-administered with ritonavir have been evaluated in healthy adult volunteers and in HIV-infected patients; no substantial differences were observed between the two groups. Lopinavir is essentially completely metabolised by CYP3A. Ritonavir inhibits the metabolism of lopinavir, thereby increasing the plasma levels of lopinavir. Across studies, administration of Kaletra 400/100 mg twice daily yields mean steady-state lopinavir plasma concentrations 15 to 20-fold higher than those of ritonavir in HIV-infected patients. The plasma levels of ritonavir are less than 7% of those obtained after the ritonavir dose of 600 mg twice daily. The *in vitro* antiviral EC_{50} of lopinavir is approximately 10-fold lower than that of ritonavir. Therefore, the antiviral activity of Kaletra is due to lopinavir.

Absorption: multiple dosing with 400/100 mg Kaletra twice daily for 2 weeks and without meal restriction produced a mean ± SD lopinavir peak plasma concentration (C_{max}) of 12.3 ± 5.4 μg/ml, occurring approximately 4 hours after administration. The mean steady-state trough concentration prior to the morning dose was 8.1 ± 5.7 μg/ml. Lopinavir AUC over a 12 hour dosing interval averaged 113.2 ± 60.5 μg•h/ml. The absolute bioavailability of lopinavir co-formulated with ritonavir in humans has not been established.

Effects of food on oral absorption*:* Administration of a single 400/100 mg dose of Kaletra tablets under fed conditions (high fat, 872 kcal, 56% from fat) compared to fasted state was associated with no significant changes in C_{max} and AUC_{inf}. Therefore, Kaletra tablets may be taken with or without food. Kaletra tablets have also shown less pharmacokinetic variability under all meal conditions compared to Kaletra soft capsules.

Distribution: at steady state, lopinavir is approximately 98 – 99% bound to serum proteins. Lopinavir binds to both alpha-1-acid glycoprotein (AAG) and albumin, however, it has a higher affinity for AAG. At steady state, lopinavir protein binding remains constant over the range of observed concentrations after 400/100 mg Kaletra twice daily, and is similar between healthy volunteers and HIV-positive patients.

Metabolism: *in vitro* experiments with human hepatic microsomes indicate that lopinavir primarily undergoes oxidative metabolism. Lopinavir is extensively metabolised by the hepatic cytochrome P450 system, almost exclusively by isozyme CYP3A. Ritonavir is a potent CYP3A inhibitor which inhibits the metabolism of lopinavir and therefore, increases plasma levels of lopinavir. A ^{14}C-lopinavir study in humans showed that 89% of the plasma radioactivity after a single 400/100 mg Kaletra dose was due to parent active substance. At least 13 lopinavir oxidative metabolites have been identified in man. The 4-oxo and 4-hydroxymetabolite epimeric pair are the major metabolites with antiviral activity, but comprise only minute amounts of total plasma radioactivity. Ritonavir has been shown to induce metabolic enzymes, resulting in the induction of its own metabolism, and likely the induction of lopinavir metabolism. Pre-dose lopinavir concentrations decline with time during multiple dosing, stabilising after approximately 10 days to 2 weeks.

Elimination: after a 400/100 mg ^{14}C-lopinavir/ritonavir dose, approximately 10.4 ± 2.3% and 82.6 ± 2.5% of an administered dose of ^{14}C-lopinavir can be accounted for in urine and faeces, respectively. Unchanged lopinavir accounted for approximately 2.2% and 19.8% of the administered dose in urine and faeces, respectively. After multiple dosing, less than 3% of the lopinavir dose is excreted unchanged in the urine. The effective (peak to trough) half-life of lopinavir over a 12 hour dosing interval averaged 5 – 6 hours, and the apparent oral clearance (CL/F) of lopinavir is 6 to 7 l/h.

Once daily dosing: the pharmacokinetics of once daily Kaletra have been evaluated in HIV-infected subjects naïve to antiretroviral treatment. Kaletra 800/200 mg was administered in combination with emtricitabine 200 mg and tenofovir DF 300 mg as part of a once daily regimen. Multiple dosing of 800/200 mg Kaletra once daily for 2 weeks without meal restriction (n=16) produced a mean ± SD lopinavir peak plasma concentration (C_{max}) of 14.8 ± 3.5 μg/ml, occurring approximately 6 hours after administration. The mean steady-state trough concentration prior to the morning dose was 5.5 ± 5.4 μg/ml. Lopinavir AUC over a 24 hour dosing interval averaged 206.5 ± 89.7 μg·h/ml.

Table 1

Virologic Response of Study Subjects at Week 48 and Week 96

	Week 48			Week 96		
	QD	BID	Difference [95% CI]	QD	BID	Difference [95% CI]
NC= Failure	257/333 (77.2%)	251/331 (75.8%)	1.3 % [-5.1, 7.8]	216/333 (64.9%)	229/331 (69.2%)	-4.3% [-11.5, 2.8]
Observed data	257/295 (87.1%)	250/280 (89.3%)	-2.2% [-7.4, 3.1]	216/247 (87.4%)	229/248 (92.3%)	-4.9% [-10.2, 0.4]

As compared to the BID regimen, the once daily dosing is associated with a reduction in the C_{min}/C_{trough} values of approximately 50%.

Special Populations

Paediatrics:

There are limited pharmacokinetic data in children below 2 years of age. The pharmacokinetics of Kaletra oral solution 300/75 mg/m² twice daily and 230/57.5 mg/m² twice daily have been studied in a total of 53 paediatric patients, ranging in age from 6 months to 12 years. The lopinavir mean steady-state AUC, C_{max}, and C_{min} were 72.6 ± 31.1 μg•h/ml, 8.2 ± 2.9 μg/ml and 3.4 ± 2.1 μg/ml, respectively after Kaletra oral solution 230/57.5 mg/m² twice daily without nevirapine (n=12), and were 85.8 ± 36.9 μg•h/ml, 10.0 ± 3.3 μg/ml and 3.6 ± 3.5 μg/ml, respectively after 300/75 mg/m² twice daily with nevirapine (n=12). The 230/57.5 mg/m² twice daily regimen without nevirapine and the 300/75 mg/m² twice daily regimen with nevirapine provided lopinavir plasma concentrations similar to those obtained in adult patients receiving the 400/100 mg twice daily regimen without nevirapine. Kaletra once daily has not been evaluated in paediatric patients.

Gender, Race and Age:

Kaletra pharmacokinetics have not been studied in the elderly. No age or gender related pharmacokinetic differences have been observed in adult patients. Pharmacokinetic differences due to race have not been identified.

Renal Insufficiency:

Kaletra pharmacokinetics have not been studied in patients with renal insufficiency; however, since the renal clearance of lopinavir is negligible, a decrease in total body clearance is not expected in patients with renal insufficiency.

Hepatic Insufficiency:

The steady state pharmacokinetic parameters of lopinavir in HIV-infected patients with mild to moderate hepatic impairment were compared with those of HIV-infected patients with normal hepatic function in a multiple dose study with lopinavir/ritonavir 400/100 mg twice daily. A limited increase in total lopinavir concentrations of approximately 30% has been observed which is not expected to be of clinical relevance (see section 4.2).

5.3 Preclinical safety data

Repeat-dose toxicity studies in rodents and dogs identified major target organs as the liver, kidney, thyroid, spleen and circulating red blood cells. Hepatic changes indicated cellular swelling with focal degeneration. While exposure eliciting these changes were comparable to or below human clinical exposure, dosages in animals were over 6-fold the recommended clinical dose. Mild renal tubular degeneration was confined to mice exposed with at least twice the recommended human exposure; the kidney was unaffected in rats and dogs. Reduced serum thyroxin led to an increased release of TSH with resultant follicular cell hypertrophy in the thyroid glands of rats. These changes were reversible with withdrawal of the active substance and were absent in mice and dogs. Coombs-negative anisocytosis and poikilocytosis were observed in rats, but not in mice or dogs. Enlarged spleens with histiocytosis were seen in rats but not other species. Serum cholesterol was elevated in rodents but not dogs, while triglycerides were elevated only in mice.

During *in vitro* studies, cloned human cardiac potassium channels (HERG) were inhibited by 30% at the highest concentrations of lopinavir/ritonavir tested, corresponding to a lopinavir exposure 7-fold total and 15-fold free peak plasma levels achieved in humans at the maximum recommended therapeutic dose. In contrast, similar concentrations of lopinavir/ritonavir demonstrated no repolarisation delay in the canine cardiac Purkinje fibres. Lower concentrations of lopinavir/ritonavir did not produce significant potassium (HERG) current blockade. Tissue distribution studies conducted in the rat did not suggest significant cardiac retention of the active substance; 72-hour AUC in heart was approximately 50% of measured plasma AUC. Therefore, it is reasonable to expect that cardiac lopinavir levels would not be significantly higher than plasma levels.

In dogs, prominent U waves on the electrocardiogram have been observed associated with prolonged PR interval and bradycardia. These effects have been assumed to be caused by electrolyte disturbance.

The clinical relevance of these preclinical data is unknown, however, the potential cardiac effects of this product in humans cannot be ruled out (see also sections 4.4 and 4.8).

In rats, embryofoetotoxicity (pregnancy loss, decreased foetal viability, decreased foetal body weights, increased frequency of skeletal variations) and postnatal developmental toxicity (decreased survival of pups) was observed at maternally toxic dosages. The systemic exposure to lopinavir/ritonavir at the maternal and developmental toxic dosages was lower than the intended therapeutic exposure in humans.

Long-term carcinogenicity studies of lopinavir/ritonavir in mice revealed a nongenotoxic, mitogenic induction of liver tumours, generally considered to have little relevance to human risk.

Carcinogenicity studies in rats revealed no tumourigenic findings. Lopinavir/ritonavir was not found to be mutagenic or clastogenic in a battery of *in vitro* and *in vivo* assays including the Ames bacterial reverse mutation assay, the mouse lymphoma assay, the mouse micronucleus test and chromosomal aberration assays in human lymphocytes.

6. PHARMACEUTICAL PARTICULARS

6.1 List of excipients

Tablet contents:

Copovidone

Sorbitan laurate

Colloidal anhydrous silica

Sodium stearyl fumarate

Film-coating:

Hypromellose

Titanium dioxide

Macrogols type 400 (Polyethylene glycol 400)

Hydroxypropyl cellulose

Talc

Colloidal anhydrous silica

Macrogols type 3350 (Polyethylene glycol 3350)

Yellow ferric oxide E172

Polysorbate 80

6.2 Incompatibilities

Not applicable.

6.3 Shelf life

3 years.

6.4 Special precautions for storage

This medicinal product does not require any special storage conditions.

6.5 Nature and contents of container

High density polyethylene (HDPE) bottles closed with propylene caps. Each bottle contains 120 tablets. Each pack contains 1 bottle (120 tablets).

Blisters consisting of PVC/fluoropolymer foil. Each carton contains 5 foil blisters each containing 8 film-coated tablets (40 tablets). Each pack contains 3 cartons (120 tablets).

6.6 Special precautions for disposal and other handling

No special requirements.

7. MARKETING AUTHORISATION HOLDER

Abbott Laboratories Limited

Queenborough

Kent ME11 5EL

United Kingdom

8. MARKETING AUTHORISATION NUMBER(S)

EU/1/01/172/004

EU/1/01/172/005

9. DATE OF FIRST AUTHORISATION/RENEWAL OF THE AUTHORISATION

Date of first authorisation: 20 March 2001

Date of last renewal: 20 March 2006

10. DATE OF REVISION OF THE TEXT

21 August 2009

Kaletra 80mg/20mg Oral Solution

(Abbott Laboratories Limited)

1. NAME OF THE MEDICINAL PRODUCT

Kaletra (80 mg + 20 mg) / ml oral solution

2. QUALITATIVE AND QUANTITATIVE COMPOSITION

Each 5 ml of Kaletra oral solution contains 400 mg of lopinavir co-formulated with 100 mg of ritonavir as a pharmacokinetic enhancer.

Name of the	Quantity per ml
- active substance	
Lopinavir	80 mg
Ritonavir	20 mg
- excipient (s)	
Alcohol (42% v/v)	356.3 mg
High fructose corn syrup	168.6 mg
Propylene glycol	152.7 mg
Glycerol	59.6 mg
Polyoxyl 40 hydrogenated castor oil	10.2 mg
Acesulfame potassium	4.1 mg

For a full list of excipients, see section 6.1.

3. PHARMACEUTICAL FORM

Oral solution

The solution is light yellow to golden.

4. CLINICAL PARTICULARS

4.1 Therapeutic indications

Kaletra is indicated for the treatment of HIV-1 infected adults and children above the age of 2 years, in combination with other antiretroviral agents.

Most experience with Kaletra is derived from the use of the product in antiretroviral therapy naïve patients. Data in heavily pretreated protease inhibitor experienced patients are limited. There are limited data on salvage therapy on patients who have failed therapy with Kaletra.

The choice of Kaletra to treat protease inhibitor experienced HIV-1 infected patients should be based on individual viral resistance testing and treatment history of patients (see sections 4.4 and 5.1).

4.2 Posology and method of administration

Kaletra should be prescribed by physicians who are experienced in the treatment of HIV infection.

Adult and adolescent use: the recommended dosage of Kaletra is 5 ml of oral solution (400/100 mg) twice daily taken with food.

Paediatric use (2 years of age and above): the recommended dosage of Kaletra is 230/57.5 mg/m² twice daily taken with food, up to a maximum dose of 400/100 mg twice daily. The 230/57.5 mg/m² dosage might be insufficient in some children when co-administered with nevirapine or efavirenz. An increase of the dose of Kaletra to 300/75 mg/m² should be considered in these patients. Dose should be administered using a calibrated oral dosing syringe.

The oral solution is the recommended option for the most accurate dosing in children based on body surface area. However, if it is judged necessary to resort to soft capsules in children, they should be used with particular caution since they are associated with less precise dosing capabilities. Therefore, children receiving soft capsules might have higher exposure (with the risk of increased toxicity) or suboptinal exposure (with the risk of insufficient efficacy). Consequently when dosing children with soft capsules, therapeutic drug monitoring may be a useful tool to ensure appropriate lopinavir exposure in an individual patient.

Paediatric Dosing Guidelines for the Dose 230/57.5 mg/m²		
Body Surface Area* (m²)	**Twice Daily Oral Solution Dose (dose in mg)**	**Twice Daily Soft Capsule Dose (dose in mg)**
0.25	0.7 ml (57.5/14.4 mg)	NA
0.40	1.2 ml (96/24 mg)	1 soft capsule (133.3/33.3 mg)
0.50	1.4 ml (115/28.8 mg)	1 soft capsule (133.3/33.3 mg)
0.75	2.2 ml (172.5/43.1 mg)	1 soft capsule (133.3/33.3 mg)
0.80	2.3 ml (184/46 mg)	2 soft capsules (266.6/66/6 mg)
1.00	2.9 ml (230/57.5 mg)	2 soft capsules (266.6/66/6 mg)
1.25	3.6 ml (287.5/71.9 mg)	2 soft capsules (266.6/66/6 mg)
1.3	3.7 ml (299/74.8 mg)	2 soft capsules (266.6/66/6 mg)
1.4	4.0 ml (322/80.5 mg)	3 soft capsules (400/100 mg)
1.5	4.3 ml (345/86.3 mg)	3 soft capsules (400/100 mg)
1.7	5 ml (402.5/100.6 mg)	3 soft capsules (400/100 mg)

* Body surface area can be calculated with the following equation

BSA (m²) = √ (Height (cm) X Weight (kg) / 3600)

Children less than 2 years of age: Kaletra is not recommended for use in children below 2 years of age due to insufficient data on safety and efficacy (see section 5.1). Paediatric patients should switch from Kaletra oral solution to soft capsules as soon as they are able to swallow the capsule formulation (see section 4.4).

Hepatic impairment: In HIV-infected patients with mild to moderate hepatic impairment, an increase of approximately 30% in lopinavir exposure has been observed but is not expected to be of clinical relevance. (see section 5.2). No data are available in patients with severe hepatic impairment. Kaletra should not be given to these patients (see section 4.3).

Renal impairment: No dose adjustment is necessary in patients with renal impairment. Caution is warranted when

Kaletra is used in patients with severe renal impairment (see section 4.4).

4.3 Contraindications

Patients with known hypersensitivity to lopinavir, ritonavir or any of the excipients.

Patients with severe hepatic insufficiency.

Kaletra contains lopinavir and ritonavir, both of which are inhibitors of the P450 isoform CYP3A. Kaletra should not be co-administered with medicinal products that are highly dependent on CYP3A for clearance and for which elevated plasma concentrations are associated with serious and/or life threatening events. These medicinal products include astemizole, terfenadine, oral midazolam (for caution on parenterally administered midazolam, see section 4.5), triazolam, cisapride, pimozide, amiodarone, ergot alkaloids (e.g. ergotamine, dihydroergotamine and ergonovine and methylergonovine) and vardenafil.

Herbal preparations containing St John's wort (*Hypericum perforatum*) must not be used while taking lopinavir and ritonavir due to the risk of decreased plasma concentrations and reduced clinical effects of lopinavir and ritonavir (see section 4.5).

Kaletra oral solution is contraindicated in children below the age of 2 years, pregnant women, patients with hepatic or renal failure and patients treated with disulfiram or metronidazole due to the potential risk of toxicity from the excipient propylene glycol (see section 4.4).

4.4 Special warnings and precautions for use

Patients with coexisting conditions

Hepatic impairment: the safety and efficacy of Kaletra has not been established in patients with significant underlying liver disorders. Kaletra is contraindicated in patients with severe liver impairment (see section 4.3). Patients with chronic hepatitis B or C and treated with combination antiretroviral therapy are at an increased risk for severe and potentially fatal hepatic adverse reactions. In case of concomitant antiviral therapy for hepatitis B or C, please refer to the relevant product information for these medicinal products.

Patients with pre-existing liver dysfunction including chronic hepatitis have an increased frequency of liver function abnormalities during combination antiretroviral therapy and should be monitored according to standard practice. If there is evidence of worsening liver disease in such patients, interruption or discontinuation of treatment should be considered.

Renal impairment: since the renal clearance of lopinavir and ritonavir is negligible, increased plasma concentrations are not expected in patients with renal impairment. Because lopinavir and ritonavir are highly protein bound, it is unlikely that they will be significantly removed by haemodialysis or peritoneal dialysis.

Haemophilia: there have been reports of increased bleeding, including spontaneous skin haematomas and haemarthrosis in patients with haemophilia type A and B treated with protease inhibitors. In some patients additional factor VIII was given. In more than half of the reported cases, treatment with protease inhibitors was continued or reintroduced if treatment had been discontinued. A causal relationship had been evoked, although the mechanism of action had not been elucidated. Haemophiliac patients should therefore be made aware of the possibility of increased bleeding.

Lipid elevations

Treatment with Kaletra has resulted in increases, sometimes marked, in the concentration of total cholesterol and triglycerides. Triglyceride and cholesterol testing is to be performed prior to initiating Kaletra therapy and at periodic intervals during therapy. Particular caution should be paid to patients with high values at baseline and with history of lipid disorders. Lipid disorders are to be managed as clinically appropriate (see also section 4.5 for additional information on potential interactions with HMG-CoA reductase inhibitors).

Pancreatitis

Cases of pancreatitis have been reported in patients receiving Kaletra, including those who developed hypertriglyceridaemia. In most of these cases patients have had a prior history of pancreatitis and/or concurrent therapy with other medicinal products associated with pancreatitis. Marked triglyceride elevation is a risk factor for development of pancreatitis. Patients with advanced HIV disease may be at risk of elevated triglycerides and pancreatitis.

Pancreatitis should be considered if clinical symptoms (nausea, vomiting, abdominal pain) or abnormalities in laboratory values (such as increased serum lipase or amylase values) suggestive of pancreatitis should occur. Patients who exhibit these signs or symptoms should be evaluated and Kaletra therapy should be suspended if a diagnosis of pancreatitis is made (see section 4.8).

Hyperglycaemia

New onset diabetes mellitus, hyperglycaemia or exacerbation of existing diabetes mellitus has been reported in patients receiving protease inhibitors. In some of these the hyperglycaemia was severe and in some cases also associated with ketoacidosis. Many patients had confounding medical conditions some of which required therapy with agents that have been associated with the development of diabetes mellitus or hyperglycaemia.

Fat redistribution & metabolic disorders

Combination antiretroviral therapy has been associated with redistribution of body fat (lipodystrophy) in HIV patients. The long-term consequences of these events are currently unknown. Knowledge about the mechanism is incomplete. A connection between visceral lipomatosis and protease inhibitors (PIs) and lipoatrophy and nucleoside reverse transcriptase inhibitors (NRTIs) has been hypothesised. A higher risk of lipodystrophy has been associated with individual factors such as older age, and with drug related factors such as longer duration of antiretroviral treatment and associated metabolic disturbances. Clinical examination should include evaluation for physical signs of fat redistribution. Consideration should be given to measurement of fasting serum lipids and blood glucose. Lipid disorders should be managed as clinically appropriate (see section 4.8).

Immune Reactivation Syndrome

In HIV-infected patients with severe immune deficiency at the time of institution of combination antiretroviral therapy (CART), an inflammatory reaction to asymtomatic or residual opportunistic pathogens may arise and cause serious clinical conditions, or aggravation of symptoms. Typically, such reactions have been observed within the first few weeks or months of initiation of CART. Relevant examples are cytomegalovirus retinitis, generalised and/or focal mycobacterial infections, and Pneumocystis carinii pneumonia. Any inflammatory symptoms should be evaluated and treatment instituted when necessary.

Osteonecrosis

Although the etiology is considered to be multifactorial (including corticosteroid use, alcohol consumption, severe immunosuppression, higher body mass index), cases of osteonecrosis have been reported particularly in patients with advanced HIV-disease and/or long-term exposure to combination antiretroviral therapy (CART). Patients should be advised to seek medical advice if they experience joint aches and pain, joint stiffness or difficulty in movement.

PR interval prolongation

Lopinavir/ritonavir has been shown to cause modest asymptomatic prolongation of the PR interval in some healthy adult subjects. Rare reports of 2nd or 3rd degree atroventricular block in patients with underlying structural heart disease and pre-existing conduction system abnormalities or in patients receiving drugs known to prolong the PR interval (such as verapamil or atazanavir) have been reported in patients receiving lopinavir/ritonavir. Kaletra should be used with caution in such patients (see section 5.1).

Interactions with medicinal products

Kaletra contains lopinavir and ritonavir, both of which are inhibitors of the P450 isoform CYP3A. Kaletra is likely to increase plasma concentrations of medicinal products that are primarily metabolised by CYP3A. These increases of plasma concentrations of co-administered medicinal products could increase or prolong their therapeutic effect and adverse events (see sections 4.3 and 4.5).

The HMG-CoA reductase inhibitors simvastatin and lovastatin are highly dependent on CYP3A for metabolism, thus concomitant use of Kaletra with simvastatin or lovastatin is not recommended due to an increased risk of myopathy including rhabdomyolysis. Caution must also be exercised and reduced doses should be considered if Kaletra is used concurrently with rosuvastatin or with atorvastatin, which is metabolised to a lesser extent by CYP3A4. If treatment with an HMG-CoA reductase inhibitor is indicated, pravastatin or fluvastatin is recommended (see section 4.5).

Particular caution must be used when prescribing Kaletra and medicinal products known to induce QT interval prolongation such as: chlorpheniramine, quinidine, erythromycin, clarithromycin. Indeed, Kaletra could increase concentrations of the co-administered medicinal products and this may result in an increase of their associated cardiac adverse events. Cardiac events have been reported with Kaletra in preclinical studies; therefore, the potential cardiac effects of Kaletra cannot be currently ruled out (see sections 4.8 and 5.3).

Co-administration of Kaletra with rifampicin is not recommended. Rifampicin in combination with Kaletra causes large decreases in lopinavir concentrations which may in turn significantly decrease the lopinavir therapeutic effect. Adequate exposure to lopinavir/ritonavir may be achieved when a higher dose of Kaletra is used but this is associated with a higher risk of liver and gastrointestinal toxicity. Therefore, this co-administration should be avoided unless judged strictly necessary (see section 4.5).

Other

Patients taking the oral solution, particularly those with renal impairment or with decreased ability to metabolise propylene glycol (e.g. those of Asian origin), should be monitored for adverse reactions potentially related to propylene glycol toxicity (i.e. seizures, stupor, tachycardia, hyperosmolarity, lactic acidosis, renal toxicity, haemolysis) (see section 4.3).

Kaletra is not a cure for HIV infection or AIDS. It does not reduce the risk of passing HIV to others through sexual contact or contamination with blood. Appropriate precautions should be taken. People taking Kaletra may still develop infections or other illnesses associated with HIV disease and AIDS.

There are limited data on salvage therapy on patients who have failed with Kaletra. There are ongoing studies to further establish the usefulness of potential salvage therapy regimens (e.g. amprenavir or saquinavir). There are currently limited data on the use of Kaletra in protease inhibitor-experienced patients.

Besides propylene glycol as described above, Kaletra oral solution contains alcohol (42% v/v) which is potentially harmful for those suffering from liver disease, alcoholism, epilepsy, brain injury or disease as well as for pregnant women and children. It may modify or increase the effects of other medicines. Kaletra oral solution contains up to 0.8 g of fructose per dose when taken according to the dosage recommendations. This may be unsuitable in hereditary fructose intolerance. Kaletra oral solution contains up to 0.3 g of glycerol per dose. Only at high inadvertent doses, it can cause headache and gastrointestinal upset. Furthermore, polyoxol 40 hydrogenated castor oil and potassium present in Kaletra oral solution may cause only at high inadvertent doses gastrointestinal upset. Patients on a low potassium diet should be cautioned.

Concomitant use of Kaletra and fluticasone or other glucocorticoids that are metabolised by CYP3A4 is not recommended unless the potential benefit of treatment outweighs the risk of systemic corticosteroid effects, including Cushing's syndrome and adrenal suppression (see section 4.5).

4.5 Interaction with other medicinal products and other forms of interaction

Kaletra contains lopinavir and ritonavir, both of which are inhibitors of the P450 isoform CYP3A *in vitro*. Co-administration of Kaletra and medicinal products primarily metabolised by CYP3A may result in increased plasma concentrations of the other medicinal product, which could increase or prolong its therapeutic and adverse reactions. Kaletra does not inhibit CYP2D6, CYP2C9, CYP2C19, CYP2E1, CYP2B6 or CYP1A2 at clinically relevant concentrations (see section 4.3).

Kaletra has been shown *in vivo* to induce its own metabolism and to increase the biotransformation of some medicinal products metabolised by cytochrome P450 enzymes and by glucuronidation. This may result in lowered plasma concentrations and potential decrease of efficacy of co-administered medicinal products.

Medicinal products that are contraindicated specifically due to the expected magnitude of interaction and potential for serious adverse events are listed in section 4.3.

Antiretroviral agents

Nucleoside/Nucleotide reverse transcriptase inhibitors (NRTIs):

Stavudine and Lamivudine: no change in the pharmacokinetics of lopinavir was observed when Kaletra was given alone or in combination with stavudine and lamivudine in clinical studies.

Didanosine: it is recommended that didanosine be administered on an empty stomach; therefore, didanosine is to be given one hour before or two hours after Kaletra (given with food). The gastroresistant formulation of didanosine should be administered at least two hours after a meal.

Zidovudine and Abacavir: Kaletra induces glucuronidation, therefore Kaletra has the potential to reduce zidovudine and abacavir plasma concentrations. The clinical significance of this potential interaction is unknown.

Tenofovir: when tenofovir disoproxil fumarate was co-administered with Kaletra, tenofovir concentrations were increased by approximately 30% with no changes noted in lopinavir or ritonavir concentrations. Higher tenofovir concentrations could potentiate tenofovir associated adverse events, including renal disorders.

Non-nucleoside reverse transcriptase inhibitors (NNRTIs):

Nevirapine: no change in the pharmacokinetics of lopinavir was apparent in healthy volunteers during nevirapine and Kaletra co-administration. Results from a study in HIV-positive paediatric patients revealed a decrease in lopinavir concentrations during nevirapine co-administration. The effect of nevirapine in HIV-positive adults is expected to be similar to that in paediatric patients and lopinavir concentrations may be decreased. The clinical significance of the pharmacokinetic interaction is unknown. No formal recommendation could be drawn on dosage adjustment when Kaletra is used in combination with nevirapine. However, based on clinical experience, Kaletra dose increase to 533/133 mg twice daily (~6.5 ml) may be considered when co-administered with nevirapine, particularly for patients in whom reduced lopinavir susceptibility is likely.

Efavirenz: when used in combination with efavirenz and two nucleoside reverse transcriptase inhibitors in multiple protease inhibitor-experienced patients, increasing the dose of Kaletra 33.3% from 400/100 mg (3 capsules) twice daily to 533/133 mg (4 capsules) twice daily yielded similar lopinavir plasma concentrations as compared to historical data of Kaletra 400/100 mg (3 capsules) twice daily.

Dosage increase of Kaletra from 400/100 mg (5 ml) twice daily to 533/133 mg (~6.5 ml) twice daily should be considered when co-administered with efavirenz. Caution is warranted since this dosage adjustment might be insufficient in some patients.

Co-administration with other HIV protease inhibitors (PIs):
Kaletra (400/100 mg twice daily) has been studied in combination with reduced doses of amprenavir, indinavir, nelfinavir and saquinavir in steady-state controlled healthy volunteer studies relative to clinical doses of each HIV protease inhibitor in the absence of ritonavir. Comparisons to published pharmacokinetic data with ritonavir-enhanced amprenavir and saquinavir regimens are also described. Additionally, the effect of additional ritonavir on the pharmacokinetics of lopinavir are discussed. Note that the historical comparisons to ritonavir-enhanced protease inhibitor regimens should be interpreted with caution (see details of combinations below). Appropriate doses of HIV-protease inhibitors in combination with Kaletra with respect to safety and efficacy have not been established. Therefore, the concomitant administration of Kaletra with PIs requires close monitoring.

Amprenavir: the concomitant use of Kaletra with amprenavir 750 mg twice daily, resulted in an increase in amprenavir AUC by 70% and of C_{min} by 4.6-fold, relative to amprenavir 1200 mg twice daily alone. On the other hand, the AUC of lopinavir decreases by 38%. A dose increase of Kaletra may be necessary but may further affect concentrations of amprenavir.

Combined with Kaletra, amprenavir concentrations were lower (approximately 30%) relative to boosted amprenavir (amprenavir 600 mg/ritonavir 100 mg) twice daily alone.

Fosamprenavir: co-administration of standard doses of lopinavir/ritonavir with fosamprenavir results in a significant reduction in amprenavir concentrations. Co-administration of increased doses of fosamprenavir 1400 mg twice daily with lopinavir/ritonavir 533/133 mg twice daily to protease inhibitor-experienced patients resulted in a higher incidence of gastrointestinal adverse events and elevations in triglycerides with the combination regimen without increases in virological efficacy, when compared with standard doses of fosamprenavir/ritonavir. Therefore, concomitant administration of these medicinal products is not recommended.

Indinavir: indinavir 600 mg twice daily in combination with Kaletra produces similar indinavir AUC, higher C_{min} (by 3.5-fold) and lower C_{max} relative to indinavir 800 mg three times daily alone. Furthermore, concentrations of lopinavir do not appear to be affected when both medicinal products, Kaletra and indinivir, are combined, based on historical comparison with Kaletra alone.

Nelfinavir: administration of nelfinavir 1000 mg twice daily in combination with Kaletra produces a similar nelfinavir C_{max} and AUC and higher C_{min} relative to nelfinavir 1250 mg twice daily alone. Additionally, concentrations of the active M8 metabolite of nelfinavir were increased.

On the other hand, lopinavir AUC was decreased by 27% during nelfinavir co-administration with Kaletra. A dose increase of Kaletra may be necessary but may further affect concentrations of nelfinavir and its active metabolite. Higher doses of Kaletra have not been studied.

Saquinavir: saquinavir 800 mg twice daily co-administered with Kaletra produces an increase of saquinavir AUC by 9.6-fold relative to saquinavir 1200 mg three times daily given alone.

Saquinavir 800 mg twice daily co-administered with Kaletra resulted in an increase of saquinavir AUC by approximately 30% relative to saquinavir/ritonavir 1000/100 mg twice daily, and produces similar exposure to those reported after saquinavir/ritonavir 400/400 mg twice daily.

When saquinavir 1200 mg twice daily was combined with Kaletra, no further increase of concentrations was noted. Furthermore, concentrations of lopinavir do not appear to be affected when both medicinal products, Kaletra and saquinavir, are combined, based on historical comparison with Kaletra alone.

Ritonavir: Kaletra co-administered with an additional 100 mg ritonavir twice daily resulted in an increase of lopinavir AUC and C_{min} of 33% and 64%, respectively, as compared to Kaletra alone.

Other medicinal products:

Acid reducing agents (omeprazole, ranitidine): in a study performed in healthy volunteers, no clinically relevant interaction has been observed when Kaletra tablets 400/100 mg twice daily was co-administered with omeprazole or with ranitidine. Kaletra can be co-administered with acid reducing agents with no dose adjustment.

Antiarrhythmics: (bepridil, systemic lidocaine and quinidine): concentrations may be increased when co-administered with Kaletra. Caution is warranted and therapeutic concentration monitoring is recommended when available.

Anticancer agents (eg vincristine, vinblastine): these agents may have their serum concentrations increased when co-administered with lopinavir/ritonavir resulting in the potential for increased adverse events usually associated with these anticancer agents.

Anticoagulants: warfarin concentrations may be affected when co-administered with Kaletra. It is recommended that INR (international normalised ratio) be monitored.

Anticonvulsants (phenobarbital, phenytoin, carbamazepine): will induce CYP3A4 and may decrease lopinavir concentrations.

In addition, co-administration of phenytoin and lopinavir/ritonavir resulted in moderate decreases in steady-state phenytoin concentrations. Phenytoin levels should be monitored when co-administering with lopinavir/ritonavir.

Bupropion: in healthy volunteers, the AUC and C_{max} of bupropion and of its active metabolite, hydroxybupropion, were decreased by about 50% when co-administered with lopinavir/ritonavir capsules 400/100 mg twice daily at steady-state. This effect may be due to induction of bupropion metabolism. Therefore, if the co-administration of lopinavir/ritonavir with bupropion is judged unavoidable, this should be done under close clinical monitoring for bupropion efficacy, without exceeding the recommended dosage, despite the observed induction.

Trazodone: in a pharmacokinetic study performed in healthy volunteers, concomitant use of low dose ritonavir (200 mg twice daily) with a single dose of trazodone led to an increase in plasma concentrations of trazodone (AUC increased by 2.4 fold). Adverse events of nausea, dizziness, hypotension and syncope were observed following co-administration of trazodone and ritonavir in this study. However, it is unknown whether the combination of lopinavir/ritonavir causes a similar increase in trazodone exposure. The combination should be used with caution and a lower dose of trazodone should be considered.

Digoxin: plasma concentrations of digoxin may be increased when co-administered with Kaletra. Caution is warranted and therapeutic drug monitoring of digoxin concentrations, if available, is recommended in case of co-administration of Kaletra and digoxin. Particular caution should be used when prescribing Kaletra in patients taking digoxin as the acute inhibitory effect of ritonavir on Pgp is expected to significantly increase digoxin levels. The increased digoxin level may lessen over time as Pgp induction develops. Initiation of digoxin in patients already taking Kaletra is expected to result in lower increase of digoxin concentrations.

Dihydropyridine calcium channel blockers: (e.g. felodipine, nifedipine, nicardipine): may have their serum concentrations increased by Kaletra.

Disulfiram, metronidazole: Kaletra oral solution contains alcohol which can produce disulfiram-like reactions when co-administered with disulfiram or other medicinal products that produce this reaction.

Lipid lowering agents: HMG-CoA reductase inhibitors which are highly dependent on CYP3A4 metabolism, such as lovastatin and simvastatin, are expected to have markedly increased plasma concentrations when co-administered with Kaletra. Since increased concentrations of HMG-CoA reductase inhibitors may cause myopathy, including rhabdomyolysis, the combination of these medicinal products with Kaletra is not recommended. Atorvastatin is less dependent on CYP3A for metabolism. When atorvastatin was given concurrently with Kaletra, a mean 4.7-fold and 5.9-fold increase in atorvastatin C_{max} and AUC, respectively, was observed. When used with Kaletra, the lowest possible dose of atorvastatin should be administered. Rosuvastatin is not dependent on CYP3A. However, when given concurrently with Kaletra a mean 5-fold and 2-fold increase in rosuvastatin C_{max} and AUC, respectively, was observed. Caution should be exercised when Kaletra is co-administered with rosuvastatin. Results from an interaction study with Kaletra and pravastatin reveal no clinically significant interaction. The metabolism of pravastatin and fluvastatin is not dependent on CYP3A4, and interactions are not expected with Kaletra. If treatment with a HMG-CoA reductase inhibitor is indicated, pravastatin or fluvastatin is recommended.

Dexamethasone: may induce CYP3A4 and may decrease lopinavir concentrations.

Phosphodiesterase inhibitors: phosphodiesterase inhibitors which are dependent on CYP3A4 metabolism, such as tadalafil and sildenafil, are expected to result in an approximately 2-fold and 11-fold increase in AUC respectively, when co-administered with ritonavir containing regimens including Kaletra and may result in an increase in PDE5 inhibitor associated adverse reactions including hypotension, synope, visual changes and prolonged erection. Particular caution must be used when prescribing sildenafil or tadalafil in patients receiving Kaletra with increased monitoring for adverse events. Co-administration of vardenafil with ritonavir containing regimens including Kaletra is expected to result in 49-fold increase in vardenafil AUC. The use of vardenafil with Kaletra is contraindicated (see section 4.3).

Cyclosporin, sirolimus (rapamycin) and tacrolimus: concentrations may be increased when co-administered with Kaletra. More frequent therapeutic concentration monitoring is recommended until plasma levels of these products have been stabilised.

Ketoconazole and itraconazole: may have serum concentrations increased by Kaletra. High doses of ketoconazole and itraconazole > 200 mg/day) are not recommended.

Voriconazole: due to the potential for reduced voriconazole concentrations, co-administration of voriconazole and low dose ritonavir (100 mg twice daily) as contained in Kaletra should be avoided unless an assessment of the benefit/risk to patient justifies the use of voriconazole.

Clarithromycin: moderate increases in clarithromycin AUC are expected when co-administered with Kaletra. For patients with renal or hepatic impairment dose reduction of clarithromycin should be considered (see section 4.4).

Buprenorphine: buprenorphine (dosed at 16 mg daily) co-administered with lopinavir/ritonavir (dosed at 400/100 mg twice daily) showed no clinically significant interaction. Kaletra can be co-administered with buprenorphine with no dose adjustment.

Methadone: Kaletra was demonstrated to lower plasma concentrations of methadone. Monitoring plasma concentrations of methadone is recommended.

Contraceptives: levels of ethinyl oestradiol were decreased when oestrogen-based oral contraceptives were co-administered with Kaletra. In case of co-administration of Kaletra with contraceptives containing ethinyl oestradiol (whatever the contraceptive formulation e.g. oral or patch), alternative methods of contraception are to be used.

Rifabutin: when rifabutin and Kaletra were co-administered for 10 days, rifabutin (parent substance and active 25-O-desacetyl metabolite) C_{max} and AUC were increased by 3.5- and 5.7-fold, respectively. On the basis of these data, a rifabutin dose reduction of 75% (i.e. 150 mg every other day or 3 times per week) is recommended when administered with Kaletra. Further reduction may be necessary.

Rifampicin: co-administration of Kaletra with rifampicin is not recommended. Rifampicin administered with Kaletra causes large decreases in lopinavir concentrations which may in turn significantly decrease the lopinavir therapeutic effect. A dose adjustment of Kaletra 400 mg/400 mg twice daily has allowed compensating for the CYP 3A4 inducer effect of rifampicin. However, such a dose adjustment might be associated with ALT/AST elevations and with increase in gastrointestinal disorders. Therefore, this co-administration should be avoided unless judged strictly necessary. If this co-administration is judged unavoidable, increased dose of Kaletra at 400 mg/400 mg twice daily may be administered with rifampicin under close safety and therapeutic drug monitoring. The Kaletra dose should be titrated upward only after rifampicin has been initiated (see section 4.4).

St John's wort: serum levels of lopinavir and ritonavir can be reduced by concomitant use of the herbal preparation St John's wort (*Hypericum perforatum)*. This is due to the induction of drug metabolising enzymes by St John's wort. Herbal preparations containing St John's wort should therefore not be combined with lopinavir and ritonavir. If a patient is already taking St John's wort, stop St John's wort and if possible check viral levels. Lopinavir and ritonavir levels may increase on stopping St John's wort. The dose of Kaletra may need adjusting. The inducing effect may persist for at least 2 weeks after cessation of treatment with St John's wort (see section 4.3).

Midazolam: midazolam is extensively metabolised by CYP3A4. Co-administration with Kaletra may cause a large increase in the concentration of this benzodiazepine. A phenotyping cocktail study in 14 healthy volunteers showed an increase of AUC by about 13 fold with oral midazolam and an increase by about 4 fold with parenteral midazolam. Therefore, Kaletra should not be co-administered with orally administered midazolam (see section 4.3), whereas caution should be used with co-administration of Kaletra and parenteral midazolam. If Kaletra is co-administered with parenteral midazolam, it should be done in an intensive care unit (ICU) or similar setting which ensures close clinical monitoring and appropriate medical management in case of respiratory depression and/or prolonged sedation. Dosage adjustment for midazolam should be considered especially if more than a single dose of midazolam is administered.

Fluticasone propionate (interaction with ritonavir): in a clinical study where ritonavir 100 mg capsules twice daily were co – administered with 50 μg intranasal fluticasone propionate (4 times daily) for seven days in healthy subjects, the fluticasone propionate plasma levels increased significantly, whereas the intrinsic cortisol levels decreased by approximately 86% (90% confidence interval 82 – 89%). Greater effects may be expected when fluticasone propionate is inhaled. Systemic corticosteroid effects including Cushing's syndrome and adrenal suppression have been reported in patients receiving ritonavir and inhaled or intranasally administered fluticasone propionate; this could also occur with other corticosteroids metabolised via the P450 3A pathway eg budesonide. Consequently, concomitant administration of Kaletra and these glucocorticoids is not recommended unless the potential benefit of treatment outweighs the risk of systemic corticosteroid effects (see section 4.4). A dose reduction of the glucocorticoid should be considered with close monitoring of local and systemic effects or a switch to a glucocorticoid, which is not a substrate for CYP3A4 (eg beclomethasone). Moreover, in case of withdrawal of glucocorticoids progressive dose reduction may have to be performed over a longer period. The effects of high fluticasone systemic exposure on ritonavir plasma levels is yet unknown.

Based on known metabolic profiles, clinically significant interactions are not expected between Kaletra and fluvastatin, dapsone, trimethoprim/sulfamethoxazole, azithromycin or fluconazole.

4.6 Pregnancy and lactation
There are no data from the use of Kaletra in pregnant women. Studies in animals have shown reproductive toxicity (see section 5.3). The potential risk for humans is unknown. Kaletra should not be used during pregnancy unless clearly necessary.

Studies in rats revealed that lopinavir is excreted in the milk. It is not known whether this medicinal product is excreted in human milk. HIV-infected women must not breast-feed their infants under any circumstances to avoid transmission of HIV.

4.7 Effects on ability to drive and use machines

No studies on the effects on the ability to drive and use machines have been performed. Patients should be informed that nausea has been reported during treatment with Kaletra (see section 4.8).

Kaletra oral solution contains approximately 42% v/v alcohol.

4.8 Undesirable effects

The safety of Kaletra has been investigated in over 1400 patients in Phase II/III clinical trials. In some studies, Kaletra was used in combination with efavirenz or nevirapine.

The most common adverse event associated with Kaletra therapy was diarrhoea and was generally of mild to moderate severity. Discontinuation due to adverse reactions was 4.5% (naïve patients) and 9% (experienced patients) over a 48 week period.

It is important to note that cases of pancreatitis have been reported in patients receiving Kaletra, including those who developed hypertriglyceridaemia. Furthermore, rare increases in PR interval have been reported during Kaletra therapy (see section 4.4: sections pancreatitis and lipid elevations).

Increased CPK, myalgia, myositis, and rarely, rhabdomyolysis have been reported with protease inhibitors, particularly in combination with nucleoside reverse transcriptase inhibitors.

Combination antiretroviral therapy has been associated with redistribution of body fat (lipodystrophy) in HIV patients including the loss of peripheral and facial subcutaneous fat, increased intra-abdominal and visceral fat, breast hypertrophy and dorsocervical fat accumulation (buffalo hump).

Combination antiretroviral therapy has been associated with metabolic abnormalities such as hypertriglyceridaemia, hypercholesterolaemia, insulin resistance, hyperglycaemia and hyperlactataemia (see section 4.4).

In HIV-infected patients with severe immune deficiency at the time of initiation of combination antiretroviral therapy (CART), an inflammatory reaction to asymptomatic or residual opportunistic infections may arise (see section 4.4).

Adult patients

Adverse reactions:

The following adverse reactions of moderate to severe intensity with possible or probable relationship to Kaletra have been reported. The adverse reactions are displayed by system organ class. Within each frequency grouping, undesirable effects are presented in order of decreasing seriousness: very common (≥1/10), common (≥ 1/100 to < 1/10, uncommon ≥ 1/1000 to < 1/100) and rare (≥ 1/10,000 to < 1/1,000).

Undesirable effects in clinical studies in adult patients

System organ class	Frequency	Adverse reaction
Investigations	Very common (Grade 3 or 4)	Blood triglycerides increased, blood cholesterol increased, gamma-glutamyltransferase increased
	Common (Grade 3 or 4)	Blood glucose increased, blood amylase increased, aspartate aminotransferase increased, alanine aminotransferase increased, liver function tests abnormal
	Uncommon	Glucose tolerance decreased, blood bilirubin increased, creatinine renal clearance decreased, lipase increased, weight increased, weight decreased, hormone level abnormal, laboratory test abnormal
	Rare	Blood alkaline phosphatase increased
Cardiac disorders	Uncommon	Myocardial infarction[1], palpitations
	Rare	Atrioventricular block
Blood and lymphatic system disorders	Uncommon	Anaemia, leucopenia, lymphadenopathy
	Rare	Splenomegaly
Nervous system disorders	Common	Headache, paresthesia
	Uncommon	Extrapyramidal disorder, migraine, facial palsy, encephalopathy, dizziness, amnesia, coordination abnormal, hypertonia, neuropathy, neuropathy peripheral, somnolence, tremor, ageusia, dysgeusia, dyskinesia
Eye disorders	Uncommon	Visual disturbance
Ear and labyrinth disorders	Uncommon	Tinnitus
	Rare	Vertigo, hyperacusis
Respiratory, thoracic and mediastinal disorders	Uncommon	Pulmonary oedema, dyspnoea, cough
Gastrointestinal disorders	Very common	Diarrhoea
	Common	Nausea, vomiting, abdominal pain, abnormal faeces, dyspepsia, flatulence, gastrointestinal disorder
	Uncommon	Haemorrhagic colitis, pancreatitis[2], enterocolitis, oesophagitis, constipation, faecal incontinence, abdominal distension, gastrooesophageal reflux disease, dry mouth, dysphagia, eructation, gastritis, mouth ulcerations, stomatitis, periodontitis
	Rare	Haemorrhoids
Renal and urinary disorders	Uncommon	Nephrolithiasis, nephritis, albuminuria, hypercalcinuria, urine abnormality
Skin and subcutaneous tissue disorders	Common	Rash, lipodystrophy acquired, acne
	Uncommon	Alopecia, eczema, dermatitis exfoliative, rash maculopapular, dermatitis allergic, dry skin, nail disorder, pruritis, seborrhoea, skin discoloration, skin ulcer, hyperhidrosis, skin striae
	Rare	Idiopathic capillaritis
Musculoskeletal and connective tissue disorders	Uncommon	Arthralgia, osteoarthritis, myalgia, back pain, arthropathy
Endocrine disorders	Uncommon	Cushing syndrome, hypothyroidism, hypogonadism male,
Metabolism and nutrition disorders	Uncommon	Diabetes mellitus, dehydration, lactic acidosis, oedema, increased appetite, obesity, anorexia, hyperglycaemia, hypocholesteremia, lipomatosis, hyperuricaemia, hypovitaminosis
	Rare	Hypophosphataemia, decreased appetite
Infections and infestations	Uncommon	Gastroenteritis, otitis media, bronchitis, sinusitis, sialadenitis, furunculosis, bacterial infection, viral infection, pharyngitis, influenza, rhinitis
	Rare	Cellulitis, folliculitis, perineal abscess
Neoplasms benign, malignant and unspecified (including cysts and polyps)	Uncommon	Benign neoplasm of skin
Vascular disorders	Uncommon	Hypertension, thrombophlebitis, deep vein thrombosis, vasculitis, varicose vein, angiopathy
General disorders and administration site conditions	Common	Asthenia, pain
	Uncommon	Chest pain, chest pain substernal, chills, pyrexia, malaise, oedema peripheral, face oedema, drug interaction, cyst
Immune system disorders	Uncommon	Drug hypersensitivity
	Rare	Immune reconstitution syndrome
Hepatobiliary disorders	Uncommon	Hepatitis, cholecystitis, hepatic steatosis, hepatomegaly, liver tenderness
Reproductive system and breast disorders	Uncommon	Amenorrhoea, menorrhagia, ejaculation disorder, erectile dysfunction, breast enlargement, gynecomastia
Psychiatric disorders	Common	Insomnia
	Uncommon	Agitation, anxiety, confusional state, depression, affect lability, abnormal dreams, decreased libido, nervousness, abnormal thinking

[1] This event had a fatal outcome.

[2] See section 4.4: pancreatitis and lipids

Paediatric patients

In children 2 years of age and older, the nature of the safety profile is similar to that seen in adults.

Undesirable effects in clinical studies in paediatric patients

Infections and infestations	Common	Viral infection
Nervous system disorders	Common	Taste perversion
Gastrointestinal disorders	Common	Constipation, vomiting, pancreatitis*
Hepatobiliary disorders	Common	Hepatomegaly
Skin and subcutaneous tissue disorders	Common	Rash, dry skin
General disorders and administration site conditions	Common	Fever
Investigations	Common (Grade 3 or 4)	Increased activated partial thromboplastin time, decreased haemoglobin, decreased platelets, increased sodium, increased potassium, increased calcium, increased bilirubin, increased SGPT/ALT, increased SGOT/AST, increased total cholesterol, increased amylase, increased uric acid, decreased sodium, decreased potassium, decreased calcium, decreased neutrophils

* see section 4.4: pancreatitis and lipids

Post marketing experience

Hepatitis, and rarely jaundice, have been reported in patients on Kaletra therapy in the presence or absence of identifiable risk factors for hepatitis.

Stevens-Johnson syndrome and erythema multiforme have been reported.

Cases of osteonecrosis have been reported, particularly in patients with generally acknowledged risk factors, advanced HIV disease or long-term exposure to combination antiretroviral therapy (CART). The frequency of this is unknown (see section 4.4).

4.9 Overdose

To date, there is limited human experience of acute overdose with Kaletra.

The adverse clinical signs observed in dogs included salivation, emesis and diarrhoea/abnormal stool. The signs of toxicity observed in mice, rats or dogs included decreased activity, ataxia, emaciation, dehydration and tremors.

There is no specific antidote for overdose with Kaletra. Treatment of overdose with Kaletra is to consist of general supportive measures including monitoring of vital signs and observation of the clinical status of the patient. If indicated, elimination of unabsorbed active substance is to be achieved by emesis or gastric lavage. Administration of activated charcoal may also be used to aid in removal of unabsorbed active substance. Since Kaletra is highly protein bound, dialysis is unlikely to be beneficial in significant removal of the active substance.

5. PHARMACOLOGICAL PROPERTIES

5.1 Pharmacodynamic properties

Pharmaco-therapeutic group: protease inhibitor, ATC code: J05AE06

Mechanism of action: Lopinavir provides the antiviral activity of Kaletra. Lopinavir is an inhibitor of the HIV-1 and HIV-2 proteases. Inhibition of HIV protease prevents cleavage of the *gag-pol* polyprotein resulting in the production of immature, non-infectious virus.

Effects on the electrocardiogram: QTcF interval was evaluated in a randomised, placebo and active (moxifloxacin 400 mg once daily) controlled crossover study in 39 healthy adults, with 10 measurements over 12 hours on Day 3. The maximum mean (95% upper confidence bound) differences in QTcF from placebo were 3.6 (6.3) and 13.1(15.8) for 400/100 mg twice daily and supratherapeutic 800/200 mg twice daily LPV/r, respectively. The induced QRS interval prolongation from 6 ms to 9.5 ms with high dose lopinavir/ritonavir (800/200 mg twice daily) contributes to QT prolongation. The two regimens resulted in exposures on Day 3 which were approximately 1.5 and 3-fold higher than those observed with recommended once daily or twice daily LPV/r doses at steady state. No subject experienced an increase in QTcF of ⩾60 msec from baseline or a QTcF interval exceeding the potentially clinically relevant threshold of 500 msec.

Modest prolongation of the PR interval was also noted in subjects receiving lopinavir/ritonavir in the same study on Day 3. The mean changes from baseline in PR interval ranged from 11.6 ms to 24.4 ms in the 12 hour interval post dose. Maximum PR interval was 286 msec and no second or third degree heart block was observed (see section 4.4).

Antiviral activity in vitro: the *in vitro* antiviral activity of lopinavir against laboratory and clinical HIV strains was evaluated in acutely infected lymphoblastic cell lines and peripheral blood lymphocytes, respectively. In the absence of human serum, the mean IC_{50} of lopinavir against five different HIV-1 laboratory strains was 19 nM. In the absence and presence of 50% human serum, the mean IC_{50} of lopinavir against HIV-1_{IIIB} in MT4 cells was 17 nM and 102 nM, respectively. In the absence of human serum, the mean IC_{50}- of lopinavir was 6.5 nM against several HIV-1 clinical isolates.

Resistance

In vitro selection of resistance:

HIV-1 isolates with reduced susceptibility to lopinavir have been selected *in vitro*. HIV-1 has been passaged *in vitro* with lopinavir alone and with lopinavir plus ritonavir at concentration ratios representing the range of plasma concentration ratios observed during Kaletra therapy. Genotypic and phenotypic analysis of viruses selected in these passages suggest that the presence of ritonavir, at these concentration ratios, does not measurably influence the selection of lopinavir-resistant viruses. Overall, the *in vitro* characterisation of phenotypic cross-resistance between lopinavir and other protease inhibitors suggest that decreased susceptibility to lopinavir correlated closely with decreased susceptibility to ritonavir and indinavir, but did not correlate closely with decreased susceptibility to amprenavir, saquinavir, and nelfinavir.

Analysis of resistance in ARV-naive patients:

In a Phase II study (M97-720) through 204 weeks of treatment, genotypic analysis of viral isolates was successfully conducted in 11 of 16 patients with confirmed HIV RNA above 400 copies/ml revealed no primary or active site mutations in protease (amino acids at positions 8, 30, 32, 46, 47, 48, 50, 82, 84 and 90) or protease inhibitor phenotypic resistance.

In a Phase III study (M98-863) of 653 patients randomised to receive stavudine plus lamivudine with either lopinavir/ritonavir or nelfinavir, 113 nelfinavir-treated subjects and 74 lopinavir/ritonavir-treated subjects had an HIV RNA above 400 copies/ml while on treatment from Week 24 through Week 96. Of these, isolates from 96 nelfinavir-treated subject and 51 lopinavir/ritonavir-treated subjects could be amplified for resistance testing. Resistance to nelfinavir, defined as the presence of the D30N or L90M mutation in protease, was observed in 41/96 (43%) subjects. Resistance to lopinavir, defined as the presence of any primary or active site mutations in protease (see above), was observed in 0/51 (0%) subjects. Lack of resistance to lopinavir was confirmed by phenotypic analysis.

Analysis of resistance in PI-experienced patients:

The selection of resistance to lopinavir in patients having failed prior protease inhibitor therapy was characterised by analysing the longitudinal isolates from 19 protease inhibitor-experienced subjects in 2 Phase II and one Phase III studies who either experienced incomplete virologic suppression or viral rebound subsequent to initial response to Kaletra and who demonstrated incremental in vitro resistance between baseline and rebound (defined as emergence of new mutations or 2-fold change in phenotypic susceptibility to lopinavir). Incremental resistance was most common in subjects whose baseline isolates had several protease inhibitor-associated mutations, but < 40-fold reduced susceptibility to lopinavir at baseline. Mutations V82A, I54V and M46I emerged most frequently. Mutations L33F, I50V and V32I combined with I47V/A were also observed. The 19 isolates demonstrated a 4.3-fold increase in IC_{50} compared to baseline isolates (from 6.2- to 43-fold, compared to wild-type virus).

Genotypic correlates of reduced phenotypic susceptibility to lopinavir in viruses selected by other protease inhibitors. The *in vitro* antiviral activity of lopinavir against 112 clinical isolates taken from patients failing therapy with one or more protease inhibitors was assessed. Within this panel, the following mutations in HIV protease were associated with reduced *in vitro* susceptibility to lopinavir: L10F/I/R/V, K20M/R, L24I, M46I/L, F53L, I54L/T/V, L63P, A71I/L/T/V, V82A/F/T, I84V and L90M. The median EC_{50} of lopinavir against isolates with 0 – 3, 4 – 5, 6 – 7 and 8 – 10 mutations at the above amino acid positions was 0.8, 2.7 13.5 and 44.0-fold higher than the EC_{50} against wild type HIV, respectively. The 16 viruses that displayed > 20-fold change in susceptibility all contained mutations at positions 10, 54, 63 plus 82 and/or 84. In addition, they contained a median of 3 mutations at amino acid positions 20, 24, 46, 53, 71 and 90. In addition to the mutations described above, mutations V32I and I47A have been observed in rebound isolates with reduced lopinavir susceptibility from protease inhibitor experienced patients receiving Kaletra therapy.

In addition to the mutations described above, mutations I47A and L76V have been observed in rebound isolates with reduced lopinavir susceptibility from patients receiving Kaletra therapy.

Conclusions regarding the relevance of particular mutations or mutational patterns are subject to change with additional data, and it is recommended to always consult current interpretation systems for analysing resistance test results.

Antiviral activity of Kaletra in patients failing protease inhibitor therapy: the clinical relevance of reduced *in vitro* susceptibility to lopinavir has been examined by assessing the virologic response to Kaletra therapy, with respect to baseline viral genotype and phenotype, in 56 patients previous failing therapy with multiple protease inhibitors. The EC_{50} of lopinavir against the 56 baseline viral isolates ranged from 0.6 to 96-fold higher than the EC_{50} against wild type HIV. After 48 weeks of treatment with Kaletra, efavirenz and nucleoside reverse transcriptase inhibitors, plasma HIV RNA ⩽ 400 copies/ml was observed in 93% (25/27), 73% (11/15), and 25% (2/8) of patients with < 10-fold, 10 to 40-fold, and > 40-fold reduced susceptibility to lopinavir at baseline, respectively. In addition, virologic response was observed in 91% (21/23), 71% (15/21) and 33% (2/6) patients with 0 – 5, 6 – 7, and 8 – 10 mutations of the above mutations in HIV protease associated with reduced *in vitro* susceptibility to lopinavir. Since these patients had not previously been exposed to either Kaletra or efavirenz, part of the response may be attributed to the antiviral activity of efavirenz, particularly in patients harbouring highly lopinavir resistant virus. The study did not contain a control arm of patients not receiving Kaletra.

Cross-resistance: Activity of other protease inhibitors against isolates that developed incremental resistance to lopinavir after Kaletra therapy in protease inhibitor experienced patients: The presence of cross resistance to other protease inhibitors was analysed in 18 rebound isolates that had demonstrated evolution of resistance to lopinavir during 3 Phase II and one Phase III studies of Kaletra in protease inhibitor-experienced patients. The median fold IC_{50} of lopinavir for these 18 isolates at baseline and rebound was 6.9- and 63-fold, respectively, compared to wild type virus. In general, rebound isolates either retained (if cross-resistant at baseline) or developed significant cross-resistance to indinavir, saquinavir and atazanavir. Modest decreases in amprenavir activity were noted with a median increase of IC_{50} from 3.7- to 8-fold in the baseline and rebound isolates, respectively. Isolates retained susceptibility to tipranavir with a median increase of IC_{50} in baseline and rebound isolates of 1.9- and 1.8–fold, respectively, compared to wild type virus. Please refer to the Aptivus Summary of Product Characteristics for additional information on the use of tipranavir, including genotypic predictors of response, in treatment of lopinavir-resistant HIV-1 infection.

Clinical pharmacodynamic data

The effects of Kaletra (in combination with other antiretroviral agents) on biological markers (plasma HIV RNA levels and CD_4 counts) have been investigated in a controlled study of Kaletra of 48 weeks duration, and in additional studies of Kaletra of 360 weeks duration.

Adult Use

Patients without prior antiretroviral therapy

Study M98-863 is a randomised, double-blind trial of 653 antiretroviral treatment naïve patients investigating Kaletra (400/100 mg twice daily) compared to nelfinavir (750 mg three times daily) plus nucleoside reverse transcriptase inhibitors. By intent to treat analysis where patients with missing values are considered virologic failures, the proportion of patients at 48 weeks with HIV RNA < 400 copies/ml in the Kaletra arm was 75% and 63% in the nelfinavir arm. Mean baseline CD_4 cell count was 259 cells/mm^3 (range: 2 to 949 cells/mm^3) and mean baseline plasma HIV-1 RNA was 4.9 log_{10} copies/ml (range: 2.6 to 6.8 log_{10} copies/ml). Through 48 weeks of therapy, the proportion of patients in the Kaletra arm with plasma RNA < 50 copies/ml was 67% and 52% in the nelfinavir arm. The mean increase from baseline in CD_4 cell count was 207 cells/mm^3 in the Kaletra arm and 195 cells/mm^3 in the nelfinavir arm. Through 48 weeks of therapy, a statistically significantly higher proportion of patients in the Kaletra arm had HIV RNA < 50 copies/ml compared to the nelfinavir arm.

Sustained virological response to Kaletra (in combination with nucleoside/nucleotide reverse transcriptase inhibitors) has been also observed in a small Phase II study (M97-720) through 360 weeks of treatment. One hundred patients were originally treated with Kaletra in the study (including 51 patients receiving 400/100 mg twice daily and 49 patients at either 200/100 mg twice daily or 400/200 mg twice daily). All patients converted to open-label Kaletra at the 400/100 mg twice daily dose between week 48 and week 72. Sixty-one patients completed the study (35 patients received the recommended 400/100 mg twice daily dose throughout the study). Through 360 weeks of treatment, the proportion of patients with HIV RNA < 400 (< 50) copies/ml was 61% (59%), and the corresponding mean increase in CD_4 cell count was 501 cells/mm^3. Thirty-nine patients (39%) discontinued the study, including 16 (16%) discontinuations due to adverse events, one of which was associated with a death.

Patients with prior antiretroviral therapy

Study M97-765 is a randomised, double-blind trial evaluating Kaletra at two dose levels (400/100 mg and 400/200 mg, both twice daily) plus nevirapine (200 mg twice daily) and two nucleoside reverse transcriptase inhibitors in 70 single protease inhibitor experienced, non-nucleoside reverse transcriptase inhibitor naïve patients. Median baseline CD_4 cell count was 349 cells/mm^3 (range 72 to 807 cells/mm^3) and median baseline plasma HIV-1 RNA was 4.0 log_{10} copies/ml (range 2.9 to 5.8 log_{10} copies/ml). By intent-to-treat analysis where patients with missing values are considered virologic failures, the proportion of patients with HIV RNA < 400 (< 50) copies/ml at 24 weeks was 75% (58%) and the mean increase from baseline in CD_4 cell count was 174 cells/mm^3 for the 36 patients receiving the 400/100 mg dose of Kaletra.

M98-957 is a randomised, open-label study evaluating Kaletra treatment at two dose levels (400/100 mg and 533/133 mg, both twice daily) plus efavirenz (600 mg once daily) and nucleoside reverse transcriptase inhibitors in 57 multiple protease inhibitor experienced, non-nucleoside reverse transcriptase inhibitor naïve patients. Between week 24 and 48, patients randomised to a dose of 400/100 mg were converted to a dose of 533/133 mg. Median baseline CD_4 cell count was 220 cells/mm^3 (range13 to 1030 cells/mm^3). By intent-to-treat analysis of both dose groups combined (n=57), where patients with missing values are considered virologic failures, the proportion of patients with HIV RNA < 400 copies/ml at 48 weeks was 65% and the mean increase from baseline CD_4 cell count was 94 cells/mm^3.

Paediatric Use

M98-940 is an open-label study of a liquid formulation of Kaletra in 100 antiretroviral naïve (44%) and experienced (56%) paediatric patients. All patients were non-nucleoside reverse transcriptase inhibitor naïve. Patients were randomised to either 230 mg lopinavir/57.5 mg ritonavir per m^2 or 300 mg lopinavir/75 mg ritonavir per m^2. Naïve patients also received nucleoside reverse transcriptase inhibitors. Experienced patients received nevirapine plus up to two nucleoside reverse transcriptase inhibitors. Safety, efficacy and pharmacokinetic profiles of the two dose regimens were assessed after 3 weeks of therapy in each patient. Subsequently, all patients were continued on the 300/75 mg per m^2 dose. Patients had a mean age of 5 years (range 6 months to 12 years) with 14 patients less than 2 years old and 6 patients one year or less. Mean baseline CD_4 cell count was 838 cells/mm^3 and mean baseline plasma HIV-1 RNA was 4.7 log_{10} copies/ml. Through 48 weeks of therapy, the proportion of patients with HIV RNA < 400 copies/ml was 84% for antiretroviral naïve patients and 75% for antiretroviral experienced patients and the mean increase from baseline in CD_4 cell count were 404 cells/mm^3 and 284 cells/mm^3 respectively.

5.2 Pharmacokinetic properties

The pharmacokinetic properties of lopinavir co-administered with ritonavir have been evaluated in healthy adult volunteers and in HIV-infected patients; no substantial differences were observed between the two groups. Lopinavir is essentially completely metabolised by CYP3A. Ritonavir inhibits the metabolism of lopinavir, thereby increasing the plasma levels of lopinavir. Across studies, administration of Kaletra 400/100 mg twice daily yields mean steady-state lopinavir plasma concentrations 15 to 20-fold higher than those of ritonavir in HIV-infected patients. The plasma levels of ritonavir are less than 7% of those obtained after the ritonavir dose of 600 mg twice daily. The *in vitro* antiviral EC_{50} of lopinavir is approximately 10-fold lower than that of ritonavir. Therefore, the antiviral activity of Kaletra is due to lopinavir.

Absorption: multiple dosing with 400/100 mg Kaletra twice daily for 2 weeks and without meal restriction produced a mean ± SD lopinavir peak plasma concentration (C_{max}) of 12.3 ± 5.4 µg/ml, occurring approximately 4 hours after administration. The mean steady-state trough concentration prior to the morning dose was 8.1 ± 5.7 µg/ml. Lopinavir AUC over a 12 hour dosing interval averaged 113.2 ± 60.5 µg•h/ml. The absolute bioavailability of lopinavir co-formulated with ritonavir in humans has not been established.

Effects of food on oral absorption: Kaletra soft capsules and liquid have been shown to be bioequivalent under nonfasting conditions (moderate fat meal). Administration of a single 400/100 mg dose of Kaletra soft capsules with a moderate fat meal (500 – 682 kcal, 22.7 –25.1% from fat) was associated with a mean increase of 48% and 23% in lopinavir AUC and C_{max}, respectively, relative to fasting. For Kaletra oral solution, the corresponding increases in lopinavir AUC and C_{max} were 80% and 54%, respectively. Administration of Kaletra with a high fat meal (872 kcal, 55.8% from fat) increased lopinavir AUC and C_{max} by 96% and 43%, respectively, for soft capsules, and 130% and 56%, respectively, for oral solution. To enhance bioavailability and minimise variability Kaletra is to be taken with food.

Distribution: at steady state, lopinavir is approximately 98 – 99% bound to serum proteins. Lopinavir binds to both alpha-1-acid glycoprotein (AAG) and albumin, however, it has a higher affinity for AAG. At steady state, lopinavir protein binding remains constant over the range of observed concentrations after 400/100 mg Kaletra twice daily, and is similar between healthy volunteers and HIV-positive patients.

Metabolism: *in vitro* experiments with human hepatic microsomes indicate that lopinavir primarily undergoes oxidative metabolism. Lopinavir is extensively metabolised by the hepatic cytochrome P450 system, almost exclusively by isozyme CYP3A. Ritonavir is a potent CYP3A inhibitor which inhibits the metabolism of lopinavir and therefore, increases plasma levels of lopinavir. A ^{14}C-lopinavir study in humans showed that 89% of the plasma radioactivity after a single 400/100 mg Kaletra dose was due to parent active substance. At least 13 lopinavir oxidative metabolites have been identified in man. The 4-oxo and 4-hydroxymetabolite epimeric pair are the major metabolites with antiviral activity, but comprise only minute amounts of total plasma radioactivity. Ritonavir has been shown to induce metabolic enzymes, resulting in the induction of its own metabolism, and likely the induction of lopinavir metabolism. Pre-dose lopinavir concentrations decline with time during multiple dosing, stabilising after approximately 10 days to 2 weeks.

Elimination: after a 400/100 mg ^{14}C-lopinavir/ritonavir dose, approximately 10.4 ± 2.3% and 82.6 ± 2.5% of an administered dose of ^{14}C-lopinavir can be accounted for in urine and faeces, respectively. Unchanged lopinavir accounted for approximately 2.2% and 19.8% of the administered dose in urine and faeces, respectively. After multiple dosing, less than 3% of the lopinavir dose is excreted unchanged in the urine. The effective (peak to trough) half-life of lopinavir over a 12 hour dosing interval averaged 5 – 6 hours, and the apparent oral clearance (CL/F) of lopinavir is 6 to 7 l/h.

Special Populations

Paediatrics:

There are limited pharmacokinetic data in children below 2 years of age. The pharmacokinetics of Kaletra 300/75 mg/m^2 twice daily and 230/57.5 mg/m^2 twice daily have been studied in a total of 53 paediatric patients, ranging in age from 6 months to 12 years. The lopinavir mean steady-state AUC, C_{max}, and C_{min} were 72.6 ± 31.1 µg•h/ml, 8.2 ± 2.9 µg/ml and 3.4 ± 2.1 µg/ml, respectively after Kaletra 230/57.5 mg/m^2 twice daily without nevirapine (n=12), and were 85.8 ± 36.9 µg•h/ml, 10.0 ± 3.3 µg/ml and 3.6 ± 3.5 µg/ml, respectively after 300/75 mg/m^2 twice daily with nevirapine (n=12). The 230/57.5 mg/m^2 twice daily regimen without nevirapine and the 300/75 mg/m^2 twice daily regimen with nevirapine provided lopinavir plasma concentrations similar to those obtained in adult patients receiving the 400/100 mg twice daily regimen without nevirapine. Kaletra soft capsules and Kaletra oral solution are bioequivalent under nonfasting conditions.

Gender, Race and Age:

Kaletra pharmacokinetics have not been studied in the elderly. No age or gender related pharmacokinetic differences have been observed in adult patients. Pharmacokinetic differences due to race have not been identified.

Renal Insufficiency:

Kaletra pharmacokinetics have not been studied in patients with renal insufficiency; however, since the renal clearance of lopinavir is negligible, a decrease in total body clearance is not expected in patients with renal insufficiency.

Hepatic Insufficiency:

The steady state pharmacokinetic parameters of lopinavir in HIV-infected patients with mild to moderate hepatic impairment were compared with those of HIV-infected patients with normal hepatic function in a multiple dose study with lopinavir/ritonavir 400/100 mg twice daily. A limited increase in total lopinavir concentrations of approximately 30% has been observed which is not expected to be of clinical relevance (see section 4.2).

5.3 Preclinical safety data

Repeat-dose toxicity studies in rodents and dogs identified major target organs as the liver, kidney, thyroid, spleen and circulating red blood cells. Hepatic changes indicated cellular swelling with focal degeneration. While exposure eliciting these changes were comparable to or below human clinical exposure, dosages in animals were over 6-fold the recommended clinical dose. Mild renal tubular degeneration was confined to mice exposed with at least twice the recommended human exposure; the kidney was unaffected in rats and dogs. Reduced serum thyroxin led to an increased release of TSH with resultant follicular cell hypertrophy in the thyroid glands of rats. These changes were reversible with withdrawal of the active substance and were absent in mice and dogs. Coombs-negative anisocytosis and poikilocytosis were observed in rats, but not in mice or dogs. Enlarged spleens with histiocytosis were seen in rats but not other species. Serum cholesterol was elevated in rodents but not dogs, while triglycerides were elevated only in mice.

During *in vitro* studies, cloned human cardiac potassium channels (HERG) were inhibited by 30% at the highest concentrations of lopinavir/ritonavir tested, corresponding to a lopinavir exposure 7-fold total and 15-fold free peak plasma levels achieved in humans at the maximum recommended therapeutic dose. In contrast, similar concentrations of lopinavir/ritonavir demonstrated no repolarisation delay in the canine cardiac Purkinje fibres. Lower concentrations of lopinavir/ritonavir did not produce significant potassium (HERG) current blockade. Tissue distribution studies conducted in the rat did not suggest significant cardiac retention of the active substance; 72-hour AUC in heart was approximately 50% of measured plasma AUC. Therefore, it is reasonable to expect that cardiac lopinavir levels would not be significantly higher than plasma levels.

In dogs, prominent U waves on the electrocardiogram have been observed associated with prolonged PR interval and bradycardia. These effects have been assumed to be caused by electrolyte disturbance.

The clinical relevance of these preclinical data is unknown, however, the potential cardiac effects of this product in humans cannot be ruled out (see also sections 4.4 and 4.8).

In rats, embryofoetotoxicity (pregnancy loss, decreased foetal viability, decreased foetal body weights, increased frequency of skeletal variations) and postnatal developmental toxicity (decreased survival of pups) was observed at maternally toxic dosages. The systemic exposure to lopinavir/ritonavir at the maternal and developmental toxic dosages was lower than the intended therapeutic exposure in humans.

Long-term carcinogenicity studies of lopinavir/ritonavir in mice revealed a nongenotoxic, mitogenic induction of liver tumours, generally considered to have little relevance to human risk. Carcinogenicity studies in rats revealed no tumourigenic findings. Lopinavir/ritonavir was not found to be mutagenic or clastogenic in a battery of *in vitro* and *in vivo* assays including the Ames bacterial reverse mutation assay, the mouse lymphoma assay, the mouse micronucleus test and chromosomal aberration assays in human lymphocytes.

6. PHARMACEUTICAL PARTICULARS

6.1 List of excipients

Oral solution contains:

alcohol (42% v/v),

high fructose corn syrup,

propylene glycol,

purified water,

glycerol,

povidone,

magnasweet-110 flavour (mixture of monoammonium glycyrrhizinate and glycerol),

vanilla flavour (containing p-hydroxybenzoic acid, p-hydroxybenzaldehyde, vanillic acid, vanillin, heliotrope, ethyl vanillin),

polyoxyl 40 hydrogenated castor oil,

cotton candy flavour (containing ethyl maltol, ethyl vanillin, acetoin, dihydrocoumarin, propylene glycol),

acesulfame potassium,

saccharin sodium,

sodium chloride,

peppermint oil,

sodium citrate,

citric acid,

menthol.

6.2 Incompatibilities

Not applicable.

6.3 Shelf life

2 years

6.4 Special precautions for storage

Store in a refrigerator (2°C - 8°C).

In use storage: If kept outside of the refrigerator, do not store above 25°C and discard any unused contents after 42 days (6 weeks). It is advised to write the date of removal from the refrigerator on the package.

Avoid exposure to excessive heat.

6.5 Nature and contents of container

Amber coloured multiple-dose polyethylene terephthalate (PET) bottles in a 60 ml size. Each pack contains 5 bottles of 60 ml (300 ml). The pack also contains 5 × 5 ml syringes with 0.1 ml graduations from 0 to 5 ml (400/100 mg).

6.6 Special precautions for disposal and other handling

No special requirements.

7. MARKETING AUTHORISATION HOLDER

Abbott Laboratories Limited

Queenborough

Kent ME11 5EL

United Kingdom

8. MARKETING AUTHORISATION NUMBER(S)

EU/1/01/172/003

9. DATE OF FIRST AUTHORISATION/RENEWAL OF THE AUTHORISATION

Date of first authorisation: 20 March 2001

Date of last renewal: 20 March 2006

10. DATE OF REVISION OF THE TEXT

21 August 2009

Kemadrin Tablets 5 mg

(GlaxoSmithKline UK)

1. NAME OF THE MEDICINAL PRODUCT

Kemadrin Tablets 5mg

2. QUALITATIVE AND QUANTITATIVE COMPOSITION

Procyclidine Hydrochloride BP 5mg per tablet

3. PHARMACEUTICAL FORM

Tablet

4. CLINICAL PARTICULARS

4.1 Therapeutic indications

Kemadrin is indicated for the treatment and symptomatic relief of all forms of Parkinson's disease e.g. idiopathic (paralysis agitans), postencephalitic and arteriosclerotic disease.

Kemadrin is also indicated for the control of extrapyramidal symptoms induced by neuroleptic drugs including pseudo-parkinsonism, acute dystonic reactions and akathisia.

4.2 Posology and method of administration

The variation in optimum dosage from one patient to another should be taken into consideration by the physician.

Dosage in adults:-

Parkinson's disease:-

Treatment is usually started at 2.5mg procyclidine three times per day, increasing by 2.5 to 5mg per day at intervals of two or three days until the optimum clinical response is achieved.

The usual maintenance dose to achieve optimal response is 15 to 30 mg procyclidine per day.

Addition of a fourth dose before retiring has been seen to be beneficial in some patients. Doses up to 60mg procyclidine have been well tolerated, and at the discretion of the attending physician dosing to this level may be appropriate.

In general younger patients or those with postencephalitic parkinsonism may require higher doses for a therapeutic response than older patients and those with arteriosclerotic parkinsonism.

Kemadrin may be combined with levodopa or amantadine in patients who are inadequately controlled on a single agent.

Neuroleptic-induced extrapyramidal symptoms:-

Treatment is usually initiated at 2.5mg procyclidine three times per day increasing by 2.5mg daily until symptoms are relieved.

The effective maintenance dose is usually 10 to 30mg procyclidine per day.

After a period of 3 to 4 months of therapy, KEMADRIN should be withdrawn and the patient observed to see whether the neuroleptic-induced extra-pyramidal symptoms recur.

If this is the case KEMADRIN should be reintroduced to avoid debilitating extra-pyramidal symptoms. Cessation of treatment periodically is to be recommended even in patients who appear to require the drug for longer periods.

Dosage in children:-

The use of Kemadrin in this age group is not recommended.

Dosage in the Elderly:-

Elderly patients may be more susceptible than younger adults to the anticholinergic effects of Kemadrin and a reduced dosage may be required (See Special Warnings and Special Precautions for Use).

Administration:-

Pharmacokinetic studies have indicated that the mean plasma elimination half life of Kemadrin is sufficient to allow twice daily administration orally or intravenously, if more convenient.

Oral administration may be better tolerated if associated with a meal.

4.3 Contraindications

Kemadrin is contra-indicated in individuals with known hypersensitivity to any component of the preparation, untreated urinary retention, closed angle glaucoma and gastro-intestinal obstruction.

4.4 Special warnings and precautions for use

As with all anticholinergics the benefit/risk ratio should be assessed when prescribing Kemadrin in patients with existing angle-closure (narrow angle) glaucoma or those considered to be predisposed to glaucoma. Cautious prescribing is also indicated in patients predisposed to obstructive disease of the gastro-intestinal tract and those with urinary symptoms associated with prostatic hypertrophy.

In a proportion of patients undergoing neuroleptic treatment, tardive dyskinesias will occur. While anticholinergic agents do not cause this syndrome, when given in combination with neuroleptics they may exacerbate the symptoms of tardive dyskinesias or reduce the threshold at which these symptoms appear in predisposed patients. In such individuals subsequent adjustment of neuroleptic therapy or reduction in anticholinergic treatment should be considered.

Patients with mental disorders occasionally experience a precipitation of a psychotic episode when procyclidine is administered for the treatment of the extrapyramidal side effects of neuroleptics.

Elderly patients, especially those on high doses of anticholinergics may be more susceptible to the adverse events associated with such therapy (See ADVERSE EVENTS). Specifically, the elderly patient may be particularly vulnerable to Central Nervous System disturbances such as confusion, impairment of cognitive function and memory, disorientation and hallucinations. These effects are usually reversible on reduction or discontinuation of anticholinergic therapy.

There is no specific information available concerning the use of procyclidine hydrochloride in patients with impaired renal or hepatic function. However, since procyclidine is metabolised in the liver and excreted via the urine care should be exercised when administering procyclidine to patients with impairment of renal or hepatic function.

Kemadrin should not be withdrawn abruptly as rebound parkinsonian symptoms may occur.

Patients with rare hereditary problems of galactose intolerance, the Lapp lactase deficiency or glucose-galactose malabsorption should not take this medicine.

Abuse

Kemadrin, along with other anticholinergic drugs, has the potential to be abused. Although the cases of abuse are rare, physicians should exercise caution in prescribing Kemadrin to patients with symptoms that may not be genuine.

4.5 Interaction with other medicinal products and other forms of interaction

Monoamine oxidase inhibitors or drugs with anticholinergic properties, such as amantadine, memantine, antihistamines, phenothiazines, tricyclic and related antidepressants, clozapine, disopyramide and nefopam may increase the anticholinergic action of procyclidine.

The use of drugs with cholinergic properties, such as tacrine, may reduce the therapeutic response to Kemadrin. Furthermore, drugs with anticholinergic properties may antagonise the effect of parasympathomimetic agents.

The concomitant use of procyclidine with some neuroleptics for the treatment of extrapyramidal symptoms has been associated with a reduction in neuroleptic plasma concentrations. However this reduction is unlikely to be associated with a significant reduction in clinical effect.

Drugs with anticholinergic properties may decrease salivation causing dry mouth and, in theory, may reduce the absorption and therefore the therapeutic effect of sublingual or buccal nitrate tablets.

Anticholinergics, including procyclidine, may reduce the efficacy of levodopa by increasing gastric emptying time, resulting in enhanced gastric degradation.

The effect of anticholinergics such as procyclidine may antagonise the gastrointestinal effects of cisapride, domperidone and metoclopramide.

Procyclidine may potentiate the vagolytic effects of quinidine.

Anticholinergics may reduce the absorption of ketoconazole.

Exposure to high environmental temperature and humidity in association with a phenothiazine/anticholinergic drug regimen has rarely resulted in hyperpyrexia.

Daily administration of paroxetine increases significantly the plasma levels of procyclidine. If anticholinergic effects are seen, the dose of procyclidine should be reduced

4.6 Pregnancy and lactation

Pregnancy:-

The safety of using Kemadrin during pregnancy has not been established. However, extensive clinical use has not given any evidence that it in any way compromises the normal course of pregnancy. Nevertheless, as with all drugs, use should be considered only when the expected clinical benefit of treatment for the mother outweighs any possible risk to the developing foetus.

Lactation:-

No information is available on the passage of procyclidine into human breast milk following administration of Kemadrin.

4.7 Effects on ability to drive and use machines

Adverse events of a neurological character such as blurred vision, dizziness, confusion and disorientation have been reported with procyclidine. Therefore, if affected, patients should be advised not to drive or operate machinery.

4.8 Undesirable effects

For this preparation there is no modern clinical documentation which can be used as support for determining the frequency of adverse reactions.

Psychiatric disorders	Uncommon (≥1/1000 and <1/100)	Agitation, anxiety, nervousness, confusion, disorientation, hallucinations.
	Rare (<1/1000)	Psychotic disorder
Nervous system disorders	Uncommon (≥1/1000 and <1/100)	Dizziness, memory impairment, impaired cognition
Eye disorders	Common (≥ 1/100)	Blurred vision
Gastrointestinal disorders	Common (≥ 1/100)	Dry mouth, constipation
	Uncommon (≥1/1000 and <1/100)	Nausea, vomiting, gingivitis
Skin and subcutaneous tissue Disorder	Uncommon (≥1/1000 and <1/100)	Rash
Renal and urinary disorders	Common (≥1/100)	Urinary retention

The main undesirable effects are those to be expected from any anticholinergic agent – these are generally reversible on reducing the dosage.

With high doses of procyclidine dizziness, mental confusion, impaired cognition and memory, disorientation, anxiety, agitation and hallucinations may occur.

4.9 Overdose

Symptoms and Signs:

Symptoms of overdosage include stimulant effects such as agitation, restlessness and confusion with severe sleeplessness lasting up to 24 hours or more. Visual and auditory hallucinations have been reported. Most subjects are euphoric but the occasional patient may be anxious and aggressive. The pupils are widely dilated and unreactive to light. In recorded cases, the disorientation has lasted 1 to 4 days and ended in a recuperative sleep. Signs of CNS depression including somnolence, reduced consciousness, and occasionally coma have been reported usually following very large overdoses.

Tachycardia has also been reported in association with cases of Kemadrin overdose.

Treatment:

If procyclidine has been ingested within the previous hour or two (or possibly longer in view of its likely effects on gastric motility) then activated charcoal should be used to reduce absorption. Gastric lavage should only be considered if clinically appropriate. Other active measures such as the use of cholinergic agents or haemodialysis are extremely unlikely to be of clinical value although if convulsions occur they should be controlled by injections of diazepam.

5. PHARMACOLOGICAL PROPERTIES

5.1 Pharmacodynamic properties

Procyclidine is a synthetic anticholinergic agent which blocks the excitatory effects of acetylcholine at the muscarinic receptor.

Idiopathic Parkinson's disease is thought to result from degeneration of neurones in the substantia nigra whose axons project and inhibit cells in the corpus striatum. Blockade by neuroleptic drugs of the dopamine released by these terminals produces a similar clinical picture. The cell bodies in the corpus striatum also receive cholinergic innervation which is excitatory.

Relief of the Parkinsonian syndrome can be achieved, either by potentiation of the dopaminergic system or blockade of the cholinergic input by anticholinergics. It is by a central action of this latter type by which procyclidine exerts its effect.

Procyclidine is particularly effective in the alleviation of rigidity. Tremor, akinesia, speech and writing difficulties, gait, sialorrhoea and drooling, sweating, oculogyric crises and depressed mood are also beneficially influenced.

5.2 Pharmacokinetic properties

Procyclidine is adequately absorbed from the gastro-intestinal tract with a bioavailability of 75% and disappears rapidly from the tissues. The relatively low clearance of 68ml/min represents a predominantly metabolic change with a small first pass effect. The mean plasma elimination half-life after both oral and intravenous administration is approximately 12 hours.

No detailed information is available on the metabolic fate of procyclidine but very little of the parent compound is excreted in the urine unchanged. When given orally about one fifth of the dose is known to be metabolised in the liver, principally by cytochrome P450 and then conjugated with glucuronic acid. This conjugate has been detected in the urine.

5.3 Preclinical safety data

Fertility:-

A three generation study in rats dosed at 40 mg/kg/day via the diet before and during pregnancy showed only that the number of viable pups was slightly decreased from the second mating. No other parameters were affected.

Teratogenicity:-

No teratogenic effects were seen in rats dosed subcutaneously with 10, 30 or 100 mg/kg/day on days 8 to 16 of pregnancy. Maternal bodyweight gain was reduced at doses of 30 or 100 mg/kg/day, and a 10% reduction in foetal weight was seen at 100 mg/kg/day

Mutagenicity:-

No data is available regarding the mutagenic potential of procyclidine hydrochloride.

Carcinogenicity:-

There is no data on the carcinogenic potential of procyclidine hydrochloride.

6. PHARMACEUTICAL PARTICULARS

6.1 List of excipients

Lactose

Sodium Starch Glycollate

Povidone

Magnesium Stearate

6.2 Incompatibilities

None

6.3 Shelf life

5 years

6.4 Special precautions for storage

Store below 25°C

6.5 Nature and contents of container

Amber glass bottles with low density polyethylene snap fit closures.

Polypropylene containers with polyethylene snap-fit lids.

Round enamelled tins with lever lids.

6.6 Special precautions for disposal and other handling

See posology and method of administration.

Administrative Data

7. MARKETING AUTHORISATION HOLDER

The Wellcome Foundation

Glaxo Wellcome House

Berkeley Avenue

Greenford

Middlesex

UB6 ONN

Trading as

GlaxoSmithKline UK

Stockley Park West

Uxbridge

Middlesex UB11 1BT

8. MARKETING AUTHORISATION NUMBER(S)

PL 00003/5255R

9. DATE OF FIRST AUTHORISATION/RENEWAL OF THE AUTHORISATION

19th September 2006

10. DATE OF REVISION OF THE TEXT

13th May 2008

11 Legal Status

POM

Kemicetine Succinate Injection

(Pharmacia Limited)

1. NAME OF THE MEDICINAL PRODUCT
Kemicetine Succinate Injection or Chloramphenicol Sodium Succinate 1.377g Injection

2. QUALITATIVE AND QUANTITATIVE COMPOSITION
Chloramphenicol sodium succinate (BP) 1.377 g
– equivalent to laevorotatory chloramphenicol 1.0 g

3. PHARMACEUTICAL FORM
Freeze dried powder for injection.

4. CLINICAL PARTICULARS
4.1 Therapeutic indications
Kemicetine (chloramphenicol) is a broad-spectrum antibiotic and is active against many gram-negative organisms, *Spirillae* and *Rickettsia*. Kemicetine should not be used for trivial infections due to the possibility of severe blood dyscrasias, which may prove fatal.

Kemicetine succinate is indicated for typhoid, meningitis caused by *H. influenzae* and other serious infections caused by bacteria susceptible to chloramphenicol. It is also indicated wherever chloramphenicol is deemed the antibiotic of choice and oral administration is not possible, or where higher than usual blood concentrations are required.

4.2 Posology and method of administration
To be given by i.v. or i.m. injection.

In order to ensure rapid attainment of high blood levels, Kemicetine succinate is best administered by i.v. injection. Where this is not possible, however, intramuscular administration may be used, although it should be borne in mind that absorption may be slow and unpredictable.

The injection should be reconstituted with Water for Injections, Sodium ChlorideInjection, or Dextrose Injection 5 %. The following dilution table may be useful for the administration of a proportion of the contents of a vial:

Concentration	Solution strength	Volume of diluent to be added	Total volume after dilution
40%	400 mg/ml	1.7 ml	2.5 ml
25%	250 mg/ml	3.2 ml	4.0 ml
20%	200 mg/ml	4.2 ml	5.0 ml

The dose administered and the concentration used is dependent on the severity of the infection. The recommended standard dosage is as follows:

Adults: The equivalent of 1 g of chloramphenicol every 6-8 hours.

Elderly: The usual adult dosage should be given subject to normal hepatic and renal function.

Children: The equivalent of 50 mg/kg chloramphenicol according to body weight, daily in divided doses every 6 hours (this dose should not be exceeded). The patient should be carefully observed for signs of toxicity.

Neonates and Premature Infants: 25 mg/kg in divided doses.

Only 10% or lower concentrations to be used. The 10% solution can be prepared by extracting 5ml of the 20% solution and adding 5ml of diluent (Water for Injections, Sodium Chloride Injection or Dextrose Injection 5%) under aseptic conditions.

The 10 % solution should be given by intravenous injection over a period of about a minute, or in a larger volume of fluid, by slow intravenous infusion. The concurrent administration of i.v. Kemicetine succinate with topical treatment has been found to be very effective in the treatment of osteomyelitic foci, abscesses, empyema and skin and urinary infections.

In exceptional cases, such as patients with septicaemia or meningitis, dosage schedule up to 100 mg/kg/day may be prescribed. However, these high doses should be decreased as soon as clinically indicated. To prevent relapses treatment should be continued after the temperature has returned to normal for 4 days in rickettsial diseases and for 8 – 10 days in typhoid fever.

4.3 Contraindications
Kemicetine succinate is contra-indicated in patients with a previous history of sensitivity and/or toxic reaction to chloramphenicol.

4.4 Special warnings and precautions for use
Kemicetine is to be administered only under the direction of a medical practitioner.

Chloramphenicol may cause severe bone marrow depression which may lead to agranulocytosis, thrombocytopenic purpura or aplastic anaemia. These effects of the haemopoietic system are usually associated with a high dose, prolonged administration, or repeated courses, but they may occur at relatively low doses.

Chloramphenicol should not be used in the treatment of any infection for which a less toxic antibiotic is available. It is also advisable to perform blood tests in the case of prolonged or repeated administration. Evidence of any detrimental effect on blood elements is an indication to discontinue therapy immediately.

The dosage of chloramphenicol should be reduced in patients with impairment of hepatic or renal function.

Because of its toxic nature it is important to monitor serum levels of this antibiotic particularly in new-born and premature infants, in the elderly, in patients with renal or hepatic disease and in those receiving other drugs with which chloramphenicol may interact.

4.5 Interaction with other medicinal products and other forms of interaction
Chloramphenicol has been shown to interact with, and enhance the effects of coumarin anticoagulants, some hypoglycaemic agents (e.g. tolbutamide) and phenytoin. When given concurrently, a dose reduction of these agents may be necessary.

Plasma concentrations of chloramphenicol may be reduced with concomitant usage of phenobarbital and rifampicin.

4.6 Pregnancy and lactation
The use of chloramphenicol is contra-indicated in pregnancy and whilst breastfeeding.

4.7 Effects on ability to drive and use machines
None stated.

4.8 Undesirable effects
The following may become apparent after chloramphenicol treatment: dryness of the mouth, nausea and vomiting, diarrhoea, urticaria, optic neuritis with blurring or temporary loss of vision, peripheral neuritis, headache and depression.

Superinfection by fungi e.g. *C. albicans* in the gastro-intestinal tract or vagina, may also occur due to the disturbance of normal bacterial flora.

Chloramphenicol may also impede the development of immunity and should therefore not be given during active immunisation.

The "Grey syndrome" may occur after administration in patients with immature hepatic metabolic capacity, i.e. infants and neonates, usually in those treated with doses substantially in excess of those recommended.

4.9 Overdose
General supportive therapy.

5. PHARMACOLOGICAL PROPERTIES
5.1 Pharmacodynamic properties
After administration chloramphenicol is rapidly released from chloramphenicol sodium succinate. Chloramphenicol is active against many gram-positive and gram negative organisms, *Spirillae* and *Rickettsia*. It acts b interfering with bacterial protein synthesis. Chloramphenicol is widely distributed in body tissues and fluids and enters the cerebrospinal fluid.

Chloramphenicol sodium succinate, free chloramphenicol and metabolites are excreted in the urine.

5.2 Pharmacokinetic properties
After intravenous administration of chloramphenicol succinate every 6 hours elimination half-lives were 4.03 hours for chloramphenicol and 2.65 hours for chloramphenicol succinate. After intravenous chloramphenicol sodium succinate, steady state peak concentrations were reached on average 18.0 minutes after cessation of the infusion.

In infants and children aged 3 days to 16 years the apparent half-life was extremely variable ranging from 1.7 to 12.0 hours.

5.3 Preclinical safety data
None stated.

6. PHARMACEUTICAL PARTICULARS
6.1 List of excipients
There are no excipients.

6.2 Incompatibilities
None stated.

6.3 Shelf life
48 months.

6.4 Special precautions for storage
Keep container in the outer carton.

6.5 Nature and contents of container
Type III colourless glass vials with grey chlorobutyl rubber bung and aluminium seal.

Pack size: 1, 20 or 25 vials.

6.6 Special precautions for disposal and other handling
To be reconstituted with Water for Injection, Sodium Chloride Injection or Dextrose Injection 5%.

7. MARKETING AUTHORISATION HOLDER
Pharmacia Limited
Ramsgate Road
Sandwich
Kent CT13 9NJ
United Kingdom

8. MARKETING AUTHORISATION NUMBER(S)
PL 00032/0341

9. DATE OF FIRST AUTHORISATION/RENEWAL OF THE AUTHORISATION
13th September 2002/ 2nd March 2009

10. DATE OF REVISION OF THE TEXT
March 2009

LEGAL CATEGORY
POM

Company Ref: KM4_0

Keppra 250,500,750 and 1000 mg film-coated Tablets, 100 mg/ml oral solution and 100 mg/ml concentrate for solution for infusion

(UCB Pharma Limited)

1. NAME OF THE MEDICINAL PRODUCT
Keppra 250 mg film-coated tablets.
Keppra 500 mg film-coated tablets.
Keppra 750 mg film-coated tablets.
Keppra 1000 mg film-coated tablets.
Keppra 100 mg/ml, oral solution.
Keppra 100 mg/ml concentrate for solution for infusion.

2. QUALITATIVE AND QUANTITATIVE COMPOSITION
Tablets:
Each film-coated tablet contains 250 mg levetiracetam, 500 mg levetiracetam, 750 mg levetiracetam & excipient colouring agent E110 or 1000 mg levetiracetam.

Oral solution:
Each ml contains 100 mg levetiracetam.

Excipients: methyl parahydroxybenzoate (E218), propyl parahydroxybenzoate (E216) and 300 mg maltitol liquid.

Concentrate for solution for infusion:
Each ml contains 100 mg of levetiracetam.

The 5 ml vial contains 500 mg of levetiracetam.

For a full list of excipients, see section 6.1.

3. PHARMACEUTICAL FORM
Film-coated tablet:
Blue, oblong, scored and debossed with the code "ucb" and "250" on one side.

Yellow, oblong, scored and debossed with the code "ucb 500" on one side.

Orange, oblong, scored and debossed with the code "ucb 750" on one side.

White, oblong, scored and debossed with the code "ucb 1000" on one side.

Oral solution:
Clear liquid.

Concentrate for solution for infusion:
Keppra concentrate is a clear, colourless, sterile solution.

4. CLINICAL PARTICULARS
4.1 Therapeutic indications
Keppra is indicated as monotherapy in the treatment of partial onset seizures with or without secondary generalisation in patients from 16 years of age with newly diagnosed epilepsy.

The daily dose is administered in two equally divided doses.

Keppra is indicated as adjunctive therapy

• in the treatment of partial onset seizures with or without secondary generalisation in adults, children and infants from 1 month of age with epilepsy. *(The concentrate for solution for infusion: is indicated for adults, adolescents and children from 4 years of age.)*

• in the treatment of myoclonic seizures in adults and adolescents from 12 years of age with Juvenile Myoclonic Epilepsy.

• in the treatment of primary generalised tonic-clonic seizures in adults and adolescents from 12 years of age with Idiopathic Generalised Epilepsy.

Oral solution
The oral solution may be diluted in a glass of water and may be taken with or without food. A graduated oral syringe, an adaptor for the syringe and instructions for use in the package leaflet are provided with Keppra.

Concentrate for solution for infusion
Keppra concentrate is an alternative for patients when oral administration is temporarily not feasible.

4.2 Posology and method of administration
Film-coated tablets
The film-coated tablets must be taken orally, swallowed with a sufficient quantity of liquid and may be taken with or without food. The daily dose is administered in two equally divided doses.

Oral solution

The oral solution may be diluted in a glass of water and may be taken with or without food. A graduated oral syringe, an adaptor for the syringe and instructions for use in the package leaflet are provided with Keppra.

The daily dose is administered in two equally divided doses.

Concentrate for solution for infusion

Keppra therapy can be initiated with either intravenous or oral administration.

Conversion to or from oral to intravenous administration can be done directly without titration. The total daily dose and frequency of administration should be maintained.

Keppra concentrate is for intravenous use only and the recommended dose must be diluted in at least 100 ml of a compatible diluent and administered intravenously as a 15-minute intravenous infusion (see section 6.6).

There is no experience with administration of intravenous levetiracetam for longer period than 4 days.

• Monotherapy

Adults and adolescents from 16 years of age

The recommended starting dose is 250 mg twice daily which should be increased to an initial therapeutic dose of 500 mg twice daily after two weeks. The dose can be further increased by 250 mg twice daily every two weeks depending upon the clinical response. The maximum dose is 1500 mg twice daily.

• Add-on therapy

Adults (≥18 years) and adolescents (12 to 17 years) weighing 50 kg or more

The initial therapeutic dose is 500 mg twice daily. This dose can be started on the first day of treatment.

Depending upon the clinical response and tolerability, the daily dose can be increased up to 1,500 mg twice daily. Dose changes can be made in 500 mg twice daily increases or decreases every two to four weeks.

Elderly (65 years and older)

Adjustment of the dose is recommended in elderly patients with compromised renal function (see "Patients with renal impairment" below).

Infants aged from 6 to 23 months, children (2 to 11 years) and adolescents (12 to 17 years) weighing less than 50 kg

The initial therapeutic dose is 10 mg/kg twice daily.

Depending upon the clinical response and tolerability, the dose can be increased up to 30 mg/kg twice daily. Dose changes should not exceed increases or decreases of 10 mg/kg twice daily every two weeks. The lowest effective dose should be used.

Dosage in children 50 kg or greater is the same as in adults.

The physician should prescribe the most appropriate pharmaceutical form and strength according to weight and dose.

Dosage recommendations for infants from 6 months of age, children and adolescents:

Weight	Starting dose: 10 mg/kg twice daily	Maximum dose: 30 mg/kg twice daily
6 kg (1)	60 mg (0.6 mL) twice daily	180 mg (1.8 mL) twice daily
10 kg (1)	100 mg (1 mL) twice daily	300 mg (3 mL) twice daily
15 kg (1)	150 mg (1.5 mL) twice daily	450 mg (4.5 mL) twice daily
20 kg (1)	200 mg (2 mL) twice daily	600 mg (6 mL) twice daily
25 kg	250 mg twice daily	750 mg twice daily
From 50 kg (2)	500 mg twice daily	1500 mg twice daily

(1) Children 20 kg or less should preferably start the treatment with Keppra 100 mg/ml oral solution.

(2) Dosage in children and adolescents 50 kg or more is the same as in adults.

A Keppra concentrate vial contains 500 mg levetiracetam in 5 ml (corresponding to 100 mg/ml).

Infants from 1 month to less than 6 months

The initial therapeutic dose is 7 mg/kg twice daily.

Depending upon the clinical response and tolerability, the dose can be increased up to 21 mg/kg twice daily. Dose changes should not exceed increases or decreases of 7 mg/kg twice daily every two weeks. The lowest effective dose should be used.

Infants should start the treatment with Keppra 100 mg/ml oral solution.

Dosage recommendations for infants less than 6 months:

Weight	Starting dose: 7 mg/kg twice daily	Maximum dose: 21 mg/kg twice daily
4 kg	28 mg (0.3 mL) twice daily	84 mg (0.85 mL) twice daily
5 kg	35 mg (0.35 mL) twice daily	105 mg (1.05 mL) twice daily
7 kg	49 mg (0.5 mL) twice daily	147 mg (1.5 mL) twice daily

Keppra concentrate for solution for infusion is not recommended for use in children below 4 years of age due to insufficient data on safety and efficacy (see section 5.2).

The physician should prescribe the most appropriate pharmaceutical form, presentation and strength according to weight and dose.

Keppra oral solution

Three presentations are available:

- A 300 ml bottle with graduated oral syringe containing up to 1000 mg levetiracetam (corresponding to 10 ml) with a graduation every 0.25 ml (corresponding to 25 mg).

- A 150 ml bottle with graduated oral syringe containing up to 300 mg levetiracetam (corresponding to 3 ml) with a graduation every 0.1 ml (corresponding to10 mg)

In order to ensure the accuracy of the dosing, the smaller bottle (150 ml) and syringe graduated from 0.1 to 3 ml per graduation of 0.1ml should be prescribed for infants older than 6 months and young children.

- A 150 ml bottle with graduated oral syringe containing up to 100 mg levetiracetam (corresponding to 1 ml) with a graduation every 0.05 ml (corresponding to 5 mg)

In order to ensure the accuracy of the dosing, the smaller bottle (150 ml) and syringe graduated from 0.05 to 1 ml per graduation of 0.05 ml should be prescribed for infants less than 6 months.

Patients with renal impairment

The daily dose must be individualised according to renal function.

For adult patients, refer to the following table and adjust the dose as indicated. To use this dosing table, an estimate of the patient's creatinine clearance (CLcr) in ml/min is needed. The CLcr in ml/min may be estimated from serum creatinine (mg/dl) determination, for adults and adolescents weighing 50 kg or more, the following formula:

$$CLcr\ (ml/min) = \frac{[140 - age\ (years)] \times weight\ (kg)}{72 \times serum\ creatinine\ (mg/dl)}\ (\times 0.85\ for\ women)$$

Then CLcr is adjusted for body surface area (BSA) as follows:

$$CLcr\ (ml/min/1.73\ m^2) = \frac{CLcr\ (ml/min)}{BSA\ subject\ (m^2)} \times 1.73$$

Dosing adjustment for adult patients with impaired renal function

Group	Creatinine clearance (ml/min/1.73m²)	Dosage and frequency
Normal	> 80	500 to 1,500 mg twice daily
Mild	50-79	500 to 1,000 mg twice daily
Moderate	30-49	250 to 750 mg twice daily
Severe	< 30	250 to 500 mg twice daily
End-stage renal disease patients undergoing dialysis (1)	-	500 to 1,000 mg once daily (2)

(1) A 750 mg loading dose is recommended on the first day of treatment with levetiracetam.

(2) Following dialysis, a 250 to 500 mg supplemental dose is recommended.

For children with renal impairment, levetiracetam dose needs to be adjusted based on the renal function as levetiracetam clearance is related to renal function. This recommendation is based on a study in adult renally impaired patients.

The CLcr in ml/min/1.73 m^2 may be estimated from serum creatinine (mg/dl) determination, for young adolescents, children and infants, using the following formula (Schwartz formula):

$$CLcr\ (ml/min/1.73\ m^2) = \frac{Height\ (cm) \times ks}{Serum\ Creatinine\ (mg/dl)}$$

ks= 0.45 in Term infants to 1 year old; ks= 0.55 in Children to less than 13 years; ks= 0.7 in adolescent male

Dosing adjustment for infants and children patients with impaired renal function

(see Table 1 on next page)

Patients with hepatic impairment

No dose adjustment is needed in patients with mild to moderate hepatic impairment. In patients with severe hepatic impairment, the creatinine clearance may underestimate the renal insufficiency. Therefore a 50 % reduction of the daily maintenance dose is recommended when the creatinine clearance is < 60 ml/min/1.73m^2.

4.3 Contraindications

Hypersensitivity to levetiracetam or other pyrrolidone derivatives or any of the excipients.

4.4 Special warnings and precautions for use

In accordance with current clinical practice, if Keppra has to be discontinued it is recommended to withdraw it gradually (*e.g.* in adults: 500 mg decreases twice daily every two to four weeks; in infants older than 6 months, children and adolescents weighing less than 50 kg: dose decrease should not exceed 10 mg/kg twice daily every two weeks; in infants (less than 6 months): dose decrease should not exceed 7 mg/kg twice daily every two weeks).

Available data in children did not suggest impact on growth and puberty. However, long term effects on learning, intelligence, growth, endocrine function, puberty and childbearing potential in children remain unknown.

An increase in seizure frequency of more than 25 % was reported in 14 % of levetiracetam treated adult and paediatric patients (4 to 16 years of age) with partial onset seizures, whereas it was reported in 26 % and 21 % of placebo treated adult and paediatric patients, respectively.

When Keppra was used to treat primary generalised tonic-clonic seizures in adults and adolescents with idiopathic generalised epilepsy, there was no effect on the frequency of absences.

The administration of Keppra to patients with renal impairment may require dose adjustment. In patients with severely impaired hepatic function, assessment of renal function is recommended before dose selection (see section 4.2).

Suicide, suicide attempt, suicidal ideation and behaviour have been reported in patients treated with anti-epileptic agents (including levetiracetam). A meta-analysis of randomized placebo-controlled trials of anti-epileptic drugs has shown a small increased risk of suicidal thoughts and behaviour. The mechanism of this risk is not known.

Therefore patients should be monitored for signs of depression and/or suicidal ideation and behaviours and appropriate treatment should be considered. Patients (and caregivers of patients) should be advised to seek medical advice should signs of depression and/or suicidal ideation or behaviour emerge.

The tablet formulation is not adapted for use in infants under the age of 6 months.

Keppra Oral Solution 100mg/ml

Keppra 100 mg/ml oral solution includes methyl parahydroxybenzoate (E218) and propyl parahydroxybenzoate (E216) which may cause allergic reactions (possibly delayed).

It also includes maltitol liquid; patients with rare hereditary problems of fructose intolerance should not take this medicine.

Concentrate for solution for infusion

This medicinal product contains 2.5 mmol (or 57 mg) sodium per maximum single dose. To be taken into consideration by patients on a controlled sodium diet.

The safety and efficacy of levetiracetam has not been thoroughly assessed in infants aged less than 1 year. Only 35 infants aged less than 1 year have been exposed in clinical studies of which only 13 were aged < 6 months.

4.5 Interaction with other medicinal products and other forms of interaction

Pre-marketing data from clinical studies conducted in adults indicate that Keppra did not influence the serum concentrations of existing antiepileptic medicinal products (phenytoin, carbamazepine, valproic acid, phenobarbital, lamotrigine, gabapentin and primidone) and that these antiepileptic medicinal products did not influence the pharmacokinetics of Keppra.

As in adults, there is no evidence of clinically significant medicinal product interactions in paediatric patients receiving up to 60 mg/kg/day levetiracetam.

A retrospective assessment of pharmacokinetic interactions in children and adolescents with epilepsy (4 to 17 years) confirmed that adjunctive therapy with orally administered levetiracetam did not influence the steady-state

Table 1 Dosing adjustment for infants and children patients with impaired renal function

Group	Creatinine clearance (ml/min/1.73m²)	Dosage and frequency	
		Infants 1 to less than 6 months	Infants 6 to 23 months, children and adolescents weighing less than 50 kg
Normal	> 80	7 to 21 mg/kg (0.07 to 0.21 ml/kg) twice daily	10 to 30 mg/kg (0.10 to 0.30 ml/kg) twice daily
Mild	50-79	7 to 14 mg/kg (0.07 to 0.14 ml/kg) twice daily	10 to 20 mg/kg (0.10 to 0.20 ml/kg) twice daily
Moderate	30-49	3.5 to 10.5 mg/kg (0.035 to 0.105 ml/kg) twice daily	5 to 15 mg/kg (0.05 to 0.15 ml/kg) twice daily
Severe	< 30	3.5 to 7 mg/kg (0.035 to 0.07 ml/kg) twice daily	5 to 10 mg/kg (0.05 to 0.10 ml/kg) twice daily
End-stage renal disease patients undergoing dialysis	–	7 to 14 mg/kg (0.07 to 0.14 ml/kg) once daily (1) (3)	10 to 20 mg/kg (0.10 to 0.20 ml/kg) once daily (2) (4)

(1) A 10.5 mg/kg (0.105 ml/kg) loading dose is recommended on the first day of treatment with levetiracetam.
(2) A 15 mg/kg (0.15 ml/kg) loading dose is recommended on the first day of treatment with levetiracetam.
(3) Following dialysis, a 3.5 to 7 mg/kg (0.035 to 0.07 ml/kg) supplemental dose is recommended.
(4) Following dialysis, a 5 to 10 mg/kg (0.05 to 0.10 ml/kg) supplemental dose is recommended.

serum concentrations of concomitantly administered carbamazepine and valproate. However, data suggested a 20% higher levetiracetam clearance in children taking enzyme-inducing antiepileptic medicinal products. Dosage adjustment is not required.

Probenecid (500 mg four times daily), a renal tubular secretion blocking agent, has been shown to inhibit the renal clearance of the primary metabolite but not of levetiracetam. Nevertheless, the concentration of this metabolite remains low. It is expected that other medicinal products excreted by active tubular secretion could also reduce the renal clearance of the metabolite. The effect of levetiracetam on probenecid was not studied and the effect of levetiracetam on other actively secreted medicinal products, *e.g.* NSAIDs, sulfonamides and methotrexate, is unknown.

Levetiracetam 1,000 mg daily did not influence the pharmacokinetics of oral contraceptives (ethinyl-estradiol and levonorgestrel); endocrine parameters (luteinizing hormone and progesterone) were not modified. Levetiracetam 2,000 mg daily did not influence the pharmacokinetics of digoxin and warfarin; prothrombin times were not modified. Co-administration with digoxin, oral contraceptives and warfarin did not influence the pharmacokinetics of levetiracetam.

No data on the influence of antacids on the absorption of levetiracetam are available.

The extent of absorption of levetiracetam was not altered by food, but the rate of absorption was slightly reduced.

No data on the interaction of levetiracetam with alcohol are available.

4.6 Pregnancy and lactation

There are no adequate data from the use of Keppra in pregnant women. Studies in animals have shown reproductive toxicity (see section 5.3). The potential risk for human is unknown.

Keppra should not be used during pregnancy unless clearly necessary.

As with other antiepileptic drugs, physiological changes during pregnancy may affect levetiracetam concentration. Decrease in levetiracetam plasma concentrations has been observed during pregnancy. This decrease is more pronounced during the third trimester (up to 60% of baseline concentration before pregnancy). Appropriate clinical management of pregnant women treated with levetiracetam should be ensured. Discontinuation of antiepileptic treatments may result in exacerbation of the disease which could be harmful to the mother and the foetus.

Levetiracetam is excreted in human breast milk. Therefore, breast-feeding is not recommended.

However, if levetiracetam treatment is needed during breastfeeding, the benefit/risk of the treatment should be weighed considering the importance of breastfeeding.

4.7 Effects on ability to drive and use machines

No studies on the effects on the ability to drive and use machines have been performed.

Due to possible different individual sensitivity, some patients might experience somnolence or other central nervous system related symptoms, especially at the beginning of treatment or following a dose increase. Therefore, caution is recommended in those patients when performing skilled tasks, *e.g.* driving vehicles or operating machinery. Patients are advised not to drive or use machines until it is established that their ability to perform such activities is not affected.

4.8 Undesirable effects

Undesirable effects that resulted from Keppra intravenous use are similar to those associated with Keppra oral use. The most frequently reported adverse reactions were dizziness, somnolence, headache and postural dizziness. Since there was limited exposure for Keppra intravenous use and since oral and intravenous formulations are bioequivalent, the safety information of Keppra intravenous will rely on Keppra oral use.

Pooled safety data from clinical studies conducted with Keppra oral formulations in adult patients with partial onset seizures showed that 46.4 % of the patients in the Keppra group and 42.2 % of the patients in the placebo group experienced undesirable effects. Serious undesirable effects were experienced in 2.4% of the patients in the Keppra and 2.0% of the patients in the placebo groups. The most commonly reported undesirable effects were somnolence, asthenia and dizziness. In the pooled safety analysis, there was no clear dose-response relationship but incidence and severity of the central nervous system related undesirable effects decreased over time.

In monotherapy 49.8 % of the subjects experienced at least one drug related undesirable effect. The most frequently reported undesirable effects were fatigue and somnolence.

A study conducted in paediatric patients (4 to 16 years) with partial onset seizures showed that 55.4 % of the patients in the Keppra group and 40.2 % of the patients in the placebo group experienced undesirable effects. Serious undesirable effects were experienced in 0.0 % of the patients in the Keppra group and 1.0 % of the patients in the placebo group. The most commonly reported undesirable effects were somnolence, hostility, nervousness, emotional lability, agitation, anorexia, asthenia and headache in the paediatric population. Safety results in paediatric patients were consistent with the safety profile of levetiracetam in adults except for behavioural and psychiatric adverse events which were more common in children than in adults (38.6% versus 18.6%). However, the relative risk was similar in children as compared to adults.

A study conducted in paediatric patients (1 month to less than 4 years) with partial onset seizures showed that 21.7 % of the patients in the Keppra group and 7.1 % of the patients in the placebo group experienced undesirable effects. No Serious undesirable effects were experienced in patients in the Keppra or Placebo group. During the long-term follow-up study N01148, the most frequent drug-related treatment-emergent adverse events in the 1m – <4y group were irritability (7.9%), convulsion (7.2%), somnolence (6.6%), psychomotor hyperactivity (3.3%), sleep disorder (3.3%), and aggression (3.3%). Safety results in paediatric patients were consistent with the safety profile of levetiracetam in older children aged 4 to 16 years.

A double-blind, placebo-controlled paediatric safety study with a non-inferiority design has assessed the cognitive and neuropsychological effects of Keppra in children 4 to 16 years of age with partial onset seizures. It was concluded that Keppra was not different (non inferior) from placebo with regard to the change from baseline of the Leiter-R Attention and Memory, Memory Screen Composite score in the per-protocol population. Results related to behavioral and emotional functioning indicated a worsening in Keppra treated patients on aggressive behavior as measured in a standardized and systematic way using a validated instrument (CBCL – Achenbach Child Behavior Checklist). However subjects, who took Keppra in the long-term open label follow-up study, did not experience a worsening, on average, in their behavioural and emotional functioning; in particular measures of aggressive behavior were not worse than baseline.

A study conducted in adults and adolescents with myoclonic seizures (12 to 65 years) showed that 33.3% of the patients in the Keppra group and 30.0% of the patients in the placebo group experienced undesirable effects that were judged to be related to treatment. The most commonly reported undesirable effects were headache and somnolence. The incidence of undesirable effects in patients with myoclonic seizures was lower than that in adult patients with partial onset seizures (33.3% versus 46.4%).

A study conducted in adults and children (4 to 65 years) with idiopathic generalised epilepsy with primary generalised tonic-clonic seizures showed that 39.2 % of the patients in the Keppra group and 29.8 % of the patients in the placebo group experienced undesirable effects that were judged to be related to treatment. The most commonly reported undesirable effect was fatigue.

Undesirable effects reported in clinical studies (adults, adolescents, children and infants > 1 month) or from post-marketing experience are listed in the following table per System Organ Class and per frequency. For clinical trials, the frequency is defined as follows: very common (≥1/10); common (≥1/100, <1/10); uncommon (≥1/1,000, <1/100); rare (≥1/10,000, <1/1,000); very rare (<1/10,000), including isolated reports. Data from post-marketing experience are insufficient to support an estimate of their incidence in the population to be treated.

- General disorders and administration site conditions

Very common: asthenia/fatigue

- Nervous system disorders

Very common: somnolence

Common: amnesia, ataxia, convulsion, dizziness, headache, hyperkinesia, tremor, balance disorder, disturbance in attention, memory impairment.

Post-marketing experience: paraesthesia

- Psychiatric disorders

Common: agitation, depression, emotional lability/mood swings, hostility/aggression, insomnia, nervousness/irritability, personality disorders, thinking abnormal

Post-marketing experience: abnormal behaviour, anger, anxiety, confusion, hallucination, psychotic disorder, suicide, suicide attempt and suicidal ideation

- Gastrointestinal disorders

Common: abdominal pain, diarrhoea, dyspepsia, nausea, vomiting

Post-marketing experience: pancreatitis

- Hepatobiliary disorders:

Post-marketing experience: hepatic failure, hepatitis, liver function test abnormal

- Metabolism and nutrition disorders

Common: anorexia, weight increase.

The risk of anorexia is higher when topiramate is coadministered with levetiracetam.

Post-marketing experience: weight loss

- Ear and labyrinth disorders

Common: vertigo

- Eye disorders

Common: diplopia, vision blurred

- Musculoskeletal and connective tissue disorders

Common: myalgia

- Injury, poisoning and procedural complications

Common: accidental injury

- Infections and infestations

Common: infection, nasopharyngitis

- Respiratory, thoracic and mediastinal disorders

Common: cough increased

- Skin and subcutaneous tissue disorders

Common: rash, eczema, pruritus

Post-marketing experience: alopecia: in several cases, recovery was observed when Keppra was discontinued.

- Blood and lymphatic system disorders

Common: thrombocytopenia

Post-marketing experience: leukopenia, neutropenia, pancytopenia (with bone marrow suppression identified in some of the cases)

4.9 Overdose

Symptoms

Somnolence, agitation, aggression, depressed level of consciousness, respiratory depression and coma were observed with Keppra overdoses.

Management of overdose

After an acute overdose, the stomach may be emptied by gastric lavage or by induction of emesis. There is no specific antidote for levetiracetam. Treatment of an overdose will be symptomatic and may include haemodialysis. The dialyser extraction efficiency is 60 % for levetiracetam and 74 % for the primary metabolite.

5. PHARMACOLOGICAL PROPERTIES

5.1 Pharmacodynamic properties

Pharmacotherapeutic group: antiepileptics, ATC code: N03AX14.

The active substance, levetiracetam, is a pyrrolidone derivative (S-enantiomer of α-ethyl-2-oxo-1-pyrrolidine acetamide), chemically unrelated to existing antiepileptic active substances.

Mechanism of action

The mechanism of action of levetiracetam still remains to be fully elucidated but appears to be different from the mechanisms of current antiepileptic medicinal products. *In vitro* and *in vivo* experiments suggest that levetiracetam does not alter basic cell characteristics and normal neurotransmission.

In vitro studies show that levetiracetam affects intraneuronal Ca2+ levels by partial inhibition of N-type Ca2+ currents and by reducing the release of Ca2+ from intraneuronal stores. In addition it partially reverses the reductions in GABA- and glycine-gated currents induced by zinc and β-carbolines. Furthermore, levetiracetam has been shown in *in vitro* studies to bind to a specific site in rodent brain tissue. This binding site is the synaptic vesicle protein 2A, believed to be involved in vesicle fusion and neurotransmitter exocytosis. Levetiracetam and related analogs show a rank order of affinity for binding to the synaptic vesicle protein 2A which correlates with the potency of their anti-seizure protection in the mouse audiogenic model of epilepsy. This finding suggests that the interaction between levetiracetam and the synaptic vesicle protein 2A seems to contribute to the antiepileptic mechanism of action of the medicinal product.

Pharmacodynamic effects

Levetiracetam induces seizure protection in a broad range of animal models of partial and primary generalised seizures without having a pro-convulsant effect. The primary metabolite is inactive.

In man, an activity in both partial and generalised epilepsy conditions (epileptiform discharge/photoparoxysmal response) has confirmed the broad spectrum pharmacological profile of levetiracetam.

Clinical experience

Adjunctive therapy in the treatment of partial onset seizures with or without secondary generalisation in adults, adolescents, children and infants from 1 month of age with epilepsy:

In adults, levetiracetam efficacy has been demonstrated in 3 double-blind, placebo-controlled studies at 1000 mg, 2000 mg, or 3000 mg/day, given in 2 divided doses, with a treatment duration of up to 18 weeks. In a pooled analysis, the percentage of patients who achieved 50% or greater reduction from baseline in the partial onset seizure frequency per week at stable dose (12/14 weeks) was of 27.7%, 31.6% and 41.3% for patients on 1000, 2000 or 3000 mg levetiracetam respectively and of 12.6% for patients on placebo.

In paediatric patients (4 to 16 years of age), levetiracetam efficacy was established in a double-blind, placebo-controlled study, which included 198 patients and had a treatment duration of 14 weeks. In this study, the patients received levetiracetam as a fixed dose of 60 mg/kg/day (with twice a day dosing).

44.6% of the levetiracetam treated patients and 19.6% of the patients on placebo had a 50% or greater reduction from baseline in the partial onset seizure frequency per week. With continued long-term treatment, 11.4% of the patients were seizure-free for at least 6 months and 7.2% were seizure-free for at least 1 year.

In paediatric patients (1 month to less than 4 years of age), levetiracetam efficacy was established in a double-blind, placebo-controlled study, which included 116 patients and had a treatment duration of 5 days. In this study, patients were prescribed 20 mg/kg, 25 mg/kg, 40 mg/kg or 50 mg/kg daily dose of oral solution based on their age titration schedule. A dose of 20 mg/kg/day titrating to 40 mg/kg/day for infants one month to less than six month and a dose of 25 mg/kg/day titrating to 50 mg/kg/day for infants and children 6 month to less than 4 years old, was use in this study. The total daily dose was administered b.i.d.

The primary measure of effectiveness was the responder rate (percent of patients with ⩾ 50% reduction from baseline in average daily partial onset seizure frequency) assessed by a blinded central reader using a 48-hour video EEG. The efficacy analysis consisted of 109 patients who had at least 24 hours of video EEG in both baseline and evaluation periods. 43.6% of the levetiracetam treated patients and 19.6% of the patients on placebo were considered as responders. The results are consistent across age group. With continued long-term treatment, 8.6% of the patients were seizure-free for at least 6 months and 7.8% were seizure-free for at least 1 year.

Monotherapy in the treatment of partial onset seizures with or without secondary generalisation in patients from 16 years of age with newly diagnosed epilepsy.

Efficacy of levetiracetam as monotherapy was established in a double-blind, parallel group, non-inferiority comparison to carbamazepine controlled release (CR) in 576 patients 16 years of age or older with newly or recently diagnosed epilepsy. The patients had to present with unprovoked partial seizures or with generalized tonic-clonic seizures only. The patients were randomized to carbamazepine CR 400 – 1200 mg/day or levetiracetam 1000 - 3000 mg/day, the duration of the treatment was up to 121 weeks depending on the response.

Six-month seizure freedom was achieved in 73.0% of levetiracetam-treated patients and 72.8% of carbamazepine-CR treated patients; the adjusted absolute difference between treatments was 0.2% (95% CI: -7.8 8.2). More than half of the subjects remained seizure free for 12 months (56.6% and 58.5% of subjects on levetiracetam and on carbamazepine CR respectively).

In a study reflecting clinical practice, the concomitant antiepileptic medication could be withdrawn in a limited number of patients who responded to levetiracetam adjunctive therapy (36 adult patients out of 69).

Adjunctive therapy in the treatment of myoclonic seizures in adults and adolescents from 12 years of age with Juvenile Myoclonic Epilepsy.

Levetiracetam efficacy was established in a double-blind, placebo-controlled study of 16 weeks duration, in patients 12 years of age and older suffering from idiopathic generalized epilepsy with myoclonic seizures in different syndromes. The majority of patients presented with juvenile myoclonic epilepsy.

In this study, levetiracetam, dose was 3000 mg/day given in 2 divided doses.

58.3% of the levetiracetam treated patients and 23.3% of the patients on placebo had at least a 50% reduction in myoclonic seizure days per week. With continued long-term treatment, 28.6% of the patients were free of myoclonic seizures for at least 6 months and 21.0% were free of myoclonic seizures for at least 1 year.

Adjunctive therapy in the treatment of primary generalised tonic-clonic seizures in adults and adolescents from 12 years of age with idiopathic generalised epilepsy.

Levetiracetam efficacy was established in a 24-week double-blind, placebo-controlled study which included adults, adolescents and a limited number of children suffering from idiopathic generalized epilepsy with primary generalized tonic-clonic (PGTC) seizures in different syndromes (juvenile myoclonic epilepsy, juvenile absence epilepsy, childhood absence epilepsy, or epilepsy with Grand Mal seizures on awakening). In this study, levetiracetam dose was 3000 mg/day for adults and adolescents or 60 mg/kg/day for children, given in 2 divided doses.

72.2% of the levetiracetam treated patients and 45.2% of the patients on placebo had a 50% or greater decrease in the frequency of PGTC seizures per week. With continued long-term treatment, 47.4% of the patients were free of tonic-clonic seizures for at least 6 months and 31.5% were free of tonic-clonic seizures for at least 1 year.

5.2 Pharmacokinetic properties

Levetiracetam is a highly soluble and permeable compound. The pharmacokinetic profile is linear with low intra- and inter-subject variability. There is no modification of the clearance after repeated administration. There is no evidence for any relevant gender, race or circadian variability. The pharmacokinetic profile is comparable in healthy volunteers and in patients with epilepsy.

Due to its complete and linear absorption, plasma levels can be predicted from the oral dose of levetiracetam expressed as mg/kg bodyweight. Therefore there is no need for plasma level monitoring of levetiracetam.

A significant correlation between saliva and plasma concentrations has been shown in adults and children (ratio of saliva/plasma concentrations ranged from 1 to 1.7 for oral tablet formulation and after 4 hours post-dose for oral solution formulation).

Adults and adolescents

Absorption

Levetiracetam is rapidly absorbed after oral administration. Oral absolute bioavailability is close to 100 %.

Peak plasma concentrations (C_{max}) are achieved at 1.3 hours after dosing. Steady-state is achieved after two days of a twice daily administration schedule.

Peak concentrations (C_{max}) are typically 31 and 43 μg/ml following a single 1,000 mg dose and repeated 1,000 mg twice daily dose, respectively.

The extent of absorption is dose-independent and is not altered by food.

Distribution

No tissue distribution data are available in humans.

Neither levetiracetam nor its primary metabolite are significantly bound to plasma proteins (< 10 %).

The volume of distribution of levetiracetam is approximately 0.5 to 0.7 l/kg, a value close to the total body water volume.

Biotransformation

Levetiracetam is not extensively metabolised in humans. The major metabolic pathway (24 % of the dose) is an enzymatic hydrolysis of the acetamide group. Production of the primary metabolite, ucb L057, is not supported by liver cytochrome P_{450} isoforms. Hydrolysis of the acetamide group was measurable in a large number of tissues including blood cells. The metabolite ucb L057 is pharmacologically inactive.

Two minor metabolites were also identified. One was obtained by hydroxylation of the pyrrolidone ring (1.6 % of the dose) and the other one by opening of the pyrrolidone ring (0.9 % of the dose).

Other unidentified components accounted only for 0.6 % of the dose.

No enantiomeric interconversion was evidenced *in vivo* for either levetiracetam or its primary metabolite.

In vitro, levetiracetam and its primary metabolite have been shown not to inhibit the major human liver cytochrome P_{450} isoforms (CYP3A4, 2A6, 2C9, 2C19, 2D6, 2E1 and 1A2), glucuronyl transferase (UGT1A1 AND UGT1A6]) and epoxide hydroxylase activities. In addition, levetiracetam does not affect the *in vitro* glucuronidation of valproic acid.

In human hepatocytes in culture, levetiracetam had little or no effect on CYP1A2, SULT1E1 or UGT1A1. Levetiracetam caused mild induction of CYP2B6 and CYP3A4. The in vitro data and in vivo interaction data on oral contraceptives, digoxin and warfarin indicate that no significant enzyme induction is expected in vivo. Therefore, the interaction of Keppra with other substances, or *vice versa,* is unlikely.

Elimination

The plasma half-life in adults was 7±1 hours and did not vary either with dose, route of administration or repeated administration. The mean total body clearance was 0.96 ml/min/kg.

The major route of excretion was via urine, accounting for a mean 95 % of the dose (approximately 93 % of the dose was excreted within 48 hours). Excretion *via* faeces accounted for only 0.3 % of the dose.

The cumulative urinary excretion of levetiracetam and its primary metabolite accounted for 66 % and 24 % of the dose, respectively during the first 48 hours.

The renal clearance of levetiracetam and ucb L057 is 0.6 and 4.2 ml/min/kg respectively indicating that levetiracetam is excreted by glomerular filtration with subsequent tubular reabsorption and that the primary metabolite is also excreted by active tubular secretion in addition to glomerular filtration. Levetiracetam elimination is correlated to creatinine clearance.

Elderly

In the elderly, the half-life is increased by about 40 % (10 to 11 hours). This is related to the decrease in renal function in this population (see section 4.2).

Children (4 to 12 years)

Following single oral dose administration (20 mg/kg) to epileptic children (6 to 12 years), the half-life of levetiracetam was 6.0 hours. The apparent body weight adjusted clearance was approximately 30 % higher than in epileptic adults.

Following repeated oral dose administration (20 to 60 mg/kg/day) to epileptic children (4 to 12 years), levetiracetam was rapidly absorbed. Peak plasma concentration was observed 0.5 to 1.0 hour after dosing. Linear and dose proportional increases were observed for peak plasma concentrations and area under the curve. The elimination half-life was approximately 5 hours. The apparent body clearance was 1.1 ml/min/kg.

Infants and children (1 month to 4 years)

Following single dose administration (20 mg/kg) of a 100 mg/ml oral solution to epileptic children (1 month to 4 years), levetiracetam was rapidly absorbed and peak plasma concentrations were observed approximately 1 hour after dosing. The pharmacokinetic results indicated that half-life was shorter (5.3 h) than for adults (7.2 h) and apparent clearance was faster (1.5 ml/min/kg) than for adults (0.96 ml/min/kg).

In the population pharmacokinetic analysis conducted in patients from 1 month to 16 years of age, body weight was significantly correlated to apparent clearance (clearance increased with an increase in body weight) and apparent volume of distribution. Age also had an influence on both parameters. This effect was pronounced for the younger infants, and subsided as age increased, to become negligible around 4 years of age.

In both population pharmacokinetic analyses, there was about a 20% increase of apparent clearance of levetiracetam when it was co-administered with an enzyme-inducing AED.

Renal impairment

The apparent body clearance of both levetiracetam and of its primary metabolite is correlated to the creatinine clearance. It is therefore recommended to adjust the maintenance daily dose of Keppra, based on creatinine clearance in patients with moderate and severe renal impairment (see section 4.2).

In anuric end-stage renal disease adult subjects the half-life was approximately 25 and 3.1 hours during interdialytic and intradialytic periods, respectively.

The fractional removal of levetiracetam was 51 % during a typical 4-hour dialysis session.

Hepatic impairment

In subjects with mild and moderate hepatic impairment, there was no relevant modification of the clearance of levetiracetam. In most subjects with severe hepatic impairment, the clearance of levetiracetam was reduced by more than 50 % due to a concomitant renal impairment (see section 4.2).

5.3 Preclinical safety data

Non-clinical data reveal no special hazard for humans based on conventional studies of safety pharmacology, genotoxicity and carcinogenicity.

Adverse effects not observed in clinical studies but seen in the rat and to a lesser extent in the mouse at exposure levels similar to human exposure levels and with possible

Table 2 Preparation and administration of Keppra concentrate

Dose	Withdrawal Volume	Volume of Diluent	Infusion Time	Frequency of administration	Total Daily Dose
250 mg	2.5 ml (half 5 ml vial)	100 ml	15 minutes	Twice daily	500 mg/day
500 mg	5 ml (one 5 ml vial)	100 ml	15 minutes	Twice daily	1000 mg/day
1000 mg	10 ml (two 5 ml vials)	100 ml	15 minutes	Twice daily	2000 mg/day
1500 mg	15 ml (three 5 ml vials)	100 ml	15 minutes	Twice daily	3000 mg/day

relevance for clinical use were liver changes, indicating an adaptive response such as increased weight and centrilobular hypertrophy, fatty infiltration and increased liver enzymes in plasma.

Two embryo-fetal development (EFD) studies were performed in rats at 400, 1200 and 3600 mg/kg/day. At 3600 mg/kg/day, in only one of the 2 EFD studies, there was a slight decrease in fetal weight associated with a marginal increase in skeletal variations/minor anomalies. There was no effect on embryomortality and no increased incidence of malformations. The NOAEL (No Observed Adverse Effect Level) was 3600 mg/kg/day for pregnant female rats (x 12 the MRHD on a mg/m2 basis) and 1200 mg/kg/day for foetuses.

Four embryo-fetal development studies were performed in rabbits covering doses of 200, 600, 800, 1200 and 1800 mg/kg/day. The dose level of 1800 mg/kg/day induced a marked maternal toxicity and a decrease in fetal weight associated with increased incidence of foetuses with cardiovascular/skeletal anomalies. The NOAEL was <200 mg/kg/day for the dams and 200 mg/kg/day for the foetuses (equal to the MRHD on a mg/m2 basis).

A peri- and post-natal development study was performed in rats with levetiracetam doses of 70, 350 and 1800 mg/kg/day. The NOAEL was ≥ 1800 mg/kg/day for the F0 females, and for the survival, growth and development of the F1 offspring up to weaning (x 6 the MRHD on a mg/m2 basis).

Neonatal and juvenile animal studies in rats and dogs demonstrated that there were no adverse effects seen in any of the standard developmental or maturation endpoints at doses up to 1800 mg/kg/day (x 6 – 17 the MRHD on a mg/m2 basis).

6. PHARMACEUTICAL PARTICULARS

6.1 List of excipients

Tablets

Keppra 250 mg, Keppra 500 mg, Keppra 750 mg, Keppra 1000 mg film coated tablets

Core: Sodium croscarmellose, Macrogol 6000, colloidal anhydrous silica, magnesium stearate.

Keppra 250 mg

Film-coating: Opadry 85F20694: Polyvinyl alcohol-part.hydrolyzed, Titanium dioxide (E171), Macrogol 3350, Talc, Indigo carmine aluminium lake (E132).

Keppra 500 mg

Film-coating: Opadry 85F32004: Polyvinyl alcohol-part.hydrolyzed, Titanium dioxide (E171), Macrogol 3350, Talc, Iron oxide yellow (E172).

Keppra 750 mg

Film-coating: Opadry 85F23452: Polyvinyl alcohol-part.hydrolyzed, Titanium dioxide (E171), Macrogol 3350, Talc, sunset yellow FCF aluminium lake (E110), Iron oxide red (E172).

Keppra 1000 mg

Film-coating: Opadry 85F18422: Polyvinyl alcohol-part.hydrolyzed, Titanium dioxide (E171), Macrogol 3350, Talc.

Keppra 100 mg/ml, oral solution

Sodium citrate, citric acid monohydrate, methyl parahydroxybenzoate (E 218), propyl parahydroxybenzoate (E 216), ammonium glycyrrhizate, glycerol (E 422), maltitol (E 965), acesulfame potassium (E 950), grape flavour, purified water.

Keppra 100 mg/ml concentrate for solution for infusion.

Sodium acetate, glacial acetic acid, sodium chloride, water for injection.

6.2 Incompatibilities

Not applicable.

Keppra 100 mg/ml concentrate for solution for infusion:

This medicinal product must not be mixed with other medicinal products except those mentioned in section 6.6.

6.3 Shelf life

Tablets:

3 years.

Oral solution:

Finished product: 2 years.

After first opening: 4 months

Keppra 100 mg/ml concentrate for solution for infusion:

Finished product: 2 years.

From a microbiological point of view, the product should be used immediately after dilution. If not used immediately, in-use storage time and conditions prior to use are the responsibility of the user and would normally not be longer than 24 hours at 2 to 8°C, unless dilution has taken place in controlled and validated aseptic conditions.

6.4 Special precautions for storage

Tablets:

No special precautions for storage.

Oral solution:

Store in original container.

Keppra 100 mg/ml concentrate for solution for infusion:

No special precautions for storage. For storage conditions of the diluted medicinal product, see section 6.3.

6.5 Nature and contents of container

Tablets:

Keppra 250 mg, Keppra 500mg, Keppra 750mg, Keppra 1000 mg film-coated tablets are packaged in aluminium/PVC blisters placed into cardboard boxes containing 20, 30, 50, 60, 100 & 200 film-coated tablets.

Oral solution:

300 ml amber glass bottle (type III) with a white child resistant closure (polypropylene) in a cardboard box also containing a 10 ml graduated oral syringe (polypropylene, polyethylene) an adaptor for the syringe (polyethylene) and a patient information leaflet.

150 ml amber glass bottle (type III) with a white child resistant closure (polypropylene) in a cardboard box also containing a 3 ml graduated oral syringe (polypropylene, polyethylene) an adaptor for the syringe (polyethylene) and a patient information leaflet.

150 ml amber glass bottle (type III) with a white child resistant closure (polypropylene) in a cardboard box also containing a 1 ml graduated oral syringe (polypropylene, polyethylene) an adaptor for the syringe (polyethylene) and a patient information leaflet.

Concentrate for solution for infusion:

Keppra 100 mg/ml concentrate for solution for infusion is packed in glass vials (type I) with Teflon faced stoppers and sealed with an aluminium/polypropylene flip off cap. The vials are placed into cartons of 10 vials. Each vial contains 5 ml of concentrate.

Not all pack sizes may be marketed.

6.6 Special precautions for disposal and other handling

Tablets and oral solution:

No special requirements.

Concentrate for solution for infusion:

One vial of Keppra concentrate contains 500 mg levetiracetam (5 ml concentrate of 100 mg/ml). See Table 2 for the recommended preparation and administration of Keppra concentrate to achieve a total daily dose of 500 mg, 1000 mg, 2000 mg, or 3000 mg in two divided doses.

Table 2. Preparation and administration of Keppra concentrate

(see Table 2 above)

This medicinal product is for single use only, any unused solution should be discarded.

Keppra concentrate was found to be physically compatible and chemically stable when mixed with the following diluents for at least 24 hours and stored in PVC bags at controlled room temperature 15-25°C.

Diluents:

- Sodium chloride (0.9%) injection
- Lactated Ringer's injection
- Dextrose 5% injection

Product with particulate matter or discoloration should not be used.

7. MARKETING AUTHORISATION HOLDER

UCB Pharma SA

Allée de la Recherche 60

B-1070 Brussels

Belgium

8. MARKETING AUTHORISATION NUMBER(S)

EU/1/00/146/004 – 250 mg film-coated tablets × 60

EU/1/00/146/010 – 500 mg film-coated tablets × 60

EU/1/00/146/017 – 750 mg film-coated tablets × 60

EU/1/00/146/024 – 1000 mg film-coated tablets × 60

EU/1/00/146/027 – 100 mg/ml oral solution – 300 ml with 10 ml syringe and adaptor

EU/1/00/146/030 – Concentrate Solution for infusion

EU/1/00/146/031 - 100 mg/ml oral solution – 150 ml with 3 ml syringe and adaptor

EU/1/00/146/032 – 100 mg/ml oral solution – 150 ml with 1 ml syringe and adaptor

9. DATE OF FIRST AUTHORISATION/RENEWAL OF THE AUTHORISATION

Date of first authorisation: 29 September 2000

Date of last renewal: 08 July 2005

10. DATE OF REVISION OF THE TEXT

September 2009

Keral

(A. Menarini Pharma U.K. S.R.L.)

1. NAME OF THE MEDICINAL PRODUCT

KERAL 25 mg film-coated tablets

2. QUALITATIVE AND QUANTITATIVE COMPOSITION

Each tablet contains: Dexketoprofen trometamol 36.9 mg corresponding to dexketoprofen 25 mg.

For a full list of excipients, see section 6.1

3. PHARMACEUTICAL FORM

Film coated tablets.

Keral 25 mg: white, round, scored film-coated tablets. The tablets can be divided into equal halves.

4. CLINICAL PARTICULARS

4.1 Therapeutic indications

Symptomatic treatment of pain of mild to moderate intensity, such as musculo-skeletal pain, dysmenorrhoea, dental pain.

4.2 Posology and method of administration

General population:

According to the nature and severity of pain, the recommended dosage is generally 12.5 mg every 4-6 hours or 25 mg every 8 hours. The total daily dose should not exceed 75 mg.

Undesirable effects may be minimised by using the lowest effective dose for the shortest duration necessary to control symptoms (see section 4.4).

KERAL tablets are not intended for long term use and the treatment must be limited to the symptomatic period.

Concomitant administration with food delays the absorption rate of the drug (see Pharmacokinetic Properties), thus in case of acute pain it is recommended that administration is at least 30 minutes before meals.

Elderly:

In elderly patients it is recommended to start the therapy at the lower end of the dosage range (50 mg total daily dose). The dosage may be increased to that recommended for the general population only after good general tolerance has been ascertained.

Hepatic dysfunction:

Patients with mild to moderate hepatic dysfunction should start therapy at reduced doses (50 mg total daily dose) and be closely monitored. KERAL tablets should not be used in patients with severe hepatic dysfunction.

Renal dysfunction:

The initial dosage should be reduced to 50 mg total daily dose in patients with mildly impaired renal function. KERAL tablets should not be used in patients with moderate to severe renal dysfunction.

Children and adolescents:

KERAL tablets have not been studied in children and adolescents. Therefore, safety and efficacy have not been established and the product should not be used in children and adolescents.

4.3 Contraindications

KERAL tablets must not be administered in the following cases:

- patients hypersensitive to dexketoprofen, to any other NSAID, or to any of the excipients of the product.
- patients in whom substances with a similar action (e.g. aspirin, or other NSAIDs) precipitate attacks of asthma, bronchospasm, acute rhinitis, or cause nasal polyps, urticaria or angioneurotic oedema.
- patients with active or suspected peptic ulcer/haemorrhage or history of recurrent peptic ulcer/haemorrhage (two or more distinct episodes of proven ulceration or bleeding) or chronic dyspepsia.
- patients with history of gastrointestinal bleeding or perforation, related to previous NSAIDs therapy
- patients who have gastrointestinal bleeding or other active bleedings or bleeding disorders.
- patients with Crohn's disease or ulcerative colitis.
- patients with a history of bronchial asthma.
- patients with severe heart failure.
- patients with moderate to severe renal dysfunction.
- patients with severely impaired hepatic function.

- patients with haemorrhagic diathesis and other coagulation disorders.

- during pregnancy and lactation period.

4.4 Special warnings and precautions for use

The safe use in children and adolescents has not been established.

Administer with caution in patients with a history of allergic conditions.

The use of Keral with concomitant other NSAIDs including cyclooxygenase-2 selective inhibitors should be avoided.

Undesirable effects may be minimised by using the minimum effective dose for the shortest duration necessary to control symptoms (see section 4.2, and GI and cardiovascular risks below).

Gastrointestinal bleeding, ulceration or perforation which can be fatal, have been reported with all NSAIDs at anytime during treatment, with or without warning symptoms or a previous history of serious gastrointestinal events. When gastrointestinal bleeding or ulceration occurs in patients receiving Keral, the treatment should be withdrawn.

The risk of gastrointestinal bleeding, ulceration or perforation is higher with increasing NSAID doses, in patients with a history of ulcer, particularly if complicated with haemorrhage or perforation (see section 4.3), and in the elderly.

Elderly: The elderly have an increased frequency of adverse reactions to NSAIDs especially gastrointestinal bleeding and perforation which may be fatal (see section 4.2).

These patients should commence treatment on the lowest dose available.

As with all NSAIDs, any history of oesophagitis, gastritis and/or peptic ulcer must be sought in order to ensure their total cure before starting treatment with dexketoprofen trometamol.

Patients with gastrointestinal symptoms or history of gastrointestinal disease should be monitored for digestive disturbances, especially gastrointestinal bleeding.

NSAIDs should be given with care to patients with a history of gastrointestinal disease (ulcerative colitis, Crohn's disease) as their condition may be exacerbated (see section 4.8 undesirable effects).

Combination therapy with protective agents (e.g. misoprostol or proton pump inhibitors) should be considered for these patients, and also for patients requiring concomitant low dose aspirin, or other drugs likely to increase gastrointestinal risk (see below and section 4.5).

Patients with a history of gastrointestinal toxicity, particularly when elderly, should report any unusual abdominal symptoms (especially gastrointestinal bleeding) particularly in the initial stages of treatment.

Caution should be advised in patients receiving concomitant medications which could increase the risk of ulceration or bleeding, such as oral corticosteroids, anticoagulants such as warfarin, selective serotonin-reuptake inhibitors or anti-platelet agents such as aspirin (see section 4.5).

All non-selective NSAIDs can inhibit platelet aggregation and prolong bleeding time via inhibition of prostaglandin synthesis. Therefore, the use of dexketoprofen trometamol in patients who are receiving other therapy that interferes with haemostasis, such as warfarin or other coumarins or heparins is not recommended (see Section 4.5).

As with all NSAIDs, it can increase plasma urea nitrogen and creatinine. As with other inhibitors of prostaglandin synthesis, it can be associated with adverse effects on the renal system which can lead to glomerular nephritis, interstitial nephritis, renal papillary necrosis, nephrotic syndrome and acute renal failure.

As with other NSAIDs, it can cause transient small increases in some liver parameters, and also significant increases in SGOT and SGPT. In case of a relevant increase in such parameters, therapy must be discontinued.

KERAL tablets should be administered with caution to patients suffering from haematopoietic disorders, systemic lupus erythematosus or mixed connective tissue disease.

As other NSAIDs, dexketoprofen can mask the symptoms of infectious diseases.

Caution should be exercised in patients with impairment of hepatic and/or renal functions as well as in patients with a history of hypertension and/or heart failure. In these patients, the use of NSAIDs may result in deterioration of renal function, fluid retention and oedema. Caution is also required in patients receiving diuretic therapy or those who could develop hypovolaemia as there is an increased risk of nephrotoxicity. Special caution should be exercised in patients with a history of cardiac disease, in particular those with previous episodes of heart failure as there is an increased risk of triggering heart failure.

Elderly patients are more likely to be suffering from impaired renal cardiovascular or hepatic function (see section 4.2).

Serious skin reactions, some of them fatal, including exfoliative dermatitis, Stevens-Johnson syndrome, and toxic epidermal necrolysis, have been reported very rarely in association with the use of NSAIDs (see section 4.8). Patients appear to be at highest risk of these reactions early in the course of therapy, the onset of the reaction occurring in the majority of cases within the first month of treatment. Keral should be discontinued at the first appearance of skin rash, mucosal lesions, or any other sign of hypersensitivity.

As with other NSAIDS, the use of dexketoprofen trometamol may impair female fertility and is not recommended in women attempting to conceive. In women who have difficulties conceiving or who are undergoing investigation of infertility, withdrawal of dexketoprofen trometamol should be considered.

Appropriate monitoring and advice are required for patients with a history of hypertension and/or mild to moderate congestive heart failure as fluid retention and oedema have been reported in association with NSAIDs therapy.

Clinical trial and epidemiological data suggest that use of some NSAIDs (particularly at high doses and in long term treatment) may be associated with a small increased risk of arterial thrombotic events (for example myocardial infarction or stroke). There are insufficient data to exclude such a risk for Dexketoprofen Trometamol.

Patients with uncontrolled hypertension, congestive heart failure, established ischaemic heart disease, peripheral arterial disease, and/or cerebrovascular disease should only be treated with Dexketoprofen Trometamol after careful consideration. Similar consideration should be made before initiating longer-term treatment of the patients with risk factors for cardiovascular disease (e.g. hypertension, hyperlipidaemia, diabetes mellitus, smoking).

4.5 Interaction with other medicinal products and other forms of interaction

The following interactions apply to non-steroidal antiinflammatory drugs (NSAIDs) in general:

Inadvisable combinations:

- Other NSAIDs, including high doses of salicylates ($\geqslant$ 3 g/day): administration of several NSAIDs together may increase the risk of gastrointestinal ulcers and bleeding, via a synergistic effect.

- Anticoagulants: NSAIDs may enhance the effects of anticoagulants, such as warfarin (see section 4.4) due to the high plasma protein binding of dexketoprofen and the inhibition of platelet function and damage to the gastroduodenal mucosa. If the combination cannot be avoided, close clinical observation and monitoring of laboratory values should be carried out.

- Heparins: increased risk of haemorrhage (due to the inhibition of platelet function and damage to the gastroduodenal mucosa). If the combination cannot be avoided, close clinical observation and monitoring of laboratory values should be carried out.

- Corticosteroids: there is an increased risk of gastrointestinal ulceration or bleeding (see section 4.4)

- Lithium (described with several NSAIDs): NSAIDs increase blood lithium levels, which may reach toxic values (decreased renal excretion of lithium). This parameter therefore requires monitoring during the initiation, adjustment and withdrawal of treatment with dexketoprofen.

- Methotrexate, used at high doses of 15 mg/week or more: increased haematological toxicity of methotrexate via a decrease in its renal clearance by antiinflammatory agents in general.

- Hydantoines and sulphonamides: the toxic effects of these substances may be increased.

Combinations requiring precautions:

- Diuretics, ACE inhibitors and angiotensin II receptor antagonists: Dexketoprofen may reduce the effect of diuretics and antihypertensive drugs. In some patients with compromised renal function (e. g. dehydrated patients or elderly patients with compromised renal function), the coadministration of agents that inhibit cyclo-oxygenase and ACE inhibitors or angiotensin II receptor antagonists may result in further deterioration of renal function, which is usually reversible. In case of combined prescription of dexketoprofen and a diuretic, it is essential to ensure that the patient is adequately hydrated and to monitor renal function at the start of the treatment (see section 4.4 Special warnings and special precautions for use).

- Methotrexate, used at low doses, less than 15 mg/week: increased haematological toxicity of methotrexate via a decrease in its renal clearance by antiinflammatory agents in general. Weekly monitoring of blood count during the first weeks of the combination. Increased surveillance in the presence of even mildly impaired renal function, as well as in the elderly.

- Pentoxyfilline: increased risk of bleeding. Increase clinical monitoring and check bleeding time more often.

- Zidovudine: risk of increased red cell line toxicity via action on reticulocytes, with severe anaemia occurring one week after the NSAID is started. Check CBC and reticulocyte count one to two weeks after starting treatment with the NSAID.

- Sulfonylureas: NSAIDs can increase the hypoglycaemic effect of sulfonylureas by displacement from plasma protein binding sites.

Associations needing to be taken into account:

- Beta-blockers: treatment with a NSAID may decrease their antihypertensive effect via inhibition of prostaglandin synthesis.

- Cyclosporin and tacrolimus: nephrotoxicity may be enhanced by NSAIDs via renal prostaglandin mediated effects. During combination therapy, renal function has to be measured.

- Thrombolytics: increased risk of bleeding.

- Anti-platelet agents and selective serotonin reuptake inhibitors (SSRIs): increased risk of gastrointestinal bleeding (see section 4.4).

- Probenecid: plasma concentrations of dexketoprofen may be increased; this interaction can be due to an inhibitory mechanism at the site of renal tubular secretion and of glucuronoconjugation and requires adjustment of the dose of dexketoprofen.

- Cardiac Glycosides: NSAIDS may increase plasma glycoside concentration.

- Mifepristone: Because of a theoretical risk that prostaglandin synthetase inhibitors may alter the efficacy of mifepristone, NSAIDS should not be used for 8-12 days after mifepristone administration.

- Quinolone antibiotics: Animal data indicate that high doses of quinolones in combination with NSAIDS can increase the risk of developing convulsions.

4.6 Pregnancy and lactation

KERAL tablets are contraindicated during pregnancy and lactation (see section 4.3).

Pregnancy

Inhibition of prostaglandin synthesis may adversely affect the pregnancy and/or the embryo/foetal development. Data from epidemiological studies raise concern about an increased risk of miscarriage and of cardiac malformation and gastroschisis after use of a prostaglandin synthesis inhibitor in early pregnancy. The absolute risk for cardiovascular malformation was increased from less than 1%, up to approximately 1.5%. The risk is believed to increase with dose and duration of therapy. In animals, administration of a prostaglandin synthesis inhibitor has been shown to result in increased pre- and post-implantation loss and embryo-foetal lethality. In addition, increased incidences of various malformations including cardiovascular, have been reported in animals given a prostaglandin synthesis inhibitor during the organogenetic period. Nevertheless, animal studies with dexketoprofen trometamol haven't shown reproductive toxicity (see 5.3). During the first and second trimester of pregnancy, dexketoprofen trometamol should not be given unless clearly necessary. If dexketoprofen trometamol is used by a woman attempting to conceive, or during the first and second trimester of pregnancy, the dose should be kept as low and duration of treatment as short as possible.

During the third trimester of pregnancy, all prostaglandin synthesis inhibitors may expose the fetus to:

- cardiopulmonary toxicity (with premature closure of the ductus arteriosus and pulmonary hypertension);

- renal dysfunction, which may progress to renal failure with oligo-hydroamniosis;

the mother and the neonate, at the end of pregnancy, to:

- possible prolongation of bleeding time, an anti-aggregating effect which may occur even at very low doses

- inhibition of uterine contractions resulting in delayed or prolonged labour.

It is not known whether dexketoprofen is excreted in human milk.

4.7 Effects on ability to drive and use machines

KERAL tablets can cause minor or moderate effects on the ability to drive or use machines due to the possibility of dizziness or drowsiness occurring.

4.8 Undesirable effects

The adverse reactions reported as at least possibly related with dexketoprofen trometamol in clinical trials, as well as the adverse reactions reported after the marketing of KERAL tablets are tabulated below, classified by system organ class and ordered by frequency:

(see Table 1 on next page)

Gastrointestinal: The most commonly-observed adverse events are gastrointestinal in nature. Peptic ulcers, perforation or gastrointestinal bleeding, sometimes fatal, particularly in the elderly, may occur (see section 4.4). Nausea, vomiting, diarrhoea, flatulence, constipation, dyspepsia, abdominal pain, melaena, haematemesis, ulcerative stomatitis, exacerbation of colitis and Crohn's disease (see section 4.4 Special warnings and precautions for use) have been reported following administration. Less frequently, gastritis has been observed.

Oedema, hypertension and cardiac failure have been reported in association with NSAIDs treatment.

As with other NSAIDS, the following undesirable effects may appear: aseptic meningitis, which might predominantly occur in patients with systemic lupus erythematosus or mixed connective tissue disease; haematological reactions (purpura, aplastic and haemolytic anaemia, and rarely agranulocytosis and medullar hypoplasia).

Bullous reactions including Stevens Johnson Syndrome and Toxic Epidermal Necrolysis (very rare).

Clinical trial and epidemiological data suggest that use of some NSAIDs (particularly at high doses and in long term treatment) may be associated with a small increased risk of

Table 1

SYSTEM ORGAN CLASS	Common (1-10%)	Uncommon (0.1-1%)	Rare (0.01-0.1%)	Very rare / Isolated reports (< 0.01%)
Blood and lymphatic system disorders				Neutropenia Thrombocytopenia
Immune system disorders				Anaphylactic reaction, including anaphylactic shock
Metabolism and nutrition disorders			Anorexia	
Psychiatric disorders		Insomnia, anxiety		
Nervous system disorders		Headache, dizziness, somnolence	Paraesthesia, syncope	
Eye disorders				Blurred vision
Ear and labyrinth disorders		Vertigo		Tinnitus
Cardiac disorders		Palpitations		Tachycardia
Vascular disorders		Flushing	Hypertension	Hypotension
Respiratory, thoracic and mediastinal disorders			Bradypnoea	Bronchospasm, dyspnoea
Gastrointestinal disorders	Nausea and/or vomiting, abdominal pain, diarrhoea, dyspepsia.	Gastritis, constipation, dry mouth, flatulence	Peptic ulcer, peptic ulcer haemorrhage or peptic ulcer perforation (see section 4.4)	Pancreatitis
Hepatobiliary disorders				Hepatocellular damage
Skin and subcutaneous tissue disorders		Rash	Urticaria, acne, sweating increased	Stevens Johnson syndrome, toxic epidermal necrolysis (Lyell's syndrome), angioneurotic oedema, facial oedema, photosensitivity reactions, pruritus
Musculoskeletal and connective tissue disorders			Back pain	
Renal and urinary disorders			Polyuria	Nephritis or nephrotic syndrome
Reproductive system and breast disorders			Menstrual disorder, prostatic disorder	
General disorders and administration site conditions		Fatigue, pain, asthenia, rigors, malaise	Peripheral oedema	
Investigations			Liver function test abnormal	

arterial thrombotic events (for example myocardial infarction or stroke) (see section 4.4).

4.9 Overdose

In case of accidental or excessive intake, immediately institute symptomatic therapy according to the patient's clinical condition. Activated charcoal should be administered if more than 5 mg/kg has been ingested by an adult or a child within an hour. Dexketoprofen trometamol may be removed by dialysis.

5. PHARMACOLOGICAL PROPERTIES

5.1 Pharmacodynamic properties

Pharmacotherapeutic group: propionic acid derivatives

ATC code: M01AE17.

Dexketoprofen trometamol is the tromethamine salt of S-(+)-2-(3-benzoylphenyl)propionic acid, an analgesic, anti-inflammatory and antipyretic drug, which belongs to the non-steroidal anti-inflammatory group of drugs (M01AE).

The mechanism of action of non-steroidal antiinflammatory drugs is related to the reduction of prostaglandin synthesis by the inhibition of cyclooxygenase pathway. Specifically, there is an inhibition of the transformation of arachidonic acid into cyclic endoperoxides, PGG_2 and PGH_2, which produce prostaglandins PGE_1, PGE_2, $PGF_{2\alpha}$ and PGD_2 and also prostacyclin PGI_2 and thromboxanes (TxA_2 and TxB_2). Furthermore, the inhibition of the synthesis of prostaglandins could affect other inflammation mediators such as kinins, causing an indirect action which would be additional to the direct action.

Dexketoprofen has been demonstrated to be an inhibitor for COX-1 and COX-2 activities in experimental animals and humans.

Clinical studies performed on several pain models demonstrated effective analgesic activity of dexketoprofen trometamol. The onset of the analgesic activity was obtained in some studies at 30 minutes post-administration. The analgesic effect persists for 4 to 6 hours.

5.2 Pharmacokinetic properties

After oral administration of dexketoprofen trometamol to humans, the Cmax is reached at 30 min (range 15 to 60 min).

The distribution half-life and elimination half-life values of dexketoprofen trometamol are 0.35 and 1.65 hours, respectively. As with other drugs with a high plasma protein binding (99%), its volume of distribution has a mean value below 0.25 l/kg. The main elimination route for dexketoprofen is glucuronide conjugation followed by renal excretion.

After administration of dexketoprofen trometamol only the S-(+) enantiomer is obtained in urine, demonstrating that no conversion to the R-(-) enantiomer occurs in humans.

In multiple-dose pharmacokinetic studies, it was observed that the AUC after the last administration is not different from that obtained following a single dose, indicating that no drug accumulation occurs.

When administered concomitantly with food, the AUC does not change, however the Cmax of dexketoprofen trometamol decreases and its absorption rate is delayed (increased tmax).

5.3 Preclinical safety data

Preclinical data revealed no special hazard for humans based on conventional studies of safety pharmacology, repeated dose toxicity, genotoxicity, toxicity to reproduction and immunopharmacology. The chronic toxicity studies carried out in mice and monkeys gave a No Observed Adverse Effect Level (NOAEL) of 3 mg/kg/day. The main adverse effect observed at high doses was gastrointestinal erosions and ulcers that developed dose-dependently.

6. PHARMACEUTICAL PARTICULARS

6.1 List of excipients

Maize starch, microcrystalline cellulose, sodium starch glycollate, glycerol distearate, hypromellose, titanium dioxide, propylene glycol, macrogol 6000.

6.2 Incompatibilities

Not applicable

6.3 Shelf life

2 years.

6.4 Special precautions for storage

Do not store above 30°C; keep the blister packs in the outer carton in order to protect from light.

6.5 Nature and contents of container

Tablets are provided in blister packs (PVC-aluminium blister)

KERAL 25 mg tablets - 4, 10, 20, 30, 50, or 500 film-coated tablets/pack

(Not all pack sizes may be marketed).

6.6 Special precautions for disposal and other handling

No special requirements.

7. MARKETING AUTHORISATION HOLDER

MENARINI INTERNATIONAL O.L.S.A.

1, Avenue de la Gare, L-1611

Luxembourg.

8. MARKETING AUTHORISATION NUMBER(S)

PL 16239/0007

9. DATE OF FIRST AUTHORISATION/RENEWAL OF THE AUTHORISATION

Date of first authorisation: 14 January 1998

Date of last renewal: 25 April 2006

10. DATE OF REVISION OF THE TEXT

March 2007

Legal Category

POM

Ketalar Injection

(Pfizer Limited)

1. NAME OF THE MEDICINAL PRODUCT

Ketalar^{TM} 10 mg/ml, 50 mg/ml, 100 mg/ml Injection

2. QUALITATIVE AND QUANTITATIVE COMPOSITION

Each 1 ml of solution contains:

Ketalar 10mg/ml Injection: ketamine hydrochloride Ph Eur equivalent to 10 mg ketamine base per ml.

Ketalar 50mg/ml Injection: ketamine hydrochloride Ph Eur equivalent to 50 mg ketamine base per ml.

Ketalar 100mg/ml Injection: ketamine hydrochloride Ph Eur equivalent to 100 mg ketamine base per ml.

3. PHARMACEUTICAL FORM

Solution for injection or infusion.

A clear solution for injection or infusion.

4. CLINICAL PARTICULARS

4.1 Therapeutic indications

Ketalar is recommended:

As an anaesthetic agent for diagnostic and surgical procedures. When used by intravenous or intramuscular injection, Ketalar is best suited for short procedures. With additional doses, or by intravenous infusion, Ketalar can be used for longer procedures. If skeletal muscle relaxation is desired, a muscle relaxant should be used and respiration should be supported.

For the induction of anaesthesia prior to the administration of other general anaesthetic agents.

To supplement other anaesthetic agents.

Specific areas of application or types of procedures:

When the intramuscular route of administration is preferred.

Debridement, painful dressings, and skin grafting in burned patients, as well as other superficial surgical procedures.

Neurodiagnostic procedures such as pneumoencephalograms, ventriculograms, myelograms, and lumbar punctures.

Diagnostic and operative procedures of the eye, ear, nose, and mouth, including dental extractions.

Note: Eye movements may persist during ophthalmological procedures.

Anaesthesia in poor-risk patients with depression of vital functions or where depression of vital functions must be avoided, if at all possible.

Orthopaedic procedures such as closed reductions, manipulations, femoral pinning, amputations, and biopsies.

Sigmoidoscopy and minor surgery of the anus and rectum, circumcision and pilonidal sinus.

Cardiac catheterization procedures.

Caesarean section; as an induction agent in the absence of elevated blood pressure.

Anaesthesia in the asthmatic patient, either to minimise the risks of an attack of bronchospasm developing, or in the presence of bronchospasm where anaesthesia cannot be delayed.

4.2 Posology and method of administration

For intravenous infusion, intravenous injection or intramuscular injection.

NOTE: All doses are given in terms of ketamine base

Adults, elderly (over 65 years) and children:

For surgery in elderly patients ketamine has been shown to be suitable either alone or supplemented with other anaesthetic agents.

Preoperative preparations

Ketalar has been safely used alone when the stomach was not empty. However, since the need for supplemental agents and muscle relaxants cannot be predicted, when preparing for elective surgery it is advisable that nothing be given by mouth for at least six hours prior to anaesthesia.

Premedication with an anticholinergic agent (e.g. atropine, hyoscine or glycopyrolate) or another drying agent should be given at an appropriate interval prior to induction to reduce ketamine-induced hypersalivation.

Midazolam, diazepam, lorazepam, or flunitrazepam used as a premedicant or as an adjunct to ketamine, have been effective in reducing the incidence of emergence reactions.

Onset and duration

As with other general anaesthetic agents, the individual response to Ketalar is somewhat varied depending on the dose, route of administration, age of patient, and concomitant use of other agents, so that dosage recommendation cannot be absolutely fixed. The dose should be titrated against the patient's requirements.

Because of rapid induction following intravenous injection, the patient should be in a supported position during administration. An intravenous dose of 2 mg/kg of bodyweight usually produces surgical anaesthesia within 30 seconds after injection and the anaesthetic effect usually lasts 5 to 10 minutes. An intramuscular dose of 10 mg/kg of bodyweight usually produces surgical anaesthesia within 3 to 4 minutes following injection and the anaesthetic effect usually lasts 12 to 25 minutes. Return to consciousness is gradual.

A. Ketalar as the sole anaesthetic agent

Intravenous Infusion

The use of Ketalar by continuous infusion enables the dose to be titrated more closely, thereby reducing the amount of drug administered compared with intermittent administration. This results in a shorter recovery time and better stability of vital signs.

A solution containing 1 mg/ml of ketamine in dextrose 5% or sodium chloride 0.9% is suitable for administration by infusion.

General Anaesthesia Induction

An infusion corresponding to 0.5 – 2 mg/kg as total induction dose.

Maintenance of anaesthesia

Anaesthesia may be maintained using a microdrip infusion of 10 - 45 microgram/kg/min (approximately 1 – 3 mg/min).

The rate of infusion will depend on the patient's reaction and response to anaesthesia. The dosage required may be reduced when a long acting neuromuscular blocking agent is used.

Intermittent Injection

Induction

Intravenous Route

The initial dose of Ketalar administered intravenously may range from 1 mg/kg to 4.5mg/kg (in terms of ketamine base). The average amount required to produce 5 to 10 minutes of surgical anaesthesia has been 2.0 mg/kg. It is recommended that intravenous administration be accomplished slowly (over a period of 60 seconds). More rapid administration may result in respiratory depression and enhanced pressor response.

Note: the 100 mg/ml concentration of ketamine should not be injected intravenously without proper dilution. It is recommended that the drug be diluted with an equal volume of either sterile water for injection, normal saline, or 5% dextrose in water.

Intramuscular Route

The initial dose of Ketalar administered intramuscularly may range from 6.5 mg/kg to 13 mg/kg (in terms of ketamine base). A low initial intramuscular dose of 4 mg/kg has been used in diagnostic manoeuvres and procedures not involving intensely painful stimuli. A dose of 10 mg/kg will usually produce 12 to 25 minutes of surgical anaesthesia.

Dosage in Hepatic Insufficiency:

Dose reductions should be considered in patients with cirrhosis or other types of liver impairment (see section 4.4 Special Warnings and Special Precautions for Use).

Maintenance of general anaesthesia

Lightening of anaesthesia may be indicated by nystagmus, movements in response to stimulation, and vocalization. Anaesthesia is maintained by the administration of additional doses of Ketalar by either the intravenous or intramuscular route.

Each additional dose is from ½ to the full induction dose recommended above for the route selected for maintenance, regardless of the route used for induction.

The larger the total amount of Ketalar administered, the longer will be the time to complete recovery.

Purposeless and tonic-clonic movements of extremities may occur during the course of anaesthesia. These movements do not imply a light plane and are not indicative of the need for additional doses of the anaesthetic.

B. Ketalar as induction agent prior to the use of other general anaesthetics

Induction is accomplished by a full intravenous or intramuscular dose of Ketalar as defined above. If Ketalar has been administered intravenously and the principal anaesthetic is slow-acting, a second dose of Ketalar may be required 5 to 8 minutes following the initial dose. If Ketalar has been administered intramuscularly and the principal anaesthetic is rapid-acting, administration of the principal anaesthetic may be delayed up to 15 minutes following the injection of Ketalar.

C. Ketalar as supplement to anaesthetic agents

Ketalar is clinically compatible with the commonly used general and local anaesthetic agents when an adequate respiratory exchange is maintained. The dose of Ketalar for use in conjunction with other anaesthetic agents is usually in the same range as the dosage stated above; however, the use of another anaesthetic agent may allow a reduction in the dose of Ketalar.

D. Management of patients in recovery

Following the procedure the patient should be observed but left undisturbed. This does not preclude the monitoring of vital signs. If, during the recovery, the patient shows any indication of emergence delirium, consideration may be given to the use of diazepam (5 to 10 mg I.V. in an adult). A hypnotic dose of a thiobarbiturate (50 to 100 mg I.V.) may be used to terminate severe emergence reactions. If any one of these agents is employed, the patient may experience a longer recovery period.

4.3 Contraindications

Ketalar is contra-indicated in persons in whom an elevation of blood pressure would constitute a serious hazard (see section 4.8 Undesirable effects). Ketamine hydrochloride is contraindicated in patients who have shown hypersensitivity to the drug or its components. Ketalar should not be used in patients with eclampsia or pre-eclampsia, severe coronary or myocardial disease, cerebrovascular accident or cerebral trauma.

4.4 Special warnings and precautions for use

To be used only in hospitals by or under the supervision of experienced medically qualified anaesthetists except under emergency conditions.

As with any general anaesthetic agent, resuscitative equipment should be available and ready for use.

Respiratory depression may occur with overdosage of Ketalar, in which case supportive ventilation should be employed. Mechanical support of respiration is preferred to the administration of analeptics.

The intravenous dose should be administered over a period of 60 seconds. More rapid administration may result in transient respiratory depression or apnoea and enhanced pressor response.

Because pharyngeal and laryngeal reflexes usually remain active, mechanical stimulation of the pharynx should be avoided unless muscle relaxants, with proper attention to respiration, are used.

Although aspiration of contrast medium has been reported during Ketalar anaesthesia under experimental conditions (Taylor, P A and Towey, R M, Brit. Med. J. 1971, 2: 688), in clinical practice aspiration is seldom a problem.

In surgical procedures involving visceral pain pathways, Ketalar should be supplemented with an agent which obtunds visceral pain.

When Ketalar is used on an outpatient basis, the patient should not be released until recovery from anaesthesia is complete and then should be accompanied by a responsible adult.

Ketalar should be used with caution in patients with the following conditions:

Use with caution in the chronic alcoholic and the acutely alcohol-intoxicated patient.

Ketamine is metabolised in the liver and hepatic clearance is required for termination of clinical effects. A prolonged duration of action may occur in patients with cirrhosis or other types of liver impairment. Dose reductions should be considered in these patients.

Since an increase in cerebrospinal fluid (CSF) pressure has been reported during Ketalar anaesthesia, Ketalar should be used with special caution in patients with preanaesthetic elevated cerebrospinal fluid pressure.

Use with caution in patients with globe injuries and increased intraocular pressure (e.g. glaucoma) because the pressure may increase significantly after a single dose of ketamine.

Use with caution in patients with neurotic traits or psychiatric illness (e.g. schizophrenia and acute psychosis).

Use in caution in patients with acute intermittent porphyria.

Use in caution in patients with seizures.

Use in caution in patients with hyperthyroidism or patients receiving thyroid replacement (increased risk of hypertension and tachycardia).

Use in caution in patients with pulmonary or upper respiratory infection (ketamine sensitises the gag reflex, potentially causing laryngospasm).

Use in caution in patients with intracranial mass lesions, a presence of head injury, or hydrocephalus.

Emergence Reaction

The psychological manifestations vary in severity between pleasant dream-like states, vivid imagery, hallucinations, nightmares or illusions and emergence delirium (often consisting of dissociative or floating sensations), In some cases these states have been accompanied by confusion, excitement, and irrational behaviour which a few patients recall as an unpleasant experience. (See section 4.8 Undesirable Effects).

Emergence delirium phenomena may occur during the recovery period. The incidence of these reactions may be reduced if verbal and tactile stimulation of the patient is minimised during the recovery period. This does not preclude the monitoring of vital signs.

Because of the substantial increase in myocardial oxygen consumption, ketamine should be used in caution in patients with hypovolemia, dehydration or cardiac disease, especially coronary artery disease (e.g. congestive heart failure, myocardial ischemia and myocardial infarction). In addition ketamine should be used with caution in patients with mild-to-moderate hypertension and tachyarrythmais.

Cardiac function should be continually monitored during the procedure in patients found to have hypertension or cardiac decompensation.

Ketalar has been reported as being a drug of abuse. If used on a daily basis for a few weeks, dependence and tolerance may develop, particularly in individuals with a history of drug abuse and dependence. Therefore the use of Ketalar should be closely supervised and it should be prescribed and administered with caution.

4.5 Interaction with other medicinal products and other forms of interaction

Prolonged recovery time may occur if barbiturates and/or narcotics are used concurrently with Ketalar.

Ketalar is chemically incompatible with barbiturates and diazepam because of precipitate formation. Therefore, these should not be mixed in the same syringe or infusion fluid.

Ketamine may potentiate the neuromuscular blocking effects of atracurium and tubocurarine including respiratory depression with apnea.

The use of halogenated anesthetics concomitantly with ketamine can lengthen the elimination half-life of ketamine and delay recovery from anesthesia. Concurrent use of ketamine (especially in high doses or when rapidly administered) with halogenated anesthetics can increase the risk of developing bradycardia, hypotension or decreased cardiac output.

The use of ketamine with other central nervous system (CNS) depressants (e.g. ethanol, phenothiazines, sedating H_1 – blockers or skeletal muscle relaxants) can potentiate CNS depression and/or increase risk of developing respiratory depression. Reduced doses of ketamine may be required with concurrent administration of other anxiolytics, sedatives and hypnotics.

Ketamine has been reported to antagonise the hypnotic effect of thiopental.

Patients taking thyroid hormones have an increased risk of developing hypertension and tachycardia when given ketamine.

Concomitant use of antihypertensive agents and ketamine increases the risk of developing hypotension.

When ketamine and theophylline are given concurrently, a clinically significant reduction in the seizure threshold is observed. Unpredictable extensor-type seizures have been reported with concurrent administration of these agents.

4.6 Pregnancy and lactation

Ketalar crosses the placenta. This should be borne in mind during operative obstetric procedures in pregnancy. With the exception of administration during surgery for abdominal delivery or vaginal delivery, no controlled clinical studies in pregnancy have been conducted. The safe use in pregnancy, and in lactation, has not been established and such use is not recommended.

4.7 Effects on ability to drive and use machines

Patients should be cautioned that driving a car, operating hazardous machinery or engaging in hazardous activities should not be undertaken for 24 hours or more after anaesthesia.

4.8 Undesirable effects

Cardiac and Vascular Disorders:

Temporary elevation of blood pressure and pulse rate is frequently observed following administration of ketamine hydrochloride. However, hypotension and bradycardia have been reported. Arrhythmias have also occurred. The median peak rise of blood pressure has ranged from 20 to 25 per cent of preanaesthetic values. Depending on the condition of the patient, this elevation of blood pressure may be considered an adverse reaction or a beneficial effect.

Respiratory, Thoracic and Mediastinal Disorders:

Depression of respiration or apnoea may occur following over rapid intravenous administration or high doses of ketamine hydrochloride. Laryngospasm and other forms of airway obstruction have occurred during ketamine hydrochloride anaesthesia. Increased salivation leading to respiratory difficulties may occur unless an antisialogogue is used.

Eye Disorders:

Diplopia and nystagmus may occur following ketamine hydrochloride administration. An elevation in intraocular pressure may also occur.

Psychiatric Disorders:

Reports suggest that ketamine produces a variety of symptoms including, but not limited to, flashbacks, hallucinations, nightmares, illusions, dysphoria, anxiety, insomnia or disorientation (often consisting of dissociative or floating sensations).

During recovery from anaesthesia the patient may experience emergence delirium, characterised by vivid dreams (pleasant or unpleasant), with or without psychomotor activity, manifested by confusion and irrational behaviour. The fact that these reactions are observed less often in the young (15 years of age or less) makes Ketalar especially useful in paediatric anaesthesia. These reactions are also less frequent in the elderly (over 65 years of age) patient. The incidence of emergence reactions is reduced as experience with the drug is gained. No residual psychological effects are known to have resulted from the use of Ketalar.

Nervous System Disorders:

In some patients, enhanced skeletal muscle tone may be manifested by tonic and clonic movements sometimes resembling seizures. These movements do not imply a light plane of anaesthesia and are not indicative of a need for additional doses of the anaesthetic.

Metabolism and Nutritional Disorders:

Anorexia has been observed; however this is not usually severe and allows the great majority of patients to take liquids by mouth shortly after regaining consciousness.

Gastro-intestinal Disorders:

Nausea and vomiting have been observed; however, these are uncommon and are not usually severe. The great majority of patients are able to take liquids by mouth shortly after regaining consciousness. Hypersalivation (see section 4.2 Posology and Method of Administration – Preoperative Preparations).

Immune System Disorders:

There have been a number of reported cases of anaphylaxis.

General Disorders and Administration Site Conditions:

Local pain and exanthema at the injection site have infrequently been reported.

Skin and Subcutaneous Tissue Disorders:

Transient erythema and/or morbilliform rash have also been reported.

4.9 Overdose

Respiratory depression can result from an overdosage of ketamine hydrochloride. Supportive ventilation should be employed. Mechanical support of respiration that will maintain adequate blood oxygen saturation and carbon dioxide elimination is preferred to administration of analeptics.

Ketalar has a wide margin of safety; several instances of unintentional administration of overdoses of Ketalar (up to 10 times that usually required) have been followed by prolonged but complete recovery.

5. PHARMACOLOGICAL PROPERTIES

5.1 Pharmacodynamic properties

Ketamine is a rapidly acting general anaesthetic for intravenous or intramuscular use with a distinct pharmacological action. Ketamine hydrochloride produces dissociative anaesthesia characterised by catalepsy, amnesia, and marked analgesia which may persist into the recovery period. Pharyngeal-laryngeal reflexes remain normal and skeletal muscle tone may be normal or can be enhanced to varying degrees. Mild cardiac and respiratory stimulation and occasionally respiratory depression occur.

Mechanism of Action:

Ketamine induces sedation, immobility, amnesia and marked analgesia. The anaesthetic state produced by ketamine has been termed "dissociative anaesthesia" in that it appears to selectively interrupt association pathways of the brain before producing somesthetic sensory blockade. It may selectively depress the thalamoneocortical system before significantly obtunding the more ancient cerebral centres and pathways (reticular-activating and limbic systems). Numerous theories have been proposed to explain the effects of ketamine, including binding to N-methyl-D-aspartate (NMDA) receptors in the CNS, interactions with opiate receptors at central and spinal sites and interaction with norepinephrine, serotonin and muscarinic cholinergic receptors. The activity on NMDA receptors may be responsible for the analgesic as well as psychiatric (psychosis) effects of ketamine. Ketamine has sympathomimetic activity resulting in tachycardia, hypertension, increased myocardial and cerebral oxygen consumption, increased cerebral blood flow and increased intracranial and intraocular pressure. Ketamine is also a potent bronchodilator. Clinical effects observed following ketamine administration include increased blood pressure, increased muscle tone (may resemble catatonia), opening of eyes (usually accompanied by nystagmus) and increased myocardial oxygen consumption.

5.2 Pharmacokinetic properties

Ketamine is rapidly distributed into perfused tissues including brain and placenta. Animal studies have shown ketamine to be highly concentrated in body fat, liver and lung. Biotransformation takes place in liver. Termination of anaesthetic is partly by redistribution from brain to other tissues and partly by metabolism. Elimination half-life is approximately 2-3 hours, and excretion renal, mostly as conjugated metabolites.

5.3 Preclinical safety data

Preclinical safety data does not add anything of further significance to the prescriber.

6. PHARMACEUTICAL PARTICULARS

6.1 List of excipients

Ketalar 10mg/ml Injection: sodium chloride, benzethonium chloride, water for injection

Ketalar 50mg/ml Injection: benzethonium chloride, water for injection

Ketalar 100mg/ml Injection: benzethonium chloride, water for injection

6.2 Incompatibilities

Ketalar is chemically incompatible with barbiturates and diazepam because of precipitate formation. Therefore, these should not be mixed in the same syringe or infusion fluid.

6.3 Shelf life

3 years

For single use only. Discard any unused product at the end of each operating session.

After dilution the solutions should be used immediately.

6.4 Special precautions for storage

Do not store above 25°C. Do not freeze. Store in the original container. Discard any unused product at the end of each operating session.

6.5 Nature and contents of container

Ketalar 10mg/ml Injection: 20 ml white neutral glass vial with rubber closure and aluminium flip-off cap containing 10 mg ketamine base per ml.

Ketalar 50mg/ml Injection: 12 ml vials containing 10 ml of solution as 50 mg ketamine base per ml.

Ketalar 100mg/ml Injection: 12 ml vials containing 10 ml of solution as 100 mg ketamine base per ml.

6.6 Special precautions for disposal and other handling

For single use only. Discard any unused product at the end of each operating session.

See Section 4.2 Posology and method of administration.

7. MARKETING AUTHORISATION HOLDER

Pfizer Limited, Sandwich, Kent CT13 9NJ, United Kingdom

8. MARKETING AUTHORISATION NUMBER(S)

PL 00057/0529, PL 00057/0530, PL 00057/0531

9. DATE OF FIRST AUTHORISATION/RENEWAL OF THE AUTHORISATION

1st July 2003

10. DATE OF REVISION OF THE TEXT

May 2009

Company Reference: KE 6_1 UK

Ketek 400mg Tablets

(sanofi-aventis)

1. NAME OF THE MEDICINAL PRODUCT

Ketek 400 mg film-coated tablets.▼

2. QUALITATIVE AND QUANTITATIVE COMPOSITION

Each film-coated tablet contains 400 mg of telithromycin.

For a full list of excipients, see section 6.1.

3. PHARMACEUTICAL FORM

Film-coated tablet.

Light orange, oblong, biconvex tablet, imprinted with H3647 on one side and 400 on the other.

4. CLINICAL PARTICULARS

4.1 Therapeutic indications

When prescribing Ketek, consideration should be given to official guidance on the appropriate use of antibacterial agents and the local prevalence of resistance (see also sections 4.4 and 5.1).

Ketek is indicated for the treatment of the following infections:

In patients of 18 years and older:

- Community-acquired pneumonia, mild or moderate (see section 4.4).
- When treating infections caused by known or suspected beta-lactam and/or macrolide resistant strains (according to history of patients or national and/or regional resistance data) covered by the antibacterial spectrum of telithromycin (see sections 4.4 and 5.1):

- Acute exacerbation of chronic bronchitis,

- Acute sinusitis

In patients of 12 years and older:

- Tonsillitis/pharyngitis caused by *Streptococcus pyogenes*, as an alternative when beta lactam antibiotics are not appropriate in countries/regions with a significant prevalence of macrolide resistant S. pyogenes, when mediated by ermTR or mefA (see sections 4.4 and 5.1).

4.2 Posology and method of administration

The recommended dose is 800 mg once a day i.e. two 400 mg tablets once a day. The tablets should be swallowed whole with a sufficient amount of water. The tablets may be taken with or without food.

Consideration may be given to taking Ketek at bedtime, to reduce the potential impact of visual disturbances and loss of consciousness (see section 4.4).

In patients of 18 years and older, according to the indication, the treatment regimen will be:

- Community-acquired pneumonia: 800 mg once a day for 7 to 10 days,

- Acute exacerbation of chronic bronchitis: 800 mg once a day for 5 days,

- Acute sinusitis: 800 mg once a day for 5 days,

- Tonsillitis/pharyngitis caused by *Streptococcus pyogenes*: 800 mg once a day for 5 days.

In patients of 12 to 18 years old, the treatment regimen will be:

- Tonsillitis/pharyngitis caused by *Streptococcus pyogenes*: 800 mg once a day for 5 days.

In the elderly:

No dosage adjustment is required in elderly patients based on age alone.

In children:

Ketek is not recommended for use in children below 12 years of age due to lack of data on safety and efficacy (see section 5.2).

Impaired renal function:

No dosage adjustment is necessary in patients with mild or moderate renal impairment. Ketek is not recommended as first choice in patients with severe renal impairment (creatinine clearance <30ml/min) or patients with both severe renal impairment and co-existing hepatic impairment, as an optimal dosage format (600 mg) is not available. If telithromycin treatment is deemed necessary, these patients may be treated with alternating daily doses of 800 mg and 400 mg, starting with the 800 mg dose.

In haemodialysed patients, the posology should be adjusted so that Ketek 800 mg is given after the dialysis session (see also section 5.2).

Impaired hepatic function:

No dosage adjustment is necessary in patients with mild, moderate, or severe hepatic impairment, unless renal function is severely impaired, however the experience in patients with impaired hepatic function is limited. Hence, Ketek should be used with caution (see also section 4.4 and 5.2).

4.3 Contraindications

Ketek is contraindicated in patients with myasthenia gravis (see section 4.4).

Hypersensitivity to the active substance, to any of the macrolide antibacterial agents, or to any of the excipients.

Ketek must not be used in patients with previous history of hepatitis and/or jaundice associated with the use of telithromycin.

Concomitant administration of Ketek and any of the following substances is contraindicated: cisapride, ergot alkaloid derivatives (such as ergotamine and dihydroergotamine), pimozide, astemizole and terfenadine (see section 4.5).

Ketek should not be used concomitantly with simvastatin, atorvastatin and lovastatin. Treatment with these agents should be interrupted during Ketek treatment (see section 4.5).

Ketek is contraindicated in patients with a history of congenital or a family history of long QT syndrome (if not excluded by ECG) and in patients with known acquired QT interval prolongation.

In patients with severely impaired renal and/or hepatic function, concomitant administration of Ketek and strong

Table 1

System organ class	Very common (≥1/10)	Common (≥1/100 to <1/10)	Uncommon (≥1/1,000 to <1/100)	Rare (≥1/10,000 to <1/1,000)	Very rare (<1/10,000)	Frequency unknown (cannot be estimated from available data)*
Cardiac disorders			Flush Palpitations	Atrial arrhythmia, hypotension, bradycardia		QT/QTc interval prolongation
Blood and the lymphatic system disorders			Eosinophilia			
Nervous system disorders		Dizziness, headache, disturbance of taste	Vertigo somnolence, nervousness, insomnia,	Transient loss of consciousness, paraesthesia	Parosmia	Cases of rapid onset of exacerbaion of myasthenia gravis have been reported (see sections 4.3 and 4.4). Ageusia, anosmia,
Eye disorders			Blurred vision	Diplopia		
Gastro-intestinal disorders	Diarrhoea	Nausea, vomiting, gastrointestinal pain, flatulence	Oral *Candida* infection, stomatitis anorexia, constipation		Pseudo-membranous colitis	Pancreatitis
Skin and subcutaneous tissue disorders			Rash, urticaria, pruritus	Eczema	Erythema multiforme	
Musculoskeletal, connective tissue					Muscle cramps	Arthralgia, myalgia
Immune system disorders						Angioneurotic oedema, anaphylactic reactions including anaphylactic shock, hyper-sensitivity.
Hepato-biliary disorders		Increase in liver enzymes (AST, ALT, alkaline phosphatase)	Hepatitis	Cholestatic jaundice		Severe hepatitis and liver failure (see section 4.4)
Reproductive system disorders		Vaginal *Candida* infection				
Psychiatric disorders						Confusion, hallucination

* postmarketing experience.

CYP3A4 inhibitors, such as protease inhibitors or ketoconazole, is contraindicated.

4.4 Special warnings and precautions for use

As with macrolides, due to a potential to increase QT interval, Ketek should be used with care in patients with coronary heart disease, a history of ventricular arrhythmias, uncorrected hypokalaemia and or hypomagnesaemia, bradycardia (<50 bpm), or during concomitant administration of Ketek with QT interval prolonging agents or potent CYP 3A4 inhibitors such as protease inhibitors and ketoconazole.

As with nearly all antibacterial agents, diarrhoea, particularly if severe, persistent and /or bloody, during or after treatment with Ketek may be caused by *pseudomembranous colitis*. If *pseudomembranous colitis* is suspected, the treatment must be stopped immediately and patients should be treated with supportive measures and/or specific therapy.

Exacerbations of myasthenia gravis have been reported in patients treated with telithromycin and sometimes occurred within a few hours of the first dose. Reports have included death and life threatening acute respiratory failure with rapid onset (see section 4.8).

Alterations in hepatic enzymes have been commonly observed in clinical studies with telithromycin. Post-marketing cases of severe hepatitis and liver failure, including fatal cases (which have generally been associated with serious underlying diseases or concomitant medications), have been reported (see section 4.8). These hepatic reactions were observed during or immediately after treatment, and in most cases were reversible after discontinuation of telithromycin.

Patients should be advised to stop treatment and contact their doctor if signs and symptoms of hepatic disease develop such as anorexia, jaundice, dark urine, pruritus or tender abdomen.

Due to limited experience, Ketek should be used with caution in patients with liver impairment (see section 5.2).

Ketek may cause visual disturbances particularly in slowing the ability to accommodate and the ability to release accommodation. Visual disturbances included blurred vision, difficulty focusing, and diplopia. Most events were mild to moderate; however, severe cases have been reported (see sections 4.7 and 4.8).

There have been post-marketing adverse event reports of transient loss of consciousness including some cases associated with vagal syndrome (see sections 4.7 and 4.8).

Consideration may be given to taking Ketek at bedtime, to reduce the potential impact of visual disturbances and loss of consciousness.

Ketek should not be used during and 2 weeks after treatment with CYP3A4 inducers (such as rifampicin, phenytoin, carbamazepine, phenobarbital, St John's wort). Concomitant treatment with these medicinal products is likely to result in subtherapeutic levels of telithromycin and therefore encompass a risk of treatment failure (see section 4.5).

Ketek is an inhibitor of CYP3A4 and should only be used under specific circumstances during treatment with other medicinal products that are metabolised by CYP3A4. Patients with concomitant treatment of pravastatin, rosuvastatin or fluvastatin should be carefully monitored for signs and symptoms of myopathy and rhabdomyolysis (see sections 4.3 and 4.5).

In areas with a high incidence of erythromycin A resistance, it is especially important to take into consideration the evolution of the pattern of susceptibility to telithromycin and other antibiotics.

In community acquired pneumonia, efficacy has been demonstrated in a limited number of patients with risk factors such as pneumococcal bacteraemia or age higher than 65 years.

Experience of treatment of infections caused by penicillin/ or erythromycin resistant *S. pneumoniae* is limited, but so far, clinical efficacy and eradication rates have been similar compared with the treatment of susceptible *S. pneumoniae*. Caution should be taken when *S. aureus* is the suspected pathogen and there is a likelihood of erythromycin resistance based on local epidemiology.

L. pneumophila is highly susceptible to telithromycin *in vitro*, however, the clinical experience of the treatment of pneumonia caused by *legionella* is limited.

As for macrolides, *H. influenzae* is classified as intermediately susceptible. This should be taken into account when treating infections caused by *H. influenzae.*

4.5 Interaction with other medicinal products and other forms of interaction

Interaction studies have only been performed in adults.

• Effect of Ketek on other medicinal product

Telithromycin is an inhibitor of CYP3A4 and a weak inhibitor of CYP2D6. In vivo studies with simvastatin, midazolam and cisapride have demonstrated a potent inhibition of intestinal CYP3A4 and a moderate inhibition of hepatic CYP3A4. The degree of inhibition with different CYP3A4 substrates is difficult to predict. Hence, Ketek should not be used during treatment with medicinal products that are CYP3A4 substrates, unless plasma concentrations of the CYP3A4 substrate, efficacy or adverse events can be closely monitored. Alternatively, interruption in the treatment with the CYP3A4 substrate should be made during treatment with Ketek.

Medicinal products with a potential to prolong QT interval

Ketek is expected to increase the plasma levels of cisapride, pimozide, astemizole and terfenadine. This could result in QT interval prolongation and cardiac arrhythmias including ventricular tachycardia, ventricular fibrillation and torsades de pointes. Concomitant administration of Ketek and any of these medicinal products is contraindicated (see section 4.3).

Caution is warranted when Ketek is administered to patients taking other medicinal products with the potential to prolong QT interval (see section 4.4).

Ergot alkaloid derivatives (such as ergotamine and dihydroergotamine)

By extrapolation from erythromycin A and josamycin, concomitant medication of Ketek and alkaloid derivatives could lead to severe vasoconstriction ("ergotism") with possibly necrosis of the extremities. The combination is contraindicated (see section 4.3).

Statins

When simvastatin was coadministered with Ketek, there was a 5.3 fold increase in simvastatin C_{max}, an 8.9 fold increase in simvastatin AUC, a 15-fold increase in simvastatin acid C_{max} and an 11-fold increase in simvastatin acid AUC. Ketek may produce a similar interaction with lovastatin and atorvastatin which are also mainly metabolized by CYP3A4. Ketek should therefore not be used concomitantly with simvastatin, atorvastatin or lovastatin (see section 4.3). Treatment with these agents should be interrupted during Ketek treatment. The exposure of pravastatin, rosuvastatin and to a lesser extent fluvastatin, may be increased due to possible involvement of transporters proteins, but this increase is expected to be lesser than interactions involving CYP3A4 inhibition. However, patients should be carefully monitored for signs and symptoms of myopathy and rhabdomyolysis when co-treated with pravastatin, rosuvastatin and fluvastatin.

Benzodiazepines

When midazolam was coadministered with Ketek, midazolam AUC was increased 2.2-fold after intravenous administration of midazolam and 6.1-fold after oral administration. The midazolam half-life was increased about 2.5-fold. Oral administration of midazolam concomitantly with Ketek should be avoided. Intravenous dosage of midazolam should be adjusted as necessary and monitoring of the patient be undertaken. The same precautions should also apply to the other benzodiazepines which are metabolized by CYP3A4, (especially triazolam but also to a lesser extent alprazolam). For those benzodiazepines which are not metabolized by CYP3A4 (temazepam, nitrazepam, lorazepam) an interaction with Ketek is unlikely.

Cyclosporin, tacrolimus, sirolimus

Due to its CYP3A4 inhibitory potential, telithromycin can increase blood concentrations of these CYP34A4 substrates. Thus, when initiating telithromycin in patients already receiving any of theses immunosuppressive agents, cyclosporin, tacrolimus or sirolimus levels must be carefully monitored and their doses decreased as necessary. When telithromycin is discontinued, cyclosporin, tacrolimus or sirolimus levels must be again carefully monitored and their dose increased as necessary.

Metoprolol

When metoprolol (a CYP2D6 substrate) was coadministered with Ketek, metropolol Cmax and AUC were increased by approximately 38%, however, there was no effect on the elimination half-life of metoprolol. The increase exposure to metoprolol may be of clinical importance in patients with heart failure treated with metoprolol. In these patients, co-administration of Ketek and metoprolol, a CYP2D6 substrate, should be considered with caution.

Digoxin

Ketek has been shown to increase the plasma concentrations of digoxin. The plasma trough levels, C_{max}, AUC and renal clearance were increased by 20 %, 73 %, 37 % and 27% respectively, in healthy volunteers. There were no significant changes in ECG parameters and no signs of digoxin toxicity were observed. Nevertheless, monitoring of serum digoxin level should be considered during concomitant administration of digoxin and Ketek.

Theophylline

There is no clinically relevant pharmacokinetic interaction of Ketek and theophylline administered as extended release formulation. However, the co-administration of both medicinal products should be separated by one hour in order to avoid possible digestive side effects such as nausea and vomiting.

Oral anticoagulants

Increased anticoagulant activity has been reported in patients simultaneously treated with anticoagulants and antibiotics, including telithromycin. The mechanisms are incompletely known. Although Ketek has no clinically relevant pharmacokinetic or pharmacodynamic interaction with warfarin after single dose administration, more frequent monitoring of prothrombin time/INR (International Normalised Ratio) values should be considered during concomitant treatment.

Oral contraceptives

There is no pharmacodynamic or clinically relevant pharmacokinetic interaction with low-dose triphasic oral contraceptives in healthy subjects.

• Effect of other medicinal products on Ketek

During concomitant administration of rifampicin and telithromycin in repeated doses, C_{max} and AUC of telithromycin were on average decreased by 79% and 86% respectively. Therefore, concomitant administration of CYP3A4 inducers (such as rifampicin, phenytoin, carbamazepine, phenobarbital, St John's wort) is likely to result in subtherapeutic levels of telithromycin and loss of effect. The induction gradually decreases during 2 weeks after cessation of treatment with CYP3A4 inducers. Ketek should not be used during and 2 weeks after treatment with CYP3A4 inducers.

Interaction studies with itraconazole and ketoconazole, two CYP3A4 inhibitors, showed that maximum plasma concentrations of telithromycin were increased respectively by 1.22 and 1.51 fold and AUC by respectively 1.54 fold and 2.0 fold. These changes in the pharmacokinetics of telithromycin do not necessitate dosage adjustment as telithromycin exposure remains within a well tolerated range. The effect of ritonavir on telithromycin has not been studied and could lead to larger increase in telithromycin exposure. The combination should be used with caution.

Ranitidine (taken 1 hour before Ketek) and antacid containing aluminium and magnesium hydroxide has no clinically relevant influence on telithromycin pharmacokinetics.

4.6 Pregnancy and lactation

There are no adequate data from the use of Ketek in pregnant women. Studies in animals have shown reproductive toxicity (see section 5.3). The potential risk for humans is unknown. Ketek should not be used during pregnancy unless clearly necessary.

Telithromycin is excreted in the milk of lactating animals, at concentrations about 5 times those of maternal plasma. Corresponding data for humans is not available. Ketek should not be used by breast-feeding women.

4.7 Effects on ability to drive and use machines

Ketek may cause undesirable effects such as visual disturbances, confusion or hallucination which may reduce the capacity for the completion of certain tasks. In addition, rare cases of transient loss of consciousness, which may be preceded by vagal symptoms, have been reported (see section 4.8). Because of potential visual difficulties or loss of consciousness, patients should attempt to minimize activities such as driving a motor vehicle, operating heavy machinery or engaging in other hazardous activities during treatment with Ketek. If patients experience visual disorders or loss of consciousness while taking Ketek, patients should not drive a motor vehicle, operate heavy machinery or engage in other hazardous activities (see sections 4.4 and 4.8).

Patients should be informed that these undesirable effects may occur as early as after the first dose of medication. Patients should be cautioned about the potential effects of these events on the ability to drive or operate machinery.

4.8 Undesirable effects

In 2461 patients treated by Ketek in phase III clinical trials, the following undesirable effects possibly or probably related to telithromycin have been reported. This is shown below.

Within each frequency grouping, undesirable effects are presented in order of decreasing seriousness.

(see Table 1 on previous page)

Visual disturbances (<1%) associated with the use of Ketek, including blurred vision, difficulty focusing and diplopia, were mostly mild to moderate. They typically occurred within a few hours after the first or second dose, recurred upon subsequent dosing, lasted several hours and were fully reversible either during therap y or following the end of treatment. These events have not been associated with signs of ocular abnormality (see sections 4.4 and 4.7).

In clinical trials the effect on QTc was small (mean of approximately 1 msec). In comparative trials, similar effects to those observed with clarithromycin were seen with an on-therapy ΔQTc>30 msec in 7.6% and 7.0% of cases, respectively. No patient in either group developed a ΔQTc>60 msec. There were no reports of TdP or other serious ventricular arrhythmias or related syncope in the clinical program and no subgroups at risk were identified.

4.9 Overdose

In the event of acute overdose the stomach should be emptied. The patients should be carefully observed and given symptomatic and supportive treatment. Adequate hydration should be maintained. Blood electrolytes (especially potassium) must be controlled. Due to the potential for the prolongation of the QT interval and increased risk of arrhythmia, ECG monitoring must take place

5. PHARMACOLOGICAL PROPERTIES

5.1 Pharmacodynamic properties

Pharmacotherapeutic group: macrolides, lincosamides and streptogramins, ATC Code: J01FA15.

Telithromycin is a semisynthetic derivative of erythromycin A belonging to the ketolides, a class of antibacterial agents related to macrolides.

Mode of action

Telithromycin inhibits protein synthesis by acting at the ribosome level.

The affinity of telithromycin for the 50S bacterial subunit of ribosome is 10 fold higher than that of erythromycin A when the strain is susceptible to erythromycin A. Against erythromycin A resistant strains, due to an MLS_B mechanism of resistance, telithromycin shows a more than 20 fold affinity compared to erythromycin A in the 50S bacterial subunit.

Telithromycin interferes with the ribosome translation at the 23S ribosomal RNA level, where it interacts with domain V and II. Furthermore, telithromycin is able to block the formation of the 50S and 30S ribosomal subunits.

Breakpoints

The recommended MIC breakpoints for telithromycin, separating susceptible organisms from intermediately susceptible organisms and intermediately susceptible organisms from resistant organisms, are: susceptible ⩽0.5 mg/l, resistant >2mg/l.

Antibacterial spectrum

The prevalence of resistance may vary geographically and with time for selected species and local information on resistance is desirable, particularly when treating severe infections. As necessary, expert advice should be sought when the local prevalence of resistance is such that the utility of the agent in at least some types of infections is questionable.

This information provides only an approximate guidance on probabilities as to whether microorganisms will be susceptible to telithromycin.

Commonly susceptible species Aerobic Gram-positive bacteria
Staphylococcus aureus methicillin susceptible (MSSA)* Lancefield group C and G (β haemolytic) streptococci *Streptococcus agalactiae* *Streptococcus pneumoniae**
Viridans group streptococci
Aerobic Gram- negative bacteria
Legionella pneumophila *Moraxella catarrhalis* *
Other
Chlamydophila pneumoniae * *Chlamydia psittaci* *Mycoplasma pneumoniae* *
Species for which acquired resistance may be a problem Aerobic Gram-positive bacteria *Staphylococcus aureus* methicillin resistant (MRSA)+ *Streptococcus pyogenes* * Aerobic Gram- negative bacteria *Haemophilus influenzae* $ * *Haemophilus parainfluenzae* $
Inherantly resistant organisms
Aerobic Gram- negative bacteria *Acinetobacter* *Enterobacteriaceae* *Pseudomonas*

* Clinical efficacy has been demonstrated for susceptible isolates in the approved clinical indications.

$ natural intermediate susceptibility

+ Among MRSA the rate of MLSBc resistant strains is more than 80%, telithromycin is not active against MLS_BC.

Resistance

Telithromycin does not induce MLS_B resistance in vitro to *Staphylococcus aureus*, *Streptococcus pneumoniae*, and *Streptococcus pyogenes*, an attribute related to its 3 keto function. Development of in vitro resistance to telithromycin due to spontaneous mutation is rare. The majority of MRSA are resistant to erythromycin A by a constitutive MLS_B mechanism.

In vitro results have shown that telithromycin is affected by the erythromycin ermB or mefA related resistance mechanisms but to lesser extent than erythromycin. While exposure to telithromycin did select for pneumococcal mutants with increased MICs, the MICs remained within the proposed susceptibility range.

For *Streptococcus pneumoniae*, there is no cross- or co-resistance between telithromycin and other antibacterial classes including erythromycin A and/or penicillin resistance.

For *Streptococcus pyogenes*, cross-resistance occurs for high-level erythromycin A resistant strains.

Effect on oral and faecal flora

In a comparative study in healthy human volunteers, telithromycin 800 mg daily and clarithromycin 500 mg twice daily for 10 days showed a similar and reversible reduction of oral and faecal flora. However, in contrast to clarithromycin, no resistant strains of alpha streptococci emerged in saliva on treatment with telithromycin.

5.2 Pharmacokinetic properties

Absorption

Following oral administration, telithromycin is fairly rapidly absorbed. A mean maximum plasma concentration of about 2 mg/l is reached within 1-3 hour after dose with once-daily dosing of telithromycin 800 mg. The absolute bioavailability is about 57 % after a single dose of 800 mg. The rate and extent of absorption is unaffected by food intake, and thus Ketek tablets can be given without regard to food.

Mean steady-state trough plasma concentrations of between 0.04 and 0.07 mg/l are reached within 3 to 4 days with once-daily dosing of telithromycin 800 mg. At steady-state AUC is approximately 1.5 fold increased compared to the single dose.

Mean peak and trough plasma concentrations at steady state in patients were 2.9±1.6 mg/l (range 0.02-7.6 mg/l) and 0.2±0.2 mg/l (range 0.010 to 1.29 mg/l), during a therapeutic 800 mg once-daily dose regimen.

Distribution

The in vitro protein binding is approximately 60 % to 70 %. Telithromycin is widely distributed throughout the body. The volume of distribution is 2.9±1.0 l/kg. Rapid distribution of telithromycin into tissues results in significantly higher telithromycin concentrations in most target tissues than in plasma. The maximum total tissue concentration in epithelial lining fluid, alveolar macrophages, bronchial mucosa, tonsils and sinus tissue were 14.9±11.4 mg/l, 318.1±231 mg/l, 3.88±1.87 mg/kg, 3.95±0.53 mg/kg and 6.96±1.58 mg/kg, respectively. The total tissue concentration 24 h after dose in epithelial lining fluid, alveolar macrophages, bronchial mucosa, tonsils and sinus tissue were 0.84±0.65 mg/l, 162±96 mg/l, 0.78±0.39 mg/kg, 0.72±0.29 mg/kg and 1.58±1.68 mg/kg, respectively. The mean maximum white blood cell concentration of telithromycin was 83±25 mg/l.

Metabolism

Telithromycin is metabolized primarily by the liver. After oral administration, two-thirds of the dose is eliminated as metabolites and one-third unchanged. The main circulating compound in plasma is telithromycin. Its principal circulating metabolite represents approximately 13 % of telithromycin AUC, and has little antimicrobial activity compared with the parent medicinal product. Other metabolites were detected in plasma, urine and faeces and represent less or equal than 3 % of plasma AUC.

Telithromycin is metabolized both by CYP450 isoenzymes and non-CYP enzymes. The major CYP450 enzyme involved in the metabolism of telithromycin is CYP3A4. Telithromycin is an inhibitor of CYP3A4 and CYP2D6, but has no or limited effect on CYP1A, 2A6, 2B6, 2C8, 2C9, 2C19 and 2E1.

Elimination

After oral administration of radiolabelled telithromycin, 76 % of the radioactivity was recovered from faeces, and 17 % from the urine. Approximately one-third of telithromycin was eliminated unchanged; 20 % in faeces and 12 % in urine. Telithromycin displays moderate non-linear pharmacokinetics. The non-renal clearance is decreased as the dose is increased. The total clearance (mean ±SD) is approximately 58±5 l/h after an intravenous administration with renal clearance accounting for about 22 % of this. Telithromycin displays a tri-exponential decay from plasma, with a rapid distribution half-life of 0.17 h. The main elimination half-life of telithromycin is 2-3 h and the terminal, less important, half-life is about 10 h at the dose 800 mg once daily.

Special populations

- Renal impairment

In a multiple-dose study, 36 subjects with varying degrees of renal impairment, a 1.4-fold increase in $C_{max,ss}$, and a 2-fold increase in AUC $(0\text{-}24)_{ss}$ at 800 mg multiple doses in the severe renally impaired group (CLCR < 30 mL/min) compared to healthy volunteers were observed and a reduced dosage of Ketek is recommended (See Section 4.2.). Based on observed data, a 600 mg daily dose is approximately equivalent with the target exposure observed in healthy subjects. Based on simulation data, an alternating daily dosing regimen of 800 mg and 400 mg in patients with severe renal impairment can approximate the AUC (0-48h) in healthy subjects receiving 800 mg once daily.

The effect of dialysis on the elimination of telithromycin has not been assessed.

- Hepatic impairment

In a single-dose study (800 mg) in 12 patients and a multiple-dose study (800 mg) in 13 patients with mild to severe hepatic insufficiency (Child Pugh Class A, B and C), the C_{max}, AUC and $t_{1/2}$ of telithromycin were similar compared to those obtained in age- and sex-matched healthy subjects. In both studies, higher renal elimination was observed in the hepatically impaired patients. Due to limited experience in patients with decreased metabolic capacity of the liver, Ketek should be used with caution in patients with hepatic impairment (see also section 4.4).

- Elderly subjects

In subjects over 65 (median 75 years), the maximum plasma concentration and AUC of telithromycin were increased approximately 2 fold compared with those achieved in young healthy adults. These changes in pharmacokinetics do not necessitate dosage adjustment.

- Paediatric patients

The pharmacokinetics of telithromycin in paediatric population less than 12 years old have not yet been studied. Limited data, obtained in paediatric patients 13 to 17 years of age, showed that telithromycin concentrations in this age group were similar to the concentrations in patients 18 to 40 years of age.

- Gender

The pharmacokinetics of telithromycin are similar between males and females.

5.3 Preclinical safety data

Repeated dose toxicity studies of 1, 3 and 6 months duration with telithromycin conducted in rat, dog and monkey showed that the liver was the principal target for toxicity with elevations of liver enzymes, and histological evidence of damage. These effects showed a tendency to regress after cessation of treatment. Plasma exposures based on free fraction of active substance, at the no observed adverse effect levels ranged from 1.6 to 13 times the expected clinical exposure.

Phospholipidosis (intracellular phospholipid accumulation) affecting a number of organs and tissues (e.g., liver, kidney, lung, thymus, spleen, gall bladder, mesenteric lymph nodes, GI-tract) has been observed in rats and dogs administered telithromycin at repeated doses of 150 mg/kg/day or more for 1 month and 20 mg/kg/day or more for 3-6 months. This administration corresponds to free active substance systemic exposure levels of at least 9 times the expected levels in human after 1 month and less than the expected level in humans after 6 months, respectively. There was evidence of reversibility upon cessation of treatment. The significance of these findings for humans is unknown.

In similarity to some macrolides, telithromycin caused a prolongation of Qtc interval in dogs and on action potential duration in rabbit Purkinje fibers in vitro. Effects were evident at plasma levels of free drug 8 to 13 times the expected clinical level. Hypokalaemia and quinidine had additive/supra-additive effects in vitro while potentiation was evident with sotalol. Telithromycin, but not its major human metabolites, had inhibitory activity on HERG and Kv1.5 channels.

Reproduction toxicity studies showed reduced gamete maturation in rat and adverse effects on fertilization. At high doses embryotoxicity was apparent and an increase in incomplete ossification and in skeletal anomalies was seen. Studies in rats and rabbits were inconclusive with respect to potential for teratogenicity, there was equivocal evidence of adverse effects on foetal development at high doses.

Telithromycin, and its principal human metabolites, were negative in tests on genotoxic potential *in vitro* and *in vivo*. No carcinogenicity studies have been conducted with telithromycin.

6. PHARMACEUTICAL PARTICULARS

6.1 List of excipients

Tablet core:

Microcrystalline cellulose

Povidone K25

Croscarmellose sodium

Magnesium stearate

Tablet coating:

Talc

Macrogol 8000

Hypromellose 6 cp

Titanium dioxide E171

Yellow iron oxide E172

Red iron oxide E172

6.2 Incompatibilities

Not applicable.

6.3 Shelf life

3 years.

6.4 Special precautions for storage

No special precautions for storage.

6.5 Nature and contents of container

Two tablets are contained in each blister cavity.

Available as packs of 10

6.6 Special precautions for disposal and other handling

No special requirements.

7. MARKETING AUTHORISATION HOLDER

Aventis Pharma S.A.

20, Avenue Raymond Aron

F-92160 ANTONY

France

8. MARKETING AUTHORISATION NUMBER(S)

EU/1/01/191/001

9. DATE OF FIRST AUTHORISATION/RENEWAL OF THE AUTHORISATION

Date of first authorisation: 9 July 2001

Date of first renewal: 9 July 2006

10. DATE OF REVISION OF THE TEXT

2 June 2009

Legal category: POM

Ketorolac 30mg/ml solution for injection (Beacon Pharmaceuticals)

(Beacon Pharmaceuticals)

1. NAME OF THE MEDICINAL PRODUCT

Ketorolac Trometamol 30mg/ml Injection Solution

2. QUALITATIVE AND QUANTITATIVE COMPOSITION

Each 1ml ampoule contains 30 mg Ketorolac trometamol

For excipients please see section 6.1

3. PHARMACEUTICAL FORM

Solution for Injection

Colourless or slightly yellowish solution in amber glass ampoules.

4. CLINICAL PARTICULARS

4.1 Therapeutic indications

Ketorolac Injection is indicated for the short-term management of moderate to severe acute post-operative pain.

4.2 Posology and method of administration

Ketorolac Injection is for administration by intramuscular or bolus intravenous injection. Bolus intravenous doses should be given over at least 15 seconds. Ketorolac Injection should not be used for epidural or spinal administration.

The time to onset of analgesic effect following both IV and IM administration is similar and is approximately 30 minutes, maximum analgesia occurs within one to two hours. Analgesia normally lasts for four to six hours.

Dosage should be adjusted according to the severity of the pain and the patient response. Undesirable effects may be minimised by using the lowest effective dose for the shortest duration necessary to control symptoms (see section 4.4).

The administration of continuous multiple daily doses of ketorolac intramuscularly or intravenously should not exceed two days because adverse events may increase with prolonged usage. There has been limited experience with dosing for longer periods since the vast majority of patients have transferred to oral medication or no longer require analgesic therapy after this time.

Adults

The recommended initial dose of Ketorolac Injection is 10mg followed by 10 to 30mg every four to six hours as required. In the initial post-operative period, Ketorolac Injection may be given as often as every two hours if needed. The lowest effective dose should be given. A total daily dose of 90mg for non-elderly and 60mg for the elderly, patients with renal impairment and patients less than 50kg should not be exceeded. The maximum duration of treatment should not exceed two days.

The dosage in patients under 50kg should be reduced.

Opioid analgesics (e.g. morphine, pethidine) may be used concomitantly, and may be required for optimal analgesic effect in the early post-operative period when pain is most severe. Ketorolac does not interfere with opioid binding and does not exacerbate opioid-related respiratory depression or sedation. When used in association with Ketorolac Injection, the daily dose of opioid is usually less than that normally required. However, opioid side-effects should still be considered, especially in day-case surgery.

Patients receiving Ketorolac Injection, and who are converted to oral Ketorolac, should receive a total combined daily dose not exceeding 90mg (60mg for the elderly, patients with renal impairment and patients less than 50kg). The oral component should not exceed 40mg on the day the change of formulation is made. Patients should be converted to oral treatment as soon as possible.

Elderly

For patients over 65 years, the lower end of the dosage range is recommended and a total daily dose of 60mg should not be exceeded (see section 4.4 Special warnings and special precautions for use).

Children

Safety and efficacy in children have not been established. Therefore, Ketorolac Injection is not recommended for use in children under 16 years of age.

Renal impairment

Ketorolac Injection should not be used in moderate to severe renal impairment and a reduced dosage given in lesser impairment (not exceeding 60mg/day IV or IM) (see section 4.3 Contra-indications).

4.3 Contraindications

- Active or previous peptic ulcer. History of upper gastrointestinal bleeding or perforation, related to previous NSAID therapy.
- suspected or confirmed cerebrovascular bleeding
- haemorrhagic diatheses, including coagulation disorders
- hypersensitivity to ketorolac trometamol or other NSAIDs and those patients in whom aspirin or other prostaglandin synthesis inhibitors induce allergic reactions (severe anaphylactic-like reactions have been observed in such patients)
- the complete or partial syndrome of nasal polyps, angioedema or bronchospasm
- concurrent treatment with other NSAIDs including cyclooxygenase 2 specific inhibitors, oxpentifylline, probenecid or lithium salts
- hypovolaemia from any cause or dehydration
- moderate or severe renal impairment (serum creatinine > 160 micromol/l)
- a history of asthma
- severe heart failure
- patients who have had operations with a high risk of haemorrhage or incomplete haemostasis
- patients on anti-coagulants including low dose heparin (2500 - 5000 units twelve hourly)
- during pregnancy, labour, delivery or lactation
- children under 16 years of age
- Ketorolac is contra-indicated as prophylactic analgesia before surgery due to inhibition of platelet aggregation and is contra-indicated intra-operatively because of the increased risk of bleeding
- patients currently receiving aspirin

4.4 Special warnings and precautions for use

Physicians should be aware that in some patients pain relief might not occur until 30 minutes or more after IV or IM administration.

Use in the elderly: in common with other NSAIDs, patients over the age of 65 years may be at an increased risk of experiencing adverse events compared to younger patients. The elderly have an increased plasma half-life and reduced plasma clearance of ketorolac, therefore a total daily dose of greater than 60mg ketorolac is not recommended.

Undesirable effects may be minimised by using the lowest effective dose for the shortest duration necessary to control symptoms (see section 4.2, and GI and cardiovascular risks below).

Gastro-intestinal effects: ketorolac can cause gastrointestinal irritation, ulcers or bleeding in patients with or without a history of previous symptoms. Elderly and debilitated patients are more prone to develop these reactions. The incidence increases with dose and duration of treatment.

A study has shown increased rates of clinically serious GI bleeding in patients < 65 years of age who received an average daily dose of > 90mg ketorolac IM as compared to those patients receiving parenteral opioids.

GI bleeding, ulceration or perforation, which can be fatal, has been reported with all NSAIDs at any time during treatment, with or without warning symptoms or a previous history of serious GI events.

The risk of GI bleeding, ulceration or perforation is higher with increasing NSAID doses, in patients with a history of ulcer, particularly if complicated with haemorrhage or perforation (see section 4.3), and in the elderly. These patients should commence on the lowest dose available.

Patients with a history of GI toxicity, particularly when elderly, should report any unusual abdominal symptoms (especially GI bleeding) particularly in the initial stages of treatment.

Caution should be advised in patients receiving concomitant medications which could increase the risk of gastrotoxicity or bleeding, such as corticosteroids, or anticoagulants such as warfarin or anti-platelet agents such as aspirin (see section 4.5).

Where GI bleeding or ulceration occurs in patients receiving Ketorolac, the treatment should be withdrawn.

Cardiovascular and cerebrovascular effects: Appropriate monitoring and advice are required for patients with a history of hypertension and/or mild to moderate congestive heart failure as fluid retention and oedema have been reported in association with NSAID therapy.

Clinical trial and epidemiological data suggest that use of some NSAIDs (particulary at high doses and in long term treatment) may be associated with a small increased risk of arterial thrombotic events (for example myocardial infarction or stroke). There are insufficient data to exclude such a risk for Ketorolac.

Patients with uncontrolled hypertension, congestive heart failure, established ischaemic heart disease, peripheral arterial disease, and/or cerebrovascular disease should only be treated with Ketorolac after careful consideration. Similar consideration should be made before initiating longer-term treatment of patients with risk factors for cardiovascular disease (e.g. hypertension, hyperlipidaemia, diabetes mellitus, smoking).

Respiratory effects: bronchospasm may be precipitated in patients with a history of asthma.

Renal effects: drugs that inhibit prostaglandin biosynthesis (including non-steroidal anti-inflammatory drugs) have been reported to cause nephrotoxicity including but not limited to: glomerular nephritis, interstitial nephritis, renal papillary necrosis, nephrotic syndrome and acute renal failure. In patients with renal, cardiac or hepatic impairment, caution is required since the use of NSAIDs may result in deterioration of renal function.

As with other drugs that inhibit prostaglandin synthesis, elevations of serum urea, creatinine and potassium have been reported with ketorolac and may occur after one dose.

Patients with impaired renal function: since ketorolac and its metabolites are excreted primarily by the kidney, patients with moderate to severe impairment of renal function (serum creatinine greater than 160 micromol/l) should not receive Ketorolac Injection. Patients with lesser renal impairment should receive a reduced dose of ketorolac (not exceeding 60mg/day IM or IV) and their renal status should be closely monitored.

Female fertility: the use of Ketorolac may impair female fertility and is not recommended in women attempting to conceive. In women who have difficulties conceiving or who are undergoing investigation for infertility, withdrawal of Ketorolac should be considered.

Caution should be observed in patients with conditions leading to a reduction in blood volume and/or renal blood flow, where renal prostaglandins have a supportive role in the maintenance of renal perfusion. In these patients, administration of an NSAID may cause a dose-dependent reduction in renal prostaglandin formation and may precipitate overt renal failure. Patients at greatest risk of this reaction are those who are volume depleted because of blood loss or severe dehydration, patients with impaired renal function, heart failure, liver dysfunction, the elderly and those taking diuretics. Discontinuation of NSAID therapy is typically followed by recovery to the pre-treatment state. Inadequate fluid/blood replacement during surgery, leading to hypovolaemia, may lead to renal dysfunction, which could be exacerbated when ketorolac is administered. Therefore, volume depletion should be corrected and close monitoring of serum urea and creatinine and urine output is recommended until the patient is normovolaemic. In patients on renal dialysis, ketorolac clearance was reduced to approximately half the normal rate and terminal half-life increased approximately three-fold.

Fluid retention and oedema have been reported with the use of ketorolac and it should therefore be used with caution in patients with cardiac decompensation, hypertension or similar conditions.

Patients with impaired hepatic function from cirrhosis do not have any clinically important changes in ketorolac clearance or terminal half-life.

Borderline elevations of one or more liver function tests may occur. These abnormalities may be transient, may remain unchanged, or may progress with continued therapy. Meaningful elevations (greater than three times normal) of serum glutamate pyruvate transaminase (SGPT/ALT) or serum glutamate oxaloacetate transaminase (SGOT/AST) occurred in controlled clinical trials in less than 1% of patients. If clinical signs and symptoms consistent with liver disease develop, or if systemic manifestations occur, ketorolac should be discontinued.

Haematological effects: patients with coagulation disorders should not receive ketorolac. Patients on anti-coagulation therapy may be at increased risk of bleeding if given ketorolac concurrently. The concomitant use of ketorolac and prophylactic low-dose heparin (2500 - 5000 units twelve hourly) has not been studied extensively and may also be associated with an increased risk of bleeding. Patients already on anti-coagulants or who require low-dose heparin should not receive ketorolac. Patients who are receiving other drug therapy that interferes with haemostasis should be carefully observed if ketorolac is administered. In controlled clinical studies, the incidence of clinically significant post-operative bleeding was less than 1%.

Ketorolac inhibits platelet aggregation and prolongs bleeding time. In patients with normal bleeding function, bleeding times were raised, but not outside the normal range of two to eleven minutes. Unlike the prolonged effects from aspirin, platelet function returns to normal within 24 to 48 hours after ketorolac is discontinued.

Post-operative wound haemorrhage has been reported in association with the immediate peri-operative use of ketorolac. Therefore, ketorolac should not be used in patients who have had operations with a high risk of haemorrhage or incomplete haemostasis. Caution should be used where strict haemostasis is critical, e.g. in cosmetic or day-case surgery. Haematomata and other signs of wound haemorrhage and epistaxis have been reported with the use of ketorolac. Physicians should be aware of the pharmacological similarity of ketorolac to other non-steroidal anti-inflammatory drugs that inhibit cyclo-oxygenase and the risk of bleeding, particularly in the elderly.

The risk of clinically serious gastro-intestinal bleeding is dose-dependent. This is particularly true in elderly patients who receive an average daily dose greater than 60mg/day of ketorolac.

Ketorolac is not an anaesthetic agent and possesses no sedative or anxiolytic properties; therefore it is not recommended as a pre-operative medication for the support of anaesthesia when these effects are required.

4.5 Interaction with other medicinal products and other forms of interaction

Ketorolac should not be used with other NSAIDs or in patients receiving aspirin because of the potential for additive side-effects.

Ketorolac is highly bound to human plasma protein (mean 99.2%) and binding is concentration-independent.

Ketorolac did not alter digoxin protein binding. In vitro studies indicated that at therapeutic concentrations of salicylate (300μg/ml) and above, the binding of ketorolac was reduced from approximately 99.2% to 97.5%. Therapeutic concentrations of digoxin, warfarin, paracetamol, phenytoin and tolbutamide did not alter ketorolac protein binding. Because ketorolac is a highly potent drug and present in low concentrations in plasma, it would not be expected to displace other protein-bound drugs significantly.

Care should be taken when administering ketorolac with anti-coagulants since co-administration may cause an enhanced anti-coagulant effect.

There is no evidence in animal or human studies that ketorolac induces or inhibits the hepatic enzymes capable of metabolising itself or other drugs. Hence ketorolac would not be expected to alter the pharmacokinetics of other drugs due to enzyme induction or inhibition mechanisms.

In normovolaemic healthy subjects, ketorolac reduces the diuretic response to frusemide by approximately 20%, so particular care should be taken in patients with cardiac decompensation.

Ketorolac and other non-steroidal anti-inflammatory drugs can reduce the anti-hypertensive effect of beta-blockers and may increase the risk of renal impairment when administered concurrently with ACE inhibitors, particularly in volume depleted patients.

NSAIDs may exacerbate cardiac failure, reduce GFR and increase plasma cardiac glycoside levels when co-administered with cardiac glycosides.

Caution is advised when methotrexate is administered concurrently, since some prostaglandin synthesis inhibiting drugs have been reported to reduce the clearance of methotrexate, and thus possibly enhance its toxicity.

Probenecid should not be administered concurrently with ketorolac because of increases in ketorolac plasma level and half-life.

As with all NSAIDs caution is advised when cyclosporin is co-administered because of the increased risk of nephrotoxicity.

NSAIDs should not be used for eight to twelve days after mifepristone administration as NSAIDs can reduce the effects of mifepristone.

As with all NSAIDs, caution should be taken when co-administering with cortico-steroids because of the increased risk of gastro-intestinal bleeding.

Patients taking quinolones may have an increased risk of developing convulsions.

Co-administration with diuretics can lead to a reduced diuretic effect, and increase the risk of nephrotoxicity of NSAIDs.

Because of an increased tendency to bleeding when oxpentifylline is administered concurrently, this combination should be avoided.

In patients receiving lithium there is a possible inhibition of renal lithium clearance, increased plasma lithium concentration and potential lithium toxicity. (See section 4.3 Contra-indications).

4.6 Pregnancy and lactation

There is no evidence of teratogenicity in rats or rabbits studied at maternally-toxic doses of ketorolac. Prolongation of the gestation period and/or delayed parturition was seen in the rat. Ketorolac and its metabolites have been shown to pass into the foetus and milk of animals. Ketorolac has been detected in human milk at low levels. Safety in human pregnancy has not been established. Congenital abnormalities have been reported in association with NSAID administration in man, however these are low in frequency and do not follow any discernible pattern. Ketorolac is therefore contra-indicated during pregnancy, labour or delivery, or in mothers who are breast-feeding.

4.7 Effects on ability to drive and use machines

Some patients may experience dizziness, drowsiness, visual disturbances, headaches, vertigo, insomnia or depression with the use of ketorolac. If patients experience these, or other similar undesirable effects, they should not drive or operate machinery.

4.8 Undesirable effects

The following side-effects have been reported.

Gastro-intestinal:

Nausea, dyspepsia, gastro-intestinal pain, gastro-intestinal bleeding, abdominal discomfort, haematemesis, gastritis, oesophagitis, diarrhoea, eructation, constipation, flatulence, fullness, melaena, peptic ulcer, non-peptic gastro-intestinal ulceration, rectal bleeding, ulcerative stomatitis, vomiting, haemorrhage, perforation, pancreatitis. Peptic ulcers, perforation or GI bleeding, sometimes fatal, particularly in the elderly, may occur (see section 4.4).

Central nervous/musculoskeletal systems:

Anxiety, drowsiness, dizziness, headache, sweating, dry mouth, nervousness, paraesthesia, functional disorders, abnormal thinking, depression, euphoria, convulsions, excessive thirst, inability to concentrate, insomnia, malaise, fatigue, stimulation, vertigo, abnormal taste and vision, optic neuritis, myalgia, abnormal dreams, hallucinations, hyperkinesia, hearing loss, tinnitus, aseptic meningitis, psychotic reactions.

Renal:

Nephrotoxicity including increased urinary frequency, oliguria, acute renal failure, hyponatraemia, hyperkalaemia, haemolytic uraemic syndrome, flank pain (with or without haematuria), raised serum urea and creatinine, interstitial nephritis, urinary retention, nephrotic syndrome.

Cardiovascular/haematological:

Flushing, bradycardia, pallor, purpura, thrombocytopenia, neutropenia, agranulocytosis, aplastic anaemia, haemolytic anaemia, hypertension, palpitations, chest pain.

Clinical trial and epidemiological data suggest that the use of some NSAIDs (particularly at high does and in long term treatment) may be associated with an increased risk of arterial thrombotic events (for example myocardial infarction or stroke) (see section 4.4).

Oedema, hypertension, and cardiac failure, have been reported in association with NSAID treatment.

Respiratory:

Dyspnoea, asthma, pulmonary oedema.

Dermatological:

Pruritus, urticaria, skin photosensitivity, Lyell's syndrome, Stevens-Johnson syndrome, exfoliative dermatitis, maculopapular rash.

Hypersensitivity reactions:

Anaphylaxis, bronchospasm, laryngeal oedema, hypotension, flushing and rash. Such reactions may occur in patients with or without known sensitivity to ketorolac or other non-steroidal anti-inflammatory drugs.

These may also occur in individuals with a history of angioedema, bronchospastic reactivity (e.g. asthma and nasal polyps). Anaphylactoid reactions, like anaphylaxis, may have a fatal outcome (see section 4.3 Contra-indications).

Bleeding:

Post-operative wound haemorrhage, haematomata, epistaxis, increased bleeding time.

Reproductive, female:

Infertility

Other:

Asthenia, oedema, weight gain, abnormalities of liver function tests, hepatitis, liver failure, jaundice, fever. Injection site pain has been reported in some patients.

4.9 Overdose

Doses of 360mg given intramuscularly over an eight hour interval for five consecutive days have caused abdominal pain and peptic ulcers that have healed after discontinuation of dosing. Two patients recovered from unsuccessful suicide attempts. One patient experienced nausea after 210mg ketorolac, and the other hyperventilation after 300mg ketorolac.

5. PHARMACOLOGICAL PROPERTIES

5.1 Pharmacodynamic properties

ATC code M01A

Ketorolac is a potent analgesic agent of the non-steroidal, anti-inflammatory class (NSAID). It is not an opioid and has no known effects on opioid receptors. Its mode of action is to inhibit the cyclo-oxygenase enzyme system and hence prostaglandin synthesis and it demonstrates a minimal anti-inflammatory effect at its analgesic dose.

5.2 Pharmacokinetic properties

Intramuscular

Following intramuscular administration, ketorolac was rapidly and completely absorbed. A mean peak plasma concentration of 2.2μg/ml occurred an average of 50 minutes after a single 30mg dose. Age, kidney and liver function affect terminal plasma half-life and mean total clearance as outlined in the table below (estimated from a single 30mg IM dose of ketorolac).

Type of subjects	Total clearance (l/hr/kg) mean (range)	Terminal half-life (hrs) mean (range)
Normal subjects (n = 54)	0.023 (0.010 - 0.046)	5.3 (3.5 - 9.2)
Patients with hepatic dysfunction (n = 7)	0.029 (0.013 - 0.066)	5.4 (2.2 - 6.9)
Patients with renal impairment (n = 25) (serum creatinine 160 - 430 micromol/l)	0.016 (0.005 - 0.043)	10.3 (5.9 - 19.2)
Renal dialysis patients (n = 9)	0.016 (0.003 - 0.036)	13.6 (8.0 - 39.1)
Healthy elderly subjects (n = 13) (mean age 72)	0.019 (0.013 - 0.034)	7.0 (4.7 - 8.6)

Intravenous

Intravenous administration of a single 10mg dose of ketorolac resulted in a mean peak plasma concentration of 2.4µg/ml at an average of 5.4 minutes after dosing. The terminal plasma elimination half-life was 5.1 hours, average volume of distribution 0.15 l/kg, and total plasma clearance 0.35ml/min/kg.

The pharmacokinetics of ketorolac in man following single or multiple doses are linear. Steady-state plasma levels are achieved after dosing every six hours for one day. No changes in clearance occurred with chronic dosing. The primary route of excretion of ketorolac and its metabolites is renal: 91.4% (mean) of a given dose being found in the urine and 6.1% (mean) in the faeces.

More than 99% of the ketorolac in plasma is protein-bound over a wide concentration range.

5.3 Preclinical safety data

An 18-month study in mice with oral doses of ketorolac trometamol at 2mg/kg/day (0.9 times human systemic exposure at the recommended IM or IV dose of 30mg qid, based on area-under-the-plasma-concentration curve [AUC]), and a 24-month study in rats at 5mg/kg/day (0.5 times the human AUC), showed no evidence of tumourigenicity.

Ketorolac trometamol was not mutagenic in the Ames test, unscheduled DNA synthesis and repair, and in forward mutation assays. Ketorolac trometamol did not cause chromosome breakage in the in vivo mouse micronucleus assay. At 1590µg/ml and at higher concentrations, ketorolac trometamol increased the incidence of chromosomal aberrations in Chinese hamster ovarian cells.

Impairment of fertility did not occur in male or female rats at oral doses of 9mg/kg (0.9 times the human AUC) and 16mg/kg (1.6 times the human AUC) of ketorolac trometamol, respectively.

6. PHARMACEUTICAL PARTICULARS

6.1 List of excipients

Ethanol, sodium chloride, sodium hydroxide and water for injections

6.2 Incompatibilities

Ketorolac Injection should not be mixed in a small volume (e.g. in a syringe) with morphine sulphate, pethidine hydrochloride, promethazine hydrochloride or hydroxyzine hydrochloride, as precipitation of ketorolac will occur.

It is compatible with normal saline, 5% dextrose, Ringer's, lactated Ringer's or Plasmacyte solutions. Compatibility of Ketorolac Injection with other drugs is unknown.

6.3 Shelf life

Two years

From a microbiological point of view, the product should be used immediately. If not used immediately, in-use storage time sand conditions prior to use are the responsibility of the user and would normally not be longer than 24 hours at 2 to 8°C, unless reconstitution/dilution has taken place in controlled and validated aseptic conditions.

6.4 Special precautions for storage

Do not store above 30°C. Keep container in the outer carton and protect from light.

6.5 Nature and contents of container

Ampoules, amber type I glass. In cartons containing either 6 or 100 ampoules.

6.6 Special precautions for disposal and other handling

There are no special instructions.

7. MARKETING AUTHORISATION HOLDER

Beacon Pharmaceutical Ltd

Tunbridge Wells

Kent TN1 1YG

8. MARKETING AUTHORISATION NUMBER(S)

PL 18157/0012

9. DATE OF FIRST AUTHORISATION/RENEWAL OF THE AUTHORISATION

30/04/2007

10. DATE OF REVISION OF THE TEXT

30/04/2007

Ketovite Liquid

(Paines & Byrne Limited)

1. NAME OF THE MEDICINAL PRODUCT

Ketovite Liquid.

2. QUALITATIVE AND QUANTITATIVE COMPOSITION

Vitamin A as palmitate (1.7 × 10^6 units/g) HSE 2500 units

Vitamin D_2 (ergocalciferol) BP 400 units

Cyanocobalamin BP 12.5 microgram

Choline chloride HSE 150.0 mg

3. PHARMACEUTICAL FORM

Oral emulsion.

4. CLINICAL PARTICULARS

4.1 Therapeutic indications

As a sugar-free therapeutic supplement for the prevention of vitamin deficiency in conditions such as galactosaemia, disaccharide intolerance, phenylketonuria and other disorders of carbohydrate or amino acid metabolism, as well as in patients who are on restricted, specialised or synthetic diets.

In order to achieve complete vitamin supplementation Ketovite Liquid should be used in conjunction with Ketovite Tablets.

4.2 Posology and method of administration

For adults, children and the elderly: 5 ml daily, by oral administration.

4.3 Contraindications

Hypersensitivity to the product. Hypercalcaemia.

4.4 Special warnings and precautions for use

The recommended dose should not be exceeded without medical advice. No other vitamin supplement containing Vitamins A and D should be taken with Ketovite Liquid except under medical supervision. The methyl parahydroxybenzoate (E218) in Ketovite Liquid may cause allergic reactions which can be delayed. Warning: do not exceed the stated dose.

4.5 Interaction with other medicinal products and other forms of interaction

Absorption of some vitamins in this preparation may be reduced in conditions of fat malabsorption or with the concurrent use of neomycin, colestyramine, liquid paraffin, aminoglycosides, aminosalicylic acid, anticonvulsants, biguanides, chloramphenicol, cimetidine, colchicine, potassium salts and methyl-dopa. Serum B_{12} concentrations may be decreased by concurrent administration of oral contraceptives.

4.6 Pregnancy and lactation

Caution should be used in pregnancy as excessive doses of Vitamin A may be teratogenic, especially when taken in the first trimester.

Large doses of Vitamin D in lactating mothers may cause hypercalcaemia in infants.

4.7 Effects on ability to drive and use machines

None known.

4.8 Undesirable effects

None, in the absence of overdosage.

4.9 Overdose

Symptoms of overdosage may include anorexia, nausea, vomiting, rough dry skin, polyuria, thirst, loss of hair, painful bones and joints as well as raised plasma and urine calcium and phosphate concentration.

No emergency procedure or antidote is applicable and symptoms are rapidly reduced upon withdrawal of the preparation.

5. PHARMACOLOGICAL PROPERTIES

5.1 Pharmacodynamic properties

The product is a multivitamin supplemental product.

5.2 Pharmacokinetic properties

The pharmacokinetics of the active substances would not differ from that of the same substance when derived naturally from oral foodstuffs.

5.3 Preclinical safety data

No relevant pre-clinical data has been generated.

6. PHARMACEUTICAL PARTICULARS

6.1 List of excipients

Methyl cellulose (methocel E4M) HSE

Saccharin BP

Methyl parahydroxybenzoate BP

Polysorbate 80 BP

Ascorbic acid BP

DL α tocopherol HSE

Terpeneless orange oil BP

Ammonia solution 0.88m HSE

Deionised water HSE

6.2 Incompatibilities

None known.

6.3 Shelf life

24 months.

6.4 Special precautions for storage

Store at 2-8°C.

6.5 Nature and contents of container

Amber glass bottle with plastic screw cap. Park sizes 100, 150 and 140.

6.6 Special precautions for disposal and other handling

Not applicable.

Administrative Data

7. MARKETING AUTHORISATION HOLDER

Paines and Byrne Ltd

Lovett House

Lovett Road

Staines

TW18 3AZ

United Kingdom

8. MARKETING AUTHORISATION NUMBER(S)

PL0051/5080R

9. DATE OF FIRST AUTHORISATION/RENEWAL OF THE AUTHORISATION

First authorisation granted 30 January 1990

Renewal granted 9 September 2005

10. DATE OF REVISION OF THE TEXT

28 January 2008

11. Legal Category

P

Ketovite Tablets

(Paines & Byrne Limited)

1. NAME OF THE MEDICINAL PRODUCT

Ketovite Tablets.

2. QUALITATIVE AND QUANTITATIVE COMPOSITION

Thiamine hydrochloride BP 1.0 mg

Riboflavin BP 1.0 mg

Pyridoxine hydrochloride 0.33 mg

Nicotinamide BP 3.3 mg

Calcium pantothenate PhEur 1.16 mg

Ascorbic acid BP 16.6 mg

Acetomenaphthone BP 1973 0.5 mg

Alpha-tocopheryl acetate BP 5.0 mg

Inositol NF XII 50.0 mg

Biotin USP 0.17 mg

Folic acid BP 0.25 mg

3. PHARMACEUTICAL FORM

Tablet

4. CLINICAL PARTICULARS

4.1 Therapeutic indications

As a therapeutic supplement for the prevention of vitamin deficiency in conditions such as galactosaemia, disaccharide intolerance, phenylketonuria and other disorders of carbohydrate or amino acid metabolism, as well as in patients who are on restricted, specialised or synthetic diets.

In order to achieve complete vitamin supplementation Ketovite Tablets should be used in conjunction with Ketovite Liquid.

4.2 Posology and method of administration

For Adults, Children and the Elderly: One tablet three times a day, by oral administration.

4.3 Contraindications

Hypersensitivity to the product.

4.4 Special warnings and precautions for use

None stated.

4.5 Interaction with other medicinal products and other forms of interaction

Pyridoxine may increase the peripheral metabolism of levodopa reducing therapeutic efficacy in patients with Parkinson's disease.

4.6 Pregnancy and lactation

The recommended dose should not be exceeded without medical advice.

4.7 Effects on ability to drive and use machines

None.

4.8 Undesirable effects

None stated.

4.9 Overdose

Large overdoses of water-soluble vitamins are readily excreted in the urine. No emergency procedure or antidote is applicable and any symptoms are rapidly reduced upon withdrawal of the preparation.

5. PHARMACOLOGICAL PROPERTIES

5.1 Pharmacodynamic properties

Multivitamin preparation.

5.2 Pharmacokinetic properties

In normal circumstances the active constituents are obtained by the same route of administration (oral) from food.

5.3 Preclinical safety data

No relevant pre-clinical data has been generated.

6. PHARMACEUTICAL PARTICULARS

6.1 List of excipients

Heavy magnesium carbonate

Magnesium stearate

Magnesium trisilicate

Stearic acid

Methylcellulose

Colloidal silicon dioxide

6.2 Incompatibilities

None.

6.3 Shelf life

Two years.

6.4 Special precautions for storage

Store at 2-8°C.

6.5 Nature and contents of container

Securitainers containing 84, 90, 100 or 500 tablets.

6.6 Special precautions for disposal and other handling

None.

Administrative Data

7. MARKETING AUTHORISATION HOLDER

Paines and Byrne Limited

Lovett House

Lovett Road

Staines

TW18 3AZ

United Kingdom

8. MARKETING AUTHORISATION NUMBER(S)

0051/5079R

9. DATE OF FIRST AUTHORISATION/RENEWAL OF THE AUTHORISATION

27 March 1987; renewed 21 January 2005

10. DATE OF REVISION OF THE TEXT

22nd December 2005

11. Legal Category

POM

Kivexa film-coated tablets

(GlaxoSmithKline UK)

1. NAME OF THE MEDICINAL PRODUCT

Kivexa 600 mg/300 mg film-coated tablets

2. QUALITATIVE AND QUANTITATIVE COMPOSITION

Each film-coated tablet contains 600 mg of abacavir (as sulfate) and 300 mg lamivudine.

Excipients

Sunset yellow (E110) 1.7 mg per tablet

For a full list of excipients see section 6.1.

3. PHARMACEUTICAL FORM

Film-coated tablet.

Orange, film-coated, modified capsule shaped tablets, debossed with GS FC2 on one side.

4. CLINICAL PARTICULARS

4.1 Therapeutic indications

Kivexa is a fixed-dose combination of two nucleoside analogues (abacavir and lamivudine). It is indicated in antiretroviral combination therapy for the treatment of Human Immunodeficiency Virus (HIV) infection in adults and adolescents from 12 years of age.

The demonstration of the benefit of the combination abacavir/lamivudine as a once daily regimen in antiretroviral therapy, is mainly based on results of one study performed in primarily asymptomatic treatment-naïve adult patients (see sections 4.4 and 5.1).

Before initiating treatment with abacavir, screening for carriage of the HLA-B*5701 allele should be performed in any HIV-infected patient, irrespective of racial origin. Abacavir should not be used in patients known to carry the HLA-B*5701 allele, unless no other therapeutic option is available in these patients, based on the treatment history and resistance testing (see section 4.4 and 4.8).

4.2 Posology and method of administration

Therapy should be prescribed by a physician experienced in the management of HIV infection.

The recommended dose of Kivexa in adults and adolescents is one tablet once daily.

Table 1

Hypersensitivity Reaction (see also section 4.8)

In clinical studies approximately 5% of subjects receiving abacavir develop a hypersensitivity reaction. Some of these cases were life-threatening and resulted in a fatal outcome despite taking precautions.

Studies have shown that carriage of the HLA-B*5701 allele is associated with a significantly increased risk of a hypersensitivity reaction to abacavir. Based on the prospective study CNA106030 (PREDICT-1), use of pre-therapy screening for the HLA-B*5701 allele and subsequently avoiding abacavir in patients with this allele significantly reduced the incidence of abacavir hypersensitivity reactions. In populations similar to that enrolled in the PREDICT-1 study, it is estimated that 48% to 61% of patients with the HLA-B*5701 allele will develop a hypersensitivity reaction during the course of abacavir treatment compared with 0% to 4% of patients who do not have the HLA-B*5701 allele.

These results are consistent with those of prior retrospective studies.

As a consequence, before initiating treatment with abacavir, screening for carriage of the HLA-B*5701 allele should be performed in any HIV-infected patient, irrespective of racial origin. Abacavir should not be used in patients known to carry the HLA-B*5701 allele, unless no other therapeutic option is available based on the treatment history and resistance testing (see section 4.1).

In any patient treated with abacavir, the clinical diagnosis of suspected hypersensitivity reaction must remain the basis of clinical decision-making. It is noteworthy that among patients with a clinically suspected hypersensitivity reaction, a proportion did not carry HLA-B*5701. Therefore, even in the absence of HLA-B*5701 allele, it is important to permanently discontinue abacavir and not rechallenge with abacavir if a hypersensitivity reaction cannot be ruled out on clinical grounds, due to the potential for a severe or even fatal reaction.

Skin patch testing was used as a research tool for the PREDICT-1 study but has no utility in the clinical management of patients and therefore should not be used in the clinical setting.

• **Clinical Description**

Hypersensitivity reactions are characterised by the appearance of symptoms indicating multi-organ system involvement. Almost all hypersensitivity reactions will have fever and/or rash as part of the syndrome.

Other signs and symptoms may include respiratory signs and symptoms such as dyspnoea, sore throat, cough, and abnormal chest x-ray findings (predominantly infiltrates, which can be localised), gastrointestinal symptoms, such as nausea, vomiting, diarrhoea, or abdominal pain, **and may lead to misdiagnosis of hypersensitivity as respiratory disease (pneumonia, bronchitis, pharyngitis), or gastroenteritis.**
Other frequently observed signs or symptoms of the hypersensitivity reaction may include lethargy or malaise and musculoskeletal symptoms (myalgia, rarely myolysis, arthralgia).

The symptoms related to this hypersensitivity reaction worsen with continued therapy and can be life- threatening. These symptoms usually resolve upon discontinuation of abacavir.

• **Clinical Management**

Hypersensitivity reaction symptoms usually appear within the first six weeks of initiation of treatment with abacavir, although these reactions **may occur at any time during therapy**. Patients should be monitored closely, especially during the first two months of treatment with abacavir, with consultation every two weeks.

Patients who are diagnosed with a hypersensitivity reaction whilst on therapy **MUST discontinue Kivexa immediately.**

Kivexa, or any other medicinal product containing abacavir (Ziagen or Trizivir), MUST NEVER be restarted in patients who have stopped therapy due to a hypersensitivity reaction.
Restarting abacavir following a hypersensitivity reaction results in a prompt return of symptoms within hours. This recurrence is usually more severe than on initial presentation, and may include life-threatening hypotension and death.

To avoid a delay in diagnosis and minimise the risk of a life-threatening hypersensitivity reaction, Kivexa must be permanently discontinued if hypersensitivity cannot be ruled out, even when other diagnoses are possible (respiratory diseases, flu-like illness, gastroenteritis or reactions to other medicinal products).

Special care is needed for those patients simultaneously starting treatment with Kivexa and other medicinal products known to induce skin toxicity (such as non-nucleoside reverse transcriptase inhibitors - NNRTIs). This is because it is currently difficult to differentiate between rashes induced by these products and abacavir related hypersensitivity reactions.

• **Management after an interruption of Kivexa therapy**

If therapy with Kivexa has been discontinued for any reason and restarting therapy is under consideration, the reason for discontinuation must be established to assess whether the patient had any symptoms of a hypersensitivity reaction. **If a hypersensitivity reaction cannot be ruled out, Kivexa or any other medicinal product containing abacavir (Ziagen or Trizivir) must not be restarted.**

Hypersensitivity reactions with rapid onset, including life-threatening reactions have occurred after restarting abacavir in patients who had only one of the key symptoms of hypersensitivity (skin rash, fever, gastrointestinal, respiratory or constitutional symptoms such as lethargy and malaise) prior to stopping abacavir. The most common isolated symptom of a hypersensitivity reaction was a skin rash. Moreover, on very rare occasions hypersensitivity reactions have been reported in patients who have restarted therapy, and who had no preceding symptoms of a hypersensitivity reaction.
In both cases if a decision is made to restart abacavir this must be done in a setting where medical assistance is readily available.

• **Essential patient information**

Prescribers must ensure that patients are fully informed regarding the following information on the hypersensitivity reaction:

- Patients must be made aware of the possibility of a hypersensitivity reaction to abacavir that may result in a life-threatening reaction or death.

- Patients developing signs or symptoms possibly linked with a hypersensitivity reaction **MUST CONTACT their doctor IMMEDIATELY.**

- Patients who are hypersensitive to abacavir should be reminded that they must never take Kivexa or any other medicinal product containing abacavir (Ziagen or Trizivir) again.

- In order to avoid restarting abacavir, patients who have experienced a hypersensitivity reaction should dispose of their remaining Kivexa tablets in their possession in accordance with the local requirements, and ask their doctor or pharmacist for advice.

- Patients who have stopped Kivexa for any reason, and particularly due to possible adverse reactions or illness, must be advised to contact their doctor before restarting.

- Patients should be advised of the importance of taking Kivexa regularly.

- Each patient should be reminded to read the Package Leaflet included in the Kivexa package.

- They should be reminded of the importance of removing the Alert Card included in the package, and keeping it with them at all times.

Kivexa should not be administered to adults or adolescents who weigh less than 40 kg because it is a fixed-dose tablet that cannot be dose reduced.

Kivexa can be taken with or without food.

Kivexa is a fixed-dose tablet and should not be prescribed for patients requiring dosage adjustments. Separate preparations of abacavir or lamivudine are available in cases where discontinuation or dose adjustment of one of the active substances is indicated. In these cases the physician should refer to the individual product information for these medicinal products.

Renal impairment: Kivexa is not recommended for use in patients with a creatinine clearance < 50 ml/min (see section 5.2).

Hepatic impairment: No data are available in patients with moderate hepatic impairment, therefore the use of Kivexa is not recommended unless judged necessary. In patients with mild and moderate hepatic impairment close monitoring is required, and if feasible, monitoring of abacavir plasma levels is recommended (see sections 4.4 and 5.2). Kivexa is contraindicated in patients with severe hepatic impairment (see section 4.3).

Elderly: No pharmacokinetic data are currently available in patients over 65 years of age. Special care is advised in this age group due to age associated changes such as the decrease in renal function and alteration of haematological parameters.

Children: Kivexa is not recommended for treatment of children less than 12 years of age as the necessary dose adjustment cannot be made.

4.3 Contraindications

Kivexa is contraindicated in patients with known hypersensitivity to the active substances or to any of the excipients. See BOXED INFORMATION ON ABACAVIR HYPERSENSITIVITY REACTIONS in section 4.4 and section 4.8.

Patients with severe hepatic impairment.

4.4 Special warnings and precautions for use

The special warnings and precautions relevant to abacavir and lamivudine are included in this section. There are no additional precautions and warnings relevant to Kivexa.

(see Table 1 on previous page)

Table 2

Abacavir hypersensitivity (see also section 4.4)

In clinical studies, approximately 5 % of subjects receiving abacavir developed a hypersensitivity reaction. In clinical studies with abacavir 600 mg once daily the reported rate of hypersensitivity remained within the range recorded for abacavir 300 mg twice daily.

Some of these hypersensitivity reactions were life-threatening and resulted in fatal outcome despite taking precautions. This reaction is characterised by the appearance of symptoms indicating multi-organ/body-system involvement.

Almost all patients developing hypersensitivity reactions will have fever and/or rash (usually maculopapular or urticarial) as part of the syndrome, however reactions have occurred without rash or fever.

The signs and symptoms of this hypersensitivity reaction are listed below. These have been identified either from clinical studies or post marketing surveillance. Those reported **in at least 10% of patients** with a hypersensitivity reaction are in bold text.

Skin	**Rash** (usually maculopapular or urticarial)
Gastrointestinal tract	**Nausea, vomiting, diarrhoea, abdominal pain**, mouth ulceration
Respiratory tract	**Dyspnoea, cough**, sore throat, adult respiratory distress syndrome, respiratory failure
Miscellaneous	**Fever, lethargy, malaise**, oedema, lymphadenopathy, hypotension, conjunctivitis, anaphylaxis
Neurological/Psychiatry	**Headache**, paraesthesia
Haematological	Lymphopenia
Liver/pancreas	**Elevated liver function tests,** hepatitis, hepatic failure
Musculoskeletal	**Myalgia**, rarely myolysis, arthralgia, elevated creatine phosphokinase
Urology	Elevated creatinine, renal failure

Some patients with hypersensitivity reactions were initially thought to have gastroenteritis, respiratory disease (pneumonia, bronchitis, pharyngitis) or a flu-like illness. This delay in diagnosis of hypersensitivity has resulted in abacavir being continued or re-introduced, leading to more severe hypersensitivity reactions or death. Therefore, the diagnosis of hypersensitivity reaction should be carefully considered for patients presenting with symptoms of these diseases.

Symptoms usually appeared within the first six weeks (median time to onset 11 days) of initiation of treatment with abacavir, although these reactions may occur at any time during therapy. Close medical supervision is necessary during the first two months, with consultations every two weeks.

It is likely that intermittent therapy may increase the risk of developing sensitisation and therefore occurrence of clinically significant hypersensitivity reactions. Consequently, patients should be advised of the importance of taking Kivexa regularly.

Restarting abacavir following a hypersensitivity reaction results in a prompt return of symptoms within hours. This recurrence of the hypersensitivity reaction was usually more severe than on initial presentation, and may include life-threatening hypotension and death. **Patients who develop this hypersensitivity reaction must discontinue Kivexa and must never be rechallenged with Kivexa, or any other medicinal product containing abacavir (Ziagen or Trizivir).**

To avoid a delay in diagnosis and minimise the risk of a life-threatening hypersensitivity reaction, abacavir must be permanently discontinued if hypersensitivity cannot be ruled out, even when other diagnoses are possible (respiratory diseases, flu-like illness, gastroenteritis or reactions to other medicinal products).

Hypersensitivity reactions with rapid onset, including life-threatening reactions have occurred after restarting abacavir in patients who had only one of the key symptoms of hypersensitivity (skin rash, fever, gastrointestinal, respiratory or constitutional symptoms such as lethargy and malaise) prior to stopping abacavir. The most common isolated symptom of a hypersensitivity reaction was a skin rash. Moreover, on very rare occasions hypersensitivity reactions have been reported in patients who have restarted therapy and who had no preceding symptoms of a hypersensitivity reaction. In both cases, if a decision is made to restart abacavir this must be done in a setting where medical assistance is readily available.

Each patient must be warned about this hypersensitivity reaction to abacavir.

Lactic acidosis: lactic acidosis, usually associated with hepatomegaly and hepatic steatosis, has been reported with the use of nucleoside analogues. Early symptoms (symptomatic hyperlactatemia) include benign digestive symptoms (nausea, vomiting and abdominal pain), non-specific malaise, loss of appetite, weight loss, respiratory symptoms (rapid and/or deep breathing) or neurological symptoms (including motor weakness). Lactic acidosis has a high mortality and may be associated with pancreatitis, liver failure, or renal failure. Lactic acidosis generally occurred after a few or several months of treatment.

Treatment with nucleoside analogues should be discontinued in the setting of symptomatic hyperlactatemia and metabolic/lactic acidosis, progressive hepatomegaly, or rapidly elevating aminotransferase levels. Caution should be exercised when administering nucleoside analogues to any patient (particularly obese women) with hepatomegaly, hepatitis or other known risk factors for liver disease and hepatic steatosis (including certain medicinal products and alcohol). Patients co-infected with hepatitis C and treated with alpha interferon and ribavirin may constitute a special risk.

Patients at increased risk should be followed closely.

Lipodystrophy: combination antiretroviral therapy has been associated with the redistribution of body fat (lipodystrophy) in HIV patients. The long-term consequences of these events are currently unknown. Knowledge about the mechanism is incomplete. A connection between visceral lipomatosis and protease inhibitors (PIs) and lipoatrophy and nucleoside reverse transcriptase inhibitors (NRTIs) has been hypothesised. A higher risk of lipodystrophy has been associated with individual factors such as older age, and with drug related factors such as longer duration of antiretroviral treatment and associated metabolic disturbances. Clinical examination should include evaluation for physical signs of fat redistribution. Consideration should be given to the measurement of fasting serum lipids and blood glucose. Lipid disorders should be managed as clinically appropriate (see section 4.8).

Pancreatitis: pancreatitis has been reported, but a causal relationship to lamivudine and abacavir is uncertain.

Clinical studies: the benefit of the combination of abacavir and lamivudine as a once daily regimen is mainly based on a study performed in combination with efavirenz, in antiretroviral-naïve adults patients (see section 5.1).

Triple nucleoside therapy: There have been reports of a high rate of virological failure, and of emergence of resistance at an early stage when abacavir and lamivudine were combined with tenofovir disoproxil fumarate as a once daily regimen.

Liver disease: if lamivudine is being used concomitantly for the treatment of HIV and HBV, additional information relating to the use of lamivudine in the treatment of hepatitis B infection is available in the Zeffix SPC.

The safety and efficacy of Kivexa has not been established in patients with significant underlying liver disorders. Kivexa is contraindicated in patients with severe hepatic impairment (see section 4.3).

Patients with chronic hepatitis B or C and treated with combination antiretroviral therapy are at an increased risk of severe and potentially fatal hepatic adverse events. In case of concomitant antiviral therapy for hepatitis B or C, please refer also to the relevant product information for these medicinal products.

If Kivexa is discontinued in patients co-infected with hepatitis B virus, periodic monitoring of both liver function tests and markers of HBV replication is recommended, as withdrawal of lamivudine may result in an acute exacerbation of hepatitis (see Zeffix SPC).

Patients with pre-existing liver dysfunction, including chronic active hepatitis have an increased frequency of liver function abnormalities during combination antiretroviral therapy, and should be monitored according to standard practice. If there is evidence of worsening liver disease in such patients, interruption or discontinuation of treatment must be considered.

Mitochondrial dysfunction: nucleoside and nucleotide analogues have been demonstrated *in vitro* and *in vivo* to cause a variable degree of mitochondrial damage. There have been reports of mitochondrial dysfunction in HIV-negative infants exposed *in utero* and/or post-natally to nucleoside analogues. The main adverse events reported are haematological disorders (anaemia, neutropenia), metabolic disorders (hyperlactatemia, hyperlipasemia). These events are often transitory. Some late-onset neurological disorders have been reported (hypertonia, convulsion, abnormal behaviour). Whether the neurological disorders are transient or permanent is currently unknown. Any child exposed *in utero* to nucleoside and nucleotide analogues, even HIV-negative children, should have clinical and laboratory follow-up and should be fully investigated for possible mitochondrial dysfunction in case of relevant signs or symptoms. These findings do not affect current national recommendations to use antiretroviral therapy in pregnant women to prevent vertical transmission of HIV.

Immune Reactivation Syndrome: in HIV-infected patients with severe immune deficiency at the time of institution of combination antiretroviral therapy (CART), an inflammatory reaction to asymptomatic or residual opportunistic pathogens may arise and cause serious clinical conditions, or aggravation of symptoms. Typically, such reactions have been observed within the first few weeks or months of initiation of CART. Relevant examples are cytomegalovirus retinitis, generalised and/or focal mycobacterial infections, and *Pneumocystis carinii* pneumonia. Any inflammatory symptoms should be evaluated and treatment instituted when necessary.

Osteonecrosis: Although the etiology is considered to be multifactorial (including corticosteroid use, alcohol consumption, severe immunosuppression, higher body mass index), cases of osteonecrosis have been reported particularly in patients with advanced HIV-disease and/or long-term exposure to combination antiretroviral therapy (CART). Patients should be advised to seek medical advice if they experience joint aches and pain, joint stiffness or difficulty in movement.

Excipients: Kivexa contains the azo colouring agent sunset yellow, which may cause allergic reactions.

Opportunistic infections: patients should be advised that Kivexa or any other antiretroviral therapy does not cure HIV infection and that they may still develop opportunistic infections and other complications of HIV infection. Therefore patients should remain under close clinical observation by physicians experienced in the treatment of these associated HIV diseases.

Transmission of HIV: patients should be advised that current antiretroviral therapy, including Kivexa, has not been proven to prevent the risk of transmission of HIV to others through sexual contact or blood contamination. Appropriate precautions should continue to be taken.

Myocardial Infarction: Observational studies have shown an association between myocardial infarction and the use of abacavir. Those studied were mainly antiretroviral experienced patients. Data from clinical trials showed limited numbers of myocardial infarction and could not exclude a small increase in risk. Overall the available data from observational cohorts and from randomised trials show some inconsistency so can neither confirm nor refute a causal relationship between abacavir treatment and the risk of myocardial infarction. To date, there is no established biological mechanism to explain a potential increase in risk. When prescribing Kivexa, action should be taken to try to minimize all modifiable risk factors (e.g. smoking, hypertension, and hyperlipidaemia).

4.5 Interaction with other medicinal products and other forms of interaction

Kivexa contains abacavir and lamivudine, therefore any interactions identified for these individually are relevant to Kivexa. Clinical studies have shown that there are no clinically significant interactions between abacavir and lamivudine.

Abacavir and lamivudine are not significantly metabolised by cytochrome P_{450} enzymes (such as CYP 3A4, CYP 2C9 or CYP 2D6) nor do they inhibit or induce this enzyme system. Therefore, there is little potential for interactions with antiretroviral protease inhibitors, non-nucleosides and other medicinal products metabolised by major P_{450} enzymes. The interactions listed below should not be considered exhaustive but are representative of the classes of medicinal products where caution should be exercised.

Interactions relevant to abacavir

Potent enzymatic inducers such as rifampicin, phenobarbital and phenytoin may via their action on UDP-glucuronyltransferases slightly decrease the plasma concentrations of abacavir.

The metabolism of abacavir is altered by concomitant consumption of ethanol resulting in an increase in AUC of abacavir of about 41%. These findings are not considered clinically significant. Abacavir has no effect on the metabolism of ethanol.

Retinoid compounds are eliminated via alcohol dehydrogenase. Interaction with abacavir is possible but has not been studied.

In a pharmacokinetic study, coadministration of 600 mg abacavir twice daily with methadone showed a 35% reduction in abacavir C_{max} and a 1 hour delay in t_{max}, but the AUC was unchanged. The changes in abacavir pharmacokinetics are not considered clinically relevant. In this study, abacavir increased the mean methadone systemic clearance by 22%. The induction of metabolizing enzymes cannot therefore be excluded. Patients being treated with methadone and abacavir should be monitored for evidence of withdrawal symptoms indicating under dosing, as occasionally methadone re-titration may be required.

Interactions relevant to lamivudine

The likelihood of metabolic interactions with lamivudine is low due to limited metabolism and plasma protein binding, and almost complete renal clearance. The possibility of interactions with other medicinal products administered concurrently with Kivexa should be considered, particularly when the main route of elimination is active renal secretion, especially via the cationic transport system e.g. trimethoprim. Other medicinal products (e.g. ranitidine, cimetidine) are eliminated only in part by this mechanism and were shown not to interact with lamivudine. The nucleoside analogues (e.g. zidovudine and didanosine) are not metabolised by this mechanism and are unlikely to interact with lamivudine.

Administration of trimethoprim/sulfamethoxazole 160 mg/800 mg results in a 40% increase in lamivudine exposure, because of the trimethoprim component. However, unless the patient has renal impairment, no dosage adjustment of lamivudine is necessary (see section 4.2). The pharmacokinetics of trimethoprim or sulfamethoxazole are not affected. When concomitant administration with co-trimoxazole is warranted, patients should be monitored clinically. Co-administration of Kivexa with high doses of co-trimoxazole for the treatment of *Pneumocystis carinii* pneumonia (PCP) and toxoplasmosis should be avoided.

Co-administration of lamivudine with intravenous ganciclovir or foscarnet is not recommended until further information is available.

Lamivudine may inhibit the intracellular phosphorylation of zalcitabine when the two medicinal products are used concurrently. Kivexa is therefore not recommended to be used in combination with zalcitabine.

4.6 Pregnancy and lactation

Kivexa is not recommended during pregnancy. The safety of abacavir and lamivudine in human pregnancy has not been established. Studies with abacavir and lamivudine in animals have shown reproductive toxicity (see section 5.3).

It is recommended that HIV-infected women do not breast-feed their infants under any circumstances in order to avoid transmission of HIV. Lamivudine is excreted in human milk at similar concentrations to those found in serum. It is expected that abacavir will also be secreted into human milk, although this has not been confirmed. It is therefore recommended that mothers do not breast-feed their babies while receiving treatment with Kivexa.

4.7 Effects on ability to drive and use machines

No studies on the effects on ability to drive and use machines have been performed. The clinical status of the patient and the adverse event profile of Kivexa should be borne in mind when considering the patient's ability to drive or operate machinery.

4.8 Undesirable effects

The adverse reactions reported for Kivexa were consistent with the known safety profiles of abacavir and lamivudine when given as separate medicinal products. For many of these adverse reactions it is unclear whether they are related to the active substance, the wide range of other medicinal products used in the management of HIV infection, or whether they are a result of the underlying disease process.

(see Table 2 on previous page)

Many of the adverse reactions listed in the table below occur commonly (nausea, vomiting, diarrhoea, fever, lethargy, rash) in patients with abacavir hypersensitivity. Therefore, patients with any of these symptoms should be carefully evaluated for the presence of this hypersensitivity reaction. If Kivexa has been discontinued in patients due to experiencing any one of these symptoms and a decision is made to restart a medicinal product containing abacavir, this must be done in a setting where medical assistance is readily available (see section 4.4). Very rarely cases of erythema multiforme, Stevens-Johnson syndrome or toxic epidermal necrolysis have been reported where abacavir hypersensitivity could not be ruled out. In such cases medicinal products containing abacavir should be permanently discontinued.

The adverse reactions considered at least possibly related to abacavir or lamivudine are listed by body system, organ class and absolute frequency. Frequencies are defined as very common (> 1/10), common (> 1/100, < 1/10), uncommon (> 1/1000, < 1/100), rare (> 1/10,000, < 1/1000), very rare (< 1/10,000).

Body system	Abacavir	Lamivudine
Blood and lymphatic systems disorders		*Uncommon:* Neutropenia and anaemia (both occasionally severe), thrombocytopenia *Very rare:* Pure red cell aplasia
Immune system disorders	*Common:* hypersensitivity	
Metabolism and nutrition disorders	*Common:* anorexia	
Nervous system disorders	*Common:* headache	*Common:* Headache, insomnia. *Very rare:* Cases of peripheral neuropathy (or paraesthesia) have been reported
Respiratory, thoracic and mediastinal disorders		*Common:* Cough, nasal symptoms
Gastrointestinal disorders	*Common:* nausea, vomiting, diarrhoea *Rare:* pancreatitis has been reported, but a causal relationship to abacavir treatment is uncertain	*Common:* Nausea, vomiting, abdominal pain or cramps, diarrhoea *Rare:* Rises in serum amylase. Cases of pancreatitis have been reported
Hepatobiliary disorders		*Uncommon:* Transient rises in liver enzymes (AST, ALT), *Rare:* Hepatitis
Skin and subcutaneous tissue disorders	*Common:* rash (without systemic symptoms) *Very rare:* erythema multiforme, Stevens-Johnson syndrome and toxic epidermal necrolysis	*Common:* Rash, alopecia
Musculoskeletal and connective tissue disorders		*Common:* Arthralgia, muscle disorders *Rare:* Rhabdomyolysis
General disorders and administration site conditions	*Common:* fever, lethargy, fatigue.	*Common:* fatigue, malaise, fever.

Cases of lactic acidosis, sometimes fatal, usually associated with severe hepatomegaly and hepatic steatosis, have been reported with the use of nucleoside analogues (see section 4.4).

Combination antiretroviral therapy has been associated with redistribution of body fat (lipodystrophy) in HIV patients including the loss of peripheral and facial subcutaneous fat, increased intra-abdominal and visceral fat, breast hypertrophy and dorsocervical fat accumulation (buffalo hump).

Combination antiretroviral therapy has been associated with metabolic abnormalities such as hypertriglyceridaemia, hypercholesterolaemia, insulin resistance, hyperglycaemia and hyperlactataemia (see section 4.4).

In HIV-infected patients with severe immune deficiency at the time of initiation of combination antiretroviral therapy, an inflammatory reaction to asymptomatic or residual opportunistic infections may arise (see section 4.4).

Cases of osteonecrosis have been reported, particularly in patients with generally acknowledged risk factors, advanced HIV disease or long-term exposure to combination antiretroviral therapy (CART). The frequency of this is unknown (see section 4.4).

4.9 Overdose

No specific symptoms or signs have been identified following acute overdose with abacavir or lamivudine, apart from those listed as undesirable effects.

If overdose occurs the patient should be monitored for evidence of toxicity (see section 4.8), and standard supportive treatment applied as necessary. Since lamivudine is dialysable, continuous haemodialysis could be used in the treatment of overdose, although this has not been studied. It is not known whether abacavir can be removed by peritoneal dialysis or haemodialysis.

5. PHARMACOLOGICAL PROPERTIES

5.1 Pharmacodynamic properties

Pharmacotherapeutic group: Antivirals for treatment of HIV infections, combinations. ATC code: J05AR02.

Mechanism of action: Abacavir and lamivudine are NRTIs, and are potent selective inhibitors of HIV-1 and HIV-2. Both abacavir and lamivudine are metabolised sequentially by intracellular kinases to the respective 5'-triphosphate (TP) which are the active moieties. Lamivudine-TP and carbovir-TP (the active triphosphate form of abacavir) are substrates for and competitive inhibitors of HIV reverse transcriptase (RT). However, their main antiviral activity is through incorporation of the monophosphate form into the viral DNA chain, resulting in chain termination. Abacavir and lamivudine triphosphates show significantly less affinity for host cell DNA polymerases.

Lamivudine has been shown to be highly synergistic with zidovudine, inhibiting the replication of HIV in cell culture. Abacavir shows synergy *in vitro* in combination with amprenavir, nevirapine and zidovudine. It has been shown to be additive in combination with didanosine, stavudine and lamivudine.

In-vitro resistance: HIV-1 resistance to lamivudine involves the development of a M184I or, more commonly, M184V amino acid change close to the active site of the viral RT.

Abacavir-resistant isolates of HIV-1 have been selected *in vitro* and are associated with specific genotypic changes in the RT codon region (codons M184V, K65R, L74V and Y115F). Viral resistance to abacavir develops relatively slowly *in vitro*, requiring multiple mutations for a clinically relevant increase in EC_{50} over wild-type virus.

In vivo resistance (Therapy-naive patients): The M184V or M184I variants arise in HIV-1 infected patients treated with lamivudine-containing antiretroviral therapy.

Isolates from most patients experiencing virological failure with a regimen containing abacavir in pivotal clinical trials showed either no NRTI-related changes from baseline (45%) or only M184V or M184I selection (45%). The overall selection frequency for M184V or M184I was high (54%), and less common was the selection of L74V (5%), K65R (1%) and Y115F (1%) (see Table). The inclusion of zidovudine in the regimen has been found to reduce the frequency of L74V and K65R selection in the presence of abacavir (with zidovudine: 0/40, without zidovudine: 15/192, 8%).

(see Table 3 on next page)

TAMs might be selected when thymidine analogs are associated with abacavir. In a meta-analysis of six clinical trials, TAMs were not selected by regimens containing abacavir without zidovudine (0/127), but were selected by regimens containing abacavir and the thymidine analogue zidovudine (22/86, 26%).

In vivo resistance (Therapy experienced patients): The M184V or M184I variants arise in HIV-1 infected patients treated with lamivudine-containing antiretroviral therapy and confer high-level resistance to lamivudine. *In vitro* data

Table 3

Therapy	Abacavir + Combivir[1]	Abacavir + lamivudine + NNRTI	Abacavir + lamivudine + PI (or PI/ritonavir)	Total
Number of Subjects	282	1094	909	2285
Number of Virological Failures	43	90	158	306
Number of On-Therapy Genotypes	40 (100%)	51 (100%)[2]	141 (100%)	232 (100%)
K65R	0	1 (2%)	2 (1%)	3 (1%)
L74V	0	9 (18%)	3 (2%)	12 (5%)
Y115F	0	2 (4%)	0	2 (1%)
M184V/I	34 (85%)	22 (43%)	70 (50%)	126 (54%)
TAMs[3]	3 (8%)	2 (4%)	4 (3%)	9 (4%)

1. Combivir is a fixed dose combination of lamivudine and zidovudine
2. Includes three non-virological failures and four unconfirmed virological failures.
3. Number of subjects with ⩾1 Thymidine Analogue Mutations (TAMs).

tend to suggest that the continuation of lamivudine in antiretroviral regimen despite the development of M184V might provide residual anti-retroviral activity (likely through impaired viral fitness). The clinical relevance of these findings is not established. Indeed, the available clinical data are very limited and preclude any reliable conclusion in the field. In any case, initiation of susceptible NRTIs should always be preferred to maintenance of lamivudine therapy. Therefore, maintaining lamivudine therapy despite emergence of M184V mutation should only be considered in cases where no other active NRTIs are available.

Clinically significant reduction of susceptibility to abacavir has been demonstrated in clinical isolates of patients with uncontrolled viral replication, who have been pre-treated with and are resistant to other nucleoside inhibitors. In a meta-analysis of five clinical trials where ABC was added to intensify therapy, of 166 subjects, 123 (74%) had M184V/I, 50 (30%) had T215Y/F, 45 (27%) had M41L, 30 (18%) had K70R and 25 (15%) had D67N. K65R was absent and L74V and Y115F were uncommon (⩽3%). Logistic regression modelling of the predictive value for genotype (adjusted for baseline plasma HIV-1RNA [vRNA], CD4+ cell count, number and duration of prior antiretroviral therapies) showed that the presence of 3 or more NRTI resistance-associated mutations was associated with reduced response at Week 4 ($p=0.015$) or 4 or more mutations at median Week 24 ($p \leqslant 0.012$). In addition, the 69 insertion complex or the Q151M mutation, usually found in combination with A62V, V75I, F77L and F116Y, cause a high level of resistance to abacavir.

(see Table 4 below)

Phenotypic resistance and cross-resistance: Phenotypic resistance to abacavir requires M184V with at least one other abacavir-selected mutation, or M184V with multiple TAMs. Phenotypic cross-resistance to other NRTIs with M184V or M184I mutation alone is limited. Zidovudine, didanosine, stavudine and tenofovir maintain their antiretroviral activities against such HIV-1 variants. The presence of M184V with K65R does give rise to cross-resistance between abacavir, tenofovir, didanosine and lamivudine, and M184V with L74V gives rise to cross-resistance between abacavir, didanosine and lamivudine. The presence of M184V with Y115F gives rise to cross-resistance between abacavir and lamivudine. Appropriate use of abacavir can be guided using currently recommended resistance algorithms.

Cross-resistance between abacavir or lamivudine and antiretrovirals from other classes e.g. PIs or NNRTIs is unlikely.

Clinical experience

Therapy-naïve patients

The combination of abacavir and lamivudine as a once daily regimen is supported by a 48 weeks multi-centre, double-blind, controlled study (CNA30021) of 770 HIV-infected, therapy-naïve adults. These were primarily asymptomatic HIV infected patients (CDC stage A). They were randomised to receive either abacavir (ABC) 600 mg once daily or 300 mg twice daily, in combination with lamivudine 300 mg once daily and efavirenz 600 mg once daily. The results are summarised in the table below:

Virological Response Based on Plasma HIV-1 RNA < 50 copies/ml at Week 48

ITT-Exposed Population

Treatment regimen	ABC once/day (N = 384)	ABC twice/day (N = 386)
Virological response	253/384 (66%)	261/386 (68%)

Similar clinical success (point estimate for treatment difference: -1.7, 95% CI -8.4, 4.9) was observed for both regimens. From these results, it can be concluded with 95% confidence that the true difference is no greater than 8.4% in favour of the twice daily regimen. This potential difference is sufficiently small to draw an overall conclusion of non-inferiority of abacavir once daily over abacavir twice daily.

There was a low, similar overall incidence of virologic failure (viral load > 50 copies/ml) in both the once and twice daily treatment groups (10% and 8% respectively). In the small sample size for genotypic analysis, there was a trend toward a higher rate of NRTI-associated mutations in the once daily versus the twice daily abacavir regimens. No firm conclusion could be drawn due to the limited data derived from this study. Long term data with abacavir used as a once daily regimen (beyond 48 weeks) are currently limited.

Therapy-experienced patients

In study CAL30001, 182 treatment-experienced patients with virologic failure were randomised and received treatment with either Kivexa once daily or abacavir 300 mg twice daily plus lamivudine 300 mg once daily, both in combination with tenofovir and a PI or an NNRTI for 48 weeks. Results indicate that the Kivexa group was non-inferior to the abacavir twice daily group, based on similar reductions in HIV-1 RNA as measured by average area under the curve minus baseline (AAUCMB, -1.65 $\log_{10}$ copies/ml versus -1.83 $\log_{10}$ copies/ml respectively, 95% CI -0.13, 0.38). Proportions with HIV-1 RNA < 50 copies/ml (50% versus 47%) and < 400 copies/ml (54% versus 57%) were also similar in each group (ITT population). However, as there were only moderately experienced patients included in this study with an imbalance in baseline viral load between the arms, these results should be interpreted with caution.

In study ESS30008, 260 patients with virologic suppression on a first line therapy regimen containing abacavir 300 mg plus lamivudine 150 mg, both given twice daily and a PI or NNRTI, were randomised to continue this regimen or switch to Kivexa plus a PI or NNRTI for 48 weeks. Results indicate that the Kivexa group was associated with a similar virologic outcome (non-inferior) compared to the abacavir plus lamivudine group, based on proportions of subjects with HIV-1 RNA < 50 copies/ml (90% and 85% respectively, 95% CI -2.7, 13.5).

Table 4

Baseline Reverse Transcriptase Mutation	Week 4 (n = 166)		
	n	**Median Change vRNA ($\log_{10}$ c/mL)**	**Percent with <400 copies/mL vRNA**
None	15	-0.96	40%
M184V alone	75	-0.74	64%
Any one NRTI mutation	82	-0.72	65%
Any two NRTI-associated mutations	22	-0.82	32%
Any three NRTI-associated mutations	19	-0.30	5%
Four or more NRTI-associated mutations	28	-0.07	11%

5.2 Pharmacokinetic properties

The fixed-dose combination tablet of abacavir/lamivudine (FDC) has been shown to be bioequivalent to lamivudine and abacavir administered separately. This was demonstrated in a single dose, 3-way crossover bioequivalence study of FDC (fasted) versus 2 × 300 mg abacavir tablets plus 2 × 150 mg lamivudine tablets (fasted) versus FDC administered with a high fat meal, in healthy volunteers (n = 30). In the fasted state there was no significant difference in the extent of absorption, as measured by the area under the plasma concentration-time curve (AUC) and maximal peak concentration (C_{max}), of each component. There was also no clinically significant food effect observed between administration of FDC in the fasted or fed state. These results indicate that FDC can be taken with or without food. The pharmacokinetic properties of lamivudine and abacavir are described below.

Absorption

Abacavir and lamivudine are rapidly and well absorbed from the gastro-intestinal tract following oral administration. The absolute bioavailability of oral abacavir and lamivudine in adults is about 83% and 80-85% respectively. The mean time to maximal serum concentrations (t_{max}) is about 1.5 hours and 1.0 hour for abacavir and lamivudine, respectively. Following a single dose of 600 mg of abacavir, the mean (CV) C_{max} is 4.26 μg/ml (28%) and the mean (CV) AUC_{∞} is 11.95 μg.h/ml (21%). Following multiple-dose oral administration of lamivudine 300 mg once daily for seven days, the mean (CV) steady-state C_{max} is 2.04 μg/ml (26%) and the mean (CV) AUC_{24} is 8.87 μg.h/ml (21%).

Distribution

Intravenous studies with abacavir and lamivudine showed that the mean apparent volume of distribution is 0.8 and 1.3 l/kg respectively. Plasma protein binding studies *in vitro* indicate that abacavir binds only low to moderately (~49%) to human plasma proteins at therapeutic concentrations. Lamivudine exhibits linear pharmacokinetics over the therapeutic dose range and displays limited plasma protein binding *in vitro* (< 36%). This indicates a low likelihood for interactions with other medicinal products through plasma protein binding displacement.

Data show that abacavir and lamivudine penetrate the central nervous system (CNS) and reach the cerebrospinal fluid (CSF). Studies with abacavir demonstrate a CSF to plasma AUC ratio of between 30 to 44%. The observed values of the peak concentrations are 9 fold greater than the IC_{50} of abacavir of 0.08 μg/ml or 0.26 μM when abacavir is given at 600 mg twice daily. The mean ratio of CSF/serum lamivudine concentrations 2-4 hours after oral administration was approximately 12%. The true extent of CNS penetration of lamivudine and its relationship with any clinical efficacy is unknown.

Metabolism

Abacavir is primarily metabolised by the liver with approximately 2% of the administered dose being renally excreted, as unchanged compound. The primary pathways of metabolism in man are by alcohol dehydrogenase and by glucuronidation to produce the 5'-carboxylic acid and 5'-glucuronide which account for about 66% of the administered dose. These metabolites are excreted in the urine.

Metabolism of lamivudine is a minor route of elimination. Lamivudine is predominately cleared by renal excretion of unchanged lamivudine. The likelihood of metabolic drug interactions with lamivudine is low due to the small extent of hepatic metabolism (5-10%).

Elimination

The mean half-life of abacavir is about 1.5 hours. Following multiple oral doses of abacavir 300 mg twice a day there is no significant accumulation of abacavir. Elimination of abacavir is via hepatic metabolism with subsequent excretion of metabolites primarily in the urine. The metabolites and unchanged abacavir account for about 83% of the administered abacavir dose in the urine. The remainder is eliminated in the faeces.

The observed lamivudine half-life of elimination is 5 to 7 hours. The mean systemic clearance of lamivudine is approximately 0.32 l/h/kg, predominantly by renal clearance (> 70%) via the organic cationic transport system. Studies in patients with renal impairment show lamivudine elimination is affected by renal dysfunction. Dose reduction is required for patients with creatinine clearance < 50 ml/min (see section 4.2).

Intracellular pharmacokinetics

In a study of 20 HIV-infected patients receiving abacavir 300 mg twice daily, with only one 300 mg dose taken prior to the 24 hour sampling period, the geometric mean terminal carbovir-TP intracellular half-life at steady-state was 20.6 hours, compared to the geometric mean abacavir plasma half-life in this study of 2.6 hours. In a crossover study in 27 HIV-infected patients, intracellular carbovir-TP exposures were higher for the abacavir 600 mg once daily regimen ($AUC_{24,ss}$ + 32 %, $C_{max24,ss}$ + 99 % and C_{trough} + 18 %) compared to the 300 mg twice daily regimen. For patients receiving lamivudine 300 mg once daily, the terminal intracellular half-life of lamivudine-TP was prolonged to 16-19 hours, compared to the plasma lamivudine half-life of 5-7 hours. In a crossover study in 60 healthy volunteers, intracellular lamivudine-TP pharmacokinetic parameters were similar ($AUC_{24,ss}$ and $C_{max24,ss}$) or lower (C_{trough} − 24 %) for the lamivudine 300 mg once daily regimen compared to the lamivudine 150 mg twice daily regimen. Overall, these data support the use of lamivudine 300 mg and abacavir 600 mg once daily for the treatment of HIV-infected patients. Additionally, the efficacy and safety of this combination given once daily has been demonstrated in a pivotal clinical study (CNA30021- See Clinical experience).

Special populations

Hepatically impaired: There are no data available on the use of Kivexa in hepatically impaired patients. Pharmacokinetic data has been obtained for abacavir and lamivudine alone.

Abacavir is metabolised primarily by the liver. The pharmacokinetics of abacavir have been studied in patients with mild hepatic impairment (Child-Pugh score 5-6) receiving a single 600 mg dose. The results showed that there was a mean increase of 1.89 fold [1.32; 2.70] in the abacavir AUC, and 1.58 [1.22; 2.04] fold in the elimination half-life. No recommendation on dosage reduction is possible in patients with mild hepatic impairment due to substantial variability of abacavir exposure.

Data obtained in patients with moderate to severe hepatic impairment show that lamivudine pharmacokinetics are not significantly affected by hepatic dysfunction.

Renally impaired: Pharmacokinetic data have been obtained for lamivudine and abacavir alone. Abacavir is primarily metabolised by the liver with approximately 2% of abacavir excreted unchanged in the urine. The pharmacokinetics of abacavir in patients with end-stage renal disease is similar to patients with normal renal function. Studies with lamivudine show that plasma concentrations (AUC) are increased in patients with renal dysfunction due to decreased clearance. Dose reduction is required for patients with creatinine clearance of < 50 ml/min.

Elderly: No pharmacokinetic data are available in patients over 65 years of age.

5.3 Preclinical safety data

With the exception of a negative *in vivo* rat micronucleus test, there are no data available on the effects of the combination of abacavir and lamivudine in animals.

Mutagenicity and carcinogenicity

Neither abacavir nor lamivudine were mutagenic in bacterial tests, but like many nucleoside analogues they show activity in the *in vitro* mammalian tests such as the mouse lymphoma assay. This is consistent with the known activity of other nucleoside analogues. The results of an *in vivo* rat micronucleus test with abacavir and lamivudine in combination were negative.

Lamivudine has not shown any genotoxic activity in the *in vivo* studies at doses that gave plasma concentrations up to 30-40 times higher than clinical plasma concentrations. Abacavir has a weak potential to cause chromosomal damage both *in vitro* and *in vivo* at high tested concentrations.

The carcinogenic potential of a combination of abacavir and lamivudine has not been tested. In long-term oral carcinogenicity studies in rats and mice, lamivudine did not show any carcinogenic potential. Carcinogenicity studies with orally administered abacavir in mice and rats showed an increase in the incidence of malignant and non-malignant tumours. Malignant tumours occurred in the preputial gland of males and the clitoral gland of females of both species, and in rats in the thyroid gland of males and in the liver, urinary bladder, lymph nodes and the subcutis of females.

The majority of these tumours occurred at the highest abacavir dose of 330 mg/kg/day in mice and 600 mg/kg/day in rats. The exception was the preputial gland tumour which occurred at a dose of 110 mg/kg in mice. The systemic exposure at the no effect level in mice and rats was equivalent to 3 and 7 times the human systemic exposure during therapy. While the carcinogenic potential in humans is unknown, these data suggest that a carcinogenic risk to humans is outweighed by the potential clinical benefit.

Repeat-dose toxicity

In toxicology studies abacavir was shown to increase liver weights in rats and monkeys. The clinical relevance of this is unknown. There is no evidence from clinical studies that abacavir is hepatotoxic. Additionally, autoinduction of abacavir metabolism or induction of the metabolism of other medicinal products hepatically metabolised has not been observed in man.

Mild myocardial degeneration in the heart of mice and rats was observed following administration of abacavir for two years. The systemic exposures were equivalent to 7 to 24 times the expected systemic exposure in humans. The clinical relevance of this finding has not been determined.

Reproductive toxicology

In reproductive toxicity studies in animals, lamivudine and abacavir were shown to cross the placenta.

Lamivudine was not teratogenic in animal studies but there were indications of an increase in early embryonic deaths in rabbits at relatively low systemic exposures, comparable to those achieved in humans. A similar effect was not seen in rats even at very high systemic exposure.

Abacavir demonstrated toxicity to the developing embryo and foetus in rats, but not in rabbits. These findings included decreased foetal body weight, foetal oedema, and an increase in skeletal variations/malformations, early intra-uterine deaths and still births. No conclusion can be drawn with regard to the teratogenic potential of abacavir because of this embryo-foetal toxicity.

A fertility study in rats has shown that abacavir and lamivudine had no effect on male or female fertility.

6. PHARMACEUTICAL PARTICULARS

6.1 List of excipients

Core:

magnesium stearate

microcrystalline cellulose

sodium starch glycollate.

Coating:

Opadry Orange YS-1-13065-A containing:

hypromellose

titanium dioxide (E171)

macrogol 400, polysorbate 80

sunset yellow aluminium lake (E110).

6.2 Incompatibilities

Not applicable.

6.3 Shelf life

3 years.

6.4 Special precautions for storage

Do not store above 30°C.

6.5 Nature and contents of container

30 tablets in opaque white (PVC/PVDC/Aluminium) blister packs and white (HDPE) bottles with child-resistant closure.

90 (3x30) tablets in opaque white (PVC/PVDC/Aluminium) blister packs.

Not all pack sizes may be marketed.

6.6 Special precautions for disposal and other handling

No special requirements.

7. MARKETING AUTHORISATION HOLDER

Glaxo Group Ltd

Greenford

Middlesex UB6 0NN

United Kingdom

8. MARKETING AUTHORISATION NUMBER(S)

EU/1/04/298/001-002

EU/1/04/298/003

9. DATE OF FIRST AUTHORISATION/RENEWAL OF THE AUTHORISATION

17 December 2004

10. DATE OF REVISION OF THE TEXT

08 June 2009

Detailed information on this medicinal product is available on the website of the European Medicines Agency (EMEA) http://www.emea.europa.eu

Klaricid 250mg Tablets

(Abbott Laboratories Limited)

1. NAME OF THE MEDICINAL PRODUCT

Klaricid **or Clarithromycin 250 mg Tablets**

2. QUALITATIVE AND QUANTITATIVE COMPOSITION

250 mg/tablet

Active: Clarithromycin

3. PHARMACEUTICAL FORM

A yellow, ovaloid fil m-coated tablet containing 250 mg of clarithromycin.

4. CLINICAL PARTICULARS

4.1 Therapeutic indications

Clarithromycin is indicated for treatment of infections caused by susceptible organisms. Indications include:

Lower respiratory tract infections for example, acute and chronic bronchitis, and pneumonia.

Upper respiratory tract infections for example, sinusitis and pharyngitis.

Clarithromycin is appropriate for initial therapy in community acquired respiratory infections and has been shown to be active *in vitro* against common and atypical respiratory pathogens as listed in the microbiology section.

Clarithromycin is also indicated in skin and soft tissue infections of mild to moderate severity.

Clarithromycin in the presence of acid suppression effected by omeprazole or lansoprazole is also indicated for the eradication of *H. pylori* in patients with duodenal ulcers. See Dosage and Administration section.

Clarithromycin is usually active against the following organisms in vitro:

Gram-positive Bacteria: *Staphylococcus aureus* (methicillin susceptible); *Streptococcus pyogenes* (Group A beta-hemolytic streptococci); alpha-hemolytic streptococci (viridans group); *Streptococcus (Diplococcus) pneumoniae; Streptococcus agalactiae; Listeria monocytogenes.*

Gram-negative Bacteria: *Haemophilus influenzae; Haemophilus parainfluenzae; Moraxella (Branhamella) catarrhalis; Neisseria gonorrhoeae; Legionella pneumophila; Bordetella pertussis; Helicobacter pylori; Campylobacter jejuni.*

Mycoplasma: *Mycoplasma pneumoniae; Ureaplasma urealyticum.*

Other Organisms: *Chlamydia trachomatis; Mycobacterium avium; Mycobacterium leprae.*

Anaerobes: Macrolide-*susceptible Bacteroides fragilis; Clostridium perfringens*; Peptococcus species; Peptostreptococcus species; *Propionibacterium acnes.*

Clarithromycin has bactericidal activity against several bacterial strains. The organisms include *Haemophilus influenzae; Streptococcus pneumoniae; Streptococcus pyogenes; Streptococcus agalactiae; Moraxella (Branhamella) catarrhalis; Neisseria gonorrhoeae; H. pylori* and Campylobacter spp.

The activity of clarithromycin against *H. pylori* is greater at neutral pH than at acid pH.

4.2 Posology and method of administration

Patients with respiratory tract/skin and soft tissue infections.

Adults: The usual dose is 250 mg twice daily for 7 days although this may be increased to 500mg twice daily for up to 14 days in severe infections.

Children older than 12 years: As for adults.

Children younger than 12 years: Use Clarithromycin Paediatric Suspension.

Eradication of *H. pylori* in patients with duodenal ulcers (Adults)

Triple Therapy (7 - 14 days)

Clarithromycin (500mg) twice daily and lansoprazole 30mg twice daily should be given with amoxycillin 1000mg twice daily for 7 - 14 days.

Triple Therapy (7 days)

Clarithromycin (500mg) twice daily and lansoprazole 30mg twice daily should be given with metronidazole 400mg twice daily for 7 days.

Triple Therapy (7 days)

Clarithromycin (500mg) twice daily and omeprazole 40mg daily should be given with amoxycillin 1000mg twice daily or metronidazole 400mg twice daily for 7 days.

Triple Therapy (10 days)

Clarithromycin (500mg) twice daily should be given with amoxycillin 1000mg twice daily and omeprazole 20mg daily for 10 days.

Dual Therapy (14 days)

The usual dose of Clarithromycin is 500 mg three times daily for 14 days. Clarithromycin should be administered with oral omeprazole 40 mg once daily. The pivotal study was conducted with omeprazole 40 mg once daily for 28 days. Supportive studies have been conducted with omeprazole 40 mg once daily for 14 days.

For further information on the dosage for omeprazole see the Astra data sheet.

Elderly: As for adults.

Renal impairment: Dosage adjustments are not usually required except in patients with severe renal impairment (creatinine clearance < 30 ml/min). If adjustment is necessary, the total daily dosage should be reduced by half, e.g. 250 mg once daily or 250 mg twice daily in more severe infections.

Clarithromycin may be given without regard to meals as food does not affect the extent of bioavailability.

4.3 Contraindications

Clarithromycin is contra-indicated in patients with known hypersensitivity to macrolide antibiotic drugs.

Clarithromycin and ergot derivatives should not be co-administered (see section 4.5).

Concomitant administration of clarithromycin and any of the following drugs is contraindicated: cisapride, pimozide and terfenadine. Elevated cisapride, pimozide and terfenadine levels have been reported in patients receiving either of these drugs and clarithromycin concomitantly. This may result in QT prolongation and cardiac arrhythmias including ventricular tachycardia, ventricular fibrillation and Torsade de Pointes. Similar effects have been observed with concomitant administration of astemizole and other macrolides.

4.4 Special warnings and precautions for use

Clarithromycin is principally excreted by the liver and kidney. Caution should be exercised in administering this antibiotic to patients with impaired hepatic or renal function.

Prolonged or repeated use of clarithromycin may result in an overgrowth of non-susceptible bacteria or fungi. If super-infection occurs, clarithromycin should be discontinued and appropriate therapy instituted.

H. pylori organisms may develop resistance to clarithromycin in a small number of patients.

There have been post-marketing reports of colchicine toxicity with concomitant use of clarithromycin and colchicine, especially in the elderly, some of which occurred in patients with renal insufficiency. Deaths have been reported in some such patients (see section 4.5).

4.5 Interaction with other medicinal products and other forms of interaction
Clarithromycin has been shown not to interact with oral contraceptives.

As with other macrolide antibiotics the use of clarithromycin in patients concurrently taking drugs metabolised by the cytochrome P450 system (eg. cilostazol, methylprednisolone, oral anticoagulants (eg warfarin), quinidine, sildenafil, ergot alkaloids, alprazolam, triazolam, midazolam, disopyramide, lovastatin, rifabutin, phenytoin, cyclosporin vinblastine, valporate and tacrolimus) may be associated with elevations in serum levels of these other drugs. Rhabdomyolysis, co-incident with the co- administration of clarithromycin, and HMG-CoA reductase inhibitors, such as lovastatin and simvastatin has been reported.

The administration of clarithromycin to patients who are receiving theophylline has been associated with an increase in serum theophylline levels and potential theophylline toxicity.

The use of clarithromycin in patients receiving warfarin may result in potentiation of the effects of warfarin. Prothrombin time should be frequently monitored in these patients. The effects of digoxin may be potentiated with concomitant administration of Klaricid **or Clarithromycin 250 mg Tablets**. Monitoring of serum digoxin levels should be considered.

Clarithromycin may potentiate the effects of carbamazepine due to a reduction in the rate of excretion.

Simultaneous oral administration of clarithromycin tablets and zidovudine to HIV infected adult patients may result in decreased steady-state zidovudine levels. This can be largely avoided by staggering the doses of Clarithromycin and zidovudine by 1 -2 hours. No such reaction has been reported in children.

Ritonavir increases the area under the curve (AUC), C_{max} and C_{min} of clarithromycin when administered concurrently. Because of the large therapeutic window for clarithromycin, no dosage reduction should be necessary in patients with normal renal function. However, for patients with renal impairment, the following dosage adjustments should be considered: For patients with CL_{CR} 30 to 60 ml/min the dose of clarithromycin should be reduced by 50%. For patients with CL_{CR} <30ml/min the dose of clarithromycin should be decreased by 75%. Doses of clarithromycin greater than 1g/day should not be coadministered with ritonavir.

Although the plasma concentrations of clarithromycin and omeprazole may be increased when they are administered concurrently, no adjustment to the dosage is necessary. At the dosages recommended, there is no clinically significant interaction between clarithromycin and lansoprazole. Increased plasma concentrations of clarithromycin may also occur when it is co-administered with Maalox or ranitidine. No adjustment to the dosage is necessary.

There have been post-marketed reports of Torsade de Points occurring with the concurrent use of clarithromycin and quinidine or disopyramide. Levels of these medications should be monitored during clarithromycin therapy.

Colchicine is a substrate for both CYP3A and the efflux transporter, P-glycoprotein (Pgp). Clarithromycin and other macrolides are known to inhibit CYP3A and Pgp. When clarithromycin and colchicine are administered together, inhibition of Pgp and/or CYP3A by clarithromycin may lead to increased exposure to colchicines. Patients should be monitored for clinical symptoms of colchicine toxicity (see Section 4.4).

Postmarketing reports indicate that co-administration of clarithromycin with ergotamine or dihydroergotamine has been associated with acute ergot toxicity characterized by vasospasm, and ischaemia of the extremities and other tissues including the central nervous system (see Section 4.3 Contra-indications).

4.6 Pregnancy and lactation
The safety of clarithromycin during pregnancy and breast feeding of infants has not been established. Clarithromycin should thus not be used during pregnancy or lactation unless the benefit is considered to outweigh the risk. Some animal studies have suggested an embryotoxic effect, but only at dose levels which are clearly toxic to mothers. Clarithromycin has been found in the milk of lactating animals and in human breast milk.

4.7 Effects on ability to drive and use machines
None known.

4.8 Undesirable effects
Clarithromycin is generally well tolerated. Side effects include nausea, dyspepsia, diarrhoea, vomiting, abdominal pain and paraesthesia. Stomatitis, glossitis, oral monilia and tongue discolouration have been reported. Other side-effects include headache, arthralgia, myalgia and allergic reactions ranging from urticaria, mild skin eruptions and angioedema to anaphylaxis have been reported. There have been reports of Stevens-Johnson syndrome / toxic epidermal necrolysis with orally administered clarithromycin.

Reports of alteration of the sense of smell, usually in conjunction with taste perversion have also been received.

There have been reports of tooth discolouration in patients treated with clarithromycin. Tooth discolouration is usually reversible with professional dental cleaning.

There have been reports of transient central nervous system side-effects including dizziness, vertigo, anxiety, insomnia, bad dreams, tinnitus, confusion, disorientation, hallucinations, psychosis and depersonalisation. There have been reports of hearing loss with clarithromycin which is usually reversible on withdrawal of therapy. Pseudomembranous colitis has been reported rarely with clarithromycin, and may range in severity from mild to life threatening. There have been rare reports of hypoglycaemia, some of which have occurred in patients on concomitant oral hypoglycaemic agents or insulin. There have been very rare reports of uveitis mainly in patients treated with concomitant rifabutin, most of these were reversible. Isolated cases of leukopenia and thrombocytopenia have been reported.

As with other macrolides, hepatic dysfunction (which is usually reversible) including altered liver function tests, hepatitis and cholestasis with or without jaundice, has been reported. Dysfunction may be severe and very rarely fatal hepatic failure has been reported.

Cases of increased serum creatinine, interstitial nephritis, renal failure, pancreatitis and convulsions have been reported rarely.

As with other macrolides, QT prolongation, ventricular tachycardia and Torsade de Pointes have been rarely reported with clarithromycin.

There have been post-marketing reports of colchicine toxicity with concomitant use of clarithromycin and colchicine, especially in the elderly, some of which occurred in patients with renal insufficiency. Deaths have been reported in some such patients (see Sections 4.4 and 4.5).

4.9 Overdose
Reports indicate that the ingestion of large amounts of clarithromycin can be expected to produce gastro-intestinal symptoms. One patient who had a history of bipolar disorder ingested 8 grams of clarithromycin and showed altered mental status, paranoid behaviour, hypokalemia and hypoxemia. Adverse reactions accompanying overdosage should be treated by gastric lavage and supportive measures. As with other macrolides, clarithromycin serum levels are not expected to be appreciably affected by haemodialysis or peritoneal dialysis.

5. PHARMACOLOGICAL PROPERTIES

5.1 Pharmacodynamic properties
Clarithromycin is a semi-synthetic derivative of erythromycin A. It exerts its antibacterial action by binding to the 50s ribosomal sub-unit of susceptible bacteria and suppresses protein synthesis. It is highly potent against a wide variety of aerobic and anaerobic gram-positive and gram-negative organisms. The minimum inhibitory concentrations (MICs) of clarithromycin are generally two-fold lower than the MICs of erythromycin.

The 14-hydroxy metabolite of clarithromycin also has antimicrobial activity. The MICs of this metabolite are equal or two-fold higher than the MICs of the parent compound, except for *H. influenzae* where the 14-hydroxy metabolite is two-fold more active than the parent compound.

Clarithromycin is usually active against the following organisms in vitro:-

Gram-positive Bacteria: *Staphylococcus aureus* (methicillin susceptible); *Streptococcus pyogenes* (Group A beta-hemolytic streptococci); alpha-hemolytic streptococci (viridans group); *Streptococcus (Diplococcus) pneumoniae; Streptococcus agalactiae; Listeria monocytogenes.*

Gram-negative Bacteria: *Haemophilus influenzae; Haemophilus parainfluenzae; Moraxella (Branhamella) catarrhalis; Neisseria gonorrhoeae; Legionella pneumophila; Bordetella pertussis; Helicobacter pylori; Campylobacter jejuni.*

Mycoplasma: *Mycoplasma pneumoniae; Ureaplasma urealyticum.*

Other Organisms: *Chlamydia trachomatis; Mycobacterium avium; Mycobacterium leprae.*

Anaerobes: Macrolide-susceptible *Bacteroides fragilis; Clostridium perfringens*; Peptococcus species; Peptostreptococcus species; *Propionibacterium acnes*.

Clarithromycin has bactericidal activity against several bacterial strains. The organisms include *Haemophilus influenzae, Streptococcus pneumoniae, Streptococcus pyogenes, Streptococcus agalactiae, Moraxella (Branhamella) catarrhalis, Neisseria gonorrhoeae, H. pylori* and Campylobacter spp.

5.2 Pharmacokinetic properties
H. pylori is associated with acid peptic disease including duodenal ulcer and gastric ulcer in which about 95% and 80% of patients respectively are infected with the agent. *H. pylori* is also implicated as a major contribution factor in the development of gastric and ulcer recurrence in such patients.

Clarithromycin has been used in small numbers of patients in other treatment regimens. Possible kinetic interactions have not been fully investigated. These regimens include:

Clarithromycin plus tinidazole and omeprazole; clarithromycin plus tetracycline, bismuth subsalicylate and ranitidine; clarithromycin plus ranitidine alone.

Clinical studies using various different *H. pylori* eradication regimens have shown that eradication of *H. pylori* prevents ulcer recurrence.

Clarithromycin is rapidly and well absorbed from the gastro-intestinal tract after oral administration of Clarithromycin tablets. The microbiologically active metabolite 14-hydroxyclarithromycin is formed by first pass metabolism. Clarithromycin may be given without regard to meals as food does not affect the extent of bioavailability of Clarithromycin tablets. Food does slightly delay the onset of absorption of clarithromycin and formation of the 14-hydroxymetabolite. The pharmacokinetics of clarithromycin are non linear; however, steady-state is attained within 2 days of dosing. At 250 mg b.i.d. 15-20% of unchanged drug is excreted in the urine. With 500 mg b.i.d. daily dosing urinary excretion is greater (approximately 36%). The 14-hydroxyclarithromycin is the major urinary metabolite and accounts for 10-15% of the dose. Most of the remainder of the dose is eliminated in the faeces, primarily via the bile. 5-10% of the parent drug is recovered from the faeces.

When clarithromycin 500 mg is given three times daily, the clarithromycin plasma concentrations are increased with respect to the 500 mg twice daily dosage.

Clarithromycin provides tissue concentrations that are several times higher than the circulating drug levels. Increased levels have been found in both tonsillar and lung tissue. Clarithromycin is 80% bound to plasma proteins at therapeutic levels.

Clarithromycin also penetrates the gastric mucus. Levels of clarithromycin in gastric mucus and gastric tissue are higher when clarithromycin is co-administered with omeprazole than when clarithromycin is administered alone.

5.3 Preclinical safety data
In acute mouse and rat studies, the median lethal dose was greater than the highest feasible dose for administration (5g/kg).

In repeated dose studies, toxicity was related to dose, duration of treatment and species. Dogs were more sensitive than primates or rats. The major clinical signs at toxic doses included emesis, weakness, reduced food consumption and weight gain, salivation, dehydration and hyperactivity. In all species the liver was the primary target organ at toxic doses. Hepatotoxicity was detectable by early elevations of liver function tests. Discontinuation of the drug generally resulted in a return to or toward normal results. Other tissues less commonly affected included the stomach, thymus and other lymphoid tissues and the kidneys. At near therapeutic doses, conjunctival injection and lacrimation occurred only in dogs. At a massive dose of 400mg/kg/day, some dogs and monkeys developed corneal opacities and/or oedema.

Fertility and reproduction studies in rats have shown no adverse effects. Teratogenicity studies in rats (Wistar (p.o.) and Spraque-Dawley (p.o. and i.v.)), New Zealand White rabbits and cynomolgous monkeys failed to demonstrate any teratogenicity from clarithromycin. However, a further similar study in Sprague-Dawley rats indicated a low (6%) incidence of cardiovascular abnormalities which appeared to be due to spontaneous expression of genetic changes. Two mouse studies revealed a variable incidence (3-30%) of cleft palate and embryonic loss was seen in monkeys but only at dose levels which were clearly toxic to the mothers.

6. PHARMACEUTICAL PARTICULARS

6.1 List of excipients
Croscarmellose sodium, starch pregelatinised, cellulose microcrystalline, silica gel, povidone, stearic acid, magnesium stearate, talc, hypromellose, hydroxypropylcellulose, propylene glycol, sorbitan monooleate, titanium dioxide, sorbic acid, vanillin, quinoline yellow E104.

6.2 Incompatibilities
None known.

6.3 Shelf life
The recommended shelf life is 24 months.

6.4 Special precautions for storage
Protect from light. Store in a dry place.

6.5 Nature and contents of container
2/14/56 tablets in a blister original pack. The blisters are packaged in a carton with a pack insert.

6.6 Special precautions for disposal and other handling
Not applicable

7. MARKETING AUTHORISATION HOLDER
Abbott Laboratories Limited

Queenborough

Kent

ME11 5EL, UK

8. MARKETING AUTHORISATION NUMBER(S)
PL 0037/0211

9. DATE OF FIRST AUTHORISATION/RENEWAL OF THE AUTHORISATION
09/04/91

10. DATE OF REVISION OF THE TEXT
September 2006

Klaricid 500

(Abbott Laboratories Limited)

1. NAME OF THE MEDICINAL PRODUCT
Klaricid 500 or **Clarithromycin 500 mg Tablets**

2. QUALITATIVE AND QUANTITATIVE COMPOSITION
500mg/tablet
Active: Clarithromycin

3. PHARMACEUTICAL FORM
A yellow, ovaloid film-coated tablet containing 500 mg of clarithromycin.

4. CLINICAL PARTICULARS

4.1 Therapeutic indications
Clarithromycin is indicated for treatment of infections caused by susceptible organisms. Indications include:

Lower respiratory tract infections for example, acute and chronic bronchitis, and pneumonia.

Upper respiratory tract infections for example, sinusitis and pharyngitis.

Clarithromycin is appropriate for initial therapy in community acquired respiratory infections and has been shown to be active in vitro against common and atypical respiratory pathogens as listed in the microbiology section.

Clarithromycin is also indicated in skin and soft tissue infections of mild to moderate severity.

Clarithromycin in the presence of acid suppression effected by omeprazole or lansoprazole is also indicated for the eradication of *H. pylori* in patients with duodenal ulcers. See Dosage and Administration section.

Clarithromycin is usually active against the following organisms *in vitro*:

Gram-positive Bacteria: *Staphylococcus aureus* (methicillin susceptible); *Streptococcus pyogenes* (Group A beta-hemolytic streptococci), alpha-hemolytic streptococci (viridans group); *Streptococcus (Diplococcus) pneumoniae; Streptococcus agalactiae; Listeria monocytogenes.*

Gram-negative Bacteria: *Haemophilus influenzae, Haemophilus parainfluenzae, Moraxella (Branhamella) catarrhalis, Neisseria gonorrhoeae; Legionella pneumophila, Bordetella pertussis, Helicobacter pylori; Campylobacter jejuni.*

Mycoplasma: *Mycoplasma pneumoniae; Ureaplasma urealyticum.*

Other Organisms: *Chlamydia trachomatis; Mycobacterium avium; Mycobacterium leprae; Mycobacterum kansasii; Mycobacterium chelonae; Mycobacterium fortuitum; Mycobacterium intracellulare.*

Anaerobes: Macrolide-susceptible *Bacteroides fragilis; Clostridium perfringens*; Peptococcus species; Peptostreptococcus species; *Propionibacterium acnes*.

Clarithromycin has bactericidal activity against several bacterial strains. The organisms include *Haemophilus influenzae, Streptococcus pneumoniae, Streptococcus pyogenes, Streptococcus agalactiae, Moraxella (Branhamella) catarrhalis, Neisseria gonorrhoeae, H. pylori* and Campylobacter spp.

The activity of clarithromycin against *H. pylori* is greater at neutral pH than at acid pH.

4.2 Posology and method of administration
Patients with respiratory tract/skin and soft tissue infections.

Adults: The usual dose is 250 mg twice daily for 7 days although this may be increased to 500mg twice daily for up to 14 days in severe infections.

Children older than 12 years: As for adults.

Children younger than 12 years: Use Clarithromycin Paediatric Suspension.

Eradication of *H. pylori* in patients with duodenal ulcers (Adults)

Triple Therapy (7 - 14 days)

Clarithromycin (500mg) twice daily and lansoprazole 30mg twice daily should be given with amoxycillin 1000mg twice daily for 7 - 14 days.

Triple Therapy (7 days)

Clarithromycin (500mg) twice daily and lansoprazole 30mg twice daily should be given with metronidazole 400mg twice daily for 7 days.

Triple Therapy (7 days)

Clarithromycin (500mg) twice daily and omeprazole 40mg daily should be given with amoxycillin 1000mg twice daily or metronidazole 400mg twice daily for 7 days.

Triple Therapy (10 days)

Clarithromycin (500mg) twice daily should be given with amoxycillin 1000mg twice daily and omeprazole 20mg daily for 10 days.

Dual Therapy (14 days)

The usual dose of Clarithromycin is 500 mg three times daily for 14 days. Clarithromycin should be administered with oral omeprazole 40 mg once daily. The pivotal study was conducted with omeprazole 40 mg once daily for 28 days. Supportive studies have been conducted with omeprazole 40 mg once daily for 14 days.

For further information on the dosage for omeprazole see the Astra data sheet.

Elderly: As for adults.

Renal impairment: Dosage adjustments are not usually required except in patients with severe renal impairment (creatinine clearance < 30 ml/min). If adjustment is necessary, the total daily dosage should be reduced by half, e.g. 250 mg once daily or 250 mg twice daily in more severe infections.

Clarithromycin may be given without regard to meals as food does not affect the extent of bioavailability.

4.3 Contraindications
Clarithromycin is contra-indicated in patients with known hypersensitivity to macrolide antibiotic drugs.

Clarithromycin and ergot derivatives should not be co-administered (see Section4.5).

Concomitant administration of clarithromycin and any of the following drugs is contraindicated: cisapride, pimozide and terfenadine. Elevated cisapride, pimozide and terfenadine levels have been reported in patients receiving either of these drugs and clarithromycin concomitantly. This may result in QT prolongation and cardiac arrhythmias including ventricular tachycardia, ventricular fibrillation and Torsade de Pointes. Similar effects have been observed with concomitant administration of astemizole and other macrolides.

4.4 Special warnings and precautions for use
Clarithromycin is principally excreted by the liver and kidney. Caution should be exercised in administering this antibiotic to patients with impaired hepatic or renal function.

Prolonged or repeated used of clarithromycin may result in an overgrowth of non-susceptible bacteria or fungi. If super-infection occurs, clarithromycin should be discontinued and appropriate therapy instituted.

H. pylori organisms may develop resistance to clarithromycin in a small number of patients.

There have been post-marketing reports of colchicine toxicity with concomitant use of clarithromycin and colchicine, especially in the elderly, some of which occurred in patients with renal insufficiency. Deaths have been reported in some such patients (see section 4.5).

4.5 Interaction with other medicinal products and other forms of interaction
Clarithromycin has been shown not to interact with oral contraceptives.

As with other macrolide antibiotics the use of clarithromycin in patients concurrently taking drugs metabolised by the cytochrome P450 system (eg. Cilostazol, methylprednisolone, oral anticoagulants (eg warfarin), quinidine, sildenafil, ergot alkaloids, alprazolam, triazolam, midazolam, disopyramide, lovastatin, rifabutin, phenytoin, cyclosporine vinblastine, valproate and tacrolimus.) may be associated with elevations in serum levels of these other drugs. Rhabdomyolysis, co-incident with the co- administration of clarithromycin, and HMG-CoA reductase inhibitors, such as lovastatin and simvastatin has been reported.

The administration of clarithromycin to patients who are receiving theophylline has been associated with an increase in serum theophylline levels and potential theophylline toxicity.

The use of clarithromycin in patients receiving warfarin may result in potentiation of the effects of warfarin. Prothrombin time should be frequently monitored in these patients. The effects of digoxin may be potentiated with concomitant administration of Clarithromycin. Monitoring of serum digoxin levels should be considered.

Clarithromycin may potentiate the effects of carbamazepine due to a reduction in the rate of excretion.

Simultaneous oral administration of clarithromycin tablets and zidovudine to HIV infected adult patients may result in decreased steady-state zidovudine levels. This can be largely avoided by staggering the doses of Clarithromycin and zidovudine by 1 -2 hours. No such reaction has been reported in children.

Ritonavir increases the area under the curve (AUC), C_{max} and C_{min} of clarithromycin when administered concurrently. Because of the large therapeutic window for clarithromycin, no dosage reduction should be necessary in patients with normal renal function. However, for patients with renal impairment, the following dosage adjustments should be considered: For patients with CL_{CR} 30 to 60 ml/min the dose of clarithromycin should be reduced by 50%. For patients with CL_{CR} <30ml/min the dose of clarithromycin should be decreased by 75%. Doses of clarithromycin greater than 1g/day should not be coadministered with ritonavir.

Although the plasma concentrations of clarithromycin and omeprazole may be increased when they are administered concurrently, no adjustment to the dosage is necessary. At the dosages recommended, there is no clinically significant interaction between clarithromycin and lansoprazole.Increased plasma concentrations of clarithromycin may also occur when it is co-administered with Maalox or ranitidine. No adjustment to the dosage is necessary.

There have been postmarketed reports of Torsade de Pointes occurring with the concurrent use of clarithromycin and quinidine or disopyramide. Levels of these medications should be monitored during clarithromycin therapy.

Colchicine is a substrate for both CYP3A and the efflux transporter, P-glycoprotein (Pgp). Clarithromycin and other macrolides are known to inhibit CYP3A and Pgp. When clarithromycin and colchicine are administered together, inhibition of Pgp and/or CYP3A by clarithromycin may lead to increased exposure to colchicine. Patients should be monitored for clinical symptoms of colchicine toxicity (see Section 4.4).

Post-marketing reports indicate that co-administration of clarithromycin with ergotamine or dihydroergotaine has been associated with acute ergot toxicity characterized by vasospasm and ischaemia of the extremities and other tissues including the central nervous system (see Section 4.3 Contra-indications).

4.6 Pregnancy and lactation
The safety of clarithromycin during pregnancy and breast feeding of infants has not been established. Clarithromycin should thus not be used during pregnancy or lactation unless the benefit is considered to outweigh the risk. Some animal studies have suggested an embryotoxic effect, but only at dose levels which are clearly toxic to mothers. Clarithromycin has been found in the milk of lactating animals and in human breast milk.

4.7 Effects on ability to drive and use machines
None known.

4.8 Undesirable effects
Clarithromycin is generally well tolerated. Side effects include nausea, dyspepsia, diarrhoea, vomiting, abdominal pain and paraesthesia. Stomatitis, glossitis, oral monilia and tongue discolouration have been reported. Other side-effects include headache, arthralgia, myalgia and allergic reactions ranging from urticaria, mild skin eruptions and angioedema to anaphylaxis have been reported. There have been reports of Stevens-Johnson syndrome / toxic epidermal necrolysis with orally administered clarithromycin.

Reports of alteration of the sense of smell, usually in conjunction with taste perversion have also been received. There have been reports of tooth discolouration in patients treated with clarithromycin. Tooth discolouration is usually reversible with professional dental cleaning.

There have been reports of transient central nervous system side-effects including dizziness, vertigo, anxiety, insomnia, bad dreams, tinnitus, confusion, disorientation, hallucinations, psychosis and depersonalisation. There have been reports of hearing loss with clarithromycin which is usually reversible on withdrawal of therapy. Pseudomembranous colitis has been reported rarely with clarithromycin, and may range in severity from mild to life threatening. There have been rare reports of hypoglycaemia, some of which have occurred in patients on concomitant oral hypoglycaemic agents or insulin. There have been very rare reports of uveitis mainly in patients treated with concomitant rifabutin, most of these were reversible. Isolated cases of leukopenia andthrombocytopenia have been reported.

As with other macrolides, hepatic dysfunction (which is usually reversible) including altered liver function tests, hepatitis and cholestasis with or without jaundice, has been reported. Dysfunction may be severe and very rarely fatal hepatic failure has been reported.

Cases of increased serum creatinine, interstitial nephritis, renal failure, pancreatitis and convulsions have been reported rarely.

As with other macrolides, QT prolongation, ventricular tachycardia and Torsade de Pointes have been rarely reported with clarithromycin.

There have been post-marketing reports of colchicine toxicity with concomitant use of clarithromycin and colchicine especially in the elderly, some of which occurred in patients with renal insufficiency. Deaths have been reported in some such patients (see Setions 4.4 and 4.5).

4.9 Overdose
Reports indicate that the ingestion of large amounts of clarithromycin can be expected to produce gastro-intestinal symptoms. One patient who had a history of bipolar disorder ingested 8 grams of clarithromycin and showed altered mental status, paranoid behaviour, hypokalemia and hypoxemia. Adverse reactions accompanying overdosage should be treated by gastric lavage and supportive measures. As with other macrolides, clarithromycin serum levels are not expected to be appreciably affected by haemodialysis or peritoneal dialysis.

5. PHARMACOLOGICAL PROPERTIES

5.1 Pharmacodynamic properties
Clarithromycin is a semi-synthetic derivative of erythromycin A. It exerts its antibacterial action by binding to the 50s ribosomal sub-unit of susceptible bacteria and suppresses protein synthesis. It is highly potent against a wide variety of aerobic and anaerobic gram-positive and gram-negative organisms. The minimum inhibitory concentrations (MICs) of clarithromycin are generally two-fold lower than the MICs of erythromycin.

The 14-hydroxy metabolite of clarithromycin also has antimicrobial activity. The MICs of this metabolite are equal or two-fold higher than the MICs of the parent compound, except for *H. influenzae* where the 14-hydroxy metabolite is two-fold more active than the parent compound.

Clarithromycin is usually active against the following organisms in vitro:-

Gram-positive Bacteria: *Staphylococcus aureus* (methicillin susceptible); *Streptococcus pyogenes* (Group A beta-hemolytic streptococci) alpha-hemolytic streptococci (viridans group); *Streptococcus (Diplococcus) pneumoniae; Streptococcus agalactiae; Listeria monocytogenes.*

Gram-negative Bacteria: *Haemophilus influenzae, Haemophilus parainfluenzae, Moraxella (Branhamella) catarrhalis, Neisseria gonorrhoeae; Legionella pneumophila, Bordetella pertussis, Helicobacter pylori; Campylobacter jejuni.*

Mycoplasma: *Mycoplasma pneumoniae; Ureaplasma urealyticum.*

Other Organisms: *Chlamydia trachomatis; Mycobacterium avium; Mycobacterium leprae; Mycobacterium kansasii; Mycobacterium chelonae; Mycobacterium fortuitum; Mycobacterium intracellulare.*

Anaerobes: Macrolide-susceptible *Bacteroides fragilis; Clostridium perfringens*; Peptococcus species; Peptostreptococcus species; *Propionibacterium acnes.*

Clarithromycin has bactericidal activity against several bacterial strains. The organisms include *Haemophilus influenzae, Streptococcus pneumoniae, Streptococcus pyogenes, Streptococcus agalactiae, Moraxella (Branhamella) catarrhalis, Neisseria gonorrhoeae, H. pylori* and Campylobacter spp.

5.2 Pharmacokinetic properties

H. pylori is associated with acid peptic disease including duodenal ulcer and gastric ulcer in which about 95% and 80% of patients respectively are infected with the agent. *H. pylori* is also implicated as a major contribution factor in the development of gastritis and ulcer recurrence in such patients.

Clarithromycin has been used in small numbers of patients in other treatment regimens. Possible kinetic interactions have not been fully investigated. These regimens include:

Clarithromycin plus tinidazole and omeprazole; clarithromycin plus tetracycline, bismuth subsalicylate and ranitidine; clarithromycin plus ranitidine alone.

Clinical studies using various different *H. pylori* eradication regimens have shown that eradication of *H. pylori* prevents ulcer recurrence.

Clarithromycin is rapidly and well absorbed from the gastro-intestinal tract after oral administration of Clarithromycin tablets. The microbiologically active metabolite 14-hydroxyclarithromycin is formed by first pass metabolism. Clarithromycin may be given without regard to meals as food does not affect the extent of bioavailability of Clarithromycin tablets. Food does slightly delay the onset of absorption of clarithromycin and formation of the 14-hydroxymetabolite. The pharmacokinetics of clarithromycin are non linear; however, steady-state is attained within 2 days of dosing. At 250 mg b.i.d. 15-20% of unchanged drug is excreted in the urine. With 500 mg b.i.d. daily dosing urinary excretion is greater (approximately 36%). The 14-hydroxyclarithromycin is the major urinary metabolite and accounts for 10-15% of the dose. Most of the remainder of the dose is eliminated in the faeces, primarily via the bile. 5-10% of the parent drug is recovered from the faeces.

When clarithromycin 500 mg is given three times daily, the clarithromycin plasma concentrations are increased with respect to the 500 mg twice daily dosage.

Clarithromycin provides tissue concentrations that are several times higher than the circulating drug levels. Increased levels have been found in both tonsillar and lung tissue. Clarithromycin is 80% bound to plasma proteins at therapeutic levels.

Clarithromycin also penetrates the gastric mucus. Levels of clarithromycin in gastric mucus and gastric tissue are higher when clarithromycin is co-administered with omeprazole than when clarithromycin is administered alone.

5.3 Preclinical safety data

In acute mouse and rat studies, the median lethal dose was greater than the highest feasible dose for administration (5g/kg).

In repeated dose studies, toxicity was related to dose, duration of treatment and species. Dogs were more sensitive than primates or rats. The major clinical signs at toxic doses included emesis, weakness, reduced food consumption and weight gain, salivation, dehydration and hyperactivity. In all species the liver was the primary target organ at toxic doses. Hepatotoxicity was detectable by early elevations of liver function tests. Discontinuation of the drug generally resulted in a return to or toward normal results. Other tissues less commonly affected included the stomach, thymus and other lymphoid tissues and the kidneys. At near therapeutic doses, conjunctival injection and lacrimation occurred only in dogs. At a massive dose of 400mg/kg/day, some dogs and monkeys developed corneal opacities and/or oedema.

Fertility and reproduction studies in rats have shown no adverse effects. Teratogenicity studies in rats (Wistar (p.o.) and Sprague-Dawley (p.o. and i.v.)), New Zealand White rabbits and cynomolgous monkeys failed to demonstrate any teratogenicity from clarithromycin. However, a further similar study in Sprague-Dawley rats indicated a low (6%) incidence of cardiovascular abnormalities which appeared to be due to spontaneous expression of genetic changes. Two mouse studies revealed a variable incidence (3-30%) of cleft palate and embryonic loss was seen in monkeys but only at dose levels which were clearly toxic to the mothers.

6. PHARMACEUTICAL PARTICULARS

6.1 List of excipients

Croscarmellose sodium, cellulose microcrystalline, silicon dioxide,

povidone, stearic acid, magnesium stearate, talc, hypromellose, hydroxypropylcellulose, propylene glycol, sorbitan monooleate, titanium dioxide, sorbic acid, vanillin, quinoline yellow E104.

6.2 Incompatibilities

None known.

6.3 Shelf life

36 months.

6.4 Special precautions for storage

Store in a dry place, protected from light.

6.5 Nature and contents of container

Tablets in a 300μ PVC/60gsm PVdC/20μ Al foil blister pack. Pack sizes are 14,20,28,42,84,168 tablets in a carton with a patient leaflet.

Tablets in HDPE bottle with a patient leaflet. Pack sizes are 100,250,500,1000 tablets.

6.6 Special precautions for disposal and other handling

Not applicable

7. MARKETING AUTHORISATION HOLDER

Abbott Laboratories Limited

Queenborough

Kent

ME11 5EL,

England

United Kingdom

8. MARKETING AUTHORISATION NUMBER(S)

PL 0037/0254

9. DATE OF FIRST AUTHORISATION/RENEWAL OF THE AUTHORISATION

24/03/94

10. DATE OF REVISION OF THE TEXT

September 2006

Klaricid Adult Sachet 250mg or Clarithromycin 250mg Granules for Oral Suspension

(Abbott Laboratories Limited)

1. NAME OF THE MEDICINAL PRODUCT

Klaricid Adult Sachet 250mg or Clarithromycin 250mg Granules for Oral Suspension

2. QUALITATIVE AND QUANTITATIVE COMPOSITION

Activemg/sachet

Clarithromycin 250.00

3. PHARMACEUTICAL FORM

Granules for oral suspension.

4. CLINICAL PARTICULARS

4.1 Therapeutic indications

Clarithromycin is indicated in the treatment of infections caused by one or more susceptible organisms. Indications include:

Lower respiratory tract infections for example, acute and chronic bronchitis, and pneumonia.

Upper respiratory tract infections for example, sinusitus and pharyngitis.

Clarithromycin is appropriate for initial therapy in community acquired respiratory infections and has been shown to be active *in vitro* against common and atypical respiratory pathogens as listed in the microbiology section.

Clarithromycin is also indicated in skin and soft tissue infections of mild to moderate severity.

Clarithromycin in the presence of acid suppression effected by lansoprazole or omeprazole is also indicated for the eradication of *H. pylori* in patients with duodenal ulcers. See Dosage and Administration section.

Clarithromycin is usually active against the following organisms *in vitro:*

Gram-positive Bacteria:*Staphylococcus aureus* (methicillin susceptible); *Streptococcus pyogenes* (Group A beta-hemolytic streptococci); alpha-hemolytic streptococci (viridans group); *Streptococcus (Diplococcus) pneumoniae; Streptococcus agalactiae; Listeria monocytogenes.*

Gram-negative Bacteria: *Haemophilus influenzae; Haemophilus parainfluenzae; Moraxella (Branhamella) catarrhalis; Neisseria gonorrhoeae; Legionella pneumophila; Bordetella pertussis; Helicobacter pylori; Campylobacter jejuni.*

Mycoplasma:*Mycoplasma pneumoniae; Ureaplasma urealyticum.*

Other Organisms:*Chlamydia trachomatis; Mycobacterium avium; Mycobacterium leprae.*

Anaerobes: Macrolide-susceptible *Bacteroides fragilis; Clostridium perfringens;* Peptococcus species; Peptostreptococcus species; *Propionibacterium acnes.*

Clarithromycin has bactericidal activity against several bacterial strains. These organisms include *Haemophilus influenzae; Streptococcus pneumoniae; Streptococcus pyogenes; Streptococcus agalactiae; Moraxella (Branhamella) catarrhalis; Neisseria gonorrhoeae; Helicobacter pylori* and Campylobacter spp.

The activity of clarithromycin against *H. pylori* is greater at neutral pH than at acid pH.

4.2 Posology and method of administration

Patients with respiratory tract/skin and soft tissue infections.

Adults: The usual dose is 250 mg twice daily for 7 days although this may be increased to 500mg twice daily for up to 14 days in severe infections.

Children older than 12 years: As for adults.

Children younger than 12 years: Use Clarithromycin Paediatric Suspension.

Eradication of *H. pylori* in patients with duodenal ulcers (Adults)

Triple Therapy (7 - 14 days)

Clarithromycin 500mg twice daily and lansoprazole 30mg twice daily should be given with amoxycillin 1000mg twice daily for 7 - 14 days.

Triple Therapy (7 days)

Clarithromycin (500mg) twice daily and lansoprazole 30mg twice daily should be given with metronidazole 400mg twice daily for 7 days.

Triple Therapy (7 days)

Clarithromycin (500mg) twice daily and omeprazole 40mg daily should be given with amoxycillin 1000mg twice daily or metronidazole 400mg twice daily for 7 days.

Triple Therapy (10 days)

Clarithromycin (500mg) twice daily should be given with amoxycillin 1000mg twice daily and omeprazole 20mg daily for 10 days.

Dual Therapy (14 days)

The usual dose of Clarithromycin is 500 mg three times daily for 14 days. Clarithromycin should be administered with oral omeprazole 40 mg once daily. The pivotal study was conducted with omeprazole 40 mg once daily for 28 days. Supportive studies have been conducted with omeprazole 40 mg once daily for 14 days.

For further information on the dosage for omeprazole see the Astra data sheet.

Elderly: As for adults.

Renal impairment: Dosage adjustments are not usually required except in patients with severe renal impairment (creatinine clearance < 30 ml/min). If adjustment is necessary, the total daily dosage should be reduced by half, e.g. 250 mg once daily or 250 mg twice daily in more severe infections.

Clarithromycin may be given without regard to meals as food does not affect the extent of bioavailability.

4.3 Contraindications

Clarithromycin is contra-indicated in patients with known hypersensitivity to macrolide antibiotic drugs.

Clarithromycin and ergot derivatives should not be co-administered (see Section 4.5).

Concomitant administration of clarithromycin and any of the following drugs is contraindicated: cisapride, pimozide and terfenadine. Elevated cisapride, pimozide and terfenadine levels have been reported in patients receiving either of these drugs and clarithromycin concomitantly. This may result in QT prolongation and cardiac arrhythmias including ventricular tachycardia, ventricular fibrillation and Torsade de Pointes. Similar effects have been observed with concomitant administration of astemizole and other macrolides.

4.4 Special warnings and precautions for use

Clarithromycin is principally excreted by the liver and kidney. Caution should be exercised in administering this antibiotic to patients with impaired hepatic or renal function.

Prolonged or repeated use of clarithromycin may result in an overgrowth of non-susceptable bacteria or fungi. If super-infection occurs, clarithromycin should be discontinued and appropriate therapy instituted.

H. pylori organisms may develop resistance to clarithromycin in a small number of patients.

There have been post-marketing reports of colchicine toxicity with concomitant use of clarithromycin and colchicine, especially in the elderly, some of which occurred in patients with renal insufficiency. Deaths have been reported ins ome such patients (see Section 4.5).

Patients with rare hereditary problems of fructose intolerance, glucose-galactose malabsorption or sucrase-isomaltase insufficiency should not take this medicine.

4.5 Interaction with other medicinal products and other forms of interaction

Clarithromycin has been shown not to interact with oral contraceptives.

As with other macrolide antibiotics the use of clarithromycin in patients concurrently taking drugs metabolised by the cytochrome P450 system (eg. cilostazol, methylprednisolone, oral anticoagulants (eg warfarin), quinidine, ergot alkaloids, alprazolam, triazolam, midazolam, disopyramide, lovastatin, rifabutin, phenytoin, cyclosporin, vinblastine valproate and tacrolimus) may be associated with elevations in serum levels of these other drugs. Rhabdomyolysis, co-incident with the co- administration of clarithromycin, and HMG-CoA reductase inhibitors, such as lovastatin and simvastatin has been reported.

The administration of clarithromycin to patients who are receiving theophylline has been associated with an increase in serum theophylline levels and potential theophylline toxicity.

The use of clarithromycin in patients receiving warfarin may result in potentiation of the effects of warfarin. Prothrombin time should be frequently monitored in these patients. The effects of digoxin may be potentiated with concomitant administration of Clarithromycin. Monitoring of serum digoxin levels should be considered.

Clarithromycin may potentiate the effects of carbamazepine due to a reduction in the rate of excretion.

Simultaneous oral administration of clarithromycin tablets and zidovudine to HIV infected adult patients may result in decreased steady-state zidovudine levels. This can be largely avoided by staggering the doses of Clarithromycin and zidovudine by 1 -2 hours. No such reaction has been reported in children.

Ritonavir increases the area under the curve (AUC), C_{max} and C_{min} of clarithromycin when administered concurrently. Because of the large therapeutic window for clarithromycin, no dosage reduction should be necessary in patients with normal renal function. However, for patients with renal impairment, the following dosage adjustments should be considered: For patients with CL_{CR} 30 to 60 ml/min the dose of clarithromycin should be reduced by 50%. For patients with CL_{CR} <30ml/min the dose of clarithromycin should be decreased by 75%. Doses of clarithromycin greater than 1g/day should not be coadministered with ritonavir.

Although the plasma concentrations of clarithromycin and omeprazole may be increased when they are administered concurrently, no adjustment to the dosage is necessary. At the dosages recommended, there is no clinically significant interaction between clarithromycin and lansoprazole. Increased plasma concentrations of clarithromycin may also occur when it is co-administered with Maalox or ranitidine. No adjustment to the dosage is necessary.

There have been post-marketed reports of Torsade de Pointes occurring with the concurrent use of clarithromycin and quinidine or disopyramide. Levels of these medications should be monitored during clarithromycin therapy.

Colchicine is a substrate for both CYP3A and the efflux transporter, P-glycoprotein (Pgp). Clarithromycin and other macrolides are known to inhibit CYP3A and Pgp. When clarithromycin and colchicine are administered together, inhibition of Pgp and/or CYP3A by clarithromycin may lead to increased exposure to colchicine. Patients should be monitored for clinical symptoms of colchicine toxicity (see Section 4.4).

Post-marketing reports indicate that co-administration of clarithromycin with ergotamine or dihydroergotamine has been associated with acute ergot toxicity characterized by vasospasm and ischaemia of the extremities and other tissues including the central nervous system (see section 4.3 Contra-indications).

4.6 Pregnancy and lactation

The safety of clarithromycin during pregnancy and breast feeding of infants has not been established. Clarithromycin should thus not be used during pregnancy or lactation unless the benefit is considered to outweigh the risk. Some animal studies have suggested an embryotoxic effect, but only at dose levels which are clearly toxic to mothers. Clarithromycin has been found in the milk of lactating animals and in human breast milk.

4.7 Effects on ability to drive and use machines

None known.

4.8 Undesirable effects

Clarithromycin is generally well tolerated. Side effects include nausea, dyspepsia, diarrhoea, vomiting, abdominal pain and paraesthesia. Stomatitis, glossitis, oral monilia and tongue discolouration have been reported. Other side-effects include headache, arthralgia, myalgia and allergic reactions ranging from urticaria, mild skin eruptions and angioedema to anaphylaxis have been reported. There have been reports of Stevens-Johnson syndrome / toxic epidermal necrolysis with orally administered clarithromycin.

Reports of alteration of the sense of smell, usually in conjunction with taste perversion have also been received. There have been reports of tooth discolouration in patients treated with clarithromycin. Tooth discolouration is usually reversible with professional dental cleaning.

There have been reports of transient central nervous system side-effects including dizziness, vertigo, anxiety, insomnia, bad dreams, tinnitus, confusion, disorientation, hallucinations, psychosis and depersonalisation. There have been reports of hearing loss with clarithromycin which is usually reversible on withdrawal of therapy. Pseudomembranous colitis has been reported rarely with clarithromycin, and may range in severity from mild to life threatening. There have been rare reports of hypoglycaemia, some of which have occurred in patients on concomitant oral hypoglycaemic agents or insulin. There have been very rare reports of uveitis mainly in patients treated with concomitant rifabutin, most of these were reversible. Isolated cases of leukopenia and thrombocytopenia have been reported.

As with other macrolides, hepatic dysfunction (which is usually reversible) including altered liver function tests, hepatitis and cholestasis with or without jaundice, has been reported. Dysfunction may be severe and very rarely fatal hepatic failure has been reported.

Cases of increased serum creatinine, interstitial nephritis and renal failure, pancreatitis and convulsions have been reported rarely.

As with other macrolides, QT prolongation, ventricular tachycardia and Torsade de Pointes have been rarely reported with clarithromycin.

There have been post-marketing reports of colchicine toxicity with concomitant use of clarithromycin and colchicine, especially in the elderly, some of which occurred in patients with renal insufficiency. Deaths have been reported in some such patients (see sections 4.4 and 4.5).

4.9 Overdose

Reports indicate that the ingestion of large amounts of clarithromycin can be expected to produce gastro-intestinal symptoms. One patient who had a history of bipolar disorder ingested 8 grams of clarithromycin and showed altered mental status, paranoid behaviour, hypokalemia and hypoxemia. Adverse reactions accompanying overdosage should be treated by gastric lavage and supportive measures. As with other macrolides, clarithromycin serum levels are not expected to be appreciably affected by haemodialysis or peritoneal dialysis.

5. PHARMACOLOGICAL PROPERTIES

5.1 Pharmacodynamic properties

Clarithromycin is a semi-synthetic derivative of erythromycin A. It exerts its antibacterial action by binding to the 50s ribosomal sub-unit of susceptible bacteria and suppresses protein synthesis. It is highly potent against a wide variety of aerobic and anaerobic gram-positive and gram-negative organisms. The minimum inhibitory concentrations (MICs) of clarithromycin are generally two-fold lower than the MICs of erythromycin.

The 14-hydroxy metabolite of clarithromycin also has antimicrobial activity. The MICs of this metabolite are equal or two-fold higher than the MICs of the parent compound, except for *H. influenzae* where the 14-hydroxy metabolite is two-fold more active than the parent compound.

Clarithromycin is usually active against the following organisms *in vitro*:-

Gram-positive Bacteria:*Staphylococcus aureus* (methicillin susceptible); *Streptococcus pyogenes* (Group A beta-hemolytic streptococci); alpha-hemolytic streptococci (viridans group); *Streptococcus (Diplococcus) pneumoniae; Streptococcus agalactiae; Listeria monocytogenes.*

Gram-negative Bacteria:*Haemophilus influenzae; Haemophilus parainfluenzae; Moraxella (Branhamella) catarrhalis; Neisseria gonorrhoeae; Legionella pneumophila; Bordetella pertussis; Helicobacter pylori; Campylobacter jejuni.*

Mycoplasma: *Mycoplasma pneumoniae; Ureaplasma urealyticum.*

Other Organisms:*Chlamydia trachomatis; Mycobacterium avium; Mycobacterium leprae; Mycobacterum Kansasaii; Mycobacterium chelonae; Mycobacterium fortuitum; Mycobacterium intracellulare.*

Anaerobes: Macrolide-susceptible *Bacteroides fragilis; Clostridium perfringens;* Peptococcus species; Peptostreptococcus species; *Propionibacterium acnes.*

Clarithromycin has bactericidal activity against several bacterial strains. The organisms include *Haemophilus influenzae; Streptococcus pneumoniae; Streptococcus pyogenes; Streptococcus agalactiae; Moraxella (Branhamella) catarrhalis; Neisseria gonorrhoeae; Helicobacter pylori* and Campylobacter spp.

5.2 Pharmacokinetic properties

Helicobacter pylori (H. pylori) is associated with acid peptic disease including duodenal ulcer and gastric ulcer in which about 95% and 80% of patients respectively are infected with the agent. *H. pylori* is also implicated as a major contribution factor in the development of gastritis and ulcer recurrence in such patients.

Clarithromycin has been used in small numbers of patients in other treatment regimens. Possible kinetic interactions have not been fully investigated. These regimens include:

Clarithromycin plus tinidazole and omeprazole; clarithromycin plus tetracycline, bismuth subsalicylate and ranitidine; clarithromycin plus ranitidine alone.

Clinical studies using various different *H. pylori* eradication regimens (including clarithromycin plus omeprazole) have shown that eradication of *H. pylori* prevents ulcer recurrence.

Clarithromycin is rapidly and well absorbed from the gastro-intestinal tract after oral administration of Clarithromycin tablets. The microbiologically active metabolite

14-hydroxyclarithromycin is formed by first pass metabolism. Clarithromycin may be given without regard to meals as food does not affect the extent of bioavailability of Clarithromycin tablets. Food does slightly delay the onset of absorption of clarithromycin and formation of the 14-hydroxymetabolite. The pharmacokinetics of clarithromycin are non linear; however, steady-state is attained within 2 days of dosing. At 250 mg b.i.d. 15-20% of unchanged drug is excreted in the urine. With 500 mg b.i.d. daily dosing urinary excretion is greater (approximately 36%). The 14-hydroxyclarithromycin is the major urinary metabolite and accounts for 10-15% of the dose. Most of the remainder of the dose is eliminated in the faeces, primarily via the bile. 5-10% of the parent drug is recovered from the faeces.

When clarithromycin (500 mg) is given three times daily, the clarithromycin plasma concentrations are increased with respect to the 500 mg twice daily dosage.

Clarithromycin provides tissue concentrations that are several times higher than the circulating drug levels. Increased levels have been found in both tonsillar and lung tissue. Clarithromycin is 80% bound to plasma proteins at therapeutic levels.

Clarithromycin also penetrates the gastric mucus. Levels of clarithromycin in gastric mucus and gastric tissue are higher when clarithromycin is co-administered with omeprazole than when clarithromycin is administered alone.

5.3 Preclinical safety data

In acute mouse and rat studies, the median lethal dose was greater than the highest feasible dose for administration (5g/kg).

In repeated dose studies, toxicity was related to dose, duration of treatment and species. Dogs were more sensitive than primates or rats. The major clinical signs at toxic doses included emesis, weakness, reduced food consumption and weight gain, salivation, dehydration and hyperactivity. In all species the liver was the primary target organ at toxic doses. Hepatotoxicity was detectable by early elevations of liver function tests. Discontinuation of the drug generally resulted in a return to or toward normal results. Other tissues less commonly affected included the stomach, thymus and other lymphoid tissues and the kidneys. At near therapeutic doses, conjunctival injection and lacrimation occurred only in dogs. At a massive dose of 400mg/kg/day, some dogs and monkeys developed corneal opacities and/or oedema.

Fertility and reproduction studies in rats have shown no adverse effects. Teratogenicity studies in rate (Wistar (p.o.) and Spraque-Dawley (p.o. and i.v.)), New Zealand White rabbits and cynomolgous monkeys failed to demonstrate any teratogenicity from clarithromycin. However, a further similar study in Sprague-Dawley rats indicated a low (6%) incidence of cardiovascular abnormalities which appeared to be due to spontaneous expression of genetic changes. Two mouse studies revealed a variable incidence (3-30%) of cleft palate, and embryonic loss was seen in monkeys but only at dose levels which were clearly toxic to the mothers.

6. PHARMACEUTICAL PARTICULARS

6.1 List of excipients

Carbopol 974P, povidone K90, water purified, hydroxypropylmethylcellulose phthalate (HP-55), castor oil, ethanol, acetone, silicon dioxide, maltodextrin, sucrose, titanium dioxide, ultrasperse modified starch, fruit of the forest flavour, myrtille flavour, ammonium glycyrrhizinate, Acesulfame K.

6.2 Incompatibilities

None known.

6.3 Shelf life

The recommended shelf life is 18 months when stored below 30°C.

6.4 Special precautions for storage

Store in a cool dry place.

6.5 Nature and contents of container

Nature of container - laminate comprising a polyethylene film with aluminium/foil.paper layers. 2 or 14 unit packs.

Contents of container - granules for oral suspension.

6.6 Special precautions for disposal and other handling

Not applicable.

7. MARKETING AUTHORISATION HOLDER

Abbott Laboratories Limited
Queenborough
Kent
ME11 5EL

8. MARKETING AUTHORISATION NUMBER(S)

0037/0272

9. DATE OF FIRST AUTHORISATION/RENEWAL OF THE AUTHORISATION

5th May 1997

10. DATE OF REVISION OF THE TEXT
14 September 2006

Klaricid IV

(Abbott Laboratories Limited)

1. NAME OF THE MEDICINAL PRODUCT
Klaricid IV **or Clarithromycin 500 mg/vial Powder for Solution for Injection**

2. QUALITATIVE AND QUANTITATIVE COMPOSITION
Active: Clarithromycin 500mg/vial

3. PHARMACEUTICAL FORM
Lyophilised powder for reconstitution to give a solution for IV administration.

4. CLINICAL PARTICULARS
4.1 Therapeutic indications
Klaricid IV **or Clarithromycin 500 mg/vial Powder for Solution for Injection** is indicated whenever parenteral therapy is required for treatment of infections caused by susceptible organisms in the following conditions;

- Lower respiratory tract infections for example, acute and chronic bronchitis, and pneumonia.

- Upper respiratory tract infections for example, sinusitis and pharyngitis.

- Skin and soft tissue infections.

4.2 Posology and method of administration
For intravenous administration only.

Intravenous therapy may be given for 2 to 5 days and should be changed to oral clarithromycin therapy when appropriate.

Adults: The recommended dosage of Klaricid IV **or Clarithromycin 500 mg/vial Powder for Solution for Injection** is 1.0 gram daily, divided into two 500mg doses, appropriately diluted as described below.

Children: At present, there are insufficient data to recommend a dosage regimen for routine use in children.

Elderly: As for adults.

Renal Impairment: In patients with renal impairment who have creatinine clearance less than 30ml/min, the dosage of clarithromycin should be reduced to one half of the normal recommended dose.

Recommended administration:

Klaricid IV **or Clarithromycin 500 mg/vial Powder for Solution for Injection** should be administered into one of the larger proximal veins as an IV infusion over 60 minutes, using a solution concentration of about 2mg/ml. Clarithromycin should not be given as a bolus or an intramuscular injection.

4.3 Contraindications
Klaricid IV **or Clarithromycin 500 mg/vial Powder for Solution for Injection** is contra-indicated in patients with known hypersensitivity to macrolide antibiotic drugs.

Clarithromycin and ergot derivatives should not be co-administered (see section 4.5).

Concomitant administration of clarithromycin and any of the following drugs is contraindicated: cisapride, pimozide and terfenadine. Elevated cisapride, pimozide and terfenadine levels have been reported in patients receiving either of these drugs and clarithromycin concomitantly. This may result in QT prolongation and cardiac arrhythmias including ventricular tachycardia, ventricular fibrillation and Torsade de Pointes. Similar effects have been observed with concomitant administration of astemizole and other macrolides.

4.4 Special warnings and precautions for use
Clarithromycin is principally excreted by the liver and kidney. Caution should be exercised in administering this antibiotic to patients with impaired hepatic and renal function.

Prolonged or repeated use of clarithromycin may result in an overgrowth of non-susceptible bacteria or fungi. If super-infection occurs, clarithromycin should be discontinued and appropriate therapy instituted.

There have been post-marketing reports of colchicine toxicity with concomitant use of clarithromycin and colchicine, especially in the elderly, some of which occurred in patients with renal insufficiency. Deaths have been reported in some such patients (see Section 4.5).

4.5 Interaction with other medicinal products and other forms of interaction
Clarithromycin has been shown not to interact with oral contraceptives.

As with other macrolide antibiotics the use of clarithromycin in patients concurrently taking drugs metabolised by the cytochrome p450 system (e.g. cilostazol, methylprednisolone, oral anticoagulants (eg warfarin), quinidine, sildenafil, ergot alkaloids, alprazolam, triazolam, midazolam, disopyramide, lovastatin, rifabutin, phenytoin, cyclosporin, vinblastine, valproate and tacrolimus) may be associated with elevations in serum levels of these other drugs. Rhabdomyolysis, co-incident with the co-administration of clarithromycin, and HMG-CoA reductase inhibitors, such as lovastatin and simvastatin has been reported.

The administration of Clarithromycin to patients who are receiving theophylline has been associated with increased serum theophylline levels and potential theophylline toxicity.

The use of Clarithromycin in patients receiving warfarin may result in a potentiation of the effects of warfarin. Prothrombin time should be frequently monitored in these patients. The effects of digoxin may be potentiated with concomitant administration of Clarithromycin. Monitoring of serum digoxin levels should be considered.

Clarithromycin may potentiate the effects of carbamazepine due to a reduction in the rate of excretion.

Simultaneous oral administration of clarithromycin tablets and zidovudine to HIV infected adults may result in decreased steady-state zidovudine concentrations. Since this interaction in adults is thought to be due to interference of clarithromycin with simultaneously administered oral zidovudine, this interaction should not be a problem when clarithromycin is administered intravenously. With oral clarithromycin, the interaction can be largely avoided by staggering the doses; see Summary of Product Characteristics for Clarithromycin tablets for further information. No similar reaction has been reported in children.

Ritonavir increases the area under the curve (AUC), C_{max} and C_{min} of clarithromycin when administered concurrently. Because of the large therapeutic window for clarithromycin, no dosage reduction should be necessary in patients with normal renal function. However, for patients with renal impairment, the following dosage adjustments should be considered: For patients with CL_{CR} 30 to 60ml/min the dose of clarithromycin should be decreased by 50%. For patients with CL_{CR} <30ml/min the dose of clarithromycin should be decreased by 75%. Doses of clarithromycin greater than 1g/day should not be coadministered with ritonavir.

There have been post-marketed reports of Torsade de Pointes occurring with the concurrent use of clarithromycin and quinidine or disopyramide. Levels of these medications should be monitored during clarithromycin therapy.

Colchicine is a substrate for both CYP3A and the efflux transporter, P-glycoprotein (Pgp). Clarithromycin and other macrolides are known to inhibit CYP3A and Pgp. When clarithromycin and colchicine are administered together, inhibition of Pgp and/or CYP3A by clarithromycin may lead to increased exposure to colchicine. Patients should be monitored for clinical symptoms of colchicine toxicity (see Section 4.4).

Post-marketing reports indicate that co-administration of clarithromycin with ergotamine or dihydroergotamine has been associated with acute ergot toxicity characterized by vasospasm and ischaemia of the extremities and other tissues including the central nervous system (see section 4.3 Contraindications).

4.6 Pregnancy and lactation
The safety of Clarithromycin during pregnancy and breast feeding of infants has not been established. Clarithromycin should thus not be used during pregnancy or lactation unless the benefit is considered to outweigh the risk. Some animal studies have suggested an embryotoxic effect but only at dose levels which are clearly toxic to mothers. Clarithromycin has been found in the milk of lactating animals and in human breast milk.

4.7 Effects on ability to drive and use machines
None reported.

4.8 Undesirable effects
The most frequently reported infusion-related adverse events in clinical studies were injection-site inflammation, tenderness, phlebitis and pain. The most common non-infusion related adverse event reported was taste perversion.

During clinical studies with oral Clarithromycin, the drug was generally well tolerated. Side-effects included nausea, vomiting, diarrhoea, dyspepsia and abdominal pain and paraesthesia. Stomatitis, glossitis and oral monilia have been reported. Other side-effects include headache, tooth and tongue discolouration, arthralgia, myalgia and allergic reactions ranging from urticaria, mild skin eruptions and angioedema to anaphylaxis have been reported. There have been reports of Stevens-Johnson syndrome/ toxic epidermal necrolysis with orally administered clarithromycin.

Reports of alteration of the sense of smell, usually in conjunction with taste perversion have also been received. There have been reports of transient central nervous system side-effects including dizziness, vertigo, anxiety, insomnia, bad dreams, tinnitus, confusion, disorientation, hallucinations, psychosis, and depersonalisation. There have been reports of hearing loss with clarithromycin which is usually reversible upon withdrawal of therapy.

Pseudomembranous colitis has been reported rarely with clarithromycin, and may range in severity from mild to life threatening.

There have been rare reports of hypoglycaemia, some of which have occurred in patients on concomitant oral hypoglycaemic agents or insulin.

There have been very rare reports of uveitis mainly in patients treated with concomitant rifabutin, most of these were reversible.

Isolated cases of leukopenia and thrombocytopenia have been reported.

As with other macrolides, hepatic dysfunction (which is usually reversible) including altered liver function tests, hepatitis and cholestasis with or without jaundice, has been reported. Dysfunction may be severe and very rarely fatal hepatic failure has been reported.

Cases of increased serum creatinine, interstitial nephritis, renal failure, pancreatitis and convulsions have been reported rarely.

As with other macrolides, QT prolongation, ventricular tachycardia and Torsade de Pointes have been rarely reported with clarithromcyin.

There have been post-marketing reports of colchicine toxicity with concomitant use of clarithromycin and colchicine, especially in the elderly, some of which occurred in patients with renal insufficiency. Deaths have been reported in some such patients (see sections 4.4 and 4.5).

4.9 Overdose
There is no experience of overdosage after IV administration of clarithromycin. However, reports indicate that the ingestion of large amounts of clarithromycin orally can be expected to produce gastro-intestinal symptoms. Adverse reactions accompanying overdosage should be treated by gastric lavage and supportive measures.

As with other macrolides, clarithromycin serum levels are not expected to be appreciably affected by haemodialysis or peritoneal dialysis.

One patient who had a history of bipolar disorder ingested 8 grams of clarithromycin and showed altered mental status, paranoid behaviour, hypokalaemia and hypoxaemia.

5. PHARMACOLOGICAL PROPERTIES
5.1 Pharmacodynamic properties
Clarithromycin is a semi-synthetic derivative of erythromycin A. It exerts its antibacterial action by binding to the 50s ribosomal sub-unit of susceptible bacteria and suppresses protein synthesis. Clarithromycin demonstrates excellent *in vitro* activity against standard strains of clinical isolates. It is highly potent against a wide variety of aerobic and anaerobic gram positive and negative organisms. The minimum inhibitory concentrations (MICs) of clarithromycin are generally two-fold lower than the MICs of erythromycin.

The 14-(R)-hydroxy metabolite of clarithromycin, formed in man by first pass metabolism also has anti-microbial activity. The MICs of this metabolite are equal to or two-fold higher than the MICs of the parent compound except for *H. influenzae* where the 14-hydroxy metabolite is two-fold more active than the parent compound.

Klaricid IV **or Clarithromycin 500 mg/vial Powder for Solution for Injection** is usually active against the following organisms in vitro:

Gram-positive Bacteria:*Staphylococcus aureus* (methicillin susceptible); *Streptococcus pyogenes* (Group A beta-haemolytic streptococci); alpha-haemolytic streptococcus (viridans group); *Streptococcus (Diplococcus) pneumoniae; Streptococcus agalactiae; Listeria monocytogenes.*

Gram-negative Bacteria:*Haemophilus influenzae, Haemophilus parainfluenzae, Moraxella (Branhamella) catarrhalis, Neisseria gonorrhoeae*; *Legionella pneumophila, Bordetella pertussis, Helicobacter pylori*; *Campylobacter jejuni.*

Mycoplasma:*Mycoplasma pneumoniae*; *Ureaplasma urealyticum.*

Other Organisms:*Chlamydia trachomatis*; *Mycobacterium avium*; *Mycobacterium leprae*; *Chlamydia pneumoniae.*

Anaerobes: Macrolide-susceptible *Bacteriodes fragilis*; *Clostridium perfringens*; Peptococcus species; Peptostreptococcus species; *Propionibacterium acnes*.

Clarithromycin has bactericidal activity against several bacterial strains. These organisms include *H. influenzae, Streptococcus pneumoniae, Streptococcus pyogenes, Streptococcus agalactiae, Morazella (Brahamella) catarrhalis, Neisseria gonorrhoeae, Helicobacter pylori* and Campylobacter spp.

The activity of clarithromycin against *H. pylori* is greater at neutral pH than at acid pH.

5.2 Pharmacokinetic properties
The microbiologically active metabolite 14-hydroxyclarithromycin is formed by first pass metabolism as indicated by lower bioavailability of the metabolite following IV administration. Following IV administration the blood levels of clarithromycin achieved are well in excess of the MIC $_{90}$s for the common pathogens and the levels of 14-hydroxyclarithromycin exceed the necessary concentrations for important pathogens, e.g. *H. influenzae.*

The pharmacokinetics of clarithromycin and the 14-hydroxy metabolite are non-linear; steady state is achieved by day 3 of IV dosing. Following a single 500mg IV dose over 60 minutes, about 33% clarithromycin and 11% 14-hydroxyclarithromycin is excreted in the urine at 24 hours.

Klaricid IV **or Clarithromycin 500 mg/vial Powder for Solution for Injection** does not contain tartrazine or other azo dyes, lactose or gluten.

5.3 Preclinical safety data
There are no pre-clinical data of relevance to the prescriber which are additional to that already included in other sections of the SPC.

6. PHARMACEUTICAL PARTICULARS

6.1 List of excipients
Lactobionic acid and Sodium Hydroxide EP.

6.2 Incompatibilities
None known. However, Klaricid IV **or Clarithromycin 500 mg/vial Powder for Solution for Injection** should only be diluted with the diluents recommended.

6.3 Shelf life
36 months unopened.

24 hours (at 5°C - 25°C) once reconstituted in 10ml water for injections.

6 hours (at 25°C) or 24 hours at (5°C) once diluted in 250ml of appropriate diluent.

6.4 Special precautions for storage
Do not store above 30° C. Store in the original container.

6.5 Nature and contents of container
15ml Ph.Eur. Type I flint glass tubing vial with a 20mm grey halobutyl siliconised lyophilisation stopper with a flip-off cap. Vials are packed in units of 1, 4 and 6. Pack size 500mg.

6.6 Special precautions for disposal and other handling
Klaricid IV **or Clarithromycin 500 mg/vial Powder for Solution for Injection** should be administered into one of the larger proximal veins as an IV infusion over 60 minutes, using a solution concentration of about 2mg/ml. Clarithromycin should not be given as a bolus or an intramuscular injection.

7. MARKETING AUTHORISATION HOLDER
Abbott Laboratories Limited
Queenborough
Kent
ME11 5EL.

8. MARKETING AUTHORISATION NUMBER(S)
PL 00037 / 0251

9. DATE OF FIRST AUTHORISATION/RENEWAL OF THE AUTHORISATION
22/09/93

10. DATE OF REVISION OF THE TEXT
07 July 2009

Klaricid Paediatric Suspension

(Abbott Laboratories Limited)

1. NAME OF THE MEDICINAL PRODUCT
Klaricid Paediatric Suspension **or Clarithromycin 125 mg/5ml Granules for Oral Suspension**

2. QUALITATIVE AND QUANTITATIVE COMPOSITION
Activemg/5ml

Clarithromycin 125

3. PHARMACEUTICAL FORM
White to off - white granules for reconstitution.

4. CLINICAL PARTICULARS

4.1 Therapeutic indications
Klaricid Paediatric Suspension **or Clarithromycin 125 mg/5ml Granules for Oral Suspension** is indicated for the treatment of infections caused by susceptible organisms. Indications include:

Lower respiratory tract infections.

Upper respiratory tract infections.

Skin and skin structure infections.

Acute otitis media.

Klaricid Paediatric Suspension **or Clarithromycin 125 mg/5ml Granules for Oral Suspension** is usually active against the following organisms *in vitro*:

Gram-positive Bacteria:*Staphylococcus aureus* (methicillin susceptible); *Streptococcus pyogenes* (Group A beta-haemolytic streptococci); alpha-haemolytic streptococci (viridans group); *Streptococcus (Diplococcus) pneumoniae*; *Streptococcus agalactiae*; *Listeria monocytogenes*.

Gram-negative Bacteria: *Haemophilus influenzae, Haemophilus parainfluenzae, Moraxella (Branhamella) catarrhalis, Neisseria gonorrhoeae; Legionella pneumophila, Bordetella pertussis, Helicobacter pylori; Campylobacter jejuni*.

Mycoplasma: *Mycoplasma pneumoniae; Ureaplasma urealyticum*.

Other Organisms:*Chlamydia trachomatis; Mycobacterium avium; Mycobacterium leprae; Chlamydia pneumoniae*.

Anaerobes: Macrolide-susceptible *Bacteroides fragilis; Clostridium perfringens; Peptococcus* species; *Peptostreptococcus* species; *Propionibacterium acnes*.

Klaricid Paediatric Suspension **or Clarithromycin 125 mg/5ml Granules for Oral Suspension** has bactericidal activity against several bacterial strains. These organisms include *H. influenzae, Streptococcus pneumoniae, Streptococcus pyogenes, Streptococcus agalactiae, Moraxella (Branhamella) catarrhalis, Neisseria gonorrhoeae, Helicobacter pylori and Campylobacter* species.

The activity of clarithromycin against *H. pylori* is greater at neutral pH than at acid pH.

4.2 Posology and method of administration
Recommended doses and dosage schedules:

The usual duration of treatment is for 5 to 10 days depending on the pathogen involved and the severity of the condition. The recommended daily dosage of Klaricid Paediatric Suspension **or Clarithromycin 125 mg/5ml Granules for Oral Suspension** in children is given in the following table and is based on a 7.5mg/kg b.i.d. dosing regime. Doses up to 500mg b.i.d. have been used in the treatment of severe infections.

KLARICID PAEDIATRIC SUSPENSION **OR CLARITHROMYCIN 125 MG/5ML GRANULES FOR ORAL SUSPENSION** DOSAGE IN CHILDREN

Dosage Based on Body Weight (kg)

Weight* (kg)	Approx Age (yrs)	Dosage (ml) bid	Dosage per 5ml teaspoonful twice daily
8-11	1 - 2	2.50	1/2
12-19	3 - 6	5.00	1.00
20-29	7 - 9	7.50	1 1/2
30-40	10 - 12	10.00	2.00

* Children < 8 kg should be dosed on a per kg basis (approx. 7.5 mg/kg bid)

Preparation for use: 140ml bottle: 74ml of water should be added to the granules in the bottle and shaken to yield 140ml of reconstituted suspension. The concentration of clarithromycin in the reconstituted suspension is 125mg per 5ml.

100 ml bottle:

53ml of water should be added to the granules in the bottle and shaken to yield 100ml of reconstituted suspension. The concentration of clarithromycin in the reconstituted suspension is 125mg per 5ml.

70 ml bottle:

37ml of water should be added to the granules in the bottle and shaken to yield 70ml of reconstituted suspension. The concentration of clarithromycin in the reconstituted suspension is 125mg per 5ml.

50 ml bottle:

27ml of water should be added to the granules in the bottle and shaken to yield 50ml of reconstituted suspension. The concentration of clarithromycin in the reconstituted suspension is 125mg per 5ml.

Sachet: After cutting along the dotted line, empty contents of sachet into a glass, half fill the sachet with cold water. Add to glass and stir thoroughly before taking.

4.3 Contraindications
Klaricid Paediatric Suspension **or Clarithromycin 125 mg/5ml Granules for Oral Suspension** is contra-indicated in patients with known hypersensitivity to macrolide antibiotic drugs and other ingredients.

Klaricid Paediatric Suspension **or Clarithromycin 125 mg/5ml Granules for Oral Suspension** and ergot derivatives should not be co-administered (see section 4.5).

Concomitant administration of clarithromycin and any of the following drugs is contraindicated: cisapride, pimozide and terfenadine. Elevated cisapride, pimozide and terfenadine levels have been reported in patients receiving either of these drugs and clarithromycin concomitantly. This may result in QT prolongation and cardiac arrhythmias including ventricular tachycardia, ventricular fibrillation and Torsade de Pointes. Similar effects have been observed with concomitant administration of astemizole and other macrolides.

4.4 Special warnings and precautions for use
Clarithromycin is principally excreted by the liver and kidneys. This antibiotic should not be administered to paediatric patients with hepatic or renal failure.

Prolonged or repeated use of clarithromycin may result in an overgrowth of non-susceptible bacteria or fungi. If super-infection occurs, clarithromycin should be discontinued and appropriate therapy instituted.

There have been post-marketing reports of colchicine toxicity with concomitant use of clarithromycin and colchicine, especially in the elderly, some of which occurred in patients with renal insufficiency. Deaths have been reported in some such patients (see section 4.5).

Patients with rare hereditary problems of fructose intolerance, glucose-galactose malabsorption or sucrase-isomaltase insufficiency should not take this medicine.

4.5 Interaction with other medicinal products and other forms of interaction
As with other macrolide antibiotics, the use of clarithromycin in patients concurrently taking drugs metabolised by the cytochrome P450 system (eg. Cilostazol, methylprednisolone, oral anticoagulants (eg warfarin), quinidine, ergot alkaloids, alprazolam, triazolam, midazolam, disopyramide, lovastatin, rifabutin, phenytoin, cyclosporin, vinblastine, valproate and tacrolimus) may be associated with elevations in serum levels of these other drugs. Rhabdomyolysis, co-incident with the co- administration of clarithromycin, and HMG-CoA reductase inhibitors, such as lovastatin and simvastatin has been reported.

The administration of clarithromycin to patients who are receiving theophylline has been associated with an increase of serum theophylline levels and potential theophylline toxicity.

The use of Klaricid Paediatric Suspension **or Clarithromycin 125 mg/5ml Granules for Oral Suspension** in patients receiving digoxin, warfarin and carbamazepine may result in potentiation of their effects due to a reduction in the rate of excretion. Prothrombin time should be frequently monitored in patients receiving warfarin. Monitoring of serum digoxin levels should be considered.

Ritonavir increases the AUC (area under the curve) of clarithromycin when administered concurrently. Because of the large therapeutic window for clarithromycin, no dosage reduction should be necessary in patients with normal renal function. However, for patients with renal impairment, the following dosage adjustments should be considered: For patients with CL_{CR} 30 to 60 ml/min the dose of clarithromycin should be reduced by 50%. For patients with CL_{CR}<30ml/min the dose of clarithromycin should be decreased by 75%. Doses of clarithromycin greater than 1g/day should not be coadministered with ritonavir.

Simultaneous oral administration of clarithromycin tablets and zidovudine to HIV-infected adult patients may result in decreased steady-state zidovudine levels. To date, this interaction does not appear to occur in paediatric HIV-infected patients taking Klaricid Paediatric Suspension **or Clarithromycin 125 mg/5ml Granules for Oral Suspension** with zidovudine or dideoxyinosine.

There have been postmarketed reports of Torsade de Points occurring with the concurrent use of clarithrtomycin and quinidine or disopyramide. Levels of these medications should be monitored during clarithromycin therapy.

Colchicine is a substrate for both CYP3A and the efflux transporter, P-glycoprotein (Pgp). Clarithromycin and other macrolides are known to inhibit CYP3A and Pgp. When clarithromycin and colchicine are administered together, inhibition of Pgp and/or CYP3A by clarithromycin may lead to increased exposure to colchicine. Patients should be monitored for clinical symptoms of colchicine toxicity (see section 4.4).

Post-marketing reports indicate that co-administration of clarithromycin with ergotamine or dihydroergotamine has been associated with acute ergot toxicity characterized by vasospasm, and ischemia of the extremeties and other tissues including the central nervous system (see section 4.3, Contraindications)

4.6 Pregnancy and lactation
The safety of clarithromycin during pregnancy and breast feeding of infants has not been established. Some animal studies have suggested an embryotoxic effect but only at dose levels which are clearly toxic to mothers. Therefore, if a patient of post-pubertal age becomes pregnant, clarithromycin should not be used during pregnancy or lactation unless the benefit outweighs the risk. Clarithromycin has been found in the milk of lactating animals and in human breast milk.

4.7 Effects on ability to drive and use machines
None known.

4.8 Undesirable effects
Clarithromycin is generally well tolerated. Side effects reported include nausea, dyspepsia, diarrhoea, vomiting, abdominal pain and paraesthesia. Stomatitis, glossitis, oral monilia and tongue discolouration have been reported.

Other side-effects include headache, arthralgia, myalgia and allergic reactions ranging from urticaria, mild skin eruptions and angioedema to anaphylaxis have been reported. There have been reports of Stevens-Johnson syndrome / toxic epidermal necrolysis with orally administered clarithromycin.

Reports of alteration of the sense of smell, usually in conjunction with taste perversion have also been received. There have been reports of tooth discolouration in patients treated with clarithromycin. Tooth discolouration is usually reversible with professional dental cleaning. There have been reports of transient central nervous system side-effects including dizziness, vertigo, anxiety, insomnia, bad dreams, tinnitus, confusion, disorientation, hallucinations, psychosis and depersonalisation. There have been reports of hearing loss with clarithromycin which is usually reversible upon withdrawal of therapy. Pseudomembranous colitis has been reported rarely with clarithromycin, and may range in severity from mild to life threatening. There have been rare reports of hypoglycaemia, some of which have occurred in patients on concomitant oral hypoglycaemic agents or insulin. There have been very rare reports of uveitis mainly in patients treated with concomitant rifabutin, most of these were reversible.

Isolated cases of leukopenia and thrombocytopenia have been reported. As with other macrolides, hepatic dysfunction (which is usually reversible) including altered liver function tests, hepatitis and cholestasis with or without jaundice, has been reported.

Dysfunction may be severe and very rarely fatal hepatic failure has been reported.

Cases of increased serum creatinine, interstitial nephritis, renal failure, pancreatitis and convulsions have been reported rarely.

As with other macrolides, QT prolongation, ventricular tachycardia and Torsade de Pointes have been rarely reported with clarithromycin.

There have been post-marketing reports of colchicine toxicity with concomitant use of clarithromycin and colchicine, especially in the elderly, some of which occurred in patients with renal insufficiency. Deaths have been reported in some such patients (see sections 4.4 and 4.5).

4.9 Overdose

Reports indicate that the ingestion of large amounts of clarithromycin can be expected to produce gastro-intestinal symptoms. Adverse reactions accompanying overdosage should be treated by gastric lavage and general supportive measures. One patient who had a history of bipolar disorder ingested 8 grams of clarithromycin and showed altered mental status, paranoid behaviour, hypokalaemia and hypoxaemia. As with other macrolides, clarithromycin serum levels are not expected to be appreciably affected by haemodialysis or peritoneal dialysis.

5. PHARMACOLOGICAL PROPERTIES

5.1 Pharmacodynamic properties

Clarithromycin is a semi-synthetic derivative of erythromycin A. It exerts its anti-bacterial action by binding to the 50s ribosomal sub-unit of susceptible bacteria and suppresses protein synthesis. Clarithromycin demonstrates excellent *in-vitro* activity against standard strains of clinical isolates. It is highly potent against a wide variety of aerobic and anaerobic gram-positive and gram-negative organisms. The minimum inhibitory concentrations (MICs) of clarithromycin are generally two-fold lower than the MICs of erythromycin.

The 14-(R)-hydroxy metabolite of clarithromycin formed in man by first pass metabolism also has anti-microbial activity. The MICs of this metabolite are equal or two-fold higher than the MICs of the parent compound, except for H.influenzae where the 14-hydroxy metabolite is two-fold more active than the parent compound. Clarithromycin is also bactericidal against several bacterial strains.

Clarithromycin is usually active against the following organisms in vitro:-

Gram-positive Bacteria:*Staphylococcus aureus* (methicillin susceptible); *Streptococcus pyogenes* (Group A beta-haemolytic streptococci); alpha-haemolytic streptococci (viridans group); *Streptococcus (Diplococcus) pneumoniae*; *Streptococcus agalactiae*; *Listeria monocytogenes*.

Gram-negative Bacteria: *Haemophilus influenzae, Haemophilus parainfluenzae, Moraxella (Branhamella) catarrhalis, Neisseria gonorrhoeae; Legionella pneumophila, Bordetella pertussis, Helicobacter pylori; Campylobacter jejuni.*

Mycoplasma: *Mycoplasma pneumoniae; Ureaplasma urealyticum.*

Other Organisms:*Chlamydia trachomatis; Mycobacterium avium; Mycobacterium leprae; Chlamydia pneumoniae.*

Anaerobes: Macrolide-susceptible *Bacteroides fragilis*; *Clostridium perfringens*; *Peptococcus* species; *Peptostreptococcus* species; *Propionibacterium acnes*.

Clarithromycin also has bactericidal activity against several bacterial strains. These organisms include *H. influenzae, Streptococcus pneumoniae, Streptococcus pyogenes, Streptococcus agalactiae, Moraxella (Brahamella) catarrhalis, Neisseria gonorrhoeae, Helicobacter pylori* and *Campylobacter* species.

5.2 Pharmacokinetic properties

Clarithromycin is rapidly and well absorbed from the gastro-intestinal tract after oral administration. The microbiologically active 14(R)-hydroxyclarithromycin is formed by first pass metabolism. Clarithromycin, may be given without regard to meals as food does not affect the extent of bioavailability. Food does slightly delay the onset of absorption of clarithromycin and formation of the 14-hydroxy metabolite. Although the pharmacokinetics of clarithromycin are non linear, steady state is attained within 2 days of dosing. 14-Hydroxyclarithromycin is the major urinary metabolite and accounts for 10-15% of the dose. Most of the remainder of the dose is eliminated in the faeces, primarily via the bile. 5-10% of the parent drug is recovered from the faeces.

Clarithromycin provides tissue concentrations that are several times higher than circulating drug level. Increased levels of clarithromycin have been found in both tonsillar and lung tissue. Clarithromycin penetrates into the middle ear fluid at concentrations greater than in the serum. Clarithromycin is 80% bound to plasma proteins at therapeutic levels.

Klaricid Paediatric Suspension **or Clarithromycin 125 mg/5ml Granules for Oral Suspension** does not contain tartrazine or other azo dyes, lactose or gluten.

5.3 Preclinical safety data

The acute oral LD_{50} values for a clarithromycin suspension administered to 3-day old mice were 1290 mg/kg for males and 1230 mg/kg for females. The LD_{50} values in 3-day old rats were 1330 mg/kg for males and 1270 mg/kg for females. For comparison, the LD_{50} of orally-administered clarithromycin is about 2700 mg/kg for adult mice and about 3000 mg/kg for adult rats. These results are consistent with other antibiotics of the penicillin group, cephalosporin group and macrolide group in that the LD_{50} is generally lower in juvenile animals than in adults.

In both mice and rats, body weight was reduced or its increase suppressed and suckling behaviour and spontaneous movements were depressed for the first few days following drug administration. Necropsy of animals that died disclosed dark-reddish lungs in mice and about 25% of the rats; rats treated with 2197 mg/kg or more of a clarithromycin suspension were also noted to have a reddish - black substance in the intestines, probably because of bleeding. Deaths of these animals were considered due to debilitation resulting from depressed suckling behaviour or bleeding from the intestines.

Pre-weaning rats (5 days old) were administered a clarithromycin suspension formulation for two weeks at doses of 0, 15, 55 and 200 mg/kg/day. Animals from the 200 mg/kg/day group had decreased body-weight gains, decreased mean haemoglobin and haematocrit values, and increased mean relative kidney weights compared to animals from the control group. Treatment-related minimal to mild multifocal vacuolar degeneration of the intrahepatic bile duct epithelium and an increased incidence of nephritic lesions were also observed in animals from this treatment group. The "no-toxic effect" dosage for this study was 55 mg/kg/day.

An oral toxicity study was conducted in which immature rats were administered a clarithromycin suspension (granules for suspension) for 6 weeks at daily dosages of 0, 15, 50 and 150 mg base/kg/day. No deaths occurred and the only clinical sign observed was excessive salivation for some of the animals at the highest dosage from 1 to 2 hours after administration during the last 3 weeks of treatment. Rats from the 150 mg/kg dose group had lower mean body weights during the first three weeks, and were observed to have decreased mean serum albumin values and increased mean relative liver weight compared to the controls. No treatment-related gross or microscopic histopathological changes were found. A dosage of 150 mg/kg/day produced slight toxicity in the treated rats and the "no effect dosage" was considered to be 50 mg/kg/day.

Juvenile beagle dogs, 3 weeks of age, were treated orally daily for four weeks with 0, 30, 100, or 300 mg/kg of clarithromycin, followed by a 4-week recovery period. No deaths occurred and no changed in the general condition of the animals were observed. Necropsy revealed no abnormalities. Upon histological examination, fatty deposition of centrilobular hepatocytes and cell infiltration of portal areas were observed by light microscopy and an increase in hepatocellular fat droplets was noted by electron microscopy in the 300 mg/kg dose group. The toxic dose in juvenile beagle dogs was considered to be greater than 300 mg/kg and the "no effect dose" 100 mg/kg.

Fertility, Reproduction and Teratogenicity

Fertility and reproduction studies have shown daily dosages of 150-160 mg/kg/day to male and female rats caused no adverse effects on the oestrus cycle, fertility, parturition and number and viability of offspring. Two teratogenicity studies in both Wistar (p.o.) and Sprague-Dawley (p.o. and i.v.) rats, one study in New Zealand white rabbits and one study in cynomolgus monkeys failed to demonstrate any teratogenicity from clarithromycin.

6. PHARMACEUTICAL PARTICULARS

6.1 List of excipients

Carbopol 974P, povidone K90, water purified, hydroxypropylmethylcellulose phthalate (HP-55), castor oil, acetone, ethanol, silicon dioxide, sucrose, xanthan gum, flavour - fruit punch, potassium sorbate, citric acid, titanium dioxide and maltodextrin

6.2 Incompatibilities

None known.

6.3 Shelf life

Bottles: The recommended shelf life is 36 months.

Once reconstituted, Klaricid Paediatric Suspension **or Clarithromycin 125 mg/5ml Granules for Oral Suspension** should be used within 14 days.

Sachets: The recommended shelf life is 18 months.

6.4 Special precautions for storage

Do not store above 25°C.

6.5 Nature and contents of container

Granules for reconstitution in a HDPE bottle. Pack sizes of 50, 70, 100 and 140ml are available.

Granules for reconstitution in paper/LDPE/Al foil/LDPE sachet. Packs of 2 sachets.

6.6 Special precautions for disposal and other handling

Not applicable

7. MARKETING AUTHORISATION HOLDER

Abbott Laboratories Limited
Queenborough
Kent, ME11 5EL

8. MARKETING AUTHORISATION NUMBER(S)

PL 0037/0264

9. DATE OF FIRST AUTHORISATION/RENEWAL OF THE AUTHORISATION

16 October 1995

10. DATE OF REVISION OF THE TEXT

14 September 2006

Klaricid Paediatric Suspension 250

(Abbott Laboratories Limited)

1. NAME OF THE MEDICINAL PRODUCT

Klaricid Paediatric Suspension 250mg/5ml **or Clarithromycin 250mg/5ml Granules for Oral Suspension**

2. QUALITATIVE AND QUANTITATIVE COMPOSITION

Activemg/5ml

Clarithromycin 250

3. PHARMACEUTICAL FORM

White to off - white granules for oral suspension.

4. CLINICAL PARTICULARS

4.1 Therapeutic indications

Klaricid Paediatric Suspension 250mg/5ml **or Clarithromycin 250mg/5ml Granules for Oral Suspension** is indicated for the treatment of infections caused by susceptible organisms. Indications include:

Lower respiratory tract infections.

Upper respiratory tract infections.

Skin and skin structure infections.

Acute otitis media.

Klaricid Paediatric Suspension 250mg/5ml **or Clarithromycin 250mg/5ml Granules for Oral Suspension** is usually active against the following organisms *in vitro*:

Gram-positive Bacteria:*Staphylococcus aureus* (methicillin susceptible); *Streptococcus pyogenes* (Group A beta-haemolytic streptococci); alpha-haemolytic streptococci (viridans group); *Streptococcus (Diplococcus) pneumoniae*; *Streptococcus agalactiae*; *Listeria monocytogenes*.

Gram-negative Bacteria: *Haemophilus influenzae*; *Haemophilus parainfluenzae*; *Moraxella (Branhamella) catarrhalis*; *Neisseria gonorrhoeae*; *Legionella pneumophila*; *Bordetella pertussis*; *Helicobacter pylori*; *Campylobacter jejuni*.

Mycoplasma: *Mycoplasma pneumoniae*; *Ureaplasma urealyticum*.

Other Organisms:*Chlamydia trachomatis*; *Mycobacterium avium*; *Mycobacterium leprae*; *Chlamydia pneumoniae*.

Anaerobes: Macrolide-susceptible *Bacteroides fragilis*; *Clostridium perfringens*; Peptococcus species; Peptostreptococcus species; *Propionibacterium acnes*.

Klaricid Paediatric Suspension 250mg/5ml **or Clarithromycin 250mg/5ml Granules for Oral Suspension** has bactericidal activity against several bacterial strains. These organisms include *H. influenzae, Streptococcus pneumoniae, Streptococcus pyogenes, Streptococcus agalactiae, Moraxella (Branhamella) catarrhalis, Neisseria gonorrhoeae, Helicobacter pylori* and Campylobacter species.

The activity of clarithromycin against *H. pylori* is greater at neutral pH than at acid pH.

4.2 Posology and method of administration

Recommended doses and dosage schedules:

The usual duration of treatment is for 5 to 10 days depending on the pathogen involved and the severity of the condition. The recommended daily dosage of Klaricid Paediatric Suspension 250mg/5ml **or Clarithromycin 250mg/5ml Granules for Oral Suspension** in children is given in the following table and is based on a 7.5mg/kg twice a day dosage regimen. Doses up to 500mg twice a day have been used in the treatment of severe infections.

KLARICID PAEDIATRIC SUSPENSION 250MG/5ML **OR CLARITHROMYCIN 250MG/5ML GRANULES FOR ORAL SUSPENSION**

DOSAGE IN CHILDREN

Dosage Based on Body Weight (kg)

Weight * (kg)	Approx Age (yrs)	Dosage twice a day (ml)	(mg)
8-11	1 - 2	1.25	62.50
12-19	3 - 6	2.5	125.00
20-29	7 - 9	3.75	187.50
30-40	10 - 12	5	250.00

* Children < 8 kg should be dosed on a per kg basis (approx. 7.5 mg/kg twice a day)

Preparation for use: 140ml bottle: 74ml of water should be added to the granules in the bottle and shaken to yield 140ml of reconstituted suspension. The concentration of clarithromycin in the reconstituted suspension is 250mg per 5ml.

100 ml bottle:

53ml of water should be added to the granules in the bottle and shaken to yield 100ml of reconstituted suspension. The concentration of clarithromycin in the reconstituted suspension is 250mg per 5ml.

70 ml bottle:

37ml of water should be added to the granules in the bottle and shaken to yield 70ml of reconstituted suspension. The concentration of clarithromycin in the reconstituted suspension is 250mg per 5ml.

50 ml bottle:

27ml of water should be added to the granules in the bottle and shaken to yield 50ml of reconstituted suspension. The concentration of clarithromycin in the reconstituted suspension is 250mg per 5ml.

4.3 Contraindications

Klaricid Paediatric Suspension 250mg/5ml **or Clarithromycin 250mg/5ml Granules for Oral Suspension** is contra-indicated in patients with known hypersensitivity to macrolide antibiotic drugs and other ingredients.

Klaricid Paediatric Suspension 250mg/5ml **or Clarithromycin 250mg/5ml Granules for Oral Suspension** and ergot derivatives should not be co-administered (see section 4.5).

Concomitant administration of clarithromycin and any of the following drugs is contraindicated: cisapride, pimozide and terfenadine. Elevated cisapride, pimozide and terfenadine levels have been reported in patients receiving either of these drugs and clarithromycin concomitantly. This may result in QT prolongation and cardiac arrhythmias including ventricular tachycardia, ventricular fibrillation and Torsade de Pointes. Similar effects have been observed with concomitant administration of astemizole and other macrolides.

4.4 Special warnings and precautions for use

Clarithromycin is principally excreted by the liver and kidneys. This antibiotic should not be administered to paediatric patients with hepatic or renal failure.

Prolonged or repeated use of clarithromycin may result in an overgrowth of non-susceptible bacteria or fungi. If super-infection occurs, clarithromycin should be discontinued and appropriate therapy instituted.

There have been post-marketing reports of colchicine toxicity with concomitant use of clarithromycin and colchicine, especially in the elderly, some of which occurred in patients with renal insufficiency. Deaths have been reported in some such patients (see section 4.5).

Patients with rare hereditary problems of fructose intolerance, glucose-galactose malabsorption or sucrase-isomaltase insufficiency should not take this medicine.

4.5 Interaction with other medicinal products and other forms of interaction

As with other macrolide antibiotics the use of clarithromycin in patients concurrently taking drugs metabolised by the cytochrome P450 system (eg. cilostazol, methylprednisolone, oral anticoagulants (e.g warfarin), quinidine, ergot alkaloids, alprazolam, triazolam, midazolam, disopyramide, lovastatin, rifabutin,phenytoin, cyclosporin, vinblastine, valproate and tacrolimus) may be associated with elevations in serum levels of these other drugs. Rhabdomyolysis, co-incident with the co- administration of clarithromycin, and HMG-CoA reductase inhibitors, such as lovastatin and simvastatin has been reported.

The administration of clarithromycin to patients who are receiving theophylline has been associated with an increase of serum theophylline levels and potential theophylline toxicity.

The use of Klaricid Paediatric Suspension 250mg/5ml **or Clarithromycin 250mg/5ml Granules for Oral Suspension** in patients receiving digoxin, warfarin and carbamazepine may result in potentiation of their effects due to a reduction in the rate of excretion. Prothrombin time should be frequently monitored in patients receiving warfarin. Monitoring of serum digoxin levels should be considered.

Ritonavir increases the AUC (area under the curve) of clarithromycin when administered concurrently. Because of the large therapeutic window for clarithromycin, no dosage reduction should be necessary in patients with normal renal function. However, for patients with renal impairment, the following dosage adjustments should be considered: For patients with CL_{CR} 30 to 60 ml/min the dose of clarithromycin should be reduced by 50%. For patients with $CL_{CR} < 30$ml/min the dose of clarithromycin should be decreased by 75%. Doses of clarithromycin greater than 1g/day should not be coadministered with ritonavir.

Simultaneous oral administration of clarithromycin tablets and zidovudine to HIV-infected adult patients may result in decreased steady-state zidovudine levels. To date, this interaction does not appear to occur in paediatric HIV-infected patients taking Klaricid Paediatric Suspension 250mg/5ml **or Clarithromycin 250mg/5ml Granules for Oral Suspension** with zidovudine or dideoxyinosine.

There have been postmarketed reports of Torsade de Points occurring with the concurrent use of clarithrtomycin and quinidine or disopyramide. Levels of these medications should be monitored during clarithromycin therapy.

Colchicine is a substrate for both CYP3A and the efflux transporter, P-glycoprotein (Pgp). Clarithromycin and other macrolides are known to inhibit CYP3A and Pgp. When clarithromycin and colchicine are administered together, inhibition of Pgp and/or CYP3A by clarithromycin may lead to increased exposure to colchicine. Patients should be monitored for clinical symptoms of colchicine toxicity (see section 4.4).

Post-marketing reports indicate that co-administration of clarithromycin with ergotamine or dihydroergotamine has been associated with acute ergot toxicity characterized by vasospasm, and ischemia of the extremeties and other tissues including the central nervous system (see section 4.3, Contraindications)

4.6 Pregnancy and lactation

The safety of clarithromycin during pregnancy and breast feeding of infants has not been established. Some animal studies have suggested an embryotoxic effect but only at dose levels which are clearly toxic to mothers. Therefore, if a patient of post-pubertal age becomes pregnant, clarithromycin should not be used during pregnancy or lactation unless the benefit outweighs the risk. Clarithromycin has been found in the milk of lactating animals and in human breast milk.

4.7 Effects on ability to drive and use machines

None known.

4.8 Undesirable effects

Clarithromycin is generally well tolerated. Side effects reported include nausea, dyspepsia, diarrhoea, vomiting and abdominal pain and paraesthesia. Stomatitis, glossitis and oral monilia and tongue discolouration have been reported. Other side-effects include headache, arthralgia, myalgia and allergic reactions ranging from urticaria, mild skin eruptions and angioedema to anaphylaxis have been reported. There have been reports of Stevens-Johnson syndrome / toxic epidermal necrolysis with orally administered clarithromycin.

Reports of alteration of the sense of smell, usually in conjunction with taste perversion have also been received. There have been reports of tooth discolouration in patients treated with clarithromycin. Tooth discolouration is usually reversible with professional dental cleaning.

There have been reports of transient central nervous system side-effects including dizziness, vertigo, anxiety, insomnia, bad dreams, tinnitus, confusion, disorientation, hallucinations, psychosis and depersonalisation. There have been reports of hearing loss with clarithromycin which is usually reversible upon withdrawal of therapy. Pseudomembranous colitis has been reported rarely with clarithromycin, and may range in severity from mild to life threatening. There have been rare reports of hypoglycaemia, some of which have occurred in patients on concomitant oral hypoglycaemic agents or insulin. There have been very rare reports of uveitis mainly in patients treated with concomitant rifabutin, most of these were reversible. Isolated cases of leukopenia andthrombocytopenia have been reported.

As with other macrolides, hepatic dysfunction (which is usually reversible) including altered liver function tests, hepatitis and cholestasis with or without jaundice, has been reported. Dysfunction may be severe and very rarely fatal hepatic failure has been reported.

Cases of increased serum creatinine, interstitial nephritis, renal failure, pancreatitis and convulsions have been reported rarely.

As with other macrolides, QT prolongation, ventricular tachycardia and Torsade de Pointes have been rarely reported with clarithromycin.

There have been post-marketing reports of colchicine toxicity with concomitant use of clarithromycin and colchicine, especially in the elderly, some of which occurred in patients with renal insufficiency. Deaths have been reported in some such patients (see sections 4.4 and 4.5).

4.9 Overdose

Reports indicate that the ingestion of large amounts of clarithromycin can be expected to produce gastro-intestinal symptoms. Adverse reactions accompanying overdosage should be treated by gastric lavage and general supportive measures. One patient who had a history of bipolar disorder ingested 8 grams of clarithromycin and showed altered mental status, paranoid behaviour, hypokalaemia and hypoxaemia. As with other macrolides, clarithromycin serum levels are not expected to be appreciably affected by haemodialysis or peritoneal dialysis.

5. PHARMACOLOGICAL PROPERTIES

5.1 Pharmacodynamic properties

Clarithromycin is a semi-synthetic derivative of erythromycin A. It exerts its anti-bacterial action by binding to the 50s ribosomal sub-unit of susceptible bacteria and suppresses protein synthesis. Clarithromycin demonstrates excellent *in-vitro* activity against standard strains of clinical isolates. It is highly potent against a wide variety of aerobic and anaerobic gram-positive and gram-negative organisms. The minimum inhibitory concentrations (MICs) of clarithromycin are generally two-fold lower than the MICs of erythromycin.

The 14-(R)-hydroxy metabolite of clarithromycin formed in man by first pass metabolism also has anti-microbial activity. The MICs of this metabolite are equal or two-fold higher than the MICs of the parent compound, except for *H.influenzae* where the 14-hydroxy metabolite is two-fold more active than the parent compound. Clarithromycin is also bactericidal against several bacterial strains.

Clarithromycin is usually active against the following organisms *in vitro*:-

Gram-positive Bacteria:*Staphylococcus aureus* (methicillin susceptible); *Streptococcus pyogenes* (Group A beta-haemolytic streptococci); alpha-haemolytic streptococci (viridans group); *Streptococcus (Diplococcus) pneumoniae*; *Streptococcus agalactiae*; *Listeria monocytogenes*.

Gram-negative Bacteria: *Haemophilus influenzae; Haemophilus parainfluenzae; Moraxella (Branhamella) catarrhalis; Neisseria gonorrhoeae; Legionella pneumophila; Bordetella pertussis; Helicobacter pylori; Campylobacter jejuni*.

Mycoplasma: *Mycoplasma pneumoniae; Ureaplasma urealyticum*.

Other Organisms:*Chlamydia trachomatis; Mycobacterium avium; Mycobacterium leprae; Chlamydia pneumoniae*.

Anaerobes: Macrolide-susceptible *Bacteroides fragilis*; *Clostridium perfringens*; Peptococcus species; Peptostreptococcus species; *Propionibacterium acnes*.

Clarithromycin also has bactericidal activity against several bacterial strains. These organisms include *H. influenzae, Streptococcus pneumoniae, Streptococcus pyogenes, Streptococcus agalactiae, Moraxella (Branhamella) catarrhalis, Neisseria gonorrhoeae, Helicobacter pylori* and Campylobacter species.

5.2 Pharmacokinetic properties

Clarithromycin is rapidly and well absorbed from the gastro-intestinal tract after oral administration. The microbiologically active 14(R)-hydroxyclarithromycin is formed by first pass metabolism. Clarithromycin may be given without regard to meals as food does not affect the extent of bioavailability. Food does slightly delay the onset of absorption of clarithromycin and formation of the 14-hydroxy metabolite. Although the pharmacokinetics of clarithromycin are non linear, steady state is attained within 2 days of dosing. 14-Hydroxyclarithromycin is the major urinary metabolite and accounts for 10-15% of the dose. Most of the remainder of the dose is eliminated in the faeces, primarily via the bile. 5-10% of the parent drug is recovered from the faeces.

Clarithromycin provides tissue concentrations that are several times higher than circulating drug level. Increased levels of clarithromycin have been found in both tonsillar and lung tissue. Clarithromycin penetrates into the middle ear fluid at concentrations greater than in the serum. Clarithromycin is 80% bound to plasma proteins at therapeutic levels.

Klaricid Paediatric Suspension 250mg/5ml **or Clarithromycin 250mg/5ml Granules for Oral Suspension** does not contain tartrazine or other azo dyes, lactose or gluten.

5.3 Preclinical safety data

In both mice and rats, body weight was reduced or its increase suppressed and suckling behaviour and spontaneous movements were depressed for the first few days following drug administration. Necropsy of animals that died disclosed dark-reddish lungs in mice and about 25% of the rats; rats treated with 2197 mg/kg or more of a clarithromycin suspension were also noted to have a reddish - black substance in the intestines, probably because of bleeding. Deaths of these animals were considered due to debilitation resulting from depressed suckling behaviour or bleeding from the intestines.

Pre-weaning rats (5 days old) were administered a clarithromycin suspension formulation for two weeks at doses of 0, 15, 55 and 200 mg/kg/day. Animals from the 200 mg/kg/day group had decreased body-weight gains, decreased mean haemoglobin and haematocrit values, and increased mean relative kidney weights compared to animals from the control group. Treatment-related minimal to mild multifocal vacuolar degeneration of the intrahepatic bile duct epithelium and an increased incidence of nephritic lesions were also observed in animals from this treatment group. The "no-toxic effect" dosage for this study was 55 mg/kg/day.

An oral toxicity study was conducted in which immature rats were administered a clarithromycin suspension (granules for suspension) for 6 weeks at daily dosages of 0, 15, 50 and 150 mg base/kg/day. No deaths occurred and the only clinical sign observed was excessive salivation for some of the animals at the highest dosage from 1 to 2 hours after administration during the last 3 weeks of treatment. Rats from the 150 mg/kg dose group had lower mean body weights during the first three weeks, and were observed to have decreased mean serum albumin values and increased mean relative liver weight compared to the controls. No treatment-related gross or microscopic histopathological changes were found. A dosage of 150 mg/kg/day produced slight toxicity in the treated rats and the "no effect dosage" was considered to be 50 mg/kg/day.

Juvenile beagle dogs, 3 weeks of age, were treated orally daily for four weeks with 0, 30, 100, or 300 mg/kg of clarithromycin, followed by a 4-week recovery period. No deaths occurred and no changes in the general condition of the animals were observed. Necropsy revealed no abnormalities. Upon histological examination, fatty deposition of centrilobular hepatocytes and cell infiltration of portal areas were observed by light microscopy and an increase in hepatocellular fat droplets was noted by electron microscopy in the 300 mg/kg dose group. The toxic dose in juvenile beagle dogs was considered to be greater than 300 mg/kg and the "no effect dose" 100 mg/kg.

Fertility, Reproduction and Teratogenicity

Fertility and reproduction studies have shown daily dosages of 150-160 mg/kg/day to male and female rats caused no adverse effects on the oestrus cycle, fertility, parturition and number and viability of offspring. Two teratogenicity studies in both Wistar (p.o.) and Sprague-Dawley (p.o. and i.v.) rats, one study in New Zealand white rabbits and one study in cynomolgus monkeys failed to demonstrate any teratogenicity from clarithromycin.

6. PHARMACEUTICAL PARTICULARS

6.1 List of excipients

Carbopol 974P, povidone K90, water purified, hypromellose phthalate (HP-55), castor oil, silicon dioxide, sucrose, xanthan gum, flavour - fruit punch, potassium sorbate, citric acid, titanium dioxide and maltodextrin.

6.2 Incompatibilities

None known.

6.3 Shelf life

The recommended shelf life of the dry granule is 24 months.

Once reconstituted, Klaricid Paediatric Suspension 250mg/5ml **or Clarithromycin 250mg/5ml Granules for Oral Suspension** should be used within 14 days.

6.4 Special precautions for storage

Do not store above 30°C. Do not refrigerate or freeze.

6.5 Nature and contents of container

Granules for reconstitution in a HDPE bottle. Pack sizes of 50, 70, 100 and 140ml are available.

6.6 Special precautions for disposal and other handling

Not applicable.

7. MARKETING AUTHORISATION HOLDER

Abbott Laboratories Limited

Queenborough

Kent

ME11 5EL

8. MARKETING AUTHORISATION NUMBER(S)

0037/0277

9. DATE OF FIRST AUTHORISATION/RENEWAL OF THE AUTHORISATION

19th May 1999

10. DATE OF REVISION OF THE TEXT

14 September 2006

Klaricid XL

(Abbott Laboratories Limited)

1. NAME OF THE MEDICINAL PRODUCT

Klaricid XL **or Clarithromycin 500 mg Modified Release Tablets**

2. QUALITATIVE AND QUANTITATIVE COMPOSITION

	mg/tablet
Active: Clarithromycin	500.00

3. PHARMACEUTICAL FORM

A yellow, ovaloid tablet containing 500mg clarithromycin in a modified-release preparation.

4. CLINICAL PARTICULARS

4.1 Therapeutic indications

Klaricid XL **or Clarithromycin 500 mg Modified Release Tablets** is indicated for treatment of infections caused by susceptible organisms. Indications include:

Lower respiratory tract infections for example, acute and chronic bronchitis, and pneumonia.

Upper respiratory tract infections for example, sinusitis and pharyngitis.

Klaricid XL **or Clarithromycin 500 mg Modified Release Tablets** is also indicated in skin and soft tissue infections of mild to moderate severity, for example folliculitis, cellulitis and erysipelas.

4.2 Posology and method of administration

Adults: The usual recommended dosage of Klaricid XL **or Clarithromycin 500 mg Modified Release Tablets** in adults is one 500mg modified-release tablet daily to be taken with food.

In more severe infections, the dosage can be increased to two 500mg modified-release tablets daily. The usual duration of treatment is 7 to 14 days.

Children older than 12 years: As for adults.

Children younger than 12 years: Use Klaricid Paediatric Suspension **or Clarithromycin 125 mg/5ml Granules for Oral Suspension**.

Klaricid XL **or Clarithromycin 500 mg Modified Release Tablets** should not be used in patients with renal impairment (creatinine clearance less than 30 mL/min). Clarithromycin immediate release tablets may be used in this patient population. (See 4.3 Contra-indications).

4.3 Contraindications

Clarithromycin is contra-indicated in patients with known hypersensitivity to macrolide antibiotic drugs.

Clarithromycin and ergot derivatives should not be co-administered (see section 4.5).

As the dose cannot be reduced from 500mg daily, Klaricid XL **or Clarithromycin 500 mg Modified Release Tablets** is contraindicated in patients with creatinine clearance less than 30 mL/min.

Concomitant administration of clarithromycin and any of the following drugs is contraindicated: cisapride, pimozide and terfenadine. Elevated cisapride, pimozide and terfenadine levels have been reported in patients receiving either of these drugs and clarithromycin concomitantly. This may result in QT prolongation and cardiac arrhythmias including ventricular fibrillation and torsade de pointes. Similar effects have been observed with concomitant administration of astemizole and other macrolides.

4.4 Special warnings and precautions for use

Clarithromycin is principally excreted by the liver and kidney. Caution should be exercised in administering this antibiotic to patients with impaired hepatic and renal function.

Prolonged or repeated used of clarithromycin may result in an overgrowth of non-susceptible bacteria or fungi. If super-infection occurs, clarithromycin should be discontinued and appropriate therapy instituted.

There have been post-marketing reports of colchicine toxicity with concomitant use of clarithromycin and colchicine, especially in the elderly, some of which occurred in patients with renal insufficiency. Deaths have been reported ins ome such patients (see Section 4.5).

Patients with rare hereditary problems of fructose intolerance, glucose-galactose malabsorption or sucrase-isomaltase insufficiency should not take this medicine.

4.5 Interaction with other medicinal products and other forms of interaction

Clarithromycin has been shown not to interact with oral contraceptives.

As with other macrolide antibiotics the use of clarithromycin in patients concurrently taking drugs metabolised by the cytochrome P450 system (eg. Cilostazol, methylprednisolone, anticoagulants (eg warfarin) quinidine, sildenafil, ergot alkaloids, alprazolam, triazolam, midazolam, disopyramide, lovastatin, rifabutin, phenytoin, cyclosporin, vinblastine, valproate and tacrolimus) may be associated with elevations in serum levels of these other drugs. Rhabdomyolysis, co-incident with the co- administration of clarithromycin, and HMG-CoA reductase inhibitors, such as lovastatin and simvastatin has been reported.

The administration of clarithromycin to patients who are receiving theophylline has been associated with an increase in serum theophylline levels and potential theophylline toxicity.

The use of clarithromycin in patients receiving warfarin may result in potentiation of the effects of warfarin. Prothrombin time should be frequently monitored in these patients.

The effects of digoxin may be potentiated with concomitant administration of clarithromycin. Monitoring of serum digoxin levels should be considered.

Clarithromycin may potentiate the effects of carbamazepine due to a reduction in the rate of excretion.

Interaction studies have not been conducted with Klaricid XL **or Clarithromycin 500 mg Modified Release Tablets** and zidovudine. If concomitant administration of clarithromycin and zidovudine is required, then an immediate release formulation of clarithromycin should be used.

There have been post-marketed reports of Torsade de Pointes occurring with the concurrent use of clarithromycin and quinidine or disopyramide. Levels of these medications should be monitored during clarithromycin therapy.

Colchicine is a substrate for both CYP3A and the efflux transporter, P-glycoprotein (Pgp). Clarithromycin and other macrolides are known to inhibit CYP3A and Pgp. When clarithromycin and colchicine are administered together, inhibition of Pgp and/or CYP3A by clarithromycin may lead to increased exposure to colchicine. Patients should be monitored for clinical symptoms of colchicine toxicity (see Section 4.4).

Post-marketing reports indicate that co-administration of clarithromycin with ergotamine or dihydroergotamine has been associated with acute ergot toxicity characterized by vasospasm and ischaemia of the extremities and other tissues including the central nervous system (see section 4.3 Contra-indications).

Ritonavir increases the area under the curve (AUC), C_{max} and C_{min} of clarithromycin when administered concurrently. Because of the large therapeutic window for clarithromycin, no dosage reduction should be necessary in patients with normal renal function. However, for patients with renal impairment an immediate release form of clarithromycin should be used. Doses of clarithromycin greater than 1g/day should not be coadministered with ritonavir.

4.6 Pregnancy and lactation

The safety of clarithromycin during pregnancy and breast feeding of infants has not been established. Clarithromycin should thus not be used during pregnancy or lactation unless the benefit is considered to outweigh the risk. Some animal studies have suggested an embryotoxic effect, but only at dose levels which are clearly toxic to mothers. Clarithromycin has been found in the milk of lactating animals and in human breast milk.

4.7 Effects on ability to drive and use machines

The medicine is unlikely to produce an effect.

4.8 Undesirable effects

Clarithromycin is generally well tolerated. Side effects include nausea, dyspepsia, diarrhoea, vomiting, abdominal pain and paraesthesia. Stomatitis, glossitis, oral monilia and tongue discolouration have been reported. Other side-effects include headache, arthralgia, myalgia and allergic reactions ranging from urticaria, mild skin eruptions and angioedema to anaphylaxis have been reported. There have been reports of Stevens-Johnson syndrome / toxic epidermal necrolysis with orally administered clarithromycin.

Reports of alteration of the sense of smell, usually in conjunction with taste perversion have also been received. There have been reports of tooth discolouration in patients treated with clarithromycin. Tooth discolouration is usually reversible with professional dental cleaning.

There have been reports of transient central nervous system side-effects including dizziness, vertigo, anxiety, insomnia, bad dreams, tinnitus, confusion, disorientation, hallucinations, psychosis and depersonalisation. There have been reports of hearing loss with clarithromycin which is usually reversible on withdrawal of therapy. Pseudomembranous colitis has been reported rarely with clarithromycin, and may range in severity from mild to life threatening. There have been rare reports of hypoglycaemia, some of which have occurred in patients on concomitant oral hypoglycaemic agents or insulin. There have been very rare reports of uveitis mainly in patients treated with concomitant rifabutin, most of these were reversible. Isolated cases of leukopenia andthrombocytopenia have been reported.

As with other macrolides, hepatic dysfunction (which is usually reversible) including altered liver function tests, hepatitis and cholestasis with or without jaundice, has been reported. Dysfunction may be severe and very rarely fatal hepatic failure has been reported.

Cases of increased serum creatinine, interstitial nephritis, renal failure, pancreatitis and convulsions have been reported rarely.

As with other macrolides, QT prolongation, ventricular tachycardia and Torsade de Pointes have been rarely reported with clarithromycin.

There have been post-marketing reports of colchicine toxicity with concomitant use of clarithromycin and colchicine, especially in the elderly, some of which occurred in patients with renal insufficiency. Deaths have been reported in some such patients (see Sections 4.4 and 4.5).

4.9 Overdose

Reports indicate that the ingestion of large amounts of clarithromycin can be expected to produce gastro-intestinal symptoms. One patient who had a history of bipolar disorder ingested 8 grams of clarithromycin and showed altered mental status, paranoid behaviour, hypokalaemia and hypoxaemia. Adverse reactions accompanying overdosage should be treated by gastric lavage and supportive measures. As with other macrolides, clarithromycin serum levels are not expected to be appreciably affected by haemodialysis or peritoneal dialysis.

5. PHARMACOLOGICAL PROPERTIES

5.1 Pharmacodynamic properties

Clarithromycin is a semi-synthetic derivative of erythromycin A. It exerts its antibacterial action by binding to the 50s ribosomal sub-unit of susceptible bacteria and suppresses protein synthesis. It is highly potent against a wide variety of aerobic and anaerobic gram-positive and gram-negative organisms. The minimum inhibitory concentrations (MICs) of clarithromycin are generally two-fold lower than the MICs of erythromycin.

The 14-hydroxy metabolite of clarithromycin also has antimicrobial activity. The MICs of this metabolite are equal or two-fold higher than the MICs of the parent compound, except for *H. influenzae* where the 14-hydroxy metabolite is two-fold more active than the parent compound.

Clarithromycin is usually active against the following organisms in vitro:

Gram-positive Bacteria: *Staphylococcus aureus* (methicillin susceptible); *Streptococcus pyogenes* (Group A beta-hemolytic streptococci); alpha-hemolytic streptococci (viridans group); *Streptococcus (Diplococcus) pneumoniae; Streptococcus agalactiae; Listeria monocytogenes.*

Gram-negative Bacteria: *Haemophilus influenza; Haemophilus parainfluenza; Moraxella (Branhamella) catarrhalis; Neisseria gonorrhoeae; Legionella pneumophila; Bordetella pertussis; Campylobacter jejuni.*

Mycoplasma: *Mycoplasma pneumoniae; Ureaplasma urealyticum.*

Other Organisms: *Chlamydia trachomatis; Mycobacterium avium; Mycobacterium leprae; Mycobacterium kansasii; Mycobacterium chelonae; Mycobacterium fortuitum; Mycobacterium intracellularis; Chlamydia pneumoniae.*

Anaerobes: *Clostridium perfringens*; Peptococcus species; Peptostreptococcus species; *Propionibacterium acnes*.

Clarithromycin has bactericidal activity against several bacterial strains. The organisms include *Haemophilus influenzae; Streptococcus pneumoniae; Streptococcus pyogenes; Streptococcus agalactiae; Moraxella (Branhamella) catarrhalis; Neisseria gonorrhoeae* and Campylobacter spp.

5.2 Pharmacokinetic properties

The kinetics of orally administered modified-release clarithromycin have been studied in adult humans and compared with clarithromycin 250mg and 500mg immediate release tablets. The extent of absorption was found to be equivalent when equal total daily doses were administered. The absolute bioavailability is approximately 50%. Little or no unpredicted accumulation was found and the metabolic disposition did not change in any species following multiple dosing. Based upon the finding of equivalent absorption the following *in vitro* and *in vivo* data are applicable to the modified-release formulation.

In vitro: Results of in vitro studies showed that the protein binding of clarithromycin in human plasma averaged about 70 % at concentrations of 0.45 - 4.5μg/mL. A decrease in binding to 41% at 45.0μg/mL suggested that the binding sites might become saturated, but this only occurred at concentrations far in excess of therapeutic drug levels.

In vivo: Clarithromycin levels in all tissues, except the central nervous system, were several times higher than the circulating drug levels. The highest concentrations were found in the liver and lung tissue, where the tissue to plasma ratios reached 10 to 20.

The pharmacokinetic behaviour of clarithromycin is non-linear. In fed patients given 500mg clarithromycin modified-release daily, the peak steady state plasma concentration of clarithromycin and 14 hydroxy clarithromycin were 1.3 and 0.48μg/mL, respectively. When the dosage was increased to 1000mg daily, these steady-state values were 2.4μg/mL and 0.67μg/mL respectively. Elimination half-lives of the parent drug and metabolite were approximately 5.3 and 7.7 hours respectively. The apparent half-lives of both clarithromycin and its hydroxylated metabolite tended to be longer at higher doses.

Urinary excretion accounted for approximately 40% of the clarithromycin dose. Faecal elimination accounts for approximately 30%.

5.3 Preclinical safety data

In repeated dose studies, clarithromycin toxicity was related to dose and duration of treatment. The primary target organ was the liver in all species, with hepatic lesions seen after 14 days in dogs and monkeys. Systemic exposure levels associated with this toxicity are not known but toxic mg/kg doses were higher than the dose recommended for patient treatment.

No evidence of mutagenic potential of clarithromycin was seen during a range of in vitro and in vivo tests.

Fertility and reproduction studies in rats have shown no adverse effects. Teratogenicity studies in rats (Wistar (p.o.) and Sprague-Dawley (p.o. and i.v.)), New Zealand White rabbits and cynomolgous monkeys failed to demonstrate any teratogenicity from clarithromycin. However, a further similar study in Sprague-Dawley rats indicated a low (6%) incidence of cardiovascular abnormalities which appeared to be due to spontaneous expression of genetic changes. Two mouse studies revealed a variable incidence (3-30%) of cleft palate and in monkeys embryonic loss was seen but only at dose levels which were clearly toxic to the mothers.

No other toxicological findings considered to be of relevance to the dose level recommended for patient treatment have been reported.

6. PHARMACEUTICAL PARTICULARS

6.1 List of excipients

Citric acid anhydrous, sodium alginate, sodium calcium alginate, lactose, povidone K30, talc, stearic acid, magnesium stearate, methyl hydroxypropylcellulose 6cps, polyethylene glycol 400, macrogol 8000, titanium dioxide (E171), sorbic acid, quinoline yellow (dye) aluminium lake (E104).

6.2 Incompatibilities

None known.

6.3 Shelf life

The shelf-life is 18 months when stored in HDPE or glass bottles and 36 months when stored in PVC/PVdC blisters.

6.4 Special precautions for storage

Do not store above 30°C Store in the original package.

6.5 Nature and contents of container

1,4,5,6,7 or 14 tablets in a blister original pack or in bottles. The blisters, of PVC/PVdC, are heat sealed with 20 micron hard tempered aluminium foil and packaged in a cardboard carton with a pack insert. The bottles, of HDPE or glass, are packaged in a cardboard carton with a pack insert.

6.6 Special precautions for disposal and other handling

Not applicable.

7. MARKETING AUTHORISATION HOLDER

Abbott Laboratories Limited

Queenborough

Kent

ME11 5EL

8. MARKETING AUTHORISATION NUMBER(S)

PL00037/0275

9. DATE OF FIRST AUTHORISATION/RENEWAL OF THE AUTHORISATION

December 1996

10. DATE OF REVISION OF THE TEXT

September 2007

KLEAN PREP 69g, sachet powders for oral solution.

(Norgine Limited)

1. NAME OF THE MEDICINAL PRODUCT

KLEAN PREP 69g, sachet powders for oral solution.

2. QUALITATIVE AND QUANTITATIVE COMPOSITION

Each sachet of KLEAN PREP contains the following active ingredients:

Macrogol 3350	59.000 g
Anhydrous Sodium Sulphate	5.685 g
Sodium Bicarbonate	1.685 g
Sodium Chloride	1.465 g
Potassium Chloride	0.7425 g

The content of electrolyte ions per sachet when made up to one litre of water is as follows:

Sodium	125 mM
Sulphate	40 mM
Chloride	35 mM
Bicarbonate	20 mM
Potassium	10 mM

For excipients, see 6.1.

3. PHARMACEUTICAL FORM

A whitish powder which, when dissolved in water, gives a clear, colourless solution for oral administration.

4. CLINICAL PARTICULARS

4.1 Therapeutic indications

For colonic lavage prior to diagnostic examination or surgical procedures requiring a clean colon, eg colonoscopy, barium enema or colonic resection.

4.2 Posology and method of administration

Adults: Each sachet should be dissolved in 1 litre of water. The usual dose is up to 4 sachets taken at a rate of 250 ml every 10 to 15 minutes until the total volume is consumed or rectal effluent is clear, or as directed by the physician.

The solutions from all 4 sachets should be drunk within 4 to 6 hours. Alternatively, administration may be divided, for example, taking 2 sachets during the evening before the examination, and the remaining 2 sachets on the morning of the examination.

If administration is by nasogastric tube, the usual rate should be 20 to 30 ml/minute.

Children: There is no recommended dosage.

Renal patients: No dosage adjustment need be made.

4.3 Contraindications

Use in patients with known or suspected gastrointestinal obstruction or perforation, ileus, gastric retention, acute intestinal or gastric ulceration, toxic colitis or toxic megacolon.

Hypersensitivity to any of the ingredients.

4.4 Special warnings and precautions for use

No solid food should be eaten for at least 2 hours before taking KLEAN PREP. The product should only be administered with caution to patients with impaired gag reflex, reflux oesophagitis or those with diminished levels of consciousness and patients with ulcerative colitis.

Unconscious, semi-conscious patients or patients prone to aspiration or regurgitation should be observed during administration especially if this is via the nasogastric route.

4.5 Interaction with other medicinal products and other forms of interaction

Oral medication taken within one hour of administration of KLEAN PREP may be flushed from the gastro-intestinal tract and not absorbed.

4.6 Pregnancy and lactation

The preparation should only be used during pregnancy and lactation if considered essential by the physician. There is no experience of use during pregnancy. The purpose and mechanisms of use should be borne in mind if the physician is considering administration.

4.7 Effects on ability to drive and use machines

There is no known effect on the ability to drive and use machines.

4.8 Undesirable effects

Nausea, abdominal fullness and bloating may be experienced. Should distension or pain arise, the rate of administration should be slowed down or temporarily stopped until symptoms subside. Abdominal cramps, vomiting and anal irritation occur less frequently.

These effects normally subside rapidly. Urticaria and allergic reactions have been reported rarely.

4.9 Overdose

In case of gross accidental overdosage, where diarrhoea is severe, conservative measures are usually sufficient; generous amounts of fluid, especially fruit juices, should be given.

5. PHARMACOLOGICAL PROPERTIES

5.1 Pharmacodynamic properties

ATC Code: A06A D

Macrogol 3350 exerts its effects by virtue of its osmotic effect in the gut, which induces a laxative effect. The electrolytes also present in the formulation ensure that there is virtually no net gain or loss of sodium, potassium or water, and thus no dehydration.

5.2 Pharmacokinetic properties

Macrogol 3350 is unchanged along the gut. It is virtually unabsorbed from the gastro-intestinal tract. Any macrogol 3350 that is absorbed is excreted via the urine.

5.3 Preclinical safety data

Preclinical studies provide evidence that macrogol 3350 has no significant systemic toxicity potential.

6. PHARMACEUTICAL PARTICULARS

6.1 List of excipients

Vanilla flavour

Aspartame.

6.2 Incompatibilities

None are known.

6.3 Shelf life

Sachets:	3 years
Solution after reconstitution:	24 hours

6.4 Special precautions for storage

Sachets: Store in a dry place. Do not store above 25°C.

6.5 Nature and contents of container

Sachets containing 69gm white powder, in a box of 4 sachets.

6.6 Special precautions for disposal and other handling

The solution should be used within 24 hours.

7. MARKETING AUTHORISATION HOLDER

Norgine Limited

Chaplin House

Widewater Place

Moorhall Road

Harefield

UXBRIDGE

Middlesex UB9 6NS

United Kingdom.

8. MARKETING AUTHORISATION NUMBER(S)

PL: 00322/0068.

9. DATE OF FIRST AUTHORISATION/RENEWAL OF THE AUTHORISATION

August 1991/March 1997.

10. DATE OF REVISION OF THE TEXT

29 April 2009

Kliofem

(Novo Nordisk Limited)

1. NAME OF THE MEDICINAL PRODUCT

Kliofem®

2. QUALITATIVE AND QUANTITATIVE COMPOSITION

Active ingredients:

Estradiol 2 mg

Norethisterone acetate 1 mg.

For excipients, see 6.1

3. PHARMACEUTICAL FORM

Film-coated tablet for oral administration.

4. CLINICAL PARTICULARS

4.1 Therapeutic indications

1 Hormone replacement therapy (HRT) for oestrogen deficiency symptoms in women more than one year after menopause.

2 Prevention of osteoporosis in postmenopausal women at high risk of future fractures who are intolerant of, or contra-indicated for, other medicinal products approved for the prevention of osteoporosis.

See also section 4.4

The experience of treating women older than 65 years is limited.

4.2 Posology and method of administration

Kliofem is a continuous combined hormone replacement product intended for use in women with an intact uterus. One tablet should be taken orally once a day without interruption, preferably at the same time every day.

For initiation and continuation of treatment of postmenopausal symptoms, the lowest effective dose for the shortest duration (see also section 4.4) should be used.

In women with amenorrhea and not taking HRT or women transferring from another continuous combined HRT product, treatment with Kliofem may be started on any convenient day. In women transferring from sequential HRT regimens, treatment should start as soon as their withdrawal bleeding has ended.

Unless there is a previous diagnosis of endometriosis, it is not recommended to add a progestogen in hysterectomised women.

If the patient has forgotten to take one tablet, the forgotten tablet should be taken within the next twelve hours. Otherwise the tablet should be discarded. Forgetting a dose may increase the likelihood of breakthrough bleeding and spotting.

4.3 Contraindications

- Known, past or suspected breast cancer.
- Known or suspected oestrogen-dependent malignant tumours (e.g. endometrial cancer).
- Undiagnosed genital bleeding.
- Untreated endometrial hyperplasia.
- Previous idiopathic or current venous thromboembolism (deep venous thrombosis, pulmonary embolism).
- Active or recent arterial thromboembolic disease (e.g. angina, myocardial infarction).
- Acute liver disease, or a history of liver disease as long as liver function tests have failed to return to normal.
- Known hypersensitivity to the active substances or any of the excipients.
- Porphyria.

4.4 Special warnings and precautions for use

For the treatment of postmenopausal symptoms, HRT should only be initiated for symptoms that adversely affect quality of life. In all cases, a careful appraisal of the risks and benefits should be undertaken at least annually and HRT should only be continued as long as the benefit outweighs the risk.

Medical examination/follow-up

Before initiating or reinstituting HRT, a complete personal and family medical history should be taken. Physical (including pelvic and breast) examination should be guided by this and by the contra-indications and warnings for use. During treatment, periodic check-ups are recommended of a frequency and nature adapted to the individual woman. Women should be advised what changes in their breasts should be reported to their doctor or nurse (see 'Breast cancer' section below). Investigations, including mammography, should be carried out in accordance with currently accepted screening practices, modified to the clinical needs of the individual.

Conditions which need supervision

If any of the following conditions are present, have occurred previously, and/or have been aggravated during pregnancy or previous hormone treatment, the patient should be closely supervised. It should be taken into account that these conditions may recur or be aggravated during treatment with Kliofem, in particular:

- Leiomyoma (uterine fibroids) or endometriosis
- A history of, or risk factors for, thromboembolic disorders (see below)
- Risk factors for oestrogen dependent tumours, e.g. 1st degree heredity for breast cancer
- Hypertension
- Liver disorders (e.g. liver adenoma)
- Diabetes mellitus with or without vascular involvement
- Cholelithiasis
- Migraine or (severe) headache
- Systemic lupus erythematosus
- A history of endometrial hyperplasia (see below)
- Epilepsy
- Asthma
- Otosclerosis

Reasons for immediate withdrawal of therapy

Therapy should be discontinued in case a contra-indication is discovered and in the following situations:

- Jaundice or deterioration in liver function
- Significant increase in blood pressure
- New onset of migraine-type headache
- Pregnancy

Endometrial hyperplasia

The risk of endometrial hyperplasia and carcinoma is increased when oestrogens are administered alone for prolonged periods (see section 4.8). The addition of a progestogen for at least 12 days per cycle in non-hysterectomised women greatly reduces this risk.

Breakthrough bleeding and spotting may occur during the first months of treatment. If breakthrough bleeding or spotting occurs after some time on therapy, or continues after treatment has been discontinued, the reason should be investigated, which may include endometrial biopsy to exclude endometrial malignancy.

Breast Cancer

A randomised placebo-controlled trial, the Women's Health Initiative study (WHI), and epidemiological studies, including the Million Women Study (MWS), have reported an increased risk of breast cancer in women taking oestrogens, oestrogen-progestogen combinations or tibolone for HRT for several years (see Section 4.8). For all HRT, an excess risk becomes apparent within a few years of use and increases with duration of intake but returns to baseline within a few (at most five) years after stopping treatment.

In the MWS, the relative risk of breast cancer with conjugated equine oestrogens (CEE) or estradiol (E2) was greater when a progestogen was added, either sequentially or continuously, and regardless of type of progestogen. There was no evidence of a difference in risk between the different routes of administration.

In the WHI study, the continuous combined conjugated equine oestrogen and medroxyprogesterone acetate (CEE + MPA) product used was associated with breast cancers that were slightly larger in size and more frequently had local lymph node metastases compared to placebo.

HRT, especially oestrogen-progestogen combined treatment, increases the density of mammographic images which may adversely affect the radiological detection of breast cancer.

Venous thromboembolism

HRT is associated with a higher relative risk of developing venous thromboembolism (VTE), i.e. deep vein thrombosis or pulmonary embolism. One randomised controlled trial and epidemiological studies found a two- to threefold higher risk for users compared with non-users. For non-users it is estimated that the number of cases of VTE that will occur over a 5 year period is about 3 per 1000 women aged 50-59 years and 8 per 1000 women aged between 60-69 years. It is estimated that in healthy women who use HRT for 5 years, the number of additional cases of VTE over a 5 year period will be between 2 and 6 (best estimate = 4) per 1000 women aged 50-59 years and between 5 and 15 (best estimate = 9) per 1000 women aged 60-69 years. The occurrence of such an event is more likely in the first year of HRT than later.

Generally recognised risk factors for VTE include a personal history or family history, severe obesity (BMI >30 kg/m^2) and systemic lupus erythematosus (SLE). There is no consensus about the possible role of varicose veins in VTE.

Patients with a history of VTE or known thrombophilic states have an increased risk of VTE. HRT may add to this risk. Personal or strong family history of thromboembolism, or recurrent spontaneous abortion, should be investigated in order to exclude a thrombophilic predisposition. Until a thorough evaluation of thrombophilic factors has been made or anticoagulant treatment initiated, use of HRT in such patients should be viewed as contraindicated. Those women already on anticoagulant treatment require careful consideration of the benefit-risk of use of HRT.

The risk of VTE may be temporarily increased with prolonged immobilisation, major trauma or major surgery. As in all postoperative patients, scrupulous attention should be given to prophylactic measures to prevent VTE following surgery. Where prolonged immobilisation is liable to follow elective surgery, particularly abdominal or orthopaedic surgery to the lower limbs, consideration should be given to temporarily stopping HRT 4 to 6 weeks earlier, if possible. Treatment should not be restarted until the woman is completely mobilised.

If VTE develops after initiating therapy, the drug should be discontinued. Patients should be told to contact their doctors immediately when they are aware of a potential thromboembolic symptom (e.g. painful swelling of a leg, sudden pain in the chest, dyspnoea).

Coronary artery disease (CAD)

There is no evidence from randomised controlled trials of cardiovascular benefit with continuous combined conjugated oestrogens and medroxyprogesterone acetate (MPA). Two large clinical trials (WHI and HERS i.e. Heart and Estrogen/progestin Replacement Study) showed a possible increased risk of cardiovascular morbidity in the first year of use and no overall benefit. For other HRT products there are only limited data from randomised controlled trials examining effects in cardiovascular morbidity or mortality. Therefore it is uncertain whether these findings also extend to other HRT products.

Stroke

One large randomised clinical trial (WHI-trial) found, as a secondary outcome, an increased risk of ischaemic stroke in healthy women during treatment with continuous combined conjugated oestrogens and MPA. For women who do not use HRT, it is estimated that the number of cases of stroke that will occur over a 5-year period is about 3 per 1000 women aged 50-59 years and 11 per 1000 women aged 60-69 years. It is estimated that for women who use conjugated oestrogens and MPA for 5 years, the number of additional cases will be between 0 and 3 (best estimate = 1) per 1000 users aged 50-59 years and between 1 and 9 (best estimate = 4) per 1000 users aged 60-69 years. It is unknown whether the increased risk also extends to other HRT products.

Ovarian cancer

Long term (at least 5-10 years) use of oestrogen-only HRT products in hysterectomised women has been associated with an increased risk of ovarian cancer in some epidemiological studies. It is uncertain whether long-term use of combined HRT confers a different risk than oestrogen-only products.

Other conditions

- Oestrogens may cause fluid retention, and therefore patients with cardiac or renal dysfunction should be carefully observed. Patients with terminal renal insufficiency should be closely observed, since it is expected that the level of circulating active ingredients in Kliofem will be increased.

- Women with pre-existing hypertriglyceridemia should be followed closely during oestrogen replacement or hormone replacement therapy, since rare cases of large increases of plasma triglycerides leading to pancreatitis have been reported with oestrogen therapy in this condition.

- Oestrogens increase thyroid binding globulin (TGB), leading to increased circulating total thyroid hormone, as measured by protein-bound iodine (PBI), T4 levels (by column or by radio-immunoassay) or T3 levels (by radio-immunoassay). T3 resin uptake is decreased, reflecting the elevated TBG. Free T4 and free T3 concentrations are unaltered. Other binding proteins may be elevated in serum, i.e. corticoid binding globulin (CBG), sex-hormone-binding globulin (SHBG) leading to increased circulating corticosteroids and sex steroids, respectively. Free or biologically active hormone concentrations are unchanged. Other plasma proteins may be increased (angiotensinogen/renin substrate, alpha-1-antitrypsin, ceruloplasmin).

- There is no conclusive evidence for improvement of cognitive function. There is some evidence from the WHI trial of increased risk of probable dementia in women who start using continuous combined CEE and MPA after the age of 65. It is unknown whether the findings apply to younger post-menopausal women or other HRT products.

- Kliofem tablets contain lactose. Patients with rare hereditary problems of galactose intolerance, the Lapp lactase deficiency or glucose-galactose malabsorption should not take this medicine.

4.5 Interaction with other medicinal products and other forms of interaction

The metabolism of oestrogens and progestogens may be increased by concomitant use of substances known to induce drug-metabolising enzymes, specifically cytochrome P450 enzymes, such as anticonvulsants (e.g. phenobarbital, phenytoin, carbamezapin) and anti-infectives (e.g. rifampicin, rifabutin, nevirapine, efavirenz).

Ritonavir and nelfinavir, although known as strong inhibitors, by contrast exhibit inducing properties when used concomitantly with steroid hormones. Herbal preparations containing St John's wort (*Hypericum perforatum*) may induce the metabolism of oestrogens and progestogens.

Clinically, an increased metabolism of oestrogens and progestogens may lead to decreased effect and changes in the uterine bleeding profile.

Drugs that inhibit the activity of hepatic microsomal drug metabolising enzymes, e.g. ketoconazole, may increase circulating levels of the active substances in Kliofem.

4.6 Pregnancy and lactation

Kliofem is not indicated during pregnancy. If pregnancy occurs during medication with Kliofem, treatment should be withdrawn immediately.

Data on a limited number of exposed pregnancies indicate adverse effects of norethisterone on the foetus. At dose levels higher than normally used in OC and HRT formulations masculinisation of female foetuses was observed. The results of most of epidemiological studies to-date have not indicated a teratogenic or foetotoxic effect when combinations of oestrogens with progestogens at dose levels relevant for Kliofem were taken inadvertently during pregnancy.

Lactation

Kliofem is not indicated during lactation.

4.7 Effects on ability to drive and use machines

No effects known.

4.8 Undesirable effects

Clinical experience:

The most frequently reported adverse events in the clinical trials with Kliofem were vaginal bleedings and breast pain/tenderness, reported in approximately 10% to 30% of patients. Vaginal bleedings usually occurred in the first months of treatment. Breast pain usually disappears after a few months of therapy. All adverse events observed in the randomised clinical trials with a higher frequency in patients treated with Kliofem or similar HRT products as compared to placebo and which on an overall judgement were considered as possibly related to treatment are presented below.

(see Table 1 on next page)

Table 1

System organ class	Very common >1/10	Common >1/100; <1/10	Uncommon >1/1,000; <1/100	Rare >1/10,000; <1/1,000
Infections and infestations		Genital candidiasis or vaginitis, see also 'Reproductive system and breast disorders'		
Immune system disorders			Hypersensitivity, see also 'Skin and subcutaneous tissue disorders'	
Metabolism and nutrition disorders		Fluid retention, see also 'General disorders and administration site conditions'		
Psychiatric disorders		Depression or depression aggravated	Nervousness	
Nervous system disorders		Headache, migraine or migraine aggravated		
Vascular disorders			Thrombophlebitis superficial	Pulmonary embolism Deep vein thrombosis See also sections 4.3 and 4.4
Gastrointestinal disorders		Nausea Abdominal pain, abdominal distension or abdominal discomfort	Flatulence or bloating	
Skin and subcutaneous tissue disorders			Alopecia, hirsutism or acne Pruritus or urticaria	
Musculoskeletal, connective tissue and bone disorders		Back pain Leg cramps		
Reproductive system and breast disorders	Breast pain or breast tenderness Vaginal haemorrhage	Breast oedema or breast enlargement Uterine fibroids aggravated or uterine fibroids re-occurrence or uterine fibroids		
General disorders and administration site conditions		Oedema peripheral	Drug ineffective	
Investigations		Weight increased		

Post-marketing experience:

In addition to the above-mentioned adverse drug reactions, those presented below have been spontaneously reported, and by an overall judgement considered possible related to Kliofem treatment. The reporting rate of these spontaneous adverse drug reactions is very rare (<1/10,000 patient years):

Neoplasms benign and malignant (incl. cysts and polyps): Endometrial cancer

Psychiatric disorders: Insomnia, anxiety, libido decreased, libido increased

Nervous system disorders: Dizziness, stroke

Eye disorders: Visual disturbances

Vascular disorders: Hypertension aggravated

Cardiac disorders: Myocardial infarction

Gastrointestinal disorders: Dyspepsia, vomiting

Hepatobiliary disorders: Gallbladder disease, cholelithiasis, cholelithiasis aggravated, cholelithiasis re-occurrence

Skin and subcutaneous tissue disorder: Seborrhoea, rash, angioneurotic oedema

Reproductive system and breast disorders: Hyperplasia endometrial, vulvovaginal pruritus

Investigations: Weight decreased, blood pressure increased

Other adverse reactions have been reported in association with oestrogen/progestogen treatment:

- Skin and subcutaneous tissue disorders: chloasma, erythema multiforme, erythema nodosum, vascular purpura.

- Probable dementia (see section 4.4).

Breast cancer

According to evidence from a large number of epidemiological studies and one randomised placebo-controlled trial, the Women's Health Initiative (WHI), the overall risk of breast cancer increases with increasing duration of HRT use in current or recent HRT users.

For *oestrogen-only* HRT, estimates of relative risk (RR) from a reanalysis of original data from 51 epidemiological studies (in which >80% of HRT use was oestrogen-only HRT) and from the epidemiological Million Women Study (MWS) are similar at 1.35 (95% CI: 1.21-1.49) and 1.30 (95% CI: 1.21-1.40), respectively.

For *oestrogen plus progestogen* combined HRT, several epidemiological studies have reported an overall higher risk for breast cancer than with oestrogens alone.

The MWS reported that, compared to never users, the use of various types of oestrogen-progestogen combined HRT was associated with a higher risk of breast cancer (RR = 2.00, 95% CI: 1.88-2.12) than use of oestrogens alone (RR = 1.30, 95% CI: 1.21-1.40) or use of tibolone (RR = 1.45, 95% CI: 1.25-1.68).

The WHI trial reported a risk estimate of 1.24 (95% CI: 1.01-1.54) after 5.6 years of use of oestrogen-progestogen combined HRT (CEE + MPA) in all users compared with placebo.

The absolute risks calculated from the MWS and the WHI trials are presented below:

The MWS has estimated, from the known average incidence of breast cancer in developed countries, that:

- For women not using HRT, about 32 in every 1000 are expected to have breast cancer diagnosed between the ages of 50 and 64 years.

- For 1000 current or recent users of HRT, the number of *additional* cases during the corresponding period will be

  - For users of *oestrogen only* replacement therapy,
    - between 0 and 3 (best estimate = 1.5) for 5 years' use
    - between 3 and 7 (best estimate = 5) for 10 years' use.
  - For users of *oestrogen plus progestogen* combined HRT,
    - between 5 and 7 (best estimate = 6) for 5 years' use
    - between 18 and 20 (best estimate = 19) for 10 years use.

The WHI trial estimated that after 5.6 years of follow-up of women between the ages of 50 and 79 years, an *additional* 8 cases of invasive breast cancer would be due to *oestrogen-progestogen combined* HRT (CEE + MPA) per 10,000 women years. According to calculations from the trial data, it is estimated that:

- For 1000 women in the placebo group,

- about 16 cases of invasive breast cancer would be diagnosed in 5 years.

- For 1000 women who used oestrogen + progestogen combined HRT (CEE + MPA), the number of additional cases would be

- between 0 and 9 (best estimate = 4) for 5 years' use.

The number of additional cases of breast cancer in women who use HRT is broadly similar for women who start HRT irrespective of age at start of use (between the ages of 45-65) (see section 4.4).

Endometrial cancer

In women with an intact uterus, the risk of endometrial hyperplasia and endometrial cancer increases with increasing duration of use of unopposed oestrogens. According to data from epidemiological studies, the best estimate of the risk is that for women not using HRT, about 5 in every 1000 are expected to have endometrial cancer diagnosed between the ages of 50 and 65. Depending on the duration of treatment and oestrogen dose, the reported increase in endometrial cancer risk among unopposed oestrogen users varies from 2- to 12-fold greater compared with non-users. Adding a progestogen to oestrogen-only therapy greatly reduces this increased risk.

4.9 Overdose

Overdosage may be manifested by nausea and vomiting. There is no specific antidote and treatment should be symptomatic.

5. PHARMACOLOGICAL PROPERTIES

5.1 Pharmacodynamic properties

ATC code: G03F A01

Oestrogen and progestogen for continuous combined HRT treatment.

Estradiol: The active ingredient, synthetic 17 beta-estradiol, is chemically and biologically identical to endogenous human estradiol. It substitutes for the loss of oestrogen production in menopausal women, and alleviates menopausal symptoms.

Oestrogens prevent bone loss following menopause or ovariectomy.

Norethisterone acetate: As oestrogens promote the growth of the endometrium, unopposed oestrogens increase the risk of endometrial hyperplasia and cancer. The addition of a progestogen greatly reduces the oestrogen-induced risk of endometrial hyperplasia in non-hysterectomised women.

Relief of menopausal symptoms is achieved during the first few weeks of treatment.

Kliofem is a continuous combined HRT given with the intention of avoiding the regular withdrawal bleeding associated with cyclic or sequential HRT. Amenorrhoea (no bleeding and spotting) was seen in 94% of the women during months 10-12 of treatment. Bleeding and/or spotting appeared in 30% of the women during the first three months of treatment and in 6% during months 10-12 of treatment.

Oestrogen deficiency at menopause is associated with an increasing bone turnover and decline in bone mass. The effect of oestrogens on the bone mineral density is dose-dependent. Protection appears to be effective for as long as treatment is continued. After discontinuation of HRT, bone mass is lost at a rate similar to that in untreated women.

Evidence from the WHI trial and meta-analysed trials shows that current use of HRT, alone or in combination with a progestogen - given to predominantly healthy women - reduces the risk of hip, vertebral, and other osteoporotic fractures. HRT may also prevent fractures in women with low bone density and/or established osteoporosis, but the evidence for that is limited.

The effects of Kliofem on bone mineral density were examined in a 2-year, randomised, double-blind, placebo-controlled trial in postmenopausal women (n=327, including 48 on Kliofem). All women received calcium supplementation 1000 mg daily. Kliofem significantly prevented bone loss at the lumbar spine, total hip, distal radius and total body in comparison with calcium supplemented placebo-treated women. In early postmenopausal women (1 to 5 years since last menses), the percentage change from baseline in bone mineral density at lumbar spine, femoral neck and femoral trochanter after 2 years of treatment with Kliofem was 5.4±0.7%, 2.9±0.8% and 5.0±0.9%, respectively. The percentage of women who maintained or gained bone mineral density during treatment with Kliofem was 91% after 2 years of treatment.

5.2 Pharmacokinetic properties

Following oral administration of 17β-estradiol in micronised form, rapid absorption from the gastrointestinal tract occurs. It undergoes extensive first-pass metabolism in the liver and other enteric organs, and reaches a peak plasma concentration of approximately 44 pg/ml (range 30-53 pg/ml) within 5-8 hours after intake of 1 Kliofem tablet. The half life of 17β-estradiol is about 12-14 hours. It circulates bound to SHBG (37%) and to albumin (61%), while only approximately 1-2% is unbound. Metabolism of 17β-estradiol occurs mainly in the liver and the gut but also in target organs and involves the formation of less active or inactive metabolites, including oestrone, catecholoestrogens and several oestrogen sulphates and glucuronides. Oestrogens are excreted with the bile, where they are hydrolysed and reabsorbed (enterohepatic circulation), and mainly in urine in biologically inactive form.

After oral administration norethisterone acetate is rapidly absorbed and transformed to norethisterone (NET). It undergoes first-pass metabolism in the liver and other enteric organs, and reaches a peak plasma concentration of approximately 9 ng/ml (range 6-11 ng/ml) within 0.5 - 1.5 hours after intake of 1mg. The terminal half-life of NET is about 8-11 hours. NET binds to SHBG (36%) and to albumin (61%). The most important metabolites are isomers of 5α-dihydro-NET and of tetrahydro-NET, which are excreted mainly in the urine as sulphate or glucuronide conjugates.

The pharmacokinetics in the elderly have not been studied.

5.3 Preclinical safety data

Acute toxicity of oestrogens is low. Because of marked differences between animal species and between animal species and humans, preclinical results possess a limited predictive value for the use of oestrogens in humans.

In experimental animals estradiol and estradiol valerate displayed an embryolethal effect at relatively low doses; malformations of the urogenital tract and feminisation of male foetuses was observed.

Norethisterone, like other progestogens, caused virilisation of female foetuses in rats and monkeys. After high doses of norethisterone embryolethal effects were observed.

Preclinical data based on conventional studies of repeated dose toxicity, genotoxicity and carcinogenic potential revealed no particular human risks beyond those discussed in other sections of the SPC.

6. PHARMACEUTICAL PARTICULARS

6.1 List of excipients

Tablet core:

Lactose monohydrate

Maize starch

Gelatin

Magnesium stearate

Film-coating:

Hypromellose (E464)

Triacetin

Talc

6.2 Incompatibilities

None known.

6.3 Shelf life

48 months (max 25°C)

6.4 Special precautions for storage

Store at room temperature (max 25°C); protect from light and moisture.

6.5 Nature and contents of container

Polypropylene/polystyrene calendar dial pack containing 28 tablets. Calendar dial packs (3 × 28 tablets) are contained within outer carton.

6.6 Special precautions for disposal and other handling

Each carton contains a patient information leaflet with instructions for use of the calendar dial pack.

7. MARKETING AUTHORISATION HOLDER

Novo Nordisk Limited

Broadfield Park, Brighton Road

Crawley, West Sussex, RH11 9RT

8. MARKETING AUTHORISATION NUMBER(S)

PL 3132/0080

9. DATE OF FIRST AUTHORISATION/RENEWAL OF THE AUTHORISATION

18/06/2008

10. DATE OF REVISION OF THE TEXT

18/06/2008

LEGAL CATEGORY

POM.

Kliovance

(Novo Nordisk Limited)

1. NAME OF THE MEDICINAL PRODUCT

Kliovance® film-coated tablets.

2. QUALITATIVE AND QUANTITATIVE COMPOSITION

Each film-coated tablet contains:

Estradiol anhydrous 1 mg (as estradiol hemihydrate) and norethisterone acetate 0.5 mg.

For excipients, see 6.1.

3. PHARMACEUTICAL FORM

Film-coated tablets.

White film-coated, round, biconvex tablets with a diameter of 6 mm. The tablets are engraved with NOVO 288 on one side and the APIS on the other.

4. CLINICAL PARTICULARS

4.1 Therapeutic indications

Hormone Replacement Therapy (HRT) for oestrogen deficiency symptoms in women more than one year after menopause.

Prevention of osteoporosis in postmenopausal women at high risk of future fractures who are intolerant of, or contraindicated for, other medicinal products approved for the prevention of osteoporosis.

The experience of treating women older than 65 years is limited.

4.2 Posology and method of administration

Kliovance is a continuous-combined hormone replacement product intended for use in women with an intact uterus. One tablet should be taken orally once a day without interruption, preferably at the same time every day.

For initiation and continuation of treatment of postmenopausal symptoms, the lowest effective dose for the shortest duration (see also section 4.4) should be used.

A switch to a higher dose combination product could be indicated if the response after three months is insufficient for satisfactory symptom relief.

In women with amenorrhea and not taking HRT or women transferring from another continuous combined HRT product, treatment with Kliovance may be started on any convenient day. In women transferring from sequential HRT regimens, treatment should start as soon as their withdrawal bleeding has ended.

If the patient has forgotten to take one tablet, the forgotten tablet is to be discarded. Forgetting a dose may increase the likelihood of breakthrough bleeding and spotting.

4.3 Contraindications

- Known, past or suspected breast cancer
- Known or suspected oestrogen-dependent malignant tumours (e.g. endometrial cancer)
- Undiagnosed genital bleeding
- Untreated endometrial hyperplasia
- Previous idiopathic or current venous thromboembolism (deep venous thrombosis, pulmonary embolism)
- Active or recent arterial thromboembolic disease (e.g. angina, myocardial infarction)
- Acute liver disease, or a history of liver disease as long as liver function tests have failed to return to normal
- Known hypersensitivity to the active substances or to any of the excipients
- Porphyria

4.4 Special warnings and precautions for use

For the treatment of postmenopausal symptoms, HRT should only be initiated for symptoms that adversely affect quality of life. In all cases, a careful appraisal of the risks and benefits should be undertaken at least annually and HRT should only be continued as long as the benefit outweighs the risk.

Medical examination/follow-up

Before initiating or reinstituting HRT, a complete personal and family medical history should be taken. Physical (including pelvic and breast) examination should be guided by this and by the contraindications and warnings for use. During treatment periodic check-ups are recommended of a frequency and nature adapted to the individual woman. Women should be advised what changes in their breasts should be reported to their doctor or nurse (please see 'Breast cancer' section below). Investigations, including mammography, should be carried out in accordance with currently accepted screening practices, modified to the clinical needs of the individual.

Conditions which need supervision

If any of the following conditions are present, have occurred previously and/or have been aggravated during pregnancy or previous hormone treatment, the patient should be closely supervised. It should be taken into account that these conditions may recur or be aggravated during treatment with Kliovance, in particular:

- Leiomyoma (uterine fibroids) or endometriosis
- A history of, or risk factors for, thromboembolic disorders (see below)
- Risk factors for oestrogen dependent tumours, e.g. 1st degree heredity for breast cancer
- Hypertension
- Liver disorders (e.g. liver adenoma)
- Diabetes mellitus with or without vascular involvement
- Cholelithiasis
- Migraine or (severe) headache
- Systemic lupus erythematosus
- A history of endometrial hyperplasia (see below)
- Epilepsy
- Asthma
- Otosclerosis

Reasons for immediate withdrawal of therapy

Therapy should be discontinued in case a contra-indication is discovered and in the following situations:

- Jaundice or deterioration in liver function
- Significant increase in blood pressure
- New onset of migraine-type headache
- Pregnancy

Endometrial hyperplasia

The risk of endometrial hyperplasia and carcinoma is increased when oestrogens are administered alone for prolonged periods (see section 4.8). The addition of a progestogen for at least 12 days per cycle in non-hysterectomised women greatly reduces this risk.

Breakthrough bleeding and spotting may occur during the first months of treatment. If breakthrough bleeding or spotting appears after some time on therapy, or continues after treatment has been discontinued, the reason should be investigated, which may include endometrial biopsy to exclude endometrial malignancy.

Breast cancer

A randomised placebo-controlled trial, the Women's Health Initiative study (WHI), and epidemiological studies, including the Million Women Study (MWS), have reported an increased risk of breast cancer in women taking oestrogens, oestrogen-progestogen combinations or tibolone for HRT for several years (see Section 4.8). For all HRT an excess risk becomes apparent within a few years of use and increases with duration of intake but returns to baseline within a few (at most five) years after stopping treatment.

In the MWS, the relative risk of breast cancer with conjugated equine oestrogens (CEE) or estradiol (E2) was greater when a progestogen was added, either sequentially or continuously, and regardless of type of progestogen. There was no evidence of a difference in the risk between the different routes of administration.

In the WHI study, the continuous combined conjugated equine oestrogen and medroxyprogesterone acetate (CEE + MPA) product used was associated with breast cancers that were slightly larger in size and more frequently had local lymph node metastases compared to placebo.

HRT, especially oetrogen-progestogen combined treatment, increases the density of mammographic images which may adversely affect the radiological detection of breast cancers.

Venous thromboembolism

HRT is associated with a higher relative risk of developing venous thromboembolism (VTE), i.e. deep vein thrombosis or pulmonary embolism. One randomised controlled trial and epidemiological studies found a two- to threefold higher risk for users compared with non-users. For non-users it is estimated that the number of cases of VTE that will occur over a 5 year period is about 3 per 1000 women aged 50-59 years and 8 per 1000 women aged between 60-69 years. It is estimated that in healthy women who use HRT for 5 years, the number of additional cases of VTE over a 5 year period will be between 2 and 6 (best estimate=4) per 1000 women aged 50-59 years and between 5 and 15 (best estimate=9) per 1000 women aged 60-69 years. The occurrence of such an event is more likely in the first year of HRT than later.

Generally recognised risk factors for VTE include a personal history or family history, severe obesity (Body Mass Index > 30 kg/m^2) and systemic lupus erythematosus (SLE). There is no consensus about the possible role of varicose veins in VTE.

Patients with a history of VTE or known thrombophilic states have an increased risk of VTE. HRT may add to this risk. Personal or strong family history of thromboembolism, or recurrent spontaneous abortion, should be investigated in order to exclude a thrombophilic predisposition. Until a thorough evaluation of thrombophilic factors has been made or anticoagulant treatment initiated, use of HRT in such patients should be viewed as contraindicated. Those women already on anticoagulant treatment require careful consideration of the benefit-risk of use of HRT.

The risk of VTE may be temporarily increased with prolonged immobilisation, major trauma or major surgery. As in all post-operative patients, scrupulous attention should be given to prophylactic measures to prevent VTE following surgery. Where prolonged immobilisation is liable to follow elective surgery, particularly abdominal or orthopaedic surgery to the lower limbs, consideration should be given to temporarily stopping HRT four to six weeks earlier, if possible. Treatment should not be restarted until the woman is completely mobilised.

If VTE develops after initiating therapy, the drug should be discontinued. Patients should be told to contact their doctors immediately when they are aware of a potential thromboembolic symptom (e.g. painful swelling of a leg, sudden pain in the chest, dyspnea).

Coronary artery disease (CAD)

There is no evidence from randomised controlled trials of cardiovascular benefit with continuous combined conjugated oestrogens and medroxyprogesterone acetate (MPA). Two large clinical trials (WHI and HERS i.e. Heart and Estrogen/progestin Replacement Study) showed a possible increased risk of cardiovascular morbidity in the first year of use and no overall benefit. For other HRT products there are only limited data from randomised controlled trials examining effects in cardiovascular morbidity or mortality. Therefore, it is uncertain whether these findings also extend to other HRT products.

Stroke

One large randomised clinical trial (WHI-trial) found, as a secondary outcome, an increased risk of ischaemic stroke in healthy women during treatment with continuous combined conjugated oestrogens and MPA. For women who do not use HRT, it is estimated that the number of cases of stroke that will occur over a 5 year period is about 3 per 1000 women aged 50-59 years and 11 per 1000 women aged 60-69 years. It is estimated that for women who use conjugated oestrogens and MPA for 5 years, the number of additional cases will be between 0 and 3 (best estimate=1) per 1000 users aged 50-59 years and between 1 and 9 (best estimate=4) per 1000 users aged 60-69 years. It is unknown whether the increased risk also extends to other HRT products.

Ovarian cancer

Long-term (at least 5-10 years) use of oestrogen-only HRT products in hysterectomised women has been associated with an increased risk of ovarian cancer in some epidemiological studies. It is uncertain whether long-term use of combined HRT confers a different risk than oestrogen-only products.

Other conditions

Oestrogens may cause fluid retention, and therefore patients with cardiac or renal dysfunction should be carefully observed. Patients with terminal renal insufficiency should be closely observed, since it is expected that the level of circulating active ingredients in Kliovance will increase.

Women with pre-existing hypertriglyceridemia should be followed closely during oestrogen replacement or hormone replacement therapy, since rare cases of large increases of plasma triglycerides leading to pancreatitis have been reported with oestrogen therapy in this condition.

Oestrogens increase thyroid binding globulin (TBG), leading to increased circulating total thyroid hormone, as measured by protein-bound iodine (PBI), T4 levels (by column or by radio-immunoassay) or T3 levels (by radio-immunoassay). T3 resin uptake is decreased, reflecting the elevated TBG. Free T4 and free T3 concentrations are unaltered. Other binding proteins may be elevated in serum, i.e. corticoid binding globulin (CBG), sex-hormone-binding globulin (SHBG) leading to increased circulating corticosteroids and sex steroids, respectively. Free or biological active hormone concentrations are unchanged. Other plasma proteins may be increased (angiotensinogen/renin substrate, alpha-I-antitrypsin, ceruloplasmin).

There is no conclusive evidence for improvement of cognitive function. There is some evidence from the WHI trial of increased risk of probable dementia in women who start using continuous combined CEE and MPA after the age of 65. It is unknown whether the findings apply to younger post-menopausal women or other HRT products.

Kliovance tablets contain lactose. Patients with rare hereditary problems of galactose intolerance, the Lapp lactase deficiency or glucose-galactose malabsorption should not take this medicine.

4.5 Interaction with other medicinal products and other forms of interaction

The metabolism of oestrogens and progestogens may be increased by concomitant use of substances known to induce drug-metabolising enzymes, specifically cytochrome P450 enzymes such as anticonvulsants (e.g. phenobarbital, phenytoin, carbamazepin) and anti-infectives (e.g. rifampicin, rifabutin, nevirapine, efavirenz).

Ritonavir and nelfinavir, although known as strong inhibitors, by contrast exhibit inducing properties when used concomitantly with steroid hormones. Herbal preparations containing St John's Wort (*Hypericum perforatum*) may induce the metabolism of oestrogens and progestogens.

Clinically, an increased metabolism of oestrogens and progestogens may lead to decreased effect and changes in the uterine bleeding profile.

Drugs that inhibit the activity of hepatic microsomal drug metabolizing enzymes e.g. ketoconazole, may increase circulating levels of the active substances in Kliovance.

4.6 Pregnancy and lactation

Kliovance is not indicated during pregnancy.

If pregnancy occurs during medication with Kliovance, treatment should be withdrawn immediately.

Data on a limited number of exposed pregnancies indicate adverse effects of norethisterone acetate on the foetus. At doses higher than normally used in OC and HRT formulations masculinisation of female foetuses was observed. The results of most epidemiological studies to date relevant to inadvertent foetal exposure to combinations of oestrogens and progestogens indicate no teratogenic or foetotoxic effect.

Lactation

Kliovance is not indicated during lactation.

4.7 Effects on ability to drive and use machines

No effects known.

4.8 Undesirable effects

Clinical experience:

The most frequently reported adverse events in the clinical trials with Kliovance were vaginal bleeding and breast pain/tenderness, reported in approximately 10% to 20% of patients. Vaginal bleeding usually occurred in the first months of treatment. Breast pain usually disappeared after a few months of therapy. All adverse events observed in the randomised clinical trials with a higher frequency in patients treated with Kliovance as compared to placebo and which on an overall judgement are possibly related to treatment are presented in the table below.

(see Table 1 on next page)

Breast cancer

According to evidence from a large number of epidemiological studies and one randomised placebo-controlled trial, the Women's Health Initiative (WHI), the overall risk of breast cancer increases with increasing duration of HRT use in current or recent HRT users.

For *oestrogen-only* HRT, estimates of relative risk (RR) from a reanalysis of original data from 51 epidemiological studies (in which >80% of HRT use was oestrogen-only HRT) and from the epidemiological Million Women Study (MWS) are similar at 1.35 (95% CI: 1.21-1.49) and 1.30 (95% CI: 1.21-1.40), respectively.

For *oestrogen plus progestogen* combined HRT, several epidemiological studies have reported an overall higher risk for breast cancer than with oestrogens alone.

The MWS reported that, compared to never users, the use of various types of oestrogen-progestogen combined HRT was associated with a higher risk of breast cancer (RR = 2.00, 95% CI: 1.88-2.12) than use of oestrogens alone (RR = 1.30, 95% CI: 1.21-1.40) or use of tibolone (RR = 1.45, 95% CI: 1.25-1.68).

The WHI trial reported a risk estimate of 1.24 (95% CI: 1.01-1.54) after 5.6 years of use of oestrogen-progestogen combined HRT (CEE + MPA) in all users compared with placebo.

The absolute risks calculated from the MWS and the WHI trial are presented below:

The MWS has estimated, from the known average incidence of breast cancer in developed countries, that:

- For women not using HRT, about 32 in every 1000 are expected to have breast cancer diagnosed between the ages of 50 and 64 years.
- For 1000 current or recent users of HRT, the number of *additional* cases during the corresponding period will be
  - For users of *oestrogen-only* replacement therapy,
    - between 0 and 3 (best estimate = 1.5) for 5 years' use
    - between 3 and 7 (best estimate = 5) for 10 years' use.
  - For users of *oestrogen plus progestogen* combined HRT,
    - between 5 and 7 (best estimate = 6) for 5 years' use
    - between 18 and 20 (best estimate = 19 for 10 years use.

The WHI trial estimated that after 5.6 years of follow-up of women between the ages of 50 and 79 years, an *additional* 8 cases of invasive breast cancer would be due to *oestrogen-progestogen combined* HRT (CEE + MPA) per 10,000 women years. According to calculations from the trial data, it is estimated that:

- For 1000 women in the placebo group,
  - about 16 cases of invasive breast cancer would be diagnosed in 5 years.
- For 1000 women who used oestrogen + progestogen combined HRT (CEE + MPA), the number of additional cases would be
  - between 0 and 9 (best estimate = 4) for 5 years' use.

The number of additional cases of breast cancer in women who use HRT is broadly similar for women who start HRT irrespective of age at start of use (between the ages of 45-65) (see section 4.4).

Endometrial cancer

In women with an intact uterus, the risk of endometrial hyperplasia and endometrial cancer increases with increasing duration of use of unopposed oestrogens. According to data from epidemiological studies, the best estimate of the risk is that for women not using HRT, about 5 in every 1000 are expected to have endometrial cancer diagnosed between the ages of 50 and 65. Depending on the duration of treatment and oestrogen dose, the reported increase in endometrial cancer risk among unopposed oestrogen users varies from 2- to 12-fold greater compared with non-users. Adding a progestogen to oestrogen-only therapy greatly reduces this increased risk.

Post marketing experience:

In addition to the above mentioned adverse drug reactions, those presented below have been spontaneously reported, and are by an overall judgement considered possibly related to Kliovance treatment. The reporting rate of these spontaneous adverse drug reactions is very rare (<1/10,000 patient years). Post-marketing experience is subject to underreporting especially with regard to trivial and well known adverse drug reactions. The presented frequencies should be interpreted in that light:

Neoplasms benign and malignant (incl. cysts and polyps): Endometrial cancer

Psychiatric disorders: Insomnia, anxiety, libido decreased, libido increased

Nervous system disorders: Dizziness

Eye disorders: Visual disturbances

Vascular disorders: Hypertension aggravated

Gastrointestinal disorders: Dyspepsia, vomiting

Hepatobiliary disorders: Gallbladder disease, cholelithiasis, cholelithiasis aggravated, cholelithiasis re-occurrence

Skin and subcutaneous tissue disorder: Seborrhoea, rash, angioneurotic oedema

Reproductive system and breast disorders: Hyperplasia endometrial, vulvovaginal pruritus

Investigations: Weight decreased, blood pressure increased

Other adverse reactions have been reported in association with oestrogen/progestogen treatment:

- Oestrogen-dependent neoplasms benign and malignant, e.g. endometrial cancer
- Venous thromboembolism, i.e. deep leg or pelvic venous thrombosis and pulmonary embolism, is more frequent among hormone replacement therapy users than among non-users. For further information, see section 4.3 Contraindications and 4.4 Special warnings and precautions for use.
- Myocardial infarction and stroke
- Skin and subcutaneous disorders: chloasma, erythema multiforme, erythema nodosum, vascular purpura
- Probable dementia (see section 4.4).

4.9 Overdose

Overdose may be manifested by nausea and vomiting. Treatment should be symptomatic.

5. PHARMACOLOGICAL PROPERTIES

5.1 Pharmacodynamic properties

ATC code G03F A01

Oestrogen and progestogen for continuous combined hormone replacement therapy (HRT).

Oestradiol: The active ingredient, synthetic 17 beta-oestradiol, is chemically and biologically identical to endogenous human oestradiol. It substitutes for the loss of oestrogen production in menopausal women, and alleviates menopausal symptoms.

Oestrogens prevent bone loss following menopause or ovariectomy.

Norethisterone acetate: As oestrogens promote the growth of the endometrium, unopposed oestrogens increase the risk of endometrial hyperplasia and cancer. The addition of a progestogen greatly reduces the oestrogen-induced risk of endometrial hyperplasia in non-hysterectomised women.

In clinical trials with Kliovance, the addition of the norethisterone acetate component enhanced the vasomotor symptom relieving effect of 17beta-estradiol.

Relief of menopausal symptoms is achieved during the first few weeks of treatment.

Kliovance is a continuous combined HRT given with the intent of avoiding the regular withdrawal bleeding associated with cyclic or sequential HRT. Amenorrhoea (no bleeding and spotting) was seen in 90% of the women during months 9-12 of treatment. Bleeding and/or spotting appeared in 27% of the women during the first three months of treatment and in 10% during months 10-12 of treatment.

Oestrogen deficiency at menopause is associated with an increasing bone turnover and decline in bone mass. The effect of oestrogens on the bone mineral density is dose-dependent. Protection appears to be effective for as long as treatment is continued. After discontinuation of HRT, bone mass is lost at a rate similar to that in untreated women.

Evidence from the WHI trial and meta-analysed trials shows that current use of HRT, alone or in combination with a progestogen – given to predominantly healthy women – reduces the risk of hip, vertebral, and other osteoporotic fractures. HRT may also prevent fractures in women with low bone density and/or established osteoporosis, but the evidence for that is limited.

The effects of Kliovance on bone mineral density were examined in two 2-year, randomised, double-blind, placebo-controlled clinical trials in postmenopausal women (n=327 in one trial, including 47 on Kliovance and 48 on Kliofem (2 mg estradiol and 1 mg norethisterone acetate); and n=135 in the other trial including 46 on Kliovance). All women received calcium supplementation ranging from 500 to 1000 mg daily. Kliovance significantly prevented bone loss at the lumbar spine, total hip, distal radius and total body in comparison with calcium supplemented placebo-treated women. In early postmenopausal women (1 to 5 years since last menses), the percentage change from

Table 1

System organ class	Very common ≥1/10	Common ≥1/100; <1/10	Uncommon ≥1/1,000; <1/100	Rare ≥1/10,000; <1/1,000
Infections and infestations		Genital candidiasis or vaginitis, see also "Reproductive system and breast disorders"		
Immune system disorders			Hypersensi-tivity, see also "Skin and subcutaneous tissue disorders"	
Metabolism and nutrition disorders		Fluid retention, see also "General disorders and administration site conditions"		
Psychiatric disorders		Depression or depression aggravated	Nervousness	
Nervous system disorders		Headache, migraine or migraine aggravated		
Vascular disorders			Thrombo phlebitis superficial	Deep venous tromboembolism Pulmonary embolism
Gastrointestinal disorders		Nausea	Abdominal pain, abdominal distension or abdominal discomfort Flatulence or bloating	
Skin and subcutaneous tissue disorders			Alopecia, hirsutism or acne Pruritus or urticaria	
Muscle-skeletal, connective tissue and bone disorders		Back pain	Leg cramps	
Reproductive system and breast disorders	Breast pain or breast tenderness Vaginal haemor-rhage	Breast oedema or breast enlargement Uterine fibroids aggravated or uterine fibroids re-occurrence or uterine fibroids		
General disorders and administration site conditions		Oedema peripheral	Drug ineffective	
Investigations		Weight increased		

baseline in bone mineral density at lumbar spine, femoral neck and femoral trochanter in patients completing 2 years of treatment with Kliovance was 4.8 ± 0.6%, 1.6 ± 0.7% and 4.3 ± 0.7% (mean ± SEM), respectively, while with the higher dose combination containing 2 mg E_2 and 1 mg NETA (Kliofem) it was 5.4 ± 0.7%, 2.9 ± 0.8% and 5.0 ± 0.9%, respectively. The percentage of women who maintained or gained bone mineral density during treatment with Kliovance and Kliofem was 87% and 91%, respectively, after 2 years of treatment. In a study conducted in postmenopausal women with a mean age of 58 years, treatment with Kliovance for 2 years increased the bone mineral density at lumbar spine by 5.9 ± 0.9%, at total hip by 4.2 ± 1.0%, at distal radius by 2.1 ± 0.6%, and at total body by 3.7 ± 0.6%.

5.2 Pharmacokinetic properties

Following oral administration of 17 beta-estradiol in micronized form, rapid absorption from the gastrointestinal tract occurs. It undergoes extensive first-pass metabolism in the liver and other enteric organs and reaches a peak plasma concentration of approximately 35 pg/ml (range 21-52 pg/ml) within 5-8 hours. The half-life of 17 beta-estradiol is about 12-14 hours. It circulates bound to SHBG (37%) and to albumin (61%), while only approximately 1-2% is unbound. Metabolism of 17 beta-estradiol, occurs mainly in the liver and gut but also in target organs, and involves the formation of less active or inactive metabolites, including oestrone, catecholoestrogens and several oestrogen sulphates and glucuronides. Oestrogens are excreted with the bile, where they are hydrolysed and reabsorbed (enterohepatic circulation), and mainly in urine in biologically inactive form.

After oral administration norethisterone acetate is rapidly absorbed and transformed to norethisterone (NET). It undergoes first-pass metabolism in the liver and other enteric organs and reaches a peak plasma concentration of approximately 3.9 ng/ml (range 1.4-6.8 ng/ml) within 0.5-1.5 hour. The terminal half-life of NET is about 8-11 hours. NET binds to SHBG (36%) and to albumin (61%). The most important metabolites are isomers of 5α-dihydro-NET and of tetrahydro-NET, which are excreted mainly in the urine as sulphate or glucuronide conjugates.

The pharmacokinetics in the elderly have not been studied.

5.3 Preclinical safety data

Acute toxicity of oestrogens is low. Because of marked differences between animal species and between animals and humans preclinical results possess a limited predictive value for the application of oestrogens in humans.

In experimental animals oestradiol or oestradiol valerate displayed an embryolethal effect already at relatively low doses; malformations of the urogenital tract and feminisation of male foetuses were observed.

Norethisterone, like other progestogens, caused virilisation of female foetuses in rats and monkeys. After high doses of norethisterone embryolethal effects were observed.

Preclinical data based on conventional studies of repeated dose toxicity, genotoxicity and carcinogenic potential revealed no particular human risks beyond those discussed in other sections of the SPC.

6. PHARMACEUTICAL PARTICULARS

6.1 List of excipients

Tablet core:

Lactose monohydrate

Maize starch

Copovidone

Talc

Magnesium stearate

Film-coating:

Hypromellose

Triacetin

Talc

6.2 Incompatibilities

Not applicable.

6.3 Shelf life

3 years.

6.4 Special precautions for storage

Do not store above 25°C. Do not refrigerate. Keep the container in the outer carton.

6.5 Nature and contents of container

The tablets are contained in calendar dial packs; each calendar dial pack contains 28 tablets.

Packs containing 3 calendar dial packs are available (3 × 28 tablets)

The calendar dial pack with 28 tablets consists of the following 3 parts:

- The base made of coloured non-transparent polypropylene
- The ring-shaped lid made of transparent polystyrene
- The centre-dial made of coloured non-transparent polystyrene

6.6 Special precautions for disposal and other handling

No special requirements.

7. MARKETING AUTHORISATION HOLDER

Novo Nordisk Limited

Broadfield Park

Brighton Road

Crawley, West Sussex

RH11 9RT

8. MARKETING AUTHORISATION NUMBER(S)

PL 03132/0125

9. DATE OF FIRST AUTHORISATION/RENEWAL OF THE AUTHORISATION

20 August 1998/20 August 2003

10. DATE OF REVISION OF THE TEXT

8 May 2007

LEGAL CATEGORY

Prescription-only medicine (POM)

Konakion MM

(Roche Products Limited)

1. NAME OF THE MEDICINAL PRODUCT

Konakion MM.

2. QUALITATIVE AND QUANTITATIVE COMPOSITION

Each Konakion MM Ampoule contains 10.0mg vitamin K_1 (phytomenadione) Ph. Eur in 1ml.

3. PHARMACEUTICAL FORM

Amber glass ampoules containing 10mg phytomenadione in 1ml. The ampoule solution is clear to slightly opalescent, pale yellow in colour and contains the active constituent in a mixed micelles vehicle of glycocholic acid and lecithin.

4. CLINICAL PARTICULARS

4.1 Therapeutic indications

Konakion MM is indicated as an antidote to anticoagulant drugs of the coumarin type in the treatment of haemorrhage or threatened haemorrhage, associated with a low blood level of prothrombin or factor VII.

4.2 Posology and method of administration

Adults:*As an antidote to anticoagulant drugs*

For potentially fatal and severe haemorrhages: Konakion MM therapy should be accompanied by a more immediate effective treatment such as transfusions of whole blood or blood clotting factors. The anticoagulant should be withdrawn and an intravenous injection of Konakion MM given slowly in a dose of 10 – 20mg. The prothrombin level should be estimated three hours later and, if the response has been inadequate, the dose should be repeated. Not more than 40mg of Konakion MM should be given intravenously in 24 hours. Coagulation profiles must be monitored on a daily basis until these have returned to acceptable levels; in severe cases more frequent monitoring is necessary and where there is no immediate efficacy, transfusion of whole blood or blood clotting factors should be used.

Less severe haemorrhage: Oral treatment with Konakion tablets may be used.

Elderly

Elderly patients tend to be more sensitive to reversal of anticoagulation with Konakion MM; dosage in this group should be at the lower end of the ranges recommended.

Instructions for infusion in adults

Konakion MM Ampoules are for intravenous injection and should be diluted with 55ml of 5% glucose before slowly infusing the product. The solution should be freshly prepared and protected from light. Konakion MM Ampoule solution should not be diluted or mixed with other injectables, but may be injected into the lower part of an infusion apparatus.

Children aged 1 to 18 years

It is advisable that a haematologist is consulted about appropriate investigation and treatment in any child in whom Konakion MM is being considered.

Likely indications for using vitamin K in children are limited and may include:

1. Children with disorders that interfere with absorption of vitamin K (chronic diarrhoea, cystic fibrosis, biliary atresia, hepatitis, coeliac disease).

2. Children with poor nutrition who are receiving broad spectrum antibiotics.

3. Liver disease.

4. Patients receiving anticoagulant therapy with warfarin in whom the INR is increased outside the therapeutic range and therefore are at risk of, or are bleeding, and those with an INR in the therapeutic range who are bleeding.

For patients on warfarin therapy, therapeutic intervention must take into consideration the reason for the child being on warfarin and whether or not anticoagulant therapy has to be continued (e.g. in a child with mechanical heart valve or repeated thromboembolic complications) as vitamin K administration is likely to interfere with anticoagulation with warfarin for 2 – 3 weeks.

It should be noted that the earliest effect seen with vitamin K treatment is at 4 – 6 hours and therefore in patients with severe haemorrhage replacement with coagulation factors may be indicated (discuss with haematologist).

Dose of vitamin K

There are few data available regarding use of Konakion MM in children over 1 year. There have been no dose ranging studies in children with haemorrhage. Suggested dosages based on clinical experience are as follows:

Haemorrhage in children: 2 – 5mg i.v.

Asymptomatic children at risk of bleeding: 1 – 5mg i.v.

Prothrombin levels should be measured 2 to 6 hours later and if the response has not been adequate, the dose may be repeated. Frequent monitoring of vitamin K dependent clotting factors is essential in these patients.

Children on warfarin therapy who need to remain anticoagulated are not included in the above dosage recommendations.

Neonates and babies

Konakion MM Paediatric should be used in these patients. (See separate prescribing information.)

4.3 Contraindications

Use in patients with a known hypersensitivity to any of the constituents.

4.4 Special warnings and precautions for use

When treating patients with severely impaired liver function, it should be borne in mind that one Konakion MM Ampoule 10mg/1ml contains 54.6mg glycocholic acid and this may have a bilirubin displacing effect.

At the time of use, the ampoule contents should be clear. Following incorrect storage, the contents may become turbid or present a phase-separation. In this case the ampoule must no longer be used.

In potentially fatal and severe haemorrhage due to overdosage of coumarin anticoagulants, intravenous injections of Konakion MM must be administered slowly and not more than 40mg should be given during a period of 24 hours. Konakion MM therapy should be accompanied by a more immediate effective treatment such as transfusion of whole blood or blood clotting factors. When patients with prosthetic heart valves are given transfusions for the treatment of severe or potentially fatal haemorrhages, fresh frozen plasma should be used.

Large doses of Konakion MM (more than 40mg per day) should be avoided if it is intended to continue with anticoagulant therapy because there is no experience with doses above this maximum of 40mg per day and higher doses may give rise to unexpected adverse events. Clinical studies have shown a sufficient decrease in the prothrombin time with the recommended dosage. If haemorrhage is severe, a transfusion of fresh whole blood may be necessary whilst awaiting the effect of the vitamin K_1.

Vitamin K_1 is not an antidote to heparin.

4.5 Interaction with other medicinal products and other forms of interaction

No significant interactions are known other than antagonism of coumarin anticoagulants.

4.6 Pregnancy and lactation

There is no specific evidence regarding the safety of Konakion MM in pregnancy but, as with most drugs, the administration during pregnancy should only occur if the benefits outweigh the risks.

4.7 Effects on ability to drive and use machines

None.

4.8 Undesirable effects

There are only few unconfirmed reports of the occurrence of possible anaphylactoid reactions after intravenous injection of Konakion MM. Very rarely, venous irritation or phlebitis has been reported in association with intravenous administration of Konakion mixed micelle solution. Injection site reactions have been reported after intramuscular injection of Konakion.

4.9 Overdose

Hypervitaminosis of vitamin K_1 is unknown.

5. PHARMACOLOGICAL PROPERTIES

5.1 Pharmacodynamic properties

Konakion MM is a synthetic preparation of vitamin K. The presence of vitamin K (i.e. vitamin K or substances with vitamin K activity) is essential for the formation within the body of prothrombin, factor VII, factor IX and factor X. Lack of vitamin K leads to an increased tendency to haemorrhage. When an antidote to an anticoagulant is necessary it is essential to use vitamin K_1 itself, as vitamin K analogues are much less effective.

In the mixed micelles solution, vitamin K_1 is solubilised by means of a physiological colloidal system, also found in the human body, consisting of lecithin and bile acid. Owing to the absence of organic solvents, the Konakion mixed micelles solution is well tolerated on intravenous administration.

5.2 Pharmacokinetic properties

In blood plasma, 90% of vitamin K_1 is bound to lipoproteins. Following an intramuscular dose of 10mg vitamin K, plasma concentrations of 10 – 20mcg/l are produced (normal range 0.4 – 1.2mcg/l). Systemic availability following intramuscular administration is about 50% and elimination half-life in plasma is approximately 1.5 – 3 hours.

5.3 Preclinical safety data

None applicable.

6. PHARMACEUTICAL PARTICULARS

6.1 List of excipients

Glycocholic acid HSE

Sodium hydroxide Ph. Eur

Lecithin (phospholipon 100) HSE

Hydrochloric acid Ph. Eur.

Water for injection Ph. Eur.

6.2 Incompatibilities

None.

6.3 Shelf life

The recommended shelf-life of Konakion MM Ampoules is 36 months.

6.4 Special precautions for storage

The recommended maximum storage temperature is 25°C. Do not use if the solution is turbid.

6.5 Nature and contents of container

Konakion MM is supplied in amber glass ampoules containing 10mg phytomenadione in 1ml. The ampoule solution is clear to slightly opalescent, pale yellow in colour and contains the active constituent in a mixed micelles vehicle of glycocholic acid and lecithin.

6.6 Special precautions for disposal and other handling

See section 4.2.

7. MARKETING AUTHORISATION HOLDER

Roche Products Limited, 6 Falcon Way, Shire Park, Welwyn Garden City, AL7 1TW, United Kingdom.

8. MARKETING AUTHORISATION NUMBER(S)

PL 0031/0254

9. DATE OF FIRST AUTHORISATION/RENEWAL OF THE AUTHORISATION

17 August 1993

10. DATE OF REVISION OF THE TEXT

September 2005

LEGAL STATUS

POM

Konakion is a registered trade mark

Item Code

Konakion MM Paediatric

(Roche Products Limited)

1. NAME OF THE MEDICINAL PRODUCT

Konakion ▼ MM Paediatric 2mg/0.2ml

2. QUALITATIVE AND QUANTITATIVE COMPOSITION

Each ampoule contains 2mg phytomenadione in 0.2ml.

3. PHARMACEUTICAL FORM

The ampoule solution is clear to slightly opalescent, pale yellow in colour and contains the active constituent in a mixed micelles vehicle of glycocholic acid and lecithin.

4. CLINICAL PARTICULARS

4.1 Therapeutic indications

Konakion MM Paediatric is indicated for the prophylaxis and treatment of vitamin K deficiency bleeding (VKDB) in neonates and infants.

Konakion MM Paediatric can be used, following specialist advice from a haematologist, as an antidote to anticoagulant drugs of the coumarin type in infants and children. For use as an antidote to anticoagulant drugs of the coumarin type in adolescents and adults, refer to Konakion MM Ampoules 10mg/ml.

4.2 Posology and method of administration

Prophylaxis of vitamin K deficiency bleeding (VKDB)

Healthy neonates of 36 weeks gestation and older:

Either:

- 1mg administered by intramuscular injection at birth or soon after birth

or

- 2mg orally at birth or soon after birth. The oral dose should be followed by a second dose of 2mg at 4-7 days.

Exclusively breast-fed babies who received oral Konakion at birth: In addition to the doses at birth and at 4-7 days, a further 2mg oral dose should be given 1 month after birth. Further monthly 2mg oral doses until formula feeding is introduced have been advised, but no safety or efficacy data exist for these additional doses.

Preterm neonates of less than 36 weeks gestation weighing 2.5kg or greater, and term neonates at special risk: 1mg IM or IV at birth or soon after birth, the size and frequency of further doses depending on coagulation status.

*Preterm neonates of less than 36 weeks gestation weighing less than 2.5kg:*0.4mg/kg (equivalent to 0.04ml/kg) IM or IV at birth or soon after birth, see dosing table below. This parenteral dose should not be exceeded (see *Special warnings and special precautions for use*). The frequency of further doses should depend on coagulation status.

CAUTION: care is required when calculating and measuring the dose in relation to the baby's weight (10x errors are common).

Dosing information for preterm babies at birth for the prophylaxis of VKDB

Weight of the baby	Dose of vitamin K at birth	Injection volume
1kg	0.4mg	0.04ml
1.5kg	0.6mg	0.06ml
2kg	0.8mg	0.08ml
2.5kg	1mg	0.1ml
Over 2.5kg	1mg	0.1ml

Therapy of early and/or late vitamin K deficiency bleeding (VKDB)

Initially 1mg IV and further doses as required, depending on clinical picture and coagulation status. Konakion therapy may need to be accompanied by a more immediate effective treatment, such as transfusion of blood or blood clotting factors to compensate for severe blood loss and delayed response to vitamin K_1.

Antidote therapy to anticoagulant drugs of the coumarin type

There have been no dose ranging studies performed to recommend a specific dose of Konakion MM Paediatric used as an antidote to anticoagulant drugs of the coumarin type in infants and children. Suggested doses are detailed below. Konakion MM Paediatric must be administered by intravenous injection in these patients. It is advisable that a haematologist is consulted about appropriate investigation and treatment in any infant or child in whom Konakion MM Paediatric is being considered.

For patients on warfarin therapy, therapeutic intervention must consider the reason for the patient being on warfarin and whether or not anticoagulant therapy has to be continued (e.g. in a patient with mechanical heart valve or repeated thrombo-embolic complications) as vitamin K administration is likely to interfere with anticoagulation with warfarin for 2 - 3 weeks. For patients continuing to receive warfarin, the suggested dose for the partial reversal of anticoagulation is 30 micrograms/kg administered by IV injection. Konakion MM Paediatric is only suitable for the administration of doses of 30 micrograms/kg in children weighing over 13 kg.

The suggested dose of vitamin K for patients requiring a complete reversal of a warfarin overdose is 250-300 micrograms/kg administered by IV injection. It should be noted that the earliest effect seen with vitamin K treatment is at 4 to 6 hours and therefore, in patients with severe haemorrhage, replacement with coagulation factor concentrates may be indicated (discuss with haematologist). Konakion MM Paediatric is only suitable for the administration of doses of 250-300 micrograms/kg in children weighing over 1.6 kg. Prothrombin time should be measured 2 to 6 hours later and if the response has not been adequate, Konakion MM Paediatric administration may be repeated. Frequent monitoring of vitamin K dependent clotting factors is essential in these patients.

Method of administration

Konakion MM Paediatric can be administered by intramuscular or intravenous injection or by oral administration depending on the indication.

Parenteral use: For the administration of injection volumes of 0.04ml (0.4mg) to 0.1ml (1mg), 0.5ml syringes with 0.01ml gradations are recommended, see section 6.6 *Instructions for use/handling*.

Administration of Konakion MM Paediatric by i.v. infusion is not recommended because Konakion MM Paediatric must not be diluted or mixed with other parenteral medications. However, Konakion MM Paediatric may be administered by injecting the dose into the lower part of an infusion set containing 5% dextrose or 0.9% sodium chloride running at ⩾ 0.7ml/minute, see section 6.2 *Incompatibilities*.

Oral use: For oral administration, oral dispensers are provided in the pack. After breaking the ampoule open, 0.2ml of solution should be withdrawn into the oral dispenser until it reaches the mark on the dispenser (0.2ml = 2mg vitamin K). Drop the contents of the dispenser directly into the baby's mouth by pressing the plunger.

4.3 Contraindications
Use in patients with a known hypersensitivity to any of the constituents.

4.4 Special warnings and precautions for use
At the time of use, the ampoule contents should be clear. Following incorrect storage, the contents may become turbid or present a phase-separation. In this case the ampoule must no longer be used.

Parenteral administration to premature babies weighing less than 2.5kg may increase the risk for the development of kernicterus (bilirubin encephalopathy).

Infants with cholestatic disease must receive Konakion MM Paediatric by intramuscular or intravenous injection since oral absorption is impaired in these patients.

Konakion MM Paediatric must be administered by intravenous injection when used as an antidote to anticoagulant drugs of the coumarin type, as intramuscular injections may result in significant bleeding in these patients.

4.5 Interaction with other medicinal products and other forms of interaction
No significant interactions are known other than antagonism of coumarin anticoagulants.

4.6 Pregnancy and lactation
Not applicable.

4.7 Effects on ability to drive and use machines
Not applicable.

4.8 Undesirable effects
There are only few unconfirmed reports on the occurrence of possible anaphylactoid reactions after IV injection of Konakion MM. Local irritation may occur at the injection site but is unlikely due to the small injection volume. Rarely, injection site reactions may occur which may be severe, including inflammation, atrophy and necrosis.

4.9 Overdose
There is no known clinical syndrome attributable to hypervitaminosis of vitamin K_1.

The following adverse events have been reported concerning overdose with use of Konakion in neonates and infants: jaundice, hyperbilirubinaemia, increase GOT and GGT, abdominal pain, constipation, soft stools, malaise, agitation and cutaneous eruption. The causality of those cannot be established. The majority of these adverse events were considered non-serious and resolved without any treatment.

Treatment of suspected overdose should be aimed at alleviating symptoms.

5. PHARMACOLOGICAL PROPERTIES

5.1 Pharmacodynamic properties
Konakion MM is a preparation of synthetic phytomenadione (vitamin K_1). The presence of vitamin K_1 is essential for the formation within the body of prothrombin, factor VII, factor IX and factor X, and of the coagulation inhibitors, protein C and protein S.

Vitamin K_1 does not readily cross the placental barrier from mother to child and is poorly excreted in breast milk.

Lack of vitamin K_1 leads to an increased tendency to haemorrhagic disease in the newborn. Vitamin K_1 administration, which promotes synthesis of the above-mentioned coagulation factors by the liver, can reverse an abnormal coagulation status due to vitamin K_1 deficiency.

5.2 Pharmacokinetic properties
In the mixed micelle solution, vitamin K_1 is solubilised by means of a physiological colloidal system consisting of lecithin and a bile acid.

Following oral administration vitamin K_1 is absorbed from the small intestine. The systemic availability following oral dosing is approximately 50%, with a wide range of inter-individual variability. Absorption is limited in the absence of bile.

After intramuscular administration vitamin K_1 release into the circulation is prolonged, i.e. the IM route acts as a depot. A single 1mg IM dose results in comparable vitamin K_1 concentrations at 1 month as two 2 mg doses (one given at birth and the other at one week).

Vitamin K_1 accumulates predominantly in the liver, is up to 90% bound to lipoproteins in the plasma and is stored in the body only for short periods of time.

Vitamin K_1 is transformed to more polar metabolites, such as phytomenadione-2,3-epoxide.

The half-life of vitamin K_1 in plasma is approximately 72 hours in neonates and about 1.5 to 3 hours in adults. Vitamin K_1 is excreted in bile and urine as the glucuronide and sulphate conjugates.

5.3 Preclinical safety data
None applicable.

6. PHARMACEUTICAL PARTICULARS

6.1 List of excipients
Glycocholic acid, lecithin, sodium hydroxide, hydrochloric acid and water.

6.2 Incompatibilities
Incompatibilities have been observed with diluted Konakion MM solution and certain siliconised syringes, therefore, Konakion MM Paediatric must not be diluted before injection.

Do not dilute with sodium chloride containing solutions as precipitation may occur, see section 4.2 *Posology and Method of Administration*.

6.3 Shelf life
3 years.

6.4 Special precautions for storage
Konakion MM Paediatric ampoule solution should be stored below 25°C and be protected from light. The solution should not be frozen. Do not use if the solution is turbid.

6.5 Nature and contents of container
Amber glass ampoules containing 2mg phytomenadione in 0.2ml. Plastic oral dispensers. Packs of 1, 5 or 10.

6.6 Special precautions for disposal and other handling
See section 4.2 *Posology and method of administration,* section 4.4 *Special warnings and precautions for use* and section 6.2 *Incompatibilities* for advice regarding the administration of Konakion MM Paediatric.

Undiluted Konakion MM Paediatric is compatible with 0.5ml syringes supplied by B. Braun.

7. MARKETING AUTHORISATION HOLDER
Roche Products Limited, 6 Falcon Way, Shire Park, Welwyn Garden City, AL7 1TW, United Kingdom.

8. MARKETING AUTHORISATION NUMBER(S)
PL 0031/0346

9. DATE OF FIRST AUTHORISATION/RENEWAL OF THE AUTHORISATION
20 June 1996

10. DATE OF REVISION OF THE TEXT
February 2007

LEGAL STATUS
POM

Konakion is a registered trade mark

Item Code

Konakion Tablets 10mg

(Roche Products Limited)

1. NAME OF THE MEDICINAL PRODUCT
Konakion Tablets 10mg

2. QUALITATIVE AND QUANTITATIVE COMPOSITION
Each Konakion Tablet contains 10mg phytomenadione (vitamin K_1).

For excipients, see 6.1.

3. PHARMACEUTICAL FORM
Round off-white sugar-coated tablets.

4. CLINICAL PARTICULARS

4.1 Therapeutic indications
Konakion is indicated in the treatment of haemorrhage or threatened haemorrhage associated with a low blood level of prothrombin or factor VII. The main indications are:

As an antidote to anticoagulant drugs of the coumarin type.

4.2 Posology and method of administration
Konakion tablets are for oral administration and should be chewed or allowed to dissolve slowly in the mouth.

Adults: As an antidote to anticoagulant drugs

For potentially fatal and severe haemorrhages: Konakion intravenous injection (see separate prescribing information).

Less severe haemorrhage: Konakion is given orally in doses of 10 - 20mg (1 to 2 tablets). The prothrombin level is estimated 8 to 12 hours later, and if the response has been inadequate, the dose should be repeated.

Lowering of prothrombin to dangerous level but no haemorrhage: A dose of 5 - 10mg Konakion orally may be given to bring the prothrombin level back to within safe limits. In such instances it is not usually necessary to discontinue the anticoagulant.

Adults: Other indications

Doses of 10 - 20mg as required.

Elderly

Elderly patients tend to be more sensitive to reversal of anticoagulation with Konakion; dosage in this group should be at the lower end of the ranges recommended.

Children

If, on the recommendation of a physician, a children's dosage is required, then it is suggested that 5 - 10mg be given.

4.3 Contraindications
Use in patients with a known hypersensitivity to any of the constituents.

4.4 Special warnings and precautions for use
Large doses of Konakion should be avoided if it is intended to continue with anticoagulant therapy.

Vitamin K_1 is not an antidote to heparin.

Konakion tablets contain glucose, sucrose and lactose (skimmed milk powder). Patients with rare galactose intolerance, Lapp lactase deficiency, fructose intolerance, glucose-galactose malabsorption or sucrase-isomaltase insufficiency should not take this medicine.

4.5 Interaction with other medicinal products and other forms of interaction
None known.

4.6 Pregnancy and lactation
There is no specific evidence regarding the safety of Konakion in pregnancy but, as with most drugs, the administration during pregnancy should only occur if the benefits outweigh the risks.

4.7 Effects on ability to drive and use machines
None known.

4.8 Undesirable effects
None known.

4.9 Overdose
Hypervitaminosis of vitamin K_1 is unknown.

5. PHARMACOLOGICAL PROPERTIES

5.1 Pharmacodynamic properties
Konakion is a synthetic preparation of vitamin K_1. The presence of vitamin K (i.e. vitamin K_1 itself or substances with vitamin K activity) is essential for the formation within the body of prothrombin, factor VII, factor IX and factor X. Lack of vitamin K leads to increased tendency to haemorrhage. When an antidote to an anticoagulant is necessary it is essential to use vitamin K_1 itself, as vitamin K analogues are much less effective.

5.2 Pharmacokinetic properties
The fat-soluble vitamin compound phytomenadione (Vitamin K_1) requires the presence of bile for its absorption from the gastro-intestinal tract. Vitamin K accumulates mainly in the liver but is stored in the body only for short periods of time. Vitamin K does not appear to cross the placenta readily and it is poorly distributed into breast milk. Phytomenadione is rapidly metabolised to more polar metabolites and is excreted in bile and urine as glucuronide and sulphate conjugates.

5.3 Preclinical safety data
None stated.

6. PHARMACEUTICAL PARTICULARS

6.1 List of excipients
Tablet core:

Silica, colloidal hydrated

Sucrose

Glucose, anhydrous

Skim Milk Powder

Cocoa

Theobroma oil

Carob Bean Gum

Glycerol

Tablet coat:

Sucrose

Rice Starch

Titanium Dioxide (E171)

Ethyl Vanillin

Acacia, Spray-Dried

Paraffin, Light Liquid

Paraffin, Hard

Talc

Carmellose sodium

6.2 Incompatibilities
Not applicable.

6.3 Shelf life
The recommended shelf life of Konakion Tablets is 5 years.

6.4 Special precautions for storage
Keep the bottle tightly closed. Store the bottle in the outer carton in order to protect from light.

6.5 Nature and contents of container
Konakion Tablets are supplied in white HDPE bottles with tamper evident snap-fit, containing 25 coated tablets or in amber glass bottles with HDPE closures and cotton-viscose pads, containing 10 coated tablets.

6.6 Special precautions for disposal and other handling
No special requirements.

7. MARKETING AUTHORISATION HOLDER
Roche Products Limited, 6 Falcon Way, Shire Park, Welwyn Garden City, AL7 1TW, United Kingdom.

8. MARKETING AUTHORISATION NUMBER(S)
PL 0031/5022R

9. DATE OF FIRST AUTHORISATION/RENEWAL OF THE AUTHORISATION
31 May 1996

10. DATE OF REVISION OF THE TEXT
September 2005

LEGAL STATUS
POM

Konakion is a registered trade mark

Kuvan 100 mg soluble tablets

(Merck Serono)

1. NAME OF THE MEDICINAL PRODUCT

Kuvan ▼ 100 mg soluble tablets

2. QUALITATIVE AND QUANTITATIVE COMPOSITION

Each soluble tablet contains 100 mg of sapropterin dihydrochloride (equivalent to 77 mg of sapropterin).

For a full list of excipients, see section 6.1.

3. PHARMACEUTICAL FORM

Soluble tablet.

Off-white to light yellow soluble tablet with "177" imprinted on one face.

4. CLINICAL PARTICULARS

4.1 Therapeutic indications

Kuvan is indicated for the treatment of hyperphenylalaninaemia(HPA) in adult and paediatric patients of 4 years of age and over with phenylketonuria (PKU) who have been shown to be responsive to such treatment (see section 4.2).

Kuvan is also indicated for the treatment of hyperphenylalaninaemia (HPA) in adult and paediatric patients with tetrahydrobiopterin (BH4) deficiency who have been shown to be responsive to such treatment (see section 4.2).

4.2 Posology and method of administration

Treatment with Kuvan must be initiated and supervised by a physician experienced in the treatment of PKU and BH4 deficiency. Kuvan should be administered with a meal as a single daily dose, at the same time each day, preferably in the morning.

Active management of dietary phenylalanine and overall protein intake while taking Kuvan is required to ensure adequate control of blood phenylalanine levels and nutritional balance.

As HPA due to either PKU or BH4 deficiency is a chronic condition, once responsiveness is demonstrated, Kuvan is intended for long-term use. However, there are limited data regarding the long-term use of Kuvan.

Posology

Kuvan is provided as 100 mg tablets. The calculated daily dose based on body weight should be rounded to the nearest multiple of 100. For instance, a calculated dose of 401 to 450 mg should be rounded down to 400 mg corresponding to 4 tablets. A calculated dose of 451 mg to 499 mg should be rounded up to 500 mg corresponding to 5 tablets.

PKU

The starting dose of Kuvan in adult and paediatric patients with PKU is 10 mg/kg body weight once daily. The dose is adjusted, usually between 5 and 20 mg/kg/day, to achieve and maintain adequate blood phenylalanine levels as defined by the physician.

BH4 deficiency

The starting dose of Kuvan in adult and paediatric patients with BH4 deficiency is 2 to 5 mg/kg body weight once daily. Doses may be adjusted up to 20 mg/kg/day. It may be necessary to divide the total daily dose into 2 or 3 administrations, distributed over the day, to optimise the therapeutic effect.

Determination of Response

It is of primary importance to initiate Kuvan treatment as early as possible to avoid the appearance of non-reversible clinical manifestations of neurological disorders in paediatric patients and cognitive deficits and psychiatric disorders in adults due to sustained elevations of blood phenylalanine.

Response to treatment is determined by a decrease in blood phenylalanine following treatment with Kuvan. Blood phenylalanine levels should be checked before initiating treatment and after 1 week of treatment with Kuvan at the recommended starting dose. If an unsatisfactory reduction in blood phenylalanine levels is observed, then the dose of Kuvan can be increased weekly to a maximum of 20 mg/kg/day, with continued weekly monitoring of blood phenylalanine levels over a one month period. The dietary phenylalanine intake should be maintained at a constant level during this period.

A satisfactory response is defined as a ≥30 percent reduction in blood phenylalanine levels or attainment of the therapeutic blood phenylalanine goals defined for an individual patient by the treating physician. Patients who fail to achieve this level of response within the described one month test period should be considered non-responsive and should not receive treatment with Kuvan.

Once responsiveness to Kuvan has been established, the dose may be adjusted within the range of 5 to 20 mg/kg/day according to response to therapy.

It is recommended that blood phenylalanine and tyrosine levels be tested one or two weeks after each dose adjustment and monitored frequently thereafter. Patients treated with Kuvan must continue a restricted phenylalanine diet and undergo regular clinical assessment (such as monitoring of blood phenylalanine and tyrosine levels, nutrient intake, and psycho-motor development).

Method of administration

The tablets should be administered as a single daily dose with a meal, to increase the absorption, and at the same time each day preferably in the morning.

Patients should be advised not to swallow the desiccant capsule found in the bottle.

The prescribed number of tablets should be placed in a glass or cup of water and stirred until dissolved. It may take a few minutes for the tablets to dissolve. To make the tablets dissolve faster they can be crushed. Small particles may be visible in the solution and will not affect the effectiveness of the medicinal product. The solution should be drunk within 15 to 20 minutes.

For doses below 100 mg, one tablet should be dissolved in 100 ml of water and the volume of solution corresponding to the prescribed dose administered. An accurate measuring device with suitable graduations should be used to ensure administration of the appropriate volume of solution.

Adults

The prescribed number of tablets should be placed in a glass or cup with 120 to 240 ml of water and stirred until dissolved.

Paediatric patients

The prescribed number of tablets should be placed in a glass or cup with up to 120 ml of water and stirred until dissolved.

Dose adjustment

Treatment with Kuvan may decrease blood phenylalanine levels below the desired therapeutic level. Adjustment of the sapropterin dose or modification of dietary phenylalanine intake may be required to achieve and maintain blood phenylalanine levels within the desired therapeutic range.

Blood phenylalanine and tyrosine levels should be tested, particularly in children, one to two weeks after each dose adjustment and monitored frequently thereafter, under the direction of the treating physician.

If inadequate control of blood phenylalanine levels is observed during treatment with Kuvan, the patient's adherence to the prescribed treatment, and diet, should be reviewed before considering an adjustment of the dose of Kuvan.

Discontinuation of Kuvan treatment should be done only under the supervision of a physician. More frequent monitoring may be required, as blood phenylalanine levels may increase. Dietary modification may be necessary to maintain blood phenylalanine levels within the desired therapeutic range.

Special populations

Kuvan has not been specifically studied in paediatric patients under 4 years of age (see section 5.1).

Safety and efficacy of Kuvan in patients above 65 years of age have not been established. Caution must be exercised when prescribing to elderly patients.

Safety and efficacy of Kuvan in patients with renal or hepatic insufficiency have not been established. Caution must be exercised when prescribing to such patients.

4.3 Contraindications

Hypersensitivity to the active substance or to any of the excipients.

4.4 Special warnings and precautions for use

Patients treated with Kuvan must continue a restricted phenylalanine diet and undergo regular clinical assessment (such as monitoring of blood phenylalanine and tyrosine levels, nutrient intake, and psycho-motor development).

Sustained or recurrent dysfunction in the phenylalanine-tyrosine-dihydroxy-L-phenylalanine (DOPA) metabolic pathway can result in deficient body protein and neurotransmitter synthesis. Prolonged exposure to low blood phenylalanine and tyrosine levels during infancy has been associated with impaired neurodevelopmental outcome. Active management of dietary phenylalanine and overall protein intake while taking Kuvan is required to ensure adequate control of blood phenylalanine and tyrosine levels and nutritional balance.

Consultation with a physician is recommended during illness as blood phenylalanine levels may increase.

There are limited data regarding the long-term use of Kuvan.

Caution is advised when sapropterin is used in patients with predisposition to convulsions. In clinical studies of patients with BH4 deficiency treated with a preparation of sapropterin, convulsions and exacerbation of convulsions was observed. This was not observed in the clinical trials of Kuvan in patients with PKU.

Sapropterin should be used with caution in patients who are receiving concomitant levodopa, as combined treatment with sapropterin may cause increased excitability and irritability.

Special populations

Kuvan has not been specifically studied in paediatric patients under 4 years of age (see section 5.1).

Safety and efficacy of Kuvan in patients above 65 years of age have not been established. Caution must be exercised when prescribing to elderly patients.

Safety and efficacy of Kuvan in patients with renal or hepatic insufficiency have not been established.

4.5 Interaction with other medicinal products and other forms of interaction

No interaction studies have been performed.

Although concomitant administration of inhibitors of dihydrofolate reductase (e.g. methotrexate, trimethoprim) has not been studied, such medicinal products may interfere with BH4 metabolism. Caution is recommended when using such agents while taking Kuvan.

BH4 is a cofactor for nitric oxide synthetase. Caution is recommended during concomitant use of Kuvan with all agents that cause vasodilation, including those administered topically, by affecting nitric oxide (NO) metabolism or action including classical NO donors (e.g. glyceryl trinitrate (GTN), isosorbide dinitrate (ISDN), sodium nitroprusside (SNP), molsidomin), phosphodiesterase type 5 (PDE-5) inhibitors and minoxidil.

Caution should be exercised when prescribing Kuvan to patients receiving treatment with levodopa, as it may cause increased excitability and irritability.

4.6 Pregnancy and lactation

For Kuvan, no clinical data on exposed pregnancies are available. Animal studies do not indicate direct or indirect harmful effects with respect to pregnancy, embryonal/foetal development, parturition or postnatal development.

Maternal blood phenylalanine levels must be strictly controlled before and during pregnancy. If maternal phenylalanine levels are not strictly controlled before and during pregnancy, this could be harmful to the mother and the foetus. Physician-supervised restriction of dietary phenylalanine intake prior to and throughout pregnancy is the first choice of treatment in this patient group.

The use of Kuvan should be considered only if strict dietary management does not adequately reduce blood phenylalanine levels. Caution must be exercised when prescribing to pregnant women.

It is not known whether sapropterin or its metabolites are excreted in human breast milk. Kuvan should not be used during breast-feeding.

4.7 Effects on ability to drive and use machines

No studies on the effects on the ability to drive and use machines have been performed.

4.8 Undesirable effects

Approximately 35% of the 579 patients who received treatment with sapropterin dihydrochloride (5 to 20 mg/kg/day) in the clinical trials for Kuvan experienced adverse reactions. The most commonly reported events are headache and rhinorrhoea.

In the pivotal clinical trials for Kuvan, the following undesirable effects have been identified.

Frequencies are defined as: Very common (≥1/10) and Common (≥1/100 to <1/10). Within each frequency grouping, undesirable effects are presented in order of decreasing seriousness.

System Organ Class	Very Common	Common
Nervous system disorders	Headache	
Respiratory, thoracic and mediastinal disorders	Rhinorrhoea	Pharyngolaryngeal pain Nasal congestion Cough
Gastrointestinal disorders		Diarrhoea Vomiting Abdominal pain
Metabolism and nutrition disorders		Hypophenylalaninemia

Additional information

Rebound, as defined by an increase in blood phenylalanine levels above pre-treatment levels, may occur upon cessation of treatment.

4.9 Overdose

Headache and dizziness have been reported after the administration of sapropterin dihydrochloride above the recommended maximum dose of 20 mg/kg/day. Treatment of overdose should be directed to symptoms.

5. PHARMACOLOGICAL PROPERTIES

5.1 Pharmacodynamic properties

Pharmacotherapeutic group: Various alimentary tract and metabolism products, ATC code: A16AX07

Mechanism of action

Hyperphenylalaninaemia (HPA) is diagnosed as an abnormal elevation in blood phenylalanine levels and is usually caused by autosomal recessive mutations in the genes encoding for phenylalanine hydroxylase enzyme (in the case of phenylketonuria, PKU) or for the enzymes involved in 6R-tetrahydrobiopterin (6R-BH4) biosynthesis or regeneration (in the case of BH4 deficiency). BH4 deficiency is a group of disorders arising from mutations or deletions in the genes encoding for one of the five enzymes involved in the biosynthesis or recycling of BH4. In both cases, phenylalanine cannot be effectively transformed into the amino acid tyrosine, leading to increased phenylalanine levels in the blood.

Sapropterin is a synthetic version of the naturally occurring 6R-BH4, which is a cofactor of the hydroxylases for phenylalanine, tyrosine and tryptophan.

The rationale for administration of Kuvan in patients with BH4-responsive PKU is to enhance the activity of the defective phenylalanine hydroxylase and thereby increase or restore the oxidative metabolism of phenylalanine sufficient to reduce or maintain blood phenylalanine levels, prevent or decrease further phenylalanine accumulation, and increase tolerance to phenylalanine intake in the diet. The rationale for administration of Kuvan in patients with BH4 Deficiency is to replace the deficient levels of BH4, thereby restoring the activity of phenylalanine hydroxylase.

Clinical efficacy

The Phase III clinical development program for Kuvan included 2, randomised placebo-controlled studies in patients with PKU. The results of these studies demonstrate the efficacy of Kuvan to reduce blood phenylalanine levels and to increase dietary phenylalanine tolerance.

In 88 subjects with poorly controlled PKU who had elevated blood phenylalanine levels at screening, sapropterin dihydrochloride 10 mg/kg/day significantly reduced blood phenylalanine levels as compared to placebo. The baseline blood phenylalanine levels for the Kuvan-treated group and the placebo group were similar, with mean ± SD baseline blood phenylalanine levels of 842.7 ± 299.6 µmol/l and 888.3 ± 323.1 µmol/l, respectively. The mean ± SD decrease from baseline in blood phenylalanine levels at the end of the 6 week study period was 235.9 ± 257.0 µmol/l for the sapropterin treated group (n=47) as compared to an increase of 2.9 ± 239.5 µmol/l for the placebo group (n=41) ($p<0.001$). For patients with baseline blood phenylalanine levels ⩾600 µmol/l, 41.9% (13/31) of those treated with sapropterin and 13.2% (5/38) of those treated with placebo had blood phenylalanine levels < 600 µmol/l at the end of the 6-week study period ($p=0.012$).

In a separate 10-week, placebo-controlled study, 45 PKU patients with blood phenylalanine levels controlled on a stable phenylalanine-restricted diet (blood phenylalanine ⩽ 480 µmol/l on enrolment) were randomized 3:1 to treatment with sapropterin dihydrochloride 20 mg/kg/day (n=33) or placebo (n=12). After 3 weeks of treatment with sapropterin dihydrochloride 20 mg/kg/day, blood phenylalanine levels were significantly reduced; the mean ± SD decrease from baseline in blood phenylalanine level within this group was 148.5 ±134.2 µmol/l ($p<0.001$). After 3 weeks, subjects in both the sapropterin and placebo treatment groups were continued on their phenylalanine-restricted diets and dietary phenylalanine intake was increased or decreased using standardized phenylalanine supplements with a goal to maintain blood phenylalanine levels at <360 µmol/l. There was a significant difference in dietary phenylalanine tolerance in the sapropterin treatment group as compared to the placebo group. The mean ± SD increase in dietary phenylalanine tolerance was 17.513 ±13.268 mg/kg/day for the group treated with sapropterin dihydrochloride 20 mg/kg/day, compared to 3.259 ± 5.291 mg/kg/day for the placebo group ($p = 0.006$). For the sapropterin treatment group, the mean ± SD total dietary phenylalanine tolerance was 38.406 ± 21.606 mg/kg/day during treatment with sapropterin dihydrochloride 20 mg/kg/day compared to 15.660 ± 7.159 mg/kg/day before treatment.

Paediatric population

Kuvan has not been specifically studied in children under 4 years of age, although the published literature indicates that more than 600 children of 0 to 4 years old with PKU, have been exposed to treatment with an un-registered preparation of BH4, including at least 35 who received therapy ⩾ 2 months. The maximum daily dose used was 20 mg/kg body weight.

Limited studies have been conducted in patients under 4 years of age with BH4 deficiency using another formulation of the same active substance (sapropterin) or an un-registered preparation of BH4.

5.2 Pharmacokinetic properties

Absorption

Sapropterin is absorbed after oral administration of the dissolved tablet, and the maximum blood concentration (C_{max}) is achieved 3 to 4 hours after dosing in the fasted state. The rate and extent of absorption of sapropterin is influenced by food. The absorption of sapropterin is higher after a high-fat, high-calorie meal as compared to fasting, resulting, in average, in 40-85% higher maximum blood concentrations achieved 4 to 5 hours after administration.

Absolute bioavailability or bioavailability for humans after oral administration is not known.

Distribution

In non-clinical studies, sapropterin was primarily distributed to the kidneys, adrenal glands, and liver as assessed by levels of total and reduced biopterin concentrations. In rats, following intravenous radiolabeled sapropterin administration, radioactivity was found to distribute in foetuses. Excretion of total biopterin in milk was demonstrated in rats by intravenous route. No increase in total biopterin concentrations in either foetuses or milk was observed in rats after oral administration of 10mg/kg sapropterin dihydrochloride.

Biotransformation

Sapropterin dihydrochloride is primarily metabolised in the liver to dihydrobiopterin and biopterin. Since sapropterin dihydrochloride is a synthetic version of the naturally occurring 6R-BH4, it can be reasonably anticipated to undergo the same metabolism, including 6R-BH4 regeneration.

Elimination

Following intravenous administration in rats, sapropterin dihydrochloride is mainly excreted in the urine. Following oral administration it is mainly eliminated through faeces while a small proportion is excreted in urine.

5.3 Preclinical safety data

Non-clinical data reveal no special hazard for humans based on conventional studies of safety pharmacology (CNS, respiratory, cardiovascular, genitourinary), and toxicity to reproduction.

An increased incidence of altered renal microscopic morphology (collecting tubule basophilia) was observed in rats following chronic oral administration of sapropterin dihydrochloride at exposures at or slightly above the maximal recommended human dose.

Sapropterin was found to be weakly mutagenic in bacterial cells and an increase in chromosome aberrations was detected in Chinese hamster lung and ovary cells. However, sapropterin has not been shown to be genotoxic in the *in vitro* test with human lymphocytes as well as in *in vivo* micronucleus mouse tests.

No tumorigenic activity was observed in an oral carcinogenicity study in mice at doses of up to 250 mg/kg/day(12.5 to 50 times the human therapeutic dose range).

Emesis has been observed in both the safety pharmacology and the repeated-dose toxicity studies. Emesis is considered to be related to the pH of the solution containing sapropterin.

No clear evidence of teratogenic activity was found in rats and in rabbits at doses of approximately 3 and 10 times the maximum recommended human dose, based on body surface area.

6. PHARMACEUTICAL PARTICULARS

6.1 List of excipients

Mannitol (E421)

Calcium hydrogen phosphate, anhydrous

Crospovidone type A

Ascorbic acid (E300)

Sodium stearyl fumarate

Riboflavin (E101)

6.2 Incompatibilities

Not applicable.

6.3 Shelf life

2 years.

6.4 Special precautions for storage

Store below 25°C.

Keep the bottle tightly closed in order to protect from moisture.

6.5 Nature and contents of container

High-density polyethylene (HDPE) bottle with child-resistant closure. The bottles are sealed with an aluminium seal. Each bottle of Kuvan contains a small plastic tube of desiccant (silica gel).

Each bottle contains 30, 120 or 240 tablets.

1 bottle per carton.

Not all pack sizes may be marketed.

6.6 Special precautions for disposal and other handling

Disposal

No special requirements.

Handling

Patients should be advised not to swallow the desiccant capsule found in the bottle.

7. MARKETING AUTHORISATION HOLDER

Merck KGaA

Frankfurter Str. 250

64293 Darmstadt

Germany

8. MARKETING AUTHORISATION NUMBER(S)

EU/1/08/481/001

EU/1/08/481/002

EU/1/08/481/003

9. DATE OF FIRST AUTHORISATION/RENEWAL OF THE AUTHORISATION

Date of the first authorisation: 2 December 2008

10. DATE OF REVISION OF THE TEXT

Detailed information on this product is available on the website of the European Medicines Agency (EMEA) http://www.emea.europa.eu.

Kytril Ampoules 1mg/1ml

(Roche Products Limited)

1. NAME OF THE MEDICINAL PRODUCT

Kytril Ampoules 1mg/1ml

2. QUALITATIVE AND QUANTITATIVE COMPOSITION

Each 1ml contains 1mg granisetron (as the hydrochloride). For excipients, see section *6.1.*

3. PHARMACEUTICAL FORM

A glass ampoule containing a sterile, clear colourless solution. The content allows withdrawal of 1ml.

Concentrate for solution for infusion or injection.

4. CLINICAL PARTICULARS

4.1 Therapeutic indications

Kytril is indicated for the prevention or treatment of nausea and vomiting induced by cytostatic therapy and for the prevention and treatment of post-operative nausea and vomiting.

4.2 Posology and method of administration

Cytostatic therapy

Children

Prevention: A single dose of 40µg/kg bodyweight (up to 3mg) should be administered as an intravenous infusion, diluted in 10 to 30ml infusion fluid and administered over five minutes. Administration should be completed prior to the start of cytostatic therapy.

Treatment: The same dose of Kytril as above should be used for treatment as prevention.

One additional dose of 40µg/kg bodyweight (up to 3mg) may be administered within a 24-hour period if required. This additional dose should be administered at least 10 minutes apart from the initial infusion.

Renally impaired

No special requirements apply.

Hepatically impaired

No special requirements apply.

Post-operative nausea and vomiting

Adults

For prevention in adults, a single dose of 1mg of Kytril should be diluted to 5ml and administered as a slow intravenous injection (over 30 seconds). Administration should be completed prior to induction of anaesthesia.

For the treatment of established post-operative nausea and vomiting in adults, a single dose of 1mg of Kytril should be diluted to 5ml and administered by slow intravenous injection (over 30 seconds).

Maximum dose and duration of treatment

Two doses (2mg) in one day.

Children

There is no experience in the use of Kytril in the prevention and treatment of post-operative nausea and vomiting in children. Kytril is not therefore recommended for the treatment of post-operative nausea and vomiting in this age group.

Elderly

As for adults.

Renally impaired

As for adults.

Hepatically impaired

As for adults.

4.3 Contraindications

Hypersensitivity to granisetron or related substances.

4.4 Special warnings and precautions for use

As Kytril may reduce lower bowel motility, patients with signs of sub-acute intestinal obstruction should be monitored following administration of Kytril.

No special precautions are required for the elderly or renally or hepatically impaired patient.

4.5 Interaction with other medicinal products and other forms of interaction

In studies in healthy subjects, no evidence of any interaction has been indicated between Kytril and cimetidine or lorazepam. No evidence of drug interactions has been observed in clinical studies conducted.

No specific interaction studies have been conducted in anaesthetised patients, but Kytril has been safely administered with commonly used anaesthetic and analgesic agents. In addition, *in vitro* human microsomal studies have shown that the cytochrome P450 sub-family 3A4 (involved in the metabolism of some of the main narcotic analgesic agents) is not modified by Kytril.

4.6 Pregnancy and lactation

Whilst animal studies have shown no teratogenic effects, there is no experience of Kytril in human pregnancy. Therefore Kytril should not be administered to women who are pregnant unless there are compelling clinical reasons. There are no data on the excretion of Kytril in breast milk. Breast feeding should therefore be discontinued during therapy.

4.7 Effects on ability to drive and use machines

There has been no evidence from human studies that Kytril has any adverse effect on alertness.

4.8 Undesirable effects

Kytril has been generally well tolerated in human studies. As reported with other drugs of this class, headache and constipation have been the most frequently noted adverse events but the majority have been mild or moderate in nature. Rare cases of hypersensitivity reaction, occasionally severe (e.g. anaphylaxis) have been reported. Other allergic reactions including minor skin rashes have also been reported. In clinical trials, transient increases in hepatic transaminases, generally within the normal range, have been seen.

Dystonias and dyskinesias have been reported with medicines in the 5-HT_3 antagonist class. Such events have been reported rarely with Kytril.

4.9 Overdose

There is no specific antidote for Kytril. In the case of overdosage, symptomatic treatment should be given. One patient has received 30mg of Kytril intravenously. The patient reported a slight headache but no other sequelae were observed.

5. PHARMACOLOGICAL PROPERTIES

5.1 Pharmacodynamic properties

Kytril is a potent anti-emetic and highly selective antagonist of 5-hydroxytryptamine (5-HT_3) receptors. Radioligand binding studies have demonstrated that Kytril has negligible affinity for other receptor types including 5-HT and dopamine D_2 binding sites.

Kytril is effective intravenously, either prophylactically or by intervention, in abolishing the retching and vomiting evoked by administration of cytotoxic drugs or by whole body X-irradiation.

Kytril is effective, intravenously, in the prevention and treatment of post-operative nausea and vomiting.

5.2 Pharmacokinetic properties

General characteristics

Distribution

Kytril is extensively distributed, with a mean volume of distribution of approximately 3L/kg; plasma protein binding is approximately 65%.

Biotransformation

Biotransformation pathways involve N-demethylation and aromatic ring oxidation followed by conjugation.

Elimination

Clearance is predominantly by hepatic metabolism. Urinary excretion of unchanged Kytril averages 12% of dose whilst that of metabolites amounts to about 47% of dose. The remainder is excreted in faeces as metabolites. Mean plasma half-life in patients is approximately nine hours, with a wide inter-subject variability.

Characteristics in patients

The plasma concentration of Kytril is not clearly correlated with anti-emetic efficacy. Clinical benefit may be conferred even when Kytril is not detectable in plasma.

In elderly subjects after single intravenous doses, pharmacokinetic parameters were within the range found for non-elderly subjects. In patients with severe renal failure, data indicate that pharmacokinetic parameters after a single intravenous dose are generally similar to those in normal subjects. In patients with hepatic impairment due to neoplastic liver involvement, total plasma clearance of an intravenous dose was approximately halved compared to patients without hepatic involvement. Despite these changes, no dosage adjustment is necessary.

5.3 Preclinical safety data

Data from two-year carcinogenicity studies have shown an increase in hepatocellular carcinoma and/or adenoma in rats and mice of both sexes given 50mg/kg (rat dosage reduced to 25mg/kg/day at week 59). Increases in hepatocellular neoplasia were also detected at 5mg/kg in male rats. In both species, drug-induced effects (hepatocellular neoplasia) were not observed in the low-dose group (1mg/kg).

In several *in vitro* and *in vivo* assays, Kytril was shown to be non-genotoxic in mammalian cells.

6. PHARMACEUTICAL PARTICULARS

6.1 List of excipients

Sodium Chloride

Water for Injection

Citric acid, monohydrate

Hydrochloric acid

Sodium hydroxide

6.2 Incompatibilities

As a general precaution, Kytril should not be mixed in solution with other drugs. Prophylactic administration of Kytril should be completed prior to the start of cytostatic therapy or induction of anaesthesia.

6.3 Shelf life

Kytril ampoules have a shelf-life of three years.

Once opened 24 hours.

6.4 Special precautions for storage

Do not store above 30°C. Keep container in the outer carton. Do not freeze.

6.5 Nature and contents of container

Kytril is supplied in clear glass ampoules in packs of five, with an outer carton.

6.6 Special precautions for disposal and other handling

Preparing the infusion

Children: To prepare the dose of 40 μg/kg, the appropriate volume is withdrawn and diluted with infusion fluid to a total volume of 10 to 30ml. Any one of the following solutions may be used:

0.9% w/v Sodium Chloride Injection BP; 0.18% w/v Sodium Chloride and 4% w/v Glucose Injection BP; 5% w/v Glucose Injection BP; Hartmann's Solution for Injection BP; Sodium Lactate Injection BP; or 10% Mannitol Injection BP. No other diluents should be used.

Ideally, intravenous infusions of Kytril should be prepared at the time of administration. After dilution (see above), or when the container is opened for the first time, the shelf-life is 24 hours when stored at ambient temperature in normal indoor illumination protected from direct sunlight. It must not be used after 24 hours. If to be stored after preparation, Kytril infusions must be prepared under appropriate aseptic conditions.

Adults: to prepare a dose of 1mg, 1ml should be withdrawn from the ampoule and diluted to 5ml with 0.9% w/v Sodium Chloride Injection BP. No other diluent should be used.

7. MARKETING AUTHORISATION HOLDER

Roche Products Limited, 6 Falcon Way, Shire Park, Welwyn Garden City, AL7 1TW, United Kingdom.

8. MARKETING AUTHORISATION NUMBER(S)

PL 00031/0595

9. DATE OF FIRST AUTHORISATION/RENEWAL OF THE AUTHORISATION

23rd October 1995/23rd October 2000.

10. DATE OF REVISION OF THE TEXT

June 2007

LEGAL STATUS

POM

Kytril is a registered trade mark

Item Code

Kytril Infusion 3mg/3ml

(Roche Products Limited)

1. NAME OF THE MEDICINAL PRODUCT

Kytril Infusion 3mg/3ml.

2. QUALITATIVE AND QUANTITATIVE COMPOSITION

Each 3ml contains 3.0mg granisetron (as the hydrochloride).

For excipients, see 6.1.

3. PHARMACEUTICAL FORM

An ampoule containing a sterile, clear, colourless or slightly straw-coloured solution equivalent to 1mg of granisetron per 1ml of solution. The content allows withdrawal of 3ml.

Concentrate for solution for infusion, or bolus injection.

4. CLINICAL PARTICULARS

4.1 Therapeutic indications

Kytril is indicated for the prevention or treatment of nausea and vomiting induced by cytostatic therapy.

4.2 Posology and method of administration

Adults

Kytril ampoules are for intravenous administration only.

3mg Kytril, which should be administered *either* in 15ml infusion fluid as an intravenous bolus over not less than 30 seconds *or* diluted in 20 to 50ml infusion fluid and administered over five minutes.

Prevention: In clinical trials, the majority of patients have required only a single dose of Kytril to control nausea and vomiting over 24 hours. Up to two additional doses of 3mg Kytril may be administered within a 24-hour period. There is clinical experience in patients receiving daily administration for up to five consecutive days in one course of therapy. Prophylactic administration of Kytril should be completed prior to the start of cytostatic therapy.

Treatment: The same dose of Kytril should be used for treatment as prevention. Additional doses should be administered at least 10 minutes apart.

Maximum daily dosage

Up to three doses of 3mg Kytril may be administered within a 24-hour period. The maximum dose of Kytril to be administered over 24 hours should not exceed 9mg.

Concomitant use of dexamethasone

The efficacy of Kytril may be enhanced by the addition of dexamethasone.

Children

Prevention: A single dose of 40 μg/kg body weight (up to 3mg) should be administered as an intravenous infusion, diluted in 10 to 30ml infusion fluid and administered over five minutes. Administration should be completed prior to the start of cytostatic therapy.

Treatment: The same dose of Kytril as above should be used for treatment as prevention.

One additional dose of 40 μg/kg body weight (up to 3mg) may be administered within a 24-hour period. This additional dose should be administered at least 10 minutes apart from the initial infusion.

Elderly

No special requirements apply to elderly patients.

Patients with renal or hepatic impairment

No special requirements apply to those patients with renal or hepatic impairment.

4.3 Contraindications

Hypersensitivity to granisetron, related substances or the excipients (see section *6.1*).

4.4 Special warnings and precautions for use

As Kytril may reduce lower bowel motility, patients with signs of sub-acute intestinal obstruction should be monitored following administration of Kytril.

No special precautions are required for the elderly or renally or hepatically impaired patient.

4.5 Interaction with other medicinal products and other forms of interaction

In studies in healthy subjects, no evidence of any interaction has been indicated between Kytril and cimetidine or lorazepam. No evidence of drug interactions has been observed in clinical studies conducted.

4.6 Pregnancy and lactation

Whilst animal studies have shown no teratogenic effects, there is no experience of Kytril in human pregnancy. Therefore Kytril should not be administered to women who are pregnant unless there are compelling clinical reasons. There are no data on the excretion of Kytril in breast milk. Breast feeding should therefore be discontinued during therapy.

4.7 Effects on ability to drive and use machines

There has been no evidence from human studies that Kytril has any adverse effect on alertness.

4.8 Undesirable effects

Kytril has been generally well tolerated in human studies. As reported with other drugs of this class, headache and constipation have been the most frequently noted adverse events but the majority have been mild or moderate in nature. Rare cases of hypersensitivity reaction, occasionally severe (e.g. anaphylaxis) have been reported. Other allergic reactions including minor skin rashes have also been reported. In clinical trials, transient increases in hepatic transaminases, generally within the normal range, have been seen.

Dystonias and dyskinesias have been reported with medicines in the 5-HT_3 antagonist class. Such events have been reported rarely with Kytril.

4.9 Overdose

There is no specific antidote for Kytril. In the case of overdosage, symptomatic treatment should be given. One patient has received 30mg of Kytril intravenously. The patient reported a slight headache but no other sequelae were observed.

5. PHARMACOLOGICAL PROPERTIES

5.1 Pharmacodynamic properties

Kytril is a potent anti-emetic and highly selective antagonist of 5-hydroxytryptamine (5-HT_3) receptors. Radioligand binding studies have demonstrated that Kytril has negligible affinity for other receptor types including 5-HT and dopamine D_2 binding sites.

Kytril is effective intravenously, either prophylactically or by intervention, in abolishing the retching and vomiting evoked by administration of cytotoxic drugs or by whole body X-irradiation.

5.2 Pharmacokinetic properties

General characteristics

Distribution

Kytril is extensively distributed, with a mean volume of distribution of approximately 3 L/kg; plasma protein binding is approximately 65%.

Biotransformation

Biotransformation pathways involve N-demethylation and aromatic ring oxidation followed by conjugation.

Elimination

Clearance is predominantly by hepatic metabolism. Urinary excretion of unchanged Kytril averages 12% of dose whilst that of metabolites amounts to about 47% of dose. The remainder is excreted in faeces as metabolites. Mean plasma half-life in patients is approximately nine hours, with a wide inter-subject variability.

Characteristics in patients

The plasma concentration of Kytril is not clearly correlated with anti-emetic efficacy. Clinical benefit may be conferred even when Kytril is not detectable in plasma.

In elderly subjects after single intravenous doses, pharmacokinetic parameters were within the range found for non-elderly subjects. In patients with severe renal failure, data indicate that pharmacokinetic parameters after a single intravenous dose are generally similar to those in normal subjects. In patients with hepatic impairment due to neoplastic liver involvement, total plasma clearance of an intravenous dose was approximately halved compared to patients without hepatic involvement. Despite these changes, no dosage adjustment is necessary.

5.3 Preclinical safety data
Data from two-year carcinogenicity studies have shown an increase in hepatocellular carcinoma and/or adenoma in rats and mice of both sexes given 50mg/kg (rat dosage reduced to 25mg/kg/day at week 59). Increases in hepatocellular neoplasia were also detected at 5mg/kg in male rats. In both species, drug-induced effects (hepatocellular neoplasia) were not observed in the low-dose group (1mg/kg).

In several *in vitro* and *in vivo* assays, Kytril was shown to be non-genotoxic in mammalian cells.

6. PHARMACEUTICAL PARTICULARS
6.1 List of excipients
Sodium Chloride

Water for Injection

Citric acid, monohydrate

Hydrochloric acid

Sodium hydroxide

6.2 Incompatibilities
As a general precaution, Kytril should not be mixed in solution with other drugs. Prophylactic administration of Kytril should be completed prior to the start of cytostatic therapy.

6.3 Shelf life
Kytril ampoules have a shelf-life of three years.

6.4 Special precautions for storage
Kytril ampoules should be stored protected from light. Do not freeze.

6.5 Nature and contents of container
Kytril is supplied in clear glass ampoules packaged in boxes of 5 or 10 ampoules.

6.6 Special precautions for disposal and other handling
Preparing the infusion
Adults: To prepare a dose of 3mg, 3ml is withdrawn from the ampoule and diluted either to 15ml with 0.9% w/v Sodium Chloride Injection BP (for bolus administration) or in infusion fluid to a total volume of 20 to 50ml in any of the following solutions: 0.9% w/v Sodium Chloride Injection BP; 0.18% w/v Sodium Chloride and 4% w/v Glucose Injection BP; 5% w/v Glucose Injection BP; Hartmann's Solution for Injection BP; Sodium Lactate Injection BP; or 10% Mannitol Injection BP (for infusion). No other diluents should be used.

Children: To prepare the dose of 40μg/kg the appropriate volume (up to 3ml) is withdrawn from the ampoule and diluted with infusion fluid (as for adults) to a total volume of 10 to 30ml.

Ideally, intravenous infusions of Kytril should be prepared at the time of administration. After dilution (see above) the shelf life is 24 hours when stored at ambient temperature in normal indoor illumination protected from direct sunlight. It must not be used after 24 hours. If to be stored after preparation, Kytril infusions must be prepared under appropriate aseptic conditions.

As a general precaution, Kytril should not be mixed in solution with other drugs.

7. MARKETING AUTHORISATION HOLDER
Roche Products Limited, 6 Falcon Way, Shire Park, Welwyn Garden City, AL7 1TW, United Kingdom.

8. MARKETING AUTHORISATION NUMBER(S)
PL 00031/0594

9. DATE OF FIRST AUTHORISATION/RENEWAL OF THE AUTHORISATION
15 October 2001

10. DATE OF REVISION OF THE TEXT
June 2007

Legal STATUS
POM

Kytril is a registered trade mark

Item Code

Kytril Tablets 1mg and 2mg

(Roche Products Limited)

1. NAME OF THE MEDICINAL PRODUCT
Kytril Tablets 1mg and 2mg.

2. QUALITATIVE AND QUANTITATIVE COMPOSITION
Each tablet contains 1mg or 2mg granisetron (as hydrochloride).

Excipients include lactose (see section *4.3 Contraindications*).

For full list of excipients, see section *6.1*.

3. PHARMACEUTICAL FORM
Film-coated Tablet.

White triangular film-coated tablets marked 'K1' or 'K2' on one side.

4. CLINICAL PARTICULARS
4.1 Therapeutic indications
Kytril tablets are indicated for the prevention of nausea and vomiting induced by cytostatic therapy.

4.2 Posology and method of administration
Adults
The dose of Kytril is 1mg twice a day or 2mg once a day during cytostatic therapy.

The first dose of Kytril should be administered within one hour before the start of cytostatic therapy.

Concomitant use of dexamethasone: The efficacy of Kytril may be enhanced by the addition of dexamethasone.

Maximum Dose and Duration of Treatment
Kytril is also available as ampoules for intravenous administration. The maximum dose of Kytril administered orally and/or intravenously over 24 hours should not exceed 9mg.

Children
There is insufficient evidence on which to base appropriate dosage regimens for children under 12 years old. Kytril Tablets are therefore not recommended in this age group.

Elderly
As for adults.

Renally Impaired
As for adults.

Hepatically Impaired
As for adults.

4.3 Contraindications
Hypersensitivity to granisetron, related substances, or the excipients (see section *6.1*).

Owing to the presence of lactose, patients with rare hereditary problems of galactose intolerance, the Lapp lactase deficiency or glucose-galactose malabsorption should not take this medicine.

4.4 Special warnings and precautions for use
As Kytril may reduce lower bowel motility, patients with signs of sub-acute intestinal obstruction should be monitored following administration of Kytril.

4.5 Interaction with other medicinal products and other forms of interaction
In studies in healthy subjects, no evidence of any interaction has been indicated between Kytril and cimetidine or lorazepam. No evidence of drug interactions has been observed in clinical studies.

4.6 Pregnancy and lactation
Whilst animal studies have shown no teratogenic effects, there is no experience of Kytril in human pregnancy. Therefore Kytril should not be administered to women who are pregnant unless there are compelling clinical reasons. There are no data on the excretion of Kytril in breast milk. Breast feeding should therefore be discontinued during therapy.

4.7 Effects on ability to drive and use machines
There has been no evidence from human studies that Kytril has any adverse effect on alertness.

4.8 Undesirable effects
Kytril has been generally well tolerated in human studies. As reported with other drugs of this class, headache and constipation have been the most frequently noted adverse events, but the majority have been mild or moderate in nature. Rare cases of hypersensitivity reaction, occasionally severe (e.g. anaphylaxis), have been reported. Other allergic reactions including minor skin rashes have also been reported. In clinical trials, transient increases in hepatic transaminases, generally within the normal range, have been seen.

Dystonias and dyskinesias have been reported with medicines in the 5-HT_3 antagonist class. Such events have been reported rarely with Kytril.

4.9 Overdose
There is no specific antidote for Kytril. In the case of overdosage, symptomatic treatment should be given. One patient has received 30mg of Kytril intravenously. The patient reported a slight headache but no other sequelae were observed.

5. PHARMACOLOGICAL PROPERTIES
5.1 Pharmacodynamic properties
Kytril is a potent anti-emetic and highly selective antagonist of 5-hydroxytryptamine (5-HT_3) receptors. Radioligand binding studies have demonstrated that Kytril has negligible affinity for other receptor types including 5-HT and dopamine D_2 binding sites.

Kytril is effective orally prophylactically in abolishing the retching and vomiting evoked by cytostatic therapy.

5.2 Pharmacokinetic properties
General Characteristics
Absorption
Absorption of Kytril is rapid and complete, though oral bioavailability is reduced to about 60% as a result of first pass metabolism. Oral bioavailability is generally not influenced by food.

Distribution
Kytril is extensively distributed, with a mean volume of distribution of approximately 3 l/kg; plasma protein binding is approximately 65%.

Biotransformation
Biotransformation pathways involve N-demethylation and aromatic ring oxidation followed by conjugation.

Elimination
Clearance is predominantly by hepatic metabolism. Urinary excretion of unchanged Kytril averages 12% of dose whilst that of metabolites amounts to about 47% of dose. The remainder is excreted in faeces as metabolites. Mean plasma half-life in patients is approximately nine hours, with a wide inter-subject variability.

The pharmacokinetics of Kytril demonstrate no marked deviations from linear pharmacokinetics at oral doses up to 2.5-fold of the recommended clinical dose.

Characteristics in Patients
The plasma concentration of Kytril is not clearly correlated with anti-emetic efficacy. Clinical benefit may be conferred even when Kytril is not detectable in plasma.

In elderly subjects after single intravenous doses, pharmacokinetic parameters were within the range found for non-elderly subjects. In patients with severe renal failure, data indicate that pharmacokinetic parameters after a single intravenous dose are generally similar to those in normal subjects. In patients with hepatic impairment due to neoplastic liver involvement, total plasma clearance of an intravenous dose was approximately halved compared to patients without hepatic involvement. Despite these changes, no dosage adjustment is necessary.

5.3 Preclinical safety data
Data from two-year carcinogenicity studies have shown an increase in hepatocellular carcinoma and/or adenoma in rats and mice of both sexes given 50mg/kg (rat dosage reduced to 25mg/kg/day at week 59). Increases in hepatocellular neoplasia were also detected at 5mg/kg in male rats. In both species, drug-induced effects (hepatocellular neoplasia) were not observed in the low-dose group (1mg/kg).

In several *in vitro* and *in vivo* assays, Kytril was shown to be non-genotoxic in mammalian cells.

6. PHARMACEUTICAL PARTICULARS
6.1 List of excipients
Microcrystalline Cellulose (E460)

Sodium Starch Glycolate

Hypromellose (E464)

Lactose monohydrate

Magnesium Stearate (E572)

Film coat:

Hypromellose (E464)

Titanium dioxide (E171)

Macrogol 400

Polysorbate 80 (E433)

6.2 Incompatibilities
None.

6.3 Shelf life
Kytril Tablets have a shelf-life of three years.

6.4 Special precautions for storage
None.

6.5 Nature and contents of container
Opaque PVC/aluminium foil blister packs packed in cartons containing 10 tablets (1mg) or 5 tablets (2mg).

6.6 Special precautions for disposal and other handling
None.

7. MARKETING AUTHORISATION HOLDER
Roche Products Limited, 6 Falcon Way, Shire Park, Welwyn Garden City, AL7 1TW, United Kingdom.

8. MARKETING AUTHORISATION NUMBER(S)
PL 00031/0591 (1mg)

PL 00031/0592 (2mg)

9. DATE OF FIRST AUTHORISATION/RENEWAL OF THE AUTHORISATION
15 September 2001

10. DATE OF REVISION OF THE TEXT
July 2007

Legal STATUS
POM

Kytril is a registered trade mark

Lacri-Lube/Refresh Night Time Eye Ointment

(Allergan Ltd)

1. NAME OF THE MEDICINAL PRODUCT
LACRI-LUBE® Eye ointment

REFRESH NIGHT TIME® Eye ointment

2. QUALITATIVE AND QUANTITATIVE COMPOSITION
No pharmacologically active ingredient is present.

For excipients, see 6.1.

3. PHARMACEUTICAL FORM
Eye ointment.

Smooth, homogeneous, off-white, preservative-free ointment.

4. CLINICAL PARTICULARS

4.1 Therapeutic indications
As adjunctive therapy to lubricate and protect the eye in conditions such as exposure keratitis, decreased corneal sensitivity, recurrent corneal erosions, keratitis sicca, ophthalmic and non-ophthalmic surgery.

4.2 Posology and method of administration
For topical ocular administration.

Pull lower eye lid down to form a pocket and apply small amount as required.

There is no variation in dosage for age.

4.3 Contraindications
Hypersensitivity to lanolin alcohols.

4.4 Special warnings and precautions for use
To avoid contamination during use, do not touch the tube tip to any surface.
If irritation, pain, redness and changes in vision occur or worsen, treatment discontinuation should be considered and a re-evaluation of the patient's condition should be made.
Contact lenses should not be worn during instillation of the drug. After instillation there should be an interval of at least 30 minutes before reinsertion.

In circumstances where concomitant topical ocular medication is necessary, there should be an interval of at least 5 minutes between the two medications. LACRI-LUBE® / REFRESH NIGHT TIME® should always be the last medication instilled.

4.5 Interaction with other medicinal products and other forms of interaction
No interactions have been observed with LACRI-LUBE® / REFRESH NIGHT TIME®. Since the constituents have a well-established medicinal use, no interactions are anticipated.

4.6 Pregnancy and lactation
The constituents of LACRI-LUBE® / REFRESH NIGHT TIME® have been used as pharmaceutical agents for many years with no untoward effects. No special precautions are therefore necessary for the use of LACRI-LUBE® / REFRESH NIGHT TIME® in pregnancy and lactation.

Women of child-bearing potential: suitable for use.

Fertility: no known implications.

4.7 Effects on ability to drive and use machines
May cause transient blurring of vision. Do not drive or use machinery unless vision is clear.

4.8 Undesirable effects
Local (ocular) effects:

Transient blurring of vision (typically lasting 1-15 minutes) may occur.

Rare (>1/10,000, <1/1,000): irritation/stinging/burning sensation,

Very rare (<1/10,000): allergic reaction, pain, hyperaemia, and conjunctivitis.

Isolated reports of oedema, and pruritus.

4.9 Overdose
Accidental topical ocular overdosage will present no hazard, apart from a transient effect on vision (see 4.7).

5. PHARMACOLOGICAL PROPERTIES

5.1 Pharmacodynamic properties
Pharmacotherapeutic group (ATC code) = *S01X A* 20.

The ingredients of LACRI-LUBE® / REFRESH NIGHT TIME® are pharmacologically inert, bland oleaginous substances for lubrication and to maintain hydration of the ocular surfaces by occlusion.

5.2 Pharmacokinetic properties
Not applicable.

5.3 Preclinical safety data
No information.

6. PHARMACEUTICAL PARTICULARS

6.1 List of excipients
White soft paraffin (white petroleum jelly)

Mineral oil

Lanolin alcohols

6.2 Incompatibilities
None known.

6.3 Shelf life
Shelf life of the medicinal product as packaged for sale = 36 months.

Shelf life after first opening of container = 1 month.

6.4 Special precautions for storage
Do not store above 25°C.

6.5 Nature and contents of container
Container: 3.5 and 5.0g per tube.

Collapsible metal tube:

Aluminium (99.5 to 99.7%) or pig tin (98.8%).

Internal coating:

Melamine-epoxy resin or epoxyphenolic liner.

Closure

Polyethylene; colourant: black.

Sealant

Darex WBC 2311D-63.5 or Valspar LO-7505.

Dispensing under medical prescription or sale from registered pharmacies.

6.6 Special precautions for disposal and other handling
Discard any unused product 1 month after first opening.

7. MARKETING AUTHORISATION HOLDER
Allergan Ltd

Marlow International

The Parkway

Marlow

Bucks

SL7 1YL

United Kingdom

8. MARKETING AUTHORISATION NUMBER(S)
PL 00426/0041

9. DATE OF FIRST AUTHORISATION/RENEWAL OF THE AUTHORISATION
23rd July 2003

10. DATE OF REVISION OF THE TEXT
1st April 2008

Lactugal

(Intrapharm Laboratories Ltd)

1. NAME OF THE MEDICINAL PRODUCT
Lactugal.

2. QUALITATIVE AND QUANTITATIVE COMPOSITION
Active Ingredient:

Lactulose Solution BP 99.897 % v/v

(Equivalent to 62.0-74.0% w/v of Lactulose).

3. PHARMACEUTICAL FORM
Oral solution. Banana Flavour

4. CLINICAL PARTICULARS

4.1 Therapeutic indications
Constipation; Hepatic encephalopathy (Portal systemic encephalopathy).

4.2 Posology and method of administration
For oral administration.

Adults:

Constipation: 15ml once or twice daily.

Hepatic Encephalopathy: Initially 30-50ml three times daily, adjust dose to produce 2 or 3 soft stools daily.

Children:

1-5 years: 5ml twice daily.

5-10 years: l0ml twice daily.

Elderly:

The normal adult dosage is appropriate.

4.3 Contraindications
Lactugal is contra-indicated where there is evidence of gastro-intestinal obstruction and to patients with galactosaemia.

4.4 Special warnings and precautions for use
There are no warnings or precautions for patients with any impaired organ function.

Lactulose should be used with caution in patients exhibiting lactose intolerance.

Due to the product's physiological mode of action it may take up to 48 hours before effects are obtained, however, the product does exhibit a 'carry over' effect which may enable the patient to reduce the dose gradually over a period of time.

Lactulose solution has a calorific value of approximately 19Kcals/5ml. As, however, only negligible amounts of lactulose are absorbed from the gastrointestinal tract the available calories will be much lower than this, and therefore, is unlikely to adversely affect diabetes.

4.5 Interaction with other medicinal products and other forms of interaction
There are no known interactions with lactulose.

4.6 Pregnancy and lactation
Wide clinical experience in combination with data from animal production studies has not revealed any embryotoxic hazards to the foetus if used in the recommended dosage during pregnancy. If drug therapy is required during pregnancy or for lactating mothers, the use of this drug is acceptable.

4.7 Effects on ability to drive and use machines
There is no evidence to show that lactulose affects driving ability.

4.8 Undesirable effects
A normal dosage of lactulose may cause mild abdominal pain and flatulence which will disappear spontaneously after a few days. High doses may provoke nausea in some patients and this can be minimised by administration with water, fruit juice or meals.

4.9 Overdose
If clinically important electrolyte disturbances occur, suitable corrective measures should be taken.

5. PHARMACOLOGICAL PROPERTIES

5.1 Pharmacodynamic properties
Lactulose is a synthetic disaccharide which is metabolised by gastro-intestinal bacterial flora to low molecular weight acids (chiefly lactic and acetic acids). There is no endogenous metabolising enzyme in the human gut.

Its mode of action in constipation is as an osmotic agent producing soft stools.

A dual mode of action is proposed for the efficacy of lactulose in Portal System Encephalopathy, relating to the metabolism of ammonia and subsequent nitrogenous toxins. The reduction in gastro-intestinal pH results in a net entrapment of ammonia in the gut lumen. Lactulose has also been shown to alter ammonia metabolism by microbial flora.

5.2 Pharmacokinetic properties
Lactulose is absorbed from the gastro-intestinal tract to 0.4 - 2% and is excreted unchanged with the urine. There are no human lactulose disaccharide enzymes; metabolism of lactulose to lactic acid occurs via gastro-intestinal microbial flora only. Due to its poor bioavailability, plasma lactulose concentrations are negligible.

There are no known changes in kinetic properties in patients with organic diseases which may alter drug disposition.

5.3 Preclinical safety data
None stated.

6. PHARMACEUTICAL PARTICULARS

6.1 List of excipients
Banana Flavour Quinoline Yellow

(17.41.0042) (E 1 04)

6.2 Incompatibilities
There are no known incompatibilities.

6.3 Shelf life
36 months from the date of manufacture.

6.4 Special precautions for storage
Store at a temperature not exceeding 20°C. Do not freeze

6.5 Nature and contents of container
Amber glass winchesters with polypropylene caps as closures. Polyethylene containers with polypropylene caps as closures.

6.6 Special precautions for disposal and other handling
There are no special storage or handling instructions for this product.

Administrative Data

7. MARKETING AUTHORISATION HOLDER
Intrapharm Laboratories Ltd

Maidstone

Kent

ME15 9QS

United Kingdom

8. MARKETING AUTHORISATION NUMBER(S)
PL 17509/0011

9. DATE OF FIRST AUTHORISATION/RENEWAL OF THE AUTHORISATION
4 September 2003

10. DATE OF REVISION OF THE TEXT

Lactulose Solution (Novartis Consumer Health)

(Novartis Consumer Health)

1. NAME OF THE MEDICINAL PRODUCT
Lactulose Liquid Ph Eur

Lactulose Liquid EP

2. QUALITATIVE AND QUANTITATIVE COMPOSITION
Lactulose 67.0% w/v

3. PHARMACEUTICAL FORM
Oral Solution

4. CLINICAL PARTICULARS
4.1 Therapeutic indications
A. Chronic constipation.

B. Chronic portal systemic encephalopathy.

4.2 Posology and method of administration
Adults

Initially:	15-30ml daily for first 2-3 days (45ml may be given in obstinate cases).
Maintenance:	10-15ml daily or according to the need of the patient

Children

Initially:	10-25ml daily for first 2-3 days.
Maintenance:	5-15ml daily or according to the need of the patient.

Dosage does not appear to be related to the age or weight of the child and should be adjusted to produce the required response.

Chronic portal systemic encephalopathy
Initially 30-50ml three times daily according to the requirements of the patient for adequate acidification of the colonic contents.

Use in the elderly
No evidence exists that elderly patients require different dosages or show different side-effects from younger patients.

4.3 Contraindications
In common with other preparations used for the treatment of constipation, Lactulose solution should not be used in patients with gastrointestinal obstruction. Lactulose solution should not be given to patients with galactosaemia or lactose intolerance.

4.4 Special warnings and precautions for use
Prolonged use of Lactulose in children may contribute to the development of dental caries. Patients should be instructed to pay careful attention to dental hygiene.

4.5 Interaction with other medicinal products and other forms of interaction
There are no known interactions involving Lactulose.

4.6 Pregnancy and lactation
Lactulose solution should be used with caution during the first trimester of pregnancy.

4.7 Effects on ability to drive and use machines
There is no evidence that Lactulose affects driving ability.

4.8 Undesirable effects
Side-effects rarely occur after the administration of Lactulose solution. Mild transient effects such as abdominal distension or cramps and flatulence, which subside after the initial stages of treatment, have occasionally been reported. High doses may provoke nausea in some patients.

This can be minimised by administration with water, fruit juice or with meals.

4.9 Overdose
No cases of intoxication due to deliberate or accidental overdosage with Lactulose solution have been reported to the company.

5. PHARMACOLOGICAL PROPERTIES
5.1 Pharmacodynamic properties
The active principle of Lactulose solution, lactulose, is neither broken down nor absorbed in the stomach and small intestine. In the colon it acts as a substrate for and promotes the growth of naturally occurring glycolytic micro-organisms, and is broken down to lactic acid. The pH of the intestinal contents is lowered, the growth of acidophilic flora is promoted and the putrefactive micro-organisms are suppressed. This reduces the formation of ammonia and amines and their absorption from the gut, thus leading to a fall in blood ammonia levels (responsible for hepatic encephalopathy). By normalising the intestinal flora Lactulose solution ensures the passage of normal stools, without excessive peristalsis.

5.2 Pharmacokinetic properties
Not appropriate.

5.3 Preclinical safety data
There are no preclinical data of relevance to the prescriber which are additional to those already included in other sections of the Summary of Product Characteristics.

6. PHARMACEUTICAL PARTICULARS
6.1 List of excipients
Other sugars (lactose, galactose, tagatose and other ketoses)

Purified water

6.2 Incompatibilities
Not applicable.

6.3 Shelf life
36 months.

6.4 Special precautions for storage
Do not store above 25°C.

6.5 Nature and contents of container
Amber glass bottles, plastic bottles (HDPE), PET bottles with polyethylene closure (polyethylene wad faced with PP. PVDC or PET lining), containing 200 ml, 300 ml, 500 ml or 1 litre of Lactulose solution.

6.6 Special precautions for disposal and other handling
Not applicable.

Administrative Data
7. MARKETING AUTHORISATION HOLDER
Novartis Consumer Health UK Limited

Trading as Novartis Consumer Health

Wimblehurst Road

Horsham

West Sussex

RH12 5AB

UK

8. MARKETING AUTHORISATION NUMBER(S)
PL 00030/0175

9. DATE OF FIRST AUTHORISATION/RENEWAL OF THE AUTHORISATION
10 April 2000

10. DATE OF REVISION OF THE TEXT
4th January 2006

Legal category
P

Lamictal Combined Tablets

(GlaxoSmithKline UK)

1. NAME OF THE MEDICINAL PRODUCT
Lamictal Tablets 25mg

Lamictal Tablets 50mg

Lamictal Tablets 100mg

Lamictal Tablets 200mg

Lamictal Dispersible 2mg

Lamictal Dispersible 5mg

Lamictal Dispersible 25mg

Lamictal Dispersible 100mg

2. QUALITATIVE AND QUANTITATIVE COMPOSITION
Lamictal Tablets containing 25mg lamotrigine.

Lamictal Tablets containing 50mg lamotrigine.

Lamictal Tablets containing 100mg lamotrigine.

Lamictal Tablets containing 200mg lamotrigine.

Lamictal Dispersible 2 mg contain 2 mg lamotrigine.

Lamictal Dispersible 5 mg contain 5 mg lamotrigine.

Lamictal Dispersible 25 mg contain 25 mg lamotrigine.

Lamictal Dispersible 100 mg contain 100 mg lamotrigine.

For excipients see section 6.1.

3. PHARMACEUTICAL FORM
Lamictal tablets 25mg are pale yellowish brown, multi-faceted, superelliptical unscored tablets, branded 'GSEC7'on one side, with '25' on the reverse.

Lamictal Tablets 50mg are pale yellowish brown, multi-faceted, superelliptical unscored tablets, branded 'GSEE1'on one side, with '50' on the reverse.

Lamictal Tablets 100mg are pale yellowish brown, multi-faceted, superelliptical unscored tablets, branded 'GSEE5'on one side, with '100' on the reverse.

Lamictal Tablets 200mg are pale yellowish brown, multi-faceted, superelliptical unscored tablets, branded 'GSEE7'on one side, with '200' on the reverse.

Lamictal Dispersible 2mg are white to off-white round tablets with a blackcurrant odour. One side has a bevelled edge and is engraved with LTG over the number 2. The other side is engraved with two overlapping super-ellipses at right angles.

Lamictal Dispersible 5mg are white elongated, biconvex, tablets with "5" on one side and "GSCL2" on the other.

Lamictal Dispersible 25mg are white, multifaceted, super elliptical tablets with "25" on one side and "GSCL5" on the other.

Lamictal Dispersible 100mg are white multifaceted, super elliptical tablets with "100" on one side and "GSCL7" on the other.

4. CLINICAL PARTICULARS
4.1 Therapeutic indications
Epilepsy: *Monotherapy in adults and children over 12 years of age:*

Simple partial seizures

Complex partial seizures

Secondarily generalised tonic-clonic seizures

Primary generalised tonic-clonic seizures

Monotherapy in children under 12 years of age is not recommended until such time as adequate information is made available from controlled trials in this particular target population.

Add-on therapy in adults and children over 2 years of age

Simple partial seizures

Complex partial seizures

Secondarily generalised tonic-clonic seizures

Primary generalised tonic-clonic seizures

Lamictal is also indicated for the treatment of seizures associated with Lennox-Gastaut Syndrome.

4.2 Posology and method of administration
Administration
Lamictal Tablets should be swallowed whole with a little water.

Lamictal Dispersible tablets may be chewed, dispersed in a small volume of water (at least enough to cover the whole tablet) or swallowed whole with a little water.

To ensure a therapeutic dose is maintained the weight of a child must be monitored and the dose reviewed as weight changes occur.

If a calculated dose of lamotrigine (e.g. for use in children and patients with hepatic impairment) does not equate to whole tablets the dose to be administered is that equal to the lower number of whole tablets.

When concomitant antiepileptic drugs are withdrawn to achieve Lamictal monotherapy or other antiepileptic drugs (AEDs)/medications are added-on to treatment regimes containing Lamictal consideration should be given to the effect this may have on lamotrigine pharmacokinetics (see 4.5 Interaction with other Medicinal Products and other Forms of Interaction).

Restarting Therapy
Prescribers should assess the need for escalation to maintenance dose when restarting lamotrigine in patients who have discontinued lamotrigine for any reason, since the risk of serious rash is associated with high initial doses and exceeding the recommended dose escalation for lamotrigine (see section 4.4). The greater the interval of time since the previous dose, the more consideration should be given to escalation to the maintenance dose. When the interval since discontinuing lamotrigine exceeds five half-lives (see section 5.2), lamotrigine should generally be escalated to the maintenance dose according to the appropriate schedule, as though initiating therapy (see section 4.2).

Dosage in monotherapy
Adults and children over 12 years (see Table 1)

The initial Lamictal dose in monotherapy is 25mg once a day for two weeks, followed by 50mg once a day for two weeks. Thereafter, the dose should be increased by a maximum of 50mg-100mg every 1-2 weeks until the optimal response is achieved. The usual maintenance dose to achieve optimal response is 100 - 200mg/day given once a day or as two divided doses. Some patients have required 500mg/day of Lamictal to achieve the desired response.

The initial dose and subsequent dose escalation should not be exceeded to minimise the risk of rash (see Special Warnings and Special Precautions for Use).

Children aged 2 to 12 years

There is insufficient evidence available from appropriate studies in children, upon which to base dosage recommendations for monotherapy use in children under the age of 12 years (see Therapeutic Indications).

Dosage in add-on therapy
Adults and children over 12 years (see Table 1)

In patients taking valproate with / without any other anti-epileptic drug (AED) the initial Lamictal dose is 25 mg every alternate day for two weeks, followed by 25 mg once a day for two weeks. Thereafter, the dose should be increased by a maximum of 25-50mg every 1-2 weeks until the optimal response is achieved. The usual maintenance dose to achieve optimal response is 100-200mg/day given once a day or in two divided doses.

In those patients taking concomitant AEDs or other medications (see section 4.5) that induce lamotrigine glucuronidation with / without other AED's (except valproate) the initial Lamictal dose is 50 mg once a day for two weeks, followed by 100 mg/day given in two divided doses for two

Table 1 Recommended treatment regimen for adults and children over 12 years of age

Treatment regimen		Weeks 1 + 2	Weeks 3 + 4	Usual Maintenance Dose
Monotherapy		25 mg (once a day)	50 mg (once a day)	100 – 200 mg (once a day or two divided doses) To achieve maintenance, doses may be increased by 50 – 100 mg every one to two weeks
Add-on therapy with valproate regardless of any concomitant medications		12.5 mg (given 25 mg on alternate days)	25 mg (once a day)	100 – 200 mg (once a day or two divided doses) To achieve maintenance, doses may be increased by 25 – 50 mg every one to two weeks
Add-on therapy without valproate	This dosage regimen should be used with: Phenytoin Carbamazepine Phenobarbital primidone or with other inducers of lamotrigine glucuronidation (see section 4.5).	50 mg (once a day)	100 mg (two divided doses)	200 – 400 mg (two divided doses) To achieve maintenance, doses may be increased by 100 mg every one to two weeks
	With oxcarbazepine without inducers or inhibitors of lamotrigine glucuronidation	25 mg (once a day)	50 mg (once a day)	100 – 200 mg (once a day or two divided doses) To achieve maintenance, doses may be increased by 50 – 100 mg every one to two weeks

Note: In patients taking AEDs where the pharmacokinetic interaction with lamotrigine is currently not known (see section 4.5), the treatment regimen as recommended for lamotrigine with concurrent valproate should be used, thereafter, the dose should be increased until optimal response is achieved.

weeks. Thereafter, the dose should be increased by a maximum of 100mg every 1-2 weeks until the optimal response is achieved. The usual maintenance dose to achieve optimal response is 200-400mg/day given in two divided doses. Some patients have required 700 mg/day of Lamictal to achieve the desired response.

In those patients taking oxcarbazepine without any other inducers or inhibitors of lamotrigine glucuronidation, the initial lamotrigine dose is 25 mg once a day for two weeks, followed by 50 mg once a day for two weeks. Thereafter, the dose should be increased by a maximum of 50 to 100 mg every one to two weeks until the optimal response is achieved. The usual maintenance dose to achieve an optimal response is 100 to 200 mg/day given once a day or as two divided doses.

Table 1 Recommended treatment regimen for adults and children over 12 years of age

(see Table 1 above)

The initial dose and subsequent dose escalation should not be exceeded to minimise the risk of rash (see Special Warnings and Special Precautions for Use).

Children aged 2 to 12 years (see Table 2)

In patients taking valproate with / without any other anti-epileptic drug (AED), the initial Lamictal dose is 0.15 mg/kg bodyweight/day given once a day for two weeks, followed by 0.3 mg/kg/day given once a day for two weeks. Thereafter, the dose should be increased by a maximum of 0.3 mg/kg every 1-2 weeks until the optimal response is achieved. The usual maintenance dose to achieve optimal response is 1-5 mg/kg/day given once a day or in two divided doses.

In those patients taking concomitantAEDs or other medications (see section 4.5) that induce lamotrigine glucuronidation with / without other AED's (except valproate) the initial Lamictal dose is 0.6 mg/kg bodyweight/day given in two divided doses for two weeks, followed by 1.2mg/kg/day for two weeks. Thereafter, the dose should be increased by a maximum of 1.2 mg/kg every 1-2 weeks until the optimal response is achieved. The usual maintenance dose to achieve optimal response is 5-15mg/kg/day given in two divided doses.

In patients taking oxcarbazepine without any inducers or inhibitors of lamotrigine glucuronidation, the initial lamotrigine dose is 0.3 mg/kg bodyweight/day given once a day or in two divided doses for two weeks, followed by 0.6 mg/kg/day given once a day or in two divided doses for two weeks. Thereafter, the dose should be increased by a maximum of 0.6 mg/kg every one to two weeks until the optimal response is achieved. The usual maintenance dose to achieve optimal response is 1 to 10 mg/kg/day given once a day or in two divided doses, with a maximum of 200 mg/day.

Table 2 Recommended treatment regimen of Lamictal for children aged 2-12 years (Total daily dose in mg/kg bodyweight/day)

(see Table 2 opposite)

The initial dose and subsequent dose escalation should not be exceeded to minimise the risk of rash (see Special Warnings and Special Precautions for Use).

It is likely that patients aged 2-6 years will require a maintenance dose at the higher end of the recommended range.

Children aged less than 2 years

There is insufficient information on the use of Lamictal in children aged less than 2 years.

Women and Hormonal Contraceptives (see sections 4.4 and 4.5)

(a) Starting lamotrigine in patients taking hormonal contraceptives

Dose escalation should follow the guidelines recommended in Table 1 above (see sections 4.4 and 4.5).

(b) Starting hormonal contraceptives in patients taking lamotrigine

For women NOT taking inducers of lamotrigine glucuronidation such as phenytoin, carbamazepine, phenobarbital, primidone or rifampicin, the maintenance dose of lamotrigine may need to be increased by as much as two-fold, according to clinical response (see sections 4.4 and 4.5). For women taking lamotrigine in addition to inducers of lamotrigine glucoronidation, adjustment may not be necessary.

(c) Stopping hormonal contraceptives in patients taking lamotrigine

For women NOT taking inducers of lamotrigine glucoronidation the maintenance dose of lamotrigine may need to be decreased by as much as 50%, according to clinical response (see sections 4.4 and 4.5).

For women taking lamotrigine in addition to inducers of lamotrigine glucuronidation, adjustment may not be necessary.

Pregnancy and *post-partum*

Dose adjustment may be necessary during pregnancy and post-partum (see section 4.6).

Elderly

No dosage adjustment from recommended schedule is required. The pharmacokinetics of lamotrigine in this age group do not differ significantly from a non-elderly population.

Hepatic Impairment

Initial, escalation and maintenance doses should generally be reduced by approximately 50% in patients with moderate (Child-Pugh grade B) and 75% in severe (Child-Pugh grade C) hepatic impairment. Escalation and maintenance doses should be adjusted according to clinical response.

4.3 Contraindications

Lamictal is contraindicated in individuals with known hypersensitivity to lamotrigine.

4.4 Special warnings and precautions for use

There have been reports of adverse skin reactions, which have generally occurred within the first 8 weeks after initiation of lamotrigine (Lamictal) treatment. The majority of rashes are mild and self limiting, however rarely, serious potentially life threatening skin rashes including Stevens Johnson syndrome (SJS) and toxic epidermal necrolysis (TEN) have been reported (see Undesirable Effects).

The approximate incidence of serious skin rashes reported as SJS in adults and children over the age of 12 is 1 in 1000. The risk in children under the age of 12 is higher than in adults. Available data from a number of studies suggest that the incidence of rashes associated with hospitalisation in children under the age of 12 is from 1 in 300 to 1 in 100 (see Undesirable Effects).

In children, the initial presentation of a rash can be mistaken for an infection; physicians should consider the possibility of a drug reaction in children that develop symptoms of rash and fever during the first eight weeks of therapy.

Additionally the overall risk of rash appears to be strongly associated with:-

- High initial doses of lamotrigine and exceeding the recommended dose escalation of lamotrigine therapy (see Posology and Method of Administration).
- Concomitant use of valproate (See Posology and Method of Administration).

Caution is also required when treating patients with a history of allergy or rash to other antiepileptic drugs as the frequency of non-serious rash after treatment with lamotrigine was approximately three times higher in these patients than in those without such history.

All patients (adults and children) who develop a rash should be promptly evaluated and lamotrigine withdrawn immediately unless the rash is clearly not drug related. Lamotrigine should not be restarted in patients with previous hypersensitivity (see section 4.3).

Rash has also been reported as part of a hypersensitivity syndrome associated with a variable pattern of systemic symptoms including fever, lymphadenopathy, facial oedema and abnormalities of the blood and liver. The syndrome shows a wide spectrum of clinical severity and may, rarely, lead to disseminated intravascular coagulation (DIC) and multiorgan failure. It is important to note that early manifestations of hypersensitivity (e.g., fever, lymphadenopathy) may be present even though rash is not evident. Patients should be warned to seek immediate medical advice if signs and symptoms develop. If such signs and symptoms are present the patient should be evaluated immediately and Lamictal discontinued if an alternative aetiology cannot be established

Table 2 Recommended treatment regimen of Lamictal for children aged 2-12 years (Total daily dose in mg/kg bodyweight/day)

Treatment regimen		Weeks 1 + 2	Weeks 3 + 4	Usual Maintenance Dose
Add-on therapy with valproate regardless of any other concomitant medication		0.15 mg/kg* (once a day)	0.3 mg/kg (once a day)	0.3 mg/kg increments every one to two weeks to achieve a maintenance dose of 1 – 5 mg/kg (once a day or two divided doses).
Add-on therapy without valproate	This dosage regimen should be used with: phenytoin carbamazepine phenobarbital primidone or with other inducers of lamotrigine glucuronidation (see section 4.5).	0.6 mg/kg (two divided doses)	1.2 mg/kg (two divided doses)	1.2 mg/kg increments every one to two weeks to achieve a maintenance dose of 5 – 15 mg/kg (two divided doses).
	With oxcarbazepine without inducers or inhibitors of lamotrigine glucuronidation	0.3 mg/kg (one or two divided doses)	0.6 mg/kg (one or two divided doses)	0.6 mg/kg increments every one to two weeks to achieve a maintenance dose of 1 - 10 mg/kg (once a day or two divided doses) to a maximum of 200 mg/day.

Note: In patients taking AEDs where the pharmacokinetic interaction with lamotrigine is currently not known (see section 4.5), the treatment regimen as recommended for lamotrigine with concurrent valproate should be used, thereafter, the dose should be increased until optimal response is achieved.

* If the calculated daily dose in patients taking valproate is 1 to 2 mg, then 2 mg lamotrigine may be taken on alternate days for the first two weeks. If the calculated daily dose in patients taking valproate is less than 1 mg, then lamotrigine should not be administered.

Specialist contraceptive advice should be given to women who are of child-bearing age. Women of child-bearing age should be encouraged to use effective alternative non-hormonal methods of contraception.

Effects of hormonal contraceptives on lamotrigine efficacy:

Systemic lamotrigine concentrations are approximately halved during co-administration of oral contraceptives. This may result in reduced seizure control in women on a stable lamotrigine dose who start an oral contraceptive, or in adverse effects following withdrawal of an oral contraceptive. Dose adjustments of lamotrigine may be required (see sections 4.2 and 4.5).

The effects of co-administration of other hormonal contraceptives and hormone replacement therapy have not been studied; they may similarly affect lamotrigine pharmacokinetic parameters.

Effects of lamotrigine on hormonal contraceptive efficacy:

An interaction study demonstrated some loss of suppression of the hypothalamic-pituitary-ovarian axis when 300mg lamotrigine was co-administered with a combined oral contraceptive (see section 4.5). The impact of these changes on ovarian ovulatory activity is unknown. However, the possibility of decreased contraceptive efficacy cannot be excluded. Therefore, women should have a review of their contraception when starting lamotrigine, and the use of alternative non-hormonal methods of contraception should be encouraged. A hormonal contraceptive should only be used as the sole method of contraception if there is no other alternative. If the oral contraceptive pill is chosen as the sole method of contraception, women should be advised to promptly notify their physician if they experience changes in menstrual pattern (e.g. breakthrough bleeding) while taking Lamictal as this may be an indication of decreased contraceptive efficacy. Women taking Lamictal should notify their physician if they plan to start or stop use of oral contraceptives or other female hormonal preparations.

As with other AEDs, abrupt withdrawal of Lamictal may provoke rebound seizures. Unless safety concerns (for example rash) require an abrupt withdrawal, the dose of Lamictal should be gradually decreased over a period of 2 weeks.

During clinical experience with lamotrigine used as add-on therapy, there have been, rarely, deaths following rapidly progressive illnesses with status epilepticus, rhabdomyolysis, multiorgan dysfunction and disseminated intravascular coagulation (DIC). The contribution of lamotrigine to these events remains to be established.

Lamictal is a weak inhibitor of dihydrofolate reductase hence there is a possibility of interference with folate metabolism during long-term therapy. However, during prolonged human dosing, lamotrigine did not induce significant changes in the haemoglobin concentration, mean corpuscular volume, or serum or red blood cell folate concentrations up to 1 year or red blood cell folate concentrations for up to 5 years.

In single dose studies in subjects with end stage renal failure, plasma concentrations of lamotrigine were not significantly altered. However, accumulation of the glucuronide metabolite is to be expected; caution should therefore be exercised in treating patients with renal failure.

In patients with severe hepatic impairment (Child-Pugh grade C) it has been shown that initial and maintenance doses should be reduced by 75%. Caution should be exercised when dosing this severely hepatically impaired population.

4.5 Interaction with other medicinal products and other forms of interaction

UDP-glucuronyl transferases have been identified as the enzymes responsible for metabolism of lamotrigine. There is no evidence that lamotrigine causes clinically significant induction or inhibition of hepatic oxidative drug-metabolising enzymes, and interactions between lamotrigine and drugs metabolised by cytochrome P450 enzymes are unlikely to occur. Lamotrigine may induce its own metabolism but the effect is modest and unlikely to have significant clinical consequences.

Table 3 Effects of other drugs on glucuronidation of lamotrigine

Drugs that significantly inhibit glucuronidation of lamotrigine	Drugs that significantly induce glucuronidation of lamotrigine	Drugs that do not significantly inhibit or induce glucuronidation of lamotrigine
Valproate	Carbamazepine	Olanzapine
	Phenytoin	Oxcarbazepine
	Primidone	
	Phenobarbital	
	Rifampicin	
	Ethinylestradiol/ levonorgestrel combination*	

* Other hormonal contraceptives and hormone replacement therapy have not been studied; they may similarly affect lamotrigine pharmacokinetic parameters.

Interactions involving AEDs (see section 4.2)

Certain antiepileptic agents which induce drug-metabolising enzymes (such as phenytoin, carbamazepine, phenobarbital and primidone) induce the glucuronidation of lamotrigine and enhance the metabolism of lamotrigine and may increase dose requirements.

Sodium valproate, which inhibits the glucuronidation of lamotrigine, reduces the metabolism of lamotrigine and increases the mean half life of lamotrigine nearly two fold.

Although changes in the plasma concentrations of other antiepileptic drugs have been reported, controlled studies have shown no evidence that lamotrigine affects the plasma concentrations of concomitant antiepileptic drugs. Evidence from in vitro studies indicates that lamotrigine does not displace other antiepileptic drugs from protein binding sites.

There have been reports of central nervous system events including headache, nausea, blurred vision, dizziness, diplopia and ataxia in patients taking carbamazepine following the introduction of lamotrigine. These events usually resolve when the dose of carbamazepine is reduced. A similar effect was seen during a study of lamotrigine and oxcarbazepine in healthy adult volunteers, but dose reduction was not investigated.

In a study in healthy adult volunteers using doses of 200 mg lamotrigine and 1200 mg oxcarbazepine, oxcarbazepine did not alter the metabolism of lamotrigine and lamotrigine did not alter the metabolism of oxcarbazepine.

Interactions involving other psychoactive agents (see section 4.2)

In a study in healthy adult volunteers, 15 mg olanzapine reduced the AUC and Cmax of lamotrigine by an average of 24% and 20%, respectively. Therefore an effect of this magnitude is generally not expected to be clinically relevant but may be important to consider in some patients. Lamotrigine at 200 mg did not affect the pharmacokinetics of olanzapine.

Interactions involving Oral Contraceptives

Effect of oral contraceptives on lamotrigine:

Systemic lamotrigine concentrations are approximately halved during co-administration of oral contraceptives. This may result in reduced seizure control after the addition of an oral contraceptive, or adverse effects following withdrawal of an oral contraceptive. Dose adjustments of lamotrigine may be required (see section 4.2).

In a study of 16 female volunteers, 30 mcg ethinylestradiol/ 150 mcg levonorgestrel in a combined oral contraceptive pill caused an approximately two-fold increase in lamotrigine oral clearance, resulting in an average 52% and 39% reduction in lamotrigine AUC and Cmax, respectively. Serum lamotrigine concentrations gradually increased during the course of the week of inactive medication (e.g. "pill-free" week), with pre-dose concentrations at the end of the week of inactive medication being, on average, approximately two-fold higher than during co-therapy.

The effect of other hormonal contraceptive products or hormone replacement therapy has not been evaluated although the effect may be similar.

Effect of lamotrigine on oral contraceptives:

Co-administration of 300mg lamotrigine in a study of 16 female volunteers had no effect on the pharmacokinetics of the ethinylestradiol component of a combined oral contraceptive pill. A modest increase in oral clearance of the levonorgestrel component was observed, resulting in an average 19% and 12% reduction in levonorgestrel AUC and Cmax, respectively. Measurement of serum follicle-stimulating hormone (FSH), luteinising hormone (LH) and estradiol during the study indicated some loss of suppression of ovarian hormonal activity, although measurement of serum progesterone indicated that there was no hormonal evidence of ovulation in any of the 16 subjects. The impact of the modest increase in levonorgestrel clearance, and the changes in serum FSH and LH, on ovarian ovulatory activity is unknown (see section 4.4). Vaginal bleeding was reported by some volunteers (see section 4.4). The effects of doses of lamotrigine other than 300mg/day have not been studied and studies with other female hormonal preparations have not been conducted.

4.6 Pregnancy and lactation

Fertility

Administration of Lamictal did not impair fertility in animal reproductive studies.

There is no experience of the effect of Lamictal on human fertility.

Pregnancy

Risk related to antiepileptic drugs in general

Specialist advice should be given to women who are of childbearing potential. The need for antiepileptic treatment should be reviewed when a woman is planning to become pregnant. Sudden discontinuation of antiepileptic therapy should be avoided as this may lead to breakthrough seizures which could have serious consequences for the woman and the unborn child.

The risk of congenital malformations is increased by a factor of 2 to 3 in the offspring of mothers treated with antiepileptics compared with the expected incidence in the general population of approximately 3%. The most frequently reported defects are cleft lip, cardiovascular malformations and neural tube defects.

Multiple antiepileptic drug therapy is associated with a higher risk of congenital malformations than monotherapy and therefore monotherapy should be used whenever possible.

Risk related to lamotrigine

Epidemiological studies involving in total approximately 2000 women exposed to lamotrigine monotherapy during pregnancy cannot exclude an increased risk for congenital malformations. One registry has reported an increased incidence of facial clefts. Other data sets have not confirmed this finding. Animal studies have shown developmental toxicity (see section 5.3).

If therapy with lamotrigine is considered necessary during pregnancy, the lowest possible therapeutic dose is recommended.

Lamotrigine has a slight inhibitory effect on dihydrofolic acid reductase and could therefore theoretically lead to an increased risk of embryofoetal damage by reducing folic acid levels. Intake of folic acid when planning pregnancy and during early pregnancy may be considered.

Physiological changes during pregnancy may affect lamotrigine levels and/or therapeutic effect. There have been reports of decreased lamotrigine plasma levels during pregnancy. Appropriate clinical management of pregnant women during lamotrigine therapy should be ensured.

Lactation

There is limited information on the use of lamotrigine in lactation. Preliminary data indicate that it passes into breast milk in concentrations usually of the order of 40-60% of the serum concentration. In a small number of infants known to have been breastfed, the serum concentrations of lamotrigine reached levels at which pharmacological effects may occur. The potential benefits of breast feeding should be weighed against the potential risk of adverse effects occurring in the infant.

4.7 Effects on ability to drive and use machines

Two volunteer studies have demonstrated that the effect of lamotrigine on fine visual motor co-ordination, eye movements, body sway and subjective sedative effects did not differ from placebo.

In clinical trials with lamotrigine adverse events of a neurological character such as dizziness and diplopia have been reported. As there is individual variation in response to all antiepileptic drug therapy patients should consult their physician on the specific issues of driving and epilepsy.

4.8 Undesirable effects

In double-blind, add-on clinical trials, skin rashes occurred in up to 10% of patients taking lamotrigine and in 5% of patients taking placebo. The skin rashes led to the withdrawal of lamotrigine treatment in 2% of patients. The rash, usually maculopapular in appearance, generally appears within eight weeks of starting treatment and resolves on withdrawal of lamotrigine (see Special Warnings and Special Precautions for Use).

Rarely, serious potentially life threatening skin rashes, including Stevens Johnson syndrome and toxic epidermal necrolysis (Lyell Syndrome) have been reported. Although the majority recover on drug withdrawal, some patients experience irreversible scarring and there have been rare cases of associated death. (See Special Warnings and Special Precautions for Use)

The approximate incidence of serious skin rashes reported as SJS in adults and children over the age of 12 is 1 in 1000. The risk in children under the age of 12 is higher than in adults. Available data from a number of studies suggest that the incidence in children under the age of 12 requiring hospitalisation due to rash ranges from 1 in 300 to 1 in 100 (see Special Warnings and Special Precautions for Use).

In children, the initial presentation of a rash can be mistaken for an infection; physicians should consider the possibility of a drug reaction in children that develop symptoms of rash and fever during the first eight weeks of therapy.

Additionally the overall risk of rash appears to be strongly associated with:-

High initial doses of lamotrigine and exceeding the recommended dose escalation of lamotrigine therapy (see Posology and Method of Administration).

Concomitant use of valproate (See Posology and Method of Administration).

All patients (adults and children) who develop a rash should be promptly evaluated and lamotrigine withdrawn immediately unless the rash is clearly not drug related.

Rash has also been reported as part of a hypersensitivity syndrome associated with a variable pattern of systemic symptoms including fever, lymphadenopathy, facial oedema and abnormalities of the blood and liver. The syndrome shows a wide spectrum of clinical severity and may, rarely, lead to disseminated intravascular coagulation (DIC) and multiorgan failure. It is important to note that early manifestations of hypersensitivity (e.g., fever, lymphadenopathy) may be present even though rash is not evident. Patients should be warned to seek immediate medical advice if signs and symptoms develop. If such signs and symptoms are present the patient should be evaluated immediately and Lamictal discontinued if an alternative aetiology cannot be established

Adverse experiences reported during Lamictal monotherapy trials include headache, tiredness, rash, nausea, dizziness, drowsiness and insomnia.

Other adverse experiences have included diplopia, blurred vision, conjunctivitis, dizziness, drowsiness, headache, tiredness, gastrointestinal disturbance (including vomiting and diarrhoea), irritability/aggression, tremor, agitation, confusion and hallucinations. Very rarely, lupus-like reactions have been reported.

There have been reports of haematological abnormalities which may or may not be associated with the hypersensitivity syndrome. These have included neutropenia, leucopenia, anaemia, thrombocytopenia, pancytopenia, and very rarely aplastic anaemia and agranulocytosis.

Movement disorders such as tics, unsteadiness, ataxia, nystagmus and tremor have also been reported. There have been reports that Lamictal may worsen parkinsonian symptoms in patients with pre-existing Parkinson's disease, and isolated reports of extrapyramidal effects and choreoathetosis in patients with this underlying condition. Very rarely, increase in seizure frequency has been reported.

Elevations of liver function tests and rare reports of hepatic dysfunction, including hepatic failure, have been reported. Hepatic dysfunction usually occurs in association with hypersensitivity reactions but isolated cases have been reported without overt signs of hypersensitivity.

Additionally, arthralgia, pain and back pain were reported commonly during the clinical development programme for lamotrigine in bipolar disorder.

4.9 Overdose
Symptoms and signs

Acute ingestion of doses in excess of 10 – 20 times the maximum therapeutic dose has been reported. Overdose has resulted in symptoms including nystagmus, ataxia, impaired consciousness and coma.

Treatment

In the event of overdosage, the patient should be admitted to hospital and given appropriate supportive therapy. Gastric lavage should be performed if indicated.

5. PHARMACOLOGICAL PROPERTIES
5.1 Pharmacodynamic properties
Mode of action

The results of pharmacological studies suggest that lamotrigine is a use-dependent blocker of voltage gated sodium channels. It produces a use- and voltage-dependent block of sustained repetitive firing in cultured neurones and inhibits pathological release of glutamate (the amino acid which plays a key role in the generation of epileptic seizures), as well as inhibiting glutamate-evoked bursts of action potentials.

Pharmacodynamics

In tests designed to evaluate the central nervous system effects of drugs, the results obtained using doses of 240 mg lamotrigine administered to healthy volunteers did not differ from placebo, whereas both 1000 mg phenytoin and 10 mg diazepam each significantly impaired fine visual motor co-ordination and eye movements, increased body sway and produced subjective sedative effects.

In another study, single oral doses of 600mg carbamazepine significantly impaired fine visual motor co-ordination and eye movements, while increasing both body sway and heart rate, whereas results with lamotrigine at doses of 150mg and 300mg did not differ from placebo.

5.2 Pharmacokinetic properties

Lamotrigine is rapidly and completely absorbed from the gut with no significant first pass metabolism. Peak plasma concentrations occur approximately 2.5 hours after oral drug administration. Time to maximum concentration is slightly delayed after food but the extent of absorption is unaffected. The pharmacokinetics are linear up to 450mg, the highest single dose tested. There is considerable inter-individual variation in steady state maximum concentrations but within an individual concentrations vary very little.

Binding to plasma proteins is about 55%. It is very unlikely that displacement from plasma proteins would result in toxicity. The volume of distribution is 0.92 to 1.22 L/kg.

The mean steady state clearance in healthy adults is 39 ± 14 mL/min. Clearance of lamotrigine is primarily metabolic with subsequent elimination of glucuronide-conjugated material in urine. Less than 10% is excreted unchanged in the urine. Only about 2% of drug-related material is excreted in faeces. Clearance and half-life are independent of dose. The mean elimination half-life in healthy adults is 24 to 35 hours. UDP-glucuronyl transferases have been identified as the enzymes responsible for metabolism of lamotrigine. In a study of subjects with Gilbert's Syndrome, mean apparent clearance was reduced by 32% compared with normal controls but the values are within the range for the general population.

Lamotrigine induces its own metabolism to a modest extent depending on dose. However, there is no evidence that lamotrigine affects the pharmacokinetics of other AEDs and data suggest that interactions between lamotrigine and drugs metabolised by cytochrome P450 enzymes are unlikely to occur.

The half-life of lamotrigine is greatly affected by concomitant medication. Mean half-life is reduced to approximately 14 hours when given with glucuronidation-inducing drugs such as carbamazepine and phenytoin and is increased to a mean of approximately 70 hours when co-administered with sodium valproate alone. (see sections 4.2 and 4.5).

Clearance adjusted for bodyweight is higher in children aged 12 years and under than in adults with the highest values in children under five years. The half-life of lamotrigine is generally shorter in children than in adults with a mean value of approximately 7 hours when given with enzyme-inducing drugs such as carbamazepine and phenytoin and increasing to mean values of 45 to 50 hours when co-administered with sodium valproate alone (see Posology and Method of Administration).

The results of pharmacokinetic studies of lamotrigine in 12 healthy elderly volunteers aged 65 to 76 years and 12 young volunteers aged 26 to 38 years following a 150mg single dose revealed that average plasma clearance was about 37% lower in the elderly. However the mean clearance in the elderly (0.39 mL/min/kg) lies within the range of the mean clearance values (0.31 to 0.65 mL/min/kg) obtained in 9 studies with non-elderly adults after single doses of 30 to 450mg. A population pharmacokinetic analysis with both young and elderly subjects (including 12 elderly volunteers from the pharmacokinetic study and 13 elderly epilepsy patients enrolled in monotherapy clinical trials) indicated that the clearance of lamotrigine did not change to a clinically relevant extent. After single doses apparent clearance decreased by 12% from 35mL/min at age 20 to 31 mL/min at 70 years. The decrease after 48 weeks of treatment was 10% from 41 to 37mL/min between the young and elderly groups. To date there have been no specific studies of lamotrigine pharmacokinetics in elderly patients with epilepsy.

There is no experience of treatment with lamotrigine of patients with renal failure. Pharmacokinetic studies using single doses in subjects with renal failure indicate that lamotrigine pharmacokinetics are little affected but plasma concentrations of the major glucuronide metabolite increase almost eight-fold due to reduced renal clearance.

A single dose pharmacokinetic study was performed in 24 subjects with various degrees of hepatic impairment and 12 healthy subjects as controls. The median apparent clearance of lamotrigine was 0.31, 0.24, 0.10 mL/min/kg in patients with Grade A, B or C (Child-Pugh Classification) hepatic impairment respectively, compared to 0.34 mL/min/kg in the healthy controls. Reduced doses should generally be used in patients with Grade B or C hepatic impairment (see 4.2 Posology and Method of Administration)

5.3 Preclinical safety data
Teratogenicity

In reproductive and developmental toxicity studies in rodents and rabbits, no teratogenic effects but reduced foetal weight and retarded skeletal ossification were observed, at exposure levels below or similar to the expected clinical exposure. Since higher exposure levels could not be tested in animals due to maternal toxicity, the teratogenic potential of lamotrigine has not been characterised above clinical exposure.

In rats, enhanced foetal as well as postnatal mortality was observed when lamotrigine was administered later during gestation (day 15-20). These effects were observed at the expected clinical exposure.

Animal experiments did not reveal impairment of fertility by lamotrigine. Lamotrigine reduced foetal folic acid levels in rats. Folic acid deficiency is assumed to be associated with an enhanced risk of congenital malformations in animals as well as in humans.

Mutagenicity

The results of a wide range of mutagenicity tests indicate that Lamictal does not present a genetic risk to man.

Carcinogenicity

Lamictal was not carcinogenic in long-term studies in the rat and the mouse.

6. PHARMACEUTICAL PARTICULARS
6.1 List of excipients

Lamictal Tablets

Lactose

Microcrystalline Cellulose

Povidone

Sodium Starch Glycollate

Iron Oxide Yellow (E172) EEC Requirements

Magnesium Stearate

Lamictal Dispersible Tablets

Calcium carbonate

Low substituted hydroxypropyl cellulose

Aluminium magnesium silicate

Sodium starch glycollate

Povidone K30

Saccharin sodium

Blackcurrant flavour

Magnesium stearate

6.2 Incompatibilities

Not applicable.

6.3 Shelf life

Lamictal Tablets 25mg	3 years.
Lamictal Tablets 50mg	3 years
Lamictal Tablets 100mg	3 years
Lamictal Tablets 200mg	3 years
Lamictal Dispersible 2mg	2 years
Lamictal Dispersible 5mg	3 years
Lamictal Dispersible 25mg	3 years
Lamictal Dispersible 100mg	3 years

6.4 Special precautions for storage

Lamictal Tablets 25mg	Store below 30°C. Keep dry.
Lamictal Tablets 50mg	Store below 30°C. Keep dry.
Lamictal Tablets 100mg	Store below 30°C. Keep dry.
Lamictal Tablets 200mg	Store below 30°C. Keep dry.
Lamictal Dispersible 2mg	No special precautions for storage
Lamictal Dispersible 5mg	Store below 30°C. Keep dry. Protect from light.
Lamictal Dispersible 25mg	Store below 30°C. Keep dry. Protect from light.
Lamictal Dispersible 100mg	Store below 30°C. Keep dry. Protect from light.

6.5 Nature and contents of container

Lamictal Tablets 25mg	PVC/Aluminium foil blister packs containing 21 or 42 tablets.
Lamictal Tablets 50mg	PVC/Aluminium foil blisters containing 42 or 56 tablets
Lamictal Tablets 100mg	PVC/Aluminium foil blisters containing 56 tablets
Lamictal Tablets 200mg	PVC /Aluminium foil blisters containing 56 tablets
Lamictal Dispersible 2mg	HDPE bottle containing 30 tablets
Lamictal Dispersible 5mg	PVC/Aluminium foil blisters containing 28 tablets
Lamictal Dispersible 25mg	PVC/Aluminium foil blisters containing 56 tablets
Lamictal Dispersible 100mg	PVC/Aluminium foil blisters containing 56 tablets

6.6 Special precautions for disposal and other handling

None

Administrative Data
7. MARKETING AUTHORISATION HOLDER

The Wellcome Foundation Ltd
Glaxo Wellcome House
Berkeley Avenue
Greenford
Middlesex UB6 0NN
Trading as
GlaxoSmithKline UK
Stockley Park West
Uxbridge
Middlesex UB11 1BT

8. MARKETING AUTHORISATION NUMBER(S)

Lamictal Tablets 25mg: PL 0003/0272
Lamictal Tablets 50mg: PL 0003/0273
Lamictal Tablets 100mg: PL 0003/0274
Lamictal Tablets 200mg: PL 0003/0297
Lamictal Dispersible 2mg: PL 0003/0375
Lamictal Dispersible 5mg: PL 0003/0346
Lamictal Dispersible 25mg: PL 0003/0347
Lamictal Dispersible 100mg: PL 0003/0348

9. DATE OF FIRST AUTHORISATION/RENEWAL OF THE AUTHORISATION

Lamictal Tablets 25mg: 27th August 1997
Lamictal Tablets 50mg: 27th August 1997
Lamictal Tablets 100mg: 27th August 1997
Lamictal Tablets 200mg: 6th September 1999
Lamictal Dispersible 2mg: 18th December 2000
Lamictal Dispersible 5mg: 6th September 1999
Lamictal Dispersible 25mg: 6th September 1999
Lamictal Dispersible 100mg: 6th September 1999

10. DATE OF REVISION OF THE TEXT

1 March 2007

11. Legal Status

POM

Lamisil Cream

(Novartis Consumer Health)

1. NAME OF THE MEDICINAL PRODUCT

LAMISIL® Cream

2. QUALITATIVE AND QUANTITATIVE COMPOSITION
Terbinafine hydrochloride 1.0% w/w

3. PHARMACEUTICAL FORM
White, smooth or almost smooth glossy cream

4. CLINICAL PARTICULARS
4.1 Therapeutic indications
Fungal infections of the skin caused by *Trichophyton* (eg. *T. Rubrum, T. Mentagrophytes, T. Verrucosum, T. Violaceum), Microsporum canis* and *Epidermophyton floccosum*.

Yeast infections of the skin, principally those caused by the genus *Candida* (eg. *C. albicans*).

Pityriasis (tinea) versicolor due to *Pityrosporum orbiculare* (also known as *Malassezia furfur*).

4.2 Posology and method of administration
LAMISIL can be applied once or twice daily. Cleanse and dry the affected areas thoroughly before application of LAMISIL. Apply the cream to the affected skin and surrounding area in a thin layer and rub in lightly. In the case of intertriginous infections (submammary, interdigital, intergluteal, inguinal) the application may be covered with a gauze strip, especially at night.

The likely durations of treatment are as follows:

Tinea corporis, cruris: 1 to 2 weeks

Tinea pedis: 1 week

Cutaneous candidiasis: 2 weeks

Pityriasis versicolor: 2 weeks

Relief of clinical symptoms usually occurs within a few days. Irregular use or premature discontinuation of treatment carries the risk of recurrence. If there are no signs of improvement after two weeks, the diagnosis should be verified.

Children

The experience with topical LAMISIL in children is still limited and its use cannot therefore be recommended.

Use in the elderly

There is no evidence to suggest that elderly patients require different dosages or experience side-effects different to those of younger patients.

Method of administration

Via the topical route.

4.3 Contraindications
Hypersensitivity to terbinafine or any of the excipients contained in the cream.

4.4 Special warnings and precautions for use
LAMISIL Cream is for external use only. Contact with the eyes should be avoided. In case of accidental contact with the eyes, rinse the eyes thoroughly with running water.

4.5 Interaction with other medicinal products and other forms of interaction
There are no known drug interactions with LAMISIL Cream.

4.6 Pregnancy and lactation
Foetal toxicity and fertility studies in animals suggest no adverse effects.

There is no clinical experience with LAMISIL Cream in pregnant women, therefore, unless the potential benefits outweigh any potential risks, LAMISIL Cream should not be administered during pregnancy.

Terbinafine is excreted in breast milk and therefore mothers should not receive LAMISIL whilst breast-feeding. Infants should also not be allowed to come into contact with any treated skin, including the breast.

4.7 Effects on ability to drive and use machines
None known.

4.8 Undesirable effects
Redness, itching or stinging occasionally occur at the site of application; however, treatment rarely has to be discontinued for this reason. This must be distinguished from allergic reactions such as pruritus, rash, bullous eruptions and hives which are very rare but require discontinuation.

4.9 Overdose
The low systemic absorption of topical terbinafine cream renders overdosage extremely unlikely. Accidental ingestion of the contents of one 30g tube of LAMISIL Cream, which contains 300mg terbinafine hydrochloride, is comparable to one LAMISIL 250mg tablet (adult oral unit dose).

No case of overdosage has been reported with LAMISIL Cream. However, should a larger amount of LAMISIL Cream be inadvertently ingested, adverse effects similar to those observed with an overdosage of LAMISIL tablets are to be expected. These include headache, nausea, epigastric pain and dizziness.

The recommended treatment of overdosage consists of eliminating the drug, primarily by the administration of activated charcoal, and giving symptomatic supportive therapy, if needed.

5. PHARMACOLOGICAL PROPERTIES
5.1 Pharmacodynamic properties
Pharmacotherapeutic group: Antifungal for topical use (ATC code D01A E15)

Terbinafine is an allylamine which has a broad spectrum of antifungal activity. At low concentrations terbinafine is fungicidal against dermatophytes, moulds and certain dimorphic fungi. The activity versus yeasts is fungicidal or fungistatic depending of the species.

Terbinafine interferes specifically with fungal sterol biosynthesis at an early step. This leads to a deficiency in ergosterol and to an intracellular accumulation of squalene, resulting in fungal cell death. Terbinafine acts by inhibition of squalene epoxidase in the fungal cell membrane. The enzyme squalene epoidase is not linked to the cytochrome P450 system.

5.2 Pharmacokinetic properties
Less than 5% of the dose is absorbed after topical application to humans; systemic exposure is therefore very slight.

5.3 Preclinical safety data
None stated

6. PHARMACEUTICAL PARTICULARS
6.1 List of excipients
Sodium hydroxide, benzyl alcohol, sorbitan monostearate, cetyl palmitate, cetyl alcohol, stearyl alcohol, polysorbate 60, isopropyl myristate, demineralised water.

6.2 Incompatibilities
None known.

6.3 Shelf life
Aluminium tube: 5 years.

Polypropylene dispenser tube: 3 years.

6.4 Special precautions for storage
None.

6.5 Nature and contents of container
Aluminium tube with membrane, with an interior coating of phenol-epoxy based lacquer, closed with a polypropylene cap, containing 15g or 30g LAMISIL Cream.

Polypropylene dispenser tube with polypropylene screw-cap closure containing 15 or 30g LAMISIL cream

6.6 Special precautions for disposal and other handling
Not applicable.

7. MARKETING AUTHORISATION HOLDER
Novartis Consumer Health UK Limited

Wimblehurst Road

Horsham

West Sussex

RH 12 5AB

United Kingdom

8. MARKETING AUTHORISATION NUMBER(S)
PL 00030/0421

9. DATE OF FIRST AUTHORISATION/RENEWAL OF THE AUTHORISATION
3 October 1990 / 18 April 2001

10. DATE OF REVISION OF THE TEXT
27th April 2009

Legal category: POM

Lamisil Once

(Novartis Consumer Health)

1. NAME OF THE MEDICINAL PRODUCT
Lamisil® Once™ 1% cutaneous solution

2. QUALITATIVE AND QUANTITATIVE COMPOSITION
Each gram contains 10 mg terbinafine (as hydrochloride).

For excipients, see section 6.1.

3. PHARMACEUTICAL FORM
Cutaneous solution.

Clear to slightly opaque viscous solution.

4. CLINICAL PARTICULARS
4.1 Therapeutic indications
Treatment for tinea pedis (athlete's foot).

4.2 Posology and method of administration
Adults 18 years of age and over: single administration.

Lamisil Once should be applied once on both feet, even if lesions are visible on one foot only. This ensures elimination of the fungi (dermatophytes) that might be found in areas of the foot where no lesions are visible.

Patients should wash and dry both feet and hands before applying the product. They should treat one foot, then the other.

Starting between the toes, patients should apply a thin layer evenly between and all around the toes, as well as cover the sole and sides of the foot for up to 1.5 cm. The product should be applied in the same way to the other foot, even if the skin looks healthy. The product should be left to dry to a film for 1-2 minutes. Patients should then wash their hands. Lamisil Once should not be massaged into skin.

For the best results, the treated area should not be washed for 24 hours after application. It is therefore recommended to apply Lamisil Once after a shower or bath and wait until the same time the following day before washing the feet again.

Patients should use the quantity they need to cover both feet as instructed above. Any unused medication is to be discarded.

Relief of clinical symptoms usually occurs within a few days. If there are no signs of improvement after one week, patients should see a doctor. There are no data on repeated treatment with Lamisil Once. Therefore a second treatment cannot be recommended within a particular episode of athlete's foot.

Children:

Lamisil Once has not been studied in the paediatric population. Its use is therefore not recommended in patients below 18 years of age.

The elderly:

There is no evidence to suggest that elderly patients require different dosages or experience side effects different from those in younger patients.

4.3 Contraindications
Hypersensitivity to terbinafine or any of the excipients (see 6.1. List of excipients).

4.4 Special warnings and precautions for use
Lamisil Once is not recommended to treat hyperkeratotic chronic plantar tinea pedis (moccasin type).

Lamisil Once is for external use only. It should not be used on the face; it may be irritating to the eyes. In case of accidental contact with the eyes, rinse eyes thoroughly with running water. Do not swallow.

In the unlikely event of allergic reaction, the film should be removed with an organic solvent such as denatured alcohol and the feet washed with warm soapy water.

Contains alcohol; keep away from naked flames

4.5 Interaction with other medicinal products and other forms of interaction
No drug interactions are known with use of topical Lamisil formulations.

4.6 Pregnancy and lactation
Animal studies did not reveal any teratogenic or embryo-foetotoxic potential of terbinafine. No cases of malformations in humans have been reported with terbinafine to date. However, since clinical experience in pregnant women is very limited, Lamisil Once should be used only if clearly indicated during pregnancy.

Terbinafine is excreted in breast milk, and therefore mothers should not receive Lamisil Once whilst breast-feeding.

4.7 Effects on ability to drive and use machines
Cutaneous application of Lamisil Once does not affect the ability to drive and use machines.

4.8 Undesirable effects
Undesirable effects include mild and transient reactions at the site of application. In very rare instances, allergic reactions may occur.

Skin and subcutaneous tissue disorders:

Very rare (<1/10,000, including isolated reports): allergic reactions such as rash, pruritus, dermatitis bullous and urticaria.

General disorders and administration site conditions

Uncommon (>1/1,000, <1/100): application site reactions such as skin dryness, skin irritation or burning sensation.

4.9 Overdose
Overdose is very unlikely to happen since the product is for single dose, cutaneous use, and the tube only contains the necessary quantity for one application. Accidental ingestion of one 4 g tube of product which contains 40 mg terbinafine is much lower than one 250 mg Lamisil tablet (oral unit dose). Should several tubes be ingested however, adverse effects similar to those observed with an overdose of Lamisil tablets (e.g. headache, nausea, epigastric pain and dizziness) are to be expected.

5. PHARMACOLOGICAL PROPERTIES
5.1 Pharmacodynamic properties
Pharmacotherapeutic group: Antifungal for topical use (ATC code D01 A E15)

Terbinafine is an allylamine which has a broad spectrum of antifungal activity in fungal infections of the skin caused by dermatophytes such as *Trichophyton* (e.g. *T. rubrum, T. mentagrophytes, T. verrucosum, T. violaceum), Microsporum canis* and *Epidermophyton floccosum*. At low concentrations terbinafine is fungicidal against dermatophytes and moulds. The activity against yeasts is fungicidal (e.g. *Pityrosporum orbiculare* or *Malassezia furfur)* or fungistatic, depending on the species.

Terbinafine interferes specifically with fungal sterol biosynthesis at an early step. This leads to a deficiency in ergosterol and to an intracellular accumulation of squalene, resulting in fungal cell death. Terbinafine acts by inhibition of squalene epoxidase in the fungal cell membrane. The enzyme squalene epoxidase is not linked to the cytochrome P450 system. Terbinafine does not influence the metabolism of hormones or other drugs.

Studies in patients have shown that a single dose application of Lamisil Once 1 % cutaneous solution on both feet demonstrated efficacy in patients with tinea pedis (athlete's foot) presenting lesions between the toes, and extending to adjacent skin areas of the sides and soles of the feet. The rate of relapse/reinfection at 3 months after treatment was low: 1 person out of 8 (12.5%).

5.2 Pharmacokinetic properties

Once applied to the skin, Lamisil Once 1 % cutaneous solution forms a film on the skin. Terbinafine in the film stays on the skin for up to 72 hours. The film quickly delivers terbinafine to the stratum corneum: at 60 minutes after application, 16 to 18% of the applied dose will be present in the stratum corneum. Delivery progressively continues and terbinafine persists in the stratum corneum for up to 13 days, at levels which are in excess of the in vitro Minimum Inhibitory Concentration for terbinafine against dermatophytes.

Systemic bioavailability is very low. An application of Lamisil Once 1 % cutaneous solution on the back, on an area of 3 times the area of both feet, resulted in exposure to terbinafine of less than 0.5% of the exposure following oral administration of a 250 mg tablet.

5.3 Preclinical safety data

In long-term studies (up to 1 year) in rats and dogs no marked toxic effects were seen in either species up to oral doses of about 100 mg/kg a day. At high oral doses, the liver and possibly also the kidneys were identified as potential target organs.

In a two-year oral carcinogenicity study in mice, no neoplastic or other abnormal findings attributable to treatment were made up to doses of 130 (males) and 156 (females) mg/kg a day. In a two-year oral carcinogenicity study in rats at the highest dose level, 69 mg/kg a day, an increased incidence of liver tumours was observed in males. The changes, which may be associated with peroxisome proliferation, have been shown to be species-specific since they were not seen in the carcinogenicity study in mice or in other studies in mice, dogs or monkeys.

During the studies of high dose oral terbinafine in monkeys, refractile irregularities were observed in the retina at the higher doses (non-toxic effect level was 50 mg/kg). These irregularities were associated with the presence of a terbinafine metabolite in ocular tissue and disappeared after drug discontinuation. There were no associated histological changes.

A standard battery of *in vitro* and *in vivo* genotoxicity tests revealed no evidence of a mutagenic or clastogenic potential for the drug.

No adverse effects on fertility or other reproduction parameters were observed in studies in rats or rabbits.

Repeated dermal administration of Lamisil Once 1 % cutaneous solution in rats and minipigs produces plasma terbinafine levels which are at least 50-100 times lower than the no-adverse-effect-levels established in terbinafine animal toxicity studies, so use of the product is not expected to produce any systemic adverse effect. Lamisil Once 1 % cutaneous solution was well tolerated in a variety of tolerability studies and did not cause sensitisation.

6. PHARMACEUTICAL PARTICULARS

6.1 List of excipients

Acrylates/octylacrylamide copolymer;

hydroxypropylcellulose;

medium chain triglycerides;

ethanol.

6.2 Incompatibilities

Not applicable.

6.3 Shelf life

3 years.

6.4 Special precautions for storage

Store in the original package. There is no special temperature precaution for storage.

6.5 Nature and contents of container

4 g aluminium laminated tube (polyethylene-aluminium-polyethylene) with a polyethylene screw cap.

6.6 Special precautions for disposal and other handling

No special requirements.

7. MARKETING AUTHORISATION HOLDER

Novartis Consumer Health, Horsham, RH12 5AB, UK

8. MARKETING AUTHORISATION NUMBER(S)

PL 00030/0213

9. DATE OF FIRST AUTHORISATION/RENEWAL OF THE AUTHORISATION

4 November 2005

10. DATE OF REVISION OF THE TEXT

23 November 2005

Legal category

P

Lanoxin 125 Tablets

(GlaxoSmithKline UK)

1. NAME OF THE MEDICINAL PRODUCT

Lanoxin 125 Tablets

2. QUALITATIVE AND QUANTITATIVE COMPOSITION

Digoxin Ph Eur 0.125 mg/tablet

3. PHARMACEUTICAL FORM

Tablet

4. CLINICAL PARTICULARS

4.1 Therapeutic indications

Lanoxin is indicated in the management of chronic cardiac failure where the dominant problem is systolic dysfunction. Its therapeutic benefit is greatest in those patients with ventricular dilatation.

Lanoxin is specifically indicated where cardiac failure is accompanied by atrial fibrillation.

Lanoxin is indicated in the management of certain supraventricular arrhythmias, particularly chronic atrial flutter and fibrillation.

4.2 Posology and method of administration

The dose of Lanoxin for each patient has to be tailored individually according to age, lean body weight and renal function. Suggested doses are intended only as an initial guide.

The difference in bioavailability between injectable Lanoxin and oral formulations must be considered when changing from one dosage form to another. For example, if patients are switched from oral to the i.v. formulation the dosage should be reduced by approximately 33 %.

Adults with chronic cardiac failure in the absence of supraventricular arrhythmia:

No loading dose is required. The usual daily dose is 125 to 250 micrograms (0.125 to 0.25 mg) for patients with normal renal function. A lower dose of 62.5 micrograms (0.0625 mg) should be considered in the elderly.

For the management of atrial fibrillation or flutter in adults and children over 10 years:

Rapid Oral Loading:

If medically appropriate, rapid digitalisation may be achieved in a number of ways, such as the following:

750 to 1500 micrograms (0.75 to 1.5 mg) as a single dose.

Where there is less urgency, or greater risk of toxicity eg. in the elderly, the oral loading dose should be given in divided doses 6 hours apart, assessing clinical response before giving each additional dose. (See *Special Warnings and Precautions for Use*).

Slow Oral Loading:

Digitalisation may be achieved more slowly with doses of 250 to 750 micrograms (0.25 to 0.75 mg) daily for 1 week followed by an appropriate maintenance dose. A clinical response should be seen within one week.

NOTE: The choice between slow and rapid oral loading depends on the clinical state of the patient and the urgency of the condition.

Maintenance Dose:

The maintenance dosage should be based upon the percentage of the peak body stores lost each day through elimination. The following formula has had wide clinical use:

$$\text{Maintenance Dose} = \text{Peak body stores} \times \frac{\%\ \text{daily loss}}{100}$$

Where:

$$\text{Peak Body Stores} = \text{Loading Dose}$$
$$\%\ \text{Daily Loss} = 14 + \text{Creatinine Clearance } (C_{cr})/5.$$

C_{cr} is creatinine clearance corrected to 70 kg body weight or 1.73 m^2 body surface area. If only serum creatinine (S_{cr}) concentrations are available, a C_{cr} (Corrected to 70 kg body weight) may be estimated in men as

$$C_{cr} = \frac{(140 - \text{age})}{S_{cr}\ (\text{in mg/100 ml})}$$

NOTE: Where serum creatinine values are obtained in micromol/l these may be converted to mg/100 ml (mg %) as follows

$$S_{cr}\ (\text{mg/100 ml}) = \frac{S_{cr}\ (\text{micromol/L}) \times 113.12}{10{,}000} = \frac{S_{cr}\ (\text{micromol/L})}{88.4}$$

Where 113.12 is the molecular weight of creatinine.

For women, this result should be multiplied by 0.85.

NOTE: These formulae cannot be used for creatinine clearance in children.

In practice, this will mean that most patients will be maintained on 0.125 to 0.25 mg digoxin daily; however in those who show increased sensitivity to the adverse effects of digoxin, a dosage of 62.5 microgram (0.0625 mg) daily or less may suffice. Conversely, some patients may require a higher dose.

Neonates, infants and children up to 10 years of age (if cardiac glycosides have not been given in the preceding two weeks):

In the newborn, particularly in the premature infant, renal clearance of digoxin is diminished and suitable dose reductions must be observed, over and above general dosage instructions.

Beyond the immediate newborn period, children generally require proportionally larger doses than adults on the basis of body weight or body surface area, as indicated in the schedule below. Children over 10 years of age require adult dosages in proportion to their body weight.

Oral Loading Dose:

This should be administered in accordance with the following schedule:

Preterm neonates < 1.5 kg	25 microgram/kg over 24 hours
Preterm neonates 1.5 to 2.5 kg	30 microgram/kg over 24 hours
Term neonates to 2 years	45 microgram/kg over 24 hours
2 to 5 years	35 microgram/kg over 24 hours
5 to 10 years	25 microgram/kg over 24 hours

The loading dose should be administered in divided doses with approximately half the total dose given as the first dose and further fractions of the total dose given at intervals of 4 to 8 hours, assessing clinical response before giving each additional dose.

Maintenance Dose:

The maintenance dose should be administered in accordance with the following schedule:

Preterm neonates:

daily dose	=	20% of 24-hour loading dose (intravenous or oral)

Term neonates and children up to 10 years

daily dose	=	25% of 24-hour loading dose (intravenous or oral)

These dosage schedules are meant as guidelines and careful clinical observation and monitoring of serum digoxin levels (see *Monitoring*) should be used as a basis for adjustment of dosage in these paediatric patients groups.

If cardiac glycosides have been given in the two weeks preceding commencement of Lanoxin therapy, it should be anticipated that optimum loading doses of Lanoxin will be less than those recommended above.

Use in the elderly:

The tendency to impaired renal function and low lean body mass in the elderly influences the pharmacokinetic of Lanoxin such that high serum digoxin levels and associated toxicity can occur quite readily, unless doses of Lanoxin lower than those in non-elderly patients are used. Serum digoxin levels should be checked regularly and hypokalaemia avoided.

Dose recommendations in renal disorder or with diuretic therapy:

See *Special Warnings and Precautions for Use*.

Monitoring:

Serum concentrations of digoxin may be expressed in conventional units of nanogram/ml (ng/ml) or SI units of nanomol/L (nmol/L). To convert ng/ml to nmol/L, multiply ng/ml by 1.28.

The serum concentration of digoxin can be determined by radioimmunoassay. Blood should be taken 6 hours or more after the last dose of Lanoxin. Several post hoc analyses of heart failure patients in the Digitalis Investigation Group trial suggest that the optimal trough digoxin serum level may be 0.5 ng/mL (0.64 nanomol/L) to 1.0 ng/mL (1.28 nanomol/L).

Digoxin toxicity is more commonly associated with serum digoxin concentration greater than 2 ng/mL. However, toxicity may occur with lower digoxin serum concentrations. In deciding whether a patient's symptoms are due to digoxin, the patients clinical state together with the serum potassium level and thyroid function are important factors.

Other glycosides, including metabolites of digoxin, can interfere with the assays that are available and one should always be wary of values which do not seem commensurate with the clinical state of the patient.

4.3 Contraindications

Lanoxin is contra-indicated in intermittent complete heart block or second degree atrioventricular block, especially if there is a history of Stokes-Adams attacks.

Lanoxin is contra-indicated in arrhythmias caused by cardiac glycoside intoxication.

Lanoxin is contra-indicated in surpraventricular arrhythmias associated with an accessory atrioventricular pathway, as in the Wolff-Parkinson-White syndrome, unless the electrophysiological characteristics of the accessory pathway and any possible deleterious effect of digoxin on these characteristics has been evaluated. If an accessory pathway is known or suspected to be present and there is no history of previous supraventricular arrhythmias, Lanoxin is similarly contra-indicated.

Lanoxin is contra-indicated in ventricular tachycardia or ventricular fibrillation.

Lanoxin is contra-indicated in hypertrophic obstructive cardiomyopathy, unless there is concomitant atrial fibrillation and heart failure but even then caution should be exercised if Lanoxin is to be used.

Lanoxin is contra-indicated in patients known to be hypersensitive to digoxin, other digitalis glycosides, or to any component of the preparation.

4.4 Special warnings and precautions for use

Arrhythmias may be precipitated by digoxin toxicity, some of which can resemble arrhythmias for which the drug could be advised. For example, atrial tachycardia with varying atrioventricular block requires care as clinically the rhythm resembles atrial fibrillation.

In some cases of sinoatrial disorder (ie. Sick Sinus Syndrome) digoxin may cause or exacerbate sinus bradycardia or cause sinoatrial block.

Determination of the serum digoxin concentration may be very helpful in making a decision to treat with further digoxin, but toxic doses of other glycosides may cross-react in the assay and wrongly suggest apparently satisfactory measurements. Observations during the temporary withholding of digoxin might be more appropriate.

In cases where cardiac glycosides have been taken in the preceding two weeks the recommendations for initial dosing of a patient should be reconsidered and a reduced dose is advised.

The dosing recommendations should be reconsidered if patients are elderly or there are other reasons for the renal clearance of digoxin being reduced. A reduction in both initial and maintenance doses should be considered.

Hypokalaemia sensitises the myocardium to the actions of cardiac glycosides.

Hypoxia, hypomagnesaemia and marked hypercalcaemia increase myocardial sensitivity to cardiac glycosides.

Administering Lanoxin to a patient with thyroid disease requires care. Initial and maintenance doses of Lanoxin should be reduced when thyroid function is subnormal. In hyperthyroidism there is relative digoxin resistance and the dose may have to be increased. During the course of treatment of thyrotoxicosis, dosage should be reduced as the thyrotoxicosis comes under control.

Patients with malabsorption syndrome or gastro-intestinal reconstructions may require larger doses of digoxin.

The risk of provoking dangerous arrhythmias with direct current cardioversion is greatly increased in the presence of digitalis toxicity and is in proportion to the cardioversion energy used.

For elective direct current cardioversion of a patient who is taking digoxin, the drug should be withheld for 24 hours before cardioversion is performed. In emergencies, such as cardiac arrest when attempting cardioversion the lowest effective energy should be applied. Direct current cardioversion is inappropriate in the treatment of arrhythmias though to be caused by cardiac glycosides.

Many beneficial effects of digoxin on arrhythmias result from a degree of atrioventricular conduction blockage. However, when incomplete atrioventricular block already exists the effects of a rapid progression in the block should be anticipated. In complete heart block the idioventricular escape rhythm may be suppressed.

The administration of digoxin in the period immediately following myocardial infarction is not contra-indicated. However, the use of inotropic drugs in some patients in this setting may result in undesirable increased in myocardial oxygen demand and ischaemia, and some retrospective follow-up studies have suggested digoxin to be associated with an increased risk of death. However, the possibility of arrhythmias arising in patients who may be hypokalaemic after myocardial infarction and are likely to be cardiologically unstable must be borne in mind. The limitations imposed thereafter on direct current cardioversion must also be remembered.

Treatment with digoxin should generally be avoided in patients with heart failure associated with cardiac amyloidosis. However, if alternative treatments are not appropriate, digoxin can be used with caution to control the ventricular rate in patients with cardiac amyloidosis and atrial fibrillation.

Digoxin can rarely precipitate vasoconstriction and therefore should be avoided in patients with myocarditis.

Patients with beri beri heart disease may fail to respond adequately to digoxin if the underlying thiamine deficiency is not treated concomitantly. There is also some published information indicating that digoxin may inhibit the uptake of thiamine in myocytes in beri beri heart disease.

Digoxin should not be used in constrictive pericarditis unless it is used to control the ventricular rate in atrial fibrillation or to improve systolic dysfunction.

Digoxin improves exercise tolerance in patients with impaired left ventricular systolic dysfunction and normal sinus rhythm. This may or may not be associated with an improved haemodynamic profile. However, the benefit of patients with supraventricular arrhythmias is most evident at rest, less evident with exercise.

In patients receiving diuretics and an ACE inhibitor, or diuretics alone, the withdrawal of digoxin has been shown to result in clinical deterioration.

The use of therapeutic doses of digoxin may cause prolongation of the PR interval and depression of the ST segment on the electrocardiogram.

Digoxin may produce false positive ST-T changes on the electrocardiogram during exercise testing. These electrophysiologic effects reflect an expected effect of the drug and are not indicative of toxicity.

Patients receiving digoxin should have their serum electrolytes and renal function (serum creatinine concentration) assessed periodically; the frequency of assessments will depend on the clinical setting.

Although many patients with chronic congestive cardiac failure benefit from acute administration of digoxin. There are some in whom it does not lead to constant, marked or lasting haemodynamic improvement. It is therefore important to evaluate the response of each patient individually when Lanoxin is continued long-term.

Patients with severe respiratory disease may have an increased myocardial sensitivity to digitalis glycosides.

Patients with rare hereditary problems of galactose intolerance, the Lapp lactose deficiency or glucose galactose malabsorption should not take this medicine.

4.5 Interaction with other medicinal products and other forms of interaction

Interactions may arise from effects on the renal excretion, tissue binding, plasma protein binding, distribution within the body, gut absorptive capacity and sensitivity to Lanoxin. Consideration of the possibility of an interaction whenever concomitant therapy is contemplated is the best precaution and a check on serum digoxin concentration is recommended when any doubt exists.

Digoxin, in association with beta-adrenoceptor blocking drugs, may increase atrio-ventricular conduction time.

Agents causing hypokalaemia or intracellular potassium deficiency may cause increased sensitivity to Digoxin; they include diuretics, lithium salts, corticosteroids and carbenoxolone.

Patients receiving Digoxin are more susceptible to the effects of suxamethonium-exacerbated hyperkalaemia.

Calcium, particularly if administered rapidly by the intravenous route, may produce serious arrhythmias in digitalized patients.

Serum levels of digoxin may be **increased** by concomitant administration of the following:

Alprazolam, amiodarone, flecainide, gentamicin, indometacin, itraconazole, prazosin, propafenone, quinidine, quinine, spironolactone, macrolide antibiotics (e.g. erythromycin and clarithromycin), tetracycline (and possibly other antibiotics), trimethoprim, propantheline, atorvastatin, ciclosporin, epoprostenol (transient) and carvedilol.

Serum levels of digoxin may be **reduced** by concomitant administration of the following:

Adrenaline (epinephrine), antacids, kaolin-pectin, some bulk laxatives, colestyramine, acarbose, salbutamol, sulfasalazine, neomycin, rifampicin, some cytostatics, phenytoin, metoclopramide, penicillamine and the herbal remedy St John's wort (*Hypericum perforatum*).

Calcium channel blocking agents may either increase or cause no change in serum digoxin levels. Verapamil, felodipine and tiapamil increase serum digoxin levels. Nifedipine and diltiazem may increase or have no effect on serum digoxin levels. Isradipine causes no change in serum digoxin levels. Angiotensin converting enzyme (ACE) inhibitors may also increase or cause no change in serum digoxin concentrations.

Milrinone does not alter steady-state serum digoxin levels.

Digoxin is a substrate of P-glycoprotein. Thus, inhibitors of P-glycoprotein may increase blood concentrations of digoxin by enhancing its absorption and/or by reducing its renal clearance (See *5.2 Pharmacokinetic Properties*).

4.6 Pregnancy and lactation

No data are available on whether or not digoxin has teratogenic effects.

There is no information available on the effect of digoxin on human fertility.

The use of digoxin in pregnancy is not contra-indicated, although the dosage and control may be less predictable in pregnant than in non-pregnant women with some requiring an increased dosage of digoxin during pregnancy. As with all drugs, use should be considered only when the expected clinical benefit of treatment to the mother outweighs any possible risk to the developing foetus.

Despite extensive antenatal exposure to digitalis preparations, no significant adverse effects have been observed in the foetus or neonate when maternal serum digoxin concentrations are maintained within the normal range. Although it has been speculated that a direct effect of digoxin on the myometrium may result in relative prematurity and low birthweight, a contributing role of the underlying cardiac disease cannot be excluded. Maternally administered digoxin has been successfully used to treat foetal tachycardia and congestive heart failure.

Adverse foetal effects have been reported in mothers with digitalis toxicity.

Although digoxin is excreted in breast milk, the quantities are minute and breast feeding is not contra-indicated.

4.7 Effects on ability to drive and use machines

Since central nervous system and visual disturbances have been reported in patients receiving Lanoxin, patients should exercise caution before driving, using machinery or participating in dangerous activities.

4.8 Undesirable effects

Adverse reactions are listed below by system organ class and frequency. Frequencies are defined as: very common (≥ 1/10), common (≥ 1/100 and < 1/10), uncommon (≥ 1/1000 and < 1/100), rare (≥ 1/10,000 and < 1/1000), very rare (< 1/10,000), including isolated reports. Very common, common and uncommon events were generally determined from clinical trial data. The incidence in placebo was taken into account. Adverse drug reactions identified through post-marketing surveillance were considered to be rare or very rare (including isolated reports).

Blood and lymphatic system disorders	
Very rare:	Thrombocytopenia
Metabolism and nutrition disorders	
Very Rare:	Anorexia
Psychiatric disorders	
Uncommon:	Depression
Very rare:	Psychosis, apathy, confusion
Nervous system disorders	
Common:	CNS disturbances, dizziness
Very rare:	Headache
Eye disorders	
Common:	Visual disturbances (blurred or yellow vision)
Cardiac disorders	
Common:	Arrhythmia, conduction disturbances, bigeminy, trigeminy, PR prolongation, sinus bradycardia
Very rare:	Supraventricular tachyarrhythmia, atrial tachycardia (with or without block), junctional (nodal) tachycardia, ventricular arrhythmia, ventricular premature contraction, ST segment depression
Gastrointestinal disorders	
Common:	Nausea, vomiting, diarrhoea
Very rare:	Intestinal ischaemia, intestinal necrosis
Skin disorders	
Common:	Skin rashes of urticarial or scarlatiniform character may be accompanied by pronounced eosinophilia
Reproductive system and breast disorders	
Very rare:	Gynaecomastia can occur with long term administration
General disorders and administration site conditions	
Very rare:	Fatigue, malaise, weakness

4.9 Overdose

The symptoms and signs of toxicity are generally similar to those described in the Undesirable Effects section but may be more frequent and can be more severe.

Signs and symptoms of digoxin toxicity become more frequent with levels above 2.0 nanograms/mL (2.56 nanomol/L) although there is considerable interindividual variation. However, in deciding whether a patient's symptoms are due to digoxin, the clinical state, together with serum electrolyte levels and thyroid function are important factors (see Dosage and Administration).

Adults

In adults without heart disease, clinical observation suggests that an overdose of digoxin of 10 to 15 mg was the dose resulting in death of half of the patients.

Cardiac manifestations

Cardiac manifestations are the most frequent and serious sign of both acute and chronic toxicity. Peak cardiac effects generally occur 3 to 6 hours following overdosage and may persist for the ensuing 24 hours or longer. Digoxin toxicity may result in almost any type of arrhythmia. Multiple rhythm disturbances in the same patient are common. These include paroxysmal atrial tachycardia with variable atrioventricular (AV) block, accelerated junctional rhythm, slow atrial fibrillation (with very little variation in the ventricular rate) and bi directional ventricular tachycardia.

Premature ventricular contractions (PVCs) are often the earliest and most common arrhythmia. Bigeminy or trigeminy also occur frequently.

Sinus bradycardia and other bradyarrhythmias are very common.

First, second, third degree heart blocks and AV dissociation are also common.

Early toxicity may only be manifested by prolongation of the PR interval.

Ventricular tachycardia may also be a manifestation of toxicity.

Cardiac arrest from asystole or ventricular fibrillation due to digoxin toxicity is usually fatal.

Hypokalaemia may contribute to toxicity (see *Warnings and Precautions*).

Non-cardiac manifestations

Acute massive digoxin overdosage can result in mild to pronounced hyperkalaemia due to inhibition of the sodium-potassium (Na+-K+) pump.

Gastrointestinal symptoms are very common in both acute and chronic toxicity. The symptoms precede cardiac manifestations in approximately half of the patients in most literature reports. Anorexia, nausea and vomiting have been reported with an incidence up to 80%. These symptoms usually present early in the course of an overdose.

Neurologic and visual manifestations occur in both acute and chronic toxicity. Dizziness, various CNS disturbances, fatigue and malaise are very common. The most frequent visual disturbance is an aberration of colour vision (predominance of yellow green). These neurological and visual symptoms may persist even after other signs of toxicity have resolved.

In chronic toxicity, non-specific extracardiac symptoms, such as malaise and weakness, may predominate.

Children

In children aged 1 to 3 years without heart disease, clinical observation suggests that an overdose of digoxin of 6 to 10 mg was the dose resulting in death in half of the patients.

Most manifestations of toxicity in children occur during or shortly after the loading phase with digoxin.

Cardiac manifestations

The same arrhythmias or combination of arrhythmias that occur in adults can occur in children. Sinus tachycardia, supraventricular tachycardia, and rapid atrial fibrillation are seen less frequently in the paediatric population.

Paediatric patients are more likely to present with an AV conduction disturbance or a sinus bradycardia.

Ventricular ectopy is less common, however in massive overdose, ventricular ectopy, ventricular tachycardia and ventricular fibrillation have been reported.

Any arrhythmia or alteration in cardiac conduction that develops in a child taking digoxin should be assumed to be caused by digoxin, until further evaluation proves otherwise.

Extracardiac manifestations

The frequent extracardiac manifestations similar to those seen in adults are gastrointestinal, CNS and visual. However, nausea and vomiting are not frequent in infants and small children.

In addition to the undesirable effects seen with recommended doses, weight loss in older age groups and failure to thrive in infants, abdominal pain due to mesenteric artery ischaemia, drowsiness and behavioural disturbances including psychotic manifestations have been reported in overdose.

Treatment

After recent ingestion, such as accidental or deliberate self-poisoning, the load available for absorption may be reduced by gastric lavage.

Patients with massive digitalis ingestion should receive large doses of activated charcoal to prevent absorption and bind digoxin in the gut during enteroenteric recirculation.

If more than 25 mg of digoxin was ingested by an adult without heart disease, death or progressive toxicity responsive only to digoxin-binding Fab antibody fragments (Digibind®) resulted. If more that 10 mg of digoxin was ingested by a child aged 1 to 3 years without heart disease, the outcome was uniformly fatal when Fab fragment treatment was not given.

Hypokalaemia should be corrected. In cases where a large amount of Lanoxin has been ingested hyperkalaemia may be present due to release of potassium from skeletal muscle. Before administering potassium in digoxin overdose the serum potassium level must be known.

Bradyarrhythmias may respond to atropine but temporary cardiac pacing may be required. Ventricular arrhythmias may respond to lignocaine or phenytoin.

Dialysis is not particularly effective in removing digoxin from the body in potentially life-threatening toxicity.

Rapid reversal of the complications that are associated with serious poisoning by digoxin, digitoxin and related glycosides has followed intravenous administration of digoxin-specific (ovine) antibody fragments (Fab) when other therapies have failed. Digibind®is the only specific treatment for digoxin toxicity.

5. PHARMACOLOGICAL PROPERTIES

5.1 Pharmacodynamic properties

Mode of Action:-

Digoxin increases contractility of the myocardium by direct activity. This effect is proportional to dose in the lower range and some effect is achieved with quite low dosing; it occurs even in normal myocardium although it is then entirely without physiological benefit. The primary action of digoxin is specifically to inhibit adenosine triphosphatase, and thus sodium-potassium (Na^+-K^+) exchange activity, the altered ionic distribution across the membrane resulting in an augmented calcium ion influx and thus an increase in the availability of calcium at the time of excitation-contraction coupling. The potency of digoxin may therefore appear considerably enhanced when the extracellular potassium concentration is low, with hyperkalaemia having the opposite effect.

Digoxin exerts the same fundamental effect of inhibition of the Na^+-K^+ exchange mechanism on cells of the autonomic nervous system, stimulating them to exert indirect cardiac activity. Increases in efferent vagal impulses result in reduced sympathetic tone and diminished impulse conduction rate through the atria and atrioventricular node. Thus, the major beneficial effect of digoxin is reduction of ventricular rate.

Indirect cardiac contractility changes also result from changes in venous compliance brought about by the altered autonomic activity and by direct venous stimulation. The interplay between direct and indirect activity governs the total circulatory response, which is not identical for all subjects. In the presence of certain supraventricular arrhythmias, the neurogenically mediated slowing of AV conduction is paramount.

The degree of neurohormonal activation occurring in patients with heart failure is associated with clinical deterioration and an increased risk of death. Digoxin reduces activation of both the sympathetic nervous system and the (renin-angiotensin) system independently of its inotropic actions, and may thus favourably influence survival. Whether this is achieved via direct sympathoinhibitory effects or by re-sensitising baroreflex mechanisms remains unclear.

5.2 Pharmacokinetic properties

Absorption

Intravenous administration of a loading dose produces an appreciable pharmacological effect within 5 to 30 minutes; this reaches a maximum in 1 to 5 hours. Upon oral administration, digoxin is absorbed from the stomach and upper part of the small intestine. When digoxin is taken after meals, the rate of absorption is slowed, but the total amount of digoxin absorbed is usually unchanged. When taken with meals high in fibre, however, the amount absorbed from an oral dose may be reduced.

Using the oral route the onset of effect occurs in 0.5 to 2 hours and reaches its maximum at 2 to 6 hours. The bioavailability of orally administered Lanoxin is approximately 63% in tablet form and 75% as paediatric elixir.

Distribution

The initial distribution of digoxin from the central to the peripheral compartment generally lasts from 6 to 8 hours. This is followed by a more gradual decline in serum digoxin concentration, which is dependent upon digoxin elimination from the body. The volume of distribution is large (Vd_{ss} = 510 litres in healthy volunteers), indicating digoxin to be extensively bound to body tissues. The highest digoxin concentrations are seen in the heart, liver and kidney, that in the heart averaging 30- fold that in the systemic circulation. Although the concentration in skeletal muscle is far lower, this store cannot be overlooked since skeletal muscle represents 40% of total body weight. Of the small proportion of digoxin circulating in plasma, approximately 25% is bound to protein.

Elimination

The major route of elimination is renal excretion of the unchanged drug.

Digoxin is a substrate for P-glycoprotein. As an efflux protein on the apical membrane of enterocytes, P-glycoprotein may limit the absorption of digoxin. P-glycoprotein in renal proximal tubules appears to be an important factor in the renal elimination of digoxin (See *4.5 Interaction with other medicinal products and other forms of interaction*).

Following intravenous administration to healthy volunteers, between 60 and 75% of a digoxin dose is recovered unchanged in the urine over a 6 day follow-up period. Total body clearance of digoxin has been shown to be directly related to renal function, and percent daily loss is thus a function of creatinine clearance, which in turn may be estimated from a stable serum creatinine. The total and renal clearances of digoxin have been found to be 193 ± 25 ml/min and 152 ± 24 mil/min in a healthy control population.

In a small percentage of individuals, orally administered digoxin is converted to cardioinactivate reduction products (digoxin reduction products or DRPs) by colonic bacteria in the gastrointestinal tract. In these subjects over 40% of the dose may be excreted as DRPs in the urine. Renal clearances of the two main metabolites, dihydrodigoxin and digoxygenin, have been found to be 79 ± 13 ml/min and 100 ± 26 ml/min respectively.

In the majority of cases however, the major route of digoxin elimination is renal excretion of the unchanged drug.

The terminal elimination half life of digoxin in patients with normal renal function is 30 to 40 hours. It is prolonged in patients with impaired renal function, and in anuric patients may be of the order of 100 hours.

In the newborn period, renal clearance of digoxin is diminished and suitable dosage adjustments must be observed. This is specially pronounced in the premature infant since renal clearance reflects maturation of renal function. Digoxin clearance has been found to be 65.6 ± 30 ml/min/1.73m^2 at 3 months, compared to only 32 ± 7 ml/min/1.73m^2 at 1 week. Beyond the immediate newborn period, children generally require proportionally larger doses than adults on the basis of body weight and body surface area.

Since most of the drug is bound to the tissues rather than circulating in the blood, digoxin is not effectively removed from the body during cardiopulmonary by-pass. Furthermore, only about 3% of a digoxin dose is removed from the body during five hours of haemodialysis.

5.3 Preclinical safety data

No data are available on whether or not digoxin has mutagenic or carcinogenic effects.

6. PHARMACEUTICAL PARTICULARS

6.1 List of excipients

Lactose Ph Eur

Starches Ph Eur

Hydrolysed Starch HSE

Magnesium Stearate Ph Eur

6.2 Incompatibilities

None known

6.3 Shelf life

Amber glass bottle: 60 months

Blister packs: 36 months

6.4 Special precautions for storage

Store below 25°C

6.5 Nature and contents of container

Amber glass bottle with low-density polyethylene snap-fit closure

Pack sizes: 28, 50, 500 tablets

Amber glass bottle with a clic-loc child resistant closure

Pack size: 56 tablets

White opaque PVC/aluminium foil blister

Pack sizes: 30, 60, 90, 120 tablets

Not all pack sizes may be marketed.

6.6 Special precautions for disposal and other handling

Not applicable.

Adminsitrative Data

7. MARKETING AUTHORISATION HOLDER

The Wellcome Foundation Limited

Greenford

Middlesex

UB6 0NN

Trading as:

GlaxoSmithKline UK

Stockley Park West

Uxbridge

Middlesex UB11 1BT

8. MARKETING AUTHORISATION NUMBER(S)

PL 0003/0102R

9. DATE OF FIRST AUTHORISATION/RENEWAL OF THE AUTHORISATION

24 April 2003

10. DATE OF REVISION OF THE TEXT

14 May 2009

11. Legal Status

POM

Lanoxin Injection

(GlaxoSmithKline UK)

1. NAME OF THE MEDICINAL PRODUCT

Lanoxin Injection.

2. QUALITATIVE AND QUANTITATIVE COMPOSITION

Digoxin 0.025 % w/v

3. PHARMACEUTICAL FORM

Solution for Injection.

4. CLINICAL PARTICULARS

4.1 Therapeutic indications

Lanoxin is indicated in the management of chronic cardiac failure where the dominant problem is systolic dysfunction. Its therapeutic benefit is greatest in those patients with ventricular dilatation.

Lanoxin is specifically indicated where cardiac failure is accompanied by atrial fibrillation.

Lanoxin is indicated in the management of certain supraventricular arrhythmias, particularly chronic atrial flutter and fibrillation.

4.2 Posology and method of administration

The dose of Lanoxin for each patient has to be tailored individually according to age, lean body weight and renal function. Suggested doses are intended only as an initial guide.

The difference in bioavailability between injectable Lanoxin and oral formulations must be considered when changing from one dosage form to another. For example, if patients are switched from oral to the i.v. formulation the dosage should be reduced by approximately 33 %.

Adults and children over 10 years of age:

Parenteral Loading:

Note: For use in patients who have not been given cardiac glycosides within the preceding two weeks.

The loading of parenteral Lanoxin is 500 to 1000 micrograms (0.5 to 1.0 mg) depending on age, lean body weight and renal function.

The loading dose should be administered in divided doses with approximately half the total dose given as the first dose and further fractions of the total dose given at intervals of 4 to 8 hours. An assessment of clinical response should be performed before giving each additional dose. Each dose should be given by intravenous infusion (*Dilution Instructions: see 6.6*) over 10 to 20 minutes.

Maintenance Dose:

The maintenance dosage should be based upon the percentage of the peak body stores lost each day through elimination. The following formula has had wide clinical use:

$$\text{Maintenance Dose} = \text{Peak body stores} \times \frac{\text{\% daily loss}}{100}$$

Where:

Peak Body Stores = Loading Dose

% Daily Loss = 14 + Creatinine Clearance (C_{cr})/5.

C_{cr} is creatinine clearance corrected to 70 kg body weight or 1.73 m^2 body surface area. If only serum creatinine (S_{cr}) concentrations are available, a C_{cr} (corrected to 70 kg body weight) may be estimated in men as

$$C_{cr} = \frac{(140 - \text{age})}{S_{cr} \text{ (in mg/100 ml)}}$$

NOTE: Where serum creatinine values are obtained in micromol/L these may be converted to mg/100 ml (mg %) as follows:

$$S_{cr} \text{ (mg/100 ml)} = \frac{S_{cr} \text{ (micromol/L)} \times 113.12}{10{,}000} = \frac{S_{cr} \text{ (micromol/L)}}{88.4}$$

Where 113.12 is the molecular weight of creatinine.

For *women*, this result should be multiplied by 0.85.

NOTE: These formulae cannot be used for creatinine clearance in children.

In practice, this will mean that most patients will be maintained on 0.125 to 0. 25 mg digoxin daily; however in those who show increased sensitivity to the adverse effects of digoxin, a dosage of 62.5 microgram (0.0625 mg) daily or less may suffice. Conversely, some patients may require a higher dose.

Neonates, infants and children up to 10 years of age (if cardiac glycosides have not been given in the preceding two weeks):

In the newborn, particularly in the premature infant, renal clearance of digoxin is diminished and suitable dose reductions must be observed, over and above general dosage instructions.

Beyond the immediate newborn period, children generally require proportionally larger doses than adults on the basis of body weight or body surface area, as indicated in the schedule below. Children over 10 years of age require adult dosages in proportion to their body weight.

Parenteral Loading:

The *parenteral loading dose* in the above groups should be administered in accordance with the following schedule:

Preterm neonates < 1.5 kg	20 microgram/kg over 24 hours
Preterm neonates 1.5 kg to 2.5 kg	30 microgram/kg over 24 hours
Term neonates to 2 years	35 microgram/kg over 24 hours
2 to 5 years	35 microgram/kg over 24 hours
5 to 10 years	25 microgram/kg over 24 hours

The loading dose should be administered in divided doses with approximately half the total dose given as the first dose and further fractions of the total dose given at intervals of 4 to 8 hours. An assessment of clinical response should be performed before giving each additional dose. Each dose should be given by intravenous infusion (*Dilution instructions: see 6.6*) over 10 to 20 minutes.

If cardiac glycosides have been given in the two weeks preceding commencement of Lanoxin therapy, it should be anticipated that optimum loading doses of Lanoxin will be less than those recommended above.

Maintenance Dose:

The maintenance dose should be administered in accordance with the following schedule:

Preterm neonates:

daily dose = 20% of 24-hour loading dose (intravenous or oral)

Term neonates and children up to 10 years:

daily dose = 25% of 24-hour loading dose (intravenous or oral)

These dosage schedules are meant as guidelines and careful clinical observation and monitoring of serum digoxin levels (see *Monitoring*) should be used as a basis for adjustment of dosage in these paediatric patient groups.

If cardiac glycosides have been given in the two weeks preceding commencement of Lanoxin therapy, it should be anticipated that optimum loading doses of Lanoxin will be less than those recommended above.

Use in the elderly:

The tendency to impaired renal function and low lean body mass in the elderly influences the pharmacokinetics of Lanoxin such that high serum digoxin levels and associated toxicity can occur quite readily, unless doses of Lanoxin lower than those in non-elderly patients are used. Serum digoxin levels should be checked regularly and hypokalaemia avoided.

Dose recommendations in renal disorder or with diuretic therapy:

See *Special Warnings and Precautions for use.*

Monitoring:

Serum concentrations of digoxin may be expressed in conventional units of nanogram/ml (ng/ml) or SI Units of nanomol/L (nmol/L). To convert ng/ml to nmol/L, multiply ng/ml by 1.28.

The serum concentration of digoxin can be determined by radioimmunoassay. Blood should be taken 6 hours or more after the last dose of Lanoxin. Several post hoc analyses of heart failure patients in the Digitalis Investigation Group trial suggest that the optimal trough digoxin serum level may be 0.5 ng/mL (0.64 nanomol/L) to 1.0 ng/mL (1.28 nanomol/L).

Digoxin toxicity is more commonly associated with serum digoxin concentration greater than 2 ng/mL. However, toxicity may occur with lower digoxin serum concentrations. In deciding whether a patient's symptoms are due to digoxin, the patient's clinical state together with the serum potassium level and thyroid function are important factors.

Other glycosides, including metabolites of digoxin, can interfere with the assays that are available and one should always be wary of values which do not seem commensurate with the clinical state of the patient.

4.3 Contraindications

Lanoxin is contra-indicated in intermittent complete heart block or second degree atrioventricular block, especially if there is a history of Stokes-Adams attacks.

Lanoxin is contra-indicated in arrhythmias caused by cardiac glycoside intoxication.

Lanoxin is contra-indicated in supraventricular arrhythmias associated with an accessory atrioventricular pathway, as in the Wolff-Parkinson-White syndrome unless the electrophysiological characteristics of the accessory pathway and any possible deleterious effect of digoxin on these characteristics has been evaluated. If an accessory pathway is known or suspected to be present and there is no history of previous supraventricular arrhythmias, Lanoxin is similarly contra-indicated.

Lanoxin is contra-indicated in ventricular tachycardia or ventricular fibrillation.

Lanoxin is contra-indicated in hypertrophic obstructive cardiomyopathy, unless there is concomitant atrial fibrillation and heart failure, but even then caution should be exercised if digoxin is to be used.

Lanoxin is contra-indicated in patients known to be hypersensitive to digoxin, other digitalis glycosides, or to any component of the preparation.

4.4 Special warnings and precautions for use

Arrhythmias may be precipitated by digoxin toxicity, some of which can resemble arrhythmias for which the drug could be advised. For example, atrial tachycardia with varying atrioventricular block requires particular care as clinically the rhythm resembles atrial fibrillation.

In some cases of sinoatrial disorder (i.e. Sick Sinus Syndrome) digoxin may cause or exacerbate sinus bradycardia or cause sinoatrial block.

Determination of the serum digoxin concentration may be very helpful in making a decision to treat with further digoxin, but toxic doses of other glycosides may cross-react in the assay and wrongly suggest apparently satisfactory measurements. Observations during the temporary withholding of digoxin might be more appropriate.

In cases where cardiac glycosides have been taken in the preceding two weeks, the recommendations for initial dosing of a patient should be reconsidered and a reduced dose is advised.

The dosing recommendations should be reconsidered if patients are elderly or there are other reasons for the renal clearance of digoxin being reduced. A reduction in both initial and maintenance doses should be considered.

Hypokalaemia sensitises the myocardium to the actions of cardiac glycosides.

Hypoxia, hypomagnesaemia and marked hypercalcaemia increase myocardial sensitivity to cardiac glycosides.

Rapid intravenous injection can cause vasoconstriction producing hypertension and/or reduced coronary flow. A slow injection rate is therefore important in hypertensive heart failure and acute myocardial infarction.

Administering Lanoxin to a patient with thyroid disease requires care. Initial and maintenance doses of Lanoxin should be reduced when thyroid function is subnormal. In hyperthyroidism there is relative digoxin resistance and the dose may have to be increased. During the course of treatment of thyrotoxicosis, dosage should be reduced as the thyrotoxicosis comes under control.

Patients with malabsorption syndrome or gastro-intestinal reconstructions may require larger doses of digoxin.

The risk of provoking dangerous arrhythmias with direct current cardioversion is greatly increased in the presence of digitalis toxicity and is in proportion to the cardioversion energy used.

For elective direct current cardioversion of a patient who is taking digoxin, the drug should be withheld for 24 hours before cardioversion is performed. In emergencies, such as cardiac arrest, when attempting cardioversion the lowest effective energy should be applied. Direct current cardioversion is inappropriate in the treatment of arrhythmias thought to be caused by cardiac glycosides.

Many beneficial effects of digoxin on arrhythmias result from a degree of atrioventricular conduction blockade. However, when incomplete atrioventricular block already exists the effects of a rapid progression in the block should be anticipated. In complete heart block the idioventricular escape rhythm may be suppressed.

The administration of digoxin in the period immediately following myocardial infarction is not contra-indicated. However, the use of inotropic drugs in some patients in this setting may result in undesirable increases in myocardial oxygen demand and ischaemia, and some retrospective follow-up studies have suggested digoxin to be associated with an increased risk of death. However, the possibility of arrhythmias arising in patients who may be hypokalaemic after myocardial infarction and are likely to be cardiologically unstable must be borne in mind. The limitations imposed thereafter on direct current cardioversion must also be remembered.

Treatment with digoxin should generally be avoided in patients with heart failure associated with cardiac amyloidosis. However, if alternative treatments are not appropriate, digoxin can be used with caution to control the ventricular rate in patients with cardiac amyloidosis and atrial fibrillation.

Digoxin can rarely precipitate vasoconstriction and therefore should be avoided in patients with myocarditis.

Patients with beri beri heart disease may fail to respond adequately to digoxin if the underlying thiamine deficiency is not treated concomitantly. There is also some published information indicating that digoxin may inhibit the uptake of thiamine in myocytes in beri beri heart disease.

Digoxin should not be used in constrictive pericarditis unless it is used to control the ventricular rate in atrial fibrillation or to improve systolic dysfunction.

Digoxin improves exercise tolerance in patients with impaired left ventricular systolic dysfunction and normal sinus rhythm. This may or may not be associated with an improved haemodynamic profile. However, the benefit of patients with supraventricular arrhythmias is most evident at rest, less evident with exercise.

In patients receiving diuretics and an ACE inhibitor, or diuretics alone, the withdrawal of digoxin has been shown to result in clinical deterioration.

The use of therapeutic doses of digoxin may cause prolongation of the PR interval and depression of the ST segment on the electrocardiogram.

Digoxin may produce false positive ST-T changes on the electrocardiogram during exercise testing. These electrophysiologic effects reflect an expected effect of the drug and are not indicative of toxicity.

Patients receiving digoxin should have their serum electrolytes and renal function (serum creatinine concentration) assessed periodically; the frequency of assessments will depend on the clinical setting.

Although many patients with chronic congestive cardiac failure benefit from acute administration of digoxin, there are some in whom it does not lead to constant, marked or lasting haemodynamic improvement. It is therefore important to evaluate the response of each patient individually when Lanoxin is continued long-term.

The intramuscular route is painful and is associated with muscle necrosis. This route cannot be recommended.

Patients with severe respiratory disease may have an increased myocardial sensitivity to digitalis glycosides.

The packs will carry the following statements:

Do not store above 25°C

Protect from light

For intravenous injection under medical supervision

Keep out of reach of children

4.5 Interaction with other medicinal products and other forms of interaction

Interactions may arise from effects on the renal excretion, tissue binding, plasma protein binding, distribution within the body, gut absorptive capacity and sensitivity to Lanoxin. Consideration of the possibility of an interaction whenever concomitant therapy is contemplated is the best precaution and a check on serum digoxin concentration is recommended when any doubt exists.

Digoxin, in association with beta-adrenoceptor blocking drugs, may increase atrio-ventricular conduction time.

Agents causing hypokalaemia or intracellular potassium deficiency may cause increased sensitivity to Digoxin; they include diuretics, lithium salts, corticosteroids and carbenoxolone.

Patients receiving Digoxin are more susceptible to the effects of suxamethonium-exacerbated hyperkalaemia.

Calcium, particularly if administered rapidly by the intravenous route, may produce serious arrhythmias in digitalized patients.

Serum levels of digoxin may be **increased** by concomitant administration of the following:

Alprazolam, amiodarone, flecainide, gentamicin, indometacin, itraconazole, prazosin, propafenone, quinidine, quinine, spironolactone, macrolide antibiotics (e.g. erythromycin and clarithromycin), tetracycline (and possibly other antibiotics), trimethoprim, propantheline, atorvastatin, ciclosporin, epoprostenol (transient) and carvedilol.

Serum levels of digoxin may be **reduced** by concomitant administration of the following:

Adrenaline (epinephrine), antacids, kaolin-pectin, some bulk laxatives, colestyramine, acarbose, salbutamol, sulfasalazine, neomycin, rifampicin, some cytostatics, phenytoin, metoclopramide, penicillamine and the herbal remedy St John's wort (*Hypericum perforatum*).

Calcium channel blocking agents may either increase or cause no change in serum digoxin levels. Verapamil, felodipine and tiapamil increase serum digoxin levels. Nifedipine and diltiazem may increase or have no effect on serum digoxin levels. Isradipine causes no change in serum digoxin levels. Angiotensin converting enzyme (ACE) inhibitors may also increase or cause no change in serum digoxin concentrations.

Milrinone does not alter steady-state serum digoxin levels.

Digoxin is a substrate of P-glycoprotein. Thus, inhibitors of P-glycoprotein may increase blood concentrations of digoxin by enhancing its absorption and/or by reducing its renal clearance (See *5.2 Pharmacokinetic Properties*).

4.6 Pregnancy and lactation

No data are available on whether or not digoxin has teratogenic effects.

There is no information available on the effect of digoxin on human fertility.

The use of digoxin in pregnancy is not contra-indicated, although the dosage and control may be less predictable in pregnant than in non-pregnant women with some requiring an increased dosage of digoxin during pregnancy. As with all drugs, use should be considered only when the expected clinical benefit of treatment to the mother outweighs any possible risk to the developing foetus.

Despite extensive antenatal exposure to digitalis preparations, no significant adverse effects have been observed in the foetus or neonate when maternal serum digoxin concentrations are maintained within the normal range. Although it has been speculated that a direct effect of digoxin in the myometrium may result in relative prematurity and low birthweight, a contributing role of the underlying cardiac disease cannot be excluded. Maternally administered digoxin has been successfully used to treat foetal tachycardia and congestive heart failure.

Adverse foetal effects have been reported in mothers with digitalis toxicity.

Although digoxin is excreted in breast milk, the quantities are minute and breast feeding is not contra-indicated.

4.7 Effects on ability to drive and use machines

Since central nervous system and visual disturbances have been reported in patients receiving Lanoxin, patients should exercise caution before driving, using machinery or participating in dangerous activities.

4.8 Undesirable effects

Adverse reactions are listed below by system organ class and frequency. Frequencies are defined as: very common ($\geqslant$ 1/10), common ($\geqslant$ 1/100 and $<$ 1/10), uncommon ($\geqslant$ 1/1000 and $<$ 1/100), rare ($\geqslant$ 1/10,000 and $<$ 1/1000), very rare ($<$ 1/10,000), including isolated reports. Very common, common and uncommon events were generally determined from clinical trial data. The incidence in placebo was taken into account. Adverse drug reactions identified through post-marketing surveillance were considered to be rare or very rare (including isolated reports).

Blood and lymphatic system disorders

Very rare: Thrombocytopaenia

Metabolism and nutrition disorders

Very Rare: Anorexia

Psychiatric disorders

Uncommon: Depression

Very rare: Psychosis, apathy, confusion

Nervous system disorders

Common: CNS disturbances, dizziness

Very rare: Headache

Eye disorders

Common: Visual disturbances (blurred or yellow vision)

Cardiac disorders

Common: Arrhythmia, conduction disturbances, bigeminy, trigeminy, PR prolongation, sinus bradycardia

Very rare: Supraventricular tachyarrhythmia, atrial tachycardia (with or without block), junctional (nodal) tachycardia, ventricular arrhythmia, ventricular premature contraction, ST segment depression

Gastrointestinal disorders

Common: Nausea, vomiting, diarrhoea

Very rare: Intestinal ischaemia, intestinal necrosis

Skin disorders

Common: Skin rashes of urticarial or scarlatiniform character may be accompanied by pronounced eosinophilia

Reproductive system and breast disorders

Very rare: Gynaecomastia can occur with long term administration

General disorders and administration site conditions

Very rare: Fatigue, malaise, weakness

4.9 Overdose

The symptoms and signs of toxicity are generally similar to those described in the Undesirable Effects section but may be more frequent and can be more severe.

Signs and symptoms of digoxin toxicity become more frequent with levels above 2.0 nanograms/mL (2.56 nanomol/L) although there is considerable interindividual variation. However, in deciding whether a patient's symtoms are due to digoxin, the clinical state, together with serum electrolyte levels and thyroid function are important factors (see *Dosage and Administration*).

Adults

In adults without heart disease, clinical observation suggests that an overdose of digoxin of 10 to 15 mg was the dose resulting in death of half of the patients.

Cardiac manifestations

Cardiac manifestations are the most frequent and serious sign of both acute and chronic toxicity. Peak cardiac effects generally occur 3 to 6 hours following overdosage and may persist for the ensuing 24 hours or longer. Digoxin toxicity may result in almost any type of arrhythmia. Multiple rhythm disturbances in the same patient are common. These include paroxysmal atrial tachycardia with variable atrioventricular (AV) block, accelerated junctional rhythm, slow atrial fibrillation (with very little variation in the ventricular rate) and bi directional ventricular tachycardia.

Premature ventricular contractions (PVCs) are often the earliest and most common arrhythmia. Bigeminy or trigeminy also occur frequently.

Sinus bradycardia and other bradyarrhythmias are very common.

First, second, third degree heart blocks and AV dissociation are also common.

Early toxicity may only be manifested by prolongation of the PR interval.

Ventricular tachycardia may also be a manifestation of toxicity.

Cardiac arrest from asystole or ventricular fibrillation due to digoxin toxicity is usually fatal.

Hypokalaemia may contribute to toxicity (see *Warnings and Precautions*).

Non-cardiac manifestations

Acute massive digoxin overdosage can result in mild to pronounced hyperkalaemia due to inhibition of the sodium-potassium (Na+-K+) pump.

Gastrointestinal symptoms are very common in both acute and chronic toxicity. The symptoms precede cardiac manifestations in approximately half of the patients in most literature reports. Anorexia, nausea and vomiting have been reported with an incidence up to 80%. These symptoms usually present early in the course of an overdose.

Neurologic and visual manifestations occur in both acute and chronic toxicity. Dizziness, various CNS disturbances, fatigue and malaise are very common. The most frequent visual disturbance is an aberration of colour vision (predominance of yellow green). These neurological and visual symptoms may persist even after other signs of toxicity have resolved.

In chronic toxicity, non-specific extracardiac symptoms, such as malaise and weakness, may predominate.

Children

In children aged 1 to 3 years without heart disease, clinical observation suggests that an overdose of digoxin of 6 to 10 mg was the dose resulting in death in half of the patients.

Most manifestations of toxicity in children occur during or shortly after the loading phase with digoxin.

Cardiac manifestations

The same arrhythmias or combination of arrhythmias that occur in adults can occur in children. Sinus tachycardia, supraventricular tachycardia, and rapid atrial fibrillation are seen less frequently in the paediatric population.

Paediatric patients are more likely to present with an AV conduction disturbance or a sinus bradycardia.

Ventricular ectopy is less common, however in massive overdose, ventricular ectopy, ventricular tachycardia and ventricular fibrillation have been reported.

Any arrhythmia or alteration in cardiac conduction that develops in a child taking digoxin should be assumed to be caused by digoxin, until further evaluation proves otherwise.

Extracardiac manifestations

The frequent extracardiac manifestations similar to those seen in adults are gastrointestinal, CNS and visual. However, nausea and vomiting are not frequent in infants and small children.

In addition to the undesirable effects seen with recommended doses, weight loss in older age groups and failure to thrive in infants, abdominal pain due to mesenteric artery ischaemia, drowsiness and behavioural disturbances including psychotic manifestations have been reported in overdose.

Treatment

After recent ingestion, such as accidental or deliberate self-poisoning, the load available for absorption may be reduced by gastric lavage.

Patients with massive digitalis ingestion should receive large doses of activated charcoal to prevent absorption and bind digoxin in the gut during enteroenteric recirculation.

If more than 25 mg of digoxin was ingested by an adult without heart disease, death or progressive toxicity responsive only to digoxin-binding Fab antibody fragments (Digibind®) resulted. If more than 10 mg of digoxin was ingested by a child aged 1 to 3 years without heart disease, the outcome was uniformly fatal when Fab fragment treatment was not given.

Hypokalaemia should be corrected. In cases where a large amount of Lanoxin has been ingested, hyperkalaemia may be present due to release of potassium from skeletal muscle. Before administering potassium in digoxin overdose the serum potassium level must be known.

Bradyarrhythmias may respond to atropine but temporary cardiac pacing may be required. Ventricular arrhythmias may respond to lignocaine or phenytoin.

Dialysis is not particularly effective in removing digoxin from the body in potentially life-threatening toxicity.

Rapid reversal of the complications that are associated with serious poisoning by digoxin, digitoxin and related glycosides has followed intravenous administration of digoxin-specific (ovine) antibody fragments (Fab) when other therapies have failed. Digibind® is the only specific treatment for digoxin toxicity.

5. PHARMACOLOGICAL PROPERTIES

5.1 Pharmacodynamic properties

Mode of Action:-

Digoxin increases contractility of the myocardium by direct activity. This effect is proportional to dose in the lower range and some effect is achieved with quite low dosing; it occurs even in normal myocardium although it is then entirely without physiological benefit. The primary action of digoxin is specifically to inhibit adenosine triphosphatase, and thus sodium-potassium (Na^+-K^+) exchange activity, the altered ionic distribution across the membrane resulting in an augmented calcium ion influx and thus an increase in the availability of calcium at the time of excitation-contraction coupling. The potency of digoxin may therefore appear considerably enhanced when the extracellular potassium concentration is low, with hyperkalaemia having the opposite effect.

Digoxin exerts the same fundamental effect of inhibition of the Na^+-K^+ exchange mechanism on cells of the autonomic nervous system, stimulating them to exert indirect cardiac activity. Increases in efferent vagal impulses result in reduced sympathetic tone and diminished impulse conduction rate through the atria and atrioventricular node. Thus, the major beneficial effect of digoxin is reduction of ventricular rate.

Indirect cardiac contractility changes also result from changes in venous compliance brought about by the altered autonomic activity and by direct venous stimulation. The interplay between direct and indirect activity governs the total circulatory response, which is not identical for all subjects. In the presence of certain supraventricular arrhythmias, the neurogenically mediated slowing of AV conduction is paramount.

The degree of neurohormonal activation occurring in patients with heart failure is associated with clinical deterioration and an increased risk of death. Digoxin reduces activation of both the sympathetic nervous system and the (renin-angiotensin) system independently of its inotropic actions, and may thus favourably influence survival. Whether this is achieved via direct sympathoinhibitory effects or by re-sensitising baroreflex mechanisms remains unclear.

5.2 Pharmacokinetic properties

Absorption

Intravenous administration of a loading dose produces an appreciable pharmacological effect within 5 to 30 minutes; this reaches a maximum in 1 to 5 hours. Upon oral administration, digoxin is absorbed from the stomach and upper part of the small intestine. When digoxin is taken after meals, the rate of absorption is slowed, but the total amount of digoxin absorbed is usually unchanged. When taken with meals high in fibre, however, the amount absorbed from an oral dose may be reduced.

Using the oral route the onset of effect occurs in 0.5 to 2 hours and reaches its maximum at 2 to 6 hours. The bioavailability of orally administered Lanoxin is approximately 63% in tablet form and 75% as paediatric elixir.

Distribution

The initial distribution of digoxin from the central to the peripheral compartment generally lasts from 6 to 8 hours. This is followed by a more gradual decline in serum digoxin concentration, which is dependent upon digoxin elimination from the body. The volume of distribution is large (Vd_{ss} = 510 litres in healthy volunteers), indicating digoxin to be extensively bound to body tissues. The highest digoxin concentrations are seen in the heart, liver and kidney, that in the heart averaging 30- fold that in the systemic circulation. Although the concentration in skeletal muscle is far lower, this store cannot be overlooked since skeletal muscle represents 40% of total body weight. Of the small proportion of digoxin circulating in plasma, approximately 25% is bound to protein.

Elimination

The major route of elimination is renal excretion of the unchanged drug.

Digoxin is a substrate for P-glycoprotein. As an efflux protein on the apical membrane of enterocytes, P-glycoprotein may limit the absorption of digoxin. P-glycoprotein in renal proximal tubules appears to be an important factor in the renal elimination of digoxin (See *4.5 Interaction with other medicinal products and other forms of interaction*).

Following intravenous administration to healthy volunteers, between 60 and 75% of a digoxin dose is recovered unchanged in the urine over a 6 day follow-up period. Total body clearance of digoxin has been shown to be directly related to renal function, and percent daily loss is thus a function of creatinine clearance, which in turn may be estimated from a stable serum creatinine. The total and renal clearances of digoxin have been found to be 193 ± 25 ml/min and 152 ± 24 mil/min in a healthy control population.

In a small percentage of individuals, orally administered digoxin is converted to cardioinactivate reduction products (digoxin reduction products or DRPs) by colonic bacteria in the gastrointestinal tract. In these subjects over 40% of the dose may be excreted as DRPs in the urine. Renal clearances of the two main metabolites, dihydrodigoxin and digoxygenin, have been found to be 79 ± 13 ml/min and 100 ± 26 ml/min respectively.

In the majority of cases however, the major route of digoxin elimination is renal excretion of the unchanged drug.

The terminal elimination half life of digoxin in patients with normal renal function is 30 to 40 hours. It is prolonged in patients with impaired renal function, and in anuric patients may be of the order of 100 hours.

In the newborn period, renal clearance of digoxin is diminished and suitable dosage adjustments must be observed. This is specially pronounced in the premature infant since renal clearance reflects maturation of renal function. Digoxin clearance has been found to be 65.6 ± 30 ml/min/1.73m^2 at 3 months, compared to only 32 ± 7 ml/min/1.73m^2 at 1 week. Beyond the immediate newborn period, children generally require proportionally larger doses than adults on the basis of body weight and body surface area.

Since most of the drug is bound to the tissues rather than circulating in the blood, digoxin is not effectively removed from the body during cardiopulmonary by-pass. Furthermore, only about 3% of a digoxin dose is removed from the body during five hours of haemodialysis.

5.3 Preclinical safety data

No data are available on whether or not digoxin has mutagenic or carcinogenic effects.

6. PHARMACEUTICAL PARTICULARS

6.1 List of excipients

Ethanol

Propylene Glycol

Citric Acid Monohydrate

Sodium phosphate anhydrous

or

Sodium phosphate

Water for Injections

6.2 Incompatibilities

None known.

6.3 Shelf life

5 years.

6.4 Special precautions for storage

Do not store above 25°C.

Store in the original container

6.5 Nature and contents of container

Neutral glass ampoules

6.6 Special precautions for disposal and other handling

Lanoxin Injection can be administered undiluted or diluted with a 4-fold or greater volume of diluent. The use of less than a 4-fold volume of diluent could lead to precipitation of digoxin.

Lanoxin Injection, 250 micrograms/ml when diluted in the ratio of 1 to 250 (i.e. One 2 ml ampoule containing 500 micrograms added to 500 ml of infusion solution) is known to be compatible with the following infusion solutions:

Sodium Chloride Intravenous Infusion, BP, 0.9% w/v

Sodium Chloride (0.18% w/v) and Glucose (4% w/v) Intravenous Infusion, BP

Glucose Intravenous Infusion, BP, 5% w/v

Chemical in-use stability has been demonstrated for up to 96 hours at ambient temperature (20-25°C).

From a microbiological point of view, the product should be used immediately. If not used immediately, in-use storage times and conditions prior to use are the responsibility of the user and would normally not be longer than 24 hours at 2 to 8°C, unless reconstitution / dilution (etc) has taken place in controlled and validated aseptic conditions.

Any unused solution should be discarded.

Ampoules are equipped with the OPC (One Point Cut) opening system and must be opened as follows:

Hold with the hand the bottom part of the ampoule as indicated in Picture 1

Put the other hand on the top of the ampoule positioning the thumb above the coloured point and press as indicated in Picture 2

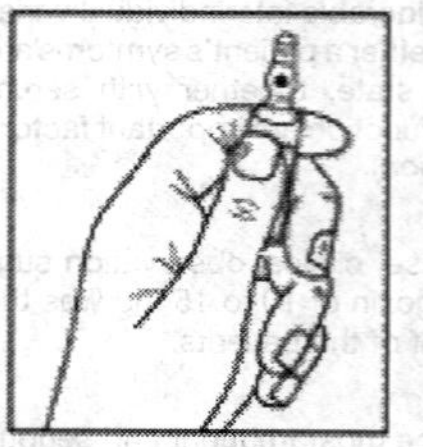

Picture 1

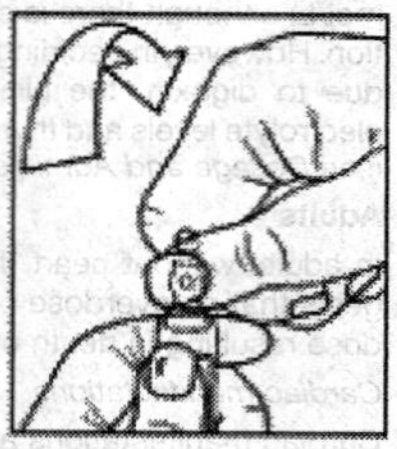

Picture 2

Administrative Data

7. MARKETING AUTHORISATION HOLDER

The Wellcome Foundation Limited

Greenford

Middlesex

UB6 0NN

Trading as:

GlaxoSmithKline UK

Stockley Park West

Uxbridge

Middlesex UB11 1BT

8. MARKETING AUTHORISATION NUMBER(S)

PL0003/5259R

9. DATE OF FIRST AUTHORISATION/RENEWAL OF THE AUTHORISATION

24 April 2003

10. DATE OF REVISION OF THE TEXT

14 May 2009

Lanoxin PG Elixir

(GlaxoSmithKline UK)

1. NAME OF THE MEDICINAL PRODUCT

Lanoxin PG Elixir

2. QUALITATIVE AND QUANTITATIVE COMPOSITION

Digoxin 0.005 % w/v

3. PHARMACEUTICAL FORM

Oral solution.

4. CLINICAL PARTICULARS

4.1 Therapeutic indications

Lanoxin is indicated in the management of chronic cardiac failure where the dominant problem is systolic dysfunction. Its therapeutic benefit is greatest in those patients with ventricular dilatation.

Lanoxin is specifically indicated where cardiac failure is accompanied by atrial fibrillation.

Lanoxin is indicated in the management of certain supraventricular arrhythmias, particularly chronic atrial flutter and fibrillation.

4.2 Posology and method of administration

The dose of Lanoxin for each patient has to be tailored individually according to age, lean body weight and renal function. Suggested doses are intended only as an initial guide.

The difference in bioavailability between injectable Lanoxin and oral formulations must be considered when changing from one dosage form to another. For example, if patients are switched from oral to the i.v. formulation the dosage should be reduced by approximately 33 %.

Lanoxin PG Elixir, 50 micrograms in 1 ml, is supplied with a graduated pipette and this should be used for measurement of all doses.

Adults with chronic cardiac failure in the absence of supraventricular arrhythmia:

No loading dose is required. The usual daily dose is 125 to 250 micrograms (0.125 to 0.25 mg) for patients with normal renal function. A lower dose of 62.5 micrograms (0.0625 mg) should be considered in the elderly.

For the management of atrial fibrillation or flutter in adults and children over 10 years:

Rapid Oral Loading:

If medically appropriate, rapid digitalisation may be achieved in a number of ways, such as the following:

750 to 1500 micrograms (0.75 to 1.5 mg) as a single dose.

Where there is less urgency, or greater risk of toxicity (e.g. in the elderly), the oral loading dose should be given in divided doses 6 hours apart, assessing clinical response before giving each additional dose (see *Special Warnings and Precautions for Use*).

Slow Oral Loading:

Digitalisation may be achieved more slowly with doses of 250 to 750 micrograms (0.25 to 0.75 mg) given daily for 1 week followed by an appropriate maintenance dose. A clinical response should be seen within one week.

NOTE: The choice between slow and rapid oral loading depends on the clinical state of the patient and the urgency of the condition.

Maintenance Dose:

The maintenance dosage should be based upon the percentage of the peak body stores lost each day through elimination. The following formula has had wide clinical use:

$$\text{Maintenance Dose} = \text{Peak body stores} \times \frac{\text{\% daily loss}}{100}$$

Where:

Peak Body Stores = Loading Dose

% Daily Loss = 14 + Creatinine Clearance (C_{cr})/5.

C_{cr} is creatinine clearance corrected to 70 kg body weight or 1.73 m^2 body surface area. If only serum creatinine (S_{cr}) concentrations are available, a C_{cr} (corrected to 70 kg body weight) maybe estimated in men as:

$$C_{cr} = \frac{(140 - \text{age})}{S_{cr}\ (\text{in mg/100 ml})}$$

NOTE: Where serum creatinine values are obtained in micromol/L. These may be converted to mg/100 ml (mg %) as follows:

$$S_{cr}\ (\text{mg/100 ml}) = \frac{S_{cr}\ (\text{micromol/L}) \times 113.12}{10{,}000} = \frac{S_{cr}\ (\text{micromol/L})}{88.4}$$

Where 113.12 is the molecular weight of creatinine.

For women, this result should be multiplied by 0.85

NOTE: These formulae cannot be used for creatinine clearance in children.

In practice, this will mean that most patients be maintained on 0.125 to 0.25 mg digoxin daily; however in those who show increased sensitivity to the adverse effects of digoxin, a dosage of 62.5 microgram (0.0625 mg) daily or less may suffice. Conversely, some patients may require a higher dose.

Neonates, infants and children up to 10 years of age (if cardiac glycosides have not been given in preceding two weeks):

In the newborn, particularly in the premature infant, renal clearance of digoxin is diminished and suitable dose reductions must be observed, over and above general dosage instructions.

Beyond the immediate newborn period, children generally require proportionally larger doses than adults on the basis of body weight or body surface area, as indicated in the schedule below. Children over 10 years of age require adult dosages in proportion to their body weight.

Oral Loading Dose:

This should be administered in accordance with the following schedule:-

Preterm neonates < 1.5 kg	25 microgram/kg over 24 hours
Preterm neonates 1.5 to 2.5 kg	30 microgram/kg over 24 hours
Term neonates to 2 years	45 microgram/kg over 24 hours
2 to 5 years	35 microgram/kg over 24 hours
5 to 10 years	25 microgram/kg over 24 hours

The loading dose should be administered in divided doses with approximately half the total dose given as the first dose and further fractions of the total dose given at intervals of 4 to 8 hours, assessing clinical response before giving each additional dose.

Maintenance Dose:

The maintenance dose should be administered in accordance with the following schedule:

Preterm neonates:

daily dose = 20% of 24-hour loading dose (intravenous or oral)

Term neonates and children up to10 years:

daily dose = 25% of 24-hour loading dose (intravenous or oral)

These dosage schedules are meant as guidelines and careful clinical observation and monitoring of serum digoxin levels (see *Monitoring*) should be used as a basis for adjustment of dosage in these paediatric patient groups.

If cardiac glycosides have been given in the two weeks preceding commencement of Lanoxin therapy, it should be anticipated that optimum loading doses of Lanoxin will be less than those recommended above.

Use in the elderly:

The tendency to impaired renal function and low lean body mass in the elderly influences the pharmacokinetics of Lanoxin such that high serum digoxin levels and associated toxicity can occur quite readily, unless doses of Lanoxin lower than those in non-elderly patients are used. Serum digoxin levels should be checked regularly and hypokalaemia avoided.

Dose recommendations in renal disorder or with diuretic therapy:

See *Special Warnings and Precautions for Use*.

Monitoring:

Serum concentrations of digoxin may be expressed in conventional units of nanogram/ml (ng/ml) or SI units of nanomol/L (nmol/L). To convert ng/ml to nmol/L, multiply ng/ml by 1.28.

The serum concentration of digoxin can be determined by radioimmunoassay. Blood should be taken 6 hours or more after the last dose of Lanoxin. Several post hoc analyses of heart failure patients in the Digitalis Investigation Group trial suggest that the optimal trough digoxin serum level may be 0.5 ng/mL (0.64 nanomol/L) to 1.0 ng/mL (1.28 nanomol/L).

Digoxin toxicity is more commonly associated with serum digoxin concentration greater than 2 ng/mL. However, toxicity may occur with lower digoxin serum concentrations. In deciding whether a patient's symptoms are due to digoxin, the patient's clinical state together with the serum potassium level and thyroid function are important factors.

Other glycosides, including metabolites of digoxin, can interfere with the assays that are available and one should always be wary of values which do not seem commensurate with the clinical state of the patient.

4.3 Contraindications

Lanoxin is contra-indicated in intermittent complete heart block or second degree atrioventricular block, especially if there is a history of Stokes-Adams attacks.

Lanoxin is contra-indicated in arrhythmias caused by cardiac glycoside intoxication.

Lanoxin is contra-indicated in supraventricular arrhythmias associated with an accessory atrioventricular pathway, as in the Wolff-Parkinson-White syndrome, unless the electrophysiological characteristics of the accessory pathway and any possible deleterious effect of digoxin on these characteristics has been evaluated. If an accessory pathway is known or suspected to be present and there is no history of previous supraventricular arrhythmias, Lanoxin is similarly contra-indicated.

Lanoxin is contra-indicated in ventricular tachycardia or ventricular fibrillation.

Lanoxin is contra-indicated in hypertrophic obstructive cardiomyopathy, unless there is concomitant atrial fibrillation and heart failure but even then caution should be exercised if Lanoxin is to be used.

Lanoxin is contra-indicated in patients known to be hypersensitive to digoxin, other digitalis glycosides, or to any component of the preparation.

4.4 Special warnings and precautions for use

Arrhythmias may be precipitated by digoxin toxicity, some of which can resemble arrhythmias for which the drug could be advised. For example, atrial tachycardia with varying atrioventricular block requires particular care as clinically the rhythm resembles atrial fibrillation.

In some cases of sinoatrial disorder (i.e. sick sinus syndrome) digoxin may cause or exacerbate sinus bradycardia or cause sinoatrial block.

Determination of the serum digoxin concentration may be very helpful in making a decision to treat with further digoxin, but toxic doses of other glycosides may cross-react in the assay and wrongly suggest apparently satisfactory measurements. Observations during the temporary withholding of digoxin may be more appropriate.

In cases where cardiac glycosides have been taken in the preceding two weeks the recommendations for initial dosing of a patient should be reconsidered and a reduced dose is advised.

The dosing recommendations should be reconsidered if patients are elderly or there are other reasons for the renal clearance of digoxin being reduced. A reduction in both initial and maintenance doses should be considered.

Hypokalaemia sensitises the myocardium to the actions of cardiac glycosides.

Hypoxia, hypomagnesaemia and marked hypercalcaemia increase myocardial sensitivity to cardiac glycosides.

Administering Lanoxin to a patient with thyroid disease requires care. Initial and maintenance doses of Lanoxin should be reduced when thyroid function is subnormal. In hyperthyroidism there is relative digoxin resistance and the dose may have to be increased. During the course of treatment of thyrotoxicosis, dosage should be reduced as the thyrotoxicosis comes under control.

Patients with malabsorption syndrome or gastro-intestinal reconstruction may require larger doses of digoxin.

The risk of provoking dangerous arrhythmias with direct current cardioversion is greatly increased in the presence of digitalis toxicity and is in proportion to the cardioversion energy used.

For elective direct current cardioversion of a patient who is taking digoxin, the drug should be withheld for 24 hours before cardioversion is performed. In emergencies, such as cardiac arrest, when attempting cardioversion the lowest effective energy should be applied. Direct current cardioversion is inappropriate in the treatment of arrhythmias thought to be caused by cardiac glycosides.

Many beneficial effects of digoxin on arrhythmias result from a degree of atrioventricular conduction blockade. However, when incomplete atrioventricular block already exists, the effects of a rapid progression in the block should be anticipated. In complete heart block the idioventricular escape rhythm may be suppressed.

The administration of digoxin in the period immediately following myocardial infarction is not contra-indicated. However, the use of inotropic drugs in some patients in this setting may result in undesirable increases in myocardial oxygen demand and ischaemia, and some retrospective follow-up studies have suggested digoxin to be associated with an increased risk of death. However, the possibility of arrhythmias arising in patients who may be hypokalaemic after myocardial infarction and are likely to be cardiologically unstable must be borne in mind. The limitations imposed thereafter on direct current cardioversion must also be remembered.

Treatment with digoxin should generally be avoided in patients with heart failure associated with cardiac amyloidosis. However, if alternative treatments are not appropriate, digoxin can be used with caution to control the ventricular rate in patients with cardiac amyloidosis and atrial fibrillation.

Digoxin can rarely precipitate vasoconstriction and therefore should be avoided in patients with myocarditis.

Patients with beri beri heart disease may fail to respond adequately to digoxin if the underlying thiamine deficiency is not treated concomitantly. There is also some published information indicating that digoxin may inhibit the uptake of thiamine in myocytes in beri beri heart disease.

Digoxin should not be used in constrictive pericarditis unless it is used to control the ventricular rate in atrial fibrillation or to improve systolic dysfunction.

Digoxin improves exercise tolerance in patients with impaired left ventricular systolic dysfunction and normal sinus rhythm. This may or may not be associated with an improved haemodynamic profile. However, the benefit of digoxin in patients with supraventricular arrythmias is most evident at rest, less evident with exercise.

In patients receiving diuretics and an ACE inhibitor, or diuretics alone, the withdrawal of digoxin has been shown to result in clinical deterioration.

The use of therapeutic doses of digoxin may cause prolongation of the PR interval and depression of the ST segment on the electrocardiogram.

Digoxin may produce false positive ST-T changes on the electrocardiogram during exercise testing. These electrophysiologic effects reflect an expected effect of the drug and are not indicative of toxicity.

Patients receiving digoxin should have their serum electrolytes and renal function (serum creatinine concentration) assessed periodically; the frequency of assessments will depend on the clinical setting.

Although many patients with chronic congestive cardiac failure benefit from acute administration of digoxin, there are some in whom it does not lead to constant, marked or lasting haemodynamic improvement. It is therefore important to evaluate the response of each patient individually when the Lanoxin is continued long-term.

Patients with severe respiratory diseases may have an increased myocardial sensitivity to digitalis glycosides.

Patients with rare hereditary problems of fructose intolerance, glucose-galactose malabsorption or sucrase-isomaltase insufficiency should not take this medicine.

4.5 Interaction with other medicinal products and other forms of interaction

Interactions may arise from effects on the renal excretion, tissue binding, plasma protein binding, distribution within the body, gut absorptive capacity and sensitivity to Lanoxin. Consideration of the possibility of an interaction whenever concomitant therapy is contemplated is the best precaution and a check on serum digoxin concentration is recommended when any doubt exists.

Digoxin, in association with beta-adrenoceptor blocking drugs, may increase atrio-ventricular conduction time.

Agents causing hypokalaemia or intracellular potassium deficiency may cause increased sensitivity to Digoxin; they include diuretics, lithium salts, corticosteroids and carbenoxolone.

Patients receiving Digoxin are more susceptible to the effects of suxamethonium-exacerbated hyperkalaemia.

Calcium, particularly if administered rapidly by the intravenous route, may produce serious arrhythmias in digitalized patients.

Serum levels of digoxin may be **increased** by concomitant administration of the following:

Alprazolam, amiodarone, flecainide, gentamicin, indometacin, itraconazole, prazosin, propafenone, quinidine, quinine, spironolactone, macrolide antibiotics (e.g. erythromycin and clarithromycin), tetracycline (and possibly other antibiotics), trimethoprim, propantheline, atorvastatin, ciclosporin, epoprostenol (transient) and carvedilol.

Serum levels of digoxin may be **reduced** by concomitant administration of the following:

Adrenaline (epinephrine), antacids, kaolin-pectin, some bulk laxatives, colestyramine, acarbose, salbutamol, sulfasalazine, neomycin, rifampicin, some cytostatics, phenytoin, metoclopramide, penicillamine and the herbal remedy St John's wort (*Hypericum perforatum*).

Calcium channel blocking agents may either increase or cause no change in serum digoxin levels. Verapamil, felodipine and tiapamil increase serum digoxin levels. Nifedipine and diltiazem may increase or have no effect on serum digoxin levels. Isradipine causes no change in serum digoxin levels. Angiotensin converting enzyme (ACE) inhibitors may also increase or cause no change in serum digoxin concentrations.

Milrinone does not alter steady-state serum digoxin levels.

Digoxin is a substrate of P-glycoprotein. Thus, inhibitors of P-glycoprotein may increase blood concentrations of digoxin by enhancing its absorption and/or by reducing its renal clearance (See *5.2 Pharmacokinetic Properties*).

4.6 Pregnancy and lactation

No data are available on whether or not digoxin has teratogenic effects.

There is no information available on the effect of digoxin on human fertility.

The use of digoxin in pregnancy is not contra-indicated, although the dosage may be less predictable in pregnant than in non-pregnant women with some requiring an increased dosage of digoxin during pregnancy. As with all drugs, use should be considered only when the expected clinical benefit of treatment to the mother outweighs any possible risk to the developing foetus.

Despite extensive antenatal exposure to digitalis preparations, no significant adverse effects have been observed in the foetus or neonate when maternal serum digoxin concentrations are maintained within the normal range. Although it has been speculated that a direct effect of digoxin n the myometrium may result in relative prematurity and low birthweight, a contributing role of the underlying cardiac disease cannot be excluded. Maternally administered digoxin has been successfully used to treat foetal tachycardia and congestive heart failure.

Adverse foetal effects have been reported in mothers with digitalis toxicity.

Although digoxin is excreted in breast milk, the quantities are minute and breast feeding is not contra-indicated.

4.7 Effects on ability to drive and use machines

Since central nervous system and visual disturbances have been reported in patients receiving Lanoxin, patients should exercise caution before driving, using machinery or participating in dangerous activities.

4.8 Undesirable effects

Adverse reactions are listed below by system organ class and frequency. Frequencies are defined as: very common (⩾ 1/10), common (⩾ 1/100 and < 1/10), uncommon (⩾ 1/1000 and < 1/100), rare (⩾ 1/10,000 and < 1/1000), very rare (< 1/10,000), including isolated reports. Very common, common and uncommon events were generally determined from clinical trial data. The incidence in placebo was taken into account. Adverse drug reactions identified through post-marketing surveillance were considered to be rare or very rare (including isolated reports).

Blood and lymphatic system disorders

Very rare:	Thrombocytopaenia

Metabolism and nutrition disorders

Very Rare:	Anorexia

Psychiatric disorders

Uncommon:	Depression
Very rare:	Psychosis, apathy, confusion

Nervous system disorders

Common:	CNS disturbances, dizziness
Very rare:	Headache

Eye disorders

Common:	Visual disturbances (blurred or yellow vision)

Cardiac disorders

Common:	Arrhythmia, conduction disturbances, bigeminy, trigeminy, PR prolongation, sinus bradycardia
Very rare:	Supraventricular tachyarrhythmia, atrial tachycardia (with or without block), junctional (nodal) tachycardia, ventricular arrhythmia, ventricular premature contraction, ST segment depression

Gastrointestinal disorders

Common:	Nausea, vomiting, diarrhoea
Very rare:	Intestinal ischaemia, intestinal necrosis

Skin disorders

Common:	Skin rashes of urticarial or scarlatiniform character may be accompanied by pronounced eosinophilia

Reproductive system and breast disorders

Very rare:	Gynaecomastia can occur with long term administration

General disorders and administration site conditions

Very rare:	Fatigue, malaise, weakness

4.9 Overdose

The symptoms and signs of toxicity are generally similar to those described in the Undesirable Effects section but may be more frequent and can be more severe.

Signs and symptoms of digoxin toxicity become more frequent with levels above 2.0 nanograms/mL (2.56 nanomol/L) although there is considerable interindividual variation. However, in deciding whether a patient's symtoms are due to digoxin, the clinical state, together with serum electrolyte levels and thyroid function are important factors (see *Dosage and Administration*).

Adults

In adults without heart disease, clinical observation suggests that an overdose of digoxin of 10 to 15 mg was the dose resulting in death of half of the patients.

Cardiac manifestations

Cardiac manifestations are the most frequent and serious sign of both acute and chronic toxicity. Peak cardiac effects generally occur 3 to 6 hours following overdosage and may persist for the ensuing 24 hours or longer. Digoxin toxicity may result in almost any type of arrhythmia. Multiple rhythm disturbances in the same patient are common. These include paroxysmal atrial tachycardia with variable atrioventricular (AV) block, accelerated junctional rhythm, slow atrial fibrillation (with very little variation in the ventricular rate) and bi directional ventricular tachycardia.

Premature ventricular contractions (PVCs) are often the earliest and most common arrhythmia. Bigeminy or trigeminy also occur frequently.

Sinus bradycardia and other bradyarrhythmias are very common.

First, second, third degree heart blocks and AV disocciation are also common.

Early toxicity may only be manifested by prolongation of the PR interval.

Ventricular tachycardia may also be a manifestation of toxicity.

Cardiac arrest from asystole or ventricular fibrillation due to digoxin toxicity is usually fatal.

Hypokalaemia may contribute to toxicity (see *Warnings and Precautions*).

Non-cardiac manifestations

Acute massive digoxin overdosage can result in mild to pronounced hyperkalaemia due to inhibition of the sodium-potassium (Na^+-K^+) pump.

Gastrointestinal symptoms are very common in both acute and chronic toxicity. The symptoms precede cardiac manifestations in approximately half of the patients in most literature reports. Anorexia, nausea and vomiting have been reported with an incidence up to 80%. These symptoms usually present early in the course of an overdose.

Neurologic and visual manifestations occur in both acute and chronic toxicity. Dizziness, various CNS disturbances, fatigue and malaise are very common. The most frequent visual disturbance is an aberration of colour vision (predominance of yellow green). These neurological and visual symptoms may persist even after other signs of toxicity have resolved.

In chronic toxicity, non-specific extracardiac symptoms, such as malaise and weakness, may predominate.

Children

In children aged 1 to 3 years without heart disease, clinical observation suggests that an overdose of digoxin of 6 to 10 mg was the dose resulting in death in half of the patients.

Most manifestations of toxicity in children occur during or shortly after the loading phase with digoxin.

Cardiac manifestations

The same arrhythmias or combination of arrhythmias that occur in adults can occur in children. Sinus tachycardia, supraventricular tachycardia, and rapid atrial fibrillation are seen less frequently in the paediatric population.

Paediatric patients are more likely to present with an AV conduction disturbance or a sinus bradycardia.

Ventricular ectopy is less common, however in massive overdose, ventricular ectopy, ventricular tachycardia and verntricular fibrillation have been reported.

Any arrhythmia or alteration in cardiac conduction that develops in a child taking digoxin should be assumed to be caused by digoxin, until further evaluation proves otherwise.

Extracardiac manifestations

The frequent extracardiac manifestations similar to those seen in adults are gastrointestinal, CNS and visual. However, nausea and vomiting are not frequent in infants and small children.

In addition to the undesirable effects seen with recommended doses, weight loss in older age groups and failure to thrive in infants, abdominal pain due to mesenteric artery ischaemia, drowsiness and behavioural disturbances including psychotic manifestations have been reported in overdose.

Treatment

After recent ingestion, such as accidental or deliberate self-poisoning, the load available for absorption may be reduced by gastric lavage.

Patients with massive digitalis ingestion should receive large doses of activated charcoal to prevent absorption and bind digoxin in the gut during enteroenteric recirculation.

If more than 25 mg of digoxin was ingested by an adult without hear disease, death or progressive toxicity responsive only to digoxin-binding Fab antibody fragments (Digibind®) resulted. If more than 10mg of digoxin was ingested by a child aged 1 to 3 years without heart disease, the outcome was uniformly fatal when Fab fragment treatment was not given.

Hypokalaemia should be corrected. In cases where a large amount of Lanoxin has been ingested hyperkalaemia may be present due to release of potassium from skeletal muscle. Before administering potassium in digoxin overdose the serum potassium level must be known.

Bradyarrhythmias may respond to atropine but temporary cardiac pacing may be required. Ventricular arrhythmias may respond to lignocaine or phenytoin.

Dialysis is not particularly effective in removing digoxin from the body in potentially life-threatening toxicity.

Rapid reversal of the complications that are associated with serious poisoning by digoxin, digitoxin and related glycosides has followed intravenous administration of digoxin-specific (ovine) antibody fragments (Fab) when other therapies have failed. Digibind is the only specific treatment for digoxin toxicity.

5. PHARMACOLOGICAL PROPERTIES

5.1 Pharmacodynamic properties

Mode of Action:-

Digoxin increases contractility of the myocardium by direct activity. This effect is proportional to dose in the lower range and some effect is achieved with quite low dosing; it occurs even in normal myocardium although it is then entirely without physiological benefit. The primary action of digoxin is specifically to inhibit adenosine triphosphatase, and thus sodium-potassium (Na^+-K^+) exchange activity, the altered ionic distribution across the membrane resulting in an augmented calcium ion influx and thus an increase in the availability of calcium at the time of excitation-contraction coupling. The potency of digoxin may therefore appear considerably enhanced when the extracellular potassium concentration is low, with hyperkalaemia having the opposite effect.

Digoxin exerts the same fundamental effect of inhibition of the Na^+-K^+ exchange mechanism on cells of the autonomic nervous system, stimulating them to exert indirect cardiac activity. Increases in efferent vagal impulses result in reduced sympathetic tone and diminished impulse conduction rate through the atria and atrioventricular node. Thus, the major beneficial effect of digoxin is reduction of ventricular rate.

Indirect cardiac contractility changes also result from changes in venous compliance brought about by the altered autonomic activity and by direct venous stimulation. The interplay between direct and indirect activity governs the total circulatory response, which is not identical for all subjects. In the presence of certain supraventricular arrhythmias, the neurogenically mediated slowing of AV conduction is paramount.

The degree of neurohormonal activation occurring in patients with heart failure is associated with clinical deterioration and an increased risk of death. Digoxin reduces activation of both the sympathetic nervous system and the (renin-angiotensin) system independently of its inotropic actions, and may thus favourably influence survival. Whether this is achieved via direct sympathoinhibitory effects or by re-sensitizing baroreflex mechanisms remains unclear.

5.2 Pharmacokinetic properties

Absorption

Intravenous administration of a loading dose produces an appreciable pharmacological effect within 5 to 30 minutes; this reaches a maximum in 1 to 5 hours. Upon oral administration, digoxin is absorbed from the stomach and upper part of the small intestine. When digoxin is taken after meals, the rate of absorption is slowed, but the total amount of digoxin absorbed is usually unchanged. When taken with meals high in fibre, however, the amount absorbed from an oral dose may be reduced.

Using the oral route the onset of effect occurs in 0.5 to 2 hours and reaches its maximum at 2 to 6 hours. The bioavailability of orally administered Lanoxin is approximately 63% in tablet form and 75% as paediatric elixir.

Distribution

The initial distribution of digoxin from the central to the peripheral compartment generally lasts from 6 to 8 hours. This is followed by a more gradual decline in serum digoxin concentration, which is dependent upon digoxin elimination from the body. The volume of distribution is large (Vd_{ss} = 510 litres in healthy volunteers), indicating digoxin to be extensively bound to body tissues. The highest digoxin concentrations are seen in the heart, liver and kidney, that in the heart averaging 30- fold that in the systemic circulation. Although the concentration in skeletal muscle is far lower, this store cannot be overlooked since skeletal muscle represents 40% of total body weight. Of the small proportion of digoxin circulating in plasma, approximately 25% is bound to protein.

Elimination

The major route of elimination is renal excretion of the unchanged drug.

Digoxin is a substrate for P-glycoprotein. As an efflux protein on the apical membrane of enterocytes, P-glycoprotein may limit the absorption of digoxin. P-glycoprotein in renal proximal tubules appears to be an important factor in the renal elimination of digoxin (See *4.5 Interaction with other medicinal products and other forms of interaction*).

Following intravenous administration to healthy volunteers, between 60 and 75% of a digoxin dose is recovered unchanged in the urine over a 6 day follow-up period. Total body clearance of digoxin has been shown to be directly related to renal function, and percent daily loss is thus a function of creatinine clearance, which in turn may be estimated from a stable serum creatinine. The total and renal clearances of digoxin have been found to be 193 ± 25 ml/min and 152 ± 24 mil/min in a healthy control population.

In a small percentage of individuals, orally administered digoxin is converted to cardioinactivate reduction products (digoxin reduction products or DRPs) by colonic bacteria in the gastrointestinal tract. In these subjects over 40% of the dose may be excreted as DRPs in the urine. Renal clearances of the two main metabolites, dihydrodigoxin and digoxygenin, have been found to be 79 ± 13 ml/min and 100 ± 26 ml/min respectively.

In the majority of cases however, the major route of digoxin elimination is renal excretion of the unchanged drug.

The terminal elimination half life of digoxin in patients with normal renal function is 30 to 40 hours. It is prolonged in patients with impaired renal function, and in anuric patients may be of the order of 100 hours.

In the newborn period, renal clearance of digoxin is diminished and suitable dosage adjustments must be observed. This is specially pronounced in the premature infant since renal clearance reflects maturation of renal function. Digoxin clearance has been found to be 65.6 ± 30 ml/min/1.73m² at 3 months, compared to only 32 ± 7 ml/min/1.73m² at 1 week. Beyond the immediate newborn period, children generally require proportionally larger doses than adults on the basis of body weight and body surface area.

Since most of the drug is bound to the tissues rather than circulating in the blood, digoxin is not effectively removed from the body during cardiopulmonary by-pass. Furthermore, only about 3% of a digoxin dose is removed from the body during five hours of haemodialysis.

5.3 Preclinical safety data
No data are available on whether or not digoxin has mutagenic or carcinogenic effects.

6. PHARMACEUTICAL PARTICULARS

6.1 List of excipients
Methyl Hydroxybenzoate Ph Eur
Sucrose Ph Eur*
Syrup BP*
Anhydrous Sodium Phosphate HSE
Citric Acid Monohydrate Ph Eur
Quinine Yellow HSE
Ethanol (96%) BP
Propylene Glycol Ph Eur
Lime Flavour No. 1 NA HSE
Purified Water Ph Eur
*These ingredients are alternatives.

6.2 Incompatibilities
None known.

6.3 Shelf life
36 months

6.4 Special precautions for storage
Store below 25°C.

6.5 Nature and contents of container
Amber glass bottle with a metal roll-on closure and a graduated polyethene dropper assembly plus cap.
Pack size: 60 ml

6.6 Special precautions for disposal and other handling
Do not dilute.

Administrative Data

7. MARKETING AUTHORISATION HOLDER
The Wellcome Foundation Limited
Greenford
Middlesex
UB6 0NN
Trading as:
GlaxoSmithKline UK
Stockley Park West
Uxbridge
Middlesex UB11 1BT

8. MARKETING AUTHORISATION NUMBER(S)
PL0003/5260R

9. DATE OF FIRST AUTHORISATION/RENEWAL OF THE AUTHORISATION
24 April 2003

10. DATE OF REVISION OF THE TEXT
14 May 2009

Lanoxin PG Tablets

(GlaxoSmithKline UK)

1. NAME OF THE MEDICINAL PRODUCT
Lanoxin PG Tablets

2. QUALITATIVE AND QUANTITATIVE COMPOSITION
Digoxin Ph Eur 0.0625 mg/tablet

3. PHARMACEUTICAL FORM
Tablet

4. CLINICAL PARTICULARS

4.1 Therapeutic indications
Lanoxin is indicated in the management of chronic cardiac failure where the dominant problem is systolic dysfunction Its therapeutic benefit is greatest in those patients with ventricular dilatation.

Lanoxin is specifically indicated where cardiac failure is accompanied by atrial fibrillation.

Lanoxin is indicated in the management of certain supraventricular arrhythmias, particularly chronic atrial flutter and fibrillation.

4.2 Posology and method of administration
The dose of Lanoxin for each patient has to be tailored individually according to age, lean body weight and renal function. Suggested doses are intended only as an initial guide.

The difference in bioavailability between injectable Lanoxin and oral formulations must be considered when changing from one dosage form to another. For example, if patients are switched from oral to the i.v. formulation the dosage should be reduced by approximately 33 %.

Adults with chronic cardiac failure in the absence of supraventricular arrhythmia:

No loading dose is required. The usual daily dose is 125 to 250 micrograms (0.125 to 0.25 mg) for patients with normal renal function. A lower dose of 62.5 micrograms (0.0625 mg) should be considered in the elderly.

For the management of atrial fibrillation or flutter in adults and children over 10 years:

Rapid Oral Loading:

If medically appropriate, rapid digitalisation may be achieved in a number of ways, such as the following:

750 to 1500 micrograms (0.75 to 1.5 mg) as a single dose.

Where there is less urgency, or greater risk of toxicity (e.g. in the elderly), the oral loading dose should be given in divided doses 6 hours apart, assessing clinical response before giving each additional dose (See *Special Warnings and Precautions for Use*).

Slow Oral Loading:

Digitalisation may be achieved more slowly with doses of 250 to 750 micrograms (0.25 to 0.75 mg) should be given daily for 1 week followed by an appropriate maintenance dose. A clinical response should be seen within one week.

NOTE: The choice between slow and rapid oral loading depends on the clinical state of the patient and the urgency of the condition.

Maintenance Dose:

The maintenance dosage should be based upon the percentage of the peak body stores lost each day through elimination. The following formula has had wide clinical use:

$$\text{Maintenance Dose} = \text{Peak body stores} \times \frac{\%\ \text{daily loss}}{100}$$

Where:

$$\text{Peak Body Stores} = \text{Loading Dose}$$
$$\%\ \text{Daily Loss} = 14 + \text{Creatinine Clearance } (C_{cr})/5.$$

C_{cr} is creatinine clearance corrected to 70 kg body weight or 1.73 m^2 body surface area. If only serum creatinine (S_{cr}) concentrations are available, a C_{cr} (corrected to 70 kg body weight) may be estimated in men as

$$C_{cr} = \frac{(140 - \text{age})}{S_{cr}\ (\text{in mg/100 ml})}$$

NOTE: Where serum creatinine values are obtained in micromol/L these may be converted to mg/100 ml (mg %) as follows:

$$S_{cr}\ (\text{mg/100 ml}) = \frac{S_{cr}\ (\text{micromol/L}) \times 113.12}{10{,}000} = \frac{S_{cr}\ (\text{micromol/L})}{88.4}$$

Where 113.12 is the molecular weight of creatinine.

For women, this result should be multiplied by 0.85.

NOTE: These formulae cannot be used for creatinine clearance in children.

In practice, this will mean that most patients will be maintained on 0.125 to 0. 25 mg digoxin daily; however in those who show increased sensitivity to the adverse effects of digoxin, a dosage of 62.5 microgram (0.0625 mg) daily or less may suffice. Conversely, some patients may require a higher dose.

Neonates, infants and children up to 10 years of age (if cardiac glycosides have not been given in the preceding two weeks):

In the newborn, particularly in the premature infant, renal clearance of digoxin is diminished and suitable dose reductions must be observed, over and above general dosage instructions.

Beyond the immediate newborn period, children generally require proportionally larger doses than adults on the basis of body weight or body surface area, as indicated in the schedule below. Children over 10 years of age require adult dosages in proportion to their body weight.

Oral loading dose:

This should be administered in accordance with the following schedule:

Preterm neonates < 1.5 kg	25 microgram/kg over 24 hours
Preterm neonates 1.5 kg to 2.5 kg	30 microgram/kg over 24 hours
Term neonates to 2 years	45 microgram/kg over 24 hours
2 to 5 years	35 microgram/kg over 24 hours
5 to 10 years	25 microgram/kg over 24 hours

The loading dose should be administered in divided doses with approximately half the total dose given as the first dose and further fractions of the total dose given at intervals of 4 to 8 hours, assessing clinical response before giving each additional dose.

Maintenance Dose:

The maintenance dose should be administered in accordance with the following schedule:

Preterm neonates:

daily dose = 20% of 24-hour loading dose (intravenous or oral)

Term neonates and children up to 10 years:

daily dose = 25% of 24-hour loading dose (intravenous or oral)

These dosage schedules are meant as guidelines and careful clinical observation and monitoring of serum digoxin levels (see *Monitoring*) should be used as a basis for adjustment of dosage in these paediatric patient groups.

If cardiac glycosides have been given in the two weeks preceding commencement of Lanoxin therapy, it should be anticipated that optimum loading doses of Lanoxin will be less than those recommended above.

Use in the elderly:

The tendency to impaired renal function and low lean body mass in the elderly influences the pharmacokinetics of Lanoxin such that high serum digoxin levels and associated toxicity can occur quite readily, unless doses of Lanoxin lower than those in non-elderly patients are used. Serum digoxin levels should be checked regularly and hypokalaemia avoided.

Dose recommendations in renal disorder or with diuretic therapy:

See *Special Warnings and Precautions for use.*

Monitoring:

Serum concentrations of digoxin may be expressed in conventional units of nanogram/ml (ng/ml) or SI units of nanomol//L (nmol/L). To convert ng/ml to nmol/L, multiply ng/ml by 1.28.

The serum concentration of digoxin can be determined by radioimmunoassay. Blood should be taken 6 hours or more after the last dose of Lanoxin. Several post hoc analyses of heart failure patients in the Digitalis Investigation Group trial suggest that the optimal trough digoxin serum level may be 0.5 ng/mL (0.64 nanomol/L) to 1.0 ng/mL (1.28 nanomol/L).

Digoxin toxicity is more commonly associated with serum digoxin concentration greater than 2 ng/mL. However, toxicity may occur with lower digoxin serum concentrations. In deciding whether a patient's symptoms are due to digoxin, the patient's clinical state together with the serum potassium level and thyroid function are important factors.

Other glycosides, including metabolites of digoxin, can interfere with the assays that are available and one should always be wary of values which do not seem commensurate with the clinical state of the patient.

4.3 Contraindications
Lanoxin is contra-indicated in intermittent complete heart block or second degree atrioventricular block, especially if there is a history of Stokes-Adams attacks.

Lanoxin is contra-indicated in arrhythmias caused by cardiac glycoside intoxication.

Lanoxin is contra-indicated in supraventricular arrhythmias associated with an accessory atrioventricular pathway, as in the Wolff-Parkinson-White Syndrome, unless the electrophysiological characteristics of the accessory pathway and any possible deleterious effect of digoxin on these characteristics has been evaluated. If an accessory pathway is known or suspected to be present and there is no history of previous supraventricular arrhythmias, Lanoxin is similarly contra-indicated.

Lanoxin is contra-indicated in ventricular tachycardia or ventricular fibrillation.

Lanoxin is contra-indicated in hypertrophic obstructive cardiomyopathy, unless there is concomitant atrial fibrillation and heart failure but even then caution should be exercised if Lanoxin is to be used.

Lanoxin is contra-indicated in patients known to be hypersensitive to digoxin, other digitalis glycosides, or to any component of the preparation.

4.4 Special warnings and precautions for use
Arrhythmias may be precipitated by digoxin toxicity, some of which can resemble arrhythmias for which the drug could be advised. For example, atrial tachycardia with varying atrioventricular block requires care, as clinically the rhythm resembles atrial fibrillation.

In some cases of sinoatrial disorder (i.e. Sick Sinus Syndrome) digoxin may cause or exacerbate sinus bradycardia or cause sinoatrial block.

Determination of the serum digoxin concentration may be very helpful in making a decision to treat with further digoxin, but toxic doses of other glycosides may cross-react in the assay and wrongly suggest apparently satisfactory measurements. Observations during the temporary withholding of digoxin might be more appropriate.

In cases where cardiac glycosides have been taken in the preceding two weeks, the recommendations for initial dosing of a patient should be reconsidered and a reduced dose is advised.

The dosing recommendations should be reconsidered if patients are elderly or there are other reasons for the renal clearance of digoxin being reduced. A reduction in both initial and maintenance doses should be considered.

Hypokalaemia sensitises the myocardium to the actions of cardiac glycosides.

Hypoxia, hypomagnesaemia and marked hypercalcaemia increase myocardial sensitivity to cardiac glycosides.

Administering Lanoxin to a patient with thyroid disease requires care. Initial and maintenance doses of Lanoxin should be reduced when thyroid function is subnormal. In hyperthyroidism there is relative digoxin resistance and the dose may have to be increased. During the course of treatment of thyrotoxicosis, dosage should be reduced as the thyrotoxicosis comes under control.

Patients with malabsorption syndrome or gastro-intestinal reconstructions may require larger doses of digoxin.

The risk of provoking dangerous arrhythmias with direct current cardioversion is greatly increased in the presence of digitalis toxicity and is in proportion to the cardioversion energy used.

For elective direct current cardioversion of a patient who is taking digoxin, the drug should be withheld for 24 hours before cardioversion is performed. In emergencies, such as cardiac arrest, when attempting cardioversion the lowest effective energy should be applied. Direct current cardioversion is inappropriate in the treatment of arrhythmias thought to be caused by cardiac glycosides.

Many beneficial effects of digoxin on arrhythmias result from a degree of atrioventricular conduction blockade. However, when incomplete atrioventricular block already exists the effects of a rapid progression in the block should be anticipated. In complete heart block the idioventricular escape rhythm may be suppressed.

The administration of digoxin in the period immediately following myocardial infarction is not contra-indicated. However, the use of inotropic drugs in some patients in this setting may result in undesirable increases in myocardial oxygen demand and ischaemia, and some retrospective follow-up studies have suggested digoxin to be associated with an increased risk of death. However, the possibility of arrhythmias arising in patients who may be hypokalaemic after myocardial infarction and are likely to be cardiologically unstable must be borne in mind. The limitations imposed thereafter on direct current cardioversion must also be remembered.

Treatment with digoxin should generally be avoided in patients with heart failure associated with cardiac amyloidosis. However, if alternative treatments are not appropriate, digoxin can be used with caution to control the ventricular rate in patients with cardiac amyloidosis and atrial fibrillation.

Digoxin can rarely precipitate vasoconstriction and therefore should be avoided in patients with myocarditis.

Patients with beri beri heart disease may fail to respond adequately to digoxin if the underlying thiamine deficiency is not treated concomitantly. There is also some published information indicating that digoxin may inhibit the uptake of thiamine in myocytes in beri beri heart disease.

Digoxin should not be used in constrictive pericarditis unless it is used to control the ventricular rate in atrial fibrillation or to improve systolic dysfunction.

Digoxin improves exercise tolerance in patients with impaired left ventricular systolic dysfunction and normal sinus rhythm. This may or may not be associated with an improved haemodynamic profile. However, the benefit of digoxin in patients with supraventricular arrythmias is most evident at rest, less evident with exercise.

In patients receiving diuretics and an ACE inhibitor, or diuretics alone, the withdrawal of digoxin has been shown to result in clinical deterioration.

The use of therapeutic doses of digoxin may cause prolongation of the PR interval and depression of the ST segment on the electrocardiogram.

Digoxin may produce false positive ST-T changes on the electrocardiogram during exercise testing. These electrophysiologic effects reflect an expected effect of the drug and are not indicative of toxicity.

Patients receiving digoxin should have their serum electrolytes and renal function (serum creatinine concentration) assessed periodically; the frequency of assessments will depend on the clinical setting.

Although many patients with chronic congestive cardiac failure benefit from acute administration of digoxin, there are some in whom it does not lead to constant, marked or lasting haemodynamic improvement. It is therefore important to evaluate the response of each patient individually when Lanoxin is continued long-term.

Patients with severe respiratory disease may have an increased myocardial sensitivity to digitalis glycosides.

Patients with rare hereditary problems of galactose intolerance, the Lapp lactose deficiency or glucose galactose malabsorption should not take this medicine.

4.5 Interaction with other medicinal products and other forms of interaction

Interactions may arise from effects on the renal excretion, tissue binding, plasma protein binding, distribution within the body, gut absorptive capacity and sensitivity to Lanoxin. Consideration of the possibility of an interaction whenever concomitant therapy is contemplated is the best precaution and a check on serum digoxin concentration is recommended when any doubt exists.

Digoxin, in association with beta-adrenoceptor blocking drugs, may increase atrio-ventricular conduction time.

Agents causing hypokalaemia or intracellular potassium deficiency may cause increased sensitivity to Digoxin; they include diuretics, lithium salts, corticosteroids and carbenoxolone.

Patients receiving Digoxin are more susceptible to the effects of suxamethonium-exacerbated hyperkalaemia.

Calcium, particularly if administered rapidly by the intravenous route, may produce serious arrhythmias in digitalized patients.

Serum levels of digoxin may be **increased** by concomitant administration of the following:

Alprazolam, amiodarone, flecainide, gentamicin, indometacin, itraconazole, prazosin, propafenone, quinidine, quinine, spironolactone, macrolide antibiotics (e.g. erythromycin and clarithromycin), tetracycline (and possibly other antibiotics), trimethoprim, propantheline, atorvastatin, ciclosporin, epoprostenol (transient) and carvedilol.

Serum levels of digoxin may be **reduced** by concomitant administration of the following:

Adrenaline (epinephrine), antacids, kaolin-pectin, some bulk laxatives, colestyramine, acarbose, salbutamol, sulfasalazine, neomycin, rifampicin, some cytostatics, phenytoin, metoclopramide, penicillamine and the herbal remedy St John's wort (*Hypericum perforatum*).

Calcium channel blocking agents may either increase or cause no change in serum digoxin levels. Verapamil, felodipine and tiapamil increase serum digoxin levels. Nifedipine and diltiazem may increase or have no effect on serum digoxin levels. Isradipine causes no change in serum digoxin levels. Angiotensin converting enzyme (ACE) inhibitors may also increase or cause no change in serum digoxin concentrations.

Milrinone does not alter steady-state serum digoxin levels.

Digoxin is a substrate of P-glycoprotein. Thus, inhibitors of P-glycoprotein may increase blood concentrations of digoxin by enhancing its absorption and/or by reducing its renal clearance (See *5.2 Pharmacokinetic Properties*).

4.6 Pregnancy and lactation

No data are available on whether or not digoxin has teratogenic effects.

There is no information available on the effect of digoxin on human fertility.

The use of digoxin in pregnancy is not contra-indicated, although the dosage and control may be less predictable in pregnant than in non-pregnant women with some requiring an increased dosage of digoxin during pregnancy. As with all drugs, use should be considered only when the expected clinical benefit of treatment to the mother outweighs any possible risk to the developing foetus.

Despite extensive antenatal exposure to digitalis preparations, no significant adverse effects have been observed in the foetus or neonate when maternal serum digoxin concentrations are maintained within the normal range. Although it has been speculated that a direct effect of digoxin on the myometrium may result in relative prematurity and low birthweight, a contributing role of the underlying cardiac disease cannot be excluded. Maternally administered digoxin has been successfully used to treat foetal tachycardia and congestive heart failure.

Adverse foetal effects have been reported in mothers with digitalis toxicity.

Although digoxin is excreted in breast milk, the quantities are minute and breast feeding is not contra-indicated.

4.7 Effects on ability to drive and use machines

Since central nervous system and visual disturbances have been reported in patients receiving Lanoxin, patients should exercise caution before driving, using machinery or participating in dangerous activities.

4.8 Undesirable effects

Adverse reactions are listed below by system organ class and frequency. Frequencies are defined as: very common ($\geqslant$ 1/10), common ($\geqslant$ 1/100 and < 1/10), uncommon ($\geqslant$ 1/1000 and < 1/100), rare ($\geqslant$ 1/10,000 and < 1/1000), very rare (< 1/10,000), including isolated reports. Very common, common and uncommon events were generally determined from clinical trial data. The incidence in placebo was taken into account. Adverse drug reactions identified through post-marketing surveillance were considered to be rare or very rare (including isolated reports).

Blood and lymphatic system disorders

Very rare: Thrombocytopenia

Metabolism and nutrition disorders

Very Rare: Anorexia

Psychiatric disorders

Uncommon: Depression

Very rare: Psychosis, apathy, confusion

Nervous system disorders

Common: CNS disturbances, dizziness

Very rare: Headache

Eye disorders

Common: Visual disturbances (blurred or yellow vision)

Cardiac disorders

Common: Arrhythmia, conduction disturbances, bigeminy, trigeminy, PR prolongation, sinus bradycardia

Very rare: Supraventricular tachyarrhythmia, atrial tachycardia (with or without block), junctional (nodal) tachycardia, ventricular arrhythmia, ventricular premature contraction, ST segment depression

Gastrointestinal disorders

Common: Nausea, vomiting, diarrhoea

Very rare: Intestinal ischaemia, intestinal necrosis

Skin disorders

Common: Skin rashes of urticarial or scarlatiniform character may be accompanied by pronounced eosinophilia

Reproductive system and breast disorders

Very rare: Gynaecomastia can occur with long term administration

General disorders and administration site conditions

Very rare: Fatigue, malaise, weakness

4.9 Overdose

The symptoms and signs of toxicity are generally similar to those described in the Undesirable Effects section but may be more frequent and can be more severe.

Signs and symptoms of digoxin toxicity become more frequent with levels above 2.0 nanograms/mL (2.56 nanomol/L) although there is considerable interindividual variation. However, in deciding whether a patient's symtoms are due to digoxin, the clinical state, together with serum electrolyte levels and thyroid function are important factors (see *Dosage and Administration*).

Adults

In adults without heart disease, clinical observation suggests that an overdose of digoxin of 10 to 15 mg was the dose resulting in death of half of the patients.

Cardiac manifestations

Cardiac manifestations are the most frequent and serious sign of both acute and chronic toxicity. Peak cardiac effects generally occur 3 to 6 hours following overdosage and may persist for the ensuing 24 hours or longer. Digoxin toxicity may result in almost any type of arrhythmia. Multiple rhythm disturbances in the same patient are common. These include paroxysmal atrial tachycardia with variable atrioventricular (AV) block, accelerated junctional rhythm, slow atrial fibrillation (with very little variation in the ventricular rate) and bi directional ventricular tachycardia.

Premature ventricular contractions (PVCs) are often the earliest and most common arrhythmia. Bigeminy or trigeminy also occur frequently.

Sinus bradycardia and other bradyarrhythmias are very common.

First, second, third degree heart blocks and AV dissociation are also common.

Early toxicity may only be manifested by prolongation of the PR interval.

Ventricular tachycardia may also be a manifestation of toxicity.

Cardiac arrest from asystole or ventricular fibrillation due to digoxin toxicity is usually fatal.

Hypokalaemia may contribute to toxicity (see *Warnings and Precautions*).

Non-cardiac manifestations

Acute massive digoxin overdosage can result in mild to pronounced hyperkalaemia due to inhibition of the sodium-potassium (Na+-K+) pump.

Gastrointestinal symptoms are very common in both acute and chronic toxicity. The symptoms precede cardiac manifestations in approximately half of the patients in most literature reports. Anorexia, nausea and vomiting have been reported with an incidence up to 80%. These symptoms usually present early in the course of an overdose.

Neurologic and visual manifestations occur in both acute and chronic toxicity. Dizziness, various CNS disturbances, fatigue and malaise are very common. The most frequent visual disturbance is an aberration of colour vision (predominance of yellow green). These neurological and visual symptoms may persist even after other signs of toxicity have resolved.

In chronic toxicity, non-specific extracardiac symptoms, such as malaise and weakness, may predominate.

Children

In children aged 1 to 3 years without heart disease, clinical observation suggests that an overdose of digoxin of 6 to 10 mg was the dose resulting in death in half of the patients.

Most manifestations of toxicity in children occur during or shortly after the loading phase with digoxin.

Cardiac manifestations

The same arrhythmias or combination of arrhythmias that occur in adults can occur in children. Sinus tachycardia, supraventricular tachycardia, and rapid atrial fibrillation are seen less frequently in the paediatric population.

Paediatric patients are more likely to present with an AV conduction disturbance or a sinus bradycardia.

Ventricular ectopy is less common, however in massive overdose, ventricular ectopy, ventricular tachycardia and verntricular fibrillation have been reported.

Any arrhythmia or alteration in cardiac conduction that develops in a child taking digoxin should be assumed to be caused by digoxin, until further evaluation proves otherwise.

Extracardiac manifestations

The frequent extracardiac manifestations similar to those seen in adults are gastrointestinal, CNS and visual. However, nausea and vomiting are not frequent in infants and small children.

In addition to the undesirable effects seen with recommended doses, weight loss in older age groups and failure to thrive in infants, abdominal pain due to mesenteric artery ischaemia, drowsiness and behavioural disturbances including psychotic manifestations have been reported in overdose.

Treatment

After recent ingestion, such as accidental or deliberate self-poisoning, the load available for absorption may be reduced by gastric lavage.

Patients with massive digitalis ingestion should receive large doses of activated charcoal to prevent absorption and bind digoxin in the gut during enteroenteric recirculation.

If more than 25 mg of digoxin was ingested by an adult without heart disease, death or progressive toxicity responsive only to digoxin-binding Fab antibody fragments (Digibind®) resulted. If more than 10 mg of digoxin was ingested by a child aged 1 to 3 years without heart disease, the outcome was uniformly fatal when Fab fragment treatment was not given.

Hypokalaemia should be corrected. In cases where a large amount of Lanoxin has been ingested, hyperkalaemia may be present due to release of potassium from skeletal muscle. Before administering potassium in digoxin overdose the serum potassium level must be known.

Bradyarrhythmias may respond to atropine but temporary cardiac pacing may be required. Ventricular arrhythmias may respond to lignocaine or phenytoin.

Dialysis is not particularly effective in removing digoxin from the body in potentially life-threatening toxicity.

Rapid reversal of the complications that are associated with serious poisoning by digoxin, digitoxin and related glycosides has followed intravenous administration of digoxin-specific (ovine) antibody fragments (Fab) when other therapies have failed. Digibind® is the only specific treatment for digoxin toxicity.

5. PHARMACOLOGICAL PROPERTIES

5.1 Pharmacodynamic properties

Mode of Action:-

Digoxin increases contractility of the myocardium by direct activity. This effect is proportional to dose in the lower range and some effect is achieved with quite low dosing; it occurs even in normal myocardium although it is then entirely without physiological benefit. The primary action of digoxin is specifically to inhibit adenosine triphosphatase, and thus sodium-potassium (Na^+-K^+) exchange activity, the altered ionic distribution across the membrane resulting in an augmented calcium ion influx and thus an increase in the availability of calcium at the time of excitation-contraction coupling. The potency of digoxin may therefore appear considerably enhanced when the extracellular potassium concentration is low, with hyperkalaemia having the opposite effect.

Digoxin exerts the same fundamental effect of inhibition of the Na^+-K^+ exchange mechanism on cells of the autonomic nervous system, stimulating them to exert indirect cardiac activity. Increases in efferent vagal impulses result in reduced sympathetic tone and diminished impulse conduction rate through the atria and atrioventricular node. Thus, the major beneficial effect of digoxin is reduction of ventricular rate.

Indirect cardiac contractility changes also result from changes in venous compliance brought about by the altered autonomic activity and by direct venous stimulation. The interplay between direct and indirect activity governs the total circulatory response, which is not identical for all subjects. In the presence of certain supraventricular arrhythmias, the neurogenically mediated slowing of AV conduction is paramount.

The degree of neurohormonal activation occurring in patients with heart failure is associated with clinical deterioration and an increased risk of death. Digoxin reduces activation of both the sympathetic nervous system and the (renin-angiotensin) system independently of its inotropic actions, and may thus favourably influence survival. Whether this is achieved via direct sympathoinhibitory effects or by re-sensitising baroreflex mechanisms remains unclear.

5.2 Pharmacokinetic properties

Absorption

Intravenous administration of a loading dose produces an appreciable pharmacological effect within 5 to 30 minutes; this reaches a maximum in 1 to 5 hours. Upon oral administration, digoxin is absorbed from the stomach and upper part of the small intestine. When digoxin is taken after meals, the rate of absorption is slowed, but the total amount of digoxin absorbed is usually unchanged. When taken with meals high in fibre, however, the amount absorbed from an oral dose may be reduced.

Using the oral route the onset of effect occurs in 0.5 to 2 hours and reaches its maximum at 2 to 6 hours. The bioavailability of orally administered Lanoxin is approximately 63% in tablet form and 75% as paediatric elixir.

Distribution

The initial distribution of digoxin from the central to the peripheral compartment generally lasts from 6 to 8 hours. This is followed by a more gradual decline in serum digoxin concentration, which is dependent upon digoxin elimination from the body. The volume of distribution is large (Vd_{ss} = 510 litres in healthy volunteers), indicating digoxin to be extensively bound to body tissues. The highest digoxin concentrations are seen in the heart, liver and kidney, that in the heart averaging 30- fold that in the systemic circulation. Although the concentration in skeletal muscle is far lower, this store cannot be overlooked since skeletal muscle represents 40% of total body weight. Of the small proportion of digoxin circulating in plasma, approximately 25% is bound to protein.

Elimination

The major route of elimination is renal excretion of the unchanged drug.

Digoxin is a substrate for P-glycoprotein. As an efflux protein on the apical membrane of enterocytes, P-glycoprotein may limit the absorption of digoxin. P-glycoprotein in renal proximal tubules appears to be an important factor in the renal elimination of digoxin (See *4.5 Interaction with other medicinal products and other forms of interaction*).

Following intravenous administration to healthy volunteers, between 60 and 75% of a digoxin dose is recovered unchanged in the urine over a 6 day follow-up period. Total body clearance of digoxin has been shown to be directly related to renal function, and percent daily loss is thus a function of creatinine clearance, which in turn may be estimated from a stable serum creatinine. The total and renal clearances of digoxin have been found to be 193 ± 25 ml/min and 152 ± 24 ml/min in a healthy control population.

In a small percentage of individuals, orally administered digoxin is converted to cardioinactivate reduction products (digoxin reduction products or DRPs) by colonic bacteria in the gastrointestinal tract. In these subjects over 40% of the dose may be excreted as DRPs in the urine. Renal clearances of the two main metabolites, dihydrodigoxin and digoxygenin, have been found to be 79 ± 13 ml/min and 100 ± 26 ml/min respectively.

In the majority of cases however, the major route of digoxin elimination is renal excretion of the unchanged drug.

The terminal elimination half life of digoxin in patients with normal renal function is 30 to 40 hours. It is prolonged in patients with impaired renal function, and in anuric patients may be of the order of 100 hours.

In the newborn period, renal clearance of digoxin is diminished and suitable dosage adjustments must be observed. This is specially pronounced in the premature infant since renal clearance reflects maturation of renal function. Digoxin clearance has been found to be 65.6 ± 30 ml/min/1.73m^2 at 3 months, compared to only 32 ± 7 ml/min/1.73m^2 at 1 week. Beyond the immediate newborn period, children generally require proportionally larger doses than adults on the basis of body weight and body surface area.

Since most of the drug is bound to the tissues rather than circulating in the blood, digoxin is not effectively removed from the body during cardiopulmonary by-pass. Furthermore, only about 3% of a digoxin dose is removed from the body during five hours of haemodialysis.

5.3 Preclinical safety data

No data are available on whether or not digoxin has mutagenic or carcinogenic effects.

6. PHARMACEUTICAL PARTICULARS

6.1 List of excipients

Lactose Ph Eur

Starches Ph Eur

Indigo Carmine HSE

Hydrolysed Starch HSE

Povidone BP

Magnesium Stearate Ph Eur

6.2 Incompatibilities

None known

6.3 Shelf life

60 months

6.4 Special precautions for storage

Store below 25°C

6.5 Nature and contents of container

Amber glass bottle with polyethylene snap fit closure

Pack sizes: 28, 50, 100, 500 tablets

15 ml amber glass bottle with a clic-loc child resistant closure

Pack size: 56 tablets

6.6 Special precautions for disposal and other handling

Not applicable

Administrative Data

7. MARKETING AUTHORISATION HOLDER

The Wellcome Foundation Limited

Greenford

Middlesex

UB6 0NN

Trading as:

GlaxoSmithKline UK

Stockley Park West

Uxbridge

Middlesex UB11 1BT

8. MARKETING AUTHORISATION NUMBER(S)

PL0003/0091R

9. DATE OF FIRST AUTHORISATION/RENEWAL OF THE AUTHORISATION

24 April 2003

10. DATE OF REVISION OF THE TEXT

14 May 2009

Lanoxin Tablets 0.25mg

(GlaxoSmithKline UK)

1. NAME OF THE MEDICINAL PRODUCT

Lanoxin Tablets 0.25 mg

2. QUALITATIVE AND QUANTITATIVE COMPOSITION

Digoxin Ph Eur 0.25 mg/tablet

3. PHARMACEUTICAL FORM

Tablet

4. CLINICAL PARTICULARS

4.1 Therapeutic indications

Lanoxin is indicated in the management of chronic cardiac failure where the dominant problem is systolic dysfunction. Its therapeutic benefit is greatest in those patients with ventricular dilatation.

Lanoxin is specifically indicated where cardiac failure is accompanied by atrial fibrillation.

Lanoxin is indicated in the management of certain supraventricular arrhythmias, particularly chronic atrial flutter and fibrillation.

4.2 Posology and method of administration

The dose of Lanoxin for each patient has to be tailored individually according to age, lean body weight and renal function. Suggested doses are intended only as an initial guide.

The difference in bioavailability between injectable Lanoxin and oral formulations must be considered when changing from one dosage form to another. For example, if patients are switched from oral to the i.v. formulation the dosage should be reduced by approximately 33 %.

Adults with chronic cardiac failure in the absence of supraventricular arrhythmia:

No loading dose is required. The usual daily dose is 125 to 250 micrograms (0.125 to 0.25 mg) for patients with normal renal function. A lower dose of 62.5 micrograms (0.0625 mg) should be considered in the elderly.

For the management of atrial fibrillation or flutter in adults and children over 10 years:

Rapid Oral Loading:

If medically appropriate, rapid digitalisation may be achieved in a number of ways, such as the following:

750 to 1500 micrograms (0.75 to 1.5 mg) as a single dose.

Where there is less urgency, or greater risk of toxicity e.g. in the elderly, the oral loading dose should be given in divided doses 6 hours apart, assessing clinical response before giving each additional dose (*See Special Warnings and Precautions for Use*).

Slow Oral Loading:

Digitalisation may be achieved more slowly with doses of 250 to 750 micrograms (0.25 to 0.75 mg) given daily for 1 week followed by an appropriate maintenance dose. A clinical response should be seen within one week.

NOTE: The choice between slow and rapid oral loading depends on the clinical state of the patient and the urgency of the condition.

Maintenance Dose:

The maintenance dosage should be based upon the percentage of the peak body stores lost each day through elimination. The following formula has had wide clinical use:

$$\text{Maintenance Dose} = \text{Peak body stores} \times \frac{\%\ \text{daily loss}}{100}$$

Where:

Peak Body Stores = Loading Dose

% Daily Loss = 14 + Creatinine Clearance (C_{cr})/5.

C_{cr} is creatinine clearance corrected to 70 kg body weight or 1.73 m^2 body surface area. If only serum creatinine (S_{cr}) concentrations are available, a C_{cr} (corrected to 70 kg body weight) may be estimated in men as

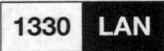

$$C_{cr} = \frac{(140 - age)}{S_{cr}\ (in\ mg/100\ ml)}$$

NOTE: Where serum creatinine values are obtained in micromol/L these may be converted to mg/100 ml (mg %) as follows:

$$S_{cr}\ (mg/100\ ml) = \frac{S_{cr}\ (micromol/L) \times 113.12}{10{,}000} = \frac{S_{cr}\ (micromol/L)}{88.4}$$

Where 113.12 is the molecular weight of creatinine.

For *women*, this result should be multiplied by 0.85.

NOTE: These formulae cannot be used for creatinine clearance in children.

In practice, this will mean that most patients will be maintained on 0.125 to 0. 25 mg digoxin daily; however in those who show increased sensitivity to the adverse effects of digoxin, a dosage of 62.5 microgram (0.0625 mg) daily or less may suffice. Conversely, some patients may require a higher dose.

Neonates, infants and children up to 10 years of age (if cardiac glycosides have not been given in the preceding two weeks):

In the newborn, particularly in the premature infant, renal clearance of digoxin is diminished and suitable dose reductions must be observed, over and above general dosage instructions.

Beyond the immediate newborn period, children generally require proportionally larger doses than adults on the basis of body weight or body surface area, as indicated in the schedule below. Children over 10 years of age require adult dosages in proportion to their body weight.

Oral loading dose:

This should be administered in accordance with the following schedule:

Preterm neonates < 1.5 kg	25 microgram/kg over 24 hours
Preterm neonates 1.5 kg to 2.5 kg	30 microgram/kg over 24 hours
Term neonates to 2 years	45 microgram/kg over 24 hours
2 to 5 years	35 microgram/kg over 24 hours
5 to 10 years	25 microgram/kg over 24 hours

The loading dose should be administered in divided doses with approximately half the total dose given as the first dose and further fractions of the total dose given at intervals of 4 to 8 hours, assessing clinical response before giving each additional dose.

Maintenance Dose:

The maintenance dose should be administered in accordance with the following schedule:

Preterm neonates:

daily dose = 20% of 24-hour loading dose (intravenous or oral)

Term neonates and children up to 10 years:

daily dose = 25% of 24-hour loading dose (intravenous or oral)

These dosage schedules are meant as guidelines and careful clinical observation and monitoring of serum digoxin levels (see *Monitoring*) should be used as a basis for adjustment of dosage in these paediatric patient groups.

If cardiac glycosides have been given in the two weeks preceding commencement of Lanoxin therapy, it should be anticipated that optimum loading doses of Lanoxin will be less than those recommended above.

Use in the elderly:

The tendency to impaired renal function and low lean body mass in the elderly influences the pharmacokinetics of Lanoxin such that high serum digoxin levels and associated toxicity can occur quite readily, unless doses of Lanoxin lower than those in non-elderly patients are used. Serum digoxin levels should be checked regularly and hypokalaemia avoided.

Dose recommendations in renal disorder or with diuretic therapy:

See *Special Warnings and Precautions for Use*.

Monitoring:

Serum concentrations of digoxin may be expressed in conventional units of nanogram/ml (ng/ml) or SI Units of nanomol/L (nmol/L). To convert ng/ml to nmol/L, multiply ng/ml by 1.28.

The serum concentration of digoxin can be determined by radioimmunoassay. Blood should be taken 6 hours or more after the last dose of Lanoxin. Several post hoc analyses of heart failure patients in the Digitalis Investigation Group trial suggest that the optimal trough digoxin serum level may be 0.5 ng/mL (0.64 nanomol/L) to 1.0 ng/mL (1.28 nanomol/L).

Digoxin toxicity is more commonly associated with serum digoxin concentration greater than 2 ng/mL. However, toxicity may occur with lower digoxin serum concentrations. In deciding whether a patient's symptoms are due to digoxin, the patient's clinical state together with the serum potassium level and thyroid function are important factors.

Other glycosides, including metabolites of digoxin, can interfere with the assays that are available and one should always be wary of values which do not seem commensurate with the clinical state of the patient.

4.3 Contraindications

Lanoxin is contra-indicated in intermittent complete heart block or second degree atrioventricular block, especially if there is a history of Stokes-Adams attacks.

Lanoxin is contra-indicated in arrhythmias caused by cardiac glycoside intoxication.

Lanoxin is contra-indicated in supraventricular arrhythmias associated with an accessory atrioventricular pathway, as in the Wolff-Parkinson-White Syndrome, unless the electrophysiological characteristics of the accessory pathway and any possible deleterious effect of digoxin on these characteristics have been evaluated. If an accessory pathway is known or suspected to be present and there is no history of previous supraventricular arrhythmias, Lanoxin is similarly contra-indicated.

Lanoxin is contra-indicated in ventricular tachycardia or ventricular fibrillation.

Lanoxin is contra-indicated in hypertrophic obstructive cardiomyopathy, unless there is concomitant atrial fibrillation and heart failure but even then caution should be exercised if Lanoxin is to be used.

Lanoxin is contra-indicated in patients known to be hypersensitive to digoxin, other digitalis glycosides, or to any component of the preparation.

4.4 Special warnings and precautions for use

Arrhythmias may be precipitated by digoxin toxicity, some of which can resemble arrhythmias for which the drug could be advised. For example, atrial tachycardia with varying atrioventricular block requires particular care as clinically the rhythm resembles atrial fibrillation.

In some cases of sinoatrial disorder (i.e. Sick Sinus Syndrome) digoxin may cause or exacerbate sinus bradycardia or cause sinoatrial block.

Determination of the serum digoxin concentration may be very helpful in making a decision to treat with further digoxin, but toxic doses of other glycosides may cross-react in the assay and wrongly suggest apparently satisfactory measurements. Observations during the temporary withholding of digoxin might be more appropriate.

In cases where cardiac glycosides have been taken in the preceding two weeks, the recommendations for initial dosing of a patient should be reconsidered and a reduced dose is advised.

The dosing recommendations should be reconsidered if patients are elderly or there are other reasons for the renal clearance of digoxin being reduced. A reduction in both initial and maintenance doses should be considered.

Hypokalaemia sensitises the myocardium to the actions of cardiac glycosides.

Hypoxia, hypomagnesaemia and marked hypercalcaemia increase myocardial sensitivity to cardiac glycosides.

Administering Lanoxin to a patient with thyroid disease requires care. Initial and maintenance doses of Lanoxin should be reduced when thyroid function is subnormal. In hyperthyroidism there is relative digoxin resistance and the dose may have to be increased. During the course of treatment of thyrotoxicosis, dosage should be reduced as the thyrotoxicosis comes under control.

Patients with malabsorption syndrome or gastro-intestinal reconstructions may require larger doses of digoxin.

The risk of provoking dangerous arrhythmias with direct current cardioversion is greatly increased in the presence of digitalis toxicity and is in proportion to the cardioversion energy used.

For elective direct current cardioversion of a patient who is taking digoxin, the drug should be withheld for 24 hours before cardioversion is performed. In emergencies, such as cardiac arrest, when attempting cardioversion the lowest effective energy should be applied. Direct current cardioversion is inappropriate in the treatment of arrhythmia thought to be caused by cardiac glycosides.

Many beneficial effects of digoxin on arrhythmias result from a degree of atrioventricular conduction blockade. However, when incomplete atrioventricular block already exists the effects of a rapid progression in the block should be anticipated. In complete heart block the idioventricular escape rhythm may be suppressed.

The administration of digoxin in the period immediately following myocardial infarction is not contra-indicated. However, the use of inotropic drugs in some patients in this setting may result in undesirable increases in myocardial oxygen demand and ischaemia, and some retrospective follow-up studies have suggested digoxin to be associated with an increased risk of death. However, the possibility of arrhythmias arising in patients who may be hypokalaemic after myocardial infarction and are likely to be cardiologically unstable must be borne in mind. The limitations imposed thereafter on direct current cardioversion must also be remembered.

Treatment with digoxin should generally be avoided in patients with heart failure associated with cardiac amyloidosis. However, if alternative treatments are not appropriate, digoxin can be used with caution to control the ventricular rate in patients with cardiac amyloidosis and atrial fibrillation.

Digoxin can rarely precipitate vasoconstriction and therefore should be avoided in patients with myocarditis.

Patients with beri beri heart disease may fail to respond adequately to digoxin if the underlying thiamine deficiency is not treated concomitantly. There is also some published information indicating that digoxin may inhibit the uptake of thiamine in myocytes in beri beri heart disease.

Digoxin should not be used in constrictive pericarditis unless it is used to control the ventricular rate in atrial fibrillation or to improve systolic dysfunction.

Digoxin improves exercise tolerance in patients with impaired left ventricular systolic dysfunction and normal sinus rhythm. This may or may not be associated with an improved haemodynamic profile. However, the benefit of patients with supraventricular arrhythmias is most evident at rest, less evident with exercise.

In patients receiving diuretics and an ACE inhibitor, or diuretics alone, the withdrawal of digoxin has been shown to result in clinical deterioration.

The use of therapeutic doses of digoxin may cause prolongation of the PR interval and depression of the ST segment on the electrocardiogram.

Digoxin may produce false positive ST-T changes on the electrocardiogram during exercise testing. These electrophysiologic effects reflect an expected effect of the drug and are not indicative of toxicity.

Patients receiving digoxin should have their serum electrolytes and renal function (serum creatinine concentration) assessed periodically; the frequency of assessments will depend on the clinical setting.

Although many patients with chronic congestive cardiac failure benefit from acute administration of digoxin, there are some in whom it does not lead to constant, marked or lasting haemodynamic improvement. It is therefore important to evaluate the response of each patient individually when Lanoxin is continued long-term.

Patients with severe respiratory disease may have an increased myocardial sensitivity to digitalis glycosides.

Patients with rare hereditary problems of galactose intolerance, the Lapp lactose deficiency or glucose galactose malabsorption should not take this medicine.

4.5 Interaction with other medicinal products and other forms of interaction

Interactions may arise from effects on the renal excretion, tissue binding, plasma protein binding, distribution within the body, gut absorptive capacity and sensitivity to Lanoxin. Consideration of the possibility of an interaction whenever concomitant therapy is contemplated is the best precaution and a check on serum digoxin concentration is recommended when any doubt exists.

Digoxin, in association with beta-adrenoceptor blocking drugs, may increase atrio-ventricular conduction time.

Agents causing hypokalaemia or intracellular potassium deficiency may cause increased sensitivity to Digoxin; they include diuretics, lithium salts, corticosteroids and carbenoxolone.

Patients receiving Digoxin are more susceptible to the effects of suxamethonium-exacerbated hyperkalaemia.

Calcium, particularly if administered rapidly by the intravenous route, may produce serious arrhythmias in digitalized patients.

Serum levels of digoxin may be **increased** by concomitant administration of the following:

Alprazolam, amiodarone, flecainide, gentamicin, indometacin, itraconazole, prazosin, propafenone, quinidine, quinine, spironolactone, macrolide antibiotics (e.g. erythromycin and clarithromycin), tetracycline (and possibly other antibiotics), trimethoprim, propantheline, atorvastatin, ciclosporin, epoprostenol (transient) and carvedilol.

Serum levels of digoxin may be **reduced** by concomitant administration of the following:

Adrenaline (epinephrine), antacids, kaolin-pectin, some bulk laxatives, colestyramine, acarbose, salbutamol, sulfasalazine, neomycin, rifampicin, some cytostatics, phenytoin, metoclopramide, penicillamine and the herbal remedy St John's wort (*Hypericum perforatum*).

Calcium channel blocking agents may either increase or cause no change in serum digoxin levels. Verapamil, felodipine and tiapamil increase serum digoxin levels. Nifedipine and diltiazem may increase or have no effect on serum digoxin levels. Isradipine causes no change in serum digoxin levels. Angiotensin converting enzyme (ACE) inhibitors may also increase or cause no change in serum digoxin concentrations.

Milrinone does not alter steady-state serum digoxin levels.

Digoxin is a substrate of P-glycoprotein. Thus, inhibitors of P-glycoprotein may increase blood concentrations of digoxin by enhancing its absorption and/or by reducing its renal clearance (See *5.2 Pharmacokinetic Properties*).

4.6 Pregnancy and lactation

No data are available on whether or not digoxin has teratogenic effects.

There is no information available on the effect of digoxin on human fertility.

The use of digoxin in pregnancy is not contra-indicated, although the dosage and control may be less predictable in pregnant than in non-pregnant women with some requiring an increased dosage of digoxin during pregnancy. As with all drugs, use should be considered only when the expected clinical benefit of treatment to the mother outweighs any possible risk to the developing foetus.

Despite extensive antenatal exposure to digitalis preparations, no significant adverse effects have been observed in the foetus or neonate when maternal serum digoxin concentrations are maintained within the normal range. Although it has been speculated that a direct effect of digoxin on the myometrium may result in relative prematurity and low birthweight, a contributing role of the underlying cardiac disease cannot be excluded. Maternally administered digoxin has been successfully used to treat foetal tachycardia and congestive heart failure.

Adverse foetal effects have been reported in mothers with digitalis toxicity.

Although digoxin is excreted in breast milk, the quantities are minute and breast feeding is not contra-indicated.

4.7 Effects on ability to drive and use machines

Since central nervous system and visual disturbances have been reported in patients receiving Lanoxin, patients should exercise caution before driving, using machinery or participating in dangerous activities.

4.8 Undesirable effects

Adverse reactions are listed below by system organ class and frequency. Frequencies are defined as: very common (≥ 1/10), common (≥ 1/100 and < 1/10), uncommon (≥ 1/1000 and < 1/100), rare (≥ 1/10,000 and < 1/1000), very rare (< 1/10,000), including isolated reports. Very common, common and uncommon events were generally determined from clinical trial data. The incidence in placebo was taken into account. Adverse drug reactions identified through post-marketing surveillance were considered to be rare or very rare (including isolated reports).

Blood and lymphatic system disorders

Very rare: Thrombocytopenia

Metabolism and nutrition disorders

Very Rare: Anorexia

Psychiatric disorders

Uncommon: Depression

Very rare: Psychosis, apathy, confusion

Nervous system disorders

Common: CNS disturbances, dizziness

Very rare: Headache

Eye disorders

Common: Visual disturbances (blurred or yellow vision)

Cardiac disorders

Common: Arrhythmia, conduction disturbances, bigeminy, trigeminy, PR prolongation, sinus bradycardia

Very rare: Supraventricular tachyarrhythmia, atrial tachycardia (with or without block), junctional (nodal) tachycardia, ventricular arrhythmia, ventricular premature contraction, ST segment depression

Gastrointestinal disorders

Common: Nausea, vomiting, diarrhoea

Very rare: Intestinal ischaemia, intestinal necrosis

Skin disorders

Common: Skin rashes of urticarial or scarlatiniform character may be accompanied by pronounced eosinophilia

Reproductive system and breast disorders

Very rare: Gynaecomastia can occur with long term administration

General disorders and administration site conditions

Very rare: Fatigue, malaise, weakness

4.9 Overdose

The symptoms and signs of toxicity are generally similar to those described in the Undesirable Effects section but may be more frequent and can be more severe.

Signs and symptoms of digoxin toxicity become more frequent with levels above 2.0 nanograms/mL (2.56 nanomol/L) although there is considerable interindividual variation. However, in deciding whether a patient's symptoms are due to digoxin, the clinical state, together with serum electrolyte levels and thyroid function are important factors (see *Dosage and Administration*).

Adults

In adults without heart disease, clinical observation suggests that an overdose of digoxin of 10 to 15 mg was the dose resulting in death of half of the patients.

Cardiac manifestations

Cardiac manifestations are the most frequent and serious sign of both acute and chronic toxicity. Peak cardiac effects generally occur 3 to 6 hours following overdosage and may persist for the ensuing 24 hours or longer. Digoxin toxicity may result in almost any type of arrhythmia. Multiple rhythm disturbances in the same patient are common. These include paroxysmal atrial tachycardia with variable atrioventricular (AV) block, accelerated junctional rhythm, slow atrial fibrillation (with very little variation in the ventricular rate) and bi directional ventricular tachycardia.

Premature ventricular contractions (PVCs) are often the earliest and most common arrhythmia. Bigeminy or trigeminy also occur frequently.

Sinus bradycardia and other bradyarrhythmias are very common.

First, second, third degree heart blocks and AV dissociation are also common.

Early toxicity may only be manifested by prolongation of the PR interval.

Ventricular tachycardia may also be a manifestation of toxicity.

Cardiac arrest from asystole or ventricular fibrillation due to digoxin toxicity is usually fatal.

Hypokalaemia may contribute to toxicity (see *Warnings and Precautions*).

Non-cardiac manifestations

Acute massive digoxin overdosage can result in mild to pronounced hyperkalaemia due to inhibition of the sodium-potassium (Na+-K+) pump.

Gastrointestinal symptoms are very common in both acute and chronic toxicity. The symptoms precede cardiac manifestations in approximately half of the patients in most literature reports. Anorexia, nausea and vomiting have been reported with an incidence up to 80%. These symptoms usually present early in the course of an overdose.

Neurologic and visual manifestations occur in both acute and chronic toxicity. Dizziness, various CNS disturbances, fatigue and malaise are very common. The most frequent visual disturbance is an aberration of colour vision (predominance of yellow green). These neurological and visual symptoms may persist even after other signs of toxicity have resolved.

In chronic toxicity, non-specific extracardiac symptoms, such as malaise and weakness, may predominate.

Children

In children aged 1 to 3 years without heart disease, clinical observation suggests that an overdose of digoxin of 6 to 10 mg was the dose resulting in death in half of the patients.

Most manifestations of toxicity in children occur during or shortly after the loading phase with digoxin.

Cardiac manifestations

The same arrhythmias or combination of arrhythmias that occur in adults can occur in children. Sinus tachycardia, supraventricular tachycardia, and rapid atrial fibrillation are seen less frequently in the paediatric population.

Paediatric patients are more likely to present with an AV conduction disturbance or a sinus bradycardia.

Ventricular ectopy is less common, however in massive overdose, ventricular ectopy, ventricular tachycardia and verntricular fibrillation have been reported.

Any arrhythmia or alteration in cardiac conduction that develops in a child taking digoxin should be assumed to be caused by digoxin, until further evaluation proves otherwise.

Extracardiac manifestations

The frequent extracardiac manifestations similar to those seen in adults are gastrointestinal, CNS and visual. However, nausea and vomiting are not frequent in infants and small children.

In addition to the undesirable effects seen with recommended doses, weight loss in older age groups and failure to thrive in infants, abdominal pain due to mesenteric artery ischaemia, drowsiness and behavioural disturbances including psychotic manifestations have been reported in overdose.

Treatment

After recent ingestion, such as accidental or deliberate self-poisoning, the load available for absorption may be reduced by gastric lavage.

Patients with massive digitalis ingestion should receive large doses of activated charcoal to prevent absorption and bind digoxin in the gut during enteroenteric recirculation.

If more than 25 mg of digoxin was ingested by an adult without heart disease, death or progressive toxicity responsive only to digoxin-binding Fab antibody fragments (Digibind®) resulted. If more than 10 mg of digoxin was ingested by a child aged 1 to 3 years without heart disease, the outcome was uniformly fatal when Fab fragment treatment was not given.

Hypokalaemia should be corrected. In cases where a large amount of Lanoxin has been ingested, hyperkalaemia may be present due to release of potassium from skeletal muscle. Before administering potassium in digoxin overdose the serum potassium level must be known.

Bradyarrhythmias may respond to atropine but temporary cardiac pacing may be required. Ventricular arrhythmias may respond to lignocaine or phenytoin.

Dialysis is not particularly effective in removing digoxin from the body in potentially life-threatening toxicity.

Rapid reversal of the complications that are associated with serious poisoning by digoxin, digitoxin and related glycosides has followed intravenous administration of digoxin-specific (ovine) antibody fragments (Fab) when other therapies have failed. Digibind® is the only specific treatment for digoxin toxicity.

5. PHARMACOLOGICAL PROPERTIES

5.1 Pharmacodynamic properties

Mode of Action:-

Digoxin increases contractility of the myocardium by direct activity. This effect is proportional to dose in the lower range and some effect is achieved with quite low dosing; it occurs even in normal myocardium although it is then entirely without physiological benefit. The primary action of digoxin is specifically to inhibit adenosine triphosphatase, and thus sodium-potassium (Na^+-K^+) exchange activity, the altered ionic distribution across the membrane resulting in an augmented calcium ion influx and thus an increase in the availability of calcium at the time of excitation-contraction coupling. The potency of digoxin may therefore appear considerably enhanced when the extracellular potassium concentration is low, with hyperkalaemia having the opposite effect.

Digoxin exerts the same fundamental effect of inhibition of the Na^+-K^+ exchange mechanism on cells of the autonomic nervous system, stimulating them to exert indirect cardiac activity. Increases in efferent vagal impulses result in reduced sympathetic tone and diminished impulse conduction rate through the atria and atrioventricular node. Thus, the major beneficial effect of digoxin is reduction of ventricular rate.

Indirect cardiac contractility changes also result from changes in venous compliance brought about by the altered autonomic activity and by direct venous stimulation. The interplay between direct and indirect activity governs the total circulatory response, which is not identical for all subjects. In the presence of certain supraventricular arrhythmias, the neurogenically mediated slowing of AV conduction is paramount.

The degree of neurohormonal activation occurring in patients with heart failure is associated with clinical deterioration and an increased risk of death. Digoxin reduces activation of both the sympathetic nervous system and the (renin-angiotensin) system independently of its inotropic actions, and may thus favourably influence survival. Whether this is achieved via direct sympathoinhibitory effects or by re-sensitising baroreflex mechanisms remains unclear.

5.2 Pharmacokinetic properties

Absorption

Intravenous administration of a loading dose produces an appreciable pharmacological effect within 5 to 30 minutes; this reaches a maximum in 1 to 5 hours. Upon oral administration, digoxin is absorbed from the stomach and upper part of the small intestine. When digoxin is taken after meals, the rate of absorption is slowed, but the total amount of digoxin absorbed is usually unchanged. When taken with meals high in fibre, however, the amount absorbed from an oral dose may be reduced.

Using the oral route the onset of effect occurs in 0.5 to 2 hours and reaches its maximum at 2 to 6 hours. The bioavailability of orally administered Lanoxin is approximately 63% in tablet form and 75% as paediatric elixir.

Distribution

The initial distribution of digoxin from the central to the peripheral compartment generally lasts from 6 to 8 hours. This is followed by a more gradual decline in serum digoxin concentration, which is dependent upon digoxin elimination from the body. The volume of distribution is large (Vd_{ss} = 510 litres in healthy volunteers), indicating digoxin to be extensively bound to body tissues. The highest digoxin concentrations are seen in the heart, liver and kidney, that in the heart averaging 30- fold that in the systemic circulation. Although the concentration in skeletal muscle is far lower, this store cannot be overlooked since skeletal muscle represents 40% of total body weight. Of the small proportion of digoxin circulating in plasma, approximately 25% is bound to protein.

Elimination

The major route of elimination is renal excretion of the unchanged drug.

Digoxin is a substrate for P-glycoprotein. As an efflux protein on the apical membrane of enterocytes, P-glycoprotein may limit the absorption of digoxin. P-glycoprotein in renal proximal tubules appears to be an important factor in the renal elimination of digoxin (See *4.5 Interaction with other medicinal products and other forms of interaction*).

Following intravenous administration to healthy volunteers, between 60 and 75% of a digoxin dose is recovered unchanged in the urine over a 6 day follow-up period. Total body clearance of digoxin has been shown to be directly related to renal function, and percent daily loss is thus a function of creatinine clearance, which in turn may be estimated from a stable serum creatinine. The total and renal clearances of digoxin have been found to be 193 ± 25 ml/min and 152 ± 24 mil/min in a healthy control population.

In a small percentage of individuals, orally administered digoxin is converted to cardioinactive reduction products (digoxin reduction products or DRPs) by colonic bacteria in the gastrointestinal tract. In these subjects over 40% of the dose may be excreted as DRPs in the urine. Renal clearances of the two main metabolites, dihydrodigoxin and digoxygenin, have been found to be 79 ± 13 ml/min and 100 ± 26 ml/min respectively.

In the majority of cases however, the major route of digoxin elimination is renal excretion of the unchanged drug.

The terminal elimination half life of digoxin in patients with normal renal function is 30 to 40 hours. It is prolonged in patients with impaired renal function, and in anuric patients may be of the order of 100 hours.

In the newborn period, renal clearance of digoxin is diminished and suitable dosage adjustments must be observed. This is specially pronounced in the premature infant since renal clearance reflects maturation of renal function. Digoxin clearance has been found to be 65.6 ± 30 ml/min/1.73m^2 at 3 months, compared to only 32 ± 7 ml/min/1.73m^2 at 1 week. Beyond the immediate newborn period, children generally require proportionally larger doses than adults on the basis of body weight and body surface area.

Since most of the drug is bound to the tissues rather than circulating in the blood, digoxin is not effectively removed from the body during cardiopulmonary by-pass. Furthermore, only about 3% of a digoxin dose is removed from the body during five hours of haemodialysis.

5.3 Preclinical safety data

No data are available on whether or not digoxin has mutagenic or carcinogenic effects.

6. PHARMACEUTICAL PARTICULARS

6.1 List of excipients

Lactose Ph Eur

Maize Starch Ph Eur

Hydrolysed Starch HSE

Magnesium Stearate Ph Eur

Rice Starch Ph Eur

6.2 Incompatibilities

None known

6.3 Shelf life

Amber glass bottle: 60 months

Blister packs: 36 months

6.4 Special precautions for storage

Store below 25°C

6.5 Nature and contents of container

Amber glass bottle and low-density polyethene snap fit closure

Pack sizes: 28, 50, 500 tablets

Amber glass bottle and a clic-loc child resistant closure

Pack size: 56 tablets

Polypropylene containers with polyethyene snap fit closures

Pack sizes: 1000, 5000 tablets

White opaque PVC/aluminium foil blister

Pack sizes: 30, 60, 90, 120 tablets

Not all pack sizes may be marketed.

6.6 Special precautions for disposal and other handling

Not applicable

Administrative Data

7. MARKETING AUTHORISATION HOLDER

The Wellcome Foundation Limited

Greenford

Middlesex

UB6 0NN

Trading as:

GlaxoSmithKline UK

Stockley Park West

Uxbridge

Middlesex UB11 1BT

8. MARKETING AUTHORISATION NUMBER(S)

PL0003/0090R

9. DATE OF FIRST AUTHORISATION/RENEWAL OF THE AUTHORISATION

24 April 2003

10. DATE OF REVISION OF THE TEXT

14 May 2009

Lantus 100 Units/ml solution for injection in a vial, cartridge and a pre-filled pen.

(sanofi-aventis)

1. NAME OF THE MEDICINAL PRODUCT

Lantus 100 Units/ml solution for injection in a vial

Lantus 100 Units/ml solution for injection in a cartridge

Lantus 100 Units/ml solution for injection in a pre-filled pen

2. QUALITATIVE AND QUANTITATIVE COMPOSITION

Each ml contains 100 Units insulin glargine (equivalent to 3.64 mg).

Each vial contains 10 ml of solution for injection, equivalent to 1000 Units.

Each cartridge contains 3 ml of solution for injection, equivalent to 300 Units.

Each OptiSet pen contains 3 ml of solution for injection, equivalent to 300 Units.

Insulin glargine is produced by recombinant DNA technology in *Escherichia coli*.

For a full list of excipients, see section 6.1.

3. PHARMACEUTICAL FORM

Solution for injection in a vial, cartridge or pre-filled pen (OptiSet).

Clear colourless solution.

4. CLINICAL PARTICULARS

4.1 Therapeutic indications

For the treatment of adults, adolescents and children of 6 years or above with diabetes mellitus, where treatment with insulin is required.

4.2 Posology and method of administration

The potency of this preparation is stated in units. These units are exclusive to Lantus and are not the same as IU or the units used to express the potency of other insulin analogues. See section 5.1 (Pharmacodynamics).

Lantus contains insulin glargine an insulin analogue with a prolonged duration of action. It should be administered once daily at any time but at the same time each day.

OptiSet delivers insulin in increments of 2 Units up to a maximum single dose of 40 Units.

The dosage and timing of dose of Lantus should be individually adjusted. In patients with type 2 diabetes mellitus, Lantus can also be given together with orally active antidiabetic medicinal products.

Children

In children efficacy and safety of Lantus have only been demonstrated when given in the evening.

Due to limited experience the efficacy and safety of Lantus have not been demonstrated in children below the age of 6 years.

Transition from other insulins to Lantus

When changing from a treatment regimen with an intermediate or long-acting insulin to a regimen with Lantus, a change of the dose of the basal insulin may be required and the concomitant antidiabetic treatment may need to be adjusted (dose and timing of additional regular insulins or fast-acting insulin analogues or the dose of oral antidiabetic agents).

To reduce the risk of nocturnal and early morning hypoglycaemia, patients who are changing their basal insulin regimen from a twice daily NPH insulin to a once daily regimen with Lantus should reduce their daily dose of basal insulin by 20-30% during the first weeks of treatment. During the first weeks the reduction should, at least partially, be compensated by an increase in mealtime insulin, after this period the regimen should be adjusted individually.

As with other insulin analogues, patients with high insulin doses because of antibodies to human insulin may experience an improved insulin response with Lantus.

Close metabolic monitoring is recommended during the transition and in the initial weeks thereafter.

With improved metabolic control and resulting increase in insulin sensitivity a further adjustment in dosage regimen may become necessary. Dose adjustment may also be required, for example, if the patient's weight or life-style changes, change of timing of insulin dose or other circumstances arise that increase susceptibility to hypo-or hyperglycaemia (see section 4.4).

Administration

Lantus is administered subcutaneously.

Lantus should not be administered intravenously. The prolonged duration of action of Lantus is dependent on its injection into subcutaneous tissue. Intravenous administration of the usual subcutaneous dose could result in severe hypoglycaemia.

There are no clinically relevant differences in serum insulin or glucose levels after abdominal, deltoid or thigh administration of Lantus. Injection sites must be rotated within a given injection area from one injection to the next.

Lantus must not be mixed with any other insulin or diluted. Mixing or diluting can change its time/action profile and mixing can cause precipitation.

For further details on handling, see section 6.6. Before using OptiSet, the Instructions for Use included in the Package Leaflet must be read carefully (see section 6.6)

Due to limited experience the efficacy and safety of Lantus could not be assessed in the following groups of patients: patients with impaired liver function or patients with moderate/severe renal impairment (see section 4.4).

4.3 Contraindications

Hypersensitivity to the active substance or to any of the excipients.

4.4 Special warnings and precautions for use

Lantus is not the insulin of choice for the treatment of diabetic ketoacidosis. Instead, regular insulin administered intravenously is recommended in such cases.

Safety and efficacy of Lantus have been established in adolescents and children of 6 years and above.

Due to limited experience the efficacy and safety of Lantus could not be assessed in children below 6 years of age, in patients with impaired liver function or in patients with moderate/severe renal impairment (see section 4.2).

In patients with renal impairment, insulin requirements may be diminished due to reduced insulin metabolism. In the elderly, progressive deterioration of renal function may lead to a steady decrease in insulin requirements.

In patients with severe hepatic impairment, insulin requirements may be diminished due to reduced capacity for gluconeogenes is and reduced insulin metabolism.

In case of insufficient glucose control or a tendency to hyper- or hypoglycaemic episodes, the patient's adherence to the prescribed treatment regimen, injection sites and proper injection technique and all other relevant factors must be reviewed before dose adjustment is considered.

Switching a patient to another type or brand of insulin should be done under strict medical supervision and may require change in dose.

Insulin administration may cause insulin antibodies to form. In rare cases, the presence of such insulin antibodies may necessitate adjustment of the insulin dose in order to correct a tendency to hyper- or hypoglycaemia. (See section 4.8)

Hypoglycaemia

The time of occurrence of hypoglycaemia depends on the action profile of the insulins used and may, therefore, change when the treatment regimen is changed. Due to more sustained basal insulin supply with Lantus, less nocturnal but more early morning hypoglycaemia can be expected.

Particular caution should be exercised, and intensified blood glucose monitoring is advisable in patients in whom hypoglycaemic episodes might be of particular clinical relevance, such as in patients with significant stenoses of the coronary arteries or of the blood vessels supplying the brain (risk of cardiac or cerebral complications of hypoglycaemia) as well as in patients with proliferative retinopathy, particularly if not treated with photocoagulation (risk of transient amaurosis following hypoglycaemia).

Patients should be aware of circumstances where warning symptoms of hypoglycaemia are diminished. The warning symptoms of hypoglycaemia may be changed, be less pronounced or be absent in certain risk groups. These include patients:

- in whom glycaemic control is markedly improved,
- in whom hypoglycaemia develops gradually,
- who are elderly,
- after transfer from animal insulin to human insulin,
- in whom an autonomic neuropathy is present,
- with a long history of diabetes,
- suffering from a psychiatric illness,
- receiving concurrent treatment with certain other medicinal products (see section 4.5).

Such situations may result in severe hypoglycaemia (and possibly loss of consciousness) prior to the patient's awareness of hypoglycaemia.

The prolonged effect of subcutaneous insulin glargine may delay recovery from hypoglycaemia.

If normal or decreased values for glycated haemoglobin are noted, the possibility of recurrent, unrecognised (especially nocturnal) episodes of hypoglycaemia must be considered.

Adherence of the patient to the dosage and dietary regimen, correct insulin administration and awareness of hypoglycaemia symptoms are essential to reduce the risk of hypoglycaemia. Factors increasing the susceptibility to hypoglycaemia require particularly close monitoring and may necessitate dose adjustment. These include:

- change in the injection area,
- improved insulin sensitivity (by, e.g., removal of stress factors),
- unaccustomed, increased or prolonged physical activity,
- intercurrent illness (e.g. vomiting, diarrhoea),
- inadequate food intake,
- missed meals,
- alcohol consumption,
- certain uncompensated endocrine disorders, (e.g. in hypothyroidism and in anterior pituitary or adrenocortical insufficiency),
- concomitant treatment with certain other medicinal products.

Intercurrent illness

Intercurrent illness requires intensified metabolic monitoring. In many cases urine tests for ketones are indicated, and often it is necessary to adjust the insulin dose. The insulin requirement is often increased. Patients with type 1 diabetes must continue to consume at least a small amount of carbohydrates on a regular basis, even if they are able to eat only little or no food, or are vomiting etc. and they must never omit insulin entirely.

Handling of the pen

Before using OptiSet, the Instructions for Use included in the Package Leaflet must be read carefully. OptiSet has to be used as recommended in these Instructions for Use (see section 6.6).

4.5 Interaction with other medicinal products and other forms of interaction

A number of substances affect glucose metabolism and may require dose adjustment of insulin glargine.

Substances that may enhance the blood-glucose-lowering effect and increase susceptibility to hypoglycaemia include oral antidiabetic agents, angiotensin converting enzyme (ACE) inhibitors, disopyramide, fibrates, fluoxetine, monoamine oxidase (MAO) inhibitors, pentoxifylline, propoxyphene, salicylates and sulfonamide antibiotics.

Substances that may reduce the blood-glucose-lowering effect include corticosteroids, danazol, diazoxide, diuretics, glucagon, isoniazid, oestrogens and progestogens, phenothiazine derivatives, somatropin, sympathomimetic agents (e.g. epinephrine [adrenaline], salbutamol, terbutaline), thyroid hormones, atypical antipsychotic medicinal products (e.g. clozapine and olanzapine) and protease inhibitors.

Beta-blockers, clonidine, lithium salts or alcohol may either potentiate or weaken the blood-glucose-lowering effect of insulin. Pentamidine may cause hypoglycaemia, which may sometimes be followed by hyperglycaemia.

In addition, under the influence of sympatholytic medicinal products such as beta-blockers, clonidine, guanethidine and reserpine, the signs of adrenergic counter-regulation may be reduced or absent.

4.6 Pregnancy and lactation

Pregnancy

For insulin glargine no clinical data on exposed pregnancies from controlled clinical trials are available. A limited number of exposed pregnancies from Post Marketing Surveillance indicate no adverse effects of insulin glargine on pregnancy or on the health of the foetus and newborn child. To date, no other relevant epidemiological data are available.

Animal studies do not indicate direct harmful effects with respect to pregnancy, embryonal /foetal development, parturition or postnatal development (see section 5.3).

The available clinical data is insufficient to exclude a risk. The use of Lantus may be considered in pregnancy, if necessary.

It is essential for patients with pre-existing or gestational diabetes to maintain good metabolic control throughout pregnancy. Insulin requirements may decrease during the first trimester and generally increase during the second and third trimesters. Immediately after delivery, insulin requirements decline rapidly (increased risk of hypoglycaemia). Careful monitoring of glucose control is essential.

Lactation

Lactating women may require adjustments in insulin dose and diet.

4.7 Effects on ability to drive and use machines

The patient's ability to concentrate and react may be impaired as a result of hypoglycaemia or hyperglycaemia or, for example, as a result of visual impairment. This may constitute a risk in situations where these abilities are of special importance (e.g. driving a car or operating machinery).

Patients should be advised to take precautions to avoid hypoglycaemia whilst driving. This is particularly important in those who have reduced or absent awareness of the warning symptoms of hypoglycaemia or have frequent episodes of hypoglycaemia. It should be considered whether it is advisable to drive or operate machinery in these circumstances.

4.8 Undesirable effects

Hypoglycaemia, in general the most frequent undesirable effect of insulin therapy, may occur if the insulin dose is too high in relation to the insulin requirement.

The following related adverse reactions from clinical investigations were listed below by system organ class and in order of decreasing incidence (very common: ⩾1/10; common: ⩾1/100 to <1/10; uncommon: ⩾1/1,000 to < 1/100; rare: ⩾1/10,000 to <1/1,000; very rare: < 1/10,000).

Within each frequency grouping, undesirable effects are presented in order of decreasing seriousness.

Metabolism and nutrition disorders

Very common: Hypoglycaemia

Severe hypoglycaemic attacks, especially if recurrent, may lead to neurological damage. Prolonged or severe hypoglycaemic episodes may be life-threatening.

In many patients, the signs and symptoms of neuroglycopenia are preceded by signs of adrenergic counter-regulation. Generally, the greater and more rapid the decline in blood glucose, the more marked is the phenomenon of counter-regulation and its symptoms.

Immune system disorders

Rare: Allergic reaction

Immediate-type allergic reactions to insulin are rare. Such reactions to insulin (including insulin glargine) or the excipients may, for example, be associated with generalised skin reactions, angio-oedema, bronchospasm, hypotension and shock, and may be life-threatening.

Insulin administration may cause insulin antibodies to form. In clinical studies, antibodies that cross-react with human insulin and insulin glargine were observed with the same frequency in both NPH-insulin and insulin glargine treatment groups. In rare cases, the presence of such insulin antibodies may necessitate adjustment of the insulin dose in order to correct a tendency to hyper- or hypoglycaemia.

Nervous system disorders

Very rare: Dysgeusia

Eyes disorders

Rare: Visual impairment

A marked change in glycaemic control may cause temporary visual impairment, due to temporary alteration in the turgidity and refractive index of the lens.

Rare: Retinopathy

Long-term improved glycaemic control decreases the risk of progression of diabetic retinopathy. However, intensification of insulin therapy with abrupt improvement in glycaemic control may be associated with temporary worsening of diabetic retinopathy. In patients with proliferative retinopathy, particularly if not treated with photocoagulation, severe hypoglycaemic episodes may result in transient amaurosis.

Skin and subcutaneous tissue disorders

As with any insulin therapy, lipodystrophy may occur at the injection site and delay local insulin absorption. Continuous rotation of the injection site within the given injection area may help to reduce or prevent these reactions.

Common: Lipohypertrophy

Uncommon: Lipoatrophy

Musculoskeletal and connective tissue disorders

Very rare: Myalgia

General disorders and administration site conditions

Common: Injection site reactions

Such reactions include redness, pain, itching, hives, swelling, or inflammation. Most minor reactions to insulins at the injection site usually resolve in a few days to a few weeks.

Rare: Oedema

Rarely, insulin may cause sodium retention and oedema particularly if previously poor metabolic control is improved by intensified insulin therapy.

Paediatric population

In general, the safety profile for patients ⩽ 18 years of age is similar to the safety profile for patients > 18 years.

The adverse event reports received from Post Marketing Surveillance included relatively more frequent injection site reactions (injection site pain, injection site reaction) and skin reactions (rash, urticaria) in patients ⩽ 18 years of age than in patients > 18 years.

No clinical study safety data are available in patients below 6 years of age.

4.9 Overdose

Symptoms

Insulin overdose may lead to severe and sometimes long-term and life-threatening hypoglycaemia.

Management

Mild episodes of hypoglycaemia can usually be treated with oral carbohydrates. Adjustments in dosage of the medicinal product, meal patterns, or physical activity may be needed.

More severe episodes with coma, seizure, or neurologic impairment may be treated with intramuscular/subcutaneous glucagon or concentrated intravenous glucose. Sustained carbohydrate intake and observation may be necessary because hypoglycaemia may recur after apparent clinical recovery.

5. PHARMACOLOGICAL PROPERTIES

5.1 Pharmacodynamic properties

Pharmacotherapeutic group: Antidiabetic agent. Insulins and analogues for injection, long-acting. ATC Code: A10A E04.

Insulin glargine is a human insulin analogue designed to have a low solubility at neutral pH. It is completely soluble at the acidic pH of the Lantus injection solution (pH 4). After injection into the subcutaneous tissue, the acidic solution is neutralised leading to formation of micro-precipitates from which small amounts of insulin glargine are continuously released, providing a smooth, peakless, predictable concentration/time profile with a prolonged duration of action.

Insulin receptor binding: Insulin glargine is very similar to human insulin with respect to insulin receptor binding kinetics. It can, therefore, be considered to mediate the same type of effect via the insulin receptor as insulin.

The primary activity of insulin, including insulin glargine, is regulation of glucose metabolism. Insulin and its analogues lower blood glucose levels by stimulating peripheral glucose uptake, especially by skeletal muscle and fat, and by inhibiting hepatic glucose production. Insulin inhibits lipolysis in the adipocyte, inhibits proteolysis and enhances protein synthesis.

In clinical pharmacology studies, intravenous insulin glargine and human insulin have been shown to be equipotent when given at the same doses. As with all insulins, the time course of action of insulin glargine may be affected by physical activity and other variables.

In euglycaemic clamp studies in healthy subjects or in patients with type 1 diabetes, the onset of action of subcutaneous insulin glargine was slower than with human NPH insulin, its effect profile was smooth and peakless, and the duration of its effect was prolonged.

The following graph shows the results from a study in patients:

(see Figure 1 below)

The longer duration of action of insulin glargine is directly related to its slower rate of absorption and supports once daily administration. The time course of action of insulin and insulin analogues such as insulin glargine may vary considerably in different individuals or within the same individual.

In a clinical study, symptoms of hypoglycaemia or counter-regulatory hormone responses were similar after intravenous insulin glargine and human insulin both in healthy volunteers and patients with type 1 diabetes.

Effects of Lantus (once daily) on diabetic retinopathy were evaluated in an open-label 5-year NPH-controlled study (NPH given bid) in 1024 type 2 diabetic patients in which progression of retinopathy by 3 or more steps on the Early Treatment Diabetic Retinopathy Study (ETDRS) scale was investigated by fundus photography. No significant difference was seen in the progression of diabetic retinopathy when Lantus was compared to NPH insulin.

5.2 Pharmacokinetic properties

In healthy subjects and diabetic patients, insulin serum concentrations indicated a slower and much more prolonged absorption and showed a lack of a peak after subcutaneous injection of insulin glargine in comparison

Figure 1

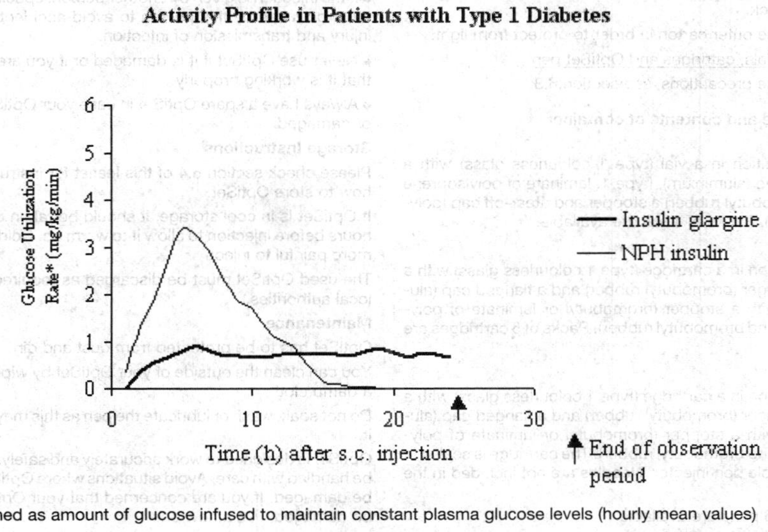

*determined as amount of glucose infused to maintain constant plasma glucose levels (hourly mean values)

to human NPH insulin. Concentrations were thus consistent with the time profile of the pharmacodynamic activity of insulin glargine. The graph above shows the activity profiles over time of insulin glargine and NPH insulin.

Insulin glargine injected once daily will reach steady state levels in 2-4 days after the first dose.

When given intravenously the elimination half-life of insulin glargine and human insulin were comparable.

In man, insulin glargine is partly degraded in the subcutaneous tissue at the carboxyl terminus of the Beta chain with formation of the active metabolites 21^A-Gly-insulin and 21^A-Gly-des-30^B-Thr-insulin. Unchanged insulin glargine and degradation products are also present in the plasma.

In clinical studies, subgroup analyses based on age and gender did not indicate any difference in safety and efficacy in insulin glargine-treated patients compared to the entire study population.

5.3 Preclinical safety data

Non-clinical data reveal no special hazard for humans based on conventional studies of safety pharmacology, repeated dose toxicity, genotoxicity, carcinogenic potential, toxicity to reproduction.

6. PHARMACEUTICAL PARTICULARS

6.1 List of excipients

10 ml vials:

Zinc chloride

m-cresol

glycerol

hydrochloric acid

Polysorbate 20

sodium hydroxide

water for injections

Cartridges or OptiSet pens:

Zinc chloride

m-cresol

glycerol

hydrochloric acid

sodium hydroxide

water for injections.

6.2 Incompatibilities

This medicinal product must not be mixed with other medicinal products. It is important to ensure that syringes do not contain traces of any other material.

6.3 Shelf life

Vials: 2 years.

Shelf-life after first use of the vial: The product may be stored for a maximum of 4 weeks not above 25°C away from direct heat or direct light. Keep the vial in the outer carton in order to protect from light.

It is recommended that the date of the first use from the vial be noted on the label.

Cartridges or OptiSet Pens: 3 years.

Shelf life after first use of the cartridge: The product may be stored for a maximum of 4 weeks not above 25°C away from direct heat or direct light. The pen containing a cartridge or the OptiSet pens in use must not be stored in the refrigerator.

The pen cap must be put back on the pen after each injection in order to protect from light.

6.4 Special precautions for storage

Unopened vials, cartridges and OptiSet pens

Store in a refrigerator (2°C-8°C).

Do not freeze.

Do not put Lantus next to the freezer compartment or a freezer pack.

Keep in the outer carton in order to protect from light.

Opened vials, catridges and OptiSet pen

For storage precautions, see section 6.3.

6.5 Nature and contents of container

Vial:

10 ml solution in a vial (type 1 colourless glass) with a flanged cap (aluminium), (type 1, laminate of polyisoprene and bromobutyl rubber) a stopper and atear-off cap (polypropylene). Packs of 1 vial are available.

Cartridge:

3 ml solution in a cartridge (type 1 colourless glass) with a black plunger (bromobutyl rubber) and a flanged cap (aluminium) with a stopper (bromobutyl or laminate of polyisoprene and bromobutyl rubber). Packs of 5 cartridges are available.

OptiSet:

3 ml solution in a cartridge (type 1 colourless glass) with a black plunger (bromobutyl rubber) and a flanged cap (aluminium) with a stopper (bromobutyl or laminate of polyisoprene and bromobutyl rubber). The cartridge is sealed in a disposable pen injector. Needles are not included in the pack.

Packs of 5 pens are available.

Handling of the pen

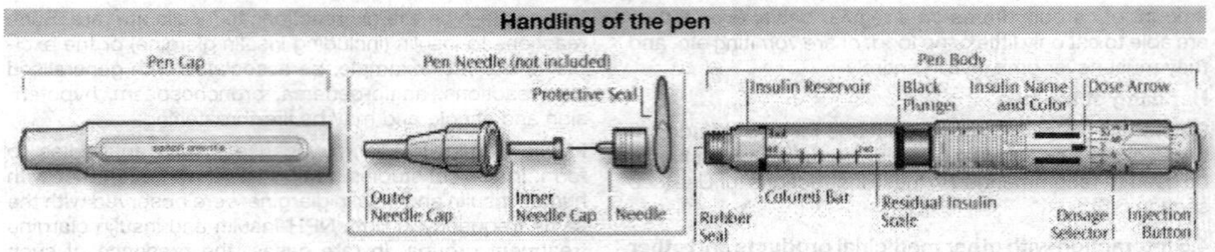

Schematic diagram of the pen

6.6 Special precautions for disposal and other handling

Vial:

Inspect the vial before use. It must only be used if the solution is clear, colourless, with no solid particles visible, and if it is of water-like consistency. Since Lantus is a solution, it does not require resuspension before use.

Insulin pen

The cartridges are to be used in conjunction with an insulin pen such as OptiPen and other pens suitable for Lantus cartridges, and as recommended in the information provided by the device manufacturer.

The manufacturer's instructions for using the pen must be followed carefully for loading the cartridge, attaching the needle, and administering the insulin injection.

If the insulin pen is damaged or not working properly (due to mechanical defects) it has to be discarded, and a new insulin pen has to be used.

If the pen malfunctions (see instructions for using the pen), the solution may be drawn from the cartridge into a syringe (suitable for an insulin with 100 Units/ml) and injected.

Cartridge

Before insertion into the pen, the cartridge must be stored at room temperature for 1 to 2 hours.

Inspect the cartridge before use. It must only be used if the solution is clear, colourless, with no solid particles visible, and if it is of water-like consistency. Since Lantus is a solution, it does not require resuspension before use.

Air bubbles must be removed from the cartridge before injection (see instructions for using the pen). Empty cartridges must not be refilled.

OptiSet

Before first use, the pen must be stored at room temperature for 1 to 2 hours.

Inspect the cartridge before use. It must only be used if the solution is clear, colourless, with no solid particles visible, and if it is of water-like consistency. Since Lantus is a solution, it does not require resuspension before use.

Empty pens must never be reused and must be properly discarded.

To prevent the possible transmission of disease, each pen must be used by one patient only.

Handling of the pen

The Instructions for Use included in the Package Leaflet must be read carefully before using OptiSet.

(see Handling of the pen above)

Important information for use of OptiSet:

- Always attach a new needle before each use. Only use needles that are compatible for use with OptiSet.
- Always perform the safety test before each injection.
- If a new OptiSet is used the initial safety test must be done with the 8 units preset by the manufacturer.
- The dosage selector can only be turned in one direction.
- Never turn the dosage selector (change the dose) after injection button has been pulled out.
- This pen is only for the patients use. It must not be shared with anyone else.
- If the injection is given by another person, special caution must be taken by this person to avoid accidental needle injury and transmission of infection.
- Never use OptiSet if it is damaged or if you are not sure that it is working properly.
- Always have a spare OptiSet in case your OptiSet is lost or damaged.

Storage Instructions

Please check section 6.4 of this leaflet for instructions on how to store OptiSet.

If OptiSet is in cool storage, it should be taken out 1 to 2 hours before injection to allow it to warm up. Cold insulin is more painful to inject.

The used OptiSet must be discarded as required by your local authorities.

Maintenance

OptiSet has to be protected from dust and dirt.

You can clean the outside of your OptiSet by wiping it with a damp cloth.

Do not soak, wash or lubricate the pen as this may damage it.

OptiSet is designed to work accurately and safely. It should be handled with care. Avoid situations where OptiSet might be damaged. If you are concerned that your OptiSet may be damaged, use a new one.

Step 1. Check the Insulin

After removing the pen cap, the label on the pen and the insulin reservoir should be checked to make sure it contains the correct insulin. The appearance of insulin should also be checked: the insulin solution must be clear, colourless, with no solid particles visible, and must have a water-like consistency. Do not use this OptiSet if the insulin is cloudy, coloured or has particles.

Step 2. Attach the needle

The needle should be carefully attached straight onto the pen.

Step 3. Perform a safety test

Prior to each injection a safety test has to be performed.

For a new and unused OptiSet, a dose of 8 units is already preset by the manufacturer for the first safety test.

In-use OptiSet, select a dose of 2 units by turning the dosage selector forward till the dose arrow points to 2. The dosage selector will only turn in one direction.

Pull out the injection button completely in order to load the dose. Never turn the dosage selector after injection button has been pulled out.

The outer and inner needle caps should be removed. Keep the outer cap to remove the used needle.

While holding the pen with the needle pointing upwards, the insulin reservoir should be tapped with the finger so that any air bubbles rise up towards the needle.

Then the injection button should be pressed all the way in.

If insulin has been expelled through the needle tip, then the pen and the needle are working properly.

If no insulin appears at the needle tip, step 3 should be repeated two more times until insulin appears at the needle tip. If still no insulin comes out, change the needle, as it might be blocked and try again. If no insulin comes out after changing the needle, the OptiSet may be damaged. Do not use this OptiSet.

Step 4. Select the dose

The dose can be set in steps of 2 units, from a minimum of 2 units to a maximum of 40 units. If a dose greater than 40 units is required, it should be given as two or more injections.

Check if you have enough insulin for the dose.

The residual insulin scale on the transparent insulin reservoir shows approximately how much insulin remains in the OptiSet. This scale must not be used to set the insulin dose.

If the black plunger is at the beginning of the coloured bar, then there are approximately 40 units of insulin available.

If the black plunger is at the end of the coloured bar, then there are approximately 20 units of insulin available.

The dosage selector should be turned forward until the dose arrow points to the required dose.

Step 5. Load the dose

The injection button should be pulled out as far as it will go in order to load the pen.

Check if the selected dose is fully loaded. Note that the injection button only goes out as far as the amount of insulin that is left in the reservoir.

The injection button allows checking the actual loaded dose. The injection button must be held out under tension during this check. The last thick line visible on the injection button shows the amount of insulin loaded. When the injection button is held out only the top part of this thick line can be seen.

Step 6. Inject the dose

The patient should be informed on the injection technique by his health care professional.

The needle should be inserted into the skin.

The injection button should be pressed all the way in. A clicking sound can be heard, which will stop when the injection button has been pressed.in completely. Then the injection button should be held down 10 seconds before withdrawing the needle from the skin. This ensures that the full dose of insulin has been delivered.

Step 7. Remove and discard the needle

The needle should be removed after each injection and discarded. This helps prevent contamination and/or infection as well as entry of air into the insulin reservoir and leakage of insulin, which can cause inaccurate dosing. Needles must not be reused.

The pen cap should be replaced on the pen.

7. MARKETING AUTHORISATION HOLDER
Sanofi-Aventis Deutschland GmbH, D-65926 Frankfurt am Main, Germany.

8. MARKETING AUTHORISATION NUMBER(S)
EU/1/00/134/012 Lantus 100 U/ml solution for injection in a 10 ml vial (1 vial/pack)

EU/1/00/134/006 Lantus 100 U/ml solution for injection in a cartridge (5 cartridges/pack)

EU/1/00/134/010 Lantus 100 U/ml OptiSet solution for injection (5 pens/pack)

9. DATE OF FIRST AUTHORISATION/RENEWAL OF THE AUTHORISATION
Date of first authorisation: 9 June 2000

Date of latest renewal: 9 June 2005

10. DATE OF REVISION OF THE TEXT
17 September 2008

Legal category: POM

Lantus 100 Units/ml solution for injection in OptiClik cartridge.

(sanofi-aventis)

1. NAME OF THE MEDICINAL PRODUCT
Lantus 100 Units/ml solution for injection in a cartridge.

2. QUALITATIVE AND QUANTITATIVE COMPOSITION
Each ml contains 100 Units insulin glargine (equivalent to 3.64 mg). Each cartridge contains 3 ml of solution for injection, equivalent to 300 Units.

Insulin glargine is produced by recombinant DNA technology in *Escherichia coli*.

For a full list of excipients, see section 6.1.

3. PHARMACEUTICAL FORM
Solution for injection in a cartridge for OptiClik.

Clear colourless solution.

4. CLINICAL PARTICULARS

4.1 Therapeutic indications
For the treatment of adults, adolescents and children of 6 years or above with diabetes mellitus, where treatment with insulin is required.

4.2 Posology and method of administration
The potency of this preparation is stated in units. These units are exclusive to Lantus and are not the same as IU or the units used to express the potency of other insulin analogues. See section 5.1 (Pharmacodynamics).

Lantus contains insulin glargine an insulin analogue with a prolonged duration of action. It should be administered once daily at any time but at the same time each day.

The dosage and timing of dose of Lantus should be individually adjusted. In patients with type 2 diabetes mellitus, Lantus can also be given together with orally active antidiabetic medicinal products.

Children
In children, efficacy and safety of Lantus have only been demonstrated when given in the evening.

Due to limited experience, the efficacy and safety of Lantus have not been demonstrated in children below the age of 6 years.

Transition from other insulins to Lantus
When changing from a treatment regimen with an intermediate or long-acting insulin to a regimen with Lantus, a change of the dose of the basal insulin may be required and the concomitant antidiabetic treatment may need to be adjusted (dose and timing of additional regular insulins or fast-acting insulin analogues or the dose of oral antidiabetic agents).

To reduce the risk of nocturnal and early morning hypoglycaemia, patients who are changing their basal insulin regimen from a twice daily NPH insulin to a once daily regimen with Lantus should reduce their daily dose of basal insulin by 20-30% during the first weeks of treatment

During the first weeks the reduction should, at least partially, be compensated by an increase in mealtime insulin, after this period the regimen should be adjusted individually.

As with other insulin analogues, patients with high insulin doses because of antibodies to human insulin may experience an improved insulin response with Lantus.

Close metabolic monitoring is recommended during the transition and in the initial weeks thereafter.

With improved metabolic control and resulting increase in insulin sensitivity a further adjustment in dosage regimen may become necessary. Dose adjustment may also be required, for example, if the patient's weight or life-style changes, change of timing of insulin dose or other circumstances arise that increase susceptibility to hypo-or hyperglycaemia (see section 4.4).

Administration
Lantus is administered subcutaneously.

Lantus should not be administered intravenously. The prolonged duration of action of Lantus is dependent on its injection into subcutaneous tissue. Intravenous administration of the usual subcutaneous dose could result in severe hypoglycaemia.

There are no clinically relevant differences in serum insulin or glucose levels after abdominal, deltoid or thigh administration of Lantus. Injection sites must be rotated within a given injection area from one injection to the next.

Lantus must not be mixed with any other insulin or diluted. Mixing or diluting can change its time/action profile and mixing can cause precipitation.

For further details on handling, see section 6.6.

Due to limited experience the efficacy and safety of Lantus could not be assessed in the following groups of patients: patients with impaired liver function or patients with moderate/severe renal impairment (see section 4.4).

4.3 Contraindications
Hypersensitivity to the active substance or to any of the excipients.

4.4 Special warnings and precautions for use
Lantus is not the insulin of choice for the treatment of diabetic ketoacidosis. Instead, regular insulin administered intravenously is recommended in such cases.

Safety and efficacy of Lantus have been established in adolescents and children of 6 years and above.

Due to limited experience the efficacy and safety of Lantus could not be assessed in children below 6 years of age, in patients with impaired liver function or in patients with moderate/severe renal impairment (see section 4.2).

In patients with renal impairment, insulin requirements may be diminished due to reduced insulin metabolism. In the elderly, progressive deterioration of renal function may lead to a steady decrease in insulin requirements.

In patients with severe hepatic impairment, insulin requirements may be diminished due to reduced capacity for gluconeogenesis and reduced insulin metabolism.

In case of insufficient glucose control or a tendency to hyper- or hypoglycaemic episodes, the patient's adherence to the prescribed treatment regimen, injection sites and proper injection technique and all other relevant factors must be reviewed before dose adjustment is considered.

Switching a patient to another type or brand of insulin should be done under strict medical supervision and may require change in dose.

Insulin administration may cause insulin antibodies to form. In rare cases, the presence of such insulin antibodies may necessitate adjustment of the insulin dose in order to correct a tendency to hyper- or hypoglycaemia. (See section 4.8)

Hypoglycaemia
The time of occurrence of hypoglycaemia depends on the action profile of the insulins used and may, therefore, change when the treatment regimen is changed. Due to more sustained basal insulin supply with Lantus, less nocturnal but more early morning hypoglycaemia can be expected.

Particular caution should be exercised, and intensified blood glucose monitoring is advisable in patients in whom hypoglycaemic episodes might be of particular clinical relevance, such as in patients with significant stenoses of the coronary arteries or of the blood vessels supplying the brain (risk of cardiac or cerebral complications of hypoglycaemia) as well as in patients with proliferative retinopathy, particularly if not treated with photocoagulation (risk of transient amaurosis following hypoglycaemia).

Patients should be aware of circumstances where warning symptoms of hypoglycaemia are diminished. The warning symptoms of hypoglycaemia may be changed, be less pronounced or be absent in certain risk groups. These include patients:

- in whom glycaemic control is markedly improved,
- in whom hypoglycaemia develops gradually,
- who are elderly,
- after transfer from animal insulin to human insulin,
- in whom an autonomic neuropathy is present,
- with a long history of diabetes,
- suffering from a psychiatric illness,
- receiving concurrent treatment with certain other medicinal products (see section 4.5).

Such situations may result in severe hypoglycaemia (and possibly loss of consciousness) prior to the patient's awareness of hypoglycaemia.

The prolonged effect of subcutaneous insulin glargine may delay recovery from hypoglycaemia.

If normal or decreased values for glycated haemoglobin are noted, the possibility of recurrent, unrecognised (especially nocturnal) episodes of hypoglycaemia must be considered.

Adherence of the patient to the dosage and dietary regimen, correct insulin administration and awareness of hypoglycaemia symptoms are essential to reduce the risk of hypoglycaemia. Factors increasing the susceptibility to hypoglycaemia require particularly close monitoring and may necessitate dose adjustment. These include:

- change in the injection area,
- improved insulin sensitivity (by, e.g., removal of stress factors),
- unaccustomed, increased or prolonged physical activity,
- intercurrent illness (e.g. vomiting, diarrhoea),
- inadequate food intake,
- missed meals,
- alcohol consumption,
- certain uncompensated endocrine disorders, (e.g. in hypothyroidism and in anterior pituitary or adrenocortical insufficiency),
- concomitant treatment with certain other medicinal products.

Intercurrent illness
Intercurrent illness requires intensified metabolic monitoring. In many cases urine tests for ketones are indicated, and often it is necessary to adjust the insulin dose. The insulin requirement is often increased. Patients with type 1 diabetes must continue to consume at least a small amount of carbohydrates on a regular basis, even if they are able to eat only little or no food, or are vomiting etc. and they must never omit insulin entirely.

4.5 Interaction with other medicinal products and other forms of interaction
A number of substances affect glucose metabolism and may require dose adjustment of insulin glargine.

Substances that may enhance the blood-glucose-lowering effect and increase susceptibility to hypoglycaemia include oral antidiabetic agents, angiotensin converting enzyme (ACE) inhibitors, disopyramide, fibrates, fluoxetine, monoamine oxidase (MAO) inhibitors, pentoxifylline, propoxyphene, salicylates and sulfonamide antibiotics.

Substances that may reduce the blood-glucose-lowering effect include corticosteroids, danazol, diazoxide, diuretics, glucagon, isoniazid, oestrogens and progestogens, phenothiazine derivatives, somatropin, sympathomimetic agents (e.g. epinephrine [adrenaline], salbutamol, terbutaline), thyroid hormones, atypical antipsychotic medicinal products (e.g. clozapine and olanzapine) and protease inhibitors.

Beta-blockers, clonidine, lithium salts or alcohol may either potentiate or weaken the blood-glucose-lowering effect of insulin. Pentamidine may cause hypoglycaemia, which may sometimes be followed by hyperglycaemia.

In addition, under the influence of sympatholytic medicinal products such as beta-blockers, clonidine, guanethidine and reserpine, the signs of adrenergic counter-regulation may be reduced or absent.

4.6 Pregnancy and lactation
Pregnancy

For insulin glargine no clinical data on exposed pregnancies from controlled clinical trials are available. A limited number of exposed pregnancies from Post Marketing Surveillance indicate no adverse effects of insulin glargine on pregnancy or on the health of the foetus and newborn child. To date, no other relevant epidemiological data are available.

Animal studies do not indicate direct harmful effects with respect to pregnancy, embryonal /foetal development, parturition or postnatal development (see section 5.3).

The available clinical data is insufficient to exclude a risk. The use of Lantus may be considered in pregnancy, if necessary.

It is essential for patients with pre-existing or gestational diabetes to maintain good metabolic control throughout pregnancy. Insulin requirements may decrease during the first trimester and generally increase during the second and third trimesters. Immediately after delivery, insulin requirements decline rapidly (increased risk of hypoglycaemia). Careful monitoring of glucose control is essential.

Lactation

Lactating women may require adjustments in insulin dose and diet.

4.7 Effects on ability to drive and use machines
The patient's ability to concentrate and react may be impaired as a result of hypoglycaemia or hyperglycaemia or, for example, as a result of visual impairment. This may constitute a risk in situations where these abilities are of special importance (e.g. driving a car or operating machinery).

Patients should be advised to take precautions to avoid hypoglycaemia whilst driving. This is particularly important in those who have reduced or absent awareness of the warning symptoms of hypoglycaemia or have frequent episodes of hypoglycaemia. It should be considered whether it is advisable to drive or operate machinery in these circumstances.

4.8 Undesirable effects
Hypoglycaemia, in general the most frequent undesirable effect of insulin therapy, may occur if the insulin dose is too high in relation to the insulin requirement.

The following related adverse reactions from clinical investigations were listed below by system organ class and in order of decreasing incidence (very common: $\geqslant 1/10$; common: $\geqslant 1/100$ to $< 1/10$; uncommon: $\geqslant 1/1{,}000$ to $< 1/100$; rare: $\geqslant 1/10{,}000$ to $< 1/1{,}000$; very rare: $< 1/10{,}000$).

Within each frequency grouping, undesirable effects are presented in order of decreasing seriousness.

Metabolism and nutrition disorders

Very common: Hypoglycaemia

Severe hypoglycaemic attacks, especially if recurrent, may lead to neurological damage. Prolonged or severe hypoglycaemic episodes may be life-threatening.

In many patients, the signs and symptoms of neuroglycopenia are preceded by signs of adrenergic counter-regulation. Generally, the greater and more rapid the decline in blood glucose, the more marked is the phenomenon of counter-regulation and its symptoms.

Immune system disorders

Rare: Allergic reaction

Immediate-type allergic reactions to insulin are rare. Such reactions to insulin (including insulin glargine) or the excipients may, for example, be associated with generalised skin reactions, angio-oedema, bronchospasm, hypotension and shock, and may be life-threatening.

Insulin administration may cause insulin antibodies to form. In clinical studies, antibodies that cross-react with human insulin and insulin glargine were observed with the same frequency in both NPH-insulin and insulin glargine treatment groups. In rare cases, the presence of such insulin antibodies may necessitate adjustment of the insulin dose in order to correct a tendency to hyper- or hypoglycaemia.

Nervous system disorders:

Very rare: Dysgeusia

Eyes disorders

Rare: Visual impairment

A marked change in glycaemic control may cause temporary visual impairment, due to temporary alteration in the turgidity and refractive index of the lens.

Rare: Retinopathy

Long-term improved glycaemic control decreases the risk of progression of diabetic retinopathy. However, intensification of insulin therapy with abrupt improvement in glycaemic control may be associated with temporary worsening of diabetic retinopathy. In patients with proliferative retinopathy, particularly if not treated with photocoagulation, severe hypoglycaemic episodes may result in transient amaurosis.

Skin and subcutaneous tissue disorders

As with any insulin therapy, lipodystrophy may occur at the injection site and delay local insulin absorption. Continuous rotation of the injection site within the given injection area may help to reduce or prevent these reactions.

Common: Lipohypertrophy

Uncommon: Lipoatrophy

Musculoskeletal and connective tissue disorders

Very rare: Myalgia

General disorders and administration site conditions

Common: Injection site reactions

Such reactions include redness, pain, itching, hives, swelling, or inflammation. Most minor reactions to insulins at the injection site usually resolve in a few days to a few weeks.

Rare: Oedema

Rarely, insulin may cause sodium retention and oedema particularly if previously poor metabolic control is improved by intensified insulin therapy.

Paediatric population

In general, the safety profile for patients ≤ 18 years of age is similar to the safety profile for patients > 18 years.

The adverse event reports received from Post Marketing Surveillance included relatively more frequent injection site reactions (injection site pain, injection site reaction) and skin reactions (rash, urticaria) in patients ≤ 18 years of age than in patients > 18 years.

No clinical study safety data are available in patients below 6 years of age.

4.9 Overdose

Symptoms

Insulin overdose may lead to severe and sometimes long-term and life-threatening hypoglycaemia.

Management

Mild episodes of hypoglycaemia can usually be treated with oral carbohydrates. Adjustments in dosage of the medicinal product, meal patterns, or physical activity may be needed.

More severe episodes with coma, seizure, or neurologic impairment may be treated with intramuscular/subcutaneous glucagon or concentrated intravenous glucose. Sustained carbohydrate intake and observation may be necessary because hypoglycaemia may recur after apparent clinical recovery.

5. PHARMACOLOGICAL PROPERTIES

5.1 Pharmacodynamic properties

Pharmacotherapeutic group: Antidiabetic agent. Insulins and analogues for injection, long-acting. ATC Code: A10A E04.

Insulin glargine is a human insulin analogue designed to have a low solubility at neutral pH. It is completely soluble at the acidic pH of the Lantus injection solution (pH 4). After injection into the subcutaneous tissue, the acidic solution is neutralised leading to formation of micro-precipitates from which small amounts of insulin glargine are continuously released, providing a smooth, peakless, predictable concentration/time profile with a prolonged duration of action.

Insulin receptor binding: Insulin glargine is very similar to human insulin with respect to insulin receptor binding kinetics. It can, therefore, be considered to mediate the same type of effect via the insulin receptor as insulin.

The primary activity of insulin, including insulin glargine, is regulation of glucose metabolism. Insulin and its analogues lower blood glucose levels by stimulating peripheral glucose uptake, especially by skeletal muscle and fat, and by inhibiting hepatic glucose production. Insulin inhibits lipolysis in the adipocyte, inhibits proteolysis and enhances protein synthesis.

In clinical pharmacology studies, intravenous insulin glargine and human insulin have been shown to be equipotent when given at the same doses. As with all insulins, the time course of action of insulin glargine may be affected by physical activity and other variables.

In euglycaemic clamp studies in healthy subjects or in patients with type 1 diabetes, the onset of action of subcutaneous insulin glargine was slower than with human NPH insulin, its effect profile was smooth and peakless, and the duration of its effect was prolonged.

The following graph shows the results from a study in patients:

(see Figure 1 below)

The longer duration of action of insulin glargine is directly related to its slower rate of absorption and supports once daily administration. The time course of action of insulin and insulin analogues such as insulin glargine may vary considerably in different individuals or within the same individual.

In a clinical study, symptoms of hypoglycaemia or counter-regulatory hormone responses were similar after intravenous insulin glargine and human insulin both in healthy volunteers and patients with type 1 diabetes.

Effects of Lantus (once daily) on diabetic retinopathy were evaluated in an open-label 5-year NPH-controlled study (NPH given bid) in 1024 type 2 diabetic patients in which progression of retinopathy by 3 or more steps on the Early Treatment Diabetic Retinopathy Study (ETDRS) scale was investigated by fundus photography. No significant difference was seen in the progression of diabetic retinopathy when Lantus was compared to NPH insulin.

5.2 Pharmacokinetic properties

In healthy subjects and diabetic patients, insulin serum concentrations indicated a slower and much more prolonged absorption and showed a lack of a peak after subcutaneous injection of insulin glargine in comparison to human NPH insulin. Concentrations were thus consistent with the time profile of the pharmacodynamic activity of insulin glargine. The graph above shows the activity profiles over time of insulin glargine and NPH insulin.

Insulin glargine injected once daily will reach steady state levels in 2-4 days after the first dose.

When given intravenously the elimination half-life of insulin glargine and human insulin were comparable.

In man, insulin glargine is partly degraded in the subcutaneous tissue at the carboxyl terminus of the Beta chain with formation of the active metabolites 21^A-Gly-insulin and 21^A-Gly-des-30^B-Thr-insulin. Unchanged insulin glargine and degradation products are also present in the plasma.

In clinical studies, subgroup analyses based on age and gender did not indicate any difference in safety and efficacy in insulin glargine-treated patients compared to the entire study population.

5.3 Preclinical safety data

Non-clinical data reveal no special hazard for humans based on conventional studies of safety pharmacology, repeated dose toxicity, genotoxicity, carcinogenic potential, toxicity to reproduction.

6. PHARMACEUTICAL PARTICULARS

6.1 List of excipients

Zinc chloride, m-cresol, glycerol, hydrochloric acid, sodium hydroxide, water for injections.

6.2 Incompatibilities

This medicinal product must not be mixed with other medicinal products. It is important to ensure that syringes do not contain traces of any other material.

6.3 Shelf life

3 years.

Shelf life after first use of the cartridge

The product may be stored for a maximum of 4 weeks not above 25°C away from direct heat or direct light. The pen containing a cartridge must not be stored in the refrigerator.

The pen cap must be put back on the pen after each injection in order to protect from light.

6.4 Special precautions for storage

Unopened cartridges

Store in a refrigerator (2°C-8°C).

Do not freeze.

Do not put Lantus next the freezer compartment or a freezer pack.

Keep the cartridge in the outer carton in order to protect from light.

In use cartridges

For storage precautions, see section 6.3.

6.5 Nature and contents of container

3 ml solution in a cartridge (type 1 colourless glass) with a black plunger (bromobutyl rubber) and a flanged cap (aluminium) with a stopper (bromobutyl or laminate of polyisoprene and bromobutyl rubber). The glass cartridge is irreversibly integrated in a transparent container and assembled to a plastic mechanism with a threaded rod at one extremity.

Packs of 5 cartridges for OptiClik are available.

6.6 Special precautions for disposal and other handling

The cartridges for OptiClik are to be used in conjunction with OptiClik only and as recommended in the information provided by the device manufacturer.

The manufacturer's instructions for using the pen must be followed carefully for loading the cartridge, attaching the needle, and administering the insulin injection.

If OptiClik is damaged or not working properly (due to mechanical defects) it has to be discarded, and a new OptiClik has to be used.

Before insertion into the pen, the cartridge must be stored at room temperature for 1 to 2 hours.

Inspect the cartridge before use. It must only be used if the cartridge is intact and the solution is clear, colourless, with no solid particles visible, and if it is of water-like consistency. Since Lantus is a solution, it does not require resuspension before use.

Air bubbles must be removed from the cartridge before injection (see instructions for using the pen). Empty cartridges must not be refilled.

Figure 1

Figure 1. Activity Profile in Patients with Type 1 Diabetes

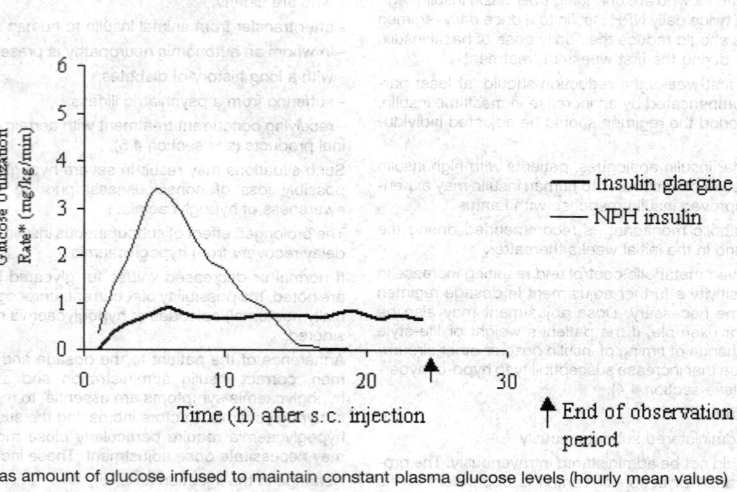

*determined as amount of glucose infused to maintain constant plasma glucose levels (hourly mean values)

If the pen malfunctions (see instructions for using the pen), the solution may be drawn from the cartridge into a syringe (suitable for an insulin with 100 Units/ml) and injected.

7. MARKETING AUTHORISATION HOLDER
Sanofi-Aventis Deutschland GmbH, D-65926 Frankfurt am Main, Germany

8. MARKETING AUTHORISATION NUMBER(S)
EU/1/00/134/025

9. DATE OF FIRST AUTHORISATION/RENEWAL OF THE AUTHORISATION
Date of first authorisation: 9 June 2000

Date of latest renewal: 9 June 2005

10. DATE OF REVISION OF THE TEXT
17th September 2008

Legal category: POM

Lantus 100 Units/ml solution for injection in SoloStar pre-filled pen

(sanofi-aventis)

1. NAME OF THE MEDICINAL PRODUCT
Lantus 100 Units/ml solution for injection in a pre-filled pen

2. QUALITATIVE AND QUANTITATIVE COMPOSITION
Each ml contains 100 Units insulin glargine (equivalent to 3.64 mg). Each pen contains 3 ml of solution for injection, equivalent to 300 Units.

Insulin glargine is produced by recombinant DNA technology in *Escherichia coli*.

For a full list of excipients, see section 6.1.

3. PHARMACEUTICAL FORM
Solution for injection in a pre-filled pen. SoloStar.

Clear colourless solution.

4. CLINICAL PARTICULARS

4.1 Therapeutic indications
For the treatment of adults, adolescents and children of 6 years or above with diabetes mellitus, where treatment with insulin is required.

4.2 Posology and method of administration
The potency of this preparation is stated in units. These units are exclusive to Lantus and are not the same as IU or the units used to express the potency of other insulin analogues. See section 5.1 (Pharmacodynamics).

Lantus contains insulin glargine an insulin analogue with a prolonged duration of action. It should be administered once daily at any time but at the same time each day.

The dosage and timing of dose of Lantus should be individually adjusted. In patients with type 2 diabetes mellitus, Lantus can also be given together with orally active antidiabetic medicinal products.

Children

In children, efficacy and safety of Lantus have only been demonstrated when given in the evening.

Due to limited experience, the efficacy and safety of Lantus have not been demonstrated in children below the age of 6 years.

Transition from other insulins to Lantus
When changing from a treatment regimen with an intermediate or long-acting insulin to a regimen with Lantus, a change of the dose of the basal insulin may be required and the concomitant antidiabetic treatment may need to be adjusted (dose and timing of additional regular insulins or fast-acting insulin analogues or the dose of oral antidiabetic agents).

To reduce the risk of nocturnal and early morning hypoglycaemia, patients who are changing their basal insulin regimen from a twice daily NPH insulin to a once daily regimen with Lantus should reduce their daily dose of basal insulin by 20-30% during the first weeks of treatment

During the first weeks the reduction should, at least partially, be compensated by an increase in mealtime insulin, after this period the regimen should be adjusted individually.

As with other insulin analogues, patients with high insulin doses because of antibodies to human insulin may experience an improved insulin response with Lantus.

Close metabolic monitoring is recommended during the transition and in the initial weeks thereafter.

With improved metabolic control and resulting increase in insulin sensitivity a further adjustment in dosage regimen may become necessary. Dose adjustment may also be required, for example, if the patient's weight or life-style changes, change of timing of insulin dose or other circumstances arise that increase susceptibility to hypo-or hyperglycaemia (see section 4.4).

Administration

Lantus is administered subcutaneously.

Lantus should not be administered intravenously. The prolonged duration of action of Lantus is dependent on its injection into subcutaneous tissue. Intravenous administration of the usual subcutaneous dose could result in severe hypoglycaemia.

There are no clinically relevant differences in serum insulin or glucose levels after abdominal, deltoid or thigh administration of Lantus. Injection sites must be rotated within a given injection area from one injection to the next.

Lantus must not be mixed with any other insulin or diluted. Mixing or diluting can change its time/action profile and mixing can cause precipitation.

Before using SoloStar, the Instructions for Use included in the Package Leaflet must be read carefully (see section 6.6).

Due to limited experience the efficacy and safety of Lantus could not be assessed in the following groups of patients: patients with impaired liver function or patients with moderate/severe renal impairment (see section 4.4).

4.3 Contraindications
Hypersensitivity to the active substance or to any of the excipients.

4.4 Special warnings and precautions for use
Lantus is not the insulin of choice for the treatment of diabetic ketoacidosis. Instead, regular insulin administered intravenously is recommended in such cases.

Safety and efficacy of Lantus have been established in adolescents and children of 6 years and above.

Due to limited experience the efficacy and safety of Lantus could not be assessed in children below 6 years of age, in patients with impaired liver function or in patients with moderate/severe renal impairment (see section 4.2).

In patients with renal impairment, insulin requirements may be diminished due to reduced insulin metabolism. In the elderly, progressive deterioration of renal function may lead to a steady decrease in insulin requirements.

In patients with severe hepatic impairment, insulin requirements may be diminished due to reduced capacity for gluconeogenesis and reduced insulin metabolism.

In case of insufficient glucose control or a tendency to hyper- or hypoglycaemic episodes, the patient's adherence to the prescribed treatment regimen, injection sites and proper injection technique and all other relevant factors must be reviewed before dose adjustment is considered.

Switching a patient to another type or brand of insulin should be done under strict medical supervision and may require change in dose.

Insulin administration may cause insulin antibodies to form. In rare cases, the presence of such insulin antibodies may necessitate adjustment of the insulin dose in order to correct a tendency to hyper- or hypoglycaemia. (See section 4.8)

Hypoglycaemia

The time of occurrence of hypoglycaemia depends on the action profile of the insulins used and may, therefore, change when the treatment regimen is changed. Due to more sustained basal insulin supply with Lantus, less nocturnal but more early morning hypoglycaemia can be expected.

Particular caution should be exercised, and intensified blood glucose monitoring is advisable in patients in whom hypoglycaemic episodes might be of particular clinical relevance, such as in patients with significant stenoses of the coronary arteries or of the blood vessels supplying the brain (risk of cardiac or cerebral complications of hypoglycaemia) as well as in patients with proliferative retinopathy, particularly if not treated with photocoagulation (risk of transient amaurosis following hypoglycaemia).

Patients should be aware of circumstances where warning symptoms of hypoglycaemia are diminished. The warning symptoms of hypoglycaemia may be changed, be less pronounced or be absent in certain risk groups. These include patients:

- in whom glycaemic control is markedly improved,
- in whom hypoglycaemia develops gradually,
- who are elderly,
- after transfer from animal insulin to human insulin,
- in whom an autonomic neuropathy is present,
- with a long history of diabetes,
- suffering from a psychiatric illness,
- receiving concurrent treatment with certain other medicinal products (see section 4.5).

Such situations may result in severe hypoglycaemia (and possibly loss of consciousness) prior to the patient's awareness of hypoglycaemia.

The prolonged effect of subcutaneous insulin glargine may delay recovery from hypoglycaemia.

If normal or decreased values for glycated haemoglobin are noted, the possibility of recurrent, unrecognised (especially nocturnal) episodes of hypoglycaemia must be considered.

Adherence of the patient to the dosage and dietary regimen, correct insulin administration and awareness of hypoglycaemia symptoms are essential to reduce the risk of hypoglycaemia. Factors increasing the susceptibility to hypoglycaemia require particularly close monitoring and may necessitate dose adjustment. These include:

- change in the injection area,
- improved insulin sensitivity (by, e.g., removal of stress factors),
- unaccustomed, increased or prolonged physical activity,
- intercurrent illness (e.g. vomiting, diarrhoea),
- inadequate food intake,
- missed meals,
- alcohol consumption,
- certain uncompensated endocrine disorders, (e.g. in hypothyroidism and in anterior pituitary or adrenocortical insufficiency),
- concomitant treatment with certain other medicinal products.

Intercurrent illness
Intercurrent illness requires intensified metabolic monitoring. In many cases urine tests for ketones are indicated, and often it is necessary to adjust the insulin dose. The insulin requirement is often increased. Patients with type 1 diabetes must continue to consume at least a small amount of carbohydrates on a regular basis, even if they are able to eat only little or no food, or are vomiting etc. and they must never omit insulin entirely.

Handling of the pen
Before using SoloStar, the Instructions for Use included in the Package Leaflet must be read carefully. SoloStar has to be used as recommended in these Instructions for Use (see section 6.6).

4.5 Interaction with other medicinal products and other forms of interaction
A number of substances affect glucose metabolism and may require dose adjustment of insulin glargine.

Substances that may enhance the blood-glucose-lowering effect and increase susceptibility to hypoglycaemia include oral antidiabetic agents, angiotensin converting enzyme (ACE) inhibitors, disopyramide, fibrates, fluoxetine, monoamine oxidase (MAO) inhibitors, pentoxifylline, propoxyphene, salicylates and sulfonamide antibiotics.

Substances that may reduce the blood-glucose-lowering effect include corticosteroids, danazol, diazoxide, diuretics, glucagon, isoniazid, oestrogens and progestogens, phenothiazine derivatives, somatropin, sympathomimetic agents (e.g. epinephrine [adrenaline], salbutamol, terbutaline), thyroid hormones, atypical antipsychotic medicinal products (e.g. clozapine and olanzapine) and protease inhibitors.

Beta-blockers, clonidine, lithium salts or alcohol may either potentiate or weaken the blood-glucose-lowering effect of insulin. Pentamidine may cause hypoglycaemia, which may sometimes be followed by hyperglycaemia.

In addition, under the influence of sympatholytic medicinal products such as beta-blockers, clonidine, guanethidine and reserpine, the signs of adrenergic counter-regulation may be reduced or absent.

4.6 Pregnancy and lactation
Pregnancy

For insulin glargin no clinical data on exposed pregnancies from controlled clinical trials are available. A limited number of exposed pregnancies from Post Marketing Surveillance indicate no adverse effects of insulin glargine on pregnancy or on the health of the foetus and newborn child. To date, no other relevant epidemiological data are available.

Animal studies do not indicate direct harmful effects with respect to pregnancy, embryonal /foetal development, parturition or postnatal development (see section 5.3).

The available clinical data is insufficient to exclude a risk. The use of Lantus may be considered in pregnancy, if necessary.

It is essential for patients with pre-existing or gestational diabetes to maintain good metabolic control throughout pregnancy. Insulin requirements may decrease during the first trimester and generally increase during the second and third trimesters. Immediately after delivery, insulin requirements decline rapidly (increased risk of hypoglycaemia). Careful monitoring of glucose control is essential.

Lactation

Lactating women may require adjustments in insulin dose and diet.

4.7 Effects on ability to drive and use machines
The patient's ability to concentrate and react may be impaired as a result of hypoglycaemia or hyperglycaemia or, for example, as a result of visual impairment. This may constitute a risk in situations where these abilities are of special importance (e.g. driving a car or operating machinery).

Patients should be advised to take precautions to avoid hypoglycaemia whilst driving. This is particularly important in those who have reduced or absent awareness of the warning symptoms of hypoglycaemia or have frequent episodes of hypoglycaemia. It should be considered whether it is advisable to drive or operate machinery in these circumstances.

4.8 Undesirable effects
Hypoglycaemia, in general the most frequent undesirable effect of insulin therapy, may occur if the insulin dose is too high in relation to the insulin requirement.

The following related adverse reactions from clinical investigations were listed below by system organ class and in order of decreasing incidence (very common: ≥1/10;

common: ⩾1/100 to <1/10; uncommon: ⩾ 1/1,000 to < 1/100; rare: ⩾1/10,000 to <1/1,000; very rare: < 1/10,000).

Within each frequency grouping, undesirable effects are presented in order of decreasing seriousness.

Metabolism and nutrition disorders

Very common: Hypoglycaemia

Severe hypoglycaemic attacks, especially if recurrent, may lead to neurological damage. Prolonged or severe hypoglycaemic episodes may be life-threatening.

In many patients, the signs and symptoms of neuroglycopenia are preceded by signs of adrenergic counter-regulation. Generally, the greater and more rapid the decline in blood glucose, the more marked is the phenomenon of counter-regulation and its symptoms.

Immune system disorders

Rare: Allergic reaction

Immediate-type allergic reactions to insulin are rare. Such reactions to insulin (including insulin glargine) or the excipients may, for example, be associated with generalised skin reactions, angio-oedema, bronchospasm, hypotension and shock, and may be life-threatening.

Insulin administration may cause insulin antibodies to form. In clinical studies, antibodies that cross-react with human insulin and insulin glargine were observed with the same frequency in both NPH-insulin and insulin glargine treatment groups. In rare cases, the presence of such insulin antibodies may necessitate adjustment of the insulin dose in order to correct a tendency to hyper- or hypoglycaemia.

Nervous system disorders:

Very rare: Dysgeusia

Eyes disorders

Rare: Visual impairment

A marked change in glycaemic control may cause temporary visual impairment, due to temporary alteration in the turgidity and refractive index of the lens.

Rare: Retinopathy

Long-term improved glycaemic control decreases the risk of progression of diabetic retinopathy. However, intensification of insulin therapy with abrupt improvement in glycaemic control may be associated with temporary worsening of diabetic retinopathy. In patients with proliferative retinopathy, particularly if not treated with photocoagulation, severe hypoglycaemic episodes may result in transient amaurosis.

Skin and subcutaneous tissue disorders

As with any insulin therapy, lipodystrophy may occur at the injection site and delay local insulin absorption. Continuous rotation of the injection site within the given injection area may help to reduce or prevent these reactions.

Common: Lipohypertrophy

Uncommon: Lipoatrophy

Musculoskeletal and connective tissue disorders

Very rare: Myalgia

General disorders and administration site conditions

Common: Injection site reactions

Such reactions include redness, pain, itching, hives, swelling, or inflammation. Most minor reactions to insulins at the injection site usually resolve in a few days to a few weeks.

Rare: Oedema

Rarely, insulin may cause sodium retention and oedema particularly if previously poor metabolic control is improved by intensified insulin therapy.

Paediatric population

In general, the safety profile for patients ⩽ 18 years of age is similar to the safety profile for patients > 18 years.

The adverse event reports received from Post Marketing Surveillance included relatively more frequent injection site reactions (injection site pain, injection site reaction) and skin reactions (rash, urticaria) in patients ⩽ 18 years of age than in patients > 18 years.

No clinical study safety data are available in patients below 6 years of age.

4.9 Overdose

Symptoms

Insulin overdose may lead to severe and sometimes long-term and life-threatening hypoglycaemia.

Management

Mild episodes of hypoglycaemia can usually be treated with oral carbohydrates. Adjustments in dosage of the medicinal product, meal patterns, or physical activity may be needed.

More severe episodes with coma, seizure, or neurologic impairment may be treated with intramuscular/subcutaneous glucagon or concentrated intravenous glucose. Sustained carbohydrate intake and observation may be necessary because hypoglycaemia may recur after apparent clinical recovery.

5. PHARMACOLOGICAL PROPERTIES

5.1 Pharmacodynamic properties

Pharmacotherapeutic group: Antidiabetic agent. Insulins and analogues for injection, long-acting. ATC Code: A10A E04.

Insulin glargine is a human insulin analogue designed to have a low solubility at neutral pH. It is completely soluble at the acidic pH of the Lantus injection solution (pH 4). After injection into the subcutaneous tissue, the acidic solution is neutralised leading to formation of micro-precipitates from which small amounts of insulin glargine are continuously released, providing a smooth, peakless, predictable concentration/time profile with a prolonged duration of action.

Insulin receptor binding: Insulin glargine is very similar to human insulin with respect to insulin receptor binding kinetics. It can, therefore, be considered to mediate the same type of effect via the insulin receptor as insulin.

The primary activity of insulin, including insulin glargine, is regulation of glucose metabolism. Insulin and its analogues lower blood glucose levels by stimulating peripheral glucose uptake, especially by skeletal muscle and fat, and by inhibiting hepatic glucose production. Insulin inhibits lipolysis in the adipocyte, inhibits proteolysis and enhances protein synthesis.

In clinical pharmacology studies, intravenous insulin glargine and human insulin have been shown to be equipotent when given at the same doses. As with all insulins, the time course of action of insulin glargine may be affected by physical activity and other variables.

In euglycaemic clamp studies in healthy subjects or in patients with type 1 diabetes, the onset of action of subcutaneous insulin glargine was slower than with human NPH insulin, its effect profile was smooth and peakless, and the duration of its effect was prolonged.

The following graph shows the results from a study in patients:

(see Figure 1 below)

The longer duration of action of insulin glargine is directly related to its slower rate of absorption and supports once daily administration. The time course of action of insulin and insulin analogues such as insulin glargine may vary considerably in different individuals or within the same individual.

In a clinical study, symptoms of hypoglycaemia or counter-regulatory hormone responses were similar after intravenous insulin glargine and human insulin both in healthy volunteers and patients with type 1 diabetes.

Effects of Lantus (once daily) on diabetic retinopathy were evaluated in an open-label 5-year NPH-controlled study (NPH given bid) in 1024 type 2 diabetic patients in which progression of retinopathy by 3 or more steps on the Early Treatment Diabetic Retinopathy Study (ETDRS) scale was investigated by fundus photography. No significant difference was seen in the progression of diabetic retinopathy when Lantus was compared to NPH insulin.

5.2 Pharmacokinetic properties

In healthy subjects and diabetic patients, insulin serum concentrations indicated a slower and much more prolonged absorption and showed a lack of a peak after subcutaneous injection of insulin glargine in comparison to human NPH insulin. Concentrations were thus consistent with the time profile of the pharmacodynamic activity of insulin glargine. The graph above shows the activity profiles over time of insulin glargine and NPH insulin.

Insulin glargine injected once daily will reach steady state levels in 2-4 days after the first dose.

When given intravenously the elimination half-life of insulin glargine and human insulin were comparable.

In man, insulin glargine is partly degraded in the subcutaneous tissue at the carboxyl terminus of the Beta chain with formation of the active metabolites 21^{A}-Gly-insulin and 21^{A}-Gly-des-30^{B}-Thr-insulin. Unchanged insulin glargine and degradation products are also present in the plasma.

In clinical studies, subgroup analyses based on age and gender did not indicate any difference in safety and efficacy in insulin glargine-treated patients compared to the entire study population.

5.3 Preclinical safety data

Non-clinical data reveal no special hazard for humans based on conventional studies of safety pharmacology, repeated dose toxicity, genotoxicity, carcinogenic potential, toxicity to reproduction.

6. PHARMACEUTICAL PARTICULARS

6.1 List of excipients

Zinc chloride

m-cresol

glycerol

hydrochloric acid

sodium hydroxide

water for injections.

6.2 Incompatibilities

This medicinal product must not be mixed with other medicinal products.

6.3 Shelf life

3 years.

Shelf life after first use of the pen

The product may be stored for a maximum of 4 weeks not above 25°C away from direct heat or direct light. Pens in use must not be stored in the refrigerator. The pen cap must be put back on the pen after each injection in order to protect from light.

6.4 Special precautions for storage

Not in-use pens

Store in a refrigerator (2°C-8°C).

Do not freeze. Do not put Lantus next to the freezer compartment or a freezer pack.

Keep the pre-filled pen in the outer carton in order to protect from light.

In use pens

For storage precautions, see section 6.3.

6.5 Nature and contents of container

3 ml solution in a cartridge (type 1 colourless glass) with a black plunger (bromobutyl rubber) and a flanged cap (aluminium) with a stopper (bromobutyl or laminate of polyisoprene and bromobutyl rubber). The cartridge is sealed in a disposable pen injector. Needles are not included in the pack.

Packs of 5 pens are available.

6.6 Special precautions for disposal and other handling

Before first use, the pen must be stored at room temperature for 1 to 2 hours.

Inspect the cartridge before use. It must only be used if the solution is clear, colourless, with no solid particles visible, and if it is of water-like consistency. Since Lantus is a solution, it does not require resuspension before use.

Empty pens must never be reused and must be properly discarded.

To prevent the possible transmission of disease, each pen must be used by one patient only.

Handling of the pen

The Instructions for Use included in the Package Leaflet must be read carefully before using SoloStar.

(see Handling of the pen on next page)

Important information for use of SoloStar:

- Before each use, a new needle must always be carefully attached and a safety test must be performed. Only use needles that are compatible for use with SoloStar.
- Special caution must be taken to avoid accidental needle injury and transmission of infection.
- Never use SoloStar if it is damaged or if you are not sure that it is working properly.
- Always have a spare SoloStar in case your SoloStar is lost or damaged.

Figure 1

Activity Profile in Patients with Type 1 Diabetes

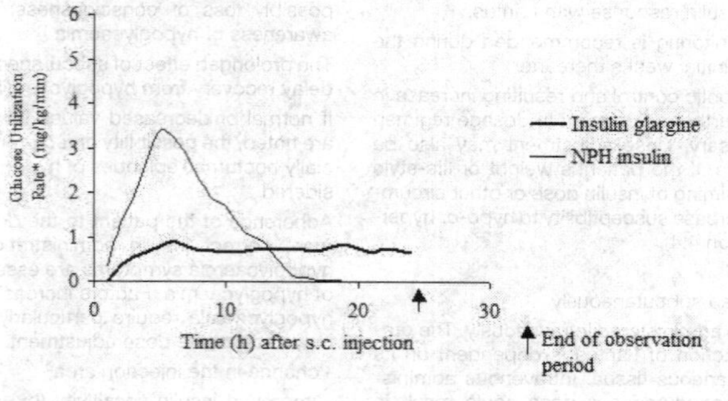

*determined as amount of glucose infused to maintain constant plasma glucose levels (hourly mean values)

Handling of the pen

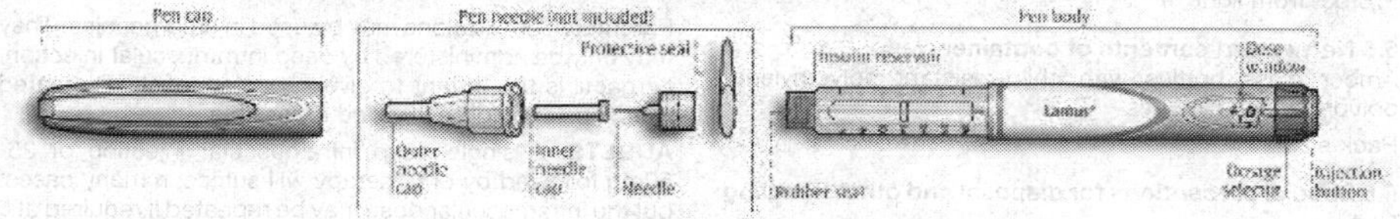

Schematic diagram of the pen

Storage Instructions

Please check section 6.4 of this leaflet for instructions on how to store SoloStar.

If SoloStar is in cool storage, it should be taken out 1 to 2 hours before injection to allow it to warm up. Cold insulin is more painful to inject.

The used SoloStar must be discarded as required by your local authorities.

Maintenance

SoloStar has to be protected from dust and dirt.

You can clean the outside of your SoloStar by wiping it with a damp cloth.

Do not soak, wash or lubricate the pen as this may damage it.

SoloStar is designed to work accurately and safely. It should be handled with care. Avoid situations where SoloStar might be damaged. If you are concerned that your SoloStar may be damaged, use a new one.

Step 1. Check the Insulin

The label on the pen should be checked to make sure it contains the correct insulin. The Lantus SoloStar is grey with a purple injection button. After removing the pen cap, the appearance of insulin should also be checked: the insulin solution must be clear, colorless, with no solid particles visible, and must have a water-like consistency.

Step 2. Attach the needle

Only needles that are compatible for use with SoloStar should be used.

A new sterile needle will be always used for each injection. After removing the cap, the needle should be carefully attached straight onto the pen.

Step 3. Perform a safety test

Prior to each injection a safety test has to be performed to ensure that pen and needle work properly and to remove air bubbles.

Select a dose of 2.

The outer and inner needle caps should be removed.

While holding the pen with the needle pointing upwards, the insulin reservoir should be tapped gently with the finger so that any air bubbles rise up towards the needle

Then the injection button should be pressed in completely.

If insulin has been expelled through the needle tip, then the pen and the needle are working properly.

If no insulin appears at the needle tip, step 3 should be repeated until insulin appears at the needle tip.

Step 4. Select the dose

The dose can be set in steps of 1 unit, from a minimum of 1 unit to a maximum of 80 units. If a dose greater than 80 units is required, it should be given as two or more injections.

The dose window must show "0" following the safety test. The dose can then be selected.

Step 5. Inject the dose

The patient should be informed on the injection technique by his health care professional.

The needle should be inserted into the skin.

The injection button should be pressed in completely. Then the injection button should be held down 10 seconds before withdrawing the needle. This ensures that the full dose of insulin has been injected.

Step 6. Remove and discard the needle

The needle should always be removed after each injection and discarded. This helps prevent contamination and/or infection, entry of air into the insulin reservoir and leakage of insulin. Needles must not be reused.

Special caution must be taken when removing and disposing the needle. Follow recommended safety measures for removal and disposal of needles (e.g. a one handed capping technique) in order to reduce the risk of accidental needle injury and transmission of infectious diseases.

The pen cap should be replaced on the pen.

7. MARKETING AUTHORISATION HOLDER

Sanofi-Aventis Deutschland GmbH, D-65926 Frankfurt am Main, Germany

8. MARKETING AUTHORISATION NUMBER(S)

EU/1/00/134/033

9. DATE OF FIRST AUTHORISATION/RENEWAL OF THE AUTHORISATION

Date of first authorisation: 9 June 2000

Date of latest renewal: 9 June 2005

10. DATE OF REVISION OF THE TEXT

17th September 2008

Legal category: POM

Lanvis Tablets

(GlaxoSmithKline UK)

1. NAME OF THE MEDICINAL PRODUCT

Lanvis Tablets

2. QUALITATIVE AND QUANTITATIVE COMPOSITION

40mg Tioguanine BP per tablet

3. PHARMACEUTICAL FORM

Tablet

4. CLINICAL PARTICULARS

4.1 Therapeutic indications

Lanvis is indicated primarily for the treatment of acute leukaemias especially acute myelogenous leukaemia and acute lymphoblastic leukaemia.

Lanvis is also used in the treatment of chronic granulocytic leukaemia.

4.2 Posology and method of administration

Route of administration: oral.

The exact dose and duration of administration will depend on the nature and dosage of other cytotoxic drugs given in conjunction with Lanvis.

Lanvis is variably absorbed following oral administration and plasma levels may be reduced following emesis or intake of food.

Lanvis can be used at various stages of treatment in short term cycles. However it is not recommended for use during maintenance therapy or similar long-term continuous treatments due to the high risk of liver toxicity (see Special Warnings and Precautions for Use and Undesirable Effects).

Adults

The usual dosage of Lanvis is between 100 and 200 mg/m^2 body surface area, per day.

Children

Similar dosages to those used in adults, with appropriate correction for body surface area, have been used.

Use in the elderly

There are no specific dosage recommendations in elderly patients (see dosage in renal or hepatic impairment).

Lanvis has been used in various combination chemotherapy schedules in elderly patients with acute leukaemia at equivalent doses to those used in younger patients.

Dosage in renal or hepatic impairment

Consideration should be given to reducing the dosage in patients with impaired hepatic or renal function.

4.3 Contraindications

In view of the seriousness of the indications there are no absolute contra-indications.

4.4 Special warnings and precautions for use

Lanvis is an active cytotoxic agent for use only under the direction of physicians experienced in the administration of such agents.

Immunisation using a live organism vaccine has the potential to cause infection in immunocompromised hosts. Therefore, immunisations with live organism vaccines are not recommended.

Hepatic Effects

Lanvis is not recommended for maintenance therapy or similar long-term continuous treatments due to the high risk of liver toxicity associated with vascular endothelial damage (see Posology and Method of Administration and Undesirable Effects). This liver toxicity has been observed in a high proportion of children receiving Lanvis as part of maintenance therapy for acute lymphoblastic leukaemia and in other conditions associated with continuous use of tioguanine. This liver toxicity is particularly prevalent in males. Liver toxicity usually presents as the clinical syndrome of hepatic veno-occlusive disease (hyperbilirubinaemia, tender hepatomegaly, weight gain due to fluid retention and ascites) or with signs of portal hypertension (splenomegaly, thrombocytopenia and oesophageal varices). Histopathological features associated with this toxicity include hepatoportal sclerosis, nodular regenerative hyperplasia, peliosis hepatis and periportal fibrosis.

Lanvis therapy should be discontinued in patients with evidence of liver toxicity as reversal of signs and symptoms of liver toxicity have been reported upon withdrawal.

Monitoring

Patients must be carefully monitored during therapy including blood cell counts and weekly liver function tests. Early indications of liver toxicity are signs associated with portal hypertension such as thrombocytopenia out of proportion with neutropenia and splenomegaly. Elevations of liver enzymes have also been reported in association with liver toxicity but do not always occur.

Haematological Effects

Treatment with Lanvis causes bone marrow suppression leading to leucopenia and thrombocytopenia. Anaemia has been reported less frequently.

Bone marrow suppression is readily reversible if Lanvis is withdrawn early enough.

There are individuals with an inherited deficiency of the enzyme thiopurine methyltransferase (TPMT) who may be unusually sensitive to the myelosuppressive effect of Lanvis and prone to developing rapid bone marrow depression following the initiation of treatment with Lanvis. This problem could be exacerbated by coadministration with drugs that inhibit TPMT, such as olsalazine, mesalazine or sulphasalzine. Some laboratories offer testing for TPMT deficiency, although these tests have not been shown to identify all patients at risk of severe toxicity. Therefore close monitoring of blood counts is still necessary.

During remission indication in acute myelogenous leukaemia the patient may frequently have to survive a period of relative bone marrow aplasia and it is important that adequate supportive facilities are available.

Patients on myelosuppressive chemotherapy are particularly susceptible to a variety of infections.

During remission induction, particularly when rapid cell lysis is occurring, adequate precautions should be taken to avoid hyperuricaemia and/or hyperuricosuria and the risk of uric acid nephropathy.

Monitoring

During remission induction, full blood counts must be carried out frequently.

The leucocyte and platelet counts continue to fall after treatment is stopped, so at the first sign of an abnormally large fall in these counts, treatment should be temporarily discontinued.

In view of its action on cellular DNA, tioguanine is potentially mutagenic and carcinogenic.

It is recommended that the handling of Lanvis tablets follows the "Guidelines for the handling of cytotoxic drugs" issued by the Royal Pharmaceutical Society of Great Britain Working Party on the handling of cytotoxic drugs.

If halving of a tablet is required, care should be taken not to contaminate the hands or inhale the drug.

Lesch-Nyhan syndrome

Since the enzyme hypoxanthine guanine phosphoribosyl transferase is responsible for the conversion of Lanvis to its active metabolite, it is possible that patients deficient in this enzyme, such as those suffering from Lesch-Nyhan Syndrome, may be resistant to the drug. Resistance to azathioprine (Imuran*) which has one of the same active metabolites as Lanvis, has been demonstrated in two children with Lesch-Nyhan Syndrome.

4.5 Interaction with other medicinal products and other forms of interaction

Vaccinations with live organism vaccines are not recommended in immunocompromised individuals (see Warnings and Precautions).

As there is *in vitro* evidence that aminosalicylate derivatives (eg. olsalazine, mesalazine or sulfasalazine) inhibit the TPMT enzyme, they should be administered with caution to patients receiving concurrent Lanvis therapy (see Special Warnings and Precautions for Use).

4.6 Pregnancy and lactation

Lanvis, like other cytotoxic agents is potentially teratogenic. There have been isolated cases where men, who have received combinations of cytotoxic agents including Lanvis, have fathered children with congenital abnormalities. Its use should be avoided whenever possible during pregnancy, particularly during the first trimester. In any individual case the potential hazard to the foetus must be balanced against the expected benefit to the mother.

As with all cytotoxic chemotherapy, adequate contraceptive precautions should be advised when either partner is receiving Lanvis.

There are no reports documenting the presence of Lanvis or its metabolites in maternal milk. It is suggested that mothers receiving Lanvis should not breast feed.

4.7 Effects on ability to drive and use machines

None known.

4.8 Undesirable effects

For this product there is a lack of modern clinical documentation which can be used as support for determining the frequency of undesirable effects. Lanvis is usually one component of combination chemotherapy and consequently it is not possible to ascribe the side effects unequivocally to this drug alone.

The following convention has been utilised for the classification of frequency of undesirable effects:- Very common ≥1/10 (≥10%), Common ≥1/100 and <1/10 (≥1% and <10%), Uncommon ≥1/1000 and <1/100 (≥0.1% and <1%), Rare ≥1/10,000 and <1/1000 (≥0.01% and <0.1%), Very rare <1/10,000 (<0.01%).

Blood and lymphatic system disorders

Very Common: Bone marrow suppression

Gastrointestinal disorders

Common: stomatitis, gastrointestinal intolerance

Rare: intestinal necrosis and perforation

Hepato-biliary disorders

Very Common: liver toxicity associated with vascular endothelial damage when Lanvis is used in maintenance or similar long term continuous therapy which is not recommended (see Dosage and Administration and Warnings and Precautions).

Usually presenting as the clinical syndrome of hepatic veno-occlusive disease (hyperbilirubinaemia, tender hepatomegaly, weight gain due to fluid retention and ascites) or signs and symptoms of portal hypertension (splenomegaly, thrombocytopenia and oesophageal varices). Elevation of liver transaminases, alkaline phosphatase and gamma glutamyl transferase and jaundice may also occur. Histopathological features associated with this toxicity include hepatoportal sclerosis, nodular regenerative hyperplasia, peliosis hepatis and periportal fibrosis.

Common: liver toxicity during short term cyclical therapy presenting as veno-occlusive disease.

Reversal of signs and symptoms of this liver toxicity has been reported upon withdrawal of short term or long term continuous therapy.

Rare: centrilobular hepatic necrosis has been reported in a few cases including patients receiving combination chemotherapy, oral contraceptives, high dose Lanvis and alcohol.

4.9 Overdose

The principal toxic effect is on the bone marrow and haematological toxicity is likely to be more profound with chronic overdosage than with a single ingestion of Lanvis. As there is no known antidote the blood picture should be closely monitored and general supportive measures, together with appropriate blood transfusion instituted if necessary.

5. PHARMACOLOGICAL PROPERTIES

5.1 Pharmacodynamic properties

Tioguanine is a sulphydryl analogue of guanine and behaves as a purine antimetabolite. It is activated to its nucleotide, thioguanylic acid. Tioguanine metabolites inhibit *de novo* purine synthesis and purine nucleotide interconversions. Tioguanine is also incorporated into nucleic acids and DNA (deoxyribonucleic acid) incorporation is claimed to contribute to the agent's cytotoxicity. Cross resistance usually exists between tioguanine and mercaptopurine, and it is not to be expected that patients resistant to one will respond to the other.

5.2 Pharmacokinetic properties

Tioguanine is extensively metabolised *in vivo*. There are two principal catabolic routes: methylation to 2-amino-6-methyl-thiopurine and deamination to 2-hydroxy-6-mercaptopurine, followed by oxidation to 6-thiouric acid.

Studies with radioactive tioguanine show that peak blood levels of total radioactivity are achieved about 8-10 hours after oral administration and decline slowly thereafter. Later studies using HPLC have shown 6-tioguanine to be the major thiopurine present for at least the first 8 hours after intravenous administration. Peak plasma concentrations of 61-118 nanomol (nmol)/ml are obtainable following intravenous administration of 1 to 1.2 g of 6-tioguanine/m^2 body surface area.

Plasma levels decay biexponentially with initial and terminal half-lives of 3 and 5.9 hours, respectively. Following oral administration of 100 mg/m2, peak levels as measured by HPLC occur at 2-4 hours and lie in the range of 0.03-0.94 micromolar (0.03-0.94 nmol/ml). Levels are reduced by concurrent food intake (as well as vomiting).

5.3 Preclinical safety data

There are no pre-clinical data of relevance to the prescriber which are additional to that already included in other sections of the SPC.

6. PHARMACEUTICAL PARTICULARS

6.1 List of excipients

Lactose	NF
Starch, potato	HSE
Acacia	NF
Stearic acid	NF
Magnesium stearate	NF
Purified water	USP

6.2 Incompatibilities

None known.

6.3 Shelf life

60 months (unopened).

6.4 Special precautions for storage

Store below 25°C

Keep dry

Protect from light

6.5 Nature and contents of container

Amber glass bottles with child-resistant polyethylene/polypropylene closures

Pack size 25

6.6 Special precautions for disposal and other handling

None

Administrative Data

7. MARKETING AUTHORISATION HOLDER

The Wellcome Foundation Limited

Glaxo Wellcome House

Berkeley Avenue

Greenford

Middlesex UB6 0NN

Trading as

GlaxoSmithKline UK

Stockley Park West

Uxbridge

Middlesex UB11 1BT

8. MARKETING AUTHORISATION NUMBER(S)

PL00003/0083

9. DATE OF FIRST AUTHORISATION/RENEWAL OF THE AUTHORISATION

29 October 1997/1 December 2008

10. DATE OF REVISION OF THE TEXT

1 December 2008

Largactil Injection

(sanofi-aventis)

1. NAME OF THE MEDICINAL PRODUCT

Largactil Injection.

2. QUALITATIVE AND QUANTITATIVE COMPOSITION

2.5% w/v chlorpromazine hydrochloride.

3. PHARMACEUTICAL FORM

Sterile solution for injection.

4. CLINICAL PARTICULARS

4.1 Therapeutic indications

Largactil injection is a phenothiazine neuroleptic. It is indicated in the following conditions:

- Schizophrenia and other psychoses (especially paranoid) mania and hypomania.

- Anxiety, psychomotor agitation, excitement, violent or dangerously impulsive behaviour. Largactil is used as an adjunct in the short-term treatment of these conditions.

- Intractable hiccup.

- Nausea and vomiting of terminal illness (where other drugs have failed or are not available).

- Induction of hypothermia is facilitated by Largactil which prevents shivering and causes vasodilation.

- Childhood schizophrenia and autism.

4.2 Posology and method of administration

Route of administration: Deep intramuscular injection.

Oral route administration should be used wherever possible.

Parenteral formulations may be used in emergencies. They may only be administered by deep intramuscular injection. Largactil is too irritant to give subcutaneously. Repeated injections should be avoided if possible.

ADULTS: A single deep intramuscular injection of 25-50mg followed by oral therapy will suffice in many cases, but the intramuscular dose may be repeated if required at 6 to 8 hour intervals. As soon as possible oral administration should be substituted.

ELDERLY: Should be started on half or even quarter of the adult dosage.

Dosage of chloropromazine in schizophrenia, other psychoses, anxiety and agitation, childhood schizophrenias and autism:

(see Table 1 below)

Hiccup, induction of hypothermia to prevent shivering:

(see Table 2 below)

Nausea and vomiting of terminal illness:

(see Table 3 on next page)

4.3 Contraindications

Known hypersensitivity to chlorpromazine or to any of the excipients. Bone marrow depression.

4.4 Special warnings and precautions for use

Largactil should be avoided in patients with liver or renal dysfunction, Parkinson's disease, hypothyroidism, cardiac failure, phaeochromocytoma, myasthenia gravis and prostate hypertrophy. It should be avoided in patients known to be hypersensitive to phenothiazines or with a history of narrow angle glaucoma or agranulocytosis. It should be used with caution in the elderly, particularly during very hot or cold weather (risk of hyper-, hypothermia). The elderly are particularly susceptible to postural hypotension.

Postural hypotension with tachycardia as well as local pain or nodule formation may occur after intramuscular administration. The patient should be kept supine and blood pressure monitored when receiving parenteral chlorpromazine. The elderly are particularly susceptible to postural hypotension.

Close monitoring is required in patients with epilepsy or a history of seizures, as phenothiazines may lower the seizure threshold.

As agranulocytosis has been reported, regular monitoring of the complete blood count is recommended. The occurrence of unexplained infections or fever may be evidence of blood dyscrasia (see section 4.8 below), and requires immediate haematological investigation.

It is imperative that treatment be discontinued in the event of unexplained fever, as this may be a sign of neuroleptic malignant syndrome (pallor, hyperthermia, autonomic dysfunction, altered consciousness, muscle rigidity). Signs of autonomic dysfunction, such as sweating and arterial instability, may precede the onset of hyperthermia and serve as early warning signs. Although neuroleptic malignant syndrome may be idiosyncratic in origin, dehydration and organic brain disease are predisposing factors.

Acute withdrawal symptoms, including nausea, vomiting and insomnia, have very rarely been reported following the abrupt cessation of high doses of neuroleptics. Relapse may also occur, and the emergence of extrapyramidal reactions has been reported. Therefore, gradual withdrawal is advisable.

Table 1 Dosage of chlopromazine in schizophrenia, other psychoses, anxiety and agitation, childhood schizophrenias and autism

Route	Adults	Children under 1 year	Children 1-5 years	Children 6-12 years	Elderly or debilitated patients
i.m.	For acute relief of symptoms 25-50 mg every 6-8 hours.	Do not use unless need is life saving.	0.5 mg/kg bodyweight every 6-8 hours. Dosage is not advised to exceed 40 mg daily.	0.5 mg/kg bodyweight every 6-8 hours. Dosage is not advised to exceed 75 mg daily.	Doses in the lower range for adults should be sufficient to control symptoms i.e. 25 mg 8 hourly.

Table 2 Hiccup, induction of hypothermia to prevent shivering

Indication	Route	Adults	Children under 1 year	Children 1-5 years	Children 6-12 years	Elderly or debilitated patients
Hiccups	i.m.	25-50 mg and if this fails 25-50 mg in 500-1000 ml sodium chloride injection by slow intravenous infusion.	No information available.			
Induction of hypothermia to prevent shivering	i.m.	25-50 mg every 6-8 hours.	Do not use.	Initial dose 0.5 to 1 mg/kg. Maintenance 0.5 mg/kg every 4-6 hours.	Initial dose 0.5 to 1 mg/kg. Maintenance 0.5 mg/kg every 4-6 hours.	No data available.

Table 3 Nausea and vomiting of terminal illness

Route	Adults	Children under 1 year	Children 1-5 years	Children 6-12 years	Elderly or debilitated patients
i.m.	25 mg initially then 25-50 mg every 3-4 hours until vomiting stops then drug to be taken orally.	Do not use unless need is life saving.	0.5 mg/kg 6-8 hourly. It is advised that maximum daily dosage should not exceed 40 mg.	0.5 mg/kg every 6-8 hours. It is advised that maximum daily dosage should not exceed 75 mg.	Not recommended.

In schizophrenia, the response to neuroleptic treatment may be delayed. If treatment is withdrawn, the recurrence of symptoms may not become apparent for some time.

Neuroleptic phenothiazines may potentiate QT interval prolongation which increases the risk of onset of serious ventricular arrhythmias of the torsade de pointes type, which is potentially fatal (sudden death). QT prolongation is exacerbated, in particular, in the presence of bradycardia, hypokalaemia, and congenital or acquired (i.e. drug induced) QT prolongation. The risk-benefit should be fully assessed before Largactil treatment is commenced. If the clinical situation permits, medical and laboratory evaluations (e.g. biochemical status and ECG) should be performed to rule out possible risk factors (e.g. cardiac disease; family history of QT prolongation: metabolic abnormalities such as hypokalaemia, hypocalcaemia or hypomagnesaemia; starvation; alcohol abuse; concomitant therapy with other drugs known to prolong the QT interval) before initiating treatment with Largactil and during the initial phase of treatment, or as deemed necessary during the treatment (see also sections 4.4 and 4.8).

Avoid concomitant treatment with other neuroleptics (see section 4.5).

Stroke: In randomised clinical trials versus placebo performed in a population of elderly patients with dementia and treated with certain atypical antipsychotic drugs, a 3-fold increase of the risk of cerebrovascular events has been observed. The mechanism of such risk increase is not known. An increase in the risk with other antipsychotic drugs or other populations of patients cannot be excluded. Largactil should be used with caution in patients with stroke risk factors.

As with all antipsychotic drugs, Largactil should not be used alone where depression is predominant. However, it may be combined with antidepressant therapy to treat those conditions in which depression and psychosis coexist.

Because of the risk of photosensitisation, patients should be advised to avoid exposure to direct sunlight (see section 4.8).

In those frequently handling preparations of phenothiazines, the greatest care must be taken to avoid contact of the drug with the skin.

4.5 Interaction with other medicinal products and other forms of interaction

Adrenaline must not be used in patients overdosed with Largactil.

The CNS depressant actions of Largactil and other neuroleptic agents may be intensified (additively) by alcohol, barbiturates and other sedatives. Respiratory depression may occur.

Anticholinergic drugs may reduce the antipsychotic effect of Largactil and the mild anticholinergic effect of Largactil may be enhanced by other anticholinergic drugs possibly leading to constipation, heat stroke, etc.

Some drugs interfere with absorption of neuroleptic agents: antacids, anti-Parkinson drugs and lithium.

Documented adverse clinically significant interactions occur with alcohol, guanethidine and hypoglycaemic agents.

Where treatment for neuroleptic-induced extrapyramidal symptoms is required, anticholinergic antiparkinsonian agents should be used in preference to levodopa, since neuroleptics antagonise the antiparkinsonian action of dopaminergics.

High doses of Largactil reduce the response to hypoglycaemic agents the dosage of which might have to be raised.

The hypotensive effect of most antihypertensive drugs especially alpha adrenoceptor blocking agents may be exaggerated by Largactil.

The action of some drugs may be opposed by Largactil; these include amphetamine, levodopa, clonidine, guanethidine and adrenaline.

Increases or decreases in the plasma concentrations of a number of drugs, e.g. propranolol Phenobarbital have been observed but were not of clinical significance.

Simultaneous administration of desferrioxamine and prochlorperazine has been observed to induce a transient metabolic encephalopathy characterised by loss of consciousness for 48-72 hours. It is possible this may occur with Largactil since it shares many of the pharmacological properties of prochlorperazine.

There is an increased risk of arrhythmias when neuroleptics are used with concomitant QT prolonging drugs (including certain antiarrhythmics, antidepressants and other antipsychotics) and drugs causing electrolyte imbalance.

There is an increased risk of agranulocytosis when neuroleptics are used concurrently with drugs with myelosuppressive potential, such as carbamazepine or certain antibiotics and cytotoxics.

In patients treated concurrently with neuroleptics and lithium, there have been rare reports of neurotoxicity.

4.6 Pregnancy and lactation

There is inadequate evidence of the safety of Largactil in human pregnancy. There is evidence of harmful effects in animals. Like other drugs it should be avoided in pregnancy unless the physician considers it essential. It may occasionally prolong labour and at such a time should be withheld until the cervix is dilated 3-4 cm. Possible adverse effects on the foetus include lethargy or paradoxical hyperexcitability, tremor and low Apgar score. Largactil may be excreted in milk, therefore breastfeeding should be suspended during treatment.

4.7 Effects on ability to drive and use machines

Patients should be warned about drowsiness during the early days of treatment and advised not to drive or operate machinery.

4.8 Undesirable effects

Generally, adverse reactions occur at low frequency; the most common reported adverse reactions are nervous system disorders.

Blood and lymphatic system disorders: A mild leucopaenia occurs in up to 30% of patients on prolonged high dosage. Agranulocytosis may occur rarely; it is not dose related.

Immune system disorders: Allergic phenomena such as angiodema, bronchospasm, and urticaria have occurred with phenothiazines but anaphylactic reactions have been exceedingly rare. In very rare cases, treatment with chlorpromazine may be associated with systemic lupus erythematosus.

Endocrine: Hyperprolactinaemia which may result in galactorrhoea, gynaecomastia, amenorrhoea and impotence.

Nervous system disorders: Acute dystonias or dyskenias, usually transitory are more common in children and young adults and usually occur within the first 4 days of treatment or after dosage increases.

Akathisia characteristically occurs after large initial doses.

Parkinsonism is more common in adults and the elderly. It usually develops after weeks or months of treatment. One or more of the following may be seen: tremor, rigidity, akinesia or other features of Parkinsonism. Commonly just tremor.

Tardive Dyskinesia: If this occurs it is usually, but not necessarily, after prolonged high dosage. It can even occur after treatment has been stopped. Dosage should therefore be kept low whenever possible.

Insomnia and agitation may occur.

Eye disorders: Ocular changes and the development of a metallic greyish-mauve coloration of exposed skin have been noted in some individuals, mainly females, who have received chlorpromazine continuously for long periods (four to eight years).

Cardiac disorders: ECG changes include QT prolongation (as with other neuroleptics), ST depression, U-Wave and T-Wave changes. Cardiac arrhythmias, including ventricular arrhythmias and atrial arrhythmias, a-v block, ventricular tachycardia, which may result in ventricular fibrillation or cardiac arrest have been reported during neuroleptic phenothiazine therapy, possibly related to dosage. Pre-existing cardiac disease, old age, hypokalaemia and concurrent tricyclic antidepressants may predispose.

There have been isolated reports of sudden death, with possible causes of cardiac origin (see section 4.4, above), as well as cases of unexplained sudden death, in patients receiving neuroleptic phenothiazines.

There have been isolated reports of sudden death, with possible causes of cardiac origin (see section 4.4, above), as well as cases of unexplained sudden death, in patients receiving neuroleptic phenothiazines.

Vascular disorders: Hypotension, usually postural, commonly occurs. Elderly or volume depleted subjects are particularly susceptible: it is more likely to occur after intramuscular administration.

Gastrointestinal disorders: dry mouth may occur.

Respiratory, thoracic and mediastinal disorders: Respiratory depression is possible in susceptible patients. Nasal stuffiness may occur.

Hepato-biliary disorders: Jaundice, usually transient, occurs in a very small percentage of patients taking chlorpromazine. A premonitory sign may be a sudden onset of fever after one to three weeks of treatment followed by the development of jaundice. Chlorpromazine jaundice has the biochemical and other characteristics of obstructive (cholestatic) jaundice and is associated with obstructions of the canaliculi by bile thrombi; the frequent presence of an accompanying eosinophilia indicates the allergic nature of this phenomenon. Liver injury, sometimes fatal, has been reported rarely in patients treated with chlorpromazine. Treatment should be withheld on the development of jaundice (see section 4.4, above).

Skin and subcutaneous tissue disorders: Contact skin sensitisation may occur rarely in those frequently handling preparations of chlorpromazine (see section 4.4, above). Skin rashes of various kinds may also be seen in patients treated with the drug. Patients on high dosage may develop photosensitivity in sunny weather and should avoid exposure to direct sunlight.

Reproductive system and breast disorders: Priapism has been very rarely reported in patients treated with chlorpromazine.

General disorders and administration site conditions: Neuroleptic malignant syndrome (hyperthermia, rigidity, autonomic dysfunction and altered consciousness) may occur (see section 4.4, above).

4.9 Overdose

Toxicity and treatment of overdosage: Symptoms of chlorpromazine overdosage include drowsiness or loss of consciousness, hypotension, tachycardia, ECG changes, ventricular arrhythmia's and hypothermia. Severe extra-pyramidal dyskinesias may occur.

If the patient is seen sufficiently soon (up to 6 hours) after ingestion of a toxic dose, gastric lavage may be attempted. Pharmacological induction of emesis is unlikely to be of any use. Activated charcoal should be given. There is no specific antidote. Treatment is supportive.

Generalised vasodilation may result in circulatory collapse; raising the patient's legs may suffice. In severe cases, volume expansion by intravenous fluids may be needed; infusion fluids should be warmed before administration in order not to aggravate hypothermia.

Positive inotropic agents such as dopamine may be tried if fluid replacement is insufficient to correct the circulatory collapse. Peripheral vasoconstriction agents are not generally recommended; avoid the use of adrenaline.

Ventricular or supraventricular tachy-arrhythmias usually respond to restoration of normal body temperature and correction of circulatory or metabolic disturbances. If persistent or life threatening, appropriate anti-arrhythmic therapy may be considered. Avoid lidocaine and, as far as possible, long acting anti-arrhythmic drugs.

Pronounced central nervous system depression requires airway maintenance or, in extreme circumstances, assisted respiration. Severe dystonic reactions usually respond to procyclidine (5-10mg) or orphenadrine (20-40mg) administered intramuscularly or intravenously. Convulsions should be treated with intravenous diazepam.

Neuroleptic malignant syndrome should be treated with cooling. Dantrolene sodium may be tried.

5. PHARMACOLOGICAL PROPERTIES

5.1 Pharmacodynamic properties

Largactil is a phenothiazine neuroleptic.

5.2 Pharmacokinetic properties

Chlorpromazine is rapidly absorbed and widely distributed in the body. It is metabolised in the liver and excreted in the urine and bile. Whilst plasma concentration of chlorpromazine itself rapidly declines excretion of chlorpromazine metabolites is very slow. The drug is highly bound to plasma protein. It readily diffuses across the placenta. Small quantities have been detected in milk from treated women. Children require smaller dosages per kg than adults.

5.3 Preclinical safety data

There are no preclinical data of relevance to the prescriber which are additional to that already included in other sections of the.

6. PHARMACEUTICAL PARTICULARS

6.1 List of excipients

Sodium sulphite anhydrous (E221), Sodium citrate, Sodium metabisulphite (E223), Sodium chloride, Water for Injections.

6.2 Incompatibilities

Largactil injection solutions have a pH of 5.0-6.5; they are incompatible with benzylpenicillin potassium, pentobarbital sodium and phenobarbital sodium.

6.3 Shelf life

The shelf life of the Largactil Injection is 60 months.

6.4 Special precautions for storage

Largactil injection should be stored protected from light. Discoloured solution should not be used.

6.5 Nature and contents of container

Largactil Injection 2.5% w/v is supplied in boxes containing 10 × 2 ml in glass ampoules.

6.6 Special precautions for disposal and other handling

None.

7. MARKETING AUTHORISATION HOLDER

Sanofi-aventis,

One Onslow Street,

Guildford,

Surrey,

GU1 4YS

8. MARKETING AUTHORISATION NUMBER(S)

PL 04425/0582

9. DATE OF FIRST AUTHORISATION/RENEWAL OF THE AUTHORISATION

24 April 2007

10. DATE OF REVISION OF THE TEXT

12 March 2009

Legal category: POM

Lariam

(Roche Products Limited)

1. NAME OF THE MEDICINAL PRODUCT

Lariam 250mg tablets

2. QUALITATIVE AND QUANTITATIVE COMPOSITION

Each tablet contains 250mg mefloquine (as 274.09mg mefloquine hydrochloride).

For excipients, see section *6.1*.

3. PHARMACEUTICAL FORM

Tablet. White to off-white cylindrical biplanar tablets, cross scored and imprinted with Roche on one face.

4. CLINICAL PARTICULARS

4.1 Therapeutic indications

Therapy and prophylaxis of malaria.

Therapy: Lariam is especially indicated for therapy of *P. falciparum* malaria in which the pathogen has become resistant to other antimalarial agents.

Following treatment of *P. vivax* malaria with Lariam, relapse prophylaxis with an 8-amino-quinoline derivative, for example primaquine, should be considered in order to eliminate parasites in the hepatic phase.

Prophylaxis: Malaria prophylaxis with Lariam is particularly recommended for travellers to malarious areas in which multiple resistant *P. falciparum* strains occur.

For current advice on geographical resistance patterns and appropriate chemoprophylaxis, current guidelines or the Malaria Reference Laboratory should be consulted, details of which can be found in the British National Formulary (BNF).

4.2 Posology and method of administration

Curative treatment

The recommended total therapeutic dose of mefloquine for non-immune patients is 20 – 25mg/kg. A lower total dose of 15mg/kg may suffice for partially immune individuals.

The recommended total therapeutic dosages of Lariam tablets relative to body weight and immune status are presented in the following table.*

	Non-immune patients	Partially immune patients
< 20kg **	¼ tablet / 2.5 – 3kg 1 tablet / 10 – 12 kg	¼ tablet / 4kg 1 tablet / 16kg
20 – 30kg	2 – 3 tablets	1¼– 2 tablets
> 30 – 45kg	3 – 4 tablets	2 – 3 tablets
> 45 – 60kg	4 – 5 tablets	3 – 4 tablets
> 60kg ***	6 tablets	4 – 6 tablets

* Splitting the total curative dosage into 2 – 3 doses (e.g. 3 + 1, 3 + 2 or 3 + 2 + 1 tablets) taken 6 – 8 hours apart may reduce the occurrence or severity of adverse events.

** Experience with Lariam in infants less than 3 months old or weighing less than 5kg is limited.

*** There is no specific experience with total dosages of more than 6 tablets in very heavy patients.

A second full dose should be given to patients who vomit less than 30 minutes after receiving the drug. If vomiting occurs 30 – 60 minutes after a dose, an additional half-dose should be given.

If a full treatment course with Lariam does not lead to improvement within 48 – 72 hours, alternative treatments should be considered. When breakthrough malaria occurs during Lariam prophylaxis, physicians should carefully evaluate which antimalarial to use for therapy.

Lariam can be given for severe acute malaria after an initial course of intravenous quinine lasting at least 2 – 3 days. Interactions leading to adverse events can largely be prevented by allowing an interval of at least 12 hours after the last dose of quinine (see section *4.5 Interaction with other medicinal products and other forms of interaction*).

In areas with multi-resistant malaria, initial treatment with artemisinin or a derivative, if available, followed by Lariam is also an option.

Malaria prophylaxis

For malaria prophylaxis the stated dose of Lariam should be given once weekly, always on the same day. Treatment should be initiated at least one week and up to 2-3 weeks before arrival in a malarious area and continued for 4 weeks after leaving (minimum treatment period 6 weeks). The maximum recommended duration of administration of Lariam is 12 months.

The following dosage schedule is given as a guide.

	Dosage
Adults and children of more than 45kg bodyweight	1 tablet
Children and adults weighing less than 45kg	
5 – 19kg	¼ tablet
20 – 30kg	½ tablet
31 – 45kg	¾ tablet

The tablets should be swallowed whole preferably after a meal with plenty of liquid.

Elderly

No specific adaptation of the usual adult dosage is required for elderly patients.

4.3 Contraindications

Prophylactic use in patients with severe impairment of liver function should be regarded for the time being as a contra-indication as no experience has been gained in such patients.

Patients with a history of psychiatric disturbances (including depression) or convulsions should not be prescribed Lariam prophylactically, as it may precipitate these conditions (see section *4.4 Special warnings anl precautions for use* and section *4.5 Interaction with other medicinal products and other forms of interaction*).

Lariam should not be administered to patients with a known hypersensitivity to mefloquine or related compounds, e.g. quinine.

Because of the danger of a potentially fatal prolongation of the QTc interval, halofantrine must not be given simultaneously with or subsequent to Lariam. No data are available where Lariam was given after halofantrine.

4.4 Special warnings and precautions for use

Women of childbearing potential travelling to malarious areas in which multiple resistant *P. falciparum* is found and who are receiving Lariam for the treatment and prophylaxis of malaria should take reliable contraceptive precautions for the entire duration of therapy and for three months after the last dose of Lariam (see section *4.6 Pregnancy and lactation*).

If psychiatric disturbances occur during prophylactic use, Lariam should be discontinued and an alternative prophylactic agent should be recommended (see section *4.3 Contraindications*).

Experience with Lariam in infants less than 3 months old or weighing less than 5kg is limited.

There is no evidence that dose adjustment is necessary for patients with renal insufficiency. However, since clinical evidence in such patients is limited, caution should be exercised when using Lariam in patients with impaired renal function.

In patients with epilepsy, mefloquine may increase the risk of convulsions. Therefore in such cases, Lariam should be used only for curative treatment and only if compelling reasons exist (see section *4.3 Contraindications* and section *4.5 Interaction with other medicinal products and other forms of interaction*).

Lariam should be taken with caution in patients suffering from cardiac conduction disorders, since transient cardiac conduction alterations have been observed during curative and preventative use.

Due to the risk of a potentially fatal prolongation of the QTc interval, halofantrine must not be given during Lariam therapy for prophylaxis or treatment of malaria, or within 15 weeks after the last dose of Lariam. Due to increased plasma concentrations and elimination half-life of mefloquine following co-administration with ketoconazole, the risk of QTc prolongation may also be expected if ketoconazole is taken during Lariam therapy for prophylaxis or treatment of malaria, or within 15 weeks after the last dose of Lariam (*see 4.5 Interaction with other Medicinal Products and other Forms of Interaction).*

Patients should not disregard the possibility that re-infection or recrudescence may occur after effective antimalarial therapy.

Patients with rare hereditary problems of galactose intolerance, the Lapp lactase deficiency or glucose-galactose malabsorption should not take this medicine.

4.5 Interaction with other medicinal products and other forms of interaction

Concomitant administration of Lariam and other related compounds (e.g. quinine, quinidine and chloroquine) may produce electrocardiographic abnormalities and increase the risk of convulsions. There is evidence that the use of halofantrine during Lariam therapy for prophylaxis or treatment of malaria, or within 15 weeks after the last dose of Lariam, causes a significant lengthening of the QTc interval (*see 4.4 Special warnings and precautions for use*). Clinically significant QTc prolongation has not been found with mefloquine alone.

This appears to be the only clinically relevant interaction of this kind with Lariam, although theoretically co-administration of other drugs known to alter cardiac conduction (e.g. anti-arrhythmic or β-adrenergic blocking agents, calcium channel blockers, antihistamines or H_1-blocking agents, tricyclic antidepressants and phenothiazines) might also contribute to a prolongation of the QTc interval.

In patients taking an anticonvulsant (e.g. valproic acid, carbamazepine, phenobarbital or phenytoin), the concomitant use of Lariam may reduce seizure control by lowering the plasma levels of the anticonvulsant. Dosage adjustments of anti-seizure medication may be necessary in some cases (see section *4.3 Contraindications* and section *4.4 Special warnings and precautions for use*).

When Lariam is taken concurrently with oral live typhoid vaccines, attenuation of immunisation cannot be excluded. Vaccinations with oral attenuated live bacteria should therefore be completed at least 3 days before the first dose of Lariam.

Other Potential Interactions

Mefloquine does not inhibit or induce the cytochrome P450 enzyme system. It is therefore not expected that the metabolism of drugs given concomitantly with mefloquine is affected. However, inhibitors or inducers of the isoenzyme CYP3A4 may modify the pharmacokinetics/metabolism of mefloquine, leading to an increase or decrease in mefloquine plasma concentrations, respectively.

Inhibitors of CYP3A4

One pharmacokinetic study in healthy volunteers showed that the co-administration of ketoconazole, a strong inhibitor of CYP3A4, increased the plasma concentrations and elimination half-life of mefloquine.

Inducers of CYP3A4

The long-term use of rifampicin, a potent inducer of CYP3A4, reduced the plasma concentrations and elimination half-life of mefloquine.

Substrates and inhibitors of P-glycoprotein

It has been shown in vitro that mefloquine is a substrate and an inhibitor of P-glycoprotein. Therefore, drug-drug interactions could also occur with drugs that are substrates, or are known to modify the expression of this transporter. The clinical relevance of these interactions is not known to date.

No other drug interactions are known. Nevertheless, the effects of Lariam on travellers receiving co-medication, particularly those on anticoagulants or antidiabetics, should be checked before departure.

4.6 Pregnancy and lactation

Lariam has been shown to be teratogenic in mice and rats and embryotoxic in rabbits. Data from a limited number of exposed pregnancies indicate no adverse effects of mefloquine on pregnancy or on the health of the foetus/newborn child. To date, no other relevant epidemiological data are available.

Lariam should not be used during pregnancy particularly in the first trimester unless the expected benefit justifies the potential risk to the foetus.

Women of childbearing potential should be advised to practice contraception during malaria prophylaxis with Lariam and for up to 3 months thereafter.

As mefloquine is secreted into the breast milk, nursing mothers should not breast-feed while taking Lariam.

4.7 Effects on ability to drive and use machines

Mefloquine can cause dizziness or disturbed sense of balance. It is consequently recommended not to drive or carry out tasks demanding fine co-ordination and spatial discrimination during treatment with mefloquine. Patients should avoid such tasks for at least 3 weeks following therapeutic use, as dizziness, a disturbed sense of balance or neuropsychiatric reactions have been reported up to three weeks after the use of Lariam.

Prophylactic use

Caution should be exercised with regard to driving, piloting aircraft and operating machines, as dizziness, a disturbed sense of balance or neuropsychiatric reactions have been reported during and up to three weeks after use of Lariam.

In a small number of patients it has been reported that dizziness or vertigo and loss of balance may continue for months after discontinuation of the drug (see section *4.8 Undesirable Effects*).

4.8 Undesirable effects

At the doses given for acute malaria, adverse reactions to Lariam may not be distinguishable from symptoms of the disease itself. The overall incidence of adverse events reported during mefloquine prophylaxis is comparable to that reported for other chemoprophylactic regimens. However, the profile of mefloquine adverse events is predominantly characterised by neuropsychological adverse events.

Because of the long half-life of mefloquine, adverse reactions to Lariam may occur or persist for more than several weeks after discontinuation of the drug. In a small number of patients, it has been reported that dizziness or vertigo and loss of balance may continue for months after discontinuation of the drug.

Patients should be advised to obtain medical advice before the next weekly dose of Lariam, if any concerning or neuropsychiatric symptoms develop. Discontinuation of Lariam should be considered, particularly if neuropsychiatric reactions occur. The need for alternative antimalarial therapy or prophylaxis can then be evaluated.

The following adverse events have been reported, although their absolute frequencies are not known (cannot be estimated from the available data):

Blood and Lymphatic System Disorders: Leucopenia or leucocystosis and thrombocytopenia.

Immune System Disorders: There have been rare reports of anaphylaxis in patients taking Lariam.

Metabolism and Nutrition Disorders: Anorexia.

Psychiatric Disorders: Sleep disorders (insomnia, abnormal dreams), agitation, restlessness, anxiety, depression, mood swings, panic attacks, confusional state, hallucinations, aggression, psychotic or paranoid reactions.

There have been rare reports of suicidal ideation and suicide, but no relationship to drug administration has been established.

Nervous System Disorders: Dizziness, loss of balance, headache and somnolence, syncope, convulsions, memory impairment, sensory and motor neuropathies (including paraesthesia, tremor and ataxia). Isolated cases of encephalopathy have been reported.

Eye Disorders: Visual disturbances.

Ear and Labyrinth Disorders: Vertigo, vestibular disorders including tinnitus and hearing impairment.

Cardiac Disorders: Tachycardia, palpitation, bradycardia, irregular heart rate, extrasystoles, other transient cardiac conduction alterations. Isolated cases of AV-block have been reported.

Vascular Disorders: Circulatory disturbances (hypotension, hypertension, flushing).

Respiratory, Thoracic and Mediastinal Disorders: Dyspnoea. Very rare cases of pneumonitis of possible allergic etiology have been reported.

Gastrointestinal Disorders: Nausea, vomiting, diarrhoea and abdominal pain, dyspepsia.

Hepatobiliary disorders: Transient elevation of transaminases.

Skin and Subcutaneous Tissue Disorders: Rash, exanthema, erythema, urticaria, pruritus, alopecia, hyperhidrosis. Isolated cases of erythema multiforme and Stevens-Johnson syndrome have been reported.

Musculoskeletal and Connective Tissue Disorders: Muscle weakness, muscle cramps, myalgia, arthralgia.

General Disorders and Administration Site Disorders: Oedema, chest pain, asthenia, malaise, fatigue, chills, pyrexia.

Studies *in vitro* and *in vivo* showed no haemolysis associated with G6PD deficiency.

4.9 Overdose

Symptoms and signs

In cases of overdosage with Lariam, the symptoms mentioned under section *4.8* (*Undesirable effects*) may be more pronounced.

Treatment

Patients should be managed by symptomatic and supportive care following Lariam overdose. There are no specific antidotes. The use of oral activated charcoal to limit mefloquine absorption may be considered within one hour of ingestion of an overdose. Monitor cardiac function (if possible by ECG) and neuropsychiatric status for at least 24 hours. Provide symptomatic and intensive supportive treatment as required, particularly for cardiovascular disorders.

5. PHARMACOLOGICAL PROPERTIES

5.1 Pharmacodynamic properties

The effectiveness of Lariam in the therapy and prophylaxis of malaria is due essentially to destruction of the asexual forms of the malarial pathogens that affect humans (*Plasmodium falciparum, P. vivax, P. malariae, P. ovale*).

Lariam is also effective against malarial parasites resistant to other antimalarials such as chloroquine and other 4-aminoquinoline derivatives, proguanil, pyrimethamine and pyrimethamine-sulphonamide combinations. However, strains of *P. falciparum* resistant to mefloquine have been reported (e.g. in parts of Indochina). Cross-resistance between mefloquine and halofantrine has been observed.

In vitro and *in vivo* studies with mefloquine showed no haemolysis associated with glucose-6-phosphate dehydrogenase deficiency.

5.2 Pharmacokinetic properties

Absorption: The maximum plasma concentration is reached within 6 to 24 hours after a single oral dose of Lariam. The level in micrograms per litre is roughly equivalent to the dose in milligrams (for example approximately 1000μg/l after a single dose of 1000mg). The presence of food significantly enhances the rate and extent of absorption.

At a dose of 250mg once weekly, maximum steady state plasma concentrations of 1000 – 2000μg/l are reached after 7 – 10 weeks. The RBC concentration is almost twice as high as the plasma level. Plasma protein binding is about 98%. Clinical experience suggests a minimal suppressive plasma concentration of mefloquine in the order of 600μg/l.

Metabolism: Mefloquine is extensively metabolised in the liver by the cytochrome P450 system. In vitro and in vivo studies strongly suggest that CYP3A4 is the major isoform involved.

Elimination: The average half-life of mefloquine in Europeans is 21 days. There is evidence that mefloquine is excreted mainly in the bile and faeces. In volunteers, urinary excretion of unchanged mefloquine and its main metabolite accounted for about 9% and 4% of the dose, respectively.

Special clinical situations: The pharmacokinetics of mefloquine may be altered in acute malaria. Pharmacokinetic differences have been observed between various ethnic populations. In practice however, these are of minor importance compared with the host immune status and sensitivity of the parasite.

Mefloquine crosses the placenta. Excretion into breast milk appears to be minimal.

5.3 Preclinical safety data

Mefloquine crosses the placenta and is teratogenic when administered to rats and mice in early gestation (see section *4.6 Pregnancy and lactation*).

6. PHARMACEUTICAL PARTICULARS

6.1 List of excipients

Microcrystalline cellulose

lactose

crospovidone

maize starch

ammonium-calcium alginate

poloxamer (polyoxyethylene-polyoxypropylene copolymer)

talc

magnesium stearate

6.2 Incompatibilities

Not applicable.

6.3 Shelf life

3 years.

6.4 Special precautions for storage

Store in the original package.

6.5 Nature and contents of container

Aluminium foil packs containing 8 tablets.

6.6 Special precautions for disposal and other handling

Not applicable.

7. MARKETING AUTHORISATION HOLDER

Roche Products Limited

6 Falcon Way

Shire Park

Welwyn Garden City

AL7 1TW

United Kingdom

8. MARKETING AUTHORISATION NUMBER(S)

PL 00031/0236

9. DATE OF FIRST AUTHORISATION/RENEWAL OF THE AUTHORISATION

5 October 1989 / 1 February 2004

10. DATE OF REVISION OF THE TEXT

27 August 2009

LEGAL STATUS

POM

Lariam is a registered trade mark

Lasilactone

(sanofi-aventis)

1. NAME OF THE MEDICINAL PRODUCT

Lasilactone

2. QUALITATIVE AND QUANTITATIVE COMPOSITION

Lasilactone contains 20mg Furosemide and 50mg Spironolactone.

For excipients, see section 6.1

3. PHARMACEUTICAL FORM

Capsule.

4. CLINICAL PARTICULARS

4.1 Therapeutic indications

Lasilactone contains a short-acting diuretic and a long-acting aldosterone antagonist. It is indicated in the treatment of resistant oedema where this is associated with secondary hyperaldosteronism; conditions include chronic congestive cardiac failure and hepatic cirrhosis.

Treatment with Lasilactone should be reserved for cases refractory to a diuretic alone at conventional doses.

This fixed ratio combination should only be used if titration with the component drugs separately indicates that this product is appropriate.

The use of Lasilactone in the management of essential hypertension should be restricted to patients with demonstrated hyperaldosteronism. It is recommended that in these patients also, this combination should only be used if titration with the component drugs separately indicates that this product is appropriate.

4.2 Posology and method of administration

For oral administration.

Adults: 1-4 capsules daily.

Children: The product is not suitable for use in children.

Elderly: Furosemide and Spironolactone may both be excreted more slowly in the elderly.

The capsules should be swallowed whole. They are best taken at breakfast and/or lunch with a generous amount of liquid (approx. 1 glass). An evening dose is not recommended, especially during initial treatment, because of the increased nocturnal output of urine to be expected in such cases.

4.3 Contraindications

Patients with hypovolaemia or dehydration (with or without accompanying hypotension). Patients with an impaired renal function and a creatinine clearance below 30ml/min per 1.73 m^2 body surface area, anuria or renal failure with anuria not responding to furosemide, renal failure as a result of poisoning by nephrotoxic or hepatotoxic agents or renal failure associated with hepatic coma, hyperkalaemia, severe hypokalaemia, severe hyponatraemia, Addison's disease and breast feeding women.

Hypersensitivity to furosemide, spironolactone, sulphonamides or sulphonamide derivatives, or any of the excipients of Lasilactone.

4.4 Special warnings and precautions for use

Spironolactone may cause vocal changes. In determining whether to initiate treatment with Lasilactone, special attention must be given to this possibility in patients whose voice is particularly important for their work (e.g., actors, singers, teachers).

Urinary output must be secured. Patients with partial obstruction of urinary outflow, for example patients with prostatic hypertrophy or impairment of micturition have an increased risk of developing acute retention and require careful monitoring.

Where indicated, steps should be taken to correct hypotension or hypovolaemia before commencing therapy.

Particularly careful monitoring is necessary in:

• patients with hypotension.

• patients who are at risk from a pronounced fall in blood pressure.

• patients where latent diabetes may become manifest or the insulin requirements of diabetic patients may increase.

• patients with gout.

• patients with hepatic cirrhosis together with impaired renal function.

• patients with hypoproteinaemia, e.g. associated with nephrotic syndrome (the effect of furosemide may be weakened and its ototoxicity potentiated). Cautious dose titration is required.

Administration of Lasilactone should be avoided in the presence of a raised serum potassium. Concomitant administration of triamterene, amiloride, potassium supplements or non-steroidal anti-inflammatory drugs is not recommended as hyperkalaemia may result.

Caution should be observed in patients liable to electrolyte deficiency. Regular monitoring of serum sodium, potassium, creatinine and glucose is generally recommended during therapy; particularly close monitoring is required in patients at high risk of developing electrolyte imbalances or in case of significant additional fluid loss. Hypovolaemia or dehydration as well as any significant electrolyte and acid-base disturbances must be corrected. This may require temporary discontinuation of Lasilactone.

Frequent checks of the serum potassium level are necessary in patients with impaired renal function and a creatinine clearance below 60ml/min per 1.73m^2 body surface area as well as in cases where Lasilactone is taken in combination with certain other drugs which may lead to an increase in potassium levels.

In patients who are at high risk for radiocontrast nephropathy, furosemide is not recommended to be used for diuresis as part of the preventative measures against radiocontrast-induced nephropathy.

Patients with rare hereditary problems of galactose intolerance, the Lapp lactase deficiency or glucose-galactose malabsorption should not take this medicine.

4.5 Interaction with other medicinal products and other forms of interaction

The dosage of concurrently administered cardiac glycosides, diuretics, anti-hypertensive agents, or other drugs with blood-pressure-lowering potential may require adjustment as a more pronounced fall in blood pressure must be anticipated if given concomitantly with Lasilactone. A marked fall in blood pressure and deterioration in renal function may be seen when ACE inhibitors or angiotensin II receptor antagonists are added to furosemide therapy, or their dose level increased. The dose of Lasilactone should be reduced for at least three days, or the drug stopped, before initiating the ACE inhibitor or angiotensin II receptor antagonist or increasing their dose.

When Lasilactone is taken in combination with potassium salts, with drugs which reduce potassium excretion, with non-steroidal anti-inflammatory drugs or with ACE inhibitors, an increase in serum potassium concentration and hyperkalaemia may occur.

The toxic effects of nephrotoxic drugs may be increased by concomitant administration of potent diuretics such as furosemide.

Lasilactone and sucralfate must not be taken within two hours of each other because sucralfate decreases the absorption of furosemide from the intestine and so reduced its effect.

In common with other diuretics, serum lithium levels may be increased when lithium is given concomitantly with Lasilactone, resulting in increased lithium toxicity, including increased risk of cardiotoxic and neurotoxic effects of lithium. Therefore, it is recommended that lithium levels are carefully monitored and where necessary the lithium dosage is adjusted in patients receiving this combination.

Certain non-steroidal anti-inflammatory agents (e.g.indometacin, acetylsalicylic acid) may attenuate the action of Lasilactone and may cause acute renal failure in cases of pre-existing hypovolaemia or dehydration.

Salicylic toxicity may be increased by Lasilactone. Lasilactone may sometimes attenuate the effects of other drugs (e.g. the effects of antidiabetics and pressor amines) and sometimes potentiate them (e.g. the effects of salicylates, theophylline and curare-type muscle relaxants).

Lasilactone may potentiate the ototoxicity of aminoglycosides and other ototoxic drugs. Since this may lead to irreversible damage, these drugs must only be used with Lasilactone if there are compelling medical reasons.

There is a risk of ototoxic effects if cisplatin and furosemide are given concomitantly. In addition, nephrotoxicity of cisplatin may be enhanced if furosemide is not given in low doses (e.g. 40 mg in patients with normal renal function) and with positive fluid balance when used to achieve forced diuresis during cisplatin treatment.

Spironolactone may cause raised digoxin levels. Some electrolyte disturbances (e.g. hypokalaemia, hypomagnesaemia) may increase the toxicity of certain other drugs (e.g. digitalis preparations and drugs inducing QT interval prolongation syndrome).

Attenuation of the effect of Lasilactone may occur following concurrent administration of phenytoin.

Concomitant administration of carbamazepine or aminoglutethimide may increase the risk of hyponatraemia.

Corticosteroids administered concurrently may cause sodium retention.

Both spironolactone and carbenoloxone may impair the action of the other substance. In this regard, liquorice in larger amounts acts in a similar manner to carbenoxolone. Corticosteroids, carbenoxolone, liquorice, B_2 sympathomimetics in large amounts, and prolonged use of laxatives, reboxetine and amphotericin may increase the risk of developing hypokalaemia.

Probenecid, methotrexate and other drugs which, like furosemide, undergo significant renal tubular secretion may reduce the effect of Lasilactone. Conversely, furosemide may decrease renal elimination of these drugs. In case of high-dose treatment (in particular, of both furosemide and the other drugs), this may lead to increased serum levels and an increased risk of adverse effects due to furosemide or the concomitant medication.

Impairment of renal function may develop in patients receiving concurrent treatment with furosemide and high doses of certain cephalosporins.

Concomitant use of ciclosporin and furosemide is associated with increased risk of gouty arthritis.

4.6 Pregnancy and lactation

Pregnancy:

Results of animal work, in general, show no hazardous effect of furosemide in pregnancy. There is clinical evidence of safety of the drug in the third trimester of human pregnancy; however, furosemide crosses the placental barrier.

Spironolactone or its metabolites may cross the placental barrier.

Lasilactone must not be used in pregnancy unless there are compelling medical reasons. Treatment during pregnancy requires monitoring of foetal growth.

Lactation:

Furosemide passes into breast milk and may inhibit lactation. Canerone, a metabolite of spironolactone, appears in breast milk and Lasilactone must therefore not be used in breast-feeding mothers. See section 4.3.

4.7 Effects on ability to drive and use machines

Reduced mental alertness may impair the ability to drive or operate dangerous machinery. This applies especially at the commencement of treatment.

4.8 Undesirable effects

Furosemide is generally well tolerated.

Bone marrow depression has been reported as a rare complication and necessitates withdrawal of treatment.

Occasionally, thrombocytopenia may occur. In rare cases, leucopenia and, in isolated cases, agranulocytosis, aplastic anaemia or haemolytic anaemia may develop. Eosinophilia is rare.

Rarely, paraesthesiae may occur.

Hepatic encephalopathy in patients with hepatocellular insufficiency may occur (see Section 4.3).

Serum calcium levels may be reduced; in very rare cases tetany has been observed. Nephrocalcinosis / Nephrolithiasis has been reported in premature infants.

Serum cholesterol and triglyceride levels may rise during furosemide treatment. During long-term therapy they will usually return to normal within six months.

Glucose tolerance may decrease with furosemide. In patients with diabetes mellitus this may lead to a deterioration of metabolic control; latent diabetes mellitus may become manifest.

Hearing disorders and tinnitus, although usually transitory, may occur in rare cases, particularly in patients with renal failure, hypoproteinaemia (e.g. in nephrotic syndrome) and/or when intravenous furosemide has been given too rapidly.

Furosemide may cause a reduction in blood pressure which, if pronounced may cause signs and symptoms such as impairment of concentration and reactions, light-headedness, sensations of pressure in the head, headache, dizziness, drowsiness, weakness, disorders of vision, dry mouth, orthostatic intolerance.

In isolated cases, intrahepatic cholestasis, an increase in liver transaminases or acute pancreatitis may develop.

The incidence of allergic reactions, such as skin rashes, photosensitivity, vasculitis, fever or interstitial nephritis, is very low, but when these occur treatment should be withdrawn. Skin and mucous membrane reactions may occasionally occur, e.g. itching, urticaria, other rashes or bullous lesions, erythema multiforme, bullous pemphigoid, exfoliative dermatitis, purpura.

As with other diuretics, electrolytes and water balance may be disturbed as a result of diuresis after prolonged therapy.

Furosemide leads to increased excretion of sodium and chloride and consequently water. In addition excretion of other electrolytes (in particular, calcium and magnesium) is increased. The two active ingredients exert opposing influences on potassium excretion. The serum potassium concentration may decrease, especially at the commencement of treatment (owing to the earlier onset of action of furosemide), although particularly as treatment is continued, the potassium concentration may increase (owing to the later onset of action of spironolactone), especially in patients with renal failure.

Symptomatic electrolyte disturbances and metabolic alkalosis may develop in the form of a gradually increasing electrolyte deficit or, e.g. where higher furosemide doses are administered to patients with normal renal function, acute severe electrolyte losses. Warning signs of electrolyte disturbances include increased thirst, headache, hypotension, confusion, muscle cramps, tetany, muscle weakness, disorders of cardiac rhythm and gastrointestinal symptoms. In the event of an irregular pulse, tiredness or muscle weakness (e.g., in the legs), particular consideration must be given to the possibility of hyperkalaemia. Pre-existing metabolic alkalosis (e.g. in decompensated cirrhosis of the liver) may be aggravated by furosemide treatment.

Disturbances in electrolyte balance, particularly if pronounced, must be corrected.

The diuretic action may lead to or contribute to hypovolaemia and dehydration, especially in elderly patients. To avert these, it is important to compensate any undesired losses of fluid (e.g., due to vomiting or diarrhoea, or to intense sweating). Severe fluid depletion may lead to haemoconcentration with a tendency for thromboses to develop.

Increased production of urine may provoke or aggravate complaints in patients with an obstruction of urinary outflow. Thus, acute retention of urine with possible secondary complications may occur for example, in patients with bladder-emptying disorders, prostatic hyperplasia or narrowing of the urethra.

If furosemide is administered to premature infants during the first weeks of life, it may increase the risk of persistence of patent ductus arteriosus.

Severe anaphylactic or anaphylactoid reactions (e.g. with shock) occur rarely.

Side-effects of a minor nature such as nausea, malaise or gastric upset (vomiting or diarrhoea) may occur but are not usually severe enough to necessitate withdrawal of treatment.

As with other diuretics, treatment with furosemide may lead to transitory increases in blood creatinine and urea levels. Serum levels of uric acid may increase and attacks of gout may occur.

Spironolactone has been reported to induce gastrointestinal intolerance. Stomach ulcers (sometimes with bleeding) have been reported rarely. Spironolactone may also cause drowsiness, headache, ataxia and mental confusion.

Because of its chemical similarity to the sex hormones, spironolactone may make the nipples more sensitive to touch. Dose dependent mastodynia and reversible gynaecomastia may occur in both sexes. Maculopapular or erythematous cutaneous eruptions have been reported rarely, as have mild androgenic manifestation such as hirsutism and menstrual irregularities. In men, potency may occasionally be impaired. Rarely, spironolactone may cause vocal changes in the form of hoarseness and (in women), deepening of the voice or (in men) increase in pitch. In some patients these vocal changes persist even after Lasilactone has been discontinued.

4.9 Overdose

The clinical picture in acute or chronic overdose depends primarily on the extent and consequences of electrolyte and fluid loss, e.g. hypovolaemia, dehydration, haemoconcentration, cardiac arrhythmias due to excessive diuresis. Symptoms of these disturbances include severe hypotension (progressing to shock), acute renal failure, thrombosis, delirious states, flaccid paralysis, apathy and confusion.

Treatment should therefore be aimed at fluid replacement and correction of the electrolyte imbalance. Together with the prevention and treatment of serious complications resulting from such disturbances and of other effects on the body (e.g., hyperkalaemia), this corrective action may necessitate general and specific intensive medical monitoring and therapeutic measures (e.g., to promote potassium elimination).

No specific antidote to furosemide is known. If ingestion has only just taken place, attempts may be made to limit further systemic absorption of the active ingredient by measures such as gastric lavage or those designated to reduce absorption (e.g. activated charcoal).

5. PHARMACOLOGICAL PROPERTIES

5.1 Pharmacodynamic properties

ATC code: CO3E B01

Furosemide: Furosemide is a diuretic acting on the Loop of Henle.

Spironolactone: Spironolactone is a competitive inhibitor of aldosterone.

5.2 Pharmacokinetic properties

Furosemide: Furosemide is a short-acting diuretic; diuresis usually commences within one hour and lasts for four to six hours.

Spironolactone: Spironolactone, a competitive inhibitor of aldosterone, increases sodium excretion whilst reducing potassium loss at the distal renal tubule. It has a slow and prolonged action, maximum response being usually attained after 2-3 days' treatment.

5.3 Preclinical safety data

Carcinogenicity: Spironolactone has been shown to produce tumours in rats when administered at high doses over a long period of time. The significance of these findings with respect to clinical use is not certain. However, the long-term use of spironolactone in young patients requires careful consideration of the benefits and the potential hazard involved.

6. PHARMACEUTICAL PARTICULARS

6.1 List of excipients

Microcrystalline cellulose

Lactose

Talc

Magnesium stearate

Sodium amylopectin glycollate

Indigotin (FD&C Blue 2)

Titanium dioxide

Gelatin

6.2 Incompatibilities

None known.

6.3 Shelf life

Four years.

6.4 Special precautions for storage

Store at ambient temperature proteced from light.

6.5 Nature and contents of container

Blister pack containing 28 capsules.

6.6 Special precautions for disposal and other handling

Not applicable.

7. MARKETING AUTHORISATION HOLDER

Sanofi-aventis

One Onslow Street

Guildford

Surrey

GU1 4YS

UK

8. MARKETING AUTHORISATION NUMBER(S)
PL 13402/0033

9. DATE OF FIRST AUTHORISATION/RENEWAL OF THE AUTHORISATION
31 December 1997.

10. DATE OF REVISION OF THE TEXT
16th June 2008

11. LEGAL CLASSIFICATION
POM

Lasix Injection 20mg/2ml

(sanofi-aventis)

1. NAME OF THE MEDICINAL PRODUCT
Lasix 20 mg /2 ml Injection

2. QUALITATIVE AND QUANTITATIVE COMPOSITION
Lasix 20 mg/2 ml Injection contains 20 mg Furosemide in 2 ml aqueous solution.

For excipients, see section 6.1

3. PHARMACEUTICAL FORM
Solution for injection.

4. CLINICAL PARTICULARS

4.1 Therapeutic indications
Lasix 20 mg/2 ml Injection is a diuretic indicated for use when a prompt and effective diuresis is required. The intravenous formulation is appropriate for use in emergencies or when oral therapy is precluded. Indications include cardiac, pulmonary, hepatic and renal oedema.

4.2 Posology and method of administration
Route of administration: intramuscular or intravenous

Intravenous furosemide must be injected or infused slowly; a rate of 4 mg per minute must not be exceeded. In patients with severe impairment of renal function (serum creatinine >5 mg/dl), it is recommended that an infusion rate of 2.5 mg per minute is not exceeded.

Intramuscular administration must be restricted to exceptional cases where neither oral nor intravenous administration are feasible. It must be noted that intramuscular injection is not suitable for the treatment of acute conditions such as pulmonary oedema.

To achieve optimum efficacy and suppress counter-regulation, a continuous furosemide infusion is generally to be preferred to repeated bolus injections. Where continuous furosemide infusion is not feasible for follow-up treatment after one or several acute bolus doses, a follow-up regimen with low doses given at short intervals (approx. 4 hours) is to be preferred to a regimen with higher bolus doses at longer intervals.

Doses of 20 to 50 mg intramuscularly or intravenously may be given initially. If larger doses are required, they should be given increasing by 20 mg increments and not given more often than every two hours. If doses greater than 50 mg are required it is recommended that they be given by slow intravenous infusion. The recommended maximum daily dose of furosemide administration is 1,500 mg.

Elderly: The dosage recommendations for adults apply, but in the elderly furosemide is generally eliminated more slowly. Dosage should be titrated until the required response is achieved.

Children: Parenteral doses for children range from 0.5 to 1.5 mg/kg body weight daily up to a maximum total daily dose of 20 mg.

4.3 Contraindications
Lasix 20 mg/2 ml Injection is contra-indicated in patients with hypovolaemia or dehydration, anuria or renal failure with anuria not responding to furosemide, renal failure as a result of poisoning by nephrotoxic or hepatotoxic agents or renal failure associated with hepatic coma, severe hypokalaemia, severe hyponatraemia, pre-comatose and comatose states associated with hepatic encephalopathy and breast feeding women.

Hypersensitivity to furosemide or any of the excipients of Lasix 20 mg/2 ml Injection. Patients allergic to sulphonamides may show cross-sensitivity to furosemide.

4.4 Special warnings and precautions for use
Urinary output must be secured. Patients with partial obstruction of urinary outflow, for example patients with prostatic hypertrophy or impairment of micturition have an increased risk of developing acute retention and require careful monitoring.

Where indicated, steps should be taken to correct hypotension or hypovolaemia before commencing therapy.

Particularly careful monitoring is necessary in:

- patients with hypotension.
- patients who are at risk from a pronounced fall in blood pressure.
- patients where latent diabetes may become manifest or the insulin requirements of diabetic patients may increase.
- patients with gout
- patients with hepatorenal syndrome
- patients with hypoproteinaemia, e.g. associated with nephritic syndrome (the effect of furosemide may be weakened and its ototoxicity potentiated). Cautious dose titration is required.
- premature infants (possible development nephrocalcinosis/nephrolithiasis; renal function must be monitored and renal ultrasonography performed).

Caution should be observed in patients liable to electrolyte deficiency. Regular monitoring of serum sodium, potassium and creatinine is generally recommended during furosemide therapy; particularly close monitoring is required in patients at high risk of developing electrolyte imbalances or in case of significant additional fluid loss. Hypovolaemia or dehydration as well as any significant electrolyte and acid-base disturbances must be corrected. This may require temporary discontinuation of furosemide.

In patients who are at high risk for radiocontrast nephropathy, furosemide is not recommended to be used for duiresis as part of the preventative measures against radiocontrast-induced nephropathy.

4.5 Interaction with other medicinal products and other forms of interaction
The dosage of concurrently administered cardiac glycosides, diuretics, anti-hypertensive agents, or other drugs with blood-pressure-lowering potential may require adjustment as a more pronounced fall in blood pressure must be anticipated if given concomitantly with furosemide. A marked fall in blood pressure and deterioration in renal function may be seen when ACE inhibitors or angiotensin II receptor antagonists are added to furosemide therapy, or their dose level increased. The dose of furosemide should be reduced for at least three days, or the drug stopped, before initiating the ACE inhibitor or angiotensin II receptor antagonist or increasing their dose.

The toxic effects of nephrotoxic drugs may be increased by concomitant administration of potent diuretics such as furosemide.

Oral furosemide and sucralfate must not be taken within 2 hours of each other because sucralfate decreases the absorption of furosemide from the intestine and so reduces its effect.

In common with other diuretics, serum lithium levels may be increased when lithium is given concomitantly with furosemide, resulting in increased lithium toxicity, including increased risk of cardiotoxic and neurotoxic effects of lithium. Therefore, it is recommended that lithium levels are carefully monitored and where necessary the lithium dosage is adjusted in patients receiving this combination.

Certain non-steroidal anti-inflammatory agents (e.g. indometacin, acetylsalicylic acid) may attenuate the action of furosemide and may cause acute renal failure in cases of pre-existing hypovolaemia or dehydration. Salicylate toxicity may be increased by furosemide. Furosemide may sometimes attenuate the effects of other drugs (e.g. the effects of anti-diabetics and of pressor amines) and sometimes potentiate them (e.g. the effects of salicylates, theophylline and curare-type muscle relaxants).

Furosemide may potentiate the ototoxicity of aminoglycosides and other ototoxic drugs. Since this may lead to irreversible damage, these drugs must only be used with furosemide if there are compelling medical reasons.

There is a risk of ototoxic effects if cisplatin and furosemide are given concomitantly. In addition, nephrotoxicity of cisplatin may be enhanced if furosemide is not given in low doses (e.g. 40 mg in patients with normal renal function) and with positive fluid balance when used to achieve forced diuresis during cisplatin treatment.

Some electrolyte disturbances (e.g. hypokalaemia, hypomagnesaemia) may increase the toxicity of certain other drugs (e.g. digitalis preparations and drugs inducing QT interval prolongation syndrome).

Attenuation of the effect of furosemide may occur following concurrent administration of phenytoin.

Concomitant administration of carbamazepine or aminoglutethimide may increase the risk of hyponatraemia.

Corticosteroids administered concurrently may cause sodium retention.

Corticosteroids, carbenoxolone, liquorice, B_2 sympathomimetics in large amounts, prolonged use of laxatives, reboxetine and amphotericin may increase the risk of developing hypokalaemia.

Probenecid, methotrexate and other drugs which, like furosemide, undergo significant renal tubular secretion may reduce the effect of furosemide. Conversely, furosemide may decrease renal elimination of these drugs. In case of high-dose treatment (in particular, of both furosemide and the other drugs), this may lead to increased serum levels and an increased risk of adverse effects due to furosemide or the concomitant medication.

Impairment of renal function may develop in patients receiving concurrent treatment with furosemide and high doses of certain cephalosporins

Concomitant use of ciclosporin and furosemide is associated with increased risk of gouty arthritis.

4.6 Pregnancy and lactation
Results of animal work, in general, show no hazardous effect of furosemide in pregnancy. There is clinical evidence of safety of the drug in the third trimester of human pregnancy; however, furosemide crosses the placental barrier. It must not be given during pregnancy unless there are compelling medical reasons. Treatment during pregnancy requires monitoring of foetal growth.

Furosemide passes into breast milk and may inhibit lactation. Women must not breast-feed if they are treated with furosemide.

4.7 Effects on ability to drive and use machines
Reduced mental alertness may impair ability to drive or operate dangerous machinery.

4.8 Undesirable effects
Lasix 20 mg/2 ml Injection is generally well tolerated.

Eosinophilia is rare.

Occasionally, thrombocytopenia may occur. In rare cases, leucopenia and, in isolated cases, agranulocytosis, aplastic anaemia or haemolytic anaemia may develop.

Bone marrow depression has been reported as a rare complication and necessitates withdrawal of treatment.

Rarely, paraesthesiae may occur.

Hepatic encephalopathy in patients with hepatocellular insufficiency may occur (see Section 4.3).

Serum calcium levels may be reduced; in very rare cases tetany has been observed. Nephrocalcinosis / Nephrolithiasis has been reported in premature infants.

Serum cholesterol and triglyceride levels may rise during furosemide treatment. During long term therapy they will usually return to normal within six months.

Glucose tolerance may decrease with furosemide. In patients with diabetes mellitus this may lead to a deterioration of metabolic control; latent diabetes mellitus may become manifest.

Hearing disorders and tinnitus, although usually transitory, may occur in rare cases, particularly in patients with renal failure, hypoproteinaemia (e.g. in nephritic syndrome) and/or when intravenous furosemide has been given too rapidly.

Furosemide may cause a reduction in blood pressure which, if pronounced may cause signs and symptoms such as impairment of concentration and reactions, light-headedness, sensations of pressure in the head, headache, dizziness, drowsiness, weakness, disorders of vision, dry mouth, orthostatic intolerance.

In isolated cases, intrahepatic cholestasis, an increase in liver transaminases or acute pancreatitis may develop.

The incidence of allergic reactions, such as skin rashes, photosensitivity, vasculitis, fever, interstitial nephritis or shock is very low, but when these occur treatment should be withdrawn. Skin and mucous membrane reactions may occasionally occur, e.g. itching, urticaria, other rashes or bullous lesions, erythema multiforme, bullous pemphigoid, exfoliative dermatitis, purpura.

As with other diuretics, electrolytes and water balance may be disturbed as a result of diuresis after prolonged therapy. Furosemide leads to increased excretion of sodium and chloride and consequently water. In addition excretion of other electrolytes (in particular potassium, calcium and magnesium) is increased. Symptomatic electrolyte disturbances and metabolic alkalosis may develop in the form of a gradually increasing electrolyte deficit or, e.g. where higher furosemide doses are administered to patients with normal renal function, acute severe electrolyte losses. Warning signs of electrolyte disturbances include increased thirst, headache, hypotension, confusion, muscle cramps, tetany, muscle weakness, disorders of cardiac rhythm and gastrointestinal symptoms. Pre-existing metabolic alkalosis (e.g. in decompensated cirrhosis of the liver) may be aggravated by furosemide treatment.

The diuretic action of furosemide may lead to or contribute to hypovolaemia and dehydration, especially in elderly patients. Severe fluid depletion may lead to haemoconcentration with a tendency for thromboses to develop.

Increased production of urine may provoke or aggravate complaints in patients with an obstruction of urinary outflow. Thus, acute retention of urine with possible secondary complications may occur, for example, in patients with bladder-emptying disorders, prostatic hyperplasia or narrowing of the urethra.

If furosemide is administered to premature infants during the first weeks of life, it may increase the risk of persistence of patent ductus arteriosus.

Severe anaphylactic or anaphylactoid reactions (e.g. with shock) occur rarely.

Side-effects of a minor nature such as nausea, malaise or gastric upset (vomiting or diarrhoea) may occur but are not usually severe enough to necessitate withdrawal of treatment.

Following intramuscular injection, local reactions such as pain may occur.

As with other diuretics, treatment with furosemide may lead to transitory increases in blood creatinine and urea levels. Serum levels of uric acid may increase and attacks of gout may occur.

4.9 Overdose
The clinical picture in acute or chronic overdose depends primarily on the extent and consequences of electrolyte and fluid loss, e.g. hypovolaemia, dehydration, haemoconcentration, cardiac arrhythmias due to excessive diuresis.

Symptoms of these disturbances include severe hypotension (progressing to shock), acute renal failure, thrombosis, delirious states, flaccid paralysis, apathy and confusion.

Treatment should therefore be aimed at fluid replacement and correction of the electrolyte imbalance. Together with the prevention and treatment of serious complications resulting from such disturbances and of other effects on the body, this corrective action may necessitate general and specific intensive medical monitoring and therapeutic measures.

No specific antidote to furosemide is known. If ingestion has only just taken place, attempts may be made to limit further systemic absorption of the active ingredient by measures such as gastric lavage or those designated to reduce absorption (e.g. activated charcoal).

5. PHARMACOLOGICAL PROPERTIES

5.1 Pharmacodynamic properties

ATC code: CO3C A01

The evidence from many experimental studies suggests that furosemide acts along the entire nephron with the exception of the distal exchange site. The main effect is on the ascending limb of the loop of Henle with a complex effect on renal circulation. Blood-flow is diverted from the juxta-medullary region to the outer cortex. The principle renal action of furosemide is to inhibit active chloride transport in the thick ascending limb. Re-absorption of sodium chloride from the nephron is reduced and a hypotonic or isotonic urine produced. It has been established that prostaglandin (PG) biosynthesis and the renin-angiotensin system are affected by furosemide administration and that furosemide alters the renal permeability of the glomerulus to serum proteins.

5.2 Pharmacokinetic properties

Furosemide is a weak carboxylic acid which exists mainly in the dissociated form in the gastrointestinal tract. Furosemide is rapidly but incompletely absorbed (60-70%) on oral administration and its effect is largely over within 4 hours. The optimal absorption site is the upper duodenum at pH 5.0. Regardless of route of administration 69-97% of activity from a radio-labelled dose is excreted in the first 4 hours after the drug is given. Furosemide is bound to plasma albumin and little biotransformation takes place. Furosemide is mainly eliminated via the kidneys (80-90%); a small fraction of the dose undergoes biliary elimination and 10-15% of the activity can be recovered from the faeces.

In renal/ hepatic impairment

Where liver disease is present, biliary elimination is reduced up to 50%. Renal impairment has little effect on the elimination rate of Lasix 20 mg/2 ml Injection, but less than 20% residual renal function increases the elimination time.

The elderly

The elimination of furosemide is delayed in the elderly where a certain degree of renal impairment is present.

New born

A sustained diuretic effect is seen in the newborn, possibly due to immature tubular function.

5.3 Preclinical safety data

Not applicable

6. PHARMACEUTICAL PARTICULARS

6.1 List of excipients

Sodium hydroxide

Sodium chloride

Water for Injection

6.2 Incompatibilities

Furosemide may precipitate out of solution in fluids of low pH (e.g. dextrose solutions).

6.3 Shelf life

60 months

6.4 Special precautions for storage

Lasix 20 mg/2 ml Injection should be stored protected from light.

6.5 Nature and contents of container

Each pack contains 5x 2ml Lasix 20 mg/2 ml Injection in amber glass ampoules.

6.6 Special precautions for disposal and other handling

Lasix 20 mg/2 ml Injection solution should not be mixed with any other drugs in the injection bottle.

7. MARKETING AUTHORISATION HOLDER

Sanofi-aventis,

One Onslow Street,

Guildford,

Surrey,

GU1 4YS,

UK

8. MARKETING AUTHORISATION NUMBER(S)

PL13402/0035

9. DATE OF FIRST AUTHORISATION/RENEWAL OF THE AUTHORISATION

31 December 1997

10. DATE OF REVISION OF THE TEXT

16th June 2008

Legal category: POM

Laxido Orange, powder for oral solution

(Galen Limited)

1. NAME OF THE MEDICINAL PRODUCT

Laxido Orange, powder for oral solution.

2. QUALITATIVE AND QUANTITATIVE COMPOSITION

Each sachet contains the following quantitative composition of active ingredients:

Macrogol 3350	13.125g
Sodium Chloride	350.7mg
Sodium Hydrogen Carbonate	178.5mg
Potassium Chloride	46.6mg

The content of electrolyte ions per sachet following reconstitution in 125ml of water is equivalent to:

Sodium	65mmol/l
Chloride	53mmol/l
Hydrogen Carbonate (Bicarbonate)	17mmol/l
Potassium	5.4mmol/l

For a full list of excipients, see section 6.1.

3. PHARMACEUTICAL FORM

Powder for oral solution. Single-dose sachet containing a free flowing white powder.

4. CLINICAL PARTICULARS

4.1 Therapeutic indications

For the treatment of chronic constipation. Laxido Orange is also effective in resolving faecal impaction, defined as refractory constipation with faecal loading of the rectum and/or colon.

4.2 Posology and method of administration

Laxido Orange is for oral use.

Chronic Constipation:

A course of treatment for chronic constipation with Laxido Orange does not normally exceed 2 weeks, although this can be repeated if required. As for all laxatives, prolonged use is not usually recommended. Extended use may be necessary in the care of patients with severe chronic or resistant constipation, secondary to multiple sclerosis or Parkinson's Disease, or induced by regular constipating medication in particular opioids and antimuscarinics.

Adults, adolescents and the elderly: 1-3 sachets daily in divided doses, according to individual response. For extended use, the dose can be adjusted down to 1 or 2 sachets daily.

Children below 12 years old: Not recommended.

Faecal Impaction:

A course of treatment for faecal impaction with Laxido Orange does not normally exceed 3 days.

Adults, adolescents and the elderly: 8 sachets daily, all of which should be consumed within a 6 hour period.

Children below 12 years old: Not recommended.

Patients with impaired cardiovascular function: For the treatment of faecal impaction the dose should be divided so that no more than 2 sachets are taken in any one hour.

Patients with renal insufficiency: No dosage change is necessary for the treatment of constipation or faecal impaction.

Administration:

Each sachet should be dissolved in 125 ml water. For use in faecal impaction, 8 sachets may be dissolved in 1 litre of water.

4.3 Contraindications

Laxido Orange is contraindicated in intestinal obstruction or perforation caused by functional or structural disorder of the gut wall, ileus and in patients with severe inflammatory conditions of the intestinal tract (e.g. ulcerative colitis, Crohn's disease and toxic megacolon).

Hypersensitivity to the active substances or any of the excipients.

4.4 Special warnings and precautions for use

The faecal impaction diagnosis should be confirmed by appropriate physical or radiological examination of the rectum and abdomen.

Mild adverse drug reactions are possible as indicated in Section 4.8. If patients develop any symptoms indicating shifts of fluids/electrolytes (e.g. oedema, shortness of breath, increasing fatigue, dehydration, cardiac failure) Laxido Orange should be stopped immediately and electrolytes measured and any abnormality should be treated appropriately.

The orange flavour in Laxido Orange contains glucose. Patients with rare glucose-galactose malabsorption should not take this medicine. The orange flavour also contains sulphur dioxide (E220), which may rarely cause severe hypersensitivity reactions and bronchospasm.

4.5 Interaction with other medicinal products and other forms of interaction

There are no known interactions of Laxido Orange with other medicinal products. However, macrogol 3350 raises the solubility of medicinal products that are soluble in alcohol and mainly insoluble in water. It is a theoretical possibility that absorption of these drugs could be reduced transiently. Therefore, other medicines should not be taken orally for one hour before and for one hour after taking Laxido Orange.

4.6 Pregnancy and lactation

There is no experience with the use of Laxido Orange during pregnancy and lactation and it should not be used during pregnancy and lactation unless clearly necessary.

4.7 Effects on ability to drive and use machines

Laxido Orange has no influence on the ability to drive and use machines.

4.8 Undesirable effects

Immune System Disorders:

Allergic reactions are possible.

Gastro-intestinal Disorders:

Potential gastro-intestinal effects that may occur include abdominal distension and pain, borborygmi and nausea. Mild diarrhoea may also occur, but normally resolves after dose reduction.

4.9 Overdose

Severe distension or pain can be treated using nasogastric aspiration. Vomiting or diarrhoea may induce extensive fluid loss, possibly leading to electrolyte disturbances that should be treated appropriately.

5. PHARMACOLOGICAL PROPERTIES

5.1 Pharmacodynamic properties

Pharmacotherapeutic group: Osmotically acting laxatives.

ATC code: A06A D65

Macrogol 3350 induces a laxative effect through its osmotic action in the gut. This product also contains electrolytes to ensure that there is no overall gain or loss of water, potassium or sodium.

Clinical studies using the listed active substances for the treatment of chronic constipation have shown that the dose required to produce normally formed stools tends to decrease over time. For most patients, the maintenance dose will be one to two sachets per day (adjusted according to individual response).

Comparative studies in faecal impaction using active controls (e.g. enemas) have not been performed. However, results from a non-comparative study have shown that, from a population of 27 adult patients, the listed combination of active substances cleared faecal impaction in 12/27 (44%) patients after one day's treatment, increasing to 23/27 (85%) following two days' treatment and 24/27 (89%) recovered at the end of three days.

5.2 Pharmacokinetic properties

Macrogol 3350 is virtually unabsorbed from the gastro-intestinal tract and is excreted, unaltered, in faeces. Any macrogol 3350 that enters the systemic circulation is excreted in urine.

5.3 Preclinical safety data

Preclinical studies provide evidence that macrogol 3350 has no significant systemic toxicity potential, although no tests of its effects on reproduction or genotoxicity have been conducted.

There are no long-term animal toxicity or carcinogenicity studies involving macrogol 3350, although there are toxicity studies using high levels of orally administered high-molecular weight macrogols that provide evidence of safety at the recommended therapeutic dose.

6. PHARMACEUTICAL PARTICULARS

6.1 List of excipients

Acesulfame Potassium (E950)

Orange Flavour

(Orange flavour contains the following constituents: natural flavouring substances and preparations, glucose, maltodextrin and sulphur dioxide [E220])

6.2 Incompatibilities

Not applicable.

6.3 Shelf life

Sachet: Two years.

Reconstituted solution: Six hours.

6.4 Special precautions for storage

Sachet: Store below 25°C.

Reconstituted solution: Store covered in a refrigerator (2°C to 8°C).

6.5 Nature and contents of container

The sachet is composed of paper, low density polyethylene and aluminium.

Sachets are packed in cartons of 2, 8, 10, 20, 30, 50 and 100.

Not all pack sizes may be marketed.

6.6 Special precautions for disposal and other handling

No special requirements.

7. MARKETING AUTHORISATION HOLDER

Galen Limited
Seagoe Industrial Estate
Craigavon
BT63 5UA
UK

8. MARKETING AUTHORISATION NUMBER(S)

PL 21590/0087.

9. DATE OF FIRST AUTHORISATION/RENEWAL OF THE AUTHORISATION

01 May 2008.

10. DATE OF REVISION OF THE TEXT

10 November 2008

Leukeran Tablets 2mg

(GlaxoSmithKline UK)

1. NAME OF THE MEDICINAL PRODUCT

Leukeran Tablets 2 mg

2. QUALITATIVE AND QUANTITATIVE COMPOSITION

Each tablet contains 2 mg of the active ingredient chlorambucil.

3. PHARMACEUTICAL FORM

Film-coated tablet

4. CLINICAL PARTICULARS

4.1 Therapeutic indications

Leukeran is indicated in the treatment of Hodgkin's disease, certain forms of non-Hodgkin's lymphoma, chronic lymphocytic leukaemia, and Waldenstrom's macroglobulinaemia.

4.2 Posology and method of administration

Adults:

Hodgkin's Disease: Used as a single agent in the palliative treatment of advanced disease a typical dosage is 0.2 mg/kg/day for 4-8 weeks. Leukeran is usually included in combination therapy and a number of regimes have been used. Leukeran has been used as an alternative to nitrogen mustard with a reduction in toxicity but similar therapeutic results.

Non-Hodgkin's Lymphoma: Used as a single agent the usual dosage is 0.1-0.2 mg/kg/day for 4-8 weeks initially, maintenance therapy is then given either by a reduced daily dosage or intermittent courses of treatment. Leukeran is useful in the management of patients with advanced diffuse lymphocytic lymphoma and those who have relapsed after radiotherapy. There is no significant difference in the overall response rate obtained with chlorambucil as a single agent and combination chemotherapy in patients with advanced non-Hodgkin's lymphocytic lymphoma.

Chronic Lymphocytic Leukaemia: Treatment with Leukeran is usually started after the patient has developed symptoms or when there is evidence of impaired bone marrow function (but not bone marrow failure) as indicated by the peripheral blood count. Initially Leukeran is given at a dosage of 0.15 mg/kg/day until the total leucocyte count has fallen to 10,000 per μL. Treatment may be resumed 4 weeks after the end of the first course and continued at a dosage of 0.1 mg/kg/day.

In a proportion of patients, usually after about 2 years of treatment, the blood leucocyte count is reduced to the normal range, enlarged spleen and lymph nodes become impalpable and the proportion of lymphocytes in the bone marrow is reduced to less than 20 per cent. Patients with evidence of bone marrow failure should first be treated with prednisolone and evidence of marrow regeneration should be obtained before commencing treatment with Leukeran. Intermittent high dose therapy has been compared with daily Leukeran but no significant difference in therapeutic response or frequency of side effects was observed between the two treatment groups.

Waldenstrom's Macroglobulinaemia: Leukeran is the treatment of choice in this indication. Starting doses of 6-12 mg daily until leucopenia occurs are recommended followed by 2-8 mg daily indefinitely.

Children:

Leukeran may be used in the management of Hodgkin's disease and non-Hodgkin's lymphomas in children. The dosage regimes are similar to those used in adults.

Use in the Elderly:

No specific studies have been carried out in the elderly, however, it may be advisable to monitor renal or hepatic function and if there is serious impairment then caution should be exercised.

4.3 Contraindications

Hypersensitivity to chlorambucil or to any of the excipients.

4.4 Special warnings and precautions for use

Continued treatment with chlorambucil should be assessed if a rash develops since there have been reports of Stevens-Johnson Syndrome in patients receiving chlorambucil (see section 4.8).

Leukeran is an active cytotoxic agent for use only under the direction of physicians experienced in the administration of such agents.

Safe Handling of Leukeran tablets:

See 6.6 Instructions for Use/Handling

Immunisation using a live organism vaccine has the potential to cause infection in immunocompromised hosts. Therefore, immunisations with live organism vaccines are not recommended.

Monitoring: Since Leukeran is capable of producing irreversible bone marrow suppression, blood counts should be closely monitored in patients under treatment.

At therapeutic dosage Leukeran depresses lymphocytes and has less effect on neutrophil and platelet counts and on haemoglobin levels. Discontinuation of Leukeran is not necessary at the first sign of a fall in neutrophils but it must be remembered that the fall may continue for 10 days or more after the last dose.

Leukeran should not be given to patients who have recently undergone radiotherapy or received other cytotoxic agents.

When lymphocytic infiltration of the bone marrow is present or the bone marrow is hypoplastic, the daily dose should not exceed 0.1 mg/kg body weight.

Children with nephrotic syndrome, patients prescribed high pulse dosing regimens and patients with a history of seizure disorder, should be closely monitored following administration of Leukeran, as they may have an increased risk of seizures.

Renal impairment:

Patients with evidence of impaired renal function should be carefully monitored as they are prone to additional myelosuppression associated with azotaemia.

Hepatic impairment:

The metabolism of Leukeran is still under investigation and consideration should be given to dose reduction in patients with gross hepatic dysfunction.

Mutagenicity and Carcinogenicity:

Leukeran has been shown to cause chromatid or chromosome damage in man.

Development of acute leukaemia after Leukeran therapy for chronic lymphocytic leukaemia has been reported. However, it was not clear whether the acute leukaemia was part of the natural history of the disease or if the chemotherapy was the cause.

A comparison of patients with ovarian cancer who received alkylating agents with those who did not, showed that the use of alkylating agents, including Leukeran, significantly increased the incidence of acute leukaemia.

Acute myelogenous leukaemia has been reported in a small proportion of patients receiving Leukeran as long term adjuvant therapy for breast cancer.

The leukaemogenic risk must be balanced against the potential therapeutic benefit when considering the use of Leukeran.

Sugar intolerances:

Patients with rare hereditary problems of glucose intolerance, the Lapp lactase deficiency or glucose-galactose malabsorption should not take this medication. Each Leukeran 2mg tablet contains 68mg of lactose.

4.5 Interaction with other medicinal products and other forms of interaction

Vaccinations with live organism vaccines are not recommended in immunocompromised individuals (see Section 4.4 Special Warnings and Precautions for use).

Patients receiving phenylbutazone may require a reduced dose of Leukeran.

4.6 Pregnancy and lactation

As with other cytotoxic agents Leukeran is potentially teratogenic. The use of Leukeran should be avoided whenever possible during pregnancy, particularly during the first trimester. In any individual case, the potential hazard to the foetus must be balanced against the expected benefit to the mother.

As with all cytotoxic chemotherapy, adequate contraceptive precautions should be advised when either partner is receiving Leukeran.

Mothers receiving Leukeran should not breast feed.

4.7 Effects on ability to drive and use machines

None known

4.8 Undesirable effects

For this product there is no modern clinical documentation which can be used as support for determining the frequency of undesirable effects. Undesirable effects may vary in their incidence depending on the dose received and also when given in combination with other therapeutic agents.

The following convention has been utilised for the classification of frequency: Very common ($\geqslant$1/10), common ($\geqslant$1/100 and $<$1/10), uncommon ($\geqslant$1/1000 and $<$1/100), rare ($\geqslant$1/10,000 and $<$1/1000) and very rare ($<$1/10,000).

Blood and lymphatic system disorders

Very common:	Leucopenia, neutropenia, thrombocytopenia, pancytopenia or bone marrow suppression.
Common:	Anaemia.
Very rare:	Irreversible bone marrow failure.

Although bone marrow suppression frequently occurs, it is usually reversible if Leukeran is withdrawn early enough.

Immune system disorders

Uncommon:	Rash.
Rare:	Allergic reactions such as urticaria and angioneurotic oedema following initial or subsequent dosing. Stevens-Johnson syndrome and toxic epidermal necrolysis. (See Skin and subcutaneous tissue disorders)

On rare occasions skin rash has been reported to progress to serious conditions including Stevens-Johnson Syndrome and toxic epidermal necrolysis.

Nervous system disorders

Common:	Seizures in children with nephrotic syndrome.
Rare:	Seizures#, focal and/or generalised in children and adults receiving therapeutic daily doses or high pulse dosing regimens of chlorambucil.
Very rare:	Movement disorders including tremor, twitching and myoclonia in the absence of convulsions. Peripheral neuropathy.
	#Patients with a history of seizure disorder may be particularly susceptible.

Respiratory, thoracic and mediastinal disorders

Very rare:	Interstitial pulmonary fibrosis, interstitial pneumonia.

Severe interstitial pulmonary fibrosis has occasionally been reported in patients with chronic lymphocytic leukaemia on long-term Leukeran therapy. However, this may be reversible on withdrawal of Leukeran.

Gastrointestinal disorders

Common:	Gastro-intestinal disturbances such as nausea and vomiting, diarrhoea and oral ulceration.

Hepatobiliary disorders

Rare:	Hepatoxicity, jaundice.

Skin and subcutaneous tissue disorders

Uncommon:	Rash.
Rare:	Allergic reactions such as urticaria and angioneurotic oedema following initial or subsequent dosing. Stevens-Johnson syndrome and toxic epidermal necrolysis. (See Immune system disorders) On rare occasions skin rash has been reported to progress to serious conditions including Stevens-Johnson syndrome and toxic epidermal necrolysis.

Renal and urinary disorders

Very rare:	Sterile cystitis.

General disorders and administration site conditions

Rare:	Drug fever.

4.9 Overdose

Reversible pancytopenia was the main finding of inadvertent overdoses of Leukeran. Neurological toxicity ranging from agitated behaviour and ataxia to multiple grand mal seizures has also occurred. As there is no known antidote the blood picture should be closely monitored and general supportive measures should be instituted, together with appropriate blood transfusion if necessary.

5. PHARMACOLOGICAL PROPERTIES

5.1 Pharmacodynamic properties

Chlorambucil is an aromatic nitrogen mustard derivative which acts as a bifunctional alkylating agent. Alkylation takes place through the formation of a highly reactive ethylenimonium radical. A probable mode of action involves cross-linkage of the ethylenimonium derivative between 2 strands of helical DNA and subsequent interference with replication.

5.2 Pharmacokinetic properties

In a study of 12 patients administered chlorambucil 0.2 mg/kg body weight orally, the mean dose adjusted maximum plasma concentration (492 ± 160 ng/ml) occurred between 0.25 and 2 hours after administration. The mean (± SD) terminal plasma elimination half-life was 1.3 ± 0.5 hours.

After oral administration of [^{14}C]-chlorambucil, maximum plasma radioactivity occurs between 40 and 70 minutes later. Studies have shown that chlorambucil disappears from the plasma with a mean terminal phase life of 1.5 hours and that its urinary excretion is low. A high level of urinary radioactivity after oral or intravenous administration of [^{14}C]-chlorambucil indicates that the drug is well absorbed after oral dosage.

The metabolism of chlorambucil in man appears to be similar to that in laboratory animals and involves S-oxidation of the butyric acid side chain. Bis-2-chlorethyl-2 (4-aminophenyl) acetic acid [phenylacetic acid mustard

(PAAM)] is a major metabolite of chlorambucil. In a study of 12 patients administered chlorambucil 0.2 mg/kg body weight orally, the mean dose adjusted-peak plasma concentration of PAAM (306 ± 73 ng/ml) was reached within 1 - 3 hours. The mean terminal elimination plasma half-life was 1.8 ± 0.4 hours. The significant contribution of PAAM to the alkylating activity of the drug was evident as the mean area under the plasma concentration time curve (AUC) of PAAM was approximately 1.33 times greater than the AUC of chlorambucil.

5.3 Preclinical safety data

Mutagenicity and Carcinogenicity

As with other cytotoxic agents chlorambucil is mutagenic in *in vitro* and *in vivo* genotoxicity tests and carcinogenic in animals and humans.

Teratogenicity

See information under 'Pregnancy and Lactation' section.

Chlorambucil has been shown to induce skeletal abnormalities in the embryos of mice and rats following a single oral administration of 4-20 mg/kg. Chlorambucil has also been shown to induce renal abnormalities in the offspring of rats following a single intraperitoneal injection of 3-6 mg/kg.

Effects on fertility

Leukeran may cause suppression of ovarian function and amenorrhoea has been reported following Leukeran therapy.

Azoospermia has been observed as a result of therapy with Leukeran although it is estimated that a total dose of at least 400 mg is necessary.

Varying degrees of recovery of spermatogenesis have been reported in patients with lymphoma following treatment with Leukeran in total doses of 400-2600 mg.

In rats, chlorambucil has been shown to damage spermatogenesis and cause testicular atrophy.

6. PHARMACEUTICAL PARTICULARS

6.1 List of excipients

Tablet Core:

Microcrystalline cellulose

Anhydrous lactose

Colloidal anhydrous silica

Stearic acid

Tablet Film Coating:

Hypromellose

Titanium dioxide

Synthetic yellow iron oxide

Synthetic red iron oxide

Macrogol

6.2 Incompatibilities

None known.

6.3 Shelf life

3 years.

6.4 Special precautions for storage

Store at 2°C - 8°C.

6.5 Nature and contents of container

Leukeran are brown film-coated, round, biconvex tablets engraved "GX EG3" on one side and "L" on the other, supplied in amber glass bottles with a child resistant closure containing 25 tablets.

6.6 Special precautions for disposal and other handling

Leukeran is an active cytotoxic agent for use only under the direction of physicians experienced in the administration of such agents.

Safe handling of Leukeran Tablets: The handling of Leukeran Tablets should follow guidelines for the handling of cytotoxic drugs according to prevailing local recommendations and/or regulations (for example, Royal Pharmaceutical Society of Great Britain Working Party on the Handling of Cytotoxic Drugs).

Provided that the outer coating of the tablet is intact, there is no risk in handling Leukeran Tablets. Leukeran Tablets should not be divided.

Administrative Data

7. MARKETING AUTHORISATION HOLDER

The Wellcome Foundation Ltd

Glaxo Wellcome House

Berkeley Avenue

Greenford

Middlesex

trading as

GlaxoSmithKline UK

Stockley Park West

Uxbridge

Middlesex UB11 1BT

8. MARKETING AUTHORISATION NUMBER(S)

PL 00003/5264R

9. DATE OF FIRST AUTHORISATION/RENEWAL OF THE AUTHORISATION

6 July 1995

10. DATE OF REVISION OF THE TEXT

02 August 2007

11. Legal Status

POM

Leustat Injection.

(Janssen-Cilag Ltd)

1. NAME OF THE MEDICINAL PRODUCT

Leustat Injection.

2. QUALITATIVE AND QUANTITATIVE COMPOSITION

LEUSTAT (cladribine) Injection is a synthetic antineoplastic agent for continuous intravenous infusion. It is a clear, colourless, sterile, preservative-free, isotonic solution. LEUSTAT Injection is available in single-use vials containing 10 mg (1 mg/ml) of cladribine, a chlorinated purine nucleoside analogue. Each millilitre of LEUSTAT Injection contains 1 mg of the active ingredient, cladribine, and 9 mg (0.15 mEq) of sodium chloride as an inactive ingredient. The solution has pH range of 5.5 to 8.0. Phosphoric acid and/or dibasic sodium phosphate may have been added to adjust the pH.

3. PHARMACEUTICAL FORM

A sterile, buffered solution in vials containing 10 mg (1 mg/ml) of cladribine for dilution and subsequent continuous intravenous infusion.

4. CLINICAL PARTICULARS

4.1 Therapeutic indications

LEUSTAT Injection is indicated for the primary or secondary treatment of patients with Hairy Cell Leukaemia (HCL).

LEUSTAT is also indicated for the treatment of patients with B-cell chronic lymphocytic leukaemia (CLL) who have not responded to, or whose disease has progressed during or after, treatment with at least one standard alkylating-agent-containing regimen.

4.2 Posology and method of administration

Usual dose:

Adults and elderly:

HCL: The recommended treatment for Hairy Cell Leukaemia is a single course of LEUSTAT given by continuous intravenous infusion for 7 consecutive days at a dose of 0.09 mg/kg/day (3.6 mg/m^2/day). Deviations from this dosage regimen are not advised. Physicians should consider delaying or discontinuing the drug if neurotoxicity or renal toxicity occurs.

CLL: In patients with CLL, the recommended treatment consists of a continuous intravenous infusion of LEUSTAT for 2 hours on days 1 to 5 of a 28 day cycle at a dose of 0.12 mg/kg/day (4.8 mg/m^2/day). The patient's response to therapy should be determined every two cycles of treatment. It is recommended that LEUSTAT Injection be administered in responding patients for 2 cycles after maximum response has occurred, up to a maximum of 6 cycles. Therapy should be discontinued after 2 cycles in non-responding patients. Response for this treatment decision is defined as a lymphocyte reduction of 50% or more, ie if lymphocyte count decreases by 50% or more, administer 2 more cycles and re-evaluate response for decision whether to continue with 2 more cycles up to a maximum of 6 cycles.

Children:

Safety and efficacy in children have not been established.

Specific risk factors predisposing to increased toxicity from LEUSTAT have not been defined. In view of the known toxicities of agents of this class, it would be prudent to proceed carefully in patients with known or suspected renal insufficiency or severe bone marrow impairment of any aetiology. Patients should be monitored closely for haematological and renal and hepatic toxicity.

Preparation and administration of intravenous solutions:

LEUSTAT Injection must be diluted with the designated diluent prior to administration. Since the product does not contain any anti-microbial preservative or bacteriostatic agent, aseptic technique and proper environmental precautions must be observed in preparation of a solution of LEUSTAT. For full details concerning preparation of an infusion solution, see 6.6 Instructions for Use/Handling.

4.3 Contraindications

LEUSTAT Injection is contra-indicated in those patients who are hypersensitive to this drug or any of its components. LEUSTAT is contra-indicated in pregnant women and nursing mothers.

4.4 Special warnings and precautions for use

LEUSTAT Injection is a potent antineoplastic agent with potentially significant toxic side effects. It should be administered under the supervision of a qualified physician experienced in the use of antineoplastic therapy.

CLL: The weight of evidence suggests that a patient whose disease has progressed while treated with fludarabine is unlikely to respond to treatment with LEUSTAT Injection and therefore use in such a patient is not recommended.

Patients should be monitored closely for infections. Patients with active infection should be treated for the underlying condition prior to receiving therapy with LEUSTAT Injection. Patients who are or who become Coombs' positive should be monitored carefully for occurrence of haemolysis.

Patients with high tumour burden or who are considered at risk for the development of hyperuricaemia as a result of tumour breakdown should receive appropriate prophylactic treatment.

4.4.1 Bone Marrow Suppression:

Suppression of bone marrow function should be anticipated. This is usually reversible and appears to be dose dependent. Severe bone marrow suppression, including neutropenia, anaemia and thrombocytopenia, has been commonly observed in patients treated with LEUSTAT, especially at high doses. At initiation of treatment, most patients in the clinical studies had haematological impairment as a manifestation of active Hairy Cell Leukaemia or Chronic Lymphocytic Leukaemia. Following treatment with LEUSTAT, further haematological impairment occurred before recovery of peripheral blood counts began. Proceed carefully in patients with severe bone marrow impairment of any aetiology since further suppression of bone marrow function should be anticipated.

HCL: During the first two weeks after treatment initiation, mean platelet count, absolute neutrophil count (ANC), and haemoglobin concentration declined and then subsequently increased with normalisation of mean counts by day 15, week 5 and week 8, respectively. The myelosuppressive effects of LEUSTAT were most notable during the first month following treatment. Forty three percent (43%) of patients received transfusions with RBCs and 13% received transfusions with platelets during month 1. Careful haematological monitoring, especially during the first 4 to 8 weeks after treatment with LEUSTAT is recommended. (See 4.8, Undesirable Effects).

CLL: During the first 2 cycles of therapy with LEUSTAT Injection, haemoglobin concentration, platelet count and absolute neutrophil count declined to a nadir usually observed in Cycle 2. There appeared to be no cumulative toxicity upon administration of further cycles of therapy. Careful haematological monitoring is recommended throughout administration of LEUSTAT Injection.

4.4.2 Neurotoxicity:

Serious neurological toxicity (including irreversible paraparesis and quadraparesis) has been reported in patients who received LEUSTAT Injection by continuous infusion at high doses (4 to 9 times the recommended dose for hairy cell leukaemia). Neurological toxicity appears to demonstrate a dose relationship; however, severe neurological toxicities have been reported rarely with the recommended dose. Physicians should consider delaying or discontinuing therapy if neurotoxicity occurs.

4.4.3 Fever/Infection:

HCL: Fever (temperature greater than or equal to 37.8°C) was associated with the use of LEUSTAT in approximately 72% (89/124) of patients. Most febrile episodes occurred during the first month. Although seventy percent (70%) of patients were treated empirically with parenteral antibiotics, less than a third of febrile events were associated with documented infection.

CLL: Pyrexia was reported in 22-24% of CLL patients during Cycle 1 of therapy with LEUSTAT Injection, and in less than 3% of patients during subsequent cycles. Forty of 123 patients (32.5%) reported at least one infection during Cycle 1. Infections that occurred in 5% or more were: respiratory infection/inflammation (8.9%), pneumonia (7.3%), bacterial infection (5.7%), and viral skin infections (5.7%). Approximately 70% of patients had at least one infection during the overall study period of 6 years, including treatment and follow-up.

Since the majority of fevers occurred in neutropenic patients, patients should be closely monitored during the first month of treatment and empirical antibiotics should be initiated as clinically indicated. Given the known myelosuppressive effects of LEUSTAT, practitioners should carefully evaluate the risks and benefits of administering this drug to patients with active infections. Since fever may be accompanied by increased fluid loss, patients should be kept well hydrated (See 4.8, Undesirable effects).

4.4.4

Rare cases of tumour lysis syndrome have been reported in patients with haematological malignancies having a high tumour burden.

4.4.5 Effect on Renal and Hepatic Function:

Acute renal insufficiency has developed in some patients receiving high doses of LEUSTAT. In addition, there are inadequate data on dosing of patients with renal or hepatic insufficiency. Until more information is available, caution is advised when administering the drug to patients with known or suspected renal or hepatic insufficiency. All patients should have their renal and hepatic function monitored regularly. (See 4.8.1.4, Effects of High Doses).

4.4.6

LEUSTAT Injection must be diluted in a designated intravenous solution prior to administration (See 6.6, Instructions for Use/Handling for full details concerning preparation of an infusion solution).

4.4.7 Laboratory Tests:

During and following treatment, the patient's haematological profile should be monitored regularly to determine the degree of haematopoietic suppression. In HCL patients, bone marrow aspiration and biopsy should be performed to confirm response to treatment with LEUSTAT after peripheral counts have normalised. Febrile events should be investigated with appropriate laboratory and radiological studies. As with other potent chemotherapeutic agents, monitoring of renal and hepatic function should be performed as clinically indicated, especially in patients with underlying kidney or liver dysfunction.

4.4.8 Carcinogenesis/Mutagenesis:

Please refer to section 5.3: Preclinical Safety Data

4.4.9 Impairment of Fertility:

When administered intravenously to Cynomolgus monkeys, LEUSTAT (cladribine) has been shown to cause suppression of rapidly generating cells, including testicular cells. The effect on human fertility is unknown.

4.4.10 Extravasation:

Should the drug accidentally be given extravenously, local tissue damage is unlikely. If extravasation occurs, the administration should be stopped immediately and restarted in another vein. Other recommended local measures include elevating the arm and applying an ice pack to reduce swelling.

4.5 Interaction with other medicinal products and other forms of interaction

Caution should be exercised if LEUSTAT Injection is administered following or in conjunction with other drugs known to cause myelosuppression. Following administration of LEUSTAT Injection, caution should be exercised before administering other immunosuppressive or myelosuppressive therapy. (See 4.4.1 and 4.8.1.2 Bone Marrow Suppression).

4.6 Pregnancy and lactation

LEUSTAT Injection is teratogenic in mice and rabbits and consequently has the potential to cause foetal harm when administered to a pregnant woman. There are no human data, but LEUSTAT Injection is contra-indicated in pregnancy.

A significant increase in foetal variations was observed in mice receiving 1.5 mg/kg/day (4.5 mg/m^2) and increased resorptions, reduced litter size and increased foetal malformations were observed when mice received 3.0 mg/kg/day (9 mg/m^2). Foetal death and malformations were observed in rabbits that received 3.0 mg/kg/day (33.0 mg/m^2). No foetal effects were seen in mice at 0.5 mg/kg/day (1.5 mg/m^2) or in rabbits at 1.0 mg/kg/day (11.0 mg/m^2).

Although there is no evidence of teratogenicity in humans due to LEUSTAT, other drugs which inhibit DNA synthesis (eg methotrexate and aminopterin) have been reported to be teratogenic in humans. LEUSTAT has been shown to be embryotoxic in mice when given at doses equivalent to the recommended dose.

It is not known whether this drug is excreted in human milk. Because it may be excreted in human milk and because there is potential for serious adverse reactions in nursing infants, LEUSTAT should not be given to a nursing mother.

4.7 Effects on ability to drive and use machines

Given the patients underlying medical condition and the safety profile of LEUSTAT Injection, caution should be exercised when a patient is performing activities requiring substantial physical well-being (See 4.8, Undesirable Effects).

4.8 Undesirable effects

4.8.1 Clinical Trial Experience

4.8.1.1 Overview:

HCL: The following safety data are based on 124 patients with HCL enrolled in the pivotal studies. Severe neutropenia was noted in 70% of patients in month 1; fever in 72% at anytime; and infection was documented in 31% of patients in month 1. Other adverse experiences reported frequently during the first 14 days after initiating treatment included: fatigue (49%), nausea (29%), rash (31%), headache (23%) and decreased appetite (23%). Most non-haematological adverse experiences were mild to moderate in severity.

During the first 14 days, events reported by greater than 5% but less than 20% of patients included:

Body as a whole:	Chills (13%), asthenia (11%), diaphoresis (11%), malaise (8%), trunk pain (7%).
Gastro-intestinal:	Vomiting (14%), constipation (14%), diarrhoea (12%), abdominal pain (8%), flatulence (7%).
Haemic/Lymphatic:	Purpura (12%), petechia (9%).
Nervous System:	Dizziness (13%), insomnia (8%), anxiety (7%).
Cardiovascular System:	Oedema (8%), tachycardia (8%), heart murmur (7%).
Respiratory System:	Abnormal breath sounds (14%), cough (12%), abnormal chest sounds (12%), shortness of breath (7%).
Skin/Subcutaneous Tissue:	Injection site reaction (15%), pruritus (9%), pain (9%), erythema (8%).
Musculoskeletal System:	Myalgia (8%).

Injection site reactions (ie redness, swelling, pain), thrombosis and phlebitis appear usually to be related to the infusion procedure and/or indwelling catheter, rather than to the medication or the vehicle.

From day 15 to the last day of follow-up, the following effects were reported in greater than 5% of patients: fatigue (14%), rash (10%), headache (7%), oedema (7%), arthralgia (7%), malaise (6%), diaphoresis (6%).

<u>CLL</u>: The following safety data are based on 124 patients with CLL enrolled in an open-label safety study. Haematological parameters declined during Cycle 1 and Cycle 2, reaching nadir values in Cycle 2; the percentage of patients having a haemoglobin level below 8.5 g/dL in Cycle 2 was 46.1%. The percentage of patients with platelet counts below 20 × 10(9)/L was 22.5% during Cycle 2. Absolute neutrophil count was below 500 × 10(6)/L in 61.8% of patients in Cycle 2. Adverse experiences reported frequently during the first 14 days after initiating treatment included: skin reaction at the injection site (22.8%), pyrexia (17.9%), fatigue (16.3%), oedema (13.8%), headache (13.0%), cough (11.4%), purpura (10.6%), diaphoresis (8.9%), diarrhoea (7.3%), nausea (6.5%), coagulation defect (6.5%), abnormal breath sounds (5.7%), pneumonia (5.7%), and abnormal chest sounds (5.7%). Adverse experiences that occurred in 5% or more of patients during the remainder of follow-up for Cycle 1 were: pyrexia (6.7%), and preterminal events (6.7%). Drug-related adverse experiences reported during cycles of therapy subsequent to Cycle 1 were limited to the following: skin reaction at medication site (22.8%), phlebitis (5.0%), bacterial skin infection (2.0%), cellulitis (1.0%), nausea (1.0%), skin pain (1.0%), and bacterial infection (1.0%). Skin reactions at the injection site were felt to be more likely related to the indwelling IV catheter and not study drug related. LEUSTAT Injection was not associated with renal or hepatic toxicities.

4.8.1.2 Bone Marrow Suppression:

HCL: Myelosuppression was frequently observed during the first month after starting treatment with LEUSTAT Injection. Neutropenia (ANC less than 500 × 10^6/L) was noted in 69% of patients, compared with 25% in whom it was present initially. Severe anaemia (haemoglobin less than 8.5 g/dL) occurred in 41.1% of patients, compared with 12% initially and thrombocytopenia (platelets less than 20 × 10^9/L) occurred in 15% of patients, compared to 5% in whom it was noted initially.

Analysis of lymphocyte subsets indicates that treatment with cladribine is associated with prolonged depression of the CD4 counts. Prior to treatment, the mean CD4 count was 766/µl. The mean CD4 count nadir, which occurred 4 to 6 months following treatment, was 272/µl. Fifteen (15) months after treatment, mean CD4 counts remained below 500/µl. CD8 counts behaved similarly, though increasing counts were observed after 9 months. There were no serious opportunistic infections reported during this time. The clinical significance of the prolonged CD4 lymphopenia is unclear.

Prolonged bone marrow hypocellularity (< 35%) was observed. It is not known whether the hypocellularity is the result of disease related marrow fibrosis or LEUSTAT Injection toxicity.

<u>CLL</u>: Patients with CLL treated with LEUSTAT Injection were more severely myelosuppressed prior to therapy than HCL patients; increased myelo-suppression was observed during Cycle 1 and Cycle 2 of therapy, reaching a nadir during Cycle 2. The percentage of patients having a haemoglobin level below 8.5 g/dL was 16.9% at baseline, 37.9% in Cycle 1, and 46.1% in Cycle 2. The percentage of patients with platelet counts below 20 × 10(9)/L was 4.0% at baseline, 20.2% during Cycle 1, and 22.5% during Cycle 2. Absolute neutrophil count was below 500 × 10(6)/L in 19.0% of patients at baseline, 56.5% in Cycle 1, 61.8% in Cycle 2, 59.3% in Cycle 3 and 55.9% in Cycle 4. There appeared to be no cumulative toxicity upon administration of multiple cycles of therapy. Marked blood chemistry abnormalities noted during the study were pre-existing, or were isolated abnormalities which resolved, or were associated with death due to the underlying disease.

4.8.1.3 Fever/Infection:

HCL: As with other agents having known immunosuppressive effects, opportunistic infections have occurred in the acute phase of treatment due to the immunosuppression mediated by cladribine. Fever was a frequently observed side effect during the first month of study.

During the first month, 12% of patients experienced severe fever (ie greater than or equal to 40°C). Documented infections were noted in fewer than one-third of all febrile episodes. Of the 124 patients treated, 11 were noted to have a documented infection in the month prior to treatment. In the month following treatment, 31% of patients had a documented infection: 13.7% of patients had bacterial infection, 6.5% had viral and 6.5% had fungal infections. Seventy percent (70%) of these patients were treated empirically with antibiotics.

During the first month, serious infections (eg septicaemia, pneumonia), were reported in 7% of all patients; the remainder were mild or moderate. During the second month, the overall rate of documented infection was 8%; these infections were mild to moderate and no severe systemic infections were seen. After the third month, the monthly incidence of infection was either less than or equal to that of the months immediately preceding LEUSTAT therapy.

CLL: During Cycle 1, 23.6% of patients experienced pyrexia, and 32.5% experienced at least one documented infection. Infections that occurred in 5% or more of the patients during Cycle 1 were: respiratory infection/inflammation (8.9%), pneumonia (7.3%), bacterial infection (5.6%), and viral skin infections (5.7%). In Cycles 2 through 9, 71.3% of the patients had at least one infection. Infections that occurred in 10% or more of patients were: pneumonia (28.7%), bacterial infection (21.8%), viral skin infection (20.8%), upper respiratory infection (12.9%), other intestinal infection/inflammation (12.9%), oral candidiasis (11.9%), urinary tract infection (11.9%), and other skin infections (11.9%). Overall, 72.4% of the patients had at least one infection during therapy with LEUSTAT Injection. Of these, 32.6% had been administered concomitant immunosuppressive therapy (prednisone).

4.8.1.4 Effects of High Doses:

In a Phase 1 study with 31 patients in which LEUSTAT Injection was administered at high doses (4 to 9 times that recommended for hairy cell leukaemia) for 7-14 days in conjunction with cyclophosphamide and total body irradiation as preparation for bone marrow transplantation, acute nephrotoxicity, delayed onset neurotoxicity, severe bone marrow suppression with neutropenia, anaemia, and thrombocytopenia and gastro-intestinal symptoms were reported.

Nephrotoxicity: Six patients (19%) developed manifestations of acute renal dysfunction/insufficiency (eg acidosis, anuria, elevated serum creatinine, etc) within 7 to 13 days after starting treatment with LEUSTAT, 5 of the affected patients required dialysis. Renal insufficiency was reversible in 2 of these patients. Evidence of tubular damage was noted at autopsy in 2 (of 4) patients whose renal function had not recovered at the time of death. Several of these patients had also been treated with other medications having known nephrotoxic potential.

Neurotoxicity: Eleven patients (35%) experienced delayed onset neurological toxicity. In the majority, this was characterised by progressive irreversible motor weakness, of the upper and/or lower extremities (paraparesis/quadraparesis), noted 35 to 84 days after starting high dose therapy.

Non-invasive neurological testing was consistent with demyelinating disease.

4.8.2 Post-marketing Experience:

The following additional adverse events have been reported since the drug became commercially available. These adverse events have been reported primarily in patients who received multiple courses of LEUSTAT Injection:

<u>Haematological</u>: bone marrow suppression with prolonged pancytopenia, including some reports of aplastic anaemia; haemolytic anaemia, which was reported in patients with lymphoid malignancies, occurring within the first few weeks following treatment; hypereosinophilia. **Rare cases of myelodysplastic syndrome have been reported.**

<u>Hepatic</u>: reversible, generally mild, increases in bilirubin and transaminases.

<u>Nervous System</u>: confusion, neuropathy, ataxia, insomnia and somnolence.

<u>Respiratory System</u>: pulmonary interstitial infiltrates, in most cases an infectious aetiology was identified.

<u>Skin/Subcutaneous: urticaria.</u>

Opportunistic infections have occurred in the acute phase of treatment due to the immunosuppression mediated by LEUSTAT Injection.

4.9 Overdose

High doses of LEUSTAT have been associated with serious neurological toxicity (including irreversible paraparesis/quadraparesis), acute nephrotoxicity, and severe bone marrow suppression resulting in neutropenia, anaemia and thrombocytopenia (See 4.4, Special Warnings and Special Precautions for Use). There is no known specific antidote to overdosage. It is not known whether the drug can be removed from the circulation by dialysis or haemofiltration. Treatment of overdosage consists of discontinuation of LEUSTAT Injection, careful observation and appropriate supportive measures.

5. PHARMACOLOGICAL PROPERTIES

5.1 Pharmacodynamic properties

LEUSTAT Injection (cladribine) is a synthetic antineoplastic agent.

Cellular Resistance and Sensitivity: The selective toxicity cladribine towards certain normal and malignant lymphocyte and monocyte populations is based on the relative activities of deoxycytidine kinase, deoxynucleotidase and adenosine deaminase. It is postulated that cells with high deoxycytidine kinase and low deoxynucleotidase activities will be selectively killed by cladribine as toxic deoxynucleotides accumulate intracellularly.

Cells containing high concentrations of deoxynucleotides are unable to properly repair single-strand DNA breaks. LEUSTAT Injection can be distinguished from other chemotherapeutic agents affecting purine metabolism in that it is cytotoxic to both actively dividing and quiescent lymphocytes and monocytes, inhibiting both DNA synthesis and repair.

5.2 Pharmacokinetic properties

When LEUSTAT Injection was given by continuous intravenous infusion over 7 days the mean steady-state serum concentration was estimated to be 5.7 ng/ml with an estimated systemic clearance of 663.5 ml/h/kg. Accumulation of LEUSTAT over the seven day treatment period was not noted.

Plasma concentrations are reported to decline multi-exponentially after intravenous infusions with terminal half-lives ranging from approximately 3-22 hours. In general, the apparent volume of distribution of cladribine is very large (mean approximately 9l/kg), indicating an extensive distribution of cladribine in body tissues. The mean half-life of cladribine in leukaemic cells has been reported to be 23 hours.

There is little information available on the metabolism or route of excretion of cladribine in man. An average of 18% of the administered dose has been reported to be excreted in urine of patients with solid tumours during a 5-day continuous intravenous infusion of 3.5-8.1 mg/m^2/day of LEUSTAT. The effect of renal and hepatic impairment on the elimination of cladribine has not been investigated in humans.

Cladribine penetrates into cerebrospinal fluid. One report indicates that concentrations are approximately 25% of those in plasma.

Cladribine is bound approximately 20% to plasma proteins.

5.3 Preclinical safety data

Carcinogenesis/Mutagenesis: No animal carcinogenicity studies have been conducted with cladribine. However, its carcinogenic potential cannot be excluded based on demonstrated genotoxicity of cladribine. Cladribine induced chromosomal effects when tested in both an *in vivo* bone marrow micronucleus assay in mice and an *in vitro* assay using CHO-WBL cells. Cladribine is mutagenic in mammalian cells in culture. Cladribine was not mutagenic to bacteria and did not induce unscheduled DNA synthesis in primary rat hepatocyte cultures.

Other preclinical safety data has been included in specific sections of SPC. However, a full tabulation is attached in Appendix 1.

6. PHARMACEUTICAL PARTICULARS

6.1 List of excipients

9.0 mg (0.15 mEq) of sodium chloride as an inactive ingredient. Phosphoric acid and/or dibasic sodium phosphate to adjust the pH to a range of 5.5 to 8.0.

6.2 Incompatibilities

Since limited compatibility data are available, adherence to the recommended diluents and infusion systems is advised.

Solutions containing LEUSTAT Injection should not be mixed with other intravenous drugs or additives or infused simultaneously via a common intravenous line, since compatibility testing has not been performed.

If the same intravenous line is used for sequential infusion of several different drugs, the line should be flushed with a compatible diluent before and after infusion of LEUSTAT (See 4.2 or 6.6).

The use of 5% dextrose as a diluent is not recommended because of increased degradation of cladribine.

6.3 Shelf life

The shelf life for LEUSTAT Injection is 3 years.

When stored in refrigerated conditions between 2° to 8°C (36° to 46°F) protected from light, unopened vials of LEUSTAT Injection are stable until the expiration date indicated on the package. Freezing does not adversely affect the solution.

If freezing occurs, thaw naturally to room temperature. DO NOT heat or microwave. Once thawed, the vial of LEUSTAT Injection is stable until expiry if refrigerated. DO NOT REFREEZE.

Once diluted, solutions containing LEUSTAT Injection should be administered promptly or stored in the refrigerator (2° to 8°C) for no more than 8 hours prior to start of administration.

6.4 Special precautions for storage

Store refrigerated at 2° to 8°C (36° to 46°F). Protect from light during storage.

6.5 Nature and contents of container

LEUSTAT Injection is supplied as a sterile, preservative-free, isotonic solution containing 10 mg (1 mg/ml) of cladribine (as 10 ml) in a single-use, flint glass 20 ml vial.

6.6 Special precautions for disposal and other handling

Preparation and administration of intravenous solutions: LEUSTAT Injection must be diluted with the designated diluent prior to administration. Since the drug product does not contain any anti-microbial preservative or bacteriostatic agent, aseptic technique and proper environmental precautions must be observed in preparation of a solution of LEUSTAT.

Parenteral drug products should be inspected visually for particulate matter and discoloration prior to administration, whenever solution and container permit. A precipitate may occur during the exposure of LEUSTAT to low temperatures; it may be resolubilised by allowing the solution to warm naturally to room temperature and by shaking vigorously. *DO NOT HEAT OR MICROWAVE.*

Care must be taken to assure the sterility of prepared solutions. Once diluted, solutions of LEUSTAT Injection should be administered promptly or stored in the refrigerator (2° to 8°C) for no more than 8 hours prior to start of administration. Vials of LEUSTAT Injection are for single-use only. Any unused portion should be discarded in an appropriate manner.

The potential hazards associated with cytotoxic agents are well established and proper precautions should be taken when handling, preparing, and administering LEUSTAT Injection. The use of disposable gloves and protective garments is recommended. If LEUSTAT Injection contacts the skin or mucous membranes, wash the involved surface immediately with copious amounts of water.

Preparation of a Single Daily Dose:

HCL: Add the calculated dose for a 24 hour period (0.09 mg/kg or 0.09 ml/kg or 3.6 mg/m^2) of LEUSTAT Injection to an infusion bag containing 100 ml to 500 ml of 0.9% sodium chloride injection (PhEur). Infuse intravenously continuously over 24 hours. Repeat daily for a total of 7 consecutive days.

CLL: Add the calculated dose for a 2 hour period (0.12 mg/kg or 4.8 mg/m^2) of LEUSTAT Injection to an infusion bag containing 100 ml to 500 ml of 0.9% sodium chloride injection (PhEur). Infuse intravenously continuously over 2 hours. Repeat daily for a total of 5 consecutive days.

The use of 5% dextrose as a diluent is not recommended because of increased degradation of cladribine. Admixtures of LEUSTAT Injection are chemically and physically stable for at least 24 hours at room temperature under normal room fluorescent light in most commonly available PVC infusion containers.

	DOSE OF LEUSTAT	RECOMMENDED DILUENT	QUANTITY OF DILUENT
HCL:			
24-hour infusion method	0.09 mg/kg/ day	0.9% sodium chloride injection, PhEur	100 ml to 500 ml
CLL:			
2-hour infusion method	0.12 mg/kg/ day	0.9% sodium chloride injection, PhEur	100 ml to 500 ml

7. MARKETING AUTHORISATION HOLDER

Janssen-Cilag Ltd

50-100 Holmers Farm Way

High Wycombe

Bucks

HP12 4EG

8. MARKETING AUTHORISATION NUMBER(S)

PL 0242/0232

9. DATE OF FIRST AUTHORISATION/RENEWAL OF THE AUTHORISATION

3 February 1995

10. DATE OF REVISION OF THE TEXT

July 2008

Levemir Cartridge 100 U/ml, Levemir Pre-filled Pen 100 U/ml

(Novo Nordisk Limited)

1. NAME OF THE MEDICINAL PRODUCT

Levemir 100 U/ml solution for injection in cartridge.

Levemir 100 U/ml solution for injection in pre-filled pen.

2. QUALITATIVE AND QUANTITATIVE COMPOSITION

1 ml of the solution contains 100 U insulin detemir* (equivalent to 14.2 mg). 1 cartridge contains 3 ml equivalent to 300 U. 1 pre-filled pen contains 3 ml equivalent to 300 U.

*Insulin detemir is produced by recombinant DNA technology in *Saccharomyces cerevisiae*.

For a full list of excipients, see section 6.1.

3. PHARMACEUTICAL FORM

Solution for injection in cartridge. Penfill.

Solution for injection in pre-filled pen. FlexPen.

Solution for injection in pre-filled pen. InnoLet.

Clear, colourless, neutral solution.

4. CLINICAL PARTICULARS

4.1 Therapeutic indications

Treatment of diabetes mellitus in adults and adolescents and children aged 6 - 17 years.

4.2 Posology and method of administration

Levemir is a long-acting insulin analogue used as a basal insulin.

Posology

In combination with oral antidiabetic medicines it is recommended to use Levemir once daily, initially at a dose of 10 U or 0.1-0.2 U/kg. The injection can be given at any time during the day, but at the same time each day. The dose of Levemir should be titrated based on individual patients' needs.

Based on study results, the following titration guideline is recommended:

Average pre-breakfast SMPG*	Levemir dose adjustment
> 10.0 mmol/L (180 mg/dL)	+ 8 U
9.1-10.0 mmol/L (163-180 mg/dL)	+ 6 U
8.1-9.0 mmol/L (145-162 mg/dL)	+ 4 U
7.1-8.0 mmol/L (127-144 mg/dL)	+ 2 U
6.1-7.0 mmol/L (109-126 mg/dL)	+ 2 U
If one SMPG measurement	
3.1-4.0 mmol/L (56-72 mg/dL)	- 2 U
< 3.1 mmol/L (< 56 mg/dL)	- 4 U

* Self Monitored Plasma Glucose

When Levemir is used as part of a basal-bolus insulin regimen Levemir should be administered once or twice daily depending on patients' needs. Dosage of Levemir should be adjusted individually.

For patients who require twice daily dosing to optimise blood glucose control, the evening dose can be administered in the evening or at bedtime. Adjustment of dosage may be necessary if patients undertake increased physical activity, change their usual diet or during concomitant illness.

Special populations

As with all insulin products, in elderly patients and patients with renal or hepatic impairment, glucose monitoring should be intensified and insulin detemir dosage adjusted on an individual basis.

Paediatric use

The efficacy and safety of Levemir were demonstrated in children and adolescents aged 6 to 17 years in studies up to 6 months (see section 5.1).

The efficacy and safety of Levemir have not been studied in children below the age of 6 years. Levemir should only be used in this age group under careful medical supervision.

Transfer from other insulin products

Transfer to Levemir from other intermediate or long-acting insulin products may require adjustment of dose and timing of administration (see section 4.4).

As with all insulin products, close glucose monitoring is recommended during the transfer and in the initial weeks thereafter.

Concomitant antidiabetic treatment may need to be adjusted (dose and/or timing of oral antidiabetic medicines or concurrent short/rapid-acting insulin products).

Method of administration

Levemir is for subcutaneous administration **only**. Levemir must not be administered intravenously, as it may result in severe hypoglycaemia. Intramuscular administration should also be avoided. Levemir is not to be used in insulin infusion pumps.

Levemir is administered subcutaneously by injection in the abdominal wall, the thigh, the upper arm, the deltoid region or the gluteal region. Injection sites should therefore always be rotated within the same region. As with all insulin products the duration of action will vary according to the dose, injection site, blood flow, temperature and level of physical activity.

Levemir Penfill is designed to be used with Novo Nordisk insulin delivery systems and NovoFine needles. Levemir Penfill, Levemir FlexPen and Levemir InnoLet are accompanied by a package leaflet with detailed instruction for use to be followed.

4.3 Contraindications

Hypersensitivity to the active substance or to any of the excipients.

4.4 Special warnings and precautions for use

Inadequate dosing or discontinuation of treatment, especially in type 1 diabetes, may lead to hyperglycaemia and diabetic ketoacidosis. Usually the first symptoms of hyperglycaemia develop gradually over a period of hours or days. They include thirst, increased frequency of urination, nausea, vomiting, drowsiness, flushed dry skin, dry mouth, loss of appetite as well as acetone odour of breath. In type 1 diabetes, untreated hyperglycaemic events eventually lead to diabetic ketoacidosis, which is potentially lethal.

Hypoglycaemia

Omission of a meal or unplanned strenuous physical exercise may lead to hypoglycaemia.

Hypoglycaemia may occur if the insulin dose is too high in relation to the insulin requirement (see sections 4.8 and 4.9).

Patients whose blood glucose control is greatly improved, e.g. by intensified insulin therapy, may experience a change in their usual warning symptoms of hypoglycaemia, and should be advised accordingly. Usual warning symptoms may disappear in patients with longstanding diabetes.

Concomitant illness, especially infections and feverish conditions, usually increases the patient's insulin requirements.

Transfer from other insulin products

Transferring a patient to another type or brand of insulin should be done under strict medical supervision. Changes in strength, brand (manufacturer), type, origin (animal, human, human insulin analogue) and/or method of manufacture (recombinant DNA versus animal source insulin) may result in the need for a change in dosage. Patients transferred to Levemir from another type of insulin may require a change in dosage from that used with their usual insulins. If an adjustment is needed, it may occur with the first dose or during the first few weeks or months.

Injection site reactions

As with any insulin therapy, injection site reactions may occur and include pain, redness, hives, inflammation, bruising, swelling and itching. Continuous rotation of the injection site within a given area may help to reduce or prevent these reactions. Reactions usually resolve in a few days to a few weeks. On rare occasions, injection site reactions may require discontinuation of Levemir.

Hypoalbuminaemia

There are limited data in patients with severe hypoalbuminaemia. Careful monitoring is recommended in these patients.

4.5 Interaction with other medicinal products and other forms of interaction

A number of medicinal products are known to interact with the glucose metabolism.

The following substances may reduce the patient's insulin requirements:

Oral antidiabetic medicinal products, monoamine oxidase inhibitors (MAOI), beta-blockers, angiotensin converting enzyme (ACE) inhibitors, salicylates, anabolic steroids and sulphonamides.

The following substances may increase the patient's insulin requirements:

Oral contraceptives, thiazides, glucocorticoids, thyroid hormones, sympathomimetics, growth hormone and danazol.

Beta-blocking agents may mask the symptoms of hypoglycaemia.

Octreotide/lanreotide may both increase or decrease insulin requirement.

Alcohol may intensify or reduce the hypoglycaemic effect of insulin.

4.6 Pregnancy and lactation

Pregnancy

There is no clinical experience with insulin detemir during pregnancy.

Animal reproduction studies have not revealed any differences between insulin detemir and human insulin regarding embryotoxicity and teratogenicity. Caution should be exercised when prescribing to pregnant women.

In general, intensified blood glucose control and monitoring of pregnant women with diabetes are recommended throughout pregnancy and when contemplating pregnancy. Insulin requirements usually fall in the first trimester and increase subsequently during the second and third trimester. After delivery, insulin requirements normally return rapidly to pre-pregnancy values.

Breast-feeding

There is no clinical experience with insulin detemir during breast-feeding. Caution should be exercised when prescribing to breast-feeding women. Breast-feeding women may require adjustments in insulin dose and diet.

4.7 Effects on ability to drive and use machines

The patient's ability to concentrate and react may be impaired as a result of hypoglycaemia. This may constitute a risk in situations where these abilities are of special importance (e.g. driving a car or operating machinery).

Patients should be advised to take precautions to avoid hypoglycaemia while driving. This is particularly important in those who have reduced or absent awareness of the warning signs of hypoglycaemia or have frequent episodes of hypoglycaemia. The advisability of driving should be considered in these circumstances.

4.8 Undesirable effects

Adverse reactions observed in patients using Levemir are mainly dose-dependent and due to the pharmacologic effect of insulin. The overall percentage of treated patients expected to experience adverse drug reactions is estimated to be 12%.

Hypoglycaemia is a common undesirable effect. It may occur if the insulin dose is too high in relation to the insulin requirement. From clinical investigations it is known that major hypoglycaemia, defined as requirement for third party intervention, occurs in approximately 6% of the patients treated with Levemir. Severe hypoglycaemia may lead to unconsciousness and/or convulsions and may result in temporary or permanent impairment of brain function or even death.

Injection site reactions are seen more frequently during treatment with Levemir than with human insulin. These reactions include pain, redness, hives, inflammation, bruising, swelling and itching at the injection site. Most of the injection site reactions are minor and of a transitory nature, i.e. they normally disappear during continued treatment in a few days to a few weeks.

Adverse reactions listed below are classified according to frequency and System Organ Class. Frequency categories are defined according to the following convention: Very common ($\geq$1/10); common ($\geq$1/100 to $<$1/10); uncommon ($\geq$1/1,000 to $\leq$1/100); rare ($\geq$1/10,000 to $\leq$1/1,000); very rare ($\leq$1/10,000), not known (cannot be estimated from the available data).

Nervous system disorders	Rare - Peripheral neuropathy Fast improvement in blood glucose control may be associated with the condition "acute painful neuropathy", which is usually reversible
Eye disorders	Uncommon - Refraction disorders Refraction anomalies may occur upon initiation of insulin therapy. These symptoms are usually of transitory nature.
	Uncommon - Diabetic retinopathy Long-term improved glycaemic control decreases the risk of progression of diabetic retinopathy. However, intensification of insulin therapy with abrupt improvement in glycaemic control may be associated with temporary worsening of diabetic retinopathy.
Metabolism and nutrition disorders	Common – Hypoglycaemia Symptoms of hypoglycaemia usually occur suddenly. They may include cold sweats, cool pale skin, fatigue, nervousness or tremor, anxiousness, unusual tiredness or weakness, confusion, difficulty in concentration, drowsiness, excessive hunger, vision changes, headache, nausea and palpitation. Severe hypoglycaemia may lead to unconsciousness and/or convulsions and may result in temporary or permanent impairment of brain function or even death.
General disorders and administration site conditions	Common - Injection site reactions Injection site reactions (pain, redness, hives, inflammation, bruising, swelling and itching) at the injection site may occur during treatment with insulin. These reactions are usually transitory and normally they disappear during continued treatment.
	Uncommon - Lipodystrophy Lipodystrophy may occur at the injection site as a consequence of failure to rotate injection sites within an area.
	Uncommon - Oedema Oedema may occur upon initiation of insulin therapy. These symptoms are usually of transitory nature.
Immune system disorders*	Common In three clinical studies with subjects treated in combination with oral antidiabetic agents a frequency of 2.2% of allergic reactions and potentially allergic reactions have been observed.
	Uncommon Allergic reactions, potentially allergic reactions, urticaria, rash and eruptions: Such symptoms may be due to generalised hypersensitivity. Other signs of generalised hypersensitivity may be itching, sweating, gastrointestinal upset, angioneurotic oedema, difficulties in breathing, palpitation and reduction in blood pressure. Generalised hypersensitivity reactions are potentially life threatening (anaphylactic reactions).

* Frequencies are uncommon in basal-bolus regimen, but common in three clinical trials in combination with oral antidiabetic medicine.

4.9 Overdose

A specific overdose for insulin cannot be defined, however, hypoglycaemia may develop over sequential stages if too high doses relative to the patient's requirement are administered:

- Mild hypoglycaemic episodes can be treated by oral administration of glucose or sugary products. It is therefore recommended that the diabetic patient always carries sugar containing products
- Severe hypoglycaemic episodes, where the patient has become unconscious, can be treated by glucagon (0.5 to 1 mg) given intramuscularly or subcutaneously by a trained person, or by glucose given intravenously by a health care professional. Glucose must also be given intravenously, if the patient does not respond to glucagon within 10 to 15 minutes. Upon regaining consciousness, administration of oral carbohydrates is recommended for the patient in order to prevent a relapse.

5. PHARMACOLOGICAL PROPERTIES

5.1 Pharmacodynamic properties

Pharmacotherapeutic group: Insulins and analogues for injection, long-acting: ATC code: A10AE05.

Mechanism of action

Insulin detemir is a soluble, long-acting insulin analogue with a prolonged duration of effect used as a basal insulin.

The blood glucose lowering effect of insulin detemir is due to the facilitated uptake of glucose following binding of insulin to receptors on muscle and fat cells and to the simultaneous inhibition of glucose output from the liver.

The time action profile of insulin detemir is statistically significantly less variable and therefore more predictable than for NPH (Neutral Protamine Hagedorn) insulin as seen from the within-subject Coefficients of Variation (CV) for the total and maximum pharmacodynamic effect in Table 1.

Table 1. Within-Subject Variability of the time action profile of insulin detemir and NPH insulin

Pharmacodynamic Endpoint	Insulin detemir CV (%)	NPH insulin CV (%)
$AUC_{GIR,0\text{-}24h}$*	27	68
GIR_{max}**	23	46

*Area under the curve ** Glucose Infusion Rate p-value < 0.001 for all comparisons with insulin detemir

The prolonged action of insulin detemir is mediated by the strong self-association of insulin detemir molecules at the injection site and albumin binding via the fatty acid side-chain. Insulin detemir is distributed more slowly to peripheral target tissues compared to NPH insulin. These combined mechanisms of protraction provide a more reproducible absorption and action profile of insulin detemir compared to NPH insulin.

(see Figure 1 on next page)

The duration of action is up to 24 hours depending on dose providing an opportunity for once or twice daily administration. If administered twice daily, steady state will occur after 2-3 dose administrations. For doses in the interval of 0.2 - 0.4 U/kg, Levemir exerts more than 50% of its maximum effect from 3-4 hours and up to approximately 14 hours after dose administration.

Dose proportionality in pharmacodynamic response (maximum effect, duration of action, total effect) is observed after subcutaneous administration.

Lower day-to-day variability in FPG was demonstrated during treatment with Levemir compared to NPH in long-term clinical trials.

Studies in patients with type 2 diabetes treated with basal insulin in combination with oral antidiabetic medicines demonstrated that glycaemic control (HbA_{1c}) with Levemir is comparable to NPH insulin and insulin glargine and associated with less weight gain, please see Table 2 below. In the study versus insulin glargine, insulin detemir was allowed to be administered once or twice daily whereas insulin glargine was to be administered once a day, 55% of the insulin detemir-treated subjects completed the 52 weeks of treatment on the twice daily regimen.

Table 2. Change in body weight after insulin treatment

(see Table 2 on next page)

In trials with the use of OAD-insulin combination therapy Levemir treatment resulted in a 61-65% lower risk of minor nocturnal hypoglycaemia compared to NPH insulin.

In long-term treatment trials in patients with type 1 diabetes, fasting plasma glucose was improved with Levemir compared with NPH insulin when given as basal/bolus therapy including in children and adolescents aged 6 to 17 years. Glycaemic control (HbA_{1c}) with Levemir is comparable to NPH insulin, with a lower risk of nocturnal hypoglycaemia and no associated weight gain.

In clinical trials using basal bolus insulin therapy, the overall rates of hypoglycaemia with Levemir and NPH insulin were similar. Analyses of nocturnal hypoglycaemia in patients with type 1 diabetes showed a significantly lower risk of minor nocturnal hypoglycaemia (able to self-treat and confirmed by capillary blood glucose less than 2.8 mmol/L or 3.1 mmol/L if expressed as plasma glucose) than with NPH

Figure 1

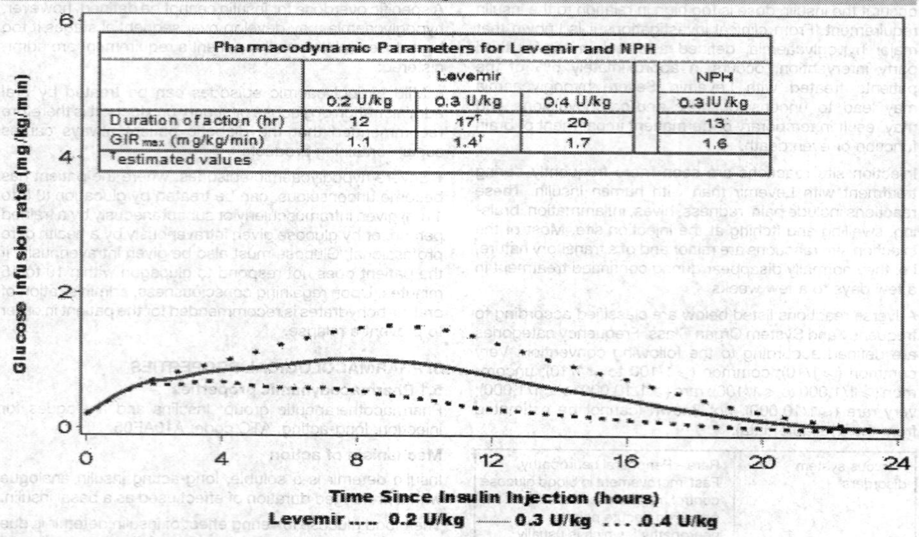

Pharmacodynamic Parameters for Levemir and NPH				
	Levemir			NPH
	0.2 U/kg	0.3 U/kg	0.4 U/kg	0.3 IU/kg
Duration of action (hr)	12	17[†]	20	13
GIR_{max} (mg/kg/min)	1.1	1.4[†]	1.7	1.6
[†]estimated values				

Figure 1: Activity profiles of Levemir in patients with type 1 diabetes.

insulin, whereas no difference was seen in type 2 diabetes. Furthermore, the overall risk of nocturnal hypoglycaemia in children and adolescents aged 6 to 17 years with type 1 diabetes was significantly lower with Levemir compared to NPH insulin.

Antibody development has been observed with the use of Levemir. However, this does not appear to have any impact on glycaemic control.

5.2 Pharmacokinetic properties

Absorption:

Maximum serum concentration is reached between 6 and 8 hours after administration. When administered twice daily, steady state serum concentrations are reached after 2-3 dose administrations. Within-patient variation in absorption is lower for Levemir than for other basal insulin preparations.

The absolute bioavailability of insulin detemir when administered subcutaneous is approximately 60%.

Distribution

An apparent volume of distribution for insulin detemir (approximately 0.1 l/kg) indicates that a high fraction of insulin detemir is circulating in the blood.

The results of the *in vitro* and *in vivo* protein binding studies suggest that there is no clinically relevant interaction between insulin detemir and fatty acids or other protein bound medicinal products.

Metabolism

Degradation of insulin detemir is similar to that of human insulin; all metabolites formed are inactive.

Elimination

The terminal half-life after subcutaneous administration is determined by the rate of absorption from the subcutaneous tissue. The terminal half-life is between 5 and 7 hours depending on the dose.

Linearity

Dose proportionality in serum concentrations (maximum concentration, extent of absorption) is observed after subcutaneous administration in the therapeutic dose range.

Special populations

Paediatric patients: The pharmacokinetic properties of insulin detemir were investigated in children (6–12 years) and adolescents (13–17 years) and compared to adults with type 1 diabetes. There was no clinically relevant difference in pharmacokinetic properties.

Elderly: There was no clinically relevant difference in pharmacokinetics of insulin detemir between elderly and young subjects.

Renal and hepatic impairment: There was no clinically relevant difference in pharmacokinetics of insulin detemir between subjects with renal or hepatic impairment and healthy subjects. As the pharmacokinetics of insulin detemir has not been studied extensively in these populations, it is advised to monitor plasma glucose closely in these populations.

Gender: There are no clinically relevant differences between genders in pharmacokinetic properties of insulin detemir.

5.3 Preclinical safety data

Non-clinical data reveal no special hazard for humans based on conventional studies of safety pharmacology, repeated dose toxicity, genotoxicity and toxicity to reproduction. Receptor affinity data and *in vitro* mitogenicity tests revealed no evidence of an increased mitogenic potential compared to human insulin.

6. PHARMACEUTICAL PARTICULARS

6.1 List of excipients

Glycerol

Phenol

Metacresol

Zinc acetate

Disodium phosphate dihydrate

Sodium chloride

Hydrochloric acid (for pH adjustment)

Sodium hydroxide (for pH adjustment)

Water for injections

6.2 Incompatibilities

Substances added to Levemir may cause degradation of insulin detemir, e.g. if the medicinal product contains thiols or sulphites. Levemir should not be added to infusion fluids.

This medicinal product must not be mixed with other medicinal products.

6.3 Shelf life

30 months.

After first opening: A maximum of 6 weeks when stored below 30°C.

6.4 Special precautions for storage

Store in a refrigerator (2°C - 8°C). Keep away from the cooling element. Do not freeze.

Keep the cartridge in the outer carton in order to protect from light.

Keep the cap on FlexPen and InnoLet in order to protect from light.

After first opening or carried as a spare: Do not refrigerate. Store below 30°C.

Levemir must be protected from excessive heat and light.

6.5 Nature and contents of container

Levemir Penfill

3 ml solution cartridge (type 1 glass) with a plunger (bromobutyl) and a stopper (bromobutyl/polyisoprene) in a carton. Pack sizes of 1, 5 and 10 cartridges. Not all pack sizes may be marketed.

Levemir FlexPen and Levemir InnoLet

3 ml solution in cartridge (type 1 glass) with a plunger (bromobutyl) and a stopper (bromobutyl/polyisoprene) contained in a pre-filled multidose disposable pen made of polypropylene. Pack sizes of 1, 5 and 10 pre-filled pens. Not all pack sizes may be marketed.

Table 2 Change in body weight after insulin treatment

Study duration	Insulin detemir once daily	Insulin detemir twice daily	NPH insulin	Insulin glargine
20 week	+0.7 kg		+1.6 kg	
26 weeks		+1.2 kg	+2.8 kg	
52 weeks	+2.3 kg	+3.7 kg		+4.0 kg

6.6 Special precautions for disposal and other handling

Levemir Penfill is for use by one person only. The cartridge must not be refilled.

Levemir FlexPen is for use by one person only. The cartridge must not be refilled.

Levemir InnoLet is for use by one person only. The cartridge must not be refilled.

Levemir must not be used if it does not appear clear and colourless.

Levemir which has been frozen must not be used.

The patient should be advised to discard the needle after each injection.

7. MARKETING AUTHORISATION HOLDER

Novo Nordisk A/S

Novo Allé

DK-2880 Bagsværd

Denmark

8. MARKETING AUTHORISATION NUMBER(S)

Levemir Penfill EU/1/04/278/001-003

Levemir FlexPen EU/1/04/278/002-006

Levemir InnoLet EU/1/04/278/003-009

9. DATE OF FIRST AUTHORISATION/RENEWAL OF THE AUTHORISATION

Date of first authorisation: 01 June 2004

Date of last renewal: 16 April 2009

10. DATE OF REVISION OF THE TEXT

04/2009

LEGAL CATEGORY

POM (Prescription Only Medicine)

Levofolinic acid 50 mg/ml Solution for injection or infusion (medac UK)

(medac GmbH)

1. NAME OF THE MEDICINAL PRODUCT

Levofolinic acid 50 mg/ml Solution for injection or infusion

2. QUALITATIVE AND QUANTITATIVE COMPOSITION

Each ml of solution contains 54.65 mg disodium levofolinate equivalent to 50 mg levofolinic acid.

Each 1 ml vial contains 54.65 mg disodium levofolinate equivalent to 50 mg levofolinic acid.

Each 4 ml vial contains 218.6 mg disodium levofolinate equivalent to 200 mg levofolinic acid.

Each 9 ml vial contains 491.85 mg disodium levofolinate equivalent to 450 mg levofolinic acid.

For a full list of excipients, see section 6.1.

3. PHARMACEUTICAL FORM

Solution for injection or infusion

Slightly yellow, clear solution.

4. CLINICAL PARTICULARS

4.1 Therapeutic indications

Disodium levofolinate is indicated

- to diminish the toxicity and counteract the action of folic acid antagonists such as methotrexate in cytotoxic therapy and overdose in adults and children;
- in combination with 5-fluorouracil in cytotoxic therapy.

4.2 Posology and method of administration

Levofolinic acid 50 mg/ml Solution for injection or infusion is administered intravenously, either undiluted by injection or by infusion after dilution (for dilution see section 6.6). **Disodium levofolinate should not be administered intrathecally.**

Disodium levofolinate in combination with 5-fluorouracil in cytotoxic therapy

The combined use of disodium levofolinate and fluorouracil is reserved for physicians experienced in the combination of folinates with 5-fluorouracil in cytotoxic therapy.

Different regimes and different dosages are used, without any dosage having been proven to be the optimal one.

The following regimes have been used in adults and elderly in the treatment of advanced or metastatic colorectal cancer and are given as examples.

There are no data on the use of these combinations in children.

Bimonthly regimen: 100 mg/m^2 levofolinic acid (= 109.3 mg/m^2 disodium levofolinate) by intravenous infusion over two hours, followed by bolus 400 mg/m^2 of 5-fluorouracil and 22-hour infusion of 5-fluorouracil (600 mg/m^2) for 2 consecutive days, every 2 weeks on days l and 2.

Weekly regimen: 10 mg/m^2 levofolinic acid (= 10.93 mg/m^2 disodium levofolinate) by bolus i.v. injection or 100 to 250 mg/m^2 levofolinic acid (= 109.3 mg/m^2 to 273.25 mg/m^2 disodium levofolinate) as i.v. infusion over a period of 2 hours plus 500 mg/m^2 5-fluorouracil as i.v. bolus injection in the middle or at the end of the disodium levofolinate infusion.

Monthly regimen: 10 mg/m^2 levofolinic acid (= 10.93 mg/m^2 disodium levofolinate) by bolus i.v. injection or 100 to 250 mg/m^2 levofolinic acid (= 109.3 mg/m^2 to 273.25 mg/m^2 disodium levofolinate) as i.v. infusion over a period of 2 hours immediately followed by 425 or 370 mg/m^2 5-fluorouracil as i.v. bolus injection during 5 consecutive days.

For the combination therapy with 5-fluorouracil, modification of the 5-fluorouracil dosage and the treatment-free interval may be necessary depending on patient condition, clinical response and dose limiting toxicity as stated in the product information of 5-fluorouracil. A reduction of disodium levofolinate dosage is not required.

The number of repeat cycles used is at the discretion of the clinician.

Disodium levofolinate rescue in methotrexate therapy

Since the disodium levofolinate rescue dosage regimen depends heavily on the posology and method of the intermediate- or high-dose methotrexate administration, the methotrexate protocol will dictate the dosage regimen of disodium levofolinate rescue. Therefore, it is best to refer to the applied intermediate or high dose methotrexate protocol for posology and method of administration of disodium levofolinate.

The following guidelines may serve as an illustration of regimens used in adults, elderly and children:

Disodium levofolinate rescue has to be performed by parenteral administration in patients with malabsorption syndromes or other gastrointestinal disorders where enteral absorption is not assured.

Dosages above 12.5-25 mg should be given parenterally due to saturable enteral absorption of disodium levofolinate.

Disodium levofolinate rescue is necessary when methotrexate is given at doses exceeding 500 mg/m^2 body surface and should be considered with doses of 100 mg - 500 mg/m^2 body surface.

Dosage and duration of disodium levofolinate rescue primarily depend on the type and dosage of methotrexate therapy, the occurrence of toxicity symptoms, and the individual excretion capacity for methotrexate. As a rule, the first dose of levofolinic acid is 7.5 mg (3-6 mg/m^2) to be given 12-24 hours (24 hours at the latest) after the beginning of methotrexate infusion. The same dose is given every 6 hours throughout a period of 72 hours. After several parenteral doses treatment can be switched over to the oral form.

In addition to levofolinic acid administration, measures to ensure the prompt excretion of methotrexate are important.

These measures include:

a. Alkalinisation of urine so that the urinary pH is greater than 7.0 before methotrexate infusion (to increase solubility of methotrexate and its metabolites).

b. Maintenance of urine output of 1800-2000 cc/m^2/24 hr by increased oral or intravenous fluids on days 2, 3 and 4 following methotrexate therapy.

c. Plasma methotrexate concentration, BUN and creatinine should be measured on days 2, 3 and 4.

These measures must be continued until the plasma methotrexate level is less than 10^{-7} molar (0.l μM).

Delayed methotrexate excretion may be seen in some patients. This may be caused by a third space accumulation (as seen in ascites or pleural effusion for example), renal insufficiency or inadequate hydration. Under such circumstances, higher doses of levofolinic acid or prolonged administration may be indicated. Patients who experience delayed early methotrexate elimination are likely to develop reversible renal failure.

Forty-eight hours after the start of the methotrexate infusion, the residual methotrexate-level should be measured. If the residual methotrexate-level is >0.5 μmol/l, disodium levofolinate dosages should be adapted according to the following table:

Residual methotrexate blood level 48 hours after the start of the methotrexate administration:	Additional levofolinic acid to be administered every 6 hours for 48 hours or until levels of methotrexate are lower than 0.05 μmol/l:
⩾ 0.5 μmol/l	7.5 mg/m^2
⩾ 1.0 μmol/l	50 mg/m^2
⩾ 2.0 μmol/l	100 mg/m^2

4.3 Contraindications

Known hypersensitivity to disodium levofolinate or to any of the excipients.

Disodium levofolinate is not suitable for the treatment of pernicious anaemia or other anaemias due to Vitamin B12 deficiency. Although haematological remissions may occur, the neurological manifestations remain progressive.

The combination of disodium levofolinate with fluorouracil is not indicated in:

- existing contraindications against fluorouracil
- severe diarrhoea.

Therapy with disodium levofolinate combined with fluorouracil must not be initiated or continued in patients who have symptoms of gastrointestinal toxicity of any severity until those symptoms have completely resolved. Patients with diarrhoea must be monitored with particular care until the diarrhoea has resolved, as rapid clinical deterioration leading to death can occur (see also sections 4.2, 4.4 and 4.5).

Regarding the use of disodium levofolinate with methotrexate or 5-fluorouracil during pregnancy and lactation, see section 4.6, "Pregnancy and Lactation" and the summaries of product characteristics for methotrexate- and 5-fluorouracil-containing medicinal products.

4.4 Special warnings and precautions for use

Disodium levofolinate should only be given intravenously, either undiluted by injection or by infusion after dilution and must not be administered intrathecally.

When levofolinic acid has been administered intrathecally following intrathecal overdose of methotrexate, death has been reported.

General

Disodium levofolinate should only be used with methotrexate or 5-fluorouracil under the direct supervision of a clinical experienced in the use of cancer chemotherapeutic agents.

Levofolinic acid treatment may mask pernicious anaemia and other anaemias resulting from vitamin B12 deficiency.

Many cytotoxic medicinal products – direct or indirect DNA synthesis inhibitors – lead to macrocytosis (hydroxycarbamide, cytarabine, mercaptopurine, thioguanine). Such macrocytosis should not be treated with levofolinic acid.

Epileptic Patients

In epileptic patients treated with phenobarbital, phenytoin, primidone, there is an increased risk of seizures due to decreased serum concentrations of anti-epileptic drugs. Clinical monitoring, possibly monitoring of the plasmatic concentrations and if necessary, dose adaptation of the anti-epileptic drug during disodium levofolinate administration and after discontinuation is recommended (see section 4.5).

Levofolinic acid/5-fluorouracil

In the combination regimen with fluorouracil, the toxicity profile of fluorouracil may be enhanced or shifted by disodium levofolinate. The most common manifestations are leucopenia, mucositis, stomatitis and/or diarrhoea which may be dose limiting. When disodium levofolinate and fluorouracil are used in combination, the fluorouracil dosage must be reduced more in cases of toxicity than when fluorouracil is used alone. Gastrointestinal toxicities are observed more commonly and may be more severe or even life threatening (particularly stomatitis and diarrhoea). In severe cases, treatment is withdrawal of fluorouracil and disodium levofolinate, and supportive intravenous therapy. Combined 5-fluorouracil/levofolinic acid treatment should neither be initiated nor maintained in patients with symptoms of gastrointestinal toxicity, regardless of the severity, until all of these symptoms have completely disappeared.

Because diarrhoea may be a sign of gastrointestinal toxicity, patients presenting with diarrhoea must be carefully monitored until the symptoms have disappeared completely, since a rapid clinical deterioration leading to death can occur. If diarrhoea and/or stomatitis occur, it is advisable to reduce the dose of 5-FU until symptoms have fully disappeared. Especially the elderly and patients with a low physical performance due to their illness are prone to these toxicities. Therefore, particular care should be taken when treating these patients.

Patients should be instructed to consult their treating physician immediately if stomatitis (mild to moderate ulcers) and/or diarrhoea (watery stools or bowel movements) two times per day occur (see also section 4.2).

Particular care should be taken in the treatment of elderly or debilitated patients or patients who have undergone preliminary radiotherapy, as these patients may be at increased risk of severe toxicity, in these patients it is recommended to begin with a reduced dosage of 5-fluorouracil.

Levofolinic acid/methotrexate

Disodium levofolinate should not be given simultaneously with an antineoplastic folic acid antagonist (e.g. methotrexate) to modify or abort clinical toxicity, as the therapeutic effect of the antagonist may be nullified except in the case of folic acid antagonist overdose (see below). For specific details on reduction of methotrexate toxicity refer to the SPC of methotrexate.

An accidental overdosage with a folate antagonist, such as methotrexate, should be treated quickly as a medical emergency. As the time interval between methotrexate administration and disodium levofolinate rescue increases, levofolinic acid effectiveness in counteracting toxicity decreases. Monitoring of the serum methotrexate concentration is essential in determining the optimal dose and duration of treatment with disodium levofolinate. Delayed methotrexate excretion may be caused by third space fluid accumulation (i.e. ascites, pleural effusion), renal insufficiency, inadequate hydration or non steroidal anti inflammatory or salicylates drug administration. Under such circumstances, higher doses of disodium levofolinate or prolonged administration may be indicated.

Disodium levofolinate has no effect on non-haematological toxicities of methotrexate such as the nephrotoxicity resulting from drug and/or metabolite precipitation in the kidney. Patients who experience delayed early methotrexate elimination are likely to develop reversible renal failure and all toxicities associated with methotrexate (please refer to the SPC for methotrexate). The presence of pre-existing or methotrexate induced renal insufficiency is potentially associated with delayed excretion of methotrexate and may increase the need for higher doses or more prolonged use of levofolinic acid.

Excessive levofolinic acid doses must be avoided since this might impair the antitumour activity of methotrexate, especially in CNS tumours where levofolinic acid accumulates after repeated courses.

Resistance to methotrexate as a result of decreased membrane transport implies also resistance to folinic acid rescue as both medicinal products share the same transport system.

The possibility that the patient is taking other medications that interact with methotrexate (e.g., medications which may interfere with methotrexate elimination or binding to serum albumin) should always be considered when laboratory abnormalities or clinical toxicities are observed.

4.5 Interaction with other medicinal products and other forms of interaction

Disodium levofolinate is an antidote of folic acid antagonists – e.g. methotrexate. Following the use of methotrexate, disodium levofolinate overdosage may lead to a loss of the effect of methotrexate therapy ("over-rescue").

Concomitant use of disodium levofolinate counteracts the antineoplastic activity of methotrexate and increases the cytotoxic effects of fluorouracil.

Life-threatening diarrhoeas have been observed if 600 mg/m^2 of fluorouracil (i.v. bolus once weekly) is given together with disodium levofolinate. When disodium levofolinate and fluorouracil are used in combination, the fluorouracil dosage must be reduced more than when fluorouracil is used alone.

Disodium levofolinate may diminish the effect of anti-epileptic substances: phenobarbital, primidone, phenytoin and succinimides, and may increase the frequency of seizures (a decrease of plasma levels of enzymatic inductor anticonvulsant drugs may be observed because the hepatic metabolism is increased as folates are one of the cofactors) (see section 4.4).

When disodium levofolinate is given in conjunction with a folic acid antagonist (e.g. cotrimoxazole, pyrimethamine) the efficacy of the folic acid antagonist may either be reduced or completely neutralised.

4.6 Pregnancy and lactation

Pregnancy

There are no adequate and well-controlled clinical studies conducted in pregnant or breast-feeding women. No formal animal reproductive toxicity studies with disodium levofolinate have been conducted. There are no indications that folinic acid induces harmful effects if administered during pregnancy. During pregnancy, methotrexate should only be administered on strict indications, where the benefits of the drug to the mother should be weighed against possible hazards to the foetus. Should treatment with methotrexate or other folate antagonists take place despite pregnancy, there are no limitations as to the use of disodium levofolinate to diminish toxicity or counteract the effects.

5-fluorouracil use is generally contraindicated during pregnancy and breast-feeding; this applies also to the combined use of disodium levofolinate with 5-fluorouracil.

Please refer also to the summaries of product characteristics for methotrexate-, other folate antagonists and 5-fluorouracil-containing medicinal products.

Lactation

It is not known whether disodium levofolinate is excreted in human milk. Disodium levofolinate alone can be used during breast feeding when considered necessary according to the therapeutic indications. However, MTX or 5-FU must not be given to breast-feeding woman because both substances are able to penetrate into breast milk. Woman must stop breast feeding before such treatment is initiated.

4.7 Effects on ability to drive and use machines

Disodium levofolinate is unlikely to affect the ability to drive or operate machines. The general condition of the patient is likely to be more significant than any drug-induced effects.

4.8 Undesirable effects

Frequencies

- Very common (⩾1/10)
- Common (⩾1/100 to <1/10)
- Uncommon (⩾1/1,000 to <1/100)
- Rare (⩾1/10,000 to <1/1,000)
- Very rare (<1/10,000), not known (cannot be estimated from the available data)

Immune system disorders	Very rare Allergic reactions including anaphylactoid reactions and urticaria

Psychiatric disorders	Rare Insomnia, agitation and depression after high doses
Gastrointestinal disorders	Rare Gastrointestinal disorders after high doses
Nervous system disorders	Rare Increase in the frequency of attacks in epileptics (see also section 4.5)
General disorders and administration site conditions	Uncommon Fever has been observed after administration of disodium levofolinate as solution for injection

Combination therapy with 5-FU:

Generally, the safety profile depends on the applied regimen of 5-FU due to enhancement of the 5-FU induced toxicities.

Monthly regimen:

Gastrointestinal disorders	Very common Vomiting and nausea
General disorders and administration site conditions	Very common Mucosal toxicities, which can be severe

No enhancement of other 5-FU induced toxicities (e.g. neurotoxicity).

Weekly regimen:

Gastrointestinal disorders	Very common Diarrhoea with higher grades of toxicity, and dehydration resulting in hospital admission for treatment and even death

4.9 Overdose

There have been no reported sequelae in patients who have received significantly more disodium levofolinate than the recommended dosage.

There is no specific antidote.

When using methotrexate, an overdosage of disodium levofolinate may result in a decrease of efficacy of methotrexate ("over-rescue").

Should overdosage of the combination of fluorouracil and Levofolinic acid 50 mg/ml Solution for injection or infusion occur, overdosage instructions for fluorouracil should be followed.

5. PHARMACOLOGICAL PROPERTIES

5.1 Pharmacodynamic properties

Pharmacotherapeutic group: Detoxifying agents for antineoplastic treatment

ATC code: V 03 AF

Folinic acid is the formyl derivative of tetrahydrofolic acid i.e. the active form of folic acid. Levofolinic acid is the biologically active l-isomer of racemic folinic acid. It is involved in various metabolic processes including purine synthesis, pyrimidine nucleotide synthesis and amino acid metabolism.

Levofolinic acid is frequently used to diminish the toxicity and counteract the action of folate antagonists, such as methotrexate. Levofolinic acid and folate antagonists share the same membrane transport carrier and compete for transport into cells, stimulating folate antagonist efflux. It also protects cells from the effects of folate antagonist by repletion of the reduced folate pool. Levofolinic acid does not require reduction by the enzyme dihydrofolate reductase. Thus it serves as a pre-reduced source of H4 folate; it can therefore bypass folate antagonist blockage of the dihydrofolate reductase and provide a source for the various coenzyme forms of folic acid.

Biochemical rationale for the combination of disodium levofolinate with fluorouracil:

Fluorouracil can inhibit DNA synthesis by binding to the enzyme thymidylate synthetase. The combination of disodium levofolinate with fluorouracil results in the formation of a stable ternary complex consisting of thymidylate synthetase, 5-fluorodeoxy-uridinemonophosphate and 5,10-methylenetetrahydrofolate.

This leads to an extended blockade of thymidylate synthetase with enhanced inhibition of DNA biosynthesis, resulting in increased cytotoxicity as compared to fluorouracil monotherapy.

5.2 Pharmacokinetic properties

Disodium levofolinate is bioequivalent with calcium levofolinate as well as with the racemate disodium folinate with respect to plasma concentrations of levofolinic acid and the main, active metabolite, 5-methyltetrahydrofolic acid after intravenous administration of the same molar dose of the active isomer.

Distribution

The protein binding of levofolinic acid is about 27%. The volume of distribution is about 17.5 litres.

Elimination

The active isomeric form levofolinic acid (l-5-formyltetrahydrofolic acid) is quickly metabolised to 5-methyltetrahydrofolic acid in the liver. It is assumed that this conversion is not linked to the presence of dihydrofolate reductase. About 20 % of an intravenous dose is excreted as unchanged levofolinic acid in urine. The clearance for levofolinic acid is about 205 ml/min. After intravenous administration, the half-life of levofolinic acid and the active metabolite, 5-methyltetrahydrofolic acid, is 0.5 hours and 6.5 hours, respectively.

5.3 Preclinical safety data

Toxicity tests on combined use with fluorouracil have not been carried out.

No further information is available of relevance to the prescriber which is not already included in other relevant sections of the SPC.

6. PHARMACEUTICAL PARTICULARS

6.1 List of excipients

Sodium hydroxide (for pH-adjustment)

Hydrochloric acid (for pH-adjustment)

Water for injections

6.2 Incompatibilities

This medicinal product must not be mixed with other medicinal products except those mentioned in section 6.6.

6.3 Shelf life

2 years

After mixing with fluorouracil or dilution with 0.9 % sodium chloride solution or 5% glucose solution (see section 6.6):

Chemical and physical in-use stability has been demonstrated for 72 hours at 20-25°C.

From a microbiological point of view the product should be used immediately. If not used immediately, in use storage times and conditions prior to use are the responsibility of the user and would normally not be longer than 24 hours at 2-8°C unless dilution has taken place in controlled and validated aseptic conditions.

6.4 Special precautions for storage

Store in a refrigerator (2°C – 8°C). Keep the vial in the outer carton in order to protect from light.

For storage conditions of the diluted medicinal product, see section 6.3.

6.5 Nature and contents of container

Colourless glass vials type I with bromobutyl rubber stoppers and aluminium flip-off caps.

Pack sizes: Vials with 1 ml, 4 ml, or 9 ml solution for injection or infusion in packs of 1 or 5 vials. Not all pack sizes may be marketed.

6.6 Special precautions for disposal and other handling

Levofolinic acid 50 mg/ml Solution for injection or infusion is administered intravenously, either undiluted by injection or by infusion after dilution. Preparation of solution for infusion must take place in aseptic conditions. The solution for injection or infusion may be diluted with 0.9% sodium chloride solution or 5% glucose solution.

Levofolinic acid 50 mg/ml is compatible with fluorouracil.

Only clear solutions without visible particles should be used.

For single use only. Any unused product should be disposed of in accordance with local requirements.

7. MARKETING AUTHORISATION HOLDER

medac

Gesellschaft für klinische

Spezialpräparate mbH

Fehlandtstraβe 3

D-20354 Hamburg

Germany

8. MARKETING AUTHORISATION NUMBER(S)

11587/0042

9. DATE OF FIRST AUTHORISATION/RENEWAL OF THE AUTHORISATION

19/03/2008

10. DATE OF REVISION OF THE TEXT

01/07/2008

Lexpec Folic Acid Oral Solution 2.5mg/5ml

(Rosemont Pharmaceuticals Limited)

1. NAME OF THE MEDICINAL PRODUCT

Lexpec 2.5mg/5ml Oral Solution

2. QUALITATIVE AND QUANTITATIVE COMPOSITION

Folic Acid 2.5mg/5ml

3. PHARMACEUTICAL FORM

Oral Solution

4. CLINICAL PARTICULARS

4.1 Therapeutic indications

1. Folate deficient megaloblastic anaemia
2. Folate deficient megaloblastic anaemia in infants
3. Malabsorption syndromes
   3.1 Tropical sprue
   3.2 Coeliac disease
   3.3 Non-tropical sprue
4. Megaloblastic anaemia in pregnancy
5. Megaloblastic anaemia associated with alcoholism
6. Megaloblastic anaemia associated with anti-convulsant therapy
7. Haemolytic anaemias e.g. Sickle Cell Anaemia

4.2 Posology and method of administration

For oral administration only.

Children:

May be given 5mg to 15mg daily, in divided doses, according to the severity of the deficiency state.

Adults:

Initial dose of 10mg to 20mg daily, in divided doses, for 14 days or until a haematopoietic response has been obtained.

Maintenance dose is 2.5mg to 10mg daily.

Prophylactic dose in pregnancy 0.5mg (1ml) daily.

Elderly:

As for adults.

4.3 Contraindications

Known hypersensitivity to folic acid.

Known hypersensitivity to hydroxybenzoate esters.

Patients with folate dependent tumours.

Patients with malignant disease, unless megaloblastic anaemia due to folic acid deficiency

4.4 Special warnings and precautions for use

If folic acid is used indiscriminately, there is a danger that patients with pernicious anaemia and other B_{12} deficiency states, despite a haematological remission, may develop irreparable neurological lesions. Therefore a full clinical diagnosis should be made before initiating treatment.

Folic acid is removed by haemodialysis.

Excipients in the Formulation

Methyl and propyl hydroxybenzoates are contained in this product which may cause allergic reactions (possibly delayed).

4.5 Interaction with other medicinal products and other forms of interaction

Folic acid has been observed to reduce plasma levels of anticonvulsants, particularly phenytoin and primidone and therefore patients should be carefully monitored by the physician and the anticonvulsant drug dose adjusted as necessary.

4.6 Pregnancy and lactation

There are no known hazards to the use of folic acid, indeed folic acid supplements are often necessary in pregnancy.

Folic acid is excreted in breast milk.

4.7 Effects on ability to drive and use machines

There are no known effects of this preparation on the ability to drive or use machines.

4.8 Undesirable effects

Allergic reactions to folic acid have been reported.

Mild gastro-intestinal upsets are rare but may occur

4.9 Overdose

No cases of acute overdosage appear to have been reported, but even extremely high doses are unlikely to cause harm to patients.

5. PHARMACOLOGICAL PROPERTIES

5.1 Pharmacodynamic properties

ATC Code: B03B B

After conversion into co-enzyme forms it is concerned in single carbon unit transfers in the synthesis of purines, pyrimidines and methionine.

5.2 Pharmacokinetic properties

About 70-80% of a 2mg oral solution of folic acid is absorbed. Larger doses are probably equally well absorbed. It is distributed into plasma and extracellular fluid. In plasma, folate is bound weakly to albumin (70%). There is a further high affinity binder for folate but this has a very low capacity and is barely detectable in normal sera. About 70% of small doses of folate (about 1mg) are retained and the rest excreted into the urine. With larger doses most is excreted into the urine. With a 5mg dose of folate, urinary excretion will be complete in about 5 hours. There is an enterohepatic circulation of folate. The retained folate is taken into cells and reduced by dihydrofolate to tetrahydrofolate. Folic acid is a relatively poor substrate for folate reduction, the normal substrate being dihydrofolate.

Folic acid itself does not occur in natural materials, it is entirely a pharmacological form of the compound. Once reduced, folate has additional glutamic acid residues added, a folate pentaglutamate being the dominant intracellular analogue. These polyglutamates are the active co-enzymes.

5.3 Preclinical safety data
Folic Acid is a drug on which extensive clinical experience has been obtained. Relevant information for the prescriber is provided elsewhere in the Summary of Product Characteristics.

6. PHARMACEUTICAL PARTICULARS

6.1 List of excipients
Mannitol (E421), glycerol (E422), methyl hydroxybenzoate (E218), ethyl hydroxybenzoate (E214), propyl hydroxybenzoate (E216), sodium dihydrogen phosphate, disodium hydrogen phosphate (E339), disodium ethylene diamine tetra acetic acid, strawberry flavour (containing propylene glycol E1520) and purified water.

6.2 Incompatibilities
None stated.

6.3 Shelf life
18 months

6.4 Special precautions for storage
Do not store above 25°C

6.5 Nature and contents of container
Bottle: Amber (Type III) glass with 125ml or 150ml capacity.

Closure: a) Aluminium, EPE wadded, roll-on pilfer-proof
b) HDPE, EPE wadded, tamper evident
c) HDPE, EPE wadded, tamper evident, child resistant.

6.6 Special precautions for disposal and other handling
Not applicable.

Administrative Data

7. MARKETING AUTHORISATION HOLDER
Rosemont Pharmaceuticals Ltd, Rosemont House, Yorkdale Industrial Park, Braithwaite Street, Leeds, LS11 9XE, UK

8. MARKETING AUTHORISATION NUMBER(S)
PL 00427/0034

9. DATE OF FIRST AUTHORISATION/RENEWAL OF THE AUTHORISATION
30.10.74

10. DATE OF REVISION OF THE TEXT
31 March 2008

Lidocaine Hydrochloride BP Laryngojet 4%
(International Medication Systems (UK) Ltd)

1. NAME OF THE MEDICINAL PRODUCT
Lidocaine Hydrochloride BP Laryngojet 4% w/v.

2. QUALITATIVE AND QUANTITATIVE COMPOSITION
Lidocaine Hydrochloride BP 160mg in 4ml.

3. PHARMACEUTICAL FORM
Sterile aqueous solution for topical application to the oral mucosa.

4. CLINICAL PARTICULARS

4.1 Therapeutic indications
For topical anaesthesia of the mucous membranes of the oropharynx, trachea, and respiratory tract, e.g. in bronchoscopy, bronchography, laryngoscopy, endotracheal intubation and biopsy in these areas.

4.2 Posology and method of administration
The lowest effective dose should be administered. The usual adult dose is 160mg (one pre-filled syringe). If less is required, the excess should be expelled before use to avoid inadvertent overdosage.

Adults: 1-5ml (40-200mg lidocaine).

Elderly: may need reduced dosage depending on physical state.

Children: up to 3mg/kg.

The solution may be sprayed, instilled (if a cavity) or applied with a swab. Anaesthesia usually occurs within 5 minutes.

4.3 Contraindications
Lidocaine is contraindicated in patients with known hypersensitivity to local anaesthetics of the amide type or in patients with porphyria.

4.4 Special warnings and precautions for use
Topical application of lidocaine should be used with caution if the mucosa in the area of application has been traumatised or sepsis is present, as absorption will be high.

Use with caution in patients with epilepsy, liver disease, congestive heart failure, marked hypoxia, severe respiratory depression, hypovolaemia or shock and in patients with any form of heart block or sinus bradycardia, or myasthenia gravis.

It should be kept in mind that absorption of aqueous drugs from the respiratory tract may often be nearly as rapid and complete as that occurring with intravenous injection. If there are likely to be high blood levels, resuscitation equipment should be available.

Anaesthesia around the oral cavity may impair swallowing and thus increase the risk of aspiration.

4.5 Interaction with other medicinal products and other forms of interaction
Propranolol and cimetidine may reduce the renal and hepatic clearance of lidocaine, thus increasing toxicity. The cardiac depressant effects of lidocaine are additive to those of other antiarrhythmic agents. Lidocaine prolongs the action of suxamethonium.

4.6 Pregnancy and lactation
The safe use of lidocaine has not been established with respect to possible adverse effects upon foetal development. Lidocaine is excreted into breast milk and so should therefore be used with caution in nursing women.

4.7 Effects on ability to drive and use machines
Not applicable.

4.8 Undesirable effects
Adverse effects are usually due to inadvertent intravenous administration or overdosage. Rarely, lidocaine may induce an allergic reaction including anaphylaxis.

The following systemic reactions have been reported in association with lidocaine:

Central nervous system: light-headedness, drowsiness, dizziness, apprehension, euphoria, tinnitus, blurred or double vision, nystagmus, vomiting, sensations of heat, cold or numbness, twitching, tremors, convulsions, unconsciousness, respiratory depression and arrest, nausea.

Cardiovascular system: hypotension, cardiovascular collapse and bradycardia which may lead to cardiac arrest.

4.9 Overdose
Symptoms: reactions due to overdose with lidocaine (high plasma levels) are systemic and involve the central nervous and cardiovascular systems. Effects include medullary depression, tonic and clonic convulsions and cardiovascular collapse.

Treatment: institute emergency resuscitative procedures and administer the drugs necessary to manage the severe reaction. For severe convulsions small increments of diazepam or an ultra-short acting barbiturate (thiopentone), or if not available, a short-acting barbiturate (pentobarbitone or quinalbarbitone), or if the patient is under anaesthesia, a short-acting muscle relaxant (suxamethonium) may be given intravenously. Patency of the airway and adequacy of ventilation must be assured.

Should circulatory depression occur vasopressors such as metaraminol may be used.

5. PHARMACOLOGICAL PROPERTIES

5.1 Pharmacodynamic properties
Lidocaine stabilises the neuronal membrane and prevents the initiation and transmission of nerve impulses, thereby effecting local anaesthetic action. The onset of action is rapid and the blockade may last from one to one and a half hours.

5.2 Pharmacokinetic properties
Lidocaine is rapidly distributed to all body tissues. About 65% is plasma bound. Lidocaine crosses the placenta and the blood brain barrier. The plasma half life is 1.6 hours. About 80% of the dose is metabolised in the liver; less than 10% is found unchanged in the urine.

5.3 Preclinical safety data
Not applicable since lidocaine has been used in clinical practice for many years and its effects in man are well known.

6. PHARMACEUTICAL PARTICULARS

6.1 List of excipients
Sodium Hydroxide NF

Water for Injection USP

6.2 Incompatibilities
None known.

6.3 Shelf life
36 months.

6.4 Special precautions for storage
Store below 25°C

6.5 Nature and contents of container
The solution is contained in a USP type I glass vial with an elastomeric closure which meets all the relevant USP specifications. The product is available as 4ml.

6.6 Special precautions for disposal and other handling
The container is specially designed for use with the IMS Laryngojet injector device.

7. MARKETING AUTHORISATION HOLDER
International Medication Systems (UK) Limited

208 Bath Road

Slough

Berkshire

SL1 3WE

UK

8. MARKETING AUTHORISATION NUMBER(S)
PL 03265/0040.

9. DATE OF FIRST AUTHORISATION/RENEWAL OF THE AUTHORISATION
Date first granted: 15 November 1977

Date renewed: 21 November 1997

10. DATE OF REVISION OF THE TEXT
June 2004

POM

Lidocaine Hydrochloride Injection BP Minijet 1%
(International Medication Systems (UK) Ltd)

1. NAME OF THE MEDICINAL PRODUCT
Lidocaine Hydrochloride Injection BP Minijet 1% w/v.

2. QUALITATIVE AND QUANTITATIVE COMPOSITION
Lidocaine Hydrochloride BP 10 mg per ml

3. PHARMACEUTICAL FORM
Sterile aqueous solution for infiltration injection or intravenous administration.

4. CLINICAL PARTICULARS

4.1 Therapeutic indications
For local anaesthesia by infiltration, intravenous regional anaesthesia and nerve blocks.

By intravenous injection for the emergency management of ventricular arrhythmias, particularly after myocardial infarction and cardiac surgery.

4.2 Posology and method of administration
For local anaesthesia:
The dosage varies depending upon the area to be anaesthetised, vascularity of the tissues, number of neuronal segments to be blocked, individual tolerance and the anaesthetic technique. The lowest dosage needed to provide anaesthesia should be administered.

Adults: the usual dose should not exceed 200 mg.

Children: the usual dose should not exceed 3 mg/kg.

For epidurals, a test dose should be administered at least 5 minutes before total dose to prevent inadvertent intravascular or subarachnoid injection.

For continuous epidural, caudal or paracervical anaesthesia, the maximal dose should not be repeated at intervals under 90 minutes.

For IV regional anaesthesia (Bier's block), the tourniquet should not be released until at least 20 minutes after administration.

For intravenous use in cardiac arrhythmias:
Adults: the usual dose is 50 to 100 mg administered intravenously under ECG monitoring. This dose may be injected at a rate of approximately 25 to 50 mg (2.5 to 5.0 ml 1% solution or 1.25 to 2.5 ml 2% solution) per minute. A sufficient period of time should be allowed to enable a slow circulation to carry the drug to the site of action. If the initial dose of 50 to 100 mg does not produce the desired response, a second dose may be given after 5 minutes. No more than 200 to 300 mg of lidocaine should be administered during a one hour period.

Following a single injection in those patients in whom arrhythmia tends to recur and who are incapable of receiving oral antiarrhythmic therapy, intravenous infusions of lidocaine may be administered at the rate of 1 to 4 mg/minute (20 to 50 mcg/kg/minute). IV infusions must be given under ECG monitoring to avoid potential overdosage and toxicity. The infusion should be terminated as soon as the patient's basic cardiac rhythm appears to be stable or at the earliest signs of toxicity. It should rarely be necessary to continue the infusion beyond 24 hours. As soon as possible, patients should be changed to an oral antiarrhythmic agent for maintenance therapy.

Children: experience with lidocaine is limited. A suggested paediatric dose is a loading dose of 0.8 to 1 mg/kg repeated if necessary up to 3-5 mg/kg, followed by continuous infusion of 10 to 50 mcg/kg/minute.

Elderly: doses may need to be reduced depending on age and physical state.

4.3 Contraindications
Lidocaine is contraindicated in patients with known hypersensitivity to local anaesthetics of the amide type and in patients with porphyria.

4.4 Special warnings and precautions for use
Constant ECG monitoring is necessary during IV administration. Resuscitative equipment and drugs should be immediately available for the management of severe adverse cardiovascular, respiratory or central nervous system effects. If severe reactions occur, lidocaine should be discontinued.

Use with caution in patients with epilepsy, liver disease, congestive heart failure, severe renal disease, marked hypoxia, severe respiratory depression, hypovolaemia or shock and in patients with any form of heart block or sinus bradycardia. Hypokalaemia, hypoxia and disorders of acid-base balance should be corrected before treatment with lidocaine begins.

4.5 Interaction with other medicinal products and other forms of interaction
Propranolol and cimetidine may reduce the renal and hepatic clearance of lidocaine, thus increasing toxicity. The cardiac depressant effects of lidocaine are additive to those of other antiarrhythmic agents. Lidocaine prolongs the action of suxamethonium.

4.6 Pregnancy and lactation
The safe use of lidocaine has not been established with respect to possible adverse effects upon foetal development. Lidocaine is excreted in breast milk and so should be used with caution in nursing women.

4.7 Effects on ability to drive and use machines
Not applicable; this preparation is intended for use only in emergencies.

4.8 Undesirable effects
Adverse effects are usually due to inadvertent intravenous administration or overdosage. Allergic reactions (including anaphylaxis) have been reported rarely.

The following systemic reactions have been reported in association with lidocaine:

Central nervous system: light-headedness, drowsiness, dizziness, apprehension, nervousness, euphoria, tinnitus, blurred or double vision, nystagmus, vomiting, sensations of heat, cold or numbness, twitching, tremors, paraesthesia, convulsions, unconsciousness, respiratory depression and arrest.

Cardiovascular system: hypotension, cardiovascular collapse and bradycardia which may lead to cardiac arrest.

4.9 Overdose
Symptoms: reactions due to overdose with lidocaine (high plasma levels) are systemic and involve the central nervous and cardiovascular systems. Effects include medullary depression, tonic and clonic convulsions and cardiovascular collapse.

Treatment: institute emergency resuscitative procedures and administer the drugs necessary to manage the severe reaction. For severe convulsions, small increments of diazepam or an ultra-short acting barbiturate (thiopentone), or if not available, a short-acting barbiturate (pentobarbitone or quinalbarbitone), or if the patient is under anaesthesia, a short-acting muscle relaxant (suxamethonium) may be given intravenously. Patency of the airway and adequacy of ventilation must be assured.

Should circulatory depression occur vasopressors such as metaraminol may be used.

5. PHARMACOLOGICAL PROPERTIES

5.1 Pharmacodynamic properties
Lidocaine stabilises the neuronal membrane and prevents the initiation and transmission of nerve impulses, thereby effecting local anaesthetic action. The onset of action is rapid and the blockade may last up to 2 hours.

In the heart, lidocaine reduces automaticity by decreasing the rate of diastolic (phase 4) depolarisation. Lidocaine is considered as a class 1b (membrane stabilising) antiarrhythmic agent. The duration of the action potential is decreased due to blockade of the sodium channel and the refractory period is shortened.

5.2 Pharmacokinetic properties
Lidocaine is rapidly distributed to all body tissues. About 65% is plasma bound. Lidocaine crosses the placenta and the blood brain barrier. The plasma half life is 1.6 hours. About 80% of the dose is metabolised in the liver; less than 10% is found unchanged in the urine.

5.3 Preclinical safety data
Not applicable since lidocaine has been used in clinical practice for many years and its effects in man are well known.

6. PHARMACEUTICAL PARTICULARS

6.1 List of excipients
Hydrochloric Acid BP
Sodium Chloride BP
Sodium Hydroxide BP
Water for Injection USP

6.2 Incompatibilities
None known.

6.3 Shelf life
3 years.

6.4 Special precautions for storage
Store below 25°C.

6.5 Nature and contents of container
The solution is contained in a USP type I glass vial with an elastomeric closure which meets all the relevant USP specifications. The product is available as a 1% solution in a 10ml vial.

6.6 Special precautions for disposal and other handling
The container is specially designed for use with the IMS Minijet injector.

7. MARKETING AUTHORISATION HOLDER
International Medication Systems (UK) Ltd
208 Bath Road
Slough
Berkshire
SL1 3WE
UK

8. MARKETING AUTHORISATION NUMBER(S)
PL 03265/0005R

9. DATE OF FIRST AUTHORISATION/RENEWAL OF THE AUTHORISATION
Date first granted: 28 February 1991
Date renewed: 29 November 1996

10. DATE OF REVISION OF THE TEXT
June 2004
POM

Lidocaine Hydrochloride Injection BP Minijet 2%
(International Medication Systems (UK) Ltd)

1. NAME OF THE MEDICINAL PRODUCT
Lidocaine Hydrochloride Injection BP Minijet 2% w/v.

2. QUALITATIVE AND QUANTITATIVE COMPOSITION
Lidocaine Hydrochloride BP 20 mg per ml

3. PHARMACEUTICAL FORM
Sterile aqueous solution for infiltration injection or intravenous administration.

4. CLINICAL PARTICULARS

4.1 Therapeutic indications
For local anaesthesia by infiltration, intravenous regional anaesthesia and nerve blocks.

By intravenous injection for the emergency management of ventricular arrhythmias, particularly after myocardial infarction and cardiac surgery.

4.2 Posology and method of administration
For local anaesthesia:

The dosage varies depending upon the area to be anaesthetised, vascularity of the tissues, number of neuronal segments to be blocked, individual tolerance and the anaesthetic technique. The lowest dosage needed to provide anaesthesia should be administered.

Adults: the usual dose should not exceed 200 mg.

Children: the usual dose should not exceed 3 mg/kg.

For epidurals, a test dose should be administered at least 5 minutes before total dose to prevent inadvertent intravascular or subarachnoid injection.

For continuous epidural, caudal or paracervical anaesthesia, the maximal dose should not be repeated at intervals under 90 minutes.

For IV regional anaesthesia (Bier's block), the tourniquet should not be released until at least 20 minutes after administration.

For intravenous use in cardiac arrhythmias:

Adults: the usual dose is 50 to 100 mg administered intravenously under ECG monitoring. This dose may be injected at a rate of approximately 25 to 50 mg (2.5 to 5.0 ml 1% solution or 1.25 to 2.5 ml 2% solution) per minute. A sufficient period of time should be allowed to enable a slow circulation to carry the drug to the site of action. If the initial dose of 50 to 100 mg does not produce the desired response, a second dose may be given after 5 minutes. No more than 200 to 300 mg of lidocaine should be administered during a one hour period.

Following a single injection in those patients in whom arrhythmia tends to recur and who are incapable of receiving oral antiarrhythmic therapy, intravenous infusions of lidocaine may be administered at the rate of 1 to 4 mg/minute (20 to 50 mcg/kg/minute). IV infusions must be given under ECG monitoring to avoid potential overdosage and toxicity. The infusion should be terminated as soon as the patient's basic cardiac rhythm appears to be stable or at the earliest signs of toxicity. It should rarely be necessary to continue the infusion beyond 24 hours. As soon as possible, patients should be changed to an oral antiarrhythmic agent for maintenance therapy.

Children: experience with lidocaine is limited. A suggested paediatric dose is a loading dose of 0.8 to 1 mg/kg repeated if necessary up to 3-5 mg/kg, followed by continuous infusion of 10 to 50 mcg/kg/minute.

Elderly: doses may need to be reduced depending on age and physical state.

4.3 Contraindications
Lidocaine is contraindicated in patients with known hypersensitivity to local anaesthetics of the amide type and in patients with porphyria.

4.4 Special warnings and precautions for use
Constant ECG monitoring is necessary during IV administration. Resuscitative equipment and drugs should be immediately available for the management of severe adverse cardiovascular, respiratory or central nervous system effects. If severe reactions occur, lidocaine should be discontinued.

Use with caution in patients with epilepsy, liver disease, congestive heart failure, severe renal disease, marked hypoxia, severe respiratory depression, hypovolaemia or shock and in patients with any form of heart block or sinus bradycardia. Hypokalaemia, hypoxia and disorders of acid-base balance should be corrected before treatment with lidocaine begins.

4.5 Interaction with other medicinal products and other forms of interaction
Propranolol and cimetidine may reduce the renal and hepatic clearance of lidocaine, thus increasing toxicity. The cardiac depressant effects of lidocaine are additive to those of other antiarrhythmic agents. Lidocaine prolongs the action of suxamethonium.

4.6 Pregnancy and lactation
The safe use of lidocaine has not been established with respect to possible adverse effects upon foetal development. Lidocaine is excreted in breast milk and so should be used with caution in nursing women.

4.7 Effects on ability to drive and use machines
Not applicable; this preparation is intended for use only in emergencies.

4.8 Undesirable effects
Adverse effects are usually due to inadvertent intravenous administration or overdosage. Allergic reactions (including anaphylaxis) have been reported rarely.

The following systemic reactions have been reported in association with lidocaine:

Central nervous system: light-headedness, drowsiness, dizziness, apprehension, nervousness, euphoria, tinnitus, blurred or double vision, nystagmus, vomiting, sensations of heat, cold or numbness, twitching, tremors, paraesthesia, convulsions, unconsciousness, respiratory depression and arrest.

Cardiovascular system: hypotension, cardiovascular collapse and bradycardia which may lead to cardiac arrest.

4.9 Overdose
Symptoms: reactions due to overdose with lidocaine (high plasma levels) are systemic and involve the central nervous and cardiovascular systems. Effects include medullary depression, tonic and clonic convulsions and cardiovascular collapse.

Treatment: institute emergency resuscitative procedures and administer the drugs necessary to manage the severe reaction. For severe convulsions, small increments of diazepam or an ultra-short acting barbiturate (thiopentone), or if not available, a short-acting barbiturate (pentobarbitone or quinalbarbitone), or if the patient is under anaesthesia, a short-acting muscle relaxant (suxamethonium) may be given intravenously. Patency of the airway and adequacy of ventilation must be assured.

Should circulatory depression occur vasopressors such as metaraminol may be used.

5. PHARMACOLOGICAL PROPERTIES

5.1 Pharmacodynamic properties
Lidocaine stabilises the neuronal membrane and prevents the initiation and transmission of nerve impulses, thereby effecting local anaesthetic action. The onset of action is rapid and the blockade may last up to 2 hours.

In the heart, lidocaine reduces automaticity by decreasing the rate of diastolic (phase 4) depolarisation. Lidocaine is considered as a class 1b (membrane stabilising) antiarrhythmic agent. The duration of the action potential is decreased due to blockade of the sodium channel and the refractory period is shortened.

5.2 Pharmacokinetic properties
Lidocaine is rapidly distributed to all body tissues. About 65% is plasma bound. Lidocaine crosses the placenta and the blood brain barrier. The plasma half life is 1.6 hours. About 80% of the dose is metabolised in the liver; less than 10% is found unchanged in the urine.

5.3 Preclinical safety data
Not applicable since lidocaine has been used in clinical practice for many years and its effects in man are well known.

6. PHARMACEUTICAL PARTICULARS

6.1 List of excipients
Hydrochloric Acid BP
Sodium Chloride BP
Sodium Hydroxide BP
Water for Injection USP

6.2 Incompatibilities
None known.

6.3 Shelf life
3 years.

6.4 Special precautions for storage
Store below 25°C.

6.5 Nature and contents of container
The solution is contained in a USP type I glass vial with an elastomeric closure which meets all the relevant USP

specifications. The product is available as a 2% solution in a 5ml vial.

6.6 Special precautions for disposal and other handling
The container is specially designed for use with the IMS Minijet injector.

7. MARKETING AUTHORISATION HOLDER
International Medication Systems (UK) Ltd
208 Bath Road
Slough
Berkshire
SL1 3WE
UK

8. MARKETING AUTHORISATION NUMBER(S)
PL 03265/0006R

9. DATE OF FIRST AUTHORISATION/RENEWAL OF THE AUTHORISATION
Date first granted: 28 February 1991
Date renewed: 29 November 1996

10. DATE OF REVISION OF THE TEXT
June 2004

11. Legal category
POM

Lipantil Micro 200

(Solvay Healthcare Limited)

1. NAME OF THE MEDICINAL PRODUCT
Lipantil® Micro 200 mg, capsules.

2. QUALITATIVE AND QUANTITATIVE COMPOSITION
Each capsule contains 200 mg fenofibrate.
For excipients, see 6.1

3. PHARMACEUTICAL FORM
Orange, hard gelatin capsule.

4. CLINICAL PARTICULARS

4.1 Therapeutic indications
Lipantil Micro 200 reduces elevated serum cholesterol and triglyceride and is of benefit in the treatment of severe dyslipidaemia in patients in whom dietary measures alone have failed to produce an adequate response. Lipantil Micro 200 is therefore indicated in appropriate cases of hyperlipidaemia (Fredrickson classification types IIa, IIb, III, IV and V).

Type	Major lipid elevated	Lipoproteins elevated
IIa	Cholesterol	LDL
IIb	Cholesterol, triglyceride	LDL, VLDL
III (rare)	Cholesterol, triglyceride	LDL and Chylomicron Remnants
IV	Triglyceride	VLDL
V (rare)	Triglyceride	Chylomicrons, VLDL

Lipantil Micro 200 should only be used in patients whose disease is unresponsive to dietary control and in whom a full investigation has been performed to define their abnormality, and where long-term risks associated with their condition warrant treatment. Other risk factors, such as hypertension and smoking, may also require management.

4.2 Posology and method of administration
Adults
The recommended initial dose is one capsule taken daily during a main meal. In elderly patients without renal impairment, the normal adult dose is recommended. Since it is less well absorbed from an empty stomach, Lipantil Micro 200 should always be taken with food. Dietary restrictions instituted before therapy should be continued.

Response to therapy should be monitored by determination of serum lipid values. Rapid reduction of serum lipid levels usually follows Lipantil Micro 200 treatment, but treatment should be discontinued if an adequate response has not been achieved within three months.

4.3 Contraindications
Lipantil Micro 200 is contra-indicated in children, in patients with severe liver dysfunction, gallbladder disease, biliary cirrhosis, severe renal disorders and in patients hypersensitive to fenofibrate or any component of this medication, known photoallergy or phototoxic reaction during treatment with fibrates or ketoprofen.

Chronic or acute pancreatitis with the exception of acute pancreatitis due to severe hypertriglyceridemia.

Use during pregnancy and lactation (see section 4.6).

4.4 Special warnings and precautions for use
Renal Impairment
In renal dysfunction the dose of fenofibrate may need to be reduced, depending on the rate of creatinine clearance. In this case, Lipantil Micro 67 (micronised fenofibrate) should be used, e.g. 2 capsules of Lipantil Micro 67 daily for creatinine clearance levels of <60 ml/min and 1 capsule of Lipantil Micro 67 daily for creatinine clearance levels of <20 ml/min.

Use of Lipantil Micro 67 is also to be preferred in elderly patients with renal impairment where dosage reduction may be required.

Serum Transaminases
Moderately elevated levels of serum transaminases may be found in some patients but rarely interfere with treatment. However, it is recommended that serum transaminases should be monitored every three months during the first twelve months of treatment. Treatment should be interrupted in the event of ALAT (SGPT) or ASAT (SGOT) elevations to more than 3 times the upper limit of the normal range or more than one hundred international units.

Pancreatitis
Pancreatitis has been reported in patients taking fenofibrate (see sections 4.3 and 4.8). This occurrence may represent a failure of efficacy in patients with severe hypertriglyceridaemia, a direct drug effect, or a secondary phenomenon mediated through biliary tract stone or sludge formation, resulting in the obstruction of the common bile duct.

Myopathy
Patients with pre-disposing factors for rhabdomyolysis, including renal impairment, hypothyroidism and high alcohol intake, may be at an increased risk of developing rhabdomyolysis.

Muscle toxicity, including very rare cases of rhabdomyolysis, has been reported with administration of fibrates and other lipid-lowering agents. The incidence of this disorder increases in cases of hypoalbuminaemia and previous renal insufficiency. Muscle toxicity should be suspected in patients presenting diffuse myalgia, myositis, muscular cramps and weakness and/or marked increases in CPK (levels exceeding 5 times the normal range). In such cases treatment with fenofibrate should be stopped.

The risk of muscle toxicity may be increased if the drug is administered with another fibrate or an HMG-CoA reductase inhibitor, especially in cases of pre-existing muscular disease. Consequently, the co-prescription of fenofibrate with a statin should be reserved to patients with severe combined dyslipidaemia and high cardiovascular risk without any history of muscular disease. This combination therapy should be used with caution and patients should be monitored closely for signs of muscle toxicity.

For hyperlipidaemic patients taking oestrogens or contraceptives containing oestrogen it should be ascertained whether the hyperlipidaemia is of primary or secondary nature (possible elevation of lipid values caused by oral oestrogen).

For patients with rare hereditary problems of galactose intolerance, the Lapp lactase deficiency or glucose-galactose malabsorption: although the amount of lactose contained in Lipantil Micro 200 mg is low, caution should be exercised in these patients (as no study has been formally conducted in this special population).

4.5 Interaction with other medicinal products and other forms of interaction
Oral Anti-coagulants
Fenofibrate enhances oral anti-coagulant effect and may increase risk of bleeding. In patients receiving oral anti-coagulant therapy, the dose of anti-coagulant should be reduced by about one-third at the commencement of treatment and then gradually adjusted if necessary according to INR (International Normalised Ratio) monitoring.

HMG-CoA reductase inhibitorsor Other Fibrates
The risk of serious muscle toxicity is increased if fenofibrate is used concomitantly with HMG-CoA reductase inhibitors or other fibrates. Such combination therapy should be used with caution and patients monitored closely for signs of muscle toxicity (see section 4.4.).

There is currently no evidence to suggest that fenofibrate affects the pharmacokinetics of simvastatin.

Cyclosporin
Some severe cases of reversible renal function impairment have been reported during concomitant administration of fenofibrate and cyclosporin. The renal function of these patients must therefore be closely monitored and the treatment with fenofibrate stopped in the case of severe alteration of laboratory parameters.

Other
No proven clinical interactions of fenofibrate with other drugs have been reported, although in vitro interaction studies suggest displacement of phenylbutazone from plasma protein binding sites. In common with other fibrates, fenofibrate induces microsomal mixed-function oxidases involved in fatty acid metabolism in rodents and may interact with drugs metabolised by these enzymes.

4.6 Pregnancy and lactation
There are no adequate data from the use of fenofibrate in pregnant women. Animal studies have not demonstrated any teratogenic effects. Embryotoxic effects have been shown at doses in the range of maternal toxicity (see section 5.3). The potential risk for humans is unknown.

There are no data on the excretion of fenofibrate and/or its metabolites into breast milk. It is therefore recommended that Lipantil Micro 200 should not be administered to women who are pregnant or are breast feeding.

4.7 Effects on ability to drive and use machines
No effect noted to date.

4.8 Undesirable effects
Adverse reactions observed during Lipantil Micro 200 treatment are not very frequent (2 - 4 % of cases): they are generally minor, transient and do not interfere with treatment.

The most commonly reported adverse reactions include:

Gastrointestinal: Digestive, gastric or intestinal disorders (abdominal pain, nausea, vomiting, diarrhoea, and flatulence) moderate in severity.

Uncommon: Pancreatitis*

Cardiovascular system
Uncommon: Thromboembolism (pulmonary embolism, deep vein thrombosis)*

Skin: Reactions such as rashes, pruritus, urticaria or photosensitivity reactions; in individual cases (even after many months of uncomplicated use) cutaneous photosensitivity may occur with erythema, vesiculation or nodulation on parts of the skin exposed to sunlight or artificial UV light (e.g. sun lamp).

Neurological disorders: Headache.

General disorders: Fatigue.

Disorders of the ear: Vertigo.

Less frequently reported adverse reactions:

Liver: Moderately elevated levels of serum transaminases may be found in some patients but rarely interfere with treatment (see also section 4.4). Episodes of hepatitis have been reported very rarely. When symptoms (e.g. jaundice, pruritus) indicative of hepatitis occur, laboratory tests are to be conducted for verification and fenofibrate discontinued, if applicable (see Special Warnings). Development of gallstones has been reported.

Muscle: As with other lipid lowering agents, cases of muscle toxicity (diffuse myalgia, myositis, muscular cramps and weakness) and very rare cases of rhabdomyolysis have been reported. These effects are usually reversible when the drug is withdrawn (see Special Warnings).

In rare cases, the following effects are reported: Sexual asthenia and alopecia. Increases in serum creatinine and urea, which are generally slight, and also a slight decrease in haemoglobin and leukocytes may be observed.

Very rare cases of interstitial pneumopathies have been reported.

* In the FIELD-study, a randomized placebo-controlled trial performed in 9795 patients with type 2 diabetes mellitus, a statistically significant increase in pancreatitis cases was observed in patients receiving fenofibrate versus patients receiving placebo (0.8% versus 0.5%; p = 0.031). In the same study, a statistically significant increase was reported in the incidence of pulmonary embolism (0.7% in the placebo group versus 1.1% in the fenofibrate group; p = 0.022) and a statistically non-significant increase in deep vein thromboses (placebo: 1.0 % [48/4900 patients] versus fenofibrate 1.4% [67/4895 patients]; p = 0.074).

4.9 Overdose
No case of overdosage has been reported. No specific antidote is known. If overdose is suspected, treat symptomatically and institute appropriate supportive measures as required. Fenofibrate cannot be eliminated by haemodialysis.

5. PHARMACOLOGICAL PROPERTIES

5.1 Pharmacodynamic properties
Serum Lipid Reducing Agents/Cholesterol and Triglyceride Reducers/Fibrates. ATC code:C10 AB 05.

Lipantil Micro 200 is a formulation containing 200mg of micronised fenofibrate; the administration of this product results in effective plasma concentrations identical to those obtained with 3 capsules of Lipantil Micro 67 containing 67mg of micronised fenofibrate.

The lipid-lowering properties of fenofibrate seen in clinical practice have been explained in vivo in transgenic mice and in human hepatocyte cultures by activation of Peroxisome Proliferator Activated Receptor type α (PPARα). Through this mechanism, fenofibrate increases lipolysis and elimination of triglyceride rich particles from plasma by activating lipoprotein lipase and reducing production of Apoprotein C-III. Activation of PPARα also induces an increase in the synthesis of Apoproteins A-I, A-II and of HDL cholesterol.

Epidemiological studies have demonstrated a positive correlation between abnormally increased serum lipid levels and an increased risk of coronary heart disease. The control of such dyslipidaemia forms the rationale for treatment with Lipantil Micro 200. However the possible beneficial and adverse long term consequences of drugs used in the management of dyslipidaemia are still the subject of scientific discussion. Therefore the presumptive beneficial effect of Lipantil Micro 200 on cardiovascular morbidity and mortality is as yet unproven.

Studies with fenofibrate on lipoprotein fractions show decreases in levels of LDL and VLDL cholesterol. HDL cholesterol levels are frequently increased. LDL and VLDL triglycerides are reduced. The overall effect is a decrease in the ratio of low and very low density lipoproteins to high density lipoproteins, which epidemiological studies have correlated with a decrease in atherogenic risk. Apolipoprotein-A and apolipoprotein-B levels are altered in parallel with HDL and LDL and VLDL levels respectively.

Regression of xanthomata has been observed during fenofibrate therapy.

Plasma uric acid levels are increased in approximately 20% of hyperlipidaemic patients, particularly in those with type IV disease. Lipantil Micro 200 has a uricosuric effect and is therefore of additional benefit in such patients.

Patients with raised levels of fibrinogen and Lp(a) have shown significant reductions in these measurements during clinical trials with fenofibrate.

5.2 Pharmacokinetic properties

Absorption

The unchanged compound is not recovered in the plasma. Fenofibric acid is the major plasma metabolite. Peak plasma concentration occurs after a mean period of 5 hours following dosing.

Mean plasma concentration is 15µg/ml for a daily dose of 200mg of micronised fenofibrate, equivalent to 3 capsules of Lipantil Micro 67.

Steady state levels are observed throughout continuous treatments.

Fenofibric acid is highly bound to plasma albumin; it can displace antivitamin K compounds from protein binding sites and may potentiate their anti-coagulant effect.

The plasma half-life of elimination of fenofibric acid is approximately 20 hours.

Metabolism and excretion

The product is mainly excreted in the urine; 70% in 24 hours and 88% in 6 days, at which time the total excretion in urine and faeces reaches 93%. Fenofibrate is mainly excreted as fenofibric acid and its derived glucuroconjugate.

Kinetic studies after administration of repeated doses show the absence of accumulation of the product.

Fenofibric acid is not eliminated during haemodialysis.

5.3 Preclinical safety data

Chronic toxicity studies have yielded no relevant information about specific toxicity of fenofibrate.

Studies on mutagenicity of fenofibrate have been negative.

In rats and mice, liver tumours have been found at high dosages, which are attributable to peroxisome proliferation. These changes are specific to small rodents and have not been observed in other animal species. This is of no relevance to therapeutic use in man.

Studies in mice, rats and rabbits did not reveal any teratogenic effect. Embryotoxic effects were observed at doses in the range of maternal toxicity. Prolongation of the gestation period and difficulties during delivery were observed at high doses. No sign of any effect on fertility has been detected.

6. PHARMACEUTICAL PARTICULARS

6.1 List of excipients

Excipients: lactose monohydrate, pregelatinised starch, sodium laurilsulfate, crospovidone and magnesium stearate.

Composition of the capsule shell: gelatin, titanium dioxide (E171), ferrous oxide (E172) and erythrosine (E127).

6.2 Incompatibilities

No effect noted to date.

6.3 Shelf life

3 years.

6.4 Special precautions for storage

Store in the original package. Do not store above 30°C.

6.5 Nature and contents of container

Pack of 10, 28, 30 capsules in blisters (PVC/Aluminium).

*Not all pack sizes may be marketed.

6.6 Special precautions for disposal and other handling

-

7. MARKETING AUTHORISATION HOLDER

Solvay Healthcare Ltd
Mansbridge Road
West End
Southampton
SO18 3JD
United Kingdom

8. MARKETING AUTHORISATION NUMBER(S)

PL 00512/0390

9. DATE OF FIRST AUTHORISATION/RENEWAL OF THE AUTHORISATION

November 1993/December 2003

10. DATE OF REVISION OF THE TEXT

July 2007

11. LEGAL CATEGORY

POM

Lipantil Micro 267

(Solvay Healthcare Limited)

1. NAME OF THE MEDICINAL PRODUCT

Lipantil®Micro 267 mg, capsules.

2. QUALITATIVE AND QUANTITATIVE COMPOSITION

Each capsule contains 267 mg fenofibrate.

For excipients, see 6.1

3. PHARMACEUTICAL FORM

Orange/ivory, hard gelatin capsule.

4. CLINICAL PARTICULARS

4.1 Therapeutic indications

Lipantil Micro 267 reduces elevated serum cholesterol and triglycerides and is of benefit in the treatment of severe dyslipidaemia in patients in whom dietary measures alone have failed to produce an adequate response. Lipantil Micro 267 is indicated in appropriate cases of dyslipidaemia (Fredrickson classification types IIa, IIb, III, IV and V).

Type	Major lipid elevated	Lipoproteins elevated
IIa	Cholesterol	LDL
IIb	Cholesterol, triglycerides	LDL, VLDL
III (rare)	Cholesterol, triglycerides	IDL and chylomicron remnants
IV	Triglyceride	VLDL
V (rare)	Triglyceride	Chylomicrons, VLDL

Lipantil Micro 267 should only be used in patients in whom a full investigation has been performed to define their abnormality. Other risk factors, such as hypertension and smoking, may also require management.

4.2 Posology and method of administration

Adults

The initial recommended dose is one capsule of Lipantil Micro 200 taken daily with food. However, in patients with severe dyslipidaemia, an increased dose of 267mg (Lipantil Micro 267), is recommended. Lipantil Micro 267 should always be taken with food, because it is less well absorbed from an empty stomach. Dietary measures instituted before therapy should be continued.

Children

This dosage is not recommended in children.

Elderly

In elderly patients without renal impairment, the normal adult dose is recommended.

Renal impairment

In renal dysfunction, the dosage may need to be reduced depending on the rate of creatinine clearance, for example:

Creatinine clearance (ml/min)	Dosage
< 60	One Lipantil Micro 140 mg capsule
< 20	One Lipantil Micro 67 mg capsule

4.3 Contraindications

Lipantil Micro 267 is contra-indicated in children, in patients with severe liver or renal dysfunction, gallbladder disease, biliary cirrhosis and in patients hypersensitive to fenofibrate or any component of this medication, known photoallergy or phototoxic reaction during treatment with fibrates or ketoprofen.

Chronic or acute pancreatitis with the exception of acute pancreatitis due to severe hypertriglyceridemia.

Use during pregnancy and lactation (see section 4.6).

4.4 Special warnings and precautions for use

In renal impairment

In renal dysfunction the dose of fenofibrate may need to be reduced, depending on the rate of creatinine clearance, (see section 4.2). Dose reduction should be considered in elderly patients with impaired renal function.

Transaminases

Moderately elevated levels of serum transaminases may be found in some patients but rarely interfere with treatment. However, it is recommended that serum transaminases should be monitored every three months during the first twelve months of treatment. Treatment should be interrupted in the event of ALAT (SGPT) or ASAT (SGOT) elevations to more than 3 times the upper limit of the normal range or more than one hundred international units.

Pancreatitis

Pancreatitis has been reported in patients taking fenofibrate (see sections 4.3 and 4.8). This occurrence may represent a failure of efficacy in patients with severe hypertriglyceridaemia, a direct drug effect, or a secondary phenomenon mediated through biliary tract stone or sludge formation, resulting in the obstruction of the common bile duct.

Myopathy

Patients with pre-disposing factors for rhabdomyolysis, including renal impairment, hypothyroidism and high alcohol intake, may be at an increased risk of developing rhabdomyolysis.

Muscle toxicity, including very rare cases of rhabdomyolysis, has been reported with administration of fibrates and other lipid-lowering agents. The incidence of this disorder increases in cases of hypoalbuminaemia and previous renal insufficiency. Muscle toxicity should be suspected in patients presenting diffuse myalgia, myositis, muscular cramps and weakness and/or marked increases in CPK (levels exceeding 5 times the normal range). In such cases treatment with fenofibrate should be stopped.

The risk of muscle toxicity may be increased if the drug is administered with another fibrate or an HMG-CoA reductase inhibitor, especially in cases of pre-existing muscular disease. Consequently, the co-prescription of fenofibrate with a statin should be reserved to patients with severe combined dyslipidaemia and high cardiovascular risk without any history of muscular disease. This combination therapy should be used with caution and patients should be monitored closely for signs of muscle toxicity.

For hyperlipidaemic patients taking oestrogens or contraceptives containing oestrogen it should be ascertained whether the hyperlipidaemia is of primary or secondary nature (possible elevation of lipid values caused by oral oestrogen).

For patients with rare hereditary problems of galactose intolerance, the Lapp lactase deficiency or glucose-galactose malabsorption: although the amount of lactose contained in Lipantil Micro 267 mg is low, caution should be exercised in these patients (as no study has been formally conducted in this special population).

4.5 Interaction with other medicinal products and other forms of interaction

Oral anti-coagulants

Fenofibrate enhances oral anti-coagulant effect and may increase risk of bleeding. In patients receiving oral anti-coagulant therapy, the dose of anti-coagulant should be reduced by about one-third at the commencement of treatment and then gradually adjusted if necessaryaccording to INR (International Normalised Ratio) monitoring.

HMG-CoA reductase inhibitorsor Other Fibrates

The risk of serious muscle toxicity is increased if fenofibrate is used concomitantly with HMG-CoA reductase inhibitors or other fibrates. Such combination therapy should be used with caution and patients monitored closely for signs of muscle toxicity (see section 4.4).

There is currently no evidence to suggest that fenofibrate affects the pharmacokinetics of simvastatin.

Cyclosporin

Some severe cases of reversible renal function impairment have been reported during concomitant administration of fenofibrate and cyclosporin. The renal function of these patients must therefore be closely monitored and the treatment with fenofibrate stopped in the case of severe alteration of laboratory parameters.

Other

No proven clinical interactions of fenofibrate with other drugs have been reported, although in vitro interaction studies suggest displacement of phenylbutazone from plasma protein binding sites. In common with other fibrates, fenofibrate induces microsomal mixed-function oxidases involved in fatty acid metabolism in rodents and may interact with drugs metabolised by these enzymes.

4.6 Pregnancy and lactation

There are no adequate data from the use of fenofibrate in pregnant women. Animal studies have not demonstrated any teratogenic effects. Embryotoxic effects have been shown at doses in the range of maternal toxicity (see section 5.3). The potential risk for humans is unknown.

There are no data on the excretion of fenofibrate and/or its metabolites into breast milk. It is therefore recommended that Lipantil Micro 267 should not be administered to women who are pregnant or are breast feeding.

4.7 Effects on ability to drive and use machines

No effect noted to date.

4.8 Undesirable effects

Fenofibrate is generally well tolerated. Adverse reactions observed during fenofibrate treatment are not very frequent; they are generally minor, transient and do not interfere with treatment.

The most commonly reported adverse reactions include:

Gastrointestinal: Digestive, gastric or intestinal disorders (abdominal pain, nausea, vomiting, diarrhoea, and flatulence) moderate in severity.

Uncommon: Pancreatitis*

Cardiovascular system

Uncommon: Thromboembolism (pulmonary embolism, deep vein thrombosis)*

Skin: Reactions such as rashes, pruritus, urticaria or photosensitivity reactions; in individual cases (even after many months of uncomplicated use) cutaneous photosensitivity may occur with erythema, vesiculation or nodulation on parts of the skin exposed to sunlight or artificial UV light (e.g. sun lamp).

Neurological disorders: Headache

General disorders: Fatigue

Disorders of the ear: Vertigo

Less frequently reported adverse reactions:

Liver: Moderately elevated levels of serum transaminases may be found in some patients but rarely interfere with treatment (see also section 4.4). Episodes of hepatitis have been reported very rarely. When symptoms (e.g. jaundice, pruritus) indicative of hepatitis occur, laboratory tests are to be conducted for verification and fenofibrate discontinued, if applicable (see Special Warnings). Development of gallstones has been reported.

Muscle: As with other lipid lowering agents, cases of muscle toxicity (diffuse myalgia, myositis, muscular cramps and weakness) and very rare cases of rhabdomyolysis have been reported. These effects are usually reversible when the drug is withdrawn (see Special Warnings).

In rare cases, the following effects are reported: Sexual asthenia and alopecia. Increases in serum creatinine and urea, which are generally slight, and also a slight decrease in haemoglobin and leukocytes may be observed.

Very rare cases of interstitial pneumopathies have been reported.

* In the FIELD-study, a randomized placebo-controlled trial performed in 9795 patients with type 2 diabetes mellitus, a statistically significant increase in pancreatitis cases was observed in patients receiving fenofibrate versus patients receiving placebo (0.8% versus 0.5%; p = 0.031). In the same study, a statistically significant increase was reported in the incidence of pulmonary embolism (0.7% in the placebo group versus 1.1% in the fenofibrate group; p = 0.022) and a statistically non-significant increase in deep vein thromboses (placebo: 1.0 % [48/4900 patients] versus fenofibrate 1.4% [67/4895 patients]; p = 0.074).

4.9 Overdose

No case of overdosage has been reported. No specific antidote is known. If overdose is suspected, treat symptomatically and institute appropriate supportive measures as required. Fenofibrate cannot be eliminated by haemodialysis.

5. PHARMACOLOGICAL PROPERTIES

5.1 Pharmacodynamic properties

Serum Lipid Reducing Agents/Cholesterol and Triglyceride Reducers/Fibrates.

ATC code: C10 AB 05

Lipantil Micro 267 is a formulation containing 267 mg of micronised fenofibrate.

The lipid lowering properties of fenofibrate seen in clinical practice have been explained in vivo in transgenic mice and in human hepatocyte cultures by activation of Peroxisome Proliferator Activated Receptor type α (PPARα). Through this mechanism, fenofibrate increases lipolysis and elimination of triglyceride-rich particles from plasma by activating lipoprotein lipase and reducing production of Apoprotein C-III. Activation of PPARα also induces an increase in the synthesis of Apoproteins A-I, A-II and of HDL cholesterol.

Epidemiological studies have demonstrated a positive correlation between increased serum lipid levels and an increased risk of coronary heart disease. The control of such dyslipidaemias forms the rationale for treatment with fenofibrate. However, the possible beneficial and adverse long-term consequences of drugs used in the management of dyslipidaemias are still the subject of scientific discussion. Therefore the presumptive beneficial effect of Lipantil Micro 267 on cardiovascular morbidity and mortality is as yet unproven.

Studies with fenofibrate consistently show decreases in levels of LDL-cholesterol. HDL-cholesterol levels are frequently increased. Triglyceride levels are also reduced. This results in a decrease in the ratio of low and very low density lipoproteins to high density lipoproteins, which has been correlated with a decrease in atherogenic risk in epidemiological studies. Apolipoprotein-A and apolipoprotein-B levels are altered in parallel with HDL and LDL and VLDL levels respectively.

Regression of xanthomata has been observed during fenofibrate therapy.

Plasma uric acid levels are increased in approximately 20% of hyperlipidaemic patients, particularly in those with type IV phenotype. Lipantil Micro 267 has a uricosuric effect and is therefore of additional benefit in such patients.

Patients with raised levels of fibrinogen and Lp(a) have shown significant reductions in these measurements during clinical trials with fenofibrate.

5.2 Pharmacokinetic properties

Absorption

The unchanged compound is not recovered in the plasma. Fenofibric acid is the major plasma metabolite. Peak plasma concentration occurs after a mean period of 5 hours following dosing.

Mean plasma concentration is 15 μg/ml for a daily dosage of 200 mg of micronised fenofibrate.

Steady state levels are observed throughout continuous treatments.

Fenofibric acid is highly bound to plasma albumin: it can displace antivitamin K compounds from the protein binding sites and potentiate their anti-coagulant effect.

Plasma half-life

The plasma half-life of elimination of fenofibric acid is approximately 20 hours.

Metabolism and excretion

The product is mainly excreted in the urine: 70% in 24 hours and 88% in 6 days, at which time total excretion in urine and faeces reaches 93%. Fenofibrate is mainly excreted as fenofibric acid and its derived glucuroconjugate.

Kinetic studies after administration of repeated doses show the absence of accumulation of the product.

Fenofibric acid is not eliminated during haemodialysis.

5.3 Preclinical safety data

Chronic toxicity studies have yielded no relevant information about specific toxicity of fenofibrate.

Studies on mutagenicity of fenofibrate have been negative.

In rats and mice, liver tumours have been found at high dosages, which are attributable to peroxisome proliferation. These changes are specific to small rodents and have not been observed in other animal species. This is of no relevance to therapeutic use in man.

Studies in mice, rats and rabbits did not reveal any teratogenic effect. Embryotoxic effects were observed at doses in the range of maternal toxicity. Prolongation of the gestation period and difficulties during delivery were observed at high doses. No sign of any effect on fertility has been detected.

6. PHARMACEUTICAL PARTICULARS

6.1 List of excipients

Excipients: lactose monohydrate, magnesium stearate, pregelatinised starch, sodium laurilsulfate, crospovidone.

Composition of the capsule shell: gelatin, titanium dioxide (E 171), yellow and red ferrous oxide (E 172).

6.2 Incompatibilities

No effect noted to date.

6.3 Shelf life

3 years.

6.4 Special precautions for storage

Store in the original package. Do not store above 30°C.

6.5 Nature and contents of container

Pack of 28, 30 capsules in blisters (PVC/Aluminium).

*Not all pack sizes may be marketed.

6.6 Special precautions for disposal and other handling

Capsules should be swallowed whole with water.

7. MARKETING AUTHORISATION HOLDER

Solvay Healthcare Ltd

Mansbridge Road

West End

Southampton

SO18 3JD

United Kingdom

8. MARKETING AUTHORISATION NUMBER(S)

PL 00512/0391

9. DATE OF FIRST AUTHORISATION/RENEWAL OF THE AUTHORISATION

3 February 1999/February 2004

10. DATE OF REVISION OF THE TEXT

July 2007

11. LEGAL CATEGORY

POM

Lipantil Micro 67

(Solvay Healthcare Limited)

1. NAME OF THE MEDICINAL PRODUCT

Lipantil® Micro 67 mg, capsules.

2. QUALITATIVE AND QUANTITATIVE COMPOSITION

Each capsule contains 67 mg fenofibrate.

For excipients, see 6.1

3. PHARMACEUTICAL FORM

Yellow, hard gelatin capsule.

4. CLINICAL PARTICULARS

4.1 Therapeutic indications

Lipantil Micro 67 reduces elevated serum cholesterol and triglycerides and is of benefit in the treatment of severe dyslipidaemia in patients in whom dietary measures alone have failed to produce an adequate response. Lipantil Micro 67 is indicated in appropriate cases of dyslipidaemia (Fredrickson classification types IIa, IIb, III, IV and V).

Type	Major lipid elevated	Lipoproteins elevated
IIa	Cholesterol	LDL
IIb	Cholesterol, triglycerides	LDL, VLDL
III (rare)	Cholesterol, triglycerides	LDL and chylomicron remnants
IV	Triglycerides	VLDL
V (rare)	Triglycerides	Chylomicrons, VLDL

Lipantil Micro 67 should only be used in patients in whom a full investigation has been performed to define their abnormality. Other risk factors, such as hypertension and smoking, may also require management.

4.2 Posology and method of administration

Adults

In adults, the recommended initial dose is 3 capsules taken daily in divided doses. Lipantil Micro 67 should always be taken with food, because it is less well absorbed from an empty stomach. Dietary measures instituted before therapy should be continued.

The response to therapy should be monitored by determination of serum lipid values and the dosage may be altered within the range 2-4 capsules of Lipantil Micro 67 daily.

Children

In children, the recommended dose is one capsule (67mg) micronised fenofibrate / day / 20kg body weight.

Elderly

In elderly patients without renal impairment, the normal adult dose is recommended.

Renal Impairment

In renal dysfunction, the dosage may need to be reduced depending on the rate of creatinine clearance, for example:

Creatinine clearance (ml/min)	Dosage
<60	Two 67mg capsules
<20	One 67mg capsule

4.3 Contraindications

Lipantil Micro 67 is contra-indicated in patients with severe liver or renal dysfunction, gallbladder disease, biliary cirrhosis and in patients hypersensitive to fenofibrate or any component of this medication, known photoallergy or phototoxic reaction during treatment with fibrates or ketoprofen.

Chronic or acute pancreatitis with the exception of acute pancreatitis due to severe hypertriglyceridemia.

Use during pregnancy and lactation (see section 4.6).

4.4 Special warnings and precautions for use

In renal impairment

In renal dysfunction the dose of fenofibrate may need to be reduced, depending on the rate of creatinine clearance, (see section 4.2). Dose reduction should be considered in elderly patients with impaired renal function.

Transaminases

Moderately elevated levels of serum transaminases may be found in some patients but rarely interfere with treatment. However, it is recommended that serum transaminases should be monitored every three months during the first twelve months of treatment. Treatment should be interrupted in the event of ALAT (SGPT) or ASAT (SGOT) elevations to more than 3 times the upper limit of the normal range or more than one hundred international units.

Pancreatitis

Pancreatitis has been reported in patients taking fenofibrate (see sections 4.3 and 4.8). This occurrence may represent a failure of efficacy in patients with severe hypertriglyceridaemia, a direct drug effect, or a secondary phenomenon mediated through biliary tract stone or sludge formation, resulting in the obstruction of the common bile duct.

Myopathy

Patients with pre-disposing factors for rhabdomyolysis, including renal impairment, hypothyroidism and high alcohol intake, may be at an increased risk of developing rhabdomyolysis.

Muscle toxicity, including very rare cases of rhabdomyolysis, has been reported with administration of fibrates and other lipid-lowering agents. The incidence of this disorder increases in cases of hypoalbuminaemia and previous renal insufficiency. Muscle toxicity should be suspected in patients presenting diffuse myalgia, myositis, muscular cramps and weakness and/or marked increases in CPK (levels exceeding 5 times the normal range). In such cases treatment with fenofibrate should be stopped.

The risk of muscle toxicity may be increased if the drug is administered with another fibrate or an HMG-CoA reductase inhibitor, especially in cases of pre-existing muscular disease. Consequently, the co-prescription of fenofibrate with a statin should be reserved to patients with severe combined dyslipidaemia and high cardiovascular risk without any history of muscular disease. This combination therapy should be used with caution and patients should be monitored closely for signs of muscle toxicity.

For hyperlipidaemic patients taking oestrogens or contraceptives containing oestrogen it should be ascertained whether the hyperlipidaemia is of primary or secondary nature (possible elevation of lipid values caused by oral oestrogen).

For patients with rare hereditary problems of galactose intolerance, the Lapp lactase deficiency or glucose-galactose malabsorption: although the amount of lactose contained in Lipantil Micro 67 mg is low, caution should be exercised in these patients (as no study has been formally conducted in this special population).

In children

Only an hereditary disease (familial hyperlipidaemia) justifies early treatment, and the precise nature of the hyperlipidaemia must be determined by genetic and laboratory investigations. It is recommended to begin treatment with controlled dietary restrictions for a period of at least 3 months. Proceeding to medicinal treatment should only be considered after specialist advice and only in severe forms with clinical signs of atherosclerosis and/or xanthomata and/or in cases where patients suffer from atherosclerotic cardiovascular disease before the age of 40.

4.5 Interaction with other medicinal products and other forms of interaction

Oral anti-coagulants

Fenofibrate enhances oral anti-coagulant effect and may increase risk of bleeding. In patients receiving oralanticoagulant therapy, the dose of anti-coagulant should be reduced by about one-third at the commencement of treatment and then gradually adjusted if necessary according to INR (International Normalised Ratio) monitoring.

HMG-CoA reductase inhibitors or Other Fibrates

The risk of serious muscle toxicity is increased if fenofibrate is used concomitantly with HMG-CoA reductase inhibitors or other fibrates. Such combination therapy should be used with caution and patients monitored closely for signs of muscle toxicity (see Section 4.4).

There is currently no evidence to suggest that fenofibrate affects the pharmacokinetics of simvastatin.

Cyclosporin

Some severe cases of reversible renal function impairment have been reported during concomitant administration of fenofibrate and cyclosporin. The renal function of these patients must therefore be closely monitored and the treatment with fenofibrate stopped in the case of severe alteration of laboratory parameters.

Other

No proven clinical interactions of fenofibrate with other drugs have been reported, although in vitro interaction studies suggest displacement of phenylbutazone from plasma protein binding sites. In common with other fibrates, fenofibrate induces microsomal mixed-function oxidases involved in fatty acid metabolism in rodents and may interact with drugs metabolised by these enzymes.

4.6 Pregnancy and lactation

There are no adequate data from the use of fenofibrate in pregnant women. Animal studies have not demonstrated any teratogenic effects. Embryotoxic effects have been shown at doses in the range of maternal toxicity (see section 5.3). The potential risk for humans is unknown.

There are no data on the excretion of fenofibrate and/or its metabolites into breast milk.

It is therefore recommended that Lipantil Micro 67 should not be administered to women who are pregnant or are breast feeding.

4.7 Effects on ability to drive and use machines

No effect noted to date.

4.8 Undesirable effects

Fenofibrate is generally well tolerated. Adverse reactions observed during fenofibrate treatment are not very frequent; they are generally minor, transient and do not interfere with treatment.

The most commonly reported adverse reactions include:

Gastrointestinal: Digestive, gastric or intestinal disorders (abdominal pain, nausea, vomiting, diarrhoea, and flatulence) moderate in severity.

Uncommon: Pancreatitis *

Cardiovascular system

Uncommon: Thromboembolism (pulmonary embolism, deep vein thrombosis)*.

Skin: Reactions such as rashes, pruritus, urticaria or photosensitivity reactions; in individual cases (even after many months of uncomplicated use) cutaneous photosensitivity may occur with erythema, vesiculation or nodulation on parts of the skin exposed to sunlight or artificial UV light (e.g. sun lamp).

Neurological disorders: Headache.

General disorders: Fatigue.

Disorders of the ear: Vertigo.

Less frequently reported adverse reactions:

Liver: Moderately elevated levels of serum transaminases may be found in somepatientsbut rarely interfere with treatment (see also section 4.4). Episodes of hepatitis have been reported very rarely. When symptoms (e.g.jaundice, pruritus) indicative of hepatitis occur, laboratory tests are to be conducted for verification and fenofibrate discontinued, if applicable (see Special Warnings). Development of gallstones has been reported.

Muscle: As with other lipid lowering agents, cases of muscle toxicity (diffuse myalgia, myositis, muscular cramps and weakness) and very rare cases of rhabdomyolysis have been reported. These effects are usually reversible when the drug is withdrawn (see Special Warnings).

In rare cases, the following effects are reported: sexual asthenia and alopecia. Increases in serum creatinine and urea, which are generally slight, and also a slight decrease in haemoglobin and leukocytes may be observed.

Very rare cases of interstitial pneumopathies have been reported.

* In the FIELD-study, a randomized placebo-controlled trial performed in 9795 patients with type 2 diabetes mellitus, a statistically significant increase in pancreatitis cases was observed in patients receiving fenofibrate versus patients receiving placebo (0.8% versus 0.5%; p = 0.031). In the same study, a statistically significant increase was reported in the incidence of pulmonary embolism (0.7% in the placebo group versus 1.1% in the fenofibrate group; p = 0.022) and a statistically non-significant increase in deep vein thromboses (placebo: 1.0 % [48/4900 patients] versus fenofibrate 1.4% [67/4895 patients]; p = 0.074).

4.9 Overdose

No case of overdosage has been reported. No specific antidote is known. If overdose is suspected, treat symptomatically and institute appropriate supportive measures as required. Fenofibrate cannot be eliminated by haemodialysis.

5. PHARMACOLOGICAL PROPERTIES

5.1 Pharmacodynamic properties

Serum Lipid Reducing Agents/Cholesterol and Triglyceride Reducers/Fibrates. ATC code:C10 AB 05.

Lipantil Micro 67 is a formulation containing 67mg of micronised fenofibrate.

The lipid-lowering properties of fenofibrate seen in clinical practice have been explained in vivo in transgenic mice and in human hepatocyte cultures by activation of Peroxisome Proliferator Activated Receptor type α (PPARα). Through this mechanism, fenofibrate increases lipolysis and elimination of triglyceride rich particles from plasma by activating lipoprotein lipase and reducing production of Apoprotein C-III. Activation of PPARα also induces an increase in the synthesis of Apoproteins A-I, A-II and of HDL cholesterol.

Epidemiological studies have demonstrated a positive correlation between increased serum lipid levels and an increased risk of coronary heart disease. The control of such dyslipidaemias forms the rationale for treatment with fenofibrate. However, the possible beneficial and adverse long-term consequences of drugs used in the hyperlipidaemias are still the subject of scientific discussion. Therefore the presumptive beneficial effect of Lipantil Micro 67 on cardiovascular morbidity and mortality is as yet unproven.

Studies with fenofibrate consistently show decreases in levels of LDL-cholesterol. HDL-cholesterol levels are frequently increased. Triglyceride levels are also reduced. This results in a decrease in the ratio of low and very low density lipoproteins to high density lipoproteins, which has been correlated with a decrease in atherogenic risk in epidemiological studies. Apolipoprotein-A and apolipoprotein-B levels are altered in parallel with HDL and LDL and VLDL levels respectively.

Regression of xanthomata has been observed during fenofibrate therapy.

Plasma uric acid levels are increased in approximately 20% of hyperlipidaemic patients, particularly in those with type IV phenotype. Lipantil Micro 67 has a uricosuric effect and is therefore of additional benefit in such patients.

Patients with raised levels of fibrinogen and Lp(a) have shown significant reductions in these measurements during clinical trials with fenofibrate.

5.2 Pharmacokinetic properties

Absorption

The unchanged compound is not recovered in the plasma. Fenofibric acid is the major plasma metabolite. Peak plasma concentration occurs after a mean period of 5 hours following dosing.

Mean plasma concentration is 15μg/ml for a daily dosage of 200mg of micronised fenofibrate, equivalent to 3 capsules of Lipantil Micro 67.

Steady state levels are observed throughout continuous treatments.

Fenofibric acid is highly bound to plasma albumin: it can displace antivitamin K compounds from the protein binding sites and potentiate their anti-coagulant effect.

Plasma half-life

The plasma half-life of elimination of fenofibric acid is approximately 20 hours.

Metabolism and excretion

The product is mainly excreted in the urine: 70% in 24 hours and 88% in 6 days, at which time total excretion in urine and faeces reaches 93%. Fenofibrate is mainly excreted as fenofibric acid and its derived glucuroconjugate.

Kinetic studies after administration of repeated doses show the absence of accumulation of the product.

Fenofibric acid is not eliminated during haemodialysis.

5.3 Preclinical safety data

Chronic toxicity studies have yielded no relevant information about specific toxicity of fenofibrate. Studies on mutagenicity of fenofibrate have been negative. In rats and mice, liver tumours have been found at high dosages, which are attributable to peroxisome proliferation. These changes are specific to small rodents and have not been observed in other animal species. This is of no relevance to therapeutic use in man. Studies in mice, rats and rabbits did not reveal any teratogenic effect. Embryotoxic effects were observed at doses in the range of maternal toxicity. Prolongation of the gestation period and difficulties during delivery were observed at high doses. No sign of any effect on fertility has been detected.

6. PHARMACEUTICAL PARTICULARS

6.1 List of excipients

Excipients: lactose monohydrate, magnesium stearate, pregelatinised starch, sodium laurilsulfate, crospovidone.

Composition of the capsule shell: gelatin, titanium dioxide (E171), quinoline yellow (E104) and erythrosine (E127).

6.2 Incompatibilities

No effect noted to date.

6.3 Shelf life

3 years.

6.4 Special precautions for storage

Store in the original package. Do not store above 30°C.

6.5 Nature and contents of container

Pack of 28,56,84,90 capsules in blisters (PVC/Aluminium).

*Not all pack sizes may be marketed.

6.6 Special precautions for disposal and other handling

Capsules should be swallowed whole with water.

7. MARKETING AUTHORISATION HOLDER

Solvay Healthcare Ltd
Mansbridge Road
West End
Southampton
SO18 3JD
United Kingdom

8. MARKETING AUTHORISATION NUMBER(S)

PL 00512/0387

9. DATE OF FIRST AUTHORISATION/RENEWAL OF THE AUTHORISATION

11 September 1997/10th September 2002

10. DATE OF REVISION OF THE TEXT

July 2007

11. LEGAL CATEGORY

POM

Lipitor 10mg, 20mg, 40mg, 80mg Tablets

(Pfizer Limited)

1. NAME OF THE MEDICINAL PRODUCT

Lipitor™ 10 mg, 20mg, 40mg, 80 mg Tablets.

2. QUALITATIVE AND QUANTITATIVE COMPOSITION

Each tablet contains 10 mg, 20mg, 40mg, or 80mg atorvastatin as atorvastatin calcium trihydrate.

For excipients see section 6.1.

3. PHARMACEUTICAL FORM

Film-coated tablets.

White, elliptical, film-coated tablets debossed '10' on one side and 'PD 155' on the other side.

White, elliptical, film-coated tablets debossed '20' on one side and 'PD 156' on the other side.

White, elliptical, film-coated tablets debossed '40' on one side and 'PD 157' on the other side.

White, elliptical, film-coated tablets debossed '80' on one side and 'PD 158' on the other side.

4. CLINICAL PARTICULARS

4.1 Therapeutic indications

Hypercholesterolaemia:

Lipitor is indicated as an adjunct to diet for reduction of elevated total cholesterol, LDL-cholesterol, apolipoprotein B, and triglycerides in adults and children aged 10 years and older with primary hypercholesterolaemia, heterozygous familial hypercholesterolaemia or combined (mixed) hyperlipidaemia when response to diet and other nonpharmacological measures is inadequate.

Lipitor also raises HDL-cholesterol and lowers the LDL/HDL and total cholesterol/HDL ratios.

Lipitor is also indicated as an adjunct to diet and other non-dietary measures in reducing elevated total cholesterol, LDL-cholesterol, and apolipoprotein B in patients with homozygous familial hypercholesterolaemia when response to these measures is inadequate.

Primary prevention in type II diabetes:

Lipitor is indicated for reducing the risk of cardiovascular events in diabetic patients with at least 1 additional risk factor, without clinically evident coronary heart disease irrespective of whether cholesterol is raised. See section 5.1.

4.2 Posology and method of administration

The patient should be placed on a standard cholesterol-lowering diet before receiving Lipitor and should continue on this diet during treatment with Lipitor. The usual starting dose is 10 mg once a day. Doses should be individualised according to baseline LDL-C levels, the goal of therapy, and patient response. Adjustment of dosage should be made at intervals of 4 weeks or more. The maximum dose is 80 mg once a day.

For patients taking interacting drugs that increase plasma exposure to atorvastatin, the starting dose should be 10 mg once a day, and a maximum dose of less than 80mg may need to be considered. In some cases a dose reduction, or where not practical, a temporary dose suspension may be considered (see Sections 4.4 and 4.5).

Doses above 20mg/day have not been investigated in patients aged <18 years. Doses may be given at any time of day with or without food.

Primary Hypercholesterolaemia and Combined (Mixed) Hyperlipidaemia

Adults:

The majority of patients are controlled with 10 mg Lipitor once a day. A therapeutic response is evident within 2 weeks, and the maximum response is usually achieved within 4 weeks. The response is maintained during chronic therapy.

Current consensus guidelines should be consulted to establish treatment goals for individual patients.

Children aged 10-17 years:

Doses above 20mg/day have not been investigated.

Heterozygous Familial Hypercholesterolaemia

Adults:

Patients should be started with Lipitor 10 mg daily. Doses should be individualised and adjusted every 4 weeks to 40 mg daily. Thereafter, either the dose may be increased to a maximum of 80 mg daily or a bile acid sequestrant (eg, colestipol) may be combined with 40 mg Lipitor.

Children aged 10-17 years:

Doses above 20mg/day and combination therapies have not been investigated.

Homozygous Familial Hypercholesterolaemia

Adults: In a compassionate-use study of patients with homozygous familial hypercholesterolaemia, most patients responded to a dose of 80 mg of Lipitor (see Section 5.1 Pharmacodynamics).

Children: Treatment experience in a paediatric population with doses of Lipitor up to 80 mg/day is limited.

Dosage in Patients With Renal Insufficiency

Renal disease has no influence on the plasma concentrations nor lipid effects of Lipitor; thus, no adjustment of dose is required.

Dosage in Patients With Hepatic Dysfunction

In patients with moderate to severe hepatic dysfunction, the therapeutic response to Lipitor is unaffected but exposure to the drug is greatly increased. Cmax increases by approximately 16 fold and AUC (0-24) by approximately 11 fold. Therefore, caution should be exercised in patients who consume substantial quantities of alcohol and/or have a history of liver disease.

Geriatric Use

Adequate treatment experience in adults age 70 or older with doses of Lipitor up to 80 mg/day has been obtained. Efficacy and safety in older patients using recommended doses is similar to that seen in the general population.

Prevention of Cardiovascular disease

In the primary prevention trials, the dose was 10mg/day (see section 5.1 for the lipid levels where this dose was found to be effective, patients with higher levels will require conventional measurement and dose titration).

4.3 Contraindications

Lipitor is contraindicated in patients with hypersensitivity to any component of this medication, active liver disease or unexplained persistent elevations of serum transaminases exceeding 3 times the upper limit of normal, during pregnancy, while breast-feeding, and in women of child-bearing potential not using appropriate contraceptive measures.

4.4 Special warnings and precautions for use

Liver Effects

Liver function tests should be performed before the initiation of treatment and periodically thereafter. Patients who develop any signs or symptoms suggestive of liver injury should have liver function tests performed. Patients who develop increased transaminase levels should be monitored until the abnormality(ies) resolve. Should an increase in ALT or AST of greater than 3 times the upper limit of normal persist, reduction of dose or withdrawal of Lipitor is recommended.

Lipitor should be used with caution in patients who consume substantial quantities of alcohol and/or have a history of liver disease.

Stroke Prevention by Aggressive Reduction in Cholesterol Levels (SPARCL)

In a post-hoc analysis of stroke subtypes in patients without CHD who had a recent stroke or TIA there was a higher incidence of haemorrhagic stroke in patients initiated on atorvastatin 80 mg compared to placebo. The increased risk was particularly noted in patients with prior haemorrhagic stroke or lacunar infarct at study entry. For patients with prior haemorrhagic stroke or lacunar infarct, the balance of risks and benefits of atorvastatin 80 mg is uncertain and the potential risk of haemorrhagic stroke should be carefully considered before initiating treatment (see Section 5.1).

Muscle effects

Treatment with HMG-CoA reductase inhibitors (statins) has been associated with the onset of myalgia, myopathy, and very rarely rhabdomyolysis. Myopathy must be considered in any patient under statin therapy presenting with unexplained muscle symptoms such as pain or tenderness, muscle weakness or muscle cramps. In such cases creatine kinase (CK) levels should be measured (see below).

Creatine phosphokinase measurement

Creatine phosphokinase (CPK) should not be measured following strenuous exercise or in the presence of any plausible alternative cause of CPK increase as this makes value interpretation difficult. If CPK levels are significantly elevated at baseline (>5 times ULN), levels should be remeasured within 5 to 7 days later to confirm the results.

Before treatment

As with other statins atorvastatin should be prescribed with caution in patients with pre-disposing factors for rhabdomyolysis. A creatine phosphokinase (CPK) level should be measured before starting treatment in the following situations:

– Renal impairment

– Hypothyroidism

– Personal or familial history of hereditary muscular disorders

– Previous history of muscular toxicity with a statin or fibrate

– Previous history of liver disease and/or where substantial quantities of alcohol are consumed

– In elderly (age > 70 years), the necessity of such measurement should be considered, according to the presence of other predisposing factors for rhabdomyolysis

In such situations, the risk of treatment should be considered in relation to possible benefit and clinical monitoring is recommended. If CPK levels are significantly elevated (>5 times ULN) at baseline, treatment should not be started.

Whilst on treatment

– If muscular pain, weakness or cramps occur whilst a patient is receiving treatment with a statin, their CPK levels should be measured. If these levels are found to be significantly elevated (> 5 times ULN), treatment should be stopped.

– If muscular symptoms are severe and cause daily discomfort, even if CPK levels are elevated to ≤ 5 times ULN, treatment discontinuation should be considered.

– If symptoms resolve and CPK levels return to normal, then re-introduction of atorvastatin or introduction of an alternative statin may be considered at the lowest dose and with close monitoring.

These CPK elevations should be considered when evaluating the possibility of myocardial infarction in the differential diagnosis of chest pain.

As with other drugs in this class, rhabdomyolysis with acute renal failure has been reported.

Children aged 10-17 years

In patients aged <18 years efficacy and safety have not been studied for treatment periods >52 weeks' duration and effects on long-term cardiovascular outcomes are unknown.

The effects of atorvastatin in children aged <10 years and premenarchal girls have not been investigated.

Long term effects on cognitive development, growth and pubertal maturation are unknown.

Risk of dose-related side effects including rhabdomyolysis is increased when atorvastatin is administered concomitantly with certain medications that may increase the plasma concentration of atorvastatin such as: ciclosporin, erythromycin, clarithromycin, itraconazole, ketoconazole, nefazodone, niacin, gemfibrozil, other fibrates or HIV-protease inhibitors. The risk of myopathy may also be increased with the concomitant use of ezetimibe. If possible alternative (non-interacting) therapies should be considered instead of these medications. In cases where co-administration of these medications with atorvastatin is only necessary for a few days, a dose reduction or where not practical, a temporary suspension of treatment with atorvastatin may be considered. If co-administration with interacting drugs is unavoidable, the starting dose of atorvastatin should be 10 mg once a day. In the case of ciclosporin, clarithromycin and itraconazole, a lower maximum dose of atorvastatin should be used (see Section 4.5). Lipid levels should be monitored to ensure that the lowest dose necessary of atorvastatin is employed.

Patients with rare hereditary problems of galactose intolerance, Lapp lactose deficiency or glucose-galactose malabsorption should not take this medicine.

Temporary suspension of atorvastatin may be appropriate during fusidic acid therapy (see Section 4.5)

4.5 Interaction with other medicinal products and other forms of interaction

The risk of myopathy during treatment with HMG-CoA reductase inhibitors is increased with concurrent administration of ciclosporin, fibrates, macrolide antibiotics including erythromycin, azole antifungals, HIV-protease inhibitors or niacin and on rare occasions has resulted in rhabdomyolysis with renal dysfunction secondary to myoglobinuria. In cases where co-administration of these medications with atorvastatin is necessary, the benefit and the risk of concurrent treatment should be carefully considered. When patients are receiving drugs that increase the plasma concentration of atorvastatin, the starting dose of atorvastatin should be 10 mg once a day. In the case of ciclosporin, clarithromycin and itraconazole, a lower maximum dose of atorvastatin should be used (see below and Section 4.2). Lipid levels should be monitored to ensure that the lowest dose necessary of atorvastatin is used. (see Section 4.4).

Transporter Inhibitors:

Atorvastatin and atorvastatin-metabolites are substrates of the OATP1B1 transporter. Concomitant administration of atorvastatin 10 mg and ciclosporin 5.2 mg/kg/day resulted in an 8.7 fold increase in atorvastatin AUC. In cases where co-administration of atorvastatin with ciclosporin is necessary, the dose of atorvastatin should not exceed 10 mg.

Clarithromycin: Clarithromycin is a known inhibitor of cytochrome P450 3A4. Co-admistration of atorvastatin 10 mg OD and clarithromycin (500 mg BID) resulted in a 4.4 fold increase in atorvastatin AUC. In cases where co-administration of clarithromycin with atorvastatin is necessary, the maintenance dose of atorvastatin should not exceed 20 mg daily. Patients who normally require 40mg or 80mg of atorvastatin should either reduce their dosage during concomitant clarithromycin treatment, or alternatively (for short courses of this antibiotic) where not practical, a temporary suspension of treatment with atorvastatin may be considered.

Erythromycin: Erythromycin is a known inhibitor of cytochrome P450 3A4. Co-administration of atorvastatin 80 mg OD and erythromycin (500 mg QID) resulted in a 33% increase in exposure to total atorvastatin activity.

Azithromycin: Co-administration of Lipitor (10 mg OD) and azithromycin (500 mg OD) did not alter the plasma concentrations of atorvastatin.

Itraconazole: Concomitant administration of atorvastatin 20 to 40 mg and itraconazole 200 mg daily resulted in a 2.5-3.3 fold increase in atorvastatin AUC. In cases where co-administration of itraconazole with atorvastatin is necessary, the maintenance dose of atorvastatin should not exceed 40 mg daily. Patients who normally require 80 mg of atorvastatin should either reduce their dosage during concomitant itraconazole treatment, or alternatively (for short courses of this antibiotic) where not practical, a temporary suspension of treatment with atorvastatin may be considered.

Protease inhibitors: Co-administration of atorvastatin and protease inhibitors, known inhibitors of cytochrome P450 3A4, was associated with an approximately two-fold increase in plasma concentrations of atorvastatin. Lipid levels should be monitored to ensure that the lowest dose necessary of atorvastatin is used.

Diltiazem hydrochloride: Co-administration of atorvastatin 40 mg with diltiazem 240 mg resulted in a 51% increase in atorvastatin AUC. After initiation of diltiazem or following dosage adjustment, lipid levels should be monitored to ensure that the lowest dose necessary of atorvastatin is used.

Ezetimibe: The use of ezetimibe alone is associated with myopathy. The risk of myopathy may therefore be increased with concomitant use of ezetimibe and atorvastatin.

Grapefruit juice: Contains one or more components that inhibit CYP3A4 and can increase plasma concentrations of drugs metabolised by CYP3A4. Intake of one 240 ml glass of grapefruit juice resulted in an increase in atorvastatin AUC of 37 % and a decreased AUC of 20.4 % for the active orthohydroxy metabolite. However, large quantities of grapefruit juice (over 1.2L daily for 5 days) increased AUC of atorvastatin 2.5 fold and AUC of active (atorvastatin and metabolites) HMG-CoA reductase inhibitors 1.3 fold. Concomitant intake of large quantities of grapefruit juice and atorvastatin is therefore not recommended.

Inducers of cytochrome P450 3A4: Concomitant administration of atorvastatin with inducers of cytochrome P450 3A4 (eg efavirenz, rifampin, St. John's Wort) can lead to variable reductions in plasma concentrations of atorvastatin. Due to the dual interaction mechanism of rifampin, (cytochrome P450 3A4 induction and inhibition of hepatocyte uptake transporter OATP1B1), simultaneous co-administration of atorvastatin with rifampin is recommended, as delayed administration of atorvastatin after administration of rifampin has been associated with a significant reduction in atorvastatin plasma concentrations.

Verapamil and Amiodarone: Interaction studies with atorvastatin and verapamil or amiodarone have not been conducted. Both verapamil and amiodarone are known to inhibit CYP3A4 activity and co-administration with atorvastatin may result in increased exposure to atorvastatin. Lipid levels should be monitored to ensure that the lowest dose necessary of atorvastatin is used.

Other concomitant therapy

Gemfibrozil/fibrates: The use of fibrates alone is occasionally associated with myopathy. The risk of atorvastatin-induced myopathy may be increased with the concomitant use of fibrates (see Section 4.4). Concomitant administration of gemfibrozil 600 mg BID resulted in a 24% increase in atorvastatin AUC.

Digoxin: When multiple doses of digoxin and 10 mg Lipitor were co-administered, steady state plasma digoxin concentrations were unaffected. However, digoxin concentrations increased approximately 20% following administration of digoxin with 80 mg Lipitor daily. Patients taking digoxin should be monitored appropriately.

Oral contraceptives: Administration of Lipitor with an oral contraceptive containing norethisterone and ethinyl oestradiol produced increases in plasma concentrations of norethisterone and ethinyl oestradiol. These increased concentrations should be considered when selecting oral contraceptive doses.

Colestipol: Plasma concentrations of atorvastatin were lower (approximately 25%) when colestipol was administered with Lipitor. However, lipid effects were greater when Lipitor and colestipol were administered together than when either drug was given alone.

Antacid: Administration of Lipitor with an oral antacid suspension containing magnesium and aluminium hydroxides decreased atorvastatin plasma concentrations approximately 35%; however, LDL-C reduction was not altered.

Warfarin: Administration of Lipitor with warfarin caused a minimal decrease in prothrombin time (mean ± SE of 1.7 ± 0.4 seconds) during the first 4 days of dosing with 80 mg Lipitor. Dosing continued for 15 days and prothrombin time returned to normal by the end of Lipitor treatment. Nevertheless, patients receiving warfarin should be closely monitored when Lipitor is added to their therapy.

Phenazone: Co-administration of multiple doses of atorvastatin and phenazone showed little or no detectable effect in the clearance of phenazone.

Cimetidine: An interaction study with cimetidine and Lipitor was conducted, and no interaction was seen.

Amlodipine: In a drug-drug interaction study in healthy subjects, co-administration of atorvastatin 80 mg and amlodipine 10 mg resulted in an 18% increase in atorvastatin AUC.

Fusidic acid: Although interaction studies with atorvastatin and fusidic acid have not been conducted, severe muscle problems such as rhabdomyolysis have been reported in post-marketing experience with this combination. Patients should be closely monitored and temporary suspension of atorvastatin treatment may be appropriate.

Other: In clinical studies in which atorvastatin was administered with antihypertensives or hypoglycaemic agents no clinically significant interactions were seen.

4.6 Pregnancy and lactation

Lipitor is contraindicated in pregnancy and while breast-feeding. Women of child-bearing potential should use appropriate contraceptive measures.

An interval of 1 month should be allowed from stopping Lipitor treatment to conception in the event of planning a pregnancy.

In animal studies atorvastatin had no effect on fertility and was not teratogenic, however, at maternally toxic doses foetal toxicity was observed in rats and rabbits. The development of the rat offspring was delayed and post-natal survival reduced during exposure of the dams to atorvastatin equivalent to 6 and 21 times that expected in man, respectively.

In rats, plasma concentrations of atorvastatin are similar to those in milk. It is not known whether this drug or its metabolites is excreted in human milk.

4.7 Effects on ability to drive and use machines

There is no pattern of reported adverse events suggesting that patients taking Lipitor will have any impairment of ability to drive and use hazardous machinery.

4.8 Undesirable effects

Adverse reactions have usually been mild and transient. Less than 2% of patients were discontinued from clinical trials due to side effects attributed to Lipitor.

The most frequent (1% or more) adverse effects associated with Lipitor therapy, in patients participating in controlled clinical studies were:

Psychiatric Disorders: insomnia

Nervous System Disorders: headache

Gastrointestinal Disorders: abdominal pain, dyspepsia, nausea, flatulence, constipation, diarrhoea

Musculoskeletal and Connective Tissue Disorders: myalgia

General Disorders and Administration Site Conditions: asthenia

Elevated serum ALT levels have been reported in 1.3% of patients receiving Lipitor. Clinically important (>3 times upper normal limit) elevations in serum ALT levels occurred in 19 of the 2483 (0.8%) patients on Lipitor. It was dose related and was reversible in all 19 patients. In 10 cases, the increase was first observed within 12 weeks of starting the treatment. Only 1 case occurred after 36 weeks and only 1 patient had symptoms suggestive of hepatitis. Treatment was discontinued in only 9 of these 19 cases.

Elevated serum CPK levels (>3 times upper normal limit) occurred in 62 of the 2452 (2.5%) patients on Lipitor compared with 3.1% with other HMG-CoA reductase inhibitors in clinical trials. Levels above 10 times the normal upper range occurred in only 11 (0.4%) Lipitor-treated patients. Only 3 (0.1%) of these 11 patients had concurrent muscle pain, tenderness, or weakness.

Adverse events that have been reported in atorvastatin clinical trials and in post marketing experience are categorised below according to system organ class and frequency. Frequencies are defined as: very common (≥10%), common (≥1% and <10%), uncommon (≥0.1% and <1%), rare (≥0.01% and <0.1%) and very rare (<0.01%).

Gastrointestinal disorders

Common: constipation, flatulence, dyspepsia, nausea, diarrhoea

Uncommon: anorexia, vomiting, pancreatitis

Blood and lymphatic system disorders

Uncommon: thrombocytopenia.

Immune system disorders

Common: allergic reactions (including anaphylaxis).

Endocrine disorders

Uncommon: alopecia, hyperglycaemia, hypoglycaemia.

Psychiatric

Common: insomnia.

Uncommon: amnesia.

Nervous system disorders

Common: headache, dizziness, paraesthesia, hypoesthesia.

Uncommon: peripheral neuropathy.

Very rare: dysgeusia.

Eye disorders

Very rare: visual disturbance.

Hepato-biliary disorders

Rare: hepatitis, cholestatic jaundice.

Very rare: hepatic failure.

Skin/Appendages

Common: Skin rash, pruritus

Uncommon: urticaria, alopecia.

Very rare: angioneurotic oedema, bullous rashes (including erythema multiforme, Stevens-Johnson syndrome and toxic epidermal necrolysis).

Ear and Labyrinth Disorders

Uncommon: tinnitus.

Very rare: hearing loss.

Musculoskeletal disorders

Common: myalgia, arthralgia.

Uncommon: myopathy, muscle cramps.

Rare: myositis, rhabdomyolysis.

Very rare: tendon rupture.

Reproductive system and breast disorders

Uncommon: impotence.

Very rare: gynecomastia.

General disorders

Common: asthenia, chest pain, back pain, fatigue.

Uncommon: malaise, weight gain.

Rare: peripheral oedema

4.9 Overdose

Specific treatment is not available for Lipitor overdosage. Should an overdose occur, the patient should be treated symptomatically and supportive measures instituted, as required. Liver function tests and serum CPK levels should be monitored. Due to extensive drug binding to plasma proteins, haemodialysis is not expected to significantly enhance atorvastatin clearance.

5. PHARMACOLOGICAL PROPERTIES

5.1 Pharmacodynamic properties

Atorvastatin is a selective, competitive inhibitor of HMG-CoA reductase, the rate-limiting enzyme responsible for the conversion of 3-hydroxy-3-methyl-glutaryl-coenzyme A to mevalonate, a precursor of sterols, including cholesterol. Triglycerides and cholesterol in the liver are incorporated into VLDL and released into the plasma for delivery to peripheral tissues. Low-density lipoprotein (LDL) is formed from VLDL and is catabolised primarily through the high affinity LDL receptor.

Atorvastatin lowers plasma cholesterol and lipoprotein levels by inhibiting HMG-CoA reductase and cholesterol synthesis in the liver and increases the number of hepatic LDL receptors on the cell surface for enhanced uptake and catabolism of LDL.

Atorvastatin reduces LDL production and the number of LDL particles. Atorvastatin produces a profound and sustained increase in LDL receptor activity coupled with a beneficial change in the quality of circulating LDL particles.

Approximately 70% of circulating inhibitory activity for HMG-CoA reductase is attributed to active metabolites (see Section 5.2 Pharmacokinetic Properties).

Atorvastatin has been shown to reduce total-C, LDL-C, apolipoprotein B, and triglycerides while producing variable increases in HDL-C in a dose-response study as shown in Table 1 below.

(see Table 1 below)

Atorvastatin produced a variable but small increase in apolipoprotein A1. However, there was no clear dose response effect.

Review of the current clinical database of 24 complete studies shows that atorvastatin increases HDL-cholesterol and reduces the LDL/HDL and total cholesterol/HDL ratios.

These results are consistent in patients with heterozygous familial hypercholesterolaemia, nonfamilial forms of hypercholesterolaemia, and mixed hyperlipidaemia, including patients with noninsulin-dependent diabetes mellitus.

Lipitor is effective in reducing LDL-C in patients with homozygous familial hypercholesterolaemia, a population that has not usually responded to lipid-lowering medication. In a compassionate use study, 41 patients aged 6 to 51 years with homozygous familial hypercholesterolaemia or with severe hypercholesterolaemia, who had ≤15% reduction in LDL-C in response to previous maximum dose combination drug therapy, received daily doses of 40 to 80 mg of Lipitor. Twenty four patients with homozygous familial hypercholesterolaemia received 80 mg Lipitor. Nineteen of these 24 patients responded with a greater than 15% reduction of LDL-C (mean 26%, range 18% to 42%).

Atherosclerosis

In the Reversing Atherosclerosis with Aggressive Lipid-Lowering Study (REVERSAL), the effect of atorvastatin 80 mg and pravastatin 40 mg on coronary atherosclerosis was assessed by intravascular ultrasound (IVUS), during angiography, in patients with coronary heart disease. In this randomized, double-blind, multicenter, controlled clinical trial, IVUS was performed at baseline and at 18 months in 502 patients. In the atorvastatin group (n=253), there was no progression of atherosclerosis evaluated by the percentage change in atheroma volume in a pre-defined target vessel with a stenosis between 20% and 50%. The median percent change, from baseline, in total atheroma volume (the primary study criteria) was -0.4% (p=0.98) in the atorvastatin group and +2.7% (p=0.001) in the pravastatin group (n=249). When compared to pravastatin, the effects of atovastatin were statistically significant (p=0.02).

In the atorvastatin group, LDL-C was reduced to a mean of 2.04 mmol/L ± 0.8 (78.9 mg/dL + 30) from baseline 3.89 mmol/L + 0.7 (150 mg/dL ± 28) and in the pravastatin group, LDL-C was reduced to a mean of 2.85 mmol/L + 0.7 (110 mg/dL ± 26) from baseline 3.89 mmol/L + 0.7 (150 mg/dL ± 26) (p<0.0001). Atorvastatin also significantly reduced mean TC by 34.1% (pravastatin: -18.4%, p<0.0001), mean TG levels by 20% (pravastatin: -6.8%, p<0.0009), and mean apolipoprotein B by 39.1% (pravastatin: -22.0%, p<0.0001). Atorvastatin increased mean HDL-C by 2.9% (pravastatin: +5.6%, p=*NS*). There was a 36.4% mean reduction in CRP in the atorvastatin group compared to a 5.2% reduction in the pravastatin group (p<0.0001).

Table 1 Dose Response in Patients with Primary Hypercholesterolaemia

Lipitor Dose (mg)	N	Total-C	LDL-C	Apo B	TG	HDL-C
Placebo	12	5	8	6	-1	-2
10	11	-30	-41	-34	-14	4
20	10	-35	-44	-36	-33	12
40	11	-38	-50	-41	-25	-3
80	11	-46	-61	-50	-27	3

Adjusted Mean % Change from Baseline

The safety and tolerability profiles of the two treatment groups were comparable.

The effect of intensive lipid lowering with atorvastatin on cardiovascular mortality and morbidity was not investigated in this 18-month study. Therefore, the clinical significance of these imaging results with regard to the primary and secondary prevention of cardiovascular events is unknown.

Heterozygous Familial Hypercholesterolaemia in Paediatric Patients

In a double-blind, placebo controlled study followed by an open-label phase, 187 boys and postmenarchal girls 10-17 years of age (mean age 14.1 years) with heterozygous familial hypercholesterolaemia (FH) or severe hypercholesterolaemia were randomised to atorvastatin (n=140) or placebo (n=47) for 26 weeks and then all received atorvastatin for 26 weeks. Inclusion in the study required 1) a baseline LDL-C level ≥4.91 mmol/l or 2) a baseline LDL-C ≥4.14 mmol/l and positive family history of FH or documented premature cardiovascular disease in a first- or second degree relative. The mean baseline LDL-C value was 5.65 mmol/l (range: 3.58-9.96 mmol/l) in the atorvastatin group compared to 5.95 mmol/l (range: 4.14-8.39 mmol/l) in placebo group. The dosage if atorvastatin (once daily) was 10mg for the first 4 weeks and up-titrated to 20mg if the LDL-C level was >3.36 mmol/l. The number of atorvastatin-treated patients who required up-titration to 20mg after Week 4 during the double-blind phase was 80 (57.1%).

Atorvastatin significantly decreased plasma levels of total-C, LDL-C, triglycerides, and apolipoprotein B during the 26 week double-blind phase (see Table 2).

(see Table 2 below)

The mean achieved LDL-C value was 3.38 mmol/l (range: 1.81-6.26 mmol/l) in the atorvastatin group compared to 5.91 mmol/l (range: 3.93-9.96 mmol/l) in the placebo group during the 26-week double-blind phase.

In this limited controlled study, there was no detectable effect on growth or sexual maturation in boys or on menstrual length in girls. Atorvastatin has not been studied in controlled clinical trials involving pre-pubertal patients or patients younger than 10 years of age. The safety and efficacy of doses above 20mg have not been studied in controlled trials in children. The long-term efficacy of atorvastatin therapy in childhood to reduce morbidity and mortality in adulthood has not been established.

Prevention of Cardiovascular Disease

In the Anglo Scandinavian Cardiac Outcomes Trial Lipid Lowering Arm (ASCOT-LLA), the effect of atorvastatin on fatal and non-fatal coronary heart disease was assessed in 10,305 hypertensive patients 40-79 years of age, with no previous myocardial infarction or treatment for angina, and with TC levels ≤ 6.5mmol/l (251 mg/dl). Additionally, all patients had at least 3 of the predefined cardiovascular risk factors: male gender, age ≥55 years, smoking, diabetes, history of CHD in a first degree relative, TC:HDL ≥ 6, peripheral vascular disease, left ventricular hypertrophy, prior cerebrovascular event, specific ECG abnormality, proteinuria/albuminuria.

In this randomised, double-blind, placebo-controlled study, patients were treated with anti-hypertensive therapy and either atorvastatin 10mg daily (n=5168) or placebo (n=5137). After 3 years treatment with amlodipine or atenolol-based regimen, mean blood pressure fell from 164.2/94.9 to 138.9/80.1 mmHg (atorvastatin) and 164.2/94.3 to 138.9/80.0 mmHg (placebo).

After a median of 3.3 years of treatment, there was a statistically significant reduction in the rate of myocardial infarction (a component of the primary endpoint), 1.2% on atorvastatin versus 2.1% on placebo.

Fatal and non-fatal ischaemic strokes tended to be lower in the atorvastatin group with a relative risk reduction of 26% (89 vs. 119 events) and an absolute risk reduction of 0.6%. The difference did not reach pre-defined levels of statistical significance.

Women constituted 20% of the trial population and a subgroup analysis did not demonstrate any benefit on the primary endpoint of coronary events (fatal CHD plus non-fatal MI) (RR 1.11, 95% CI 0.58-2.13).

In the Collaborative Atorvastatin Diabetes Study (CARDS), the effect of atorvastatin on fatal and nonfatal cardiovascular disease was assessed in 2838 patients with type 2 diabetes 40-75 years of age, without prior history of cardiovascular disease and with LDL ≤4.14 mmol/l (160 mg/dl) and TG ≤ 6.78mmol/l (600mg/dl). Additionally, all patients had at least 1 of the following risk factors: hypertension, current smoking, retinopathy, microalbuminuria or macroalbuminuria.

In this randomised, double-blind, multi-centre, placebo-controlled trial, patients were treated with either atorvastatin 10 mg daily (n=1428) or placebo (n=1410) for a median follow-up of 3.9 years.

The absolute and relative risk reduction effect of atorvastatin is as follows:

(see Table 3 below)

Although the relative risk reduction in the primary end-point was similar between men and women, the absolute benefit for the women was less since the primary event rate on placebo was approximately 1/3 of the male event rate.

Recurrent Stroke

In the Stroke Prevention by Aggressive Reduction in Cholesterol Levels (SPARCL) study, the effect of atorvastatin 80 mg daily or placebo on stroke was evaluated in 4731 patients who had a stroke or transient ischemic attack (TIA) within the preceding 6 months and no history of coronary heart disease (CHD). Patients were 60% male, 21-92 years of age (average age 63 years) and had an average baseline LDL of 133 mg/dl (3.4 mmol/l). The mean LDL-C was 73 mg/dl (1.9 mmol/l) during treatment with atorvastatin and 129 mg/dL (3.3 mmol/L) during treatment with placebo. Median follow-up was 4.9 years.

Atorvastatin 80 mg reduced the risk of the primary end-point of fatal or non-fatal stroke by 15% (HR 0.85; 95% CI, 0.72-1.00; p=0.05 or 0.84; 95% CI, 0.71-0.99; p=0.03 after adjustment for baseline factors) compared to placebo. All cause mortality was 9.1% (216/2365) for atorvastatin versus 8.9% (211/2366) for placebo.

In a post-hoc analysis, atorvastatin 80 mg reduced the incidence of ischemic stroke (218/2365, 9.2% vs. 274/2366, 11.6%, p=0.01) and increased the incidence of haemorrhagic stroke (55/2365, 2.3% vs. 33/2366, 1.4%, p=0.02) compared to placebo.

- The risk of haemorrhagic stroke was increased in patients who entered the study with prior haemorrhagic stroke (7/45 for atorvastatin versus 2/48 for placebo; HR 4.06; 95% CI, 0.84-19.57) and the risk of ischemic stroke was similar between groups (3/45 for atorvastatin versus 2/48 for placebo; HR 1.64; 95% CI, 0.27-9.82).
- The risk of haemorrhagic stroke was increased in patients who entered the study with prior lacunar infarct (20/708 for atorvastatin versus 4/701 for placebo; HR 4.99; 95% CI, 1.71-14.61), but the risk of ischemic stroke was also decreased in these patients (79/708 for atorvastatin versus 102/701 for placebo; HR 0.76; 95% CI, 0.57-1.02). It is possible that the net risk of stroke is increased in patients with prior lacunar infarct who receive atorvastatin 80 mg/day.

All cause mortality was 15.6% (7/45) for atorvastatin versus 10.4% (5/48) in the subgroup of patients with prior haemorrhagic stroke. All cause mortality was 10.9% (77/708) for atorvastatin versus 9.1% (64/701) for placebo in the subgroup of patients with prior lacunar infarct.

Table 2 Lipid Lowering effects of atorvastatin in adolescent boys and girls with heterozygous familial hypercholesterolaemia or severe hypocholesterolaemia (mean percent change from baseline at endpoint in intention- to-treat-population)

DOSAGE	N	Total-C	LDL-C	HDL-C	TG	Apo B
Placebo	47	-1.5	-0.4	-1.9	1.0	0.7
Atorvastatin	140	-31.4	-39.6	2.8	-12.0	-34.0

Table 3 The absolute and relative risk reduction effect of atorvastatin

Event	Relative Risk Reduction (%)	Absolute Risk Reduction[1] (%)	No of events (atorvastatin vs.placebo)	p-value
Major cardiovascular events (fatal and non-fatal AMI, silent MI, acute CHD death, unstable angina, CABG, PTCA, revascularisation, stroke)	37%	3.2%	83 vs. 127	0.001
MI (fatal and non-fatal AMI, silent MI)	42%	1.9%	38 vs. 64	0.007
Strokes (Fatal and non-fatal)	48%	1.3%	21 vs. 39	0.016

[1]Based on difference in crude events rates occurring over a median follow-up of 3.9 years.

AMI= acute myocardial infarction; CABG= coronary artery bypass graft; CHD=coronary heart disease; MI=myocardial infarction; PTCA=percutaneous transluminal coronary angioplasty.

5.2 Pharmacokinetic properties

Pharmacokinetics and Drug Metabolism

Absorption: Atorvastatin is rapidly absorbed after oral administration; maximum plasma concentrations occur within 1 to 2 hours. Extent of absorption increases in proportion to atorvastatin dose. Lipitor tablets are bioequivalent to atorvastatin solutions. The absolute bioavailability of atorvastatin is approximately 12% and the systemic availability of HMG-CoA reductase inhibitory activity is approximately 30%. The low systemic availability is attributed to presystemic clearance in gastrointestinal mucosa and/or hepatic first-pass metabolism.

Distribution: Mean volume of distribution of atorvastatin is approximately 381 L. Atorvastatin is ≥98% bound to plasma proteins.

Metabolism: Atorvastatin is metabolised by cytochrome P450 3A4 to ortho- and parahydroxylated derivatives and various beta-oxidation products. In vitro, inhibition of HMG-CoA reductase by ortho- and parahydroxylated metabolites is equivalent to that of atorvastatin. Approximately 70% of circulating inhibitory activity for HMG-CoA reductase is attributed to active metabolites.

Excretion: Atorvastatin and atorvastatin metabolites are substrates of P-glycoprotein (see section 4.5). Atorvastatin is eliminated primarily in bile following hepatic and/or extrahepatic metabolism. However, the drug does not appear to undergo significant enterohepatic recirculation. Mean plasma elimination half-life of atorvastatin in humans is approximately 14 hours. The half-life of inhibitory activity for HMG-CoA reductase is approximately 20 to 30 hours due to the contribution of active metabolites.

Special Populations

Geriatric: Plasma concentrations of atorvastatin are higher in healthy elderly subjects than in young adults while the lipid effects were comparable to those seen in younger patient populations.

Paediatric: Pharmacokinetic data in the paediatric population are not available.

Gender: Concentrations of atorvastatin in women differ (approximately 20% higher for Cmax and 10% lower for AUC) from those in men. These differences were of no clinical significance, resulting in no clinically significant differences in lipid effects among men and women.

Renal Insufficiency: Renal disease has no influence on the plasma concentrations or lipid effects of atorvastatin.

Hepatic Insufficiency: Plasma concentrations of atorvastatin are markedly increased (approximately 16-fold in Cmax and 11-fold in AUC) in patients with chronic alcoholic liver disease (Childs-Pugh B).

5.3 Preclinical safety data

Atorvastatin was not carcinogenic in rats. The maximum dose used was 63-fold higher than the highest human dose (80 mg/day) on a mg/kg body-weight basis and 8 to 16-fold higher based on AUC(0-24) values as determined by total inhibitory activity. In a 2-year study in mice, incidences of hepatocellular adenoma in males and hepatocellular carcinomas in females were increased at the maximum dose used, and the maximum dose used was 250-fold higher than the highest human dose on a mg/kg body-weight basis. Systemic exposure was 6- to 11-fold higher based on AUC(0-24). Atorvastatin did not demonstrate mutagenic or clastogenic potential in 4 in vitro tests with and without metabolic activation and in 1 in vivo assay.

6. PHARMACEUTICAL PARTICULARS

6.1 List of excipients

The 10-, 20-, and 40-mg dosage forms each contain the following excipients:

Calcium carbonate, E170
Microcrystalline cellulose, E460
Lactose monohydrate
Croscarmellose sodium
Polysorbate 80, E433
Hydroxypropyl cellulose, E463
Magnesium stearate, E572
Opadry White YS-1-7040 (containing hypromellose, E464, macrogol 8000, titanium dioxide, E171 and talc, E553b)
Simeticone Emulsion (containing simeticone, E900, macrogol stearate and sorbic acid, E200, water)
Candelilla wax

The 80-mg dosage form contains the following excipients:

Calcium carbonate, E170
Microcrystalline cellulose, E460
Lactose monohydrate
Croscarmellose sodium
Polysorbate 80, E433
Hydroxypropyl cellulose, E463
Magnesium stearate, E572
Opadry White YS-1-7040 (containing hypromellose, E464, macrogol 8000, titanium dioxide, E171 and talc, E553b)
Simeticone Emulsion (containing simeticone, E900, macrogol stearate and sorbic acid, E200, water)

6.2 Incompatibilities
Not applicable.

6.3 Shelf life
Three Years.

6.4 Special precautions for storage
No special precautions for storage.

6.5 Nature and contents of container
Foil/foil blisters consisting of a polyamide/aluminium foil/polyvinyl chloride unit-dose blister and a paper/polyester/aluminium foil/vinyl heat-seal coated backing or an aluminium foil/vinyl heat-seal coated backing.

Lipitor is supplied in packs of 28 tablets.

6.6 Special precautions for disposal and other handling
No special instructions needed.

7. MARKETING AUTHORISATION HOLDER
Pfizer Ireland Pharmaceuticals
Pottery Road
Dun Laoghaire
Co Dublin
Ireland

8. MARKETING AUTHORISATION NUMBER(S)
Lipitor 10mg PL 16051/0001
Lipitor 20mg PL 16051/0002
Lipitor 40mg PL 16051/0003
Lipitor 80mg PL 16051/0005

9. DATE OF FIRST AUTHORISATION/RENEWAL OF THE AUTHORISATION
Lipitor 10mg, 20mg, and 40mg Tablets: 8 September 1997
Lipitor 80mg Tablets: 15 August 2000

10. DATE OF REVISION OF THE TEXT
September 2008

11. LEGAL CATEGORY
POM

REF: LR_ 11_0

Lipobase
(Astellas Pharma Ltd)

1. NAME OF THE MEDICINAL PRODUCT
Lipobase.

2. QUALITATIVE AND QUANTITATIVE COMPOSITION
Lipobase contains no active ingredient.

3. PHARMACEUTICAL FORM
Cream.

4. CLINICAL PARTICULARS
4.1 Therapeutic indications
For use where it is desired by the physician to reduce gradually the topical dosage of Locoid Lipocream. It may also be used where a continuously alternating application of the active product and the base is required e.g. in prophylactic therapy. Application of the Lipobase is also recommended where it is felt by the physician that the use of a bland emollient base is preferable to the cessation of therapy with the active product. Lipobase may also be used as a diluent for the active product in those cases where dilution is regarded as necessary by the prescriber. Lipobase may also be used other than in conjunction with a topical corticosteroid for its emollient action, and for the treatment of mild skin lesions such as pruritus or dry, scaly skin, where topical corticosteroid is not warranted.

4.2 Posology and method of administration
For adults, children and the elderly: Lipobase may be used either by replacing an application of the active product or alternating the application of the active product and the base, gradually diminishing the application of the active product until therapy ceases, or by the application of the product for its emollient action.

4.3 Contraindications
None stated.

4.4 Special warnings and precautions for use
A small number of people may be hypersensitive (allergic) to the constituents of Lipobase.

Cetostearyl alcohol may cause local skin reactions (e.g. contact dermatitis).

Methyl parahydroxybenzoate may cause allergic skin reactions (possibly delayed).

4.5 Interaction with other medicinal products and other forms of interaction
None stated.

4.6 Pregnancy and lactation
None stated.

4.7 Effects on ability to drive and use machines
None stated.

4.8 Undesirable effects
None stated.

4.9 Overdose
None stated.

5. PHARMACOLOGICAL PROPERTIES
5.1 Pharmacodynamic properties
The product acts topically as an emollient cream.

5.2 Pharmacokinetic properties
Topical administration with no pharmacologically active constituents.

5.3 Preclinical safety data
No relevant preclinical safety data has been generated.

6. PHARMACEUTICAL PARTICULARS
6.1 List of excipients
Cetostearyl alcohol
Macrogol cetostearyl ether
Light liquid paraffin
White soft paraffin
Methyl parahydroxybenzoate
Sodium citrate, anhydrous
Citric acid, anhydrous
Purified water

6.2 Incompatibilities
None stated.

6.3 Shelf life
30g, 50g, 100g and 200g packs, 3 years.
200g and 500g packs, 2 years

6.4 Special precautions for storage
Do not store above 25°C.

6.5 Nature and contents of container
Collapsible aluminium tube with plastic screw cap containing 30 g, 50 g, 100 g or 200 g; and pump dispenser containing 200 g or 500 g.

6.6 Special precautions for disposal and other handling
Not applicable.

7. MARKETING AUTHORISATION HOLDER
Astellas Pharma Ltd
Lovett House
Lovett Road
Staines
TW18 3AZ
United Kingdom

8. MARKETING AUTHORISATION NUMBER(S)
PL0166/0125

9. DATE OF FIRST AUTHORISATION/RENEWAL OF THE AUTHORISATION
First authorisation granted 19 February 1985
Renewal granted 23 January 2001.

10. DATE OF REVISION OF THE TEXT
7th February 2007

11. Legal category
P

Liquifilm Tears
(Allergan Ltd)

1. NAME OF THE MEDICINAL PRODUCT
Liquifilm Tears 1.4% w/v eye drops, solution

2. QUALITATIVE AND QUANTITATIVE COMPOSITION
Polyvinyl alcohol 1.4% w/v

Excipient: Benzalkonium chloride 0.005% w/v

For a full list of excipients, see section 6.1.

3. PHARMACEUTICAL FORM
Eye drops, solution

A clear, colourless solution.

4. CLINICAL PARTICULARS
4.1 Therapeutic indications
As an ocular lubricant for the relief of dry eye and dry eye symptoms.

4.2 Posology and method of administration
Dosage schedule: One to two drops as required or directed for all ages.

Route of administration: Topical instillation into conjunctival sac.

4.3 Contraindications
Hypersensitivity to the active substance or to any of the excipients.

Not for use with soft contact lenses.

4.4 Special warnings and precautions for use
If irritation, pain, redness and changes in vision occur or worsen or persist for more than 72 hours, treatment should be discontinued and a new assessment considered.

To avoid contamination, the dropper tip should not be allowed to touch the eye or any other surface.

Contact lenses should be removed before each application and may be reinserted after 15 minutes.

Liquifilm Tears contain benzalkonium chloride which is irritant to the eye and could cause discolouration of soft lenses. Avoid contact with soft contact lenses. Remove contact lenses before Liquifilm Tears is used and wait for at least 15 minutes before reinsertion.

Concomitant ocular medication should be administered 15 minutes prior to the instillation of Liquifilm Tears.

4.5 Interaction with other medicinal products and other forms of interaction
No interaction studies have been performed.

4.6 Pregnancy and lactation
The constituents of Liquifilm Tears have been used as pharmaceutical agents for many years with no untoward effects. No special precautions are necessary for the use of Liquifilm Tears in pregnancy and lactation.

4.7 Effects on ability to drive and use machines
No studies on the effects on the ability to drive and use machines have been performed.

Based upon the information available, Liquifilm Tears has no or negligible influence on the ability to drive and use machines. However, it may cause transient blurring of vision. Do not drive or use hazardous machinery unless vision is clear.

4.8 Undesirable effects
The following undesirable effects have been reported since Liquifilm Tears was marketed.

Frequency:

Not known: the incidence cannot be determined from available information.

Eye disorders:

Not known: Eye irritation, eye pain, ocular hyperaemia, lacrimation increased, foreign body sensation, eye pruritus.

Immune system disorders:

Not known: hypersensitivity

4.9 Overdose
No case of overdose has been reported.

5. PHARMACOLOGICAL PROPERTIES
5.1 Pharmacodynamic properties
Pharmacotherapeutic group: Artificial tears and other indifferent preparations, ATC code: S01AX20.

Not applicable. Liquifilm Tears contains no pharmacologically active ingredient.

5.2 Pharmacokinetic properties
Not applicable. Liquifilm Tears contains no pharmacologically active ingredient.

5.3 Preclinical safety data
The constituents of Liquifilm Tears have been used safely in pharmaceutical products for many years. Topical administration in animal studies showed no untoward effects.

6. PHARMACEUTICAL PARTICULARS
6.1 List of excipients
Sodium chloride
Sodium phosphate dibasic
Sodium phosphate monobasic
Benzalkonium chloride
Edetate disodium
Hydrochloric acid or sodium hydroxide (to adjust pH)
Purified water

6.2 Incompatibilities
None known.

6.3 Shelf life
24 months unopened.

Discard 28 days after opening.

6.4 Special precautions for storage
Do not store above 25°C. Do not refrigerate or freeze.

6.5 Nature and contents of container
Low density polyethylene (LDPE) bottle and tip and medium impact polystyrene (MIPS) screw cap. Safety seal to ensure integrity of the container.

Liquifilm Tears is available in 15ml bottles.

6.6 Special precautions for disposal and other handling
No special requirements.

7. MARKETING AUTHORISATION HOLDER
Allergan Ltd
Marlow International
The Parkway
Marlow
Bucks
SL7 1YL
UK

8. MARKETING AUTHORISATION NUMBER(S)
PL 00426/0009R

9. DATE OF FIRST AUTHORISATION/RENEWAL OF THE AUTHORISATION
Date of first authorisation: 19th September 1974

Date of latest renewal: 10th October 2005

10. DATE OF REVISION OF THE TEXT
15 July 2009

Liquifilm Tears Preservative Free

(Allergan Ltd)

1. NAME OF THE MEDICINAL PRODUCT
Liquifilm® Tears Preservative Free

or

Refresh Ophthalmic™

2. QUALITATIVE AND QUANTITATIVE COMPOSITION
Polyvinyl alcohol 1.4% w/v.

3. PHARMACEUTICAL FORM
Eye drops, solution

4. CLINICAL PARTICULARS

4.1 Therapeutic indications
Symptomatic relief of dry eye and symptomatic relief of eye irritation associated with deficient tear production.

4.2 Posology and method of administration
Ensure container is intact. Twist off tab and apply eye-drops.

Dosage schedule: Apply one or two drops in each eye as needed, or as directed. No special dosage for the elderly or for children.

Route of administration: Ocular instillation.

4.3 Contraindications
Hypersensitivity to the active substance polyvinyl alcohol or any of the other excipients.

4.4 Special warnings and precautions for use
If irritation, pain, redness and changes in vision occur or worsen, treatment should be discontinued and a new assessment considered.

To avoid contamination, the dropper tip should not be allowed to touch the eye or any other surface.

Contact lenses should be removed before each application and may be reinserted after 15 minutes.

Concomitant ocular medication should be administered 15 minutes prior to the instillation of Liquifilm Tears Preservative Free or Refresh Ophthalmic.

4.5 Interaction with other medicinal products and other forms of interaction
No interaction studies have been performed.

4.6 Pregnancy and lactation
The constituents of Liquifilm Tears Preservative Free or Refresh Ophthalmic have been used as pharmaceutical agents for many years with no untoward effects. No special precautions are necessary for the use of Liquifilm Tears Preservative Free or Refresh Ophthalmic in pregnancy and lactation.

4.7 Effects on ability to drive and use machines
Liquifilm Tears Preservative Free or Refresh Ophthalmic has minor or moderate influence on the ability to drive and use machines as it may cause transient blurring of vision. Do not drive or use hazardous machinery unless vision is clear.

4.8 Undesirable effects
Liquifilm Tears Preservative Free or Refresh Ophthalmic may cause transient stinging or irritation on instillation.

The frequency of the following undesirable effects is not known (cannot be estimated from the available data).

Eye disorders

- Eye irritation
- Eye pain
- Ocular hyperaemia
- Vision blurred
- Eye pruritus
- Foreign body sensation
- Eye discharge
- Hypersensitivity

4.9 Overdose
No case of overdose has been reported. Accidental overdose will not present any hazard.

5. PHARMACOLOGICAL PROPERTIES

5.1 Pharmacodynamic properties
Liquifilm® Tears Preservative Free / or Refresh Ophthalmic™ exerts a mechanical, not a pharmacological action. The viscosity enhancing agent is polyvinyl alcohol and the lubricating-enhancing agent is povidone.

5.2 Pharmacokinetic properties
Not applicable

5.3 Preclinical safety data
The constituents of Liquifilm® Tears Preservative Free / or Refresh Ophthalmic™ have been used safely in pharmaceutical products for many years. Topical administration in animals studies showed no untoward effects.

6. PHARMACEUTICAL PARTICULARS

6.1 List of excipients
Povidone

Sodium chloride

Sodium hydroxide or hydrochloric acid (to adjust pH)

Purified water

6.2 Incompatibilities
None known.

6.3 Shelf life
24 months (unopened).

Do not store opened container.

6.4 Special precautions for storage
Store at 25°C or below.

6.5 Nature and contents of container
Low density polyethylene unit dose vials containing 0.4 ml of Liquifilm® Tears Preservative Free / or Refresh Ophthalmic™

Cartons contain 2, 5, 10, 15, 30 or 50 units per pack.

6.6 Special precautions for disposal and other handling
Ensure container is intact. Twist off tab and apply eye-drops.

7. MARKETING AUTHORISATION HOLDER
Allergan Limited

Marlow International

The Parkway

Marlow

Bucks, SL7 1YL

UK

8. MARKETING AUTHORISATION NUMBER(S)
PL 00426/0063

9. DATE OF FIRST AUTHORISATION/RENEWAL OF THE AUTHORISATION
14th August 2003

10. DATE OF REVISION OF THE TEXT
23rd July 2008

Liskonum Tablets

(GlaxoSmithKline UK)

1. NAME OF THE MEDICINAL PRODUCT
Liskonum™ Tablets

2. QUALITATIVE AND QUANTITATIVE COMPOSITION
Liskonum Tablets are available in one strength. Each tablet contains 450 mg lithium carbonate (12.2 mmol Li^+) in controlled-release form.

3. PHARMACEUTICAL FORM
White, oblong, film-coated tablets, with convex faces and a breakline on both sides.

4. CLINICAL PARTICULARS

4.1 Therapeutic indications
Liskonum is a controlled-release tablet, designed to reduce fluctuations in serum lithium levels and the likelihood of adverse reactions.

It is indicated for the treatment of acute episodes of mania or hypomania and for the prophylaxis of recurrent manic-depressive illness.

4.2 Posology and method of administration
Dosage:

Adults only: Liskonum should be given twice a day.

Treatment of acute mania or hypomania

Patients should be started on one or one-and-a-half tablets twice a day. Dosage should then be adjusted to achieve a serum lithium level of 0.8 to a maximum of 1.5 mmol/l. Serum concentration of lithium should be measured after four to seven days' treatment and then at least once a week until dosage has remained constant for four weeks. When the acute symptoms have been controlled, recommendations for prophylaxis should be followed.

Prophylaxis: The usual starting dosage is one tablet twice a day. Dosage should then be adjusted until a serum level of 0.5 to 1.0 mmol/l is maintained. Serum concentration of lithium should be measured after four to seven days' treatment and then every week until dosage has remained constant for four weeks. Frequency of monitoring may then be gradually decreased to a minimum of once every two months, but should be increased following any situation where changes in lithium levels are possible (see Section 4.4).

Blood samples for measurement of serum lithium concentration should be taken just before a dose is due and not less than 12 hours after the previous dose.

Levels of more than 2 mmol/l *must* be avoided.

Elderly: Use with caution. Start with half a tablet twice a day and adjust serum levels to the lower end of the above ranges (see also Section 4.4).

The full prophylactic effect of lithium may not be evident for six to 12 months, and treatment should be continued through any recurrence of the illness.

Children: Not recommended for use in children under 12 years of age

Administration:

Oral.

Planned Discontinuation of Liskonum

Gradual withdrawal of lithium (over a period of at least 2 weeks) is recommended, as it may delay recurrence of the patient's underlying symptoms.

Discontinuation of Liskonum due to toxicity

On the first sign of toxicity, treatment should be immediately discontinued (see Section 4.4).

4.3 Contraindications
Do not use in patients with a history of hypersensitivity to lithium, impaired renal function, cardiac disease, or untreated hypothyroidism. Lithium should not be given to patients with low body sodium levels, including, for example, dehydrated patients, those on low sodium diets, or those with Addison's disease.

4.4 Special warnings and precautions for use
Vomiting, diarrhoea, intercurrent infection, fluid deprivation and drugs likely to upset electrolyte balance, such as diuretics, may all reduce lithium excretion and thereby precipitate intoxication; reduction of dosage may be required. Use with care in elderly patients as lithium excretion may also be reduced.

The possibility of hypothyroidism and of renal dysfunction arising during prolonged treatment should be borne in mind and periodic assessments made.

Histological changes (including tubulointerstitial nephropathy) have been reported after long-term treatment with lithium. These changes may lead to impaired renal function. It is unclear if these changes are always reversible on stopping lithium. It is advisable to monitor renal function periodically.

Patients should be warned of the symptoms of impending intoxication (see Section 4.8), of the urgency of immediate action should these symptoms appear, and also of the need to maintain a constant and adequate salt and water intake. Outpatients should be warned to take their medication at the stipulated time. If a dose is missed, the patient should wait until the next scheduled time of dosing. A double dose to make up for the dose that has been missed should not be taken. Treatment should be discontinued immediately on the first signs of toxicity, which include cardiovascular, renal, neurological and gastrointestinal events (see Section 4.8). Acute renal failure has been reported rarely with lithium toxicity.

Patients with the rare hereditary galactose intolerance, lactase deficiency or glucose-galactose malabsorption should not take Liskonum.

Lithium should be used with particular care in the elderly since this group may be particularly susceptible to toxicity due to decreasing renal function and hence elimination *(see Dosage and Administration)*.

4.5 Interaction with other medicinal products and other forms of interaction
Interactions which increase lithium concentrations:

- Metronidazole
- Non-steroidal anti-inflammatory drugs, including selective cyclo-oxygenase (COX) II inhibitors (monitor serum lithium concentrations more frequently if NSAID therapy is initiated or discontinued)
- ACE inhibitors
- Angiotensin II receptor antagonists.
- Diuretics (thiazides show a paradoxical antidiuretic effect resulting in possible water retention and lithium intoxication)

Interactions which decrease serum lithium concentrations:

- Urea
- Xanthines
- Sodium bicarbonate containing products
- Diuretics (carbonic anhydrase inhibitors)

Interactions causing neurotoxicity:

- Neuroleptics (particularly haloperidol at higher dosages)
- Carbamazepine
- Methyldopa
- Selective Serotonin Re-uptake Inhibitors (e.g. fluvoxamine and fluoxetine) as this combination may precipitate a serotonergic syndrome.
- Calcium channel blockers
- Tri-cyclic antidepressants

Lithium may prolong the effects of neuromuscular blocking agents.

4.6 Pregnancy and lactation
Lithium crosses the placental barrier. In animal studies, lithium has been reported to interfere with fertility, gestation and foetal development. There is epidemiological evidence that the drug may be harmful in human pregnancy. Lithium therapy should not be used during pregnancy, especially during the first trimester, unless considered

essential. In certain cases where a severe risk to the patient could exist if treatment were to be stopped, lithium has been continued during pregnancy. If given, however, serum levels should be measured frequently because of the changes in renal function associated with pregnancy and parturition.

Since adequate human data on use during lactation and adequate animal reproduction studies are not available, bottle feeding is advisable.

4.7 Effects on ability to drive and use machines

As lithium may cause disturbances of the CNS, patients should be warned of the possible hazards when driving or operating machinery.

4.8 Undesirable effects

Initial therapy: Fine tremor of the hands, polyuria thirst and nausea may occur.

The frequency classifications for these adverse reactions cannot be accurately estimated from the available clinical trial data.

Blood and lymphatic system disorders: Leukocytosis

Endocrine disorders: Euthyroid goitre, hypothyroidism, hyperthyroidism, hyperparathyroidism

Metabolism and nutrition disorders: Hyperglycemia, hypercalcemia, weight gain, anorexia, polydipsia

Psychiatric disorders: Hallucinations, somnolence, memory loss

Nervous system disorders: Tremor, ataxia, peripheral sensorimotor neuropathy, hyperactive deep tendon reflexes, extrapyramidal symptoms, seizures, slurred speech, dizziness, vertigo, giddiness, nystagmus, stupor, coma, pseudotumor cerebri, dysgeusia, myasthenia gravis

Eye disorders: Scotomata, blurred vision

Cardiac disorders: Cardiac arrhythmia, of which bradycardia due to sinus node dysfunction is most frequent, and oedema. ECG changes: reversible flattening and inversion of T-waves.

Vascular disorders: Peripheral circulatory collapse, hypotension, Raynaud's phenomena

Gastrointestinal disorders: Nausea, vomiting, diarrhoea, gastritis, excessive salivation, dry mouth

Skin and subcutaneous tissue disorders: Alopecia, folliculitis, pruritus, psoriasis exacerbation, rash and other signs of skin hypersensitivity, acneiform eruptions, papular skin disorder

Musculoskeletal and connective tissue disorders: Muscle weakness, arthralgia, myalgia

Renal and urinary disorders: Symptoms of nephrogenic diabetes insipidus, and after long-term therapy, histological renal changes (including tubulointerstitial nephropathy) and impaired renal function

Reproductive system and breast disorders: Sexual dysfunction

General disorders and administration site conditions: Oedema, dazed feeling

Intoxication (see 4.4): Cardiovascular events e.g. QT/QTc prolongation. Gastrointestinal events e.g. vomiting, diarrhoea. Neurological events e.g. drowsiness, lack of coordination and/or a coarse tremor of the extremities and lower jaw may occur, especially with serum levels above the therapeutic range. Ataxia, giddiness, blurred vision, dysarthria, tinnitus, muscle hyperirritability, choreoathetoid movements peripheral neuropathy, hypoactive or absent deep tendon reflexes, and toxic psychosis have also been described.

If any of the above symptoms appear, treatment should be stopped immediately and arrangements made for serum lithium measurement.

4.9 Overdose

The toxic concentrations for lithium are close to the therapeutic concentrations. Any overdose in a patient who has been taking chronic lithium therapy should be regarded as potentially serious. A single acute overdose usually carries low risk and patients tend to show mild symptoms only, irrespective of their serum lithium concentration. However more severe symptoms may occur after a delay if lithium elimination is reduced because of renal impairment, particularly if a slow-release preparation has been taken.

If an acute overdose has been taken by a patient on chronic lithium therapy, this can lead to serious toxicity occurring even after a modest overdose as the extravascular tissues are already saturated with lithium.

Symptoms

The onset of symptoms may be delayed, with peak effects not occurring for as long as 24 hours, especially in patients who are not receiving chronic lithium therapy, or following the use of a sustained release preparation.

Mild: Nausea, diarrhoea, vomiting, blurred vision, polyuria, light headedness, fine resting tremor, first degree heart block, muscular weakness and drowsiness.

Moderate: Increasing confusion, blackouts, fasciculation and increased deep tendon reflexes, myoclonic twitches and jerks, ataxia, choreoathetoid movements, urinary and faecal incontinence, increasing restlessness followed by stupor. Hypernatraemia.

Severe: Coma, convulsions, cerebellar signs, cardiac dysrhythmias including sino-atrial block, sinus and junctional bradycardia. Hypotension or rarely hypertension, circulatory collapse and renal failure.

Management

There is no known antidote. Supportive and symptomatic treatment should be initiated. Correction of electrolyte balance and fluid resuscitation is critical Gut decontamination is not useful for chronic accumulation. Whole bowel irrigation may be helpful in patients ingesting large quantities of slow-release preparation.

NOTE: activated charcoal does not adsorb lithium.

Haemodialysis is the treatment of choice for severe poisoning and should be considered in all patients with marked neurological features. It is the most efficient method of lowering lithium concentrations rapidly but substantial rebound increases can be expected when dialysis is stopped, and prolonged, or repeated treatments may be required. It should be considered also in acute, acute on chronic or chronic overdose in patients with severe symptoms regardless of serum lithium concentration; discuss with your local poisons service.

NOTE: Clinical improvement generally takes longer than reduction of serum lithium concentrations regardless of the method used.

5. PHARMACOLOGICAL PROPERTIES

5.1 Pharmacodynamic properties

Lithium carbonate is used as a source of lithium ions. The mechanism by which it exerts its effect in affective disorders is not known but may be related to inhibition of neurotransmitter receptor mediated processes involving beta-adrenoceptors. It is used in the treatment of acute episodes of mania or hypomania and for prophylaxis of recurrent manic depressive illness.

5.2 Pharmacokinetic properties

Lithium is readily absorbed from the gastrointestinal tract, and is distributed throughout the body over a period of several hours. Lithium is excreted almost exclusively in the kidneys but can also be detected in sweat and saliva. It is not bound to plasma proteins. It crosses the placenta, and is excreted in breast milk. The half-life of non-sustained lithium varies considerably, but generally is considered to be about 12 to 24 hours following a single dose. It is however increased for example in those with renal impairment and with age, and may increase significantly during long-term therapy.

5.3 Preclinical safety data

Not applicable

6. PHARMACEUTICAL PARTICULARS

6.1 List of excipients

Povidone
Maize Starch
Lactose
Gelatin
Calcium
Carboxymethylcellulose
Talcum (E553Cb)
Calcium Arachinate
Titanium Dioxide (E171)
Magnesium Stearate (E572)
Polyethylene Glycol 6000
Eudragit E12.5

6.2 Incompatibilities

Not applicable.

6.3 Shelf life

Liskonum Tablets have a shelf-life of five years.

6.4 Special precautions for storage

Store below 25°C.

6.5 Nature and contents of container

Opaque Blister Packs (OP) of 60 (6 × 10) tablets.

6.6 Special precautions for disposal and other handling

Tablets may be halved but should not be chewed or broken up.

Administrative Data

7. MARKETING AUTHORISATION HOLDER

Smith Kline & French Laboratories Limited

Great West Road

Brentford

Middlesex TW8 9GS

Trading as:

GlaxoSmithKline UK,

Stockley Park West,

Uxbridge,

Middlesex, UB11 1BT

8. MARKETING AUTHORISATION NUMBER(S)

PL 0002/0083

9. DATE OF FIRST AUTHORISATION/RENEWAL OF THE AUTHORISATION

29.09.02

10. DATE OF REVISION OF THE TEXT

July 2009

Loceryl 0.25% Cream

(Galderma (U.K) Ltd)

1. NAME OF THE MEDICINAL PRODUCT

Loceryl 0.25% cream

2. QUALITATIVE AND QUANTITATIVE COMPOSITION

Loceryl cream contains 0.25% w/w amorolfine in the form of hydrochloride. Amorolfine is chemically described as *cis*-4-[(RS)-3[4-(1,1-Dimethylpropyl)phenyl]-2-methylpropyl]-2,6-dimethylmorpholine.

Amorolfine hydrochloride HSE 0.279 w/w

(equivalent to 0.25% w/w base)

3. PHARMACEUTICAL FORM

Cream.

4. CLINICAL PARTICULARS

4.1 Therapeutic indications

Dermatomyces caused by dermatophytes: tinea pedis (athlete's foot), tinea cruris, tinea inguinalis, tinea corporis, tinea manuum. Pityriasis versicolor.

4.2 Posology and method of administration

Dermatomycoses

Cream: To be applied to affected skin areas once daily following cleansing (in the evening).

The treatment should be continued without interruption until clinical cure, and for 3 - 5 days thereafter. The required duration of treatment depends on the species of fungi and on the localisation of the infection. In general, treatment should be continued for at least two to three weeks. With foot mycoses, up to six weeks of therapy may be necessary.

Elderly

There are no specific dosage recommendations for use in elderly patients.

Children

There are no specific dosage recommendations for children owing to the lack of clinical experience available to date.

4.3 Contraindications

Loceryl cream must not be reused by patients who have shown hypersensitivity to the treatment.

No experience exists of use during pregnancy and nursing, therefore, the use of Loceryl should be avoided during pregnancy and lactation.

4.4 Special warnings and precautions for use

Avoid contact of Loceryl cream with eyes, ears and mucous membranes.

This medicinal product contains stearyl alcohol which may cause local skin reaction (e.g. contact dermatitis)

4.5 Interaction with other medicinal products and other forms of interaction

There are no specific studies involving concomitant treatment with other topical medicines. Use of nail varnish or artificial nails should be avoided during treatment.

4.6 Pregnancy and lactation

Reproductive toxicology studies showed no evidence of teratogenicity in laboratory animals but embryotoxicity was observed at high oral doses. The systemic absorption of amorolfine during and after topical administration is very low and therefore the risk to the human foetus appears to be negligible. However, because there is no relevant experience Loceryl should be avoided during pregnancy and breast feeding.

4.7 Effects on ability to drive and use machines

None.

4.8 Undesirable effects

Adverse drug reactions are rare and mostly mild in nature.

System Organ Class	Frequency	Adverse drug reaction
Skin and subcutaneous tissue disorders	Rare (≥1/10 000, ≤ 1/1000)	Skin Irritation, erythema, pruritus, skin burning sensation
	Very rare (≤ 1/10000)	Contact dermatitis

4.9 Overdose

Accidental oral Ingestion

Loceryl is for topical use. In the event of accidental oral ingestion, an appropriate method of gastric emptying may be used.

5. PHARMACOLOGICAL PROPERTIES

5.1 Pharmacodynamic properties

Loceryl is a topical antimycotic. Amorolfine belongs to a new chemical class, and its fungicidal action is based on an alteration of the fungal cell membrane targeted primarily on sterol biosynthesis. The ergosterol content is reduced, and at the same time unusual sterically nonplanar sterols accumulate.

Amorolfine is a broad spectrum antimycotic. It is highly active (MIC < 2mcg/ml) *in vitro* against

yeasts:Candida, Cryptococcus, Malassezia

dermatophytes: Trichophyton, Microsporum, Epidermophyton

moulds: Hendersonula, Alternaria, Scopulariopsis

dematiacea: Cladosporium, Fonsecaea, Wangiella

dimorphic fungi: Coccidioides, Histoplasma, Sporothrix

With the exception of *Actinomyces*, bacteria are not sensitive to amorolfine. *Propionibacterium acnes* is only slightly sensitive.

5.2 Pharmacokinetic properties
Amorolfine from cream penetrates into the stratum corneum. Nevertheless, systemic absorption is extremely low during and after therapeutic use.

5.3 Preclinical safety data
None stated.

6. PHARMACEUTICAL PARTICULARS
6.1 List of excipients
Polyoxyl 40 stearate, stearyl alcohol, paraffin liquid, white soft paraffin, carbomer, sodium hydroxide, disodium edetate, 2 phenoxyethanol.

6.2 Incompatibilities
None.

6.3 Shelf life
3 years.

6.4 Special precautions for storage
Loceryl cream should be stored below 30°C.

6.5 Nature and contents of container
20g collapsible aluminium tube, sealed with an aluminium membrane and fitted with a plastic screw cap.

6.6 Special precautions for disposal and other handling
No special instructions.

7. MARKETING AUTHORISATION HOLDER
Galderma (UK) Limited
Meridien House
69-71 Clarendon Road
Watford
Herts.
WD17 1DS
UK

8. MARKETING AUTHORISATION NUMBER(S)
PL 10590/0041

9. DATE OF FIRST AUTHORISATION/RENEWAL OF THE AUTHORISATION
April 1999

10. DATE OF REVISION OF THE TEXT
August 2006
Loceryl is a registered trade mark

Loceryl Nail Lacquer 5%

(Galderma (U.K) Ltd)

1. NAME OF THE MEDICINAL PRODUCT
Loceryl Nail Lacquer 5%.

2. QUALITATIVE AND QUANTITATIVE COMPOSITION
Loceryl nail lacquer contains 5% w/v amorolfine in the form of hydrochloride. Amorolfine is chemically described as *cis*-4-[(RS)-3[4-(1,1-Dimethylpropyl)phenyl]-2-methylpropyl]-2,6-dimethylmorpholine.

Amorolfine hydrochloride HSE 6.40 w/w

3. PHARMACEUTICAL FORM
Lacquer.

4. CLINICAL PARTICULARS
4.1 Therapeutic indications
Onychomycoses caused by dermatophytes, yeasts and moulds.

4.2 Posology and method of administration
The nail lacquer should be applied to the affected finger or toe nails once weekly. Twice weekly application may prove beneficial in some cases.

The patient should apply the nail lacquer as follows:

1. Before the first application of Loceryl, it is essential that the affected areas of nail (particularly the nail surfaces) should be filed down as thoroughly as possible using the nail file supplied. The surface of the nail should then be cleansed and degreased using a cleaning pad (as supplied). Before repeat application of Loceryl, the affected nails should be filed down again as required, following cleansing with a cleaning pad to remove any remaining lacquer.

Caution: Nail files used for affected nails must not be used for healthy nails.

2. With one of the reusable applicators supplied, apply the nail lacquer to the entire surface of the affected nails and allow it to dry. After use, clean the applicator with the same cleaning pad used before for nail cleaning. Keep the bottle tightly closed.

For each nail to be treated, dip the applicator into the nail lacquer without wiping off any of the lacquer on the bottle neck.

Caution: When working with organic solvents (thinners, white spirit, etc.) wear impermeable gloves in order to protect the Loceryl lacquer on the nails.

Treatment should be continued without interruption until the nail is regenerated and the affected areas are finally cured. The required frequency and duration of treatment depends essentially on intensity and localisation of the infection. In general, it is six months (finger nails) and nine to twelve months (toe nails). A review of the treatment is recommended at intervals of approximately three months.

Co-existent tinea pedis should be treated with an appropriate antimycotic cream.

Elderly

There are no specific dosage recommendations for use in elderly patients.

Children

There are no specific dosage recommendations for children owing to the lack of clinical experience available to date.

4.3 Contraindications
Loceryl nail lacquer must not be reused by patients who have shown hypersensitivity to the treatment.

No experience exists of use during pregnancy and nursing, therefore, the use of Loceryl should be avoided during pregnancy and lactation.

4.4 Special warnings and precautions for use
Avoid contact of the lacquer with eyes, ears and mucous membranes.

4.5 Interaction with other medicinal products and other forms of interaction
There are no specific studies involving concomitant treatment with other topical medicines.

Use of nail varnish or artificial nails should be avoided during treatment.

4.6 Pregnancy and lactation
Reproductive toxicology studies showed no evidence of teratogenicity in laboratory animals but embryotoxicity was observed at high oral doses. The systemic absorption of amorolfine during and after topical administration is very low and therefore the risk to the human foetus appears to be negligible. However, because there is no relevant experience, Loceryl should be avoided during pregnancy and breast feeding.

4.7 Effects on ability to drive and use machines
None.

4.8 Undesirable effects
Adverse drug reactions are rare. Nail disorders (e.g. nail discoloration, broken nails, brittle nails) may occur. These reactions can also be linked to the onychomycosis itself.

System Organ Class	Frequency	Adverse drug reaction
Skin and subcutaneous tissue disorders	Rare (⩾ 1/10000, ⩽ 1/1000)	Nail disorder, nail discoloration, onychoclasis
	Very rare (⩽ 1/10000)	Skin burning sensation, contact dermatitis

4.9 Overdose
Accidental oral ingestion
Loceryl is for topical use. In the event of accidental oral ingestion, an appropriate method of gastric emptying may be used.

5. PHARMACOLOGICAL PROPERTIES
5.1 Pharmacodynamic properties
Loceryl is a topical antimycotic. Amorolfine belongs to a new chemical class, and its fungicidal action is based on an alteration of the fungal cell membrane targeted primarily on sterol biosynthesis. The ergosterol content is reduced, and at the same time unusual sterically nonplanar sterols accumulate.

Amorolfine is a broad spectrum antimycotic. It is highly active (MIC < 2mcg/ml) *in vitro* against

yeasts:Candida, Cryptococcus, Malassezia

dermatophytes: Trichophyton, Microsporum, Epidermophyton

moulds: Hendersonula, Alternaria, Scopulariopsis

dematiacea: Cladosporium, Fonsecaea, Wangiella

dimorphic fungi: Coccidioides, Histoplasma, Sporothrix

With the exception of *Actinomyces*, bacteria are not sensitive to amorolfine. *Propionibacterium acnes* is only slightly sensitive.

5.2 Pharmacokinetic properties
Amorolfine from nail lacquer penetrates into and diffuses through the nail plate and is thus able to eradicate poorly accessible fungi in the nail bed. Systemic absorption of the active ingredient is very low with this type of application.

Following prolonged use of Loceryl Nail Lacquer, there is no indication of drug accumulation in the body.

5.3 Preclinical safety data
None stated.

6. PHARMACEUTICAL PARTICULARS
6.1 List of excipients
Ammonio methacrylate copolymer A, triacetin, butyl acetate, ethyl acetate, ethanol absolute.

6.2 Incompatibilities
None.

6.3 Shelf life
3 years.

6.4 Special precautions for storage
Loceryl nail lacquer should be stored below 30°C. Protect from heat. Keep bottle tightly closed after use.

6.5 Nature and contents of container
Amber glass container with screw thread and plastic screw closure.

Pack Sizes: 2.5 ml (1 × 2.5 ml)
5.0 ml (1 × 5.0 ml)
7.5 ml (1 × 2.5 ml & 1 × 5.0 ml)
10.0 ml (2 × 5.0 ml)

All packs contain cleansing swabs, spatulas and nail files.

6.6 Special precautions for disposal and other handling
No special instructions.

7. MARKETING AUTHORISATION HOLDER
Galderma (UK) Limited
Meridien House
69-71 Clarendon Road
Watford
Herts.
WD17 1DS
UK

8. MARKETING AUTHORISATION NUMBER(S)
PL 10590/0042

9. DATE OF FIRST AUTHORISATION/RENEWAL OF THE AUTHORISATION
April 1999

10. DATE OF REVISION OF THE TEXT
August 2006
Loceryl Nail Lacquer is a registered trade mark

Locoid Cream

(Astellas Pharma Ltd)

1. NAME OF THE MEDICINAL PRODUCT
LOCOID CREAM

2. QUALITATIVE AND QUANTITATIVE COMPOSITION
Contains 0.1% w/w hydrocortisone butyrate.

For excipients, see 6.1

3. PHARMACEUTICAL FORM
Cream

White to practically white cream.

4. CLINICAL PARTICULARS
4.1 Therapeutic indications
The product is recommended for clinical use in the treatment of conditions responsive to topical corticosteroids e.g. eczema, dermatitis and psoriasis.

Topical corticosteroids are not generally indicated in psoriasis but may be acceptable in psoriasis excluding widespread plaque psoriasis provided warnings are given, see section 4.4 Special warnings and special precautions for use.

4.2 Posology and method of administration
For topical application.

Dosage: To be applied evenly and sparingly no more than twice daily.

Application may be made under occlusion in the more resistant lesions such as thickened psoriatic plaques on elbows and knees.

Adults and the Elderly: The same dose is used for adults and the elderly, as clinical evidence would indicate that no special dosage regimen is necessary in the elderly.

Children: Long term treatment should be avoided where possible.

Infants: Therapy should be limited if possible to a maximum of seven days.

4.3 Contraindications
Hypersensitivity to hydrocortisone or to any of the ingredients of the cream.

This preparation is contraindicated in the presence of untreated viral or fungal infections, tubercular or syphilitic lesions, peri-oral dermatitis, acne vulgaris and rosacea and in bacterial infections unless used in connection with appropriate chemotherapy.

4.4 Special warnings and precautions for use
Although generally regarded as safe, even for long-term administration in adults, there is a potential for adverse effects if over used in infancy. Extreme caution is required in dermatoses of infancy including napkin eruption. In such

Table 1 Undesirable effects

System Organ Class	Rare >/10,000, </1000	Very rare </10,000	Not known
Immune system disorders			Hypersensitivity
Endocrine disorders		Adrenal suppression	
Skin and subcutaneous tissue disorders	Skin atrophy, often irreversible, with thinning of the epidermis Telangiectasia Skin striae Pustular acne Perioral dermatitis Rebound effect Skin depigmentation Dermatitis and eczema, including contact dermatitis		

patients courses of treatment should not normally exceed 7 days.

Application under occlusion should be restricted to dermatoses involving limited areas.

As with all corticosteroids, application to the face, flexures and other areas of thin skin may cause skin atrophy and increased absorption and should be avoided.

Topical corticosteroids may be hazardous in psoriasis for a number of reasons including rebound relapses following development of tolerance, risk of generalised pustular psoriasis and local and systemic toxicity due to impaired barrier function of the skin. Steroids may have a place in psoriasis of the scalp and chronic plaque psoriasis of the hands and feet. Careful patient supervision is important.

Keep away from the eyes

The cetostearyl alcohol may cause local skin reactions (e.g contact dermatitis) and the butyl and propyl parahydroxybenzoate may cause allergic reactions which can be delayed.

4.5 Interaction with other medicinal products and other forms of interaction

None known.

4.6 Pregnancy and lactation

There is inadequate evidence of safety in human pregnancy. Topical administration of corticosteroids to pregnant animals can cause abnormalities of foetal development including cleft palate and intra-uterine growth retardation. There may therefore be a very small risk of such effects in the human foetus. Theoretically, there is the possibility that if maternal systemic absorption occurred the infant's adrenal function could be affected.

The use of topical corticosteroids during lactation is unlikely to present a hazard to infants being breast-fed.

4.7 Effects on ability to drive and use machines

None known.

4.8 Undesirable effects

(see Table 1 above)

4.9 Overdose

Excessive use under occlusive dressings may produce adrenal suppression. No special procedures or antidote. Treat any adverse effects symptomatically.

5. PHARMACOLOGICAL PROPERTIES

5.1 Pharmacodynamic properties

Hydrocortisone butyrate is a potent topical corticosteroid.

5.2 Pharmacokinetic properties

The topical activity has been demonstrated *in vivo* using the McKenzie-Stoughton test.

5.3 Preclinical safety data

No preclinical safety data have been generated.

6. PHARMACEUTICAL PARTICULARS

6.1 List of excipients

Cetostearyl alcohol, Macrogol Cetostearyl ether, Light Liquid Paraffin, White Soft Paraffin, Butyl parahydroxybenzoate, Propyl parahydroxybenzoate, Citric Acid (anhydrous), Sodium Citrate (anhydrous), Purified Water.

6.2 Incompatibilities

None stated.

6.3 Shelf life

3 years

6.4 Special precautions for storage

Do not store above 25°C. Do not refrigerate or freeze.

6.5 Nature and contents of container

Collapsible aluminium tubes containing either 30 G, 50 G, 100 G or 200G. Packed in a carton.

6.6 Special precautions for disposal and other handling

No special requirements.

7. MARKETING AUTHORISATION HOLDER

Astellas Pharma Ltd

Lovett House

Lovett Road

Staines

TW18 3AZ

United Kingdom

8. MARKETING AUTHORISATION NUMBER(S)

PL 00166/0058R

9. DATE OF FIRST AUTHORISATION/RENEWAL OF THE AUTHORISATION

First authorised 28 September 1973, renewed 19 December 2003.

10. DATE OF REVISION OF THE TEXT

15 July 2009

11. LEGAL CATEGORY

POM

Locoid Crelo

(Astellas Pharma Ltd)

1. NAME OF THE MEDICINAL PRODUCT

LOCOID CRELO

2. QUALITATIVE AND QUANTITATIVE COMPOSITION

Contains 0.1% w/w hydrocortisone butyrate.

For excipients, see 6.1

3. PHARMACEUTICAL FORM

Topical emulsion.

4. CLINICAL PARTICULARS

4.1 Therapeutic indications

The product is recommended for clinical use in the treatment of conditions responsive to topical corticosteroids, e.g. eczema, dermatitis and psoriasis. The product is intended for topical application especially to the scalp or hirsute skin.

Topical corticosteroids are not generally indicated in psoriasis but may be acceptable in psoriasis excluding widespread plaque psoriasis provided warnings are given, see section 4.4 Special warnings and special precautions for use.

4.2 Posology and method of administration

For topical application.

Dosage: To be applied evenly and sparingly no more than twice daily.

Adults and the Elderly: The same dose is used for adults and the elderly, as clinical evidence would indicate that no special dosage regimen is necessary in the elderly.

Children: Long term treatment should be avoided where possible.

Infants: Therapy should be limited if possible to a maximum of seven days.

The formulation of the product makes it suitable for use in both scaly lesions and for moist, weeping lesions.

4.3 Contraindications

Hypersensitivity to hydrocortisone or to any of the ingredients of the lotion.

This preparation is contraindicated in the presence of untreated viral or fungal infections, tubercular or syphilitic lesions, peri-oral dermatitis, acne vulgaris and rosacea and in bacterial infections unless used in connection with appropriate chemotherapy.

4.4 Special warnings and precautions for use

Although generally regarded as safe, even for long-term administration in adults, there is a potential for adverse effects if over used in infancy. Extreme caution is required in dermatoses of infancy including napkin eruption. In such patients, courses of treatment should not normally exceed 7 days.

As with all corticosteroids, application to the face, flexures and other areas of thin skin may cause skin atrophy and increased absorption and should be avoided.

Topical corticosteroids may be hazardous in psoriasis for a number of reasons including rebound relapses following development of tolerance, risk of generalised pustular psoriasis and local and systemic toxicity due to impaired barrier function of the skin. Steroids may have a place in psoriasis of the scalp and chronic plaque psoriasis of the hands and feet. Careful patient supervision is important.

Keep away from the eyes.

The cetostearyl alcohol and butylhydroxytoluene may cause local skin reactions (e.g. contact dermatitis). The propylene glycol may cause skin irritation. The butylhydroxytoluene may cause irritation to the eyes and mucous membranes

(e.g. nose). The propyl and butyl parahydroxybenzoate may cause allergic reactions which can be delayed.

4.5 Interaction with other medicinal products and other forms of interaction

None known.

4.6 Pregnancy and lactation

There is inadequate evidence of safety in human pregnancy. Topical administration of corticosteroids to pregnant animals can cause abnormalities of foetal development including cleft palate and intra-uterine growth retardation. There may therefore be a very small risk of such effects in the human foetus.

Theoretically, there is the possibility that if maternal systemic absorption occurred the infant's adrenal function could be affected.

The use of topical corticosteroids during lactation is unlikely to present a hazard to infants being breast-fed.

4.7 Effects on ability to drive and use machines

None known.

4.8 Undesirable effects

(see Table 1 below)

4.9 Overdose

Excessive use under occlusive dressings may produce adrenal suppression. No special procedures or antidote. Treat any adverse effects symptomatically.

5. PHARMACOLOGICAL PROPERTIES

5.1 Pharmacodynamic properties

The active constituent, hydrocortisone butyrate, is an established topical corticosteroid, equi-efficacious with those corticosteroids classified as potent.

5.2 Pharmacokinetic properties

In human in-vivo studies, the potency of this form of active ingredient has been shown to be of the same order as other topical corticosteroids classed as potent. The active ingredient metabolises to hydrocortisone and butyric acid.

5.3 Preclinical safety data

The well-established use of hydrocortisone 17-butyrate topical preparations over many years does not warrant further safety evaluation studies in animals.

6. PHARMACEUTICAL PARTICULARS

6.1 List of excipients

Macrogol cetostearyl ether

Cetostearyl Alcohol

White soft paraffin

Hard paraffin

Borage oil

Butylhydroxytoluene

Propyleneglycol

Sodium citrate

Anhydrous citric acid

Propyl parahydroxybenzoate

Butyl hydroxybenzoate

Purified water

Table 1 Undesirable effects

System Organ Class	Rare >/10,000, </1000	Very rare </10,000	Not known
Immune system disorders			Hypersensitivity
Endocrine disorders		Adrenal suppression	
Skin and subcutaneous tissue disorders	Skin atrophy, often irreversible, with thinning of the epidermis Telangiectasia Skin striae Pustular acne Perioral dermatitis Rebound effect Skin depigmentation Dermatitis and eczema, including contact dermatitis		

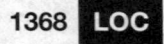

6.2 Incompatibilities
None known.

6.3 Shelf life
2 years.

6.4 Special precautions for storage
Do not store above 25°C.

6.5 Nature and contents of container
White opaque low density polyethylene bottles of 15, 25, 30, 50 and 100 g capacity, equipped with a natural low density polyethylene dropper applicator, closed with a white polypropylene screw cap.

6.6 Special precautions for disposal and other handling
No special requirements.

7. MARKETING AUTHORISATION HOLDER
Astellas Pharma Ltd
Lovett House
Lovett Road
Staines
TW18 3AZ
United Kingdom

8. MARKETING AUTHORISATION NUMBER(S)
PL0166/0170.

9. DATE OF FIRST AUTHORISATION/RENEWAL OF THE AUTHORISATION
23 May 1995 / 19th December 2003

10. DATE OF REVISION OF THE TEXT
15 July 2009

11. LEGAL CATEGORY
POM

Locoid Lipocream

(Astellas Pharma Ltd)

1. NAME OF THE MEDICINAL PRODUCT
LOCOID LIPOCREAM

2. QUALITATIVE AND QUANTITATIVE COMPOSITION
Contains 0.1% w/w hydrocortisone butyrate.

For excipients, see 6.1

3. PHARMACEUTICAL FORM
Cream

4. CLINICAL PARTICULARS

4.1 Therapeutic indications
The product is recommended for clinical use in the treatment of conditions responsive to topical corticosteroids e.g. eczema, dermatitis and psoriasis.

Topical corticosteroids are not generally indicated in psoriasis but may be acceptable in psoriasis excluding widespread plaque psoriasis provided warnings are given; see section 4.4 Special warnings and special precautions for use.

4.2 Posology and method of administration
For topical application.

Dosage: To be applied evenly and sparingly no more than twice daily

Application may be made under occlusion in the more resistant lesions such as thickened psoriatic plaques on elbows and knees.

Adults and the Elderly: The same dose is used for adults and the elderly, as clinical evidence would indicate that no special dosage regimen is necessary in the elderly.

Children: Long term treatment should be avoided where possible.

Infants: Therapy should be limited if possible to a maximum of seven days.

Due to the formulation of the base the product may be used both for dry scaly lesions and for moist or weeping lesions.

4.3 Contraindications
Hypersensitivity to hydrocortisone or to any of the ingredients of the cream.

This preparation is contraindicated in the presence of untreated viral or fungal infections, tubercular or syphilitic lesions, peri-oral dermatitis, acne vulgaris and rosacea and in bacterial infections unless used in connection with appropriate chemotherapy.

4.4 Special warnings and precautions for use
Although generally regarded as safe, even for long-term administration in adults, there is a potential for adverse effects if over used in infancy. Extreme caution is required in dermatoses of infancy including napkin eruption. In such patients courses of treatment should not normally exceed 7 days.

Application under occlusion should be restricted to dermatoses involving limited areas.

As with all corticosteroids, application to the face, flexures and other areas of thin skin may cause skin atrophy and increased absorption and should be avoided.

Topical corticosteroids may be hazardous in psoriasis for a number of reasons including rebound relapses following development of tolerance, risk of generalised pustular psoriasis and local and systemic toxicity due to impaired barrier function of the skin. Steroids may have a place in psoriasis of the scalp and chronic plaque psoriasis of the hands and feet. Careful patient supervision is important.

Keep away from the eyes.

The cetostearyl alcohol may cause local skin reactions (e.g. contact dermatitis) and the propyl parahydroxybenzoate may cause allergic reactions which can be delayed.

4.5 Interaction with other medicinal products and other forms of interaction
None known.

4.6 Pregnancy and lactation
There is inadequate evidence of safety in human pregnancy. Topical administration of corticosteroids to pregnant animals can cause abnormalities of foetal development including cleft palate and intra-uterine growth retardation. There may therefore be a very small risk of such effects in the human foetus. Theoretically, there is the possibility that if maternal systemic absorption occurred the infant's adrenal function could be affected.

The use of topical corticosteroids during lactation is unlikely to present a hazard to infants being breast-fed.

4.7 Effects on ability to drive and use machines
None known.

4.8 Undesirable effects
(see Table 1 below)

4.9 Overdose
Excessive use under occlusive dressings may produce adrenal suppression. No special procedures or antidote. Treat any adverse effects symptomatically

5. PHARMACOLOGICAL PROPERTIES

5.1 Pharmacodynamic properties
The active substance, hydrocortisone butyrate, is an established topical corticosteroid, equi-efficacious with those corticosteroids classified as potent.

5.2 Pharmacokinetic properties
In human in-vivo studies the potency of this formulation has been shown to be of the same order as other topical corticosteroids classified as potent. The active substance metabolises to hydrocortisone and butyric acid.

5.3 Preclinical safety data
No relevant pre-clinical safety data have been generated

6. PHARMACEUTICAL PARTICULARS

6.1 List of excipients
Macrogol cetostearyl ether
Cetostearyl alcohol
White soft paraffin
Light liquid paraffin
Sodium citrate anhydrous E331
Citric acid anhydrous E330
Propyl parahydroxybenzoate E216
Benzyl alcohol
Purified water

Table 1 Undesirable effects

System Organ Class	Rare >/10,000, </1000	Very rare </10,000	Not known
Immune system disorders			Hypersensitivity
Endocrine disorders		Adrenal suppression	
Skin and subcutaneous tissue disorders	Skin atrophy, often irreversible, with thinning of the epidermis Telangiectasia Skin striae Pustular acne Perioral dermatitis Rebound effect Skin depigmentation Dermatitis and eczema, including contact dermatitis		

6.2 Incompatibilities
None stated.

6.3 Shelf life
Three years

6.4 Special precautions for storage
Do not store above 25°C. Do not refrigerate or freeze.

6.5 Nature and contents of container
Collapsible aluminium tube with plastic screw cap containing 15g, 30g, 50g or 100 g.

6.6 Special precautions for disposal and other handling
No special requirements.

7. MARKETING AUTHORISATION HOLDER
Astellas Pharma Ltd
Lovett House
Lovett Road
Staines
TW18 3AZ
United Kingdom

8. MARKETING AUTHORISATION NUMBER(S)
PL 0166/0112

9. DATE OF FIRST AUTHORISATION/RENEWAL OF THE AUTHORISATION
First authorised 3 May 1983; renewed 19 December 2003.

10. DATE OF REVISION OF THE TEXT
15 July 2009

11. LEGAL CATEGORY
POM

Locoid Ointment

(Astellas Pharma Ltd)

1. NAME OF THE MEDICINAL PRODUCT
LOCOID OINTMENT

2. QUALITATIVE AND QUANTITATIVE COMPOSITION
Contains 0.1% w/w hydrocortisone butyrate.

For excipients, see 6.1

3. PHARMACEUTICAL FORM
Ointment.

Translucent, light grey to whitish, soft fatty ointment.

4. CLINICAL PARTICULARS

4.1 Therapeutic indications
The product is recommended for clinical use in the treatment of conditions responsive to topical corticosteroids e.g. eczema, dermatitis and psoriasis.

Topical corticosteroids are not generally indicated in psoriasis but may be acceptable in psoriasis excluding widespread plaque psoriasis provided warnings are given, see section 4.4 Special warnings and special precautions for use.

4.2 Posology and method of administration
For topical application.

Dosage: To be applied evenly and sparingly no more than twice daily.

Application may be made under occlusion in the more resistant lesions such as thickened psoriatic plaques on elbows and knees.

Adults and the Elderly: The same dose is used for adults and the elderly, as clinical evidence would indicate that no special dosage regimen is necessary in the elderly.

Children: Long term treatment should be avoided where possible.

Infants: Therapy should be limited if possible to a maximum of seven days.

4.3 Contraindications
Hypersensitivity to hydrocortisone or to any of the ingredients of the ointment.

This preparation is contraindicated in the presence of untreated viral or fungal infections, tubercular or syphilitic lesions, peri-oral dermatitis, acne vulgaris and rosacea and in bacterial infections unless used in connection with appropriate chemotherapy.

4.4 Special warnings and precautions for use
Although generally regarded as safe, even for long-term administration in adults, there is a potential for adverse effects if over used in infancy. Extreme caution is required in dermatoses of infancy including napkin eruption. In such patients courses of treatment should not normally exceed 7 days.

Application under occlusion should be restricted to dermatoses involving limited areas.

As with all corticosteroids, application to the face, flexures and other areas of thin skin may cause skin atrophy and increased absorption and should be avoided.

Topical corticosteroids may be hazardous in psoriasis for a number of reasons including rebound relapses following development of tolerance, risk of generalised pustular psoriasis and local and systemic toxicity due to impaired barrier

Table 1 Undesirable effects

System Organ Class	Rare >/10,000, </1000	Very rare </10,000	Not known
Immune system disorders			Hypersensitivity
Endocrine disorders		Adrenal suppression	
Skin and subcutaneous tissue disorders	Skin atrophy, often irreversible, with thinning of the epidermis Telangiectasia Skin striae Pustular acne Perioral dermatitis Rebound effect Skin depigmentation Dermatitis and eczema, including contact dermatitis		

function of the skin. Steroids may have a place in psoriasis of the scalp and chronic plaque psoriasis of the hands and feet. Careful patient supervision is important.

Keep away from the eyes.

4.5 Interaction with other medicinal products and other forms of interaction

None known.

4.6 Pregnancy and lactation

There is inadequate evidence of safety in human pregnancy. Topical administration of corticosteroids to pregnant animals can cause abnormalities of foetal development including cleft palate and intra-uterine growth retardation. There may therefore be a very small risk of such effects in the human foetus.

Theoretically, there is the possibility that if maternal systemic absorption occurred the infant's adrenal function could be affected.

The use of topical corticosteroids during lactation is unlikely to present a hazard to infants being breast-fed.

4.7 Effects on ability to drive and use machines

None known.

4.8 Undesirable effects

(see Table 1 above)

4.9 Overdose

Excessive use under occlusive dressings may produce adrenal suppression. No special procedures or antidote. Treat any adverse effects symptomatically.

5. PHARMACOLOGICAL PROPERTIES

5.1 Pharmacodynamic properties

Hydrocortisone butyrate is a potent topical corticosteroid.

5.2 Pharmacokinetic properties

The topical activity has been demonstrated *in vivo* using the McKenzie-Stoughton test.

5.3 Preclinical safety data

No preclinical safety data have been generated.

6. PHARMACEUTICAL PARTICULARS

6.1 List of excipients

Polyethylene oleogel (liquid paraffin, polyethylene)

6.2 Incompatibilities

None stated.

6.3 Shelf life

5 years

6.4 Special precautions for storage

Do not store above 25°C.

6.5 Nature and contents of container

Collapsible aluminium tubes containing either 30 G, 50 G, 100 G or 200G. Packed in a carton.

6.6 Special precautions for disposal and other handling

No special requirements.

7. MARKETING AUTHORISATION HOLDER

Astellas Pharma Ltd

Lovett House

Lovett Road

Staines

TW18 3AZ

United Kingdom

8. MARKETING AUTHORISATION NUMBER(S)

PL 00166/0059R

9. DATE OF FIRST AUTHORISATION/RENEWAL OF THE AUTHORISATION

First authorised 28 September 1973, renewed 19 December 2003.

10. DATE OF REVISION OF THE TEXT

15 July 2009

11. LEGAL CATEGORY

POM

Locoid Scalp Lotion

(Astellas Pharma Ltd)

1. NAME OF THE MEDICINAL PRODUCT

LOCOID SCALP LOTION

2. QUALITATIVE AND QUANTITATIVE COMPOSITION

Contains 0.1% w/v hydrocortisone butyrate.

For excipients, see 6.1

3. PHARMACEUTICAL FORM

Cutaneous solution.

Clear, colourless solution.

4. CLINICAL PARTICULARS

4.1 Therapeutic indications

The product is recommended for clinical use in the treatment of scalp conditions responsive to topical corticosteroids e.g. eczema, dermatitis and psoriasis.

Topical corticosteroids are not generally indicated in psoriasis but may be acceptable in psoriasis excluding widespread plaque psoriasis provided warnings are given; see section 4.4 Special warnings and special precautions for use.

4.2 Posology and method of administration

For topical application to the scalp.

Dosage: To be applied evenly and sparingly no more than twice daily

Adults and the Elderly: The same dose is used for adults and the elderly, as clinical evidence would indicate that no special dosage regimen is necessary in the elderly.

Children: Long term treatment should be avoided where possible.

Infants: Therapy should be limited if possible to a maximum of seven days.

4.3 Contraindications

Hypersensitivity to hydrocortisone or to any of the ingredients of the lotion.

This preparation is contraindicated in the presence of untreated viral or fungal infections, tubercular or syphilitic lesions, peri-oral dermatitis, acne vulgaris and rosacea and in bacterial infections unless used in connection with appropriate chemotherapy.

4.4 Special warnings and precautions for use

Although generally regarded as safe, even for long-term administration in adults, there is a potential for adverse effects if over used in infancy. Extreme caution is required in dermatoses of infancy. In such patients courses of treatment should not normally exceed 7 days.

As with all corticosteroids, application to the face, flexures and other areas of thin skin may cause skin atrophy and increased absorption and should be avoided.

Topical corticosteroids may be hazardous in psoriasis for a number of reasons including rebound relapses following development of tolerance, risk of generalised pustular psoriasis and local and systemic toxicity due to impaired barrier function of the skin. Steroids may have a place in psoriasis of the scalp and chronic plaque psoriasis of the hands and feet. Careful patient supervision is important.

Keep away from eyes.

4.5 Interaction with other medicinal products and other forms of interaction

None known.

4.6 Pregnancy and lactation

There is inadequate evidence of safety in human pregnancy. Topical administration of corticosteroids to pregnant animals can cause abnormalities of foetal development including cleft palate and intra-uterine growth retardation. There may therefore be a very small risk of such effects in the human foetus.

Theoretically, there is the possibility that if maternal systemic absorption occurred the infant's adrenal function could be affected.

The use of topical corticosteroids during lactation is unlikely to present a hazard to infants being breast-fed.

4.7 Effects on ability to drive and use machines

None known.

4.8 Undesirable effects

(see Table 1 below)

4.9 Overdose

Excessive use under occlusive dressings may produce adrenal suppression. No special procedures or antidote. Treat any adverse effects symptomatically.

5. PHARMACOLOGICAL PROPERTIES

5.1 Pharmacodynamic properties

Hydrocortisone butyrate is a potent topical corticosteroid.

5.2 Pharmacokinetic properties

The topical activity has been demonstrated *in vivo* using the McKenzie-Stoughton test.

5.3 Preclinical safety data

No preclinical safety data have been generated.

6. PHARMACEUTICAL PARTICULARS

6.1 List of excipients

Isopropyl alcohol, glycerol (85%), Povidone K90, anhydrous citric acid, anhydrous sodium citrate, purified water.

6.2 Incompatibilities

None stated.

6.3 Shelf life

2 years

6.4 Special precautions for storage

Do not store above 25°C.

6.5 Nature and contents of container

Plastic, dropper-necked screw cap vial.

Pack sizes: 30 ml and 100 ml.

6.6 Special precautions for disposal and other handling

No special requirements.

7. MARKETING AUTHORISATION HOLDER

Astellas Pharma Ltd

Lovett House

Lovett Road

Staines

TW18 3AZ

United Kingdom

8. MARKETING AUTHORISATION NUMBER(S)

PL 00166/0060R

9. DATE OF FIRST AUTHORISATION/RENEWAL OF THE AUTHORISATION

First authorised 28 September 1973; renewed 19 December 2003.

10. DATE OF REVISION OF THE TEXT

15 July 2009

11. LEGAL CATEGORY

POM

Table 1 Undesirable effects

System Organ Class	Rare >/10,000, </1000	Very rare </10,000	Not known
Immune system disorders			Hypersensitivity
Endocrine disorders		Adrenal suppression	
Skin and subcutaneous tissue disorders	Skin atrophy, often irreversible, with thinning of the epidermis Telangiectasia Skin striae Pustular acne Perioral dermatitis Rebound effect Skin depigmentation Dermatitis and eczema, including contact dermatitis		

Loestrin 20

(Galen Limited)

1. NAME OF THE MEDICINAL PRODUCT
Loestrin 20.

2. QUALITATIVE AND QUANTITATIVE COMPOSITION
Each Loestrin 20 tablet contains:

Norethisterone acetate	Ph Eur	1mg
Ethinylestradiol	Ph Eur	0.02mg

3. PHARMACEUTICAL FORM
Blue convex film coated tablet.

4. CLINICAL PARTICULARS

4.1 Therapeutic indications
For the prevention of pregnancy in women who elect to use oral contraceptives. The efficacy of any contraceptive method, except sterilisation, depends upon the reliability with which it is used. Correct and consistent use of methods can result in lower failure rates.

4.2 Posology and method of administration
For oral use.

One Loestrin 20 tablet should be taken daily at approximately the same time of day for three weeks, starting on the first day of menstrual bleeding and then an interval of one week allowed before commencing the second course of tablets. If starting on the fourth day of the cycle or later, additional contraceptive precautions should be used for the first seven days. Second and subsequent courses should be taken for three weeks with one week without tablets between courses. Thus each new course of tablets is always started on the same day of the week. It is important that the tablets are taken as directed and should be taken without regard to menstrual bleeding except in the initial cycle.

Missed pills

If a tablet is not taken at the usual time, it must be taken as soon as possible and the next tablet taken at the normal time. If the delay exceeds twelve hours, additional contraception (barriers and spermicides) should be used for the next 7 days whilst continuing to take Loestrin. Additionally, if pills have been missed during the last 7 days of a pack, there should be no break before the next pack is started.

Gastrointestinal upset

Vomiting or diarrhoea may reduce efficacy by preventing full absorption. Barriers and spermicides should therefore be used during and for 7 days after recovery and if these 7 days overrun the end of a pack, the next pack should be started without a break. In this case, a withdrawal bleed should not be expected until the end of the second pack. If the patient does not have a withdrawal bleed at the end of the second pack, she must return to the doctor to exclude the possibility of pregnancy.

Changing from another 21 day combined oral contraceptive to Loestrin

The first Loestrin tablet should be taken on the first day immediately after the end of the previous oral contraceptive course. Additional contraception is not required. A withdrawal bleed should not be expected until the end of the first Loestrin pack.

Changing from an everyday (ED) 28 day combined oral contraceptive to Loestrin

The first tablet of Loestrin should be taken on the day immediately after the day on which the last active pill in the ED pack has been taken. The remaining (inactive) tablets in the ED pack should be discarded. Additional contraception is not required. A withdrawal bleed should not be expected until the end of the first pack of Loestrin.

Changing from a progestogen-only-pill (POP) to Loestrin

The first tablet of Loestrin should be taken on the first day of menstruation, even if the POP for that day has already been taken. The remaining tablets in the POP pack should be discarded. Additional contraception is not required.

Post-partum and post-abortum use

After pregnancy combined oral contraception can be started in non-lactating women 21 days after a vaginal delivery, provided that the patient is fully ambulant and there are no puerperal complications.

If the pill is started later than 21 days after delivery, then barriers and spermicides should be used until oral contraception is started and for the first 7 days of pill-taking. If unprotected intercourse has taken place after 21 days post partum, then oral contraception should not be started until the first menstrual bleed after childbirth.

After a miscarriage or abortion, oral contraceptives may be started immediately.

4.3 Contraindications

1) Known or suspected pregnancy and lactation.

2) History of confirmed venous thromboembolism (VTE), family history of idiopathic VTE and other known risk factors for VTE.

3) Ischaemic heart disease, severe hypertension or coagulation abnormalities.

4) Liver disease including disorders of hepatic excretion e.g. Dubin-Johnson or Rotor syndromes, infective hepatitis (until liver function returns to normal), known or suspected disorders of lipid metabolism, porphyria, liver adenoma or carcinoma, gallstones or jaundice with prior pill use.

5) Sickle cell anaemia.

6) Known or suspected carcinoma of the breast or estrogen dependent neoplasms.

7) Undiagnosed abnormal vaginal bleeding.

8) History during pregnancy of idiopathic jaundice, severe pruritus, chorea, herpes or deterioration of otosclerosis.

9) Focal, severe or crescendo migraine or transient cerebral ischaemic attacks without headaches.

Figure 1 Estimated cumulative numbers of breast cancers per 10,000 women diagnosed in 5 years of use and up to 10 years after stopping COCs, compared with numbers of breast cancers diagnosed in 10,000 women who had never used COCs

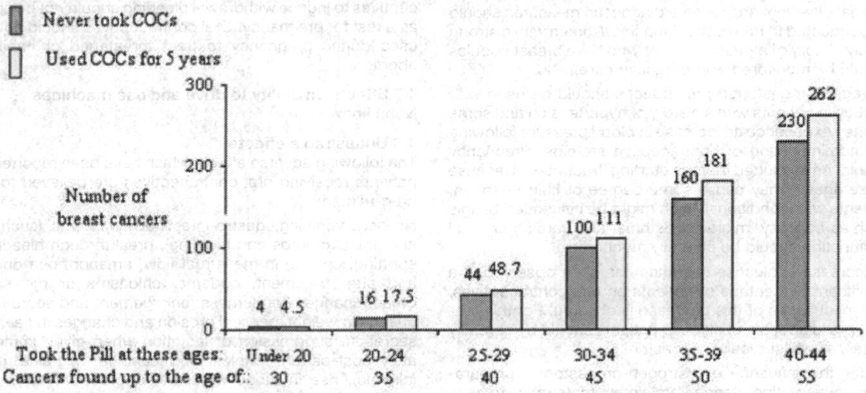

4.4 Special warnings and precautions for use

The following information is principally based on studies in patients who used oral contraceptives with higher concentrations of estrogens and progestogens than those in common use today. The effect of long-term use of the oral contraceptives with lower concentrations of both estrogens and progestogens remains to be determined. The efficacy of any contraceptive method, except sterilisation, depends upon the reliability with which it is used. Correct and consistent use of such methods can result in lower failure rates.

Thrombo-embolism

An increased risk of thromboembolic disease (VTE) associated with the use of oral contraceptives is well established but is smaller than that associated with pregnancy, which has been estimated at 60 cases per 100,000 pregnancies. Some epidemiological studies have reported a greater risk of VTE for women using combined oral contraceptives containing desogestrel or gestodene (the so-called 'third generation' pills) than for women using pills containing levonorgestrel or norethisterone (the so-called 'second generation' pills).

The spontaneous incidence of VTE in healthy, non-pregnant women (not taking any oral contraceptive) is about 5 cases per 100,000 per year. The incidence in users of second generation pills is about 15 per 100,000 women per year of use. The incidence in third generation pills is about 25 cases per 100,000 women per year of use; this excess incidence has not been satisfactorily explained by bias or confounding. The risk of venous thromboembolism is highest during the first year a combined oral contraceptive is taken. This increased risk applies to the first time ever combined oral contraceptive use is begun rather than each time a woman starts a new type of combined oral contraceptive. The level of all these risks of VTE increases with age and is likely to be further increased in women with other known risk factors for VTE such as obesity. The suitability of combined oral contraceptives for patients with any of these risk factors should be discussed with the patient before a final decision is taken.

The physician should be alert to the earliest manifestations of these disorders (thrombophlebitis, cerebrovascular disorders, pulmonary embolism and retinal thrombosis). Should any of these occur or be suspected, Loestrin should be discontinued immediately.

Cigarette smoking increases the risk of serious cardiovascular side effects from oral contraceptive use. This risk increases with age and with heavy smoking (15 or more cigarettes a day) and is quite marked in women over 35 years of age. Women who use oral contraceptives should be strongly advised not to smoke.

Hepatic tumours

Benign hepatic tumours have been associated with oral contraceptive usage. Malignant hepatic tumours have also been reported on rare occasions in long term users of oral contraceptives. A hepatic tumour should be considered in the differential diagnosis when upper abdominal pain, enlarged liver or signs of intra-abdominal haemorrhage occur.

Ovarian, endometrial, cervical and breast cancer

Numerous epidemiological studies have been reported on the risks of ovarian, endometrial, cervical and breast cancer in women using combined oral contraceptives. The evidence is clear that combined oral contraceptives offer substantial protection against both ovarian and endometrial cancer.

An increased risk of cervical cancer in long term users of combined oral contraceptives has been reported in some studies, but there continues to be controversy about the extent to which this is attributable to the confounding effects of sexual behaviour and other factors.

A meta-analysis from 54 epidemiological studies reported that there is a slightly increased relative risk (RR = 1.24) of having breast cancer diagnosed in women who are currently using combined oral contraceptives (COCs). The observed pattern of increased risk may be due to an earlier diagnosis of breast cancer in COC users, the biological effects of COCs or, a combination of both. The additional breast cancers diagnosed in current users of COCs, or in women who have used COCs in the last ten years, are more likely to be localised to the breast than in those women who have never used COCs.

Breast cancer is rare among women under 40 years of age, whether or not they take COCs. Whilst this background risk increases with age, the excess number of breast cancer diagnoses in current and recent COC users is small in relation to the overall risk of breast cancer (see bar chart).

The most important risk factor for breast cancer in COC users is the age women discontinue the COC; the older the age at stopping, the more breast cancers are diagnosed. Duration of use is less important and the excess risk gradually disappears during the course of the ten years after stopping COC use, such that by 10 years there appears to be no excess.

The possible increase in risk of breast cancer should be discussed with the user and weighed against the benefits of COCs taking into account the evidence that they offer substantial protection against the risk of developing certain other cancers (e.g. ovarian and endometrial cancer).

Estimated cumulative numbers of breast cancers per 10,000 women diagnosed in 5 years of use and up to 10 years after stopping COCs, compared with numbers of breast cancers diagnosed in 10,000 women who had never used COCs

(see Figure 1 above)

Reasons for stopping Loestrin immediately

1) Occurrence of migraine in patients who have never previously suffered from it. Any unusually frequent or severe headaches.

2) Any kind of visual disturbance e.g. proptosis or diplopia and migraine.

3) Suspicion of thrombosis or infarction.

4) Combined oral contraceptives should be stopped at least six weeks before elective surgery and during and following prolonged immobilisation e.g. after accidents, etc.

5) Loestrin should be discontinued if the patient becomes jaundiced or has a significant rise in blood pressure.

6) Patients with a history of depression should be carefully observed and the drug discontinued if the depression recurs to a serious degree.

7) Since the safety of Loestrin in pregnancy has not been demonstrated, it is recommended that for any patient who has missed a period, the absence of pregnancy should be established before continuing the contraceptive regimen.

8) Clear exacerbation of conditions known to be capable of deteriorating during oral contraception or pregnancy.

Assessment of women prior to starting oral contraceptives (and at regular intervals thereafter) should include a personal and family medical history of each woman. Physical examination should be guided by this and by the contra-indications (section 4.3) and warnings (section 4.4) for this product. The frequency and nature of these assessments should be based upon relevant guidelines and should be adapted to the individual woman, but should include measurement of blood pressure and, if judged appropriate by the clinician, breast, abdominal and pelvic examination including cervical cytology.

In case of undiagnosed, persistent or recurrent abnormal vaginal bleeding, appropriate diagnostic measures should be conducted to rule out malignancy. Women with a strong family history of breast cancer or who have breast nodules should be monitored with particular care.

Estrogen-progestogen preparations should be used with caution in patients with a history of hypertension and some women experience an increase in blood pressure following the administration of contraceptive steroids. Pregnancy should be excluded before starting treatment. Because these agents may cause some degree of fluid retention, patients with conditions which might be influenced by this such as epilepsy, migraine, asthma, and cardiac or renal dysfunction should be carefully monitored.

A decrease in glucose tolerance has been observed in a significant percentage of patients on oral contraceptives. The mechanism of this decrease is obscure. For this reason, pre-diabetic and diabetic patients should be carefully observed whilst receiving Loestrin.

Under the influence of estrogen-progestogen preparations, pre-existing uterine fibroleiomyomata may increase in size. Loestrin may mask the onset of the climacteric.

The following conditions also require careful consideration: multiple sclerosis, porphyria, tetany, disturbed liver function, gallstones, cardiovascular disease, renal disease, chloasma or any disease that is prone to worsen during pregnancy. The deterioration or first appearance of any of these conditions may indicate that the oral contraceptive should be stopped. Contact lens wearers who develop visual changes or changes to lens tolerance should be assessed by an optometrist.

Interference with laboratory tests

The following laboratory results may be altered by the use of oral contraceptives: hepatic function (increased sulphobromophthalein retention and other tests); thyroid function (increased thyroid binding globulin (TBG) leading to increased circulating total thyroid hormone as measured by protein-bound iodine (PBI), T4 by column or by radioimmunoassay. Free T3 resin uptake is decreased, reflecting the elevated TBG. Free T4 concentration is unaltered); haematological tests (increased prothrombin and factors VII, VIII, IX and X, decreased antithrombin 3 and increased adrenaline induced platelet aggregation); measurement of pregnanediol excretion (reduced). Other binding proteins may be elevated in the serum, sex-binding globulins are increased, triglycerides may be increased and serum folate levels may be depressed. Therefore, if such tests are abnormal in a patient taking Loestrin, it is recommended that they be repeated after Loestrin has been withdrawn for two months. The pathologist should be advised of the administration of Loestrin when relevant specimens are submitted. Any influence of prolonged administration of Loestrin on pituitary, ovarian, adrenal, hepatic and uterine functions is unknown at present.

4.5 Interaction with other medicinal products and other forms of interaction

Effects of other drugs on oral contraceptives

The effectiveness of combined oral contraceptives may be considerably reduced by interaction with drugs that induce hepatic enzyme activity e.g. carbamazepine, griseofulvin, phenytoin, phenobarbital, primidone and rifampicin. Other drugs suspected of having the capacity to reduce the efficacy of oral contraceptives include ampicillin and other broad-spectrum antibiotics.

Additional contraceptive precautions should be taken whilst taking enzyme inducing drugs and some antibiotics and for at least seven days after stopping them. If these seven days run beyond the end of the packet, the new packet should be started immediately without a break. Rifampicin is such a potent inducer that even if the course lasts for less than 7 days, the additional contraceptive precautions should be continued for at least 4 weeks after stopping it.

The herbal remedy St. John's Wort *(Hypericum perforatum)* should not be taken concomitantly with this medicine as this could potentially lead to a loss of contraceptive effect.

Ascorbic acid and paracetamol may increase plasma ethinylestradiol concentrations, possibly by inhibition of conjugation.

Administration of atorvastatin concomitantly with oral contraceptives containing ethinylestradiol and norethisterone acetate increased AUC values for norethisterone and ethinylestradiol by approximately 30% and 20% respectively.

Effects of oral contraceptives on other drugs:

Oral contraceptive combinations containing ethinylestradiol may inhibit the metabolism of other compounds. Increased plasma concentrations of ciclosporin, prednisolone and theophylline have been reported with concomitant administration of oral contraceptives. In addition, oral contraceptives may induce conjugation of other compounds. Decreased plasma concentrations of paracetamol have been noted when administered with oral contraceptives.

4.6 Pregnancy and lactation

Loestrin is not recommended for use during pregnancy, suspected pregnancy and in lactating mothers. Studies do not suggest a teratogenic effect, particularly in so far as cardiac anomalies and limb reduction defects are concerned, when oral contraceptives are taken inadvertently during early pregnancy. The administration of oral contraceptives to induce withdrawal bleeding should not be used as a test for pregnancy. Oral contraceptives should not be used during pregnancy to treat threatened or habitual abortion.

4.7 Effects on ability to drive and use machines

None known.

4.8 Undesirable effects

The following adverse effects which have been reported in patients receiving oral contraceptives are believed to be drug-related:

Nausea, vomiting, gastro-intestinal symptoms (such as abdominal cramps and bloating), breakthrough bleeding, spotting, change in menstrual flow, amenorrhoea during and after treatment, oedema, chloasma or melasma, breast changes (tenderness, enlargement and secretion), change in weight, cervical erosion and changes in cervical secretion, suppression of lactation when given immediately post-partum, cholestatic jaundice, migraine, rash (allergic), rise in blood pressure, depression, thromboembolic disorders, temporary infertility after discontinuation of treatment, reduced tolerance to carbohydrates, vaginal candidiasis, change in corneal curvature (steepening) and intolerance to contact lenses.

Although the following adverse effects have been reported in women taking oral contraceptives, an association has been neither confirmed nor refuted: prolonged amenorrhoea after discontinuing oral contraceptives, pre-menstrual like syndrome, headache, nervousness, dizziness, fatigue, cataract, backache, hirsutism, loss of scalp hair, erythema multiforme, erythema nodusum, haemorrhagic eruption, itching, changes in appetite, cystitis-like syndrome, vaginitis, porphyria, impaired renal function, haemolytic uraemic syndrome, Budd-Chiari syndrome, acne, changes in libido and colitis.

Menstrual changes

Breakthrough bleeding and spotting are sometimes encountered, especially during the first three months of use. Non-hormonal causes should be considered and adequate diagnostic measures taken to rule out malignancy or pregnancy in the event of breakthrough bleeding, as in the case of any abnormal vaginal bleeding. If pathology has been excluded, time or a change to another formulation may solve the problem.

4.9 Overdose

The usual effects in children are nausea and drowsiness. Slight vaginal bleeding occasionally occurs in girls. In view of the low toxicity following overdosage with oral contraceptives, it is suggested that treatment should be conservative.

5. PHARMACOLOGICAL PROPERTIES

5.1 Pharmacodynamic properties

Loestrin achieves its contraceptive effect primarily by inhibition of ovulation through gonadotrophin suppression. It is possible that other sites of action such as changes in cervical mucus and in the endometrium may contribute to the efficacy of combined oral contraceptives.

5.2 Pharmacokinetic properties

Ethinylestradiol is rapidly and almost completely absorbed and peak serum levels are usually attained within an hour of oral administration. At this time, the majority of drug is already conjugated, largely as the sulphate. These conjugates have a primary serum half-life of approximately 7 hours and a terminal half-life of 48 hours and are excreted in urine and faeces.

Norethisterone acetate undergoes rapid absorption with peak serum concentrations occurring at one hour after oral administration. Less than 5% is cleared as unchanged norethisterone; glucuronide and sulphate conjugates are excreted in urine and faeces. The terminal half-life for norethisterone conjugates has been estimated at 70 hours (range: 42 - 84 hours).

5.3 Preclinical safety data

The results of the preclinical tests do not add anything of further significance to the prescriber.

6. PHARMACEUTICAL PARTICULARS

6.1 List of excipients

Lactose, sucrose, maize starch, talc, powdered acacia, magnesium stearate, industrial methylated spirit*, purified water*, dichloromethane*, propylene glycol*, hypromellose 15, carnauba wax, E104, E127, E132, E171 and hydroxypropylcellulose.

* Not present in final product

6.2 Incompatibilities

None known.

6.3 Shelf life

3 years.

6.4 Special precautions for storage

Do not store above 30°C. Store in the outer carton.

6.5 Nature and contents of container

Printed aluminium foil blister strip contained in a cardboard carton together with a product leaflet. Supplied in packs of 21 and 63 tablets.

6.6 Special precautions for disposal and other handling

No special instructions needed.

7. MARKETING AUTHORISATION HOLDER

Galen Limited

Seagoe Industrial Estate

Craigavon

BT63 5UA

UK.

8. MARKETING AUTHORISATION NUMBER(S)

PL 21590/0083.

9. DATE OF FIRST AUTHORISATION/RENEWAL OF THE AUTHORISATION

03 April 1974/10 February 2009.

10. DATE OF REVISION OF THE TEXT

10 February 2009.

Loestrin 30

(Galen Limited)

1. NAME OF THE MEDICINAL PRODUCT

Loestrin 30.

2. QUALITATIVE AND QUANTITATIVE COMPOSITION

Each Loestrin 30 tablet contains:

Norethisterone acetate	Ph Eur	1.5mg
Ethinylestradiol Ph Eur	Ph Eur	0.03mg

3. PHARMACEUTICAL FORM

Pale green convex film coated tablet.

4. CLINICAL PARTICULARS

4.1 Therapeutic indications

For the prevention of pregnancy in women who elect to use oral contraceptives. The efficacy of any contraceptive method, except sterilisation, depends upon the reliability with which it is used. Correct and consistent use of methods can result in lower failure rates.

4.2 Posology and method of administration

For oral use.

One Loestrin 30 tablet should be taken daily at approximately the same time of day for three weeks, starting on the first day of menstrual bleeding and then an interval of one week allowed before commencing the second course of tablets. If starting on the fourth day of the cycle or later, additional contraceptive precautions should be used for the first seven days. Second and subsequent courses should be taken for three weeks with one week without tablets between courses. Thus each new course of tablets is always started on the same day of the week. It is important that the tablets are taken as directed and should be taken without regard to menstrual bleeding except in the initial cycle.

Missed pills

If a tablet is not taken at the usual time, it must be taken as soon as possible and the next tablet taken at the normal time. If the delay exceeds twelve hours, additional contraception (barriers and spermicides) should be used for the next 7 days whilst continuing to take Loestrin. Additionally, if pills have been missed during the last 7 days of a pack, there should be no break before the next pack is started.

Gastrointestinal upset

Vomiting or diarrhoea may reduce efficacy by preventing full absorption. Barriers and spermicides should therefore be used during and for 7 days after recovery and if these 7 days overrun the end of a pack, the next pack should be started without a break. In this case, a withdrawal bleed should not be expected until the end of the second pack. If the patient does not have a withdrawal bleed at the end of the second pack, she must return to the doctor to exclude the possibility of pregnancy.

Changing from another 21 day combined oral contraceptive to Loestrin

The first Loestrin tablet should be taken on the first day immediately after the end of the previous oral contraceptive course. Additional contraception is not required. A withdrawal bleed should not be expected until the end of the first Loestrin pack.

Changing from an everyday (ED) 28 day combined oral contraceptive to Loestrin

The first tablet of Loestrin should be taken on the day immediately after the day on which the last active pill in the ED pack has been taken. The remaining (inactive) tablets in the ED pack should be discarded. Additional contraception is not required. A withdrawal bleed should not be expected until the end of the first pack of Loestrin.

Changing from a progestogen-only-pill (POP) to Loestrin

The first tablet of Loestrin should be taken on the first day of menstruation, even if the POP for that day has already been taken. The remaining tablets in the POP pack should be discarded. Additional contraception is not required.

Post-partum and post-abortum use

After pregnancy combined oral contraception can be started in non-lactating women 21 days after a vaginal delivery, provided that the patient is fully ambulant and there are no puerperal complications.

If the pill is started later than 21 days after delivery, then barriers and spermicides should be used until oral contraception is started and for the first 7 days of pill-taking. If unprotected intercourse has taken place after 21 days post partum, then oral contraception should not be started until the first menstrual bleed after childbirth.

After a miscarriage or abortion, oral contraceptives may be started immediately.

4.3 Contraindications

1) Known or suspected pregnancy and lactation.

2) History of confirmed venous thromboembolism (VTE), family history of idiopathic VTE and other known risk factors for VTE.

3) Ischaemic heart disease, severe hypertension or coagulation abnormalities.

4) Liver disease including disorders of hepatic excretion e.g. Dubin-Johnson or Rotor syndromes, infective hepatitis (until liver function returns to normal), known or suspected disorders of lipid metabolism, porphyria, liver adenoma or carcinoma, gallstones or jaundice with prior pill use.

5) Sickle cell anaemia.

6) Known or suspected carcinoma of the breast or estrogen dependent neoplasms.

7) Undiagnosed abnormal vaginal bleeding.

8) History during pregnancy of idiopathic jaundice, severe pruritus, chorea, herpes or deterioration of otosclerosis.

9) Focal, severe or crescendo migraine or transient cerebral ischaemic attacks without headaches.

4.4 Special warnings and precautions for use

The following information is principally based on studies in patients who used oral contraceptives with higher concentrations of estrogens and progestogens than those in common use today. The effect of long-term use of the oral contraceptives with lower concentrations of both estrogens and progestogens remains to be determined. The efficacy of any contraceptive method, except sterilisation, depends upon the reliability with which it is used. Correct and consistent use of such methods can result in lower failure rates.

Thrombo-embolism

An increased risk of thromboembolic disease (VTE) associated with the use of oral contraceptives is well established but is smaller than that associated with pregnancy, which has been estimated at 60 cases per 100,000 pregnancies. Some epidemiological studies have reported a greater risk of VTE for women using combined oral contraceptives containing desogestrel or gestodene (the so-called 'third generation' pills) than for women using pills containing levonorgestrel or norethisterone (the so-called 'second generation' pills).

The spontaneous incidence of VTE in healthy, non-pregnant women (not taking any oral contraceptive) is about 5 cases per 100,000 per year. The incidence in users of second generation pills is about 15 per 100,000 women per year of use. The incidence in third generation pills is about 25 cases per 100,000 women per year of use; this excess incidence has not been satisfactorily explained by bias or confounding. The risk of venous thromboembolism is highest during the first year a combined oral contraceptive is taken. This increased risk applies to the first time ever combined oral contraceptive use is begun rather than each time a woman starts a new type of combined oral contraceptive. The level of all these risks of VTE increases with age and is likely to be further increased in women with other known risk factors for VTE such as obesity. The suitability of combined oral contraceptives for patients with any of these risk factors should be discussed with the patient before a final decision is taken.

The physician should be alert to the earliest manifestations of these disorders (thrombophlebitis, cerebrovascular disorders, pulmonary embolism and retinal thrombosis). Should any of these occur or be suspected, Loestrin should be discontinued immediately.

Cigarette smoking increases the risk of serious cardiovascular side effects from oral contraceptive use. This risk increases with age and with heavy smoking (15 or more cigarettes a day) and is quite marked in women over 35 years of age. Women who use oral contraceptives should be strongly advised not to smoke.

Hepatic tumours

Benign hepatic tumours have been associated with oral contraceptive usage. Malignant hepatic tumours have also been reported on rare occasions in long term users of oral contraceptives. A hepatic tumour should be considered in the differential diagnosis when upper abdominal pain, enlarged liver or signs of intra-abdominal haemorrhage occur.

Ovarian, endometrial, cervical and breast cancer

Numerous epidemiological studies have been reported on the risks of ovarian, endometrial, cervical and breast cancer in women using combined oral contraceptives. The evidence is clear that combined oral contraceptives offer substantial protection against both ovarian and endometrial cancer.

An increased risk of cervical cancer in long term users of combined oral contraceptives has been reported in some

Figure 1 Estimated cumulative numbers of breast cancers per 10,000 women diagnosed in 5 years of use and up to 10 years after stopping COCs, compared with numbers of breast cancers diagnosed in 10,000 women who had never used COCs

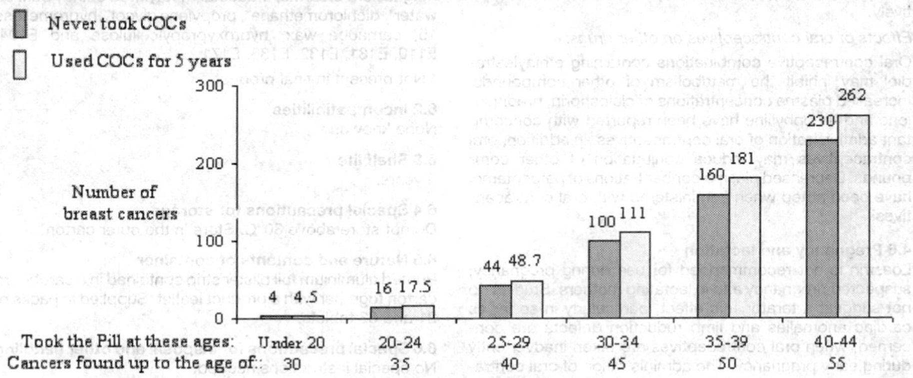

studies, but there continues to be controversy about the extent to which this is attributable to the confounding effects of sexual behaviour and other factors.

A meta-analysis from 54 epidemiological studies reported that there is a slightly increased relative risk (RR = 1.24) of having breast cancer diagnosed in women who are currently using combined oral contraceptives (COCs). The observed pattern of increased risk may be due to an earlier diagnosis of breast cancer in COC users, the biological effects of COCs or, a combination of both. The additional breast cancers diagnosed in current users of COCs, or in women who have used COCs in the last ten years, are more likely to be localised to the breast than in those women who have never used COCs.

Breast cancer is rare among women under 40 years of age, whether or not they take COCs. Whilst this background risk increases with age, the excess number of breast cancer diagnoses in current and recent COC users is small in relation to the overall risk of breast cancer (see bar chart).

The most important risk factor for breast cancer in COC users is the age women discontinue the COC; the older the age at stopping, the more breast cancers are diagnosed. Duration of use is less important and the excess risk gradually disappears during the course of the ten years after stopping COC use, such that by 10 years there appears to be no excess.

The possible increase in risk of breast cancer should be discussed with the user and weighed against the benefits of COCs taking into account the evidence that they offer substantial protection against the risk of developing certain other cancers (e.g. ovarian and endometrial cancer).

Estimated cumulative numbers of breast cancers per 10,000 women diagnosed in 5 years of use and up to 10 years after stopping COCs, compared with numbers of breast cancers diagnosed in 10,000 women who had never used COCs

(see Figure 1 above)

Reasons for stopping Loestrin immediately

1) Occurrence of migraine in patients who have never previously suffered from it. Any unusually frequent or severe headaches.

2) Any kind of visual disturbance e.g. proptosis or diplopia and migraine.

3) Suspicion of thrombosis or infarction.

4) Combined oral contraceptives should be stopped at least six weeks before elective surgery and during and following prolonged immobilisation e.g. after accidents, etc.

5) Loestrin should be discontinued if the patient becomes jaundiced or has a significant rise in blood pressure.

6) Patients with a history of depression should be carefully observed and the drug discontinued if the depression recurs to a serious degree.

7) Since the safety of Loestrin in pregnancy has not been demonstrated, it is recommended that for any patient who has missed a period, the absence of pregnancy should be established before continuing the contraceptive regimen.

8) Clear exacerbation of conditions known to be capable of deteriorating during oral contraception or pregnancy.

Assessment of women prior to starting oral contraceptives (and at regular intervals thereafter) should include a personal and family medical history of each woman. Physical examination should be guided by this and by the contraindications (section 4.3) and warnings (section 4.4) for this product. The frequency and nature of these assessments should be based upon relevant guidelines and should be adapted to the individual woman, but should include measurement of blood pressure and, if judged appropriate by the clinician, breast, abdominal and pelvic examination including cervical cytology.

In case of undiagnosed, persistent or recurrent abnormal vaginal bleeding, appropriate diagnostic measures should be conducted to rule out malignancy. Women with a strong family history of breast cancer or who have breast nodules should be monitored with particular care.

Estrogen-progestogen preparations should be used with caution in patients with a history of hypertension and some women experience an increase in blood pressure following the administration of contraceptive steroids. Pregnancy should be excluded before starting treatment. Because these agents may cause some degree of fluid retention, patients with conditions which might be influenced by this such as epilepsy, migraine, asthma, and cardiac or renal dysfunction should be carefully monitored.

A decrease in glucose tolerance has been observed in a significant percentage of patients on oral contraceptives. The mechanism of this decrease is obscure. For this reason, pre-diabetic and diabetic patients should be carefully observed whilst receiving Loestrin.

Under the influence of estrogen-progestogen preparations, pre-existing uterine fibroleiomyomata may increase in size. Loestrin may mask the onset of the climacteric.

The following conditions also require careful consideration: multiple sclerosis, porphyria, tetany, disturbed liver function, gallstones, cardiovascular disease, renal disease, chloasma or any disease that is prone to worsen during pregnancy. The deterioration or first appearance of any of these conditions may indicate that the oral contraceptive should be stopped. Contact lens wearers who develop visual changes or changes to lens tolerance should be assessed by an optometrist.

Interference with laboratory tests

The following laboratory results may be altered by the use of oral contraceptives: hepatic function (increased sulphobromophthalein retention and other tests); thyroid function (increased thyroid binding globulin (TBG) leading to increased circulating total thyroid hormone as measured by protein-bound iodine (PBI), T4 by column or by radioimmunoassay. Free T3 resin uptake is decreased, reflecting the elevated TBG. Free T4 concentration is unaltered); haematological tests (increased prothrombin and factors VII, VIII, IX and X, decreased antithrombin 3 and increased adrenaline induced platelet aggregation); measurement of pregnanediol excretion (reduced). Other binding proteins may be elevated in the serum, sex-binding globulins are increased, triglycerides may be increased and serum folate levels may be depressed. Therefore, if such tests are abnormal in a patient taking Loestrin, it is recommended that they be repeated after Loestrin has been withdrawn for two months. The pathologist should be advised of the administration of Loestrin when relevant specimens are submitted. Any influence of prolonged administration of Loestrin on pituitary, ovarian, adrenal, hepatic and uterine functions is unknown at present.

4.5 Interaction with other medicinal products and other forms of interaction

Effects of other drugs on oral contraceptives

The effectiveness of combined oral contraceptives may be considerably reduced by interaction with drugs that induce hepatic enzyme activity e.g. carbamazepine, griseofulvin, phenytoin, phenobarbital, primidone and rifampicin. Other drugs suspected of having the capacity to reduce the efficacy of oral contraceptives include ampicillin and other broad-spectrum antibiotics.

Additional contraceptive precautions should be taken whilst taking enzyme inducing drugs and some antibiotics and for at least seven days after stopping them. If these seven days run beyond the end of the packet, the new packet should be started immediately without a break. Rifampicin is such a potent inducer that even if the course lasts for less than 7 days, the additional contraceptive precautions should be continued for at least 4 weeks after stopping it.

The herbal remedy St. John's Wort *(Hypericum perforatum)* should not be taken concomitantly with this medicine as this could potentially lead to a loss of contraceptive effect.

Ascorbic acid and paracetamol may increase plasma ethinylestradiol concentrations, possibly by inhibition of conjugation.

Administration of atorvastatin concomitantly with oral contraceptives containing ethinylestradiol and norethisterone acetate increased AUC values for norethisterone and ethinylestradiol by approximately 30% and 20% respectively.

Effects of oral contraceptives on other drugs:

Oral contraceptive combinations containing ethinylestradiol may inhibit the metabolism of other compounds. Increased plasma concentrations of ciclosporin, prednisolone and theophylline have been reported with concomitant administration of oral contraceptives. In addition, oral contraceptives may induce conjugation of other compounds. Decreased plasma concentrations of paracetamol have been noted when administered with oral contraceptives.

4.6 Pregnancy and lactation

Loestrin is not recommended for use during pregnancy, suspected pregnancy and in lactating mothers. Studies do not suggest a teratogenic effect, particularly in so far as cardiac anomalies and limb reduction defects are concerned, when oral contraceptives are taken inadvertently during early pregnancy. The administration of oral contraceptives to induce withdrawal bleeding should not be used as a test for pregnancy. Oral contraceptives should not be used during pregnancy to treat threatened or habitual abortion.

4.7 Effects on ability to drive and use machines

None known.

4.8 Undesirable effects

The following adverse effects which have been reported in patients receiving oral contraceptives are believed to be drug-related:

Nausea, vomiting, gastro-intestinal symptoms (such as abdominal cramps and bloating), breakthrough bleeding, spotting, change in menstrual flow, amenorrhoea during and after treatment, oedema, chloasma or melasma, breast changes (tenderness, enlargement and secretion), change in weight, cervical erosion and changes in cervical secretion, suppression of lactation when given immediately post-partum, cholestastic jaundice, migraine, rash (allergic), rise in blood pressure, depression, thrombo-embolic disorders, temporary infertility after discontinuation of treatment, reduced tolerance to carbohydrates, vaginal candidiasis, change in corneal curvature (steepening) and intolerance to contact lenses.

Although the following adverse effects have been reported in women taking oral contraceptives, an association has been neither confirmed nor refuted: prolonged amenorrhoea after discontinuing oral contraceptives, pre-menstrual like syndrome, headache, nervousness, dizziness, fatigue, cataract, backache, hirsutism, loss of scalp hair, erythema multiforme, erythema nodusum, haemorrhagic eruption, itching, changes in appetite, cystitis-like syndrome, vaginitis, porphyria, impaired renal function, haemolytic uraemic syndrome, Budd-Chiari syndrome, acne, changes in libido and colitis.

Menstrual changes

Breakthrough bleeding and spotting are sometimes encountered, especially during the first three months of use. Non-hormonal causes should be considered and adequate diagnostic measures taken to rule out malignancy or pregnancy in the event of breakthrough bleeding, as in the case of any abnormal vaginal bleeding. If pathology has been excluded, time or a change to another formulation may solve the problem.

4.9 Overdose

The usual effects in children are nausea and drowsiness. Slight vaginal bleeding occasionally occurs in girls. In view of the low toxicity following overdosage with oral contraceptives, it is suggested that treatment should be conservative.

5. PHARMACOLOGICAL PROPERTIES

5.1 Pharmacodynamic properties

Loestrin achieves its contraceptive effect primarily by inhibition of ovulation through gonadotrophin suppression. It is possible that other sites of action such as changes in cervical mucus and in the endometrium may contribute to the efficacy of combined oral contraceptives.

5.2 Pharmacokinetic properties

Ethinylestradiol is rapidly and almost completely absorbed and peak serum levels are usually attained within an hour of oral administration. At this time, the majority of drug is already conjugated, largely as the sulphate. These conjugates have a primary serum half-life of approximately 7 hours and a terminal half-life of 48 hours and are excreted in urine and faeces.

Norethisterone acetate undergoes rapid absorption with peak serum concentrations occurring at one hour after oral administration. Less than 5% is cleared as unchanged norethisterone; glucuronide and sulphate conjugates are excreted in urine and faeces. The terminal half-life for norethisterone conjugates has been estimated at 70 hours (range: 42 - 84 hours).

5.3 Preclinical safety data

The results of the preclinical tests do not add anything of further significance to the prescriber.

6. PHARMACEUTICAL PARTICULARS

6.1 List of excipients

Lactose, sucrose, maize starch, talc, powdered acacia, magnesium stearate, industrial methylated spirit*, purified water*, dichloromethane*, propylene glycol*, hypromellose 15, carnauba wax, hydroxypropylcellulose and E104, E110, E131, E132, E133, E171.

* Not present in final product

6.2 Incompatibilities

None known.

6.3 Shelf life

3 years.

6.4 Special precautions for storage

Do not store above 30°C. Store in the outer carton.

6.5 Nature and contents of container

Printed aluminium foil blister strip contained in a cardboard carton together with a product leaflet. Supplied in packs of 21 and 63 tablets.

6.6 Special precautions for disposal and other handling

No special instructions needed.

7. MARKETING AUTHORISATION HOLDER

Galen Limited

Seagoe Industrial Estate

Craigavon

BT63 5UA

UK.

8. MARKETING AUTHORISATION NUMBER(S)

PL 21590/0084.

9. DATE OF FIRST AUTHORISATION/RENEWAL OF THE AUTHORISATION

03 April 1974/11 February 2009.

10. DATE OF REVISION OF THE TEXT

11 February 2009.

Lofepramine 70mg tablets (Merck Serono Ltd)

(Merck Serono)

1. NAME OF THE MEDICINAL PRODUCT

Lofepramine 70mg tablets

2. QUALITATIVE AND QUANTITATIVE COMPOSITION

Lofepramine hydrochloride 76.10mg/tablet

equivalent to lofepramine base 70mg/tablet

3. PHARMACEUTICAL FORM

Oral tablet

4. CLINICAL PARTICULARS

4.1 Therapeutic indications

The treatment of symptoms of depressive illness

4.2 Posology and method of administration

Route of administration:

Oral

Recommended dosage:

The usual dose is 70mg twice daily (140mg) or three times daily (210mg) depending upon patient response.

Children: Not recommended

Elderly: May respond to lower doses in some cases

4.3 Contraindications

Lofepramine should not be used in patients hypersensitive to dibenzazepines, in mania, severe liver impairment and/or severe renal impairment, heart block, cardiac arrhythmias or during the recovery phase following a myocardial infarction.

Lofepramine should not be administered with or within 2 weeks of cessation of therapy with monoamine oxidase inhibitors (see Section 4.5)

Use of lofepramine with amiodarone should be avoided (see Section 4.5).

Use of lofepramine with terfenadine should be avoided (see Section 4.5).

4.4 Special warnings and precautions for use

Suicide/suicidal thoughts or clinical worsening

Depression is associated with an increased risk of suicidal thoughts, self harm and suicide (suicide-related events). This risk persists until significant remission occurs. As improvement may not occur during the first few weeks or more of treatment, patients should be closely monitored until such improvement occurs. It is general clinical experience that the risk of suicide may increase in the early stages of recovery.

Other psychiatric conditions for which Lofepramine is prescribed can also be associated with an increased risk of suicide-related events. In addition, these conditions may be co-morbid with major depressive disorder. The same precautions observed when treating patients with major depressive disorder should therefore be observed when treating patients with other psychiatric disorders.

Patients with a history of suicide-related events, or those exhibiting a significant degree of suicidal ideation prior to commencement of treatment are known to be at greater risk of suicidal thoughts or suicide attempts, and should receive careful monitoring during treatment. A meta-analysis of placebo-controlled clinical trials of antidepressant drugs in adult patients with psychiatric disorders showed an increased risk of suicidal behaviour with antidepressants compared to placebo in patients less than 25 years old.

Close supervision of patients and in particular those at high risk should accompany drug therapy especially in early treatment and following dose changes. Patients (and caregivers of patients) should be alerted about the need to monitor for any clinical worsening, suicidal behaviour or thoughts and unusual changes in behaviour and to seek medical advice immediately if these symptoms present.

It should be remembered that severely depressed patients are at risk of suicide. An improvement in depression may not occur immediately upon initiation of treatment, therefore the patient should be closely monitored until symptoms improve.

Lofepramine may lower the convulsion threshold, therefore it should be used with extreme caution in patients with a history of epilepsy or recent convulsions or other predisposing factors, or during withdrawal from alcohol or other drugs with anticonvulsant properties.

Concurrent electroconvulsive therapy should only be undertaken with careful supervision.

Caution is needed in patients with hyperthyroidism, or during concomitant treatment with thyroid preparations, since aggravation of unwanted cardiac effects may occur.

Lofepramine should be used with caution in patients with cardiovascular disease, impaired liver function, impaired renal function, blood dyscrasias or porphyria.

Caution is called for where there is a history of prostatic hypertrophy, narrow angle glaucoma or increased intra-ocular pressure, because of lofepramine's anticholinergic properties.

In chronic constipation, tricyclic antidepressants may cause paralytic ileus, particularly in elderly and bedridden patients.

Care should be exercised in patients with tumours of the adrenal medulla (e.g. phaeochromocytoma, neuroblastoma) in whom tricyclic antidepressants may provoke anti-hypertensive crises.

Blood pressure should be checked before initiating treatment because individuals with hypertension, or an unstable circulation, may react to lofepramine with a fall in blood pressure.

Anaesthetics may increase the risks of arrhythmias and hypotension (see Interactions), therefore before local or general anaesthesia, the anaesthetist should be informed that the patient has been taking lofepramine.

Lofepramine should be used with caution where there is a history of mania. Psychotic symptoms may be aggravated. There have also been reports of hypomanic or manic episodes during a depressive phase in patients with cyclic affective disorders receiving tricyclic antidepressants.

Abrupt withdrawal of lofepramine should be avoided if possible.

4.5 Interaction with other medicinal products and other forms of interaction

MAO Inhibitors: Lofepramine should not be administered with or within 2 weeks of cessation of therapy with monoamine oxidase inhibitors. (See Section 4.3). It should be introduced cautiously using a low initial dose and the effects monitored.

SSRI Inhibitors: Co-medication may lead to additive effects on the serotonergic system. Fluvoxamine and fluoxetine may also increase plasma concentrations of lofepramine resulting in a lowered convulsion threshold and seizures.

Anti-arrhythmic drugs: There is an increased risk of ventricular arrhythmias if lofepramine is given with drugs which prolong the Q-T interval e.g. disopyramide, procainamide, propafenone, quinidine and amiodarone. Concomitant use with amiodarone should be avoided (See Section 4.3)

Sympathomimetic drugs: Lofepramine should not be given with sympathomimetic agents (e.g. adrenalin, ephedrine, isoprenaline, noradrenaline, phenylephedrine, phenylpropanolamine) since their cardiovascular effects may be potentiated.

CNS depressants: Lofepramine's effects may be potentiated when administered with CNS depressant substances e.g. barbiturates, general anaesthetics and alcohol. If surgery is necessary, the anaesthetist should be informed that a patient is being so treated because of the increased risk of arrhythmias and hypotension.

Neuroleptics: There is an increased risk of arrythmias; there may be an increased plasma level of the tricyclic antidepressant, a lowered convulsion threshold and seizures.

Adrenergic neurone blockers: Lofepramine may decrease or abolish the antihypertensive effects of some adrenergic neurone blocking drugs eg guanethidine, betanidine, reserpine, clonidine and a-methyl-dopa. Antihypertensives of a different type eg diuretics, vasodilators or β-blockers should be given therefore where patients require co-medication for hypertension.

Anticoagulants: Lofepramine may inhibit hepatic metabolism leading to an enhancement of anticoagulant effect. Careful monitoring of plasma prothrombin is advised.

Anti-cholinergic agents: Lofepramine may potentiate the effects of these drugs (e.g. phenothiazine, antiparkinson agents, antihistamines, atropine, beperiden) on the central nervous system, eye, bowel and bladder.

Analgesics: There is an increased risk of ventricular arrhythmias.

Anti-epileptics: Antagonism can lead to a lowering of the convulsive threshold. Plasma levels of some tricyclic antidepressants, and therefore the therapeutic effect, may be reduced.

Calcium channel blockers: diltiazem and verapamil increase the plasma concentration of lofepramine.

Diuretics: There is an increased risk of postural hypotension.

Rifampicin: The metabolism of lofepramine is accelerated by rifampicin leading to a reduced plasma concentration

Digitalis glycosides: With digitalis glycosides there is a higher risk of arrhythmias.

Sotalol: The risk of ventricular arrhythmias associated with sotalol is increased.

Cimetidine: Cimetidine can increase the plasma concentration of lofepramine.

Clonidine: The effect of antihypertensive agents of the clonidine type can be weakened.

Altretamine: There is a risk of severe postural hypotension when co-administered with tricyclic antidepressants

Disulfiram and alprazolam: Co-medication with either disulfiram or alprazolam may require a reduction in the dose of lofepramine

Nitrates: The effectiveness of sublingual nitrates may be reduced where the tricyclic antidepressant's anticholinergic effect has lead to dryness of the mouth

Ritonavir: There may be an increased plasma concentration of lofepramine.

Thyroid hormone therapy: During concomitant treatment, there may be aggravation of unwanted cardiac effects.

Oral contraceptives: Oestrogens and progestogens may antagonise the therapeutic effect of tricyclic antidepressants whilst the latter's side effects may be exacerbated due to an increased plasma concentration.

4.6 Pregnancy and lactation

The safety of lofepramine for use during pregnancy has not been established and there is evidence of harmful effects in pregnancy in animals when high doses are given. Lofepramine has been shown to be excreted in breast milk. The administration of lofepramine in pregnancy and during breast feeding therefore is not advised unless there are compelling medical reasons.

4.7 Effects on ability to drive and use machines

As with other antidepressants, ability to drive a car and operate machinery may be affected, especially in conjunction with alcohol.

Therefore caution should be exercised initially until the individual reaction to treatment is known.

4.8 Undesirable effects

The following side effects have been reported with lofepramine:

Cases of suicidal ideation and suicidal behaviours have been reported during lofepramine therapy or early after discontinuation (see section 4.4)

Cardiovascular: hypotension, tachycardia, cardiac conduction disorders, increase in cardiac insufficiency, arrhythmias.

CNS & Neuromuscular: dizziness, sleep disturbances, agitation, confusion, headache, malaise, paraesthesia; rarely, drowsiness, hypomania and convulsions; very rarely, uncoordinated movement.

Anticholinergic: dryness of mouth, constipation, disturbances of accommodation, urinary hesitancy, urinary retention, sweating and tremor, induction of glaucoma; rarely, impairment of the sense of taste; very rarely, tinnitus.

Urinogenital: testicular disorders eg pain

Allergic: skin rash, allergic skin reactions, "photosensitivity reactions", facial oedema; rarely, cutaneous bleeding, inflammation of mucosal membranes.

Gastrointestinal: nausea, vomiting.

Endocrine: rarely, hyponatraemia (inappropriate secretion of antidiuretic hormone), interference with sexual function, changes of blood sugar level, gynaecomastia, galactorrhoea.

Haematological/biochemical: rarely, bone marrow depression including isolated reports of: agranulocytosis, eosinophilia, granulocytopenia, leucopenia, pancytopenia, thrombocytopenia.

Increases in liver enzymes, sometimes progressing to clinical hepatitis and jaundice, have been reported in some patients, usually occurring within the first 3 months of starting therapy.

The following adverse effects have been encountered in patients under treatment with tricyclic antidepressants and should therefore be considered as theoretical hazards of lofepramine even in the absence of substantiation: psychotic manifestations, including mania and paranoid delusions may be exacerbated during treatment with tricyclic antidepressants; withdrawal symptoms may occur on abrupt cessation of therapy and include insomnia, irritability and excessive perspiration; adverse effects such as withdrawal symptoms, respiratory depression and agitation have been reported in neonates whose mothers have taken tricyclic antidepressants during the last trimester of pregnancy.

4.9 Overdose

The treatment of overdosage is symptomatic and supportive. It should include immediate gastric lavage and routine close monitoring of cardiac function.

5. PHARMACOLOGICAL PROPERTIES

5.1 Pharmacodynamic properties

Lofepramine is a tricyclic antidepressant. It exerts its therapeutic effect by blocking the uptake of noradrenaline by the nerve cell thus increasing the amine in the synaptic cleft and hence the effect on the receptors. There is evidence to suggest that serotonin may also be involved. Other pharmacological effects are due to anti-cholinergic activity, but less sedation is observed than with other tricyclics.

5.2 Pharmacokinetic properties

Lofepramine is a tertiary amine, similar in structure to imipramine but with improved lipophilicity and lower base strength. It is readily absorbed when given orally. From the plasma it is distributed throughout the body notably to the brain, lungs, liver and kidney. It is metabolised in the liver by cleavage of the p-chlorophenacyl group from the lofepramine molecule leaving desmethylimipramine (DMI).

The latter is pharmacologically active. The p-chlorobenzoyl portion is mainly metabolised to p-chlorobenzoic acid which is then conjugated with glycine. The conjugate is excreted mostly in the urine. DMI has been found excreted in the faeces. In a study of protein binding capability it has been found that lofepramine is up to 99% protein bound.

5.3 Preclinical safety data

N/A

6. PHARMACEUTICAL PARTICULARS

6.1 List of excipients

Excipients

Lactose

Corn starch

L(+) ascorbic acid

Talcum

Glycerol

Glycerol monostearate

Ethylene dinitriletetra acetic acid disodium salt (dihydrate) [titriplex III]

Dimethicone

Silicone dioxide

Hydroxypropyl methyl cellulose

Coating

1,2-Propanediol

Hydroxypropyl methyl cellulose

Ponceau 4R aluminium lake E124

Talc

Titanium dioxide

Indigotine lake E132

6.2 Incompatibilities

None

6.3 Shelf life

3 years

6.4 Special precautions for storage

Protect from light and moisture. Store in the original package.

6.5 Nature and contents of container

Containers

1. PVDC/Al foil blister calendar packs containing 28, 56, 1008 or 2016 tablets

2. Polypropylene containers containing 56, 250, 500 or 1000 tablets

3. Amber glass bottles containing 56 tablets

6.6 Special precautions for disposal and other handling

None

7. MARKETING AUTHORISATION HOLDER

Merck Serono Ltd
Bedfont Cross
Stanwell Road
Feltham
Middlesex
TW14 8NX,
United Kingdom

8. MARKETING AUTHORISATION NUMBER(S)

11648/0011

9. DATE OF FIRST AUTHORISATION/RENEWAL OF THE AUTHORISATION

30 July 1982/ 1 December 1998

10. DATE OF REVISION OF THE TEXT

19 February 2008

Lomont 70mg/5ml Oral Suspension

(Rosemont Pharmaceuticals Limited)

1. NAME OF THE MEDICINAL PRODUCT

Lomont 70mg/5ml Oral Suspension

2. QUALITATIVE AND QUANTITATIVE COMPOSITION

Active Ingredient	Per 5ml
Lofepramine Hydrochloride,	76.1mg
(equivalent to Lofepramine base)	70mg

3. PHARMACEUTICAL FORM

A white to pale yellow/orange suspension with odour of Cherry.

4. CLINICAL PARTICULARS

4.1 Therapeutic indications

For the treatment of symptoms of depressive illness.

4.2 Posology and method of administration

Adults: The usual dose 70mg twice daily (140mg) or three times daily (210mg) depending upon patient response.

Elderly: Elderly patients may respond to lower doses in some cases.

Children: Not recommended

4.3 Contraindications

Lofepramine should not be used in patients hypersensitive to dibenzazepines, in mania, severe liver impairment and/ or severe renal impairment, heart block, cardiac arrhythmias, or during the recovery phase following a myocardial infarction.

Lofepramine should not be administered with or within 2 weeks of cessation of therapy with monoamine oxidase inhibitors (see Section 4.5).

Use of lofepramine with amiodarone should be avoided (see Section 4.5).

Use of lofepramine with terfenadine should be avoided (see Section 4.5).

4.4 Special warnings and precautions for use

It should be remembered that severely depressed patients are at risk of suicide. An improvement in depression may not occur immediately upon initiation of treatment, therefore the patient should be closely monitored until symptoms improve.

Lofepramine may lower the convulsion threshold, therefore it should be used with extreme caution in patients with a history of epilepsy or recent convulsions or other predisposing factors, or during withdrawal from alcohol or other drugs with anticonvulsant properties.

Concurrent electroconvulsive therapy should only be undertaken with careful supervision.

Lofepramine should be used with caution where there is a history of mania. Psychotic symptoms may be aggravated. There have also been reports of hypomanic or manic episodes during a depressive phase in patients with cyclic affective disorders receiving tricyclic antidepressants.

Lofepramine should be used with caution in patients with cardiovascular disease, impaired liver or renal function, narrow angle glaucoma, symptoms suggestive of prostatic hypertrophy, blood dyscrasias or porphyria.

Caution is needed in patients with hyperthyroidism, or during concomitant treatment with thyroid preparations, since aggravation of unwanted cardiac effects may occur.

In chronic constipation, tricyclic antidepressants may cause paralytic ileus, particularly in elderly and bedridden patients.

Care should be exercised in patients with tumours of the adrenal medulla (eg phaeochromocytoma, neuroblastoma) in whom tricyclic antidepressants may provoke hypertensive crises.

Blood pressure should be checked before initiating treatment because individuals with hypertension, or an unstable circulation, may react to lofepramine with a fall in blood pressure.

Anaesthetics may increase the risks of arrhythmias and hypotension (see Interactions), therefore before local or general anaesthesia, the anaesthetist should be informed that the patient has been taking lofepramine.

Hyponatraemia (usually in the elderly and possibly due to inappropriate secretion of antidiuretic hormone) has been associated with all types of antidepressants and should be considered in all patients who develop drowsiness, confusion or convulsions while taking lofepramine.

Abrupt withdrawal of lofepramine should be avoided if possible.

Suicide/suicidal thoughts or clinical worsening

Depression is associated with an increased risk of suicidal thoughts, self harm and suicide (suicide-related events).

This risk persists until significant remission occurs. As improvement may not occur during the first few weeks or more of treatment, patients should be closely monitored until such improvement occurs. It is general clinical experience that the risk of suicide may increase in the early stages of recovery.

Patients with a history of suicide-related events, or those exhibiting a significant degree of suicidal ideation prior to commencement of treatment are known to be at greater risk of suicidal thoughts or suicide attempts, and should receive careful monitoring during treatment. A meta-analysis of placebo-controlled clinical trials of antidepressant drugs in adult patients with psychiatric disorders showed an increased risk of suicidal behaviour with antidepressants compared to placebo in patients less than 25 years old.

Close supervision of patients and in particular those at high risk should accompany drug therapy especially in early treatment and following dose changes. Patients (and care-givers of patients) should be alerted about the need to monitor for any clinical worsening, suicidal behaviour or thoughts and unusual changes in behaviour and to seek medical advice immediately if these symptoms present.

Excipient Warnings

This product contains 10%v/v ethanol, i.e. up to 395mg per dose equivalent to 10ml of beer or 4ml of wine per dose. It is harmful for those suffering from alcoholism. It should be taken into account in pregnant or lactating women, children and high-risk groups such as patients with liver disease or epilepsy. It may modify or increase the effect of other medicines. The amount of alcohol in this product may impair the ability to drive or use machines.

This product also contains liquid maltitol and sorbitol. Patients with rare hereditary problems of fructose intolerance should not take this medicine.

Methyl and propyl hydroxybenzoates are contained in this product which may cause allergic reactions (possibly delayed).

4.5 Interaction with other medicinal products and other forms of interaction

Lofepramine should not be administered concurrently with or within 2 weeks of cessation of therapy of monamine oxidase inhibitors. It should then be introduced cautiously using a low initial dosage.

SSRI Inhibitors: co-medication may lead to additive effects on the serotonergic system. Fluvoxamine and fluoxetine may also increase plasma concentrations of lofepramine resulting in a lowered convulsion threshold and seizures.

Anti-arrhythmic drugs: There is an increased risk of ventricular arrhythmias if lofepramine is given with drugs which prolong the Q-T interval e.g. disopyramide, procainamide, propafenone, quinidine and amiodarone. Concomitant use with amiodarone should be avoided (See Section 4.3)

Neuroleptics: There is an increased risk of arrhythmias; there may be an increased plasma level of the tricyclic antidepressant, a lowered convulsion threshold and seizures.

Lofepramine should not be given with sympathomimetic agents (cardiovascular effects may be potentiated), central nervous depressants including alcohol or thyroid hormone therapy since its effects may be potentiated.

Lofepramine may decrease the antihypertensive effect of adrenergic neurone-blocking drugs; it is therefore advisable to review this form of antihypertensive therapy during treatment.

Anaesthetics given during tricyclic antidepressant therapy may increase the risk of arrhythmias and hypotension. If surgery is necessary, the anaesthetist should be informed that a patient is being so treated. Barbiturates may increase the rate of metabolism.

Possible interactions between lofepramine and warfarin, leading to an enhancement of anticoagulant effect, have been reported rarely. Careful monitoring of plasma prothrombin is advised.

Anti-cholinergic agents: Lofepramine may potentiate the effects of these drugs (e.g. phenothiazine, antiparkinson agents, antihistamines, atropine, beperiden) on the central nervous system, eye, bowel and bladder.

Analgesics: There is an increased risk of ventricular arrhythmias.

Anti-epileptics: Antagonism can lead to a lowering of the convulsive threshold. Plasma levels of some tricyclic antidepressants, and therefore the therapeutic effect, may be reduced.

Calcium channel blockers: diltiazem and verapamil increase the plasma concentration of lofepramine.

Diuretics: There is an increased risk of postural hypotension.

Terfenadine: There is an increased risk of ventricular arrhythmias therefore concomitant use should be avoided.

Rifampicin: The metabolism of lofepramine is accelerated by rifampicin leading to a reduced plasma concentration

Digitalis glycosides: With digitalis glycosides there is a higher risk of arrhythmias.

Sotalol: The risk of ventricular arrhythmias associated with sotalol is increased.

Cimetidine: Cimetidine can increase the plasma concentration of lofepramine.

Clonidine: The effect of antihypertensive agents of the clonidine type can be weakened.

Altretamine: There is a risk of severe postural hypotension when co-administered with tricyclic antidepressants

Disulfiram and alprazolam: Co-medication with either disulfiram or alprazolam may require a reduction in the dose of lofepramine.

Nitrates: The effectiveness of sublingual nitrates may be reduced where the tricyclic antidepressant's anticholinergic effect has lead to dryness of the mouth.

Ritonavir: There may be an increased plasma concentration of lofepramine.

Oral contraceptives: Oestrogens and progestogens may antagonise the therapeutic effect of tricyclic antidepressants whilst the latter's side effects may be exacerbated due to an increased plasma concentration.

4.6 Pregnancy and lactation

The safety of Lofepramine for use during pregnancy has not been established and there is evidence of harmful effects in pregnancy in animals when high doses are given. Lofepramine has been shown to be excreted in breast milk. The administration of Lofepramine in pregnancy and during breast feeding therefore, is not advised unless there are compelling medical reasons.

Adverse effects such as withdrawal symptoms, respiratory depression and agitation have been reported in neonates whose mothers have taken tricyclic antidepressants during the last trimester of pregnancy.

4.7 Effects on ability to drive and use machines

Ability to drive a car and operate machinery may be affected. Therefore caution should be exercised initially until the individual reaction to treatment is known.

4.8 Undesirable effects

Lofepramine has been shown to be well tolerated and side-effects, when they occur, tend to be mild. Comparative clinical trials have shown that Lofepramine is associated with a low incidence of anticholinergic side effects. The following side effects have been reported with Lofepramine:

Cardiovascular: Hypotension, tachycardia, cardiac conduction disorders, increase in cardiac insufficiency, arrhythmias.

CNS and Neuromuscular: Dizziness, sleep disturbances, agitation, confusion, headache, malaise, paraesthesia; rarely, drowsiness, hypomania and convulsions (See section 4.4 Special Warnings and Precautions for Use); very rarely, uncoordinated movement.

Anticholinergic: Dryness of mouth, constipation, disturbances of accommodation, urinary hesitancy, urinary retention, sweating and tremor, induction of glaucoma; rarely, impairment of the sense of taste; very rarely, tinnitus.

Urinogenital: Testicular disorders e.g. pain.

Allergic: Skin rash, allergic skin reactions, photosensitivity reactions, facial oedema; rarely, cutaneous bleeding, inflammation of mucosal membranes.

Gastro-intestinal: Nausea, vomiting

Endocrine: Rarely, hyponatraemia (inappropriate secretion of antidiuretic hormone), interference with sexual function, changes of blood sugar level, gynaecomastia, galactorrhoea.

Haematological/ biochemical: Rarely, bone marrow depression including isolated report of: agranulocytosis, eosinophilia, granuloctyopenia, leucopenia, pancytopenia, thrombocytopenia. Increases in liver enzymes, sometimes progressing to clinical hepatitis and jaundice, have been observed in some patients, usually occurring within the first three months of starting therapy. There have been a small number of reports of jaundice. These reactions are reversible on cessation of therapy.

The following adverse effects have been encountered in patients under treatment with tricyclic antidepressants and should therefore be considered as theoretical hazards of Lofepramine even in the absence of substantiation: psychotic manifestations including mania and paranoid delusions may be exacerbated during treatment with tricyclic antidepressants; withdrawal symptoms may occur on abrupt cessation of therapy and include insomnia, irritability and excessive perspiration; adverse effects such as withdrawal symptoms, respiratory depression and agitation have been reported in neonates whose mothers have taken tricyclic antidepressants during the last trimester of pregnancy.

Cases of suicidal ideation and suicidal behaviours have been reported during lofepramine therapy or early after treatment discontinuation (see section 4.4).

4.9 Overdose

Treatment of overdosage is symptomatic and supportive. It should include immediate gastric lavage and routine close monitoring of cardiac function. Reports of overdosage with Lofepramine, with quantities ranging from 0.7g up to 6.72g, have shown no serious sequelae directly attributable to the drug.

5. PHARMACOLOGICAL PROPERTIES

5.1 Pharmacodynamic properties

Lofepramine inhibits the re-uptake of monoamines in peripheral adrenergic nerves. Lofepramine produces a lesser increase in heart rate than that produced by Amitriptyline when administered to normal individuals.

5.2 Pharmacokinetic properties

Lofepramine is rapidly absorbed with peak plasma concentration being reached within 1 hour and having a plasma half-life of 5 hours. In common with Imipramine, Lofepramine appears to undergo significant presystemic metabolism.

Plasma protein binding is approximately 99%. After oral administration higher concentrations of Lofepramine and its metabolites can be found in blood, lungs, liver, kidney and brain.

Almost all of the drug is metabolized before excretion, which is mainly in the urine and in faeces. Lofepramine is metabolized by N-dealkylation, hydroxylation and glucuronidation. It is extensively metabolized to its principal metabolite, desmethylimipramine, on first pass through the liver. During chronic administration, the plasma level of desmethylimipramine is typically three times greater than that of lofepramine, except in the first few hours following administration of each dose, during which time the plasma level of the parent drug can exceed that of its metabolite. Desipramine, which is also an antidepressant is converted to 2-hydroxydesipramine in the liver. Both compounds are excreted mainly in the urine as glucuronides, but also by biliary excretion in the faeces. Less than 5% is excreted unchanged in the urine over 24 hours.

Neither renal disease or old age has any appreciable effect on the kinetics of desipramine. Elimination may be reduced and bioavailability increased in hepatic disease.

5.3 Preclinical safety data

Lofepramine Hydrochloride is a well established active substance.

Lofepramine, like other tricyclic antidepressants, has been shown to inhibit the neuronal uptake of noradrenaline and to potentiate serotonergic transmission.

The safety of Lofepramine for use during pregnancy has not been established and there is evidence of harmful effects in pregnancy in animals when high doses are given. Lofepramine has been shown to be excreted in breast milk. The administration of Lofepramine in pregnancy and breast feeding therefore, is not advised unless there are compelling medical reasons.

Adverse effects such as withdrawal symptoms, respiratory depression and agitation have been reported in neonates whose mothers have taken tricyclic antidepressants during the last trimester of pregnancy.

The toxological data available in the published literature on lofepramine have not revealed any hazards, which are likely to occur at the usual oral therapeutic dosage. The excipients in the formulation would not be anticipated to influence the pharmacology or toxicology of the drug.

6. PHARMACEUTICAL PARTICULARS

6.1 List of excipients

Purified water, sodium ascorbate, sorbitol solution 70% (non-crystallising), liquid maltitol, methyl hydroxybenzoate, propyl hydroxybenzoate, propylene glycol, ethanol (absolute), colloidal silicon dioxide (aerosil) and cherry flavour 28T7704.

6.2 Incompatibilities

None known

6.3 Shelf life

24 months

6.4 Special precautions for storage

Store between 4°C and 25°C. Protect from light.

6.5 Nature and contents of container

150ml, 200ml or 300ml amber (type III) glass bottles

Closures: - 1) Aluminium, EPE wadded, roll-on, pilfer-proof, or 2) HDPE, EPE wadded, tamper evident or 3) HDPE EPE wadded, tamper evident child resistant.

6.6 Special precautions for disposal and other handling

Keep out of the reach of children. Shake before use.

Administrative Data

7. MARKETING AUTHORISATION HOLDER

Rosemont Pharmaceuticals Ltd
Rosemont House
Yorkdale Industrial Park
Braithwaite Street
Leeds
LS11 9XE

8. MARKETING AUTHORISATION NUMBER(S)

0427/0094

9. DATE OF FIRST AUTHORISATION/RENEWAL OF THE AUTHORISATION

1 February 1996

10. DATE OF REVISION OF THE TEXT

02 February 2009

Lomustine "medac" 40 mg

(medac GmbH)

1. NAME OF THE MEDICINAL PRODUCT
Lomustine "medac" 40 mg

2. QUALITATIVE AND QUANTITATIVE COMPOSITION
Lomustine (CCNU) 40 mg per capsule

3. PHARMACEUTICAL FORM
Hard capsule

4. CLINICAL PARTICULARS

4.1 Therapeutic indications
As palliative or supplementary treatment, usually in combination with radiotherapy and/or surgery as part of multiple drug regimens in:

Brain tumours (primary or metastatic)

Lung tumours (especially oat-cell carcinoma)

Hodgkin's disease (resistant to conventional combination chemotherapy)

Malignant melanoma (metastatic)

Lomustine "medac" may also be of value as second-line treatment in Non-Hodgkin's lymphoma, myelomatosis, gastrointestinal tumours, carcinoma of the kidney, the testis, the ovary, the cervix uteri and the breast.

4.2 Posology and method of administration
Dosage

Adults:

Lomustine "medac" is given by mouth. The recommended dose in patients with normally functioning bone marrow receiving Lomustine "medac" as their only chemotherapy is 120-130 mg/m^2 as a single dose every six to eight weeks (or as a divided dose over 3 days, e.g. 40 mg/m^2/day).

Dosage is reduced if:

(i) Lomustine "medac" is being given as part of a drug regimen which includes other marrow-depressant drugs, and

(ii) In the presence of leucopenia below 3,000/mm^3 or thrombocytopenia below 75,000/mm^3.

Marrow depression after Lomustine "medac" is sustained longer than after nitrogen mustards and recovery of white cell and platelet counts may not occur for six weeks or more. Blood elements depressed below the above levels should be allowed to recover to 4,000/mm^3 (WBC) and 100,000/mm^3 (platelets) before repeating Lomustine "medac" dosage.

Children:
Until further data is available, administration of Lomustine "medac" to children with malignancies other than brain tumours should be restricted to specialised centres and exceptional situations. Dosage in children, like that in adults, is based on body surface area (120 - 130 mg/m^2 every six to eight weeks, with the same qualifications as apply to adults).

Route of Administration:
Lomustine "medac" is given by mouth.

4.3 Contraindications
Lomustine can cause birth defects. Men and women are recommended to take contraceptive precautions during therapy with lomustine and for 6 months after treatment. Men should be informed about the risk for an irreversible infertility due to treatment with lomustine.

Lomustine "medac" should not be administered to patients who are pregnant or to mothers who are breast feeding.

Other contraindications are:

(i) Previous hypersensitivity to nitrosoureas;

(ii) Previous failure of the tumor to respond to other nitrosoureas;

(iii) Severe bone-marrow depression;

(iv) Severe renal impairment;

(v) Coeliac disease or wheat allergy.

4.4 Special warnings and precautions for use
Patients receiving Lomustine "medac" chemotherapy should be under the care of doctors experienced in cancer treatment. Blood counts should be carried out before starting the drug and at frequent intervals (preferably weekly) during treatment. Treatment and dosage is governed principally by the haemoglobin, white cell count and platelet count. Liver and kidney function should also be assessed periodically.

4.5 Interaction with other medicinal products and other forms of interaction
Lomustine "medac" use in combination with theophylline or with the H_2-receptor antagonist cimetidine may potentiate bone marrow toxicity. Cross resistance with other nitrosoureas is usual, but cross resistance with conventional alkylating agents is unusual.

Pre-treatment with phenobarbital can lead to a reduced antitumour effect of lomustine due to an accelerated elimination caused by induction of microsomal liver enzyms.

4.6 Pregnancy and lactation
Lomustine is contraindicated in women who are pregnant and mothers who are breast feeding.

4.7 Effects on ability to drive and use machines
Lomustine "medac" capsules can impair the ability to drive and use machines, e.g. because of nausea and vomiting.

4.8 Undesirable effects
Haematological

The principal adverse effect is marrow toxicity of a delayed or prolonged nature. Thrombocytopenia appears about four weeks after a dose of Lomustine "medac" and lasts one or two weeks at a level around 80-100,000/mm^3. Leucopenia appears after six weeks and persists for one or two weeks at about 4 - 5,000/mm^3.

The haematological toxicity may be cumulative, leading to successively lower white cell and platelet counts with successive doses of the drug.

Gastrointestinal

Nausea and vomiting usually occur four to six hours after a full single dose of Lomustine "medac" and last for 24-48 hours, followed by anorexia for two or three days. The effects are less troublesome if the 6 weekly dose is divided into three doses given on each of the first three days of the six week period. Gastrointestinal tolerance is usually good, however, if prophylactic antiemetics are given (e. g. metoclopramide or chlorpromazine). Disorders of liver function have been reported commonly. They are mild in most cases. In rare cases a cholestatic jaundice occurs. Transient elevation of liver enzymes (SGOT, SGPT, LDH or alkaline phosphatase) are occasionally observed.

More rarely patients are troubled by stomatitis and diarrhoea.

Neurologic system

Mild neurologic symptoms, like e.g. apathy, disorientation, confusion and stuttering can occur uncommonly in combination therapy with other antineoplastic drugs or radiation.

Pulmonary system

Interstitial pneumonia or lung fibrosis have been reported rarely.

Renal system

Renal failure has been reported in single cases after prolonged treatment with lomustine reaching a high cumulative total dose. Therefore it is recommended not to exceed a maximum cumulative total lomustine dose of 1000 mg/m^2.

Other Side Effects

Loss of scalp hair has been reported rarely.

In single cases an irreversible vision loss has been reported after a combined therapy of lomustine with radiation.

4.9 Overdose
Symptoms

Symptoms of overdosage with Lomustine "medac" will probably include bone-marrow toxicity, haematological toxicity, nausea and vomiting.

Emergency Procedures

Overdosage should be treated immediately by gastric lavage.

Antidote

There is no specific antidote to overdosage with Lomustine "medac". Treatment should be symptomatic and supportive. Appropriate blood product replacement should be given as clinically required.

5. PHARMACOLOGICAL PROPERTIES

5.1 Pharmacodynamic properties
The mode of action is believed to be partly as an alkylating agent and partly by inhibition of several steps in the synthesis of nucleic acid and inhibition of the repair of single strand breaks in DNA chains.

5.2 Pharmacokinetic properties
Lomustine "medac" is readily absorbed from the intestinal tract. A maximum plasma concentration of 0.5-2 ng/ml is reached after 3 hours following an oral dose of 30-100 mg/m^2.

The plasma-disappearance of the chloroethyl-group follows by a single phased course with a half-life of 72 hours. The cyclohexyl-group disappears according to a twofold plasma-disappearance with half-lives of 4 hours (t ½α) and 50 hours (t ½β). After oral application of radioactive marked lomustine the blood-brain-barrier is passed. Approximately 15 to 30 % of the measured radioactivity in the plasma can be detected in the cerebrospinal fluid.

Lomustine "medac" is rapidly metabolised and metabolites are excreted mainly via the kidneys. Lomustine "medac" cannot be detected in its active form in the urine at any time.

5.3 Preclinical safety data
None available.

6. PHARMACEUTICAL PARTICULARS

6.1 List of excipients
Capsule Contents:

Lactose

Wheat Starch

Talc

Magnesium Stearate

Capsule Shell:

Gelatin

Indigo carmine E132

Titanium Dioxide E171

6.2 Incompatibilities
None stated.

6.3 Shelf life
3 years as packaged for sale.

6.4 Special precautions for storage
Do not store above 25°C.

Store in the original container protected from light and moisture.

6.5 Nature and contents of container
Securitainers containing 20 capsules.

6.6 Special precautions for disposal and other handling
None.

7. MARKETING AUTHORISATION HOLDER
medac - Gesellschaft fuer klinische Spezialpraeparate mbH

Fehlandtstrasse 3

20354 Hamburg, Germany

8. MARKETING AUTHORISATION NUMBER(S)
PL 11587/0003

9. DATE OF FIRST AUTHORISATION/RENEWAL OF THE AUTHORISATION
25/08/2006

10. DATE OF REVISION OF THE TEXT
25/08/2006

Loniten Tablets 2.5 mg, 5 mg and 10mg

(Pharmacia Limited)

1. NAME OF THE MEDICINAL PRODUCT
Loniten Tablets 2.5 mg, 5 mg and 10mg

2. QUALITATIVE AND QUANTITATIVE COMPOSITION
Each Loniten Tablet contains 2.5 mg, 5 mg or 10 mg minoxidil USP.

3. PHARMACEUTICAL FORM
Tablet

4. CLINICAL PARTICULARS

4.1 Therapeutic indications
Loniten is indicated for the treatment of severe hypertension.

It should not be used as the sole agent to initiate therapy. It is a peripheral vasodilator and should be given in conjunction with a diuretic, to control salt and water retention, and a beta-adrenergic blocking agent, or appropriate substitute, to control reflex tachycardia.

4.2 Posology and method of administration
Oral Administration

Adults and Patients over 12 years of age: An initial daily dose of 5 mg, which may be given as a single or divided dosage, is recommended. This dose may first be increased to 10 mg daily and subsequent increases should be by increments of 10 mg in the daily dose. Dosage adjustments should be made at intervals of not less than three days, until optimum control of blood pressure is achieved. It is seldom necessary to exceed 50 mg per day although, in exceptional circumstances, doses up to 100 mg per day have been used. Twice-daily dosage is satisfactory. Where diastolic pressure reduction of less than 30 mm Hg is required, once daily dosing has been reported as effective.

Dosage requirements may be lower in dialysis patients. Minoxidil is removed from the blood by dialysis, but its pharmacological action, once established is not reversed. Therefore haemodialysis patients should take Loniten either after or at least two hours before dialysis.

Children: For patients of 12 years of age or under, the initial dose should be 200 micrograms per kilogram (0.2 mg/kg) given as a single or divided daily dosage. Incremental increases of 100 - 200 micrograms per kilogram (0.1-0.2 mg/kg) in the daily dose are recommended at intervals of not less than three days until optimum blood pressure control has been achieved, or the maximum daily dose of 1.0 mg/kg has been reached.

Rapid reduction of blood pressure: Under hospital monitoring conditions, rapid reduction of blood pressure can be achieved using continuous blood pressure monitoring and incremental doses of 5 mg every six hours.

Concomitant antihypertensive therapy: It is recommended that, where possible, antihypertensive therapy, other than a beta-adrenergic blocking agent and a diuretic be discontinued before Loniten treatment is started. It is recognised that some antihypertensive agents should not be abruptly discontinued. These drugs should be gradually discontinued during the first week of Loniten treatment.

Loniten causes sodium retention and if used alone can result in several hundred milli-equivalents of salt being retained together with a corresponding volume of water.

Therefore, in all patients who are not on dialysis, Loniten must be given in conjunction with a diuretic in sufficient dosage to maintain salt and water balance. Examples of the daily dosages of diuretics commonly used when starting therapy with Loniten include:

1. Hydrochlorothiazide (100 mg) - or other thiazides at equi-effective dosage.

2. Chlortalidone (100 mg).

3. Furosemide (80 mg).

If excessive water retention results in a weight gain of more than 3 pounds when a thiazide or chlortalidone is being used, diuretic therapy should be changed to furosimide, the dose of which may be increased in accordance with the patient's requirements. Diuretic dosage in children should be proportionally less in relation to weight.

Patients will require a sympathetic nervous system suppressant to limit a Loniten-induced rise in heart rate. The preferred agent is a beta-blocker equivalent to an adult propranolol dosage of 80 - 160 mg/day. Higher doses may be required when pre-treated patients have an increase in heart rate exceeding 20 beats per minute or when simultaneous introduction causes an increase exceeding 10 beats per minute. When beta-blockers are contra-indicated, alternatives such as methyldopa may be used instead and should be started 24 hours prior to Loniten.

Elderly patients: At present there are no extensive clinical studies with minoxidil in patients over age 65. There is data indicating that elevated systolic and diastolic pressures are important risk factors for cardiovascular disease in individuals over age 65. However, elderly patients may be sensitive to the blood pressure lowering effect of minoxidil and thus caution is urged in initiating therapy as orthostatic hypotension may occur. It is suggested that 2.5 mg per day be used as the initial starting dose in patients over 65 years of age.

4.3 Contraindications

Loniten is contra-indicated in patients with a phaeochromocytoma.

4.4 Special warnings and precautions for use

If used alone, Loniten can cause a significant retention of salt and water leading to positive physical signs such as oedema, and to clinical deterioration of some patients with heart failure. Diuretic treatment alone, or in combination with restricted salt intake is, therefore, necessary for all patients taking Loniten.

Patients who have had myocardial infarction should only be treated with Loniten after a stable post-infarction state has been established.

The physician should bear in mind that if not controlled by sympathetic suppressants, the rise in cardiac rate and output that follows the use of potent vasodilators may induce anginal symptoms in patients with undiagnosed coronary artery disease, or may aggravate pre-existing angina pectoris.

The effect of Loniten may be additive to concurrent antihypertensive agents. The interaction of Loniten with sympathetic-blocking agents such as guanethidine or betanidine may produce excessive blood pressure reduction and/or orthostasis.

Hypertrichosis occurs in most patients treated with Loniten and all patients should be warned of this possibility before starting therapy. Spontaneous reversal to the pre-treatment state can be expected one to three months after cessation of therapy.

Soon after starting Loniten therapy approximately 60% of patients exhibit ECG alterations in the direction and magnitude of their T waves. Large changes may encroach on the ST segment, unaccompanied by evidence of ischaemia. These asymptomatic changes usually disappear with continuing Loniten treatment. The ECG reverts to the pre-treatment state if Loniten is discontinued.

Pericardial effusion has been detected in patients treated with a Loniten-containing regime. A cause and effect relationship has not been established. Most effusions have either been present before Loniten was given, or occurred among uraemic patients. However, it is suggested that Loniten-treated patients should be periodically monitored for signs or symptoms of pericardial effusion and appropriate therapy instituted if necessary.

Salt and water retention in excess of 2 to 3 pounds may diminish the effectiveness of Loniten. Patients should, therefore, be carefully instructed about compliance with diuretic therapy and a detailed record of body weight should be maintained.

4.5 Interaction with other medicinal products and other forms of interaction

The effect of Loniten may be additive to concurrent antihypertensive agents. The interaction of Loniten with sympathetic-blocking agents such as guanethidine or betanidine may produce excessive blood pressure reduction and/or orthostasis.

4.6 Pregnancy and lactation

The safety of Loniten in pregnancy remains to be established. Minoxidil has been shown to reduce the conception rate in rats and to show evidence of increased fetal absorption in rabbits. There was no evidence of teratogenic effects in rats and rabbits. Minoxidil has been reported to be secreted in breast milk. Therefore, breast-feeding should not be undertaken while a patient is on Loniten Tablets.

4.7 Effects on ability to drive and use machines

No adverse effects reported

4.8 Undesirable effects

Most patients receiving Loniten experience a diminution of pre-existing side-effects attributable to their disease or previous therapy. New events or side-effects likely to increase include peripheral oedema, associated with or independent of weight gain; increases in heart rate; hypertrichosis; and a temporary rise in creatinine and blood urea nitrogen. Gastro-intestinal intolerance, rash and breast tenderness are infrequently reported side-effects of Loniten therapy.

4.9 Overdose

If exaggerated hypotension is encountered, it is most likely to occur in association with residual sympathetic nervous system blockade (guanethidine-like effects or alpha-adrenergic blockade). Recommended treatment is intravenous administration of normal saline. Sympathomimetic drugs, such as noradrenaline or adrenaline, should be avoided because of their excessive cardiac-stimulating action. Phenylephrine, angiotensin II and vasopressin, which reverse the effect of Loniten, should be used only if inadequate perfusion of a vital organ is evident.

5. PHARMACOLOGICAL PROPERTIES

5.1 Pharmacodynamic properties

Minoxidil is an antihypertensive agent which acts predominantly by causing direct peripheral vasodilation of the arterioles.

5.2 Pharmacokinetic properties

About 90% of an oral dose of minoxidil has been reported to associated from the GI tract.

Following oral administration the maximum hypotensive effect usually occurs after 2-3 hours. The action may persist for up to 75 hours. The plasma half life is about 4.2 hours.

Minoxidil is not bound to plasma proteins. It is extensively metabolised in the liver primarily by conjugation with glucuronic acid and is excreted in the urine mainly in the form of metabolites.

6. PHARMACEUTICAL PARTICULARS

6.1 List of excipients

Lactose hydrous, microcrystalline cellulose, starch, colloidal silicon dioxide and magnesium stearate.

6.2 Incompatibilities

None

6.3 Shelf life

Shelf-life of the medicinal product as packaged for sale: 36 months.

6.4 Special precautions for storage

Store below 25°C.

6.5 Nature and contents of container

High density polyethylene (HDPE) bottles with LDPE caps. Each bottle contains 100 tablets.

20-25 micron aluminium foil/250 micron opaque pvc blister. Pack contains 60 tablets.

6.6 Special precautions for disposal and other handling

No special requirements.

7. MARKETING AUTHORISATION HOLDER

Pharmacia Limited, Ramsgate Road, Sandwich, CT13 9NJ, UK

8. MARKETING AUTHORISATION NUMBER(S)

PL 0032/0064 2.5mg

PL 0032/0065 5 mg

PL 0032/0066 10 mg

9. DATE OF FIRST AUTHORISATION/RENEWAL OF THE AUTHORISATION

24 May 1995.

10. DATE OF REVISION OF THE TEXT

January 2008

LEGAL CATEGORY

POM

Company Ref: LN 3_0

Lopid 300mg Capsules & 600mg Film-coated Tablets

(Pfizer Limited)

1. NAME OF THE MEDICINAL PRODUCT

Lopid® 300mg Capsules

Lopid™ 600mg Film-coated Tablets

2. QUALITATIVE AND QUANTITATIVE COMPOSITION

Each capsule contains 300 mg gemfibrozil.

Each film-coated tablet contains 600mg gemfibrozil.

For excipients, see 6.1.

3. PHARMACEUTICAL FORM

Lopid 300mg capsules: A fine white powder contained in a hard gelatin capsule with a white opaque body and maroon cap, radially imprinted 'Lopid 300' on each capsule half.

Lopid 600mg film-coated tablets: A white, elliptical, film-coated tablet embossed with 'LOPID' on one side.

4. CLINICAL PARTICULARS

4.1 Therapeutic indications

Lopid is indicated as an adjunct to diet and other non-pharmacological treatment (e.g. exercise, weight reduction) for the following:

Treatment of dyslipidemia

Mixed dyslipidaemia characterised by hypertriglyceridaemia and/or low HDL-cholesterol. Primary hypercholesterolaemia, particularly when a statin is considered inappropriate or is not tolerated.

Primary prevention

Reduction of cardiovascular morbidity in males with increased non-HDL cholesterol and at high risk for a first cardiovascular event, particularly when a statin is considered inappropriate or is not tolerated (see section 5.1).

4.2 Posology and method of administration

Prior to initiating gemfibrozil, other medical problems such as hypothyroidism and diabetes mellitus must be controlled as best as possible and patients should be placed on a standard lipid-lowering diet, which should be continued during treatment. Lopid should be taken orally.

Adult

The dose range is 900 mg to 1200 mg daily.

The only dose with documented effect on morbidity is 1200 mg daily.

The 1200 mg dose is taken as 600 mg twice daily, half an hour before breakfast and half an hour before the evening meal.

The 900 mg dose is taken as a single dose half an hour before the evening meal.

Elderly (over 65 years old)

As for adults

Children and adolescents

Gemfibrozil therapy has not been investigated in children. Due to the lack of data the use of Lopid in children is not recommended.

Renal impairment

In patients with mild to moderate renal impairment (Glomerular filtration rate 50 - 80 and 30 - < 50 ml/min/1.73 m^2, respectively), start treatment at 900 mg daily and assess renal function before increasing dose. Lopid should not be used in patients with severely impaired renal function (see section 4.3).

Hepatic impairment

Gemfibrozil is contraindicated in hepatic impairment (see section 4.3).

4.3 Contraindications

Hypersensitivity to gemfibrozil or any of the excipients.

Hepatic impairment.

Severe renal impairment.

History of/or pre-existing gall bladder or biliary tract disease, including gallstones

Concomitant use of repaglinide (see section 4.5).

Patients with previous history of photoallergy or phototoxic reaction during treatment with fibrates.

4.4 Special warnings and precautions for use

Muscle disorders (myopathy/rhabdomyolysis)

There have been reports of myositis, myopathy and markedly elevated creatine phosphokinase associated with gemfibrozil. Rhabdomyolysis has also been reported rarely.

Muscle damage must be considered in any patient presenting with diffuse myalgia, muscle tenderness and/or marked increase in muscle CPK levels (>5x ULN); under these conditions treatment must be discontinued.

Concomitant HMG CoA reductase inhibitors

The risk of muscle damage may be increased in the event of combination with an HMG-CoA reductase inhibitor. Pharmacokinetic interactions may also be present (see also section 4.5) and dosage adjustments may be necessary.

The benefit of further alterations in lipid levels by the combined use of gemfibrozil and HMG-CoA reductase inhibitors should be carefully weighed against the potential risks of such combinations and clinical monitoring is recommended.

A creatine phosphokinase (CPK) level should be measured before starting such a combination in patients with predisposing factors for rhabdomyolysis as follows:

- renal impairment
- hypothyroidism
- alcohol abuse
- age > 70 years
- personal or family history of hereditary muscular disorders

• previous history of muscular toxicity with another fibrate or HMG-CoA reductase inhibitor

In most subjects who have had an unsatisfactory lipid response to either drug alone, the possible benefits of combined therapy with HMG-CoA reductase inhibitors and gemfibrozil does not outweigh the risks of severe myopathy, rhabdomylosis and acute renal failure.

Use in patients with gallstone formation

Gemfibrozil may increase cholesterol excretion into the bile raising the potential for gallstone formation. Cases of cholelithiasis have been reported with gemfibrozil therapy. If cholelithiasis is suspected, gallbladder studies are indicated. Gemfibrozil therapy should be discontinued if gallstones are found.

Monitoring serum lipids

Periodic determinations of serum lipids are necessary during treatment with gemfibrozil. Sometimes a paradoxical increase of (total and LDL) cholesterol can occur in patients with hypertriglyceridaemia. If the response is insufficient after 3 months of therapy at recommended doses treatment should be discontinued and alternative treatment methods considered.

Monitoring liver function

Elevated levels of ALAT, ASAT, alkaline phosphatase, LDH, CK and bilirubin have been reported. These are usually reversible when gemfibrozil is discontinued. Therefore liver function tests should be performed periodically. Gemfibrozil therapy should be terminated if abnormalities persist.

Monitoring blood counts

Periodic blood count determinations are recommended during the first 12 months of gemfibrozil administration. Anaemia, leucopenia, thrombocytopenia, eosinophilia and bone marrow hypoplasia have been reported rarely (see section 4.8).

Interactions with other medicinal products (see also sections 4.3 and 4.5).

Concomitant use with CYP2C8, CYP2C9, CYP2C19, CYP1A2, UGTA1 and UGTA3 substrates.

The interaction profile of gemfibrozil is complex resulting in increased exposure of many medicinal products if administered concomitantly with gemfibrozil.

Gemfibrozil potently inhibits CYP2C8, CYP2C9, CYP2C19, CYP1A2, UGTA1 and UGTA3 enzymes (see section 4.5)

Concomitant use with hypoglycaemic agents

There have been reports of hypoglycaemic reactions after concomitant use with gemfibrozil and hypoglycaemic agents (oral agents and insulin). Monitoring of glucose levels is recommended.

Concomitant oral anticoagulants

Gemfibrozil may potentiate the effects of oral anticoagulants, which necessitates careful monitoring of the anticoaglant dosing. Caution should be exercised when anticoagulants are given in conjunction with gemfibrozil. The dosage of the anticoagulant may need to be reduced to maintain desired prothrombin time levels (see Section 4.5.)

4.5 Interaction with other medicinal products and other forms of interaction

The interaction profile of gemfibrozil is complex. In vivo studies indicate that gemfibrozil is a potent inhibitor of CYP2C8 (an enzyme important for the metabolism of e.g. repaglinide, rosiglitazone and paclitaxel). In vitro studies have shown that gemfibrozil is a strong inhibitor of CYP2C9 (an enzyme involved in the metabolism of e.g. warfarin and glimepiride), but also of CYP 2C19, CYP1A2 and UGTA1 and UGTA3 (see Section 4.4).

Repaglinide

The combination of gemfibrozil with repaglinide is contraindicated (see Section 4.3). Concomitant administration has resulted in 8-fold increase in repaglinide plasma concentration probably by inhibition of the CYP2C8 enzyme, resulting in hypoglycaemic reactions.

Rosiglitazone

The combination of gemfibrozil with rosiglitazone should be approached with caution. Co-administration with rosiglitazone has resulted in 2.3-fold increase in rosiglitazone systemic exposure, probably by inhibition of the CYP2C8 isozyme (see section 4.4).

HMG CoA reductase inhibitors

The combined use of gemfibrozil and a statin should generally be avoided (see section 4.4). The use of fibrates alone is occasionally associated with myopathy. An increased risk of muscle related adverse events, including rhabdomyolysis, has been reported when fibrates are co-administered with statins.

Gemfibrozil has also been reported to influence the pharmacokinetics of simvaststin, lovastatin, pravastatin and rosuvastatin. Gemfibrozil caused an almost 3-fold increased in AUC of simvastatin acid possibly due to inhibition of glucoronidation via UGTA1 and UGTA3, and a 3-fold increase in pravastatin AUC which may be due to interference with transport proteins. One study indicated that the co-administration of a single rosuvastatin dose of 80 mg to healthy volunteers on gemfibrozil (600 mg twice daily) resulted in a 2.2-fold increase in mean C_{max} and a 1.9-fold increase in mean AUC of rosuvastatin.

Oral anticoagulants

Gemfibrozil may potentiate the effects of oral anticoagulants, which necessitates careful monitoring of the anticoagulant dosing (see section 4.4).

Bexarotene

Concomitant administration of gemfibrozil with bexarotene is not recommended. A population analysis of plasma bexarotene concentrations in patients with cutaneous T-cell lymphoma (CTCL) indicated that concomitant administration of gemfibrozil resulted in substantial increases in plasma concentrations of bexarotene.

Bile Acid – Binding Resins

Reduced bioavailability of gemfibrozil may result when given simultaneously with resin-granule drugs such as colestipol. Administration of the products two hours or more apart is recommended.

Gemfibrozil is highly bound to plasma proteins and there is potential for displacement interactions with other drugs.

4.6 Pregnancy and lactation

Pregnancy

There are no adequate data on use of Lopid in pregnant women. Animal studies are insufficiently clear to allow conclusions to be drawn on pregnancy and foetal development (see section 5.3). The potential risk for humans is unknown. Lopid should not be used during pregnancy unless it is clearly necessary.

Lactation

There are no data on excretion of gemfibrozil in milk. Lopid should not be used when breast feeding.

4.7 Effects on ability to drive and use machines

No studies on the effects on the ability to drive and use machines have been performed. In isolated cases dizziness and visual disturbances can occur which may negatively influence driving.

4.8 Undesirable effects

Most commonly reported adverse reactions are of gastro-intestinal character and are seen in approximately 7% of the patients. These adverse reactions do not usually lead to discontinuation of the treatment.

Adverse reactions are ranked according to frequency using the following convention: Very common (>1/10), Common (>1/100, <1/10), Uncommon (>1/1,000, <1/100), Rare (>1/10,000, <1/1,000), Very rare (<1/10,000), including isolated reports:

Platelet, bleeding and clotting disorders

Rare: thrombocytopenia.

Red blood cell disorders

Rare: severe anaemia. Self-limiting, mild haemoglobin and haematocrit decrease have been observed on initiating gemfibrozil therapy.

White cell and reticuloendothelial system disorders

Rare: leucopoenia, eosinophilia, bone marrow hypoplasia. Self-limiting, white cell decrease has been observed on initiating gemfibrozil therapy.

Central and peripheral nervous system

Common: vertigo, headache.

Rare: dizziness, somnolence, paresthesia, peripheral neuritis, depression, decreased libido.

Vision disorders

Rare: blurred vision.

Heart rate and rhythm disorders

Uncommon: atrial fibrillation.

Gastro-intestinal system disorders

Very common: dyspepsia.

Common: abdominal pain, diarrhoea, flatulence, nausea, vomiting, constipation.

Rare: pancreatitis, acute appendicitis.

Liver and biliary system disorders

Rare: cholestatic jaundice, disturbed liver function, hepatitis, cholelithiasis, cholecystitis.

Skin and appendages disorders

Common: eczema, rash.

Rare: exfoliative dermatitis, dermatitis, pruritus, alopecia.

Musculoskeletal disorders

Rare: arthralgia, synovitis, myalgia, myopathy, myasthenia, painful extremities and myositis accompanied by increase in creatine kinase (CK), rhabdomyolysis.

Urinary system disorders

Rare: impotence.

Body as a whole-general disorders

Common: fatigue.

Rare: photosensitivity, angioedema, laryngeal edema, urticaria.

4.9 Overdose

Overdose has been reported. Symptoms reported with overdosage were abdominal cramps, abdominal LFT's, diarrhoea, increased CPK, joint muscle pain, nausea and vomiting. The patients fully recovered. Symptomatic supportive measures should be taken if overdose occurs.

5. PHARMACOLOGICAL PROPERTIES

5.1 Pharmacodynamic properties

Pharmacotherapeutic group: Serum-lipid lowering agent

Chemical subgroup: Fibrates

ATC code: C10A B04

Gemfibrozil is a non-halogenated phenoxypentanoic acid. Gemfibrozil is a lipid regulating agent which regulates lipid fractions.

Gemfibrozil's mechanism of action has not been definitively established. In man, gemfibrozil stimulates the peripheral lipolysis of triglyceride rich lipoproteins such as VLDL and cholymicrons (by stimulation of LPL). Gemfibrozil also inhibits synthesis of VLDL in the liver. Gemfibrozil increases the HDL_2 and HDL_3 subfractions as well as apolipoprotein A-I and A-II.

Animal studies suggest that the turnover and removal of cholesterol from the liver is increased by gemfibrozil.

In the Helsinki Heart Study, which was a large placebo-controlled study with 4081 male subjects, 40 to 55 years of age, with primary dyslipidaemia (predominantly raised non-HDL cholesterol +/- hypertriglyceridaemia), but no previous history of coronary heart disease, gemfibrozil 600 mg twice daily, produced a significant reduction in total plasma triglycerides, total and low density lipoprotein cholesterol and a significant increase in high density lipoprotein cholesterol. The cumulative rate of cardiac end-points (cardiac death and non-fatal myocardial infarction) during a 5 year follow-up was 27.3/1000 in the gemfibrozil group (56 subjects) and 41.4/1000 in the placebo group (84 subjects) showing a relative risk reduction of 34.0% (95% confidence interval 8.2 to 52.6, $p<0.02$) and an absolute risk reduction of 1.4% in the gemfibrozil group compared to placebo. There was a 37% reduction in non-fatal myocardial infarction and a 26% reduction in cardiac deaths. The number of deaths from all causes was, however, not different (44 in the gemfibrozil group and 43 in the placebo group). Diabetes patients and patients with severe lipid fraction deviations showed a 68% and 71% reduction of CHD endpoints, respectively.

5.2 Pharmacokinetic properties

Absorption

Gemfibrozil is well absorbed from the gastro-intestinal tract after oral administration with a bioavailability close to 100%. As the presence of food alters the bioavailability slightly gemfibrozil should be taken 30 minutes before a meal. Peak plasma levels occur in one to two hours. After administration of 600 mg twice daily a C_{max} in the range 15 to 25 mg/ml is obtained.

Distribution

Volume of distribution at steady state is 9-13 l. The plasma protein binding of gemfibrozil and its main metabolite are at least 97%.

Biotransformation

Gemfibrozil undergoes oxidation of a ring methyl group to form successively a hydroxymethyl and a carboxyl metabolite (the main metabolite). This metabolite has a low activity compared to the mother compound gemfibrozil and an elimination half-life of approximately 20 hours.

The enzymes involved in the metabolism of gemfibrozil are not known. The interaction profile of gemfibrozil is complex (see sections 4.3, 4.4 and 4.5). In vitro and in vivo studies have shown that gemfibrozil inhibits CYP2C8, CYP2C9, CYP2C19, CYP1A2, UGTA1 and UGTA3.

Elimination

Gemfibrozil is eliminated mainly by metabolism. Approximately 70% of the administered human dose is excreted in the urine, mainly as conjugates of gemfibrozil and its metabolites. Less than 6% of the dose is excreteed unchanged in the urine. Six percent of the dose is found in faeces. The total clearance of gemfibrozil is in the range 100 to 160 ml/min, and the elimination half-life is in the range 1.3 to 1.5 hours. The pharmacokinetics is linear within the therapeutic dose range.

Special patient groups

No pharmacokinetic studies have been performed in patients with impaired hepatic function.

There are limited data on patients with mild, moderate and non-dialysed severe renal impairment. The limited data support the use of up to 1200 mg a day in patients with mild to moderate renal failure not receiving another lipid lowering drug.

5.3 Preclinical safety data

In a 2-year study of gemfibrozil, subcapsular bilateral cataracts occurred in 10%, and unilateral in 6.3%, of male rats treated at 10 times the human dose.

In a mouse carcinogenicity study at dosages corresponding to 0.1 and 0.7 times the clinical exposure (based on AUC), there were no significant differences from controls in the incidence of tumors. In a rat carcinogenicity study at dosages corresponding to 0.2 and 1.3 times the clinical exposure (based on AUC), the incidence of benign liver nodules and liver carcinomas was significantly increased in high dose males, and the incidence of liver carcinomas increased also in the low dose males, but this increase was not statistically significant.

Liver tumours induced by gemfibrozil and other fibrates in small rodents are generally considered to be related to the extensive proliferation of peroxisomes in these species and, consequently, of minor clinical relevance.

In the male rat, gemfibrozil also induced benign Leydig cell tumors. The clinical relevance of this finding is minimal.

In reproductive toxicity studies, administration of gemfibrozil at approximately 2 times the human dose (based on body surface area) to male rats for 10 weeks resulted in decreased fertility. Fertility was restored after a drug-free period of 8 weeks. Gemfibrozil was not teratogenic in either rats or rabbits. Administration of 1 and 3 times the human dose (based on body surface area) of gemfibrozil to female rabbits during organogenesis caused a dose-related decrease in litter size. Administration of 0.6 and 2 times the human dose (based on body surface area) of gemfibrozil to female rats from gestation Day 15 through weaning caused dose-related decreases in birth weight and suppression of pup growth during lactation. Maternal toxicity was observed in both species and the clinical relevance of decreases in rabbit litter size and rat pup weight is uncertain.

6. PHARMACEUTICAL PARTICULARS

6.1 List of excipients

Polysorbate on silica, maize starch, titanium dioxide (E171), gelatin, erythrosine (E127), indigo carmine (E132), shellac, black iron oxide (E172) and propylene glycol.

6.2 Incompatibilities

None Known.

6.3 Shelf life

3 years

6.4 Special precautions for storage

Lopid 300mg capsules: Do not store above 30°C.

Lopid 600 film-coated tablets: Do not store above 25°C

6.5 Nature and contents of container

Not all pack sizes may be marketed

Securitainer with tamper evident polyethylene cap containing 100 capsules.

Tampertainer bottle with a white tamper evident cap containing 100 capsules.

Aluminium foil blister strips supplied in packs of 100 or 112 capsules.

6.6 Special precautions for disposal and other handling

No special instructions needed.

7. MARKETING AUTHORISATION HOLDER

Pfizer Limited

Ramsgate Road

Sandwich

Kent CT13 9NJ

United Kingdom

8. MARKETING AUTHORISATION NUMBER(S)

Lopid 300mg capsules: PL 00057/0534

Lopid 600mg film-coated tablets: PL 00057/0535

9. DATE OF FIRST AUTHORISATION/RENEWAL OF THE AUTHORISATION

05/12/2005

10. DATE OF REVISION OF THE TEXT

July 2007

Ref: LP8_0 UK

Loron 520

(Roche Products Limited)

1. NAME OF THE MEDICINAL PRODUCT

Loron 520

2. QUALITATIVE AND QUANTITATIVE COMPOSITION

Each Loron 520 tablet contains 520mg disodium clodronate.

3. PHARMACEUTICAL FORM

Film-coated tablets for oral administration.

4. CLINICAL PARTICULARS

4.1 Therapeutic indications

Loron is indicated for the management of osteolytic lesions, hypercalcaemia and bone pain associated with skeletal metastases in patients with carcinoma of the breast or multiple myeloma. Loron 520 is also indicated for the maintenance of clinically acceptable serum calcium levels in patients with hypercalcaemia of malignancy initially treated with an intravenous infusion of disodium clodronate.

4.2 Posology and method of administration

Adults

The recommended dose is 2 tablets (1040mg disodium clodronate) daily. If necessary, the dosage may be increased but should not exceed a maximum of 4 tablets (2080mg disodium clodronate) daily.

The tablets may be taken as a single dose or in two equally divided doses if necessary to improve gastrointestinal tolerance. Loron tablets should be swallowed with a little fluid, but not milk, at least one hour before or one hour after food.

The oral bioavailability of bisphosphonates is poor. Bioequivalence studies have shown appreciable differences in bioavailability between different oral formulations of disodium clodronate, as well as marked inter and intra patient variability. Dose adjustment may be required if the formulation is changed.

Elderly

No special dosage recommendations.

Children

Safety and efficacy in children has not been established.

Use in renal impairment

In patients with renal insufficiency with creatinine clearance between 10 and 30ml/min, the daily dose should be reduced to one half the recommended adult dose. Serum creatinine should be monitored during therapy. Disodium clodronate is contra-indicated in patients with creatinine clearance below 10ml/min.

4.3 Contraindications

Hypersensitivity to disodium clodronate. Acute, severe inflammatory conditions of the gastrointestinal tract. Pregnancy and lactation. Renal failure with creatinine clearance below 10ml/min, except for short term use in the presence of purely functional renal insufficiency caused by elevated serum calcium levels. Concomitant use of other bisphosphonates.

4.4 Special warnings and precautions for use

No information is available on the potential carcinogenicity of disodium clodronate, but patients have been treated in clinical trials for up to 2 years. The duration of the treatment is therefore at the discretion of the physician, according to the status of the underlying malignancy.

It is recommended that appropriate monitoring of renal function with serum creatinine be carried out during treatment. Serum calcium and phosphate should be monitored periodically. Monitoring of liver enzymes and white cells is advised (see side effects).

Osteonecrosis of the jaw, generally associated with tooth extraction and/or local infection (including osteomyelitis) has been reported in patients with cancer receiving treatment regimens including primarily intravenously administered bisphosphonates. Many of these patients were also receiving chemotherapy and corticosteroids. Osteonecrosis of the jaw has also been reported in patients with osteoporosis receiving oral bisphosphonates.

A dental examination with appropriate preventive dentistry should be considered prior to treatment with bisphosphonates in patients with concomitant risk factors (e.g. cancer, chemotherapy, radiotherapy, corticosteroids, poor oral hygiene).

While on treatment, these patients should avoid invasive dental procedures if possible. For patients who develop osteonecrosis of the jaw while on bisphosphonate therapy, dental surgery may exacerbate the condition. For patients requiring dental procedures, there are no data available to suggest whether discontinuation of bisphosphonate treatment reduces the risk of osteonecrosis of the jaw. Clinical judgement of the treating physician should guide the management plan of each patient based on individual benefit/risk assessment.

4.5 Interaction with other medicinal products and other forms of interaction

No other bisphosphonate drugs should be given with Loron tablets.

The calcium-lowering action of clodronate can be potentiated by the administration of aminoglycosides either concomitantly or one to several weeks apart. Severe hypocalcaemia has been observed in some cases. Hypomagnesaemia may also occur simultaneously. Patients receiving NSAID's in addition to disodium clodronate have developed renal dysfunction. However, a synergistic action has not been established. There is no evidence from clinical experience that sodium clodronate interacts with other medication, such as steroids, diuretics, calcitonin, non NSAID analgesics, or chemotherapeutic agents. Calcium rich foods, mineral supplements and antacids may impair absorption.

4.6 Pregnancy and lactation

There are insufficient data either from animal studies or from experience in humans of the effects of disodium clodronate on the embryo and foetus. No studies have been conducted on excretion in breast milk. Consequently, disodium clodronate is contraindicated in pregnancy and lactation.

4.7 Effects on ability to drive and use machines

No known effects which would impair alertness.

4.8 Undesirable effects

Patients may experience a mild gastrointestinal upset, usually in the form of nausea or mild diarrhoea. The symptoms may respond to the use of a twice daily dosage regime rather than a single dose. It is not normally required to withdraw therapy or to provide medication to control these effects. Asymptomatic hypocalcaemia has been noted rarely. A reversible elevation of serum parathyroid hormone may occur. In a small proportion of patients, a mild, reversible increase in serum lactate dehydrogenase and a modest transient leucopenia have been reported although these may have been associated with concurrent chemotherapy. Renal dysfunction, including renal failure has been reported. Hypersensitivity reactions have been mainly confined to the skin: pruritus, urticaria and rarely exfoliative dermatitis. However, bronchospasm has been precipitated in patients with or without a previous history of asthma.

4.9 Overdose

Symptoms and signs: There is no experience of acute overdosage in humans. The development of hypocalcaemia is possible for up to 2 or 3 days following the overdosage.

Treatment: Serum calcium should be monitored and oral or parenteral calcium supplementation may be required. Acute overdosage may be associated with gastrointestinal symptoms such as nausea and vomiting. Treatment should be symptomatic.

5. PHARMACOLOGICAL PROPERTIES

5.1 Pharmacodynamic properties

Disodium clodronate is a bisphosphonate which has a high affinity to bone. It is mainly the portion of the dose adsorbed to bone which is pharmacologically active. The pharmacological effect of disodium clodronate is to suppress osteoclast mediated bone resorption as judged by bone histology and decreases in serum calcium, urine calcium and urinary excretion of hydroxyproline, without adversely affecting mineralisation.

5.2 Pharmacokinetic properties

Oral bioavailability is in the order of 2%.

Disodium clodronate is not metabolised. The volume of distribution is approximately 0.3L/kg. Elimination from serum is rapid, 75% of the dose is recovered unchanged in urine within 24 hours.

The elimination kinetics best fit a 3 compartment model. The first two compartments have relatively short half-lives. The third compartment is probably the skeleton. Elimination half life is approximately 12 - 13 hours.

5.3 Preclinical safety data

Disodium clodronate shows relatively little toxicity either on single oral administration or after daily oral administration for a period of up to 6 months. In rats, a dose of 200mg/kg/day in the chronic toxicity test is at the limit of tolerability. In dogs, 40mg/kg/day chronically is within the tolerated range.

On daily administration of 500mg/kg for 6 weeks to rats, signs of renal failure with a clear rise in BUN, and initial liver parenchymal reaction with rises of SGOT, SGPT and AP occurred. No significant haematological changes were found in the toxicological investigations.

Investigations for mutagenic properties did not show any indication of mutagenic potency.

Reproduction toxicology investigations did not provide any indication of peri and post natal disorders, teratogenic damage or disorders of fertility.

It is not known if disodium clodronate passes into the mother's milk or through the placenta.

6. PHARMACEUTICAL PARTICULARS

6.1 List of excipients

Loron 520 tablets also contain:

Core

Disodium clodronate, talc, maize starch, microcrystalline cellulose, magnesium stearate, sodium starch glycollate.

Coating

Methylhydroxypropylcellulose, poly(meth) acrylic acid esters (Eudragit NE 30D), polyoxyethylene alkyl ether (Macrogol 1000), lactose monohydrate, talc, titanium dioxide (E171), polysorbate 80, sodium citrate.

6.2 Incompatibilities

Not applicable.

6.3 Shelf life

PVC/aluminium blister packs: 5 years.

6.4 Special precautions for storage

None.

6.5 Nature and contents of container

PVC/aluminium blister packs containing 10 or 60 tablets.

6.6 Special precautions for disposal and other handling

No special instructions.

7. MARKETING AUTHORISATION HOLDER

Roche Products Limited

6 Falcon Way

Shire Park

Welwyn Garden City

AL7 1TW, United Kingdom

8. MARKETING AUTHORISATION NUMBER(S)

PL 00031/0521

9. DATE OF FIRST AUTHORISATION/RENEWAL OF THE AUTHORISATION

1 July 1999

10. DATE OF REVISION OF THE TEXT

16 July 2009

11 LEGAL CATEGORY

POM

Loron is a registered trade mark

Losec Capsules 10mg, 20mg & 40mg

(AstraZeneca UK Limited)

1. NAME OF THE MEDICINAL PRODUCT

Losec Capsules 10mg.

Losec Capsules 20mg.

Losec Capsules 40mg.

2. QUALITATIVE AND QUANTITATIVE COMPOSITION

Each capsule contains omeprazole 10, 20 or 40 mg.

For excipients, see 6.1.

3. PHARMACEUTICAL FORM

Hard gelatin capsules.

Losec Capsules 10mg: hard gelatin capsules with an opaque pink body, marked 10 and an opaque pink cap marked A/OS in black ink. Each capsule contains omeprazole 10mg as enteric coated granules, with an aqueous based coating.

Losec Capsules 20mg: hard gelatin capsules with an opaque pink body, marked 20 and an opaque reddish-brown cap marked A/OM in black ink. Each capsule contains omeprazole 20mg as enteric coated granules, with an aqueous based coating.

Losec Capsules 40mg: hard gelatin capsules with an opaque reddish-brown body, marked 40 and an opaque reddish-brown cap marked A/OL in black ink. Each capsule contains omeprazole 40mg as enteric coated granules, with an aqueous based coating

4. CLINICAL PARTICULARS

4.1 Therapeutic indications

Treatment of oesophageal reflux disease. In reflux oesophagitis the majority of patients are healed after 4 weeks. Symptom relief is rapid.

Treatment of duodenal and benign gastric ulcers including those complicating NSAID therapy.

Relief of associated dyspeptic symptoms.

Helicobacter pylori eradication: Omeprazole should be used in combination with antibiotics for eradication of *Helicobacter pylori* (*Hp*) in peptic ulcer disease.

Prophylaxis of acid aspiration.

Zollinger-Ellison syndrome.

For 10 and 20mg Capsules only:

Relief of reflux-like symptoms (e.g. heartburn) and/or ulcer-like symptoms (e.g. epigastric pain) associated with acid-related dyspepsia.

Treatment and prophylaxis of NSAID-associated benign gastric ulcers, duodenal ulcers and gastroduodenal erosions in patients with a previous history of gastroduodenal lesions who require continued NSAID treatment.

Children over 1 year of age and ⩾ 10 kg: Reflux oesophagitis. Symptomatic treatment of heartburn and acid regurgitation in gastroesophageal reflux disease.

4.2 Posology and method of administration

Adults

Oesophageal reflux disease including reflux oesophagitis

The usual dosage is 20 mg Losec once daily. The majority of patients are healed after 4 weeks. For those patients not fully healed after the initial course, healing usually occurs during a further 4-8 weeks treatment.

Losec has also been used in a dose of 40 mg once daily in patients with reflux oesophagitis refractory to other therapy. Healing usually occurred within 8 weeks. Patients can be continued at a dosage of 20 mg once daily.

Acid reflux disease

For long-term management Losec 10 mg once daily is recommended, increasing to 20 mg if symptoms return.

Duodenal and benign gastric ulcers

The usual dose is 20 mg Losec once daily. The majority of patients with duodenal ulcer are healed after 4 weeks. The majority of patients with benign gastric ulcer are healed after 8 weeks. In severe or recurrent cases the dose may be increased to 40 mg Losec daily. Long-term therapy for patients with a history of recurrent duodenal ulcer is recommended at a dosage of 20 mg Losec once daily.

For prevention of relapse in patients with duodenal ulcer the recommended dose is Losec 10 mg once daily, increasing to 20 mg once daily, if symptoms return.

The following groups are at risk from recurrent ulcer relapse: those with *Helicobacter pylori* infection, younger patients (<60 years), those whose symptoms persist for more than one year and smokers. These patients will require initial long-term therapy with Losec 20 mg once daily, reducing to 10 mg once daily, if necessary.

Helicobacter pylori (Hp) **eradication regimens in peptic ulcer disease**

Losec is recommended at a dose of 40 mg once daily or 20 mg twice daily in association with antimicrobial agents as detailed below:

Triple therapy regimens in duodenal ulcer disease:

Losec and the following antimicrobial combinations:

Amoxicillin 500 mg and metronidazole 400 mg both three times a day for one week

or

Clarithromycin 250 mg and metronidazole 400 mg (or tinidazole 500 mg) both twice a day for one week

or

Amoxicillin 1 g and clarithromycin 500 mg both twice a day for one week.

Dual therapy regimens in duodenal ulcer disease:

Losec and amoxicillin 750 mg to 1 g twice daily for two weeks. Alternatively, Losec and clarithromycin 500 mg three times a day for two weeks.

Dual therapy regimens in gastric ulcer disease:

Losec and amoxicillin 750 mg to 1 g twice daily for two weeks.

In each regimen if symptoms return and the patient is *Hp* positive, therapy may be repeated or one of the alternative regimens can be used; if the patient is *Hp* negative then see dosage instructions for acid reflux disease.

To ensure healing in patients with active peptic ulcer disease, see further dosage recommendations for duodenal and benign gastric ulcer.

Prophylaxis of acid aspiration

For patients considered to be at risk of aspiration of the gastric contents during general anaesthesia, the recommended dosage is Losec 40 mg on the evening before surgery followed by Losec 40 mg 2-6 hours prior to surgery.

Zollinger-Ellison syndrome

The recommended initial dosage is 60 mg Losec once daily. The dosage should be adjusted individually and treatment continued as long as clinically indicated. More than 90% of patients with severe disease and inadequate response to other therapies have been effectively controlled on doses of 20-120 mg daily. With doses above 80 mg daily, the dose should be divided and given twice daily.

For 10 and 20mg Capsules only:

Acid-related dyspepsia

The usual dosage is Losec 10 mg or 20 mg once daily for 2-4 weeks depending on the severity and persistence of symptoms.

Patients who do not respond after 4 weeks or who relapse shortly afterwards, should be investigated.

For the treatment of NSAID-associated gastric ulcers, duodenal ulcers or gastroduodenal erosions

The recommended dosage of Losec is 20 mg once daily. Symptom resolution is rapid and in most patients healing occurs within 4 weeks. For those patients who may not be fully healed after the initial course, healing usually occurs during a further 4 weeks treatment.

For the prophylaxis of NSAID-associated gastric ulcers, duodenal ulcers, gastroduodenal erosions and dyspeptic symptoms in patients with a previous history of gastroduodenal lesions who require continued NSAID treatment

The recommended dosage of Losec is 20 mg once daily.

Elderly

Dose adjustment is not required in the elderly.

Children

Reflux oesophagitis

The treatment time is 4–8 weeks.

Symptomatic treatment of heartburn and acid regurgitation in gastroesophageal reflux disease

The treatment time is 2-4 weeks. If symptom control has not been achieved after 2-4 weeks the patient should be investigated further.

The dosage recommendations are as follows:

Age	Weight	Dosage
⩾ 1 year of age	10-20 kg	10 mg once daily. The dosage can be increased to 20 mg once daily if needed
⩾ 2 years of age	> 20 kg	20 mg once daily. The dosage can be increased to 40 mg once daily if needed.

Children over 4 years of age

In combination with antibiotics in treatment of duodenal ulcer caused by Helicobacter pylori. When selecting appropriate combination therapy consideration should be given to official local guidance regarding bacterial resistance, duration of treatment (most commonly 7 days but sometimes up to 14 days), and appropriate use of antibacterial agents. The treatment should be supervised by a specialist.

Weight	Dosage
15-⩽30 kg	Combination with two antibiotics: Losec 10 mg, amoxicillin 25mg/kg body weight and clarithromycin 7.5 mg/kg body weight are all administered together 2 times daily for 1 week
30-⩽40 kg	Combination with two antibiotics: Losec 20 mg, amoxicillin 750 mg and clarithromycin 7.5 mg/kg body weight are all administered 2 times daily for 1 week.
>40 kg	Combination with two antibiotics: Losec 20 mg, amoxicillin 1 g and clarithromycin 500 mg are all administered 2 times daily for 1 week.

Impaired renal function

Dose adjustment is not required in patients with impaired renal function.

Impaired hepatic function

As bioavailability and half-life can increase in patients with impaired hepatic function, the dose requires adjustment with a maximum daily dose of 20 mg.

For patients (including children aged 1 year and above who can drink or swallow semi-solid food) who are unable to swallow Losec Capsules

The capsules may be opened and the contents swallowed directly with half a glass of water or suspended in 10 ml of non-carbonated water, any fruit juice with a pH less than 5 e.g. apple, orange, pineapple, or in applesauce or yoghurt and swallowed after gentle mixing. The dispersion should be taken immediately or within 30 minutes. Stir just before drinking and rinse it down with half a glass of water. Alternatively the actual capsules may be sucked and then swallowed with half a glass of water. There is no evidence to support the use of sodium bicarbonate buffer as a delivery form. It is important that the contents of the capsules should not be crushed or chewed.

4.3 Contraindications

Known hypersensitivity to omeprazole or to any of the other constituents of the formulation.

When gastric ulcer is suspected, the possibility of malignancy should be excluded before treatment with Losec is instituted, as treatment may alleviate symptoms and delay diagnosis.

Omeprazole like other PPIs should not be administered with atazanavir (see section 4.5).

4.4 Special warnings and precautions for use

Decreased gastric acidity due to any means, including proton pump inhibitors, increases gastric counts of bacteria normally present in the gastrointestinal tract. Treatment with acid-reducing drugs may lead to a slightly increased risk of gastrointestinal infections such as *Salmonella* and *Campylobacter*.

Some children with chronic illnesses may require long-term treatment although it is not recommended.

Patients with rare hereditary problems of galactose intolerance, the Lapp lactase deficiency or glucose-galactose malabsorption should not take this medicine.

4.5 Interaction with other medicinal products and other forms of interaction

Due to the decreased intragastric acidity the absorption of ketoconazole or itraconazole may be reduced during omeprazole treatment as it is during treatment with other acid secretion inhibitors.

As Losec is metabolised in the liver through cytochrome P450 it can prolong the elimination of diazepam, phenytoin, warfarin and other vitamin K antagonists which are in part substrates for this enzyme.

Monitoring of patients receiving phenytoin is recommended and a reduction of the phenytoin dose may be necessary. However concomitant treatment with Losec 20 mg daily did not change the blood concentration of phenytoin in patients on continuous treatment with phenytoin. In patients receiving warfarin or other vitamin K antagonists, monitoring of INR is recommended and a reduction of the warfarin (or other vitamin K antagonist) dose may be necessary. Concomitant treatment with Losec 20 mg daily did, however, not change coagulation time in patients on continuous treatment with warfarin.

Plasma concentrations of omeprazole and clarithromycin are increased during concomitant administration. This is considered to be a useful interaction during *H. pylori* eradication. There is no interaction with metronidazole or amoxicillin. These antimicrobials are used together with omeprazole for eradication of *Helicobacter pylori* .

There is no evidence of an interaction with phenacetin, theophylline, caffeine, propranolol, metoprolol, ciclosporin, lidocaine, quinidine, estradiol, or antacids. The absorption of Losec is not affected by alcohol or food.

There is no evidence of an interaction with piroxicam, diclofenac or naproxen. This is considered useful when patients are required to continue these treatments.

Simultaneous treatment with omeprazole and digoxin in healthy subjects lead to a 10% increase in the bioavailability of digoxin as a consequence of the increased intragastric pH.

Co-administration of omeprazole (40mg once daily) with atazanavir 300 mg/ritonavir 100mg to healthy volunteers resulted in a substantial reduction in atazanavir exposure (approximately 75% decrease in AUC, Cmax, and Cmin). Increasing the atazanavir dose to 400mg did not compensate for the impact of omeprazole on atazanavir exposure. PPIs including omeprazole should not be co-administered with atazanavir (see section 4.3)

Concomitant administration of omeprazole and tacrolimus may increase the serum levels of tacrolimus.

Concomitant administration of omeprazole and a CYP2C19 and CYP3A4 inhibitor, voriconazole, resulted in more than doubling of the omeprazole exposure. Omeprazole (40 mg once daily) increased voriconazole (a CYP2C19 substrate) C_{max} and AUC_{τ} by 15% and 41%, respectively. A dose adjustment of omeprazole is not regularly required in either of these situations. However, dose adjustment should be considered in patients with severe hepatic impairment and if long-term treatment is indicated.

4.6 Pregnancy and lactation

Pregnancy

The analysis of the results from three epidemiological studies has revealed no evidence of adverse events of omeprazole on pregnancy or on the health of the foetus/newborn child. Losec can be used during pregnancy.

Lactation

Omeprazole is excreted in breast milk but is not likely to influence the child when therapeutic doses are used.

4.7 Effects on ability to drive and use machines

No effects are foreseen.

4.8 Undesirable effects

Losec is well tolerated and adverse reactions have generally been mild and reversible. The following have been reported as adverse events in clinical trials or reported from routine use, but in many cases a relationship to treatment with omeprazole has not been established.

The following definitions of frequencies are used:

Common	≥1/100
Uncommon	≥1/1000 and < 1/100
Rare	< 1/1000

Common	*Central and peripheral nervous system*	Headache
	Gastrointestinal	Diarrhoea, constipation, abdominal pain, nausea/vomiting and flatulence
Uncommon	*Central and peripheral nervous system*	Dizziness, paraesthesia, light headedness, feeling faint, somnolence, insomnia and vertigo
	Hepatic	Increased liver enzymes
	Skin	Rash, dermatitis and/or pruritus. urticaria
	Other	Malaise
Rare	*Central and peripheral nervous system*	Reversible mental confusion, agitation, aggression, depression and hallucinations, predominantly in severely ill patients
	Endocrine	Gynaecomastia
	Gastrointestinal	Dry mouth, stomatitis and gastrointestinal candidiasis
	Haematological	Leukopenia, thrombocytopenia, agranulocytosis and pancytopenia
	Hepatic	Encephalopathy in patients with pre-existing severe liver disease; hepatitis with or without jaundice, hepatic failure
	Musculoskeletal	Arthritic and myalgic symptoms and muscular weakness
	Reproductive system and breast disorders	Impotence
	Skin	Photosensitivity, bullous eruption, erythema multiforme, Stevens-Johnson syndrome, toxic epidermal necrolysis (TEN), alopecia
	Other	Hypersensitivity reactions e.g. angioedema, fever, broncho-spasm, interstitial nephritis and anaphylactic shock. Increased sweating, peripheral oedema, blurred vision, taste disturbance and hyponatraemia

The safety of omeprazole has been assessed in a total of 310 children aged 0 to 16 years with acid-related disease. There are limited long term safety data from 46 children who received maintenance therapy of omeprazole during a clinical study for severe erosive oesophagitis for up to 749 days. The adverse event profile was generally the same as for adults in short- as well as in long-term treatment. There are no long term data regarding the effects of omeprazole treatment on puberty and growth.

4.9 Overdose

Rare reports have been received of overdosage with omeprazole. In the literature, doses of up to 560 mg have been described and occasional reports have been received when single oral doses have reached up to 2400 mg omeprazole (120 times the usual recommended clinical dose). Nausea, vomiting, dizziness, abdominal pain, diarrhoea and headache have been reported from overdosage with omeprazole. Also apathy, depression and confusion have been described in single cases.

The symptoms described in connection to omeprazole overdosage have been transient, and no serious outcome due to omeprazole has been reported. The rate of elimination was unchanged (first order kinetics) with increased doses and no specific treatment has been needed.

5. PHARMACOLOGICAL PROPERTIES

5.1 Pharmacodynamic properties

Losec reduces gastric acid secretion through a unique mechanism of action. It is a specific inhibitor of the gastric proton pump in the parietal cell. It is rapidly acting and produces reversible control of gastric acid secretion with once daily dosing.

Oral dosing with 20 mg Losec once daily provides for rapid and effective inhibition of gastric acid secretion with maximum effect being achieved within 4 days of treatment. In duodenal ulcer patients, a mean decrease of approximately 80% in 24 hour intragastric acidity is then maintained, with the mean decrease in peak acid output after pentagastrin stimulation being about 70%, 24 hours after dosing with Losec.

Clinical data for omeprazole in the prophylaxis of NSAID induced gastroduodenal lesions are derived from clinical studies of up to 6 months duration.

Helicobacter pylori (*Hp*) is associated with acid peptic disease including duodenal ulcer (DU) and gastric ulcer (GU) in which about 95% and 80% of patients respectively are infected with this bacterium. *Hp* is implicated as a major contributing factor in the development of gastritis and ulcers in such patients. Recent evidence also suggests a causative link between *Hp* and gastric carcinoma.

Omeprazole has been shown to have a bactericidal effect on *Hp in vitro*.

Eradication of *Hp* with omeprazole and antimicrobials is associated with rapid symptom relief, high rates of healing of any mucosal lesions, and long-term remission of peptic ulcer disease thus reducing complications such as gastrointestinal bleeding as well as the need for prolonged antisecretory treatment.

In recent clinical data in patients with acute peptic ulcer omeprazole *Hp* eradication therapy improved patients' quality of life.

During long-term treatment an increased frequency of gastric glandular cysts have been reported. These changes are a physiological consequence of pronounced inhibition of acid secretion. The cysts are benign and appear to be reversible. No other treatment related mucosal changes have been observed in patients treated continuously with omeprazole for periods up to 5 years.

Paediatric data

In a non-controlled study in children (1 to 16 years of age) with severe reflux oesophagitis, omeprazole at doses of 0.7 to 1.4 mg/kg improved oesophagitis level in 90 % of the cases and significantly reduced reflux symptoms. In a single-blind study, children aged 0-24 months with clinically diagnosed GERD were treated with 0.5, 1.0 or 1.5 mg omeprazole/kg. The frequency of vomiting/regurgitation episodes decreased by 50 % after 8 weeks of treatment irrespective of the dose.

Eradication of Helicobacter pylori in children:

A randomised, double blind clinical study (Héliot study) has concluded to the efficacy and an acceptable safety for omeprazole associated to two antibiotics (amoxicillin and clarithromycin) in the treatment of Helicobacter pylori infection in children of 4 years old and above with a gastritis: Helicobacter pylori eradication rate: 74.2% (23/31 patients) with omeprazole + amoxicillin + clarithromycin versus 9.4% (3/32 patients) with amoxicillin + clarithromycin. However, there was no evidence of clinical benefit demonstrated regarding dyspeptic symptoms. This study does not support any information for children aged less than 4 years old.

Site and mechanism of action

Omeprazole is a weak base and is concentrated and converted to the active form in the acid environment of the intracellular canaliculi within the parietal cell, where it inhibits the enzyme H^+, K^+-ATPase - the proton pump. This effect on the final step of the gastric acid formation process is dose-dependent and provides for effective inhibition of both basal acid secretion and stimulated acid secretion irrespective of the stimulus.

All pharmacodynamic effects observed are explained by the effect of omeprazole on acid secretion.

5.2 Pharmacokinetic properties

Absorption and distribution

Omeprazole is acid labile and is administered orally as enteric-coated granules in capsules. Absorption takes place in the small intestine and is usually completed within 3-6 hours. The systemic bioavailability of omeprazole from a single oral dose of Losec is approximately 35%. After repeated once-daily administration, the bioavailability increases to about 60%. Concomitant intake of food has no influence on the bioavailability. The plasma protein binding of omeprazole is about 95%.

Elimination and metabolism

The average half-life of the terminal phase of the plasma concentration-time curve is approximately 40 minutes. There is no change in half-life during treatment. The inhibition of acid secretion is related to the area under the plasma concentration-time curve (AUC) but not to the actual plasma concentration at a given time.

Omeprazole is entirely metabolised mainly in the liver. Identified metabolites in plasma are the sulphone, the sulphide and hydroxy-omeprazole, these metabolites have no significant effect on acid secretion. About 80% of the metabolites are excreted in the urine and the rest in the faeces. The two main urinary metabolites are hydroxy-omeprazole and the corresponding carboxylic acid.

The systemic bioavailability of omeprazole is not significantly altered in patients with reduced renal function. The area under the plasma concentration-time curve is increased in patients with impaired liver function, but no tendency to accumulation of omeprazole has been found.

Children

During treatment with the recommended doses to children from the age of 1 year, similar plasma concentrations were obtained as compared to adults. In children younger than 6 months, clearance of omeprazole is low due to low capacity to metabolise omeprazole.

5.3 Preclinical safety data

Animal Toxicology

Gastric ECL-cell hyperplasia and carcinoids, have been observed in life-long studies in rats treated with omeprazole or subjected to partial fundectomy. These changes are the result of sustained hypergastrinaemia secondary to acid inhibition, and not from a direct effect of any individual drug.

6. PHARMACEUTICAL PARTICULARS

6.1 List of excipients

Mannitol, hyprolose, cellulose microcrystalline, lactose anhydrous, sodium laurilsulfate, disodium hydrogen phosphate dihydrate, hypromellose, methacrylic acid copolymer, macrogol, red iron oxide (E172), titanium dioxide (E171), gelatin and magnesium stearate.

6.2 Incompatibilities

None known.

6.3 Shelf life

3 years.

Bottles: 3 month in-use shelf-life

6.4 Special precautions for storage

Do not store above 30°C.

Blisters: Store in the original container.

Bottles: Keep the container tightly closed.

6.5 Nature and contents of container

Losec Capsules are provided in high density polyethylene bottles with tamper-proof child-resistant lids containing integral desiccant. Packs of 5, 7, 14, 28 Capsules

or

Losec Capsules are provided in Aluminium-PVC/Aluminium foil blister packs. Packs of 7, 14 and 28 capsules.

Not all pack sizes may be marketed.

6.6 Special precautions for disposal and other handling

The cap should be replaced firmly after use.

To be dispensed in original containers.

7. MARKETING AUTHORISATION HOLDER

AstraZeneca UK Ltd.,
600 Capability Green,
Luton, LU1 3LU, UK.

8. MARKETING AUTHORISATION NUMBER(S)

PL 17901/0132

PL 17901/0133

PL 17901/0134

9. DATE OF FIRST AUTHORISATION/RENEWAL OF THE AUTHORISATION

14th May 2002

10. DATE OF REVISION OF THE TEXT

19th February 2008

Losec I.V. Injection 40mg

(AstraZeneca UK Limited)

1. NAME OF THE MEDICINAL PRODUCT

Losec® I.V. Injection 40 mg

2. QUALITATIVE AND QUANTITATIVE COMPOSITION

a) Each vial of powder for solution for injection contains omeprazole sodium 42.6 mg, equivalent to omeprazole 40 mg. After reconstitution, 1 ml contains omeprazole sodium 4.26 mg, equivalent to 4.00 mg omeprazole.

b) Each ampoule contains 10 ml of solvent for injection

For excipients, see 6.1.

3. PHARMACEUTICAL FORM

Powder and solvent for solution for injection.

4. CLINICAL PARTICULARS

4.1 Therapeutic indications

Prophylaxis of acid aspiration.

In patients who are unable to take oral therapy for the short-term treatment (up to 5 days) of reflux oesophagitis, duodenal and benign gastric ulcers, including those complicating NSAID therapy e.g. perioperative use.

4.2 Posology and method of administration

Dosage

Adults only

Prophylaxis of acid aspiration: Losec 40 mg to be given slowly (over a period of 5 minutes) as an intravenous injection, one hour before surgery.

Treatment in patients where oral therapy is inappropriate e.g. in severely ill patients with either reflux oesophagitis, duodenal ulcer or gastric ulcer: Losec 40 mg given as an intravenous injection once daily is recommended for up to 5 days.

Clinical experience in Zollinger-Ellison syndrome is limited (see section 5.1 Pharmacodynamic properties).

Administration

Losec powder and solvent for solution for injection is for intravenous administration **only** and must **not** be given by any other route.

Losec powder and solvent for solution for injection should only be dissolved in the solvent provided. No other solvents for I.V. injection should be used.

After reconstitution outside validated aseptic conditions, use within 4 hours of preparation and any unused portion should be discarded.

The duration of administration should be over 5 minutes.

Use in the elderly

Dosage adjustment is not necessary.

Use in children

There is limited experience of use in children.

Impaired renal function

Dose adjustment is not required in patients with impaired renal function.

Impaired hepatic function

As half-life is increased in patients with impaired hepatic function, the dose requires adjustment and a daily dose of 10 mg–20 mg may be sufficient.

4.3 Contraindications

Known hypersensitivity to any of the constituents of the formulation.

Omeprazole like other PPIs should not be administered with atazanavir (see section 4.5).

4.4 Special warnings and precautions for use

When gastric ulcer is suspected, the possibility of malignancy should be excluded before treatment with Losec is instituted, as treatment may alleviate symptoms and delay diagnosis.

Decreased gastric acidity due to any means including proton pump inhibitors, increases gastric counts of bacteria normally present in the gastrointestinal tract. Treatment with acid-reducing drugs may lead to a slightly increased risk of gastrointestinal infections, such as *Salmonella* and *Campylobacter*.

4.5 Interaction with other medicinal products and other forms of interaction

Due to the decreased intragastric acidity, the absorption of ketoconazole or itraconazole may be reduced during omeprazole therapy as it is during treatment with other acid secretion inhibitors.

As omeprazole is metabolised in the liver through cytochrome P450 it can prolong the elimination of diazepam, phenytoin, warfarin and other vitamin K antagonists, which are in part substrates for this enzyme.

Monitoring of patients receiving phenytoin is recommended and a reduction of the phenytoin dose may be necessary when Losec is added to treatment. However, concomitant treatment with Losec 20 mg orally daily, did not change the blood concentration of phenytoin in patients on continuous treatment with phenytoin. In patients receiving warfarin or other vitamin K antagonists, monitoring of INR is recommended and a reduction of the warfarin (or other vitamin K antagonist) dose may be necessary. Concomitant treatment with Losec 20 mg orally daily, did not change coagulation time in patients on continuous treatment with warfarin.

Plasma concentrations of omeprazole and clarithromycin are increased during concomitant oral administration. There is no interaction with metronidazole or amoxicillin. These antimicrobials are used together with omeprazole for eradication of *Helicobacter pylori* .

There is no evidence of an interaction with phenacetin, theophylline, caffeine, propranolol, metoprolol, ciclosporin, lidocaine, quinidine, estradiol, or antacids when Losec is given orally. The absorption of Losec given orally is not affected by alcohol or food.

There is no evidence of an interaction with piroxicam, diclofenac or naproxen, this is considered useful when patients are required to continue these treatments.

Simultaneous treatment with omeprazole and digoxin in healthy subjects led to a 10% increase in the bioavailability of digoxin as a consequence of the increased intragastric pH.

Interaction with other drugs also metabolised via the cytochrome P450 system cannot be excluded.

Co-administration of omeprazole (40mg once daily) with atazanavir 300 mg/ritonavir 100mg to healthy volunteers resulted in a substantial reduction in atazanavir exposure (approximately 75% decrease in AUC, Cmax, and Cmin). Increasing the atazanavir dose to 400mg did not compensate for the impact of omeprazole on atazanavir exposure. PPIs including omeprazole should not be co-administered with atazanavir (see section 4.3)

Concomitant administration of omeprazole and tacrolimus may increase the serum levels of tacrolimus.

Concomitant administration of omeprazole and a CYP2C19 and CYP3A4 inhibitor, voriconazole, resulted in more than doubling of the omeprazole exposure. Omeprazole (40 mg once daily) increased voriconazole (a CYP2C19 substrate) C_{max} and AUC_{τ} by 15% and 41%, respectively. A dose adjustment of omeprazole is not regularly required in either of these situations. However, dose adjustment should be considered in patients with severe hepatic impairment and if long-term treatment is indicated.

4.6 Pregnancy and lactation

Use in pregnancy

The analysis of the results from three epidemiological studies has revealed no evidence of adverse events of omeprazole on pregnancy or on the health of the foetus/newborn child. Losec can be used during pregnancy.

Use in lactation

Omeprazole is excreted in breast milk but is not likely to influence the child when therapeutic doses are used.

4.7 Effects on ability to drive and use machines

No effects are foreseen.

4.8 Undesirable effects

Losec is well tolerated and adverse reactions have generally been mild and reversible. The following have been reported as adverse events in clinical trials or reported from routine use, but in many cases a relationship to treatment with omeprazole has not been established.

The following definitions of frequencies are used:

Common - $\geq$ 1/100

Uncommon - $\geq$ 1/1000 and $<$ 1/100

Rare - $<$ 1/1000

Common	*Central and peripheral nervous system*	Headache
	Gastrointestinal	Diarrhoea, constipation, abdominal pain, nausea/vomiting and flatulence
Uncommon	*Central and peripheral nervous system*	Dizziness, paraesthesia, somnolence, insomnia and vertigo
	Hepatic	Increased liver enzymes
	Skin	Rash, dermatitis and/or pruritus, urticaria
	Other	Malaise
Rare	*Central and peripheral nervous system*	Reversible mental confusion, agitation, aggression, depression and hallucinations, predominantly in severely ill patients
	Endocrine	Gynaecomastia
	Gastrointestinal	Dry mouth, stomatitis and gastrointestinal candidiasis
	Haematological	Leukopenia, thrombocytopenia, agranulocytosis and pancytopenia
	Hepatic	Encephalopathy in patients with pre-existing severe liver disease; hepatitis with or without jaundice, hepatic failure, increased liver enzymes
	Musculoskeletal	Arthritic and myalgic symptoms and muscular weakness
	Reproductive system and breast disorders	Impotence
	Skin	Photosensitivity, bullous eruption erythema multiforme, Stevens-Johnson syndrome, toxic epidermal necrolysis (TEN), alopecia
	Other	Hypersensitivity reactions e.g. angioedema, fever, broncho-spasm, interstitial nephritis and anaphylactic shock. Increased sweating, peripheral oedema, blurred vision, taste disturbance and hyponatraemia

Isolated cases of irreversible visual impairment have been reported in critically ill patients who have received Losec Intravenous Injection, particularly at high doses, however no causal relationship has been established.

4.9 Overdose

Intravenous doses of up to 270 mg on a single day and up to 650 mg over a three-day period have been given in clinical trials without any dose-related adverse effects.

5. PHARMACOLOGICAL PROPERTIES

5.1 Pharmacodynamic properties

Omeprazole reduces gastric acid secretion through a unique mechanism of action. It is a specific inhibitor of the gastric proton pump in the parietal cell. It is rapidly acting and produces reversible control of gastric acid secretion with once daily dosing.

Intravenous administration of omeprazole results in an immediate reduction of intragastric acidity and a mean decrease over 24 hours of approximately 90% in patients with duodenal ulcer disease. A single 40 mg i.v. dose has similar effect on intragastric acidity over a 24 hour period as repeated oral dosing with 20 mg once daily. A higher dose of 60 mg i.v. twice daily has been used in a clinical study in patients with Zollinger-Ellison syndrome.

Site and mechanism of action

Omeprazole is a weak base and is concentrated and converted to the active form in the acid environment of the intracellular canaliculi within the parietal cell, where it inhibits the enzyme H^+, K^+,-ATPase–the proton pump. This effect on the final step of the gastric acid formation process is dose-dependent and provides for effective inhibition of both basal acid secretion and stimulated acid secretion irrespective of the stimulus.

All pharmacodynamic effects observed are explained by the effect of omeprazole on acid secretion. No tachyphylaxis has been observed during treatment with omeprazole.

5.2 Pharmacokinetic properties

Distribution

The apparent volume of distribution in healthy subjects is approximately 0.3 L/kg and a similar value is also seen in patients with renal insufficiency. In the elderly and in patients with hepatic insufficiency, the volume of distribution is slightly decreased. The plasma protein binding of omeprazole is about 95%.

Metabolism and excretion

The average half-life of the terminal phase of the plasma concentration-time curve following i.v. administration of omeprazole is approximately 40 minutes; the total plasma clearance is 0.3 to 0.6 L/min. There is no change in half-life during treatment.

Omeprazole is completely metabolised by the cytochrome P450 system, mainly in the liver. The major part of its metabolism is dependent on the polymorphically expressed, specific isoform CYP2C19 (S-mephenytoin hydroxylase), responsible for the formation of hydroxyomeprazole, the major metabolite in plasma.

No metabolite has been found to have any effect on gastric acid secretion. Almost 80% of an intravenously given dose is excreted as metabolites in the urine, and the remainder is found in the faeces, primarily originating from biliary secretion.

Elimination of omeprazole is unchanged in patients with reduced renal function. The elimination half-life is increased in patients with impaired liver function, but omeprazole has not shown any accumulation with once daily oral dosing.

5.3 Preclinical safety data

Animal Toxicology

Gastric ECL-cell hyperplasia and carcinoids, have been observed in life-long studies in rats treated with omeprazole or subjected to partial fundectomy. These changes are the result of sustained hypergastrinaemia secondary to acid inhibition, and not from a direct effect of any individual drug.

6. PHARMACEUTICAL PARTICULARS

6.1 List of excipients

a) Vial: Sodium hydroxide.

b) Ampoule: Macrogol 400, Citric acid monohydrate and Water for Injections.

6.2 Incompatibilities

No other drugs should be mixed with reconstituted Losec I.V. Injection solution.

6.3 Shelf life

Unopened packs: 2 years.

Reconstituted solution: 4 hours.

6.4 Special precautions for storage

Do not store above 25°C. Keep the containers in outer carton.

6.5 Nature and contents of container

Combination pack consisting of a clear, Type I, glass vial containing omeprazole sodium 42.6 mg with grey bromobutyl rubber stopper, white polypropylene cap with aluminium frame and a clear, Type I, (OPC) glass ampoule containing solvent for intravenous administration, both packed together in a plastic tray in a hard cardboard box.

6.6 Special precautions for disposal and other handling

The entire contents of the vial should be completely dissolved with the 10 ml of solvent provided in the ampoule. No other solvents for I.V. injection should be used.

Use on one patient during one treatment only.

Do not use if any particles are present in the reconstituted solution.

Chemical and physical in-use stability of the reconstituted product has been shown for 4 hours when stored at 25°C.

From a microbiological point of view, once opened and reconstituted the product may be stored for a maximum of 4 hours at 25°C. Other in-use storage times and conditions are the responsibility of the user.

Any unused portion should be discarded.

Preparation:

NOTE: Stages 1 to 5 should be done in immediate sequence.

With a syringe draw 10 ml of solvent from the ampoule.

Add approximately 5 ml of the solvent to the vial with freeze-dried omeprazole.

Withdraw as much air as possible from the vial back into the syringe in order to reduce positive pressure. This will make it easier to add the remaining solvent.

Add the remaining solvent into the vial, make sure that the syringe is empty.

Rotate and shake the vial to ensure all the freeze-dried omeprazole has dissolved.

7. MARKETING AUTHORISATION HOLDER

AstraZeneca UK Ltd.,

600 Capability Green,

Luton, LU1 3LU, UK.

8. MARKETING AUTHORISATION NUMBER(S)

PL 17901/0135

9. DATE OF FIRST AUTHORISATION/RENEWAL OF THE AUTHORISATION

18th June 2002

10. DATE OF REVISION OF THE TEXT

28th January 2008

Losec Infusion 40mg

(AstraZeneca UK Limited)

1. NAME OF THE MEDICINAL PRODUCT

Losec® Infusion 40 mg

2. QUALITATIVE AND QUANTITATIVE COMPOSITION

Each vial of powder for solution for infusion contains Omeprazole Sodium 42.6 mg equivalent to Omeprazole 40 mg.

For excipients, see 6.1

3. PHARMACEUTICAL FORM

Powder for solution for infusion.

4. CLINICAL PARTICULARS

4.1 Therapeutic indications

Prophylaxis of acid aspiration.

In patients who are unable to take oral therapy for the short-term treatment (up to 5 days) of reflux oesophagitis, duodenal and benign gastric ulcers, including those complicating NSAID therapy e.g. perioperative use.

4.2 Posology and method of administration

Dosage

Adults only

Prophylaxis of acid aspiration: Losec 40 mg given as an intravenous infusion to be completed one hour before surgery.

Treatment in patients where oral therapy is inappropriate e.g. in severely ill patients with either reflux oesophagitis, duodenal ulcer or gastric ulcer: Losec 40 mg given as an intravenous infusion once daily is recommended for up to 5 days.

The i.v. infusion produces an immediate decrease in intragastric acidity and a mean decrease over 24 hours of approximately 90%.

Clinical experience in Zollinger-Ellison syndrome is limited (see section 5.1 Pharmacodynamic properties).

Administration

Losec powder for solution for infusion is for intravenous administration **only** and must **not** be given by any other route.

Losec powder for solution for infusion should only be dissolved in either 100 ml normal saline for infusion or 100 ml 5% dextrose for infusion. No other solutions for i.v. infusion should be used.

After reconstitution from a microbiological point of view, use immediately (i.e. within 3 hours) and any unused portion should be discarded.

The duration of administration should be 20–30 minutes.

Use in the elderly

Dosage adjustment is not necessary.

Use in children

There is limited experience of use in children.

Impaired renal function

Dose adjustment is not required in patients with impaired renal function.

Impaired hepatic function

As half-life is increased in patients with impaired hepatic function, the dose requires adjustment and a daily dose of 10 mg–20 mg may be sufficient.

4.3 Contraindications

Known hypersensitivity to omeprazole or to any of the other constituents of the formulation.

Omeprazole like other PPIs should not be administered with atazanavir (see section 4.5).

4.4 Special warnings and precautions for use

When gastric ulcer is suspected the possibility of malignancy should be excluded before treatment with Losec is instituted, as treatment may alleviate symptoms and delay diagnosis.

Decreased gastric acidity due to any means including proton pump inhibitors, increases gastric counts of bacteria normally present in the gastrointestinal tract. Treatment with acid-reducing drugs may lead to a slightly increased risk of gastrointestinal infections, such as *Salmonella* and *Campylobacter*.

4.5 Interaction with other medicinal products and other forms of interaction

Due to the decreased intragastric acidity, the absorption of ketoconazole or itraconazole may be reduced during omeprazole therapy as it is during treatment with other acid secretion inhibitors.

As omeprazole is metabolised in the liver through cytochrome P450 it can prolong the elimination of diazepam, phenytoin, warfarin and other vitamin K antagonists, which are in part substrates for this enzyme.

Monitoring of patients receiving phenytoin, is recommended and a reduction of the phenytoin dose may be necessary. However, concomitant treatment with Losec 20 mg orally daily did not change the blood concentration of phenytoin in patients on continuous treatment with phenytoin. In patients receiving warfarin or other vitamin K antagonists, monitoring of INR is recommended and a reduction of the warfarin (or other vitamin K antagonist) dose may be necessary. Concomitant treatment with Losec 20 mg orally daily did not change coagulation time in patients on continuous treatment with warfarin.

Plasma concentrations of omeprazole and clarithromycin are increased during concomitant oral administration. There is no interaction with metronidazole or amoxicillin. These antimicrobials are used together with omeprazole for eradication of *Helicobacter pylori* .

There is no evidence of an interaction with phenacetin, theophylline, caffeine, propranolol, metoprolol, ciclosporin, lidocaine, quinidine, estradiol, or antacids when Losec is given orally. The absorption of Losec given orally is not affected by alcohol or food.

There is no evidence of an interaction with piroxicam, diclofenac or naproxen, this is considered useful when patients are required to continue these treatments.

Simultaneous treatment with omeprazole and digoxin in healthy subjects led to a 10% increase in the bioavailability of digoxin as a consequence of the increased intragastric pH.

Interaction with other drugs also metabolised via the cytochrome P450 system cannot be excluded.

Co-administration of omeprazole (40mg once daily) with atazanavir 300 mg/ritonavir 100mg to healthy volunteers resulted in a substantial reduction in atazanavir exposure (approximately 75% decrease in AUC, Cmax, and Cmin). Increasing the atazanavir dose to 400mg did not compensate for the impact of omeprazole on atazanavir exposure. PPIs including omeprazole should not be co-administered with atazanavir (see section 4.3)

Concomitant administration of omeprazole and tacrolimus may increase the serum levels of tacrolimus.

Concomitant administration of omeprazole and a CYP2C19 and CYP3A4 inhibitor, voriconazole, resulted in more than doubling of the omeprazole exposure. Omeprazole (40 mg once daily) increased voriconazole (a CYP2C19 substrate) C_{max} and AUC_{τ} by 15% and 41%, respectively. A dose adjustment of omeprazole is not regularly required in either of these situations. However, dose adjustment should be considered in patients with severe hepatic impairment and if long-term treatment is indicated.

4.6 Pregnancy and lactation

Use in pregnancy

The analysis of the results from three epidemiological studies has revealed no evidence of adverse events of omeprazole on pregnancy or on the health of the fetus/newborn child. Losec can be used during pregnancy.

Use in lactation

Omeprazole is excreted in breast milk but is not likely to influence the child when therapeutic doses are used.

4.7 Effects on ability to drive and use machines

No effects are foreseen.

4.8 Undesirable effects

Losec is well tolerated and adverse reactions have generally been mild and reversible. The following have been reported as adverse events in clinical trials or reported from routine use, but in many cases a relationship to treatment with omeprazole has not been established.

The following definitions of frequencies are used:

Common $\geq$ 1/100

Uncommon $\geq$ 1/1000 and $<$ 1/100

Rare $<$ 1/1000

Common	*Central and peripheral nervous system*	Headache
	Gastrointestinal	Diarrhoea, constipation, abdominal pain, nausea/vomiting and flatulence
Uncommon	*Central and peripheral nervous system*	Dizziness, paraesthesia, light-headedness, feeling faint, somnolence, insomnia and vertigo
	Hepatic	Increased liver enzymes
	Skin	Rash, dermatitis and/or pruritus, urticaria
	Other	Malaise
Rare	*Central and peripheral nervous system*	Reversible mental confusion, agitation, aggression, depression and hallucinations, predominantly in severely ill patients
	Endocrine	Gynaecomastia
	Gastrointestinal	Dry mouth, stomatitis and gastrointestinal candidiasis
	Haematological	Leukopenia, thrombocytopenia, agranulocytosis and pancytopenia
	Hepatic	Encephalopathy in patients with pre-existing severe liver disease; hepatitis with or without jaundice, hepatic failure increased liver enzymes
	Musculoskeletal	Arthritic and myalgic symptoms and muscular weakness
	Reproductive system and breast disorders	Impotence
	Skin	Photosensitivity, erythema multiforme, Stevens-Johnson syndrome, toxic epidermal necrolysis (TEN), alopecia

	Other	Hypersensitivity reactions e.g. angioedema, fever, bronchospasm, interstitial nephritis and anaphylactic shock. Increased sweating, peripheral oedema, blurred vision, taste disturbance and hyponatraemia

Isolated cases of irreversible visual impairment have been reported in critically ill patients who have received Losec Intravenous Injection, particularly at high doses, however no causal relationship has been established.

4.9 Overdose

Intravenous doses of up to 270 mg on a single day and up to 650 mg over a three-day period have been given in clinical trials without any dose-related adverse effects.

5. PHARMACOLOGICAL PROPERTIES

5.1 Pharmacodynamic properties

Omeprazole reduces gastric acid secretion through a unique mechanism of action. It is a specific inhibitor of the gastric proton pump in the parietal cell. It is rapidly acting and produces reversible control of gastric acid secretion with once daily dosing.

Intravenous administration of omeprazole results in an immediate reduction of intragastric acidity and a mean decrease over 24 hours of approximately 90% in patients with duodenal ulcer disease. A single 40 mg i.v. dose has similar effect on intragastric acidity over a 24 hour period as repeated oral dosing with 20 mg once daily. A higher dose of 60 mg i.v. twice daily has been used in a clinical study in patients with Zollinger-Ellison syndrome.

Site and mechanism of action

Omeprazole is a weak base and is concentrated and converted to the active form in the acid environment of the intracellular canaliculi within the parietal cell, where it inhibits the enzyme H^+, K^+,-ATPase–the proton pump. This effect on the final step of the gastric acid formation process is dose-dependent and provides for effective inhibition of both basal acid secretion and stimulated acid secretion irrespective of the stimulus.

All pharmacodynamic effects observed are explained by the effect of omeprazole on acid secretion. No tachyphylaxis has been observed during treatment with omeprazole.

5.2 Pharmacokinetic properties

Distribution

The apparent volume of distribution in healthy subjects is approximately 0.3 L/kg and a similar value is also seen in patients with renal insufficiency. In the elderly and in patients with hepatic insufficiency, the volume of distribution is slightly decreased. The plasma protein binding of omeprazole is about 95%.

Metabolism and excretion

The average half-life of the terminal phase of the plasma concentration-time curve following i.v. administration of omeprazole is approximately 40 minutes; the total plasma clearance is 0.3 to 0.6 L/min. There is no change in half-life during treatment.

Omeprazole is completely metabolised by the cytochrome P450 system, mainly in the liver. The major part of its metabolism is dependent on the polymorphically expressed, specific isoform CYP2C19 (S-mephenytoin hydroxylase), responsible for the formation of hydroxyomeprazole, the major metabolite in plasma.

No metabolite has been found to have any effect on gastric acid secretion. Almost 80% of an intravenously given dose is excreted as metabolites in the urine, and the remainder is found in the faeces, primarily originating from biliary secretion.

Elimination of omeprazole is unchanged in patients with reduced renal function. The elimination half-life is increased in patients with impaired liver function, but omeprazole has not shown any accumulation with once daily oral dosing.

5.3 Preclinical safety data

Animal Toxicology

Gastric ECL-cell hyperplasia and carcinoids, have been observed in life-long studies in rats treated with omeprazole or subjected to partial fundectomy. These changes are the result of sustained hypergastrinaemia secondary to acid inhibition, and not from a direct effect of any individual drug.

6. PHARMACEUTICAL PARTICULARS

6.1 List of excipients

Sodium hydroxide and disodium edetate.

6.2 Incompatibilities

No other drugs should be mixed with reconstituted Losec Infusion solution.

6.3 Shelf life

Unopened pack: 2 years.

After reconstitution in normal saline at 25°C: 12 hours.

After reconstitution in 5% dextrose at 25°C: 3 hours

For additional information, see section 6.6

6.4 Special precautions for storage

Do not store above 25°C. Keep container in outer carton.

6.5 Nature and contents of container

Pack of 5, clear, Type I, glass 10 ml vials each containing omeprazole sodium 42.6 mg with grey bromobutyl stopper, blue polypropylene cap and golden aluminium frame.

6.6 Special precautions for disposal and other handling

The entire contents of each vial should be dissolved in approximately 5 ml and then immediately diluted to 100 ml. Normal saline for infusion or 5 % dextrose for infusion should be used. No other solutions for i.v. infusion should be used.

Use on one patient during one treatment only.

Do not use if any particles are present in the reconstituted solution.

Chemical and physical in use stability of the product has been shown for 12 hours when dissolved in normal saline and 3 hours in 5% dextrose when stored at 25°C.

From a microbiological point of view, the product should be used immediately (i.e. within 3 hours).

Any unused portion should be discarded.

Preparation:

1. With a syringe draw approximately 5 ml of infusion solution from the infusion bottle or bag.

2. Add the infusion solution to the vial with the freeze-dried omeprazole, mix thoroughly making sure all omeprazole is dissolved.

3. Draw the omeprazole solution back into the syringe.

4. Transfer the solution in the infusion bottle or bag.

5. Repeat 1–4 to make sure all omeprazole is transferred from the vial into the infusion bottle or bag.

Alternative preparation for infusions in flexible containers:

1. Use a double-ended transfer needle and attach to the injection membrane of the infusion bag. Connect the other needle-end from the vial with freeze-dried omeprazole.

2. Dissolve the omeprazole substance by pumping the infusion solution back and forward between the infusion bag and the vial.

3. Make sure all omeprazole is dissolved.

(see diagrams below)

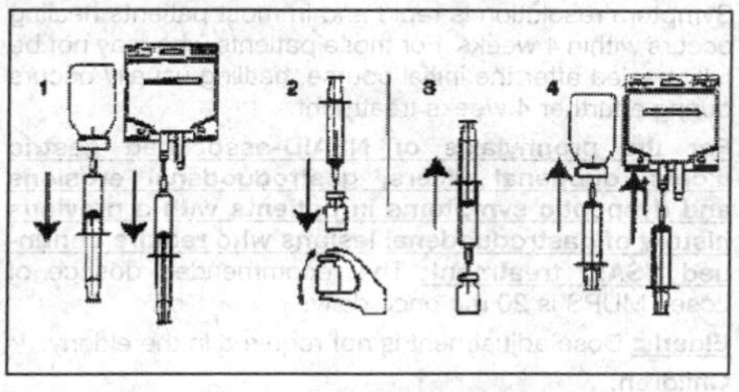

7. MARKETING AUTHORISATION HOLDER

AstraZeneca UK Ltd.,

600 Capability Green,

Luton, LU1 3LU, UK.

8. MARKETING AUTHORISATION NUMBER(S)

PL 17901/0136

9. DATE OF FIRST AUTHORISATION/RENEWAL OF THE AUTHORISATION

14th May 2002

10. DATE OF REVISION OF THE TEXT

28th January 2008

Losec IV Injection Solvent

(AstraZeneca UK Limited)

1. NAME OF THE MEDICINAL PRODUCT

Solvent for Losec® i.v. Injection 40 mg.

2. QUALITATIVE AND QUANTITATIVE COMPOSITION

Each ampoule contains 10ml of solvent for injection

For excipients, see 6.1.

3. PHARMACEUTICAL FORM

Solvent for solution for injection

4. CLINICAL PARTICULARS

4.1 Therapeutic indications

To be used as a Solvent for i.v. injection with 1 vial of powder for injection which contains Omeprazole sodium 42.6mg, equivalent to Omeprazole 40mg

4.2 Posology and method of administration

Dosage and Administration

The intravenous solution is obtained by dissolving the lyophilised omeprazole in the solvent provided. No other solvent should be used and the solution must be given by intravenous injection and not added to any other solutions for injection. The injection should be given slowly over a period of 5 minutes. The solution should be used within 4 hours of preparation.

Use in the Elderly:

Dosage adjustment is not necessary.

Use in Children:

There is limited experience of use in children.

4.3 Contraindications

Known hypersensitivity macrogol 400 and citric acid monohydrate.

4.4 Special warnings and precautions for use

None stated

4.5 Interaction with other medicinal products and other forms of interaction

None stated

4.6 Pregnancy and lactation

None stated

4.7 Effects on ability to drive and use machines

None stated

4.8 Undesirable effects

None stated

4.9 Overdose

None stated

5. PHARMACOLOGICAL PROPERTIES

5.1 Pharmacodynamic properties

None stated

5.2 Pharmacokinetic properties

Macrogols entering the systemic circulation are predominantly excreted unchanged in the urine, low molecular-weight macrogols may be partly metabolised.

5.3 Preclinical safety data

Citric acid and macrogols are commonly used in pharmaceutical preparations, no addition information is necessary.

6. PHARMACEUTICAL PARTICULARS

6.1 List of excipients

Macrogol 400, Citric acid monohydrate and water for injections.

6.2 Incompatibilities

None known.

6.3 Shelf life

Unopened pack: 2 years.

Reconstituted solution: 4 hours.

6.4 Special precautions for storage

Do not store above 25°C. Keep container in outer carton.

6.5 Nature and contents of container

A clear, Type I (OPC) glass ampoule containing solvent for intravenous administration, packed in a plastic tray with a glass vial in a hard cardboard box.

6.6 Special precautions for disposal and other handling

The solvent in the ampoule is used to reconstitute lyophilised powder to provide a solution for i.v. injection.

Use on one patient during one treatment only.

DO NOT USE if any particles are present in the reconstituted solution.

From a microbiological point of view, once opened and reconstituted the product may be stored for a maximum of 4 hours at 25°C. Other in-use storage times and conditions are the responsibility of the user.

Any unused portion should be discarded.

Preparation:

NOTE: Stages 1 to 5 should be done in immediate sequence.

1. With a syringe draw 10ml of solvent from the ampoule.

2. Add approximately 5ml of the solvent to the vial with the lyophilised powder.

3. Withdraw as much air as possible from the vial back into the syringe in order to reduce positive pressure. This will make it easier to add the remaining solvent.

4. Add the remaining solvent into the vial, make sure that the syringe is empty.

5. Rotate and shake the vial to ensure all the lyophilised powder has been dissolved.

7. MARKETING AUTHORISATION HOLDER

AstraZeneca UK Ltd,

600 Capability Green,

Luton, LU1 3LU, UK.

8. MARKETING AUTHORISATION NUMBER(S)

PL 17901/0167

9. DATE OF FIRST AUTHORISATION/RENEWAL OF THE AUTHORISATION

18th June 2002/7th June 2006

10. DATE OF REVISION OF THE TEXT

7th June 2006

Losec MUPS Tablets 10mg, 20mg & 40mg

(AstraZeneca UK Limited)

1. NAME OF THE MEDICINAL PRODUCT
Losec MUPS® Tablets 10 mg.

Losec MUPS® Tablets 20 mg.

Losec MUPS® Tablets 40 mg.

2. QUALITATIVE AND QUANTITATIVE COMPOSITION
Each tablet contains 10.3, 20.6 or 41.3 mg of omeprazole magnesium equivalent to 10, 20 or 40 mg omeprazole respectively.

For excipients, see 6.1

3. PHARMACEUTICAL FORM
Film coated tablet

LOSEC MUPS® tablets 10mg: Light-pink, oblong, biconvex, film-coated tablets engraved with on one side and 10mg on the other side. Each tablet contains omeprazole magnesium 10.3mg as enteric coated pellets.

LOSEC MUPS® tablets 20mg: Pink, oblong, biconvex, film-coated tablets engraved with on one side and 20mg on the other side. Each tablet contains omeprazole magnesium 20.6mg as enteric coated pellets.

LOSEC MUPS® tablets 40mg: A red-brown, oblong, biconvex, film-coated tablet with a score and engraved with on one side and 40mg on the other side. Each tablet contains omeprazole magnesium 41.3mg as enteric coated pellets.

4. CLINICAL PARTICULARS
4.1 Therapeutic indications
Treatment of oesophageal reflux disease. In reflux oesophagitis the majority of patients are healed after 4 weeks. Symptom relief is rapid.

Treatment of duodenal and benign gastric ulcers including those complicating NSAID therapy.

Relief of associated dyspeptic symptoms.

Helicobacter pylori eradication: Omeprazole should be used in combination with antibiotics for eradication of *Helicobacter pylori* (*Hp*) in peptic ulcer disease.

Prophylaxis of acid aspiration.

Zollinger-Ellison syndrome.

10 mg and 20 mg tablets only:

Relief of reflux-like symptoms (e.g. heartburn) and/or ulcer-like symptoms (e.g. epigastric pain) associated with acid-related dyspepsia.

Treatment and prophylaxis of NSAID-associated benign gastric ulcers, duodenal ulcers and gastroduodenal erosions in patients with a previous history of gastroduodenal lesions who require continued NSAID treatment.

Children over 1 year of age and ⩾ 10 kg: Reflux oesophagitis. Symptomatic treatment of heartburn and acid regurgitation in gastroesophageal reflux disease.

4.2 Posology and method of administration
Dosage

Adults

Oesophageal reflux disease including reflux oesophagitis: The usual dosage is 20 mg Losec MUPS once daily. The majority of patients are healed after 4 weeks. For those patients not fully healed after the initial course, healing usually occurs during a further 4–8 weeks treatment.

Losec MUPS can also been used at a dose of 40 mg once daily in patients with reflux oesophagitis refractory to other therapy. Healing usually occurs within 8 weeks. Patients can be continued at a dosage of 20 mg once daily.

Acid reflux disease: For long-term management, Losec MUPS 10mg once daily is recommended, increasing to 20mg if symptoms return.

Duodenal and benign gastric ulcers: The usual dose is 20 mg Losec MUPS once daily. The majority of patients with duodenal ulcer are healed after 4 weeks. The majority of patients with benign gastric ulcer are healed after 8 weeks. In severe or recurrent cases the dose may be increased to 40 mg Losec MUPS daily. Long-term therapy for patients with a history of recurrent duodenal ulcer is recommended at a dosage of 20 mg Losec MUPS once daily.

For prevention of relapse in patients with duodenal ulcer the recommended dose is Losec MUPS 10 mg, once daily, increasing to 20 mg, once daily if symptoms return.

The following groups are at risk from recurrent ulcer relapse: those with *Helicobacter pylori* infection, younger patients (<60 years), those whose symptoms persist for more than one year and smokers. These patients will require initial long-term therapy with Losec MUPS 20 mg once daily, reducing to 10 mg once daily, if necessary.

***Helicobacter pylori* (*Hp*) eradication regimens in peptic ulcer disease:** Losec MUPS is recommended at a dose of 40 mg once daily or 20 mg twice daily in association with antimicrobial agents as detailed below:

Triple therapy regimens in duodenal ulcer disease:
Losec MUPS and the following antimicrobial combinations:

Amoxicillin 500 mg and metronidazole 400 mg both three times a day for one week

or

Clarithromycin 250 mg and metronidazole 400 mg (or tinidazole 500 mg) both twice a day for one week

or

Amoxicillin 1 g and clarithromycin 500 mg both twice a day for one week.

Dual therapy regimens in duodenal ulcer disease:
Losec MUPS and amoxicillin 750 mg to 1 g twice daily for two weeks. Alternatively Losec MUPS and clarithromycin 500mg three times a day for two weeks.

Dual therapy regimens in gastric ulcer disease:
Losec MUPS and amoxicillin 750mg to 1g twice daily for two weeks

In each regimen if symptoms return and the patient is *Hp* positive, therapy may be repeated or one of the alternative regimens can be used; if the patient is *Hp* negative then see dosage instructions for acid reflux disease.

To ensure healing in patients with active peptic ulcer disease, see further dosage recommendations for duodenal and benign gastric ulcer.

Prophylaxis of acid aspiration: For patients considered to be at risk of aspiration of the gastric contents during general anaesthesia, the recommended dosage is Losec MUPS 40 mg on the evening before surgery followed by Losec MUPS 40 mg 2–6 hours prior to surgery.

Zollinger-Ellison syndrome: The recommended initial dosage is 60 mg Losec MUPS once daily. The dosage should be adjusted individually and treatment continued as long as clinically indicated. More than 90% of patients with severe disease and inadequate response to other therapies have been effectively controlled on doses of 20–120 mg daily. With doses above 80 mg daily, the dose should be divided and given twice daily.

10 mg and 20 mg tablets only:

Acid-related dyspepsia: The usual dosage is Losec MUPS 10 mg or 20 mg once daily for 2–4 weeks depending on the severity and persistence of symptoms. Patients who do not respond after 4 weeks or who relapse shortly afterwards, should be investigated.

For the treatment of NSAID-associated gastric ulcers, duodenal ulcers or gastroduodenal erosions: The recommended dosage of Losec MUPS is 20 mg once daily. Symptom resolution is rapid and in most patients healing occurs within 4 weeks. For those patients who may not be fully healed after the initial course, healing usually occurs during a further 4 weeks treatment.

For the prophylaxis of NSAID-associated gastric ulcers, duodenal ulcers, gastroduodenal erosions and dyspeptic symptoms in patients with a previous history of gastroduodenal lesions who require continued NSAID treatment: The recommended dosage of Losec MUPS is 20 mg once daily.

Elderly: Dose adjustment is not required in the elderly.

Children:

Reflux oesophagitis

The treatment time is 4–8 weeks.

Symptomatic treatment of heartburn and acid regurgitation in gastroesophageal reflux disease

The treatment time is 2-4 weeks. If symptom control has not been achieved after 2-4 weeks the patient should be investigated further.

The dosage recommendations are as follows:

Age	Weight	Dosage
⩾ 1 year of age	10-20 kg	10 mg once daily The dosage can be increased to 20 mg once daily if needed.
⩾ 2 years of age	> 20 kg	20 mg once daily The dosage can be increased to 40 mg once daily if needed

Children over 4 years of age

In combination with antibiotics in treatment of duodenal ulcer caused by Helicobacter pylori. When selecting appropriate combination therapy consideration should be given to official local guidance regarding bacterial resistance, duration of treatment (most commonly 7 days but sometimes up to 14 days), and appropriate use of antibacterial agents. The treatment should be supervised by a specialist.

Weight	Dosage
15-⩽30 kg	Combination with two antibiotics: Losec Mups 10 mg, amoxicillin 25mg/kg body weight and clarithromycin 7,5 mg/kg body weight are all administered together 2 times daily for 1 week
30-⩽40 kg	Combination with two antibiotics: Losec Mups 20 mg, amoxicillin 750 mg and clarithromycin 7.5 mg/kg body weight are all administered 2 times daily for 1 week.
>40 kg	Combination with two antibiotics: Losec Mups 20 mg, amoxicillin 1 g and clarithromycin 500 mg are all administered 2 times daily for 1 week.

Impaired renal function: Dose adjustment is not required in patients with impaired renal function.

Impaired hepatic function: As bioavailability and half-life can increase in patients with impaired hepatic function, the dose requires adjustment with a maximum daily dose of 20 mg.

For patients (including children aged 1 year and above who can drink or swallow semi-solid food) who are unable to swallow Losec MUPS tablets: The tablets may be dispersed in 10 ml of non-carbonated water and then suspended in a small amount of any fruit juice with a pH less than 5 e.g. apple, orange, pineapple or in apple-sauce or yoghurt after gentle mixing. Do not use milk or carbonated water. The dispersion should be taken immediately or within 30 minutes. Stir the dispersion just before drinking and rinse it down with half a glass of water. There is no evidence to support the use of sodium bicarbonate buffer as a delivery form. It is important that the tablets should not be crushed or chewed.

4.3 Contraindications
Known hypersensitivity to omeprazole or to any of the other constituents of the formulation.

When gastric ulcer is suspected, the possibility of malignancy should be excluded before treatment with Losec MUPS is instituted, as treatment may alleviate symptoms and delay diagnosis.

Omeprazole like other PPIs should not be administered with atazanavir (see section 4.5).

4.4 Special warnings and precautions for use
When treatment with Losec MUPS tablets is instituted, patients on previous Losec capsules therapy should be monitored for any reports of 'flare up' of disease symptoms.

Decreased gastric acidity due to any means including proton pump inhibitors, increases gastric counts of bacteria normally present in the gastrointestinal tract. Treatment with acid-reducing drugs may lead to slightly increased risk of gastrointestinal infections such as *Salmonella* or *Campylobacter*.

Some children with chronic illnesses may require long-term treatment although it is not recommended.

4.5 Interaction with other medicinal products and other forms of interaction
Due to the decreased intragastric acidity, the absorption of ketoconazole or itraconazole may be reduced during omeprazole treatment as it is during treatment with other acid secretion inhibitors.

As omeprazole it is metabolised in the liver through cytochrome P450 it can prolong the elimination of diazepam, phenytoin, warfarin and other vitamin K antagonists which are in part substrates for this enzyme.

Monitoring of patients receiving phenytoin is recommended and a reduction of the phenytoin dose may be necessary. However concomitant treatment with omeprazole 20 mg daily did not change the blood concentration of phenytoin in patients on continuous treatment with phenytoin. In patients receiving warfarin or other vitamin K antagonists, monitoring of INR is recommended and a reduction of the warfarin (or other vitamin K antagonist) dose maybe necessary. Concomitant treatment with omeprazole 20 mg daily did, however, not change coagulation time in patients on continuous treatment with warfarin.

Plasma concentrations of omeprazole and clarithromycin are increased during concomitant administration. This is considered to be a useful interaction during *H. pylori* eradication. There is no interaction with metronidazole or amoxicillin. These antimicrobials are used together with omeprazole for eradication of *Helicobacter pylori* .

There is no evidence of an interaction with phenacetin, theophylline, caffeine, propranolol, metoprolol, cyclosporin, lidocaine, quinidine, estradiol or antacids. The absorption of omeprazole is not affected by alcohol or food.

There is no evidence of an interaction with piroxicam, diclofenac or naproxen. This is considered useful when patients are required to continue these treatments.

Simultaneous treatment with omeprazole and digoxin in healthy subjects lead to a 10% increase in the bioavailability of digoxin as a consequence of the increased intragastric pH.

Co-administration of omeprazole (40mg once daily) with atazanavir 300 mg/ritonavir 100mg to healthy volunteers resulted in a substantial reduction in atazanavir exposure (approximately 75% decrease in AUC, Cmax, and Cmin). Increasing the atazanavir dose to 400mg did not compensate for the impact of omeprazole on atazanavir exposure. PPIs including omeprazole should not be co-administered with atazanavir (see section 4.3)

Concomitant administration of omeprazole and tacrolimus may increase the serum levels of tacrolimus.

Concomitant administration of omeprazole and a CYP2C19 and CYP3A4 inhibitor, voriconazole, resulted in more than doubling of the omeprazole exposure. Omeprazole (40 mg once daily) increased voriconazole (a CYP2C19 substrate) C_{max} and AUC_{τ} by 15% and 41%, respectively. A dose adjustment of omeprazole is not regularly required in either of these situations. However, dose adjustment should be considered in patients with severe hepatic impairment and if long-term treatment is indicated.

4.6 Pregnancy and lactation

Pregnancy

Results from three prospective epidemiological studies indicate no adverse effects of omeprazole on pregnancy or on the health of the foetus/newborn child. Losec can be used during pregnancy.

Lactation

Omeprazole is excreted in breast milk but is not likely to influence the child when therapeutic doses are used.

4.7 Effects on ability to drive and use machines

No effects are foreseen.

4.8 Undesirable effects

Omeprazole is well tolerated and adverse reactions have generally been mild and reversible. The following have been reported as adverse events in clinical trials or reported from routine use, but in many cases a relationship to treatment with omeprazole has not been established.

The following definitions of frequencies are used:

Common $\geq$ 1/100

Uncommon $\geq$ 1/1000 and < 1/100

Rare < 1/1000

Common	*Central and peripheral nervous system*	Headache
	Gastrointestinal	Diarrhoea, constipation, abdominal pain, nausea/vomiting and flatulence
Uncommon	*Central and peripheral nervous system*	Dizziness, paraesthesia, light headedness, feeling faint, somnolence, insomnia and vertigo
	Hepatic	Increased liver enzymes
	Skin	Rash, dermatitis and/or pruritus, urticaria
	Other	Malaise
Rare	*Central and peripheral nervous system*	Reversible mental confusion, agitation, aggression, depression and hallucinations, predominantly in severely ill patients
	Endocrine	Gynaecomastia
	Gastrointestinal	Dry mouth, stomatitis and gastrointestinal candidiasis
	Haematological	Leukopenia, thrombocytopenia, agranulocytosis and pancytopenia
	Hepatic	Encephalopathy in patients with pre-existing severe liver disease, hepatitis with or without jaundice, hepatic failure
	Musculoskeletal	Arthritic and myalgic symptoms and muscular weakness
	Reproductive system and breast disorders	Impotence
	Skin	Photosensitivity, bullous eruption erythema multiforme, Stevens-Johnson syndrome, toxic epidermal necrolysis (TEN), alopecia
	Other	Hypersensitivity reactions e.g. angioedema, fever, bronchospasm, interstitial nephritis and anaphylactic shock [3]. Increased sweating, peripheral oedema, blurred vision, taste disturbance and hyponatraemia

The safety of omeprazole has been assessed in a total of 310 children aged 0 to 16 years with acid-related disease. There are limited long term safety data from 46 children who received maintenance therapy of omeprazole during a clinical study for severe erosive oesophagitis for up to 749 days. The adverse event profile was generally the same as for adults in short- as well as in long-term treatment. There are no long term data regarding the effects of omeprazole treatment on puberty and growth.

4.9 Overdose

Rare reports have been received of overdosage with omeprazole. In the literature, doses of up to 560 mg have been described and occasional reports have been received when single oral doses have reached up to 2400 mg omeprazole (120 times the usual recommended clinical dose). Nausea, vomiting, dizziness, abdominal pain, diarrhoea and headache have been reported from overdosage with omeprazole. Also apathy, depression and confusion have been described in single cases.

The symptoms described in connection to omeprazole overdosage have been transient, and no serious outcome due to omeprazole has been reported. The rate of elimination was unchanged (first order kinetics) with increased doses and no specific treatment has been needed.

5. PHARMACOLOGICAL PROPERTIES

5.1 Pharmacodynamic properties

Omeprazole reduces gastric acid secretion through a unique mechanism of action. It is a specific inhibitor of the gastric proton pump in the parietal cell. It is rapidly acting and produces reversible control of gastric acid secretion with once daily dosing.

Oral dosing with 20 mg Losec MUPS once daily, provides for rapid and effective inhibition of gastric acid secretion with maximum effect being achieved within 4 days of treatment. In duodenal ulcer patients, a mean decrease of approximately 80% in 24 hour intragastric acidity is then maintained, with the mean decrease in peak acid output after pentagastrin stimulation being about 70%, 24 hours after dosing with omeprazole.

Clinical data for omeprazole in the prophylaxis of NSAID induced gastroduodenal lesions are derived from clinical studies of up to 6 months duration.

Helicobacter pylori (*Hp*) is associated with acid peptic disease including duodenal ulcer (DU) and gastric ulcer (GU) in which about 95% and 80% of patients respectively are infected with this bacterium. *Hp* is implicated as a major contributing factor in the development of gastritis and ulcers in such patients. Recent evidence also suggests a causative link between *Hp* and gastric carcinoma.

Omeprazole has been shown to have a bactericidal effect on *Hp in vitro*.

Eradication of *Hp* with omeprazole and antimicrobials is associated with rapid symptom relief, high rates of healing of any mucosal lesions, and long-term remission of peptic ulcer disease thus reducing complications such as gastro-intestinal bleeding as well as the need for prolonged anti-secretory treatment.

In clinical data in patients with acute peptic ulcer, omeprazole *Hp* eradication therapy improved patients' quality of life.

During long-term treatment an increased frequency of gastric glandular cysts have been reported. These changes are a physiological consequence of pronounced inhibition of acid secretion. The cysts are benign and appear to be reversible. No other treatment-related mucosal changes have been observed in patients treated continuously with omeprazole for periods up to 5 years.

Paediatric data

In a non-controlled study in children (1 to 16 years of age) with severe reflux oesophagitis, omeprazole at doses of 0.7 to 1.4 mg/kg improved oesophagitis level in 90 % of the cases and significantly reduced reflux symptoms. In a single-blind study, children aged 0-24 months with clinically diagnosed GERD were treated with 0.5, 1.0 or 1.5 mg omeprazole/kg. The frequency of vomiting/regurgitation episodes decreased by 50 % after 8 weeks of treatment irrespective of the dose.

Eradication of Helicobacter pylori in children:

A randomised, double blind clinical study (Héliot study) has concluded to the efficacy and an acceptable safety for omeprazole associated to two antibiotics (amoxicillin and clarithromycin) in the treatment of Helicobacter pylori infection in children of 4 years old and above with a gastritis: Helicobacter pylori eradication rate: 74.2% (23/31 patients) with omeprazole + amoxicillin + clarithromycin versus 9.4% (3/32 patients) with amoxicillin + clarithromycin. However, there was no evidence of clinical benefit demonstrated regarding dyspeptic symptoms. This study does not support any information for children aged less than 4 years old.

<u>**Site and mechanism of action**</u>

Omeprazole is a weak base and is concentrated and converted to the active form in the acid environment of the intracellular canaliculi within the parietal cell, where it inhibits the enzyme H^+, K^+-ATPase–the proton pump. This effect on the final step of the gastric acid formation process is dose-dependent and provides for effective inhibition of both basal acid secretion and stimulated acid secretion irrespective of the stimulus.

All pharmacodynamic effects observed are explained by the effect of omeprazole on acid secretion.

5.2 Pharmacokinetic properties

<u>**Absorption and distribution**</u>

Omeprazole and omeprazole magnesium are acid labile and are administered orally as enteric-coated granules in capsules or tablets. Bioequivalence between Losec® Capsules and Losec MUPS® Tablets based on the omeprazole plasma concentration-time curve (AUC) has been demonstrated. Absorption of omeprazole takes place in the small intestine and is usually completed within 3–6 hours. The systemic bioavailability of omeprazole from a single oral dose of omeprazole is approximately 35%. After repeated once daily administration, the bioavailability increases to about 60%. Concomitant intake of food has no influence on the bioavailability. The plasma protein binding of omeprazole is about 95%.

<u>**Metabolism and elimination**</u>

The average half-life of the terminal phase of the plasma concentration-time curve is approximately 40 minutes. There is no change in half-life during treatment. The inhibition of acid secretion is related to the area under the plasma concentration-time curve (AUC) but not to the actual plasma concentration at a given time.

Omeprazole is entirely metabolised, mainly in the liver. Identified metabolites in plasma are the sulphone, the sulphide and hydroxy-omeprazole, these metabolites have no significant effect on acid secretion. About 80% of the metabolites are excreted in the urine and the rest in the faeces. The two main urinary metabolites are hydroxy-omeprazole and the corresponding carboxylic acid.

The systemic bioavailability of omeprazole is not significantly altered in patients with reduced renal function. The area under the plasma concentration-time curve is increased in patients with impaired liver function, but no tendency to accumulation of omeprazole has been found.

<u>**Children:**</u> During treatment with the recommended doses to children from the age of 1 year, similar plasma concentrations were obtained as compared to adults. In children younger than 6 months, clearance of omeprazole is low due to low capacity to metabolise omeprazole.

5.3 Preclinical safety data

<u>**Animal Toxicology**</u>

Gastric ECL-cell hyperplasia and carcinoids, have been observed in life-long studies in rats treated with omeprazole or subjected to partial fundectomy.

These changes are the result of sustained hypergastrinaemia secondary to acid inhibition, and not from a direct effect of any individual drug.

6. PHARMACEUTICAL PARTICULARS

6.1 List of excipients

Microcrystalline cellulose

glycerol monostearate

hydroxypropylcellulose

hypromellose

magnesium stearate

methylacrylic acid – ethyl acrylate co-polymer (1:1) dispersion 30 per cent

sugar spheres

synthetic paraffin

macrogol

polysorbate

crospovidone

sodium stearyl fumarate

sodium hydroxide*

talc

triethyl citrate

iron oxide

titanium dioxide.

* May be added as a pH adjuster

6.2 Incompatibilities

None known.

6.3 Shelf life

3 years.

6.4 Special precautions for storage

Do not store above 25°C.

Store in the original container.

6.5 Nature and contents of container

Losec MUPS Tablets are provided in press-through Aluminium-Polyamide-PVC/Aluminium foil calendarised blister packs. Packs of 7, 14, 28, 56 and 560 tablets.

Not all pack sizes may be marketed.

6.6 Special precautions for disposal and other handling

To be dispensed in original containers.

7. MARKETING AUTHORISATION HOLDER

AstraZeneca UK Ltd.,

600 Capability Green,

Luton, LU1 3LU, UK.

8. MARKETING AUTHORISATION NUMBER(S)

PL 17901/0137

PL 17901/0138

PL 17901/0139

9. DATE OF FIRST AUTHORISATION/RENEWAL OF THE AUTHORISATION

14th May 2002/7th June 2006

10. DATE OF REVISION OF THE TEXT

19th February 2008

Lumigan

(Allergan Ltd)

1. NAME OF THE MEDICINAL PRODUCT

LUMIGAN 0.3 mg/ml eye drops, solution

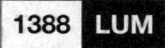

2. QUALITATIVE AND QUANTITATIVE COMPOSITION

One ml of solution contains 0.3 mg bimatoprost.

Excipient: benzalkonium chloride 0.05 mg/ml.

For a full list of excipients, see section 6.1.

3. PHARMACEUTICAL FORM

Eye drops, solution.

Colourless to slightly yellow solution.

4. CLINICAL PARTICULARS

4.1 Therapeutic indications

Reduction of elevated intraocular pressure in chronic open-angle glaucoma and ocular hypertension in adults (as monotherapy or as adjunctive therapy to beta-blockers).

4.2 Posology and method of administration

The recommended dose is one drop in the affected eye(s) once daily, administered in the evening. The dose should not exceed once daily as more frequent administration may lessen the intraocular pressure lowering effect.

If more than one topical ophthalmic medicinal product is being used, each one should be administered at least 5 minutes apart.

Use in children and adolescents (under the age of 18):

LUMIGAN is not recommended for use in children below 18 years, due to a lack of data on safety and efficacy (see sections 5.1 and 5.2).

Use in hepatic and renal impairment:

LUMIGAN has not been studied in patients with renal or moderate to severe hepatic impairment and should therefore be used with caution in such patients. In patients with a history of mild liver disease or abnormal alanine aminotransferase (ALT), aspartate aminotransferase (AST) and/or bilirubin at baseline, LUMIGAN had no adverse effect on liver function over 24 months.

4.3 Contraindications

Hypersensitivity to the active substance or to any of the excipients.

4.4 Special warnings and precautions for use

Before treatment is initiated, patients should be informed of the possibility of eyelash growth, darkening of the eyelid skin and increased iris pigmentation since these have been observed during treatment with LUMIGAN. Some of these changes may be permanent, and may lead to differences in appearance between the eyes when only one eye is treated. The change in iris pigmentation occurs slowly and may not be noticeable for several months or years. At 12 months, the incidence was 1.5% and did not increase following 3 years treatment (see section 4.8). Periorbital tissue pigmentation has been reported to be reversible in some patients.

LUMIGAN contains the preservative benzalkonium chloride, which may be absorbed by soft contact lenses. Contact lenses should be removed prior to instillation and may be reinserted 15 minutes following administration.

Benzalkonium chloride, which is commonly used as a preservative in ophthalmic products, has been reported to cause punctate keratopathy and/or toxic ulcerative keratopathy. Since LUMIGAN contains benzalkonium chloride, monitoring is required with frequent or prolonged use in dry eye patients or where the cornea is compromised.

LUMIGAN has not been studied in patients with compromised respiratory function and should therefore be used with caution in such patients. In clinical studies, in those patients with a history of a compromised respiratory function, no significant untoward respiratory effects have been seen.

LUMIGAN has not been studied in patients with heart block more severe than first degree or uncontrolled congestive heart failure.

LUMIGAN has not been studied in patients with inflammatory ocular conditions, neovascular, inflammatory, angle-closure glaucoma, congenital glaucoma or narrow-angle glaucoma.

Cystoid macular oedema has been uncommonly reported (≥1/1000 to <1/100) following treatment with LUMIGAN and should therefore be used with caution in patients with known risk factors for macular oedema (e.g. aphakic patients, pseudophakic patients with a torn posterior lens capsule).

4.5 Interaction with other medicinal products and other forms of interaction

No interaction studies have been performed.

No interactions are anticipated in humans, since systemic concentrations of bimatoprost are extremely low (less than 0.2 ng/ml) following ocular dosing. Bimatoprost is biotransformed by any of multiple enzymes and pathways, and no effects on hepatic drug metabolising enzymes were observed in preclinical studies.

In clinical studies, LUMIGAN was used concomitantly with a number of different ophthalmic beta-blocking agents without evidence of interactions.

Concomitant use of LUMIGAN and antiglaucomatous agents other than topical beta-blockers has not been evaluated during adjunctive glaucoma therapy.

4.6 Pregnancy and lactation

Pregnancy

There are no adequate data from the use of bimatoprost in pregnant women. Animal studies have shown reproductive toxicity at high maternotoxic doses (see section 5.3).

LUMIGAN should not be used during pregnancy unless clearly necessary.

Lactation

It is unkown whether bimatoprost is excreted in human breast milk. Animal studies have shown excretion of bimatoprost in breast milk. A decision on whether to continue/discontinue breast-feeding or to continue/discontinue therapy with LUMIGAN should be made taking into account the benefit of breast-feeding to the child and the benefit of LUMIGAN therapy to the woman.

4.7 Effects on ability to drive and use machines

LUMIGAN has negligible influence on the ability to drive and use machines. As with any ocular treatment, if transient blurred vision occurs at instillation, the patient should wait until the vision clears before driving or using machinery.

4.8 Undesirable effects

In clinical studies, over 1800 patients have been treated with LUMIGAN. On combining the data from phase III monotherapy and adjunctive LUMIGAN usage, the most frequently reported treatment-related adverse events were: growth of eyelashes in up to 45% in the first year with the incidence of new reports decreasing to 7% at 2 years and 2% at 3 years, conjunctival hyperaemia (mostly trace to mild and thought to be of a non-inflammatory nature) in up to 44% in the first year with the incidence of new reports decreasing to 13% at 2 years and 12% at 3 years and ocular pruritus in up to 14% of patients in the first year with the incidence of new reports decreasing to 3% at 2 years and 0% at 3 years. Less than 9% of patients discontinued due to any adverse event in the first year with the incidence of additional patient discontinuations being 3% at both 2 and 3 years.

The following undesirable effects definitely, probably or possibly related to treatment were reported during clinical trials with LUMIGAN. Most were ocular, mild to moderate, and none was serious:

Very common (≥1/10); common (≥1/100 to <1/10); uncommon (≥1/1,000 to <1/100); rare (≥1/10,000 to <1/1,000); very rare (<1/10,000) and not known (cannot be estimated from available data) undesirable effects are presented according to System Organ Class in Table 1. Within each frequency grouping, undesirable effects are presented in order of decreasing seriousness.

System Organ class	Frequency	Undesirable effect
Nervous system disorders	common	headache
	uncommon	dizziness
Eye disorders	very common	conjunctival hyperaemia, ocular pruritus, growth of eyelashes
	common	superficial punctate keratitis, corneal erosion, ocular burning, ocular irritation, allergic conjunctivitis, blepharitis, worsening of visual acuity, asthenopia, conjunctival oedema, foreign body sensation, ocular dryness, eye pain, photophobia, tearing, eye discharge, visual disturbance, increased iris pigmentation, eyelash darkening.
	uncommon	retinal haemorrhage, uveitis, cystoid macular oedema, iritis, blepharospasm, eyelid retraction
	not known	enophthalmos
Vascular disorders	common	hypertension
Gastrointestinal disorders	uncommon	nausea
Skin and subcutaneous tissue disorders	common	eyelid erythema, eyelid pruritus, pigmentation of periocular skin
	uncommon	eyelid oedema, hirsutism.
General disorders and administration site conditions	uncommon	asthenia
Investigations	common	liver function test abnormal

4.9 Overdose

No case of overdose has been reported, and is unlikely to occur after ocular administration.

If overdosage occurs, treatment should be symptomatic and supportive. If LUMIGAN is accidentally ingested, the following information may be useful: in two-week oral rat and mouse studies, doses up to 100 mg/kg/day did not produce any toxicity. This dose expressed as mg/m^2 is at least 70-times higher than the accidental dose of one bottle of LUMIGAN in a 10 kg child.

5. PHARMACOLOGICAL PROPERTIES

5.1 Pharmacodynamic properties

Pharmacotherapeutic group: other antiglaucoma preparations;

ATC code: S01EE03

The mechanism of action by which bimatoprost reduces intraocular pressure in man is by increasing aqueous humour outflow through the trabecular meshwork and enhancing uveoscleral outflow. Reduction of the intraocular pressure starts approximately 4 hours after the first administration and maximum effect is reached within approximately 8 to 12 hours. The duration of effect is maintained for at least 24 hours.

Bimatoprost is a potent ocular hypotensive agent. It is a synthetic prostamide, structurally related to prostaglandin $F_{2\alpha}$ ($PGF_{2\alpha}$), that does not act through any known prostaglandin receptors. Bimatoprost selectively mimics the effects of newly discovered biosynthesised substances called prostamides. The prostamide receptor, however, has not yet been structurally identified.

During 12 months' monotherapy treatment in adults, versus timolol, mean change from baseline in morning (08:00) intraocular pressure ranged from -7.9 to -8.8 mm Hg. At any visit, the mean diurnal IOP values measured over the 12-month study period differed by no more than 1.3 mmHg throughout the day and were never greater than 18.0 mmHg.

In a 6-month clinical study, versus latanoprost, a statistically superior reduction in morning mean IOP (ranging from -7.6 to -8.2 mmHg for bimatoprost versus –6.0 to –7.2 mmHg for latanoprost) was observed at all visits throughout the study. Conjunctival hyperaemia, growth of eyelashes, and eye pruritus were statistically significantly higher with bimatoprost than with latanoprost, however, the discontinuation rates due to adverse events were low with no statistically significant difference.

Compared to treatment with beta-blocker alone, adjunctive therapy with beta-blocker and bimatoprost lowered mean morning (08:00) intraocular pressure by -6.5 to -8.1 mmHg.

Limited experience is available with the use in patients with open-angle glaucoma with pseudoexfoliative and pigmentary glaucoma, and chronic angle-closure glaucoma with patent iridotomy.

No clinically relevant effects on heart rate and blood pressure have been observed in clinical trials.

5.2 Pharmacokinetic properties

Bimatoprost penetrates the human cornea and sclera well *in vitro*. After ocular administration, the systemic exposure of bimatoprost is very low with no accumulation over time. After once daily ocular administration of one drop of 0.03% bimatoprost to both eyes for two weeks, blood concentrations peaked within 10 minutes after dosing and declined to below the lower limit of detection (0.025 ng/ml) within 1.5 hours after dosing. Mean C_{max} and AUC $_{0\text{-}24hrs}$ values were similar on days 7 and 14 at approximately 0.08 ng/ml and 0.09 ng•hr/ml respectively, indicating that a steady bimatoprost concentration was reached during the first week of ocular dosing.

Bimatoprost is moderately distributed into body tissues and the systemic volume of distribution in humans at steady-state was 0.67 l/kg. In human blood, bimatoprost resides mainly in the plasma. The plasma protein binding of bimatoprost is approximately 88%.

Bimatoprost is the major circulating species in the blood once it reaches the systemic circulation following ocular dosing. Bimatoprost then undergoes oxidation, N-deethylation and glucuronidation to form a diverse variety of metabolites.

Bimatoprost is eliminated primarily by renal excretion, up to 67% of an intravenous dose administered to healthy adult volunteers was excreted in the urine, 25% of the dose was excreted via the faeces. The elimination half-life, determined after intravenous administration, was approximately 45 minutes; the total blood clearance was 1.5 l/hr/kg.

Characteristics in elderly patients:

After twice daily dosing, the mean $AUC_{0\text{-}24hr}$ value of 0.0634 ng•hr/ml bimatoprost in the elderly (subjects 65 years or older) were significantly higher than 0.0218 ng•hr/

ml in young healthy adults. However, this finding is not clinically relevant as systemic exposure for both elderly and young subjects remained very low from ocular dosing. There was no accumulation of bimatoprost in the blood over time and the safety profile was similar in elderly and young patients.

5.3 Preclinical safety data
Effects in non-clinical studies were observed only at exposures considered sufficiently in excess of the maximum human exposure indicating little relevance to clinical use.

Monkeys administered ocular bimatoprost concentrations of ⩾0.03% daily for 1 year had an increase in iris pigmentation and reversible dose-related periocular effects characterised by a prominent upper and/or lower sulcus and widening of the palpebral fissure. The increased iris pigmentation appears to be caused by increased stimulation of melanin production in melanocytes and not by an increase in melanocyte number. No functional or microscopic changes related to the periocular effects have been observed, and the mechanism of action for the periocular changes is unknown.

Bimatoprost was not mutagenic or carcinogenic in a series of *in vitro* and *in vivo* studies.

Bimatoprost did not impair fertility in rats up to doses of 0.6 mg/kg/day (approximately 103-times the intended human exposure). In embryo/foetal developmental studies abortion, but no developmental effects were seen in mice and rats at doses that were at least 860-times or 1700-times higher than the dose in humans, respectively. These doses resulted in systemic exposures of at least 33- or 97-times higher, respectively, than the intended human exposure. In rat peri/postnatal studies, maternal toxicity caused reduced gestation time, foetal death, and decreased pup body weights at ⩾0.3 mg/kg/day (at least 41-times the intended human exposure). Neurobehavioural functions of offspring were not affected.

6. PHARMACEUTICAL PARTICULARS
6.1 List of excipients
Benzalkonium chloride
Sodium chloride
Sodium phosphate dibasic heptahydrate
Citric acid monohydrate
Hydrochloric acid or sodium hydroxide (to adjust pH)
Purified water

6.2 Incompatibilities
Not applicable.

6.3 Shelf life
2 years.

Chemical and physical in-use stability has been demonstrated for 28 days at 25°C.

From a microbiological point of view, the in-use storage times and conditions are the responsibility of the user and would normally not be longer than 28 days at 25°C.

6.4 Special precautions for storage
This medicinal product does not require any special storage conditions.

6.5 Nature and contents of container
White opaque low density polyethylene bottles with polystyrene screw cap. Each bottle has a fill volume of 3 ml.

The following pack sizes are available: cartons containing 1 or 3 bottles of 3 ml. Not all pack sizes may be marketed.

6.6 Special precautions for disposal and other handling
No special requirements.

7. MARKETING AUTHORISATION HOLDER
Allergan Pharmaceuticals Ireland
Castlebar Road
Westport
Co. Mayo
Ireland

8. MARKETING AUTHORISATION NUMBER(S)
EU/1/02/205/001-002

9. DATE OF FIRST AUTHORISATION/RENEWAL OF THE AUTHORISATION
08 March 2002 / 20 February 2007

10. DATE OF REVISION OF THE TEXT
02 September 2009

Lustral

(Pfizer Limited)

1. NAME OF THE MEDICINAL PRODUCT
LUSTRAL™

2. QUALITATIVE AND QUANTITATIVE COMPOSITION
Each tablet contains Sertraline hydrochloride equivalent to 50 mg or 100 mg sertraline.

3. PHARMACEUTICAL FORM
Film-coated tablet

50mg white, capsular shaped, film-coated scored tablets coded 'ZLT-50' on one side and 'PFIZER' on the other.

100mg white, capsular shaped, film-coated tablets coded 'ZLT-100' on one side and 'PFIZER' on the other.

4. CLINICAL PARTICULARS
4.1 Therapeutic indications
Lustral is indicated for the treatment of symptoms of depressive illness, including accompanying symptoms of anxiety. Following satisfactory response, continuation with Lustral therapy is effective in preventing relapse of the initial episode of depression or recurrence of further depressive episodes, including accompanying symptoms of anxiety.

Lustral is also indicated for the treatment of obsessive compulsive disorder (OCD). Following initial response, Lustral has been associated with sustained efficacy, safety and tolerability in up to two years treatment of OCD.

Lustral is also indicated for the treatment of paediatric patients with OCD.

Clinical trials in PTSD demonstrated efficacy in female patients but no evidence of efficacy was seen in males. Treatment with Lustral cannot normally therefore be recommended for male patients with PTSD. A therapeutic trial in males might on occasion be justified, but treatment should subsequently be withdrawn unless there is clear evidence of therapeutic benefit.

4.2 Posology and method of administration
Lustral should be given as a single daily dose. Lustral tablets can be administered with or without food.

Adults

Depression (including accompanying symptoms of anxiety): The starting dose is 50mg daily and the usual antidepressant dose is 50mg daily. In some patients, doses higher than 50mg may be required.

Obsessive Compulsive Disorder: The starting dose is 50mg daily, and the therapeutic dose range is 50-200mg daily.

Post-Traumatic Stress Disorder: Treatment for PTSD should be initiated at 25mg/day. After one week, the dose should be increased to 50mg once daily. PTSD is a heterogeneous illness and some patient groups fulfilling the criteria for PTSD do not appear to be responsive to treatment with Lustral. Dosing should be reviewed periodically by the prescribing physician to determine response to therapy and treatment should be withdrawn if there is no clear evidence of efficacy.

Depression (including accompanying symptoms of anxiety), OCD and PTSD: In some patients doses higher than 50mg daily may be required. In patients with incomplete response but good toleration at lower doses, dosage adjustments should be made in 50mg increments over a period of weeks to a maximum of 200mg daily.

Once optimal therapeutic response is achieved the dose should be reduced, depending on therapeutic response, to the lowest effective level. Dosage during prolonged maintenance therapy should be kept at the lowest effective level, with subsequent adjustments depending on therapeutic response. The onset of therapeutic effect may be seen within 7 days, although 2-4 weeks (and even longer in OCD) are usually necessary for full activity. A longer treatment period, even beyond 12 weeks in some cases, may be required in the case of a therapeutic trial in PTSD.

Use in children aged 6-17 years with OCD Treatment should only be *initiated* by specialists. The safety and efficacy of Lustral has been established in paediatric OCD patients (aged 6-17). The administration of Lustral to paediatric OCD patients (aged 13-17) should commence at 50 mg/day. Therapy for paediatric OCD patients (aged 6-12) should commence at 25mg/day increasing to 50mg/day after 1 week. Subsequent doses may be increased in case of lack of response in 50mg/day increments up to 200mg/day as needed. However, the generally lower body weights of children compared to adults should be taken into consideration in advancing the dose from 50mg, in order to avoid excessive dosing. Given the 24 hour elimination half-life of sertraline, dose changes should not occur at intervals of less than 1 week.

Children aged less than six years Lustral is not recommended in children under six years of age since safety and efficacy have not been established. See also 'Pharmacological Properties'.

Use in the elderly No special precautions are required. The usual adult dose is recommended. Several hundred elderly patients have participated in clinical studies with Lustral. The pattern and incidence of adverse reactions in the elderly is similar to that in younger patients.

Lustral tablets are for oral administration only.

4.3 Contraindications
Lustral is contra-indicated in patients with a known hypersensitivity to sertraline.

Monoamine oxidase inhibitors: Cases of serious and sometimes fatal reactions have been reported in patients receiving an SSRI in combination with a monoamine oxidase inhibitor (MAOI), including the selective MAOI selegiline and the reversible MAOI (RIMA) moclobemide and in patients who have recently discontinued an SSRI and have been started on a MAOI.

Some cases presented with features resembling serotonin syndrome. Symptoms of a drug interaction with a MAOI include: hyperthermia, rigidity, myoclonus, autonomic instability with possible rapid fluctuations of vital signs, mental status changes that include confusion, irritability and extreme agitation progressing to delirium and coma.

Lustral should not be used in combination with a MAOI. Lustral may be started 14 days after discontinuing treatment with an irreversible MAOI and at least one day after discontinuing treatment with the reversible MAOI (RIMA), moclobemide. At least 14 days should elapse after discontinuing Lustral treatment before starting a MAOI or RIMA.

Use in hepatic impairment: There is insufficient clinical experience in patients with significant hepatic dysfunction and accordingly Lustral should not be used in such patients.

Concomitant use in patients taking pimozide is contra-indicated (see section 4.5 - Interaction with Other Medicaments and Other Forms of Interaction.

4.4 Special warnings and precautions for use
Monoamine oxidase inhibitors See 'Contra-indications'.

Use in patients with renal or hepatic impairment As with many other medications, sertraline should be used with caution in patients with renal and hepatic impairment (see 'Contra-indications').

Since sertraline is extensively metabolised, excretion of unchanged drug in urine is a minor route of elimination. In patients with mild to moderate renal impairment (creatinine clearance 20-50ml/min) or severe renal impairment (creatinine clearance <20ml/min), single dose pharmacokinetic parameters were not significantly different compared with controls. However, steady state pharmacokinetics of sertraline have not been adequately studied in this patient population and caution is advised when treating patients with renal impairment.

Sertraline is extensively metabolised by the liver. A multiple dose pharmacokinetic study in subjects with mild, stable cirrhosis demonstrated a prolonged elimination half-life and approximately three-fold greater AUC and C_{max} in comparison with normal subjects. There were no significant differences in plasma protein binding observed between the two groups. The use of sertraline in patients with hepatic disease should be approached with caution. A lower or less frequent dose should be used in patients with hepatic impairment.

Diabetes In patients with diabetes, treatment with an SSRI may alter glycaemic control, possibly due to improvement of depressive symptoms. Insulin and/or oral hypoglycaemic dosage may be needed to be adjusted.

Seizures Seizures are a potential risk with antidepressant or antiobsessional drugs. The drug should be discontinued in any patient who develops seizures. Lustral should be avoided in patients with unstable epilepsy and patients with controlled epilepsy should be carefully monitored. Lustral should be discontinued if there is an increase in seizure frequency.

Electroconvulsive therapy (ECT) Since there is little clinical experience of concurrent administration of Lustral and ECT, caution is advisable.

Mania Lustral should be used with caution in patients with a history of mania/hypomania. Lustral should be discontinued in any patient entering a manic phase.

Suicide/suicidal thoughts or clinical worsening
Depression is associated with an increased risk of suicidal thoughts, self harm and suicide (suicide-related events). This risk persists until significant remission occurs. As improvement may not occur during the first few weeks or more of treatment, patients should be closely monitored until such improvement occurs. It is general clinical experience that the risk of suicide may increase in the early stages of recovery.

Other psychiatric conditions for which Lustral is prescribed can also be associated with an increased risk of suicide-related events. In addition, these conditions may be co-morbid with major depressive disorder. The same precautions observed when treating patients with major depressive disorder should therefore be observed when treating patients with other psychiatric disorders.

Patients with a history of suicide-related events, or those exhibiting a significant degree of suicidal ideation prior to commencement of treatment are known to be at greater risk of suicidal thoughts or suicide attempts, and should receive careful monitoring during treatment. A meta-analysis of placebo-controlled clinical trials of antidepressant drugs in adult patients with psychiatric disorders showed an increased risk of suicidal behaviour with antidepressants compared to placebo in patients less than 25 years old.

Close supervision of patients and in particular those at high risk should accompany drug therapy especially in early treatment and following dose changes. Patients (and caregivers of patients) should be alerted about the need to monitor for any clinical worsening, suicidal behaviour or thoughts and unusual changes in behaviour and to seek medical advice immediately if these symptoms present.

Haemorrhage There have been reports of cutaneous bleeding abnormalities such as ecchymoses and purpura with SSRIs.

Caution is advised in patients taking SSRIs, particularly in concomitant use with drugs known to affect platelet function (*e.g.* atypical antipsychotics and phenothiazines, most tricyclic antidepressants, aspirin and non-steroidal anti-inflammatory drugs (NSAIDs)) as well as in patients with a history of bleeding disorders.

Use in the elderly Several hundred elderly patients have participated in clinical studies with Lustral. The pattern and incidence of adverse reactions in the elderly is similar to that in younger patients.

Use in children and adolescents under 18 years of age More than 250 paediatric OCD patients have been exposed to Lustral in completed and ongoing studies. The safety profile of Lustral in these paediatric studies is comparable to that observed in the adult OCD studies. The efficacy of Lustral in paediatric patients with depression or panic disorder has not been demonstrated in controlled trials. Safety and effectiveness in paediatric patients below the age of 6 have not been established.

Lustral should not be used in the treatment of children and adolescents under the age of 18 years, except for patients with OCD. Suicide-related behaviours (suicide attempt and suicidal thoughts) and hostility (predominantly aggression, oppositional behaviour and anger) were more frequently observed in clinical trials among children and adolescents treated with antidepressants compared to those treated with placebo. If, based on clinical need, a decision to treat is nevertheless taken, the patient should be carefully monitored for the appearance of suicidal symptoms. In addition, long-term safety data in children and adolescents concerning growth, maturation and cognitive and behavioural development are lacking.

4.5 Interaction with other medicinal products and other forms of interaction

Monoamine oxidase inhibitors See 'Contra-indications'.

Centrally active medication Caution is advised if Lustral is administered with other centrally active medication. In particular, SSRIs have the potential to interact with tricyclic antidepressants leading to an increase in plasma levels of the tricyclic antidepressant. A possible mechanism for this interaction is the inhibitory effect of SSRIs on the CYP2D6 isoenzyme. There is variability among the SSRIs in the extent to which they inhibit the activity of CYP2D6. The clinical significance of this depends on the extent of inhibition and the therapeutic index of the co-administered drug. In formal interaction studies, chronic dosing with sertraline 50mg daily showed minimal elevation (mean 23-37%) of steady state plasma desipramine levels (a marker of CYP2D6 isoenzyme activity).

Pimozide – Increased pimozide levels have been demonstrated in a study of a single low dose pimozide (2mg) with sertraline coadministration. These increased levels were not associated with any changes in ECG. While the mechanism of this interaction is unknown, due to the narrow therapeutic index of pimozide, concomitant of pimozide and sertraline is contra-indicated.

Alcohol In 11 healthy subjects administered Lustral (200mg daily) for 9 days, there was no adverse effect on cognitive or psychomotor performance relative to placebo, following a single dose of 500mg/kg alcohol. However, the concomitant use of Lustral and alcohol in depressed patients is not recommended.

Lithium and Tryptophan In placebo-controlled trials in normal volunteers, the co-administration of Lustral and lithium did not significantly alter lithium pharmacokinetics.

Co-administration of Lustral with lithium did result in an increase in tremor relative to placebo, indicating a possible pharmacodynamic interaction. There have been other reports of enhanced effects when SSRIs have been given with lithium or tryptophan and therefore the concomitant use of SSRIs with these drugs should be undertaken with caution.

Serotonergic drugs There is limited controlled experience regarding the optimal timing of switching from other antidepressant or antiobsessional drugs to Lustral. Care and prudent medical judgement should be exercised when switching, particularly from long-acting agents. The duration of washout period which should intervene before switching from one selective serotonin reuptake inhibitor (SSRI) to another has not been established.

Until further data are available, serotonergic drugs, such as tramadol, sumatriptan or fenfluramine, should not be used concomitantly with Lustral, due to a possible enhancement of 5-HT associated effects.

St John's Wort Concomitant use of the herbal remedy St John's wort (Hypericum perforatum) in patients receiving SSRIs should be avoided since there is a possibility of serotonergic potentiation.

Drugs that affect platelet function, such as NSAIDs See 'Special warnings and special precautions for use (*Haemorrhage*)'.

Other drug interactions Since Lustral is bound to plasma proteins, the potential of Lustral to interact with other plasma protein bound drugs should be borne in mind.

Formal drug interaction studies have been performed with Lustral. Co-administration of Lustral (200mg daily) with diazepam or tolbutamide resulted in small, statistically significant changes in some pharmacokinetic parameters. Co-administration with cimetidine caused a substantial decrease in sertraline clearance. The clinical significance of these changes is unknown. Lustral had no effect on the beta-adrenergic blocking ability of atenolol. No interaction with Lustral (200mg daily) was observed with glibenclamide or digoxin.

Co-administration of Lustral (200mg daily) with warfarin resulted in a small but statistically significant increase in prothrombin time, the clinical significance of which is unknown. Accordingly, prothrombin time should be carefully monitored when Lustral therapy is initiated or stopped.

Lustral (200mg daily), did not potentiate the effects of carbamazepine, haloperidol or phenytoin on cognitive and psychomotor performance in healthy subjects.

4.6 Pregnancy and lactation

Pregnancy Although animal studies did not provide any evidence of teratogenicity, the safety of Lustral during human pregnancy has not been established. As with all drugs Lustral should only be used in pregnancy if the potential benefits of treatment to the mother outweigh the possible risks to the developing foetus.

In a retrospective case-control study the risk for developing persistent pulmonary hypertension in the newborn (PPHN) was approximately six-fold higher for infants exposed to SSRIs after the 20th week of gestation compared to infants who had not been exposed. There is currently no corroborative evidence regarding the risk of PPHN following exposure to SSRIs in pregnancy.

Lactation Lustral is known to be excreted in breast milk. Its effects on the nursing infant have not yet been established. If treatment with Lustral is considered necessary, discontinuation of breast feeding should be considered.

4.7 Effects on ability to drive and use machines

Clinical pharmacology studies have shown that Lustral has no effect on psychomotor performance. However, since antidepressant or antiobsessional drugs may impair the abilities required to perform potentially hazardous tasks such as driving a car or operating machinery, the patient should be cautioned accordingly. Lustral should not be administered with benzodiazepines or other tranquillizers in patients who drive or operate machinery.

4.8 Undesirable effects

Side-effects which occurred significantly more frequently with sertraline than placebo in multiple dose studies were: nausea, diarrhoea/loose stools, anorexia, dyspepsia, tremor, dizziness, insomnia, somnolence, increased sweating, dry mouth and sexual dysfunction (principally ejaculatory delay in males).

The side-effect profile commonly observed in double-blind, placebo-controlled studies in patients with OCD and PTSD was similar to that observed in patients with depression.

In paediatric OCD patients, side-effects which occurred significantly more frequently with sertraline than placebo were: headache, insomnia, agitation, anorexia, tremor. Most were of mild to moderate severity.

Cases of suicidal ideation and suicidal behaviours have been reported during Lustral therapy or early after treatment discontinuation (see section 4.4)

Post-marketing spontaneous reports include the following:

Cardiovascular Blood pressure disturbances including postural hypotension, tachycardia.

Eye disorders Abnormal vision.

Gastro-intestinal Vomiting, abdominal pain.

Nervous system Amnesia, headache, drowsiness, movement disorders, paraesthesia, hypoaesthesia, depressive symptoms, hallucinations, aggressive reaction, agitation, anxiety, psychosis, depersonalisation, nervousness, panic reaction and signs and symptoms associated with serotonin syndrome which include fever, rigidity, confusion, agitation, diaphoresis, tachycardia, hypertension and diarrhoea.

There have also been reports of manic reaction, although this phenomenon may be part of the underlying disease.

Convulsions (Seizures) Lustral should be discontinued in any patient who develops seizures (See 'Special warnings and special precautions for use').

Musculoskeletal Arthralgia, myalgia.

Hepatic/pancreatic Rarely, pancreatitis and serious liver events (including hepatitis, jaundice and liver failure). Asymptomatic elevations in serum transaminases (SGOT and SGPT) have been reported in association with sertraline administration (0.8 – 1.3%), with an increased risk associated with the 200mg daily dose. The abnormalities usually occurred within the first 1 to 9 weeks of drug treatment and promptly diminished upon drug discontinuation.

Renal & urinary disorders Urinary retention.

Reproductive Hyperprolactinemia, galactorrhoea, menstrual irregularities, anorgasmy.

Skin and allergic reactions Rash (including rare reports of erythema multiforme, photosensitivity), angioedema, ecchymoses, pruritus and anaphylactoid reactions.

Metabolic Rare cases of hyponatremia have been reported and appeared to be reversible when sertraline was discontinued. Some cases were possibly due to the syndrome of inappropriate antidiuretic hormone secretion. The majority of reports were associated with older patients, and patients taking diuretics or other medications.

Haematologic There have been rare reports of altered platelet function and/or abnormal clinical laboratory results in patients taking sertraline. While there have been reports of thrombocytopenia, abnormal bleeding or purpura in several patients taking sertraline, it is unclear whether sertraline had a causative role. See also 'Special warnings and special precautions for use'.

General Malaise.

Other Withdrawal reactions have been reported with Lustral. Common symptoms include dizziness, paraesthesia, headache, anxiety and nausea. Abrupt discontinuation of treatment with Lustral should be avoided. The majority of symptoms experienced on withdrawal of Lustral are non-serious and self-limiting.

Adverse events from paediatric Clinical Trials

Lustral has been evaluated in paediatric MDD patients aged 6 – 17 years in two 10 week placebo controlled studies (n=364) and one 24 week open label study. Evidence of efficacy was not adequately demonstrated in the individual studies, however, there was evidence of efficacy in a planned combined study analysis.

The following adverse events were observed in clinical trials in children and adolescents (aged 6 –17 years old) with major depressive disorder and occurred at a frequency of at least 2% and at least twice that of placebo: Anorexia (5.3% vs 1.1%), Dry mouth (2.1% vs 0.5%), Hyperkinesia (2.6% vs 0.5%), Tremor (2.1% vs 0%), Urinary Incontinence (2.1% vs 0%), Diarrhoea (9.5% vs 1.6%), Vomiting (4.2% vs 1.1%) and Agitation (6.3% vs 1.1%). In the trials there were a total of 17 discontinuations due to adverse events (9%) from sertraline and 4 (2.1%) from placebo. The most common reasons for discontinuation, due to adverse events, whether or not related to sertraline, were aggressive reaction (1.6%), agitation (1.6%) and suicidal ideation (1.6%), hyperkinesias (1.1%), suicide attempt (1.1%) and aggravated depression (1.1%).

In the safety analysis, events of suicide attempt were reported in the same number of patients in sertraline (2/189, 1.1%) and placebo (2/184, 1.1%) with an incidence of suicide attempts in sertraline-treated subjects of 1.1% (2 attempts in 2/189 subjects) versus 1.6% in placebo-treated subjects (3 attempts in 2/184 subjects). Suicidal ideation was reported by 3 sertraline treated patients (1.6%) and no placebo treated patients. No causal relationship to sertraline has been established, however, owing to the inherent risk of suicide attempt in patients with MDD, it is recommended to be attentive to the occurrence of suicidal thoughts.

4.9 Overdose

On the evidence available, Lustral has a wide margin of safety in overdose. Overdoses of Lustral alone of up to 8g have been reported. Deaths involving overdoses of Lustral in combination with other drugs and/or alcohol have been reported. Therefore, any overdosage should be treated aggressively.

Symptoms of overdose include serotonin-mediated side-effects such as somnolence, gastrointestinal disturbances (such as nausea and vomiting), tachycardia, tremor, agitation and dizziness. Less frequently reported was coma.

No specific therapy is recommended and there are no specific antidotes to Lustral. Establish and maintain an airway, ensure adequate oxygenation and ventilation. Activated charcoal, which may be used with sorbitol, may be as or more effective than emesis or lavage, and should be considered in treating overdose. Cardiac and vital signs monitoring is recommended along with general symptomatic and supportive measures. Due to the large volume of distribution of sertraline, forced diuresis, dialysis, haemoperfusion and exchange transfusion are unlikely to be of benefit.

5. PHARMACOLOGICAL PROPERTIES

5.1 Pharmacodynamic properties

Sertraline is a potent and specific inhibitor of neuronal serotonin (5-HT) uptake *in vitro* and *in vivo*, but is without affinity for muscarinic, serotonergic, dopaminergic, adrenergic, histaminergic, GABA or benzodiazepine receptors.

Sertraline is devoid of stimulant, sedative or anticholinergic activity or cardiotoxicity in animals.

Unlike tricyclic antidepressants, no weight gain is observed with treatment for depression.

Lustral has not been observed to produce physical or psychological dependence.

Lustral has been evaluated in paediatric OCD patients aged 6 to 17 in a 12 week placebo-controlled study. Therapy for paediatric OCD patients (aged 6-12) commenced at 25mg/day increasing to 50mg/day after 1 week. Side-effects which occurred significantly more frequently with sertraline than placebo were: headache, insomnia, agitation [6-12 years]; insomnia, anorexia, tremor [13-17 years]. There is limited evidence of efficacy and safety beyond 12 weeks of treatment.

5.2 Pharmacokinetic properties

Sertraline exhibits dose proportional pharmacokinetics over a range of 50-200mg. After oral administration of sertraline in man, peak blood levels occur at about 4.5 - 8.4 hours. Daily doses of sertraline achieve steady-state after one week. Sertraline has a plasma half-life of approximately 26 hours with a mean half-life for young and elderly adults ranging from 22-36 hours. Sertraline is approximately 98% bound to plasma proteins. The principal metabolite, N-desmethylsertraline, is inactive in *in vivo* models of depression and has a half-life of approximately 62-104 hours. Sertraline and N-desmethylsertraline are both extensively metabolised in man and the resultant metabolites excreted in faeces and urine in equal amounts. Only a small amount (<0.2%) of unchanged sertraline is excreted in the urine.

The pharmacokinetics of sertraline in paediatric OCD patients have been shown to be comparable with adults (although paediatric patients metabolise sertraline with slightly greater efficiency). However, lower doses may be advisable for paediatric patients given their lower body weights (especially 6-12 years), in order to avoid excessive plasma levels.

A clear relationship between sertraline concentration and the magnitude of therapeutic response has not been established.

The pharmacokinetics of sertraline in elderly patients are similar to younger adults.

Food does not significantly change the bioavailability of Lustral tablets.

5.3 Preclinical safety data

Extensive chronic safety evaluation studies in animals show that sertraline is generally well tolerated at doses that are appreciable multiples of those that are clinically effective.

6. PHARMACEUTICAL PARTICULARS

6.1 List of excipients

Sertraline tablets include the following inert ingredients:

Tablet cores:

calcium hydrogen phosphate

microcrystalline cellulose

hydroxypropylcellulose

sodium starch glycollate

magnesium stearate

Film coating:

Opadry® White

- titanium dioxide (E171)
- hypromellose
- macrogol 400
- polysorbate-80

Opadry® Clear

- hypromellose
- macrogol 400
- macrogol 6000

6.2 Incompatibilities

None.

6.3 Shelf life

5 years.

6.4 Special precautions for storage

None

6.5 Nature and contents of container

Lustral is available as:

Calendar packs of 28 tablets. Aluminium/PVC blister strips, 14 tablets/strip, 2 strips in a carton box.

6.6 Special precautions for disposal and other handling

No special requirements.

7. MARKETING AUTHORISATION HOLDER

Pfizer Limited

Ramsgate Road

Sandwich

Kent CT13 9NJ

United Kingdom

8. MARKETING AUTHORISATION NUMBER(S)

Lustral Tablets 50mg PL 0057/0308

Lustral Tablets 100mg PL 0057/0309

9. DATE OF FIRST AUTHORISATION/RENEWAL OF THE AUTHORISATION

08/01/2009

10. DATE OF REVISION OF THE TEXT

January 2009

LU 27_0 UK

Luveris 75 IU

(Merck Serono)

1. NAME OF THE MEDICINAL PRODUCT

Luveris 75 IU powder and solvent for solution for injection.

2. QUALITATIVE AND QUANTITATIVE COMPOSITION

One vial contains 75 IU of lutropin alfa (recombinant human luteinising hormone {LH}). Lutropin alfa is produced in genetically engineered Chinese hamster ovary (CHO) cells.

For a full list of excipients, see section 6.1.

3. PHARMACEUTICAL FORM

Powder and solvent for solution for injection.

Appearance of the powder: white lyophilised pellet

Appearance of the solvent: clear colourless solution

The pH of the reconstituted solution is 7.5 - 8.5.

4. CLINICAL PARTICULARS

4.1 Therapeutic indications

Luveris in association with a follicle stimulating hormone (FSH) preparation is recommended for the stimulation of follicular development in women with severe Luteinising Hormone (LH) and FSH deficiency. In clinical trials these patients were defined by an endogenous serum LH level <1.2 IU/l.

4.2 Posology and method of administration

Treatment with Luveris should be initiated under the supervision of a physician experienced in the treatment of fertility problems. Self-administration of this medicinal product should only be performed by patients who are well-motivated, adequately trained and with access to expert advice.

In LH and FSH deficient women, the objective of lutropin alfa therapy in association with FSH is to develop a single mature Graafian follicle from which the oocyte will be liberated after the administration of human chorionic gonadotrophin (hCG). Luveris should be given as a course of daily injections simultaneously with FSH. Since these patients are amenorrhoeic and have low endogenous oestrogen secretion, treatment can commence at any time.

Luveris should be adminstered concomitantly with follitropin alfa.

Treatment should be tailored to the individual patient's response as assessed by measuring follicle size by ultrasound and oestrogen response. A recommended regimen commences at 75 IU of lutropin alfa (ie. one vial of Luveris) daily with 75-150 IU FSH.

If an FSH dose increase is deemed appropriate, dose adaptation should preferably be after 7-14 day intervals and preferably by 37.5 IU-75 IU increments. It may be acceptable to extend the duration of stimulation in any one cycle to up to 5 weeks.

When an optimal response is obtained, a single injection of 250 microgram of r-hCH or 5,000 IU to 10,000 IU hCG should be administered 24-48 hours after the last lutropin alfa and FSH injections. The patient is recommended to have coitus on the day of, and on the day following, hCG administration.

Alternatively, intrauterine insemination (IUI) may be performed.

Luteal phase support may be considered since lack of substances with luteotrophic activity (LH/hCG) after ovulation may lead to premature failure of the corpus luteum.

If an excessive response is obtained, treatment should be stopped and hCG withheld. Treatment should recommence in the next cycle at a dose of FSH lower than that of the previous cycle.

Luveris is intended for subcutaneous use. The powder should be reconstituted, immediately prior to use, with the solvent provided.

4.3 Contraindications

Luveris is contraindicated in patients with:

- hypersensitivity to gonadotrophins or to any of the excipients.
- ovarian, uterine, or mammary carcinoma;
- tumours of the hypothalamus and pituitary gland;
- ovarian enlargement or ovarian cyst unrelated to polycystic ovarian disease and of unknown origin;
- gynaecological haemorrhages of unknown origin

Luveris must not be used when a condition exists which would make a normal pregnancy impossible, such as:

- primary ovarian failure
- malformations of sexual organs incompatible with pregnancy
- fibroid tumours of the uterus incompatible with pregnancy

4.4 Special warnings and precautions for use

Before starting treatment, the couple's infertility should be assessed as appropriate and putative contraindications for pregnancy evaluated. In addition, patients should be evaluated for hypothyroidism, adrenocortical deficiency, hyperprolactinemia and pituitary or hypothalamic tumours, and appropriate specific treatment given.

Patients undergoing stimulation of follicular growth are at an increased risk of developing hyperstimulation in view of possible excessive oestrogen response and multiple follicular development.

Ovarian hyperstimulation syndrome (OHSS) can become a serious medical event characterised by large ovarian cysts which are prone to rupture. Excessive ovarian response seldom gives rise to significant hyperstimulation unless hCG is administered to induce ovulation. It is therefore prudent to withhold hCG in such cases and advise the patient to refrain from coitus or use barrier methods for at least 4 days.

Careful monitoring of ovarian response, based on ultrasound is recommended prior to and during stimulation therapy, especially in patients with polycystic ovaries.

In patients undergoing induction of ovulation, the incidence of multiple pregnancies and births is increased compared with natural conception.

When significant risk of OHSS or multiple pregnancies is assumed, treatment discontinuation is advised.

To minimise the risk of OHSS or of multiple pregnancy, ultrasound scans as well as oestradiol measurements are recommended. In anovulation the risk of OHSS is increased by a serum oestradiol level > 900 pg/ml (3300 pmol/l) and by the presence of more than 3 follicles of 14 mm or more in diameter.

Adherence to recommended lutropin alfa and FSH posology and regimen of administration and careful monitoring of therapy will minimise the incidence of ovarian hyperstimulation and multiple pregnancy.

In clinical trials, the medicinal product has been shown to increase the ovarian sensitivity to follitropin alfa. If an FSH dose increase is deemed appropriate, dose adaptation should preferably be at 7-14 day intervals and preferably with 37.5-75 IU increments.

In clinical trials, there have been no reports of hypersensitivity to lutropin alfa.

The incidence of pregnancy wastage by miscarriage or abortion is higher in patients undergoing stimulation of follicular growth for ovulation induction than in the normal population.

Women with a history of tubal disease are at risk of ectopic pregnancy, whether the pregnancy is obtained by spontaneous conception or with fertility treatments. The prevalence of ectopic pregnancy after IVF was reported to be 2 to 5%, as compared to 1 to 1.5% in the general population.

There have been reports of ovarian and other reproductive system neoplasms, both benign and malignant, in women who have undergone multiple drug regimens for infertility treatment. It is not yet established whether or not treatment with gonadotrophins increases the baseline risk of these tumours in infertile women.

The prevalence of congenital malformations after ART may be slightly higher than after spontaneous conceptions. This could be due to parental factors (e.g. maternal age, genetics), ART procedures and multiple pregnancies.

In women with generally recognised risk factors for thrombo-embolic events, such as personal or family history, treatment with gonadotrophins may further increase the risk. In these women, the benefits of gonadotrophin administration need to be weighed against the risks. It should be noted however, that pregnancy itself, as well as OHSS, also carries an increased risk of thrombo-embolic events.

4.5 Interaction with other medicinal products and other forms of interaction

No interaction studies have been performed with lutropin alfa.

Luveris should not be administered as a mixture with other medicinal products, in the same injection, except follitropin alfa for which studies have shown that co-administration does not significantly alter the activity, stability, pharmacokinetic nor pharmacodynamic properties of the active substances.

4.6 Pregnancy and lactation

Luveris should not be administered during pregnancy or lactation.

4.7 Effects on ability to drive and use machines

No studies on the effects on the ability to drive or use machines have been performed.

4.8 Undesirable effects

General description

Lutropin alfa is used for the stimulation of follicular development in association with follitropin alfa. In this context, it is difficult to attribute undesirable effects to any one of the substances used.

In a clinical trial, mild and moderate injection site reactions (bruising, pain, redness, itching or swelling) were reported in 7.4% and 0.9% of the injections, respectively. No severe injection site reactions were reported. To date no systemic allergic reactions have been reported following Luveris administration.

Ovarian hyperstimulation syndrome was observed in less than 6% of patients treated with Luveris. No severe ovarian hyperstimulation syndrome was reported (section 4.4).

In rare instances, adnexal torsion (a complication of ovarian enlargement), and haemoperitoneum have been associated with human menopausal gonadotrophin therapy. Although these adverse reactions were not observed, there is the possibility that they may also occur with Luveris.

Ectopic pregnancy may also occur, especially in women with a history of prior tubal disease.

Adverse reactions

The following convention was used for the frequency (events/ no. of patients): very common (≥1/10), common (≥1/100 to <1/10), uncommon (≥1/1,000 to <1/100), rare (≥1/10,000 to <1/1,000), very rare (<1/10,000), not known (cannot be estimated from the available data).

After best evidence assessment, the following undesirable effects may be observed after administration of Luveris. Within each frequency grouping, undesirable effects are presented in order of decreasing seriousness.

System Organ Class	Common	Very rare
Gastrointestinal disorders	Nausea, abdominal pain, pelvic pain	
Vascular disorders		Thromboembolism, usually associated with severe ovarian hyperstimulation syndrome (OHSS)
General disorders and administration site conditions	Headache, somnolence, injection site reaction	
Reproductive system and breast disorders	Ovarian hyperstimulation syndrome, ovarian cyst, breast pain	

4.9 Overdose

The effects of an overdose of lutropin alfa are unknown, nevertheless there is a possibility that ovarian hyperstimulation syndrome may occur, which is further described in section 4.4.

Single doses of up to 40,000 IU of lutropin alfa have been administered to healthy female volunteers without serious adverse reactions and were well tolerated.

5. PHARMACOLOGICAL PROPERTIES

5.1 Pharmacodynamic properties

Pharmacotherapeutic group: gonadotrophins. ATC code: G03G A07

Lutropin alfa is a recombinant human luteinising hormone, a glycoprotein composed of non-covalently bound α- and β-subunits. Luteinising hormone binds on the ovarian theca (and granulosa) cells and testicular Leydig cells, to a receptor shared with human chorionic gonadotrophin hormone (hCG). This LH/CG transmembrane receptor is a member of the super-family of G protein-coupled receptors; specifically, it has a large extra-cellular domain. *In vitro* the affinity binding of recombinant hLH to the LH/CG receptor on Leydig tumour cells (MA-10) is between that for hCG and that of pituitary hLH, but within the same order of magnitude.

In the ovaries, during the follicular phase, LH stimulates theca cells to secrete androgens, which will be used as the substrate by granulosa cell aromatase enzyme to produce oestradiol, supporting FSH-induced follicular development. At mid-cycle, high levels of LH trigger corpus luteum formation and ovulation. After ovulation, LH stimulates progesterone production in the corpus luteum by increasing the conversion of cholesterol to pregnenolone.

In the stimulation of follicular development in anovulatory women deficient in LH and FSH, the primary effect resulting from administration of lutropin alfa is an increase in oestradiol secretion by the follicles, the growth of which is stimulated by FSH.

In clinical trials, patients were defined by an endogenous serum LH level < 1.2 IU/l as measured in a central laboratory. However, it should be taken into account that there are variations between LH measurements performed in different laboratories.

In these trials the ovulation rate per cycle was 70-75%.

5.2 Pharmacokinetic properties

The pharmacokinetics of lutropin alfa have been studied in pituitary desensitised female volunteers from 75 IU up to 40,000 IU.

The pharmacokinetic profile of lutropin alfa is similar to that of urinary-derived hLH. Following intravenous administration, lutropin alfa is rapidly distributed with an initial half-life of approximately one hour and eliminated from the body with a terminal half-life of about 10-12 hours. The steady state volume of distribution is around 10-14 l. Lutropin alfa shows linear pharmacokinetics, as assessed by AUC which is directly proportional to the dose administered. Total clearance is around 2 l/h, and less than 5% of the dose is excreted in the urine. The mean residence time is approximately 5 hours.

Following subcutaneous administration, the absolute bioavailability is approximately 60%; the terminal half-life is slightly prolonged. The lutropin alfa pharmacokinetics following single and repeated administration of Luveris are comparable and the accumulation ratio of lutropin alfa is minimal. There is no pharmacokinetic interaction with follitropin alfa when administered simultaneously.

5.3 Preclinical safety data

Non clinical data reveal no special hazard for humans based on conventional studies of safety pharmacology, repeated dose toxicity, genotoxicity, carcinogenic potential. As expected from the heterologous protein nature of the hormone, lutropin alfa raised an antibody response in experimental animals after a period that reduced the measurable serum LH levels but did not fully prevent its biological action. No signs of toxicity due to the development of antibodies to lutropin alfa were observed.

At doses of 10 IU/kg/day and greater, repeated administration of lutropin alfa to pregnant rats and rabbits caused impairment of reproductive function including resorption of foetuses and reduced body weight gain of the dams. However, drug-related teratogenesis was not observed in either animal model.

Other studies have shown that lutropin alfa is not mutagenic.

6. PHARMACEUTICAL PARTICULARS

6.1 List of excipients

Sucrose

Disodium phosphate dihydrate

Sodium dihydrogen phosphate monohydrate

Polysorbate 20

Phosphoric acid, concentrated (for pH adjustment)

Sodium hydroxide (for pH adjustment)

Methionine

Nitrogen

Solvent: Water for injection

6.2 Incompatibilities

This medicinal product must not be mixed with other medicinal products except those mentioned in section 6.6.

6.3 Shelf life

3 years.

6.4 Special precautions for storage

Do not store above 25°C. Store in the original package in order to protect from light.

6.5 Nature and contents of container

The powder is packaged in 3 ml neutral colourless glass (type I) vials. The vials are sealed with bromobutyl stoppers protected by aluminium seal rings and flip-off caps. The solvent is packaged either in 2 or 3 ml neutral colourless glass (type I) vials with a Teflon-coated rubber stopper or in 2 ml neutral colourless glass (type I) ampoules.

The product is supplied in packs of 1, 3 or 10 vials with the corresponding number of solvent vials or ampoules. Not all pack sizes may be marketed.

6.6 Special precautions for disposal and other handling

For immediate and single use following first opening and reconstitution.

The powder must be reconstituted with the solvent before use by gentle swirling.

The reconstituted solution should not be administered if it contains particles or is not clear.

Luveris may be mixed with follitropin alfa and co-administered as a single injection.

In this case Luveris should be reconstituted first and then used to reconstitute the follitropin alfa powder.

In order to avoid the injection of large volumes, one vial of Luveris can be reconstituted together with one or two ampoule(s)/vial(s) of follitropin alfa, 37.5 IU, 75 IU or 150 IU, in 1 ml of solvent.

Any unused product or waste material should be disposed of in accordance with local requirements.

7. MARKETING AUTHORISATION HOLDER

Merck Serono Europe Limited,
56 Marsh Wall,
London E14 9TP
United Kingdom

8. MARKETING AUTHORISATION NUMBER(S)

EU/1/00/155/001
EU/1/00/155/002
EU/1/00/155/003
EU/1/00/155/004
EU/1/00/155/005
EU/1/00/155/006

9. DATE OF FIRST AUTHORISATION/RENEWAL OF THE AUTHORISATION

Date of first authorisation: 29th November 2000.

Date of last renewal: 30th November 2005.

10. DATE OF REVISION OF THE TEXT

July 2009

Lyrica Capsules

(Pfizer Limited)

1. NAME OF THE MEDICINAL PRODUCT

LYRICA▼ 25 mg hard capsules
LYRICA▼ 50 mg hard capsules
LYRICA▼ 75 mg hard capsules
LYRICA▼ 100 mg hard capsules
LYRICA▼ 150 mg hard capsules
LYRICA▼ 200 mg hard capsules
LYRICA▼ 225 mg hard capsules
LYRICA▼ 300 mg hard capsules

2. QUALITATIVE AND QUANTITATIVE COMPOSITION

Each hard capsule contains 25 mg, 50 mg, 75 mg, 100 mg, 150 mg, 200 mg, 225 mg or 300 mg of pregabalin.

Excipients:

[25mg] Each hard capsule contains 35mg lactose monohydrate.

[50mg] Each hard capsule also contains 70 mg lactose monohydrate.

[75mg] Each hard capsule also contains 8.25 mg lactose monohydrate.

[100mg] Each hard capsule also contains 11 mg lactose monohydrate.

[150mg] Each hard capsule also contains 16.50 mg lactose monohydrate.

[200mg] Each hard capsule also contains 22 mg lactose monohydrate.

[225mg] Each hard capsule also contains 24.75 mg lactose monohydrate.

[300mg] Each hard capsule also contains 33 mg lactose monohydrate.

For a full list of excipients, see section 6.1.

3. PHARMACEUTICAL FORM

Hard capsule

25 mg capsule: White hard gelatine capsule, marked "Pfizer" on the cap and "PGN 25" on the body with black ink.

50 mg capsule: White hard gelatine capsule, marked "Pfizer" on the cap and "PGN 50" on the body with black ink. The body is also marked with a black band.

75 mg capsule: White and orange hard gelatine capsule, marked "Pfizer" on the cap and "PGN 75" on the body with black ink.

100 mg capsule: Orange hard gelatine capsules, marked "Pfizer" on the cap and "PGN 100" on the body with black ink.

150 mg capsule: White hard gelatine capsule, marked "Pfizer" on the cap and "PGN 150" on the body with black ink.

200 mg capsule: Light orange hard gelatine capsules, marked "Pfizer" on the cap and "PGN 200" on the body with black ink.

225 mg capsule: White and orange hard capsule, marked "Pfizer" on the cap and "PGN 225" on the body with black ink.

300 mg capsule: White and orange hard gelatine capsule, marked "Pfizer" on the cap and "PGN 300" on the body with black ink.

4. CLINICAL PARTICULARS

4.1 Therapeutic indications

Neuropathic pain

Lyrica is indicated for the treatment of peripheral and central neuropathic pain in adults.

Epilepsy

Lyrica is indicated as adjunctive therapy in adults with partial seizures with or without secondary generalisation.

Generalised Anxiety Disorder

LYRICA is indicated for the treatment of Generalised Anxiety Disorder (GAD) in adults.

4.2 Posology and method of administration

The dose range is 150 to 600 mg per day given in either two or three divided doses.

Lyrica may be taken with or without food.

Neuropathic pain

Pregabalin treatment can be started at a dose of 150 mg per day. Based on individual patient response and tolerability, the dosage may be increased to 300 mg per day after an interval of 3 to 7 days, and if needed, to a maximum dose of 600 mg per day after an additional 7-day interval.

Epilepsy

Pregabalin treatment can be started with a dose of 150 mg per day. Based on individual patient response and tolerability, the dosage may be increased to 300 mg per day after 1 week. The maximum dosage of 600 mg per day may be achieved after an additional week.

Generalised Anxiety Disorder

The dose range is 150 to 600 mg per day given as two or three divided doses. The need for treatment should be reassessed regularly.

Pregabalin treatment can be started with a dose of 150 mg per day. Based on individual patient response and tolerability, the dosage may be increased to 300 mg per day after 1 week. Following an additional week the dosage may be increased to 450 mg per day. The maximum dosage of 600 mg per day may be achieved after an additional week.

Discontinuation of pregabalin

In accordance with current clinical practice, if pregabalin has to be discontinued it is recommended this should be done gradually over a minimum of 1 week independent of the indication (see section 4.8).

Patients with renal impairment

Pregabalin is eliminated from the systemic circulation primarily by renal excretion as unchanged drug. As

Formula 1

$$CL_{cr}(ml/min) = \left[\frac{1.23 \times [140 - age(years)] \times weight(kg)}{serum\ creatinine\ (\mu mol/l)}\right] (\times 0.85 \text{ for female patients})$$

pregabalin clearance is directly proportional to creatinine clearance (see section 5.2), dosage reduction in patients with compromised renal function must be individualised according to creatinine clearance (CLcr), as indicated in Table 1 determined using the following formula:

(see Formula 1 above)

Pregabalin is removed effectively from plasma by haemodialysis (50% of drug in 4 hours). For patients receiving haemodialysis, the pregabalin daily dose should be adjusted based on renal function. In addition to the daily dose, a supplementary dose should be given immediately following every 4-hour haemodialysis treatment (see Table 1).

Table 1. Pregabalin dosage adjustment based on renal function

(see Table 1)

Use in patients with hepatic impairment

No dosage adjustment is required for patients with hepatic impairment (see section 5.2).

Use in children and adolescents

Lyrica is not recommended for use in children below the age of 12 years and adolescents (12 - 17 years of age) due to insufficient data on safety and efficacy (see section 5.3).

Use in the elderly (over 65 years of age)

Elderly patients may require a dose reduction of pregabalin due to a decreased renal function (see patients with renal impairment).

4.3 Contraindications

Hypersensitivity to the active substance or to any of the excipients.

4.4 Special warnings and precautions for use

In accordance with current clinical practice, some diabetic patients who gain weight on pregabalin treatment may need to adjust hypoglycaemic medications.

There have been reports in the postmarketing experience of hypersensitivity reactions, including cases of angioedema. Pregabalin should be discontinued immediately if symptoms of angioedema, such as facial, perioral, or upper airway swelling occur.

Pregabalin treatment has been associated with dizziness and somnolence, which could increase the occurrence of accidental injury (fall) in the elderly population. There have also been post marketing reports of loss of consciousness, confusion and mental impairment. Therefore, patients should be advised to exercise caution until they are familiar with the potential effects of the medication.

In controlled studies, a higher proportion of patients treated with pregabalin reported blurred vision than did patients treated with placebo which resolved in a majority of cases with continued dosing. In the clinical studies where ophthalmologic testing was conducted, the incidence of visual acuity reduction and visual field changes was greater in pregabalin-treated patients than in placebo-treated patients; the incidence of fundoscopic changes was greater in placebo-treated patients (See section 5.1).

In the postmarketing experience, visual adverse reactions have also been reported, including vision loss, visual blurring or other changes of visual acuity, many of which were transient. Discontinuation of pregabalin may result in resolution or improvement of these visual symptoms.

Cases of renal failure have been reported and discontinuation of pregabalin did show reversibility of this adverse effect.

There are insufficient data for the withdrawal of concomitant antiepileptic medicinal products, once seizure control with pregabalin in the add-on situation has been reached, in order to reach monotherapy on pregabalin.

After discontinuation of short-term and long-term treatment with pregabalin withdrawal symptoms have been observed in some patients. The following events have been mentioned: insomnia, headache, nausea, diarrhoea, flu syndrome, nervousness, depression, pain, sweating and dizziness. The patient should be informed about this at the start of the treatment.

Concerning discontinuation of long-term treatment of pregabalin there are no data of the incidence and severity of withdrawal symptoms in relation to duration of use and dosage of pregabalin.

There have been post-marketing reports of congestive heart failure in some patients receiving pregabalin. These reactions are mostly seen in elderly cardiovascular compromised patients during pregabalin treatment for a neuropathic indication. Pregabalin should be used with caution in these patients. Discontinuation of pregabalin may resolve the reaction.

Patients with rare hereditary problems of galactose intolerance, the Lapp lactase deficiency or glucose-galactose malabsorption should not take this medicine.

In the treatment of central neuropathic pain due to spinal cord injury the incidence of adverse events in general, CNS adverse events and especially somnolence was increased. This may be attributed to an additive effect due to concomitant medication (e.g. anti-spasticity agents) needed for this condition. This should be considered when prescribing pregabalin in this condition.

Suicidal ideation and behaviour have been reported in patients treated with anti-epileptic agents in several indications. A meta-analysis of randomised placebo controlled trials of anti-epileptic drugs has also shown a small increased risk of suicidal ideation and behaviour. The mechanism of this risk is not known and the available data do not exclude the possibility of an increased risk for pregabalin.

Therefore patients should be monitored for signs of suicidal ideation and behaviours and appropriate treatment should be considered. Patients (and caregivers of patients) should be advised to seek medical advice should signs of suicidal ideation or behaviour emerge.

4.5 Interaction with other medicinal products and other forms of interaction

Since pregabalin is predominantly excreted unchanged in the urine, undergoes negligible metabolism in humans (<2% of a dose recovered in urine as metabolites), does not inhibit drug metabolism *in vitro*, and is not bound to plasma proteins, it is unlikely to produce, or be subject to, pharmacokinetic interactions.

Accordingly, in *in vivo* studies no clinically relevant pharmacokinetic interactions were observed between pregabalin and phenytoin, carbamazepine, valproic acid, lamotrigine, gabapentin, lorazepam, oxycodone or ethanol. Population pharmacokinetic analysis indicated that oral antidiabetics, diuretics, insulin, phenobarbital, tiagabine and topiramate had no clinically significant effect on pregabalin clearance.

Co-administration of pregabalin with the oral contraceptives norethisterone and/or ethinyl oestradiol does not influence the steady-state pharmacokinetics of either substance.

Pregabalin may potentiate the effects of ethanol and lorazepam. In controlled clinical trials, multiple oral doses of pregabalin co-administered with oxycodone, lorazepam, or ethanol did not result in clinically important effects on respiration. In the postmarketing experience, there are reports of respiratory failure and coma in patients taking pregabalin and other CNS depressant medications. Pregabalin appears to be additive in the impairment of cognitive and gross motor function caused by oxycodone.

No specific pharmacodynamic interaction studies were conducted in elderly volunteers. Interaction studies have only been performed in adults.

4.6 Pregnancy and lactation

There are no adequate data on the use of pregabalin in pregnant women.

Studies in animals have shown reproductive toxicity (see section 5.3). The potential risk to humans is unknown. Lyrica should not be used during pregnancy unless clearly necessary (if the benefit to the mother clearly outweighs the potential risk to the foetus). Effective contraception must be used in women of child bearing potential.

It is not known if pregabalin is excreted in the breast milk of humans; however, it is present in the milk of rats. Therefore, breast-feeding is not recommended during treatment with pregabalin.

4.7 Effects on ability to drive and use machines

Lyrica may have minor or moderate influence on the ability to drive and use machines. Lyrica may cause dizziness and somnolence and therefore may influence the ability to drive or use machines. Patients are advised not to drive, operate complex machinery or engage in other potentially hazardous activities until it is known whether this medication affects their ability to perform these activities.

4.8 Undesirable effects

The pregabalin clinical programme involved over 8900 patients who were exposed to pregabalin, of who over 5600 were in double-blind placebo controlled trials. The most commonly reported adverse reactions were dizziness and somnolence. Adverse reactions were usually mild to moderate in intensity. In all controlled studies, the discontinuation rate due to adverse reactions was 12% for patients receiving pregabalin and 5% for patients receiving placebo. The most common adverse reactions resulting in discontinuation from pregabalin treatment groups were dizziness and somnolence.

In the table below all adverse reactions, which occurred at an incidence greater than placebo and in more than one patient, are listed by class and frequency (very common (> 1/10), common (> 1/100, < 1/10), uncommon (>1/1000, <1/100) and rare (<1/1000)). Within each frequency grouping, undesirable effects are presented in order of decreasing seriousness.

The adverse reactions listed may also be associated with the underlying disease and / or concomitant medications.

In the treatment of central neuropathic pain due to spinal cord injury the incidence of adverse events in general, CNS adverse events and especially somnolence was increased (see 4.4)

Additional reactions reported from post-marketing experience are included as Unknown frequency in italics in the list below.

Body System	**Adverse drug reactions**
Infections and Infestations	
Uncommon	Nasopharyngitis
Blood and lymphatic system disorders	
Rare	Neutropenia
Immune system disorders	
Frequency not known	Hypersensitivity, angioedema, allergic reaction
Metabolism and nutrition disorders	
Common	Appetite increased
Uncommon	Anorexia, hypoglycaemia
Psychiatric disorders	
Common	Euphoric mood, confusion, irritability, libido decreased, disorientation, insomnia
Uncommon	Hallucination, panic attack, restlessness, agitation, depression, depressed mood, mood swings, depersonalisation, word finding difficulty, abnormal dreams, libido increased, anorgasmia, apathy
Rare	Disinhibition, elevated mood,
Nervous system disorders	
Very Common	Dizziness, somnolence

Table 1 Pregabalin dosage adjustment based on renal function

Creatinine Clearance (CL_{cr}) (ml/min)	Total Pregabalin Daily dose *		Dose Regimen
	Starting dose (mg/day)	Maximum dose (mg/day)	
⩾ 60	150	600	BID or TID
⩾30 - <60	75	300	BID or TID
⩾15 - <30	25 – 50	150	Once Daily or BID
< 15	25	75	Once Daily
Supplementary dosage following haemodialysis (mg)			
	25	100	Single dose⁺

TID = Three divided doses

BID = Two divided doses

* Total daily dose (mg/day) should be divided as indicated by dose regimen to provide mg/dose

⁺ Supplementary dose is a single additional dose

Common	Ataxia, coordination abnormal, tremor, dysarthria, memory impairment, disturbance in attention, paraesthesia, sedation, balance disorder, lethargy
Uncommon	Syncope, stupor, myoclonus, psychomotor hyperactivity, ageusia, dyskinesia, dizziness postural, intention tremor, nystagmus, cognitive disorder, speech disorder, hyporeflexia, hypoaesthesia, amnesia, hyperaesthesia, burning sensation
Rare	Hypokinesia, parosmia, dysgraphia
Frequency not known	*Loss of consciousness, mental impairment, headache*
Eye disorders	
Common	Vision blurred, diplopia
Uncommon	Visual disturbance, eye swelling, visual field defect, visual acuity reduced, eye pain, asthenopia, dry eye, lacrimation increased
Rare	Peripheral vision loss, oscillopsia, altered visual depth perception, photopsia, eye irritation, mydriasis, strabismus, visual brightness
Frequency not known	*Vision loss, keratitis*
Ear and labyrinth disorders	
Common	Vertigo
Uncommon	Hyperacusis
Cardiac disorders	
Uncommon	Tachycardia, atrioventricular block first degree
Rare	Sinus tachycardia, sinus arrhythmia, sinus bradycardia
Frequency not known	*Congestive heart failure, QT prolongation*
Vascular disorders	
Uncommon	Flushing, hot flushes, hypotension, hypertension
Rare	Peripheral coldness,
Respiratory, thoracic and mediastinal disorders	
Uncommon	Dyspnoea, nasal dryness
Rare	Epistaxis, throat tightness, nasopharyngitis, cough, nasal congestion, rhinitis, snoring
Gastrointestinal disorders	
Common	Vomiting, dry mouth, constipation, flatulence
Uncommon	Abdominal distension, gastrooesophageal reflux disease, salivary hypersecretion, hypoaesthesia oral
Rare	Ascites, pancreatitis, dysphagia
Frequency not known	*Swollen tongue, diarrhoea, nausea*
Skin and subcutaneous tissue disorders	
Uncommon	Rash papular, sweating
Rare	Urticaria, cold sweat
Frequency not known	*Stevens Johnson syndrome, Pruritus*
Musculoskeletal and connective tissue disorders	
Uncommon	Muscle twitching, joint swelling, muscle cramp, myalgia, arthralgia, back pain, pain in limb, muscle stiffness
Rare	Rhabdomyolysis, cervical spasm, neck pain
Renal and urinary disorders	
Uncommon	Urinary incontinence, dysuria
Rare	Renal failure, oliguria
Frequency not known	*Urinary retention*
Reproductive system and breast disorders	
Common	Erectile dysfunction
Uncommon	Ejaculation delayed, sexual dysfunction
Rare	Amenorrhoea, breast discharge, breast pain, dysmenorrhoea, hypertrophy breast
General disorders and administration site conditions	
Common	Gait abnormal, feeling drunk, fatigue, oedema peripheral, oedema,
Uncommon	Fall, chest tightness, asthenia, thirst, pain, feeling abnormal, chills
Rare	Anasarca, pyrexia,
Frequency not known	*Face oedema*
Investigations	
Common	Weight increased
Uncommon	Blood creatine phosphokinase increased, alanine aminotransferase increased, aspartate aminotransferase increased, platelet count decreased
Rare	Blood glucose increased, blood potassium decreased, white blood cell count decreased, blood creatinine increased, weight decreased

After discontinuation of short-term and long-term treatment with pregabalin withdrawal symptoms have been observed in some patients. The following events have been mentioned: insomnia, headache, nausea, diarrhoea, flu syndrome, nervousness, depression, pain, sweating and dizziness. The patient should be informed about this at the start of the treatment.

Concerning discontinuation of long-term treatment of pregabalin there are no data of the incidence and severity of withdrawal symptoms in relation to duration of use and dosage of pregabalin.

4.9 Overdose

In overdoses up to 15 g, no unexpected adverse reactions were reported.

In the post-marketing experience, the most commonly reported adverse events observed when pregabalin was taken in overdose included somnolence, confusional state, agitation, and restlessness.

Treatment of pregabalin overdose should include general supportive measures and may include haemodialysis if necessary (see section 4.2 Table 1).

5. PHARMACOLOGICAL PROPERTIES

5.1 Pharmacodynamic properties

Pharmacotherapeutic group: Antiepileptics, ATC code: N03AX16

The active substance, pregabalin, is a gamma-aminobutyric acid analogue ((S)-3-(aminomethyl)-5-methylhexanoic acid).

Mechanism of action

Pregabalin binds to an auxiliary subunit (α_2-δ protein) of voltage-gated calcium channels in the central nervous system, potently displacing [^{3}H]-gabapentin.

Clinical experience

Neuropathic pain

Efficacy has been shown in studies in diabetic neuropathy and post herpetic neuralgia and spinal cord injury. Efficacy has not been studied in other models of neuropathic pain.

Pregabalin has been studied in 10 controlled clinical studies of up to 13 weeks with twice a day dosing (BID) and up to 8 weeks with three times a day (TID) dosing. Overall, the safety and efficacy profiles for BID and TID dosing regimens were similar.

In clinical trials up to 12 weeks for both peripheral and central neuropathic pain, a reduction in pain was seen by week 1 and was maintained throughout the treatment period.

In controlled clinical trials in peripheral neuropathic pain 35% of the pregabalin treated patients and 18% of the patients on placebo had a 50% improvement in pain score. For patients not experiencing somnolence, such an improvement was observed in 33% of patients treated with pregabalin and 18% of patients on placebo. For patients who experienced somnolence the responder rates were 48% on pregabalin and 16% on placebo.

In the controlled clinical trial in central neuropathic pain 22% of the Pregabalin treated patients and 7% of the patients on placebo had a 50% improvement in pain score.

Epilepsy

Pregabalin has been studied in 3 controlled clinical studies of 12 week duration with either twice a day dosing (BID) or three times a day (TID) dosing. Overall, the safety and efficacy profiles for BID and TID dosing regimens were similar.

A reduction in seizure frequency was observed by Week 1.

Generalised Anxiety Disorder

Pregabalin has been studied in 6 controlled studies of 4-6 week duration, an elderly study of 8 week duration and a long-term relapse prevention study with a double blind relapse prevention phase of 6 months duration.

Relief of the symptoms of GAD as reflected by the Hamilton Anxiety Rating Scale (HAM-A) was observed by Week 1.

In controlled clinical trials (4-8 week duration) 52% of the pregabalin treated patients and 38% of the patients on placebo had at least a 50% improvement in HAM-A total score from baseline to endpoint.

In controlled studies, a higher proportion of patients treated with pregabalin reported blurred vision than did patients treated with placebo which resolved in a majority of cases with continued dosing. Ophthamologic testing (including visual acuity testing, formal visual field testing and dilated funduscopic examination) was conducted in over 3600 patients within controlled clinical trials. In these patients, visual acuity was reduced in 6.5% of patients treated with pregabalin, and 4.8% of placebo-treated patients. Visual field changes were detected in 12.4% of pregabalin-treated, and 11.7% of placebo-treated patients. Funduscopic changes were observed in 1.7% of pregabalin-treated and 2.1% of placebo-treated patients.

5.2 Pharmacokinetic properties

Pregabalin steady-state pharmacokinetics are similar in healthy volunteers, patients with epilepsy receiving anti-epileptic drugs and patients with chronic pain.

Absorption:

Pregabalin is rapidly absorbed when administered in the fasted state, with peak plasma concentrations occurring within 1 hour following both single and multiple dose administration. Pregabalin oral bioavailability is estimated to be ⩾90% and is independent of dose. Following repeated administration, steady state is achieved within 24 to 48 hours. The rate of pregabalin absorption is decreased when given with food resulting in a decrease in C_{max} by approximately 25-30% and a delay in t_{max} to approximately 2.5 hours. However, administration of pregabalin with food has no clinically significant effect on the extent of pregabalin absorption.

Distribution:

In preclinical studies, pregabalin has been shown to cross the blood brain barrier in mice, rats, and monkeys. Pregabalin has been shown to cross the placenta in rats and is present in the milk of lactating rats. In humans, the apparent volume of distribution of pregabalin following oral administration is approximately 0.56 l/kg. Pregabalin is not bound to plasma proteins.

Metabolism:

Pregabalin undergoes negligible metabolism in humans. Following a dose of radiolabelled pregabalin, approximately 98% of the radioactivity recovered in the urine was unchanged pregabalin. The N-methylated derivative of pregabalin, the major metabolite of pregabalin found in urine, accounted for 0.9% of the dose. In preclinical studies, there was no indication of racemisation of pregabalin S-enantiomer to the R-enantiomer.

Elimination:

Pregabalin is eliminated from the systemic circulation primarily by renal excretion as unchanged drug.

Pregabalin mean elimination half-life is 6.3 hours. Pregabalin plasma clearance and renal clearance are directly proportional to creatinine clearance (see section 5.2 Renal impairment).

Dosage adjustment in patients with reduced renal function or undergoing haemodialysis is necessary (see Section 4.2 Table 1).

Linearity / non-linearity:

Pregabalin pharmacokinetics are linear over the recommended daily dose range. Inter-subject pharmacokinetic variability for pregabalin is low (<20%). Multiple dose pharmacokinetics are predictable from single-dose data. Therefore, there is no need for routine monitoring of plasma concentrations of pregabalin.

Pharmacokinetics in special patient groups

Gender

Clinical trials indicate that gender does not have a clinically significant influence on the plasma concentrations of pregabalin.

Renal impairment

Pregabalin clearance is directly proportional to creatinine clearance. In addition, pregabalin is effectively removed from plasma by haemodialysis (following a 4 hour haemodialysis treatment plasma pregabalin concentrations are reduced by approximately 50%). Because renal elimination is the major elimination pathway, dosage reduction in patients with renal impairment and dosage supplementation following haemodialysis is necessary (see section 4.2 Table 1).

Hepatic impairment

No specific pharmacokinetic studies were carried out in patients with impaired liver function. Since pregabalin does not undergo significant metabolism and is excreted predominantly as unchanged drug in the urine, impaired liver function would not be expected to significantly alter pregabalin plasma concentrations.

Elderly (over 65 years of age)

Pregabalin clearance tends to decrease with increasing age. This decrease in pregabalin oral clearance is consistent with decreases in creatinine clearance associated with increasing age. Reduction of pregabalin dose may be required in patients who have age related compromised renal function (see section 4.2 Table 1).

5.3 Preclinical safety data

In conventional safety pharmacology studies in animals, pregabalin was well-tolerated at clinically relevant doses. In repeated dose toxicity studies in rats and monkeys CNS effects were observed, including hypoactivity, hyperactivity and ataxia. An increased incidence of retinal atrophy commonly observed in aged albino rats was seen after long term exposure to pregabalin at exposures ≥ 5 times the mean human exposure at the maximum recommended clinical dose.

Pregabalin was not teratogenic in mice, rats or rabbits. Foetal toxicity in rats and rabbits occurred only at exposures sufficiently above human exposure. In prenatal/postnatal toxicity studies, pregabalin induced offspring developmental toxicity in rats at exposures >2 times the maximum recommended human exposure.

Pregabalin is not genotoxic based on results of a battery of *in vitro* and *in vivo* tests.

Two-year carcinogenicity studies with pregabalin were conducted in rats and mice. No tumours were observed in rats at exposures up to 24 times the mean human exposure at the maximum recommended clinical dose of 600 mg/day. In mice, no increased incidence of tumours was found at exposures similar to the mean human exposure, but an increased incidence of haemangiosarcoma was observed at higher exposures. The non-genotoxic mechanism of pregabalin-induced tumour formation in mice involves platelet changes and associated endothelial cell proliferation. These platelet changes were not present in rats or in humans based on short term and limited long term clinical data. There is no evidence to suggest an associated risk to humans.

In juvenile rats the types of toxicity do not differ qualitatively from those observed in adult rats. However, juvenile rats are more sensitive. At therapeutic exposures, there was evidence of CNS clinical signs of hyperactivity and bruxism and some changes in growth (transient body weight gain suppression). Effects on the oestrus cycle were observed at 5-fold the human therapeutic exposure.

Reduced acoustic startle response was observed in juvenile rats 1-2 weeks after exposure at >2 times the human therapeutic exposure. Nine weeks after exposure, this effect was no longer observable.

6. PHARMACEUTICAL PARTICULARS

6.1 List of excipients

Capsule content:

Lactose monohydrate

Maize starch

Talc

Capsule shell:

Gelatin

Titanium Dioxide (E171)

Sodium Laurilsulphate

Silica, colloidal anhydrous

Purified water

75 mg, 100 mg, 200 mg, 225 mg and 300 mg shells only:

Red Iron Oxide (E172)

Printing Ink:

Shellac

Black Iron Oxide (E172)

Propylene Glycol

Potassium Hydroxide

6.2 Incompatibilities

Not applicable.

6.3 Shelf life

3 years.

6.4 Special precautions for storage

This medicinal product does not require any special storage conditions

6.5 Nature and contents of container

PVC/Aluminium blisters containing 14, 21, 56, 84 or 112 (2 × 56) hard capsules.

100 × 1 hard capsules in PVC/Aluminium perforated unit dose blisters.

HDPE bottle containing 200 hard capsules.

100 hard capsule PVC/Aluminium blister pack (non-perforated)

Not all pack sizes may be marketed

6.6 Special precautions for disposal and other handling

No special requirements.

7. MARKETING AUTHORISATION HOLDER

Pfizer Limited,

Ramsgate Road,

Sandwich,

Kent

CT13 9NJ

UK

8. MARKETING AUTHORISATION NUMBER(S)

EU/1/04/279/001-005

EU/1/04/279/026

EU/1/04/279/036

9. DATE OF FIRST AUTHORISATION/RENEWAL OF THE AUTHORISATION

Date of first authorisation: 06/07/2004

Date of last renewal: 29/05/2009

10. DATE OF REVISION OF THE TEXT

20th August 2009

Detailed information on this product is available on the website of the European Medicines Agency (EMEA) http://www.emea.europa.eu/

11. LEGAL CATEGORY

POM

Lyrinel XL prolonged release tablet

(Janssen-Cilag Ltd)

1. NAME OF THE MEDICINAL PRODUCT

Lyrinel XL 5 mg prolonged release tablet

Lyrinel XL 10 mg prolonged release tablet

2. QUALITATIVE AND QUANTITATIVE COMPOSITION

Each prolonged release tablet contains 5 mg of oxybutynin hydrochloride

Each prolonged release tablet contains 10 mg of oxybutynin hydrochloride

For excipients, see Section 6.1.

3. PHARMACEUTICAL FORM

Prolonged release tablet.

Lyrinel XL 5 mg: Round yellow coloured tablet printed with "5 XL" on one side in black ink.

Lyrinel XL 10 mg: Round pink coloured tablet printed with "10 XL" on one side in black ink.

4. CLINICAL PARTICULARS

4.1 Therapeutic indications

Adults and Elderly

For the symptomatic treatment of urge incontinence and/or increased urinary frequency associated with urgency as may occur in patients with unstable bladder.

Children over the age of 6 years

The symptomatic treatment of detrusor hyperreflexia secondary to a neurogenic condition.

4.2 Posology and method of administration

Dosage

Adults and Elderly

Starting dose: the recommended starting dose is one 5 mg tablet once daily.

Maintenance dose/dose adjustment: In order to achieve a maintenance dose giving an optimal balance of efficacy and tolerability, after at least one week on 5 mg daily, the dose may be increased to 10 mg once daily, with subsequent incremental increases or decreases of 5 mg/day. There should be an interval of at least one week between dose changes.

Maximum dose: in patients requiring a higher dose, the total daily dose should not exceed 20 mg.

For patients currently taking oxybutynin immediate release, clinical judgement should be exercised in selecting the appropriate dose of Lyrinel XL. The dosage should be adjusted to the minimum dose that achieves an optimal balance of efficacy and tolerability, taking into account the current immediate-release dose.

Children over the age of 6 years

Initial dose of 5 mg once a day increased in 5 mg increments up to a maximum of 15 mg once a day.

Lyrinel XL is not recommended for use in children below age of 6 years, due to a lack of data on safety and efficacy (see sections 5.1 and 5.2).

Method of administration

Lyrinel XL must be swallowed whole with the aid of liquid, and must not be chewed, divided, or crushed.

Patients should be advised that the tablet membrane may pass through the gastrointestinal tract unchanged. This has no bearing on the efficacy of the product.

Lyrinel XL may be administered with or without food (see section 5.2).

4.3 Contraindications

- Hypersensitivity to oxybutynin or any of the excipients
- Narrow-angle glaucoma or shallow anterior chamber
- Myasthenia gravis
- Urinary retention
- Gastrointestinal obstructive disorder, paralytic ileus or intestinal atony
- Severe ulcerative colitis
- Toxic megacolon
- Urinary frequency and nocturia due to heart or renal failure
- Porphyria

4.4 Special warnings and precautions for use

Oxybutynin is associated with anticholinergic central nervous system (CNS) effects (see section 4.8 Undesirable Effects). Patients should be monitored for signs of anticholinergic CNS effects, particularly in the first few months after beginning treatment or increasing the dose. If a patient experiences anticholinergic CNS effects, dose reduction or drug discontinuation should be considered.

Oxybutynin should be given with caution in patients with the following conditions:

- hepatic or renal impairment
- clinically significant bladder outflow obstruction since anticholinergic drugs may aggravate bladder outflow and cause retention (see section 4.3)
- gastrointestinal motility disorders (see section 4.3)
- gastroesophageal reflux and/or who are currently taking drugs (such as bisphosphonates) that can cause or exacerbate esophagitis
- pre-existing dementia treated with cholinesterase inhibitors due to risk of aggravation of symptoms.

Oxybutynin should be used with caution in the frail elderly who may be more sensitive to the effects of oxybutynin.

If urinary tract infection is present, an appropriate antibacterial therapy should be started.

Oxybutynin may aggravate the symptoms of hyperthyroidism, congestive heart failure, cardiac arrhythmia, tachycardia, hypertension and prostatic hypertrophy.

When oxybutynin is used in patients with fever or in high environmental temperatures, this can cause heat prostration, or heat stroke, due to decreased sweating.

Patients with rare hereditary problems of galactose intolerance, the Lapp lactase deficiency or glucose-galactose malabsorption should not take this medicine.

Oxybutynin may lead to decreased salivary secretions, which could result in tooth caries, periodontitis, or oral candidiasis.

As oxybutynin may trigger angle-closure glaucoma, visual acuity and intraocular pressure should be monitored periodically during therapy. Patients should be advised to seek advice immediately if they are aware of a sudden loss of visual acuity.

4.5 Interaction with other medicinal products and other forms of interaction

The concomitant use of oxybutynin with other anticholinergic medicinal products or drugs with anticholinergic activity, such as amantadine and other anticholinergic antiparkinsonian drugs (e.g. biperiden, levodopa), antihistamines, antipsychotics (e.g. phenothiazines, butyrophenones, clozapine), quinidine, tricyclic antidepressants, atropine and related compounds like atropinic antispasmodics, dipyridamole, may increase the frequency or severity of dry mouth, constipation and drowsiness.

Anticholinergic agents may potentially alter the absorption of some concomitantly administered drugs due to anticholinergic effects on gastrointestinal motility. They may also antagonize the gastrointestinal prokinetic effects of metoclopramide and domperidone. However, the interaction between prokinetics and oxybutynin has not been established.

Sublingual nitrates may fail to dissolve under the tongue owing to dry mouth, resulting in reduced therapeutic effect.

Oxybutynin is metabolised by cytochrome P450 isoenzyme CYP3A4. Mean oxybutynin chloride concentrations were approximately 2 fold higher when Lyrinel XL was administered with ketoconazole, a potent CYP3A4 inhibitor. Other inhibitors of cytochrome P450 3A4 enzyme system, such as antimycotic agents (e.g. itraconazole and fluconazole) or macrolide antibiotics (e.g. erythromycin), may alter oxybutynin pharmacokinetics. The clinical relevance of such potential interaction is not known. Caution should be used when such drugs are co-administered.

Table 1

	Very Common ⩾ 1/10	Common ⩾ 1/100 to < 1/10	Uncommon ⩾ 1/1,000 to < 1/100	Rare ⩾ 1/10,000 to < 1/1000	Not Known*
Infections and infestations		urinary tract infection, cystitis, pharyngitis, nasopharyngitis, upper respiratory tract infection, bronchitis, sinusitis			
Blood and Lymphatic system disorders:				leukopenia, thrombocytopenia	
Immune System Disorders				hypersensitivity	
Metabolism & Nutrition Disorders			anorexia, dehydration, hyperglycaemia	appetite increased	
Psychiatric disorders		insomnia, depression, nervousness, confusional state	anxiety, abnormal dreams		hallucinations, night terror, psychotic disorder, agitation, memory impairment
Nervous System Disorders		somnolence, headache, dizziness, dysgeusia	paraesthesia, vertigo	hypertonia, tremor, tinnitus	convulsions
Eye disorders		vision blurred, dry eye, kerato-conjunctivitis sicca	conjunctivitis	diplopia, glaucoma, photophobia	
Cardiac disorders		palpitations		atrial arrhythmia, bradycardia, bundle branch block, nodal arrhythmia, supraventricular extrasystoles	arrhythmia tachycardia
Vascular disorders		hypertension	vasodilatation, migraine	hypotension, phlebitis, ecchymosis	flushing
Respiratory, thoracic and mediastinal disorders		nasal dryness, mucosal dryness, cough, pharyngo-laryngeal pain, dry throat	rhinitis, hoarseness, epistaxis, dyspnoea	laryngitis, laryngeal oedema, respiratory disorder, sputum increased	
Gastrointestinal Disorders	dry mouth	constipation, diarrhoea, nausea, dyspepsia, abdominal pain, flatulence, gastroesophageal reflux disease, loose stools, vomiting	dysphagia, mouth ulceration, abdominal distension, glossitis, stomatitis	faecal abnormality, oesophageal stenosis acquired, gastritis, gastroenteritis viral, hernia, rectal disorder, gastric atony, tongue disorder, tongue oedema	
Skin and subcutaneous tissue disorders		dry skin, pruritus	acne, urticaria, face oedema, alopecia, eczema, nail disorder, skin discolouration, anhidrosis	hair disorder, rash maculo-papular, granuloma, sweating increased, photosensitivity reaction	rash
Musculoskeletal and connective tissue disorders		pain in extremity, back pain, arthralgia	muscle cramps, myalgia	arthritis	
Renal and urinary disorders		micturition disorder, residual urine volume, urinary retention, dysuria, urinary hesitation	urinary frequency, urinary tract disorder, haematuria, nocturia, pyuria, micturition urgency	urinary incontinence, urine abnormal, urogenital disorder	impotence, erectile dysfunction
Reproductive system and breast disorders			breast pain, vaginitis	vulvovaginal disorder, uterine cervical disorder, genital discharge	
General disorders and administration site conditions		asthenia, oedema peripheral, fatigue, chest pain	pain, thirst, oedema	rigor, pyrexia, influenza like illness, malaise, pelvic pain	
Investigations		blood pressure increased	electro-cardiogram abnormal, blood urea increased, blood creatinine increased	blood alkaline phosphatase increased, blood lactase dehydrogenase increased, blood aspartate, aminotransferase increased, blood alanine aminotransferase increased	
Injury, poisoning and procedural complications					fall

*Cannot be estimated from the available clinical data.

4.6 Pregnancy and lactation

Pregnancy

There are no adequate data on the use of oxybutynin in pregnant women. Studies in animals have shown minor reproductive toxicity (see section 5.3). Lyrinel XL should only be used during pregnancy if the expected benefit outweighs the risk.

Lactation

When oxybutynin is used during lactation, a small amount is excreted in the mother's milk. Breast feeding while using oxybutynin is therefore not recommended.

4.7 Effects on ability to drive and use machines

As oxybutynin may produce drowsiness or blurred vision, patients should be cautioned regarding activities requiring mental alertness such as driving, operating machinery or performing hazardous work while taking this drug.

4.8 Undesirable effects

The table below reflects the data obtained with Lyrinel XL in clinical trials and from postmarketing experience. In clinical trials with Lyrinel XL (n=1006), adverse events were associated mainly with the anticholinergic actions of oxybutynin. Adverse events were generally dose related. As with other oxybutynin formulations, dry mouth was the most frequently reported adverse reaction. However, in clinical studies, dry mouth has been less frequently reported with Lyrinel XL than with oxybutynin immediate release formulations. For patients who required final doses of 5 or 10 mg of Lyrinel XL, the relative incidence of dry mouth that occurred at any dose level was 1.8 times lower compared with patients who required final doses > 10 mg.

(see Table 1 above)

Undesirable effects noted with other oxybutynin hydrochloride formulations:

In addition, cyclopegia, mydriasis and suppression of lactation have been reported with the use of other oxybutynin hydrochloride formulations.

4.9 Overdose

The symptoms of overdose with oxybutynin progress from an intensification of the usual CNS disturbances (from restlessness and excitement to psychotic behaviour), circulatory changes (flushing, fall in blood pressure, circulatory failure etc.), respiratory failure, paralysis and coma.

Measures to be taken are:

1) administration of activated charcoal

2) physostigmine by slow intravenous injection:

Adults: 0.5 to 2.0 mg i.v. slowly, repeated after 5 minutes if necessary, up to a maximum of 5 mg.

Fever should be treated symptomatically with tepid sponging or ice packs.

In pronounced restlessness or excitation, diazepam 10 mg may be given by intravenous injection. Tachycardia may be treated with intravenous propranolol and urinary retention managed by bladder catheterisation.

In the event of progression of curare-like effects to paralysis of the respiratory muscles, mechanical ventilation will be required.

The continuous release of oxybutynin from Lyrinel XL should be considered in the treatment of overdose. Patients should be monitored for at least 24 hours.

5. PHARMACOLOGICAL PROPERTIES

5.1 Pharmacodynamic properties

Pharmacotherapeutic group: urinary antispasmodic, ATC code: G04B D04.

Mechanism of action: oxybutynin acts as a competitive antagonist of acetylcholine at post-ganglionic muscarinic receptors, resulting in relaxation of bladder smooth muscle.

Pharmacodynamic effects: in patients with overactive bladder, characterized by detrusor muscle instability or hyperreflexia, cystometric studies have demonstrated that oxybutynin increases maximum urinary bladder capacity and increases the volume to first detrusor contraction. Oxybutynin thus decreases urinary urgency and frequency of both incontinence episodes and voluntary urination.

Oxybutynin is a racemic (50:50) mixture of R- and S-isomers. Antimuscarinic activity resides predominantly in the R-isomer. The R-isomer of oxybutynin shows greater selectivity for the M_1 and M_3 muscarinic subtypes (predominant in bladder detrusor muscle and parotid gland) compared to the M_2 subtype (predominant in cardiac tissue). The active metabolite, N-desethyloxybutynin, has pharmacological activity on the human detrusor muscle that is similar to that of oxybutynin *in vitro* studies, but has a greater binding affinity for parotid tissue than oxybutynin. The free base form of oxybutynin is pharmacologically equivalent to oxybutynin hydrochloride.

Children over the age of 6 years: in children with detrusor hyperreflexia secondary to a neurogenic condition, oxybutynin, in combination with clean intermittent urinary catheterisation, has been shown in open uncontrolled studies to increase mean urine volume per catherisation, increase maximum cystometric capacity and decrease mean detrusor pressure at maximum cystometric capacity.

5.2 Pharmacokinetic properties

Following the first dose of Lyrinel XL, oxybutynin plasma concentrations rise for 4 to 6 hours; thereafter, concentrations are maintained for up to 24 hours, thus reducing the fluctuations between peak and trough concentrations associated with oxybutynin immediate release formulations.

The relative bioavailabilities of R-oxybutynin and S-oxybutynin from Lyrinel XL are 156% and 187% respectively, compared with oxybutynin immediate release. After a 10 mg single dose of Lyrinel XL, the peak plasma concentrations of R-oxybutynin and S-oxybutynin, achieved after 12.7±5.4 and 11.8±5.3 hours respectively, are 1.0±0.6 and 1.8±1.0 ng/ml, and the plasma concentration time profiles of both enantiomers are similar in shape. The elimination half-life is 13.2±10.3 hours for R-oxybutynin and 12.4±6.1 hours for S-oxybutynin.

Steady state oxybutynin plasma concentrations are achieved by Day 3 of repeated Lyrinel XL dosing, with no observed change in oxybutynin and desethyloxybutynin pharmacokinetic parameters over time.

Pharmacokinetic parameters of oxybutynin and desethyloxybutynin (C_{max} and AUC) are dose proportional following administration of 5-20 mg of Lyrinel XL.

The pharmacokinetics of Lyrinel XL were similar in all patients studied, irrespective of gender or age and are unaffected by food intake.

Limited data suggest that the pharmacokinetics of Lyrinel XL is similar in adults and children aged 8 years and above. The pharmacokinetics of Lyrinel XL have not been investigated in patients with renal or hepatic insufficiency.

Oxybutynin is extensively metabolised by the liver, primarily by the cytochrome P450 enzyme system, particularly CYP3A4 found mostly in the liver and gut wall. Absolute bioavailability of immediate release oxybutynin has been estimated to be 2-11%. Following intravenous administration of 5 mg oxybutynin, clearance and volume of distribution were estimated to be 26 L/h and 193 L, respectively. Less than 0.1% of the administered dose is excreted unchanged in the urine. Its metabolic products include phenylcyclohexylglycolic acid, which is pharmacologically inactive, and desethyloxybutynin, which is pharmacologically active. Following Lyrinel XL administration, area under the plasma concentration profiles of R- and S-desethyloxybutynin are 73% and 92% respectively of those observed with oxybutynin immediate release formulations.

The binding of oxybutynin to plasma proteins is unknown.

5.3 Preclinical safety data

Preclinical data reveal no special hazard for humans based on studies of acute toxicity, repeat dose toxicity, genotoxicity, carcinogenic potential and local toxicity. In a fertility study of subcutaneous oxybutynin injections in rats, female fertility was impaired while no effect was noted in male animals. In a rabbit embryotoxicity study, organ anomalies were observed in the presence of maternal toxicity at a dose of 0.4 mg/kg/day subcutaneously. The relevance to human safety is unknown.

6. PHARMACEUTICAL PARTICULARS

6.1 List of excipients

5 mg

Butylhydroxytoluene (E321), cellulose acetate, hypromellose, macrogol 3350, magnesium stearate, polyethylene oxide, sodium chloride, black iron oxide (E172), ferric oxide yellow (E172) and lactose anhydrous.

Film coat: ferric oxide yellow (E172), hypromellose, macrogol 400, polysorbate 80 and titanium dioxide (E171).

Printing Ink: black iron oxide (E172), hypromellose, and propylene glycol.

10 mg

Butylhydroxytoluene (E321), cellulose acetate, hypromellose, macrogol 3350, magnesium stearate, polyethylene oxide, sodium chloride, black iron oxide (E172), ferric oxide red (E172) and lactose anhydrous.

Film coat: ferric oxide red (E172), hypromellose, macrogol 400, polysorbate 80 and titanium dioxide (E171).

Printing Ink: black iron oxide (E172), hypromellose and propylene glycol.

6.2 Incompatibilities

Not applicable.

6.3 Shelf life

Lyrinel XL 5: 2 years

Lyrinel XL 10: 18 months

6.4 Special precautions for storage

Keep the container tightly closed in order to protect from moisture. Do not store above 25°C.

6.5 Nature and contents of container

High density polyethylene bottles with child resistant closure (polypropylene) and desiccant.

Pack sizes 3, 7, 10, 14, 30, 50, 60, 90 or 100 tablets.

Not all pack sizes may be marketed.

6.6 Special precautions for disposal and other handling

No special requirements.

7. MARKETING AUTHORISATION HOLDER

Janssen-Cilag Limited

50-100 Holmers Farm Way

High Wycombe

Buckinghamshire

HP12 4EG

UK

8. MARKETING AUTHORISATION NUMBER(S)

PL 0242/0385

PL 0242/0386

9. DATE OF FIRST AUTHORISATION/RENEWAL OF THE AUTHORISATION

1 August 2002

10. DATE OF REVISION OF THE TEXT

02 April 2009

Lysovir 100mg Capsules

(Alliance Pharmaceuticals)

1. NAME OF THE MEDICINAL PRODUCT

Lysovir 100mg Capsules

2. QUALITATIVE AND QUANTITATIVE COMPOSITION

Amantadine hydrochloride PhEur 100 mg.

3. PHARMACEUTICAL FORM

Capsule.

Reddish-brown hard gelatin capsules, printed SYMM in white on both the cap and body.

4. CLINICAL PARTICULARS

4.1 Therapeutic indications

Prophylaxis and treatment of signs and symptoms of infection caused by influenza A virus. It is suggested that Lysovir be given to patients suffering from clinical influenza in which complications might be expected to occur. In addition, Lysovir is recommended prophylactically in cases particularly at risk. This can include those with chronic respiratory disease or debilitating conditions, the elderly and those living in crowded conditions. It can also be used for individuals in families where influenza has already been diagnosed, for control of institutional outbreaks or for those in essential services who are unvaccinated or when vaccination is unavailable or contra-indicated.

Lysovir does not completely prevent the host immune response to influenza A infection, so individuals who take this drug still develop immune responses to the natural disease or vaccination and may be protected when later exposed to antigenically related viruses. Lysovir may also be used in post-exposure prophylaxis in conjunction with inactivated vaccine during an outbreak until protective antibodies develop, or in patients who are not expected to have a substantial antibody response (immunosuppression).

4.2 Posology and method of administration

Treatment: It is advisable to start treating influenza as early as possible and to continue for 4 to 5 days. When amantadine is started within 48 hours of symptoms appearing, the duration of fever and other effects is reduced by one or two days and the inflammatory reaction of the bronchial tree that usually accompanies influenza resolves more quickly. **Prophylaxis:** Treat daily for as long as protection from infection is required. In most instances this is expected to be for 6 weeks. When used with inactivated influenza A vaccine, amantadine is continued for 2 to 3 weeks following inoculation.

Adults: 100mg daily for the recommended period.

Children aged 10-15 years: 100mg daily for the recommended period.

Children under 10 years of age: Dosage not established.

Adults over 65 years of age: Plasma amantadine concentrations are influenced by renal function. In elderly patients, the elimination half-life is longer and renal clearance of the compound is diminished in comparison to young people. A daily dose of less than 100mg, or 100mg given at intervals of greater than one day, may be appropriate.

*In patients with **renal impairment*** the dose of amantadine should be reduced. This can be achieved by either reducing the total daily dose, or by increasing the dosage interval in accordance with the creatinine clearance. For example,

Creatinine clearance (ml/min)	Dose
< 15	Lysovir contra-indicated.
15 – 35	100mg every 2 to 3 days.
> 35	100mg every day

The above recommendations are for guidance only and physicians should continue to monitor their patients for signs of unwanted effects.

4.3 Contraindications

Known hypersensitivity to amantadine or any of the excipients. Individuals subject to convulsions. A history of gastric ulceration. Severe renal disease. Pregnancy.

4.4 Special warnings and precautions for use

Lysovir should be used with caution in patients with confusional or hallucinatory states or underlying psychiatric disorders, in patients with liver or kidney disorders, and those suffering from, or who have a history of, cardiovascular disorders. Caution should be applied when prescribing Lysovir with other medications having an effect on the CNS (See Section 4.5, Interactions with other medicaments and other forms of interaction).

Lysovir should not be stopped abruptly in patients who are treated concurrently with neuroleptics. There have been isolated reports of precipitation or aggravation of neuroleptic malignant syndrome or neuroleptic-induced catatonia following the withdrawal of amantadine in patients taking neuroleptic agents. A similar syndrome has also been reported rarely following withdrawal of amantadine and other anti-Parkinson agents in patients who were not taking concurrent psychoactive medication.

Resistance to amantadine occurs during serial passage of influenza virus strains *in vitro* or *in vivo* in the presence of the drug. Apparent transmission of drug-resistant viruses may have been the cause of failure of prophylaxis and treatment in household contacts and in nursing-home patients. However, there is no evidence to date that the resistant virus produces a disease that is in any way different from that produced by sensitive viruses.

As some individuals have attempted suicide with amantadine, prescriptions should be written for the smallest quantity consistent with good patient management.

Peripheral oedema (thought to be due to an alteration in the responsiveness of peripheral vessels) may occur in some patients during chronic treatment (not usually before 4 weeks) with amantadine. This should be taken into account in patients with congestive heart failure.

4.5 Interaction with other medicinal products and other forms of interaction

Concurrent administration of amantadine and anticholinergic agents or levodopa may increase confusion, hallucinations, nightmares, gastro-intestinal disturbances, or other atropine-like side effects (see Section 4.9 ''Overdose''). Psychotic reactions have been observed in patients receiving amantadine and levodopa.

In isolated cases, worsening of psychotic symptoms has been reported in patients receiving amantadine and concomitant neuroleptic medication.

Concurrent administration of amantadine and drugs or substances (e.g. alcohol) acting on the CNS may result in additive CNS toxicity. Close observation is recommended (see Section 4.9 ''Overdose'').

There have been isolated reports of a suspected interaction between amantadine and combination diuretics (hydrochlorothiazide + potassium sparing diuretics). One or both of the components apparently reduce the clearance of amantadine, leading to higher plasma concentrations and toxic effects (confusion, hallucinations, ataxia, myoclonus).

4.6 Pregnancy and lactation

Amantadine-related complications during pregnancy have been reported. Lysovir is contra-indicated during pregnancy and in women wishing to become pregnant.

Amantadine passes into breast milk. Undesirable effects have been reported in breast-fed infants. Nursing mothers should not take Lysovir.

4.7 Effects on ability to drive and use machines

Patients should be warned of the potential hazards of driving or operating machinery if they experience side effects such as dizziness or blurred vision. If taken concomitantly with other products affecting the CNS, additive adverse effects could be seen.

4.8 Undesirable effects

Amantadine's undesirable effects are often mild and transient, usually appearing within the first 2 to 4 days of treatment and promptly disappearing 24 to 48 hours after discontinuation. A direct relationship between dose and incidence of side effects has not been demonstrated, although there seems to be a tendency towards more frequent undesirable effects (particularly affecting the CNS) with increasing doses.

The side effects reported after the pivotal clinical studies in influenza in over 1200 patients receiving amantadine at 100mg daily were mostly mild, transient, and equivalent to placebo. Only 7% of subjects reported adverse events, many being similar to the effects of influenza itself. The most commonly reported effects were gastro-intestinal disturbances (anorexia, nausea), CNS effects (loss of concentration, dizziness, agitation, nervousness, depression, insomnia, fatigue, weakness), or myalgia.

Side effects reported after higher doses or chronic use, in addition to those already stated, include:

Frequency estimates: frequent $> 10\%$, occasional 1%-10%, rare 0.001%-1%, isolated cases $< 0.001\%$.

Central nervous system: Occasional: anxiety, elevation of mood, lightheadedness, headache, lethargy, hallucinations, nightmares, ataxia, slurred speech, blurred vision. Hallucinations, confusion and nightmares are more common when amantadine is administered concurrently with anticholinergic agents or when the patient has an underlying psychiatric disorder. Rare: confusion, disorientation, psychosis, tremor, dyskinesia, convulsions, neuroleptic malignant-like syndrome. Delirium, hypomanic state and mania have been reported but their incidence cannot be readily deduced from the literature. *Cardiovascular system:* Frequent: oedema of ankles, livedo reticularis (usually after very high doses or use over many months). Occasional: palpitations, orthostatic hypotension. Isolated cases: heart insufficiency/failure. *Blood*: Isolated cases: leucopenia, reversible elevation of liver enzymes. *Gastrointestinal tract:* Occasional: dry mouth, anorexia, nausea, vomiting, constipation. Rare: diarrhoea. *Skin and appendages:* Occasional: diaphoresis. Rare: exanthema. Isolated cases: photosensitisation. *Sense organs*: Rare: corneal lesions, e.g. punctate subepithelial opacities which might be associated with superficial punctate keratitis, corneal epithelial oedema, and markedly reduced visual acuity. *Urogenital tract:* Rare: urinary retention, urinary incontinence.

4.9 Overdose

Signs and symptoms: *Neuromuscular* disturbances and symptoms of acute psychosis are prominent. *Central nervous system:* Hyperreflexia, motor restlessness, convulsions, extrapyramidal signs, torsion spasms, dystonic posturing, dilated pupils, confusion, disorientation, delirium, visual hallucinations. *Respiratory system:* hyperventilation, pulmonary oedema, respiratory distress, including adult respiratory distress syndrome. *Cardiovascular system*: sinus tachycardia, arrhythmia. *Gastrointestinal system*: nausea, vomiting, dry mouth. *Renal function*: urine retention, renal dysfunction, including increase in BUN and decreased creatinine clearance.

Overdose from combined drug treatment: the effects of anticholinergic drugs are increased by amantadine. Acute psychotic reactions (which may be identical to those of atropine poisoning) may occur when large doses of anticholinergic agents are used. Where alcohol or central nervous stimulants have been taken at the same time, the signs and symptoms of acute poisoning with amantadine may be aggravated and/or modified.

Management: There is no specific antidote. Induction of vomiting and/or gastric aspiration (and lavage if patient is conscious), activated charcoal or saline cathartic may be used if judged appropriate. Since amantadine is excreted mainly unchanged in the urine, maintenance of renal function and copious diuresis (forced diuresis if necessary) are effective ways to remove it from the blood stream. Acidification of the urine favours its excretion. Haemodialysis does not remove significant amounts of amantadine.

Monitor the blood pressure, heart rate, ECG, respiration and body temperature, and treat for possible hypotension and cardiac arhythmias, as necessary. *Convulsions and excessive motor restlessness*: administer anticonvulsants such as diazepam iv, paraldehyde im or per rectum, or phenobarbital im. *Acute psychotic symptoms, delirium, dystonic posturing, myoclonic manifestations*: physostigmine by slow iv infusion (1mg doses in adults, 0.5mg in children) repeated administration according to the initial response and the subsequent need, has been reported. *Retention of urine*: bladder should be catheterised; an indwelling catheter can be left in place for the time required.

5. PHARMACOLOGICAL PROPERTIES

5.1 Pharmacodynamic properties

Amantadine specifically inhibits the replication of influenza A viruses at low concentrations. If using a sensitive plaque-reduction assay, human influenza viruses, including H_1N_1, H_2N_2 and H_3N_2 subtypes, are inhibited by $\leqslant 0.4 \mu g/ml$ of amantadine. Amantadine inhibits an early stage in viral replication by blocking the proton pump of the M_2 protein in the virus. This has two actions; it stops the virus uncoating and inactivates newly synthesised viral haemagglutinin. Effects on late replicative steps have been found for representative avian influenza viruses.

Data from tests with representative strains of influenza A virus indicate that Lysovir is likely to be active against previously unknown strains, and could be used in the early stages of an epidemic, before a vaccine against the causative strain is generally available.

5.2 Pharmacokinetic properties

Absorption: Amantadine is absorbed slowly but almost completely. Peak plasma concentrations of approximately 250ng/ml and 500ng/ml are attained within 3 to 4 hours after single oral administration of 100mg and 200mg amantadine, respectively. Following repeated administration of 200mg daily, the steady-state plasma concentration settles at 300ng/ml within 3 days.

Distribution: Amantadine accumulates after several hours in nasal secretions and crosses the blood-brain barrier (this has not been quantified). *In vitro*, 67% is bound to plasma proteins, with a substantial amount bound to red blood cells. The concentration in erythrocytes in normal healthy volunteers is 2.66 times the plasma concentration. The apparent volume of distribution is 5 to 10L/kg, suggesting extensive tissue binding. This declines with increasing doses. The concentrations in the lung, heart, kidney, liver and spleen are higher than in the blood.

Biotransformation: Amantadine is metabolised to a minor extent, principally by N-acetylation.

Elimination: The drug is eliminated in healthy young adults with a mean plasma elimination half-life of 15 hours (10 to 31 hours). The total plasma clearance is about the same as renal clearance (250ml/min). The renal amantadine clearance is much higher than the creatinine clearance, suggesting renal tubular secretion. After 4 to 5 days, 90% of the dose appears unchanged in urine. The rate is considerably influenced by urinary pH: a rise in pH brings about a fall in excretion.

Characteristics in special patient populations:

Elderly patients: compared with healthy young adults, the half-life may be doubled and renal clearance diminished. Tubular secretion diminishes more than glomerular filtration in the elderly. In elderly patients with renal impairment, repeated administration of 100mg daily for 14 days raised the plasma concentration into the toxic range.

Renal impairment: amantadine may accumulate in renal failure, causing severe side effects. The rate of elimination from plasma correlates to creatinine clearance divided by body surface area, although total renal elimination exceeds this value (possibly due to tubular secretion). The effects of reduced kidney function are dramatic: a reduction of creatinine clearance to 40ml/min may result in a five-fold increase in elimination half-life. The urine is the almost exclusive route of excretion, even with renal failure, and amantadine may persist in the plasma for several days. Haemodialysis does not remove significant amounts of amantadine, possibly due to extensive tissue binding.

5.3 Preclinical safety data

Reproductive toxicity studies were performed in rats and rabbits. In rat oral doses of 50 and 100 mg/kg proved to be teratogenic. This is 33-fold the recommended dose of 100mg for influenza. The maximum recommended dose, of 400mg in Parkinson's disease, is less than 6mg/kg.

There are no other pre-clinical data of relevance to the prescriber, which are additional to those already included in other sections of the Summary of Product Characteristics.

6. PHARMACEUTICAL PARTICULARS

6.1 List of excipients

Lactose, povidone, magnesium stearate. Capsule shell: gelatin, titanium dioxide (E171), red iron oxide (E172). White printing ink: Opacode S-1-7020 containing, Shellac, I.M.S. 74 OP, purified water, soya lecithin (E322), 2-ethoxyethanol, antifoam DC 1510, titanium dioxide (E171).

6.2 Incompatibilities

None known.

6.3 Shelf life

Five years.

6.4 Special precautions for storage

Store in the original package.

6.5 Nature and contents of container

PVC/PVdC blister packs of 5 or 14 capsules.

6.6 Special precautions for disposal and other handling

None.

7. MARKETING AUTHORISATION HOLDER

Alliance Pharmaceuticals Ltd

Avonbridge House, Bath Road

Chippenham, Wiltshire SN15 2BB

8. MARKETING AUTHORISATION NUMBER(S)

PL16853/0035

9. DATE OF FIRST AUTHORISATION/RENEWAL OF THE AUTHORISATION

January 2000

10. DATE OF REVISION OF THE TEXT

4th February 2009

Mabthera 100mg and 500mg concentrate for solution for infusion

(Roche Products Limited)

1. NAME OF THE MEDICINAL PRODUCT

MabThera 100 mg (10 mg/ml) concentrate for solution for infusion

MabThera 500 mg (10 mg/ml) concentrate for solution for infusion

2. QUALITATIVE AND QUANTITATIVE COMPOSITION

Each solution contains 10 mg/ml of Rituximab.

Each single-use vial containing 100 mg of Rituximab.

Each single-use vial containing 500 mg of Rituximab.

Rituximab is a genetically engineered chimeric mouse/human monoclonal antibody representing a glycosylated immunoglobulin with human IgG1 constant regions and murine light-chain and heavy-chain variable region sequences. The antibody is produced by mammalian (Chinese hamster ovary) cell suspension culture and purified by affinity chromatography and ion exchange, including specific viral inactivation and removal procedures.

For a full list of excipients, see section 6.1.

3. PHARMACEUTICAL FORM

Concentrate for solution for infusion.

Clear, colourless liquid.

4. CLINICAL PARTICULARS

4.1 Therapeutic indications

Non-Hodgkin's lymphoma (NHL)

MabThera is indicated for the treatment of previously untreated patients with stage III-IV follicular lymphoma in combination with chemotherapy.

MabThera maintenance therapy is indicated for patients with relapsed/refractory follicular lymphoma responding to induction therapy with chemotherapy with or without MabThera.

MabThera monotherapy is indicated for treatment of patients with stage III-IV follicular lymphoma who are chemoresistant or are in their second or subsequent relapse after chemotherapy.

MabThera is indicated for the treatment of patients with CD20 positive diffuse large B cell non-Hodgkin's lymphoma in combination with CHOP (cyclophosphamide, doxorubicin, vincristine, prednisolone) chemotherapy.

Chronic lymphocytic leukaemia (CLL)

MabThera in combination with chemotherapy is indicated for the treatment of patients with previously untreated and relapsed/refractory chronic lymphocytic leukaemia.

Only limited data are available on efficacy and safety for patients previously treated with monoclonal antibodies including MabThera or patients refractory to previous MabThera plus chemotherapy.

See section 5.1 for further information.

Rheumatoid arthritis

MabThera in combination with methotrexate is indicated for the treatment of adult patients with severe active rheumatoid arthritis who have had an inadequate response or intolerance to other disease-modifying anti-rheumatic drugs (DMARD) including one or more tumour necrosis factor (TNF) inhibitor therapies.

4.2 Posology and method of administration

MabThera infusions should be administered under the close supervision of an experienced physician, and in an environment where full resuscitation facilities are immediately available.

Posology

Non-Hodgkin's lymphoma

Dosage adjustments during treatment

No dose reductions of MabThera are recommended. When MabThera is given in combination with chemotherapy, standard dose reductions for the chemotherapeutic medicinal products should be applied.

Follicular non-Hodgkin's lymphoma

Combination therapy

The recommended dose of MabThera in combination with chemotherapy for induction treatment of previously untreated or relapsed/ refractory patients with follicular NHL is: 375 mg/m^2 body surface area per cycle, for up to 8 cycles.

Mabthera should be administered on day 1 of each chemotherapy cycle, after intravenous administration of the glucocorticoid component of the chemotherapy if applicable.

Monotherapy/Maintenance

The recommended dose of MabThera used as a maintenance treatment for patients with relapsed/refractory follicular NHL who have responded to induction treatment with chemotherapy, with or without MabThera is: 375 mg/m^2 body surface area once every 3 months until disease progression or for a maximum period of two years.

The recommended dose of MabThera monotherapy used as induction treatment for adult patients with stage III-IV follicular lymphoma who are chemoresistant or are in their second or subsequent relapse after chemotherapy is: 375 mg/m^2 body surface area, administered as an intravenous infusion once weekly for four weeks.

For retreatment with MabThera monotherapy for patients who have responded to previous treatment with MabThera monotherapy for relapsed/refractory follicular NHL, the recommended dose is: 375 mg/m^2 body surface area, administered as an intravenous infusion once weekly for four weeks (see section 5.1).

Diffuse large B cell non-Hodgkin's lymphoma

MabThera should be used in combination with CHOP chemotherapy. The recommended dosage is 375 mg/m^2 body surface area, administered on day 1 of each chemotherapy cycle for 8 cycles after intravenous infusion of the glucocorticoid component of CHOP. Safety and efficacy of MabThera have not been established in combination with other chemotherapies in diffuse large B cell non-Hodgkin's lymphoma.

Chronic lymphocytic leukaemia

Prophylaxis with adequate hydration and administration of uricostatics starting 48 hours prior to start of therapy is recommended for CLL patients to reduce the risk of tumour lysis syndrome. For CLL patients whose lymphocyte counts are $> 25 \times 10^9$/L it is recommended to administer prednisone/prednisolone 100 mg intravenous shortly before infusion with MabThera to decrease the rate and severity of acute infusion reactions and/or cytokine release syndrome.

The recommended dosage of MabThera in combination with chemotherapy for previously untreated and relapsed/refractory patients is 375 mg/m^2 body surface area administered on day 0 of the first treatment cycle followed by 500 mg/m^2 body surface area administered on day 1 of each subsequent cycle for 6 cycles in total. The chemotherapy should be given after MabThera infusion.

Rheumatoid arthritis

A course of MabThera consists of two 1000 mg intravenous infusions. The recommended dosage of MabThera is 1000 mg by intravenous infusion followed by a second 1000 mg intravenous infusion two weeks later.

Disease activity should be regularly monitored. There are limited clinical data on the safety and efficacy of further courses of therapy with MabThera. In a small observational cohort, approximately 600 patients with evidence of continued disease activity received 2-5 repeated courses of treatment 6-12 months after the previous course. (See sections 4.8 and 5.1).

Human anti chimeric antibodies (HACA) develop in some patients after the first course of MabThera (see section 5.1). The presence of HACA may be associated with the worsening of infusion or allergic reactions after the second infusion of subsequent courses. Furthermore, in one case with HACA, failure to deplete B-cells after receipt of further treatment courses has been observed. Thus, the benefit/risk balance of therapy with MabThera should be carefully considered before administering subsequent courses of Mabthera. If a repeat course of treatment is considered it should not be given at an interval less than 16 weeks.

Background therapy with glucocorticoids, salicylates, non-steroidal anti-inflammatory drugs, or analgesics can be continued during treatment with MabThera.

Rheumatoid arthritis patients should receive treatment with 100 mg intravenous methylprednisolone 30 minutes prior to MabThera to decrease the rate and severity of acute infusion reactions (see method of administration).

First infusion of each course

The recommended initial rate for infusion is 50 mg/hr; after the first 30 minutes, it can be escalated in 50 mg/hr increments every 30 minutes, to a maximum of 400 mg/hr.

Second infusion of each course

Subsequent doses of MabThera can be infused at an initial rate of 100 mg/hr, and increased by 100 mg/hr increments at 30 minutes intervals, to a maximum of 400 mg/hr.

Special populations

Paediatric use

MabThera is not recommended for use in children and adolescents due to a lack of data on safety and efficacy.

Elderly

No dose adjustment is required in elderly patients (aged > 65 years).

Method of Administration

Premedication with glucocorticoids should be considered if MabThera is not given in combination with glucocorticoid-containing chemotherapy for treatment of non-Hodgkin's lymphoma and chronic lymphocytic leukaemia.

Premedication consisting of an anti-pyretic and an anti-histaminic, e.g. paracetamol and diphenhydramine, should always be administered before each infusion of MabThera.

First infusion

The recommended initial rate for infusion is 50 mg/hr; after the first 30 minutes, it can be escalated in 50 mg/hr increments every 30 minutes, to a maximum of 400 mg/hr.

Subsequent infusions

Subsequent doses of MabThera can be infused at an initial rate of 100 mg/hr, and increased by 100 mg/hr increments at 30 minutes intervals, to a maximum of 400 mg/hr.

The prepared MabThera solution should be administered as an intravenous infusion through a dedicated line. It should not be administered as an intravenous push or bolus.

Patients should be closely monitored for the onset of cytokine release syndrome (see section 4.4). Patients who develop evidence of severe reactions, especially severe dyspnoea, bronchospasm or hypoxia should have the infusion interrupted immediately. Patients with non-Hodgkin's lymphoma should then be evaluated for evidence of tumour lysis syndrome including appropriate laboratory tests and, for pulmonary infiltration, with a chest x-ray. In all patients, the infusion should not be restarted until complete resolution of all symptoms, and normalisation of laboratory values and chest x-ray findings. At this time, the infusion can be initially resumed at not more than one-half the previous rate. If the same severe adverse reactions occur for a second time, the decision to stop the treatment should be seriously considered on a case by case basis.

Mild or moderate infusion-related reactions (section 4.8) usually respond to a reduction in the rate of infusion. The infusion rate may be increased upon improvement of symptoms.

4.3 Contraindications

Contraindications for use in non-Hodgkin's lymphoma and chronic lymphocytic leukaemia

Hypersensitivity to the active substance or to any of the excipients or to murine proteins.

Active, severe infections (see section 4.4).

Contraindications for use in rheumatoid arthritis

Hypersensitivity to the active substance or to any of the excipients or to murine proteins.

Active, severe infections (see section 4.4).

Severe heart failure (New York Heart Association Class IV) or severe, uncontrolled cardiac disease.

4.4 Special warnings and precautions for use

Progressive Multifocal Leukoencephalopathy

Use of MabThera maybe associated with an increased risk of Progressive Multifocal Leukoencephalopathy (PML). Patients must be monitored at regular intervals for any new or worsening neurological symptoms or signs that may be suggestive of PML. If PML is suspected, further dosing must be suspended until PML has been excluded. The clinician should evaluate the patient to determine if the symptoms are indicative of neurological dysfunction, and if so, whether these symptoms are possibly suggestive of PML. Consultation with a Neurologist should be considered as clinically indicated.

If any doubt exists, further evaluation, including MRI scan preferably with contrast, CSF testing for JC Viral DNA and repeat neurological assessments, should be considered.

The physician should be particularly alert to symptoms suggestive of PML that the patient may not notice (e.g. cognitive, neurological or psychiatric symptoms). Patients should also be advised to inform their partner or caregivers about their treatment, since they may notice symptoms that the patient is not aware of.

If a patient develops PML the dosing of MabThera must be permanently discontinued.

Following reconstitution of the immune system in immunocompromised patients with PML, stabilisation or improved outcome has been seen. It remains unknown if early detection of PML and suspension of MabThera therapy may lead to similar stabilisation or improved outcome.

Non-Hodgkin's lymphoma and chronic lymphocytic leukaemia

Patients with a high tumour burden or with a high number ($\geq 25 \times 10^9$/l) of circulating malignant cells such as patients with CLL, who may be at higher risk of especially severe cytokine release syndrome, should only be treated with extreme caution. These patients should be very closely monitored throughout the first infusion. Consideration should be given to the use of a reduced infusion rate for the first infusion in these patients or a split dosing over two days during the first cycle and any subsequent cycles of the lymphocyte count is still $> 25 \times 10^9$/L.

Severe cytokine release syndrome is characterised by severe dyspnoea, often accompanied by bronchospasm and hypoxia, in addition to fever, chills, rigors, urticaria, and angioedema. This syndrome may be associated with some features of ***tumour lysis syndrome*** such as hyperuricaemia, hyperkalaemia, hypocalcaemia, hyperphosphataemia, acute renal failure, elevated Lactate dehydrogenase (LDH) and may be associated with acute respiratory failure and death. The acute respiratory failure may be accompanied by events such as pulmonary interstitial infiltration or oedema, visible on a chest x-ray. The syndrome frequently manifests itself within one or two hours of initiating the first infusion. Patients with a history of pulmonary insufficiency or those with pulmonary tumour infiltration may be at greater risk of poor outcome and should be treated with increased caution. Patients who develop severe cytokine release syndrome should have their infusion interrupted immediately (see section 4.2) and should receive aggressive symptomatic treatment. Since initial improvement of clinical symptoms may be followed by deterioration, these patients should be closely monitored until tumour lysis syndrome and pulmonary infiltration have been resolved or ruled out. Further treatment of patients after complete resolution of signs and symptoms has rarely resulted in repeated severe cytokine release syndrome.

Infusion related adverse reactions including cytokine release syndrome (see section 4.8) accompanied by hypotension and bronchospasm have been observed in 10 % of patients treated with MabThera. These symptoms are usually reversible with interruption of MabThera infusion and administration of an anti-pyretic, an antihistaminic, and, occasionally, oxygen, intravenous saline or bronchodilators, and glucocorticoids if required. Please see cytokine release syndrome above for severe reactions.

Anaphylactic and other hypersensitivity reactions have been reported following the intravenous administration of proteins to patients. In contrast to cytokine release syndrome, true hypersensitivity reactions typically occur within minutes after starting infusion. Medicinal products for the treatment of hypersensitivity reactions, e.g., epinephrine (adrenaline), antihistamines and glucocorticoids, should be available for immediate use in the event of an allergic reaction during administration of MabThera. Clinical manifestations of anaphylaxis may appear similar to clinical manifestations of the cytokine release syndrome (described above). Reactions attributed to hypersensitivity have been reported less frequently than those attributed to cytokine release.

Since hypotension may occur during MabThera infusion, consideration should be given to withholding anti-hypertensive medicines 12 hours prior to the MabThera infusion.

Angina pectoris, or cardiac arrhythmias such as atrial flutter and fibrillation heart failure or myocardial infarction have occurred in patients treated with MabThera. Therefore patients with a history of cardiac disease and/or cardiotoxic chemotherapy should be monitored closely.

Although MabThera is not myelosuppressive in monotherapy, caution should be exercised when considering treatment of patients with neutrophils $< 1.5 \times 10^9$/l and/or platelet counts $< 75 \times 10^9$/l as clinical experience in this population is limited. MabThera has been used in 21 patients who underwent autologous bone marrow transplantation and other risk groups with a presumable reduced bone marrow function without inducing myelotoxicity.

Consideration should be given to the need for regular full blood counts, including platelet counts, during monotherapy with MabThera. When MabThera is given in combination with CHOP or CVP (cyclophosphamide, vincristine, and prednisone) chemotherapy, regular full blood counts should be performed according to usual medical practice.

Serious infections, including fatalities, can occur during therapy with MabThera (see section 4.8). MabThera should not be administered to patients with an active, severe infection (eg. tuberculosis, sepsis and opportunistic infections, see section 4.3).

Physicians should exercise caution when considering the use of MabThera in patients with a history of recurring or chronic infections or with underlying conditions which may further predispose patients to serious infection (see section 4.8).

Cases of hepatitis B reactivation have been reported in subjects receiving MabThera including fulminant hepatitis with fatal outcome. The majority of these subjects were also exposed to cytotoxic chemotherapy. Limited information from one study in relapsed/refractory CLL patients suggest that MabThera treatment may also worsen the outcome of primary hepatitis B infections. Hepatitis B virus (HBV) screening should be considered for high risk patients before initiation of treatment with MabThera. Carriers of hepatitis B and patients with a history of hepatitis B should be closely monitored for clinical and laboratory signs of active HBV infection during and for several months following MabThera therapy.

Very rare cases of Progressive Multifocal Leukoencephalopathy (PML) have been reported during post-marketing use of MabThera in NHL and CLL (see section 4.8). The majority of patients had received rituximab in combination with chemotherapy or as part of a haematopoietic stem cell transplant.

The safety of immunisation with live viral vaccines, following MabThera therapy has not been studied for NHL and CLL patients and vaccination with live virus vaccines is not recommended. Patients treated with MabThera may receive non-live vaccinations. However, with non-live vaccines response rates may be reduced. In a non-randomised study, patients with relapsed low-grade NHL who received MabThera monotherapy when compared to healthy untreated controls had a lower rate of response to vaccination with tetanus recall antigen (16% vs. 81%) and Keyhole Limpet Haemocyanin (KLH) neoantigen (4% vs. 69% when assessed for >2-fold increase in antibody titre). For CLL patients similar results are assumable considering similarities between both diseases but this has not been investigated in clinical trials

Mean pre-therapeutic antibody titres against a panel of antigens (Streptococcus pneumoniae, influenza A, mumps, rubella, varicella) were maintained for at least 6 months after treatment with MabThera.

Rheumatoid arthritis

Infusion reactions

MabThera is associated with infusion reactions, which may be related to release of cytokines and/or other chemical mediators. Premedication with intravenous glucocorticoid significantly reduced the incidence and severity of these events (see section 4.8).

Most infusion events reported were mild to moderate in severity. The proportion of affected patients decreases with subsequent infusions. The reactions reported were usually reversible with a reduction in rate, or interruption, of MabThera infusion and administration of an anti-pyretic, an antihistamine, and, occasionally, oxygen, intravenous saline or bronchodilators, and glucocorticoids if required. In most cases, the infusion can be resumed at a 50 % reduction in rate (e.g. from 100 mg/h to 50 mg/h) when symptoms have completely resolved.

Anaphylactic and other hypersensitivity reactions have been reported following the intravenous administration of proteins, including MabThera, to patients. Medicinal products for the treatment of hypersensitivity reactions, e.g., epinephrine (adrenaline), antihistamines and glucocorticoids, should be available for immediate use in the event of an allergic reaction during administration of MabThera. The presence of HACA may be associated with worsening infusion or allergic reactions after the second infusion of subsequent courses (see section 5.1).

In clinical studies 10/990 (1 %) patients with rheumatoid arthritis who received a first infusion of MabThera at any dose experienced a serious reaction during the infusion (see section 4.8).

There are no data on the safety of MabThera in patients with moderate heart failure (NYHA class III) or severe, uncontrolled cardiovascular disease. In patients treated with MabThera, the occurrence of pre-existing ischaemic cardiac conditions becoming symptomatic, such as angina pectoris, has been observed, as well as atrial fibrillation and flutter. Therefore, in patients with a known cardiac history, the risk of cardiovascular complications resulting from infusion reactions should be considered before treatment with MabThera and patients closely monitored during administration. Since hypotension may occur during MabThera infusion, consideration should be given to withholding anti-hypertensive medications 12 hours prior to the MabThera infusion.

Infections

Serious infections, including fatalities, can occur during therapy with MabThera (see section 4.8). MabThera should not be administered to patients with an active, severe infection (eg. tuberculosis, sepsis and opportunistic infections, see section 4.3) or severely immunocompromised patients (eg. in hypogammaglobulinaemia or where levels of CD4 or CD8 are very low). Physicians should exercise caution when considering the use of MabThera in patients with a history of recurring or chronic infections or with underlying conditions which may further predispose patients to serious infection (see section 4.8).

Patients reporting signs and symptoms of infection following MabThera therapy should be promptly evaluated and treated appropriately. Before giving a subsequent course of MabThera treatment, patients should be re-evaluated for any potential risk for infections.

Very rare cases of Progressive Multifocal Leukoencephalopathy (PML) have been reported following use of MabThera for the treatment of rheumatoid arthritis and autoimmune diseases including Systemic Lupus Erythematosus (SLE) and Vasculitis. These cases involved patients with multiple risk factors for PML, including the underlying disease and long-term immunosuppressive therapy or chemotherapy.

In patients with non-Hodgkin's lymphoma receiving rituximab in combination with cytotoxic chemotherapy, very rare cases of hepatitis B reactivation have been reported (see non-Hodgkin's lymphoma).

Immunisation

Physicians should review the patient's vaccination status and follow current immunisation guidelines prior to MabThera therapy. Vaccination should be completed at least 4 weeks prior to first administration of MabThera.

The safety of immunisation with live viral vaccines following MabThera therapy has not been studied. Therefore vaccination with live virus vaccines is not recommended whilst on MabThera or whilst peripherally B cell depleted.

Patients treated with MabThera may receive non-live vaccinations. However, response rates to non-live vaccines may be reduced. In a randomised study, patients with RA treated with MabThera and methotrexate had comparable response rates to tetanus recall antigen (39% vs. 42%), reduced rates to pneumococcal polysaccharide vaccine (43% vs 82% to at least 2 pneumococcal antibody serotypes), and KLH neoantigen (47% vs. 93%), when given 6 months after MabThera as compared to patients only receiving methotrexate. Should non-live vaccinations be required whilst receiving MabThera therapy, these should be completed at least 4 weeks prior to commencing the next course of MabThera

In the overall experience of MabThera repeat treatment over one year, the proportions of patients with positive antibody titres against S. pneumoniae, influenza, mumps, rubella, varicella and tetanus toxoid were generally similar to the proportions at baseline.

Concomitant/sequential use of other DMARDs

The concomitant use of MabThera and antirheumatic therapies other than those specified under the rheumatoid arthritis indication and posology is not recommended.

There are limited data from clinical trials to fully assess the safety of the sequential use of other DMARDs (including TNF inhibitors and other biologics) following MabThera (see section 4.5). The available data indicate that the rate of clinically relevant infection is unchanged when such therapies are used in patients previously treated with MabThera, however patients should be closely observed for signs of infection if biologic agents and/or DMARDs are used following MabThera therapy.

Malignancy

Immunomodulatory drugs may increase the risk of malignancy. On the basis of limited experience with MabThera in rheumatoid arthritis patients (see section 4.8) a possible risk for the development of solid tumours cannot be excluded at this time, although present data do not seem to suggest any increased risk.

4.5 Interaction with other medicinal products and other forms of interaction

Currently, there are limited data on possible drug interactions with MabThera.

In CLL patients, co-administration with MabThera did not appear to have an effect on the pharmacokinetics of fludarabine or cyclophosphamide. In addition, there was no apparent effect of fludarabine and cyclophosphamide on the pharmacokinetics of rituximab.

Co-administration with methotrexate had no effect on the pharmacokinetics of MabThera in rheumatoid arthritis patients.

Patients with human anti-mouse antibody or human anti-chimeric antibody (HAMA/HACA) titres may have allergic or hypersensitivity reactions when treated with other diagnostic or therapeutic monoclonal antibodies.

In a cohort of patients with rheumatoid arthritis, 280 patients received subsequent therapy with other DMARDs, of whom 185 received biologic DMARD following MabThera. In these patients the rate of clinically relevant infection while on MabThera was 6.99 per 100 patient years compared to 5.49 per 100 patients years following treatment with the biologic DMARD.

4.6 Pregnancy and lactation

Pregnancy

IgG immunoglobulins are known to cross the placental barrier.

B cell levels in human neonates following maternal exposure to MabThera have not been studied in clinical trials. There are no adequate and well-controlled data from studies in pregnant women, however transient B-cell depletion and lymphocytopenia have been reported in some infants born to mothers exposed to rituximab during pregnancy. For these reasons MabThera should not be administered to pregnant women unless the possible benefit outweighs the potential risk.

Due to the long retention time of rituximab in B cell depleted patients, women of childbearing potential should use effective contraceptive methods during treatment and for 12 months following MabThera therapy.

Developmental toxicity studies performed in cynomolgus monkeys revealed no evidence of embryotoxicity in utero. New born offspring of maternal animals exposed to MabThera were noted to have depleted B cell populations during the post natal phase.

Lactation

Whether rituximab is excreted in human milk is not known. However, because maternal IgG is excreted in human milk, and rituximab was detectable in milk from lactating monkeys, women should not breastfeed while treated with MabThera and for 12 months following MabThera treatment.

4.7 Effects on ability to drive and use machines

No studies on the effects of MabThera on the ability to drive and use machines have been performed, although the

Table 1 ADRs reported in clinical trials or during postmarketing surveillance in patients with NHL and CLL disease treated with MabThera monotherapy/maintenance or in combination with chemotherapy

System Organ Class	Very Common	Common	Uncommon	Unknown
Infections and infestations	bacterial infections, viral infections, +bronchitis	sepsis, +pneumonia, +febrile infection, +herpes zoster, +respiratory tract infection, fungal infections, infections of unknown aetiology, +acute bronchitis, +sinusitis, hepatitis B[1]		serious viral infection[2],
Blood and lymphatic system disorders	neutropenia, leucopenia, +febrile neutropenia, +thrombocytopenia	anaemia, +pancytopenia, +granulocytopenia	coagulation disorders, aplastic anaemia, haemolytic anaemia, lymphadenopathy	late neutropenia[3], transient increase in serum IgM levels[3]
Immune system disorders	infusion related reactions, angioedema	hypersensitivity		tumour lysis syndrome[4], cytokine release syndrome[4], serum sickness, anaphylaxis
Metabolism and nutrition disorders		hyperglycaemia, weight decrease, peripheral oedema, face oedema, increased LDH, hypocalcaemia		
Psychiatric disorders			depression, nervousness,	
Nervous system disorders		paraesthesia, hypoaesthesia, agitation, insomnia, vasodilatation, dizziness, anxiety	dysgeusia	cranial neuropathy, peripheral neuropathy facial nerve palsy[5], loss of other senses[5]
Eye disorders		lacrimation disorder, conjunctivitis		severe vision loss[5]
Ear and labyrinth disorders		tinnitus, ear pain		hearing loss[5]
Cardiac disorders		+myocardial infarction[4 and 6], arrhythmia, +atrial fibrillation, tachycardia, +cardiac disorder	+left ventricular failure, +supraventricular tachycardia, +ventricular tachycardia, +angina, +myocardial ischaemia, bradycardia,	heart failure[4 and 6], severe cardiac events[4 and 6]
Vascular disorders		hypertension, orthostatic hypotension, hypotension		vasculitis (predominately cutaneous), leukocytoclastic vasculitis
Respiratory, thoracic and mediastinal disorders		bronchospasm[4], respiratory disease, chest pain, dyspnoea, increased cough, rhinitis	asthma, bronchiolitis obliterans, lung disorder, hypoxia	respiratory failure[4], pulmonary infiltrates, interstitial pneumonitis
Gastrointestinal disorders	nausea	vomiting, diarrhoea, abdominal pain, dysphagia, stomatitis, constipation, dyspepsia, anorexia, throat irritation	abdominal enlargement	gastro-intestinal perforation[7]
Skin and subcutaneous tissue disorders	pruritus, rash, +alopecia	urticaria, sweating, night sweats, +skin disorder		severe bullous skin reactions, toxic epidermal necrolysis[7]
Musculoskeletal, connective tissue and bone disorders		hypertonia, myalgia, arthralgia, back pain, neck pain, pain		
Renal and urinary disorders				renal failure[4]
General disorders and administration site conditions	fever, chills, asthenia, headache	tumour pain, flushing, malaise, cold syndrome, +fatigue, +shivering, +multi-organ failure[4]	pain at the infusion site	
Investigations	decreased IgG levels			

For each term, the frequency count was based on reactions of all grades (from mild to severe), except for terms marked with "+" where the frequency count was based only on severe (≥ grade 3 NCI common toxicity criteria) reactions. Only the highest frequency observed in the trials is reported

[1] includes reactivation and primary infections; frequency based on R-FC regimen in relapsed/refractory CLL

[2] see also section infection below

[3] see also section haematologic adverse reactions below

[4] see also section infusion-related reactions below. Rarely fatal cases reported

[5] signs and symptoms of cranial neuropathy. Occurred at various times up to several months after completion of MabThera therapy

[6] observed mainly in patients with prior cardiac condition and/or cardiotoxic chemotherapy and were mostly associated with infusion-related reactions

[7] includes fatal cases

pharmacological activity and adverse events reported to date do not indicate that such an effect is likely.

4.8 Undesirable effects

Experience from non-Hodgkin's lymphoma and chronic lymphocytic leukaemia.

The overall safety profile of MabThera in non-Hodgkin's lymphoma and chronic lymphocytic leukaemia is based on data from patients from clinical trials and from post-marketing surveillance. These patients were treated either with MabThera monotherapy (as induction treatment or maintenance treatment following induction treatment) or in combination with chemotherapy.

The most frequently observed adverse drug reactions (ADRs) in patients receiving MabThera were infusion-related reactions which occurred in the majority of patients during the first infusion. The incidence of infusion-related symptoms decreases substantially with subsequent infusions and is less than 1% after eight doses of MabThera.

Infectious events (predominantly bacterial and viral) occurred in approximately 30-55 % of patients during clinical trials in patients with NHL and in 30-50 % of patients during clinical trial in patients with CLL.

The most frequent reported or observed serious adverse drug reactions were:

- Infusion-related reactions (including cytokine-release syndrome, tumour-lysis syndrome), see section 4.4.
- Infections, see section 4.4.
- Cardiovascular events, see section 4.4.

Other serious ADRs reported include hepatitis B reactivation and PML (see section 4.4.).

The frequencies of ADRs reported with MabThera alone or in combination with chemotherapy are summarised in the tables below. Within each frequency grouping, undesirable effects are presented in order of decreasing seriousness. Frequencies are defined as very common (≥ 1/10), common (≥ 1/100 to < 1/10) and uncommon (≥ 1/1,000 to < 1/100). The ADRs identified only during post-marketing surveillance, and for which a frequency could not be estimated, are listed under "unknown".

Table 1 ADRs reported in clinical trials or during postmarketing surveillance in patients with NHL and CLL disease treated with MabThera monotherapy/maintenance or in combination with chemotherapy

(see Table 1 above)

The following terms have been reported as adverse events during clinical trials, however, were reported at a similar or lower incidence in the MabThera-arms compared to control arms: haematotoxicity, neutropenic infection, urinary tract infection, sensory disturbance, pyrexia.

Infusion-related reactions

Signs and symptoms suggestive of an infusion-related reaction were reported in more than 50 % of patients in clinical trials, and were predominantly seen during the first infusion, usually in the first one to two hours. These symptoms mainly comprised fever, chills and rigors. Other symptoms included flushing, angioedema, bronchospasm, vomiting, nausea, urticaria/rash, fatigue, headache, throat irritation, rhinitis, pruritus, pain, tachycardia, hypertension, hypotension, dyspnoea, dyspepsia, asthenia and features of tumour lysis syndrome. Severe infusion-related reactions (such as bronchospasm, hypotension) occurred in up to 12 % of the cases. Additional reactions reported in some cases were myocardial infarction, atrial fibrillation and pulmonary oedema and acute reversible thrombocytopenia. Exacerbations of pre-existing cardiac conditions such as angina pectoris or congestive heart failure or severe cardiac events (heart failure, myocardial infarction, atrial fibrillation), pulmonary oedema, multi-organ failure, tumour lysis syndrome, cytokine release syndrome, renal failure, and respiratory failure were reported at lower or unknown frequencies. The incidence of infusion-related symptoms decreased substantially with subsequent infusions and is <1 % of patients by the eighth cycle of MabThera (-containing) treatment.

Infections

MabThera induces B-cell depletion in about 70-80 % of patients, but was associated with decreased serum immunoglobulins only in a minority of patients.

Localised candida infections as well as Herpes zoster was reported at a higher incidence in the MabThera-containing arm of randomised studies. Severe infections were reported in about 4 % of patients treated with MabThera monotherapy. Higher frequencies of infections overall, including grade 3 or 4 infections, were observed during

MabThera maintenance treatment up to 2 years when compared to observation. There was no cumulative toxicity in terms of infections reported over a 2-year treatment period. In addition, other serious viral infections either new, reactivated or exacerbated, some of which were fatal, have been reported with MabThera treatment. The majority of patients had received MabThera in combination with chemotherapy or as part of a haematopoetic stem cell transplant. Examples of these serious viral infections are infections caused by the herpes viruses (Cytomegalovirus, Varicella Zoster Virus and Herpes Simplex Virus), JC virus (progressive multifocal leukoencephalopathy (PML)) and hepatitis C virus. Cases of hepatitis B reactivation, have been reported, the majority of which were in subjects receiving MabThera in combination with cytotoxic chemotherapy. In patients with relapsed/refractory CLL, the incidence of grade 3 / 4 hepatitis B infection (reactivation and primary infection) was 2 % in R-FC vs 0 % FC. Progression of Kaposi's sarcoma has been observed in rituximab-exposed patients with pre-existing Kaposi's sarcoma. These cases occurred in non-approved indications and the majority of patients were HIV positive.

Haematologic Adverse Reactions

In clinical trials with MabThera monotherapy given for 4 weeks, haematological abnormalities occurred in a minority of patients and were usually mild and reversible. Severe (grade 3/4) neutropenia was reported in 4.2 %, anaemia in 1.1 % and thrombocytopenia in 1.7 % of the patients. During MabThera maintenance treatment for up to 2 years, leucopenia (5 % vs 2 %, grade 3/4) and neutropenia (10 % vs 4 %, grade 3/4) were reported at a higher incidence when compared to observation. The incidence of thrombocytopenia was low (<1, grade 3/4 %) and was not different between treatment arms. In studies with MabThera in combination with chemotherapy, grade 3/4 leucopenia (R-CHOP 88 % vs CHOP 79 %, R-FC 23 % vs FC 12 %), neutropenia (R-CVP 24 % vs. CVP 14 %; R-CHOP 97 % vs. CHOP 88 %, R-FC 30 % vs FC 19 % in previously untreated CLL), pancytopenia (R-FC 3 % vs FC 1 % in previously untreated CLL) were usually reported with higher frequencies when compared to chemotherapy alone. However, the higher incidence of neutropenia in patients treated with MabThera and chemotherapy was not associated with a higher incidence of infections and infestations compared to patients treated with chemotherapy alone and the neutropenia was not prolonged in the MabThera group. There were no differences reported for the incidence of anaemia. Some cases of late neutropenia occurring more than four weeks after the last infusion of MabThera were reported. In the CLL first-line study, Binet stage C patients experienced more adverse events in the R-FC arm compared to the FC arm (R-FC 83% vs FC 71%).

In the relapsed/refractory CLL study, grade 3/4 thrombocytopenia was reported in 11 % of patients in the R-FC group compared to 9 % of patients in the FC group.

In studies of MabThera in patients with Waldenstrom's macroglobulinaemia, transient increases in serum IgM levels have been observed following treatment initiation, which may be associated with hyperviscosity and related symptoms. The transient IgM increase usually returned to at least baseline level within 4 months.

Cardiovascular reactions

Cardiovascular reactions during clinical trials with MabThera monotherapy were reported in 18.8 % of patients with the most frequently reported events being hypotension and hypertension. Cases of grade 3 or 4 arrhythmia (including ventricular and supraventricular tachycardia) and angina pectoris during infusion were reported. During maintenance treatment, the incidence of grade 3/4 cardiac disorders was comparable between patients treated with MabThera and observation. Cardiac events were reported as serious adverse events (including atrial fibrillation, myocardial infarction, left ventricular failure, myocardial ischaemia) in 3 % of patients treated with MabThera compared to <1 % on observation. In studies evaluating MabThera in combination with chemotherapy, the incidence of grade 3 and 4 cardiac arrhythmias, predominantly supraventricular arrhythmias such as tachycardia and atrial flutter/fibrillation, was higher in the R-CHOP group (14 patients, 6.9 %) as compared to the CHOP group (3 patients, 1.5 %). All of these arrhythmias either occurred in the context of a MabThera infusion or were associated with predisposing conditions such as fever, infection, acute myocardial infarction or pre-existing respiratory and cardiovascular disease. No difference between the R-CHOP and CHOP group was observed in the incidence of other grade 3 and 4 cardiac events including heart failure, myocardial disease and manifestations of coronary artery disease. In CLL, the overall incidence of grade 3 or 4 cardiac disorders was low both in the first-line study (4 % R-FC, 3 % FC) and in the relapsed/refractory study (4 % R-FC, 4 % FC).

Neurologic events

During the treatment period, four patients (2 %) treated with R-CHOP, all with cardiovascular risk factors, experienced thromboembolic cerebrovascular accidents during the first treatment cycle. There was no difference between the treatment groups in the incidence of other thromboembolic events. In contrast, three patients (1.5 %) had cerebrovascular events in the CHOP group, all of which occurred during the follow-up period. In CLL, the overall incidence of grade 3 or 4 nervous system disorders was low both in the first-line study (4 % R-FC, 4 % FC) and in the relapsed/refractory study (3 % R-FC, 3 % FC).

Gastrointestinal Disorders

Gastrointestinal perforation in some cases leading to death has been observed in patients receiving MabThera for treatment of non Hodgkin's lymphoma. In the majority of these cases, MabThera was administered with chemotherapy.

IgG levels

In the clinical trial evaluating MabThera maintenance treatment, median IgG levels were below the lower limit of normal (LLN) (< 7 g/L) after induction treatment in both the observation and the MabThera groups. In the observation group, the median IgG level subsequently increased to above the LLN, but remained constant in the MabThera group. The proportion of patients with IgG levels below the LLN was about 60 % in the MabThera group throughout the 2 year treatment period, while it decreased in the observation group (36 % after 2 years).

Patient subpopulations MabThera monotherapy

Elderly patients (⩾ 65 years):

The incidence of ADRs of all grades and grade 3 /4 ADR was similar in elderly patients compared to younger patients (<65 years).

Bulky disease

There was a higher incidence of grade 3/4 ADRs in patients with bulky disease than in patients without bulky disease (25.6 % vs. 15.4 %). The incidence of ADRs of any grade was similar in these two groups.

Re-treatment

The percentage of patients reporting ADRs upon re-treatment with further courses of MabThera was similar to the percentage of patients reporting ADRs upon initial exposure (any grade and grade 3/4 ADRs).

Patient subpopulations – MabThera combination therapy

Elderly patients (⩾ 65 years)

The incidence of grade 3/4 blood and lymphatic adverse events was higher in elderly patients compared to younger patients (<65 years), with previously untreated or relapsed/refractory CLL.

Experience from rheumatoid arthritis

The overall safety profile of MabThera in rheumatoid arthritis is based on data from patients from clinical trials and from post-marketing surveillance.

The clinical efficacy of MabThera, given together with methotrexate was studied in three double blind controlled clinical trials (one phase III two phase II trials) in patients with rheumatoid arthritis. More than 1000 patients received at least one treatment course and were followed for periods ranging from 6 months to over 3 years; nearly 600 patients received two or more courses of treatment during the follow up period.

Patients received 2 × 1000 mg of MabThera separated by an interval of two weeks; in addition to methotrexate (10-25 mg/week). MabThera infusions were administered after an intravenous infusion of 100 mg methylprednisolone; patients also received treatment with oral prednisone for 15 days. ADRs, which occurred with at least a 2 % difference compared to the control arm and more frequently by patients who had received at least one infusion of MabThera than among patients that had received placebo in the phase III trial and the combined population included in phase II studies, are listed in the Table below. Frequencies are defined as very common (⩾1/10) and common (⩾1/100 to <1/10). Within each frequency grouping, undesirable effects are presented in order of decreasing seriousness.

The most frequent adverse reactions considered due to receipt of 2x1000 mg MabThera in Phase II and III studies were acute infusion reactions. Infusion reactions occurred in 15 % patients following the first infusion of rituximab and 5 % in placebo patients. Infusion reactions decreased to 2 % following the second infusion in both rituximab and placebo groups. The safety information collected during post marketing experience reflects the expected adverse reaction profile as seen in clinical trials for MabThera (see section 4.4).

Table 2 Summary of Adverse Drug Reactions Reported in Clinical Trials or During Postmarketing Surveillance Occurring in Patients with Rheumatoid Arthritis receiving MabThera

(see Table 2 below)

The following terms have been reported as adverse events during clinical trials, however, were reported at a similar incidence in the MabThera-arms compared to control arms: lower respiratory tract infections/pneumonia, abdominal pain upper, muscle spasms and asthenia.

Multiple Courses

The limited clinical trial data on multiple courses of treatment of RA patients seem to be associated with a similar ADR profile to that observed following first exposure. However, worsening of infusion or allergic reactions and failure to B cell deplete following rituximab cannot be excluded in HACA positive patients after repeated exposure to rituximab on the basis of available data. The incidence of acute infusion reactions following subsequent treatment courses was generally lower than the incidence following the first infusion of MabThera.

Infusion-related reactions

Symptoms suggesting an acute infusion reaction (e.g.pruritus, fever, urticaria/rash, chills, pyrexia, rigors, sneezing, angioneurotic oedema, throat irritation, cough and bronchospasm, with or without associated hypotension or hypertension) were observed in 79/540 (15 %) patients following their first exposure to MabThera; In a study comparing the effect of glucocorticoid regimen, these events were observed in 5/149 (3 %) of patients following their first rituximab placebo infusion and 42/192 (22 %) of patients receiving their first infusion of 1000 mg rituximab. Premedication with intravenous glucocorticoid significantly reduced the incidence and severity of these events. Of the patients who received 1000 mg rituximab without premeditation with glucocorticoids, 18/65 (28 %) experienced an acute infusion reaction, compared with 24/127 (19 %) in patients given intravenous glucocorticoid premeditation, respectively.

Infections

The rate of infection was approximately 0.9 per patient year in MabThera treated patients. The infections consisted mostly of upper respiratory tract infections and urinary tract infections. The incidence of clinically significant infection, some of which were fatal, was 0.05 per patient year in MabThera treated patients.

Cases of Progressive Multifocal Leukoencephalopathy with fatal outcome have been reported following use of MabThera for the treatment of autoimmune diseases. This includes Rheumatoid Arthritis and off-label autoimmune diseases, including Systemic Lupus Erythematosus (SLE) and Vasculitis. All the reported cases had multiple risk factors for PML, including either the underlying disease and or long-term immunosuppressive therapy or chemotherapy.

Malignancies

The clinical data, particularly the number of repeated courses, are too limited to assess the potential incidence of malignancies following exposure to rituximab, although

Table 2 Summary of Adverse Drug Reactions Reported in Clinical Trials or During Postmarketing Surveillance Occurring in Patients with Rheumatoid Arthritis receiving MabThera

System Organ Class	Very Common	Common	Uncommon
Infections and Infestations	any infection, upper respiratory tract infection	urinary tract infections	
Immune System Disorders General disorders and administration site conditions	*Infusion related reactions (nausea, chills, rhinitis, urticaria hot flush) hypertension, rash, pyrexia, pruritus, throat irritation and hypotension		*Infusion related reactions (generalised oedema, bronchospasm, wheezing, laryngeal oedema, angioneurotic oedema, generalised pruritus, anaphylaxis, anaphylactoid reaction)
Metabolism and Nutritional Disorders		hypercholesterolaemia	
Nervous System disorders		Paraesthesia, migraine	
Gastrointestinal Disorders		dyspepsia	
Musculo skeletal disorders		arthralgia / musculoskeletal pain, osteoarthritis	

*Reactions occurring during or within 24 hours of infusion. See also infusion-related reactions below. Infusion related reactions may occur as a result of hypersensitivity and/or to the mechanism of action.

present data do not seem to suggest any increased risk. Long-term safety evaluations are ongoing.

Cardiovascular

Cardiac events were observed in 11 % patients in clinical studies with MabThera. In placebo controlled studies, serious cardiac events were reported equally in MabThera and placebo treated patients (2 %).

4.9 Overdose

There has been no experience of overdose in human clinical trials. However, single doses higher than 1000 mg have not been tested in controlled clinical trials.

5. PHARMACOLOGICAL PROPERTIES

5.1 Pharmacodynamic properties

Pharmacotherapeutic group: monoclonal antibodies, ATC code: L01X C02

Rituximab binds specifically to the transmembrane antigen, CD20, a non-glycosylated phosphoprotein, located on pre-B and mature B lymphocytes. The antigen is expressed on > 95 % of all B cell non-Hodgkin's lymphomas.

CD20 is found on both normal and malignant B cells, but not on haematopoietic stem cells, pro-B cells, normal plasma cells or other normal tissue. This antigen does not internalise upon antibody binding and is not shed from the cell surface. CD20 does not circulate in the plasma as a free antigen and, thus, does not compete for antibody binding.

The Fab domain of rituximab binds to the CD20 antigen on B lymphocytes and the Fc domain can recruit immune effector functions to mediate B cell lysis. Possible mechanisms of effector-mediated cell lysis include complement-dependent cytotoxicity (CDC) resulting from C1q binding, and antibody-dependent cellular cytotoxicity (ADCC) mediated by one or more of the Fcγ receptors on the surface of granulocytes, macrophages and NK cells. Rituximab binding to CD 20 antigen on B lymphocytes has also been demonstrated to induce cell death via apoptosis.

Peripheral B cell counts declined below normal following completion of the first dose of MabThera. In patients treated for haematological malignancies, B cell repletion began within 6 months of treatment returning to normal levels between 9 and 12 months after completion of therapy. In rheumatoid arthritis patients, immediate depletion of B cells in the peripheral blood was observed following two infusions of 1000 mg MabThera separated by a 14 day interval. Peripheral blood B cell counts begin to increase from week 24 and evidence for repopulation is observed in the majority of patients by week 40, whether MabThera was administered as monotherapy or in combination with methotrexate.

Clinical Experience in Non-Hodgkin's lymphoma and in chronic lymphocytic leukaemia

Follicular non-Hodgkin's lymphoma

Monotherapy

Initial treatment, weekly for 4 doses

In the pivotal study, 166 patients with relapsed or chemoresistant low-grade or follicular B cell NHL received 375 mg/m^2 of MabThera as an intravenous infusion once weekly for four weeks. The overall response rate (ORR) in the intent-to-treat (ITT) population was 48 % ($CI_{95\,\%}$ 41 % - 56 %) with a 6 % complete response (CR) and a 42 % partial response (PR) rate. The projected median time to progression (TTP) for responding patients was 13.0 months. In a subgroup analysis, the ORR was higher in patients with IWF B, C, and D histological subtypes as compared to IWF A subtype (58 % vs. 12 %), higher in patients whose largest lesion was < 5 cm vs.> 7 cm in greatest diameter (53 % vs. 38 %), and higher in patients with chemosensitive relapse as compared to chemoresistant (defined as duration of response < 3 months) relapse (50 % vs. 22 %). ORR in patients previously treated with autologous bone marrow transplant (ABMT) was 78 % versus 43 % in patients with no ABMT. Neither age, sex, lymphoma grade, initial diagnosis, presence or absence of bulky disease, normal or high LDH nor presence of extranodal disease had a statistically significant effect (Fisher's exact test) on response to MabThera. A statistically significant correlation was noted between response rates and bone marrow involvement. 40 % of patients with bone marrow involvement responded compared to 59 % of patients with no bone marrow involvement (p=0.0186). This finding was not supported by a stepwise logistic regression analysis in which the following factors were identified as prognostic factors: histological type, bcl-2 positivity at baseline, resistance to last chemotherapy and bulky disease.

Initial treatment, weekly for 8 doses

In a multi-centre, single-arm study, 37 patients with relapsed or chemoresistant, low grade or follicular B cell NHL received 375 mg/m^2 of MabThera as intravenous infusion weekly for eight doses. The ORR was 57 % (95% Confidence interval (CI); 41 % – 73 %; CR 14 %, PR 43 %) with a projected median TTP for responding patients of 19.4 months (range 5.3 to 38.9 months).

Initial treatment, bulky disease, weekly for 4 doses

In pooled data from three studies, 39 patients with relapsed or chemoresistant, bulky disease (single lesion ≥ 10 cm in diameter), low grade or follicular B cell NHL received 375 mg/m2 of MabThera as intravenous infusion weekly for four doses. The ORR was 36 % (CI95 % 21 % – 51 %; CR 3 %, PR 33 %) with a median TTP for responding patients of 9.6 months (range 4.5 to 26.8 months).

Re-treatment, weekly for 4 doses

In a multi-centre, single-arm study, 58 patients with relapsed or chemoresistant low grade or follicular B cell NHL, who had achieved an objective clinical response to a prior course of MabThera, were re-treated with 375 mg/m^2 of MabThera as intravenous infusion weekly for four doses. Three of the patients had received two courses of MabThera before enrollment and thus were given a third course in the study. Two patients were re-treated twice in the study. For the 60 re-treatments on study, the ORR was 38 % ($CI_{95\,\%}$ 26 % – 51 %; 10 % CR, 28 % PR) with a projected median TTP for responding patients of 17.8 months (range 5.4 – 26.6). This compares favourably with the TTP achieved after the prior course of MabThera (12.4 months).

Initial treatment, in combination with chemotherapy

In an open-label randomised trial, a total of 322 previously untreated patients with follicular lymphoma were randomised to receive either CVP chemotherapy (cyclophosphamide 750 mg/m^2, vincristine 1.4 mg/m^2 up to a maximum of 2 mg on day 1, and prednisolone 40 mg/m^2/day on days 1 - 5) every 3 weeks for 8 cycles or MabThera 375 mg/m^2 in combination with CVP (R-CVP). MabThera was administered on the first day of each treatment cycle. A total of 321 patients (162 R-CVP, 159 CVP) received therapy and were analysed for efficacy. The median follow up of patients was 53 months. R-CVP led to a significant benefit over CVP for the primary endpoint, time to treatment failure (27 months vs. 6.6 months, p < 0.0001, log-rank test). The proportion of patients with a tumour response (CR, CRu, PR) was significantly higher (p< 0.0001 Chi-Square test) in the R-CVP group (80.9 %) than the CVP group (57.2 %). Treatment with R-CVP significantly prolonged the time to disease progression or death compared to CVP, 33.6 months and 14.7 months, respectively (p < 0.0001, log-rank test). The median duration of response was 37.7 months in the R-CVP group and was 13.5 months in the CVP group (p < 0.0001, log-rank test).

The difference between the treatment groups with respect to overall survival showed a significant clinical difference (p=0.029, log-rank test stratified by centre): survival rates at 53 months were 80.9 % for patients in the R-CVP group compared to 71.1 % for patients in the CVP group

Results from three other randomised trials using MabThera in combination with chemotherapy regimen other than CVP (CHOP, MCP, CHVP/Interferon-α) have also demonstrated significant improvements in response rates, time-dependent parameters as well as in overall survival. Key results from all four studies are summarised in table 3.

Table 3 Summary of key results from four phase III randomised studies evaluating the benefit of MabThera with different chemotherapy regimens in follicular lymphoma

(see Table 3 below)

Maintenance therapy

In a prospective, open label, international, multi-centre, phase III trial, 465 patients with relapsed/refractory follicular NHL were randomised in a first step to induction therapy with either CHOP (cyclophosphamide, doxorubicin, vincristine, prednisolone; n=231) or MabThera plus CHOP (R-CHOP, n=234). The two treatment groups were well balanced with regard to baseline characteristics and disease status. A total of 334 patients achieving a complete or partial remission following induction therapy were randomised in a second step to MabThera maintenance therapy (n=167) or observation (n=167). MabThera maintenance treatment consisted of a single infusion of MabThera at 375 mg/m^2 body surface area given every 3 months until disease progression or for a maximum period of two years.

The final efficacy analysis included all patients randomised to both parts of the study. After a median observation time of 31 months for patients randomised to the induction phase, R-CHOP significantly improved the outcome of patients with relapsed/refractory follicular NHL when compared to CHOP (see Table 4).

Table 4 Induction phase: overview of efficacy results for CHOP vs R-CHOP (31 months median observation time)

(see Table 4 below)

For patients randomised to the maintenance phase of the trial, the median observation time was 28 months from maintenance randomisation. Maintenance treatment with MabThera led to a clinically relevant and statistically significant improvement in the primary endpoint, PFS, (time from maintenance randomisation to relapse, disease progression or death) when compared to observation alone (p< 0.0001 log-rank test). The median PFS was 42.2 months in the MabThera maintenance arm compared to 14.3 months in the observation arm. Using a cox regression analysis, the risk of experiencing progressive disease or death was reduced by 61 % with MabThera maintenance treatment when compared to observation (95 % CI; 45 %-72 %). Kaplan-Meier estimated progression-free rates at 12 months were 78 % in the MabThera maintenance group vs 57 % in the observation group. An analysis of overall survival confirmed the significant benefit of MabThera maintenance over observation (p=0.0039 log-rank test).

Table 3 Summary of key results from four phase III randomised studies evaluating the benefit of MabThera with different chemotherapy regimens in follicular lymphoma

Study	Treatment, n	Median FU, months	ORR, %	CR, %	Median TTF/PFS/EFS mo	OS rates, %
M39021	CVP, 159 R-CVP, 162	53	57 81	10 41	Median TTP: 14.7 33.6 P<0.0001	53-months 71.1 80.9 p=0.029
GLSG'00	CHOP, 205 R-CHOP, 223	18	90 96	17 20	Median TTF: 2.6 years Not reached p < 0.001	18-months 90 95 p = 0.016
OSHO-39	MCP, 96 R-MCP, 105	47	75 92	25 50	Median PFS: 28.8 Not reached p < 0.0001	48-months 74 87 p = 0.0096
FL2000	CHVP-IFN, 183 R-CHVP-IFN, 175	42	85 94	49 76	Median EFS: 36 Not reached p < 0.0001	42-months 84 91 p = 0.029

EFS – Event Free Survival

TTP – Time to progression or death

PFS – Progression-Free Survival

TTF – Time to Treatment Failure

OS rates – survival rates at the time of the analyses

Table 4 Induction phase: overview of efficacy results for CHOP vs R-CHOP (31 months median observation time)

	CHOP	R-CHOP	p-value	Risk Reduction[1)]
Primary Efficacy				
ORR[2)]	74 %	87 %	0.0003	na
CR[2)]	16 %	29 %	0.0005	na
PR[2)]	58 %	58 %	0.9449	na

[1)] Estimates were calculated by hazard ratios

[2)] Last tumour response as assessed by the investigator. The "primary" statistical test for "response" was the trend test of CR versus PR versus non-response (p < 0.0001)

Abbreviations: NA, not available; ORR: overall response rate; CR: complete response; PR: partial response

Table 5 Maintenance phase: overview of efficacy results MabThera vs. observation (28 months median observation time)

Efficacy Parameter	Kaplan-Meier Estimate of Median Time to Event (Months)			Risk Reduction
	Observation (N = 167)	MabThera (N=167)	Log-Rank p value	
Progression-free survival (PFS)	*14.3*	*42.2*	*<0.0001*	*61 %*
Overall Survival	*NR*	*NR*	*0.0039*	*56 %*
Time to new lymphoma treatment	*20.1*	*38.8*	*<0.0001*	*50 %*
Disease-free survival[a]	*16.5*	*53.7*	*0.0003*	*67 %*
Subgroup Analysis				
PFS				
CHOP	*11.6*	*37.5*	*<0.0001*	*71 %*
R-CHOP	*22.1*	*51.9*	*0.0071*	*46 %*
CR	*14.3*	*52.8*	*0.0008*	*64 %*
PR	*14.3*	*37.8*	*<0.0001*	*54 %*
OS				
CHOP	*NR*	*NR*	*0.0348*	*55 %*
R-CHOP	*NR*	*NR*	*0.0482*	*56 %*

NR: not reached; [a]: only applicable to patients achieving a CR

MabThera maintenance treatment reduced the risk of death by 56 % (95 % CI; 22 %-75 %).

Table 5 Maintenance phase: overview of efficacy results MabThera vs. observation (28 months median observation time)

(see Table 5 above)

The benefit of MabThera maintenance treatment was confirmed in all subgroups analysed, regardless of induction regimen (CHOP or R-CHOP) or quality of response to induction treatment (CR or PR) (table 5). MabThera maintenance treatment significantly prolonged median PFS in patients responding to CHOP induction therapy (median PFS 37.5 months vs 11.6 months, p< 0.0001) as well as in those responding to R-CHOP induction (median PFS 51.9 months vs 22.1 months, p=0.0071). Although subgroups were small, MabThera maintenance treatment provided a significant benefit in terms of overall survival for both patients responding to CHOP and patients responding to R-CHOP, although longer follow-up is required to confirm this observation.

Diffuse large B cell non-Hodgkin's lymphoma

In a randomised, open-label trial, a total of 399 previously untreated elderly patients (age 60 to 80 years) with diffuse large B cell lymphoma received standard CHOP chemotherapy (cyclophosphamide 750 mg/m^2, doxorubicin 50 mg/m^2, vincristine 1.4 mg/m^2 up to a maximum of 2 mg on day 1, and prednisolone 40 mg/m^2/day on days 1-5) every 3 weeks for eight cycles, or MabThera 375 mg/m^2 plus CHOP (R-CHOP). MabThera was administered on the first day of the treatment cycle.

The final efficacy analysis included all randomised patients (197 CHOP, 202 R-CHOP), and had a median follow-up duration of approximately 31 months. The two treatment groups were well balanced in baseline disease characteristics and disease status. The final analysis confirmed that R-CHOP treatment was associated with a clinically relevant and statistically significant improvement in the duration of event-free survival (the primary efficacy parameter; where events were death, relapse or progression of lymphoma, or institution of a new anti-lymphoma treatment) (p = 0.0001). Kaplan Meier estimates of the median duration of event-free survival were 35 months in the R-CHOP arm compared to 13 months in the CHOP arm, representing a risk reduction of 41 %. At 24 months, estimates for overall survival were 68.2 % in the R-CHOP arm compared to 57.4 % in the CHOP arm. A subsequent analysis of the duration of overall survival, carried out with a median follow-up duration of 60 months, confirmed the benefit of R-CHOP over CHOP treatment (p=0.0071), representing a risk reduction of 32 %.

The analysis of all secondary parameters (response rates, progression-free survival, disease-free survival, duration of response) verified the treatment effect of R-CHOP compared to CHOP. The complete response rate after cycle 8 was 76.2 % in the R-CHOP group and 62.4 % in the CHOP group (p=0.0028). The risk of disease progression was reduced by 46 % and the risk of relapse by 51 %.

In all patients subgroups (gender, age, age adjusted IPI, Ann Arbor stage, ECOG, β2 microglobulin, LDH, albumin, B symptoms, bulky disease, extranodal sites, bone marrow involvement), the risk ratios for event-free survival and overall survival (R-CHOP compared with CHOP) were less than 0.83 and 0.95 respectively. R-CHOP was associated with improvements in outcome for both high- and low-risk patients according to age adjusted IPI.

Clinical laboratory findings

Of 67 patients evaluated for human anti-mouse antibody (HAMA), no responses were noted. Of 356 patients evaluated for HACA, 1.1 % (4 patients) were positive.

Chronic lymphocytic leukaemia

In two open-label randomised trials, a total of 817 previously untreated patients and 552 patients with relapsed/refractory CLL were randomised to receive either FC chemotherapy (fludarabine 25 mg/m^2, cyclophosphamide 250 mg/m^2, days 1-3) every 4 weeks for 6 cycles or MabThera in combination with FC (R-FC). MabThera was administered at a dosage of 375 mg/m^2 during the first cycle one day prior to chemotherapy and at a dosage of 500 mg/m^2 on day 1 of each subsequent treatment cycle. Patients were excluded from the study in relapsed/refractory CLL if they had previously been treated with monoclonal antibodies or if they were refractory (defined as failure to achieve a partial remission for at least 6 months) to fludarabine or any nucleoside analogue. A total of 810 patients (403 R-FC, 407 FC) for the first-line study (Table 6a and Table 6b) and 552 patients (276 R-FC, 276 FC) for the relapsed/refractory study (Table 7) were analysed for efficacy.

In the first-line study, the median progression-free survival (primary endpoint) was 40 months in the R-FC group and 32 months in the FC group (p < 0.0001, log-rank test). The analysis of overall survival showed an improved survival in favour of the R-FC arm (p=0.0427, log-rank test), however longer follow-up is needed to confirm this observation. The benefit in terms of PFS was consistently observed in most patient subgroups analysed according to disease risk at baseline.

Table 6a First-line treatment of chronic lymphocytic leukaemia

Overview of efficacy results for MabThera plus FC vs. FC alone (20.7 months median observation time)

(see Table 6a below)

Table 6b First-line treatment of chronic lymphocytic leukaemia

Progression-Free Survival according to Binet stage (ITT)

(see Table 6b below)

In the relapsed/refractory study, the median progression-free survival (primary endpoint) was 30.6 months in the R-FC group and 20.6 months in the FC group (p=0.0002, log-rank test). The benefit in terms of PFS was observed in almost all patient subgroups analysed according to disease risk at baseline. A slight but not significant improvement in overall survival was reported in the R-FC compared to the FC arm.

Table 7 Treatment of relapsed/refractory chronic lymphocytic leukaemia - overview of efficacy results for MabThera plus FC vs. FC alone (25.3 months median observation time)

(see Table 7 on next page)

Results from other supportive studies using MabThera in combination with other chemotherapy regimens (including CHOP, FCM, PC, PCM, bendamustine and cladribine) for the treatment of previously untreated and/or relapsed/refractory CLL patients have also demonstrated high overall response rates with benefit in terms of PFS rates, albeit with modestly higher toxicity (especially myelotoxicity). These studies support the use of MabThera with any chemotherapy.

Data in approximately 180 patients pre-treated with MabThera have demonstrated clinical benefit (including CR) and are supportive for MabThera re-treatment.

Clinical Experience in Rheumatoid Arthritis

The efficacy and safety of MabThera in alleviating the symptoms and signs of rheumatoid arthritis was demonstrated in three randomised, controlled, double-blind, multicentre studies.

Study 1 was a double blind comparative study which included 517 patients that had experienced an inadequate response or intolerance to one or more TNF inhibitor therapies. Eligible patients had active rheumatoid arthritis for at least 6 months, diagnosed according to the criteria of the American College of Rheumatology (ACR), with swollen joint count (SJC) (8 (66 joint count)), and tender joint count (TJC) (8 (68 joint count)) and elevated CRP or ESR. The primary endpoint was the percent of patients who achieved an ACR20 response at week 24. Patients received two 1000 mg intravenous infusions of MabThera, each following an intravenous infusion of 100 mg methylprednisone and separated by an interval of 15 days. All patients received concomitant oral methotrexate (10-25 mg/week) and 60 mg oral prednisone on days 2-7 and 30 mg on days

Table 6a First-line treatment of chronic lymphocytic leukaemia
Overview of efficacy results for MabThera plus FC vs. FC alone (20.7 months median observation time)

Efficacy Parameter	Kaplan-Meier Estimate of Median Time to Event (Months)			Risk Reduction
	FC (N = 407)	R-FC (N=403)	Log-Rank p value	
Progression-free survival (PFS)	*32.2*	*39.8*	*<0.0001*	*44%*
Overall Survival	*NR*	*NR*	*0.0427*	*36%*
Event Free Survival	*31.1*	*39.8*	*<0.0001*	*45%*
Response rate (CR, nPR, or PR)	*72.7%*	*86.1%*	*<0.0001*	*n.a.*
CR rates	*17.2%*	*36.0%*	*<0.0001*	*n.a.*
*Duration of response**	*34.7*	*40.2*	*0.0040*	*39%*
*Disease free survival (DFS)***	*NR.*	*NR*	*0.7882*	*7%*
Time to new treatment	*NR.*	*NR*	*0.0052*	*35%*

Response rate and CR rates analysed using Chi-squared Test.

*: only applicable to patients achieving a CR, nPR, PR; NR: not reached n.a. not applicable

**: only applicable to patients achieving a CR;

Table 6b First-line treatment of chronic lymphocytic leukaemia
Progression-Free Survival according to Binet stage (ITT)

Progression-free survival (PFS)	Number of patients		Hazard Ratio (95% CI)	p-value (Wald test, not adjusted)
	FC	R-FC		
Binet A	*22*	*18*	*0.13 (0.03; 0.61)*	*0.0093*
Binet B	*257*	*259*	*0.45 (0.32; 0.63)*	*<0.0001*
Binet C	*126*	*125*	*0.88 (0.58; 1.33)*	*0.5406*

CI: Confidence Interval

Table 7 Treatment of relapsed/refractory chronic lymphocytic leukaemia - overview of efficacy results for MabThera plus FC vs. FC alone (25.3 months median observation time)

Efficacy Parameter	Kaplan-Meier Estimate of Median Time to Event (Months)			Risk Reduction
	FC (N = 276)	R-FC (N=276)	Log-Rank p value	
Progression-free survival (PFS)	*20.6*	*30.6*	*0.0002*	*35%*
Overall Survival	*51.9*	*NR*	*0.2874*	*17%*
Event Free Survival	*19.3*	*28.7*	*0.0002*	*36%*
Response rate (CR, nPR, or PR)	*58.0%*	*69.9%*	*0.0034*	*n.a.*
CR rates	*13.0%*	*24.3%*	*0.0007*	*n.a.*
*Duration of response **	*27.6*	*39.6*	*0.0252*	*31%*
*Disease free survival (DFS)***	*42.2*	*39.6*	*0.8842*	*-6%*
Time to new CLL treatment	*34.2*	*NR*	*0.0024*	*35%*

Response rate and CR rates analysed using Chi-squared Test.

*: only applicable to patients achieving a CR, nPR, PR; NR: not reached n.a. not applicable

**: only applicable to patients achieving a CR;

Table 8 Cross-Study Comparison of ACR Responses at Week 24 (ITT Population)

	ACR Response	Placebo+MTX	Rituximab+MTX
Study 1		N= 201	N= 298
	ACR20	36 (18%)	153 (51%)[1]
	ACR50	11 (5%)	80 (27%)[1]
	ACR70	3 (1%)	37 (12%)[1]
Study 2		N= 143	N= 185
	ACR20	45 (31%)	96 (52%)[2]
	ACR50	19 (13%)	61 (33%)[2]
	ACR70	6 (4%)	28 (15%)[2]
Study 3		N= 40	N= 40
	ACR20	15 (38%)	28 (70%)[3]
	ACR50	5 (13%)	17 (43%)[3]
	ACR70	2 (5%)	9 (23%)[3]

[1] $p \leqslant 0.0001$; [2] $p \leqslant 0.001$; [3] $p < 0.05$

MTX – Methotrexate

8-14 following the first infusion. Patients were followed beyond week 24 for long term endpoints, including radiographic assessment at 56 weeks. During this time, 81 % of patients, from the original placebo group received rituximab between weeks 24 an 56, under an open label extension study protocol.

Study 2 was a randomised, double-blind, double-dummy, controlled, 3 × 3 multifactorial study which compared two different dose levels of rituximab given with or without one of two peri infusional corticosteroid regimens in combination with weekly methotrexate in patients with active rheumatoid arthritis which had not responded to treatment with 1 to 5 other DMARDs.

Study 3 was a double-blind, double-dummy, controlled study evaluating rituximab monotherapy, and rituximab in combination with either cyclophosphamide or methotrexate in patients with active rheumatoid arthritis which had not responded to one or more prior DMARDs

The comparator group in all three studies was weekly methotrexate (10-25 mg weekly).

Disease activity outcomes

In all three studies, rituximab 2 × 1000 mg significantly increased the proportion of patients achieving at least a 20 % improvement in ACR score compared with patients treated with methotrexate alone (Table 8). The treatment effect was similar in patients independent of rheumatoid factor status, age, gender, body surface area, race, number of prior treatments or disease status.

Clinically and statistically significant improvement was also noted on all individual components of the ACR response (tender and swollen joint counts, patient and physician global assessment, disability index scores (HAQ), pain assessment and C-Reactive Proteins (mg/dL).

Table 8 Cross-Study Comparison of ACR Responses at Week 24 (ITT Population)

(see Table 8 above)

In study 3, the ACR20 response in patients treated with rituximab alone was 65 % compared with 38 % on methotrexate alone (p=0.025).

Rituximab treated patients had a significantly greater reduction in disease activity score (DAS28) than patients treated with methotrexate alone (Mean change in DAS28 from baseline -1.9 vs -0.4, p<0.0001, respectively). A good to moderate European League Against Rheumatism (EULAR) response was achieved by significantly more rituximab treated patients compared to patients treated with methotrexate alone (Table 10).

Radiographic response

In Study 1, conducted in patients with inadequate response or intolerance to one or more TNF inhibitor therapies, structural joint damage was assessed radiographically and expressed as change in modified total Sharp score and its components, the erosion score and joint space narrowing score. Patients originally receiving rituximab/MTX demonstrated significantly less radiographic progression than patients originally receiving methotrexate alone at 56 weeks. Of the patients originally receiving methotrexate alone, 81% received rituximab either as rescue between weeks 16-24 or in the extension trial, before week 56. A higher proportion of patients receiving the original rituximab/MTX treatment also had no erosive progression over 56 weeks (Table 9).

Table 9 Radiographic mean changes over 56 weeks in Study 1

	Placebo+MTX	Rituximab +MTX 2 × 1g
Study 1	(n = 184)	(n = 273)
Total Sharp score	2.31	1.00 p=0.0046
Erosion Score	1.32	0.59 p=0.0114
Joint Space narrowing score	0.99	0.41 p=0.0006
Proportion of patients with no erosive progression over 56 weeks	52%	61% p=0.0494

Quality of life outcomes

Significant reductions in disability index (HAQ-DI), fatigue (FACIT-F) (Table 10), and improvement in both the physical and mental health domains of the SF-36 were observed in patients treated with rituximab compared to patients treated with methotrexate alone (SF-36 Physical 5.8 vs 0.9, SF-36 Mental 4.7 vs 1.3, respectively, Study 1).

Table 10 Disease Activity and Quality of Life Outcomes at Week 24 in Study 1

(see Table 10 on next page)

At week 24, in all three studies, the proportion of rituximab treated patients showing a clinically relevant improvement in HAQ-DI (defined as an individual total score decrease of > 0.25) was higher than among patients receiving methotrexate alone.

Laboratory evaluations

A total of 96/1039 (9.2 %) patients with rheumatoid arthritis tested positive for HACA in clinical studies following therapy with MabThera. The emergence of HACA was not associated with clinical deterioration or with an increased risk of reactions to subsequent infusions in the majority of patients. The presence of HACA may be associated with worsening of infusion or allergic reactions after the second infusion of subsequent courses. Furthermore, in one case with HACA, failure to deplete B cells after receipt of further treatment courses has been observed.

In 675 patients in clinical studies, the following shifts in antinuclear antibody (ANA) status were observed before and after rituximab: 26 % ANA negative to positive and 32 % ANA positive to negative. There was no evidence of new onset autoimmune disease.

In rheumatoid factor (RF) positive patients, marked decreases were observed in rheumatoid factor concentrations following treatment with rituximab in all three studies (range 45-64 %).

Hyperuricaemia (grade 3/4) occurred in 143/950 (15 %) patients, with the majority post-infusion on days 1 and/or 15. It was not associated with any clinical symptoms, and none of these patients developed evidence of renal disease.

Plasma total immunoglobulin concentrations, total lymphocytes counts, and white cells generally remained within normal limits following MabThera treatment, with the exception of a transient drop in white cells counts over the first four weeks following therapy. Titres of Ig G antigen specific antibody to mumps, rubella, varicella, tetanus toxoid, influenza and streptococcus pneumococci remained stable over 24 weeks following exposure to MabThera in rheumatoid arthritis patients.

Multiple course therapy

Following completion of the 24-week double blind comparative study period, patients were permitted to enroll into an open-label long term follow up study. Patients received subsequent courses of MabThera as needed according to the treating clinician's assessment of disease activity and irrespective of the peripheral B lymphocyte count. The time interval between courses was variable, with the majority of patients receiving further therapy 6-12 months after the previous course. Some patients required even less frequent retreatment. The response to further therapy was at least the same magnitude as that following the initial treatment course, as evidenced by the change from baseline DAS28. Mean change in DAS28 from original baseline: first course -2.18, second course -2.75.

5.2 Pharmacokinetic properties

Non-Hodgkin's lymphoma

Based on a population pharmacokinetic analysis in 298 NHL patients who received single or multiple infusions of rituximab as a single agent or in combination with CHOP therapy (applied rituximab doses ranged from 100 to 500 mg/m^2), the typical population estimates of nonspecific clearance (CL_1), specific clearance (CL_2) likely contributed by B cells or tumour burden, and central compartment volume of distribution (V_1) were 0.14 L/day, 0.59 L/day, and 2.7 L, respectively. The estimated median terminal elimination half-life of rituximab was 22 days (range, 6.1 to 52 days). Baseline CD19-positive cell counts and size of measurable tumour lesions contributed to some of the variability in CL_2 of rituximab in data from 161 patients given 375 mg/m^2 as an intravenous infusion for 4 weekly doses. Patients with higher CD19-positive cell counts or tumour lesions had a higher CL_2. However, a large component of inter-individual variability remained for CL_2 after correction for CD19-positive cell counts and tumour lesion size. V_1 varied by body surface area (BSA) and CHOP therapy. This variability in V_1 (27.1% and 19.0%) contributed by the range in BSA (1.53 to 2.32 m^2) and concurrent CHOP therapy, respectively, were relatively small. Age, gender and WHO performance status had no effect on the pharmacokinetics of rituximab. This analysis suggests that dose adjustment of rituximab with any of the tested covariates is not expected to result in a meaningful reduction in its pharmacokinetic variability.

Rituximab, administered as an intravenous infusion at a dose of 375 mg/m^2 at weekly intervals for 4 doses to 203 patients with NHL naive to rituximab, yielded a mean C_{max} following the fourth infusion of 486 µg/mL (range, 77.5 to 996.6 µg/mL). Rituximab was detectable in the serum of patients 3 – 6 months after completion of last treatment.

Upon administration of rituximab at a dose of 375 mg/m^2 as an intravenous infusion at weekly intervals for 8 doses to 37 patients with NHL, the mean C_{max} increased with each

Table 10 Disease Activity and Quality of Life Outcomes at Week 24 in Study 1

Week 24 reponse: Change from baseline	Placebo+MTX[1] N= 201 mean (SD)	Rituximab+MTX[1] N= 298 mean (SD) switch	p-value
EULAR Good/moderate	22%	65%	
HAQ[2]	-0.1 (0.5)	-0.4 (0.6)	<0.0001
FACIT-F[3]	-0.5 (9.8)	-9.1 (11.3)	<0.0001

[1] MTX· [2] Health assessment questionnaire (HAQ),[3] Functional assessment of chronic illness therapy (FACIT-F)

successive infusion, spanning from a mean of 243 μg/mL (range, 16 – 582 μg/mL) after the first infusion to 550 μg/mL (range, 171 – 1177 μg/mL) after the eighth infusion.

The pharmacokinetic profile of rituximab when administered as 6 infusions of 375 mg/m^2 in combination with 6 cycles of CHOP chemotherapy was similar to that seen with rituximab alone.

Chronic lymphocytic leukaemia

Rituximab was administered as an IV infusion at a first-cycle dose of 375 mg/m^2 increased to 500 mg/m^2 each cycle for 5 doses in combination with fludarabine and cyclophosphamide in CLL patients. The mean C_{max} (N=15) was 408 μg/mL (range, 97 – 764 μg/mL) after the fifth 500 mg/m^2 infusion and the mean terminal half-life was 32 days (range, 14 – 62 days).

Rheumatoid arthritis

Following two intravenous infusions of rituximab at a dose of 1000 mg, two weeks apart, the mean terminal half-life was 20.8 days (range, 8.58 to 35.9 days), mean systemic clearance was 0.23 L/day (range, 0.091 to 0.67 L/day), and mean steady-state distribution volume was 4.6 L (range, 1.7 to 7.51 L). Population pharmacokinetic analysis of the same data gave similar mean values for systemic clearance and half-life, 0.26 L/day and 20.4 days, respectively. Population pharmacokinetic analysis revealed that BSA and gender were the most significant covariates to explain inter-individual variability in pharmacokinetic parameters. After adjusting for BSA, male subjects had a larger volume of distribution and a faster clearance than female subjects. The gender- related pharmacokinetic differences are not considered to be clinically relevant and dose adjustment is not required. Following the intravenous administration of 500 and 1000 mg doses of rituximab on two occasions, two weeks apart, mean Cmax values were 183 μg/mL (range, 81.8 to 279 μg/mL) and 370 μg/mL (212 to 637 μg/mL), and mean half-lives were 17.9 days (range, 12.3 to 31.3 days) and 19.7 days (range, 12.3 to 34.6 days), respectively. No pharmacokinetic data are available in patients with hepatic or renal impairment. No pharmacokinetic data are available for patients receiving multiple courses of therapy. The pharmacokinetic (PK) parameters in the anti-TNF inadequate responder population, following the same dosage regimen (2 × 1000 mg, iv, 2 weeks apart), were similar with a mean maximum serum concentration of 369 μg/mL and a mean terminal half-life of 19.2 days.

5.3 Preclinical safety data

Rituximab has shown to be highly specific to the CD20 antigen on B cells. Toxicity studies in cynomolgus monkeys have shown no other effect than the expected pharmacological depletion of B cells in peripheral blood and in lymphoid tissue.

Developmental toxicity studies have been performed in cynomolgus monkeys at dosages up to 100 mg/kg (treatment on gestation days 20-50) and have revealed no evidence of toxicity to the foetus due to rituximab. However, dose-dependent pharmacologic depletion of B cells in the lymphoid organs of the foetuses was observed, which persisted post natally and was accompanied by a decrease in IgG level in the newborn animals affected. B cell counts returned to normal in these animals within 6 months of birth and did not compromise the reaction to immunisation.

No long-term animal studies have been performed to establish the carcinogenic potential of rituximab, or to determine its effects on fertility in males or females. Standard tests to investigate mutagenicity have not been carried out, since such tests are not relevant for this molecule. However, due to its character it is unlikely that rituximab has any mutagenic potential.

6. PHARMACEUTICAL PARTICULARS

6.1 List of excipients

Sodium citrate

Polysorbate 80

Sodium chloride

Sodium hydroxide

Hydrochloric acid

Water for injections

6.2 Incompatibilities

No incompatibilities between MabThera and polyvinyl chloride or polyethylene bags or infusion sets have been observed.

6.3 Shelf life

30 months

The prepared infusion solution of MabThera is physically and chemically stable for 24 hours at 2°C - 8°C and subsequently 12 hours at room temperature.

From a microbiological point of view, the prepared infusion solution should be used immediately. If not used immediately, in-use storage times and conditions prior to use are the responsibility of the user and would normally not be longer than 24 hours at 2 °C – 8 °C, unless dilution has taken place in controlled and validated aseptic conditions.

6.4 Special precautions for storage

Store in a refrigerator (2 °C – 8 °C). Keep the container in the outer carton in order to protect from light.

For storage conditions of the diluted medicinal product, see section 6.3.

6.5 Nature and contents of container

Clear Type I glass vials with butyl rubber stopper containing 100 mg of rituximab in 10 ml. Packs of 2 vials.

Clear Type I glass vials with butyl rubber stopper containing 500 mg of rituximab in 50 ml. Packs of 1 vial.

6.6 Special precautions for disposal and other handling

MabThera is provided in sterile, preservative-free, non-pyrogenic, single use vials.

Aseptically withdraw the necessary amount of MabThera, and dilute to a calculated concentration of 1 to 4 mg/ml rituximab into an infusion bag containing sterile, pyrogen-free sodium chloride 9 mg/ml (0.9 %) solution for injection or 5 % D-Glucose in water. For mixing the solution, gently invert the bag in order to avoid foaming. Care must be taken to ensure the sterility of prepared solutions. Since the medicinal product does not contain any anti-microbial preservative or bacteriostatic agents, aseptic technique must be observed. Parenteral medicinal products should be inspected visually for particulate matter and discoloration prior to administration.

Any unused product or waste material should be disposed of in accordance with local requirements.

7. MARKETING AUTHORISATION HOLDER

Roche Registration Limited

6 Falcon Way

Shire Park

Welwyn Garden City

AL7 1TW

United Kingdom

8. MARKETING AUTHORISATION NUMBER(S)

EU/1/98/067/001

EU/1/98/067/002

9. DATE OF FIRST AUTHORISATION/RENEWAL OF THE AUTHORISATION

Date of first authorisation: 2 June 1998

Date of last renewal: 20 May 2008

10. DATE OF REVISION OF THE TEXT

21st August 2009

Detailed information on this medicinal product is available on the website of the European Medicines Agency (EMEA) http://www.emea.europa.eu/

Mackenzies Smelling Salts

(Actavis UK Ltd)

1. NAME OF THE MEDICINAL PRODUCT

MACKENZIES SMELLING SALTS

2. QUALITATIVE AND QUANTITATIVE COMPOSITION

Contains not less than 8.698g Ammonia Liquor 880/890 and 0.5g Eucalyptus Oil BP

3. PHARMACEUTICAL FORM

White granules.

4. CLINICAL PARTICULARS

4.1 Therapeutic indications

1) Traditionally used for the symptomatic relief of catarrh and head colds.

4.2 Posology and method of administration

Posology

Inhale vapour through nostrils as required.

Do not use for children under 3 months of age.

Method of Administration

Inhalant.

4.3 Contraindications

Do not use for children under 3 months of age.

4.4 Special warnings and precautions for use

None known.

The product labelling includes the following statements:

Not to be taken.

If symptoms persist consult your doctor.

Keep out of the reach and sight of children.

4.5 Interaction with other medicinal products and other forms of interaction

None known.

4.6 Pregnancy and lactation

No special precautions are considered necessary.

4.7 Effects on ability to drive and use machines

None known.

4.8 Undesirable effects

None known.

4.9 Overdose

No special requirements are anticipated.

5. PHARMACOLOGICAL PROPERTIES

5.1 Pharmacodynamic properties

ATC code: R01A X

Ammonia is employed in the product as a reflex stimulant.

Eucalyptus oil is an essential oil.

5.2 Pharmacokinetic properties

Not applicable.

5.3 Preclinical safety data

There are no pre-clinical data of relevance to the prescriber which are additional to that already included in other sections of the SPC.

6. PHARMACEUTICAL PARTICULARS

6.1 List of excipients

Also contains glycerol, soft soap, tapioca, water.

6.2 Incompatibilities

None known.

6.3 Shelf life

Shelf-life

Three years from the date of manufacture.

Shelf-life after dilution/reconstitution

Not applicable.

Shelf-life after first opening

Not applicable.

6.4 Special precautions for storage

Store in a cool place.

6.5 Nature and contents of container

The product container is a uniquely-shaped amber glass bottle with black polypropylene cap with foil wad or black urea formaldehyde cap with polycone.

Pack size: 17ml

6.6 Special precautions for disposal and other handling

Not applicable.

Administrative Data

7. MARKETING AUTHORISATION HOLDER

Name or style and permanent address of registered place of business of the holder of the Marketing Authorisation:

Actavis UK Limited

(Trading style: Actavis)

Whiddon Valley

BARNSTAPLE

N Devon EX32 8NS

8. MARKETING AUTHORISATION NUMBER(S)

PL 0142/5010 R

9. DATE OF FIRST AUTHORISATION/RENEWAL OF THE AUTHORISATION

16.10.86 (Product Licence of Right issued: 27.7.73)

Renewed: 14.5.92; 11.7.97

10. DATE OF REVISION OF THE TEXT

March 2007

Macugen 0.3 mg solution for injection

(Pfizer Limited)

1. NAME OF THE MEDICINAL PRODUCT

Macugen® 0.3 mg solution for injection

2. QUALITATIVE AND QUANTITATIVE COMPOSITION

A single dose pre-filled syringe delivers 1.65 mg pegaptanib sodium, corresponding to 0.3 mg of the free acid form of the oligonucleotide, in a nominal volume of 90 microlitres.

For a full list excipients, see section 6.1.

3. PHARMACEUTICAL FORM

Solution for injection.

The solution is clear and colourless.

4. CLINICAL PARTICULARS

4.1 Therapeutic indications

Macugen is indicated for the treatment of neovascular (wet) age-related macular degeneration (AMD) (see section 5.1).

4.2 Posology and method of administration

FOR INTRAVITREAL USE ONLY.

Treatment with Macugen is for intravitreal injection only and should be administered by ophthalmologists experienced in intravitreal injections.

Macugen 0.3 mg should be administered once every six weeks (9 injections per year) by intravitreal injection into the affected eye.

Macugen should be inspected visually for particulate matter and discoloration prior to administration (see section 6.6).

The injection procedure should be carried out under aseptic conditions, which includes the use of surgical hand disinfection, sterile gloves, a sterile drape and a sterile eyelid speculum (or equivalent) and the availability of sterile paracentesis (if required). The patient's medical history for hypersensitivity reactions should be carefully evaluated prior to performing the intravitreal procedure (see section 4.4). Adequate anaesthesia and a broad-spectrum topical microbicide should be administered prior to the injection.

Following the injection, transient increases in intraocular pressure were seen in Macugen treated patients. Therefore, the perfusion of the optic nerve head and intraocular pressure should be monitored. Moreover patients should be closely monitored for endophthalmitis in the two weeks following the injection. Patients should be instructed to report any symptoms suggestive of endophthalmitis without delay (see section 4.4).

After 2 consecutive injections of Macugen, if a patient does not demonstrate a treatment benefit (loss of less than 15 letters of visual acuity) at the 12-week visit, consideration should be given to stopping or withholding Macugen therapy.

Specific patient groups:

Hepatic impairment:

Macugen has not been studied in patients with hepatic impairment.

However, no special considerations are needed in this population (see section 5.2)

Renal insufficiency:

Macugen has not been adequately studied in patients with creatinine clearance < 20 ml/min. No special considerations are needed in patients with creatinine clearance above 20 ml/min (see section 5.2).

Children and adolescents:

Macugen has not been studied in patients below the age of 18 years. Use in children and adolescents is therefore not recommended.

Elderly patients:

No special considerations are needed.

Gender:

No special considerations are needed.

4.3 Contraindications

Active or suspected ocular or periocular infection.

Known hypersensitivity to the active substance or to any of the excipients.

4.4 Special warnings and precautions for use

As expected with intravitreal injections, transient increases in intraocular pressure may be seen. Therefore, the perfusion of the optic nerve head should be verified and elevation of intraocular pressure should be managed appropriately post injection.

Immediate (on the day of injection) and delayed intravitreous haemorrhages may occur following pegaptanib injections.

Intravitreal injection procedures are associated with a risk of endophthalmitis; in Macugen clinical trials, the incidence of endophthalmitis was 0.1% per injection.

Cases of anaphylaxis/anaphylactoid reactions, including angioedema, have been observed within several hours after the pegaptanib intravitreal administration procedure in the post-marketing experience. A direct relationship to Macugen or any of the various medications administered as part of the injection preparation procedure, or to other factors has not been established in these cases.

4.5 Interaction with other medicinal products and other forms of interaction

Drug interaction studies have not been conducted with Macugen. Pegaptanib is metabolised by nucleases and therefore cytochrome P450 mediated drug interactions are unlikely.

Two early clinical studies conducted in patients who received Macugen alone and in combination with PDT (photodynamic therapy) revealed no apparent difference in the plasma pharmacokinetics of pegaptanib.

4.6 Pregnancy and lactation

Pegaptanib has not been studied in pregnant women. Animal studies are insufficient, but have shown reproductive toxicity at high systemic exposure levels (see section 5.3). The potential risk to humans is unknown. The systemic exposure to pegaptanib is expected to be very low after ocular administration. Nevertheless, Macugen should be used during pregnancy only if the potential benefit to the mother justifies the potential risk to the foetus.

It is not known whether Macugen is excreted in human milk. Macugen is not recommended during breast-feeding.

4.7 Effects on ability to drive and use machines

Patients may experience temporary visual blurring after receiving Macugen by intravitreal injection. They should not drive or use machines until this has resolved

4.8 Undesirable effects

Macugen was administered to 892 patients in controlled studies for one year (total number of injections = 7545, mean number of injections/patient = 8.5) at doses of 0.3, 1.0 and 3.0 mg. All three doses shared a similar safety profile. In the 295 patients who were treated with the recommended dose of 0.3 mg for one year (total number of injections = 2478, mean number of injections/patient = 8.4), 84% of the patients experienced an adverse event attributed by the investigators as being related to the injection procedure, 3% of the patients experienced a Serious Adverse Event potentially related to the injection procedure, and 1% experienced an adverse event potentially related to the injection procedure that led to study treatment discontinuation. Twenty seven percent (27%) of the patients experienced an adverse event attributed by the investigators as being related to the study drug. Two patients (0.7%) experienced Serious Adverse Events potentially related to study drug. One of these patients had an aortic aneurysm; the other had a retinal detachment and retinal haemorrhage, which led to discontinuation of treatment.

Serious ocular Adverse Events reported in Macugen treated patients included endophthalmitis (12 cases, 1%), retinal haemorrhage (3 cases, <1%), vitreous haemorrhage (2 cases, <1%) and retinal detachment (4 cases, < 1%).

The safety data described below summarise all procedure and drug potentially related adverse events in the 295 patients in the 0.3 mg treatment group. The adverse reactions are listed by system organ class and frequency (very common (≥1/10), common (≥1/100 and <1/10), and uncommon (≥1/1000 and <1/100).

Psychiatric disorders

uncommon	nightmare, depression

Nervous system disorders

common	headache

Eye disorders

These ocular adverse reactions were considered potentially related to treatment with Macugen (either injection procedure or due to Macugen), and for the most part were considered related to the injection procedure.

very common	anterior chamber inflammation, eye pain, increased intraocular pressure, punctate keratitis, vitreous floaters and vitreous opacities
common	abnormal sensation in eye, cataract, conjunctival haemorrhage, conjunctival hyperaemia, conjunctival oedema, conjunctivitis, corneal dystrophy, corneal epithelium defect, corneal epithelium disorder, corneal oedema, dry eye, endophthalmitis, eye discharge, eye inflammation, eye irritation, eye pruritus, eye redness, eye swelling, eyelid oedema, lacrimation increased, macular degeneration, mydriasis, ocular discomfort, ocular hypertension, periorbital haematoma, photophobia, photopsia, retinal haemorrhage, vision blurred, visual acuity reduced, visual disturbance, vitreous detachment, and vitreous disorder
uncommon	asthenopia, blepharitis, conjunctivitis allergic, corneal deposits, eye haemorrhage, eyelids pruritus, keratitis, vitreous haemorrhage, pupillary reflex impaired, corneal abrasion, retinal exudates, eyelid ptosis, retinal scar, chalazion, corneal erosion, decreased intraocular pressure, injection site reaction, injection site vesicles, retinal detachment, corneal disorder, retinal artery occlusion, retinal tear, ectropion, eye movement disorder, eyelid irritation, hyphaema, pupillary disorder, iris disorder, ocular icterus, anterior uveitis, deposit eye, iritis, optic nerve cupping, pupillary deformity, retinal vein occlusion, and vitreous prolapse

Ear and labyrinth disorders

uncommon	deafness, Meniere's disease aggravated, vertigo

Cardiac disorders

uncommon	palpitations

Vascular disorders

uncommon	hypertension, aortic aneurysm

Respiratory, thoracic and mediastinal disorders

common	rhinorrhea
uncommon	nasopharyngitis

Gastrointestinal disorders

uncommon	vomiting, dyspepsia

Skin and subcutaneous tissue disorders

uncommon	contact dermatitis, eczema, hair colour changes, rash, pruritus, night sweats

Musculoskeletal and connective tissue disorders

uncommon	back pain

General disorders and administration site conditions

uncommon	fatigue, rigors, tenderness, chest pain, influenza like illness

Investigations

uncommon	increased gamma-glutamyltransferase activity

Injury, poisoning and procedural complications

uncommon	abrasion

Three hundred seventy four (374) patients received continuous treatment with Macugen for up to 2 years (128 at 0.3 mg, 126 at 1 mg, and 120 at 3 mg). The overall safety data were consistent with the Year 1 safety data, and no new safety signals emerged. In the 128 patients who were treated with the recommended dose of 0.3 mg for up to 2 years (total number of injections in second year = 913, mean number of injections in the second year = 6.9), there was no evidence of increased in frequency of adverse events compared to those seen during the first year.

Post-Marketing Experience: Rare cases of anaphylaxis/anaphylactoid reactions, including angioedema, have been reported in patients within several hours after administration of pegaptanib along with various medications administered as part of the injection preparation procedure (see sections 4.2 and 4.4).

4.9 Overdose

Overdosage with Macugen has not been reported in clinical trials.

5. PHARMACOLOGICAL PROPERTIES

5.1 Pharmacodynamic properties

Pharmacotherapeutic group: Ocular Vascular Disorder Agent, ATC code: S01LA03.

Pegaptanib is a pegylated modified oligonucleotide that binds with high specificity and affinity to extracellular Vascular Endothelial Growth Factor ($VEGF_{165}$) inhibiting its activity. VEGF is a secreted protein that induces angiogenesis, vascular permeability and inflammation, all of which are thought to contribute to the progression of the neovascular (wet) form of AMD. $VEGF_{165}$ is the VEGF isoform preferentially involved in pathological ocular neovascularisation. The selective inhibition in animals with pegaptanib proved as effective at suppressing pathological neovascularisation as pan-VEGF inhibition, however pegaptanib spared the normal vasculature whereas pan-VEGF inhibition did not.

Reductions in the growth of mean total lesion size, choroidal neovascularisation (CNV size), and fluorescein leak size, have been shown in patients with AMD treated with Macugen.

Pegaptanib was studied in two controlled, double-masked, and identically designed randomised studies (EOP1003; EOP1004) in patients with neovascular AMD. A total of 1190 patients were treated (892 pegaptanib, 298 sham (control)) with a median age of 77 years. Patients received a mean of between 8.4-8.6 treatments out of possible 9 total across all treatment arms in the first year.

Patients were randomised to receive sham or 0.3 mg, 1 mg or 3 mg pegaptanib administered as intravitreal injections every 6 weeks for 48 weeks. Verteporfin photodynamic therapy (PDT) was permitted in patients with predominantly classic lesions at the discretion of the investigators.

The two trials enrolled patients, including all neovascular AMD lesion subtypes (25% predominantly classic, 39% occult with no classic and 36% minimally classic), lesion sizes up to 12 disc areas, of which up to 50% could be comprised of subretinal haemorrhage and/or up to 25% fibrotic scar or atrophic damage. Patients had up to one prior PDT and baseline visual acuity in the study eye between 20/40 and 20/320.

At one year, pegaptanib 0.3 mg exhibited a statistically significant treatment benefit for the primary efficacy endpoint; proportion of patients losing less than 15 letters of visual acuity (prespecified pooled analysis, pegaptanib 0.3 mg 70% versus Sham 55%, p = 0.0001; EOP 1003 pegaptanib 0.3 mg 73% versus Sham 59%, p = 0.0105; EOP1004 pegaptanib 0.3 mg 67% versus Sham 52%, p = 0.0031).

(see Figure 1 on next page)

Pegaptanib 0.3mg showed treatment benefit regardless of baseline lesion subtype, lesion size and visual acuity as

Figure 1

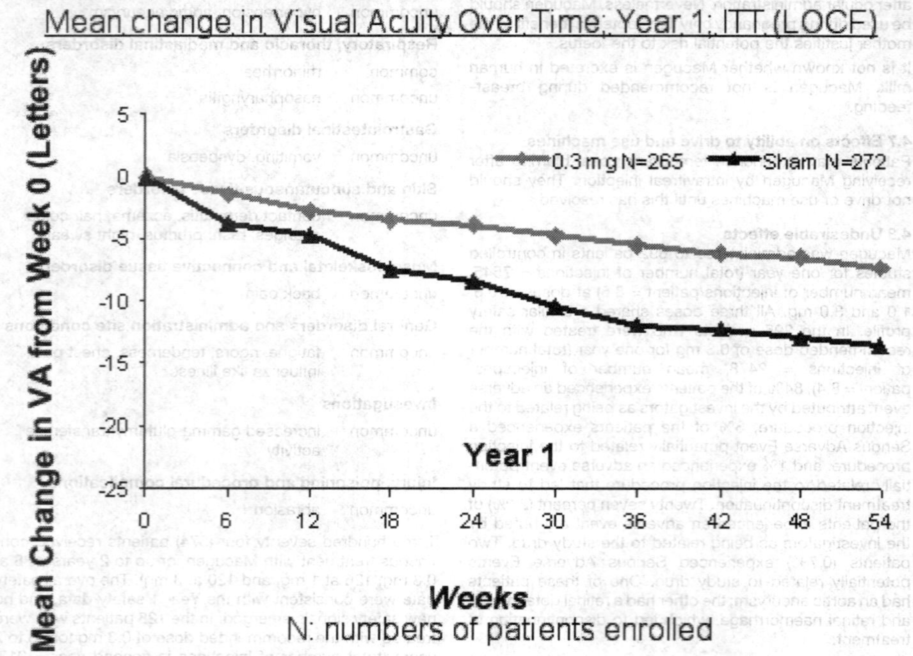

Table 1

Summary of Mean Changes in Visual Acuity from Baseline to Weeks 6, 12, 54 and 102 (LOCF)						
	EOP 1003			*EOP 1004*		
	0.3-0.3	0.3-discontinued	Sham-sham/ sham+ discontinued	0.3-0.3	0.3-discontinued	Sham-sham/ sham+ discontinued
N	67	66	54	66	66	53
Mean change in VA Week 6	-1.9	-0.0	-4.4	-1.9	-2.0	-3.4
Mean change in VA Week 12	-4.3	-2.0	-4.8	-2.8	-2.2	-4.7
Mean change in VA Week 54	-9.6	-4.3	-11.7	-8.0	-7.6	-15.6
Mean change in VA Week 102	-10.8	-9.7	-13.1	-8.0	-12.7	-21.1

well as age, gender, iris pigmentation and prior and/or baseline PDT usage.

At the end of the first year (week 54), 1053 patients were re-randomized to either continue or discontinue treatment through week 102.

On average, the treatment benefit was maintained at 102 weeks with continuing preservation of visual acuity for patients re-randomized to continue pegaptanib. Patients who were re-randomized to discontinue pegaptanib after one year, lost visual acuity during the second year.

(see Table 1 above)

Data over a two-year period indicate that Macugen treatment should be initiated as early as possible. In advanced disease the initiation and continuation of Macugen therapy should consider the potential for useful vision in the eye.

Macugen therapy administered to both eyes concurrently has not been studied.

The safety and efficacy of Macugen beyond two years has not been demonstrated.

5.2 Pharmacokinetic properties

Absorption:

In animals, pegaptanib is slowly absorbed into the systemic circulation from the eye after intravitreal administration. The rate of absorption from the eye is the rate-limiting step in the disposition of pegaptanib in animals and is likely to be in humans. In humans, the average ± standard deviation apparent plasma half-life of pegaptanib after a 3 mg (10-times the recommended dose) monocular dose is 10 ± 4 days.

A mean maximum plasma concentration of about 80 ng/ml occurs within 1 to 4 days after a 3 mg monocular dose in humans. The mean area under the plasma concentration-time curve (AUC) is about 25 µg•hr/ml at this dose. Pegaptanib does not accumulate in the plasma when administered intravitreally every 6 weeks. At doses below 0.5 mg/eye, pegaptanib plasma concentrations do not likely exceed 10 ng/ml.

The absolute bioavailability of pegaptanib after intravitreal administration has not been assessed in humans, but is approximately 70-100% in rabbits, dogs and monkeys.

In animals that received doses of pegaptanib up to 0.5 mg/eye to both eyes, plasma concentrations were 0.03% to 0.15% of those in the vitreous humour.

Distribution/Metabolism/Excretion:

In mice, rats, rabbits, dogs and monkeys, pegaptanib distributes primarily into plasma volume and is not extensively distributed to peripheral tissues after intravenous administration. Twenty-four hours after intravitreous administration of a radiolabeled dose of pegaptanib to both eyes of rabbits, radioactivity was mainly distributed in vitreous humour, retina and aqueous humour. After intravitreal and intravenous administrations of radiolabeled pegaptanib to rabbits, the highest concentrations of radioactivity (excluding the eye for the intravitreal dose) were obtained in the kidney. In rabbits, the component nucleotide, 2'-fluorouridine is found in plasma and urine after single radiolabeled pegaptanib intravenous and intravitreal doses. Pegaptanib is metabolised by endo- and exonucleases. In rabbits, pegaptanib is eliminated as parent drug and metabolites primarily in the urine.

Special populations:

Pegaptanib pharmacokinetics is similar in female and male patients and within the age range 50 to 90 years.

Pegaptanib sodium has not been adequately studied in patients with creatinine clearance below 20 ml/min. A decrease in creatinine clearance down to 20 ml/min may be associated with up to a 2.3-fold increase in pegaptanib AUC. No special considerations are needed in patients with creatinine clearance above 20 ml/min who are treated with the recommended dose of pegaptanib sodium 0.3 mg.

Pegaptanib pharmacokinetics have not been studied in patients with hepatic impairment. The systemic exposure is expected to be within a well tolerated range in patients with hepatic impairment, as a 10 fold higher dose (3 mg/eye) was well tolerated.

5.3 Preclinical safety data

Non-clinical data revealed no special hazard for humans based on conventional studies of safety pharmacology, repeated dose toxicity and genotoxicity. There are no studies on the carcinogenic potential of pegaptanib.

Pegaptanib produced no maternal toxicity and no evidence of teratogenicity or foetal mortality in mice at intravenous doses of 1 to 40 mg/kg/day. Reduced body weight (5%) and minimal delayed ossification in forepaw phalanges were observed, only at exposure levels based on AUC of over 300 fold greater than that expected in humans. These finding are therefore considered to be of limited clinical relevance. In the 40 mg/kg/day group, pegaptanib concentrations in the amniotic fluid were 0.05% of the maternal plasma levels. There are no reproductive toxicity studies in rabbits.

No data are available to evaluate male or female mating or fertility indices.

6. PHARMACEUTICAL PARTICULARS

6.1 List of excipients

Sodium chloride

Monobasic sodium phosphate monohydrate

Dibasic sodium phosphate heptahydrate

Sodium hydroxide

Hydrochloric acid

Water for injections

6.2 Incompatibilities

In the absence of compatibility studies, this medicinal product must not be mixed with other medicinal products.

6.3 Shelf life

18 months

6.4 Special precautions for storage

Store in a refrigerator (2°C - 8°C). Do not freeze.

6.5 Nature and contents of container

Macugen is supplied in a single dose pack.

Each pack contains a pouch in a carton containing a 1 ml pre-filled syringe, Type 1 glass, sealed with an elastomeric plunger stopper and a pre-attached plunger rod, held by a plastic clip. The syringe has a pre-attached polycarbonate plastic luer lock adaptor and the tip is sealed with an elastomeric tip cap.

The pack is supplied without a needle.

6.6 Special precautions for disposal and other handling

Macugen is for single use only. If the solution appears cloudy, particles are observed or if there is evidence of damage to the syringe, or if the plastic clip is missing or not attached to the syringe, Macugen should not be used.

Prior to the administration, the syringe should be removed from the plastic clip and the tip cap removed. A 27 or 30 G × ½ inch needle should be attached to the luer lock adaptor, to allow the administration of the product.

The syringe should be checked with the needle pointing up regarding the presence of bubbles. If there are bubbles, the syringe should be gently tapped with a finger until the bubbles rise to the top of the syringe. Then, the plunger should be slowly pushed up to force the bubbles out of the syringe. The plunger stopper should not be pulled back.

The last rib of the plunger stopper (closest to the plunger rod) should not be pushed past the dose line printed on the syringe. Immediately prior to administration this last rib of the plunger should be aligned with the dose line to ensure the delivery of the appropriate dose. At this point, the entire content of the syringe should be injected.

Macugen should be stored in a refrigerator. The solution to be injected should reach room temperature before injecting. Macugen should be discarded if kept at room temperature for more than two weeks. To prevent contamination, the Macugen syringe should not be removed from the pouch until the patient has been prepared for injection.

Any unused product or waste material should be disposed of in accordance with local requirements.

7. MARKETING AUTHORISATION HOLDER

Pfizer Limited

Ramsgate Road

Sandwich, Kent

CT13 9NJ

United Kingdom

8. MARKETING AUTHORISATION NUMBER(S)

EU/1/05/325/002

9. DATE OF FIRST AUTHORISATION/RENEWAL OF THE AUTHORISATION

31 January 2006

10. DATE OF REVISION OF THE TEXT

10/2008

11. LEGAL CATEGORY

POM

Ref: MC 5_0

Detailed information on this medicinal product is available on the website of the European Medicines Agency (EMEA): http://www.emea.europa.eu/

Madopar Capsules

(Roche Products Limited)

1. NAME OF THE MEDICINAL PRODUCT

Madopar 50 mg/12.5 mg Hard Capsules

Madopar 100 mg/25 mg Hard Capsules

Madopar 200 mg/50 mg Hard Capsules

2. QUALITATIVE AND QUANTITATIVE COMPOSITION

Madopar 50 mg/12.5 mg: Each capsule contains 50.0 mg Levodopa and 12.5 mg Benserazide (as benserazide hydrochloride).

Madopar 100 mg/25 mg: Each capsule contains 100.0 mg Levodopa and 25 mg Benserazide (as benserazide hydrochloride).

Madopar 200 mg/50 mg: Each capsule contains 200.0 mg Levodopa and 50 mg Benserazide (as benserazide hydrochloride).

For excipients, see section 6.1

3. PHARMACEUTICAL FORM

Capsules, hard.

Madopar 50 mg/12.5 mg: Light grey opaque body and a powder blue opaque cap, imprinted with the name 'Roche' in black ink on both sides.

Madopar 100 mg/25 mg: Pale pink opaque body and a powder blue opaque cap, imprinted with the name 'Roche' in black ink on both sides.

Madopar 200 mg/50 mg: Light brown opaque body and a powder blue opaque cap, imprinted with the name 'Roche' in black ink on both sides.

4. CLINICAL PARTICULARS

4.1 Therapeutic indications

Parkinsonism - idiopathic post-encephalitic.

Previous neurosurgery is not a contra-indication to Madopar.

4.2 Posology and method of administration

Dosage and administration are variable and no more than a guide can be given.

Adults

Patients not previously treated with levodopa

The recommended initial dose is one capsule or dispersible tablet of Madopar 50 mg/12.5 mg three or four times daily. If the disease is at an advanced stage, the starting dose should be one capsule or dispersible tablet of Madopar 100 mg/25 mg three times daily.

The daily dosage should then be increased by one capsule or dispersible tablet of Madopar 100 mg/25 mg, or their equivalent, once or twice weekly until a full therapeutic effect is obtained, or side-effects supervene.

In some elderly patients, it may suffice to initiate treatment with one capsule or dispersible tablet of Madopar 50 mg/12.5 mg once or twice daily, increasing by one capsule or dispersible tablet every third or fourth day.

The effective dose usually lies within the range of four to eight capsules or dispersible tablets of Madopar 100 mg/25 mg (two to four capsules of Madopar 200 mg/50 mg) daily in divided doses, most patients requiring no more than six capsules or dispersible tablets of Madopar 100 mg/25 mg daily.

Optimal improvement is usually seen in one to three weeks but the full therapeutic effect of Madopar may not be apparent for some time. It is advisable, therefore, to allow several weeks to elapse before contemplating dosage increments above the average dose range. If satisfactory improvement is still not achieved, the dose of Madopar may be increased but with caution. It is rarely necessary to give more than ten capsules or dispersible tablets of Madopar 100 mg /25 mg (five capsules of Madopar 200 mg/50 mg) per day.

Treatment should be continued for at least six months before failure is concluded from the absence of a clinical response.

Madopar 50 mg/12.5 mg capsules or dispersible tablets may be used to facilitate adjustment of dosage to the needs of the individual patient. Patients who experience fluctuations in response may be helped by dividing the dosage into smaller, more frequent doses with the aid of Madopar 50 mg/12.5 mg capsules or dispersible tablets without, however, altering the total daily dose.

Madopar 200 mg/50 mg capsules are only for maintenance therapy once the optimal dosage has been determined using Madopar 100 mg/25 mg capsules or dispersible tablets.

Patients previously treated with levodopa

The following procedure is recommended: Levodopa alone should be discontinued and Madopar started on the following day. The patient should be initiated on a total of one less Madopar 100 mg/25 mg capsule or dispersible tablet daily than the total number of 500 mg levodopa tablets or capsules previously taken (for example, if the patient had previously taken 2g levodopa daily, then he should start on three capsules or dispersible tablets Madopar 100 mg/25 mg daily on the following day). Observe the patient for one week and then, if necessary, increase the dosage in the manner described for new patients.

Patients previously treated with other levodopa/decarboxylase inhibitor combinations

Previous therapy should be withdrawn for 12 hours. In order to minimise the potential for any effects of levodopa withdrawal, it may be beneficial to discontinue previous therapy at night and institute Madopar therapy the following morning. The initial Madopar dose should be one capsule or dispersible tablet of Madopar 50 mg/12.5 mg three or four times daily. This dose may then be increased in the manner described for patients not previously treated with levodopa.

Other anti-Parkinsonian drugs may be given with Madopar. Existing treatment with other anti-Parkinsonian drugs, e.g. anticholinergics or amantadine, should be continued during initiation of Madopar therapy. However, as treatment with Madopar proceeds and the therapeutic effect becomes apparent, the dosage of the other drugs may need to be reduced or the drugs gradually withdrawn.

Elderly

Although there may be an age-related decrease in tolerance to levodopa in the elderly, Madopar appears to be well-tolerated and side-effects are generally not troublesome.

Children

Not to be given to patients under 25 years of age: therefore, no dosage recommendations are made for the administration of Madopar to children.

Madopar capsules are for oral administration. They should be taken with, or immediately after, meals.

4.3 Contraindications

Madopar must not be given to patients with known hypersensitivity to levodopa or benserazide.

Madopar is contra-indicated in narrow-angle glaucoma (it may be used in wide-angle glaucoma provided that the intra-ocular pressure remains under control); severe psychoneuroses or psychoses; severe endocrine, renal, hepatic or cardiac disorders.

It should not be given in conjunction with, or within 2 weeks of withdrawal of, monoamine oxidase (MAO) inhibitors, except selective MAO-B inhibitors (e.g. selegiline) or selective MAO-A inhibitors (e.g. moclobemide).

It should not be given to patients under 25 years of age.

It should not be given to pregnant women or to women of childbearing potential in the absence of adequate contraception. If pregnancy occurs in a woman taking Madopar, the drug must be discontinued.

Suspicion has arisen that levodopa may activate a malignant melanoma. Therefore, Madopar should not be used in persons who have a history of, or who may be suffering from, a malignant melanoma.

4.4 Special warnings and precautions for use

When other drugs must be given in conjunction with Madopar, the patient should be carefully observed for unusual side-effects or potentiating effects.

In the event of general anaesthesia being required, Madopar therapy may be continued as long as the patient is able to take fluids and medication by mouth. If therapy is temporarily interrupted, the usual daily dosage may be administered as soon as the patient is able to take oral medication. Whenever therapy has been interrupted for longer periods, dosage should again be adjusted gradually; however, in many cases the patient can rapidly be returned to his previous therapeutic dosage.

If a patient has to undergo emergency surgery, when Madopar has not been withdrawn, anaesthesia with halothane should be avoided.

There have been occasional reports of a neuroleptic malignant-like syndrome, involving hyperthermia, on abrupt withdrawal of levodopa preparations. Sudden discontinuation of Madopar, without close supervision, or "drug holidays" should therefore be avoided.

Pyridoxine (vitamin B_6) may be given with Madopar since the presence of a decarboxylase inhibitor protects against the peripheral levodopa transformation facilitated by pyridoxine.

Levodopa has been associated with somnolence and episodes of sudden sleep onset. Sudden onset of sleep during daily activities, in some cases without awareness or warning signs, has been reported very rarely. Patients must be informed of this and advised to exercise caution while driving or operating machines during treatment with levodopa. Patients who have experienced somnolence and/or an episode of sudden sleep onset must refrain from driving or operating machines. Furthermore a reduction of dosage or termination of therapy may be considered.

Pathological gambling, increased libido and hypersexuality have been reported in patients treated with dopamine agonists and/or levodopa for Parkinson's disease.

Care should be taken when using Madopar in the following circumstances: in endocrine, renal, pulmonary or cardiovascular disease, particularly where there is a history of myocardial infarction or arrhythmia; psychiatric disturbances (e.g. depression); hepatic disorder; peptic ulcer; osteomalacia; where sympathomimetic drugs may be required (e.g. bronchial asthma), due to possible potentiation of the cardiovascular effects of levodopa; where antihypertensive drugs are being used, due to possible increased hypotensive action.

Periodic evaluation of hepatic, haemopoietic, renal and cardiovascular functions is advised.

Patients with diabetes should undergo frequent blood sugar tests and the dosage of anti-diabetic agents should be adjusted to blood sugar levels.

Patients who improve on Madopar therapy should be advised to resume normal activities gradually as rapid mobilisation may increase the risk of injury.

4.5 Interaction with other medicinal products and other forms of interaction

Ferrous sulphate decreases the maximum plasma concentration and the AUC of levodopa by 30 - 50%. The pharmacokinetic changes observed during co-treatment with ferrous sulphate appeared to be clinically significant in some but not all patients.

Opioids and drugs which interfere with central amine mechanisms, such as rauwolfia alkaloids (reserpine), tetrabenazine (Nitoman), metoclopramide, phenothiazines, thioxanthenes, butyrophenones, amphetamines and papaverine, should be avoided where possible. If, however, their administration is considered essential, extreme care should be exercised and a close watch kept for any signs of potentiation, antagonism or other interactions and for unusual side-effects. Metoclopramide has been shown to increase the rate of levodopa absorption.

Co-administration of the anticholinergic drug trihexyphenidyl with Madopar reduces the rate, but not the extent, of levodopa absorption.

Combination with other anti-Parkinsonian agents (anticholinergics, amantadine, dopamine agonists) is permissible, though both the desired and undesired effects of treatment may be intensified. It may be necessary to reduce the dosage of Madopar or the other substance. When initiating an adjuvant treatment with a COMT inhibitor, a reduction of the dosage of Madopar may be necessary. Anticholinergics should not be withdrawn abruptly when Madopar therapy is instituted, as levodopa does not begin to take effect for some time.

There have been rare reports of possible antagonism of levodopa by diazepam. Isolated cases of hypertensive crisis have been reported with concomitant use of tricyclic antidepressants. Madopar must not be given in conjunction with MAO inhibitors (see section *4.3 Contra-indications*)

Use with antihypertensive agents may increase the hypotensive response, while sympathomimetics may increase the cardiovascular side-effects of levodopa.

Levodopa may interfere chemically with several diagnostic laboratory tests including those for glucose, ketone bodies or catecholamines in urine and for glucose or uric acid in blood. Levodopa therapy has been reported to inhibit the response to protirelin in tests of thyroid function. Coombs' tests may give a false-positive result in patients taking Madopar.

4.6 Pregnancy and lactation

Madopar is contra-indicated in pregnancy and in women of childbearing potential in the absence of adequate contraception, since there is evidence of harmful effects in studies in pregnant rabbits and the benserazide component has been found to be associated with skeletal malformations in the rat. If pregnancy occurs in a woman taking Madopar, the drug must be discontinued. Patients taking Madopar should not breast-feed their infants.

4.7 Effects on ability to drive and use machines

Patients being treated with levodopa and presenting with somnolence and/or sudden sleep episodes must be informed to refrain from driving or engaging in activities where impaired alertness may put themselves or others at risk of serious injury or death (e.g. operating machines) until such recurrent episodes and somnolence have resolved (see Section *4.4*).

4.8 Undesirable effects

Gastrointestinal:

- Anorexia, nausea, vomiting, diarrhoea (less commonly than with levodopa) mainly occurring in the early stages of treatment. May be controlled by taking Madopar with some food or liquid or increasing the dose slowly.

- Gastro-intestinal bleeding has been reported with levodopa therapy.

- Isolated cases of loss or alterations of taste.

Skin:

- rarely allergic reactions such as pruritus and rash.

Cardiovascular:

- Occasional reports of cardiac arrhythmias and orthostatic hypotension (less frequently than with levodopa alone). Orthostatic disorders usually improve following dosage reduction.

Haematological:

- Rare cases of haemolytic anaemia, transient leucopenia and thrombocytopenia.

Neuropsychiatric:

- Psychiatric disturbances are common in Parkinsonian patients, including those treated with levodopa, including mild elation, anxiety, agitation, insomnia, drowsiness, depression, aggression, delusions, hallucinations, temporal disorientation and "unmasking" of psychoses.

- Levodopa is associated with somnolence and has been associated very rarely with excessive daytime somnolence and sudden sleep onset episodes.

- Patients treated with dopamine agonists and/or levodopa for treatment of Parkinson's disease, especially at high doses, have been reported as exhibiting signs of pathological gambling, increased libido and hypersexuality, generally reversible upon reduction of the dose of treatment discontinuation.

- Involuntary movements (e.g. choreiform or athetotic, oral dyskinesias, "paddling" foot) are common, particularly on long-term administration. These are usually dose-dependant and may disappear or become tolerable after dose adjustment.

Laboratory abnormalities:

- Transient rises in SGOT, SGPT and alkaline phosphatase values have been noted.

- Increase of gamma-Glutamyltransferase has been reported.

- Serum uric acid and blood urea nitrogen levels are occasionally increased.

Others:

- Flushing and sweating have been reported with levodopa.

- Urine passed during treatment may be altered in colour; usually red-tinged, this will turn dark on standing. These changes are due to metabolites and are no cause for concern.

Tolerance to Madopar varies widely between patients and is often related to the rate of dosage increases. With long-term administration, fluctuations in the therapeutic response may be encountered. They include "freezing" episodes, end-of-dose deterioration and the so-called "on-off" effect. Patients may be helped by dosage reduction or by giving smaller and more frequent doses.

4.9 Overdose

Symptoms and signs

Symptoms and signs of overdosage are qualitatively similar to the side-effects of Madopar in therapeutic doses but may be of greater severity.

Overdose may lead to cardiovascular side effects (e.g. cardiac arrhythmias), psychiatric disturbances (e.g. confusion and insomnia), gastro-intestinal effects (e.g. nausea and vomiting) and abnormal involuntary movements (see section 4.8)

Treatment

Monitor the patient's vital signs and institute supportive measures as indicated by the patient's clinical state. In particular patients may require symptomatic treatment for cardiovascular effects (e.g. antiarrhythmics) or central nervous system effects (e.g. respiratory stimulants, neuroleptics).

5. PHARMACOLOGICAL PROPERTIES

5.1 Pharmacodynamic properties

Madopar is an anti-Parkinsonian agent. Levodopa is the metabolic precursor of dopamine. The latter is severely depleted in the striatum, pallidum and substantia nigra of Parkinsonian patients and it is considered that administration of levodopa raises the level of available dopamine in these centres. However, conversion of levodopa into dopamine by the enzyme dopa decarboxylase also takes place in extracerebral tissues. As a consequence the full therapeutic effect may not be obtained and side-effects occur.

Administration of a peripheral decarboxylase inhibitor, which blocks the extracerebral decarboxylation of levodopa, in conjunction with levodopa has significant advantages; these include reduced gastro-intestinal side-effects, a more rapid response at the initiation of therapy and a simpler dosage regimen. Madopar is a combination of levodopa and benserazide in the ratio 4:1 which in clinical trials has been shown to be the most satisfactory.

Like every replacement therapy, chronic treatment with Madopar will be necessary.

5.2 Pharmacokinetic properties

Absorption

Low levels of endogenous levodopa are detectable in predose blood samples. After oral administration of Madopar, levodopa and benserazide are rapidly absorbed, mainly in the upper regions of the small intestine and absorption there is independent of the site. Interaction studies indicate that a higher proportion of levodopa is absorbed when administered in combination with benserazide, compared with levodopa administered alone. Maximum plasma concentrations of levodopa are reached approximately one hour after ingestion of Madopar. The absolute bioavailability of levodopa from standard Madopar is approximately 98%.

The maximum plasma concentration of levodopa and the extent of absorption (AUC) increase proportionally with dose (50 - 200mg levodopa). The peak levodopa plasma concentration is 30% lower and occurs later when Madopar is administered after a standard meal. Food intake generally reduces the extent of levodopa absorption by 15% but this can be variable.

Distribution

Levodopa crosses the blood-brain barrier by a saturable transport system. It is not bound to plasma proteins. Benserazide does not cross the blood-brain barrier at therapeutic doses. Benserazide is concentrated mainly in the kidneys, lungs, small intestine and liver.

Metabolism

The 2 major routes of metabolism of levodopa are decarboxylation to form dopamine, which in turn is converted to a minor degree to norepinephrine and to a greater extent, to inactive metabolites, and O-methylation, forming 3-O-methyldopa, which has an elimination half-life of approximately 15 hours and accumulates in patients receiving therapeutic doses of Madopar. Decreased peripheral decarboxylation of levodopa when it is administered with benserazide is reflected in higher plasma levels of levodopa and 3-O-methyldopa.

Benserazide is hydroxylated to trihydroxybenzylhydrazine in the intestinal mucosa and the liver. This metabolite is a potent inhibitor of the aromatic amino acid decarboxylase.

Elimination

In the presence of the peripheral decarboxylase inhibitor, benserazide, the elimination half-life of levodopa is approximately 1.5 hours. In elderly patients the elimination half-life is slightly (25%) longer. Clearance of levodopa is 430ml/min.

Benserazide is almost entirely eliminated by metabolism. The metabolites are mainly excreted in the urine (64%) and to a small extent in faeces (24%).

5.3 Preclinical safety data

See section *4.6 Pregnancy and lactation*.

6. PHARMACEUTICAL PARTICULARS

6.1 List of excipients

Capsule contents:

Microcrystalline cellulose (E460)

Povidone (E1201)

Talc (E553b)

Magnesium stearate (E572)

Mannitol (E421)

Capsule shell:

Gelatin

Indigo carmine (E132)

Titanium dioxide (E171)

Iron oxide (E172)

Printing Ink:

Black iron oxide (E172)

6.2 Incompatibilities

None known

6.3 Shelf life

3 years.

6.4 Special precautions for storage

Do not store above 25°C. Store in the original package. Keep bottle tightly closed.

6.5 Nature and contents of container

Madopar 50 mg/12.5 mg and Madopar 100 mg/25 mg: Amber glass bottles with HDPE cap and integral desiccant containing 100 capsules.

Madopar 200 mg/50 mg: Amber glass bottles with polyethylene closure with integrated desiccant containing 100 capsules.

6.6 Special precautions for disposal and other handling

No special requirements.

7. MARKETING AUTHORISATION HOLDER

Roche Products Limited, 6 Falcon Way, Shire Park, Welwyn Garden City, AL7 1TW, United Kingdom.

8. MARKETING AUTHORISATION NUMBER(S)

Madopar 50 mg/12.5 mg: PL 00031/0125

Madopar 100 mg/25 mg: PL 00031/0073R

Madopar 200 mg/50 mg: PL 00031/0074

9. DATE OF FIRST AUTHORISATION/RENEWAL OF THE AUTHORISATION

Madopar 50 mg/12.5 mg: Date of last renewal: 14 July 2002

Madopar 100 mg/25 mg: Date of last renewal: 5 July 2003

Madopar 200 mg/50 mg: Date of last renewal: 6 July 2003

10. DATE OF REVISION OF THE TEXT

April 2009

Madopar is a registered trade mark

Madopar CR Capsules 125

(Roche Products Limited)

1. NAME OF THE MEDICINAL PRODUCT

Madopar CR 100 mg/25 mg Prolonged Release Hard Capsules

2. QUALITATIVE AND QUANTITATIVE COMPOSITION

Each capsule contains 100.0mg Levodopa and 25mg Benserazide (as benserazide hydrochloride)

For excipients see section 6.1

3. PHARMACEUTICAL FORM

Prolonged-release capsules, hard.

Light blue opaque body and dark green opaque cap imprinted with ROCHE in red.

4. CLINICAL PARTICULARS

4.1 Therapeutic indications

Treatment of all stages of Parkinson's disease. Patients with fluctuations related to levodopa plasma concentrations or timing of dose, e.g. end of dose deterioration or wearing-off effects, are more likely to benefit from switching to Madopar CR.

4.2 Posology and method of administration

Adults, including the elderly

Dosage and administration are very variable and must be titrated to the needs of the individual patient.

Madopar CR capsules must always be swallowed whole, preferably with a little water. They may be taken with or without food but antacid preparations should be avoided.

In patients with nocturnal immobility, positive effects have been reported after gradually increasing the last evening dose to two Madopar CR 100mg/25mg capsules on retiring.

Patients not currently treated with levodopa

In patients with mild to moderate disease, the initial recommended dose is one capsule of Madopar CR three times daily with meals. Higher doses, in general, of Madopar CR will be required than with conventional levodopa-decarboxylase inhibitor combinations as a result of the reduced bioavailability. The initial dosages should not exceed 600mg per day of levodopa.

Some patients may require a supplementary dose of conventional Madopar, or Madopar Dispersible, together with the first morning dose of Madopar CR to compensate for the more gradual onset of the CR formulation.

In cases of poor response to Madopar CR at total daily doses of Madopar CR plus any supplementary conventional Madopar corresponding to 1200mg levodopa, administration of Madopar CR should be discontinued and alternative therapy considered.

Patients currently treated with levodopa

Madopar CR should be substituted for the standard levodopa-decarboxylase inhibitor preparation by one capsule Madopar CR 100mg/25mg per 100mg levodopa. For example, where a patient previously received daily doses of 200mg levodopa with a decarboxylase inhibitor, then therapy should be initiated with two capsules Madopar CR 100mg/25mg. Therapy should continue with the same frequency of doses as previously.

With Madopar CR, on average, a 50% increase in daily levodopa dosage compared with previous therapy has been found to be appropriate. The dosage should be titrated every 2 to 3 days using dosage increments of Madopar CR 100mg/25mg capsules and a period of up to 4 weeks should be allowed for optimisation of dosage.

Patients already on levodopa therapy should be informed that their condition may deteriorate initially until the optimal dosage regimen has been found. Close medical supervision of the patient is advisable during the initial period whilst adjusting the dosage.

Children

Not to be given to patients under 25 years of age: therefore, no dosage recommendations are made for the administration of Madopar CR to children.

4.3 Contraindications

Madopar must not be given to patients with known hypersensitivity to levodopa or benserazide.

Madopar is contra-indicated in narrow-angle glaucoma (it may be used in wide-angle glaucoma provided that the intra-ocular pressure remains under control); severe psychoneuroses or psychoses; severe endocrine, renal, hepatic or cardiac disorders.

It should not be given in conjunction with, or within 2 weeks of withdrawal of, monoamine oxidase (MAO) inhibitors, except selective MAO-B inhibitors (e.g. selegiline) or selective MAO-A inhibitors (e.g. moclobemide).

It should not be given to patients under 25 years of age.

It should not be given to pregnant women or to women of childbearing potential in the absence of adequate contraception. If pregnancy occurs in a woman taking Madopar, the drug must be discontinued.

Suspicion has arisen that levodopa may activate a malignant melanoma. Therefore, Madopar should not be used in persons who have a history of, or who may be suffering from, a malignant melanoma.

4.4 Special warnings and precautions for use

When other drugs must be given in conjunction with Madopar, the patient should be carefully observed for unusual side-effects or potentiating effects.

In the event of general anaesthesia being required, Madopar therapy may be continued as long as the patient is able to take fluids and medication by mouth. If therapy is temporarily interrupted, the usual daily dosage may be administered as soon as the patient is able to take oral medication. Whenever therapy has been interrupted for longer periods, dosage should again be adjusted gradually; however, in many cases the patient can rapidly be returned to his previous therapeutic dosage.

If a patient has to undergo emergency surgery, when Madopar has not been withdrawn, anaesthesia with halothane should be avoided.

There have been occasional reports of a neuroleptic malignant-like syndrome, involving hyperthermia, on abrupt withdrawal of levodopa preparations. Sudden discontinuation of Madopar, without close supervision, or "drug holidays" should therefore be avoided.

Pyridoxine (vitamin B_6) may be given with Madopar since the presence of a decarboxylase inhibitor protects against the peripheral levodopa transformation facilitated by pyridoxine.

Levodopa has been associated with somnolence and episodes of sudden sleep onset. Sudden onset of sleep during daily activities, in some cases without awareness or warning signs, has been reported very rarely. Patients must be informed of this and advised to exercise caution while driving or operating machines during treatment with levodopa. Patients who have experienced somnolence and/or an episode of sudden sleep onset must refrain from driving or operating machines. Furthermore a reduction of dosage or termination of therapy may be considered.

Pathological gambling, increased libido and hypersexuality have been reported in patients treated with dopamine agonists and/or levodopa for Parkinson's disease.

Care should be taken when using Madopar in the following circumstances: in endocrine, renal, pulmonary or cardiovascular disease, particularly where there is a history of myocardial infarction or arrhythmia; psychiatric disturbances (e.g. depression); hepatic disorder; peptic ulcer; osteomalacia; where sympathomimetic drugs may be required (e.g. bronchial asthma), due to possible potentiation of the cardiovascular effects of levodopa; where antihypertensive drugs are being used, due to possible increased hypotensive action.

Periodic evaluation of hepatic, haemopoietic, renal and cardiovascular functions is advised.

Patients who improve on Madopar therapy should be advised to resume normal activities gradually as rapid mobilisation may increase the risk of injury.

Patients with diabetes should undergo frequent blood sugar tests and the dosage of antidiabetic agents should be adjusted to blood sugar levels.

4.5 Interaction with other medicinal products and other forms of interaction

Ferrous sulphate decreases the maximum plasma concentration and the AUC of levodopa by 30 – 50%. The pharmacokinetic changes observed during co-treatment with ferrous sulphate appeared to be clinically significant in some but not all patients.

Opioids and drugs which interfere with central amine mechanisms, such as rauwolfia alkaloids (reserpine), tetrabenazine (Nitoman), metoclopramide, phenothiazines, thioxanthenes, butyrophenones, amphetamines and papaverine, should be avoided where possible. If, however, their administration is considered essential, extreme care should be exercised and a close watch kept for any signs of potentiation, antagonism or other interactions and for unusual side-effects. Metoclopramide has been shown to increase the rate of levodopa absorption.

Combination with other anti-Parkinsonian agents (anticholinergics, amantadine, dopamine agonists) is permissible, though both the desired and undesired effects of treatment may be intensified. It may be necessary to reduce the dosage of Madopar or the other substance. When initiating an adjuvant treatment with a COMT inhibitor, a reduction of the dosage of Madopar may be necessary. Anticholinergics should not be withdrawn abruptly when Madopar therapy is instituted, as levodopa does not begin to take effect for some time.

There have been rare reports of possible antagonism of levodopa by diazepam. Isolated cases of hypertensive crisis have been reported with concomitant use of tricyclic antidepressants. Madopar must not be given in conjunction with MAO inhibitors (see section *4.3*).

Use with antihypertensive agents may increase the hypotensive response, while sympathomimetics may increase the cardiovascular side-effects of levodopa.

Levodopa may interfere chemically with several diagnostic laboratory tests including those for glucose, ketone bodies, or catecholamines in urine and for glucose or uric acid in blood. Levodopa therapy has been reported to inhibit the response to protirelin in tests of thyroid function. Coombs' tests may give a false-positive result in patients taking Madopar.

When Madopar CR is given with antacid preparations the bioavailability of levodopa is reduced, in comparison with conventional Madopar.

4.6 Pregnancy and lactation

Madopar is contra-indicated in pregnancy and in women of childbearing potential in the absence of adequate contraception.

Since there is evidence of harmful effects in studies in pregnant rabbits and the benserazide component has been found to be associated with skeletal malformations in the rat. If pregnancy occurs in a woman taking Madopar, the drug must be discontinued. Patients taking Madopar should not breast-feed their infants.

4.7 Effects on ability to drive and use machines

Patients being treated with levodopa and presenting with somnolence and /or sudden sleep episodes must be informed to refrain from driving or engaging in activities where impaired alertness may put themselves or others at risk of serious injury or death (e.g. operating machines) until such recurrent episodes and somnolence have resolved (see Section 4.4).

4.8 Undesirable effects

Gastro-intestinal:

– Anorexia, nausea, vomiting, diarrhoea (less commonly than with levodopa) mainly occurring in the early stages of treatment may be controlled by taking Madopar with some food or liquid or increasing the dose slowly.

– Gastro-intestinal bleeding has been reported with levodopa therapy.

– Isolated cases of loss or alterations of taste.

Skin:

– Rarely allergic reactions such as pruritus and rash.

Cardiovascular:

– Occasional reports of cardiac arrhythmias and orthostatic hypotension (less frequently than with levodopa alone). Orthostatic disorders usually improve following dosage reduction.

Haematological:

– Rare cases of haemolytic anaemia, transient leucopenia and thrombocytopenia.

Neuropsychiatric:

– Psychiatric disturbances are common in Parkinsonian patients, including those treated with levodopa, including mild elation, anxiety, agitation, insomnia, drowsiness, depression, aggression, delusions, hallucinations, temporal disorientation and "unmasking" of psychoses.

– Levodopa is associated with somnolence and has been associated very rarely with excessive daytime somnolence and sudden sleep onset episodes.

– Patients treated with dopamine agonists and/or levodopa for treatment of Parkinson's disease, especially at high doses, have been reported as exhibiting signs of pathological gambling, increased libido and hypersexuality, generally reversible upon reduction of the dose of treatment discontinuation.

– Involuntary movements (e.g. choreiform or athetotic, oral dyskinesias, "paddling" foot) are common, particularly on long-term administration. These are usually dose-dependent and may disappear or become tolerable after dose adjustment.

Laboratory abnormalities:

– Transient rises in SGOT, SGPT and alkaline phosphatase values have been noted.

– Increase of gamma-Glutamyltransferase has been reported.

– Serum uric acid and blood urea nitrogen levels are occasionally increased.

Others:

– Flushing and sweating have been reported with levodopa.

– Urine passed during treatment may be altered in colour; usually red-tinged, this will turn dark on standing. These changes are due to metabolites and are no cause for concern.

Tolerance to Madopar varies widely between patients and is often related to the rate of dosage increases.

4.9 Overdose

Symptoms and signs

Symptoms and signs of overdosage are qualitatively similar to the side-effects of Madopar in therapeutic doses but may be of greater severity.

Overdose may lead to cardiovascular side effects (e.g. cardiac arrhythmias), psychiatric disturbances (e.g. confusion and insomnia), gastro-intestinal effects (e.g. nausea and vomiting) and abnormal involuntary movements (see section 4.8).

If a patient has taken an overdose of Madopar CR, occurrence of symptoms and signs may be delayed due to delayed absorption of the active substances from the stomach.

Treatment

Monitor the patient's vital signs and institute supportive measures as indicated by the patient's clinical state. In particular patients may require symptomatic treatment for cardiovascular effects (e.g. antiarrhythmics) or central nervous system effects (e.g. respiratory stimulants, neuroleptics).

In addition, for Madopar CR further absorption should be prevented using an appropriate method.

5. PHARMACOLOGICAL PROPERTIES

5.1 Pharmacodynamic properties

Madopar is an anti-Parkinsonian agent. Levodopa is the metabolic precursor of dopamine. The latter is severely depleted in the striatum, pallidum and substantia nigra of Parkinsonian patients and it is considered that administration of levodopa raises the level of available dopamine in these centres. However, conversion of levodopa into dopamine by the enzyme dopa decarboxylase also takes place in extracerebral tissues. As a consequence the full therapeutic effect may not be obtained and side-effects occur.

Administration of a peripheral decarboxylase inhibitor, which blocks the extracerebral decarboxylation of levodopa, in conjunction with levodopa has significant advantages; these include reduced gastro-intestinal side-effects, a more rapid response at the initiation of therapy and a simpler dosage regimen. Madopar consists of levodopa and the peripheral decarboxylase inhibitor benserazide in the ratio 4:1 which in clinical trials has been shown to be the most satisfactory combination.

Like every replacement therapy, chronic treatment with Madopar will be necessary.

5.2 Pharmacokinetic properties

Madopar CR is a controlled-release form which provides more prolonged, but lower, peak plasma concentrations of levodopa than standard Madopar or other conventional formulations of levodopa.

Absorption

The active ingredients of Madopar CR are released slowly in the stomach and the maximum levodopa plasma concentration is reached approximately 3 hours after ingestion. The plasma concentration-time curve for levodopa shows a longer "half-duration" (= time-span when plasma concentrations are equal to or higher than half the maximum concentration) than that of standard Madopar, which indicates pronounced controlled-release properties. Madopar CR bioavailability is approximately 60% that of standard Madopar and is not affected by food. Maximum plasma concentrations of levodopa are not affected by food but occur later (five hours) after postprandial administration. Co-administration of an antacid with Madopar CR reduces the extent of levodopa absorption by 32%.

Distribution

Levodopa crosses the blood-brain barrier by a saturable transport system. It is not bound to plasma proteins. Benserazide does not cross the blood-brain barrier at therapeutic doses. Benserazide is concentrated mainly in the kidneys, lungs, small intestine and liver.

Metabolism

The 2 major routes of metabolism of levodopa are decarboxylation to form dopamine, which in turn is converted to a minor degree to norepinephrine and to a greater extent, to inactive metabolites, and O-methylation, forming 3-O-methyldopa, which has an elimination half-life of approximately 15 hours and accumulates in patients receiving therapeutic doses of Madopar. Decreased peripheral decarboxylation of levodopa when it is administered with benserazide is reflected in higher plasma levels of levodopa and 3-O-methyldopa.

Benserazide is hydroxylated to trihydroxybenzylhydrazine in the intestinal mucosa and the liver. This metabolite is a potent inhibitor of the aromatic amino acid decarboxylase.

Elimination

In the presence of the peripheral decarboxylase inhibitor, benserazide, the elimination half-life of levodopa is approximately 1.5 hours. In elderly patients the elimination half-life is slightly (25%) longer. Clearance of levodopa is 430 ml/min.

Benserazide is almost entirely eliminated by metabolism. The metabolites are mainly excreted in the urine (64%) and to a small extent in faeces (24%).

5.3 Preclinical safety data

Not applicable

6. PHARMACEUTICAL PARTICULARS

6.1 List of excipients

Capsule contents:

Hypromellose (E464)

Hydrogenated vegetable oil

Calcium phosphate (E341)

Mannitol (E421)

Talc (E553b)

Povidone (E1201)

Magnesium stearate (E572)

Capsule shell:

Gelatin

Indigo carmine (E132)

Titanium dioxide (E171)

Yellow iron oxide (E172)

Printing ink:

Red iron oxide (E172)

6.2 Incompatibilities

Not applicable

6.3 Shelf life

3 years.

6.4 Special precautions for storage

Do not store above 25°C. Store in the original package. Keep bottle tightly closed.

6.5 Nature and contents of container

Amber glass bottles with polyethylene closure and integrated desiccant containing 100 capsules.

6.6 Special precautions for disposal and other handling

No special requirements.

7. MARKETING AUTHORISATION HOLDER
Roche Products Limited, 6 Falcon Way, Shire Park, Welwyn Garden City, AL7 1TW, United Kingdom.

8. MARKETING AUTHORISATION NUMBER(S)
PL 00031/0227

9. DATE OF FIRST AUTHORISATION/RENEWAL OF THE AUTHORISATION
Date of last renewal: 26 April 2004

10. DATE OF REVISION OF THE TEXT
April 2009

Madopar is a registered trade mark

Madopar Dispersible

(Roche Products Limited)

1. NAME OF THE MEDICINAL PRODUCT
Madopar 50 mg/12.5 mg Dispersible Tablets

Madopar 100 mg/25 mg Dispersible Tablets

2. QUALITATIVE AND QUANTITATIVE COMPOSITION
Madopar 50 mg/12.5 mg: Each tablet contains 50mg Levodopa and 12.5mg Benserazide (as benserazide hydrochloride).

Madopar 100 mg/25 mg: Each tablet contains 100.0 mg Levodopa and 25 mg Benserazide (as benserazide hydrochloride).

For excipients, see section 6.1

3. PHARMACEUTICAL FORM
Dispersible tablet.

Madopar 50 mg/12.5 mg: Round white tablets with Roche 62.5 imprinted on one face and a single break bar on the other.

Madopar 100 mg/25 mg: Round white tablets with Roche 125 imprinted on one face and a single break bar on the other.

4. CLINICAL PARTICULARS

4.1 Therapeutic indications
Parkinsonism - idiopathic, post-encephalitic. Previous neurosurgery is not a contra-indication to Madopar. Patients requiring a more rapid onset of action, e.g. patients suffering from early morning or afternoon akinesia, or who exhibit "delayed on" or "wearing off" phenomena, are more likely to benefit from Madopar Dispersible.

4.2 Posology and method of administration
Dosage and administration are variable and no more than a guide can be given.

Adults

Patients not previously treated with levodopa

The recommended initial dose is one capsule or dispersible tablet of Madopar 50 mg/12.5 mg three or four times daily. If the disease is at an advanced stage, the starting dose should be one capsule or dispersible tablet of Madopar 100 mg/25 mg three times daily.

The daily dosage should then be increased by one capsule or dispersible tablet of Madopar 100 mg/25 mg, or their equivalent, once or twice weekly until a full therapeutic effect is obtained, or side-effects supervene.

In some elderly patients, it may suffice to initiate treatment with one capsule or dispersible tablet of Madopar 50 mg/12.5 mg once or twice daily, increasing by one capsule or dispersible tablet every third or fourth day.

The effective dose usually lies within the range of four to eight capsules or dispersible tablets of Madopar 100 mg/25 mg (two to four capsules of Madopar 200 mg/50 mg) daily in divided doses, most patients requiring no more than six capsules or dispersible tablets of Madopar 100 mg/25 mg daily.

Optimal improvement is usually seen in one to three weeks but the full therapeutic effect of Madopar may not be apparent for some time. It is advisable, therefore, to allow several weeks to elapse before contemplating dosage increments above the average dose range. If satisfactory improvement is still not achieved, the dose of Madopar may be increased but with caution. It is rarely necessary to give more than ten capsules or dispersible tablets of Madopar 100 mg/25 mg (five capsules of Madopar 200 mg/50 mg) per day.

Treatment should be continued for at least six months before failure is concluded from the absence of a clinical response.

Madopar 50 mg/12.5 mg capsules or dispersible tablets may be used to facilitate adjustment of dosage to the needs of the individual patient. Patients who experience fluctuations in response may be helped by dividing the dosage into smaller, more frequent doses with the aid of Madopar 50 mg/12.5 mg capsules or dispersible tablets without, however, altering the total daily dose.

Madopar 200 mg/50 mg capsules are only for maintenance therapy once the optimal dosage has been determined using Madopar 100 mg/25 mg capsules or dispersible tablets.

Patients previously treated with levodopa

The following procedure is recommended: Levodopa alone should be discontinued and Madopar started on the following day. The patient should be initiated on a total of one less Madopar 100 mg/25 mg capsule or dispersible tablet daily than the total number of 500 mg levodopa tablets or capsules previously taken (for example, if the patient had previously taken 2g levodopa daily, then he should start on three capsules or dispersible tablets Madopar 100 mg/25 mg daily on the following day). Observe the patient for one week and then, if necessary, increase the dosage in the manner described for new patients.

Patients previously treated with other levodopa/decarboxylase inhibitor combinations

Previous therapy should be withdrawn for 12 hours. In order to minimise the potential for any effects of levodopa withdrawal, it may be beneficial to discontinue previous therapy at night and institute Madopar therapy the following morning. The initial Madopar dose should be one capsule or dispersible tablet of Madopar 50 mg/12.5 mg three or four times daily. This dose may then be increased in the manner described for patients not previously treated with levodopa.

Other anti-Parkinsonian drugs may be given with Madopar. Existing treatment with other anti-Parkinsonian drugs, e.g. anticholinergics or amantadine, should be continued during initiation of Madopar therapy. However, as treatment with Madopar proceeds and the therapeutic effect becomes apparent, the dosage of the other drugs may need to be reduced or the drugs gradually withdrawn.

Elderly

Although there may be an age-related decrease in tolerance to levodopa in the elderly, Madopar appears to be well-tolerated and side effects are generally not troublesome.

Children

Not to be given to patients under 25 years of age, therefore, no dosage recommendations are made for the administration of Madopar to children.

Madopar capsules and dispersible tablets are for oral administration. They should be taken with, or immediately after, meals.

Madopar dispersible tablets may be swallowed whole or dispersed in at least 25ml water per tablet. They may be taken in dilute orange squash (at least 25ml per tablet) if preferred. However, orange juice should not be used. Madopar dispersible tablets are particularly suitable for patients who dislike taking capsules or have difficulty in swallowing solid dosage forms.

4.3 Contraindications
Madopar must not be given to patients with known hypersensitivity to levodopa or benserazide.

Madopar is contra-indicated in narrow-angle glaucoma (it may be used in wide-angle glaucoma provided that the intra-ocular pressure remains under control); severe psychoneuroses or psychoses; severe endocrine, renal, hepatic or cardiac disorders.

It should not be given in conjunction with, or within 2 weeks of withdrawal of, monoamine oxidase (MAO) inhibitors, except selective MAO-B inhibitors (e.g. selegiline) or selective MAO-A inhibitors (e.g. moclobemide).

It should not be given to patients under 25 years of age.

It should not be given to pregnant women or to women of childbearing potential in the absence of adequate contraception. If pregnancy occurs in a woman taking Madopar, the drug must be discontinued.

Suspicion has arisen that levodopa may activate a malignant melanoma. Therefore, Madopar should not be used in persons who have a history of, or who may be suffering from, a malignant melanoma.

4.4 Special warnings and precautions for use
When other drugs must be given in conjunction with Madopar, the patient should be carefully observed for unusual side-effects or potentiating effects.

In the event of general anaesthesia being required, Madopar therapy may be continued as long as the patient is able to take fluids and medication by mouth. If therapy is temporarily interrupted, the usual daily dosage may be administered as soon as the patient is able to take oral medication. Whenever therapy has been interrupted for longer periods, dosage should again be adjusted gradually; however, in many cases the patient can rapidly be returned to his previous therapeutic dosage.

If a patient has to undergo emergency surgery, when Madopar has not been withdrawn, anaesthesia with halothane should be avoided.

There have been occasional reports of a neuroleptic malignant-like syndrome, involving hyperthermia, on abrupt withdrawal of levodopa preparations. Sudden discontinuation of Madopar, without close supervision, or "drug holidays" should therefore be avoided.

Pyridoxine (vitamin B_6) may be given with Madopar since the presence of a decarboxylase inhibitor protects against the peripheral levodopa transformation facilitated by pyridoxine.

Levodopa has been associated with somnolence and episodes of sudden sleep onset. Sudden onset of sleep during daily activities, in some cases without awareness or warning signs, has been reported very rarely. Patients must be informed of this and advised to exercise caution while driving or operating machines during treatment with levodopa. Patients who have experienced somnolence and/or an episode of sudden sleep onset must refrain from driving or operating machines. Furthermore a reduction of dosage or termination of therapy may be considered.

Pathological gambling, increased libido and hypersexuality have been reported in patients treated with dopamine agonist and/or levodopa for Parkinson's disease.

Care should be taken when using Madopar in the following circumstances: In endocrine, renal, pulmonary or cardiovascular disease, particularly where there is a history of myocardial infarction or arrhythmia; psychiatric disturbances (e.g. depression); hepatic disorder; peptic ulcer; osteomalacia; where sympathomimetic drugs may be required (e.g. bronchial asthma), due to possible potentiation of the cardiovascular effects of levodopa; where antihypertensive drugs are being used, due to possible increased hypotensive action.

Periodic evaluation of hepatic, haemopoietic, renal and cardiovascular functions is advised.

Patients with diabetes should undergo frequent blood sugar tests and the dosage of anti-diabetic agents should be adjusted to blood sugar levels.

Patients who improve on Madopar therapy should be advised to resume normal activities gradually as rapid mobilisation may increase the risk of injury.

4.5 Interaction with other medicinal products and other forms of interaction
Ferrous sulphate decreases the maximum plasma concentration and the AUC of levodopa by 30 - 50%. The pharmacokinetic changes observed during co-treatment with ferrous sulphate appeared to be clinically significant in some but not all patients.

Opioids and drugs which interfere with central amine mechanisms, such as rauwolfia alkaloids (reserpine), tetrabenazine (Nitoman), metoclopramide, phenothiazines, thioxanthenes, butyrophenones, amphetamines and papaverine, should be avoided where possible. If, however, their administration is considered essential, extreme care should be exercised and a close watch kept for any signs of potentiation, antagonism or other interactions and for unusual side-effects. Metoclopramide has been shown to increase the rate of levodopa absorption.

Co-administration of the anticholinergic drug trihexyphenidyl with Madopar reduces the rate, but not the extent, of levodopa absorption.

Combination with other anti-Parkinsonian agents (anticholinergics, amantadine, dopamine agonists) is permissible, though both the desired and undesired effects of treatment may be intensified. It may be necessary to reduce the dosage of Madopar or the other substance. When initiating an adjuvant treatment with a COMT inhibitor, a reduction of the dosage of Madopar may be necessary. Anticholinergics should not be withdrawn abruptly when Madopar therapy is instituted, as levodopa does not begin to take effect for some time.

There have been rare reports of possible antagonism of levodopa by diazepam. Isolated cases of hypertensive crisis have been reported with concomitant use of tricyclic antidepressants. Madopar must not be given in conjunction with MAO inhibitors (see section *4.3 Contra-indications*)

Use with antihypertensive agents may increase the hypotensive response, while sympathomimetics may increase the cardiovascular side-effects of levodopa.

Levodopa may interfere chemically with several diagnostic laboratory tests including those for glucose, ketone bodies or catecholamines in urine and for glucose or uric acid in blood. Levodopa therapy has been reported to inhibit the response to protirelin in tests of thyroid function. Coombs' tests may give a false-positive result in patients taking Madopar.

4.6 Pregnancy and lactation
Madopar is contra-indicated in pregnancy and in women of childbearing potential in the absence of adequate contraception, since there is evidence of harmful effects in studies in pregnant rabbits and the benserazide component has been found to be associated with skeletal malformations in the rat. If pregnancy occurs in a woman taking Madopar, the drug must be discontinued. Patients taking Madopar should not breast-feed their infants.

4.7 Effects on ability to drive and use machines
Patients being treated with levodopa and presenting with somnolence and/or sudden sleep episodes must be informed to refrain from driving or engaging in activities where impaired alertness may put themselves or others at risk of serious injury or death (e.g. operating machines) until such recurrent episodes and somnolence have resolved (see Section *4.4*).

4.8 Undesirable effects

Gastrointestinal:

- Anorexia, nausea, vomiting, diarrhoea (less commonly than with levodopa) mainly occurring in the early stages of treatment. May be controlled by taking Madopar with some food or liquid or increasing the dose slowly.
- Gastro-intestinal bleeding has been reported with levodopa therapy.
- Isolated cases of loss or alterations of taste.

Skin:

- Rarely allergic reactions such as pruritus and rash.

Cardiovascular:

- Occasional reports of cardiac arrhythmias and orthostatic hypotension (less frequently than with levodopa alone). Orthostatic disorders usually improve following dosage reduction.

Haematological:

- Rare cases of haemolytic anaemia, transient leucopenia and thrombocytopenia.

Neuropsychiatric:

- Psychiatric disturbances are common in Parkinsonian patients, including those treated with levodopa, including mild elation, anxiety, agitation, insomnia, drowsiness, depression, aggression, delusions, hallucinations, temporal disorientation and "unmasking" of psychoses.

- Levodopa is associated with somnolence and has been associated very rarely with excessive daytime somnolence and sudden sleep onset episodes.

- Patients treated with dopamine agonists and/or levodopa for treatment of Parkinson's disease, especially at high doses, have been reported as exhibiting signs of pathological gambling, increased libido and hypersexuality, generally reversible upon reduction of the dose of treatment discontinuation.

- Involuntary movements (e.g. choreiform or athetotic, oral dyskinesias, "paddling" foot) are common, particularly on long-term administration. These are usually dose-dependant and may disappear or become tolerable after dose adjustment.

Laboratory abnormalities:

- Transient rises in SGOT, SGPT and alkaline phosphatase values have been noted.

- Increase of gamma-Glutamyltransferase has been reported.

- Serum uric acid and blood urea nitrogen levels are occasionally increased.

Others:

- Flushing and sweating have been reported with levodopa.

- Urine passed during treatment may be altered in colour; usually red-tinged, this will turn dark on standing. These changes are due to metabolites and are no cause for concern.

Tolerance to Madopar varies widely between patients and is often related to the rate of dosage increases. With long-term administration, fluctuations in the therapeutic response may be encountered. They include "freezing" episodes, end-of-dose deterioration and the so-called "on-off" effect. Patients may be helped by dosage reduction or by giving smaller and more frequent doses.

4.9 Overdose

Symptoms and Signs

Symptoms and signs of overdosage are qualitatively similar to the side-effects of Madopar in therapeutic doses but may be of greater severity.

Overdose may lead to cardiovascular side effects (e.g. cardiac arrhythmias), psychiatric disturbances (e.g. confusion and insomnia), gastro-intestinal effects (e.g. nausea and vomiting) and abnormal involuntary movements (see section 4.8).

Treatment

Monitor the patient's vital signs and institute supportive measures as indicated by the patient's clinical state. In particular patients may require symptomatic treatment for cardiovascular effects (e.g. antiarrhythmics) or central nervous system effects (e.g. respiratory stimulants, neuroleptics).

5. PHARMACOLOGICAL PROPERTIES

5.1 Pharmacodynamic properties

Madopar is an anti-Parkinsonian agent. Levodopa is the metabolic precursor of dopamine. The latter is severely depleted in the striatum, pallidum and substantia nigra of Parkinsonian patients and it is considered that administration of levodopa raises the level of available dopamine in these centres. However, conversion of levodopa into dopamine by the enzyme dopa decarboxylase also takes place in extracerebral tissues. As a consequence the full therapeutic effect may not be obtained and side-effects occur.

Administration of a peripheral decarboxylase inhibitor, which blocks the extracerebral decarboxylation of levodopa, in conjunction with levodopa has significant advantages; these include reduced gastro-intestinal side-effects, a more rapid response at the initiation of therapy and a simpler dosage regimen. Madopar is a combination of levodopa and benserazide in the ratio 4:1 which in clinical trials has been shown to be the most satisfactory.

Like every replacement therapy, chronic treatment with Madopar will be necessary.

5.2 Pharmacokinetic properties

Absorption

Low levels of endogenous levodopa are detectable in predose blood samples. After oral administration of Madopar, levodopa and benserazide are rapidly absorbed, mainly in the upper regions of the small intestine and absorption there is independent of the site. Interaction studies indicate that a higher proportion of levodopa is absorbed when administered in combination with benserazide, compared with levodopa administered alone. Maximum plasma concentrations of levodopa are reached approximately one hour after ingestion of Madopar. The absolute bioavailability of levodopa from standard Madopar is approximately 98%.

The maximum plasma concentration of levodopa and the extent of absorption (AUC) increase proportionally with dose (50 – 200mg levodopa). The peak levodopa plasma concentration is 30% lower and occurs later when Madopar is administered after a standard meal. Food intake generally reduces the extent of levodopa absorption by 15% but this can be variable.

Distribution

Levodopa crosses the blood-brain barrier by a saturable transport system. It is not bound to plasma proteins. Benserazide does not cross the blood-brain barrier at therapeutic doses. Benserazide is concentrated mainly in the kidneys, lungs, small intestine and liver.

Metabolism

The 2 major routes of metabolism of levodopa are decarboxylation to form dopamine, which in turn is converted to a minor degree to norepinephrine and to a greater extent, to inactive metabolites, and O-methylation, forming 3-O-methyldopa, which has an elimination half-life of approximately 15 hours and accumulates in patients receiving therapeutic doses of Madopar. Decreased peripheral decarboxylation of levodopa when it is administered with benserazide is reflected in higher plasma levels of levodopa and 3-O-methyldopa.

Benserazide is hydroxylated to trihydroxybenzylhydrazine in the intestinal mucosa and the liver. This metabolite is a potent inhibitor of the aromatic amino acid decarboxylase.

Elimination

In the presence of the peripheral decarboxylase inhibitor, benserazide, the elimination half-life of levodopa is approximately 1.5 hours. In elderly patients the elimination half-life is slightly (25%) longer. Clearance of levodopa is 430ml/min.

Benserazide is almost entirely eliminated by metabolism. The metabolites are mainly excreted in the urine (64%) and to a small extent in faeces (24%).

5.3 Preclinical safety data

None stated

6. PHARMACEUTICAL PARTICULARS

6.1 List of excipients

Citric acid, anhydrous (E330)

Pregelantised starch

Microcrystalline cellulose (E460)

Magnesium stearate (E572)

6.2 Incompatibilities

None known

6.3 Shelf life

3 years.

6.4 Special precautions for storage

Do not store above 25°C. Store in the original package. Keep bottle tightly closed.

6.5 Nature and contents of container

Amber glass bottles with HDPE cap with integral desiccant, containing 100 dispersible tablets.

6.6 Special precautions for disposal and other handling

No special requirements.

7. MARKETING AUTHORISATION HOLDER

Roche Products Limited, 6 Falcon Way, Shire Park, Welwyn Garden City, AL7 1TW, United Kingdom.

8. MARKETING AUTHORISATION NUMBER(S)

Madopar 50 mg/12.5 mg: PL 00031/0220

Madopar 100 mg/25 mg: PL 00031/0221

9. DATE OF FIRST AUTHORISATION/RENEWAL OF THE AUTHORISATION

Date of last renewal: 18 May 2002

10. DATE OF REVISION OF THE TEXT

April 2009

Madopar is a registered trade mark

Magnesium Sulphate Injection 50%

(UCB Pharma Limited)

1. NAME OF THE MEDICINAL PRODUCT

Magnesium Sulphate Injection 50%

2. QUALITATIVE AND QUANTITATIVE COMPOSITION

Magnesium Sulphate BP 50% w/v

3. PHARMACEUTICAL FORM

Sterile solution for parenteral use.

4. CLINICAL PARTICULARS

4.1 Therapeutic indications

Treatment of magnesium deficiency where the oral route of administration may be inappropriate, which may be due to malabsorption syndromes, chronic alcoholism, malnutrition, severe diarrhoea or patients on total parenteral nutrition.

4.2 Posology and method of administration

Magnesium sulphate injection may be administered by intramuscular or intravenous routes. For intravenous administration, a concentration of 20% or less should be used; the rate of injection not exceeding 1.5ml/minute of a 10% solution or its equivalent.

Adults

The dosage should be individualised according to patient's needs and responses.

Mild magnesium deficiency

1g intramuscularly every 6 hours for 4 doses.

Severe magnesium deficiency

Up to 250mg/kg intramuscularly given over 4 hours or 5g/litre of infusion solution intravenously over 3 hours.

Children

It is recommended that the solution be diluted to 20% w/v prior to intramuscular injection.

Elderly

No special recommendations.

4.3 Contraindications

Magnesium sulphate is contraindicated in patients with heart block, myocardial damage or impaired renal function.

4.4 Special warnings and precautions for use

Magnesium sulphate must be used with caution in patients suspected of or known to have renal impairment.

4.5 Interaction with other medicinal products and other forms of interaction

Administer with caution to patients receiving digitalis glycosides. Effects of neuromuscular blocking agents may be enhanced. Magnesium sulphate should not be administered concomitantly with high doses of barbiturates, opioids or hypnotics due to the risk of respiratory depression.

Concomitant use of nifedipine may very rarely lead to a calcium ion imbalance and could result in abnormal muscle function.

4.6 Pregnancy and lactation

Safety in human pregnancy and during breastfeeding has not been established, therefore, as with all drugs it is not advisable to administer magnesium sulphate during pregnancy or breastfeeding unless considered essential, and it must be administered under medical supervision.

4.7 Effects on ability to drive and use machines

None known.

4.8 Undesirable effects

Hypermagnesaemia characterised by flushing, thirst, hypotension, drowsiness, nausea, vomiting, confusion, loss of tendon reflexes due to neuromuscular blockade, muscle weakness, respiratory depression, cardiac arrhythmias, coma and cardiac arrest.

There is a risk of respiratory depression if magnesium sulphate is administered concomitantly with high doses of barbiturates, opioids or hypnotics (see 'Interactions').

4.9 Overdose

Symptoms: Hypermagnesaemia characterised by flushing, thirst, hypotension, drowsiness, nausea, vomiting, confusion, loss of tendon reflexes due to neuromuscular blockade, muscle weakness, respiratory depression, cardiac arrhythmias, coma and cardiac arrest.

Treatment: Maintain respiration with 10% calcium gluconate administered intravenously in a dose of 10-20ml. If renal function is normal adequate fluids should be given to assist removal of magnesium from the body. Dialysis may be necessary in patients with renal impairment or severe hypermagnesaemia.

5. PHARMACOLOGICAL PROPERTIES

5.1 Pharmacodynamic properties

Magnesium is the second most abundant cation in intracellular fluid and is an essential body electrolyte. Magnesium is a factor in a number of enzyme systems, and is involved in neurochemical transmission and muscular excitability.

Parenterally administered magnesium sulphate exerts a depressant effect on the central nervous system and acts peripherally to produce vasodilation.

5.2 Pharmacokinetic properties

Following intravenous administration, the onset of action is immediate and the duration approximately 30 minutes. Following intramuscular administration the onset of action occurs after approximately one hour and the duration of action is 3-4 hours.

Magnesium sulphate is excreted by the kidneys with small amounts being excreted in breast milk and saliva.

5.3 Preclinical safety data

None stated.

6. PHARMACEUTICAL PARTICULARS

6.1 List of excipients

Sodium hydroxide BP

Sulphuric acid BP

Water for injections HSE

6.2 Incompatibilities

Magnesium sulphate is incompatible with alkali hydroxides (forming insoluble magnesium hydroxide), alkali carbonates (forming insoluble magnesium carbonate) and salicylates. Streptomycin sulphate and tetramycin sulphate activity is inhibited by magnesium ions.

6.3 Shelf life

36 months.

6.4 Special precautions for storage

Store below 25°C.

6.5 Nature and contents of container

Neutral Type I glass ampoules containing 2ml, 4ml or 40ml, supplied in packs of 1, 5 or 10 units.

Not all pack sizes may be marketed.

6.6 Special precautions for disposal and other handling

None stated.

7. MARKETING AUTHORISATION HOLDER

UCB Pharma Limited

208 Bath Road

Slough

Berkshire

SL1 3 WE

UK

8. MARKETING AUTHORISATION NUMBER(S)

PL 00039/5903R

9. DATE OF FIRST AUTHORISATION/RENEWAL OF THE AUTHORISATION

2 June 1987 / 3 September 1997

10. DATE OF REVISION OF THE TEXT

June 2005

POM

Magnesium Sulphate Injection BP Minijet 50% w/v

(International Medication Systems (UK) Ltd)

1. NAME OF THE MEDICINAL PRODUCT

Magnesium Sulphate Injection BP Minijet 50% solution for injection.

2. QUALITATIVE AND QUANTITATIVE COMPOSITION

Magnesium Sulphate Heptahydrate 500mg per ml, equivalent to 2mmol magnesium ions per ml.

The product is available as a vial containing Magnesium Sulphate Heptahydrate 2g in 4ml

For excipients, see section 6.1.

3. PHARMACEUTICAL FORM

Solution for injection.

A clear, colourless solution practically free from visible particles.

4. CLINICAL PARTICULARS

4.1 Therapeutic indications

Treatment of magnesium deficiency where the oral route of administration may be inappropriate.

4.2 Posology and method of administration

Magnesium sulphate injection may be administered by intramuscular or intravenous routes. For intravenous administration, a concentration of 20% or less should be used; the rate of injection not exceeding 1.5ml/minute of a 10% solution or its equivalent.

Magnesium Sulphate Injection Minijet 50% may be diluted as needed in either 5% dextrose solution or in 0.9% saline solution.

Dosage should be reduced in renal impairment. Plasma magnesium concentrations should be monitored throughout therapy.

Adults

The dosage should be individualised according to patient's needs and responses.

To treat refractory ventricular fibrillation in the presence of hypomagnesaemia, treat with 8mmol (4ml) intravenously.

Mild magnesium deficiency

1g intramuscularly every 6 hours for 4 doses.

Severe magnesium deficiency

Up to 250mg/kg intramuscularly given over 4 hours or 5g/ litre of infusion solution intravenously over 3 hours.

Children

It is recommended that the solution be diluted to 20% w/v prior to intramuscular injection.

Elderly

No special recommendations except in renal impairment, see above.

4.3 Contraindications

Hypersensitivity to magnesium and it salts. Magnesium sulphate is contraindicated in patients with renal failure.

4.4 Special warnings and precautions for use

Magnesium sulphate must be used with caution in patients suspected of or known to have renal impairment. Magnesium Sulphate should not be used in hepatic coma if there is a risk of renal failure.

4.5 Interaction with other medicinal products and other forms of interaction

Administer with caution to patients receiving digitalis glycosides. Magnesium sulphate should not be administered concomitantly with high doses of barbiturates, opioids or hypnotics due to the risk of respiratory depression.

The action of non-depolarising muscle relaxants such as tubocurarine is potentiated and prolonged by parenteral magnesium salts.

Profound hypotension has been reported with concomitant use of nifedipine.

4.6 Pregnancy and lactation

Safety in human pregnancy and during breastfeeding has not been established, therefore, as with all drugs it is not advisable to administer magnesium sulphate during pregnancy or breastfeeding unless considered essential, and it must be administered under medical supervision.

4.7 Effects on ability to drive and use machines

No studies on the effects on the ability to drive and use machines have been performed.

4.8 Undesirable effects

There is a risk of respiratory depression if magnesium sulphate is administered concomitantly with high doses of barbiturates, opioids or hypnotics (see 'Interactions').

4.9 Overdose

Symptoms: Hypermagnesaemia characterised by flushing, thirst, hypotension, drowsiness, confusion, loss of tendon reflexes due to neuromuscular blockade, muscle weakness, respiratory depression, cardiac arrhythmias, coma and cardiac arrest.

Treatment: Maintain respiration with 10% calcium gluconate administered intravenously in a dose of 10-20ml. If renal function is normal adequate fluids should be given to assist removal of magnesium from the body. Dialysis may be necessary in patients with renal impairment or severe hypermagnesaemia.

5. PHARMACOLOGICAL PROPERTIES

5.1 Pharmacodynamic properties

Pharmacotherapeutic group: Mineral Supplements, ATC code: A12CC 02.

Magnesium is the second most abundant cation in intracellular fluid and is an essential body electrolyte. Magnesium is a factor in a number of enzyme systems, and is involved in neurochemical transmission and muscular excitability.

Parenterally administered magnesium sulphate exerts a depressant effect on the central nervous system and acts peripherally to produce vasodilation.

5.2 Pharmacokinetic properties

Following intravenous administration, the onset of action is immediate and the duration approximately 30 minutes. Following intramuscular administration the onset of action occurs after approximately one hour and the duration of action is 3-4 hours.

Magnesium sulphate is excreted by the kidneys with small amounts being excreted in breast milk and saliva.

5.3 Preclinical safety data

Preclinical data reveal no special hazard for humans based on conventional studies of safety pharmacology, repeated dose toxicity, genotoxicity, carcinogenic potential, toxicity to reproduction.

6. PHARMACEUTICAL PARTICULARS

6.1 List of excipients

Sulphuric acid

Sodium hydroxide

Water for injections

6.2 Incompatibilities

Magnesium sulphate is incompatible with alkali hydroxides (forming insoluble magnesium hydroxide), alkali carbonates (forming insoluble magnesium carbonate) and salicylates. Streptomycin sulphate and tetramycin sulphate activity is inhibited by magnesium ions.

6.3 Shelf life

2 years

Discard any unused solution immediately after first use.

From a microbiological point of view, the product should be used immediately. If not used immediately, in-use storage times and conditions prior to use are the responsibility of the user and would normally not be longer than 24 hours at 2 to 8°C, unless dilution has taken place in controlled and validated aseptic conditions.

6.4 Special precautions for storage

This medicinal product does not require any special storage conditions.

6.5 Nature and contents of container

The solution is contained in a type I glass vial with an elastomeric closure and a plastic vial cap. The product is available as 4ml.

An IMS Minijet®injector is supplied in the carton.

6.6 Special precautions for disposal and other handling

The container is specially designed for use with the IMS Minijet injector.

See 4.2 Posology for information regarding the dilution of this product.

7. MARKETING AUTHORISATION HOLDER

International Medications Systems (UK) Limited

208 Bath Road

Slough

Berkshire

SL1 3 WE

United Kingdom

8. MARKETING AUTHORISATION NUMBER(S)

PL 03265/0077

9. DATE OF FIRST AUTHORISATION/RENEWAL OF THE AUTHORISATION

26th November 2004

10. DATE OF REVISION OF THE TEXT

Malarone

(GlaxoSmithKline UK)

1. NAME OF THE MEDICINAL PRODUCT

Malarone 250 mg/100 mg film-coated tablets

2. QUALITATIVE AND QUANTITATIVE COMPOSITION

Each Malarone tablet contains 250 mg atovaquone and 100 mg proguanil hydrochloride.

For a full list of excipients, see section 6.1.

3. PHARMACEUTICAL FORM

Film coated tablet.

Round, biconvex, pink tablets engraved 'GX CM3' on one side.

4. CLINICAL PARTICULARS

4.1 Therapeutic indications

Malarone is a fixed dose combination of atovaquone and proguanil hydrochloride which acts as a blood schizonticide and also has activity against hepatic schizonts of *Plasmodium falciparum*. It is indicated for:

Prophylaxis of *Plasmodium falciparum* malaria.

Treatment of acute, uncomplicated *Plasmodium falciparum* malaria.

Because Malarone is effective against drug sensitive and drug resistant *P. falciparum* it is especially recommended for prophylaxis and treatment of *P. falciparum* malaria where the pathogen may be resistant to other antimalarials.

Official guidelines and local information on the prevalence of resistance to antimalarial drugs should be taken into consideration. Official guidelines will normally include WHO and public health authorities' guidelines.

4.2 Posology and method of administration

Method of administration

The daily dose should be taken with food or a milky drink (to ensure maximum absorption) at the same time each day.

If patients are unable to tolerate food, Malarone should be administered, but systemic exposure of atovaquone will be reduced. In the event of vomiting within 1 hour of dosing a repeat dose should be taken.

Posology

Prophylaxis:

Prophylaxis should

- commence 24 or 48 hours prior to entering a malaria-endemic area,
- continue during the period of the stay, **which should not exceed 28 days**,
- continue for 7 days after leaving the area.

In residents (semi-immune subjects) of endemic areas, the safety and effectiveness of Malarone has been established in studies of up to 12 weeks.

Dosage in Adults

One Malarone tablet daily.

Malarone tablets are not recommended for malaria prophylaxis in persons under 40kg bodyweight.

Treatment

Dosage in Adults

Four Malarone tablets as a single dose for three consecutive days.

Dosage in Children

11-20 kg bodyweight. One tablet daily for three consecutive days.

21-30 kg bodyweight. Two tablets as a single dose for three consecutive days.

31-40 kg bodyweight. Three tablets as a single dose for three consecutive days.

>40 kg bodyweight. Dose as for adults.

Dosage in the Elderly

A pharmacokinetic study indicates that no dosage adjustments are needed in the elderly (See Section 5.2).

Dosage in Hepatic Impairment

A pharmacokinetic study indicates that no dosage adjustments are needed in patients with mild to moderate hepatic impairment. Although no studies have been conducted in patients with severe hepatic impairment, no special precautions or dosage adjustment are anticipated (See Section 5.2).

Dosage in Renal Impairment

Pharmacokinetic studies indicate that no dosage adjustments are needed in patients with mild to moderate renal impairment. In patients with severe renal impairment (creatine clearance <30 mL/min) alternatives to Malarone for treatment of acute *P. falciparum* malaria should be recommended whenever possible (See Sections 4.4 and 5.2). For prophylaxis of *P. falciparum* malaria in patients with several renal impairments see Section 4.3.

4.3 Contraindications

Hypersensitivity to the active substances or to any of the excipients.

Malarone is contraindicated for prophylaxis of *P. falciparum* malaria in patients with severe renal impairment (creatine clearance <30 mL/min).

4.4 Special warnings and precautions for use

The safety and effectiveness of Malarone (atovaquone 250 mg/proguanil hydrochloride 100 mg tablets) for prophylaxis of malaria in patients who weigh less than 40kg has not been established.

Persons taking Malarone for prophylaxis or treatment of malaria should take a repeat dose if they vomit within 1 hour of dosing. In the event of diarrhoea, normal dosing should be continued. Absorption of atovaquone may be reduced in patients with diarrhoea or vomiting, but diarrhoea or vomiting was not associated with reduced efficacy in clinical trials of Malarone for malaria prophylaxis. However, as with other antimalarial agents, subjects with diarrhoea or vomiting should be advised to continue to comply with personal protection measures (repellants, bednets).

In patients with acute malaria who present with diarrhoea or vomiting, alternative therapy should be considered. If Malarone is used to treat malaria in these patients, parasitaemia should be closely monitored.

The safety and effectiveness of Malarone (atovaquone 250 mg/proguanil hydrochloride 100 mg tablets) for treatment of malaria in paediatric patients who weigh less than 11 kg has not been established.

Malarone has not been evaluated for the treatment of cerebral malaria or other severe manifestations of complicated malaria including hyperparasitaemia, pulmonary oedema or renal failure.

Occasionally, severe allergic reactions (including anaphylaxis) have been reported in patients taking Malarone. If patients experience an allergic reaction (see section 4.8) Malarone should be discontinued promptly and appropriate treatment initiated.

Parasite relapse occurred commonly when *P. vivax* malaria was treated with Malarone alone. Travellers with intense exposure to *P. vivax* or *P. ovale*, and those who develop malaria caused by either of these parasites, will require additional treatment with a drug that is active against hypnozoites.

In the event of recrudescent infections due to *P. falciparum* after treatment with Malarone, or failure of chemoprophylaxis, patients should be treated with a different blood schizonticide.

Parasitaemia should be closely monitored in patients receiving concurrent metoclopramide or tetracycline (see section 4.5).

The concomitant administration of Malarone and rifampicin or rifabutin is not recommended (see section 4.5).

In patients with severe renal impairment (creatinine clearance <30 mL/min) alternatives to Malarone for treatment of acute *P. falciparum* malaria should be recommended whenever possible (see sections 4.2, 4.3 and 5.2).

4.5 Interaction with other medicinal products and other forms of interaction

Proguanil may potentiate the anticoagulant effect of warfarin and other coumarin based anticoagulants. The mechanism of this potential drug interaction has not been established. Caution is advised when initiating or withdrawing malaria prophylaxis or treatment with atovaquone-proguanil in patients on continuous treatment with coumarin based anticoagulants.

Concomitant treatment with metoclopramide and tetracycline has been associated with significant decreases in plasma concentrations of atovaquone (see section 4.4).

Concomitant administration of atovaquone and indinavir results in a decrease in the C_{min} of indinavir (23% decrease; 90% CI 8-35%). Caution should be exercised when prescribing atovaquone with indinavir due to the decrease in the trough levels of indinavir.

Concomitant administration of rifampicin or rifabutin is known to reduce atovaquone levels by approximately 50% and 34%, respectively. (see section 4.4).

Atovaquone is highly protein bound (>99%) but does not displace other highly protein bound drugs *in vitro*, indicating significant drug interactions arising from displacement are unlikely.

4.6 Pregnancy and lactation

The safety of atovaquone and proguanil hydrochloride when administered concurrently for use in human pregnancy has not been established and the potential risk is unknown.

Animal studies showed no evidence for teratogenicity of the combination. The individual components have shown no effects on parturition or pre- and post-natal development. Maternal toxicity was seen in pregnant rabbits during a teratogenicity study (see section 5.3). The use of Malarone in pregnancy should only be considered if the expected benefit to the mother outweighs any potential risk to the foetus.

The proguanil component of Malarone acts by inhibiting parasitic dihydrofolate reductase. There are no clinical data indicating that folate supplementation diminishes drug efficacy. For women of childbearing age receiving folate supplements to prevent neural tube birth defects, such supplements should be continued while taking Malarone.

Lactation

The atovaquone concentrations in milk, in a rat study, were 30% of the concurrent atovaquone concentrations in maternal plasma. It is not known whether atovaquone is excreted in human milk.

Proguanil is excreted in human milk in small quantities.

Malarone should not be taken by breast-feeding women.

4.7 Effects on ability to drive and use machines

Dizziness has been reported. Patients should be warned that if affected they should not drive, operate machinery or take part in activities where this may put themselves or others at risk.

4.8 Undesirable effects

The following table provides a summary of adverse reactions reported with Malarone, atovaquone or proguanil in clinical trials and spontaneous post-marketing reports. The following convention is used for the classification of frequency: very common (≥1/10); common (≥1/100 to <1/10); uncommon (≥1/1,000 to <1/100); not known (cannot be estimated from the available data).

In clinical trials of atovaquone-proguanil for treatment of malaria, the most commonly reported adverse events, independent of attributability, were abdominal pain, headache, anorexia, nausea, vomiting, diarrhoea and coughing, and were generally reported in a similar proportion of patients receiving atovaquone-proguanil or a comparator antimalarial drug.

In clinical trials of atovaquone-proguanil for prophylaxis of malaria, the most commonly reported adverse events, independent of attributability, were headache, abdominal pain and diarrhoea, and were reported in a similar proportion of subjects receiving atovaquone-proguanil or placebo.

(see Table 1 below)

4.9 Overdose

No case of overdose has been reported. In cases of suspected overdosage symptomatic and supportive therapy should be given as appropriate.

5. PHARMACOLOGICAL PROPERTIES

5.1 Pharmacodynamic properties

Pharmacotherapeutic group: Antimalarials, ATC Code: P01B B51

Mode of Action

The constituents of Malarone, atovaquone and proguanil hydrochloride, interfere with two different pathways involved in the biosynthesis of pyrimidines required for nucleic acid replication. The mechanism of action of atovaquone against *P. falciparum* is via inhibition of mitochondrial electron transport, at the level of the cytochrome bc_1 complex, and collapse of mitochondrial membrane potential. One mechanism of action of proguanil, via its metabolite cycloguanil, is inhibition of dihydrofolate reductase, which disrupts deoxythymidylate synthesis. Proguanil also has antimalarial activity independent of its metabolism to cycloguanil, and proguanil, but not cycloguanil, is able to potentiate the ability of atovaquone to collapse mitochondrial membrane potential in malaria parasites. This latter mechanism may explain the synergy seen when atovaquone and proguanil are used in combination.

Microbiology

Atovaquone has potent activity against *Plasmodium* spp (*in vitro* IC_{50} against *P. falciparum* 0.23-1.4 ng/mL).

Atovaquone is not cross-resistant with any other antimalarial drugs in current use. Among more than 30 *P. falciparum* isolates, *in vitro* resistance was detected against chloroquine (41% of isolates), quinine (32% of isolates), mefloquine (29% of isolates), and halofantrine (48% of isolates) but not atovaquone (0% of isolates).

The antimalarial activity of proguanil is exerted via the primary metabolite cycloguanil (*in vitro* IC_{50} against various *P. falciparum* strains of 4-20 ng/mL; some activity of proguanil and another metabolite, 4-chlorophenylbiguanide, is seen *in vitro* at 600-3000 ng/mL).

Table 1

System Organ Class	Very Common	Common	Uncommon	Unknown
Blood and lymphatic disorders		Anaemia[1] Neutropenia[2]		Pancytopenia in patients with severe renal impairment[4]
Immune system disorders		Allergic reactions		Angioedema[3] Anaphylaxis[3] Vasculitis[4]
Metabolism and nutrition disorders		Hyponatraemia[2] Anorexia[1]	Elevated amylase levels[2]	
Psychiatric disorders		Abnormal dreams[1] Depression[1]	Anxiety[1]	Panic attack[3] Crying[3] Hallucinations[3] Nightmares[3]
Nervous system disorders	Headache[1]	Insomnia[1] Dizziness[1]		Seizure[3]
Cardiac disorders			Palpatations[1]	Tachycardia[3]
Gastrointestinal disorders	Nausea[2] Vomiting[1] Diarrhoea[1] Abdominal pain[1]		Stomatitis[1]	Gastric intolerance[4] Oral ulceration[4]
Hepatobiliary disorders		Elevated liver enzymes[2,5]		Hepatitis[3] Cholestasis[4]
Skin and subcutaneous tissue disorders		Rash[1]	Hair loss[1] Urticaria[1]	Stevens-Johnson Syndrome[3] Erythema multiforme[3] Blister[3] Skin exfoliation[3]
General disorders and administration site conditions		Fever[1]		
Respiratory, thoracic and mediastinal disorders		Cough[1]		

1. Frequency calculated from Malarone clinical trials

2. Frequency taken from atovaquone label. Patients participating in clinical trials with atovaquone have received higher doses and have often had complications of advance Human Immunodeficiency Virus (HIV) disease. Therefore, the causal relationship between the adverse experiences and atovaquone is difficult to evaluate. These events may have been seen at a lower frequency or not at all in clinical trials with atovaquone-proguanil.

3. Observed from post-marketing spontaneous reports and the frequency is therefore unknown

4. Observed with proguanil and the frequency is therefore unknown.

5. Clinical trial data for atovaquone-proguanil indicated that abnormalities in liver function tests were reversible and not associated with untoward clinical events.

In *in vitro* studies of *P. falciparum* the combination of atovaquone and proguanil was shown to be synergistic. This enhanced efficacy was also demonstrated in clinical studies in both immune and non-immune patients.

5.2 Pharmacokinetic properties

There are no pharmacokinetic interactions between atovaquone and proguanil at the recommended dose. In clinical trials, where children have received Malarone dosed by bodyweight, trough levels of atovaquone, proguanil and cycloguanil in children are generally within the range observed in adults.

Absorption

Atovaquone is a highly lipophilic compound with low aqueous solubility. In HIV-infected patients, the absolute bioavailability of a 750 mg single dose of atovaquone tablets taken with food is 23% with an inter-subject variability of about 45%.

Dietary fat taken with atovaquone increases the rate and extent of absorption, increasing AUC 2-3 times and C_{max} 5 times over fasting. Patients are recommended to take Malarone tablets with food or a milky drink (see section 4.2).

Proguanil hydrochloride is rapidly and extensively absorbed regardless of food intake.

Distribution

Apparent volume of distribution of atovaquone and proguanil is a function of bodyweight.

Atovaquone is highly protein bound (>99%) but does not displace other highly protein bound drugs *in vitro*, indicating significant drug interactions arising from displacement are unlikely.

Following oral administration, the volume of distribution of atovaquone in adults and children is approximately 8.8 L/kg.

Proguanil is 75% protein bound. Following oral administration, the volume of distribution of proguanil in adults and children ranged from 20 to 42 L/kg.

In human plasma the binding of atovaquone and proguanil was unaffected by the presence of the other.

Metabolism

There is no evidence that atovaquone is metabolised and there is negligible excretion of atovaquone in urine with the parent drug being predominantly (>90%) eliminated unchanged in faeces.

Proguanil hydrochloride is partially metabolised, primarily by the polymorphic cytochrome P450 isoenzyme 2C19, with less than 40% being excreted unchanged in the urine. Its metabolites, cycloguanil and 4-chlorophenylbiguanide, are also excreted in the urine.

During administration of Malarone at recommended doses proguanil metabolism status appears to have no implications for treatment or prophylaxis of malaria.

Elimination

The elimination half life of atovaquone is about 2-3 days in adults and 1-2 days in children.

The elimination half lives of proguanil and cycloguanil are about 12-15 hours in both adults and children.

Oral clearance for atovaquone and proguanil increases with increased bodyweight and is about 70% higher in an 80 kg subject relative to a 40 kg subject. The mean oral clearance in paediatric and adult patients weighing 10 to 80 kg ranged from 0.8 to 10.8 L/h for atovaquone and from 15 to 106 L/h for proguanil.

Pharmacokinetics in the elderly

There is no clinically significant change in the average rate or extent of absorption of atovaquone or proguanil between elderly and young patients. Systemic availability of cycloguanil is higher in the elderly compared to the young patients (AUC is increased by 140% and C_{max} is increased by 80%), but there is no clinically significant change in its elimination half life (see section 4.2).

Pharmacokinetics in renal impairment

In patients with mild to moderate renal impairment, oral clearance and/or AUC data for atovaquone, proguanil and cycloguanil are within the range of values observed in patients with normal renal function.

Atovaquone C_{max} and AUC are reduced by 64% and 54%, respectively, in patients with severe renal impairment.

In patients with severe renal impairment, the elimination half lives for proguanil ($t_{½}$ 39h) and cycloguanil ($t_{½}$ 37 h) are prolonged, resulting in the potential for drug accumulation with repeated dosing (see sections 4.2 and 4.4).

Pharmacokinetics in hepatic impairment

In patients with mild to moderate hepatic impairment there is no clinically significant change in exposure to atovaquone when compared to healthy patients.

In patients with mild to moderate hepatic impairment there is an 85% increase in proguanil AUC with no change in elimination half life and there is a 65-68% decrease in C_{max} and AUC for cycloguanil.

No data are available in patients with severe hepatic impairment (see section 4.2).

5.3 Preclinical safety data

Repeat dose toxicity:

Findings in repeat dose toxicity studies with atovaquone-proguanil hydrochloride combination were entirely proguanil related and were observed at doses providing no significant margin of exposure in comparison with the expected clinical exposure. As proguanil has been used extensively and safely in the treatment and prophylaxis of malaria at doses similar to those used in the combination, these findings are considered of little relevance to the clinical situation.

Reproductive toxicity studies:

In rats and rabbits there was no evidence of teratogenicity for the combination. No data are available regarding the effects of the combination on fertility or pre- and post-natal development, but studies on the individual components of Malarone have shown no effects on these parameters. In a rabbit teratogenicity study using the combination, unexplained maternal toxicity was found at a systemic exposure similar to that observed in humans following clinical use.

Mutagenicity:

A wide range of mutagenicity tests have shown no evidence that atovaquone or proguanil have mutagenic activity as single agents.

Mutagenicity studies have not been performed with atovaquone in combination with proguanil.

Cycloguanil, the active metabolite of proguanil, was also negative in the Ames test, but was positive in the Mouse Lymphoma assay and the Mouse Micronucleus assay. These positive effects with cycloguanil (a dihydrofolate antagonist) were significantly reduced or abolished with folinic acid supplementation.

Carcinogencity:

Oncogenicity studies of atovaquone alone in mice showed an increased incidence of hepatocellular adenomas and carcinomas. No such findings were observed in rats and mutagenicity tests were negative. These findings appear to be due to the inherent susceptibility of mice to atovaquone and are considered of no relevance in the clinical situation.

Oncogenicity studies on proguanil alone showed no evidence of carcinogenicity in rats and mice.

Oncogenicity studies on proguanil in combination with atovaquone have not been performed.

6. PHARMACEUTICAL PARTICULARS

6.1 List of excipients

Core

Poloxamer 188

Microcrystalline Cellulose

Low-substituted Hydroxypropyl Cellulose

Povidone K30

Sodium Starch Glycollate (Type A)

Magnesium Stearate

Coating

Hypromellose

Titanium Dioxide E171

Iron Oxide Red E172

Macrogol 400

Polyethylene Glycol 8000

6.2 Incompatibilities

Not applicable.

6.3 Shelf life

5 years.

6.4 Special precautions for storage

This medicinal product does not require any special storage conditions.

6.5 Nature and contents of container

PVC aluminium foil blister pack/s containing 12 tablets.

6.6 Special precautions for disposal and other handling

No special requirements.

7. MARKETING AUTHORISATION HOLDER

Glaxo Wellcome UK Ltd, trading as GlaxoSmithKline UK.

Stockley Park West

Uxbridge

Middlesex

UB11 1BT

8. MARKETING AUTHORISATION NUMBER(S)

PL 10949/0258

9. DATE OF FIRST AUTHORISATION/RENEWAL OF THE AUTHORISATION

Date of first authorisation: 21 October 1996.

Date of first renewal: 19 October 2006.

10. DATE OF REVISION OF THE TEXT

02 September 2009

Malarone Paediatric Tablets

(GlaxoSmithKline UK)

1. NAME OF THE MEDICINAL PRODUCT

Malarone paediatric 62.5mg/25 mg film-coated tablets.

2. QUALITATIVE AND QUANTITATIVE COMPOSITION

Each Malarone paediatric tablet contains 62.5 mg atovaquone and 25 mg proguanil hydrochloride.

For a full list of excipients, see section 6.1.

3. PHARMACEUTICAL FORM

Film-coated tablet.

Round biconvex, pink tablets engraved 'GX CG7' on one side.

4. CLINICAL PARTICULARS

4.1 Therapeutic indications

Malarone paediatric tablets contain a fixed dose combination of atovaquone and proguanil hydrochloride, which acts as a blood schizontocide and also has activity against hepatic schizonts of *Plasmodium falciparum*. They are indicated for:

Prophylaxis of *P. falciparum* malaria in individuals weighing 11-40 kg.

Treatment of acute, uncomplicated *P. falciparum* malaria in children weighing ⩾5 kg and <11 kg.

For treatment of acute, uncomplicated *P. falciparum* malaria in individuals weighing 11-40 kg please refer to the Summary of Product Characteristics for Malarone tablets.

M alarone may be active against *P. falciparum* that are resistant to one or more other antimalarial agents. Therefore, Malarone may be particularly suitable for prophylaxis and treatment against *P. falciparum* infections in areas where this species is known to be commonly resistant to one or more other antimalarial agents and also for treatment of patients infected with *P. falciparum* malaria whilst in these areas.

Official guidelines and local information on the prevalence of resistance to antimalarial drugs should be taken into consideration. Official guidelines will normally include WHO and public health authorities' guidelines.

4.2 Posology and method of administration

Method of administration

The daily dose should be taken once daily with food or a milky drink (to ensure maximum absorption) at the same time each day.

If patients are unable to tolerate food Malarone paediatric tablets should be administered, but systemic exposure of atovaquone will be reduced. In the event of vomiting within 1-hour of dosing a repeat dose should be taken.

Malarone paediatric tablets should preferably be swallowed whole. If difficulties are encountered when dosing young children, the tablets may be crushed and mixed with food or a milky drink just prior to administration.

Posology

The dosage for the prophylaxis and treatment of acute, uncomplicated *P. falciparum* malaria in children is based on body weight.

Prophylaxis

Dosage in individuals weighing 11-40 kg

(see Table 1 on next page)

The safety and effectiveness of Malarone paediatric tablets for prophylaxis of malaria in children who weigh less than 11 kg has not been established.

Prophylaxis should

- commence 24 or 48 hours prior to entering a malaria-endemic area,
- continue during the period of the stay, which should not exceed 28 days,
- continue for 7 days after leaving the area.

The safety and effectiveness of Malarone paediatric tablets have been established in studies of up to 12 weeks in residents (semi-immune) of endemic areas. (see section 5.1).

Treatment

Dosage in individuals weighing 5-11 kg

(see Table 2 on next page)

The safety and effectiveness of Malarone paediatric tablets for the treatment of malaria in children who weigh less than 5 kg has not been established.

For individuals who weigh 11 kg or more, the first choice for the treatment of acute, uncomplicated *P. falciparum* malaria is Malarone tablets (250/100 mg). Please consult the Malarone tablets SmPC for the recommended dosage for this weight range. Malarone tablets are four-times the strength of Malarone paediatric tablets.

In circumstances when sufficient Malarone tablets are not available, then Malarone paediatric tablets may be used.

Dosage in Hepatic Impairment

There are no studies in children with hepatic impairment. However, a pharmacokinetic study in adults indicates that no dosage adjustments are needed in patients with mild to moderate hepatic impairment. Although no studies have been conducted in patients with severe hepatic impairment, no special precautions or dosage adjustment are anticipated (see section 5.2).

Dosage in Renal Impairment

There are no studies in children with renal impairment. However, pharmacokinetic studies in adults indicate that no dosage adjustments are needed in those with mild to

Table 1 Dosage in individuals weighing 5-11 kg

	Dosage/day		
Body Weight Range (kg)	Atovaquone (mg)	Proguanil (mg)	No of Tablets
11-20	62.5	25	One Malarone paediatric tablet
21-30	125	50	Two Malarone paediatric tablets
31-40	187.5	75	Three Malarone paediatric tablet
>40	250	100	Subjects of >40 kg should receive ONE Malarone 250/100 mg tablet daily

Table 2 Dosage in individuals weighing 5-11 kg

	Dosage/day		
Body Weight Range (kg)	Atovaquone (mg)	Proguanil (mg)	Dosage Regimen
5-8	125	50	Two Malarone paediatric tablets daily for 3 consecutive days
9-10	187.5	75	Three Malarone paediatric tablets daily for 3 consecutive days.

moderate renal impairment. Due to the lack of information regarding appropriate dosing, Malarone is contraindicated for the prophylaxis of malaria in adults and children with severe renal impairment (creatinine clearance <30 mL/min; see sections 4.3 and 5.2).

4.3 Contraindications

Hypersensitivity to the active substances or to any of the excipients.

Malarone paediatric tablets are contraindicated for prophylaxis of *P. falciparum* malaria in patients with severe renal impairment (creatinine clearance <30 mL.min).

4.4 Special warnings and precautions for use

Individuals taking Malarone paediatric tablets for prophylaxis or treatment of malaria should take a repeat dose if they vomit within 1-hour of dosing. In the event of diarrhoea, normal dosing should be continued. Absorption of atovaquone may be reduced in individuals with diarrhoea or vomiting, but diarrhoea or vomiting was not associated with reduced efficacy in clinical trials of Malarone for malaria prophylaxis in adults. However, as with other antimalarial agents, individuals with diarrhoea or vomiting should be advised to continue to comply with personal protection measures (repellants, bednets).

The safety and effectiveness of Malarone paediatric tablets for the prophylaxis of malaria in children who weigh less than 11 kg and the treatment of malaria in children who weigh less than 5 kg have not been established.

Malarone paediatric tablets are not indicated for the treatment of acute uncomplicated *P. falciparum* malaria in individuals weighing 11-40 kg. Malarone tablets (250/100 mg) should be used in these individuals (see section 4.2).

Occasionally, severe allergic reactions (including anaphylaxis) have been reported in patients taking Malarone. If patients experience an allergic reaction (see section 4.8) Malarone should be discontinued promptly and appropriate treatment initiated.

Parasite relapse occurred commonly when *P. vivax* malaria was treated with Malarone alone. Travellers with intense exposure to *P. vivax* or *P. ovale*, and those who develop malaria caused by either of these parasites, will require additional treatment with a drug that is active against hypnozoites.

In the event of failure of chemoprophylaxis with Malarone paediatric tablets, individuals should be treated with a different blood schizonticide.

4.5 Interaction with other medicinal products and other forms of interaction

Proguanil may potentiate the anticoagulant effect of warfarin and other coumarin based anticoagulants. The mechanism of this potential drug interaction has not been established. Caution is advised when initiating or withdrawing malaria prophylaxis or treatment with atovaquone-proguanil in patients on continuous treatment with coumarin based anticoagulants.

Metoclopramide and tetracycline have been associated with significant decreases in plasma concentrations of atovaquone when administered concomitantly. Although some children have received concomitant Malarone and metoclopramide in clinical trials without any evidence of decreased protection against malaria, the possibility of a clinically significant drug interaction cannot be ruled out.

Concomitant administration of atovaquone and indinavir results in a decrease in the C_{min} of indinavir (23% decrease; 90% CI 8-35%). Caution should be exercised when prescribing atovaquone with indinavir due to the decrease in the trough levels of indinavir.

Concomitant administration of Malarone with rifampicin or rifabutin should be avoided due to the reduction in plasma levels of atovaquone by approximately 50% and 34%, respectively.

Atovaquone is highly protein bound (>99%) but does not displace other highly protein bound drugs *in vitro*, indicating significant drug interactions arising from displacement are unlikely.

4.6 Pregnancy and lactation

The safety of atovaquone and proguanil hydrochloride when administered concurrently for use in human pregnancy has not been established and the potential risk is unknown.

Animal studies showed no evidence for teratogenicity of the combination. The individual components have shown no effects on parturition or pre- and post-natal development. Maternal toxicity was seen in pregnant rabbits during a teratogenicity study (see section 5.3). The use of Malarone paediatric tablets in pregnancy should only be considered if the expected benefit to the mother outweighs any potential risk to the foetus.

Proguanil acts by inhibiting parasitic dihydrofolate reductase. There are no clinical data indicating that folate supplementation diminishes drug efficacy. For women of childbearing age receiving folate supplements to prevent neural tube birth defects, such supplements should be continued while taking Malarone paediatric tablets.

Lactation

The atovaquone concentrations in milk, in a rat study, were 30% of the concurrent atovaquone concentrations in maternal plasma. It is not known whether atovaquone is excreted in human milk.

Proguanil is excreted in human milk in small quantities.

Malarone paediatric tablets should not be taken by breast-feeding women.

4.7 Effects on ability to drive and use machines

There have been no studies to investigate the effect of Malarone paediatric tablets on driving performance or the ability to operate machinery but a detrimental effect on such activities is not predicted from the pharmacology of the component drugs.

4.8 Undesirable effects

In clinical trials of Malarone paediatric tablets for prophylaxis of malaria, 357 children or adolescents 11 to ⩽40 kg body weight received Malarone paediatric tablets. Most of these were residents of endemic areas and took Malarone paediatric tablets for about 12 weeks. The rest were travelling to endemic areas, and most took Malarone paediatric tablets for 2-4 weeks.

Open label clinical studies investigating the treatment of children weighing between ⩾5 kg and <11 kg have indicated that the safety profile is similar to that in children weighing between 11 kg and 40 kg, and adults.

There are limited long term safety data in children. In particular, the long-term effects of Malarone on growth, puberty and general development have not been studied.

In clinical trials, commonly reported (greater than 1/100) adverse events included abdominal pain, diarrhoea, fever, nausea, vomiting and headache. However, in placebo controlled trials all these events occurred at similar rates in the Malarone and placebo groups.

The following table provides a summary of adverse reactions reported with Malarone, atovaquone or proguanil in clinical trials and spontaneous post-marketing reports. The following convention is used for the classification of frequency: very common (⩾1/10); common (⩾1/100 to <1/10); uncommon (⩾1/1,000 to <1/100); not known (cannot be estimated from the available data).

In clinical trials of atovaquone-proguanil for treatment of malaria, the most commonly reported adverse events, independent of attributability, were abdominal pain, headache, anorexia, nausea, vomiting, diarrhoea and coughing, and were generally reported in a similar proportion of patients receiving atovaquone-proguanil or a comparator antimalarial drug.

In clinical trials of atovaquone-proguanil for prophylaxis of malaria, the most commonly reported adverse events, independent of attributability, were headache, abdominal pain and diarrhoea, and were reported in a similar proportion of subjects receiving atovaquone-proguanil or placebo.

(see Table 3 on next page)

4.9 Overdose

No case of overdose has been reported. In cases of suspected overdosage, symptomatic and supportive therapy should be given as appropriate.

5. PHARMACOLOGICAL PROPERTIES

5.1 Pharmacodynamic properties

Pharmacotherapeutic group: Antimalarials, ATC code: P01B B51

Mode of Action

The constituents of Malarone paediatric tablets, atovaquone and proguanil hydrochloride, interfere with two different pathways involved in the biosynthesis of pyrimidines required for nucleic acid replication. The mechanism of action of atovaquone against *P. falciparum* is via inhibition of mitochondrial electron transport, at the level of the cytochrome bc_1 complex, and collapse of mitochondrial membrane potential. One mechanism of action of proguanil, via its metabolite cycloguanil, is inhibition of dihydrofolate reductase, which disrupts deoxythymidylate synthesis. Proguanil also has antimalarial activity independent of its metabolism to cycloguanil. Proguanil, but not cycloguanil, is able to potentiate the ability of atovaquone to collapse mitochondrial membrane potential in malaria parasites. This latter mechanism may contribute to the antimalarial synergy seen when atovaquone and proguanil are used in combination.

Microbiology

Atovaquone has activity against *Plasmodium* spp (*in vitro* IC_{50} against *P. falciparum* 0.23-1.43 ng/mL).

Cross-resistance between atovaquone and antimalarial agents of other drug classes was not detected among more than 30 *P. falciparum* isolates that demonstrated resistance *in vitro* to one or more of chloroquine (41% of isolates), quinine (32% of isolates), mefloquine (29% of isolates), and halofantrine (48% of isolates).

The IC_{50} of the primary metabolite of proguanil-cycloguanil against various *P. falciparum* strains was 4-20 ng/mL; some activity of proguanil and another metabolite, 4-chlorophenylbiguanide, is seen *in vitro* at 600-3000 ng/mL).

The combination of atovaquone and proguanil was shown to be synergistic against *P. falciparum in vitro*. The combination was more effective than either drug alone in clinical studies of the treatment of malaria in both immune and non-immune patients.

Clinical Efficacy

Prophylaxis

The efficacy in non-immune paediatric travellers has not been directly established, but may be assumed through extrapolation by the results on safety and efficacy in studies of up to 12 weeks in paediatric residents (semi-immune) of endemic areas, and from results of safety and efficacy in both semi-immune and non-immune adults.

Data in the paediatric population are available from two trials that primarily evaluated the safety of Malarone paediatric tablets in (non-immune) travellers to endemic areas. In these trials, a total of 93 travellers weighing <40 kg were given Malarone and 93 received another prophylactic antimalarial regimen (81 chloroquine/proguanil and 12 mefloquine). The majority of travellers went to Africa and the mean duration of stay was between 2-3 weeks. There were no cases of malaria recorded in any subjects who took part in these studies.

Treatment

An open-label, randomised, parallel-group trial was undertaken in Gabon in 200 children weighing ⩾5 kg and <11 kg with confirmed, uncomplicated *P. falciparum* malaria. Treatment was with Malarone paediatric tablets or amodiaquine suspension. In the intent-to-treat population, the 28-day cure rate was 87% in the Malarone group (87/100 subjects). In the per-protocol population, the 28-day cure rate was 95% in the Malarone group (87/92 subjects). The parasitological cure rates for the Malarone group were 88% and 95% for the ITT and PP populations, respectively.

5.2 Pharmacokinetic properties

There are no pharmacokinetic interactions between atovaquone and proguanil at the recommended doses.

In prophylaxis clinical trials where children have received Malarone dosed by bodyweight, trough levels of atovaquone, proguanil and cycloguanil in children are generally within the range observed in adults (see following table).

Trough Plasma Concentrations [Mean ± SD, (range)] of Atovaquone, Proguanil and Cycloguanil during Prophylaxis with Malarone in Children* and Adults

(see Table 4 on next page)

Table 3

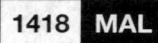

System Organ Class	Very Common	Common	Uncommon	Unknown
Blood and lymphatic disorders		Anaemia[1] Neutropenia[2]		Pancytopenia in patients with severe renal impairment[4]
Immune system disorders		Allergic reactions		Angioedema[4] Anaphylaxis[3] Vasculitis[4]
Metabolism and nutrition disorders		Hyponatraemia[2] Anorexia[1]	Elevated amylase levels[2]	
Psychiatric disorders		Abnormal dreams[1] Depression[1]	Anxiety[1]	Panic attack[3] Crying[3] Hallucination[3] Nightmares[3]
Nervous system disorders	Headache[1]	Insomnia[1] Dizziness[1]		Seizure[3]
Cardiac disorders			Palpitations[1]	Tachycardia[3]
Gastrointestinal disorders	Nausea[2] Vomiting[1] Diarrhoea[1] Abdominal pain[1]		Stomatitis[1]	Gastric intolerance[4] Oral ulceration[4]
Hepatobiliary disorders		Elevated liver enzymes[2]		Hepatitis[3] Cholestasis[4]
Skin and subcutaneous tissue disorders		Pruritus[1] Rash[1]	Hair loss[1] Urticaria[1]	Stevens-Johnson syndrome[3] Erythema multiforme[3] Blister[3] Skin exfoliation[3]
General disorders and administration site conditions		Fever[1]		
Respiratory, thoracic and mediastinal disorders		Cough[1]		

1. Frequency calculated from Malarone clinical trials
2. Frequency taken from atovaquone label. Patients participating in clinical trials with atovaquone have received higher doses and have often had complications of advance Human Immunodeficiency Virus (HIV) disease. Therefore, the causal relationship between the adverse experiences and atovaquone is difficult to evaluate. These events may have been seen at a lower frequency or not at all in clinical trials with atovaquone-proguanil.
3. Observed from post-marketing spontaneous reports and the frequency is therefore unknown
4. Observed with proguanil and the frequency is therefore unknown.
5. Clinical trial data for atovaquone-proguanil indicated that abnormalities in liver function tests were reversible and not associated with untoward clinical events

Table 4

Atovaquone: Proguanil HCl Daily Dose	62.5 mg:25 mg	125 mg:50 mg	187.5 mg:75 mg	250mg:100 mg
[Weight Category]	[11-20 kg]	[21-30 kg]	[31-40 kg]	Adult (>40 kg)
Atovaquone (μg/mL)	2.2 ± 1.1 (0.2-5.8)	3.2 ± 1.8 (0.2-10.9)	4.1 ± 1.8 (0.7-8.8)	2.1 + 1.2 (0.1-5.7)
No. Subjects	*n=87*	*n=88*	*n=76*	*n=100*
Proguanil (ng/mL)	12.3 ± 14.4 (<5.0-14.3)	18.8 ± 11.2 (<5.0-87.0)	26.8 ± 17.1 (5.1-55.9)	26.8 ± 14.0 (5.2-73.2)
No. Subjects	*n=72*	*n=83*	*n=75*	*n=95*
Cycloguanil (ng/mL)	7.7 ± 7.2 (<5.0-43.5)	8.1 ± 6.3 (<5.0-44.1)	8.7 ± 7.3 (6.4-17.0)	10.9 + 5.6 (5.0-37.8)
No. Subjects	*n=58*	*n=69*	*n=66*	*n=95*

* Pooled data from two studies

Absorption

Atovaquone is a highly lipophilic compound with low aqueous solubility. Although there are no atovaquone bioavailability data in healthy subjects, in HIV-infected patients the absolute bioavailability of a 750 mg single dose of atovaquone tablets taken with food is 21% (90% CI: 17% - 27%).

Dietary fat taken with atovaquone increases the rate and extent of absorption, increasing AUC 2-3 times and C_{max} 5 times over fasting. Patients are recommended to take Malarone paediatric tablets with food or a milky drink (see section 4.2).

Proguanil hydrochloride is rapidly and extensively absorbed regardless of food intake.

Distribution

Apparent volume of distribution of atovaquone and proguanil is a function of bodyweight.

Atovaquone is highly protein bound (>99%) but does not displace other highly protein bound drugs *in vitro*, indicating significant drug interactions arising from displacement are unlikely.

Following oral administration, the volume of distribution of atovaquone and proguanil is approximately 8.8 L/kg.

Proguanil is 75% protein bound. Following oral administration, the volume of distribution of proguanil in adults and children (>5 kg) ranged from 20 to 79 L/kg.

In human plasma the binding of atovaquone and proguanil was unaffected by the presence of the other.

Metabolism

There is no evidence that atovaquone is metabolised, and there is negligible excretion of atovaquone in urine with the parent drug being predominantly (>90%) eliminated unchanged in faeces.

Proguanil hydrochloride is partially metabolised, primarily by the polymorphic cytochrome P450 isoenzyme 2C19, with less than 40% being excreted unchanged in the urine. Its metabolites, cycloguanil and 4-chlorophenylbiguanide, are also excreted in the urine.

During administration of Malarone at recommended doses proguanil metabolism status appears to have no implications for treatment or prophylaxis of malaria.

Elimination

The elimination half life of atovaquone is 1-2 days in children.

The elimination half lives of proguanil and cycloguanil are each about 12-15 hours in children.

Oral clearance for atovaquone and proguanil increases with increased body weight and is about 70% higher in a 40 kg subject relative to a 20 kg subject. The mean oral clearance in paediatric and adult patients weighing 5 to 40 kg ranged from 0.5 to 6.3 L/h for atovaquone and from 8.7 to 64 L/h for proguanil.

Pharmacokinetics in renal impairment

There are no studies in children with renal impairment.

In adult patients with mild to moderate renal impairment, oral clearance and/or AUC data for atovaquone, proguanil and cycloguanil are within the range of values observed in patients with normal renal function.

Atovaquone C_{max} and AUC are reduced by 64% and 54%, respectively, in adult patients with severe renal impairment (<30 mL/min/1.73 m^2).

In adult patients with severe renal impairment, the elimination half lives for proguanil ($t_{½}$ 39 hours) and cycloguanil ($t_{½}$ 37 hours) are prolonged, resulting in the potential for drug accumulation with repeated dosing (see sections 4.2 and 4.4).

Pharmacokinetics in hepatic impairment

There are no studies in children with hepatic impairment.

In adult patients with mild to moderate hepatic impairment, there is no clinically significant change in exposure to atovaquone when compared to healthy patients.

In adult patients with mild to moderate hepatic impairment there is an 85% increase in proguanil AUC, with no change in elimination half life, and there is a 65-68% decrease in C_{max} and AUC for cycloguanil.

No data are available in adult patients with severe hepatic impairment (see section 4.2).

5.3 Preclinical safety data

Repeat dose toxicity:

Findings in repeat dose toxicity studies with atovaquone-proguanil hydrochloride combination were entirely proguanil-related and were observed at doses providing no significant margin of exposure in comparison with the expected clinical exposure. However, as proguanil has been used extensively and safely in the treatment and prophylaxis of malaria at doses similar to those used in the combination, these findings are considered of little relevance to the clinical situation.

Reproductive toxicity studies:

In rats and rabbits there was no evidence of teratogenicity for the combination. No data are available regarding the effects of the combination on fertility or pre- and post-natal development, but studies on the individual components of Malarone paediatric tablets have shown no effects on these parameters. In a rabbit teratogenicity study using the combination, unexplained maternal toxicity was found at a systemic exposure similar to that observed in humans following clinical use.

Mutagenicity:

A wide range of mutagenicity tests have shown no evidence that atovaquone or proguanil have mutagenic activity as single agents.

Mutagenicity studies have not been performed with atovaquone in combination with proguanil.

Cycloguanil, the active metabolite of proguanil, was also negative in the Ames test, but was positive in the Mouse Lymphoma assay and the Mouse Micronucleus assay. These positive effects with cycloguanil (a dihydrofolate antagonist) were significantly reduced or abolished with folinic acid supplementation.

Carcinogenicity:

Oncogenicity studies of atovaquone alone in mice showed an increased incidence of hepatocellular adenomas and carcinomas. No such findings were observed in rats and mutagenicity tests were negative. These findings appear to be due to the inherent susceptibility of mice to atovaquone and are considered of no relevance in the clinical situation.

Oncogenicity studies on proguanil alone showed no evidence of carcinogenicity in rats and mice.

Oncogenicity studies on proguanil in combination with atovaquone have not been performed.

6. PHARMACEUTICAL PARTICULARS

6.1 List of excipients

Core

Poloxamer 188

Microcrystalline Cellulose

Low-substituted Hydroxypropyl Cellulose

Povidone K30

Sodium Starch Glycollate (Type A)

Magnesium Stearate

Coating

Hypromellose

Titanium Dioxide E171

Iron Oxide Red E172

Macrogol 400

Polyethylene Glycol 8000

6.2 Incompatibilities

Not applicable.

6.3 Shelf life

5 years.

6.4 Special precautions for storage

This medicinal product does not require any special storage conditions.

6.5 Nature and contents of container
PVC aluminium foil blister pack containing 12 tablets.

6.6 Special precautions for disposal and other handling
No special requirements.

7. MARKETING AUTHORISATION HOLDER
Glaxo Wellcome UK Ltd. Trading as GlaxoSmithKline UK,
Stockley Park West
Uxbridge
Middlesex
UB11 1BT

8. MARKETING AUTHORISATION NUMBER(S)
PL 10949/0363

9. DATE OF FIRST AUTHORISATION/RENEWAL OF THE AUTHORISATION
Date of first authorisation: 15 July 2002
Date of latest renewal: 14 July 2007

10. DATE OF REVISION OF THE TEXT
18 August 2009

Marcain Heavy, 0.5% solution for injection.

(AstraZeneca UK Limited)

1. NAME OF THE MEDICINAL PRODUCT
Marcain Heavy, 0.5% solution for injection.

2. QUALITATIVE AND QUANTITATIVE COMPOSITION
Bupivacaine Hydrochloride BP 5.28 mg/ml equivalent to 5 mg/ml bupivacaine hydrochloride anhydrous.

For excipients, see 6.1.

3. PHARMACEUTICAL FORM
Solution for injection.

Clear, colourless solution.

4. CLINICAL PARTICULARS
4.1 Therapeutic indications
Intrathecal (subarachnoid) spinal anaesthesia for surgery (urological and lower limb surgery lasting 2–3 hours, abdominal surgery lasting 45–60 minutes).

Bupivacaine is a long-acting anaesthetic agent of the amide type. Marcain Heavy has a rapid onset of action and long duration. The duration of analgesia in the T_{10}–T_{12} segments is 2–3 hours.

Marcain Heavy produces a moderate muscular relaxation of the lower extremities lasting 2–2.5 hours. The motor blockade of the abdominal muscles makes the solution suitable for performance of abdominal surgery lasting 45–60 minutes. The duration of the motor blockade does not exceed the duration of analgesia. The cardiovascular effects of Marcain Heavy are similar or less than those seen with other spinal agents. Bupivacaine 5 mg/ml with glucose 80 mg/ml is exceptionally well tolerated by all tissues with which it comes in contact.

4.2 Posology and method of administration
Route of administration: For intrathecal injection.

The doses recommended below should be regarded as a guide for use in the average adult.

Intrathecal anaesthesia for surgery:

2-4ml (10-20mg bupivacaine hydrochloride).

The dose should be reduced in the elderly and in patients in the late stages of pregnancy, see Section 4.4.

The spread of anaesthesia obtained with Marcain Heavy depends on several factors including the volume of solution and the position of the patient during and following the injection.

When injected at the L_3–L_4 intervertebral space, with the patient in the sitting position, 3 ml of Marcain Heavy spreads to the T_7–T_{10} spinal segments. With the patient receiving the injection in the horizontal position and then turned supine, the blockade spreads to T_4–T_7 spinal segments. It should be understood that the level of spinal anaesthesia achieved with any local anaesthetic can be unpredictable in a given patient.

The recommended site of injection is below L3.

The effects of injections of Marcain Heavy exceeding 4 ml have not yet been studied and such volumes can therefore not be recommended.

4.3 Contraindications
Hypersensitivity to local anaesthetics of the amide type or to any of the excipients.

Intrathecal anaesthesia, regardless of the local anaesthetic used, has its own contraindications, which include:

- Active disease of the central nervous system such as meningitis, poliomyelitis, intracranial haemorrhage, subacute combined degeneration of the cord due to pernicious anaemia and cerebral and spinal tumours.
- Spinal stenosis and active disease (e.g. spondylitis, tuberculosis, tumour) or recent trauma (e.g. fracture) in the vertebral column.
- Septicaemia.
- Pyogenic infection of the skin at or adjacent to the site of lumbar puncture.
- Cardiogenic or hypovolaemic shock.
- Coagulation disorders or ongoing anticoagulation treatment.

4.4 Special warnings and precautions for use
Intrathecal anaesthesia should only be undertaken by clinicians with the necessary knowledge and experience.

Regional anaesthetic procedures should always be performed in a properly equipped and staffed area. Resuscitative equipment and drugs should be immediately available and the anaesthetist should remain in constant attendance.

Intravenous access, e.g. an i.v. infusion, should be in place before starting the intrathecal anaesthesia. The clinician responsible should take the necessary precautions to avoid intravascular injection and be appropriately trained and familiar with the diagnosis and treatment of side effects, systemic toxicity and other complications. If signs of acute systemic toxicity or total spinal block appear, injection of the local anaesthetic should be stopped immediately, see sections 4.8 & 4.9.

Like all local anaesthetic drugs, bupivacaine may cause acute toxicity effects on the central nervous and cardiovascular systems, if utilised for local anaesthetic procedures resulting in high blood concentrations of the drug. This is especially the case after unintentional intravascular administration or injection into highly vascular areas.

Ventricular arrhythmia, ventricular fibrillation, sudden cardiovascular collapse and death have been reported in connection with high systemic concentrations of bupivacaine. Should cardiac arrest occur, a successful outcome may require prolonged resuscitative efforts. High systemic concentrations are not expected with doses normally used for intrathecal anaesthesia.

There is an increased risk of high or total spinal blockade, resulting in cardiovascular and respiratory depression, in the elderly and in patients in the late stages of pregnancy. The dose should therefore be reduced in these patients.

Intrathecal anaesthesia with any local anaesthetic can cause hypotension and bradycardia which should be anticipated and appropriate precautions taken. These may include preloading the circulation with crystalloid or colloid solution. If hypotension develops it should be treated with a vasopressor such as ephedrine 10–15 mg intravenously. Severe hypotension may result from hypovolaemia due to haemorrhage or dehydration, or aortocaval occlusion in patients with massive ascites, large abdominal tumours or late pregnancy. Marked hypotension should be avoided in patients with cardiac decompensation.

Patients with hypovolaemia due to any cause can develop sudden and severe hypotension during intrathecal anaesthesia.

Intrathecal anaesthesia can cause intercostal paralysis and patients with pleural effusions may suffer respiratory embarrassment. Septicaemia can increase the risk of intraspinal abscess formation in the postoperative period.

Neurological injury is a rare consequence of intrathecal anaesthesia and may result in paraesthesia, anaesthesia, motor weakness and paralysis. Occasionally these are permanent.

Before treatment is instituted, consideration should be taken if the benefits outweigh the possible risks for the patient.

Patients in poor general condition due to ageing or other compromising factors such as partial or complete heart conduction block, advanced liver or renal dysfunction require special attention, although regional anaesthesia may be the optimal choice for surgery in these patients.

Patients treated with anti-arrhythmic drugs class III (e.g. amiodarone) should be kept under close surveillance and ECG monitoring considered, since cardiac effects may be additive. (See section 4.5)

4.5 Interaction with other medicinal products and other forms of interaction
Bupivacaine should be used with caution in patients receiving other local anaesthetics or agents structurally related to amide-type local anaesthetics, e.g. certain anti-arrhythmics, such as lidocaine and mexiletine, since the systemic toxic effects are additive.

Specific interaction studies with bupivacaine and anti-arrhythmic drugs class III (e.g. amiodarone) have not been performed, but caution is advised (see also section 4.4).

4.6 Pregnancy and lactation
There is no evidence of untoward effects in human pregnancy. In large doses, there is evidence of decreased pup survival in rats and an embryological effect in rabbits if Marcain is administered in pregnancy. Marcain should not therefore be given in early pregnancy unless the benefits are considered to outweigh the risks.

It should be noted that the dose should be reduced in patients in the late stages of pregnancy, see section 4.4.

Bupivacaine enters the mother's milk, but in such small quantities that there is generally no risk of affecting the child at therapeutic dose levels.

4.7 Effects on ability to drive and use machines
Besides the direct anaesthetic effect, local anaesthetics may have a very mild effect on mental function and co-ordination even in the absence of overt CNS toxicity and may temporarily impair locomotion and alertness.

4.8 Undesirable effects
4.8.1 General
The adverse reaction profile for Marcain Heavy is similar to those for other long acting local anaesthetics used for intrathecal anaesthesia.

Table of Adverse Drug Reactions

Very Common (>1/10)	*Cardiac disorders:*	Hypotension, bradycardia
	Gastrointestinal disorders:	Nausea
Common (>1/100 <1/10)	*Nervous system disorders:*	Postdural puncture headache
	Gastrointestinal disorders:	Vomiting
	Renal and urinary disorders:	Urinary retention, urinary incontinence
Uncommon (>1/1000 <1/100)	*Nervous system disorders:*	Paraesthesia, paresis, dysaesthesia
	Musculoskeletal, connective tissue and bone disorders:	Muscle weakness, back pain
Rare (<1/1000)	*Cardiac disorders:*	Cardiac arrest
	Immune system disorders:	Allergic reactions, anaphylactic shock
	Nervous system disorders:	Total unintentional spinal block, paraplegia, paralysis, neuropathy, arachnoiditis
	Respiratory disorders:	Respiratory depression

Adverse reactions caused by the drug *per se* are difficult to distinguish from the physiological effects of the nerve block (e.g. decrease in blood pressure, bradycardia, temporary urinary retention), events caused directly (e.g. spinal haematoma) or indirectly (e.g. meningitis, epidural abcess) by needle puncture or events associated to cerebrospinal leakage (e.g. postdural puncture headache).

4.8.2 Acute systemic toxicity
Marcain Heavy, used as recommended, is not likely to cause blood levels high enough to cause systemic toxicity. However, if other local anaesthetics are concomitantly administered, toxic effects are additive and may cause systemic toxic reactions.

Systemic toxicity is rarely associated with spinal anaesthesia but might occur after accidental intravascular injection. Systemic adverse reactions are characterised by numbness of the tongue, light-headedness, dizziness and tremors, followed by convulsions and cardiovascular disorders.

4.8.3 Treatment of acute systemic toxicity
No treatment is required for milder symptoms of systemic toxicity but if convulsions occur then it is important to ensure adequate oxygenation and to arrest the convulsions if they last more than 15–30 seconds. Oxygen should be given by face mask and the respiration assisted or controlled if necessary. Convulsions can be arrested by injection of thiopental 100–150 mg intravenously or with diazepam 5–10 mg intravenously. Alternatively, succinylcholine 50–100 mg intravenously may be given but only if the clinician has the ability to perform endotracheal intubation and to manage a totally paralysed patient.

High or total spinal blockade causing respiratory paralysis should be treated by ensuring and maintaining a patent airway and giving oxygen by assisted or controlled ventilation.

Hypotension should be treated by the use of vasopressors, e.g. ephedrine 10–15 mg intravenously and repeated until the desired level of arterial pressure is reached. Intravenous fluids, both electrolytes and colloids, given rapidly can also reverse hypotension.

4.9 Overdose
Marcain Heavy, used as recommended, is not likely to cause blood levels high enough to cause systemic toxicity. However, if other local anaesthetics are concomitantly administered, toxic effects are additive and may cause systemic toxic reactions. (See section 4.8.2 and 4.8.3).

5. PHARMACOLOGICAL PROPERTIES
5.1 Pharmacodynamic properties
Pharmacotherapeutic group (ATC code): N01B B01

Bupivacaine is a long acting local anaesthetic agent of the amide type.

Moderate muscular relaxation of lower extremities.

Motor blockade of the abdominal muscles.

Marcain Heavy is hyperbaric and its initial spread in the intrathecal space is affected by gravity.

5.2 Pharmacokinetic properties
Rapid onset of action and long duration i.e. T_{10}–T_{12} segments – duration 2–3 hours.

Muscular relaxation of lower extremities lasts 2–2.5 hours.

Blockade of the abdominal muscles lasts 45–60 minutes. The duration of motor blockade does not exceed duration of analgesia.

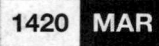

5.3 Preclinical safety data
Bupivacaine hydrochloride is a well-established active ingredient.

6. PHARMACEUTICAL PARTICULARS

6.1 List of excipients
Glucose anhydrous, sodium hydroxide and water for injections.

6.2 Incompatibilities
None known.

6.3 Shelf life
3 years.

6.4 Special precautions for storage
Do not store above 25°C.

6.5 Nature and contents of container
4 ml sterile wrapped glass ampoules or One Point Cut ampoules.

6.6 Special precautions for disposal and other handling
The solution should be used immediately after opening of the ampoule. Any remaining solution should be discarded.

7. MARKETING AUTHORISATION HOLDER
AstraZeneca UK Ltd.,

600 Capability Green,

Luton, LU1 3LU, UK.

8. MARKETING AUTHORISATION NUMBER(S)
PL 17901/0142

9. DATE OF FIRST AUTHORISATION/RENEWAL OF THE AUTHORISATION
20th September 2004

10. DATE OF REVISION OF THE TEXT
4th July 2008

Marcain Polyamp Steripack 0.25% and 0.5%

(AstraZeneca UK Limited)

1. NAME OF THE MEDICINAL PRODUCT
Marcain Polyamp Steripack 0.25%.
Marcain Polyamp Steripack 0.5%.

2. QUALITATIVE AND QUANTITATIVE COMPOSITION
Marcain Polyamp Steripack 0.25% contains Bupivacaine Hydrochloride BP 2.64mg/ml equivalent to bupivacaine hydrochloride anhydrous 2.5mg/ml.

Marcain Polyamp Steripack 0.5% contains Bupivacaine Hydrochloride BP 5.28mg/ml equivalent to bupivacaine hydrochloride anhydrous 5.0mg/ml.

3. PHARMACEUTICAL FORM
Injection.

4. CLINICAL PARTICULARS

4.1 Therapeutic indications
Marcain 0.25% and 0.5% solutions are used for the production of local anaesthesia by percutaneous infiltration, peripheral nerve block(s) and central neural block (caudal or epidural), that is, for specialist use in situations where prolonged anaesthesia is required. Because sensory nerve block is more marked than motor block, Marcain is especially useful in the relief of pain, e.g. during labour.

A list of indications and the suggested dose and strength of solution appropriate for each are shown in the table below.

4.2 Posology and method of administration
The utmost care should be taken to prevent an accidental intravascular injection, always including careful aspiration. For epidural anaesthesia, a test dose of 3-5ml of bupivacaine containing adrenaline should be administered, since an intravascular injection of adrenaline will be quickly recognised by an increase in heart rate. Verbal contact and repeated measurement of heart rate should be maintained throughout a period of 5 minutes following the test dose. Aspiration should be repeated prior to administration of the total dose. The main dose should be injected slowly, 25-50mg/min, in incremental doses under constant contact with the patient. If mild toxic symptoms occur, the injection should be stopped immediately.

When prolonged blocks are used, either by continuous infusion or by repeated bolus administration, the risks of reaching a toxic plasma concentration or inducing a local neural injury must be considered.

The dosage varies and depends upon the area to be anaesthetised, the vascularity of the tissues, the number of neuronal segments to be blocked, individual tolerance and the technique of anaesthesia used. The lowest dosage needed to provide effective anaesthesia should be administered. For most indications, the duration of anaesthesia with Marcain solutions is such that a single dose is sufficient.

The maximum dosage must be determined by evaluating the size and physical status of the patient and considering the usual rate of systemic absorption from a particular injection site. Experience to date indicates a single dose of up to 150mg bupivacaine hydrochloride. Doses of up to 50mg 2-hourly may subsequently be used. A total dose of up to 500 mg bupivacaine over 24 hours, which does not include the initial bolus dose, has been used routinely for many years without reports of toxicity. The dosages in the following table are recommended as a guide for use in the average adult. For young, elderly or debilitated patients, these doses should be reduced.

(see Table 1 below)

4.3 Contraindications
Bupivacaine hydrochloride solutions are contra-indicated in patients with hypersensitivity to local anaesthetic agents of the amide type or to any of the excipients.

Solutions of bupivacaine hydrochloride are contra-indicated for intravenous regional anaesthesia (Bier's-block).

Epidural anaesthesia, regardless of the local anaesthetic used, has its own contra-indications which include:

Active disease of the central nervous system such as meningitis, poliomyelitis, intracranial haemorrhage, subacute combined degeneration of the cord due to pernicious anaemia and cerebral and spinal tumours; tuberculosis of the spine; pyogenic infection of the skin at or adjacent to the site of lumbar puncture; cardiogenic or hypovolaemic shock; coagulation disorders or ongoing anticoagulation treatment.

4.4 Special warnings and precautions for use
There have been reports of cardiac arrest during the use of bupivacaine for epidural anaesthesia or peripheral nerve blockade where resuscitative efforts have been difficult, and were required to be prolonged before the patient responded. However, in some instances resuscitation has proven impossible despite apparently adequate preparation and appropriate management.

Like all local anaesthetic drugs, bupivacaine may cause acute toxicity effects on the central nervous and cardiovascular systems if utilised for local anaesthetic procedures resulting in high blood concentrations of the drug. This is especially the case after unintentional intravascular administration. Ventricular arrhythmia, ventricular fibrillation, sudden cardiovascular collapse and death have been reported in connection with high systemic concentrations of bupivacaine.

Major peripheral nerve blocks may require the administration of a large volume of local anaesthetic in areas of high vascularity, often close to large vessels where there is an increased risk of intravascular injection and/or systemic absorption. This may lead to high plasma concentrations.

Before any nerve block is attempted, intravenous access for resuscitation purposes should be established. Clinicians should have received adequate and appropriate training in the procedure to be performed and should be familiar with the diagnosis and treatment of side effects, systemic toxicity or other complications (see 4.9).

Adequate resuscitation equipment should be available whenever local or general anaesthesia is administered. The clinician responsible should take the necessary precautions to avoid intravascular injection (see 4.2).

Overdosage or accidental intravenous injection may give rise to toxic reactions.

Injection of repeated doses of bupivacaine hydrochloride may cause significant increases in blood levels with each repeated dose due to slow accumulation of the drug. Tolerance varies with the status of the patient.

Debilitated, elderly or acutely ill patients should be given reduced doses commensurate with their physical status.

Patients treated with anti-arrhythmic drugs class III (e.g. amiodarone) should be under close surveillance and ECG monitoring, since cardiac effects may be additive.

Only in rare cases have amide local anaesthetics been associated with allergic reactions (in most severe instances anaphylactic shock).

Patients allergic to ester-type local anaesthetic drugs (procaine, tetracaine, benzocaine, etc.) have not shown cross-sensitivity to agents of the amide type such as bupivacaine.

Local anaesthetics should be used with caution for epidural anaesthesia in patients with impaired cardiovascular function since they may be less able to compensate for functional changes associated with the prolongation of A-V conduction produced by these drugs.

Since bupivacaine is metabolised in the liver, it should be used cautiously in patients with liver disease or with reduced liver blood flow.

The physiological effects generated by a central neural blockade are more pronounced in the presence of hypotension. Patients with hypovolaemia due to any cause can develop sudden and severe hypotension during epidural anaesthesia. Epidural anaesthesia should therefore be avoided or used with caution in patients with untreated hypovolaemia or significantly impaired venous return.

Epidural anaesthesia with any local anaesthetic can cause hypotension and bradycardia which should be anticipated and appropriate precautions taken. These may include pre-loading the circulation with crystalloid or colloid solution. If hypotension develops it should be treated with a vasopressor such as ephedrine 10-15mg intravenously. Severe hypotension may result from hypovolaemia due to haemorrhage or dehydration, or aorto-caval occlusion in patients with massive ascites, large abdominal tumours or late pregnancy. Marked hypotension should be avoided in patients with cardiac decompensation.

Patients with hypovolaemia due to any cause can develop sudden and severe hypotension during epidural anaesthesia.

Epidural anaesthesia can cause intercostal paralysis and patients with pleural effusions may suffer respiratory embarrassment. Septicaemia can increase the risk of intraspinal abscess formation in the postoperative period.

Paracervical block may have a greater adverse effect on the foetus than other nerve blocks used in obstetrics. Due to the systemic toxicity of bupivacaine special care should be taken when using bupivacaine for paracervical block.

Small doses of local anaesthetics injected into the head and neck, including retrobulbar, dental and stellate ganglion blocks, may produce systemic toxicity due to inadvertent intra-arterial injection.

Retrobulbar injections may very rarely reach the cranial subarachnoid space causing serious/severe reactions, including temporary blindness, cardiovascular collapse, apnoea, convulsions.

Retro- and peribulbar injections of local anaesthetics carry a low risk of persistent ocular muscle dysfunction. The primary causes include trauma and/or local toxic effects on muscles and/or nerves. The severity of such tissue reactions is related to the degree of trauma, the concentration of the local anaesthetic and the duration of exposure of the tissue to the local anaesthetic. For this reason, as with all local anaesthetics, the lowest effective concentration and dose of local anaesthetic should be used.

4.5 Interaction with other medicinal products and other forms of interaction
Bupivacaine should be used with caution in patients receiving other local anaesthetics or agents structurally related to amide-type local anaesthetics, e.g. certain anti-arrhythmics, such as lidocaine, since the systemic toxic effects are additive.

Table 1

TYPE OF BLOCK	% CONC.	EACH DOSE		MOTOR BLOCK*
		ML	MG	
LOCAL INFILTRATION	0.25	UP TO 60	UP TO 150	-
LUMBAR EPIDURAL				
SURGICAL OPERATIONS	0.5	10 TO 20	50 TO 100	MODERATE TO COMPLETE
ANALGESIA IN LABOUR	0.5	6 to 12	30 TO 60	MODERATE TO COMPLETE
	0.25	6 to 12	15 TO 30	MINIMAL
CAUDAL EPIDURAL				
SURGICAL operations	0.5	15 TO 30	75 TO 150	MODERATE TO COMPLETE
CHILDREN (AGED UP TO 10 YEARS):				
UP TO LOWER THORACIC (T10)	0.25	0.3 - 0.4 ml/kg	0.75 - 1.0 mg/kg	
UP TO MID-THORACIC (T6)	0.25	0.4 - 0.6 ML/KG	1.0 - 1.5 MG/KG	
IF TOTAL AMOUNT GREATER THAN 20ML REDUCE CONCENTRATION TO 0.2%.				
ANALGESIA IN LABOUR	0.5	10 TO 20	50 TO 100	MODERATE TO COMPLETE
	0.25	10 TO 20	25 TO 50	MODERATE
PERIPHERAL NERVES	0.5	UP TO 30	UP TO 150	MODERATE TO COMPLETE
	0.25	UP TO 60	UP TO 150	SLIGHT TO MODERATE
SYMPATHETIC BLOCKS	0.25	20 TO 50	50 TO 125	-

* With continuous (intermittent) techniques, repeat doses increase the degree of motor block. The first repeat dose of 0.5% may produce complete motor block for intra-abdominal surgery.

Specific interaction studies with bupivacaine and anti-arrhythmic drugs class III (e.g. amiodarone) have not been performed, but caution should be advised. (see also 4.4)

4.6 Pregnancy and lactation

There is no evidence of untoward effects in human pregnancy. In large doses there is evidence of decreased pup survival in rats and an embryological effect in rabbits if Marcain is administered in pregnancy. Marcain should not therefore be given in early pregnancy unless the benefits are considered to outweigh the risks.

Foetal adverse effects due to local anaesthetics, such as foetal bradycardia, seem to be most apparent in paracervical block anaesthesia. Such effects may be due to high concentrations of anaesthetic reaching the foetus. (see also Section 4.4)

Bupivacaine enters the mother's milk, but in such small quantities that there is no risk of affecting the child at therapeutic dose levels.

4.7 Effects on ability to drive and use machines

Besides the direct anaesthetic effect, local anaesthetics may have a very mild effect on mental function and co-ordination even in the absence of overt CNS toxicity, and may temporarily impair locomotion and alertness.

4.8 Undesirable effects

Serious systemic adverse reactions are rare, but may occur in connection with overdosage (see also Section 4.9) or unintentional intravascular injection.

Bupivacaine causes systemic toxicity similar to that observed with other local anaesthetic agents. It is caused by high plasma concentrations as a result of excessive dosage, rapid absorption or, most commonly, inadvertent intravascular injection. Pronounced acidosis or hypoxia may increase the risk and severity of toxic reactions. Such reactions involve the central nervous system and the cardiovascular system. CNS reactions are characterised by numbness of the tongue, light-headedness, dizziness, blurred vision and muscle twitch, followed by drowsiness, convulsions, unconsciousness and possibly respiratory arrest.

Cardiovascular reactions are related to depression of the conduction system of the heart and myocardium leading to decreased cardiac output, heart block, hypotension, bradycardia and sometimes ventricular arrhythmias, including ventricular tachycardia, ventricular fibrillation and cardiac arrest. Usually these will be preceded or accompanied by major CNS toxicity, i.e. convulsions, but in rare cases cardiac arrest has occurred without prodromal CNS effects.

Epidural anaesthesia itself can cause adverse reactions regardless of the local anaesthetic agent used. These include hypotension and bradycardia due to sympathetic blockade and/or vasovagal fainting.

In severe cases cardiac arrest may occur.

Accidental sub-arachnoid injection can lead to very high spinal anaesthesia possibly with apnoea and severe hypotension.

Neurological damage is a rare but well recognised consequence of regional and particularly epidural and spinal anaesthesia. It may be due to several causes, e.g. direct injury to the spinal cord or spinal nerves, anterior spinal artery syndrome, injection of an irritant substance, or an injection of a non-sterile solution. These may result in localised areas of paraesthesia or anaesthesia, motor weakness, loss of sphincter control and paraplegia. Occasionally these are permanent.

Hepatic dysfunction, with reversible increases of SGOT, SGPT, alkaline phosphates and bilirubin, has been observed following repeated injections or long-term infusions of bupivacaine. If signs of hepatic dysfunction are observed during treatment with bupivacaine, the drug should be discontinued.

4.9 Overdose

4.9.1 Acute Systemic Toxicity

Central nervous system toxicity is a graded response with symptoms and signs of escalating severity. The first symptoms are usually light-headedness, circumoral paraesthesia, numbness of the tongue, hyperacusis, tinnitus and visual disturbances.

Dysarthria, muscular twitching or tremors are more serious and precede the onset of generalised convulsions. These signs must not be mistaken for a neurotic behaviour. Unconsciousness and grand mal convulsions may follow which may last from a few seconds to several minutes. Hypoxia and hypercarbia occur rapidly following convulsions due to the increased muscular activity, together with the interference with respiration. In severe cases apnoea may occur. Acidosis, hyperkalaemia and hypoxia increase and extend the toxic effects of local anaesthetics.

Recovery is due to redistribution of the local anaesthetic drug from the central nervous system and subsequent metabolism and excretion. Recovery may be rapid unless large amounts of the drug have been injected.

Cardiovascular system toxicity may be seen in severe cases and is generally preceded by signs of toxicity in the central nervous system. In patients under heavy sedation or receiving a general anaesthetic, prodromal CNS symptoms may be absent.

Hypotension, bradycardia, arrhythmia and even cardiac arrest may occur as a result of high systemic concentrations of local anaesthetics, but in rare cases cardiac arrest has occurred without prodromal CNS effects.

4.9.2 Treatment of Acute Toxicity

If signs of acute systemic toxicity appear, injection of the local anaesthetic should be immediately stopped.

Treatment of a patient with systemic toxicity consists of arresting convulsions and ensuring adequate ventilation with oxygen, if necessary by assisted or controlled ventilation (respiration). If convulsions occur they must be treated promptly by intravenous injection of thiopentone 100 to 200mg or diazepam 5 to 10mg. Alternatively succinylcholine 50mg - 100mg i.v. may be used providing the clinician is capable of performing endotracheal intubation and managing a fully paralysed patient.

Once convulsions have been controlled and adequate ventilation of the lungs ensured, no other treatment is generally required

Cardiac arrest due to bupivacaine can be resistant to electrical defibrillation and resuscitation must be continued energetically for a prolonged period.

High or total spinal blockade causing respiratory paralysis and hypotension during epidural anaesthesia should be treated by ensuring and maintaining a patent airway and giving oxygen by assisted or controlled ventilation.

Hypotension should be treated by the use of vasopressors, e.g. ephedrine 10-15mg intravenously and repeated until the desired level of arterial pressure is reached. Intravenous fluids, both electrolytes and colloids, given rapidly can also reverse hypotension.

5. PHARMACOLOGICAL PROPERTIES

5.1 Pharmacodynamic properties

Bupivacaine is a potent amide local anaesthetic with a prolonged duration of action. It affects sensory nerves more than motor nerves and is ideal for producing analgesia without motor blockade.

5.2 Pharmacokinetic properties

In adults, the terminal half-life of bupivacaine is 3.5 hours. The maximum blood concentration varies with the site of injection and is highest after intercostal nerve blockade.

Total dose, rather than concentration, is an important determinant of peak blood levels.

Bupivacaine is biodegraded in the liver and only 6% is excreted unchanged in the urine.

5.3 Preclinical safety data

Bupivacaine hydrochloride is a well established active ingredient.

6. PHARMACEUTICAL PARTICULARS

6.1 List of excipients

Sodium chloride, sodium hydroxide and water for injections.

6.2 Incompatibilities

None stated.

6.3 Shelf life

24 months.

6.4 Special precautions for storage

Store below 30°C.

6.5 Nature and contents of container

10ml and 20ml polypropylene ampoules (Steripack). Cartons contain 5 or 10 ampoules.

6.6 Special precautions for disposal and other handling

For single use only. Discard any unused solution.

7. MARKETING AUTHORISATION HOLDER

AstraZeneca UK Ltd.,

600 Capability Green,

Luton, LU1 3LU, UK.

8. MARKETING AUTHORISATION NUMBER(S)

Marcain Polyamp Steripack 0.25% - PL 17901/0144

Marcain Polyamp Steripack 0.5% - PL 17901/0145

9. DATE OF FIRST AUTHORISATION/RENEWAL OF THE AUTHORISATION

4th June 2002

10. DATE OF REVISION OF THE TEXT

4th March 2005

Matrifen

(Nycomed UK Ltd)

1. NAME OF THE MEDICINAL PRODUCT

Matrifen, 12 micrograms/hour Transdermal patch

Matrifen, 25 micrograms/hour Transdermal patch

Matrifen, 50 micrograms/hour Transdermal patch

Matrifen, 75 micrograms/hour Transdermal patch

Matrifen, 100 micrograms/hour Transdermal patch

2. QUALITATIVE AND QUANTITATIVE COMPOSITION

Matrifen 12 micrograms/hour: Each transdermal patch contains 1.38 mg fentanyl in a patch of 4.2 cm^2 and releases fentanyl 12 micrograms/hour

Matrifen 25 micrograms/hour: Each transdermal patch contains 2.75 mg fentanyl in a patch of 8.4 cm^2 and releases fentanyl 25 micrograms/hour

Matrifen 50 micrograms/hour: Each transdermal patch contains 5.50 mg fentanyl in a patch of 16.8 cm^2 and releases fentanyl 50 micrograms/hour

Matrifen 75 micrograms/hour: Each transdermal patch contains 8.25 mg fentanyl in a patch of 25.2 cm^2 and releases fentanyl 75 micrograms/hour

Matrifen 100 micrograms/hour: Each transdermal patch contains 11.0 mg fentanyl in a patch of 33.6 cm^2 and releases fentanyl 100 micrograms/hour

For a full list of excipients, see section 6.1.

3. PHARMACEUTICAL FORM

Transdermal patch.

Rectangular, translucent patch on a removable protective film. The protective film is larger than the patch.

The patches are equipped with a coloured imprint with trade name, active substance and strength:

Matrifen 12 micrograms/hour patch: brown imprint

Matrifen 25 micrograms/hour patch: red imprint

Matrifen 50 micrograms/hour patch: green imprint

Matrifen 75 micrograms/hour patch: light blue imprint

Matrifen 100 micrograms/hour patch: grey imprint

4. CLINICAL PARTICULARS

4.1 Therapeutic indications

Severe chronic pain, which can be adequately managed only with opioid analgesics.

4.2 Posology and method of administration

Fentanyl transdermal patches release the active substance over 72 hours. The fentanyl release rate is 12, 25, 50, 75 and 100 microgram/hour and the corresponding active surface area is 4.2, 8.4, 16.8, 25.2 and 33.6 cm^2.

The required fentanyl dosage is adjusted individually and should be assessed regularly after each administration.

Choice of initial dosage

The dosage level of fentanyl is based upon the previous use of opioids and takes into account the possible development of tolerance, concomitant medicinal treatment, the patient's general state of health and the degree of severity of the disorder.

The initial dosage should not exceed 25 micrograms/hour when the opioid response pattern for the pain condition is not fully known.

Changing from other opioid treatment

When changing over from oral or parenteral opioids to fentanyl treatment, the initial dosage should be calculated as follows:

1. The quantity of analgesics required over the last 24 hours should be determined.

2. The obtained sum should be converted to correspond the oral morphine dosage using Table 1.

3. The corresponding fentanyl dosage should be determined using Table 2.

Table 1: Equianalgesic efficacy of medicinal products

All i.m. and oral dosages given in the table are equivalent in analgesic effect to 10 mg morphine administered intramuscularly.

Name of medicinal product	Equianalgesic dosage (mg)	
	i.m.*	Oral
Morphine	10	30 (assuming repeated administration)**
		60 (assuming a single dose or occasional doses)
Hydromorphone	1.5	7.5
Methadone	10	20
Oxycodone	10-15	20-30
Levorphanol	2	4
Oxymorphine	1	10 (rectal)
Diamorphine	5	60
Pethidine	75	-
Codeine	-	200
Buprenorphine	0.4	0.8 (sublingual)
Ketobemidone	10	30

* Based on studies conducted with single doses, in which the i.m. dosage of each above-mentioned agent was

compared with morphine in order to achieve an equivalent efficacy. Oral dosages are the recommended dosages when changing from parenteral to oral administration.

** The efficacy ratio of 3:1 for morphine i.m./oral dosages is based upon a study conducted in patients suffering from chronic pain.

Table 2: Recommended initial dose of Matrifen based upon daily oral morphine dose

Peroral morphine dose per 24-hours (mg/day)	Dose of Matrifen transdermal patch micrograms/hour
< 135	25
135-224	50
225-314	75
315-404	100
405-494	125
495-584	150
585-674	175
675-764	200
765-854	225
855-944	250
945-1034	275
1035-1124	300

Conversion schemes are based on clinical trials. Schemes based on other trials have been found useful in clinical practice and may be used.

The initial evaluation of the maximum analgesic effect of Matrifen should not be made before the patch has been worn for 24 hours. This is due to the gradual increase in serum fentanyl concentrations during the first 24 hours after application of the patch. Previous treatment with opioids should therefore be phased out gradually from the time of the first patch application until analgesic efficacy with Matrifen is attained.

Dose titration and maintenance therapy

The patch should be replaced every 72 hours. The dose should be titrated individually until analgesic efficacy is attained. In patients who experience a marked decrease in the period 48-72 hours after application, replacement of fentanyl after 48 hours may be necessary. The dose 12 micrograms/hour is appropriate for dose titration in the lower dosage area. If analgesia is insufficient at the end of the initial application period, the dose may be increased after 3 days, until the desired effect is obtained for each patient. Additional dose adjustment should normally be performed in 12 micrograms/hour or 25 micrograms/hour increments, although the supplementary analgesic requirements and pain status of the patient should be taken into account. More than one patch may be used for dose adjustments and for doses greater than 100 micrograms/hour. Patients may require periodic supplemental doses of a short-acting analgesic for breakthrough pain. Additional or alternative methods of analgesia or alternative administration of opioids should be considered when the Matrifen dose exceeds 300 micrograms/hour.

Withdrawal symptoms have been reported when changing from long-term treatment with Morphine to transdermal fentanyl despite adequate analgesic efficacy. In case of withdrawal symptoms it is recommended to treat those with short-acting Morphine in low doses.

Discontinuation of Matrifen

If discontinuation of the patch is necessary, any replacement with other opioids should be gradual, starting at a low dose and increasing slowly. This is because fentanyl levels fall gradually after the patch is removed; it takes at least 17 hours for the fentanyl serum concentration to decrease by 50% (see section 5.2). As a general rule, the discontinuation of opioid analgesia should be gradual, in order to prevent withdrawal symptoms (nausea, vomiting, diarrhea, anxiety and muscular tremor).

Use in elderly patients

Elderly or cachectic patients should be observed carefully and the dose reduced if necessary (see section 4.4).

Use in patients with hepatic or renal impairment

Patients with impaired hepatic or renal function should carefully be observed for symptoms of an overdosage and the dose should possibly be reduced (see section 4.4).

Use in febrile patients

Dose adjustment may be necessary in patients during episodes of fever (see section 4.4).

Method of administration

For transdermal use.

Fentanyl transdermal patch should be applied to non-irritated and non-irradiated skin on a flat surface of the torso or upper arm. Hair at the application site (hairless area is preferred) should be clipped (not shaved) prior to system application. If the site requires to be cleansed prior to application of the patch, this should be done with water. Soaps, oils, lotions, alcohol or any other agent that might irritate the skin or alter its characteristics should not be used. The skin should be completely dry before application of the patch.

Since the transdermal patch is protected outwardly by a waterproof covering foil, it may also be worn when taking a short shower.

Fentanyl transdermal patch is to be attached as soon as the pack has been opened. Following removal of the protective layer, the transdermal patch should be pressed firmly in place with the palm of the hand for approximately 30 seconds, making sure the contact is complete, especially around the edges. An additional fixing of the transdermal patch may be necessary. Fentanyl transdermal patch should be worn continuously for 72 hours after which the transdermal patch is replaced. A new transdermal patch should always be applied to a different site from the previous one. The same application site may be re-used only after an interval of at least 7 days.

The transdermal patch should not be divided or cut (see section 4.4)

For disposal instructions see section 6.6.

Use in children

Method of administration

In young children the upper back is the preferred location to apply the patch, to minimize the potential of the child removing the patch.

Posology

Matrifen should be administered only to **opioid-tolerant paediatric patients (ages 2 to 16 years)** who are already receiving at least 30 mg oral morphine equivalent per day. To convert paediatric patients from oral or parenteral opioids to Matrifen, refer to Equianalgesic potency conversion (Table 1), and Recommended initial Matrifen dose based upon daily oral morphine dose (Table 3).

Table 3: Recommended initial dose of Matrifen based upon daily oral morphine dose [1]

Peroral morphine dose per 24-hours (mg/day)	Dose of Matrifen transdermal patch micrograms/hour
For paediatric patients[2] 30-44	For paediatric patients[2] 12
45-134	25

[1] Conversion schemes are based on clinical trials.
[2] Conversion to Matrifen doses greater than 25 micrograms/hour is the same for adult and paediatric patients.

For children who receive more than 90 mg oral morphine a day, only limited information is currently available from clinical trials. In the paediatric studies, the required fentanyl trandermal patch dose was calculated conservatively: 30 mg to 45 mg oral morphine per day or its equivalent opioid dose was replaced by one fentanyl 12 microgram/hour patch. It should be noted that this conversion schedule for children only applies to the switch from oral morphine (or its equivalent) to fentanyl patches. The conversion schedule could not be used to convert from fentanyl into other opioids, as overdose could then occur.

The analgesic effect of the first dose of Matrifen patches will not be optimal within the first 24 hours. Therefore during the first 12 hours after switching to Matrifen, the patients should be given the previous regular dose of analgesics. In the next 12 hours, these analgesics should be provided based on clinical need.

Since peak fentanyl levels occur after 12 to 24 hours of treatment, monitoring of the patient for adverse events, which may include hypoventilation, is recommended for at least 48 hours after initiation of Matrifen therapy or up-titration of the dose (see also section 4.4 Special warnings and precautions for use).

Dose titration and maintenance.

If the analgesic effect of Matrifen is insufficient, supplementary morphine or another short-duration opioid should be administered. Depending on the additional analgesic needs and the pain status of the child, it may be decided to use more patches. Dose adjustments should be done in 12 micrograms/hour step.

4.3 Contraindications

Hypersensitivity to the active substance or to any of the excipients.

The product should not be used for treatment of acute or postoperative pain, because of the lack of opportunity for dose titration in the short term and the possibility of life-threatening respiratory depression.

Severe impairment of the central nervous system.

Concomitant use of MAO-inhibitors or within 14 days after discontinuation of MAO-inhibitors.

4.4 Special warnings and precautions for use

The product should be used only as part of an integrated treatment of pain in cases where the patient is adequately assessed medically, socially and psychologically.

After exhibiting a serious adverse reaction a patient should be monitored for 24 hours following removal of a transdermal patch due to the half life of fentanyl (see section 5.2).

Both unused and used Fentanyl transdermal patches should be kept out of reach and sight of children.

The transdermal patch should not be divided or cut as the quality, efficacy and safety have not been established for divided patches.

Respiratory depression

As with all potent opioids some patients may experience respiratory depression with the fentanyl transdermal patch, and patients must be observed for this effect. Respiratory depression may persist beyond the removal of the patch. The incidence of respiratory depression increases as the fentanyl dose is increased. CNS active drugs may worsen the respiratory depression (see section 4.5). Fentanyl should be used only with caution and at lower dose in patients with existing respiratory depression.

If a patient is to undergo measures that fully remove the sensation of pain (e.g. regional analgesia), it is advisable to prepare for the possibility of respiratory depression. Before such measures are carried out, the fentanyl dosage should be reduced or a changeover should be made to rapid- or short-acting opioid medication.

Chronic pulmonary disease

In patients with chronic obstructive or other pulmonary diseases fentanyl may have more severe adverse effects, in such patients opioids may decrease respiratory drive and increase airway resistance.

Drug dependence

Tolerance and physical and psychological dependence may develop upon repeated administration of opioids, but is rare in treatment of cancer related pain.

Increased intracranial pressure

Matrifen should be used with caution in patients who may be particularly susceptible to the intracranial effects of CO2 retention such as those with evidence of increased intracranial pressure, impaired consciousness or coma. Fentanyl should be used with caution in patients in whom a cerebral tumour has been detected.

Cardiac disease

Fentanyl may produce bradycardia. Matrifen should therefore be administered with caution to patients with bradyarrhythmias.

Opioids may cause hypotonia, specially in patients with hypovolemia. Caution should therefore be taken in treatment of patients with hypotonia and/or patients with hypovolemia.

Impaired liver function

Fentanyl is metabolised to inactive metabolites in the liver, so patients with hepatic disease might have a delayed elimination. Patients with hepatic impairment should be observed carefully and the dose reduced if necessary.

Renal impairment

Less than 10% of fentanyl is excreted unchanged by the kidneys, and unlike morphine, there are no known active metabolites eliminated by the kidneys. Data obtained with intravenous fentanyl in patients with renal failure suggest that the volume of distribution of fentanyl may be changed by dialysis. This may affect serum concentrations. If patients with renal impairment receive transdermal fentanyl they should be observed carefully for signs of fentanyl toxicity and the dose reduced if necessary.

Patients with fever/external heat

Patients with fever should be monitored very closely for opioid side effects and if necessary the fentanyl dosage should be adjusted (see section 4.2). Patients should also be advised to avoid exposing the Fentanyl transdermal patch application site to direct external heat sources such as heating pads, hot water bottles, electric blankets, heat lamps or hot whirlpool spa baths while wearing the patch, since there is potential for temperature dependent increases in release of fentanyl from the patch.

The transdermal patch must always be removed before taking a sauna. Sauna bathing is possible only when replacing a transdermal patch (at intervals of 72 hours). A new transdermal patch is to be applied to cool, very dry skin.

Elderly Patients

Data from intravenous studies with fentanyl suggest that elderly patients may have reduced clearance, a prolonged half-life and they may be more sensitive to the drug than younger patients. Elderly, cachectic, or debilitated patients should be observed carefully for signs of fentanyl toxicity and the dose reduced if necessary.

Others

Non-epileptic (myo)clonic reactions can occur.

Caution should be exercised when treating patients with myasthenia gravis.

Children

Matrifen should not be administered to **opioid naïve paediatric patients** (see section 4.2 Posology and method of administration). The potential for serious or life-threatening hypoventilation exists regardless of the dose of Matrifen transdermal system administered (see Tables 1 and 3 in section 4.2 Posology and method of administration).

Fentanyl transdermal patch was not studied in children under 2 years of age. Matrifen should be administered only to opioid-tolerant children age 2 years or older (see section

4.2 Posology and method of administration). Matrifen should not be used in children under 2 years of age.

To guard against accidental ingestion by children, use caution when choosing the application site for Matrifen (see section 4.2 Posology and method of administration) and monitor adhesion of the patch closely.

Used transdermal patches

High quantities of fentanyl remain in the transdermal patches even after use. Due to safety and environmental reasons used transdermal patches, as well as any unused transdermal patches should be disposed of according to the instructions given in section 6.6.

4.5 Interaction with other medicinal products and other forms of interaction

The concomitant use of barbituric acid derivatives should be avoided, since the respiratory depressing effect of fentanyl may be increased.

The concomitant use of other CNS depressants, including opioids, anxiolytics and tranquilizers, hypnotics, general anaesthetics, phentiazines, skeletal muscle relaxants, sedating antihistamines and alcoholic beverages may produce additive depressant effects; hypoventilation, hypotonia and profound sedation or coma may occur. Therefore, the use of any of the above mentioned concomitant drugs requires observation of the patient.

MAO-inhibitors have been reported to increase the effect of narcotic analgesics, specially in patients with cardiac failure. Therefore, fentanyl should not be used within 14 days after discontinuation of treatment with MAO-inhibitors.

Fentanyl, a high clearance drug, is rapidly and extensively metabolised mainly by CYP3A4. Itraconazole (a potent CYP3A4 inhibitor) at 200 mg/day given orally for four days had no significant effect on the pharmacokinetics of intravenous fentanyl. Increased plasma concentrations were, however, observed in individual subjects. Oral administration of ritonavir (one of the most potent CYP3A4 inhibitors) reduced the clearance of intravenous fentanyl by two thirds and doubled the half-life. Concomitant use of potent CYP3A4-inhibitors (e.g. ritonavir, ketoconazol, itraconazol, macrolide antibiotics) with transdermally administered fentanyl may result in increased plasma concentrations of fentanyl. This may increase or prolong both the therapeutic effects and the adverse reactions, which may cause severe respiratory depression. In such cases increased care and observation of the patient should be undertaken. Combined use of ritonavir or other potent CYP3A4-inhibitors with transdermal fentanyl is not recommended, unless the patient is carefully observed.

Although pentazocine or buprenorphine have an analgesic effect, they partially antagonize some effects of fentanyl (e.g. analgesia) and may induce withdrawal symptoms in opioids dependants.

4.6 Pregnancy and lactation

The safety of fentanyl transdermal patches in pregnancy has not been established. Studies in animals have shown reproductive toxicity (see section 5.3). The potential risk for humans is unknown.

Fentanyl should only be used during pregnancy when clearly necessary.

Long-term treatment during pregnancy may cause withdrawal symptoms in the newborn child. Fentanyl should not be used during labour and delivery (including caesarean section) since fentanyl passes the placenta and may cause respiratory depression in the foetus or in the newborn child.

Fentanyl is excreted into breast milk and may cause sedation and respiratory depression in the breast-fed child. Breast-feeding should therefore be discontinued for at least 72 hours after the last administration of Matrifen.

4.7 Effects on ability to drive and use machines

Fentanyl transdermal patches have major influence on the ability to drive and use machines. This has to be expected especially at the beginning of treatment, at any change of dosage as well as in connection with alcohol or tranquilizers. Patients stabilized on a specific dosage will not necessarily be restricted. Therefore, patients should consult their physician as to whether driving or use of machines is permitted.

4.8 Undesirable effects

The following frequencies are used for the description of the occurrence of adverse reactions:

Very common (>1/10), Common (>1/100, <1/10), Uncommon (>1/1000, <1/100), Rare (>1/10,000, <1/1000), Very rare (<1/10,000) including isolated reports.

The most serious adverse reaction of fentanyl is respiratory depression.

Psychiatric disorders

Very common: Somnolence

Common: Sedation, confusion, depression, anxiety, nervousness, hallucinations, lowered appetite

Uncommon: Euphoria, amnesia, sleeplessness, agitation

Very rare: Delusions, asthenia, disorder of sexual functions

Nervous system disorders

Very common: Drowsiness, headache

Uncommon: Tremor, paresthesia, speech disturbances

Very rare: Ataxia, non-epileptic myoclonial reactions

Eye disorders

Rare: Amblyopia

Cardiac disorders

Uncommon: Bradycardia, tachycardia, hypotonia, hypertonia

Rare: Arrhythmia, vasodilatation

Respiratory, thoracic and mediastinal disorders

Uncommon: Dyspnea, hypoventilation

Very rare: Respiratory depression, apnea, hemoptysis, lung obstruction, pharyngitis and laryngospasm

Gastrointestinal disorders

Very common: Nausea, vomiting, constipation

Common: Xerostomia, dyspepsia

Uncommon: Diarrhea

Rare: Hiccups

Very rare: Ileus, painful flatulence

Immune system disorders

Very rare: Anaphylaxis

Skin and subcutaneous tissue disorders

Very common: Sweating, pruritus

Common: Skin reaction at the application site

Uncommon: Rash, erythema

Rash erythema and pruritus will usually disappear within one day after the patch has been removed.

Renal and urinary disorders

Uncommon: Urinary retention

Very rare: Oliguria, pain in the bladder

General disorders

Rare: Oedema, feeling cold

Other adverse reactions

Tolerance, physical and psychological dependence can develop during long-term use of fentanyl. Opioid withdrawal symptoms (for instance: nausea, vomiting, diarrhea, anxiety and shivering) may occur in patients after switching from previously prescribed opioid analgesics to fentanyl transdermal patch.

The adverse event profile in children and adolescents treated with fentanyl transdermal patch was similar to that observed in adults. No risk was identified in the paediatric population beyond that expected with the use of opioids for the relief of pain associated with serious illness and there does not appear to be any paediatric-specific risk associated with fentanyl trandermal patch use in children as young as 2 years old when used as directed. Very common adverse events reported in paediatric clinical trials were fever, vomiting and nausea.

4.9 Overdose

Symptoms

The symptoms of fentanyl overdose are an extension of its pharmacological actions, e.g. lethargy, coma respiratory depression with Cheyne-Stokes respiration and/or cyanosis. Other symptoms may be hypothermia, decreased muscle tonus, bradycardia, hypotonia. Signs of toxicity are deep sedation, ataxia, miosis, convulsions and respiratory depression, which is the main symptom.

Treatment

For management of respiratory depression immediate countermeasures should be started, including removing the patch and physically or verbally stimulating the patient. These actions can be followed by administration of a specific opioid antagonist such as naloxone.

A starting dose of 0.4 – 2 mg naloxone hydrochloride i.v. is recommended for adults. If needed, a similar dose can be given every 2 or 3 minutes, or be administered as continued infusion as 2 mg in 500 ml isotonic sodium chloride solution (0.9 %) or 5% dextrose solution (0.004 mg/ml). The infusion rate should be adjusted according to previous bolus injections and the individual response of the patient. If intravenous administration is impossible, naloxone hydrochloride can also be given intramuscularly or subcutaneously. Following intramuscular or subcutaneous administration the onset of action will be slower compared with intravenous administration. Intramuscular administration will give a more prolonged effect than intravenous administration. Respiratory depression due to overdose can persist longer than the effect of the opioid antagonist. Reversing the narcotic effect can give rise to acute pain and release of catecholamines. Intensive care unit treatment is important, if required by the patient's clinical condition. If severe or persistent hypotension occurs, hypovolemia should be considered, and the condition should be managed with appropriate parenteral fluid therapy.

5. PHARMACOLOGICAL PROPERTIES

5.1 Pharmacodynamic properties

Pharmacotherapeutic group: Analgesics, opioids

ATC code: N02AB03

Matrifen is a transdermal patch that provides continuous delivery of fentanyl. Fentanyl is an opioid analgesic with affinity mainly to the μ-receptor. The predominant pharmacological effects are pain relief and sedation. Patients not previously treated with opioids will have pain relief at a fentanyl concentration between 0.3 and 1.5 ng/ml. In this group of patients the frequency of adverse effects will increase at serum concentrations above 2 ng/ml. Both the lowest effective fentanyl concentration and the concentration causing adverse reactions will increase with the development of increasing tolerance. Development of tolerance varies considerably between individual subjects.

5.2 Pharmacokinetic properties

The fentanyl transdermal patch provides systemic delivery over the 72 hour administration period.

Absorption: After the first patch application serum fentanyl concentrations increase gradually, generally levelling off between 12 and 24 hours and remaining relatively constant for the remainder of the 72-hour application period. By the second 72-hour application, a steady- state serum concentration is reached and is maintained during subsequent applications of the patch of the same size. The absorption of fentanyl may differ somewhat between different application sites. A somewhat lower (approximately 25%) fentanyl absorption has been observed in studies with healthy volunteers after the patch has been applied on the chest compared with the upper arm and the back.

Distribution: The plasma protein binding for fentanyl is 84 %.

Biotransformation: Fentanyl shows linear kinetics and is metabolized primarily in the liver via CYP3A4. The major metabolite, norfentanyl, is inactive.

Elimination: After the fentanyl patch is removed, serum fentanyl concentrations decline gradually falling approximately 50% in 13-22 hours in adults or 22-25 hours in children. Continued absorption of fentanyl from the skin accounts for a slower disappearance of the drug from the serum than is seen after an intravenous infusion. Around 75% of fentanyl is excreted into the urine, mostly as metabolites, with less than 10% as unchanged drug. About 9% of the dose is recovered in the faeces, primarily as metabolites.

Pharmacokinetics in special groups

Impaired hepatic or renal function could cause increased serum concentrations. Elderly, cachectic or generally impaired patients may have a lower fentanyl clearance, which could cause a longer terminal half life for the compound (see section 4.2 and 4.4).

Children

Adjusting for body weight, clearance (L/hr/Kg) in paediatric patients appears to be 82 % higher in children 2 to 5 years old and 25 % higher in children 6 to 10 years old when compared to children 11 to 16 years old, who are likely to have the same clearance as adults. These findings have been taken into consideration in determining the dosing recommendations for paediatric patients.

5.3 Preclinical safety data

Non-clinical data reveal no special hazard for humans based on conventional studies of safety pharmacology, repeated dose toxicity and genotoxicity. Animal studies have shown reduced fertility and increased mortality in rat foetuses. Teratogenic effects have, however, not been demonstrated.

Mutagenicity testing in bacteria and in rodents yielded negative results. As well as other opioids fentanyl showed mutagenic effects in vitro in mammalian cells. A mutagenic risk in therapeutic condition seems unlikely since effects were induced only in very high concentrations.

Long-term carcinogenicity studies have not been performed.

6. PHARMACEUTICAL PARTICULARS

6.1 List of excipients

Dipropylene glycol

Hydroxypropyl cellulose

Dimeticone

Silicone adhesives (amine resistant)

Release membrane, ethylenvinylacetate (EVA)

Backing film, polyethylene terephthalate film (PET)

Removable protective film, fluoropolymercoated polyester film

Printing ink

6.2 Incompatibilities

Not applicable

6.3 Shelf life

2 years

6.4 Special precautions for storage

This medicinal product does not require any special storage conditions.

6.5 Nature and contents of container

Each patch is packed in a heat-sealed pouch made of paper, aluminium and polyacrylonitrile (PAN).

Pack sizes:

1, 2, 3, 4, 5, 8, 10, 16 and 20 patches

Not all pack sizes may be marketed

6.6 Special precautions for disposal and other handling

High quantities of fentanyl remain in the transdermal patches even after use. Used transdermal patches should be folded with the adhesive surfaces inwards, so the release membrane is not exposed, and due to safety and environmental reasons, discarded according to local requirements or returned to the pharmacy. Any unused medicinal product should be discarded according to local requirements or returned to the pharmacy.

There are no safety and pharmacokinetic data available for other application sites.

7. MARKETING AUTHORISATION HOLDER

Nycomed UK Ltd
Three Globeside Business Park
Fieldhouse Lane
Marlow
Bucks
SL7 1HZ
UK

8. MARKETING AUTHORISATION NUMBER(S)

12 microgram/hour: PL 20810/0004
25 microgram/hour: PL 20810/0005
50 microgram/hour: PL 20810/0006
75 microgram/hour: PL 20810/0007
100 microgram/hour: PL 20810/0008

9. DATE OF FIRST AUTHORISATION/RENEWAL OF THE AUTHORISATION

21/12/2006

10. DATE OF REVISION OF THE TEXT

10/11/2008

Legal category
POM/CD2

Maxalt 5mg, 10mg Tablets, Maxalt Melt 10mg Oral Lyophilisates

(Merck Sharp & Dohme Limited)

1. NAME OF THE MEDICINAL PRODUCT

MAXALT® 5 mg Tablets
MAXALT® 10 mg Tablets
MAXALT® Melt 10 mg oral lyophilisates

2. QUALITATIVE AND QUANTITATIVE COMPOSITION

Maxalt 5mg

Each tablet contains 7.265 mg of rizatriptan benzoate (corresponding to 5 mg of the rizatriptan).

Excipients: lactose 30.25 mg in the 5 mg tablet.

Maxalt 10mg

Each tablet contains 14.53 mg of rizatriptan benzoate (corresponding to 10 mg of the rizatriptan).

Excipients: lactose 60.5 mg in the 10 mg tablet.

Maxalt Melt 10mg

Each oral lyophilisate contains 14.53 mg of rizatriptan benzoate (corresponding to 10 mg of the rizatriptan).

Excipients: aspartame 3.75 mg in the 10 mg oral lyophylisate.

For a full list of excipients see section 6.1.

3. PHARMACEUTICAL FORM

Tablets

5 mg tablets are pale pink, capsule-shaped, coded MSD on one side and 266 on the other.

10 mg tablets are pale pink, capsule-shaped, coded MAXALT on one side and MSD 267 on the other.

Oral lyophilisates

10 mg oral lyophilisates are white to off-white, round with a modified square on one side, with a peppermint flavour.

4. CLINICAL PARTICULARS

4.1 Therapeutic indications

Acute treatment of the headache phase of migraine attacks, with or without aura.

4.2 Posology and method of administration

General

'Maxalt' should not be used prophylactically.

The oral tablets should be swallowed whole with liquid.

Effects of food: The absorption of rizatriptan is delayed by approximately 1 hour when administered together with food. Therefore, onset of effect may be delayed when rizatriptan is administered in the fed state. (See also 5.2 'Pharmacokinetic properties', *Absorption*).

'Maxalt' Melt oral lyophilisates need not be taken with liquid.

The oral lyophilisate is packaged in a blister within an outer aluminium sachet. Patients should be instructed not to remove the blister from the outer sachet until just prior to dosing. The blister pack should then be peeled open with dry hands and the oral lyophilisate placed on the tongue, where it will dissolve and be swallowed with the saliva.

The oral lyophilisate can be used in situations in which liquids are not available, or to avoid the nausea and vomiting that may accompany the ingestion of tablets with liquids.

Adults 18 years of age and older

The recommended dose is 10 mg.

Redosing: doses should be separated by at least two hours; no more than two doses should be taken in any 24-hour period.

- for headache recurrence within 24 hours: if headache returns after relief of the initial attack, one further dose may be taken. The above dosing limits should be observed.

- after non-response: the effectiveness of a second dose for treatment of the same attack, when an initial dose is ineffective, has not been examined in controlled trials. Therefore, if a patient does not respond to the first dose, a second dose should not be taken for the same attack.

Clinical studies have shown that patients who do not respond to treatment of an attack are still likely to respond to treatment for subsequent attacks.

Some patients should receive the lower (5 mg) dose of 'Maxalt', in particular the following patient groups:

– patients on propranolol. Administration of rizatriptan should be separated by at least two hours from administration of propranolol. (See section 4.5)

– patients with mild or moderate renal insufficiency.

– patients with mild to moderate hepatic insufficiency.

Doses should be separated by at least two hours; no more than two doses should be taken in any 24-hour period.

Paediatric patients

Children (under 12 years of age)

The use of 'Maxalt' in patients under 12 years of age is not recommended. There are no data available on the use of rizatriptan in children under 12 years of age.

Tablets: adolescents (12-17 years of age)

The use of 'Maxalt' Tablets in patients under 18 years of age is not recommended. In a placebo controlled study, the efficacy of 'Maxalt' Tablets (5 mg) was not superior to placebo. The efficacy of 'Maxalt' in patients under 18 years of age has not been established.

Oral lyophilisates: adolescents (12-17 years of age)

The use of 'Maxalt' Melt oral lyophilisates in patients under 18 years of age is not recommended. Safety and effectiveness of 'Maxalt' Melt oral lyophilisates in paediatric patients have not been evaluated.

Patients older than 65 years

The safety and effectiveness of rizatriptan in patients older than 65 years have not been systematically evaluated.

4.3 Contraindications

Hypersensitivity to rizatriptan or to any of the excipients.

Concurrent administration of monoamine oxidase (MAO) inhibitors or use within two weeks of discontinuation of MAO inhibitor therapy. (See section 4.5)

'Maxalt' is contra-indicated in patients with severe hepatic or severe renal insufficiency.

'Maxalt' is contra-indicated in patients with a previous cerebrovascular accident (CVA) or transient ischaemic attack (TIA).

Moderately severe or severe hypertension, or untreated mild hypertension.

Established coronary artery disease, including ischaemic heart disease (angina pectoris, history of myocardial infarction, or documented silent ischaemia), signs and symptoms of ischaemic heart disease, or Prinzmetal's angina.

Peripheral vascular disease.

Concomitant use of rizatriptan and ergotamine, ergot derivatives (including methysergide), or other 5-$HT_{1B/1D}$ receptor agonists. (See section 4.5).

4.4 Special warnings and precautions for use

'Maxalt' should only be administered to patients in whom a clear diagnosis of migraine has been established. 'Maxalt' should not be administered to patients with basilar or hemiplegic migraine.

'Maxalt' should not be used to treat 'atypical' headaches, i.e. those that might be associated with potentially serious medical conditions, (e.g. CVA, ruptured aneurysm) in which cerebrovascular vasoconstriction could be harmful.

Rizatriptan can be associated with transient symptoms including chest pain and tightness which may be intense and involve the throat (see section 4.8). Where such symptoms are thought to indicate ischaemic heart disease, no further dose should be taken and appropriate evaluation should be carried out.

As with other 5-$HT_{1B/1D}$ receptor agonists, rizatriptan should not be given, without prior evaluation, to patients in whom unrecognised cardiac disease is likely or to patients at risk for coronary artery disease (CAD) [e.g. patients with hypertension, diabetics, smokers or users of nicotine substitution therapy, men over 40 years of age, post-menopausal women, patients with bundle branch block, and those with strong family history for CAD]. Cardiac evaluations may not identify every patient who has cardiac disease and, in very rare cases, serious cardiac events have occurred in patients without underlying cardiovascular disease when 5-HT_1 agonists have been administered. Those in whom CAD is established should not be given 'Maxalt'. (See section 4.3)

5-$HT_{1B/1D}$ receptor agonists have been associated with coronary vasospasm. In rare cases, myocardial ischaemia or infarction have been reported with 5-$HT_{1B/1D}$ receptor agonists including 'Maxalt' (see section 4.8)

Other 5-$HT_{1B/1D}$ agonists, (e.g. sumatriptan) should not be used concomitantly with 'Maxalt'. (See section 4.5).

It is advised to wait at least six hours following use of rizatriptan before administering ergotamine-type medications, (e.g. ergotamine, dihydro-ergotamine or methysergide). At least 24 hours should elapse after the administration of an ergotamine-containing preparation before rizatriptan is given. Although additive vasospastic effects were not observed in a clinical pharmacology study in which 16 healthy males received oral rizatriptan and parenteral ergotamine, such additive effects are theoretically possible, (see section 4.3)

Serotonin syndrome (including altered mental status, autonomic instability and neuromuscular abnormalities) has been reported following concomitant treatment with triptans and selective serotonin reuptake inhibitors (SSRIs) or serotonin noradrenaline reuptake inhibitors (SNRIs). These reactions can be severe. If concomitant treatment with rizatriptan and an SSRI or SNRI is clinically warranted, appropriate observation of the patient is advised, particularly during treatment initiation, with dose increases, or with addition of another serotonergic medication (see section 4.5).

Undesirable effects may be more common during concomitant use of triptans (5-$HT_{1B/1D}$ agonists) and herbal preparations containing St John's wort (*Hypericum perforatum*).

Angioedema (e.g. facial oedema, tongue swelling and pharyngeal oedema) may occur in patients treated with triptans, among which rizatriptan. If angioedema of the tongue or pharynx occurs, the patient should be placed under medical supervision until symptoms have resolved. Treatment should promptly be discontinued and replaced by an agent belonging to another class of drugs.

The quantity of lactose in each tablet is as follows: 30.25 mg in the 5 mg tablet and 60.50 mg in the 10 mg tablet. Patients with rare hereditary problems of galactose intolerance, the Lapp lactase deficiency or glucose-galactose malabsorption should not take this medicine.

Phenylketonurics: Phenylketonuric patients should be informed that phenylalanine may be harmful. 'Maxalt' Melt oral lyophilisates contain aspartame (which contains phenylalanine). Each 10 mg oral lyophilisate contains 3.75 mg aspartame.

The potential for interaction should be considered when rizatriptan is administered to patients taking CYP 2D6 substrates (see section 4.5)

Medication overuse headache (MOH)

Prolonged use of any painkiller for headaches can make them worse. If this situation is experienced or suspected, medical advice should be obtained and treatment should be discontinued. The diagnosis of MOH should be suspected in patients who have frequent or daily headaches despite (or because of) the regular use of headache medications.

4.5 Interaction with other medicinal products and other forms of interaction

Ergotamine, ergot derivatives (including methysergide), other 5 HT $_{1B/1D}$ receptor agonists: Due to an additive effect, the concomitant use of rizatriptan and ergotamine, ergot derivatives (including methysergide), or other 5 HT $_{1B/1D}$ receptor agonists (e.g. sumatriptan, zolmitriptan, naratriptan) increase the risk of coronary artery vasoconstriction and hypertensive effects. This combination is contraindicated (see section 4.3).

Monoamine oxidase inhibitors: Rizatriptan is principally metabolised via monoamine oxidase, 'A' subtype (MAO-A). Plasma concentrations of rizatriptan and its active N-monodesmethyl metabolite were increased by concomitant administration of a selective, reversible MAO-A inhibitor. Similar or greater effects are expected with non-selective, reversible (e.g. linezolid) and irreversible MAO inhibitors. Due to a risk of coronary artery vasoconstriction and hypertensive episodes, administration of 'Maxalt' to patients taking inhibitors of MAO is contraindicated. (See section 4.3)

Beta-blockers: Plasma concentrations of rizatriptan may be increased by concomitant administration of propranolol. This increase is most probably due to first-pass metabolic interaction between the two drugs, since MAO-A plays a role in the metabolism of both rizatriptan and propranolol. This interaction leads to a mean increase in AUC and C_{max} of 70-80%. In patients receiving propranolol, the 5 mg dose of 'Maxalt' should be used. (See section 4.2)

In a drug-interaction study, nadolol and metoprolol did not alter plasma concentrations of rizatriptan.

Selective Serotonin Reuptake Inhibitors (SSRIs) /Serotonin Norepinephrine Reuptake Inhibitors (SNRIs) and Serotonin Syndrome: There have been reports describing patients with symptoms compatible with serotonin syndrome (including altered mental status, autonomic instability and neuromuscular abnormalities) following the use of selective serotonin reuptake inhibitors (SSRIs) or serotonin noradrenaline reuptake inhibitors (SNRIs) and triptans (see section 4.4).

In vitro studies indicate that rizatriptan inhibits cytochrome P450 2D6 (CYP 2D6). Clinical interaction data are not available. The potential for interaction should be considered when rizatriptan is administered to patients taking CYP 2D6 substrates.

4.6 Pregnancy and lactation

Use during pregnancy

The safety of rizatriptan for the use in human pregnancy has not been established. Animal studies do not indicate harmful effects at dose levels that exceed therapeutic dose levels with respect to the development of the embryo or foetus, or the course of gestation, parturition and post-natal development.

Because animal reproductive and developmental studies are not always predictive of human response, 'Maxalt' should be used during pregnancy only if clearly needed.

Use during lactation

Studies in rats indicated that very high milk transfer of rizatriptan occurred. Transient, very slight decreases in pre-weaning pup body weights were observed only when the mother's systemic exposure was well in excess of the maximum exposure level for humans. No data exist in humans.

Therefore, caution should be exercised when administering rizatriptan to women who are breast-feeding. Infant exposure should be minimised by avoiding breast-feeding for 24 hours after treatment.

4.7 Effects on ability to drive and use machines

Migraine or treatment with 'Maxalt' may cause somnolence in some patients. Dizziness has also been reported in some patients receiving 'Maxalt'. Patients should, therefore, evaluate their ability to perform complex tasks during migraine attacks and after administration of 'Maxalt'.

4.8 Undesirable effects

'Maxalt' (as the tablet and oral lyophilisate formulation) was evaluated in over 3,600 patients for up to one year in controlled clinical studies. The most common side effects evaluated in clinical studies were dizziness, somnolence, and asthenia/fatigue. The following side effects have been evaluated in clinical studies and/or reported in post-marketing experience:

(Very common [$\geqslant$ 1/10]; Common [$\geqslant$ 1/100, $<$1/10]; Uncommon: [$\geqslant$ 1/1000, $<$1/100]; Rare [$\geqslant$ 1/10,000 $<$1/1,000]; Very rare [$\leqslant$ 1/10000], not known [cannot be estimated from the available data]).

Immune system disorders:

Not known: hypersensitivity reaction, anaphylaxis/anaphylactoid reaction.

Psychiatric disorders:

Uncommon: disorientation, insomnia, nervousness.

Nervous system disorders:

Common: dizziness, somnolence, paresthesia, headache, hypaesthesia, decreased mental acuity, tremor.

Uncommon: ataxia, vertigo.

Rare: syncope, dysgeusia/bad taste, serotonin syndrome.

Not known: seizure.

Eye disorders:

Uncommon: blurred vision.

Cardiac disorders:

Common: palpitation, tachycardia.

Rare: Myocardial ischaemia or infarction, cerebrovascular accident. Most of these adverse reactions have been reported in patients with risk factors predictive of coronary artery disease.

Vascular disorders:

Common: hot flushes/flashes.

Uncommon: hypertension.

Not known: peripheral vascular ischaemia.

Respiratory, thoracic and mediastinal disorders:

Common: pharyngeal discomfort, dyspnoea.

Rare: wheezing.

Gastro-intestinal disorders:

Common: nausea, dry mouth, vomiting, diarrhoea.

Uncommon: thirst, dyspepsia.

Skin and subcutaneous tissue disorders:

Common: flushing, sweating.

Uncommon: pruritus, urticaria.

Rare: angioedema (e.g. facial oedema, tongue swelling, pharyngeal oedema), rash, toxic epidermal necrolysis (for angioedema see also section 4.4).

Musculoskeletal and connective tissue disorders:

Common: regional heaviness.

Uncommon: neck pain, regional tightness, stiffness, muscle weakness.

Rare: facial pain.

General disorders and administration site conditions:

Common: asthenia/fatigue, pain in abdomen or chest.

4.9 Overdose

Rizatriptan 40 mg (administered as either a single tablet dose or as two doses with a two-hour interdose interval) was generally well tolerated in over 300 patients; dizziness and somnolence were the most common drug-related adverse effects.

In a clinical pharmacology study in which 12 subjects received rizatriptan, at total cumulative doses of 80 mg (given within four hours), two subjects experienced syncope and/or bradycardia. One subject, a female aged 29 years, developed vomiting, bradycardia, and dizziness beginning three hours after receiving a total of 80 mg rizatriptan (administered over two hours). A third-degree AV block, responsive to atropine, was observed an hour after the onset of the other symptoms. The second subject, a 25 year-old male, experienced transient dizziness, syncope, incontinence, and a five-second systolic pause (on ECG monitor) immediately after a painful venipuncture. The venipuncture occurred two hours after the subject had received a total of 80 mg rizatriptan (administered over four hours).

In addition, based on the pharmacology of rizatriptan, hypertension or other more serious cardiovascular symptoms could occur after overdosage. Gastro-intestinal decontamination, (e.g. gastric lavage followed by activated charcoal) should be considered in patients suspected of an overdose with 'Maxalt'. Clinical and electrocardiographic monitoring should be continued for at least 12 hours, even if clinical symptoms are not observed.

The effects of haemo- or peritoneal dialysis on serum concentrations of rizatriptan are unknown.

5. PHARMACOLOGICAL PROPERTIES

5.1 Pharmacodynamic properties

Mechanism of action: Selective serotonin ($5HT_{1B/1D}$) agonists

Pharmacotherapeutic group: ATC-code: N02C C04

Rizatriptan binds selectively with high affinity to human $5\text{-}HT_{1B}$ and $5\text{-}HT_{1D}$ receptors and has little or no effect or pharmacological activity at $5\text{-}HT_2$, $5\text{-}HT_3$; adrenergic alpha$_1$, alpha$_2$ or beta; D_1, D_2, dopaminergic, histaminic H_1; muscarinic; or benzodiazepine receptors.

The therapeutic activity of rizatriptan in treating migraine headache may be attributed to its agonist effects at $5\text{-}HT_{1B}$ and $5\text{-}HT_{1D}$ receptors on the extracerebral intracranial blood vessels that are thought to become dilated during an attack and on the trigeminal sensory nerves that innervate them. Activation of these $5\text{-}HT_{1B}$ and $5\text{-}HT_{1D}$ receptors may result in constriction of pain-producing intracranial blood vessels and inhibition of neuropeptide release that leads to decreased inflammation in sensitive tissues and reduced central trigeminal pain signal transmission.

Pharmacodynamic effects

Tablets

The efficacy of 'Maxalt' Tablets in the acute treatment of migraine attacks was established in four multicentre, placebo-controlled trials that included over 2,000 patients who received 'Maxalt' 5 or 10 mg for up to one year. Headache relief occurred as early as 30 minutes following dosing, and response rates, (i.e. reduction of moderate or severe headache pain to no or mild pain) two hours after treatment were 67-77% with the 10 mg tablet, 60-63% with the 5 mg tablet, and 23-40% with placebo. Although patients who did not respond to initial treatment with 'Maxalt' were not redosed for the same attack, they were still likely to respond to treatment for a subsequent attack. 'Maxalt' reduced the functional disability and relieved the nausea, photophobia, and phonophobia associated with migraine attacks.

'Maxalt' remains effective in treating menstrual migraine, i.e. migraine that occurs within 3 days before or after the onset of menses.

Oral lyophilisates

The efficacy of 'Maxalt' Melt oral lyophilisates in the acute treatment of migraine attacks was established in two multicentre, randomised, placebo-controlled trials that were similar in design to the trials of 'Maxalt' Tablets. In one study (n=311), by two hours post-dosing, relief rates in patients treated with 'Maxalt' Melt oral lyophilisates were approximately 66% for rizatriptan 5 mg and 10 mg, compared to 47% in the placebo group. In a larger study (n=547), by two hours post-dosing, relief rates were 59% in patients treated with 'Maxalt' Melt oral lyophilisates 5 mg, and 74% after 10 mg, compared to 28% in the placebo group. 'Maxalt' Melt oral lyophilisates also relieved the disability, nausea, photophobia, and phonophobia which accompanied the migraine episodes. A significant effect on pain relief was observed as early as 30 minutes post-dosing in one of the two clinical trials for the 10 mg dose (see section 5.2 *Absorption*).

Based on studies with the oral tablet, rizatriptan remains effective in treating menstrual migraine, i.e. migraine that occurs within 3 days before or after the onset of menses.

'Maxalt' Melt oral lyophilisates enables migraine patients to treat their migraine attacks without having to swallow liquids. This may allow patients to administer their medication earlier, for example, when liquids are not available, and to avoid possible worsening of GI symptoms by swallowing liquids.

5.2 Pharmacokinetic properties

Absorption

Rizatriptan is rapidly and completely absorbed following oral administration.

Tablets: The mean oral bioavailability of the tablet is approximately 40-45%, and mean peak plasma concentrations (C_{max}) are reached in approximately 1-1.5 hours (T_{max}). Administration of an oral tablet dose with a high-fat breakfast had no effect on the extent of rizatriptan absorption, but absorption was delayed for approximately one hour.

Oral lyophilisates: The mean oral bioavailability of the oral lyophilisate is approximately 40-45%, and mean peak plasma concentrations (C_{max}) are reached in approximately 1.6-2.5 hours (T_{max}). The time to maximum plasma concentration following administration of rizatriptan as the oral lyophilisate formulation is delayed by 30-60 minutes relative to the tablet.

Effect of food: The effect of food on the absorption of rizatriptan from the oral lyophilisate has not been studied. For the rizatriptan tablets, T_{max} is delayed by approximately 1 hour when the tablets are administered in the fed state. A further delay in the absorption of rizatriptan may occur when the oral lyophilisate is administered after meals. (See section 4.2).

Distribution

Rizatriptan is minimally bound (14%) to plasma proteins. The volume of distribution is approximately 140 litres in male subjects, and 110 litres in female subjects.

Biotransformation

The primary route of rizatriptan metabolism is via oxidative deamination by monoamine oxidase-A (MAO-A) to the indole acetic acid metabolite, which is not pharmacologically active. N-monodesmethyl-rizatriptan, a metabolite with activity similar to that of parent compound at the $5\text{-}HT_{1B/1D}$ receptors, is formed to a minor degree, but does not contribute significantly to the pharmacodynamic activity of rizatriptan. Plasma concentrations of N-monodesmethyl-rizatriptan are approximately 14% of those of parent compound, and it is eliminated at a similar rate. Other minor metabolites include the N-oxide, the 6-hydroxy compound, and the sulphate conjugate of the 6-hydroxy metabolite. None of these minor metabolites is pharmacologically active. Following oral administration of ^{14}C-labelled rizatriptan, rizatriptan accounts for about 17% of circulating plasma radioactivity.

Elimination

Following intravenous administration, AUC in men increases proportionally and in women near-proportionally with the dose over a dose range of 10-60 µg/kg. Following oral administration, AUC increases near-proportionally with the dose over a dose range of 2.5-10 mg. The plasma half-life of rizatriptan in males and females averages 2-3 hours. The plasma clearance of rizatriptan averages about 1,000-1,500 ml/min in males and about 900-1,100 ml/min in females; about 20-30% of this is renal clearance. Following an oral dose of ^{14}C-labelled rizatriptan, about 80% of the radioactivity is excreted in urine, and about 10% of the dose is excreted in faeces. This shows that the metabolites are excreted primarily via the kidneys.

Consistent with its first pass metabolism, approximately 14% of an oral dose is excreted in urine as unchanged rizatriptan while 51% is excreted as indole acetic acid metabolite. No more than 1% is excreted in urine as the active N-monodesmethyl metabolite.

If rizatriptan is administered according to the maximum dosage regimen, no drug accumulation in the plasma occurs from day to day.

Characteristics in patients

The following data are based on studies with the oral tablet formulation.

Patients with a migraine attack: A migraine attack does not affect the pharmacokinetics of rizatriptan.

Gender: The AUC of rizatriptan (10 mg orally) was about 25% lower in males as compared to females, C_{max} was 11% lower, and T_{max} occurred at approximately the same time. This apparent pharmacokinetic difference was of no clinical significance.

Elderly: The plasma concentrations of rizatriptan observed in elderly subjects (age range 65 to 77 years) after tablet administration were similar to those observed in young adults.

Hepatic impairment (Child-Pugh's score 5-6): Following oral tablet administration in patients with hepatic impairment caused by mild alcoholic cirrhosis of the liver, plasma concentrations of rizatriptan were similar to those seen in young male and female subjects. A significant increase in AUC (50%) and C_{max} (25%) was observed in patients with moderate hepatic impairment (Child-Pugh's score 7). Pharmacokinetics were not studied in patients with Child-Pugh's score >7 (severe hepatic impairment).

Renal impairment: In patients with renal impairment (creatinine clearance 10-60 ml/min/1.73 m^2), the AUC of rizatriptan after tablet administration was not significantly different from that in healthy subjects. In haemodialysis patients (creatinine clearance <10 ml/min/1.73 m^2), the AUC for rizatriptan was approximately 44% greater than that in patients with normal renal function. The maximal plasma concentration of rizatriptan in patients with all degrees of renal impairment was similar to that in healthy subjects.

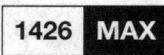

5.3 Preclinical safety data
Preclinical data indicate no risk for humans based on conventional studies of repeat dose toxicity, genotoxicity, carcinogenic potential, reproductive and developmental toxicity, safety pharmacology, and pharmacokinetics and metabolism.

6. PHARMACEUTICAL PARTICULARS
6.1 List of excipients
Tablets: Lactose monohydrate, microcrystalline cellulose (E460a), pregelatinised corn starch, ferric oxide red (E 172), and magnesium stearate (E572).

Oral lyophilisates: Gelatin, mannitol (E421), glycine, aspartame (E951), peppermint flavour and maltodextrin.

6.2 Incompatibilities
Not applicable.

6.3 Shelf life
3 years.

6.4 Special precautions for storage
Do not store above 30°C.

6.5 Nature and contents of container
Maxalt 5 mg and 10 mg tablets: All aluminium blister push through, packs of 2, 3, 6, 12 or 18 tablets.

Maxalt Melt 10 mg tablets: Aluminium/PVC/PVDC blister with one oral lyophilisate within an aluminium sachet. Packs with 2, 3, 6, 12 or 18 oral lyophilisates.

Not all pack sizes may be marketed.

6.6 Special precautions for disposal and other handling
Any unused product or waste material should be disposed of in accordance with local requirements.

7. MARKETING AUTHORISATION HOLDER
Merck Sharp & Dohme Limited
Hertford Road, Hoddesdon, Hertfordshire EN11 9BU, UK

8. MARKETING AUTHORISATION NUMBER(S)

Tablet 5 mg	PL 0025/0369
Tablet 10 mg	PL 0025/0370
Oral lyophilisate 10 mg	PL 0025/0372

9. DATE OF FIRST AUTHORISATION/RENEWAL OF THE AUTHORISATION
Date of first authorisation: June 1998.

Date of last renewal: 11 February 2008.

10. DATE OF REVISION OF THE TEXT
29 October 2008

LEGAL CATEGORY
POM

® denotes registered trademark of Merck & Co., Inc., Whitehouse Station, NJ, USA.

SPC.MXT/M.08.UK.2868 (R2) F.T. 29.10.08

Maxtrex Tablets 10 mg

(Pharmacia Limited)

1. NAME OF THE MEDICINAL PRODUCT
Maxtrex Tablets 10.0 mg

2. QUALITATIVE AND QUANTITATIVE COMPOSITION
Each tablet contains methotrexate Ph. Eur. 10.0 mg.

For excipients, see 6.1.

3. PHARMACEUTICAL FORM
Tablet.

'Capsule-shaped', uncoated, convex deep yellow tablets marked with 'M10' on one side and scored on the other.

4. CLINICAL PARTICULARS
4.1 Therapeutic indications
Methotrexate is a folic acid antagonist and is classified as an antimetabolite cytotoxic agent.

Methotrexate has been used to produce regression in a wide range of neoplastic conditions including acute leukaemias, non-Hodgkin's lymphoma, soft-tissue and osteogenic sarcomas, and solid tumours particularly breast, lung, head and neck, bladder, cervical, ovarian, and testicular carcinoma.

Methotrexate has also been used in the treatment of severe, uncontrolled psoriasis which is not responsive to other therapy.

4.2 Posology and method of administration
Method of Administration: Oral.

Dosage for cancer treatment:

A test dose of 5 - 10 mg parenterally is recommended, one week prior to therapy to detect idiosyncratic adverse events. Single doses, not exceeding 30 mg/m^2, on not more than 5 consecutive days. A rest period of at least two weeks is recommended between treatments, in order to allow the bone marrow to return to normal.

Doses in excess of 100 mg are usually given parenterally, when the injectable preparation should be used. Doses in excess of 70 mg/m^2 should not be administered without leucovorin rescue (folinic acid rescue) or assay of serum methotrexate levels 24 - 48 hours after dosing.

If methotrexate is administered in combination chemotherapy regimens, the dosage should be reduced, taking into consideration any overlapping toxicity of the other drug components.

Dosage for psoriasis:

For the treatment of severe psoriasis 10 - 25 mg orally, once weekly, is recommended. Dosage should be adjusted according to the patient's response and the haematological toxicity.

4.3 Contraindications
Methotrexate is contra-indicated in the presence of severe/significant renal or significant hepatic impairment, liver disease including fibrosis, cirrhosis, recent or active hepatitis; active infectious disease; and overt or laboratory evidence of immunodeficiency syndrome(s) and serious anaemia, leucopenia or thrombocytopenia. Maxtrex should not be used concomitantly with drugs with antifolate properties (see section 4.5, Interactions with other Medicinal Products and other forms of Interaction). Methotrexate is teratogenic and should not be given during pregnancy or to mothers who are breast feeding (see Section 4.6., Pregnancy and Lactation).

Following administration to a man or woman conception should be avoided by using an effective contraceptive method for at least 3 months after using Maxtrex Tablets 10mg (see Section 4.4, Special Warnings and Special Precautions for Use).

Patients with a known allergic hypersensitivity to methotrexate or any of the excipients should not receive methotrexate.

4.4 Special warnings and precautions for use
Methotrexate should be used with extreme caution in patients with haematological depression, renal impairment, diarrhoea, ulcerative disorders of the GI tract and psychiatric disorders. Hepatic toxicity has been observed, usually associated with chronic hepatic disease. Renal lesions may develop if the urinary flow is impeded and urinary pH is low, especially if large doses have been administered.

The administration of low doses of methotrexate for prolonged periods may give rise, in particular, to hepatic toxicity.

Particular care and possible cessation of treatment are indicated if stomatitis or GI toxicity occurs as haemorrhagic enteritis and intestinal perforation may result.

Reversible eosinophilic pulmonary reactions and treatment-resistant, interstitial fibrosis may occur, particularly after long-term treatment.

Liver function should be closely monitored. If hepatic function abnormalities develop, methotrexate dosing should be suspended for at least two weeks. It is only appropriate to restart methotrexate provided the abnormalities return to normal and the re-exposure is deemed appropriate. Renal function should be closely monitored before, during and after treatment. Reduce dose of methotrexate in patients with renal impairment. High doses may cause the precipitation of methotrexate or its metabolites in the renal tubules. A high fluid throughput and alkalinisation of the urine to pH 6.5 – 7 by oral or intravenous administration of sodium bicarbonate (5x625mg tablets every three hours) is recommended as a preventative measure.

Haematopoietic suppression caused by methotrexate may occur abruptly and with apparently safe dosages. Full blood counts should be closely monitored before, during and after treatment. If a clinically significant drop in white cell or platelet count develops, methotrexate therapy should be withdrawn immediately and appropriate supportive therapy given (see section 4.8, Undesirable Effects). Patients should be advised to report all symptoms or signs suggestive of infection.

Malignant lymphomas may occur in patients receiving low dose methotrexate, in which case therapy must be discontinued. Failure of the lymphoma to show signs of spontaneous regression requires the initiation of cytotoxic therapy.

Methotrexate has been shown to be teratogenic; it has been reported to cause foetal death and/or congenital abnormalities. Therefore, it is not recommended in women of childbearing potential unless the benefits can be expected to outweigh the considered risks. If this drug is used during pregnancy for antineoplastic indications, or if the patient becomes pregnant while taking this drug, the patient should be appraised of the potential hazard to the foetus.

Following administration to a man or woman conception should be avoided by using an effective contraceptive method for at least 3 months after using Maxtrex Tablets 10mg (see section 4.3, Contraindications).

Methotrexate has some immunosuppressive activity and therefore the immunological response to concurrent vaccination may be decreased. In addition, concomitant use of a live vaccine could cause severe antigenic reaction.

Methotrexate should only be used by clinicians that are familiar with the various characteristics of the drug and its mode of action. Before beginning methotrexate therapy or reinstituting methotrexate after a rest period, a chest x-ray, assessment of renal function, liver function and blood elements should be made by history, physical examination and laboratory tests. This will include a routine examination of lymph nodes and patients should report any unusual swelling to the doctor.

Patients receiving low-dose methotrexate should:

- Have a full blood count and renal and liver function tests before starting treatment. These should be repeated weekly until therapy is stabilised, thereafter patients should be monitored every 2-3 months throughout treatment.
- Patients should report all symptoms and signs suggestive of infection, especially sore throat.

If acute methotrexate toxicity occurs, patients may require treatment with folinic acid.

The disappearance of methotrexate from plasma should be monitored, if possible. This is recommended in particular when high, or very high doses are administered in order to permit calculation of an adequate dose of leucovorin (folinic acid) rescue.

Patients with pleural effusions and ascites should be drained prior to initiation of methotrexate therapy. A chest x-ray is recommended prior to initiation of methotrexate therapy or treatment should be withdrawn.

Methotrexate given concomitantly with radiotherapy may increase the risk of soft tissue necrosis and osteonecrosis.

Acute or chronic pneumonitis, often associated with blood eosinophilia, may occur and deaths have been reported. Symptoms typically include dyspnoea, cough (especially a dry productive cough) and fever for which patients should be monitored at each follow-up visit. Patients should be informed of the risk of pneumonitis and advised to contact their doctor immediately should they develop persistent cough or dyspnoea.

Methotrexate should be withdrawn from patients with pulmonary symptoms, and a thorough investigation should be made to exclude infection. If methotrexate induced lung disease is suspected, treatment with corticosteroids should be initiated and treatment with methotrexate should not be restarted.

Lung manifestations of RA and other connective tissue disorders are recognised to occur. In patients with RA, the physician should be specifically alerted to the potential for methotrexate induced adverse effects on the pulmonary system.

4.5 Interaction with other medicinal products and other forms of interaction
Methotrexate is immunosuppressive and may therefore reduce immunological response to concurrent vaccination. Severe antigenic reactions may occur if a live vaccine is given concurrently.

Methotrexate is extensively protein bound and may displace, or be displaced by, other acidic drugs. The concurrent administration of agents such as p-aminobenzoic acid, chloramphenicol, diphenylhydantoins, acidic anti-inflammatory agents, salicylates, sulphonamides, tetracyclines, thiazide diuretics, probenicid, sulfinpyrazone or oral hypoglycaemics will decrease the methotrexate transport function of renal tubules, thereby reducing excretion and almost certainly increasing methotrexate toxicity. Methotrexate dosage should be monitored if concomitant treatment with NSAIDs is commenced, as concomitant use of NSAID's has been associated with fatal methotrexate toxicity. Concomitant administration of folate antagonists such as trimethoprim, co-trimoxazole and nitrous oxide should be avoided. Hepatic and nephrotoxic drugs should be avoided.

Acitretin (a treatment for psoriasis) is metabolised to eretinate. Methotrexate levels may be increased by eretinate and severe hepatitis has been reported following concomitant use.

Vitamin preparations containing folic acid or its derivatives may alter response to methotrexate.

4.6 Pregnancy and lactation
Methotrexate is contra-indicated in pregnancy. Methotrexate affects spermatogenesis and oogenesis and may therefore decrease fertility. This effect appears to be reversible after discontinuation of therapy. Patients and their partners should be advised to avoid pregnancy until 3 months after cessation of methotrexate therapy.

Patients should not breast feed whilst taking methotrexate.

Methotrexate causes embryotoxicity, abortion and foetal defects in humans. Therefore, the possible risks of effects on reproduction should be discussed with patients of child bearing potential (see section 4.4, Special Warnings and Special Precautions for Use and section 4.3, Contraindications).

4.7 Effects on ability to drive and use machines
None known.

4.8 Undesirable effects
In general, the incidence and severity of side effects are considered to be dose-related. Adverse reactions for the various systems are as follows:

Skin:

Stevens-Johnson Syndrome, epidermal necrolysis, erythematous rashes, pruritus, urticaria, photosensitivity, pigmentary changes, alopecia, ecchymosis, telangiectasia, acne, furunculosis. Lesions of psoriasis may be aggravated by concomitant exposure to ultraviolet radiation. Skin ulceration in psoriatic patients and rarely painful erosion of psoriatic plaques has been reported. The recall phenomenon has been reported in both radiation and solar damaged skin.

Haematopoietic:

Bone marrow depression is most frequently manifested by leucopenia, thrombocytopenia (which are usually reversible) and anaemia, or any combination may occur. Infection or hypogammaglobulinaemia has been reported.

Alimentary System:

Mucositis (most frequently stomatitis although gingivitis, pharyngitis and even enteritis, intestinal ulceration and bleeding) may occur. In rare cases the effect of Methotrexate on the intestinal mucosa has led to malabsorption or toxic megacolon. Nausea, anorexia and vomiting and/or diarrhoea may also occur.

Hepatic:

Hepatic toxicity resulting in significant elevations of liver enzymes, acute liver atrophy, necrosis, fatty metamorphosis, periportal fibrosis or cirrhosis or death may occur, usually following chronic administration.

Urogenital System:

Renal failure and uraemia may follow methotrexate administration, particularly after high doses or prolonged administration. Vaginitis, vaginal ulcers, cystitis, haematuria and nephropathy have also been reported. Methotrexate can decrease fertility. This effect appears to be reversible after discontinuation of therapy (see section 4.6, Pregnancy and Lactation).

Pulmonary System:

Infrequently an acute or chronic interstitial pneumonitis, often associated with blood eosinophilia, may occur and deaths have been reported. Acute pulmonary oedema has also been reported after oral and intrathecal use. Pulmonary fibrosis is rare. A syndrome consisting of pleuritic pain and pleural thickening has been reported following high doses.

In the treatment of rheumatoid arthritis, methotrexate induced lung disease is a potentially serious adverse drug reaction which may occur acutely at any time during therapy. It is not always fully reversible. Pulmonary symptoms (especially a dry, non productive cough) may require interruption of treatment and careful investigation.

Central Nervous System:

Headaches, drowsiness, ataxia and blurred vision have occurred following low doses of methotrexate, transient subtle cognitive dysfunction, mood alteration, or unusual cranial sensations have been reported occasionally. Aphasia, paresis, hemiparesis, and convulsions have also occurred following administration of higher doses.

There have been reports of leucoencephalopathy following intravenous methotrexate in high doses, or low doses following cranial-spinal radiation.

Other reports include eye irritation, malaise, undue fatigue, vasculitis, sepsis, arthralgia/myalgia, chills and fever, dizziness, loss of libido/impotence and decreased resistance to infection. Also opportunistic infections such as herpes zoster. Osteoporosis, abnormal (usually "megaloblastic") red cell morphology, precipitation of diabetes, other metabolic changes, and sudden death in relation to or attributed to the use of methotrexate.

Although very rare, anaphylactic reactions to methotrexate have been reported.

Acute or chronic interstitial pneumonitis, often associated with blood eosinophila, may occur and deaths have been reported (see Section 4.4, Special Warnings and Special Precautions for Use).

4.9 Overdose

Leucovorin is a specific antidote for methotrexate and, following accidental overdosage, should be administered within one hour at a dosage equal to, or greater than, the methotrexate dose. It may be administered by i.v. bolus or infusion. Further doses may be required. The patient should be observed carefully and blood transfusions, renal dialysis and reverse barrier nursing may be necessary.

In cases of massive overdose, hydration and urinary alkalisation may be necessary to prevent precipitation of methotrexate and/or its metabolites in the renal tubules. Neither haemodialysis nor peritoneal dialysis has been shown to improve methotrexate elimination. Effective clearance of methotrexate has been reported with acute, intermittent haemodialysis using a high flux dialyser.

5. PHARMACOLOGICAL PROPERTIES

5.1 Pharmacodynamic properties

Methotrexate is a folic acid antagonist and its major site of action is the enzyme dihydrofolate reductase. Its main effect is inhibition of DNA synthesis but it also acts directly both on RNA and protein synthesis. Methotrexate is a phase specific substance, the main effect being directed during the S-phase of cell division.

The inhibition of dihydrofolate reductase can be circumvented by the use of leucovorin (folinic acid; citrovorum factor) and protection of normal tissues can be carried out by properly timed administration of leucovorin calcium.

5.2 Pharmacokinetic properties

When given in low doses, methotrexate is rapidly absorbed from the GI tract giving plasma concentrations equivalent to those achieved after i.v. administration. Higher doses are less well absorbed. About 50% has been shown to be protein bound. Biphasic and triphasic plasma clearance has been shown. The majority of the dose is excreted within 24 hours in the urine mainly as unchanged drug.

5.3 Preclinical safety data

No further preclinical safety data are available.

6. PHARMACEUTICAL PARTICULARS

6.1 List of excipients

Maize starch

Lactose

Pregelatinised starch

Polysorbate 80

Microcrystalline cellulose

Magnesium stearate

Purified water

6.2 Incompatibilities

None stated.

6.3 Shelf life

60 months.

6.4 Special precautions for storage

None stated.

6.5 Nature and contents of container

White high density polyethylene container with high density polyethylene screw closure containing 100 tablets.

6.6 Special precautions for disposal and other handling

None.

7. MARKETING AUTHORISATION HOLDER

Pharmacia Limited

Ramsgate Road

Sandwich

Kent

CT13 9NJ

United Kingdom

8. MARKETING AUTHORISATION NUMBER(S)

PL 0032/0342

9. DATE OF FIRST AUTHORISATION/RENEWAL OF THE AUTHORISATION

17 July 2002

10. DATE OF REVISION OF THE TEXT

August 2008

Legal category: POM

Version Number: MX 3_0

Maxtrex Tablets 2.5 mg

(Pharmacia Limited)

1. NAME OF THE MEDICINAL PRODUCT

Maxtrex Tablets 2.5 mg.

2. QUALITATIVE AND QUANTITATIVE COMPOSITION

Each tablet contains methotrexate Ph. Eur. 2.5 mg.

For excipients, see 6.1

3. PHARMACEUTICAL FORM

Round, uncoated, convex deep yellow tablets marked with 'M2.5' on one side.

4. CLINICAL PARTICULARS

4.1 Therapeutic indications

Methotrexate is a folic acid antagonist and is classified as an antimetabolite cytotoxic agent.

Methotrexate is used in the treatment of adults with severe, active, classical or definite rheumatoid arthritis who are unresponsive or intolerant to conventional therapy.

Methotrexate has also been used in the treatment of severe, uncontrolled psoriasis, which is not responsive to other therapy.

Methotrexate has been used to produce regression in a wide range of neoplastic conditions including acute leukaemias, non-Hodgkin's lymphoma, soft-tissue and osteogenic sarcomas, and solid tumours particularly breast, lung, head and neck, bladder, cervical, ovarian, and testicular carcinoma.

4.2 Posology and method of administration

Method of Administration: Oral

Dosage and Administration with reference to Rheumatoid arthritis and Psoriasis

Dosage for Rheumatoid arthritis

Adults:

In adults with severe, active, classical or definite rheumatoid arthritis who are unresponsive or intolerant to conventional therapy 7.5 mg orally once weekly or divided oral doses of 2.5 mg at 12 hour intervals for 3 doses (7.5 mg) as a course once weekly. The schedule may be adjusted gradually to achieve an optimal response but should not exceed a total weekly dose of 20 mg. Once response has been achieved, the schedule should be reduced to the lowest possible effective dose.

Elderly:

Methotrexate should be used with extreme caution in elderly patients, a reduction in dosage should be considered.

Children:

Safety and effectiveness in children have not been established, other than in cancer chemotherapy.

Dosage for psoriasis:

For the treatment of severe psoriasis 10 - 25 mg orally, once weekly, is recommended. Dosage should be adjusted according to the patient's response and the haematological toxicity.

Dosage for cancer treatment:

A test dose of 5 - 10 mg parenterally is recommended, one week prior to therapy to detect idiosyncratic adverse events. Single doses, not exceeding 30 mg/m^2, on not more than 5 consecutive days. A rest period of at least two weeks is recommended between treatments, in order to allow the bone marrow to return to normal.

Doses in excess of 100 mg are usually given parenterally, when the injectable preparation should be used. Doses in excess of 70 mg/m^2 should not be administered without leucovorin rescue (folinic acid rescue) or assay of serum methotrexate levels 24 - 48 hours after dosing.

If methotrexate is administered in combination chemotherapy regimens, the dosage should be reduced, taking into consideration any overlapping toxicity of the other drug components.

4.3 Contraindications

Methotrexate is contra-indicated in the presence of severe/significant renal or significant hepatic impairment. Liver disease including fibrosis, cirrhosis, recent or active hepatitis; active infectious disease; and overt or laboratory evidence of immunodeficiency syndrome(s). Serious cases of anaemia, leucopenia or thrombocytopenia. Maxtrex should not be used concomitantly with drugs with antifolate properties (eg co-trimoxazole). Methotrexate is teratogenic and should not be given during pregnancy or to mothers who are breast feeding.

Following administration to a man or woman conception should be avoided by using an effective contraceptive method for at least 3 months after using Maxtrex Tablets 2.5mg (see section 4.4, Special Warnings).

Patients with a known allergic hypersensitivity to methotrexate should not receive methotrexate.

4.4 Special warnings and precautions for use

Methotrexate should be used with extreme caution in patients with haematological depression, renal impairment, diarrhoea, and ulcerative disorders of the GI tract and psychiatric disorders. Hepatic toxicity has been observed, usually associated with chronic hepatic disease. The administration of low doses of methotrexate for prolonged periods may give rise, in particular, to hepatic toxicity. Liver function should be closely monitored. If hepatic function abnormalities develop, methotrexate dosing should be suspended for at least two weeks. It is only appropriate to restart methotrexate provided the abnormalities return to normal and the re-exposure is deemed appropriate

Particular care and possible cessation of treatment are indicated if stomatitis or GI toxicity occurs as haemorrhagic enteritis and intestinal perforation may result.

Reversible eosinophilic pulmonary reactions and treatment-resistant, interstitial fibrosis may occur, particularly after long-term treatment.

Renal lesions may develop if the urinary flow is impeded and urinary pH is low, especially if large doses have been administered. Renal function should be closely monitored before, during and after treatment. Reduce dose of methotrexate in patients with renal impairment. High doses may cause the precipitation of methotrexate or its metabolites in the renal tubules. A high fluid throughput and alkalinisation of the urine to pH 6.5 – 7 by oral or intravenous administration of sodium bicarbonate (5x625mg tablets every three hours) is recommended as a preventative measure.

Haematopoietic suppression caused by Methotrexate may occur abruptly and with apparently safe dosages. Full blood counts should be closely monitored before, during and after treatment. If a clinically significant drop in white cell or platelet count develops, methotrexate therapy should be withdrawn immediately and appropriate supportive therapy given (see Undesirable Effects section). Patients should be advised to report all symptoms or signs suggestive of infection.

Malignant lymphomas may occur in patients receiving low dose methotrexate, in which case therapy must be discontinued. Failure of the lymphoma to show signs of spontaneous regression requires the initiation of cytotoxic therapy.

Methotrexate has been shown to be teratogenic; it has been reported to cause foetal death and/or congenital abnormalities. Therefore, it is not recommended in women of childbearing potential unless the benefits can be expected to outweigh the considered risks. If this drug is used during pregnancy for antineoplastic indications, or if the patient becomes pregnant while taking this drug, the patient should be appraised of the potential hazard to the foetus.

Following administration to a man or woman conception should be avoided by using an effective contraceptive method for at least 3 months after using Maxtrex Tablets 2.5mg (see section 4.3, Contraindications).

Methotrexate has some immunosuppressive activity and therefore the immunological response to concurrent vaccination may be decreased. In addition, concomitant use of a live vaccine could cause severe antigenic reaction.

Methotrexate should only be used by clinicians that are familiar with the various characteristics of the drug and its mode of action. Before beginning Methotrexate therapy or reinstituting Methotrexate after a rest period, a chest x-ray, assessment of renal function, liver function and blood elements should be made by history, physical examination and laboratory tests. This will include a routine examination of lymph nodes and patients should report any unusual swelling to the doctor.

Patients receiving low-dose methotrexate should:

- Have a full blood count and renal and liver function tests before starting treatment. These should be repeated weekly until therapy is stabilised, thereafter patients should be monitored every 2-3 months throughout treatment.
- Patients should report all symptoms and signs suggestive of infection, especially sore throat.

If acute methotrexate toxicity occurs, patients may require treatment with folinic acid.

The disappearance of methotrexate from plasma should be monitored, if possible. This is recommended in particular when high, or very high doses are administered in order to permit calculation of an adequate dose of leucovorin (folinic acid) rescue.

Patients with pleural effusions and ascites should be drained prior to initiation of methotrexate therapy or treatment should be withdrawn.

When to perform a liver biopsy in rheumatoid arthritis patients has not been established either in terms of a cumulative Methotrexate dose or duration of therapy.

Pleuropulmonary manifestation of rheumatoid arthritis has been reported in the literature. In patients with rheumatoid arthritis, the physician should be specifically alerted to the potential for Methotrexate induced adverse effects in the pulmonary system. Patients should be advised to contact their physicians immediately should they develop a cough or dyspnoea (see Undesirable Effects section).

Methotrexate given concomitantly with radiotherapy may increase the risk of soft tissue necrosis and osteonecrosis.

Acute or chronic interstitial pneumonitis, often associated with blood eosinophilia, may occur and deaths have been reported. Symptoms typically include dyspnoea, cough (especially a dry non-productive cough) and fever for which patients should be monitored at each follow-up visit. Patients should be informed of the risk of pneumonitis and advised to contact their doctor immediately should they develop persistent cough or dyspnoea.

Methotrexate should be withdrawn from patients pulmonary symptoms, and a thorough investigation should be made to exclude infection. If methotrexate induced lung disease is suspected, treatment with corticosteroids should be initiated and treatment with methotrexate should not be restarted.

Lung manifestations of RA and other connective tissue disorders are recognised to occur. In patients with RA, the physician should be specifically alerted to the potential for methotrexate induced adverse effects on the pulmonary system.

4.5 Interaction with other medicinal products and other forms of interaction

Methotrexate is immunosuppressive and may therefore reduce immunological response to concurrent vaccination. Severe antigenic reactions may occur if a live vaccine is given concurrently.

Methotrexate is extensively protein bound and may displace, or be displaced by, other acidic drugs. The concurrent administration of agents such as p-aminobenzoic acid, chloramphenicol, diphenylhydantoins, acidic anti-inflammatory agents, salicylates, sulphonamides, tetracyclines, thiazide diuretics, probenicid or sulfinpyrazone or oral hypoglycaemics will decrease the methotrexate transport function of renal tubules, thereby reducing excretion and almost certainly increasing methotrexate toxicity. Methotrexate dosage should be monitored if concomitant treatment with NSAID's is commenced, as concomitant use of NSAID's has been associated with fatal methotrexate toxicity. Concomitant administration of folate antagonists such as trimethoprim, cotrimoxazole and nitrous oxide should be avoided. Hepatic and nephrotoxic drugs should be avoided.

Acitretin (a treatment for psoriasis) is metabolised to eretinate. Methotrexate levels may be increased by eretinate and severe hepatitis has been reported following concomitant use.

Vitamin preparations containing folic acid or its derivatives may alter response to Methotrexate.

4.6 Pregnancy and lactation

Methotrexate is contra-indicated in pregnancy. Methotrexate affects spermatogenesis and oogenesis and may therefore decrease fertility. This effect appears to be reversible after discontinuation of therapy. Patients and their partners should be advised to avoid pregnancy until 3 months after cessation of methotrexate therapy.

Patients should not breast feed whilst taking methotrexate.

Methotrexate causes embryotoxicity, abortion and foetal defects in humans. Therefore, the possible risks of effects on reproduction should be discussed with patients of child bearing potential (see Special Warnings sections).

4.7 Effects on ability to drive and use machines

None known.

4.8 Undesirable effects

In general, the incidence and severity of side effects are considered to be dose-related. Adverse reactions for the various systems are as follows:

Skin:

Stevens-Johnson Syndrome, epidermal necrolysis, erythematous rashes, pruritus, urticaria, photosensitivity, pigmentary changes, alopecia, ecchymosis, telangiectasia, acne, furunculosis. Lesions of psoriasis may be aggravated by concomitant exposure to ultraviolet radiation. Skin ulceration in psoriatic patients and rarely painful erosion of psoriatic plaques has been reported. The recall phenomenon has been reported in both radiation and solar damaged skin.

Haematopoietic:

Bone marrow depression is most frequently manifested by leucopenia, thrombocytopenia (which are usually reversible) and anaemia, or any combination may occur. Infection or Hypogammaglobulinaemia has been reported.

Alimentary System:

Mucositis (most frequently stomatitis although gingivitis, pharyngitis and even enteritis, intestinal ulceration and bleeding) may occur. In rare cases the effect of Methotrexate on the intestinal mucosa has led to malabsorption or toxic megacolon. Nausea, anorexia and vomiting and/or diarrhoea may also occur.

Hepatic:

Hepatic toxicity resulting in significant elevations of liver enzymes, acute liver atrophy, necrosis, fatty metamorphosis, periportal fibrosis or cirrhosis or death may occur, usually following chronic administration.

Urogenital System:

Renal failure and uraemia may follow Methotrexate administration, particularly after high doses or prolonged administration. Vaginitis, vaginal ulcers, cystitis, haematuria and nephropathy have also been reported. Methotrexate can decrease fertility. This effect appears to be reversible after discontinuation of therapy (see Pregnancy and Lactation section).

Pulmonary System:

Infrequently an acute or chronic interstitial pneumonitis, often associated with blood eosinophilia, may occur and deaths have been reported. Acute pulmonary oedema has also been reported after oral and intrathecal use. Pulmonary fibrosis is rare. A syndrome consisting of pleuritic pain and pleural thickening has been reported following high doses.

In the treatment of rheumatoid arthritis, Methotrexate induced lung disease is a potentially serious adverse drug reaction which may occur acutely at any time during therapy. It is not always fully reversible. Pulmonary symptoms (especially a dry, non productive cough) may require interruption of treatment and careful investigation.

Acute or chronic interstitial pneumonitis, often associated with blood eosinophilia, may occur and deaths have been reported (see Section 4.4 Warnings and Precautions for Use).

Central Nervous System:

Headaches, drowsiness, ataxia and blurred vision have occurred following low doses of Methotrexate, transient subtle cognitive dysfunction, mood alteration, or unusual cranial sensations have been reported occasionally. Aphasia, paresis, hemiparesis, and convulsions have also occurred following administration of higher doses.

There have been reports of leucoencephalopathy following intravenous Methotrexate in high doses, or low doses following cranial-spinal radiation.

Other reports include eye irritation, malaise, undue fatigue, vasculitis, sepsis, arthralgia/myalgia, chills and fever, dizziness, loss of libido/impotence and decreased resistance to infection. Also opportunistic infections such as herpes zoster. Osteoporosis, abnormal (usually "megaloblastic") red cell morphology, precipitation of diabetes, other metabolic changes, and sudden death in relation to or attributed to the use of Methotrexate.

Although very rare, anaphylactic reactions to methotrexate have been reported.

4.9 Overdose

Leucovorin is a specific antidote for methotrexate and, following accidental overdosage, should be administered within one hour at a dosage equal to, or greater than, the methotrexate dose. It may be administered by i.v. bolus or infusion. Further doses may be required. The patient should be observed carefully and blood transfusions, renal dialysis and reverse barrier nursing may be necessary.

In cases of massive overdose, hydration and urinary alkalisation may be necessary to prevent precipitation of methotrexate and/or its metabolites in the renal tubules. Neither haemodialysis nor peritoneal dialysis has been shown to improve methotrexate elimination. Effective clearance of methotrexate has been reported with acute, intermittent haemodialysis using a high flux dialyser.

5. PHARMACOLOGICAL PROPERTIES

5.1 Pharmacodynamic properties

Methotrexate is a folic acid antagonist and its major site of action is the enzyme dihydrofolate reductase. Its main effect is inhibition of DNA synthesis but it also acts directly both on RNA and protein synthesis. Methotrexate is a phase specific substance, the main effect being directed during the S-phase of cell division.

The inhibition of dihydrofolate reductase can be circumvented by the use of leucovorin (folinic acid; citrovorum factor) and protection of normal tissues can be carried out by properly timed administration of leucovorin calcium.

5.2 Pharmacokinetic properties

When given in low doses, methotrexate is rapidly absorbed from the GI tract giving plasma concentrations equivalent to those achieved after i.v. administration. Higher doses are less well absorbed. About 50% has been shown to be protein bound. Biphasic and triphasic plasma clearance has been shown. The majority of the dose is excreted within 24 hours in the urine mainly as unchanged drug.

5.3 Preclinical safety data

No further preclinical safety data are available.

6. PHARMACEUTICAL PARTICULARS

6.1 List of excipients

Maize starch

Lactose

Pregelatinised starch

Polysorbate 80

Microcrystalline cellulose

Magnesium stearate

Purified water

6.2 Incompatibilities

None stated.

6.3 Shelf life

60 months.

6.4 Special precautions for storage

None.

6.5 Nature and contents of container

White high density polyethylene container with high density polyethylene screw closure.

Pack size: 100 tablets

6.6 Special precautions for disposal and other handling

None stated.

Administrative Data

7. MARKETING AUTHORISATION HOLDER

Pharmacia Limited

Ramsgate Road

Sandwich

Kent

CT13 9NJ

UK

8. MARKETING AUTHORISATION NUMBER(S)

PL 00032/0343

9. DATE OF FIRST AUTHORISATION/RENEWAL OF THE AUTHORISATION

13/08/2002

10. DATE OF REVISION OF THE TEXT

August 2008

Legal Category: **POM**

Version Number: **MX 3_0**

Medac Disodium Pamidronate 3 mg/ml, sterile concentrate

(medac GmbH)

1. NAME OF THE MEDICINAL PRODUCT

Medac Disodium Pamidronate 3 mg/ml, sterile concentrate

2. QUALITATIVE AND QUANTITATIVE COMPOSITION

Each ml sterile concentrate contains 3 mg pamidronate disodium as pamidronic acid 2.527 mg.

1 vial with 5 ml sterile concentrate contains 15 mg pamidronate disodium.

1 vial with 10 ml sterile concentrate contains 30 mg pamidronate disodium.

1 vial with 20 ml sterile concentrate contains 60 mg pamidronate disodium.

1 vial with 30 ml sterile concentrate contains 90 mg pamidronate disodium.

For a full list of excipients, see section 6.1.

3. PHARMACEUTICAL FORM

Sterile concentrate.

Clear and colourless solution, free from visible particles.

4. CLINICAL PARTICULARS

4.1 Therapeutic indications

Treatment of conditions associated with increased osteoclast activity:

– Tumour-induced hypercalcaemia

– Osteolytic lesions in patients with bone metastases associated with breast cancer

– Multiple myeloma stage III

4.2 Posology and method of administration

Medac Disodium Pamidronate 3 mg/ml is a sterile concentrate and must therefore always be diluted in a calcium-free infusion solution (0.9 % sodium chloride or 5 % glucose) before use. The resulting solution must be infused slowly (see also section 4.4).

For information concerning compatibility with infusion solutions, see section 6.6.

The infusion rate should never exceed 60 mg/hour (1 mg/min), and the concentration of pamidronate disodium in the infusion solution should not exceed 90 mg/250 ml. A dose of 90 mg must usually be administered as a 2 hour infusion in a 250 ml solution for infusion. In patients with multiple myeloma and patients with tumour induced hypercalcaemia, it is recommended that the infusion rate does not exceed 90 mg in 500 ml over 4 hours. In order to minimise local reactions at the infusion site, the cannula should be inserted carefully into a relatively large vein.

Pamidronate disodium should be given under the supervision of a physician with the facilities to monitor the clinical and biochemical effects.

Children and adolescents (< 18 years):

There is not enough clinical experience available for the use of pamidronate disodium in children and adolescents (< 18 years) (see section 4.4).

Use only freshly prepared and clear dilutions!

Tumour-induced hypercalcaemia:

It is recommended that patients be rehydrated with 0.9% w/v sodium chloride solution before or and during treatment (see section 4.4).

The total dose of pamidronate disodium to be used for a treatment course depends on the patient's initial serum calcium levels. The following guidelines are derived from clinical data on uncorrected calcium values. However, doses within the ranges given are also applicable for calcium values corrected for serum protein or albumin in rehydrated patients.

(see Table 1 below)

The total dose of pamidronate disodium may be administered either in a single infusion or in multiple infusions over 2-4 consecutive days. The maximum dose per treatment course is 90 mg for both initial and repeat courses.

Higher doses did not improve clinical response.

A significant decrease in serum calcium is generally observed 24-48 hours after administration of pamidronate disodium, and normalisation is usually achieved within 3 to 7 days. If normocalcaemia is not achieved within this time, a further dose may be given. The duration of the response may vary from patient to patient, and treatment can be repeated whenever hypercalcaemia recurs. Clinical experience to date suggests that pamidronate disodium may become less effective as the number of treatments increases.

Osteolytic lesions in multiple myeloma:

The recommended dose is 90 mg every 4 weeks.

Osteolytic lesions in bone metastases associated with breast cancer:

The recommended dose is 90 mg every 4 weeks. This dose may also be administered at 3 weekly intervals to coincide with chemotherapy if desired.

Treatment should be continued until there is evidence of a substantial decrease in a patient's general performance status.

(see Table 2 below)

Renal Impairment:

Medac Disodium Pamidronate 3 mg/ml should not be administered to patients with severe renal impairment (creatinine clearance < 30 ml/min) unless in case of life-threatening tumour induced hypercalcaemia where the benefit outweighs the potential risk (see also section 4.4 and 5.2).

Dose adjustment is not necessary in mild (creatinine clearance 61-90 ml/min) to moderate renal impairment (creatinine clearance 30-60 ml/min). In such patients, the infusion rate should not exceed 90 mg/4h (approximately 20-22 mg/h).

As with other intravenous bisphosphonates, monitoring of renal function is recommended, for instance, measurements of serum creatinine prior to each dose of pamidronate disodium. In patients receiving pamidronate disodium for bone metastases who show evidence of deterioration in renal function, treatment with pamidronate disodium should be withheld until renal function returns to within 10 % of the baseline value.

Liver impairment:

There are no published data for the use of pamidronate disodium in patients with hepatic impairment available. Therefore no specific recommendations can be given for Pamidronate disodium in such patients (see section 5.2).

4.3 Contraindications

Known or suspected hypersensitivity to pamidronate disodium or other bisphosphonates or to any of the excipients.

Breast feeding is contra-indicated (see also section 4.6).

4.4 Special warnings and precautions for use

Warnings

Medac Disodium Pamidronate 3 mg/ml is a sterile concentrate and must therefore always be diluted and then given as a slow intravenous infusion (see section 4.2). Medac Disodium Pamidronate 3 mg/ml should be given only as an intravenous infusion.

The medicinal product contains 0.65 mmol sodium per maximum dose (90 mg). To be taken into consideration by patients on a controlled sodium diet.

Do not co-administer Medac Disodium Pamidronate 3 mg/ml with other bisphosphonates. If other calcium lowering agents are used in conjunction with pamidronate disodium, significant hypocalcaemia may result.

Convulsions have been occurred in some patients with tumour-induced hypercalcaemia due to electrolyte changes associated with this condition and its effective treatment.

Precautions

Serum electrolytes, calcium and phosphate should be monitored following initiation of therapy with Medac Disodium Pamidronate 3 mg/ml. Patients with anaemia, leukopenia or thrombocytopenia should have regular haematology assessments.

Patients who have undergone thyroid surgery may be particularly susceptible to develop hypocalcaemia due to relative hypoparathyroidism.

Although pamidronate is excreted unchanged by the kidneys, the medicinal product has been used without apparent increase in adverse effects in patients with significantly elevated plasma creatinine levels (including patients undergoing renal replacement therapy with both haemodialysis and peritoneal dialysis). However, experience with pamidronate disodium in patients with severe renal impairment (serum creatinine >440 micromol/l, or 5 mg/dl in TIH [Tumour-induced hypercalcaemia] patients; 180 micromol/l, or 2 mg/dl in multiple myeloma patients) is limited. If clinical judgement determines that the potential benefits outweigh the risk in such cases, Medac Disodium Pamidronate 3 mg/ml should be used cautiously and renal function carefully monitored.

Fluid balance (urine output, daily weights) should also be followed carefully. There is very little experience of the use of pamidronate disodium in patients receiving haemodialysis.

No specific recommendation on patients with severe liver impairment can be given as there are no clinical data available.

Patients should have standard laboratory (serum creatinine and BUN [blood urea nitrogen]) and clinical renal function parameters periodically evaluated, especially those receiving frequent pamidronate disodium infusions over a prolonged period of time, and those with pre-existing renal disease or a predisposition to renal impairment (e.g. patients with multiple myeloma and/or tumour-induced hypercalcaemia). If there is deterioration of renal function during pamidronate therapy, the infusion must be stopped. Deterioration of renal function (including renal failure) has been reported following long-term treatment with pamidronate disodium in patients with multiple myeloma. However, underlying disease progression and/or concomitant complications were also present and therefore a causal relationship with pamidronate disodium is unproven.

It is essential in the initial treatment of tumour induced hypercalcaemia that intravenous rehydration be instituted to restore urine output. Patients should be hydrated adequately throughout treatment but overhydration must be avoided. In patients with cardiac disease, especially in the elderly, additional saline overload may precipitate cardiac failure (left ventricular failure or congestive heart failure). Fever (influenza-like symptoms) may also contribute to this deterioration.

The safety and efficacy of pamidronate disodium in children and adolescents (< 18 years) has not been established.

Osteonecrosis of the jaw

Osteonecrosis of the jaw has been reported in patients with cancer receiving treatment regimens including Pamidronate. Osteonecrosis of the jaw has multiple well documented risk factors including cancer, concomitant therapies (e.g., chemotherapy, radiotherapy, corticosteroids) and co-morbid conditions (e.g., anemia, coagulopathies, infection, pre-existing oral disease).

The majority of reported cases have been associated with dental procedures such as tooth extraction. Many of these patients were also receiving chemotherapy or corticosteroids and had signs of local infection including osteomyelitis.

A dental examination with appropriate advice should be considered prior to treatment with Pamidronate.

While on treatment, these patients should avoid invasive dental procedures if possible. For patients who develop osteonecrosis of the jaw while on Pamidronate therapy, dental surgery may exacerbate the condition. For patients requiring dental procedures, there are no data available to suggest whether discontinuation of Pamidronate treatment reduces the risk of osteonecrosis of the jaw. Clinical judgement of the treating physician should guide the management plan of each patient based on individual benefit/risk assessment.

4.5 Interaction with other medicinal products and other forms of interaction

Pamidronate disodium has been administered concomitantly with commonly used anti-tumour medicinal products without significant interactions.

Medac Disodium Pamidronate 3 mg/ml should not be used concomitantly with other bisphosphonates (see also section 4.4).

Concomitant use of other bisphosphonates, other antihypercalcaemic agents and calcitonin may lead to hypocalcaemia with associated clinical symptoms (paraesthesia, tetany, hypotension).

In patients with severe hypercalcaemia, pamidronate disodium has been successfully combined with both calcitonin and mithramycin to accelerate and potentiate the calcium lowering effect.

Caution is warranted when pamidronate disodium is used with other potentially nephrotoxic medicinal products.

4.6 Pregnancy and lactation

Use in pregnancy:

There are no adequate data from the use of pamidronate disodium in pregnant women. There is no unequivocal evidence for teratogenicity in animal studies. Pamidronate may pose a risk to the foetus/newborn child through its pharmacological action on calcium homeostasis. When administered during the whole period of gestation in animals, pamidronate can cause bone mineralization disorder especially of long bones resulting in angular distortion.

Table 1

Initial plasma calcium level		Recommended total dose of pamidronate disodium	Concentration of solution for infusion	Maximum infusion rate
(mmol/l)	(mg %) (mg/100ml)	(mg)	mg/ml	mg/h
< 3.0	< 12.0	15-30	30/125	22,5
3.0-3.5	12.0-14.0	30-60	30/125 60/250	22,5
3.5-4.0	14.0-16.0	60-90	60/250 90/500	22,5
> 4.0	>16.0	90	90/500	22,5

Table 2

Indication	Treatment scheme	Solution for infusion (mg/ml	Infusion rate (mg/h)
Bone metastases Multiple Myeloma	90 mg/2h every 4 weeks 90 mg/4h every 4 weeks	90/ 250 90/ 500	45 22,5

The potential risk for humans is unknown. Therefore, pamidronate disodium should not be used during pregnancy except in cases of life-threatening hypercalcaemia.

Use in lactation:

It is unknown whether Medac Disodium Pamidronate 3 mg/ml is excreted in human breast milk. Animal studies have shown excretion of pamidronate disodium in breast milk and a risk to the breast-fed child cannot be excluded.

Therefore, breast-feeding is contraindicated in women treated with pamidronate disodium (see also section 4.3).

4.7 Effects on ability to drive and use machines

Pamidronate disodium has minor or moderate influence on the ability to drive and use machines.

Patients should be warned that in rare cases somnolence and/or dizziness may occur following pamidronate disodium infusion, in which case they should not drive, operate potentially dangerous machinery, or engage in other activities that may be hazardous because of decreased alertness.

4.8 Undesirable effects

Adverse reactions to pamidronate disodium are usually mild and transient. The most common (>1/10) symptomatic adverse reactions are influenza-like symptoms and mild fever. This mild fever (an increase in body temperature of 1-2 °C) usually occurs within the first 48 hours as a first-dose, dose-related, self-limiting reaction, often without further concomitant symptoms, and usually lasts no longer than 24 hours.

Acute "influenza-like" reactions usually occur only with the first pamidronate infusion. Local soft tissue inflammation at the infusion site occurs commonly (>1/100, <1/10), especially at the highest dose.

Osteonecrosis primarily involving the jaws has been reported rarely (see 4.4. "Precautions").

Symptomatic hypocalcaemia is very rare (<1/10,000).

When the effects of zoledronate (4 mg) and pamidronate (90 mg) were compared in one clinical trial, the number of atrial fibrillation adverse events was higher in the pamidronate group (12/556, 2.2%) than in the zoledronate group (3/563, 0.5%). Previously, it has been observed in a clinical trial, investigating patients with postmenopausal osteoporosis, that zoledronic acid treated patients (5 mg) had an increased rate of atrial fibrillation serious adverse events compared to placebo (1.3% compared to 0.6%). The mechanism behind the increased incidence of atrial fibrillation in association with zoledronic acid and pamidronate treatment is unknown.

Frequency estimate:

Very common (>1/10)

Common (>1/100, <1/10)

Uncommon (>1/1,000, <1/100)

Rare (>1/10,000, <1/1,000)

Very rare (<1/10,000), including isolated reports

Not known (cannot be estimated from the available data)

(see Table 3 below)

Many of the above listed undesirable effects may have been related to the underlying disease.

4.9 Overdose

Patients who have received doses higher than those recommended should be carefully monitored. In the event of clinically significant hypocalcaemia with paraesthesia, tetany and hypotension, reversal may be achieved with an infusion of calcium gluconate. Acute hypocalcaemia is not expected to occur with pamidronate since plasma calcium levels fall progressively for several days after treatment.

There is no available information for overdose of pamidronate disodium.

5. PHARMACOLOGICAL PROPERTIES

5.1 Pharmacodynamic properties

Pharmacotherapeutic group: Medicinal products affecting bone structure and mineralisation, Bisphosphonates

ATC: M05 BA 03

Pamidronate disodium, active substance of Medac Disodium Pamidronate 3 mg/ml, is a potent inhibitor of osteoclastic bone resorption. It binds strongly to hydroxyapatite crystals and inhibits the formation and dissolution of these crystals in vitro. Inhibition of osteoclastic bone resorption in vivo may be at least partly due to binding of the medicinal product to the bone mineral.

Pamidronate suppresses the accession of osteoclast precursors onto the bone and the so induced transformation to mature absorbing osteoclasts. However, the local and direct antiresorptive effect of bone-bound biphosphonate appears to be the predominant mode of action *in vitro* and *in vivo*.

Experimental studies have demonstrated that pamidronate inhibits tumour-induced osteolysis when given prior to or at the time of inoculation or transplantation with tumour cells. Biochemical changes reflecting the inhibitory effect of pamidronate disodium on tumour-induced hypercalcaemia, are characterised by a decrease in serum calcium and phosphate and secondarily by decreases in urinary excretion of calcium, phosphate and hydroxyproline. A dose of 90mg achieves normocalcaemia in more than 90% of patients.

The normalisation of the plasma-calcium-level can also normalise the plasma-parathyroid-hormon-level in adequately rehydrated patients.

Serum levels of parathyroid hormone-related protein (PTHrP) inversely correlate with response to pamidronate. Medicinal products that inhibit tubular reabsorption of calcium or PTHrP secretion may help in patients who do not respond to pamidronate.

Hypercalcaemia can lead to a depletion in the volume of extracellular fluid and a reduction in the glomerular filtration rate (GFR). By controlling hypercalcaemia, pamidronate disodium improves GFR and lowers elevated serum creatinine levels in most patients.

When used in addition to systemic antineoplastic therapy pamidronate reduces skeletal complications of non-vertebral fracture, radiotherapy / surgery for bone complications and increases the time to first skeletal event.

Pamidronate may also reduce bone pain in about 50% women with advanced breast cancer and clinically evident bone metastases. In women with abnormal bone scans but normal plain radiographs pain should be the primary guide to treatment.

Pamidronate has been shown to reduce pain, decrease the number of pathological fractures and the need for radiotherapy, correct hypercalcaemia and improve Quality of Life in patients with advanced multiple myeloma.

A meta-analysis of bisphosphonates in >1100 patients with multiple myeloma showed the NNT (number of patients needed to treat) to prevent one vertebral fracture was 10 and NNT to prevent one patient experiencing pain was 11 with best effects seen with pamidronate and clodronate.

5.2 Pharmacokinetic properties

General characteristics:

Pamidronate has a strong affinity for calcified tissues, and total elimination of pamidronate from the body is not observed within the time-frame of experimental studies. Calcified tissues are therefore regarded as site of "apparent elimination".

Absorption:

Pamidronate disodium is given by intravenous infusion. By definition, absorption is complete at the end of the infusion.

Distribution:

Plasma concentrations of pamidronate rise rapidly after the start of an infusion and fall rapidly when the infusion is stopped. The apparent distribution half-life in plasma is about 0.8 hours. Apparent steady-state concentrations are therefore achieved with infusions of more than about 2-3 hours duration. Peak plasma pamidronate concentrations of about 10 nmol/ml are achieved after an intravenous infusion of 60 mg given over 1 hour.

A similar percentage (approximately 50%) of the dose is retained in the body after administration of different doses (30-90 mg) of pamidronate disodium independent of infusion time (4 or 24 hours) Thus the accumulation of pamidronate in bone is not capacity-limited, and is dependent solely on the total cumulative dose administered. The percentage of circulating pamidronate bound to plasma proteins is relatively low (less than 50 %) and increases when calcium concentrations are pathologically elevated.

Elimination:

Pamidronate does not appear to be eliminated by biotransformation. After an intravenous infusion, about 20-55 % of the dose is recovered in the urine within 72 hours as unchanged pamidronate. Within the time-frame of experimental studies the remaining fraction of the dose is retained in the body. From the urinary elimination of pamidronate, two decay phases with apparent half-lives of about 1.6 and 27 hours, can be observed. The total plasma and renal clearance has been reported to be 88-254 ml/min and 38-60 ml/min, respectively. The apparent plasma clearance is about 180 ml/min. The apparent renal clearance is about 54 ml/min, and there is a tendency for the renal clearance to correlate with creatinine clearance.

Characteristics in patients:

Hepatic and metabolic clearance of pamidronate are insignificant. Impairment of liver function is therefore not expected to influence the pharmacokinetics of pamidronate disodium, although as there are no clinical data available in patients with severe liver impairment, no specific recommendations can be given for this patient population. Medac Disodium Pamidronate 3 mg/ml displays little potential for drug-drug interactions both at the metabolic level and at the level of protein binding (see section 5.2 above).

A pharmacokinetic study conducted in patients with cancer showed no differences in plasma AUC of pamidronate between patients with normal renal function and patients with mild to moderate renal impairment. In patients with severe renal impairment (creatinine clearance < 30 ml/min), the AUC of pamidronate was approximately 3 times higher than in patients with normal renal function (creatinine clearance > 90 ml/min).

5.3 Preclinical safety data

In pregnant rats, pamidronate has been shown to cross the placenta and accumulate in foetal bone in a manner similar

Table 3

Blood and lymphatic system disorders	Common (>1/100, <1/10) Lymphopenia Uncommon (>1/1,000, <1/100) Anaemia, leukopenia Very rare (<1/10,000), including isolated reports Thrombocytopenia
Immune system disorders	Uncommon (>1/1,000, <1/100) Hypersensitivity including anaphylactic reactions, bronchospasm, dyspnoea, angioneurotic oedema Very rare (<1/10,000), including isolated reports Anaphylactic shock, reactivation of herpes simplex and herpes zoster
Metabolism and nutrition disorders	Very common (>1/10) Hypocalcaemia, hypophosphataemia Common (>1/100, <1/10) Hypomagnesaemia Uncommon (>1/1,000, <1/100) Hyperkalaemia, hypokalaemia, hypernatraemia Very rare (<1/10,000), including isolated reports Hypernatraemia with confusional state
Nervous system disorders	Common (>1/100, <1/10) Headache Uncommon (>1/1,000, <1/100) Agitation, confusional state, dizziness, insomnia, somnolence, lethargy Very rare (<1/10,000), including isolated reports Seizures, visual hallucinations, symptomatic hypocalcaemia (paraesthesia, tetany, muscle cramps)
Eye disorders	Uncommon (>1/1,000, <1/100) Uveitis (iritis, iridocyclitis), scleritis, episcleritis, conjunctivitis, Very rare (<1/10,000), including isolated reports Xanthopsia, orbital inflammation
Cardiac disorders / Vascular disorders	Uncommon (>1/1,000, <1/100) Hypertension Very rare (<1/10,000), including isolated reports Hypotension, heart disease aggravated (left ventricular failure / congestive cardial failure) with dyspnoea, pulmonary oedema due to fluid overload Not known (cannot be estimated from the available data) Atrial fibrillation
Gastrointestinal disorders	Common (>1/100, <1/10) Nausea, vomiting Uncommon (>1/1,000, <1/100) Abdominal pain, anorexia, diarrhoea, constipation, dyspepsia Very rare (<1/10,000), including isolated reports Gastritis
Skin and subcutaneous tissue disorders	Uncommon (>1/1,000, <1/100) Rash, pruritus
Musculoskeletal and connective tissue disorders	Common (>1/100, <1/10) Transient bone pain, arthralgia, myalgia Uncommon (>1/1,000, <1/100) Muscle cramp Rare (>1/10,000, <1/1,000) Osteonecrosis primarily involving the jaws
Renal and urinary disorders	Rare (>1/10,000, <1/1,000) Focal segmental glomerulosclerosis including the collapsing variant, nephrotic syndrome, renal tubular disorder, glomerulonephropathy, tubulointerstitial nephritis Very rare (<1/10,000), including isolated reports Renal function aggravated in patients with multiple myeloma, haematuria, renal failure acute, renal function aggravated in patients with pre-existing renal disease.
General disorders and administration site conditions	Very common (>1/10) Fever and influenza like symptoms sometimes accompanied by malaise, rigors, fatigue and flushing Common (>1/100, <1/10) Infusion site reactions like infusion site pain, infusion site rash, infusion site swelling, infusion site induration, infusion site phlebitis, thrombophlebitis, general body pain
Investigations	Very rare (<1/10,000), including isolated reports Liver function test abnormal, blood creatinine increased, blood urea increased

to that observed in adult animals. Pamidronate disodium has been shown to increase the length of gestation and parturition in rats resulting in an increasing pup mortality when given orally at daily doses of 60 mg/kg (approximately equivalent to 1.2 mg/kg intravenously) and above (0.7 times the highest recommended human dose for a single intravenous infusion).

There was no unequivocal evidence for teratogenicity in studies with intravenous administration of pamidronate disodium to pregnant rats, although high doses (12 and 15 mg/kg/day) were associated with maternal toxicity and foetal developmental abnormalities (foetal oedema and shortened bones) and doses of 6 mg/kg and above with reduced ossification. Lower intravenous pamidronate disodium doses (1-6 mg/kg/day) interfered (pre-partum distress and fetotoxicity) with normal parturition in the rat. These effects: foetal developmental abnormalities, prolonged parturition and reduced survival rate of pups were probably caused by a decrease in maternal serum calcium levels.

Only low intravenous doses have been investigated in pregnant rabbits, because of maternal toxicity, but the highest dose used (1.5 mg/kg/day) was associated with an increased resorption rate and reduced ossification. However there was no evidence for teratogenicity.

The toxicity of pamidronate is characterised by direct (cytotoxic) effects on organs with a copious blood supply such as the stomach, lungs and kidneys. In animal studies with intravenous administration, renal tubular lesions were the prominent and consistent untoward effects of treatment.

Carcinogenesis and Mutagenesis:

Pamidronate disodium by daily oral administration was not carcinogenic in an 80 week or a 104 week study in mice.

Pamidronate disodium showed no genotoxic activity in a standard battery of assays for gene mutations and chromosomal damage.

6. PHARMACEUTICAL PARTICULARS

6.1 List of excipients

Sodium hydroxide (for pH adjustment)

Hydrochloric acid (for pH adjustment)

Water for Injections

6.2 Incompatibilities

Pamidronate will form complexes with divalent cations and should not be added to calcium-containing intravenous solutions.

The medicinal product should not be mixed with other products except those mentioned in section 6.6.

Solutions of pamidronate disodium are not soluble in lipophilic nutrition solutions, e. g. soya-bean oil.

6.3 Shelf life

Unopened vial: 4 years

Shelf life after dilution in 5 % glucose solution or in 0,9 % sodium chloride solution:

chemical and physical in-use stability has been demonstrated for 96 hours at 25°C.

From a microbiological point of view, the product should be used immediately. If not used immediately, in use storage times and conditions prior to use are the responsibility of the user and would normally not be longer than 24 hours at 2 to 8°C, unless dilution has taken place in controlled and validated aseptic conditions.

6.4 Special precautions for storage

This medicinal product does not require any special storage conditions.

6.5 Nature and contents of container

Colourless 5 ml/10 ml/20 ml/30 ml glass vials (Ph. Eur., Type 1) and bromobutylrubber stoppers (Ph. Eur., Type 1).

Pack sizes:

1, 4 or 10 vials containing 5 ml sterile concentrate

1, 4 or 10 vials containing 10 ml sterile concentrate

1, 4 or 10 vials containing 20 ml sterile concentrate

1, 4 or 10 vials containing 30 ml sterile concentrate

Not all pack sizes may be marketed.

6.6 Special precautions for disposal and other handling

Must be diluted with 5% glucose solution or 0.9% sodium chloride solution prior to administration.

The concentration of pamidronate disodium in the infusion solution should not exceed 90 mg/250 ml.

Do not use solution if particles are present.

Any portion of the contents remaining after use should be discarded.

Medac Disodium Pamidronate 3 mg/ml, sterile concentrate is for single use only.

The diluted solution for infusion should be visually inspected and only clear solutions practically free from particles should be used.

7. MARKETING AUTHORISATION HOLDER

medac

Gesellschaft für klinische Spezialpraeparate mbH

Fehlandtstraβe 3

D-20354 Hamburg

8. MARKETING AUTHORISATION NUMBER(S)

PL 11587/0027

9. DATE OF FIRST AUTHORISATION/RENEWAL OF THE AUTHORISATION

2004-09-07

10. DATE OF REVISION OF THE TEXT

2009-01-22

MEDIJEL GEL

(DDD Limited)

1. NAME OF THE MEDICINAL PRODUCT

MEDIJEL GEL

2. QUALITATIVE AND QUANTITATIVE COMPOSITION

Lidocaine Hydrochloride BP 0.66% w/w

Aminoacridine Hydrochloride BP 1968 0.05% w/w

3. PHARMACEUTICAL FORM

Oral Gel

4. CLINICAL PARTICULARS

4.1 Therapeutic indications

The quick, effective relief from the pain of common mouth ulcers, soreness of gums and denture rubbing. Medijel Gel is administered directly onto the affected area with a clean finger or small pad of cotton wool.

4.2 Posology and method of administration

The gel should be applied directly to the affected area(s) with a clean finger or small pad of cotton wool. If necessary application may be repeated after 20 minutes.

Each dose is approximately 300mg, i.e. 2mg of Lidocaine Hydrochloride and 0.15mg of Aminoacridine Hydrochloride. Medijel Gel can be used as directed for adults and children.

4.3 Contraindications

Hypersensitivity to the active substances or to any other of the ingredients.

Contains sucrose. Patients with rare hereditary problems of fructose intolerance, glucose-galactose malabsorption or sucrase-isomaltase insufficiency should not take this medicine.

4.4 Special warnings and precautions for use

If symptoms persist longer than 7 days following the use of the product a doctor or dentist should be consulted.

4.5 Interaction with other medicinal products and other forms of interaction

None stated.

4.6 Pregnancy and lactation

The safety of Medijel Gel during pregnancy and lactation has not been established, but is considered not to constitute a hazard.

4.7 Effects on ability to drive and use machines

None stated.

4.8 Undesirable effects

Hypersensitivity reactions to Lidocaine have been reported on rare occasions.

4.9 Overdose

Maximum safe dosage for a 70kg adult is 750mg for Lidocaine (Goodman & Gilman, page 313). A tube of Medijel Gel contains 82.5mg of Lidocaine hydrochloride - overdose is not a problem.

5. PHARMACOLOGICAL PROPERTIES

5.1 Pharmacodynamic properties

Lidocaine Hydrochloride is well documented in Martindale 28th Edition Page 900-904 and Goodman & Gilman, Chapter 15 and pages 767-770.

Lidocaine Hydrochloride was first introduced in 1948 and is one of the most widely used local anaesthetics, producing more prompt, more intense, longer lasting and more extensive anaesthesia than does an equal concentration of procaine (Peak anaesthesia within 2-5 minutes). Local anaesthetics are drugs that block nerve conduction when applied locally to nerve tissue in appropriate concentrations. They have good powers of penetration and their action is reversible. Their use is followed by complete recovery in nerve function with no evidence of structural damage to nerve fibres or cells.

Aminoacridine Hydrochloride is a slow acting disinfectant. It exerts germicidal action against bacteria and fungi. It is also used as a surgical and endodontic irrigant and to treat local infections of the ear, mouth and throat. Its exact mode of action is not known but it involves disruption of certain metabolic pathways.

5.2 Pharmacokinetic properties

Lidocaine is readily absorbed through mucous membranes. They exert their effects in the form of the nonionised base. Lidocaine undergoes first-pass metabolism in the liver and bioavailability is low after administration by mouth. It is rapidly de-ethylated to the active metabolite monoethylglycinexylidide and then hydrolysed by amidases to various compounds, including glycineexylidide which has reduced activity but a longer elimination half-life. Less than 10% of a dose is excreted unchanged via the kidneys. The metabolic products are excreted in the urine.

Aminoacridine Hydrochloride if administered systematically is rapidly eliminated through the kidney (0.2 grams being eliminated from the blood in 30 minutes). (Medijel Gel dose 0.15mg Aminoacridine hydrochloride).

5.3 Preclinical safety data

There are no pre-clinical data of relevance to the prescriber which are additional to that already included in other sections of the SPC.

6. PHARMACEUTICAL PARTICULARS

6.1 List of excipients

Glycerol, Hydroxypolyethoxydodecane HSE, Alcohol 96% v/v, Carbomer, Sucrose, Saccharin Sodium, Peppermint Oil, Ethyl vanillin, Di-isopropanolamine 90% aqueous, Purified Water

6.2 Incompatibilities

None encountered.

6.3 Shelf life

48 months.

6.4 Special precautions for storage

Do not store above 25°C.

6.5 Nature and contents of container

Aluminium tube with membrane seal and spiked polyethylene cap.

6.6 Special precautions for disposal and other handling

N/A

7. MARKETING AUTHORISATION HOLDER

DDD LIMITED

94, Rickmansworth Road, Watford, Hertfordshire, United Kingdom, WDI8 7JJ.

8. MARKETING AUTHORISATION NUMBER(S)

PL 0133/5000R Legal Status: GSL

9. DATE OF FIRST AUTHORISATION/RENEWAL OF THE AUTHORISATION

Date of last renewal: 20/05/03

10. DATE OF REVISION OF THE TEXT

November 2007

MEDIJEL PASTILLES

(DDD Limited)

1. NAME OF THE MEDICINAL PRODUCT

MEDIJEL PASTILLES

2. QUALITATIVE AND QUANTITATIVE COMPOSITION

Lignocaine Hydrochloride BP	0.25 % w/w
Aminacrine Hydrochloride BP 1968	0.025 %w/w

3. PHARMACEUTICAL FORM

Soft Pastille

4. CLINICAL PARTICULARS

4.1 Therapeutic indications

The quick effective relief from the pain of common mouth ulcers, soreness of gums and denture rubbing.

4.2 Posology and method of administration

Place pastille against affected area and let it dissolve slowly. Repeat as necessary.

Each pastille weighs approximately 1.2g, i.e. 3mg of Lignocaine Hydrochloride and 0.3mg of Aminacrine Hydrochloride.

Medijel Pastilles can be used as directed for adults and children.

4.3 Contraindications

Hypersensitivity to the active substances or to any other of the ingredients.

Contains sucrose and glucose. Patients with rare hereditary problems of fructose intolerance, glucose-galactose malabsorption or sucrase-isomaltase insufficiency should not take this medicine.

4.4 Special warnings and precautions for use

If symptoms persist longer than 7 days following the use of the product, a doctor or dentist should be consulted.

4.5 Interaction with other medicinal products and other forms of interaction

None stated.

4.6 Pregnancy and lactation

The safety of Medijel Pastilles during pregnancy and lactation has not been established, but is considered not to constitute a hazard.

4.7 Effects on ability to drive and use machines

None stated.

4.8 Undesirable effects

Hypersensitivity reactions to Lignocaine have been reported on rare occasions.

4.9 Overdose

Maximum safe dosage for a 70kg adult is 750mg for Lignocaine (Goodman & Gilman, page 313). A pack of Medijel pastilles contains approximately 75mg of Lignocaine Hydrochloride - overdose is not a problem.

5. PHARMACOLOGICAL PROPERTIES

5.1 Pharmacodynamic properties

Lignocaine Hydrochloride is well documented in Martindale 28th Edition page 900 - 904 and Goodman & Gilman, chapter 15 and pages 767 - 770.

Lignocaine Hydrochloride was first introduced in 1948 and is one of the most widely used local anaesthetics. However, it produces more prompt, more intense, longer lasting and more extensive anaesthesia than does an equal concentration of procaine (Peak anaesthesia within 2-5 minutes). Local anaesthetics are drugs that block nerve conduction when applied locally to nerve tissue in appropriate concentrations. They have good powers of penetration and their action is reversible. Their use is followed by complete recovery in nerve function with no evidence of structural damage to nerve fibres or cells.

Aminacrine Hydrochloride is a slow acting disinfectant. It exerts germicidal action against bacteria and fungi. It is also used as a surgical and endodontic irrigant and to treat local infections of the ear, mouth and throat. Its exact mode of action is not known but it involves disruption of certain metabolic pathways.

5.2 Pharmacokinetic properties

Lignocaine is readily absorbed through mucous membranes. They exert their effects in the form of the non-ionised base. Lignocaine undergoes first-pass metabolism in the liver and bioavailablity is low after administration by mouth. It is rapidly de-ethylated to the active metabolite monoethylglycinexylidide and then hydrolysed by amidases to various compounds, including glycineexylidide which has reduced activity but a longer elimination half-life. Less than 10% of a dose is excreted unchanged via the kidneys. The metabolic products are excreted in the urine.

Aminacrine Hydrochloride if administered systematically is rapidly eliminated through the kidney (0.2 g being eliminated from the blood in 30 minutes. Medijel Pastilles dose 0.15mg Aminacrine Hydrochloride).

5.3 Preclinical safety data

There are no pre-clinical data of relevance to the prescriber which are additional to that already included in other sections of the SPC.

6. PHARMACEUTICAL PARTICULARS

6.1 List of excipients

Hydroxypolyethoxydodecane HSE, Gelatin BP, Liquid Glucose BPC 1963, Sucrose EP,

Peppermint Oil BP, Levomenthol BP, Ethyl VanillinNF, Standard Green SE142,

Dextrose Monhydrate BP, Water (potable)

6.2 Incompatibilities

None encountered.

6.3 Shelf life

48 months.

6.4 Special precautions for storage

No special storage conditions.

6.5 Nature and contents of container

Aluminium Foil/Polyethylene laminate within coated boxboard carton.

6.6 Special precautions for disposal and other handling

None.

7. MARKETING AUTHORISATION HOLDER

DDD Limited

94, Rickmansworth Road

Watford, Hertfordshire

United Kingdom

WDI8 7JJ

8. MARKETING AUTHORISATION NUMBER(S)

PL 0133/5001R Legal Status: Pharmacy Only

9. DATE OF FIRST AUTHORISATION/RENEWAL OF THE AUTHORISATION

Date of first authorisation: 1972

10. DATE OF REVISION OF THE TEXT

August 2009

Medinol Over 6 Paracetamol Oral Suspension BP 250mg/5ml.

(SSL International plc)

1. NAME OF THE MEDICINAL PRODUCT

Medinol Over 6 Paracetamol Oral Suspension.

2. QUALITATIVE AND QUANTITATIVE COMPOSITION

Paracetamol BP 250mg/5ml.

3. PHARMACEUTICAL FORM

Oral suspension.

4. CLINICAL PARTICULARS

4.1 Therapeutic indications

For the relief of mild to moderate pain including headache, migraine, neuralgia, toothache and sore throat. Symptomatic relief of rheumatic aches and pains. Symptomatic relief of influenza, feverishness and colds.

4.2 Posology and method of administration

Oral. To be taken four times daily. Do not repeat doses more frequently than every four hours.

Adults, the elderly and children over 12 years of age: two to four 5ml spoonfuls. Children 6 to 12 years: one to two 5ml spoonfuls. Not to be given to children under 6 years of age. Do not take more than 4 doses in 24 hours

4.3 Contraindications

Should be used with caution in patients with impaired kidney or liver function. Hypersensitivity to paracetamol and/or other constituents.

4.4 Special warnings and precautions for use

Care is advised in the administration of paracetamol to patients with severe renal or severe hepatic impairment and in those with non-cirrhotic alcoholic liver disease. The hazards of overdose are greater in those with alcoholic liver disease. If pain or fever persists for more than 3 days, consult your doctor. Prolonged use without medical supervision may be harmful. Do not exceed the stated dose. Keep out of the reach of children.

The labels state: Do not give with any other paracetamol-containing products. Immediate medical advice should be sought in the event of an overdose, even if the child seems well.

The leaflet states: Immediate medical advice should be sought in the event of an overdose, even if the child seems well, because of the risk of delayed serious liver damage.

4.5 Interaction with other medicinal products and other forms of interaction

Alcohol, barbiturates, anticonvulsants and tricyclic antidepressants may increase hepatotoxicity of paracetamol, particularly after an overdose. Paracetamol may increase the half life of chloramphenicol. The speed of absorption of paracetamol may be increased by metoclopramide or domperidone and absorption reduced by cholestyramine. The anticoagulant effect of warfarin and other coumarins may be enhanced by prolonged regular use of paracetamol with increased risk of bleeding.

4.6 Pregnancy and lactation

Epidemiological studies in human pregnancy have shown no effects due to paracetamol used in the recommended dosage. However, paracetamol should be avoided in pregnancy unless considered essential by the physician.

Paracetamol is excreted in breast milk but not in a clinically significant amount. Available published data do not contraindicate breast feeding.

4.7 Effects on ability to drive and use machines

None known.

4.8 Undesirable effects

Adverse effects of paracetamol are rare but hypersensitivity including skin rash may occur. There have been reports of blood dyscrasias including thrombocytopaenia and agranulocytosis, and of acute pancreatitis.

4.9 Overdose

Symptoms of overdosage in the first 24 hours are pallor, nausea, vomiting, anorexia, and abdominal pain. Liver damage may become apparent 12 to 48 hours after ingestion. Abnormalities of glucose metabolism and metabolic acidosis may occur. In severe poisoning, hepatic failure may progress to encephalopathy, coma and death. Acute renal failure with acute tubular necrosis may develop even in the absence of severe liver damage. Cardiac arrhythmias have been reported. Liver damage is likely in adults who have taken 10g or more of paracetamol. It is considered that excess quantities of a toxic metabolite (usually adequately detoxified by gluthathione when normal doses of paracetamol are ingested), become irreversibly bound to liver tissue.

Treatment: Immediate treatment is essential in the management of a paracetamol overdose. Despite a lack of significant early symptoms, patients should be referred to hospital urgently for immediate medical attention and any patient who has ingested around 7.5g or more of paracetamol in the preceding 4 hours should undergo gastric lavage. Administration of oral methionine or intravenous N-acetylcysteine, which may have a beneficial effect up to at least 48 hours after the overdose, may be required. General supportive measures must be available.

5. PHARMACOLOGICAL PROPERTIES

5.1 Pharmacodynamic properties

Paracetamol has analgesic and antipyretic properties.

5.2 Pharmacokinetic properties

Paracetamol is readily absorbed from the gastrointestinal tract with peak plasma concentrations occurring 30 minutes to 2 hours after ingestion. It is metabolised in the liver and excreted in the urine mainly as the glucuronide and sulphate conjugates. The elimination half-life varies from 1 to 4 hours.

5.3 Preclinical safety data

There are no pre-clinical data of relevance to the prescriber that are additional to that already included in other sections of the Summary of Product Characteristics.

6. PHARMACEUTICAL PARTICULARS

6.1 List of excipients

Sodium Methylhydroxybenzoate; Sodium Propylhydroxybenzoate; Sodium Saccharin; Sodium Cyclamate 1968; Tragacanth; Lycasin 80/55; Strawberry Flavour PFW 500253E; Purified Water.

6.2 Incompatibilities

None known.

6.3 Shelf life

36 months.

6.4 Special precautions for storage

Store below 25°C.

6.5 Nature and contents of container

Amber glass sirop bottle with tamper evident cap fitted with polycone liner, containing 100 or 200ml of product.

6.6 Special precautions for disposal and other handling

Not applicable.

7. MARKETING AUTHORISATION HOLDER

Cupal Ltd. Venus, 1 Old Park Lane, Trafford Park, Manchester, M41 7HA

8. MARKETING AUTHORISATION NUMBER(S)

PL 0338/0069.

9. DATE OF FIRST AUTHORISATION/RENEWAL OF THE AUTHORISATION

10th November 1989 / 16/05/96

10. DATE OF REVISION OF THE TEXT

July 2006

Medinol Paediatric Paracetamol Oral Suspension BP 120mg/5ml

(SSL International plc)

1. NAME OF THE MEDICINAL PRODUCT

Medinol Paediatric Paracetamol Oral Suspension BP 120mg/5ml.

2. QUALITATIVE AND QUANTITATIVE COMPOSITION

Paracetamol 120mg/5ml.

3. PHARMACEUTICAL FORM

Oral suspension

4. CLINICAL PARTICULARS

4.1 Therapeutic indications

For the relief of pain and to relieve or reduce fever.

4.2 Posology and method of administration

Route of administration: oral

To be taken four times daily.

Do not repeat dose more frequently than every four hours.

Infants under 3 months: on doctors advice only (10mg/kg).

A 2.5ml dose is suitable for babies who develop a fever following vaccination at 2 months. In all other cases use only under medical supervision.

Infants 3 months to 1 year: half to one 5ml spoonful (60-120mg).

Children 1-6 years: one or two 5ml spoonfuls (120-240mg).

Children over 6 years: two or four 5ml spoonfuls (240-480mg).

Do not give more than four doses in 24 hours.

Not to be given to infants under 3 months except on medical advice.

4.3 Contraindications

Hypersensitivity to paracetamol and/or other constituents. Impaired kidney and liver function.

4.4 Special warnings and precautions for use

1. If pain or fever persists for more than 3 days consult a doctor.

2. Prolonged use without medical supervision may be harmful.

3. Do not give with other product containing paracetamol concurrently.

4. If your baby was born prematurely and is less than 3 months old consult your doctor before use.

5. In cases of accidental overdose seek medical attention immediately.

6. Care is advised in the administration of paracetamol to patients with severe renal or severe hepatic impairment. The hazards of overdose are greater in those with (non-cirrhotic) alcoholic liver disease.

7. Keep out of the reach of children.

8. Do not exceed the stated dose.

4.5 Interaction with other medicinal products and other forms of interaction
Cholestyramine may reduce absorption of paracetamol. Metoclopramide and domperidone may accelerate absorption of paracetamol. Alcohol, barbiturates, anticonvulsants and tricyclic antidepressants may increase the hepatoxicity of paracetamol particularly after an overdose. The anticoagulant effect of warfarin and other coumarins may be enhanced by prolonged regular use of paracetamol with increased risk of bleeding; occasional doses have no significant effect.

4.6 Pregnancy and lactation
Epidemiological studies in human pregnancy have shown no ill effects due to paracetamol used in the recommended dosage, but patients should follow the advice of their doctor regarding its use. Paracetamol is excreted in breast milk but not in a clinically significant amount. Available published data do not contraindicate breast-feeding. This product may, therefore, be taken during pregnancy and lactation.

4.7 Effects on ability to drive and use machines
None stated.

4.8 Undesirable effects
Adverse effects of paracetamol are rare but hypersensitivity including skin rash may occur. There have been reports of blood dyscrasias including thrombocytopaenia and agranulocytosis, but these were not necessarily causally related to paracetamol. If given in therapeutic doses side effects are rare. Haematological reactions have been reported. Most reports of adverse reactions to paracetamol relate to overdosage with the drug.

4.9 Overdose
Symptoms of paracetamol overdosage in the first 24 hours are pallor, nausea, vomiting, anorexia and abdominal pain. Liver damage may become apparent 12 to 48 hours after ingestion. Abnormalities of glucose metabolism and metabolic acidosis may occur. In severe poisoning, hepatic failure may progress to encephalopathy, coma and death. Acute renal failure with acute tubular necrosis may develop even in the absence of severe liver damage. Cardiac arrhythmias and pancreatitis have been reported. Liver damage is possible in adults who have taken 10g or more of paracetamol.

Treatment: Immediate treatment is essential in the management of paracetamol overdose. Despite a lack of significant early symptoms, patients should be referred to hospital urgently for immediate medical attention and any patient who has ingested around 7.5g or more of paracetamol in the preceding 4 hours should undergo gastric lavage. General supportive measures must be available. After gastric lavage a suitable antidote such as acetylcysteine or methionine should be given. Acetylcysteine is given by intravenous infusion in an initial dose of 150mg/kg body weight over 15 minutes, followed by 50mg/kg over 4 hours and then by 100mg/kg over the next 16 hours. Alternatively, methionine 2.5g may be given by mouth every four hours to a total of 4 doses. The blood paracetamol levels should be monitored to determine whether further therapy is necessary.

In severe poisoning, hepatic failure may progress to encephalopathy, coma and death.

5. PHARMACOLOGICAL PROPERTIES
5.1 Pharmacodynamic properties
Analgesic/antipyretic.

5.2 Pharmacokinetic properties
Not applicable

5.3 Preclinical safety data
None stated

6. PHARMACEUTICAL PARTICULARS
6.1 List of excipients
Methylhydroxybenzoate; Propylhydroxybenzoate; Sodium Saccharin; Sodium Cyclamate 1968; Tragacanth; Lycasin; Strawberry Flavour PFW 500253E; Water.

6.2 Incompatibilities
None stated.

6.3 Shelf life
36 months unopened.

6.4 Special precautions for storage
Avoid extremes of temperatures.

6.5 Nature and contents of container
Amber glass sirop or winchester bottle with tamper evident cap with fitted polycone liner containing 50, 70, 100, 140, 150 or 200ml of product. The 70ml and 140ml size will also be cartoned. 30ml universal amber glass bottle fitted with a child-resistant cap containing 20, 25 or 30ml of product. Amber glass winchester bottle with polypropylene cap with EPE wad containing 500 or 1000ml of product.

A 2.5ml syringe measuring device may also be included with each pack of suspension.

5ml CE marked polystyrene measuring spoon supplied with product.

6.6 Special precautions for disposal and other handling
Not applicable.

7. MARKETING AUTHORISATION HOLDER
Cupal Ltd., Venus, 1 Old Park Lane, Trafford Park, Manchester, M41 7HA.

8. MARKETING AUTHORISATION NUMBER(S)
PL 0338/0033.

9. DATE OF FIRST AUTHORISATION/RENEWAL OF THE AUTHORISATION
10th February 1977 / 12th February 1992.

10. DATE OF REVISION OF THE TEXT
19/07/06

Medinol Under 6 Paracetamol Oral Suspension BP 120mg/5ml

(SSL International plc)

1. NAME OF THE MEDICINAL PRODUCT
Medinol Under 6 Paracetamol Oral Suspension BP 120mg/5ml.

2. QUALITATIVE AND QUANTITATIVE COMPOSITION
Paracetamol 120mg/5ml

3. PHARMACEUTICAL FORM
Oral suspension.

4. CLINICAL PARTICULARS
4.1 Therapeutic indications
For the relief of pain and to relieve or reduce fever.

4.2 Posology and method of administration
Route of administration: oral

To be taken four times daily.

Do not repeat dose more frequently than every four hours.

Infants under 3 months: on doctors advice only (10mg/kg).

A 2.5ml dose is suitable for babies who develop a fever following vaccination at 2 months. In all other cases use only under medical supervision.

Infants 3 months to 1 year: half to one 5ml spoonful (60-120mg).

Children 1-6 years: one or two 5ml spoonfuls (120-240mg).

Children over 6 years: two or four 5ml spoonfuls (240-480mg).

Do not give more than four doses in 24 hours.

Not to be given to infants under 3 months except on medical advice.

4.3 Contraindications
Hypersensitivity to paracetamol and/or other constituents. Impaired kidney and liver function.

4.4 Special warnings and precautions for use
1. If pain or fever persists for more than 3 days consult a doctor.

2. Prolonged use without medical supervision may be harmful.

3. Do not give with other product containing paracetamol concurrently.

4. If your baby was born prematurely and is less than 3 months old consult your doctor before use.

5. In cases of accidental overdose seek medical attention immediately.

6. Care is advised in the administration of paracetamol to patients with severe renal or severe hepatic impairment. The hazards of overdose are greater in those with (non-cirrhotic) alcoholic liver disease.

7. Keep out of the reach of children.

8. Do not exceed the stated dose.

4.5 Interaction with other medicinal products and other forms of interaction
Cholestyramine may reduce absorption of paracetamol. Metoclopramide and domperidone may accelerate absorption of paracetamol. Alcohol, barbiturates, anticonvulsants and tricyclic antidepressants may increase the hepatoxicity of paracetamol particularly after an overdose. The anticoagulant effect of warfarin and other coumarins may be enhanced by prolonged regular use of paracetamol with increased risk of bleeding; occasional doses have no significant effect.

4.6 Pregnancy and lactation
Epidemiological studies in human pregnancy have shown no ill effects due to paracetamol used in the recommended dosage, but patients should follow the advice of their doctor regarding its use. Paracetamol is excreted in breast milk but not in a clinically significant amount. Available published data do not contraindicate breast-feeding. This product may, therefore, be taken during pregnancy and lactation.

4.7 Effects on ability to drive and use machines
None stated.

4.8 Undesirable effects
Adverse effects of paracetamol are rare but hypersensitivity including skin rash may occur. There have been reports of blood dyscrasias including thrombocytopaenia and agranulocytosis, but these were not necessarily causally related to paracetamol. If given in therapeutic doses side effects are rare. Haematological reactions have been reported. Most reports of adverse reactions to paracetamol relate to overdosage with the drug.

4.9 Overdose
Symptoms of paracetamol overdosage in the first 24 hours are pallor, nausea, vomiting, anorexia and abdominal pain. Liver damage may become apparent 12 to 48 hours after ingestion. Abnormalities of glucose metabolism and metabolic acidosis may occur. In severe poisoning, hepatic failure may progress to encephalopathy, coma and death. Acute renal failure with acute tubular necrosis may develop even in the absence of severe liver damage. Cardiac arrhythmias and pancreatitis have been reported. Liver damage is possible in adults who have taken 10g or more of paracetamol.

Treatment: Immediate treatment is essential in the management of paracetamol overdose. Despite a lack of significant early symptoms, patients should be referred to hospital urgently for immediate medical attention and any patient who has ingested around 7.5g or more of paracetamol in the preceding 4 hours should undergo gastric lavage. General supportive measures must be available. After gastric lavage a suitable antidote such as acetylcysteine or methionine should be given. Acetylcysteine is given by intravenous infusion in an initial dose of 150mg/kg body weight over 15 minutes, followed by 50mg/kg over 4 hours and then by 100mg/kg over the next 16 hours. Alternatively, methionine 2.5g may be given by mouth every four hours to a total of 4 doses. The blood paracetamol levels should be monitored to determine whether further therapy is necessary.

In severe poisoning, hepatic failure may progress to encephalopathy, coma and death.

5. PHARMACOLOGICAL PROPERTIES
5.1 Pharmacodynamic properties
Analgesic/antipyretic

5.2 Pharmacokinetic properties
Not applicable.

5.3 Preclinical safety data
None stated.

6. PHARMACEUTICAL PARTICULARS
6.1 List of excipients
Methylhydroxybenzoate; Propylhydroxybenzoate; Sodium Saccharin; Sodium Cyclamate 1968; Tragacanth; Lycasin; Strawberry Flavour PFW 500253E; Water.

6.2 Incompatibilities
None stated

6.3 Shelf life
36 months unopened.

6.4 Special precautions for storage
Avoid extremes of temperatures.

6.5 Nature and contents of container
Amber glass sirop or winchester bottle with tamper evident cap with fitted polycone liner containing 50, 70, 100, 140, 150 or 200ml of product. The 70ml and 140ml size will also be cartoned. 30ml universal amber glass bottle fitted with a child-resistant cap containing 20, 25 or 30ml of product. Amber glass winchester bottle with polypropylene cap with EPE wad containing 500 or 1000ml of product.

A 2.5ml syringe measuring device may also be included with each pack of suspension.

5ml CE marked polystyrene measuring spoon supplied with product.

6.6 Special precautions for disposal and other handling
Not applicable.

7. MARKETING AUTHORISATION HOLDER
Cupal Ltd., Venus, 1 Old Park Lane, Trafford Park, Manchester, M41 7HA.

8. MARKETING AUTHORISATION NUMBER(S)
PL 0338/0033.

9. DATE OF FIRST AUTHORISATION/RENEWAL OF THE AUTHORISATION
10th February 1977 / 12th February 1992.

10. DATE OF REVISION OF THE TEXT
19/07/06

Medised for Children

(SSL International plc)

1. NAME OF THE MEDICINAL PRODUCT
Medised For Children

2. QUALITATIVE AND QUANTITATIVE COMPOSITION
Paracetamol 120mg/5ml

Diphenhydramine HCl 12.5mg/5ml

3. PHARMACEUTICAL FORM
Oral solution.

Clear to pale pink liquid.

4. CLINICAL PARTICULARS

4.1 Therapeutic indications

For the treatment of mild to moderate pain including teething pain, headache, sore throat, aches and pains.

Symptomatic relief of influenza and feverish colds and the associated symptoms of runny nose and sneezing.

4.2 Posology and method of administration

Route of Administration: Oral.

Recommended Doses and Dosage Schedules:

6 years to under 12 years: 10ml-20ml (2-4 teaspoonful) 3 times daily.

Medised is contraindicated in children under 6 years of age (see section 4.3)

Parents or carers should seek medical attention if the child's condition deteriorates during treatment.

4.3 Contraindications

Do not take if you are hypersensitive to paracetamol, and/ or any other constituents.

Large doses of antihistamines may precipitate fits in epileptics.

Do not take if you are currently taking monoamine inhibitors (MAOIs) or within 14 days of stopping treatment with MAOIs.

Not to be used in children under the age of 6 years.

4.4 Special warnings and precautions for use

Do not exceed the stated dose. Immediate medical advice should be sought in the event of an overdose, even if you feel well because of the risk of delayed, serious liver damage.

Do not take with any other paracetamol-containing products, or cough and cold medicines.

Dose should not be repeated more frequently than 4 hour intervals.

Not more than 4 doses should be taken in 24 hours.

Dosage should not be continued for more than three days without consulting a doctor.

This product should be administered with caution to patients with known renal or hepatic impairment, prostatic hypertrophy, urinary retention, or susceptibility to angle-closure glaucoma. The hazards of overdose are greater in those with alcoholic liver disease.

The product may cause drowsiness. This product should not be used to sedate a child.

Keep out of the reach of children.

4.5 Interaction with other medicinal products and other forms of interaction

The speed of absorption of paracetamol may be increased by metoclopramide or domperidone and absorption reduced by cholestyramine.

The anticoagulant effect of warfarin and other coumarins may be enhanced by prolonged regular daily use of paracetamol with increased risk of bleeding.

May enhance the sedative effects of CNS depressants including barbiturates, hypnotics, opioid analgesics, anxiolytic sedatives, antipsychotics and alcohol.

May have an additive muscarinic actions with other drugs, such as atropine and some antidepressants.

Not to be used in patients taking MAOIs or within 14 days of stopping treatment as there is a risk of serotonin syndrome.

4.6 Pregnancy and lactation

Safety in pregnancy has not been established.

Epidemiological studies in human pregnancy have shown no effects due to paracetamol used in the recommended dosage, but patients should follow the advice of their doctor regarding its use. Paracetamol is excreted in breast milk, but not a clinically significant amount.

Available published data does not contraindicate breast-feeding.

4.7 Effects on ability to drive and use machines

May cause drowsiness. If affected do not drive or operate machinery.

4.8 Undesirable effects

Common side effects

CNS effects: Drowsiness (usually diminishes within a few days), paradoxical stimulation, headache, psychomotor impairment.

Antimuscarinic effects: Urinary retention, dry mouth, blurred vision, gastrointestinal disturbances, thickened respiratory tract secretions

Rare side effects:

Hypotenstion, extrapyramidal effects, dizziness, confusion, depression, sleep disturbances, tremor, convulsions, palpitation, arrhythmia, hypersensitivity reactions (including skin rash), blood disorders and liver dysfunction.

There have been a few reports of blood dyscrasias including thrombocytopenia and agranulocytosis but these were not necessarily causally related to paracetamol.

4.9 Overdose

The features of overdose are: sedation, pallor, nausea, vomiting, diarrhoea, anorexia, and abdominal pain; liver damage may become apparent within 12 to 48 hours. In some children overdose may cause cerebral stimulation resulting in convulsions and hyperpyrexia.

Abnormalities of glucose metabolism and metabolic acidosis may occur. In severe poisoning, hepatic failure may progress to encephalopathy, coma and death. Acute renal failure with acute tubular necrosis may develop even in the absence of severe liver damage. Cardiac arrhythmias and pancreatitis have been reported.

Liver damage is likely in adults who have taken 10g or more of paracetamol. It is considered that excess quantities of a toxic metabolite (usually adequately detoxified by glutathione when normal doses of paracetamol are ingested), become irreversibly bound to liver tissue.

Immediate treatment is essential in the management of paracetamol overdose. Despite a lack of significant early symptoms, patients should be referred to hospital urgently for immediate medical attention and any patient who has ingested around 7.5g or more of paracetamol in the preceding four hours should undergo gastric lavage. Administration of oral methionine or intravenous N-acetylcysteine which may have a beneficial effect up to at least 48 hours after the overdose, may be required. General supportive measures must be available.

5. PHARMACOLOGICAL PROPERTIES

5.1 Pharmacodynamic properties

Paracetamol is an antipyretic and analgesic. Diphenhydramine HCl is an antihistamine with anti-cholinergic, anti-emetic, anti-allergic and sedative effects.

5.2 Pharmacokinetic properties

Paracetamol and diphenhydramine HCl are both readily absorbed from the gastrointestinal tract. Both are widely distributed throughout the body. Both are metabolised in the liver and excreted in the urine. As Medised Infant is a solution, absorption of actives is rapid following oral ingestion.

5.3 Preclinical safety data

Paracetamol and diphenhydramine HCl are well established drug substances whose preclinical profiles have been investigated and are thoroughly established.

6. PHARMACEUTICAL PARTICULARS

6.1 List of excipients

Macrogol 4000

Glycerol

Propylene Glycol

Sorbitol Solution (non crystallising) 70%

Lycasin 80/55 (Maltitol Solution)

Sodium Cyclamate

Sodium Saccharin

Nipasept (Methylhydroxybenzoate, Ethylhydroxybenzoate and Parahydroxybenzoate)

Strawberry Flavour 513805E

Sugar Module 555049E

Water, purified

6.2 Incompatibilities

Not applicable.

6.3 Shelf life

36 months.

6.4 Special precautions for storage

Do not store above 25°C.

Do not refrigerate.

Keep container in outer carton.

6.5 Nature and contents of container

Amber type III glass bottle and plastic clic loc cap with pulp stearan wadding. 20ml, 30ml, 70ml, 100ml, 140ml and 200ml.

All pack sizes except the 20ml have a 5ml plastic spoon.

6.6 Special precautions for disposal and other handling

None.

7. MARKETING AUTHORISATION HOLDER

SSL International Plc

Venus

1 Old Park Lane

Trafford Park

Manchester

M41 7HA

UK

8. MARKETING AUTHORISATION NUMBER(S)

PL 17905/0090

9. DATE OF FIRST AUTHORISATION/RENEWAL OF THE AUTHORISATION

13/09/99

10. DATE OF REVISION OF THE TEXT

September 2009

Medrone Tablets 100mg

(Pharmacia Limited)

1. NAME OF THE MEDICINAL PRODUCT

Medrone® Tablets 100 mg.

2. QUALITATIVE AND QUANTITATIVE COMPOSITION

Each Medrone Tablet contains 100 mg methylprednisolone Ph. Eur.

3. PHARMACEUTICAL FORM

Tablet

4. CLINICAL PARTICULARS

4.1 Therapeutic indications

Medrone is a potent corticosteroid with an anti-inflammatory activity at least five times that of hydrocortisone. An enhanced separation of glucocorticoid and mineralocorticoid effect results in a reduced incidence of sodium and water retention.

Medrone is indicated for conditions requiring glucocorticoid activity such as:-

1. Collagen diseases/arteritis

Systemic lupus erythematosus

Systemic dermatomyositis (polymyositis)

Rheumatic fever with severe carditis

Giant cell arteritis/polymyalgia rheumatica

2. Dermatological diseases

Pemphigus vulgaris

3. Allergic states

Bronchial asthma

4. Respiratory diseases

Pulmonary sarcoid

5. Haematological disorders

Idiopathic thrombocytopenic purpura

Haemolytic anaemia (autoimmune)

6. Neoplastic diseases

Leukaemia (acute and lymphatic)

Malignant lymphoma

7. Gastro-intestinal diseases

Crohn's disease

8. Miscellaneous

Tuberculous meningitis (with appropriate antituberculous chemotherapy)

Transplantation

4.2 Posology and method of administration

The dosage recommendations shown in the table below are suggested initial daily doses and are intended as guides. The average total daily dose recommended may be given either as a single dose or in divided doses (excepting in alternate day therapy when the minimum effective daily dose is doubled and given every other day at 8.00 a.m.). It is envisaged that the 100 mg tablet will be used for high initial daily or alternate day doses in acute situations, with tapering of dosage achieved by using the 16 mg tablet.

Undesirable effects may be minimised by using the lowest effective dose for the minimum period (see Special warnings and special precautions for use).

The initial suppressive dose level may vary depending on the condition being treated. As soon as a satisfactory clinical response is obtained, the daily dose should be reduced gradually, either to termination of treatment in the case of acute conditions or to the minimal effective maintenance dose level in the case of chronic conditions. In chronic conditions it is important that the reduction in dosage from initial to maintenance dose levels be accomplished as clinically appropriate.

In alternate-day therapy, the minimum daily corticoid requirement is doubled and administered as a single dose every other day at 8.00 a.m. Dosage requirements depend on the condition being treated and response of the patient.

Elderly patients: Treatment of elderly patients, particularly if long-term, should be planned bearing in mind the more serious consequences of the common side-effects of corticosteroids in old age and close clinical supervision is required (see Special warnings and special precautions for use).

Children: In general, dosage for children should be based upon clinical response and is at the discretion of the clinician. Treatment should be limited to the minimum dosage for the shortest period of time. If possible, treatment should be administered as a single dose on alternate days (see Special warnings and special precautions for use).

Dosage Recommendations:

Indications	Recommended initial daily dosage
Systemic lupus erythematosus	20 - 100 mg
Systemic dermatomyositis	48 mg
Acute rheumatic fever	48 mg until ESR normal for one week.
Giant cell arteritis/ polymyalgia rheumatica	64 mg
Pemphigus vulgaris	80 - 360 mg

Bronchial asthma	up to 64 mg single dose/ alternate day up to 100 mg maximum.
Pulmonary sarcoid	32 - 48 mg on alternate days.
Haematological disorders and leukaemias	16 - 100 mg
Malignant lymphoma	16 - 100 mg
Crohn's disease	up to 48 mg per day in acute episodes.
Organ transplantation	up to 3.6 mg/kg/day

4.3 Contraindications

Medrone is contra-indicated where there is known hypersensitivity to components and in systemic fungal infection unless specific anti-infective therapy is employed.

4.4 Special warnings and precautions for use

Warnings and Precautions:

1. A Patient Information Leaflet is provided in the pack by the manufacturer.

2. Undesirable effects may be minimised by using the lowest effective dose for the minimum period, and by administering the daily requirement as a single morning dose or whenever possible as a single morning dose on alternative days. Frequent patient review is required to appropriately titrate the dose against disease activity (see Posology and method of administration).

3. Adrenal cortical atrophy develops during prolonged therapy and may persist for months after stopping treatment. In patients who have received more than physiological doses of systemic corticosteroids (approximately 6 mg methylprednisolone) for greater than 3 weeks, withdrawal should not be abrupt. How dose reduction should be carried out depends largely on whether the disease is likely to relapse as the dose of systemic corticosteroids is reduced. Clinical assessment of disease activity may be needed during withdrawal. If the disease is unlikely to relapse on withdrawal of systemic corticosteroids, but there is uncertainty about HPA suppression, the dose of systemic corticosteroid may be reduced rapidly to physiological doses. Once a daily dose of 6 mg methylprednisolone is reached, dose reduction should be slower to allow the HPA-axis to recover.

Abrupt withdrawal of systemic corticosteroid treatment, which has continued up to 3 weeks is appropriate if it considered that the disease is unlikely to relapse. Abrupt withdrawal of doses up to 32 mg daily of methylprednisolone for 3 weeks is unlikely to lead to clinically relevant HPA-axis suppression, in the majority of patients. In the following patient groups, gradual withdrawal of systemic corticosteroid therapy should be *considered* even after courses lasting 3 weeks or less:

- Patients who have had repeated courses of systemic corticosteroids, particularly if taken for greater than 3 weeks.
- When a short course has been prescribed within one year of cessation of long-term therapy (months or years).
- Patients who may have reasons for adrenocortical insufficiency other than exogenous corticosteroid therapy.
- Patients receiving doses of systemic corticosteroid greater than 32 mg daily of methylprednisolone.
- Patients repeatedly taking doses in the evening.

4. Since mineralocorticoid secretion may be impaired, salt and/or a mineralocorticoid should be administered concurrently.

5. Patients should carry 'Steroid Treatment' cards which give clear guidance on the precautions to be taken to minimise risk and which provide details of prescriber, drug, dosage and the duration of treatment.

6. Corticosteroids may mask some signs of infection, and new infections may appear during their use. Suppression of the inflammatory response and immune function increases the susceptibility to fungal, viral and bacterial infections and their severity. The clinical presentation may often be atypical and may reach an advanced stage before being recognised.

7. Chickenpox is of serious concern since this normally minor illness may be fatal in immunosuppressed patients. Patients (or parents of children) without a definite history of chickenpox should be advised to avoid close personal contact with chickenpox or herpes zoster and if exposed they should seek urgent medical attention. Passive immunization with varicella/zoster immunoglobin (VZIG) is needed by exposed non-immune patients who are receiving systemic corticosteroids or who have used them within the previous 3 months; this should be given within 10 days of exposure to chickenpox. If a diagnosis of chickenpox is confirmed, the illness warrants specialist care and urgent treatment. Corticosteroids should not be stopped and the dose may need to be increased.

8. Exposure to measles should be avoided. Medical advice must be sought immediately if exposure occurs. Prophylaxis with normal intramuscular immunoglobulin may be needed.

9. Live vaccines should not be given to individuals with impaired immune responsiveness. The antibody response to other vaccines may be diminished.

10. The use of Medrone in active tuberculosis should be restricted to those cases of fulminating or disseminated tuberculosis in which the corticosteroid is used for the management of the disease in conjunction with an appropriate antituberculous regimen. If corticosteroids are indicated in patients with latent tuberculosis or tuberculin reactivity, close observation is necessary as reactivation of the disease may occur. During prolonged corticosteroid therapy, these patients should receive chemoprophylaxis.

11. Care should be taken for patients receiving cardioactive drugs such as digoxin because of steroid induced electrolyte disturbance/potassium loss (see Undesirable effects).

Special precautions:

Particular care is required when considering the use of systemic corticosteroids in patients with the following conditions and frequent patient monitoring is necessary.

1. Osteoporosis (post-menopausal females are particularly at risk).
2. Hypertension or congestive heart failure.
3. Existing or previous history of severe affective disorders (especially previous steroid psychosis).
4. Diabetes mellitus (or a family history of diabetes).
5. History of tuberculosis.
6. Glaucoma (or a family history of glaucoma).
7. Previous corticosteroid-induced myopathy.
8. Liver failure or cirrhosis.
9. Renal insufficiency.
10. Epilepsy.
11. Peptic ulceration.
12. Fresh intestinal anastomoses.
13. Predisposition to thrombophlebitis.
14. Abscess or other pyogenic infections.
15. Ulcerative colitis.
16. Diverticulitis.
17. Myasthenia gravis.
18. Ocular herpes simplex, for fear of corneal perforation.
19. Hypothyroidism.
20. Recent myocardial infarction (myocardial rupture has been reported).
21. Kaposi's sarcoma has been reported to occur in patients receiving corticosteroid therapy. Discontinuation of corticosteroids may result in clinical remission.
22. Patients and/or carers should be warned that potentially severe psychiatric adverse reactions may occur with systemic steroids (see section 4.8). Symptoms typically emerge within a few days or weeks of starting treatment. Risks may be higher with high doses/systemic exposure (see also section 4.5 Interaction with Other Medicaments and Other Forms of Interaction that can increase the risk of side effects), although dose levels do not allow prediction of the onset, type, severity or duration of reactions. Most reactions recover after either dose reduction or withdrawal, although specific treatment may be necessary. Patients/carers should be encouraged to seek medical advice if worrying psychological symptoms develop, especially if depressed mood or suicidal ideation is suspected. Patients/carers should be alert to possible psychiatric disturbances that may occur either during or immediately after dose tapering/withdrawal of systemic steroids, although such reactions have been reported infrequently.

Particular care is required when considering the use of systemic corticosteroids in patients with existing or previous history of severe affective disorders in themselves or in their first degree relatives. These would include depressive or manic-depressive illness and previous steroid psychosis.

Use in children: Corticosteroids cause growth retardation in infancy, childhood and adolescence. Treatment should be limited to the minimum dosage for the shortest possible time. In order to minimise suppression of the hypothalamo-pituitary-adrenal axis and growth retardation, treatment should be administered where possible as a single dose on alternate days.

Use in the elderly: The common adverse effects of systemic corticosteroids may be associated with more serious consequences in old age, especially osteoporosis, hypertension, hypokalaemia, diabetes, susceptibility to infection and thinning of the skin. Close clinical supervision is required to avoid life-threatening reactions.

4.5 Interaction with other medicinal products and other forms of interaction

1. Convulsions have been reported with concurrent use of methylprednisolone and cyclosporin. Since concurrent administration of these agents results in a mutual inhibition of metabolism, it is possible that convulsions and other adverse effects associated with the individual use of either drug may be more apt to occur.

2. Drugs that induce hepatic enzymes, such as rifampicin, rifabutin, carbamazepine, phenobarbitone, phenytoin, primidone, and aminoglutethimide enhance the metabolism of corticosteroids and its therapeutic effects may be reduced.

3. Drugs which inhibit the CYP3A4 enzyme, such as cimetidine, erythromycin, ketoconazole, itraconazole, diltiazem and mibefradil, may decrease the rate of metabolism of corticosteroids and hence increase the serum concentration.

4. Steroids may reduce the effects of anticholinesterases in myasthenia gravis. The desired effects of hypoglycaemic agents (including insulin), anti-hypertensives and diuretics are antagonised by corticosteroids, and the hypokalaemic effects of acetazolamide, loop diuretics, thiazide diuretics and carbenoxolone are enhanced.

5. The efficacy of coumarin anticoagulants may be enhanced by concurrent corticosteroid therapy and close monitoring of the INR or prothrombin time is required to avoid spontaneous bleeding.

6. The renal clearance of salicylates is increased by corticosteroids and steroid withdrawal may result in salicylate intoxication. Salicylates and non-steroidal anti-inflammatory agents should be used cautiously in conjunction with corticosteroids in hypothrombinaemia.

7. Steroids have been reported to interact with neuromuscular blocking agents such as pancuronium with partial reversal of the neuromuscular block.

4.6 Pregnancy and lactation

Pregnancy

The ability of corticosteroids to cross the placenta varies between individual drugs, however, methylprednisolone does cross the placenta.

Administration of corticosteroids to pregnant animals can cause abnormalities of foetal development including cleft palate, intra-uterine growth retardation and affects on brain growth and development. There is no evidence that corticosteroids result in an increased incidence of congenital abnormalities, such as cleft palate in man, however, when administered for long periods or repeatedly during pregnancy, corticosteroids may increase the risk of intra-uterine growth retardation. Hypoadrenalism may, in theory, occur in the neonate following prenatal exposure to corticosteroids but usually resolves spontaneously following birth and is rarely clinically important. As with all drugs, corticosteroids should only be prescribed when the benefits to the mother and child outweigh the risks. When corticosteroids are essential, however, patients with normal pregnancies may be treated as though they were in the non-gravid state.

Lactation

Corticosteroids are excreted in small amounts in breast milk, however, doses of up to 40 mg daily of methylprednisolone are unlikely to cause systemic effects in the infant. Infants of mothers taking higher doses than this may have a degree of adrenal suppression, but the benefits of breastfeeding are likely to outweigh any theoretical risk.

4.7 Effects on ability to drive and use machines

None stated.

4.8 Undesirable effects

The incidence of predictable undesirable side-effects associated with the use of corticosteroids, including hypothalamic-pituitary-adrenal suppression correlates with the relative potency of the drug, dosage, timing of administration and duration of treatment (see Special warnings and special precautions for use).

GASTRO-INTESTINAL - Dyspepsia, peptic ulceration with perforation and haemorrhage, abdominal distension, oesophageal ulceration, oesophageal candidiasis, acute pancreatitis, perforation of bowel, gastric haemorrhage.

Increases in alanine transaminase (ALT, SGPT) aspartate transaminase (AST, SGOT) and alkaline phosphatase have been observed following corticosteroid treatment. These changes are usually small, not associated with any clinical syndrome and are reversible upon discontinuation.

ANTI-INFLAMMATORY AND IMMUNOSUPPRESSIVE EFFECTS - Increased susceptibility and severity of infections with suppression of clinical symptoms and signs, opportunistic infections, may suppress reactions to skin tests, recurrence of dormant tuberculosis (see Special warnings and special precautions for use).

MUSCULOSKELETAL - Proximal myopathy, osteoporosis, vertebral and long bone fractures, avascular osteonecrosis, tendon rupture, muscle weakness.

FLUID AND ELECTROLYTE DISTURBANCE - Sodium and water retention, hypertension, hypokalaemic alkalosis, potassium loss, congestive heart failure in susceptible patients.

DERMATOLOGICAL - Impaired healing, skin atrophy, bruising, striae, telangiectasia, acne, petechiae and ecchymosis. Kaposi's sarcoma has been reported in patients receiving corticosteroid therapy.

ENDOCRINE/METABOLIC - Suppression of the hypothalamo-pituitary-adrenal axis, growth suppression in infancy, childhood and adolescence, menstrual irregularity and amenorrhoea. Cushingoid facies, hirsutism, weight gain, impaired carbohydrate tolerance with increased requirement for antidiabetic therapy, negative nitrogen and calcium balance. Increased appetite.

NEUROPSYCHIATRIC - A wide range of psychiatric reactions including affective disorders (such as irritable, euphoric, depressed and labile mood psychological dependence and suicidal thoughts), psychotic reactions (including mania, delusions, hallucinations and aggravation of schizophrenia), behavioural disturbances, irritability, anxiety, sleep disturbances, seizures and cognitive dysfunction including confusion and amnesia have been reported for all corticosteroids. Reactions are common and may occur in both adults and children. In adults, the frequency of severe reactions was estimated to be 5-6%. Psychological effects have been reported on withdrawal of corticosteroids; the frequency is unknown. Increased intra-cranial pressure with papilloedema in children (pseudotumour cerebri) has been reported, usually after treatment withdrawal of methylprednisolone.

OPHTHALMIC - Increased intra-ocular pressure, glaucoma, papilloedema with possible damage to the optic nerve, cataracts, corneal or scleral thinning, exacerbation of ophthalmic viral or fungal disease, exophthalmos.

CARDIOVASCULAR – Myocardial rupture following a myocardial infarction.

GENERAL - Leucocytosis, hypersensitivity reactions including anaphylaxis, thrombo-embolism, nausea, malaise, persistent hiccups with high dose corticosteroids.

WITHDRAWAL SYMPTOMS - Too rapid a reduction of corticosteroid dosage following prolonged treatment can lead to acute adrenal insufficiency, hypotension and death (see Special warnings and special precautions for use).

A 'withdrawal syndrome' may also occur including, fever, myalgia, arthralgia, rhinitis, conjunctivitis, painful itchy skin nodules and loss of weight.

4.9 Overdose

Administration of Medrone should not be discontinued abruptly but tailed off over a period of time. Appropriate action should be taken to alleviate the symptoms produced by any side-effect that may become apparent. It may be necessary to support the patient with corticosteroids during any further period of trauma occurring within two years of overdosage.

There is no clinical syndrome of acute overdose with Medrone. Methylprednisolone is dialysable.

5. PHARMACOLOGICAL PROPERTIES

5.1 Pharmacodynamic properties

Methylprednisolone is a potent anti-inflammatory steroid. It has greater anti-inflammatory potency than prednisolone and less tendency than prednisolone to induce sodium and water retention. The relative potency of methylprednisolone to hydrocortisone is at least four to one.

5.2 Pharmacokinetic properties

The mean elimination half-life ranges from 2.4 to 3.5 hours in normal, healthy adults and appears to be independent of the route of administration.

Methylprednisolone is metabolised in the liver to inactive metabolites, the major ones being 20 b-hydroxymethylprednisolone and 20 b-hydroxy-a-methylprednisolone.

Methylprednisolone clearance is altered by concurrent administration of troleandomycin, erythromycin, rifampicin, anticonvulsants and theophylline. No dosing adjustments are necessary in renal failure. Methylprednisolone is haemodialyzable.

5.3 Preclinical safety data

–

6. PHARMACEUTICAL PARTICULARS

6.1 List of excipients

Methylcellulose, sodium starch glycolate, microcrystalline cellulose, magnesium stearate and E132.

6.2 Incompatibilities

None stated.

6.3 Shelf life

48 months.

6.4 Special precautions for storage

Store below 25°C.

6.5 Nature and contents of container

Amber glass bottle with LDPE cap and bulb or HDPE screw cap - each bottle contains 20, 25, 30 or 100 25, 30 or 100 tablets

6.6 Special precautions for disposal and other handling

No special requirements.

7. MARKETING AUTHORISATION HOLDER

Pharmacia Limited

Ramsgate Road

Sandwich

Kent CT13 9NJ

UK

8. MARKETING AUTHORISATION NUMBER(S)

PL 0032/0145

9. DATE OF FIRST AUTHORISATION/RENEWAL OF THE AUTHORISATION

1st February 2005

10. DATE OF REVISION OF THE TEXT

3rd April 2008

LEGAL CATEGORY

POM

Ref: MDD 3_0 UK

Medrone Tablets 16mg

(Pharmacia Limited)

1. NAME OF THE MEDICINAL PRODUCT

Medrone Tablets 16 mg.

2. QUALITATIVE AND QUANTITATIVE COMPOSITION

Each Medrone Tablet contains 16 mg methylprednisolone Ph. Eur.

3. PHARMACEUTICAL FORM

Tablet

4. CLINICAL PARTICULARS

4.1 Therapeutic indications

Medrone is indicated for conditions requiring glucocorticoid activity such as:-

1. Endocrine disorders

Primary and secondary adrenal insufficiency

Congenital adrenal hyperplasia

2. Rheumatic disorders

Rheumatoid arthritis

Juvenile chronic arthritis

Ankylosing spondylitis

3. Collagen diseases/arteritis

Systemic lupus erythematosus

Systemic dermatomyositis (polymyositis)

Rheumatic fever with severe carditis

Giant cell arteritis/polymyalgia rheumatica

4. Dermatological diseases

Pemphigus vulgaris

5. Allergic states

Severe seasonal and perennial allergic rhinitis

Drug hypersensitivity reactions

Serum sickness

Allergic contact dermatitis

Bronchial asthma

6. Ophthalmic diseases

Anterior uveitis (iritis, iridocyclitis)

Posterior uveitis

Optic neuritis

7. Respiratory diseases

Pulmonary sarcoid

Fulminating or disseminated tuberculosis (with appropriate anti-tuberculous chemotherapy)

Aspiration of gastric contents

8. Haematological disorders

Idiopathic thrombocytopenic purpura

Haemolytic anaemia (autoimmune)

9. Neoplastic diseases

Leukaemia (acute and lymphatic)

Malignant lymphoma

10. Gastro-intestinal diseases

Ulcerative colitis

Crohn's disease

11. Miscellaneous

Tuberculous meningitis (with appropriate anti-tuberculous chemotherapy)

Transplantation

4.2 Posology and method of administration

The dosage recommendations shown in the table below are suggested initial daily doses and are intended as guides. The average total daily dose recommended may be given either as a single dose or in divided doses (excepting in alternate day therapy when the minimum effective daily dose is doubled and given every other day at 8.00 am).

Undesirable effects may be minimised by using the lowest effective dose for the minimum period (see Special warnings and special precautions for use).

The initial suppressive dose level may vary depending on the condition being treated. This is continued until a satisfactory clinical response is obtained, a period usually of three to seven days in the case of rheumatic diseases (except for acute rheumatic carditis), allergic conditions affecting the skin or respiratory tract and ophthalmic diseases. If a satisfactory response is not obtained in seven days, re-evaluation of the case to confirm the original diagnosis should be made. As soon as a satisfactory clinical response is obtained, the daily dose should be reduced gradually, either to termination of treatment in the case of acute conditions (e.g. seasonal asthma, exfoliative dermatitis, acute ocular inflammations) or to the minimal effective maintenance dose level in the case of chronic conditions (e.g. rheumatoid arthritis, systemic lupus erythematosus, bronchial asthma, atopic dermatitis). In chronic conditions, and in rheumatoid arthritis especially, it is important that the reduction in dosage from initial to maintenance dose levels be accomplished as clinically appropriate. Decrements of not more than 2 mg at intervals of 7 - 10 days are suggested. In rheumatoid arthritis, maintenance steroid therapy should be at the lowest possible level.

In alternate-day therapy, the minimum daily corticoid requirement is doubled and administered as a single dose every other day at 8.00 am. Dosage requirements depend on the condition being treated and response of the patient.

Elderly patients: Treatment of elderly patients, particularly if long-term, should be planned bearing in mind the more serious consequences of the common side-effects of corticosteroids in old age, particularly osteoporosis, diabetes, hypertension, susceptibility to infection and thinning of skin (see Special warnings and special precautions for use).

Children: In general, dosage for children should be based upon clinical response and is at the discretion of the physician. Treatment should be limited to the minimum dosage for the shortest period of time. If possible, treatment should be administered as a single dose on alternate days (see Special warnings and special precautions for use).

Dosage Recommendations:

Indications	Recommended initial daily dosage
Rheumatoid arthritis	
severe	12 – 16 mg
moderately severe	8 – 12 mg
moderate	4 – 8 mg
children	4 - 8 mg
Systemic dermatomyositis	48 mg
Systemic lupus erythematosus	20 - 100 mg
Acute rheumatic fever	48 mg until ESR normal for one week.
Allergic diseases	12 - 40 mg
Bronchial asthma	up to 64 mg single dose/ alternate day up to 100 mg maximum.
Ophthalmic diseases	12 - 40 mg
Haematological disorders and leukaemias	16 - 100 mg
Malignant lymphoma	16 - 100 mg
Ulcerative colitis	16 - 60 mg
Crohn's disease	up to 48 mg per day in acute episodes.
Organ transplantation	up to 3.6 mg/kg/day
Pulmonary sarcoid	32 - 48 mg on alternate days.
Giant cell arteritis/ polymyalgia rheumatica	64 mg
Pemphigus vulgaris	80 - 360 mg

4.3 Contraindications

Medrone is contra-indicated where there is known hypersensitivity to components and in systemic infection unless specific anti-infective therapy is employed.

4.4 Special warnings and precautions for use

Warnings and precautions:

1. A Patient Information Leaflet is provided in the pack by the manufacturer.

2. Undesirable effects may be minimised by using the lowest effective dose for the minimum period, and by administering the daily requirement as a single morning dose or whenever possible as a single morning dose on alternative days. Frequent patient review is required to appropriately titrate the dose against disease activity (see Posology and method of administration).

3. Adrenal cortical atrophy develops during prolonged therapy and may persist for months after stopping treatment. In patients who have received more than physiological doses of systemic corticosteroids (approximately 6 mg methylprednisolone) for greater than 3 weeks, withdrawal should not be abrupt. How dose reduction should be carried out depends largely on whether the disease is likely to relapse as the dose of systemic corticosteroids is reduced. Clinical assessment of disease activity may be needed during withdrawal. If the disease is unlikely to relapse on withdrawal of systemic corticosteroids, but there is uncertainty about HPA suppression, the dose of systemic corticosteroid may be reduced rapidly to physiological doses. Once a daily dose of 6 mg methylprednisolone is reached, dose reduction should be slower to allow the HPA-axis to recover.

Abrupt withdrawal of systemic corticosteroid treatment, which has continued up to 3 weeks is appropriate if it considered that the disease is unlikely to relapse. Abrupt withdrawal of doses up to 32 mg daily of methylprednisolone for 3 weeks is unlikely to lead to clinically relevant HPA-axis suppression, in the majority of patients. In the following patient groups, gradual withdrawal of systemic corticosteroid therapy should be ***considered*** even after courses lasting 3 weeks or less:

- Patients who have had repeated courses of systemic corticosteroids, particularly if taken for greater than 3 weeks.
- When a short course has been prescribed within one year of cessation of long-term therapy (months or years).
- Patients who may have reasons for adrenocortical insufficiency other than exogenous corticosteroid therapy.
- Patients receiving doses of systemic corticosteroid greater than 32 mg daily of methylprednisolone.
- Patients repeatedly taking doses in the evening.

4. Since mineralocorticoid secretion may be impaired, salt and/or a mineralocorticoid should be administered concurrently.

5. Patients should carry 'Steroid Treatment' cards which give clear guidance on the precautions to be taken to minimise risk and which provide details of prescriber, drug, dosage and the duration of treatment.

6. Corticosteroids may mask some signs of infection, and new infections may appear during their use. Suppression of the inflammatory response and immune function increases the susceptibility to fungal, viral and bacterial infections and their severity. The clinical presentation may often be atypical and may reach an advanced stage before being recognised.

7. Chickenpox is of serious concern since this normally minor illness may be fatal in immunosuppressed patients. Patients (or parents of children) without a definite history of chickenpox should be advised to avoid close personal contact with chickenpox or herpes zoster and if exposed they should seek urgent medical attention. Passive immunization with varicella/zoster immunoglobulin (VZIG) is needed by exposed non-immune patients who are receiving systemic corticosteroids or who have used them within the previous 3 months; this should be given within 10 days of exposure to chickenpox. If a diagnosis of chickenpox is confirmed, the illness warrants specialist care and urgent treatment. Corticosteroids should not be stopped and the dose may need to be increased.

8. Exposure to measles should be avoided. Medical advice must be sought immediately if exposure occurs. Prophylaxis with normal intramuscular immunoglobulin may be needed.

9. Live vaccines should not be given to individuals with impaired immune responsiveness. The antibody response to other vaccines may be diminished.

10. The use of Medrone in active tuberculosis should be restricted to those cases of fulminating or disseminated tuberculosis in which the corticosteroid is used for the management of the disease in conjunction with an appropriate antituberculous regimen. If corticosteroids are i ndicated in patients with latent tuberculosis or tuberculin reactivity, close observation is necessary as reactivation of the disease may occur. During prolonged corticosteroid therapy, these patients should receive chemoprophylaxis.

11. Care should be taken for patients receiving cardioactive drugs such as digoxin because of steroid induced electrolyte disturbance/potassium loss (see Undesirable effects).

Special precautions:

Particular care is required when considering the use of systemic corticosteroids in patients with the following conditions and frequent patient monitoring is necessary.

1. Osteoporosis (post-menopausal females are particularly at risk).
2. Hypertension or congestive heart failure.
3. Existing or previous history of severe affective disorders (especially previous steroid psychosis).
4. Diabetes mellitus (or a family history of diabetes).
5. History of tuberculosis.
6. Glaucoma (or a family history of glaucoma).
7. Previous corticosteroid-induced myopathy.
8. Liver failure or cirrhosis.
9. Renal insufficiency.
10. Epilepsy.
11. Peptic ulceration.
12. Fresh intestinal anastomoses.
13. Predisposition to thrombophlebitis.
14. Abscess or other pyogenic infections.
15. Ulcerative colitis.
16. Diverticulitis.
17. Myasthenia gravis.
18. Ocular herpes simplex, for fear of corneal perforation.
19. Hypothyroidism.
20. Recent myocardial infarction (myocardial rupture has been reported).
21. Kaposi's sarcoma has been reported to occur in patients receiving corticosteroid therapy. Discontinuation of corticosteroids may result in clinical remission.
22. Patients and/or carers should be warned that potentially severe psychiatric adverse reactions may occur with systemic steroids (see section 4.8). Symptoms typically emerge within a few days or weeks of starting treatment. Risks may be higher with high doses/systemic exposure (see also section 4.5 Interaction with Other Medicaments and Other Forms of Interaction that can increase the risk of side effects), although dose levels do not allow prediction of the onset, type, severity or duration of reactions. Most reactions recover after either dose reduction or withdrawal, although specific treatment may be necessary. Patients/carers should be encouraged to seek medical advice if worrying psychological symptoms develop, especially if depressed mood or suicidal ideation is suspected. Patients/carers should be alert to possible psychiatric disturbances that may occur either during or immediately after dose tapering/withdrawal of systemic steroids, although such reactions have been reported infrequently.

Particular care is required when considering the use of systemic corticosteroids in patients with existing or previous history of severe affective disorders in themselves or in their first degree relatives. These would include depressive or manic-depressive illness and previous steroid psychosis.

Use in children: Corticosteroids cause growth retardation in infancy, childhood and adolescence. Treatment should be limited to the minimum dosage for the shortest possible time. In order to minimise suppression of the hypothalamo-pituitary-adrenal axis and growth retardation, treatment should be administered where possible as a single dose on alternate days.

Use in the elderly: The common adverse effects of systemic corticosteroids may be associated with more serious consequences in old age, especially osteoporosis, hypertension, hypokalaemia, diabetes, susceptibility to infection and thinning of the skin. Close clinical supervision is required to avoid life-threatening reactions.

4.5 Interaction with other medicinal products and other forms of interaction

1. Convulsions have been reported with concurrent use of methylprednisolone and ciclosporin. Since concurrent administration of these agents results in a mutual inhibition of metabolism, it is possible that convulsions and other adverse effects associated with the individual use of either drug may be more apt to occur.

2. Drugs that induce hepatic enzymes, such as rifampicin, rifabutin, carbamazepine, phenobarbitone, phenytoin, primidone, and aminoglutethimide enhance the metabolism of corticosteroids and its therapeutic effects may be reduced.

3. Drugs which inhibit the CYP3A4 enzyme, such as cimetidine, erythromycin, ketoconazole, itraconazole, diltiazem and mibefradil, may decrease the rate of metabolism of corticosteroids and hence increase the serum concentration.

4. Steroids may reduce the effects of anticholinesterases in myasthenia gravis. The desired effects of hypoglycaemic agents (including insulin), anti-hypertensives and diuretics are antagonised by corticosteroids, and the hypokalaemic effects of acetazolamide, loop diuretics, thiazide diuretics and carbenoxolone are enhanced.

5. The efficacy of coumarin anticoagulants may be enhanced by concurrent corticosteroid therapy and close monitoring of the INR or prothrombin time is required to avoid spontaneous bleeding.

6. The renal clearance of salicylates is increased by corticosteroids and steroid withdrawal may result in salicylate intoxication. Salicylates and non-steroidal anti-inflammatory agents should be used cautiously in conjunction with corticosteroids in hypothrombinaemia.

7. Steroids have been reported to interact with neuromuscular blocking agents such as pancuronium with partial reversal of the neuromuscular block.

4.6 Pregnancy and lactation

Pregnancy

The ability of corticosteroids to cross the placenta varies between individual drugs, however, methylprednisolone does cross the placenta.

Administration of corticosteroids to pregnant animals can cause abnormalities of foetal development including cleft palate, intra-uterine growth retardation and effects on brain growth and development. There is no evidence that corticosteroids result in an increased incidence of congenital abnormalities, such as cleft palate in man, however, when administered for long periods or repeatedly during pregnancy, corticosteroids may increase the risk of intra-uterine growth retardation. Hypoadrenalism may, in theory, occur in the neonate following prenatal exposure to corticosteroids but usually resolves spontaneously following birth and is rarely clinically important. As with all drugs, corticosteroids should only be prescribed when the benefits to the mother and child outweigh the risks. When corticosteroids are essential, however, patients with normal pregnancies may be treated as though they were in the non-gravid state.

Lactation

Corticosteroids are excreted in small amounts in breast milk, however, doses of up to 40 mg daily of methylprednisolone are unlikely to cause systemic effects in the infant. Infants of mothers taking higher doses than this may have a degree of adrenal suppression, but the benefits of breast-feeding are likely to outweigh any theoretical risk.

4.7 Effects on ability to drive and use machines

None stated.

4.8 Undesirable effects

The incidence of predictable undesirable side-effects associated with the use of corticosteroids, including hypothalamic-pituitary-adrenal suppression correlates with the relative potency of the drug, dosage, timing of administration and duration of treatment (see Special warnings and special precautions for use).

GASTRO-INTESTINAL - Dyspepsia, peptic ulceration with perforation and haemorrhage, abdominal distension, oesophageal ulceration, oesophageal candidiasis, acute pancreatitis, perforation of bowel, gastric haemorrhage.

Increases in alanine transaminase (ALT, SGPT) aspartate transaminase (AST, SGOT) and alkaline phosphatase have been observed following corticosteroid treatment. These changes are usually small, not associated with any clinical syndrome and are reversible upon discontinuation.

ANTI-INFLAMMATORY AND IMMUNOSUPPRESSIVE EFFECTS - Increased susceptibility and severity of infections with suppression of clinical symptoms and signs, opportunistic infections, may suppress reactions to skin tests, recurrence of dormant tuberculosis (see Special warnings and special precautions for use).

MUSCULOSKELETAL - Proximal myopathy, osteoporosis, vertebral and long bone fractures, avascular osteonecrosis, tendon rupture, muscle weakness.

FLUID AND ELECTROLYTE DISTURBANCE - Sodium and water retention, hypertension, hypokalaemic alkalosis, potassium loss, congestive heart failure in susceptible patients.

DERMATOLOGICAL - Impaired healing, skin atrophy, bruising, striae, telangiectasia, acne, petechiae and ecchymosis. Kaposi's sarcoma has been reported in patients receiving corticosteroid therapy.

ENDOCRINE/METABOLIC - Suppression of the hypothalamo-pituitary-adrenal axis, growth suppression in infancy, childhood and adolescence; menstrual irregularity and amenorrhoea. Cushingoid facies, hirsutism, weight gain, impaired carbohydrate tolerance with increased requirement for antidiabetic therapy, negative nitrogen and calcium balance. Increased appetite.

NEUROPSYCHIATRIC - A wide range of psychiatric reactions including affective disorders (such as irritable, euphoric, depressed and labile mood psychological dependence and suicidal thoughts), psychotic reactions (including mania, delusions, hallucinations and aggravation of schizophrenia), behavioural disturbances, irritability, anxiety, sleep disturbances, seizures and cognitive dysfunction including confusion and amnesia have been reported for all corticosteroids. Reactions are common and may occur in both adults and children. In adults, the frequency of severe reactions was estimated to be 5-6%. Psychological effects have been reported on withdrawal of corticosteroids; the frequency is unknown. Increased intra-cranial pressure with papilloedema in children (pseudotumour cerebri) has been reported, usually after treatment withdrawal of methylprednisolone.

OPHTHALMIC - Increased intra-ocular pressure, glaucoma, papilloedema with possible damage to the optic nerve, cataracts, corneal or scleral thinning, exacerbation of ophthalmic viral or fungal disease, exophthalmos.

CARDIOVASCULAR – Myocardial rupture following myocardial infarction.

GENERAL - Leucocytosis, hypersensitivity reactions including anaphylaxis, thrombo-embolism, nausea, malaise, persistent hiccups with high doses of corticosteroids.

WITHDRAWAL SYMPTOMS - Too rapid a reduction of corticosteroid dosage following prolonged treatment can lead to acute adrenal insufficiency, hypotension and death (see Special warnings and special precautions for use).

A 'withdrawal syndrome' may also occur including, fever, myalgia, arthralgia, rhinitis, conjunctivitis, painful itchy skin nodules and loss of weight.

4.9 Overdose

Administration of Medrone should not be discontinued abruptly but tailed off over a period of time. Appropriate action should be taken to alleviate the symptoms produced by any side-effect that may become apparent. It may be necessary to support the patient with corticosteroids during any further period of trauma occurring within two years of overdosage.

There is no clinical syndrome of acute overdose with Medrone. Methylprednisolone is dialysable.

5. PHARMACOLOGICAL PROPERTIES

5.1 Pharmacodynamic properties

Medrone is a potent corticosteroid with an anti-inflammatory activity at least five times that of hydrocortisone. An enhanced separation of glucocorticoid and mineralocorticoid effect results in a reduced incidence of sodium and water retention.

5.2 Pharmacokinetic properties

Corticosteroids are absorbed from the gastro-intestinal tract. In the circulation they are extensively bound to plasma proteins and are metabolised mainly in the liver but also in the kidney and are excreted in the urine.

The half-life of methylprednisolone has been reported to be slightly longer than that of prednisolone.

5.3 Preclinical safety data

–

6. PHARMACEUTICAL PARTICULARS

6.1 List of excipients

Lactose, sucrose, maize starch, mineral oil and calcium stearate.

6.2 Incompatibilities

None stated.

6.3 Shelf life

Bottles - 60 months

Blister packs - 36 months.

6.4 Special precautions for storage

Store below 25°C.

6.5 Nature and contents of container

High density polyethylene bottles with tamper evident caps. Each bottle contains 14 tablets.

20-25 micron hard tempered aluminium foil/lacquer, 250 micron opaque polyvinyl chloride film blister. Pack contains 30 tablets.

6.6 Special precautions for disposal and other handling

No special requirements.

7. MARKETING AUTHORISATION HOLDER

Pharmacia Ltd

Ramsgate Road

Sandwich

Kent

CT13 9NJ

UK

8. MARKETING AUTHORISATION NUMBER(S)

PL 0032/0024R

9. DATE OF FIRST AUTHORISATION/RENEWAL OF THE AUTHORISATION

1st February 2005

10. DATE OF REVISION OF THE TEXT

3rd April 2008

Legal category: POM

Ref: MDC 3_0 UK

Medrone Tablets 2mg, 4mg

(Pharmacia Limited)

1. NAME OF THE MEDICINAL PRODUCT

Medrone Tablets 2 mg.

Medrone Tablets 4 mg

2. QUALITATIVE AND QUANTITATIVE COMPOSITION

Medrone Tablets 2mg: each tablet contains 2 mg methylprednisolone Ph. Eur.

Medrone Tablets 4mg: each tablet contains 4 mg methylprednisolone Ph. Eur.

3. PHARMACEUTICAL FORM

Tablet

4. CLINICAL PARTICULARS

4.1 Therapeutic indications

Medrone is indicated for conditions requiring glucocorticoid activity such as:-

1. Endocrine disorders

Primary and secondary adrenal insufficiency

Congenital adrenal hyperplasia

2. Rheumatic disorders

Rheumatoid arthritis

Juvenile chronic arthritis

Ankylosing spondylitis

3. Collagen diseases/arteritis

Systemic lupus erythematosus

Systemic dermatomyositis (polymyositis)

Rheumatic fever with severe carditis

Giant cell arteritis/polymyalgia rheumatica

4. Dermatological diseases

Pemphigus vulgaris

5. Allergic states

Severe seasonal and perennial allergic rhinitis

Drug hypersensitivity reactions

Serum sickness

Allergic contact dermatitis

Bronchial asthma

6. Ophthalmic diseases

Anterior uveitis (iritis, iridocyclitis)

Posterior uveitis

Optic neuritis

7. Respiratory diseases

Pulmonary sarcoid

Fulminating or disseminated tuberculosis (with appropriate anti-tuberculous chemotherapy)

Aspiration of gastric contents

8. Haematological disorders

Idiopathic thrombocytopenic purpura

Haemolytic anaemia (autoimmune)

9. Neoplastic diseases

Leukaemia (acute and lymphatic)

Malignant lymphoma

10. Gastro-intestinal diseases

Ulcerative colitis

Crohn's disease

11. Miscellaneous

Tuberculous meningitis (with appropriate anti-tuberculous chemotherapy)

Transplantation

4.2 Posology and method of administration

The dosage recommendations shown in the table below are suggested initial daily doses and are intended as guides. The average total daily dose recommended may be given either as a single dose or in divided doses (excepting in alternate day therapy when the minimum effective daily dose is doubled and given every other day at 8.00 am).

Undesirable effects may be minimised by using the lowest effective dose for the minimum period (see Special warnings and special precautions for use).

The initial suppressive dose level may vary depending on the condition being treated. This is continued until a satisfactory clinical response is obtained, a period usually of three to seven days in the case of rheumatic diseases (except for acute rheumatic carditis), allergic conditions affecting the skin or respiratory tract and ophthalmic diseases. If a satisfactory response is not obtained in seven days, re-evaluation of the case to confirm the original diagnosis should be made. As soon as a satisfactory clinical response is obtained, the daily dose should be reduced gradually, either to termination of treatment in the case of acute conditions (e.g. seasonal asthma, exfoliative dermatitis, acute ocular inflammations) or to the minimal effective maintenance dose level in the case of chronic conditions (e.g. rheumatoid arthritis, systemic lupus erythematosus, bronchial asthma, atopic dermatitis). In chronic conditions, and in rheumatoid arthritis especially, it is important that the reduction in dosage from initial to maintenance dose levels be accomplished as clinically appropriate. Decrements of not more than 2 mg at intervals of 7 - 10 days are suggested. In rheumatoid arthritis, maintenance steroid therapy should be at the lowest possible level.

In alternate-day therapy, the minimum daily corticoid requirement is doubled and administered as a single dose every other day at 8.00 am. Dosage requirements depend on the condition being treated and response of the patient.

Elderly patients: Treatment of elderly patients, particularly if long-term, should be planned bearing in mind the more serious consequences of the common side-effects of corticosteroids in old age, particularly osteoporosis, diabetes, hypertension, susceptibility to infection and thinning of skin (see Special warnings and special precautions for use).

Children: In general, dosage for children should be based upon clinical response and is at the discretion of the physician. Treatment should be limited to the minimum dosage for the shortest period of time. If possible, treatment should be administered as a single dose on alternate days (see Special warnings and special precautions for use).

Dosage Recommendations:

Indications	Recommended initial daily dosage
Rheumatoid arthritis	
severe	12 – 16 mg
moderately severe	8 – 12 mg
moderate	4 – 8 mg
children	4 - 8 mg
Systemic dermatomyositis	48 mg
Systemic lupus erythematosus	20 - 100 mg
Acute rheumatic fever	48 mg until ESR normal for one week.
Allergic diseases	12 - 40 mg
Bronchial asthma	up to 64 mg single dose/ alternate day up to 100 mg maximum.
Ophthalmic diseases	12 - 40 mg
Haematological disorders and leukaemias	16 - 100 mg
Malignant lymphoma	16 - 100 mg
Ulcerative colitis	16 - 60 mg
Crohn's disease	up to 48 mg per day in acute episodes.
Organ transplantation	up to 3.6 mg/kg/day
Pulmonary sarcoid	32 - 48 mg on alternate days.
Giant cell arteritis/ polymyalgia rheumatica	64 mg
Pemphigus vulgaris	80 - 360 mg

4.3 Contraindications

Medrone is contra-indicated where there is known hypersensitivity to components and in systemic infection unless specific anti-infective therapy is employed.

4.4 Special warnings and precautions for use

Warnings and precautions:

1. A Patient Information Leaflet is provided in the pack by the manufacturer.

2. Undesirable effects may be minimised by using the lowest effective dose for the minimum period, and by administering the daily requirement as a single morning dose or whenever possible as a single morning dose on alternative days. Frequent patient review is required to appropriately titrate the dose against disease activity (see Posology and method of administration).

3. Adrenal cortical atrophy develops during prolonged therapy and may persist for months after stopping treatment. In patients who have received more than physiological doses of systemic corticosteroids (approximately 6 mg methylprednisolone) for greater than 3 weeks, withdrawal should not be abrupt. How dose reduction should be carried out depends largely on whether the disease is likely to relapse as the dose of systemic corticosteroids is reduced. Clinical assessment of disease activity may be needed during withdrawal. If the disease is unlikely to relapse on withdrawal of systemic corticosteroids, but there is uncertainty about HPA suppression, the dose of systemic corticosteroid may be reduced rapidly to physiological doses. Once a daily dose of 6 mg methylprednisolone is reached, dose reduction should be slower to allow the HPA-axis to recover.

Abrupt withdrawal of systemic corticosteroid treatment, which has continued up to 3 weeks is appropriate if it considered that the disease is unlikely to relapse. Abrupt withdrawal of doses up to 32 mg daily of methylprednisolone for 3 weeks is unlikely to lead to clinically relevant HPA-axis suppression, in the majority of patients. In the following patient groups, gradual withdrawal of systemic corticosteroid therapy should be ***considered*** even after courses lasting 3 weeks or less:

- Patients who have had repeated courses of systemic corticosteroids, particularly if taken for greater than 3 weeks.
- When a short course has been prescribed within one year of cessation of long-term therapy (months or years).
- Patients who may have reasons for adrenocortical insufficiency other than exogenous corticosteroid therapy.
- Patients receiving doses of systemic corticosteroid greater than 32 mg daily of methylprednisolone.
- Patients repeatedly taking doses in the evening.

4. Since mineralocorticoid secretion may be impaired, salt and/or a mineralocorticoid should be administered concurrently.

5. Patients should carry 'Steroid Treatment' cards which give clear guidance on the precautions to be taken to minimise risk and which provide details of prescriber, drug, dosage and the duration of treatment.

6. Corticosteroids may mask some signs of infection, and new infections may appear during their use. Suppression of the inflammatory response and immune function increases the susceptibility to fungal, viral and bacterial infections and their severity. The clinical presentation may often be atypical and may reach an advanced stage before being recognised.

7. Chickenpox is of serious concern since this normally minor illness may be fatal in immunosuppressed patients. Patients (or parents of children) without a definite history of chickenpox should be advised to avoid close personal contact with chickenpox or herpes zoster and if exposed they should seek urgent medical attention. Passive immunization with varicella/zoster immunoglobulin (VZIG) is needed by exposed non-immune patients who are receiving systemic corticosteroids or who have used them within the previous 3 months; this should be given within 10 days of exposure to chickenpox. If a diagnosis of chickenpox is confirmed, the illness warrants specialist care and urgent treatment. Corticosteroids should not be stopped and the dose may need to be increased.

8. Exposure to measles should be avoided. Medical advice must be sought immediately if exposure occurs.

Prophylaxis with normal intramuscular immunoglobulin may be needed.

9. Live vaccines should not be given to individuals with impaired immune responsiveness. The antibody response to other vaccines may be diminished.

10. The use of Medrone in active tuberculosis should be restricted to those cases of fulminating or disseminated tuberculosis in which the corticosteroid is used for the management of the disease in conjunction with an appropriate antituberculous regimen. If corticosteroids are indicated in patients with latent tuberculosis or tuberculin reactivity, close observation is necessary as reactivation of the disease may occur. During prolonged corticosteroid therapy, these patients should receive chemoprophylaxis.

11. Care should be taken for patients receiving cardioactive drugs such as digoxin because of steroid induced electrolyte disturbance/potassium loss (see Undesirable effects).

Special precautions:

Particular care is required when considering the use of systemic corticosteroids in patients with the following conditions and frequent patient monitoring is necessary.

1. Osteoporosis (post-menopausal females are particularly at risk).
2. Hypertension or congestive heart failure.
3. Existing or previous history of severe affective disorders (especially previous steroid psychosis).
4. Diabetes mellitus (or a family history of diabetes).
5. History of tuberculosis.
6. Glaucoma (or a family history of glaucoma).
7. Previous corticosteroid-induced myopathy.
8. Liver failure or cirrhosis.
9. Renal insufficiency.
10. Epilepsy.
11. Peptic ulceration.
12. Fresh intestinal anastomoses.
13. Predisposition to thrombophlebitis.
14. Abscess or other pyogenic infections.
15. Ulcerative colitis.
16. Diverticulitis.
17. Myasthenia gravis.
18. Ocular herpes simplex, for fear of corneal perforation.
19. Hypothyroidism.
20. Recent myocardial infarction (myocardial rupture has been reported).
21. Kaposi's sarcoma has been reported to occur in patients receiving corticosteroid therapy. Discontinuation of corticosteroids may result in clinical remission.
22. Patients and/or carers should be warned that potentially severe psychiatric adverse reactions may occur with systemic steroids (see section 4.8). Symptoms typically emerge within a few days or weeks of starting treatment. Risks may be higher with high doses/systemic exposure (see also section 4.5 Interaction with Other Medicaments and Other Forms of Interaction that can increase the risk of side effects), although dose levels do not allow prediction of the onset, type, severity or duration of reactions. Most reactions recover after either dose reduction or withdrawal, although specific treatment may be necessary. Patients/carers should be encouraged to seek medical advice if worrying psychological symptoms develop, especially if depressed mood or suicidal ideation is suspected. Patients/carers should be alert to possible psychiatric disturbances that may occur either during or immediately after dose tapering/withdrawal of systemic steroids, although such reactions have been reported infrequently.

Particular care is required when considering the use of systemic corticosteroids in patients with existing or previous history of severe affective disorders in themselves or in their first degree relatives. These would include depressive or manic-depressive illness and previous steroid psychosis.

Use in children: Corticosteroids cause growth retardation in infancy, childhood and adolescence. Treatment should be limited to the minimum dosage for the shortest possible time. In order to minimise suppression of the hypothalamo-pituitary-adrenal axis and growth retardation, treatment should be administered where possible as a single dose on alternate days.

Use in the elderly: The common adverse effects of systemic corticosteroids may be associated with more serious consequences in old age, especially osteoporosis, hypertension, hypokalaemia, diabetes, susceptibility to infection and thinning of the skin. Close clinical supervision is required to avoid life-threatening reactions.

4.5 Interaction with other medicinal products and other forms of interaction

1. Convulsions have been reported with concurrent use of methylprednisolone and ciclosporin. Since concurrent administration of these agents results in a mutual inhibition of metabolism, it is possible that convulsions and other adverse effects associated with the individual use of either drug may be more apt to occur.

2. Drugs that induce hepatic enzymes, such as rifampicin, rifabutin, carbamazepine, phenobarbitone, phenytoin, primidone, and aminoglutethimide enhance the metabolism of corticosteroids and its therapeutic effects may be reduced.

3. Drugs which inhibit the CYP3A4 enzyme, such as cimetidine, erythromycin, ketoconazole, itraconazole, diltiazem and mibefradil, may decrease the rate of metabolism of corticosteroids and hence increase the serum concentration.

4. Steroids may reduce the effects of anticholinesterases in myasthenia gravis. The desired effects of hypoglycaemic agents (including insulin), anti-hypertensives and diuretics are antagonised by corticosteroids, and the hypokalaemic effects of acetazolamide, loop diuretics, thiazide diuretics and carbenoxolone are enhanced.

5. The efficacy of coumarin anticoagulants may be enhanced by concurrent corticosteroid therapy and close monitoring of the INR or prothrombin time is required to avoid spontaneous bleeding.

6. The renal clearance of salicylates is increased by corticosteroids and steroid withdrawal may result in salicylate intoxication. Salicylates and non-steroidal anti-inflammatory agents should be used cautiously in conjunction with corticosteroids in hypothrombinaemia.

7. Steroids have been reported to interact with neuromuscular blocking agents such as pancuronium with partial reversal of the neuromuscular block.

4.6 Pregnancy and lactation

Pregnancy

The ability of corticosteroids to cross the placenta varies between individual drugs, however, methylprednisolone does cross the placenta.

Administration of corticosteroids to pregnant animals can cause abnormalities of foetal development including cleft palate, intra-uterine growth retardation and effects on brain growth and development. There is no evidence that corticosteroids result in an increased incidence of congenital abnormalities, such as cleft palate in man, however, when administered for long periods or repeatedly during pregnancy, corticosteroids may increase the risk of intra-uterine growth retardation. Hypoadrenalism may, in theory, occur in the neonate following prenatal exposure to corticosteroids but usually resolves spontaneously following birth and is rarely clinically important. As with all drugs, corticosteroids should only be prescribed when the benefits to the mother and child outweigh the risks. When corticosteroids are essential, however, patients with normal pregnancies may be treated as though they were in the non-gravid state.

Lactation

Corticosteroids are excreted in small amounts in breast milk, however, doses of up to 40 mg daily of methylprednisolone are unlikely to cause systemic effects in the infant. Infants of mothers taking higher doses than this may have a degree of adrenal suppression, but the benefits of breast-feeding are likely to outweigh any theoretical risk.

4.7 Effects on ability to drive and use machines

None stated.

4.8 Undesirable effects

The incidence of predictable undesirable side-effects associated with the use of corticosteroids, including hypothalamic-pituitary-adrenal suppression correlates with the relative potency of the drug, dosage, timing of administration and duration of treatment (see Special warnings and special precautions for use).

GASTRO-INTESTINAL - Dyspepsia, peptic ulceration with perforation and haemorrhage, abdominal distension, oesophageal ulceration, oesophageal candidiasis, acute pancreatitis, perforation of bowel, gastric haemorrhage.

Increases in alanine transaminase (ALT, SGPT) aspartate transaminase (AST, SGOT) and alkaline phosphatase have been observed following corticosteroid treatment. These changes are usually small, not associated with any clinical syndrome and are reversible upon discontinuation.

ANTI-INFLAMMATORY AND IMMUNOSUPPRESSIVE EFFECTS - Increased susceptibility and severity of infections with suppression of clinical symptoms and signs, opportunistic infections, may suppress reactions to skin tests, recurrence of dormant tuberculosis (see Special warnings and special precautions for use).

MUSCULOSKELETAL - Proximal myopathy, osteoporosis, vertebral and long bone fractures, avascular osteonecrosis, tendon rupture, muscle weakness.

FLUID AND ELECTROLYTE DISTURBANCE - Sodium and water retention, hypertension, hypokalaemic alkalosis, potassium loss, congestive heart failure in susceptible patients.

DERMATOLOGICAL - Impaired healing, skin atrophy, bruising, striae, telangiectasia, acne, petechiae and ecchymosis. Kaposi's sarcoma has been reported in patients receiving corticosteroid therapy.

ENDOCRINE/METABOLIC - Suppression of the hypothalamo-pituitary-adrenal axis, growth suppression in infancy, childhood and adolescence; menstrual irregularity and amenorrhoea. Cushingoid facies, hirsutism, weight gain, impaired carbohydrate tolerance with increased requirement for antidiabetic therapy, negative nitrogen and calcium balance. Increased appetite.

NEUROPSYCHIATRIC - A wide range of psychiatric reactions including affective disorders (such as irritable, euphoric, depressed and labile mood psychological dependence and suicidal thoughts), psychotic reactions (including mania, delusions, hallucinations and aggravation of schizophrenia), behavioural disturbances, irritability, anxiety, sleep disturbances, seizures and cognitive dysfunction including confusion and amnesia have been reported for all corticosteroids. Reactions are common and may occur in both adults and children. In adults, the frequency of severe reactions was estimated to be 5-6%. Psychological effects have been reported on withdrawal of corticosteroids; the frequency is unknown. Increased intra-cranial pressure with papilloedema in children (pseudotumour cerebri) has been reported, usually after treatment withdrawal of methylprednisolone.

OPHTHALMIC - Increased intra-ocular pressure, glaucoma, papilloedema with possible damage to the optic nerve, cataracts, corneal or scleral thinning, exacerbation of ophthalmic viral or fungal disease, exophthalmos.

CARDIOVASCULAR – Myocardial rupture following myocardial infarction.

GENERAL - Leucocytosis, hypersensitivity reactions including anaphylaxis, thrombo-embolism, nausea, malaise, persistent hiccups with high doses of corticosteroids.

WITHDRAWAL SYMPTOMS - Too rapid a reduction of corticosteroid dosage following prolonged treatment can lead to acute adrenal insufficiency, hypotension and death (see Special warnings and special precautions for use).

A 'withdrawal syndrome' may also occur including, fever, myalgia, arthralgia, rhinitis, conjunctivitis, painful itchy skin nodules and loss of weight.

4.9 Overdose

Administration of Medrone should not be discontinued abruptly but tailed off over a period of time. Appropriate action should be taken to alleviate the symptoms produced by any side-effect that may become apparent. It may be necessary to support the patient with corticosteroids during any further period of trauma occurring within two years of overdosage.

There is no clinical syndrome of acute overdose with Medrone. Methylprednisolone is dialysable.

5. PHARMACOLOGICAL PROPERTIES

5.1 Pharmacodynamic properties

Medrone is a potent corticosteroid with an anti-inflammatory activity at least five times that of hydrocortisone. An enhanced separation of glucocorticoid and mineralocorticoid effect results in a reduced incidence of sodium and water retention.

5.2 Pharmacokinetic properties

Corticosteroids are absorbed from the gastro-intestinal tract. In the circulation they are extensively bound to plasma proteins and are metabolised mainly in the liver but also in the kidney and are excreted in the urine.

The half-life of methylprednisolone has been reported to be slightly longer than that of prednisolone.

5.3 Preclinical safety data

None.

6. PHARMACEUTICAL PARTICULARS

6.1 List of excipients

Medrone Tablets 2mg: Lactose, rose colour, sucrose, maize starch and calcium stearate.

Medrone Tablets 4mg: Lactose, sucrose, maize starch and calcium stearate.

6.2 Incompatibilities

None stated.

6.3 Shelf life

Bottles - 60 months

Blister packs - 36 months.

6.4 Special precautions for storage

Store below 25°C.

6.5 Nature and contents of container

20-25 micron hard tempered aluminium foil/lacquer, 250 micron opaque polyvinyl chloride film blister. Pack contains 30 tablets.

6.6 Special precautions for disposal and other handling

No special requirements.

7. MARKETING AUTHORISATION HOLDER

Pharmacia Ltd

Ramsgate Road

Sandwich

Kent

CT13 9NJ

UK

8. MARKETING AUTHORISATION NUMBER(S)

Medrone Tablets 2mg: PL 0032/5017R

Medrone Tablets 4mg: PL 0032/5018R

9. DATE OF FIRST AUTHORISATION/RENEWAL OF THE AUTHORISATION

1st February 2005

10. DATE OF REVISION OF THE TEXT
3rd April 2008

Legal category
POM

Ref: MD 3_0 UK

Menadiol Diphosphate Tablets 10mg (Cambridge Laboratories)

(Cambridge Laboratories)

1. NAME OF THE MEDICINAL PRODUCT
Menadiol Diphosphate Tablets 10mg

2. QUALITATIVE AND QUANTITATIVE COMPOSITION
Each tablet contains 10mg of Menadiol Diphosphate (as Menadiol Sodium Diphosphate USP).

3. PHARMACEUTICAL FORM
Tablets.

The tablets are round, white to pale pink with CL 1L3 imprinted on one face and a single break bar on the other.

4. CLINICAL PARTICULARS

4.1 Therapeutic indications
For the treatment of haemorrhage or threatened haemorrhage associated with a low blood level of prothrombin or factor vii. The main indication is obstructive jaundice (before and after surgery).

4.2 Posology and method of administration
Menadiol Diphosphate Tablets 10mg are for oral administration.

Adults

Usual therapeutic dose: 10-40mg daily

Children

If, on the recommendation of a physician, a children's dosage is required, it is suggested that 5-20mg daily be given.

The elderly

Recommendations for use in the elderly do not differ from those for other adults.

4.3 Contraindications
Administration to neonates, infants or to mothers in the pre- and post-natal periods.

4.4 Special warnings and precautions for use
None.

4.5 Interaction with other medicinal products and other forms of interaction
Large doses of menadiol sodium diphosphate may decrease patient sensitivity to anticoagulants.

4.6 Pregnancy and lactation
There is evidence of hazard if menadiol sodium diphosphate is used in human pregnancy. It is known to be associated with a small risk of haemolytic anaemia, hyperbilirubinaemia and kernicterus in the infant if administered to the mother in late pregnancy or during labour. Menadiol sodium diphosphate is therefore contra-indicated during late pregnancy.

4.7 Effects on ability to drive and use machines
None known.

4.8 Undesirable effects
Menadiol sodium diphosphate may induce haemolysis (especially in the newborn infant) in the presence of erythrocyte glucose-6-phosphate dehydrogenase deficiency or low concentrations of alpha-tocopherol in the blood.

4.9 Overdose
No information is available.

5. PHARMACOLOGICAL PROPERTIES

5.1 Pharmacodynamic properties
Menadiol sodium diphosphate is a water-soluble vitamin K analogue. The presence of vitamin K is essential for the formation within the body of prothrombin, factor VII, factor IX and factor X. Lack of vitamin K leads to increased tendency to haemorrhage.

5.2 Pharmacokinetic properties
Menadione is absorbed from the gastro-intestinal tract without being dependent upon the presence of bile salts. Vitamin K is rapidly metabolised and excreted by the body.

5.3 Preclinical safety data
There are no pre-clinical data of relevance to the prescriber which are additional to that already included in other sections of the SPC.

6. PHARMACEUTICAL PARTICULARS

6.1 List of excipients
Lactose

Maize starch

Talc

Magnesium stearate

6.2 Incompatibilities
No information is available.

6.3 Shelf life
Three years.

6.4 Special precautions for storage
Recommended maximum storage temperature 30°C.

Protect from light.

6.5 Nature and contents of container
White HDPE bottles containing 100 tablets.

6.6 Special precautions for disposal and other handling
None.

Administrative Data

7. MARKETING AUTHORISATION HOLDER
Cambridge Laboratories Limited

Deltic House

Kingfisher Way

Silverlink Business Park

Wallsend

Tyne & Wear

NE28 9NX

8. MARKETING AUTHORISATION NUMBER(S)
PL 12070/0007

9. DATE OF FIRST AUTHORISATION/RENEWAL OF THE AUTHORISATION
30 April 1992

10. DATE OF REVISION OF THE TEXT
March 2002

Meningitec in pre-filled syringe

(Wyeth Pharmaceuticals)

1. NAME OF THE MEDICINAL PRODUCT
Meningitec suspension for injection in pre-filled syringe

Meningococcal serogroup C oligosaccharide conjugate vaccine (adsorbed).

2. QUALITATIVE AND QUANTITATIVE COMPOSITION
One dose (0.5ml) contains:

Neisseria meningitidis (strain C11)

Serogroup C oligosaccharide.................. 10 micrograms

Conjugated to *Corynebacterium diphtheriae*

CRM_{197} carrier protein....... approximately 15 micrograms

Adsorbed on aluminium phosphate ... 0.125 mg Al^{3+}

For a full list of excipients, see section 6.1.

3. PHARMACEUTICAL FORM
Suspension for injection, in pre-filled syringe. After shaking, the vaccine is a homogeneous, white suspension.

4. CLINICAL PARTICULARS

4.1 Therapeutic indications
Active immunisation of children from 2 months of age, adolescents and adults for the prevention of invasive disease caused by *Neisseria meningitidis* serogroup C.

The use of Meningitec should be determined on the basis of official recommendations.

4.2 Posology and method of administration

Posology
There are no data on the use of different Meningococcal serogroup C conjugate vaccines within the primary series or for boosting. Whenever possible, the same vaccine should be used throughout.

Primary immunisation

Infants up to the age of 12 months: two doses, each of 0.5 mL, the first dose given not earlier than 2 months of age and with an interval of at least 2 months between doses.

Children over the age of 12 months, adolescents and adults: a single dose of 0.5 mL.

The timing of the doses should be in accordance with official recommendations.

Booster doses

It is recommended that a booster dose should be given after completion of the primary immunisation series in infants. The timing of this dose should be in accordance with available official recommendations. Information on responses to booster doses and on co-administration with other childhood vaccines is given in sections 5.1 and 4.5, respectively.

The need for booster doses in subjects primed with a single dose (i.e. aged 12 months or more when first immunised) has not yet been established.

Method of administration
Meningitec is for intramuscular injection, preferably in the anterolateral thigh in infants and in the deltoid region in older children, adolescents and adults. Meningitec should not be injected in the gluteal area.

Avoid injection into or near nerves and blood vessels.

The vaccine must not be administered intravenously (see section 4.4). The safety and immunogenicity of administration via the intradermal or subcutaneous routes have not been evaluated.

Separate injection sites should be used if more than one vaccine is being administered (see section 4.5). This vaccine must not be mixed with other vaccines in the same syringe.

4.3 Contraindications
• Hypersensitivity to the active substances or to any of the excipients.

• Hypersensitivity to any vaccine containing diphtheria toxoid or non-toxic diphtheria toxin protein.

• Hypersensitivity after previous administration of Meningitec.

• As with other vaccines, the administration of Meningitec should be postponed in subjects suffering from an acute severe febrile illness.

4.4 Special warnings and precautions for use
As with all injectable vaccines, appropriate medical treatment and supervision should always be readily available in case of a rare anaphylactic/anaphylactic event following the administration of the vaccine (see section 4.8 Undesirable effects).

As with any intramuscular injection, the vaccine should be given with caution to individuals with thrombocytopenia or any coagulation disorder or to those receiving anticoagulation therapy.

Meningitec will only confer protection against serogroup C of *Neisseria meningitidis* and may not completely prevent meningococcal serogroup C disease. It will not protect against other groups of *Neisseria meningitidis* or other organisms that cause meningitis or septicaemia. In the event of petechiae and/or purpura following vaccination (see section 4.8), the aetiology should be thoroughly investigated. Both infective and non-infective causes should be considered.

Although symptoms of meningism such as neckpain/stiffness or photophobia have been reported there is no evidence that the vaccine causes meningococcal C meningitis. Clinical alertness to the possibility of co-incidental meningitis should therefore be maintained.

Consideration should be given to the risk of *Neisseria meningitidis* serogroup C disease in a given population and the perceived benefits of immunisation before the institution of a widespread immunisation programme.

No data on the applicability of the vaccine to outbreak control are available.

The safety and immunogenicity have not been established in infants below the age of two months (see section 5.1 pharmacodynamic properties).

There are limited data on safety and immunogenicity of the vaccine in the adult population and there are no data in adults aged 65 years and older (see section 5.1).

Limited data are available on the use of Meningitec in immunodeficient subjects. In individuals with impaired immune responsiveness (whether due to the use of immunosuppressive therapy, a genetic defect, human immunodeficiency virus (HIV) infection, or other causes) the expected immune response to meningococcal serogroup C conjugate vaccines may not be obtained. The implications for the actual degree of protection against infection are unknown, since this will depend also on whether the vaccine has elicited an immunological memory response. Individuals with complement deficiencies and individuals with functional or anatomical asplenia may mount an immune response to meningococcal serogroup C conjugate vaccines; however, the degree of protection that would be afforded is unknown.

The potential risk of apnoea and the need for respiratory monitoring for 48-72h should be considered when administering the primary immunisation series to very premature infants (born ⩽ 28 weeks of gestation) and particularly for those with a previous history of respiratory immaturity. As the benefit of vaccination is high in this group of infants, vaccination should not be withheld or delayed.

Immunisation with this vaccine does not substitute for routine diphtheria vaccination.

Meningitec SHOULD UNDER NO CIRCUMSTANCES BE ADMINISTERED INTRAVENOUSLY.

4.5 Interaction with other medicinal products and other forms of interaction
Meningitec must not be mixed with other vaccines in the same syringe. Separate injection sites should be used if more than one vaccine is being administered.

Administration of Meningitec at the same time as (but, for injected vaccines, at a different injection site) the following vaccines did not reduce the immunological response to any of these other antigens in clinical trials:

Oral Polio vaccine (OPV); Inactivated Polio vaccine (IPV); Hepatitis B vaccine (HBV); diphtheria and tetanus vaccine alone (D or T), in combination (DT or dT), or in combination with whole cell or acellular Pertussis vaccine (DTwP or DTaP); *Haemophilus influenzae* type b conjugate vaccine (Hib alone or in combination with other antigens) or combined Measles, Mumps, and Rubella vaccine (MMR).

Minor variations in geometric mean antibody concentrations (GMCs) or titres (GMTs) were observed between studies; however, the clinical significance, if any, of these observations is not established.

Data that support concomitant administration of Meningitec and an acellular Pertussis vaccine (i.e. DTaP) or an Inactivated Polio vaccine (IPV) are derived from studies in which subjects received either Meningitec or the same meningococcal serogroup C conjugate as in Meningitec combined with an investigational pneumococcal conjugate vaccine and from a study of concomitant administration with the Infanrix Hexa paediatric combination vaccine (DTaP-HBV-IPV/Hib).

In various studies with different vaccines, concomitant administration of meningococcal serogroup C conjugates with combinations containing acellular pertussis components (with or without inactivated polio viruses, hepatitis B surface antigen or Hib conjugates) has been shown to result in lower SBA GMTs compared to separate administrations or to co-administration with whole cell pertussis vaccines. The proportions reaching SBA titres of at least 1:8 or 1:128 are not affected. At present, the potential implications of these observations for the duration of protection are not known.

In a clinical trial that compared separate with concomitant administrations of Meningitec (two doses at 2 and 6 months and a booster dose at approximately 12 months) and Prevenar (pneumococcal conjugate 7-valent vaccine; three doses at 2, 3.5, 6 months and a booster dose at approximately 12 months) there was no evidence of immune interference between the two conjugate vaccines after the primary series or after the booster doses.

4.6 Pregnancy and lactation

Pregnancy

There are no clinical data on the use of meningococcal serogroup C conjugate vaccine in pregnant women. Animal studies are insufficient with respect to effects on pregnancy and embryonal/foetal development, parturition and postnatal development (see 5.3. Preclinical safety data). The potential risk for humans is unknown.

Nevertheless, considering the severity of meningococcal serogroup C disease, pregnancy should not preclude vaccination when the risk of exposure is clearly defined.

Lactation

The risk-benefit relationship should also be examined before making the decision as to whether immunise during lactation.

4.7 Effects on ability to drive and use machines

No studies on the effects on the ability to drive and use machines have been performed.

Some of the effects mentioned under section 4.8 (Undesirable effects) such as dizziness and somnolence may affect the ability to drive or operate machinery.

4.8 Undesirable effects

Note: the following descriptions of frequency have been defined as: Very common (⩾10%); Common (⩾1% and <10%); Uncommon (⩾0.1% and <1%); Rare (⩾0.01% and <0.1%); Very rare (<0.01%), not known (cannot be estimated from the available data).

Adverse Reactions from Clinical Trials

Adverse reactions reported across all age groups are provided below. Adverse reactions were collected on the day of vaccination and the following three days. The majority of reactions were self-limiting and resolved within the follow-up period.

In all age groups injection site reactions (including redness, swelling and tenderness/pain) were very common. However, these were not usually clinically significant. Redness or swelling of at least 3 cm and tenderness interfering with movement for more than 48 hours was infrequent where studied. Transient injection site tenderness was reported in 70% of adults during clinical trials.

Fever of at least 38.0°C was common in infants and toddlers and very common in pre-school children, but did not usually exceed 39.1°C, particularly in older age groups.

In infants and toddlers crying was common after vaccination while drowsiness, impaired sleeping, anorexia, diarrhoea and vomiting were very common. Irritability was very common in infants and in toddlers and common in children aged between 3.5 and 6 years. There was no evidence that these were related to Meningitec rather than concomitant vaccines, particularly DTP.

In trials that evaluated three-dose schedules (2, 3 and 4 months or 2, 4 and 6 months) in infants, rates of adverse events did not increase with successive doses with the exception of fever ⩾38°C. However, it should be noted that infants received other scheduled vaccines concomitantly with Meningitec in these studies.

Myalgia was common in adults. Somnolence was commonly reported in children between 3.5 and 6 years of age and in adults. Headache was common in children between 3.5 and 6 years of age and was very common in adults.

Adverse reactions reported across all age groups are provided below.

General Disorders and Administration Site Conditions:

Very common: Injection site reactions (e.g. redness, swelling, pain/tenderness)

Common: Fever ⩾ 38°C

Additional reactions reported in infants (first year of life) and toddlers (second year of life) are provided below.

Metabolism and Nutrition disorders:

Very common: Anorexia

Psychiatric Disorders:

Very common: Irritability

Common: Crying

Nervous System Disorders:

Very common: Drowsiness, impaired sleeping

Gastrointestinal Disorders:

Very common: Vomiting, diarrhoea

Additional reactions reported in older age groups including adults (4 to 60 years) included:

Psychiatric Disorders:

Common: Irritability (children between 3.5 and 6 years of age)

Nervous System Disorders:

Very common: Headache (adults)

Common: Somnolence, headache (children between 3.5 and 6 years of age)

Musculoskeletal, Connective Tissue and Bone Disorders:

Common: Myalgia (adults)

Adverse Reactions from Post Marketing Surveillance (for all age groups)

These frequencies are based on spontaneous reporting rates and have been calculated using number of reports and number of doses distributed.

Blood and Lymphatic System Disorders:

Very rare: Lymphadenopathy

Immune System Disorders:

Very rare: Anaphylactoid/anaphylactic reactions including shock, hypersensitivity reactions including bronchospasm, facial oedema and angioedema

Nervous System Disorders:

Very rare: Dizziness, faints, seizures (convulsions) including febrile seizures and seizures in patients with pre-existing seizure disorders, hypoaesthesia, paraesthesia and hypotonia (including hypotonic-hyporesponsive episode [HHE])

There have been very rare reports of seizures following Meningitec vaccination; individuals have usually rapidly recovered. Some of the reported seizures may have been faints. The reporting rate of seizures was below the background rate of epilepsy in children. In infants seizures were usually associated with fever and were likely to be febrile convulsions.

There have been very rare spontaneous reports of hypotonic-hyporesponsive episode (HHE), a condition characterised by hypotonia and reduced responsiveness in association with pallor or cyanosis, in temporal association with the administration of meningococcal serogroup C conjugate vaccine. In most cases, meningococcal serogroup C conjugate vaccine was administered concomitantly with other vaccines, the majority of which were pertussis-containing vaccines.

Gastrointestinal Disorders:

Very rare: Vomiting, nausea, abdominal pain

Skin and Subcutaneous Tissue Disorders:

Very rare: Rash, urticaria, pruritus, erythema multiforme, Stevens-Johnson syndrome

Musculoskeletal, Connective Tissue and Bone Disorders:

Very rare: Arthralgia

Renal and Urinary Disorders:

Relapse of nephrotic syndrome has been reported in association with Meningococcal serogroup C conjugate vaccines.

Very rarely, petechiae and/or purpura have been reported following immunisation (see also section 4.4).

Apnoea in very premature infants (⩽ 28 weeks of gestation) (see section 4.4).

4.9 Overdose

There have been reports of overdose with Meningitec, including cases of administration of a higher than recommended dose at one visit, cases of subsequent doses administered closer than recommended to the previous dose, and cases in which the recommended total number of doses has been exceeded. Most individuals were asymptomatic. In general, adverse events reported with overdosage have also been reported with recommended single doses of Meningitec.

5. PHARMACOLOGICAL PROPERTIES

5.1 Pharmacodynamic properties

Pharmacotherapeutic group: *Meningococcal vaccines*, ATC code: *J07AH07*

Immunogenicity

No prospective efficacy trials have been performed.

Serological correlates for protection have not been definitively established for conjugated meningococcal C vaccines; these are under study.

The serum bactericidal antibody (SBA) assay referenced in the text below, used rabbit serum as a source of complement.

Primary Series in Infants

Two doses in infants provided SBA antibody titres (using baby rabbit complement) ⩾1:8 in 98-99.5% of infants, as shown in the Table below. A two-dose infant schedule primed for a memory response to a booster dose given at 12 months of age.

% of subjects achieving ⩾1:8 SBA titres (GMT)		
STUDY with Meningitec given at age	AFTER 2ND DOSE	AFTER 12-MONTH booster
2, 3, 4 months with concomitant DTwP-Hib and OPV	98% (766) n=55	(Not studied)
3, 5, 7 months given alone	99.5% (1591)# n=214	(Not studied)
2, 4, 6 months with concomitant DTaP-HBV-IPV/Hib*	99.5% (1034)# n=218	(Not studied)
3, 5 months administered as 9vPnC-MnCC with concomitant DTaP-IPV/Hib	98.2% (572) n=56	100% (1928) n=23 (9vPnC-MnCC booster)
		100% (2623) n=28 (Meningitec+23vPnPS booster)

* See section 4.5

measured at two months after the second dose

MnCC = meningococcal serogroup C conjugate vaccine (which is the active component in Meningitec)

DTwP = whole cell pertussis vaccine with diphtheria and tetanus toxoids

OPV = oral polio virus vaccine

DTaP-IPV/Hib = acellular pertussis components, diphtheria and tetanus toxoids, inactivated polioviruses and a Hib conjugate (tetanus toxoid carrier protein)

DTaP-HBV-IPV/Hib = as above plus recombinant hepatitis B surface antigen in a hexavalent formulation

9v-PnC-MnCC = investigational 9-valent pneumococcal conjugate vaccine (not licensed) formulated with meningococcal serogroup C conjugate vaccine (which is the active component in Meningitec)

23vPnPS = 23-valent pneumococcal polysaccharide vaccine

Immunogenicity of a single primary dose in toddlers

91% of 75 toddlers of 13 months of age developed SBA titers ⩾ 1/8 and 89% of these 75 subjects showed a four-fold increase over their pre-vaccination antibody titre after receiving a single dose of Meningitec.

Immunogenicity of a single primary dose in adults

All the 15 adults of 18-60 years who received a single dose of Meningitec achieved SBA titers ⩾ 1/8 and a four-fold rise in antibody titre.

There are no data in adults aged 65 years and older.

Post-marketing surveillance following an immunisation campaign in the UK

Estimates of vaccine effectiveness from the UK's routine immunisation programme (using various quantities of three meningococcal serogroup C conjugate vaccines) covering the period from introduction at the end of 1999 to March 2004 have demonstrated the need for a booster dose after completion of the primary series (three doses administered at 2, 3 and 4 months).

Within one year of completion of the primary series, vaccine effectiveness in the infant cohort was estimated at 93% (95% CI: 67, 99). However, more than one year after completion of the primary series, there was clear evidence of waning protection. Estimates of effectiveness based on a small number of cases to date indicate that there may also be waning protection in children who received a single priming dose as toddlers. Effectiveness in all other age groups (up to 18 years) primed with a single dose has so far remained around 90% or more within and more than one year after vaccination.

5.2 Pharmacokinetic properties

Evaluation of pharmacokinetic properties is not required for vaccines.

5.3 Preclinical safety data

Female mice were immunised intramuscularly with twice the clinical dose of meningococcal serogroup C conjugate vaccine, either prior to mating or during the gestation period. Gross necropsy of viscera was performed on each mouse. All mice survived to either delivery or caesarean-section. No adverse clinical signs were present in any mouse and no parameters that were evaluated were affected by administration of the vaccine, in either the adult or foetal mice.

6. PHARMACEUTICAL PARTICULARS

6.1 List of excipients

Sodium chloride

Water for injections.

6.2 Incompatibilities

In the absence of compatibility studies, this medicinal product must not be mixed with other medicinal products.

6.3 Shelf life

2 years

6.4 Special precautions for storage

Store in a refrigerator (2°C – 8°C). Do not freeze. Discard if the vaccine has been frozen.

Store in the original package.

6.5 Nature and contents of container

0.5 ml of suspension in a pre-filled syringe (type I glass) with a plunger stopper ((latex-free gray butyl rubber) and a protective-tip cap (latex-free gray butyl rubber). Pack sizes of 1 and 10 pre-filled syringes with or without needle, and a multipack of 2 packs of 10 pre-filled syringes without needle.

Not all pack sizes may be marketed.

6.6 Special precautions for disposal and other handling

Upon storage, a white deposit and clear supernatant can be observed.

The vaccine should be well shaken in order to obtain a homogeneous white suspension and visually inspected for any foreign particulate matter and/or variation of physical aspect prior to administration. If this is observed, discard the vaccine.

Any unused product or waste material should be disposed of in accordance with local requirements.

7. MARKETING AUTHORISATION HOLDER

John Wyeth & Brother Limited

Huntercombe Lane South

Taplow, Maidenhead

Berkshire SL6 0PH

United Kingdom

8. MARKETING AUTHORISATION NUMBER(S)

PL 00011/0496

9. DATE OF FIRST AUTHORISATION/RENEWAL OF THE AUTHORISATION

19 September 2007

10. DATE OF REVISION OF THE TEXT

24 July 2009

Detailed information on this medicinal product is available on the website of www.emc.medicines.org.uk

Menitorix

(GlaxoSmithKline UK)

1. NAME OF THE MEDICINAL PRODUCT

Menitorix – Powder and solvent for solution for injection

Haemophilus type b and *Meningococcal* group C conjugate vaccine

2. QUALITATIVE AND QUANTITATIVE COMPOSITION

After reconstitution, each 0.5 ml dose contains:

Haemophilus type b polysaccharide (polyribosylribitol phosphate)	5 micrograms
conjugated to tetanus toxoid as carrier protein	12.5 micrograms
Neisseria meningitidis group C (strain C11) polysaccharide	5 micrograms
conjugated to tetanus toxoid as carrier protein	5 micrograms

For a full list of excipients, see section 6.1.

3. PHARMACEUTICAL FORM

Powder and solvent for solution for injection

White powder and a clear colourless solvent.

4. CLINICAL PARTICULARS

4.1 Therapeutic indications

Active immunization of infants from the age of 2 months and toddlers up to the age of 2 years for the prevention of invasive diseases caused by *Haemophilus influenzae* type b (Hib) and *Neisseria meningitidis* group C (MenC).

See also section 4.4.

4.2 Posology and method of administration

Posology

Primary vaccination in infants from 2 months up to 12 months of age:

Three doses, each of 0.5 ml, should be given with an interval of at least 1 month between doses.

There are no data on the use of Menitorix for one or two doses of the primary vaccination course and other Hib and/or MenC conjugate vaccines for other dose(s). It is recommended that infants who receive Menitorix for the first dose should also receive this vaccine for the second and third doses of the primary vaccination course.

Booster vaccination:

After primary vaccination in infancy, booster doses of Hib and MenC must be administered. In children who received an acellular pertussis combination vaccine containing Hib in the primary infant immunisation series the Hib booster dose should be given before the age of 2 years.

A single (0.5 ml) dose of Menitorix may be used to boost immunity to Hib and MenC in children who have previously completed a primary immunisation series with Menitorix or with other Hib or MenC conjugate vaccines. The timing of the booster dose should be in accordance with available official recommendations and should usually be given from the age of 12 months onwards and before the age of 2 years.

Menitorix is not recommended for use in children above 2 years of age due to lack of data on safety and efficacy.

Long-term immunogenicity data following the use of Menitorix as a primary and booster vaccination are not yet available (see section 5.1).

Menitorix should be given by intramuscular injection only, preferably in the anterolateral thigh region. In children 12 to 24 months of age, the vaccine may be administered in the deltoid region. (see also sections 4.4 and 4.5)

Menitorix should under no circumstances be administered intravascularly, intradermally or subcutaneously.

4.3 Contraindications

Hypersensitivity to the active substances, including tetanus toxoid, or to any of the excipients (see sections 2 and 6.1).

Hypersensitivity reaction after previous administration of Menitorix.

Acute severe febrile illness. The presence of a minor infection is not a contraindication for vaccination.

4.4 Special warnings and precautions for use

As with all injectable vaccines, appropriate medical treatment and supervision should always be readily available in case of a rare anaphylactic event following the administration of the vaccine.

Vaccination should be preceded by a review of the medical history (especially with regard to previous vaccination and possible occurrence of undesirable events) and a clinical examination.

The vaccine should be given with caution to individuals with thrombocytopenia or any coagulation disorder. No data are available on subcutaneous administration of Menitorix, therefore the possibility of any toxicity or reduced efficacy that might occur with this route of administration is unknown.

Menitorix will only confer protection against *Haemophilus influenzae* type b and *Neisseria meningitidis* group C. As for any vaccine, Menitorix may not completely protect against the infections it is intended to prevent in every vaccinated individual. There are no data available on administration of Menitorix in toddlers not already primed with Hib and MenC conjugates.

No data are available on the use of Menitorix in immunodeficient subjects. In individuals with impaired immune responsiveness (whether due to the use of immunosuppressive therapy, a genetic defect, human immunodeficiency virus (HIV) infection, or other causes) a protective immune response to Hib and MenC conjugate vaccines may not be obtained. Individuals with complement deficiencies and individuals with functional or anatomical asplenia may mount an immune response to Hib and MenC conjugate vaccines; however the degree of protection that would be afforded is unknown.

There are no data available on the use of Menitorix in infants who were born prematurely. Therefore the degree of protection that would be afforded is unknown.

Although symptoms of meningism such as neck pain/stiffness or photophobia have been reported following administration of other MenC conjugate vaccines, there is no evidence that MenC conjugate vaccines cause meningitis. Clinical alertness to the possibility of co-incidental meningitis should be maintained.

The potential risk of apnoea and the need for respiratory monitoring for 48-72h should be considered when administering the primary immunisation series to very premature infants (born ≤ 28 weeks of gestation) and particularly for those with a previous history of respiratory immaturity. As the benefit of the vaccination is high in this group of infants, vaccination should not be withheld or delayed.

Immunisation with this vaccine does not substitute for routine tetanus immunisation.

Since Hib capsular polysaccharide antigen is excreted in the urine, a positive urine antigen test can be observed within 1-2 weeks following vaccination. Other diagnostic tests, not based on the detection of the capsular antigen in urine, should be used to confirm Hib disease during this period.

4.5 Interaction with other medicinal products and other forms of interaction

Menitorix must not be mixed with any other vaccine in the same syringe.

Different injectable vaccines should always be given at different injection sites.

In various studies with licensed monovalent meningococcal group C conjugate vaccines, concomitant administration with combinations containing diphtheria, tetanus and acellular pertussis components (with or without inactivated polio viruses, hepatitis B surface antigen or Hib conjugate [e.g. DTPa-HBV-IPV-Hib*]), has been shown to result in lower serum bactericidal antibody (SBA) geometric mean titres (GMT) compared to separate administrations or to co-administration with whole cell pertussis vaccines. The proportions reaching SBA titres of at least 1:8 are not affected. At present, the potential implications of these observations for the duration of protection are not known.

In clinical trials of primary vaccination series, Menitorix was administered concomitantly (into opposite thighs) with a DTPa-HBV-IPV vaccine. Responses to all the co-administered antigens were satisfactory and were similar to those achieved in control groups that received DTPa-HBV-IPV-Hib* concomitantly with a MenC conjugate vaccine (MenCC) or DTPa-HBV-IPV* concomitantly with a Hib conjugate vaccine and no MenCC. The immune response to the Hib and MenC components of Menitorix was only assessed in primary vaccination clinical studies that employed co-administration with DTPa-IPV* or DTPa-HBV-IPV* vaccines.

In a trial of primary vaccination, concomitant administration of an investigational vaccine containing the same amount of conjugated Hib and MenC saccharides as in Menitorix with DTPa-HBV-IPV* and a licensed pneumococcal saccharide conjugated vaccine (the three injections were made into anatomically distant sites) gave similar immune responses to the seven pneumococcal serotypes as achieved in a group that received DTPa-HBV-IPV* concomitantly with Hib (conjugated to tetanus toxoid) and a licensed pneumococcal saccharide conjugated vaccine.

There are no data on concomitant use of Menitorix with whole cell pertussis and oral poliomyelitis vaccines, however, no interference is expected.

In a trial of booster vaccination against Hib and MenC, Menitorix was administered concomitantly (into opposite thighs) with a first dose of combined measles, mumps and rubella (MMR) vaccine. Compared to the two control groups that received either Menitorix or MMR alone the immune responses to the antigens in both vaccines were not affected by concomitant administration. See sections 4.8 and 5.1.

*GlaxoSmithKline combination vaccine

4.6 Pregnancy and lactation

Menitorix is not intended for use in adults. Information on the safety of the vaccine when used during pregnancy or lactation is not available.

4.7 Effects on ability to drive and use machines

Not relevant.

4.8 Undesirable effects

- Clinical trials

In clinical trials, Menitorix was administered as a 3-dose primary series (N=1,171) or as a booster (N=991) dose. When Menitorix was administered as a 3-dose primary vaccination course, a DTPa-HBV-IPV* vaccine (N=796) or a DTPa-IPV* vaccine (N=375) was administered concomitantly.

Adverse reactions occurring during these studies were mostly reported within 48 hours following vaccination.

In two clinical trials (N=578), Menitorix was administered concomitantly with Measles, Mumps, Rubella (MMR) vaccine. In one of these trials, the incidences of adverse reactions observed in subjects (N=102) who received Menitorix concomitantly with MMR* were similar to those observed in the group who received MMR alone (N=91) or Menitorix alone (N=104). (see sections 4.5 and 5.1)

Adverse reactions considered as being at least possibly related to vaccination have been categorised by frequency as follows.

Very common (≥1/10)

Common (≥1/100, <1/10)

Uncommon (≥1/1,000, <1/100)

Rare (≥1/10,000, <1/1,000)

Very rare (<1/10,000)

Not known (cannot be estimated from the available data)

Within each frequency grouping, undesirable effects are presented in order of decreasing seriousness.

Psychiatric disorders:

very common: irritability

uncommon: crying

Nervous system disorders:

very common: drowsiness

Gastrointestinal disorders:

very common: appetite lost

uncommon: diarrhoea, vomiting

Skin and subcutaneous tissue disorders:

uncommon: dermatitis atopic

rare: rash

Table 1

Antibody		2-3-4 month schedule	
		After two doses N=93	After three doses N=330†
Anti-PRP	⩾0.15 micrograms/ml	96.8%	100.0%
	⩾1 micrograms/ml	76.3%	97.3%
	GMC (micrograms/ml)	3.40	11.18
rSBA-MenC	⩾1:8	100.0%	98.8%
	⩾1:32	98.9%	97.9%
	⩾1:128	98.9%	92.4%
	GMT	679.6	685.5

N= Number of subjects with available results

%= percentage of subjects with titres equal to or above the cut-off

PRP= polyribosylribitol phosphate

rSBA-MenC= serum bactericidal antibodies against meningococcal polysaccharide C using rabbit complement

GMC or GMT= geometric mean antibody concentration or titre

†= subjects ≤ 18 weeks of age at time of third Menitorix dose

Table 2

Antibody		2-4-6 month schedule	
		After two doses N=111	After three doses N=111
Anti-PRP	⩾0.15 micrograms/ml	96.4%	100.0%
	⩾1 micrograms/ml	74.8%	97.3%
	GMC (micrograms/ml)	3.26	12.84
rSBA-MenC	⩾1:8	100.0%	100.0%
	⩾1:32	100.0%	100.0%
	⩾1:128	96.4%	99.1%
	GMT	847.2	2467.1

N= number of subjects with available results

%= percentage of subjects with titres equal to or above the cut-off

PRP= polyribosylribitol phosphate

rSBA-MenC= serum bactericidal antibodies against meningococcal polysaccharide C using rabbit complement

GMC or GMT= geometric mean antibody concentration or titre

General disorders and administration site conditions:

very common: fever (rectal ⩾ 38°C), swelling, pain, redness

common: injection site reaction

uncommon: fever (rectal > 39.5°C), malaise

• Post-marketing experience

The following adverse events have been reported after administration of Menitorix:

Blood and lymphatic system disorders:

Lymphadenopathy

Nervous system disorders:

Febrile seizures, hypotonia, headache, dizziness

Respiratory, thoracic and mediastinal disorders:

Apnoea in very premature infants (= 28 weeks of gestation) (see section 4.4)

Immune system disorders:

Allergic reactions (including urticaria and anaphylactoid reactions)

• Other possible side effects:

The following have not been reported in association with administration of Menitorix but have occurred very rarely during routine use of licensed meningococcal group C conjugate vaccines:

Severe skin reactions), collapse or shock-like state (hypotonic-hyporesponsiveness episode), faints, seizures in patients with pre-existing seizure disorders, hypoaesthesia, paraesthesia, relapse of nephrotic syndrome, arthralgia, petechiae and/or purpura.

*GlaxoSmithKline combination vaccine

4.9 Overdose

No case of overdose has been reported.

5. PHARMACOLOGICAL PROPERTIES

5.1 Pharmacodynamic properties

Pharmacotherapeutic group: bacterial vaccines ATC code: J07AG53

Primary vaccination course

Clinical studies have evaluated the antibody responses at one month after two doses and after completion of a 3-dose primary vaccination course of Menitorix (co-administered with DTPa-HBV-IPV or DTPa-IPV vaccines) given at approximately 2, 3, 4 months or 2, 4, 6 months to 814 infants.

Percentages of subjects with antibody titres ≥ assay cut-off one month after primary vaccination with Menitorix co-administered with DTPa-IPV* or DTPa-HBV-IPV* vaccines were as follows:

(see Table 1 above)

(see Table 2 avove)

Antibody persistence has been demonstrated for Hib in three clinical trials (N=217) with 98.2% of subjects having an anti-PRP concentration of ⩾ 0.15 micrograms/ml at 11-18 months of age i.e. at 7-14 months following completion of a 3-dose primary series with Menitorix.

In three clinical trials (N=209), 92.3% of subjects had an SBA-MenC titre ⩾ 1/8 at 11–18 months of age, i.e. at 7-14 months following completion of a 3-dose primary series with Menitorix. All subjects responded immunologically to a challenge dose of 10 micrograms of unconjugated group C meningococcal polysaccharide with a thirty-three-fold increase in SBA titres demonstrating the immune memory induced by the primary vaccination course.

Booster vaccination

Percentages of subjects with antibody titres ≥ assay cut-off one month after booster vaccination with Menitorix alone or co-administered with DTPa-HBV-IPV* vaccine were as follows:

(see Table 3 below)

Percentages of subjects with antibody titres ⩾ assay cut-off one month after booster vaccination with Menitorix co-administered with measles-mumps-rubella vaccine (MMR)* were as follows:

(see Table 4 on next page)

Antibody levels have been measured at 18 months after the administration of a booster dose of Menitorix at age 14 Months to subjects who had been primed in infancy with either Menitorix at 2, 4 and 6 months of age or with NeisVac-C at 2, 4 months of age (and a DTPa/Hib containing vaccine at 2, 4, 6 months of age). SBA-MenC results are available for 177 subjects, anti-PRP results for 178 subjects. Overall, 92.7% of 177 subjects had SBA-MenC titres of at least 1:8 and 99.4% of the 178 subjects had anti-PRP antibody concentrations of at least 0.15 μg/ml. In the Menitorix primed and boosted group 49/56 (87.5%) of the subjects had SBA-MenC titers of at least 1:8 and 56/56 (100%) had anti-PRP antibody concentrations of at least 0.15 μg/ml. In the group primed with NeisVac-C 115/121 (95%) had SBA-MenC titers of at least 1:8 and 121/122 (99.2%) had anti-PRP antibody concentrations of at least 0.15 μg/ml. There were no significant differences between the two groups in the proportions with SBA-MenC titers of at least 1:8 or anti-PRP antibody concentrations of at least 0.15μg /ml.

Post-marketing surveillance following an immunisation campaign in the UK

Estimates of vaccine effectiveness from the UK's routine immunisation programme (using various quantities of three meningococcal group C conjugate vaccines) covering the period from introduction at the end of 1999 to March 2004 demonstrated the need for a booster dose after completion of the primary series (three doses administered at 2, 3 and 4 months). Within one year of completion of the primary series, vaccine effectiveness in the infant cohort was estimated at 93% (95% confidence intervals 67-99). However, more than one year after completion of the primary series, there was clear evidence of waning protection.

Up to 2007, the overall estimates of effectiveness in age cohorts from 1-18 years that received a single dose of meningococcal group C conjugate vaccine during the initial catch-up vaccination programme in the UK fall between 83 and 100%. The data show no significant fall in effectiveness within these age cohorts when comparing time periods less than a year or one year or more since immunisation.

*GlaxoSmithKline combination vaccine

Table 3

	Primary vaccination history		
	Subjects primed with 3 doses of Menitorix* N=123	Subjects primed with 2 doses of NeisVac-C** N=167	Subjects primed with 3 doses of Meningitec** or Menjugate** N=96
Anti-PRP antibodies			
⩾0.15 micrograms/ml	100.0%	100.0%	100.0%
⩾1 micrograms/ml	100.0%	98.8%	99.0%
GMC micrograms/ml	56.72	77.15	30.27
rSBA-MenC			
⩾1:8	100.0%	99.4%	98.9%
⩾1:32	100.0%	99.4%	97.9%
⩾1:128	99.2%	99.4%	92.6%
GMT	4172.5	11710.5	685.0

N= number of subjects with available results

PRP= polyribosylribitol phosphate

rSBA-MenC= serum bactericidal antibodies against meningococcal polysaccharide C using rabbit complement

GMC or GMT= geometric mean antibody concentration or titre

%= percentage of subjects with titres equal to or above the cut-off

*= co-administered with DTPa-HBV-IPV

**= co-administered with DTPa-Hib-TT containing vaccines

Table 4

	Primary vaccination history		
	Subjects primed with 3 doses of Menitorix* N= 349	Subjects primed with 3 doses of Meningitec + Pediacel N= 115	Subjects primed with 3 doses of licensed Meningitec** or Menjugate** N= 96
Anti-PRP antibodies			
⩾0.15 micrograms/ml	100%	100%	100%
⩾1 micrograms/ml	100%	100%	97.9%
GMC (micrograms/ml)	93.19	44.27	37.17
rSBA-MenC			
⩾1:8	99.1%	95.6%	98.9%
⩾1:32	98.8%	94.7%	96.8%
⩾1:128	97.7%	86.0%	89.5%
GMT	2193.7	477.9	670.2

N= number of subjects with available results
PRP= polyribosylribitol phosphate
rSBA-MenC= serum bactericidal antibodies against meningococcal polysaccharide C using rabbit complement
GMC or GMT= geometric mean antibody concentration or titre
%= percentage of subjects with titres equal to or above the cut-off
*= co-administered with DTPa-HBV-IPV
**= co-administered with DTPa-Hib-TT containing vaccines

5.2 Pharmacokinetic properties
Evaluation of pharmacokinetic properties is not required for vaccines.

5.3 Preclinical safety data
Preclinical data reveal no special hazard for humans based on conventional studies of safety pharmacology and single and repeated dose toxicity studies.

6. PHARMACEUTICAL PARTICULARS
6.1 List of excipients
Powder:
Trometamol
Sucrose
Solvent:
Sodium chloride
Water for injections

6.2 Incompatibilities
In the absence of compatibility studies, this medicinal product must not be mixed with other medicinal products.

6.3 Shelf life
3 years.

After reconstitution, the vaccine should be administered promptly or kept in the refrigerator (2°C – 8°C). If it is not used within 24 hours, it should be discarded.

Experimental data show that the reconstituted vaccine could also be kept to 24 hours at ambient temperature (25°C). If it is not used within 24 hours, it should be discarded.

6.4 Special precautions for storage
Store in a refrigerator (2°C – 8°C).

Do not freeze

Store in the original package in order to protect from light.

6.5 Nature and contents of container
Powder in a vial (type I glass) with a stopper (butyl rubber),

0.5 ml of solvent in a pre-filled syringe (type I glass) with a plunger stopper (butyl rubber) with or without separate needles in the following pack sizes:

- pack size of 1 vial of powder plus 1 pre-filled syringe of solvent with 2 separate needles or without needles

- pack size of 10 vials of powder plus 10 pre-filled syringes of solvent with 2 separate needles or without needles

Not all pack sizes may be marketed.

6.6 Special precautions for disposal and other handling
The reconstituted vaccine should be inspected visually for any foreign particulate matter and/or variation of physical aspect prior to administration. In the event of either being observed, discard the vaccine.

The vaccine must be reconstituted by adding the entire contents of the pre-filled syringe of solvent to the vial containing the powder. After the addition of the solvent, the mixture should be well shaken until the powder is completely dissolved in the solvent.

The reconstituted vaccine is a clear and colourless solution. Inject the entire contents of the vial.

Any unused product or waste material should be disposed of in accordance with local requirements.

7. MARKETING AUTHORISATION HOLDER
SmithKline Beecham plc

Trading as:

GlaxoSmithKline UK

Stockley Park West, Uxbridge

Middlesex, UB11 1BT

8. MARKETING AUTHORISATION NUMBER(S)
PL10592/0217

9. DATE OF FIRST AUTHORISATION/RENEWAL OF THE AUTHORISATION
19 December 2005

10. DATE OF REVISION OF THE TEXT
4 May 2009

Menopur
(Ferring Pharmaceuticals Ltd)

1. NAME OF THE MEDICINAL PRODUCT
MENOPUR®

2. QUALITATIVE AND QUANTITATIVE COMPOSITION
Active ingredient
Each vial with dry substance contains highly purified menotrophin (human menopausal gonadotrophin, HMG) corresponding to 75 IU human follicle stimulating hormone (FSH) and 75 IU human luteinising hormone (LH).

3. PHARMACEUTICAL FORM
Powder for injection; and solvent for parenteral use.

4. CLINICAL PARTICULARS
4.1 Therapeutic indications
Treatment of female and male infertility in the following groups of patients:

- Anovulatory women: MENOPUR can be used to stimulate follicle development in amenorrhoeic patients. Clomiphene (or a similar ovulation inducing agent which influences steroid feed-back mechanisms) is the preferred treatment for women with a variety of menstrual cycle disturbances, including luteal phase insufficiency with anovulatory cycles and with normal prolactin, and also amenorrhoeic patients with evidence of endogenous oestrogen production but normal prolactin and normal gonadotrophin levels. Non-responders may then be selected for menotrophin therapy.

- Women undergoing superovulation within a medically assisted fertilisation programme: MENOPUR can be used to induce multiple follicular development in patients undergoing an assisted conception technique such as in-vitro fertilisation (IVF).

- Hypogonadotrophic hypogonadism in men: MENOPUR may be given in combination with human chorionic gonadotrophin (e.g. Choragon) for the stimulation of spermatogenesis. Patients with primary testicular failure are usually unresponsive.

4.2 Posology and method of administration
Anovulatory infertility:
Menotrophin is administered to induce follicular maturation and is followed by treatment with chorionic gonadotrophin to stimulate ovulation and corpus luteum formation.

The dosage and schedule of treatment must be determined according to the needs of each patient. Response is monitored by studying the patient's urinary oestrogen excretion or by ultrasound visualisation of follicles. Menotrophin may be given daily by either intramuscular or subcutaneous injection to provide a dose of 75 to 150 units of FSH and 75 to 150 units of LH, and gradually adjusted if necessary until an adequate response is achieved, followed after 1 or 2 days by chorionic gonadotrophin. In menstruating patients, treatment should be started within the first 7 days of the menstrual cycle. The treatment course should be abandoned if no response is seen in 3 weeks. This treatment cycle may be repeated at least twice more if necessary. Alternatively, three equal doses of menotrophin, each providing 225 to 375 units of FSH with 225 to 375 units of LH, may be given on alternate days followed by chorionic gonadotrophin one week after the first dose.

In the daily therapy schedule, the dose is gradually increased until oestrogen levels start to rise. The effective dose is then maintained until adequate pre-ovulatory oestrogen levels are reached. If oestrogen levels rise too rapidly, the dose should be decreased.

As a measure of follicle maturity the following values can be taken:

- total urinary oestrogen: 75 - 150 micrograms (270 - 540 nmol)/24 hours

- plasma 17 beta-oestradiol: 400 - 800 picograms/ml (1500 - 3000 pmol/L).

When adequate pre-ovulatory oestrogen levels have been reached, administration of MENOPUR is stopped, and ovulation may then be induced by administering human chorionic gonadotrophin at a dose of 5000 - 10000 IU.

Women undergoing superovulation in IVF or other assisted conception techniques:
In in-vitro fertilisation procedures or other assisted conception techniques menotrophin is used in conjunction with chorionic gonadotrophin and sometimes also clomiphene citrate or a gonadorelin agonist. Stimulation of follicular growth is produced by menotrophin in a dose providing 75 to 300 units of FSH with 75 to 300 units of LH daily. Treatment with menotrophin, either alone or in conjunction with clomiphene or a gonadorelin agonist, is continued until an adequate response is obtained and the final injection of menotrophin is followed 1 or 2 days later with up to 10000 units of chorionic gonadotrophin.

Maturation of follicles is monitored by measurement of oestrogen levels, ultrasound and/or clinical evaluation of oestrogen activity. It is recommended there should be at least 3 follicles greater than 17mm in diameter with 17 beta-oestradiol levels of at least 3500 pmol/L (920 picograms/ml). Egg maturation occurs by administration of human chorionic gonadotrophin in a dose of 5000-10000 IU, 30 - 40 hours after the last MENOPUR injection. Human chorionic gonadotrophin should not be administered if these criteria have not been met. Egg retrieval is carried out 32 - 36 hours after the human chorionic gonadotrophin injection.

Male infertility:
Spermatogenesis is stimulated with chorionic gonadotrophin (1000 – 2000 IU two to three times a week) and then menotrophin is given in a dose of 75 or 150 units of FSH with 75 or 150 units of LH two or three times weekly. Treatment should be continued for at least 3 or 4 months.

Children:
Not recommended for use in children.

Elderly:
Not recommended for use in the elderly.

Method of Administration:
By intramuscular or subcutaneous use.

The dry substance must be reconstituted with the diluent prior to use.

4.3 Contraindications
Men and Women
MENOPUR is contraindicated in men and women with:

- Tumours of the pituitary or hypothalamic glands

- Hypersensitivity to the active substance or any of the excipients used in the formulation (see section 6.1)

Men
- Tumours in the testes
- Prostate carcinoma

Women
- Ovarian, uterine or mammary carcinoma
- Pregnancy and lactation
- Gynaecological haemorrhage of unknown aetiology
- Ovarian cysts or enlarged ovaries not due to polycystic ovarian disease.

In the following situations treatment outcome is unlikely to be favourable, and therefore MENOPUR should not be administered:

- Primary ovarian failure
- Malformation of sexual organs incompatible with pregnancy
- Fibroid tumours of the uterus incompatible with pregnancy

- Structural abnormalities in which a satisfactory outcome cannot be expected, for example, tubal occlusion (unless superovulation is to be induced for IVF), ovarian dysgenesis, absent uterus or premature menopause.

4.4 Special warnings and precautions for use

MENOPUR is a potent gonadotropic substance capable of causing mild to severe adverse reactions, and should only be used by physicians who are thoroughly familiar with infertility problems and their management.

In the treatment of female infertility, ovarian activity should be checked (by ultrasound and plasma 17 beta-oestradiol measurement) prior to MENOPUR administration. During treatment, these tests and urinary oestrogen measurement should be carried out at regular intervals, until stimulation occurs. Close supervision is imperative during treatment. See "posology and administration" for optimum response levels of urinary oestrogen and plasma 17 beta-oestradiol. Values below these ranges may indicate inadequate follicular development.

There is considerable inter-patient variability in response to menotrophin administration, with a poor response to menotrophin in some patients. The lowest effective dose in relation to the treatment objective should be used.

The first injection of MENOPUR should be performed under direct medical supervision.

Before starting treatment, the couple's infertility should be assessed as appropriate and putative contraindications for pregnancy evaluated. In particular, patients should be evaluated for hypothyroidism, adrenocortical deficiency, hyperprolactinemia and pituitary or hypothalamic tumours, and appropriate specific treatment given.

Patients undergoing stimulation of follicular growth, whether in the frame of a treatment for anovulatory infertility or ART procedures may experience ovarian enlargement or develop hyperstimulation. Adherence to recommended MENOPUR dosage and regimen of administration, and careful monitoring of therapy will minimise the incidence of such events. Acute interpretation of the indices of follicle development and maturation requires a physician who is experienced in the interpretation of the relevant tests.

Ovarian Hyperstimulation Syndrome (OHSS)

OHSS is a medical event distinct from uncomplicated ovarian enlargement. OHSS is a syndrome that can manifest itself with increasing degrees of severity. It comprises marked ovarian enlargement, high serum sex steroids, and an increase in vascular permeability which can result in an accumulation of fluid in the peritoneal, pleural and rarely, in the pericardial cavities.

The severe form OHSS may be life-threatening and is characterised by large ovarian cysts (prone to rupture), acute abdominal pain, ascites, very often hydrothorax and occasionally thromboembolic phenomena. Other symptoms that may be observed include: abdominal distension, severe ovarian enlargement, weight gain, dyspnoea, oliguria and gastrointestinal symptoms including nausea, vomiting and diarrhoea. Clinical evaluation may reveal hypovolaemia, haemoconcentration, electrolyte imbalances, haemoperitoneum, pleural effusions and acute pulmonary distress.

If urinary oestrogen levels exceed 540 nmol (150 micrograms)/24 hours, or if plasma 17 beta-oestradiol levels exceed 3000 pmol/L (800 picograms/ml), or if there is any steep rise in values, there is an increased risk of hyperstimulation and MENOPUR treatment should be immediately discontinued and human chorionic gonadotrophin withheld. Ultrasound will reveal any excessive follicular development and unintentional hyperstimulation. In the event of hyperstimulation, the patient should refrain from sexual intercourse or to use barrier contraception methods for at least 4 days. OHSS may progress rapidly (within 24 hours to several days) to become a serious medical event, therefore patients should be followed for at least two weeks after the hCG administration.

If during ultrasound, several mature follicles are visualised, human chorionic gonadotrophin should not be given as there is a risk of multiple ovulation and the occurrence of hyperstimulation syndrome.

Adherence to recommended MENOPUR dosage, regimen of administration and careful monitoring of therapy will minimise the incidence of ovarian hyperstimulation and multiple pregnancy (see sections 4.2 and 4.8). Patients undergoing superovulation may be at an increased risk of developing hyperstimulation in view of the excessive oestrogen response and multiple follicular development. In ART, aspiration of all follicles prior to ovulation may reduce the occurrence of hyperstimulation.

OHSS may be more severe and more protracted if pregnancy occurs. Most often, OHSS occurs after hormonal treatment has been discontinued and reaches its maximum at about seven to ten days following treatment. Usually, OHSS resolves spontaneously with the onset of menses.

If severe OHSS occurs, gonadotrophin treatment should be stopped if still ongoing, the patient hospitalised and specific therapy for OHSS started.

This syndrome occurs with higher incidence in patients with polycystic ovarian disease.

Multiple pregnancy

Multiple pregnancy, especially high order, carries an increased risk of adverse maternal and perinatal outcomes.

In patients undergoing ART procedures the risk of multiple pregnancy is related mainly to the number of embryos replaced, their quality and the age of the patient.

The patient should be advised of the potential risk of multiple births before starting treatment.

Pregnancy wastage

The incidence of pregnancy wastage by miscarriage or abortion is higher in patients undergoing stimulation of follicular growth for ART procedures than in the normal population.

Ectopic pregnancy

Women with a history of tubal disease are at risk of ectopic pregnancy, whether the pregnancy is obtained by spontaneous conception or with fertility treatment. The prevalence of ectopic pregnancy after IVF has been reported to be 2 to 5%, as compared to 1 to 1.5% in the general population.

Reproductive system neoplasms

There have been reports of ovarian and other reproductive system neoplasms, both benign and malignant, in women who have undergone multiple drug regimens for infertility treatment. It is not yet established if treatment with gonadotrophins increases the baseline risk of these tumours in infertile women.

Congenital malformation

The prevalence of congenital malformations after ART may be slightly higher than after spontaneous conceptions. This is thought to be due to differences in parental characteristics (e.g. maternal age, sperm characteristics) and multiple pregnancies.

Thromboembolic events

In women with generally recognised risk factors for thromboembolic events, such as personal or family history, treatment with gonadotrophins may further increase the risk. In these women, the benefits of gonadotrophin administration need to be weighed against the risks. It should be noted however, that pregnancy itself also carries an increased risk of thromboembolic events.

4.5 Interaction with other medicinal products and other forms of interaction

No drug/drug interaction studies have been conducted with MENOPUR in humans.

Although there is no controlled clinical experience, it is expected that the concomitant use of MENOPUR and clomiphene citrate may enhance the follicular response. When using GnRH agonist for pituitary desensitization, a higher dose of MENOPUR may be necessary to achieve adequate follicular response.

4.6 Pregnancy and lactation

MENOPUR should not be given during pregnancy or to lactating mothers.

4.7 Effects on ability to drive and use machines

None known.

4.8 Undesirable effects

The most frequently reported adverse drug reactions during treatment with MENOPUR in clinical trials are ovarian hyperstimulation, abdominal pain, headache, enlarged abdomen, inflammation at the injection site, pain at the injection site and nausea, with an incidence rate between 2% and 7%. The table below displays the main adverse drug reactions in women treated with MENOPUR in clinical trials according to body system and frequency.

Body System	Frequency	Adverse Drug Reaction
Central/peripheral nervous system disorders	Common (>1/100 <1/10)	Headache
Gastro-intestinal disorders	Common (>1/100 <1/10)	Abdominal pain, enlarged abdomen, nausea and vomiting
Female reproductive disorders	Common (>1/100 <1/10)	Ovarian hyperstimulation
Application site disorders	Common (>1/100 <1/10)	Inflammation at injection site, pain at injection site
Vascular (extracardiac) disorders	Uncommon (>1/1,000 <1/100)	Deep vein thrombosis

In very rare cases, long term use of menotrophin can lead to the formation of antibodies making treatment ineffectual.

Very rare cases of allergic reactions, localised or generalised, and delayed-type hypersensitivity have been reported after treatment with gonadotrophin containing products.

4.9 Overdose

The acute toxicity of menotrophin has been shown to be very low. However, too high a dosage for more than one day may lead to hyperstimulation, which is categorised as mild, moderate or severe. Symptoms of overdosage usually appear 3 - 6 days after treatment with human chorionic gonadotrophin.

Mild hyperstimulation - Symptoms include some abdominal swelling and pain, ovaries enlarged to about 5cm diameter. Therapy - rest; careful observation and symptomatic relief. Ovarian enlargement declines rapidly.

Moderate hyperstimulation - Symptoms include more pronounced abdominal distension and pain, nausea, vomiting, occasional diarrhoea, ovaries enlarged up to 12cm diameter. Therapy - bed rest; close observation especially in the case of conception occurring, to detect any progression to severe hyperstimulation.

Pelvic examination of enlarged ovaries should be gentle in order to avoid rupture of the cysts. Symptoms subside spontaneously over 2 - 3 weeks.

Severe hyperstimulation - This is a rare but serious complication - symptoms include pronounced abdominal distension and pain, ascites, pleural effusion, decreased blood volume, reduced urine output, electrolyte imbalance and sometimes shock, ovaries enlarge to in excess of 12cm diameter. Therapy - hospitalisation; treatment should be conservative and concentrate on restoring blood volume and preventing shock. Acute symptoms subside over several days and ovaries return to normal over 20 - 40 days if conception does not occur - symptoms may be prolonged if conception occurs.

5. PHARMACOLOGICAL PROPERTIES

5.1 Pharmacodynamic properties

Menotrophin is a gonadotrophin extracted from the urine of postmenopausal women and having both luteinising hormone and follicle stimulating hormone activity. It is given by intramuscular or subcutaneous injection in the treatment of male and female infertility.

Menotrophin (HMG) directly affects the ovaries and the testes. HMG has a gametropic and steroidogenic effect.

In the ovaries, the FSH-component in HMG induces an increase in the number of growing follicles and stimulates their development. FSH increases the production of oestradiol in the granulosa cells by aromatising androgens that originate in the Theca cells under the influence of the LH-component.

In the testes, FSH induces the transformation of premature to mature Sertoli cells. It mainly causes the maturation of the seminal canals and the development of the spermatozoa. However, a high concentration of androgens within the testes is necessary and can be attained by a prior treatment using hCG.

5.2 Pharmacokinetic properties

HMG is not effective when taken orally and is injected either intramuscularly or subcutaneously. The biological effectiveness of HMG is mainly due to its FSH content. The pharmacokinetics of HMG following intramuscular or subcutaneous administration show great individual variation. The maximum serum level of FSH is reached approximately 18 hours after intramuscular injection and 12 hours after subcutaneous injection. After that, the serum level decreases by a half-life of approximately 55 hours following intramuscular administration and 50 hours following subcutaneous administration.

Excretion of HMG, following administration, is predominantly renal.

5.3 Preclinical safety data

Toxic effects caused by HMG are unknown in humans.

There is no evidence of teratogenic, mutagenic or carcinogenic activity of HMG. Antibodies against HMG can be built up in single cases following repeated cyclical administration of HMG, causing the treatment to be ineffectual.

6. PHARMACEUTICAL PARTICULARS

6.1 List of excipients

Dry substance: lactose, polysorbate 20, sodium hydroxide and hydrochloric acid for pH-adjustment.

Solvent: isotonic sodium chloride solution, dilute hydrochloric acid for pH adjustment.

6.2 Incompatibilities

None known.

6.3 Shelf life

Two years as packaged for sale.

The reconstituted product should be used immediately and any remaining solution should be discarded.

6.4 Special precautions for storage

Protect from light. Store at a temperature not exceeding 25°C.

6.5 Nature and contents of container

Dry substance: 2ml glass vial

6.6 Special precautions for disposal and other handling

The dry substance must be reconstituted with the diluent prior to use.

Use immediately after reconstitution.

7. MARKETING AUTHORISATION HOLDER

Ferring Pharmaceuticals Limited

The Courtyard

Waterside Drive

Langley

Berkshire SL3 6EZ

United Kingdom

8. MARKETING AUTHORISATION NUMBER(S)

MENOPUR PL 03194/0074

Sodium Chloride Solution for Injections 0.9% w/v PL 03194/0060

9. DATE OF FIRST AUTHORISATION/RENEWAL OF THE AUTHORISATION

19 November 2004

10. DATE OF REVISION OF THE TEXT

November 2005

11. LEGAL CATEGORY

POM

Merbentyl Syrup

(sanofi-aventis)

1. NAME OF THE MEDICINAL PRODUCT

Merbentyl Syrup

2. QUALITATIVE AND QUANTITATIVE COMPOSITION

Dicycloverine Hydrochloride 10mg

3. PHARMACEUTICAL FORM

Syrup

4. CLINICAL PARTICULARS

4.1 Therapeutic indications

Merbentyl is a smooth muscle antispasmodic primarily indicated for treatment of functional conditions involving smooth muscle spasm of the gastrointestinal tract. The commonest of these are irritable colon (mucous colitis, spastic colon).

4.2 Posology and method of administration

Adults

One to two 5ml spoonfuls (10 - 20mg) three times daily before or after meals.

Children (2-12 years):

One 5ml spoonful (10mg) three times daily.

Children (6 months - 2 years)

5 - 10mg three or four times daily, 15 minutes before feeds. Do not exceed a daily dose of 40mg. If it is necessary to dilute Merbentyl Syrup this may be done using Syrup or if diluted immediately prior to use with water.

4.3 Contraindications

Known idiosyncrasy to dicycloverine hydrochloride. Infants under 6 months of age.

Patients with rare hereditary problems of fructose intolerance, glucose galactose malabsorption or sucrase-isomaltase insufficiency should not take this medicine.

4.4 Special warnings and precautions for use

Products containing dicycloverine hydrochloride should be used with caution in any patient with or suspected of having glaucoma or prostatic hypertrophy. Use with care in patients with hiatus hernia associated with reflux oesophagitis because anticholinergic drugs may aggravate the condition. There are reports of infants, 3 months of age and under, administered dicycloverine hydrochloride syrup who have evidenced respiratory symptoms (breathing difficulty, shortness of breath, breathlessness, respiratory collapse, apnoea) as well as seizures, syncope, asphyxia, pulse rate fluctuations, muscular hypotonia and coma. The above symptoms have occurred within minutes of ingestion and lasted 20-30 minutes. The symptoms were reported in association with dicycloverine hydrochloride syrup therapy but the cause and effect relationship has neither been disproved or proved. The timing and nature of the reactions suggest that they were a consequence of local irritation and/or aspiration, rather than to a direct pharmacological effect. Although no causal relationship between these effects, observed in infants and dicycloverine administration has been established, dicycloverine hydrochloride is contra-indicated in infants under 6 months of age.

4.5 Interaction with other medicinal products and other forms of interaction

None stated.

4.6 Pregnancy and lactation

Epidemiological studies in pregnant women with products containing dicycloverine hydrochloride (at doses up to 40mg/day) have not shown that dicycloverine hydrochloride increases the risk of foetal abnormalities if administered during the first trimester of pregnancy. Reproduction studies have been performed in rats and rabbits at doses of up to 100 times the maximum recommended dose (based on 60mg per day for an adult person) and have revealed no evidence of impaired fertility or harm to the foetus due to dicycloverine. Since the risk of teratogenicity cannot be excluded with absolute certainty for any product, the drug should be used during pregnancy only if clearly needed.

It is not known whether dicycloverine is secreted in human milk. Because many drugs are excreted in human milk, caution should be exercised when dicycloverine is administered to a nursing mother.

4.7 Effects on ability to drive and use machines

None stated.

4.8 Undesirable effects

Side-effects seldom occur with Merbentyl. However, in susceptible individuals, dry mouth, thirst and dizziness may occur. On rare occasions, fatigue, sedation, blurred vision, rash, constipation, anorexia, nausea and vomiting, headache and dysuria have also been reported.

4.9 Overdose

Symptoms of Merbentyl overdosage are headache, dizziness, nausea, dry mouth, difficulty in swallowing, dilated pupils and hot dry skin. Treatment may include emetics, gastric lavage and symptomatic therapy if indicated.

5. PHARMACOLOGICAL PROPERTIES

5.1 Pharmacodynamic properties

Dicycloverine hydrochloride relieves smooth muscle spasm of the gastrointestinal tract.

Animal studies indicate that this action is achieved via a dual mechanism;

(1) a specific anticholinergic effect (antimuscarinic at the ACh-receptor sites) and

(2) a direct effect upon smooth muscle (musculotropic).

5.2 Pharmacokinetic properties

After a single oral 20mg dose of dicycloverine hydrochloride in volunteers, peak plasma concentration reached a mean value of 58ng/ml in 1 to 1.5 hours. ^{14}C labelled studies demonstrated comparable bioavailability from oral and intravenous administration. The principal route of elimination is via the urine.

5.3 Preclinical safety data

None stated.

6. PHARMACEUTICAL PARTICULARS

6.1 List of excipients

Invert Syrup Medium

Citric Acid Monohydrate

Sodium Benzoate

Raspberry Flavour

Wild Cherry Bark Flavour

Blackcurrant Essence

Vanilla Essence

Purified water

6.2 Incompatibilities

None stated.

6.3 Shelf life

3 years.

6.4 Special precautions for storage

Do not store above 25°C. Should be stored and dispensed in amber glass bottles.

6.5 Nature and contents of container

Type III, EP amber glass bottles sealed with a polyethylene screw cap equiped with a polyethylene seal and pilferproof closure.

Pack size: 1 bottle containing 120ml syrup.

6.6 Special precautions for disposal and other handling

None stated.

7. MARKETING AUTHORISATION HOLDER

Sanofi-aventis

One Onslow Street

Guildford

Surrey, GU1 4YS, UK

8. MARKETING AUTHORISATION NUMBER(S)

PL 04425/0047

9. DATE OF FIRST AUTHORISATION/RENEWAL OF THE AUTHORISATION

Date of first authorisation: 13th July 1983

Date of renewal: 31 July 2001

10. DATE OF REVISION OF THE TEXT

December 2006

Legal category: POM

Merbentyl Tablets

(sanofi-aventis)

1. NAME OF THE MEDICINAL PRODUCT

Merbentyl 10mg Tablets

Merbentyl 20mg Tablets

2. QUALITATIVE AND QUANTITATIVE COMPOSITION

Dicycloverine hydrochloride 10mg or 20mg

3. PHARMACEUTICAL FORM

Tablets

4. CLINICAL PARTICULARS

4.1 Therapeutic indications

Smooth muscle antispasmodic primarily indicated for treatment of functional conditions involving smooth muscle spasm of the gastrointestinal tract.

4.2 Posology and method of administration

Route of administration: Oral

10mg and 20mg tablets:

Adults and children over 12 years: 10-20mg three times daily before or after meals.

10mg tablets only:

Children (2-12 years): 10mg three times daily.

4.3 Contraindications

Known idiosyncrasy to dicycloverine hydrochloride.

4.4 Special warnings and precautions for use

Products containing dicycloverine hydrochloride should be used with caution in any patient with or suspected of having glaucoma or prostatic hypertrophy. Use with care in patients with hiatus hernia associated with reflux oesophagitis because anticholinergic drugs may aggravate the condition.

4.5 Interaction with other medicinal products and other forms of interaction

None stated.

4.6 Pregnancy and lactation

Epidemiological studies in pregnant women with products containing dicycloverine hydrochloride (at doses up to 40mg/day) have not shown that dicycloverine hydrochloride increases the risk of foetal abnormalities if administered during the first trimester of pregnancy. Reproduction studies have been performed in rats and rabbits at doses of up to 100 times the maximum recommended dose (based on 60mg per day for an adult person) and have revealed no evidence of impaired fertility or harm to the foetus due to dicycloverine. Since the risk of teratogenicity cannot be excluded with absolute certainty for any product, the drug should be used during pregnancy only if clearly needed.

It is not known whether dicycloverine is secreted in human milk. Because many drugs are excreted in human milk, caution should be exercised when dicycloverine is administered to a nursing mother.

4.7 Effects on ability to drive and use machines

None stated.

4.8 Undesirable effects

Side-effects seldom occur with Merbentyl tablets. However, in susceptible individuals, dry mouth, thirst and dizziness may occur. On rare occasions, fatigue, sedation, blurred vision, rash, constipation, anorexia, nausea and vomiting, headache and dysuria have also been reported.

4.9 Overdose

Symptoms of Merbentyl overdosage are headache, dizziness, nausea, dry mouth, difficulty in swallowing, dilated pupils and hot dry skin. Treatment may include emetics, gastric lavage and symptomatic therapy if indicated.

5. PHARMACOLOGICAL PROPERTIES

5.1 Pharmacodynamic properties

Dicycloverine hydrochloride relieves smooth muscle spasm of the gastrointestinal tract.

Animal studies indicate that this action is achieved via a dual mechanism;

(1) a specific anticholinergic effect (antimuscarinic at the ACh-receptor sites) and

(2) a direct effect upon smooth muscle (musculotropic).

5.2 Pharmacokinetic properties

After a single oral 20mg dose of dicycloverine hydrochloride in volunteers, peak plasma concentration reached a mean value of 58ng/ml in 1 to 1.5 hours. ^{14}C labelled studies demonstrated comparable bioavailability from oral and intravenous administration. The principal route of elimination is via the urine.

5.3 Preclinical safety data

None stated.

6. PHARMACEUTICAL PARTICULARS

6.1 List of excipients

Lactose

Calcium Hydrogen Phosphate

Icing Sugar*

Maize Starch

Glucose Liquid**

Magnesium Stearate

Purified Water

* mixture of Sucrose 97%

Starch 3%

** equivalent to 4.8mg Glucose Solids

6.2 Incompatibilities

None stated.

6.3 Shelf life
5 years.

6.4 Special precautions for storage
Do not store above 25°C.

6.5 Nature and contents of container
Container: opaque blue 250 micron PVC blisters with aluminium foil 20 micron

Pack size 10mg tablets: 100 tablets.

Pack size 20mg tablets: 84 tablets

6.6 Special precautions for disposal and other handling
None stated.

7. MARKETING AUTHORISATION HOLDER
Sanofi-aventis
One Onslow Street
Guildford
Surrey, GU1 4YS, UK

8. MARKETING AUTHORISATION NUMBER(S)
Merbentyl 10mg PL 04425/0035
Merbentyl 20mg PL 04425/0081

9. DATE OF FIRST AUTHORISATION/RENEWAL OF THE AUTHORISATION
Date of first authorisation: Merbentyl 10mg - 27th September 1982

Merbentyl 20mg - 13 February 1986

Date of renewal: Merbentyl 10mg - 14th April 1994

Merbentyl 20mg - 13 February 1991

10. DATE OF REVISION OF THE TEXT
November 2006

Legal category: POM

Meronem IV 500mg & 1g

(AstraZeneca UK Limited)

1. NAME OF THE MEDICINAL PRODUCT
Meronem IV.

2. QUALITATIVE AND QUANTITATIVE COMPOSITION

Vial for IV injection or infusion	Meronem	Meronem
	500mg	1000 mg
Active ingredient:		
Meropenem trihydrate	570 mg	1140 mg
equivalent to anhydrous meropenem	500 mg	1000 mg

For excipients, see 6.1.

3. PHARMACEUTICAL FORM
Powder for solution for injection or infusion.

4. CLINICAL PARTICULARS
4.1 Therapeutic indications
Meronem IV is indicated for treatment, in adults and children, of the following infections caused by single or multiple bacteria sensitive to meropenem.

- Pneumonias and nosocomial pneumonias
- Urinary tract infections
- Intra-abdominal infections
- Gynaecological infections, such as endometritis.
- Skin and skin structure infections
- Meningitis
- Septicaemia
- Empiric treatment, for presumed infections in adult patients with febrile neutropenia, used as monotherapy or in combination with anti-viral or anti-fungal agents.

Meronem has proved efficacious alone or in combination with other antimicrobial agents in the treatment of polymicrobial infections.

Intravenous meropenem has been used effectively in patients with cystic fibrosis and chronic lower respiratory tract infections, either as monotherapy or in combination with other antibacterial agents. Eradication of the organism was not always established.

There is no experience in paediatric patients with neutropenia or primary or secondary immunodeficiency.

4.2 Posology and method of administration
Adults
The dosage and duration of therapy shall be established depending on type and severity of infection and the condition of the patient.

The recommended daily dosage is as follows:-

500 mg IV every 8 hours in the treatment of pneumonia, UTI, gynaecological infections such as endometritis, skin and skin structure infections.

1 g IV every 8 hours in the treatment of nosocomial pneumonias, peritonitis, presumed infections in neutropenic patients, septicaemia.

In cystic fibrosis, doses up to 2 g every 8 hours have been used; most patients have been treated with 2 g every 8 hours.

In meningitis the recommended dosage is 2 g every 8 hours.

As with other antibiotics, particular caution is recommended in using meropenem as monotherapy in critically ill patients with known or suspected *Pseudomonas aeruginosa* lower respiratory tract infection.

Regular sensitivity testing is recommended when treating *Pseudomonas aeruginosa* infection.

Dosage Schedule for Adults with Impaired Renal Function

Dosage should be reduced in patients with creatinine clearance less than 51 ml/min, as scheduled below.

Table 1

Creatinine Clearance (ml/min)	Dose (based on unit doses of 500 mg, 1 g, 2 g)	Frequency
26 to50	one unit dose	every 12 hours
10 to25	one-half unit dose	every 12 hours
<10	one-half unit dose	every 24 hours

Meropenem is cleared by haemodialysis; if continued treatment with Meronem is necessary, it is recommended that the unit dose (based on the type and severity of infection) is administered at the completion of the haemodialysis procedure to restore therapeutically effective plasma concentrations.

There is no experience with the use of Meronem in patients under peritoneal dialysis.

Dosage in Adults with Hepatic Insufficiency
No dosage adjustment is necessary in patients with hepatic insufficiency (see Section 4.4).

Elderly Patients
No dosage adjustment is required for the elderly with normal renal function or creatinine clearance values above 50 ml/min.

Children
For children over 3 months and up to 12 years of age the recommended dose is 10 to 20 mg/kg every 8 hours depending on type and severity of infection, susceptibility of the pathogen and the condition of the patient. In children over 50 kg weight, adult dosage should be used.

For children aged 4 to 18 years with cystic fibrosis, doses ranging from 25 to 40 mg/kg every 8 hours have been used to treat acute exacerbations of chronic lower respiratory tract infections.

In meningitis the recommended dose is 40 mg/kg every 8 hours.

There is no experience in children with renal impairment.

Method of Administration
Meronem IV can be given as an intravenous bolus injection over approximately 5 minutes or by intravenous infusion over approximately 15 to 30 minutes using the specific available presentations.

Meronem IV to be used for bolus intravenous injection should be constituted with sterile Water for Injections (5 ml per 250 mg meropenem). This provides an approximate concentration of 50 mg/ml. Constituted solutions are clear, and colourless or pale yellow.

Meronem IV for intravenous infusion may be constituted with compatible infusion fluids (50 to 200 ml) (see Sections 6.2 and 6.4).

4.3 Contraindications
Meronem is contraindicated in patients who have demonstrated hypersensitivity to this product.

4.4 Special warnings and precautions for use
There is some clinical and laboratory evidence of partial cross-allergenicity between other carbapenems and beta-lactam antibiotics, penicillins and cephalosporins. As with all beta-lactam antibiotics, rare hypersensitivity reactions have been reported (see Section 4.8). Before initiating therapy with meropenem, careful inquiry should be made concerning previous hypersensitivity reactions to beta-lactam antibiotics. Meronem should be used with caution in patients with such a history. If an allergic reaction to meropenem occurs, the drug should be discontinued and appropriate measures taken.

Use of Meronem in patients with hepatic disease should be made with careful monitoring of transaminase and bilirubin levels.

As with other antibiotics, overgrowth of non-susceptible organisms may occur and, therefore, continuous monitoring of each patient is necessary.

Use in infections caused by meticillin resistant staphylococci is not recommended.

Rarely, pseudomembranous colitis has been reported on Meronem as with practically all antibiotics and may vary in severity from slight to life-threatening. Therefore, antibiotics should be prescribed with care for individuals with a history of gastro-intestinal complaints, particularly colitis.

It is important to consider the diagnosis of pseudomembranous colitis in the case of patients who develop diarrhoea in association with the use of Meronem. Although studies indicate that a toxin produced by *Clostridium difficile* is one of the main causes of antibiotic-associated colitis, other causes should be considered.

The co-administration of Meronem with potentially nephrotoxic drugs should be considered with caution. For dosage see Section 4.2.

Meronem may reduce serum valproic acid levels. Subtherapeutic levels may be reached in some patients.

Paediatric use
Efficacy and tolerability in infants under 3 months old have not been established; therefore, Meronem is not recommended for use below this age. There is no experience in children with altered hepatic or renal function.

4.5 Interaction with other medicinal products and other forms of interaction
Probenecid competes with meropenem for active tubular secretion and thus inhibits the renal excretion, with the effect of increasing the elimination half-life and plasma concentration of meropenem. As the potency and duration of action of Meronem dosed without probenecid are adequate, the co-administration of probenecid with Meronem is not recommended.

The potential effect of Meronem on the protein binding of other drugs or metabolism has not been studied. The protein binding of Meronem is low (approximately 2%) and therefore no interactions with other compounds based on displacement from plasma proteins would be expected.

Meronem may reduce serum valproic acid levels. Subtherapeutic levels may be reached in some patients.

Meronem has been administered concomitantly with other medications without adverse pharmacological interactions. However, no other specific data regarding potential drug interactions is available (apart from probenecid as mentioned above).

4.6 Pregnancy and lactation
Pregnancy
The safety of Meronem in human pregnancy has not been evaluated. Animal studies have not shown any adverse effect on the developing foetus. The only adverse effect observed in animal reproductive studies was an increased incidence of abortions in monkeys at 13 times the expected exposure in man. Meronem should not be used in pregnancy unless the potential benefit justifies the potential risk to the foetus. In every case, it should be used under the direct supervision of the physician.

Lactation
Meropenem is detectable at very low concentrations in animal breast milk. Meronem should not be used in breast-feeding women unless the potential benefit justifies the potential risk to the baby.

4.7 Effects on ability to drive and use machines
No data are available, but it is not anticipated that Meronem will affect the ability to drive and use machines.

4.8 Undesirable effects

Frequency	System Order Class	MedDRA Term
Meronem is generally well tolerated. Adverse events rarely lead to cessation of treatment. Serious adverse events are rare.		
Common (≥1% and < 10%)	Blood and lymphatic system disorders[1]	Thrombocythaemia.
	Nervous system disorders	Headache.
	Gastrointestinal disorders	Nausea, Vomiting, Diarrhoea, Abdominal Pain.
	Hepato-biliary disorders	Increases in serum Transaminases, Alkaline Phosphatase, Lactic Dehydrogenase.
	Skin and subcutaneous tissue disorders	Rash, Pruritis
	General disorders and administration site conditions	Inflammation, Pain.

Uncommon (⩾0.1% and <1 %)	Blood and lymphatic system disorders	Eosinophilia, Thrombocytopenia
	Hepato-biliary disorders	Increases in Bilirubin
Rare (⩾0.01% and <0.1%)	Nervous system disorders	Convulsions[2]
Not known	Blood and lymphatic system disorders	Leucopenia, Neutropenia, Agranulocytosis, Haemolytic Anaemia.
	Immune system disorders	Angioedema, Manifestations of Anaphylaxis
	Nervous system disorders	Paraesthesia
	Gastrointestinal disorders	Pseudomembranous Colitis
	Skin and subcutaneous tissue disorders	Urticaria, Erythema Multiforme, Steven-Johnson Syndrome, Toxic Epidermal Necrolysis.
	General disorders and administration site conditions	Thrombophlebitis, Oral and Vaginal Candidiasis.

[1] A positive direct or indirect Coombs test may develop in some subjects; there have been reports of reduction in partial thromboplastin time.

[2]For convulsions, the incidence is calculated on exposures in patients with infections other than meningitis.

4.9 Overdose

Accidental overdosage could occur during therapy, particularly in patients with renal impairment. Limited post-marketing experience indicates that adverse events following overdosage are consistent with the adverse event profile described in section 4.8. Treatment of overdosage should be symptomatic. In normal individuals, rapid renal elimination will occur; in subjects with renal impairment, haemodialysis will remove meropenem and its metabolite.

5. PHARMACOLOGICAL PROPERTIES

5.1 Pharmacodynamic properties

Meropenem is a carbapenem antibiotic for parenteral use, that is relatively stable to human dehydropeptidase-1 (DHP-1) and therefore does not require the addition of an inhibitor of DHP-1.

Meropenem exerts its bactericidal action by interfering with vital bacterial cell wall synthesis. The ease with which it penetrates bacterial cell walls, its high level of stability to all serine beta-lactamases and its marked affinity for the Penicillin Binding Proteins (PBPs) explain the potent bactericidal action of meropenem against a broad spectrum of aerobic and anaerobic bacteria. Minimum bactericidal concentrations (MBC) are commonly the same as the minimum inhibitory concentrations (MIC). For 76% of the bacteria tested, the MBC:MIC ratios were 2 or less.

Meropenem is stable in susceptibility tests and these tests can be performed using normal routine methods. In vitro tests show that meropenem acts synergistically with various antibiotics. It has been demonstrated both in vitro and in vivo that meropenem has a post-antibiotic effect.

A single set of meropenem susceptibility criteria are recommended based on pharmacokinetics and correlation of clinical and microbiological outcomes with zone diameter and minimum inhibitory concentrations (MIC) of the infecting organisms.

Table 2

CATEGORISATION	METHOD OF ASSESSMENT	
	Zone Diameter (mm)	**MIC breakpoints (mg/L)**
Susceptible	⩾ 14	⩽ 4
Intermediate	12 to 13	8
Resistant	⩽ 11	⩾ 16

The in vitro antibacterial spectrum of meropenem includes the majority of clinically significant Gram-positive and Gram-negative, aerobic and anaerobic strains of bacteria, as shown below:

Gram-positive aerobes:

Bacillus spp., Corynebacterium diphtheriae, Enterococcus faecalis, Enterococcus liquifaciens, Enterococcus avium, Listeria monocytogenes, Lactobacillus spp., Nocardia asteroides, Staphylococcus aureus (penicillinase negative and positive), *Staphylococci-coagulase-negative;* including, *Staphylococcus epidermidis, Staphylococcus saprophyticus, Staphylococcus capitis, Staphylococcus cohnii, Staphylococcus xylosus, Staphylococcus warneri, Staphylococcus hominis, Staphylococcus simulans, Staphylococcus intermedius, Staphylococcus sciuri, Staphylococcus lugdunensis, Streptococcus pneumoniae* (penicillin susceptible and resistant), *Streptococcus agalactiae, Streptococcus pyogenes, Streptococcus equi, Streptococcus bovis, Streptococcus mitis, Streptococcus mitior, Streptococcus milleri, Streptococcus sanguis, Streptococcus viridans, Streptococcus salivarius, Streptococcus morbillorum, Streptococcus Group G, Streptococcus Group F, Rhodococcus equi.*

Gram-negative aerobes:

Achromobacter xylosoxidans, Acinetobacter anitratus, Acinetobacter lwoffii, Acinetobacter baumannii, Aeromonas hydrophila, Aeromonas sorbria, Aeromonas caviae, Alcaligenes faecalis, Bordetella bronchiseptica, Brucella melitensis, Campylobacter coli, Campylobacter jejuni, Citrobacter freundii, Citrobacter diversus, Citrobacter koseri, Citrobacter amalonaticus, Enterobacter aerogenes, Enterobacter (Pantoea) agglomerans, Enterobacter cloacae, Enterobacter sakazakii, Escherichia coli, Escherichia hermannii, Gardnerella vaginalis, Haemophilus influenzae (including beta-lactamase positive and ampicillin resistant strains), *Haemophilus parainfluenzae, Haemophilus ducreyi, Helicobacter pylori, Neisseria meningitidis, Neisseria gonorrhoeae* (including beta-lactamase positive, penicillin resistant and spectinomycin resistant strains), *Hafnia alvei, Klebsiella pneumoniae, Klebsiella aerogenes, Klebsiella ozaenae, Klebsiella oxytoca, Moraxella (Branhamella) catarrhalis, Morganella morganii, Proteus mirabilis, Proteus vulgaris, Proteus penneri, Providencia rettgeri, Providencia stuartii, Providencia alcalifaciens, Pasteurella multocida, Plesiomonas shigelloides, Pseudomonas aeruginosa, Pseudomonas putida, Pseudomonas alcaligenes, Burkholderia (Pseudomonas) cepacia, Pseudomonas fluorescens, Pseudomonas stutzeri, Pseudomonas pseudomallei, Pseudomonas acidovorans, Salmonella spp.* including *Salmonella enteritidis/typhi, Serratia marcescens, Serratia liquefaciens, Serratia rubidaea, Shigella sonnei, Shigella flexneri, Shigella boydii, Shigella dysenteriae, Vibrio cholerae, Vibrio parahaemolyticus, Vibrio vulnificus, Yersinia enterocolitica.*

Anaerobic bacteria:

Actinomyces odontolyticus, Actinomyces meyeri, Bacteroides-Prevotella-Porphyromonas spp., Bacteroides fragilis, Bacteroides vulgatus, Bacteroides variabilis, Bacteroides pneumosintes, Bacteroides coagulans, Bacteroides uniformis, Bacteroides distasonis, Bacteroides ovatus, Bacteroides thetaiotaomicron, Bacteroides eggerthii, Bacteroides capsillosis, Prevotella buccalis, Prevotella corporis, Bacteroides gracilis, Prevotella melaninogenica, Prevotella intermedia, Prevotella bivia, Prevotella splanchnicus, Prevotella oralis, Prevotella disiens, Prevotella rumenicola, Bacteroides ureolyticus, Prevotella oris, Prevotella buccae, Prevotella denticola, Bacteroides levii, Porphyromonas asaccharolytica, Bifidobacterium spp., Bilophila wadsworthia, Clostridium perfringens, Clostridium bifermentans, Clostridium ramosum, Clostridium sporogenes, Clostridium cadaveris, Clostridium sordellii, Clostridium butyricum, Clostridium clostridiiformis, Clostridium innocuum, Clostridium subterminale, Clostridium tertium, Eubacterium lentum, Eubacterium aerofaciens, Fusobacterium mortiferum, Fusobacterium necrophorum, Fusobacterium nucleatum, Fusobacterium varium, Mobiluncus curtisii, Mobiluncus mulieris, Peptostreptococcus anaerobius, Peptostreptococcus micros, Peptostreptococcus saccharolyticus, Peptococcus saccharolyticus, Peptostreptococcus asaccharolyticus, Peptostreptococcus magnus, Peptostreptococcus prevotii, Propionibacterium acnes, Propionibacterium avidum, Propionibacterium granulosum.

Stenotrophomonas maltophilia, Enterococcus faecium and methicillin-resistant staphylococci have been found to be resistant to meropenem.

5.2 Pharmacokinetic properties

A 30 minute intravenous infusion of a single dose of Meronem in healthy volunteers results in peak plasma levels of approximately 11 microgram/ml for the 250 mg dose, 23 microgram/ml for the 500 mg dose and 49 microgram/ml for the 1g dose.

However, there is no absolute pharmacokinetic proportionality with the administered dose both as regards Cmax and AUC. Furthermore, a reduction in plasma clearance from 287 to 205 ml/min for the range of dosage 250 mg to 2 g has been observed.

A 5 minute intravenous bolus injection of Meronem in healthy volunteers results in peak plasma levels of approximately 52 microgram/ml for the 500 mg dose and 112 microgram/ml for the 1g dose.

Intravenous infusions of 1 g over 2 minutes, 3 minutes and 5 minutes were compared in a three-way crossover trial. These durations of infusion resulted in peak plasma levels of 110, 91 and 94 microgram/ml, respectively.

After an IV dose of 500 mg, plasma levels of meropenem decline to values of 1 microgram/ml or less, 6 hours after administration.

When multiple doses are administered at 8 hourly intervals to subjects with normal renal function, accumulation of meropenem does not occur.

In subjects with normal renal function, meropenem's elimination half-life is approximately 1 hour.

Plasma protein binding of meropenem is approximately 2%.

Approximately 70% of the administered dose is recovered as unchanged meropenem in the urine over 12 hours, after which little further urinary excretion is detectable. Urinary concentrations of meropenem in excess of 10 microgram/ml are maintained for up to 5 hours after the administration of a 500 mg dose. No accumulation of meropenem in plasma or urine was observed with regimens using 500 mg administered every 8 hours or 1 g administered every 6 hours in volunteers with normal renal function.

The only metabolite of meropenem is microbiologically inactive.

Meropenem penetrates well into most body fluids and tissues including cerebrospinal fluid of patients with bacterial meningitis, achieving concentrations in excess of those required to inhibit most bacteria.

Studies in children have shown that the pharmacokinetics of Meronem in children are similar to those in adults. The elimination half-life for meropenem was approximately 1.5 to 2.3 hours in children under the age of 2 years and the pharmacokinetics are linear over the dose range of 10 to 40 mg/kg.

Pharmacokinetic studies in patients with renal insufficiency have shown the plasma clearance of meropenem correlates with creatinine clearance. Dosage adjustments are necessary in subjects with renal impairment.

Pharmacokinetic studies in the elderly have shown a reduction in plasma clearance of meropenem which correlated with age-associated reduction in creatinine clearance.

Pharmacokinetic studies in patients with liver disease have shown no effects of liver disease on the pharmacokinetics of meropenem.

5.3 Preclinical safety data

Animal studies indicate that meropenem is well tolerated by the kidney. In animal studies meropenem has shown nephrotoxic effects, only at high dose levels (500 mg/kg).

Effects on the CNS; convulsions in rats and vomiting in dogs, were seen only at high doses (>2000 mg/kg).

For an IV dose the LD_{50} in rodents is greater than 2000 mg/kg. In repeat dose studies (up to 6 months) only minor effects were seen including a small decrease in red cell parameters and an increase in liver weight in dogs treated with doses of 500 mg/kg.

There was no evidence of mutagenic potential in the 5 tests conducted and no evidence of reproductive and teratogenic toxicity in studies at the highest possible doses in rats and monkeys; the no effect dose level of a (small) reduction in F_1 body weight in rat was 120 mg/kg. There was an increased incidence of abortions at 500 mg/kg in a preliminary study in monkeys.

There was no evidence of increased sensitivity to meropenem in juveniles compared to adult animals. The intravenous formulation was well tolerated in animal studies.

The sole metabolite of meropenem had a similar profile of toxicity in animal studies.

6. PHARMACEUTICAL PARTICULARS

6.1 List of excipients

Meronem for IV injection and infusion includes the excipient anhydrous sodium carbonate.

6.2 Incompatibilities

Meronem should not be mixed with or added to other drugs.

Meronem is compatible with the following infusion fluids:

0.9% Sodium Chloride solution

5% or 10% Glucose solution

5% Glucose solution with 0.02% Sodium Bicarbonate

5% Glucose solution with 0.9% Sodium Chloride

5% Glucose with 0.225% Sodium Chloride solution

5% Glucose with 0.15% Potassium Chloride solution

Mannitol 2.5% or 10% solution.

6.3 Shelf life

Meronem has a shelf life of 4 years.

6.4 Special precautions for storage

Do not store above 30°C.

Do not freeze.

It is recommended to use freshly prepared solutions of Meronem for IV injection and infusion. Reconstituted product should be used immediately and must be stored for no longer than 24 hours under refrigeration, only if necessary.

Diluent	Hours Stable up to	
	25°C	4°C
Solutions (1 to 20 mg/ml) prepared with:		
* 0.9% sodium chloride	8	48
* 5% glucose	3	14

* 5% glucose and 0.225% sodium chloride	3	14
* 5% glucose and 0.9% sodium chloride	3	14
* 5% glucose and 0.15% potassium chloride	3	14
* 2.5% or 10% mannitol intravenous infusion	3	14
* 10% glucose	2	8
* 5% glucose and 0.02% sodium bicarbonate intravenous infusion	2	8

Solutions of Meronem should not be frozen.

6.5 Nature and contents of container

Type 1 glass vials closed with halobutilic rubber stopper and sealed with an aluminium cap.

Packs for intravenous administration

Pack of 10 vials containing 500 mg or 1 g meropenem.

6.6 Special precautions for disposal and other handling

Refer to Section 4.2 "Posology and method Administration" above. Standard aseptic technique should be employed during constitution. Shake constituted solution before use.

All vials are for single use only.

7. MARKETING AUTHORISATION HOLDER

AstraZeneca UK Limited

600 Capability Green,

Luton, LU1 3LU, UK.

8. MARKETING AUTHORISATION NUMBER(S)

Meronem IV 500 mg – PL17901/0029

Meronem IV 1 g – PL17901/0030

9. DATE OF FIRST AUTHORISATION/RENEWAL OF THE AUTHORISATION

11 May 2001

10. DATE OF REVISION OF THE TEXT

5th July 2007

Metalyse

(Boehringer Ingelheim Limited)

1. NAME OF THE MEDICINAL PRODUCT

Metalyse 8,000 units

Powder and solvent for solution for injection

Metalyse 10,000 units

Powder and solvent for solution for injection

2. QUALITATIVE AND QUANTITATIVE COMPOSITION

Metalyse 8,000 units

1 vial contains 8,000 units (40 mg) tenecteplase.

1 prefilled syringe contains 8 ml water for injections.

Metalyse 10,000 units

1 vial contains 10,000 units (50 mg) tenecteplase.

1 prefilled syringe contains 10 ml water for injections.

The reconstituted solution contains 1,000 units (5 mg) tenecteplase per ml.

Potency of tenecteplase is expressed in units (U) by using a reference standard which is specific for tenecteplase and is not comparable with units used for other thrombolytic agents.

Tenecteplase is a recombinant fibrin-specific plasminogen activator.

For a full list of excipients, see section 6.1.

3. PHARMACEUTICAL FORM

Powder and solvent for solution for injection.

The powder is white to off-white.

4. CLINICAL PARTICULARS

4.1 Therapeutic indications

Metalyse is indicated for the thrombolytic treatment of suspected myocardial infarction with persistent ST elevation or recent left Bundle Branch Block within 6 hours after the onset of acute myocardial infarction (AMI) symptoms.

4.2 Posology and method of administration

Metalyse should be prescribed by physicians experienced in the use of thrombolytic treatment and with the facilities to monitor that use.

Treatment with Metalyse should be initiated as soon as possible after onset of symptoms.

Metalyse should be administered on the basis of body weight, with a maximum dose of 10,000 units (50 mg tenecteplase). The volume required to administer the correct dose can be calculated from the following scheme:

(see Table 1 below)

The required dose should be administered as a single intravenous bolus over approximately 10 seconds.

A pre-existing intravenous line may be used for administration of Metalyse in 0.9% sodium chloride solution only. Metalyse is incompatible with dextrose solution.

No other medicinal product should be added to the injection solution.

Metalyse is not recommended for use in children (below 18 years) due to a lack of data on safety and efficacy.

Adjunctive therapy

Antithrombotic adjunctive therapy with platelet inhibitors and anticoagulants should be administered according to the current relevant treatment guidelines for the management of patients with ST-elevation myocardial infarction.

Unfractionated heparin and enoxaparin have been used as antithrombotic adjunctive therapy in clinical studies with Metalyse.

Acetylsalicylic acid should be initiated as soon as possible after symptom onset and continued with lifelong treatment unless it is contraindicated.

4.3 Contraindications

Metalyse is contraindicated in the following situations because thrombolytic therapy is associated with a higher risk of bleeding:

- Significant bleeding disorder either at present or within the past 6 months
- Patients with current concomitant oral anticoagulant therapy (INR> 1.3)
- Any history of central nervous system damage (i.e. neoplasm, aneurysm, intracranial or spinal surgery)
- Known haemorrhagic diathesis
- Severe uncontrolled hypertension
- Major surgery, biopsy of a parenchymal organ, or significant trauma within the past 2 months
- (this includes any trauma associated with the current AMI)
- Recent trauma to the head or cranium
- Prolonged cardiopulmonary resuscitation > 2 minutes) within the past 2 weeks
- Acute pericarditis and/or subacute bacterial endocarditis
- Acute pancreatitis
- Severe hepatic dysfunction, including hepatic failure, cirrhosis, portal hypertension (oesophageal varices) and active hepatitis
- Active peptic ulceration
- Arterial aneurysm and known arterial/venous malformation
- Neoplasm with increased bleeding risk
- Any known history of haemorrhagic stroke or stroke of unknown origin
- Known history of ischaemic stroke or transient ischaemic attack in the preceding 6 months
- Dementia
- Hypersensitivity to the active substance tenecteplase and to any of the excipients

4.4 Special warnings and precautions for use

Bleeding

The most common complication encountered during Metalyse therapy is bleeding. The concomitant use of heparin anticoagulation may contribute to bleeding. As fibrin is lysed during Metalyse therapy, bleeding from recent puncture site may occur. Therefore, thrombolytic therapy requires careful attention to all possible bleeding sites (including catheter insertion sites, arterial and venous puncture sites, cutdown sites and needle puncture sites). The use of rigid catheters as well as intramuscular injections and non-essential handling of the patient should be avoided during treatment with Metalyse.

Most frequently haemorrhage at the injection site, and occasionally genitourinary and gingival bleeding were observed.

Should serious bleeding occur, in particular cerebral haemorrhage, concomitant heparin administration should be terminated immediately. Administration of protamine should be considered if heparin has been administered within 4 hours before the onset of bleeding. In the few patients who fail to respond to these conservative measures, judicious use of transfusion products may be indicated. Transfusion of cryoprecipitate, fresh frozen plasma, and platelets should be considered with clinical and laboratory reassessment after each administration. A target fibrinogen level of 1 g/l is desirable with cryoprecipitate infusion. Antifibrinolytic agents are available as a last alternative. In the following conditions, the risk of Metalyse therapy may be increased and should be weighed against the anticipated benefits:

- Systolic blood pressure > 160 mm Hg
- Cerebrovascular disease
- Recent gastrointestinal or genitourinary bleeding (within the past 10 days)
- High likelihood of left heart thrombus, e.g., mitral stenosis with atrial fibrillation
- Any known recent (within the past 2 days) intramuscular injection
- Advanced age, i.e. over 75 years
- Low body weight < 60 kg

Arrhythmias

Coronary thrombolysis may result in arrhythmias associated with reperfusion. It is recommended that antiarrhythmic therapy for bradycardia and/or ventricular tachyarrhythmias (pacemaker, defibrillator) be available when Metalyse is administered.

GPIIb/IIIa antagonists

Concomitant use of GPIIb/IIIa antagonists increases bleeding risk.

Re-administration

Since at present there is no experience with re-administration of Metalyse, the re-administration is not recommended. However, no antibody formation to the tenecteplase molecule has been observed. If an anaphylactoid reaction occurs, the injection should be discontinued immediately and appropriate therapy should be initiated. In any case, tenecteplase should not be re-administered before assessment of haemostatic factors like fibrinogen, plasminogen and alpha2-antiplasmin.

Primary Percutaneous Coronary Intervention (PCI)

If primary PCI is scheduled according to the current relevant treatment guidelines, Metalyse as administered in the ASSENT-4 PCI study (see section 5.1) should not be given.

4.5 Interaction with other medicinal products and other forms of interaction

No formal interaction studies with Metalyse and medicinal products commonly administered in patients with AMI have been performed. However, the analysis of data from more than 12,000 patients treated during phase I, II and III did not reveal any clinically relevant interactions with medicinal products commonly used in patients with AMI and concomitantly used with Metalyse.

Medicinal products that affect coagulation or those that alter platelet function (e.g. ticlopidine, clopidogrel, LMWH) may increase the risk of bleeding prior to, during or after Metalyse therapy.

Comcomitant use of GPIIb/IIIa antagonists increased the bleeding risk.

4.6 Pregnancy and lactation

No experience in pregnant women is available for tenecteplase. Because animal studies (see also section 5.3) have shown a high risk of vaginal bleeding presumably from the placenta and of pregnancy loss, the benefit of treatment has to be evaluated against the potential risks which may aggravate an acute life-threatening situation.

It is not known if tenecteplase is excreted into breast milk. Breast milk should be discarded within the first 24 hours after thrombolytic therapy.

4.7 Effects on ability to drive and use machines

Not relevant.

4.8 Undesirable effects

Haemorrhage is a very common undesirable effect associated with the use of tenecteplase. The type of haemorrhage is predominantly superficial at the injection site. Ecchymoses are observed commonly but usually do not require any specific action. Death and permanent disability are reported in patients who have experienced stroke (including intracranial bleeding) and other serious bleeding episodes.

Within each frequency grouping, undesirable effects are presented in order of decreasing seriousness: Very

Table 1

Patients' body weight category (kg)	Tenecteplase (U)	Tenecteplase (mg)	Corresponding volume of reconstituted solution (ml)
< 60	6,000	30	6
⩾ 60 to < 70	7,000	35	7
⩾ 70 to < 80	8,000	40	8
⩾ 80 to < 90	9,000	45	9
⩾ 90	10,000	50	10

For details see section 6.6: Special precautions for disposal common (> 1/10), common (> 1/100, < 1/10), uncommon (> 1/1,000, < 1/100), rare (> 1/10,000, < 1/1,000), very rare (< 1/10,000)

Immune system disorders

Uncommon: Anaphylactoid reactions (including rash, urticaria, bronchospasm, laryngeal oedema)

Nervous system disorders

Uncommon: Intracranial haemorrhage (such as cerebral haemorrhage, cerebral haematoma, haemorrhagic stroke, haemorrhagic transformation of stroke, intracranial haematoma, subarachnoid haemorrhage) including associated symptoms as somnolence, aphasia, hemiparesis, convulsion

Eye disorders

Very rare: Eye haemorrhage

Cardiac disorders

Very common: Reperfusion arrhythmias (such as asystole, accelerated idioventricular arrhythmia, arrhythmia, extrasystoles, atrial fibrillation, atrioventricular block I° to complete, bradycardia, tachycardia, ventricular arrhythmia, ventricular fibrillation, ventricular tachycardia) occur in close temporal relationship to treatment with tenecteplase. Reperfusion arrhythmias may lead to cardiac arrest, can be life threatening and may require the use of conventional antiarrhythmic therapies

Rare: Haemopericardium

Vascular disorders

Very common: Bleeding

Uncommon: Embolism (thrombotic embolisation)

Respiratory, thoracic and mediastinal disorders

Common: Epistaxis

Uncommon: Pulmonary haemorrhage

Gastrointestinal disorders

Common: Gastrointestinal haemorrhage (such as gastric haemorrhage, gastric ulcer haemorrhage, haemorrhage rectum, haematemesis, melaena, mouth haemorrhage), nausea, vomiting

Uncommon: Retroperitoneal haemorrhage (such as retroperitoneal haematoma)

Skin and subcutaneous tissue disorders

Common: Ecchymosis

Renal and urinary disorders

Common: Urogenital haemorrhage (such as haematuria, haemorrhage urinary tract)

General disorders and administration site conditions

Very common: Superficial bleeding, normally from punctures or damaged blood vessels

Investigations

Very common: Decreased blood pressure

Common: Increased body temperature

Injury, poisoning and procedural complications

Very rare: Fat embolisation (cholesterol crystal embolism), which may lead to corresponding consequences in the organs concerned

As with other thrombolytic agents, the following events have been reported as sequelae of myocardial infarction and/or thrombolytic administration:

- very common > 1/10): hypotension, heart rate and rhythm disorders, angina pectoris
- common > 1/100, < 1/10): recurrent ischaemia, heart failure, reinfarction, cardiogenic shock, pericarditis, pulmonary oedema
- uncommon > 1/1,000, < 1/100): cardiac arrest, mitral insufficiency, pericardial effusion, venous thrombosis, cardiac tamponade, myocardial rupture
- rare > 1/10,000, < 1/1,000): pulmonary embolism

These cardiovascular events can be life-threatening and may lead to death.

4.9 Overdose

In the event of overdose there may be an increased risk of bleeding. In case of severe prolonged bleeding substitution therapy may be considered (plasma, platelets), see also section 4.4.

5. PHARMACOLOGICAL PROPERTIES

5.1 Pharmacodynamic properties

Pharmacotherapeutic group: antithrombotic agents, ATC code: B01A D11

Mechanism of action

Tenecteplase is a recombinant fibrin-specific plasminogen activator that is derived from native t-PA by modifications at three sites of the protein structure. It binds to the fibrin component of the thrombus (blood clot) and selectively converts thrombus-bound plasminogen to plasmin, which degrades the fibrin matrix of the thrombus. Tenecteplase has a higher fibrin specificity and greater resistance to inactivation by its endogenous inhibitor (PAI-1) compared to native t-PA.

Pharmacodynamic effects

After administration of tenecteplase dose dependent consumption of α2-antiplasmin (the fluid-phase inhibitor of plasmin) with consequent increase in the level of systemic plasmin generation have been observed. This observation is consistent with the intended effect of plasminogen activation. In comparative studies a less than 15% reduction in fibrinogen and a less than 25% reduction in plasminogen were observed in subjects treated with the maximum dose of tenecteplase (10,000 U, corresponding to 50 mg), whereas alteplase caused an approximately 50% decrease in fibrinogen and plasminogen levels. No clinically relevant antibody formation was detected at 30 days.

Clinical effects

Patency data from the phase I and II angiographic studies suggest that tenecteplase, administered as a single intravenous bolus, is effective in dissolving blood clots in the infarct-related artery of subjects experiencing an AMI on a dose related basis.

A large scale mortality trial (ASSENT II) in approx. 17,000 patients showed that tenecteplase is therapeutically equivalent to alteplase in reducing mortality (6.2% for both treatments, at 30 days, upper limit of the 95% CI for the relative risk ratio 1.124) and that the use of tenecteplase is associated with a significantly lower incidence of non-intracranial bleedings (26.4% vs. 28.9%, p=0.0003). This translates into a significantly lower need of transfusions (4.3% vs. 5.5%, p=0.0002). Intracranial haemorrhage occurred at a rate of 0.93% vs. 0.94% for tenecteplase and alteplase, respectively.

Coronary patency and limited clinical outcome data showed that AMI patients have been successfully treated later than 6 hours after symptom onset.

The ASSENT-4 PCI study was designed to show if in 4000 patients with large myocardial infarctions pre-treatment with full dose tenecteplase and concomitant single bolus of up to 4,000 IU unfractionated heparin administered prior to primary Percutaneous Coronary Intervention (PCI) to be performed within 60 to 180 minutes leads to better outcomes than primary PCI alone. The trial was prematurely terminated with 1667 randomised patients due to a numerically higher mortality in the facilitated PCI group receiving tenecteplase. The occurrence of the primary endpoint, a composite of death or cardiogenic shock or congestive heart failure within 90 days, was significantly higher in the group receiving the exploratory regimen of tenecteplase followed by routine immediate PCI: 18.6% (151/810) compared to 13.4% (110/819) in the PCI only group, p=0.0045. This significant difference between the groups for the primary endpoint at 90 days was already present in-hospital and at 30 days.

Numerically all of the components of the clinical composite endpoint were in favour of the PCI only regimen: death: 6.7% vs. 4.9% p=0.14; cardiogenic shock: 6.3% vs. 4.8% p=0.19; congestive heart failure: 12.0% vs. 9.2% p=0.06 respectively. The secondary endpoints re-infarction and repeat target vessel revascularisation were significantly increased in the group pre-treated with tenecteplase: re-infarction: 6.1% vs. 3.7% p=0.0279; repeat target vessel revascularisation: 6.6% vs. 3.4% p=0.0041.

The following adverse events occurred more frequently with tenecteplase prior to PCI: intracranial haemorrhage: 1% vs. 0% p=0.0037; stroke: 1.8% vs. 0% p<0.0001; major bleeds: 5.6% vs. 4.4% p=0.3118; minor bleeds: 25.3% vs. 19.0% p=0.0021; blood transfusions: 6.2% vs. 4.2% p=0.0873; abrupt vessel closure: 1.9% vs. 0.1% p=0.0001.

5.2 Pharmacokinetic properties

Tenecteplase is an intravenously administered, recombinant protein that activates plasminogen. Tenecteplase is cleared from circulation by binding to specific receptors in the liver followed by catabolism to small peptides. Binding to hepatic receptors is, however, reduced compared to native t-PA, resulting in a prolonged half-life. Data on tissue distribution and elimination were obtained in studies with radioactively labeled tenecteplase in rats. The main organ to which tenecteplase distributed was the liver. It is not known whether and to what extent tenecteplase binds to plasma proteins in humans.

After single intravenous bolus injection of tenecteplase in patients with acute myocardial infarction, tenecteplase antigen exhibits biphasic elimination from plasma. There is no dose dependence of tenecteplase clearance in the therapeutic dose range. The initial, dominant half life is 24 ± 5.5 (mean +/-SD) min, which is 5 times longer than native t-PA. The terminal half-life is 129 ± 87 min, and plasma clearance is 119 ± 49 ml/min.

Increasing body weight resulted in a moderate increase of tenecteplase clearance, and increasing age resulted in a slight decrease of clearance. Women exhibit in general lower clearance than men, but this can be explained by the generally lower body weight of women.

The effect of renal and hepatic dysfunction on pharmacokinetics of tenecteplase in humans is not known. There is no specific experience to guide the adjustment to tenecteplase dose in patients with hepatic and severe renal insufficiency. However, based on animal data it is not expected that renal dysfunction will affect the pharmacokinetics.

5.3 Preclinical safety data

Intravenous single dose administration in rats, rabbits and dogs resulted only in dose-dependent and reversible alterations of the coagulation parameters with local haemorrhage at the injection site, which was regarded as a consequence of the pharmacodynamic effect of tenecteplase. Multiple-dose toxicity studies in rats and dogs confirmed these above-mentioned observations, but the study duration was limited to two weeks by antibody formation to the human protein tenecteplase, which resulted in anaphylaxis.

Safety pharmacology data in cynomolgus monkeys revealed reduction of blood pressure followed by changes of ECG, but these occurred at exposures that were considerably higher than the clinical exposure.

With regard to the indication and the single dose administration in humans, reproductive toxicity testing was limited to an embryotoxicity study in rabbits as a sensitive species. Tenecteplase induced total litter deaths during the mid-embryonal period. When tenecteplase was given during the mid- or late-embryonal period maternal animals showed vaginal bleeding on the day after the first dose. Secondary mortality was observed 1-2 days later. Data on the foetal period are not available.

Mutagenicity and carcinogenicity are not expected for this class of recombinant proteins and genotoxicity and carcinogenicity testing were not necessary.

No local irritation of the blood vessel was observed after intravenous, intra-arterial or paravenous administration of the final formulation of tenecteplase.

6. PHARMACEUTICAL PARTICULARS

6.1 List of excipients

Powder:

L-arginine

Phosphoric acid

Polysorbate 20.

Solvent:

Water for injections

6.2 Incompatibilities

Metalyse is incompatible with dextrose infusion solutions.

6.3 Shelf life

Shelf life as packaged for sale

2 years

Reconstituted solution

Chemical and physical in-use stability has been demonstrated for up to 24 hours at 2-8° C and 8 hours at 30° C.

From a microbiological point of view, the product should be used immediately after reconstitution. If not used immediately, in-use storage times and conditions prior to use are the responsibility of the user and would normally not be longer than 24 hours at 2-8° C.

6.4 Special precautions for storage

Do not store above 30° C. Keep the container in the outer carton.

For storage conditions of the reconstituted medicinal product, see section 6.3.

6.5 Nature and contents of container

20 ml glass vial type I, with a coated (B2-42) grey rubber stopper and a flip off cap filled with powder for solution for injection.

10 ml plastic syringe pre-filled with 8 ml or 10 ml of water for injections for reconstitution.

Sterile vial adapter.

Sterile needle for single use.

6.6 Special precautions for disposal and other handling

Metalyse should be reconstituted by adding the complete volume of water for injections from the pre-filled syringe to the vial containing the powder for injection.

1. Ensure that the appropriate vial size is chosen according to the body weight of the patient.

(see Table 2 on next page)

2. Check that the cap of the vial is still intact.

3. Remove the flip-off cap from the vial.

4. Remove the tip-cap from the syringe. Then immediately screw the pre-filled syringe on the vial adapter and penetrate the vial stopper in the middle with the spike of the vial adapter.

5. Add the water for injections into the vial by pushing the syringe plunger down slowly to avoid foaming.

6. Reconstitute by swirling gently.

7. The reconstituted preparation results in a colourless to pale yellow, clear solution. Only clear solution without particles should be used.

8. Directly before the solution will be administered, invert the vial with the syringe still attached, so that the syringe is below the vial.

9. Transfer the appropriate volume of reconstituted solution of Metalyse into the syringe, based on the patient's weight.

10. Disconnect the syringe from the vial adapter.

11. Metalyse is to be administered to the patient, intravenously in about 10 seconds. It should not be administered in a line containing dextrose.

12. Any unused solution should be discarded.

Alternatively the reconstitution can be performed with the included needle.

Table 2

Patients' body weight category (kg)	Volume of reconstituted solution (ml)	Tenecteplase (U)	Tenecteplase (mg)
< 60	6	6,000	30
≥ 60 to < 70	7	7,000	35
≥ 70 to < 80	8	8,000	40
≥ 80 to < 90	9	9,000	45
≥ 90	10	10,000	50

7. MARKETING AUTHORISATION HOLDER

Boehringer Ingelheim International GmbH

Binger Strasse 173

D-55216 Ingelheim am Rhein

Germany

8. MARKETING AUTHORISATION NUMBER(S)

EU/1/00/169/005

EU/1/00/169/006

9. DATE OF FIRST AUTHORISATION/RENEWAL OF THE AUTHORISATION

Date of first authorisation: 23 February 2001

Date of last renewal: 23 February 2006

10. DATE OF REVISION OF THE TEXT

March 2007

M10/B/SPC/7

Meted Shampoo

(Alliance Pharmaceuticals)

1. NAME OF THE MEDICINAL PRODUCT

Meted 3% & 5% w/w Shampoo

2. QUALITATIVE AND QUANTITATIVE COMPOSITION

Salicylic acid USP 3.0% w/w

Colloidal sulphur HSE 6.25% w/w

(equivalent to sulphur 5.0% w/w)

3. PHARMACEUTICAL FORM

Shampoo

4. CLINICAL PARTICULARS

4.1 Therapeutic indications

For the relief of itching, irritation, redness, flaking and/or scaling due to dandruff, seborrhoeic dermatitis, or psoriasis of the scalp.

4.2 Posology and method of administration

For topical administration.

Adults:

The hair should be thoroughly wetted and sufficient Meted Shampoo applied to produce an abundant lather. The hair should be rinsed and the procedure repeated.

Use at least twice weekly or as directed by a physician.

Children:

As for adults.

Elderly:

As for adults.

4.3 Contraindications

Meted Shampoo is contra-indicated in persons with a sensitivity to any of the ingredients.

4.4 Special warnings and precautions for use

Avoid contact with the eyes. If shampoo gets into the eyes rinse thoroughly with water.

If the condition worsens or does not improve after regular use of the product as directed, consult a physician.

Excessive prolonged use may result in symptoms of salicylism.

4.5 Interaction with other medicinal products and other forms of interaction

None known.

4.6 Pregnancy and lactation

No limitations to the use of Meted Shampoo during pregnancy or lactation are known.

Safety has not been established in either humans or animals during pregnancy and lactation. However, with the small amounts of salicylic acid absorbed transdermally from Meted it is unlikely that use will cause any adverse effects.

4.7 Effects on ability to drive and use machines

None known.

4.8 Undesirable effects

There have been no reports of adverse effects following the use of Meted Shampoo. However, salicylic acid is a mild irritant and may cause dermatitis.

As with other topical preparations containing salicylic acid prolonged use may result in symptoms of salicylism.

4.9 Overdose

There is no evidence of systemic absorption following the use of this shampoo. There are no reports available of its ingestion.

Early symptoms are ringing in the ear tinnitus with deafness, epistaxis, nausea, vomiting, sensitivity and dryness of the mucous membranes. If this occurs treatment must be stopped immediately.

5. PHARMACOLOGICAL PROPERTIES

5.1 Pharmacodynamic properties

Sulphur is a keratolytic and mild antiseptic. Salicylic acid has keratolytic and fungicidal properties.

5.2 Pharmacokinetic properties

There is no evidence of systemic absorption of sulphur or salicylic acid following use of Meted Shampoo.

5.3 Preclinical safety data

None presented.

6. PHARMACEUTICAL PARTICULARS

6.1 List of excipients

Magnesium aluminium silicate

Hypromellose

Panthenol

Sodium laureth sulphate

Sodium cocoyl sarcosinate

Cocamido propyl betaine

Fragrance - 430 015

Purified water

6.2 Incompatibilities

None known.

6.3 Shelf life

36 months.

6.4 Special precautions for storage

Do not store above 30°C.

6.5 Nature and contents of container

Meted Shampoo is supplied in a white HDPE bottle with a white polypropylene screw cap. Each bottle contains either 30ml or 120ml of Meted Shampoo.

6.6 Special precautions for disposal and other handling

For external use only.

Keep out of reach of children.

7. MARKETING AUTHORISATION HOLDER

Alliance Pharmaceuticals Ltd

Avonbridge House

Bath Road

Chippenham

Wiltshire

SN15 2BB

8. MARKETING AUTHORISATION NUMBER(S)

PL 16853/0072

9. DATE OF FIRST AUTHORISATION/RENEWAL OF THE AUTHORISATION

1st July 1999

10. DATE OF REVISION OF THE TEXT

February 2009

Metenix 5 Tablets

(sanofi-aventis)

1. NAME OF THE MEDICINAL PRODUCT

Metenix 5 Tablets

2. QUALITATIVE AND QUANTITATIVE COMPOSITION

Metolazone 5 mg

3. PHARMACEUTICAL FORM

Tablet

4. CLINICAL PARTICULARS

4.1 Therapeutic indications

Metenix 5 is a diuretic for use in the treatment of mild and moderate hypertension. Metenix 5 may be used in conjunction with non-diuretic antihypertensive agents and, in these circumstances, it is usually possible to achieve satisfactory control of blood pressure with a reduced dose of the non-diuretic agent. Patients who have become resistant to therapy with these agents may respond to the addition of Metenix 5 to their antihypertensive regimen.

Metenix 5 may also be used for the treatment of cardiac, renal and hepatic oedema, ascites or toxaemia of pregnancy.

4.2 Posology and method of administration

Route of administration: Oral

Hypertension: The recommended initial dose in mild and moderate hypertension is 5 mg daily. After three to four weeks, the dose may be reduced if necessary to 5 mg on alternate days as maintenance therapy.

Oedema: In oedematous conditions, the normal recommended dose is 5-10 mg daily, given as a single dose. In resistant conditions, this may be increased to 20 mg daily or above. However, no more than 80 mg should be given in any 24-hour period.

Children: There is insufficient knowledge of the effects of Metenix 5 in children for any dosage recommendations to be made.

Elderly: Metolazone may be excreted more slowly in the elderly.

4.3 Contraindications

Metenix 5 is contra-indicated in electrolyte deficiency states, anuria, coma or pre-comatose states associated with liver cirrhosis; also in patients with known allergy or hypersensitivity to metolazone.

4.4 Special warnings and precautions for use

Because of the antihypertensive effects of metolazone the dosage of concurrently administered non-diuretic antihypertensive agents may need to be reduced.

Caution should be exercised during Metenix 5 therapy in patients liable to electrolyte deficiency.

Chloride deficit, hyponatraemia and a low salt syndrome may also occur, particularly when the patient is also on a diet with restricted salt intake. Hypomagnesaemia has been reported as a consequence of prolonged diuretic therapy.

Prolonged therapy with Metenix 5 may result in hypokalaemia. Serum potassium levels should be determined at regular intervals and, if necessary, potassium supplementation should be instituted.

Fluid and electrolyte balance should be carefully monitored during therapy especially if Metenix 5 is used concurrently with other diuretics. In particular, Metenix 5 may potentiate the diuresis produced by furosemide and, if the two agents are used concurrently, patients should be carefully monitored.

4.5 Interaction with other medicinal products and other forms of interaction

The dosage of concurrently administered cardiac glycosides may require adjustment. Metenix 5 may aggravate the increased potassium excretion associated with steroid therapy or diseases such as cirrhosis or severe ischaemic heart disease. Latent diabetes may become manifest or the insulin requirements of diabetic patients may increase.

Non steroidal anti-inflammatory drugs (e.g. Indometacin, Sulindac) may attenuate the action of Metolazone.

Prolongation of bleeding time has been reported during concomitant administration of Metenix and warfarin.

4.6 Pregnancy and lactation

There is little evidence of safety of the drug in human pregnancy, but it has been in wide, general use for many years without apparent ill consequence, animal studies having shown no hazard.

If Metenix 5 is given to nursing mothers, metolazone may be present in the breast milk.

4.7 Effects on ability to drive and use machines

None known.

4.8 Undesirable effects

Metenix 5 is generally well tolerated. There have been occasional reports of headache, anorexia, vomiting, abdominal discomfort, muscle cramps and dizziness. There have been isolated reports of urticaria, leucopenia, tachycardia, chills and chest pain.

Hyperuricaemia or azotaemia may occur during treatment with Metenix 5, particularly in patients with impaired renal function. On rare occasions, clinical gout has been reported.

4.9 Overdose

In cases of overdose there is a danger of dehydration and electrolyte depletion. Treatment should therefore be aimed at fluid replacement and correction of the electrolyte imbalance.

5. PHARMACOLOGICAL PROPERTIES

5.1 Pharmacodynamic properties

Metolazone is a substituted quinazolinone diuretic.

5.2 Pharmacokinetic properties

Diuresis and saluresis begin within one hour of administration of Metenix 5 tablets, reaching a maximum in two hours and continuing for 12-24 hours according to dosage.

5.3 Preclinical safety data
None applicable.

6. PHARMACEUTICAL PARTICULARS

6.1 List of excipients
Microcrystalline cellulose, magnesium stearate, F D and C blue no 2 lake (E132)

6.2 Incompatibilities
None.

6.3 Shelf life
5 years.

6.4 Special precautions for storage
Metenix 5 tablets should be stored protected from light, in the original container or in containers similar to those of the manufacturer.

6.5 Nature and contents of container
Blister pack of 100 tablets.

6.6 Special precautions for disposal and other handling
None.

Administrative Data

7. MARKETING AUTHORISATION HOLDER
Sanofi-aventis
One Onslow Street
Guildford
Surrey, GU1 4YS, UK

8. MARKETING AUTHORISATION NUMBER(S)
PL 04425/0212

9. DATE OF FIRST AUTHORISATION/RENEWAL OF THE AUTHORISATION
5 November 2001

10. DATE OF REVISION OF THE TEXT
November 2006

Legal Category
POM

Metformin Hydrochloride 500mg/5ml Oral Solution

(Rosemont Pharmaceuticals Limited)

1. NAME OF THE MEDICINAL PRODUCT
Metformin Hydrochloride 500mg/5ml Oral Solution

2. QUALITATIVE AND QUANTITATIVE COMPOSITION
Metformin Hydrochloride 500mg/5ml

Excipients: Sodium methyl parahydroxybenzoate (E219), sodium propyl parahydroxybenzoate (E217), maltilol liquid (E965), acesulfame potassium (E950) and propylene glycol (E1520).

For a full list of excipients, see section 6.1.

3. PHARMACEUTICAL FORM
Oral Solution

Clear brown liquid.

4. CLINICAL PARTICULARS

4.1 Therapeutic indications
Treatment of type 2 diabetes mellitus, particularly in overweight patients, when dietary management and exercise alone does not result in adequate glycaemic control.

• In adults, Metformin Hydrochloride Oral Solution may be used as monotherapy or in combination with other oral anti-diabetic agents or with insulin.

• In children from 10 years of age and adolescents, Metformin Hydrochloride Oral Solution may be used as monotherapy or in combination with insulin.

A reduction of diabetic complications has been shown in overweight type 2 diabetic adult patients treated with metformin as first-line therapy after diet failure (see 5.1. Pharmacodynamic properties).

4.2 Posology and method of administration
Adults:
Monotherapy and combination with other oral antidiabetic agents:

• The usual starting dose is one 5ml spoonful (500mg) 2 or 3 times daily given during or after meals.

• After 10 to 15 days the dose should be adjusted on the basis of blood glucose measurements. A slow increase of dose may improve gastrointestinal tolerability. The maximum recommended dose of metformin is 3g (six 5ml spoonfuls) daily.

• If transfer from another oral antidiabetic agent is intended: discontinue the other agent and initiate metformin at the dose indicated above.

Combination with insulin:

Metformin and insulin may be used in combination therapy to achieve better blood glucose control. Metformin is given at the usual starting dose of one 5ml spoonful (500mg) 2-3 times daily, while insulin dosage is adjusted on the basis of blood glucose measurements.

Elderly:
Due to the potential for decreased renal function in elderly subjects, the metformin dosage should be adjusted based on renal function. Regular assessment of renal function is necessary (see section 4.4).

Children and adolescents:
Monotherapy and combination with insulin

• Metformin Hydrochloride Oral Solution can be used in children from 10 years of age and adolescents.

• The usual starting dose is one 5ml spoonful (500mg) once daily, given during meals or after meals.

• After 10 to 15 days the dose should be adjusted on the basis of blood glucose measurements. A slow increase of dose may improve gastrointestinal tolerability. The maximum recommended dose of metformin is 2g (four 5ml spoonfuls) daily, taken as 2 or 3 divided doses.

4.3 Contraindications
• Hypersensitivity to metformin hydrochloride or any of the excipients.

• Diabetic ketoacidosis, diabetic pre-coma.

• Renal failure or renal dysfunction (creatinine clearance < 60mL/min).

• Acute conditions with the potential to alter renal function such as:
o dehydration
o severe infection
o shock
o Intravascular administration of iodinated contrast agents (see 4.4 Warnings and special precautions for use).

• Acute or chronic disease which may cause tissue hypoxia such as:
o cardiac or respiratory failure
o recent myocardial infarction
o shock

• Hepatic insufficiency, acute alcohol intoxication, alcoholism

• Lactation

4.4 Special warnings and precautions for use
Lactic acidosis

Lactic acidosis is a rare, but serious (high mortality in the absence of prompt treatment), metabolic complication that can occur due to metformin accumulation. Reported cases of lactic acidosis in patients on metformin have occurred primarily in diabetic patients with significant renal failure. The incidence of lactic acidosis can and should be reduced by assessing also other associated risk factors such as poorly controlled diabetes, ketosis, prolonged fasting, excessive alcohol intake, hepatic insufficiency and any condition associated with hypoxia.

Diagnosis:

Lactic acidosis is characterised by acidotic dyspnoea, abdominal pain and hypothermia followed by coma. Diagnostic laboratory findings are decreased blood pH, plasma lactate levels above 5mmol/L, and an increased anion gap and lactate/pyruvate ratio. If metabolic acidosis is suspected, metformin should be discontinued and the patient should be hospitalised immediately (see section 4.9).

Renal function

As metformin is excreted by the kidney, serum creatinine levels should be determined before initiating treatment and regularly thereafter:

• at least annually in patients with normal renal function.

• at least two to four times a year in patients with serum creatinine levels at the upper limit of normal and in elderly subjects.

Decreased renal function in elderly subjects is frequent and asymptomatic. Special caution should be exercised in situations where renal function may become impaired, for example when initiating antihypertensive therapy or diuretic therapy and when starting therapy with an NSAID.

Administration of iodinated contrast agent

As the intravascular administration of iodinated contrast materials in radiologic studies can lead to renal failure, metformin should be discontinued prior to, or at the time of the test and not reinstituted until 48 hours afterwards, and only after renal function has been re-evaluated and found to be normal.

Surgery

Metformin hydrochloride should be discontinued 48 hours before elective surgery with general anaesthesia and should not be usually resumed earlier than 48 hours afterwards.

Children and adolescents

The diagnosis of type 2 diabetes mellitus should be confirmed before treatment with metformin is initiated.

No effect of metformin on growth and puberty has been detected during controlled clinical studies of one year duration but no long term data on these specific points are available. Therefore, a careful follow-up of the effect of metformin on these parameters in metformin-treated children, especially pre-pubescent children is recommended.

Children aged between 10 and 12 years:

Only 15 subjects aged between 10 and 12 years were included in the controlled clinical studies conducted in children and adolescents. Although metformin efficacy and safety in children below 12 did not differ from efficacy and safety in older children, particular caution is recommended when prescribing to children aged between 10 and 12 years.

Other precautions

All patients should continue their diet with a regular distribution of carbohydrate intake during the day. Overweight patients should continue their energy-restricted diet.

The usual laboratory tests for diabetes monitoring should be performed regularly.

Metformin alone never causes hypoglycaemia, although caution is advised when it is used in combination with insulin or sulphonylureas.

Excipient warnings

This product contains:

• Parahydroxybenzoates. These may cause allergic reactions (possibly delayed).

• Liquid maltitol. Patients with rare hereditary problems of fructose intolerance should not take this medicine.

• Sodium - 5.3mg per 5ml dose. This should be taken into consideration for patients on a controlled sodium diet.

• Potassium - 14.5mg per 5ml dose. This should be taken into consideration for patients with reduced kidney function or patients on controlled potassium diets.

4.5 Interaction with other medicinal products and other forms of interaction
Concomitant use not recommended
Alcohol
Increased risk of lactic acidosis in acute alcohol intoxication, particularly in case of:
- fasting or malnutrition
- hepatic insufficiency

Avoid consumption of alcohol and alcohol-containing medications.

Iodinated contrast agents (see section 4.4)

Intravascular administration of iodinated contrast agents may lead to renal failure, resulting in metformin accumulation and a risk of lactic acidosis.

Metformin should be discontinued prior to, or at the time of the test and not reinstituted until 48 hours afterwards, and only after renal function has been re-evaluated and found to be normal.

Combinations requiring precautions for use

Glucocorticoids (systemic and local routes), beta-2-agonists, and diuretics have intrinsic hyperglycaemic activity. Inform the patient and perform more frequent blood glucose monitoring, especially at the beginning of treatment. If necessary, adjust the dosage of the antidiabetic drug during therapy with the other drug and upon its discontinuation.

ACE-inhibitors may decrease the blood glucose levels. If necessary, adjust the dosage of the antidiabetic drug during therapy with the other drug and upon its discontinuation.

4.6 Pregnancy and lactation
To date, no relevant epidemiological data are available. Animal studies do not indicate harmful effects with respect to pregnancy, embryonal or foetal development, parturition or postnatal development (see also section 5.3).

When the patient plans to become pregnant and during pregnancy, diabetes should not be treated with metformin but insulin should be used to maintain blood glucose levels as close to normal as possible in order to lower the risk of foetal malformations associated with abnormal blood glucose levels.

Metformin is excreted into milk in lactating rats. Similar data are not available in humans and a decision should be made whether to discontinue nursing or to discontinue metformin, taking into account the importance of the compound to the mother.

4.7 Effects on ability to drive and use machines
Metformin Hydrochloride Oral Solution monotherapy does not cause hypoglycaemia and therefore has no effect on the ability to drive or to use machines.

However, patients should be alerted to the risk of hypoglycaemia when metformin is used in combination with other antidiabetic agents (sulphonylureas, insulin, repaglinide).

4.8 Undesirable effects
The following undesirable effects may occur under treatment with metformin. Frequencies are defined as follows: very common >1/10; common >1/100, <1/10; uncommon >1/1,000, <1/100; rare >1/10,000, <1/1,000; very rare <1/10,000 and isolated reports.

Metabolism and nutrition disorders:

Very rare: Decrease of vitamin B12 absorption with decrease of serum levels during long-term use of metformin. Consideration of such aetiology is recommended if a patient presents with megaloplastic anaemia.

Very rare: Lactic acidosis (see 4.4. Special warnings and precautions for use).

Nervous system disorders:

Common: Taste disturbance

Gastrointestinal disorders:

Very common: Gastrointestinal disorders such as nausea, vomiting, diarrhoea, abdominal pain and loss of appetite. These undesirable effects occur most frequently during initiation of therapy and resolve spontaneously in most cases. To prevent them, it is recommended that metformin be taken in 2 or 3 daily doses during or after meals. A slow increase of the dose may also improve gastrointestinal tolerability.

Hepatobiliary disorders:

Isolated reports: Liver function tests abnormalities or hepatitis resolving upon metformin discontinuation.

Skin and subcutaneous tissue disorders:

Very rare: Skin reactions such as erythema, pruritus, urticaria

In published and post marketing data and in controlled clinical studies in a limited paediatric population aged 10-16 years treated during 1 year, adverse event reporting was similar in nature and severity to that reported in adults.

4.9 Overdose

Hypoglycaemia has not been seen with metformin doses of up to 85g, although lactic acidosis has occurred in such circumstances. High overdose or concomitant risks of metformin may lead to lactic acidosis. Lactic acidosis is a medical emergency and must be treated in hospital. The most effective method to remove lactate and metformin is haemodialysis.

5. PHARMACOLOGICAL PROPERTIES

5.1 Pharmacodynamic properties

Pharmacotherapeutic group: Oral blood glucose lowering drugs, Biguanides

ATC Code: A10B A02

Metformin is a biguanide with antihyperglycaemic effects, lowering both basal and postprandial plasma glucose. It does not stimulate insulin secretion and therefore does not produce hypoglycaemia.

Metformin may act via 3 mechanisms:

(1) reduction of hepatic glucose production by inhibiting gluconeogenesis and glycogenolysis (2) in muscle, by increasing insulin sensitivity, improving peripheral glucose uptake and utilisation (3) and delay of intestinal glucose absorption.

Metformin stimulates intracellular glycogen synthesis by acting on glycogen synthase.

Metformin increases the transport capacity of all types of membrane glucose transporters (GLUT).

In humans, independently of its action on glycaemia, metformin has favourable effects on lipid metabolism. This has been shown at therapeutic doses in controlled, medium-term or long-term clinical studies: metformin reduces total cholesterol, LDL cholesterol and triglyceride levels.

Clinical efficacy:

The prospective randomised (UKPDS) study has established the long-term benefit of intensive blood glucose control in type 2 diabetes.

Analysis of the results for overweight patients treated with metformin after failure of diet alone showed:

- a significant reduction of the absolute risk of any diabetes-related complication in the metformin group (29.8 events/1000 patient-years) versus diet alone (43.3 events/1000 patient-years), p=0.0023, and versus the combined sulphonylurea and insulin monotherapy groups (40.1 events/1000 patient-years), p=0.0034.
- a significant reduction of the absolute risk of diabetes-related mortality: metformin 7.5 events/1000 patient-years, diet alone 12.7 events/1000 patient-years, p=0.017;
- a significant reduction of the absolute risk of overall mortality: metformin 13.5 events/1000 patient-years versus diet alone 20.6 events/1000 patient-years (p=0.011), and versus the combined sulphonylurea and insulin monotherapy groups 18.9 events/1000 patient-years (p=0.021);
- a significant reduction in the absolute risk of myocardial infarction: metformin 11 events/1000 patient-years, diet alone 18 events/1000 patient-years (p=0.01)

For metformin used as second-line therapy, in combination with a sulphonylurea, benefit regarding clinical outcome has not been shown.

In type 1 diabetes, the combination of metformin and insulin has been used in selected patients, but the clinical benefit of this combination has not been formally established.

Controlled clinical studies in a limited paediatric population aged 10-16 years treated during 1 year demonstrated a similar response in glycaemic control to that seen in adults.

5.2 Pharmacokinetic properties

Absorption:

After an oral dose of metformin, Tmax is reached in 2.5 hours. Absolute bioavailability is approximately 50-60% in healthy subjects. After an oral dose, the non-absorbed fraction recovered in faeces was 20-30%.

After oral administration, metformin absorption is saturable and incomplete. It is assumed that the pharmacokinetics of metformin absorption are non-linear.

At the usual metformin doses and dosing schedules, steady state plasma concentrations are reached within 24 to 48 hours and are generally less than 1 μg/ml. In controlled clinical trials, maximum metformin plasma levels (Cmax) did not exceed 4 μg/ml, even at maximum doses.

Food decreases the extent and slightly delays the absorption of metformin. Following administration of a dose of 850 mg, a 40% lower plasma peak concentration, a 25% decrease in AUC (area under the curve) and a 35 minute prolongation of time to peak plasma concentration were observed. The clinical relevance of these decreases is unknown.

Distribution:

Plasma protein binding is negligible. Metformin partitions into erythrocytes. The blood peak is lower than the plasma peak and appears at approximately the same time. The red blood cells most likely represent a secondary compartment of distribution. The mean Vd ranged between 63-276 L.

Metabolism:

Metformin is excreted unchanged in the urine. No metabolites have been identified in humans.

Elimination:

Renal clearance of metformin is > 400 ml/min, indicating that metformin is eliminated by glomerular filtration and tubular secretion. Following an oral dose, the apparent terminal elimination half-life is approximately 6.5 hours.

When renal function is impaired, renal clearance is decreased in proportion to that of creatinine and thus the elimination half-life is prolonged, leading to increased levels of metformin in plasma.

Paediatrics:

Single dose study: After single doses of metformin 500 mg, paediatric patients have shown similar pharmacokinetic profile to that observed in healthy adults.

Multiple dose study: Data are restricted to one study. After repeated doses of 500 mg BID for 7 days in paediatric patients the peak plasma concentration (Cmax) and systemic exposure (AUC0-t) were reduced by approximately 33% and 40%, respectively compared to diabetic adults who received repeated doses of 500 mg BID for 14 days. As the dose is individually titrated based on glycaemic control, this is of limited clinical relevance.

5.3 Preclinical safety data

Preclinical data reveal no special hazard for humans based on conventional studies on safety pharmacology, repeated dose toxicity, genotoxicity, carcinogenic potential, toxicity reproduction.

6. PHARMACEUTICAL PARTICULARS

6.1 List of excipients

Sodium Methyl parahydroxybenzoate (E219)

Sodium Propyl parahydroxybenzoate (E217)

Sodium Dihydrogen Phosphate Dihydrate

Di-sodium Hydrogen Phosphate Anhydrous (E339)

Liquid Maltitol (E965)

Acesulfame potassium (E950)

Caramel (E150)

Peppermint Flavour (containing propylene glycol, isopropyl alcohol and pulegone)

Peach Flavour (containing propylene glycol and isopropyl alcohol)

Purified Water

6.2 Incompatibilities

None known.

6.3 Shelf life

12 months unopened

28 days opened

6.4 Special precautions for storage

Do not store above 25°C.

6.5 Nature and contents of container

Amber (Type III) glass bottles

Closures: HDPE, EPE wadded, tamper evident, child resistant closure

Pack Size: 150ml

6.6 Special precautions for disposal and other handling

Any unused product or waste material should be disposed of in accordance with local requirements.

7. MARKETING AUTHORISATION HOLDER

Rosemont Pharmaceuticals Ltd

Rosemont House

Yorkdale Industrial Park

Braithwaite Street

Leeds

LS11 9XE

UK

8. MARKETING AUTHORISATION NUMBER(S)

PL 00427/0139

9. DATE OF FIRST AUTHORISATION/RENEWAL OF THE AUTHORISATION

10/07/2007

10. DATE OF REVISION OF THE TEXT

10/07/2007

Methionine Tablets 250mg (UCB Pharma Ltd)

(UCB Pharma Limited)

1. NAME OF THE MEDICINAL PRODUCT

Methionine Tablets 250mg

2. QUALITATIVE AND QUANTITATIVE COMPOSITION

Methionine (DL) 250 mg

3. PHARMACEUTICAL FORM

Tablet

4. CLINICAL PARTICULARS

4.1 Therapeutic indications

Methionine is given, by mouth, for the treatment of paracetamol overdose if n-acetyl cysteine is not available or if the patient cannot tolerate n-acetyl cysteine.

4.2 Posology and method of administration

Paracetamol Overdose: Give within 10 hours of paracetamol ingestion, subsequent to any emesis being induced.

Adults and the elderly: 2.5g (10 tablets) every 4 hours to a maximum of 10g

Children (up to 6 years): 1g (4 tablets) every 4 hours to a maximum of 4g

Children (6 years and over): As adult dose

4.3 Contraindications

Methionine should not be used for the treatment of paracetamol overdosage if more than 10 hours have elapsed since the time of the overdose.

Do not use in patients with metabolic acidosis.

4.4 Special warnings and precautions for use

Use methionine with care in patients with established liver disease as hepatic encephalopathy may be precipitated.

Use with caution in patients with schizophrenia as daily methionine doses of 10 to 20g have been reported to precipitate acute exacerbation of symptoms in such patients.

4.5 Interaction with other medicinal products and other forms of interaction

The anti-parkinsonism effects of levodopa may be reduced by methionine, especially if large doses of methionine are given.

4.6 Pregnancy and lactation

The safety, in human pregnancy or during lactation, of the ingestion of higher levels of methionine than would normally be encountered in the diet, has not been established. Methionine should only be used during pregnancy or lactation if the benefit of its use has been weighed against any potential risks.

4.7 Effects on ability to drive and use machines

Patients should be advised that methionine may cause drowsiness and their ability to drive or operate machinery may be affected.

4.8 Undesirable effects

Oral doses of methionine may cause nausea, vomiting, drowsiness and irritability. Daily doses of 6 to 20g can cause neurological changes and precipitate Encephalopathy in patients with heptic cirrhosis especially if portal hypertension is present.

4.9 Overdose

Overdosage with methionine may be associated with the appearance of the above mentioned side-effects (nausea, vomiting, drowsiness, irritability). As methionine forms part of the normal diet, no specific recommendations for treatment of overdose are available. General support measures may be appropriate.

5. PHARMACOLOGICAL PROPERTIES

5.1 Pharmacodynamic properties

Methionine is an essential amino acid that plays a vital role in intermediary metabolism. It is the primary donor of methyl groups for biosynthetic reactions but must first be converted to s-adenosylmethionine, its active moiety. It is then involved in the transmethylation of nucleic acids, proteins, lipids and other metabolites and in the synthesis of choline. Methionine is converted to cysteine, a precursor of glutathione, in the liver. Methionine is thought to prevent liver damage in paracetamol overdose by facilitating glutathione synthesis. Methionine has a lipotropic action which prevents the development of fatty liver and it also stimulates pancreatic insulin release.

5.2 Pharmacokinetic properties

Adsorption: Methionine is absorbed from the gastro-intestinal tract. Absorption is unpredictable in patients who are vomiting.

Half-Life: Not known

Distribution: Not known

Metabolism: Methionine is metabolised via s-adenosylmethionine to homocysteine. About 80% is further converted to cystathionine, cysteine, taurine and inorganic sulphate.

Excretion: Methionine is excreted in the urine as an inorganic sulphate.

5.3 Preclinical safety data

None stated

6. PHARMACEUTICAL PARTICULARS

6.1 List of excipients

Alginic acid

Starch maize

Tragacanth powdered

Magnesium stearate

Talc

Coating:

Acacia syrup solution

Talc

Light calcium carbonate

Acacia mucilage

Titanium dioxide 1700 ansteads

Opaglos AG 7350 containing:

Beeswax white

Carnauba wax yellow

Polysorbate 20

Sorbic acid (E200)

Purified water

Opacode S-1-8100HV Black containing:

Industrial Methylated Spirits

Shellac (E904)

Iron Oxide Black (E172)

Purified Water

2-Ethoxyethanol

Soya Lecithin MC Thin (E322)

Antifoam DC 1510

6.2 Incompatibilities

None known

6.3 Shelf life

36 months

6.4 Special precautions for storage

Store at room temperature

6.5 Nature and contents of container

Pigmented polypropylene container with tamper-evident closure of low density polyethylene. Containers hold either 50, 200 or 250 tablets

6.6 Special precautions for disposal and other handling

None stated

7. MARKETING AUTHORISATION HOLDER

UCB Pharma Ltd

208 Bath Road

Slough

Berkshire

SL1 3WE

8. MARKETING AUTHORISATION NUMBER(S)

PL 00039/0553

9. DATE OF FIRST AUTHORISATION/RENEWAL OF THE AUTHORISATION

4 July 2005

10. DATE OF REVISION OF THE TEXT

July 2005

Metoject 10 mg/ml solution for injection, pre-filled syringe

(medac GmbH)

1. NAME OF THE MEDICINAL PRODUCT

Metoject 10 mg/ml solution for injection, pre-filled syringe

2. QUALITATIVE AND QUANTITATIVE COMPOSITION

1 ml of solution contains 10 mg methotrexate (as methotrexate disodium).

1 pre-filled syringe of 0.75 ml contains 7.5 mg methotrexate

1 pre-filled syringe of 1 ml contains 10 mg methotrexate

1 pre-filled syringe of 1.5 ml contains 15 mg methotrexate

1 pre-filled syringe of 2 ml contains 20 mg methotrexate

1 pre-filled syringe of 2.5 ml contains 25 mg methotrexate

For excipients, see 6.1.

3. PHARMACEUTICAL FORM

Solution for injection in pre-filled syringe.

Clear, yellow solution.

4. CLINICAL PARTICULARS

4.1 Therapeutic indications

Metoject is indicated for the treatment of:

- Severe, active rheumatoid arthritis in adult patients where treatment with disease modifying antirheumatic drugs (DMARD) is indicated.

4.2 Posology and method of administration

Metoject should only be prescribed by physicians and administered by health professionals, who are familiar with the various characteristics of the medicinal product and its mode of action. Metoject is injected once weekly.

Careful monitoring should be undertaken after the first dose of methotrexate to exclude idiosyncratic hypersensitivity reactions.

Dosage in adult patients with rheumatoid arthritis:

The recommended initial dose is 7.5 mg of methotrexate once weekly, administered either subcutaneously, intramuscularly or intravenously. Depending on the individual activity of the disease and tolerability by the patient, the dose may be increased gradually by 2.5 mg per week. A weekly dose of 25 mg should not be exceeded. However, doses exceeding 20 mg/week can be associated with significant increase in toxicity, especially bone marrow suppression. Response to treatment can be expected after approximately 4 -8 weeks. Upon achieving the therapeutically desired result, the dose should be reduced gradually to the lowest possible effective maintenance dose.

Patients with renal impairment:

Metoject should be used with caution in patients with impaired renal function. The dose should be adjusted as follows:

Creatinine clearance (ml/min)

> 50 100%

20-50 50%

< 20 Metoject must not be used

Patients with hepatic impairment:

Methotrexate should be administered with great caution to patients with significant current or previous liver disease, especially if due to alcohol. If bilirubin is > 5 mg/dl (85.5 µmol/l), methotrexate is contraindicated.

Use in elderly patients:

Dose reduction should be considered in elderly patients due to reduced liver and kidney function as well as lower folate reserves which occurs with increased age.

Duration and method of administration

Metoject solution for injection can be given by intramuscular, intravenous or subcutaneous route.

The overall duration of the treatment is decided by the physician.

Note:

If changing from oral to parenteral administration a reduction of the dose may be required due to the variable bioavailability of methotrexate after oral administration.

Folic acid or folinic acid supplementation may be considered according to current treatment guidelines.

4.3 Contraindications

Metoject is contra-indicated in the case of:

- hypersensitivity to methotrexate or to any of the excipients,

- severe liver insufficiency (see also 4.2 Posology and method of administration),

- alcohol abuse,

- severe renal insufficiency (creatinine clearance less than 20 ml/min., see also 4.2 Posology and method of administration),

- pre-existing blood dycrasias, such as bone marrow hypoplasia, leukopenia, thrombocytopenia, or significant anaemia,

- severe acute or chronic infections such as tuberculosis and HIV

- ulcers of the oral cavity and known active gastrointestinal ulcer disease,

- pregnancy, breast-feeding (see also 4.6 Pregnancy and lactation).

- concurrent vaccination with live vaccines

- immunodeficiency syndromes

4.4 Special warnings and precautions for use

Patients have to be clearly informed, that Metoject must be administered once a week, not every day.

Patients undergoing therapy should be subject to appropriate supervision so that signs of possible toxic effects or adverse reactions may be detected and evaluated with minimal delay. Therefore methotrexate should only be administered by, or under the supervision of, physicians whose knowledge and experience includes the use of antimetabolite therapy. Because of the possibility of severe or even fatal toxic reactions, the patient should be fully informed of the risks involved and the recommended safety measures. However, doses exceeding 20 mg/week can be associated with significant increase in toxicity, especially bone marrow suppression.

Recommended examinations and safety measures:

Before beginning methotrexate therapy or re-instituting methotrexate therapy after a rest period:

Complete blood count with differential blood count and platelets, liver enzymes, bilirubin, serum albumin, chest x-ray and renal function tests. If clinically indicated, tuberculosis and hepatitis should be excluded.

During therapy (at least once a month during the first six months and every three months thereafter):

An increased monitoring frequency should be considered also when the dose is increased.

1. Examination of the mouth and throat for mucosal changes.

2. Complete blood count with differential blood count and platelets. Haemopoietic suppression caused by methotrexate may occur abruptly and with apparently safe dosages. Any profound drop in white-cell or platelet counts indicate immediate withdrawal of the medicinal product and appropriate supportive therapy. Patients should be advised to report all signs and symptoms suggestive of infection. Patients simultaneously taking haematotoxic medicinal products (e.g. leflunomide) should be monitored closely with blood count and platelets.

3. Liver function tests: Particular attention should be given to the appearance of liver toxicity. Treatment should not be instituted or should be discontinued if any abnormality of liver function tests, or liver biopsy, is present or develops during therapy. Such abnormalities should return to normal within two weeks after which treatment may be recommenced at the discretion of the physician. There is no evidence to support use of a liver biopsy to monitor hepatic toxicity in rheumatological indications.

However, due to the hepatotoxic potential of Methotrexate the need of a liver biopsy should be evaluated for risk patients with long-term use of methotrexate. Risk factors are:

Primary:

- Excessive prior alcohol consumption

- Persistent elevation of liver enzymes

- Anamnestical liver diseases

- Hereditary liver diseases

Monitoring of liver enzymes in serum: Temporary increases in transaminases to twice or three times of the upper limit of normal have been reported by patients at a frequency of 13 – 20 %. In the case of a constant increase in liver enzymes, a reduction of the dose or discontinuation of therapy should be taken into consideration.

Due to its potentially toxic effect on the liver, additional hepatotoxic medicinal products should not be taken during treatment with methotrexate *unless clearly necessary*, and the consumption of alcohol should be avoided or minimized (see 4.5 Interactions with other medicinal products and other forms of interaction.). Closer monitoring of liver enzymes should be exercised in patients taking other hepatotoxic medicinal products concomitantly (e.g. leflunomide). This is also required during simultaneous administration of haematotoxic medicinal products (e.g. leflunomide).

4. Renal function should be monitored by renal function tests and urinanalysis (see also 4.2 and 4.3):

As methotrexate is eliminated mainly by renal route, increased serum concentrations are to be expected in the case of renal insufficiency, which may result in severe undesirable effects.

Where renal function may be compromised (e.g. in the elderly), monitoring should take place more frequently. This applies in particular, when medicinal products are administered concomitantly, which affect the elimination of methotrexate, cause kidney damage (e.g. non-steroidal anti-inflammatory medicinal products) or which can potentially lead to impairment of blood formation. Dehydration may also intensify the toxicity of methotrexate.

5. Respiratory system: Acute or chronic interstitial pneumonitis, often associated with blood eosinophilia, may occur and deaths have been reported. Symptoms typically include dyspnoea, cough (especially a dry non-productive cough) and fever for which patients should be monitored at each follow-up visit. Patients should be informed of the risk of pneumonitis and advised to contact their doctor immediately should they develop persistent cough or dyspnoea.

Methotrexate should be withdrawn from patients with pulmonary symptoms and a thorough investigation (including chest x-ray) should be made to exclude infection. If methotrexate induced lung disease is suspected treatment with corticosteroids should be initiated and treatment with methotrexate should not be restarted.

Pulmonary affection requires a quick diagnosis and discontinuation of methotrexate therapy. Pneumonitis can occur at all dosages.

6. Methotrexate may, due to its effect on the immune system, impair the response to vaccination and affect the results of immunological tests. Particular caution is also needed in the presence of inactive, chronic infections (e.g. herpes zoster, tuberculosis, hepatitis B or C) due to possible activation. Concurrent vaccination using live vaccines should not be carried out.

Malignant lymphomas may occur in patients receiving low dose methotrexate, in which case therapy must be discontinued. Failure of the lymphoma to show signs of spontaneous regression requires the initiation of cytotoxic therapy.

Pleural effusions and ascites should be drained prior to initiation of methotrexate treatment.

Diarrhoea and ulcerative stomatitis can be toxic effects and require interruption of therapy, otherwise haemorrhagic enteritis and death from intestinal perforation may occur.

Vitamin preparations or other products containing folic acid, folinic acid or their derivatives may decrease the effectiveness of methotrexate.

This medicinal product contains less than 1 mmol sodium (23 mg) per dose and is i.e. essentially 'sodium-free'.

4.5 Interaction with other medicinal products and other forms of interaction

Alcohol, hepatotoxic medicinal products, haematotoxic medicinal products

The probability of methotrexate exhibiting a hepatotoxic effect is increased by regular alcohol consumption and when other hepatotoxic medicinal products are taken at the same time (see 4.4 Special warnings and precautions for use.). Patients taking other hepatotoxic medicinal products concomitantly (e.g. leflunomide) should be monitored with special care. This is also required during simultaneous administration of haematotoxic medicinal products (e.g. leflunomide). The incidence of pancytopenia and hepatotoxicity can be increased when leflunomide is combined with methotrexate.

Combined treatment with methotrexate and retinoids like acitretin or etretinate increases the risk of hepatotoxicity.

Oral antibiotics

Oral antibiotics like tetracyclines, chloramphenicol, and non-absorbable broad-spectrum antibiotics can interfere with the enterohepatic circulation of methotrexate, due to inhibition of the intestinal flora or suppression of the bacterial metabolism.

Antibiotics

Antibiotics, like penicillines, glycopeptides, sulfonamides, ciprofloxacin and cefalotin can, in individual cases, reduce the renal clearance of methotrexate, so that increased serum concentrations of methotrexate with simultaneous haematological and gastro-intestinal toxicity may occur.

Medicinal products with high plasma protein binding

Methotrexate is plasma protein bound and may be displaced by other protein bound drugs such as salicylates, hypoglycaemics, diuretics, sulphonamides, diphenylhydantoins, tetracyclines, chloramphenicol and p-aminobenzoic acid, and the acidic anti-inflammatory agents, which can lead to increased toxicity when used concurrently.

Probenecid, weak organic acids, pyrazoles and non-steroidal anti-inflammatory agents

Probenecid, weak organic acids such as loop diuretics, and pyrazoles (phenylbutazone) can reduce the elimination of methotrexate. Hence, higher serum concentrations can be expected, inducing higher haematological toxicity. There is also a risk of increased toxicity when low dose methotrexate and non steroidal anti-inflammatory medicinal products or salicylates are combined.

Medicinal products with adverse reactions on the bone marrow

In the case of medication with medicinal products, which may cause bone marrow depression (e.g. sulphonamides, trimethoprim-sulphamethoxazole, chloramphenicol, pyrimethamine), attention should be paid to the possibility of pronounced impairment of blood formation.

Medicinal products which may cause folate deficiency

The concomitant administration of products which may cause folate deficiency (e. g. sulphonamides, trimethoprim-sulphamethoxazole, nitrous oxide) can lead to increased methotrexate toxicity. Particular care is therefore advisable in the presence of existing folic acid deficiency.

Products containing folic acid or folinic acid

Vitamin preparations or other products containing folic acid, folinic acid or their derivatives may decrease the effectiveness of methotrexate.

Other anti-rheumatic medicinal products

An increase in the toxic effects of methotrexate is, in general, not to be expected when Metoject is administered simultaneously with other anti-rheumatic medicinal products (e. g. gold compounds, penicillamine, hydroxychloroquine, sulphasalazine, azathioprin, cyclosporin).

Sulphasalazine

The combination of methotrexate and sulphasalazine may increase the efficacy of methotrexate, but at the same time induce more undesirable effects, due to the inhibition of folic acid synthesis by sulphasalazine. However, such undesirable effects have only been observed in rare individual cases in the course of several studies.

Proton-pump inhibitors

A concomitant administration of proton-pump inhibitors like omeprazole or pantoprazole can lead to interactions: Concomitant administration of methotrexate and omeprazole has led to delayed renal elimination of methotrexate. In combination with pantoprazole inhibited renal elimination of the metabolite 7-hydroxymethotrexate with myalgia and shivering was reported in one case.

Caffeine- or theophylline-containing beverages

An excessive consumption of caffeine- or theophylline-containing beverages (coffee, caffeine-containing softdrinks, tea) should be avoided during methotrexate therapy.

4.6 Pregnancy and lactation

Metoject is contra-indicated during pregnancy (see 4.3 Contra-indications).

In animal studies methotrexate has shown reproductive toxicity, especially during the first trimester (see 5.3 Preclinical safety data).

Methotrexate has been shown to be teratogenic to humans; it has been reported to cause foetal death and/ or congenital abnormalities.

Exposure of a limited number of pregnant women (42) resulted in an increased incidence (1:14) of malformations (cranial, cardiovascular and extremities). If methotrexate is discontinued prior to conception, normal pregnancies have been reported.

Pregnancy should be excluded before treatment with Metoject is initiated.

Women must not get pregnant during methotrexate therapy. Therefore, patients of a sexually mature age (women and men) must use effective contraception during treatment with Metoject and at least 6 months thereafter.

The possible risks of effects on reproduction should be discussed with patients of childbearing potential, and their partners should be advised appropriately.

In case of women getting pregnant during therapy, medical counselling about the risk of adverse reactions for the child associated with methotrexate therapy should be sought.

Methotrexate has been reported to cause defective oogenesis, defective spermatogenesis, oligospermia, infertility, menstrual dysfunction and amenorrhoea in humans, during and for a period after cessation of therapy.

Lactation: Methotrexate is excreted in breast milk in such concentrations that there is a risk for the infant, and accordingly, breastfeeding should be discontinued prior to and throughout administration.

4.7 Effects on ability to drive and use machines

Central nervous symptoms such as tiredness and dizziness can occur during treatment, Metoject has minor or moderate influence on the ability to drive and use machines.

4.8 Undesirable effects

The most relevant undesirable effects are suppression of the haematopoetic system and gastrointestinal disorders.

The following headings are used to organise the undesirable effects in order of frequency:

Very common (> 1/10), common (> 1/100; < 1/10), uncommon (> 1/1,000; < 1/100), rare (> 1/10,000; < 1/ 1,000) and very rare (< 1/10,000).

Gastrointestinal disorders

Very common: Stomatitis, dyspepsia, nausea, reduced appetite.

Common: Oral ulcers, diarrhoea.

Uncommon: Pharyngitis, enteritis, vomiting.

Rare: Gastrointestinal ulcers, malabsorption.

Very rare: Hematemesis, hematorrhea, toxic megacolon.

Skin disorders

Common: Exanthema, erythema, pruritus.

Uncommon: Photosensitisation, loss of hair, increase in rheumatic nodules, herpes zoster, vasculitis, herpetiform eruptions of the skin, urticaria.

Rare: Increased pigmentation, acne, ecchymosis.

Very rare: Stevens-Johnson syndrome, toxic epidermal necrolysis (Lyell's syndrome), increased pigmentary changes of the nails, acute paronychia, furunculosis, telangiectasia.

General disorders and administration site conditions

Very common: Local skin reactions (burning sensation, redness) of injection site following intramuscular or subcutaneous administration. Most of these reactions are of mild degree.

Rare: Allergic reactions, anaphylactic shock, allergic vasculitis, fever, conjunctivitis, infection, sepsis, wound-healing impairment, hypogammaglobulinaemia.

Very rare: Local damage (formation of sterile abscess, lipodystrophy) of injection site following intramuscular or subcutaneous administration

Metabolism and nutrition disorders

Uncommon: Precipitation of diabetes.

Nervous system disorders

Common: Headache, tiredness, drowsiness.

Uncommon: Dizziness, confusion, depression, cognitive dysfunction.

Very rare: Impaired vision, pain, muscular asthenia or paresthesia in the extremities, changes in sense of taste (metallic taste), convulsions, meningism, paralysis.

Eye disorders

Rare: Visual disturbances

Very rare: Retinopathy

Hepatobiliary disorders

Very common: Elevated transaminases.

Uncommon: Cirrhosis, liver atrophy, periportal fibrosis and fatty degeneration of the liver.

Cardiac disorders and vascular disorders

Rare: Pericarditis, pericardial effusion, pericardial tamponade, hypotension, thromboembolic events.

Respiratory disorders

Common: Pneumonia, interstitial alveolitis/pneumonitisoften associated with eosinophilia;symptoms indicating potentially severe lung injury (interstitial pneumonitis) are: dry, non-productive cough, dyspnoea and fever.

Rare: Pulmonary fibrosis, pneumocystis carinii pneumonia, dyspnoea and bronchial asthma, pleural effusion

Blood disorders

Common: Leukopenia, anaemia, thrombocytopenia.

Uncommon: Pancytopenia.

Very rare: Agranulocytosis, severe courses of bone marrow depression.

Renal, urinary and reproductive system disorders

Uncommon: Inflammation and ulceration of the urinary bladder or vagina, renal impairment, disturbed micturition.

Rare: Renal failure, oliguria, anuria, electrolyte disturbances.

Very rare: Reduced libido, impotence, oligospermia, defective oogenesis, defective spermatogenesis, infertility, menstruation disturbances, vaginal discharge.

Musculosceletal and connective tissue disorders

Uncommon: Arthralgia, myalgia, osteoporosis.

Neoplasms

Very rare: There have been reports of individual cases of lymphoma which subsided in a number of cases once treatment with methotrexate had been discontinued. In a recent study, it could not be established that methotrexate therapy increases the incidence of lymphomas.

The appearance and degree of severity of undesirable effects depends on the dosage level and the frequency of administration. However, as severe undesirable effects can occur even at lower doses, it is indispensable that patients are monitored regularly by the doctor at short intervals.

4.9 Overdose

a) Symptoms of overdosage

Toxicity of methotrexate mainly affect the haematopoietic system.

b) Treatment measures in the case of overdosage

Calcium folinate is the specific antidote for neutralising the toxic undesirable effects of methotrexate.

In cases of accidental overdose, a dose of calcium folinate equal to or higher than the offending dose of methotrexate should be administered intravenously or intramuscularly within one hour. Early monitoring of methotrexate levels is recommended for dosage adjustment. Dosing should be continued until the serum levels of methotrexate are below 10^{-7} mol/l.

In cases of massive overdose, hydration and urinary alkalisation may be necessary to prevent precipitation of methotrexate and/or its metabolites in the renal tubules. Neither haemodialysis nor peritoneal dialysis have been shown to improve methotrexate elimination. Effective clearance of methotrexate has been reported with acute, intermittent haemodialysis using high flux techniques.

5. PHARMACOLOGICAL PROPERTIES

5.1 Pharmacodynamic properties

Pharmacotherapeutic group: Folic acid antagonist.

ATC code: L01BA01

Methotrexate is a folic acid antagonist which belongs to the class of cytotoxic agents known as antimetabolites. It acts by the competitive inhibition of the enzyme dihydrofolate reductase and thus inhibits DNA synthesis. It has not yet been clarified as to whether the efficacy of methotrexate in the management of chronic polyarthritis is due to an anti-inflammatory or immunosuppressive effect, and to which extent a methotrexate-induced increase in extracellular adenosine concentration at inflamed sites contributes to these effects.

5.2 Pharmacokinetic properties

Approximately 50 % of methotrexate is bound to serum proteins. Upon distribution into body tissues, high concentrations of polyglutamates are found in the liver, kidneys and spleen in particular, which can retain for weeks or months. When administered in small doses, methotrexate passes into the liquor in minimal amounts. The terminal half-life is on average 6 - 7 hours and demonstrates considerable variation (3 - 17 hours). The half-life can be prolonged to 4 times the normal length in patients who possess a third distribution space (pleural effusion, ascites).

Approx. 10 % of the administered methotrexate dose is metabolised intrahepatically. The principle metabolite is 7-hydroxymethotrexate.

Excretion takes places, mainly in unchanged form, primarily via glomerular filtration and active secretion in the proximal tubulus.

Approx. 5 - 20 % of methotrexate and 1 - 5 % of 7-hydroxymethotrexate are eliminated via the bile. There is a pronounced enterohepatic reuptake.

In the case of renal insufficiency, elimination is delayed significantly. It is not known whether hepatic insufficiency causes reduced methotrexate elimination.

5.3 Preclinical safety data

Animal studies show that methotrexate impairs fertility, is embryo- and foetotoxic and teratogenic. Methotrexate is mutagenic *in vivo* and *in vitro*. As conventional carcinogenicity studies have not been performed and data from chronic toxicity studies in rodents are inconsistent, methotrexate is not classifiable as to its carcinogenicity to humans.

6. PHARMACEUTICAL PARTICULARS

6.1 List of excipients

Sodium chloride

Sodium hydroxide for pH adjustment

Water for injection

6.2 Incompatibilities

Compatibility with other parenteral products has not been studied. Therefore, this medicinal product must not be mixed with other medicinal products or diluents.

6.3 Shelf life

2 years.

6.4 Special precautions for storage

Do not store above 25 °C. Keep the pre-filled syringes in the outer carton.

6.5 Nature and contents of container

Nature of container:

Fill volumes: Pre-filled syringes containing 0.75 ml, 1 ml, 1.5 ml, 2 ml or 2.5 ml solution

Syringe sizes: Pre-filled syringe (colourless glass, type I) of 1 ml, 2.25 ml and 3 ml, with or without injection needle adapter and elastomeric tip cap, plunger stoppers of chlorobutyl rubber (type I) and polystyrene rods inserted on the stopper to form the syringe plunger.

Pack sizes:

1, 5, 10 or 30 syringes.

All pack sizes are available with graduation, with and without injection needles.

6.6 Special precautions for disposal and other handling

Handling and disposal must be consistent with that of other cytotoxic preparations in accordance with local requirements. Pregnant health care personnel should not handle and/or administer Metoject.

Methotrexate must not come into contact with the skin or mucosa. In the event of contamination, the affected area must be rinsed immediately with ample amount of water.

For single use only. Any unused solution should be discarded.

7. MARKETING AUTHORISATION HOLDER

medac

Gesellschaft fuer klinische Spezialpraeparate mbH

Fehlandtstrasse 3

D-20354 Hamburg

8. MARKETING AUTHORISATION NUMBER(S)

PL 11587/0031

9. DATE OF FIRST AUTHORISATION/RENEWAL OF THE AUTHORISATION

07/07/2006

10. DATE OF REVISION OF THE TEXT

07/07/2006

Metoject 50 mg/ml solution for injection

(medac GmbH)

1. NAME OF THE MEDICINAL PRODUCT

Metoject 50 mg/ml solution for injection

2. QUALITATIVE AND QUANTITATIVE COMPOSITION

1 ml of solution contains 50 mg methotrexate (as methotrexate disodium).

1 pre-filled syringe of 0.15 ml contains 7.5 mg methotrexate.

1 pre-filled syringe of 0.20 ml contains 10 mg methotrexate.

1 pre-filled syringe of 0.30 ml contains 15 mg methotrexate.

1 pre-filled syringe of 0.40 ml contains 20 mg methotrexate.

1 pre-filled syringe of 0.50 ml contains 25 mg methotrexate.

For a full list of excipients, see section 6.1.

3. PHARMACEUTICAL FORM

Solution for injection, in pre-filled syringe.

Clear, yellow-brown solution.

4. CLINICAL PARTICULARS

4.1 Therapeutic indications

Metoject 50 mg/ml is indicated for the treatment of

– active rheumatoid arthritis in adult patients,

– severe recalcitrant disabling psoriasis, which is not adequately responsive to other forms of therapy such as phototherapy, PUVA, and retinoids, and severe psoriatic arthritis in adult patients.

4.2 Posology and method of administration

Metoject 50 mg/ml should only be prescribed by physicians, who are familiar with the various characteristics of the medicinal product and its mode of action. Metoject 50 mg/ml is injected once weekly.

The patient is to be explicitly informed about the unusual fact of administration once weekly. It is advisable to determine a fixed, appropriate weekday as day of injection.

Methotrexate elimination is reduced in patients with a third distribution space (ascites, pleural effusions). Such patients require especially careful monitoring for toxicity, and require dose reduction or, in some cases, discontinuation of methotrexate administration (see section 5.2 and 4.4).

Dosage in adult patients with rheumatoid arthritis:

The recommended initial dose is 7.5 mg of methotrexate **once weekly**, administered either subcutaneously, intramuscularly or intravenously. Depending on the individual activity of the disease and tolerability by the patient, the initial dose may be increased gradually by 2.5 mg per week. A weekly dose of 25 mg should not be exceeded. However, doses exceeding 20 mg/week are associated with significant increase in toxicity, especially bone marrow suppression. Response to treatment can be expected after approximately 4 – 8 weeks. Upon achieving the therapeutically desired result, the dose should be reduced gradually to the lowest possible effective maintenance dose.

Dosage in patients with psoriasis vulgaris and psoriatic arthritis:

It is recommended that a test dose of 5 – 10 mg should be administered parenterally, one week prior to therapy to detect idiosyncratic adverse reactions. The recommended initial dose is 7.5 mg of methotrexate once weekly, administered either subcutaneously, intramuscularly or intravenously. The dose is to be increased gradually but should not, in general, exceed a weekly dose of 25 mg of methotrexate. Doses exceeding 20 mg per week can be associated with significant increase in toxicity, especially bone marrow suppression. Response to treatment can generally be expected after approximately 2 – 6 weeks. Upon achieving the therapeutically desired result, the dose should be reduced gradually to the lowest possible effective maintenance dose.

Patients with renal impairment:

Metoject 50 mg/ml should be used with caution in patients with impaired renal function. The dose should be adjusted as follows:

Creatinine clearance (ml/min)	Dose
> 50	100 %
20 – 50	50 %
< 20	Metoject 50 mg/ml must not be used

See section 4.3

Patients with hepatic impairment:

Methotrexate should be administered with great caution, if at all, to patients with significant current or previous liver disease, especially if due to alcohol. If bilirubin is > 5 mg/dl (85.5 μmol/l), methotrexate is contraindicated.

For a full list of contraindications, see section 4.3.

Use in elderly patients:

Dose reduction should be considered in elderly patients due to reduced liver and kidney function as well as lower folate reserves which occur with increased age.

Use in patient with a third distribution space (pleural effusions, ascitis):

As the half-life of Methotrexate can be prolonged to 4 times the normal length in patients who possess a third distribution space dose reduction or, in some cases, discontinuation of methotrexate administration may be required (see section 5.2 and 4.4).

Duration and method of administration:

The medicinal is for single use only.

Metoject 50 mg/ml solution for injection can be given by intramuscular, intravenous or subcutaneous route (in children and adolescents only subcutaneous or intramuscular).

The overall duration of the treatment is decided by the physician.

Note:

If changing from oral to parenteral administration a reduction of the dose may be required due to the variable bioavailability of methotrexate after oral administration.

Folic acid supplementation may be considered according to current treatment guidelines.

4.3 Contraindications

Metoject 50 mg/ml is contraindicated in the case of

– hypersensitivity to methotrexate or to any of the excipients,

– liver insufficiency (see section 4.2),

– alcohol abuse,

– severe renal insufficiency (creatinine clearance less than 20 ml/min., see section 4.2 and section 4.4),

– pre-existing blood dyscrasias, such as bone marrow hypoplasia, leukopenia, thrombocytopenia, or significant anaemia,

– serious, acute or chronic infections such as tuberculosis, HIV or other immunodeficiency syndromes,

– ulcers of the oral cavity and known active gastrointestinal ulcer disease,

– pregnancy, breast-feeding (see section 4.6),

– concurrent vaccination with live vaccines.

4.4 Special warnings and precautions for use

Patients must be clearly informed that the therapy has to be applicated **once a week**, not every day.

Patients undergoing therapy should be subject to appropriate supervision so that signs of possible toxic effects or adverse reactions may be detected and evaluated with minimal delay. Therefore methotrexate should be only administered by, or under the supervision of physicians whose knowledge and experience includes the use of antimetabolite therapy. Because of the possibility of severe or even fatal toxic reactions, the patient should be fully informed by the physician of the risks involved and the recommended safety measures.

Recommended examinations and safety measures

Before beginning or reinstituting methotrexate therapy after a rest period:

Complete blood count with differential blood count and platelets, liver enzymes, bilirubin, serum albumin, chest x-ray and renal function tests. If clinically indicated, exclude tuberculosis and hepatitis.

During therapy (at least once a month during the first six months and every three months thereafter):

An increased monitoring frequency should be considered also when the dose is increased.

1. Examination of the mouth and throat for mucosal changes

2. Complete blood count with differential blood count and platelets. Haemopoietic suppression caused by methotrexate may occur abruptly and with apparently safe dosages. Any profound drop in white-cell or platelet counts indicates immediate withdrawal of the medicinal product and appropriate supportive therapy. Patients should be advised to report all signs and symptoms suggestive of infection. Patients taking simultaneous administration of haematotoxic medicinal products (e.g. leflunomide) should be monitored closely with blood count and platelets.

3. Liver function tests: Particular attention should be given to the appearance of liver toxicity. Treatment should not be instituted or should be discontinued if any abnormality of liver function tests, or liver biopsy, is present or develops during therapy. Such abnormalities should return to normal within two weeks after which treatment may be recommenced at the discretion of the physician. There is no evidence to support use of a liver biopsy to monitor hepatic toxicity in rheumatological indications.

For psoriasis patients the need for a liver biopsy prior to and during therapy is controversial. Further research is needed to establish whether serial liver chemistry tests or propeptide of type III collagen can detect hepatotoxicity sufficiently. The evaluation should be performed case by case and differentiate between patients with no risk factors and patients with risk factors such as excessive prior alcohol consumption, persistent elevation of liver enzymes, history of liver disease, family history of inheritable liver disease, diabetes mellitus, obesity, and history of significant exposure to hepatotoxic drugs or chemicals and prolonged Methotrexate treatment or cumulative doses of 1.5 g or more.

Check of liver-related enzymes in serum: Temporary increases in transaminases to twice or three times of the upper limit of normal have been reported by patients at a frequency of 13 – 20 %. In the case of a constant increase in liver-related enzymes, a reduction of the dose or discontinuation of therapy should be taken into consideration.

Due to its potentially toxic effect on the liver, additional hepatotoxic medicinal products should not be taken during treatment with methotrexate *unless clearly necessary* and the consumption of alcohol should be avoided or greatly reduced (see section 4.5). Closer monitoring of liver enzymes should be exercised in patients taking other hepatotoxic medicinal products concomitantly (e.g. leflunomide). The same should be taken into account with the simultaneous administration of haematotoxic medicinal products (e.g. leflunomide).

4. Renal function should be monitored by renal function tests and urinanalysis (see sections 4.2 and 4.3).

As methotrexate is eliminated mainly by renal route, increased serum concentrations are to be expected in the case of renal insufficiency, which may result in severe undesirable effects.

Where renal function may be compromised (e.g. in the elderly), monitoring should take place more frequently. This applies in particular, when medicinal products are administered concomitantly, which affect the elimination of methotrexate, cause kidney damage (e.g. non-steroidal anti-inflammatory medicinal products) or which can potentially lead to impairment of blood formation. Dehydration may also intensify the toxicity of methotrexate.

5. Assessment of respiratory system: Alertness for symptoms of lung function impairment and, if necessary lung function test. Pulmonary affection requires a quick diagnosis and discontinuation of methotrexate. Pulmonary symptoms (especially a dry, non-productive cough) or a non-specific pneumonitis occurring during methotrexate

therapy may be indicative of a potentially dangerous lesion and require interruption of treatment and careful investigation. Acute or chronic interstitial pneumonitis, often associated with blood eosinophilia, may occur and deaths have been reported. Although clinically variable, the typical patient with methotrexate-induced lung disease presents with fever, cough, dyspnoea, hypoxemia, and an infiltrate on chest X-ray, infection needs to be excluded. Pulmonary affection requires a quick diagnosis and discontinuation of methotrexate therapy. This lesion can occur at all dosages.

6. Methotrexate may, due to its effect on the immune system, impair the response to vaccination results and affect the result of immunological tests. Particular caution is also needed in the presence of inactive, chronic infections (e.g. herpes zoster, tuberculosis, hepatitis B or C) for reasons of eventual activation. Vaccination using live vaccines must not be carried out under methotrexate therapy.

Malignant lymphomas may occur in patients receiving low dose methotrexate, in which case therapy must be discontinued. Failure of the lymphoma to show signs of spontaneous regression requires the initiation of cytotoxic therapy.

Concomitant administration of folate antagonists such as trimethoprim/sulphamethoxazole has been reported to cause an acute megaloblastic pancytopenia in rare instances.

Radiation induced dermatitis and sun-burn can reappear under methotrexate therapy (recall-reaction). Psoriatic lesions can exacerbate during UV-irradiation and simultaneous administration of methotrexate.

Methotrexate elimination is reduced in patients with a third distribution space (ascites, pleural effusions). Such patients require especially careful monitoring for toxicity, and require dose reduction or, in some cases, discontinuation of methotrexate administration. Pleural effusions and ascites should be drained prior to initiation of methotrexate treatment (see section 5.2).

Diarrhoea and ulcerative stomatitis can be toxic effects and require interruption of therapy, otherwise haemorrhagic enteritis and death from intestinal perforation may occur.

Vitamin preparations or other products containing folic acid, folinic acid or their derivatives may decrease the effectiveness of methotrexate.

For the treatment of psoriasis, methotrexate should be restricted to severe recalcitrant, disabling psoriasis which is not adequately responsive to other forms to other forms of therapy, but only when the diagnosis has been established by biopsy and/or after dermatological consultation.

This medicinal product contains less than 1 mmol sodium (23 mg) per dose, i.e. essentially "sodium-free".

The absence of pregnancy should be confirmed before Metoject 50 mg/ml is administered. Methotrexate causes embryotoxicity, abortion and foetal defects in humans. Methotrexate affects spermatogenesis and oogenesis during the period of its administration which may result in decreased fertility. These effects appear to be reversible on discontinuing therapy. Effective contraception in men and women should be performed during treatment and for at least six months thereafter. The possible risks of effects on reproduction should be discussed with patients of child-bearing potential and their partners should be advised appropriately (see section 4.6).

4.5 Interaction with other medicinal products and other forms of interaction

Alcohol, hepatotoxic medicinal products, haematotoxic medicinal products

The probability of methotrexate exhibiting a hepatotoxic effect is increased by regular alcohol consumption and when other hepatotoxic medicinal products are taken at the same time (see section 4.4). Patients taking other hepatotoxic medicinal products concomitantly (e.g. leflunomide) should be monitored with special care. The same should be taken into account with the simultaneous administration of haematotoxic medicinal products (e.g. leflunomide, azathioprine, retinoids, sulfasalazine). The incidence of pancytopenia and hepatotoxicity can be increased when leflunomide is combined with methotrexate.

Combined treatment with methotrexate and retinoids like acitretin or etretinate increases the risk of hepatotoxicity.

Oral antibiotics

Oral antibiotics like tetracyclines, chloramphenicol, and non-absorbable broad-spectrum antibiotics can interfere with the enterohepatic circulation, by inhibition of the intestinal flora or suppression of the bacterial metabolism.

Antibiotics

Antibiotics, like penicillines, glycopeptides, sulfonamides, ciprofloxacin and cefalotin can, in individual cases, reduce the renal clearance of methotrexate, so that increased serum concentrations of methotrexate with simultaneous haematological and gastro-intestinal toxicity may occur.

Medicinal products with high plasma protein binding

Methotrexate is plasma protein bound and may be displaced by other protein bound drugs such as salicylates, hypoglycaemics, diuretics, sulphonamides, diphenylhydantoins, tetracyclines, chloramphenicol and p-aminobenzoic acid, and the acidic anti-inflammatory agents, which can lead to increased toxicity when used concurrently.

Probenecid, weak organic acids, pyrazoles and non-steroidal anti-inflammatory agents

Probenecid, weak organic acids such as loop diuretics, and pyrazoles (phenylbutazone) can reduce the elimination of methotrexate and higher serum concentrations may be assumed inducing higher haematological toxicity. There is also a possibility of increased toxicity when low dose methotrexate and non steroidal anti-inflammatory medicinal products or salicylates are combined.

Medicinal products with adverse reactions on the bone marrow

In the case of medication with medicinal products, which may have adverse reactions on the bone marrow (e.g. sulphonamides, trimethoprim-sulphamethoxazole, chloramphenicol, pyrimethamine); attention should be paid to the possibility of pronounced impairment of blood formation.

Medicinal products which cause folate deficiency

The concomitant administration of products which cause folate deficiency (e.g. sulphonamides, trimethoprim-sulphamethoxazole) can lead to increased methotrexate toxicity. Particular care is therefore advisable in the presence of existing folic acid deficiency.

Products containing folic acid or folinic acid

Vitamin preparations or other products containing folic acid, folinic acid or their derivatives may decrease the effectiveness of methotrexate.

Other antirheumatic medicinal products

An increase in the toxic effects of methotrexate is, in general, not to be expected when Metoject 50 mg/ml is administered simultaneously with other antirheumatic medicinal products (e.g. gold compounds, penicillamine, hydroxychloroquine, sulphasalazine, azathioprin, ciclosporin).

Sulphasalazine

Although the combination of methotrexate and sulphasalazine can cause an increase in efficacy of methotrexate and as a result more undesirable effects due to the inhibition of folic acid synthesis through sulphasalazine, such undesirable effects have only been observed in rare individual cases in the course of several studies.

Mercaptopurine

Methotrexate increases the plasma levels of mercaptopurine. The combination of methotrexate and mercaptopurine may therefore require dose adjustment.

Proton-pump inhibitors

A concomitant administration of proton-pump inhibitors like omeprazole or pantoprazole can lead to interactions: Concomitant administration of methotrexate and omeprazole has led to delayed renal elimination of methotrexate. In combination with pantoprazole inhibited renal elimination of the metabolite 7-hydroxymethotrexate with myalgia and shivering was reported in one case.

Theophylline

Methotrexate may decrease the clearance of theophylline; theophylline levels should be monitored when used concurrently with methotrexate.

Caffeine- or theophylline-containing beverages

An excessive consumption of caffeine- or theophylline-containing beverages (coffee, caffeine-containing soft drinks, black tea) should be avoided during methotrexate therapy.

4.6 Pregnancy and lactation

Metoject 50 mg/ml is contraindicated during pregnancy (see section 4.3). In animal studies, methotrexate has shown reproductive toxicity (see section 5.3). Methotrexate has been shown to be teratogenic to humans; it has been reported to cause foetal death and/or congenital abnormalities. Exposure of a limited number of pregnant women (42) resulted in an increased incidence (1:14) of malformations (cranial, cardiovascular and extremital). If methotrexate is discontinued prior to conception, normal pregnancies have been reported. Women must not get pregnant during methotrexate therapy. In case of women getting pregnant during therapy medical counselling about the risk of adverse reactions for the child associated with methotrexate therapy should be sought. Therefore, patients of a sexually mature age (women and men) must use effective contraception during treatment with Metoject 50 mg/ml and at least 6 months thereafter (see section 4.4).

In women of child-bearing age, any existing pregnancy must be excluded with certainty by taking appropriate measures, e.g. pregnancy test, prior to initiating therapy.

As methotrexate can be genotoxic, all women who wish to become pregnant are advised to consult a genetic counselling centre, if possible, already prior to therapy, and men should seek advice about the possibility of sperm preservation before starting therapy.

Lactation: Methotrexate is excreted in breast milk in such concentrations that there is a risk for the infant, and accordingly, breast-feeding should be discontinued prior to and throughout administration.

4.7 Effects on ability to drive and use machines

Central nervous symptoms such as tiredness and dizziness can occur during treatment, Metoject 50 mg/ml has minor or moderate influence on the ability to drive and use machines.

4.8 Undesirable effects

The most relevant undesirable effects are suppression of the haematopoietic system and gastrointestinal disorders.

The following headings are used to organise the undesirable effects in order of frequency:

Very common (≥ 1/10), common (≥ 1/100 to < 1/10), uncommon (≥ 1/1,000 to < 1/100), rare (≥ 1/10,000 to < 1/1,000), very rare (< 1/10,000), not known (cannot be estimated from the available data)

Gastrointestinal disorders

Very common: Stomatitis, dyspepsia, nausea, loss of appetite.

Common: Oral ulcers, diarrhoea.

Uncommon: Pharyngitis, enteritis, vomiting.

Rare: Gastrointestinal ulcers.

Very rare: Haematemesis, haematorrhea, toxic megacolon.

Skin and subcutaneous tissue disorders

Common: Exanthema, erythema, pruritus.

Uncommon: Photosensitisation, loss of hair, increase in rheumatic nodules, herpes zoster, vasculitis, herpetiform eruptions of the skin, urticaria.

Rare: Increased pigmentation, acne, ecchymosis.

Very rare: Stevens-Johnson syndrome, toxic epidermal necrolysis (Lyell's syndrome), increased pigmentary changes of the nails, acute paronychia, furunculosis, telangiectasia.

General disorders and administration site conditions

Rare: Allergic reactions, anaphylactic shock, allergic vasculitis, fever, conjunctivitis, infection, sepsis, wound-healing impairment, hypogammaglobulinaemia.

Very rare: Local damage (formation of sterile abscess, lipodystrophy) of injection site following intramuscular or subcutaneous administration.

Metabolism and nutrition disorders

Uncommon: Precipitation of diabetes mellitus.

Nervous system disorders

Common: Headache, tiredness, drowsiness.

Uncommon: Dizziness, confusion, depression.

Very rare: Impaired vision, pain, muscular asthenia or paraesthesia in the extremities, changes in sense of taste (metallic taste), convulsions, meningism, paralysis.

Eye disorders

Rare: Visual disturbances.

Very rare: Retinopathy.

Hepatobiliary disorders (see section 4.4)

Very common: Elevated transaminases.

Uncommon: Cirrhosis, fibrosis and fatty degeneration of the liver, decrease in serum albumin.

Rare: Acute hepatitis.

Very rare: Hepatic failure.

Cardiac disorders

Rare: Pericarditis, pericardial effusion, pericardial tamponade.

Vascular disorders

Rare: Hypotension, thromboembolic events.

Respiratory, thoracic and mediastinal disorders

Common: Pneumonia, interstitial alveolitis/pneumonitis often associated with eosinophilia. Symptoms indicating potentially severe lung injury (interstitial pneumonitis) are: dry, not productive cough, short of breath and fever.

Rare: Pulmonary fibrosis, *Pneumocystis carinii* pneumonia, shortness of breath and bronchial asthma, pleural effusion.

Blood and lymphatic system disorders

Common: Leukopenia, anaemia, thrombopenia.

Uncommon: Pancytopenia.

Very rare: Agranulocytosis, severe courses of bone marrow depression.

Renal and urinary disorders

Uncommon: Inflammation and ulceration of the urinary bladder, renal impairment, disturbed micturition.

Rare: Renal failure, oliguria, anuria, electrolyte disturbances.

Reproductive system and breast disorders

Uncommon: Inflammation and ulceration of the vagina.

Very rare: Loss of libido, impotence, gynaecomastia, oligospermia, impaired menstruation, vaginal discharge.

Musculoskeletal and connective tissue disorders

Uncommon: Arthralgia, myalgia, osteoporosis.

Neoplasms benign, malignant and unspecified (including cysts and polyps)

Very rare: There have been reports of individual cases of lymphoma which subsided in a number of cases once treatment with methotrexate had been discontinued. In a recent study, it could not be established that methotrexate therapy increases the incidence of lymphomas.

The appearance and degree of severity of undesirable effects depends on the dosage level and the frequency of administration. However, as severe undesirable effects can occur even at lower doses, it is indispensable that patients are monitored regularly by the doctor at short intervals.

When methotrexate is given by the intramuscular route, local undesirable effects (burning sensation) or damage (formation of sterile abscess, destruction of fatty tissue) at the site of injection can occur commonly. Subcutaneous application of methotrexate is locally well tolerated. Only mild local skin reactions were observed, decreasing during therapy.

4.9 Overdose

a) Symptoms of overdosage

Toxicity of methotrexate mainly affects the haematopoietic system.

b) Treatment measures in the case of overdosage

Calcium folinate is the specific antidote for neutralising the toxic undesirable effects of methotrexate.

In cases of accidental overdose, a dose of calcium folinate equal to or higher than the offending dose of methotrexate should be administered intravenously or intramuscularly within one hour and dosing continued until the serum levels of methotrexate are below 10^{-7} mol/l.

In cases of massive overdose, hydration and urinary alkalisation may be necessary to prevent precipitation of methotrexate and/or its metabolites in the renal tubules. Neither haemodialysis nor peritoneal dialysis has been shown to improve methotrexate elimination. Effective clearance of methotrexate has been reported with acute, intermittent haemodialysis using a high flux dialyser.

5. PHARMACOLOGICAL PROPERTIES

5.1 Pharmacodynamic properties

Pharmacotherapeutic group: Folic acid analogues

ATC code: L01BA01

Antirheumatic medicinal product for the treatment of chronic, inflammatory rheumatic diseases.

Methotrexate is a folic acid antagonist which belongs to the class of cytotoxic agents known as antimetabolites. It acts by the competitive inhibition of the enzyme dihydrofolate reductase and thus inhibits DNA synthesis. It has not yet been clarified, as to whether the efficacy of methotrexate, in the management of psoriasis, psoriasis arthritis and chronic polyarthritis, is due to an anti-inflammatory or immunosuppressive effect and to which extent a methotrexate-induced increase in extracellular adenosine concentration at inflamed sites contributes to these effects.

5.2 Pharmacokinetic properties

Following oral administration, methotrexate is absorbed from the gastrointestinal tract. In case of low-dosed administration (dosages between 7.5 mg/m^2 and 80 mg/m^2 body surface area), the mean bioavailability is approx. 70 %, but considerable interindividual and intraindividual deviations are possible (25 – 100 %). Maximum serum concentrations are achieved after 1 – 2 hours.

Bioavailability of subcutaneous, intravenous and intramuscular injection is comparable and nearly 100 %.

Approximately 50 % of methotrexate is bound to serum proteins. Upon being distributed into body tissues, high concentrations in the form of polyglutamates are found in the liver, kidneys and spleen in particular, which can be retained for weeks or months. When administered in small doses, methotrexate passes into the liquor in minimal amounts. The terminal half-life is on average 6 – 7 hours and demonstrates considerable variation (3 – 17 hours). The half-life can be prolonged to 4 times the normal length in patients who possess a third distribution space (pleural effusion, ascites).

Approx. 10 % of the administered methotrexate dose is metabolised intrahepatically. The principle metabolite is 7-hydroxymethotrexate.

Excretion takes places, mainly in unchanged form, primarily renal via glomerular filtration and active secretion in the proximal tubulus.

Approx. 5 – 20 % methotrexate and 1 – 5 % 7-hydroxymethotrexate are eliminated biliary. There is pronounced enterohepatic circulation.

In the case of renal insufficiency, elimination is delayed significantly. Impaired elimination with regard to hepatic insufficiency is not known.

5.3 Preclinical safety data

Animal studies show that methotrexate impairs fertility, is embryo- and foetotoxic and teratogenic. Methotrexate is mutagenic *in vivo* and *in vitro*. As conventional carcinogenicity studies have not been performed and data from chronic toxicity studies in rodents are inconsistent, methotrexate is considered **not classifiable** as to its carcinogenicity to humans.

6. PHARMACEUTICAL PARTICULARS

6.1 List of excipients

Sodium chloride

Sodium hydroxide for pH adjustment

Water for injections

6.2 Incompatibilities

In the absence of compatibility studies, this medicinal product must not be mixed with other medicinal products.

6.3 Shelf life

18 months.

6.4 Special precautions for storage

Store below 25 °C. Keep the pre-filled syringes in the outer carton in order to protect from light.

6.5 Nature and contents of container

Nature of container:

Pre-filled syringes of colourless glass (type I) of 1 ml capacity with embedded injection needle. Plunger stoppers of chlorobutyl rubber (type I) and polystyrene rods inserted on the stopper to form the syringe plunger

or

Pre-filled syringes of colourless glass (type I) of 1 ml capacity with enclosed injection needle. Plunger stoppers of chlorobutyl rubber (type I) and polystyrene rods inserted on the stopper to form the syringe plunger.

Pack sizes:

Pre-filled syringes containing 0.15 ml, 0.20 ml, 0.30 ml, 0.40 ml, or 0.50 ml solution are available in packs of 1, 4, 6, 12 and 24 syringes with embedded s.c. injection needle and alcohol pads.

and

Pre-filled syringes containing 0.15 ml, 0.20 ml, 0.30 ml, 0.40 ml, or 0.50 ml solution are available in packs of 1, 4, 6, 12 and 24 syringes with enclosed s.c. injection needle and alcohol pads.

All pack sizes are available with graduation marks.

Not all pack sizes may be marketed.

6.6 Special precautions for disposal and other handling

The manner of handling and disposal must be consistent with that of other cytotoxic preparations in accordance with local requirements. Pregnant health care personnel should not handle and/or administer Metoject 50 mg/ml.

Methotrexate should not come into contact with the skin or mucosa. In the event of contamination, the affected area must be rinsed immediately with ample amount of water.

For single use only.

Any unused product or waste should be disposed of in accordance with local requirements.

7. MARKETING AUTHORISATION HOLDER

medac

Gesellschaft für klinische Spezialpräparate mbH

Fehlandtstraβe 3

20354 Hamburg

Germany

8. MARKETING AUTHORISATION NUMBER(S)

PL 11587/0046

9. DATE OF FIRST AUTHORISATION/RENEWAL OF THE AUTHORISATION

21/11/2008

10. DATE OF REVISION OF THE TEXT

21/11/2008

Metopirone Capsules 250 mg

(Alliance Pharmaceuticals)

1. NAME OF THE MEDICINAL PRODUCT

Metopirone® Capsules 250mg

2. QUALITATIVE AND QUANTITATIVE COMPOSITION

Metyrapone BP 250mg.

3. PHARMACEUTICAL FORM

Yellowish-white, oblong, opaque, soft gelatin capsules printed 'CIBA' on one side and 'LN' on the other in brown ink.

4. CLINICAL PARTICULARS

4.1 Therapeutic indications

A diagnostic aid in the differential diagnosis of ACTH-dependent Cushing's syndrome. The management of patients with Cushing's syndrome.

In conjunction with glucocorticosteroids in the treatment of resistant oedema due to increased aldosterone secretion in patients suffering from cirrhosis, nephrosis and congestive heart failure.

4.2 Posology and method of administration

Adults:

The capsules should be taken with milk or after a meal, to minimise nausea and vomiting, which can lead to impaired absorption.

For use as a diagnostic aid: the patient must be hospitalised. Urinary 17-oxygenic steroid excretion is measured over 24 hours on each of 4 consecutive days. The first 2 days serve as a control period. On the third day, 750mg Metopirone (3 capsules) must be given at four-hourly intervals to give a total of 6 doses (ie 4.5g). Maximum urine steroid excretion may occur on the fourth day. If urinary steroid excretion increases in response to Metopirone, this suggests the high levels of circulatory cortisol are due to adrenocortical hyperplasia following excessive ACTH production rather than a cortisol-producing adrenal tumour.

For therapeutic use: for the management of Cushing's syndrome, the dosage must be adjusted to meet the patient's requirements; a daily dosage from 250mg to 6g may be required to restore normal cortisol levels.

For the treatment of resistant oedema: The usual daily dose of 3g (12 capsules) should be given in divided doses in conjunction with a glucocorticoid.

Children: Children should be given a smaller amount based upon 6 four-hourly doses of 15mg/kg, with a minimum dose of 250mg every four hours.

Elderly: Clinical evidence would indicate that no special dosage regimen is necessary.

4.3 Contraindications

Primary adrenocorticol insufficiency. Hypersensitivity to Metopirone or to any of the excipients. Pregnancy.

4.4 Special warnings and precautions for use

In relation to use as a diagnostic aid: anticonvulsants (eg phenytoin, barbiturates), anti-depressants and neuroleptics (eg amitriptyline, chlorpromazine), hormones that affect the hypothalamo-pituitary axis and anti-thyroid agents may influence the results of the Metopirone test. If these drugs cannot be withdrawn, the necessity of carrying out the Metopirone test should be reviewed.

If adrenocortical or anterior pituitary function is more severely compromised than indicated by the results of the test, Metopirone may trigger transient adrenocortical insufficiency. This can be rapidly corrected by giving appropriate doses of corticosteroids.

Long-term treatment with Metopirone can cause hypertension as the result of excessive secretion of desoxycorticosterone.

The ability of the adrenal cortex to respond to exogenous ACTH should be demonstrated before Metopirone is employed as a test, as Metopirone may induce acute adrenal insufficiency in patients with reduced adrenal secretory capacity, as well as in patients with gross hypopituitarism.

Patients with liver cirrhosis often show a delayed response to Metopirone, due to liver damage delaying the metabolism of cortisol.

In cases of thyroid hypofunction, urinary steroid levels may rise very slowly, or not at all, in response to Metopirone.

4.5 Interaction with other medicinal products and other forms of interaction

In some cases concomitant medication may affect the results of the Metopirone test (see Section 4.4, Special warnings and precautions for use).

4.6 Pregnancy and lactation

No data are available from animal reproduction studies. Metopirone should not be administered during pregnancy since the drug can impair the biosynthesis of foetal-placental steroids. It is not known whether metyrapone passes into the breast milk, therefore nursing mothers should refrain from breast-feeding their infants during treatment with Metopirone.

4.7 Effects on ability to drive and use machines

Patients should be warned of the potential hazards of driving or operating machinery if they experience side effects such as dizziness and sedation.

4.8 Undesirable effects

Gastrointestinal tract: Occasional: nausea, vomiting. Rare: abdominal pain.

Central nervous system: Occasional: dizziness, sedation, headache.

Cardiovascular system: Occasional: hypotension.

Skin: Rare: allergic skin reactions.

Endocrine system: Rare: hypoadrenalism, hirsutism.

4.9 Overdose

Signs and symptoms: The clinical picture of acute Metopirone poisoning is characterised by gastrointestinal symptoms and acute adrenocortical insufficiency. Laboratory findings: hyponatraemia, hypochloraemia, hyperkalaemia. In patients under treatment with insulin or oral antidiabetics, the signs and symptoms of acute poisoning with Metopirone may be aggravated or modified.

Treatment: There is no specific antidote. Gastric lavage and forced emesis should be employed to reduce the absorption of the drug. In addition to general measures, a large dose of hydrocortisone should be administered at once, together with iv saline and glucose. This should be repeated as necessary in accordance with the patient's clinical condition. For a few days, blood pressure and fluid and electrolyte balance should be monitored.

5. PHARMACOLOGICAL PROPERTIES

5.1 Pharmacodynamic properties

Metopirone inhibits the enzyme responsible for the 11β-hydroxylation stage in the biosynthesis of cortisol and to a lesser extent, aldosterone. The fall in plasma concentration of circulating glucocorticoids stimulates ACTH secretion, via the feedback mechanism which accelerates steroid biosynthesis. As a result, 11-desoxycortisol, the precursor of cortisol, is released into the circulation, metabolised by the liver and excreted in the urine. Unlike cortisol, 11-desoxycortisol does not suppress ACTH secretion and its urinary metabolites may be measured.

These metabolites can easily be determined by measuring urinary 17-hydroxycorticosteroids (17-OHCS) or 17-ketogenic steroids (17-KGS). Metopirone is used as a diagnostic test on the basis of these properties, with plasma 11-desoxycortisol and urinary 17-OHCS measured as an index of pituitary ACTH responsiveness. Metopirone may also suppress biosynthesis of aldosterone, resulting in mild natriuresis.

5.2 Pharmacokinetic properties

Metyrapone is rapidly absorbed and eliminated from the plasma. Peak plasma levels usually occur one hour after ingestion of Metopirone; after a dose of 750mg Metopirone, plasma drug levels average 3.7μg/ml. Plasma drug levels decrease to a mean value of 0.5μg/ml 4 hours after dosing. The half-life of elimination of Metopirone from the plasma is 20 to 26 minutes.

Metyrapol, the reduced form of metyrapone, is the main active metabolite. Eight hours after a single oral dose, the ratio of metyrapone to metyrapol in the plasma is 1:1.5. Metyrapol takes about twice as long as metyrapone to be eliminated in the plasma.

Seventy-two hours after a first daily dose of 4.5g Metopirone (750mg every 4 hours), 5.3% of the total dose was excreted in the urine as metyrapone (9.2% in free form and 90.8% conjugated with glucuronic acid), and 38.5% in the form of metyrapol (8.1% in free form and 91.9% conjugated with glucuronic acid).

5.3 Preclinical safety data

There are no pre-clinical data of relevance to the prescriber which are additional to those already included in other sections of the Summary of Product Characteristics.

6. PHARMACEUTICAL PARTICULARS

6.1 List of excipients

Capsule contents: Glycerin, polyethylene glycol 400, polyethylene glycol 4000 and water. Capsule shell: Sodium ethylparaben, ethyl vanillin, gelatin, glycerin 85%, p-methoxy acetophenone, sodium propylparaben and titanium oxide (E171).

6.2 Incompatibilities

None stated.

6.3 Shelf life

5 years

6.4 Special precautions for storage

Protect from moisture and heat. Store below 30°C.

6.5 Nature and contents of container

High density polyethylene bottles of 100 capsules.

6.6 Special precautions for disposal and other handling

None stated.

Administrative Details

7. MARKETING AUTHORISATION HOLDER

Alliance Pharmaceuticals Ltd
Avonbridge House
Bath Road
Chippenham
Wiltshire
SN15 2BB

8. MARKETING AUTHORISATION NUMBER(S)

PL16853/0010

9. DATE OF FIRST AUTHORISATION/RENEWAL OF THE AUTHORISATION

June 1998

10. DATE OF REVISION OF THE TEXT

February 2005

11. Legal status

POM

Alliance, Alliance Pharmaceuticals and associated devices are registered Trademarks of Alliance Pharmaceuticals Ltd.

Metrogel

(Galderma (U.K) Ltd)

1. NAME OF THE MEDICINAL PRODUCT

Metrogel

2. QUALITATIVE AND QUANTITATIVE COMPOSITION

Metronidazole BP 0.75%.

3. PHARMACEUTICAL FORM

Aqueous gel for cutaneous use.

4. CLINICAL PARTICULARS

4.1 Therapeutic indications

For the treatment of acute inflammatory exacerbation of rosacea.

For the deodorisation of the smell associated with malodorous fungating tumours.

4.2 Posology and method of administration

For the treatment of rosacea:

Adults and elderly:

Apply to the affected skin of the face in a thin film twice daily for a period of eight to nine weeks. Thereafter, further applications may be necessary depending upon the severity of the condition.

Children:

Not recommended.

For the deodorisation of malodorous fungating tumours:

Adults and elderly:

Clean the wound thoroughly. Apply the gel over the complete area and cover with a non-adherent dressing. Use once or twice daily as necessary.

Children:

Not recommended.

4.3 Contraindications

Contraindicated in individuals with a history of hypersensitivity to Metronidazole, or other ingredients of the formulation.

4.4 Special warnings and precautions for use

Metrogel has been reported to cause lacrimation of the eyes, therefore, contact with the eyes should be avoided. If a reaction suggesting local irritation occurs patients should be directed to use the medication less frequently, discontinue use temporarily or discontinue use until further instructions. Metronidazole is a nitroimidazole and should be used with care in patients with evidence of, or history of, blood dyscrasia. Exposure of treated sites to ultraviolet or strong sunlight should be avoided during use of metronidazole.

Unnecessary and prolonged use of this medication should be avoided.

4.5 Interaction with other medicinal products and other forms of interaction

Interaction with systemic medication is unlikely because absorption of metronidazole following cutaneous application of Metrogel is low. Oral metronidazole has been reported to potentiate the effect of warfarin and other coumarin anticoagulants, resulting in a prolongation of prothrombin time. The effect of topical metronidazole on prothrombin is not known. However, very rare cases of modification of the INR values have been reported with concomitant use of Metrogel and coumarin anticoagulants.

4.6 Pregnancy and lactation

The safety of metronidazole in pregnancy and lactation had not been adequately established. The gel should therefore not be used in these circumstances unless the physician considers it essential. Medication should be stopped if pregnancy occurs.

4.7 Effects on ability to drive and use machines

None.

4.8 Undesirable effects

Because of the minimal absorption of metronidazole and consequently its insignificant plasma concentration after topical administration, the adverse experiences reported with the oral form of the drug have not been reported with Metrogel. Adverse reactions reported with Metrogel have been only local and mild, and include skin discomfort (burning and stinging), erythema, pruritis, skin irritation, worsening of rosacea, nausea, metallic taste and tingling or numbness of the extremities, and watery eyes if applied too closely to this area.

4.9 Overdose

No data exists about overdosage in humans. Acute oral toxicity studies with a topical gel formulation containing 0.75% w/w metronidazole in rats have shown no toxic action with doses of up to 5 g of finished product per kilogram body weight, the highest dose used. This dose is equivalent to the oral intake of 12 tubes of 30g packaging Metrogel for an adult weighing 72 kg, and 2 tubes of Metrogel for a child weighing 12 kg.

5. PHARMACOLOGICAL PROPERTIES

5.1 Pharmacodynamic properties

The etiology of rosacea is unknown although a variety of hypotheses have been reported.

5.2 Pharmacokinetic properties

The systemic concentration of Metronidazole following the topical administration of 1 g of a 0.75% Metronidazole gel to 10 patients with rosacea ranged from 25 ng/ml (limit of detection), to 66 mg/ml with a mean Cmax of 40.6 ng/ml.

The corresponding mean Cmax following the oral administration of a solution containing 30 mg of metronidazole was 850 ng/ml (equivalent to 212 ng/ml if dose corrected. The mean Tmax for the topical formulation was 6.0 hours compared to 0.97 hours for the oral solution.

5.3 Preclinical safety data

Metronidazole is a well established pharmaceutical active ingredient and to the subject of pharmacopoeial monograph in both the BP and Ph.Eur.

6. PHARMACEUTICAL PARTICULARS

6.1 List of excipients

Bronopol BP,
Hydroxybenzoic acid esters HSE,
Hydroxyethylcellulose HSE,
Propylene glycol Ph.Eur,
Phosphoric acid Ph.Eur,
Purified water Ph.Eur.

6.2 Incompatibilities

None known

6.3 Shelf life

2 years.

6.4 Special precautions for storage

Store between 15°C and 25°C in a dry place.

6.5 Nature and contents of container

Tube: Internally lacquered, membrane sealed aluminium.

Cap: low density polyethylene

Pack sizes available: 25 g and 40 g.

6.6 Special precautions for disposal and other handling

There are no special instructions for use/handling.

7. MARKETING AUTHORISATION HOLDER

Galderma (UK) Limited
Meridien House
69-71 Clarendon Road
Watford
Herts.
WD17 1DS
UK

8. MARKETING AUTHORISATION NUMBER(S)

PL 10590/0035

9. DATE OF FIRST AUTHORISATION/RENEWAL OF THE AUTHORISATION

27 February 1998

10. DATE OF REVISION OF THE TEXT

February 2006

11. Legal category

POM

Metvix 160 mg/g cream

(Galderma (U.K) Ltd)

1. NAME OF THE MEDICINAL PRODUCT

Metvix 160 mg/g cream.

2. QUALITATIVE AND QUANTITATIVE COMPOSITION

Metvix cream contains 160 mg/g of methyl aminolevulinate (as hydrochloride) equivalent to 16.0% of methyl aminolevulinate (as hydrochloride).

The excipients include cetostearyl alcohol (40 mg/g), methyl parahydroxybenzoate (E 218; 2 mg/g), propyl parahydroxybenzoate (E 216; 1 mg/g) and arachis oil (30 mg/g).

For excipients, see 6.1.

3. PHARMACEUTICAL FORM

Cream.

The colour is cream to pale yellow.

4. CLINICAL PARTICULARS

4.1 Therapeutic indications

Treatment of thin or non-hyperkeratotic and non-pigmented actinic keratoses on the face and scalp when other therapies are considered less appropriate.

Only for treatment of superficial and/or nodular basal cell carcinoma unsuitable for other available therapies due to possible treatment related morbidity and poor cosmetic outcome; such as lesions on the mid-face or ears, lesions on severely sun damaged skin, large lesions, or recurrent lesions.

Treatment of squamous cell carcinoma *in situ* (Bowen's disease) when surgical excision is considered less appropriate.

4.2 Posology and method of administration

Adults (including the elderly)

For treatment of actinic keratoses (AK) one session of photodynamic therapy should be administered. Treated lesions should be evaluated after three months and if needed, treatment should be repeated with a second therapy session. For treatment of basal cell carcinoma (BCC) and Bowen's disease two sessions should be administered with an interval of one week between sessions. Before applying Metvix cream, the lesion surface should be prepared to remove scales and crusts and roughen the surface of the lesions. Nodular BCC lesions are often covered by an intact epidermal keratin layer which should be removed. Exposed tumour material should be removed gently without any attempt to excise beyond the tumour margins.

Apply a layer of Metvix cream (about 1 mm thick) by using a spatula to the lesion and the surrounding 5-10 mm of normal skin. Cover the treated area with an occlusive dressing for 3 hours.

Remove the dressing, and clean the area with saline and immediately expose the lesion to red light with a continuous spectrum of 570-670 nm and a total light dose of 75 J/cm^2 at the lesion surface. Red light with a narrower spectrum giving the same activation of accumulated porphyrins may be used. The light intensity at the lesion surface should not exceed 200 mW/cm^2.

Only CE marked lamps should be used, equipped with necessary filters and/or reflecting mirrors to minimize exposure to heat, blue light and UV radiation. It is important to ensure that the correct light dose is administered. The light dose is determined by factors such as the size of the light field, the distance between lamp and skin surface and illumination time. These factors vary with lamp type, and the lamp should be used according to the user manual. The light dose delivered should be monitored if a suitable detector is available.

Patient and operator should adhere to safety instructions provided with the light source. During illumination patient and operator should wear protective goggles which correspond to the lamp light spectrum.

Healthy untreated skin surrounding the lesion does not need to be protected during illumination.

Multiple lesions may be treated during the same treatment session.

Lesion responses should be assessed after three months, and at this response evaluation, lesion sites showing non-complete response may be retreated if desired. It is recommended that the response of BCC and Bowen's disease lesions be confirmed by histological examination of biopsy material. Subsequently, close long term clinical monitoring of BCC and Bowen's disease is recommended, with histology if necessary.

Children and adolescents:

There is no experience of treating patients below the age of 18 years.

4.3 Contraindications

Hypersensitivity to the active substance or to any of the excipients which includes arachis oil.

Morpheaform basal cell carcinoma.

Porphyria.

4.4 Special warnings and precautions for use

Metvix should only be administered in the presence of a physician, a nurse or other health care professionals trained in the use of photodynamic therapy with Metvix.

Metvix is not recommended during pregnancy (see 4.6).

Thick (hyperkeratotic) actinic keratoses should not be treated with Metvix. There is no experience of treating lesions which are pigmented, highly infiltrating or located on the genitalia with Metvix cream. There is no experience of treating Bowen's disease lesions larger than 40 mm. As with cryotherapy and 5-FU therapy of Bowen's disease, response rates of large lesions (>20 mm in diameter) are lower than those of small lesions. There is no experience of treating Bowen's disease in transplant patients on immunosuppressive therapy or in patients with a history of arsenic exposure.

Methyl aminolevulinate may cause sensitization by skin contact resulting in application site eczema or allergic contact dermatitis. The excipient cetostearyl alcohol may cause local skin reactions (e.g. contact dermatitis), methyl- and propyl parahydroxybenzoate (E218, E216) may cause allergic reactions (possibly delayed).

Any UV-therapy should be discontinued before treatment. As a general precaution, sun exposure of the treated lesion sites and surrounding skin should be avoided for about 2 days following treatment.

Direct eye contact with Metvix cream should be avoided.

4.5 Interaction with other medicinal products and other forms of interaction

No specific interaction studies have been performed with methyl aminolevulinate.

4.6 Pregnancy and lactation

Pregnancy

For methyl aminolevulinate, no clinical data on exposed pregnancies are available. Reproductive toxicity studies in animals have not been performed. Metvix is not recommended during pregnancy (see 4.4).

Lactation

The amount of methyl aminolevulinate excreted into human breast milk following topical administration of Metvix cream is not known. In the absence of clinical experience, breast-feeding should be discontinued for 48 hours after application of Metvix cream.

4.7 Effects on ability to drive and use machines

Not applicable.

4.8 Undesirable effects

a) Approximately 60 % of patients experience reactions localised to the treatment site that are attributable to toxic effects of the photodynamic therapy (phototoxicity) or to preparation of the lesion.

The most frequent symptoms are painful and burning skin sensation typically beginning during illumination or soon after and lasting for a few hours with resolving on the day of treatment. The symptoms are usually of mild or moderate severity and rarely require early termination of illumination. The most frequent signs of phototoxicity are erythema and scab. The majority are of mild or moderate severity and persist for 1 to 2 weeks or occasionally longer.

Repeated treatment with Metvix is associated reduced frequency and severity of local phototoxic reactions.

b) The incidence of adverse reactions in a clinical trial population of 932 patients receiving the standard treatment regimen, is shown in the table below.

Body system (MedDRA)	Frequency*	Adverse reaction
Nervous system disorders	Common	Paraesthesia, headache
Eye disorders	Uncommon	Eye swelling, eye pain
Vascular disorders	Uncommon	Wound haemorrhage
Gastrointestinal disorders	Uncommon	Nausea
Skin and subcutaneous tissue disorders	Very common	Pain of skin, skin burning sensation, scab, erythema
	Common	Skin infection, skin ulcer, skin oedema, skin swelling, blister, skin hemorrhage, pruritus, skin exfoliation, skin warm
	Uncommon	Urticaria, rash, skin irritation, photosensitivity reaction, skin hypopigmentation, skin hyperpigmentation, heat rash, skin discomfort
General disorders and administration site conditions	Common	Application site discharge, feeling hot
	Uncommon	Fatigue

* Very common adverse reactions: Adverse reactions occurring in ⩾1/10) of patients.

Common adverse reactions: Adverse reactions occurring in ⩾1/100, <1/10 of patients.

Uncommon adverse reactions: Adverse reactions occurring in ⩾1/1000, ⩽1/100 of patients.

Adverse reactions reported by more than two patients in the clinical studies are included.

Application site eczema and allergic contact dermatitis have been described in post-marketing reports. Most cases were localised to the treatment area and were not severe; rarely erythema and swelling have been more extensive.

A study conducted in immunocompromised organ transplant recipients did not identify any safety concern in this population, adverse events being similar to those reported in trials in immunocompetent patients.

4.9 Overdose

The severity of local phototoxic reactions such as erythema, pain and burning sensation may increase in case of prolonged application time or very high light intensity.

5. PHARMACOLOGICAL PROPERTIES

5.1 Pharmacodynamic properties

Pharmacotherapeutic group:

Antineoplastic agent, ATC Code: L01X D03

Mechanism of Action:

After topical application of methyl aminolevulinate, porphyrins accumulate intracellularly in the treated skin lesions. The intracellular porphyrins (including PpIX) are photoactive, fluorescing compounds and, upon light activation in the presence of oxygen, singlet oxygen is formed which causes damage to cellular compartments, in particular the mitochondria. Light activation of accumulated porphyrins leads to a photochemical reaction and thereby phototoxicity to the light-exposed target cells.

5.2 Pharmacokinetic properties

In vitro dermal absorption of radiolabelled methyl aminolevulinate applied to human skin has been studied. After 24 hours the mean cumulative absorption through human skin was 0.26 % of the administered dose. A skin depot containing 4.9 % of the dose was formed. No corresponding studies in human skin with damage similar to actinic keratosis lesions and additionally roughened surface or without stratum corneum were performed.

In humans, a higher degree of accumulation of porphyrins in lesions compared to normal skin has been demonstrated with Metvix cream. After application of the cream for 3 hours and subsequent illumination with non-coherent light of 570-670 nm wavelength and a total light dose of 75 J/cm^2, complete photobleaching occurs with levels of porphyrins returning to pre-treatment values.

5.3 Preclinical safety data

Preclinical studies on general toxicity and genotoxicity studies in the presence or absence of photoactivation, do not indicate potential risks for man. Carcinogenicity studies or studies on the reproductive function have not been performed with methyl aminolevulinate.

6. PHARMACEUTICAL PARTICULARS

6.1 List of excipients

Self-emulsifying glyceryl monostearate
cetostearyl alcohol
poloxyl 40 stearate
methyl parahydroxybenzoate (E 218)
propyl parahydroxybenzoate (E 216)
disodium edetate
glycerol
white soft paraffin
cholesterol
isopropyl myristate
arachis oil
refined almond oil
oleyl alcohol
purified water.

6.2 Incompatibilities

Not applicable.

6.3 Shelf life

Unopened: 18 months.

1 week after first opening of the container.

6.4 Special precautions for storage

Store at 2 °C - 8 °C (in a refrigerator).

6.5 Nature and contents of container

Aluminium tube with internal protective lacquer and a latex seal. Screw cap of HDPE.

Metvix cream is supplied in a tube containing 2 g cream.

6.6 Special precautions for disposal and other handling

No special requirements.

7. MARKETING AUTHORISATION HOLDER

Galderma (UK) Ltd
Meridien House
69-71 Clarendon Road
Watford
Herts
WD17 1DS
UK

8. MARKETING AUTHORISATION NUMBER(S)

PL 10590/0048

9. DATE OF FIRST AUTHORISATION/RENEWAL OF THE AUTHORISATION

20/07/2006

10. DATE OF REVISION OF THE TEXT

24/07/2008

Mezavant XL 1200mg, gastro-resistant, prolonged release tablets

(Shire Pharmaceuticals Limited)

1. NAME OF THE MEDICINAL PRODUCT

Mezavant XL 1200mg, gastro-resistant, prolonged release tablets.

2. QUALITATIVE AND QUANTITATIVE COMPOSITION

Each tablet contains 1200mg mesalazine.

For a full list of excipients, see section 6.1.

3. PHARMACEUTICAL FORM

Gastro-resistant, prolonged release tablets.

Red-brown, ellipsoidal, film-coated tablet, debossed on one side with S476.

4. CLINICAL PARTICULARS

4.1 Therapeutic indications

For the induction of clinical and endoscopic remission in patients with mild to moderate, active ulcerative colitis. For maintenance of remission.

4.2 Posology and method of administration

Mezavant XL is intended for once daily, oral administration. The tablets must not be crushed or chewed and should be taken with food.

Adults, including the elderly (>65 years)

For induction of remission: 2.4 to 4.8g (two to four tablets) should be taken once daily. The highest dose of 4.8g/day is recommended for patients not responding to lower doses of mesalazine. When using the highest dose (4.8g/day), the effect of the treatment should be evaluated at 8 weeks.

For maintenance of remission: 2.4g (two tablets) should be taken once daily.

Children and adolescents:

Mezavant XL is not recommended for use in children below the age of 18 years due to a lack of data on safety and efficacy.

Specific studies have not been performed to investigate Mezavant XL in patients with hepatic or renal impairment (see sections 4.3 and 4.4).

4.3 Contraindications

History of hypersensitivity to salicylates (including mesalazine) or any of the excipients of Mezavant XL.

Severe renal impairment (GFR <30ml/min/1.73m2) and/or severe hepatic impairment.

4.4 Special warnings and precautions for use

Reports of renal impairment, including minimal change nephropathy, and acute / chronic interstitial nephritis have been associated with preparations containing mesalazine and pro-drugs of mesalazine. Mezavant XL should be used with caution in patients with confirmed mild to moderate renal impairment. It is recommended that all patients have an evaluation of renal function prior to initiation of therapy and at least twice a year, whilst on treatment.

Patients with chronic lung function impairment, especially asthma, are at risk of hypersensitivity reactions and should be closely monitored.

Following mesalazine treatment, serious blood dyscrasias have been reported rarely. If the patient develops unexplained bleeding, bruising, purpura, anaemia, fever or sore throat, haematological investigations should be performed. If there is suspicion of blood dyscrasia, treatment should be terminated. (See sections 4.5 and 4.8).

Mesalazine induced cardiac hypersensitivity reactions (myo- and pericarditis) have been reported rarely with other mesalazine containing preparations. Caution should be used in prescribing this medication to patients with conditions predisposing to the development of myo- or pericarditis. If such hypersensitivity reaction is suspected, products containing mesalazine must not be reintroduced.

Mesalazine has been associated with an acute intolerance syndrome that may be difficult to distinguish from a flare of inflammatory bowel disease. Although the exact frequency of occurrence has not been determined, it has occurred in 3% of patients in controlled clinical trials of mesalazine or sulphasalazine. Symptoms include cramping, acute abdominal pain and bloody diarrhoea, sometimes fever, headache and rash. If acute intolerance syndrome is suspected, prompt withdrawal is required and products containing mesalazine must not be reintroduced.

There have been reports of increased liver enzyme levels in patients taking preparations containing mesalazine. Caution is recommended if Mezavant XL is administered to patients with hepatic impairment.

Caution should be exercised when treating patients allergic to sulphasalazine due to the potential risk of cross sensitivity reactions between sulphasalazine and mesalazine.

Organic or functional obstruction in the upper gastrointestinal tract may delay onset of action of the product.

4.5 Interaction with other medicinal products and other forms of interaction

No investigations have been performed on interactions between Mezavant XL and other drugs. However, there have been reports of interactions between other mesalazine containing products and other drugs.

Caution is recommended for the concomitant use of mesalazine with known nephrotoxic agents, including non-steroidal anti-inflammatory drugs (NSAIDs) and azathioprine as these may increase the risk of renal adverse reactions.

Mesalazine inhibits thiopurine methyltransferase. In patients receiving azathioprine or 6-mercaptopurine, caution is recommended for concurrent use of mesalazine as this can increase the potential for blood dyscrasias (see sections 4.4 and 4.8).

Administration with coumarin-type anticoagulants e.g. warfarin, could result in decreased anticoagulant activity. Prothrombin time should be closely monitored if this combination is essential.

Mezavant XL is recommended to be administered with food (see sections 4.2 and 5.2).

4.6 Pregnancy and lactation

Pregnancy

Limited experience with mesalazine in pregnancy does not indicate an increased risk of drug induced congenital malformations. Mesalazine crosses the placental barrier, but provides foetal concentrations much lower than those seen with adult therapeutic use. Animal studies do not indicate harmful effects of mesalazine in pregnancy, embryonal/ foetal development, parturition or postnatal development. Mesalazine should be used during pregnancy only when clearly indicated. Caution should be exercised when using high doses of mesalazine.

Lactation

Mesalazine is excreted in breast milk at low concentration. Acetylated form of mesalazine is excreted in breast milk at higher concentration. Caution should be exercised if using Mesalazine while breast-feeding and only if the benefit outweighs the risks. Sporadically acute diarrhoea has been reported in breast fed infants.

Fertility

Data on mesalazine show no sustained effect on male fertility.

4.7 Effects on ability to drive and use machines

No studies on the effects on the ability to drive and use machines have been performed. Mezavant XL is considered to have negligible influence on these abilities.

4.8 Undesirable effects

Approximately 14% of subjects experienced treatment emergent adverse drug reactions (ADRs) associated with Mezavant XL. During maintenance treatment, there are no novel events with incidence >1%. The majority of events were transient, and mild or moderate in severity. No individual ADR was reported at a frequency greater than 10%.

The most commonly reported ADRs during acute treatment were flatulence, nausea or headache, which were not dose related and occurred in less than 3% of patients receiving Mezavant XL.

Other events reported with Mezavant XL were less frequent and the incidences are presented below:

Blood and lymphatic system disorders Uncommon (>0.1% and <1%): Decreased platelet count
Nervous system disorders Common (>1% and <10%): Headache Uncommon (>0.1% and <1%): Dizziness, Somnolence, Tremor
Ear and labyrinth disorders Uncommon (>0.1% and <1%): Ear pain
Cardiac disorders Uncommon (>0.1% and <1%): Tachycardia
Vascular disorders Uncommon (>0.1% and <1%): Hypertension, Hypotension
Respiratory, thoracic and mediastinal disorders Uncommon (>0.1% and <1%): Pharyngolaryngeal pain
Gastrointestinal disorders Common (>1% and <10%): Flatulence, nausea Uncommon (>0.1% and <1%): Abdominal distension, Abdominal pain, Colitis, Diarrhoea, Dyspepsia, Pancreatitis, Rectal polyp, Vomiting
Hepatobiliary disorders Uncommon (>0.1% and <1%): Increased alanine aminotransferase, Abnormal liver function test
Skin and subcutaneous tissue disorders Uncommon (>0.1% and <1%): Acne, Alopecia, Prurigo, Pruritis, Rash, Urticaria
Musculoskeletal, connective tissue and bone disorders Uncommon (>0.1% and <1%): Arthralgia, Back pain
General disorders and administrative site disorders Uncommon (>0.1% and <1%): Asthenia, Face oedema, Fatigue, Pyrexia

Mesalazine has also been associated with the following events:

Blood and lymphatic system disorders Agranulocytosis, Aplastic anaemia, Leukopenia, Neutropenia, Pancytopenia, Thrombocytopenia.
Nervous system disorders Neuropathy
Cardiac disorders Myocarditis, Pericarditis
Respiratory, thoracic and mediastinal disorders Allergic alveolitis, Bronchospasm
Hepatobiliary disorders Cholelithiasis, Hepatitis
Skin and subcutaneous tissue disorders Angioedema
Musculoskeletal, connective tissue and bone disorders Systemic-lupus erythematosus-like syndrome, Myalgia
Renal & urinary disorders Interstitial nephritis, Nephrotic syndrome

Mesalazine induced nephrotoxicity should be suspected in patients developing renal dysfunction during treatment.

See also Section 4.4 Special Warnings and Precautions for Use.

4.9 Overdose

No case of overdose has been reported.

Mezavant XL is an aminosalicylate, and signs of salicylate toxicity include tinnitus, vertigo, headache, confusion, drowsiness, pulmonary oedema, dehydration as a result of sweating, diarrhoea and vomiting, hypoglycaemia, hyperventilation, disruption of electrolyte balance and blood-pH and hyperthermia.

Although there has been no direct experience with Mezavant XL, conventional therapy for salicylate toxicity may be beneficial in the event of acute overdosage. Hypoglycaemia, fluid and electrolyte imbalance should be corrected by the administration of appropriate therapy. Adequate renal function should be maintained.

5. PHARMACOLOGICAL PROPERTIES

5.1 Pharmacodynamic properties

Pharmacotherapeutic group: Aminosalicylic acid and similar agents

ATC code: A07E C02

Mesalazine is an aminosalicylate. The mechanism of action of mesalazine is not fully understood, but appears to be topical. Mucosal production of arachidonic acid metabolites, both through the cyclooxygenase and lipoxygenase pathways, is increased in patients with chronic inflammatory bowel disease, and it is possible that mesalazine diminishes inflammation by blocking cyclooxygenase and inhibiting prostaglandin production in the colon. Recent data also suggests that mesalazine can inhibit the activation of NFκB, a nuclear transcription factor that regulates the transcription of many genes for pro-inflammatory proteins, which has led to the suggestion that this action may underpin the drug's effects.

The Mezavant XL tablet contains a core of mesalazine 1.2g formulated in a multi-matrix system. This system is coated with methacrylic acid copolymers, Type A and Type B, which are designed to dissolve at pH 7 and above, facilitating the extended delivery of effective concentrations of mesalazine through the entire colon with limited systemic absorption.

Mezavant XL was investigated in two similarly designed, Phase III, placebo controlled studies in 623 randomised patients with mild to moderate, active Ulcerative Colitis. Mezavant XL 2.4g/day and 4.8g/day administered with food achieved statistical superiority over placebo in terms of the number of patients achieving remission from Ulcerative Colitis after 8 weeks treatment. Using the Ulcerative Colitis Disease Activity Index (UC-DAI), remission was defined as a UC-DAI score of <1 with a score of 0 for rectal bleeding and stool frequency and at least a 1-point reduction in sigmoidoscopy score from baseline. Study 302, included a comparator, mesalazine modified release 2.4g/day (0.8g administered in 3 divided doses), as an internal reference arm. On the primary variable of remission, the following results were achieved:

(see Table 1 on next page)

5.2 Pharmacokinetic properties

The mechanism of action of mesalazine (5-ASA) is considered to be topical, and therefore the clinical efficacy of Mezavant XL does not correlate with the pharmacokinetic profile. A major pathway of clearance of mesalazine is via metabolism to N-acetyl-5-aminosalicylic acid (Ac-5-ASA), which is pharmacologically inactive.

Absorption:

Gamma-scintigraphy studies have shown that a single dose of Mezavant XL 1.2g passed rapidly and intact through the upper gastrointestinal tract of fasted healthy volunteers. Scintigraphic images showed a trail of radiolabelled tracer through the colon, indicating that mesalazine had spread throughout this region of the gastrointestinal tract.

In a single and multiple dose pharmacokinetic study of Mezavant XL 2.4 and 4.8g administered with standard meals in 56 healthy volunteers, approximately 24% of the dose was absorbed; plasma concentrations of mesalazine were detectable after 4 hours and were maximal by 8 hours after the single dose. At steady state (achieved generally by 2 days after dosing), 5-ASA accumulation was 1.1- to 1.4- fold for the 2.4g and 4.8g dose, respectively, above that expected on the basis of single dose pharmacokinetics. At the highest dose level, 4.8g QD, the mean maximum plasma concentration of mesalazine was 5280 ± 3146 ng/mL and mean area under the plasma concentration-time curve within a dosage interval was 49 559 ± 23 780 ng.h/mL.

Accumulation of Ac-5-ASA was below what was expected based on single dose pharmacokinetics, i.e., 0.9- and 0.7-fold for a 2.4 or 4.8g Mezavant XL dose, respectively. This effect is likely to be due to a lower drug:metabolite ratio at higher dose and at steady-state, due to saturation of 5-ASA metabolism.

After a single dose of Mezavant XL, total systemic exposure of 5-ASA appeared to increase slightly more than dose proportionately, with area under the plasma concentration-time curve increasing approximately 2.5- fold for a 2-fold dose increase from 2.4g to 4.8g. However there was no evidence of supra-proportionality seen at steady state.

In a food interaction study in 34 healthy volunteers, the administration of a single dose of Mezavant XL 4.8g with a high fat meal resulted in delayed and further prolonged

Table 1

Study 301 (n=262#)				
	Placebo	Mezavant XL 2.4g/day in two divided doses	Mezavant XL 4.8g/day once daily	
% patients in remission	12.9	34.1*	29.2*	
Study 302 (n=341#)				
	Placebo	Mezavant XL 2.4g/day once daily	Mezavant XL 4.8g/day once daily	Mesalazine modified release 2.4g/day in three divided doses
% patients in remission	22.1	40.5*	41.2*	32.6[NS]

#Based on the ITT population; * Statistically different from placebo ($p<0.025$); NSNot significant (>0.05)

absorption. Under these conditions, mesalazine plasma levels were detectable after approximately 6 hours, and maximum plasma levels were reached after approximately 24 hours. Following a single dose of Mezavant XL 4.8g, detectable levels of mesalazine remain in plasma up to the last sampling time, 72 hours post-dose.

Additionally, systemic exposure was reduced under fed conditions, although the effect in females was less pronounced than in males.

Distribution:

Mesalazine has a relatively small volume of distribution of approximately 18L. Mesalazine is 43% bound and N-acetyl-5-aminosalicylic 78 - 83% bound to plasma proteins when in vitro plasma concentrations are up to 2.5μg/mL and up to 10μg/mL respectively.

Biotransformation:

The only major metabolite of mesalazine is N-acetyl-5-aminosalicylic acid, which is pharmacologically inactive. Its formation is brought about by N-acetyltransferase-1 activity in the liver and intestinal mucosal cells. This enzyme is not known to be subject to genetic polymorphism.

Elimination:

Elimination of absorbed mesalazine is mainly via the renal route following metabolism to N-acetyl-5-aminosalicylic acid (acetylation). However, there is also limited excretion of the parent drug in urine. Following Mezavant XL 2.4g or 4.8g once daily, on average, 2-3% of the dose was excreted unchanged in the urine after 24 hours, compared with 13-17% for N-acetyl-5-aminosalicylic acid.

Although the half-lives of pure mesalazine and N-acetyl-5-aminosalicylic acid are short (approximately 40 minutes and 70 minutes respectively), the apparent half-lives after administration of Mezavant XL 2.4g and 4.8g were absorption rate-limited as a result of the extended release profile, being on average 6-7 hours and 10-13 hours, respectively.

Special patient populations:

There are no data in patients with renal or hepatic impairment taking Mezavant XL. In patients with renal impairment, the resultant decrease in the rate of elimination and increased systemic concentration of mesalazine may constitute an increased risk of nephrotoxic adverse reactions (see section 4.4).

In different clinical studies with Mezavant XL, mesalazine plasma AUC in females appeared up to 2-fold higher than in males.

Based on limited pharmacokinetic data, 5-ASA and Ac-5-ASA pharmacokinetics appear comparable between Caucasian and Hispanic subjects.

Pharmacokinetics data have not been investigated in elderly people.

5.3 Preclinical safety data

Effects in nonclinical studies were observed only at exposures considered sufficiently in excess of the maximum human exposure indicating little relevance to clinical use.

6. PHARMACEUTICAL PARTICULARS

6.1 List of excipients

Tablet core:

Carmellose sodium

Carnauba Wax

Stearic Acid

Silica, Colloidal Hydrated

Sodium Starch Glycolate

Talc

Magnesium Stearate

Film-coating:

Talc

Methacrylic Acid Copolymer Type A, Type B

Triethylcitrate

Titanium Dioxide (E171)

Red Ferric Oxide (E172)

Macrogol 6000

6.2 Incompatibilities

Not applicable.

6.3 Shelf life

2 years.

6.4 Special precautions for storage

Store below 25°C.

Store in the original package

6.5 Nature and contents of container

Tablets are packed in polyamide/aluminium/PVC foil blister packs with aluminium push-through foil.

Packs contain 60 tablets.

6.6 Special precautions for disposal and other handling

No special requirements.

7. MARKETING AUTHORISATION HOLDER

Shire Pharmaceutical Contracts Ltd

Hampshire International Business Park

Chineham

Basingstoke

Hampshire

RG24 8EP

United Kingdom

8. MARKETING AUTHORISATION NUMBER(S)

PL 08081/0040

9. DATE OF FIRST AUTHORISATION/RENEWAL OF THE AUTHORISATION

19/01/2007

10. DATE OF REVISION OF THE TEXT

19/01/2007

LEGAL CATEGORY

POM

Mezolar Matrix Transdermal Patches

(Sandoz Limited)

1. NAME OF THE MEDICINAL PRODUCT

Mezolar Matrix 12 microgram/hour transdermal patch

Mezolar Matrix 25 microgram/hour transdermal patch

Mezolar Matrix 50 microgram/hour transdermal patch

Mezolar Matrix 75 microgram/hour transdermal patch

Mezolar Matrix 100 microgram/hour transdermal patch

2. QUALITATIVE AND QUANTITATIVE COMPOSITION

Mezolar Matrix 12 microgram/hour transdermal patch:

One transdermal patch (5.25 cm^2 absorption surface area) contains 2.89 mg fentanyl equivalent to a release rate of the active substance of 12 microgram/hour.

Mezolar Matrix 25 microgram/hour transdermal patch:

One transdermal patch (10.5 cm^2 absorption surface area) contains 5.78 mg fentanyl equivalent to a release rate of the active substance of 25 microgram/hour.

Mezolar Matrix 50 microgram/hour transdermal patch:

One transdermal patch (21 cm^2 absorption surface area) contains 11.56 mg fentanyl equivalent to a release rate of the active substance of 50 microgram/hour.

Mezolar Matrix 75 microgram/hour transdermal patch:

One transdermal patch (31.5 cm^2 absorption surface area) contains 17.34 mg fentanyl equivalent to a release rate of the active substance of 75 microgram/hour.

Mezolar Matrix 100 microgram/hour transdermal patch:

One transdermal patch (42 cm^2 absorption surface area) contains 23.12 mg fentanyl equivalent to a release rate of the active substance of 100 microgram/hour.

Excipient: Soya-bean oil, refined

Mezolar Matrix 12 microgram/hour transdermal patch: 2.89 mg

Mezolar Matrix 25 microgram/hour transdermal patch: 5.78 mg

Mezolar Matrix 50 microgram/hour transdermal patch: 11.56 mg

Mezolar Matrix 75 microgram/hour transdermal patch: 17.34 mg

Mezolar Matrix 100 microgram/hour transdermal patch: 23.12 mg

For a full list of excipients, see section 6.1.

3. PHARMACEUTICAL FORM

Transdermal patch

Transparent rounded oblong transdermal patch, consisting of a protective film (to be removed prior to application of the patch) and two functional layers: one self-adhesive matrix layer containing fentanyl and a carrier film impermeable to water.

4. CLINICAL PARTICULARS

4.1 Therapeutic indications

Severe chronic pain which can be adequately managed only with opioid analgesics.

4.2 Posology and method of administration

Mezolar Matrix 12 microgram/hour transdermal patches release fentanyl over 72 hours. The fentanyl release rate is 12 microgram/hour and the corresponding active surface area is 5.25 cm^2.

Mezolar Matrix 25 micrograms/hour transdermal patches release fentanyl over 72 hours. The fentanyl release rate is 25 microgram/hour and the corresponding active surface area is 10.5 cm^2.

Mezolar Matrix 50 microgram/hour transdermal patches release fentanyl over 72 hours. The fentanyl release rate is 50 microgram/hour and the corresponding active surface area is 21 cm^2.

Mezolar Matrix 75 microgram/hour transdermal patches release fentanyl over 72 hours. The fentanyl release rate is 75 microgram/hour and the corresponding active surface area is 31.5 cm^2.

Mezolar Matrix 100 microgram/hour transdermal patches release fentanyl over 72 hours. The fentanyl release rate is 100 microgram/hour and the corresponding active surface area is 42 cm^2.

The required fentanyl dosage is adjusted individually and should be assessed regularly after each administration.

Choice of initial dosage

The dosage level of fentanyl is based upon the previous use of opioids and takes into account the possible development of tolerance, concomitant medicinal treatment, the patient's general state of health and the degree of severity of the disorder.

In patients who have not previously received strong opioids, the initial dosage should not exceed 12-25 microgram/hour.

Changing from other opioid treatment

When changing over from oral or parenteral opioids to fentanyl treatment, the initial dosage should be calculated as follows:

1. The quantity of analgesics required over the last 24 hours should be determined.

2. The obtained sum should be converted to the corresponding oral morphine dosage using Table 1.

3. The corresponding fentanyl dosage should be determined using Table 2.

Table 1: Equianalgesic efficacy of medicinal products

All intramuscular (i.m.) and oral dosages given in the table are equivalent in analgesic effect to 10 mg morphine administered intramuscularly.

Name of medicinal product	Equianalgesic dosage (mg)	
	i.m.*	Oral
Morphine	10	30 (assuming repeated administration)** 60 (assuming a single dose or occasional doses)
Hydromorphone	1.5	7.5
Methadone	10	20
Oxycodone	10-15	20-30
Levorphanol	2	4
Oxymorphine	1	10 (rectal)
Diamorphine	5	60
Pethidine	75	
Codeine	130	200
Buprenorphine	0.4	0.8 (sublingual)
Ketobemidone	10	30

* Based on studies conducted with single doses, in which the i.m. dosage of each above-mentioned agent was compared with morphine in order to achieve an equivalent efficacy. Oral dosages are the recommended dosages when changing from parenteral to oral administration.

** The efficacy ratio of 3:1 for morphine i.m./oral dosages is based upon a study conducted in patients suffering from chronic pain.

*Table 2: Recommended dosage of Mezolar Matrix transdermal patches based upon the oral daily morphine dosage**

Oral morphine (mg/24 h)	Dosage of Mezolar Matrix transdermal patches (µg/h)
For paediatric patients **	
30-44	12
45-134	25
For adults	
<135	25
135-224	50
225-314	75
315-404	100
405-494	125
495-584	150
585-674	175
675-764	200
765-854	225
855-944	250
945-1034	275
1035-1124	300

* Conversion schemes are based on clinical trials. Schemes based on other trials have been found useful in clinical practice and may be used.

** Conversion to Mezolar Matrix transdermal patch doses greater than 25 microgram/hour is the same for adult and paediatric patients.

The initial evaluation of the maximum analgesic effect of Mezolar Matrix transdermal patch should not be made before the patch has been worn for 24 hours. This is due to the gradual increase in serum fentanyl concentrations during the first 24 hours after application of the patch.

In the first 12 hours after changing to Mezolar Matrix transdermal patch the patient continues to receive the previous analgesic at the previous dose; over the next 12 hours this analgesic is administered according to need.

Dose titration and maintenance therapy

The patch should be replaced every 72 hours. The dose should be titrated individually until analgesic efficacy is attained. In patients who experience a marked decrease in the period 48-72 hours after application, replacement of Mezolar Matrix transdermal patch after 48 hours may be necessary. The dose 12 microgram/hour is appropriate for dose titration in the lower dosage area. If analgesia is insufficient at the end of the initial application period, the dose may be increased after 3 days, until the desired effect is obtained for each patient. Additional dose adjustment should normally be performed in 12 microgram/hour or 25 microgram/hour increments, although the supplementary analgesic requirements and pain status of the patient should be taken into account. More than one patch may be used for dose adjustments and for doses greater than 100 microgram/hour. Patients may require periodic supplemental doses of a short-acting analgesic for breakthrough pain (e. g. morphine). Additional or alternative methods of analgesia or alternative administration of opioids should be considered when the transdermal fentanyl dose exceeds 300 microgram/hour.

Withdrawal symptoms have been reported when changing from long-term treatment with morphine to transdermal fentanyl despite adequate analgesic efficacy. In case of withdrawal symptoms it is recommended to treat those with short-acting morphine in low doses.

Change or discontinuation of therapy

If discontinuation of the patch is necessary, any replacement with other opioids should be gradual, starting at a low dose and increasing slowly. This is because fentanyl levels fall gradually after the patch is removed; it takes at least 17 hours for the fentanyl serum concentration to decrease by 50 % (see section 5.2). As a general rule, the discontinuation of opioid analgesia should be gradual, in order to prevent withdrawal symptoms (such as nausea, vomiting, diarrhoea, anxiety and muscular tremor).

Use in elderly patients

Elderly or cachectic patients should be observed carefully for symptoms of an overdosage and the dose reduced if necessary (see section 4.4 and 5.2).

Use in children

Mezolar Matrix transdermal patch should not be used in children under 2 years of age.

Mezolar Matrix transdermal patch should be administered only to opioid-tolerant paediatric patients (ages 2 to 16 years) who are already receiving at least 30 mg oral morphine equivalents per day. To convert paediatric patients from oral or parenteral opioids to Mezolar Matrix transdermal patch, refer to Table 1 and Table 2.

For children who receive more than 90 mg oral morphine a day, only limited information is currently available from clinical trials. In the paediatric studies, the required fentanyl transdermal patch dose was calculated conservatively: 30 mg to 45 mg oral morphine per day or its equivalent opioid dose was replaced by one fentanyl transdermal patch 12 microgram/hour. It should be noted that this conversion schedule for children only applies to the switch from oral morphine (or its equivalent) to fentanyl transdermal patches. The conversion schedule could not be used to convert from fentanyl transdermal patches into other opioids, as overdose could than occur.

The analgesic effect of the first dose of Mezolar Matrix transdermal patch will not be optimal within the first 24 hours. Therefore, during the first 12 hours after switching to Mezolar Matrix transdermal patch, the patient should be given the previous regular dose of analgesics. In the next 12 hours, these analgesics should be provided based on clinical need.

Since peak fentanyl levels occur after 12 to 24 hours of treatment, monitoring of the paediatric patient for adverse events, which may include hypoventilation, is recommended for at least 48 hours after initiation of Mezolar Matrix transdermal patch therapy or up-titration of the dose (see also section 4.4).

Dose titration and maintenance therapy

If the analgesic effect of Mezolar Matrix transdermal patch is insufficient, supplementary morphine or another short-duration opioid should be administered. Depending on the additional analgesic needs and the pain status of the child, it may be decided to use more patches. Dose adjustments should be done in 12 microgram/hour steps.

Use in patients with hepatic or renal impairment

Patients with impaired hepatic or renal function should carefully be observed for symptoms of an overdosage and the dose should possibly be reduced (see section 4.4).

Use in febrile patients

Dose adjustment may be necessary in patients during episodes of fever (see section 4.4).

Method of administration

For transdermal use.

Mezolar Matrix transdermal patch should be applied to non-irritated and non-irradiated skin on a flat surface of the torso or upper arm.

For use in children: There are no safety and pharmacokinetic data available for other application sites.

In young children, the upper back is the preferred location to apply the patch, to minimize the potential of the child removing the patch.

Hair at the application site (hairless area is preferred) should be clipped (not shaved) prior to system application. If the site requires to be cleansed prior to application of the patch, this should be done with water. Soaps, oils, lotions, alcohol or any other agent that might irritate the skin or alter its characteristics should not be used. The skin should be completely dry before application of the patch.

Since the transdermal patch is protected outwardly by a waterproof covering foil, it may also be worn when taking a shower.

Mezolar Matrix transdermal patch is to be attached as soon as the pack has been opened. Following removal of the protective layer, the transdermal patch should be pressed firmly in place with the palm of the hand for approximately 30 seconds, making sure the contact is complete, especially around the edges. Mezolar Matrix transdermal patch should be worn continuously for 72 hours after which the transdermal patch is replaced. A new transdermal patch should always be applied to a different site from the previous one. The same application site may be re-used only after an interval of at least 7 days.

If residues remain on the skin after removal of the patch, these can be cleaned off with soap and plenty of water. In no case should alcohol or other solvents be used for cleansing as these could penetrate the skin due to the effect of the patch.

The transdermal patch should not be divided, as no data are available with regard to this.

4.3 Contraindications

- Hypersensitivity to the active substance, colophonium resin (hydrogenated), soya, peanuts or to any of the excipients
- Acute or postoperative pain, because of the lack of opportunity for dose titration in the short term and the possibility of life-threatening respiratory depression
- Severe impairment of the central nervous system
- Concomitant use of MAO-inhibitors or within 14 days after discontinuation of MAO-inhibitors (see section 4.5)

4.4 Special warnings and precautions for use

The product should be used only as part of an integrated treatment of pain in cases where the patient is adequately assessed medically, socially and psychologically.

After exhibiting a serious adverse reaction a patient should be monitored for 24 hours following removal of a transdermal patch due to the half life of fentanyl (see section 5.2).

Mezolar Matrix transdermal patch must be used only on the skin of the person for whom it has been medically prescribed. In isolated cases, the patch has become attached to the skin of another person after close body contact. The patch should be removed immediately in such cases.

Respiratory depression

As with all potent opioids some patients may experience respiratory depression with the Mezolar Matrix transdermal patch, and patients must be observed for this effect. Respiratory depression may persist beyond the removal of the patch. The incidence of respiratory depression increases as the fentanyl dose is increased (see section 4.9). CNS active substances may worsen the respiratory depression (see section 4.5). Fentanyl should be used only with caution and at lower dose in patients with existing respiratory depression.

If a patient is to undergo measures that fully remove the sensation of pain (e.g. regional analgesia), it is advisable to prepare for the possibility of respiratory depression. Before such measures are carried out, the fentanyl dosage should be reduced or a changeover should be made to rapid- or short-acting opioid medication.

Chronic pulmonary disease

In patients with chronic obstructive or other pulmonary diseases fentanyl may have more severe adverse reactions; in such patients opioids may decrease respiratory drive and increase airway resistance.

Drug dependence

Tolerance and physical and psychological dependence may develop upon repeated administration of opioids, but is rare in treatment of cancer related pain. As for other opioids, the risk for dependence is greatly increased for patients with a known history of medicinal or illegal drug dependence or alcoholism. If treatment with Mezolar Matrix transdermal patch is considered appropriate for a patient with increased risk for dependence particularly careful medical supervision is necessary.

Increased intracranial pressure

Fentanyl should be used with caution in patients who may be particularly susceptible to the intracranial effects of carbon dioxide retention such as those with evidence of increased intracranial pressure, impaired consciousness or coma. Fentanyl should be used with caution in patients with brain tumours.

Cardiac disease

Fentanyl may produce bradycardia. Mezolar Matrix transdermal patch should therefore be administered with caution to patients with bradyarrhythmias.

Opioids may cause hypotension, especially in patients with hypovolemia. Caution should therefore be taken in treatment of patients with hypotension and/or patients with hypovolemia.

Impaired liver function

Fentanyl is metabolised to inactive metabolites in the liver, so patients with hepatic disease might have a delayed elimination. Patients with hepatic impairment should be observed carefully and the dose reduced if necessary.

Renal impairment

Less than 10 % of fentanyl is excreted unchanged by the kidneys, and unlike morphine, there are no known active metabolites eliminated by the kidneys. Data obtained with intravenous fentanyl in patients with renal failure suggest that the volume of distribution of fentanyl may be changed by dialysis. This may affect serum concentrations. If patients with renal impairment receive transdermal fentanyl they should be observed carefully for signs of fentanyl toxicity and the dose reduced if necessary.

Patients with fever/external heat

A pharmacokinetic model suggests that the fentanyl concentration in the blood possibly rises by a third if the skin temperature rises to 40 °C. Consequently, patients with fever should be monitored very closely for opioid side effects and if necessary the fentanyl dosage should be adjusted (see section 4.2). Patients should also be advised to avoid exposing the Mezolar Matrix transdermal patch application site to direct external heat sources such as heating pads, hot water bottles, electric blankets, heated waterbeds, heat lamps, hot whirlpool spa baths and intense sunbathing while wearing the patch, since there is potential for temperature dependent increases in release of fentanyl from the patch.

The transdermal patch must always be removed before taking a sauna. Sauna bathing is possible only when replacing a transdermal patch (at intervals of 72 hours). A new transdermal patch is to be applied to cool, very dry skin.

Elderly Patients

Data from intravenous studies with fentanyl suggest that elderly patients may have reduced clearance, a prolonged half-life and they may be more sensitive to the drug than younger patients. Elderly, cachectic, or debilitated patients should be observed carefully for signs of fentanyl toxicity and the dose reduced if necessary.

Children

Mezolar Matrix transdermal patch should not be administered to opioid naïve paediatric patients (see section 4.2). The potential for serious or life-threatening hypoventilation exists regardless of the dose of transdermal fentanyl administered (see Tables 1 and 2 in section 4.2).

Transdermal fentanyl was not studied in children under 2 years of age. Mezolar Matrix transdermal patch should be administered only to opioid-tolerant children age 2 years or older (see section 4.2). Mezolar Matrix transdermal patch should not be used in children under 2 years of age.

To guard against accidental ingestion by children, caution should be used when choosing the application site for Mezolar Matrix transdermal patch (see section 4.2) and the adhesion of the patch should be monitored closely.

Others

Non-epileptic (myo)clonic reactions can occur.

Caution should be exercised when treating patients with myasthenia gravis.

For disposal instructions see section 6.6.

4.5 Interaction with other medicinal products and other forms of interaction

The concomitant use of barbituric acid derivatives should be avoided, since the respiratory depressing effect of fentanyl may be increased.

The concomitant use of other CNS depressants, including opioids, anxiolytics and tranquilisers, hypnotics, general anaesthetics, phenothiazines, skeletal muscle relaxants, sedating antihistamines and alcoholic beverages may produce additive depressant effects; hypoventilation, hypotension and profound sedation or coma may occur. Therefore, the use of any of the above mentioned concomitant medicinal products and active substances requires observation of the patient.

MAO-inhibitors have been reported to increase the effect of narcotic analgesics, especially in patients with cardiac failure. Therefore, fentanyl should not be used within 14 days after discontinuation of treatment with MAO-inhibitors (see section 4.3).

Fentanyl, a high clearance active substance, is rapidly and extensively metabolised mainly by CYP3A4.

Itraconazole (a potent CYP3A4 inhibitor) at 200 mg/day given orally for four days had no significant effect on the pharmacokinetics of intravenous fentanyl. Increased plasma concentrations were, however, observed in individual subjects. Oral administration of ritonavir (one of the most potent CYP3A4 inhibitors) reduced the clearance of intravenous fentanyl by two thirds and doubled the half-life. Concomitant use of potent CYP3A4-inhibitors (e.g. ritonavir, ketoconazole, itraconazole, some macrolide antibiotics) with transdermally administered fentanyl may result in increased plasma concentrations of fentanyl. This may increase or prolong both the therapeutic effects and the adverse reactions, which may cause severe respiratory depression. In such cases increased care and observation of the patient should be undertaken. Combined use of ritonavir or other potent CYP3A4-inhibitors with transdermal fentanyl is not recommended, unless the patient is carefully observed.

Although pentazocine or buprenorphine have an analgesic effect, they partially antagonize some effects of fentanyl (e.g. analgesia) and may induce withdrawal symptoms in opioid dependants.

4.6 Pregnancy and lactation

The safety of fentanyl in pregnancy has not been established. Studies in animals have shown reproductive toxicity (see section 5.3). The potential risk for humans is unknown. Fentanyl should only be used during pregnancy when clearly necessary.

Long-term treatment during pregnancy may cause withdrawal symptoms in the new born infant.

Fentanyl should not be used during labour and delivery (including caesarean section) since fentanyl passes the placenta and may cause respiratory depression in the foetus or in the new-born infant.

Fentanyl is excreted into breast milk and may cause sedation and respiratory depression in the breast-fed infant. Breast-feeding should therefore be discontinued for at least 72 hours after the removal of Mezolar Matrix transdermal patch.

4.7 Effects on ability to drive and use machines

Fentanyl has major influence on the ability to drive and use machines. This has to be expected especially at the beginning of treatment, at any change of dosage as well as in connection with alcohol or tranquilisers. Patients stabilised on a specific dosage will not necessarily be restricted. Therefore, patients should consult their physician as to whether driving or use of machines is permitted.

4.8 Undesirable effects

The adverse event profile in children and adolescents treated with transdermal fentanyl was similar to that observed in adults. No risk was identified in the paediatric population beyond that expected with the use of opioids for the relief of pain associated with serious illness and there does not appear to be any paediatric-specific risk associated with transdermal fentanyl use in children as young as 2 years old when used as directed. Very common adverse events reported in paediatric clinical trials were fever, vomiting, and nausea.

The following frequencies are used for the description of the occurrence of adverse reactions:

Very common: ⩾ 1/10

Common: ⩾ 1/100 - < 1/10

Uncommon: ⩾ 1/1,000 - < 1/100

Rare: ⩾ 1/10,000 - < 1/1,000

Very rare: < 1/10,000, not known (cannot be estimated from the available data)

The most serious undesirable effect of fentanyl is respiratory depression.

Cardiac disorders

Uncommon: Tachycardia, bradycardia

Rare: Arrhythmia

Nervous system disorders

Very common: Drowsiness, headache

Uncommon: Tremor, paraesthesia, speech disturbances

Very rare: Ataxia, non-epileptic myoclonal reactions

Eye disorders

Rare: Amblyopia

Respiratory, thoracic and mediastinal disorders

Uncommon: Dyspnoea, hypoventilation

Very rare: Respiratory depression, apnoea, haemoptysis, lung obstruction, pharyngitis

Gastrointestinal disorders

Very common: Nausea, vomiting, constipation

Common: Xerostomia, dyspepsia

Uncommon: Diarrhoea

Rare: Hiccups

Very rare: Painful flatulence, ileus

Renal and urinary disorders

Uncommon: Urinary retention

Very rare: Oliguria, pain in the bladder

Skin and subcutaneous tissue disorders

Very common: Sweating, pruritus

Uncommon: Rash, erythema

Rash, erythema and pruritus will usually disappear within one day after the patch has been removed.

Vascular disorders

Uncommon: Hypertension, hypotension

Rare: Vasodilatation

General disorders and administration site conditions

Common: Skin reactions at the application site

Rare: Oedema, sensation of cold

Immune system disorders

Very rare: Anaphylaxis, laryngospasm

Psychiatric disorders

Very common: Somnolence.

Common: Sedation, confusion, depression, anxiety, nervousness, hallucinations, lowered appetite

Uncommon: Euphoria, amnesia, sleeplessness, agitation

Very rare: Delusions, states of excitement, asthenia, disorder of sexual function, withdrawal symptoms

Some of these adverse events may also be attributable to the underlying disorder or to other treatment measures.

Other adverse reactions

Tolerance, physical and psychological dependence can develop during long-term use of fentanyl.

Opioid withdrawal symptoms (for instance nausea, vomiting, diarrhea, anxiety and shivering) may occur in some patients after switching from previously prescribed opioid analgesics to fentanyl transdermal patch or after abrupt discontinuation of therapy.

In very rare cases, soya-bean oil, refined can cause allergic reactions.

4.9 Overdose

Symptoms

The symptoms of fentanyl overdose are an extension of its pharmacological actions, e.g. lethargy, coma, respiratory depression with Cheyne-Stokes respiration and/or cyanosis. Other symptoms may be hypothermia, decreased muscle tonus, bradycardia and hypotension. Signs of toxicity are deep sedation, ataxia, miosis, convulsions and respiratory depression, which is the main symptom.

Treatment

For management of respiratory depression immediate countermeasures should be started, including removing the patch and physically or verbally stimulating the patient. These actions can be followed by administration of a specific opioid antagonist such as naloxone.

A starting dose of 0.4-2 mg naloxone hydrochloride intravenously is recommended for adults. If needed, a similar dose can be given every 2 or 3 minutes, or be administered as continued infusion as 2 mg in 500 ml sodium chloride 9 mg/ml solution (0.9 %) or glucose 0.004 mg/ml solution (5 %). The infusion rate should be adjusted according to previous bolus injections and the individual response of the patient. If intravenous administration is impossible, naloxone hydrochloride can also be given intramuscularly or subcutaneously. Following intramuscular or subcutaneous administration the onset of action will be slower compared with intravenous administration. Intramuscular administration will give a more prolonged effect than intravenous administration. Respiratory depression due to overdose can persist longer than the effect of the opioid antagonist. Reversing the narcotic effect can give rise to acute pain and release of catecholamines. Intensive care unit treatment is important, if required by the patient's clinical condition. If severe or persistent hypotension occurs, hypovolemia should be considered, and the condition should be managed with appropriate parenteral fluid therapy.

5. PHARMACOLOGICAL PROPERTIES

5.1 Pharmacodynamic properties

Pharmacotherapeutic group: analgesics; opioids; phenylpiperidine derivatives

ATC Code: N02AB03

Mezolar Matrix transdermal patch is a transdermal patch that provides continuous delivery of fentanyl. Fentanyl is an opioid analgesic with affinity mainly to the μ-receptor. The predominant pharmacological effects are pain relief and sedation. Patients not previously treated with opioids will have pain relief at a fentanyl concentration between 0.3 and 1.5 ng/ml. In this group of patients the frequency of adverse reactions will increase at serum concentrations above 2 ng/ml. Both the lowest effective fentanyl concentration and the concentration causing adverse reactions will increase with the development of increasing tolerance. Development of tolerance varies considerably between individual subjects.

The safety of transdermal fentanyl was evaluated in three open-label trials in 293 paediatric patients with chronic pain, 2 years of age through to 18 years of age, of which 66 children were aged to 2 to 6 years. In these studies, 30 mg to 45 mg oral morphine per day was replaced by one fentanyl 12 microgram/hour transdermal patch. Starting dose of 25 microgram/hour and higher were used by 181 patients who had been on prior daily opioid doses of at least 45 mg per dose of oral morphine.

5.2 Pharmacokinetic properties

Following administration of Mezolar Matrix transdermal patch, fentanyl is continuously absorbed through the skin over a period of 72 hours. Due to the polymer matrix and the diffusion of fentanyl through the skin layers, the release rate remains relatively constant.

Absorption

After the first application of Mezolar Matrix transdermal patch, serum fentanyl concentrations increase gradually, generally levelling off between 12 and 24 hours, and remaining relatively constant for the remainder of the 72-hour application period. The serum fentanyl concentrations attained are dependant on the Mezolar Matrix transdermal patch size. For all practical purposes by the second 72-hour application, a steady state serum concentration is reached and is maintained during subsequent applications of a patch of the same size.

Distribution

The plasma protein binding for fentanyl is 84 %.

Biotransformation

Fentanyl shows linear kinetics and is metabolized primarily in the liver via CYP3A4. The major metabolite, norfentanyl, is inactive.

Elimination

When treatment with Fentanyl transdermal patches is withdrawn, serum fentanyl concentrations decline gradually, falling approximately 50 % in 13-22 hours in adults or 22-25 hours in children, respectively. Continued absorption of fentanyl from the skin accounts for a slower reduction in serum concentration than is seen after an intravenous infusion.

Around 75 % of fentanyl is excreted into the urine, mostly as metabolites, with less than 10 % as unchanged active substance. About 9 % of the dose is recovered in the faeces, primarily as metabolites.

Pharmacokinetics in special groups

Adjusting for body weight, clearance (l/hour/kg) in paediatric patients appears to be 82 % higher in children 2 to 5 years old and 25 % higher in children 6 to 10 years old when compared to children 11 to 16 years old, who are likely to have the same clearance as adults. These findings have been taken into consideration in determining the dosing recommendations for paediatric patients.

Elderly and debilitated patients may have reduced clearance of fentanyl leading to prolonged terminal half life. In patients with renal or hepatic impairment, clearance of fentanyl may be altered because of changes of plasma proteins and metabolic clearance resulting in increased serum concentrations (see section 4.2 and 4.4).

5.3 Preclinical safety data

Non-clinical data reveal no special hazard for humans based on conventional studies of safety pharmacology, repeated dose toxicity and genotoxicity.

Animal studies have shown reduced fertility and increased mortality in rat foetuses. Teratogenic effects have, however, not been demonstrated.

Mutagenicity testing in bacteria and in rodents yielded negative results. As well as other opioids fentanyl showed mutagenic effects in vitro in mammalian cells. A mutagenic risk in therapeutic condition seems unlikely since effects were induced only in very high concentrations.

Long-term carcinogenicitystudies have not been performed.

6. PHARMACEUTICAL PARTICULARS

6.1 List of excipients

Protective film:

Poly(ethylene terephthalate) foil, siliconised

Self-adhesive matrix layer:

Colophonium resin (hydrogenated)

Poly(2-ethylhexyl acrylate-co-vinyl acetate)

Soya-bean oil, refined

Water-impermeable cover film: Poly(ethylene terephthalate)

6.2 Incompatibilities
Not applicable.

6.3 Shelf life
2 years

6.4 Special precautions for storage
Store in the original package.

6.5 Nature and contents of container
The transdermal patches are individually packed in sachets made of paper/PE/Al/PE.

Packs with 3, 5, 7, 10, 14 and 20 transdermal patches.

Hospital packs with 5 transdermal patches.

Not all pack sizes may be marketed.

6.6 Special precautions for disposal and other handling
Significant quantities of fentanyl remain in the transdermal patches even after use. Used transdermal patches should be folded with the adhesive surfaces inwards and due to safety and environmental reasons, discarded safely or whenever possible returned to the pharmacy. Any unused medicinal product should be discarded safely or returned to the pharmacy.

7. MARKETING AUTHORISATION HOLDER
Sandoz Ltd

37 Woolmer Way

Bordon

Hants

GU35 9QE

United Kingdom

8. MARKETING AUTHORISATION NUMBER(S)
PL 04416/0823

PL 04416/0824

PL 04416/0825

PL 04416/0826

PL 04416/0827

9. DATE OF FIRST AUTHORISATION/RENEWAL OF THE AUTHORISATION
11/08/2007

10. DATE OF REVISION OF THE TEXT
06/2008

Micardis 20mg, 40mg and 80mg tablets

(Boehringer Ingelheim Limited)

1. NAME OF THE MEDICINAL PRODUCT
Micardis 20 mg tablets

Micardis 40 mg tablets

Micardis 80 mg tablets

2. QUALITATIVE AND QUANTITATIVE COMPOSITION
Each tablet contains 20 mg or 40 mg or 80 mg telmisartan.

Excipients:

Each 20 mg tablet contains 84 mg sorbitol (E420).

Each 40 mg tablet contains 169 mg sorbitol (E420).

Each 80 mg tablet contains 338 mg sorbitol (E420).

For a full list of excipients, see section 6.1.

3. PHARMACEUTICAL FORM
Tablet

20 mg:

White round tablets engraved with the code number '50H' on one side and the company logo on the other side.

40 mg:

White oblong tablets engraved with the code number '51H' on one side and the company logo on the other side.

80 mg:

White oblong tablets engraved with the code number '52H' on one side and the company logo on the other side.

4. CLINICAL PARTICULARS

4.1 Therapeutic indications
Treatment of essential hypertension in adults.

4.2 Posology and method of administration
The usually effective dose is 40 mg once daily. Some patients may already benefit at a daily dose of 20 mg. In cases where the target blood pressure is not achieved, the dose of telmisartan can be increased to a maximum of 80 mg once daily. Alternatively, telmisartan may be used in combination with thiazide-type diuretics such as hydrochlorothiazide, which has been shown to have an additive blood pressure lowering effect with telmisartan. When considering raising the dose, it must be borne in mind that the maximum antihypertensive effect is generally attained four to eight weeks after the start of treatment (see section 5.1).

Telmisartan may be taken with or without food.

Renal impairment:No posology adjustment is required for patients with mild to moderate renal impairment. Limited experience is available in patients with severe renal impairment or haemodialysis. A lower starting dose of 20 mg is recommended in these patients (see section 4.4).

Hepatic impairment: In patients with mild to moderate hepatic impairment, the posology should not exceed 40 mg once daily (see section 4.4).

Elderly

No dose adjustment is necessary for elderly patients.

Paediatric patients

Micardis is not recommended for use in children below 18 years due to a lack of data on safety and efficacy.

4.3 Contraindications

• Hypersensitivity to the active substance or to any of the excipients (see section 6.1)

• Second and third trimesters of pregnancy (see sections 4.4 and 4.6)

• Biliary obstructive disorders

• Severe hepatic impairment

4.4 Special warnings and precautions for use
Pregnancy:

Angiotensin II receptor antagonists should not be initiated during pregnancy. Unless continued angiotensin II receptor antagonist therapy is considered essential, patients planning pregnancy should be changed to alternative antihypertensive treatments which have an established safety profile for use in pregnancy. When pregnancy is diagnosed, treatment with angiotensin II receptor antagonists should be stopped immediately, and, if appropriate, alternative therapy should be started (see sections 4.3 and 4.6).

Hepatic impairment:

Micardis is not to be given to patients with cholestasis, biliary obstructive disorders or severe hepatic impairment (see section 4.3) since telmisartan is mostly eliminated with the bile. These patients can be expected to have reduced hepatic clearance for telmisartan. Micardis should be used only with caution in patients with mild to moderate hepatic impairment.

Renovascular hypertension:

There is an increased risk of severe hypotension and renal insufficiency when patients with bilateral renal artery stenosis or stenosis of the artery to a single functioning kidney are treated with medicinal products that affect the renin-angiotensin-aldosterone system.

Renal impairment and kidney transplantation:

When Micardis is used in patients with impaired renal function, periodic monitoring of potassium and creatinine serum levels is recommended. There is no experience regarding the administration of Micardis in patients with recent kidney transplantation.

Intravascular hypovolaemia:

Symptomatic hypotension, especially after the first dose of Micardis, may occur in patients who are volume and/or sodium depleted by vigorous diuretic therapy, dietary salt restriction, diarrhoea, or vomiting. Such conditions should be corrected before the administration of Micardis. Volume and/or sodium depletion should be corrected prior to administration of Micardis.

Dual blockade of the renin-angiotensin-aldosterone system: As a consequence of inhibiting the renin-angiotensin-aldosterone system, hypotension and changes in renal function (including acute renal failure) have been reported in susceptible individuals, especially if combining medicinal products that affect this system. Dual blockade of the renin-angiotensin-aldosterone system (e.g. by adding an ACE-inhibitor to an angiotensin II receptor antagonist) is therefore not recommended in patients with already controlled blood pressure and should be limited to individually defined cases with close monitoring of renal function.

Other conditions with stimulation of the renin-angiotensin-aldosterone system:

In patients whose vascular tone and renal function depend predominantly on the activity of the renin-angiotensin-aldosterone system (e.g. patients with severe congestive heart failure or underlying renal disease, including renal artery stenosis), treatment with medicinal products that affect this system such as telmisartan has been associated with acute hypotension, hyperazotaemia, oliguria, or rarely acute renal failure (see section 4.8).

Primary aldosteronism:

Patients with primary aldosteronism generally will not respond to antihypertensive medicinal products acting through inhibition of the renin-angiotensin system. Therefore, the use of telmisartan is not recommended.

Aortic and mitral valve stenosis, obstructive hypertrophic cardiomyopathy:

As with other vasodilators, special caution is indicated in patients suffering from aortic or mitral stenosis, or obstructive hypertrophic cardiomyopathy.

Hyperkalaemia:

The use of medicinal products that affect the renin-angiotensin-aldosterone system may cause hyperkalaemia.

In the elderly, in patients with renal insufficiency, in diabetic patients, in patients concomitantly treated with other medicinal products that may increase potassium levels, and/or in patients with intercurrent events, hyperkalaemia may be fatal.

Before considering the concomitant use of medicinal products that affect the renin-angiotensin-aldosterone system, the benefit risk ratio should be evaluated.

The main risk factors for hyperkalaemia to be considered are:

- Diabetes mellitus, renal impairment, age (>70 years)

- Combination with one or more other medicinal products that affect the renin-angiotensin-aldosterone system and/or potassium supplements. Medicinal products or therapeutic classes of medicinal products that may provoke hyperkalaemia are salt substitutes containing potassium, potassium-sparing diuretics, ACE inhibitors, angiotensin II receptor antagonists, non steroidal anti-inflammatory medicinal products (NSAIDs, including selective COX-2 inhibitors), heparin, immunosuppressives (cyclosporin or tacrolimus), and trimethoprim.

- Intercurrent events, in particular dehydratation, acute cardiac decompensation, metabolic acidosis, worsening of renal function, sudden worsening of the renal condition (e.g. infectious diseases), cellular lysis (e.g. acute limb ischemia, rhabdomyolysis, extend trauma).

Close monitoring of serum potassium in at risk patients is recommended (see section 4.5).

Sorbitol:

This medicinal product contains sorbitol (E420). Patients with rare hereditary problems of fructose intolerance should not take Micardis.

Ethnic differences:

As observed for angiotensin converting enzyme inhibitors, telmisartan and the other angiotensin II receptor antagonists are apparently less effective in lowering blood pressure in black people than in non-blacks, possibly because of higher prevalence of low-renin states in the black hypertensive population.

Other:

As with any antihypertensive agent, excessive reduction of blood pressure in patients with ischaemic cardiopathy or ischaemic cardiovascular disease could result in a myocardial infarction or stroke.

4.5 Interaction with other medicinal products and other forms of interaction
Interaction studies have only been performed in adults.

As with other medicinal products acting on the renin-angiotensin-aldosterone system, telmisartan may provoke hyperkalaemia (see section 4.4). The risk may increase in case of treatment combination with other medicinal products that may also provoke hyperkalaemia (salt substitutes containing potassium, potassium-sparing diuretics, ACE inhibitors, angiotensin II receptor antagonists, non steroidal anti-inflammatory medicinal products (NSAIDs, including selective COX-2 inhibitors), heparin, immunosuppressives (cyclosporin or tacrolimus), and trimethoprim).

The occurrence of hyperkalaemia depends on associated risk factors. The risk is increased in case of the above-mentioned treatment combinations. The risk is particularly high in combination with potassium sparing-diuretics, and when combined with salt substitutes containing potassium. A combination with ACE inhibitors or NSAIDs, for example, presents a lesser risk provided that precautions for use are strictly followed.

Concomitant use not recommended

Potassium sparing diuretics or potassium supplements:

Angiotensin II receptor antagonists such as telmisartan, attenuate diuretic induced potassium loss. Potassium sparing diuretics e.g. spirinolactone, eplerenone, triamterene, or amiloride, potassium supplements, or potassium-containing salt substitutes may lead to a significant increase in serum potassium. If concomitant use is indicated because of documented hypokalaemia, they should be used with caution and with frequent monitoring of serum potassium.

Lithium:

Reversible increases in serum lithium concentrations and toxicity have been reported during concomitant administration of lithium with angiotensin converting enzyme inhibitors, and with angiotensin II receptor antagonists, including telmisartan. If use of the combination proves necessary, careful monitoring of serum lithium levels is recommended.

Concomitant use requiring caution

Non-steroidal anti-inflammatory medicinal products:

NSAIDs (i.e. acetylsalicylic acid at anti-inflammatory dosage regimens, COX-2 inhibitors and non-selective NSAIDs) may reduce the antihypertensive effect of angiotensin II receptor antagonists.

In some patients with compromised renal function (e.g. dehydrated patients or elderly patients with compromised renal function), the co-administration of angiotensin II receptor antagonists and agents that inhibit cyclo-oxygenase may result in further deterioration of renal function, including possible acute renal failure, which is usually reversible. Therefore, the combination should be administered with caution, especially in the elderly. Patients should be adequately hydrated and consideration should be given to monitoring of renal function after initiation of concomitant therapy and periodically thereafter.

In one study the co-administration of telmisartan and ramipril led to an increase of up to 2.5 fold in the AUC_{0-24} and C_{max} of ramipril and ramiprilat. The clinical relevance of this observation is not known.

Diuretics (thiazide or loop diuretics):

Prior treatment with high dose diuretics such as furosemide (loop diuretic) and hydrochlorothiazide (thiazide diuretic) may result in volume depletion, and in a risk of hypotension when initiating therapy with telmisartan.

To be taken into account with concomitant use

Other antihypertensive agents:

The blood pressure lowering effect of telmisartan can be increased by concomitant use of other antihypertensive medicinal products.

Based on their pharmacological properties it can be expected that the following medicinal products may potentiate the hypotensive effects of all antihypertensives including telmisartan: Baclofen, amifostine. Furthermore, orthostatic hypotension may be aggravated by alcohol, barbiturates, narcotics, or antidepressants.

Corticosteroïds (systemic route):

Reduction of the antihypertensive effect.

4.6 Pregnancy and lactation

Pregnancy:

> The use of angiotensin II receptor antagonists is not recommended during the first trimester of pregnancy (see section 4.4). The use of angiotensin II receptor antagonists is contraindicated during the second and third trimester of pregnancy (see sections 4.3 and 4.4).

There are no adequate data from the use of Micardis in pregnant women. Studies in animals haveshown reproductive toxicity (see section 5.3).

Epidemiological evidence regarding the risk of teratogenicity following exposure to ACE inhibitors during the first trimester of pregnancy has not been conclusive; however a small increase in risk cannot be excluded. Whilst there is no controlled epidemiological data on the risk with angiotensin II receptor antagonists, similar risks may exist for this class of drugs. Unless continued angiotensin II receptor antagonist therapy is considered essential, patients planning pregnancy should be changed to alternative antihypertensive treatments which have an established safety profile for use in pregnancy. When pregnancy is diagnosed, treatment with angiotensin II receptor antagonists should be stopped immediately, and, if appropriate, alternative therapy should be started.

Exposure to angiotensin II receptor antagonist therapy during the second and third trimesters is known to induce human fetotoxicity (decreased renal function, oligohydramnios, skull ossification retardation) and neonatal toxicity (renal failure, hypotension, hyperkalaemia). (See section 5.3).

Should exposure to angiotensin II receptor antagonists have occurred from the second trimester of pregnancy, ultrasound check of renal function and skull is recommended.

Infants whose mothers have taken angiotensin II receptor antagonists should be closely observed for hypotension (see sections 4.3 and 4.4).

Lactation:

Because no information is available regarding the use of Micardis during breast-feeding, Micardis is not recommended and alternative treatments with better established safety profiles during breast-feeding are preferable, especially while nursing a newborn or preterm infant.

4.7 Effects on ability to drive and use machines

No studies on the effects on the ability to drive and use machines have been performed. However, when driving vehicles or operating machinery it should be taken into account that dizziness or drowsiness may occasionally occur when taking antihypertensive therapy.

4.8 Undesirable effects

The overall incidence of adverse events reported with telmisartan (41.4 %) was usually comparable to placebo (43.9 %) in placebo controlled trials. The incidence of adverse events was not dose related and showed no correlation with gender, age or race of the patients.

The adverse drug reactions listed below have been accumulated from all clinical trials in patients treated with telmisartan for hypertension or in patients 50 years or older at high risk of cardiovascular events.

Adverse reactions have been ranked under headings of frequency using the following convention:

very common (≥1/10); common (≥1/100 to <1/10); uncommon (≥1/1,000 to <1/100); rare (≥1/10,000 to <1/1,000); very rare (<1/10,000), not known (cannot be estimated from the available data).

Within each frequency grouping, adverse reactions are presented in order of decreasing seriousness.

Infections and infestations	
Rare:	Upper respiratory tract infection including pharyngitis and sinusitis
Not known:	Urinary tract infection including cystitis, sepsis including fatal outcome*
Blood and the lymphatic system disorders	
Rare:	Anaemia, thrombocytopenia
Not known:	Eosinophilia
Immune system disorders	
Not known:	Hypersensitivity, anaphylactic reaction
Metabolism and nutrition disorders	
Uncommon:	Hyperkalaemia
Psychiatric disorders	
Rare:	Anxiety, depression
Nervous system disorders	
Uncommon:	Syncope, insomnia
Eye disorders	
Rare:	Abnormal vision
Ear and labyrinth disorders	
Uncommon:	Vertigo
Cardiac disorders	
Rare:	Tachycardia
Not known:	Bradycardia
Vascular disorders	
Uncommon:	Hypotension
Rare:	Orthostatic hypotension
Respiratory, thoracic and mediastinal disorders	
Uncommon:	Dyspnoea
Gastrointestinal disorders	
Uncommon:	Abdominal pain, diarrhoea, dry mouth, dyspepsia, flatulence
Rare:	Stomach upset, vomiting
Hepato-biliary disorders	
Rare:	Hepatic function abnormal/liver disorder
Skin and subcutaneous tissue disorders	
Uncommon:	Hyperhidrosis, pruritus
Rare:	Erythema, angioedema, urticaria
Not known:	Drug eruption, toxic skin eruption, rash, eczema
Muscoloskeletal and connective tissue disorders	
Uncommon:	Myalgia
Rare:	Arthralgia, back pain (e.g. sciatica), muscle cramps, pain in limb, weakness
Not known:	Tendonitis
Renal and urinary disorders	
Uncommon:	Renal impairment including acute renal failure
General disorders and administration site conditions	
Uncommon:	Chest pain
Rare:	Influenza-like illness
Not known:	Drug ineffective
Investigations	
Rare:	Blood uric acid increased, blood creatinine increased, hepatic enzyme increased, blood creatine phosphokinase increased
Not known:	Haemoglobin decreased

*In the PRoFESS trial, an increased incidence of sepsis was observed with telmisartan compared with placebo. The event may be a chance finding or related to a mechanism currently not known (see section 5.1).

4.9 Overdose

There is limited information available with regard to overdose in humans.

Symptoms: The most prominent manifestations of telmisartan overdose were hypotension and tachycardia; bradycardia dizziness, increase in serum creatinine, and acute renal failure have also been reported.

Treatment: Telmisartan is not removed by haemodialysis. The patient should be closely monitored, and the treatment should be symptomatic and supportive. Management depends on the time since ingestion and the severity of the symptoms. Suggested measures include induction of emesis and / or gastric lavage. Activated charcoal may be useful in the treatment of overdosage. Serum electrolytes and creatinine should be monitored frequently. If hypotension occurs, the patient should be placed in a supine position, with salt and volume replacement given quickly.

5. PHARMACOLOGICAL PROPERTIES

5.1 Pharmacodynamic properties

Pharmacotherapeutic group: Angiotensin II Antagonists, plain, ATC Code: C09CA07.

Mechanism of action:

Telmisartan is an orally active and specific angiotensin II receptor (type AT_1) antagonist. Telmisartan displaces angiotensin II with very high affinity from its binding site at the AT_1 receptor subtype, which is responsible for the known actions of angiotensin II. Telmisartan does not exhibit any partial agonist activity at the AT_1 receptor. Telmisartan selectively binds the AT_1 receptor. The binding is long-lasting. Telmisartan does not show affinity for other receptors, including AT_2 and other less characterised AT receptors. The functional role of these receptors is not known, nor is the effect of their possible overstimulation by angiotensin II, whose levels are increased by telmisartan. Plasma aldosterone levels are decreased by telmisartan. Telmisartan does not inhibit human plasma renin or block ion channels. Telmisartan does not inhibit angiotensin converting enzyme (kininase II), the enzyme which also degrades bradykinin. Therefore it is not expected to potentiate bradykinin-mediated adverse effects.

In human, an 80 mg dose of telmisartan almost completely inhibits the angiotensin II evoked blood pressure increase. The inhibitory effect is maintained over 24 hours and still measurable up to 48 hours.

Clinical efficacy and safety:

After the first dose of telmisartan, the antihypertensive activity gradually becomes evident within 3 hours. The maximum reduction in blood pressure is generally attained 4 to 8 weeks after the start of treatment and is sustained during long-term therapy.

The antihypertensive effect persists constantly over 24 hours after dosing and includes the last 4 hours before the next dose as shown by ambulatory blood pressure measurements. This is confirmed by trough to peak ratios consistently above 80 % seen after doses of 40 and 80 mg of telmisartan in placebo controlled clinical studies. There is an apparent trend to a dose relationship to a time to recovery of baseline systolic blood pressure (SBP). In this respect data concerning diastolic blood pressure (DBP) are inconsistent.

In patients with hypertension telmisartan reduces both systolic and diastolic blood pressure without affecting pulse rate. The contribution of the medicinal product's diuretic and natriuretic effect to its hypotensive activity has still to be defined. The antihypertensive efficacy of telmisartan is comparable to that of agents representative of other classes of antihypertensive medicinal products (demonstrated in clinical trials comparing telmisartan to amlodipine, atenolol, enalapril, hydrochlorothiazide, and lisinopril).

Upon abrupt cessation of treatment with telmisartan, blood pressure gradually returns to pre-treatment values over a period of several days without evidence of rebound hypertension.

The incidence of dry cough was significantly lower in patients treated with telmisartan than in those given angiotensin converting enzyme inhibitors in clinical trials directly comparing the two antihypertensive treatments.

In the "Prevention Regimen For Effectively avoiding Second Strokes" (PRoFESS) trial in patients 50 years and older, who recently experienced stroke, an increased incidence of sepsis was noted for telmisartan compared with placebo, 0.70 % vs. 0.49 % [RR 1.43 (95 % confidence interval 1.00 - 2.06)]; the incidence of fatal sepsis cases was increased for patients taking telmisartan (0.33 %) vs. patients taking placebo (0.16 %) [RR 2.07 (95 % confidence interval 1.14 - 3.76)]. The observed increased occurrence rate of sepsis associated with the use of telmisartan may be either a chance finding or related to a mechanism not currently known.

Beneficial effects of telmisartan on mortality and cardiovascular morbidity are currently unknown.

5.2 Pharmacokinetic properties

Absorption:

Absorption of telmisartan is rapid although the amount absorbed varies. The mean absolute bioavailability for telmisartan is about 50 %. When telmisartan is taken with food, the reduction in the area under the plasma concentration-time curve ($AUC_{0-\infty}$) of telmisartan varies from approximately 6 % (40 mg dose) to approximately 19 % (160 mg dose). By 3 hours after administration, plasma concentrations are similar whether telmisartan is taken fasting or with food.

Linearity/non-linearity:

The small reduction in AUC is not expected to cause a reduction in the therapeutic efficacy. There is no linear relationship between doses and plasma levels. C_{max} and to a lesser extent AUC increase disproportionately at doses above 40 mg.

Distribution:

Telmisartan is largely bound to plasma protein (>99.5 %), mainly albumin and alpha-1 acid glycoprotein. The mean steady state apparent volume of distribution (V_{dss}) is approximately 500 l.

Metabolism:

Telmisartan is metabolised by conjugation to the glucuronide of the parent compound. No pharmacological activity has been shown for the conjugate.

Elimination:

Telmisartan is characterised by biexponential decay pharmacokinetics with a terminal elimination half-life of >20 hours. The maximum plasma concentration (C_{max}) and, to a smaller extent, the area under the plasma concentration-time curve (AUC), increase disproportionately with dose. There is no evidence of clinically relevant accumulation of telmisartan taken at the recommended dose. Plasma concentrations were higher in females than in males, without relevant influence on efficacy.

After oral (and intravenous) administration, telmisartan is nearly exclusively excreted with the faeces, mainly as unchanged compound. Cumulative urinary excretion is <1 % of dose. Total plasma clearance (Cl_{tot}) is high (approximately 1,000 ml/min) compared with hepatic blood flow (about 1,500 ml/min).

Special Populations

Gender effects:

Differences in plasma concentrations were observed, with C_{max} and AUC being approximately 3- and 2-fold higher, respectively, in females compared to males.

Elderly patients:

The pharmacokinetics of telmisartan do not differ between the elderly and those younger than 65 years.

Patients with renal impairment:

In patients with mild to moderate and severe renal impairment, doubling of plasma concentrations was observed. However, lower plasma concentrations were observed in patients with renal insufficiency undergoing dialysis. Telmisartan is highly bound to plasma protein in renal-insufficient patients and cannot be removed by dialysis. The elimination half-life is not changed in patients with renal impairment.

Patients with hepatic impairment:

Pharmacokinetic studies in patients with hepatic impairment showed an increase in absolute bioavailability up to nearly 100 %. The elimination half-life is not changed in patients with hepatic impairment.

5.3 Preclinical safety data

In preclinical safety studies, doses producing exposure comparable to that in the clinical therapeutic range caused reduced red cell parameters (erythrocytes, haemoglobin, haematocrit), changes in renal haemodynamics (increased blood urea nitrogen and creatinine), as well as increased serum potassium in normotensive animals. In dogs, renal tubular dilation and atrophy were observed. Gastric mucosal injury (erosion, ulcers or inflammation) also was noted in rats and dogs. These pharmacologically-mediated undesirable effects, known from preclinical studies with both angiotensin converting enzyme inhibitors and angiotensin II receptor antagonists, were prevented by oral saline supplementation.

In both species, increased plasma renin activity and hypertrophy/hyperplasia of the renal juxtaglomerular cells were observed. These changes, also a class effect of angiotensin converting enzyme inhibitors and other angiotensin II receptor antagonists, do not appear to have clinical significance.

There is no evidence of a teratogenic effect, but animal studies indicated some hazardous potential of telmisartan to the postnatal development of the offspring such as lower body weight, delayed eye opening, and higher mortality.

There was no evidence of mutagenicity and relevant clastogenic activity in *in vitro* studies and no evidence of carcinogenicity in rats and mice.

6. PHARMACEUTICAL PARTICULARS

6.1 List of excipients

Povidone (K25)

Meglumine

Sodium hydroxide

Sorbitol (E420)

Magnesium stearate.

6.2 Incompatibilities

Not applicable.

6.3 Shelf life

20 mg tablets: 3 years

40 mg and 80 mg tablets: 4 years

6.4 Special precautions for storage

This medicinal product does not require any special storage conditions. Store in the original package in order to protect from moisture.

6.5 Nature and contents of container

20 mg:

Aluminium/aluminium blisters (PA/Al/PVC/Al or PA/PA/Al/PVC/Al). One blister contains 7 tablets.

40 and 80 mg:

Aluminium/aluminium blisters (PA/Al/PVC/Al or PA/PA/Al/PVC/Al). One blister contains 7 or 10 tablets.

Pack sizes:

20 mg, 40 mg and 80 mg tablets:

Blister with 14, 28, 56 and 98 tablets

40 mg and 80 mg tablets only:

Blister with 30, 84 and 90 tablets or perforated unit dose blisters with 28 × 1 tablets

Not all pack sizes may be marketed.

6.6 Special precautions for disposal and other handling

No special requirements.

7. MARKETING AUTHORISATION HOLDER

Boehringer Ingelheim International GmbH

Binger Str. 173

D-55216 Ingelheim am Rhein

Germany

8. MARKETING AUTHORISATION NUMBER(S)

Micardis 20 mg tablets:

EU/1/98/090/009 (14 tablets)

EU/1/98/090/010 (28 tablets)

EU/1/98/090/011 (56 tablets)

EU/1/98/090/012 (98 tablets)

Micardis 40 mg tablets:

EU/1/98/090/001 (14 tablets)

EU/1/98/090/002 (28 tablets)

EU/1/98/090/003 (56 tablets)

EU/1/98/090/004 (98 tablets)

EU/1/98/090/013 (28 × 1 tablets)

EU/1/98/090/015 (84 tablets)

EU/1/98/090/017 (30 tablets)

EU/1/98/090/019 (90 tablets)

Micardis 80 mg tablets:

EU/1/98/090/005 (14 tablets)

EU/1/98/090/006 (28 tablets)

EU/1/98/090/007 (56 tablets)

EU/1/98/090/008 (98 tablets)

EU/1/98/090/014 (28 × 1 tablets)

EU/1/98/090/016 (84 tablets)

EU/1/98/090/018 (30 tablets)

EU/1/98/090/020 (90 tablets)

9. DATE OF FIRST AUTHORISATION/RENEWAL OF THE AUTHORISATION

Date of first authorisation: 16 December 1998

Date of last renewal: 16 December 2008

10. DATE OF REVISION OF THE TEXT

29th May 2009

LEGAL CATEGORY

POM

MicardisPlus 40/12.5 mg tablets and 80/12.5 mg tablets

(Boehringer Ingelheim Limited)

1. NAME OF THE MEDICINAL PRODUCT

MicardisPlus 40 mg/12.5 mg tablets

MicardisPlus 80mg/12.5 mg tablets

2. QUALITATIVE AND QUANTITATIVE COMPOSITION

Each tablet contains 40 mg telmisartan and 12.5 mg hydrochlorothiazide or 80 mg telmisartan and 12.5 mg hydrochlorothiazide.

Excipients (40 mg): Each tablet contains 112 mg of lactose monohydrate and 169 mg sorbitol (E420).

Excipients (80 mg): Each tablet contains 112 mg of lactose monohydrate and 338 mg sorbitol (E420).

For a full list of excipients, see section 6.1.

3. PHARMACEUTICAL FORM

Tablet.

Red and white oval shaped two layer tablet engraved with the company logo and the code 'H4' or 'H8'.

4. CLINICAL PARTICULARS

4.1 Therapeutic indications

Treatment of essential hypertension.

MicardisPlus fixed dose combination (40 mg telmisartan/12.5 mg hydrochlorothiazide) is indicated in patients whose blood pressure is not adequately controlled on telmisartan alone.

4.2 Posology and method of administration

Adults

MicardisPlus should be taken once daily with liquid, with or without food in patients whose blood pressure is not adequately controlled by telmisartan alone. Individual dose titration with each of the two components is recommended before changing to the fixed dose combination. When clinically appropriate, direct change from monotherapy to the fixed combination may be considered.

- MicardisPlus 40 mg/12.5 mg may be administered in patients whose blood pressure is not adequately controlled by Micardis 40 mg
- MicardisPlus 80 mg/12.5 mg may be administered in patients whose blood pressure is not adequately controlled by Micardis 80 mg

Renal impairment: Periodic monitoring of renal function is advised (see section 4.4).

Hepatic impairment: In patients with mild to moderate hepatic impairment the posology should not exceed MicardisPlus 40 mg/12.5 mg once daily. MicardisPlus is not indicated in patients with severe hepatic impairment. Thiazides should be used with caution in patients with impaired hepatic function (see section 4.4).

Elderly: No dosage adjustment is necessary.

Children and adolescents: MicardisPlus is not recommended for use in children below 18 years due to a lack of data on safety and efficacy.

4.3 Contraindications

- Hypersensitivity to any of the active substances or to any of the excipients (see section 6.1).
- Hypersensitivity to other sulphonamide-derived substances (since hydrochlorothiazide is a sulphonamide-derived medicinal product).
- Second and third trimesters of pregnancy (see sections 4.4 and 4.6).
- Cholestasis and biliary obstructive disorders.
- Severe hepatic impairment.
- Severe renal impairment (creatinine clearance < 30 ml/min).
- Refractory hypokalaemia, hypercalcaemia.

4.4 Special warnings and precautions for use

Pregnancy

Angiotensin II receptor antagonists should not be initiated during pregnancy. Unless continued angiotensin II receptor antagonist therapy is considered essential, patients planning pregnancy should be changed to alternative anti-hypertensive treatments which have an established safety profile for use in pregnancy. When pregnancy is diagnosed, treatment with angiotensin II receptor antagonists should be stopped immediately, and, if appropriate, alternative therapy should be started (see sections 4.3 and 4.6).

Hepatic impairment: MicardisPlus should not be given to patients with cholestasis, biliary obstructive disorders or severe hepatic insufficiency (see section 4.3) since telmisartan is mostly eliminated with the bile. These patients can be expected to have reduced hepatic clearance for telmisartan.

In addition, MicardisPlus should be used with caution in patients with impaired hepatic function or progressive liver disease, since minor alterations of fluid and electrolyte balance may precipitate hepatic coma. There is no clinical experience with MicardisPlus in patients with hepatic impairment.

Renovascular hypertension: There is an increased risk of severe hypotension and renal insufficiency when patients with bilateral renal artery stenosis or stenosis of the artery to a single functioning kidney are treated with medicinal products that affect the renin-angiotensin-aldosterone system.

Renal impairment and kidney transplantation: MicardisPlus should not be used in patients with severe renal impairment (creatinine clearance <30 ml/min) (see section 4.3). There is no experience regarding the administration of MicardisPlus in patients with recent kidney transplantation. Experience with MicardisPlus is modest in the patients with mild to moderate renal impairment, therefore periodic monitoring of potassium, creatinine and uric acid serum levels is recommended. Thiazide diuretic-associated azotaemia may occur in patients with impaired renal function.

Intravascular hypovolaemia: Symptomatic hypotension, especially after the first dose, may occur in patients who are volume and/or sodium depleted by vigorous diuretic therapy, dietary salt restriction, diarrhoea or vomiting. Such conditions should be corrected before the administration of MicardisPlus.

Other conditions with stimulation of the renin-angiotensin-aldosterone system: In patients whose vascular tone and renal function depend predominantly on the activity of the renin-angiotensin-aldosterone system (e.g. patients with severe congestive heart failure or underlying renal disease, including renal artery stenosis), treatment with medicinal products that affect this system has been associated with acute hypotension, hyperazotaemia, oliguria, or rarely acute renal failure (see section 4.8).

Primary aldosteronism: Patients with primary aldosteronism generally will not respond to antihypertensive medicinal products acting through inhibition of the renin-angiotensin system. Therefore, the use of MicardisPlus is not recommended.

Aortic and mitral valve stenosis, obstructive hypertrophic cardiomyopathy: As with other vasodilators, special caution is indicated in patients suffering from aortic or mitral stenosis, or obstructive hypertrophic cardiomyopathy.

Metabolic and endocrine effects: Thiazide therapy may impair glucose tolerance. In diabetic patients dosage adjustments of insulin or oral hypoglycaemic agents may be required. Latent diabetes mellitus may become manifest during thiazide therapy.

An increase in cholesterol and triglyceride levels has been associated with thiazide diuretic therapy; however, at the 12.5 mg dose contained in MicardisPlus, minimal or no effects were reported.

Hyperuricaemia may occur or frank gout may be precipitated in some patients receiving thiazide therapy.

Electrolyte imbalance: As for any patient receiving diuretic therapy, periodic determination of serum electrolytes should be performed at appropriate intervals.

Thiazides, including hydrochlorothiazide, can cause fluid or electrolyte imbalance (including hypokalaemia, hyponatraemia and hypochloraemic alkalosis). Warning signs of fluid or electrolyte imbalance are dryness of mouth, thirst, asthenia, lethargy, drowsiness, restlessness, muscle pain or cramps, muscular fatigue, hypotension, oliguria, tachycardia, and gastrointestinal disturbances such as nausea or vomiting (see section 4.8).

- Hypokalaemia

Although hypokalaemia may develop with the use of thiazide diuretics, concurrent therapy with telmisartan may reduce diuretic-induced hypokalaemia. The risk of hypokalaemia is greater in patients with cirrhosis of liver, in patients experiencing brisk diuresis, in patients who are receiving inadequate oral intake of electrolytes and in patients receiving concomitant therapy with corticosteroids or Adrenocorticotropic hormone (ACTH) (see section 4.5).

- Hyperkalaemia

Conversely, due to the antagonism of the angiotensin II (AT_1) receptors by the telmisartan component of MicardisPlus, hyperkalaemia might occur. Although clinically significant hyperkalaemia has not been documented with MicardisPlus, risk factors for the development of hyperkalaemia include renal insufficiency and/or heart failure, and diabetes mellitus. Potassium-sparing diuretics, potassium supplements or potassium-containing salt substitutes should be co-administered cautiously with MicardisPlus (see section 4.5).

- Hyponatraemia and hypochloraemic alkalosis

There is no evidence that MicardisPlus would reduce or prevent diuretic-induced hyponatraemia. Chloride deficit is generally mild and usually does not require treatment.

- Hypercalcaemia

Thiazides may decrease urinary calcium excretion and cause an intermittent and slight elevation of serum calcium in the absence of known disorders of calcium metabolism. Marked hypercalcaemia may be evidence of hidden hyperparathyroidism. Thiazides should be discontinued before carrying out tests for parathyroid function.

- Hypomagnesaemia

Thiazides have been shown to increase the urinary excretion of magnesium, which may result in hypomagnesaemia (see section 4.5).

Sorbitol and Lactose Monohydrate: This medicinal product contains lactose monohydrate and sorbitol. Patients with rare hereditary problems of fructose intolerance and/or with rare hereditary problems of galactose intolerance, the Lapp lactase deficiency or glucose-galactose malabsorption should not take this medicine.

Ethnic differences: As with all other angiotensin II receptor antagonists, telmisartan is apparently less effective in lowering blood pressure in black patients than in non blacks, possibly because of higher prevalence of low renin states in the black hypertensive population.

Other: As with any antihypertensive agent, excessive reduction of blood pressure in patients with ischaemic cardiopathy or ischaemic cardiovascular disease could result in a myocardial infarction or stroke.

General: Hypersensitivity reactions to hydrochlorothiazide may occur in patients with or without a history of allergy or bronchial asthma, but are more likely in patients with such a history.

Exacerbation or activation of systemic lupus erythematosus has been reported with the use of thiazide diuretics.

Cases of photosensitivity reactions have been reported with thiazide diuretics (see section 4.8). If a photosensitivity reaction occurs during treatment, it is recommended to stop the treatment. If a re-administration of the diuretic is deemed necessary, it is recommended to protect exposed areas to the sun or to artificial UVA.

4.5 Interaction with other medicinal products and other forms of interaction

Interaction studies have only been performed in adults.

Lithium: Reversible increases in serum lithium concentrations and toxicity have been reported during concomitant administration of lithium with angiotensin converting enzyme inhibitors. Rare cases have also been reported with angiotensin II receptor antagonists (including MicardisPlus). Co-administration of lithium and MicardisPlus is not recommended (see section 4.4). If this combination proves essential, careful monitoring of serum lithium level is recommended during concomitant use.

Medicinal products associated with potassium loss and hypokalaemia (e.g. other kaliuretic diuretics, laxatives, corticosteroids, ACTH, amphotericin, carbenoxolone, penicillin G sodium, salicylic acid and derivatives): If these substances are to be prescribed with the hydrochlorothiazide-telmisartan combination, monitoring of potassium plasma levels is advised. These medicinal products may potentiate the effect of hydrochlorothiazide on serum potassium (see section 4.4).

Medicinal products that may increase potassium levels or induce hyperkalaemia (e.g. ACE inhibitors, potassium-sparing diuretics, potassium supplements, salt substitutes containing potassium, cyclosporin or other medicinal products such as heparin sodium): If these medicinal products are to be prescribed with the hydrochlorothiazide-telmisartan combination, monitoring of potassium plasma levels is advised. Based on the experience with the use of other medicinal products that blunt the renin-angiotensin system, concomitant use of the above medicinal products may lead to increases in serum potassium and is, therefore, not recommended (see section 4.4).

Medicinal products affected by serum potassium disturbances: Periodic monitoring of serum potassium and ECG is recommended when MicardisPlus is administered with these medicinal products affected by serum potassium disturbances (e.g. digitalis glycosides, antiarrhythmics) and the following torsades de pointes inducing medicinal products (which include some antiarrhythmics), hypokalaemia being a predisposing factor to torsades de pointes.

- class Ia antiarrythmics (e.g. quinidine, hydroquinidine, disopyramide)

- class III antiarrythmics (e.g. amiodarone, sotalol, dofetilide, ibutilide)

- some antipsychotics (e.g. thioridazine, chlorpromazine, levomepromazine, trifluoperazine, cyamemazine, sulpiride, sultopride, amisulpride, tiapride, pimozide, haloperidol, droperidol)

- others (e.g. bepridil, cisapride, diphemanil, erythromycin IV, halofantrin, mizolastin, pentamidine, sparfloxacine, terfenadine, vincamine IV.)

Digitalis glycosides: Thiazide-induced hypokalaemia or hypomagnesaemia favours the onset of digitalis-induced arrhythmia (see section 4.4).

Other antihypertensive agents: Telmisartan may increase the hypotensive effect of other antihypertensive agents.

Antidiabetic medicinal products (oral agents and insulin): Dosage adjustment of the antidiabetic medicinal products may be required (see section 4.4).

Metformin: Metformin should be used with precaution: risk of lactic acidosis induced by a possible functional renal failure linked to hydrochlorothiazide.

Cholestyramine and colestipol resins: Absorption of hydrochlorothiazide is impaired in the presence of anionic exchange resins.

Non-steroidal anti-inflammatory medicinal products: NSAIDs (i.e. acetylsalicylic acid at anti-inflammatory dosage regimens, COX-2 inhibitors and non-selective NSAIDs) may reduce the diuretic, natriuretic and antihypertensive effects of thiazide diuretics and the antihypertensive effects of angiotensin II receptor antagonists.

In some patients with compromised renal function (e.g. dehydrated patients or elderly patients with compromised renal function) the co-administration of angiotensin II receptor antagonists and agents that inhibit cyclo-oxygenase may result in further deterioration of renal function, including possible acute renal failure, which is usually reversible. Therefore the combination should be administered with caution, especially in the elderly. Patients should be adequately hydrated and consideration should be given to monitoring of renal function after initiation of concomitant therapy and periodically thereafter.

Pressor amines (e.g. noradrenaline): The effect of pressor amines may be decreased.

Nondepolarizing skeletal muscle relaxants (e.g. tubocurarine): The effect of nondepolarizing skeletal muscle relaxants may be potentiated by hydrochlorothiazide.

Medicinal products used in the treatment for gout (e.g. probenecid, sulfinpyrazone and allopurinol): Dosage adjustment of uricosuric medications may be necessary as hydrochlorothiazide may raise the level of serum uric acid. Increase in dosage of probenecid or sulfinpyrazone may be necessary. Co-administration of thiazide may increase the incidence of hypersensitivity reactions of allopurinol.

Calcium salts: Thiazide diuretics may increase serum calcium levels due to the decreased excretion. If calcium supplements must be prescribed, serum calcium levels should be monitored and calcium dosage adjusted accordingly.

Beta-blockers and diazoxide: The hyperglycaemic effect of beta-blockers and diazoxide may be enhanced by thiazides.

Anticholinergic agents (e.g. atropine, biperiden) may increase the bioavailability of thiazide-type diuretics by decreasing gastrointestinal motility and stomach emptying rate.

Amantadine: Thiazides may increase the risk of adverse effects caused by amantadine.

Cytotoxic agents (e.g. cyclophosphamide, methotrexate): Thiazides may reduce the renal excretion of cytotoxic medicinal products and potentiate their myelosuppressive effects.

Based on their pharmacological properties it can be expected that the following medicinal products may potentiate the hypotensive effects of all antihypertensives including telmisartan: Baclofen, amifostine.

Furthermore, orthostatic hypotension may be aggravated by alcohol, barbiturates, narcotics or antidepressants.

4.6 Pregnancy and lactation

Pregnancy:

> The use of angiotensin II receptor antagonists is not recommended during the first trimester of pregnancy (see section 4.4). The use of angiotensin II receptor antagonists is contraindicated during the second and third trimesters of pregnancy (see sections 4.3 and 4.4).

There are no adequate data from the use of MicardisPlus in pregnant women. Studies in animals have shown reproductive toxicity (see section 5.3).

Epidemiological evidence regarding the risk of teratogenicity following exposure to ACE inhibitors during the first trimester of pregnancy has not been conclusive; however a small increase in risk cannot be excluded. Whilst there is no controlled epidemiological data on the risk with angiotensin II receptor antagonists, similar risks may exist for this class of drugs. Unless continued angiotensin II receptor antagonist therapy is considered essential, patients planning pregnancy should be changed to alternative antihypertensive treatments which have an established safety profile for use in pregnancy. When pregnancy is diagnosed, treatment with angiotensin II receptor antagonists should be stopped immediately, and, if appropriate, alternative therapy should be started.

Exposure to angiotensin II receptor antagonist therapy during the second and third trimesters is known to induce human fetotoxicity (decreased renal function, oligohydramnios, skull ossification retardation) and neonatal toxicity (renal failure, hypotension, hyperkalaemia). (See section 5.3).

Should exposure to angiotensin II receptor antagonists have occurred from the second trimester of pregnancy, ultrasound check of renal function and skull is recommended.

Infants whose mothers have taken angiotensin II receptor antagonists should be closely observed for hypotension (see sections 4.3 and 4.4).

Thiazides cross the placental barrier and appear in cord blood. They may cause foetal electrolyte disturbances and possibly other reactions that have occurred in the adults. Cases of neonatal thrombocytopenia, of foetal or neonatal jaundice have been reported with maternal thiazide therapy.

Lactation:

Because no information is available regarding the use of MicardisPlus during breast-feeding, MicardisPlus is not recommended and alternative treatments with better established safety profiles during breast-feeding are preferable, especially while nursing a newborn or preterm infant. Thiazides appear in human milk and may inhibit lactation.

4.7 Effects on ability to drive and use machines

No studies on the effect on the ability to drive and use machines have been performed. However, when driving vehicles or operating machinery it should be taken into account that dizziness or drowsiness may occasionally occur when taking antihypertensive therapy.

4.8 Undesirable effects

Fixed Dose Combination

The overall incidence of adverse events reported with MicardisPlus was comparable to those reported with telmisartan alone in randomised controlled trials involving 1471 patients randomised to receive telmisartan plus hydrochlorothiazide (835) or telmisartan alone (636). Dose-relationship of undesirable effects was not established and they showed no correlation with gender, age or race of the patients.

Adverse reactions reported in all clinical trials and occurring more frequently ($p \leq 0.05$) with telmisartan plus hydrochlorothiazide than with placebo are shown below according to system organ class. Adverse reactions known to occur with each component given singly but which have not been seen in clinical trials may occur during treatment with MicardisPlus.

Adverse reactions have been ranked under headings of frequency using the following convention:

very common (≥1/10); common (≥1/100 to <1/10); uncommon (≥1/1,000 to <1/100); rare (≥1/10,000 to <1/1,000); very rare (<1/10,000), not known (cannot be estimated from the available data).

Within each frequency grouping, adverse reactions are presented in order of decreasing seriousness.

Infections and infestations	
Rare: Not known:	Bronchitis Pharyngitis, sinusitis
Metabolism and nutrition disorders	
Uncommon: Rare:	Hypokalaemia, Hyperuricaemia, hyponatraemia

Psychiatric disorders	
Uncommon: Rare:	Anxiety Depression
Nervous system disorders	
Common: Uncommon: Rare:	Dizziness Syncope, paraesthesia Insomnia, sleep disorders
Eye disorders	
Rare:	Visual disturbance, vision blurred
Ear and labyrinth disorders	
Uncommon:	Vertigo
Cardiac disorders	
Uncommon:	Tachycardia, arrhythmias
Vascular disorders	
Uncommon:	Hypotension, orthostatic hypotension
Respiratory, thoracic and mediastinal disorders	
Uncommon: Rare:	Dyspnoea Respiratory distress (including pneumonitis and pulmonary oedema)
Gastrointestinal disorders	
Uncommon: Rare: Not known:	Diarrhoea, dry mouth, flatulence, Abdominal pain, constipation, dyspepsia, vomiting Gastritis
Hepatobiliary disorders	
Rare:	Abnormal hepatic function/liver disorder
Skin and subcutaneous tissue disorders	
Rare:	Angioedema, erythema, pruritus, rash, hyperhidrosis, urticaria
Muscoloskeletal, connective tissue and bone disorders	
Uncommon: Rare:	Back pain, muscle spasms, myalgia Arthralgia, muscle cramps, pain in limb
Reproductive system and breast disorders	
Uncommon:	Erectile dysfunction
General disorders and administration site conditions	
Uncommon: Rare:	Chest pain Influenza-like illness, pain
Investigations	
Uncommon: Rare:	Blood uric acid increased Blood creatinine increased, blood creatine phosphokinase increased, hepatic enzyme increased

Additional information on individual components

Undesirable effects previously reported with one of the individual components may be potential undesirable effects with MicardisPlus, even if not observed in clinical trials with this product.

Telmisartan:

Undesirable effects occurred with similar frequency in placebo and telmisartan treated patients.

The overall incidence of adverse events reported with telmisartan (41.4 %) was usually comparable to placebo (43.9 %) in placebo controlled trials. The following adverse drug reactions listed below have been accumulated from all clinical trials in patients treated with telmisartan for hypertension or in patients 50 years or older at high risk of cardiovascular events.

Adverse reactions of unknown frequency reported with the use of telmisartan alone include:

Infections and infestations	
Not known:	Upper respiratory tract infection, urinary tract infection including cystitis, sepsis including fatal outcome*
Blood and lymphatic system disorders	
Not known:	Eosinophilia, anaemia, thrombocytopenia
Immune system disorders	
Not known:	Hypersensitivity, anaphylactic reactions
Metabolism and nutrition disorders	
Not known:	Hyperkalaemia
Cardiac disorders	
Not known:	Bradycardia
Gastrointestinal disorders	
Not known:	Stomach discomfort
Skin and subcutaneous tissue disorders	
Not known:	Eczema, drug eruption, toxic skin eruption
Musculoskeletal, connective tissue and bone disorders	
Not known:	Arthrosis, tendon pain
Renal and urinary disorders	
Not known:	Renal dysfunction, renal impairment (including acute renal failure)
General disorders and administration site conditions	
Not known:	Asthenia, drug ineffective
Investigations	
Not known:	Haemoglobin decreased

*In the PRoFESS trial, an increased incidence of sepsis was observed with telmisartan compared with placebo. The event may be a chance finding or related to a mechanism currently not known (see section 5.1).

Hydrochlorothiazide:

Hydrochlorothiazide may cause or exacerbate hypovolaemia which could lead to electrolyte imbalance (see section 4.4).

Adverse reactions of unknown frequency reported with the use of hydrochlorothiazide alone include:

Infections and infestations	
Not known:	Sialoadenitis
Blood and lymphatic system disorders	
Not known:	Anaemia aplastic, haemolytic anaemia, bone marrow failure, leukopenia, neutropenia, agranulocytosis, thrombocytopenia
Immune system disorders	
Not known:	Anaphylactic reactions, hypersensitivity
Endocrine disorders	
Not known:	Diabetes mellitus inadequate control
Metabolism and nutrition disorders	
Not known:	Anorexia, appetite decreased, electrolyte imbalance, hypercholesterolaemia, hyperglycaemia, hypovolaemia
Psychiatric disorders	
Not known:	Restlessness
Nervous system disorders	
Not known:	Light-headedness
Eye disorders	
Not known	Xanthopsia
Vascular disorders	
Not known:	Vasculitis necrotizing
Gastrointestinal disorders	
Not known:	Pancreatitis, stomach discomfort
Hepatobiliary disorders	
Not known:	Jaundice hepatocellular, jaundice cholestatic
Skin and subcutaneous tissue disorders	
Not known:	Lupus-like syndrome, photosensitivity reactions, skin vasculitis, toxic epidermal necrolysis
Musculoskeletal, connective tissue and bone disorders	
Not known:	Weakness
Renal and urinary disorders	
Not known:	Nephritis interstitial, renal dysfunction, glycosuria
General disorders and administration site conditions	
Not known:	Pyrexia
Investigations	
Not known:	Triglycerides increased

4.9 Overdose

There is limited information available for telmisartan with regard to overdose in humans. The degree to which hydrochlorothiazide is removed by haemodialysis has not been established.

Symptoms: The most prominent manifestations of telmisartan overdose were hypotension and tachycardia; bradycardia, dizziness, vomiting, increase in serum creatinine, and acute renal failure have also been reported. Overdose with hydrochlorothiazide is associated with electrolyte depletion (hypokalaemia, hypochloraemia) and hypovolaemia resulting from excessive diuresis. The most common signs and symptoms of overdose are nausea and somnolence. Hypokalaemia may result in muscle spasms and/or accentuate arrhythmia associated with the concomitant use of digitalis glycosides or certain anti-arrhythmic medicinal products.

Treatment: Telmisartan is not removed by haemodialysis. The patient should be closely monitored, and the treatment should be symptomatic and supportive. Management depends on the time since ingestion and the severity of the symptoms. Suggested measures include induction of emesis and/or gastric lavage. Activated charcoal may be useful in the treatment of overdose. Serum electrolytes and creatinine should be monitored frequently. If hypotension occurs, the patient should be placed in a supine position, with salt and volume replacements given quickly.

5. PHARMACOLOGICAL PROPERTIES

5.1 Pharmacodynamic properties

Pharmacotherapeutic group: Angiotensin II receptor antagonists and diuretics, ATC code: C09DA07

MicardisPlus is a combination of an angiotensin II receptor antagonist, telmisartan, and a thiazide diuretic, hydrochlorothiazide. The combination of these ingredients has an additive antihypertensive effect, reducing blood pressure to a greater degree than either component alone. MicardisPlus once daily produces effective and smooth reductions in blood pressure across the therapeutic dose range.

Telmisartan is an orally effective and specific angiotensin II receptor subtype 1 (AT_1) antagonist. Telmisartan displaces angiotensin II with very high affinity from its binding site at the AT_1 receptor subtype, which is responsible for the known actions of angiotensin II. Telmisartan does not exhibit any partial agonist activity at the AT_1 receptor. Telmisartan selectively binds the AT_1 receptor. The binding is long-lasting. Telmisartan does not show affinity for other receptors, including AT_2 and other less characterised AT receptors. The functional role of these receptors is not known, nor is the effect of their possible overstimulation by angiotensin II, whose levels are increased by telmisartan. Plasma aldosterone levels are decreased by telmisartan. Telmisartan does not inhibit human plasma renin or block ion channels. Telmisartan does not inhibit angiotensin converting enzyme (kininase II), the enzyme which also degrades bradykinin. Therefore, it is not expected to potentiate bradykinin-mediated adverse effects.

An 80 mg dose of telmisartan administered to healthy volunteers almost completely inhibits the angiotensin II evoked blood pressure increase. The inhibitory effect is maintained over 24 hours and still measurable up to 48 hours.

After the first dose of telmisartan, the antihypertensive activity gradually becomes evident within 3 hours. The maximum reduction in blood pressure is generally attained 4-8 weeks after the start of treatment and is sustained during long-term therapy. The antihypertensive effect persists constantly over 24 hours after dosing and includes the last 4 hours before the next dose as shown by ambulatory blood pressure measurements. This is confirmed by measurements made at the point of maximum effect and immediately prior to the next dose (through to peak ratios consistently above 80 % after doses of 40 and 80 mg of telmisartan in placebo controlled clinical studies).

In patients with hypertension telmisartan reduces both systolic and diastolic blood pressure without affecting pulse rate. The antihypertensive efficacy of telmisartan is comparable to that of agents representative of other classes of antihypertensive medicinal products (demonstrated in clinical trials comparing telmisartan to amlodipine, atenolol, enalapril, hydrochlorothiazide, and lisinopril).

Upon abrupt cessation of treatment with telmisartan, blood pressure gradually returns to pre-treatment values over a period of several days without evidence of rebound hypertension.

The incidence of dry cough was significantly lower in patients treated with telmisartan than in those given angiotensin converting enzyme inhibitors in clinical trials directly comparing the two antihypertensive treatments.

In the "Prevention Regimen For Effectively avoiding Second Strokes" (PRoFESS) trial in patients 50 years and older, who recently experienced stroke, an increased incidence of sepsis was noted for telmisartan compared with placebo, 0.70 % vs. 0.49 % [RR 1.43 (95 % confidence interval 1.00 - 2.06)]; the incidence of fatal sepsis cases was increased for patients taking telmisartan (0.33 %) vs. patients taking placebo (0.16 %) [RR 2.07 (95 % confidence interval 1.14 - 3.76)]. The observed increased occurrence rate of sepsis associated with the use of telmisartan may be either a chance finding or related to a mechanism not currently known.

The effects of telmisartan on mortality and cardiovascular morbidity are currently unknown.

Hydrochlorothiazide is a thiazide diuretic. The mechanism of the antihypertensive effect of thiazide diuretics is not fully known. Thiazides have an effect on the renal tubular mechanisms of electrolyte reabsorption, directly increasing excretion of sodium and chloride in approximately equivalent amounts. The diuretic action of hydrochlorothiazide reduces plasma volume, increases plasma renin activity, increases aldosterone secretion, with consequent increases in urinary potassium and bicarbonate loss, and decreases in serum potassium. Presumably through blockade of the renin-angiotensin-aldosterone system, co-administration of telmisartan tends to reverse the potassium loss associated with these diuretics. With hydrochlorothiazide, onset of diuresis occurs in 2 hours, and peak effect occurs at about 4 hours, while the action persists for approximately 6-12 hours.

Epidemiological studies have shown that long-term treatment with hydrochlorothiazide reduces the risk of cardiovascular mortality and morbidity.

The effects of Fixed Dose Combination of telmisartan/HCTZ on mortality and cardiovascular morbidity are currently unknown.

5.2 Pharmacokinetic properties

Concomitant administration of hydrochlorothiazide and telmisartan does not appear to affect the pharmacokinetics of either substance in healthy subjects.

Absorption: Telmisartan: Following oral administration peak concentrations of telmisartan are reached in 0.5 – 1.5 h after dosing. The absolute bioavailability of telmisartan at 40 mg and 160 mg was 42 % and 58 %, respectively. Food slightly reduces the bioavailability of telmisartan with a reduction in the area under the plasma concentration time curve (AUC) of about 6 % with the 40 mg tablet and about 19 % after a 160 mg dose. By 3 hours after administration plasma concentrations are similar whether telmisartan is taken fasting or with food. The small reduction in AUC is not expected to cause a reduction in the therapeutic efficacy. The pharmacokinetics of orally administered telmisartan are non-linear over doses from 20 – 160 mg with greater than proportional increases of plasma concentrations (C_{max} and AUC) with increasing doses. Telmisartan does not accumulate significantly in plasma on repeated administration.

Hydrochlorothiazide: Following oral administration of MicardisPlus peak concentrations of hydrochlorothiazide are reached in approximately 1.0 – 3.0 hours after dosing. Based on cumulative renal excretion of hydrochlorothiazide the absolute bioavailability was about 60 %.

Distribution: Telmisartan is highly bound to plasma proteins (>99.5 %) mainly albumin and alpha l- acid glycoprotein. The apparent volume of distribution for telmisartan is approximately 500 litres indicating additional tissue binding.

Hydrochlorothiazide is 68 % protein bound in the plasma and its apparent volume of distribution is 0.83 – 1.14 l/kg.

Biotransformation and elimination: Telmisartan: Following either intravenous or oral administration of ^{14}C-labelled telmisartan most of the administered dose (>97 %) was eliminated in faeces via biliary excretion. Only minute amounts were found in urine. Telmisartan is metabolised by conjugation to form a pharmacologically inactive acylglucuronide. The glucuronide of the parent compound is the only metabolite that has been identified in humans. After a single dose of ^{14}C-labelled telmisartan the glucuronide represents approximately 11 % of the measured radioactivity in plasma. The cytochrome P450 isoenzymes are not involved in the metabolism of telmisartan. Total plasma clearance of telmisartan after oral administration is >1500 ml/min. Terminal elimination half-life was >20 hours.

Hydrochlorothiazide: Hydrochlorothiazide is not metabolised in man and is excreted almost entirely as unchanged substance in urine. About 60 % of the oral dose is eliminated as unchanged substance within 48 hours. Renal clearance is about 250 – 300 ml/min. The terminal elimination half-life of hydrochlorothiazide is 10 – 15 hours.

Special populations

Elderly patients: Pharmacokinetics of telmisartan do not differ between the elderly and those younger than 65 years.

Gender: Plasma concentrations of telmisartan are generally 2 – 3 times higher in females than in males. In clinical trials however, no significant increases in blood pressure response or in the incidence of orthostatic hypotension were found in women. No dosage adjustment is necessary. There was a trend towards higher plasma concentrations of hydrochlorothiazide in female than in male subjects. This is not considered to be of clinical relevance.

Patients with renal impairment: Renal excretion does not contribute to the clearance of telmisartan. Based on modest experience in patients with mild to moderate renal impairment (creatinine clearance of 30 – 60 ml/min, mean about 50 ml/min) no dosage adjustment is necessary in patients with decreased renal function. Telmisartan is not removed from blood by haemodialysis. In patients with impaired renal function the rate of hydrochlorothiazide elimination is reduced. In a typical study in patients with a mean creatinine clearance of 90 ml/min the elimination half-life of hydrochlorothiazide was increased. In functionally anephric patients the elimination half-life is about 34 hours.

Patients with hepatic impairment: Pharmacokinetic studies in patients with hepatic impairment showed an increase in absolute bioavailability up to nearly 100 %. The elimination half-life is not changed in patients with hepatic impairment.

5.3 Preclinical safety data

In preclinical safety studies performed with co-administration of telmisartan and hydrochlorothiazide in normotensive rats and dogs, doses producing exposure comparable to that in the clinical therapeutic range caused no additional findings not already observed with administration of either substance alone. The toxicological findings observed appear to have no relevance to human therapeutic use.

Toxicological findings also well known from preclinical studies with angiotensin converting enzyme inhibitors and angiotensin II receptor antagonists were: a reduction of red cell parameters (erythrocytes, haemoglobin, haematocrit), changes of renal haemodynamics (increased blood urea nitrogen and creatinine), increased plasma renin activity, hypertrophy/hyperplasia of the juxtaglomerular cells and gastric mucosal injury. Gastric lesions could be prevented/ameliorated by oral saline supplementation and group housing of animals. In dogs renal tubular dilation and atrophy were observed. These findings are considered to be due to the pharmacological activity of telmisartan.

Telmisartan showed no evidence of mutagenicity and relevant clastogenic activity in in vitro studies and no evidence of carcinogenicity in rats and mice. Studies with hydrochlorothiazide have shown equivocal evidence for a genotoxic or carcinogenic effect in some experimental models. However, the extensive human experience with hydrochlorothiazide has failed to show an association between its use and an increase in neoplasms.

For the foetotoxic potential of the telmisartan/hydrochlorothiazide combination see section 4.6.

6. PHARMACEUTICAL PARTICULARS

6.1 List of excipients

Lactose monohydrate

Magnesium stearate

Maize starch

Meglumine

Microcrystalline cellulose

Povidone (K25)

Red ferric oxide (E172)

Sodium hydroxide

Sodium starch glycollate (type A)

Sorbitol (E420).

6.2 Incompatibilities

Not applicable.

6.3 Shelf life

3 years

6.4 Special precautions for storage

This medicinal product does not require any special storage conditions. Store in the original package in order to protect from moisture.

6.5 Nature and contents of container

Aluminium/aluminium blisters (PA/Al/PVC/Al or PA/PA/Al/PVC/Al). One blister contains 7 or 10 tablets.

Pack sizes: Blister with 14, 28, 30, 56, 84, 90, or 98 tablets or perforated unit dose blisters with 28 × 1 tablets.

Not all pack sizes may be marketed.

6.6 Special precautions for disposal and other handling

Occasionally, the outer layer of the blister pack has been observed to separate from the inner layer between the blister pockets. No action needs to be taken if this is observed.

7. MARKETING AUTHORISATION HOLDER

Boehringer Ingelheim International GmbH

Binger Str. 173

D-55216 Ingelheim am Rhein

Germany

8. MARKETING AUTHORISATION NUMBER(S)

EU/1/02/213/001-005

EU/1/02/213/006-010

EU/1/02/213/011

EU/1/02/213/012

EU/1/02/213/013-014

EU/1/02/213/015-016

9. DATE OF FIRST AUTHORISATION/RENEWAL OF THE AUTHORISATION

Date of first authorisation:19 April 2002

Date of last renewal: 19 April 2007

10. DATE OF REVISION OF THE TEXT

29th May 2009

Legal Category

POM

MicardisPlus 80 mg/25 mg Tablets

(Boehringer Ingelheim Limited)

1. NAME OF THE MEDICINAL PRODUCT

MicardisPlus 80 mg/25 mg tablets

2. QUALITATIVE AND QUANTITATIVE COMPOSITION

Each tablet contains 80 mg telmisartan and 25 mg hydrochlorothiazide.

Excipients: Each tablet contains 99 mg of lactose monohydrate and 338 mg sorbitol (E420).

For a full list of excipients, see section 6.1.

3. PHARMACEUTICAL FORM

Tablet.

Yellow and white oval shaped tablet engraved with the company logo and the code 'H9'.

4. CLINICAL PARTICULARS

4.1 Therapeutic indications

Treatment of essential hypertension.

MicardisPlus fixed dose combination (80 mg telmisartan/25 mg hydrochlorothiazide) is indicated in patients whose blood pressure is not adequately controlled on MicardisPlus 80 mg/12.5 mg (80 mg telmisartan/12.5 mg hydrochlorothiazide) or patients who have been previously stabilised on telmisartan and hydrochlorothiazide given separately.

4.2 Posology and method of administration

Adults

MicardisPlus should be taken once daily with liquid, with or without food in patients whose blood pressure is not adequately controlled by telmisartan alone. Individual dose titration with each of the two components is recommended before changing to the fixed dose combination. When clinically appropriate, direct change from monotherapy to the fixed combination may be considered o

- MicardisPlus 80 mg/25 mg may be administered in patients whose blood pressure is not adequately controlled by MicardisPlus 80 mg/12.5 mg or in patients who have been previously stabilised on telmisartan and hydrochlorothiazide given separately.

MicardisPlus is also available at the dose strengths 40 mg/12.5 mg and 80 mg/ 12.5 mg

Renal impairment: Periodic monitoring of renal function is advised (see section 4.4).

Hepatic impairment: In patients with mild to moderate hepatic impairment the posology should not exceed MicardisPlus 40 mg/12.5 mg once daily. MicardisPlus is not indicated in patients with severe hepatic impairment. Thiazides should be used with caution in patients with impaired hepatic function (see section 4.4).

Elderly: No dosage adjustment is necessary.

Children and adolescents: MicardisPlus is not recommended for use in children below 18 years due to a lack of data on safety and efficacy.

4.3 Contraindications

- Hypersensitivity to any of the active substances or to any of the excipients (see section 6.1).
- Hypersensitivity to other sulphonamide-derived substances (since hydrochlorothiazide is a sulphonamide-derived medicinal product).
- Second and third trimesters of pregnancy (see section s 4.4 and 4.6).
- Cholestasis and biliary obstructive disorders.

• Severe hepatic impairment.

• Severe renal impairment (creatinine clearance <30 ml/min).

• Refractory hypokalaemia, hypercalcaemia.

4.4 Special warnings and precautions for use

Pregnancy

Angiotensin II receptor antagonists should not be initiated during pregnancy. Unless continued angiotensin II receptor antagonist therapy is considered essential, patients planning pregnancy should be changed to alternative antihypertensive treatments which have an established safety profile for use in pregnancy. When pregnancy is diagnosed, treatment with angiotensin II receptor antagonists should be stopped immediately, and, if appropriate, alternative therapy should be started (see sections 4.3 and 4.6).

Hepatic impairment: MicardisPlus should not be given to patients with cholestasis, biliary obstructive disorders or severe hepatic insufficiency (see section 4.3) since telmisartan is mostly eliminated with the bile. These patients can be expected to have reduced hepatic clearance for telmisartan.

In addition, MicardisPlus should be used with caution in patients with impaired hepatic function or progressive liver disease, since minor alterations of fluid and electrolyte balance may precipitate hepatic coma. There is no clinical experience with MicardisPlus in patients with hepatic impairment.

Renovascular hypertension: There is an increased risk of severe hypotension and renal insufficiency when patients with bilateral renal artery stenosis or stenosis of the artery to a single functioning kidney are treated with medicinal products that affect the renin-angiotensin-aldosterone system.

Renal impairment and kidney transplantation: MicardisPlus should not be used in patients with severe renal impairment (creatinine clearance <30 ml/min) (see section 4.3). There is no experience regarding the administration of MicardisPlus in patients with recent kidney transplantation. Experience with MicardisPlus is modest in the patients with mild to moderate renal impairment, therefore periodic monitoring of potassium, creatinine and uric acid serum levels is recommended. Thiazide diuretic-associated azotaemia may occur in patients with impaired renal function.

Intravascular hypovolaemia: Symptomatic hypotension, especially after the first dose, may occur in patients who are volume and/or sodium depleted by vigorous diuretic therapy, dietary salt restriction, diarrhoea or vomiting. Such conditions should be corrected before the administration of MicardisPlus.

Other conditions with stimulation of the renin-angiotensin-aldosterone system: In patients whose vascular tone and renal function depend predominantly on the activity of the renin-angiotensin-aldosterone system (e.g. patients with severe congestive heart failure or underlying renal disease, including renal artery stenosis), treatment with medicinal products that affect this system has been associated with acute hypotension, hyperazotaemia, oliguria, or rarely acute renal failure (see section 4.8).

Primary aldosteronism: Patients with primary aldosteronism generally will not respond to antihypertensive medicinal products acting through inhibition of the renin-angiotensin system. Therefore, the use of MicardisPlus is not recommended.

Aortic and mitral valve stenosis, obstructive hypertrophic cardiomyopathy: As with other vasodilators, special caution is indicated in patients suffering from aortic or mitral stenosis, or obstructive hypertrophic cardiomyopathy.

Metabolic and endocrine effects: Thiazide therapy may impair glucose tolerance. In diabetic patients dosage adjustments of insulin or oral hypoglycaemic agents may be required. Latent diabetes mellitus may become manifest during thiazide therapy.

An increase in cholesterol and triglyceride levels has been associated with thiazide diuretic therapy; however, at the 12.5 mg dose contained in MicardisPlus, minimal or no effects were reported.

Hyperuricaemia may occur or frank gout may be precipitated in some patients receiving thiazide therapy.

Electrolyte imbalance: As for any patient receiving diuretic therapy, periodic determination of serum electrolytes should be performed at appropriate intervals.

Thiazides, including hydrochlorothiazide, can cause fluid or electrolyte imbalance (including hypokalaemia, hyponatraemia, and hypochloraemic alkalosis). Warning signs of fluid or electrolyte imbalance are dryness of mouth, thirst, asthenia, lethargy, drowsiness, restlessness, muscle pain or cramps, muscular fatigue, hypotension, oliguria, tachycardia, and gastrointestinal disturbances such as nausea or vomiting (see section 4.8).

- Hypokalaemia

Although hypokalaemia may develop with the use of thiazide diuretics, concurrent therapy with telmisartan may reduce diuretic-induced hypokalaemia. The risk of hypokalaemia is greater in patients with cirrhosis of liver, in patients experiencing brisk diuresis, in patients who are receiving inadequate oral intake of electrolytes and in patients receiving concomitant therapy with corticosteroids or Adrenocorticotropic hormone (ACTH) (see section 4.5).

- Hyperkalaemia

Conversely, due to the antagonism of the angiotensin II (AT_1) receptors by the telmisartan component of MicardisPlus, hyperkalaemia might occur. Although clinically significant hyperkalaemia has not been documented with MicardisPlus, risk factors for the development of hyperkalaemia include renal insufficiency and/or heart failure, and diabetes mellitus. Potassium-sparing diuretics, potassium supplements or potassium-containing salt substitutes should be co-administered cautiously with MicardisPlus (see section 4.5).

- Hyponatraemia and hypochloraemic alkalosis

There is no evidence that MicardisPlus would reduce or prevent diuretic-induced hyponatraemia. Chloride deficit is generally mild and usually does not require treatment.

- Hypercalcaemia

Thiazides may decrease urinary calcium excretion and cause an intermittent and slight elevation of serum calcium in the absence of known disorders of calcium metabolism. Marked hypercalcaemia may be evidence of hidden hyperparathyroidism. Thiazides should be discontinued before carrying out tests for parathyroid function.

- Hypomagnesaemia

Thiazides have been shown to increase the urinary excretion of magnesium, which may result in hypomagnesaemia (see section 4.5).

Sorbitol and Lactose Monohydrate: This medicinal product contains lactose monohydrate and sorbitol. Patients with rare hereditary problems of fructose intolerance and/or with rare hereditary problems of galactose intolerance, the Lapp lactase deficiency or glucose-galactose malabsorption should not take this medicine.

Ethnic differences: As with all other angiotensin II receptor antagonists, telmisartan is apparently less effective in lowering blood pressure in black patients than in non blacks, possibly because of higher prevalence of low renin states in the black hypertensive population.

Other: As with any antihypertensive agent, excessive reduction of blood pressure in patients with ischaemic cardiopathy or ischaemic cardiovascular disease could result in a myocardial infarction or stroke.

General: Hypersensitivity reactions to hydrochlorothiazide may occur in patients with or without a history of allergy or bronchial asthma, but are more likely in patients with such a history.

Exacerbation or activation of systemic lupus erythematosus has been reported with the use of thiazide diuretics.

Cases of photosensitivity reactions have been reported with thiazide diuretics (see section 4.8). If a photosensitivity reaction occurs during treatment, it is recommended to stop the treatment. If a re-administration of the diuretic is deemed necessary, it is recommended to protect exposed areas to the sun or to artificial UVA.

4.5 Interaction with other medicinal products and other forms of interaction

Interaction studies have only been performed in adults.

Lithium: Reversible increases in serum lithium concentrations and toxicity have been reported during concomitant administration of lithium with angiotensin converting enzyme inhibitors. Rare cases have also been reported with angiotensin II receptor antagonists (including MicardisPlus). Co-administration of lithium and MicardisPlus is not recommended (see section 4.4). If this combination proves essential, careful monitoring of serum lithium level is recommended during concomitant use.

Medicinal products associated with potassium loss and hypokalaemia (e.g. other kaliuretic diuretics, laxatives, corticosteroids, ACTH, amphotericin, carbenoxolone, penicillin G sodium, salicylic acid and derivatives): If these substances are to be prescribed with the hydrochlorothiazide-telmisartan combination, monitoring of potassium plasma levels is advised. These medicinal products may potentiate the effect of hydrochlorothiazide on serum potassium (see section 4.4).

Medicinal products that may increase potassium levels or induce hyperkalaemia (e.g. ACE inhibitors, potassium-sparing diuretics, potassium supplements, salt substitutes containing potassium, cyclosporin or other medicinal products such as heparin sodium): If these medicinal products are to be prescribed with the hydrochlorothiazide-telmisartan combination, monitoring of potassium plasma levels is advised. Based on the experience with the use of other medicinal products that blunt the renin- angiotensin system, concomitant use of the above medicinal products may lead to increases in serum potassium and is, therefore, not recommended (see section 4.4).

Medicinal products affected by serum potassium disturbances: Periodic monitoring of serum potassium and ECG is recommended when MicardisPlus is administered with medicinal products affected by serum potassium disturbances (e.g. digitalis glycosides, antiarrhythmics) and the following torsades de pointes inducing medicinal products (which include some antiarrhythmics), hypokalaemia being a predisposing factor to torsades de pointes.

- class Ia antiarrythmics (e.g. quinidine, hydroquinidine, disopyramide)

- class III antiarrythmics (e.g. amiodarone, sotalol, dofetilide, ibutilide)

- some antipsychotics (e.g. thioridazine, chlorpromazine, levomepromazine, trifluoperazine, cyamemazine, sulpiride, sultopride, amisulpride, tiapride, pimozide, haloperidol, droperidol)

- others (e.g. bepridil, cisapride, diphemanil, erythromycin IV, halofantrin, mizolastin, pentamidine, sparfloxacine, terfenadine, vincamine IV.)

Digitalis glycosides: Thiazide-induced hypokalaemia or hypomagnesaemia favours the onset of digitalis-induced arrhythmia (see section 4.4).

Other antihypertensive agents: Telmisartan may increase the hypotensive effect of other antihypertensive agents.

Antidiabetic medicinal products (oral agents and insulin): Dosage adjustment of the antidiabetic medicinal products may be required (see section 4.4).

Metformin: Metformin should be used with precaution: risk of lactic acidosis induced by a possible functional renal failure linked to hydrochlorothiazide.

Cholestyramine and colestipol resins: Absorption of hydrochlorothiazide is impaired in the presence of anionic exchange resins.

Non-steroidal anti-inflammatory medicinal products: NSAIDs (i.e. acetylsalicylic acid at anti-inflammatory dosage regimens, COX-2 inhibitors and non-selective NSAIDs) may reduce the diuretic, natriuretic and antihypertensive effects of thiazide diuretics and the antihypertensive effects of angiotensin II receptor antagonists.

In some patients with compromised renal function (e.g. dehydrated patients or elderly patients with compromised renal function) the co-administration of angiotensin II receptor antagonists and agents that inhibit cyclo-oxygenase may result in further deterioration of renal function, including possible acute renal failure, which is usually reversible. Therefore the combination should be administered with caution, especially in the elderly. Patients should be adequately hydrated and consideration should be given to monitoring of renal function after initiation of concomitant therapy and periodically thereafter.

Pressor amines (e.g. noradrenaline): The effect of pressor amines may be decreased.

Nondepolarizing skeletal muscle relaxants (e.g. tubocurarine): The effect of nondepolarizing skeletal muscle relaxants may be potentiated by hydrochlorothiazide.

Medicinal products used in the treatment for gout (e.g. probenecid, sulfinpyrazone and allopurinol): Dosage adjustment of uricosuric medications may be necessary as hydrochlorothiazide may raise the level of serum uric acid. Increase in dosage of probenecid or sulfinpyrazone may be necessary. Co-administration of thiazide may increase the incidence of hypersensitivity reactions of allopurinol.

Calcium salts: Thiazide diuretics may increase serum calcium levels due to the decreased excretion. If calcium supplements must be prescribed, serum calcium levels should be monitored and calcium dosage adjusted accordingly.

Beta-blockers and diazoxide: The hyperglycaemic effect of beta-blockers and diazoxide may be enhanced by thiazides.

Anticholinergic agents (e.g. atropine, biperiden) may increase the bioavailability of thiazide-type diuretics by decreasing gastrointestinal motility and stomach emptying rate.

Amantadine: Thiazides may increase the risk of adverse effects caused by amantadine.

Cytotoxic agents (e.g. cyclophosphamide, methotrexate): Thiazides may reduce the renal excretion of cytotoxic medicinal products and potentiate their myelosuppressive effects.

Based on their pharmacological properties it can be expected that the following medicinal product may potentiate the hypotensive effects of all antihypertensives including telmisartan: Baclofen, amifostine.

Furthermore, orthostatic hypotension may be aggravated by alcohol, barbiturates, narcotics or antidepressants.

4.6 Pregnancy and lactation

Pregnancy:

The use of angiotensin II receptor antagonists is not recommended during the first trimester of pregnancy (see section 4.4). The use of angiotensin II receptor antagonists is contraindicated during the second and third trimesters of pregnancy (see sections 4.3 and 4.4).

There are no adequate data from the use of MicardisPlus in pregnant women. Studies in animals have shown reproductive toxicity (see section 5.3).

Epidemiological evidence regarding the risk of teratogenicity following exposure to ACE inhibitors during the first trimester of pregnancy has not been conclusive; however a small increase in risk cannot be excluded. Whilst there is no controlled epidemiological data on the risk with angiotensin II receptor antagonists, similar risks may exist for this class of drugs. Unless continued angiotensin II receptor antagonist therapy is considered essential, patients planning pregnancy should be changed to alternative antihypertensive treatments which have an established safety profile for use in pregnancy. When pregnancy is diagnosed, treatment with angiotensin II receptor antagonists should be stopped immediately, and, if appropriate, alternative therapy should be started.

Exposure to angiotensin II receptor antagonist therapy during the second and third trimesters is known to induce human fetotoxicity (decreased renal function, oligohydramnios, skull ossification retardation) and neonatal toxicity (renal failure, hypotension, hyperkalaemia). (See section 5.3).

Should exposure to angiotensin II receptor antagonists have occurred from the second trimester of pregnancy, ultrasound check of renal function and skull is recommended.

Infants whose mothers have taken angiotensin II receptor antagonists should be closely observed for hypotension (see sections 4.3 and 4.4).

Thiazides cross the placental barrier and appear in cord blood. They may cause foetal electrolyte disturbances and possibly other reactions that have occurred in the adults. Cases of neonatal thrombocytopenia, of foetal or neonatal jaundice have been reported with maternal thiazide therapy.

Lactation:

Because no information is available regarding the use of MicardisPlus during breast-feeding, MicardisPlus is not recommended and alternative treatments with better established safety profiles during breast-feeding are preferable, especially while nursing a newborn or preterm infant. Thiazides appear in human milk and may inhibit lactation.

4.7 Effects on ability to drive and use machines

No studies on the effect on the ability to drive and use machines have been performed. However, when driving vehicles or operating machinery it should be taken into account that dizziness or drowsiness may occasionally occur when taking antihypertensive therapy.

4.8 Undesirable effects

Fixed Dose Combination

The overall incidence and pattern of adverse events reported with MicardisPlus 80 mg/25 mg was comparable with MicardisPlus 80 mg/12.5 mg. A dose-relationship of undesirable effects was not established and they showed no correlation with gender, age or race of the patients.

Adverse reactions reported in all clinical trials and occurring more frequently ($p \leq 0.05$) with telmisartan plus hydrochlorothiazide than with placebo are shown below according to system organ class. Adverse reactions known to occur with each component given singly but which have not been seen in clinical trials may occur during treatment with MicardisPlus.

Adverse reactions have been ranked under headings of frequency using the following convention:

very common ($\geq 1/10$); common ($\geq 1/100$ to $< 1/10$); uncommon ($\geq 1/1,000$ to $< 1/100$); rare ($\geq 1/10,000$ to $< 1/1,000$); very rare ($< 1/10,000$), not known (cannot be estimated from the available data).

Within each frequency grouping, adverse reactions are presented in order of decreasing seriousness.

Infections and infestations	
Rare:	Bronchitis
Not known:	Pharyngitis, sinusitis
Metabolism and nutrition disorders	
Uncommon:	Hypokalaemia,
Rare:	Hyperuricaemia, hyponatraemia
Psychiatric disorders	
Uncommon:	Anxiety
Rare:	Depression
Nervous system disorders	
Common:	Dizziness
Uncommon:	Syncope, paraesthesia
Rare:	Insomnia, sleep disorders
Eye disorders	
Rare:	Visual disturbance, vision blurred
Ear and labyrinth disorders	
Uncommon:	Vertigo
Cardiac disorders	
Uncommon:	Tachycardia, arrhythmias
Vascular disorders	
Uncommon:	Hypotension, orthostatic hypotension
Respiratory, thoracic and mediastinal disorders	
Uncommon:	Dyspnoea
Rare:	Respiratory distress (including pneumonitis and pulmonary oedema)
Gastrointestinal disorders	
Uncommon:	Diarrhoea, dry mouth, flatulence
Rare:	Abdominal pain, constipation, dyspepsia, vomiting
Not known:	Gastritis
Hepatobiliary disorders	
Rare:	Abnormal hepatic function/liver disorder
Skin and subcutaneous tissue disorders	
Rare:	Angioedema, erythema, pruritus, rash, hyperhidrosis, urticaria
Muscoloskeletal, connective tissue and bone disorders	
Uncommon:	Back pain, muscle spasms, myalgia
Rare:	Arthralgia, muscle cramps, pain in limb
Reproductive system and breast disorders	
Uncommon:	Erectile dysfunction
General disorders and administration site conditions	
Uncommon:	Chest pain
Rare:	Influenza-like illness, pain
Investigations	
Uncommon:	Blood uric acid increased
Rare:	Blood creatinine increased, blood creatine phosphokinase increased, hepatic enzyme increased

Additional information on individual components

Undesirable effects previously reported with one of the individual components may be potential undesirable effects with MicardisPlus, even if not observed in clinical trials with this product.

Telmisartan:

Undesirable effects occurred with similar frequency in placebo and telmisartan treated patients.

The overall incidence of adverse events reported with telmisartan (41.4 %) was usually comparable to placebo (43.9 %) in placebo controlled trials. The following adverse drug reactions listed below have been accumulated from all clinical trials in patients treated with telmisartan for hypertension or in patients 50 years or older at high risk of cardiovascular events.

Adverse reactions of unknown frequency reported with the use of telmisartan alone include:

Infections and infestations	
Not known:	Upper respiratory tract infection, urinary tract infection including cystitis, sepsis including fatal outcome*
Blood and lymphatic system disorders	
Not known:	Eosinophilia, anaemia, thrombocytopenia
Immune system disorders	
Not known:	Hypersensitivity, anaphylactic reactions
Metabolism and nutrition disorders	
Not known:	Hyperkalaemia
Cardiac disorders	
Not known:	Bradycardia
Gastrointestinal disorders	
Not known:	Stomach discomfort
Skin and subcutaneous tissue disorders	
Not known:	Eczema, drug eruption, toxic skin eruption
Musculoskeletal, connective tissue and bone disorders	
Not known:	Arthrosis, tendon pain
Renal and urinary disorders	
Not known:	Renal dysfunction, renal impairment (including acute renal failure)
General disorders and administration site conditions	
Not known:	Asthenia, drug ineffective
Investigations	
Not known:	Haemoglobin decreased

*In the PRoFESS trial, an increased incidence of sepsis was observed with telmisartan compared with placebo. The event may be a chance finding or related to a mechanism currently not known (see section 5.1).

Hydrochlorothiazide:

Hydrochlorothiazide may cause or exacerbate hypovolaemia which could lead to electrolyte imbalance (see section 4.4).

Adverse reactions of unknown frequency reported with the use of hydrochlorothiazide alone include:

Infections and infestations	
Not known:	Sialoadenitis
Blood and lymphatic system disorders	
Not known:	Anaemia aplastic, haemolytic anaemia, bone marrow failure, leukopenia, neutropenia, agranulocytosis, thrombocytopenia
Immune system disorders	
Not known:	Anaphylactic reactions, hypersensitivity
Endocrine disorders	
Not known:	Diabetes mellitus inadequate control
Metabolism and nutrition disorders	
Not known:	Anorexia, appetite decreased, electrolyte imbalance, hypercholesterolaemia, hyperglycaemia, hypovolaemia
Psychiatric disorders	
Not known:	Restlessness
Nervous system disorders	
Not known:	Light-headedness
Eye disorders	
Not known:	Xanthopsia
Vascular disorders	
Not known:	Vasculitis necrotizing
Gastrointestinal disorders	
Not known:	Pancreatitis, stomach discomfort
Hepatobiliary disorders	
Not known:	Jaundice hepatocellular, jaundice cholestatic
Skin and subcutaneous tissue disorders	
Not known:	Lupus-like syndrome, photosensitivity reactions, skin vasculitis, toxic epidermal necrolysis
Musculoskeletal, connective tissue and bone disorders	
Not known:	Weakness
Renal and urinary disorders	
Not known:	Nephritis interstitial, renal dysfunction, glycosuria
General disorders and administration site conditions	
Not known:	Pyrexia
Investigations	
Not known:	Triglycerides increased

4.9 Overdose

There is limited information available for telmisartan with regard to overdose in humans. The degree to which hydrochlorothiazide is removed by haemodialysis has not been established.

Symptoms: The most prominent manifestations of telmisartan overdose were hypotension and tachycardia; bradycardia, dizziness, vomiting, increase in serum creatinine, and acute renal failure have also been reported. Overdose with hydrochlorothiazide is associated with electrolyte depletion (hypokalaemia, hypochloraemia) and hypovolaemia resulting from excessive diuresis. The most common signs and symptoms of overdose are nausea and somnolence. Hypokalaemia may result in muscle spasms and/or accentuate arrhythmia associated with the concomitant use of digitalis glycosides or certain anti-arrhythmic medicinal products.

Treatment: Telmisartan is not removed by haemodialysis. The patient should be closely monitored, and the treatment should be symptomatic and supportive. Management depends on the time since ingestion and the severity of the symptoms. Suggested measures include induction of emesis and/or gastric lavage. Activated charcoal may be useful in the treatment of overdose. Serum electrolytes and creatinine should be monitored frequently. If hypotension occurs, the patient should be placed in a supine position, with salt and volume replacements given quickly.

5. PHARMACOLOGICAL PROPERTIES

5.1 Pharmacodynamic properties

Pharmacotherapeutic group: Angiotensin II receptor antagonists and diuretics, ATC code: C09DA07

MicardisPlus is a combination of an angiotensin II receptor antagonist, telmisartan, and a thiazide diuretic, hydrochlorothiazide. The combination of these ingredients has an additive antihypertensive effect, reducing blood pressure to a greater degree than either component alone. MicardisPlus once daily produces effective and smooth reductions in blood pressure across the therapeutic dose range.

Telmisartan is an orally effective and specific angiotensin II receptor subtype 1 (AT_1) antagonist. Telmisartan displaces angiotensin II with very high affinity from its binding site at the AT_1 receptor subtype, which is responsible for the known actions of angiotensin II. Telmisartan does not exhibit any partial agonist activity at the AT_1 receptor. Telmisartan selectively binds the AT_1 receptor. The binding is long-lasting. Telmisartan does not show affinity for other receptors, including AT_2 and other less characterised AT receptors. The functional role of these receptors is not known, nor is the effect of their possible overstimulation by angiotensin II, whose levels are increased by telmisartan. Plasma aldosterone levels are decreased by telmisartan. Telmisartan does not inhibit human plasma renin or block ion channels. Telmisartan does not inhibit angiotensin converting enzyme (kininase II), the enzyme which also degrades bradykinin. Therefore, it is not expected to potentiate bradykinin-mediated adverse effects.

An 80 mg dose of telmisartan administered to healthy volunteers almost completely inhibits the angiotensin II evoked blood pressure increase. The inhibitory effect is maintained over 24 hours and still measurable up to 48 hours.

After the first dose of telmisartan, the antihypertensive activity gradually becomes evident within 3 hours. The maximum reduction in blood pressure is generally attained 4-8 weeks after the start of treatment and is sustained during long-term therapy. The antihypertensive effect persists constantly over 24 hours after dosing and includes the last 4 hours before the next dose as shown by ambulatory blood pressure measurements. This is confirmed by measurements made at the point of maximum effect and immediately prior to the next dose (through to peak ratios consistently above 80 % after doses of 40 and 80 mg of telmisartan in placebo controlled clinical studies).

In patients with hypertension telmisartan reduces both systolic and diastolic blood pressure without affecting pulse rate. The antihypertensive efficacy of telmisartan is comparable to that of agents representative of other classes of antihypertensive medicinal products (demonstrated in clinical trials comparing telmisartan to amlodipine, atenolol, enalapril, hydrochlorothiazide, and lisinopril).

In a double-blind controlled clinical trial (n=687 patients evaluated for efficacy) in non-responders to the 80 mg/12.5 mg combination, an incremental blood pressure lowering effect of the 80 mg/25 mg combination compared to continued treatment with the 80 mg/12.5 mg combination of 2.7/1.6 mm Hg (SBP/DBP) was demonstrated (difference in adjusted mean changes from baseline). In a follow-up trial with the 80 mg/25 mg combination, blood pressure was further decreased (resulting in an overall reduction of 11.5/9.9 mm Hg (SBP/DBP).

In a pooled analysis of two similar 8 week double-blind placebo-controlled clinical trials vs. valsartan/hydrochlorothiazide 160 mg/25 mg (n=2121 patients evaluated for efficacy) a significantly greater blood pressure lowering effect of 2.2/1.2 mm Hg (SBP/DBP) was demonstrated (difference in adjusted mean changes from baseline, respectively) in favour of telmisartan/hydrochlorothiazide 80 mg/25 mg combination.

Upon abrupt cessation of treatment with telmisartan, blood pressure gradually returns to pre-treatment values over a period of several days without evidence of rebound hypertension.

The incidence of dry cough was significantly lower in patients treated with telmisartan than in those given angiotensin converting enzyme inhibitors in clinical trials directly comparing the two antihypertensive treatments.

In the "Prevention Regimen For Effectively avoiding Second Strokes" (PRoFESS) trial in patients 50 years and older, who recently experienced stroke, an increased incidence of sepsis was noted for telmisartan compared with placebo, 0.70 % vs. 0.49 % [RR 1.43 (95 % confidence interval 1.00 - 2.06)]; the incidence of fatal sepsis cases was increased for patients taking telmisartan (0.33 %) vs. patients taking placebo (0.16 %) [RR 2.07 (95 % confidence interval 1.14 - 3.76)]. The observed increased occurrence rate of sepsis associated with the use of telmisartan may be either a chance finding or related to a mechanism not currently known.

The effects of telmisartan on mortality and cardiovascular morbidity are currently unknown.

Hydrochlorothiazide is a thiazide diuretic. The mechanism of the antihypertensive effect of thiazide diuretics is not fully known. Thiazides have an effect on the renal tubular mechanisms of electrolyte reabsorption, directly increasing excretion of sodium and chloride in approximately equivalent amounts. The diuretic action of hydrochlorothiazide reduces plasma volume, increases plasma renin activity, increases aldosterone secretion, with consequent increases in urinary potassium and bicarbonate loss, and decreases in serum potassium. Presumably through blockade of the renin-angiotensin-aldosterone system, co-administration of telmisartan tends to reverse the potassium loss associated with these diuretics. With hydrochlorothiazide, onset of diuresis occurs in 2 hours, and peak effect occurs at about 4 hours, while the action persists for approximately 6-12 hours.

Epidemiological studies have shown that long-term treatment with hydrochlorothiazide reduces the risk of cardiovascular mortality and morbidity.

The effects of Fixed Dose Combination of telmisartan/HCTZ on mortality and cardiovascular morbidity are currently unknown.

5.2 Pharmacokinetic properties

Concomitant administration of hydrochlorothiazide and telmisartan does not appear to affect the pharmacokinetics of either substance in healthy subjects.

Absorption: Telmisartan: Following oral administration peak concentrations of telmisartan are reached in 0.5 – 1.5 h after dosing. The absolute bioavailability of telmisartan at 40 mg and 160 mg was 42 % and 58 %, respectively. Food slightly reduces the bioavailability of telmisartan with a reduction in the area under the plasma concentration time curve (AUC) of about 6 % with the 40 mg tablet and about 19 % after a 160 mg dose. By 3 hours after administration plasma concentrations are similar whether telmisartan is taken fasting or with food. The small reduction in AUC is not expected to cause a reduction in the therapeutic efficacy. The pharmacokinetics of orally administered telmisartan are non-linear over doses from 20 – 160 mg with greater than proportional increases of plasma concentrations (C_{max} and AUC) with increasing doses. Telmisartan does not accumulate significantly in plasma on repeated administration.

Hydrochlorothiazide: Following oral administration of MicardisPlus peak concentrations of hydrochlorothiazide are reached in approximately 1.0 – 3.0 hours after dosing. Based on cumulative renal excretion of hydrochlorothiazide the absolute bioavailability was about 60 %.

Distribution: Telmisartan is highly bound to plasma proteins (>99.5 %) mainly albumin and alpha I- acid glycoprotein. The apparent volume of distribution for telmisartan is approximately 500 litres indicating additional tissue binding.

Hydrochlorothiazide is 68 % protein bound in the plasma and its apparent volume of distribution is 0.83 – 1.14 1/kg.

Biotransformation and elimination: Telmisartan: Following either intravenous or oral administration of ^{14}C-labelled telmisartan most of the administered dose (>97 %) was eliminated in faeces via biliary excretion. Only minute amounts were found in urine. Telmisartan is metabolised by conjugation to form a pharmacologically inactive acylglucuronide. The glucuronide of the parent compound is the only metabolite that has been identified in humans. After a single dose of ^{14}C-labelled telmisartan the glucuronide represents approximately 11 % of the measured radioactivity in plasma. The cytochrome P450 isoenzymes are not involved in the metabolism of telmisartan. Total plasma clearance of telmisartan after oral administration is >1500 ml/min. Terminal elimination half-life was >20 hours.

Hydrochlorothiazide: Hydrochlorothiazide is not metabolised in man and is excreted almost entirely as unchanged substance in urine. About 60 % of the oral dose is eliminated as unchanged substance within 48 hours. Renal clearance is about 250 – 300 ml/min. The terminal elimination half-life of hydrochlorothiazide is 10 – 15 hours.

Special populations

Elderly patients: Pharmacokinetics of telmisartan do not differ between the elderly and those younger than 65 years.

Gender: Plasma concentrations of telmisartan are generally 2 – 3 times higher in females than in males. In clinical trials however, no significant increases in blood pressure response or in the incidence of orthostatic hypotension were found in women. No dosage adjustment is necessary. There was a trend towards higher plasma concentrations of hydrochlorothiazide in female than in male subjects. This is not considered to be of clinical relevance.

Patients with renal impairment: Renal excretion does not contribute to the clearance of telmisartan. Based on modest experience in patients with mild to moderate renal impairment (creatinine clearance of 30 – 60 ml/min, mean about 50 ml/min) no dosage adjustment is necessary in patients with decreased renal function. Telmisartan is not removed from blood by haemodialysis. In patients with impaired renal function the rate of hydrochlorothiazide elimination is reduced. In a typical study in patients with a mean creatinine clearance of 90 ml/min the elimination half-life of hydrochlorothiazide was increased. In functionally anephric patients the elimination half-life is about 34 hours.

Patients with hepatic impairment: Pharmacokinetic studies in patients with hepatic impairment showed an increase in absolute bioavailability up to nearly 100 %. The elimination half-life is not changed in patients with hepatic impairment.

5.3 Preclinical safety data

No additional preclinical studies have been performed with the Fixed Dose Combination product 80 mg/25 mg. Previous preclinical safety studies performed with co-administration of telmisartan and hydrochlorothiazide in normotensive rats and dogs, in doses producing exposure comparable to that in the clinical therapeutic range, caused no additional findings not already observed with administration of either substance alone. The toxicological findings observed appear to have no relevance to human therapeutic use.

Toxicological findings also well known from preclinical studies with angiotensin converting enzyme inhibitors and angiotensin II receptor antagonists were: a reduction of red cell parameters (erythrocytes, haemoglobin, haematocrit), changes of renal haemodynamics (increased blood urea nitrogen and creatinine), increased plasma renin activity, hypertrophy/hyperplasia of the juxtaglomerular cells and gastric mucosal injury. Gastric lesions could be prevented/ameliorated by oral saline supplementation and group housing of animals. In dogs renal tubular dilation and atrophy were observed. These findings are considered to be due to the pharmacological activity of telmisartan.

Telmisartan showed no evidence of mutagenicity and relevant clastogenic activity in in vitro studies and no evidence of carcinogenicity in rats and mice. Studies with hydrochlorothiazide have shown equivocal evidence for a genotoxic or carcinogenic effect in some experimental models. However, the extensive human experience with hydrochlorothiazide has failed to show an association between its use and an increase in neoplasms.

For the foetotoxic potential of the telmisartan/hydrochlorothiazide combination see section 4.6.

6. PHARMACEUTICAL PARTICULARS

6.1 List of excipients

Lactose monohydrate

Magnesium stearate

Maize starch

Meglumine

Microcrystalline cellulose

Povidone (K25)

Yellow ferric oxide (E172)

Sodium hydroxide

Sodium starch glycollate (type A)

Sorbitol (E420).

6.2 Incompatibilities

Not applicable.

6.3 Shelf life

3 years

6.4 Special precautions for storage

This medicinal product does not require any special storage conditions. Store in the original package in order to protect from moisture.

6.5 Nature and contents of container

Aluminium/aluminium blisters (PA/Al/PVC/Al or PA/PA/Al/PVC/Al). One blister contains 7 or 10 tablets.

Pack sizes: blister with 14, 28, 30, 56, 90, or 98 tablets or perforated unit dose blisters with 28 × 1 tablets

Not all pack sizes may be marketed.

6.6 Special precautions for disposal and other handling

Occasionally, the outer layer of the blister pack has been observed to separate from the inner layer between the blister pockets. No action needs to be taken if this is observed.

7. MARKETING AUTHORISATION HOLDER

Boehringer Ingelheim International GmbH

Binger Str. 173

D-55216 Ingelheim am Rhein

Germany

8. MARKETING AUTHORISATION NUMBER(S)

EU/1/02/213/017-023

9. DATE OF FIRST AUTHORISATION/RENEWAL OF THE AUTHORISATION

Date of first authorisation:19 April 2002

Date of last renewal: 19 April 2007

10. DATE OF REVISION OF THE TEXT

29th May 2009

Legal Category

POM

Micralax Micro-Enema

(UCB Pharma Limited)

1. NAME OF THE MEDICINAL PRODUCT

Micralax Micro-enema

2. QUALITATIVE AND QUANTITATIVE COMPOSITION

Sodium alkylsulphoacetate 0.90% w/v; sodium citrate BP 9.0% w/v

3. PHARMACEUTICAL FORM

A colourless viscous liquid

4. CLINICAL PARTICULARS

4.1 Therapeutic indications

Micralax is indicated whenever an enema is necessary to relieve constipation: in dyschezia, especially in bedridden patients; in geriatrics, paediatrics and obstetrics; and in preparation for X-ray examination, proctoscopy and sigmoidoscopy.

4.2 Posology and method of administration

Adults and children aged 3 years and over: Administer the contents of one micro-enema rectally, inserting the full length of the nozzle. No lubricant is needed as a drop of the mixture is sufficient.

4.3 Contraindications

Do not use in patients with inflammatory bowel disease.

4.4 Special warnings and precautions for use

None.

4.5 Interaction with other medicinal products and other forms of interaction

None.

4.6 Pregnancy and lactation

No special recommendations.

4.7 Effects on ability to drive and use machines

None.

4.8 Undesirable effects
No side effects have been reported. Excessive use may cause diarrhoea and fluid loss, which should be treated symptomatically.

4.9 Overdose
Not applicable.

5. PHARMACOLOGICAL PROPERTIES

5.1 Pharmacodynamic properties
Micralax combines the action of sodium citrate, a peptidising agent which can displace bound water present in the faeces; sorbitol, which enhances this action, and sodium alkylsulphoacetate, a wetting agent.

5.2 Pharmacokinetic properties
Not applicable.

5.3 Preclinical safety data
Not applicable.

6. PHARMACEUTICAL PARTICULARS

6.1 List of excipients
Sorbitol Solution 70% w/v BP, Glycerin PhEur, Sorbic Acid BP and Purified Water PhEur.

6.2 Incompatibilities
None.

6.3 Shelf life
60 months.

6.4 Special precautions for storage
Store at a temperature not exceeding 25°C.

6.5 Nature and contents of container
Polythene micro-enema tubes, capped, and with elongated nozzles.

6.6 Special precautions for disposal and other handling
Micralax usually works within 5 to 15 minutes, so make sure you are near a toilet before using it.

Always use a fresh tube of Micralax every time.

1. Lie down on your side with your knees drawn up towards your tummy or, if you prefer, sit on the toilet.

2. Pull or twist the black cap off the tube.

3. If you want to lubricate the nozzle before inserting it, squeeze a drop of liquid out onto the nozzle.

4. Insert the full length of the nozzle into your back passage.

5. Gently squeeze the tube until it is empty.

6. **Keep squeezing**
the tube as you pull the nozzle out of your back passage. This is to stop the medicine being drawn back into the tube.

7. Wait for the laxative to work (5-15 minutes)

7. MARKETING AUTHORISATION HOLDER
UCB Pharma Limited
208 Bath Road
Slough
Berkshire
SL1 3WE
UK

8. MARKETING AUTHORISATION NUMBER(S)
PL 00039/0368

9. DATE OF FIRST AUTHORISATION/RENEWAL OF THE AUTHORISATION
28 June 1991/28 May 1997

10. DATE OF REVISION OF THE TEXT
June 2005
P

Micronor Oral Contraceptive Tablets

(Janssen-Cilag Ltd)

1. NAME OF THE MEDICINAL PRODUCT
Micronor Oral Contraceptive Tablets

2. QUALITATIVE AND QUANTITATIVE COMPOSITION
Each tablet contains norethisterone 0.35 mg.

3. PHARMACEUTICAL FORM
Small, round, white tablet, engraved C035 on both faces.

4. CLINICAL PARTICULARS

4.1 Therapeutic indications
Oral contraceptive.

4.2 Posology and method of administration
For oral administration.

Adults:
Tablet intake from the first pack is started on the first day of menstruation; no extra contraceptive precautions are necessary.

One tablet is taken at the same time each day, every day of the year, whether menstruation occurs or not.

Elderly:
Not applicable.

Children:
Not recommended.

4.3 Contraindications
- Existing thrombophlebitis
- Existing thrombo-embolic disorders
- Cerebrovascular disease or a past history of this condition
- Myocardial infarction or a past history of this condition
- Markedly impaired liver function
- Known or suspected hormone dependent neoplasia
- Known or suspected carcinoma of the breast
- Undiagnosed abnormal genital tract bleeding
- Known or suspected pregnancy
- Cholestatic jaundice of pregnancy or jaundice with prior pill use
- Hepatic adenomas or carcinomas

4.4 Special warnings and precautions for use
There is a general opinion, based on statistic evidence, that users of combined oral contraceptives (ie oestrogen plus progestogen) experience more often than non-users various disorders of the circulation of blood, including strokes (blood clots in, and haemorrhages from, the blood vessels of the brain), heart attacks (coronary thromboses) and blood clots obstructing the arteries of the lungs (pulmonary emboli). There may not be a full recovery from such disorders and it should be realised that in a few cases they may be fatal.

To date no association between these disorders and progestogen-only oral contraceptives (such as Micronor Oral Contraceptive Tablets) has been shown. However there is a risk that the users of such progestogen only oral contraceptives will (like users of the combined oral contraceptive) be exposed to an increased risk of suffering from these disorders.

Reasons for stopping oral contraceptives immediately
- Early manifestations of thrombotic or thrombo-embolic disorders, thrombophlebitis
- Cerebrovascular disorders (including haemorrhage)
- Myocardial infarction
- Pulmonary embolism
- Gradual or sudden, partial or complete loss of vision
- Proptosis or diplopia
- Onset or aggravation of migraine or development of headaches of a new pattern which are recurrent, persistent or severe
- Papilloedema or any evidence of retinal vascular lesions
- During periods of immobility (eg after accidents)
- Pregnancy
- Manifestations of liver tumours

Assessment of women prior to starting oral contraceptives (and at regular intervals thereafter) should include a personal and family medical history of each woman. Physical examination should be guided by this and by the contraindications (Section 4.3) and warnings (Section 4.4) for this product. The frequency and nature of these assessments should be based upon relevant guidelines and should be adapted to the individual woman, but should include measurement of blood pressure and, if judged appropriate by the clinician, breast, abdominal and pelvic examination including cervical cytology.

Because of a possible increased risk of post surgery thrombo-embolic complications in oral contraceptive users, therapy should be discontinued six weeks prior to elective surgery.

When Micronor is administered during the post-partum period, the increased risk of thrombo-embolic disease associated with the post-partum period must be considered.

The following are some of the medical conditions reported to be influenced by the combined pill, and may be affected by Micronor. The physician will have to exercise medical judgement to commence, continue or discontinue therapy as appropriate. The worsening or first appearance of any of these conditions may indicate that Micronor should be discontinued.

1. Pre-existing uterine fibromyomata may increase in size.

2. A decrease in glucose tolerance in a significant number of women.

3. An increase in blood pressure in a small but significant number of women.

4. Cholestatic jaundice. Patients with a history of cholestatic jaundice of pregnancy are more likely to develop cholestatic jaundice during oral contraceptive therapy.

5. Amenorrhoea during and after oral contraceptive therapy. Temporary infertility after discontinuation of treatment.

6. Depression.

7. Fluid retention. Conditions which might be influenced by this factor including epilepsy, migraine, asthma, cardiac or renal dysfunction.

8. Varicose veins.

9. Multiple sclerosis.

10. Porphyria.

11. Tetany.

12. Intolerance to contact lenses.

Or any condition that is prone to worsening during pregnancy.

Ectopic pregnancy
Pregnancies in progestogen-only pill (POP) users are more likely to be ectopic than are pregnancies occurring in the general population, since POPs offer less protection against ectopic pregnancy than against intra-uterine pregnancy.

Changing from another oral contraceptive
Start Micronor on the day following completion of the previous oral contraceptive pack without a break (or, in the case of the ED pill, omitting the inactive pills). No extra contraceptive precautions are required.

Post-partum administration
Micronor can be started on the 21st day after childbirth. This will ensure the patient is protected immediately. If there is any delay in taking the first dose, contraception may not be established until 7 days after the first tablet has been taken. In these circumstances, patients should be advised that extra contraceptive precautions (non-hormonal methods) are necessary.

After miscarriage or abortion
Patients can take Micronor on the day after miscarriage or abortion, in which case no additional contraceptive precautions are required.

Missed tablets
If a tablet is missed within 3 hours of the correct dosage time, then the missed tablet should be taken as soon as possible; this will ensure that contraceptive protection is maintained. If one (for longer than 3 hours) or more tablets are missed, it is recommended that the patient takes the last missed tablet as soon as possible and continues to take the rest of the tablets as usual. Additional means of contraception (non-hormonal) should be used for the next seven days.

If the patient does not have a period within 45 days of her last period, Micronor should be discontinued and pregnancy should be excluded.

Vomiting and diarrhoea
Additional contraceptive measures (non-hormonal) should be employed during the period of gastro-intestinal upset and for the next seven days.

Laboratory tests
The following laboratory determinations may be altered in patients using oral contraceptives.

Hepatic: increased BSP retention and other tests.

Coagulation: increased prothrombin, factors VII, VIII, IX and X, decreased antithrombin III, increased platelet aggregability.

Endocrine: increased PBI and butanol extractable protein-bound iodine and decreased T3 uptake, increased blood glucose levels.

Other: increased phospholipids and triglycerides, decreased serum folate values and disturbance in tryptophan metabolism, decreased pregnanediol excretion, reduced response to metapyrone test.

These tests usually return to pre-therapy values after discontinuing oral contraceptive use. However, the physician should be aware that these altered determinations may mask an underlying disease.

4.5 Interaction with other medicinal products and other forms of interaction
Reduced efficacy and increased incidence of breakthrough bleeding have been associated with concomitant use of oral contraceptives and rifampicin. A similar association has been suggested with oral contraceptives and barbiturates, phenytoin sodium, ampicillin, tetracyclines and griseofulvin.

The herbal remedy St John's wort *(Hypericum perforatum)* should not be taken concomitantly with this medicine as this could potentially lead to a loss of contraceptive effect.

4.6 Pregnancy and lactation
Masculinisation of the female foetus has occurred when progesterones have been used in pregnant women, although this has been observed at doses much higher than that contained in Micronor. Pregnancy should be ruled out before continuing administration of Micronor to patients who have gone 45 days without a menstrual period.

A small fraction of the active ingredient in oral contraceptives has been identified in the milk of mothers receiving these drugs. The effects, if any, on the breast-fed child have not been determined. If possible the use of oral contraceptives should be deferred until the infant is weaned.

4.7 Effects on ability to drive and use machines
Not applicable

4.8 Undesirable effects
Side effects are usually self-limiting and of relatively short duration. Amongst the symptoms reported are:
- Headaches/migraine

- Nausea
- Vomiting
- Breast changes
- Change in weight
- Changes in libido
- Chloasma
- Breakthrough bleeding and spotting
- Rash
- Depression
- Irregular cycle length (particularly in early cycles of therapy). It is important that patients should be advised that whilst on Micronor therapy they may experience that variation in cycle length and that they should continue taking a tablet every day whether they have a period or not. However, patients should be advised to discontinue Micronor and to consult their doctor if they have gone 45 days without having a period.

Malignant hepatic tumours have been reported on rare occasions in long-term users of oral contraceptives. Benign hepatic tumours have also been associated with oral contraceptive use. A hepatic tumour should be considered in the differential diagnosis when upper abdominal pain, enlarged liver or signs of intra-abdominal haemorrhage occur.

A meta-analysis from 54 epidemiological studies reported that there is a slightly increased relative risk of having breast cancer diagnosed in women who are currently using oral contraceptives (OCs). The observed pattern of increased risk may be due to an earlier diagnosis of breast cancer in OC users, the biological effects of OCs or a combination of both. The additional breast cancers diagnosed in current users of OCs or in women who have used OCs in the last 10 years are more likely to be localised to the breast than those in women who have never used OCs.

Breast cancer is rare among women under 40 years of age whether or not they take OCs. Whilst the background risk increases with age, the excess number of breast cancer diagnoses in current and recent progesterone-only pill (POP) users is small in relation to the overall risk of breast cancer, possibly of similar magnitude to that associated with combined OCs. However, for POPs, the evidence is based on much smaller populations of users and so is less conclusive than that for combined OCs.

The most important risk factor for breast cancer in POP users is the age women discontinue the POP; the older the age at stopping, the more breast cancers are diagnosed. Duration of use is less important and the excess risk gradually disappears during the course of the 10 years after stopping POP use, such that by 10 years there appears to be no excess.

The evidence suggests that compared with never-users, among 10,000 women who use POPs for up to five years but stop by age 20, there would be much less than one extra case of breast cancer diagnosed up to 10 years afterwards. For those stopping by age 30 after 5 years use of the POP, there would be an estimated 2-3 extra cases (additional to the 44 cases of breast cancer per 10,000 women in this age group never exposed to oral contraceptives). For those stopping by age 40 after 5 years use, there would be an estimated 10 extra cases diagnosed up to 10 years afterwards (additional to the 160 cases of breast cancer per 10,000 never-exposed women in this age group).

It is important to inform patients that users of all contraceptive pills appear to have a small increase in the risk of being diagnosed with breast cancer, compared with non-users of oral contraceptives, but that this has to be weighed against the known benefits.

4.9 Overdose
Serious ill effects have not been reported following acute ingestion of large doses of oral contraceptives by young children. Overdosage may cause nausea and withdrawal bleeding may occur in females. An appropriate method of gastric emptying may be used if considered desirable.

5. PHARMACOLOGICAL PROPERTIES
5.1 Pharmacodynamic properties
Micronor Oral Contraceptive Tablets have a progestational effect on the endometrium and the cervical mucus.

5.2 Pharmacokinetic properties
Norethisterone is absorbed from the gastro-intestinal tract and metabolised in the liver. To obtain maximal contraceptive effectiveness, the tablets should be taken at the same time each day, every day.

5.3 Preclinical safety data
No relevant information additional to that contained elsewhere in the Summary of Product Characteristics.

6. PHARMACEUTICAL PARTICULARS
6.1 List of excipients
Lactose
Magnesium stearate
Pregelatinised starch

6.2 Incompatibilities
Not applicable.

6.3 Shelf life
36 months.

6.4 Special precautions for storage
Store at room temperature (below 25°C).
Protect from light.

6.5 Nature and contents of container
PVC/aluminium foil blister strips with or without a card wallet in cardboard carton, containing either 42, 2 × 42, 3 × 28, 1 × 28 or 100 × 28 tablets.

6.6 Special precautions for disposal and other handling
Not applicable.

7. MARKETING AUTHORISATION HOLDER
Janssen-Cilag Ltd
50-100 Holmers Farm Way
High Wycombe
Buckinghamshire
HP12 4EG
UK

8. MARKETING AUTHORISATION NUMBER(S)
0242/0234

9. DATE OF FIRST AUTHORISATION/RENEWAL OF THE AUTHORISATION
Date of First Authorisation: 1 October 1995
Renewal of Authorisation: 4 December 2008

10. DATE OF REVISION OF THE TEXT
11 February 2009
Legal category POM

Midrid Capsules 15s
(Manx Healthcare)

1. NAME OF THE MEDICINAL PRODUCT
Midrid Capsules

2. QUALITATIVE AND QUANTITATIVE COMPOSITION
Paracetamol 325.0mg
Isometheptene mucate 65.0mg

3. PHARMACEUTICAL FORM
Capsule

4. CLINICAL PARTICULARS
4.1 Therapeutic indications
In the treatment of migraine and other vascular headaches

4.2 Posology and method of administration
For oral administration
Adults: 2 capsules at once, then 1 capsule every hour until relief obtained up to a maximum of 5 capsules within a 12 hour period
Children: Not recommended

4.3 Contraindications
Severe cardiac, hepatic or renal impairment, severe hypertension, glaucoma. Patients on monoamine oxidase inhibitor therapy. Porphyria. Hypersensitivity to paracetamol and/or other constituents.

4.4 Special warnings and precautions for use
Cardiovascular disease, diabetes mellitus, hyperthyroidism. When used in patients with high spinal cord lesions, isometheptene, like other sympathomimetics may cause autonomic dysreflexia.

Care is advised in the administration of this product to patients with renal or hepatic impairment. The hazards of paracetamol overdose are greater in those with non-cirrhotic alcoholic liver disease.

Do not exceed the recommended dose
If symptoms persist, consult your doctor
Keep out of the sight and reach of children
Patient information leaflet warning
Immediate medical advice should be sought in the event of an overdose, even if you feel well, because of the risk of delayed, serious liver damage.
Label warning
Do not take with any other paracetamol-containing products. Immediate medical advice should be sought in the event of an overdose, even if you feel well.

4.5 Interaction with other medicinal products and other forms of interaction
On theoretical grounds, care should be taken with patients receiving cardiac glycosides, quinidine, anti-hypertensives and tricyclic antidepressants. Alcohol reduces liver capacity to deal with paracetamol. Cholestyramine reduces absorption of paracetamol. Metoclopramide and domperidone accelerate absorption of paracetamol. May interact with chloramphenicol, causing increased plasma levels.

The anticoagulant effect of warfarin and other coumarins may be enhanced by prolonged regular use of paracetamol with increased risk of bleeding; occasional doses have no significant effect.

There is an increased risk of toxicity with bromocriptine and isometheptene.

There is an increased risk of a hypertensive crisis when sympathomimetics are given with MAOIs.

4.6 Pregnancy and lactation
There is no evidence of the product's safety in human pregnancy nor is there evidence from animal work that it is free from hazard. Avoid in pregnancy and lactation.

4.7 Effects on ability to drive and use machines
No information

4.8 Undesirable effects
Transient dizziness may appear in hypersensitive patients. This can usually be eliminated by reducing the dose. Circulatory disturbances may occur.

Adverse effects of paracetamol are rare but hypersensitivity reactions including skin rashes may occur. Anaphylaxis, angioedema, urticaria and very rare cases of fixed drug eruption have been reported. There have been reports of blood dyscrasias including thrombocytopenia, purpura and agranulocytosis, but these were not necessarily causally related to paracetamol.

Blood disorders have also been reported with isometheptene containing products.

4.9 Overdose
Liver damage is possible in adults who have taken 10g or more of paracetamol.

Ingestion of 5g or more of paracetamol may lead to liver damage if the patient has risk factors (see below).

Risk factors
If the patient

a. is on long term treatment with carbamazepine, phenobarbitone, phenytoin, primidone, rifampicin, St John's Wort or other drugs that induce liver enzymes

or

b. regularly consumes ethanol in excess of recommended amounts

or

c. is likely to be glutathione deplete eg eating disorders, cystic fibrosis, HIV infection, starvation, cachexia

Symptoms
Symptoms of paracetamol overdosage in the first 24 hours are pallor, nausea, vomiting, anorexia and abdominal pain. Liver damage may become apparent 12 to 48 hours after ingestion. Abnormalities of glucose metabolism and metabolic acidosis may occur. In severe poisoning, hepatic failure may progress to encephalopathy, haemorrhage, hypoglycaemia, cerebral oedema and death. Acute renal failure with acute tubular necrosis, strongly suggested by loin pain, haematuria and proteinuria, may develop even in the absence of severe liver damage. Cardiac arrhythmias and pancreatitis have been reported.

Management
Immediate treatment is essential in the management of paracetamol overdosage. Despite a lack of significant early symptoms, patients should be referred to hospital urgently for immediate medical attention. Symptoms may be limited to nausea or vomiting and may not reflect the severity of overdose or the risk of organ damage. Management should be in accordance with established treatment guidelines, see BNF overdose section.

Treatment with activated charcoal should be considered if the overdose has been taken within 1 hour. Plasma paracetamol concentration should be measured at 4 hours or later after ingestion (earlier concentrations are unreliable). Treatment with N-acetylcysteine may be used up to 24 hours after ingestion of paracetamol, however, the maximum protective effect is obtained up to 8 hours post-ingestion. The effectiveness of the antidote declines sharply after this time. If required the patient should be given intravenous N-acetylcysteine, in line with the established dosage schedule. If vomiting is not a problem, oral methionine may be a suitable alternative for remote areas, outside hospital. Management of patients who present with serious hepatic dysfunction beyond 24 hr from ingestion should be discussed with the NPIS or a liver unit.

5. PHARMACOLOGICAL PROPERTIES
5.1 Pharmacodynamic properties
Paracetamol is an effective analgesic and antipyretic agent but has only weak anti-inflammatory properties. Its mechanism of action is not fully understood as it is only a weak inhibitor of prostaglandin biosynthesis, but it has been suggested that it is more effective against enzymes in the CNS than those in the periphery. The drug has no effect on the cardiovascular and respiratory systems, and it does not cause gastric irritation or bleeding like salicylates.

5.2 Pharmacokinetic properties
Isometheptene mucate is rapidly excreted in man. Excretion peaks at 2-6 hours after dosing.

Paracetamol is readily absorbed from the gastrointestinal tract with peak plasma concentrations occurring about 30 minutes to 2 hours after ingestion. It is metabolised in the liver and excreted in the urine mainly as the glucuronide and sulphate conjugates. Less than 5% is excreted as unchanged paracetamol. The elimination half life varies from about 1 to 4 hours. Plasma-protein blinding is negligible at usual therapeutic concentrations but increases with increasing concentrations.

A minor hydroxylated metabolite, which is usually produced in very small amounts by mixed-function oxidases in the liver and which is usually detoxified by conjugation with liver glutathione, may accumulate following paracetamol overdosage and cause liver damage.

5.3 Preclinical safety data
There are no other data of relevance to the prescriber which are not included on the SPC

6. PHARMACEUTICAL PARTICULARS

6.1 List of excipients
Microcrystalline cellulose
Talc
Colloidal silicon dioxide
Purified water
Capsule shell:
Gelatin
Water
Titanium dioxide
Erythrosine
Quinoline yellow
Indigotine
Printing ink Opacode black S-1-8100HV

6.2 Incompatibilities
Not applicable

6.3 Shelf life
3 years

6.4 Special precautions for storage
Do not store above 25°C

6.5 Nature and contents of container
Strips of 5 or 15 capsules
Blister packs of 5, 10, 15, 20 and 30 capsules

6.6 Special precautions for disposal and other handling
None

7. MARKETING AUTHORISATION HOLDER
Manx Healthcare Ltd
Taylor Group House
Wedgnock Lane
Warwick
CV34 5YA
United Kingdom

8. MARKETING AUTHORISATION NUMBER(S)
PL 14251/0021

9. DATE OF FIRST AUTHORISATION/RENEWAL OF THE AUTHORISATION
22 September 2004 / 19 December 2007

10. DATE OF REVISION OF THE TEXT
April 2008

Midrid Capsules 30s

(Manx Healthcare)

1. NAME OF THE MEDICINAL PRODUCT
Midrid Capsules

2. QUALITATIVE AND QUANTITATIVE COMPOSITION
Paracetamol 325.0mg
Isometheptene mucate 65.0mg

3. PHARMACEUTICAL FORM
Capsule

4. CLINICAL PARTICULARS

4.1 Therapeutic indications
In the treatment of migraine and other vascular headaches

4.2 Posology and method of administration
For oral administration

Adults: 2 capsules at once, then 1 capsule every hour until relief obtained up to a maximum of 5 capsules within a 12 hour period

Children: Not recommended

4.3 Contraindications
Severe cardiac, hepatic or renal impairment, severe hypertension, glaucoma. Patients on monoamine oxidase inhibitor therapy. Porphyria. Hypersensitivity to paracetamol and/or other constituents.

4.4 Special warnings and precautions for use
Cardiovascular disease, diabetes mellitus, hyperthyroidism. When used in patients with high spinal cord lesions, isometheptene, like other sympathomimetics may cause autonomic dysreflexia.

Care is advised in the administration of this product to patients with renal or hepatic impairment. The hazards of paracetamol overdose are greater in those with non-cirrhotic alcoholic liver disease.

Do not exceed the recommended dose

If symptoms persist, consult your doctor

Keep out of the sight and reach of children

Patient information leaflet warning

Immediate medical advice should be sought in the event of an overdose, even if you feel well, because of the risk of delayed, serious liver damage.

Label warning

Do not take with any other paracetamol-containing products. Immediate medical advice should be sought in the event of an overdose, even if you feel well.

4.5 Interaction with other medicinal products and other forms of interaction
On theoretical grounds, care should be taken with patients receiving cardiac glycosides, quinidine, anti-hypertensives and tricyclic antidepressants. Alcohol reduces liver capacity to deal with paracetamol. Cholestyramine reduces absorption of paracetamol. Metoclopramide and domperidone accelerate absorption of paracetamol. May interact with chloramphenicol, causing increased plasma levels.

The anticoagulant effect of warfarin and other coumarins may be enhanced by prolonged regular use of paracetamol with increased risk of bleeding; occasional doses have no significant effect.

There is an increased risk of toxicity with bromocriptine and isometheptene.

There is an increased risk of a hypertensive crisis when sympathomimetics are given with MAOIs.

4.6 Pregnancy and lactation
There is no evidence of the product's safety in human pregnancy nor is there evidence from animal work that it is free from hazard. Avoid in pregnancy and lactation.

4.7 Effects on ability to drive and use machines
No information

4.8 Undesirable effects
Transient dizziness may appear in hypersensitive patients. This can usually be eliminated by reducing the dose. Circulatory disturbances may occur.

Adverse effects of paracetamol are rare but hypersensitivity reactions including skin rashes may occur. Anaphylaxis, angioedema, urticaria and very rare cases of fixed drug eruption have been reported. There have been reports of blood dyscrasias including thrombocytopenia, purpura and agranulocytosis, but these were not necessarily causally related to paracetamol.

Blood disorders have also been reported with isometheptene containing products.

4.9 Overdose
Liver damage is possible in adults who have taken 10g or more of paracetamol.

Ingestion of 5g or more of paracetamol may lead to liver damage if the patient has risk factors (see below).

Risk factors

If the patient

a. is on long term treatment with carbamazepine, phenobarbitone, phenytoin, primidone, rifampicin, St John's Wort or other drugs that induce liver enzymes

or

b. regularly consumes ethanol in excess of recommended amounts

or

c. is likely to be glutathione deplete eg eating disorders, cystic fibrosis, HIV infection, starvation, cachexia

Symptoms

Symptoms of paracetamol overdosage in the first 24 hours are pallor, nausea, vomiting, anorexia and abdominal pain. Liver damage may become apparent 12 to 48 hours after ingestion. Abnormalities of glucose metabolism and metabolic acidosis may occur. In severe poisoning, hepatic failure may progress to encephalopathy, haemorrhage, hypoglycaemia, cerebral oedema and death. Acute renal failure with acute tubular necrosis, strongly suggested by loin pain, haematuria and proteinuria, may develop even in the absence of severe liver damage. Cardiac arrhythmias and pancreatitis have been reported.

Management

Immediate treatment is essential in the management of paracetamol overdosage. Despite a lack of significant early symptoms, patients should be referred to hospital urgently for immediate medical attention. Symptoms may be limited to nausea or vomiting and may not reflect the severity of overdose or the risk of organ damage. Management should be in accordance with established treatment guidelines, see BNF overdose section.

Treatment with activated charcoal should be considered if the overdose has been taken within 1 hour. Plasma paracetamol concentration should be measured at 4 hours or later after ingestion (earlier concentrations are unreliable). Treatment with N-acetylcysteine may be used up to 24 hours after ingestion of paracetamol, however, the maximum protective effect is obtained up to 8 hours post-ingestion. The effectiveness of the antidote declines sharply after this time. If required the patient should be given intravenous N-acetylcysteine, in line with the established dosage schedule. If vomiting is not a problem, oral methionine may be a suitable alternative for remote areas, outside hospital. Management of patients who present with serious hepatic dysfunction beyond 24 hr from ingestion should be discussed with the NPIS or a liver unit.

5. PHARMACOLOGICAL PROPERTIES

5.1 Pharmacodynamic properties
Paracetamol is an effective analgesic and antipyretic agent but has only weak anti-inflammatory properties. Its mechanism of action is not fully understood as it is only a weak inhibitor of prostaglandin biosynthesis, but it has been suggested that it is more effective against enzymes in the CNS than those in the periphery. The drug has no effect on the cardiovascular and respiratory systems, and it does not cause gastric irritation or bleeding like salicylates.

5.2 Pharmacokinetic properties
Isometheptene mucate is rapidly excreted in man. Excretion peaks at 2-6 hours after dosing.

Paracetamol is readily absorbed from the gastrointestinal tract with peak plasma concentrations occurring about 30 minutes to 2 hours after ingestion. It is metabolised in the liver and excreted in the urine mainly as the glucuronide and sulphate conjugates. Less than 5% is excreted as unchanged paracetamol. The elimination half life varies from about 1 to 4 hours. Plasma-protein blinding is negligible at usual therapeutic concentrations but increases with increasing concentrations.

A minor hydroxylated metabolite, which is usually produced in very small amounts by mixed-function oxidases in the liver and which is usually detoxified by conjugation with liver glutathione, may accumulate following paracetamol overdosage and cause liver damage.

5.3 Preclinical safety data
There are no other data of relevance to the prescriber which are not included on the SPC

6. PHARMACEUTICAL PARTICULARS

6.1 List of excipients
Microcrystalline cellulose
Talc
Colloidal silicon dioxide
Purified water
Capsule shell:
Gelatin
Water
Titanium dioxide
Erythrosine
Quinoline yellow
Indigotine
Printing ink Opacode black S-1-8100HV

6.2 Incompatibilities
Not applicable

6.3 Shelf life
3 years

6.4 Special precautions for storage
Do not store above 25°C

6.5 Nature and contents of container
Securitainers of 100 capsules
Strips of 5 or 15 capsules
Blister packs of 5, 10, 15, 20 and 30 capsules

6.6 Special precautions for disposal and other handling
None

7. MARKETING AUTHORISATION HOLDER
Manx Healthcare Ltd
Taylor Group House
Wedgnock Lane
Warwick
CV34 5YA
United Kingdom

8. MARKETING AUTHORISATION NUMBER(S)
PL 14251/0020

9. DATE OF FIRST AUTHORISATION/RENEWAL OF THE AUTHORISATION
18 May 2004 / 19 December 2007

10. DATE OF REVISION OF THE TEXT
April 2008

Migard

(A. Menarini Pharma U.K. S.R.L.)

1. NAME OF THE MEDICINAL PRODUCT
MIGARD 2.5 mg film-coated tablets

2. QUALITATIVE AND QUANTITATIVE COMPOSITION
Each film-coated tablet contains 2.5 mg of frovatriptan (as succinate monohydrate).

Excipients: approximately 100 mg of lactose per tablet.

For a full list of excipients, see section 6.1.

3. PHARMACEUTICAL FORM
Film-coated tablet.

Round biconvex white film-coated tablet, debossed with "m" on one side and "2.5" on the other.

4. CLINICAL PARTICULARS

4.1 Therapeutic indications

Acute treatment of the headache phase of migraine attacks with or without aura.

4.2 Posology and method of administration

General

Frovatriptan should be taken as early as possible after the onset of a migraine attack but it is also effective when taken at a later stage. Frovatriptan should not be used prophylactically. The tablets should be swallowed whole with water.

If a patient does not respond to the first dose of frovatriptan, a second dose should not be taken for the same attack, since no benefit has been shown.

Frovatriptan may be used for subsequent migraine attacks.

Adults (18 to 65 years of age)

The recommended dose of frovatriptan is 2.5 mg.

If the migraine recurs after initial relief, a second dose may be taken, providing there is an interval of at least 2 hours between the two doses.

The total daily dose should not exceed 5 mg per day.

Children and adolescents (under 18 years)

There are no data of the use of frovatriptan in children and adolescents. Therefore, its use in this age group is not recommended.

Elderly (over 65 years)

Frovatriptan data in patients over 65 years remain limited. Therefore, its use in this category of patients is not recommended.

Renal impairment

No dosage adjustment is required in patients with renal impairment (see 5.2 Pharmacokinetic properties).

Hepatic impairment

No dosage adjustment is required in patients with mild to moderate hepatic impairment (see 5.2 Pharmacokinetic properties). Frovatriptan is contraindicated in patients with severe hepatic impairment (see 4.3 Contra-indications).

4.3 Contraindications

- hypersensitivity to frovatriptan or to any of the excipients.
- patients with a history of myocardial infarction, ischaemic heart disease, coronary vasospasm (e.g. Prinzmetal's angina), peripheral vascular disease, patients presenting with symptoms or signs compatible with ischaemic heart disease.
- Moderately severe or severe hypertension, uncontrolled mild hypertension.
- previous cerebrovascular accident (CVA) or transient ischaemic attack (TIA).
- severe hepatic impairment (Child-Pugh C).
- Concomitant administration of frovatriptan with ergotamine or ergotamine derivatives (including méthysergide) or other 5-hydroxytryptamine (5-HT_1) receptor agonists.

4.4 Special warnings and precautions for use

Frovatriptan should only be used where a clear diagnosis of migraine has been established.

Frovatriptan is not indicated for the management of hemiplegic, basilar or ophthalmoplegic migraine.

As with other treatments of migraine attack, it is necessary to exclude other, potentially serious, neurological conditions before treating the headache of patients without a previous diagnosis of migraine, or migraine patients presenting with atypical symptoms. It should be noted that migraineurs present an increased risk of certain cerebral vascular events (eg CVA or TIA).

The safety and efficacy of frovatriptan administered during the aura phase, before the headache phase of migraine, has not been established.

As for other 5-HT_1 receptor agonists, frovatriptan must not be administered to patients at risk of coronary artery disease (CAD), including heavy smokers or users of nicotine substitution therapy without a prior cardiovascular evaluation (see 4.3 Contra-indications). Specific attention should be given to post- menopausal women and men over 40 years of age presenting with these risk factors.

However, cardiac evaluations may not identify every patient who has cardiac disease. In very rare cases serious cardiac events have occurred in patients with no underlying cardio-vascular disease when taking 5-HT_1 receptor agonists.

Frovatriptan administration can be associated with transient symptoms including chest pain or tightness which may be intense and involve the throat. (see 4.8 Undesirable effects).

Where such symptoms are thought to indicate ischaemic heart disease no further doses of frovatriptan should be taken and additional investigations should be carried out.

It is advised to wait 24 hours following the use of frovatriptan before administering an ergotamine- type medication. At least 24 hours should be elapse after administration of an ergotamine-containing preparation before frovatriptan is given (see 4.3 Contra-indications and 4.5 Interactions with other medicinal products and other forms of interactions).

In case of too frequent use (repeated administration several days in a row corresponding to a misuse of the product), the active substance can accumulate leading to an increase of the side-effects.

Prolonged use of any type of painkiller for headaches can make them worse. If this situation is experienced or suspected, medical advice should be obtained and treatment should be discontinued. The possibility of MOH should be taken into consideration in patients who have frequent or daily headaches despite (or because of) the regular use of headache medications.

Do not exceed the recommended dose of frovatriptan.

This medicinal product contains lactose, therefore patients with rare hereditary problems of galactose intolerance, the Lapp lactase deficiency or glucose-galactose malabsorption should not take this medicine.

Undesirable effects may be more common during concomitant use of triptans (5HT agonists) and herbal preparations containing St John's Wort (Hypericum perforatum).

4.5 Interaction with other medicinal products and other forms of interaction

<u>CONCOMITANT USE CONTRAINDICATED</u>

Ergotamine and ergotamine derivatives (including méthysergide) and other 5 HT1 agonists

Risks of hypertension and coronary artery constriction due to additive vasospastic effects when used concomitantly for the same migraine attack (see 4.3 Contraindications).

Effects can be additive. It is recommended to wait at least 24 hours after administration of ergotamine-type medication before administering frovatriptan. Conversely it is recommended to wait 24 hours after frovatriptan administration before administering an ergotamine-type medication (see 4.4 Special warnings and precautions for use).

<u>CONCOMITANT USE NOT RECOMMENDED</u>

Monoamine Oxidase Inhibitors

Frovatriptan is not a substrate for MAO-A, however a potential risk of serotonin syndrome or hypertension cannot be excluded (see 5.2 Pharmacokinetic Properties).

<u>CONCOMITANT USE REQUIRING CAUTION</u>

Selective serotonin-reuptake inhibitors (citalopram, fluoxetine, fluvoxamine, paroxetine, sertraline)

Potential risk of hypertension, coronary vasoconstriction or serotonin syndrome.

Strict adherence to the recommended dose is an essential factor to prevent this syndrome.

Methylergometrine

Risks of hypertension, coronary artery constriction.

Fluvoxamine

Fluvoxamine is a potent inhibitor of cytochrome CYP1A2 and has been shown to increase the blood levels of frovatriptan by 27-49%.

Oral contraceptives

In female subjects taking oral contraceptives, concentrations of frovatriptan were 30% higher than in females not taking oral contraceptives. No increased incidence in the adverse event profile was reported.

Hypericum perforatum (St. John wort) (oral route)

As with other triptans the risk of the occurence of serotonin syndrome may be increased.

4.6 Pregnancy and lactation

<u>Pregnancy</u>

The safety of frovatriptan in pregnant women has not been established.

Studies in animals have shown reproductive toxicity (see 5.3 Preclinical safety data). The potential risk for humans is unknown. Frovatriptan should not be used during pregnancy unless clearly necessary.

<u>Lactation</u>

Frovatriptan and/or its metabolites are excreted in the milk of lactating rats with the maximum concentration in milk being four-fold higher than maximum blood levels. Although it is not known whether frovatriptan or its metabolites are excreted in human breast milk, the administration of frovatriptan to women who are breastfeeding is not recommended, unless is clearly needed. In this case, a 24 hours interval must be observed.

4.7 Effects on ability to drive and use machines

No studies on the effects on the ability to drive and use machines have been performed.

Migraine or treatment with frovatriptan may cause somnolence. Patients should be advised to evaluate their ability to perform complex tasks such as driving during migraine attacks and following administration of frovatriptan.

4.8 Undesirable effects

Frovatriptan has been administered to over 2700 patients at the recommended dose of 2.5 mg and the most common side effects (< 10%) include dizziness, fatigue, paraesthesia, headache and vascular flushing. The undesirable effects reported in clinical trials with frovatriptan were transient, generally mild to moderate and resolved spontaneously. Some of the symptoms reported as undesirable effects may be associated symptoms of migraine.

The table below shows all the adverse reactions that are considered to be related to treatment with 2.5 mg frovatriptan and showed a greater incidence than with placebo in the 4 placebo controlled trials. They are listed in decreasing incidence by body-system.

(see Table 1 on next page)

In two open long-term clinical studies the observed effects were not different from those listed above.

There have been post-marketing reports of hypersensitivity reactions of unknown frequency, including cutaneous disorders and anaphylaxis.

4.9 Overdose

There is limited data on overdose with frovatriptan tablets. The maximum single oral dose of frovatriptan given to male and female patients with migraine was 40 mg (16 times the recommended clinical dose of 2.5 mg) and the maximum single dose given to healthy male subjects was 100 mg (40 times the recommended clinical dose). Both were not associated with side effects other than those mentioned in section 4.8. However, one post-marketing serious case of coronary vasospasm has been reported, following intake of 4 times the recommended dose of frovatriptan on three consecutive days, in a patient taking migraine prophylactic treatment with a tricyclic antidepressant. The patient recovered.

There is no specific antidote for frovatriptan. The elimination half-life of frovatriptan is approximately 26 hours (5.2. Pharmacokinetic properties).

The effects of haemodialysis or peritoneal dialysis on serum concentrations of frovatriptan are unknown.

Treatment

In case of overdose with frovatriptan, the patient should be monitored closely for at least 48 hours and be given any necessary supportive therapy.

5. PHARMACOLOGICAL PROPERTIES

5.1 Pharmacodynamic properties

Pharmacotherapeutic group: selective 5-HT_1 receptor agonists (N: central nervous system)

ATC code: N02C C07

Frovatriptan is a selective agonist for 5-HT receptors, which shows high affinity for 5-HT_{1B} and 5-HT_{1D} binding sites in radioligand assays and exhibits potent agonist effects at 5-HT_{1B} and 5-HT_{1D} receptors in functional bioassays. It exhibits marked selectivity for 5-$HT_{1B/1D}$ receptors and has no significant affinity for 5-HT_2, 5-HT_3, 5-HT_4, 5-HT_6, α- adrenoreceptors, or histamine receptors. Frovatriptan has no significant affinity for benzodiazepine binding sites.

Frovatriptan is believed to act selectively on extracerebral, intracranial arteries to inhibit the excessive dilatation of these vessels in migraine. At clinically relevant concentrations, frovatriptan produced constriction of human isolated cerebral arteries with little or no effect on isolated human coronary arteries.

The clinical efficacy of frovatriptan for treatment of migraine headache and accompanying symptoms was investigated in three multicenter placebo controlled studies. In these studies frovatriptan 2.5 mg was consistently superior to placebo in terms of headache response at 2 and 4 hours post-dosing and time to first response. Pain relief (reduction from moderate-or severe headache to no or mild pain) after 2 hours was 37-46% for frovatriptan and 21-27% for placebo.

Complete pain relief after 2 hours was 9-14% for frovatriptan and 2-3% for placebo. Maximum efficacy with frovatriptan is reached in 4 hours.

In a clinical study comparing frovatriptan 2.5 mg with sumatriptan 100 mg, the efficacy of frovatriptan 2.5 mg was slightly lower than that of sumatriptan 100 mg at 2 hours and 4 hours. The frequency of undesirable events was slightly lower with frovatriptan 2.5 mg compared to sumatriptan 100 mg. No study comparing frovatriptan 2.5 mg and sumatriptan 50 mg has been carried out.

In elderly subjects in good health, transient changes in systolic arterial pressure (within normal limits) have been observed in some subjects, following a single oral dose of frovatriptan 2.5 mg.

5.2 Pharmacokinetic properties

Absorption

After administration of a single oral 2.5 mg dose to healthy subjects, the mean maximum blood concentration of frovatriptan (C_{max}), reached between 2 and 4 hours, was 4.2 ng/mL in males and 7.0 ng/mL in females. The mean area under the curve (AUC) was 42.9 and 94.0 ng.h/mL for males and females respectively.

The oral bioavailability was 22% in males and 30% in females. The pharmacokinetics of frovatriptan were similar between healthy subjects and migraine patients and there was no difference in pharmacokinetic parameters in the patients during a migraine attack or between attacks.

Frovatriptan displayed generally linear pharmacokinetics over the dose range used in clinical studies (1 mg to 40 mg).

Food had no significant effect on the bioavailability of frovatriptan, but delayed t_{max} slightly by approximately 1 hour.

Table 1

System organ class	Very common ≥ 1/10	Common ≥1/100 <1/10	Uncommon ≥1/1000 <1/100	Rare ≥1/10,000 <1/1000	Very rare < 1/10,000	Not known
Blood and the lymphatic system disorders				Lymphadenopathy		
Metabolism and nutrition disorders			Dehydration,	Hypoglycaemia		
Psychiatric disorders			Anxiety, insomnia, confusional state, nervousness, agitation, depression, depersonalisation	Abnormal dreams, personality disorder		
Nervous system disorders		Dizziness, paraesthesia, headache, somnolence, dysaesthesia, hypoaesthesia	Dysgeusia, tremor, disturbance in attention, lethargy, hyperaesthesia, sedation, vertigo, involuntary muscle contractions	Amnesia, Hypertonia, Hypotonia, hyporeflexia, movement disorder		
Eye disorders		Visual disturbance	Eye pain, eye irritation, photophobia	Night blindness		
Ear and labyrinth disorders			Tinnitus, ear pain	Ear discomfort, ear disorder, ear pruritus, hyperacusis		
Cardiac disorders			Palpitations, tachycardia	Bradycardia		
Vascular disorders		Flushing	Peripheral coldness, Hypertension			
Respiratory, thoracic and mediastinal disorders		Throat tightness	Rhinitis, sinusitis, pharingolaringeal pain	Epistaxis, hiccups, hyperventilation, respiratory disorder, throat irritation		
Gastrointestinal disorders		Nausea, dry-mouth, dyspepsia, abdominal pain	Diarrhoea, dysphagia, flatulence, stomach discomfort, abdominal distension	Constipation, eructation, gastroesophageal reflux disease, irritable bowel syndrome, lip blister, lip pain, oesophageal spasm, oral mucosal blistering, peptic ulcer, salivary gland pain, stomatitis, toothache		
Skin and subcutaneous tissue disorders		Hyperhidrosis	Pruritus	Erithema, piloerection, purpura, urticaria		
Musculoskeletal, connective tissue and bone disorders			Musculoskeletal stiffness, musculoskeletal pain, pain in extremity, back pain, arthralgia			
Renal and urinary disorders			Pollakiuria, polyuria	Nocturia, renal pain		
Reproductive system and breast disorders				Breast tenderness		
General disorders and administration site conditions		Fatigue, chest discomfort	Chest pain, feeling hot, temperature intolerance, pain, asthaenia, thirst, sluggishness, energy increased, malaise	Pyrexia		
Investigations				Blood bilirubin increased, blood calcium decreased, urine analysis abnormal		
Injury and poisoning				Bite		

Distribution

The steady state volume of distribution of frovatriptan following intravenous administration of 0.8 mg was 4.2 L/kg in males and 3.0 L/kg in females.

Binding of frovatriptan to serum proteins was low (approximately 15%). Reversible binding to blood cells at steady state was approximately 60% with no difference between males and females. The blood: plasma ratio was about 2:1 at equilibrium.

Metabolism

Following oral administration of radiolabelled frovatriptan 2.5 mg to healthy male subjects, 32% of the dose was recovered in urine and 62% in faeces. Radiolabelled compounds excreted in urine were unchanged frovatriptan, hydroxy frovatriptan, N-acetyl desmethyl frovatriptan, hydroxy N-acetyl desmethyl frovatriptan, and desmethyl frovatriptan, together with several other minor metabolites. Desmethyl frovatriptan had about 3-fold lower affinity at 5-HT1 receptors than the parent compound. N-acetyl desmethyl frovatriptan had negligible affinity at 5-HT1 receptors. The activity of other metabolites has not been studied.

The results of in vitro studies have provided strong evidence that CYP1A2 is the cytochrome P450 isoenzyme primarily involved in the metabolism of frovatriptan. Frovatriptan does not inhibit or induce CYP1A2 in vitro.

Frovatriptan is not an inhibitor of human monoamine oxidase (MAO) enzymes or cytochrome P450 isozymes and therefore has little potential for drug-drug interactions (see 4.5 Interactions with other medicinal products and other forms of interactions). Frovatriptan is not a substrate for MAO.

Elimination

The elimination of frovatriptan is biphasic with a distribution phase prevailing between 2 and 6 hours. Mean systemic clearance was 216 and 132 mL/min in males and females, respectively. Renal clearance accounted for 38% (82 mL/min) and 49% (65 mL/min) of total clearance in males and females, respectively. The terminal elimination half-life is approximately 26 hours, irrespective of the sex of the subjects, however the terminal elimination phase only becomes dominant after about 12 hours.

Gender

AUC and C_{max} values for frovatriptan are lower (by approximately 50%) in males than in females. This is due, at least in part, to the concomitant use of oral contraceptives. Based on the efficacy or safety of the 2.5 mg dose in clinical use, dosage adjustment with respect to gender is not necessary (See 4.2 Posology and method of administration).

Elderly

In healthy elderly subjects (65 to 77 years) AUC is increased by 73% in males and by 22% in females, compared to younger subjects (18 to 37 years). There was no difference in t_{max} or $t_{1/2}$ between the two populations (see 4.2 Posology and method of administration).

Renal impairment

Systemic exposure to frovatriptan and its $t_{1/2}$ were not significantly different in male and female subjects with renal impairment (creatinine clearance 16 - 73 mL/min), compared to that in healthy subjects.

Hepatic impairment

Following oral administration in male and female subjects aged 44 to 57, with mild or moderate hepatic impairment (Child-Pugh grades A and B), mean blood concentrations of frovatriptan were within the range observed in healthy young and elderly subjects. There is no pharmacokinetic or clinical experience with frovatriptan in subjects with severe hepatic impairment (See 4.3 Contra-indications).

5.3 Preclinical safety data

During toxicity studies after single or repeated administration, preclinical effects were only observed at exposure levels in excess of the maximum exposure level in man.

Standard genotoxicity studies did not reveal a clinically relevant genotoxic potential of frovatriptan.

Frovatriptan was foetotoxic in rats, but in rabbits foetotoxicity was observed only at maternally toxic dose levels.

Frovatriptan was not potentially carcinogenic in standard rodent carcinogenicity studies and in p53 (+/-) mouse studies at exposures considerably higher than anticipated in humans.

6. PHARMACEUTICAL PARTICULARS

6.1 List of excipients

Tablet core

Lactose, anhydrous

Microcrystalline cellulose

Silica, colloidal anhydrous

Sodium starch glycollate (Type A)

Magnesium stearate

Film Coat

Opadry white:

Hypromellose (E 464)

Titanium dioxide (E 171)

Lactose, anhydrous

Macrogol 3000

Triacetin

6.2 Incompatibilities

Not applicable

6.3 Shelf life
Blister: 3 years

Bottle: 2 years

6.4 Special precautions for storage
Do not store above 30°C.

Blister: store in the original package.

Bottle: keep the container tightly closed.

6.5 Nature and contents of container
Child-proof HDPE bottles containing 30 tablets.

PVC/PE/ACLAR/Aluminium blister packs with 1, 2, 3, 4, 6 and 12 tablets.

Not all pack sizes may be marketed.

6.6 Special precautions for disposal and other handling
No special requirements.

7. MARKETING AUTHORISATION HOLDER
Menarini International Operations Luxembourg S.A.

1, Avenue de la Gare

L-1611, Luxembourg.

8. MARKETING AUTHORISATION NUMBER(S)
PL 16239/0017

9. DATE OF FIRST AUTHORISATION/RENEWAL OF THE AUTHORISATION
7th October 2002/13th February 2008

10. DATE OF REVISION OF THE TEXT
July 2008

Legal Category
POM

MigraMax

(Cephalon Limited)

1. NAME OF THE MEDICINAL PRODUCT
Migramax 900mg/10mg Powder for oral solution

2. QUALITATIVE AND QUANTITATIVE COMPOSITION
Active ingredients Per sachet

DL-lysine acetylsalicylate 1,620mg

equivalent to acetylsalicylic acid 900mg

Metoclopramide (INN) hydrochloride EP 10.54mg

equivalent in terms of the anhydrous substance to: 10mg

3. PHARMACEUTICAL FORM
Sachet containing powder for oral solution

4. CLINICAL PARTICULARS

4.1 Therapeutic indications
MigraMax is indicated for the treatment of migraine-associated symptoms such as headache, nausea and vomiting.

4.2 Posology and method of administration
For oral administration only.

MigraMax must be dissolved completely in some water before taking.

Renal and hepatic insufficiency

Caution should be exercised in significant renal or hepatic impairment. Metoclopramide is metabolised in the liver and eliminated mainly via the kidney. A dose reduction may be necessary.

Adults (aged 20 years and older) and elderly: One sachet should be taken at the first warning of a migraine attack. A second sachet may be taken two hours later if the symptoms have not resolved. Do not exceed three sachets in a 24 hour period.

Migramax should not be given to patients under 20 years of age (see Section 4.4).

4.3 Contraindications

- Hypersensitivity to metoclopramide, salicylates or any of the components.
- Not recommended for patients under 20 years of age in view of the particular risk of dystonic reactions in young adults and children with metoclopramide.
- Active, chronic or recurrent gastric or duodenal ulcers.
- Congenital or acquired bleeding disorders; obstruction, haemorrhage or perforation of the GI tract.
- Known or suspected phaeochromocytoma.
- Third trimester of pregnancy.
- Metoclopramide should not be used in the immediate post-operative period (up to 3-4 days) following pyloroplasty or gut anastomosis, as vigorous gastro intestinal contractions may adversely affect healing.

4.4 Special warnings and precautions for use
If vomiting persists the patient should be reassessed to exclude the possibility of an underlying disorder e.g. cerebral irritation.

As salicylates may induce asthma attacks in susceptible individuals MigraMax should be avoided in patients at risk of developing sensitivity reactions. These include individuals with asthma or rhinitis, a history of atopy or nasal polyps, and also patients who have been sensitive to other salicylates or NSAIDs.

Use with caution in patients with a history of gastroduodenal ulcer or GI haemorrhage, or with significant hepatic impairment, gout, menorrhagia, or epilepsy. Care should be taken in patients using intra-uterine contraceptive devices and patients who have a high alcohol intake.

There is a possible association between aspirin and Reye's syndrome when given to children with a fever. Reye's syndrome is a very rare disease which affects the brain and liver, and can be fatal. For this reason aspirin should not be given to children under 12 years and should be avoided up to and including 16 years of age if feverish. MigraMax is contraindicated in patients under 20 years of age (see section 4.3).

As total clearance of metoclopramide is reduced and elimination prolonged in patients with renal failure use in patients with significant degrees of renal impairment should be approached with caution.

Metoclopramide may induce an acute hypertensive response in patients with phaeochromocytoma.

Extrapyramidal disorders, drowsiness, decreased level of consciousness, confusion and hallucination occur more frequently when high doses of metoclopramide are used (see adverse reactions).

Young adults and the elderly should be treated with care as they are at increased risk of extrapyramidal reactions.

Symptomatic treatment of extrapyramidal reactions may be necessary (benzodiazepines or anticholinergic anti-parkinsonian drugs).

Neuroleptic Malignant Syndrome (NMS), a potentially fatal symptom complex with hyperthermia, muscle rigidity, extrapyramidal symptoms, altered mental status and autonomic dysfunction, may occur. The management of NMS should include 1) immediate discontinuation of the product, 2) intensive symptomatic treatment and medical monitoring, and 3) treatment of any concomitant serious medical problems for which specific treatments are available.

Methaemoglobinemia has been reported with metoclopramide. In case of methaemoglobinemia, MigraMax should be immediately and permanently discontinued and appropriate measures initiated.

Metoclopramide is not recommended in epileptic patients as benzamides may decrease the epileptic threshold.

Care should be exercised when using MIGAMAX SACHETS in patients with a history of atopy (including asthma) or porphyria.

4.5 Interaction with other medicinal products and other forms of interaction

Metoclopramide-related interactions

Alcohol:

Alcohol potentiates the sedative effect of metoclopramide

Anticholinergics and morphine derivatives:

Anticholinergics and morphine derivatives antagonise the effects of metoclopramide on gastrointestinal motility.

CNS depressants (morphine derivatives, hypnotics, anxiolytics, sedative H1 antihistamines, sedative antidepressants, barbiturates, clonidine and related):

Combination of CNS depressants with metoclopramide may result in potentiation of sedative effects.

Antipsychotics:

Combination of antipsychotics with metoclopramide may result in potentiation of extrapyramidal effects.

Due to the promotion of gastric emptying and normal peristalsis (see section 5.1) caused by metoclopramide, the absorption of certain drugs may be modified:

Digoxin:

Metoclopramide decreased the gastric absorption of digoxin. Therefore, dose adjustment may be required.

Ciclosporin:

Metoclopramide increases ciclosporin bioavailability. Dose adjustment may be required. In one study, dosing requirements for ciclosporin were reported to be reduced by 20% when metoclopramide was administered concomitantly. To avoid toxicity, careful monitoring of ciclosporin plasma concentration is required.

Levodopa:

Levodopa and metoclopramide have a mutual antagonism. Concomitant use should be avoided.

Salicylate-related interactions

Anti-coagulants:

Salicylates may enhance the effects of anti-coagulants.

Oral anti-diabetic agents:

Salicylates may enhance the effects of oral anti-diabetic agents.

Anti-epileptics:

Salicylates may enhance the effects of phenytoin, sodium valproate.

Antimetabolites:

Salicylates may enhance the effects of methotrexate

Immunomodulating agents:

Salicylates may inhibit the action of alpha interferon

Salicylates may interact with other NSAIDs, antacids and glucorticosteroids, which may lower blood salicylate concentration during treatment and result in high levels when treatment is stopped.

The effects of diuretics and uricosurics may also be affected by salicylates.

Other anti-platelet drugs

Salicylates may increase risk of bleeding with clopidogrel and ticlopidine.

Leukotriene antagonists

Aspirin may increase plasma concentration of zafirlukast

Mifepristone

Based on theoretical grounds, mifepristone may interact with salicylates.

4.6 Pregnancy and lactation
Although teratogenic effects of acetylsalicylic acid have been recorded in animals, no such effects have been observed in humans.

No teratogenic effects have been observed with metoclopramide: data on pregnant patients (> 1000) indicate no malformative nor foeto/ neonatal toxicity during 1rst trimester of pregnancy. A limited amount of data on pregnant patients (> 300) indicate no neonatal toxicity in other trimesters. Animal studies do not indicate reproductive toxicity.

In the third trimester, the use of prostaglandin synthesis inhibitors such as acetylsalicylic acid may expose the foetus to premature closure of the ductus arteriosus. MigraMax is therefore contra-indicated during the third trimester. Like all drugs avoid use in the first and second trimester unless the physician believes the benefits outweigh the risk.

MigraMax is not recommended during lactation because acetylsalicylic acid and metoclopramide are excreted in breast milk and adverse reactions in the breast-fed baby cannot be excluded. A decision should be made whether to discontinue breast-feeding or to abstain from Migramax treatment.

4.7 Effects on ability to drive and use machines
MigraMax may cause drowsiness. This effect can be potentiated by CNS depressants or alcohol. If affected, patients should not drive or operate machinery.

4.8 Undesirable effects

Nervous system and psychiatric disorders

The following reactions, sometimes associated, occur more frequently when high doses are used:

- Extrapyramidal symptoms: acute dystonia and dyskinesia, Parkinsonian syndrome, akathisia may occur even following administration of a single dose of the drug particularly in young adults and the elderly (see section 4.4 Special warnings and precautions for use).

Extrapyramidal reactions include spasm of the facial muscles, trismus, rhythmic protrusion of the tongue, a bulbar type of speech, spasm of extraocular muscles including oculogyric crises, unnatural positioning of the head and shoulders and opisthotonos. There may be a generalised increase in muscle tone. The majority of reactions occur within 36 hours of starting treatment and the effects usually disappear within 24 hours of withdrawal of the drug. Should treatment of a dystonic reaction be required, a benzodazepine or an anticholinergic anti-Parkinsonian drug may be used.

Drowsiness, decreased level of consciousness, confusion, hallucination.

Other reactions may occur:

- Tardive dyskinesia, particularly in elderly patients and during or after prolonged treatment.
- Metoclopramide may cause lethargy, insomnia, dizziness
- Depression
- Restlessness, anxiety
- Seizures
- Neuroleptic malignant syndrome.

Endocrine disorders

Hyperprolactinaemia with amenorrhea, galactorrhea, gynaecomastia.

Blood and Lymphatic system disorders

Metoclopramide may cause:

- Methaemoglobinaemia which could be related to NADH cytochrome b5 reductase deficiency (see section 4.4 Special warnings and precautions for use).
- Sulfhaemoglobinaemia, mainly with concomitant administration of high doses of sulfur-releasing drugs.
- Aspirin may increase bleeding time, decrease platelet adhesiveness, and in large doses cause hypothrombinaemia. It may cause other blood disorders, including thrombocytopenia, iron deficiency or haemolytic anaemia and rarely agranulocytosis.

Cardiac and Vascular disorders

Bradycardia and heart block have been reported with metoclopramide, particularly the intravenous formulation.

Gastrointestinal disorders

Diarrhoea, flatulence The most common side effects occurring with therapeutic doses of salicylates are gastrointestinal disturbances such as gastric irritation with blood loss, nausea, dyspepsia, vomiting and gastric ulceration. The gastro-intestinal haemorrhaging is occasionally severe but in most cases blood loss is not significant.

General disorders and administration site conditions

Very rarely hypersensitivity, including anaphylaxis has been reported. Salicylates may induce hypersensitivity especially in those individuals with asthma or rhinitis, and a history of atopy or nasal polyps. The observed hypersensitivity reactions include anaphylaxis, urticara and bronchospasm.

Asthenia

Ear and labyrinth disorders

Tinnitus

Renal and urinary disorders

Other reported effects of salicylates include urate kidney stones.

4.9 Overdose

In cases of overdose, toxic reactions are mainly ascribable to aspirin.

Salicylate poisoning is usually associated with plasma concentrations >350 mg/L (2.5 mmol/L). Most adult deaths occur in patients whose concentrations exceed 700 mg/L (95.1 mmol/L). Single doses less than 100 mg/kg are unlikely to cause serious poisoning.

Symptoms

Common features include vomiting, dehydration, tinnitus, vertigo, deafness, sweating, warm extremities with bounding pulses, increased respiratory rate and hyperventilation. Some degree of acid-base disturbance is present in most cases. A mixed respiratory alkalosis and metabolic acidosis with normal or high arterial pH (normal or reduced hydrogen ion concentration) is usual in adults and children over the age of 4 years. In children aged 4 years or less, a dominant metabolic acidosis with low arterial pH (raised hydrogen ion concentration) is common. Acidosis may increase salicylate transfer across the blood brain barrier. Uncommon features include haematemesis, hyperpyrexia, hypoglycaemia, hypokalaemia, thrombocytopaenia, increased INR/PTR, intravascular coagulation, renal failure and non-cardiac pulmonary oedema.

Central nervous system features including confusion, disorientation, coma and convulsions are less common in adults than in children.

Management

Give activated charcoal if an adult presents within one hour of ingestion of more than 250 mg/kg. The plasma salicylate concentration should be measured, although the severity of poisoning cannot be determined from this alone and the clinical and biochemical features must be taken into account. Elimination is increased by urinary alkalinisation, which is achieved by the administration of 1.26% sodium bicarbonate. The urine pH should be monitored. Correct metabolic acidosis with intravenous 8.4% sodium bicarbonate (first check serum potassium). Forced diuresis should not be used since it does not enhance salicylate excretion and may cause pulmonary oedema. Haemodialysis is the treatment of choice for severe poisoning and should be considered in patients with plasma salicylate concentrations >700 mg/L (5.1 mmol/L), or lower concentrations associated with severe clinical or metabolic features. Patients under 10 years or over 70 have increased risk of salicylate toxicity and may require dialysis at an earlier stage.

Metoclopramide overdose may cause extrapyramidal disorders and drowsiness, decreased level of consciousness, confusion, hallucinations and convulsions.

Treatment for extrapyramidal disorders caused by metoclopramide overdose is symptomatic (benzodiazepines in children and/or anticholinergic anti-parkinsonian drugs in adults).

5. PHARMACOLOGICAL PROPERTIES

5.1 Pharmacodynamic properties

The pharmacological properties of this product are those of the two active ingredients i.e. an analgesic and an antiemetic.

Acetylsalcylic acid has analgesic, antipyretic and anti-inflammatory properties. It inhibits prostaglandin synthesis so that the prostaglandin-induced sensitivity of peripheral nerve endings to kinins and other mediators of pain and inflammation is reduced. Acetylsalicylic acid also exerts a powerful inhibition on platelet aggregation by blocking thromboxane A2 synthesis in the platelets.

Metoclopramide is an effective anti-emetic, although its exact mechanism(s) of action is not fully established. It is a cholinergic agonist acting peripherally to enhance the action of acetylcholine at muscarinic synapses and in the CNS by blocking dopamine receptors in the chemoreceptor trigger zone for vomiting.

Local effects include the promotion of gastric emptying and normal peristalsis, impairment of which are a common feature of migraine attacks.

5.2 Pharmacokinetic properties

Lysine acetylsalicylate

Absorption of lysine acetylsalicylate as a solution is rapid in healthy subjects. Lysine acetylsalicylate dissociates into lysine and acetylsalicylic acid which is rapidly hydrolysed to salicylic acid. The plasma peak of acetylsalicylic acid is achieved within 20 minutes.

Plasma salicylates are essentially bound to plasma proteins and are converted to inactive metabolites in the liver. Salicylic acid and its metabolites are excreted via the kidneys. Clearance increases with increasing urinary pH. The elimination half-life of salicylic acid is dose-dependent owing to the saturable nature of salicylic acid conjugation and ranges from as little as 2 hours after a single dose of 500 mg, lengthening to as long as 20 hours in overdosage.

Metoclopramide

The plasma peak of metoclopramide is reached within an average time of 40 minutes following oral administration. Peak plasma concentrations are 32 and 70 g/L for 10 and 20 mg doses.

Bioavailability is 80% following oral administration. Inter-individual variations are related to a 20% first-pass effect. Metoclopramide is rapidly and extensively distributed in tissues. The volume of distribution is 2.2 - 3.4 l/kg. Metoclopramide has a low degree of binding to plasma proteins (30%). The plasma elimination half-life of metoclopramide is 5 - 6 hours. Total clearance is 0.4 - 0.7 l/min.

Metoclopramide is only partially metabolised in humans; urinary excretion occurs essentially as the unchanged and sulphoconjugated compounds (50% of the dose administered).

Renal insufficiency significantly reduces the clearance of metoclopramide and increases the plasma elimination half-life.

Combination

When administered as an oral solution, lysine acetylsalicylate and metoclopramide are rapidly absorbed.

In subjects not suffering from migraine, plasma concentrations of total salicylates, acetylsalicylic acid and metoclopramide do not differ from those recorded following both drugs administered singly.

The elimination half-life of salicylates and metoclopramide is unaffected in subjects suffering from migraine receiving the two drugs in combination compared with normal subjects.

5.3 Preclinical safety data

No data of therapeutic relevance.

6. PHARMACEUTICAL PARTICULARS

6.1 List of excipients

Aspartame

Glycine

Lemon flavour (essential oil of lemon absorbed on a maltodextrin substrate)

6.2 Incompatibilities

No known major incompatibilities

6.3 Shelf life

1 year

6.4 Special precautions for storage

Store at or below 25°C.

6.5 Nature and contents of container

Pack sizes: Carton containing 2 sachets

Carton containing 6 sachets

Carton containing 20 sachets

MigraMax is packaged in sachets made of a paper-polyethylene-aluminium complex, containing one unit dose and heat-sealed.

6.6 Special precautions for disposal and other handling

Consult the patient leaflet before use.

Do not use after the stated expiry date on the sachet or carton.

To be taken orally when the powder is completely dissolved.

7. MARKETING AUTHORISATION HOLDER

Sanofi-Synthelabo Limited (or trading as Sanofi-aventis)

One Onslow Street

Guildford

Surrey

GU1 4YS

UK

or trading as

Lorex Synthelabo

or

Sanofi-Synthelabo

PO Box 597

Guildford

Surrey

8. MARKETING AUTHORISATION NUMBER(S)

PL 11723/0310

9. DATE OF FIRST AUTHORISATION/RENEWAL OF THE AUTHORISATION

29 May 2001

10. DATE OF REVISION OF THE TEXT

June 2009

Legal Classification

POM

Mildison Lipocream

(Astellas Pharma Ltd)

1. NAME OF THE MEDICINAL PRODUCT

MILDISON LIPOCREAM

2. QUALITATIVE AND QUANTITATIVE COMPOSITION

Contains 1% w/w hydrocortisone.

For excipients, see 6.1

3. PHARMACEUTICAL FORM

Cream.

White or practically white smooth cream.

4. CLINICAL PARTICULARS

4.1 Therapeutic indications

Eczema and dermatitis of all types including atopic eczema, otitis externa, primary irritant and allergic dermatitis, intertrigo, prurigo nodularis, seborrhoeic dermatitis, and insect bite reactions.

4.2 Posology and method of administration

For topical application.

For Adults, Children, and the Elderly:

Apply a small quantity only sufficient to cover the affected area two or three times a day. Due to the formulation of the base the product may be used both for dry scaly lesions and for moist or weeping lesions.

Children and infants: Long term treatment should be avoided. Courses should be limited to seven days where possible.

4.3 Contraindications

Hypersensitivity to hydrocortisone or to any of the ingredients of the cream.

This preparation is contraindicated in the presence of untreated viral or fungal infections, tubercular or syphilitic lesions, peri-oral dermatitis, acne vulgaris and rosacea and in bacterial infections unless used in connection with appropriate chemotherapy.

4.4 Special warnings and precautions for use

Although generally regarded as safe even for long term administration in adults there is a potential for overdosage in infancy. Extreme caution is required in dermatoses of infancy including napkin eruption. In such patients courses of treatment should not normally exceed seven days.

As with all corticosteroids, application to the face, flexures and other areas of thin skin may cause skin atrophy and increased absorption and should be avoided.

Keep away from eyes.

4.5 Interaction with other medicinal products and other forms of interaction

None known.

4.6 Pregnancy and lactation

There is inadequate evidence of safety in human pregnancy. Topical administration of corticosteroids to pregnant animals can cause abnormalities of foetal development including cleft palate and intra-uterine growth retardation. There may therefore be a very small risk of such effects in the human foetus. Theoretically, there is the possibility that if maternal systemic absorption occurred the infant's adrenal function could be affected.

The use of topical corticosteroids during lactation is unlikely to present a hazard to infants being breast-fed.

4.7 Effects on ability to drive and use machines

None known.

4.8 Undesirable effects

Local atrophic changes may occur, particularly in skin folds, intertriginous areas or in nappy areas in young children where moist conditions favour hydrocortisone absorption. Systemic absorption from such sites may be sufficient to produce hypercorticism and suppression of the pituitary adrenal axis after prolonged treatment. This effect is more likely to occur in infants and children and if occlusive dressings are used or large areas of skin treated. Napkins may act as occlusive dressings.

The cetostearyl alcohol may cause local skin reactions (e.g. contact dermatitis) and the methyl parahydroxybenzoate may cause allergic reactions which can be delayed.

4.9 Overdose

Excessive use, especially under occlusive dressings or over a long period of time, may produce adrenal suppression. No special procedures or antidote. Treat any adverse effects symptomatically

5. PHARMACOLOGICAL PROPERTIES

5.1 Pharmacodynamic properties

The active ingredient, hydrocortisone, is a well-established corticosteroid with the pharmacological actions of a corticosteroid classified as mildly potent.

5.2 Pharmacokinetic properties
In human in-vivo studies the potency of this formulation has been demonstrated as being of the same order as other widely available formulations of hydrocortisone 1%.

5.3 Preclinical safety data
No relevant pre-clinical safety data has been generated.

6. PHARMACEUTICAL PARTICULARS

6.1 List of excipients
Cetostearyl alcohol
Macrogol Cetostearyl Ether
Light Liquid paraffin
White soft paraffin
Methyl parahydroxybenzoate
Sodium citrate anhydrous
Citric acid anhydrous
Purified water

6.2 Incompatibilities
None stated.

6.3 Shelf life
Three years

6.4 Special precautions for storage
Do not store above 25°C.

6.5 Nature and contents of container
Collapsible membrane-necked internally coated aluminium tubes with a polyethylene screw cap containing 10 g, 15 g, 30 g, or 100 g.

6.6 Special precautions for disposal and other handling
No special requirements.

7. MARKETING AUTHORISATION HOLDER
Astellas Pharma Ltd
Lovett House
Lovett Road
Staines
TW18 3AZ
United Kingdom

8. MARKETING AUTHORISATION NUMBER(S)
PL 0166/0131

9. DATE OF FIRST AUTHORISATION/RENEWAL OF THE AUTHORISATION
First authorised 23 September 1987; renewed 21 December 2004.

10. DATE OF REVISION OF THE TEXT
4 November 2005

11. LEGAL CATEGORY
POM

Minodiab 5

(Pharmacia Limited)

1. NAME OF THE MEDICINAL PRODUCT
Minodiab 5 mg Tablets

2. QUALITATIVE AND QUANTITATIVE COMPOSITION
Glipizide 5.0 mg

3. PHARMACEUTICAL FORM
White biconvex tablets.

4. CLINICAL PARTICULARS

4.1 Therapeutic indications
Glipizide is indicated as an adjunct to diet and exercise to improve glycemic control in adults with type 2 diabetes mellitus.

4.2 Posology and method of administration
Route of administration Oral

As for any hypoglycaemic agent, dosage must be adapted for each individual case.

Short term administration of glipizide may be sufficient during periods of transient loss of control in patients usually controlled well on diet.

In general, glipizide should be given shortly before a meal to achieve the greatest reduction in post-prandial hyperglycaemia.

Initial Dose
The recommended starting dose is 5 mg, given before breakfast or the midday meal. Mild diabetics, geriatric patients or those with liver disease may be started on 2.5 mg.

Titration
Dosage adjustments should ordinarily be in increments of 2.5 to 5 mg, as determined by blood glucose response. At least several days should elapse between titration steps. The maximum recommended single dose is 15 mg. If this is not sufficient, splitting the daily dosage may prove effective. Doses above 15 mg should ordinarily be divided.

Maintenance
Some patients may be effectively controlled on a once-a-day regimen. Total daily dosage above 15 mg should ordinarily be divided.

The maximum recommended daily dosage is 20 mg.

Use in Children
Safety and effectiveness in children have not been established.

Use in Elderly and in High Risk Patients
In elderly patients, debilitated or malnourished patients and patients with an impaired renal or hepatic function, the initial and maintenance dosing should be conservative to avoid hypoglycaemic reactions (see Initial Dose and Special Warnings and Special Precautions for Use sections).

Patients Receiving Other Oral Hypoglycaemic Agents
As with other sulphonylurea class hypoglycaemics, no transition period is necessary when transferring patients to glipizide. Patients should be observed carefully (1-2 weeks) for hypoglycaemia when being transferred from longer half-life sulphonylureas (e.g. chlorpropamide) to glipizide due to potential overlapping of drug effect.

4.3 Contraindications
Glipizide is contraindicated in patients with:

1. Hypersensitivity to glipizide, other sulphonylureas or sulphonamides, or any excipients in the tablets;
2. Insulin-dependent diabetes, diabetic ketoacidosis, diabetic coma;
3. Severe renal or hepatic insufficiency;
4. Patients treated with miconazole (see 4.5 Interactions);
5. Pregnancy and lactation

4.4 Special warnings and precautions for use
Hypoglycaemia
All sulphonylurea drugs are capable of producing severe hypoglycaemia. Renal or hepatic insufficiency may cause elevated blood levels of glipizide and the latter may also diminish gluconeogenic capacity, both of which increase the risk of serious hypoglycaemic reactions. Elderly, debilitated or malnourished patients and those with adrenal or pituitary insufficiency are particularly susceptible to the hypoglycaemic action of glucose-lowering drugs.

Hypoglycaemia may be difficult to recognise in the elderly, and in people who are taking beta-adrenergic blocking drugs (see interactions). Hypoglycaemia is more likely to occur when caloric- intake is deficient, after severe or prolonged exercise, when alcohol is ingested, or when more than one glucose-lowering drug is used.

Loss of control of blood glucose
When a patient stabilised on a diabetic regimen is exposed to stress such as fever, trauma, infection, or surgery, a loss of control may occur. At such times, it may be necessary to discontinue glipizide and administer insulin.

The effectiveness of any oral hypoglycaemic drug, including glipizide, in lowering blood glucose to a desired level decreases in many patients over a period of time, which may be due to progression of the severity of diabetes or to diminished responsiveness to the drug. This phenomenon is known as secondary failure, to distinguish it from primary failure in which the drug is ineffective in an individual patient when first given. Adequate adjustment of dose and adherence to diet should be assessed before classifying a patient as a secondary failure.

Renal and Hepatic Disease
The pharmacokinetics and/or pharmacodynamics of glipizide may be affected in patients with impaired renal or hepatic function. If hypoglycaemia should occur in such patients, it may be prolonged and appropriate management should be instituted.

Information for Patients
Patients should be informed of the potential risks and advantages of glipizide and of alternative modes of therapy. They should also be informed about the importance of adherence to dietary instructions, of a regular exercise program, and of regular testing of urine and/or blood glucose.

The risks of hypoglycaemia, its symptoms and treatment, and conditions that predispose to its development should be explained to patients and responsible family members. Primary and secondary failure should also be explained.

Laboratory Tests
Blood and urine glucose should be monitored periodically. Measurement of glycosylated haemoglobin may be useful.

4.5 Interaction with other medicinal products and other forms of interaction
The following products are likely to increase the hypoglycaemic effect:

- **Contraindicated combinations**

Miconazole: increase in hypoglycaemic effect, possibly leading to symptoms of hypoglycaemia or even coma.

- **Inadvisable combinations**

Nonsteroidal anti-inflammatory agents (NSAIDS) e.g. phenylbutazone: increase in hypoglycaemic effect of sulphonylureas (displacement of sulphonylurea binding to plasma proteins and/or decrease in sulphonylurea elimination).

Alcohol: increase in hypoglycaemic reaction which can lead to hypoglycaemic coma.

- **Combinations requiring precaution**

Fluconazole: increase in the half-life of the sulphonylurea, possibly giving rise to symptoms of hypoglycaemia.

Voriconazole: Although not studied, voriconazole may increase the plasma levels of sulfonylureas, (e.g. tolbutamide, glipizide and glyburide) and therefore cause hypoglycaemia. Careful monitoring of blood glucose is recommended during co-administration.

Salicylates (acetylsalicylic acid): increase in hypoglycaemic effect by high doses of acetylsalicylic acid (hypoglycaemic action of the acetylsalicylic acid).

Beta-blockers: all beta-blockers mask some of the symptoms of hypoglycaemia, i.e. palpitations and tachycardia. Most non cardioselective beta-blockers increase the incidence and severity of hypoglycaemia.

Angiotensin converting enzyme inhibitors: the use of angiotensin converting enzyme inhibitors may lead to an increased hypoglycaemic effect in diabetic patients treated with sulphonylureas.

Cimetidine: the use of cimetidine may be associated with a reduction in post prandial blood glucose in patients treated with glipizide.

The hypoglycaemic action of sulphonylureas in general may also be potentiated by monoamine oxidase inhibitors and drugs that are highly protein bound, such as sulfonamides, chloramphenicol, probenecid, coumarins and fibrates.

When such drugs are administered to (or withdrawn from) a patient receiving glipizide, the patient should be observed closely for hypoglycaemia (or loss of control).

The following products could lead to hyperglycaemia:

- **Inadvisable combinations**

Danazol: diabetogenic effect of danazol. If it cannot be avoided, warn the patient and step up self monitoring of blood glucose and urine. Possibly adjust the dosage of antidiabetic agent during treatment with danazol and after its discontinuation.

- **Combinations requiring precaution**

Phenothiazines (e.g. chlorpromazine) at high doses (> 100 mg per day of chlorpromazine): elevation in blood glucose (reduction in insulin release).

Corticosteroids: elevation in blood glucose.

Sympathomimetics (e.g. ritodrine, salbutamol, terbutaline): elevation in blood glucose due to beta-2-adrenoceptor stimulation. *Progestogens*: diabetogenic effects of high-dose progestogens. Warn the patient and step up self-monitoring of blood glucose and urine. Possibly adjust the dosage of antidiabetic agent during treatment with the neuroleptics, corticoids or progestogen and after discontinuation.

Other drugs that may produce hyperglycaemia and lead to a loss of control include the thiazides and other diuretics, thyroid products, oestrogens, oral contraceptives, phenytoin, nicotinic acid, calcium channel blocking drugs, and isoniazid.

When such drugs are withdrawn from a patient receiving glipizide, the patient should be observed closely for hypoglycaemia.

4.6 Pregnancy and lactation
Pregnancy
Glipizide is contraindicated in pregnancy.

Glipizide was found to be mildly fetotoxic in rat reproductive studies. No teratogenic effects were found in rat or rabbit studies.

Prolonged severe hypoglycaemia (4 to 10 days) has been reported in neonates born to mothers who were receiving a sulphonylurea drug at the time of delivery.

Because recent information suggests that abnormal blood glucose levels during pregnancy are associated with a higher incidence of congenital abnormalities, many experts recommend that insulin be used during pregnancy to maintain blood glucose levels as close to normal as possible.

Lactation
No data are available on secretion into breast milk. Therefore glipizide is contraindicated in lactation.

4.7 Effects on ability to drive and use machines
The effect of glipizide on the ability to drive or operate machinery has not been studied. However, there is no evidence to suggest that glipizide may affect these abilities. Patients should be aware of the symptoms of hypoglycaemia and be careful about driving and the use of machinery, especially when optimum stabilisation has not been achieved, for example during the change-over from other medications or during irregular use.

4.8 Undesirable effects
The majority of side effects have been dose related, transient, and have responded to dose reduction or withdrawal of the medication. However, clinical experience thus far has shown that, as with other sulphonylureas, some side effects associated with hypersensitivity may be severe and deaths have been reported in some instances.

Hypoglycaemia
See Special Warnings and Special Precautions for Use and Overdose sections.

Gastrointestinal
Gastrointestinal complaints include nausea, diarrhoea, constipation and gastralgia. They appear to be dose related and usually disappear on division or reduction of dosage.

Dermatologic

Allergic skin reactions including erythema, morbilliform or maculopapular reactions, urticaria, pruritus and eczema have been reported. They frequently disappear with continued therapy. However, if they persist, the drug should be discontinued. As with other sulphonylureas, photosensitivity reactions have been reported.

Miscellaneous

Confusion, dizziness, drowsiness, headache, tremor, and visual disturbances have each been reported in patients treated with glipizide. They are usually transient and do not require discontinuance of therapy; however, they may also be symptoms of hypoglycaemia.

Laboratory Test

The pattern of laboratory test abnormalities observed with glipizide is similar to that for other sulphonylureas. Occasional mild to moderate elevations of SGOT, LDH, alkaline phosphatase, BUN and creatinine were noted. The relationship of these abnormalities to glipizide is uncertain, and they have rarely been associated with clinical symptoms.

Hepatic disorder

Cholestatic jaundice, impaired hepatic function, and hepatitis have been reported. Discontinue treatment if cholestatic jaundice occurs.

Haematologic Reactions

Leucopenia, agranulocytosis, thrombocytopenia, haemolytic anaemia, aplastic anaemia and pancytopenia have been reported.

Metabolic Reactions

Hepatic porphyria and porphyria cutanea tarda have been reported. Disulfiram-like reactions have been reported with other sulphonylureas.

Endocrine Reactions

Hyponatraemia has been reported.

4.9 Overdose

There is no well documented experience with glipizide overdosage.

Overdosage of sulphonylureas including glipizide can produce glycaemia. Mild hypoglycaemic symptoms without loss of consciousness or neurologic findings should be treated actively with oral glucose and adjustments in drug dosage and/or meal patterns. Close monitoring should continue until the physician is assured that the patient is out of danger. Severe hypoglycaemic reactions with coma, seizure, or other neurological impairment occur infrequently, but constitute medical emergencies requiring immediate hospitalisation. If hypoglycaemic coma is diagnosed or suspected, the patient should be given a rapid intravenous injection of concentrated (50%) glucose solution. This should be followed by a continuous infusion of a more dilute (10%) glucose solution at a rate that will maintain the blood glucose at a level above 100 mg/dL (5.55 mmol/L). Patients should be closely monitored for a minimum of 48 hours and depending on the status of the patient at this time the physician should decide whether further monitoring is required. Clearance of glipizide from plasma may be prolonged in persons with liver disease. Because of the extensive protein binding of glipizide, dialysis is unlikely to be of benefit.

5. PHARMACOLOGICAL PROPERTIES

5.1 Pharmacodynamic properties

Glipizide is an oral blood glucose lowering drug of the sulphonylurea class. The primary mode of action of glipizide is the stimulation of insulin secretion from the beta-cells of pancreatic islet tissue. Stimulation of insulin secretion by glipizide in response to a meal is of major importance. Fasting insulin levels are not elevated even on long-term glipizide administration, but the post-prandial insulin response continues to be enhanced after at least 6 months of treatment. The insulinotropic response to a meal occurs within 30 minutes after oral dose of glipizide in diabetic patients, but elevated insulin levels do not persist beyond the time of the meal challenge. There is also increasing evidence that extrapancreatic effects involving potentiation of insulin action form a significant component of the activity of glipizide.

Blood sugar control persists for up to 24 hours after a single dose of glipizide, even though plasma levels have declined to a small fraction of peak levels by that time (see "Pharmacokinetics" below).

5.2 Pharmacokinetic properties

Gastrointestinal absorption of glipizide in man is uniform, rapid and essentially complete. Peak plasma concentrations occur 1-3 hours after a single oral dose. The half-life of elimination ranges from 2-4 hours in normal subjects, whether given intravenously or orally. The metabolic and excretory patterns are similar with the two routes of administration, indicating that first-pass metabolism is not significant. Glipizide does not accumulate in plasma on repeated oral administration. Total absorption and disposition of an oral dose was unaffected by food in normal volunteers, but absorption was delayed by about 40 minutes. Thus, glipizide was more effective when administered about 30 minutes before, rather than with, a test meal in diabetic patients. Protein binding was studied in serum from volunteers who received either oral or intravenous glipizide and found to be 98-99% one hour after either route of administration. The apparent volume of distribution of glipizide after intravenous administration was 11 litres, indicative of localisation within the extracellular fluid compartment. In mice, no glipizide or metabolites were detectable autoradiographically in the brain or spinal cord of males or females, nor in the foetuses of pregnant females. In another study, however, very small amounts of radioactivity were detected in the foetuses of rats given labelled drug.

The metabolism of glipizide is extensive and occurs mainly in the liver. The primary metabolites are inactive hydroxylation products and polar conjugates and are excreted mainly in the urine. Less than 10% unchanged glipizide is found in urine.

5.3 Preclinical safety data

Acute toxicity studies showed no specific susceptibility. The acute oral toxicity of glipizide was extremely low in all species tested (LD50 greater than 4 g/kg). Chronic toxicity tests in rats and dogs at doses up to 8.0 mg/kg did not show any evidence of toxic effects.

A 20-month study in rats and an 18-month study in mice at doses up to 75 times the maximum human dose revealed no evidence of drug related carcinogenicity. Bacterial and in vivo mutagenicity tests were uniformly negative. Studies in rats of both sexes at doses up to 75 times the human dose showed no effects on fertility.

6. PHARMACEUTICAL PARTICULARS

6.1 List of excipients

Microcrystalline cellulose Ph. Eur.

Starch Ph. Eur.

Stearic acid HSE

Lactose Ph. Eur.

6.2 Incompatibilities

None stated.

6.3 Shelf life

12 months.

6.4 Special precautions for storage

None.

6.5 Nature and contents of container

Blister strips containing 28 or 60 tablets

6.6 Special precautions for disposal and other handling

None.

Administrative Data

7. MARKETING AUTHORISATION HOLDER

Pharmacia Limited

Ramsgate Road,

Sandwich,

Kent, CT13 9NJ

United Kingdom.

8. MARKETING AUTHORISATION NUMBER(S)

Minodiab 5 - PL 00032/0319

9. DATE OF FIRST AUTHORISATION/RENEWAL OF THE AUTHORISATION

Minodiab 5 - 5th April 2002

10. DATE OF REVISION OF THE TEXT

July 2009

Company Ref: MG 5_0

Mirapexin ▼ 0.7 mg tablets

(Boehringer Ingelheim Limited)

1. NAME OF THE MEDICINAL PRODUCT

MIRAPEXIN ▼ 0.7 mg tablets

2. QUALITATIVE AND QUANTITATIVE COMPOSITION

MIRAPEXIN 0.7 mg tablets contain 0.7 mg of pramipexole base (as 1.0 mg of pramipexole dihydrochloride monohydrate).

Please note:

Pramipexole doses as published in the literature refer to the salt form.

Therefore, doses will be expressed in terms of both pramipexole base and pramipexole salt (in brackets).

For a full list of excipients, see section 6.1.

3. PHARMACEUTICAL FORM

Tablet

All tablets are white and have a code embossed.

Strength (mg salt)	Appearance
0.125	flat, round, 6 mm diameter, no score
0.25	flat, oval, 7.86 × 5.63 mm, scores on both sides
0.5	flat, oval, 10.59 × 7.59 mm, scores on both sides
1.0	flat, round, 9 mm diameter, scores on both sides
1.5	flat, round, 11 mm diameter, scores on both sides

All tablets can be divided into equal halves (with the exception of the 0.088/0.125 mg tablet).

4. CLINICAL PARTICULARS

4.1 Therapeutic indications

MIRAPEXIN is indicated for treatment of the signs and symptoms of idiopathic Parkinson's disease, alone (without levodopa) or in combination with levodopa, i.e. over the course of the disease, through to late stages when the effect of levodopa wears off or becomes inconsistent and fluctuations of the therapeutic effect occur (end of dose or "on off" fluctuations).

MIRAPEXIN is indicated for symptomatic treatment of moderate to severe idiopathic Restless Legs Syndrome in dosages up to 0.54 mg of base (0.75 mg of salt) (see section 4.2).

4.2 Posology and method of administration

Parkinson's disease

The tablets should be taken orally, swallowed with water, and can be taken either with or without food. The daily dosage is administered in equally divided doses 3 times a day.

Initial treatment:

Dosages should be increased gradually from a starting-dose of 0.264 mg of base (0.375 mg of salt) per day and then increased every 5 - 7 days. Providing patients do not experience intolerable side-effects, the dosage should be titrated to achieve a maximal therapeutic effect.

(see Table 1a on next page)

If a further dose increase is necessary the daily dose should be increased by 0.54 mg base (0.75 mg salt) at weekly intervals up to a maximum dose of 3.3 mg of base (4.5 mg of salt) per day.

However, it should be noted that the incidence of somnolence is increased at doses higher than 1.5 mg/ day (see section 4.8).

Maintenance treatment:

The individual dose should be in the range of 0.264 mg of base (0.375 mg of salt) to a maximum of 3.3 mg of base (4.5 mg of salt) per day. During dose escalation in three pivotal studies, efficacy was observed starting at a daily dose of 1.1 mg of base (1.5 mg of salt). Further dose adjustments should be done based on the clinical response and the occurrence of undesirable effects. In clinical trials approximately 5% of patients were treated at doses below 1.1 mg (1.5 mg of salt). In advanced Parkinson's disease, doses higher than 1.1 mg (1.5 mg of salt) per day can be useful in patients where a reduction of the levodopa therapy is intended. It is recommended that the dosage of levodopa is reduced during both the dose escalation and the maintenance treatment with MIRAPEXIN, depending on reactions in individual patients.

Treatment discontinuation:

Abrupt discontinuation of dopaminergic therapy can lead to the development of aneuroleptic malignant syndrome. Therefore, pramipexole should be tapered off at a rate of 0.54 mg of base (0.75 mg of salt) per day until the daily dose has been reduced to 0.54 mg of base (0.75 mg of salt). Thereafter the dose should be reduced by 0.264 mg of base (0.375 mg of salt) per day (see section 4.4).

Dosing in patients with renal impairment:

The elimination of pramipexole is dependent on renal function. The following dosage schedule is suggested for initiation of therapy:

Patients with a creatinine clearance above 50 ml/min require no reduction in daily dose.

In patients with a creatinine clearance between 20 and 50 ml/min, the initial daily dose of MIRAPEXIN should be administered in two divided doses, starting at 0.088 mg of base (0.125 mg of salt) twice a day (0.176 mg of base/ 0.25 mg of salt daily).

In patients with a creatinine clearance less than 20 ml/min, the daily dose of MIRAPEXIN should be administered in a single dose, starting at 0.088 mg of base (0.125 mg of salt) daily.

If renal function declines during maintenance therapy, reduce MIRAPEXIN daily dose by the same percentage as the decline in creatinine clearance, i.e. if creatinine clearance declines by 30%, then reduce the MIRAPEXIN daily dose by 30%. The daily dose can be administered in two divided doses if creatinine clearance is between 20 and 50 ml/min, and as a single daily dose if creatinine clearance is less than 20 ml/min.

Dosing in patients with hepatic impairment

Dose adjustment in patients with hepatic failure is probably not necessary, as approx. 90% of absorbed active substance is excreted through the kidneys. However, the potential influence of hepatic insufficiency on MIRAPEXIN pharmacokinetics has not been investigated.

Restless Legs Syndrome

The tablets should be taken orally, swallowed with water, and can be taken either with or without food.

The recommended starting dose of MIRAPEXIN is 0.088 mg of base (0.125 mg of salt) taken once daily

Table 1a

Ascending – Dose Schedule of MIRAPEXIN				
Week	Dosage (mg of base)	Total Daily Dose (mg of base)	Dosage (mg of salt)	Total Daily Dose (mg of salt)
1	3 × 0.088	0.264	3 × 0.125	0.375
2	3 × 0.18	0.54	3 × 0.25	0.75
3	3 × 0.35	1.1	3 × 0.5	1.50

2-3 hours before bedtime. For patients requiring additional symptomatic relief, the dose may be increased every 4-7 days to a maximum of 0.54 mg of base (0.75 mg of salt) per day (as shown in the table below).

Dose Schedule of MIRAPEXIN		
Titration Step	Once Daily Evening Dose (mg of base)	Once Daily Evening Dose (mg of salt)
1	0.088	0.125
2*	0.18	0.25
3*	0.35	0.50
4*	0.54	0.75
* if needed		

As long-term efficacy of MIRAPEXIN in the treatment of RLS has not been sufficiently tested, patient's response should be evaluated after 3 months treatment and the need for treatment continuation should be reconsidered. If treatment is interrupted for more than a few days it should be re-initiated by dose titration carried out as above.

Treatment discontinuation

Since daily dose for the treatment of Restless Legs Syndrome will not exceed 0.54 mg of base (0.75 mg of salt) MIRAPEXIN can be discontinued without tapering off. Rebound (worsening of symptoms after abrupt discontinuation of treatment) can not be excluded.

Dosing in patients with renal impairment

The elimination of pramipexole is dependent on renal function. Patients with a creatinine clearance above 20 mL/min require no reduction in daily dose.

The use of MIRAPEXIN has not been studied in hemodialysis patients, or in patients with severe renal impairment.

Dosing in patients with hepatic impairment

Dose adjustment in patients with hepatic failure is not required, as approx. 90% of absorbed active substance is excreted through the kidneys.

Dosing in children and adolescents

MIRAPEXIN is not recommended for use in children and adolescents below 18 years due to a lack of data on safety and efficacy.

4.3 Contraindications

Hypersensitivity to the active substance or to any of the excipients.

4.4 Special warnings and precautions for use

When prescribing MIRAPEXIN in a patient with Parkinson's disease with renal impairment a reduced dose is suggested in line with section 4.2.

Hallucinations

Hallucinations are known as a side-effect of treatment with dopamine agonists and levodopa. Patients should be informed that (mostly visual) hallucinations can occur.

Dyskinesia

In advanced Parkinson's disease, in combination treatment with levodopa, dyskinesia can occur during the initial titration of MIRAPEXIN. If they occur, the dose of levodopa should be decreased.

Sudden onset of sleep and somnolence

MIRAPEXIN has been associated with somnolence and episodes of sudden sleep onset, particularly in patients with Parkinson's disease. Sudden onset of sleep during daily activities, in some cases without awareness or warning signs, has been reported uncommonly. Patients must be informed of this and advised to exercise caution while driving or operating machines during treatment with MIRAPEXIN. Patients who have experienced somnolence and/or an episode of sudden sleep onset must refrain from driving or operating machines. Furthermore a reduction of dosage or termination of therapy may be considered. Because of possible additive effects, caution should be advised when patients are taking other sedating medicinal products or alcohol in combination with pramipexole (see section 4.7 and section 4.8).

Impulse control disorders and compulsive behaviours

Pathological gambling, increased libido and hypersexuality have been reported in patients treated with dopamine agonists for Parkinson's disease, including MIRAPEXIN. Furthermore, patients and caregivers should be aware of the fact that other behavioural symptoms of impulse control disorders and compulsions such as binge eating and compulsive shopping can occur. Dose reduction/tapered discontinuation should be considered.

Patients with psychotic disorders

Patients with psychotic disorders should only be treated with dopamine agonists if the potential benefits outweigh the risks. Coadministration of antipsychotic medicinal products with pramipexole should be avoided (see section 4.5).

Ophthalmologic monitoring

Ophthalmologic monitoring is recommended at regular intervals or if vision abnormalities occur.

Severe cardiovascular disease

In case of severe cardiovascular disease, care should be taken. It is recommended to monitor blood pressure, especially at the beginning of treatment, due to the general risk of postural hypotension associated with dopaminergic therapy.

Neuroleptic malignant syndrome

Symptoms suggestive of neuroleptic malignant syndrome have been reported with abrupt withdrawal of dopaminergic therapy (see section 4.2.).

Augmentation

Reports in the literature indicate that treatment of Restless Legs Syndrome with dopaminergic medicinal products can result in augmentation. Augmentation refers to the earlier onset of symptoms in the evening (or even the afternoon), increase in symptoms, and spread of symptoms to involve other extremities. The controlled trials of MIRAPEXIN in patients with Restless Legs Syndrome were generally not of sufficient duration to adequately capture augmentation phenomena. The frequency of augmentation after longer use of MIRAPEXIN and the appropriate management of these events have not been evaluated in controlled clinical trials.

4.5 Interaction with other medicinal products and other forms of interaction

Plasma protein binding

Pramipexole is bound to plasma proteins to a very low (< 20%) extent, and little biotransformation is seen in man. Therefore, interactions with other medicinal products affecting plasma protein binding or elimination by biotransformation are unlikely. As anticholinergics are mainly eliminated by biotransformation, the potential for an interaction is limited, although an interaction with anticholinergics has not been investigated. There is no pharmacokinetic interaction with selegiline and levodopa.

Inhibitors/competitors of active renal elimination pathway

Cimetidine reduced the renal clearance of pramipexole by approximately 34%, presumably by inhibition of the cationic secretory transport system of the renal tubules. Therefore, medicinal products that are inhibitors of this active renal elimination pathway or are eliminated by this pathway, such as cimetidine and amantadine, may interact with pramipexole resulting in reduced clearance of either or both medicinal products. Reduction of the pramipexole dose should be considered when these medicinal products are administered concomitantly with MIRAPEXIN.

Combination with levodopa

When MIRAPEXIN is given in combination with levodopa, it is recommended that the dosage of levodopa is reduced and the dosage of other anti-parkinsonian medicinal products is kept constant while increasing the dose of MIRAPEXIN.

Because of possible additive effects, caution should be advised when patients are taking other sedating medicinal products or alcohol in combination with pramipexole.

Antipsychotic medicinal products

Coadministration of antipsychotic medicinal products with pramipexole should be avoided (see section 4.4), e.g. if antagonistic effects can be expected.

4.6 Pregnancy and lactation

The effect on pregnancy and lactation has not been investigated in humans. Pramipexole was not teratogenic in rats and rabbits, but was embryotoxic in the rat at maternotoxic doses (see section 5.3). MIRAPEXIN should not be used during pregnancy unless clearly necessary, i.e. if the potential benefit justifies the potential risk to the foetus.

As MIRAPEXIN treatment inhibits secretion of prolactin in humans, inhibition of lactation is expected.

The excretion of MIRAPEXIN into breast milk has not been studied in women. In rats, the concentration of active substance-related radioactivity was higher in breast milk than in plasma.

In the absence of human data, MIRAPEXIN should not be used during breast-feeding. However, if its use is unavoidable, breast-feeding should be discontinued.

4.7 Effects on ability to drive and use machines

MIRAPEXIN can have a major influence on the ability to drive and use machines.

Hallucinations or somnolence can occur.

Patients being treated with MIRAPEXIN and presenting with somnolence and/or sudden sleep episodes must be informed to refrain from driving or engaging in activities where impaired alertness may put themselves or others at risk of serious injury or death (e.g. operating machines) until such recurrent episodes and somnolence have resolved (see also sections 4.4, 4.5 and 4.8).

4.8 Undesirable effects

Expected adverse events

The following adverse reactions are expected under the use of MIRAPEXIN: abnormal dreams, amnesia, behavioural symptoms of impulse control disorders and compulsions such as binge eating, compulsive shopping, hypersexuality and pathological gambling; confusion, constipation, delusion, dizziness, dyskinesia, dyspnoea, fatigue, hallucinations, headache, hyperkinesias, hyperphagia, hypotension, insomnia, libido disorders, nausea, paranoia, peripheral oedema, pneumonia, pruritus, rash and other hypersensitivity; restlessness, somnolence, sudden onset of sleep, syncope, visual disturbance including vision blurred and visual acuity reduced, vomiting, weight decrease, weight increase.

Based on the analysis of pooled placebo-controlled trials, comprising a total of 1923 patients on MIRAPEXIN and 1354 patients on placebo, adverse drug reactions were frequently reported for both groups. 63% of patients on MIRAPEXIN and 52% of patients on placebo reported at least one adverse drug reaction.

Tables 1 and 2 display the frequency of adverse drug reactions from placebo-controlled clinical trials in Parkinson's disease and Restless Legs Syndrome. The adverse drug reactions reported in these tables are those events that occurred in 0.1% or more of patients treated with MIRAPEXIN and were reported significantly more often in patients taking MIRAPEXIN than placebo, or where the event was considered clinically relevant. However, the majority of common adverse drug reactions were mild to moderate, they usually start early in therapy, and most tended to disappear even as therapy was continued.

Within the system organ classes, adverse reactions are listed under headings of frequency (number of patients expected to experience the reaction), using the following categories: very common (≥ 1/10); common (≥ 1/100, < 1/10); uncommon (≥ 1/1,000, < 1/100); rare (≥ 1/10,000, < 1/1,000); very rare (< 1/10,000); not known (cannot be estimated from the available data).

Parkinson's disease, most common adverse events

The most commonly (≥ 5%) reported adverse drug reactions in patients with Parkinson's disease more frequent with MIRAPEXIN treatment than with Placebo were nausea, dyskinesia, hypotension, dizziness, somnolence, insomnia, constipation, hallucination, headache and fatigue. The incidence of somnolence is increased at doses higher than 1.5 mg/day (see section 4.2). More frequent adverse drug reactions in combination with levodopa were dyskinesia. Hypotension may occur at the beginning of treatment, especially if MIRAPEXIN is titrated too fast.

Table 1: Parkinson's disease

System Organ Class	Adverse Drug Reaction
Infections and infestations	
Uncommon	pneumonia
Psychiatric disorders	
Common	abnormal dreams, behavioural symptoms of impulse control disorders and compulsions; confusion, hallucinations, insomnia, restlessness
Uncommon	compulsive shopping, delusion, hypersexuality, libido disorder, paranoia, pathological gambling
Not known	binge eating, hyperphagia
Nervous system disorders	
Very common	dizziness, dyskinesia, somnolence
Common	amnesia, headache
Uncommon	hyperkinesia, sudden onset of sleep, syncope
Eye disorders	
Common	visual disturbance including vision blurred and visual acuity reduced

Vascular disorders	
Very common	hypotension
Respiratory, thoracic, and mediastinal disorders	
Uncommon	dyspnoea
Gastrointestinal disorders	
Very common	nausea
Common	constipation, vomiting
Skin and subcutaneous tissue disorders	
Uncommon	hypersensitivity, pruritus, rash
General disorders and administration site conditions	
Common	fatigue, peripheral oedema
Investigations	
Common	weight decrease
Uncommon	weight increase

Restless Legs Syndrome, most common adverse events

The most commonly (⩾ 5%)reported adverse drug reactions in patients with Restless Legs Syndrome treated with MIRAPEXIN were nausea, headache, dizziness and fatigue. Nausea and fatigue were more often reported in female patients treated with MIRAPEXIN (20.8% and 10.5%, respectively) compared to males (6.7% and 7.3%, respectively).

Table 2: Restless Legs Syndrome

System Organ Class	Adverse Drug Reaction
Infections and infestations	
Not known	pneumonia
Psychiatric disorders	
Common	abnormal dreams, insomnia
Uncommon	confusion, hallucinations, libido disorder, restlessness
Not known	behavioural symptoms of impulse control disorders and compulsions such as binge eating, compulsive shopping, hypersexuality, and pathological gambling; delusion, hyperphagia, paranoia
Nervous system disorders	
Common	dizziness, headache, somnolence
Uncommon	sudden onset of sleep, syncope
Not known	amnesia, dyskinesia, hyperkinesia
Eye disorders	
Uncommon	visual disturbance including vision blurred and visual acuity reduced
Vascular disorders	
Uncommon	hypotension
Respiratory, thoracic, and mediastinal disorders	
Uncommon	dyspnoea
Gastrointestinal disorders	
Very common	nausea
Common	constipation, vomiting
Skin and subcutaneous tissue disorders	
Uncommon	hypersensitivity, pruritus, rash
General disorders and administration site conditions	
Common	fatigue
Uncommon	peripheral oedema
Investigations	
Uncommon	weight decrease, weight increase

Somnolence

MIRAPEXIN is associated with somnolence (8.6%) and has been associated uncommonly with excessive daytime somnolence and sudden sleep onset episodes (0.1%). See also section 4.4.

Libido disorders

MIRAPEXIN may be associated with libido disorders (increased (0.1%) or decreased (0.4%)).

Impulse control disorders and compulsive behaviours

Patients treated with dopamine agonists for Parkinson's disease, including MIRAPEXIN, especially at high doses, have been reported as exhibiting signs of pathological gambling, increased libido and hypersexuality, generally reversible upon reduction of the dose or treatment discontinuation. See also section 4.4.

In a cross-sectional, retrospective screening and case-control study including 3090 Parkinson's disease patients, 13.6% of all patients receiving dopaminergic or non-dopaminergic treatment had symptoms of an impulse control disorder during the past six months. Manifestations observed include pathological gambling, compulsive shopping, binge eating, and compulsive sexual behaviour (hypersexuality). Possible independent risk factors for impulse control disorders included dopaminergic treatments and higher doses of dopaminergic treatment, younger age (⩽ 65 years), not being married and self-reported family history of gambling behaviours.

4.9 Overdose

There is no clinical experience with massive overdosage. The expected adverse events would be those related to the pharmacodynamic profile of a dopamine agonist, including nausea, vomiting, hyperkinesia, hallucinations, agitation and hypotension. There is no established antidote for overdosage of a dopamine agonist. If signs of central nervous system stimulation are present, a neuroleptic agent may be indicated. Management of the overdose may require general supportive measures, along with gastric lavage, intravenous fluids, administration of activated charcoal and electrocardiogram monitoring.

5. PHARMACOLOGICAL PROPERTIES

5.1 Pharmacodynamic properties

Pharmacotherapeutic group: dopamine agonists, ATC code: N04BC05

Pramipexole is a dopamine agonist that binds with high selectivity and specificity to the D2 subfamily of dopamine receptors of which it has a preferential affinity to D_3 receptors, and has full intrinsic activity.

Pramipexole alleviates Parkinsonian motor deficits by stimulation of dopamine receptors in the striatum. Animal studies have shown that pramipexole inhibits dopamine synthesis, release, and turnover.

The mechanism of action of pramipexole as treatment for Restless Legs Syndrome is unknown. Neuropharmacological evidence suggests primary dopaminergic system involvement.

In human volunteers, a dose-dependent decrease in prolactin was observed.

Clinical trials in Parkinson's disease

In patients MIRAPEXIN alleviates signs and symptoms of idiopathic Parkinson's disease.

Controlled clinical trials included approximately 2100 patients of Hoehn and Yahr stages I – IV. Out of these, approximately 900 were in more advanced stages, received concomitant levodopa therapy, and suffered from motor complications.

In early and advanced Parkinson's disease, efficacy of MIRAPEXIN in the controlled clinical trials was maintained for approximately six months. In open continuation trials lasting for more than three years there were no signs of decreasing efficacy. In a controlled double blind clinical trial of 2 year duration, initial treatment with pramipexole significantly delayed the onset of motor complications, and reduced their occurrence compared to initial treatment with levodopa. This delay in motor complications with pramipexole should be balanced against a greater improvement in motor function with levodopa (as measured by the mean change in UPDRS-score). The overall incidence of hallucinations and somnolence was generally higher in the escalation phase with the pramipexole group. However there was no significant difference during the maintenance phase. These points should be considered when initiating pramipexole treatment in patients with Parkinson's disease.

Clinical trials in Restless Legs Syndrome

The efficacy of MIRAPEXIN was evaluated in four placebo-controlled clinical trials in approximately 1000 patients with moderate to very severe idiopathic Restless Legs Syndrome. Efficacy was demonstrated in controlled trials in patients treated for up to 12 weeks. Maintenance of effect has not been sufficiently tested.

The mean change from baseline in the Restless Legs Syndrome Rating Scale (IRLS) and the Clinical Global Impression-Improvement (CGI-I) were the primary efficacy outcome measures. For both primary endpoints statistically significant differences have been observed for the pramipexole dose groups 0.25 mg, 0.5 mg and 0.75 mg in comparison to placebo. After 12 weeks of treatment the baseline IRLS score improved from 23.5 to 14.1 points for placebo and from 23.4 to 9.4 points for pramipexole (doses combined). The adjusted mean difference was -4.3 points (CI 95% -6.4; -2.1 points, p-value <0.0001). CGI-I responder rates (improved, very much improved) were 51.2% and 72.0% for placebo and pramipexole respectively (difference 20% CI 95%: 8.1%; 31.8%, $p<0.0005$). Efficacy was observed with 0.088 mg of base (0.125 mg of salt) per day after the first week of treatment.

In a placebo-controlled polysomnography study over 3 weeks MIRAPEXIN significantly reduced the number of periodic limb movements during time in bed.

5.2 Pharmacokinetic properties

Pramipexole is rapidly and completely absorbed following oral administration. The absolute bioavailability is greater than 90% and the maximum plasma concentrations occur between 1 and 3 hours. Concomitant administration with food did not reduce the extent of pramipexole absorption, but the rate of absorption was reduced. Pramipexole shows linear kinetics and a small inter-patient variation of plasma levels.

In humans, the protein binding of pramipexole is very low (< 20%) and the volume of distribution is large (400 l). High brain tissue concentrations were observed in the rat (approx. 8-fold compared to plasma).

Pramipexole is metabolised in man only to a small extent.

Renal excretion of unchanged pramipexole is the major route of elimination. Approximately 90% of ^{14}C-labelled dose is excreted through the kidneys while less than 2% is found in the faeces. The total clearance of pramipexole is approximately 500 ml/min and the renal clearance is approximately 400 ml/min. The elimination half-life ($t_{½}$) varies from 8 hours in the young to 12 hours in the elderly.

5.3 Preclinical safety data

Repeated dose toxicity studies showed that pramipexole exerted functional effects, mainly involving the CNS and female reproductive system, and probably resulting from an exaggerated pharmacodynamic effect of pramipexole.

Decreases in diastolic and systolic pressure and heart rate were noted in the minipig, and a tendency to an hypotensive effect was discerned in the monkey.

The potential effects of pramipexole on reproductive function have been investigated in rats and rabbits. Pramipexole was not teratogenic in rats and rabbits but was embryotoxic in the rat at maternally toxic doses. Due to the selection of animal species and the limited parameters investigated, the adverse effects of pramipexole on pregnancy and male fertility have not been fully elucidated.

Pramipexole was not genotoxic. In a carcinogenicity study, male rats developed Leydig cell hyperplasia and adenomas, explained by the prolactin-inhibiting effect of pramipexole. This finding is not clinically relevant to man. The same study also showed that, at doses of 2 mg/kg (of salt) and higher, pramipexole was associated with retinal degeneration in albino rats. The latter finding was not observed in pigmented rats, nor in a 2-year albino mouse carcinogenicity study or in any other species investigated.

6. PHARMACEUTICAL PARTICULARS

6.1 List of excipients

Mannitol,

maize starch,

anhydrous colloidal silica,

povidone K 25,

magnesium stearate

6.2 Incompatibilities

Not applicable

6.3 Shelf life

3 years

6.4 Special precautions for storage

Do not store above 30°C.

Store in the original package in order to protect from light.

6.5 Nature and contents of container

10 tablets per aluminium blister strips

Cartons containing 3 or 10 blister strips (30 or 100 tablets)

Not all pack sizes may be marketed

6.6 Special precautions for disposal and other handling

No special requirements

7. MARKETING AUTHORISATION HOLDER

Boehringer Ingelheim International GmbH

D-55216 Ingelheim am Rhein

Germany

8. MARKETING AUTHORISATION NUMBER(S)

EU/1/97/051/005-006

9. DATE OF FIRST AUTHORISATION/RENEWAL OF THE AUTHORISATION

Date of first authorisation: 23 February 1998

Date of Renewal of the authorisation: 23 February 2008

10. DATE OF REVISION OF THE TEXT

17 April 2009

Mircera solution for injection in pre-filled syringe

(Roche Products Limited)

1. NAME OF THE MEDICINAL PRODUCT

MIRCERA▼ 30 micrograms/0.3 ml solution for injection in pre-filled syringe

MIRCERA▼ 40 micrograms/0.3 ml solution for injection in pre-filled syringe

MIRCERA▼ 50 micrograms/0.3 ml solution for injection in pre-filled syringe

MIRCERA▼ 60 micrograms/0.3 ml solution for injection in pre-filled syringe

MIRCERA▼ 75 micrograms/0.3 ml solution for injection in pre-filled syringe

MIRCERA▼ 100 micrograms/0.3 ml solution for injection in pre-filled syringe

MIRCERA▼ 120 micrograms/0.3 ml solution for injection in pre-filled syringe

MIRCERA▼ 150 micrograms/0.3 ml solution for injection in pre-filled syringe

MIRCERA▼ 200 micrograms/0.3 ml solution for injection in pre-filled syringe

MIRCERA▼ 250 micrograms/0.3 ml solution for injection in pre-filled syringe

MIRCERA▼ 360 micrograms/0.6 ml solution for injection in pre-filled syringe

MIRCERA▼ 400 micrograms/0.6 ml solution for injection in pre-filled syringe

MIRCERA▼ 600 micrograms/0.6 ml solution for injection in pre-filled syringe

MIRCERA▼ 800 micrograms/0.6 ml solution for injection in pre-filled syringe

2. QUALITATIVE AND QUANTITATIVE COMPOSITION

One pre-filled syringe contains 30 micrograms of methoxy polyethylene glycol-epoetin beta* at a concentration of 100 micrograms/ml. The strength indicates the quantity of the protein moiety of the methoxy polyethylene glycol-epoetin beta molecule without consideration of the glycosylation.

One pre-filled syringe contains 40 micrograms of methoxy polyethylene glycol-epoetin beta* at a concentration of 133 micrograms/ml. The strength indicates the quantity of the protein moiety of the methoxy polyethylene glycol-epoetin beta molecule without consideration of the glycosylation.

One pre-filled syringe contains 50 micrograms of methoxy polyethylene glycol-epoetin beta* at a concentration of 167 micrograms/ml. The strength indicates the quantity of the protein moiety of the methoxy polyethylene glycol-epoetin beta molecule without consideration of the glycosylation.

One pre-filled syringe contains 60 micrograms of methoxy polyethylene glycol-epoetin beta* at a concentration of 200 micrograms/ml. The strength indicates the quantity of the protein moiety of the methoxy polyethylene glycol-epoetin beta molecule without consideration of the glycosylation.

One pre-filled syringe contains 75 micrograms of methoxy polyethylene glycol-epoetin beta* at a concentration of 250 micrograms/ml. The strength indicates the quantity of the protein moiety of the methoxy polyethylene glycol-epoetin beta molecule without consideration of the glycosylation.

One pre-filled syringe contains 100 micrograms of methoxy polyethylene glycol-epoetin beta* at a concentration of 333 micrograms/ml. The strength indicates the quantity of the protein moiety of the methoxy polyethylene glycol-epoetin beta molecule without consideration of the glycosylation.

One pre-filled syringe contains 120 micrograms of methoxy polyethylene glycol-epoetin beta* at a concentration of 400 micrograms/ml. The strength indicates the quantity of the protein moiety of the methoxy polyethylene glycol-epoetin beta molecule without consideration of the glycosylation.

One pre-filled syringe contains 150 micrograms of methoxy polyethylene glycol-epoetin beta* at a concentration of 500 micrograms/ml. The strength indicates the quantity of the protein moiety of the methoxy polyethylene glycol-epoetin beta molecule without consideration of the glycosylation.

One pre-filled syringe contains 200 micrograms of methoxy polyethylene glycol-epoetin beta* at a concentration of 667 micgrograms/ml. The strength indicates the quantity of the protein moiety of the methoxy polyethylene glycol-epoetin beta molecule without consideration of the glycosylation.

One pre-filled syringe contains 250 micrograms of methoxy polyethylene glycol-epoetin beta* at a concentration of 833 micrograms/ml. The strength indicates the quantity of the protein moiety of the methoxy polyethylene glycol-epoetin beta molecule without consideration of the glycosylation.

One pre-filled syringe contains 360 micrograms of methoxy polyethylene glycol-epoetin beta*at a concentration of 600 micrograms/ml. The strength indicates the quantity of the protein moiety of the methoxy polyethylene glycol-epoetin beta molecule without consideration of the glycosylation.

One pre-filled syringe contains 400 micrograms of methoxy polyethylene glycol-epoetin beta* at a concentration of 667 micrograms/ml. The strength indicates the quantity of the protein moiety of the methoxy polyethylene glycol-epoetin beta molecule without consideration of the glycosylation.

One pre-filled syringe contains 600 micrograms of methoxy polyethylene glycol-epoetin beta* at a concentration of 1000 micrograms/ml. The strength indicates the quantity of the protein moiety of the methoxy polyethylene glycol-epoetin beta molecule without consideration of the glycosylation.

One pre-filled syringe contains 800 micrograms of methoxy polyethylene glycol-epoetin beta* at a concentration of 1333 micrograms/ml. The strength indicates the quantity of the protein moiety of the methoxy polyethylene glycol-epoetin beta molecule without consideration of the glycosylation.

*Protein produced by recombinant DNA technology in Chinese Hamster Ovary (CHO) cells and covalently conjugated to a linear methoxy-polyethylene glycol (PEG).

The potency of methoxy polyethene glycol-epoetin beta should not be compared to the potency of another pegylated or non-pegylated protein of the same therapeutic class. For more information, see section 5.1.

For a full list of excipients, see section 6.1.

3. PHARMACEUTICAL FORM

Solution for injection (injection).

The solution is clear and colourless to slightly yellowish.

4. CLINICAL PARTICULARS

4.1 Therapeutic indications

Treatment of symptomatic anaemia associated with chronic kidney disease (CKD).

The safety and efficacy of MIRCERA therapy in other indications has not been established.

4.2 Posology and method of administration

Treatment of symptomatic anaemia in adult chronic kidney disease patients

Treatment with MIRCERA has to be initiated under the supervision of a physician experienced in the management of patients with renal impairment.

Anaemia symptoms and sequelae may vary with age, gender, and overall burden of disease; a physician's evaluation of the individual patient's clinical course and condition is necessary. MIRCERA should be administered either subcutaneously or intravenously in order to increase haemoglobin to not greater than 12 g/dl (7.45 mmol/l). Subcutaneous use is preferable in patients who are not receiving haemodialysis to avoid puncture of peripheral veins.

MIRCERA can be injected subcutaneously in the abdomen, arm or thigh. All three injection sites are equally suitable.

Due to intra-patient variability, occasional individual haemoglobin values for a patient above and below the desired haemoglobin level may be observed. Haemoglobin variability should be addressed through dose management, with consideration for the haemoglobin target range of 10 g/dl (6.21 mmol/l) to 12 g/dl (7.45 mmol/l). A sustained haemoglobin level of greater than 12 g/dl (7.45 mmol/l) should be avoided; guidance for appropriate dose adjustment for when haemoglobin values exceeding 12 g/dl (7.45 mmol/l) are observed are described below.

A rise in haemoglobin of greater than 2 g/dl (1.24 mmol/l) over a four-week period should be avoided. If it occurs, appropriate dose adjustment should be made as provided.

Patients should be monitored closely to ensure that the lowest approved dose of MIRCERA is used to provide adequate control of the symptoms of anaemia.

It is recommended that haemoglobin is monitored every two weeks until stabilized and periodically thereafter.

Patients not currently treated with an erythropoiesis stimulating agent (ESA):

The recommended starting dose is 0.6 microgram/kg body weight, administered once every two weeks as a single intravenous or subcutaneous injection in order to increase haemoglobin levels to greater than 10 g/dl (6.21 mmol/l).

The dose may be increased by approximately 25% of the previous dose if the rate of rise in haemoglobin is less than 1.0 g/dl (0.621 mmol/l) over a month. Further increases of approximately 25% may be made at monthly intervals until the individual target haemoglobin level is obtained.

If the rate of rise in haemoglobin is greater than 2 g/dl (1.24 mmol/l) in one month or if the haemoglobin level is increasing and approaching 12 g/dl (7.45 mmol/l), the dose is to be reduced by approximately 25%. If the haemoglobin level continues to increase, therapy should be interrupted until the haemoglobin level begins to decrease, at which point therapy should be restarted at a dose approximately 25% below the previously administered dose. After dose interruption a haemoglobin decrease of approximately 0.35 g/dl (0.22 mmol/l) per week is expected. Dose adjustments should not be made more frequently than once a month.

If the haemoglobin concentration above 10 g/dl (6.21 mmol/l) is reached for the individual patient, MIRCERA may be administered once-monthly using the dose equal to twice the previous once-every-two-weeks dose.

Patients currently treated with an ESA:

Patients currently treated with an ESA can be switched to MIRCERA administered once a month as a single intravenous or subcutaneous injection. The starting dose of methoxy polyethylene glycol-epoetin beta is based on the calculated previous weekly dose of darbepoetin alfa or epoetin at the time of substitution as described in Table 1. The first injection should start at the next scheduled dose of the previously administered darbepoetin alfa or epoetin.

Table 1: MIRCERA starting doses

Previous weekly darbepoetin alfa intravenous or subcutaneous dose (microgram/week)	Previous weekly epoetin intravenous or subcutaneous dose (IU/week)	Monthly MIRCERA intravenous or subcutaneous dose (microgram/once monthly)
<40	<8000	120
40-80	8000-16000	200
>80	>16000	360

If a dose adjustment is required to maintain the target haemoglobin concentration above 10 g/dl (6.21 mmol/l), the monthly dose may be increased by approximately 25%.

If the rate of rise in haemoglobin is greater than 2 g/dl (1.24 mmol/l) over a month or if the haemoglobin level is increasing and approaching 12 g/dl (7.45 mmol/l), the dose is to be reduced by approximately 25%. If the haemoglobin level continues to increase, therapy should be interrupted until the haemoglobin level begins to decrease, at which point therapy should be restarted at a dose approximately 25% below the previously administered dose. After dose interruption a haemoglobin decrease of approximately 0.35 g/dl (0.22 mmol/l) per week is expected. Dose adjustments should not be made more frequently than once a month.

Since the treatment experience is limited in patients on peritoneal dialysis, regular haemoglobin monitoring and strict adherence to dose adjustment guidance is recommended in these patients.

Treatment interruption

Treatment with MIRCERA is normally long-term. However, it can be interrupted at any time, if necessary.

Missed dose

If one dose of MIRCERA is missed, the missed dose is to be administered as soon as possible and administration of MIRCERA is to be restarted at the prescribed dosing frequency.

Paediatric use

MIRCERA is not recommended for use in children and adolescents below 18 years due to a lack of safety and efficacy data.

Elderly patients

In clinical studies 24% of patients treated with MIRCERA were aged 65 to 74 years, while 20% were aged 75 years and over. No dose adjustment is required in patients aged 65 years or older.

Patients with hepatic impairment

No adjustments of the starting dose nor of the dose modification rules are required in patients with hepatic impairment (see section 5.2).

4.3 Contraindications

Hypersensitivity to the active substance or to any of the excipients.

Uncontrolled hypertension.

4.4 Special warnings and precautions for use

Supplementary iron therapy is recommended for all patients with serum ferritin values below 100 microgram/l or with transferrin saturation below 20%. To ensure effective erythropoiesis, iron status has to be evaluated for all patients prior to and during treatment.

Failure to respond to MIRCERA therapy should prompt for a search for causative factors. Deficiencies of iron, folic acid or vitamin B12 reduce the effectiveness of ESAs and should therefore be corrected. Intercurrent infections, inflammatory or traumatic episodes, occult blood loss, haemolysis, severe aluminium toxicity, underlying haematologic diseases, or bone marrow fibrosis may also compromise the erythropoietic response. A reticulocyte count should be considered as part of the evaluation. If all the conditions mentioned are excluded and the patient has a sudden drop of haemoglobin associated with reticulocytopenia and anti-erythropoietin antibodies, examination of the bone marrow for the diagnosis of Pure Red Cell Aplasia (PRCA) should be considered. In case PRCA is diagnosed, therapy with MIRCERA must be discontinued and patients should not be switched to another ESA.

Pure Red Cell Aplasia caused by anti-erythropoietin antibodies has been reported in association with ESAs. These antibodies have been shown to cross-react with all ESAs, and patients suspected or confirmed to have antibodies to erythropoietin should not be switched to MIRCERA.

Haemoglobin concentration: In patients with chronic kidney disease, maintenance haemoglobin concentration should not exceed the upper limit of the target haemoglobin concentration recommended in section 4.2. In clinical trials, an increased risk of death and serious cardiovascular events was observed when erythropoiesis stimulating agents (ESAs) were administered to target a haemoglobin of greater than 12 g/dl (7.5 mmol/l).

Controlled clinical trials have not shown significant benefits attributable to the administration of epoetins when haemoglobin concentration is increased beyond the level necessary to control symptoms of anaemia and to avoid blood transfusion.

Blood pressure monitoring: As with other ESAs, blood pressure may rise during treatment with MIRCERA. Blood pressure should be adequately controlled in all patients before, at initiation of, and during treatment with MIRCERA. If high blood pressure is difficult to control by medical treatment or dietary measures, the dose must be reduced or administration discontinued (see section 4.2).

Effect on tumour growth: MIRCERA, like other ESAs, is a growth factor that primarily stimulates red blood cell production. Erythropoietin receptors may be expressed on the surface of a variety of tumour cells. As with all growth factors, there is a concern that ESAs could stimulate the growth of any type of malignancy. Two controlled clinical studies in which epoetins were administered to patients with various cancers including head and neck cancers, and breast cancer, have shown an unexplained excess mortality.

MIRCERA is not approved for the treatment of anaemia in patients with cancer.

The safety and efficacy of MIRCERA therapy has not been established in patients with haemoglobinopathies, seizures, bleeding or a recent history of bleeding requiring transfusions or with platelet levels greater than 500 × 10^9/l. Therefore, caution should be used in these patients.

Misuse of MIRCERA by healthy people may lead to an excessive increase in haemoglobin. This may be associated with life-threatening cardiovascular complications.

4.5 Interaction with other medicinal products and other forms of interaction

No interaction studies have been performed. There is no evidence that MIRCERA alters the metabolism of other medicinal products.

4.6 Pregnancy and lactation

Pregnancy:

There are no data from the use of MIRCERA in pregnant women.

Animal studies do not indicate direct harmful effects with respect to pregnancy, embryofoetal development, parturition or postnatal development but indicate a class-related reversible reduction in foetal weight (see section 5.3). Caution should be exercised when prescribing to pregnant women.

Lactation:

It is unknown whether methoxy polyethylene glycol-epoetin beta is excreted in human breast milk. One animal study has shown excretion of methoxy polyethylene glycol-epoetin beta in maternal milk. A decision on whether to continue or discontinue breast-feeding or to continue or discontinue therapy with MIRCERA should be made taking into account the benefit of breast-feeding to the child and the benefit of MIRCERA therapy to the woman.

4.7 Effects on ability to drive and use machines

MIRCERA has no or negligible influence on the ability to drive and use machines.

4.8 Undesirable effects

The safety data base from clinical trials comprised 2'737 CKD patients, including 1'789 patients treated with MIRCERA and 948 with another ESA. Approximately 6% of patients treated with MIRCERA are expected to experience adverse reactions. The most frequent reported adverse reaction was hypertension (common).

The frequencies are defined as follows:

very common (≥1/10); common (≥1/100 to <1/10); uncommon (≥1/1,000 to <1/100); rare (≥1/10,000 to <1/1,000); very rare (<1/10,000)

Table 2: Adverse reactions attributed to the treatment with MIRCERA in controlled clinical trials in CKD patients

System organ class	Frequency	Adverse reaction
Nervous system disorders	Uncommon	Headache
Nervous system disorders	Rare	Hypertensive encephalopathy
Skin and subcutaneous tissue disorders	Rare	Rash, maculo-papular
Injury, poisoning and procedural complications	Uncommon	Vascular access thrombosis
Vascular disorders	Common	Hypertension
Vascular disorders	Rare	Hot flush
Immune system disorders	Rare	Hypersensitivity

All other events attributed to MIRCERA were reported with rare frequency and the majority were mild to moderate in severity. These events were consistent with comorbidities known in the population.

During treatment with MIRCERA, a slight decrease in platelet counts remaining within the normal range was observed in clinical studies.

Platelet counts below 100 × 10^9/l were observed in 7% of patients treated with MIRCERA and 4% of patients treated with other ESAs.

4.9 Overdose

The therapeutic range of MIRCERA is wide. Individual responsiveness must be considered when treatment is initiated. Overdose can result in manifestations of an exaggerated pharmacodynamic effect, e.g. excessive erythropoiesis. In case of excessive haemoglobin levels, treatment with MIRCERA should be temporarily discontinued (see section 4.2). If clinically indicated, phlebotomy may be performed.

5. PHARMACOLOGICAL PROPERTIES

5.1 Pharmacodynamic properties

Pharmacotherapeutic group: Other antianaemic preparations, ATC code: B03XA03

Methoxy polyethylene glycol-epoetin beta, the active substance of MIRCERA, is a continuous erythropoietin receptor activator that shows a different activity at the receptor level characterized by a slower association to and faster dissociation from the receptor, a reduced specific activity *in vitro* with an increased activity *in vivo*, as well as an increased half-life, in contrast to erythropoietin. The average molecular mass is approximately 60 kDa of which the protein moiety plus the carbohydrate part constitutes approximately 30 kDa.

MIRCERA stimulates erythropoiesis by interaction with the erythropoietin receptor on progenitor cells in the bone marrow. As primary growth factor for erythroid development, the natural hormone erythropoietin is produced in the kidney and released into the bloodstream in response to hypoxia. In responding to hypoxia, the natural hormone erythropoietin interacts with erythroid progenitor cells to increase red cell production.

Data from correction studies show that the haemoglobin response rates in the MIRCERA group at the end of the correction period were high (93.3% and 97.5% in the studies in patients on dialysis and not on dialysis, respectively) and comparable to comparators (91.3% and 96.3%, respectively). The median time to response was 43 days in the MIRCERA arm and 29 days in the comparator arm, with increases of haemoglobin within the first 6 weeks of 0.2 g/dl/week and 0.3 g/dl/week, respectively.

Four randomised controlled studies were performed in dialysis patients treated with darbepoetin alfa or epoetin at the time of enrollment. Patients were randomized to stay on their treatment at the time of enrollment or to be switched to MIRCERA in order to maintain stable haemoglobin levels. At the evaluation period (week 29-36), the mean and median level of haemoglobin in patients treated with MIRCERA was virtually identical to their baseline haemoglobin level.

Erythropoietin is a growth factor that primarily stimulates red cell production. Erythropoietin receptors may be expressed on the surface of a variety of tumour cells.

Survival and tumour progression have been examined in five large controlled studies involving a total of 2'833 patients, of which four were double-blind placebo-controlled studies and one was an open-label study. Two of the studies recruited patients who were being treated with chemotherapy. The target haemoglobin concentration in two studies was >13 g/dl; in the remaining three studies it was 12-14 g/dl. In the open-label study there was no difference in overall survival between patients treated with recombinant human erythropoietin and controls. In the four placebo-controlled studies the hazard ratios for overall survival ranged between 1.25 and 2.47 in favour of controls. These studies have shown a consistent unexplained statistically significant excess mortality in patients who have anaemia associated with various common cancers who received recombinant human erythropoietin compared to controls. Overall survival outcome in the trials could not be satisfactorily explained by differences in the incidence of thrombosis and related complications between those given recombinant human erythropoietin and those in the control group.

A systematic review has also been performed involving more than 9'000 cancer patients participating in 57 clinical trials. Meta-analysis of overall survival data produced a hazard ratio point estimate of 1.08 in favour of controls (95% CI: 0.99, 1.18; 42 trials and 8'167 patients). An increased relative risk of thromboembolic events (RR 1.67, 95% CI: 1.35, 2.06, 35 trials and 6'769 patients) was observed in patients treated with recombinant human erythropoietin. There is therefore consistent evidence to suggest that there may be significant harm to patients with cancer who are treated with recombinant human erythropoietin. The extent to which these outcomes might apply to the administration of recombinant human erythropoietin to patients with cancer, treated with chemotherapy to achieve haemoglobin concentrations less than 13 g/dl, is unclear because few patients with these characteristics were included in the data reviewed.

5.2 Pharmacokinetic properties

The pharmacokinetics of methoxy polyethylene glycol-epoetin beta were studied in healthy volunteers and in anaemic patients with CKD including patients on dialysis and not on dialysis.

Following subcutaneous administration to CKD patients not on dialysis, the maximum serum concentrations of methoxy polyethylene glycol-epoetin beta were observed 95 hours (median value) after administration. The absolute bioavailability of methoxy polyethylene glycol-epoetin beta after subcutaneous administration was 54%. The observed terminal elimination half-life was 142 hours in CKD patients not on dialysis.

Following subcutaneous administration to CKD patients on dialysis, the maximum serum concentrations of methoxy polyethylene glycol-epoetin beta were observed 72 hours (median value) after administration. The absolute bioavailability of methoxy polyethylene glycol-epoetin beta after subcutaneous administration was 62% and the observed terminal elimination half-life was 139 hours in CKD patients on dialysis.

Following intravenous administration to CKD patients on dialysis, the total systemic clearance was 0.494 ml/h per kg. The elimination half-life after intravenous administration of methoxy polyethylene glycol-epoetin beta is 134 hours.

A comparison of serum concentrations of methoxy polyethylene glycol-epoetin beta measured before and after haemodialysis in 41 CKD patients showed that haemodialysis has no effect on the pharmacokinetics of this medicinal product.

An analysis in 126 CKD patients showed no pharmacokinetic difference between patients on dialysis and patients not on dialysis.

In a single dose study, after intravenous administration, the pharmacokinetics of methoxy polyethylene glycol-epoetin beta are similar in patients with severe hepatic impairment as compared to healthy subjects (see section 4.2).

5.3 Preclinical safety data

Non-clinical data show no special hazard for humans based on conventional studies of cardiovascular safety pharmacology, repeat dose toxicity and reproductive toxicity.

The carcinogenic potential of methoxy polyethylene glycol-epoetin beta has not been evaluated in long-term animal studies. It did not induce a proliferative response in non-haematological tumor cell lines *in vitro*. In a six-month rat toxicity study no tumorigenic or unexpected mitogenic responses were observed in non-haematological tissues. In addition, using a panel of human tissues, the *in vitro* binding of methoxy polyethylene glycol-epoetin beta was only observed in target cells (bone marrow progenitor cells).

No significant placental transfer of methoxy polyethylene glycol-epoetin beta was observed in the rat, and studies in animals have not shown any harmful effect on pregnancy, embryofoetal development, parturition or postnatal development. There was however a class-related reversible reduction in foetal weight and a decrease in postnatal body-weight gain of offspring at the doses causing exaggerated pharmacodynamic effects in mothers. Physical, cognitive, or sexual developments in the offspring of mothers receiving methoxy polyethylene glycol-epoetin beta during gestation and lactation were not affected. When methoxy polyethylene glycol-epoetin beta was administered subcutaneously to male and female rats prior to and during mating, reproductive performance, fertility, and sperm assessment parameters were not affected.

6. PHARMACEUTICAL PARTICULARS

6.1 List of excipients

Sodium dihydrogen phosphate monohydrate

Sodium sulphate

Mannitol (E421)

Methionine

Poloxamer 188

Water for injections

6.2 Incompatibilities

In the absence of compatibility studies, this medicinal product must not be mixed with other medicinal products.

6.3 Shelf life

3 years

6.4 Special precautions for storage

Store in a refrigerator (2°C – 8°C)

Do not freeze

Keep the pre-filled syringe in the outer carton in order to protect from light

The end-user may remove the medicinal product from refrigeration for storage at a room temperature not above 30°C for one single period of 1 month. Once removed from the refrigerator the medicinal product must be used within this period.

6.5 Nature and contents of container

Pre-filled syringe (type I glass) with laminated plunger stopper (bromobutyl rubber material) and tip cap (bromobutyl rubber material) and a needle 27G1/2. Pack size of 1.

6.6 Special precautions for disposal and other handling

The pre-filled syringe is ready for use. The sterile pre-filled syringe does not contain any preservative and is to be used for a single injection only. Only one dose should be administered per syringe. Only solutions which are clear, colourless to slightly yellowish and free of visible particles must be injected.

Do not shake.

Allow the pre-filled syringe to reach room temperature before injecting.

Any unused medicinal product or waste material should be disposed of in accordance with local requirements.

7. MARKETING AUTHORISATION HOLDER

Roche Registration Limited
6 Falcon Way
Shire Park
Welwyn Garden City
AL7 1TW
United Kingdom

8. MARKETING AUTHORISATION NUMBER(S)

EU/1/07/400/008 - MIRCERA 50 micrograms/0.3 ml solution for injection in pre-filled syringe.

EU/1/07/400/009 - MIRCERA 75 micrograms/0.3 ml solution for injection in pre-filled syringe.

EU/1/07/400/010 - MIRCERA 100 micrograms/0.3 ml solution for injection in pre-filled syringe.

EU/1/07/400/011 - MIRCERA 150 micrograms/0.3 ml solution for injection in pre-filled syringe.

EU/1/07/400/012 - MIRCERA 200 micrograms/0.3 ml solution for injection in pre-filled syringe.

EU/1/07/400/013 - MIRCERA 250 micrograms/0.3 ml solution for injection in pre-filled syringe.

EU/1/07/400/014 - MIRCERA 400 micrograms/0.6 ml solution for injection in pre-filled syringe.

EU/1/07/400/015 - MIRCERA 600 micrograms/0.6 ml solution for injection in pre-filled syringe.

EU/1/07/400/016 - MIRCERA 800 micrograms/0.6 ml solution for injection in pre-filled syringe.

EU/1/07/400/017 - MIRCERA 30 micrograms/0.3 ml solution for injection in pre-filled syringe.

EU/1/07/400/018 - MIRCERA 40 micrograms/0.3 ml solution for injection in pre-filled syringe.

EU/1/07/400/019 - MIRCERA 60 micrograms/0.3 ml solution for injection in pre-filled syringe.

EU/1/07/400/020 - MIRCERA 120 micrograms/0.3 ml solution for injection in pre-filled syringe.

EU/1/07/400/021 - MIRCERA 360 micrograms/0.6 ml solution for injection in pre-filled syringe.

9. DATE OF FIRST AUTHORISATION/RENEWAL OF THE AUTHORISATION

20 July 2007

10. DATE OF REVISION OF THE TEXT

7th April 2009

Detailed information on this medicinal product is available on the website of the European Medicines Agency (EMEA) http://www.emea.europa.eu/

Mitomycin-C Kyowa, 2mg, 10mg, 20mg or 40mg powder for solution for injection.

(Kyowa Hakko Kirin UK Ltd)

1. NAME OF THE MEDICINAL PRODUCT

Mitomycin-C Kyowa, 2mg, powder for solution for injection.

Mitomycin-C Kyowa, 10mg, powder for solution for injection.

Mitomycin-C Kyowa, 20mg, powder for solution for injection.

Mitomycin-C Kyowa, 40mg, powder for solution for injection.

2. QUALITATIVE AND QUANTITATIVE COMPOSITION

Mitomycin C 2, 10, 20 or 40mg

For excipients, see 6.1

3. PHARMACEUTICAL FORM

Powder for solution for injection.

Blue-purple crystalline powder.

4. CLINICAL PARTICULARS

4.1 Therapeutic indications

Antimitotic and Cytotoxic

Recommended for certain types of cancer in combination with other drugs or after primary therapy has failed. It has been successfully used to improve subjective and objective symptoms in a wide range of neoplastic conditions.

1. As a single agent in the treatment of superficial bladder cancer. In addition it has been shown that post-operative instillations of Mitomycin-C can reduce recurrence rates in newly diagnosed patients with superficial bladder cancer.

2. As a single agent and in combination with other drugs in metastatic breast cancer.

3. In combination with other agents in advanced squamous cell carcinoma of the uterine cervix.

4. It shows a degree of activity as part of combination therapy in carcinoma of the stomach, pancreas and lung (particularly non-small cell).

5. It shows a degree of activity as a single agent and in combination in liver cancer when given by the intra-arterial route.

6. It has a possible role in combination with other cytotoxic drugs in colo-rectal cancer.

7. It shows a degree of activity as a single agent or part of combination therapy in cancer of the head and neck.

8. It shows a degree of activity as a single agent in cancer of the prostate.

9. It has a possible role in skin cancer.

10. It has a degree of activity in leukaemia and non-solid tumours.

11. It has a possible role in sarcomas.

12. It has been successfully used in combination with surgery, pre-operatively (oesophageal squamous cell carcinoma) and post-operatively (gastric cancer).

13. It has shown to be effective when used in combination with radiotherapy.

4.2 Posology and method of administration

Intravenous administration

Intravenously, the dose should be given as slowly as possible and with great care in order to avoid extravasation.

The usual dose is in the range of 4 – 10mg (0.06-0.15mg/kg) given at 1 – 6 weekly intervals depending on whether other drugs are given in combination and on bone marrow recovery.

In a number of combination schedules, the dose is 10mg/m² of body surface area, the course being repeated at intervals for as long as required. A course ranging from 40-80mg (0.58 –1.2mg/kg) is often required for a satisfactory response when used alone or in combination. A higher dosage course may be given when used alone or as part of a particular combination schedule and total cumulative doses exceeding 2mg/kg have been given.

Intra-arterial administration

For administration into specific tissues, Mitomycin-C Kyowa can be given by the intra-arterial route directly into the tumours.

Dose reductions

Because of cumulative myelosuppression, patients should be fully re-evaluated after each course and the dose reduced if the patient has experienced any toxic effects. Doses greater than 0.6mg/kg have not been shown to be more effective and are more toxic than lower doses.

Disease progression

If disease progression continues after two courses of treatment, the drug should be stopped since the chances of response are minimal.

Use in patients with bladder tumours

In the treatment of superficial bladder tumours the usual dose is 20-40mg dissolved in 20-40ml of diluent, instilled into the bladder through a urethral catheter, weekly or three times a week for a total of 20 doses. The dose should be retained by the patient for a minimum of one hour. During this one-hour period the patient should be rotated every 15 minutes to ensure that the Mitomycin-C comes into contact with all areas of the bladder urothelium.

When the bladder is emptied in the voiding process, care must be taken to ensure that no contamination occurs locally in the groin and genitalia areas.

In the prevention of recurrent superficial bladder tumours, various doses have been used. These include 20mg in 20ml of diluent every two weeks and 40mg in 40ml of diluent monthly or three monthly. The dose is instilled into the bladder through a urethral catheter.

In both cases, the dose should be adjusted in accordance with the age and condition of the patient.

4.3 Contraindications

Patients who have demonstrated a hypersensitive or idiosyncratic reaction to Mitomycin-C Kyowa or any of the components of the product in the past. Thrombocytopenia, coagulation disorders and increased bleeding tendency.

4.4 Special warnings and precautions for use

Mitomycin-C Kyowa should be administered under the supervision of a physician experienced in cytotoxic cancer chemotherapy.

Local ulceration and cellulitis may be caused by tissue extravasation during intravenous injection and utmost care should be taken in administration. If extravasation occurs, it is recommended that the area is immediately infiltrated with sodium bicarbonate 8.4% solution, followed by an injection of 4mg dexamethasone. A systemic injection of 200mg of Vitamin B6 may be of some value in promoting the regrowth of tissues that have been damaged.

Patients should be carefully monitored with frequent laboratory testing (haematological test, liver function test, renal function test, etc.) paying particular attention to peripheral blood count including platelet count. No repeat dose should be given unless the leucocyte count is above 3.0×10^9/L or more and the platelet count is 90×10^9/L or more. The nadir is usually around four weeks after treatment and toxicity is usually cumulative, with increasing risk after each course of treatment. Serious adverse reactions such as bone marrow depression may occur. If any abnormality is observed, appropriate measures such as reduction of the dose and suspension of administration should be taken.

Extravascular leakage may cause induration or necrosis at the injection site. Intraarterial administration may cause skin disorders such as pain, redness, erythema, blisters, erosion and ulceration which may lead to skin/muscle necrosis. Since the influx of the drug solution into other sites than the targeted site in the administration to the hepatic artery may cause gastroduodenal ulcer, haemorrhage, perforation, etc, the location of the end of the catheter and drug distribution area should be confirmed photographically or by other means, paying attention to possible deviation or shift of the catheter and infusion rate. Administration should be discontinued and appropriate measures should be taken, if any of such symptoms develops.

Severe renal toxicity has occasionally been reported after treatment and renal function should be monitored before starting treatment and again after each course.

Mitomycin-C Kyowa should be administered with care in children and patients with the following:

- Hepatic or renal dysfunction as adverse reactions may be enhanced
- Bone marrow depression and bleeding tendency as these may be exacerbated
- Infections as these may be aggravated due to bone marrow depression
- Varicella as fatal systemic disorders may occur

In case administration of this drug is required in children or patients with reproductive possibility, potential effects on gonad should be considered. The safety of Mitomycin-C injection in children has not been established. Special attention should be paid to the manifestation of adverse reactions when administered in children.

Elderly patients often have reduced physiological function, bone marrow depression, which may be protracted, so administer Mitomycin-C Kyowa with caution in this population while closely monitoring patient's condition.

Occurrence of acute leukaemia (in some cases following preleukaemic phase) and myelodysplastic syndrome has been reported in the patients treated with Mitomycin-C Kyowa concomitantly with other antineoplastic agents.

4.5 Interaction with other medicinal products and other forms of interaction

Mitomycin-C Kyowa should be administered with care when it is coadministered with other antineoplastic agents or irradiation. The adverse reactions of each drug may be enhanced, for example bone marrow depression. With vinca alkaloids adverse reactions of shortness of breath and bronchospasm may be enhanced.

4.6 Pregnancy and lactation

Mitomycin-C Kyowa should not normally be administrated to patients who are pregnant, who may possibly be pregnant or to mothers who are breast-feeding. Teratological changes have been noted in animal studies.

4.7 Effects on ability to drive and use machines

Generalised weakness and lethargy have been reported on rare occasions. If affected, patients should be advised not to drive or operate machinery.

4.8 Undesirable effects

The main adverse reactions collected from literature were leucopenia in 130 (40.2%) of 323 patients, thrombocytopenia in 75 (24.7%) of 304 patients, anorexia in 58 (21.8%) of 266 patients, nausea/vomiting in 41 (15.4%) of 266 patients, malaise in 15 (5.6%) of 266 patients, weight loss in 18 (5.5%) of 329 patients, bleeding tendency in 12 (3.6%) of 329 patients and anaemia in 10 (3.0%) of 329 patients.

Nausea and vomiting are sometimes experienced immediately after treatment, but these are usually mild and of short duration. Pulmonary toxicities such as pulmonary oedema, interstitial pneumonia and pulmonary fibrosis, accompanied by fever, coughing, dyspnoea, abnormal x-ray findings and eosinophilia have been reported. Skin toxicity may occur in a small proportion of patients, with side effects such as alopecia (although this is less frequent and less severe than with certain other cytotoxic agents). Bleeding, rashes and mouth ulcers have been reported.

Shock or anaphylactoid reaction may occur, patients should be carefully observed. If symptoms such as itching, rash, hot flush, sweating, dyspnoea and decreased blood pressure occur, treatment should be immediately discontinued and appropriate measures should be taken.

Administration related Undesirable Effects

Cystitis, atrophy of the bladder, contracted bladder (pollakiuria, dysuria), and calcinosis have been reported when given by intravesical instillation.

Administration to the hepatic artery may cause liver and biliary tract disorders such as cholecystitis, cholangitis (also sclerosing), biloma, bile duct necrosis and parenchymatous liver disorder. Drug distribution area should be confirmed photographically or by other means, and treatment should be discontinued and appropriate measures taken if any abnormal signs are noted.

The following administration related adverse reactions have also been reported: vascular pain, phlebitis, thrombus, induration or necrosis at the injection site, pain, redness erythema, blisters, erosion and ulceration which may lead to skin/muscle necrosis.

Other reported effects, not already described in the text above, include the following:

Infections and Infestations
Bacterial, viral or fungal infections, sepsis and septic shock
Neoplasms benign and malignant
Myelodysplastic syndrome, acute myeloid leukaemia, acute leukaemia
Blood and lymphatic system disorders
Bone marrow depression, pancytopenia, neutropenia, granulocytopenia, febrile neutropenia, erythropenia, microangiopathic haemolytic anaemia, haemolytic uraemic syndrome, thrombotic thrombocytopenic purpura.
Immune system disorders
Hypersensitivity
Vascular disorders
Flushing, hypertension
Respiratory and mediastinal disorders
Respiratory disorders such as interstitial lung disease, bronchospasm, pneumonitis,
Gastrointestinal disorders
Diarrhoea, constipation, abdominal discomfort, stomatitis
Hepatobiliary disorders
Parenchymatous liver disorder, cholecystitis, jaundice
Skin and subcutaneous tissue disorders
Rash, pruritus
Renal and urinary disorders
Acute renal failure, renal disorder, cystitis, haematuria, proteinuria, serious nephropathy, albuminuria
General disorders
Pyrexia, chills, malaise, injection site phlebitis, oedema, generalised weakness and lethargy

4.9 Overdose
In the unlikely event of accidental overdosage then an increase in the more common side effects should be expected, such as fever, nausea, vomiting and myelosuppression. Appropriate supportive measures should be instituted.

5. PHARMACOLOGICAL PROPERTIES

5.1 Pharmacodynamic properties
ATC Code: L01D

Pharmacotherapeutic group: Other cytotoxic antibiotics

Mitomycin-C Kyowa is an antitumour antibiotic that is activated in the tissues to an alkylating agent which disrupts deoxyribonucleic acid (DNA) in cancer cells by forming a complex with DNA and also acts by inhibiting division of cancer cells by interfering with the biosynthesis of DNA.

5.2 Pharmacokinetic properties
In vivo, Mitomycin-C Kyowa is rapidly cleared from the serum after intravenous administration. The time required to reduce the serum concentration by 50% after a 30mg bolus injection is 17 minutes. After injection of 30mg, 20mg or 10mg intravenously, the maximal serum concentrations were 2.4 mcg/ml, 1.7 mcg/ml and 0.52mcg/ml respectively. Clearance is effected primarily by metabolism in the liver, but metabolism occurs in other tissues as well. The rate of clearance is inversely proportional to the maximal serum concentration because, it is thought, of saturation of the degradative pathways. Approximately 10% of a dose of Mitomycin-C Kyowa is excreted unchanged in the urine. Since metabolic pathways are saturated at relatively low doses, the percentage dose excreted in the urine increases with increasing dose. In children, the excretion of intravenously administered Mitomycin-C Kyowa is similar to that in adults.

5.3 Preclinical safety data
There are no preclinical data of relevance to the prescriber which are additional to that already included elsewhere in the SPC.

6. PHARMACEUTICAL PARTICULARS

6.1 List of excipients
Sodium Chloride Ph.Eur.

6.2 Incompatibilities
Not known

6.3 Shelf life
Four years from the date of manufacture.

After reconstitution, the solution is chemically and physically stable for 24 hours when protected from light and stored in a cool place. Do not refrigerate.

From a microbiological point of view, the product should be used immediately. If not used immediately, in-use storage times and conditions prior to use are the responsibility of the user.

6.4 Special precautions for storage
Store in the original package.

The reconstituted solution should be protected from light and stored in a cool place (See Section 6.3).

6.5 Nature and contents of container
Mitomycin-C Kyowa is contained within a colourless, type I or III glass vial with a rubber stopper and an aluminium seal.

The vials are packaged into cardboard cartons containing 1, 5 or 10 vials.

6.6 Special precautions for disposal and other handling
The contents of the vial should be reconstituted with Water for Injection or saline, at least 5ml for the 2mg, at least 10ml for the 10mg, at least 20ml for the 20mg and at least 40ml for the 40mg vial.

Mitomycin-C Kyowa should not be allowed to come into contact with the skin. If it does, it should be washed several times with 8.4% sodium bicarbonate solution, followed by soap and water. Hand creams and emollients should not be used as they may assist the penetration of the drug into the epidermal tissue.

In the event of contact with the eye, it should be rinsed several times with saline solution. It should then be observed for several days for evidence of corneal damage. If necessary, appropriate treatment should be instituted.

7. MARKETING AUTHORISATION HOLDER
Kyowa Hakko Kirin UK Ltd
258 Bath Road
Slough
Berkshire
SL1 4DX

8. MARKETING AUTHORISATION NUMBER(S)
PL 12196/0001, PL 12196/0002, PL 12196/0003

9. DATE OF FIRST AUTHORISATION/RENEWAL OF THE AUTHORISATION
26th November 1992

10. DATE OF REVISION OF THE TEXT
April 2009

Mivacron Injection 2 mg/ml

(GlaxoSmithKline UK)

1. NAME OF THE MEDICINAL PRODUCT
Mivacron Injection 2mg/ml

2. QUALITATIVE AND QUANTITATIVE COMPOSITION
Mivacurium chloride 2.14mg in each 1ml of product

3. PHARMACEUTICAL FORM
Liquid for injection

4. CLINICAL PARTICULARS

4.1 Therapeutic indications
Mivacron is a highly selective, short-acting, non-depolarising neuromuscular blocking agent with a fast recovery profile. Mivacron is used as an adjunct to general anaesthesia to relax skeletal muscles and to facilitate tracheal intubation and mechanical ventilation.

This formulation contains no antimicrobial preservative and is intended for single patient use.

4.2 Posology and method of administration
Use By Injection In Adults

Mivacron is administered by intravenous injection. The mean dose required to produce 95% suppression of the adductor pollicis single twitch response to ulnar nerve stimulations (ED_{95}) is 0.07 mg/kg (range 0.06 to 0.09) in adults receiving narcotic anaesthesia.

The recommended bolus dose range for healthy adults is 0.07-0.25 mg/kg. The duration of neuromuscular blockade is related to the dose. Doses of 0.07, 0.15, 0.20 and 0.25 mg/kg produce clinically effective block for approximately 13, 16, 20 and 23 minutes respectively.

Doses of up to 0.15 mg/kg may be administered over 5 to 15 seconds. Higher doses should be administered over 30 seconds in order to minimise the possibility of occurrence of cardiovascular effects.

The following dose regimens are recommended for tracheal intubation:

I A dose of 0.2 mg/kg, administered over 30 seconds, produces good to excellent conditions for tracheal intubation within 2 to 2.5 minutes.

II A dose of 0.25 mg/kg administered as a divided dose (0.15 mg/kg followed 30 seconds later by 0.1 mg/kg) produces good to excellent conditions for tracheal intubation within 1.5 to 2.0 minutes of completion of administration of the first dose portion.

With Mivacron, significant train-of-four fade is not seen during onset. It is often possible to intubate the trachea before complete abolition of the train-of-four response of the adductor pollicis muscle has occurred.

Full block can be prolonged by maintenance doses of Mivacron. Doses of 0.1 mg/kg administered during narcotic anaesthesia each provide approximately 15 minutes of additional clinically effective block. Successive supplementary doses do not give rise to accumulation of neuromuscular blocking effect.

The neuromuscular blocking action of Mivacron is potentiated by isoflurane or enflurane anaesthesia. If steady-state anaesthesia with isoflurane or enflurane has been established, the recommended initial Mivacron dose should be reduced by up to 25%. Halothane appears to have only a minimal potentiating effect on Mivacron and dose reduction of Mivacron is probably not necessary.

Once spontaneous recovery is underway it is complete in approximately 15 minutes and is independent of the dose of Mivacron administered.

The neuromuscular block produced by Mivacron can be reversed with standard doses of anticholinesterase agents. However, because spontaneous recovery after Mivacron is rapid, a reversal may not be routinely required as it shortens recovery time by only 5-6 minutes.

Use as an Infusion in Adults

Continuous infusion of Mivacron may be used to maintain neuromuscular block. Upon early evidence of spontaneous recovery from an initial Mivacron dose, an infusion rate of 8 to 10 micrograms/kg/min (0.5 to 0.6 mg/kg/hr) is recommended.

The initial infusion rate should be adjusted according to the patient's response to peripheral nerve stimulation and clinical criteria. Adjustments of the infusion rate should be made and should be increments of approximately 1 microgram/kg/min (0.06 mg/kg/hr). In general, a given rate should be maintained for at least 3 minutes before a rate change is made. On average, an infusion rate of 6 to 7 micrograms/kg/minute will maintain neuromuscular block within the range of 89% to 99% for extended periods in adults receiving narcotic anaesthesia. During steady-state isoflurane or enflurane anaesthesia, reduction in the infusion rate by up to 40% should be considered. A study has shown that the mivacurium infusion rate requirement should be reduced by up to 50% with sevoflurane. With halothane, smaller reductions in infusion rate may be required.

Spontaneous recovery after Mivacron infusion is independent of the duration of infusion and comparable to recovery reported for single doses.

Continuous infusion of Mivacron has not been associated with the development of tachyphylaxis or cumulative neuromuscular blockade.

Table 1

Age	Dose for Tracheal Intubation	Time to Maximum Neuromuscular Block (min)	Duration of Clinically Effective Block (min)
2 - 6 months[A]	0.15 mg/kg	1.4	9
7 months - 12 years[B]	0.2 mg/kg	1.7	9

[A]Data obtained during halothane anaesthesia.
[B]Data obtained during halothane or narcotic anaesthesia.

Table 2

Age	Maintenance Dose	Duration of Clinically Effective Block (min)	Average Infusion Rate Required to Maintain 89-99% Neuromuscular Block
2 months - 12 years[A]	0.1 mg/kg	6 - 9	11 – 14 μg/kg/min (0.7 - 0.9 mg/kg/hr)

[A]Data obtained during halothane or narcotic anaesthesia.

Mivacron (2 mg/ml) may be used undiluted for infusion.

Mivacron is compatible with the following infusion fluids.

Sodium chloride intravenous infusion (0.9% w/v)

Glucose intravenous infusion (5% w/v)

Sodium chloride (0.18% w/v) and glucose (4% w/v) intravenous infusion

Lactated Ringer's Injection USP

When diluted with the listed infusion solutions in the proportion of 1 plus 3 (i.e. to give 0.5 mg/ml) Mivacron injection has been shown to be chemically and physically stable for at least 48 hours at 30°C. However, since the product contains no antimicrobial preservative, dilution should be carried out immediately prior to use, administration should commence as soon as possible thereafter, and any remaining solution should be discarded.

Doses in Infants and Children Aged 2 Months - 12 Years

Mivacron has a faster onset, shorter clinically effective duration of action and more rapid spontaneous recovery profile in infants and children than in adults.

The ED_{95} in infants aged 2 to 6 months is approximately 0.07 mg/kg; and in infants and children aged 7 months to 12 years is approximately 0.1 mg/kg.

Pharmacodynamic data for recommended initial doses in infants and children are summarised in the following table:

(see Table 1 on previous page)

Since maximum block is usually achieved within 2 minutes following administration of these doses, tracheal intubation should be possible within this time.

Infants and children generally require more frequent maintenance doses and higher infusion rate than adults. Pharmacodynamic data for maintenance doses are summarised in the table below together with recommended infusion rates:

(see Table 2 on previous page)

The neuromuscular blocking action of mivacurium is potentiated by inhalational agents. A study has shown that the mivacurium infusion rate requirement should be reduced by up to 70% with sevoflurane in children aged 2 – 12 years.

Once spontaneous recovery is underway, it is complete in approximately 10 minutes.

Dose in Neonates and Infants Under 2 Months of Age

No dose recommendation for neonates and infants under 2 months of age can be made until further information becomes available.

Dose in the Elderly

In elderly patients receiving single bolus doses of Mivacron, the onset time, duration of action and recovery rate may be extended relative to younger patients by 20 to 30%. Elderly patients may also require decreased infusion rates or smaller or less frequent maintenance bolus doses.

Dose in Patients with Cardiovascular Disease

In patients with clinically significant cardiovascular disease, the initial dose of Mivacron should be administered over 60 seconds. Mivacron has been administered in this way with minimal haemodynamic effects to patients undergoing cardiac surgery.

Dose in Patients with Reduced Renal Function

In patients with end-stage renal failure the clinically effective duration of block produced by 0.15 mg/kg is approximately 1.5 times longer than in patients with normal renal function. Subsequently, dosage should be adjusted according to individual clinical response.

Prolonged and intensified neuromuscular blockade may also occur in patients with acute or chronic renal failure as a result of reduced levels of plasma cholinesterase (see section 4.4 Special Warnings and Precautions for Use).

Dose in Patients with Reduced Hepatic Function

In patients with end-stage liver failure the clinically effective duration of block produced by 0.15 mg/kg is approximately three times longer than in patients with normal hepatic function. This prolongation is related to the markedly reduced plasma cholinesterase activity seen in these patients. Subsequently, dosage should be adjusted according to individual clinical response.

Dose in Patients with Reduced Plasma Cholinesterase Activity

Mivacurium is metabolised by plasma cholinesterase. Plasma cholinesterase activity may be diminished in the presence of genetic abnormalities of plasma cholinesterase (e.g. patients heterozygous or homozygous for the atypical plasma cholinesterase gene), in various pathological conditions (see section 4.4 Special Warnings and Precautions for Use) and by the administration of certain drugs (see interactions with other medicaments). The possibility of prolonged neuromuscular block following administration of Mivacron must be considered in patients with reduced plasma cholinesterase activity. Mild reductions (i.e. within 20% of the lower limit of the normal range) are not associated with clinically significant effects on duration (See Contra-indications and Special Warnings and Precautions for information about use in patients who are homozygous or heterozygous for the plasma cholinesterase gene).

Dose in Obese Patients

In obese patients (those weighing 30% or more above their ideal bodyweight for height), the initial dose of Mivacron should be based upon ideal bodyweight and not actual bodyweight.

Instructions to open the ampoule

Ampoules are equipped with the OPC (One Point Cut) opening system and must be opened following the below instructions:

1. hold with the hand the bottom part of the ampoule as indicated in picture 1

2. put the other hand on the top of the ampoule positioning the thumb above the coloured point and press as indicated in picture 2

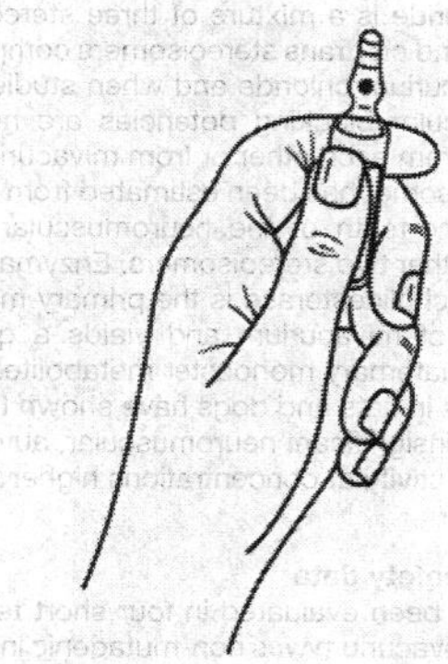

Picture 1

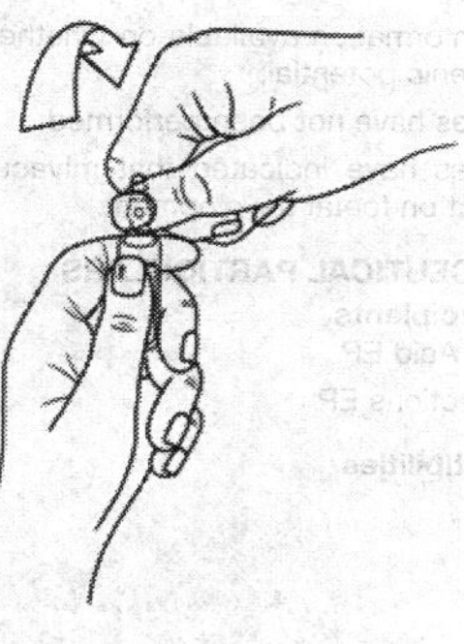

Picture 2

Monitoring

In common with all neuromuscular blocking agents, monitoring of neuromuscular function is recommended during the use of Mivacron in order to individualise dosage requirements.

4.3 Contraindications

Mivacron should not be administered to patients known to have allergic hypersensitivity to the drug.

Mivacron is contraindicated in pregnancy since there is no information on the use of Mivacron in pregnant women.

Mivacron is contraindicated in patients known or suspected of being homozygous for the atypical plasma cholinesterase gene (see "special warnings and precautions for use" section).

4.4 Special warnings and precautions for use

In common with all the other neuromuscular blocking agents, Mivacron paralyses the respiratory muscles as well as the other skeletal muscles but has no effect on consciousness. Mivacron should be administered only by or under close supervision of an experienced anaesthetist with adequate facilities for endotracheal intubation and artificial ventilation.

Prolonged and intensified neuromuscular blockade following mivacurium may occur secondary to reduced plasma cholinesterase activity in the following states or pathological conditions:

- Physiological variation as in pregnancy and the puerperium (see Pregnancy and Lactation).
- Genetically determined abnormalities of plasma cholinesterase (see below and Contraindications).
- Severe generalised tetanus, tuberculosis and other severe or chronic infections.
- Chronic debilitating disease, malignancy, chronic anaemia and malnutrition.
- Myxoedema and collagen diseases.
- Decompensated heart disease.
- Peptic ulcer.
- Burns (see below).
- End-stage hepatic failure, (see Dosage and Administration).
- Acute, chronic or end-stage renal failure (see Dosage and Administration).
- Iatrogenic: following plasma exchange, plasmapheresis, cardiopulmonary bypass, and as a result of concomitant drug therapy (see Interactions).

In common with suxamethonium/succinylcholine, adult and paediatric patients homozygous for the atypical plasma cholinesterase gene (1 in 2500 patients) are extremely sensitive to the neuromuscular blocking effect of Mivacurium. In three such adults patients, a small dose of 0.03 mg/kg (approximately the ED_{10-20} in genotypically normal patients) produced complete neuromuscular block for 26 to 128 minutes.

In patients heterozygous for the atypical plasma cholinesterase gene, the clinically effective duration of block of mivacurium 0.15 mg/kg is approximately 10 min longer than in control patients.

Once spontaneous recovery had begun, neuromuscular block in these patients was antagonised with conventional doses of neostigmine.

Patients with burns may develop resistance to non-depolarising neuromuscular blocking agents and require increased doses. However such patients may also have reduced plasma cholinesterase activity, requiring dose reduction.

Consequently burn patients should be given a test dose of 0.015-0.020 mg/kg Mivacron followed by appropriate dosing guided by monitoring of block with a nerve stimulator.

Caution should be exercised in administering Mivacron to patients with a history suggestive of an increased sensitivity to the effects of histamine e.g. asthma. If Mivacron is used in this group of patients it should be administered over 60 seconds.

High rates of cross-sensitivity (greater than 50%) between neuromuscular blocking agents have been reported. Therefore, where possible, before administering mivacurium, hypersensitivity to other neuromuscular blocking agents should be excluded. Mivacurium should only be used when absolutely essential in susceptible patients. Patients who experience a hypersensitivity reaction under general anaesthesia should be tested subsequently for hypersensitivity to other neuromuscular blockers.

Mivacron should be administered over a period of 60 seconds to patients who may be unusually sensitive to falls in arterial blood pressure, for example those who are hypovolaemic.

In adults, doses of Mivacron > 0.2 mg/kg ($>3 \times$ ED95) have been associated with histamine release when administered by rapid bolus injection. However, the slower administration of the 0.2 mg/kg Mivacron dose and the divided administration of the 0.25 mg/kg Mivacron dose minimised the cardiovascular effects of these doses. Cardiovascular safety did not appear to be compromised in children given a rapid bolus dose of 0.2 mg/kg in clinical studies.

Mivacron does not have significant vagal or ganglion blocking properties in the recommended dosage range. Recommended doses of Mivacron consequently have no clinically significant effects on heart rate and will not counteract the bradycardia produced by many anaesthetic agents or by vagal stimulation during surgery.

In common with other non-depolarising neuromuscular blocking agents, increased sensitivity to mivacurium can be expected in patients with Myasthenia Gravis, other forms of neuromuscular disease and cachectic patients. Severe acid base or electrolyte abnormalities may increase or reduce sensitivity to mivacurium.

Mivacron solution is acidic (approximately pH 4.5) and should not be mixed in the same syringe or administered simultaneously through the same needle as highly alkaline solutions (e.g. barbiturate solutions). It has been shown to be compatible with some commonly used peri-operative drugs supplied as acidic solutions e.g. Fentanyl, Alfentanil, Sufentanil, Droperidol and Midazolam. Where other anaesthetic agents are administered through the same indwelling needle or cannula as used for Mivacron, and compatibility has not been demonstrated, it is recommended that each drug is flushed through with physiological saline.

Studies in malignant hyperthermia-susceptible pigs, indicated that Mivacron does not trigger this syndrome. Mivacron has not been studied in malignant hyperthermia-susceptible patients.

No data are available on the long-term use of Mivacron in patients undergoing mechanical ventilation in the intensive care unit.

Reversal of Neuromuscular Block: as with other neuromuscular blocking agents, evidence of spontaneous recovery should be observed prior to administration of reversal agent (e.g. neostigmine). The use of a peripheral nerve stimulator to evaluate recovery prior to and following reversal of neuromuscular block is strongly recommended.

Pharmaceutical Precautions

Since no antimicrobial preservative is included, Mivacron must be used under full aseptic conditions and any dilution carried out immediately before use. Any unused solution in open ampoules should be discarded.

Mivacron injection is acidic (approximately pH 4.5) and should not be mixed with highly alkaline solutions (e.g. barbiturates). Mivacron has been shown to be compatible with some commonly used peri-operative drugs supplied as acidic solutions. Where such agents are administered through the same indwelling needle or cannula as used for Mivacron injection, and compatibility has not been demonstrated, it is recommended that each drug is flushed through with physiological saline.

The pack will contain the following statements:

Store below 25°C.

Do not freeze.

Protect from light.

Any portion of the contents remaining after use should be discarded.

Keep out of reach of children.

4.5 Interaction with other medicinal products and other forms of interaction

The neuromuscular block produced by Mivacron may be increased by the concomitant use of inhalational anaesthetics such as enflurane, isoflurane, sevoflurane and halothane.

Mivacron has been safely administered following succinylcholine facilitated intubation. Evidence of spontaneous recovery from succinylcholine should be observed prior to administration of Mivacron.

In common with all non-depolarising neuromuscular blocking agents, the magnitude and/or duration of non-depolarising neuromuscular block may be increased and infusion requirements may be reduced as a result of interaction with; antibiotics, including the aminoglycosides, polymyxins, Spectinomycin, tetracyclines, Lincomycin and Clindamycin; anti-arrhythmic drugs: Propranolol, calcium channel blockers, lidocaine, Procainamide and Quinidine, diuretics: furosemide and possibly thiazides, Mannitol and Acetazolamide, magnesium salts, ketamine, lithium salts, ganglion blocking drugs: Trimetaphan, Hexamethonium.

Drugs that may reduce plasma cholinesterase activity may also prolong the neuromuscular blocking action of Mivacron. These include anti-mitotic drugs, monoamine oxidase inhibitors, ecothiophate iodine, pancuronium, organophosphates, anticholinesterases, certain hormones, bambuterol.

Rarely, certain drugs may aggravate or unmask latent Myasthenia Gravis or actually induce a Myasthenic syndrome: increased sensitivity to Mivacron would be consequent on such a development. Such drugs include various antibiotics, beta-blockers. (Propranolol, Oxprenolol), antiarrhythmic drugs (Procainamide, Quinidine), antirheumatic drugs (Chloroquine, D-Pencillamine), Trimetaphan, Chlorpromazine, Steroids, Phenytoin and Lithium.

The administration of combinations of non-depolarising neuromuscular blocking agents in conjunction with Mivacron may produce a degree of neuromuscular blockade in excess of that which might be expected from an equipotent total dose of Mivacron. Any synergistic effect may vary between different drug combinations.

A depolarising muscle relaxant such as suxamethonium chloride should not be administered to prolong the neuromuscular blocking effects of non-depolarising agents, as this may result in a prolonged and complex block which can be difficult to reverse with anticholinesterase drugs.

4.6 Pregnancy and lactation

Plasma cholinesterase levels decrease during pregnancy. Mivacurium has been used to maintain neuromuscular block during Caesarean section, but due to the reduced levels of plasma cholinesterase, dosage adjustments to the infusion rate were necessary. A further reduction in the infusion rate may also be required during Caesarean section in patients pre-treated with $MgSO_4$, due to the potentiating effects of Mg^{2+}.

It is not known whether mivacurium is excreted in human milk.

4.7 Effects on ability to drive and use machines

This precaution is not relevant to the use of mivacurium. Mivacurium will always be used in combination with a general anaesthetic and therefore the usual precautions relating to performance of tasks following general anaesthesia apply.

4.8 Undesirable effects

Associated with the use of Mivacron there have been reports of skin flushing, erythema, urticaria, hypotension, transient tachycardia or bronchospasm which have been attributed to histamine release. These effects are dose related and more common following initial doses of $\geq$0.2 mg/kg or more when given rapidly and are reduced if Mivacron is injected over 30 to 60 seconds or in divided doses over 30 seconds.

Very rarely, severe anaphylactic or anaphylactoid reactions have been reported in patients receiving Mivacron in conjunction with one or more anaesthetic agents.

4.9 Overdose

Prolonged muscle paralysis and its consequences are the main signs of overdosage with neuromuscular blocking agents. However, the risk of haemodynamic side-effects especially decreases in blood pressure, may be increased.

It is essential to maintain a patent airway together with assisted positive pressure ventilation until spontaneous respiration is adequate. Full sedation will be required since consciousness is not impaired. Recovery may be hastened by the administration of anticholinesterase agents accompanied by atropine or glycopyrrolate, once evidence of spontaneous recovery is present. Cardiovascular support may be provided by proper positioning of the patient and administration of fluids or vasopressor agents as required.

5. PHARMACOLOGICAL PROPERTIES

5.1 Pharmacodynamic properties

Mivacurium is a short-acting, non-depolarising skeletal muscle relaxant which is hydrolysed by plasma cholinesterase. Mivacurium binds competitively with cholinergic receptors on the motor end-plate to prevent the action of acetylcholine, resulting in a blockade of neuromuscular transmission. This is rapidly reversed by the administration of the cholinesterase inhibitors, neostigmine and edrophonium.

5.2 Pharmacokinetic properties

Mivacurium chloride is a mixture of three stereoisomers, the trans-trans and cis-trans stereoisomers comprise 92% to 96% of mivacurium chloride and when studied in cats their neuromuscular blocking potencies are not significantly different from each other or from mivacurium chloride. The cis-cis isomer has been estimated from studies in cats to have one-tenth of the neuromuscular blocking potency of the other two stereoisomers. Enzymatic hydrolysis by plasma cholinesterase is the primary mechanism for inactivation of mivacurium and yields a quaternary alcohol and a quaternary monoester metabolite. Pharmacological studies in cats and dogs have shown that metabolites possess insignificant neuromuscular, autonomic or cardiovascular activity at concentrations higher than seen in man.

5.3 Preclinical safety data

Mivacurium has been evaluated in four short term mutagenicity tests. Mivacurium was non-mutagenic in the Ames salmonella assay, the mouse lymphoma assay, the human lymphocyte assay and the *in vivo* rat bone marrow cytogenetic assay.

There is no information available on whether Mivacurium has carcinogenic potential.

Fertility studies have not been performed.

Animal studies have indicated that mivacurium has no adverse effect on foetal development.

6. PHARMACEUTICAL PARTICULARS

6.1 List of excipients

Hydrochloric Acid EP

Water for Injections EP

6.2 Incompatibilities

None known

6.3 Shelf life

18 months

6.4 Special precautions for storage

Store below 25°C. Do not freeze. Protect from light.

6.5 Nature and contents of container

Neutral glass ampoules containing 5ml or 10ml of product.

6.6 Special precautions for disposal and other handling

No special instructions are required.

Administrative Data

7. MARKETING AUTHORISATION HOLDER

The Wellcome Foundation Ltd:

Berkeley Avenue

Greenford

Middlesex UB6 0NN

Trading as

Glaxo Wellcome and/or GlaxoSmithKline UK

Stockley Park West

Uxbridge

Middlesex UB11 1BT

8. MARKETING AUTHORISATION NUMBER(S)

PL 00003/0325

9. DATE OF FIRST AUTHORISATION/RENEWAL OF THE AUTHORISATION

21st January 2009

10. DATE OF REVISION OF THE TEXT

9th March 2009

11. Legal Status

POM

Mixtard 30 100 IU/ml, Mixtard 30 Penfill 100 IU/ml, Mixtard 30 InnoLet 100 IU/ml

(Novo Nordisk Limited)

1. NAME OF THE MEDICINAL PRODUCT

Mixtard 30 100 IU/ml suspension for injection in a vial

Mixtard 30 Penfill 100 IU/ml suspension for injection in a cartridge

Mixtard 30 InnoLet 100 IU/ml suspension for injection in a pre-filled pen

2. QUALITATIVE AND QUANTITATIVE COMPOSITION

Insulin human, rDNA (produced by recombinant DNA technology in *Saccharomyces cerevisiae*).

1 ml contains 100 IU of insulin human

1 vial contains 10 ml equivalent to 1000 IU

1 cartridge contains 3 ml equivalent to 300 IU

1 pre-filled pen contains 3 ml equivalent to 300 IU

One IU (International Unit) corresponds to 0.035 mg of anhydrous human insulin.

Mixtard is a mixture of dissolved insulin and isophane (NPH) insulin.

Mixtard 30 consists of 30% dissolved insulin and 70% isophane insulin.

For a full list of excipients, see section 6.1.

3. PHARMACEUTICAL FORM

Suspension for injection in a vial.

Suspension for injection in a cartridge.

Suspension for injection in a pre-filled pen.

Cloudy, white, aqueous suspension.

4. CLINICAL PARTICULARS

4.1 Therapeutic indications

Treatment of diabetes mellitus.

4.2 Posology and method of administration

Mixtard is a dual-acting insulin. It is a biphasic formulation containing fast-acting and long-acting insulin.

Premixed insulin products are usually given once or twice daily when a rapid initial effect together with a more prolonged effect is desired.

Dosage

Dosage is individual and determined in accordance with the needs of the patient. The individual insulin requirement is usually between 0.3 and 1.0 IU/kg/day. The daily insulin requirement may be higher in patients with insulin resistance (e.g. during puberty or due to obesity) and lower in patients with residual, endogenous insulin production.

In patients with diabetes mellitus optimised glycaemic control delays the onset of late diabetic complications. Close blood glucose monitoring is recommended.

An injection should be followed within 30 minutes by a meal or snack containing carbohydrates.

Dosage adjustment

Concomitant illness, especially infections and feverish conditions, usually increases the patient's insulin requirement.

Renal or hepatic impairment may reduce insulin requirement.

Adjustment of dosage may also be necessary if patients change physical activity or their usual diet.

Dosage adjustment may be necessary when transferring patients from one insulin preparation to another (see section 4.4).

Administration

For subcutaneous use. Insulin suspensions are never to be administered intravenously.

Mixtard is administered subcutaneously in the thigh or abdominal wall. If convenient, the gluteal region or the deltoid region may also be used.

Subcutaneous injection into the abdominal wall ensures a faster absorption than from other injection sites.

Injection into a lifted skin fold minimises the risk of unintended intramuscular injection.

The needle should be kept under the skin for at least 6 seconds to make sure the entire dose is injected.

Injection sites should be rotated within an anatomic region in order to avoid lipodystrophy.

The vials are for use with insulin syringes with a corresponding unit scale.

The cartridges are designed to be used with Novo Nordisk delivery systems (durable devices for repeated use) and NovoFine needles. Detailed instruction accompanying the delivery system must be followed.

Mixtard InnoLet is designed to be used with NovoFine short cap needles of 8 mm or shorter in length. The needle box is marked with an **S.**

InnoLet delivers 1-50 units in increments of 1 unit.

The pens should be primed before injection so that the dose selector returns to zero and a drop of insulin appears at the needle tip.

The dose is set by turning the selector, which returns to zero during the injection.

Mixtard is accompanied by a package leaflet with detailed instruction for use to be followed.

4.3 Contraindications

Hypersensitivity to the active substance or to any of the excipients (see section 6.1).

Hypoglycaemia

4.4 Special warnings and precautions for use

Inadequate dosage or discontinuation of treatment, especially in type 1 diabetes, may lead to **hyperglycaemia**.

Usually the first symptoms of hyperglycaemia set in gradually, over a period of hours or days. They include thirst, increased frequency of urination, nausea, vomiting, drowsiness, flushed dry skin, dry mouth, loss of appetite as well as acetone odour of breath.

In type 1 diabetes, untreated hyperglycaemic events eventually lead to diabetic ketoacidosis, which is potentially lethal.

Hypoglycaemia may occur if the insulin dose is too high in relation to the insulin requirement (see sections 4.8 and 4.9).

Omission of a meal or unplanned, strenuous physical exercise may lead to hypoglycaemia.

Patients whose blood glucose control is greatly improved e.g. by intensified insulin therapy, may experience a change in their usual warning symptoms of hypoglycaemia and should be advised accordingly.

Usual warning symptoms may disappear in patients with long-standing diabetes.

Transferring a patient to another type or brand of insulin should be done under strict medical supervision. Changes in strength, brand (manufacturer), type (fast-, dual-, long-acting insulin etc.), origin (animal, human or analogue insulin) and/or method of manufacture (recombinant DNA versus animal source insulin) may result in a need for a change in dosage.

If an adjustment is needed when switching the patients to Mixtard, it may occur with the first dose or during the first several weeks or months.

As with any insulin therapy, injection site reactions may occur and include pain, itching, hives, swelling and inflammation. Continuous rotation of the injection site within a given area may help to reduce or prevent these reactions. Reactions usually resolve in a few days to a few weeks. On rare occasions.injection site reactions may require discontinuation of Mixtard.

A few patients who have experienced hypoglycaemic reactions after transfer from animal source insulin have reported that early warning symptoms of hypoglycaemia were less pronounced or different from those experienced with their previous insulin.

Before travelling between different time zones, the patient should be advised to consult the physician, since this may mean that the patient has to take insulin and meals at different times.

Insulin suspensions are not to be used in insulin infusion pumps.

Mixtard contains metacresol, which may cause allergic reactions.

4.5 Interaction with other medicinal products and other forms of interaction

A number of medicinal products are known to interact with glucose metabolism. The physician must therefore take possible interactions into account and should always ask his patients about any medicinal products they take.

The following substances may reduce insulin requirement:

Oral hypoglycaemic agents (OHA), monoamine oxidase inhibitors (MAOI), non-selective beta-blocking agents, angiotensin converting enzyme (ACE) inhibitors, salicylates, alcohol, anabolic steroids and sulphonamides.

The following substances may increase insulin requirement:

Oral contraceptives, thiazides, glucocorticoids, thyroid hormones and beta-sympathomimetics, growth hormone and danazol.

Beta-blocking agents may mask the symptoms of hypoglycaemia and delay recovery from hypoglycaemia.

Octreotide/lanreotide may both decrease and increase insulin requirement.

Alcohol may intensify and prolong the hypoglycaemic effect of insulin.

4.6 Pregnancy and lactation

There are no restrictions on treatment of diabetes with insulin during pregnancy, as insulin does not pass the placental barrier.

Both hypoglycaemia and hyperglycaemia, which can occur in inadequately controlled diabetes therapy, increase the risk of malformations and death *in utero*. Intensified control in the treatment of pregnant women with diabetes is therefore recommended throughout pregnancy and when contemplating pregnancy.

Insulin requirements usually fall in the first trimester and subsequently increase during the second and third trimesters.

After delivery, insulin requirements return rapidly to pre-pregnancy values.

Insulin treatment of the nursing mother presents no risk to the baby. However, the Mixtard dosage may need to be adjusted.

4.7 Effects on ability to drive and use machines

The patient's ability to concentrate and react may be impaired as a result of hypoglycaemia. This may constitute a risk in situations where these abilities are of special importance (e.g. driving a car or operating machinery).

Patients should be advised to take precautions to avoid hypoglycaemia whilst driving. This is particularly important in those who have reduced or absent awareness of the warning signs of hypoglycaemia or have frequent episodes of hypoglycaemia. The advisability of driving should be considered in these circumstances.

4.8 Undesirable effects

As for other insulin products, in general, hypoglycaemia is the most frequently occurring undesirable effect. It may occur if the insulin dose is too high in relation to the insulin requirement. In clinical trials and during marketed use the frequency varies with patient population and dose regimens. Therefore, no specific frequency can be presented. Severe hypoglycaemia may lead to unconsciousness and/or convulsions and may result in temporary or permanent impairment of brain function or even death.

Frequencies of adverse drug reactions from clinical trials, that are considered related to Mixtard are listed below. The frequencies are defined as: uncommon ($\geq$1/1000, $<$ 1/100). Isolated spontaneous cases are presented as very rare defined as $<$ 1/10,000 including isolated reports.

Within each frequency grouping, undesirable effects are presented in order of decreasing seriousness.

<u>Nervous system disorders</u>

Uncommon – Peripheral neuropathy

Fast improvement in blood glucose control may be associated with a condition termed "acute painful neuropathy", which is usually reversible.

<u>Eye disorders</u>

Very rare – Refraction disorders

Refraction anomalies may occur upon initiation of insulin therapy. These symptoms are usually of transitory nature.

Uncommon – Diabetic retinopathy

Long-term improved glycaemic control decreases the risk of progression of diabetic retinopathy. However, intensification of insulin therapy with abrupt improvement in glycaemic control may be associated with temporary worsening of diabetic retinopathy.

<u>Skin and subcutaneous tissue disorders</u>

Uncommon – Lipodystrophy

Lipodystrophy may occur at the injection site as a consequence of failure to rotate injection sites within an area.

<u>General disorders and administration site conditions</u>

Uncommon – Injection site reactions

Injection site reactions (redness, swelling, itching, pain and haematoma at the injection site) may occur during treatment with insulin. Most reactions are transitory and disappear during continued treatment.

Uncommon – Oedema

Oedema may occur upon initiation of insulin therapy. These symptoms are usually of transitory nature.

<u>Immune system disorders</u>

Uncommon – Urticaria, rash

Very rare – Anaphylactic reactions

Symptoms of generalised hypersensitivity may include generalised skin rash, itching, sweating, gastrointestinal upset, angioneurotic oedema, difficulties in breathing, palpitation, reduction in blood pressure and fainting/loss of consciousness. Generalised hypersensitivity reactions are potentially life threatening.

4.9 Overdose

A specific overdose of insulin cannot be defined. However, hypoglycaemia may develop over sequential stages:

• Mild hypoglycaemic episodes can be treated by oral administration of glucose or sugary products. It is therefore recommended that the diabetic patients carry some sugar lumps, sweets, biscuits or sugary fruit juice.

• Severe hypoglycaemic episodes, where the patient has become unconscious, can be treated by glucagon (0.5 to 1 mg) given intramuscularly or subcutaneously by a person who has received appropriate instruction, or by glucose given intravenously by a medical professional. Glucose must also be given intravenously, if the patient does not respond to glucagon within 10 to 15 minutes.

Upon regaining consciousness, administration of oral carbohydrate is recommended for the patient in order to prevent relapse.

5. PHARMACOLOGICAL PROPERTIES

5.1 Pharmacodynamic properties

Pharmacotherapeutic group: Insulins and analogues for injection, intermediate-acting combined with fast-acting, insulin (human). ATC code: A10A D01.

The blood glucose lowering effect of insulin is due to the facilitated uptake of glucose following binding of insulin to receptors on muscle and fat cells and to the simultaneous inhibition of glucose output from the liver.

Mixtard is a dual-acting insulin.

Onset of action is within ½ hour, reaches a maximum effect within 2-8 hours and the entire time of duration is up to 24 hours.

5.2 Pharmacokinetic properties

Insulin in the blood stream has a half-life of a few minutes. Consequently, the time-action profile of an insulin preparation is determined solely by its absorption characteristics.

This process is influenced by several factors (e.g. insulin dosage, injection route and site, thickness of subcutaneous fat, type of diabetes). The pharmacokinetics of insulins is therefore affected by significant intra- and inter-individual variation.

<u>Absorption</u>

The absorption profile is due to the product being a mixture of insulin products with fast and protracted absorption respectively. The maximum plasma concentration of the fast-acting insulin is reached within 1.5-2.5 hours after subcutaneous administration.

<u>Distribution</u>

No profound binding to plasma proteins, except circulating insulin antibodies (if present) has been observed.

<u>Metabolism</u>

Human insulin is reported to be degraded by insulin protease or insulin-degrading enzymes and possibly protein disulfide isomerase. A number of cleavage (hydrolysis) sites on the human insulin molecule have been proposed; none of the metabolites formed following the cleavage are active.

<u>Elimination</u>

The terminal half-life is determined by the rate of absorption from the subcutaneous tissue. The terminal half-life ($t_{½}$) is therefore a measure of the absorption rather than of the elimination per se of insulin from plasma (insulin in the blood stream has a $t_{½}$ of a few minutes). Trials have indicated a $t_{½}$ of about 5-10 hours.

5.3 Preclinical safety data

Non-clinical data reveal no special hazard for humans based on conventional studies of safety pharmacology, repeated dose toxicity, genotoxicity, carcinogenic potential, toxicity to reproduction.

6. PHARMACEUTICAL PARTICULARS

6.1 List of excipients

Zinc chloride

Glycerol

Metacresol

Phenol

Disodium phosphate dihydrate

Sodium hydroxide (for pH adjustment)

Hydrochloric acid (for pH adjustment)

Protamine sulphate

Water for injections

6.2 Incompatibilities

Insulin products should only be added to compounds with which it is known to be compatible.

Insulin suspensions should not be added to infusion fluids.

6.3 Shelf life

30 months when stored between 2°C-8°C.

Mixtard 30:

6 weeks when used or stored at room temperature (below 25°C).

Mixtard 30 Penfill, Mixtard 30 InnoLet:

6 weeks when used or carried as a spare (below 30°).

6.4 Special precautions for storage

Before use: store in a refrigerator (2°C - 8°C).

Do not store them in or too near the freezer section or cooling element.

Do not freeze.

Mixtard 30:

During use: do not refrigerate. Do not store above 25°C.

Keep the vial in the outer carton in order to protect from light.

Protect from excessive heat and sunlight.

Mixtard 30 Penfill:

During use: do not refrigerate. Do not store above 30°C.

Keep the cartridge in the outer carton in order to protect from light.

Protect from excessive heat and sunlight.

Mixtard 30 InnoLet

During use: do not refrigerate. Do not store above 30°C.

Keep the pen cap on in order to protect the insulin from light.

Protect from excessive heat and sunlight.

6.5 Nature and contents of container

10 ml glass vial (type 1) closed with a bromobutyl/polyisoprene rubber stopper and a protective tamper-proof cap.

Pack size: 1 vial × 10 ml.

3 ml glass cartridge (type 1) with a bromobutyl rubber plunger and a bromobutyl/polyisoprene rubber stopper. The cartridge contains a glass ball to facilitate the re-suspension.

Pack size: 5 cartridges × 3 ml.

Pre-filled pen (multidose disposable pen) comprising a pen injector with a cartridge (3 ml). The cartridge is made of glass (type 1), containing a bromobutyl rubber plunger and a bromobutyl/polyisoprene rubber stopper. The cartridge contains a glass ball to facilitate the re-suspension. The pen injector is made of plastic.

Pack size: 5 pre-filled pens × 3 ml.

6.6 Special precautions for disposal and other handling
Cartridges and pens should only be used in combination with products that are compatible with them and allow the cartridge and pen to function safely and effectively.

Mixtard Penfill and Mixtard InnoLet are for single person use only. The container must not be refilled.

Insulin preparations, which have been frozen, must not be used.

After removing Mixtard vial, Mixtard Penfill or Mixtard InnoLet from the refrigerator it is recommended to allow the vial, Penfill or InnoLet to reach room temperature (not above 25°C) before resuspending the insulin as instructed for first time use.

Insulin suspensions should not be used if they do not appear uniformly white and cloudy after re-suspension.

Any unused product or waste material should be disposed of in accordance with local requirements.

7. MARKETING AUTHORISATION HOLDER
Novo Nordisk A/S

Novo Allé

DK-2880 Bagsværd

Denmark

8. MARKETING AUTHORISATION NUMBER(S)

Mixtard 30 100 IU/ml:	EU/1/02/231/003
Mixtard 30 Penfill 100 IU/ml:	EU/1/02/231/012
Mixtard 30 InnoLet 100 IU/ml:	EU/1/02/231/031

9. DATE OF FIRST AUTHORISATION/RENEWAL OF THE AUTHORISATION
Date of first authorisation: 07 October 2002

Date of last renewal: 18 October 2007

10. DATE OF REVISION OF THE TEXT
09/2007

Legal Status
POM

Mizollen 10 mg modified- release film-coated tablets

(sanofi-aventis)

1. NAME OF THE MEDICINAL PRODUCT
Mizollen 10 mg modified- release film-coated tablets

2. QUALITATIVE AND QUANTITATIVE COMPOSITION
Mizolastine 10mg per tablet

For a full list of excipients, see section 6.1

3. PHARMACEUTICAL FORM
Modified-release film-coated tablet

Oblong, white tablets with a scored line on one side and a mark "MZI 10" on the reverse side.

4. CLINICAL PARTICULARS

4.1 Therapeutic indications
Mizolastine is a long-acting H_1 -antihistamine indicated for the symptomatic relief of seasonal allergic rhinoconjunctivitis (hay fever), perennial allergic rhinoconjunctivitis and urticaria.

4.2 Posology and method of administration
Adults, including the elderly, and children 12 years of age and over:

The recommended daily dose is one 10mg tablet.

4.3 Contraindications
Hypersensitivity to the active ingredient or to any of the excipients.

Concomitant administration with macrolide antibiotics or systemic imidazole antifungals.

Significantly impaired hepatic function.

Clinically significant cardiac disease or a history of symptomatic arrhythmias.

Patients with known or suspected QT prolongation or with electrolyte imbalance, in particular hypokalaemia.

Clinically significant bradycardia.

Drugs known to prolong the QT interval, such as Class I and III anti- arrhythmics.

4.4 Special warnings and precautions for use
Mizolastine has a weak potential to prolong the QT interval in a few individuals. The degree of prolongation is modest and has not been associated with cardiac arrhythmias.

The elderly may be particularly susceptible to the sedative effects of mizolastine and the potential effects of the drug on cardiac repolarisation.

Due to the presence of lactose, patients with rare hereditary problems of galactose intolerance, the Lapp lactase deficiency or glucose-galactose malabsorption should not take this medicine.

4.5 Interaction with other medicinal products and other forms of interaction
Although the bioavailability of mizolastine is high and the drug is principally metabolised by glucuronidation, systemically administered ketoconazole and erythromycin moderately increase the plasma concentration of mizolastine and their concurrent use is contraindicated.

Concurrent use of other potent inhibitors or substrates of hepatic oxidation (cytochrome P450 3A4) with mizolastine should be approached with caution. These would include cimetidine, ciclosporin, and nifedipine.

Alcohol: In studies with mizolastine, no potentiation of the sedation and the alteration in performance caused by alcohol has been observed.

4.6 Pregnancy and lactation
The safety of mizolastine for use in human pregnancy has not been established. The evaluation of experimental animal studies does not indicate direct or indirect harmful effects with respect to the development of the embryo or foetus, the course of gestation and peri- and post-natal development. However, as with all drugs, mizolastine should be avoided in pregnancy, particularly during the first trimester.

Mizolastine is excreted into breast milk, therefore its use by lactating women is not recommended.

4.7 Effects on ability to drive and use machines
Most patients taking mizolastine may drive or perform tasks requiring concentration. However, in order to identify sensitive people who have unusual reactions to drugs, it is advisable to check the individual response before driving or performing complicated tasks.

4.8 Undesirable effects
•Gastro-intestinal disorders:
Common: dry mouth, diarrhoea, abdominal pain (including dyspepsia), nausea

• Central nervous system disorders and psychiatric disorders:
Common: drowsiness often transient, headache, dizziness

Uncommon: anxiety and depression

• Liver disorders
Uncommon: raised liver enzymes

• Haematological disorders
Very rare: low neutrophil count

• Body as a whole
Common: asthenia often transient, increased appetite associated with weight gain.

Very rare: allergic reactions including anaphylaxis, angioedema, generalised rash/urticaria, pruritus and hypotension

• Cardiovascular disorders
Uncommon: hypotension, tachycardia, palpitations

Very rare: vasovagal attack

• Musculoskeletal disorders
Uncommon: arthralgia and myalgia

There were reports of bronchospasm and aggravation of asthma but in view of the high frequency of asthma in the patient population being treated, a causal relationship remains uncertain.

Treatment with certain antihistamines has been associated with QT interval prolongation increasing the risk of serious cardiac arrhythmias in susceptible subjects.

Minor changes in blood sugar and electrolytes have been observed rarely. The clinical significance of these changes in otherwise healthy individuals remains unclear. Patients at risk (diabetics, those susceptible to electrolyte imbalance and cardiac arrhythmias) should be monitored periodically.

4.9 Overdose
In cases of overdosage, general symptomatic surveillance with cardiac monitoring including QT interval and cardiac rhythm for at least 24 hours is recommended, along with standard measures to remove any unabsorbed drug.

Studies in patients with renal insufficiency suggest that haemodialysis does not increase clearance of the drug.

5. PHARMACOLOGICAL PROPERTIES

5.1 Pharmacodynamic properties
Antihistamines for systemic use (ATC code: R06AX25)

Mizolastine possesses antihistamine and antiallergic properties due to a specific and selective antagonism of peripheral histamine H_1 receptors. It has also been shown to inhibit histamine release from mast cells (at 0.3 mg/kg orally) and the migration of neutrophils (at 3 mg/kg orally) in animal models of allergic reactions.

In man, histamine-induced wheal and flare studies have shown that mizolastine 10 mg is a rapid, potent (80 % inhibition after 4 hrs) and sustained (24hr) antihistamine. No tachyphylaxis occurred after long-term administration.

In both preclinical and clinical studies, no anticholinergic effect has been demonstrated.

5.2 Pharmacokinetic properties
Following oral administration mizolastine is rapidly absorbed. Peak plasma concentration is reached at a median time of 1.5 hours.

Bioavailability is 65% and linear kinetics have been demonstrated.

The mean elimination half-life is 13.0 hours with plasma protein binding of 98.4%.

In hepatic insufficiency the absorption of mizolastine is slower and the distribution phase longer, with a resulting moderate increase in AUC of 50%.

The principal metabolic pathway is glucuronidation of the parent compound. The cytochrome P_{450} 3A4 enzyme system is involved in one of the additional metabolic pathways with formation of the hydroxylated metabolites of mizolastine. None of the identified metabolites contribute to the pharmacological activity of mizolastine.

An increase in mizolastine plasma levels, observed with systemic ketoconazole and erythromycin, led to concentrations equivalent to those obtained after a 15 to 20 mg dose of mizolastine alone.

In studies carried out in healthy volunteers, no clinically significant interaction has been recorded with food, warfarin, digoxin, theophylline, lorazepam, or diltiazem.

5.3 Preclinical safety data
Pharmacological studies in several species have shown an effect on cardiac repolarisation at doses in excess of 10-20 times the therapeutic dose. In conscious dogs, mizolastine has shown pharmacological interactions with ketoconazole at the electrocardiographic level at 70 times the therapeutic dose.

6. PHARMACEUTICAL PARTICULARS

6.1 List of excipients
Core:

Hydrogenated castor oil

Lactose monohydrate

Microcrystalline cellulose

Tartaric acid

Povidone

Anhydrous colloidal silica

Magnesium stearate.

Film-coating:

Hypromellose

Titanium dioxide (E171)

Propylene glycol.

6.2 Incompatibilities
Not applicable.

6.3 Shelf life
2 years in blisters.

6.4 Special precautions for storage
Do not store above 25°C. Store in the original package.

6.5 Nature and contents of container
Aluminium/PVC blisters: Packs of 30 tablets.

6.6 Special precautions for disposal and other handling
Tablets should not be taken if they become discoloured

7. MARKETING AUTHORISATION HOLDER
Sanofi-aventis

One Onslow Street

Guildford

Surrey

GU1 4YS

UK

8. MARKETING AUTHORISATION NUMBER(S)
PL 11723/0318

9. DATE OF FIRST AUTHORISATION/RENEWAL OF THE AUTHORISATION
7 March 2003

10. DATE OF REVISION OF THE TEXT
26 March 2009

Legal Category: POM

Mobic 15mg Tablets

(Boehringer Ingelheim Limited)

1. NAME OF THE MEDICINAL PRODUCT
Mobic 15 mg tablets

2. QUALITATIVE AND QUANTITATIVE COMPOSITION
Meloxicam 15.0 mg

Excipient(s): Lactose monohydrate

For a full list of excipients, see section 6.1.

3. PHARMACEUTICAL FORM
Tablet

Light yellow round scored tablet with the logotype of the company on one side and a score with 77C/77C on the other side.

4. CLINICAL PARTICULARS

4.1 Therapeutic indications
- Short-term symptomatic treatment of exacerbations of osteoarthrosis.

- Long term symptomatic treatment of rheumatoid arthritis or ankylosing spondylitis.

4.2 Posology and method of administration
Oral use

The total daily amount should be taken as a single dose, with water or another liquid, during a meal.

Undesirable effects may be minimised by using the lowest effective dose for the shortest duration necessary to control symptoms (see section 4.4). The patient's need for symptomatic relief and response to therapy should be re-evaluated periodically, especially in patients with osteoarthritis.

- Exacerbations of osteoarthrosis: 7.5 mg/day (half a 15 mg tablet).

If necessary, in the absence of improvement, the dose may be increased to 15 mg/day (one 15 mg tablet).

- Rheumatoid arthritis, ankylosing spondylitis: 15 mg/day (one 15 mg tablet).

(see also section 'Special populations' below)

According to the therapeutic response, the dose may be reduced to 7.5 mg/day (half a 15 mg tablet).

DO NOT EXCEED THE DOSE OF 15 MG/DAY.

Special populations

Elderly patients and patients with increased risks for adverse reaction (see section 5.2):

The recommended dose for long term treatment of rheumatoid arthritis and ankylosing spondylitis in elderly patients is 7.5 mg per day. Patients with increased risks for adverse reactions should start treatment with 7.5 mg per day (see section 4.4).

Renal impairment (see section 5.2):

In dialysis patients with severe renal failure, the dose should not exceed 7.5 mg per day.

No dose reduction is required in patients with mild to moderate renal impairment (i.e. patients with a creatinine clearance of greater than 25 ml/min). (For patients with non-dialysed severe renal failure, see section 4.3)

Hepatic impairment (see section 5.2):

No dose reduction is required in patients with mild to moderate hepatic impairment (For patients with severely impaired liver function, see section 4.3).

Children and adolescents:

Mobic 15 mg tablets is contraindicated in children and adolescents aged under 16 years (see section 4.3).

This medicinal product exists in other dosages, which may be more appropriate.

4.3 Contraindications

This medicinal product is contra-indicated in the following situations:

- third trimester of pregnancy (see section 4.6 'Pregnancy and lactation');
- children and adolescents aged under 16 years;
- hypersensitivity to meloxicam or to one of the excipients or hypersensitivity to substances with a similar action, e.g. NSAIDs, aspirin. Meloxicam should not be given to patients who have developed signs of asthma, nasal polyps, angioneurotic edema or urticaria following the administration of aspirin or other NSAIDs;
- history of gastrointestinal bleeding or perforation, related to previous NSAIDs therapy;
- active, or history of recurrent peptic ulcer/haemorrhage (two or more distinct episodes of proven ulceration or bleeding);
- severely impaired liver function;
- non-dialysed severe renal failure;
- gastrointestinal bleeding, history of cerebrovascular bleeding or other bleeding disorders;
- severe heart failure.

4.4 Special warnings and precautions for use

Undesirable effects may be minimised by using the lowest effective dose for the shortest duration necessary to control symptoms (see section 4.2, and GI and cardiovascular risks below).

The recommended maximum daily dose should not be exceeded in case of insufficient therapeutic effect, nor should an additional NSAID be added to the therapy because this may increase the toxicity while therapeutic advantage has not been proven. The use of meloxicam with concomitant NSAIDs including cyclooxygenase-2 selective inhibitors should be avoided.

Meloxicam is not appropriate for the treatment of patients requiring relief from acute pain.

In the absence of improvement after several days, the clinical benefit of the treatment should be reassessed.

Any history of oesophagitis, gastritis and/or peptic ulcer must be sought in order to ensure their total cure before starting treatment with meloxicam. Attention should routinely be paid to the possible onset of a recurrence in patients treated with meloxicam and with a past history of this type.

Gastrointestinal effects

GI bleeding, ulceration or perforation, which can be fatal, has been reported with all NSAIDs at anytime during treatment, with or without warning symptoms or a previous history of serious GI events.

The risk of GI bleeding, ulceration or perforation is higher with increasing NSAID doses, in patients with a history of ulcer, particularly if complicated with haemorrhage or perforation (see section 4.3), and in the elderly. These patients should commence treatment on the lowest dose available. Combination therapy with protective agents (e.g. misoprostol or proton pump inhibitors) should be considered for these patients, and also for patients requiring concomitant low dose aspirin, or other drugs likely to increase gastrointestinal risk (see below and 4.5).

Patients with a history of GI toxicity, particularly when elderly, should report any unusual abdominal symptoms (especially GI bleeding) particularly in the initial stages of treatment.

Caution is advised in patients receiving concomitant medications which could increase the risk of ulceration or bleeding, such as heparin as curative treatment or given in geriatrics, anticoagulants such as warfarin, or other non steroidal anti-inflammatory drugs, including acetylsalicylic acid given at anti-inflammatory doses (⩾ 1g as single intake or ⩾ 3g as total daily amount) (see section 4.5).

When GI bleeding or ulceration occurs in patients receiving meloxicam, the treatment should be withdrawn.

NSAIDs should be given with care to patients with a history of gastrointestinal disease (ulcerative colitis, Crohn's disease) as these conditions may be exacerbated (see section 4.8 – undesirable effects).

Cardiovascular and cerebrovascular effects

Appropriate monitoring and advice are required for patients with a history of hypertension and/or mild to moderate congestive heart failure as fluid retention and oedema have been reported in association with NSAID therapy.

Clinical monitoring of blood pressure for patients at risk is recommended at baseline and especially during treatment initiation with meloxicam.

Clinical trial and epidemiological data suggest that use of some NSAIDs including meloxicam (particularly at high doses and in long term treatment) may be associated with a small increased risk of arterial thrombotic events (for example myocardial infarction or stroke). There are insufficient data to exclude such a risk for meloxicam.

Patients with uncontrolled hypertension, congestive heart failure, established ischaemic heart disease, peripheral arterial disease, and/or cerebrovascular disease should only be treated with meloxicam after careful consideration. Similar consideration should be made before initiating longer-term treatment of patients with risk factors for cardiovascular disease (e.g. hypertension, hyperlipidaemia, diabetes mellitus, smoking).

Skin reactions

Serious skin reactions, some of them fatal, including exfoliative dermatitis, Stevens-Johnson syndrome, and toxic epidermal necrolysis, have been reported very rarely in association with the use of NSAIDs (see 4.8). Patients appear to be at highest risk of these reactions early in the course of therapy, the onset of the reaction occurring in the majority of cases within the first month of treatment. Meloxicamshould be discontinued at the first appearance of skin rash, mucosal lesions, or any other sign of hypersensitivity.

Parameters of liver and renal function

As with most NSAIDs, occasional increases in serum transaminase levels, increases in serum bilirubin or other liver function parameters, as well as increases in serum creatinine and blood urea nitrogen and other laboratory disturbances, have been reported. The majority of these instances involved transitory and slight abnormalities. Should any such abnormality prove significant or persistent, the administration of Meloxicam should be stopped and appropriate investigations undertaken.

Functional renal failure

NSAIDs, by inhibiting the vasodilating effect of renal prostaglandins, may induce a functional renal failure by reduction of glomerular filtration. This adverse event is dose-dependant. At the beginning of the treatment, or after dose increase, careful monitoring of diuresis and renal function is recommended in patients with the following risk factors:

- Elderly
- Concomitant treatments such as ACE inhibitors, angiotensin-II antagonists, sartans, diuretics (see section 4.5. Interaction with other medicinal products and other forms of interaction)
- Hypovolemia (whatever the cause)
- Congestive heart failure
- Renal failure
- Nephrotic syndrome
- Lupus nephropathy
- Severe hepatic dysfunction (serum albumin <25 g/l or Child-Pugh score ⩾10)

In rare instance NSAIDs may be the cause of interstitial nephritis, glomerulonephritis, renal medullary necrosis or nephrotic syndrome.

The dose of meloxicam in patients with end-stage renal failure on haemodialysis should not be higher than 7.5 mg. No dose reduction is required in patients with mild or moderate renal impairment (i.e. in patients with a creatinine clearance of greater than 25 ml/min).

Sodium, potassium and water retention

Induction of sodium, potassium and water retention and interference with the natriuretic effects of diuretics may occur with NSAIDs. Furthermore, a decrease of the antihypertensive effect of antihypertensive drugs can occur (see section 4.5). Consequently, oedema, cardiac failure or hypertension may be precipitated or exacerbated in susceptible patients as a result. Clinical monitoring is therefore necessary for patients at risk (see sections 4.2 and 4.3).

Hyperkalaemia

Hyperkalaemia can be favoured by diabetes or concomitant treatment known to increase kalaemia (see section 4.5). Regular monitoring of potassium values should be performed in such cases.

Other warnings and precautions

Adverse reactions are often less well tolerated in elderly, fragile or weakened individuals, who therefore require careful monitoring. As with other NSAIDs, particular caution is required in the elderly, in whom renal, hepatic and cardiac functions are frequently impaired. The elderly have an increased frequency of adverse reactions to NSAIDs especially gastrointestinal bleeding and perforation which may be fatal (see section 4.2).

Meloxicam, as any other NSAID may mask symptoms of an underlying infectious disease.

The use of meloxicam, as with any drug known to inhibit cyclooxygenase / prostaglandin synthesis, may impair fertility and is not recommended in women attempting to conceive. In women who have difficulties conceiving, or who are undergoing investigation of infertility, withdrawal of meloxicam should be considered.

Mobic 15 mg tablets contain lactose. Patients with rare hereditary problems of galactose intolerance, the Lapp-lactase deficiency or glucose-galactose malabsorption should not take this medicine.

4.5 Interaction with other medicinal products and other forms of interaction

Interaction studies have only been performed in adults.

Pharmacodynamic Interactions:

Other non steroidal anti-inflammatory drugs (NSAIDs) and acetylsalicylic acid ≥ 3g/d:

combination (see section 4.4) with other non steroidal anti-inflammatory drugs, including acetylsalicylic acid given at anti-inflammatory doses (⩾ 1g as single intake or ⩾ 3g as total daily amount) is not recommended.

Corticosteroids (e.g. Glucocorticoids):

The concomitant use with corticosteroids requests caution because of an increased risk of bleeding or gastrointestinal ulceration.

anticoagulant or heparin administered in geriatrics or at curative doses:

Considerably increased risk of bleeding, via inhibition of platelet function and damage to the gastroduodenal mucosa. NSAIDs may enhance the effects of anti-coagulants, such as warfarin (see section 4.4). The concomitant use of NSAIDs and anticoagulants or heparin administered in geriatrics or at curative dose is not recommended (see section 4.4).

In remaining cases of heparin use caution is necessary due to an increased bleeding risk.

Careful monitoring of the INR is required if it proves impossible to avoid such combination.

Thrombolytics and antiplatelet drugs:

Increased risk of bleeding, via inhibition of platelet function and damage to the gastroduodenal mucosa.

Selective serotonin reuptake inhibitors (SSRIs):

Increased risk of gastrointestinal bleeding.

Diuretics, ACE inhibitors and Angiotensin-II Antagonists:

NSAIDs may reduce the effect of diuretics and other antihypertensive drugs. In some patients with compromised renal function (e.g. dehydrated patients or elderly patients with compromised renal function) the co-administration of an ACE inhibitor or Angiotensin-II antagonists and agents that inhibit cyclo-oxygenase may result in further deterioration of renal function, including possible acute renal failure, which is usually reversible. Therefore, the combination should be administered with caution, especially in the elderly. Patients should be adequately hydrated and consideration should be given to monitoring of renal function after initiation of concomitant therapy, and periodically thereafter (see also section 4.4).

Other antihypertensive drugs (e.g. Beta-blockers):

As for the latter, a decrease of the antihypertensive effect of beta-blockers (due to inhibition of prostaglandins with vasodilatory effect) can occur.

Calcineurin inhibitors (e.g. cyclosporin, tacrolimus):

Nephrotoxicity of *calcineurin inhibitors* may be enhanced by NSAIDs via renal prostaglandin mediated effects. During combined treatment renal function is to be measured. A careful monitoring of the renal function is recommended, especially in the elderly.

Intrauterine devices:

NSAIDs have been reported to decrease the efficacy of intrauterine devices.

A decrease of the efficacy of intrauterine devices by NSAIDs has been previously reported but needs further confirmation.

Pharmacokinetic Interactions: Effect of meloxicam on the pharmacokinetics of other drugs

Lithium:

NSAIDs have been reported to increase blood lithium levels (via decreased renal excretion of lithium), which may reach toxic values. The concomitant use of lithium and NSAIDs is not recommended (see section 4.4). If this combination appears necessary, lithium plasma concentrations should be monitored carefully during the initiation, adjustment and withdrawal of meloxicam treatment.

Methotrexate:

NSAIDs can reduce the tubular secretion of methotrexate thereby increasing the plasma concentrations of methotrexate. For this reason, for patients on high dosages of methotrexate (more than 15 mg/week) the concomitant use of NSAIDs is not recommended (see section 4.4).

The risk of an interaction between NSAID preparations and methotrexate, should be considered also in patients on low dosage of methotrexate, especially in patients with impaired renal function. In case combination treatment is necessary blood cell count and the renal function should be monitored. Caution should be taken in case both NSAID and methotrexate are given within 3 days, in which case the plasma level of methotrexate may increase and cause increased toxicity.

Although the pharmacokinetics of methotrexate (15mg/week) were not relevantly affected by concomitant meloxicam treatment, it should be considered that the haematological toxicity of methotrexate can be amplified by treatment with NSAID drugs (see above). (See section 4.8)

Pharmacokinetic Interactions: Effect of other drugs on the pharmacokinetics of meloxicam

Cholestyramine:

Cholestyramine accelerates the elimination of meloxicam by interrupting the enterohepatic circulation so that clearance for meloxicam increases by 50% and the half-life decreases to 13±3 hrs. This interaction is of clinical significance.

No clinically relevant pharmacokinetic drug-drug interactions were detected with respect to the concomitant administration of antacids, cimetidine and digoxin.

4.6 Pregnancy and lactation

Pregnancy

Inhibition of prostaglandin synthesis may adversely affect the pregnancy and/or the embryo/foetal development. Data from epidemiological studies suggest an increased risk of miscarriage and of cardiac malformation and gastroschisis after use of a prostaglandin synthesis inhibitor in early pregnancy. The absolute risk for cardiovascular malformation was increased from less than 1%, up to approximately 1.5 %. The risk is believed to increase with dose and duration of therapy. In animals, administration of a prostaglandin synthesis inhibitor has been shown to result in increased pre- and post-implantation loss and embryo-foetal lethality. In addition, increased incidences of various malformations, including cardiovascular, have been reported in animals given a prostaglandin synthesis inhibitor during the organogenetic period.

During the first and second trimester of pregnancy, meloxicam should not be given unless clearly necessary. If meloxicam is used by a woman attempting to conceive, or during the first and second trimester of pregnancy, the dose should be kept as low and duration of treatment as short as possible.

During the third trimester of pregnancy, all prostaglandin synthesis inhibitors may expose

* the foetus to:

• cardiopulmonary toxicity (with premature closure of the ductus arteriosus and pulmonary hypertension).

• renal dysfunction, which may progress to renal failure with oligo-hydroamniosis.

* the mother and the neonate, at the end of pregnancy, to:

• possible prolongation of bleeding time, an anti-aggregating effect which may occur even at very low doses.

• inhibition of uterine contractions resulting in delayed or prolonged labour.

Consequently, meloxicam is contraindicated during the third trimester of pregnancy.

Lactation

While no specific experience exists for meloxicam, NSAIDs are known to pass into mother's milk. Administration therefore is not recommended in women who are breastfeeding.

4.7 Effects on ability to drive and use machines

There are no specific studies of the ability to drive and use machinery. However, on the basis of the pharmacodynamic profile and reported adverse drug reactions, meloxicam is likely to have no or negligible influence on these abilities. However, when visual disturbances or drowsiness, vertigo or other central nervous system disturbances occur, it is advisable to refrain from driving and operating machinery.

4.8 Undesirable effects

a) General Description

Clinical trial and epidemiological data suggest that use of some NSAIDs (particularly at high doses and in long term treatment) may be associated with a small increased risk of arterial thrombotic events (for example myocardial infarction or stroke) (see section 4.4).

Oedema, hypertension, and cardiac failure, have been reported in association with NSAID treatment.

The most commonly-observed adverse events are gastrointestinal in nature. Peptic ulcers, perforation or GI bleeding, sometimes fatal, particularly in the elderly, may occur (see section 4.4). Nausea, vomiting, diarrhoea, flatulence, constipation, dyspepsia, abdominal pain, melaena, haematemesis, ulcerative stomatitis, exacerbation of colitis and Crohn's disease (see section 4.4 - Special warnings and precautions for use) have been reported following administration. Less frequently, gastritis has been observed.

The frequencies of adverse drug reactions given below are based on corresponding occurrences of reported adverse events in 27 clinical trials with a treatment duration of at least 14 days. The information is based on clinical trials involving 15197 patients who have been treated with daily oral doses of 7.5 or 15 mg meloxicam tablets or capsules over a period of up to one year.

Adverse drug reactions that have come to light as a result of reports received in relation to administration of the marketed product are included.

Adverse reactions have been ranked under headings of frequency using the following convention:

Very common (≥1/10); common (≥1/100 to <1/10); uncommon (≥1/1,000 to <1/100); rare (≥1/10,000 to <1/1.000); very rare (<1/10,000), not known (cannot be estimated from the available data)

b) Table of adverse reactions

Blood and lymphatic system disorders

Uncommon:	Anaemia
Rare:	Blood count abnormal (including differential white cell count), leukopenia, thrombocytopenia

Very rare cases of agranulocytosis have been reported (see section c).

Immune system disorders

Uncommon:	Allergic reactions other than anaphylactic or anaphylactoid reactions
Not known:	Anaphylactic reaction, anaphylactoid reaction

Psychiatric disorders

Rare:	Mood altered, nightmares
Not known:	Confusional state, disorientation

Nervous system disorders

Common:	Headache
Uncommon:	Dizziness, somnolence

Eye disorders

Rare:	Visual disturbance including vision blurred; conjunctivitis

Ear and labyrinth disorders

Uncommon:	Vertigo
Rare:	Tinnitus

Cardiac disorders

Rare:	Palpitations

Cardiac failure has been reported in association with NSAID treatment.

Vascular disorders

Uncommon:	Blood pressure increased (see section 4.4), flushing

Respiratory, thoracic and mediastinal disorders

Rare:	Asthma in individuals allergic to aspirin or other NSAIDs

Gastrointestinal disorders

Very common:	Dyspepsia, nausea, vomiting, abdominal pain, constipation, flatulence, diarrhoea
Uncommon:	Occult or macroscopic gastrointestinal haemorrhage, stomatitis, gastritis, eructation
Rare:	Colitis, gastroduodenal ulcer, oesophagitis
Very rare:	Gastrointestinal perforation

Gastrointestinal haemorrhage, ulceration or perforation may sometimes be severe and potentially fatal, especially in elderly (see section 4.4).

Hepatobiliary disorders

Uncommon:	Liver function disorder (e.g. raised transaminases or bilirubin)
Very rare:	Hepatitis

Skin and subcutaneous tissue disorders

Uncommon:	Angioedema, pruritus, rash
Rare:	Stevens-Johnson syndrome, toxic epidermal necrolysis, urticaria
Very rare:	Dermatitis bullous, erythema multiforme
Not known:	Photosensitivity reaction

Renal and urinary disorders

Uncommon:	Sodium and water retention, hyperkalaemia (see section 4.4. Special warnings and special precautions for use and section 4.5.), renal function test abnormal (increased serum creatinine and/or serum urea)
Very rare:	Acute renal failure in particular in patients with risk factors (see section 4.4.)

General disorders and administration site conditions

Uncommon:	Oedema including oedema of the lower limbs.

c) Information Characterising Individual Serious and/or Frequently Occurring Adverse Reactions

Very rare cases of agranulocytosis have been reported in patients treated with meloxicam and other potentially myelotoxic drugs (see section 4.5).

d) Adverse reactions which have not been observed yet in relation to the product, but which are generally accepted as being attributable to other compounds in the class

Organic renal injury probably resulting in acute renal failure: very rare cases of interstitial nephritis, acute tubular necrosis, nephrotic syndrome, and papillary necrosis have been reported (see section 4.4).

4.9 Overdose

Symptoms following acute NSAID overdose are usually limited to lethargy, drowsiness, nausea, vomiting and epigastric pain, which are generally reversible with supportive care. Gastrointestinal bleeding can occur. Severe poisoning may result in hypertension, acute renal failure, hepatic dysfunction, respiratory depression, coma, convulsions, cardiovascular collapse and cardiac arrest. Anaphylactoid reactions have been reported with therapeutic ingestion of NSAIDs and may occur following an overdose.

Patients should be managed with symptomatic and supportive care following an NSAID overdose. Accelerated removal of meloxicam by 4 g oral doses of cholestyramine given three times a day was demonstrated in a clinical trial.

5. PHARMACOLOGICAL PROPERTIES

5.1 Pharmacodynamic properties

Pharmacotherapeutic group: Non Steroidal Anti-Inflammatory agent, Oxicams

ATC Code: M01AC06

Meloxicam is a non-steroidal anti-inflammatory drug (NSAID) of the oxicam family, with anti-inflammatory, analgesic and antipyretic properties.

The anti-inflammatory activity of meloxicam has been proven in classical models of inflammation. As with other NSAIDs, its precise mechanism of action remains unknown. However, there is at least one common mode of action shared by all NSAIDs (including Meloxicam): inhibition of the biosynthesis of prostaglandins, known inflammation mediators.

5.2 Pharmacokinetic properties

Absorption

Meloxicam is well absorbed from the gastrointestinal tract, which is reflected by a high absolute bioavailability of 89% following oral administration (capsule). Tablets, oral suspension and capsules were shown to be bioequivalent.

Following single dose administration of meloxicam, mean maximum plasma concentrations are achieved within 2 hours for the suspension and within 5-6 hours with solid oral dosage forms (capsules and tablets).

With multiple dosing, steady state conditions were reached within 3 to 5 days. Once daily dosing leads to drug plasma concentrations with a relatively small peak-trough fluctuation in the range of 0.4 - 1.0 μg/mL for 7.5 mg doses and 0.8 - 2.0 μg/mL for 15 mg doses, respectively (C_{min} and C_{max} at steady state, respectively). Maximum plasma concentrations of meloxicam at steady state are achieved within five to six hours for the tablet, capsule and the oral suspension, respectively. Extent of absorption for meloxicam following oral administration is not altered by concomitant food intake.

Distribution

Meloxicam is very strongly bound to plasma proteins, essentially albumin (99%). Meloxicam penetrates into synovial fluid to give concentrations approximately half of those in plasma.

Volume of distribution is low, on average 11 L. Interindividual variation is the order of 30-40%.

Biotransformation

Meloxicam undergoes extensive hepatic biotransformation. Four different metabolites of meloxicam were identified in urine, which are all pharmacodynamically inactive. The major metabolite, 5'-carboxymeloxicam (60% of dose), is formed by oxidation of an intermediate metabolite 5'- hydroxymethylmeloxicam, which is also excreted to a lesser extent (9% of dose). In vitro studies suggest that CYP 2C9 plays an important role in this metabolic pathway, with a minor contribution from the CYP 3A4 isoenzyme. The patient's peroxidase activity is probably responsible for the other two metabolites, which account for 16% and 4% of the administered dose respectively.

Elimination

Meloxicam is excreted predominantly in the form of metabolites and occurs to equal extents in urine and faeces. Less than 5% of the daily dose is excreted unchanged in faeces, while only traces of the parent compound are excreted in urine.

The mean elimination half-life is about 20 hours. Total plasma clearance amounts on average 8 mL/min.

Linearity/non-linearity

Meloxicam demonstrates linear pharmacokinetics in the therapeutic dose range of 7.5 mg 15 mg following per oral or intramuscular administration.

Special populations

Hepatic/renal Insufficiency:

Neither hepatic, nor mild to moderate renal insufficiencies have a substantial effect on meloxicam pharmacokinetics. In terminal renal failure, the increase in the volume of distribution may result in higher free meloxicam concentrations, and a daily dose of 7.5 mg must not be exceeded (see section 4.2).

Elderly:

Mean plasma clearance at steady state in elderly subjects was slightly lower than that reported for younger subjects.

5.3 Preclinical safety data

The toxicological profile of meloxicam has been found in preclinical studies to be identical to that of NSAIDs: gastrointestinal ulcers and erosions, renal papillary necrosis at high doses during chronic administration in two animal species.

Oral reproductive studies in the rat have shown a decrease of ovulations and inhibition of implantations and embryotoxic effects (increase of resorptions) at maternotoxic dose levels at 1mg/kg and higher. Studies of toxicity on reproduction in rats and rabbits did not reveal teratogenicity up to oral doses of 4 mg/kg in rats and 80 mg/kg in rabbits.

The affected dose levels exceeded the clinical dose (7.5-15 mg) by a factor of 10 to 5-fold on a mg/kg dose basis (75 kg person). Fetotoxic effects at the end of gestation, shared by all prostaglandin synthesis inhibitors, have been described. No evidence has been found of any mutagenic effect, either in vitro or in vivo. No carcinogenic risk has been found in the rat and mouse at doses far higher than those used clinically.

6. PHARMACEUTICAL PARTICULARS

6.1 List of excipients

Sodium citrate, lactose monohydrate, microcrystalline cellulose, povidone, anhydrous colloidal silica, crospovidone, magnesium stearate.

6.2 Incompatibilities

Not applicable

6.3 Shelf life

3 years

6.4 Special precautions for storage

Store in the original package, in order to protect from moisture.

6.5 Nature and contents of container

PVC/PVDC/Aluminium blister, boxes of 1, 2, 7, 10, 14, 15, 20, 28, 30, 50, 60, 100, 140, 280, 300, 500, 1,000 tablets.

Not all pack sizes may be marketed.

6.6 Special precautions for disposal and other handling

No special requirements

Any unused product or waste material should be disposed of in accordance with local requirements.

7. MARKETING AUTHORISATION HOLDER

Boehringer Ingelheim International GmbH

D-55216 Ingelheim am Rhein

Germany

8. MARKETING AUTHORISATION NUMBER(S)

PL 14598/0003

9. DATE OF FIRST AUTHORISATION/RENEWAL OF THE AUTHORISATION

30/09/2005

10. DATE OF REVISION OF THE TEXT

30/04/2009

LEGAL CATEGORY

POM

Modecate Concentrate Injection 100mg/ml

(sanofi-aventis)

1. NAME OF THE MEDICINAL PRODUCT

Modecate Concentrate Injection 100mg/ml.

2. QUALITATIVE AND QUANTITATIVE COMPOSITION

The product contains Fluphenazine Decanoate BP 100mg/ml.

3. PHARMACEUTICAL FORM

Intramuscular injection for administration to human beings.

4. CLINICAL PARTICULARS

4.1 Therapeutic indications

For the treatment and maintenance of schizophrenic patients and those with paranoid psychoses.

While Modecate concentrate injection has been shown to be effective in acute states, it is particularly useful in the maintenance treatment of chronic patients who are unreliable at taking their oral medication, and also of those who do not absorb their oral phenothiazine adequately.

4.2 Posology and method of administration

Dosage and Administration

Adults

It is recommended that patients be stabilised on the injection in hospital.

Recommended dosage regimes for all indications:

A. Patients without previous exposure to a depot fluphenazine formulation:

Initially 0.125ml ie. 12.5mg (0.0625ml ie 6.25mg for patients over 60) by deep intramuscular injection into the gluteal region.

The onset of action generally appears between 24 and 72 hours after injection and the effects of the drug on psychotic symptoms become significant within 48 to 96 hours. Subsequent injections and the dosage interval are determined in accordance with the patient's response. When administered as maintenance therapy, a single injection may be effective in controlling schizophrenic symptoms for up to four weeks or longer.

It is desirable to maintain as much flexibility in the dose as possible to achieve the best therapeutic response with the least side-effects; most patients are successfully maintained within the dose range 0.125ml (12.5mg) to 1ml (100mg) given at a dose interval of 2 to 5 weeks.

Patients previously maintained on oral fluphenazine:

It is not possible to predict the equivalent dose of depot formulation in view of the wide variability of individual response.

B. Patients previously maintained on depot fluphenazine:

Patients who have suffered a relapse following cessation of depot fluphenazine therapy may be restarted on the same dose (as they were receiving formerly), although the frequency of injections may need to be increased in the early weeks of treatment until satisfactory control is obtained.

Elderly:

Elderly patients may be particularly susceptible to extra-pyramidal reactions. Therefore reduced maintenance dosage may be required and a smaller initial dose (See above).

Children:

Not recommended for children.

*Where a very small volume/low concentration of fluphenazine is required patients may be transferred to the equivalent dose of Modecate Injection 25mg/ml on the basis that 1ml Modecate Concentrate (100mg/ml) is equivalent to 4ml Modecate Injection.

Note

The dosage should not be increased without close supervision and it should be noted that there is a variability in individual response.

The response to antipsychotic drug treatment may be delayed. If drugs are withdrawn, recurrence of symptoms may not become apparent for several weeks or months.

Route of administration: Intramuscular.

4.3 Contraindications

The product is contraindicated in the following cases:

Comatose states

Marked cerebral atherosclerosis

Phaeochromocytoma

Renal failure

Liver failure

Severe cardiac insufficiency

Severely depressed states

Existing blood dyscrasias

History of hypersensitivity to any of the ingredients

4.4 Special warnings and precautions for use

Caution should be exercised with the following:

Liver disease

Renal impairment

Cardiac arrhythmias, cardiac disease

Thyrotoxicosis

Severe respiratory disease

Epilepsy, conditions predisposing to epilepsy (eg. alcohol withdrawal or brain damage)

Parkinson's disease

Patients who have shown hypersensitivity to other phenothiazines

Personal or family history of narrow angle glaucoma

In very hot weather

The elderly, particularly if frail or at risk of hypothermia

Hypothyroidism

Myasthenia gravis

Prostatic hypertrophy

Patients with known or with a family history of cardiovascular disease should receive ECG screening, and monitoring and correction of electrolyte balance prior to treatment with fluphenazine.

Acute withdrawal symptoms, including nausea, vomiting, sweating and insomnia have been described after abrupt cessation of antipsychotic drugs. Recurrence of psychotic symptoms may also occur, and the emergence of involuntary movement disorders (such as akathisia, dystonia and dyskinesia) has been reported. Therefore, gradual withdrawal is advisable.

Psychotic patients on large doses of phenothiazines who are undergoing surgery should be watched carefully for hypotension. Reduced amounts of anaesthetics or central nervous system depressants may be necessary.

Fluphenazine should be used with caution in patients exposed to organophosphorus insecticides

Neuroleptic drugs elevate prolactin levels, and an increase in mammary neoplasms has been found in rodents after chronic administration. However, studies to date have not shown an association between chronic administration of these drugs and human mammary tumours.

As with any phenothiazine, the physician should be alert to the possibility of "silent pneumonias" in patients receiving long-term fluphenazine.

4.5 Interaction with other medicinal products and other forms of interaction

The possibility should be borne in mind that phenothiazines may:

1. Increase the central nervous system depression produced by drugs such as alcohol, general anaesthetics, hypnotics, sedatives or strong analgesics.

2. Antagonise the action of adrenaline and other sympathomimetic agents and reverse the blood-pressure lowering effects of adrenergic-blocking agents such as guanethidine and clonidine.

3. Impair: the anti-parkinsonian effect of L-dopa; the effect of anti-convulsants; metabolism of tricyclic antidepressants; the control of diabetes.

4. Increase the effect of anticoagulants and antidepressants.

5. Interact with lithium.

Anticholinergic effects may be enhanced by anti-parkinsonian or other anticholinergic drugs.

Phenothiazines may enhance: the absorption of corticosteroids, digoxin, and neuromuscular blocking agents. Fluphenazine is metabolised by P450 2D6 and is itself an inhibitor of this drug metabolising enzyme. The plasma concentrations and the effects of fluphenazine may therefore be increased and prolonged by drugs that are either the substrates or inhibitors of this P450 isoform, possibly resulting in severe hypotension, cardiac arrhythmias or CNS side effects. Examples of drugs which are substrates or inhibitors of cytochrome P450 2D6 include anti-arrhythmics, certain antidepressants including SSRIs and tricyclics, certain antipsychotics, β-blockers, protease inhibitors, opiates, cimetidine and ecstasy (MDMA). This list is not exhaustive.

Concomitant use of barbiturates with phenothiazines may result in reduced serum levels of both drugs, and an increased response if one of the drugs is withdrawn.

The effect of fluphenazine on the QT interval is likely to be potentiated by concurrent use of other drugs that also prolong the QT interval. Therefore, concurrent use of these drugs and fluphenazine is contraindicated. Examples include certain anti-arrhythmics, such as those of Class 1A (such as quinidine, disopyramide and procainamide) and Class III (such as amiodarone and sotalol), tricyclic antidepressants (such as amitriptyline); certain tetracyclic antidepressants (such as maprotiline); certain antipsychotic medications (such as phenothiazines and pimozide); certain antihistamines (such as terfenadine); lithium, quinine, pentamidine and sparfloxacin. This list is not exhaustive.

Electrolyte imbalance, particularly hypokalaemia, greatly increases the risk of QT interval prolongation. Therefore, concurrent use of drugs that cause electrolyte imbalance should be avoided.

Concurrent use of MAO inhibitors may increase sedation, constipation, dry mouth and hypotension.

Owing to their adrenolytic action, phenothiazines may reduce the pressor effect of adrenergic vasoconstrictors (i.e. ephedrine, phenylephrine).

Phenylpropanolamine has been reported to interact with phenothiazines and cause ventricular arrhythmias.

Concurrent use of phenothiazines and ACE inhibitors or angiotensin II antagonists may result in severe postural hypotension.

Concurrent use of thiazide diuretics may cause hypotension. Diuretic-induced hypokalaemia may potentiate phenothiazine-induced cardiotoxicity.

Clonidine may decrease the antipsychotic activity of phenothiazines.

Methyldopa increases the risk of extrapyramidal side effects with phenothiazines.

The hypotensive effect of calcium channel blockers is enhanced by concurrent use of antipsychotic drugs.

Phenothiazines may predispose to metrizamide-induced seizures.

Concurrent use of phenothiazines and amfetamine/anorectic agents may produce antagonistic pharmacological effects.

Concurrent use of phenothiazines and cocaine may increase the risk of acute dystonia.

There have been rare reports of acute Parkinsonism when an SSRI has been used in combination with a phenothiazine.

Phenothiazines may impair the action of anti-convulsants. Serum levels of phenytoin may be increased or decreased.

Phenothiazines inhibit glucose uptake into cells, and hence may affect the interpretation of PET studies using labelled glucose.

4.6 Pregnancy and lactation

Use in pregnancy: The safety for the use of this drug during pregnancy has not been established; therefore, the possible hazards should be weighed against the potential benefits when administering this drug to pregnant patients.

Nursing mothers: Breast feeding is not recommended during treatment with depot fluphenazines, owing to the possibility that fluphenazine is excreted in the breast milk.

4.7 Effects on ability to drive and use machines

The use of this drug may impair the mental and physical abilities required for driving a car or operating heavy machinery.

4.8 Undesirable effects

Side effects: Acute dystonic reactions occur infrequently, as a rule within the first 24-48 hours, although delayed reactions may occur. In susceptible individuals they may occur after only small doses. These may include such dramatic manifestations as oculogyric crises and opisthotonos. They are rapidly relieved by intravenous administration of an anti-parkinsonian agent such as procyclidine.

Parkinsonian-like states may occur particularly between the second and fifth days after each injection, but often decrease with subsequent injection. These reactions may be reduced by using smaller doses more frequently, or by the concomitant use of anti-parkinsonian drugs such as trihexyphenidyl, benzatropine or procyclidine. Anti-parkinsonian drugs should not be prescribed routinely, because of the possible risks of aggravating anti-cholinergic side effects or precipitating toxic confusional states, or of impairing therapeutic efficacy.

With careful monitoring of the dose the number of patients requiring anti-parkinsonian drugs can be minimised.

Tardive Dyskinesia: As with all antipsychotic agents, tardive dyskinesia may appear in some patients on long term therapy or may occur after drug therapy has been discontinued. The risk seems to be greater in elderly patients on high dose therapy, especially females. The symptoms are persistent and in some patients appear to be irreversible.

The syndrome is characterised by rhythmical involuntary movements of the tongue, face, mouth or jaw (eg. protrusion of tongue, puffing of cheeks, puckering of mouth, chewing movements). Sometimes these may be accompanied by involuntary movements of the extremities. There is no known effective treatment for tardive dyskinesia: anti-parkinsonian agents usually do not alleviate the symptoms of this syndrome. It is suggested that all antipsychotic agents be discontinued if these symptoms appear. Should it be necessary to reinstitute treatment, or increase the dosage of the agent, or switch to a different antipsychotic agent, the syndrome may be masked. It has been reported that fine vermicular movements of the tongue may be an early sign of the syndrome and if the medication is stopped at that time, the syndrome may not develop.

Other Undesirable Effects: As with other phenothiazines, drowsiness, lethargy, blurred vision, dryness of the mouth, constipation, urinary hesitancy or incontinence, mild hypotension, impairment of judgement and mental skills, and epileptiform attacks are occasionally seen.

Headache, nasal congestion, vomiting, agitation, excitement and insomnia, and hyponatraemia have also been observed during phenothiazine therapy.

Blood dyscrasias have rarely been reported with phenothiazine derivatives. Blood counts should be performed if the patient develops signs of persistent infection. Transient leucopenia and thrombocytopenia have been reported. Antinuclear antibodies and SLE have been reported very rarely.

Jaundice has rarely been reported. Transient abnormalities of liver function tests may occur in the absence of jaundice.

A transient rise in serum cholesterol has been reported rarely in patients on oral fluphenazine.

Abnormal skin pigmentation and lens opacities have sometimes been seen following long-term administration of high doses of phenothiazines.

Phenothiazines are known to cause photosensitivity reactions but this has not been reported for fluphenazine. Skin rashes, hypersensitivity and anaphylactic reactions have occasionally been reported.

Elderly patients may be more susceptible to the sedative and hypotensive effects.

The effects of phenothiazines on the heart are dose-related. ECG changes with prolongation of the QT interval and T-Wave changes have been reported commonly in patients treated with moderate to high dosage; they have been reported to precede serious arrhythmias, including ventricular tachycardia and fibrillation, which have also occurred after overdosage. Sudden, unexpected and unexplained deaths have been reported in hospitalised psychotic patients receiving phenothiazines.

Phenothiazines may impair body temperature regulation. Elderly or hypothyroid patients may be particularly susceptible to hypothermia. The hazard of hyperpyrexia may be increased by especially hot or humid weather, or by drugs such as anti-parkinsonian agents, which impair sweating.

Rare occurrences of neuroleptic malignant syndrome (NMS) have been reported in patients on neuroleptic therapy. The syndrome is characterised by hyperthermia, together with some or all of the following: muscular rigidity, autonomic instability (labile blood pressure, tachycardia, diaphoresis), akinesia, and altered consciousness, sometimes progressing to stupor or coma. Leucocytosis, elevated CPK, liver function abnormalities, and acute renal failure may also occur. Neuroleptic therapy should be discontinued immediately and vigorous symptomatic treatment implemented since the syndrome is potentially fatal.

Hormonal effects of phenothiazines include hyperprolactinaemia, which may cause galactorrhoea, gynaecomastia and oligomenorrhoea or amenorrhoea. Sexual function may be impaired, and false results may be observed with pregnancy tests. Syndrome of inappropriate anti-diuretic hormone secretion has also been observed.

Oedema has been reported with phenothiazine medication.

4.9 Overdose

Overdosage should be treated symptomatically and supportively, extrapyramidal reactions will respond to oral or parenteral anti-parkinsonian drugs such as procyclidine or benzatropine. In cases of severe hypotension, all procedures for the management of circulatory shock should be instituted, eg. vasoconstrictors and/or intravenous fluids. However, only the vasoconstrictors metaraminol or noradrenaline should be used, as adrenaline may further lower the blood pressure through interaction with the phenothiazine.

5. PHARMACOLOGICAL PROPERTIES

5.1 Pharmacodynamic properties

Fluphenazine decanoate is an ester of the potent neuroleptic fluphenazine, a phenothiazine derivative of the piperazine type. The ester is slowly absorbed from the intramuscular site of injection and is then hydrolysed in the plasma to the active therapeutic agent, fluphenazine.

Extrapyramidal reactions are not uncommon, but fluphenazine does not have marked sedative or hypotensive properties.

5.2 Pharmacokinetic properties

Plasma level profiles of fluphenazine following intramuscular injection have shown half-lives of plasma clearance ranging from 2.5 - 16 weeks, emphasising the importance of adjusting dose and interval to the individual requirements of each patient. The slow decline of plasma levels in most patients means that a reasonably stable plasma level can usually be achieved with injections spaced at 2 - 4 week intervals.

5.3 Preclinical safety data

Not applicable.

6. PHARMACEUTICAL PARTICULARS

6.1 List of excipients

Benzyl alcohol and sesame oil.

6.2 Incompatibilities

None.

6.3 Shelf life

2 years.

6.4 Special precautions for storage

Store below 25°C. Protect from direct sunlight.

6.5 Nature and contents of container

Clear type I glass ampoules containing 0.5ml (packs of 10) and 1ml

(packs of 5).

6.6 Special precautions for disposal and other handling

For intramuscular administration only.

7. MARKETING AUTHORISATION HOLDER

Sanofi-aventis

One Onslow Street

Guildford

Surrey

GU1 4YS

8. MARKETING AUTHORISATION NUMBER(S)

PL 04425/0575

9. DATE OF FIRST AUTHORISATION/RENEWAL OF THE AUTHORISATION

9 March 2009

10. DATE OF REVISION OF THE TEXT

9 March 2009

LEGAL CATEGORY

POM

Modecate Injection 25mg/ml

(sanofi-aventis)

1. NAME OF THE MEDICINAL PRODUCT

Modecate Injection 25mg/ml.

2. QUALITATIVE AND QUANTITATIVE COMPOSITION

The product contains Fluphenazine Decanoate BP 25mg/ml.

3. PHARMACEUTICAL FORM

Intramuscular injection for administration to human beings.

4. CLINICAL PARTICULARS

4.1 Therapeutic indications

For the treatment and maintenance of schizophrenic patients and those with paranoid psychoses.

While Modecate injection has been shown to be effective in acute states, it is particularly useful in the maintenance treatment of chronic patients who are unreliable at taking their oral medication, and also of those who do not absorb their oral phenothiazine adequately.

4.2 Posology and method of administration

Dosage and Administration

Adults

It is recommended that patients be stabilised on the injection in hospital.

Recommended dosage regimes for all indications:

A. Patients without previous exposure to a depot fluphenazine formulation:

Initially 0.5ml ie 12.5mg (0.25 ml ie 6.25mg for patients over 60) by deep intramuscular injection into the gluteal region.

The onset of action generally appears between 24 and 72 hours after injection and the effects of the drug on psychotic symptoms become significant within 48 to 96 hours. Subsequent injections and the dosage interval are determined in accordance with the patient's response. When administered as maintenance therapy, a single injection may be effective in controlling schizophrenic symptoms for up to four weeks or longer.

It is desirable to maintain as much flexibility in the dose as possible to achieve the best therapeutic response with the least side-effects; most patients are successfully maintained within the dose range 0.5ml (12.5mg) to 4.0ml (100mg) given at a dose interval of 2 to 5 weeks.

Patients previously maintained on oral fluphenazine:

It is not possible to predict the equivalent dose of depot formulation in view of the wide variability of individual response.

B. Patients previously maintained on depot fluphenazine:

Patients who have suffered a relapse following cessation of depot fluphenazine therapy may be restarted on the same dose, although the frequency of injections may need to be increased in the early weeks of treatment until satisfactory control is obtained.

Elderly:

Elderly patients may be particularly susceptible to extrapyramidal reactions, sedative and hypotensive effects. In order to avoid this, a reduced maintenance dosage may be required and a smaller initial dose (see above).

Children:

Not recommended for children.

* Where a smaller volume of injection is desirable, patients may be transferred directly to the equivalent dose of Modecate Concentrate injection on the basis that 1ml Modecate Concentrate injection is equivalent to 4ml Modecate injection.

Note:

The dosage should not be increased without close supervision and it should be noted that there is a variability in individual response.

The response to antipsychotic drug treatment may be delayed. If drugs are withdrawn, recurrence of symptoms may not become apparent for several weeks or months.

Route of administration: Intramuscular.

4.3 Contraindications

The product is contraindicated in the following cases.

Comatose states

Marked cerebral atherosclerosis

Phaeochromocytoma

Renal failure

Liver failure

Severe cardiac insufficiency

Severely depressed states

Existing blood dyscrasias

History of hypersensitivity to any of the ingredients.

4.4 Special warnings and precautions for use

Caution should be exercised with the following:

Liver disease

Renal impairment

Cardiac arrhythmias, cardiac disease

Thyrotoxicosis

Severe respiratory disease

Epilepsy, conditions predisposing to epilepsy (eg. alcohol withdrawal or brain damage)

Parkinson's disease

Patients who have shown hypersensitivity to other phenothiazines

Personal or family history of narrow angle glaucoma

In very hot weather

The elderly, particularly if frail or at risk of hypothermia

Hypothyroidism

Myasthenia gravis

Prostatic hypertrophy.

Patients with known or with a family history of cardiovascular disease should receive ECG screening, and monitoring and correction of electrolyte balance prior to treatment with fluphenazine.

Acute withdrawal symptoms, including nausea, vomiting, sweating and insomnia have been described after abrupt cessation of antipsychotic drugs. Recurrence of psychotic symptoms may also occur, and the emergence of involuntary movement disorders (such as akathisia, dystonia and dyskinesia) has been reported. Therefore, gradual withdrawal is advisable.

Psychotic patients on large doses of phenothiazines who are undergoing surgery should be watched carefully for hypotension. Reduced amounts of anaesthetics or central nervous system depressants may be necessary.

Fluphenazine should be used with caution in patients exposed to organophosphorus insecticides

Neuroleptic drugs elevate prolactin levels, and an increase in mammary neoplasms has been found in rodents after chronic administration. However, studies to date have not shown an association between chronic administration of these drugs and human mammary tumours.

As with any phenothiazine, the physician should be alert to the possibility of "silent pneumonias" in patients receiving long-term fluphenazine.

4.5 Interaction with other medicinal products and other forms of interaction

The possibility should be borne in mind that phenothiazines may:

1 Increase the central nervous system depression produced by drugs such as alcohol, general anaesthetics, hypnotics, sedatives or strong analgesics.

2 Antagonise the action of adrenaline and other sympathomimetic agents and reverse the blood-pressure lowering effects of adrenergic-blocking agents such as guanethidine and clonidine.

3 Impair: the anti-parkinsonian effect of L-dopa; the effect of anti-convulsants; metabolism of tricyclic antidepressants; the control of diabetes.

4 Increase the effect of anticoagulants and antidepressants.

5 Interact with lithium.

Anticholinergic effects may be enhanced by anti-parkinsonian or other anticholinergic drugs.

Phenothiazines may enhance: the absorption of corticosteroids, digoxin, and neuromuscular blocking agents.

Fluphenazine is metabolised by P450 2D6 and is itself an inhibitor of this drug metabolising enzyme. The plasma concentrations and the effects of fluphenazine may therefore be increased and prolonged by drugs that are either the substrates or inhibitors of this P450 isoform, possibly resulting in severe hypotension, cardiac arrhythmias or CNS side effects. Examples of drugs which are substrates or inhibitors of cytochrome P450 2D6 include anti-arrhythmics, certain antidepressants including SSRIs and tricyclics, certain antipsychotics, β-blockers, protease inhibitors, opiates, cimetidine and ecstasy (MDMA). This list is not exhaustive.

Concomitant use of barbiturates with phenothiazines may result in reduced serum levels of both drugs, and an increased response if one of the drugs is withdrawn.

The effect of fluphenazine on the QT interval is likely to be potentiated by concurrent use of other drugs that also prolong the QT interval. Therefore, concurrent use of these drugs and fluphenazine is contraindicated. Examples include certain anti-arrhythmics, such as those of Class 1A (such as quinidine, disopyramide and procainamide) and Class III (such as amiodarone and sotalol), tricyclic antidepressants (such as amitriptyline); certain tetracyclic antidepressants (such as maprotiline); certain antipsychotic medications (such as phenothiazines and pimozide); certain antihistamines (such as terfenadine); lithium, quinine, pentamidine and sparfloxacin. This list is not exhaustive.

Electrolyte imbalance, particularly hypokalaemia, greatly increases the risk of QT interval prolongation. Therefore, concurrent use of drugs that cause electrolyte imbalance should be avoided.

Concurrent use of MAO inhibitors may increase sedation, constipation, dry mouth and hypotension.

Owing to their adrenolytic action, phenothiazines may reduce the pressor effect of adrenergic vasoconstrictors (i.e. ephedrine, phenylephrine).

Phenylpropanolamine has been reported to interact with phenothiazines and cause ventricular arrhythmias.

Concurrent use of phenothiazines and ACE inhibitors or angiotensin II antagonists may result in severe postural hypotension.

Concurrent use of thiazide diuretics may cause hypotension. Diuretic-induced hypokalaemia may potentiate phenothiazine-induced cardiotoxicity.

Clonidine may decrease the antipsychotic activity of phenothiazines.

Methyldopa increases the risk of extrapyramidal side effects with phenothiazines.

The hypotensive effect of calcium channel blockers is enhanced by concurrent use of antipsychotic drugs.

Phenothiazines may predispose to metrizamide-induced seizures.

Concurrent use of phenothiazines and amfetamine/anorectic agents may produce antagonistic pharmacological effects.

Concurrent use of phenothiazines and cocaine may increase the risk of acute dystonia.

There have been rare reports of acute Parkinsonism when an SSRI has been used in combination with a phenothiazine.

Phenothiazines may impair the action of anti-convulsants. Serum levels of phenytoin may be increased or decreased.

Phenothiazines inhibit glucose uptake into cells, and hence may affect the interpretation of PET studies using labelled glucose.

4.6 Pregnancy and lactation

Use in pregnancy: The safety for the use of this drug during pregnancy has not been established; therefore, the possible hazards should be weighed against the potential benefits when administering this drug to pregnant patients.

Nursing mothers: Breast feeding is not recommended during treatment with depot fluphenazines, owing to the possibility that fluphenazine may be excreted in the breast milk.

4.7 Effects on ability to drive and use machines

The use of this drug may impair the mental and physical abilities required for driving a car or operating heavy machinery.

4.8 Undesirable effects

Side Effects: Acute dystonic reactions occur infrequently, as a rule within the first 24-48 hours, although delayed reactions may occur. In susceptible individuals they may occur after only small doses. These may include such dramatic manifestations as oculogyric crises and opisthotonos. They are rapidly relieved by intravenous administration of an anti-parkinsonian agent such as procyclidine.

Parkinsonian-like states may occur particularly between the second and fifth days after each injection, but often decrease with subsequent injection. These reactions may be reduced by using smaller doses more frequently, or by the concomitant use of anti-parkinsonian drugs such as trihexyphenidyl, benzatropine or procyclidine. Anti-parkinsonian drugs should not be prescribed routinely, because of the possible risks of aggravating anti-cholinergic side effects or precipitating toxic confusional states, or of impairing therapeutic efficacy.

With careful monitoring of the dose the number of patients requiring anti-parkinsonian drugs can be minimised.

Tardive Dyskinesia: As with all antipsychotic agents, tardive dyskinesia may appear in some patients on long term therapy or may occur after drug therapy has been discontinued. The risk seems to be greater in elderly patients on high dose therapy, especially females. The symptoms are persistent and in some patients appear to be irreversible.

The syndrome is characterised by rhythmical involuntary movements of the tongue, face, mouth or jaw (eg protrusion of tongue, puffing of cheeks, puckering of mouth, chewing movements). Sometimes these may be accompanied by involuntary movements of the extremities. There is no known effective treatment for tardive dyskinesia: anti-parkinsonian agents usually do not alleviate the symptoms of this syndrome. It is suggested that all antipsychotic agents be discontinued if these symptoms appear. Should it be necessary to reinstitute treatment, or increase the dosage of the agent, or switch to a different antipsychotic agent, the syndrome may be masked. It has been reported that fine vermicular movements of the tongue may be an early sign of the syndrome and if the medication is stopped at that time, the syndrome may not develop.

Other Undesirable Effects: As with other phenothiazines, drowsiness, lethargy, blurred vision, dryness of the mouth, constipation, urinary hesitancy or incontinence, mild hypotension, impairment of judgement and mental skills, and epileptiform attacks are occasionally seen.

Headache, nasal congestion, vomiting, agitation, excitement, insomnia and hyponatraemia have also been observed during phenothiazine therapy.

Blood dyscrasias have rarely been reported with phenothiazine derivatives. Blood counts should be performed if the patient develops signs of persistent infection. Transient leucopenia and thrombocytopenia have been reported. Antinuclear antibodies and SLE have been reported very rarely.

Jaundice has rarely been reported. Transient abnormalities of liver function tests may occur in the absence of jaundice.

A transient rise in serum cholesterol has been reported rarely in patients on oral fluphenazine.

Abnormal skin pigmentation and lens opacities have sometimes been seen following long-term administration of high doses of phenothiazines.

Phenothiazines are known to cause photosensitivity reactions but this has not been reported for fluphenazine. Skin rashes, hypersensitivity and anaphylactic reactions have occasionally been reported.

Elderly patients may be more susceptible to the sedative and hypotensive effects.

The effects of phenothiazines on the heart are dose-related. ECG changes with prolongation of the QT interval and T-Wave changes have been reported commonly in patients treated with moderate to high dosage; they have been reported to precede serious arrhythmias, including ventricular tachycardia and fibrillation, which have also occurred after overdosage. Sudden, unexpected and unexplained deaths have been reported in hospitalised psychotic patients receiving phenothiazines.

Phenothiazines may impair body temperature regulation. Elderly or hypothyroid patients may be particularly susceptible to hypothermia. The hazard of hyperpyrexia may be increased by especially hot or humid weather, or by drugs such as anti-parkinsonian agents, which impair sweating.

Rare occurrences of neuroleptic malignant syndrome (NMS) have been reported in patients on neuroleptic therapy. The syndrome is characterised by hyperthermia, together with some or all of the following: muscular rigidity, autonomic instability (labile blood pressure, tachycardia, diaphoresis), akinesia, and altered consciousness, sometimes progressing to stupor or coma. Leucocytosis, elevated CPK, liver function abnormalities, and acute renal failure may also occur. Neuroleptic therapy should be discontinued immediately and vigorous symptomatic treatment implemented since the syndrome is potentially fatal.

Hormonal effects of phenothiazines include hyperprolactinaemia, which may cause galactorrhoea, gynaecomastia and oligomenorrhoea or amenorrhoea. Sexual function may be impaired, and false results may be observed with pregnancy tests. Syndrome of inappropriate anti-diuretic hormone secretion has also been observed.

Oedema has been reported with phenothiazine medication.

4.9 Overdose

Overdosage should be treated symptomatically and supportively, extrapyramidal reactions will respond to oral or parenteral anti-parkinsonian drugs such as procyclidine or benzatropine. In cases of severe hypotension, all procedures for the management of circulatory shock should be instituted, eg vasoconstrictors and/or intravenous fluids. However, only the vasoconstrictors metaraminol or noradrenaline should be used, as adrenaline may further lower the blood pressure through interaction with the phenothiazine.

5. PHARMACOLOGICAL PROPERTIES

5.1 Pharmacodynamic properties

Fluphenazine decanoate is an ester of the potent neuroleptic fluphenazine, a phenothiazine derivative of the piperazine type. The ester is slowly absorbed from the intramuscular site of injection and is then hydrolysed in the plasma to the active therapeutic agent, fluphenazine.

Extrapyramidal reactions are not uncommon, but fluphenazine does not have marked sedative or hypotensive properties.

5.2 Pharmacokinetic properties

Plasma level profiles of fluphenazine following intramuscular injection have shown half-lives of plasma clearance ranging from 2.5-16 weeks, emphasising the importance of adjusting dose and interval to the individual requirements of each patient. The slow decline of plasma levels in most patients means that a reasonably stable plasma level can usually be achieved with injections spaced at 2-4 week intervals.

5.3 Preclinical safety data

Not applicable.

6. PHARMACEUTICAL PARTICULARS

6.1 List of excipients

Benzyl alcohol and sesame oil.

6.2 Incompatibilities

None.

6.3 Shelf life

2 years.

The in use shelf life for the 10ml vial is 28 days

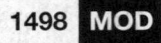

6.4 Special precautions for storage
Store below 25°C. Protect from direct sunlight.

6.5 Nature and contents of container
Type I Glass ampoules containing 0.5, 1 and 2ml.

6.6 Special precautions for disposal and other handling
For intramuscular administration only.

7. MARKETING AUTHORISATION HOLDER
Sanofi-aventis
One Onslow Street
Guildford
Surrey
GU1 4YS
UK

8. MARKETING AUTHORISATION NUMBER(S)
PL 04425/0386

9. DATE OF FIRST AUTHORISATION/RENEWAL OF THE AUTHORISATION
19 March 2009

10. DATE OF REVISION OF THE TEXT
19 March 2009

Legal category: POM

Moduret 25

(Merck Sharp & Dohme Limited)

1. NAME OF THE MEDICINAL PRODUCT
MODURET® 25

2. QUALITATIVE AND QUANTITATIVE COMPOSITION
Each tablet of Moduret 25 contains amiloride hydrochloride equivalent to 2.5 mg anhydrous amiloride hydrochloride and 25 mg hydrochlorothiazide.

3. PHARMACEUTICAL FORM
Off-white, diamond-shaped tablets, with a break-line and marked with identification number '923'.

4. CLINICAL PARTICULARS

4.1 Therapeutic indications
Potassium-conserving diuretic and anti-hypertensive for the treatment of patients with congestive heart failure, hypertension, or hepatic cirrhosis with ascites and oedema, in whom potassium depletion might be anticipated.

4.2 Posology and method of administration

Hypertension:

Initially one Moduret 25 tablet given once a day. If necessary increase to two Moduret 25 tablets given once a day or in divided doses.

Congestive heart failure:

Initially one tablet of Moduret 25 a day, subsequently adjusted if required, but not exceeding four Moduret 25 tablets a day. Optimal dosage is determined by the diuretic response and the plasma potassium level. Once an initial diuresis has been achieved, reduction in dosage may be attempted for maintenance therapy. Maintenance therapy may be on an intermittent basis.

Hepatic cirrhosis with ascites:

Initiate therapy with a low dose. A single daily dose of two Moduret 25 tablets may be increased gradually until there is an effective diuresis. Dosage should not exceed four Moduret 25 tablets a day. Maintenance dosages may be lower than those required to initiate diuresis; dosage reduction should therefore be attempted when the patient's weight is stabilised. A gradual weight reduction is especially desirable in cirrhotic patients to reduce the likelihood of untoward reactions associated with diuretic therapy.

Paediatric use:

Moduret 25 is not recommended for children. (See 4.3 'Contraindications').

Use in elderly:

Particular caution is needed in the elderly because of their susceptibility to electrolyte imbalance; the dosage should be carefully adjusted to renal function and clinical response.

4.3 Contraindications
Hyperkalaemia (plasma potassium over 5.5 mmol/l); other potassium-conserving diuretics. Potassium supplements or potassium-rich food (except in severe and/or refractory cases of hypokalaemia under careful monitoring); concomitant use with spironolactone or triamterene; anuria; acute renal failure, severe progressive renal disease, severe hepatic failure, precoma associated with hepatic cirrhosis, Addison's disease, hypercalcaemia, concurrent lithium therapy, diabetic nephropathy; patients with blood urea over 10 mmol/l, patients with diabetes mellitus, or those with serum creatinine over 130 μmol/l in whom serum electrolyte and blood urea levels cannot be monitored carefully and frequently. Prior hypersensitivity to amiloride hydrochloride, hydrochlorothiazide or other sulphonamide derived drugs. In renal impairment, use of a potassium - conserving agent may result in rapid development of hyperkalaemia. Because the safety of amiloride hydrochloride for use in children has not been established, Moduret 25 is not recommended for children. For 'Use in pregnancy' and 'Use in breast-feeding mothers', see 'Pregnancy and Lactation'.

4.4 Special warnings and precautions for use
Hyperkalaemia has been observed in patients receiving amiloride hydrochloride, either alone or with other diuretics, particularly in the aged or in hospital patients with hepatic cirrhosis or congestive heart failure with renal involvement, who were seriously ill, or were undergoing vigorous diuretic therapy. Such patients should be carefully observed for clinical, laboratory, and ECG evidence of hyperkalaemia (not always associated with an abnormal ECG).

Neither potassium supplements nor a potassium-rich diet should be used with Moduret 25 except under careful monitoring in severe and/or refractory cases of hypokalaemia.

Some deaths have been reported in this group of patients.

Treatment of hyperkalaemia: Should hyperkalaemia develop, discontinue treatment immediately and, if necessary, take active measures to reduce the plasma potassium to normal.

Impaired renal function: Renal function should be monitored because the use of Moduret 25 in impaired renal function may result in the rapid development of hyperkalaemia. Thiazide diuretics become ineffective when creatinine clearance falls below 30 ml/min.

Electrolyte imbalance: Although the likelihood of electrolyte imbalance is reduced by Moduret 25, careful check should be kept for such signs of fluid and electrolyte imbalance as hyponatraemia, hypochloraemic alkalosis, hypokalaemia and hypomagnesaemia.

It is particularly important to make serum and urine electrolyte determinations when the patient is vomiting excessively or receiving parenteral fluids. Warning signs or symptoms of fluid or electrolyte imbalance include: dryness of the mouth, weakness, lethargy, drowsiness, restlessness, seizures, confusion, muscle pains or cramps, muscular fatigue, hypotension, oliguria, tachycardia, and gastro-intestinal disturbances such as nausea and vomiting.

Hypokalaemia may develop, especially as a result of brisk diuresis, after prolonged therapy or when severe cirrhosis is present. Hypokalaemia can sensitise or exaggerate the response of the heart to the toxic effects of digitalis (e.g. increased ventricular irritability).

Diuretic-induced hyponatraemia is usually mild and asymptomatic. It may become severe and symptomatic in a few patients who will then require immediate attention and appropriate treatment.

Thiazides may decrease urinary calcium excretion. Thiazides may cause intermittent and slight elevation of serum calcium in the absence of known disorders of calcium metabolism. Therapy should be discontinued before carrying out tests for parathyroid function.

Uraemia may be precipitated or increased by hydrochlorothiazide. Cumulative effects of the drug may develop in patients with impaired renal function. If increasing uraemia and oliguria develop during treatment of renal disease, Moduret 25 should be discontinued.

Hepatic disease: Thiazides should be used with caution in patients with impaired hepatic function or progressive liver disease (see 4.3 'Contraindications'), since minor alterations of fluid and electrolyte balance may precipitate hepatic coma.

Metabolic: Hyperuricaemia may occur, or gout may be precipitated or aggravated, in certain patients receiving thiazides. Thiazides may impair glucose tolerance. Diabetes mellitus may be precipitated or aggravated by therapy with Moduret 25 (see 4.3 'Contraindications'). Dosage adjustment of antidiabetic agents, including insulin, may be required.

Increases in cholesterol and triglyceride levels may be associated with thiazide diuretic therapy.

To minimise the risk of hyperkalaemia in diabetic or suspected diabetic patients, the status of renal function should be determined before initiating therapy with Moduret 25. Therapy should be discontinued at least three days before giving a glucose tolerance test. Potassium-conserving therapy should be initiated only with caution in severely ill patients in whom metabolic or respiratory acidosis may occur, e.g. patients with cardiopulmonary disease or patients with inadequately controlled diabetes.

Shifts in acid-base balance alter the balance of extracellular/intracellular potassium, and the development of acidosis may be associated with rapid increases in plasma potassium.

Sensitivity reactions: The possibility that thiazides may activate or exacerbate systemic lupus erythematosus has been reported.

4.5 Interaction with other medicinal products and other forms of interaction
Lithium generally should not be given with diuretics. Diuretic agents reduce the renal clearance of lithium and add a high risk of lithium toxicity. Refer to the prescribing information for lithium preparations before use of such preparations.

Non-Steroidal Anti-Inflammatory Drugs: In some patients the administration of a non-sterdoidal anti-inflammatory agent can reduce the diuretic, natriuretic and antihypertensive effects of diuretics. Concomitant administration of non-steroidal anti-inflammatory drugs (NSAIDs) and potassium-sparing agents, including amiloride hydrochloride may cause hyperkalaemia and renal failure particularly in elderly patients. Therefore when amiloride hydrochloride is used concomitantly with NSAIDs, renal function and serum potassium levels should be carefully monitored.

Amiloride Hydrochloride

When amiloride hydrochloride is administered concomitantly with an ACE inhibitor, angiotensin II receptor antagonist, ciclosporin or tacrolimus the risk of hyperkalaemia may be increased. Therefore, if concomitant use of these agents is indicated because of demonstrated hypokalaemia, they should be used with caution and with frequent monitoring of serum potassium.

Hydrochlorothiazide

When given concurrently, the following drugs may interact with thiazide diuretics:

Alcohol, barbiturates or narcotics: Co-administration may potentiate orthostatic hypotension. **Oral and parenteral antidiabetic drugs** may require adjustment of dosage with concurrent use. Moduret 25 can act synergistically with chlorpropamide to increase the risk of hyponatraemia. **Other antihypertensive drugs** may have an additive effect. Therefore the dosage of these agents, especially adrenergic-blockers, may need to be reduced when Moduret 25 is added to the regimen. Diuretic therapy should, be discontinued for 2-3 days prior to initiation of therapy with an ACE inhibitor to reduce the likelihood of first dose hypotension. **Cholestyramine and colestipol resins**: absorption of hydrochlorothiazide is impaired in the presence of anionic exchange resins. Single doses of either cholestyramine or colestipol resins bind the hydrochlorothiazide and reduce its absorption from the gastrointestinal tract by up to 85 and 43 percent, respectively. When cholestyramine is given 4 hours after the hydrochlorothiazide, the absorption of hydrochlorothiazide is reduced by 30 to 35 percent. **Corticosteroids or ACTH** may intensify any thiazide-induced electrolyte depletion, particularly hypokalaemia. **Pressor-amines such as epinephrine (adrenaline)** may show decreased arterial responsiveness when used with Moduret 25 but this reaction is not enough to preclude their therapeutic usefulness. **Non-depolarising muscle relaxants such as tubocurarine** may possibly interact with Moduret 25 to increase muscle relaxation. **Drug/laboratory tests:** Because thiazides may affect calcium metabolism, Moduret 25 may interfere with tests for parathyroid function.

4.6 Pregnancy and lactation
Use in pregnancy: The routine use of diuretics in otherwise healthy pregnant women with or without mild oedema is not indicated, because they may be associated with hypovolaemia, increased blood viscosity, and decreased placental perfusion. Diuretics do not prevent the development of toxaemia of pregnancy and there is no satisfactory evidence that they are useful for its treatment.

Since thiazides cross the placental barrier and appear in cord blood, use where pregnancy is present or suspected requires that the benefits of the drug be weighed against possible hazards to the foetus. These hazards include foetal or neonatal jaundice, thrombocytopenia, bone marrow depression and possibly other side effects that have occurred in the adult.

Use in breast-feeding mothers: Although it is not known whether amiloride hydrochloride is excreted in human milk, it is known that thiazides do appear in breast milk. If use of the drug combination is deemed essential, the patient should stop breast-feeding.

4.7 Effects on ability to drive and use machines
Infrequently, patients may experience weakness, fatigue, dizziness, stupor and vertigo. Should any of these occur, the patient should be cautioned not to drive or operate machinery.

4.8 Undesirable effects
Although minor side effects are relatively common, significant side effects are infrequent.

Reported side effects are generally associated with diuresis, thiazide therapy, or with the underlying disease.

No increase in the risk of adverse reactions has been seen over those of the individual components.

The following side effects have been reported with Moduret 25:

Body as a whole: headache, weakness, fatigue, malaise, chest pain, back pain, syncope.

Cardiovascular: arrhythmias, tachycardia, digitalis toxicity, orthostatic hypotension, angina pectoris.

Digestive: anorexia, nausea, vomiting, diarrhoea, constipation, abdominal pain, GI bleeding, appetite changes, abdominal fullness, flatulence, thirst, hiccups.

Metabolic: elevated plasma potassium levels (above 5.5 mmol/l), electrolyte imbalance, hyponatraemia (see 4.4 'special warnings and precautions for use'), gout, dehydration, symptomatic hyponatraemia.

Integumentary: rash, pruritis, flushing, diaphoresis.

Musculoskeletal: leg ache, muscle cramps, joint pain.

Nervous: dizziness, vertigo, paraesthesiae, stupor.

Psychiatric: insomnia, nervousness, mental confusion, depression, sleepiness.

Respiratory: dyspnoea.

Special senses: bad taste, visual disturbance, nasal congestion.

Urogenital: impotence, dysuria, nocturia, incontinence, renal dysfunction including renal failure.

Additional side effects that have been reported with the individual components and may be potential side effects of Moduret 25 are listed below:

Amiloride:

Body as a whole: neck/shoulder ache, pain in extremities.

Digestive: abnormal liver function, activation of probable pre-existing peptic ulcer, dyspepsia, jaundice.

Integumentary: dry mouth, alopecia.

Nervous: tremors, encephalopathy.

Haematological: aplastic anaemia, neutropenia.

Cardiovascular: one patient with partial heart block developed complete heart block, palpitation.

Psychiatric: decreased libido, somnolence.

Respiratory: cough.

Special senses: tinnitus, increased intra-ocular pressure.

Urogenital: polyuria, urinary frequency, bladder spasm.

Hydrochlorothiazide:

Body as a whole: anaphylactic reaction, fever.

Cardiovascular: necrotising angiitis (vasculitis, cutaneous vasculitis).

Digestive: jaundice (intrahepatic cholestatic jaundice), pancreatitis, cramping, gastric irritation.

Endocrine/Metabolic: glycosuria, hyperglycaemia, hyperuricaemia, hypokalaemia.

Integumentary: photosensitivity, sialadenitis, urticaria, toxic epidermal necrolysis.

Haematological: agranulocytosis, aplastic anaemia, haemolytic anaemia, leucopenia, purpura, thrombocytopenia.

Psychiatric: restlessness.

Renal: interstitial nephritis.

Respiratory: respiratory distress, including pneumonitis, pulmonary oedema.

Special senses: transient blurred vision, xanthopsia.

4.9 Overdose

No specific data are available on overdosage with Moduret 25. No specific antidote is available, and it is not known whether the drug is dialysable.

Treatment should be symptomatic and supportive. Therapy should be discontinued and the patient watched closely. Emesis should be induced and/or gastric lavage performed. The most common signs and symptoms of overdosage with amiloride hydrochloride are dehydration and electrolyte imbalance. Blood pressure should be monitored and corrected where necessary. If hyperkalaemia occurs, active measures should be taken to reduce the plasma potassium levels.

Electrolyte depletion (hypokalaemia, hypochloraemia, hyponatraemia) and dehydration are the most common signs and symptoms of hydrochlorothiazide overdosage. If digitalis has been administered, hypokalaemia may accentuate cardiac arrhythmias.

The plasma half-life of hydrochlorothiazide is 5.6 hours with a subsequent longer terminal half-life; the plasma half-life of amiloride is about six hours.

5. PHARMACOLOGICAL PROPERTIES

5.1 Pharmacodynamic properties

Moduret 25 provides diuretic and antihypertensive activity (principally due to the hydrochlorothiazide component), while acting through the amiloride components to prevent excessive potassium loss that may occur in patients receiving a thiazide diuretic. Due to this latter component, the urinary excretion of magnesium is less with Moduret 25 than with a thiazide or loop diuretic used alone. The onset of the diuretic action of Moduret 25 is within 1 to 2 hours and this action appears to be sustained for approximately 24 hours.

5.2 Pharmacokinetic properties

Amiloride hydrochloride usually begins to act within 2 hours after an oral dose. Its effect on electrolyte excretion reaches a peak between 6 and 10 hours and lasts about 24 hours. Peak plasma levels are obtained in 3 to 4 hours and the plasma half-life varies from 6 to 9 hours. Effects on electrolytes increase with single doses of amiloride hydrochloride up to approximately 15 mg.

Amiloride hydrochloride is not metabolised by the liver but is excreted unchanged by the kidneys. About 50 percent of a 20 mg dose of amiloride hydrochloride is excreted in the urine and 40 percent in the stool within 72 hours. Amiloride hydrochloride has little effect on glomerular filtration rate or renal blood flow. Because amiloride hydrochloride is not metabolised by the liver, drug accumulation is not anticipated in patients with hepatic dysfunction, but accumulation can occur if the hepatorenal syndrome develops.

The onset of the diuretic action of hydrochlorothiazide occurs in 2 hours and the peak action in about 4 hours. Diuretic activity lasts about 6 to 12 hours. Hydrochlorothiazide is eliminated rapidly by the kidney.

The mechanism of the antihypertensive effect of thiazides may be related to the excretion and redistribution of body sodium. Hydrochlorothiazide usually does not cause clinically important changes in normal blood pressure.

5.3 Preclinical safety data

No further information.

6. PHARMACEUTICAL PARTICULARS

6.1 List of excipients

Calcium Hydrogen Phosphate E341

Guar Gum

Lactose

Magnesium Stearate E572

Maize Starch

Pregelatinised Maize Starch

6.2 Incompatibilities

Not applicable.

6.3 Shelf life

3 Years.

6.4 Special precautions for storage

Store in a dry place below 25°C, protected from light.

6.5 Nature and contents of container

Calendar pack of 28 tablets or bottles of 100 tablets.

6.6 Special precautions for disposal and other handling

Not applicable.

7. MARKETING AUTHORISATION HOLDER

Merck Sharp & Dohme Limited

Hertford Road

Hoddesdon

Hertfordshire

EN11 9BU

United Kingdom

8. MARKETING AUTHORISATION NUMBER(S)

PL 0025/0178

9. DATE OF FIRST AUTHORISATION/RENEWAL OF THE AUTHORISATION

10 December 1982 / 23 March 2005

10. DATE OF REVISION OF THE TEXT

March 2009

LEGAL CATEGORY

POM

® denotes registered trademark of Merck & Co., Inc., Whitehouse Station, NJ, USA.

SPC.MUE-T25.08.UK.2989

Moduretic

(Merck Sharp & Dohme Limited)

1. NAME OF THE MEDICINAL PRODUCT

MODURETIC® Tablets

2. QUALITATIVE AND QUANTITATIVE COMPOSITION

Amiloride hydrochloride equivalent to 5 mg anhydrous amiloride hydrochloride and 50 mg hydrochlorothiazide.

3. PHARMACEUTICAL FORM

Tablets.

Peach-coloured, half-scored, diamond shaped tablet, marked 'MSD 917'.

4. CLINICAL PARTICULARS

4.1 Therapeutic indications

Potassium-conserving diuretic and antihypertensive.

'Moduretic' is indicated in patients with: hypertension, congestive heart failure, hepatic cirrhosis with ascites and oedema. In hypertension, 'Moduretic' may be used alone or in conjunction with other antihypertensive agents.

'Moduretic' is intended for the treatment of patients in whom potassium depletion might be suspected or anticipated. The presence of amiloride hydrochloride minimises the likelihood of potassium loss during vigorous diuresis for long-term maintenance therapy. The combination is thus indicated especially in conditions where potassium balance is particularly important.

4.2 Posology and method of administration

Hypertension: Initially half a 'Moduretic' tablet given once a day. If necessary, increase to one 'Moduretic' tablet given once a day or in divided doses.

Congestive heart failure: Initially half a 'Moduretic' tablet a day, subsequently adjusted if required, but not exceeding two 'Moduretic' tablets a day. Optimal dosage is determined by the diuretic response and the plasma potassium level. Once an initial diuresis has been achieved, reduction in dosage may be attempted for maintenance therapy. Maintenance therapy may be on an intermittent basis.

Hepatic cirrhosis with ascites: Initiate therapy with a low dose. A single daily dose of one 'Moduretic' tablet may be increased gradually until there is an effective diuresis. Dosage should not exceed two 'Moduretic' tablets a day. Maintenance dosages may be lower than those required to initiate diuresis; dosage reduction should therefore be attempted when the patient's weight is stabilised. A gradual weight reduction is especially desirable in cirrhotic patients to reduce the likelihood of untoward reactions associated with diuretic therapy.

Paediatric use: 'Moduretic' is not recommended for children under 18 years as safety and efficacy have not been established (see 4.3 'Contraindications').

Use in the elderly: Particular caution is needed in the elderly because of their susceptibility to electrolyte imbalance; the dosage should be carefully adjusted to renal function and clinical response.

4.3 Contraindications

Hyperkalaemia (plasma potassium over 5.5 mmol/l); other potassium-conserving diuretics. Potassium supplements or potassium-rich food (except in severe and/or refractory cases of hypokalaemia under careful monitoring); concomitant use with spironolactone or triamterene; anuria; acute renal failure, severe progressive renal disease, severe hepatic failure, precoma associated with hepatic cirrhosis, Addison's disease, hypercalcaemia, concurrent lithium therapy, diabetic nephropathy; patients with blood urea over 10 mmol/l, patients with diabetes mellitus, or those with serum creatinine over 130 μmol/l in whom serum electrolyte and blood urea levels cannot be monitored carefully and frequently. Prior hypersensitivity to amiloride hydrochloride, hydrochlorothiazide or other sulphonamide-derived drugs. Because the safety of amiloride hydrochloride for use in children has not been established, 'Moduretic' is not recommended for children under 18 years of age. For use in pregnancy and breast-feeding mothers, see 4.6 'Pregnancy and lactation'.

4.4 Special warnings and precautions for use

Hyperkalaemia has been observed in patients receiving amiloride hydrochloride, either alone or with other diuretics, particularly in the aged or in hospital patients with hepatic cirrhosis or congestive heart failure with renal involvement, who were seriously ill, or were undergoing vigorous diuretic therapy. Such patients should be carefully observed for clinical, laboratory, and ECG evidence of hyperkalaemia (not always associated with an abnormal ECG).

Neither potassium supplements nor a potassium-rich diet should be used with 'Moduretic' except under careful monitoring in severe and/or refractory cases of hypokalaemia.

Some deaths have been reported in this group of patients.

Treatment of hyperkalaemia: Should hyperkalaemia develop, discontinue treatment immediately and, if necessary, take active measures to reduce the plasma potassium to normal.

Impaired renal function: Renal function should be monitored because the use of 'Moduretic' in impaired renal function may result in the rapid development of hyperkalaemia. Thiazide diuretics become ineffective when creatinine levels fall below 30 ml/min.

Electrolyte imbalance: Although the likelihood of electrolyte imbalance is reduced by 'Moduretic', careful check should be kept for such signs of fluid and electrolyte imbalance as hyponatraemia, hypochloraemic alkalosis, hypokalaemia and hypomagnesaemia. It is particularly important to make serum and urine electrolyte determinations when the patient is vomiting excessively or receiving parenteral fluids. Warning signs or symptoms of fluid or electrolyte imbalance include: dryness of the mouth, weakness, lethargy, drowsiness, restlessness, seizures, confusion, muscle pains or cramps, muscular fatigue, hypotension, oliguria, tachycardia, and gastro-intestinal disturbances such as nausea and vomiting.

Hypokalaemia may develop, especially as a result of brisk diuresis, after prolonged therapy or when severe cirrhosis is present. Hypokalaemia can sensitise or exaggerate the response of the heart to the toxic effects of digitalis (e.g. increased ventricular irritability).

Diuretic-induced hyponatraemia is usually mild and asymptomatic. It may become severe and symptomatic in a few patients who will then require immediate attention and appropriate treatment.

Thiazides may decrease urinary calcium excretion. Thiazides may cause intermittent and slight elevation of serum calcium in the absence of known disorders of calcium metabolism. Therapy should be discontinued before carrying out tests for parathyroid function.

Azotaemia may be precipitated or increased by hydrochlorothiazide. Cumulative effects of the drug may develop in patients with impaired renal function. If increasing azotaemia and oliguria develop during treatment of renal disease, 'Moduretic' should be discontinued.

Hepatic disease: Thiazides should be used with caution in patients with impaired hepatic function or progressive liver disease (see 4.3 'Contraindications'), since minor alterations of fluid and electrolyte balance may precipitate hepatic coma.

Metabolic: Hyperuricaemia may occur, or gout may be precipitated or aggravated, in certain patients receiving thiazides. Thiazides may impair glucose tolerance. Diabetes mellitus may be precipitated or aggravated by therapy with 'Moduretic' (see 4.3 'Contraindications'). Dosage adjustment of antidiabetic agents, including insulin, may be required.

Increases in cholesterol and triglyceride levels may be associated with thiazide diuretic therapy.

To minimise the risk of hyperkalaemia in diabetic or suspected diabetic patients, the status of renal function should be determined before initiating therapy with 'Moduretic'. Therapy should be discontinued at least three days before giving a glucose tolerance test. Potassium-conserving therapy should be initiated only with caution in severely ill patients in whom metabolic or respiratory acidosis may occur, e.g. patients with cardiopulmonary disease or patients with inadequately controlled diabetes.

Shifts in acid-base balance alter the balance of extracellular/intracellular potassium, and the development of acidosis may be associated with rapid increases in plasma potassium.

Sensitivity reactions: The possibility that thiazides may activate or exacerbate systemic lupus erythematosus has been reported.

4.5 Interaction with other medicinal products and other forms of interaction

Lithium generally should not be given with diuretics. Diuretic agents reduce the renal clearance of lithium and add a high risk of lithium toxicity. Refer to the prescribing information for lithium preparations before use of such preparations.

Non-Steroidal Anti-inflammatory Drugs: In some patients the administration of a non-steroidal anti-inflammatory agent can reduce the diuretic, natriuretic and antihypertensive effects of diuretics. Concomitant administration of non-steroidal anti-inflammatory drugs (NSAIDs) and potassium-sparing agents, including amiloride hydrochloride, may cause hyperkalaemia and renal failure, particularly in elderly patients. Therefore, when amiloride hydrochloride is used concomitantly with NSAIDs, renal function and serum potassium levels should be carefully monitored.

Amiloride Hydrochloride

When amiloride hydrochloride is administered concomitantly with an angiotensin-converting enzyme inhibitor, angiotensin II receptor antagonist, trilostane, ciclosporin or tacrolimus, the risk of hyperkalaemia may be increased. Therefore, if concomitant use of these agents is indicated because of demonstrated hypokalaemia, they should be used with caution and with frequent monitoring of serum potassium.

Hydrochlorothiazide

When given concurrently, the following drugs may interact with thiazide diuretics:

Alcohol, barbiturates or narcotics: Co-administration may potentiate orthostatic hypotension. **Oral and parenteral antidiabetic drugs** may require adjustment of dosage with concurrent use. 'Moduretic' can act synergistically with chlorpropamide to increase the risk of hyponatraemia. **Other antihypertensive drugs** may have an additive effect. Therefore the dosage of these agents, especially adrenergic-blockers, may need to be reduced when 'Moduretic' is added to the regimen. Diuretic therapy should be discontinued for 2-3 days prior to initiation of therapy with an ACE inhibitor to reduce the likelihood of first dose hypotension. **Cholestyramine and colestipol resins:** absorption of hydrochlorothiazide is impaired in the presence of anionic exchange resins. Single doses of either cholestyramine or colestipol resins bind the hydrochlorothiazide and reduce its absorption from the gastrointestinal tract by up to 85 and 43 percent, respectively. When cholestyramine is given 4 hours after the hydrochlorothiazide, the absorption of hydrochlorothiazide is reduced by 30 to 35 percent. **Corticosteroids or ACTH** may intensify any thiazide-induced electrolyte depletion, particularly hypokalaemia. **Pressor amines such as epinephrine (adrenaline)** may show decreased arterial responsiveness when used with 'Moduretic' but this reaction is not enough to preclude their therapeutic usefulness. **Non-depolarising muscle relaxants such as tubocurarine** may possibly interact with 'Moduretic' to increase muscle relaxation.

Drug/laboratory tests: Because thiazides may affect calcium metabolism, 'Moduretic' may interfere with tests for parathyroid function.

4.6 Pregnancy and lactation

Use in pregnancy: The routine use of diuretics in otherwise healthy pregnant women with or without mild oedema is not indicated, because they may be associated with hypovolaemia, increased blood viscosity, and decreased placental perfusion. Diuretics do not prevent the development of toxaemia of pregnancy and there is no satisfactory evidence that they are useful for its treatment.

Since thiazides cross the placental barrier and appear in cord blood, use where pregnancy is present or suspected requires that the benefits of the drug be weighed against possible hazards to the foetus. These hazards include foetal or neonatal jaundice, thrombocytopenia, bone marrow depression, and possibly other side effects that have occurred in the adult.

Use in breast-feeding mothers: Although it is not known whether amiloride hydrochloride is excreted in human milk, it is known that thiazides do appear in breast milk. If use of the drug combination is deemed essential, the patient should stop breast-feeding.

4.7 Effects on ability to drive and use machines

Infrequently, patients may experience weakness, fatigue, dizziness, stupor and vertigo. Should any of these occur, the patient should be cautioned not to drive or operate machinery.

4.8 Undesirable effects

Although minor side effects are relatively common, significant side effects are infrequent.

Reported side effects are generally associated with diuresis, thiazide therapy, or with the underlying disease.

No increase in the risk of adverse reactions has been seen over those of the individual components.

The following side effects have been reported with 'Moduretic':

Body as a whole: headache, weakness, fatigue, malaise, chest pain, back pain, syncope.

Cardiovascular: arrhythmias, tachycardia, digitalis toxicity, orthostatic hypotension, angina pectoris.

Digestive: anorexia, nausea, vomiting, diarrhoea, constipation, abdominal pain, GI bleeding, appetite changes, abdominal fullness, flatulence, thirst, hiccups.

Metabolic: elevated plasma potassium levels (above 5.5 mmol/l), electrolyte imbalance, hyponatraemia (see 4.4 'Special warnings and precautions for use'), gout, dehydration, symptomatic hyponatraemia.

Integumentary: rash, pruritus, flushing, diaphoresis.

Musculoskeletal: leg ache, muscle cramps, joint pain.

Nervous: dizziness, vertigo, paraesthesiae, stupor.

Psychiatric: insomnia, nervousness, mental confusion, depression, sleepiness.

Respiratory: dyspnoea.

Special senses: bad taste, visual disturbance, nasal congestion.

Urogenital: impotence, dysuria, nocturia, incontinence, renal dysfunction including renal failure.

Additional side effects that have been reported with the individual components and may be potential side effects of 'Moduretic' are listed below:

Amiloride:

Body as a whole: neck/shoulder ache, pain in extremities.

Digestive: abnormal liver function, activation of probable pre-existing peptic ulcer, dyspepsia, jaundice.

Integumentary: dry mouth, alopecia.

Nervous: tremors, encephalopathy.

Haematological: aplastic anaemia, neutropenia.

Cardiovascular: one patient with partial heart block developed complete heart block, palpitation.

Psychiatric: decreased libido, somnolence.

Respiratory: cough.

Special senses: tinnitus, increased intra-ocular pressure.

Urogenital: polyuria, urinary frequency, bladder spasm.

Hydrochlorothiazide:

Body as a whole: anaphylactic reaction, fever.

Cardiovascular: necrotising angiitis (vasculitis, cutaneous vasculitis.)

Digestive: jaundice (intrahepatic cholestatic jaundice), pancreatitis, cramping, gastric irritation.

Endocrine/Metabolic: glycosuria, hyperglycaemia, hyperuricaemia, hypokalaemia.

Integumentary: photosensitivity, sialadenitis, urticaria, toxic epidermal necrolysis.

Haematological: agranulocytosis, aplastic anaemia, haemolytic anaemia, leucopenia, purpura, thrombocytopenia.

Psychiatric: restlessness.

Renal: interstitial nephritis.

Respiratory: respiratory distress, including pneumonitis, pulmonary oedema.

Special senses: transient blurred vision, xanthopsia.

4.9 Overdose

No specific data are available on overdosage with 'Moduretic'. No specific antidote is available, and it is not known whether the drug is dialysable.

Treatment should be symptomatic and supportive. Therapy should be discontinued and the patient watched closely. Emesis should be induced and/or gastric lavage performed. The most common signs and symptoms of overdosage with amiloride hydrochloride are dehydration and electrolyte imbalance. Blood pressure should be monitored and corrected where necessary. If hyperkalaemia occurs, active measures should be taken to reduce the plasma potassium levels.

Electrolyte depletion (hypokalaemia, hypochloraemia, hyponatraemia) and dehydration are the most common signs and symptoms of hydrochlorothiazide overdosage. If digitalis has been administered, hypokalaemia may accentuate cardiac arrhythmias.

5. PHARMACOLOGICAL PROPERTIES

5.1 Pharmacodynamic properties

Hydrochlorothiazide is a diuretic with antihypertensive properties. It acts by inhibiting the renal tubular reabsorption of sodium and chloride ions, which are excreted with an accompanying volume of water. Potassium excretion is also promoted.

Amiloride hydrochloride is a potassium-sparing diuretic. It also promotes the excretion of sodium and chloride, but it reduces the excretion of potassium.

5.2 Pharmacokinetic properties

About 70% of an oral dose of hydrochlorothiazide is absorbed. It has a plasma half life of 5.6 to 14.8 hours. It is excreted unchanged in the urine. It crosses the placental barrier and is secreted in breast milk.

About 50% of an oral dose of amiloride hydrochloride is absorbed. It has a plasma half life of about 6 to 9 hours, but its effects may persist for up to 48 hours after a single dose. It is excreted unchanged in the urine and faeces.

5.3 Preclinical safety data

No relevant data.

6. PHARMACEUTICAL PARTICULARS

6.1 List of excipients

Calcium hydrogen phosphate

Guar gum

Lactose

Magnesium stearate

Maize starch

Pregelatinised maize starch

Sunset yellow aluminium lake E110

6.2 Incompatibilities

None known.

6.3 Shelf life

3 years.

6.4 Special precautions for storage

Store in a dry place below 25°C.

6.5 Nature and contents of container

White opaque polypropylene HDPE or glass bottles containing 30, 50, 100 or 500 tablets.

PVC blister packs, lidded with aluminium foil containing 28 tablets.

6.6 Special precautions for disposal and other handling

None.

7. MARKETING AUTHORISATION HOLDER

Merck Sharp & Dohme Limited

Hertford Road, Hoddesdon, Hertfordshire EN11 9BU, UK

8. MARKETING AUTHORISATION NUMBER(S)

PL 0025/5016R

9. DATE OF FIRST AUTHORISATION/RENEWAL OF THE AUTHORISATION

6 November 1989 / 23 March 2005

10. DATE OF REVISION OF THE TEXT

March 2009

LEGAL CATEGORY

POM

SPC.MUE-T.08.UK.2990

Molipaxin 50mg and 100mg Capsules

(sanofi-aventis)

1. NAME OF THE MEDICINAL PRODUCT

Molipaxin 50mg Capsules

Molipaxin 100mg Capsules

2. QUALITATIVE AND QUANTITATIVE COMPOSITION

Trazodone hydrochloride 50mg or 100mg per capsule.

For excipients see 6.1

3. PHARMACEUTICAL FORM

Capsules.

4. CLINICAL PARTICULARS

4.1 Therapeutic indications

Anxiety, depression, mixed anxiety and depression.

4.2 Posology and method of administration

Route of administration: Oral.

DEPRESSION:

Adults:

Initially 150mg/day in divided doses after food or as a single dose on retiring.

This may be increased up to 300mg/day in a single or divided doses. The major portion of a divided dose to be taken on retiring. The dose may be further increased to 600mg/day in divided doses in hospitalised patients.

Elderly:

For very elderly or frail patients initially 100mg/day in divided doses or as a single night-time dose. This may be increased, under supervision, according to efficacy and tolerance. It is unlikely that 300mg/day will be exceeded.

Children:

There are insufficient data to recommend the use of Molipaxin in children.

DEPRESSION ACCOMPANIED BY ANXIETY:

As for depression.

ANXIETY:

75mg/day increasing to 300mg/day as necessary.

Tolerability may be improved by taking Molipaxin after food.

4.3 Contraindications

Known sensitivity to trazodone and any of the excipients.

4.4 Special warnings and precautions for use

Suicide/suicidal thoughts or clinical worsening

Depression is associated with an increased risk of suicidal thoughts, self harm and suicide (suicide-related events). This risk persists until significant remission occurs. As improvement may not occur during the first few weeks or more of treatment, patients should be closely monitored until such improvement occurs. It is general clinical experience that the risk of suicide may increase in the early stages of recovery.

Other psychiatric conditions for which Molipaxin is prescribed can also be associated with an increased risk of suicide-related events. In addition, these conditions may be co-morbid with major depressive disorder. The same precautions observed when treating patients with major depressive disorder should therefore be observed when treating patients with other psychiatric disorders.

Patients with a history of suicide-related events, or those exhibiting a significant degree of suicidal ideation prior to commencement of treatment are known to be at greater risk of suicidal thoughts or suicide attempts, and should receive careful monitoring during treatment. A meta-analysis of placebo-controlled clinical trials of antidepressant drugs in adult patients with psychiatric disorders showed an increased risk of suicidal behaviour with antidepressants compared to placebo in patients less than 25 years old.

Close supervision of patients and in particular those at high risk should accompany drug therapy especially in early treatment and following dose changes. Patients (and caregivers of patients) should be alerted about the need to monitor for any clinical worsening, suicidal behaviour or thoughts and unusual changes in behaviour and to seek medical advice immediately if these symptoms present.

Care should be exercised when administering Molipaxin to patients suffering epilepsy, avoiding in particular, abrupt increases or decreases in dosage.

Molipaxin should be administered with care in patients with severe hepatic, renal or cardiac disease.

Potent CYP3A4 inhibitors may lead to increases in trazodone serum levels. See section 4.5 for further information.

4.5 Interaction with other medicinal products and other forms of interaction

In vitro drug metabolism studies suggest that there is a potential for drug interactions when Molipaxin is given with potent CYP3A4 inhibitors such as erythromycin, ketoconazole, itraconazole, ritonavir, indinavir, and nefazodone. It is likely that potent CYP3A4 inhibitors may lead to substantial increases in trazodone plasma concentrations with the potential for adverse effects. Exposure to ritonavir during initiation or resumption of treatment in patients receiving Molipaxin will increase the potential for excessive sedation, cardiovascular, and gastrointestinal effects. If Molipaxin is used with a potent CYP3A4 inhibitor, a lower dose of Molipaxin should be considered. However, the co-administration of Molipaxin and potent CYP3A4 inhibitors should be avoided where possible.

Carbamazepine reduced plasma concentrations of trazodone when coadministered. Patients should be closely monitored to see if there is a need for an increased dose of Molipaxin when taken with carbamazepine.

Although no untoward effects have been reported, Molipaxin may enhance the effects of muscle relaxants and volatile anaesthetics. Similar considerations apply to combined administration with sedative and anti-depressant drugs, including alcohol. Molipaxin has been well tolerated in depressed schizophrenic patients receiving standard phenothiazine therapy and also in depressed parkinsonian patients receiving therapy with levodopa.

Possible interactions with monoamine oxidase inhibitors have occasionally been reported. Although some clinicians do give both concurrently, we do not recommend concurrent administration with MAOIs, or within two weeks of stopping treatment with these compounds. Nor do we recommend giving MAOIs within one week of stopping Molipaxin

Since Molipaxin is only a very weak inhibitor of noradrenaline re-uptake and does not modify the blood pressure response to tyramine, interference with the hypotensive action of guanethidine-like compounds is unlikely. However, studies in laboratory animals suggest that Molipaxin may inhibit most of the acute actions of clonidine. In the case of other types of antihypertensive drug, although no clinical interactions have been reported, the possibility of potentiation should be considered.

Concurrent use with Molipaxin may result in elevated serum levels of digoxin or phenytoin. Monitoring of serum levels should be considered in these patients.

4.6 Pregnancy and lactation

Although studies in animals have not shown any direct teratogenic effect, the safety of Molipaxin in human pregnancy has not been established. On basic principles, therefore, its use during the first trimester should be avoided.

The possibility of Molipaxin being excreted in the milk should also be considered in nursing mothers.

4.7 Effects on ability to drive and use machines

As with all other drugs acting on the central nervous system, patients should be warned against the risk of handling machinery and driving.

4.8 Undesirable effects

Cases of suicidal ideation and suicidal behaviours have been reported during Molipaxin therapy or early after treatment discontinuation (see section 4.4).

Molipaxin is a sedative antidepressant and drowsiness, sometimes experienced during the first days of treatment, usually disappears on continued therapy.

Anticholinergic-like symptoms do occur but the incidence is similar to placebo.

The following symptoms, most of which are commonly reported in cases of untreated depression, have also been recorded in small numbers of patients receiving Molipaxin therapy: dizziness, headache, nausea and vomiting, weakness, decreased alertness, weight loss, tremor, dry mouth, bradycardia, tachycardia, postural hypotension, oedema, constipation, diarrhoea, blurred vision, restlessness, confusional states, insomnia and skin rash.

Blood dyscrasias, including agranulocytosis, thrombocytopenia and anaemia, have been reported on rare occasions. Adverse effects on hepatic function, including jaundice and hepatocellular damage, sometimes severe, have been rarely reported. Should such effects occur, Molipaxin should be discontinued immediately.

As with other drugs with alpha-adrenolytic activity, Molipaxin has very rarely been associated with priapism. This may be treated with an intracavernosum injection of an alpha-adrenergic agent such as adrenaline or metaraminol. However there are reports of Trazodone-induced priapism which have required surgical intervention or led to permanent sexual dysfunction. Patients developing this suspected adverse reaction should cease Molipaxin immediately.

In contrast to the tricyclic antidepressants, Molipaxin is devoid of anticholinergic activity. Consequently, troublesome side effects such as dry mouth, blurred vision and urinary hesitancy have occurred no more frequently than in patients receiving placebo therapy. This may be of importance when treating depressed patients who are at risk from conditions such as glaucoma, urinary retention and prostatic hypertrophy.

Studies in animals have shown that Molipaxin is less cardiotoxic than the tricyclic antidepressants, and clinical studies suggest that the drug may be less likely to cause cardiac arrhythmias in man. Clinical studies in patients with pre-existing cardiac disease indicate that Trazodone may be arrhythmogenic in some patients in that population. Arrhythmias identified include isolated premature ventricular contractions, ventricular couplets, and short episodes (3-4 beats) of ventricular tachycardia.

There have been occasional reports of serotonin syndrome and convulsions associated with the use of Molipaxin, especially when associated with other psychotropic drugs. Neuroleptic malignant syndrome may, very rarely, arise in the course of treatment with Molipaxin.

Hyponatraemia has been reported in association with treatment with this product. Fluid and electrolyte status should be monitored in symptomatic patients.

Molipaxin has had no effect on arterial blood pCO_2 or pO_2 levels in patients with severe respiratory insufficiency due to chronic bronchial or pulmonary disease.

4.9 Overdose

FEATURES OF TOXICITY

The most frequently reported reactions to overdose have included drowsiness, dizziness, nausea and vomiting. In more serious cases coma, tachycardia, hypotension, hyponatraemia, convulsions and respiratory failure have been reported. Cardiac features may include bradycardia, QT prolongation and torsade de pointes. Symptoms may appear 24 hours or more after overdose.

Overdoses of Molipaxin in combination with other antidepressants may cause serotonin syndrome.

MANAGEMENT

There is no specific antidote to trazodone. Activated charcoal should be considered in adults who have ingested more than 1 g trazodone, or in children who have ingested more than 150 mg trazodone within 1 hour of presentation. Alternatively, in adults, gastric lavage may be considered within 1 hour of ingestion of a potentially life-threatening overdose.

Observe for at least 6 hours after ingestion (or 12 hours if a sustained release preparation has been taken). Monitor BP, pulse and GCS. Monitor oxygen saturation if GCS is reduced. Cardiac monitoring is appropriate in symptomatic patients.

Single brief convulsions do not require treatment. Control frequent or prolonged convulsions with intravenous diazepam (0.1-0.3 mg/kg body weight) or lorazepam (4 mg in an adult and 0.05 mg/kg in a child). If these measures do not control the fits, an intravenous infusion of phenytoin may be useful. Give oxygen and correct acid base and metabolic disturbances as required.

Treatment should be symptomatic and supportive in the case of hypotension and excessive sedation. If severe hypotension persists consider use of inotropes, eg dopamine or dobutamine

5. PHARMACOLOGICAL PROPERTIES

5.1 Pharmacodynamic properties

ATC code: N06A X05. Other antidepressants.

Molipaxin is a potent antidepressant. It also has anxiety reducing activity. Molipaxin is a triazolopyridine derivative chemically unrelated to known tricyclic, tetracyclic and other antidepressant agents. It has negligible effect on noradrenaline re-uptake mechanisms. Whilst the mode of action of Molipaxin is not known precisely, its antidepressant activity may concern noradrenergic potentiation by mechanisms other than uptake blockade. A central antiserotonin effect may account for the drug's anxiety reducing properties.

5.2 Pharmacokinetic properties

Trazodone is rapidly absorbed from the gastro-intestinal tract and extensively metabolised. Paths of metabolism of Trazodone include n-oxidation and hydroxylation. The metabolic m-chlorophenylpiperazine is active. Trazodone is excreted in the urine almost entirely in the form of its metabolites, either in free or in conjugated form. The elimination of Trazodone is biphasic, with a terminal elimination half-life of 5 to 13 hours. Trazodone is excreted in breast milk.

There was an approximate two-fold increase in terminal phase half-life and significantly higher plasma concentrations of Trazodone in 10 subjects aged 65 to 74 years compared with 12 subjects aged 23 to 30 years following a 100mg dose of Trazodone. It was suggested that there is an age-related reduction in the hepatic metabolism of Trazodone.

In vitro studies in human liver microsomes show that trazodone is metabolised by cytochrome P4503A4 (CYP3A4) to form m-chlorophenylpiperazine. Whilst significant, the role of this pathway in the total clearance of trazodone *in vivo* has not been fully determined.

5.3 Preclinical safety data

None stated.

6. PHARMACEUTICAL PARTICULARS

6.1 List of excipients

Lactose

Magnesium stearate

Gelatin

Titanium dioxide E171

Erythrosine E127

Indigo Carmine E132

Red iron oxide E172

Yellow iron oxide E172

Ink (1028 (S-1-27794) or 1014 (SW-9008) Black)

6.2 Incompatibilities

None stated.

6.3 Shelf life

60 months.

6.4 Special precautions for storage

Blister packs: Store below 30°C in a dry place.

6.5 Nature and contents of container

50mg: PVdC coated 250μm PVC blisters sealed with 20μm aluminium foil: contents 84 capsules.

100mg: PVdC coated 250μm PVC blisters sealed with 20μm aluminium foil: contents

56 capsules.

6.6 Special precautions for disposal and other handling

Not applicable.

7. MARKETING AUTHORISATION HOLDER

Sanofi-aventis

One Onslow Street

Guildford

Surrey

GU1 4YS

UK

8. MARKETING AUTHORISATION NUMBER(S)

50mg: PL 04425/0609

100mg: PL 04425/0180

9. DATE OF FIRST AUTHORISATION/RENEWAL OF THE AUTHORISATION

26 August 2009

10. DATE OF REVISION OF THE TEXT
26 August 2009

LEGAL STATUS
POM

Molipaxin Liquid 50mg/5ml

(sanofi-aventis)

1. NAME OF THE MEDICINAL PRODUCT
Molipaxin™ Liquid (50mg/5ml)

2. QUALITATIVE AND QUANTITATIVE COMPOSITION
Each 5ml contains 50mg of Trazodone hydrochloride.

For excipients, see 6.1.

3. PHARMACEUTICAL FORM
Clear, colourless solution with an orange odour and taste.

4. CLINICAL PARTICULARS

4.1 Therapeutic indications
Relief of symptoms in all types of depression including depression accompanied by anxiety.

Symptoms of depression likely to respond in the first week of treatment include depressed mood, insomnia, anxiety, somatic symptoms and hypochondriasis.

4.2 Posology and method of administration
Route of administration: Oral.

Adults:

Starting dose is 150mg/day in divided doses after food or as a single dose before retiring. This may be increased to 300mg/day, the major portion of which is preferably taken on retiring. In hospitalised patients dosage may be further increased to 600mg/day.

Children:

There are insufficient data to recommend the use of Molipaxin in children.

Elderly or Frail:

For elderly or very frail patients initial starting dose 100mg/day in divided doses or as a single night-time dose. This may be increased, under supervision, according to efficacy and tolerance. Doses above 300mg/day are unlikely to be required.

Tolerability may be improved by taking Molipaxin after food.

In conformity with current psychiatric opinion, it is suggested that Molipaxin be continued for several months after remission. Cessation of Molipaxin treatment should be gradual.

4.3 Contraindications
Known sensitivity to trazodone or to any of the excipients.

4.4 Special warnings and precautions for use
Suicide/suicidal thoughts or clinical worsening

Depression is associated with an increased risk of suicidal thoughts, self harm and suicide (suicide-related events). This risk persists until significant remission occurs. As improvement may not occur during the first few weeks or more of treatment, patients should be closely monitored until such improvement occurs. It is general clinical experience that the risk of suicide may increase in the early stages of recovery.

Other psychiatric conditions for which Molipaxin is prescribed can also be associated with an increased risk of suicide-related events. In addition, these conditions may be co-morbid with major depressive disorder. The same precautions observed when treating patients with major depressive disorder should therefore be observed when treating patients with other psychiatric disorders.

Patients with a history of suicide-related events, or those exhibiting a significant degree of suicidal ideation prior to commencement of treatment are known to be at greater risk of suicidal thoughts or suicide attempts, and should receive careful monitoring during treatment. A meta-analysis of placebo-controlled clinical trials of antidepressant drugs in adult patients with psychiatric disorders showed an increased risk of suicidal behaviour with antidepressants compared to placebo in patients less than 25 years old.

Close supervision of patients and in particular those at high risk should accompany drug therapy especially in early treatment and following dose changes. Patients (and caregivers of patients) should be alerted about the need to monitor for any clinical worsening, suicidal behaviour or thoughts and unusual changes in behaviour and to seek medical advice immediately if these symptoms present.

Molipaxin should be administered with care in patients with severe hepatic, renal or cardiac disease.

Care should be exercised when administering Molipaxin to patients suffering epilepsy, avoiding in particular, abrupt increases or decreases in dosage.

Potent CYP3A4 inhibitors may lead to increases in trazodone serum levels. See section 4.5 for further information.

4.5 Interaction with other medicinal products and other forms of interaction
In vitro drug metabolism studies suggest that there is a potential for drug interactions when Molipaxin is given with potent CYP3A4 inhibitors such as erythromycin, ketoconazole, itraconazole, ritonavir, indinavir, and nefazodone. It is likely that potent CYP3A4 inhibitors may lead to substantial increases in trazodone plasma concentrations with the potential for adverse effects. Exposure to ritonavir during initiation or resumption of treatment in patients receiving Molipaxin will increase the potential for excessive sedation, cardiovascular, and gastrointestinal effects. If Molipaxin is used with a potent CYP3A4 inhibitor, a lower dose of Molipaxin should be considered. However, the co-administration of Molipaxin and potent CYP3A4 inhibitors should be avoided where possible.

Carbamazepine reduced plasma concentrations of trazodone when coadministered. Patients should be closely monitored to see if there is a need for an increased dose of Molipaxin when taken with carbamazepine.

Although no untoward effects have been reported, Molipaxin may enhance the effects of muscle relaxants and volatile anaesthetics. Similar considerations apply to combined administration with sedative and anti-depressant drugs, including alcohol.

Molipaxin has been well tolerated in depressed schizophrenic patients receiving standard phenothiazine therapy and also in depressed parkinsonian patients receiving therapy with levodopa.

Possible interactions with monoamine oxidase inhibitors have occasionally been reported. Although some clinicians do give both concurrently, we do not recommend concurrent administration with MAOIs, or within two weeks of stopping treatment with these compounds. Nor do we recommend giving MAOIs within one week of stopping Molipaxin.

Since Molipaxin is only a very weak inhibitor of noradrenaline re-uptake and does not modify the blood pressure response to tyramine, interference with the hypotensive action of guanethidine-like compounds is unlikely. However, studies in laboratory animals suggest that Molipaxin may inhibit most of the acute actions of clonidine. In the case of other types of antihypertensive drug, although no clinical interactions have been reported, the possibility of potentiation should be considered.

Concurrent use with Molipaxin may result in elevated serum levels of digoxin or phenytoin. Monitoring of serum levels should be considered in these patients.

Molipaxin has had no effect on arterial blood pCO_2 or pO_2 levels in patients with severe respiratory insufficiency due to chronic bronchial or pulmonary disease.

4.6 Pregnancy and lactation
Although studies in animals have not shown any direct teratogenic effect, the safety of Molipaxin in human pregnancy has not been established. On basic principles, therefore, its use during the first trimester should be avoided.

The possibility of Molipaxin being excreted in the milk should also be considered in nursing mothers.

Molipaxin should only be administered during pregnancy and lactation if considered essential by the physician.

4.7 Effects on ability to drive and use machines
As with all other drugs acting on the central nervous system, patients should be warned against the risk of handling machinery and driving.

4.8 Undesirable effects
Cases of suicidal ideation and suicidal behaviours have been reported during Molipaxin therapy or early after treatment discontinuation (see section 4.4).

Molipaxin is a sedative antidepressant and drowsiness, sometimes experienced during the first days of treatment, usually disappears on continued therapy.

Anticholinergic-like symptoms do occur but the incidence is similar to placebo.

The following symptoms, most of which are commonly reported in cases of untreated depression, have also been recorded in small numbers of patients receiving Molipaxin therapy: dizziness, headache, nausea and vomiting, weakness, decreased alertness, weight loss, tremor, dry mouth, bradycardia, tachycardia, postural hypotension, oedema, constipation, diarrhoea, blurred vision, restlessness, confusional states, insomnia and skin rash.

Blood dyscrasias, including agranulocytosis, thrombocytopenia and anaemia, have been reported on rare occasions. Adverse effects on hepatic function, including jaundice and hepatocellular damage, sometimes severe, have been rarely reported. Should such effects occur, Molipaxin should be discontinued immediately.

As with other drugs with alpha-adrenolytic activity, Molipaxin has very rarely been associated with priapism. This may be treated with an intracavernosum injection of an alpha-adrenergic agent such as adrenaline or metaraminol. However there are reports of Trazodone-induced priapism which have required surgical intervention or led to permanent sexual dysfunction. Patients developing this suspected adverse reaction should cease Molipaxin immediately.

In contrast to the tricyclic antidepressants, Molipaxin is devoid of anticholinergic activity. Consequently, troublesome side effects such as dry mouth, blurred vision and urinary hesitancy have occurred no more frequently than in patients receiving placebo therapy. This may be of importance when treating depressed patients who are at risk from conditions such as glaucoma, urinary retention and prostatic hypertrophy.

Studies in animals have shown that Molipaxin is less cardiotoxic than the tricyclic antidepressants, and clinical studies suggest that the drug may be less likely to cause cardiac arrhythmias in man. Clinical studies in patients with pre-existing cardiac disease indicate that Molipaxin may be arrhythmogenic in some patients in that population. Arrhythmias identified include isolated premature ventricular contractions, ventricular couplets, and short episodes (3-4 beats) of ventricular tachycardia.

There have been occasional reports of serotonin syndrome and convulsions associated with the use of Molipaxin, especially when associated with other psychotropic drugs. Neuroleptic malignant syndrome may, very rarely, arise in the course of treatment with Molipaxin.

Hyponatraemia has been reported in association with treatment with this product. Fluid and electrolyte status should be monitored in symptomatic patients.

Molipaxin has had no effect on arterial blood pCO_2 or pO_2 levels in patients with severe respiratory insufficiency due to chronic bronchial or pulmonary disease.

4.9 Overdose
FEATURES OF TOXICITY

The most frequently reported reactions to overdose have included drowsiness, dizziness, nausea and vomiting. In more serious cases coma, tachycardia, hypotension, hyponatraemia, convulsions and respiratory failure have been reported. Cardiac features may include bradycardia, QT prolongation and torsade de pointes. Symptoms may appear 24 hours or more after overdose.

Overdoses of Molipaxin in combination with other antidepressants may cause serotonin syndrome.

MANAGEMENT

There is no specific antidote to trazodone. Activated charcoal should be considered in adults who have ingested more than 1 g trazodone, or in children who have ingested more than 150 mg trazodone within 1 hour of presentation. Alternatively, in adults, gastric lavage may be considered within 1 hour of ingestion of a potentially life-threatening overdose.

Observe for at least 6 hours after ingestion (or 12 hours if a sustained release preparation has been taken). Monitor BP, pulse and GCS. Monitor oxygen saturation if GCS is reduced. Cardiac monitoring is appropriate in symptomatic patients.

Single brief convulsions do not require treatment. Control frequent or prolonged convulsions with intravenous diazepam (0.1-0.3 mg/kg body weight) or lorazepam (4 mg in an adult and 0.05 mg/kg in a child). If these measures do not control the fits, an intravenous infusion of phenytoin may be useful. Give oxygen and correct acid base and metabolic disturbances as required.

Treatment should be symptomatic and supportive in the case of hypotension and excessive sedation. If severe hypotension persists consider use of inotropes, eg dopamine or dobutamine

5. PHARMACOLOGICAL PROPERTIES

5.1 Pharmacodynamic properties
ATC code: N06A X05. Other antidepressants.

Trazodone is a triazolopyridine derivative which differs chemically from other currently available antidepressants. Although Trazodone bears some resemblance to the benzodiazepines, phenothiazines and tricyclic antidepressants, its pharmacological profile differs from each of these classes of drugs. The basic idea for the development of Trazodone was the hypothesis that depression involves an imbalance of the mechanism responsible for the emotional integration of unpleasant experiences. Consequently, new animal models of depression consisting of responses to unpleasant or noxious stimuli, instead of the current tests related to the aminergic theory of depression, were used in studying the drug. Trazodone inhibits serotonin uptake into rat brain synaptosomes and by rat platelets at relatively high concentrations and inhibits brain uptake of noradrenaline *in vitro* only at very high concentrations. It possesses antiserotonin-adrenergic blocking and analgesic effects. The anticholinergic activity of Trazodone is less than that of the tricyclic antidepressants in animal studies and this has been confirmed in therapeutic trials in depressed patients.

The electroencephalographic profile of Trazodone in humans is distinct from that of the tricyclic antidepressants or the benzodiazepines, although bearing some resemblance to these agents in its effect in certain wavebands. Studies of the cardiovascular effects of Trazodone in humans, His bundle and surface electrocardiograms in dogs, and experience with overdosage in man indicate that Trazodone is less liable than imipramine to cause important adverse effects on the heart. However, studies in depressed patients with significant cardiac impairment suggest that Trazodone may aggravate existing ventricular arrhythmias in a small undefined subgroup of such patients.

5.2 Pharmacokinetic properties
Peak plasma concentrations are attained about 1.5 hours after oral administration of Trazodone. Absorption is delayed and somewhat enhanced by food. The area under

the plasma concentration-time curve is directly proportional to dosage after oral administration of 25 to 100mg. Trazodone is extensively metabolised, less than 1% of an oral dose being excreted unchanged in the urine. The main route of elimination is via the kidneys with 70 to 75% of an oral dose being recovered in the urine within the first 72 hours of ingestion. The elimination half-life for unchanged drug has been reported to be about 7 hours.

In vitro studies in human liver microsomes show that trazodone is metabolised by cytochrome P4503A4 (CYP3A4) to form m-chlorophenylpiperazine. Whilst significant, the role of this pathway in the total clearance of trazodone in vivo has not been fully determined.

5.3 Preclinical safety data
None stated.

6. PHARMACEUTICAL PARTICULARS

6.1 List of excipients
Glycerol, sorbitol, benzoic acid, saccharin sodium, orange flavour FC 901775, sodium hydroxide solution 1N, purified water and nitrogen.

6.2 Incompatibilities
None stated.

6.3 Shelf life
18 Months

6.4 Special precautions for storage
Store below 25°C and protect from light.

6.5 Nature and contents of container
Type III PhEur, 125ml amber glass bottle, sealed with a polyethylene screw cap with polypropylene seal and tamper evident closure, containing 120ml of solution.

6.6 Special precautions for disposal and other handling
None.

7. MARKETING AUTHORISATION HOLDER
Sanofi-aventis
One Onslow Street
Guildford
Surrey
GU1 4YS
UK

8. MARKETING AUTHORISATION NUMBER(S)
PL 04425/0326

9. DATE OF FIRST AUTHORISATION/RENEWAL OF THE AUTHORISATION
1st September 2009

10. DATE OF REVISION OF THE TEXT
1st September 2009

LEGAL CLASSIFICATION
POM

Molipaxin Tablets 150mg

(sanofi-aventis)

1. NAME OF THE MEDICINAL PRODUCT
Molipaxin 150mg Tablets

2. QUALITATIVE AND QUANTITATIVE COMPOSITION
Tablet containing 150mg of Trazodone Hydrochloride.

For excipients, see 6.1

3. PHARMACEUTICAL FORM
Tablets.

4. CLINICAL PARTICULARS

4.1 Therapeutic indications
Relief of symptoms in all types of depression including depression accompanied by anxiety.

4.2 Posology and method of administration
Route of administration: Oral.

Depression:

a) Adults:

Initially 150mg/day in divided doses after food or as a single dose on retiring.

This may be increased up to 300mg/day in a single or divided doses. The major portion of a divided dose to be taken on retiring. The dose may be further increased to 600mg/day in divided doses in hospitalised patients.

b) Elderly:

For very elderly or frail patients initially 100mg/day in divided doses or as a single night-time dose. This may be increased, under supervision, according to efficacy and tolerance. It is unlikely that 300mg/day will be exceeded.

Depression accompanied by anxiety:

As for depression.

Anxiety:

75mg/day increasing to 300mg/day as necessary.

Tolerability may be improved by taking Molipaxin after food.

4.3 Contraindications
Known sensitivity to trazodone and any of the excipients.

4.4 Special warnings and precautions for use
Suicide/suicidal thoughts or clinical worsening

Depression is associated with an increased risk of suicidal thoughts, self harm and suicide (suicide-related events). This risk persists until significant remission occurs. As improvement may not occur during the first few weeks or more of treatment, patients should be closely monitored until such improvement occurs. It is general clinical experience that the risk of suicide may increase in the early stages of recovery.

Other psychiatric conditions for which Molipaxin is prescribed can also be associated with an increased risk of suicide-related events. In addition, these conditions may be co-morbid with major depressive disorder. The same precautions observed when treating patients with major depressive disorder should therefore be observed when treating patients with other psychiatric disorders.

Patients with a history of suicide-related events, or those exhibiting a significant degree of suicidal ideation prior to commencement of treatment are known to be at greater risk of suicidal thoughts or suicide attempts, and should receive careful monitoring during treatment. A meta-analysis of placebo-controlled clinical trials of antidepressant drugs in adult patients with psychiatric disorders showed an increased risk of suicidal behaviour with antidepressants compared to placebo in patients less than 25 years old.

Close supervision of patients and in particular those at high risk should accompany drug therapy especially in early treatment and following dose changes. Patients (and caregivers of patients) should be alerted about the need to monitor for any clinical worsening, suicidal behaviour or thoughts and unusual changes in behaviour and to seek medical advice immediately if these symptoms present.

Care should be exercised when administering Molipaxin to patients suffering epilepsy, avoiding in particular, abrupt increases or decreases in dosage.

Molipaxin should be administered with care in patients with severe hepatic, renal or cardiac disease.

Potent CYP3A4 inhibitors may lead to increases in trazodone serum levels. See section 4.5 for further information.

4.5 Interaction with other medicinal products and other forms of interaction
In vitro drug metabolism studies suggest that there is a potential for drug interactions when Molipaxin is given with potent CYP3A4 inhibitors such as erythromycin, ketoconazole, itraconazole, ritonavir, indinavir, and nefazodone. It is likely that potent CYP3A4 inhibitors may lead to substantial increases in trazodone plasma concentrations with the potential for adverse effects. Exposure to ritonavir during initiation or resumption of treatment in patients receiving Molipaxin will increase the potential for excessive sedation, cardiovascular, and gastrointestinal effects. If Molipaxin is used with a potent CYP3A4 inhibitor, a lower dose of Molipaxin should be considered. However, the co-administration of Molipaxin and potent CYP3A4 inhibitors should be avoided where possible.

Carbamazepine reduced plasma concentrations of trazodone when coadministered. Patients should be closely monitored to see if there is a need for an increased dose of Molipaxin when taken with carbamazepine.

Although no untoward effects have been reported, Molipaxin may enhance the effects of muscle relaxants and volatile anaesthetics. Similar considerations apply to combined administration with sedative and anti-depressant drugs, including alcohol. Molipaxin has been well tolerated in depressed schizophrenic patients receiving standard phenothiazine therapy and also in depressed parkinsonian patients receiving therapy with levodopa.

Possible interactions with monoamine oxidase inhibitors have occasionally been reported. Although some clinicians do give both concurrently, we do not recommend concurrent administration with MAOIs, or within two weeks of stopping treatment with these compounds. Nor do we recommend giving MAOIs within one week of stopping Molipaxin.

Since Molipaxin is only a very weak inhibitor of noradrenaline re-uptake and does not modify the blood pressure response to tyramine, interference with the hypotensive action of guanethidine-like compounds is unlikely. However, studies in laboratory animals suggest that Molipaxin may inhibit most of the acute actions of clonidine. In the case of other types of antihypertensive drug, although no clinical interactions have been reported, the possibility of potentiation should be considered.

Concurrent use with Molipaxin may result in elevated serum levels of digoxin or phenytoin. Monitoring of serum levels should be considered in these patients.

4.6 Pregnancy and lactation
Although studies in animals have not shown any direct teratogenic effect, the safety of Molipaxin in human pregnancy has not been established. On basic principles, therefore, its use during the first trimester should be avoided.

The possibility of Molipaxin being excreted in the milk should also be considered in nursing mothers.

4.7 Effects on ability to drive and use machines
As with all other drugs acting on the central nervous system, patients should be warned against the risk of handling machinery and driving.

4.8 Undesirable effects
Cases of suicidal ideation and suicidal behaviours have been reported during Molipaxin therapy or early after treatment discontinuation (see section 4.4).

Molipaxin is a sedative antidepressant and drowsiness, sometimes experienced during the first days of treatment, usually disappears on continued therapy.

Anticholinergic-like symptoms do occur but the incidence is similar to placebo.

The following symptoms, most of which are commonly reported in cases of untreated depression, have also been recorded in small numbers of patients receiving Molipaxin therapy: dizziness, headache, nausea and vomiting, weakness, decreased alertness, weight loss, tremor, dry mouth, bradycardia, tachycardia, postural hypotension, oedema, constipation, diarrhoea, blurred vision, restlessness, confusional states, insomnia and skin rash.

Blood dyscrasias, including agranulocytosis, thrombocytopenia and anaemia, have been reported on rare occasions. Adverse effects on hepatic function, including jaundice and hepatocellular damage, sometimes severe, have been rarely reported. Should such effects occur, Molipaxin should be discontinued immediately.

As with other drugs with alpha-adrenolytic activity, Molipaxin has very rarely been associated with priapism. This may be treated with an intracavernosum injection of an alpha-adrenergic agent such as adrenaline or metaraminol. However there are reports of Trazodone-induced priapism which have required surgical intervention or led to permanent sexual dysfunction. Patients developing this suspected adverse reaction should cease Molipaxin immediately.

In contrast to the tricyclic antidepressants, Molipaxin is devoid of anticholinergic activity. Consequently, troublesome side effects such as dry mouth, blurred vision and urinary hesitancy have occurred no more frequently than in patients receiving placebo therapy. This may be of importance when treating depressed patients who are at risk from conditions such as glaucoma, urinary retention and prostatic hypertrophy.

Studies in animals have shown that Molipaxin is less cardiotoxic than the tricyclic antidepressants, and clinical studies suggest that the drug may be less likely to cause cardiac arrhythmias in man. Clinical studies in patients with pre-existing cardiac disease indicate that Trazodone may be arrhythmogenic in some patients in that population. Arrhythmias identified include isolated premature ventricular contractions, ventricular couplets, and short episodes (3-4 beats) of ventricular tachycardia.

There have been occasional reports of serotonin syndrome and convulsions associated with the use of Molipaxin, especially when associated with other psychotropic drugs. Neuroleptic malignant syndrome may, very rarely, arise in the course of treatment with Molipaxin.

Hyponatraemia has been reported in association with treatment with this product. Fluid and electrolyte status should be monitored in symptomatic patients.

Molipaxin has had no effect on arterial blood pCO_2 or pO_2 levels in patients with severe respiratory insufficiency due to chronic bronchial or pulmonary disease.

4.9 Overdose
FEATURES OF TOXICITY

The most frequently reported reactions to overdose have included drowsiness, dizziness, nausea and vomiting. In more serious cases coma, tachycardia, hypotension, hyponatraemia, convulsions and respiratory failure have been reported. Cardiac features may include bradycardia, QT prolongation and torsade de pointes. Symptoms may appear 24 hours or more after overdose.

Overdoses of Molipaxin in combination with other antidepressants may cause serotonin syndrome.

MANAGEMENT

There is no specific antidote to trazodone. Activated charcoal should be considered in adults who have ingested more than 1 g trazodone, or in children who have ingested more than 150 mg trazodone within 1 hour of presentation. Alternatively, in adults, gastric lavage may be considered within 1 hour of ingestion of a potentially life-threatening overdose.

Observe for at least 6 hours after ingestion (or 12 hours if a sustained release preparation has been taken). Monitor BP, pulse and GCS. Monitor oxygen saturation if GCS is reduced. Cardiac monitoring is appropriate in symptomatic patients.

Single brief convulsions do not require treatment. Control frequent or prolonged convulsions with intravenous diazepam (0.1-0.3 mg/kg body weight) or lorazepam (4 mg in an adult and 0.05 mg/kg in a child). If these measures do not control the fits, an intravenous infusion of phenytoin may be useful. Give oxygen and correct acid base and metabolic disturbances as required.

Treatment should be symptomatic and supportive in the case of hypotension and excessive sedation. If severe hypotension persists consider use of inotropes, eg dopamine or dobutamine

5. PHARMACOLOGICAL PROPERTIES

5.1 Pharmacodynamic properties
ATC code: N06A X05. Other antidepressants.

Molipaxin is a potent antidepressant. It also has anxiety reducing activity. Molipaxin is a triazolopyridine derivative chemically unrelated to known tricyclic, tetracyclic and other antidepressant agents. It has negligible effect on noradrenaline re-uptake mechanisms. Whilst the mode of action of Molipaxin is not known precisely, its antidepressant activity may concern noradrenergic potentiation by mechanisms other than uptake blockade. A central anti-serotonin effect may account for the drug's anxiety reducing properties.

5.2 Pharmacokinetic properties
Trazodone is rapidly absorbed from the gastro-intestinal tract and extensively metabolised. Paths of metabolism of Trazodone include n-oxidation and hydroxylation. The metabolic m-chlorophenylpiperazine is active. Trazodone is excreted in the urine almost entirely in the form of its metabolites, either in free or in conjugated form. The elimination of Trazodone is biphasic, with a terminal elimination half-life of 5 to 13 hours. Trazodone is excreted in breast milk.

There was an approximate two-fold increase in terminal phase half-life and significantly higher plasma concentrations of Trazodone in 10 subjects aged 65 to 74 years compared with 12 subjects aged 23 to 30 years following a 100mg dose of Trazodone. It was suggested that there is an age-related reduction in the hepatic metabolism of Trazodone.

In vitro studies in human liver microsomes show that trazodone is metabolised by cytochrome P4503A4 (CYP3A4) to form m-chlorophenylpiperazine. Whilst significant, the role of this pathway in the total clearance of trazodone in vivo has not been fully determined.

5.3 Preclinical safety data
None stated.

6. PHARMACEUTICAL PARTICULARS
6.1 List of excipients
The tablets also contain lactose, calcium hydrogen phosphate, microcrystalline cellulose, maize starch, sodium starch glycollate, povidone and magnesium stearate. The film coating contains hydroxypropyl methyl cellulose, propylene glycol, red iron oxide E172 and titanium dioxide.

6.2 Incompatibilities
None stated.

6.3 Shelf life
36 months.

6.4 Special precautions for storage
Blister packs: Store in a dry place below 30°C.

6.5 Nature and contents of container
Blister packs: pack size 28

6.6 Special precautions for disposal and other handling
None.

7. MARKETING AUTHORISATION HOLDER
Sanofi-aventis

One Onslow Street

Guildford

Surrey

GU1 4YS

UK

8. MARKETING AUTHORISATION NUMBER(S)
PL 00109/0133

9. DATE OF FIRST AUTHORISATION/RENEWAL OF THE AUTHORISATION
16 April 1997

10. DATE OF REVISION OF THE TEXT
5 March 2008

LEGAL CLASSIFICATION
POM

Morhulin Ointment (Actavis UK Ltd)

(Actavis UK Ltd)

1. NAME OF THE MEDICINAL PRODUCT
Morhulin Ointment

2. QUALITATIVE AND QUANTITATIVE COMPOSITION
Morhulin Ointment contains:

Zinc Oxide BP 38.0% w/w

Cod Liver Oil BP 11.4% w/w

3. PHARMACEUTICAL FORM
Ointment

4. CLINICAL PARTICULARS
4.1 Therapeutic indications
The treatment of minor wounds, minor excoriations, pressure sores, varicose ulcers, eczema and napkin rash.

4.2 Posology and method of administration
Adults, Children and the Elderly

Directions for use in wounds requiring a dressing.

The ointment should be applied thinly to clean dressing material, sufficient to cover the affected area and an area of healthy skin extending beyond the affected part. The dressing should then be pressed gently on to the wound.

Directions for use in superficial wounds:

The ointment can be used directly, one to three times a day.

4.3 Contraindications
Hypersensitivity to any of the ingredients.

4.4 Special warnings and precautions for use
If symptoms persist, the doctor should be consulted. For external use only.

4.5 Interaction with other medicinal products and other forms of interaction
None known.

4.6 Pregnancy and lactation
Medicines should be avoided during pregnancy unless the anticipated benefits outweigh the risks.

4.7 Effects on ability to drive and use machines
None stated.

4.8 Undesirable effects
In rare cases, rashes may occur.

4.9 Overdose
In the case of deliberate or accidental ingestion of large quantities of Morhulin Ointment, symptomatic and supportive treatment should be provided.

5. PHARMACOLOGICAL PROPERTIES
5.1 Pharmacodynamic properties
Cod Liver Oil promotes the healing of wounds. The oil contains glyceryl ethers which have a direct action on tissues of mesenchymal origin which may explain the healing properties of Cod Liver Oil. Cod Liver Oil also contains Vitamin A which contributes to its healing effects. Zinc Oxide accelerates the removal of necrotic tissue from skin ulcers and has an established value in the treatment of minor skin wounds.

5.2 Pharmacokinetic properties
Morhulin Ointment is applied topically to the affected area.

5.3 Preclinical safety data
Not applicable

6. PHARMACEUTICAL PARTICULARS
6.1 List of excipients
Liquid Paraffin BP

Yellow Soft Paraffin BP

Lanolin Anhydrous BP

Castor Oil BP

Diluted Sodium Hypochlorite Solution NF

6.2 Incompatibilities
None known.

6.3 Shelf life
Two years.

6.4 Special precautions for storage
Store at or below 25°C in a dry place.

6.5 Nature and contents of container
a) Lacquered aluminium tube with white polypropylene flowerpot cap (20G).

b) Plain aluminium tube with polyethylene flowerpot cap (50G).

c) White polyethylene jar with white polyethylene wadless cap (350G).

6.6 Special precautions for disposal and other handling
None stated.

7. MARKETING AUTHORISATION HOLDER
Actavis Group PTC ehf

Reykjavíkurvegi 76-78

220 Hafnarfjordur

Iceland.

8. MARKETING AUTHORISATION NUMBER(S)
PL 30306/0079

9. DATE OF FIRST AUTHORISATION/RENEWAL OF THE AUTHORISATION
15th January 2003

10. DATE OF REVISION OF THE TEXT

Morphine Sulphate Injection BP 10mg in 1ml, 15mg in 1ml & 30mg in 1ml

(UCB Pharma Limited)

1. NAME OF THE MEDICINAL PRODUCT
Morphine Sulphate Injection BP 10mg in1ml, 15mg in 1ml or 30mg in 1ml.

2. QUALITATIVE AND QUANTITATIVE COMPOSITION
Morphine Sulphate Injection BP 10mg, 15mg or 30mg in 1ml.

3. PHARMACEUTICAL FORM
Sterile aqueous solution for parenteral administration to human beings.

4. CLINICAL PARTICULARS
4.1 Therapeutic indications
Morphine is used for the symptomatic relief of severe pain; relief of dyspnoea of left ventricular failure and pulmonary oedema; pre-operative use.

4.2 Posology and method of administration
The injection may be given by the intravenous, intramuscular or subcutaneous route.

Adults: The dosage should be based on the severity of the pain and the response and tolerance of the patient. The usual adult subcutaneous or intramuscular dose is 10mg every 4 hours if necessary, but may range from 5mg to 20mg.

The usual adult intravenous dose is 2.5mg to 15mg not more than 4 hourly, where necessary, but dosage and dosing interval must be titrated against the patient's response and adjustments made until analgesia is achieved.

Elderly: Because of the depressant effect on respiration, caution is necessary when giving morphine to the elderly and reduced doses may be required.

Children: Use in children is not recommended.

4.3 Contraindications
Respiratory depression, obstructive airways disease, concurrent treatment with monoamine oxidase inhibitors or within two weeks of their discontinuation of treatment with them.

Known morphine sensitivity, or sensitivity to any of the ingredients. Cerebral oedema, head injuries, coma, convulsive disorders and raised intracranial pressure, biliary colic and acute alcoholism.

Administration of morphine is contra-indicated in patients with phaeochromocytoma or those at risk of paralytic ileus.

4.4 Special warnings and precautions for use
Morphine should be administered with care to patients with hypotension, asthma, hypothyroidism, decreased respiratory reserve, hepatic and renal impairment, adrenocortical insufficiency, prostatic hypertrophy, shock, inflammatory or obstructive bowel disease or myasthenia gravis, and to patients with a history of drug abuse.

4.5 Interaction with other medicinal products and other forms of interaction
Concurrent administration of other CNS depressants, including hypnotics and anxiolytics, may potentiate the sedative effects.

Morphine should not be administered to patients receiving monoamine oxidase inhibitors (see section 4.3).

Anticholinergic agents such as atropine antagonise morphine-induced respiratory depression and can partially reverse biliary spasm but are additive to the gastro-intestinal and urinary tract effects. Consequently, severe constipation and urinary retention may occur during intensive anticholinergic-analgesic therapy.

Morphine sulphate should not be used for premedication when ciprofloxacin is given for surgical prophylaxis as serum levels of ciprofloxacin are reduced and adequate cover may not be obtained during surgery.

4.6 Pregnancy and lactation
Pregnancy: Since morphine rapidly crosses the placental barrier, it is not advised to administer morphine during labour because of the risk of respiratory depression in the new born infant.

As with all drugs it is not advisable to administer morphine during pregnancy.

Lactation: Only small amounts of morphine are secreted in breast milk and the quantity that may reach the neonate via breast milk is probably insufficient to cause major problems of dependence or adverse effects. However, caution is advised on the use of morphine in breast-feeding patient and the benefit must outweigh the risk to the infant. If breast feeding is continued, the infant should be observed for possible adverse effects.

4.7 Effects on ability to drive and use machines
Morphine may cause drowsiness. If this occurs the patient should not be allowed to drive or operate machinery.

4.8 Undesirable effects
Morphine may cause nausea, vomiting, constipation, drowsiness, confusion, dry mouth, sweating, facial flushing, vertigo, bradycardia, palpitations, tachycardia, orthostatic hypotension, hypothermia, restlessness, hallucinations, headache, changes of mood and miosis, muscle rigidity with high doses, decreased libido or potency. Micturition may be difficult and there may be ureteric or biliary spasm. There is also an antidiuretic effect. These effects are more likely to occur in ambulant patients.

Raised intracranial pressure occurs in some patients. Morphine has been reported to increase liver enzymes as a result of spasm of the sphincter of Oddi.

Allergic reactions including urticaria, pruritus, rash, contact dermatitis, bronchospasm, angioedema and anaphylactic reactions may occasionally occur. Pain and irritation may occur on injection.

Larger doses of morphine may produce respiratory depression and hypotension with circulatory failure and deepening coma. Death may occur from respiratory failure.

Morphine may produce physical and psychological dependence.

4.9 Overdose
Symptoms of serious overdose include respiratory depression and hypotension with circulatory failure, deepening coma, hypothermia, convulsions especially in infants and children and rhabdomyolosis progressing to renal failure.

Treatment with specific antidote Naloxone is used to rapidly counteract the severe respiratory depression and coma produced by excessive doses of morphine.

5. PHARMACOLOGICAL PROPERTIES
5.1 Pharmacodynamic properties
Morphine is a narcotic analgesic obtained from opium, which acts mainly on the central nervous system and smooth muscle.

5.2 Pharmacokinetic properties
Absorption: Variably absorbed after oral administration; rapidly absorbed after subcutaneous or intramuscular administration.

Blood concentration: After an oral dose of 10mg as the sulphate, peak serum concentrations of free morphine of about 10ng/ml are attained in 15 to 60 minutes; after an intramuscular dose of 10mg, peak serum concentrations of 70 to 80ng/ml are attained in 10 to 20 minutes; after an intravenous dose of 10mg, serum concentrations of about 60ng/ml are obtained in 15 minutes falling to 30ng/ml after 30 minutes and to 10ng/ml after 3 hours; subcutaneous doses give similar concentrations to intramuscular doses at 15 minutes but remain slightly higher during the following 3 hours; serum concentrations measured soon after administration correlate closely with the ages of the subjects studied and are increased in the aged.

Half life: Serum half life in the period 10 minutes to 6 hours following intravenous administration, 2 to 3 hours; serum half life in the period 6 hours onwards, 10 to 44 hours.

Distribution: Widely distributed throughout the body, mainly in the kidneys, liver, lungs and spleen; lower concentrations appear in the brain and muscles; morphine crosses the placenta and traces are secreted in sweat and milk; protein binding, about 35% bound to albumin and to immunoglobulins at concentrations within the therapeutic range.

Metabolic reactions: Mainly glucuronic acid conjugation to form morphine-3 and 6-glucuronides, with sulphate conjugation. N-demethylation, 0-methylation and N-oxide glucuronide formation occurs in the intestinal mucosa and liver; N-demethylation occurs to a greater extent after oral than parenteral administration; the 0-methylation pathway to form codeine has been challenged and codeine and norcodeine metabolites in urine may be formed from codeine impurities in the morphine sample studied.

Excretion: After an oral dose, about 60% is excreted in the urine in 24 hours, with about 3% excreted as free morphine in 48 hours; after parenteral dose, about 90% is excreted in 24 hours, with about 10% as free morphine, 65 to 70% as conjugated morphine, 1% as normorphine and 3% as normorphine glucuronide; after administration of large doses to addicts about 0.1% of a dose is excreted as norcodeine; urinary excretion of morphine appears to be pH dependent to some extent: as the urine becomes more acid more free morphine is excreted and as the urine becomes more alkaline more of the glucuronide conjugate is excreted; up to 10% of a dose may be excreted in the bile.

5.3 Preclinical safety data
None available

6. PHARMACEUTICAL PARTICULARS
6.1 List of excipients
Sodium metabisulphite
Sodium hydroxide (as in solution)
Sulphuric acid (as in solution)
Water for injection

6.2 Incompatibilities
Morphine salts may be precipitated in alkaline solution.

6.3 Shelf life
3 years

6.4 Special precautions for storage
Store below 25°C and protect from light.

6.5 Nature and contents of container
Ceramically printed, ring snap ampoule manufactured from white neutral glass type 1, conforming to European Pharmacopoeia test for hydrolytic resistance containing morphine sulphate injection 10mg in 1ml, packed in cartons of 5 or 10 ampoules; 15mg in 1ml packed in cartons of 5 or 10 ampoules or 30mg in 1ml packed in cartons of 5 or 10 ampoules and 60mg in 2ml, packed in cartons of 5 ampoules.

Ring snap ampoule manufactured from white neutral glass type 1 conforming to European Pharmacopoeia test for hydrolytic resistance to which will be attached an adhesive vinyl label after filling containing morphine sulphate injection 10mg in 1ml, packed in cartons of 5 or 10 ampoules; 15mg in 1ml packed in cartons of 5 or 10 ampoules or 300mg in 10ml, packed in cartons of 1 ampoule.

6.6 Special precautions for disposal and other handling
None

7. MARKETING AUTHORISATION HOLDER
UCB Pharma Limited
208 Bath Road
Slough
Berkshire
SL1 3WE
UK

8. MARKETING AUTHORISATION NUMBER(S)
10mg/ml: PL 00039/5681R
15mg/ml PL 00039/5682R
30mg/ml: PL 00039/5684R

9. DATE OF FIRST AUTHORISATION/RENEWAL OF THE AUTHORISATION
10mg/ml: 17 May 1982 / 15 September 1997
15mg/ml: 17 May 1982 / 20 August 1997
30mg/ml: 14 May 1982 / 20 August 1997

10. DATE OF REVISION OF THE TEXT
June 2005

Morphine Sulphate Injection BP Minijet 1mg/ml (International Medication Systems)

(International Medication Systems (UK) Ltd)

1. NAME OF THE MEDICINAL PRODUCT
Morphine Sulphate Injection BP Minijet™

2. QUALITATIVE AND QUANTITATIVE COMPOSITION
Morphine Sulphate 1 mg/ml
For excipients, see 6.1.

3. PHARMACEUTICAL FORM
Sterile aqueous solution for intravenous, intramuscular or subcutaneous injection.

4. CLINICAL PARTICULARS
4.1 Therapeutic indications
For intravenous, intramuscular or subcutaneous injection.

For the relief of moderate to severe pain such as in myocardial infarction, severe injuries, neoplastic disease, surgery, renal colic, terminal disease and other conditions where non-narcotic analgesia has failed.

Morphine is effective in the control of post-operative pain and anxiety.

Morphine may be used for its sedative effect in the management of the severe dyspnoea in terminal lung cancer or other terminal respiratory disease.

Morphine should be used as a sedative or hypnotic generally only when pain relief and sedation are required. It is used in pre-anaesthetic medication for surgery, where it reduces anxiety and also the amount of anaesthetic required.

For open-heart surgery, especially in high risk patients with cardiac disease, morphine may be used to produce anaesthesia.

4.2 Posology and method of administration
The dose and dosing regimen should be tailored to the individual patient's needs.

Adults and children over 12 years:

Intramuscular or subcutaneous administration

5-20 mg every 4 hours as necessary, dependent upon the patient's response and cause of pain.

For the relief of pain and as pre-anaesthetic, the usual dose is 10mg every 4 hours depending on the severity of the condition and the patient's response. The usual individual dose range is 5-15mg. The usual daily dose range is 12-120mg.

Intravenous administration

Acute pain:

2 to 15mg by slow intravenous injection.

or

Loading dose as above, followed by 2.5 - 5mg every hour by infusion. If using Patient Controlled Analgesia (PCA), bolus doses of 1 - 2mg may be given with a lock out of 5 - 20 minutes. A commonly applied dose limit used in PCA is 30mg in 4 hours, although some patients may require higher doses.

or

Frequent small doses (eg 1 -3 mg every 5 minutes) reaching a maximum cumulative dose of 2 - 3mg/kg. (This is the preferred regimen for patients with myocardial infarction.)

Chronicpain:

Loading doses of 15mg or more. Maintenance doses for infusion are in the range 0.8 - 80mg/hour, although higher maintenance doses of 150-200mg/hour may be required.

Similar doses have been given by subcutaneous infusion.

Open heart surgery

Large doses (0.5 - 3mg/kg) may be administered intravenously by slow continuous infusion as the sole anaesthetic agent.

Elderly:

Morphine should be administered with caution in the elderly and a reduced starting dose titrated to provide optimal pain relief.

Children under 12 years:

Intramuscular or subcutaneous administration:

Up to 1 month: 150mcg/kg every 4 hours
1-12 months: 200mcg/kg every 4 hours
1-5 years: 2.5-5mg every 4 hours
6-12 years: 5-10mg every 4 hours

Slow intravenous infusion:

Up to 6 months: up to 10mcg/kg/hour with respiratory support. Bolus injection to be avoided.

6 months - 12 years: 10-30mcg/kg/hour. A loading dose of 100-200mcg/kg may be given initially with bolus top-up doses of 50-100mcg/kg every 4 hours.

Subcutaneous infusion:

6 months - 12 years: 30-60mcg/kg/hour. For the relief of pain in terminal disease.

4.3 Contraindications
Morphine is contraindicated in patients with obstructive airways disease; respiratory depression; known morphine sensitivity; sensitivity to any of the other ingredients; head injuries; coma; convulsive disorders and raised intracranial pressure; biliary colic; acute alcoholism; cerebral oedema; concurrent treatment with monoamine oxidase inhibitors or within two weeks of their discontinuation of treatment with them; phaeochromocytoma and those at risk of paralytic ileus.

4.4 Special warnings and precautions for use
Morphine is a potent medicine but with considerable potential for harmful effect, including addiction. It should be used only if other drugs with fewer hazards are inadequate, and with the recognition that it may possibly mask significant manifestations of disease which should be identified for proper diagnosis and treatment. Dependence may occur after 1-2 weeks of treatment.

Morphine should be given with caution where there is a reduced respiratory reserve as in emphysema, chronic cor pulmonale, kyphoscoliosis and excessive obesity. Opiates should also be used cautiously in patients with cardiac arrhythmias, myasthenia gravis or inflammatory or obstructive bowel disorders.

Morphine should be administered with caution or in reduced doses to patients with hypothyroidism, adrenocortical insufficiency, impaired kidney or liver function, prostatic hypertrophy or shock.

Morphine should be given with great care to infants, especially neonates. Dosage should be reduced in elderly and debilitated patients.

4.5 Interaction with other medicinal products and other forms of interaction
Monoamine oxidase inhibitors markedly potentiate the action of morphine; morphine should not be administered to patients receiving monoamine oxidase inhibitors (see section 4.3).

The depressant effects of morphine may be potentiated and prolonged by central nervous system depressants such as alcohol, anaesthetics, analgesics, antihistamines, barbiturates, narcotics, phenothiazines, sedatives, hypnotics and tricyclic antidepressants.

Chlorpromazine and some other phenothiazines appear to enhance the sedative action but diminish the analgesic effect of morphine. The use of tricyclic antidepressants, aspirin and other NSAIDs may increase the extent of pain relief of morphine. They also increase the risks of adverse effects.

Anticholinergic agents such as atropine antagonise morphine-induced respiratory depression and can partially reverse biliary spasm but are additive to the gastro-intestinal and urinary tract effects. Consequently, severe constipation and urinary retention may occur during intensive anticholinergic-analgesic therapy.

Morphine Sulphate should not be used for pre-medication when ciprofloxacin is given for surgical prophylaxis as serum levels of ciprofloxacin are reduced and adequate cover may not be obtained during surgery.

4.6 Pregnancy and lactation
There is inadequate evidence of safety in human pregnancy. Morphine is known to cross the placenta and it may cause respiratory depression by this route. It is not advised to administer morphine during pregnancy or during labour. It may reduce uterine contractions, cause respiratory depression in the foetus and neonate, and may have significant effects on the foetal heart rate.

Only small amounts of morphine are secreted in breast milk and the quantity that may reach the neonate via breast milk is probably insufficient to cause major problems of dependence or adverse effects. However, caution is advised on the use of morphine in breast-feeding patient and the benefit must outweigh the risk to the infant. If breast feeding is continued, the infant should be observed for possible adverse effects.

4.7 Effects on ability to drive and use machines
Morphine may cause drowsiness. Patients receiving morphine should not drive or operate machinery.

4.8 Undesirable effects
The commonest side effects are nausea, vomiting, constipation, drowsiness and confusion. Psychological and physical dependence may occur. Other side effects include bronchospasm, angioedema, urinary retention, ureteric or biliary spasm, dry mouth, sweating, rash, facial flushing, vertigo, tachycardia, bradycardia, palpitations, orthostatic hypotension, hypothermia, restlessness, mood change, hallucinations, seizures (adults and children) and miosis, headache and allergic reactions (including anaphylaxis) and decreased libido or potency. Raised intracranial pressure occurs in some patients. Muscle rigidity may occur with high doses.

Morphine has been reported to increase liver enzymes as a result of spasm of the sphincter of Oddi.

Large doses can produce respiratory depression, hypotension with circulatory failure and coma. Convulsions may occur in children and infants. Rhabdomyolysis may progress to renal failure. Death may occur from respiratory depression or from pulmonary oedema after overdose.

Urticaria, pruritus, hypotension and flushing may be caused by a morphine dose-related histamine release. Contact dermatitis may occur. Pain at the site of the injection has been reported.

4.9 Overdose
Symptoms: respiratory depression, pin-point pupils and coma. In addition, shock, reduced body temperature and hypotension may occur. In mild overdose, symptoms include nausea and vomiting, tremor, miosis, dysphoria, hypothermia, hypotension, confusion and sedation. In acute poisoning, respiratory collapse and death may occur.

Treatment: the patient must be given respiratory support and the specific antagonist, naloxone, should be administered at a dose of 0.4-2.0 mg intravenously. This dose should be repeated at 2-3 minute intervals if improvement is not achieved, up to a total of 10 mg. Fluid and electrolyte levels should be maintained.

5. PHARMACOLOGICAL PROPERTIES
5.1 Pharmacodynamic properties
ATC Code: N02A A01
Morphine is the principle alkaloid of opium and is a potent analgesic. It exerts its primary effects on the central nervous system and smooth muscle. Pharmacological effects include analgesia, drowsiness, alteration in mood, reduction in body temperature, dose-related respiratory depression, interference with adrenocortical response to stress (at high doses) and a reduction in peripheral resistance with little or no effect on cardiac index and miosis. Morphine, as other opioids, acts as an agonist interacting with stereospecific and saturable binding sites/receptors in the brain, spinal cord and other tissues.

Morphine acts on the cough centre to suppress coughing and also directly stimulates the chemoreceptor trigger zone in the medulla to produce nausea and vomiting. Morphine provokes the release of histamine.

5.2 Pharmacokinetic properties
After subcutaneous or intramuscular injection, morphine is readily absorbed into the blood. Peak analgesia occurs 50-90 minutes after SC injection, 30-60 minutes after IM and 20 minutes after IV infusion. The effect persists for up to 4-5 hours.

Most of the morphine dose is conjugated with glucoronide in the liver (first pass effect), resulting in morphine-3-glucoronide (inactive) and morphine-6-glucuronide (active). Other active metabolites are formed in small amounts.

About 35% of the dose is protein bound. Morphine can cross the placenta and blood-brain barrier and its metabolites have been detected in the cerebrospinal fluid. Morphine is distributed throughout the body, mainly into skeletal muscle, kidneys, liver, intestinal tract, lungs and spleen.

The mean plasma elimination half life for morphine is 1.5-2.0 hours and for the 3-glucuronide ranges from 2.5-7.0 hours.

Approximately 90% of a parenteral dose of morphine appears in the urine within 24 hours, primarily as the product of glucuronide conjugation with only a small amount as the unchanged drug. 7-10% is excreted in the bile and eliminated in the faeces.

5.3 Preclinical safety data
Not applicable, since morphine sulphate has been used in clinical practice for many years and its effects on man are well known.

6. PHARMACEUTICAL PARTICULARS
6.1 List of excipients
Disodium edetate

Sodium metabisulphite

Water for Injection

6.2 Incompatibilities
Morphine salts may be precipitated in alkaline solution. Compatibility should be checked before admixture with other drugs.

6.3 Shelf life
24 months.

6.4 Special precautions for storage
Do not store above 25°C. Protect from light.

6.5 Nature and contents of container
The solution is contained in a Type I USP glass vial with a rubber closure which meets all the relevant USP specifications for elastomeric closures.

The following volumes are available:

Morphine Sulphate Injection 1mg/ml: 2ml (Minijet™)

10ml (Minijet™)

6.6 Special precautions for disposal and other handling
The 2ml and 10ml containers are designed for use with the IMS Minijet™ injector.

7. MARKETING AUTHORISATION HOLDER
International Medication Systems (UK) Ltd

208 Bath Road

Slough

Berkshire

SL1 3WE

UK

8. MARKETING AUTHORISATION NUMBER(S)
PL 03265/0037

9. DATE OF FIRST AUTHORISATION/RENEWAL OF THE AUTHORISATION
Date first granted: 14 March 1978

Date renewed: 12 October 2002

10. DATE OF REVISION OF THE TEXT
February 2005

POM

Motens Tablets 4mg
(Boehringer Ingelheim Limited)

1. NAME OF THE MEDICINAL PRODUCT
Motens® 4 mg Tablets.

2. QUALITATIVE AND QUANTITATIVE COMPOSITION
Tablets containing lacidipine 4 mg.

Excipient: Lactose 255.25 mg per tablet.

For full list of excipients, see 6.1.

3. PHARMACEUTICAL FORM
Film coated tablets.

4. CLINICAL PARTICULARS
4.1 Therapeutic indications
MOTENS is indicated for the treatment of hypertension either alone or in combination with other antihypertensive agents, including β-adrenoceptor antagonists, diuretics, and ACE-inhibitors.

4.2 Posology and method of administration
Adults:

The treatment of hypertension should be adapted to the severity of the condition, and according to the individual response.

The recommended initial dose is 2 mg once daily. The dose may be increased to 4 mg (and then, if necessary, to 6 mg) after adequate time has been allowed for the full pharmacological effect to occur. In practice, this should not be less than 3 to 4 weeks. Daily doses above 6 mg have not been shown to be significantly more effective.

MOTENS should be taken at the same time each day, preferably in the morning.

Treatment with MOTENS may be continued indefinitely.

Patients with hepatic impairment:

Lacidipine is metabolised primarily by the liver and therefore in patients with hepatic impairment, the bioavailability of MOTENS may be increased and the hypotensive effect enhanced. These patients should be carefully monitored, and in severe cases, a dose reduction may be necessary.

Patients with kidney disease:

As MOTENS is not cleared by the kidneys, the dose does not require modification in patients with kidney disease.

Use in children:

No experience has been gained with MOTENS in children.

4.3 Contraindications
MOTENS tablets are contraindicated in patients with known hypersensitivity to any ingredient of the preparation. MOTENS should only be used with great care in patients with a previous allergic reaction to another dihydropyridine because there is a theoretical risk of cross-reactivity.

As with other calcium antagonists, MOTENS should be discontinued in patients who develop cardiogenic shock and unstable angina. In addition, dihydropyridines have been shown to reduce coronary arterial blood-flow in patients with aortic stenosis and in such patients MOTENS is contraindicated.

MOTENS should not be used during or within one month of a myocardial infarction.

In case of rare hereditary conditions that may be incompatible with an excipient of the product (please refer to section 4.4 Special Warnings and Precautions for Use) the use of the product is contraindicated.

4.4 Special warnings and precautions for use
In specialised studies MOTENS has been shown neither to affect the spontaneous function of the sinoatrial (SA) node nor to cause prolonged conduction within the atrioventricular (AV) node. However, the theoretical potential for a calcium antagonist to affect the activity of the SA and AV nodes should be noted, and care should be taken in patients with pre-existing abnormalities. As has been reported with certain dihydropyridine calcium channel antagonists, MOTENS should be used with caution in patients with congenital or documented acquired QT prolongation. MOTENS should also be used with caution in patients treated concomitantly with medications known to prolong the QT interval such as class I and III antiarrhythmics, tricyclic antidepressants, certain antipsychotics, antibiotics and antihistaminic agents.

There is no evidence that MOTENS is useful for secondary prevention of myocardial infarction.

In healthy volunteers, patients and pre-clinical studies, MOTENS did not inhibit myocardial contractility. But as with other calcium antagonists, MOTENS should be used with caution in patients with poor cardiac reserve.

The efficacy and safety of MOTENS in the treatment of malignant hypertension has not been established.

Caution should be exercised in patients with hepatic impairment because the antihypertensive effect may be increased.

There is no evidence that MOTENS impairs glucose tolerance or alters diabetic control.

This product contains 255.25 mg lactose. Patients with rare hereditary problems of galactose intolerance, the Lapp lactase deficiency or glucose-galactose malabsorption should not take this medicine.

4.5 Interaction with other medicinal products and other forms of interaction
Co-administration of MOTENS with other agents recognised to have a hypotensive effect including antihypertensive agents (e.g. diuretics, β-adrenoceptor antagonists or ACE-inhibitors) may have an additive hypotensive effect.

The plasma concentration of MOTENS may be increased by simultaneous administration of cimetidine.

As with other dihydropyridines, MOTENS should not be taken with grapefruit juice as bioavailability may be altered.

MOTENS is highly protein-bound (>95%) to albumin and α_1-glycoprotein.

No specific pharmacodynamic interaction problems have been identified in studies with common antihypertensive agents or with digoxin, tolbutamide or warfarin.

Lacidipine is known to be metabolised by cytochrome CYP3A4 and, therefore, significant inhibitors and inducers of CYP3A4 administered concurrently may interact with the metabolism and elimination of lacidipine.

4.6 Pregnancy and lactation
Although some dihydropyridine compounds have been found to be teratogenic in animals, data in the rat and rabbit for MOTENS provide no evidence of a teratogenic effect. Using doses far above the therapeutic range, in animals MOTENS shows evidence of maternal toxicity resulting in increased pre- and post-implantation losses and possibly delayed ossification. Evidence from experimental animals has indicated that administration of MOTENS results in prolongation of gestational period and prolonged and difficult labour as a consequence of relaxation of uterine muscle. Milk transfer studies in animals have shown that lacidipine (or its metabolites) are likely to be excreted into breast milk. There is, however, no clinical experience of MOTENS in pregnancy and lactation. Accordingly, MOTENS should not be used during pregnancy or lactation.

4.7 Effects on ability to drive and use machines
MOTENS may cause dizziness. Patients should be warned not to drive or operate machinery if they experience dizziness or related symptoms.

4.8 Undesirable effects
MOTENS is generally well tolerated. Some individuals may experience minor side effects which are related to its known pharmacological action of peripheral vasodilation. Such effects, indicated by a hash (#), are usually transient and usually disappear with continued administration of MOTENS at the same dosage.

Adverse events have been ranked under headings of frequency using the following convention:

Very common	≥1/10
Common	≥1/100, <1/10
Uncommon	≥1/1000, <1/100
Rare	≥1/10000, <1/1000
Very rare	<1/10000
Not known	Cannot be estimated from the available data

<u>Nervous system disorders:</u>

Dizziness#	common
Tremor	very rare
Headache#	common

Cardiac disorders:

Angina pectoris	uncommon

As with other dihydropyridines aggravation of underlying angina pectoris has been reported in a small number of individuals, especially at the start of treatment. This is more likely to happen in patients with symptomatic ischaemic heart disease. MOTENS should be discontinued under medical supervision in patients who develop unstable angina.

Palpitations#	common
Vascular disorders:	
Flushing#	common
Gastrointestinal disorders:	
Stomach discomfort	common
Nausea	common
Gingival hyperplasia	uncommon
Skin and subcutaneous tissue disorders:	
Angioedema	rare
Urticaria	rare
Rash	common
Erythema	common
Pruritus	common
Renal and urinary disorders:	
Polyuria	common
General disorders and administration site conditions:	
Asthenia	common
Oedema#	common
Investigations:	
Blood alkaline phosphatase increased	common

Muscle cramps and disturbances of mood have also been reported rarely.

4.9 Overdose

Symptoms:

There have been no recorded cases of MOTENS overdosage. The expected symptoms could comprise prolonged peripheral vasodilation associated with hypotension and tachycardia. Bradycardia or prolonged AV conduction could occur.

Therapy:

There is no specific antidote. Standard general measures for monitoring cardiac function and appropriate supportive and therapeutic measures should be used.

5. PHARMACOLOGICAL PROPERTIES

5.1 Pharmacodynamic properties

MOTENS is a specific and potent calcium antagonist with a predominant selectivity for calcium channels in the vascular smooth muscle. Its main action is to dilate peripheral arterioles, reducing peripheral vascular resistance and lowering blood pressure.

In a study of ten patients with a renal transplant, MOTENS has been shown to prevent an acute decrease in renal plasma flow and glomerular filtration rate about six hours after administering oral cyclosporin. During the trough phase of cyclosporin treatment, there was no difference in renal plasma flow and glomerular filtration rate between patients with or without MOTENS.

Following the oral administration of 4 mg lacidipine to volunteer subjects, a minimal prolongation of QTc interval has been observed (mean QTcF increase between 3.44 and 9.60 ms in young and elderly volunteers). This was not associated with any adverse clinical effects or cardiac arrhythmias on monitoring.

5.2 Pharmacokinetic properties

MOTENS is a highly lipophilic compound; it is rapidly absorbed from the gastrointestinal tract following oral dosing. Absolute bioavailability averages about 10% due to extensive first-pass metabolism in the liver.

Peak plasma concentrations are reached between 30 and 150 minutes. The drug is eliminated primarily by hepatic metabolism (involving cytochrome P450 CYP3A4). There is no evidence that MOTENS causes either induction or inhibition of hepatic enzymes.

The principal metabolites possess little, if any, pharmacodynamic activity.

Approximately 70% of the administered dose is eliminated as metabolites in the faeces and the remainder as metabolites in the urine.

The average terminal half-life of MOTENS ranges from between 13 and 19 hours at steady state.

5.3 Preclinical safety data

In acute toxicity studies, MOTENS has shown a wide safety margin.

In repeated dose toxicological studies, findings in animals, related to the safety profile of MOTENS in man, were reversible and reflected the pharmacodynamic effect of MOTENS.

No data of clinical relevance have been gained from *in vivo* and *in vitro* studies on reproduction toxicity, genetic toxicity or oncogenicity.

6. PHARMACEUTICAL PARTICULARS

6.1 List of excipients

Tablet core:

Lactose (monohydrate)

Lactose (spray-dried)

Povidone K30

Magnesium stearate

Film coating:

Titanium Dioxide (E 171)

Methylhydroxypropylcellulose

6.2 Incompatibilities

None known.

6.3 Shelf life

24 months

6.4 Special precautions for storage

Do not store above 30°C.

MOTENS is light sensitive. MOTENS tablets should, therefore, be stored in the original container and should not be removed from their foil pack until required for administration.

Keep out of the reach of children.

6.5 Nature and contents of container

Cartons containing 7, 14 and 28 tablets packed in blister strips.

[The 7 tablet pack is not currently marketed.]

6.6 Special precautions for disposal and other handling

No special requirements.

7. MARKETING AUTHORISATION HOLDER

Boehringer Ingelheim Limited

Ellesfield Avenue

Bracknell

Berkshire

RG12 8YS

United Kingdom

8. MARKETING AUTHORISATION NUMBER(S)

PL 00015/0189

9. DATE OF FIRST AUTHORISATION/RENEWAL OF THE AUTHORISATION

29 April 1993

10. DATE OF REVISION OF THE TEXT

June 2009

Legal category

POM

Motifene 75mg

(Daiichi Sankyo UK Limited)

1. NAME OF THE MEDICINAL PRODUCT

Motifene

2. QUALITATIVE AND QUANTITATIVE COMPOSITION

Capsules containing 75 mg diclofenac sodium. Each capsule contains 25 mg diclofenac as enteric coated pellets and 50 mg diclofenac as sustained release pellets.

3. PHARMACEUTICAL FORM

Hard gelatin capsules (size 2) with light blue opaque cap and colourless transparent body marked in white print "D75M".

4. CLINICAL PARTICULARS

4.1 Therapeutic indications

Motifene is indicated for the treatment of rheumatoid arthritis; osteoarthrosis; low back pain; acute musculo-skeletal disorders and trauma such as periarthritis (especially frozen shoulder), tendinitis, tenosynovitis, bursitis, sprains, strains and dislocations; relief of pain in fractures; ankylosing spondylitis; acute gout; control of pain and inflammation in orthopaedic, dental and other minor surgery.

4.2 Posology and method of administration

For oral administration.

The capsules should be swallowed whole with a liberal quantity of liquid.

To be taken preferably with or after food.

Undesirable effects may be minimised by using the lowest effective dose for the shortest duration necessary to control symptoms (see section 4.4).

Adults:

One capsule daily. Dose may be increased to two capsules daily if necessary. The first dose should be taken in the morning with breakfast and the second if required 8-12 hours later.

Children:

Not for use in children.

Elderly:

The elderly are at increased risk of the serious consequences of adverse reactions. If an NSAID is considered necessary, the lowest effective dose should be used and for the shortest possible duration. The patient should be monitored regularly for GI bleeding during NSAID therapy.

4.3 Contraindications

- Hypersensitivity to any of the constituents.
- Previous hypersensitivity reactions (eg asthma, urticaria, angioedema or rhinitis) in response to ibuprofen, aspirin or other non-steroidal anti-inflammatory drugs.
- Severe hepatic, renal and cardiac failure (See section 4.4 – Special warnings and precautions for use).
- During the last trimester of pregnancy (See section 4.6 – Pregnancy and lactation).
- Active or previous peptic ulcer.
- History of upper gastrointestinal bleeding or perforation, related to previous NSAID therapy.
- Use with concomitant NSAIDs including cyclooxygenase-2 specific inhibitors (See section 4.5 - Interactions).

4.4 Special warnings and precautions for use

In all patients:

Undesirable effects may be minimised by using the lowest effective dose for the shortest duration necessary to control symptoms (see section 4.2, and GI and cardiovascular risks below).

Elderly:

The elderly have an increased frequency of adverse reactions to NSAIDs especially gastrointestinal bleeding and perforation which may be fatal (See section 4.2 – Posology and administration).

Respiratory disorders:

Caution is required if administered to patients suffering from, or with a previous history of, bronchial asthma since NSAIDs have been reported to precipitate bronchospasm in such patients.

Renal and Hepatic Impairment:

The administration of an NSAID may cause a dose dependent reduction in prostaglandin formation and precipitate renal failure. Patients at greatest risk of this reaction are those with impaired renal function, cardiac impairment, liver dysfunction, those taking diuretics and the elderly. Renal function should be monitored in these patients (See section 4.3 – Contraindications).

Cardiovascular and cerebrovascular effects:

Appropriate monitoring and advice are required for patients with a history of hypertension and/or mild to moderate congestive heart failure as fluid retention and oedema have been reported in association with NSAID therapy.

Clinical trial and epidemiological data suggest that use of diclofenac, particularly at high dose (150 mg daily) and in long term treatment may be associated with a small increased risk of arterial thrombotic events (for example myocardial infarction or stroke).

Patients with uncontrolled hypertension, congestive heart failure, established ischaemic heart disease, peripheral arterial disease, and/or cerebrovascular disease should only be treated with diclofenac after careful consideration. Similar consideration should be made before initiating longer-term treatment of patients with risk factors for cardiovascular events (eg hypertension, hyperlipidaemia, diabetes mellitus, smoking).

Gastrointestinal bleeding, ulceration and perforation:

GI bleeding, ulceration or perforation, which can be fatal, has been reported with all NSAIDs at any time during treatment, with or without warning symptoms or a previous history of serious GI events.

Patients with a history of GI toxicity, particularly when elderly, should report any unusual abdominal symptoms (especially GI bleeding) particularly in the initial stages of treatment.

Caution should be advised in patients receiving concomitant medications which could increase the risk of gastrotoxicity or bleeding, such as corticosteroids, or anticoagulants such as warfarin or anti-platelet agents such as aspirin (See section 4.5 – Interactions).

When GI bleeding or ulceration occurs in patients receiving Motifene, the treatment should be withdrawn.

NSAIDs should be given with care to patients with a history of gastrointestinal disease (ulcerative colitis, Crohn's disease) as these conditions may be exacerbated (See section 4.8 – Undesirable effects).

SLE and mixed connective tissue disease:

In patients with systemic lupus erythematosus (SLE) and mixed connective tissue disorders there may be an increased risk of aseptic meningitis (See section 4.8 – Undesirable effects).

Female fertility:

The use of Motifene may impair female fertility and is not recommended in women attempting to conceive. In women who have difficulties conceiving or who are undergoing investigation of infertility, withdrawal of Motifene should be considered.

Motifene, in common with other NSAIDs, can reversibly inhibit platelet aggregation.

4.5 Interaction with other medicinal products and other forms of interaction

Other analgesics: Avoid concomitant use of two or more NSAIDs (including aspirin) as this may increase the risk of adverse effects (See section 4.3 – Contraindications).

Anti-hypertensives: Reduced anti-hypertensive effect.

Diuretics: Reduced diuretic effect. Diuretics can increase the risk of nephrotoxicity of NSAIDs. Concomitant treatment with potassium-sparing diuretics may be associated with increased serum potassium levels, hence serum potassium should be monitored.

Cardiac glycosides: NSAIDs may exacerbate cardiac failure, reduced GFR (Glomerular Filtration Rate) and increase plasma glycoside levels.

Lithium: Decreased elimination of lithium.

Methotrexate: Decreased elimination of methotrexate.

Caution should be exercised if NSAIDs and methotrexate are administered within 24 hours of each other.

Ciclosporin: Increased risk of nephrotoxicity.

Mifepristone: NSAIDs should not be used for 8-12 days after mifepristone administration as NSAIDs can reduce the effect of mifepristone.

Corticosteroids: Increased risk of GI bleeding (See section 4.4 – Special warnings and precautions for use).

Anti-coagulants: NSAIDs may enhance the effects of anti-coagulants, such as warfarin (See section 4.4 – Special warnings and precautions for use).

Quinolone antibiotics: Animal data indicate that NSAIDs can increase the risk of convulsions associated with quinolone antibiotics. Patients taking NSAIDs and quinolones may have an increased risk of developing convulsions.

Tacrolimus: Possible increased risk of nephrotoxicity when NSAIDs are given with tacrolimus.

Pharmacodynamic studies have shown no potentiation of oral hypoglycaemic drugs, but caution and adequate monitoring are nevertheless advised.

4.6 Pregnancy and lactation

Pregnancy:

Congenital abnormalities have been reported in association with NSAID administration in man, however these are low in frequency and do not appear to follow any discernible pattern.

In view of the known effects of NSAIDs on the foetal cardiovascular system (risk of closure of the ductus arteriosus), use in the last trimester of pregnancy is contra-indicated.

The onset of labour may be delayed and the duration increased with an increased bleeding tendency in both mother and child (See section 4.3 – Contraindications).

NSAIDs should not be used during the first two trimesters of pregnancy or labour unless the potential benefit to the patient outweighs the potential risk to the foetus.

Lactation:

Following oral doses of 50 mg every 8 hours, traces of active substance have been detected in breast milk. Motifene should therefore be avoided in patients who are breast-feeding.

4.7 Effects on ability to drive and use machines

Patients who experience dizziness, drowsiness, fatigue and visual disturbances while taking NSAIDs should not drive or operate machinery.

4.8 Undesirable effects

If serious side-effects occur, Motifene should be withdrawn.

Gastrointestinal tract: The most commonly observed adverse events are gastrointestinal in nature. Peptic ulcers, perforation or GI bleeding (sometimes fatal, particularly in the elderly) may occur (See section 4.4 – Special warnings and precautions for use).

Nausea, vomiting, diarrhoea, flatulence, constipation, dyspepsia, abdominal pain, melaena, haematemesis, ulcerative stomatitis, exacerbation of colitis and Crohn's disease (See section 4.4 – Special warnings and precautions for use) have been reported following administration. Less frequently, gastritis has been observed.

Hypersensitivity: Hypersensitivity reactions have been reported following treatment with NSAIDs. These may consist of:

(a) non-specific allergic reactions and anaphylaxis

(b) respiratory reactivity comprising asthma, aggravated asthma, bronchospasm or dyspnoea

(c) assorted skin disorders, including rashes of various types, pruritus, urticaria, purpura, angiodema and, more rarely, exfoliative and bullous dermatoses (including epidermal necrolysis and erythema multiforme).

Cardiovascular: Oedema has been reported in association with NSAID treatment.

Other adverse events reported less commonly include:

Renal: Nephrotoxicity in various forms, including interstitial nephritis, nephrotic syndrome, renal failure and urinary abnormalities (e.g. haematuria).

Hepatic: Abnormal liver function, hepatitis (in isolated cases fulminant) and jaundice.

Neurological and special senses: Disturbances of vision (blurred vision, diplopia), optic neuritis, headache, paraesthesia, reports of aseptic meningitis (especially in patients with existing auto-immune disorders, such as lupus erythematosus, mixed connective tissue disease) with symptoms such as stiff neck, headache, nausea, vomiting, fever or disorientation (See section 4.4), depression, confusion, hallucinations, tinnitus, dizziness, vertigo, malaise, fatigue and drowsiness.

Isolated cases of memory disturbance, disorientation, impaired hearing, insomnia, irritability, convulsions, anxiety, nightmares, tremor, psychotic reactions.

Dermatological: Photosensitivity reactions, rashes, skin eruptions, urticaria.

Isolated cases of bullous eruptions, eczema, erythema multiforme, Stevens-Johnson syndrome, Lyell's syndrome, loss of hair.

Haematological: Thrombocytopenia, neutropenia, leucopenia, agranulocytosis, haemolytic anaemia, aplastic anaemia.

Clinical trial and epidemiological data suggest that use of diclofenac, particularly at high doses (150 mg daily) and in long term treatment may be associated with a small increased risk of arterial thrombotic events (for example myocardial infarction or stroke) (see section 4.4).

4.9 Overdose

Symptoms:

Symptoms include headache, nausea, vomiting, epigastric pain, gastrointestinal bleeding, rarely diarrhoea, disorientation, excitation, coma, drowsiness, dizziness, tinnitus, fainting and occasionally convulsions. In cases of significant poisoning, acute renal failure and liver damage are possible.

Treatment:

Management of acute poisoning with NSAIDs essentially consists of supportive and symptomatic measures.

Within one hour of ingestion of a potentially toxic amount, activated charcoal should be considered. Alternatively, in adults, gastric lavage should be considered within one hour of ingestion of a potentially life-threatening overdose.

Good urine output should be ensured.

Renal and liver function should be closely monitored.

Patients should be closely monitored for at least four hours after ingestion of potentially toxic amounts.

Frequent or prolonged convulsions should be treated with intravenous diazepam.

Other measures may be indicated by the patient's clinical condition. Specific therapies such as forced diureses; dialysis or haemoperfusion are probably of no help in eliminating NSAIDs due to their high rate of protein binding and extensive metabolism.

5. PHARMACOLOGICAL PROPERTIES

5.1 Pharmacodynamic properties

Motifene is a non-steroidal agent with marked analgesic/anti-inflammatory properties.

It is an inhibitor of prostaglandin synthetase (cyclo-oxygenase).

5.2 Pharmacokinetic properties

Diclofenac sodium is rapidly absorbed from the gut and is subject to first-pass metabolism. Therapeutic plasma concentrations occur about ½ hour after administration of Motifene. The active substance is 99.7% protein bound and the plasma half-life for the terminal elimination phase is 1-2 hours. Approximately 60% of the administered dose is excreted via the kidneys in the form of metabolites and less than 1% in unchanged form. The remainder of the dose is excreted via the bile in metabolised form.

Following rapid gastric passage, the enteric coated pellet component of Motifene ensures quick availability of the active component in the blood stream. The sustained release pellets cause a delayed release of the active component, which means one single daily dose is usually sufficient.

5.3 Preclinical safety data

Not applicable

6. PHARMACEUTICAL PARTICULARS

6.1 List of excipients

Enteric Coated Pellets:

Microcrystalline cellulose, polyvidone, colloidal anhydrous silica, methacrylic acid copolymer type C, sodium hydroxide, propylene glycol, talc, isopropanol, purified water.

Sustained Release Pellets:

Microcrystalline cellulose, polyvidone, colloidal anhydrous silica, poly (ethyl acrylate, methyl methacrylate, trimethylammonio, ethyl methacrylate chloride), dibutyl phthalate, talc, isopropanol, acetone.

Capsule Shell:

Indigotine E132, titanium dioxide E171, purified water, gelatin.

Capsule Body:

Gelatin, ink: containing shellac (USP/NF), soy lecithin (food grade) (USP), antifoam DC 1510, titanium dioxide E171, industrial methylated spirit, purified water, N-butyl alcohol.

6.2 Incompatibilities

None known.

6.3 Shelf life

5 years.

6.4 Special precautions for storage

Store below 25°C.

6.5 Nature and contents of container

The capsules are blister packed in PVC/PDVC and aluminium foil and are packed into folding cardboard cartons.

Motifene is available in 2, 4, 28, 56s.

6.6 Special precautions for disposal and other handling

Not applicable.

7. MARKETING AUTHORISATION HOLDER

Daiichi Sankyo UK Limited
Chiltern Place
Chalfont Park
Gerrards Cross
Buckinghamshire
SL9 0BG
UK

8. MARKETING AUTHORISATION NUMBER(S)

PL 08265/0003

9. DATE OF FIRST AUTHORISATION/RENEWAL OF THE AUTHORISATION

5 August 1994/9 September 2004

10. DATE OF REVISION OF THE TEXT

5 February 2008

Movelat Cream/Movelat Relief Cream

(Genus Pharmaceuticals)

1. NAME OF THE MEDICINAL PRODUCT

Movelat Cream/Movelat Relief Cream

2. QUALITATIVE AND QUANTITATIVE COMPOSITION

Mucopolysaccharide polysulphate (MPS) 0.2% w/w

Salicylic acid 2.0% w/w

3. PHARMACEUTICAL FORM

Topical Cream.

4. CLINICAL PARTICULARS

4.1 Therapeutic indications

Movelat/Movelat Relief is a mild to moderate anti-inflammatory and analgesic topical preparation for the symptomatic relief of muscular pain and stiffness, sprains and strains and pain due to rheumatic and non-serious arthritic conditions.

4.2 Posology and method of administration

Adults, the elderly and children over 12 years of age:

Two to six inches (5 -15 cm) to be massaged to the affected area up to four times a day.

Children:

The use of Movelat/Movelat Relief is contra-indicated in children under 12 years of age.

4.3 Contraindications

Not to be used on large areas of skin, broken or sensitive skin or on mucous membranes. Not to be used on children under 12 years of age. Not to be used in individuals with a known sensitivity to any active or inactive component of the formulation.

Hypersensitivity to aspirin or other non-steroidal anti-inflammatory drugs (including when taken by mouth) especially where associated with a history of asthma.

4.4 Special warnings and precautions for use

For external use only. The stated dose should not be exceeded. If the condition persists or worsens, consult a Doctor. Although systemic absorption of topical salicylate is much less than for oral dosage forms, the side effects of salicylates are theoretically possible.

Consult a doctor before use if pregnant, breast-feeding, asthmatic or on any prescribed medicines.

Some people may experience discomfort, particularly those with sensitive skin or if used in hot weather or after a bath. Wash hands immediately after use.

Discontinue use if excessive irritation or other unwanted effects occur.

4.5 Interaction with other medicinal products and other forms of interaction

Although no adequately controlled interaction studies have been undertaken, it is possible that excessive use of topical salicylates may increase the effect of coumarin anticoagulants. It is therefore advisable that caution be exercised with patients who are taking coumarin anticoagulants.

4.6 Pregnancy and lactation

Do not use during the first trimester or during late pregnancy. As with most medicines, patients must seek the doctor's advice before using if they are pregnant or breast feeding.

4.7 Effects on ability to drive and use machines
None.

4.8 Undesirable effects
Allergic skin reactions (which may include redness, burning sensation or rashes) may occur in individuals sensitive to salicylates.

4.9 Overdose
Following accidental ingestion of Movelat/Movelat Relief, individuals may present with the symptoms of salicylate poisoning (hyperventilation, tinnitus, deafness, vasodilation, sweating). The stomach should be emptied and plasma salicylate, plasma pH and electrolytes should be monitored. Forced alkaline diuresis may be required if the plasma salicylate levels are in excess of 500 mg/litre (3.6 mmol/litre) in adults or 300 mg/litre (2.2 mmol/litre) in children.

5. PHARMACOLOGICAL PROPERTIES

5.1 Pharmacodynamic properties
The Mucopolysaccharide polysulphate component of Movelat/Movelat Relief is recognised as having:

A weak inhibitory effect of PGE_2 synthesis and an indirect effect on LTB_4 production based on *in vitro* studies.

Anti-coagulant activity: as a heparinoid.

Thrombolytic activity: through potentiation of urokinase activity.

Anti-exudatory activity: through inhibition of hyaluronidase.

Salicylic acid is employed in the formulation of Movelat/Movelat Relief for its keratolytic activity.

5.2 Pharmacokinetic properties
Radiochemical studies of absorption following cutaneous application of mucopolysaccharide polysulphate have shown that between 0.3 and 4% of the mucopolysaccharide is absorbed by tissues other than at the site of application within the first eight hours. Typically between 1.7% and 4.6% will be absorbed within two to four days. Animal studies have also shown that mucopolysaccharide is bound intracellularly within the subcutis. Peak serum concentrations following cutaneous application are below the threshold of physiological relevance for coagulation.

Mucopolysaccharide is excreted in the urine partly unchanged and partly as depolymerized, shorter chain length molecules.

The plasma level of salicylic acid following cutaneous application of Movelat/Movelat Relief has been shown to remain constant at approximately 0.2 µg/ml even after repeated dosing. The total excretion of salicylate reaches a constant figure of approximately 12 mg/day. Over a seven-day period, approximately 6.9% of the administered dose is excreted renally, primarily as salicylic acid.

5.3 Preclinical safety data
None stated.

6. PHARMACEUTICAL PARTICULARS

6.1 List of excipients
Glycerol 85%
Stearic acid
Anhydrous eucerine
Myristyl alcohol
Emulsifying cetostearyl alcohol
Ethanolamine
Thymol
Isopropyl alcohol
Purified water

6.2 Incompatibilities
None.

6.3 Shelf life
5 years.

6.4 Special precautions for storage
Store below 25°C.

6.5 Nature and contents of container
Lacquered aluminium tubes.

Pack sizes: 14, 40, 50, 80, 100 g

6.6 Special precautions for disposal and other handling
Not applicable.

7. MARKETING AUTHORISATION HOLDER
Genus Pharmaceuticals Limited
T/A Genus Pharmaceuticals
Park View House
65 London Road
Newbury
Berkshire RG14 1JN
United Kingdom

8. MARKETING AUTHORISATION NUMBER(S)
PL 06831/0176

9. DATE OF FIRST AUTHORISATION/RENEWAL OF THE AUTHORISATION
24/05/2006

10. DATE OF REVISION OF THE TEXT
23 July 2008

Movelat Gel/ Movelat Relief Gel

(Genus Pharmaceuticals)

1. NAME OF THE MEDICINAL PRODUCT
Movelat Gel
Movelat Relief Gel
Movelat Relief Sport Gel

2. QUALITATIVE AND QUANTITATIVE COMPOSITION
Mucopolysaccharide polysulphate (MPS) 0.2% w/w
Salicylic acid 2.0% w/w

3. PHARMACEUTICAL FORM
Topical Gel.

4. CLINICAL PARTICULARS

4.1 Therapeutic indications
Movelat/Movelat Relief/Movelat Relief Sport is a mild to moderate anti-inflammatory and analgesic topical preparation for the symptomatic relief of muscular pain and stiffness, sprains and strains and pain due to rheumatic and non-serious arthritic conditions.

4.2 Posology and method of administration
Adults, the elderly and children over 12 years of age:
Two to six inches (5 -15 cm) to be applied to the affected area up to four times a day.
Children:
The use of Movelat/Movelat Relief/Movelat Relief Sport is contra-indicated in children under 12 years of age.

4.3 Contraindications
Not to be used on large areas of skin, broken or sensitive skin or on mucous membranes. Not to be used on children under 12 years of age. Not to be used in individuals with a known sensitivity to any active or inactive component of the formulation.

Hypersensitivity to aspirin or other non-steroidal anti-inflammatory drugs (including when taken by mouth) especially where associated with a history of asthma.

4.4 Special warnings and precautions for use
For external use only. The stated dose should not be exceeded. If the condition persists or worsens, consult a Doctor. Although systemic absorption of topical salicylate is much less than for oral dosage forms, the side effects of salicylates are theoretically possible.

Consult a doctor before use if pregnant, breast-feeding, asthmatic or on any prescribed medicines.

Some people may experience discomfort, particularly those with sensitive skin or if used in hot weather or after a bath. Wash hands immediately after use.

Discontinue use if excessive irritation or other unwanted effects occur.

4.5 Interaction with other medicinal products and other forms of interaction
Although no adequately controlled interaction studies have been undertaken, it is possible that excessive use of topical salicylates may increase the effect of coumarin anticoagulants. It is therefore advisable that caution be exercised with patients who are taking coumarin anticoagulants.

4.6 Pregnancy and lactation
Do not use during the first trimester or during late pregnancy. As with most medicines, patients must seek the doctor's advice before using if they are pregnant or breast feeding.

4.7 Effects on ability to drive and use machines
None.

4.8 Undesirable effects
Allergic skin reactions (which may include redness, burning sensation or rashes) may occur in individuals sensitive to salicylates.

4.9 Overdose
Following accidental ingestion of Movelat/Movelat Relief/Movelat Relief Sport, individuals may present with the symptoms of salicylate poisoning (hyperventilation, tinnitus, deafness, vasodilation, sweating). The stomach should be emptied and plasma salicylate, plasma pH and electrolytes should be monitored. Forced alkaline diuresis may be required if the plasma salicylate levels are in excess of 500 mg/litre (3.6 mmol/litre) in adults or 300 mg/litre (2.2 mmol/litre) in children.

5. PHARMACOLOGICAL PROPERTIES

5.1 Pharmacodynamic properties
The Mucopolysaccharide polysulphate component of Movelat/Movelat Relief/Movelat Relief Sport is recognised as having:

A weak inhibitory effect of PGE_2 synthesis and an indirect effect on LTB_4 production based on *in vitro* studies.

Anti-coagulant activity: as a heparinoid.

Thrombolytic activity: through potentiation of urokinase activity.

Anti-exudatory activity: through inhibition of hyaluronidase.

Salicylic acid is employed in the formulation of Movelat/Movelat Relief/Movelat Relief Sport for its keratolytic activity.

5.2 Pharmacokinetic properties
Radiochemical studies of absorption following cutaneous application of mucopolysaccharide polysulphate have shown that between 0.3 and 4% of the mucopolysaccharide is absorbed by tissues other than at the site of application within the first eight hours. Typically between 1.7% and 4.6% will be absorbed within two to four days. Animal studies have also shown that mucopolysaccharide is bound intracellularly within the subcutis. Peak serum concentrations following cutaneous application are below the threshold of physiological relevance for coagulation.

Mucopolysaccharide is excreted in the urine partly unchanged and partly as depolymerized, shorter chain length molecules.

The plasma level of salicylic acid following cutaneous application of Movelat/Movelat Relief/Movelat Relief Sport has been shown to remain constant at approximately 0.2 µg/ml even after repeated dosing. The total excretion of salicylate reaches a constant figure of approximately 12 mg/day. Over a seven-day period, approximately 6.9% of the administered dose is excreted renally, primarily as salicylic acid.

5.3 Preclinical safety data
None stated.

6. PHARMACEUTICAL PARTICULARS

6.1 List of excipients
Isopropyl alcohol
Monoethanolamine
Carbomer (Carbopol 940)
Disodium edetate (Titriplex III)
Polyethylene glyceryl-oleate (Tagat O)
Rosemary oil
Purified water

6.2 Incompatibilities
None.

6.3 Shelf life
5 years.

6.4 Special precautions for storage
Store below 25°C.

6.5 Nature and contents of container
Lacquered aluminium tubes.

Pack sizes: 14, 40, 50, 80, 100 g

6.6 Special precautions for disposal and other handling
Not applicable.

7. MARKETING AUTHORISATION HOLDER
Genus Pharmaceuticals Limited
T/A Genus Pharmaceuticals
Park View House
65 London Road
Newbury
Berkshire RG14 1JN
United Kingdom

8. MARKETING AUTHORISATION NUMBER(S)
PL 06831/0177

9. DATE OF FIRST AUTHORISATION/RENEWAL OF THE AUTHORISATION
24/05/2006

10. DATE OF REVISION OF THE TEXT
23 July 2008

Movicol 13.8g sachet, powder for oral solution

(Norgine Limited)

1. NAME OF THE MEDICINAL PRODUCT
MOVICOL® 13.8g sachet, powder for oral solution

2. QUALITATIVE AND QUANTITATIVE COMPOSITION
Each sachet of MOVICOL contains the following active ingredients:

Macrogol 3350	13.125 g
Sodium chloride	350.7 mg
Sodium bicarbonate	178.5 mg
Potassium chloride	46.6 mg

The content of electrolyte ions per sachet when made up to 125 ml of solution is as follows:

Sodium	65 mmol/l
Chloride	53 mmol/l
Potassium	5.4 mmol/l
Bicarbonate	17 mmol/l

For excipients, see *Section* 6.1

3. PHARMACEUTICAL FORM
Powder for oral solution. Free flowing white powder.

4. CLINICAL PARTICULARS

4.1 Therapeutic indications

For the treatment of chronic constipation. MOVICOL is also effective in resolving faecal impaction, defined as refractory constipation with faecal loading of the rectum and/or colon.

4.2 Posology and method of administration

Chronic constipation

A course of treatment for constipation with MOVICOL does not normally exceed 2 weeks, although this can be repeated if required.

As for all laxatives, prolonged use is not usually recommended. Extended use may be necessary in the care of patients with severe chronic or resistant constipation, secondary to multiple sclerosis or Parkinson's Disease, or induced by regular constipating medication in particular opioids and antimuscarinics.

Adults, adolescents and the elderly: 1 –3 sachets daily in divided doses, according to individual response.

For extended use, the dose can be adjusted down to 1 or 2 sachets daily.

Children below 12 years old: Not recommended. Alternative MOVICOL products are available for children.

__Faecal impaction__

A course of treatment for faecal impaction with MOVICOL does not normally exceed 3 days.

Adults, adolescents and the elderly: 8 sachets daily, all of which should be consumed within a 6 hour period.

Children below 12 years old: Not recommended. Alternative MOVICOL products are available for children.

Patients with impaired cardiovascular function: For the treatment of faecal impaction the dose should be divided so that no more than 2 sachets are taken in any one hour.

Patients with renal insufficiency: No dosage change is necessary for the treatment of constipation or faecal impaction.

__Administration__

Each sachet should be dissolved in 125 ml water. For use in faecal impaction 8 sachets may be dissolved in 1 litre of water.

4.3 Contraindications

Intestinal perforation or obstruction due to structural or functional disorder of the gut wall, ileus, severe inflammatory conditions of the intestinal tract, such as Crohn's disease and ulcerative colitis and toxic megacolon.

Hypersensitivity to the active ingredients or to any of the excipients.

4.4 Special warnings and precautions for use

Diagnosis of impaction/faecal loading of the rectum should be confirmed by physical or radiological examination of the abdomen and rectum.

Mild adverse drug reactions are possible as indicated in Section 4.8. If patients develop any symptoms indicating shifts of fluids/electrolytes (e.g. oedema, shortness of breath, increasing fatigue, dehydration, cardiac failure) MOVICOL should be stopped immediately and electrolytes measured and any abnormality should be treated appropriately.

4.5 Interaction with other medicinal products and other forms of interaction

No clinical interactions with other medicinal products have been reported. Macrogol raises the solubility of medicinal products that are soluble in alcohol and relatively insoluble in water. There is therefore a theoretical possibility that the absorption of such medicinal products could be transiently reduced.

4.6 Pregnancy and lactation

There is no experience of the use of MOVICOL during pregnancy and lactation and it should only be used if considered essential by the physician.

4.7 Effects on ability to drive and use machines

MOVICOL has no influence on the ability to drive and use machines.

4.8 Undesirable effects

Abdominal distension and pain, borborygmi and nausea, attributable to the expansion of the contents of the intestinal tract can occur. Mild diarrhoea which usually responds to dose reduction. Allergic reactions are a possibility.

4.9 Overdose

Severe pain or distension can be treated by nasogastric aspiration. Extensive fluid loss by diarrhoea or vomiting may require correction of electrolyte disturbances.

5. PHARMACOLOGICAL PROPERTIES

5.1 Pharmacodynamic properties

Pharmacotherapeutic group: Osmotically acting laxatives.

ATC code: A06A D65

Macrogol 3350 acts by virtue of its osmotic action in the gut, which induces a laxative effect. Macrogol 3350 increases the stool volume, which triggers colon motility via neuromuscular pathways. The physiological consequence is an improved propulsive colonic transportation of the softened stools and a facilitation of the defaecation. Electrolytes combined with macrogol 3350 are exchanged across the intestinal barrier (mucosa) with serum electrolytes and excreted in faecal water without net gain or loss of sodium, potassium and water.

For the indication of faecal impaction controlled comparative studies have not been performed with other treatments (e.g. enemas). In a non-comparative study in 27 adult patients, MOVICOL cleared the faecal impaction in 12/27 (44%) after 1 day's treatment; 23/27 (85%) after 2 days' treatment and 24/27 (89%) at the end of 3 days.

Clinical studies in the use of MOVICOL in chronic constipation have shown that the dose needed to produce normal formed stools tends to reduce over time. Many patients respond to between 1 and 2 sachets a day, but this dose should be adjusted depending on individual response.

5.2 Pharmacokinetic properties

Macrogol 3350 is unchanged along the gut. It is virtually unabsorbed from the gastro-intestinal tract. Any macrogol 3350 that is absorbed is excreted via the urine.

5.3 Preclinical safety data

Preclinical studies provide evidence that macrogol 3350 has no significant systemic toxicity potential, although no tests of its effects on reproduction or genotoxicity have been conducted.

There are no long-term animal toxicity or carcinogenicity studies involving macrogol 3350, although there are toxicity studies using high levels of orally administered high molecular macrogols that provide evidence of safety at the recommended therapeutic dose.

6. PHARMACEUTICAL PARTICULARS

6.1 List of excipients

Acesulfame potassium(E950)

Lime and lemon flavour*

(Lime and lemon flavour contains the following constituents: acacia solids, maltodextrin, lime oil, lemon oil, citral, citric acid and water).

6.2 Incompatibilities

None are known.

6.3 Shelf life

3 years.

Reconstituted solution: 6 hours.

6.4 Special precautions for storage

Sachet: Do not store above 25°C.

Reconstituted solution: Store at 2 - 8°C (in a refrigerator and covered).

6.5 Nature and contents of container

Sachet: laminate consisting of four layers: low density polyethylene, aluminium, low density polyethylene and paper.

Pack sizes: boxes of 2, 6, 8, 10, 20, 30, 50, 60 or 100 sachets. Not all pack sizes may be marketed.

6.6 Special precautions for disposal and other handling

Any unused solution should be discarded within 6 hours.

7. MARKETING AUTHORISATION HOLDER

Norgine Limited
Chaplin House
Widewater Place
Moorhall Road
Harefield
Uxbridge
Middlesex UB9 6NS
United Kingdom

8. MARKETING AUTHORISATION NUMBER(S)

PL 00322/0070

9. DATE OF FIRST AUTHORISATION/RENEWAL OF THE AUTHORISATION

18th December 1995 / 18th December 2005

10. DATE OF REVISION OF THE TEXT

March 2007

Legal Category:

P

MOVICOL Chocolate 13.9g sachet, powder for oral solution

(Norgine Limited)

1. NAME OF THE MEDICINAL PRODUCT

MOVICOL Chocolate 13.9g sachet, powder for oral solution

2. QUALITATIVE AND QUANTITATIVE COMPOSITION

Each sachet of MOVICOL Chocolate contains the following active ingredients:

Macrogol 3350	13.1250g
Sodium Chloride	0.3507g
Sodium Hydrogen Carbonate	0.1785g
Potassium Chloride	0.0317g

The content of electrolyte ions per sachet when made up to 125 ml of solution is as follows:

Sodium	65 mmol/l
Chloride	51 mmol/l
Potassium	5.4 mmol/l
Hydrogen Carbonate	17 mmol/l

The content of electrolyte ions per sachet when made up to 125 ml of solution is as follows:

For a full list of excipients, see section 6.1.

3. PHARMACEUTICAL FORM

Powder for oral solution. White to light brown free flowing powder.

4. CLINICAL PARTICULARS

4.1 Therapeutic indications

For the treatment of chronic constipation in adults and children above the age of 12. MOVICOL Chocolate is also effective in resolving faecal impaction, defined as refractory constipation with faecal loading of the rectum and/or colon.

4.2 Posology and method of administration

__Chronic Constipation__

A course of treatment for constipation with MOVICOL Chocolate does not normally exceed two weeks, although this can be repeated if required.

As for all laxatives, prolonged use is not usually recommended. Extended use may be necessary in the care of patients with severe chronic or resistant constipation, secondary to multiple sclerosis or Parkinson's Disease, or induced by regular constipating medication, in particular opioids and antimuscarinics.

Adults, adolescents and elderly: 1-3 sachets daily in divided doses, according to individual response.

For extended use, the dose can be adjusted down to 1 or 2 sachets daily.

Children under 12 years of age: Not recommended. Alternative MOVICOL products are available for children.

__Faecal impaction__

A course of treatment for faecal impaction with MOVICOL Chocolate does not normally exceed 3 days.

Adults, adolescents and the elderly: 8 sachets daily, all of which should be consumed within a 6 hour period.

Children under 12 years of age: Not recommended. Alternative MOVICOL products are available for children.

Patients with impaired cardiovascular function: For the treatment of faecal impaction the dose should be divided so that no more than two sachets are taken in any one hour.

Patients with renal insufficiency: No dosage change is necessary for treatment of either constipation or faecal impaction.

__Administration__

Each sachet should be dissolved in 125ml water. For use in faecal impaction 8 sachets may be dissolved in 1 litre of water.

4.3 Contraindications

Intestinal perforation or obstruction due to structural or functional disorder of the gut wall, ileus, severe inflammatory conditions of the intestinal tract, such as Crohn's disease and ulcerative colitis and toxic megacolon.

Hypersensitivity to the active ingredients or to any of the excipients.

4.4 Special warnings and precautions for use

Diagnosis of impaction/ faecal loading of the rectum should be confirmed by physical or radiological examination of the abdomen and rectum.

If patients develop any symptoms indicating shifts of fluid/electrolytes (e.g. oedema, shortness of breath, increasing fatigue, dehydration, cardiac failure) MOVICOL Chocolate should be stopped immediately and electrolytes measured, and any abnormality should be treated appropriately.

4.5 Interaction with other medicinal products and other forms of interaction

No clinical interactions with other medicinal products have been reported. Macrogol raises the solubility of medicinal products that are soluble in alcohol and relatively insoluble in water (i.e. substances that have a hydrophilic and a hydrophobic pole in their molecular structure). There is therefore a theoretical possibility that the absorption of such medicinal products could be transiently reduced.

4.6 Pregnancy and lactation

There is no experience of the use of MOVICOL Chocolate during pregnancy and lactation and it should only be used if considered essential by the physician.

4.7 Effects on ability to drive and use machines

MOVICOL Chocolate has no influence on the ability to drive and use machines.

4.8 Undesirable effects

The frequency of adverse reactions to MOVICOL from post marketing data is defined using the following MEDRA convention:

Very common ($\geq$ 1/10); common ($\geq$ 1/100, $<$ 1/10); uncommon ($\geq$ 1/1,000, $<$ 1/100); rare ($\geq$ 1/10,000,

< 1/1,000); very rare (< 1/10,000), not known (cannot be estimated from the available data).

Adverse reactions to MOVICOL are very rare.

- Gastrointestinal disorders

Very rare: Abdominal pain attributable to the expansion of the contents of the intestinal tract, diarrhoea which usually responds to dose reduction, flatulence, vomiting, nausea,

- Immune system disorders

Very rare: allergic reactions, allergic rash, anaphylactic events,

- Skin and subcutaneous tissue disorders

Very rare: pruritis, exanthema

4.9 Overdose
Severe pain or distension can be treated by nasogastric aspiration. Extensive fluid loss by diarrhoea or vomiting may require correction of electrolyte disturbances.

5. PHARMACOLOGICAL PROPERTIES

5.1 Pharmacodynamic properties
Pharmacotherapeutic group: Osmotically acting laxatives

ATC code: A06A D65

Macrogols are long linear polymers, also known as polyethylene glycols

Macrogol 3350 acts by virtue of its osmotic action in the gut, which induces a laxative effect. Macrogol 3350 increases the water content and hence the stool volume, which triggers colon motility via neuromuscular pathways. The physiological consequence is an improved propulsive colonic transportation of the softened stools and a facilitation of the defaecation. Electrolytes combined with macrogol 3350 are exchanged across the intestinal barrier (mucosa) with serum electrolytes and excreted in faecal water without net gain or loss of sodium, potassium and water.

For the indication of faecal impaction controlled comparative studies have not been performed with other treatments (e.g. enemas). In a non-comparative study in 27 adult patients, MOVICOL (parent product) cleared the faecal impaction in 12/27 (44%) after 1 day's treatment; 23/27 (85%) after 2 days' treatment and 24/27 (89%) at the end of 3 days.

Clinical studies in the use of MOVICOL (parent product) in chronic constipation have shown that the dose needed to produce normal formed stools tends to reduce over time. Many patients respond to between 1 and 2 sachets a day, but this dose should be adjusted depending on individual response.

5.2 Pharmacokinetic properties
Macrogol 3350 is unchanged along the gut. It is virtually unabsorbed from the gastro-intestinal tract. Any macrogol 3350 that is absorbed is excreted via the urine.

5.3 Preclinical safety data
Preclinical studies provide evidence that macrogol 3350 has no significant systemic toxicity potential, although no tests of its effects on reproduction or genotoxicity have been conducted.

There are no long-term animal toxicity or carcinogenicity studies involving macrogol 3350, although there are toxicity studies using high levels of orally administered high molecular macrogols that provide evidence of safety at the recommended therapeutic dose.

6. PHARMACEUTICAL PARTICULARS

6.1 List of excipients
Acesulfame Potassium (E950)

Chocolate Flavour (contains maltodextrin, acacia gum E414, vegetable oils and fats, propylene glycol E1520, and ethyl alcohol)

6.2 Incompatibilities
None are known.

6.3 Shelf life
3 years

Reconstituted solution: 6 hours.

6.4 Special precautions for storage
Sachet: Do not store above 25°C.

Reconstituted solution: Store at 2-8°C (in a refrigerator and keep covered).

6.5 Nature and contents of container
Sachet: laminate consisting of four layers: low density polyethylene, aluminium, low density polyethylene and paper.

Pack sizes: boxes of 20 or 30 sachets.

Not all pack sizes may be marketed.

6.6 Special precautions for disposal and other handling
Any unused solution should be discarded within 6 hours.

7. MARKETING AUTHORISATION HOLDER
Norgine Ltd,

Chaplin House, Widewater Place,

Moorhall Road,

Harefield, Uxbridge,

Middlesex, UB9 6NS,

United Kingdom

8. MARKETING AUTHORISATION NUMBER(S)
PL 00322/0086

9. DATE OF FIRST AUTHORISATION/RENEWAL OF THE AUTHORISATION
Date of first authorisation: 21st August 2008

10. DATE OF REVISION OF THE TEXT
21st August 2008

11 LEGAL CATEGORY
Pharmacy only

11. DOSIMETRY
Not applicable

MOVICOL Paediatric Plain 6.9 g sachet, powder for oral solution

(Norgine Limited)

1. NAME OF THE MEDICINAL PRODUCT
MOVICOL Paediatric Plain 6.9 g sachet, powder for oral solution.

2. QUALITATIVE AND QUANTITATIVE COMPOSITION
Each sachet of MOVICOL Paediatric Plain contains the following active ingredients:

Macrogol 3350	6.563 g
Sodium Chloride	175.4 mg
Sodium Bicarbonate	89.3 mg
Potassium Chloride	25.1 mg

The content of electrolyte ions per sachet when made up to 62.5 ml of solution is as follows:

Sodium	65 mmol/l
Chloride	53 mmol/l
Potassium	5.4 mmol/l
Bicarbonate	17 mmol/l

3. PHARMACEUTICAL FORM
Powder for oral solution.

Free flowing white powder.

4. CLINICAL PARTICULARS

4.1 Therapeutic indications
For the treatment of chronic constipation in children 2 to 11 years of age.

For the treatment of faecal impaction in children from the age of five years, defined as refractory constipation with faecal loading of the rectum and/or colon.

4.2 Posology and method of administration

Chronic constipation

The usual starting dose is 1 sachet daily for children aged 2 to 6 years, and 2 sachets daily for children aged 7 – 11 years. The dose should be adjusted up or down as required to produce regular soft stools. If the dose needs increasing this is best done every second day. The maximum dose needed does not normally exceed 4 sachets a day.

Treatment of children with chronic constipation needs to be or a prolonged period (a least 6 – 12 months). However, safety and efficacy of MOVICOL Paediatric Plain has only been proved for a period of up to three months. Treatment should be stopped gradually and resumed if constipation recurs.

Faecal impaction

A course of treatment for faecal impaction with MOVICOL Paediatric Plain is for up to 7 days as follows:

Daily dosage regimen:

(see Table 1)

The daily number of sachets should be taken in divided doses, all consumed within a 12 hour period. The above dosage regimen should be stopped once disimpaction has occurred. An indicator of disimpaction is the passage of a large volume of stools. After disimpaction it is recommended that the child follows an appropriate bowel management program to prevent reimpaction (dosing for prevention of re-impaction should be as for patients with chronic constipation; see above).

MOVICOL Paediatric Plain is not recommended for children below five years of age for the treatment of faecal impaction, or in children below two years of age for the treatment of chronic constipation. For patients of 12 years and older it is recommended to use MOVICOL.

Patients with impaired cardiovascular function:

There are no clinical data for this group of patients. Therefore MOVICOL Paediatric Plain is not recommended for treating faecal impaction in children with impaired cardiovascular function.

Patients with renal insufficiency:

There are no clinical data for this group of patients. Therefore MOVICOL Paediatric Plain is not recommended for treating faecal impaction in children with impaired renal function.

Administration

Each sachet should be dissolved in 62.5 ml (quarter of a glass) of water. The correct number of sachets may be reconstituted in advance and kept covered and refrigerated for up to 24 hours. For example, for use in faecal impaction, 12 sachets can be made up into 750 ml of water.

4.3 Contraindications
Intestinal perforation or obstruction due to structural or functional disorder of the gut wall, ileus, severe inflammatory conditions of the intestinal tract, such as Crohn's disease and ulcerative colitis and toxic megacolon.

Hypersensitivity to the active substances.

4.4 Special warnings and precautions for use
Diagnosis of faecal impaction/faecal loading of the rectum should be confirmed by the physical or radiological examination of the abdomen and rectum.

Rarely symptoms indicating shifts of fluid/electrolytes e.g. oedema, shortness of breath, increasing fatigue, dehydration and cardiac failure have been reported in adults when using preparations containing macrogol. If this occurs MOVICOL Paediatric Plain should be stopped immediately, electrolytes measured, and any abnormality should be treated appropriately.

When used in high doses to treat faecal impaction this medicinal product should be administered with caution to patients with impaired gag reflex, reflux oesophagitis or diminished levels of consciousness.

MOVICOL solution when reconstituted has no calorific value.

4.5 Interaction with other medicinal products and other forms of interaction
Medicinal products in solid dose form taken within one hour of administration of large volumes of macrogol preparations (as used when treating faecal impaction) may be flushed from the gastrointestinal tract and not absorbed.

No clinical interactions with other medicinal products have been reported. Macrogol raises the solubility of medicinal products that are soluble in alcohol and relatively insoluble in water. There is therefore a theoretical possibility that the absorption of such medicinal products could be transiently altered.

4.6 Pregnancy and lactation
There are no data on the use of MOVICOL Paediatric Plain during pregnancy and lactation and it should only be used if considered essential by the physician.

4.7 Effects on ability to drive and use machines
MOVICOL Paediatric Plain has no influence on the ability to drive and use machines.

4.8 Undesirable effects
The frequency of the adverse reactions listed below is defined using the following convention: very common (>1/10); common (>1/100, <1/10); uncommon (>1/1,000, <1/100); rare (>1/10,000, <1/1,000); and very rare (<1/10,000).

Chronic Constipation Indication:

Gastrointestinal disorders:

Very common: abdominal pain, borborygmi, diarrhoea or loose stools which normally respond to a reduction in dose.

Common: nausea, mild vomiting, abdominal distension, flatulence, perianal inflammation and soreness.

Immune system disorders:

Rare: allergic reactions

Faecal Impaction Indication:

Gastrointestinal disorders:

Very common: mild vomiting, abdominal distension and pain which are attributable to the expansion of the contents of the intestinal tract, perianal inflammation and soreness.

Vomiting may be resolved if the dose is reduced or delayed.

Common: borborygmi, nausea and mild diarrhoea.

Immune system disorders:

Rare: allergic reactions.

4.9 Overdose
Severe abdominal pain or distension can be treated by nasogastric aspiration. Extensive fluid loss by diarrhoea or

Table 1 Daily dosage regimen

Number of MOVICOL Paediatric Plain sachets							
Age (years)	Day 1	Day 2	Day 3	Day 4	Day 5	Day 6	Day 7
5 - 11	4	6	8	10	12	12	12

vomiting may require correction of electrolyte disturbances.

5. PHARMACOLOGICAL PROPERTIES

5.1 Pharmacodynamic properties

Pharmacotherapeutic group: Osmotically acting laxatives

ATC code: A06A D65

Macrogol 3350 acts by virtue of its osmotic action in the gut, which induces a laxative effect. Macrogol 3350 increases the stool volume, which triggers colon motility via neuromuscular pathways. The physiological consequence is an improved propulsive colonic transportation of the softened stools and a facilitation of the defaecation. Electrolytes combined with macrogol 3350 are exchanged across the intestinal barrier (mucosa) with serum electrolytes and excreted in faecal water without net gain or loss of sodium, potassium and water.

In an open study of MOVICOL in chronic constipation, weekly defaecation frequency was increased from 1.3 at baseline to 6.7, 7.2 and 7.1 at weeks 2, 4 and 12 respectively. In a study comparing MOVICOL and lactulose as maintenance therapy after disimpaction, weekly stool frequency at the last visit was 9.4 (SD 4.46) in the MOVICOL group compared with 5.9 (SD 4.29). In the lactulose group 7 children re-impacted (23%) compared with no children in the MOVICOL group.

For the indication of faecal impaction comparative studies have not been performed with other treatments (e.g. enemas). In a non-comparative study in 63 children, MOVICOL (Paediatric) cleared the faecal impaction in the majority of patients within 3 - 7 days of treatment. For the 5 - 11 years age group the average total number of sachets of MOVICOL Paediatric required was 47.2.

5.2 Pharmacokinetic properties

Macrogol 3350 is unchanged along the gut. It is virtually unabsorbed from the gastrointestinal tract. Any macrogol 3350 that is absorbed is excreted via the urine.

5.3 Preclinical safety data

Preclinical studies provide evidence that macrogol 3350 has no significant systemic toxicity potential, although no tests of its effects on reproduction or genotoxicity have been conducted.

There are no long-term animal toxicity or carcinogenicity studies involving macrogol 3350, although there are toxicity studies using high levels of orally administered high molecular macrogols that provide evidence of safety at the recommended therapeutic dose.

6. PHARMACEUTICAL PARTICULARS

6.1 List of excipients

None.

6.2 Incompatibilities

None are known.

6.3 Shelf life

3 years.

Reconstituted solution: 24 hours

6.4 Special precautions for storage

Sachet: Do not store above 25°C.

Reconstituted solution: Store in a refrigerator (2°C - 8°C) and covered.

6.5 Nature and contents of container

Sachet: laminate consisting of four layers: low density polyethylene (LDPE), aluminium, LDPE and paper.

Pack sizes: boxes of 6, 8, 10, 20, 30, 40, 50, 60 or 100 sachets.

Not all pack sizes may be marketed.

6.6 Special precautions for disposal and other handling

Any unused solution should be discarded within 24 hours.

7. MARKETING AUTHORISATION HOLDER

Norgine Pharmaceuticals Limited

Chaplin House

Widewater Place

Moorhall Road, Harefield

UXBRIDGE, Middlesex

UB9 6NS, United Kingdom

8. MARKETING AUTHORISATION NUMBER(S)

PL 20011/0005

9. DATE OF FIRST AUTHORISATION/RENEWAL OF THE AUTHORISATION

24 September 2003

10. DATE OF REVISION OF THE TEXT

March 2008

Legal Category:
POM

MOVICOL Plain 13.7g sachet, powder for oral solution

(Norgine Limited)

1. NAME OF THE MEDICINAL PRODUCT

MOVICOL Plain 13.7g sachet, powder for oral solution

2. QUALITATIVE AND QUANTITATIVE COMPOSITION

Each sachet of MOVICOL Plain contains the following active ingredients:

Macrogol 3350	13.1250 g
Sodium Chloride	0.3508 g
Sodium Hydrogen Carbonate	0.1786 g
Potassium Chloride	0.0502 g

The content of electrolyte ions per sachet when made up to 125 ml of solution is as follows:

Sodium	65 mmol/l
Chloride	53 mmol/l
Potassium	5.4 mmol/l
Hydrogen Carbonate	17 mmol/l

For excipients, see Section 6.1.

3. PHARMACEUTICAL FORM

Powder for oral solution. Free flowing white powder.

4. CLINICAL PARTICULARS

4.1 Therapeutic indications

For the treatment of chronic constipation. MOVICOL Plain is also effective in resolving faecal impaction, defined as refractory constipation with faecal loading of the rectum and/or colon.

4.2 Posology and method of administration
Chronic Constipation

A course of treatment for constipation with MOVICOL Plain does not normally exceed two weeks, although this can be repeated if required.

As for all laxatives, prolonged use is not usually recommended. Extended use may be necessary in the care of patients with severe chronic or resistant constipation, secondary to multiple sclerosis or Parkinson's Disease, or induced by regular constipating medication, in particular opioids and antimuscarinics.

Adults, adolescents and the elderly: 1-3 sachets daily in divided doses, according to individual response.

For extended use, the dose can be adjusted down to 1 or 2 sachets daily.

Children (below 12 years old): Not recommended. Alternative MOVICOL products are available for children.

Faecal impaction

A course of treatment for faecal impaction with MOVICOL Plain does not normally exceed 3 days.

Adults, adolescents and the elderly: 8 sachets daily, all of which should be consumed within a 6 hour period.

Children (below 12 years old): Not recommended. Alternative MOVICOL products are available for children.

Patients with impaired cardiovascular function: For the treatment of faecal impaction the dose should be divided so that no more than two sachets are taken in any one hour.

Patients with renal insufficiency: No dosage change is necessary for treatment of either constipation or faecal impaction.

Administration

Each sachet should be dissolved in 125ml water. For use in faecal impaction 8 sachets may be dissolved in 1 litre water.

4.3 Contraindications

Intestinal perforation or obstruction due to structural or functional disorder of the gut wall, ileus, severe inflammatory conditions of the intestinal tract, such as Crohn's disease and ulcerative colitis and toxic megacolon.

Hypersensitivity to the active ingredients or to any of the excipients.

4.4 Special warnings and precautions for use

Diagnosis of impaction/faecal loading of the rectum should be confirmed by physical or radiological examination of the abdomen and rectum.

Mild adverse drug reactions are possible as indicated in Section 4.8. If patients develop any symptoms indicating shifts of fluid/electrolytes (e.g. oedema, shortness of breath, increasing fatigue, dehydration, cardiac failure) MOVICOL Plain should be stopped immediately and electrolytes measured, and any abnormality should be treated appropriately.

4.5 Interaction with other medicinal products and other forms of interaction

No clinical interactions with other medicinal products have been reported. Macrogol raises the solubility of medicinal products that are soluble in alcohol and relatively insoluble in water. There is therefore a theoretical possibility that the absorption of such medicinal products could be transiently reduced.

4.6 Pregnancy and lactation

There is no experience of the use of MOVICOL Plain during pregnancy and lactation and it should only be used if considered essential by the physician.

4.7 Effects on ability to drive and use machines

MOVICOL Plain has no influence on the ability to drive and use machines.

4.8 Undesirable effects

Abdominal distension and pain, borborygmi and nausea, attributable to the expansion of the contents of the intestinal tract can occur. Mild diarrhoea which usually responds to dose reduction. Allergic reactions are a possibility.

4.9 Overdose

Severe pain or distension can be treated by nasogastric aspiration. Extensive fluid loss by diarrhoea or vomiting may require correction of electrolyte disturbances.

5. PHARMACOLOGICAL PROPERTIES

5.1 Pharmacodynamic properties

Pharmacotherapeutic group: Osmotically acting laxatives.

ATC code: A06A D65

Macrogol 3350 acts by virtue of its osmotic action in the gut, which induces a laxative effect. Macrogol 3350 increases the stool volume, which triggers colon motility via neuromuscular pathways. The physiological consequence is an improved propulsive colonic transportation of the softened stools and a facilitation of the defaecation. Electrolytes combined with macrogol 3350 are exchanged across the intestinal barrier (mucosa) with serum electrolytes and excreted in faecal water without net gain or loss of sodium, potassium and water.

For the indication of faecal impaction controlled comparative studies have not been performed with other treatments (e.g. enemas). In a non-comparative study in 27 adult patients, MOVICOL cleared the faecal impaction in 12/27 (44%) after 1 day's treatment; 23/27 (85%) after 2 days' treatment and 24/27 (89%) at the end of 3 days.

Clinical studies in the use of MOVICOL in chronic constipation have shown that the dose needed to produce normal formed stools tends to reduce over time. Many patients respond to between 1 and 2 sachets a day, but this dose should be adjusted depending on individual response.

5.2 Pharmacokinetic properties

Macrogol 3350 is unchanged along the gut. It is virtually unabsorbed from the gastro-intestinal tract. Any macrogol 3350 that is absorbed is excreted via the urine.

5.3 Preclinical safety data

Preclinical studies provide evidence that macrogol 3350 has no significant systemic toxicity potential, although no tests of its effects on reproduction or genotoxicity have been conducted.

There are no long-term animal toxicity or carcinogenicity studies involving macrogol 3350, although there are toxicity studies using high levels of orally administered high molecular macrogols that provide evidence of safety at the recommended therapeutic dose.

6. PHARMACEUTICAL PARTICULARS

6.1 List of excipients

None

6.2 Incompatibilities

None are known.

6.3 Shelf life

3 years.

Reconstituted solution: 6 hours.

6.4 Special precautions for storage

Sachet: Do not store above 25°C.

Reconstituted solution: Store at 2-8°C (in a refrigerator and covered)

6.5 Nature and contents of container

Each sachet contains 13.7 g of powder.

Sachet: laminate consisting of four layers: low density polyethylene, aluminium, low density polyethylene and paper.

Pack sizes: boxes of 6, 8, 10, 20, 30, 40, 50, 60 or 100 sachets.

Not all pack sizes may be marketed

6.6 Special precautions for disposal and other handling

Any unused solution should be discarded within 6 hours

7. MARKETING AUTHORISATION HOLDER

Norgine BV

Hogehilweg 7

1101 CA Amsterdam ZO

The Netherlands

8. MARKETING AUTHORISATION NUMBER(S)

PL 20142/0004

9. DATE OF FIRST AUTHORISATION/RENEWAL OF THE AUTHORISATION

12 September 2006

10. DATE OF REVISION OF THE TEXT

May 2008

MOVICOL-Half

(Norgine Limited)

1. NAME OF THE MEDICINAL PRODUCT

MOVICOL-Half 6.9g sachet, powder for oral solution

2. QUALITATIVE AND QUANTITATIVE COMPOSITION

Each sachet of MOVICOL-Half contains the following active ingredients:

Macrogol 3350	6.563g
Sodium Chloride	175.4 mg
Sodium Bicarbonate	89.3 mg
Potassium Chloride	23.3 mg

The content of electrolyte ions per sachet when made up to 62.5 ml of solution is as follows:

Sodium	65 mmol/l
Chloride	53 mmol/l
Potassium	5.4 mmol/l
Bicarbonate	17 mmol/l

For excipients, see 6.1.

3. PHARMACEUTICAL FORM

Powder for oral solution.

Free flowing white powder.

4. CLINICAL PARTICULARS

4.1 Therapeutic indications

Chronic Constipation

For the treatment of chronic constipation in adults, adolescents and the elderly.

Faecal Impaction

For resolving faecal impaction in adults, adolescents and the elderly Faecal impaction is defined as refractory constipation with faecal loading of the rectum and/or colon confirmed by physical or radiological examination of the abdomen and rectum.

4.2 Posology and method of administration

Chronic Constipation

A course of treatment for constipation with MOVICOL-Half does not normally exceed two weeks, although this can be repeated if required.

As for all laxatives, prolonged use is not usually recommended. Extended use may be necessary in the care of patients with severe chronic or resistant constipation, secondary to multiple sclerosis or Parkinson's Disease, or induced by regular constipating medication, in particular opioids and antimuscarinics.

Adults, adolescents and elderly

2 - 6 sachets daily in divided doses, according to individual response.

For extended use, the dose can be adjusted down to 2 - 4 sachets daily.

Faecal Impaction

Adults, adolescents and elderly

A course of treatment for faecal impaction with MOVICOL-Half does not normally exceed 3 days.

Dosage is 16 sachets daily, all of which should be consumed within a 6 hour period.

The above dosage regimen should be stopped once disimpaction has occurred. An indicator of disimpaction is the passage of a large volume of stools. After disimpaction it is recommended that the patient follows an appropriate bowel management programme to prevent reimpaction.

This dosage regimen is based on one clinical trial.

Children (below 12 years of age): Not recommended.

Patients with impaired cardiovascular function

For the treatment of faecal impaction the dose should be divided so that no more than four sachets are taken in any one hour.

Patients with renal insufficiency

No dosage change is necessary for treatment of either constipation or faecal impaction.

Administration

Each sachet should be dissolved in 62.5ml water. For use in faecal impaction the correct number of sachets can be reconstituted in advance and kept covered and refrigerated for up to 6 hours. For example 16 sachets can be made up into one litre of water.

4.3 Contraindications

Intestinal perforation or obstruction due to structural or functional disorder of the gut wall, ileus, severe inflammatory conditions of the intestinal tract, such as Crohn's disease and ulcerative colitis and toxic megacolon.

Known hypersensitivity to any of the active substances or excipients.

4.4 Special warnings and precautions for use

Mild adverse drug reactions are possible as indicated in Section 4.8. If patients develop any symptoms indicating shifts of fluid/electrolytes (e.g. oedema, shortness of breath, increasing fatigue, dehydration, cardiac failure) MOVICOL-Half should be stopped immediately and electrolytes measured, and any abnormality should be treated appropriately.

4.5 Interaction with other medicinal products and other forms of interaction

Medication in solid dose form taken within one hour of administration of large volumes of macrogol preparations may be flushed from the gastrointestinal tract and not absorbed.

Clinical interactions with other drugs have been reported extremely rarely. No specific reactions with individual drugs or classes of drugs have been observed.

Macrogol raises the solubility of medicinal products that are soluble in alcohol and relatively insoluble in water. There is therefore a theoretical possibility that the absorption of such medicinal products could be transiently reduced.

4.6 Pregnancy and lactation

There is no experience of the use of MOVICOL-Half during pregnancy and lactation and it should only be used if considered essential by the physician.

4.7 Effects on ability to drive and use machines

There is no effect on the ability to drive and use machines.

4.8 Undesirable effects

Reactions related to the gastrointestinal tract are the most common to occur. These may include:

Abdominal pain

Nausea

Borborygmi

Diarrhoea

Abdominal distension

Vomiting

Flatulence

Anal discomfort

These reactions may occur as a consequence of expansion of the contents of the gastrointestinal tract, and an increase in motility due to the pharmacologic effects of MOVICOL-Half. Mild diarrhoea usually responds to dose reduction.

Allergic reactions, including anaphylaxis. Other symptoms of allergic reactions include pruritus, urticaria and dyspnoea.

4.9 Overdose

Severe pain or distension can be treated by nasogastric aspiration. Extensive fluid loss by diarrhoea or vomiting may require correction of electrolyte disturbances.

5. PHARMACOLOGICAL PROPERTIES

5.1 Pharmacodynamic properties

ATC code: A06A D

Macrogol 3350 acts by virtue of its osmotic action in the gut, which induces a laxative effect. Macrogol 3350 increases the stool volume, which triggers colon motility via neuromuscular pathways. The physiological consequence is an improved propulsive colonic transportation of the softened stools and a facilitation of the defaecation. Electrolytes combined with macrogol 3350 are exchanged across the intestinal barrier (mucosa) with serum electrolytes and excreted in faecal water without net gain or loss of sodium, potassium and water.

For the indication of faecal impaction comparative studies have not been performed with other treatments (e.g. enemas). In a non-comparative study in 27 adult patients, MOVICOL 13.8g cleared the faecal impaction in 12/27 (44%) after 1 day's treatment; 23/27 (85%) after 2 days' treatment and 24/27 (89%) at the end of 3 days.

Clinical studies in the use of MOVICOL in chronic constipation have shown that the dose needed to produce normal formed stools tends to reduce over time. Many patients respond to between 2-4 sachets of MOVICOL-Half per day, but this dose should be adjusted depending on individual response.

5.2 Pharmacokinetic properties

Macrogol 3350 is unchanged along the gut. It is virtually unabsorbed from the gastro-intestinal tract. Any macrogol 3350 that is absorbed is excreted via the urine.

5.3 Preclinical safety data

Preclinical studies provide evidence that macrogol 3350 has no significant systemic toxicity potential, although no tests of its effects on reproduction or genotoxicity have been conducted.

There are no long-term animal toxicity or carcinogenicity studies involving macrogol 3350, although there are toxicity studies using high levels of orally administered high molecular macrogols that provide evidence of safety at the recommended therapeutic dose.

6. PHARMACEUTICAL PARTICULARS

6.1 List of excipients

Acesulfame K (E950)

Lime and Lemon Flavour

6.2 Incompatibilities

None are known.

6.3 Shelf life

The shelf life of the sachets is 3 years.

Discard any solution not used within 6 hours.

6.4 Special precautions for storage

Sachet: Do not store above 25°C.

Solution: Store at 2 - 8°C (refrigerated and covered)

6.5 Nature and contents of container

6.9g sachets contained in boxes of 6, 8, 10, 20, 30, 40, 50, 60 or 100 sachets.

6.6 Special precautions for disposal and other handling

None.

7. MARKETING AUTHORISATION HOLDER

Norgine Limited

Chaplin House

Widewater Place

Moorhall Road, Harefield

UXBRIDGE, Middlesex

UB9 6NS, United Kingdom

8. MARKETING AUTHORISATION NUMBER(S)

PL 00322/0080

9. DATE OF FIRST AUTHORISATION/RENEWAL OF THE AUTHORISATION

16th October 2002

10. DATE OF REVISION OF THE TEXT

Approved: January 2009

Legal Category: **P**

MOVIPREP, powder for oral solution in sachets

(Norgine Limited)

1. NAME OF THE MEDICINAL PRODUCT

MOVIPREP, powder for oral solution in sachets

2. QUALITATIVE AND QUANTITATIVE COMPOSITION

The ingredients of MOVIPREP are contained in two separate sachets.

Sachet A contains the following active substances:

Macrogol 3350	100 g
Sodium sulphate anhydrous	7.500 g
Sodium chloride	2.691 g
Potassium chloride	1.015 g

Sachet B contains the following active substances:

Ascorbic acid	4.700 g
Sodium ascorbate	5.900 g

The concentration of electrolyte ions when both sachets are made up to one litre of solution is as follows:

Sodium	181.6 mmol/l (of which not more than 56.2 mmol is absorbable)
Sulphate	52.8 mmol/l
Chloride	59.8 mmol/l
Potassium	14.2 mmol/l
Ascorbate	29.8 mmol/l

This product contains 0.233 g of aspartame per sachet A.

For a full list of excipients, see section 6.1.

3. PHARMACEUTICAL FORM

Powder for oral solution.

Free flowing white to yellow powder in Sachet A.

Free flowing white to light brown powder in Sachet B.

4. CLINICAL PARTICULARS

4.1 Therapeutic indications

For bowel cleansing prior to any clinical procedures requiring a clean bowel e.g. bowel endoscopy or radiology.

4.2 Posology and method of administration

Adults and elderly: A course of treatment consists of two litres of MOVIPREP. It is strongly recommended that one litre of clear liquid, which may include water, clear soup, fruit juice without pulp, soft drinks, tea and/or coffee without milk, is also taken during the course of treatment.

A litre of MOVIPREP consists of one 'Sachet A' and one 'Sachet B' dissolved together in one litre of water. This reconstituted solution should be drunk over a period of one to two hours. This should be repeated with a second litre of MOVIPREP.

This course of treatment can be taken:

either divided as one litre of MOVIPREP in the evening before and one litre of MOVIPREP in the early morning of the day of the clinical procedure,

- or, in the evening preceding the clinical procedure.

There should be at least one hour between the end of intake of fluid (MOVIPREP or clear liquid) and the start of colonoscopy.

No solid food should be taken from the start of the course of treatment until after the clinical procedure.

Children: Not recommended for use in children below 18 years of age, as MOVIPREP has not been studied in the paediatric population.

4.3 Contraindications

Do not use in patients with known or suspected:

- gastrointestinal obstruction or perforation

- disorders of gastric emptying (e.g. gastroparesis)
- ileus
- phenylketonuria (due to presence of aspartame)
- glucose-6-phosphate dehydrogenase deficiency (due to presence of ascorbate)
- hypersensitivity to any of the ingredients
- toxic megacolon which complicates severe inflammatory conditions of the intestinal tract including Crohn's disease and ulcerative colitis.

Do not use in unconscious patients.

4.4 Special warnings and precautions for use

Diarrhoea is an expected effect resulting from the use of MOVIPREP.

MOVIPREP should be administered with caution to fragile patients in poor health or patients with serious clinical impairment such as:

- impaired gag reflex, or with a tendency to aspiration or regurgitation
- impaired consciousness
- severe renal insufficiency (creatinine clearance <30 ml/min)
- cardiac impairment (NYHA grade III or IV)
- dehydration
- severe acute inflammatory disease

The presence of dehydration should be corrected before the use of MOVIPREP.

Semi-conscious patients or patients prone to aspiration or regurgitation should be closely observed during administration, especially if this is via a nasogastric route.

If patients develop any symptoms indicating shifts of fluid/electrolytes (e.g. oedema, shortness of breath, increasing fatigue, cardiac failure), plasma electrolytes should be measured and any abnormality treated appropriately.

In debilitated fragile patients, patients with poor health, those with clinically significant renal impairment and those at risk of electrolyte imbalance, the physician should consider performing a baseline and post-treatment electrolyte and renal function test.

If patients experience symptoms such as severe bloating, abdominal distention, abdominal pain or any other reaction which makes it difficult to continue the preparation, they may slow down or temporarily stop consuming MOVIPREP and should consult their doctor.

4.5 Interaction with other medicinal products and other forms of interaction

Oral medication should not be taken within one hour of administration of MOVIPREP as it may be flushed from the gastro-intestinal tract and not absorbed. The therapeutic effect of drugs with a narrow therapeutic index or short half-life may be particularly affected.

4.6 Pregnancy and lactation

There are no data on the use of MOVIPREP during pregnancy or lactation and it should only be used if considered essential by the physician.

4.7 Effects on ability to drive and use machines

There is no known effect on the ability to drive and use machines.

4.8 Undesirable effects

The frequency of adverse reactions to MOVIPREP is defined using the following convention:

Very common ≥ 1/10 (≥ 10%);

Common ≥ 1/100, < 1/10 (≥ 1% < 10%);

Uncommon ≥ 1/1,000, < 1/100 (≥ 0.1% < 1%);

Rare ≥ 1/10,000, < 1/1,000 (≥ 0.01% < 0.1%);

Very rare < 1/10,000 (< 0.01%).

Diarrhoea is an expected outcome of bowel preparation. Due to the nature of the intervention, undesirable effects occur in the majority of patients during the process of bowel preparation. Whilst these vary between preparations, nausea, vomiting, bloating, abdominal pain, anal irritation and sleep disturbance commonly occur in patients undergoing bowel preparation.

As with other macrogol containing products, allergic reactions including rash, urticaria, oedema and anaphylaxis are a possibility.

Data from clinical studies are available in a population of 591 patients treated with MOVIPREP in which undesirable effect data were actively elicited.

Body System	Adverse drug reaction
Metabolism and nutrition disorders:	
Common:	hunger
Uncommon	hypophosphatemia
Psychiatric disorders:	
Common	sleep disorder
Nervous system disorders:	
Common	dizziness
Uncommon	headache
Gastrointestinal disorders:	
Very common	abdominal pain, nausea, abdominal distension, anal discomfort
Common	vomiting, dyspepsia
Uncommon	dysphagia
General disorders and administration site conditions:	
Very common	malaise, thirst
Common	rigors
Uncommon	discomfort
Investigations:	
Uncommon	blood bicarbonate decreased:, blood calcium decreased:, hypercalcaemia:, blood chloride decreased:, blood chloride increased:, blood phosphorus decreased:, liver function tests abnormal

4.9 Overdose

In case of gross accidental overdosage, where diarrhoea is severe, conservative measures are usually sufficient; generous amounts of fluid, especially fruit juices, should be given. In the rare event of overdose provoking severe metabolic derangement, intravenous rehydration may be used.

5. PHARMACOLOGICAL PROPERTIES

5.1 Pharmacodynamic properties

Pharmacotherapeutic group: A06A D

Macrogol 3350, sodium sulphate and high doses of ascorbic acid exert an osmotic action in the gut, which induce a laxative effect. Macrogol 3350 increases the stool volume, which triggers colon motility via neuromuscular pathways. The physiological consequence is a propulsive colonic transportation of the softened stools. The electrolytes present in the formulation as well as the supplementary clear liquid intake ensure that there are no clinically significant variations of sodium, potassium or water, and thus no dehydration risk.

5.2 Pharmacokinetic properties

Macrogol 3350 is unchanged along the gut. It is virtually unabsorbed from the gastro-intestinal tract. Any macrogol 3350 that is absorbed is excreted via the urine

Ascorbic acid is absorbed mainly at the small intestine level by a mechanism of active transport, which is sodium dependent and saturable. There is an inverse relationship between the ingested dose and the percentage of the absorbed dose. For oral doses between 30 and 180 mg an amount of about 70-85 % of the dose is absorbed. Following oral intake of up to 12 g ascorbic acid, it is known that only 2 g is absorbed.

After high oral doses of ascorbic acid and when plasma concentrations exceed 14 mg/litre, the absorbed ascorbic acid is mainly eliminated unchanged in the urine.

5.3 Preclinical safety data

Pre-clinical studies provide evidence that macrogol 3350, ascorbic acid and sodium sulphate have no significant systemic toxicity potential.

6. PHARMACEUTICAL PARTICULARS

6.1 List of excipients

Aspartame (E951)

Acesulfame Potassium (E950)

Lemon flavour containing maltodextrin, citral, lemon oil, lime oil, xanthan gum, vitamin E.

6.2 Incompatibilities

Not applicable

6.3 Shelf life

Sachets	3 years
Reconstituted solution	24 hours

6.4 Special precautions for storage

Sachets: Store below 25°C. Store in the original package.

Reconstituted Solution: Store below 25°C. The solution may be refrigerated. Keep the solution covered.

6.5 Nature and contents of container

A paper / low density polyethylene / aluminium / low density polyethylene sachet containing 112 g of powder ('sachet A') and a paper / low density polyethylene / aluminium / low density polyethylene sachet containing 11 g of powder ('sachet B'). Both sachets are contained in a transparent bag. One pack of MOVIPREP contains a single treatment of two bags.

Pack sizes of 1, 10, 40, 80, 160 and 320 packs of a single treatment. Hospital packs of 40 single treatments. Not all pack sizes may be marketed.

6.6 Special precautions for disposal and other handling

Reconstitution of MOVIPREP in water may take up to 5 minutes and is best performed by adding the powder to the mixing vessel first followed by the water. The patient should wait until all the powder has dissolved before drinking the solution.

After reconstitution in water, MOVIPREP consumption may begin immediately or if preferred it may be cooled before use.

7. MARKETING AUTHORISATION HOLDER

Norgine BV

Hogehilweg 7, 1101CA

Amsterdam ZO

The Netherlands

8. MARKETING AUTHORISATION NUMBER(S)

PL: 20142/0005

9. DATE OF FIRST AUTHORISATION/RENEWAL OF THE AUTHORISATION

19/01/2006

10. DATE OF REVISION OF THE TEXT

27/03/2007

Legal Category: **P**

MST Continus suspensions 20, 30, 60, 100 and 200 mg

(Napp Pharmaceuticals Limited)

1. NAME OF THE MEDICINAL PRODUCT

MST® CONTINUS® suspension 20, 30, 60, 100 and 200 mg.

2. QUALITATIVE AND QUANTITATIVE COMPOSITION

Morphine equivalent to Morphine Sulphate 20, 30, 60, 100 and 200 mg.

For excipients see 6.1.

3. PHARMACEUTICAL FORM

Pink granules.

Prolonged release granules for oral suspension.

4. CLINICAL PARTICULARS

4.1 Therapeutic indications

For the prolonged relief of severe and intractable pain.

4.2 Posology and method of administration

Route of administration: Oral.

20, 30 & 60 mg strengths: The contents of one sachet should be mixed with at least 10 ml water or sprinkled on to soft food, for example yogurt.

100 mg strength: The contents of one sachet should be mixed with at least 20 ml water or sprinkled on to soft food, for example yogurt.

200 mg strength: The contents of one sachet should be mixed with at least 30 ml water or sprinkled on to soft food, for example yogurt.

The controlled release granules must be suspended whole and ingested immediately, but not be broken, chewed or crushed. The administration of broken, chewed or crushed morphine granules leads to a rapid release and absorption of a potentially fatal dose of morphine (see section 4.9, Overdose).

MST CONTINUS suspension should be used at 12-hourly intervals. The dosage is dependent upon the severity of the pain, the patient's age and previous history of analgesic requirements.

Adults:

A patient presenting with severe pain, uncontrolled by weaker opioids (e.g. dihydrocodeine) should normally be started on 30 mg 12-hourly. Patients previously on normal release oral morphine should be given the same total daily dose as MST CONTINUS suspension but in divided doses at 12-hourly intervals.

Increasing severity of pain will require an increased dosage of the suspension. Higher doses should be made, where possible in 30-50% increments as required. The correct dosage for any individual patient is that which is sufficient to control pain with no, or tolerable, side effects for a full 12 hours. It is recommended that the 200 mg strength is reserved for patients who have already been titrated to a stable analgesic dose using lower strengths of morphine or other opioid preparations.

Patients receiving MST CONTINUS suspension in place of parenteral morphine should be given a sufficiently increased dosage to compensate for any reduction in analgesic effects associated with oral administration. Usually such increased requirement is of the order of

100%. In such patients individual dose adjustments are required.

Children:

The use of MST CONTINUS suspension in children has not been extensively evaluated. For children with severe cancer pain, a starting dose in the range of 0.2 to 0.8 mg morphine per kg bodyweight 12-hourly is recommended. Doses should then be titrated as for adults.

Post-operative pain

MST CONTINUS suspension is not recommended in the first 24 hours post-operatively or until normal bowel function has returned; thereafter it is suggested that the following dosage schedule be observed at the physician's discretion:

(a) MST CONTINUS suspension 20 mg 12-hourly to patients under 70 kg

(b) MST CONTINUS suspension 30 mg 12-hourly to patients over 70 kg

(c) Elderly - a reduction in dosage may be advisable in the elderly

(d) Children - not recommended

Supplemental parenteral morphine may be given if required but with careful attention to the total dosages of morphine, and bearing in mind the prolonged effects of morphine in this controlled release formulation.

4.3 Contraindications

Hypersensitivity to any of the constituents.

Respiratory depression, head injury, paralytic ileus, 'acute abdomen', delayed gastric emptying, obstructive airways disease, known morphine sensitivity, acute hepatic disease, concurrent administration of monoamine oxidase inhibitors or within two weeks of discontinuation of their use. Children under one year of age. Pre-operative administration of MST CONTINUS suspension is not recommended.

4.4 Special warnings and precautions for use

As with all narcotics a reduction in dosage may be advisable in the elderly, in hypothyroidism and in patients with significantly impaired renal or hepatic function. Use with caution in patients with impaired respiratory function, convulsive disorders, acute alcoholism, delirium tremens, raised intracranial pressure, hypotension with hypovolaemia, severe cor pulmonale, patients with a history of substance abuse, diseases of the biliary tract, pancreatitis, inflammatory bowel disorders, prostatic hypertrophy, adrenocortical insufficiency and opiate dependent patients.

Morphine may lower the seizure threshold in patients with a history of epilepsy.

Should paralytic ileus be suspected or occur during use, MST CONTINUS suspension should be discontinued immediately. Patients about to undergo additional pain relieving procedures (e.g. surgery, plexus blockade) should not receive MST CONTINUS suspension for 24 hours prior to the intervention. If further treatment with MST CONTINUS suspension is indicated, then the dosage should be adjusted to the new post-operative requirement.

MST CONTINUS suspension should be used with caution post-operatively, and following abdominal surgery as morphine impairs intestinal motility and should not be used until the physician is assured of normal bowel function. MST CONTINUS Suspension is not recommended preoperatively or within the first 24 hours post operatively.

It is not possible to ensure bio-equivalence between different brands of controlled release morphine products. Therefore, it should be emphasised that patients, once titrated to an effective dose, should not be changed from MST CONTINUS preparations to other slow, sustained or controlled release morphine or other potent narcotic analgesic preparations without retitration and clinical assessment.

The major risk of opioid excess is respiratory depression.

The patient may develop tolerance to the drug with chronic use and require progressively higher doses to maintain pain control. Prolonged use of this product may lead to physical dependence and a withdrawal syndrome may occur upon abrupt cessation of therapy. When a patient no longer requires therapy with morphine, it may be advisable to taper the dose gradually to prevent symptoms of withdrawal.

Morphine has an abuse profile similar to other strong agonist opioids. Morphine may be sought and abused by people with latent or manifest addiction disorders. The product should be used with particular care in patients with a history of alcohol and drug abuse.

Abuse of oral dosage forms by parenteral administration can be expected to result in serious adverse events which may be fatal.

The excipient Ponceau 4R may cause allergic reactions.

4.5 Interaction with other medicinal products and other forms of interaction

Morphine potentiates the effects of tranquillisers, anaesthetics, phenothiazines, hypnotics, sedatives, alcohol, muscle relaxants and antihypertensives. Interactive effects resulting in respiratory depression, hypotension, profound sedation, or coma may result if these drugs are taken in combination with the usual doses of morphine.

Medicinal products that block the action of acetylcholine, for example antihistamines, anti-parkinsonians and anti-emetics, may interact with morphine to potentiate anticholinergic adverse events.

Concurrent administration of antacids may result in a more rapid release of morphine than otherwise expected; dosing should therefore be separated by a minimum of two hours. Cimetidine inhibits the metabolism of morphine.

Monoamine oxidase inhibitors are known to interact with narcotic analgesics producing CNS excitation or depression with hyper- or hypotensive crisis. Morphine should not be co administered with monoamine oxidase inhibitors or within two weeks of such therapy.

Plasma concentrations of morphine may be reduced by rifampicin.

Although there are no pharmacokinetic data available for concomitant use of ritonavir with morphine, ritonavir induces the hepatic enzymes responsible for the glucuronidation of morphine, and may possibly decrease plasma concentrations of morphine.

Mixed agonist/antagonist opioid analgesics (e.g. buprenorphine, nalbuphine, pentazocine) should not be administered to a patient who has received a course of therapy with a pure opioid agonist analgesic.

4.6 Pregnancy and lactation

MST CONTINUS suspension is not recommended during pregnancy and labour due to the risk of neonatal respiratory depression. Administration to nursing mothers is not recommended as morphine is excreted in breast milk. Withdrawal symptoms may be observed in the newborn of mothers undergoing chronic treatment.

4.7 Effects on ability to drive and use machines

Morphine may modify the patient's reactions to a varying extent depending on the dosage and susceptibility. If affected, patients should not drive or operate machinery.

4.8 Undesirable effects

In normal doses, the commonest side effects of morphine are nausea, vomiting, constipation and drowsiness. With chronic therapy, nausea and vomiting are unusual with MST CONTINUS suspension but should they occur the suspension can be readily combined with an anti-emetic if required. Constipation may be treated with appropriate laxatives.

Common (incidence of ⩾ 1%) and Uncommon (incidence of ⩽ 1%) adverse drug reactions are listed in the table below:

Undesirable Effects	Common (⩾ 1%)	Uncommon (⩽ 1%)
Immune system disorders		Allergic reaction Anaphylactic reaction Anaphylactoid reaction
Psychiatric disorders	Confusion Insomnia Thinking disturbances	Agitation Drug dependence Dysphoria Euphoria Hallucinations Mood altered
Nervous system disorders	Headache Involuntary muscle contractions Myoclonus Somnolence	Convulsions Hypertonia Paraesthesia Syncope Vertigo
Eye disorders		Miosis Visual disturbance
Cardiac disorders		Bradycardia Palpitations Tachycardia
Vascular disorders		Facial flushing Hypotension Hypertension
Respiratory, thoracic and mediastinal disorders	Bronchospasm Cough decreased	Pulmonary oedema Respiratory depression
Gastrointestinal disorders	Abdominal pain Anorexia Constipation Dry mouth Dyspepsia Exacerbation of pancreatitis Nausea Vomiting	Gastrointestinal disorders Ileus Colic Taste perversion
Hepatobiliary disorders		Biliary pain Increased hepatic enzymes
Skin and subcutaneous tissue disorders	Hyperhidrosis Rash	Urticaria
Renal and urinary disorders		Ureteric spasm Urinary retention
Reproductive system and breast disorders		Amenorrhea Decreased libido Erectile dysfunction
General disorders and administration site conditions	Asthenia Pruritus	Drug tolerance Drug withdrawal syndrome Malaise Peripheral oedema

The effects of morphine have led to its abuse and dependence may develop with regular, inappropriate use. This is not a major concern in the treatment of patients with severe pain.

4.9 Overdose

Signs of morphine toxicity and overdosage are pin-point pupils, skeletal muscle flaccidity, bradycardia, respiratory depression and hypotension. Circulatory failure and deepening coma may occur in more severe cases. Overdosage can result in death. Rhabdomyolosis progressing to renal failure has been reported in opioid overdosage.

Crushing and taking contents of a controlled release dosage form leads to the release of the morphine in an immediate fashion; this might result in a fatal overdose.

Treatment of morphine overdosage

Primary attention should be given to the establishment of a patent airway and institution of assisted or controlled ventilation.

The pure opioid agonists are specific antidotes against the effects of opioid overdose. Other supportive measures should be employed as needed.

In the case of massive overdosage, administer naloxone 0.8 mg intravenously. Repeat at 2-3 minute intervals as necessary, or by an infusion of 2 mg in 500 ml of normal saline or 5% dextrose (0.004 mg/ml).

The infusion should be run at a rate related to the previous bolus doses administered and should be in accordance with the patient's response. However, because the duration of action of naloxone is relatively short, the patient must be carefully monitored until spontaneous respiration is reliably re-established. MST CONTINUS suspension will continue to release and add to the morphine load for up to 12 hours after administration and the management of morphine overdosage should be modified accordingly.

For less severe overdosage, administer naloxone 0.2 mg intravenously followed by increments of 0.1 mg every 2 minutes if required.

Naloxone should not be administered in the absence of clinically significant respiratory or circulatory depression secondary to morphine overdosage.

Naloxone should be administered cautiously to persons who are known, or suspected, to be physically dependent on morphine. In such cases, an abrupt or complete reversal of opioid effects may precipitate an acute withdrawal syndrome.

Gastric contents may need to be emptied as this can be useful in removing unabsorbed drug, particularly when a modified release formulation has been taken.

5. PHARMACOLOGICAL PROPERTIES

5.1 Pharmacodynamic properties

Pharmacotherapeutic group: Natural opium alkaloid.

ATC Code: N02A 01

Morphine acts as an agonist at opiate receptors in the CNS, particularly mu and, to a lesser extent, kappa receptors. Mu receptors are thought to mediate supraspinal analgesia, respiratory depression and euphoria, and kappa receptors, spinal analgesia, miosis and sedation.

Central Nervous System

The principal actions of therapeutic value of morphine are analgesia and sedation (i.e., sleepiness and anxiolysis).

Morphine produces respiratory depression by direct action on brain stem respiratory centers.

Morphine depresses the cough reflex by direct effect on the cough center in the medulla. Antitussive effects may occur with doses lower than those usually required for analgesia.

Morphine causes miosis, even in total darkness. Pinpoint pupils are a sign of narcotic overdose but are not pathognomonic (e.g., pontine lesions of hemorrhagic or ischemic origin may produce similar findings). Marked mydriasis rather than miosis may be seen with hypoxia in the setting of morphine overdose.

Gastrointestinal Tract and Other Smooth Muscle

Morphine causes a reduction in motility associated with an increase in smooth muscle tone in the antrum of the stomach and duodenum. Digestion of food in the small intestine is delayed and propulsive contractions are decreased. Propulsive peristaltic waves in the colon are decreased, while tone is increased to the point of spasm resulting in constipation.

Morphine generally increases smooth muscle tone, especially the sphincters of the gastrointestinal and biliary tracts. Morphine may produce spasm of the sphincter of Oddi, thus raising intrabiliary pressure.

Cardiovascular System

Morphine may produce release of histamine with or without associated peripheral vasodilation. Manifestations of histamine release and/or peripheral vasodilation may include pruritus, flushing, red eyes, sweating, and/or orthostatic hypotension.

Endocrine System

Opioids may influence the hypothalamic-pituitary-adrenal or -gonadal axes. Some changes that can be seen include an increase in serum prolactin, and decreases in plasma cortisol, oestrogen and testosterone in association with inappropriately low or normal ACTH, LH or FSH levels. Clinical symptoms may be manifest from these hormonal changes.

Other Pharmacologic Effects

In vitro and animal studies indicate various effects of natural opioids, such as morphine, on components of the immune system; the clinical significance of these findings is unknown.

5.2 Pharmacokinetic properties

Morphine is bound to a cationic exchange resin and drug release is effected when morphine is displaced by ions in the gastrointestinal tract. Morphine is well absorbed and adequate plasma morphine levels are achieved following the recommended dosage regimen. However, first-pass metabolism occurs in the liver. In a single-dose study in healthy volunteers, the systemic availability of morphine from MST CONTINUS suspension 30 mg was equivalent to that from an immediate release solution 30 mg (mean 91%, 95% CI 81-102%) and from MST CONTINUS tablet 30 mg (mean 101%, 95% CI 93-109%). The suspension provided a retarded plasma profile which was comparable to that of the MST CONTINUS tablet.

5.3 Preclinical safety data

There are no pre-clinical data of relevance to the prescriber which are additional to that already included in other sections of the SPC.

6. PHARMACEUTICAL PARTICULARS

6.1 List of excipients

Dowex 50WX8 100-200 mesh cationic exchange resin

Xylitol

Xanthan gum

Raspberry flavour

Ponceau 4R (E124)

6.2 Incompatibilities

Not Applicable

6.3 Shelf life

2 years.

6.4 Special precautions for storage

Do not store above 25°C.

6.5 Nature and contents of container

Pack type: Surlyn lined, laminated aluminium foil sachets coated with polyethylene and clay coated Kraft paper.

Pack size: Boxboard cartons of 30 sachets.

6.6 Special precautions for disposal and other handling

The contents of the sachet should be added to water or sprinkled onto soft food, e.g. yogurt (see 4.2 Posology and method of administration).

Administrative Data

7. MARKETING AUTHORISATION HOLDER

Napp Pharmaceuticals Limited

Cambridge Science Park

Milton Road

Cambridge

CB4 0GW

United Kingdom

8. MARKETING AUTHORISATION NUMBER(S)

PL 16950/0030-0034

9. DATE OF FIRST AUTHORISATION/RENEWAL OF THE AUTHORISATION

14 January 1994//19 November 2006

10. DATE OF REVISION OF THE TEXT

18.02.2008

11. LEGAL CATEGORY

CD (Sch 2), POM

MST Continus tablets 5 mg, 10 mg, 15 mg, 30 mg, 60 mg, 100 mg, 200 mg

(Napp Pharmaceuticals Limited)

1. NAME OF THE MEDICINAL PRODUCT

MST® CONTINUS® tablets 5 mg, 10 mg, 15 mg, 30 mg, 60 mg, 100 mg, 200 mg.

2. QUALITATIVE AND QUANTITATIVE COMPOSITION

Tablets containing Morphine Sulphate 5 mg, 10 mg, 15 mg, 30 mg, 60 mg, 100 mg, 200 mg.

3. PHARMACEUTICAL FORM

Prolonged release, film-coated, biconvex tablets marked with the NAPP logo on one side and the strength of the preparation on the other.

MST CONTINUS tablets 5 mg are white.

MST CONTINUS tablets 10 mg are golden brown.

MST CONTINUS tablets 15 mg are green.

MST CONTINUS tablets 30 mg are purple.

MST CONTINUS tablets 60 mg are orange.

MST CONTINUS tablets 100 mg are grey.

MST CONTINUS tablets 200 mg are teal green.

4. CLINICAL PARTICULARS

4.1 Therapeutic indications

For the prolonged relief of severe and intractable pain. MST CONTINUS tablets 5 mg, 10 mg, 15 mg and 30 mg are additionally indicated for the relief of post-operative pain.

4.2 Posology and method of administration

Route of administration:

Oral.

MST CONTINUS tablets should be swallowed whole and not broken, chewed or crushed. The administration of broken, chewed or crushed tablets may lead to a rapid release and absorption of a potentially fatal dose of morphine sulphate (see section 4.9, Overdose).

MST CONTINUS tablets should be used at 12-hourly intervals. The dosage is dependent upon the severity of the pain, the patient's age and previous history of analgesic requirements.

Adults:

A patient presenting with severe pain, uncontrolled by weaker opioids (e.g. dihydrocodeine) should normally be started on 30 mg 12-hourly. Patients previously on normal release oral morphine should be given the same total daily dose as MST CONTINUS tablets but in divided doses at 12-hourly intervals.

Increasing severity of pain will require an increased dosage of the tablets. Higher doses should be made, where possible in 30-50% increments as required. The correct dosage for any individual patient is that which is sufficient to control pain with no, or tolerable, side effects for a full 12 hours. It is recommended that the 200 mg strength is reserved for patients who have already been titrated to a stable analgesic dose using lower strengths of morphine sulphate or other opioid preparations.

Patients receiving MST CONTINUS tablets in place of parenteral morphine sulphate should be given a sufficiently increased dosage to compensate for any reduction in analgesic effects associated with oral administration. Usually such increased requirement is of the order of 100%. In such patients individual dose adjustments are required.

Children:

For children with severe cancer pain, a starting dose in the range of 0.2 to 0.8 mg morphine sulphate per kg bodyweight 12-hourly is recommended. Doses should then be titrated as for adults.

Post-operative pain:

MST CONTINUS tablets are not recommended in the first 24 hours post-operatively or until normal bowel function has returned; thereafter it is suggested that the following dosage schedule be observed at the physician's discretion:

(a) MST CONTINUS tablets 20 mg 12-hourly to patients under 70 kg

(b) MST CONTINUS tablets 30 mg 12-hourly to patients over 70 kg

(c) Elderly - a reduction in dosage may be advisable in the elderly

(d) Children - not recommended.

Supplemental parenteral morphine sulphate may be given if required but with careful attention to the total dosages of morphine sulphate, and bearing in mind the prolonged effects of morphine sulphate in this prolonged release formulation.

4.3 Contraindications

Respiratory depression, head injury, paralytic ileus, 'acute abdomen', delayed gastric emptying, obstructive airways disease, hypersensitivity to any of the tablet constituents, acute hepatic disease, concurrent administration of monoamine oxidase inhibitors or within two weeks of discontinuation of their use. Children under one year of age.

Not recommended for pre-operative use or for the first 24 hours post-operatively.

4.4 Special warnings and precautions for use

As with all narcotics a reduction in dosage may be advisable in the elderly, in hypothyroidism and in patients with significantly impaired renal or hepatic function. Use with caution in patients with impaired respiratory function, convulsive disorders, acute alcoholism, delirium tremens, raised intracranial pressure, hypotension with hypovolaemia, severe cor pulmonale, patients with a history of substance abuse, opiate dependent patients, diseases of the biliary tract, pancreatitis, inflammatory bowel disorders, prostatic hypertrophy and adrenocortical insufficiency.

Morphine sulphate may lower the seizure threshold in patients with a history of epilepsy.

Should paralytic ileus be suspected or occur during use, MST CONTINUS tablets should be discontinued immediately. As with all morphine sulphate preparations, patients about to undergo additional pain relieving procedures (e.g. surgery, plexus blockade) should not receive MST CONTINUS tablets for 24 hours prior to the intervention. If further treatment with MST CONTINUS tablets is indicated then the dosage should be adjusted to the new post-operative requirement.

As with all oral morphine sulphate preparations, MST CONTINUS tablets should be used with caution post-operatively and following abdominal surgery, as morphine sulphate impairs intestinal motility and should not be used until the physician is assured of normal bowel function.

The major risk of opioid excess is respiratory depression.

The patient may develop tolerance to the drug with chronic use and require progressively higher doses to maintain pain control. Prolonged use of this product may lead to physical dependence and a withdrawal syndrome may occur upon abrupt cessation of therapy. When a patient no longer requires therapy with morphine sulphate, it may be advisable to taper the dose gradually to prevent symptoms of withdrawal.

Morphine sulphate has an abuse profile similar to other strong agonist opioids. Morphine sulphate may be sought and abused by people with latent or manifest addiction disorders. The product should be used with particular care in patients with a history of alcohol and drug abuse.

The prolonged release tablets must be swallowed whole, and not broken, chewed, dissolved or crushed. The administration of broken, chewed or crushed tablets may lead to a rapid release and absorption of a potentially fatal dose of morphine sulphate (see section 4.9).

It is not possible to ensure bioequivalence between different brands of prolonged release morphine sulphate products. Therefore, it should be emphasised that patients, once titrated to an effective dose, should not be changed from MST CONTINUS preparations to other slow, sustained or prolonged release morphine sulphate or other potent narcotic analgesic preparations without retitration and clinical assessment.

4.5 Interaction with other medicinal products and other forms of interaction

Morphine sulphate potentiates the effects of tranquillisers, anaesthetics, phenothiazines, hypnotics, sedatives, alcohol, muscle relaxants and antihypertensives.

Morphine sulphate should not be co-administered with monoamine oxidase inhibitors or within two weeks of such therapy. Interactive effects resulting in respiratory depression, hypotension, profound sedation, or coma may result if these drugs are taken in combination with the usual doses of morphine sulphate

Medicinal products that block the action of acetylcholine, for example antihistamines, anti-parkinsons and anti-emetics, may interact with morphine sulphate to potentiate anticholinergic adverse events.

Cimetidine inhibits the metabolism of morphine sulphate.

Plasma concentrations of morphine sulphate may be reduced by rifampicin.

Although there are no pharmacokinetic data available for concomitant use of ritonavir with morphine sulphate, ritonavir induces the hepatic enzymes responsible for the glucuronidation of morphine sulphate, and may possibly decrease plasma concentrations of morphine sulphate.

4.6 Pregnancy and lactation

MST CONTINUS tablets are not recommended during pregnancy and labour due to the risk of neonatal respiratory depression. Administration to nursing mothers is not recommended as morphine sulphate is excreted in breast milk. Withdrawal symptoms may be observed in the newborn of mothers undergoing chronic treatment.

4.7 Effects on ability to drive and use machines

Morphine sulphate may modify the patient's reactions to a varying extent depending on the dosage and susceptibility. If affected, patients should not drive or operate machinery.

4.8 Undesirable effects

In normal doses, the commonest side effects of morphine sulphate are nausea, vomiting, constipation and drowsiness. With chronic therapy, nausea and vomiting are unusual with MST CONTINUS tablets but should they occur the tablets can be readily combined with an anti-emetic if required. Constipation may be treated with appropriate laxatives.

Common (incidence of $>1\%$) and Uncommon (incidence of $< 1\%$) adverse drug reactions are listed in the table below:

Undesirable Effects	Common ($\geq 1\%$)	Uncommon ($\leq 1\%$)
Immune system disorders		Allergic reaction Anaphylactic reaction Anaphylactoid reaction

Psychiatric disorders	Confusion Insomnia Thinking disturbances	Agitation Drug dependence Dysphoria Euphoria Hallucinations Mood altered
Nervous system disorders	Headache Involuntary muscle contractions Myoclonus Somnolence	Convulsions Hypertonia Paraesthesia Syncope Vertigo
Eye disorders		Miosis Visual disturbance
Cardiac disorders		Bradycardia Palpitations Tachycardia
Vascular disorders		Facial flushing Hypotension Hypertension
Respiratory, thoracic and mediastinal disorders	Bronchospasm Cough decreased	Pulmonary oedema Respiratory depression
Gastrointestinal disorders	Abdominal pain Anorexia Constipation Dry mouth Dyspepsia Nausea Vomiting	Gastrointestinal disorders Ileus Taste perversion
Hepatobiliary disorders	Exacerbation of pancreatitis	Biliary pain Increased hepatic enzymes
Skin and subcutaneous tissue disorders	Hyperhidrosis Rash	Urticaria
Renal and urinary disorders		Ureteric spasm Urinary retention
Reproductive system and breast disorders		Amenorrhea Decreased libido Erectile dysfunction
General disorders and administration site conditions	Asthenia Pruritus	Drug tolerance Drug withdrawal syndrome Malaise Peripheral oedema

The effects of morphine sulphate have led to its abuse and dependence may develop with regular, inappropriate use. This is not a major concern in the treatment of patients with severe pain.

4.9 Overdose

Signs of morphine sulphate toxicity and overdosage are pin-point pupils, skeletal muscle flaccidity, bradycardia, respiratory depression and hypotension. Circulatory failure and deepening coma may occur in more severe cases. Overdosage can result in death. Rhabdomyolysis progressing to renal failure has been reported in opioid overdosage.

Crushing and taking the contents of a prolonged release dosage form may lead to the release of morphine sulphate in an immediate fashion; this might result in a fatal overdose.

Treatment of morphine sulphate overdosage:

Primary attention should be given to the establishment of a patent airway and institution of assisted or controlled ventilation.

The pure opioid antagonists are specific antidotes against the effects of opioid overdose. Other supportive measures should be employed as needed.

In the case of massive overdosage, administer naloxone 0.8 mg intravenously. Repeat at 2-3 minute intervals as necessary, or by an infusion of 2 mg in 500 ml of normal saline or 5% dextrose (0.004 mg/ml).

The infusion should be run at a rate related to the previous bolus doses administered and should be in accordance with the patient's response. However, because the duration of action of naloxone is relatively short, the patient must be carefully monitored until spontaneous respiration is reliably re-established. MST CONTINUS tablets will continue to release and add to the morphine sulphate load for up to 12 hours after administration and the management of morphine sulphate overdosage should be modified accordingly.

For less severe overdosage, administer naloxone 0.2 mg intravenously followed by increments of 0.1 mg every 2 minutes if required.

Naloxone should not be administered in the absence of clinically significant respiratory or circulatory depression secondary to morphine sulphate overdosage. Naloxone should be administered cautiously to persons who are known, or suspected, to be physically dependent on morphine sulphate. In such cases, an abrupt or complete reversal of opioid effects may precipitate an acute withdrawal syndrome.

Gastric contents may need to be emptied as this can be useful in removing unabsorbed drug, particularly when a prolonged release formulation has been taken.

5. PHARMACOLOGICAL PROPERTIES

5.1 Pharmacodynamic properties

Pharmacotherapeutic group: natural opium alkaloid ATC code: N02A A01

Morphine sulphate acts as an agonist at opiate receptors in the CNS, particularly Mu and, to a lesser extent, Kappa receptors. Mu receptors are thought to mediate supraspinal analgesia, respiratory depression and euphoria, and Kappa receptors, spinal analgesia, miosis and sedation.

Central Nervous System

The principal actions of therapeutic value of morphine sulphate are analgesia and sedation (i.e., sleepiness and anxiolysis). Morphine sulphate produces respiratory depression by direct action on brain stem respiratory centers.

Morphine sulphate depresses the cough reflex by direct effect on the cough centre in the medulla. Antitussive effects may occur with doses lower than those usually required for analgesia. Morphine sulphate causes miosis, even in total darkness. Pinpoint pupils are a sign of narcotic overdose but are not pathognomonic (e.g., pontine lesions of haemorrhagic or ischaemic origin may produce similar findings). Marked mydriasis rather than miosis may be seen with hypoxia in the setting of morphine sulphate overdose.

Gastrointestinal Tract and Other Smooth Muscle

Morphine sulphate causes a reduction in motility associated with an increase in smooth muscle tone in the antrum of the stomach and duodenum. Digestion of food in the small intestine is delayed and propulsive contractions are decreased. Propulsive peristaltic waves in the colon are decreased, while tone is increased to the point of spasm resulting in constipation. Morphine sulphate generally increases smooth muscle tone, especially the sphincters of the gastrointestinal and biliary tracts. Morphine sulphate may produce spasm of the sphincter of Oddi, thus raising intrabiliary pressure.

Cardiovascular System

Morphine sulphate may produce release of histamine with or without associated peripheral vasodilation. Manifestations of histamine release and/or peripheral vasodilation may include pruritus, flushing, red eyes, sweating, and/or orthostatic hypotension.

Endocrine System

Opioids may influence the hypothalamic-pituitary-adrenal or -gonadal axes. Some changes that can be seen include an increase in serum prolactin, and decreases in plasma cortisol and testosterone in association with inappropriately low or normal ACTH, LH or FSH levels. Some premenopausal women may have low oestrogen levels. Clinical symptoms may be manifest from these hormonal changes.

Other Pharmacological Effects

In vitro and animal studies indicate various effects of natural opioids, such as morphine sulphate, on components of the immune system; the clinical significance of these findings is unknown.

5.2 Pharmacokinetic properties

Morphine sulphate is well absorbed from MST CONTINUS tablets and, in general, peak plasma concentrations are achieved 1-5 hours following administration. The availability is complete when compared to an equivalent dose of immediate release oral solution. Morphine sulphate is subject to a significant first-pass effect which results in a lower bioavailability when compared to an equivalent intravenous dose.

The major metabolic transformation of morphine sulphate is glucuronidation to morphine sulphate-3-glucuronide and morphine sulphate-6-glucuronide which then undergo renal excretion. These metabolites are excreted in bile and may be subject to hydrolysis and subsequent reabsorption.

Patients are titrated to appropriate pain control using the wide range of strengths of MST CONTINUS tablets. Consequently, there is a large inter-patient variation in required dosage, the minimum dosage being 5 mg 12-hourly, and a dose of 5.6 g 12-hourly has been recorded.

5.3 Preclinical safety data

There are no pre-clinical data of relevance to the prescriber which are additional to that already included in other sections of the SPC.

6. PHARMACEUTICAL PARTICULARS

6.1 List of excipients

Tablet core:

Hydroxyethylcellulose Ph Eur

Purified Water Ph Eur

Cetostearyl Alcohol BP

Magnesium Stearate Ph Eur

Purified TalcPh Eur

Lactose Anhydrous (except for 100 mg and 200 mg tablets)NF

Hypromellose (E464) Ph Eur

Macrogol Ph Eur

The following tablets have the colourants listed below:

10 mg - Iron oxide (E172), Titanium dioxide (E171)

15 mg - Iron oxide (E172), brilliant blue (E133), quinoline yellow (E104), indigo carmine (E132) Titanium dioxide (E171)

30 mg - Erythrosine (E127), indigo carmine (E132), sunset yellow (E110), Titanium dioxide (E171)

60 mg - Erythrosine (E127), quinoline yellow (E104), sunset yellow (E110), Titanium dioxide (E171)

100 mg - Iron oxide (E172), indigo carmine (E132), Titanium dioxide (E171)

200 mg - Brilliant blue (E133), quinoline yellow (E104), Titanium dioxide (E171.

6.2 Incompatibilities

None stated.

6.3 Shelf life

Five years.

6.4 Special precautions for storage

Do not store above 25°C.

6.5 Nature and contents of container

Aluminium foil-backed PVdC/PVC blister packs. Pack size 60 tablets.

6.6 Special precautions for disposal and other handling

None.

7. MARKETING AUTHORISATION HOLDER

Napp Pharmaceuticals Limited

Cambridge Science Park

Milton Road

Cambridge CB4 0GW

8. MARKETING AUTHORISATION NUMBER(S)

PL 16950/0035-0041

9. DATE OF FIRST AUTHORISATION/RENEWAL OF THE AUTHORISATION

1 May 1999

10. DATE OF REVISION OF THE TEXT

April 2008

11 LEGAL CATEGORY

CD (Sch 2), POM

® MST, MST CONTINUS, CONTINUS, NAPP and the NAPP devices are Registered Trade Marks.

Mucodyne Capsules, Syrup and Paediatric Syrup

(sanofi-aventis)

1. NAME OF THE MEDICINAL PRODUCT

Mucodyne Capsules 375 mg

Mucodyne Syrup 250 mg/5 ml

Mucodyne Paediatric Syrup 125 mg

2. QUALITATIVE AND QUANTITATIVE COMPOSITION

Capsules: Carbocisteine 375 mg

Syrup: Carbocisteine 250 mg/5 ml

Paediatric Syrup: Carbocisteine 125 mg/5 ml.

For a full list of excipients, see section 6.1.

3. PHARMACEUTICAL FORM

Capsules: Size 1, yellow capsules printed 'Mucodyne 375' in black.

Syrup: A clear amber syrup smelling of rum and slightly of cinnamon.

Paediatric Syrup: Clear, red syrup.

4. CLINICAL PARTICULARS

4.1 Therapeutic indications

Carbocisteine is a mucolytic agent for the adjunctive therapy of respiratory tract disorders characterised by excessive, viscous mucus, including chronic obstructive airways disease.

4.2 Posology and method of administration

Capsules and syrup:

Adults including the elderly:

Dosage is based upon an initial daily dosage of 2250mg carbocisteine in divided doses, reducing to 1500mg daily in divided doses when a satisfactory response is obtained e.g. two capsules three times a day reducing to one capsule four times a day, for normal syrup 15ml tds. reducing to 10ml tds.

Children:

The capsule and syrup formulations are not recommended for children. The normal daily dosage is 20mg/kg bodyweight in divided doses. It is recommended that this is achieved with Mucodyne Paediatric Syrup.

Mucodyne capsules and Syrup are for oral administration.

Paediatric Syrup:

Children 5 - 12 years: 10 ml three times daily.

Children 2 - 5 years: 2.5 - 5 ml four times daily.

Mucodyne Paediatric Syrup is for oral administration.

4.3 Contraindications
Capsules and Syrup: Active peptic ulceration.

Paediatric syrup: None.

4.4 Special warnings and precautions for use
None stated.

4.5 Interaction with other medicinal products and other forms of interaction
None stated.

4.6 Pregnancy and lactation
Although tests in mammalian species have revealed no teratogenic effects, Mucodyne is not recommended during the first trimester of pregnancy.

Use in lactation: Effects not known.

4.7 Effects on ability to drive and use machines
None stated.

4.8 Undesirable effects
Capsules, Syrup and Paediatric Syrup:
Immune System Disorders

There have been reports of anaphylactic reactions and fixed drug eruption.

Skin and subcutaneous tissue disorders

There have been reports of skin rashes and allergic skin eruptions.

Capsules and Syrup:
Gastrointestinal disorders

There have been rare reports of gastrointestinal bleeding occurring during treatment with Mucodyne.

4.9 Overdose
Gastric lavage may be beneficial, followed by observation. Gastrointestinal disturbance is the most likely symptom of Mucodyne overdosage.

5. PHARMACOLOGICAL PROPERTIES
5.1 Pharmacodynamic properties
Carbocisteine (S-carboxymethyl L-cysteine) has been shown in normal and bronchitic animal models to affect the nature and amount of mucus glycoprotein which is secreted by the respiratory tract. An increase in the acid:-neutral glycoprotein ratio of the mucus and a transformation of serous cells to mucus cells is known to be the initial response to irritation and will normally be followed by hypersecretion. The administration of carbocisteine to animals exposed to irritants indicates that the glycoprotein that is secreted remains normal; administration after exposure indicates that return to the normal state is accelerated. Studies in humans have demonstrated that carbocisteine reduces goblet cell hyperplasia. Carbocisteine can therefore be demonstrated to have a role in the management of disorders characterised by abnormal mucus.

5.2 Pharmacokinetic properties
Carbocisteine is rapidly absorbed from the GI tract. In an 'in-house' study, at steady state (7 days) Mucodyne capsules 375mg given as 2 capsules t.d.s. to healthy volunteers gave the following pharmacokinetic parameters:

Plasma Determinations	Mean	Range
T Max (Hr)	2.0	1.0-3.0
T½ (Hr)	1.87	1.4-2.5
K_{EL} (Hr^{-1})	0.387	0.28-0.50
$AUC_{0-7.5}$ ($mcg.Hr.ml^{-1}$)	39.26	26.0-62.4
Derived Pharmacokinetic Parameters		
*CL_S ($L.Hr^{-1}$)	20.2	-
CL_S ($ml.min^{-1}$)	331	-
V_D (L)	105.2	-
V_D ($L.Kg^{-1}$)	1/75	-
*Calculated from dose for day 7 of study		

5.3 Preclinical safety data
No additional data of relevance to the prescriber.

6. PHARMACEUTICAL PARTICULARS
6.1 List of excipients
Capsules: Magnesium stearate (E572), Silica, anhydrous collodial (E551), Lactose monohydrate (spray dried), Sodium lauril sulphate, Size 1 yellow opaque gelatin capsules containing quinoline yellow (E104), sunset yellow (E110) and titanium dioxide (E171).

Syrup: Methyl parahydroxybenzoate (E218), Sucrose, Caramel powder (E150), Aromatic Elixir (containing ethyl alcohol, rum and aromatic rum flavour), Cinnamon oil, Sodium hydroxide, Purified water.

Paediatric syrup: Sucrose, Sodium methyl parahydroxybenzoate, Vanillin

Raspberry flavour, Cherry flavour, Red Ponceau 4R (E124), Sodium hydroxide (E524), Hydrochloric acid (E507), Purified water

6.2 Incompatibilities
Capsules and Paediatric syrup: None stated.

Syrup: Mixture with linctus of pholcodine causes precipitation of carbocisteine from solution.

6.3 Shelf life
36 months.

6.4 Special precautions for storage
Capsules: Do not store above 25°C.

Syrup and Paediatric Syrup: Do not store above 25°C. Dilution may be effected with unpreserved syrup BP but diluted preparations should not be kept for more than 14 days.

6.5 Nature and contents of container
Capsules: Blister packs of 120 capsules.

Syrup: 300ml Clear Glass (Ph Eur Type III) bottle. Polypropylene cap with polyethylene liner. Graduated polypropylene beaker

Paediatric Syrup: Clear Glass Type III bottle with a White Polypropylene child-resistant cap and Polyethylene liner, containing 300 ml (with graduated Polypropylene measuring beaker) and a tamper evident band.

6.6 Special precautions for disposal and other handling
None stated.

7. MARKETING AUTHORISATION HOLDER
Sanofi-aventis
One Onslow Street
Guildford
Surrey
GU1 4YS
UK

8. MARKETING AUTHORISATION NUMBER(S)
Capsules: PL 04425/0203
Syrup: PL 04425/0204
Paediatric Syrup: PL 04425/0205

9. DATE OF FIRST AUTHORISATION/RENEWAL OF THE AUTHORISATION
Capsules: 7 February 2009
Syrup: 30 April 2003
Paediatric Syrup: 23 February 2004

10. DATE OF REVISION OF THE TEXT
Capsules: February 2009
Syrup: 8 December 2008
Paediatric Syrup: 14 November 2008

LEGAL CLASSIFICATION
POM

MultiHance

(Bracco UK Limited)

1. NAME OF THE MEDICINAL PRODUCT
MultiHance, 0.5 M solution for injection

2. QUALITATIVE AND QUANTITATIVE COMPOSITION
1 ml of solution for injection contains: gadobenic acid 334 mg (0.5M) as the dimeglumine salt.

[Gadobenate dimeglumine 529 mg = gadobenic acid 334 mg + meglumine 195 mg].

For excipients, see 6.1.

3. PHARMACEUTICAL FORM
Solution for injection

Clear aqueous solution filled into colourless glass vials.

Osmolality at 37°C: 1.97 osmol/kg

Viscosity at 37°C: 5.3 mPa.s

4. CLINICAL PARTICULARS
4.1 Therapeutic indications
This medicinal product is for diagnostic use only.

MultiHance is a paramagnetic contrast agent for use in diagnostic magnetic resonance imaging (MRI) indicated for:

• MRI of the liver for the detection of focal liver lesions in patients with known or suspected primary liver cancer (eg. hepatocellular carcinoma) or metastatic disease.

• MRI of the brain and spine where it improves the detection of lesions and provides diagnostic information additional to that obtained with unenhanced MRI.

• Contrast-enhanced MR- angiography where it improves the diagnostic accuracy for detecting clinically significant steno-occlusive vascular disease in patients with suspected or known vascular disease of the abdominal or peripheral arteries.

4.2 Posology and method of administration
MRI of the liver: the recommended dose of MultiHance injection in adult patients is 0.05 mmol/kg body weight. This corresponds to 0.1 mL/kg of the 0.5 M solution.

MRI of the brain and spine: the recommended dose of MultiHance injection in adult patients is 0.1 mmol/kg body weight. This corresponds to 0.2 mL/kg of the 0.5 M solution.

MRA: the recommended dose of MultiHance injection in adult patients is 0.1 mmol/kg body weight. This corresponds to 0.2 mL/kg of the 0.5 M solution.

MultiHance should be drawn up into the syringe immediately before use and should not be diluted. Any unused product should be discarded and not be used for other MRI examinations.

To minimise the potential risks of soft tissue extravasation of MultiHance, it is important to ensure that the i.v. needle or cannula is correctly inserted into a vein.

Liver and Brain and Spine: the product should be administered intravenously either as a bolus or slow injection (10 mL/min.).

MRA: the product should be administered intravenously as a bolus injection, either manually or using an automatic injector system.

The injection should be followed by a saline flush.

Post-contrast imaging acquisition:

Liver	Dynamic imaging:	Immediately following bolus injection.
	Delayed imaging:	between 40 and 120 minutes following the injection, depending on the individual imaging needs.
Brain and Spine	up to 60 minutes after the administration.	
MRA	immediately after the administration, with scan delay calculated on the basis of test bolus or automatic bolus detection technique. If an automatic contrast detection pulse sequence is not used for bolus timing, then a test bolus injection ≤2 mL of the agent should be used to calculate the appropriate scan delay.	

The safety and efficacy of MultiHance have not been established in patients under 18 years old. Therefore, use of MultiHance in this patient group cannot be recommended.

4.3 Contraindications
MultiHance is contra-indicated in patients with hypersensitivity to any of the ingredients.

MultiHance should not be used in patients with a history of allergic or adverse reactions to other gadolinium chelates.

4.4 Special warnings and precautions for use
The safety and efficacy of MultiHance have not been established in patients under 18 years old. Therefore, use of MultiHance in this patient group cannot be recommended.

Patients should be kept under close supervision for 15 minutes following the injection as the majority of severe reactions occur at this time. The patient should remain in the hospital environment for one hour after the time of injection.

The accepted general safety procedures for Magnetic Resonance Imaging, in particular the exclusion of ferromagnetic objects, for example cardiac pace-makers or aneurysm clips, are also applicable when MultiHance is used.

Caution is advised in patients with cardiovascular disease.

The use of diagnostic contrast media, such as MultiHance, should be restricted to hospitals or clinics staffed for intensive care emergencies and where cardiopulmonary resuscitation equipment is readily available.

Small quantities of benzyl alcohol (<0.2%) may be released by gadobenate dimeglumine during storage. Thus MultiHance should not be used in patients with a history of sensitivity to benzyl alcohol.

As with other gadolinium-chelates, a contrast-enhanced MRI should not be performed within 7 hours of a MultiHance-enhanced MRI examination to allow for clearance of MultiHance from the body.

Impaired renal function

There have been reports of Nephrogenic Systemic Fibrosis (NSF) associated with use of some gadolinium-containing contrast agents in patients with severe renal impairment (GFR<30ml/min/1.73m^2). As there is a possibility that NSF may occur with MultiHance, it should be avoided in patients with acute or chronic severe renal impairment (GFR<30ml/min/1.73m^2) and in patients with acute renal insufficiency of any severity due to the hepato-renal syndrome or in the perioperative liver transplantation period unless the diagnostic information is essential and cannot be obtained through other means.

The risk for the development of NSF in patients with moderate renal impairment is unknown, therefore MultiHance should be used with caution in patients with moderate renal impairment (GFR 30-59ml/min/1.73m^2).

All patients should be screened, in particular patients over the age of 65, for renal dysfunction by obtaining a history and/or laboratory tests.

Haemodialysis shortly after MultiHance administration may be useful at removing MultiHance from the body. There is no evidence to support the initiation of haemodialysis for prevention or treatment of NSF in patients not already undergoing haemodialysis.

4.5 Interaction with other medicinal products and other forms of interaction

Interaction studies with other medicinal products were not carried out during the clinical development of MultiHance. However no drug interactions were reported during the clinical development programme.

4.6 Pregnancy and lactation

There are no adequate data for the use of gadobenate dimeglumine in pregnant women. Studies in animals have shown reproductive toxicity (see section 5.3). The potential risk for humans is unknown.

MultiHance should not be used during pregnancy unless clearly necessary.

Although it is not known to what extent gadobenate dimeglumine is excreted in human milk, it is known from animal experiments that minimal amounts, less than 0.5% of the administered dose were transferred via milk from mother to neonates. Although the clinical relevance of this observation is unknown, breast-feeding should be discontinued prior to the administration of MultiHance and should not be recommenced until at least 24 hours after the administration of MultiHance.

4.7 Effects on ability to drive and use machines

On the basis of the pharmacokinetic and pharmacodynamic profiles, no or negligible influence is expected with the use of MultiHance on the ability to drive or use machines.

4.8 Undesirable effects

The following adverse events were seen during the clinical development of MultiHance among 2637 adult subjects. There were no adverse reactions with a frequency greater than 2%.

(see Table 1 below)

Laboratory abnormalities cited above include hypochromic anaemia, leukocytosis, leukopenia, basophilia, hypoproteinaemia, hypocalcaemia, hyperkalaemia, hyperglycaemia or hypoglycaemia, albuminuria, glycosuria, haematuria, hyperlipidaemia, hyperbilirubinaemia, serum iron increased, and increases in serum transaminases, alkaline phosphatase, lactic dehydrogenase, and in serum creatinine and were reported in equal or less than 0.4% of patients following the administration of MultiHance. However these findings were mostly seen in patients with evidence of pre-existing impairment of hepatic function or pre-existing metabolic disease.

The majority of these events were non-serious, transient and spontaneously resolved without residual effects. There was no evidence of any correlation with age, gender or dose administered.

In marketed use, adverse reactions were reported in fewer than 0.1 % of patients.

Most commonly reported were: nausea, vomiting, signs and symptoms of hypersensitivity reactions including anaphylactic shock, anaphylactoid reactions, angioedema, laryngeal spasm and rash.

Injection site reactions due to extravasation of the contrast medium leading to local pain or burning sensations, swelling and blistering have been reported.

Isolated cases of NSF have been reported with MultiHance in patients co-administered other gadolinium-containing contrast agents (see Section 4.4).

4.9 Overdose

There have been no cases of overdose reported. Therefore, the signs and symptoms of overdosage have not been characterised. Doses up to 0.4 mmol/kg were administered to healthy volunteers, without any serious adverse events. However, doses exceeding the specific approved dosage are not recommended. In the event of overdosage, the patient should be carefully monitored and treated symptomatically.

MultiHance has been shown to be dialysable.

5. PHARMACOLOGICAL PROPERTIES

5.1 Pharmacodynamic properties

Pharmacotherapeutic group: paramagnetic contrast media, ATC code V08CA08

In liver imaging, MultiHance may detect lesions not visualised in pre-contrast enhanced MRI examination of patients with known or suspected hepatocellular cancer or metastatic disease. The nature of the lesions visualised after contrast enhancement with MultiHance has not been verified by pathological anatomical investigation. Furthermore, where the effect on patient management was assessed, the visualisation of post-contrast-enhanced lesions was not always associated with a change in the patient management.

The gadolinium chelate, gadobenate dimeglumine, shortens longitudinal (T1), and, to a lesser extent, transversal (T2) relaxation times of tissue water protons.

The relaxivities of gadobenate dimeglumine in aqueous solution are $r_1 = 4.39$ and $r_2 = 5.56\ mM^{-1}s^{-1}$ at 20 MHz.

Gadobenate dimeglumine experiences a strong increase in relaxivity on going from aqueous solution to solutions containing serum proteins, r_1 and r_2 values were 9.7 and 12.5 respectively in human plasma.

Table 1

System organ classes	Common (≥ 1/100, < 1/10)	Uncommon (≥ 1/1,000, < 1/100)	Rare (≥ 1/10,000, < 1/1,000)
Infections and infestations		Nasopharyngitis	
Nervous system disorders	Headache	Paraesthesia, dizziness, syncope, parosmia	Hyperaesthesia, tremor, intracranial hypertension, hemiplegia
Eye disorders			Conjunctivitis
Ear and labyrinth disorders			Tinnitus
Cardiac disorders		Tachycardia, atrial fibrillation, first-degree atrioventricular block, ventricular extrasystoles, sinus bradycardia,	Arrhythmia, myocardial ischaemia, prolonged PR interval
Vascular disorders		Hypertension, hypotension	
Respiratory, thoracic and mediastinal disorders		Rhinitis,	Dyspnoea N.O.S., laryngospasm, wheezing, pulmonary congestion, pulmonary oedema
Gastrointestinal disorders	Nausea	Dry mouth, taste perversion, diarrhoea, vomiting, dyspepsia, salivation, abdominal pain	Constipation, faecal incontinence, necrotising pancreatitis
Skin & subcutaneous tissue disorders		Pruritus, rash, face oedema, urticaria, sweating	
Musculoskeletal, connective tissue and bone disorders		Back pain, myalgia	
Renal and urinary disorders			Urinary incontinence, urinary urgency
General disorders and administration site conditions	Injection Site Reaction, feeling hot	Asthenia, fever, chills, chest pain, pain, injection site pain, injection site extravasation	injection site inflammation
Investigations		Abnormal laboratory tests, abnormal ECG, prolonged QT	

In the liver MultiHance provides strong and persistent signal intensity enhancement of normal parenchyma on T1-weighted imaging. The signal intensity enhancement persists at high level for at least two hours after the administration of doses of either 0.05 or 0.10 mmol/kg. Contrast between focal liver lesions and normal parenchyma is observed almost immediately after bolus injection (up to 2-3 minutes) on T1-weighted dynamic imaging. Contrast tends to decrease at later time points because of non-specific lesion enhancement. However, progressive wash-out of MultiHance from the lesions and persistent signal intensity enhancement of normal parenchyma are considered to result in enhanced lesion detection and a lower detection threshold for lesion site between 40 and 120 minutes after MultiHance administration.

Data from pivotal Phase II and Phase III studies in patients with liver cancer indicate that, compared with other reference imaging modalities (e.g. intraoperative ultrasonography, computed tomographic angio-portography, CTAP, or computed tomography following intra-arterial injection of iodized oil), with MultiHance enhanced MRI scans there was a mean sensitivity of 95% and a mean specificity of 80% for detection of liver cancer or metastasis in patients with a high suspicion of these conditions.

In MRI of the brain and spine, MultiHance enhances normal tissues lacking a blood-brain barrier, extra axial tumours and regions in which the blood-brain-barrier has broken down. In the pivotal phase III clinical trials in this indication, off-site readers reported an improvement in level of diagnostic information in 32-69% of images with MultiHance, and 35-69% of images with the active comparator.

In MRA, MultiHance improves image quality by increasing blood signal to noise ratio as a result of blood T1 shortening, reduces motion artifacts by shortening scan times and eliminates flow artifacts. In the phase III clinical trials in MRA of arteries extending from the supra-aortic territory to the pedal circulation, off-site readers reported an improvement in diagnostic accuracy ranging from 8% to 28% for the detection of clinically significant steno-occlusive disease (i.e. stenosis of >51% or >60% depending on the vascular territory) with MultiHance-enhanced images compared to time of flight (TOF) MRA, on the basis of conventional angiographic findings.

5.2 Pharmacokinetic properties

Modelling of the human pharmacokinetics was well described using a biexponential decay model. The apparent distribution and elimination half-times range from 0.085 to 0.117 h and from 1.17 to 1.68 respectively. The apparent total volume of distribution, ranging from 0.170 to 0.248 L/kg body weight, indicates that the compound is distributed in plasma and in the extracellular space.

Gadobenate ion is rapidly cleared from plasma and is eliminated mainly in urine and to a lesser extent in bile. Total plasma clearance, ranging from 0.098 to 0.133 L/h kg body weight, and renal clearance, ranging from 0.082 to 0.104 L/h kg body weight, indicate that the compound is predominantly eliminated by glomerular filtration. Plasma concentration and area under the curve (AUC) values show statistically significant linear dependence on the administered dose. Gadobenate ion is excreted unchanged in urine in amounts corresponding to 78%-94% of the injected dose within 24 hours. Between 2% and 4% of the dose is recovered in the faeces.

Gadobenate ion does not cross the intact blood-brain barrier and, therefore, does not accumulate in normal brain or in lesions that have a normal blood-brain barrier. However, disruption of the blood-brain barrier or abnormal vascularity allows gadobenate ion penetration into the lesion.

5.3 Preclinical safety data

Preclinical data reveal no special hazard for humans based on conventional studies of safety pharmacology, repeated dose toxicity, genotoxicity, carcinogenic potential.

Indeed, preclinical effects were observed only at exposures considered sufficiently in excess of the maximum human exposure indicating little relevance to clinical use.

Animal experiments revealed a poor local tolerance of MultiHance, especially in case of accidental paravenous application where severe local reaction, such as necrosis and eschars, could be observed.

Local tolerance in case of accidental intra-arterial application has not been investigated, so that it is particularly important to ensure that the i.v. needle or cannula is correctly inserted into a vein (see section 4.2).

Pregnancy and lactation

In animal studies no untoward effects on the embryonic or foetal development were exerted by daily intravenous administration of gadobenate dimeglumine in rats. Also, no adverse effects on physical and behavioural development were observed in the offspring of rats. However, after repeated daily dosing in rabbit, isolated cases of skeletal variations and two cases of visceral malformations were reported.

6. PHARMACEUTICAL PARTICULARS

6.1 List of excipients

Water for injections.

6.2 Incompatibilities

MultiHance should not be admixed with any other drug.

6.3 Shelf life
3 years

From a microbiological point of view, the product should be used immediately after drawing into the syringe.

6.4 Special precautions for storage
Do not freeze.

6.5 Nature and contents of container
5 mL, 10 mL, 15 mL and 20 mL of a clear aqueous solution filled into colourless type I glass vials with elastomeric closures, aluminium sealing crimps and polypropylene caps.

Not all pack sizes may be marketed.

6.6 Special precautions for disposal and other handling
MultiHance should be drawn up into the syringe immediately before use and should not be diluted.

Before use, examine the product to assure that the container and closure have not been damaged, the solution is not discoloured and no particulate matter is present.

When MultiHance is used in conjunction with an injector system, the connecting tubes to the patient and the relevant disposable parts should be disposed after each patient examination. Any additional instructions from the respective equipment manufacturer must also be adhered to.

For single use only. Any unused product should be discarded.

7. MARKETING AUTHORISATION HOLDER
Bracco spa

Via Egidio Folli

20134 – Milan - Italy

8. MARKETING AUTHORISATION NUMBER(S)
PL 06099/006 (UK)

PA 729/2/1 (Ireland)

9. DATE OF FIRST AUTHORISATION/RENEWAL OF THE AUTHORISATION
Date of first authorisation: 22 July 1997

Date of last renewal: 21 July 2007

10. DATE OF REVISION OF THE TEXT
1 November 2007

MultiHance PFS

(Bracco UK Limited)

1. NAME OF THE MEDICINAL PRODUCT
MultiHance 529 mg/ml solution for injection in pre-filled syringe

2. QUALITATIVE AND QUANTITATIVE COMPOSITION
1 ml of solution for injection contains: gadobenic acid 334 mg (0.5 mmol) as dimeglumine salt. [Gadobenate dimeglumine 529 mg = gadobenic acid 334 mg + meglumine 195 mg].

10 ml of solution for injection contain: gadobenic acid 3340 mg (0.5 mmol) as dimeglumine salt. [gadobenate dimeglumine 5290 mg = gadobenic acid 3340 mg + meglumine 1950 mg]

15 ml of solution for injection contain: gadobenic acid 5010 mg (0.5 mmol) as dimeglumine salt. [gadobenate dimeglumine 7935= gadobenic acid 5010 mg + meglumine 2925]

20 ml of solution for injection contain: gadobenic acid 6680 mg (0.5 mmol) as dimeglumine salt. [gadobenate dimeglumine 10580 mg = gadobenic acid 6680 mg + meglumine 3900]

For a full list of excipients, see Section 6.1'.

3. PHARMACEUTICAL FORM
Solution for injection in a pre-filled syringe.

Clear, colourless to slightly yellow, aqueous solution.

Osmolality at 37°C: 1.97 osmol/kg

Viscosity at 37°C: 5.3 mPa.s

pH: 6.9-7.3

4. CLINICAL PARTICULARS
4.1 Therapeutic indications
This medicinal product is for diagnostic use only.

MultiHance is a paramagnetic contrast agent for use in diagnostic magnetic resonance imaging (MRI) indicated for:

• MRI of the liver for the detection of focal liver lesions in patients with known or suspected primary liver cancer (eg. hepatocellular carcinoma) or metastatic disease.

• MRI of the brain and spine where it improves the detection of lesions and provides diagnostic information additional to that obtained with unenhanced MRI.

4.2 Posology and method of administration
MRI of the liver: the recommended dose of MultiHance in adult patients is 0.05 mmol/kg body weight. This corresponds to 0.1 mL/kg of the 0.5 M solution.

MRI of the brain and spine: the recommended dose of MultiHance in adult patients is 0.1 mmol/kg body weight. This corresponds to 0.2 mL/kg of the 0.5 M solution.

MultiHance should be used immediately after opening and should not be diluted. Any unused product should be discarded and not be used for other MRI examinations.

To use the syringe, the threaded tip of the plunger rod clockwise should be screwed into the plunger and pushed forward a few millimetres to break any friction between the plunger and syringe barrel.

Whilst holding syringe erect (with the nozzle cap upwards), the nozzle cap should be removed aseptically from the tip of the syringe and either a sterile, disposable needle or 5/6 tubing with a compatible luer lock should be attached using a push-twist action.

While still holding the syringe erect, the plunger should be pushed forward until all the air is evacuated and the fluid either appears at the tip of the needle or the tubing is completely filled.

The injection should be completed following the usual aspiration procedure.

To minimise the potential risks of soft tissue extravasation of MultiHance, it is important to ensure that the i.v. needle or cannula is correctly inserted into a vein.

The product should be administered intravenously either as a bolus or slow injection (10 mL/min.).

The injection should be followed by a flush of sodium chloride 9 mg/ml (0.9%) solution for injection.

<u>Post-contrast imaging acquisition:</u>

<u>Liver</u>	<u>Dynamic imaging:</u>	<u>Immediately following bolus injection.</u>
	<u>Delayed imaging:</u>	between 40 and 120 minutes following the injection, depending on the individual imaging needs.
<u>Brain and Spine</u>	up to 60 minutes after the administration.	

The safety and efficacy of MultiHance have not been established in patients under 18 years old. Therefore, use of MultiHance in this patient group cannot be recommended.

4.3 Contraindications
MultiHance is contra-indicated in patients with hypersensitivity to the active substance or to any of the excipients.

MultiHance should not be used in patients with a history of allergic or adverse reactions to other gadolinium chelates.

4.4 Special warnings and precautions for use
Patients should be kept under close supervision for 15 minutes following the injection as the majority of severe reactions occur at this time. The patient should remain in the hospital environment for one hour after the time of injection.

The accepted general safety procedures for Magnetic Resonance Imaging, in particular the exclusion of ferromagnetic objects, for example cardiac pace-makers or aneurysm clips, are also applicable when MultiHance is used.

Caution is advised in patients with cardiovascular disease.

The use of diagnostic contrast media, such as MultiHance, should be restricted to hospitals or clinics staffed for intensive care emergencies and where cardiopulmonary resuscitation equipment is readily available.

Small quantities of benzyl alcohol (<0.2%) may be released by gadobenate dimeglumine during storage. Thus MultiHance should not be used in patients with a history of sensitivity to benzyl alcohol.

As with other gadolinium-chelates, a contrast-enhanced MRI should not be performed within 7 hours of a MultiHance-enhanced MRI examination to allow for clearance of MultiHance from the body.

Impaired renal function

There have been reports of Nephrogenic Systemic Fibrosis (NSF) associated with use of some gadolinium-containing contrast agents in patients with severe renal impairment (GFR <30ml/min/1.73m^2). As there is a possibility that NSF may occur with MultiHance, it should be avoided in patients with acute or chronic severe renal impairment (GFR <30ml/min/1.73m^2) and in patients with acute renal insufficiency of any severity due to the hepato-renal syndrome or in the perioperative liver transplantation period unless the diagnostic information is essential and cannot be obtained through other means.

The risk for the development of NSF in patients with moderate renal impairment is unknown, therefore MultiHance should be used with caution in patients with moderate renal impairment (GFR 30-59ml/min/1.73m^2).

All patients should be screened, in particular patients over the age of 65, for renal dysfunction by obtaining a history and/or laboratory tests.

Haemodialysis shortly after MultiHance administration may be useful at removing MultiHance from the body. There is no evidence to support the initiation of haemodialysis for prevention or treatment of NSF in patients not already undergoing haemodialysis.

4.5 Interaction with other medicinal products and other forms of interaction
No interaction studies have been performed during the clinical development of MultiHance. However no drug interactions were reported during the clinical development programme.

4.6 Pregnancy and lactation
There are no adequate data for the use of gadobenate dimeglumine in pregnant women. Studies in animals have shown reproductive toxicity (see section 5.3). The potential risk for humans is unknown.

MultiHance should not be used during pregnancy unless clearly necessary.

Although it is not known to what extent gadobenate dimeglumine is excreted in human milk, it is known from animal experiments that minimal amounts, less than 0.5% of the administered dose were transferred via milk from mother to new-born infants. Although the clinical relevance of this observation is unknown, breast-feeding should be discontinued prior to the administration of MultiHance and should not be recommenced until at least 24 hours after the administration of MultiHance.

4.7 Effects on ability to drive and use machines
On the basis of the pharmacokinetic and pharmacodynamic profiles, no or negligible influence is expected with the use of MultiHance on the ability to drive or use machines.

4.8 Undesirable effects
The following adverse events were seen during the clinical development of MultiHance among 2637 adult subjects. There were no adverse reactions with a frequency greater than 2%.

(see Table 1 on next page)

Laboratory abnormalities cited above include hypochromic anaemia, leukocytosis, leukopenia, basophilia, hypoproteinaemia, hypocalcaemia, hyperkalaemia, hyperglycaemia or hypoglycaemia, albuminuria, glycosuria, haematuria, hyperlipidaemia, hyperbilirubinaemia, serum iron increased, and increases in serum transaminases, alkaline phosphatase, lactic dehydrogenase, and in serum creatinine and were reported in equal or less than 0.4% of patients following the administration of MultiHance. However these findings were mostly seen in patients with evidence of pre-existing impairment of hepatic function or pre-existing metabolic disease.

The majority of these events were non-serious, transient and spontaneously resolved without residual effects. There was no evidence of any correlation with age, gender or dose administered.

<u>In marketed use</u>, adverse reactions were reported in fewer than 0.1 % of patients.

Most commonly reported were: nausea, vomiting, signs and symptoms of hypersensitivity reactions including anaphylactic shock, anaphylactoid reactions, angioedema, laryngeal spasm and rash.

Injection site reactions due to extravasation of the contrast medium leading to local pain or burning sensations, swelling and blistering have been reported.

Isolated cases of NSF have been reported with MultiHance in patients co-administered other gadolinium-containing contrast agents (see Section 4.4).

4.9 Overdose
There have been no cases of overdose reported. Therefore, the signs and symptoms of overdosage have not been characterised. Doses up to 0.4 mmol/kg were administered to healthy volunteers, without any serious adverse events. However, doses exceeding the specific approved dosage are not recommended. In the event of overdosage, the patient should be carefully monitored and treated symptomatically.

MultiHance has been shown to be dialysable.

5. PHARMACOLOGICAL PROPERTIES
5.1 Pharmacodynamic properties
Pharmacotherapeutic group: paramagnetic contrast media ATC code V08CA08

<u>In liver imaging</u>, MultiHance may detect lesions not visualised in pre-contrast enhanced MRI examination of patients with known or suspected hepatocellular cancer or metastatic disease. The nature of the lesions visualised after contrast enhancement with MultiHance has not been verified by pathological anatomical investigation. Furthermore, where the effect on patient management was assessed, the visualisation of post-contrast-enhanced lesions was not always associated with a change in the patient management.

The gadolinium chelate, gadobenate dimeglumine, shortens longitudinal (T1), and, to a lesser extent, transversal (T2) relaxation times of tissue water protons.

The relaxivities of gadobenate dimeglumine in aqueous solution are r_1 = 4.39 and r_2 = 5.56 mM^{-1}s^{-1} at 20 MHz.

Gadobenate dimeglumine experiences a strong increase in relaxivity on going from aqueous solution to solutions containing serum proteins, r_1 and r_2 values were 9.7 and 12.5 respectively in human plasma.

In the liver MultiHance provides strong and persistent signal intensity enhancement of normal parenchyma on T1-weighted imaging. The signal intensity enhancement

Table 1

System organ classes	Common (≥1/100, <1/10)	Uncommon (≥1/1,000, <1/100)	Rare (≥1/10,000, <1/1,000)
Infections and infestations		Nasopharyngitis	
Nervous system disorders	Headache	Paraesthesia, dizziness, syncope, parosmia	Hyperaesthesia, tremor, intracranial hypertension, hemiplegia
Eye disorders			Conjunctivitis
Ear and labyrinth disorders			Tinnitus
Cardiac disorders		Tachycardia, atrial fibrillation, first-degree atrioventricular block, ventricular extrasystoles, sinus bradycardia,	Arrhythmia, myocardial ischaemia, prolonged PR interval
Vascular disorders		Hypertension, hypotension	
Respiratory, thoracic and mediastinal disorders		Rhinitis,	Dyspnoea N.O.S., laryngospasm, wheezing, pulmonary congestion, pulmonary oedema
Gastrointestinal disorders	Nausea	Dry mouth, taste perversion, diarrhoea, vomiting, dyspepsia, salivation, abdominal pain	Constipation, faecal incontinence, necrotising pancreatitis
Skin & subcutaneous tissue disorders		Pruritus, rash, face oedema, urticaria, sweating	
Musculoskeletal, connective tissue and bone disorders		Back pain, myalgia	
Renal and urinary disorders			Urinary incontinence, urinary urgency
General disorders and administration site conditions	Injection Site Reaction, feeling hot	Asthenia, fever, chills, chest pain, pain, injection site pain, injection site extravasation	injection site inflammation
Investigations		Abnormal laboratory tests, abnormal ECG, prolonged QT	

persists at high level for at least two hours after the administration of doses of either 0.05 or 0.10 mmol/kg. Contrast between focal liver lesions and normal parenchyma is observed almost immediately after bolus injection (up to 2-3 minutes) on T1-weighted dynamic imaging. Contrast tends to decrease at later time points because of non-specific lesion enhancement. However, progressive wash-out of MultiHance from the lesions and persistent signal intensity enhancement of normal parenchyma are considered to result in enhanced lesion detection and a lower detection threshold for lesion site between 40 and 120 minutes after MultiHance administration.

Data from pivotal Phase II and Phase III studies in patients with liver cancer indicate that, compared with other reference imaging modalities (e.g. intraoperative ultrasonography, computed tomographic angio-portography, CTAP, or computed tomography following intra-arterial injection of iodized oil), with MultiHance enhanced MRI scans there was a mean sensitivity of 95% and a mean specificity of 80% for detection of liver cancer or metastasis in patients with a high suspicion of these conditions.

In MRI of the brain and spine, MultiHance enhances normal tissues lacking a blood-brain barrier, extra axial tumours and regions in which the blood-brain-barrier has broken down. In the pivotal phase III clinical trials in this indication, off-site readers reported an improvement in level of diagnostic information in 32-69% of images with MultiHance, and 35-69% of images with the active comparator.

5.2 Pharmacokinetic properties

Modelling of the human pharmacokinetics was well described using a biexponential decay model. The apparent distribution and elimination half-times range from 0.085 to 0.117 h and from 1.17 to 1.68 respectively. The apparent total volume of distribution, ranging from 0.170 to 0.248 L/kg body weight, indicates that the compound is distributed in plasma and in the extracellular space.

Gadobenate ion is rapidly cleared from plasma and is eliminated mainly in urine and to a lesser extent in bile. Total plasma clearance, ranging from 0.098 to 0.133 L/h kg body weight, and renal clearance, ranging from 0.082 to 0.104 L/h kg body weight, indicate that the compound is predominantly eliminated by glomerular filtration. Plasma concentration and area under the curve (AUC) values show statistically significant linear dependence on the administered dose. Gadobenate ion is excreted unchanged in urine in amounts corresponding to 78%-94% of the injected dose within 24 hours. Between 2% and 4% of the dose is recovered in the faeces.

Gadobenate ion does not cross the intact blood-brain barrier and, therefore, does not accumulate in normal brain or in lesions that have a normal blood-brain barrier. However, disruption of the blood-brain barrier or abnormal vascularity allows gadobenate ion penetration into the lesion.

5.3 Preclinical safety data

Non-clinical data reveal no special hazard for humans based on conventional studies of safety pharmacology, repeated dose toxicity, genotoxicity, carcinogenic potential.

Indeed, preclinical effects were observed only at exposures considered sufficiently in excess of the maximum human exposure indicating little relevance to clinical use.

Animal experiments revealed a poor local tolerance of MultiHance, especially in case of accidental paravenous application where severe local reaction, such as necrosis and eschars, could be observed.

Local tolerance in case of accidental intra-arterial application has not been investigated, so that it is particularly important to ensure that the i.v. needle or cannula is correctly inserted into a vein (see section 4.2).

Pregnancy and lactation

In animal studies no untoward effects on the embryonic or foetal development were exerted by daily intravenous administration of gadobenate dimeglumine in rats. Also, no adverse effects on physical and behavioural development were observed in the offspring of rats. However, after repeated daily dosing in rabbit, isolated cases of skeletal variations and two cases of visceral malformations were reported.

6. PHARMACEUTICAL PARTICULARS

6.1 List of excipients

Water for injections.

6.2 Incompatibilities

This medicinal product must not be mixed with other medicinal products.

6.3 Shelf life

3 years

From a microbiological point of view, the product should be used immediately after opening.

6.4 Special precautions for storage

Do not freeze.

6.5 Nature and contents of container

10, 15 and 20 mL solution filled into a transparent plastic (cyclic polyolefin) syringe with chlorobutyl rubber plunger and tip cap.

Not all pack sizes may be marketed.

6.6 Special precautions for disposal and other handling

For single use only.

Before use, examine the product to assure that the container and closure have not been damaged, the solution is not discoloured and no particulate matter is present.

Any unused product or waste material should be disposed of in accordance with local requirements.

7. MARKETING AUTHORISATION HOLDER

(Company) Name: Bracco SpA

Address: via Egidio Folli 50 -20134 Milan

Country: Italy

8. MARKETING AUTHORISATION NUMBER(S)

PL 06099/0012

9. DATE OF FIRST AUTHORISATION/RENEWAL OF THE AUTHORISATION

19/02/2008

10. DATE OF REVISION OF THE TEXT

19/02/2008

MXL capsules 30 mg, 60 mg, 90 mg, 120 mg, 150 mg, 200 mg

(Napp Pharmaceuticals Limited)

1. NAME OF THE MEDICINAL PRODUCT

MXL® 30 mg, 60 mg, 90 mg, 120 mg, 150 mg, 200 mg prolonged release capsules.

2. QUALITATIVE AND QUANTITATIVE COMPOSITION

Capsules containing morphine sulphate 30 mg, 60 mg, 90 mg, 120 mg, 150 mg, 200 mg.

For excipients, see 6.1.

3. PHARMACEUTICAL FORM

Capsules, prolonged release

Hard gelatin capsules containing white to off white multi-particulates.

MXL capsules 30 mg are size 4, light blue capsules marked MS OD30.

MXL capsules 60 mg are size 3, brown capsules marked MS OD60.

MXL capsules 90 mg are size 2, pink capsules marked MS OD90.

MXL capsules 120 mg are size 1, olive capsules marked MS OD120.

MXL capsules 150 mg are size 1, blue capsules marked MS OD150.

MXL capsules 200 mg are size 0, rust capsules marked MS OD200

4. CLINICAL PARTICULARS

4.1 Therapeutic indications

The prolonged relief of severe and intractable pain.

4.2 Posology and method of administration

Route of administration

Oral.

The capsules may be swallowed whole or opened and the contents sprinkled on to soft cold food. The capsules and contents should not be crushed or chewed. ***MXL*** capsules should be used at 24-hourly intervals. The dosage is dependent upon the severity of the pain, the patient's age and previous history of analgesic requirements.

Adults and elderly

Patients presenting with severe uncontrolled pain, who are not currently receiving opioids, should have their dose requirements calculated through the use of immediate release morphine, where possible, before conversion to ***MXL*** capsules.

Patients presenting in pain, who are currently receiving weaker opioids should be started on:

a) 60 mg ***MXL*** capsule once-daily if they weigh over 70 kg.

b) 30 mg ***MXL*** capsule once-daily if they weigh under 70 kg, are frail or elderly.

Increasing severity of pain will require an increased dosage of ***MXL*** capsules using 30 mg, 60 mg, 90 mg, 120 mg, 150 mg or 200 mg alone or in combination to achieve pain relief. Higher doses should be made, where appropriate in 30% - 50% increments as required. The correct dosage for any individual patient is that which controls the pain with no or tolerable side effects for a full 24 hours.

Patients receiving ***MXL*** capsules in place of parenteral morphine should be given a sufficiently increased dosage to compensate for any reduction in analgesic effects associated with oral administration. Usually such increased requirement is of the order of 100%. In such patients individual dose adjustments are required.

Children aged 1 year and above

The use of ***MXL*** capsules in children has not been extensively evaluated.

For severe and intractable pain in cancer a starting dose in the range of 0.4 to 1.6 mg morphine per kg bodyweight daily is recommended. Doses should be titrated in the normal way as for adults.

4.3 Contraindications

Hypersensitivity to any of the constituents.

Respiratory depression, head injury, paralytic ileus, acute abdomen, delayed gastric emptying, obstructive airways disease, known morphine sensitivity, acute hepatic disease, concurrent administration of monoamine oxidase inhibitors (MAOIs) or within two weeks of discontinuation of their use. Not recommended during pregnancy or for pre-operative use or for the first 24 hours post-operatively. Children under one year of age.

4.4 Special warnings and precautions for use

As with all narcotics, a reduction in dosage may be advisable in the elderly, in hypothyroidism, in renal and chronic hepatic disease. Use with caution in patients with impaired respiratory function, convulsive disorders, acute alcoholism, delirium tremens, raised intracranial pressure, hypotension with hypovolaemia, severe cor pulmonale, opioid dependent patients, patients with a history of substance abuse, diseases of the biliary tract, pancreatitis, inflammatory bowel disorders, prostatic hypertrophy and adrenocortical insufficiency. ***MXL*** capsules should not be used where there is a possibility of paralytic ileus occurring. Should paralytic ileus be suspected or occur during use, ***MXL*** capsules should be discontinued immediately. As with all morphine preparations, patients who are to undergo cordotomy or other pain relieving surgical procedures should not receive ***MXL*** capsules for 24 hours prior to surgery. If further treatment with ***MXL*** capsules is then indicated the dosage should be adjusted to the new post-operative requirement.

It is not possible to ensure bio-equivalence between different brands of controlled release morphine products. Therefore, it should be emphasised that patients, once titrated to an effective dose should not be changed from ***MXL*** capsules to other slow, sustained or controlled release morphine or other potent narcotic analgesic preparations without retitration and clinical assessment.

The major risk of opioid excess is respiratory depression.

The patient may develop tolerance to the drug with chronic use and require progressively higher doses to maintain pain control. Prolonged use of this product may lead to physical dependence and a withdrawal syndrome may occur upon abrupt cessation of therapy. When a patient no longer requires therapy with morphine, it may be advisable to taper the dose gradually to prevent symptoms of withdrawal.

Morphine has an abuse profile similar to other strong agonist opioids. Morphine may be sought and abused by people with latent or manifest addiction disorders. The development of psychological dependence to opioid analgesics in properly managed patients with pain has been reported to be rare. However, data are not available to establish the true incidence of psychological dependence in chronic pain patients. The product should be used with particular care in patients with a history of alcohol and drug abuse.

The controlled release granules must be swallowed whole, and not broken, chewed, dissolved or crushed. The administration of broken, chewed or crushed morphine granules leads to a rapid release and absorption of a potentially fatal dose of morphine (see section 4.9).

Morphine may lower the seizure threshold in patients with a history of epilepsy.

4.5 Interaction with other medicinal products and other forms of interaction

Morphine should be used with caution in patients who are concurrently receiving other central nervous system depressants including sedatives or hypnotics, general anesthetics, phenothiazines, other tranquilizers, muscle relaxants, antihypertensives and alcohol. Interactive effects resulting in respiratory depression, hypotension, profound sedation, or coma may result if these drugs are taken in combination with the usual doses of morphine. Morphine should not be co-administered with monoamine oxidase inhibitors or within two weeks of such therapy.

Mixed agonist/antagonist opioid analgesics (e.g. buprenorphine, nalbuphine, pentazocine) should not be administered to a patient who has received a course of therapy with a pure opioid agonist analgesic.

Cimetidine inhibits the metabolism of morphine.

Plasma concentrations of morphine may be reduced by rifampicin.

Although there are no pharmacokinetic data available for concomitant use of ritonavir with morphine, ritonavir induces the hepatic enzymes responsible for the glucuronidation of morphine, and may possibly decrease plasma concentrations of morphine.

4.6 Pregnancy and lactation

MXL capsules are not recommended for use in pregnancy and labour due to the risk of neonatal respiratory depression. Administration to nursing mothers is not recommended as morphine is excreted in breast milk. Withdrawal symptoms may be observed in the newborn of mothers undergoing chronic treatment.

4.7 Effects on ability to drive and use machines

Morphine may modify the patient's reactions to a varying extent depending on the dosage and individual susceptibility. If affected, patients should not drive or operate machinery.

4.8 Undesirable effects

In normal doses, the commonest side effects of morphine are nausea, vomiting, constipation and drowsiness. With chronic therapy, nausea and vomiting are unusual with ***MXL*** capsules but should they occur the capsules can be readily combined with an anti-emetic if required. Constipation may be treated with appropriate laxatives.

Common (incidence of ⩾ 1% and Uncommon (incidence of ⩽ 1%) adverse drug reactions are listed in the table below:

Undesirable Effects	Common (⩾ 1%)	Uncommon (⩽ 1%)
Immune system disorders		Allergic reaction Anaphylactic reaction Anaphylactoid reaction
Psychiatric disorders	Confusion Insomnia Thinking disturbances	Agitation Drug dependence Dysphoria Euphoria Hallucinations Mood altered
Nervous system disorders	Headache Involuntary muscle contractions Myoclonus Somnolence	Convulsions Hypertonia Paraesthesia Syncope Vertigo
Eye disorders		Miosis Visual disturbance
Cardiac disorders		Bradycardia Palpitations Hypertension Tachycardia
Vascular disorders		Facial flushing Hypotension
Respiratory, thoracic and mediastinal disorders	Bronchospasm Cough decreased	Pulmonary oedema Respiratory depression
Gastrointestinal disorders	Abdominal pain Anorexia Constipation Dry mouth Dyspepsia Nausea Vomiting	Gastrointestinal disorders Ileus Taste perversion
Hepatobiliary disorders	Exacerbation of pancreatitis	Biliary pain Increased hepatic enzymes
Skin and subcutaneous tissue disorders	Hyperhidrosis Rash	Urticaria
Renal and urinary disorders		Ureteric spasm Urinary retention
Reproductive system and breast disorders		Amenorrhea Decreased libido Erectile dysfunction
General disorders and administration site conditions	Asthenia Pruritus	Drug tolerance Drug withdrawal syndrome Malaise Peripheral oedema

The effects of morphine have led to its abuse and dependence may develop with regular, inappropriate use. This is not a major concern in the treatment of patients with severe pain.

4.9 Overdose

Signs of morphine toxicity and overdosage are drowsiness, pin-point pupils, skeletal muscle flaccidity, bradycardia, respiratory depression and hypotension. Circulatory failure and deepening coma may occur in more severe cases. Overdosage can result in death. Rhabdomyolysis progressing to renal failure has been reported in opioid overdosage.

Crushing and taking the contents of a controlled release dosage form leads to the release of the morphine in an immediate fashion; this might result in a fatal overdose.

Treatment of morphine overdosage:

Primary attention should be given to the establishment of a patent airway and institution of assisted or controlled ventilation.

The pure opioid antagonists are specific antidotes against the effects of opioid overdose. Other supportive measures should be employed as needed.

In the case of massive overdosage, administer naloxone 0.8 mg intravenously. Repeat at 2-3 minute intervals as necessary, or by an infusion of 2 mg in 500 ml of normal saline or 5% dextrose (0.004 mg/ml).

The infusion should be run at a rate related to the previous bolus doses administered and should be in accordance with the patient's response. However, because the duration of action of naloxone is relatively short, the patient must be carefully monitored until spontaneous respiration is reliably re-established. ***MXL*** capsules will continue to release and add to the morphine load for up to 24 hours after administration and the management of morphine overdosage should be modified accordingly.

For less severe overdosage, administer naloxone 0.2 mg intravenously followed by increments of 0.1 mg every 2 minutes if required.

Naloxone should not be administered in the absence of clinically significant respiratory or circulatory depression secondary to morphine overdosage. Naloxone should be administered cautiously to persons who are known, or suspected, to be physically dependent on morphine. In such cases, an abrupt or complete reversal of opioid effects may precipitate an acute withdrawal syndrome.

Gastric contents may need to be emptied as this can be useful in removing unabsorbed drug, particularly when a modified release formulation has been taken.

5. PHARMACOLOGICAL PROPERTIES

5.1 Pharmacodynamic properties

Pharmacotherapeutic group: natural opium alkaloid

ATC code: N02A A01

Morphine acts as an agonist at opiate receptors in the CNS particularly mu and to a lesser extent kappa receptors. mu receptors are thought to mediate supraspinal analgesia, respiratory depression and euphoria and kappa receptors, spinal analgesia, miosis and sedation.

Central Nervous System

The principal actions of therapeutic value of morphine are analgesia and sedation (i.e., sleepiness and anxiolysis). Morphine produces respiratory depression by direct action on brain stem respiratory centres.

Morphine depresses the cough reflex by direct effect on the cough centre in the medulla. Antitussive effects may occur with doses lower than those usually required for analgesia.

Morphine causes miosis, even in total darkness. Pinpoint pupils are a sign of narcotic overdose but are not pathognomonic (e.g., pontine lesions of haemorrhagic or ischaemic origin may produce similar findings). Marked mydriasis rather than miosis may be seen with hypoxia in the setting of morphine overdose.

Gastrointestinal Tract and Other Smooth Muscle

Morphine causes a reduction in motility associated with an increase in smooth muscle tone in the antrum of the stomach and duodenum. Digestion of food in the small intestine is delayed and propulsive contractions are decreased. Propulsive peristaltic waves in the colon are decreased, while tone is increased to the point of spasm resulting in constipation.

Morphine generally increases smooth muscle tone, especially the sphincters of the gastrointestinal and biliary tracts. Morphine may produce spasm of the sphincter of Oddi, thus raising intrabiliary pressure.

Cardiovascular System

Morphine may produce release of histamine with or without associated peripheral vasodilation. Manifestations of histamine release and/or peripheral vasodilation may include pruritus, flushing, red eyes, sweating, and/or orthostatic hypotension.

Endocrine System

Opioids may influence the hypothalamic-pituitary-adrenal or -gonadal axes. Some changes that can be seen include an increase in serum prolactin, and decreases in plasma cortisol, oestrogen and testosterone in association with inappropriately low or normal ACTH, LH or FSH levels. Clinical symptoms may be manifest from these hormonal changes.

Other Pharmacological Effects

In vitro and animal studies indicate various effects of natural opioids, such as morphine, on components of the immune system; the clinical significance of these findings is unknown.

5.2 Pharmacokinetic properties

Morphine is well absorbed from the capsules and, in general, peak plasma concentrations are achieved 2-6 hours following administration. The availability is complete when compared to an immediate release oral solution or ***MST CONTINUS*** tablets. The pharmacokinetics of morphine are linear across a very wide dose range. Morphine is subject to a significant first-pass effect which results in a lower bioavailability when compared to an equivalent intravenous or intramuscular dose.

The major metabolic transformation of morphine is glucuronidation to morphine-3-glucuronide and morphine-6-glucuronide which then undergo renal excretion. These metabolites are excreted in bile and may be subject to hydrolysis and subsequent reabsorption.

Because of the high inter-patient variation in morphine pharmacokinetics, and in analgesic requirements, the daily dosage in individual patients must be titrated to achieve appropriate pain control. Daily doses of up to 11.2 g have been recorded from twelve-hourly ***MST CONTINUS*** tablets. For this reason the capsules have been formulated in strengths of 30 mg, 60 mg, 90 mg, 120 mg, 150 mg and 200 mg.

5.3 Preclinical safety data

There are no pre-clinical data of relevance to the prescriber which are additional to that already included in other sections of the SPC.

6. PHARMACEUTICAL PARTICULARS

6.1 List of excipients

Hydrogenated vegetable Oil BP

Macrogol 6000 Ph Eur.

Talc Ph Eur.

Magnesium stearate Ph Eur.

Capsule shells

Gelatin (containing sodium dodecylsulphate)

The following colours are also present:

30 mg: indigo carmine (E132), titanium dioxide (E171);

60 mg: indigo carmine (E132), titanium dioxide (E171), iron oxide (E172);

90 mg: erythrosine (E127), titanium dioxide (E171), iron oxide (E172);

120 mg: indigo carmine (E132), titanium dioxide (E171), iron oxide (E172);

150 mg: erythrosine (E127), indigo carmine (E132), titanium dioxide (E171), iron oxide (E172);

200 mg: titanium dioxide (E171), iron oxide (E172).

Printing ink

Shellac DAB 10

Iron oxide, black (E172)

Propylene glycol

6.2 Incompatibilities

Not applicable

6.3 Shelf life

2 years

6.4 Special precautions for storage

Do not store above 25°C.

6.5 Nature and contents of container

PVdC (⩾ 40 gsm) coated PVC (250 μm) blister strip with aluminium backing foil. The blister strips will be enclosed in a cardboard box. Each box will contain 28 capsules.

6.6 Special precautions for disposal and other handling

No special requirements

7. MARKETING AUTHORISATION HOLDER

Napp Pharmaceuticals Ltd

Cambridge Science Park

Milton Road

Cambridge CB4 0GW

8. MARKETING AUTHORISATION NUMBER(S)

PL 16950/0042-47

9. DATE OF FIRST AUTHORISATION/RENEWAL OF THE AUTHORISATION

29 March 1996/ 29 March 2006

10. DATE OF REVISION OF THE TEXT

September 2009

11 Legal Category

CD (Sch 2), POM

Mycamine 50mg and 100mg powder for solution for infusion

(Astellas Pharma Ltd)

1. NAME OF THE MEDICINAL PRODUCT

Mycamine®▼ 50 mg powder for solution for infusion

Mycamine®▼ 100 mg powder for solution for infusion

2. QUALITATIVE AND QUANTITATIVE COMPOSITION

Each vial contains 50 mg micafungin (as sodium).

After reconstitution each ml contains 10 mg micafungin (as sodium).

Each vial contains 100 mg micafungin (as sodium).

After reconstitution each ml contains 20 mg micafungin (as sodium).

Excipients:

Each 50 mg vial contains 200 mg lactose.

Each 100 mg vial contains 200 mg lactose.

For a full list of excipients, see section 6.1.

3. PHARMACEUTICAL FORM

Powder for solution for infusion.

White compact powder.

4. CLINICAL PARTICULARS

4.1 Therapeutic indications

Mycamine is indicated for:

Adults, adolescents ⩾ 16 years of age and elderly:

- Treatment of invasive candidiasis.
- Treatment of oesophageal candidiasis in patients for whom intravenous therapy is appropriate.
- Prophylaxis of Candida infection in patients undergoing allogeneic haematopoietic stem cell transplantation or patients who are expected to have neutropenia (absolute neutrophil count < 500 cells / μl) for 10 or more days.

Children (including neonates) and adolescents < 16 years of age:

- Treatment of invasive candidiasis.
- Prophylaxis of Candida infection in patients undergoing allogeneic haematopoietic stem cell transplantation or patients who are expected to have neutropenia (absolute neutrophil count < 500 cells / μl) for 10 or more days.

The decision to use Mycamine should take into account a potential risk for the development of liver tumours (see section 4.4). Mycamine should therefore only be used if other antifungals are not appropriate.

4.2 Posology and method of administration

Consideration should be given to official/national guidance on the appropriate use of antifungal agents.

Treatment with Mycamine should be initiated by a physician experienced in the management of fungal infections.

Specimens for fungal culture and other relevant laboratory studies (including histopathology) should be obtained prior to therapy to isolate and identify causative organism(s). Therapy may be instituted before the results of the cultures and other laboratory studies are known. However, once these results become available, antifungal therapy should be adjusted accordingly.

The dose regimen of Mycamine depends on the body weight of the patient as given in the following tables:

Use in adults, adolescents ⩾ 16 years of age and elderly

Indication		
	Body weight > 40 kg	Body weight ⩽ 40 kg
Treatment of invasive candidiasis	100 mg/day*	2 mg/kg/day*
Treatment of oesophageal candidiasis	150 mg/day	3 mg/kg/day
Prophylaxis of *Candida* infection	50 mg/day	1 mg/kg/day

*If the patient's response is inadequate, e.g. persistence of cultures or if clinical condition does not improve, the dose may be increased to 200 mg/day in patients weighing > 40 kg or 4 mg/kg/day in patients ⩽ 40 kg.

Treatment duration

Invasive candidiasis: The treatment duration of *Candida* infection should be a minimum of 14 days. The antifungal treatment should continue for at least one week after two sequential negative blood cultures have been obtained and ***after*** resolution of clinical signs and symptoms of infection.

Oesophageal candidiasis: For the treatment of oesophageal candidiasis, Mycamine should be administered for at least one week after resolution of clinical signs and symptoms.

Prophylaxis of *Candida* infections: For prophylaxis of *Candida* infection, Mycamine should be administered for at least one week after neutrophil recovery.

Use in children (including neonates) and adolescents < 16 years of age

Indication		
	Body weight > 40 kg	Body weight ⩽ 40 kg
Treatment of invasive candidiasis	100 mg/day*	2 mg/kg/day*
Prophylaxis of *Candida* infection	50 mg/day	1 mg/kg/day

*If the patient's response is inadequate, e.g. persistence of cultures or if clinical condition does not improve, the dose may be increased to 200 mg/day in patients weighing > 40 kg or 4 mg/kg/day in patients weighing ⩽ 40 kg.

Treatment duration

Invasive candidiasis: The treatment duration of *Candida* infection should be a minimum of 14 days. The antifungal treatment should continue for at least one week after two sequential negative blood cultures have been obtained and ***after*** resolution of clinical signs and symptoms of infection.

Prophylaxis of *Candida* infections: For prophylaxis of *Candida* infection, Mycamine should be administered for at least one week after neutrophil recovery. Experience with Mycamine in patients less than 2 years of age is limited.

Gender/Race

No dose adjustment is necessary based on gender or race (see section 5.2).

Use in patients with hepatic impairment

No dose adjustment is necessary in patients with mild or moderate hepatic impairment (see section 5.2). There are currently no data available for the use of Mycamine in patients with severe hepatic impairment and its use is not recommended in these patients (see section 4.4).

Use in patients with renal impairment

No dose adjustment is necessary in patients with renal impairment (see section 5.2).

After reconstitution and dilution, the solution should be administered by intravenous infusion over approximately 1 hour. More rapid infusions may result in more frequent histamine mediated reactions.

For reconstitution instructions see section 6.6.

4.3 Contraindications

Hypersensitivity to the active substance or to any of the excipients.

4.4 Special warnings and precautions for use

Hepatic effects:
The development of foci of altered hepatocytes (FAH) and hepatocellular tumours after a treatment period of 3 months or longer were observed in rats. The assumed threshold for tumour development in rats is approximately in the range of clinical exposure. The relevance of this finding for the therapeutic use in patients can not be excluded. Liver function should be carefully monitored during micafungin treatment. To minimise the risk of adaptive regeneration and potentially subsequent liver tumour formation, early discontinuation in the presence of significant and persistent elevation of ALT/AST is recommended. Micafungin treatment should be conducted on a careful risk/benefit basis, particularly in patients having severe liver function impairment or chronic liver diseases known to represent preneoplastic conditions, such as advanced liver fibrosis, cirrhosis, viral hepatitis, neonatal liver disease or congenital enzyme defects, or receiving a concomitant therapy including hepatotoxic and/or genotoxic properties.

Micafungin treatment was associated with significant impairment of liver function (increase of ALT, AST or total bilirubin > 3 times ULN) in both healthy volunteers and patients. In some patients more severe hepatic dysfunction, hepatitis, or hepatic failure including fatal cases have been reported. Paediatric patients < 1 year of age might be more prone to liver injury (see section 4.8).

There are insufficient data on the pharmacokinetics of micafungin in patients with severe hepatic impairment (see section 5.2).

During administration of micafungin, anaphylactoid reactions including shock may occur. If these reactions occur, micafungin infusion should be discontinued and appropriate treatment administered.

Rare cases of haemolysis including acute intravascular haemolysis or haemolytic anaemia have been reported in patients treated with micafungin. Patients who develop clinical or laboratory evidence of haemolysis during micafungin therapy should be monitored closely for evidence of worsening of these conditions and evaluated for the risk/benefit of continuing micafungin therapy.

Micafungin may cause kidney problems, renal failure, and abnormal renal function test. Patients should be closely monitored for worsening of renal function.

The incidence of some adverse reactions was higher in paediatric patients than in adult patients (see section 4.8).

This medicinal product for intravenous use contains lactose. Patients with rare hereditary problems of galactose intolerance, the Lapp lactase deficiency or glucose-galactose malabsorption should not take this medicine.

4.5 Interaction with other medicinal products and other forms of interaction

Micafungin has a low potential for interactions with medicines metabolised via CYP3A mediated pathways.

Drug interaction studies in healthy human subjects were conducted to evaluate the potential for interaction between micafungin and mycophenolate mofetil, ciclosporin, tacrolimus, prednisolone, sirolimus, nifedipine, fluconazole, ritonavir, rifampicin, itraconazole, voriconazole and amphotericin B. In these studies, no evidence of altered pharmacokinetics of micafungin was observed. No micafungin dose adjustments are necessary when these medicines are administered concomitantly. Exposure (AUC) of itraconazole, sirolimus and nifedipine was slightly increased in the presence of micafungin (22%, 21% and 18% respectively).

Patients receiving sirolimus, nifedipine or itraconazole in combination with Mycamine should be monitored for sirolimus, nifedipine or itraconazole toxicity and the sirolimus, nifedipine or itraconazole dosage should be reduced if necessary.

4.6 Pregnancy and lactation

There are no data from the use of micafungin in pregnant women. In animal studies micafungin crossed the placental barrier and reproductive toxicity was seen (see section 5.3). The potential risk for humans is unknown.

Mycamine should not be used during pregnancy unless clearly necessary.

It is not known whether micafungin is excreted in human breast milk. Animal studies have shown excretion of micafungin in breast milk. A decision on whether to continue/discontinue breast-feeding or to continue/discontinue

Table 1

System Organ Class	Common ≥ 1/100 to < 1/10	Uncommon ≥ 1/1,000 to < 1/100	Rare ≥ 1/10,000 to < 1/1,000	Not known (frequency cannot be estimated from available data)
Blood and lymphatic system disorders	leukopenia, neutropenia, anaemia	pancytopenia, thrombocytopenia, eosinophilia, hypoalbuminaemia	haemolytic anaemia, haemolysis (see section 4.4)	
Immune system disorders		anaphylactic / anaphylactoid reaction (see section 4.4), hypersensitivity		
Endocrine disorders		hyperhidrosis		
Metabolism and nutritional disorders	hypokalaemia, hypomagnesaemia, hypocalcaemia	hyponatraemia, hyperkalaemia, hypophosphataemia, anorexia		
Psychiatric disorders		insomnia, anxiety, confusion		
Nervous system disorders	headache	somnolence, tremor, dizziness, dysgeusia		
Cardiac disorders		tachycardia, palpitations, bradycardia		
Vascular disorders	phlebitis	hypotension, hypertension, flushing		shock
Respiratory, thoracic and mediastinal disorders		dyspnoea		
Gastrointestinal disorders	nausea, vomiting, diarrhoea, abdominal pain	dyspepsia, constipation		
Hepatobiliary disorders	blood alkaline phosphatase increased, aspartate aminotransferase increased, alanine aminotransferase increased, blood bilirubin increased (including hyperbilirubinaemia), liver function test abnormal	hepatic failure (see section 4.4), gamma-glutamyltransferase increased, jaundice, cholestasis, hepatomegaly, hepatitis		hepatocellular damage including fatal cases (see section 4.4)
Skin and subcutaneous tissue disorders	rash	urticaria, pruritus, erythema		
Renal and urinary disorders		blood creatinine increased, blood urea increased, renal failure aggravated		renal impairment (see section 4.4), acute renal failure
General disorders and administration site conditions	pyrexia, rigors	injection site thrombosis, infusion site inflammation, injection site pain, peripheral oedema		
Investigations		blood lactate dehydrogenase increased		

therapy with Mycamine should be made taking into account the benefit of breast-feeding to the child and the benefit of Mycamine therapy to the mother.

Testicular toxicity was observed in animal studies (see section 5.3). Micafungin may have the potential to affect male fertility in humans.

4.7 Effects on ability to drive and use machines

No studies on the effects on the ability to drive and use machines have been performed. However, adverse reactions may occur, which may influence the ability to drive and use machines (see section 4.8).

4.8 Undesirable effects

The safety profile of micafungin is based on 3028 patients treated with micafungin in clinical studies: 2.002 patients with *Candida* infections (including candidaemia, invasive candidiasis and oesophageal candidiasis), 375 with invasive aspergillosis (primarily refractory infections) and 651 for prophylaxis of systemic fungal infections.

The patients treated with micafungin in clinical studies represent a critically ill patient population that requires multiple medicinal products including antineoplastic chemotherapy, potent systemic immunosuppressants and broad spectrum antibiotics. These patients had a wide variety of complex underlying conditions such as haematological malignancies and HIV-infection or were transplant recipients and/or treated in intensive care. Patients treated prophylactically with micafungin were those undergoing haematopoetic stem cell transplantation (HSCT) who were at high risk for fungal infections.

Overall 32.2% of the patients experienced adverse drug reactions. The most frequently reported adverse reactions were nausea (2.8%), blood alkaline phosphatase increased (2.7%), phlebitis (2.5%, primarily in HIV infected patients with peripheral lines), vomiting (2.5%), and aspartate aminotransferase increased (2.3%). No clinically significant differences were seen when the safety data were analysed by gender or race.

In the following table adverse reactions are listed by system organ class and MedDRA preferred term. Within each frequency grouping, undesirable effects are presented in order of decreasing seriousness.

(see Table 1 above)

Possible allergic-like symptoms

Symptoms such as rash and rigors have been reported in clinical studies. The majority were of mild to moderate intensity and not treatment limiting. Serious reactions (e.g. anaphylactoid reaction 0.2%, 6/3028) were uncommonly reported during therapy with micafungin and only in patients with serious underlying conditions (e.g. advanced AIDS, malignancies) requiring multiple co-medications.

Hepatic adverse reactions

The overall incidence of hepatic adverse reactions in the patients treated with micafungin in clinical studies was 8.6% (260/3028). The majority of hepatic adverse reactions were mild and moderate. Most frequent reactions were increase in AP (2.7%), AST (2.3%), ALT (2.0%), blood bilirubin (1.6%) and liver function test abnormal (1.5%). Few patients (1.1%; 0.4% serious) discontinued treatment due to a hepatic event. Cases of serious hepatic dysfunction occurred uncommonly (see section 4.4).

Injection-site reactions

None of the injection-site adverse reactions were treatment limiting.

Paediatric patients

The incidence of some adverse reactions (listed in the table below) was higher in paediatric patients than in adult patients. Additionally, paediatric patients < 1 year of age experienced about two times more often an increase in ALT, AST and AP than older paediatric patients (see section 4.4). The most likely reason for these differences were different underlying conditions compared with adults or older paediatric patients observed in clinical studies. At the time of entering the study, the proportion of paediatric patients with neutropenia was several-fold higher than in adult patients (40.2% and 7.3% of children and adults, respectively), as well as allogeneic HSCT (29.4% and 13.4%, respectively) and haematological malignancy (29.1% and 8.7%, respectively).

Blood and lymphatic system disorders	
common	thrombocytopenia
Cardiac disorders	
common	tachycardia
Vascular disorders	
common	hypertension, hypotension
Hepatobiliary disorders	
common	hyperbilirubinaemia, hepatomegaly
Renal and urinary disorders	
common	acute renal failure, blood urea increased

4.9 Overdose

Repeated daily doses up to 8 mg/kg (maximum total dose 896 mg) in adult patients have been administered in clinical trials with no reported dose-limiting toxicity. One case of mis-dosage of 7.8 mg/kg/day for 7 days was reported in a newborn patient. No adverse reactions associated with this high dose were noted.

There is no experience with overdoses of micafungin. In case of overdose, general supportive measures and symptomatic treatment should be administered. Micafungin is highly protein-bound and not dialysable.

5. PHARMACOLOGICAL PROPERTIES

5.1 Pharmacodynamic properties

Pharmacotherapeutic group: Other antimycotics for systemic use, ATC code: J02AX05

Mode of action

Micafungin non-competitively inhibits the synthesis of 1,3-β-D-glucan, an essential component of the fungal cell wall. 1,3-β-D-glucan is not present in mammalian cells.

Micafungin exhibits fungicidal activity against most *Candida* species and prominently inhibits actively growing hyphae of *Aspergillus* species.

PK/PD relationship

An additive or synergistic pharmacodynamic interaction of micafungin and amphotericin B was found in a mouse model of pulmonary aspergillosis (immunosuppression with hydrocortisone, intranasal infection with Aspergillus fumigatus).

Mechanism(s) of resistance

As for all antimicrobial agents, cases of reduced susceptibility and resistance have been reported and cross-resistance with other echinocandins cannot be excluded. Reduced susceptibility to echinocandins has been associated with mutations in the Fks1 gene coding for a major subunit of glucan synthase.

Breakpoints

Susceptibility testing was performed with modifications according to the Clinical and Laboratory Standards Institute (CLSI) methods M27-A2 (*Candida* species) and M38-A (*Aspergillus* species), respectively. To date, standardised techniques for susceptibility testing for 1,3-β-D-glucan synthesis inhibitors have not been established and results of susceptibility testing do not necessarily correlate with clinical outcome.

Although no MIC breakpoints for echinocandins have been established, a MIC of ≤ 2 mg/l encompasses > 99% of all clinical isolates of Candida spp. without bisecting any species group and represents a concentration that is easily maintained throughout the dosing interval. Infections due to Candida spp. in this MIC range are likely to respond to therapy.

The prevalence of resistance may vary geographically and with time for selected species and local information on resistance is desirable, particularly when treating severe infections. This information is only a guide to the probabilities of whether micro-organisms will be susceptible to micafungin or not. Where applicable the information on the European range of acquired resistance for the individual micro-organisms is indicated in brackets.

Commonly susceptible species [MIC ranges in Europe, mg/l]
Candida albicans [0.007 - 0.25]
Candida glabrata [0.007 - 0.12]
Candida tropicalis [0.007 - 0.12]
Candida krusei [0.015 - 0.12]
Candida kefyr [0.03 - 0.06]
Candida parapsilosis [0.12 - 2]
Candida guilliermondii [0.5]
Candida lusitaniae [0.12 - 0.25]
Candida spp. [0.015 - 0.5]
incl. *C. famata, C. dubliniensis, C. lipolytica, C. pelliculosa, C. rugosa, C. stellatoidea and C. zeylanoides)*

Aspergillus fumigatus *Aspergillus flavus* *Aspergillus niger* *Aspergillus terreus* *Aspergillus nidulans* *Aspergillus versicolor*
The mycelial form of dimorphic fungi (e.g. *Histoplasma capsulatum, Blastomyces dermatitidis, Coccidioides immitis*)
Species for which acquired resistance may be a problem
None
Inherently resistant organisms
Cryptococcus spp. *Pseudallescheria* spp. *Scedosporium* spp. *Fusarium* spp. *Trichosporon* spp. *Zygomycetes* spp.

Information from clinical studies

Candidaemia and Invasive Candidiasis: Micafungin (100 mg/day or 2 mg/kg/day) was as effective as and better tolerated than liposomal amphotericin B (3 mg/kg) as first-line treatment of candidaemia and invasive candidiasis in a randomised, double-blind, multinational non-inferiority study. Micafungin and liposomal amphotericin B were received for a median duration of 15 days (range, 4 to 42 days in adults; 12 to 42 days in children).

Non-inferiority was proven for adult patients, and similar findings were demonstrated for the paediatric subpopulations (including neonates and premature infants). Efficacy findings were consistent, independent of the infective *Candida* species, primary site of infection and neutropenic status (see Table). Micafungin demonstrated a smaller mean peak decrease in estimated glomerular filtration rate during treatment (p<0.001) and a lower incidence of infusion-related reactions (p=0.001) than liposomal amphotericin B.

Overall Treatment Success in the Per Protocol Set, Invasive Candidiasis Study

(see Table 2 below)

Oesophageal Candidiasis: In a randomised, double-blind study of micafungin versus fluconazole in the first-line treatment of oesophageal candidiasis, 518 patients received at least a single dose of study drug. The median treatment duration was 14 days and the median average daily dose was 150 mg for micafungin (N=260) and 200 mg for fluconazole (N=258). An endoscopic grade of 0 (endoscopic cure) at the end of treatment was observed for 87.7% (228/260) and 88.0% (227/258) of patients in the micafungin and fluconazole groups, respectively (95% CI for difference: [-5.9%, 5.3%]). The lower limit of the 95% CI was above the predefined non-inferiority margin of -10%, proving non-inferiority. The nature and incidence of adverse events were similar between treatment groups.

Prophylaxis: Micafungin was more effective than fluconazole in preventing invasive fungal infections in a population of patients at high risk of developing a systemic fungal infection (patients undergoing haematopoietic stem cell transplantation [HSCT] in a randomised, double-blind, multicentre study). Treatment success was defined as the absence of a proven, probable, or suspected systemic fungal infection through the end of therapy and absence of a proven or probable systemic fungal infection through the end of study. Most patients (97%, N=882) had neutropenia at baseline (< 200 neutrophils/µL). Neutropenia persisted for a median of 13 days. There was a fixed daily dose of 50 mg (1.0 mg/kg) for micafungin and 400 mg (8 mg/kg) for fluconazole. The mean period of treatment was 19 days for micafungin and 18 days for fluconazole in the adult population (N=798) and 23 days for both treatment arms in the paediatric population (N=84).

The rate of treatment success was statistically significantly higher for micafungin than fluconazole (1.6% *versus* 2.4% breakthrough infections). Breakthrough *Aspergillus* infections were observed in 1 *versus* 7 patients, and proven or probable breakthrough *Candida* infections were observed in 4 *versus* 2 patients in the micafungin and fluconazole groups, respectively. Other breakthrough infections were caused by *Fusarium* (1 and 2 patients, respectively) and *Zygomycetes* (1 and 0 patients, respectively). The nature and incidence of adverse reactions were similar between treatment groups.

5.2 Pharmacokinetic properties

Absorption

Micafungin is an intravenously administered medication. Pharmacokinetics are linear over the daily dose range of 12.5 mg to 200 mg and 3 mg/kg to 8 mg/kg. There is no evidence of systemic accumulation with repeated administration and steady-state is generally reached within 4 to 5 days.

Distribution

Following intravenous administration concentrations of micafungin show a biexponential decline. The drug is rapidly distributed into tissues.

In systemic circulation, micafungin is highly bound to plasma protein (> 99%), primarily to albumin. Binding to albumin is independent of micafungin concentration (10-100 µg/ml).

The volume of distribution at steady state (Vss) was approximately 18-19 litres.

Metabolism

Unchanged micafungin is the principal circulating compound in systemic circulation. Micafungin has been shown to be metabolised to several compounds; of these M-1 (catechol form), M-2 (methoxy form of M-1) and M-5 (hydroxylation at the side chain) of micafungin have been detected in systemic circulation. Exposure to these metabolites is low and metabolites do not contribute to the overall efficacy of micafungin.

Even though micafungin is a substrate for CYP3A *in vitro*, hydroxylation by CYP3A is not a major pathway for micafungin metabolism *in vivo*.

Elimination and excretion

The mean terminal half-life is approximately 10-17 hours and stays consistent across doses up to 8 mg/kg and after single and repeated administration. Total clearance was 0.15-0.3 ml/min/kg in healthy subjects and adult patients and is independent of dose after single and repeated administration.

Following a single intravenous dose of ^{14}C-micafungin (25 mg) to healthy volunteers, 11.6% of the radioactivity was recovered in the urine and 71.0% in the faeces over 28 days. These data indicate that elimination of micafungin is primarily non-renal. In plasma, metabolites M-1 and M-2 were detected only at trace concentrations and metabolite M-5, the more abundant metabolite, accounted for a total of 6.5% relative to parent compound.

Special populations

Paediatric patients: In paediatric patients AUC values were dose proportional over the dose range of 0.5-4 mg/kg. Clearance was influenced by age, with mean values of clearance in younger children (2-11 years) being approximately 1.3 -fold greater than those in older children (12-17 years). Older children had mean clearance values similar to those determined in adult patients. Mean clearance in premature infants (gestational age approximately 26 weeks) is approximately 5-fold greater than in adults.

Elderly: When administered as a single 1-hour infusion of 50 mg the pharmacokinetics of micafungin in the elderly (aged 66-78 years) were similar to those in young (20-24 years) subjects. No dose adjustment is necessary for the elderly.

Patients with hepatic impairment: In a study performed in patients with moderate hepatic impairment (Child-Pugh score 7-9), (n=8), the pharmacokinetics of micafungin did not significantly differ from those in healthy subjects (n=8). Therefore, no dose adjustment is necessary for patients with mild to moderate hepatic impairment. The pharmacokinetics of micafungin has not been studied in patients with severe hepatic insufficiency.

Patients with renal impairment: Severe renal impairment (Glomerular Filtration Rate [GFR] < 30 ml/min) did not significantly affect the pharmacokinetics of micafungin. No dose adjustment is necessary for patients with renal impairment.

Gender/Race: Gender and race (Caucasian, Black and Oriental) did not significantly influence the pharmacokinetic parameters of micafungin. No dose adjustment of micafungin is required based on gender or race.

5.3 Preclinical safety data

The development of foci of altered hepatocytes (FAH) and hepatocellular tumours in rats was dependent on both dose and duration of micafungin treatment. FAH recorded after treatment for 13 weeks or longer persisted after a 13-week withdrawal period and developed into hepatocellular tumours following a treatment free period which covered the life span of rats. No standard carcinogenicity studies have been conducted but the development of FAH was assessed in female rats after up to 20 and 18 months after cessation of a 3 and 6 month treatment, respectively. In both studies increased incidences/numbers of hepatocellular tumours were observed after the 18 and 20 month treatment free period in the high dose group of 32 mg/kg/day as well as in a lower dose group (although not statistically significant). The plasma exposure at the assumed threshold for tumour development in rats (i.e. the dose where no FAH and liver tumours were detected) was in the same range as the clinical exposure. The relevance of the hepatocarcinogenic potential of micafungin for the human therapeutic use is not known.

The toxicology of micafungin following repeated intravenous dosing in rats and/or dogs showed adverse responses in liver, urinary tract, red blood cells, and male reproductive organs. The exposure levels at which these effects did not occur (NOAEL) were in the same range as the clinical exposure or lower. Consequently, the occurrence of these adverse responses may be expected in human clinical use of micafungin.

In standard safety pharmacology tests, cardiovascular and histamine releasing effects of micafungin were evident and appeared to be time above threshold dependent. Prolongation of infusion time reducing the plasma concentration peak appeared to reduce these effects.

In repeated dose toxicity studies in rat signs of hepatotoxicity consisted of increased liver enzymes and degenerative changes of hepatocytes which were accompanied by signs of compensatory regeneration. In dog, liver effects consisted of increased weight and centrilobular hypertrophy, no degenerative changes of hepatocytes were observed.

In rats, vacuolation of the renal pelvic epithelium as well as vacuolation and thickening (hyperplasia) of the bladder epithelium were observed in 26-week repeat dose studies.

Table 2 Overall Treatment Success in the Per Protocol Set, Invasive Candidiasis Study

	Micafungin		Liposomal Amphotericin B		% Difference [95% CI]
	N	n (%)	N	n (%)	
Adult Patients					
Overall Treatment Success	202	181 (89.6)	190	170 (89.5)	0.1 [-5.9, 6.1] †
Overall Treatment Success by Neutropenic Status					
Neutropenia at baseline	24	18 (75.0)	15	12 (80.0)	0.7 [-5.3, 6.7] ‡
No neutropenia at baseline	178	163 (91.6)	175	158 (90.3)	
Paediatric Patients					
Overall Treatment Success	48	35 (72.9)	50	38 (76.0)	-2.7 [-17.3, 11.9] §
< 2 years old	26	21 (80.8)	31	24 (77.4)	
Premature Infants	10	7 (70.0)	9	6 (66.7)	
Neonates (0 days to < 4 weeks)	7	7 (100)	5	4 (80)	
2 to 15 years old	22	14 (63.6)	19	14 (73.7)	
Adults and Children Combined, Overall Treatment Success by *Candida* Species					
Candida albicans	102	91 (89.2)	98	89 (90.8)	
Non-*albicans* species ¶: all	151	133 (88.1)	140	123 (87.9)	
C. tropicalis	59	54 (91.5)	51	49 (96.1)	
C. parapsilosis	48	41 (85.4)	44	35 (79.5)	
C. glabrata	23	19 (82.6)	17	14 (82.4)	
C. krusei	9	8 (88.9)	7	6 (85.7)	

† Micafungin rate minus the liposomal amphotericin B rate, and 2-sided 95% confidence interval for the difference in overall success rate based on large sample normal approximation.

‡ Adjusted for neutropenic status; primary endpoint.

§ The paediatric population was not sized to test for non-inferiority.

¶ Clinical efficacy was also observed (< 5 patients) in the following *Candida* species: *C. guilliermondii, C. famata, C. lusitaniae, C. utilis, C. inconspicua* and *C. dubliniensis*.

Table 3 Preparation of the solution for infusion

Dose (mg)	Mycamine vial to be used (mg/vial)	Volume of sodium chloride (0.9%) or glucose (5%) to be added per vial	Volume (concentration) of reconstituted powder	Standard infusion (added up to 100 ml) Final concentration
50	1 × 50	5 ml	approx. 5 ml (10 mg/ml)	0.5 mg/ml
100	1 × 100	5 ml	approx. 5 ml (20 mg/ml)	1.0 mg/ml
150	1 × 100 + 1 × 50	5 ml	approx. 10 ml	1.5 mg/ml
200	2 × 100	5 ml	approx. 10 ml	2.0 mg/ml

In a second 26-week study hyperplasia of transitional cells in the urinary bladder occurred with a much lower incidence. These findings showed reversibility over a follow-up period of 18 months. The duration of micafungin dosing in these rat studies (6 months) exceeds the usual duration of micafungin dosing in patients (see section 5.1).

Micafungin haemolysed rabbit blood *in vitro*. In rats, signs of haemolytic anaemia were observed after repeated bolus injection of micafungin. In repeat dose studies in dogs, haemolytic anaemia was not observed.

In reproductive and developmental toxicity studies, reduced birth weight of the pups was noted. One abortion occurred in rabbits at 32 mg/kg/day. Male rats treated intravenously for 9 weeks showed vacuolation of the epididymal ductal epithelial cells, increased epididymis weights and reduced number of sperm cells (by 15%), however, in studies of 13 and 26 weeks duration these changes did not occur. In adult dogs, atrophy of seminiferous tubules with vacuolation of the seminiferous epithelium and decreased sperm in the epididymides were noted after prolonged treatment (39 weeks) but not after 13 weeks of treatment. In juvenile dogs, 39 weeks treatment did not induce lesions in the testis and epididymides in a dose dependent manner at the end of treatment but after a treatment free period of 13 weeks a dose dependent increase in these lesions were noted in the treated recovery groups. No impairment of male or female fertility was observed in the fertility and early embryonic development study in rats.

Micafungin was not mutagenic or clastogenic when evaluated in a standard battery of *in vitro* and *in vivo* tests, including an *in vitro* study on unscheduled DNA synthesis using rat hepatocytes.

6. PHARMACEUTICAL PARTICULARS

6.1 List of excipients

Lactose monohydrate

Citric acid anhydrous (to adjust the pH)

Sodium hydroxide (to adjust the pH)

6.2 Incompatibilities

This medicinal product must not be mixed or co-infused with other medicinal products except those mentioned in section 6.6.

6.3 Shelf life

Unopened vial: 3 years.

Reconstituted concentrate in vial:

Chemical and physical in-use stability has been demonstrated for up to 48 hours at 25°C when reconstituted with sodium chloride 9 mg/ml (0.9%) solution for infusion or glucose 50 mg/ml (5%) solution for infusion.

Diluted infusion solution:

Chemical and physical in-use stability has been demonstrated for 96 hours at 25°C when protected from light when diluted with sodium chloride 9 mg/ml (0.9%) solution for infusion or glucose 50 mg/ml (5%) solution for infusion.

Mycamine contains no preservatives. From a microbiological point of view, the reconstituted and diluted solutions should be used immediately. If not used immediately, in-use storage times and conditions prior to use are the responsibility of the user and would normally not be longer than 24 hours at 2 to 8°C, unless the reconstitution and dilution have taken place in controlled and validated aseptic conditions.

6.4 Special precautions for storage

Unopened vials: This medicinal product does not require any special storage conditions.

For storage conditions of the reconstituted and diluted medicinal product, see section 6.3.

6.5 Nature and contents of container

10 ml Type I glass vial with an isobutylene-isoprene (Teflon-laminated) rubber stopper and a flip-off cap. The vial is wrapped with an UV-protective film.

Supplied in packs of 1 vial.

6.6 Special precautions for disposal and other handling

Any unused product or waste material should be disposed of in accordance with local requirements.

Mycamine must not be mixed or co-infused with other medicinal products except those mentioned below. Using aseptic techniques at room temperature, Mycamine is reconstituted and diluted as follows:

1. The plastic cap must be removed from the vial and the stopper disinfected with alcohol.

2. Five ml of sodium chloride 9 mg/ml (0.9%) solution for infusion or glucose 50 mg/ml (5%) solution for infusion (taken from a 100 ml bottle/bag) should be aseptically and slowly injected into each vial along the side of the inner wall. Although the concentrate will foam, every effort should be made to minimise the amount of foam generated. A sufficient number of vials of Mycamine must be reconstituted to obtain the required dose in mg (see table below).

3. The vial should be rotated gently. DO NOT SHAKE. The powder will dissolve completely. The concentrate should be used immediately. The vial is for single use only. Therefore, please discard unused reconstituted concentrate immediately.

4. All of the reconstituted concentrate should be withdrawn from each vial and returned into the infusion bottle/bag from which it was originally taken. The diluted infusion solution should be used immediately. Chemical and physical in-use stability has been demonstrated for 96 hours at 25°C when protected from light and diluted as described above.

5. The infusion bottle/bag should be gently inverted to disperse the diluted solution but NOT agitated in order to avoid foaming. Do not use if the solution is cloudy or has precipitated.

6. The infusion bottle/bag containing the diluted infusion solution should be inserted into a closable opaque bag for protection from light.

Preparation of the solution for infusion

(see Table 3 above)

After reconstitution and dilution, the solution should be administered by intravenous infusion over approximately 1 hour.

7. MARKETING AUTHORISATION HOLDER

Astellas Pharma Europe B.V.

Elisabethhof 19

2353 EW Leiderdorp

Netherlands

8. MARKETING AUTHORISATION NUMBER(S)

EU/1/08/448/001

EU/1/08/448/002

9. DATE OF FIRST AUTHORISATION/RENEWAL OF THE AUTHORISATION

Date of first authorisation: 25/04/2008

10. DATE OF REVISION OF THE TEXT

29th September 2008

11. LEGAL CATEGORY

POM

Detailed information on this medicinal product is available on the website of the European Medicines Agency (EMEA) http://www.emea.europa.eu/.

Mycobutin

(Pharmacia Limited)

1. NAME OF THE MEDICINAL PRODUCT

Mycobutin.

2. QUALITATIVE AND QUANTITATIVE COMPOSITION

Rifabutin INN 150.0 mg

3. PHARMACEUTICAL FORM

Opaque, red-brown, hard gelatin capsules Size N°. 0 containing 150 mg rifabutin in transparent PVC/Al blisters or in amber glass bottles.

The capsules are for oral administration.

4. CLINICAL PARTICULARS

4.1 Therapeutic indications

Mycobutin is indicated for:

- the prophylaxis of *M. avium intracellulare complex* (MAC) infections in patients with HIV disease with CD4 counts lower than 75 cells/mcl

- the treatment of non-tuberculous mycobacterial disease (such as that caused by MAC and M. xenopi)

- pulmonary tuberculosis

4.2 Posology and method of administration

Mycobutin can be administered as a single, daily, oral dose at any time independently of meals.

Adults

- prophylaxis of *M. avium intracellulare complex* (MAC) infections in patients with HIV disease with CD4 counts lower than 75 cells/mcl:

o 300 mg (2 capsules) as a single agent.

- treatment of non-tuberculous mycobacterial disease:

o 450 - 600 mg (3 - 4 capsules) in combination regimens for up to 6 months after negative cultures are obtained.

o When Mycobutin is given in association with clarithromycin (or other macrolides) and/or fluconazole (or related compounds) the Mycobutin dosage may need to be reduced to 300 mg (see Section 4.5).

- treatment of pulmonary tuberculosis:

o 150 - 450 mg (1 - 3 capsules) in combination regimens for at least 6 months.

In accordance with the commonly accepted criteria for the treatment of mycobacterial infections, Mycobutin should always be given in combination with other anti-mycobacterial drugs not belonging to the family of rifamycins.

Children

There are inadequate data to support the use of Mycobutin in children at the present time.

Elderly

No specific recommendations for dosage alterations in the elderly are suggested.

4.3 Contraindications

Mycobutin is contra-indicated in patients with a history of hypersensitivity to rifabutin or other rifamycins (eg rifampicin).

Due to insufficient clinical experience in pregnant and breast-feeding women and in children, Mycobutin should not be used in these patients.

4.4 Special warnings and precautions for use

Before starting Mycobutin prophylaxis, patients should be assessed to ensure that they do not have active disease caused by pulmonary tuberculosis or other mycobacteria.

Prophylaxis against MAC infection may need to be continued throughout the patient's lifetime.

Mycobutin may impart a red-orange colour to the urine and possibly to skin and body secretions. Contact lenses, especially soft, may be permanently stained.

Mild hepatic impairment does not require a dose modification. Mycobutin should be used with caution in cases of severe liver insufficiency. Mild to moderate renal impairment does not require any dosage adjustment.

Severe renal impairment (creatinine clearance below 30 ml/min) requires a dosage reduction of 50%.

It is recommended that white blood cell and platelet counts and liver enzymes be monitored periodically during treatment.

Because of the possibility of occurrence of uveitis, patients should be carefully monitored when rifabutin is given in combination with clarithromycin (or other macrolides) and/or fluconazole (and related compounds). If such an event occurs, the patient should be referred to an ophthalmologist and, if considered necessary, Mycobutin treatment should be suspended.

Uveitis associated with Mycobutin must be distinguished from other ocular complications of HIV.

Clostridium difficile associated diarrhoea (CDAD) has been reported with use of nearly all antibacterial agents, including rifabutin, and may range in severity from mild diarrhoea to fatal colitis. Treatment with antibacterial agents alters the normal flora of the colon leading to overgrowth of *C. difficile*.

C. difficile produces toxins A and B which contribute to the development of CDAD. Hypertoxin producing strains of *C. difficile* cause increased morbidity and mortality, as these infections can be refractory to antimicrobial therapy and may require colectomy. CDAD must be considered in all patients who present with diarrhoea following antibiotic use. Careful medical history is necessary since CDAD has been reported to occur over two months after the administration of antibacterial agents.

4.5 Interaction with other medicinal products and other forms of interaction

Rifabutin has been shown to induce the enzymes of the cytochrome P450 3A subfamily and therefore may affect the pharmacokinetic behaviour of drugs metabolised by the enzymes belonging to this subfamily. Upward adjustment of the dosage of such drugs may be required when administered with Mycobutin.

Similarly, Mycobutin might reduce the activity of analgesics, anticoagulants, corticosteroids, cyclosporin, digitalis (although not digoxin), oral hypoglycaemics, narcotics, phenytoin and quinidine.

Clinical studies have shown that Mycobutin does not affect the pharmacokinetics of didanosine (DDI), and isoniazid (however, for the latter refer also to undesirable effects). On the basis of the above metabolic considerations no significant interaction may be expected with ethambutol, theophylline, sulphonamides, pyrazinamide and zalcitabine (DDC).

As p-aminosalicylic acid has been shown to impede GI absorption of rifamycins it is recommended that when it and Mycobutin are both to be administered they be given with an interval of 8 - 12 hours.

The following table provides details of the possible effects of co-administration, on rifabutin and the co-administered drug, and risk-benefit statement.

(see Table 1 opposite)

4.6 Pregnancy and lactation

Due to lack of data in pregnant women, as a precautionary measure, Mycobutin should not be administered to pregnant women or those breast-feeding children even though in experimental animal studies the drug was not teratogenic.

Mycobutin may interact with oral contraceptives (see Section 4.5).

4.7 Effects on ability to drive and use machines

There have been no reports of adverse effects on ability to drive and use machines.

4.8 Undesirable effects

The tolerability of Mycobutin in multiple drug regimens was assessed in both immunocompetent and immunocompromised patients, suffering from tuberculosis and non-tuberculous mycobacteriosis in long term studies with daily dosages up to 600 mg.

Bearing in mind that Mycobutin was often given in these studies as part of a multi-drug regimen it is not possible to define with certainty a drug-event relationship. Treatment discontinuation was necessary only in a very few cases. The most commonly reported adverse events were primarily related to:

- the gastro-intestinal system, such as nausea, vomiting, increase of liver enzymes, jaundice;
- the blood and lymphatic system, such as leucopoenia, neutropenia, thrombocytopenia and anaemia, where the frequency and severity of haematologic reactions could be increased by combined administration of isoniazid;
- the musculo-skeletal system: arthralgia and myalgia.

Also, fever, rash and rarely other hypersensitivity reactions such as eosinophilia, bronchospasm and shock might occur as has been seen with other antibiotics.

In addition, mild to severe, reversible uveitis has been reported. The risk appears to be low, when Mycobutin is used at 300 mg as monotherapy in MAC prophylaxis, but increases when Mycobutin is administered at higher doses in combination with clarithromycin (or other macrolides) for MAC treatment (see Section 4.4). The possible role of fluconazole (and related compounds) has not been established yet.

Asymptomatic corneal opacities have been reported after long term therapy.

Pseudojaundice (yellow skin discolouration with normal plasma bilirubin) has been reported with high doses of rifabutin.

Flu-like syndrome, chest pressure or pain with dyspnoea and rarely hepatitis and haemolysis.

Clostridium difficile diarrhoea has been reported rarely.

4.9 Overdose

Gastric lavage and diuretic treatment should be carried out. Supportive care and symptomatic treatment should be administered.

5. PHARMACOLOGICAL PROPERTIES

5.1 Pharmacodynamic properties

In vitro activity of rifabutin against laboratory strains and clinical isolates of *M. tuberculosis* has been shown to be very high. *In vitro* studies carried out so far have shown that from one-third to half of *M.tuberculosis* strains resistant to rifampicin are susceptible to rifabutin, indicating that cross-resistance between the two antibiotics is incomplete.

The *in vivo* activity of rifabutin on experimental infections caused by *M. tuberculosis* was about 10 times greater than that of rifampicin in agreement with the *in vitro* findings.

Rifabutin was seen to be active against non-tuberculous (atypical) mycobacteria including *M. avium-intracellulare* (MAC), *in vitro* as well as in experimental infections caused by these pathogens in mice with induced immuno-deficiency.

5.2 Pharmacokinetic properties

In man, rifabutin is rapidly absorbed and maximum plasma concentrations are reached around 2-4 hours after oral administration. The pharmacokinetics of rifabutin is linear after single administration of 300, 450, and 600 mg to healthy volunteers. With these doses, C max is in the range of 0.4-0.7 μg/ml. Plasma concentrations are maintained above the MIC values for *M. tuberculosis* up to about 30 hours from administration.

Rifabutin is widely distributed in various animal organs with the exception of the brain. In particular, in human lung tissue the concentrations measured up to 24 hours after dosing were about 5-10 times higher than the plasma levels.

Table 1

Coadministered drugs	Effect on rifabutin	Effect on co-administered drug	Comments
ANTIVIRALS			
Indinavir	20% increase in AUC.	32% decrease in AUC.	
Saquinavir	No data.	40% decrease in AUC.	
Ritonavir	4-fold increase in AUC, 2.5-fold increase in Cmax	No data	Due to this multifold increase in rifabutin concentrations and the subsequent risk of side effects, patients requiring both rifabutin and a protease inhibitor, other protease inhibitors should be considered.
Zidovudine	No significant change in kinetics	Approx. 32% decrease in Cmax and AUC.	A large clinical study has shown that these changes are of no clinical relevance.
ANTIFUNGALS			
Fluconazole	82% increase in AUC.	No significant change in steady-state plasma concentrations	
Itraconazole	No data.	70-75% decrease in Cmax and AUC.	A case report indicates an increase in rifabutin serum levels in the presence of itraconazole.
Ketoconazole/ miconazole	No data.	No data.	Co-administered medications, such as ketoconazole, that competitively inhibit the Cyt P450IIIA activity may increase circulating drug levels of rifabutin.
ANTI-PCP (Pneumocystis carinii pneumonia)			
Dapsone	No data.	Approximately 27%-40% decrease in AUC.	Study conducted in HIV infected patients (rapid and slow acetylators)
Sulfamethoxazole-Trimethoprim	No significant change in Cmax and AUC.	Approx. 15-20% decrease in AUC.	In another study, only trimethoprim (not sulfamethoxazole had 14% decrease in AUC and 6% in Cmax but were not considered clinically significant.
ANTI-MAC (Mycobacterium avium intracellulare complex)			
Clarithromycin	Approx. 77% increase in AUC.	Approx. 50% decrease in AUC.	Study conducted in HIV infected patients
OTHER			
Methadone	No data.	No significant effect.	No apparent effect of rifabutin on either peak levels of methadone or systemic exposure based upon AUC. Rifabutin kinetics not evaluated.
Oral contraceptives	No data.	No data.	Contraceptive cover may not be adequate during concomitant therapy with rifabutin, therefore, patients should be advised to use other methods of contraception.
Tacrolimus	No data.	No data.	Rifabutin decreases tacrolimus trough blood levels.

The intracellular penetration of rifabutin is very high as demonstrated by intracellular/extracellular concentration ratios which ranged from 9 in neutrophils to 15 in monocytes, both obtained from human sources.

The high intracellular concentration is likely to play a crucial role in sustaining the efficacy of rifabutin against intracellular pathogens such as mycobacteria.

Rifabutin and its metabolites are eliminated mainly by the urinary route. The $t_{½}$ of rifabutin in man is approximately 35-40 hours.

5.3 Preclinical safety data

Preclinical safety studies of rifabutin indicate a good safety margin in rodents and in monkeys.

In repeated dose studies, target organs were identified at doses producing blood levels higher than those achieved with recommended doses for human therapy. The main target organs are liver and, to a lesser degree, erythrocytes.

Rifabutin did not show any teratogenic, mutagenic or carcinogenic potential.

6. PHARMACEUTICAL PARTICULARS

6.1 List of excipients

Microcrystalline cellulose

Sodium lauryl sulphate

Magnesium stearate

Silica gel

6.2 Incompatibilities

None known

6.3 Shelf life

24 months at room temperature.

6.4 Special precautions for storage

None

6.5 Nature and contents of container

Transparent PVC/Al blisters in cardboard cartons containing 30 capsules or amber glass bottles containing 30 or 100 capsules.

6.6 Special precautions for disposal and other handling

There are no special instructions for handling.

Administrative Data

7. MARKETING AUTHORISATION HOLDER

Pharmacia Limited
Ramsgate Road
Sandwich
Kent CT13 9NJ
United Kingdom

8. MARKETING AUTHORISATION NUMBER(S)

PL 00032/0320

9. DATE OF FIRST AUTHORISATION/RENEWAL OF THE AUTHORISATION

15th January 2003.

10. DATE OF REVISION OF THE TEXT

June 2009

Ref: MY_3_0

Mydrilate 0.5% Eye Drops

(Intrapharm Laboratories Ltd)

1. NAME OF THE MEDICINAL PRODUCT

Mydrilate 0.5 % Eye Drops.

2. QUALITATIVE AND QUANTITATIVE COMPOSITION

Cyclopentolate Hydrochloride BP 0.5 % w/v.

3. PHARMACEUTICAL FORM
Eye drops.

4. CLINICAL PARTICULARS

4.1 Therapeutic indications

(i) Diagnostic purposes for fundoscopy and cycloplegic refraction.

(ii) Dilating the pupil in inflammatory conditions of the iris and uveal tract.

4.2 Posology and method of administration

(i) Refraction / Fundoscopy

Adults (and the elderly):

One drop of 0.5 % solution instilled into the eye, repeated after 15 minutes if necessary, approximately 40 minutes before examination.

Deeply pigmented eyes may require the use of a 1 % solution.

NB: Maximum effect is reached after 30-60 minutes.

Children 6-16 years:

One drop of 1 % solution instilled into the eye, repeated after 15 minutes if necessary, approximately 40 minutes before examination.

Children under 6 years:

One or two drops of 1 % solution instilled into the eye, repeated after 15 minutes if necessary, approximately 40 minutes before examination.

(ii) For Uveitis, Iritis and Iridocyclitis:

Adults and the elderly:

One or two drops of 0.5 % solution instilled into the eye up to 4 times daily or as required.

Deeply pigmented eyes may require the use of a 1 % solution.

Children:

At the discretion of the physician

Do not use during the first three months of life due to possible association between the cycloplegia produced and the development of amblyopia and also the increased risks of systemic toxicity in neonates.

Cycloplegia following administration is quick in onset and short-lived. Maximal cycloplegia is achieved within 15 - 45 minutes of instillation and lasts on average about 20 minutes. Recovery normally takes place in about 4 hours, but very occasionally some effect persists for up to 24 hours.

Mydriasis is produced very rapidly and an average pupil diameter of 7 mm is usually reached 15 - 30 minutes after instillation of one drop of 0.5 % solution. Complete recovery from the mydriatic effect generally occurs spontaneously in not more than 20 hours.

No specific information on the use of this product in the elderly is available. Clinical trials have included patients over 65 years and no adverse reactions specific to this age group have been reported.

4.3 Contraindications

(i) Use in narrow-angle glaucoma or those with a tendency towards glaucoma e.g. patients with a shallow anterior chamber.

(ii) Hypersensitivity to cyclopentolate hydrochloride, benzalkonium chloride or any other components of the formulation.

(iii) This preparation contains benzalkonium chloride and should not be used whilst soft contact lenses are being worn.

(iv) Use in patients with paralytic ileus.

(v) Use in children with organic brain syndromes, including congenital or neuro-developmental abnormalities, particularly those predisposing to epileptic seizures.

4.4 Special warnings and precautions for use

Because of the risk of precipitating angle-closure glaucoma in the elderly and others prone to raised intraocular pressure, an estimate of the depth of the anterior chamber should be made before use, particularly if therapy is likely to be intense or protracted.

Caution should be observed when drugs of this group are administered to patients with prostatic enlargement, coronary insufficiency or cardiac failure, or ataxia. Atropine-like effects have been reported as side-effects.

Extreme caution is advised for use in children and individuals susceptible to belladonna alkaloids because of the increased risk of systemic toxicity.

Patients should be warned of the oral toxicity of this preparation, and advised to wash their hands after use. If accidentally swallowed, patients should be advised to seek medical attention.

Use with caution in an inflamed eye as the hyperaemia greatly increases the rate of systemic absorption through the conjunctiva.

To reduce systemic absorption the lacrimal sac should be compressed at the medial canthus by digital pressure for at least two minutes after instillation of the drops.

4.5 Interaction with other medicinal products and other forms of interaction

The effects of anti-muscarinic agents may be enhanced by the concomitant administration of other drugs with anti-muscarinic properties such as some antihistamines, butyrophenones, phenothiazines, tricyclic antidepressants and amantadine.

4.6 Pregnancy and lactation

There is insufficient evidence as to drug safety in pregnancy and lactation. This product should not be used during pregnancy unless it is considered essential by a physician.

4.7 Effects on ability to drive and use machines

May cause blurred vision, difficulty in focusing and sensitivity to light. Patients should be warned not to drive or engage in other hazardous activities (including climbing ladders and scaffolding) unless vision is clear. Complete recovery from the effects of Mydrilate Eye Drops may take up to 24 hours.

4.8 Undesirable effects

(i) Local:

Increased intraocular pressure, transient stinging, and sensitivity to light secondary to pupillary dilation. Prolonged administration may lead to local irritation, hyperaemia, oedema and conjunctivitis.

(ii) Systemic:

Systemic anticholinergic toxicity is manifested by dryness of the mouth, flushing, dryness of the skin, bradycardia followed by tachycardia with palpitations and arrhythmias, urinary urgency, difficulty and retention, reduction in the tone and motility of the gastrointestinal tract leading to constipation.

(iii) Vomiting, giddiness and staggering may occur, a rash may be present in children, abdominal distension in infants. Psychotic reactions, behavioural disturbances and cardio-respiratory collapse may occur in children.

4.9 Overdose

Systemic toxicity may occur following topical use, particularly in children. It is manifested by flushing and dryness of the skin (a rash may be present in children), blurred vision, a rapid and irregular pulse, fever, abdominal distension in infants, convulsions and hallucinations and the loss of neuromuscular co-ordination.

Treatment is supportive (there is no evidence that physostigmine is superior to supportive management). In infants and small children the body surface must be kept moist. If accidentally ingested, induce emesis or perform gastric lavage.

5. PHARMACOLOGICAL PROPERTIES

5.1 Pharmacodynamic properties

Cyclopentolate is an anti-muscarinic agent used topically in the eye as a mydriatic and cycloplegic. The effects are similar to those of atropine, but with a more rapid onset and a shorter duration of action.

5.2 Pharmacokinetic properties

None stated.

5.3 Preclinical safety data

None stated.

6. PHARMACEUTICAL PARTICULARS

6.1 List of excipients

Boric acid

Potassium chloride

Benzalkonium chloride solution

Purified water.

6.2 Incompatibilities

None stated.

6.3 Shelf life

2 years.

6.4 Special precautions for storage

Store at 2-8 C. Refrigerate, do not freeze. Protect from light.

Do not dilute or dispense from any container other than the original bottle. Discard one month after opening.

6.5 Nature and contents of container

5 ml dropper bottle of 0.5 % solution.

Bottle: LE 6601 PH (LDPE)

Natural colour

Cap Melochem ™

White colour

6.6 Special precautions for disposal and other handling

When using the product for the first time, screw down firmly to pierce the seal at the tip of the plastic nozzle.

7. MARKETING AUTHORISATION HOLDER

Intrapharm Laboratories Ltd

60 Boughton Lane

Maidstone

Kent

ME15 9QS

United Kingdom

8. MARKETING AUTHORISATION NUMBER(S)

17509/0007

9. DATE OF FIRST AUTHORISATION/RENEWAL OF THE AUTHORISATION

17 December 1999

10. DATE OF REVISION OF THE TEXT

June 2003

11. Legal category

POM

Mydrilate 1.0% Eye Drops

(Intrapharm Laboratories Ltd)

1. NAME OF THE MEDICINAL PRODUCT

Mydrilate 1.0 % Eye Drops

2. QUALITATIVE AND QUANTITATIVE COMPOSITION

Cyclopentolate Hydrochloride BP 1.0 % w/v.

3. PHARMACEUTICAL FORM

Eye drops.

4. CLINICAL PARTICULARS

4.1 Therapeutic indications

(i) Diagnostic purposes for fundoscopy and cycloplegic refraction.

(ii) Dilating the pupil in inflammatory conditions of the iris and uveal tract.

4.2 Posology and method of administration

(i) Refraction / Fundoscopy

Adults (and the elderly):

One drop of 0.5 % solution instilled into the eye, repeated after 15 minutes if necessary, approximately 40 minutes before examination.

Deeply pigmented eyes may require the use of a 1 % solution.

NB: Maximum effect is reached after 30-60 minutes.

Children 6-16 years:

One drop of 1 % solution instilled into the eye, repeated after 15 minutes if necessary, approximately 40 minutes before examination.

Children under 6 years:

One or two drops of 1 % solution instilled into the eye, repeated after 15 minutes if necessary, approximately 40 minutes before examination.

(ii) For Uveitis, Iritis and Iridocyclitis:

Adults and the elderly:

One or two drops of 0.5 % solution instilled into the eye up to 4 times daily or as required.

Deeply pigmented eyes may require the use of a 1 % solution.

Children:

At the discretion of the physician

Do not use during the first three months of life due to possible association between the cycloplegia produced and the development of amblyopia and also the increased risks of systemic toxicity in neonates.

Cycloplegia following administration is quick in onset and short-lived. Maximal cycloplegia is achieved within 15 - 45 minutes of instillation and lasts on average about 20 minutes. Recovery normally takes place in about 4 hours, but very occasionally some effect persists for up to 24 hours.

Mydriasis is produced very rapidly and an average pupil diameter of 7 mm is usually reached 15 - 30 minutes after instillation of one drop of 0.5 % solution. Complete recovery from the mydriatic effect generally occurs spontaneously in not more than 20 hours.

No specific information on the use of this product in the elderly is available. Clinical trials have included patients over 65 years and no adverse reactions specific to this age group have been reported.

4.3 Contraindications

(i) Use in narrow-angle glaucoma or those with a tendency towards glaucoma e.g. patients with a shallow anterior chamber.

(ii) Hypersensitivity to cyclopentolate hydrochloride, benzalkonium chloride or any other components of the formulation.

(iii) This preparation contains benzalkonium chloride and should not be used whilst soft contact lenses are being worn.

(iv) Use in patients with paralytic ileus.

(v) Use in children with organic brain syndromes, including congenital or neuro-developmental abnormalities, particularly those predisposing to epileptic seizures.

4.4 Special warnings and precautions for use

Because of the risk of precipitating angle-closure glaucoma in the elderly and others prone to raised intraocular pressure, an estimate of the depth of the anterior chamber should be made before use, particularly if therapy is likely to be intense or protracted.

Caution should be observed when drugs of this group are administered to patients with prostatic enlargement, coronary insufficiency or cardiac failure, or ataxia. Atropine-like effects have been reported as side-effects.

Extreme caution is advised for use in children and individuals susceptible to belladonna alkaloids because of the increased risk of systemic toxicity.

Patients should be warned of the oral toxicity of this preparation, and advised to wash their hands after use. If accidentally swallowed, patients should be advised to seek medical attention.

Use with caution in an inflamed eye as the hyperaemia greatly increases the rate of systemic absorption through the conjunctiva.

To reduce systemic absorption the lacrimal sac should be compressed at the medial canthus by digital pressure for at least two minutes after instillation of the drops.

4.5 Interaction with other medicinal products and other forms of interaction

The effects of anti-muscarinic agents may be enhanced by the concomitant administration of other drugs with anti-muscarinic properties such as some antihistamines, butyrophenones, phenothiazines, tricyclic antidepressants and amantadine.

4.6 Pregnancy and lactation

There is insufficient evidence as to drug safety in pregnancy and lactation. This product should not be used during pregnancy unless it is considered essential by a physician.

4.7 Effects on ability to drive and use machines

May cause blurred vision, difficulty in focusing and sensitivity to light. Patients should be warned not to drive or engage in other hazardous activities (including climbing ladders and scaffolding) unless vision is clear. Complete recovery from the effects of Mydrilate Eye Drops may take up to 24 hours.

4.8 Undesirable effects

(i) Local:

Increased intraocular pressure, transient stinging, and sensitivity to light secondary to pupillary dilation. Prolonged administration may lead to local irritation, hyperaemia, oedema and conjunctivitis.

(ii) Systemic:

Systemic anticholinergic toxicity is manifested by dryness of the mouth, flushing, dryness of the skin, bradycardia followed by tachycardia with palpitations and arrhythmias, urinary urgency, difficulty and retention, reduction in the tone and motility of the gastrointestinal tract leading to constipation.

(iii) Vomiting, giddiness and staggering may occur, a rash may be present in children, abdominal distension in infants. Psychotic reactions, behavioural disturbances and cardio-respiratory collapse may occur in children.

4.9 Overdose

Systemic toxicity may occur following topical use, particularly in children. It is manifested by flushing and dryness of the skin (a rash may be present in children), blurred vision, a rapid and irregular pulse, fever, abdominal distension in infants, convulsions and hallucinations and the loss of neuromuscular co-ordination.

Treatment is supportive (there is no evidence that physostigmine is superior to supportive management). In infants and small children the body surface must be kept moist. If accidentally ingested, induce emesis or perform gastric lavage.

5. PHARMACOLOGICAL PROPERTIES

5.1 Pharmacodynamic properties

Cyclopentolate is an anti-muscarinic agent used topically in the eye as a mydriatic and cycloplegic. The effects are similar to those of atropine, but with a more rapid onset and a shorter duration of action.

5.2 Pharmacokinetic properties

None stated.

5.3 Preclinical safety data

None stated.

6. PHARMACEUTICAL PARTICULARS

6.1 List of excipients

Boric acid

Potassium chloride

Benzalkonium chloride solution

Purified water.

6.2 Incompatibilities

None stated.

6.3 Shelf life

2 years.

6.4 Special precautions for storage

Store at 2-8°C. Refrigerate, do not freeze. Protect from light. Do not dilute or dispense from any container other than the original bottle. Discard one month after opening.

6.5 Nature and contents of container

5 ml dropper bottle of 1.0 % solution.

Bottle:	LE 6601 PH (LDPE) Natural colour
Cap:	Melochem White colour

6.6 Special precautions for disposal and other handling

When using the product for the first time, screw down the cap firmly on the bottle to pierce the seal at the tip of the plastic nozzle and unscrew the cap for use.

7. MARKETING AUTHORISATION HOLDER

Intrapharm Laboratories Ltd

60 Boughton Lane

Maidstone

Kent

ME15 9QS

United Kingdom

8. MARKETING AUTHORISATION NUMBER(S)

PL 17509/0008

9. DATE OF FIRST AUTHORISATION/RENEWAL OF THE AUTHORISATION

8 August 2001

10. DATE OF REVISION OF THE TEXT

June 2003

11. Legal category

POM

Myleran film coated tablets 2mg

(GlaxoSmithKline UK)

1. NAME OF THE MEDICINAL PRODUCT

Myleran film coated tablets 2 mg

2. QUALITATIVE AND QUANTITATIVE COMPOSITION

Each 2 mg tablet contains 2 mg of the active substance busulfan

3. PHARMACEUTICAL FORM

Film coated tablet

Myleran 2 mg tablets are white, film-coated, round, biconvex tablets engraved "GXEF3" on one side and "M" on the other.

4. CLINICAL PARTICULARS

4.1 Therapeutic indications

Myleran is indicated as conditioning treatment prior to haematopoietic progenitor cell transplantation in patients when the combination of high dose busulfan and cyclophosphamide is considered the best available option.

Myleran is indicated for the palliative treatment of the chronic phase of chronic granulocytic leukaemia.

Myleran is effective in producing prolonged remission in polycythaemia vera, particularly in cases with marked thrombocytosis.

Myleran may be useful in selected cases of essential thrombocythaemia and myelofibrosis.

4.2 Posology and method of administration

General:

Myleran tablets are usually given in courses or administered continuously. The dose must be adjusted for the individual patient under close clinical and haematological control. Should a patient require an average daily dose of less than the content of the available Myleran tablets, this can be achieved by introducing one or more busulfan free days between treatment days. The tablets should not be divided (see 6.6 Instructions for Use/Handling).

• Obese

Dosing based on body surface area or adjusted ideal body weight should be considered in the obese (see Pharmacokinetics).

The relevant literature should be consulted for full details of treatment schedules.

Conditioning prior to haematopoietic progenitor cell transplantation

When bulsulfan is used as a conditioning treatment prior to haematopoietic progenitor cell transplantation, drug level monitoring is recommended.

Populations

• Adults

The recommended dose of busulfan in adult patients is 1 mg/kg every 6 hours for four days, starting seven days prior to transplantation. 60 mg/kg per day of cyclophosphamide is usually given for two days commencing 24 h after the final dose of Busulfan (see Warnings and Precautions and Interactions).

• Children less than 18 years of age

Busulfan can be administered in accordance to local protocols up to a maximum dose of 37.5 mg/m^2 every 6 hours for 4 days, starting seven days prior to transplantation. The dosing of cyclophosphamide is the same as for adults.

Chronic granulocytic leukaemia

Induction in Adults

Treatment is usually initiated as soon as the condition is diagnosed. The dose is 0.06 mg/kg/day, with an initial daily maximum of 4 mg, which may be given as a single dose.

There is individual variation in the response to Myleran and in a small proportion of patients the bone marrow may be extremely sensitive. (See 4.4 Special Warnings and Precautions for Use).

The blood count must be monitored at least weekly during the induction phase and it may be helpful to plot counts on semilog graph paper.

The dose should be increased only if the response is inadequate after three weeks.

Treatment should be continued until the total leucocyte count has fallen to between 15 and 25 $\times$ 10^9 per litre (typically 12 to 20 weeks). Treatment may then be interrupted, following which a further fall in the leucocyte count may occur over the next two weeks. Continued treatment at the induction dose after this point or following depression of the platelet count to below 100 $\times$ 10^9 per litre is associated with a significant risk of prolonged and possibly irreversible bone marrow aplasia.

Maintenance in adults:

Control of the leukaemia may be achieved for long periods without further Myleran treatment; further courses are usually given when the leucocyte count rises to 50 $\times$ 10^9 per litre, or symptoms return.

Some clinicians prefer to give continuous maintenance therapy. Continuous treatment is more practical when the duration of unmaintained remissions is short.

The aim is to maintain a leucocyte count of 10 to 15 $\times$ 10^9 per litre and blood counts must be performed at least every 4 weeks. The usual maintenance dosage is on average 0.5 to 2 mg/day, but individual requirements may be much less. Should a patient require an average daily dose of less than the content of one tablet, the maintenance dose may be adjusted by introducing one or more Busulfan free days between treatment days.

Note: Lower doses of Myleran should be used if it is administered in conjunction with other cytotoxic agents. (See also 4.8 Undesirable Effects and 4.5 Interactions with other Medicaments and other forms of Interaction).

Children:

Chronic granulocytic leukaemia is rare in the paediatric age group. Busulfan may be used to treat Philadelphia chromosome positive (Ph' positive) disease, but the Ph' negative juvenile variant responds poorly.

Polycythaemia vera

The usual dose is 4 to 6 mg daily, continued for 4 to 6 weeks, with careful monitoring of the blood count, particularly the platelet count.

Further courses are given when relapse occurs; alternatively, maintenance therapy may be given using approximately half the induction dose.

If the polycythaemia is controlled primarily by venesection, short courses of Myleran may be given solely to control the platelet count.

Myelofibrosis

The usual initial dose is 2 to 4 mg daily.

Very careful haematological control is required because of the extreme sensitivity of the bone marrow in this condition.

Essential thrombocythaemia

The usual dose is 2 to 4 mg per day.

Treatment should be interrupted if the total leucocyte count falls below 5 $\times$ 10^9 per litre or the platelet count below 500 $\times$ 10^9 per litre.

4.3 Contraindications

Myleran should not be used in patients whose disease has demonstrated resistance to busulfan.

Myleran should not be given to patients who have previously suffered a hypersensitivity reaction to the busulfan or any other component of the preparation.

4.4 Special warnings and precautions for use

Myleran is an active cytotoxic agent for use only under the direction of physicians experienced in the administration of such agents.

Immunisation using a live organism vaccine has the potential to cause infection in immunocompromised hosts. Therefore, immunisations with live organism vaccines are not recommended.

Myleran should be discontinued if lung toxicity develops (See 4.8 Undesirable Effects).

Myleran should not generally be given in conjunction with or soon after radiotherapy.

Myleran is ineffective once blast transformation has occurred.

If anaesthesia is required in patients with possible pulmonary toxicity, the concentration of inspired oxygen should be kept as low as safely as possible and careful attention given to post-operative respiratory care.

Hyperuricaemia and/or hyperuricosuria are not uncommon in patients with chronic granulocytic leukaemia and should be corrected before starting treatment with Myleran. During treatment, hyperuricaemia and the risk of uric acid nephropathy should be prevented by adequate prophylaxis, including adequate hydration and the use of allopurinol.

Conventional dose Treatment

Patients co-administered itraconazole or metronidazole with conventional dose Busulfan should be monitored closely for signs of Busulfan toxicity. Weekly measurements of blood counts are recommended when co-administering these drugs (see Interactions).

Monitoring:

Careful attention must be paid to monitoring the blood counts throughout treatment to avoid the possibility of excessive myelosuppression and the risk of irreversible bone marrow aplasia (see also 4.8 Undesirable Effects).

High-dose Treatment:

If high-dose Myleran is prescribed, patients should be given prophylactic anticonvulsant therapy, preferably with a benzodiazepine rather than phenytoin.

Concomitant administration of itraconazole or metronidazole with high-dose busulfan has been reported to be associated with an increased risk of busulfan toxicity (see Interactions). Co-administration of metronidazole and high dose busulfan is not recommended. Co-administration of itraconazole with high dose busulfan should be at the discretion of the prescribing physician and should be based on a risk/benefit assessment.

A reduced incidence of hepatic veno-occlusive disease and other regimen-related toxicities have been observed in patients treated with high-dose Myleran and cyclophosphamide when the first dose of cyclophosphamide has been delayed for > 24 hours after the last dose of Busulfan.

Safe Handling of Myleran Tablets:

See 6.6 Instructions for Use/Handling

Myleran is genotoxic in non-clinical studies (see Section 5.3 Preclinical Safety Data).

Mutagenicity:

Various chromosome aberrations have been noted in cells from patients receiving busulfan.

Carcinogenicity:

On the basis of human studies, Myleran was considered by the International Agency for Research on cancer to show sufficient evidence for carcinogenicity. The World Health Association has concluded that there is a causal relationship between Myleran exposure and cancer.

Widespread epithelial dysplasia has been observed in patients treated with long-term Myleran, with some of the changes resembling precancerous lesions.

A number of malignant tumours have been reported in patients who have received Myleran treatment.

The evidence is growing that Myleran, in common with other alkylating agents, is leukaemogenic. In a controlled prospective study in which 2 years' Myleran treatment was given as an adjuvant to surgery for lung cancer, long-term follow-up showed an increased incidence of acute leukaemia compared with the placebo-treated group. The incidence of solid tumours was not increased.

Although acute leukaemia is probably part of the natural history of polycythaemia vera, prolonged alkylating agent therapy may increase the incidence.

Very careful consideration should be given to the use of busulfan for the treatment of polycythaemia vera and essential thrombocythaemia in view of the drug's carcinogenic potential. The use of busulfan for these indications should be avoided in younger or asymptomatic patients. If the drug is considered necessary treatment courses should be kept as short as possible.

4.5 Interaction with other medicinal products and other forms of interaction

Vaccinations with live organism vaccines are not recommended in immunocompromised individuals (see Warnings and Precautions).

The effects of other cytotoxics producing pulmonary toxicity may be additive.

The administration of phenytoin to patients receiving high-dose Myleran may result in a decrease in the myeloblative effect.

In patients receiving high-dose Busulfan it has been reported that co-administration of itraconazole decreases clearance of Busulfan by approximately 20% with corresponding increases in plasma Busulfan levels. Metronidazole has been reported to increase trough levels of Busulfan by approximately 80%. Fluconazole had no effect on Busulfan clearance. Consequently, high-dose Busulfan in combination with itraconazole or metronidazole is reported to be associated with an increased risk of Busulfan toxicity (see Warnings and Precautions).

A reduced incidence of hepatic veno-occlusive disease and other regimen-related toxicities have been observed in patients treated with high-dose Myleran and cyclophosphamide when the first dose of cyclophosphamide has been delayed for > 24 hours after the last dose of busulfan.

4.6 Pregnancy and lactation

Pregnancy:

As with all cytotoxic chemotherapy, adequate contraceptive precautions should be advised when either partner is receiving Myleran.

The use of Myleran should be avoided during pregnancy whenever possible. In animal studies (see section 5.3 Preclinical Safety Data) it has the potential for teratogenic effects, whilst exposure during the latter half of pregnancy resulted in impairment of fertility in offspring. In every individual case the expected benefit of treatment to the mother must be weighed against the possible risk to the foetus.

A few cases of congenital abnormalities, not necessarily attributable to busulfan, have been reported and third trimester exposure may be associated with impaired intra-uterine growth. However, there have also been many reported cases of apparently normal children born after exposure to Myleran *in utero*, even during the first trimester.

Lactation:

It is not known whether Myleran or its metabolites are excreted in human breast milk. Mothers receiving Myleran should not breast-feed their infants.

4.7 Effects on ability to drive and use machines

There are no data on the effect of Busulfan on driving performance or the ability to operate machinery. A detrimental effect on these activities cannot be predicted from the pharmacology of the drug.

4.8 Undesirable effects

For this product there is no modern clinical documentation which can be used as support for determining the frequency of undesirable effects. Undesirable effects may vary in their incidence depending on the dose received and also when given in combination with other therapeutic agents.

The following convention has been utilised for the classification of frequency: Very common (⩾1/10), common (⩾1/100 and <1/10), uncommon (⩾1/1000 and <1/100), rare (⩾1/10,000 and <1/1000) and very rare (<1/10,000).

Neoplasms benign, malignant and unspecified (including cysts and polyps)

Common: Secondary acute leukaemia (see Warnings and Precautions; Carcinogenicity).

Blood and lymphatic system disorders

Very common: Dose-related bone marrow depression, manifest as leucopenia and particularly thrombocytopenia.

Rare: Aplastic anaemia

Aplastic anaemia (sometimes irreversible) has been reported rarely, typically following long-term conventional doses and also high doses of Busulfan.

Nervous system disorders

Rare: Convulsions at high dose (see 4.5 Interaction with Other Medicinal Products and Other Forms of Interaction, and 4.4 Special Warnings and Special Precautions for Use).

Very rare: Myasthenia gravis.

Eye disorders

Rare: Lens changes and cataracts, which may be bilateral; corneal thinning reported after bone marrow transplantation preceded by high-dose Busulfan treatment.

Cardiac disorders

Common: Cardiac tamponade in patients with thalassaemia receiving high-dose Busulfan.

Respiratory, thoracic and mediastinal disorders

Very common: Idiopathic pneumonia syndrome following high dose use.

Common: Interstitial pneumonitis following long term conventional dose use.

Pulmonary toxicity after either high or conventional dose treatment typically presents with non-specific non-productive cough, dyspnoea and hypoxia with evidence of abnormal pulmonary physiology. Other cytotoxic agents may cause additive lung toxicity (see 4.5 Interactions). It is possible that subsequent radiotherapy can augment subclinical lung injury caused by busulfan. Once pulmonary toxicity is established the prognosis is poor despite busulfan withdrawal and there is little evidence that corticosteroids are helpful

Idiopathic pneumonia syndrome is a non-infectious diffuse pneumonia which usually occurs within three months of high dose Busulfan conditioning prior to allogeneic or autologous haemopoietic transplant. Diffuse alveolar haemorrhage may also be detected in some cases after broncholavage. Chest X-rays or CT scans show diffuse or non-specific focal infiltrates and biopsy shows interstitial pneumonitis and diffuse alveolar damage and sometimes fibrosis.

Interstitial pneumonitis may occur following conventional dose use and lead to pulmonary fibrosis. This usually occurs after prolonged treatment over a number of years. The onset is usually insidious but may also be acute. Histological features include atypical changes of the alveolar and bronchiolar epithelium and the presence of giant cells with large hyperchromatic nuclei. The lung pathology may be complicated by superimposed infections. Pulmonary ossification and dystrophic calcification have also been reported.

Gastrointestinal disorders

Very common: Gastro-intestinal effects such as nausea and vomiting, diarrhoea and oral ulceration at high-dose.

Rare: Gastro-intestinal effects such as nausea and vomiting, diarrhoea and oral ulceration at conventional dose, may possibly be ameliorated by using divided doses.

Hepatobiliary disorders

Very common: Hyperbilirubinaemia, jaundice, hepatic veno-occlusive disease (see Special Warnings and Precautions for Use and Interaction with Other Medicinal Products and Other Forms of Interaction) and centrilobular sinusoidal fibrosis with hepatocellular atrophy and necrosis

Rare: Cholestatic jaundice and liver function abnormalities, at conventional dose. Centrilobular sinusoidal fibrosis.

Busulfan is not generally considered to be significantly hepatotoxic at normal therapeutic doses. However, retrospective review of postmortem reports of patients who had been treated with low-dose busulfan for at least two years for chronic granulocytic leukaemia showed evidence of centrilobular sinusoidal fibrosis.

Skin and subcutaneous tissue disorders

Common: Alopecia at high-dose.

Hyperpigmentation (see also General disorders and administration site conditions).

Rare: Alopecia at conventional dose, skin reactions including urticaria, erythema multiformae, erythema nodosum, porphyria cutanea tarda, an allopurinol-type rash and excessive dryness and fragility of the skin with complete anhydrosis, dryness of oral mucous membranes and cheilosis, Sjorgen's syndrome. An increased cutaneous radiation effect in patients receiving radiotherapy soon after high-dose Busulfan.

Hyperpigmentation occurs, particularly inthose with a dark complexion. It is often most marked on the neck, upper trunk, nipples, abdomen and palmar creases. This may also occur as part of a clinical syndrome (see General disorders and administration site conditions).

Renal and urinary disorders

Common: Haemorrhagic cystitis at high dose in combination with cyclophosphamide.

Reproductive system and breast disorders

Very common: Ovarian suppression and amenorrhoea with menopausal symptoms in pre-menopausal patients at high-dose; severe and persistent ovarian failure, including failure to achieve puberty after administration to young girls and pre-adolescents at high-dose

Sterility, azoospermia and testicular atrophy in male patients receiving Busulfan.

Uncommon: Ovarian suppression and amenorrhoea with menopausal symptoms in pre-menopausal patients at conventional dose. In very rare cases, recovery of ovarian function has been reported with continuing treatment.

Very rare: Gynecomastia.

Studies of busulfan treatment in animals have shown reproductive toxicity (see Section 5.3).

General disorders and administration site conditions

Very rare: Clinical syndrome# (weakness, severe fatigue, anorexia, weight loss, nausea and vomiting and hyperpigmentation of the skin) resembling adrenal insufficiency (Addison's disease) but without biochemical evidence of adrenal suppression, mucous membrane hyperpigmentation or hair loss.

(See Skin and subcutaneous tissue disorders)

Rare: Widespread dysplasia of epithelia.

Seen in a few cases following prolonged Busulfan therapy. The syndrome has sometimes resolved when busulfan has been withdrawn.

Many histological and cytological changes have been observed in patients treated with busulfan, including widespread dysplasia affecting uterine cervical, bronchial and other epithelia. Most reports relate to long-term treatment but transient epithelial abnormalities have been observed following short-term, high-dose treatment.

4.9 Overdose

Symptoms and signs:

The acute dose-limiting toxicity of Myleran in man is myelosuppression (see 4.8 Undesirable Effects).

The main effect of chronic overdose is bone marrow depression and pancytopenia.

Treatment:

There is no known antidote to Myleran. Haemoialysis should be considered in the management of overdose as there is one report of successful haemodialysis of Busulfan.

Appropriate supportive treatment should be given during the period of haematological toxicity.

5. PHARMACOLOGICAL PROPERTIES

5.1 Pharmacodynamic properties

Busulfan (1,4-butanediol dimethanesulfonate) is a bifunctional alkylating agent. Binding to DNA is believed to play a role in its mode of action and di-guanyl derivaties have been isolated but interstrand crosslinking has not been conclusively demonstrated.

The basis for the uniquely selective effect of busulfan on granulocytopoiesis is not fully understood. Although not curative, Myleran is very effective in reducing the total granulocyte mass, relieving the symptoms of disease and improving the clinical state of the patient. Myleran has been shown to be superior to splenic irradiation when judged by survival times and maintenance of haemoglobin levels and is as effective in controlling spleen size.

5.2 Pharmacokinetic properties

Absorption:

The bioavailability of oral Busulfan shows large intra-individual variations ranging from 47% to 103% (mean 68%) in adults.

The area under the curve (AUC) and peak plasma concentrations (C_{max}) of Busulfan have been shown to be linearly dose dependent. Following administration of a single 2 mg oral dose of Busulfan, the AUC and C_{max} of Busulfan were 125±17 nanograms.h/ml and 28±5 nanograms/ml respectively.

A lag time between Busulfan administration and detection in the plasma of up to 2 h has been reported.

High-dose Treatment:

Drug was assayed either using gas liquid chromatography with electron capture detection or by high-performance liquid chromatography (HPLC).

Following oral administration of high dose Busulfan (1 mg/kg every 6 h for 4 days), AUC and C_{max} in adults are highly variable but have been reported to be 8260 nanograms.h/ml (range 2484 to 21090) and 1047 nanograms/ml (range 295 to 2558) respectively when measured by HPLC and 6135 nanograms.h/ml (range 3978 to 12304) and 1980 nanograms/ml (range 894 to 3800) respectively using gas chromatography.

Distribution:

Busulfan is reported to have a volume of distribution of 0.64±0.12 L/kg in adults.

Busulfan given in high doses has recently been shown to enter the cerebrospinal fluid (CSF) in concentrations comparable to those found in plasma, with a mean CSF:plasma ration of 1.3:1. The saliva:plasma distribution of Busulfan was 1.1:1.

The level of busulfan bound reversibly to plasma proteins has been variably reported to be insignificant or approximately 55%. Irreversible binding of drug to blood cells and plasma proteins has been reported to be 47% and 32%, respectively.

Metabolism:

Busulfan metabolism involves a reaction with glutathione, which occurs via the liver and is mediated by glutathione-S-transferase.

The urinary metabolites of busulfan have been identified as 3-hydroxysulpholane, tetrahydrothiophene 1-oxide and sulpholane, in patients treated with high-dose Busulfan. Very little busulfane is excreted unchanged in the urine.

Elimination:

Busulfan has a mean elimination half life of between 2.3 and 2.8 h. Adult patients have demonstrated a clearance of busulfan of 2.4 to 2.6 ml/min/kg. The elimination half life of busulfan has been reported to decrease upon repeat dosing suggesting that busulfan potentially increases its own metabolism.

Very little (1 to 2%) busulfan is excreted unchanged in the urine.

Special Patient Populations:

Children

The bioavailability of oral busulfan shows large intra-individual variation ranging from 22% to 120% (mean 80%) in children.

Plasma clearance is reported to be 2 to 4 times higher in children than in adults when receiving 1 mg/kg every 6 h for 4 days. Dosing children according to body surface area has been shown to give AUC and C_{max} values similar to those seen in adults. The area under the curve has been shown to be half that of adults in children under the age of 15 years and a quarter of that of adults in children under 3 years of age.

Busulfan is reported to have a volume of distribution of 1.15±0.52 L/kg in children.

When busulfan is administered at a dose of 1 mg/kg every 6 h for 4 days, the CSF:plasma ratio has been shown to be 1.02:1. However, when administered at a dose of 37.5 mg/m^2 every 6 h for 4 days the ratio was 1.39:1.

Obese Patients

Obesity has been reported to increase busulfan clearance. Dosing based on body surface area or adjusted ideal bodyweight should be considered in the obese.

5.3 Preclinical safety data

Busulfan has been shown to be mutagenic in various experimental systems, including bacteria, fungi, *Drosophila* and cultured mouse lymphoma cells.

In vivo cytogenetic studies in rodents have shown an increased incidence of chromosome aberrations in both germ cells and somatic cells after Busulfan treatment.

Carcinogenicity:

There is limited evidence from preclinical studies that Myleran is carcinogenic in animals (see 4.4 Special Warnings and Precautions for Use).

Teratogenicity:

There is evidence form animal studies that busulfan produces foetal abnormalities and adverse effects on offspring, including defects of the musculo-skeletal system, reduced body weight and size, impairment of gonad development and effects on fertility.

Fertility:

Busulfan interferes with spermatogenesis in experimental animals. Limited studies in female animals indicate busulfan has a marked and irreversible effect on fertility through oocyte depletion.

6. PHARMACEUTICAL PARTICULARS

6.1 List of excipients

2 mg Tablets:

Tablet core: Anhydrous lactose

Pregelatinised starch

Magnesium stearate

Tablet coating: Hypromellose

Titanium dioxide

Triacetin

6.2 Incompatibilities

None known

6.3 Shelf life

3 years

6.4 Special precautions for storage

Do not store above25°C

6.5 Nature and contents of container

Myleran tablets are supplied in amber glass bottles with a child resistant closure containing 25 or 100 tablets.

6.6 Special precautions for disposal and other handling

Safe handling of Myleran tablets:

The tablets should not be divided and provided the outer coating is intact, there is no risk in handling Myleran tablets.

Handlers of Myleran tablets should follow guidelines for the handling of cytotoxic drugs.

Disposal:

Myleran tablets surplus to requirements should be destroyed in a manner appropriate for the destruction of dangerous substances.

Administrative Data

7. MARKETING AUTHORISATION HOLDER

The Wellcome Foundation Ltd trading as GlaxoSmithKline UK

Glaxo Wellcome House Stockley Park West

Berkeley Avenue Uxbridge

Greenford Middlesex UB11 1BT

Middlesex UB6 ONN

8. MARKETING AUTHORISATION NUMBER(S)

PL0003/5112R

9. DATE OF FIRST AUTHORISATION/RENEWAL OF THE AUTHORISATION

23 January 2003

10. DATE OF REVISION OF THE TEXT

23 October 2006

Myocet

(Cephalon Limited)

1. NAME OF THE MEDICINAL PRODUCT

Myocet ▼ 50 mg powder and pre-admixtures for concentrate for liposomal dispersion for infusion

2. QUALITATIVE AND QUANTITATIVE COMPOSITION

Liposome–encapsulated doxorubicin–citrate complex corresponding to 50 mg doxorubicin HCl. For a full list of excipients, see section 6.1.

3. PHARMACEUTICAL FORM

Powder and pre-admixtures for concentrate for liposomal dispersion for infusion

Myocet is supplied as a three-vial system:

Myocet doxorubicin HCl (a red lyophilised powder),

Myocet liposomes (a white to off-white, opaque and homogeneous solution),

Myocet buffer (a clear colourless solution).

4. CLINICAL PARTICULARS

4.1 Therapeutic indications

Myocet, in combination with cyclophosphamide, is indicated for the first line treatment of metastatic breast cancer in women.

4.2 Posology and method of administration

The use of Myocet should be confined to units specialised in the administration of cytotoxic chemotherapy and should only be administered under the supervision of a physician experienced in the use of chemotherapy.

Dosage When Myocet is administered in combination with cyclophosphamide (600 mg/m^2) the initial recommended dose of Myocet is 60-75 mg/m^2 every three weeks.

Administration Myocet must be reconstituted and further diluted prior to administration (see section 6.6). A final concentration of between 0.4 to 1.2 mg/ml doxorubicin HCl, is required. Myocet is administered by intravenous infusion over a period of 1 hour.

Myocet must not be administered by the intramuscular or subcutaneous route or as a bolus injection.

Paediatric patients The safety and efficacy of Myocet has not yet been established in paediatric patients (below 18 years of age).

Elderly patients Safety and efficacy of Myocet have been assessed in 61 patients with metastatic breast cancer, age 65 and over. Data from randomised controlled clinical trials show that the efficacy and cardiac safety of Myocet in this population was comparable to that observed in patients less than 65 years old.

Use in patients with impaired hepatic function As metabolism and excretion of doxorubicin occurs primarily by the hepatobiliary route, evaluation of hepatobiliary function should be performed before and during therapy with Myocet.

Based on limited data in patients with liver metastases, it is recommended that the initial dose of Myocet is reduced in accordance with the following table

Liver function tests	Dose
Bilirubin < ULN and normal AST	Standard dose of 60 - 75mg/m^2
Bilirubin < ULN and raised AST	Consider a 25% dose reduction
Bilirubin > ULN but < 50 μmol/l	50% dose reduction
Bilirubin > 50 μmol/l	75% dose reduction

If possible, Myocet should be avoided in patients with bilirubin > 50 μmol/l as the recommendation is based mainly on extrapolations.

For dose reductions due to other toxicity, see section 4.4.

Use in patients with impaired renal function Doxorubicin is metabolised largely by the liver and excreted in the bile. Therefore dose modification is not required for patients with renal function impairment.

4.3 Contraindications

Hypersensitivity to the active substance, to the pre-admixtures or to any of the excipients.

4.4 Special warnings and precautions for use

Myelosuppression Therapy with Myocet causes myelosuppression. Myocet should not be administered to individuals with absolute neutrophil counts (ANC) lower than 1,500 cells/μl or platelets less than 100,000/μl prior to the next cycle. Careful haematological monitoring (including white blood cell and platelet count, and haemoglobin) should be performed during therapy with Myocet.

Haematological as well as other toxicity may require dose reductions or delays. The following dosage modifications are recommended during therapy and should be performed in parallel for both Myocet and cyclophosphamide. Dosing subsequent to a dose reduction is left to the discretion of the physician in charge of the patient.

(see Table 1a on next page)

If myelotoxicity delays treatment to greater than 35 days after the first dose of the previous cycle, then consideration should be given to stopping treatment.

	Mucositis	
Grade	**Symptoms**	**Modification**
1	Painless ulcers, erythema, or mild soreness.	None
2	Painful erythema, oedema or ulcers but can eat.	Wait one week and if the symptoms improve redose at 100% dose
3	Painful erythema, oedema or ulcers and cannot eat	Wait one week and if symptoms improve redose at 25% dose reduction
4	Requires parenteral or enteral support	Wait one week and if symptoms improve redose at 50% dose reduction

For dose reduction of Myocet due to liver function impairment, see section 4.2.

Cardiac toxicity Doxorubicin and other anthracyclines can cause cardiotoxicity. The risk of toxicity rises with increasing cumulative doses of those medicinal products and is higher in individuals with a history of cardiomyopathy, or mediastinal irradiation or pre-existing cardiac disease.

Analyses of cardiotoxicity in clinical trials have shown a statistically significant reduction in cardiac events in patients treated with Myocet compared to patients treated with conventional doxorubicin at the same dose in mg. The full clinical relevance of these findings is currently unclear.

Table 1a

	Haematological Toxicity		
Grade	**Nadir ANC (cells/µl)**	**Nadir Platelet Count (cells/µl)**	**Modification**
1	1500 – 1900	75,000 – 150,000	None
2	1000 – Less than 1500	50,000 – Less than 75,000	None
3	500 – 999	25,000 – Less than 50,000	Wait until ANC 1500 or more and/or platelets 100,000 or more then redose at 25% dose reduction
4	Less than 500	Less than 25,000	Wait until ANC 1500 and/or platelets 100,000 or more then redose at 50% dose reduction

In a phase III study in combination with cyclophosphamide (CPA) comparing Myocet (60 mg/m^2) + CPA (600 mg/m^2) versus doxorubicin (60 mg/m^2) + CPA (600 mg/m^2), 6% versus 21% of patients, respectively, developed a significant decrease in left ventricular ejection fraction (LVEF). In a phase III study comparing single-agent Myocet (75 mg/m^2) versus single-agent doxorubicin (75 mg/m^2), 12% versus 27% of patients, respectively developed a significant decrease in LVEF. The corresponding figures for congestive heart failure (CHF), which was less accurately assessed, were 0% for Myocet + CPA versus 3% for doxorubicin + CPA, and 2% for Myocet versus 8% for doxorubicin. The median lifetime cumulative dose of Myocet in combination with CPA to a cardiac event was > 1260 mg/m^2, compared to 480 mg/m^2 for doxorubicin combination with CPA.

There is no experience with Myocet in patients with a history of cardiovascular disease, e.g. myocardial infarction within 6 months prior to treatment. Thus, caution should be exercised in patients with impaired cardiac function. The cardiac function of the patients treated concomitantly with Myocet and trastuzumab must be appropriately monitored as described below.

The total dose of Myocet should also take into account any previous, or concomitant, therapy with other cardiotoxic compounds, including anthracyclines and anthraquinones.

Before initiation of Myocet therapy a measurement of left ventricular ejection fraction (LVEF) is routinely recommended, either by Multiple Gated Arteriography (MUGA) or by echocardiography. These methods should also be applied routinely during Myocet treatment. The evaluation of left ventricular function is considered mandatory before each additional administration of Myocet once a patient exceeds a lifetime cumulative anthracycline dose of 550 mg/m^2 or whenever cardiomyopathy is suspected. If LVEF has decreased substantially from baseline e.g. by > 20 points to a final value > 50% or by > 10 points to a final value of < 50%, the benefit of continued therapy must be carefully evaluated against the risk of producing irreversible cardiac damage. However, the most definitive test for anthracycline myocardial injury, i.e., endomyocardial biopsy, should be considered.

All patients receiving Myocet should also routinely undergo ECG monitoring. Transient ECG changes such as T-wave flattening, S-T segment depression and benign arrhythmias are not considered mandatory indications for the cessation of Myocet therapy. However, reduction of the QRS complex is considered more indicative of cardiac toxicity.

Congestive heart failure due to cardiomyopathy may occur suddenly, and may also be encountered after discontinuation of therapy.

Injection site reactions Myocet should be considered an irritant and precautions should be taken to avoid extravasation. If extravasation occurs, the infusion should be immediately terminated. Ice may be applied to the affected area for approximately 30 minutes. Subsequently, the Myocet infusion should be restarted in a different vein than that in which the extravasation has occurred. Note that Myocet may be administered through a central or peripheral vein. In the clinical program, there were nine cases of accidental extravasation of Myocet, none of which were associated with severe skin damage, ulceration or necrosis.

Infusion associated reactions

When infused rapidly acute reactions associated with liposomal infusions have been reported.

Reported symptoms have included flushing, dyspnoea, fever, facial swelling, headache, back pain, chills, tightness in the chest and throat, and/or hypotension. These acute phenomena may be avoided by using a 1-hour infusion time.

Other

For precautions regarding the use of Myocet with other medicinal products, see section 4.5.

Efficacy and safety of Myocet in the adjuvant treatment of breast cancer have not been determined.

The importance of apparent differences in tissue distribution between Myocet and conventional doxorubicin has not been elucidated with respect to long-term antitumour efficacy.

4.5 Interaction with other medicinal products and other forms of interaction

Specific drug compatibility studies have not been performed with Myocet. Myocet is likely to interact with substances that are known to interact with conventional doxorubicin. Plasma levels of doxorubicin and its metabolite, doxorubicinol, may be increased when doxorubicin is administered with cyclosporin, verapamil, paclitaxel or other agents that inhibit P-glycoprotein (P-Gp). Interactions with doxorubicin have also been reported for streptozocin, phenobarbital, phenytoin and warfarin. Studies of the effect of Myocet on other substances are also lacking. However, doxorubicin may potentiate the toxicity of other antineoplastic agents. Concomitant treatment with other substances reported to be cardiotoxic or with cardiologically active substances (e.g. calcium antagonists) may increase the risk for cardiotoxicity. Concomitant therapy with other liposomal or lipid-complexed substances or intravenous fat emulsions could change the pharmacokinetic profile of Myocet.

4.6 Pregnancy and lactation

Due to the known cytotoxic, mutagenic and embryotoxic properties of doxorubicin, Myocet should not be used during pregnancy unless clearly necessary. Women of childbearing potential should use an effective contraceptive during treatment with Myocet and up to 6 months following discontinuation of therapy. Women receiving Myocet should not breastfeed.

4.7 Effects on ability to drive and use machines

Myocet has been reported to cause dizziness. Patients who suffer from this should avoid driving and operating machinery.

4.8 Undesirable effects

Clinical Program

Adverse drug reactions (ADR) data obtained from 323 patients with metastatic breast cancer in three randomised phase III trials of Myocet as a single agent and in combination with Cyclophosphamide (CPA) have been provided in Table 1 as pooled data. Treatment cycles were every three weeks in each trial and G-CSF was used in 38-56% of the cycles.

Table 1: Adverse reactions from pooled study results of three randomised Phase III clinical trials of Myocet as a single agent and in combination with Cyclophosphamide (CPA). (n=323)

System Organ Class	Frequency (as percentage)	Adverse Reactions 1,2
Infections and Infestations		**Infection**
	40	(All Grades)
	8	(Grade ⩾3)
		Neutropenic Fever 3
	11	ANC < 500 & fever >38 °C 3,4
	9	ANC > 500 & fever > 38 °C 3,4
Blood and Lymphatic System Disorders		**Neutropenia**
	94	<2000/µl
	64	<500/µl
	6	<500/µl for ⩾ 7 days
		Thrombocytopenia
	62	<100,000/µl
	7	<20,000/µl
		Anaemia
	89	<11 g/dl
	23	<8 g/dl
Gastrointestinal Disorders		**Nausea/Vomiting**
	85	(All Grades)
	15	(Grade ⩾3)
		Stomatitis/ Mucositis
	44	(All Grades)
	6	(Grade ⩾3)
		Diarrhoea
	26	(All Grades)
	2	(Grade ⩾3)
Skin and Subcutaneous Tissue Disorders	86	**Alopecia -** Pronounced
		Skin Related Toxicities (e.g. rash, dry skin)
	11	(All Grades)
	0	(Grade ⩾3)
General Disorders and Administration Site Conditions		**Fatigue/Malaise/ Asthenia**
	49	(All Grades)
	7	(Grade ⩾3)
		Injection Site Toxicity
	7	(All Grades)
	0	(Grade ⩾3)

[1] Incidence of the adverse reaction considered at least possibly related by the investigator, from pooled clinical trials involving 323 patients taking the medicinal product.

[2] all adverse reactions have been ranked by frequency within each system organ class.

[3] with IV antibiotics and/or hospitalisation

[4] absolute neutrophil counts (ANC)

The following clinically relevant grade 3/4 adverse reactions with an incidence of < 5% were also observed from clinical trials involving 948 patients with solid tumours. AIDS patients with Kaposi's sarcoma were not included.

Incidence of less than 5% (Grade 3 or 4, possibly, probably, or definitely related):

Infections and Infestations: fever, Herpes Zoster, injection site infection, sepsis **Blood and Lymphatic System Disorders:** leukopenia, lymphopenia, neutropenic sepsis, purpura **Metabolism and Nutrition Disorders:** anorexia, dehydration, hypokalaemia, hyperglycaemia **Psychiatric Disorders:** agitation **Nervous System Disorders:** abnormal gait, dysphonia, insomnia, somnolence **Cardiac Disorders:** arrhythmia, cardiomyopathy, congestive cardiac failure, pericardial effusion **Vascular Disorders:** hot flushes, hypotension **Respiratory, Thoracic and Mediastinal Disorders:** chest pain, dyspnoea, epistaxis, haemoptysis, pharyngitis, pleural effusion, pneumonitis **Gastrointestinal Disorders:** constipation, gastric ulcer, oesophagitis **Hepato-Biliary Disorders:** increased hepatic transaminases, increased alkaline phosphatase, increased serum bilirubin, jaundice **Musculoskeletal, Connective Tissue and Bone Disorders:** back pain, muscle weakness, myalgia **Skin and Subcutaneous Tissue Disorders:** folliculitis, nail disorder, pruritus, **Renal and Urinary Disorders:** haemorrhagic cystitis, oliguria **General Disorders and Administration Site Conditions:** dizziness, headache, injection site reaction, pain, rigors, weight loss

Post-Marketing

Relevant adverse reactions obtained from post marketing surveillance have been tabulated in Table 2.

Table 2: Adverse reactions obtained from post-marketing surveillance (4.5 years data).

System Organ Class	Adverse Reactions
Blood and Lymphatic System Disorders	**Pancytopenia**

4.9 Overdose

Acute overdose with Myocet will worsen toxic side effects. Treatment of acute overdose should focus on supportive care for expected toxicity and may include hospitalisation, antibiotics, platelet and granulocyte transfusions and symptomatic treatment of mucositis.

5. PHARMACOLOGICAL PROPERTIES

5.1 Pharmacodynamic properties

Pharmaco-therapeutic group*:* Cytotoxic agents (anthracyclines and related substances), ATC code: L01DB01 The active substance in Myocet is doxorubicin HCl. Doxorubicin may exert its antitumour and toxic effects by a number of mechanisms including inhibition of topoisomerase II,

Table 3 Antitumour efficacy summary for combination and single-agent studies

	Myocet/CPA (60/600 mg/m^2) (n=142)	Dox 60/CPA (60/600 mg/m^2) (n=155)	Myocet/CPA (75/600 mg/m^2) (n=80)	Epi/CPA (75/600 mg/m^2) (n=80)	Myocet (75 mg/m^2) (n=108)	Dox (75 mg/m^2) (n=116)
Tumour response rate Relative Risk (95% C.I.) Median PFS (months)[a] Risk Ratio (95% C.I.)	43% 43% 1.01 (0.78-1.31)	5.1 5.5 1.03 (0.80-1.34)	46% 39% 1.19 (0.83-1.72)	7.7 5.6 1.52 (1.06-2.20)	26% 26%1.00 (0.64-1.56)	2.9 3.2 0.87 (0.66-1.16)

intercalation with DNA and RNA polymerases, free radical formation and membrane binding. Liposomal-encapsulated compared with conventional doxorubicin was not found more active in doxorubicin resistant cell lines *in vitro*. In animals, liposome-encapsulated doxorubicin reduced the distribution to heart and gastrointestinal mucosa compared with conventional doxorubicin, while antitumoural efficacy in experimental tumours was maintained.

Myocet (60 mg/m^2) + CPA (600 mg/m^2) was compared with conventional doxorubicin + CPA (at the same doses) and Myocet (75 mg/m^2) + CPA (600 mg/m^2) was compared to epirubicin + CPA (at the same doses). In a third trial, Myocet (75 mg/m^2) monotherapy was compared with conventional doxorubicin monotherapy (at the same dose). Findings regarding response rate and progression-free survival are provided in Table 3.

Table 3

Antitumour efficacy summary for combination and single-agent studies

(see Table 3 above)

Abbreviations: PFS, progression-free survival; Dox, doxorubicin; Epi, epirubicin; Relative Risk, comparator taken as reference; Risk Ratio, Myocet taken as reference [a] Secondary endpoint

5.2 Pharmacokinetic properties

The plasma pharmacokinetics for total doxorubicin in patients receiving Myocet shows a high degree of inter-patient variability. In general however, the plasma levels of total doxorubicin are substantially higher with Myocet than with conventional doxorubicin, while the data indicate that peak plasma levels of free (not liposome-encapsulated) doxorubicin are lower with Myocet than with conventional doxorubicin. Available pharmacokinetic data preclude conclusions regarding the relationship between plasma levels of total/free doxorubicin and its influence on the efficacy/safety of Myocet. The clearance of total doxorubicin was 5.1 ± 4.8 l/h and the volume of distribution at steady state (V_d) was

56.6 ± 61.5 l whereas after conventional doxorubicin, clearance and V_d were 46.7 ± 9.6 l/h and 1,451 ± 258 l, respectively. The major circulating metabolite of doxorubicin, doxorubicinol, is formed via aldo-keto-reductase. The peak levels of doxorubicinol occur in the plasma later with Myocet than with conventional doxorubicin.

The pharmacokinetics of Myocet have not been specifically studied in patients with renal insufficiency. Doxorubicin is known to be eliminated in large part by the liver. A dose reduction of Myocet has been shown to be appropriate in patients with impaired hepatic function (see section 4.2 for dosage recommendations).

Substances that inhibit P-glycoprotein (P-Gp) have been shown to alter the disposition of doxorubicin and doxorubicinol (see also section 4.5).

5.3 Preclinical safety data

Studies of genotoxicity, carcinogenicity and reproductive toxicity of Myocet have not been performed but doxorubicin is known to be both mutagenic and carcinogenic and may cause toxicity to reproduction.

6. PHARMACEUTICAL PARTICULARS

6.1 List of excipients

Myocet doxorubicin HCl

lactose Myocet liposomes

egg phosphatidylcholine

cholesterol

citric acid

sodium hydroxide

water for injections Myocet buffer

sodium carbonate

water for injections

6.2 Incompatibilities

This medicinal product must not be mixed with other medicinal products except those mentioned in section 6.6.

6.3 Shelf life

18 months

Chemical and physical in-use stability after reconstitution has been demonstrated for up to 8 hours at 25°C, and for up to 5 days at 2°C – 8°C.

From a microbiological point of view, the product should be used immediately. If not used immediately, in-use storage times and conditions prior to use are the responsibility of the user and would normally not be longer than 24 hours at 2°C – 8°C, unless reconstitution and dilution has taken place in controlled and validated aseptic conditions.

6.4 Special precautions for storage

Store in a refrigerator (2°C – 8°C).

6.5 Nature and contents of container

Myocet is available in cartons containing 2 sets of the three constituents. Sodium chloride for injection 0.9%, needed to dissolve doxorubicin HCl, is not provided in the package.

Myocet doxorubicin HCl Type I glass vials containing 50 mg of doxorubicin HCl lyophilised powder, sealed with grey butyl rubber stoppers and orange flip-off aluminium seals.

Myocet liposomes Type I flint glass tubing vials containing not less than 1.9 ml of liposomes, sealed with siliconised grey stopper and green flip-off aluminium seals.

Myocet buffer Glass vials containing not less than 3 ml of buffer, sealed with siliconised grey stopper and blue aluminium flip-off seals.

6.6 Special precautions for disposal and other handling

Preparation of Myocet ASEPTIC TECHNIQUE MUST BE STRICTLY OBSERVED THROUGHOUT HANDLING OF MYOCET SINCE NO PRESERVATIVE IS PRESENT.

Caution should be exercised in the handling and preparation of Myocet. The use of gloves is required

Step 1. Set up

Two alternative heating methods can be used: a Techne DB-3 Dri Block heater or a water bath:

Turn on the Techne DB-3 Dri Block heater and set the controller to 75-76°C. Verify the temperature set point by checking the thermometer(s) on each heat block insert.

If using a water bath, turn on the water bath and allow it to equilibrate at 58°C (55-60°C). Verify the temperature set point by checking the thermometer.

(Please note that whilst the control settings on the water bath and heat block are set to different levels the temperature of the vial contents are in the same range (55-60°C)).

Remove the carton of Myocet constituents from the refrigerator.

Step 2. Reconstitute doxorubicin HCl

Withdraw 20 ml sodium chloride for injection (0.9%), *preservative free*, (not provided in the package), and inject into each Myocet doxorubicin HCl, intended for preparation.

• Shake well in the inverted position to ensure doxorubicin is fully dissolved.

Step 3. Heat in water bath or dry heat block

Heat the reconstituted Myocet doxorubicin HCl vial in the Techne DB-3 Dri Block heater with the thermometer in the block reading (75-76°C) for 10 minutes (not to exceed 15 minutes). If using the water bath heat the Myocet doxorubicin HCl vial with the thermometer temperature reading 55-60°C for 10 minutes (not to exceed 15 minutes).

• While heating proceed to step 4

Step 4. Adjust Ph of liposomes

Withdraw 1.9 ml of Myocet liposomes. Inject into Myocet buffer vial to adjust the Ph of liposomes. Pressure build-up may require venting.

• Shake well.

Step 5. Add Ph-adjusted liposomes to doxorubicin

Using syringe, withdraw the entire vial contents of Ph-adjusted liposomes from the Myocet buffer vial.

Remove the reconstituted Myocet doxorubicin HCl vial from the water bath or dry heat block. SHAKE VIGOROUSLY. Carefully insert a pressure-venting device equipped with a hydrophobic filter. Then IMMEDIATELY (within 2 minutes) inject Ph-adjusted liposomes into vial of heated reconstituted Myocet doxorubicin HCl. Remove venting device.

SHAKE VIGOROUSLY.

WAIT FOR A MINIMUM OF 10 MINUTES BEFORE USING, KEEPING THE MEDICINE AT ROOM TEMPERATURE.

The Techne DB-3 Dri Block Heater is fully validated for use in the constitution of Myocet. Three inserts, each with two 43.7mm openings per insert must be used. To ensure correct temperature control the use of a 35mm immersion thermometer is recommended.

The resulting reconstituted preparation of Myocet contains 50 mg of doxorubicin HCl/25 ml of liposomal dispersion (2 mg/ml).

After reconstitution the finished product must be further diluted in 0.9% (w/v) sodium chloride for injection, or 5% (w/v) glucose for injection to a final volume of 40 ml to 120 ml per 50 mg reconstituted Myocet so that a final concentration of 0.4 to 1.2 mg/ml doxorubicin is obtained.

Once constituted, the liposomal dispersion for infusion containing liposome-encapsulated doxorubicin should be a red orange opaque homogeneous dispersion. All parenteral solutions should be inspected visually for particulate matter and discoloration prior to administration. Do not use the preparation if foreign particulate matter is present.

Procedure for proper disposal

Any unused product or waste material should be disposed of in accordance with local requirements.

7. MARKETING AUTHORISATION HOLDER

Cephalon Europe 5 Rue Charles Martigny 94700 Maisons Alfort France

8. MARKETING AUTHORISATION NUMBER(S)

EU/1/00/141/001

9. DATE OF FIRST AUTHORISATION/RENEWAL OF THE AUTHORISATION

13-07-2000/13-07-2005

10. DATE OF REVISION OF THE TEXT

November 2008

Myocrisin Injection 10%

(sanofi-aventis)

1. NAME OF THE MEDICINAL PRODUCT

Myocrisin injection 10%

2. QUALITATIVE AND QUANTITATIVE COMPOSITION

In terms of the active ingredient (BAN rINN if appropriate)

Sodium aurothiomalate 50 mg in 0.5 ml (10.0% w/v)

3. PHARMACEUTICAL FORM

Injection

4. CLINICAL PARTICULARS

4.1 Therapeutic indications

Myocrisin is used in the management of active progressive rheumatoid arthritis and progressive juvenile chronic arthritis especially if polyarticular or seropositive.

4.2 Posology and method of administration

Do not use a darkened solution (more than pale yellow).

Myocrisin should be administered only by deep intramuscular injection followed by gentle massage of the area. The patient should remain under medical observation for a period of 30 minutes after drug administration.

Adults

An initial test dose of 10 mg should be given in the first week followed by weekly doses of 50 mg until signs of remission occur. At this point 50 mg doses should be given at two week intervals until full remission occurs. With full remission the interval between injections should be increased progressively to three, four and then, after 18 months to 2 years, to six weeks.

If after reaching a total dose of 1 g (excluding the test dose), no major improvement has occurred and the patient has not shown any signs of gold toxicity, six 100 mg injections may be administered at weekly intervals. If no sign of remission occurs after this time other forms of treatment are to be considered.

Elderly

There are no specific dosage recommendations. Elderly patients should be monitored with extra caution.

Children: Progressive juvenile chronic arthritis:

Weekly doses of 1 mg/kg should be given but not exceeding a maximum weekly dose of 50 mg. Depending on urgency, this dose may be preceded by a smaller test dose such as 1/10 or 1/5 of the full dose for 2-3 weeks. Continue weekly doses until signs of remission appear then increase the intervals between injections to two weeks. With full remission increase the interval to three then four weeks. In the absence of signs of remission after twenty weeks consider raising the dose slightly or changing to another therapy.

Treatment should be continued for six months. Response can be expected at the 300-500 mg level. If patients respond, maintenance therapy should be continued with the dosage administered over the previous 2-4 weeks, for 1-5 years.

4.3 Contraindications

Pregnancy (see section 4.6).

Myocrisin is contraindicated in patients with gross renal or hepatic disease, a history of blood dyscrasias, exfoliative dermatitis or systemic lupus erythematosus.

The absolute contraindications should be positively excluded before considering gold therapy.

4.4 Special warnings and precautions for use

As with other gold preparations, reactions which resemble anaphylactoid effects have been reported. These effects may occur after any course of therapy within the first ten minutes following drug administration (see administration).

If anaphylactoid effects are observed, treatment with Myocrisin should be discontinued (see section 4.8).

Myocrisin should be administered with extra caution in the elderly and in patients with a history of urticaria, eczema or colitis. Extra caution should also be exercised if phenylbutazone or oxyphenbutazone are administered concurrently.

Before starting treatment and again before each injection, the urine should be tested for protein, the skin inspected for rash and a full blood count performed, including a numerical platelet count (not an estimate) and the readings plotted. Blood dyscrasias are most likely to occur when between 400 mg and 1 g of gold have been given, or between the 10th and 20th week of treatment, but can also occur with much lower doses or after only 2-4 weeks of therapy (see section 4.8).

The presence of albuminuria, pruritus or rash, or an eosinophilia, are indications of developing toxicity (see section 4.8). The Myocrisin should be withheld for one or two weeks until all signs have disappeared when the course may be restarted on a test dose followed by a decreased frequency of gold injections.

A complaint of sore throat, glossitis, buccal ulceration and/or easy bruising or bleeding, demands an immediate blood count, followed if indicated, by appropriate treatment for agranulocytosis, aplastic anaemia and/or thrombocytopenia (see section 4.8). Every patient treated with Myocrisin should be warned to report immediately the appearance of pruritus, metallic taste, sore throat or tongue, buccal ulceration or easy bruising, purpura, epistaxis, bleeding gums, menorrhagia or diarrhoea (see section 4.8).

4.5 Interaction with other medicinal products and other forms of interaction

Concurrent gold administration may exacerbate aspirin-induced hepatic dysfunction. Caution should be exercised if phenylbutazone or oxyphenbutazone are administered concurrently.

Caution is needed in patients treated concomitantly with sodium aurothiomalate and angiotensin-converting enzyme inhibitors due to an increased risk of severe anaphylactoid reaction in these patients.

4.6 Pregnancy and lactation

The safety of Myocrisin in the foetus and the newborn has not been established. Female patients receiving Myocrisin should be instructed to avoid pregnancy. Pregnant patients should not be treated with Myocrisin. Lactating mothers under treatment with Myocrisin excrete significant amounts of gold in their breast milk and should not breast feed their infants.

4.7 Effects on ability to drive and use machines

None.

4.8 Undesirable effects

Blood dyscrasias including thrombocytopenia, pancytopenia, agranulocytosis, aplastic anaemia, leucopenia & neutropenia have been reported (see section 4.4).

Anaphylactic/Anaphylactoid reactions have been reported, symptoms of which may include weakness, flushing, hypotension, tachycardia, dyspnoea, palpitations, abdominal pain, shock and possibly collapse (see section 4.4).

Hepatotoxicity with cholestatic jaundice is a rare complication which may occur early in the course of treatment. It subsides on withdrawing Myocrisin. A rare but severe form of enterocolitis has been described.

Diffuse unilateral or bilateral pulmonary fibrosis very rarely occurs. This progressive condition usually responds to drug withdrawal and steroid therapy. An annual x-ray is recommended and attention should be paid to unexplained breathlessness and dry cough.

Side effects may be largely avoided by the indicated careful titration of dosage. Minor reactions, usually manifest as skin rashes and pruritus are the most frequent and commonly benign, but as such reactions may be the forerunners of severe gold toxicity they must never be treated lightly. Other indicators of developing toxicity could be the presence of albuminuria or an eosinophilia (see section 4.4).

Severe skin reactions that have been reported include exfoliative dermatitis and bullous eruptions. Irreversible skin pigmentation (chrysiasis) can occur in sun-exposed areas after prolonged treatment with Myocrisin. Rare reports of alopecia exist. Nephrotic syndrome has been rarely reported.

Neurological manifestations of gold toxicity including very rare cases of peripheral neuropathy, Guillain-Barré syndrome and encephalopathy have been observed.

4.9 Overdose

Minor side effects resolve spontaneously on withdrawal of Myocrisin. Symptomatic treatment of pruritus with antihistamines may be helpful. Major skin lesions and serious blood dyscrasias demand hospital admission when dimercaprol or penacillamine may be used to enhance gold excretion. Fresh blood and/or platelet transfusions, corticosteroids and androgenic steroids may be required in the management of severe blood dyscrasias.

5. PHARMACOLOGICAL PROPERTIES

5.1 Pharmacodynamic properties

The precise mode of action of sodium aurothiomalate is not yet known. Treatment with gold has been shown to be accompanied by a fall in ESR and C-reactive protein, an increase in serum histidine and sulphydryl levels and a reduction in serum immunoglobulins, rheumatoid factor titres and Clq-binding activity.

Numerous experimental observations have been recorded including physico-chemical changes in collagen and interference with complement activation, gammaglobulin aggregation, prostaglandin biosynthesis, inhibition of cathepsin and production of superoxide radicals by activated polymophonuclear leucocytes.

5.2 Pharmacokinetic properties

Sodium aurothiomalate is absorbed readily after intramuscular injection and becomes bound to plasma proteins. With doses of 50 mg weekly the steady-state serum concentration of gold is about 3 to 5 microgram per ml. It is widely distributed and accumulates in the body. Concentrations in synovial fluid have been shown to be similar or slightly less than those in plasma. Sodium aurothiomalate is mainly excreted in the urine with smaller amounts in the faeces. The serum half-life of gold clearance is about 5 or 6 days but after a course of treatment, gold may be found in the urine for up to a year or more owing to its presence in deep body compartments.

Gold has been detected in the foetus following administration of sodium aurothiomalate to the mother. Gold has been detected in the breast fed child where the mother has received sodium aurothiomalate.

5.3 Preclinical safety data

No additional pre-clinical data of relevance to the prescriber.

6. PHARMACEUTICAL PARTICULARS

6.1 List of excipients

Phenylmercuric nitrate

Water for Injections

6.2 Incompatibilities

None known.

6.3 Shelf life

36 months

6.4 Special precautions for storage

Store below 25°C. Protect from light.

6.5 Nature and contents of container

Carton containing 10 sealed glass ampoules each containing 0.5ml injection solution.

6.6 Special precautions for disposal and other handling

None stated.

7. MARKETING AUTHORISATION HOLDER

Sanofi-aventis

One Onslow Street

Guildford

Surrey, GU1 4YS, UK

8. MARKETING AUTHORISATION NUMBER(S)

PL04425/0389

9. DATE OF FIRST AUTHORISATION/RENEWAL OF THE AUTHORISATION

19 December 2005

10. DATE OF REVISION OF THE TEXT

November 2006

Legal Category

POM

Myocrisin Injection 2%

(sanofi-aventis)

1. NAME OF THE MEDICINAL PRODUCT

Myocrisin injection 2%

2. QUALITATIVE AND QUANTITATIVE COMPOSITION

In terms of the active ingredient (BAN rINN if appropriate)

Sodium aurothiomalate 10 mg in 0.5 ml (2.0% w/v)

3. PHARMACEUTICAL FORM

Injection

4. CLINICAL PARTICULARS

4.1 Therapeutic indications

Myocrisin is used in the management of active progressive rheumatoid arthritis and progressive juvenile chronic arthritis especially if polyarticular or seropositive.

4.2 Posology and method of administration

Do not use a darkened solution (more than pale yellow).

Myocrisin should be administered only by deep intramuscular injection followed by gentle massage of the area. The patient should remain under medical observation for a period of 30 minutes after drug administration.

Adults

An initial test dose of 10 mg should be given in the first week followed by weekly doses of 50 mg until signs of remission occur. At this point 50 mg doses should be given at two week intervals until full remission occurs. With full remission the interval between injections should be increased progressively to three, four and then, after 18 months to 2 years, to six weeks.

If after reaching a total dose of 1 g (excluding the test dose), no major improvement has occurred and the patient has not shown any signs of gold toxicity, six 100 mg injections may be administered at weekly intervals. If no sign of remission occurs after this time other forms of treatment are to be considered.

Elderly

There are no specific dosage recommendations. Elderly patients should be monitored with extra caution

Children: Progressive juvenile chronic arthritis:

Weekly doses of 1 mg/kg should be given but not exceeding a maximum weekly dose of 50 mg. Depending on urgency, this dose may be preceded by a smaller test dose such as 1/10 or 1/5 of the full dose for 2-3 weeks. Continue weekly doses until signs of remission appear then increase the intervals between injections to two weeks. With full remission increase the interval to three then four weeks. In the absence of signs of remission after twenty weeks consider raising the dose slightly or changing to another therapy.

Treatment should be continued for six months. Response can be expected at the 300-500 mg level. If patients respond, maintenance therapy should be continued with the dosage administered over the previous 2-4 weeks, for 1-5 years.

4.3 Contraindications

Pregnancy (see section 4.6)

Myocrisin is contraindicated in patients with gross renal or hepatic disease, a history of blood dyscrasias, exfoliative dermatitis or systemic lupus erythematosus.

The absolute contraindications should be positively excluded before considering gold therapy.

4.4 Special warnings and precautions for use

As with other gold preparations, reactions which resemble anaphylactoid effects have been reported. These effects may occur after any course of therapy within the first ten minutes following drug administration (see administration). If anaphylactoid effects are observed, treatment with Myocrisin should be discontinued (see section 4.8).

Myocrisin should be administered with extra caution in the elderly and in patients with a history of urticaria, eczema or colitis. Extra caution should also be exercised if phenylbutazone or oxyphenbutazone are administered concurrently.

Before starting treatment and again before each injection, the urine should be tested for protein, the skin inspected for rash and a full blood count performed, including a numerical platelet count (not an estimate) and the readings plotted. Blood dyscrasias are most likely to occur when between 400 mg and 1 g of gold have been given, or between the 10th and 20th week of treatment, but can also occur with much lower doses or after only 2-4 weeks of therapy (see section 4.8).

The presence of albuminuria, pruritus or rash, or an eosinophilia, are indications of developing toxicity **(see section 4.8).** The Myocrisin should be withheld for one or two weeks until all signs have disappeared when the course may be restarted on a test dose followed by a decreased frequency of gold injections.

A complaint of sore throat, glossitis, buccal ulceration and/or easy bruising or bleeding, demands an immediate blood count, followed if indicated, by appropriate treatment for agranulocytosis, aplastic anaemia and/or thrombocytopenia (see section 4.8). Every patient treated with Myocrisin should be warned to report immediately the appearance of pruritus, metallic taste, sore throat or tongue, buccal ulceration or easy bruising, purpura, epistaxis, bleeding gums, menorrhagia or diarrhoea (see section 4.8).

4.5 Interaction with other medicinal products and other forms of interaction

Concurrent gold administration may exacerbate aspirin-induced hepatic dysfunction. Caution should be exercised if phenylbutazone or oxyphenbutazone are administered concurrently.

Caution is needed in patients treated concomitantly with sodium aurothiomalate and angiotensin-converting enzyme inhibitors due to an increased risk of severe anaphylactoid reaction in these patients.

4.6 Pregnancy and lactation

The safety of Myocrisin in the foetus and the newborn has not been established. Female patients receiving Myocrisin should be instructed to avoid pregnancy. Pregnant patients should not be treated with Myocrisin. Lactating mothers under treatment with Myocrisin excrete significant amounts of gold in their breast milk and should not breast feed their infants.

4.7 Effects on ability to drive and use machines

None

4.8 Undesirable effects

Blood dyscrasias including thrombocytopenia, pancytopenia, agranulocytosis, aplastic anaemia, leucopenia & neutropenia have been reported (see section 4.4).

Anaphylactic/Anaphylactoid reactions have been reported, symptoms of which may include weakness, flushing, hypotension, tachycardia, dyspnoea, palpitations, abdominal pain, shock and possibly collapse (see section 4.4).

Hepatotxicity with cholestatic jaundic is a rare complication which may occur early in the course of treatment. It subsides on withdrawing Myocrisin. A rare but severe form of enterocolitis has been described.

Diffuse unilateral or bilateral pulmonary fibrosis very rarely occurs. This progressive condition usually responds to drug withdrawal and steroid therapy. An annual x-ray is recommended and attention should be paid to unexplained breathlessness and dry cough.

Side effects may be largly avoided by the indicated careful titration of dosage. Minor reactions, usually manifest as skin rashes and pruritus are the most frequent and commonly benign, but as such reactions may be the forerunners of severe gold toxicity they must never be treated lightly. Other indicators of developing toxicity could be the presence of albuminuria or an eosinophilia (see section 4.4)

Severe skin reactions that have been reported include exfoliative dermatitis and bullous eruptions. Irreversible skin pigmentation (chrysiasis) can occur in sun-exposed areas after prolonged treatment with Myocrisin. Rare reports of alopecia exist. Nephrotic syndrome has been rarely reported.

Neurological manifestations of gold toxicity including very rare cases of peripheral neuropathy, Guillain-Barré syndrome and encephalopathy have been observed.

4.9 Overdose

Minor side effects resolve spontaneously on withdrawal of Myocrisin. Symptomatic treatment of pruritus with antihistamines may be helpful. Major skin lesions and serious blood dyscrasias demand hospital admission when dimercaprol or penacillamine may be used to enhance gold excretion. Fresh blood and/or platelet transfusions, corticosteroids and androgenic steroids may be required in the management of severe blood dyscasias.

5. PHARMACOLOGICAL PROPERTIES

5.1 Pharmacodynamic properties

The precise mode of action of sodium aurothiomalate is not yet known. Treatment with gold has been shown to be accompanied by a fall in ESR and C-reactive protein, an increase in serum histidine and sulphydryl levels and a reduction in serum immunoglobulins, rheumatoid factor titres and Clq-binding activity.

Numerous experimental observations have been recorded including physico-chemical changes in collagen and interference with complement activation, gammaglobulin aggregation, prostaglandin biosythesis, inhibition of cathepsin and production of superoxide radicals by activated polymophonuclear leucocytes.

5.2 Pharmacokinetic properties

Sodium aurothiomalate is absorbed readily after intramuscular injection and becomes bound to plasma proteins. With doses of 50 mg weekly the steady-state serum concentration of gold is about 3 to 5 microgram per ml. It is widely distributed and accumulates in the body. Concentrations in synovial fluid have been shown to be similar or slightly less than those in plasma. Sodium aurothiomalate is mainly excreted in the urine with smaller amounts in the faeces. The serum half-life of gold clearance is about 5 or 6 days but after a course of treatment, gold may be found in the urine for up to a year or more owing to its presence in deep body compartments.

Gold has been detected in the foetus following administration of sodium aurothiomalate to the mother. Gold has been detected in the breast fed child where the mother has received sodium aurothiomalate.

5.3 Preclinical safety data

No additional pre-clinical data of relevance to the prescriber.

6. PHARMACEUTICAL PARTICULARS

6.1 List of excipients

Phenylmercuric nitrate

Water for Injections

6.2 Incompatibilities

None known

6.3 Shelf life

36 months

6.4 Special precautions for storage

Store below 25°C. Protect from light

6.5 Nature and contents of container

Carton containing 10 sealed glass ampoules each containing 0.5ml injection solution.

6.6 Special precautions for disposal and other handling

None stated

7. MARKETING AUTHORISATION HOLDER

Sanofi-aventis

One Onslow Street

Guildford

Surrey

GU1 4YS

UK

8. MARKETING AUTHORISATION NUMBER(S)

PL04425/0387

9. DATE OF FIRST AUTHORISATION/RENEWAL OF THE AUTHORISATION

6th December 2006

10. DATE OF REVISION OF THE TEXT

9th January 2007

11 LEGAL CLASSIFICATION

POM

Nalcrom

(sanofi-aventis)

1. NAME OF THE MEDICINAL PRODUCT
Nalcrom™

2. QUALITATIVE AND QUANTITATIVE COMPOSITION
in terms of the active ingredient (INN) name

The active component per capsule is:

Sodium Cromoglicate 100.0mg

3. PHARMACEUTICAL FORM
Nalcrom is presented as a hard gelatin capsule with a colourless, transparent cap and body, printed in black 'SODIUM CROMOGLICATE 100 mg' and containing a white powder.

4. CLINICAL PARTICULARS

4.1 Therapeutic indications
Nalcrom is indicated for food allergy (where adequate investigations have been performed to determine sensitivity to one or more ingested allergens) in conjunction with restriction of main causative allergens.

4.2 Posology and method of administration
Nalcrom must be administered orally

Adults (including the elderly)

Initial dose: 2 capsules four times daily before meals

Children (2 - 14 years)

Initial dose: 1 capsule four times daily before meals

For adults (including the elderly) and children, if satisfactory control is not achieved within two to three weeks, the dosage may be doubled but should not exceed 40 mg/Kg/day.

Maintenance dose: Once a therapeutic response has been achieved, the dose may be reduced to the minimum required to maintain the patient free from symptoms.

4.3 Contraindications
Nalcrom is contraindicated in patients with a known sensitivity to sodium cromoglicate.

4.4 Special warnings and precautions for use
None stated

4.5 Interaction with other medicinal products and other forms of interaction
None known.

4.6 Pregnancy and lactation
As with all medication caution should be exercised especially during the first trimester of pregnancy. Cumulative experience with sodium cromoglicate suggests that it has no adverse effects on foetal development. It should only be used in pregnancy where there is a clear need.

It is not known whether sodium cromoglicate is excreted in the breast milk but on the basis of its physico-chemical properties this is considered unlikely. There is no information to suggest that the use of sodium cromoglicate has any undesirable effects on the baby.

4.7 Effects on ability to drive and use machines
None known.

4.8 Undesirable effects
Nausea, skin rashes and joint pains have been reported in a few cases.

4.9 Overdose
As Nalcrom is only absorbed to a minimum extent, no action other than medical supervision should be necessary.

5. PHARMACOLOGICAL PROPERTIES

5.1 Pharmacodynamic properties
Sodium cromoglicate inhibits the release from mast cells of mediators of the allergic reaction. In gastrointestinal allergy the release of mediators can result in gastrointestinal symptoms or may allow absorption of antigenic material leading to systemic allergic reactions.

5.2 Pharmacokinetic properties
Not applicable

5.3 Preclinical safety data
Animal studies have shown that sodium cromoglicate has a very low order of local or systemic toxicity.

6. PHARMACEUTICAL PARTICULARS

6.1 List of excipients
Purified Water

No 2 hard gelatin capsules

Black ink containing:

Water

Ethyl alcohol

Iso-propyl alcohol

Propylene alcohol

N-butyl alcohol

Shellac

Ammonium hydroxide

Potassium hydroxide

Iron oxide black (E172)

6.2 Incompatibilities
None stated.

6.3 Shelf life
60 months

6.4 Special precautions for storage
Store in a dry place.

6.5 Nature and contents of container
An aluminium can with aluminium screw cap containing 100 capsules or an HDPE bottle with screw cap containing 100 capsules.

6.6 Special precautions for disposal and other handling
Instructions for use are supplied with each pack.

7. MARKETING AUTHORISATION HOLDER
Sanofi-aventis

One Onslow Street

Guildford

Surrey, GU1 4YS, UK

8. MARKETING AUTHORISATION NUMBER(S)
PL 04425/0370

9. DATE OF FIRST AUTHORISATION/RENEWAL OF THE AUTHORISATION
1st May 2005

10. DATE OF REVISION OF THE TEXT
November 2006

11. LEGAL CATEGORY
POM

Naloxone Hydrochloride Injection, Minijet. (International Medication Systems)

(International Medication Systems (UK) Ltd)

1. NAME OF THE MEDICINAL PRODUCT
Naloxone Hydrochloride Injection, Minijet®, Solution for Injection.

2. QUALITATIVE AND QUANTITATIVE COMPOSITION
Naloxone hydrochloride (as dihydrate) 0.4mg/ml.

3. PHARMACEUTICAL FORM
Solution for injection.

4. CLINICAL PARTICULARS

4.1 Therapeutic indications
Naloxone is indicated for the treatment of respiratory depression induced by natural and synthetic opioids, such as codeine, diamorphine, levorphanol, methadone, morphine, concentrated opium alkaloid hydrochlorides and propoxyphene. It is also useful for the treatment of respiratory depression caused by opioid agonist/ antagonists nalbuphine and pentazocine. Naloxone is also used for the diagnosis of suspected acute opioid overdose.

4.2 Posology and method of administration
Naloxone hydrochloride may be administered by IV, IM or SC injection or IV infusion.

Adults:

Naloxone may be diluted for intravenous infusion in normal saline or 5% dextrose solutions. The addition of 2 mg of naloxone in 500 ml of either solution provides a concentration of 4 µg /ml. Infusion should be commenced as soon as practicable after preparation of the mixture in order to reduce microbiological hazards. Preparations not used within 24 hours should be discarded. The rate of administration should be titrated in accordance with the patient's response. Parenteral drug products should be inspected visually for particulate matter and discolouration prior to administration whenever solution and container permit.

Naloxone hydrochloride may be used postoperatively to reverse central depression resulting from the use of opioids during surgery. The usual dosage is 100 - 200 µg IV given at 2 to 3 minute intervals to obtain optimum respiratory response while maintaining adequate analgesia. Additional doses may be necessary at one to two hour intervals depending on the response of the patient and the dosage and duration of action of the opioid administered.

For the treatment of known opioid overdosage or as an aid in the diagnosis of suspected opioid overdosage, the usual initial adult dosage of naloxone hydrochloride is 400 - 2000 µg IV, administered at 2 to 3 minute intervals if necessary. If no response is observed after a total of 10 mg of the drug has been administered, the depressive condition may be caused by a drug or disease process not responsive to naloxone. When the IV route cannot be used, the drug may be administered by IM or SC injection.

Children:

The usual initial dose in children is 10 µg / kg bodyweight given IV. If the dose does not result in the desired degree of clinical improvement, a subsequent dose of 100 µg / kg body weight may be administered. If the IV route of administration is not available, naloxone may be administered IM or SC in divided doses. If necessary naloxone can be diluted with sterile water for injection.

Opioid - induced depression in neonates resulting from the administration of opioid analgesics to the mother during labour may be reversed by administering naloxone hydrochloride 10 µg / kg body weight to the infant by IM, IV or SC injections, repeated at intervals of 2 to 3 minutes if necessary. Alternatively, a single IM dose of about 60 µg / kg may be given at birth for a more prolonged action.

Elderly:

In elderly patients with pre-existing cardiovascular disease or in those receiving potentially cardiotoxic drugs, naloxone should be used with caution since serious adverse cardiovascular effects such as ventricular tachycardia and fibrillation have occurred in postoperative patients following administration of naloxone.

4.3 Contraindications
Naloxone is contraindicated in patients with known hypersensitivity to the drug.

4.4 Special warnings and precautions for use
It should be administered with caution to patients who have received large doses of opioids or to those physically dependent on opioids since too rapid reversal may precipitate an acute withdrawal syndrome in such patients. When naloxone hydrochloride is used in the management of acute opioid overdosage, other resuscitation measures should be readily available. A withdrawal syndrome may also be precipitated in newborn infants of opioid-dependent mothers.

Following the use of opioids during surgery, excessive dosage of naloxone hydrochloride should be avoided, because it may cause excitement, increase in blood pressure and clinically important reversal of analgesia. A reversal of opioid effects achieved too rapidly may induce nausea, vomiting, sweating or tachycardia.

Naloxone should be also used with caution in patients with preexisting cardiovascular disease or in those receiving potentially cardiotoxic drugs, since serious adverse cardiovascular effects such as ventricular tachycardia and fibrillation have occurred in postoperative patients following administration of naloxone.

Patients who have responded to naloxone should be carefully monitored, since the duration of action of some opioids may exceed that of naloxone.

4.5 Interaction with other medicinal products and other forms of interaction
No drug or chemical agent should be added to naloxone unless its effect on the chemical and physical stability of the solution has first been established.

4.6 Pregnancy and lactation
Reproductive studies in mice and rats using naloxone hydrochloride dosage up to 1000 times the usual human dosage have not revealed evidence of impaired fertility or harm to the foetus. There are no adequate and controlled studies using the drug in pregnant women. Naloxone hydrochloride should be used only when clearly needed. Since it is not known whether naloxone hydrochloride is distributed into breast milk, the drug should be used with caution in nursing women.

4.7 Effects on ability to drive and use machines
Not applicable.

4.8 Undesirable effects
Abrupt reversal of narcotic depression may result in nausea, vomiting, sweating, tachycardia, hyperventilation, increased blood pressure and tremulousness.

In postoperative patients, larger than necessary dosages of naloxone may result in significant reversal of analgesia and in excitement.

Hypotension, hypertension, ventricular tachycardia and fibrillation, hyperventilation and pulmonary oedema have been associated with the use of naloxone postoperatively. Seizures have occurred on rare occasions following the administration of naloxone, but a causal relationship to the drug has not been established.

4.9 Overdose
There have been no reports of acute overdosage due to naloxone hydrochloride.

5. PHARMACOLOGICAL PROPERTIES
5.1 Pharmacodynamic properties
Naloxone hydrochloride is a semisynthetic (N-allylnoroxy-morphine hydrochloride) opioid antagonist which is derived from thebaine. When administered in usual doses to patients who have not recently received opioids, naloxone exerts little or no pharmacologic effect. Even extremely high doses of the drug (10 times the usual therapeutic dose) produces insignificant analgesia, only slight drowsiness and no respiratory depression, psychotomimetic effects, circulatory changes or miosis.

In patients who have received large doses of diamorphine or other analgesic drugs with morphine-like effects, naloxone antagonises most of the effects of the opioid. There is an increase in respiratory rate and minute volume, arterial p CO_2 decreases toward normal and blood pressure returns to normal if depressed. Naloxone antagonises mild respiratory depression cause by small doses of opioids. Because the duration of action of naloxone is generally shorter than that of the opioid, the effects of the opioid may return as the effects of naloxone dissipates. Naloxone antagonises opioid-induced sedation or sleep. Reports are conflicting on whether or not the drug modifies opioid-induced excitement or siezures.

Naloxone does not produce tolerance or physical or psychological dependence. However, 0.4 mg of naloxone hydrochloride administered SC will precipitate potentially severe withdrawal symptoms in patients physically dependent on opioids or pentazocine. The precise mechanism of action of the opioid antagonist effects of naloxone is not known. Naloxone is thought to act as a competitive antagonist at μ, K or σ opioid receptors in the central nervous system. It is thought that the drug has the highest affinity for the μ receptor.

5.2 Pharmacokinetic properties
Naloxone has an onset of action within 1 to 2 minutes following IV administration and within 2 to 5 minutes following SC or IM administration. The duration of action depends on the dose and route of administration and is more prolonged following IM administration than after IV administration. In one study, the duration of action was 45 minues following IV administration of naloxone hydrochloride 0.4 mg/70 kg.

Following administration of 35 or 70 μg of naloxone hydrochloride in the umbilical vein in neonates in one study, peak plasma naloxone concentrations occurred within 40 minutes and were 4 - 5.4 ng/ml and 9.2 - 20.2 ng/ml, respectively. After IM administration of 0.2 mg to neonates in the same study, peak plasma naloxone concentrations of 11.3 - 34.7 ng/ml occurred within 0.5 - 2 hours.

Following parenteral administration, naloxone is rapidly distributed into body tissues and fluids. In rats, high concentrations are observed in the brain, kidney, spleen, lungs, heart and skeletal muscles. In humans, the drug readily crosses the placenta. It is not known whether naloxone is distributed into milk.

The plasma half-life of naloxone has been reported to be 60 to 90 minutes in adults and about 3 hours in neonates.

Naloxone is rapidly metabolised in the liver, principally by conjugation with glucuronic acid. The major metabolite is naloxone-3-glucuronide. Naloxone also undergoes N-dealkylation and reduction of the 6-keto group followed by conjugation. Limited studies with radiolabeled naloxone indicated that 25 - 40% IV doses of the drug is excreted as metabolites in urine in 6 hours, about 50% in 24 hours and 60 - 70% in 72 hours.

5.3 Preclinical safety data
Not applicable since naloxone has been used in clinical practice for many years and its effects in man are well known.

6. PHARMACEUTICAL PARTICULARS
6.1 List of excipients
Sodium Chloride

Hydrochloric Acid

Water for Injection

6.2 Incompatibilities
Naloxone should not be mixed with preparations containing bisulphite, metabisulphite, long-chain or high molecular anions or any solution having an alkaline pH.

6.3 Shelf life
1ml: 3 years

2ml: 2 years

5ml: 2 years

6.4 Special precautions for storage
Do not store above 25°C.

6.5 Nature and contents of container
The solution is contained in a Type I USP glass vial with a rubber closure which meets all the relevent USP specifications for elastomeric closures. The product is available as 1ml, 2ml or 5ml.

6.6 Special precautions for disposal and other handling
The container is specially designed for use with the IMS Minijet® injector, fitted with either a Luer lock / Clave connector or in addition, for the 1ml vial only, an integral 21ga × 1.5 inch needle.

7. MARKETING AUTHORISATION HOLDER
International Medication Systems (UK) Ltd

208 Bath Road

Slough

Berkshire

SL1 3WE

UK

8. MARKETING AUTHORISATION NUMBER(S)
PL 03265/0071

9. DATE OF FIRST AUTHORISATION/RENEWAL OF THE AUTHORISATION
Date first granted: 29 September 1986

Date renewed: 24 June 1999

10. DATE OF REVISION OF THE TEXT
August 2007

POM

Napratec OP

(Pharmacia Limited)

1. NAME OF THE MEDICINAL PRODUCT
NAPRATEC™ OP

2. QUALITATIVE AND QUANTITATIVE COMPOSITION
Napratec is a combination pack containing 56 Naproxen 500mg tablets and 56 Cytotec (misoprostol) 200mcg tablets.

For excipients, see 6.1

3. PHARMACEUTICAL FORM
Tablet

Naproxen 500mg tablets are yellow, oblong and engraved 'NXN500' with a breakline on one side and CP on the reverse.

Cytotec is a white/off-white hexagonal tablet, scored on both sides, engraved SEARLE 1461 on one side.

4. CLINICAL PARTICULARS
4.1 Therapeutic indications
Napratec combination pack is indicated for use for patients who require Naproxen 500mg twice daily and Cytotec 200mcg twice daily.

Naproxen is indicated for the treatment of rheumatoid arthritis, osteoarthritis (degenerative arthritis) and ankylosing spondylitis.

Cytotec is indicated for the prophylaxis of nonsteroidal anti-inflammatory drug (NSAID)-induced gastroduodenal ulceration.

4.2 Posology and method of administration
For oral administration

Adults

1 tablet of Naproxen and 1 tablet of Cytotec to be taken together twice daily with or after food.

Elderly

Studies indicate that although total plasma concentration of naproxen is unchanged, the unbound plasma fraction of naproxen is increased in the elderly.

With Cytotec the usual dosage may be used in the elderly.

Napratec should only be used in those patients for whom 500mg naproxen twice daily is appropriate and in whom no reduction of naproxen dosage is necessary (see also sections on renal and hepatic impairment).

The elderly are at an increased risk of the serious consequences of adverse reactions. The patient should be monitored regularly for GI bleeding during NSAID therapy.

Renal Impairment

As the final pathway for the elimination of naproxen metabolites is largely (95%) by urinary excretion via glomerular filtration it should be used with great caution in patients with impaired renal function and the monitoring of serum creatinine and/or creatinine clearance is advised in these patients. Naproxen is not recommended in patients having a baseline creatinine clearance of less than 20ml/minute.

Certain patients, specifically those whose renal blood flow is compromised, such as in extracellular volume depletion, cirrhosis of the liver, sodium restriction, congestive heart failure, and pre-existing renal disease, should have renal function assessed before and during naproxen therapy. Some elderly patients in whom impaired renal function may be expected could also fall within this category. Where there is a possibility of accumulation of naproxen metabolites, such patients may not be suitable to receive naproxen 500mg twice daily.

With Cytotec no dosage alteration is necessary in patients with impaired renal function.

Hepatic Impairment

Chronic alcoholic liver disease and probably also other forms of cirrhosis reduce the total plasma concentration of naproxen, but the plasma concentration of unbound naproxen is increased.

With Cytotec no dosage alteration is necessary in patients with impaired hepatic function.

Children

Napratec is not recommended.

Undesirable effects may be minimised by using the lowest effective dose for the shortest duration necessary to control symptoms (see section 4.4).

4.3 Contraindications
Use in Pregnancy and Lactation

Napratec is contraindicated in pregnancy and lactation (see section 4.6)

This medicine is also contraindicated in patients planning to become pregnant.

Napratec is contraindicated in patients with a known hypersensitivity to naproxen, or to misoprostol or to any of the excipients.

As the potential exists with naproxen for cross-sensitivity to aspirin and other nonsteroidal anti-inflammatory drugs, Napratec should not be administered to patients in whom aspirin, ibuprofen and other NSAIDs induce asthma, rhinitis, urticaria or angioedema.

As Napratec is a "prevention pack" it should not be used for treating arthritis in patients with active gastric or duodenal ulceration / haemorrhage. Such patients may be treated with a healing dose of Cytotec, 800 micrograms daily in divided doses with meals, and the NSAID continued or discontinued at the physician's discretion.

Use in pre-menopausal women

Napratec should not be used in pre-menopausal women unless the patient is at high risk of complications from NSAID-induced ulceration. In such patients it is advised that Napratec should only be used if the patient:

- takes effective contraceptive measures
- has been advised of the risks of taking the product if pregnant

Napratec is contraindicated in patients with severe heart failure, hepatic failure and renal failure (see section 4.4).

4.4 Special warnings and precautions for use
Precautions

Undesirable effects may be minimised by using the lowest effective dose for the shortest duration necessary to control symptoms (see section 4.2, and GI and cardiovascular risks below).

The use of Naproxen with concomitant NSAIDs including cyclooxygenase-2 selective inhibitors should be avoided (see section 4.5).

Naproxen, in common with other NSAIDs, decreases platelet aggregation and prolongs bleeding time. This effect should be considered when bleeding times are determined.

Elderly:

The elderly have an increased frequency of adverse reactions to NSAIDs especially gastrointestinal bleeding and perforation which may be fatal (see section 4.2)

Respiratory disorders:

Caution is required if administered to patients suffering from, or with a previous history of, bronchial asthma or allergic disease since NSAIDs have been reported to precipitate bronchospasm in such patients.

Cardiovascular, Renal and Hepatic Impairment:

The administration of an NSAID may cause a dose dependent reduction in prostaglandin formation and precipitate renal failure. Patients at greatest risk of this reaction are those with impaired renal function, cardiac impairment, liver dysfunction, those taking diuretics and the elderly. Renal function should be monitored in these patients (see also section 4.3).

Mild peripheral oedema has been observed in a few patients receiving naproxen. Although sodium retention has not been reported in metabolic studies, it is possible that patients with questionable or compromised cardiac function may be at a greater risk when taking naproxen.

Cardiovascular and cerebrovascular effects:

Appropriate monitoring and advice are required for patients with a history of hypertension and/or mild to moderate congestive heart failure as fluid retention and oedema have been reported in association with NSAID therapy.

Clinical trial and epidemiological data suggest that use of coxibs and some NSAIDs (particularly at high doses and in long term treatment) may be associated with a small increased risk of arterial thrombotic events (for example myocardial infarction or stroke). Although data suggest that the use of naproxen (1000 mg daily) may be associated with a lower risk, some risk cannot be excluded.

Patients with uncontrolled hypertension, congestive heart failure, established ischaemic heart disease, peripheral arterial disease, and/or cerebrovascular disease should only be treated with naproxen after careful consideration. Similar consideration should be made before initiating longer-term treatment of patients with risk factors for cardiovascular events (e.g. hypertension, hyperlipidaemia, diabetes mellitus, smoking).

Gastrointestinal bleeding, ulceration and perforation:

Gastrointestinal bleeding, ulceration or perforation, which can be fatal, has been reported with all NSAIDs at any time during treatment, with or without warning symptoms or a previous history of serious GI events. When GI bleeding or ulceration occurs in patients receiving Napratec OP, the treatment should be withdrawn. The risk of GI bleeding, ulceration or perforation is higher with increasing NSAID doses, in patients with a history of ulcer, particularly if complicated with haemorrhage or perforation and in the elderly.

Patients with a history of GI toxicity, particularly if complicated when elderly, should report any unusual abdominal symptoms (especially GI bleeding) particularly in the initial stages of treatment.

Caution should be advised in patients receiving concomitant medications which could increase the risk of ulceration or bleeding, such as oral corticosteroids, anticoagulants such as warfarin, selective serotonin-reuptake inhibitors or anti-platelet agents such as aspirin. (see section 4.5)

NSAIDs should be given with care to patients with a history of gastrointestinal disease (ulcerative colitis, Crohn's disease) as these conditions may be exacerbated (see section 4.8).

SLE and mixed connective tissue disease:

In patients with systemic lupus erythematosus (SLE) and mixed connective tissue disorders there may be an increased risk of aseptic meningitis (see section 4.8)

Dermatological:

Serious skin reactions, some of them fatal, including exfoliative dermatitis, Stevens-Johnson syndrome, and toxic epidermal necrolysis, have been reported very rarely in association with use of NSAID (see section 4.8). Patients appear to be at highest risk for these reactions early in the course of therapy: onset of the reaction occurring in the majority of cases within the first month of treatment. Napratec should be discontinued at the first appearance of skin rash, mucosal lesions, or any other sign of hypersensitivity.

Sporadic abnormalities in laboratory tests (e.g. liver function tests) have occurred in patients on naproxen, but no definite trend was seen in any test indicating toxicity.

Cytotec should be used with caution in disease states where hypotension might precipitate severe complications, e.g. cerebrovascular disease, coronary artery disease or severe peripheral vascular disease including hypertension.

Patients with rare hereditary problems of galactose intolerance, the Lapp lactase deficiency or glucose-galactose malabsorption should not take this medicine.

4.5 Interaction with other medicinal products and other forms of interaction

Drug Interactions

Due to the high plasma protein binding of naproxen, patients simultaneously receiving hydantoins, anti-coagulants or a highly protein-bound sulphonamide should be observed for signs of over dosage of these drugs. No interactions have been observed in clinical studies with naproxen and anti-coagulants or sulphonylureas, but caution is nevertheless advised since interaction has been seen with other non-steroidal agents of this class.

Diuretics: NSAIDs may attenuate the natriuretic efficacy of diuretics due to inhibition of intrarenal synthesis of prostaglandins. NSAIDs may also cause a reduced diuretic effect. Diuretics can increase the risk of nephrotoxicity of NSAIDs.

Ciclosporin: Because of their effect on renal prostaglandins, cyclo-oxygenase inhibitors such as naproxen can increase the nephrotoxicity of ciclosporin

Other analgesics including cyclooxygenase-2-selective inhibitors: Avoid concomitant use of two or more NSAIDs (including aspirin) as this may increase the risk of adverse events (see section 4.4).

Lithium: NSAIDs including naproxen have been reported to increase steady state plasma lithium levels. It is recommended that these are monitored whenever initiating, adjusting or discontinuing naproxen products.

Cardiac glycosides: Concomitant administration of Naproxen with cardiac glycosides may exacerbate cardiac failure, reduce GFR and increase plasma glycoside levels.

Anti-hypertensives: Concomitant administration of naproxen with beta-blockers may reduce their antihypertensive effect.

Corticosteroids: Concomitant administration of naproxen with corticosteroids increases the risk of gastrointestinal ulceration or bleeding (see section 4.4) and may increase the frequency of side effects generally.

Quinolone antibiotics: Animal data indicate that NSAIDs can increase the risk of convulsions associated with quinolone antibiotics. Patients taking NSAIDs and quinolones may have an increased risk of developing convulsions.

Probenecid: Increases naproxen plasma levels and extends its plasma half-life considerably.

Methotrexate: Caution is advised when methotrexate is administered concurrently because of possible enhancement of its toxicity since naproxen, among other NSAIDs, has been reported to induce the tubular secretion of methotrexate in an animal model.

Mifepristone: NSAIDs should not be used for 8 – 12 days after mifepristone administration as NSAIDs can reduce the effect of mifepristone.

Anti-coagulants: NSAIDs may enhance the effects of anticoagulatnts, such as warfarin (see section 4.4).

Anti-platelet agents and selective serotonin reuptake inhibitors (SSRIs): Increased risk of gastrointestinal bleeding (see section 4.4).

Tacrolimus: Possible increased risk of nephrotoxicity when NSAIDs are given with tacrolimus.

Zidovudine: Increased risk of haematological toxicity when NSAIDs are given with zidovudine. There is evidence of an increased risk of haemarthroses and haematoma in HIV(+) haemophiliacs receiving concurrent treatment with zidovudine and ibuprofen.

Naproxen therapy should be temporarily withdrawn before adrenal function tests are performed as it may artificially interfere with some tests for 17-ketogenic steroids. Similarly, naproxen may interfere with some assays of urinary 5-hydroxyindoleacetic acid.

Cytotec is predominantly metabolised via fatty acid oxidising systems and has shown no adverse effect on the hepatic microsomal mixed function oxidase (P450) enzyme system. No drug interactions have been attributed to Cytotec, and in specific studies, no clinically significant pharmacokinetic or pharmacodynamic interaction has been demonstrated with antipyrine, diazepam, propranolol or NSAIDs.

4.6 Pregnancy and lactation

Napratec is contraindicated in pregnancy and lactation. The product is contraindicated in pregnancy on the basis that Cytotec is contraindicated in pregnancy or women planning a pregnancy as it increases uterine tone and contractions in pregnancy which may cause partial or complete expulsion of the products of conception.

Teratology studies with naproxen in rats and rabbits at dose levels equivalent on a human multiple basis to those which have produced foetal abnormality with certain other NSAIDs, e.g. aspirin, have not produced evidence of foetal damage with naproxen. As with other drugs of this type, naproxen delays parturition in animals (the relevance of this finding to human patients is unknown) and also affects the human foetal cardiovascular system (closure of the ductus arteriosus).

4.7 Effects on ability to drive and use machines

Dizziness, drowsiness, fatigue, visual disturbances or headaches are possible undesirable effects after taking NSAIDs. If affected, patients should not drive or operate machinery.

4.8 Undesirable effects

Naproxen:

Gastrointestinal: The most commonly-observed adverse events are gastrointestinal in nature. Peptic ulcers, perforation or gastrointestinal bleeding, sometimes fatal, particularly in the elderly may occur. Nausea, vomiting, diarrhoea, flatulence, constipation, dyspepsia, abdominal pain or discomfort and epigastric distress, melaena, haematemesis, ulcerative stomatitis, exacerbation of colitis and Crohn's disease (see section 4.4) have been reported following administration. The more serious reaction, colitis, may occasionally occur. Less frequently, gastritis has been observed. Pancreatitis has been reported very rarely.

Naproxen also causes gastrointestinal bleeding and gastric and duodenal ulceration, the consequences of which may be haemorrhage and perforation. The inclusion of Cytotec in the combination pack is to prevent naproxen-induced gastric and duodenal ulceration.

Hypersensitivity and Dermatological: Non-specific allergic reactions and anaphylaxis, respiratory tract reactivity comprising asthma, aggravated asthma, bronchospasm or dyspnoea, assorted skin disorders including rashes of various types, pruritus, purpura, urticaria, angio-oedema. Anaphylactic reactions to naproxen and naproxen sodium formulations; eosinophilic pneumonitis, alopecia, photosensitivity reactions and more rarely epidermolysis bullosa, epidermal necrolysis, erythema multiforme, pseudoporphyria, Stevens Johnson syndrome and toxic epidermal necrolysis (very rare).

Cardiovascular and cerebrovascular:

Oedema, hypertension, and cardiac failure, have been reported in association with NSAID treatment.

Clinical trial and epidemiological data suggest that use of some NSAIDs (particularly at high doses and in long term treatment) may be associated with a small increased risk of arterial thrombotic events (for example myocardial infarction or stroke) (see section 4.4).

Neurological and special senses: Headache, visual disturbances, insomnia, optic neuritis, paraesthesia, inability to concentrate, cognitive dysfunction, reports of aseptic meningitis (especially in patients with existing auto-immune disorders, such as systemic lupus erythematosus, mixed connective tissue disease) with symptoms such as stiff neck, headache, nausea, vomiting, fever or disorientation (see section 4.4), depression, confusion, hallucinations, tinnitus, hearing impairment, vertigo, dizziness, malaise, fatigue and drowsiness.

Renal: As a class NSAIDs have been associated with renal pathology including nephropathy, papillary necrosis, interstitial nephritis, nephrotic syndrome and renal failure.

Hepatic: Abnormal liver function, fatal hepatitis and jaundice.

Haematological: Thrombocytopenia, neutropenia, granulocytopenia, agranulocytosis, aplastic anaemia and haemolytic anaemia may occur rarely.

Other: Mild peripheral oedema, vasculitis, and haematuria.

Cytotec:

Gastrointestinal: Diarrhoea has been reported and is occasionally severe and prolonged, and may require withdrawal of the drug. It can be minimised by taking Cytotec with food and by avoiding the use of predominantly magnesium-containing antacids when an antacid is required. Abdominal pain with or without associated dyspepsia can follow Cytotec therapy. Other gastrointestinal adverse effects reported include dyspepsia, flatulence, nausea and vomiting.

Female Reproductive System: Menorrhagia, vaginal bleeding and intermenstrual bleeding have been reported in both pre- and post-menopausal women.

Other Adverse Effects: Skin rashes have been reported. Dizziness has been infrequently reported.

4.9 Overdose

Naproxen:

Symptoms - Symptoms include drowsiness, heartburn, indigestion, nausea, vomiting, headache, epigastric pain, gastrointestinal bleeding, rarely diarrhoea, disorientataion, excitation, coma, dizziness, tinnitus, fainting, occasionally convulsions. A few patients have experienced seizures, but it is not clear whether these were naproxen-related or not. In cases of significant poisoning acute renal failure and liver damage are possible. It is not known what dose of the drug would be life-threatening.

Therapeutic measures - In the event of overdosage with naproxen, the stomach may be emptied and usual supportive measures employed.

- Patients should be treated symptomatically as required.
- Within one hour of ingestion of a potential toxic amount, activated charcoal should be considered. Animal studies indicate that the prompt administration of activated charcoal in adequate amounts would tend to reduce markedly the absorption of the drug. Alternatively, in adult, gastric lavage should be considered within one hour of ingestion of a potentially life-threatening overdose.
- Good urine output should be insured.
- Renal and liver function should be closely monitored
- Patients should be observed for at least four hours after ingestion of potentially toxic amounts
- Frequent or prolonged convulsions should be treated with intravenous diazepam
- Other measures may be indicated by the patient's clinical condition.

Haemodialysis does not decrease the plasma concentration of naproxen because of the high degree of protein binding. However, haemodialysis may still be appropriate in a patient with renal failure who has taken naproxen.

Cytotec:

Intensification of pharmacological and adverse effects may occur with overdose. In the event of overdosage with Cytotec, symptomatic and supportive therapy should be given as appropriate.

5. PHARMACOLOGICAL PROPERTIES

5.1 Pharmacodynamic properties

Naproxen is a non-steroidal anti-inflammatory drug with well-documented properties, i.e. analgesic, antipyretic and anti-inflammatory.

Misoprostol is a synthetic prostaglandin E_1 analogue which enhances several of the factors that maintain gastroduodenal mucosal integrity.

5.2 Pharmacokinetic properties

Naproxen is readily absorbed from the GI tract. Peak plasma concentrations are obtained 2-4 hours after ingestion. At therapeutic concentrations, naproxen is more than 98% bound to plasma proteins and has an elimination half-life of between 12-15 hours.

Misoprostol is rapidly absorbed following oral administration with peak plasma levels of the active metabolite (misoprostol acid) occurring after about 30 minutes. The plasma elimination half-life of misoprostol acid is 20-40 minutes.

Increases in C_{max} and AUC for misoprostol acid have been observed when co-administered with naproxen in a single dose study. These changes are not thought to be clinically significant since the higher values are still well within the variation seen after 200 micrograms misoprostol in other studies. No accumulation of misoprostol acid in plasma occurs after repeated dosing of 400 micrograms twice daily.

5.3 Preclinical safety data

Naproxen causes gastric erosions when given orally or subcutaneously to fasting rats. There is no evidence of mutagenicity or carcinogenicity when administered to rats in studies of two years duration. There is no evidence of teratogenicity in mice, rats or rabbits.

Misoprostol in multiples of the recommended therapeutic dose in animals has produced gastric mucosal hyperplasia. This characteristic response to E-series prostaglandins reverts to normal on discontinuation of the compound.

6. PHARMACEUTICAL PARTICULARS

6.1 List of excipients

Naproxen 500mg tablets contain: Lactose, maize starch, povidone, sodium starch glycolate, magnesium stearate, yellow lake CLF 3076 (E104 and E172).

Cytotec 200mcg tablets contain: microcrystalline cellulose, sodium starch glycolate, hydrogenated castor oil and hypromellose.

6.2 Incompatibilities

Not applicable.

6.3 Shelf life

3 years

6.4 Special precautions for storage

Do not store above 30°C. Store in the original package.

6.5 Nature and contents of container

Combination pack containing 8 × 7 day blisters containing 56 Naproxen 500mg tablets and 56 Cytotec 200mcg tablets in cold-formed aluminium blisters.

6.6 Special precautions for disposal and other handling

No special requirements.

7. MARKETING AUTHORISATION HOLDER

Pharmacia Limited
Ramsgate Road
Sandwich
Kent, CT13 9NJ
United Kingdom

8. MARKETING AUTHORISATION NUMBER(S)

PL 00032/0486

9. DATE OF FIRST AUTHORISATION/RENEWAL OF THE AUTHORISATION

26 June 2002

10. DATE OF REVISION OF THE TEXT

February 2009

11. LEGAL CATEGORY

POM

Ref: NA4_0 UK

Naprosyn 250mg and 500mg Tablets

(Roche Products Limited)

1. NAME OF THE MEDICINAL PRODUCT

Naprosyn 250mg Tablets

Naprosyn 500mg Tablets

2. QUALITATIVE AND QUANTITATIVE COMPOSITION

Naprosyn 250mg Tablets: Each tablet contains 250mg naproxen

Naprosyn 500mg Tablets: Each tablet contains 500mg naproxen

For excipients, see 6.1.

3. PHARMACEUTICAL FORM

Tablet.

Naprosyn 250mg Tablets:

Round, yellow uncoated tablet embossed "NPR LE 250" on one face and with a breakline on the other.

Naprosyn 500mg Tablets:

Oval, yellow uncoated tablet embossed "NPR LE 500" on one face with a breakline on the other.

4. CLINICAL PARTICULARS

4.1 Therapeutic indications

Adults:

Treatment of rheumatoid arthritis, osteoarthrosis (degenerative arthritis), ankylosing spondylitis, acute gout, acute musculoskeletal disorders and dysmenorrhoea.

Children:

Juvenile rheumatoid arthritis

4.2 Posology and method of administration

Route of administration

For oral administration.

To be taken preferably with or after food.

Undesirable effects may be minimised by using the lowest effective dose for the shortest duration necessary to control symptoms (see section 4.4).

Adults

Rheumatoid arthritis, osteoarthritis and ankylosing spondylitis

500mg to 1g taken in 2 doses at 12-hour intervals or alternatively, as a single administration. In the following cases a loading dose of 750mg or 1g per day for the acute phase is recommended:

a) In patients reporting severe night-time pain/or morning stiffness.

b) In patients being switched to Naprosyn from a high dose of another anti-rheumatic compound.

c) In osteoarthrosis where pain is the predominant symptom.

Acute gout

750mg at once then 250mg every 8 hours until the attack has passed.

Acute musculoskeletal disorders and dysmenorrhoea

500mg initially followed by 250mg at 6 - 8 hour intervals as needed, with a maximum daily dose after the first day of 1250mg.

Elderly

Studies indicate that although total plasma concentration of naproxen is unchanged, the unbound plasma fraction of naproxen is increased in the elderly. The implication of this finding for Naprosyn dosing is unknown. As with other drugs used in the elderly it is prudent to use the lowest effective dose and for the shortest duration possible as elderly patients are more prone to adverse events. The patient should be monitored regularly for GI bleeding during NSAID therapy. For the effect of reduced elimination in the elderly refer to Section 4.4.

Children (over 5 years)

For juvenile rheumatoid arthritis: 10mg/kg/day taken in 2 doses at 12-hour intervals. Naprosyn is not recommended for use in any other indication in children under 16 years of age.

Renal/hepatic impairment

A lower dose should be considered in patients with renal or hepatic impairment. Naprosyn is contraindicated in patients with baseline creatinine clearance less than 30 ml/minute because accumulation of naproxen metabolites has been seen in patients with severe renal failure or those on dialysis (see section 4.3).

Treatment should be reviewed at regular intervals and discontinued if no benefit is seen or intolerance occurs.

4.3 Contraindications

Active or history of peptic ulceration or active gastrointestinal bleeding (two or more distinct episodes of proven ulceration or bleeding). History of gastrointestinal bleeding or perforation, related to previous NSAIDs therapy.

Hypersensitivity to naproxen, naproxen sodium, or any of the excipients. Since the potential exists for cross-sensitivity reactions, Naprosyn should not be given to patients in whom aspirin or other non-steroidal anti-inflammatory/analgesic drugs induce the syndrome of asthma, rhinitis, nasal polyps or urticaria. These reactions have the potential of being fatal. Severe anaphylactic-like reactions to naproxen have been reported in such patients.

Severe renal, hepatic or heart failure.

Naproxen is contraindicated during the last trimester of pregnancy (see Section 4.6).

4.4 Special warnings and precautions for use

Undesirable effects may be minimised by using the lowest effective dose for the shortest duration necessary to control symptoms (see section 4.2 and GI and cardiovascular risks below). Patients treated with NSAIDs long-term should undergo regular medical supervision to monitor for adverse events.

Elderly and/or debilitated patients are particularly susceptible to the adverse effects of NSAIDs, especially gastrointestinal bleeding and perforation, which may be fatal. Prolonged use of NSAIDs in these patients is not recommended. Where prolonged therapy is required, patients should be reviewed regularly.

The antipyretic and anti-inflammatory activities of Naprosyn may reduce fever and inflammation, thereby diminishing their utility as diagnostic signs.

Bronchospasm may be precipitated in patients suffering from, or with a history of, bronchial asthma or allergic disease.

As with other non-steroidal anti-inflammatory drugs, elevations of one or more liver function tests may occur. Hepatic abnormalities may be the result of hypersensitivity rather than direct toxicity. Severe hepatic reactions, including jaundice and hepatitis (some cases of hepatitis have been fatal) have been reported with this drug as with other non-steroidal anti-inflammatory drugs. Cross reactivity has been reported.

Naproxen decreases platelet aggregation and prolongs bleeding time. This effect should be kept in mind when bleeding times are determined.

Although sodium retention has not been reported in metabolic studies, it is possible that patients with questionable or compromised cardiac function may be at a greater risk when taking Naprosyn.

Gastrointestinal bleeding, ulceration and perforation

GI bleeding, ulceration or perforation, which can be fatal, has been reported with all NSAIDs at anytime during treatment, with or without warning symptoms or a previous history of serious GI events.

The risk of GI bleeding, ulceration or perforation is higher with increasing NSAID doses, in patients with a history of ulcer, particularly if complicated with haemorrhage or perforation (see section 4.3), and in the elderly. These patients should commence treatment on the lowest dose available.

Combination therapy with protective agents (e.g. misoprostol or proton pump inhibitors) should be considered for these patients, and also for patients requiring concomitant low dose aspirin, or other drugs likely to increase gastrointestinal risk (see section 4.5).

Patients with a history of GI toxicity, particularly when elderly, should report any unusual abdominal symptoms (especially GI bleeding) particularly in the initial stages of treatment.

Caution should be advised in patients receiving concomitant medications which could increase the risk of ulceration or bleeding, such as oral corticosteroid, anticoagulants such as warfarin, selective serotonin-reuptake inhibitors or anti-platelet agents such as aspirin (see Section 4.5).

When GI bleeding or ulceration occurs in patients receiving Naprosyn, the treatment should be withdrawn.

NSAIDs should be given with care to patients with a history of gastrointestinal disease (ulcerative colitis, Crohn's disease) as these conditions may be exacerbated (see Section 4.8).

Renal Effects

There have been reports of impaired renal function, renal failure, acute interstitial nephritis, haematuria, proteinuria, renal papillary necrosis and occasionally nephrotic syndrome associated with naproxen.

Renal failure linked to reduced prostaglandin production

The administration of an NSAID may cause a dose dependent reduction in prostaglandin formation and precipitate renal failure. Patients at greatest risk of this reaction are those with impaired renal function, cardiac impairment, liver dysfunction, those taking diuretics and the elderly. Renal function should be monitored in these patients (see also Section 4.3).

Use in patients with impaired renal function

As naproxen is eliminated to a large extent (95%) by urinary excretion via glomerular filtration, it should be used with great caution in patients with impaired renal function and the monitoring of serum creatinine and/or creatinine clearance is advised in these patients. Naprosyn is contraindicated in patients having a baseline creatinine clearance of less than 30ml/minute.

Haemodialysis does not decrease the plasma concentration of naproxen because of the high degree of protein binding.

Certain patients, specifically those whose renal blood flow is compromised, such as in extracellular volume depletion, cirrhosis of the liver, sodium restriction, congestive heart failure, and pre-existing renal disease, should have renal function assessed before and during Naprosyn therapy. Some elderly patients in whom impaired renal function may be expected, as well as patients using diuretics, may also fall within this category. A reduction in daily dosage should be considered to avoid the possibility of excessive accumulation of naproxen metabolites in these patients.

Use in patients with impaired liver function

Chronic alcoholic liver disease and probably also other forms of cirrhosis reduce the total plasma concentration of naproxen, but the plasma concentration of unbound naproxen is increased. The implication of this finding for Naprosyn dosing is unknown but it is prudent to use the lowest effective dose.

Haematological

Patients who have coagulation disorders or are receiving drug therapy that interferes with haemostasis should be carefully observed if naproxen-containing products are administered.

Patients at high risk of bleeding or those on full anti-coagulation therapy (e.g. dicoumarol derivatives) may be at increased risk of bleeding if given naproxen-containing products concurrently.

Anaphylactic (anaphylactoid) reactions

Hypersensitivity reactions may occur in susceptible individuals. Anaphylactic (anaphylactoid) reactions may occur both in patients with and without a history of hypersensitivity or exposure to aspirin, other non-steroidal anti-inflammatory drugs or naproxen-containing products. They may also occur in individuals with a history of angio-oedema, bronchospastic reactivity (e.g. asthma), rhinitis and nasal polyps.

Anaphylactoid reactions, like anaphylaxis, may have a fatal outcome.

Steroids

If steroid dosage is reduced or eliminated during therapy, the steroid dosage should be reduced slowly and the patients must be observed closely for any evidence of adverse effects, including adrenal insufficiency and exacerbation of symptoms of arthritis.

Ocular effects

Studies have not shown changes in the eye attributable to naproxen administration. In rare cases, adverse ocular disorders including papillitis, retrobulbar optic neuritis and papilloedema, have been reported in users of NSAIDs including naproxen, although a cause-and-effect relationship cannot be established; accordingly, patients who develop visual disturbances during treatment with naproxen-containing products should have an ophthalmological examination.

Cardiovascular and cerebrovascular effects

Appropriate monitoring and advice are required for patients with a history of hypertension and/or mild to moderate congestive heart failure as fluid retention and oedema have been reported in association with NSAID therapy.

Clinical trial and epidemiological data suggest that use of coxibs and some NSAIDs (particularly at high doses and in long term treatment) may be associated with a small increased risk of arterial thrombotic events (for example myocardial infarction or stroke). Although data suggest that the use of naproxen (1000mg daily) may be associated with a lower risk, some risk cannot be excluded.

Patients with uncontrolled hypertension, congestive heart failure, established ischaemic heart disease, peripheral arterial disease, and/or cerebrovascular disease should only be treated with naproxen after careful consideration. Similar consideration should be made before initiating longer-term treatment of patients with risk factors for cardiovascular events (e.g. hypertension, hyperlipidaemia, diabetes mellitus, smoking).

SLE and mixed connective tissue disease

In patients with systemic lupus erythematosus (SLE) and mixed connective tissue disorders there may be an increased risk of aseptic meningitis (see Section 4.8).

Dermatological

Serious skin reactions, some of them fatal, including exfoliative dermatitis, Stevens-Johnson syndrome, and toxic epidermal necrolysis, have been reported very rarely in association with the use of NSAIDs (see 4.8). Patients appear to be at highest risk for these reactions early in the course of therapy: the onset of the reactions occurring in the majority of cases within the first month of treatment. Naprosyn should be discontinued at the first appearance of skin rash, mucosal lesions, or any other sign of hypersensitivity.

Precautions related to fertility

The use of naproxen, as with any drug known to inhibit cyclooxygenase/prostaglandin synthesis, may impair fertility and is not recommended in women attempting to conceive. In women who have difficulty conceiving or are undergoing investigation of infertility, withdrawal of naproxen should be considered.

Combination with other NSAIDs

The combination of naproxen-containing products and other NSAIDs, including cyclooxygenase-2 selective inhibitors, is not recommended, because of the cumulative risks of inducing serious NSAID-related adverse events.

4.5 Interaction with other medicinal products and other forms of interaction

Concomitant administration of antacid or colestyramine can delay the absorption of naproxen but does not affect its extent. Concomitant administration of food can delay the absorption of naproxen, but does not affect its extent.

It is considered unsafe to take NSAIDs in combination with anti-coagulants such as warfarin or heparin unless under direct medical supervision, as NSAIDs may enhance the effects of anti-coagulants (see Section 4.4).

Other analgesics including cyclooxygenase-2 selective inhibitors: Avoid concomitant use of two or more NSAIDs (including aspirin) as this may increase the risk of adverse effects (see Section 4.4).

Due to the high plasma protein binding of naproxen, patients simultaneously receiving hydantoins, anticoagulants, other NSAIDs, aspirin or a highly protein-bound sulphonamide should be observed for signs of overdosage of these drugs. Patients simultaneously receiving Naprosyn and a hydantoin, sulphonamide or sulphonylurea should be observed for adjustment of dose if required. No interactions have been observed in clinical studies with naproxen and anticoagulants or sulphonylureas, but caution is nevertheless advised since interaction has been seen with other non-steroidal agents of this class.

Caution is advised when Naprosyn is co-administered with diuretics as there can be a decreased diuretic effect. The natriuretic effect of furosemide has been reported to be inhibited by some drugs of this class. Diuretics can increase the risk of nephrotoxicity of NSAIDs.

Inhibition of renal lithium clearance leading to increases in plasma lithium concentrations has also been reported.

Naproxen and other non-steroidal anti-inflammatory drugs can reduce the anti-hypertensive effect of anti-hypertensives and may increase the risk of renal impairment associated with the use of ACE inhibitors.

Probenecid given concurrently increases naproxen plasma levels and extends its half-life considerably.

Caution is advised where methotrexate is given concurrently because of possible enhancement of its toxicity, since naproxen, among other non-steroidal anti-inflammatory drugs, has been reported to reduce the tubular secretion of methotrexate in an animal model.

NSAIDs may exacerbate cardiac failure, reduce GFR and increase plasma cardiac glycoside levels when co-administered with cardiac glycosides.

As with all NSAIDs caution is advised when ciclosporin is co-administered because of the increased risk of nephrotoxicity.

NSAIDs should not be used for 8 - 12 days after mifepristone administration as NSAIDs can reduce the effects of mifepristone.

As with all NSAIDs, caution should be taken when co-administering with cortico-steroids because of the increased risk of gastrointestinal ulceration or bleeding.

Animal data indicate that NSAIDs can increase the risk of convulsions associated with quinolone antibiotics. Patients taking quinolones may have an increased risk of developing convulsions.

There is an increased risk of gastrointestinal bleeding (see Section 4.4) when anti-platelet agents and selective serotonin reuptake inhibitors (SSRIs) are combined with NSAIDs.

There is a possible risk of nephrotoxicity when NSAIDs are given with tacrolimus.

There is an increased risk of haematological toxicity when NSAIDs are given with zidovudine. There is evidence of an increased risk of haemarthroses and haematoma in HIV(+) haemophiliacs receiving concurrent treatment with zidovudine and ibuprofen.

It is suggested that Naprosyn therapy be temporarily discontinued 48 hours before adrenal function tests are performed, because naproxen may artifactually interfere with some tests for 17-ketogenic steroids. Similarly, naproxen may interfere with some assays of urinary 5-hydroxyindoleacetic acid.

4.6 Pregnancy and lactation

Pregnancy

Congenital abnormalities have been reported in association with NSAID administration in man; however, these are low in frequency and do not appear to follow any discernible pattern. As with other drugs of this type, naproxen produces delay in parturition in animals and also affects the human foetal cardiovascular system (closure of ductus arteriosus). Use of Naprosyn in the last trimester of pregnancy is contraindicated (see Section 4.3). NSAIDs should not be used during the first two trimesters of pregnancy, unless the potential benefit to the patient outweighs the potential risk to the foetus.

Labour and delivery

Naproxen containing products are not recommended in labour and delivery because, through its prostaglandin synthesis inhibitory effect, naproxen may adversely affect foetal circulation and inhibit contractions, with an increased bleeding tendency in both mother and child.

Nursing mothers

Naproxen has been found in the milk of lactating women. The use of Naprosyn should be avoided in patients who are breast-feeding.

See Section 4.4 regarding female fertility.

4.7 Effects on ability to drive and use machines

Some patients may experience drowsiness, dizziness, vertigo, insomnia, fatigue, visual disturbances or depression with the use of Naprosyn. If patients experience these or similar undesirable effects, they should not drive or operate machinery.

4.8 Undesirable effects

The following adverse events have been reported with NSAIDs and with naproxen.

Gastrointestinal disorders: The most commonly observed adverse events are gastrointestinal in nature. Heartburn, nausea, vomiting, constipation, diarrhoea, flatulence, dyspepsia, abdominal discomfort and epigastric distress. More serious reactions which may occur are gastro-intestinal bleeding, which is sometimes fatal, particularly in the elderly (see section 4.4), peptic ulceration, perforation, non-peptic gastro-intestinal ulceration, melaena, haematemesis, stomatitis, ulcerative stomatitis, exacerbation of ulcerative colitis and Crohn's disease (see section 4.4), oesophagitis, gastritis and pancreatitis.

Blood and lymphatic system disorders: Neutropenia, thrombocytopenia, granulocytopenia including agranulocytosis, eosinophilia, leucopenia, aplastic anaemia and haemolytic anaemia.

Immune system disorders: Hypersensitivity reactions have been reported following treatment with NSAIDs in patients with, or without, a history of previous hypersensitivity reactions to NSAIDs. These may consist of (a) non-specific allergic reactions and anaphylaxis (b) respiratory tract reactivity comprising asthma, aggravated asthma, bronchospasm or dyspnoea, or (c) assorted skin disorders, including rashes of various types, pruritus, urticaria, purpura, angio-oedema and more rarely exfoliative and bullous dermatoses (including epidermal necrolysis and erythema multiforme).

Metabolic and nutrition disorders: hyperkalaemia.

Psychiatric disorders: Insomnia, dream abnormalities, depression, confusion and hallucinations.

Nervous system disorders: Convulsions, dizziness, headache, lightheadedness, drowsiness, paraesthesia, retrobulbar optic neuritis, inability to concentrate and cognitive dysfunction have been reported. Aseptic meningitis (especially in patients with existing auto-immune disorders, such as systemic lupus erythematosus, mixed connective tissue disease), with symptoms such as stiff neck, headache, nausea, vomiting, fever or disorientation (see section 4.4).

Eye Disorders: Visual disturbances, corneal opacity, papillitis and papilloedema.

Ear and Labyrinth disorders: Tinnitus, hearing disturbances including impairment and vertigo.

Cardiac disorders: Oedema, palpitations, cardiac failure and congestive heart failure have been reported.

Clinical trial and epidemiological data suggest that use of coxibs and some NSAIDs (particularly at high doses and in long term treatment) may be associated with a small increased risk of arterial thrombotic events (for example myocardial infarction or stroke) (see section 4.4).

Vascular disorders: Hypertension, vasculitis.

Respiratory, thoracic and mediastinal disorders: Dyspnoea, asthma, eosinophilic pneumonitis and pulmonary oedema.

Hepatobiliary disorders: Jaundice, fatal hepatitis and abnormal liver function tests.

Skin and subcutaneous tissue disorders: Skin rashes including fixed drug eruption, itching (pruritus), urticaria, ecchymoses, purpura, sweating. Alopecia, erythema multiforme, Stevens Johnson syndrome, erythema nodosum, lichen planus, pustular reaction, SLE, epidermal necrolysis, very rarely toxic epidermal necrolysis, photosensitivity reactions (including cases in which skin resembles porphyria cutanea tarda "pseudoporphyria") or epidermolysis bullosa-like reactions which may occur rarely.

If skin fragility, blistering or other symptoms suggestive of pseudoporphyria occur, treatment should be discontinued and the patient monitored.

Musculoskeletal and connective tissue disorders: Myalgia and muscle weakness.

Renal and urinary disorders: Including, but not limited to, glomerular nephritis, interstitial nephritis, nephrotic syndrome, haematuria, raised serum creatinine, renal papillary necrosis and renal failure.

Reproductive system and breast disorders: Female infertility.

General disorders and administration site conditions: Thirst, pyrexia, fatigue and malaise.

4.9 Overdose

Symptoms include headache, heartburn, nausea, vomiting, epigastric pain, gastrointestinal bleeding, rarely diarrhoea, disorientation, excitation, drowsiness, dizziness, tinnitus, fainting. In cases of significant poisoning acute renal failure and liver damage are possible.

Respiratory depression and coma may occur after the ingestion of NSAIDs but are rare.

In one case of naproxen overdose, transient prolongation of the prothrombin time due to hypothrombinaemia may have been due to selective inhibition of the synthesis of vitamin-K dependent clotting factors.

A few patients have experienced seizures, but it is not known whether these were naproxen-related or not. It is not known what dose of the drug would be life-threatening.

Patients should be treated symptomatically as required. Within one hour of ingestion of a potentially toxic amount activated charcoal should be considered. Alternatively in adults gastric lavage should be considered within one hour of ingestion of a potentially life-threatening overdose.

Good urine output should be ensured.

Renal and liver function should be closely monitored.

Patients should be observed for at least four hours after ingestion of potentially toxic amounts.

Frequent or prolonged convulsions should be treated with intravenous diazepam.

Other measures may be indicated by the patient's clinical condition.

Haemodialysis does not decrease the plasma concentration of naproxen because of the high degree of protein binding. However, haemodialysis may still be appropriate in a patient with renal failure who has taken naproxen.

5. PHARMACOLOGICAL PROPERTIES

5.1 Pharmacodynamic properties

Naproxen is a non-steroidal anti-inflammatory analgesic compound with antipyretic properties as has been demonstrated in classical animal test systems. Naproxen exhibits its anti-inflammatory effect even in adrenalectomised animals, indicating that its action is not mediated through the pituitary-adrenal axis.

Naproxen inhibits prostaglandin synthetase (as do other NSAIDs). As with other NSAIDs, however, the exact mechanism of its anti-inflammatory action is not known.

5.2 Pharmacokinetic properties

Naproxen is completely absorbed from the gastro-intestinal tract, and peak plasma levels are reached in 2 to 4 hours. Naproxen is present in the blood mainly as unchanged drug, extensively bound to plasma proteins. The plasma half-life is between 12 and 15 hours, enabling a steady state to be achieved within 3 days of initiation of therapy on a twice daily dose regimen. The degree of absorption is not significantly affected by either foods or most antacids. Excretion is almost entirely via the urine, mainly as conjugated naproxen, with some unchanged drug. Metabolism in children is similar to that in adults. Chronic alcoholic liver disease reduces the total plasma concentration of naproxen but the concentration of unbound naproxen increases. In the elderly, the unbound plasma concentration of naproxen is increased although total plasma concentration is unchanged.

5.3 Preclinical safety data

Carcinogenicity

Naproxen was administered with food to Sprague-Dawley rats for 24 months at doses of 8, 16 and 24mg/kg/day. Naproxen was not carcinogenic in rats.

Mutagenicity

Mutagenicity was not seet in *Salmonella typhimurium* (5 cell lines), *Sachharomyces cerevisisae* (1 cell line), and mouse lymphoma tests.

Fertility

Naproxen did not affect the fertility of rats when administered orally at doses of 30mg/kg/day to males and 20mg/kg/day to females.

Teratogenicity

Naproxen was not teratogenic when administered orally at does of 20mg/kg/day during organogenesis to rats and rabbits.

Perinatal/Postnatal Reproduction

Oral administration of naproxen to pregnant rats at doses of 2, 10 and 20mg/kg/day during the third trimester of pregnancy resulted in difficult labour. These are know effects of this class of compounds and were demonstrated in pregnant rats with aspirin and indometacin.

6. PHARMACEUTICAL PARTICULARS

6.1 List of excipients

Povidone

Croscarmellose sodium

Magnesium stearate

Iron oxide E 172

6.2 Incompatibilities

None stated.

6.3 Shelf life

60 months.

6.4 Special precautions for storage

Store below 30°C.

Bottles: Store in the original package.

Blisters: Keep blister in the outer carton.

6.5 Nature and contents of container

Naprosyn 250 and 500 are supplied in polypropylene securitainers with LDPE closures or polypropylene bottles with foil induction seals and polypropylene screw closures or amber glass bottles with metal closures fitted with an expanded polythene wad, containing 50, 60, 120, 250 and 500 tablets.

Clear or opaque PVC blister packaging with aluminium lidding in cartons, containing 2, 4, 56, 60 and 112 Naprosyn 250, or 2, 4, 56, 60 Naprosyn 500 tablets.

6.6 Special precautions for disposal and other handling

None given.

Administrative Data

7. MARKETING AUTHORISATION HOLDER

Roche Products Limited

6 Falcon Way

Shire Park

Welwyn Garden City

AL7 1TW

United Kingdom

8. MARKETING AUTHORISATION NUMBER(S)

Naprosyn 250mg Tablets: PL 0031/0471

Naprosyn 500mg Tablets: PL 0031/0484

9. DATE OF FIRST AUTHORISATION/RENEWAL OF THE AUTHORISATION

Naprosyn 250mg Tablets: 09 February 2009

Naprosyn 500mg Tablets: 09 February 2009

10. DATE OF REVISION OF THE TEXT

February 2009

Legal Status: POM

Naprosyn is a registered trade mark

Item Code

Naprosyn EC 250mg and 500mg Tablets

(Roche Products Limited)

1. NAME OF THE MEDICINAL PRODUCT

Naprosyn EC 250mg Tablets

Naprosyn EC 375mg Tablets

Naprosyn EC 500mg Tablets

2. QUALITATIVE AND QUANTITATIVE COMPOSITION

Naprosyn EC 250mg Tablets:

Each tablet contains 250mg naproxen.

Naprosyn EC 375mg Tablets:

Each tablet contains 375mg naproxen.

Naprosyn EC 500mg Tablets:

Each tablet contains 500mg naproxen.

For excipients, see 6.1.

3. PHARMACEUTICAL FORM

Gastro-resistant film-coated tablets.

Naprosyn EC 250mg Tablets:

Round white tablet marked 'NPR EC 250' in black ink on one side.

Naprosyn EC 375mg Tablets:

White, oval convex tablet marked 'NPR EC 375' in black ink on one side.

Naprosyn EC 500mg Tablets:

Capsule shaped, white tablet marked 'NPR EC 500' in black ink on one side.

4. CLINICAL PARTICULARS

4.1 Therapeutic indications

Naprosyn EC is indicated for the treatment of rheumatoid arthritis, osteoarthrosis (degenerative arthritis), ankylosing spondylitis, acute musculoskeletal disorders (such as sprains and strains, direct trauma, lumbosacral pain, cervical spondylitis, tenosynovitis and fibrositis) and dysmenorrhoea.

4.2 Posology and method of administration

For oral administration.

To be taken preferably with or after food.

Undesirable effects may be minimised by using the lowest effective dose for the shortest duration necessary to control symptoms (see section 4.4).

Adults

Naprosyn EC tablets should be swallowed whole and not broken or crushed.

Therapy should be started at the lowest recommended dose, especially in the elderly.

Rheumatoid arthritis, osteoarthritis and ankylosing spondylitis

The usual dose is 500mg to 1g daily taken in 2 doses at 12-hour intervals. Where 1g per day is needed either one 500mg tablet twice daily or two 500mg tablets in a single administration (morning or evening) is recommended. In the following cases a loading dose of 750mg or 1g per day for the acute phase is recommended:

a) In patients reporting severe night-time pain/or morning stiffness.

b) In patients being switched to Naprosyn from a high dose of another anti-rheumatic compound.

c) In osteoarthrosis where pain is the predominant symptom.

Acute musculoskeletal disorders and dysmenorrhoea

500mg initially followed by 250mg at 6 - 8 hour intervals as needed, with a maximum daily dose after the first day of 1250mg.

Elderly

Studies indicate that although total plasma concentration of naproxen is unchanged, the unbound plasma fraction of naproxen is increased in the elderly. The implication of this finding for Naprosyn EC dosing is unknown. As with other drugs used in the elderly it is prudent to use the lowest effective dose and for the shortest possible duration as elderly patients are more prone to adverse events. The patient should be monitored regularly for GI bleeding during NSAID therapy. For the effect of reduced elimination in the elderly see section 4.4.

Children

Naprosyn EC is not recommended for use in children under 16 years of age.

Renal/hepatic impairment

A lower dose should be considered in patients with renal or hepatic impairment. Naprosyn is contraindicated in patients with baseline creatinine clearance less than 30 ml/minute because accumulation of naproxen metabolites has been seen in patients with severe renal failure or those on dialysis (see section 4.3).

Treatment should be reviewed at regular intervals and discontinued if no benefit is seen.

4.3 Contraindications

Active or history of peptic ulceration or active gastrointestinal bleeding (two or more distinct episodes of proven ulceration or bleeding). History of gastrointestinal bleeding or perforation, related to previous NSAIDs therapy.

Hypersensitivity to naproxen, naproxen sodium, or any of the excipients. Since the potential exists for cross-sensitivity reactions, Naprosyn EC should not be given to patients in whom aspirin or other non-steroidal anti-inflammatory/analgesic drugs induce asthma, rhinitis, nasal polyps or urticaria. These reactions have the potential of being fatal. Severe anaphylactic-like reactions to naproxen have been reported in such patients.

Severe renal, hepatic or heart failure

Naproxen EC is contraindicated during the last trimester of pregnancy (see Section 4.6).

4.4 Special warnings and precautions for use

Undesirable effects may be minimised by using the lowest effective dose for the shortest duration necessary to control symptoms (see section 4.2 and GI and cardiovascular risks below. Patients treated with NSAIDs long-term should undergo regular medical supervision to monitor for adverse events.

Elderly and/or debilitated patients are particularly susceptible to the adverse events of NSAIDs, especially gastrointestinal bleeding and perforation, which may be fatal. Prolonged use of NSAIDs in these patients is not recommended. Where prolonged therapy is required, patients should be reviewed regularly.

The antipyretic and anti-inflammatory activities of Naprosyn EC may reduce fever and inflammation, thereby diminishing their utility as diagnostic signs.

Bronchospasm may be precipitated in patients suffering from, or with a history of, bronchial asthma or allergic disease.

As with other non-steroidal anti-inflammatory drugs, elevations of one or more liver function tests may occur. Hepatic abnormalities may be the result of hypersensitivity rather than direct toxicity. Severe hepatic reactions, including jaundice and hepatitis (some cases of hepatitis have been fatal) have been reported with this drug as with other non-steroidal anti-inflammatory drugs. Cross reactivity has been reported.

Naproxen decreases platelet aggregation and prolongs bleeding time. This effect should be kept in mind when bleeding times are determined.

Although sodium retention has not been reported in metabolic studies, it is possible that patients with questionable or compromised cardiac function may be at a greater risk when taking Naprosyn EC.

Gastrointestinal bleeding, ulceration and perforation

GI bleeding, ulceration or perforation, which can be fatal, has been reported with all NSAIDs at anytime during treatment, with or without warning symptoms or a previous history of serious GI events.

The risk of GI bleeding, ulceration or perforation is higher with increasing NSAID doses, in patients with a history of ulcer, particularly if complicated with haemorrhage or perforation (see section 4.3), and in the elderly. These patients should commence treatment on the lowest dose available. Combination therapy with protective agents (e.g. misoprostol or proton pump inhibitors) should be considered for these patients, and also for patients requiring concomitant low dose aspirin, or other drugs likely to increase gastrointestinal risk (see section 4.5).

Patients with a history of GI toxicity, particularly when elderly, should report any unusual abdominal symptoms (especially GI bleeding) particularly in the initial stages of treatment.

Caution should be advised in patients receiving concomitant medications which could increase the risk of ulceration or bleeding, such as oral corticosteroid, anticoagulants such as warfarin, selective serotonin-reuptake inhibitors or anti-platelet agents such as aspirin (see Section 4.5).

When GI bleeding or ulceration occurs in patients receiving Naprosyn, the treatment should be withdrawn.

NSAIDs should be given with care to patients with a history of gastrointestinal disease (ulcerative colitis, Crohn's disease) as these conditions may be exacerbated (see Section 4.8).

Renal Effects

There have been reports of impaired renal function, renal failure, acute interstitial nephritis, haematuria, proteinuria, renal papillary necrosis and occasionally nephrotic syndrome associated with naproxen.

Renal failure linked to reduced prostaglandin production

The administration of an NSAID may cause a dose dependent reduction in prostaglandin formation and precipitate renal failure. Patients at greatest risk of this reaction are those with impaired renal function, cardiac impairment, liver dysfunction, those taking diuretics and the elderly. Renal function should be monitored in these patients (see also Section 4.3).

Use in patients with impaired renal function

As naproxen is eliminated to a large extent (95%) by urinary excretion via glomerular filtration, it should be used with great caution in patients with impaired renal function and the monitoring of serum creatinine and/or creatinine clearance is advised in these patients. Naprosyn EC is contraindicated in patients having a baseline creatinine clearance of less than 30ml/minute.

Haemodialysis does not decrease the plasma concentration of naproxen because of the high degree of protein binding.

Certain patients, specifically those whose renal blood flow is compromised, because of extracellular volume depletion, cirrhosis of the liver, sodium restriction, congestive heart failure, and pre-existing renal disease, should have renal function assessed before and during Naprosyn EC therapy. Some elderly patients in whom impaired renal function may be expected, as well as patients using diuretics, may also fall within this category. A reduction in daily dosage should be considered to avoid the possibility of excessive accumulation of naproxen metabolites in these patients.

Use in patients with impaired liver function

Chronic alcoholic liver disease and probably also other forms of cirrhosis reduce the total plasma concentration of naproxen, but the plasma concentration of unbound naproxen is increased. The implication of this finding for Naprosyn EC dosing is unknown but it is prudent to use the lowest effective dose.

Haematological

Patients who have coagulation disorders or are receiving drug therapy that interferes with haemostasis should be carefully observed if naproxen-containing products are administered.

Patients at high risk of bleeding or those on full anti-coagulation therapy (e.g. dicoumarol derivatives) may be at increased risk of bleeding if given naproxen-containing products concurrently.

Anaphylactic (anaphylactoid) reactions

Hypersensitivity reactions may occur in susceptible individuals. Anaphylactic (anaphylactoid) reactions may occur both in patients with and without a history of hypersensitivity or exposure to aspirin, other non-steroidal anti-inflammatory drugs or naproxen-containing products. They may also occur in individuals with a history of angio-oedema, bronchospastic reactivity (e.g. asthma), rhinitis and nasal polyps.

Anaphylactoid reactions, like anaphylaxis, may have a fatal outcome.

Steroids

If steroid dosage is reduced or eliminated during therapy, the steroid dosage should be reduced slowly and the patients must be observed closely for any evidence of adverse effects, including adrenal insufficiency and exacerbation of symptoms of arthritis.

Ocular effects

Studies have not shown changes in the eye attributable to naproxen administration. In rare cases, adverse ocular disorders including papillitis, retrobulbar optic neuritis and papilloedema, have been reported in users of NSAIDs including naproxen, although a cause-and-effect relationship cannot be established; accordingly, patients who develop visual disturbances during treatment with naproxen-containing products should have an ophthalmological examination.

Cardiovascular and cerebrovascular effects

Appropriate monitoring and advice are required for patients with a history of hypertension and/or mild to moderate congestive heart failure as fluid retention and oedema have been reported in association with NSAID therapy.

Clinical trial and epidemiological data suggest that use of coxibs and some NSAIDs (particularly at high doses and in long term treatment) may be associated with a small increased risk of arterial thrombotic events (for example myocardial infarction or stroke). Although data suggest that the use of naproxen (1000mg daily) may be associated with a lower risk, some risk cannot be excluded.

Patients with uncontrolled hypertension, congestive heart failure, established ischaemic heart disease, peripheral arterial disease, and/or cerebrovascular disease should only be treated with naproxen after careful consideration. Similar consideration should be made before initiating longer-term treatment of patients with risk factors for cardiovascular events (e.g. hypertension, hyperlipidaemia, diabetes mellitus, smoking).

SLE and mixed connective tissue disease

In patients with systemic lupus erythematosus (SLE) and mixed connective tissue disorders there may be an increased risk of aseptic meningitis (see Section 4.8).

Dermatological

Serious skin reactions, some of them fatal, including exfoliative dermatitis, Stevens-Johnson syndrome, and toxic epidermal necrolysis, have been reported very rarely in association with the use of NSAIDs (see 4.8). Patients appear to be at highest risk for these reactions early in the course of therapy: the onset of the reactions occurring in the majority of cases within the first month of treatment. Naprosyn should be discontinued at the first appearance of skin rash, mucosal lesions, or any other sign of hypersensitivity.

Precautions related to fertility

The use of naproxen, as with any drug known to inhibit cyclooxygenase/prostaglandin synthesis, may impair fertility and is not recommended in women attempting to conceive. In women who have difficulty conceiving or are undergoing investigation of infertility, withdrawal of naproxen should be considered.

Combination with other NSAIDs

The combination of naproxen-containing products and other NSAIDs, including cyclooxygenase-2 selective inhibitors is not recommended, because of the cumulative risks of inducing serious NSAID-related adverse events.

4.5 Interaction with other medicinal products and other forms of interaction

Concomitant administration of antacid or colestyramine can delay the absorption of naproxen but does not affect its extent. Concomitant administration of food can delay the absorption of naproxen, but does not affect its extent.

Due to the high plasma protein binding of naproxen, patients simultaneously receiving hydantoins, anticoagulants, other NSAIDs, aspirin or a highly protein-bound sulphonamide should be observed for signs of overdosage of these drugs. Patients simultaneously receiving Naprosyn EC and a hydantoin, sulphonamide or sulphonylurea should be observed for adjustment of dose if required.

It is considered unsafe to take NSAIDs in combination with anti-coagulants such as warfarin or heparin unless under direct medical supervision, as NSAIDs may enhance the effects of anti-coagulants (see section 4.4).

Other analgesics including cyclooxygenase-2 selective inhibitors: Avoid concomitant use of two or more NSAIDs (including aspirin) as this may increase the risk of adverse effects (see Section 4.4).

No interactions have been observed in clinical studies with naproxen and anticoagulants or sulphonylureas, but caution is nevertheless advised since interaction has been seen with other non-steroidal agents of this class.

Caution is advised when Naprosyn EC is co-administered with diuretics as there can be a decreased diuretic effect. The natriuretic effect of furosemide has been reported to be inhibited by some drugs of this class. Diuretics can increase the risk of nephrotoxicity of NSAIDs.

Inhibition of renal lithium clearance leading to increases in plasma lithium concentrations has also been reported.

Naproxen and other non-steroidal anti-inflammatory drugs can reduce the anti-hypertensive effect of anti-hypertensives and may increase the risk of renal impairment associated with the use of ACE-inhibitors.

Probenecid given concurrently increases naproxen plasma levels and extends its half-life considerably.

Caution is advised where methotrexate is administered concurrently because of possible enhancement of its toxicity, since naproxen, in common with other non-steroidal anti-inflammatory drugs, has been reported to reduce the tubular secretion of methotrexate in an animal model.

NSAIDs may exacerbate cardiac failure, reduce GFR and increase plasma cardiac glycoside levels when co-administered with cardiac glycosides.

As with all NSAIDs caution is advised when ciclosporin is co-administered because of the increased risk of nephrotoxicity.

NSAIDs should not be used for 8 - 12 days after mifepristone administration as NSAIDs can reduce the effects of mifepristone.

As with all NSAIDs, caution should be taken when co-administering with corticosteroids because of the increased risk of gastrointestinal ulceration or bleeding.

Animal data indicate that NSAIDs can increase the risk of convulsions associated with quinolone antibiotics. Patients taking quinolones may have an increased risk of developing convulsions.

There is an increased risk of gastrointestinal bleeding (see Section 4.4) when anti-platelet agents and selective serotonin reuptake inhibitors (SSRIs) are combined with NSAIDs.

There is a possible risk of nephrotoxicity when NSAIDs are given with tacrolimus.

There is an increased risk of haematological toxicity when NSAIDs are given with zidovudine. There is evidence of an increased risk of haemarthroses and haematoma in HIV(+) haemophiliacs receiving concurrent treatment with zidovudine and ibuprofen.

It is suggested that Naprosyn EC therapy be temporarily discontinued 48 hours before adrenal function tests are performed, because naproxen may artifactually interfere with some tests for 17-ketogenic steroids. Similarly, naproxen may interfere with some assays of urinary 5-hydroxyindoleacetic acid.

4.6 Pregnancy and lactation

Pregnancy

Congenital abnormalities have been reported in association with NSAID administration in man; however, these are low in frequency and do not appear to follow any discernible pattern. As with other drugs of this type, naproxen produces delay in parturition in animals and also affects the human foetal cardiovascular system (closure of ductus arteriosus). Use of Naprosyn EC in the last trimester of pregnancy is contraindicated (see Section 4.3). NSAIDs should not be used during the first two trimesters of pregnancy, unless the potential benefit to the patient outweighs the potential risk to the foetus.

Labour and delivery

Naproxen containing products are not recommended in labour and delivery because, through its prostaglandin synthesis inhibitory effect, naproxen may adversely affect foetal circulation and inhibit contractions with an increased bleeding tendency in both mother and child.

Nursing mothers

Naproxen has been found in the milk of lactating women. The use of Naprosyn EC should therefore be avoided in patients who are breast-feeding.

See Section 4.4 regarding female fertility.

4.7 Effects on ability to drive and use machines

Some patients may experience drowsiness, dizziness, vertigo, insomnia, fatigue, visual disturbances or depression with the use of Naprosyn. If patients experience these or similar undesirable effects, they should not drive or operate machinery.

4.8 Undesirable effects

The following adverse events have been reported with NSAIDs and with naproxen.

Gastrointestinal disorders: The most commonly observed adverse events are gastrointestinal in nature. Heartburn, nausea, vomiting, constipation, diarrhoea, flatulence, dyspepsia, abdominal discomfort and epigastric distress. More serious reactions which may occur are gastro-intestinal bleeding, which is sometimes fatal, particularly in the elderly (see section 4.4), peptic ulceration, perforation, non-peptic gastro-intestinal ulceration, melaena, haematemesis, stomatitis, ulcerative stomatitis, exacerbation of ulcerative colitis and Crohn's disease (see section 4.4), oesophagitis, gastritis and pancreatitis.

Blood and lymphatic system disorders: Neutropenia, thrombocytopenia, granulocytopenia including agranulocytosis, eosinophilia, leucopenia, aplastic anaemia and haemolytic anaemia.

Immune system disorders: Hypersensitivity reactions have been reported following treatment with NSAIDs in patients with, or without, a history of previous hypersensitivity reactions to NSAIDs. These may consist of (a) non-specific allergic reactions and anaphylaxis (b) respiratory tract reactivity comprising asthma, aggravated asthma, bronchospasm or dyspnoea, or (c) assorted skin disorders, including rashes of various types, pruritus, urticaria, purpura, angio-oedema and more rarely exfoliative and bullous dermatoses (including epidermal necrolysis and erythema multiforme).

Metabolic and nutrition disorders: hyperkalaemia.

Psychiatric disorders: Insomnia, dream abnormalities, depression, confusion and hallucinations.

Nervous system disorders: Convulsions, dizziness, headache, lightheadedness, drowsiness, paraesthesia, retrobulbar optic neuritis, inability to concentrate and cognitive dysfunction have been reported. Aseptic meningitis (especially in patients with existing auto-immune disorders, such as systemic lupus erythematosus, mixed connective tissue disease), with symptoms such as stiff neck, headache, nausea, vomiting, fever or disorientation (see section 4.4).

Eye Disorders: Visual disturbances, corneal opacity, papillitis and papilloedema.

Ear and Labyrinth disorders: Tinnitus, hearing disturbances including impairment and vertigo.

Cardiac disorders: Oedema, palpitations, cardiac failure and congestive heart failure have been reported.

Clinical trial and epidemiological data suggest that use of coxibs and some NSAIDs (particularly at high doses and in long term treatment) may be associated with a small increased risk of arterial thrombotic events (for example myocardial infarction or stroke) (see section 4.4).

Vascular disorders: Hypertension, vasculitis.

Respiratory, thoracic and mediastinal disorders: Dyspnoea, asthma, eosinophilic pneumonitis and pulmonary oedema.

Hepatobiliary disorders: Jaundice, fatal hepatitis and abnormal liver function tests.

Skin and subcutaneous tissue disorders: Skin rashes including fixed drug eruption, itching (pruritus), urticaria, ecchymoses, purpura, sweating. Alopecia, erythema multiforme, Stevens Johnson syndrome, erythema nodosum, lichen planus, pustular reaction, SLE, epidermal necrolysis, very rarely toxic epidermal necrolysis, photosensitivity reactions (including cases in which skin resembles porphyria cutanea tarda "pseudoporphyria") or epidermolysis bullosa-like reactions which may occur rarely.

If skin fragility, blistering or other symptoms suggestive of pseudoporphyria occur, treatment should be discontinued and the patient monitored.

Musculoskeletal and connective tissue disorders: Myalgia and muscle weakness.

Renal and urinary disorders: Including, but not limited to, glomerular nephritis, interstitial nephritis, nephrotic syndrome, haematuria, raised serum creatinine, renal papillary necrosis and renal failure.

Reproductive system and breast disorders: Female infertility.

General disorders and administration site conditions: Thirst, pyrexia, fatigue and malaise.

4.9 Overdose

Symptoms include headache, heartburn, nausea, vomiting, epigastric pain, gastrointestinal bleeding, rarely diarrhoea, disorientation, excitation, drowsiness, dizziness, tinnitus, fainting. In cases of significant poisoning acute renal failure and liver damage are possible.

Respiratory depression and coma may occur after the ingestion of NSAIDs but are rare.

In one case of naproxen overdose, transient prolongation of the prothrombin time due to hypotrhrombinaemia may have been due to selective inhibition of the synthesis of vitamin-K dependent clotting factors.

A few patients have experienced seizures, but it is not known whether these were naproxen-related or not. It is not known what dose of the drug would be life-threatening.

Patients should be treated symptomatically as required. Within one hour of ingestion of a potentially toxic amount activated charcoal should be considered. Alternatively in adults gastric lavage should be considered within one hour of ingestion of a potentially life-threatening overdose.

Good urine output should be ensured.

Renal and liver function should be closely monitored.

Patients should be observed for at least four hours after ingestion of potentially toxic amounts.

Frequent or prolonged convulsions should be treated with intravenous diazepam.

Other measures may be indicated by the patient's clinical condition.

Haemodialysis does not decrease the plasma concentration of naproxen because of the high degree of protein binding. However, haemodialysis may still be appropriate in a patient with renal failure who has taken naproxen.

5. PHARMACOLOGICAL PROPERTIES

5.1 Pharmacodynamic properties

Naproxen has been shown to have anti-inflammatory, analgesic and antipyretic properties when tested in classical animal test systems. It exhibits its anti-inflammatory effect even in adrenalectomised animals, indicating that its action is not mediated through the pituitary-adrenal axis. It inhibits prostaglandin synthetase, as do other non-steroidal anti-inflammatory agents. As with other agents, however, the exact mechanism of its anti-inflammatory action is not known.

5.2 Pharmacokinetic properties

Naproxen is completely absorbed from the gastro-intestinal tract, and peak plasma levels are reached in 2 to 4 hours. Naproxen is present in the blood mainly as unchanged drug, extensively bound to plasma proteins. The plasma half-life is between 12 and 15 hours, enabling a steady state to be achieved within 3 days of initiation of therapy on a twice daily dose regimen. The degree of absorption is not significantly affected by either foods or most antacids. Excretion is almost entirely via the urine, mainly as conjugated naproxen, with some unchanged drug. Metabolism in children is similar to that in adults. Chronic alcoholic liver disease reduces the total plasma concentration of naproxen but the concentration of unbound naproxen increases. In the elderly, the unbound plasma concentration of naproxen is increased although total plasma concentration is unchanged.

When naproxen is administered in the enteric-coated form, the peak plasma levels are delayed compared to those seen with standard tablets. However, the mean areas under the plasma concentration-time curves, and hence bioavailability, are equivalent. The tablets, therefore, perform as one would anticipate for a drug which does not disintegrate until it reaches the small intestine, where dissolution is rapid and complete.

5.3 Preclinical safety data

Carcinogenicity

Naproxen was administered with food to Sprague-Dawley rats for 24 months at doses of 8, 16 and 24mg/kg/day. Naproxen was not carcinogenic in rats.

Mutagenicity

Mutagenicity was not seen in *Salmonella typhimurium* (5 cell lines), *Sachharomyces cerevisisae* (1 cell line), and mouse lymphoma tests.

Fertility

Naproxen did not affect the fertility of rats when administered orally at doses of 30mg/kg/day to males and 20mg/kg/day to females.

Teratogenicity

Naproxen was not teratogenic when administered orally at does of 20mg/kg/day during organogenesis to rats and rabbits.

Perinatal/Postnatal Reproduction

Oral administration of naproxen to pregnant rats at doses of 2, 10 and 20mg/kg/day during the third trimester of pregnancy resulted in difficult labour. These are know effects of this class of compounds and were demonstrated in pregnant rats with aspirin and indometacin.

6. PHARMACEUTICAL PARTICULARS

6.1 List of excipients

Tablet Core

Povidone

Croscarmellose sodium

Magnesium stearate

Tablet Coating

Methacrylic acid copolymer

Purified talc

Sodium hydroxide

Triethyl citrate

Simethicone emulsion

Printing Ink

Iron oxide, black

Shellac

Propylene glycol

6.2 Incompatibilities

None known.

6.3 Shelf life

36 months.

6.4 Special precautions for storage

Store below 30°C.

Bottles: Store in the original package

Blisters: Keep blister in the outer carton

6.5 Nature and contents of container

Polypropylene, polyethylene or glass bottles containing 50, 60, 100 or 250 tablets.

Clear or opaque PVC blister with aluminium lidding in cartons containing 2, 4, 10 or 56 tablets.

6.6 Special precautions for disposal and other handling

None applicable.

Administrative Data

7. MARKETING AUTHORISATION HOLDER

Roche Products Limited

6 Falcon Way

Shire Park

Welwyn Garden City

AL7 1TW

United Kingdom

8. MARKETING AUTHORISATION NUMBER(S)

Naprosyn EC 250mg Tablets: PL 0031/0467

Naprosyn EC 375mg Tablets: PL 0031/0468

Naprosyn EC 500mg Tablets: PL 0031/0469

9. DATE OF FIRST AUTHORISATION/RENEWAL OF THE AUTHORISATION

Naprosyn EC 250mg Tablets: 09 February 2009

Naprosyn EC 375mg Tablets: 09 February 2009

Naprosyn EC 500mg Tablets: 09 February 2009

10. DATE OF REVISION OF THE TEXT

February 2009

LEGAL STATUS

POM

Naprosyn is a registered trade mark

Item Code

Naramig Tablets 2.5mg

(GlaxoSmithKline UK)

1. NAME OF THE MEDICINAL PRODUCT

Naramig Tablets 2.5mg

2. QUALITATIVE AND QUANTITATIVE COMPOSITION

Tablets containing 2.5mg of naratriptan as naratriptan hydrochloride.

3. PHARMACEUTICAL FORM

Tablets

4. CLINICAL PARTICULARS

4.1 Therapeutic indications

Naramig Tablets are indicated for the acute treatment of migraine attacks with or without aura.

4.2 Posology and method of administration

Naramig Tablets are recommended as monotherapy for the acute treatment of a migraine attack.

Naramig Tablets should not be used prophylactically.

Naramig Tablets should be swallowed whole with water.

Adults (18-65 years of age)

The recommended dose of Naramig Tablets is a single 2.5mg tablet.

The total dose should not exceed two 2.5mg tablets in any 24 hour period.

If symptoms of migraine should recur, following an initial response, a second dose may be taken provided that there is a minimum interval of four hours between the two doses.

If a patient does not respond to a first dose of Naramig Tablets a second dose should not be taken for the same attack, as it is unlikely to be of benefit. However Naramig Tablets may be used for subsequent migraine attacks.

Adolescents (12-17 years of age)

Efficacy of Naramig Tablets at single doses of 0.25, 1.0 and 2.5mg was not demonstrated to be greater than placebo in a placebo-controlled study in adolescents (12 to 17 years). Therefore, the use of Naramig Tablets in patients under 18 years of age is not recommended.

Children (under 12 years of age)

There are no data available on the use of naratriptan in children under 12 years of age therefore its use in this age group is not recommended.

Elderly (over 65 years of age)

The safety and effectiveness of naratriptan in individuals over age 65 have not been evaluated and therefore, its use in this age group can not be recommended. There is a moderate decrease in clearance with age (see Pharmacokinetics).

Renal Impairment

Naramig should be used with caution in patients with renal impairment. The maximum dose in any 24 hour treatment period is a single 2.5mg tablet. The use of Naramig is contraindicated in patients with severe renal impairment (creatinine clearance < 15mL/min)

(See Contraindications and Pharmacokinetics).

Hepatic Impairment

Naramig should be used with caution in patients with hepatic impairment. The maximum dose in any 24 hour treatment period is a single 2.5mg tablet. The use of Naramig is contraindicated in patients with severe hepatic impairment (Child-Pugh grade C)

(See Contraindications and Pharmacokinetics).

4.3 Contraindications

Hypersensitivity to any component of the preparation.

As with other 5-hydroxytryptamine1 (5-HT1) receptor agonists naratriptan should not be used in patients who have had a myocardial infarction or have ischaemic heart disease, or Prinzmetal's angina/coronary vasospasm, peripheral vascular disease or patients who have symptoms or signs consistent with ischaemic heart disease.

Naratriptan should not be administered to patients with a history of cerebrovascular accident (CVA) or transient ischaemic attack (TIA).

The use of naratriptan in patients with uncontrolled hypertension is contraindicated.

The concomitant administration of ergotamine, derivatives or ergotamine (including methysergide) or/and any triptan/5-hydroxytryptamine$_1$ (5-HT$_1$) receptor agonist with naratriptan is contraindicated (see Section 4.5).

Naratriptan is contraindicated in patients with severely impaired renal or hepatic function.

4.4 Special warnings and precautions for use

Naratriptan should only be used where there is a clear diagnosis of migraine.

Naratriptan is not indicated for use in the management of hemiplegic, basilar or ophthalmoplegic migraine.

As with other acute migraine therapies, before treating headaches in patients not previously diagnosed as migraineurs, and in migraineurs who present with atypical symptoms, care should be taken to exclude other potentially serious neurological conditions. It should be noted that migraineurs may be at risk of certain cerebrovascular events (eg. CVA or TIA).

As with other 5-HT1 receptor agonists, naratriptan should not be given to patients in whom unrecognised cardiac disease is likely without a prior evaluation for underlying cardiovascular disease. Such patients include postmenopausal women, males over 40 and patients with risk factors for coronary artery disease.

If symptoms consistent with ischaemic heart disease occur appropriate evaluation should be carried out (See Section 4.8).

Serotonin syndrome (including altered mental status, autonomic instability and neuromuscular abnormalities) has been reported following concomitant treatment with triptans and selective serotonin reuptake inhibitors (SSRIs)/serotonin noradrenaline reuptake inhibitors (SNRIs). If concomitant treatment with naratriptan and an SSRI/SNRI is clinically warranted, appropriate observation of the patient is advised (see Section 4.5).

Naratriptan contains a sulphonamide component therefore there is a theoretical risk of a hypersensitivity reaction in patients with known hypersensitivity to sulphonamides.

The recommended dose of naratriptan should not be exceeded.

Prolonged use of any type of painkiller for headaches can make them worse. If thissituation is experienced or suspected, medical advice should be obtained and treatment should be discontinued. The diagnosis of MOH should be suspected in patients who have frequent or daily headaches despite (or because of) the regular use of headache medications.

Undesirable effects may be more common during concomitant use of triptans and herbal preparations containing St John's Wort (*Hypericum perforatum*).

4.5 Interaction with other medicinal products and other forms of interaction

Serotonin syndrome (including altered mental status, autonomic instability and neuromuscular abnormalities) has been reported following concomitant treatment with triptans and SSRIs/SNRIs (see Section 4.4).

There is no evidence of a pharmacokinetic interaction with β-blockers, tricyclic antidepressants, selective serotonin reuptake inhibitors, alcohol or food.

Co-administration of naratriptan with ergotamine, dihydroergotamine, or sumatriptan did not result in clinically significant effects on blood pressure, heart rate or ECG or affect naratriptan exposure. However, an increased risk of coronary vasospasm is a theoretical possibility and concomitant administration with preparations containing ergotamine or another triptan/5-HT1 receptor agonist is contraindicated (see section 4.3).

Naratriptan does not inhibit monoamine oxidase enzymes; therefore interactions with monoamine oxidase inhibitors are not anticipated. In addition, the limited metabolism of naratriptan and the wide range of cytochrome P450 isoenzymes involved suggest that significant drug interactions with naratriptan are unlikely (see Pharmacokinetics).

4.6 Pregnancy and lactation

The safe use of naratriptan in pregnant women has not been established. Evaluation of experimental animal studies does not indicate any direct teratogenic effects or harmful effects on peri- and postnatal development.

Because animal reproduction studies are not always predictive of human response administration of naratriptan should only be considered if the expected benefit to the mother is greater than any possible risk to the foetus.

Naratriptan and/or drug related metabolites are secreted into the milk of lactating rats. Caution should be exercised when considering administration of naratriptan to nursing women.

4.7 Effects on ability to drive and use machines

Caution is recommended in patients performing skilled tasks (e.g. driving or operating machinery) as drowsiness may occur as a result of migraine. Drowsiness was no more apparent with naratriptan than with placebo in clinical trials.

4.8 Undesirable effects

At therapeutic doses of naratriptan the incidence of side effects reported in clinical trials was similar to placebo. Some of the symptoms may be part of the migraine attack.

Undesirable effects are ranked under headings of frequency using the following convention: Very common ($\geq$1/10), common ($\geq$1/100 and $<$1/10), uncommon ($\geq$1/1,000 and $<$1/100), rare ($\geq$1/10,000 and $<$1/1,000) and very rare ($<$1/10,000).

Immune system disorders

Rare: Hypersensitivity reactions ranging from cutaneous hypersensitivity to rare cases of anaphylaxis.

Nervous system disorders

Common: Tingling. This is usually of short duration, may be severe and may affect any part of the body including the chest or throat. Dizziness and drowsiness.

Eye disorders

Uncommon: Visual disturbance.

Cardiac disorders

Uncommon: Bradycardia, tachycardia, palpitations.

Very Rare: Coronary artery vasospasm, transient ischaemic ECG changes, angina and myocardial infarction have been reported very rarely (see Contraindications and Warnings and Precautions).

Vascular disorders

Very rare: Peripheral vascular ischaemia.

Gastrointestinal

Common: Nausea and vomiting.

Rare: Ischaemic colitis.

General disorders and administration site conditions:

The following symptoms are usually of short duration, may be severe and may affect any part of the body including the chest or throat:

Common: Pain, sensations of heat. Malaise/fatigue.

Uncommon: Sensations of heaviness, pressure or tightness.

4.9 Overdose

There is limited experience of accidental overdosage with naratriptan. However, there is no evidence to suggest that overdose is associated with adverse events other than those described above (see section 4.8 Undesirable Effects).

It is unknown what effect haemodialysis or peritoneal dialysis has on the plasma concentrations of naratriptan.

Treatment

If overdosage with naratriptan occurs, the patient should be monitored for at least 24 hours and standard supportive treatment applied as required.

5. PHARMACOLOGICAL PROPERTIES

5.1 Pharmacodynamic properties

Naratriptan has been shown to be a selective agonist for 5 hydroxytryptamine1 (5-HT$_1$) receptors mediating vascular contraction. This receptor is found predominantly in intracranial (cerebral and dural) blood vessels. Naratriptan has high affinity for human cloned 5-HT$_{1B}$ and 5-HT$_{1D}$ receptors, the human 5-HT$_{1B}$ receptor is thought to correspond to the vascular 5-HT$_1$ receptor mediating contraction of intracranial blood vessels. Naratriptan has little or no effect at other 5-HT receptor (5-HT$_2$, 5-HT$_3$, 5-HT$_4$ and 5-HT$_7$) subtypes.

In animals, naratriptan selectively constricts the carotid arterial circulation. This circulation supplies blood to the extracranial and intracranial tissues such as the meninges, and dilatation and/or oedema formation in these vessels is thought to be the underlying mechanism of migraine in man. In addition, experimental evidence suggests that naratriptan inhibits trigeminal nerve activity. Both these actions may contribute to the anti-migraine action of naratriptan in humans.

In man, a meta-analysis of BP recordings in 15 studies showed that the population average maximum increases in systolic and diastolic blood pressure after a 2.5mg dose of naratriptan tablets would be less than 5mmHg and 3mmHg respectively. The blood pressure response was unaffected by age, weight, hepatic or renal impairment.

5.2 Pharmacokinetic properties

Absorption, distribution, metabolism and elimination

Following oral administration, naratriptan is rapidly absorbed with maximum plasma concentrations observed at 2-3 hours. After administration of a 2.5mg naratriptan tablet Cmax is approximately 8.3ng/mL (95% CI: 6.5 to 10.5ng/mL) in women and 5.4ng/mL (95% CI: 4.7 to 6.1ng/mL) in men.

The oral bioavailability is 74% in women and 63% in men with no differences in efficacy and tolerability in clinical use. Therefore a gender related dose adjustment is not required.

Naratriptan is distributed in a volume of 170L. Plasma protein binding is low (29%).

The mean elimination half-life ($t_{1/2}$) is 6 hours.

Mean clearance after intravenous administration was 470mL/min in men and 380mL/min in women. Renal clearance is similar in men and women at 220mL/min and is higher than the glomerular filtration rate suggesting that naratriptan is actively secreted in the renal tubules. Naratriptan is predominantly excreted in the urine with 50% of the dose recovered as unchanged naratriptan and 30% recovered as inactive metabolites. In vitro naratriptan was metabolised by a wide range of cytochrome P450 isoenzymes. Consequently significant metabolic drug interactions with naratriptan are not anticipated (see Interactions).

Special Patient Populations

Elderly

In healthy elderly subjects (n=12), clearance was decreased by 26% when compared to healthy young subjects (n=12) in the same study (See Posology and method of administration).

Gender

The naratriptan AUC and Cmax were approximately 35% lower in males compared to females however, with no differences in efficacy and tolerability in clinical use.

Therefore a gender related dose adjustment is not required (see Posology and method of administration).

Renal Impairment

Renal excretion is the major route for the elimination of naratriptan. Accordingly exposure to naratriptan may be increased in patients with renal disease.

In a study in male and female renally impaired patients (creatinine clearance 18 to 115mL/min; n=15) matched for sex, age and weight with healthy subjects (n=8), renally impaired patients had an approximately 80% increase in $t_{1/2}$ and an approximately 50% reduction in clearance (See Posology and method of administration).

Hepatic Impairment

The liver plays a lesser role in the clearance of orally administered naratriptan. In a study in male and female hepatically impaired patients (Child-Pugh grade A or B n=8) matched for sex, age and weight with healthy subjects who received oral naratriptan, hepatically impaired patients had an approximately 40% increase in $t_{1/2}$ and an approximately 30% reduction in clearance (See Posology and method of administration).

5.3 Preclinical safety data

No clinically relevant findings were observed in preclinical studies.

6. PHARMACEUTICAL PARTICULARS

6.1 List of excipients

Tablet core

Microcrystalline cellulose

Anhydrous lactose

Croscarmellose sodium

Magnesium stearate

Film coat

Methylhydroxypropylcellulose

Titanium dioxide (E171)

Triacetin

Iron oxide yellow (E172)

Indigo carmine aluminium lake (E132)

6.2 Incompatibilities

None reported

6.3 Shelf life

36 months

6.4 Special precautions for storage

Store below 30°C.

6.5 Nature and contents of container

2, 4, 6 or 12 tablets in a double foil blister pack

Not all pack sizes may be marketed

6.6 Special precautions for disposal and other handling

None

Administrative Data

7. MARKETING AUTHORISATION HOLDER

Glaxo Wellcome UK Ltd, trading as GlaxoSmithKline UK
Stockley Park West,
Uxbridge,
Middlesex. UB11 1BT

8. MARKETING AUTHORISATION NUMBER(S)

PL 10949/0273

9. DATE OF FIRST AUTHORISATION/RENEWAL OF THE AUTHORISATION

28 April 2002

10. DATE OF REVISION OF THE TEXT

29 October 2008

11. Legal Status

POM

Naropin 10 mg/ml solution for injection

(AstraZeneca UK Limited)

1. NAME OF THE MEDICINAL PRODUCT

Naropin®10 mg/ml solution for injection

2. QUALITATIVE AND QUANTITATIVE COMPOSITION

Naropin® 10 mg/ml:

1 ml solution for injection contains ropivacaine hydrochloride monohydrate equivalent to 10 mg ropivacaine hydrochloride.

1 ampoule of 10 ml or 20 ml solution for injection contains ropivacaine hydrochloride monohydrate equivalent to 100 mg and 200 mg ropivacaine hydrochloride respectively.

For excipients, see section 6.1.

3. PHARMACEUTICAL FORM

Solution for injection for perineural and epidural administration (10–20 ml).

Clear, colourless solution.

4. CLINICAL PARTICULARS

4.1 Therapeutic indications

Naropin is indicated for:

1. Surgical anaesthesia

- Epidural blocks for surgery, including Caesarean section.
- Major nerve blocks.
- Field blocks.

2. Acute pain management

- Continuous epidural infusion or intermittent bolus administration during postoperative or labour pain.
- Field blocks.

4.2 Posology and method of administration

Naropin should only be used by, or under the supervision of, clinicians experienced in regional anaesthesia.

Posology

Adults and children above 12 years of age:

The following table is a guide to dosage for the more commonly used blocks. The smallest dose required to produce an effective block should be used. The clinician's experience and knowledge of the patient's physical status are of importance when deciding the dose.

(see Table 1 on next page)

In general, surgical anaesthesia (e.g. epidural administration) requires the use of the higher concentrations and doses. The Naropin 10 mg/ml formulation is recommended for epidural anaesthesia in which a complete motor block is essential for surgery. For analgesia (e.g. epidural administration for acute pain management) the lower concentrations and doses are recommended.

Method of administration

Careful aspiration before and during injection is recommended to prevent intravascular injection. When a large dose is to be injected, a test dose of 3–5 ml lidocaine (lignocaine) with adrenaline (epinephrine) (Xylocaine® 2% with Adrenaline (epinephrine) 1:200,000) is recommended. An inadvertent intravascular injection may be recognised by a temporary increase in heart rate and an accidental intrathecal injection by signs of a spinal block.

Aspiration should be performed prior to and during administration of the main dose, which should be injected slowly or in incremental doses, at a rate of 25–50 mg/min, while closely observing the patient's vital functions and maintaining verbal contact. If toxic symptoms occur, the injection should be stopped immediately.

In epidural block for surgery, single doses of up to 250 mg ropivacaine have been used and well tolerated.

In brachial plexus block a single dose of 300 mg has been used in a limited number of patients and was well tolerated.

When prolonged blocks are used, either through continuous infusion or through repeated bolus administration, the risks of reaching a toxic plasma concentration or inducing local neural injury must be considered. Cumulative doses up to 675 mg ropivacaine for surgery and postoperative analgesia administered over 24 hours were well tolerated in adults, as were postoperative continuous epidural

Table 1

	Conc.	Volume	Dose	Onset	Duration
	mg/ml	ml	mg	minutes	hours
Surgical anaesthesia					
Lumbar Epidural Administration					
Surgery	7.5	15–25	113–188	10–20	3–5
	10	15–20	150–200	10–20	4–6
Caesarean section	7.5	15–20	113–150[1]	10–20	3–5
Thoracic Epidural Administration					
To establish block for postoperative pain relief	7.5	5–15 (depending on the level of injection)	38–113	10–20	n/a[2]
Major Nerve Block*					
Brachial plexus block	7.5	30–40	225–300[3]	10–25	6–10
Field Block	7.5	1–30	7.5–225	1–15	2–6
(e.g. minor nerve blocks and infiltration)					
Acute pain management					
Lumbar Epidural Administration					
Bolus	2	10–20	20–40	10–15	0.5–1.5
Intermittent injections (top up) (e.g. labour pain management)	2	10–15 (minimum interval 30 minutes)	20–30		
Continuous infusion e.g. labour pain	2	6–10 ml/h	12–20 mg/h	n/a[2]	n/a[2]
Postoperative pain management	2	6–14 ml/h	12–28 mg/h	n/a[2]	n/a[2]
Thoracic Epidural Administration					
Continuous infusion (postoperative pain management)	2	6–14 ml/h	12–28 mg/h	n/a[2]	n/a[2]
Field Block					
(e.g. minor nerve blocks and infiltration)	2	1–100	2–200	1–5	2–6
Peripheral nerve block (Femoral or interscalene block)					
Continuous infusion or intermittent injections (e.g. postoperative pain management)	2	5–10 ml/h	10–20 mg/h	n/a	n/a

The doses in the table are those considered to be necessary to produce a successful block and should be regarded as guidelines for use in adults. Individual variations in onset and duration occur. The figures in the column 'Dose' reflect the expected average dose range needed. Standard textbooks should be consulted for both factors affecting specific block techniques and individual patient requirements.

* With regard to major nerve block, only for brachial plexus block a dose recommendation can be given. For other major nerve blocks lower doses may be required. However, there is presently no experience of specific dose recommendations for other blocks.

(1) Incremental dosing should be applied, the starting dose of about 100 mg (97.5 mg = 13 ml; 105 mg = 14 ml) to be given over 3–5 minutes. Two extra doses, in total an additional 50mg, may be administered as needed.

(2) n/a = not applicable

(3) The dose for a major nerve block must be adjusted according to site of administration and patient status. Interscalene and supraclavicular brachial plexus blocks may be associated with a higher frequency of serious adverse reactions, regardless of the local anaesthetic used, (see section 4.4. Special warnings and special precautions for use).

infusions at rates up to 28 mg/hour for 72 hours. In a limited number of patients, higher doses of up to 800 mg/day have been administered with relatively few adverse reactions.

For treatment of postoperative pain, the following technique can be recommended: Unless preoperatively instituted, an epidural block with Naropin 7.5 mg/ml is induced via an epidural catheter. Analgesia is maintained with Naropin 2 mg/ml infusion. Infusion rates of 6–14 ml (12–28 mg) per hour provide adequate analgesia with only slight and non-progressive motor block in most cases of moderate to severe postoperative pain. The maximum duration of epidural block is 3 days. However, close monitoring of analgesic effect should be performed in order to remove the catheter as soon as the pain condition allows it. With this technique a significant reduction in the need for opioids has been observed.

In clinical studies an epidural infusion of Naropin 2 mg/ml alone or mixed with fentanyl 1-4 μg/ml has been given for postoperative pain management for up to 72 hours. The combination of Naropin and fentanyl provided improved pain relief but caused opioid side effects. The combination of Naropin and fentanyl has been investigated only for Naropin 2 mg/ml.

When prolonged peripheral nerve blocks are applied, either through continuous infusion or through repeated injections, the risks of reaching a toxic plasma concentration or inducing local neural injury must be considered. In clinical studies, femoral nerve block was established with 300 mg Naropin 7.5 mg/ml and interscalene block with 225 mg Naropin 7.5 mg/ml, respectively, before surgery. Analgesia was then maintained with Naropin 2 mg/ml. Infusion rates or intermittent injections of 10–20 mg per hour for 48 hours provided adequate analgesia and were well tolerated.

Concentrations above 7.5 mg/ml Naropin have not been documented for Caesarean section.

4.3 Contraindications

Hypersensitivity to ropivacaine or to other local anaesthetics of the amide type.

General contraindications related to epidural anaesthesia, regardless of the local anaesthetic used, should be taken into account.

Intravenous regional anaesthesia.

Obstetric paracervical anaesthesia.

Hypovolaemia.

4.4 Special warnings and precautions for use

Regional anaesthetic procedures should always be performed in a properly equipped and staffed area. Equipment and drugs necessary for monitoring and emergency resuscitation should be immediately available. Patients receiving major blocks should be in an optimal condition and have an intravenous line inserted before the blocking procedure. The clinician responsible should take the necessary precautions to avoid intravascular injection (see section 4.2 Posology and method of administration) and be appropriately trained and familiar with diagnosis and treatment of side effects, systemic toxicity and other complications (see section 4.8 Undesirable effects and 4.9 Overdose) such as inadvertent subarachnoid injection, which may produce a high spinal block with apnoea and hypotension. Convulsions have occurred most often after brachial plexus block and epidural block. This is likely to be the result of either accidental intravascular injection or rapid absorption from the injection site.

Caution is required to prevent injections in inflamed areas.

Cardiovascular

Patients treated with anti-arrhythmic drugs class III (eg, amiodarone) should be under close surveillance and ECG monitoring considered, since cardiac effects may be additive.

There have been rare reports of cardiac arrest during the use of Naropin for epidural anaesthesia or peripheral nerve blockade, especially after unintentional accidental intravascular administration in elderly patients and in patients with concomitant heart disease. In some instances, resuscitation has been difficult. Should cardiac arrest occur, prolonged resuscitative efforts may be required to improve the possibility of a successful outcome.

Head and neck blocks

Certain local anaesthetic procedures, such as injections in the head and neck regions, may be associated with a higher frequency of serious adverse reactions, regardless of the local anaesthetic used.

Major peripheral nerve blocks

Major peripheral nerve blocks may imply the administration of a large volume of local anaesthetic in highly vascularized areas, often close to large vessels where there is an increased risk of intravascular injection and/or rapid systemic absorption, which can lead to high plasma concentrations.

Hypersensitivity

A possible cross–hypersensitivity with other amide–type local anaesthetics should be taken into account.

Hypovolaemia

Patients with hypovolaemia due to any cause can develop sudden and severe hypotension during epidural anaesthesia, regardless of the local anaesthetic used.

Patients in poor general health

Patients in poor general condition due to ageing or other compromising factors such as partial or complete heart conduction block, advanced liver disease or severe renal dysfunction require special attention, although regional anaesthesia is frequently indicated in these patients.

Patients with hepatic and renal impairment

Ropivacaine is metabolised in the liver and should therefore be used with caution in patients with severe liver disease; repeated doses may need to be reduced due to delayed elimination. Normally there is no need to modify the dose in patients with impaired renal function when used for single dose or short-term treatment. Acidosis and reduced plasma protein concentration, frequently seen in patients with chronic renal failure, may increase the risk of systemic toxicity.

Acute porphyria

Naropin® solution for injection and infusion is possibly porphyrinogenic and should only be prescribed to patients with acute porphyria when no safer alternative is available. Appropriate precautions should be taken in the case of vulnerable patients, according to standard textbooks and/or in consultation with disease area experts.

Excipients with recognised action/effect

This medicinal product contains maximum 3.7 mg sodium per ml. To be taken into consideration by patients on a controlled sodium diet.

Prolonged administration

Prolonged administration of ropivacaine should be avoided in patients concomitantly treated with strong CYP1A2 inhibitors, such as fluvoxamine and enoxacin, see section 4.5.

4.5 Interaction with other medicinal products and other forms of interaction

Naropin should be used with caution in patients receiving other local anaesthetics or agents structurally related to amide-type local anaesthetics, e.g. certain antiarrhythmics, such as lidocaine and mexiletine, since the systemic toxic effects are additive. Simultaneous use of Naropin with general anaesthetics or opioids may potentiate each others (adverse) effects. Specific interaction studies with ropivacaine and anti-arrhythmic drugs class III (e.g. amiodarone) have not been performed, but caution is advised (see also section 4.4 Special warnings and precautions for use).

Cytochrome P450 (CYP) 1A2 is involved in the formation of 3-hydroxy-ropivacaine, the major metabolite. *In vivo*, the plasma clearance of ropivacaine was reduced by up to 77% during co-administration of fluvoxamine, a selective and potent CYP1A2 inhibitor. Thus strong inhibitors of CYP1A2, such as fluvoxamine and enoxacin given concomitantly during prolonged administration of Naropin, can interact with Naropin. Prolonged administration of ropivacaine should be avoided in patients concomitantly treated with strong CYP1A2 inhibitors, see also section 4.4.

In vivo, the plasma clearance of ropivacaine was reduced by 15% during co-administration of ketoconazole, a selective and potent inhibitor of CYP3A4. However, the inhibition of this isozyme is not likely to have clinical relevance.

In vitro, ropivacaine is a competitive inhibitor of CYP2D6 but does not seem to inhibit this isozyme at clinically attained plasma concentrations.

4.6 Pregnancy and lactation

Pregnancy

Apart from epidural administration for obstetrical use, there are no adequate data on the use of ropivacaine in human pregnancy. Experimental animal studies do not indicate direct or indirect harmful effects with respect to pregnancy, embryonal/fœtal development, parturition or postnatal development (see section 5.3 Preclinical safety data).

Lactation

There are no data available concerning the excretion of ropivacaine into human milk.

4.7 Effects on ability to drive and use machines

No data are available. Depending on the dose, local anaesthetics may have a minor influence on mental function and co-ordination even in the absence of overt CNS toxicity and may temporarily impair locomotion and alertness.

4.8 Undesirable effects

General

The adverse reaction profile for Naropin is similar to those for other long acting local anaesthetics of the amide type. Adverse drug reactions should be distinguished from the physiological effects of the nerve block itself e.g. a decrease in blood pressure and bradycardia during spinal/epidural block.

Table of adverse drug reactions

Within each system organ class, the ADRs have been ranked under the headings of frequency, most frequent reactions first.

Very common (>1/10)	*Vascular Disorders*	Hypotension
	Gastrointestinal Disorders	Nausea
Common (>1/100)	*Nervous System Disorders*	Headache, paraesthesia, dizziness
	Cardiac Disorders	Bradycardia, tachycardia
	Vascular Disorders	Hypertension
	Gastrointestinal Disorders	Vomiting
	Renal and Urinary Disorders	Urinary retention
	General Disorder and Administration Site Conditions	Temperature elevation, rigor, back pain
Uncommon (>1/1,000)	*Psychiatric Disorders*	Anxiety
	Nervous System Disorders	Symptoms of CNS toxicity (convulsions, grand mal convulsions, seizures, light headedness, circumoral paraesthesia, numbness of the tongue, hyperacusis, tinnitus, visual disturbances, dysarthria, muscular twitching, tremor)*, Hypoaesthesia.
	Vascular Disorders	Syncope
	Respiratory, Thoracic and Mediastinal Disorders	Dyspnoea
	General Disorders and Administration Site Conditions	Hypothermia
Rare (>1/10,000)	*Cardiac Disorders*	Cardiac arrest, cardiac arrhythmias
	General Disorder and Administration Site Conditions	Allergic reactions (anaphylactic reactions, angioneurotic oedema and urticaria)

* These symptoms usually occur because of inadvertent intravascular injection, overdose or rapid absorption, see section 4.9

Class-related adverse drug reactions:

Neurological complications

Neuropathy and spinal cord dysfunction (e.g. anterior spinal artery syndrome, arachnoiditis, cauda equina), which may result in rare cases of permanent sequelae, have been associated with regional anaesthesia, regardless of the local anaesthetic used.

Total spinal block

Total spinal block may occur if an epidural dose is inadvertently administered intrathecally.

Acute systemic toxicity

Systemic toxic reactions primarily involve the central nervous system (CNS) and the cardiovascular system (CVS). Such reactions are caused by high blood concentration of a local anaesthetic, which may appear due to (accidental) intravascular injection, overdose or exceptionally rapid absorption from highly vascularized areas, see also section 4.4. CNS reactions are similar for all amide local anaesthetics, while cardiac reactions are more dependent on the drug, both quantitatively and qualitatively.

Central nervous system toxicity

Central nervous system toxicity is a graded response with symptoms and signs of escalating severity. Initially symptoms such as visual or hearing disturbances, perioral numbness, dizziness, light-headedness, tingling and paraesthesia are seen. Dysarthria, muscular rigidity and muscular twitching are more serious and may precede the onset of generalised convulsions. These signs must not be mistaken for neurotic behaviour. Unconsciousness and grand mal convulsions may follow, which may last from a few seconds to several minutes. Hypoxia and hypercarbia occur rapidly during convulsions due to the increased muscular activity, together with the interference with respiration. In severe cases even apnoea may occur. The respiratory and metabolic acidosis increases and extends the toxic effects of local anaesthetics.

Recovery follows the redistribution of the local anaesthetic drug from the central nervous system and subsequent metabolism and excretion. Recovery may be rapid unless large amounts of the drug have been injected.

Cardiovascular system toxicity

Cardiovascular toxicity indicates a more severe situation. Hypotension, bradycardia, arrhythmia and even cardiac arrest may occur as a result of high systemic concentrations of local anaesthetics. In volunteers the intravenous infusion of ropivacaine resulted in signs of depression of conductivity and contractility.

Cardiovascular toxic effects are generally preceded by signs of toxicity in the central nervous system, unless the patient is receiving a general anaesthetic or is heavily sedated with drugs such as benzodiazepines or barbiturates.

In children, early signs of local anaesthetic toxicity may be difficult to detect since they may not be able to verbally express them. See also section 4.4.

Treatment of acute systemic toxicity

See section 4.9 Overdose.

4.9 Overdose

Symptoms:

Accidental intravascular injections of local anaesthetics may cause immediate (within seconds to a few minutes) systemic toxic reactions. In the event of overdose, peak plasma concentrations may not be reached for one to two hours, depending on the site of the injection, and signs of toxicity may thus be delayed. (See section 4.8 Acute systemic toxicity, Central nervous system toxicity and Cardiovascular system toxicity).

Treatment

If signs of acute systemic toxicity appear, injection of the local anaesthetic should be stopped immediately and CNS symptoms (convulsions, CNS depression) must promptly be treated with appropriate airway/respiratory support and the administration of anticonvulsant drugs.

If circulatory arrest should occur, immediate cardiopulmonary resuscitation should be instituted. Optimal oxygenation and ventilation and circulatory support as well as treatment of acidosis are of vital importance.

If cardiovascular depression occurs (hypotension, bradycardia), appropriate treatment with intravenous fluids, vasopressor, and or inotropic agents should be considered. Children should be given doses commensurate with age and weight.

Should cardiac arrest occur, a successful outcome may require prolonged resuscitative efforts.

5. PHARMACOLOGICAL PROPERTIES

5.1 Pharmacodynamic properties

Pharmacotherapeutic group: Anaesthetics, local, Amides

ATC code: N01B B09

Ropivacaine is a long-acting, amide-type local anaesthetic with both anaesthetic and analgesic effects. At high doses Naropin produces surgical anaesthesia, while at lower doses it produces sensory block with limited and non-progressive motor block.

The mechanism is a reversible reduction of the membrane permeability of the nerve fibre to sodium ions. Consequently the depolarisation velocity is decreased and the excitable threshold increased, resulting in a local blockade of nerve impulses.

The most characteristic property of ropivacaine is the long duration of action. Onset and duration of the local anaesthetic efficacy are dependent upon the administration site and dose, but are not influenced by the presence of a vasoconstrictor (e.g. adrenaline (epinephrine)). For details concerning the onset and duration of action of Naropin, see table under posology and method of administration.

Healthy volunteers exposed to intravenous infusions tolerated ropivacaine well at low doses and with expected CNS symptoms at the maximum tolerated dose. The clinical experience with this drug indicates a good margin of safety when adequately used in recommended doses.

5.2 Pharmacokinetic properties

Ropivacaine has a chiral center and is available as the pure S-(-)-enantiomer. It is highly lipid-soluble. All metabolites have a local anaesthetic effect but of considerably lower potency and shorter duration than that of ropivacaine.

The plasma concentration of ropivacaine depends upon the dose, the route of administration and the vascularity of the injection site. Ropivacaine follows linear pharmacokinetics and the C_{max} is proportional to the dose.

Ropivacaine shows complete and biphasic absorption from the epidural space with half-lives of the two phases of the order of 14 min and 4 h in adults. The slow absorption is the rate-limiting factor in the elimination of ropivacaine, which explains why the apparent elimination half-life is longer after epidural than after intravenous administration.

Ropivacaine has a mean total plasma clearance in the order of 440 ml/min, a renal clearance of 1 ml/min, a volume of distribution at steady state of 47 litres and a terminal half-life of 1.8 h after iv administration. Ropivacaine has an intermediate hepatic extraction ratio of about 0.4. It is mainly bound to α_1- acid glycoprotein in plasma with an unbound fraction of about 6%.

An increase in total plasma concentrations during continuous epidural infusion has been observed, related to a postoperative increase of α_1- acid glycoprotein.

Variations in unbound, i.e. pharmacologically active, concentration have been much less than in total plasma concentration.

Ropivacaine readily crosses the placenta and equilibrium in regard to unbound concentration will be rapidly reached. The degree of plasma protein binding in the foetus is less than in the mother, which results in lower total plasma concentrations in the foetus than in the mother.

Ropivacaine is extensively metabolised, predominantly by aromatic hydroxylation. In total, 86% of the dose is excreted in the urine after intravenous administration, of which only about 1% relates to unchanged drug. The major metabolite is 3-hydroxy-ropivacaine, about 37% of which is excreted in the urine, mainly conjugated. Urinary excretion of 4-hydroxy-ropivacaine, the N-dealkylated metabolite and the 4-hydroxy-dealkylated accounts for 1–3%. Conjugated and unconjugated 3-hydroxy-ropivacaine shows only detectable concentrations in plasma.

There is no evidence of *in vivo* racemisation of ropivacaine.

5.3 Preclinical safety data

Based on conventional studies of safety pharmacology, single and repeated dose toxicity, reproduction toxicity, mutagenic potential and local toxicity, no hazards for humans were identified other than those which can be expected on the basis of the pharmacodynamic action of high doses of ropivacaine (e.g. CNS signs, including convulsions, and cardiotoxicity).

6. PHARMACEUTICAL PARTICULARS

6.1 List of excipients

Sodium chloride

Hydrochloric acid

Sodium hydroxide

Water for injection

6.2 Incompatibilities

In alkaline solutions precipitation may occur as ropivacaine shows poor solubility at pH > 6

6.3 Shelf life

3 years.

Shelf life after first opening:

From a microbiological point of view, the product should be used immediately. If not used immediately, in-use storage times and conditions prior to use are the responsibility of the user and would normally not be longer than 24 hours at 2–8°C.

6.4 Special precautions for storage

Do not store above 30°C. Do not freeze.

For storage after opening, see section 6.3.

6.5 Nature and contents of container

10 ml polypropylene ampoules (Polyamp) in packs of 5 and 10.

10 ml polypropylene ampoules (Polyamp) in sterile blister packs of 5 and 10.

20 ml polypropylene ampoules (Polyamp) in packs of 5 and 10.

20 ml polypropylene ampoules (Polyamp) in sterile blister packs of 5 and 10.

The polypropylene ampoules (Polyamp) are specially designed to fit Luer lock and Luer fit syringes.

6.6 Special precautions for disposal and other handling

Naropin products are preservative-free and are intended for single use only. Discard any unused solution.

The intact container must not be re-autoclaved. A blistered container should be chosen when a sterile outside is required.

7. MARKETING AUTHORISATION HOLDER

AstraZeneca UK Ltd.,

600 Capability Green,

Luton, LU1 3LU, UK.

8. MARKETING AUTHORISATION NUMBER(S)

PL 17901/0150

9. DATE OF FIRST AUTHORISATION/RENEWAL OF THE AUTHORISATION

Date of first authorisation: 3rd October 1995

Date of last renewal: 15th September 2005

10. DATE OF REVISION OF THE TEXT

15th August 2008

Naropin 2 mg/ml solution for injection

(AstraZeneca UK Limited)

1. NAME OF THE MEDICINAL PRODUCT

Naropin®2 mg/ml solution for injection

2. QUALITATIVE AND QUANTITATIVE COMPOSITION

Naropin® 2 mg/ml:

1 ml solution for injection contains ropivacaine hydrochloride monohydrate equivalent to 2 mg ropivacaine hydrochloride.

1 ampoule of 10 ml or 20 ml solution for injection contains ropivacaine hydrochloride monohydrate equivalent to 20 mg and 40 mg ropivacaine hydrochloride respectively.

For excipients, see section 6.1.

3. PHARMACEUTICAL FORM

Solution for injection for perineural and epidural administration (10–20 ml).

Clear, colourless solution.

4. CLINICAL PARTICULARS

4.1 Therapeutic indications

Naropin is indicated for:

1. Surgical anaesthesia

- Epidural blocks for surgery, including Caesarean section.
- Major nerve blocks.
- Field blocks.

2. Acute pain management

- Continuous epidural infusion or intermittent bolus administration during postoperative or labour pain.
- Field blocks.
- Continuous peripheral nerve block via a continuous infusion or intermittent bolus injections, e.g. postoperative pain management

3. Acute pain management in paediatrics

(per- and postoperative)

- Caudal epidural block in neonates, infants and children up to and including 12 years.
- Continuous epidural infusion in neonates, infants and children up to and including 12 years.

4.2 Posology and method of administration

Naropin should only be used by, or under the supervision of, clinicians experienced in regional anaesthesia.

Posology

Adults and children above 12 years of age:

The following table is a guide to dosage for the more commonly used blocks. The smallest dose required to produce an effective block should be used. The clinician's experience and knowledge of the patient's physical status are of importance when deciding the dose.

(see Table 1 opposite)

In general, surgical anaesthesia (e.g. epidural administration) requires the use of the higher concentrations and doses. The Naropin 10 mg/ml formulation is recommended for epidural anaesthesia in which a complete motor block is essential for surgery. For analgesia (e.g. epidural administration for acute pain management) the lower concentrations and doses are recommended.

Method of administration

Careful aspiration before and during injection is recommended to prevent intravascular injection. When a large dose is to be injected, a test dose of 3–5 ml lidocaine (lignocaine) with adrenaline (epinephrine) (Xylocaine® 2% with Adrenaline (epinephrine) 1:200,000) is recommended. An inadvertent intravascular injection may be recognised by a temporary increase in heart rate and an accidental intrathecal injection by signs of a spinal block.

Aspiration should be performed prior to and during administration of the main dose, which should be injected slowly or in incremental doses, at a rate of 25–50 mg/min, while closely observing the patient's vital functions and maintaining verbal contact. If toxic symptoms occur, the injection should be stopped immediately.

In epidural block for surgery, single doses of up to 250 mg ropivacaine have been used and well tolerated.

In brachial plexus block a single dose of 300 mg has been used in a limited number of patients and was well tolerated.

When prolonged blocks are used, either through continuous infusion or through repeated bolus administration, the risks of reaching a toxic plasma concentration or inducing local neural injury must be considered. Cumulative doses up to 675 mg ropivacaine for surgery and postoperative analgesia administered over 24 hours were well tolerated in adults, as were postoperative continuous epidural infusions at rates up to 28 mg/hour for 72 hours. In a limited number of patients, higher doses of up to 800 mg/day have been administered with relatively few adverse reactions.

For treatment of postoperative pain, the following technique can be recommended: Unless preoperatively instituted, an epidural block with Naropin 7.5 mg/ml is induced via an epidural catheter. Analgesia is maintained with Naropin 2 mg/ml infusion. Infusion rates of 6–14 ml (12–28 mg) per hour provide adequate analgesia with only slight and non-progressive motor block in most cases of moderate to severe postoperative pain. The maximum duration of epidural block is 3 days. However, close monitoring of analgesic effect should be performed in order to remove the catheter as soon as the pain condition allows it. With this technique a significant reduction in the need for opioids has been observed.

In clinical studies an epidural infusion of Naropin 2 mg/ml alone or mixed with fentanyl 1-4 μg/ml has been given for postoperative pain management for up to 72 hours. The combination of Naropin and fentanyl provided improved pain relief but caused opioid side effects. The combination of Naropin and fentanyl has been investigated only for Naropin 2 mg/ml.

When prolonged peripheral nerve blocks are applied, either through continuous infusion or through repeated injections, the risks of reaching a toxic plasma concentration or inducing local neural injury must be considered. In clinical studies, femoral nerve block was established with 300 mg Naropin 7.5 mg/ml and interscalene block with 225 mg Naropin 7.5 mg/ml, respectively, before surgery. Analgesia was then maintained with Naropin 2 mg/ml. Infusion rates or intermittent injections of 10–20 mg per hour for 48 hours provided adequate analgesia and were well tolerated.

Concentrations above 7.5 mg/ml Naropin have not been documented for Caesarean section.

Paediatric patients 0 up to and including 12 years of age:

(see Table 2 on next page)

Method of Administration

Careful aspiration before and during injection is recommended to prevent intravascular injection. The patient's vital functions should be observed closely during the injection. If toxic symptoms occur, the injection should be stopped immediately.

A single caudal epidural injection of ropivacaine 2 mg/ml produces adequate postoperative analgesia below T12 in the majority of patients when a dose of 2 mg/kg is used in a volume of 1 ml/kg. The volume of the caudal epidural injection may be adjusted to achieve a different distribution of sensory block, as recommended in standard textbooks. In children above 4 years of age, doses up to 3 mg/kg of a concentration of ropivacaine 3 mg/ml have been studied. However, this concentration is associated with a higher incidence of motor block.

Fractionation of the calculated local anaesthetic dose is recommended, whatever the route of administration.

The use of ropivacaine in premature children has not been documented.

4.3 Contraindications

Hypersensitivity to ropivacaine or to other local anaesthetics of the amide type.

General contraindications related to epidural anaesthesia, regardless of the local anaesthetic used, should be taken into account.

Intravenous regional anaesthesia.

Table 1

	Conc.	Volume	Dose	Onset	Duration
	mg/ml	ml	mg	minutes	hours
Surgical anaesthesia					
Lumbar Epidural Administration					
Surgery	7.5	15–25	113–188	10–20	3–5
	10	15–20	150–200	10–20	4–6
Caesarean section	7.5	15–20	113–150(1)	10–20	3–5
Thoracic Epidural Administration					
To establish block for postoperative pain relief	7.5	5–15 (depending on the level of injection)	38–113	10–20	n/a(2)
Major Nerve Block*					
Brachial plexus block	7.5	30–40	225–300(3)	10–25	6–10
Field Block	7.5	1–30	7.5–225	1–15	2–6
(e.g. minor nerve blocks and infiltration)					
Acute pain management					
Lumbar Epidural Administration					
Bolus	2	10–20	20–40	10–15	0.5–1.5
Intermittent injections (top up) (e.g. labour pain management)	2	10–15 (minimum interval 30 minutes)	20–30		
Continuous infusion e.g. labour pain	2	6–10 ml/h	12–20 mg/h	n/a(2)	n/a(2)
Postoperative pain management	2	6–14 ml/h	12–28 mg/h	n/a(2)	n/a(2)
Thoracic Epidural Administration					
Continuous infusion (postoperative pain management)	2	6–14 ml/h	12–28 mg/h	n/a(2)	n/a(2)
Field Block					
(e.g. minor nerve blocks and infiltration)	2	1–100	2–200	1–5	2–6
Peripheral nerve block (Femoral or interscalene block)					
Continuous infusion or intermittent injections (e.g. postoperative pain management)	2	5–10 ml/h	10–20 mg/h	n/a	n/a

The doses in the table are those considered to be necessary to produce a successful block and should be regarded as guidelines for use in adults. Individual variations in onset and duration occur. The figures in the column 'Dose' reflect the expected average dose range needed. Standard textbooks should be consulted for both factors affecting specific block techniques and individual patient requirements.

* With regard to major nerve block, only for brachial plexus block a dose recommendation can be given. For other major nerve blocks lower doses may be required. However, there is presently no experience of specific dose recommendations for other blocks.

(1) Incremental dosing should be applied, the starting dose of about 100 mg (97.5 mg = 13 ml; 105 mg = 14 ml) to be given over 3–5 minutes. Two extra doses, in total an additional 50mg, may be administered as needed.

(2) n/a = not applicable

(3) The dose for a major nerve block must be adjusted according to site of administration and patient status. Interscalene and supraclavicular brachial plexus blocks may be associated with a higher frequency of serious adverse reactions, regardless of the local anaesthetic used, (see section 4.4. Special warnings and special precautions for use).

Table 2 Paediatric patients 0 up to and including 12 years of age

	Conc.	Volume	Dose
	mg/ml	ml/kg	mg/kg
ACUTE PAIN MANAGEMENT			
(per and postoperative)			
Single Caudal Epidural Block			
Blocks below T12, in children with a body weight up to 25 kg	2.0	1	2
Continuous Epidural Infusion			
In children with a body weight up to 25 kg			
0 up to 6 months			
Bolus dose[a]	2.0	0.5–1	1–2
Infusion up to 72 hours	2.0	0.1 mL/kg/h	0.2 mg/kg/h
6 up to 12 months			
Bolus dose[a]	2.0	0.5–1	1–2
Infusion up to 72 hours	2.0	0.2 mL/kg/h	0.4 mg/kg/h
1 to 12 years			
Bolus dose[b]	2.0	1	2
Infusion up to 72 hours	2.0	0.2 mL/kg/h	0.4 mg/kg/h

The dose in the table should be regarded as guidelines for use in paediatrics. Individual variations occur. In children with a high body weight, a gradual reduction of the dosage is often necessary and should be based on the ideal body weight. The volume for single caudal epidural block and the volume for epidural bolus doses should not exceed 25 mL in any patient. Standard textbooks should be consulted for factors affecting specific block techniques and for individual patient requirements.

a Doses in the low end of the dose interval are recommended for thoracic epidural blocks while doses in the high end are recommended for lumbar or caudal epidural blocks.

b Recommended for lumbar epidural blocks. It is good practice to reduce the bolus dose for thoracic epidural analgesia.

Obstetric paracervical anaesthesia.

Hypovolaemia.

4.4 Special warnings and precautions for use

Regional anaesthetic procedures should always be performed in a properly equipped and staffed area. Equipment and drugs necessary for monitoring and emergency resuscitation should be immediately available. Patients receiving major blocks should be in an optimal condition and have an intravenous line inserted before the blocking procedure. The clinician responsible should take the necessary precautions to avoid intravascular injection (see section 4.2 Posology and method of administration) and be appropriately trained and familiar with diagnosis and treatment of side effects, systemic toxicity and other complications (see section 4.8 Undesirable effects and 4.9 Overdose) such as inadvertent subarachnoid injection, which may produce a high spinal block with apnoea and hypotension. Convulsions have occurred most often after brachial plexus block and epidural block. This is likely to be the result of either accidental intravascular injection or rapid absorption from the injection site.

Caution is required to prevent injections in inflamed areas.

Cardiovascular

Patients treated with anti-arrhythmic drugs class III (eg, amiodarone) should be under close surveillance and ECG monitoring considered, since cardiac effects may be additive.

There have been rare reports of cardiac arrest during the use of Naropin for epidural anaesthesia or peripheral nerve blockade, especially after unintentional accidental intravascular administration in elderly patients and in patients with concomitant heart disease. In some instances, resuscitation has been difficult. Should cardiac arrest occur, prolonged resuscitative efforts may be required to improve the possibility of a successful outcome.

Head and neck blocks

Certain local anaesthetic procedures, such as injections in the head and neck regions, may be associated with a higher frequency of serious adverse reactions, regardless of the local anaesthetic used.

Major peripheral nerve blocks

Major peripheral nerve blocks may imply the administration of a large volume of local anaesthetic in highly vascularized areas, often close to large vessels where there is an increased risk of intravascular injection and/or rapid systemic absorption, which can lead to high plasma concentrations.

Hypersensitivity

A possible cross–hypersensitivity with other amide–type local anaesthetics should be taken into account.

Hypovolaemia

Patients with hypovolaemia due to any cause can develop sudden and severe hypotension during epidural anaesthesia, regardless of the local anaesthetic used.

Patients in poor general health

Patients in poor general condition due to ageing or other compromising factors such as partial or complete heart conduction block, advanced liver disease or severe renal dysfunction require special attention, although regional anaesthesia is frequently indicated in these patients.

Patients with hepatic and renal impairment

Ropivacaine is metabolised in the liver and should therefore be used with caution in patients with severe liver disease; repeated doses may need to be reduced due to delayed elimination. Normally there is no need to modify the dose in patients with impaired renal function when used for single dose or short-term treatment. Acidosis and reduced plasma protein concentration, frequently seen in patients with chronic renal failure, may increase the risk of systemic toxicity.

Acute porphyria

Naropin® solution for injection and infusion is possibly porphyrinogenic and should only be prescribed to patients with acute porphyria when no safer alternative is available. Appropriate precautions should be taken in the case of vulnerable patients, according to standard textbooks and/ or in consultation with disease area experts.

Excipients with recognised action/effect

This medicinal product contains maximum 3.7 mg sodium per ml. To be taken into consideration by patients on a controlled sodium diet.

Prolonged administration

Prolonged administration of ropivacaine should be avoided in patients concomitantly treated with strong CYP1A2 inhibitors, such as fluvoxamine and enoxacin, see section 4.5.

Paediatric patients

Neonates may need special attention due to immaturity of metabolic pathways. The larger variations in plasma concentrations of ropivacaine observed in clinical trials in neonates suggest that there may be an increased risk of systemic toxicity in this age group, especially during continuous epidural infusion. The recommended doses in neonates are based on limited clinical data. When ropivacaine is used in this patient group, regular monitoring of systemic toxicity (e.g. by signs of CNS toxicity, ECG, SpO_2) and local neurotoxicity (e.g. prolonged recovery) is required, which should be continued after ending infusion, due to a slow elimination in neonates.

4.5 Interaction with other medicinal products and other forms of interaction

Naropin should be used with caution in patients receiving other local anaesthetics or agents structurally related to amide-type local anaesthetics, e.g. certain antiarrhythmics, such as lidocaine and mexiletine, since the systemic toxic effects are additive. Simultaneous use of Naropin with general anaesthetics or opioids may potentiate each others (adverse) effects. Specific interaction studies with ropivacaine and anti-arrhythmic drugs class III (e.g. amiodarone) have not been performed, but caution is advised (see also section 4.4 Special warnings and precautions for use).

Cytochrome P450 (CYP) 1A2 is involved in the formation of 3-hydroxy-ropivacaine, the major metabolite. *In vivo*, the plasma clearance of ropivacaine was reduced by up to 77% during co-administration of fluvoxamine, a selective and potent CYP1A2 inhibitor. Thus strong inhibitors of CYP1A2, such as fluvoxamine and enoxacin given concomitantly during prolonged administration of Naropin, can interact with Naropin. Prolonged administration of ropivacaine should be avoided in patients concomitantly treated with strong CYP1A2 inhibitors, see also section 4.4.

In vivo, the plasma clearance of ropivacaine was reduced by 15% during co-administration of ketoconazole, a selective and potent inhibitor of CYP3A4. However, the inhibition of this isozyme is not likely to have clinical relevance.

In vitro, ropivacaine is a competitive inhibitor of CYP2D6 but does not seem to inhibit this isozyme at clinically attained plasma concentrations.

4.6 Pregnancy and lactation

Pregnancy

Apart from epidural administration for obstetrical use, there are no adequate data on the use of ropivacaine in human pregnancy. Experimental animal studies do not indicate direct or indirect harmful effects with respect to pregnancy, embryonal/foetal development, parturition or postnatal development (see section 5.3 Preclinical safety data).

Lactation

There are no data available concerning the excretion of ropivacaine into human milk.

4.7 Effects on ability to drive and use machines

No data are available. Depending on the dose, local anaesthetics may have a minor influence on mental function and co-ordination even in the absence of overt CNS toxicity and may temporarily impair locomotion and alertness.

4.8 Undesirable effects

General

The adverse reaction profile for Naropin is similar to those for other long acting local anaesthetics of the amide type. Adverse drug reactions should be distinguished from the physiological effects of the nerve block itself e.g. a decrease in blood pressure and bradycardia during spinal/epidural block.

Table of adverse drug reactions

Within each system organ class, the ADRs have been ranked under the headings of frequency, most frequent reactions first.

Very common (>1/10)	*Vascular Disorders*	Hypotension[a]
	Gastrointestinal Disorders	Nausea
Common (>1/100)	*Nervous System Disorders*	Headache, paraesthesia, dizziness
	Cardiac Disorders	Bradycardia, tachycardia
	Vascular Disorders	Hypertension
	Gastrointestinal Disorders	Vomiting[b]
	Renal and Urinary Disorders	Urinary retention
	General Disorder and Administration Site Conditions	Temperature elevation, rigor, back pain
Uncommon (>1/1,000)	*Psychiatric Disorders*	Anxiety
	Nervous System Disorders	Symptoms of CNS toxicity (convulsions, grand mal convulsions, seizures, light headedness, circumoral paraesthesia, numbness of the tongue, hyperacusis, tinnitus, visual disturbances, dysarthria, muscular twitching, tremor)*, Hypoaesthesia.
	Vascular Disorders	Syncope
	Respiratory, Thoracic and Mediastinal Disorders	Dyspnoea
	General Disorders and Administration Site Conditions	Hypothermia
Rare (>1/10,000)	*Cardiac Disorders*	Cardiac arrest, cardiac arrhythmias
	General Disorder and Administration Site Conditions	Allergic reactions (anaphylactic reactions, angioneurotic oedema and urticaria)

[a] Hypotension is less frequent in children (>1/100).

[b] Vomiting is more frequent in children (>1/10).

* These symptoms usually occur because of inadvertent intravascular injection, overdose or rapid absorption, see section 4.9

Class-related adverse drug reactions:

Neurological complications

Neuropathy and spinal cord dysfunction (e.g. anterior spinal artery syndrome, arachnoiditis, cauda equina), which may result in rare cases of permanent sequelae, have been associated with regional anaesthesia, regardless of the local anaesthetic used.

Total spinal block

Total spinal block may occur if an epidural dose is inadvertently administered intrathecally.

Acute systemic toxicity

Systemic toxic reactions primarily involve the central nervous system (CNS) and the cardiovascular system (CVS). Such reactions are caused by high blood concentration of a local anaesthetic, which may appear due to (accidental) intravascular injection, overdose or exceptionally rapid absorption from highly vascularized areas, see also section

4.4. CNS reactions are similar for all amide local anaesthetics, while cardiac reactions are more dependent on the drug, both quantitatively and qualitatively.

Central nervous system toxicity

Central nervous system toxicity is a graded response with symptoms and signs of escalating severity. Initially symptoms such as visual or hearing disturbances, perioral numbness, dizziness, light-headedness, tingling and paraesthesia are seen. Dysarthria, muscular rigidity and muscular twitching are more serious and may precede the onset of generalised convulsions. These signs must not be mistaken for neurotic behaviour. Unconsciousness and grand mal convulsions may follow, which may last from a few seconds to several minutes. Hypoxia and hypercarbia occur rapidly during convulsions due to the increased muscular activity, together with the interference with respiration. In severe cases even apnoea may occur. The respiratory and metabolic acidosis increases and extends the toxic effects of local anaesthetics.

Recovery follows the redistribution of the local anaesthetic drug from the central nervous system and subsequent metabolism and excretion. Recovery may be rapid unless large amounts of the drug have been injected.

Cardiovascular system toxicity

Cardiovascular toxicity indicates a more severe situation. Hypotension, bradycardia, arrhythmia and even cardiac arrest may occur as a result of high systemic concentrations of local anaesthetics. In volunteers the intravenous infusion of ropivacaine resulted in signs of depression of conductivity and contractility.

Cardiovascular toxic effects are generally preceded by signs of toxicity in the central nervous system, unless the patient is receiving a general anaesthetic or is heavily sedated with drugs such as benzodiazepines or barbiturates.

In children, early signs of local anaesthetic toxicity may be difficult to detect since they may not be able to verbally express them. See also section 4.4.

Treatment of acute systemic toxicity

See section 4.9 Overdose.

4.9 Overdose

Symptoms:

Accidental intravascular injections of local anaesthetics may cause immediate (within seconds to a few minutes) systemic toxic reactions. In the event of overdose, peak plasma concentrations may not be reached for one to two hours, depending on the site of the injection, and signs of toxicity may thus be delayed. (See section 4.8 Acute systemic toxicity, Central nervous system toxicity and Cardiovascular system toxicity).

Treatment

If signs of acute systemic toxicity appear, injection of the local anaesthetic should be stopped immediately and CNS symptoms (convulsions, CNS depression) must promptly be treated with appropriate airway/respiratory support and the administration of anticonvulsant drugs.

If circulatory arrest should occur, immediate cardiopulmonary resuscitation should be instituted. Optimal oxygenation and ventilation and circulatory support as well as treatment of acidosis are of vital importance.

If cardiovascular depression occurs (hypotension, bradycardia), appropriate treatment with intravenous fluids, vasopressor, and or inotropic agents should be considered. Children should be given doses commensurate with age and weight.

Should cardiac arrest occur, a successful outcome may require prolonged resuscitative efforts.

5. PHARMACOLOGICAL PROPERTIES

5.1 Pharmacodynamic properties

Pharmacotherapeutic group: Anaesthetics, local, Amides

ATC code: N01B B09

Ropivacaine is a long-acting, amide-type local anaesthetic with both anaesthetic and analgesic effects. At high doses it produces surgical anaesthesia, while at lower doses it produces sensory block with limited and non-progressive motor block.

The mechanism is a reversible reduction of the membrane permeability of the nerve fibre to sodium ions. Consequently the depolarisation velocity is decreased and the excitable threshold increased, resulting in a local blockade of nerve impulses.

The most characteristic property of ropivacaine is the long duration of action. Onset and duration of the local anaesthetic efficacy are dependent upon the administration site and dose, but are not influenced by the presence of a vasoconstrictor (e.g. adrenaline (epinephrine)). For details concerning the onset and duration of action, see table under posology and method of administration.

Healthy volunteers exposed to intravenous infusions tolerated ropivacaine well at low doses and with expected CNS symptoms at the maximum tolerated dose. The clinical experience with this drug indicates a good margin of safety when adequately used in recommended doses.

5.2 Pharmacokinetic properties

Ropivacaine has a chiral center and is available as the pure S-(-)-enantiomer. It is highly lipid-soluble. All metabolites have a local anaesthetic effect but of considerably lower potency and shorter duration than that of ropivacaine.

The plasma concentration of ropivacaine depends upon the dose, the route of administration and the vascularity of the injection site. Ropivacaine follows linear pharmacokinetics and the C_{max} is proportional to the dose.

Ropivacaine shows complete and biphasic absorption from the epidural space with half-lives of the two phases of the order of 14 min and 4 h in adults. The slow absorption is the rate-limiting factor in the elimination of ropivacaine, which explains why the apparent elimination half-life is longer after epidural than after intravenous administration. Ropivacaine shows a biphasic absorption from the caudal epidural space also in children.

Ropivacaine has a mean total plasma clearance in the order of 440 ml/min, a renal clearance of 1 ml/min, a volume of distribution at steady state of 47 litres and a terminal half-life of 1.8 h after iv administration. Ropivacaine has an intermediate hepatic extraction ratio of about 0.4. It is mainly bound to α_1-acid glycoprotein in plasma with an unbound fraction of about 6%.

An increase in total plasma concentrations during continuous epidural and interscalene infusion has been observed, related to a postoperative increase of α_1-acid glycoprotein.

Variations in unbound, i.e. pharmacologically active, concentration have been much less than in total plasma concentration.

Since ropivacaine has an intermediate to low hepatic extraction ratio, its rate of elimination should depend on the unbound plasma concentration. A postoperative increase in AAG will decrease the unbound fraction due to increased protein binding, which will decrease the total clearance and result in an increase in total plasma concentrations, as seen in the paediatric and adult studies. The unbound clearance of ropivacaine remains unchanged as illustrated by the stable unbound concentrations during postoperative infusion. It is the unbound plasma concentration that is related to systemic pharmacodynamic effects and toxicity.

Ropivacaine readily crosses the placenta and equilibrium in regard to unbound concentration will be rapidly reached. The degree of plasma protein binding in the foetus is less than in the mother, which results in lower total plasma concentrations in the foetus than in the mother.

Ropivacaine is extensively metabolised, predominantly by aromatic hydroxylation. In total, 86% of the dose is excreted in the urine after intravenous administration, of which only about 1% relates to unchanged drug. The major metabolite is 3-hydroxy-ropivacaine, about 37% of which is excreted in the urine, mainly conjugated. Urinary excretion of 4-hydroxy-ropivacaine, the N-dealkylated metabolite (PPX) and the 4-hydroxy-dealkylated accounts for 1–3%. Conjugated and unconjugated 3-hydroxy-ropivacaine shows only detectable concentrations in plasma.

A similar pattern of metabolites has been found in children above one year.

There is no evidence of *in vivo* racemisation of ropivacaine.

Paediatrics

The pharmacokinetics of ropivacaine was characterized in a pooled population PK analysis on data in 192 children between 0 and 12 years. Unbound ropivacaine and PPX clearance and ropivacaine unbound volume of distribution depend on both body weight and age up to the maturity of liver function, after which they depend largely on body weight. The maturation of unbound ropivacaine clearance appears to be complete by the age of 3 years, that of PPX by the age of 1 year and unbound ropivacaine volume of distribution by the age of 2 years. The PPX unbound volume of distribution only depends on body weight. As PPX has a longer half-life and a lower clearance, it may accumulate during epidural infusion.

Unbound ropivacaine clearance (Cl_u) for ages above 6 months has reached values within the range of those in adults. Total ropivacaine clearance (CL) values displayed in the table below are those not affected by the postoperative increase in AAG.

Estimates of pharmacokinetic parameters derived from the pooled paediatric population PK analysis

(see Table 3 below)

The simulated mean unbound maximal plasma concentration (Cu_{max}) after a single caudal block tended to be higher in neonates and the time to Cu_{max} (t_{max}) decreased with an increase in age. Simulated mean unbound plasma concentrations at the end of a 72 h continuous epidural infusion at recommended dose rates also showed higher levels in neonates as compared to those in infants and children. See also section 4.4.

Simulated mean and observed range of unbound Cu_{max} after a single caudal block

(see Table 4 below)

At 6 months, the breakpoint for change in the recommended dose rate for continuous epidural infusion, unbound ropivacaine clearance has reached 34% and unbound PPX 71% of its mature value. The systemic exposure is higher in neonates and also somewhat higher in infants between 1 and 6 months compared to older children, which is related to the immaturity of their liver function. However, this is partly compensated for by the recommended 50% lower dose rate for continuous infusion in infants below 6 months.

Simulations on the sum of unbound plasma concentrations of ropivacaine and PPX, based on the PK parameters and their variance in the population analysis, indicate that for a single caudal block the recommended dose must be increased by a factor of 2.7 in the youngest group and a factor of 7.4 in the 1–10 year group in order for the upper prediction 90% confidence interval limit to touch the threshold for systemic toxicity. Corresponding factors for the continuous epidural infusion are 1.8 and 3.8 respectively.

5.3 Preclinical safety data

Based on conventional studies of safety pharmacology, single and repeated dose toxicity, reproduction toxicity, mutagenic potential and local toxicity, no hazards for humans were identified other than those which can be expected on the basis of the pharmacodynamic action of high doses of ropivacaine (e.g. CNS signs, including convulsions, and cardiotoxicity).

6. PHARMACEUTICAL PARTICULARS

6.1 List of excipients

Sodium chloride

Hydrochloric acid

Sodium hydroxide

Water for injection

6.2 Incompatibilities

In alkaline solutions precipitation may occur as ropivacaine shows poor solubility at pH > 6

Table 3 Estimates of pharmacokinetic parameters derived from the pooled paediatric population PK analysis

Age Group	BW[a] kg	Clu[b] (L/h/kg)	Vu[c] (L/kg)	CL[d] (L/h/kg)	$t_{1/2}$[e] (h)	$t_{1/2ppx}$[f] (h)
Newborn	3.27	2.40	21.86	0.096	6.3	43.3
1m	4.29	3.60	25.94	0.143	5.0	25.7
6m	7.85	8.03	41.71	0.320	3.6	14.5
1y	10.15	11.32	52.60	0.451	3.2	13.6
4y	16.69	15.91	65.24	0.633	2.8	15.1
10y	32.19	13.94	65.57	0.555	3.3	17.8

[a] Median bodyweight for respective age from WHO database.

[b] Unbound ropivacaine clearance

[c] Ropivacaine unbound volume of distribution

[d] Total ropivacaine clearance

[e] Ropivacaine terminal half life

[f] PPX terminal half life

Table 4 Simulated mean and observed range of unbound Cu_{max} after a single caudal block

Age group	Dose (mg/kg)	Cu_{max}[a] (mg/L)	t_{max}[b] (h)	Cu_{max}[c] (mg/L)
0-1m	2.00	0.0582	2.00	0.05-0.08 (n=5)
1-6m	2.00	0.0375	1.50	0.02-0.09 (n=18)
6-12m	2.00	0.0283	1.00	0.01-0.05 (n=9)
1-10y	2.00	0.0221	0.50	0.01-0.05 (n=60)

[a] Unbound maximal plasma concentration

[b] Time to unbound maximal plasma concentration

[c] Observed and dose-normalised unbound maximal plasma concentration

6.3 Shelf life

3 years.

Shelf life after first opening:

From a microbiological point of view, the product should be used immediately. If not used immediately, in-use storage times and conditions prior to use are the responsibility of the user and would normally not be longer than 24 hours at 2–8°C.

6.4 Special precautions for storage

Do not store above 30°C. Do not freeze.

For storage after opening, see section 6.3.

6.5 Nature and contents of container

10 ml polypropylene ampoules (Polyamp) in packs of 5 and 10.

10 ml polypropylene ampoules (Polyamp) in sterile blister packs of 5 and 10.

20 ml polypropylene ampoules (Polyamp) in packs of 5 and 10.

20 ml polypropylene ampoules (Polyamp) in sterile blister packs of 5 and 10.

The polypropylene ampoules (Polyamp) are specially designed to fit Luer lock and Luer fit syringes.

6.6 Special precautions for disposal and other handling

Naropin products are preservative-free and are intended for single use only. Discard any unused solution.

The intact container must not be re-autoclaved. A blistered container should be chosen when a sterile outside is required.

7. MARKETING AUTHORISATION HOLDER

AstraZeneca UK Ltd.,

600 Capability Green,

Luton, LU1 3LU, UK.

8. MARKETING AUTHORISATION NUMBER(S)

PL 17901/0151

9. DATE OF FIRST AUTHORISATION/RENEWAL OF THE AUTHORISATION

Date of first authorisation: 3rd October 1995

Date of last renewal: 15th September 2005

10. DATE OF REVISION OF THE TEXT

15th August 2008

Naropin 2 mg/ml solution for infusion

(AstraZeneca UK Limited)

1. NAME OF THE MEDICINAL PRODUCT

Naropin® 2 mg/ml solution for infusion

2. QUALITATIVE AND QUANTITATIVE COMPOSITION

Naropin® 2 mg/ml:

1 ml solution for infusion contains ropivacaine hydrochloride monohydrate equivalent to 2 mg ropivacaine hydrochloride.

1 bag of 100 or 200 ml solution for infusion contains ropivacaine hydrochloride monohydrate equivalent to 200 mg and 400 mg ropivacaine hydrochloride respectively.

For excipients, see section 6.1.

3. PHARMACEUTICAL FORM

Solution for infusion for perineural and epidural administration (100 and 200 ml).

Clear, colourless solution.

4. CLINICAL PARTICULARS

4.1 Therapeutic indications

Naropin is indicated for:

1. Surgical anaesthesia

- Epidural blocks for surgery, including Caesarean section.
- Major nerve blocks.
- Field blocks.

2. Acute pain management

- Continuous epidural infusion or intermittent bolus administration during postoperative or labour pain.
- Field blocks.
- Continuous peripheral nerve block via a continuous infusion or intermittent bolus injections, e.g. postoperative pain management

3. Acute pain management in paediatrics:

(per- and postoperative)

- Caudal epidural block in neonates, infants and children up to and including 12 years.
- Continuous epidural infusion in neonates, infants and children up to and including 12 years.

4.2 Posology and method of administration

Naropin should only be used by, or under the supervision of, clinicians experienced in regional anaesthesia.

Posology

Adults and children above 12 years of age:

The following table is a guide to dosage for the more commonly used blocks. The smallest dose required to produce an effective block should be used. The clinician's experience and knowledge of the patient's physical status are of importance when deciding the dose.

Table 1

	Conc.	Volume	Dose	Onset	Duration
	mg/ml	ml	mg	minutes	hours
Surgical anaesthesia					
Lumbar Epidural Administration					
Surgery	7.5	15–25	113–188	10–20	3–5
	10	15–20	150–200	10–20	4–6
Caesarean section	7.5	15–20	113–150(1)	10–20	3–5
Thoracic Epidural Administration					
To establish block for postoperative pain relief	7.5	5–15 (depending on the level of injection)	38–113	10–20	n/a(2)
Major Nerve Block*					
Brachial plexus block	7.5	30–40	225–300(3)	10–25	6–10
Field Block	7.5	1–30	7.5–225	1–15	2–6
(e.g. minor nerve blocks and infiltration)					
Acute pain management					
Lumbar Epidural Administration					
Bolus	2	10–20	20–40	10–15	0.5–1.5
Intermittent injections (top up) (e.g. labour pain management)	2	10–15 (minimum interval 30 minutes)	20–30		
Continuous infusion e.g. labour pain	2	6–10 ml/h	12–20 mg/h	n/a(2)	n/a(2)
Postoperative pain management	2	6–14 ml/h	12–28 mg/h	n/a(2)	n/a(2)
Thoracic Epidural Administration					
Continuous infusion (postoperative pain management)	2	6–14 ml/h	12–28 mg/h	n/a(2)	n/a(2)
Field Block					
(e.g. minor nerve blocks and infiltration)	2	1–100	2–200	1–5	2–6
Peripheral nerve block (Femoral or interscalene block)					
Continuous infusion or intermittent injections (e.g. postoperative pain management)	2	5–10 ml/h	10–20 mg/h	n/a	n/a

The doses in the table are those considered to be necessary to produce a successful block and should be regarded as guidelines for use in adults. Individual variations in onset and duration occur. The figures in the column 'Dose' reflect the expected average dose range needed. Standard textbooks should be consulted for both factors affecting specific block techniques and individual patient requirements.

* With regard to major nerve block, only for brachial plexus block a dose recommendation can be given. For other major nerve blocks lower doses may be required. However, there is presently no experience of specific dose recommendations for other blocks.

(1) Incremental dosing should be applied, the starting dose of about 100 mg (97.5 mg = 13 ml; 105 mg = 14 ml) to be given over 3–5 minutes. Two extra doses, in total an additional 50mg, may be administered as needed.

(2) n/a = not applicable

(3) The dose for a major nerve block must be adjusted according to site of administration and patient status. Interscalene and supraclavicular brachial plexus blocks may be associated with a higher frequency of serious adverse reactions, regardless of the local anaesthetic used, (see section 4.4. Special warnings and special precautions for use).

(see Table 1 above)

In general, surgical anaesthesia (e.g. epidural administration) requires the use of the higher concentrations and doses. The Naropin 10 mg/ml formulation is recommended for epidural anaesthesia in which a complete motor block is essential for surgery. For analgesia (e.g. epidural administration for acute pain management) the lower concentrations and doses are recommended.

Method of administration

Careful aspiration before and during injection is recommended to prevent intravascular injection. When a large dose is to be injected, a test dose of 3–5 ml lidocaine (lignocaine) with adrenaline (epinephrine) (Xylocaine® 2% with Adrenaline (epinephrine) 1:200,000) is recommended. An inadvertent intravascular injection may be recognised by a temporary increase in heart rate and an accidental intrathecal injection by signs of a spinal block.

Aspiration should be performed prior to and during administration of the main dose, which should be injected slowly or in incremental doses, at a rate of 25–50 mg/min, while closely observing the patient's vital functions and maintaining verbal contact. If toxic symptoms occur, the injection should be stopped immediately.

In epidural block for surgery, single doses of up to 250 mg ropivacaine have been used and well tolerated.

In brachial plexus block a single dose of 300 mg has been used in a limited number of patients and was well tolerated.

When prolonged blocks are used, either through continuous infusion or through repeated bolus administration, the risks of reaching a toxic plasma concentration or inducing local neural injury must be considered. Cumulative doses up to 675 mg ropivacaine for surgery and postoperative analgesia administered over 24 hours were well tolerated in adults, as were postoperative continuous epidural infusions at rates up to 28 mg/hour for 72 hours. In a limited number of patients, higher doses of up to 800 mg/day have been administered with relatively few adverse reactions.

For treatment of postoperative pain, the following technique can be recommended: Unless preoperatively instituted, an epidural block with Naropin 7.5 mg/ml is induced via an epidural catheter. Analgesia is maintained with Naropin 2 mg/ml infusion. Infusion rates of 6–14 ml (12–28 mg) per hour provide adequate analgesia with only slight and non-progressive motor block in most cases of moderate to severe postoperative pain. The maximum duration of epidural block is 3 days. However, close monitoring of analgesic effect should be performed in order to remove the catheter as soon as the pain condition allows it. With this technique a significant reduction in the need for opioids has been observed.

In clinical studies an epidural infusion of Naropin 2 mg/ml alone or mixed with fentanyl 1-4 μg/ml has been given for postoperative pain management for up to 72 hours. The combination of Naropin and fentanyl provided improved pain relief but caused opioid side effects. The combination of Naropin and fentanyl has been investigated only for Naropin 2 mg/ml.

Table 2 Paediatric patients 0 up to and including 12 years of age

	Conc.	Volume	Dose
	mg/ml	ml/kg	mg/kg
ACUTE PAIN MANAGEMENT			
(per and postoperative)			
Single Caudal Epidural Block Blocks below T12, in children with a body weight up to 25 kg	2.0	1	2
Continuous Epidural Infusion In children with a body weight up to 25 kg			
0 up to 6 months Bolus dose[a] Infusion up to 72 hours	 2.0 2.0	 0.5–1 0.1 mL/kg/h	 1–2 0.2 mg/kg/h
6 up to 12 months Bolus dose[a] Infusion up to 72 hours	 2.0 2.0	 0.5–1 0.2 mL/kg/h	 1–2 0.4 mg/kg/h
1 to 12 years Bolus dose[b] Infusion up to 72 hours	 2.0 2.0	 1 0.2 mL/kg/h	 2 0.4 mg/kg/h

The dose in the table should be regarded as guidelines for use in paediatrics. Individual variations occur. In children with a high body weight, a gradual reduction of the dosage is often necessary and should be based on the ideal body weight. The volume for single caudal epidural block and the volume for epidural bolus doses should not exceed 25 mL in any patient. Standard textbooks should be consulted for factors affecting specific block techniques and for individual patient requirements.

a Doses in the low end of the dose interval are recommended for thoracic epidural blocks while doses in the high end are recommended for lumbar or caudal epidural blocks.

b Recommended for lumbar epidural blocks. It is good practice to reduce the bolus dose for thoracic epidural analgesia.

When prolonged peripheral nerve blocks are applied, either through continuous infusion or through repeated injections, the risks of reaching a toxic plasma concentration or inducing local neural injury must be considered. In clinical studies, femoral nerve block was established with 300 mg Naropin 7.5 mg/ml and interscalene block with 225 mg Naropin 7.5 mg/ml, respectively, before surgery. Analgesia was then maintained with Naropin 2 mg/ml. Infusion rates or intermittent injections of 10–20 mg per hour for 48 hours provided adequate analgesia and were well tolerated.

Concentrations above 7.5 mg/ml Naropin have not been documented for Caesarean section.

Paediatric patients 0 up to and including 12 years of age:

(see Table 2 above)

Method of Administration

Careful aspiration before and during injection is recommended to prevent intravascular injection. The patient's vital functions should be observed closely during the injection. If toxic symptoms occur, the injection should be stopped immediately.

A single caudal epidural injection of ropivacaine 2 mg/ml produces adequate postoperative analgesia below T12 in the majority of patients when a dose of 2 mg/kg is used in a volume of 1 ml/kg. The volume of the caudal epidural injection may be adjusted to achieve a different distribution of sensory block, as recommended in standard textbooks. In children above 4 years of age, doses up to 3 mg/kg of a concentration of ropivacaine 3 mg/ml have been studied. However, this concentration is associated with a higher incidence of motor block.

Fractionation of the calculated local anaesthetic dose is recommended, whatever the route of administration.

The use of ropivacaine in premature children has not been documented.

4.3 Contraindications

Hypersensitivity to ropivacaine or to other local anaesthetics of the amide type.

General contraindications related to epidural anaesthesia, regardless of the local anaesthetic used, should be taken into account.

Intravenous regional anaesthesia.

Obstetric paracervical anaesthesia.

Hypovolaemia.

4.4 Special warnings and precautions for use

Regional anaesthetic procedures should always be performed in a properly equipped and staffed area. Equipment and drugs necessary for monitoring and emergency resuscitation should be immediately available. Patients receiving major blocks should be in an optimal condition and have an intravenous line inserted before the blocking procedure. The clinician responsible should take the necessary precautions to avoid intravascular injection (see section 4.2 Posology and method of administration) and be appropriately trained and familiar with diagnosis and treatment of side effects, systemic toxicity and other complications (see section 4.8 Undesirable effects and 4.9 Overdose) such as inadvertent subarachnoid injection, which may produce a high spinal block with apnoea and hypotension. Convulsions have occurred most often after brachial plexus block and epidural block. This is likely to be the result of either accidental intravascular injection or rapid absorption from the injection site.

Caution is required to prevent injections in inflamed areas.

Cardiovascular

Patients treated with anti-arrhythmic drugs class III (eg, amiodarone) should be under close surveillance and ECG monitoring considered, since cardiac effects may be additive.

There have been rare reports of cardiac arrest during the use of Naropin for epidural anaesthesia or peripheral nerve blockade, especially after unintentional accidental intravascular administration in elderly patients and in patients with concomitant heart disease. In some instances, resuscitation has been difficult. Should cardiac arrest occur, prolonged resuscitative efforts may be required to improve the possibility of a successful outcome.

Head and neck blocks

Certain local anaesthetic procedures, such as injections in the head and neck regions, may be associated with a higher frequency of serious adverse reactions, regardless of the local anaesthetic used.

Major peripheral nerve blocks

Major peripheral nerve blocks may imply the administration of a large volume of local anaesthetic in highly vascularized areas, often close to large vessels where there is an increased risk of intravascular injection and/or rapid systemic absorption, which can lead to high plasma concentrations.

Hypersensitivity

A possible cross–hypersensitivity with other amide–type local anaesthetics should be taken into account.

Hypovolaemia

Patients with hypovolaemia due to any cause can develop sudden and severe hypotension during epidural anaesthesia, regardless of the local anaesthetic used.

Patients in poor general health

Patients in poor general condition due to ageing or other compromising factors such as partial or complete heart conduction block, advanced liver disease or severe renal dysfunction require special attention, although regional anaesthesia is frequently indicated in these patients.

Patients with hepatic and renal impairment

Ropivacaine is metabolised in the liver and should therefore be used with caution in patients with severe liver disease; repeated doses may need to be reduced due to delayed elimination. Normally there is no need to modify the dose in patients with impaired renal function when used for single dose or short-term treatment. Acidosis and reduced plasma protein concentration, frequently seen in patients with chronic renal failure, may increase the risk of systemic toxicity.

Acute porphyria

Naropin® solution for injection and infusion is possibly porphyrinogenic and should only be prescribed to patients with acute porphyria when no safer alternative is available. Appropriate precautions should be taken in the case of vulnerable patients, according to standard textbooks and/or in consultation with disease area experts.

Excipients with recognised action/effect

This medicinal product contains maximum 3.7 mg sodium per ml. To be taken into consideration by patients on a controlled sodium diet.

Prolonged administration

Prolonged administration of ropivacaine should be avoided in patients concomitantly treated with strong CYP1A2 inhibitors, such as fluvoxamine and enoxacin, see section 4.5.

Paediatric patients

Neonates may need special attention due to immaturity of metabolic pathways. The larger variations in plasma concentrations of ropivacaine observed in clinical trials in neonates suggest that there may be an increased risk of systemic toxicity in this age group, especially during continuous epidural infusion. The recommended doses in neonates are based on limited clinical data. When ropivacaine is used in this patient group, regular monitoring of systemic toxicity (e.g. by signs of CNS toxicity, ECG, SpO_2) and local neurotoxicity (e.g. prolonged recovery) is required, which should be continued after ending infusion, due to a slow elimination in neonates.

4.5 Interaction with other medicinal products and other forms of interaction

Naropin should be used with caution in patients receiving other local anaesthetics or agents structurally related to amide-type local anaesthetics, e.g. certain antiarrhythmics, such as lidocaine and mexiletine, since the systemic toxic effects are additive. Simultaneous use of Naropin with general anaesthetics or opioids may potentiate each others (adverse) effects. Specific interaction studies with ropivacaine and anti-arrhythmic drugs class III (e.g. amiodarone) have not been performed, but caution is advised (see also section 4.4 Special warnings and precautions for use).

Cytochrome P450 (CYP) 1A2 is involved in the formation of 3-hydroxy-ropivacaine, the major metabolite. *In vivo*, the plasma clearance of ropivacaine was reduced by up to 77% during co-administration of fluvoxamine, a selective and potent CYP1A2 inhibitor. Thus strong inhibitors of CYP1A2, such as fluvoxamine and enoxacin given concomitantly during prolonged administration of Naropin, can interact with Naropin. Prolonged administration of ropivacaine should be avoided in patients concomitantly treated with strong CYP1A2 inhibitors, see also section 4.4.

In vivo, the plasma clearance of ropivacaine was reduced by 15% during co-administration of ketoconazole, a selective and potent inhibitor of CYP3A4. However, the inhibition of this isozyme is not likely to have clinical relevance.

In vitro, ropivacaine is a competitive inhibitor of CYP2D6 but does not seem to inhibit this isozyme at clinically attained plasma concentrations.

4.6 Pregnancy and lactation

Pregnancy

Apart from epidural administration for obstetrical use, there are no adequate data on the use of ropivacaine in human pregnancy. Experimental animal studies do not indicate direct or indirect harmful effects with respect to pregnancy, embryonal/fœtal development, parturition or postnatal development (see section 5.3 Preclinical safety data).

Lactation

There are no data available concerning the excretion of ropivacaine into human milk.

4.7 Effects on ability to drive and use machines

No data are available. Depending on the dose, local anaesthetics may have a minor influence on mental function and co-ordination even in the absence of overt CNS toxicity and may temporarily impair locomotion and alertness.

4.8 Undesirable effects

General

The adverse reaction profile for Naropin is similar to those for other long acting local anaesthetics of the amide type. Adverse drug reactions should be distinguished from the physiological effects of the nerve block itself e.g. a decrease in blood pressure and bradycardia during spinal/epidural block.

Table of adverse drug reactions

Within each system organ class, the ADRs have been ranked under the headings of frequency, most frequent reactions first.

Very common (>1/10)	*Vascular Disorders*	Hypotension[a]
	Gastrointestinal Disorders	Nausea
Common (>1/100)	*Nervous System Disorders*	Headache, paraesthesia, dizziness
	Cardiac Disorders	Bradycardia, tachycardia
	Vascular Disorders	Hypertension
	Gastrointestinal Disorders	Vomiting[b]
	Renal and Urinary Disorders	Urinary retention
	General Disorder and Administration Site Conditions	Temperature elevation, rigor, back pain
Uncommon (>1/1,000)	*Psychiatric Disorders*	Anxiety

	Nervous System Disorders	Symptoms of CNS toxicity (convulsions, grand mal convulsions, seizures, light headedness, circumoral paraesthesia, numbness of the tongue, hyperacusis, tinnitus, visual disturbances, dysarthria, muscular twitching, tremor)*, Hypoaesthesia.
	Vascular Disorders	Syncope
	Respiratory, Thoracic and Mediastinal Disorders	Dyspnoea
	General Disorders and Administration Site Conditions	Hypothermia
Rare (>1/10,000)	*Cardiac Disorders*	Cardiac arrest, cardiac arrhythmias
	General Disorder and Administration Site Conditions	Allergic reactions (anaphylactic reactions, angioneurotic oedema and urticaria)

[a] Hypotension is less frequent in children (>1/100).

[b] Vomiting is more frequent in children (>1/10).

[*] These symptoms usually occur because of inadvertent intravascular injection, overdose or rapid absorption, see section 4.9

Class-related adverse drug reactions:

Neurological complications

Neuropathy and spinal cord dysfunction (e.g. anterior spinal artery syndrome, arachnoiditis, cauda equina), which may result in rare cases of permanent sequelae, have been associated with regional anaesthesia, regardless of the local anaesthetic used.

Total spinal block

Total spinal block may occur if an epidural dose is inadvertently administered intrathecally.

Acute systemic toxicity

Systemic toxic reactions primarily involve the central nervous system (CNS) and the cardiovascular system (CVS). Such reactions are caused by high blood concentration of a local anaesthetic, which may appear due to (accidental) intravascular injection, overdose or exceptionally rapid absorption from highly vascularized areas, see also section 4.4. CNS reactions are similar for all amide local anaesthetics, while cardiac reactions are more dependent on the drug, both quantitatively and qualitatively.

Central nervous system toxicity

Central nervous system toxicity is a graded response with symptoms and signs of escalating severity. Initially symptoms such as visual or hearing disturbances, perioral numbness, dizziness, light-headedness, tingling and paraesthesia are seen. Dysarthria, muscular rigidity and muscular twitching are more serious and may precede the onset of generalised convulsions. These signs must not be mistaken for neurotic behaviour. Unconsciousness and grand mal convulsions may follow, which may last from a few seconds to several minutes. Hypoxia and hypercarbia occur rapidly during convulsions due to the increased muscular activity, together with the interference with respiration. In severe cases even apnoea may occur. The respiratory and metabolic acidosis increases and extends the toxic effects of local anaesthetics.

Recovery follows the redistribution of the local anaesthetic drug from the central nervous system and subsequent metabolism and excretion. Recovery may be rapid unless large amounts of the drug have been injected.

Cardiovascular system toxicity

Cardiovascular toxicity indicates a more severe situation. Hypotension, bradycardia, arrhythmia and even cardiac arrest may occur as a result of high systemic concentrations of local anaesthetics. In volunteers the intravenous infusion of ropivacaine resulted in signs of depression of conductivity and contractility.

Cardiovascular toxic effects are generally preceded by signs of toxicity in the central nervous system, unless the patient is receiving a general anaesthetic or is heavily sedated with drugs such as benzodiazepines or barbiturates.

In children, early signs of local anaesthetic toxicity may be difficult to detect since they may not be able to verbally express them. See also section 4.4.

Treatment of acute systemic toxicity

See section 4.9 Overdose.

4.9 Overdose

Symptoms:

Accidental intravascular injections of local anaesthetics may cause immediate (within seconds to a few minutes) systemic toxic reactions. In the event of overdose, peak plasma concentrations may not be reached for one to two hours, depending on the site of the injection, and signs of toxicity may thus be delayed. (See section 4.8 Acute systemic toxicity, Central nervous system toxicity and Cardiovascular system toxicity).

Treatment

If signs of acute systemic toxicity appear, injection of the local anaesthetic should be stopped immediately and CNS symptoms (convulsions, CNS depression) must promptly be treated with appropriate airway/respiratory support and the administration of anticonvulsant drugs.

If circulatory arrest should occur, immediate cardiopulmonary resuscitation should be instituted. Optimal oxygenation and ventilation and circulatory support as well as treatment of acidosis are of vital importance.

If cardiovascular depression occurs (hypotension, bradycardia), appropriate treatment with intravenous fluids, vasopressor, and or inotropic agents should be considered. Children should be given doses commensurate with age and weight.

Should cardiac arrest occur, a successful outcome may require prolonged resuscitative efforts.

5. PHARMACOLOGICAL PROPERTIES

5.1 Pharmacodynamic properties

Pharmacotherapeutic group: Anaesthetics, local, Amides

ATC code: N01B B09

Ropivacaine is a long-acting, amide-type local anaesthetic with both anaesthetic and analgesic effects. At high doses it produces surgical anaesthesia, while at lower doses it produces sensory block with limited and non-progressive motor block.

The mechanism is a reversible reduction of the membrane permeability of the nerve fibre to sodium ions. Consequently the depolarisation velocity is decreased and the excitable threshold increased, resulting in a local blockade of nerve impulses.

The most characteristic property of ropivacaine is the long duration of action. Onset and duration of the local anaesthetic efficacy are dependent upon the administration site and dose, but are not influenced by the presence of a vasoconstrictor (e.g. adrenaline (epinephrine)). For details concerning the onset and duration of action, see table under posology and method of administration.

Healthy volunteers exposed to intravenous infusions tolerated ropivacaine well at low doses and with expected CNS symptoms at the maximum tolerated dose. The clinical experience with this drug indicates a good margin of safety when adequately used in recommended doses.

5.2 Pharmacokinetic properties

Ropivacaine has a chiral center and is available as the pure S-(-)-enantiomer. It is highly lipid-soluble. All metabolites have a local anaesthetic effect but of considerably lower potency and shorter duration than that of ropivacaine.

The plasma concentration of ropivacaine depends upon the dose, the route of administration and the vascularity of the injection site. Ropivacaine follows linear pharmacokinetics and the C_{max} is proportional to the dose.

Ropivacaine shows complete and biphasic absorption from the epidural space with half-lives of the two phases of the order of 14 min and 4 h in adults. The slow absorption is the rate-limiting factor in the elimination of ropivacaine, which explains why the apparent elimination half-life is longer after epidural than after intravenous administration. Ropivacaine shows a biphasic absorption from the caudal epidural space also in children.

Ropivacaine has a mean total plasma clearance in the order of 440 ml/min, a renal clearance of 1 ml/min, a volume of distribution at steady state of 47 litres and a terminal half-life of 1.8 h after iv administration. Ropivacaine has an intermediate hepatic extraction ratio of about 0.4. It is mainly bound to α_1-acid glycoprotein in plasma with an unbound fraction of about 6%.

An increase in total plasma concentrations during continuous epidural and interscalene infusion has been observed, related to a postoperative increase of α_1-acid glycoprotein.

Variations in unbound, i.e. pharmacologically active, concentration have been much less than in total plasma concentration.

Since ropivacaine has an intermediate to low hepatic extraction ratio, its rate of elimination should depend on the unbound plasma concentration. A postoperative increase in AAG will decrease the unbound fraction due to increased protein binding, which will decrease the total clearance and result in an increase in total plasma concentrations, as seen in the paediatric and adult studies. The unbound clearance of ropivacaine remains unchanged as illustrated by the stable unbound concentrations during postoperative infusion. It is the unbound plasma concentration that is related to systemic pharmacodynamic effects and toxicity.

Ropivacaine readily crosses the placenta and equilibrium in regard to unbound concentration will be rapidly reached. The degree of plasma protein binding in the foetus is less than in the mother, which results in lower total plasma concentrations in the foetus than in the mother.

Ropivacaine is extensively metabolised, predominantly by aromatic hydroxylation. In total, 86% of the dose is excreted in the urine after intravenous administration, of which only about 1% relates to unchanged drug. The major metabolite is 3-hydroxy-ropivacaine, about 37% of which is excreted in the urine, mainly conjugated. Urinary excretion of 4-hydroxy-ropivacaine, the N-dealkylated metabolite (PPX) and the 4-hydroxy-dealkylated accounts for 1–3%. Conjugated and unconjugated 3-hydroxy-ropivacaine shows only detectable concentrations in plasma.

A similar pattern of metabolites has been found in children above one year.

There is no evidence of *in vivo* racemisation of ropivacaine.

Paediatrics

The pharmacokinetics of ropivacaine was characterized in a pooled population PK analysis on data in 192 children between 0 and 12 years. Unbound ropivacaine and PPX clearance and ropivacaine unbound volume of distribution depend on both body weight and age up to the maturity of liver function, after which they depend largely on body weight. The maturation of unbound ropivacaine clearance appears to be complete by the age of 3 years, that of PPX by the age of 1 year and unbound ropivacaine volume of distribution by the age of 2 years. The PPX unbound volume of distribution only depends on body weight. As PPX has a longer half-life and a lower clearance, it may accumulate during epidural infusion.

Unbound ropivacaine clearance (Cl_u) for ages above 6 months has reached values within the range of those in adults. Total ropivacaine clearance (CL) values displayed in the table below are those not affected by the postoperative increase in AAG.

Estimates of pharmacokinetic parameters derived from the pooled paediatric population PK analysis

(see Table 3 below)

Table 3 Estimates of pharmacokinetic parameters derived from the pooled paediatric population PK analysis

Age Group	BW^a kg	Clu^b (L/h/kg)	Vu^c (L/kg)	CL^d (L/h/kg)	$t_{1/2}^{e}$ (h)	$t_{1/2ppx}^{f}$ (h)
Newborn	3.27	2.40	21.86	0.096	6.3	43.3
1m	4.29	3.60	25.94	0.143	5.0	25.7
6m	7.85	8.03	41.71	0.320	3.6	14.5
1y	10.15	11.32	52.60	0.451	3.2	13.6
4y	16.69	15.91	65.24	0.633	2.8	15.1
10y	32.19	13.94	65.57	0.555	3.3	17.8

[a] Median bodyweight for respective age from WHO database.

[b] Unbound ropivacaine clearance

[c] Ropivacaine unbound volume of distribution

[d] Total ropivacaine clearance

[e] Ropivacaine terminal half life

[f] PPX terminal half life

Table 4 Simulated mean and observed range of unbound Cu_{max} after a single caudal block

Age group	Dose (mg/kg)	Cu_{max}^{a} (mg/L)	t_{max}^{b} (h)	Cu_{max}^{c} (mg/L)
0-1m	2.00	0.0582	2.00	0.05-0.08 (n=5)
1-6m	2.00	0.0375	1.50	0.02-0.09 (n=18)
6-12m	2.00	0.0283	1.00	0.01-0.05 (n=9)
1-10y	2.00	0.0221	0.50	0.01-0.05 (n=60)

[a] Unbound maximal plasma concentration

[b] Time to unbound maximal plasma concentration

[c] Observed and dose-normalised unbound maximal plasma concentration

The simulated mean unbound maximal plasma concentration (Cu_{max}) after a single caudal block tended to be higher in neonates and the time to Cu_{max} (t_{max}) decreased with an increase in age. Simulated mean unbound plasma concentrations at the end of a 72 h continuous epidural infusion at recommended dose rates also showed higher levels in neonates as compared to those in infants and children. See also section 4.4.

Simulated mean and observed range of unbound Cu_{max} after a single caudal block

(see Table 4 on previous page)

At 6 months, the breakpoint for change in the recommended dose rate for continuous epidural infusion, unbound ropivacaine clearance has reached 34% and unbound PPX 71% of its mature value. The systemic exposure is higher in neonates and also somewhat higher in infants between 1 and 6 months compared to older children, which is related to the immaturity of their liver function. However, this is partly compensated for by the recommended 50% lower dose rate for continuous infusion in infants below 6 months.

Simulations on the sum of unbound plasma concentrations of ropivacaine and PPX, based on the PK parameters and their variance in the population analysis, indicate that for a single caudal block the recommended dose must be increased by a factor of 2.7 in the youngest group and a factor of 7.4 in the 1–10 year group in order for the upper prediction 90% confidence interval limit to touch the threshold for systemic toxicity. Corresponding factors for the continuous epidural infusion are 1.8 and 3.8 respectively.

5.3 Preclinical safety data

Based on conventional studies of safety pharmacology, single and repeated dose toxicity, reproduction toxicity, mutagenic potential and local toxicity, no hazards for humans were identified other than those which can be expected on the basis of the pharmacodynamic action of high doses of ropivacaine (e.g. CNS signs, including convulsions, and cardiotoxicity).

6. PHARMACEUTICAL PARTICULARS

6.1 List of excipients

Sodium chloride

Hydrochloric acid

Sodium hydroxide

Water for injection

6.2 Incompatibilities

Compatibilities with other solutions than those mentioned in section 6.6 have not been investigated. In alkaline solutions precipitation may occur as ropivacaine shows poor solubility at pH > 6

6.3 Shelf life

2 years.

Shelf life after first opening:

From a microbiological point of view, the product should be used immediately. If not used immediately, in-use storage times and conditions prior to use are the responsibility of the user and would normally not be longer than 24 hours at 2–8°C.

For mixtures, see section 6.6.

6.4 Special precautions for storage

Do not store above 30°C. Do not freeze.

For storage after opening, see section 6.3.

6.5 Nature and contents of container

100 ml polypropylene bags (Polybag) in sterile blister packs of 5.

200 ml polypropylene bags (Polybag) in sterile blister packs of 5.

6.6 Special precautions for disposal and other handling

Naropin products are preservative-free and are intended for single use only. Discard any unused solution.

The intact container must not be re-autoclaved. A blistered container should be chosen when a sterile outside is required.

Naropin solution for infusion in plastic infusion bags (Polybag) is chemically and physically compatible with the following drugs:

Concentration of Naropin: 1–2 mg/ml	
Additive	**Concentration***
Fentanyl citrate	1–10 microgram/ml
Sufentanil citrate	0.4–4 microgram/ml
Morphine sulphate	20–100 microgram/ml
Clonidine hydrochloride	5–50 microgram/ml

* The concentration ranges stated in the table are wider than those used in clinical practice. Epidural infusions of Naropin/sufentanil citrate, Naropin/morphine sulphate and Naropin/clonidine hydrochloride have not been evaluated in clinical studies.

The mixtures are chemically and physically stable for 30 days at 20 to 30°C. From a microbiological point of view, the mixtures should be used immediately. If not used immediately, in-use storage times and conditions prior to use are the responsibility of the user and would normally not be longer than 24 hours at 2 to 8°C.

7. MARKETING AUTHORISATION HOLDER

AstraZeneca UK Ltd.,

600 Capability Green,

Luton, LU1 3LU, UK.

8. MARKETING AUTHORISATION NUMBER(S)

PL 17901/0149

9. DATE OF FIRST AUTHORISATION/RENEWAL OF THE AUTHORISATION

Date of first authorisation: 3rd October 1995

Date of last renewal: 15th September 2005

10. DATE OF REVISION OF THE TEXT

15th August 2008

Naropin 7.5 mg/ml solution for injection

(AstraZeneca UK Limited)

1. NAME OF THE MEDICINAL PRODUCT

Naropin® 7.5 mg/ml solution for injection

2. QUALITATIVE AND QUANTITATIVE COMPOSITION

Naropin® 7.5 mg/ml:

1 ml solution for injection contains ropivacaine hydrochloride monohydrate equivalent to 7.5 mg ropivacaine hydrochloride.

1 ampoule of 10 ml or 20 ml solution for injection contains ropivacaine hydrochloride monohydrate equivalent to 75 mg and 150 mg ropivacaine hydrochloride respectively.

For excipients, see section 6.1.

3. PHARMACEUTICAL FORM

Solution for injection for perineural and epidural administration (10–20 ml).

Clear, colourless solution.

4. CLINICAL PARTICULARS

4.1 Therapeutic indications

Naropin is indicated for:

1. Surgical anaesthesia

- Epidural blocks for surgery, including Caesarean section.
- Major nerve blocks.
- Field blocks.

2. Acute pain management

- Continuous epidural infusion or intermittent bolus administration during postoperative or labour pain.
- Field blocks.

4.2 Posology and method of administration

Naropin should only be used by, or under the supervision of, clinicians experienced in regional anaesthesia.

Posology

Adults and children above 12 years of age:

The following table is a guide to dosage for the more commonly used blocks. The smallest dose required to produce an effective block should be used. The clinician's experience and knowledge of the patient's physical status are of importance when deciding the dose.

(see Table 1 on next page)

In general, surgical anaesthesia (e.g. epidural administration) requires the use of the higher concentrations and doses. The Naropin 10 mg/ml formulation is recommended for epidural anaesthesia in which a complete motor block is essential for surgery. For analgesia (e.g. epidural administration for acute pain management) the lower concentrations and doses are recommended.

Method of administration

Careful aspiration before and during injection is recommended to prevent intravascular injection. When a large dose is to be injected, a test dose of 3–5 ml lidocaine (lignocaine) with adrenaline (epinephrine) (Xylocaine® 2% with Adrenaline (epinephrine) 1:200,000) is recommended. An inadvertent intravascular injection may be recognised by a temporary increase in heart rate and an accidental intrathecal injection by signs of a spinal block.

Aspiration should be performed prior to and during administration of the main dose, which should be injected slowly or in incremental doses, at a rate of 25–50 mg/min, while closely observing the patient's vital functions and maintaining verbal contact. If toxic symptoms occur, the injection should be stopped immediately.

In epidural block for surgery, single doses of up to 250 mg ropivacaine have been used and well tolerated.

In brachial plexus block a single dose of 300 mg has been used in a limited number of patients and was well tolerated.

When prolonged blocks are used, either through continuous infusion or through repeated bolus administration, the risks of reaching a toxic plasma concentration or inducing local neural injury must be considered. Cumulative doses up to 675 mg ropivacaine for surgery and postoperative analgesia administered over 24 hours were well tolerated in adults, as were postoperative continuous epidural infusions at rates up to 28 mg/hour for 72 hours. In a limited number of patients, higher doses of up to 800 mg/day have been administered with relatively few adverse reactions.

For treatment of postoperative pain, the following technique can be recommended: Unless preoperatively instituted, an epidural block with Naropin 7.5 mg/ml is induced via an epidural catheter. Analgesia is maintained with Naropin 2 mg/ml infusion. Infusion rates of 6–14 ml (12–28 mg) per hour provide adequate analgesia with only slight and non-progressive motor block in most cases of moderate to severe postoperative pain. The maximum duration of epidural block is 3 days. However, close monitoring of analgesic effect should be performed in order to remove the catheter as soon as the pain condition allows it. With this technique a significant reduction in the need for opioids has been observed.

In clinical studies an epidural infusion of Naropin 2 mg/ml alone or mixed with fentanyl 1-4 μg/ml has been given for postoperative pain management for up to 72 hours. The combination of Naropin and fentanyl provided improved pain relief but caused opioid side effects. The combination of Naropin and fentanyl has been investigated only for Naropin 2 mg/ml.

When prolonged peripheral nerve blocks are applied, either through continuous infusion or through repeated injections, the risks of reaching a toxic plasma concentration or inducing local neural injury must be considered. In clinical studies, femoral nerve block was established with 300 mg Naropin 7.5 mg/ml and interscalene block with 225 mg Naropin 7.5 mg/ml, respectively, before surgery. Analgesia was then maintained with Naropin 2 mg/ml. Infusion rates or intermittent injections of 10–20 mg per hour for 48 hours provided adequate analgesia and were well tolerated.

Concentrations above 7.5 mg/ml Naropin have not been documented for Caesarean section.

4.3 Contraindications

Hypersensitivity to ropivacaine or to other local anaesthetics of the amide type.

General contraindications related to epidural anaesthesia, regardless of the local anaesthetic used, should be taken into account.

Intravenous regional anaesthesia.

Obstetric paracervical anaesthesia.

Hypovolaemia.

4.4 Special warnings and precautions for use

Regional anaesthetic procedures should always be performed in a properly equipped and staffed area. Equipment and drugs necessary for monitoring and emergency resuscitation should be immediately available. Patients receiving major blocks should be in an optimal condition and have an intravenous line inserted before the blocking procedure. The clinician responsible should take the necessary precautions to avoid intravascular injection (see section 4.2 Posology and method of administration) and be appropriately trained and familiar with diagnosis and treatment of side effects, systemic toxicity and other complications (see section 4.8 Undesirable effects and 4.9 Overdose) such as inadvertent subarachnoid injection, which may produce a high spinal block with apnoea and hypotension. Convulsions have occurred most often after brachial plexus block and epidural block. This is likely to be the result of either accidental intravascular injection or rapid absorption from the injection site.

Caution is required to prevent injections in inflamed areas.

Cardiovascular

Patients treated with anti-arrhythmic drugs class III (eg, amiodarone) should be under close surveillance and ECG monitoring considered, since cardiac effects may be additive.

There have been rare reports of cardiac arrest during the use of Naropin for epidural anaesthesia or peripheral nerve blockade, especially after unintentional accidental intravascular administration in elderly patients and in patients with concomitant heart disease. In some instances, resuscitation has been difficult. Should cardiac arrest occur, prolonged resuscitative efforts may be required to improve the possibility of a successful outcome.

Head and neck blocks

Certain local anaesthetic procedures, such as injections in the head and neck regions, may be associated with a higher frequency of serious adverse reactions, regardless of the local anaesthetic used.

Major peripheral nerve blocks

Major peripheral nerve blocks may imply the administration of a large volume of local anaesthetic in highly vascularized areas, often close to large vessels where there is an increased risk of intravascular injection and/or rapid systemic absorption, which can lead to high plasma concentrations.

Hypersensitivity

A possible cross–hypersensitivity with other amide–type local anaesthetics should be taken into account.

Hypovolaemia

Patients with hypovolaemia due to any cause can develop sudden and severe hypotension during epidural anaesthesia, regardless of the local anaesthetic used.

Table 1

	Conc.	Volume	Dose	Onset	Duration
	mg/ml	ml	mg	minutes	hours
Surgical anaesthesia					
Lumbar Epidural Administration					
Surgery	7.5	15–25	113–188	10–20	3–5
	10	15–20	150–200	10–20	4–6
Caesarean section	7.5	15–20	113–150(1)	10–20	3–5
Thoracic Epidural Administration					
To establish block for postoperative pain relief	7.5	5–15 (depending on the level of injection)	38–113	10–20	n/a(2)
Major Nerve Block*					
Brachial plexus block	7.5	30–40	225–300(3)	10–25	6–10
Field Block	7.5	1–30	7.5–225	1–15	2–6
(e.g. minor nerve blocks and infiltration)					
Acute pain management					
Lumbar Epidural Administration					
Bolus	2	10–20	20–40	10–15	0.5–1.5
Intermittent injections (top up) (e.g. labour pain management)	2	10–15 (minimum interval 30 minutes)	20–30		
Continuous infusion e.g. labour pain	2	6–10 ml/h	12–20 mg/h	n/a(2)	n/a(2)
Postoperative pain management	2	6–14 ml/h	12–28 mg/h	n/a(2)	n/a(2)
Thoracic Epidural Administration					
Continuous infusion (postoperative pain management)	2	6–14 ml/h	12–28 mg/h	n/a(2)	n/a(2)
Field Block					
(e.g. minor nerve blocks and infiltration)	2	1–100	2–200	1–5	2–6
Peripheral nerve block (Femoral or interscalene block)					
Continuous infusion or intermittent injections (e.g. postoperative pain management)	2	5–10 ml/h	10–20 mg/h	n/a	n/a

The doses in the table are those considered to be necessary to produce a successful block and should be regarded as guidelines for use in adults. Individual variations in onset and duration occur. The figures in the column 'Dose' reflect the expected average dose range needed. Standard textbooks should be consulted for both factors affecting specific block techniques and individual patient requirements.

* With regard to major nerve block, only for brachial plexus block a dose recommendation can be given. For other major nerve blocks lower doses may be required. However, there is presently no experience of specific dose recommendations for other blocks.

(1) Incremental dosing should be applied, the starting dose of about 100 mg (97.5 mg = 13 ml; 105 mg = 14 ml) to be given over 3–5 minutes. Two extra doses, in total an additional 50mg, may be administered as needed.

(2) n/a = not applicable

(3) The dose for a major nerve block must be adjusted according to site of administration and patient status. Interscalene and supraclavicular brachial plexus blocks may be associated with a higher frequency of serious adverse reactions, regardless of the local anaesthetic used, (see section 4.4. Special warnings and special precautions for use).

Patients in poor general health

Patients in poor general condition due to ageing or other compromising factors such as partial or complete heart conduction block, advanced liver disease or severe renal dysfunction require special attention, although regional anaesthesia is frequently indicated in these patients.

Patients with hepatic and renal impairment

Ropivacaine is metabolised in the liver and should therefore be used with caution in patients with severe liver disease; repeated doses may need to be reduced due to delayed elimination. Normally there is no need to modify the dose in patients with impaired renal function when used for single dose or short-term treatment. Acidosis and reduced plasma protein concentration, frequently seen in patients with chronic renal failure, may increase the risk of systemic toxicity.

Acute porphyria

Naropin® solution for injection and infusion is possibly porphyrinogenic and should only be prescribed to patients with acute porphyria when no safer alternative is available. Appropriate precautions should be taken in the case of vulnerable patients, according to standard textbooks and/ or in consultation with disease area experts.

Excipients with recognised action/effect

This medicinal product contains maximum 3.7 mg sodium per ml. To be taken into consideration by patients on a controlled sodium diet.

Prolonged administration

Prolonged administration of ropivacaine should be avoided in patients concomitantly treated with strong CYP1A2 inhibitors, such as fluvoxamine and enoxacin, see section 4.5.

4.5 Interaction with other medicinal products and other forms of interaction

Naropin should be used with caution in patients receiving other local anaesthetics or agents structurally related to amide-type local anaesthetics, e.g. certain antiarrhythmics, such as lidocaine and mexiletine, since the systemic toxic effects are additive. Simultaneous use of Naropin with general anaesthetics or opioids may potentiate each others (adverse) effects. Specific interaction studies with ropivacaine and anti-arrhythmic drugs class III (e.g. amiodarone) have not been performed, but caution is advised (see also section 4.4 Special warnings and precautions for use).

Cytochrome P450 (CYP) 1A2 is involved in the formation of 3-hydroxy-ropivacaine, the major metabolite. *In vivo*, the plasma clearance of ropivacaine was reduced by up to 77% during co-administration of fluvoxamine, a selective and potent CYP1A2 inhibitor. Thus strong inhibitors of CYP1A2, such as fluvoxamine and enoxacin given concomitantly during prolonged administration of Naropin, can interact with Naropin. Prolonged administration of ropivacaine should be avoided in patients concomitantly treated with strong CYP1A2 inhibitors, see also section 4.4.

In vivo, the plasma clearance of ropivacaine was reduced by 15% during co-administration of ketoconazole, a selective and potent inhibitor of CYP3A4. However, the inhibition of this isozyme is not likely to have clinical relevance.

In vitro, ropivacaine is a competitive inhibitor of CYP2D6 but does not seem to inhibit this isozyme at clinically attained plasma concentrations.

4.6 Pregnancy and lactation

Pregnancy

Apart from epidural administration for obstetrical use, there are no adequate data on the use of ropivacaine in human pregnancy. Experimental animal studies do not indicate direct or indirect harmful effects with respect to pregnancy, embryonal/fœtal development, parturition or postnatal development (see section 5.3 Preclinical safety data).

Lactation

There are no data available concerning the excretion of ropivacaine into human milk.

4.7 Effects on ability to drive and use machines

No data are available. Depending on the dose, local anaesthetics may have a minor influence on mental function and co-ordination even in the absence of overt CNS toxicity and may temporarily impair locomotion and alertness.

4.8 Undesirable effects

General

The adverse reaction profile for Naropin is similar to those for other long acting local anaesthetics of the amide type. Adverse drug reactions should be distinguished from the physiological effects of the nerve block itself e.g. a decrease in blood pressure and bradycardia during spinal/epidural block.

Table of adverse drug reactions

Within each system organ class, the ADRs have been ranked under the headings of frequency, most frequent reactions first.

Very common (>1/10)	*Vascular Disorders*	Hypotension
	Gastrointestinal Disorders	Nausea
Common (>1/100)	*Nervous System Disorders*	Headache, paraesthesia, dizziness
	Cardiac Disorders	Bradycardia, tachycardia
	Vascular Disorders	Hypertension
	Gastrointestinal Disorders	Vomiting
	Renal and Urinary Disorders	Urinary retention
	General Disorder and Administration Site Conditions	Temperature elevation, rigor, back pain
Uncommon (>1/1,000)	*Psychiatric Disorders*	Anxiety
	Nervous System Disorders	Symptoms of CNS toxicity (convulsions, grand mal convulsions, seizures, light headedness, circumoral paraesthesia, numbness of the tongue, hyperacusis, tinnitus, visual disturbances, dysarthria, muscular twitching, tremor)*, Hypoaesthesia.
	Vascular Disorders	Syncope
	Respiratory, Thoracic and Mediastinal Disorders	Dyspnoea
	General Disorders and Administration Site Conditions	Hypothermia
Rare (>1/10,000)	*Cardiac Disorders*	Cardiac arrest, cardiac arrhythmias
	General Disorder and Administration Site Conditions	Allergic reactions (anaphylactic reactions, angioneurotic oedema and urticaria)

* These symptoms usually occur because of inadvertent intravascular injection, overdose or rapid absorption, see section 4.9

Class-related adverse drug reactions:

Neurological complications

Neuropathy, and spinal cord dysfunction (e.g. anterior spinal artery syndrome, arachnoiditis, cauda equina), which may result in rare cases of permanent sequelae, have been associated with regional anaesthesia, regardless of the local anaesthetic used.

Total spinal block

Total spinal block may occur if an epidural dose is inadvertently administered intrathecally.

Acute systemic toxicity

Systemic toxic reactions primarily involve the central nervous system (CNS) and the cardiovascular system (CVS). Such reactions are caused by high blood concentration of a local anaesthetic, which may appear due to (accidental) intravascular injection, overdose or exceptionally rapid absorption from highly vascularized areas, see also section 4.4. CNS reactions are similar for all amide local anaesthetics, while cardiac reactions are more dependent on the drug, both quantitatively and qualitatively.

Central nervous system toxicity

Central nervous system toxicity is a graded response with symptoms and signs of escalating severity. Initially symptoms such as visual or hearing disturbances, perioral numbness, dizziness, light-headedness, tingling and paraesthesia are seen. Dysarthria, muscular rigidity and muscular twitching are more serious and may precede the onset of generalised convulsions. These signs must not be mistaken for neurotic behaviour. Unconsciousness and grand mal convulsions may follow, which may last from a few seconds to several minutes. Hypoxia and hypercarbia occur rapidly during convulsions due to the increased muscular activity, together with the interference with respiration. In severe cases even apnoea may occur. The respiratory and metabolic acidosis increases and extends the toxic effects of local anaesthetics.

Recovery follows the redistribution of the local anaesthetic drug from the central nervous system and subsequent metabolism and excretion. Recovery may be rapid unless large amounts of the drug have been injected.

Cardiovascular system toxicity

Cardiovascular toxicity indicates a more severe situation. Hypotension, bradycardia, arrhythmia and even cardiac arrest may occur as a result of high systemic concentrations of local anaesthetics. In volunteers the intravenous infusion of ropivacaine resulted in signs of depression of conductivity and contractility.

Cardiovascular toxic effects are generally preceded by signs of toxicity in the central nervous system, unless the patient is receiving a general anaesthetic or is heavily sedated with drugs such as benzodiazepines or barbiturates.

In children, early signs of local anaesthetic toxicity may be difficult to detect since they may not be able to verbally express them. See also section 4.4.

Treatment of acute systemic toxicity

See section 4.9 Overdose.

4.9 Overdose

Symptoms:

Accidental intravascular injections of local anaesthetics may cause immediate (within seconds to a few minutes) systemic toxic reactions. In the event of overdose, peak plasma concentrations may not be reached for one to two hours, depending on the site of the injection, and signs of toxicity may thus be delayed. (See section 4.8 Acute systemic toxicity, Central nervous system toxicity and Cardiovascular system toxicity).

Treatment

If signs of acute systemic toxicity appear, injection of the local anaesthetic should be stopped immediately and CNS symptoms (convulsions, CNS depression) must promptly be treated with appropriate airway/respiratory support and the administration of anticonvulsant drugs.

If circulatory arrest should occur, immediate cardiopulmonary resuscitation should be instituted. Optimal oxygenation and ventilation and circulatory support as well as treatment of acidosis are of vital importance.

If cardiovascular depression occurs (hypotension, bradycardia), appropriate treatment with intravenous fluids, vasopressor, and or inotropic agents should be considered. Children should be given doses commensurate with age and weight.

Should cardiac arrest occur, a successful outcome may require prolonged resuscitative efforts.

5. PHARMACOLOGICAL PROPERTIES

5.1 Pharmacodynamic properties

Pharmacotherapeutic group: Anaesthetics, local, Amides

ATC code: N01B B09

Ropivacaine is a long-acting, amide-type local anaesthetic with both anaesthetic and analgesic effects. At high doses Naropin produces surgical anaesthesia, while at lower doses it produces sensory block with limited and non-progressive motor block.

The mechanism is a reversible reduction of the membrane permeability of the nerve fibre to sodium ions. Consequently the depolarisation velocity is decreased and the excitable threshold increased, resulting in a local blockade of nerve impulses.

The most characteristic property of ropivacaine is the long duration of action. Onset and duration of the local anaesthetic efficacy are dependent upon the administration site and dose, but are not influenced by the presence of a vasoconstrictor (e.g. adrenaline (epinephrine)). For details concerning the onset and duration of action of Naropin, see table under posology and method of administration.

Healthy volunteers exposed to intravenous infusions tolerated ropivacaine well at low doses and with expected CNS symptoms at the maximum tolerated dose. The clinical experience with this drug indicates a good margin of safety when adequately used in recommended doses.

5.2 Pharmacokinetic properties

Ropivacaine has a chiral center and is available as the pure S-(-)-enantiomer. It is highly lipid-soluble. All metabolites have a local anaesthetic effect but of considerably lower potency and shorter duration than that of ropivacaine.

The plasma concentration of ropivacaine depends upon the dose, the route of administration and the vascularity of the injection site. Ropivacaine follows linear pharmacokinetics and the C_{max} is proportional to the dose.

Ropivacaine shows complete and biphasic absorption from the epidural space with half-lives of the two phases of the order of 14 min and 4 h in adults. The slow absorption is the rate-limiting factor in the elimination of ropivacaine, which explains why the apparent elimination half-life is longer after epidural than after intravenous administration.

Ropivacaine has a mean total plasma clearance in the order of 440 ml/min, a renal clearance of 1 ml/min, a volume of distribution at steady state of 47 litres and a terminal half-life of 1.8 h after iv administration. Ropivacaine has an intermediate hepatic extraction ratio of about 0.4. It is mainly bound to α_1- acid glycoprotein in plasma with an unbound fraction of about 6%.

An increase in total plasma concentrations during continuous epidural infusion has been observed, related to a postoperative increase of α_1- acid glycoprotein.

Variations in unbound, i.e. pharmacologically active, concentration have been much less than in total plasma concentration.

Ropivacaine readily crosses the placenta and equilibrium in regard to unbound concentration will be rapidly reached. The degree of plasma protein binding in the foetus is less than in the mother, which results in lower total plasma concentrations in the foetus than in the mother.

Ropivacaine is extensively metabolised, predominantly by aromatic hydroxylation. In total, 86% of the dose is excreted in the urine after intravenous administration, of which only about 1% relates to unchanged drug. The major metabolite is 3-hydroxy-ropivacaine, about 37% of which is excreted in the urine, mainly conjugated. Urinary excretion of 4-hydroxy-ropivacaine, the N-dealkylated metabolite and the 4-hydroxy-dealkylated accounts for 1–3%. Conjugated and unconjugated 3-hydroxy-ropivacaine shows only detectable concentrations in plasma.

There is no evidence of *in vivo* racemisation of ropivacaine.

5.3 Preclinical safety data

Based on conventional studies of safety pharmacology, single and repeated dose toxicity, reproduction toxicity, mutagenic potential and local toxicity, no hazards for humans were identified other than those which can be expected on the basis of the pharmacodynamic action of high doses of ropivacaine (e.g. CNS signs, including convulsions, and cardiotoxicity).

6. PHARMACEUTICAL PARTICULARS

6.1 List of excipients

Sodium chloride

Hydrochloric acid

Sodium hydroxide

Water for injection

6.2 Incompatibilities

In alkaline solutions precipitation may occur as ropivacaine shows poor solubility at pH > 6

6.3 Shelf life

3 years.

Shelf life after first opening:

From a microbiological point of view, the product should be used immediately. If not used immediately, in-use storage times and conditions prior to use are the responsibility of the user and would normally not be longer than 24 hours at 2–8°C.

6.4 Special precautions for storage

Do not store above 30°C. Do not freeze.

For storage after opening, see section 6.3.

6.5 Nature and contents of container

10 ml polypropylene ampoules (Polyamp) in packs of 5 and 10.

10 ml polypropylene ampoules (Polyamp) in sterile blister packs of 5 and 10.

20 ml polypropylene ampoules (Polyamp) in packs of 5 and 10.

20 ml polypropylene ampoules (Polyamp) in sterile blister packs of 5 and 10.

The polypropylene ampoules (Polyamp) are specially designed to fit Luer lock and Luer fit syringes.

6.6 Special precautions for disposal and other handling

Naropin products are preservative-free and are intended for single use only. Discard any unused solution.

The intact container must not be re-autoclaved. A blistered container should be chosen when a sterile outside is required.

7. MARKETING AUTHORISATION HOLDER

AstraZeneca UK Ltd.,

600 Capability Green,

Luton, LU1 3LU, UK.

8. MARKETING AUTHORISATION NUMBER(S)

PL 17901/0152

9. DATE OF FIRST AUTHORISATION/RENEWAL OF THE AUTHORISATION

Date of first authorisation: 3rd October 1995

Date of last renewal: 15th September 2005

10. DATE OF REVISION OF THE TEXT

15th August 2008

Nasacort Nasal Spray

(sanofi-aventis)

1. NAME OF THE MEDICINAL PRODUCT

NASACORT 55 micrograms/dose, nasal spray, suspension.

2. QUALITATIVE AND QUANTITATIVE COMPOSITION

Triamcinolone acetonide

Bottles of NASACORT contain 16.5 g of suspension (with 9.075 mg triamcinolone acetonide). Each actuation delivers 55 micrograms triamcinolone acetonide.

Excipient: benzalkonium chloride (15 micrograms/actuation).

For a full list of excipients, see section 6.1.

3. PHARMACEUTICAL FORM

Nasal spray, suspension.

It is an unscented, thixotropic suspension of microcrystalline triamcinolone acetonide in an aqueous medium.

4. CLINICAL PARTICULARS

4.1 Therapeutic indications

NASACORT is indicated for the treatment of symptoms of seasonal and perennial allergic rhinitis.

4.2 Posology and method of administration

NASACORT is for nasal use only.

Patients aged 12 years and over: The recommended starting dose is 220 micrograms as 2 sprays in each nostril once daily. Once symptoms are controlled patients can be maintained on 110 micrograms (1 spray in each nostril once daily).

Paediatric patients aged 6 to 12 years: The recommended dose is 110 micrograms as 1 spray in each nostril once daily. In patients with more severe symptoms, a dose of 220 micrograms may be used. But once symptoms are controlled, patients should be maintained on the lowest effective dose.

Until further evidence is available, continuous use beyond 3 months in children under 12 years is not recommended.

It is important to shake the bottle gently before each use.

Each actuation delivers 55 micrograms triamcinolone acetonide from the nose piece to the patient (estimated from *in vitro* testing) after an initial priming of 5 sprays until a fine mist is achieved. NASACORT will remain adequately primed for 2 weeks. If the product is unused for more than 2 weeks, then it can be adequately reprimed with one spray. The nozzle should be pointed away from you while you are doing this.

After using the spray: Wipe the nozzle carefully with a clean tissue or handkerchief, and replace the dust-cap.

If the spray does not work and it may be blocked, clean it as follows. NEVER try to unblock it or enlarge the tiny spray hole with a pin or other sharp object because this will destroy the spray mechanism.

The nasal spray should be cleaned at least once a week or more often if it gets blocked.

TO CLEAN THE SPRAY

1. Remove the dust-cap and the spray nozzle only* (pull off).

2. Soak the dust-cap and spray nozzle in warm water for a few minutes, and then rinse under cold running tap water.

3. Shake or tap off the excess water and allow to air-dry.

4. Re-fit the spray nozzle.

5. Prime the unit as necessary until a fine mist is produced and use as normal.

* Part as indicated on diagram below,

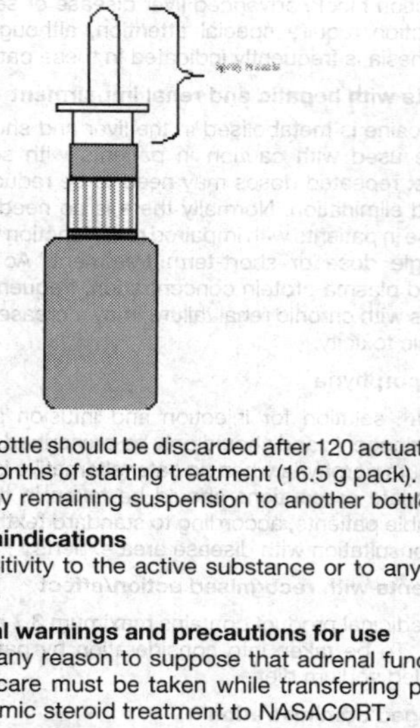

Also, the bottle should be discarded after 120 actuations or within 2 months of starting treatment (16.5 g pack). Do not transfer any remaining suspension to another bottle.

4.3 Contraindications

Hypersensitivity to the active substance or to any of the excipients.

4.4 Special warnings and precautions for use

If there is any reason to suppose that adrenal function is impaired, care must be taken while transferring patients from systemic steroid treatment to NASACORT.

In clinical studies with NASACORT administered intranasally, the development of localised infections of the nose and pharynx with Candida albicans has rarely occurred. When such an infection develops it may require treatment with appropriate local therapy and temporary discontinuance of treatment with NASACORT.

Because of the inhibitory effect of corticosteroids on wound healing in patients who have experienced recent nasal septal ulcers, nasal surgery or trauma, NASACORT should be used with caution until healing has occurred.

Systemic effects of nasal corticosteroids may occur, particularly at high doses prescribed for prolonged periods.

Treatment with higher than recommended doses may result in clinically significant adrenal suppression. If there is evidence for higher than recommended doses being used then additional systemic corticosteroid cover should be considered during periods of stress or elective surgery.

As experience with NASACORT in children under 6 years of age is limited, use in this age group is not recommended.

Growth retardation has been reported in children receiving nasal corticosteroids at licensed doses.

It is recommended that the height of children receiving prolonged treatment with nasal corticosteroids is regularly monitored. If growth is slowed, therapy should be reviewed with the aim of reducing the dose of nasal corticosteroid, if possible, to the lowest dose at which effective control of symptoms is maintained. In addition, consideration should be given to referring the patient to a paediatric specialist.

4.5 Interaction with other medicinal products and other forms of interaction
No interactions with other medicaments are known.

4.6 Pregnancy and lactation
Clinical experience in pregnant women is limited. In animal studies, corticosteroids have been shown to induce teratogenic effects. Triamcinolone acetonide may pass into human breast milk. Triamcinolone acetonide should not be administered during pregnancy or lactation unless the therapeutic benefit to the mother is considered to outweigh the potential risk to the foetus/baby.

4.7 Effects on ability to drive and use machines
NASACORT has no known effect on the ability to drive and operate machines.

4.8 Undesirable effects
The most commonly reported adverse reactions are rhinitis, headache and pharyngitis.

Respiratory disorders: epistaxis, nasal irritation, dry mucous membrane, naso-sinus congestion and sneezing; rarely, nasal septal perforations

In clinical trials, these adverse reactions with the exception of epistaxis, were reported at approximately the same or lower incidence as placebo treated patients.

Skin or subcutaneous disorders: rarely allergic reactions including rash, urticaria, pruritus and facial oedema.

Systemic effects of nasal corticosteroids may occur, particularly when prescribed at high doses for prolonged periods.

4.9 Overdose
Like any other nasally administered corticosteroid, acute overdosing with NASACORT is unlikely in view of the total amount of active ingredient present. In the event that the entire contents of the bottle were administered all at once, via either oral or nasal application, clinically significant systemic adverse events would most likely not result. The patient may experience some gastrointestinal upset if taken orally.

5. PHARMACOLOGICAL PROPERTIES

5.1 Pharmacodynamic properties
Pharmacotherapeutic group: nasal corticosteroid, ATC code: R 01 AD.

Triamcinolone acetonide is a more potent derivative of triamcinolone and is approximately 8 times more potent than prednisone. Although the precise mechanism of corticosteroid antiallergic action is unknown, corticosteroids are very effective in the treatment of allergic diseases in man.

NASACORT does not have an immediate effect on allergic signs and symptoms. An improvement in some patient symptoms may be seen within the first day of treatment with NASACORT and relief may be expected in 3 to 4 days. When NASACORT is prematurely discontinued symptoms may not recur for several days.

In clinical studies performed in adults and children at doses up to 440 mcg/day intranasally, no suppression of the Hypothalamic-Pituitary-Adrenal (HPA) axis has been observed.

5.2 Pharmacokinetic properties
Single dose intranasal administration of 220 micrograms of NASACORT in normal adult subjects and in adult patients with allergic rhinitis demonstrated low absorption of triamcinolone acetonide. The mean peak plasma concentration was approximately 0.5 ng/ml (range 0.1 to 1 ng/ml) and occurred at 1.5 hours post dose. The mean plasma drug concentration was less than 0.06 ng/ml at 12 hours and below the assay detection limit at 24 hours. The average terminal half life was 3.1 hours. Dose proportionality was demonstrated in normal subjects and in patients following a single intranasal dose of 110 micrograms or 220 micrograms NASACORT. Following multiple doses in paediatric patients, plasma drug concentrations, AUC, Cmax and Tmax were similar to those values observed in adult patients.

5.3 Preclinical safety data
In preclinical studies, only effects typical of glucocorticoids were observed.

Like other corticosteroids, triamcinolone acetonide (administered by inhalation or other routes) has been shown to be teratogenic in rats and rabbits, resulting in cleft palate and/or internal hydrocephaly and axial skeletal defects. Teratogenic effects, including CNS and cranial malformations, have also been observed in non-human primates.

No evidence of mutagenicity was detected in in vitro gene mutation tests.

Carcinogenicity assays in rodents show no increase in the incidence of individual tumour types.

6. PHARMACEUTICAL PARTICULARS

6.1 List of excipients
- microcrystalline cellulose
- carmellose sodium (Avicel CL-611),
- polysorbate 80,
- purified water,
- anhydrous glucose,
- benzalkonium chloride,
- disodium edentate
- hydrochloric acid or sodium hydroxide (for pH-adjustment).

6.2 Incompatibilities
Not applicable

6.3 Shelf life
Unopened: 2 years.

After first opening: 2 months

6.4 Special precautions for storage
Do not store above 25°C.

6.5 Nature and contents of container
NASACORT is contained in a 20 ml high density polyethylene (HDPE) bottle fitted with a metered-dose spray pump unit. Bottles of NASACORT contain 16.5 g of suspension, providing 120 actuations.

6.6 Special precautions for disposal and other handling
No special requirements.

7. MARKETING AUTHORISATION HOLDER
Sanofi-aventis
One Onslow Street
Guildford
Surrey GU1 4YS
UK

8. MARKETING AUTHORISATION NUMBER(S)
PL 04425/0287

9. DATE OF FIRST AUTHORISATION/RENEWAL OF THE AUTHORISATION
19th January 2007

10. DATE OF REVISION OF THE TEXT
March 2007
Legal Category: POM

Naseptin Nasal Cream

(Alliance Pharmaceuticals)

1. NAME OF THE MEDICINAL PRODUCT
Naseptin Nasal Cream

2. QUALITATIVE AND QUANTITATIVE COMPOSITION
Chlorhexidine dihydrochloride PhEur 0.1% w/w and neomycin sulphate PhEur 0.5% w/w.

3. PHARMACEUTICAL FORM
A smooth white cream with a fatty odour.

4. CLINICAL PARTICULARS

4.1 Therapeutic indications
Eradication of nasal infection with, and carriage of, Staphylococci.

4.2 Posology and method of administration
For nasal application only.

A small amount of Naseptin is placed on the little finger and applied to the inside of each nostril.

For prophylaxis: Naseptin is applied as above, twice daily, to prevent patients from becoming carriers and to inhibit the dispersion of Staphylococci.

For eradication of infection: Naseptin is applied four times daily for 10 days to eliminate organisms from the nares.

Children and elderly patients: There are no special dosage recommendations for either children or elderly patients.

4.3 Contraindications
Patients who have previously shown a hypersensitivity reaction to neomycin or chlorhexidine, although such reactions are extremely rare.

4.4 Special warnings and precautions for use
For nasal application only. Keep out of the eyes and ears.

Naseptin contains Arachis oil (peanut oil) and should not be taken/applied by patients known to be allergic to peanut. As there is a possible relationship between allergy to peanut and allergy to Soya, patients with Soya allergy should also avoid Naseptin.

Irritative skin reactions can occasionally occur. Prolonged use of neomycin can lead to skin sensitisation, ototoxicity and nephrotoxicity.

4.5 Interaction with other medicinal products and other forms of interaction
None known.

4.6 Pregnancy and lactation
Chlorhexidine and neomycin cannot be detected in the blood following application of Naseptin and its use is unlikely to have any effect on the foetus or on breast feeding.

4.7 Effects on ability to drive and use machines
None known.

4.8 Undesirable effects
Irritative skin reactions can occasionally occur.

Topical application of neomycin preparations can lead to skin sensitisation in a small number of patients. Prolonged use of neomycin can lead to ototoxicity and nephrotoxicity. Therefore, use with caution in children, elderly patients and patients with impaired hearing.

4.9 Overdose
Accidental ingestion of the contents of a Naseptin tube is unlikely to have any adverse effects on the patient.

5. PHARMACOLOGICAL PROPERTIES

5.1 Pharmacodynamic properties
Chlorhexidine is effective against a wide range of Gram negative and Gram positive vegetative bacteria, yeasts, dermatophyte fungi and lipophilic viruses. It is inactive against bacterial spores except at elevated temperatures.

Neomycin is a rapidly bactericidal aminoglycoside antibiotic effective against Gram positive organisms including staphylococci and a wide range of Gram negative organisms. Strains of *Pseudomonas aeruginosa* are resistant to neomycin, as are fungi and viruses.

5.2 Pharmacokinetic properties
Because of its cationic nature, chlorhexidine binds strongly to the skin, mucosa and other tissues and is thus very poorly absorbed. No detectable blood levels have been found in man following oral use and percutaneous absorption, if it occurs at all, is insignificant.

Neomycin is either not absorbed or is absorbed only minimally through intact skin. Any neomycin which is absorbed will be rapidly excreted by the kidneys in an unchanged state.

5.3 Preclinical safety data
There are no pre-clinical data of relevance to the prescriber which are additional to those already included in other sections of the Summary of Product Characteristics.

6. PHARMACEUTICAL PARTICULARS

6.1 List of excipients
Arachis oil, cetostearyl alcohol, cetostearyl alcohol/ethylene oxide condensate, purified water.

6.2 Incompatibilities
Hypochlorite bleaches may cause brown stains to develop in fabrics which have previously been in contact with preparations containing chlorhexidine.

Chlorhexidine is incompatible with soap and other anionic agents.

6.3 Shelf life
3 years.

6.4 Special precautions for storage
Store below 30°C.

6.5 Nature and contents of container
Collapsible, internally lacquered aluminium tubes of 15g with white food-grade polypropylene screw caps.

6.6 Special precautions for disposal and other handling
For nasal application only.

Administrative Data

7. MARKETING AUTHORISATION HOLDER
Alliance Pharmaceuticals Ltd
Avonbridge House
Bath Road
Chippenham
Wiltshire
SN15 2BB

8. MARKETING AUTHORISATION NUMBER(S)
PL16853/0024

9. DATE OF FIRST AUTHORISATION/RENEWAL OF THE AUTHORISATION
August 1999

10. DATE OF REVISION OF THE TEXT
13th March 2009

11. Legal Status

POM

Alliance, Alliance Pharmaceuticals and associated devices are registered Trademarks of Alliance Pharmaceuticals Ltd.

Natrilix

(Servier Laboratories Limited)

1. NAME OF THE MEDICINAL PRODUCT

NATRILIX 2.5 mg Tablets

2. QUALITATIVE AND QUANTITATIVE COMPOSITION

One tablet contains 2.5 mg Indapamide hemihydrate

Excipient: 57.5mg lactose monohydrate

For a full list of excipients, see section 6.1

3. PHARMACEUTICAL FORM

Tablet

White, round, biconvex, film-coated tablets.

4. CLINICAL PARTICULARS

4.1 Therapeutic indications

For the treatment of essential hypertension. Natrilix may be used as sole therapy or combined with other antihypertensive agents.

4.2 Posology and method of administration

Adults:

The dosage is one tablet, containing 2.5 mg indapamide hemihydrate, daily, to be taken in the morning. The action of Natrilix® is progressive and the reduction in blood pressure may continue and not reach a maximum until several months after the start of therapy. A larger dose than 2.5 mg Natrilix® daily is not recommended as there is no appreciable additional antihypertensive effect but a diuretic effect may become apparent. If a single daily tablet of Natrilix® does not achieve a sufficient reduction in blood pressure, another antihypertensive agent may be added; those which have been used in combination with Natrilix® include beta-blockers, ACE inhibitors, methyldopa, clonidine and other adrenergic blocking agents. The co-administration of Natrilix® with diuretics which may cause hypokalaemia is not recommended.

There is no evidence of rebound hypertension on withdrawal of Natrilix®.

Renal failure: (see sections 4.3 and 4.4)

In severe renal failure (creatinine clearance below 30 ml/min), treatment is contraindicated.

Thiazide and related diuretics are fully effective only when renal function is normal or only minimally impaired.

Elderly(see section 4.4):

In the elderly, the plasma creatinine must be adjusted in relation to age, weight and gender. Elderly patients can be treated with NATRILIX SR when renal function is normal or only minimally impaired.

Patients with hepatic impairment (see sections 4.3 and 4.4):

In severe hepatic impairment, treatment is contraindicated.

Children and adolescents:

NATRILIX 2.5mg is not recommended for use in children and adolescents due to a lack of data on safety and efficacy.

4.3 Contraindications

- Hypersensitivity to indapamide, to other sulfonamides or to any of the excipients.

- Severe renal failure.

- Hepatic encephalopathy or severe impairment of liver function.

- Hypokalaemia.

4.4 Special warnings and precautions for use

Special warnings

When liver function is impaired, thiazide-related diuretics may cause hepatic encephalopathy, particularly in case of electrolyte imbalance. Administration of the diuretic must be stopped immediately if this occurs.

Photosensitivity:

Cases of photosensitivity reactions have been reported with thiazides and thiazide-related diuretics (see section 4.8). If photosensitivity reaction occurs during treatment, it is recommended to stop the treatment. If a re-administration of the diuretic is deemed necessary, it is recommended to protect exposed areas to the sun or to artificial UVA.

Excipients:

Patients with rare hereditary problems of galactose intolerance, the Lapp lactase deficiency or glucose-galactose malabsorption should not take this medicine.

Special precautions for use

- Water and electrolyte balance:

• Plasma sodium:

This must be measured before starting treatment, then at regular intervals subsequently. Any diuretic treatment may cause hyponatraemia, sometimes with very serious consequences. The fall in plasma sodium may be asymptomatic initially and regular monitoring is therefore essential, and should be even more frequent in the elderly and cirrhotic patients (see sections 4.8 and 4.9).

• Plasma potassium:

Potassium depletion with hypokalaemia is the major risk of thiazide and related diuretics. The risk of onset of hypokalaemia (< 3.4 mmol/l) must be prevented in certain high risk populations, *i.e.* the elderly, malnourished and/or polymedicated, cirrhotic patients with oedema and ascites, coronary artery disease and cardiac failure patients. In this situation, hypokalaemia increases the cardiac toxicity of digitalis preparations and the risks of arrhythmias.

Individuals with a long QT interval are also at risk, whether the origin is congenital or iatrogenic. Hypokalaemia, as well as bradycardia, is then a predisposing factor to the onset of severe arrhythmias, in particular, potentially fatal *torsades de pointes*.

More frequent monitoring of plasma potassium is required in all the situations indicated above. The first measurement of plasma potassium should be obtained during the first week following the start of treatment.

Detection of hypokalaemia requires its correction.

• Plasma calcium:

Thiazide and related diuretics may decrease urinary calcium excretion and cause a slight and transitory rise in plasma calcium. Frank hypercalcaemia may be due to previously unrecognised hyperparathyroidism.

Treatment should be withdrawn before the investigation of parathyroid function.

- Blood glucose:

Monitoring of blood glucose is important in diabetics, in particular in the presence of hypokalaemia.

- Uric acid:

Tendency to gout attacks may be increased in hyperuricaemic patients.

- Renal function and diuretics:

Thiazide and related diuretics are fully effective only when renal function is normal or only minimally impaired (plasma creatinine below levels of the order of 25 mg/l, *i.e.* 220 µmol/l in an adult). In the elderly, this plasma creatinine must be adjusted in relation to age, weight and gender.

Hypovolaemia, secondary to the loss of water and sodium induced by the diuretic at the start of treatment causes a reduction in glomerular filtration. This may lead to an increase in blood urea and plasma creatinine. This transitory functional renal insufficiency is of no consequence in individuals with normal renal function but may worsen preexisting renal insufficiency.

- Athletes:

The attention of athletes is drawn to the fact that this medicinal product contains a drug substance, which may give a positive reaction in doping tests.

4.5 Interaction with other medicinal products and other forms of interaction

Combinations that are not recommended:

Lithium:

Increased plasma lithium with signs of overdosage, as with a salt-free diet (decreased urinary lithium excretion). However, if the use of diuretics is necessary, careful monitoring of plasma lithium and dose adjustment are required.

Combinations requiring precautions for use:

Torsades de pointes-inducing drugs:

- class Ia antiarrhythmics (quinidine, hydroquinidine, disopyramide),

- class III antiarrhythmics (amiodarone, sotalol, dofetilide, ibutilide),

- some antipsychotics:

phenothiazines (chlorpromazine, cyamemazine, levomepromazine, thioridazine, trifluoperazine),

benzamides (amisulpride, sulpiride, sultopride, tiapride)

butyrophenones (droperidol, haloperidol)

others: bepridil, cisapride, diphemanil, erythromycin IV, halofantrine, mizolastine, pentamidine, sparfloxacin, moxifloxacin, vincamine IV.

Increased risk of ventricular arrhythmias, particularly *torsades de pointes* (hypokalaemia is a risk factor).

Monitor for hypokalaemia and correct, if required, before introducing this combination. Clinical, plasma electrolytes and ECG monitoring.

Use substances which do not have the disadvantage of causing torsades de pointes in the presence of hypokalaemia.

N.S.A.I.Ds. (systemic route) including COX-2 selective inhibitors, high dose salicylic acid (≥ 3 g/day):

Possible reduction in the antihypertensive effect of indapamide.

Risk of acute renal failure in dehydrated patients (decreased glomerular filtration). Hydrate the patient; monitor renal function at the start of treatment.

Angiotensin converting enzyme (A.C.E.) inhibitors:

Risk of sudden hypotension and/or acute renal failure when treatment with an A.C.E. is initiated in the presence of preexisting sodium depletion (particularly in patients with renal artery stenosis).

In hypertension, when prior diuretic treatment may have caused sodium depletion, it is necessary:

- either to stop the diuretic 3 days before starting treatment with the A.C.E. inhibitor, and restart a hypokalaemic diuretic if necessary;

- or give low initial doses of the A.C.E. inhibitor and increase the dose gradually.

In congestive heart failure, start with a very low dose of A.C.E. inhibitor, possibly after a reduction in the dose of the concomitant hypokalaemic diuretic.

In all cases, monitor renal function (plasma creatinine) during the first weeks of treatment with an A.C.E. inhibitor.

Other compounds causing hypokalaemia: amphotericin B (IV), gluco- and mineralo-corticoids (systemic route), tetracosactide, stimulant laxatives:

Increased risk of hypokalaemia (additive effect).

Monitoring of plasma potassium and correction if required. Must be particularly borne in mind in case of concomitant digitalis treatment. Use non-stimulant laxatives.

Baclofen:

Increased antihypertensive effect.

Hydrate the patient; monitor renal function at the start of treatment.

Digitalis preparations:

Hypokalaemia predisposing to the toxic effects of digitalis.

Monitoring of plasma potassium and ECG and, if necessary, adjust the treatment.

Combinations to be taken into consideration:

Potassium-sparing diuretics (amiloride, spironolactone, triamterene):

Whilst rational combinations are useful in some patients, hypokalaemia (particularly in patients with renal failure or diabetes) or hyperkalaemia may still occur. Plasma potassium and ECG should be monitored and, if necessary, treatment reviewed.

Metformin:

Increased risk of metformin induced lactic acidosis due to the possibility of functional renal failure associated with diuretics and more particularly with loop diuretics. Do not use metformin when plasma creatinine exceeds 15 mg/l (135 µmol/l) in men and 12 mg/l (110 µmol/l) in women.

Iodinated contrast media:

In the presence of dehydration caused by diuretics, increased risk of acute renal failure, in particular when large doses of iodinated contrast media are used.

Rehydration before administration of the iodinated compound.

Imipramine-like antidepressants, neuroleptics:

Antihypertensive effect and increased risk of orthostatic hypotension increased (additive effect).

Calcium (salts):

Risk of hypercalcaemia resulting from decreased urinary elimination of calcium.

Ciclosporin, tacrolimus:

Risk of increased plasma creatinine without any change in circulating cyclosporin levels, even in the absence of water/sodium depletion.

Corticosteroids, tetracosactide (systemic route):

Decreased antihypertensive effect (water/sodium retention due to corticosteroids).

4.6 Pregnancy and lactation

Pregnancy:

As a general rule, the administration of diuretics should be avoided in pregnant women and should never be used to treat physiological oedema of pregnancy. Diuretics can cause foetoplacental ischaemia, with a risk of impaired foetal growth.

Lactation:

Breast-feeding is inadvisable (Indapamide is excreted in human milk).

4.7 Effects on ability to drive and use machines

Indapamide does not affect vigilance but different reactions in relation with the decrease in blood pressure may occur in individual cases, especially at the start of the treatment or when another antihypertensive agent is added.

As a result the ability to drive vehicles or to operate machinery may be impaired.

4.8 Undesirable effects

The majority of adverse reactions concerning clinical or laboratory parameters are dose-dependent.

Thiazide-related diuretics, including indapamide, may cause the following undesirable effects ranked under the following frequency:

Very common (>1/10); common (>1/100, <1/10); uncommon (>1/1000, <1/100); rare (>1/10000, <1/1000), very rare (<1/10000), not known (cannot be estimated from the available data).

Blood and the lymphatic system disorders:

Very rare: thrombocytopenia, leucopenia, agranulocytosis, aplastic anaemia, haemolytic anaemia

Nervous system disorders:

Rare: vertigo, fatigue, headache, paresthesia

Cardiac disorders:

Very rare: arrhythmia, hypotension.

Gastrointestinal disorders:

Uncommon: vomiting

Rare: nausea, constipation, dry mouth

Very rare: pancreatitis

Renal and urinary disorders:

Very rare: renal failure

Hepato-biliary disorders:

Very rare: abnormal hepatic function

Not known: possibility of onset of hepatic encephalopathy in case of hepatic insufficiency (see sections 4.3 and 4.4)

Skin and subcutaneous tissue disorders:

Hypersensitivity reactions, mainly dermatological, in subjects with a predisposition to allergic and asthmatic reactions:

- Common: maculopapular rashes
- Uncommon: purpura
- Very rare: angioneurotic oedema and/or urticaria, toxic epidermic necrolysis, Steven Johnson syndrome

Not known: possible worsening of pre-existing acute disseminated lupus erythematosus.

Cases of photosensitivity reactions have been reported (see section 4.4).

Laboratory parameters:

During clinical trials, hypokalaemia (plasma potassium <3.4 mmol/l) was seen in 10 % of patients and < 3.2 mmol/l in 4 % of patients after 4 to 6 weeks treatment. After 12 weeks treatment, the mean fall in plasma potassium was 0.23 mmol/l.

Very rare: Hypercalcaemia

Not known:

- Potassium depletion with hypokalaemia, particularly serious in certain high risk populations (see section 4.4).
- Hyponatraemia with hypovolaemia responsible for dehydration and orthostatic hypotension. Concomitant loss of chloride ions may lead to secondary compensatory metabolic alkalosis: the incidence and degree of this effect are slight.

Increase in plasma uric acid and blood glucose during treatment: appropriateness of these diuretics must be very carefully weighed in patients with gout or diabetes.

4.9 Overdose

Indapamide has been found free of toxicity at up to 40 mg, *i.e.* 27 times the therapeutic dose.

Signs of acute poisoning take the form above all of water/electrolyte disturbances (hyponatraemia, hypokalaemia). Clinically, possibility of nausea, vomiting, hypotension, cramps, vertigo, drowsiness, confusion, polyuria or oliguria possibly to the point of anuria (by hypovolaemia).

Initial measures involve the rapid elimination of the ingested substance(s) by gastric wash-out and/or administration of activated charcoal, followed by restoration of water/electrolyte balance to normal in a specialised centre.

5. PHARMACOLOGICAL PROPERTIES

5.1 Pharmacodynamic properties

Pharmacotherapeutic group: Sulfonamides, plain

ATC code: C 03 BA 11

Natrilix® (indapamide) is a non-thiazide sulphonamide with an indole ring, belonging to the diuretic family. At the dose of 2.5 mg per day Natrilix® exerts a prolonged antihypertensive activity in hypertensive human subjects.

Dose-effect studies have demonstrated that, at the dose of 2.5 mg per day, the antihypertensive effect is maximal and the diuretic effect is sub-clinical.

At this antihypertensive dose of 2.5 mg per day, Natrilix® reduces vascular hyperreactivity to noradrenaline in hypertensive patients and decreases total peripheral resistance and arteriolar resistance.

The implication of an extrarenal mechanism of action in the antihypertensive effect is demonstrated by maintenance of its antihypertensive efficacy in functionally anephric hypertensive patients.

The vascular mechanism of action of Natrilix® involves:

- a reduction in the contractility of vascular smooth muscle due to a modification of transmembrane ion exchanges, essentially calcium;
- vasodilatation due to stimulation of the synthesis of prostaglandin PGE_2 and the vasodilator and platelet anti-aggregant prostacyclin PGI_2;
- potentiation of the vasodilator action of bradykinin.

It has also been demonstrated that in the short-, medium- and long-term, in hypertensive patients, Natrilix®:

- reduces left ventricular hypertrophy;
- does not appear to alter lipid metabolism: triglycerides, LDL-cholesterol and HDL-cholesterol;
- does not appear to alter glucose metabolism, even in diabetic hypertensive patients. Normalisation of blood pressure and a significant reduction in microalbuminuria have been observed after prolonged administration of Natrilix® in diabetic hypertensive subjects.

Lastly, the co-prescription of Natrilix® with other antihypertensives (beta-blockers, calcium channel blockers, angiotensin converting enzyme inhibitors) results in an improved control of hypertension with an increased percentage of responders compared to that observed with single-agent therapy.

5.2 Pharmacokinetic properties

Indapamide is rapidly and completely absorbed after oral administration. Peak blood levels are obtained after 1 to 2 hours.

Indapamide is concentrated in the erythrocytes and is 79% bound to plasma protein and to erythrocytes. It is taken up by the vascular wall in smooth vascular muscle according to its high lipid solubility. 70% of a single oral dose is eliminated by the kidneys and 23% by the gastrointestinal tract. Indapamide is metabolised to a marked degree with 7% of the unchanged product found in the urine during the 48 hours following administration. Elimination half-life (β phase) of indapamide is approximately 15 - 18 hours.

5.3 Preclinical safety data

No findings in the preclinical testing which could be of relevance for the prescriber.

6. PHARMACEUTICAL PARTICULARS

6.1 List of excipients

Tablet

Lactose monohydrate,

maize starch,

magnesium stearate,

talc,

povidone.

Tablet Coating:

glycerol,

white beeswax,

sodium lauryl sulphate,

methylhydroxypropylcellulose,

polyoxyethylene glycol 6000,

magnesium stearate,

titanium dioxide.

6.2 Incompatibilities

Not applicable

6.3 Shelf life

5 years.

6.4 Special precautions for storage

This medicinal product does not require any special storage conditions.

6.5 Nature and contents of container

30 tablet pack: 1 blister strip (PVC / Aluminium) of 30 tablets per carton.

60 tablet pack: 2 blister strips (PVC / Aluminium) of 30 tablets per carton.

6.6 Special precautions for disposal and other handling

No special requirements

7. MARKETING AUTHORISATION HOLDER

Servier Laboratories Ltd

Gallions, Wexham Springs

Framewood Road, Wexham

Slough

SL3 6RJ

8. MARKETING AUTHORISATION NUMBER(S)

PL 0093/0022

9. DATE OF FIRST AUTHORISATION/RENEWAL OF THE AUTHORISATION

20 December 1977

10. DATE OF REVISION OF THE TEXT

01/2008

Natrilix SR

(Servier Laboratories Limited)

1. NAME OF THE MEDICINAL PRODUCT

NATRILIX® SR 1.5 mg Tablets

2. QUALITATIVE AND QUANTITATIVE COMPOSITION

Indapamide: 1.5 mg per prolonged-release film-coated tablet

Excipient: 124.5 mg lactose monohydrate

For a full list of excipients, see section 6.1.

3. PHARMACEUTICAL FORM

Prolonged-release tablet.

White, round, film-coated tablet.

4. CLINICAL PARTICULARS

4.1 Therapeutic indications

Essential hypertension.

4.2 Posology and method of administration

Oral use.

One tablet per 24 hours, preferably in the morning, to be swallowed whole with water and not chewed.

At higher doses the antihypertensive action of indapamide is not enhanced but the saluretic effect is increased.

Renal failure (see sections 4.3 and 4.4):

In severe renal failure (creatinine clearance below 30 ml/min), treatment is contraindicated.

Thiazide and related diuretics are fully effective only when renal function is normal or only minimally impaired.

Elderly (see section 4.4):

In the elderly, the plasma creatinine must be adjusted in relation to age, weight and gender. Elderly patients can be treated with NATRILIX SR when renal function is normal or only minimally impaired.

Patients with hepatic impairment (see sections 4.3 and 4.4):

In severe hepatic impairment, treatment is contraindicated.

Children and adolescents:

NATRILIX SR is not recommended for use in children and adolescents due to a lack of data on safety and efficacy.

4.3 Contraindications

- Hypersensitivity to indapamide, to other sulfonamides or to any of the excipients.
- Severe renal failure.
- Hepatic encephalopathy or severe impairment of liver function.
- Hypokalaemia.

4.4 Special warnings and precautions for use

Special warnings

When liver function is impaired, thiazide-related diuretics may cause hepatic encephalopathy, particularly in case of electrolyte imbalance. Administration of the diuretic must be stopped immediately if this occurs.

Photosensitivity:

Cases of photosensitivity reactions have been reported with thiazides and thiazide-related diuretics (see section 4.8). If photosensitivity reaction occurs during treatment, it is recommended to stop the treatment. If a re-administration of the diuretic is deemed necessary, it is recommended to protect exposed areas to the sun or to artificial UVA.

Excipients:

Patients with rare hereditary problems of galactose intolerance, the Lapp lactase deficiency or glucose-galactose malabsorption should not take this medicine.

Special precautions for use

- Water and electrolyte balance:

- Plasma sodium:

This must be measured before starting treatment, then at regular intervals subsequently. Any diuretic treatment may cause hyponatraemia, sometimes with very serious consequences. The fall in plasma sodium may be asymptomatic initially and regular monitoring is therefore essential, and should be even more frequent in the elderly and cirrhotic patients (see sections 4.8 and 4.9).

- Plasma potassium:

Potassium depletion with hypokalaemia is the major risk of thiazide and related diuretics. The risk of onset of hypokalaemia (< 3.4 mmol/l) must be prevented in certain high risk populations, *i.e.* the elderly, malnourished and/or polymedicated, cirrhotic patients with oedema and ascites, coronary artery disease and cardiac failure patients. In this situation, hypokalaemia increases the cardiac toxicity of digitalis preparations and the risks of arrhythmias.

Individuals with a long QT interval are also at risk, whether the origin is congenital or iatrogenic. Hypokalaemia, as well as bradycardia, is then a predisposing factor to the onset of severe arrhythmias, in particular, potentially fatal *torsades de pointes*.

More frequent monitoring of plasma potassium is required in all the situations indicated above. The first measurement of plasma potassium should be obtained during the first week following the start of treatment.

Detection of hypokalaemia requires its correction.

- Plasma calcium:

Thiazide and related diuretics may decrease urinary calcium excretion and cause a slight and transitory rise in plasma calcium. Frank hypercalcaemia may be due to previously unrecognised hyperparathyroidism.

Treatment should be withdrawn before the investigation of parathyroid function.

- Blood glucose:

Monitoring of blood glucose is important in diabetics, in particular in the presence of hypokalaemia.

- Uric acid:

Tendency to gout attacks may be increased in hyperuricaemic patients.

- Renal function and diuretics:

Thiazide and related diuretics are fully effective only when renal function is normal or only minimally impaired (plasma creatinine below levels of the order of 25 mg/l, *i.e.*

220 µmol/l in an adult). In the elderly, this plasma creatinine must be adjusted in relation to age, weight and gender.

Hypovolaemia, secondary to the loss of water and sodium induced by the diuretic at the start of treatment causes a reduction in glomerular filtration. This may lead to an increase in blood urea and plasma creatinine. This transitory functional renal insufficiency is of no consequence in individuals with normal renal function but may worsen preexisting renal insufficiency.

- Athletes:

The attention of athletes is drawn to the fact that this medicinal product contains a drug substance, which may give a positive reaction in doping tests.

4.5 Interaction with other medicinal products and other forms of interaction

Combinations that are not recommended:

Lithium:

Increased plasma lithium with signs of overdosage, as with a salt-free diet (decreased urinary lithium excretion). However, if the use of diuretics is necessary, careful monitoring of plasma lithium and dose adjustment are required.

Combinations requiring precautions for use:

Torsades de pointes-inducing drugs:

- class Ia antiarrhythmics (quinidine, hydroquinidine, disopyramide),

- class III antiarrhythmics (amiodarone, sotalol, dofetilide, ibutilide),

- some antipsychotics:

phenothiazines (chlorpromazine, cyamemazine, levomepromazine, thioridazine, trifluoperazine),

benzamides (amisulpride, sulpiride, sultopride, tiapride)

butyrophenones (droperidol, haloperidol)

others: bepridil, cisapride, diphemanil, erythromycin IV, halofantrine, mizolastine, pentamidine, sparfloxacin, moxifloxacin, vincamine IV.

Increased risk of ventricular arrhythmias, particularly *torsades de pointes* (hypokalaemia is a risk factor).

Monitor for hypokalaemia and correct, if required, before introducing this combination. Clinical, plasma electrolytes and ECG monitoring.

Use substances which do not have the disadvantage of causing torsades de pointes in the presence of hypokalaemia.

N.S.A.I.Ds. (systemic route) including COX-2 selective inhibitors, high dose salicylic acid (⩾ 3 g/day):

Possible reduction in the antihypertensive effect of indapamide.

Risk of acute renal failure in dehydrated patients (decreased glomerular filtration). Hydrate the patient; monitor renal function at the start of treatment.

Angiotensin converting enzyme (A.C.E.) inhibitors:

Risk of sudden hypotension and/or acute renal failure when treatment with an A.C.E. is initiated in the presence of preexisting sodium depletion (particularly in patients with renal artery stenosis).

In hypertension, when prior diuretic treatment may have caused sodium depletion, it is necessary:

- either to stop the diuretic 3 days before starting treatment with the A.C.E. inhibitor, and restart a hypokalaemic diuretic if necessary;

- or give low initial doses of the A.C.E. inhibitor and increase the dose gradually.

In congestive heart failure, start with a very low dose of A.C.E. inhibitor, possibly after a reduction in the dose of the concomitant hypokalaemic diuretic.

In all cases, monitor renal function (plasma creatinine) during the first weeks of treatment with an A.C.E. inhibitor.

Other compounds causing hypokalaemia: amphotericin B (IV), gluco- and mineralo-corticoids (systemic route), tetracosactide, stimulant laxatives:

Increased risk of hypokalaemia (additive effect).

Monitoring of plasma potassium and correction if required. Must be particularly borne in mind in case of concomitant digitalis treatment. Use non-stimulant laxatives.

Baclofen:

Increased antihypertensive effect.

Hydrate the patient; monitor renal function at the start of treatment.

Digitalis preparations:

Hypokalaemia predisposing to the toxic effects of digitalis.

Monitoring of plasma potassium and ECG and, if necessary, adjust the treatment.

Combinations to be taken into consideration:

Potassium-sparing diuretics (amiloride, spironolactone, triamterene):

Whilst rational combinations are useful in some patients, hypokalaemia (particularly in patients with renal failure or diabetes) or hyperkalaemia may still occur. Plasma potassium and ECG should be monitored and, if necessary, treatment reviewed.

Metformin:

Increased risk of metformin induced lactic acidosis due to the possibility of functional renal failure associated with diuretics and more particularly with loop diuretics. Do not use metformin when plasma creatinine exceeds 15 mg/l (135 µmol/l) in men and 12 mg/l (110 µmol/l) in women.

Iodinated contrast media:

In the presence of dehydration caused by diuretics, increased risk of acute renal failure, in particular when large doses of iodinated contrast media are used.

Rehydration before administration of the iodinated compound.

Imipramine-like antidepressants, neuroleptics:

Antihypertensive effect and increased risk of orthostatic hypotension increased (additive effect).

Calcium (salts):

Risk of hypercalcaemia resulting from decreased urinary elimination of calcium.

Ciclosporin, tacrolimus:

Risk of increased plasma creatinine without any change in circulating cyclosporin levels, even in the absence of water/sodium depletion.

Corticosteroids, tetracosactide (systemic route):

Decreased antihypertensive effect (water/sodium retention due to corticosteroids).

4.6 Pregnancy and lactation

Pregnancy:

As a general rule, the administration of diuretics should be avoided in pregnant women and should never be used to treat physiological oedema of pregnancy. Diuretics can cause foetoplacental ischaemia, with a risk of impaired foetal growth.

Lactation:

Breast-feeding is inadvisable (Indapamide is excreted in human milk).

4.7 Effects on ability to drive and use machines

Indapamide does not affect vigilance but different reactions in relation with the decrease in blood pressure may occur in individual cases, especially at the start of the treatment or when another antihypertensive agent is added.

As a result the ability to drive vehicles or to operate machinery may be impaired.

4.8 Undesirable effects

The majority of adverse reactions concerning clinical or laboratory parameters are dose-dependent.

Thiazide-related diuretics, including indapamide, may cause the following undesirable effects ranked under the following frequency:

Very common (>1/10); common (>1/100, <1/10); uncommon (>1/1000, <1/100); rare (>1/10000, <1/1000), very rare (<1/10000), not known (cannot be estimated from the available data).

Blood and the lymphatic system disorders:

Very rare: thrombocytopenia, leucopenia, agranulocytosis, aplastic anaemia, haemolytic anaemia

Nervous system disorders:

Rare: vertigo, fatigue, headache, paresthesia

Cardiac disorders:

Very rare: arrhythmia, hypotension.

Gastrointestinal disorders:

Uncommon: vomiting

Rare: nausea, constipation, dry mouth

Very rare: pancreatitis

Renal and urinary disorders:

Very rare: renal failure

Hepato-biliary disorders:

Very rare: abnormal hepatic function

Not known: possibility of onset of hepatic encephalopathy in case of hepatic insufficiency (see sections 4.3 and 4.4)

Skin and subcutaneous tissue disorders:

Hypersensitivity reactions, mainly dermatological, in subjects with a predisposition to allergic and asthmatic reactions:

- Common: maculopapular rashes

- Uncommon: purpura

- Very rare: angioneurotic oedema and/or urticaria, toxic epidermic necrolysis, Steven Johnson syndrome

Not known: possible worsening of pre-existing acute disseminated lupus erythematosus.

Cases of photosensitivity reactions have been reported (see section 4.4).

Laboratory parameters:

During clinical trials, hypokalaemia (plasma potassium <3.4 mmol/l) was seen in 10 % of patients and < 3.2 mmol/l in 4 % of patients after 4 to 6 weeks treatment. After 12 weeks treatment, the mean fall in plasma potassium was 0.23 mmol/l.

Very rare: Hypercalcaemia

Not known:

- Potassium depletion with hypokalaemia, particularly serious in certain high risk populations (see section 4.4).

- Hyponatraemia with hypovolaemia responsible for dehydration and orthostatic hypotension. Concomitant loss of chloride ions may lead to secondary compensatory metabolic alkalosis: the incidence and degree of this effect are slight.

- Increase in plasma uric acid and blood glucose during treatment: appropriateness of these diuretics must be very carefully weighed in patients with gout or diabetes.

4.9 Overdose

Indapamide has been found free of toxicity at up to 40 mg, *i.e.* 27 times the therapeutic dose.

Signs of acute poisoning take the form above all of water/electrolyte disturbances (hyponatraemia, hypokalaemia). Clinically, possibility of nausea, vomiting, hypotension, cramps, vertigo, drowsiness, confusion, polyuria or oliguria possibly to the point of anuria (by hypovolaemia).

Initial measures involve the rapid elimination of the ingested substance(s) by gastric wash-out and/or administration of activated charcoal, followed by restoration of water/electrolyte balance to normal in a specialised centre.

5. PHARMACOLOGICAL PROPERTIES

5.1 Pharmacodynamic properties

Pharmacotherapeutic group: Sulfonamides, plain

ATC code: C 03 BA 11

Indapamide is a sulphonamide derivative with an indole ring, pharmacologically related to thiazide diuretics, which acts by inhibiting the reabsorption of sodium in the cortical dilution segment. It increases the urinary excretion of sodium and chlorides and, to a lesser extent, the excretion of potassium and magnesium, thereby increasing urine output and having an antihypertensive action.

Phase II and III studies using monotherapy have demonstrated an antihypertensive effect lasting 24 hours. This was present at doses where the diuretic effect was of mild intensity.

The antihypertensive activity of indapamide is related to an improvement in arterial compliance and a reduction in arteriolar and total peripheral resistance.

Indapamide reduces left ventricular hypertrophy.

Thiazide and related diuretics have a plateau therapeutic effect beyond a certain dose, while adverse effects continue to increase. The dose should not be increased if treatment is ineffective.

It has also been shown, in the short-, mid- and long-term in hypertensive patients, that indapamide:

. does not interfere with lipid metabolism: triglycerides, LDL-cholesterol and HDL-cholesterol;

. does not interfere with carbohydrate metabolism, even in diabetic hypertensive patients.

5.2 Pharmacokinetic properties

Indapamide 1.5 mg is supplied in a prolonged release dosage based on a matrix system in which the drug substance is dispersed within a support which allows sustained release of indapamide.

Absorption:

The fraction of indapamide released is rapidly and totally absorbed via the gastrointestinal digestive tract.

Eating slightly increases the rapidity of absorption but has no influence on the amount of the drug absorbed.

Peak serum level following a single dose occurs about 12 hours after ingestion, repeated administration reduces the variation in serum levels between 2 doses. Intra-individual variability exists.

Distribution:

Binding of indapamide to plasma proteins is 79%.

The plasma elimination half-life is 14 to 24 hours (mean 18 hours).

Steady state is achieved after 7 days.

Repeated administration does not lead to accumulation.

Metabolism:

Elimination is essentially urinary (70% of the dose) and faecal (22%) in the form of inactive metabolites.

High risk individuals:

Pharmacokinetic parameters are unchanged in renal failure patients.

5.3 Preclinical safety data

The highest doses administered orally to different animal species (40 to 8000 times the therapeutic dose) have shown an exacerbation of the diuretic properties of indapamide. The major symptoms of poisoning during acute toxicity studies with indapamide administered intravenously or intraperitoneally were related to the pharmacological action of indapamide, *i.e.* bradypnoea and peripheral vasodilation.

Indapamide has been tested negative concerning mutagenic and carcinogenic properties.

6. PHARMACEUTICAL PARTICULARS

6.1 List of excipients

Tablet:

Silica, colloidal anhydrous

Hypromellose

Lactose monohydrate

Magnesium stearate

Povidone

Film-coating:

Glycerol

Hypromellose

Macrogol 6000

Magnesium stearate

Titanium dioxide

6.2 Incompatibilities
Not applicable

6.3 Shelf life
2 years.

6.4 Special precautions for storage
Store below 30°C.

6.5 Nature and contents of container
10, 14, 15, 20, 30, 50, 60, 90, 100 tablets in blisters (PVC/aluminium).

Not all pack sizes may be marketed.

6.6 Special precautions for disposal and other handling
No special requirements

7. MARKETING AUTHORISATION HOLDER
Les Laboratoires Servier

22 rue Garnier

92200 Neuilly Sur Seine

France

8. MARKETING AUTHORISATION NUMBER(S)
PL 05815/0010

9. DATE OF FIRST AUTHORISATION/RENEWAL OF THE AUTHORISATION
9th January 1996/25th February 2007 (MRP)

10. DATE OF REVISION OF THE TEXT
March 2008

Navelbine 10 mg / ml concentrate for solution for infusion

(Pierre Fabre Limited)

1. NAME OF THE MEDICINAL PRODUCT
NAVELBINE 10 mg / ml concentrate for solution for infusion

2. QUALITATIVE AND QUANTITATIVE COMPOSITION
Vinorelbine 10 mg/ml as vinorelbine tartrate

Each 1ml vial contains 10 mg Vinorelbine as vinorelbine tartrate

Each 4ml vial contains 40 mg Vinorelbine as vinorelbine tartrate

Each 5ml vial contains 50 mg Vinorelbine as vinorelbine tartrate

For a full list of excipients, see section 6.1

3. PHARMACEUTICAL FORM
Concentrate for solution for infusion.

NAVELBINE is a clear colourless to pale yellow solution with a pH range from 3.3 to 3.8.

4. CLINICAL PARTICULARS

4.1 Therapeutic indications
- As a single agent or in combination for the first line treatment of stage 3 or 4 non small cell lung cancer.

- Treatment of advanced breast cancer stage 3 and 4 relapsing after or refractory to an anthracycline containing regimen.

4.2 Posology and method of administration
FOR INTRAVENOUS USE ONLY AFTER APPROPRIATE DILUTION.

The use of intrathecal route is contra-indicated: see section 4.4

NAVELBINE must only be administered by the intravenous route as an infusion over 5 – 10 minutes.

Instructions for use and handling: see section 6.6.

Administration
- It is recommended to infuse NAVELBINE over 5 to 10 minutes after dilution in a 50 ml infusion bag with sodium chloride 9 mg/ml (0.9%) solution for injection or in 5% glucose solution for injection.

- Administration should always be followed with at least 250 ml of a normal saline infusion to flush the vein.

- The infusion time of 5 to 10 minutes must be followed as the risk of venous irritation is increased if the infusion exposure time is increased.

- It is vital to ensure that the cannula is accurately placed in the vein before starting to infuse Navelbine. If the drug extravasates into the surrounding tissue during the administration considerable local irritation may occur. In this case, the administration should be stopped, the vein flushed with 0.9 % sodium chloride solution and the remaining dose administered in another vein.

The management of any extravasation should be according to local hospital guidelines and policies.

In adults:
NAVELBINE is usually given at 25-30mg/m^2 weekly.

__Advanced non-small cell lung cancer and advanced breast cancer__
- In monotherapy the usual dose given is 25-30 mg/m^2 once weekly.

- In combination chemotherapy the usual dose (25-30 mg/m^2) is usually maintained, while the frequency of administration is reduced e.g. day 1 and 5 every 3 weeks or day 1 and 8 every 3 weeks according to treatment protocol.

Administration in the elderly
Clinical experience has not detected any significant differences among elderly patients with regard to the response rate, although greater sensitivity in some of these patients cannot be excluded. Age does not modify the pharmacokinetics of vinorelbine: see section 5.2.

Administration in patients with liver insufficiency
For patients presenting with severe liver impairment (bilirubin > 2xUNL and/or transaminases > 5xUNL), it is suggested that the dose be reduced by 33% and the haematological parameters closely monitored since the maximum dose which was evaluated in this subset of patients was 20 mg/m^2: see sections: 4.4;: 5.2.

Administration in patients with renal insufficiency
Given the minor renal excretion, there is no pharmacokinetic justification for reducing the dose of Navelbine in patients with renal insufficiency: see section 4.4:

Administration in children
Navelbine is not recommended for use in children due to a lack of data on safety and efficacy: see section 5.1.

4.3 Contraindications
- Known hypersensitivity to vinorelbine or other vinca alkaloids, or to any of the excipients.

- Neutrophil count < 1500/mm^3 or severe infection current or recent (within 2 weeks)

- Platelet count < 75000/mm^3

- In combination with yellow fever vaccine: see section 4.5

- Pregnancy: see section 4.6

- Lactation: see section 4.6

4.4 Special warnings and precautions for use
Special warnings
NAVELBINE must only be administered by the intravenous route as an infusion over 5 – 10 minutes.

The use of intrathecal route is contra-indicated.

NAVELBINE should be administered under the supervision of a physician experienced in the use of chemotherapy.

The risk of venous irritation is increased if the infusion exposure time exceeds the recommendation time of 5 to 10 minutes.

Since inhibition of the hematopoietic system is the main risk associated with NAVELBINE, close haematological monitoring should be undertaken during treatment (determination of haemoglobin level and the leukocyte, neutrophil and platelet counts on the day of each new administration).

The dose limiting adverse reaction is mainly neutropenia. This effect is non-cumulative, having its nadir between 7 and 14 days after the administration and is rapidly reversible within 5 to 7 days. If the neutrophil count is below 1500/mm^{3}and/or the platelet count is below 75,000/mm^3, then the treatment should be delayed until recovery.

If patients present signs or symptoms suggestive of infection, a prompt investigation should be carried out.

Precautions for use
Special care should be taken when prescribing for patients with history of ischemic heart disease: see section 4.8.

The pharmacokinetics of NAVELBINE is not modified in patients presenting moderate or severe liver impairment: see section 5.2.

For dosage adjustment in this specific patient group, see section 4.2.

As there is a low level of renal excretion there is no pharmacokinetic rationale for reducing the dose of NAVELBINE in patients with impaired kidney function: see sections 4.2, 5.2.

NAVELBINE should not be given concomitantly with radiotherapy if the treatment field includes the liver.

This product is specifically contra-indicated with yellow fever vaccine and its concomitant use with other live attenuated vaccines is not recommended.

Caution must be exercised when combining Navelbine and strong inhibitors or inducers of CYP3A4: see section 4.5, and its combination with phenytoin (like all cytotoxics) and with itraconazole (like all vinca alkaloids) is not recommended.

All contact with the eyes should be strictly avoided. There is a risk of severe irritation and even corneal ulceration if the drug is sprayed under pressure. Immediate washing of the eye with normal saline solution should be undertaken if any contact occurs.

4.5 Interaction with other medicinal products and other forms of interaction
Concomitant use contraindicated
__Yellow fever vaccine__: as with all cytotoxics, risk of fatal generalised vaccine disease: see section 4.3.

Concomitant use not recommended
__Live attenuated vaccines__: (for yellow fever vaccine, see concomitant use contraindicated) as with all cytotoxics, risk of generalised vaccine disease, possibly fatal. This risk is increased in patients already immunodepressed by their underlying disease. It is recommended to use an inactivated vaccine when one exists (e.g. poliomyelitis): see section 4.4

__Phenytoin__: as with all cytotoxics, risk of exacerbation of convulsions resulting from the decrease of phenytoin digestive absorption by cytotoxic drug or risk of toxicity enhancement or loss of efficacy of the cytotoxic drug due to increased hepatic metabolism by phenytoin.

__Itraconazole__: as with all vinca-alkaloids, increased neurotoxicity of vinca-alkaloids due to the decrease of their hepatic metabolism.

Concomitant use to take into consideration
__Cisplatin__: There is no mutual pharmacokinetic interaction when combining NAVELBINE with cisplatin over several cycles of treatment. However, the incidence of granulocytopenia associated with NAVELBINE use in combination with cisplatin is higher than associated with NAVELBINE single agent.

__Mitomycin C__: as with all vinca-alkaloids, increased risk of pulmonary toxicity Caution is advised when using vinorelbine and mitomycin C simultaneously.

The combination of NAVELBINE with other drugs with known bone marrow toxicity is likely to exacerbate the myelosuppressive adverse effects.

As CYP 3A4 is mainly involved in the metabolism of vinorelbine, combination with strong inhibitors of this isoenzyme (e.g. azole antifungals such as ketoconazole and itraconazole) could increase blood concentrations of vinorelbine and combination with strong inducers of this isoenzyme (e.g. rifampicin, phenytoin) could decrease blood concentrations of vinorelbine.

__Anticoagulant treatment__: as with all cytotoxics, the frequency of INR (International Normalised Ratio) monitoring should be increased due to the potential interaction with oral anticoagulants and increased variability of coagulation in patients with cancer.

4.6 Pregnancy and lactation
Pregnancy:

Navelbine is suspected to cause serious birth effects when administered during pregnancy: see section 5.3.

Navelbine is contraindicated in pregnancy: see section 4.3.

In case of a vital indication for treatment with Navelbine during pregnancy a medical consultation concerning the risk of harmful effects for the child should be conducted. If pregnancy occurs during treatment genetic counselling should be offered.

Women of child-bearing potential

Women of child-bearing potential have to use effective contraception during treatment and up to 3 months after treatment: see section 4.3.

Lactation:

It is unknown whether Navelbine is excreted in human breast milk. The excretion of Navelbine in milk has not been studied in animal studies.

A risk to the suckling can not be excluded therefore breast feeding must be discontinued before starting treatment with Navelbine: see section 4.3.

Fertility:

Men being treated with Navelbine are advised not to father a child during and up to 3 months after treatment: see section 4.3.

4.7 Effects on ability to drive and use machines
No studies on the effects on the ability to drive and use machines have been performed.

On the basis of the vinorelbine pharmacodynamic profile, Navelbine is unlikely to impair the ability to drive or operate machinery. However, caution is necessary in patients treated with Navelbine considering some side effects of the drug: see section 4.8.

4.8 Undesirable effects
Adverse reactions reported as more than isolated cases are listed below, by system organ class and by the MedRA frequency. Additional Adverse reactions from Post Marketing experience has been added according to the MedDRA classification with the frequency *Not known.*

Very common	>1/10
Common	>1/100, <1/10
Uncommon	>1/1,000, <1/100
Rare	>1/10,000, <1/1,000
Very rare	<1/10,000), including isolated reports
Not known	Post marketing reports

__See table of adverse reactions__

The most commonly reported adverse drug reactions are bone marrow depression with neutropenia, anaemia, neurologic disorders, gastrointestinal toxicity with nausea,

Table 1

System organ class (MedDRA classification)	Very common (⩾ 1/10)	Common (⩾ 1/100 and <1/10)	Uncommon (⩾ 1/1,000, ⩽ 1/100)	Rare (> 1/10,000, ⩽ 1/1,000)	Very Rare (<1/10,000	Not known
Infections and infestations		Infection viral, bacterial, or fungal	Severe sepsis with other visceral failure Septicaemia		Complicated septicaemia Septicaemia fatal	
Blood and lymphatic system disorders	Bone marrow depression Neuropenia Anaemia	Thrombocytopenia				Febrile neutropenia
Immune system disorders						Systemic allergic reactions
Endocrine disorders						Inappropriate antidiuretic hormone secretion (SIADH)
Metabolism and nutrition disorders				Severe hyponatraemia		Anorexia
Nervous system disorders	Neurologic disorders Weakness of the lower extremities		Severe paresthesias			
Cardiac disorders				Ischemic heart disease Angina pectoris Myocardial infarction	Tachycardia Palpitations Heart rhythm disorders	
Vascular disorders			Hypotension, Hypertension Flushing Peripheral coldness	Severe hypotension, Collapse		
Respiratory system, thoracic and mediastinal disorders			Dyspnoea Bronchospasm	Interstitial pneumopathy		
Gastrointestinal disorders	Stomatitis, Nausea Vomiting, Constipation	Diarrhoea		Paralytic ileus Pancreatitis		
Hepatobiliary disorders	Transient elevations of liver function tests					
Skin and subcutaneous tissue disorders	Alopecia			Generalized cutaneous reactions		
Musculoskeletal and connective tissue disorders		Arthralgia including jaw pain and myalgia				
General disorders and administration site conditions:	Reactions at injection site as: Erythema Burning pain Vein discoloration Local phlebitis	Fatigue, Fever, Pain at different sites, Chest pain and Pain at tumour site		Local necrosis		

vomiting, stomatitis and constipation, Transient elevations of liver function tests, alopecia and local phlebitis.

Infections and infestations

Common: Infection bacterial, viral or fungal at different sites.

Uncommon: Septicaemia [very rarely fatal].

Blood and lymphatic system disorders:

Very Common: Bone marrow depression resulting mainly in neutropenia reversible within 5 to 7 days and noncumulative over time.

- Anaemia

Common: Thrombocytopenia.

Not known: Febrile neutropenia

Immune system disorders

Not known: Systemic allergic reactions as anaphylaxis, anaphylactic shock or anaphylactoïd type reaction.

Endocrine disorders

Not known: Inappropriate antidiuretic hormone secretion (SIADH)

Metabolism and nutrition disorders

Rare: Severe hyponatraemia

Not known: Anorexia

Nervous system disorders

Very Common: Neurologic disorders including loss of deep tendon reflexes.

- Weakness of the lower extremities has been reported after a prolonged chemotherapy.

Uncommon: Severe paresthesias with sensory and motor symptoms. These effects are generally reversible upon discontinuation of treatment.

Cardiac disorders

Rare: Ischemic heart disease: angina pectoris, myocardial infarction.

Very rare: Tachycardia, palpitation and heart rhythm disorders.

Vascular disorders

Uncommon: Hypotension.

- Hypertension.

- Flushing and peripheral coldness.

Rare: Severe hypotension

- Collapse.

Respiratory system, thoracic and mediastinal disorders

Uncommon: Dyspnoea and bronchospasm may occur in association with Navelbine treatment.

Rare: Interstitial pneumonopathies have been reported in particular in patients treated with Navelbine in combination with mitomycin.

Gastrointestinal disorders

Very Common: Stomatitis.

- Nausea and vomiting

- Constipation

Common: Diarrhoea.

Rare: Paralytic ileus, treatment may be resumed after recovery of normal bowel mobility.

- Pancreatitis.

Hepatobiliary disorders

Very common: Transient elevations of liver function tests without clinical symptoms were reported.

Skin and subcutaneous tissue disorders

Very common: Alopecia, usually mild in nature, may occur

Rare: Generalized cutaneous reactions

Musculoskeletal and connective tissue disorders

Common: Arthralgia including jaw pain and myalgia.

General disorders and administration site conditions

Very common: Reactions at the injection site may include erythema, burning pain, vein discoloration and local phlebitis

Common: Fatigue, fever, pain at different sites including chest pain and pain at the tumour site.

Rare: Local necrosis has been observed. Proper positioning of the cannula in the vein before starting to infuse Navelbine followed by liberal flushing of the vein can limit these effects.

(see Table 1 above)

4.9 Overdose

Symptoms

Overdosage with Navelbine could produce bone marrow hypoplasia sometimes associated with infection, fever and paralytic ileus.

Emergency procedure

General supportive measures together with blood transfusion and broad spectrum antibiotic therapy should be instituted as deemed necessary by the physician.

Antidote

There is no known antidote for overdosage of NAVELBINE.

5. PHARMACOLOGICAL PROPERTIES

5.1 Pharmacodynamic properties

Pharmacotherapeutic group: Vinca alkaloïds and analogues

ATC Code: L01C A04

NAVELBINE is an antineoplastic drug of the vinca alkaloid family but unlike all the other vinca alkaloids, the catharantine moiety of vinorelbine has been structurally modified. At the molecular level, it acts on the dynamic equilibrium of tubulin in the microtubular apparatus of the cell. It inhibits tubulin polymerization and binds preferentially to mitotic microtubules, affecting axonal microtubules at high concentrations only. The induction of tubulin spiralization is less than that produced by vincristine.

NAVELBINE blocks mitosis at G2-M, causing cell death in interphase or at the following mitosis.

Safety and efficacy of Navelbine in paediatric patients have not been established. Clinical data from a single- arm study in 46 patients with recurrent solid tumours, including rhabdomyosarcoma / undifferentiated sarcoma, neuroblastoma, and CNS tumours, at doses similar to those used in adults showed no meaningful clinical activity. Toxicities were similar to those reported in adult patients: see section 4.2.

5.2 Pharmacokinetic properties

Pharmacokinetic parameters of vinorelbine were evaluated in blood.

Table 2 List of excipients

EXCIPIENTS	FORMULATION		
	10 mg / 1 ml	40 mg / 4 ml	50 mg / 5 ml
Water for injections (ml) qs	1.00	4.00	5.00
Nitrogen qs	Inert filling	Inert filling	Inert filling

Distribution

The steady-state volume of distribution is large, on average 21.2 l/h/kg (range: 7.5-39.7 l/h/kg), which indicates extensive tissue distribution.

Vinorelbine has high affinity for platelets and lymphocytes. Binding to plasma protein is low (13.5%). However, vinorelbine binds strongly to blood cells and especially to platelets (78%) of the total blood-bound vinorelbine was associated with platelets and 4.8% of the total blood-bound vinorelbine was associated with lymphocytes.

There is significant uptake of vinorelbine in the lungs, as assessed by surgical lung biopsies, which showed concentrations up to 300-fold higher than in serum. Vinorelbine is not found in the central nervous system.

Biotransformation

All metabolites of vinorelbine are formed by CYP 3A4 isoform of cytochromes P450, except 4-O-deacetylvinorelbine likely to be formed by carboxylesterases. 4-O-deacetylvinorelbine is the only active metabolite and the main one observed in blood.

Neither sulfate nor glucuronide conjugates are found.

Elimination

The mean terminal half-life of vinorelbine is around 40 hours. Blood clearance is high, approaching hepatic blood flow, and is 0.72 l/h/kg on average (range: 0.32 – 1.26 l/h/kg).

Renal elimination is low (< 20% of the intravenous dose administered) and consists mostly in parent compound. Biliary excretion is the predominant elimination route of unchanged vinorelbine, which is the main recovered compound, and its metabolites.

Special patient groups

Renal impairment

The effects of renal dysfunction on the pharmacokinetics of vinorelbine have not been studied. However, dose reduction in case of reduced renal function is not indicated due to the low renal elimination.

Liver impairment

A first study has reported the effects of liver impairment on vinorelbine pharmacokinetics. This study was performed in patients with liver metastases due to breast cancer, and concluded that a change in mean clearance of vinorelbine was only observed when more than 75% of the liver is involved.

A phase I pharmacokinetic dose-adjusted study was conducted in cancer patients with liver dysfunction: 6 patients with moderate dysfunction (Bilirubin $\leq$ 2 $\times$ UNL and Transaminases $\leq$ 5 $\times$ UNL) treated up to 25 mg/m^2 and 8 patients with severe dysfunction (Bilirubin > 2 $\times$ UNL and/or Transaminases > 5 $\times$ UNL) treated up to 20 mg/m^2. Mean total clearance in these two subsets of patients was similar to that in patients with normal hepatic function. Therefore, the pharmacokinetics of vinorelbine is not modified in patients presenting moderate or severe liver impairment. Nevertheless, in a conservative approach it is suggested that the dose be reduced by 33% and the haematological parameters closely monitored in patient with severe liver impairment since the maximum dose which was given in this subset of patients was 20 mg/m^2.

Elderly patients

A study with Navelbine in elderly patients ($\geqslant$ 70 years) with NSCLC demonstrated that pharmacokinetics of vinorelbine were not influenced by age. However, since elderly patients are frail, caution should be exercised when increasing the dose of Navelbine: see section 4.2

Pharmacokinetic / pharmacodynamic relationships

A strong relationship has been demonstrated between vinorelbine blood exposure and of leucocytes or PMNs decreases.

5.3 Preclinical safety data

Mutagenic and carcinogenic potential

The interaction of NAVELBINE with the spindle apparatus during mitosis can cause an incorrect distribution of chromosomes. In animal studies NAVELBINE induced aneuploidy and polyploidy. It is therefore to be assumed that NAVELBINE can also cause mutagenic effects (induction of aneuploidy) in man.

The carcinogenicity studies, in which NAVELBINE was administered only once every two weeks in order to avoid the toxic effects of the drug, are negative.

Reproductive toxicity

In animal reproductive studies NAVELBINE was embryo- and feto-lethal and teratogenic.

The NOEL in the rat was 0.26 mg/kg every 3 days.

Following peri/postnatal administration in the rat at doses of 1.0 mg/kg every 3 days i.v., retarded weight gain was found in the offspring up to the 7th week of life.

Safety pharmacology

Bibliographic review concerning the tolerance of vinca alkaloids on the cardiovascular system shows the occurrence of some cardiac events (such as angina, myocardial infarction), but the incidence of these is low.

Haemodynamic and electrocardiographic studies on animals have been carried out by Pierre Fabre Médicament Laboratories; no haemodynamic effects have been found using a maximal tolerated dose in dogs, however only some non significant disturbances of repolarization were found for all vinca alkaloids tested. No effect on the cardiovascular system has been detected using repeated doses (study 39 weeks) of NAVELBINE on primates.

6. PHARMACEUTICAL PARTICULARS

6.1 List of excipients

(see Table 2 above)

6.2 Incompatibilities

- NAVELBINE should not be diluted in alkaline solutions (risk of precipitation)

This medicinal product must not be mixed with other medicinal products except those mentioned in section 6.6

6.3 Shelf life

Vial before opening:

3 years.

After dilution:

After diluting NAVELBINE in sodium chloride 9 mg/ml (0.9%) solution for injection or in glucose solution for injection 5%, chemical and physical in-use stability has been demonstrated for 8 days at room temperature (20°C ± 5°C) or in the refrigerator (2°C - 8°C) protected from light, in neutral glass bottle, PVC and vinyl acetate bags.

From a microbiological point of view, the product should be used immediately. If not used immediately, in use storage times and conditions prior to use are under the responsibility of the user and would normally not be longer than 24 hours at 2° - 8°C, unless preparation has taken place in controlled and validated aseptic conditions.

6.4 Special precautions for storage

Store in a refrigerator at 2° C - 8° C

Do not freeze

Store in the original container in order to protect from light.

Diluted solution: see section 6.3.

6.5 Nature and contents of container

The drug is distributed in clear glass vials (type I) of appropriated volume closed by a butyl or chlorobutyl stopper. The stopper is covered with a crimped-on aluminium cap equipped with a polypropylene seal.

Vials of 1, 4 and 5 ml.

Boxes containing 10 vials for each strength:

10 mg / 1 ml

40 mg / 4 ml

50 mg / 5 ml

Not all pack sizes may be marketed

6.6 Special precautions for disposal and other handling

Handling and Use

The preparation and administration of Navelbine should be carried out by trained staff and as with all cytotoxic agents, precautions should be taken to avoid exposing staff during pregnancy.

Caution should be exercised in handling and preparing the Navelbine solution:

- Suitable eye protection, disposable gloves, face mask and disposable apron should be worn.

- Eventual spillage or leakage should be mopped up wearing protective gloves.

- All contact with the eye should be strictly avoided: risk of severe irritation and even corneal ulceration if the drug is sprayed under pressure. Immediate liberal washing of the eye with normal saline solution should be undertaken if any contact occurs.

- On completion, any exposed surface should be thoroughly cleaned and hands and face washed.

Preparation of the solution for infusion

Navelbine must be diluted prior to administration in a 50 ml volume of sodium chloride 9 mg/ml (0.9 %) solution for injection or in 5 % glucose solution for injection.

In case of polychemotherapy, Navelbine should not be mixed with other agents

There is no content / container incompatibility between Navelbine and neutral glass bottle, PVC bag, vinyl acetate bag or infusion set with PVC tubing.

The intra-thecal route is contraindicated: see sections 4.2 and 4.4

NAVELBINE must only be administered by the intravenous route as an infusion.

For further instructions on administration: see section 4.2.

Disposal

Any unused product or waste material should be disposed of in accordance with local requirements.

7. MARKETING AUTHORISATION HOLDER

PIERRE FABRE Ltd

Hyde Abbey House

23 Hyde Street

Winchester

Hampshire SO23 7DR

UNITED KINGDOM

8. MARKETING AUTHORISATION NUMBER(S)

PL 00603/0028

9. DATE OF FIRST AUTHORISATION/RENEWAL OF THE AUTHORISATION

Date of First Authorisation 10 May 1996

Date of last renewal: 10 May 2002

10. DATE OF REVISION OF THE TEXT

03 June 2009

Navelbine 80mg Soft Capsule

(Pierre Fabre Limited)

1. NAME OF THE MEDICINAL PRODUCT

NAVELBINE 80 mg soft capsule

2. QUALITATIVE AND QUANTITATIVE COMPOSITION

Each soft capsule contains 80mg vinorelbine as tartrate

For a full list of excipients, see section 6.1

3. PHARMACEUTICAL FORM

Soft capsule

Pale yellow soft capsule printed N80

4. CLINICAL PARTICULARS

4.1 Therapeutic indications

As a single agent or in combination for:

- The first line treatment of stage 3 or 4 non small cell lung cancer.
- The treatment of advanced breast cancer stage 3 and 4 relapsing after or refractory to an anthracycline containing regimen.

4.2 Posology and method of administration

Navelbine must be given strictly by the oral route.

Navelbine should be swallowed with water without chewing or sucking the capsule. It is recommended to take the capsule with some food.

In adult patients

As a single agent, the recommended regimen is:

First three administrations

60mg/m^2 of body surface area, administered once weekly

Subsequent administrations

Beyond the third administration, it is recommended to increase the dose of Navelbine to 80mg/m^2 once weekly except in those patients for whom the neutrophil count dropped once below 500/mm^3 or more than once between 500 and 1000/mm^3 during the first three administrations at 60mg/m^2.

(see Table 1 on next page)

Dose modification

For any administration planned to be given at 80mg/m^2, if the neutrophil count is below 500/mm^3 or more than once between 500 and 1000 / mm^3 the administration should be delayed until recovery and the dose reduced from 80 to 60mg/mm^3 per week during the 3 following administrations.

(see Table 2 on next page)

It is possible to re-escalate the dose from 60 to 80 mg/m^2 per week if the neutrophil count did not drop below 500/mm^3 or more than once between 500 and 1000/mm^3 during 3 administrations given at 60 mg/m^2 according to the rules previously defined for the first 3 administrations.

If the neutrophil count is below 1500 /mm^3 and/or the platelet count is between 75000 and 100000/mm^3, then the treatment should be delayed until recovery

For combination regimens, the dose and schedule will be adapted to the treatment protocol.

Based on clinical studies, the oral dose of 80 mg/m^2 was demonstrated to correspond to 30 mg/m^2 of the iv form and 60 mg/m^2 to 25 mg/m^2.

This has been the base for combination regimens alternating iv and oral forms improving patient convenience.

Table 1

Neutrophil count during the first 3 administrations of 60 mg/m²/week	Neutrophils > 1000	Neutrophils ≥ 500 and < 1000 (1 episode)	Neutrophils ≥ 500 and < 1000 (2 episodes)	Neutrophils < 500
Recommended dose starting with the 4th administration	80	80	60	60

Table 2

Neutrophil count beyond the 4th administration of 80 mg/m²/week	Neutrophils > 1000	Neutrophils ≥ 500 and < 1000 (1 episode)	Neutrophils ≥ 500 and < 1000 (2 episodes)	Neutrophils < 500
Recommended dose Starting with the next administration	80	60		

Capsules of different strengths (20, 30, 80 mg) are available in order to choose the adequate combination for the right dosage.

The following table gives the dose required for appropriate ranges of body surface area (BSA).

	60 mg/m²	80 mg/m²
BSA (m²)	Dose (mg)	Dose (mg)
0.95 to 1.04	60	80
1.05 to 1.14	70	90
1.15 to 1.24	70	100
1.25 to 1.34	80	100
1.35 to 1.44	80	110
1.45 to 1.54	90	120
1.55 to 1.64	100	130
1.65 to 1.74	100	140
1.75 to 1.84	110	140
1.85 to 1.94	110	150
≥ 1.95	120	160

Even for patients with BSA ≥ 2 m² the total dose should never exceed 120 mg per week at 60 mg/m² and 160 mg per week at 80 mg/m².

Administration in the elderly

Clinical experience has not detected any significant differences among elderly patients with regard to the response rate, although greater sensitivity in some of these patients cannot be excluded. Age does not modify the pharmacokinetics of vinorelbine: see section 5.2.

Administration in children

Navelbine is not recommended for use in children due to a lack of data on safety and efficacy. Administration is therefore not recommended: see section 5.1

Administration in patients with liver insufficiency

Navelbine can be administered at the standard dose of 60 mg/m²/week in patients with mild liver impairment (bilirubin < 1.5 × ULN, and ALAT and/or ASAT from 1.5 to 2.5 × ULN). In patients with moderate liver impairment (bilirubin from 1.5 to 3 × ULN, whatever the levels of ALAT and ASAT), Navelbine should be administered at a dose of 50 mg/m²/week. The administration of Navelbine in patients with severe hepatic impairment is contra-indicated: see sections 4.3, 4.4, 5.2.

Administration in patients with renal insufficiency

Given the minor renal excretion, there is no pharmacokinetic justification for reducing the dose of Navelbine in patients with serious renal insufficiency: see sections 4.4, 5.2.

Administration

Navelbine is to be administered orally.

Navelbine must be swallowed whole with water, without chewing, sucking or dissolving the capsule.

It is recommended to administer the capsule with some food.

Specific instructions must be observed for administration of Navelbine: see section 6.6

4.3 Contraindications

- Known hypersensitivity to vinorelbine or other vinca alkaloids or to any of the constituents.
- Disease significantly affecting absorption
- Previous significant surgical resection of stomach or small bowel.
- Neutrophil count below 1500/mm3 or severe infection current or recent (within 2 weeks).
- Severe hepatic insufficiency not related to the tumoural process
- Pregnancy: see section 4.6
- Lactation: see section 4.6
- Patients requiring long-term oxygen therapy

4.4 Special warnings and precautions for use

<u>Special warnings</u>

NAVELBINE soft capsules should be prescribed by a physician experienced in the use of chemotherapy

If the patient chews or sucks the capsule by error, proceed to mouth rinses with water or preferably a normal saline solution.

In the event of the capsule being cut or damaged, the liquid content is an irritant, and so may cause damage if in contact with skin, mucosa or eyes. Damaged capsules should not be swallowed and should be returned to the pharmacy or to the doctor in order to be properly destroyed. If any contact occurs, immediate thorough washing with water or preferably with normal saline solution should be undertaken.

In the case of vomiting within a few hours after drug intake, never repeat the administration of this dose. Supportive treatment (such as metoclopramide) may reduce the occurrence of this.

Close haematological monitoring should be undertaken during treatment (determination of haemoglobin level and the leucocyte, neutrophil and platelet counts on the day of each new administration).

Dosing should be determined by haematological status

- If the neutrophil count is below 1500 /mm³ and/or the platelet count is between 75,000 and 100,000/mm³ then the treatment should be delayed until recovery.

- For dose escalation from 60 to 80 mg/m² per week, after the third administration: see section 4.2.

- For the administrations given at 80mg/m², if the neutrophil count is below 500/mm³ or more than once between 500 and 1000 /mm³, the administration should not only be delayed but also reduced to 60mg/m² per week. It is possible to re-escalate the dose from 60 to 80 mg/m² per week: see section 4.2.

During clinical trials where treatments were initiated at 80 mg/m², a few patients developed severe neutropenic complications. Therefore it is highly recommended that the starting dose should be 60 mg/m² escalating to 80 mg/m² if the dose is tolerated as described in section 4.2.

If patients present signs or symptoms suggestive of infection, a prompt investigation should be carried out.

Because of the presence of Sorbitol, patients with rare hereditary problems of fructose intolerance should not take this medicine.

<u>**Special precautions for use**</u>

Special care should be taken when prescribing for patients with history of ischemic heart disease.

Navelbine should not be given concomitantly with radiotherapy if the treatment field includes the liver.

Oral Navelbine was studied in patients with liver impairment at the following doses:

- 60 mg/m² in 7 patients with mild liver impairment (bilirubin < 1.5 × ULN, and ALAT and/or ASAT from 1.5 to 2.5 × ULN);
- 50 mg/m² in 6 patients with moderate liver impairment (bilirubin from 1.5 to 3 × ULN, whatever the levels of ALAT and ASAT).

Total clearance of vinorelbine was neither modified between mild and moderate liver impairment nor was it altered in hepatically impaired patients when compared with clearance in patients with normal liver function. Oral Navelbine was not studied in patients with severe hepatic impairment therefore its use is contra-indicated in these patients: see sections 4.2, 4.3, 5.2.

As there is a low level of renal excretion there is no pharmacokinetic rationale for reducing Navelbine dose in patients with impaired kidney function.

4.5 Interaction with other medicinal products and other forms of interaction

Concomitant use contraindicated

<u>Yellow fever vaccine</u>: as with all cytotoxics, risk of fatal generalised vaccine disease: see section 4.3.

Concomitant use not recommended

<u>Live attenuated vaccines</u>: (for yellow fever vaccine, see concomitant use contraindicated) as with all cytotoxics, risk of generalised vaccine disease, possibly fatal. This risk is increased in patients already immunodepressed by their underlying disease. It is recommended to use an inactivated vaccine when one exists (e.g. poliomyelitis): see section 4.4

<u>Phenytoin</u>: as with all cytotoxics, risk of exacerbation of convulsions resulting from the decrease of phenytoin digestive absorption by cytotoxic drug or risk of toxicity enhancement or loss of efficacy of the cytotoxic drug due to increased hepatic metabolism by phenytoin.

<u>Itraconazole</u>: as with all vinca-alkaloids, increased neurotoxicity of vinca-alkaloids due to the decrease of their hepatic metabolism.

Concomitant use to take into consideration

<u>Cisplatin</u>: There is no mutual pharmacokinetic interaction when combining NAVELBINE with cisplatin over several cycles of treatment. However, the incidence of granulocytopenia associated with NAVELBINE use in combination with cisplatin is higher than associated with NAVELBINE single agent.

<u>Mitomycin C</u>: as with all vinca-alkaloids, increased risk of pulmonary toxicity Caution is advised when using vinorelbine and mitomycin C simultaneously.

The combination of NAVELBINE with other drugs with known bone marrow toxicity is likely to exacerbate the myelosuppressive adverse effects.

As CYP 3A4 is mainly involved in the metabolism of vinorelbine, combination with strong inhibitors of this isoenzyme (e.g. azole antifungals such as ketoconazole and itraconazole) could increase blood concentrations of vinorelbine and combination with strong inducers of this isoenzyme (e.g. rifampicin, phenytoin) could decrease blood concentrations of vinorelbine.

<u>Anticoagulant treatment</u>: as with all cytotoxics, the frequency of INR (International Normalised Ratio) monitoring should be increased due to the potential interaction with oral anticoagulants and increased variability of coagulation in patients with cancer.

Food does not modify the pharmacokinetics of vinorelbine.

4.6 Pregnancy and lactation

Pregnancy

Navelbine is suspected to cause serious birth effects when administered during pregnancy: see section 5.3.

Navelbine is contra-indicated in pregnancy: see section 4.3.

In case of a vital indication for treatment with Navelbine during pregnancy a medical consultation concerning the risk of harmful effects for the child should be conducted. If pregnancy occurs during treatment genetic counseling should be offered.

Women of child-bearing potential

Women of child-bearing potential must use effective contraception during treatment and up to 3 months after treatment: see section 4.3

Lactation

It is unknown whether vinorelbine is excreted in human breast milk.

The excretion of vinorelbine in milk has not been studied in animal studies.

A risk to the suckling child cannot be excluded therefore breast feeding must be discontinued before starting treatment with Navelbine: see section 4.3.

Fertility

Men and women being treated with Navelbine are advised not to conceive a child during and up to 3 months after treatment: see section 4.3.

4.7 Effects on ability to drive and use machines

No studies on the effects on the ability to drive and use machines have been performed but on the basis of the pharmacodynamic profile vinorelbine does not affect the ability to drive and use machines. However, caution is necessary in patients treated with vinorelbine considering some adverse effects of the drug: see section 4.8.

4.8 Undesirable effects

The overall reported incidence of undesirable effects was determined from clinical studies in 138 patients (76 patients with non small cell lung cancer and 62 patients with breast cancer) who received the recommended regimen of Navelbine soft capsules (first three administrations at 60mg/m²/week followed by 80mg/m²/week).

The most common undesirable effects are gastro-intestinal.

<u>Haematopoietic system</u>

- Neutropenia is the dose limiting toxicity. Grade 1-2 neutropenia was seen in 21 % of patients. Grade 3 neutropenia (neutrophil count between 1000 and 500/mm³) was observed in 18.8 % of patients. Grade 4 neutropenia (< 500/mm³) was reported in 23.2 % of patients and was associated with fever over 38°C in 3.0 % of patients. Infections were observed in 15.9 % of patients but were severe in only 5.8 % of them.
- Anaemia was very common but usually mild to moderate (72.5 % of patients with grade 1 or 2, 4.3 % with grade 3, 0.7 % with grade 4).
- Thrombocytopenia might occur but was seldom severe (8 % of patients with grade 1-2).

<u>Gastro-intestinal System</u>

Gastrointestinal adverse events were reported and included: nausea (71 % grade 1-2, 8.1 % grade 3, 0.6 % grade 4), vomiting (55.8 % grade 1-2, 4.3 % grade 3, 2.9 %

grade 4) and diarrhoea (44.2 % grade1-2), 2.9 % grade 3, 2.2 % grade 4) and anorexia (29.7 % with grade 1-2, 6.5 % with grade 3, 1.5 % with grade 4). Symptoms of severe intensity were infrequently observed.

Supportive treatment (such as metoclopramide) may reduce their occurrence.

Stomatitis usually mild to moderate occurred in 8.7 % (grade 1-2) of patients.

Oesophagitis was seen in 4.3 % of patients (grade 3 in 0.7 %).

Peripheral and Central Nervous System

• Peripheral:

Neurosensory disorders were generally limited to loss of tendon reflexes in 8 % (grade 1-2) of patients and infrequently severe. One patient presented partially reversible grade 3 ataxia.

Neuromotor disorders were seen in 8 % of patients (2.2 % of patients with grade 3).

• Gastro-intestinal autonomic nervous system:

Neuroconstipation was seen in 9.4 % of patients (8 % grade 1-2) and rarely progressed to paralytic ileus (1.4%). One episode of fatal paralytic ileus was reported. Prescription of laxatives may be appropriate in patients with prior history of constipation and/or who received concomitant treatment with morphine or morphinomimetics.

Skin

Alopecia may appear progressively with an extended course of treatment.

Alopecia, usually mild in nature, may occur in 25.4 % of patients (24 % grade 1-2, 1.4 % grade 3).

Other adverse effects

Fatigue (19.5 % of patients with grade 1-2, 6.7 % with grade 3), fever (9.4 % with grade 1-2), arthralgia including jaw pain/ myalgia (10.7 % with grade 1-2), pain including pain at the tumour site (5.8 % with grade 1-2) have been experienced by patients receiving Navelbine soft capsules.

In addition, it cannot be ruled out that the following effects may be observed with the use of oral vinorelbine as with other vinca alkaloids:

Cardiovascular System

There have been rare reports of ischemic cardiac disease (angina pectoris, myocardial infarction).

Liver

Transient elevations of liver function tests without clinical symptoms were reported.

Respiratory system

As with other vinca alkaloids, the intravenous administration of Navelbine has been associated with dyspnea, bronchospasm and rare cases of interstitial pneumopathy in particular in patients treated with Navelbine injectable solution in combination with mitomycin.

Skin

Rarely vinca alkaloids may produce generalized cutaneous reactions.

4.9 Overdose

Symptoms

Overdosage with Navelbine soft capsules could produce bone marrow hypoplasia sometimes associated with infection, fever, paralytic ileus and hepatic disorders.

Emergency procedure

General supportive measures together with blood transfusion, growth factors, and broad spectrum antibiotic therapy should be instituted as deemed necessary by the physician.

Antidote

There is no known antidote for overdosage of Navelbine.

5. PHARMACOLOGICAL PROPERTIES

5.1 Pharmacodynamic properties

Pharmacotherapeutic group: Vinca alkaloids and analogues (ATC Code: L01C A04)

Navelbine is a antineoplastic drug of the vinca alkaloid family but unlike all the other vinca alkaloids, the catharantine moiety of vinorelbine has been structurally modified. At the molecular level, it acts on the dynamic equilibrium of tubulin in the microtubular apparatus of the cell. It inhibits tubulin polymerization and binds preferentially to mitotic microtubules, affecting axonal microtubules at high concentrations only. The induction of tubulin spiralization is less than that produced by vincristine.

Navelbine blocks mitosis at G2-M, causing cell death in interphase or at the following mitosis.

Safety and efficacy of Navelbine in paediatric patients have not been established. Clinical data from a single-arm study in 46 paediatric patients with recurrent solid tumours, including rhabdomyosarcoma/undifferentiated sarcoma, neuroblastoma, and CNS tumours, at doses similar to those used in adults, showed no meaningful clinical activity. Toxicities were similar to those reported in adult patients: see section 4.2.

5.2 Pharmacokinetic properties

Pharmacokinetic parameters of vinorelbine were evaluated in blood.

Absorption

After oral administration, vinorelbine is rapidly absorbed and the T_{max} is reached between 1.5 to 3 h with a blood concentration peak (C_{max}) of approximately 130 ng/ml after a dose of 80 mg/m^2.

The absolute bioavailability is approximately 40% and a simultaneous intake of food does not alter the exposure to vinorelbine.

Oral vinorelbine at 60 and 80 mg/m^2 leads to blood exposure comparable to that achieved with intravenous vinorelbine at 25 and 30 mg/m^2, respectively.

The blood exposure to vinorelbine increases proportionally with the dose up to 100mg/m^2. Interindividual variability of the exposure is similar after administration by intravenous and oral routes.

Distribution

The steady-state volume of distribution is large, on average 21.2 l/kg (range: 7.5 - 39.7 l/kg), which indicates extensive tissue distribution.

Binding to plasma proteins is weak (13.5%), vinorelbine binds strongly to blood cells and especially to platelets (78%).

There is a significant uptake of vinorelbine in lungs, as assessed by pulmonary surgical biopsies which showed concentration up to a 300- fold higher concentration than in serum. Vinorelbine is not found in the central nervous system.

Biotransformation

All metabolites of vinorelbine are formed by CYP 3A4 isoform of cytochromes P450, except 4-O-deacetylvinorelbine likely to be formed by carboxylesterases. 4-O-deacetylvinorelbine is the only active metabolite and the main one observed in blood.

Neither sulfate nor glucuronide conjugates are found.

Elimination

The mean terminal half-life of vinorelbine is around 40 hours. Blood clearance is high, approaching hepatic blood flow, and is 0.72 l/h/kg (range: 0.32-1.26 l/h/kg).

Renal elimination is low (<5 % of the dose administered) and consists mostly in parent compound. Biliary excretion is the predominant elimination route of both unchanged vinorelbine, which is the main recovered compound, and its metabolites.

Special patients groups

Renal and liver impairment:

The effects of renal dysfunction on the pharmacokinetics of vinorelbine have not been studied. However, dose reduction in case of reduced renal function is not indicated with vinorelbine due to the low level of renal elimination.

Pharmacokinetics of orally administered vinorelbine were not modified after administration of 60 mg/m^2 in patients with mild liver impairment (bilirubin $< 1.5 \times$ ULN, and ALAT and/or ASAT from 1.5 to 2.5 $\times$ ULN) and of 50 mg/m^2 in 6 patients with moderate liver impairment (bilirubin from 1.5 to 3 $\times$ ULN, whatever the levels of ALAT and ASAT). Total clearance of vinorelbine was neither modified between mild and moderate impairment nor was it altered in hepatically impaired patients when compared with clearance in patients with normal liver function.

No data is available for patients with severe liver impairment therefore Navelbine is contra-indicated in these patients: see sections 4.2, 4.3 and 4.4.

Elderly patients

A study with oral vinorelbine in elderly patients ($\geqslant$ 70 years) with NSCLC demonstrated that pharmacokinetics of vinorelbine were not influenced by age. However, since elderly patients are frail, caution should be exercised when increasing the dose of Navelbine soft capsule: see section 4.2.

Pharmacokinetics/Pharmacodynamic relationships

A strong relationship has been demonstrated between blood exposure and depletion of leucocytes or PMNs.

5.3 Preclinical safety data

Preclinical data reveal no special hazard for humans based on conventional studies of repeated dose toxicity and carcinogenic potential.

It is assumed that Navelbine® can cause mutagenic effects (induction of aneuploidy) in man.

In animal reproductive studies, Navelbine was embryo-foeto-lethal and teratogenic.

No haemodynamic effects were found in dogs receiving vinorelbine at maximal tolerated dose; only some minor, non significant disturbances of repolarisation were found as with other vinca alkaloids tested. No effect on the cardiovascular system was observed in primates receiving repeated doses of vinorelbine over 39 weeks.

6. PHARMACEUTICAL PARTICULARS

6.1 List of excipients

Fill solution:

Ethanol, anhydrous

Water, purified

Glycerol

Macrogol 400

Shell capsule:

Gelatin

Glycerol 85 %

Sorbitol / Sorbitan (Anidrisorb 85/70)

Yellow iron oxide E172

Titanium dioxide E171

Triglycerides, medium chain

Phosal 53 MCT (Phosphatidylcholine; Glycerides; Ethanol, anhydrous)

Edible printing ink:

Cochineal extract E120

Hypromellose

Propylene glycol

6.2 Incompatibilities

Not applicable

6.3 Shelf life

The shelf life of the medicinal product as packaged for sale is 2 years for Navelbine soft capsules 80 mg.

6.4 Special precautions for storage

Store at 2° C - 8° C (in a refrigerator). Store in the original container.

6.5 Nature and contents of container

Peel-push PVC/PVDC/ aluminium blister.

Pack size: 1 capsule

6.6 Special precautions for disposal and other handling

Any unused product or waste material should be disposed of in accordance with local requirements.

Instructions for use/handling

To open the packaging:

1. Cut the blister along the black dotted line
2. Peel the soft plastic foil off
3. Push the capsule through the aluminium foil.

7. MARKETING AUTHORISATION HOLDER

PIERRE FABRE Limited

Hyde Abbey House

23 Hyde Street

Winchester Hampshire S023 7DR

United Kingdom

8. MARKETING AUTHORISATION NUMBER(S)

PL 00603/0032

9. DATE OF FIRST AUTHORISATION/RENEWAL OF THE AUTHORISATION

31st March 2005

10. DATE OF REVISION OF THE TEXT

28 August 2009

Nebilet 5mg Tablets

(A. Menarini Pharma U.K. S.R.L.)

1. NAME OF THE MEDICINAL PRODUCT

NEBILET® 5 mg tablets

2. QUALITATIVE AND QUANTITATIVE COMPOSITION

Each Nebilet tablet contains 5 mg of nebivolol (as nebivolol hydrochloride):

2.5 mg of SRRR-nebivolol (or d-nebivolol) and 2.5 mg of RSSS-nebivolol (or l-nebivolol).

Excipients: amongst others lactose monohydrate (see section 4.4 and 6.1).

For a full list of excipients, see section 6.1.

3. PHARMACEUTICAL FORM

Tablets.

White, round, cross-scored tablets. The tablets can be divided in equal quarters.

4. CLINICAL PARTICULARS

4.1 Therapeutic indications

Hypertension

Treatment of essential hypertension.

Chronic heart failure (CHF)

Treatment of stable mild and moderate chronic heart failure in addition to standard therapies in elderly patients $\geq$ 70 years.

4.2 Posology and method of administration

Hypertension

Adults

The dose is one tablet (5 mg) daily, preferably at the same time of the day. Tablets may be taken with meals.

The blood pressure lowering effect becomes evident after 1-2 weeks of treatment. Occasionally, the optimal effect is reached only after 4 weeks.

Combination with other antihypertensive agents

Beta-blockers can be used alone or concomitantly with other antihypertensive agents. To date, an additional antihypertensive effect has been observed only when Nebilet 5 mg is combined with hydrochlorothiazide 12.5-25 mg.

Patients with renal insufficiency

In patients with renal insufficiency, the recommended starting dose is 2.5 mg daily. If needed, the daily dose may be increased to 5 mg.

Patients with hepatic insufficiency

Data in patients with hepatic insufficiency or impaired liver function are limited. Therefore the use of Nebilet in these patients is contra-indicated.

Elderly

In patients over 65 years, the recommended starting dose is 2.5 mg daily. If needed, the daily dose may be increased to 5 mg. However, in view of the limited experience in patients above 75 years, caution must be exercised and these patients monitored closely.

Children and adolescents

No studies have been conducted in children and adolescents. Therefore, use in children and adolescents is not recommended.

Chronic heart failure (CHF)

The treatment of stable chronic heart failure has to be initiated with a gradual uptitration of dosage until the optimal individual maintenance dose is reached.

Patients should have stable chronic heart failure without acute failure during the past six weeks. It is recommended that the treating physician should be experienced in the management of chronic heart failure.

For those patients receiving cardiovascular drug therapy including diuretics and/or digoxin and/or ACE inhibitors and/or angiotensin II antagonists, dosing of these drugs should be stabilised during the past two weeks prior to initiation of Nebilet treatment.

The initial uptitration should be done according to the following steps at 1-2 weekly intervals based on patient tolerability:

1.25 mg nebivolol, to be increased to 2.5 mg nebivolol once daily, then to 5 mg once daily and then to 10 mg once daily.

The maximum recommended dose is 10 mg nebivolol once daily.

Initiation of therapy and every dose increase should be done under the supervision of an experienced physician over a period of at least 2 hours to ensure that the clinical status (especially as regards blood pressure, heart rate, conduction disturbances, signs of worsening of heart failure) remains stable.

Occurrence of adverse events may prevent all patients being treated with the maximum recommended dose. If necessary, the dose reached can also be decreased step by step and reintroduced as appropriate.

During the titration phase, in case of worsening of the heart failure or intolerance, it is recommended first to reduce the dose of nebivolol, or to stop it immediately if necessary (in case of severe hypotension, worsening of heart failure with acute pulmonary oedema, cardiogenic shock, symptomatic bradycardia or AV block).

Treatment of stable chronic heart failure with nebivolol is generally a long-term treatment.

The treatment with nebivolol is not recommended to be stopped abruptly since this might lead to a transitory worsening of heart failure. If discontinuation is necessary, the dose should be gradually decreased divided into halves weekly.

Tablets may be taken with meals.

Patients with renal insufficiency

No dose adjustment is required in mild to moderate renal insufficiency since uptitration to the maximum tolerated dose is individually adjusted. There is no experience in patients with severe renal insufficiency (serum creatinine $\geqslant$ 250μmol/L). Therefore, the use of nebivolol in these patients is not recommended.

Patients with hepatic insufficiency

Data in patients with hepatic insufficiency are limited. Therefore the use of Nebilet in these patients is contra-indicated.

Elderly

No dose adjustment is required since uptitration to the maximum tolerated dose is individually adjusted.

Children and adolescents

No studies have been conducted in children and adolescents. Therefore, use in children and adolescents is not recommended.

4.3 Contraindications

- Hypersensitivity to the active substance or to any of the excipients.

- Liver insufficiency or liver function impairment.

- Acute heart failure, cardiogenic shock or episodes of heart failure decompensation requiring i.v. inotropic therapy.

In addition, as with other beta-blocking agents, Nebilet is contra-indicated in:

- sick sinus syndrome, including sino-atrial block.
- second and third degree heart block (without a pacemaker).
- history of bronchospasm and bronchial asthma.
- untreated phaeochromocytoma.
- metabolic acidosis.
- bradycardia (heart rate < 60 bpm prior to start therapy).
- hypotension (systolic blood pressure < 90 mmHg).
- severe peripheral circulatory disturbances.

4.4 Special warnings and precautions for use

See also 4.8 Undesirable effects.

The following warnings and precautions apply to beta-adrenergic antagonists in general.

Anaesthesia

Continuation of beta blockade reduces the risk of arrhythmias during induction and intubation. If beta blockade is interrupted in preparation for surgery, the beta-adrenergic antagonist should be discontinued at least 24 hours beforehand.

Caution should be observed with certain anaesthetics that cause myocardial depression. The patient can be protected against vagal reactions by intravenous administration of atropine.

Cardiovascular

In general, beta-adrenergic antagonists should not be used in patients with untreated congestive heart failure (CHF), unless their condition has been stabilised.

In patients with ischaemic heart disease, treatment with a beta-adrenergic antagonist should be discontinued gradually, i.e. over 1-2 weeks. If necessary replacement therapy should be initiated at the same time, to prevent exacerbation of angina pectoris.

Beta-adrenergic antagonists may induce bradycardia: if the pulse rate drops below 50-55 bpm at rest and/or the patient experiences symptoms that are suggestive of bradycardia, the dosage should be reduced.

Beta-adrenergic antagonists should be used with caution:

- in patients with peripheral circulatory disorders (Raynaud's disease or syndrome, intermittent claudication), as aggravation of these disorders may occur;
- in patients with first degree heart block, because of the negative effect of beta-blockers on conduction time;
- in patients with Prinzmetal's angina due to unopposed alphareceptor mediated coronary artery vasoconstriction: beta-adrenergic antagonists may increase the number and duration of anginal attacks.

Combination of nebivolol with calcium channel antagonists of the verapamil and diltiazem type, with Class I antiarrhythmic drugs, and with centrally acting antihypertensive drugs is generally not recommended, for details please refer to section 4.5.

Metabolic/Endocrinological

Nebilet does not affect glucose levels in diabetic patients. Care should be taken in diabetic patients however, as nebivolol may mask certain symptoms of hypoglycaemia (tachycardia, palpitations).

Beta-adrenergic blocking agents may mask tachycardic symptoms in hyperthyroidism. Abrupt withdrawal may intensify symptoms.

Respiratory

In patients with chronic obstructive pulmonary disorders, beta-adrenergic antagonists should be used with caution as airway constriction may be aggravated.

Other

Patients with a history of psoriasis should take beta-adrenergic antagonists only after careful consideration.

Beta-adrenergic antagonists may increase the sensitivity to allergens and the severity of anaphylactic reactions.

The initiation of Chronic Heart Failure treatment with nebivolol necessitates regular monitoring. For the posology and method of administration please refer to section 4.2. Treatment discontinuation should not be done abruptly unless clearly indicated. For further information please refer to section 4.2.

This medicinal product contains lactose. Patients with rare hereditary problems of galactose intolerance, the Lapp lactase deficiency or glucose-galactose malapsorption should not take this medicinal product.

4.5 Interaction with other medicinal products and other forms of interaction

Pharmacodynamic interactions:

The following interactions apply to beta-adrenergic antagonists in general.

Combinations not recommended:

Class I antiarrhythmics (quinidine, hydroquinidine, cibenzoline, flecainide, disopyramide, lidocaine, mexiletine, propafenone): effect on atrio-ventricular conduction time may be potentiated and negative inotropic effect increased (see section 4.4).

Calcium channel antagonists of verapamil/diltiazem type: negative influence on contractility and atrio-ventricular conduction. Intravenous administration of verapamil in patients with β-blocker treatment may lead to profound hypotension and atrio-ventricular block (see section 4.4).

Centrally-acting antihypertensives (clonidine, guanfacin, moxonidine, methyldopa, rilmenidine): concomitant use of centrally acting antihypertensive drugs may worsen heart failure by a decrease in the central sympathetic tonus (reduction of heart rate and cardiac output, vasodilation) (see section 4.4). Abrupt withdrawal, particularly if prior to beta-blocker discontinuation, may increase risk of "rebound hypertension".

Combinations to be used with caution

Class III antiarrhythmic drugs (Amiodarone): effect on atrio-ventricular conduction time may be potentiated.

Anaesthetics - volatile halogenated: concomitant use of beta-adrenergic antagonists and anaesthetics may attenuate reflex tachycardia and increase the risk of hypotension (see section 4.4). As a general rule, avoid sudden withdrawal of beta-blocker treatment. The anaesthesiologist should be informed when the patient is receiving Nebilet.

Insulin and oral antidiabetic drugs: although nebivolol does not affect glucose level, concomitant use may mask certain symptoms of hypoglycaemia (palpitations, tachycardia).

Combinations to be considered

Digitalis glycosides: concomitant use may increase atrio-ventricular conduction time. Clinical trials with nebivolol have not shown any clinical evidence of an interaction. Nebivolol does not influence the kinetics of digoxin.

Calcium antagonists of the dihydropyridine type (amlodipine, felodipine, lacidipine, nifedipine, nicardipine, nimodipine, nitrendipine): concomitant use may increase the risk of hypotension, and an increase in the risk of a further deterioration of the ventricular pump function in patients with heart failure cannot be excluded.

Antipsychotics, antidepressants (tricyclics, barbiturates and phenothiazines): concomitant use may enhance the hypothensive effect of the beta-blockers (additive effect).

Non steroidal anti-inflammatory drugs (NSAID): no effect on the blood pressure lowering effect of nebivolol.

Sympathicomimetic agents: concomitant use may counteract the effect of beta-adrenergic antagonists. Beta-adrenergic agents may lead to unopposed alpha-adrenergic activity of sympathicomimetic agents with both alpha- and beta-adrenergic effects (risk of hypertension, severe bradycardia and heart block).

Pharmacokinetic interactions:

As nebivolol metabolism involves the CYP2D6 isoenzyme, co-administration with substances inhibiting this enzyme, especially paroxetine, fluoxetine, thioridazine and quinidine may lead to increased plasma levels of nebivolol associated with an increased risk of excessive bradycardia and adverse events.

Co-administration of cimetidine increased the plasma levels of nebivolol, without changing the clinical effect. Co-administration of ranitidine did not affect the pharmacokinetics of nebivolol. Provided Nebilet is taken with the meal, and an antacid between meals, the two treatments can be co-prescribed.

Combining nebivolol with nicardipine slightly increased the plasma levels of both drugs, without changing the clinical effect. Co-administration of alcohol, furosemide or hydrochlorothiazide did not affect the pharmacokinetics of nebivolol. Nebivolol does not affect the pharmacokinetics and pharmacodynamics of warfarin.

4.6 Pregnancy and lactation

Use in pregnancy

Nebivolol has pharmacological effects that may cause harmful effects on pregnancy and/or the foetus/newborn. In general, beta-adrenoceptor blockers reduce placental perfusion, which has been associated with growth retardation, intrauterine death, abortion or early labour. Adverse effects (e.g. hypoglycaemia and bradycardia) may occur in the foetus and newborn infant. If treatment with beta-adrenoceptor blockers is necessary, $beta_1$-selective adrenoceptor blockers are preferable.

Nebivolol should not be used during pregnancy unless clearly necessary. If treatment with nebivolol is considered necessary, the uteroplacental blood flow and the foetal growth should be monitored. In case of harmful effects on pregnancy or the foetus alternative treatment should be considered. The newborn infant must be closely monitored. Symptoms of hypoglycaemia and bradycardia are generally to be expected within the first 3 days.

Use in lactation

Animal studies have shown that nebivolol is excreted in breast milk. It is not known whether this drug is excreted in human milk. Most beta-blockers, particularly lipophilic compounds like nebivolol and its active metabolites, pass into breast milk although to a variable extent. Therefore, breastfeeding is not recommended during administration of nebivolol.

4.7 Effects on ability to drive and use machines

No studies on the effects of Nebilet on the ability to drive and use machines have been performed. Pharmacodynamic studies have shown that Nebilet 5 mg does not affect psychomotor function. When driving vehicles or operating machines it should be taken into account that dizziness and fatigue may occasionally occur.

4.8 Undesirable effects

Adverse events are listed separately for hypertension and CHF because of differences in the background diseases.

Hypertension

The adverse reactions reported, which are in most of the cases of mild to moderate intensity, are tabulated below, classified by system organ class and ordered by frequency:

(see Table 1 below)

The following adverse reactions have also been reported with some beta adrenergic antagonists: hallucinations, psychoses, confusion, cold/cyanotic extremities, Raynaud phenomenon, dry eyes, and oculo-mucocutaneous toxicity of the practolol-type.

Chronic heart failure

Data on adverse reactions in CHF patients are available from one placebo-controlled clinical trial involving 1067 patients taking nebivolol and 1061 patients taking placebo. In this study, a total of 449 nebivolol patients (42.1%) reported at least possibly causally related adverse reactions compared to 334 placebo patients (31.5%). The most commonly reported adverse reactions in nebivolol patients were bradycardia and dizziness, both occurring in approximately 11% of patients. The corresponding frequencies among placebo patients were approximately 2% and 7%, respectively.

The following incidences were reported for adverse reactions (at least possibly drug-related) which are considered specifically relevant in the treatment of chronic heart failure:

- Aggravation of cardiac failure occurred in 5.8 % of nebivolol patients compared to 5.2% of placebo patients.
- Postural hypotension was reported in 2.1% of nebivolol patients compared to 1.0% of placebo patients.
- Drug intolerance occurred in 1.6% of nebivolol patients compared to 0.8% of placebo patients.
- First degree atrio-ventricular block occurred in 1.4% of nebivolol patients compared to 0.9% of placebo patients.
- Oedema of the lower limb were reported by 1.0% of nebivolol patients compared to 0.2% of placebo patients.

4.9 Overdose

No data are available on overdosage with Nebilet.

Symptoms

Symptoms of overdosage with beta-blockers are: bradycardia, hypotension, bronchospasm and acute cardiac insufficiency.

Treatment

In case of overdosage or hypersensitivity, the patient should be kept under close supervision and be treated in an intensive care ward. Blood glucose levels should be checked. Absorption of any drug residues still present in the gastro-intestinal tract can be prevented by gastric lavage and the administration of activated charcoal and a laxative. Artificial respiration may be required. Bradycardia or extensive vagal reactions should be treated by administering atropine or methylatropine. Hypotension and shock should be treated with plasma/plasma substitutes and, if necessary, catecholamines. The beta-blocking effect can be counteracted by slow intravenous administration of isoprenaline hydrochloride, starting with a dose of approximately 5 µg/minute, or dobutamine, starting with a dose of 2.5 µg/minute, until the required effect has been obtained. In refractory cases isoprenaline can be combined with dopamine. If this does not produce the desired effect either, intravenous administration of glucagon 50-100 µg/kg i.v. may be considered. If required, the injection should be repeated within one hour, to be followed -if required- by an i.v. infusion of glucagon 70 µg/kg/h. In extreme cases of treatment-resistant bradycardia, a pacemaker may be inserted.

5. PHARMACOLOGICAL PROPERTIES

5.1 Pharmacodynamic properties

Pharmacotherapeutic group: Beta blocking agent, selective.

ATC code: C07AB12

Nebivolol is a racemate of two enantiomers, SRRR-nebivolol (or d-nebivolol) and RSSS-nebivolol (or l-nebivolol). It combines two pharmacological activities:

- It is a competitive and selective beta-receptor antagonist: this effect is attributed to the SRRR-enatiomer (d-enantiomer).
- It has mild vasodilating properties due to an interaction with the L-arginine/nitric oxide pathway.

Single and repeated doses of nebivolol reduce heart rate and blood pressure at rest and during exercise, both in normotensive subjects and in hypertensive patients. The antihypertensive effect is maintained during chronic treatment.

At therapeutic doses, nebivolol is devoid of alpha-adrenergic antagonism.

During acute and chronic treatment with nebivolol in hypertensive patients systemic vascular resistance is decreased. Despite heart rate reduction, reduction in cardiac output during rest and exercise may be limited due to an increase in stroke volume. The clinical relevance of these haemodynamic differences as compared to other beta1 receptor antagonists has not been fully established.

In hypertensive patients, nebivolol increases the NO-mediated vascular response to acetylcholine (ACh) which is reduced in patients with endothelial dysfunction.

In a mortality–morbidity, placebo-controlled trial performed in 2128 patients ⩾ 70 years (median age 75.2 years) with stable chronic heart failure with or without impaired left ventricular ejection fraction (mean LVEF: 36 ± 12.3%, with the following distribution: LVEF less than 35% in 56% of patients, LVEF between 35% and 45% in 25% of patients and LVEF greater than 45% in 19% of patients) followed for a mean time of 20 months, nebivolol, on top of standard therapy, significantly prolonged the time to occurrence of deaths or hospitalisations for cardiovascular reasons (primary end-point for efficacy) with a relative risk reduction of 14% (absolute reduction: 4.2%). This risk reduction developed after 6 months of treatment and was maintained for all treatment duration (median duration: 18 months). The effect of nebivolol was independent from age, gender, or left ventricular ejection fraction of the population on study. The benefit on all cause mortality did not reach statistical significance in comparison to placebo (absolute reduction: 2.3%).

A decrease in sudden death was observed in nebivolol treated patients (4.1% vs 6.6%, relative reduction of 38%).

In vitro and in vivo experiments in animals showed that Nebivolol has no intrinsic sympathicomimetic activity.

In vitro and in vivo experiments in animals showed that at pharmacological doses nebivolol has no membrane stabilising action.

In healthy volunteers, nebivolol has no significant effect on maximal exercise capacity or endurance.

5.2 Pharmacokinetic properties

Both nebivolol enantiomers are rapidly absorbed after oral administration. The absorption of nebivolol is not affected by food; nebivolol can be given with or without meals.

Nebivolol is extensively metabolised, partly to active hydroxy-metabolites. Nebivol is metabolised via alicyclic and aromatic hydroxylation, N-dealkylation and glucuronidation; in addition, glucuronides of the hydroxy-metabolites are formed. The metabolism of nebivolol by aromatic hydroxylation is subject to the CYP2D6 dependent genetic oxidative polymorphism. The oral bioavailability of nebivolol averages 12% in fast metabolisers and is virtually complete in slow metabolisers. At steady state and at the same dose level, the peak plasma concentration of unchanged nebivolol is about 23 times higher in poor metabolisers than in extensive metabolisers. When unchanged drug plus active metabolites are considered, the difference in peak plasma concentrations is 1.3 to 1.4 fold. Because of the variation in rates of metabolism, the dose of Nebilet should always be adjusted to the individual requirements of the patient: poor metabolisers therefore may require lower doses.

In fast metabolisers, elimination half-lives of the nebivolol enantiomers average 10 hours. In slow metabolisers, they are 3-5 times longer. In fast metabolisers, plasma levels of the RSSS-enantiomer are slightly higher than for the SRRR-enantiomer. In slow metabolisers, this difference is larger. In fast metabolisers, elimination half-lives of the hydroxymetabolites of both enantiomers average 24 hours, and are about twice as long in slow metabolisers.

Steady-state plasma levels in most subjects (fast metabolisers) are reached within 24 hours for nebivolol and within a few days for the hydroxy-metabolites.

Plasma concentrations are dose-proportional between 1 and 30 mg. The pharmacokinetics of nebivolol are not affected by age.

In plasma, both nebivolol enantiomers are predominantly bound to albumin.

Plasma protein binding is 98.1% for SRRR-nebivolol and 97.9% for RSSS-nebivolol.

One week after administration, 38% of the dose is excreted in the urine and 48% in the faeces. Urinary excretion of unchanged nebivolol is less than 0.5% of the dose.

5.3 Preclinical safety data

Preclinical data reveal no special hazard for humans based on conventional studies of genotoxicity and carcinogenic potential.

6. PHARMACEUTICAL PARTICULARS

6.1 List of excipients

Polysorbate 80

Hypromellose

Lactose monohydrate

Maize starch

Croscarmellose sodium,

Microcrystalline cellulose

Colloidal anhydrous silica

Magnesium stearate

6.2 Incompatibilities

Not applicable

6.3 Shelf life

3 years.

6.4 Special precautions for storage

This medicinal product does not require any special storage precautions.

6.5 Nature and contents of container

Tablets are provided in blister packs (PVC/aluminium blister).

Pack sizes of 7, 14, 28, 30, 50, 56, 90, 100, 500 tablets

(Not all pack sizes may be marketed)

6.6 Special precautions for disposal and other handling

No special requirements.

7. MARKETING AUTHORISATION HOLDER

Menarini International Operations Luxembourg S.A.

1, Avenue de la Gare,

L-1611 Luxembourg

8. MARKETING AUTHORISATION NUMBER(S)

PL 16239/0013

9. DATE OF FIRST AUTHORISATION/RENEWAL OF THE AUTHORISATION

Date of first authorisation: 4th January 1999

Date of last renewal: 18 October 2005

Table 1

SYSTEM ORGAN CLASS	Common (≥1/100 to < 1/10)	Uncommon (≥1/1,000 to ⩽1/100)	Very Rare (⩽1/10,000)	Not Known
Immune system disorders				angioneurotic oedema, hypersensitivity
Psychiatric disorders		nightmares; depression		
Nervous system disorders	headache, dizziness, paraesthesia		syncope	
Eye disorders		impaired vision		
Cardiac disorders		bradycardia, heart failure, slowed AV conduction/AV-block		
Vascular disorders		hypotension, (increase of) intermittent claudication		
Respiratory, thoracic and mediastinal disorders	dyspnoea	bronchospasm		
Gastrointestinal disorders	constipation, nausea, diarrhoea	dyspepsia, flatulence, vomiting		
Skin and subcutaneous tissue disorders		pruritus, rash erythematous	psoriasis aggravated	
Reproductive system and breast disorders		impotence		
General disorders and administration site conditions	tiredness, oedema			

10. DATE OF REVISION OF THE TEXT
August 2007

Legal category
POM

Neo-Cytamen Injection 1000mcg

(UCB Pharma Limited)

1. NAME OF THE MEDICINAL PRODUCT
Neo-Cytamen Injection 1000mcg

2. QUALITATIVE AND QUANTITATIVE COMPOSITION
Hydroxocobalamin chloride 1.027mg equivalent to 1.0 mg Hydroxocobalamin.

For excipients, see 6.1

3. PHARMACEUTICAL FORM
Solution for injection.

4. CLINICAL PARTICULARS

4.1 Therapeutic indications
Addisonian pernicious anaemia.

Prophylaxis and treatment of other macrocytic anaemias associated with vitamin B_{12} deficiency.

Tobacco amblyopia and Leber's optic atrophy.

4.2 Posology and method of administration
Route of administration: Intramuscular.

Adults and Children

Addisonian pernicious anaemia and other macrocytic anaemias without neurological involvement:

Initially: 250 to 1000mcg intramuscularly on alternate days for one to two weeks, then 250mcg weekly until the blood count is normal.

Maintenance: 1000mcg every two to three months.

Addisonian pernicious anaemia and other macrocytic anaemias with neurological involvement:

Initially: 1000mcg on alternate days as long as improvement is occurring.

Maintenance: 1000mcg every two months.

Prophylaxis of macrocytic anaemia associated with vitamin B_{12} deficiency resulting from gastrectomy, some malabsorption syndromes and strict vegetarianism:

1000mcg every two to three months.

Tobacco amblyopia and Leber's optic atrophy:

Initially: 1000mcg or more daily by intramuscular injection for two weeks. Then twice weekly as long as improvement is occurring.

Maintenance: 1000mcg monthly.

4.3 Contraindications
Hypersensitivity to any ingredient of the preparation.

Hydroxocobalamin should not be used for treatment of megaloblastic anaemia of pregnancy unless vitamin B12 deficiency has been demonstrated.

4.4 Special warnings and precautions for use
Precautions:

The dosage schemes given above are usually satisfactory, but regular examination of the blood is advisable. If megaloblastic anaemia fails to respond to hydroxocobalamin, folate metabolism should be investigated. Doses in excess of 10mcg daily may produce a haematological response in patients with folate deficiency. Indiscriminate administration may mask the true diagnosis. The haematological and neurological state should be monitored regularly to ensure adequacy of therapy. Cardiac arrhythmias secondary to hypokalaemia during initial therapy have been reported. Plasma potassium should therefore be monitored during this period. Platelet count should be monitored during the first weeks of use in megaloblastic anaemia due to the possible occurrence of reactive thrombocytosis.

4.5 Interaction with other medicinal products and other forms of interaction
Chloramphenicol-treated patients may respond poorly to hydroxocobalamin. Serum concentrations of hydroxocobalamin may be lowered by oral contraceptives but this interaction is unlikely to have clinical significance. Antimetabolites and most antibiotics invalidate vitamin B_{12} assays by microbiological techniques.

4.6 Pregnancy and lactation
Hydroxocobalamin should not be used for the treatment of megaloblastic anaemia of pregnancy unless vitamin B_{12} deficiency has been demonstrated. Hydroxocobalamin is secreted into breast milk but this is unlikely to harm the infant, and may be beneficial if the mother and infant are vitamin B_{12} deficient.

4.7 Effects on ability to drive and use machines
None stated.

4.8 Undesirable effects
The following effects have been reported and are listed below by body system:

Blood and lymphatic system disorders

Reactive thrombocytosis can occur during the first weeks of use in megaloblastic anaemia.

Cardiovascular disorders:

Arrhythmias secondary to hypokalaemia.

Disorders of the immune system:

Hypersensitivity reactions including skin reactions (e.g. rash, itching) and exceptionally anaphylaxis.

Gastro intestinal disorders:

Nausea, vomiting, diarrhoea.

General disorders:

Fever, chills, hot flushing, dizziness, malaise, pain. Injection site reactions including injection site pain, injection site erythema, injection site pruritus, injection site induration, and injection site swelling.

Neurological disorders:

Headache, sensory abnormalities such as paraesthesiae. Tremor.

Renal and unrinary disorders:

Chromaturia

Skin and subcutaneous tissue disorders:

Acneiform and bullous eruptions.

4.9 Overdose
Treatment is unlikely to be needed in cases of overdosage.

5. PHARMACOLOGICAL PROPERTIES

5.1 Pharmacodynamic properties
Hydroxocobalamin is one of the forms of vitamin B_{12}.

5.2 Pharmacokinetic properties
An intramuscular injection of hydroxocobalamin produces higher serum levels than the same dose of cyanocobalamin, and these levels are well maintained.

After injection of hydroxocobalamin, 90% of a 100 microgram dose and 30% of a 1000 microgram dose are retained. Vitamin B12 is extensively bound to specific plasma proteins called transcobalamins; transcobalamin II appears to be involved in the rapid transport of the cobalamins to tissues. Vitamin B12 is stored in the liver, excreted in the bile, and undergoes extensive enterohepatic recycling; part of an administered dose is excreted in the urine, most of it in the first 8 hours; urinary excretion, however, accounts for only a small fraction in the reduction of total body stores acquired by dietary means. Vitamin B12 diffuses across the placenta and also appears in breast milk.

5.3 Preclinical safety data
None stated.

6. PHARMACEUTICAL PARTICULARS

6.1 List of excipients
Sodium chloride, acetic acid, Water for Injections.

6.2 Incompatibilities
None.

6.3 Shelf life
36 months.

6.4 Special precautions for storage
Protect from light. Do not store above 25°C.

6.5 Nature and contents of container
1ml glass ampoules in packs of 5.

6.6 Special precautions for disposal and other handling
Not applicable.

7. MARKETING AUTHORISATION HOLDER
UCB Pharma Limited

208 Bath Road

Slough

Berkshire

SL1 3WE

UK

8. MARKETING AUTHORISATION NUMBER(S)
PL 00039/0405

9. DATE OF FIRST AUTHORISATION/RENEWAL OF THE AUTHORISATION
14 October 1992 / October 1997 / October 2002

10. DATE OF REVISION OF THE TEXT
September 2008

POM

Neorecormon Multidose Powder and Solvent for Solution for Injection

(Roche Products Limited)

1. NAME OF THE MEDICINAL PRODUCT
NeoRecormon Multidose 50,000 IU Lyophilisate and solvent for solution for injection (5000 IU/ml)

NeoRecormon Multidose 100,000 IU Lyophilisate and solvent for solution for injection (20,000 IU/ml)

2. QUALITATIVE AND QUANTITATIVE COMPOSITION
One vial contains 50,000 international units (IU) corresponding to 415 micrograms epoetin beta* (recombinant human erythropoietin).

One ampoule contains 10 ml solvent (water for injections with benzyl alcohol and benzalkonium chloride as preservatives).

One ml of reconstituted solution contains 5000 IU epoetin beta.

One vial contains 100,000 international units (IU) corresponding to 830 micrograms epoetin beta* (recombinant human erythropoietin).

One ampoule contains 5 ml solvent (water for injections with benzyl alcohol and benzalkonium chloride as preservatives).

One ml of reconstituted solution contains 20,000 IU epoetin beta.

* produced in Chinese Hamster Ovary cells (CHO) by recombinant DNA technology

Excipients:

Phenylalanine (up to 5.0 mg/vial)

Sodium (less than 1 mmol per dose)

Benzyl alcohol (up to 40 mg per multidose solvent ampoule)

For a full list of excipients, see section 6.1.

3. PHARMACEUTICAL FORM
Lyophilisate and solvent for solution for injection.

White lyophilisate and clear, colourless solvent.

4. CLINICAL PARTICULARS

4.1 Therapeutic indications
- Treatment of symptomatic anaemia associated with chronic renal failure (CRF) in adult and paediatric patients.

- Treatment of symptomatic anaemia in adult patients with non-myeloid malignancies receiving chemotherapy.

- Increasing the yield of autologous blood from patients in a pre-donation programme.

Its use in this indication must be balanced against the reported increased risk of thromboembolic events. Treatment should only be given to patients with moderate anaemia (Hb 10 - 13 g/dl [6.21 - 8.07 mmol/l], no iron deficiency) if blood conserving procedures are not available or insufficient when the scheduled major elective surgery requires a large volume of blood (4 or more units of blood for females or 5 or more units for males).

4.2 Posology and method of administration
Therapy with NeoRecormon should be initiated by physicians experienced in the above mentioned indications. As anaphylactoid reactions were observed in isolated cases, it is recommended that the first dose be administered under medical supervision.

This multidose preparation can be used for several patients. To avoid the risk of cross-infection always follow aseptic techniques and use disposable sterile syringes and needles for each administration. Please check that only one vial of NeoRecormon Multidose is in use (i.e. reconstituted) at any one time.

The reconstituted product is a colourless, clear to slightly opalescent solution.

For instructions on reconstitution of the product before administration, see section 6.6.

Treatment of symptomatic anaemia in adult and paediatric chronic renal failure patients:

Anaemia symptoms and sequelae may vary with age, gender, and overall burden of disease; a physician's evaluation of the individual patient's clinical course and condition is necessary. NeoRecormon should be administered either subcutaneously or intravenously in order to increase haemoglobin to not greater than 12 g/dl (7.5 mmol/l). Subcutaneous use is preferable in patients who are not receiving haemodialysis to avoid puncture of peripheral veins. In case of intravenous administration, the solution should be injected over approx. 2 minutes, e.g. in haemodialysis patients via the arterio-venous fistula at the end of dialysis.

Due to intra-patient variability, occasional individual haemoglobin values for a patient above and below the desired haemoglobin level may be observed. Haemoglobin variability should be addressed through dose management, with consideration for the haemoglobin target range of 10 g/dl (6.2 mmol/l) to 12 g/dl (7.5 mmol/l). A sustained haemoglobin level of greater than 12 g/dl (7.5 mmol/l) should be avoided; guidance for appropriate dose adjustment for when haemoglobin values exceeding 12 g/dl (7.5 mmol/l) are observed are described below.

A rise in haemoglobin of greater than 2 g/dl (1.25 mmol/l) over a four week period should be avoided. If it occurs, appropriate dose adjustment should be made as provided. If the rate of rise in haemoglobin is greater than 2 g/dl (1.25 mmol/l) in one month or if the haemoglobin level is increasing and approaching 12 g/dl (7.45 mmol/l), the dose is to be reduced by approximately 25 %. If the haemoglobin level continues to increase, therapy should be interrupted until the haemoglobin level begins to decrease, at which point therapy should be restarted at a dose approximately 25 % below the previously administered dose.

Patients should be monitored closely to ensure that the lowest approved dose of NeoRecormon is used to provide adequate control of the symptoms of anaemia.

In the presence of hypertension or existing cardiovascular, cerebrovascular or peripheral vascular diseases, the weekly increase in Hb and the target Hb should be determined individually taking into account the clinical picture.

Treatment with NeoRecormon is divided into two stages.

1. Correction phase

- Subcutaneous administration:

The initial dosage is 3 × 20 IU/kg body weight per week. The dosage may be increased every 4 weeks by 3 × 20 IU/kg per week if the increase of Hb is not adequate (< 0.25 g/dl per week).

The weekly dose can also be divided into daily doses.

- Intravenous administration:

The initial dosage is 3 × 40 IU/kg per week. The dosage may be raised after 4 weeks to 80 IU/kg - three times per week - and by further increments of 20 IU/kg if needed, three times per week, at monthly intervals.

For both routes of administration, the maximum dose should not exceed 720 IU/kg per week.

2. Maintenance phase

To maintain an Hb of between 10 and 12 g/dl, the dosage is initially reduced to half of the previously administered amount. Subsequently, the dose is adjusted at intervals of one or two weeks individually for the patient (maintenance dose).

In the case of subcutaneous administration, the weekly dose can be given as one injection per week or in divided doses three or seven times per week. Patients who are stable on a once weekly dosing regimen may be switched to once every two weeks administration. In this case dose increases may be necessary.

Results of clinical studies in children have shown that, on average, the younger the patients, the higher the NeoRecormon doses required. Nevertheless, the recommended dosing schedule should be followed as the individual response cannot be predicted.

Treatment with NeoRecormon is normally a long-term therapy. It can, however, be interrupted, if necessary, at any time. Data on the once weekly dosing schedule are based on clinical studies with a treatment duration of 24 weeks.

Treatment of symptomatic chemotherapy-induced anaemia in cancer patients:

NeoRecormon should be administered by the subcutaneous route to patients with anaemia (e.g. haemoglobin concentration ⩽ 10g/dl (6.2 mmol/l)). Anaemia symptoms and sequelae may vary with age, gender, and overall burden of disease; a physician's evaluation of the individual patient's clinical course and condition is necessary.

The weekly dose can be given as one injection per week or in divided doses 3 to 7 times per week.

The recommended initial dose is 30,000 IU per week (corresponding to approximately 450 IU/kg body weight per week, based on an average weighted patient).

Due to intra-patient variability, occasional individual haemoglobin values for a patient above and below the desired haemoglobin level may be observed. Haemoglobin variability should be addressed through dose management, with consideration for the haemoglobin target range of 10 g/dl (6.2 mmol/l) to 12 g/dl (7.5 mmol/l). A sustained haemoglobin level of greater than 12 g/dl (7.5 mmol/l) should be avoided; guidance for appropriate dose adjustment for when haemoglobin values exceeding 12 g/dl (7.5 mmol/l) are observed are described below.

If, after 4 weeks of therapy, the haemoglobin value has increased by at least 1 g/dl (0.62 mmol/l), the current dose should be continued. If the haemoglobin value has not increased by at least 1 g/dl (0.62 mmol/l), a doubling of the weekly dose should be considered. If, after 8 weeks of therapy, the haemoglobin value has not increased by at least 1 g/dl (0.62 mmol/l), response is unlikely and treatment should be discontinued.

The therapy should be continued up to 4 weeks after the end of chemotherapy.

The maximum dose should not exceed 60,000 IU per week.

Once the therapeutic objective for an individual patient has been achieved, the dose should be reduced by 25 to 50 % in order to maintain haemoglobin at that level. Appropriate dose titration should be considered.

If the haemoglobin exceeds 12 g/dl (7.5 mmol/l), the dose should be reduced by approximately 25 to 50 %. Treatment with NeoRecormon should be temporarily discontinued if haemoglobin levels exceed 13 g/dl (8.1 mmol/l). Therapy should be reinitiated at approximately 25 % lower than the previous dose after haemoglobin levels fall to 12 g/dl (7.5 mmol/l) or below.

If the rise in haemoglobin is greater than 2 g/dl (1.3 mmol/l) in 4 weeks, the dose should be reduced by 25 to 50 %.

Patients should be monitored closely to ensure that the lowest approved dose of NeoRecormon is used to provide adequate control of the symptoms of anaemia.

Treatment for increasing the amount of autologous blood:

The reconstituted solution is administered intravenously over approx. 2 minutes or subcutaneously.

NeoRecormon is administered twice weekly over 4 weeks. On those occasions where the patient's PCV allows blood donation, i.e. PCV ⩾ 33 %, NeoRecormon is administered at the end of blood donation.

Figure 1

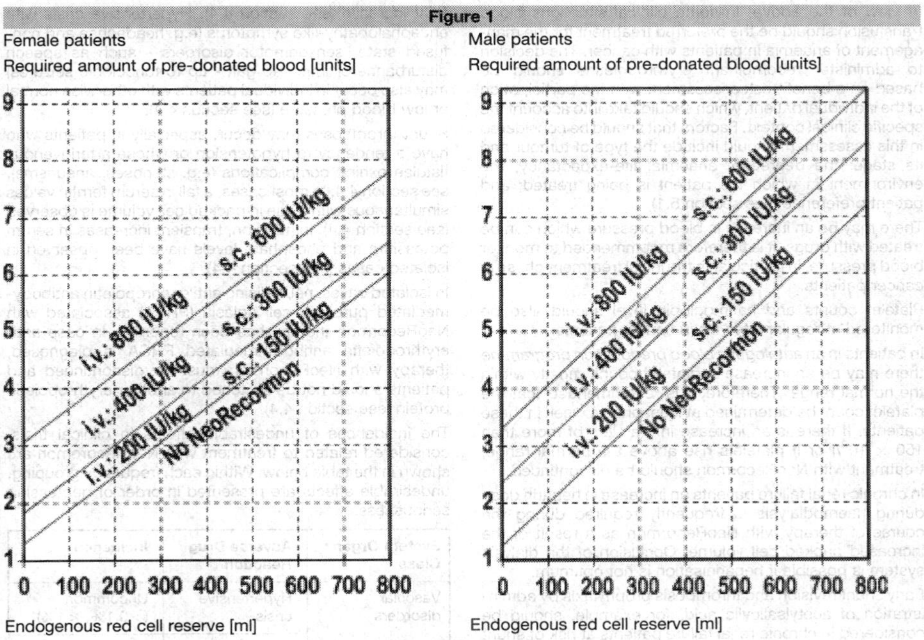

During the entire treatment period, a PCV of 48 % should not be exceeded.

The dosage must be determined by the surgical team individually for each patient as a function of the required amount of pre-donated blood and the endogenous red cell reserve:

1. The required amount of pre-donated blood depends on the anticipated blood loss, use of blood conserving procedures and the physical condition of the patient.

This amount should be that quantity which is expected to be sufficient to avoid homologous blood transfusions.

The required amount of pre-donated blood is expressed in units whereby one unit in the nomogram is equivalent to 180 ml red cells.

2. The ability to donate blood depends predominantly on the patient's blood volume and baseline PCV. Both variables determine the endogenous red cell reserve, which can be calculated according to the following formula.

Endogenous red cell reserve = blood volume [ml] × (PCV - 33) ÷ 100

Women: blood volume [ml] = 41 [ml/kg] × body weight [kg] + 1200 [ml]

Men: blood volume [ml] = 44 [ml/kg] × body weight [kg] + 1600 [ml]

(body weight ⩾ 45 kg)

The indication for NeoRecormon treatment and, if given, the single dose should be determined from the required amount of pre-donated blood and the endogenous red cell reserve according to the following graphs.

(see Figure 1 above)

The single dose thus determined is administered twice weekly over 4 weeks. The maximum dose should not exceed 1600 IU/kg body weight per week for intravenous or 1200 IU/kg per week for subcutaneous administration.

4.3 Contraindications

Hypersensitivity to the active substance or any of the excipients.

Poorly controlled hypertension.

In the indication "increasing the yield of autologous blood": myocardial infarction or stroke in the month preceding treatment, unstable angina pectoris, increased risk of deep venous thrombosis such as history of venous thromboembolic disease.

NeoRecormon Multidose contains benzyl alcohol as a preservative and must therefore not be given to infants or young children up to three years old.

4.4 Special warnings and precautions for use

NeoRecormon should be used with caution in the presence of refractory anaemia with excess blasts in transformation, epilepsy, thrombocytosis, and chronic liver failure. Folic acid and vitamin B_{12} deficiencies should be ruled out as they reduce the effectiveness of NeoRecormon.

In order to ensure effective erythropoiesis, iron status should be evaluated for all patients prior to and during treatment and supplementary iron therapy may be necessary and conducted in accordance with therapeutic guidelines.

Severe aluminium overload due to treatment of renal failure may compromise the effectiveness of NeoRecormon.

The indication for NeoRecormon treatment of nephrosclerotic patients not yet undergoing dialysis should be defined individually, as a possible acceleration of progression of renal failure cannot be ruled out with certainty.

Pure red cell aplasia caused by neutralising anti-erythropoietin antibodies has been reported in association with erythropoietin therapy, including NeoRecormon. These antibodies have been shown to cross-react with all erythropoietic proteins, and patients suspected or confirmed to have neutralising antibodies to erythropoietin should not be switched to NeoRecormon (see section 4.8).

In *chronic renal failure* patients an increase in blood pressure or aggravation of existing hypertension, especially in cases of rapid PCV increase can occur. These increases in blood pressure can be treated with medicinal products. If blood pressure rises cannot be controlled by drug therapy, a transient interruption of NeoRecormon therapy is recommended. Particularly at beginning of therapy, regular monitoring of the blood pressure is recommended, including between dialyses. Hypertensive crisis with encephalopathy-like symptoms may occur and require the immediate attention of a physician and intensive medical care. Particular attention should be paid to sudden stabbing migraine like headaches as a possible warning sign.

In *chronic renal failure* patients there may be a moderate dose-dependent rise in the platelet count within the normal range during treatment with NeoRecormon, especially after intravenous administration. This regresses during the course of continued therapy. It is recommended that the platelet count be monitored regularly during the first 8 weeks of therapy.

In patients with chronic renal failure, maintenance haemoglobin concentration should not exceed the upper limit of the target haemoglobin concentration recommended in section 4.2. In clinical trials, an increased risk of death and serious cardiovascular events was observed when erythropoiesis stimulating agents (ESAs) were administered to target a haemoglobin of greater than 12 g/dl (7.5 mmol/l).

Controlled clinical trials have not shown significant benefits attributable to the administration of epoetins when haemoglobin concentration is increased beyond the level necessary to control symptoms of anaemia and to avoid blood transfusion.

Effect on tumour growth

Epoetins are growth factors that primarily stimulate red blood cell production. Erythropoietin receptors may be expressed on the surface of a variety of tumour cells. As with all growth factors, there is a concern that epoetins could stimulate the growth of tumours. In several controlled studies, epoetins have not been shown to improve overall survival or decrease the risk of tumour progression in patients with anaemia associated with cancer.

In controlled clinical studies, use of NeoRecormon and other erythropoiesis-stimulating agents (ESAs) have shown:

- shortened time to tumour progression in patients with advanced head and neck cancer receiving radiation therapy when administered to target a haemoglobin of greater than 14 g/dl (8.7 mmol/l),

- shortened overall survival and increased deaths attributed to disease progression at 4 months in patients with metastatic breast cancer receiving chemotherapy when administered to target a haemoglobin of 12-14 g/dl (7.5-8.7 mmol/l),

- increased risk of death when administered to target a haemoglobin of 12 g/dl (7.5 mmol/l) in patients with active malignant disease receiving neither chemotherapy nor radiation therapy. ESAs are not indicated for use in this patient population.

In view of the above, in some clinical situations blood transfusion should be the preferred treatment for the management of anaemia in patients with cancer. The decision to administer recombinant erythropoietins should be based on a benefit-risk assessment with the participation of the individual patient, which should take into account the specific clinical context. Factors that should be considered in this assessment should include the type of tumour and its stage; the degree of anaemia; life-expectancy; the environment in which the patient is being treated; and patient preference (see section 5.1)

There may be an increase in blood pressure which can be treated with drugs. It is therefore recommended to monitor blood pressure, in particular in the initial treatment phase in cancer patients.

Platelet counts and haemoglobin level should also be monitored at regular intervals in cancer patients.

In patients in an *autologous blood predonation programme* there may be an increase in platelet count, mostly within the normal range. Therefore, it is recommended that the platelet count be determined at least once a week in these patients. If there is an increase in platelets of more than 150 × 10^9/l or if platelets rise above the normal range, treatment with NeoRecormon should be discontinued.

In chronic renal failure patients an increase in heparin dose during haemodialysis is frequently required during the course of therapy with NeoRecormon as a result of the increased packed cell volume. Occlusion of the dialysis system is possible if heparinisation is not optimum.

Early shunt revision and thrombosis prophylaxis by administration of acetylsalicylic acid, for example, should be considered in chronic renal failure patients at risk of shunt thrombosis.

Serum potassium and phosphate levels should be monitored regularly during NeoRecormon therapy. Potassium elevation has been reported in a few uraemic patients receiving NeoRecormon, though causality has not been established. If an elevated or rising potassium level is observed then consideration should be given to ceasing NeoRecormon administration until the level has been corrected.

For use of NeoRecormon in an autologous predonation programme, the official guidelines on principles of blood donation must be considered, in particular:

- only patients with a PCV ≥ 33 % (haemoglobin ≥ 11 g/dl [6.83 mmol/l]) should donate;
- special care should be taken with patients below 50 kg weight;
- the single volume drawn should not exceed approx. 12 % of the patient's estimated blood volume.

Treatment should be reserved for patients in whom it is considered of particular importance to avoid homologous blood transfusion taking into consideration the risk/benefit assessment for homologous transfusions.

Misuse by healthy persons may lead to an excessive increase in packed cell volume. This may be associated with life-threatening complications of the cardiovascular system.

NeoRecormon Multidose contains up to 5.0 mg phenylalanine/vial as an excipient. Therefore this should be taken into consideration in patients affected with severe forms of phenylketonuria.

NeoRecormon in reconstituted multidose solution contains benzyl alcohol which may cause toxic reactions and anaphylactoid reactions in infants and children up to 3 years old.

This medicinal product contains less than 1 mmol sodium (23 mg) per dose, i.e. essentially "sodium-free".

4.5 Interaction with other medicinal products and other forms of interaction

The clinical results obtained so far do not indicate any interaction of NeoRecormon with other medicinal products.

Animal experiments revealed that epoetin beta does not increase the myelotoxicity of cytostatic medicinal products like etoposide, cisplatin, cyclophosphamide, and fluorouracil.

4.6 Pregnancy and lactation

For epoetin beta no clinical data on exposed pregnancies are available. Animal studies do not indicate direct or indirect harmful effects with respect to pregnancy, embryonal/foetal development, parturition or postnatal development (see 5.3).

Caution should be exercised when prescribing to pregnant women.

4.7 Effects on ability to drive and use machines

NeoRecormon has no influence on the ability to drive and use machines.

4.8 Undesirable effects

Based on results from clinical trials including 1725 patients approximately 8 % of patients treated with NeoRecormon are expected to experience adverse reactions.

- Anaemic patients with chronic renal failure

The most frequent adverse reaction during treatment with NeoRecormon is an increase in blood pressure or aggravation of existing hypertension, especially in cases of rapid PCV increase (see section 4.4). Hypertensive crisis with encephalopathy-like symptoms (e.g. headaches and confused state, sensorimotor disorders - such as speech disturbance or impaired gait - up to tonoclonic seizures) may also occur in individual patients with otherwise normal or low blood pressure (see section 4.4).

Shunt thromboses may occur, especially in patients who have a tendency to hypotension or whose arteriovenous fistulae exhibit complications (e.g. stenoses, aneurisms), see section 4.4. In most cases, a fall in serum ferritin values simultaneous with a rise in packed cell volume is observed (see section 4.4). In addition, transient increases in serum potassium and phosphate levels have been observed in isolated cases (see section 4.4).

In isolated cases, neutralising anti erythropoietin antibody-mediated pure red cell aplasia (PRCA) associated with NeoRecormon therapy has been reported. In case anti-erythropoietin antibody-mediated PRCA is diagnosed, therapy with NeoRecormon must be discontinued and patients should not be switched to another erythropoietic protein (see section 4.4).

The incidences of undesirable effects in clinical trials, considered related to treatment with NeoRecoromon are shown in the table below. Within each frequency grouping, undesirable effects are presented in order of decreasing seriousness.

System Organ Class	Adverse Drug Reaction	Incidence
Vascular disorders	Hypertensive crisis	Uncommon (>0.1%, <1%)
	Hypertension	Common (>1%, <10%)
Nervous system disorders	Headache	Common (>1%, <10%)
Blood and the lymphatic system disorders	Shunt thrombosis	Rare (>0.01%, <0.1%)
	Thrombocytosis	Very rare (<0.01%)

- Patients with cancer

Epoetin beta treatment-related headache and hypertension which can be treated with drugs are common (>1%, <10%) (see section 4.4).

In some patients, a fall in serum iron parameters is observed (see section 4.4).

Clinical studies have shown a higher frequency of thromboembolic events in cancer patients treated with NeoRecormon compared to untreated controls or placebo. In patients treated with NeoRecormon, this incidence is 7 % compared to 4 % in controls; this is not associated with any increase in thromboembolic mortality compared with controls.

The incidences of undesirable effects in clinical trials, considered related to treatment with NeoRecoromon are shown in the table below. Within each frequency grouping, undesirable effects are presented in order of decreasing seriousness.

System Organ Class	Adverse Drug Reaction	Incidence
Vascular disorders	Hypertension	Common (>1%, <10%)
Blood and the lymphatic system disorders	Thromboembolic event	Common (>1%, <10%)
Nervous system disorders	Headache	Common (>1%, <10%)

- Patients in an autologous blood predonation programme

Patients in an autologous blood predonation programme have been reported to show a slightly higher frequency of thromboembolic events. However, a causal relationship with treatment with NeoRecormon could not be established.

In placebo controlled trials temporary iron deficiency was more pronounced in patients treated with NeoRecormon than in controls (see section 4.4).

The incidences of undesirable effects in clinical trials, considered related to treatment with NeoRecoromon are shown in the table below. Within each frequency grouping, undesirable effects are presented in order of decreasing seriousness.

System Organ Class	Adverse Drug Reaction	Incidence
Nervous system disorders	Headache	Common (>1%, <10%)

- All indications

Rarely (≥1/10.000 to ≤1/1.000), epoetin beta treatment-related skin reactions such as rash, pruritus, urticaria or injection site reactions may occur. In very rare cases (≤1/10.000), epoetin beta treatment-related anaphylactoid reactions have been reported. However, in controlled clinical studies no increased incidence of hypersensitivity reactions was found.

In very rare cases (≤1/10.000), particularly when starting treatment, epoetin beta treatment-related flu-like symptoms such as fever, chills, headaches, pain in the limbs, malaise and/or bone pain have been reported. These reactions were mild or moderate in nature and subsided after a couple of hours or days.

4.9 Overdose

The therapeutic margin of NeoRecormon is very wide. Even at very high serum levels no symptoms of poisoning have been observed.

5. PHARMACOLOGICAL PROPERTIES

5.1 Pharmacodynamic properties

Pharmacotherapeutic group: antianaemic, ATC code: B03XA

Epoetin beta is identical in its amino acid and carbohydrate composition to erythropoietin that has been isolated from the urine of anaemic patients.

Erythropoietin is a glycoprotein that stimulates the formation of erythrocytes from its committed progenitors. It acts as a mitosis stimulating factor and differentiation hormone.

The biological efficacy of epoetin beta has been demonstrated after intravenous and subcutaneous administration in various animal models *in vivo* (normal and uraemic rats, polycythaemic mice, dogs). After administration of epoetin beta, the number of erythrocytes, the Hb values and reticulocyte counts increase as well as the ^{59}Fe-incorporation rate.

An increased ^{3}H-thymidine incorporation in the erythroid nucleated spleen cells has been found *in vitro* (mouse spleen cell culture) after incubation with epoetin beta.

Investigations in cell cultures of human bone marrow cells showed that epoetin beta stimulates erythropoiesis specifically and does not affect leucopoiesis. Cytotoxic actions of epoetin beta on bone marrow or on human skin cells were not detected.

After single dose administration of epoetin beta no effects on behaviour or locomotor activity of mice and circulatory or respiratory function of dogs were observed.

Erythropoietin is a growth factor that primarily stimulates red cell production. Erythropoietin receptors may be expressed on the surface of a variety of tumour cells.

Survival and tumour progression have been examined in five large controlled studies involving a total of 2833 patients, of which four were double-blind placebo-controlled studies and one was an open-label study. Two of the studies recruited patients who were being treated with chemotherapy. The target haemoglobin concentration in two studies was > 13 g/dl; in the remaining three studies it was 12-14 g/dl. In the open-label study there was no difference in overall survival between patients treated with recombinant human erythropoietin and controls. In the four placebo-controlled studies the hazard ratios for overall survival ranged between 1.25 and 2.47 in favour of controls. These studies have shown a consistent unexplained statistically significant excess mortality in patients who have anaemia associated with various common cancers who received recombinant human erythropoietin compared to controls. Overall survival outcome in the trials could not be satisfactorily explained by differences in the incidence of thrombosis and related complications between those given recombinant human erythropoietin and those in the control group.

An individual patient data based meta-analysis, which included data from all 12 controlled clinical studies in anaemic cancer patients conducted with NeoRecormon (n=2301), showed an overall hazard ratio point estimate for survival of 1.13 in favour of controls (95 % CI 0.87, 1.46). In patients with baseline haemoglobin ≤ 10 g/dl (n=899), the hazard ratio point estimate for survival was 0.98 (95 % CI 0.68 to 1.40). An increased relative risk for thromboembolic events was observed in the overall population (RR 1.62, 95 % CI: 1.13, 2.31).

A systematic review has also been performed involving more than 9000 cancer patients participating in 57 clinical trials. Meta-analysis of overall survival data produced a hazard ratio point estimate of 1.08 in favour of controls (95 % CI: 0.99, 1.18; 42 trials and 8167 patients). An increased relative risk of thromboembolic events (RR 1.67, 95 % CI: 1.35, 2.06, 35 trials and 6769 patients) was observed in patients treated with recombinant human erythropoietin. There is therefore consistent evidence to suggest that there may be significant harm to patients with cancer who are treated with recombinant human erythropoietin. The extent to which these outcomes might apply to the administration of recombinant human erythropoietin to patients with cancer, treated with chemotherapy to achieve haemoglobin concentrations less than 13 g/dl, is unclear because few patients with these characteristics were included in the data reviewed.

In very rare cases, neutralising anti-erythropoietin antibodies with or without pure red cell aplasia (PRCA) occurred during rHuEPO therapy.

5.2 Pharmacokinetic properties

Pharmacokinetic investigations in healthy volunteers and uraemic patients show that the half-life of intravenously administered epoetin beta is between 4 and 12 hours and that the distribution volume corresponds to one to two times the plasma volume. Analogous results have been found in animal experiments in uraemic and normal rats.

After subcutaneous administration of epoetin beta to uraemic patients, the protracted absorption results in a serum concentration plateau, whereby the maximum concentration is reached after an average of 12 - 28 hours. The terminal half-life is higher than after intravenous administration, with an average of 13 - 28 hours.

Bioavailability of epoetin beta after subcutaneous administration is between 23 and 42 % as compared with intravenous administration.

5.3 Preclinical safety data

Non-clinical data reveal no special hazard for humans based on conventional studies of safety pharmacology, repeated dose toxicity, genotoxicity, and toxicity to reproduction.

A carcinogenicity study with homologous erythropoietin in mice did not reveal any signs of proliferative or tumourigenic potential.

6. PHARMACEUTICAL PARTICULARS

6.1 List of excipients

Lyophilisate:

Urea,

Sodium chloride,

Polysorbate 20,

Sodium dihydrogen phosphate,

Disodium hydrogen phosphate,

Calcium chloride,

Glycine,

L-Leucine,

L-Isoleucine,

L-Threonine,

L-Glutamic acid,

L-Phenylalanine.

Solvent:

Benzyl alcohol,

Benzalkonium chloride,

Water for injections.

6.2 Incompatibilities

This medicinal product must not be mixed with other medicinal products except those mentioned in section 6.6. (content of accompanying solvent ampoule).

6.3 Shelf life

3 years.

Chemical and physical in-use stability of the reconstituted solution has been demonstrated for one month at 2°C - 8°C. From a microbiological point of view, once opened, the reconstituted solution may be stored for maximum of one month at 2°C - 8°C. Other in-use storage times and conditions are the responsibility of the user.

6.4 Special precautions for storage

Store in a refrigerator (2°C – 8°C).

Keep the vial in the outer carton, in order to protect from light.

For the purpose of ambulatory use, the patient may remove the unreconstituted product from the refrigerator and store it at room temperature (not above 25°C) for one single period of up to 5 days.

Leaving the reconstituted solution outside the refrigerator should be limited to the time necessary for preparing the injections.

For storage conditions of the reconstituted medicinal product see section 6.3.

6.5 Nature and contents of container

Lyophilisate (50,000 IU) for solution for injection in a vial (type I glass) with a stopper (teflonised rubber) and 10 ml of solvent in an ampoule (type I glass), with one reconstitution and withdrawal device with one needle (21G2), and one disposable syringe (polypropylene and polyethylene) (10 ml).

Lyophilisate (100,000 IU) for solution for injection in a vial (type 1 glass) with a stopper (teflonised rubber) and 5 ml of solvent in an ampoule (type 1 glass), with one reconstitution and withdrawal device with one needle (21G2) and one disposable syringe (polypropylene and polyethylene) (5 ml).

6.6 Special precautions for disposal and other handling

NeoRecormon Multidose is supplied as a lyophilisate for solution for injection in vials. This is dissolved with the contents of the accompanying solvent ampoule by means of a reconstitution and withdrawal device according to the instructions given below. Only solutions which are clear or slightly opalescent, colourless and practically free of visible particles may be injected. Do not use glass materials for injection, use only plastic materials.

This is a multidose preparation from which different single doses can be withdrawn over a period of 1 month after dissolution. To avoid the risk of contamination of the contents always observe aseptic techniques (i.e. use disposable sterile syringes and needles to administer each dose) and strictly follow the handling instructions below. Before withdrawing each dose disinfect the rubber seal of the withdrawal device with alcohol to prevent contamination of the contents by repeated needle insertions.

<u>Preparation of NeoRecormon Multidose solution</u>

(1) Take the vial with the freeze-dried substance out of the package. Write the date of reconstitution and expiry on the label (expiry is 1 month after reconstitution).

(2) Remove the plastic cap from the vial.

(3) Disinfect the rubber seal with alcohol.

(4) Take the reconstitution and withdrawal device (which allows sterile air exchange) out of the blister and remove the protective cover from the spike.

(5) Attach the device to the vial until the snap lock clicks home.

(6) Put the green needle on the syringe contained in the package and remove the needle cover.

(7) Hold the OPC (One-Point-Cut) ampoule with the blue point upwards. Shake or tap the ampoule to get any fluid in the stem into the body of the ampoule. Take hold of the stem and snap off away from you. Withdraw <u>all the solvent</u> into the syringe. Disinfect the rubber seal of the device with alcohol.

(8) Penetrate the seal with the needle to a depth of about 1 cm and slowly inject the solvent into the vial. Then disconnect the syringe (with needle) from the device.

(9) Swirl the vial gently until the lyophilisate has dissolved. Do not shake. Check that the solution is clear, colourless and practically free from particles. Put the protective cap on the top of the device.

(10) Before and after reconstitution NeoRecormon Multidose must be stored at +2° to +8°C (refrigerator).

<u>Preparation of a single injection</u>

(1) Before withdrawing each dose disinfect the rubber seal of the device with alcohol.

(2) Place a 26G needle onto an appropriate single-use syringe (max.1 ml).

(3) Remove the needle cover and insert the needle through the rubber seal of the device. Withdraw NeoRecormon solution into the syringe, expel air from the syringe into the vial and adjust the amount of NeoRecormon solution in the syringe to the dose prescribed. Then disconnect the syringe (with needle) from the device.

(4) Replace the needle by a new one (the new needle should have the size which you normally use for injections).

(5) Remove the needle cover and carefully expel air from the needle by holding the syringe vertically and gently pressing the plunger upwards until a bead of liquid appears at the needle tip.

For subcutaneous injection, clean the skin at the site of injection using an alcohol wipe. Form a skin fold by pinching the skin between the thumb and the forefinger. Hold the syringe near to the needle and insert the needle into the skin with a quick, firm action. Inject NeoRecormon solution. Withdraw the needle quickly and apply pressure over the injection site with a dry, sterile pad.

Any unused product or waste material should be disposed of in accordance with local requirements.

7. MARKETING AUTHORISATION HOLDER

Roche Registration Limited

6 Falcon Way

Shire Park

Welwyn Garden City

AL7 1TW

United Kingdom

8. MARKETING AUTHORISATION NUMBER(S)

NeoRecormon Multidose 50,000 IU Lyophilisate and solvent for solution for injection: EU/1/97/031/019

NeoRecormon Multidose 100,000 IU Lyophilisate and solvent for solution for injection: EU/1/97/031/020

9. DATE OF FIRST AUTHORISATION/RENEWAL OF THE AUTHORISATION

Date of the first authorisation: 16 July 1997

Date of the last renewal: 16 July 2007

10. DATE OF REVISION OF THE TEXT

23 October 2008

Detailed information on this medicinal product is available on the website of the European Medicines Agency (EMEA) http://www.emea.europa.eu/

NeoRecormon Powder and Solvent for Solution for Injection in Cartridge

(Roche Products Limited)

1. NAME OF THE MEDICINAL PRODUCT

NeoRecormon 10,000 IU Lyophilisate and solvent for solution for injection in cartridge (10,000 IU/ml)

NeoRecormon 20,000 IU Lyophilisate and solvent for solution for injection in cartridge (20,000 IU/ml)

NeoRecormon 60,000 IU Lyophilisate and solvent for solution for injection in cartridge (60,000 IU/ml)

2. QUALITATIVE AND QUANTITATIVE COMPOSITION

One cartridge contains 10,000 international units (IU) corresponding to 83 micrograms epoetin beta* (recombinant human erythropoietin) and 1 ml solvent (water for injections with benzyl alcohol and benzalkonium chloride as preservatives).

One ml solution for injection contains 10,000 IU epoetin beta.

One cartridge contains 20,000 international units (IU) corresponding to 166 micrograms epoetin beta* (recombinant human erythropoietin) and 1 ml solvent (water for injections with benzyl alcohol and benzalkonium chloride as preservatives).

One ml solution for injection contains 20,000 IU epoetin beta.

One cartridge contains 60,000 international units (IU) corresponding to 498 micrograms epoetin beta* (recombinant human erythropoietin) and 1 ml solvent (water for injections with benzyl alcohol and benzalkonium chloride as preservatives).

One ml solution for injection contains 60,000 IU epoetin beta.

* produced in Chinese Hamster Ovary cells (CHO) by recombinant DNA technology

Excipients:

Phenylalanine (up to 0.5 mg/cartridge)

Sodium (less than 1 mmol/cartridge)

Benzyl alcohol (up to 4 mg/cartridge)

For a full list of excipients, see section 6.1.

3. PHARMACEUTICAL FORM

Lyophilisate and solvent for solution for injection.

White lyophilisate and clear, colourless solvent.

4. CLINICAL PARTICULARS

4.1 Therapeutic indications

- Treatment of symptomatic anaemia associated with chronic renal failure (CRF) in adult and paediatric patients.
- Treatment of symptomatic anaemia in adult patients with non-myeloid malignancies receiving chemotherapy.
- Increasing the yield of autologous blood from patients in a pre-donation programme.

Its use in this indication must be balanced against the reported increased risk of thromboembolic events. Treatment should only be given to patients with moderate anaemia (Hb 10 - 13 g/dl [6.21 - 8.07 mmol/l], no iron deficiency) if blood conserving procedures are not available or insufficient when the scheduled major elective surgery requires a large volume of blood (4 or more units of blood for females or 5 or more units for males).

4.2 Posology and method of administration

Therapy with NeoRecormon should be initiated by physicians experienced in the above mentioned indications. As anaphylactoid reactions were observed in isolated cases, it is recommended that the first dose be administered under medical supervision.

The reconstituted product is a colourless, clear to slightly opalescent solution.

For instructions on reconstitution of the product before administration, see section 6.6.

The prepared solution is administered subcutaneously.

<u>Treatment of symptomatic anaemia in adult and paediatric chronic renal failure patients:</u>

Anaemia symptoms and sequelae may vary with age, gender, and overall burden of disease; a physician's evaluation of the individual patient's clinical course and condition is necessary. NeoRecormon should be administered subcutaneously in order to increase haemoglobin to not greater than 12 g/dl (7.5 mmol/l).

Due to intra-patient variability, occasional individual haemoglobin values for a patient above and below the desired haemoglobin level may be observed. Haemoglobin variability should be addressed through dose management, with consideration for the haemoglobin target range of 10 g/dl (6.2 mmol/l) to 12 g/dl (7.5 mmol/l). A sustained haemoglobin level of greater than 12 g/dl (7.5 mmol/l) should be avoided; guidance for appropriate dose adjustment for when haemoglobin values exceeding 12 g/dl (7.5 mmol/l) are observed are described below.

A rise in haemoglobin of greater than 2 g/dl (1.25 mmol/l) over a four week period should be avoided. If it occurs, appropriate dose adjustment should be made as provided. If the rate of rise in haemoglobin is greater than 2 g/dl (1.25 mmol/l) in one month or if the haemoglobin level is increasing and approaching 12 g/dl (7.45 mmol/l), the dose is to be reduced by approximately 25 %. If the haemoglobin level continues to increase, therapy should be interrupted until the haemoglobin level begins to decrease, at which point therapy should be restarted at a dose approximately 25 % below the previously administered dose.

Patients should be monitored closely to ensure that the lowest approved dose of NeoRecormon is used to provide adequate control of the symptoms of anaemia.

In the presence of hypertension or existing cardiovascular, cerebrovascular or peripheral vascular diseases, the weekly increase in Hb and the target Hb should be determined individually taking into account the clinical picture.

Treatment with NeoRecormon is divided into two stages.

1. <u>Correction phase</u>

The initial dosage is 3 × 20 IU/kg body weight per week. The dosage may be increased every 4 weeks by 3 × 20

IU/kg per week if the increase of Hb is not adequate (< 0.25 g/dl per week).

The weekly dose can also be divided into daily doses.

The maximum dose should not exceed 720 IU/kg per week.

2. Maintenance phase

To maintain an Hb of between 10 and 12 g/dl, the dosage is initially reduced to half of the previously administered amount. Subsequently, the dose is adjusted at intervals of one or two weeks individually for the patient (maintenance dose).

The weekly dose can be given as one injection per week or in divided doses three or seven times per week. Patients who are stable on a once weekly dosing regimen may be switched to once every two weeks administration. In this case dose increases may be necessary.

Results of clinical studies in children have shown that, on average, the younger the patients, the higher the NeoRecormon doses required. Nevertheless, the recommended dosing schedule should be followed as the individual response cannot be predicted.

Treatment with NeoRecormon is normally a long-term therapy. It can, however, be interrupted, if necessary, at any time. Data on the once weekly dosing schedule are based on clinical studies with a treatment duration of 24 weeks.

Treatment of symptomatic chemotherapy-induced anaemia in cancer patients:

NeoRecormon should be administered by the subcutaneous route to patients with anaemia (e.g. haemoglobin concentration ⩽ 10g/dl (6.2 mmol/l)). Anaemia symptoms and sequelae may vary with age, gender, and overall burden of disease; a physician's evaluation of the individual patient's clinical course and condition is necessary.

The weekly dose can be given as one injection per week or in divided doses 3 to 7 times per week.

The recommended initial dose is 30,000 IU per week (corresponding to approximately 450 IU/kg body weight per week, based on an average weighted patient).

Due to intra-patient variability, occasional individual haemoglobin values for a patient above and below the desired haemoglobin level may be observed. Haemoglobin variability should be addressed through dose management, with consideration for the haemoglobin target range of 10 g/dl (6.2 mmol/l) to 12 g/dl (7.5 mmol/l). A sustained haemoglobin level of greater than 12 g/dl (7.5 mmol/l) should be avoided; guidance for appropriate dose adjustment for when haemoglobin values exceeding 12 g/dl (7.5 mmol/l) are observed are described below.

If, after 4 weeks of therapy, the haemoglobin value has increased by at least 1 g/dl (0.62 mmol/l), the current dose should be continued. If the haemoglobin value has not increased by at least 1 g/dl (0.62 mmol/l), a doubling of the weekly dose should be considered. If, after 8 weeks of therapy, the haemoglobin value has not increased by at least 1 g/dl (0.62 mmol/l), response is unlikely and treatment should be discontinued.

The therapy should be continued up to 4 weeks after the end of chemotherapy.

The maximum dose should not exceed 60,000 IU per week.

Once the therapeutic objective for an individual patient has been achieved, the dose should be reduced by 25 to 50 % in order to maintain haemoglobin at that level. Appropriate dose titration should be considered.

If the haemoglobin exceeds 12 g/dl (7.5 mmol/l), the dose should be reduced by approximately 25 to 50 %. Treatment with NeoRecormon should be temporarily discontinued if haemoglobin levels exceed 13 g/dl (8.1 mmol/l). Therapy should be reinitiated at approximately 25 % lower than the previous dose after haemoglobin levels fall to 12 g/dl (7.5 mmol/l) or below.

If the rise in haemoglobin is greater than 2 g/dl (1.3 mmol/l) in 4 weeks, the dose should be reduced by 25 to 50 %.

Patients should be monitored closely to ensure that the lowest approved dose of NeoRecormon is used to provide adequate control of the symptoms of anaemia.

Treatment for increasing the amount of autologous blood:

NeoRecormon is administered twice weekly over 4 weeks. On those occasions where the patient's PCV allows blood donation, i.e. PCV ⩾ 33 %, NeoRecormon is administered at the end of blood donation.

During the entire treatment period, a PCV of 48 % should not be exceeded.

The dosage must be determined by the surgical team individually for each patient as a function of the required amount of pre-donated blood and the endogenous red cell reserve:

1. The required amount of pre-donated blood depends on the anticipated blood loss, use of blood conserving procedures and the physical condition of the patient.

This amount should be that quantity which is expected to be sufficient to avoid homologous blood transfusions.

The required amount of pre-donated blood is expressed in units whereby one unit in the nomogram is equivalent to 180 ml red cells.

Figure 1

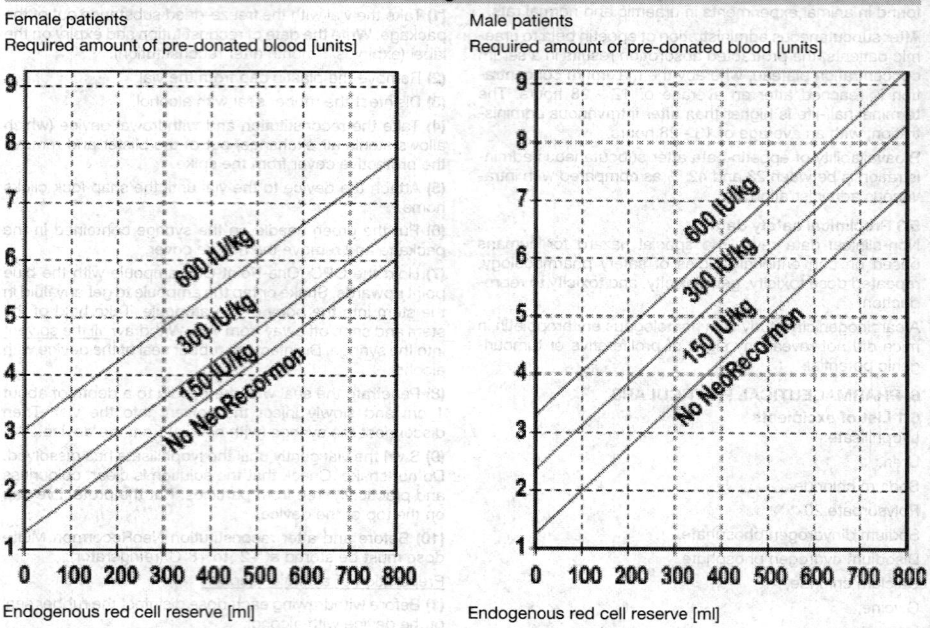

2. The ability to donate blood depends predominantly on the patient's blood volume and baseline PCV. Both variables determine the endogenous red cell reserve, which can be calculated according to the following formula.

Endogenous red cell reserve = blood volume [ml] × (PCV - 33) ÷ 100

Women: blood volume [ml] = 41 [ml/kg] × body weight [kg] + 1200 [ml]

Men: blood volume [ml] = 44 [ml/kg] × body weight [kg] + 1600 [ml]

(body weight ⩾ 45 kg)

The indication for NeoRecormon treatment and, if given, the single dose should be determined from the required amount of pre-donated blood and the endogenous red cell reserve according to the following graphs.

(see Figure 1 above)

The single dose thus determined is administered twice weekly over 4 weeks. The maximum dose should not exceed 1200 IU/kg body weight per week.

4.3 Contraindications

Hypersensitivity to the active substance or any of the excipients.

Poorly controlled hypertension.

In the indication "increasing the yield of autologous blood ": myocardial infarction or stroke in the month preceding treatment, unstable angina pectoris, increased risk of deep venous thrombosis such as history of venous thromboembolic disease.

NeoRecormon in cartridge contains benzyl alcohol as a preservative and must therefore not be given to infants or young children up to three years old.

4.4 Special warnings and precautions for use

NeoRecormon should be used with caution in the presence of refractory anaemia with excess blasts in transformation, epilepsy, thrombocytosis, and chronic liver failure. Folic acid and vitamin B_{12} deficiencies should be ruled out as they reduce the effectiveness of NeoRecormon.

In order to ensure effective erythropoiesis, iron status should be evaluated for all patients prior to and during treatment and supplementary iron therapy may be necessary and conducted in accordance with therapeutic guidelines.

Severe aluminium overload due to treatment of renal failure may compromise the effectiveness of NeoRecormon.

The indication for NeoRecormon treatment of nephrosclerotic patients not yet undergoing dialysis should be defined individually, as a possible acceleration of progression of renal failure cannot be ruled out with certainty.

Pure red cell aplasia caused by neutralising anti-erythropoietin antibodies has been reported in association with erythropoietin therapy, including NeoRecormon. These antibodies have been shown to cross-react with all erythropoietic proteins, and patients suspected or confirmed to have neutralising antibodies to erythropoietin should not be switched to NeoRecormon (see section 4.8).

In *chronic renal failure* patients an increase in blood pressure or aggravation of existing hypertension, especially in cases of rapid PCV increase can occur. These increases in blood pressure can be treated with medicinal products. If blood pressure rises cannot be controlled by drug therapy, a transient interruption of NeoRecormon therapy is recommended. Particularly at beginning of therapy, regular monitoring of the blood pressure is recommended, including between dialyses. Hypertensive crisis with encephalopathy-like symptoms may occur and require the immediate attention of a physician and intensive medical care. Particular attention should be paid to sudden stabbing migraine like headaches as a possible warning sign.

In *chronic renal failure* patients there may be a moderate dose-dependent rise in the platelet count within the normal range during treatment with NeoRecormon, especially after intravenous administration. This regresses during the course of continued therapy. It is recommended that the platelet count be monitored regularly during the first 8 weeks of therapy.

In patients with chronic renal failure, maintenance haemoglobin concentration should not exceed the upper limit of the target haemoglobin concentration recommended in section 4.2. In clinical trials, an increased risk of death and serious cardiovascular events was observed when erythropoiesis stimulating agents (ESAs) were administered to target a haemoglobin of greater than 12 g/dl (7.5 mmol/l).

Controlled clinical trials have not shown significant benefits attributable to the administration of epoetins when haemoglobin concentration is increased beyond the level necessary to control symptoms of anaemia and to avoid blood transfusion.

Effect on tumour growth

Epoetins are growth factors that primarily stimulate red blood cell production. Erythropoietin receptors may be expressed on the surface of a variety of tumour cells. As with all growth factors, there is a concern that epoetins could stimulate the growth of tumours. In several controlled studies, epoetins have not been shown to improve overall survival or decrease the risk of tumour progression in patients with anaemia associated with cancer.

In controlled clinical studies, use of NeoRecormon and other erythropoiesis-stimulating agents (ESAs) have shown:

- shortened time to tumour progression in patients with advanced head and neck cancer receiving radiation therapy when administered to target a haemoglobin of greater than 14 g/dl (8.7 mmol/l),

- shortened overall survival and increased deaths attributed to disease progression at 4 months in patients with metastatic breast cancer receiving chemotherapy when administered to target a haemoglobin of 12-14 g/dl (7.5-8.7 mmol/l),

- increased risk of death when administered to target a haemoglobin of 12 g/dl (7.5 mmol/l) in patients with active malignant disease receiving neither chemotherapy nor radiation therapy. ESAs are not indicated for use in this patient population.

In view of the above, in some clinical situations blood transfusion should be the preferred treatment for the management of anaemia in patients with cancer. The decision to administer recombinant erythropoietins should be based on a benefit-risk assessment with the participation of the individual patient, which should take into account the specific clinical context. Factors that should be considered in this assessment should include the type of tumour and its stage; the degree of anaemia; life-expectancy; the environment in which the patient is being treated; and patient preference (see section 5.1)

There may be an increase in blood pressure which can be treated with drugs. It is therefore recommended to monitor blood pressure, in particular in the initial treatment phase in cancer patients.

Platelet counts and haemoglobin level should also be monitored at regular intervals in cancer patients.

In patients in an *autologous blood predonation programme* there may be an increase in platelet count, mostly within the normal range. Therefore, it is recommended that the platelet count be determined at least once a week in these patients. If there is an increase in platelets of more than 150 × 10^9/l or if platelets rise above the normal range, treatment with NeoRecormon should be discontinued.

In chronic renal failure patients an increase in heparin dose during haemodialysis is frequently required during the course of therapy with NeoRecormon as a result of the increased packed cell volume. Occlusion of the dialysis system is possible if heparinisation is not optimum.

Early shunt revision and thrombosis prophylaxis by administration of acetylsalicylic acid, for example, should be considered in chronic renal failure patients at risk of shunt thrombosis.

Serum potassium and phosphate levels should be monitored regularly during NeoRecormon therapy. Potassium elevation has been reported in a few uraemic patients receiving NeoRecormon, though causality has not been established. If an elevated or rising potassium level is observed then consideration should be given to ceasing NeoRecormon administration until the level has been corrected.

For use of NeoRecormon in an autologous predonation programme, the official guidelines on principles of blood donation must be considered, in particular:

- only patients with a PCV ⩾ 33 % (haemoglobin ⩾ 11 g/dl [6.83 mmol/l]) should donate;
- special care should be taken with patients below 50 kg weight;
- the single volume drawn should not exceed approx. 12 % of the patient's estimated blood volume.

Treatment should be reserved for patients in whom it is considered of particular importance to avoid homologous blood transfusion taking into consideration the risk/benefit assessment for homologous transfusions.

Misuse by healthy persons may lead to an excessive increase in packed cell volume. This may be associated with life-threatening complications of the cardiovascular system.

NeoRecormon in cartridge contains up to 0.5 mg phenylalanine/cartridge as an excipient. Therefore this should be taken into consideration in patients affected with severe forms of phenylketonuria.

NeoRecormon in cartridge contains up to 4 mg benzyl alcohol which may cause toxic reactions and anaphylactoid reactions in infants and children up to 3 years old.

This medicinal product contains less than 1 mmol sodium (23 mg) per cartridge, i.e. essentially "sodium-free".

4.5 Interaction with other medicinal products and other forms of interaction

The clinical results obtained so far do not indicate any interaction of NeoRecormon with other medicinal products.

Animal experiments revealed that epoetin beta does not increase the myelotoxicity of cytostatic medicinal products like etoposide, cisplatin, cyclophosphamide, and fluorouracil.

4.6 Pregnancy and lactation

For epoetin beta no clinical data on exposed pregnancies are available. Animal studies do not indicate direct or indirect harmful effects with respect to pregnancy, embryonal/foetal development, parturition or postnatal development (see 5.3).

Caution should be exercised when prescribing to pregnant women.

4.7 Effects on ability to drive and use machines

NeoRecormon has no influence on the ability to drive and use machines.

4.8 Undesirable effects

Based on results from clinical trials including 1725 patients approximately 8 % of patients treated with NeoRecormon are expected to experience adverse reactions.

- Anaemic patients with chronic renal failure

The most frequent adverse reaction during treatment with NeoRecormon is an increase in blood pressure or aggravation of existing hypertension, especially in cases of rapid PCV increase (see section 4.4). Hypertensive crisis with encephalopathy-like symptoms (e.g. headaches and confused state, sensorimotor disorders - such as speech disturbance or impaired gait - up to tonoclonic seizures) may also occur in individual patients with otherwise normal or low blood pressure (see section 4.4).

Shunt thromboses may occur, especially in patients who have a tendency to hypotension or whose arteriovenous fistulae exhibit complications (e.g. stenoses, aneurisms), see section 4.4. In most cases, a fall in serum ferritin values simultaneous with a rise in packed cell volume is observed (see section 4.4). In addition, transient increases in serum potassium and phosphate levels have been observed in isolated cases (see section 4.4).

In isolated cases, neutralising anti erythropoietin antibody-mediated pure red cell aplasia (PRCA) associated with NeoRecormon therapy has been reported. In case anti-erythropoietin antibody-mediated PRCA is diagnosed, therapy with NeoRecormon must be discontinued and patients should not be switched to another erythropoietic protein (see section 4.4).

The incidences of undesirable effects in clinical trials, considered related to treatment with NeoRecoromon are shown in the table below. Within each frequency grouping, undesirable effects are presented in order of decreasing seriousness.

System Organ Class	Adverse Drug Reaction	Incidence
Vascular disorders	Hypertensive crisis Hypertension	Uncommon (>0.1%, <1%) Common (>1%, <10%)
Nervous system disorders	Headache	Common (>1%, <10%)
Blood and the lymphatic system disorders	Shunt thrombosis Thrombocytosis	Rare (>0.01%, <0.1%) Very rare (<0.01%)

- Patients with cancer

Epoetin beta treatment-related headache and hypertension which can be treated with drugs are common (>1%, <10%) (see section 4.4).

In some patients, a fall in serum iron parameters is observed (see section 4.4).

Clinical studies have shown a higher frequency of thromboembolic events in cancer patients treated with NeoRecormon compared to untreated controls or placebo. In patients treated with NeoRecormon, this incidence is 7 % compared to 4 % in controls; this is not associated with any increase in thromboembolic mortality compared with controls.

The incidences of undesirable effects in clinical trials, considered related to treatment with NeoRecoromon are shown in the table below. Within each frequency grouping, undesirable effects are presented in order of decreasing seriousness.

System Organ Class	Adverse Drug Reaction	Incidence
Vascular disorders	Hypertension	Common (>1%, <10%)
Blood and the lymphatic system disorders	Thromboembolic event	Common (>1%, <10%)
Nervous system disorders	Headache	Common (>1%, <10%)

- Patients in an autologous blood predonation programme

Patients in an autologous blood predonation programme have been reported to show a slightly higher frequency of thromboembolic events. However, a causal relationship with treatment with NeoRecormon could not be established.

In placebo controlled trials temporary iron deficiency was more pronounced in patients treated with NeoRecormon than in controls (see section 4.4).

The incidences of undesirable effects in clinical trials, considered related to treatment with NeoRecoromon are shown in the table below. Within each frequency grouping, undesirable effects are presented in order of decreasing seriousness.

System Organ Class	Adverse Drug Reaction	Incidence
Nervous system disorders	Headache	Common (>1%, <10%)

- All indications

Rarely (⩾1/10.000 to ⩽1/1.000), epoetin beta treatment-related skin reactions such as rash, pruritus, urticaria or injection site reactions may occur. In very rare cases (⩽1/10.000), epoetin beta treatment-related anaphylactoid reactions have been reported. However, in controlled clinical studies no increased incidence of hypersensitivity reactions was found.

In very rare cases (⩽1/10.000), particularly when starting treatment, epoetin beta treatment-related flu-like symptoms such as fever, chills, headaches, pain in the limbs, malaise and/or bone pain have been reported. These reactions were mild or moderate in nature and subsided after a couple of hours or days.

4.9 Overdose

The therapeutic margin of NeoRecormon is very wide. Even at very high serum levels no symptoms of poisoning have been observed.

5. PHARMACOLOGICAL PROPERTIES

5.1 Pharmacodynamic properties

Pharmacotherapeutic group: antianaemic, ATC code: B03XA

Epoetin beta is identical in its amino acid and carbohydrate composition to erythropoietin that has been isolated from the urine of anaemic patients.

Erythropoietin is a glycoprotein that stimulates the formation of erythrocytes from its committed progenitors. It acts as a mitosis stimulating factor and differentiation hormone.

The biological efficacy of epoetin beta has been demonstrated after intravenous and subcutaneous administration in various animal models *in vivo* (normal and uraemic rats, polycythaemic mice, dogs). After administration of epoetin beta, the number of erythrocytes, the Hb values and reticulocyte counts increase as well as the ^{59}Fe-incorporation rate.

An increased ^{3}H-thymidine incorporation in the erythroid nucleated spleen cells has been found *in vitro* (mouse spleen cell culture) after incubation with epoetin beta.

Investigations in cell cultures of human bone marrow cells showed that epoetin beta stimulates erythropoiesis specifically and does not affect leucopoiesis. Cytotoxic actions of epoetin beta on bone marrow or on human skin cells were not detected.

After single dose administration of epoetin beta no effects on behaviour or locomotor activity of mice and circulatory or respiratory function of dogs were observed.

Erythropoietin is a growth factor that primarily stimulates red cell production. Erythropoietin receptors may be expressed on the surface of a variety of tumour cells.

Survival and tumour progression have been examined in five large controlled studies involving a total of 2833 patients, of which four were double-blind placebo-controlled studies and one was an open-label study. Two of the studies recruited patients who were being treated with chemotherapy. The target haemoglobin concentration in two studies was >13 g/dl; in the remaining three studies it was 12-14 g/dl. In the open-label study there was no difference in overall survival between patients treated with recombinant human erythropoietin and controls. In the four placebo-controlled studies the hazard ratios for overall survival ranged between 1.25 and 2.47 in favour of controls. These studies have shown a consistent unexplained statistically significant excess mortality in patients who have anaemia associated with various common cancers who received recombinant human erythropoietin compared to controls. Overall survival outcome in the trials could not be satisfactorily explained by differences in the incidence of thrombosis and related complications between those given recombinant human erythropoietin and those in the control group.

An individual patient data based meta-analysis, which included data from all 12 controlled clinical studies in anaemic cancer patients conducted with NeoRecormon (n=2301), showed an overall hazard ratio point estimate for survival of 1.13 in favour of controls (95 % CI 0.87, 1.46). In patients with baseline haemoglobin ⩽ 10 g/dl (n=899), the hazard ratio point estimate for survival was 0.98 (95 % CI 0.68 to 1.40). An increased relative risk for thromboembolic events was observed in the overall population (RR 1.62, 95 % CI: 1.13, 2.31).

A systematic review has also been performed involving more than 9000 cancer patients participating in 57 clinical trials. Meta-analysis of overall survival data produced a hazard ratio point estimate of 1.08 in favour of controls (95 % CI: 0.99, 1.18; 42 trials and 8167 patients). An increased relative risk of thromboembolic events (RR 1.67, 95 % CI: 1.35, 2.06, 35 trials and 6769 patients) was observed in patients treated with recombinant human erythropoietin. There is therefore consistent evidence to suggest that there may be significant harm to patients with cancer who are treated with recombinant human erythropoietin. The extent to which these outcomes might apply to the administration of recombinant human erythropoietin to patients with cancer, treated with chemotherapy to achieve haemoglobin concentrations less than 13 g/dl, is unclear because few patients with these characteristics were included in the data reviewed.

In very rare cases, neutralising anti-erythropoietin antibodies with or without pure red cell aplasia (PRCA) occurred during rHuEPO therapy.

5.2 Pharmacokinetic properties

Pharmacokinetic investigations in healthy volunteers and uraemic patients show that the half-life of intravenously administered epoetin beta is between 4 and 12 hours and that the distribution volume corresponds to one to two times the plasma volume. Analogous results have been found in animal experiments in uraemic and normal rats.

After subcutaneous administration of epoetin beta to uraemic patients, the protracted absorption results in a serum concentration plateau, whereby the maximum concentration is reached after an average of 12 - 28 hours. The terminal half-life is higher than after intravenous administration, with an average of 13 - 28 hours.

Bioavailability of epoetin beta after subcutaneous administration is between 23 and 42 % as compared with intravenous administration.

5.3 Preclinical safety data

Non-clinical data reveal no special hazard for humans based on conventional studies of safety pharmacology, repeated dose toxicity, genotoxicity, and toxicity to reproduction.

A carcinogenicity study with homologous erythropoietin in mice did not reveal any signs of proliferative or tumourigenic potential.

6. PHARMACEUTICAL PARTICULARS

6.1 List of excipients

Lyophilisate:

Urea,

Sodium chloride,

Polysorbate 20,

Sodium dihydrogen phosphate,

Disodium hydrogen phosphate,

Calcium chloride,

Glycine,

L-Leucine,

L-Isoleucine,

L-Threonine,

L-Glutamic acid,

L-Phenylalanine.

Solvent:

Benzyl alcohol,

Benzalkonium chloride,

Water for injections.

6.2 Incompatibilities

NeoRecormon in cartridge should only be used with the Reco-Pen. In the absence of compatibility studies, this medicinal product should not be mixed with other medicinal products.

6.3 Shelf life

2 years.

Chemical and physical in-use stability of the reconstituted solution has been demonstrated for one month at 2°C-8°C. From a microbiological point of view, once opened, the reconstituted solution may be stored for maximum of one month at 2°C-8°C. Other in-use storage times and conditions are the responsibility of the user.

6.4 Special precautions for storage

Store in a refrigerator (2°C – 8°C).

Keep the cartridge in the outer carton, in order to protect from light.

For the purpose of ambulatory use, the patient may remove the cartridge not yet inserted into the Reco-Pen from the refrigerator and store it at room temperature (not above 25°C) for one single period of up to 5 days.

After insertion into the Reco-Pen, the cooling chain may only be interrupted for administration of the product.

For storage conditions of the reconstituted medicinal product see section 6.3.

6.5 Nature and contents of container

Lyophilisate (10,000 IU) and solvent (1 ml) for solution for injection in two-chamber cartridge for Reco-Pen (type I glass) with front disk made of rubber material of pharmaceutical quality and with stoppers (teflonised rubber). Pack sizes of 1 or 3.

Lyophilisate (20,000 IU) and solvent (1 ml) for solution for injection in two-chamber cartridge for Reco-Pen (type I glass) with front disk made of rubber material of pharmaceutical quality and with stoppers (teflonised rubber). Pack sizes of 1 or 3.

Lyophilisate (60,000 IU) and solvent (1 ml) for solution for injection in two-chamber cartridge for Reco-Pen (type I glass) with front disk made of rubber material of pharmaceutical quality and with stoppers (teflonised rubber). Pack sizes of 1 or 3.

Not all pack sizes may be marketed.

6.6 Special precautions for disposal and other handling

This NeoRecormon presentation is a two-chamber cartridge containing lyophilisate for solution for injection and preserved solution. The ready-to-use solution is prepared by inserting the cartridge into the Reco-Pen. Prior to this a needle should be attached to the Reco-Pen. Only solutions which are clear or slightly opalescent, colourless and practically free of visible particles may be injected.

Please observe the instructions for use which are delivered with the Reco-Pen.

Any unused product or waste material should be disposed of in accordance with local requirements.

7. MARKETING AUTHORISATION HOLDER

Roche Registration Limited

6 Falcon Way

Shire Park

Welwyn Garden City

AL7 1TW

United Kingdom

8. MARKETING AUTHORISATION NUMBER(S)

NeoRecormon 10,000 IU Lyophilisate and solvent for solution for injection in cartridge: EU/1/97/031/021 - 022

NeoRecormon 20,000 IU Lyophilisate and solvent for solution for injection in cartridge: EU/1/97/031/023 - 024

NeoRecormon 60,000 IU Lyophilisate and solvent for solution for injection in cartridge: EU/1/97/031/039 - 040

9. DATE OF FIRST AUTHORISATION/RENEWAL OF THE AUTHORISATION

10,000 and 20,000 IU:	Date of the first authorisation: 16 July 1997 Date of the last renewal: 16 July 2007
60,000 IU:	Date of the first authorisation: 10 February 2000 Date of the last renewal: 16 July 2007

10. DATE OF REVISION OF THE TEXT

23 October 2008

Detailed information on this medicinal product is available on the website of the European Medicines Agency (EMEA) http://www.emea.europa.eu/

Neorecormon Solution for Injection in Pre-Filled Syringe

(Roche Products Limited)

1. NAME OF THE MEDICINAL PRODUCT

NeoRecormon solution for injection in pre-filled syringe

2. QUALITATIVE AND QUANTITATIVE COMPOSITION

One pre-filled syringe with 0.3 ml solution for injection contains 500 international units (IU) corresponding to 4.15 micrograms epoetin beta* (recombinant human erythropoietin).

One ml solution for injection contains 1667 IU epoetin beta.

One pre-filled syringe with 0.3 ml solution for injection contains 1000 international units (IU) corresponding to 8.3 micrograms epoetin beta* (recombinant human erythropoietin).

One ml solution for injection contains 3333 IU epoetin beta.

One pre-filled syringe with 0.3 ml solution for injection contains 2000 international units (IU) corresponding to 16.6 micrograms epoetin beta* (recombinant human erythropoietin).

One ml solution for injection contains 6667 IU epoetin beta.

One pre-filled syringe with 0.3 ml solution for injection contains 3000 international units (IU) corresponding to 24.9 micrograms epoetin beta* (recombinant human erythropoietin).

One ml solution for injection contains 10,000 IU epoetin beta.

One pre-filled syringe with 0.3 ml solution for injection contains 4000 international units (IU) corresponding to 33.2 micrograms epoetin beta* (recombinant human erythropoietin).

One ml solution for injection contains 13,333 IU epoetin beta.

One pre-filled syringe with 0.3 ml solution for injection contains 5000 international units (IU) corresponding to 41.5 micrograms epoetin beta* (recombinant human erythropoietin).

One ml solution for injection contains 16,667 IU epoetin beta.

One pre-filled syringe with 0.3 ml solution for injection contains 6000 international units (IU) corresponding to 49.8 micrograms epoetin beta* (recombinant human erythropoietin).

One ml solution for injection contains 20,000 IU epoetin beta.

One pre-filled syringe with 0.6 ml solution for injection contains 10,000 international units (IU) corresponding to 83 micrograms epoetin beta* (recombinant human erythropoietin).

One ml solution for injection contains 16,667 IU epoetin beta.

One pre-filled syringe with 0.6 ml solution for injection contains 20,000 international units (IU) corresponding to 166 micrograms epoetin beta* (recombinant human erythropoietin).

One ml solution for injection contains 33,333 IU epoetin beta.

One pre-filled syringe with 0.6 ml solution for injection contains 30,000 international units (IU) corresponding to 250 micrograms epoetin beta* (recombinant human erythropoietin).

One ml solution for injection contains 50,000 IU epoetin beta.

* produced in Chinese Hamster Ovary cells (CHO) by recombinant DNA technology

Excipients:

Phenylalanine (up to 0.3 mg/syringe)

Sodium (less than 1 mmol/syringe)

For a full list of excipients, see section 6.1.

3. PHARMACEUTICAL FORM

Solution for injection.

Colourless, clear to slightly opalescent solution.

4. CLINICAL PARTICULARS

4.1 Therapeutic indications

- Treatment of symptomatic anaemia associated with chronic renal failure (CRF) in adult and paediatric patients.

- Prevention of anaemia of prematurity in infants with a birth weight of 750 to 1500 g and a gestational age of less than 34 weeks.

- Treatment of symptomatic anaemia in adult patients with non-myeloid malignancies receiving chemotherapy.

- Increasing the yield of autologous blood from patients in a pre-donation programme.

Its use in this indication must be balanced against the reported increased risk of thromboembolic events. Treatment should only be given to patients with moderate anaemia (Hb 10 - 13 g/dl [6.21 - 8.07 mmol/l], no iron deficiency) if blood conserving procedures are not available or insufficient when the scheduled major elective surgery requires a large volume of blood (4 or more units of blood for females or 5 or more units for males).

4.2 Posology and method of administration

Therapy with NeoRecormon should be initiated by physicians experienced in the above mentioned indications. As anaphylactoid reactions were observed in isolated cases, it is recommended that the first dose be administered under medical supervision.

The NeoRecormon pre-filled syringe is ready for use. Only solutions which are clear or slightly opalescent, colourless and practically free of visible particles may be injected.

NeoRecormon in pre-filled syringe is a sterile but unpreserved product. Under no circumstances should more than one dose be administered per syringe; the medicinal product is for single use only.

Treatment of symptomatic anaemia in adult and paediatric chronic renal failure patients:

Anaemia symptoms and sequelae may vary with age, gender, and overall burden of disease; a physician's evaluation of the individual patient's clinical course and condition is necessary. NeoRecormon should be administered subcutaneously in order to increase haemoglobin to not greater than 12 g/dl (7.5 mmol/l). Subcutaneous use is preferable in patients who are not receiving haemodialysis to avoid puncture of peripheral veins. In case of intravenous administration, the solution should be injected over approx. 2 minutes, e.g. in haemodialysis patients via the arterio-venous fistula at the end of dialysis.

Due to intra-patient variability, occasional individual haemoglobin values for a patient above and below the desired haemoglobin level may be observed. Haemoglobin variability should be addressed through dose management, with consideration for the haemoglobin target range of 10 g/dl (6.2 mmol/l) to 12 g/dl (7.5 mmol/l). A sustained haemoglobin level of greater than 12 g/dl (7.5 mmol/l) should be avoided; guidance for appropriate dose adjustment for when haemoglobin values exceeding 12 g/dl (7.5 mmol/l) are observed are described below.

A rise in haemoglobin of greater than 2 g/dl (1.25 mmol/l) over a four week period should be avoided. If it occurs, appropriate dose adjustment should be made as provided. If the rate of rise in haemoglobin is greater than 2 g/dl (1.25 mmol/l) in one month or if the haemoglobin level is increasing and approaching 12 g/dl (7.45 mmol/l), the dose is to be reduced by approximately 25%. If the haemoglobin level continues to increase, therapy should be interrupted until the haemoglobin level begins to decrease, at which point therapy should be restarted at a dose approximately 25% below the previously administered dose.

Patients should be monitored closely to ensure that the lowest approved dose of NeoRecormon is used to provide adequate control of the symptoms of anaemia.

In the presence of hypertension or existing cardiovascular, cerebrovascular or peripheral vascular diseases, the weekly increase in Hb and the target Hb should be determined individually taking into account the clinical picture.

Treatment with NeoRecormon is divided into two stages.

1. Correction phase

- Subcutaneous administration:

The initial dosage is 3 × 20 IU/kg body weight per week. The dosage may be increased every 4 weeks by 3 × 20 IU/kg per week if the increase of Hb is not adequate (< 0.25 g/dl per week).

The weekly dose can also be divided into daily doses.

- Intravenous administration:

The initial dosage is 3 × 40 IU/kg per week. The dosage may be raised after 4 weeks to 80 IU/kg - three times per week - and by further increments of 20 IU/kg if needed, three times per week, at monthly intervals.

For both routes of administration, the maximum dose should not exceed 720 IU/kg per week.

2. Maintenance phase

To maintain an Hb of between 10 and 12 g/dl, the dosage is initially reduced to half of the previously administered amount. Subsequently, the dose is adjusted at intervals of one or two weeks individually for the patient (maintenance dose).

In the case of subcutaneous administration, the weekly dose can be given as one injection per week or in divided doses three or seven times per week. Patients who are stable on a once weekly dosing regimen may be switched to once every two weeks administration. In this case dose increases may be necessary.

Results of clinical studies in children have shown that, on average, the younger the patients, the higher the NeoRecormon doses required. Nevertheless, the recommended dosing schedule should be followed as the individual response cannot be predicted.

Treatment with NeoRecormon is normally a long-term therapy. It can, however, be interrupted, if necessary, at any time. Data on the once weekly dosing schedule are based on clinical studies with a treatment duration of 24 weeks.

Prevention of anaemia of prematurity:

The solution is administered subcutaneously at a dose of 3 × 250 IU/kg b.w. per week. Treatment with NeoRecormon should start as early as possible, preferably by day 3 of life. Premature infants who have already been transfused by the start of treatment with NeoRecormon are not likely to benefit as much as untransfused infants. The treatment should last for 6 weeks.

Treatment of symptomatic chemotherapy-induced anaemia in cancer patients:

NeoRecormon should be administered by the subcutaneous route to patients with anaemia (e.g. haemoglobin concentration ⩽ 10g/dl (6.2 mmol/l)). Anaemia symptoms and sequelae may vary with age, gender, and overall burden of disease; a physician's evaluation of the individual patient's clinical course and condition is necessary.

The weekly dose can be given as one injection per week or in divided doses 3 to 7 times per week.

The recommended initial dose is 30,000 IU per week (corresponding to approximately 450 IU/kg body weight per week, based on an average weighted patient).

Due to intra-patient variability, occasional individual haemoglobin values for a patient above and below the desired haemoglobin level may be observed. Haemoglobin variability should be addressed through dose management, with consideration for the haemoglobin target range of 10 g/dl (6.2 mmol/l) to 12 g/dl (7.5 mmol/l). A sustained haemoglobin level of greater than 12 g/dl (7.5 mmol/l) should be avoided; guidance for appropriate dose adjustment for when haemoglobin values exceeding 12 g/dl (7.5 mmol/l) are observed are described below.

If, after 4 weeks of therapy, the haemoglobin value has increased by at least 1 g/dl (0.62 mmol/l), the current dose should be continued. If the haemoglobin value has not increased by at least 1 g/dl (0.62 mmol/l), a doubling of the weekly dose should be considered. If, after 8 weeks of therapy, the haemoglobin value has not increased by at least 1 g/dl (0.62 mmol/l), response is unlikely and treatment should be discontinued.

The therapy should be continued up to 4 weeks after the end of chemotherapy.

The maximum dose should not exceed 60,000 IU per week.

Once the therapeutic objective for an individual patient has been achieved, the dose should be reduced by 25 to 50 % in order to maintain haemoglobin at that level.

Appropriate dose titration should be considered.

If the haemoglobin exceeds 12 g/dl (7.5 mmol/l), the dose should be reduced by approximately 25 to 50 %. Treatment with NeoRecormon should be temporarily discontinued if haemoglobin levels exceed 13 g/dl (8.1 mmol/l). Therapy should be reinitiated at approximately 25 % lower than the previous dose after haemoglobin levels fall to 12 g/dl (7.5 mmol/l) or below.

If the rise in haemoglobin is greater than 2 g/dl (1.3 mmol/l) in 4 weeks, the dose should be reduced by 25 to 50 %.

Patients should be monitored closely to ensure that the lowest approved dose of NeoRecormon is used to provide adequate control of the symptoms of anaemia.

Treatment for increasing the amount of autologous blood:

The solution is administered intravenously over approx. 2 minutes or subcutaneously.

NeoRecormon is administered twice weekly over 4 weeks. On those occasions where the patient's PCV allows blood donation, i.e. PCV ⩾ 33 %, NeoRecormon is administered at the end of blood donation.

During the entire treatment period, a PCV of 48 % should not be exceeded.

The dosage must be determined by the surgical team individually for each patient as a function of the required amount of pre-donated blood and the endogenous red cell reserve:

1. The required amount of pre-donated blood depends on the anticipated blood loss, use of blood conserving procedures and the physical condition of the patient.

This amount should be that quantity which is expected to be sufficient to avoid homologous blood transfusions.

The required amount of pre-donated blood is expressed in units whereby one unit in the nomogram is equivalent to 180 ml red cells.

Figure 1

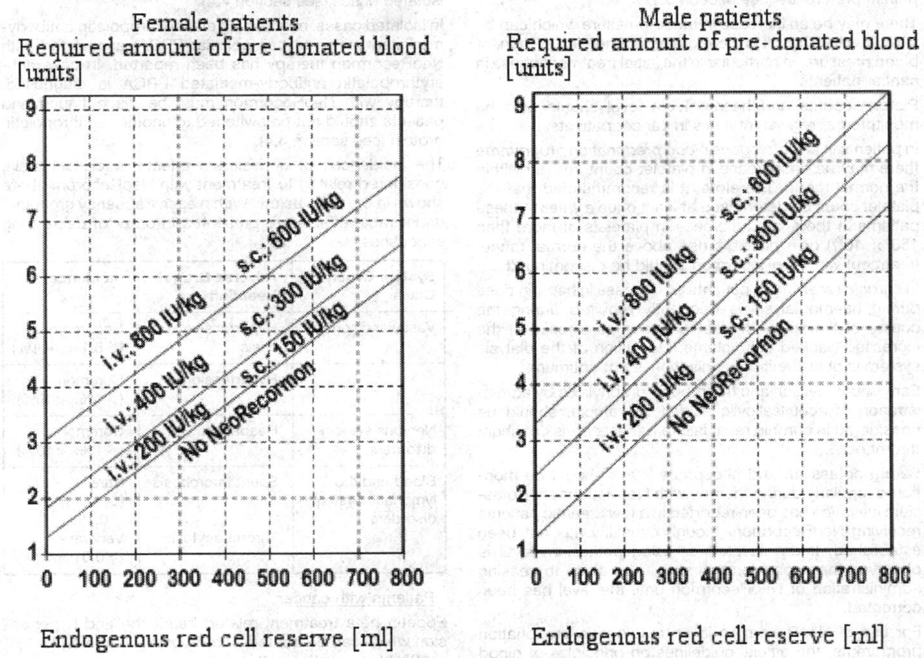

2. The ability to donate blood depends predominantly on the patient's blood volume and baseline PCV. Both variables determine the endogenous red cell reserve, which can be calculated according to the following formula.

Endogenous red cell reserve = blood volume [ml] × (PCV - 33) ÷ 100

Women: blood volume [ml] = 41 [ml/kg] × body weight [kg] + 1200 [ml]

Men: blood volume [ml] = 44 [ml/kg] × body weight [kg] + 1600 [ml]

(body weight ⩾ 45 kg)

The indication for treatment with NeoRecormon and, if given, the single dose should be determined from the required amount of pre-donated blood and the endogenous red cell reserve according to the following graphs.

(see Figure 1 above)

The single dose thus determined is administered twice weekly over 4 weeks. The maximum dose should not exceed 1600 IU/kg body weight per week for intravenous or 1200 IU/kg per week for subcutaneous administration.

4.3 Contraindications

Hypersensitivity to the active substance or any of the excipients.

Poorly controlled hypertension.

In the indication "increasing the yield of autologous blood": myocardial infarction or stroke in the month preceding treatment, unstable angina pectoris, increased risk of deep venous thrombosis such as history of venous thromboembolic disease.

4.4 Special warnings and precautions for use

NeoRecormon should be used with caution in the presence of refractory anaemia with excess blasts in transformation, epilepsy, thrombocytosis, and chronic liver failure. Folic acid and vitamin B_{12} deficiencies should be ruled out as they reduce the effectiveness of NeoRecormon.

In order to ensure effective erythropoiesis, iron status should be evaluated for all patients prior to and during treatment and supplementary iron therapy may be necessary and conducted in accordance with therapeutic guidelines.

Severe aluminium overload due to treatment of renal failure may compromise the effectiveness of NeoRecormon.

The indication for treatment with NeoRecormon of nephrosclerotic patients not yet undergoing dialysis should be defined individually, as a possible acceleration of progression of renal failure cannot be ruled out with certainty.

Pure red cell aplasia caused by neutralising anti-erythropoietin antibodies has been reported in association with erythropoietin therapy, including NeoRecormon. These antibodies have been shown to cross-react with all erythropoietic proteins, and patients suspected or confirmed to have neutralising antibodies to erythropoietin should not be switched to NeoRecormon (see section 4.8).

In *chronic renal failure* patients an increase in blood pressure or aggravation of existing hypertension, especially in cases of rapid PCV increase can occur. These increases in blood pressure can be treated with medicinal products. If blood pressure rises cannot be controlled by drug therapy, a transient interruption of NeoRecormon therapy is recommended. Particularly at beginning of therapy, regular monitoring of the blood pressure is recommended, including between dialyses. Hypertensive crisis with encephalopathy-like symptoms may occur and require the immediate attention of a physician and intensive medical care. Particular attention should be paid to sudden stabbing migraine like headaches as a possible warning sign.

In *chronic renal failure* patients there may be a moderate dose-dependent rise in the platelet count within the normal range during treatment with NeoRecormon, especially after intravenous administration. This regresses during the course of continued therapy. It is recommended that the platelet count be monitored regularly during the first 8 weeks of therapy.

In patients with chronic renal failure, maintenance haemoglobin concentration should not exceed the upper limit of the target haemoglobin concentration recommended in section 4.2. In clinical trials, an increased risk of death and serious cardiovascular events was observed when erythropoiesis stimulating agents (ESAs) were administered to target a haemoglobin of greater than 12 g/dl (7.5 mmol/l).

Controlled clinical trials have not shown significant benefits attributable to the administration of epoetins when haemoglobin concentration is increased beyond the level necessary to control symptoms of anaemia and to avoid blood transfusion.

In premature infants there may be a slight rise in platelet counts, particularly up to day 12 – 14 of life, therefore platelets should be monitored regularly.

Effect on tumour growth

Epoetins are growth factors that primarily stimulate red blood cell production. Erythropoietin receptors may be expressed on the surface of a variety of tumour cells. As with all growth factors, there is a concern that epoetins could stimulate the growth of tumours. In several controlled studies, epoetins have not been shown to improve overall survival or decrease the risk of tumour progression in patients with anaemia associated with cancer.

In controlled clinical studies, use of NeoRecormon and other erythropoiesis-stimulating agents (ESAs) have shown:

- shortened time to tumour progression in patients with advanced head and neck cancer receiving radiation therapy when administered to target a haemoglobin of greater than 14 g/dl (8.7 mmol/l),

- shortened overall survival and increased deaths attributed to disease progression at 4 months in patients with metastatic breast cancer receiving chemotherapy when administered to target a haemoglobin of 12-14 g/dl (7.5-8.7 mmol/l),

- increased risk of death when administered to target a haemoglobin of 12 g/dl (7.5 mmol/l) in patients with active malignant disease receiving neither chemotherapy nor radiation therapy. ESAs are not indicated for use in this patient population.

In view of the above, in some clinical situations blood transfusion should be the preferred treatment for the management of anaemia in patients with cancer. The decision to administer recombinant erythropoietins should be based on a benefit-risk assessment with the participation of the individual patient, which should take into account the specific clinical context. Factors that should be considered in this assessment should include the type of tumour and its stage; the degree of anaemia; life-expectancy; the environment in which the patient is being treated; and patient preference (see section 5.1)

There may be an increase in blood pressure which can be treated with drugs. It is therefore recommended to monitor blood pressure, in particular in the initial treatment phase in cancer patients.

Platelet counts and haemoglobin level should also be monitored at regular intervals in cancer patients.

In patients in an *autologous blood predonation programme* there may be an increase in platelet count, mostly within the normal range. Therefore, it is recommended that the platelet count be determined at least once a week in these patients. If there is an increase in platelets of more than 150×10^9/l or if platelets rise above the normal range, treatment with NeoRecormon should be discontinued.

In *chronic renal failure* patients an increase in heparin dose during haemodialysis is frequently required during the course of therapy with NeoRecormon as a result of the increased packed cell volume. Occlusion of the dialysis system is possible if heparinisation is not optimum.

Early shunt revision and thrombosis prophylaxis by administration of acetylsalicylic acid, for example, should be considered in chronic renal failure patients at risk of shunt thrombosis.

Serum potassium and phosphate levels should be monitored regularly during therapy with NeoRecormon. Potassium elevation has been reported in a few uraemic patients receiving NeoRecormon, though causality has not been established. If an elevated or rising potassium level is observed then consideration should be given to ceasing administration of NeoRecormon until the level has been corrected.

For use of NeoRecormon in an autologous predonation programme, the official guidelines on principles of blood donation must be considered, in particular:

- only patients with a PCV ⩾ 33 % (haemoglobin ⩾ 11 g/dl [6.83 mmol/l]) should donate;

- special care should be taken with patients below 50 kg weight;

- the single volume drawn should not exceed approx. 12 % of the patient's estimated blood volume.

Treatment should be reserved for patients in whom it is considered of particular importance to avoid homologous blood transfusion taking into consideration the risk/benefit assessment for homologous transfusions.

Misuse by healthy persons may lead to an excessive increase in packed cell volume. This may be associated with life-threatening complications of the cardiovascular system.

NeoRecormon in pre-filled syringe contains up to 0.3 mg phenylalanine/syringe as an excipient. Therefore this should be taken into consideration in patients affected with severe forms of phenylketonuria.

This medicinal product contains less than 1 mmol sodium (23 mg) per syringe, i.e. essentially "sodium-free".

4.5 Interaction with other medicinal products and other forms of interaction

The clinical results obtained so far do not indicate any interaction of NeoRecormon with other medicinal products.

Animal experiments revealed that epoetin beta does not increase the myelotoxicity of cytostatic medicinal products like etoposide, cisplatin, cyclophosphamide, and fluorouracil.

4.6 Pregnancy and lactation

For epoetin beta no clinical data on exposed pregnancies are available. Animal studies do not indicate direct or indirect harmful effects with respect to pregnancy, embryonal/foetal development, parturition or postnatal development (see 5.3).

Caution should be exercised when prescribing to pregnant women.

4.7 Effects on ability to drive and use machines

NeoRecormon has no influence on the ability to drive and use machines.

4.8 Undesirable effects

Based on results from clinical trials including 1725 patients approximately 8 % of patients treated with NeoRecormon are expected to experience adverse reactions.

- Anaemic patients with chronic renal failure

The most frequent adverse reaction during treatment with NeoRecormon is an increase in blood pressure or aggravation of existing hypertension, especially in cases of rapid PCV increase (see section 4.4). Hypertensive crisis with encephalopathy-like symptoms (e.g. headaches and confused state, sensorimotor disorders - such as speech disturbance or impaired gait - up to tonoclonic seizures) may also occur in individual patients with otherwise normal or low blood pressure (see section 4.4).

Shunt thromboses may occur, especially in patients who have a tendency to hypotension or whose arteriovenous fistulae exhibit complications (e.g. stenoses, aneurisms), see section 4.4. In most cases, a fall in serum ferritin values simultaneous with a rise in packed cell volume is observed (see section 4.4). In addition, transient increases in serum potassium and phosphate levels have been observed in isolated cases (see section 4.4).

In isolated cases, neutralising anti erythropoietin antibody-mediated pure red cell aplasia (PRCA) associated with NeoRecormon therapy has been reported. In case anti-erythropoietin antibody-mediated PRCA is diagnosed, therapy with NeoRecormon must be discontinued and patients should not be switched to another erythropoietic protein (see section 4.4).

The incidences of undesirable effects in clinical trials, considered related to treatment with NeoRecoromon are shown in the table below. Within each frequency grouping, undesirable effects are presented in order of decreasing seriousness.

System Organ Class	Adverse Drug Reaction	Incidence
Vascular disorders	Hypertensive crisis	Uncommon (>0.1%, <1%)
	Hypertension	Common (>1%, <10%)
Nervous system disorders	Headache	Common (>1%, <10%)
Blood and the lymphatic system disorders	Shunt thrombosis	Rare (>0.01%, <0.1%)
	Thrombocytosis	Very rare (<0.01%)

- Patients with cancer

Epoetin beta treatment-related headache and hypertension which can be treated with drugs are common (>1%, <10%) (see section 4.4).

In some patients, a fall in serum iron parameters is observed (see section 4.4).

Clinical studies have shown a higher frequency of thromboembolic events in cancer patients treated with NeoRecormon compared to untreated controls or placebo. In patients treated with NeoRecormon, this incidence is 7 % compared to 4 % in controls; this is not associated with any increase in thromboembolic mortality compared with controls.

The incidences of undesirable effects in clinical trials, considered related to treatment with NeoRecoromon are shown in the table below. Within each frequency grouping, undesirable effects are presented in order of decreasing seriousness.

System Organ Class	Adverse Drug Reaction	Incidence
Vascular disorders	Hypertension	Common (>1%, <10%)
Blood and the lymphatic system disorders	Thromboembolic event	Common (>1%, <10%)
Nervous system disorders	Headache	Common (>1%, <10%)

- Patients in an autologous blood predonation programme

Patients in an autologous blood predonation programme have been reported to show a slightly higher frequency of thromboembolic events. However, a causal relationship with treatment with NeoRecormon could not be established.

In placebo controlled trials temporary iron deficiency was more pronounced in patients treated with NeoRecormon than in controls (see section 4.4).

The incidences of undesirable effects in clinical trials, considered related to treatment with NeoRecoromon are shown in the table below. Within each frequency grouping, undesirable effects are presented in order of decreasing seriousness.

System Organ Class	Adverse Drug Reaction	Incidence
Nervous system disorders	Headache	Common (>1%, <10%)

- Premature infants

A fall in serum ferritin values is very common (>10%) (see section 4.4).

- All indications

Rarely (⩾1/10.000 to ⩽1/1.000), epoetin beta treatment-related skin reactions such as rash, pruritus, urticaria or injection site reactions may occur. In very rare cases (⩽1/10.000), epoetin beta treatment-related anaphylactoid reactions have been reported. However, in controlled clinical studies no increased incidence of hypersensitivity reactions was found.

In very rare cases (⩽1/10.000), particularly when starting treatment, epoetin beta treatment-related flu-like symptoms such as fever, chills, headaches, pain in the limbs, malaise and/or bone pain have been reported. These reactions were mild or moderate in nature and subsided after a couple of hours or days.

4.9 Overdose

The therapeutic margin of NeoRecormon is very wide. Even at very high serum levels no symptoms of poisoning have been observed.

5. PHARMACOLOGICAL PROPERTIES

5.1 Pharmacodynamic properties

Pharmacotherapeutic group: antianaemic, ATC code: B03XA

Epoetin beta is identical in its amino acid and carbohydrate composition to erythropoietin that has been isolated from the urine of anaemic patients.

Erythropoietin is a glycoprotein that stimulates the formation of erythrocytes from its committed progenitors. It acts as a mitosis stimulating factor and differentiation hormone.

The biological efficacy of epoetin beta has been demonstrated after intravenous and subcutaneous administration in various animal models *in vivo* (normal and uraemic rats, polycythaemic mice, dogs). After administration of epoetin beta, the number of erythrocytes, the Hb values and reticulocyte counts increase as well as the ^{59}Fe-incorporation rate.

An increased ^{3}H-thymidine incorporation in the erythroid nucleated spleen cells has been found *in vitro* (mouse spleen cell culture) after incubation with epoetin beta.

Investigations in cell cultures of human bone marrow cells showed that epoetin beta stimulates erythropoiesis specifically and does not affect leucopoiesis. Cytotoxic actions of epoetin beta on bone marrow or on human skin cells were not detected.

After single dose administration of epoetin beta no effects on behaviour or locomotor activity of mice and circulatory or respiratory function of dogs were observed.

Erythropoietin is a growth factor that primarily stimulates red cell production. Erythropoietin receptors may be expressed on the surface of a variety of tumour cells.

Survival and tumour progression have been examined in five large controlled studies involving a total of 2833 patients, of which four were double-blind placebo-controlled studies and one was an open-label study. Two of the studies recruited patients who were being treated with chemotherapy. The target haemoglobin concentration in two studies was >13 g/dl; in the remaining three studies it was 12-14 g/dl. In the open-label study there was no difference in overall survival between patients treated with recombinant human erythropoietin and controls. In the four placebo-controlled studies the hazard ratios for overall survival ranged between 1.25 and 2.47 in favour of controls. These studies have shown a consistent unexplained statistically significant excess mortality in patients who have anaemia associated with various common cancers who received recombinant human erythropoietin compared to controls. Overall survival outcome in the trials could not be satisfactorily explained by differences in the incidence of thrombosis and related complications between those given recombinant human erythropoietin and those in the control group.

An individual patient data based meta-analysis, which included data from all 12 controlled clinical studies in anaemic cancer patients conducted with NeoRecormon (n=2301), showed an overall hazard ratio point estimate for survival of 1.13 in favour of controls (95 % CI 0.87, 1.46). In patients with baseline haemoglobin ⩽ 10 g/dl (n=899), the hazard ratio point estimate for survival was 0.98 (95 % CI 0.68 to 1.40). An increased relative risk for thromboembolic events was observed in the overall population (RR 1.62, 95% CI: 1.13, 2.31).

A systematic review has also been performed involving more than 9000 cancer patients participating in 57 clinical trials. Meta-analysis of overall survival data produced a hazard ratio point estimate of 1.08 in favour of controls (95 % CI: 0.99, 1.18; 42 trials and 8167 patients). An increased relative risk of thromboembolic events (RR 1.67, 95% CI: 1.35, 2.06, 35 trials and 6769 patients) was observed in patients treated with recombinant human erythropoietin. There is therefore consistent evidence to suggest that there may be significant harm to patients with cancer who are treated with recombinant human erythropoietin. The extent to which these outcomes might apply to the administration of recombinant human erythropoietin to patients with cancer, treated with chemotherapy to achieve haemoglobin concentrations less than 13 g/dl, is unclear because few patients with these characteristics were included in the data reviewed.

In very rare cases, neutralising anti-erythropoietin antibodies with or without pure red cell aplasia (PRCA) occurred during rHuEPO therapy.

5.2 Pharmacokinetic properties

Pharmacokinetic investigations in healthy volunteers and uraemic patients show that the half-life of intravenously administered epoetin beta is between 4 and 12 hours and that the distribution volume corresponds to one to two times the plasma volume. Analogous results have been found in animal experiments in uraemic and normal rats.

After subcutaneous administration of epoetin beta to uraemic patients, the protracted absorption results in a serum concentration plateau, whereby the maximum concentration is reached after an average of 12 - 28 hours. The terminal half-life is higher than after intravenous administration, with an average of 13 - 28 hours.

Bioavailability of epoetin beta after subcutaneous administration is between 23 and 42 % as compared with intravenous administration.

5.3 Preclinical safety data

Non-clinical data reveal no special hazard for humans based on conventional studies of safety pharmacology, repeated dose toxicity, genotoxicity, and toxicity to reproduction.

A carcinogenicity study with homologous erythropoietin in mice did not reveal any signs of proliferative or tumourigenic potential.

6. PHARMACEUTICAL PARTICULARS

6.1 List of excipients

Urea,

Sodium chloride,

Polysorbate 20,

Sodium dihydrogen phosphate dihydrate,

Disodium phosphate dodecahydrate,

Calcium chloride dihydrate,

Glycine,

L-Leucine,

L-Isoleucine,

L-Threonine,

L-Glutamic acid,

L-Phenylalanine,

Water for injections.

6.2 Incompatibilities

In the absence of compatibility studies, this medicinal product should not be mixed with other medicinal products.

6.3 Shelf life

2 years.

6.4 Special precautions for storage

Store in a refrigerator (2°C – 8°C).

Keep the pre-filled syringe in the outer carton, in order to protect from light.

For the purpose of ambulatory use, the patient may remove the product from the refrigerator and store it at room temperature (not above 25°C) for one single period of up to 3 days.

6.5 Nature and contents of container

500 IU, 1000 IU:

0.3 ml of solution in pre-filled syringe (Type I glass) with a tip cap and a plunger stopper (teflonised rubber) with a needle 30G1/2.

Pack sizes of 1 or 6

2000 IU, 3000 IU, 4000 IU, 5000 IU, 6000 IU:

0.3 ml of solution in pre-filled syringe (Type 1 glass) with a tip cap and a plunger stopper (teflonised rubber) with a needle of 27G1/2.

Pack sizes of 1 or 6

10,000 IU, 20,000IU:

0.6 ml of solution in pre-filled syringe (Type I glass) with a tip cap and a plunger stopper (teflonised rubber) with a needle 27G1/2. (4 pre-filled syringes and 4 needles for 30,000 IU).

Pack sizes of 1 or 6

30,000IU:

0.6 ml of solution in pre-filled syringe (Type I glass) with a tip cap and a plunger stopper (teflonised rubber) with a needle 27G1/2.

Pack sizes of 1 or 4

Not all pack sizes may be marketed.

6.6 Special precautions for disposal and other handling

First wash your hands!

1. Remove one syringe from the pack and check that the solution is clear, colourless and practically free from visible particles. Remove the cap from the syringe.

2. Remove one needle from the pack, fix it on the syringe and remove the protective cap from the needle.

3. Expel air from the syringe and needle by holding the syringe vertically and gently pressing the plunger upwards. Keep pressing the plunger until the amount of NeoRecormon in the syringe is as prescribed.

4. Clean the skin at the site of injection using an alcohol wipe. Form a skin fold by pinching the skin between thumb and forefinger. Hold the syringe barrel near to the needle, and insert the needle into the skin fold with a quick, firm action. Inject the NeoRecormon solution. Withdraw the needle quickly and apply pressure over the injection site with a dry, sterile pad.

This medicinal product is for single use only. Any unused product or waste material should be disposed of in accordance with local requirements.

7. MARKETING AUTHORISATION HOLDER

Roche Registration Limited

6 Falcon Way

Shire Park

Welwyn Garden City

AL7 1TW

United Kingdom

8. MARKETING AUTHORISATION NUMBER(S)

NeoRecormon 500 IU solution for injection in pre-filled syringe:

EU/1/97/031/025 - 026

NeoRecormon 1000 IU solution for injection in pre-filled syringe:

EU/1/97/031/027 - 028

NeoRecormon 2000 IU solution for injection in pre-filled syringe:

EU/1/97/031/029 - 030

NeoRecormon 3000 IU solution for injection in pre-filled syringe:

EU/1/97/031/031 - 032

NeoRecormon 4000 IU solution for injection in pre-filled syringe:

EU/1/97/031/041 - 042

NeoRecormon 5000 IU solution for injection in pre-filled syringe:

EU/1/97/031/033 - 034

NeoRecormon 6000 IU solution for injection in pre-filled syringe:

EU/1/97/031/043 - 044

NeoRecormon 10,000 IU solution for injection in pre-filled syringe:

EU/1/97/031/035 - 036

NeoRecormon 20,000 IU solution for injection in pre-filled syringe:

EU/1/97/031/037 - 038

NeoRecormon 30,000 IU solution for injection in pre-filled syringe:

EU/1/97/031/045 - 046

9. DATE OF FIRST AUTHORISATION/RENEWAL OF THE AUTHORISATION

500, 1000, 2000, 3000, 5000, 10,000 20,000 IU:

Date of the first authorisation: 2 April 1998

Date of the last renewal: 16 July 2007

4000, 6000 IU:

Date of the first authorisation: 10 February 2000

Date of the last renewal: 16 July 2007

30,000 IU:

Date of the first authorisation: 23 February 2004

Date of the last renewal: 16 July 2007

10. DATE OF REVISION OF THE TEXT

23 October 2008

Detailed information on this medicinal product is available on the website of the European Medicines Agency (EMEA) http://www.emea.europa.eu/

Neostigmine Bromide Tablets

(Cambridge Laboratories)

1. NAME OF THE MEDICINAL PRODUCT

Neostigmine Bromide Tablets

2. QUALITATIVE AND QUANTITATIVE COMPOSITION

Each tablet contains 15 mg Neostigmine Bromide Ph.Eur.

3. PHARMACEUTICAL FORM

Tablets

4. CLINICAL PARTICULARS

4.1 Therapeutic indications

Myasthenia gravis; paralytic ileus; post-operative urinary retention.

4.2 Posology and method of administration

Neostigmine bromide has a slower onset of effect when given orally than when given parenterally, but the duration of action is longer and the intensity of action more uniform.

To facilitate change of treatment from one route of administration to another, the following doses are approximately equivalent in effect:

0.5 mg intravenously = 1-1.5 mg intramuscularly or subcutaneously = 15 mg orally.

Myasthenia gravis

Adults: Doses of 15 to 30 mg by mouth are given at intervals throughout the day when maximum strength is needed (for example, on rising and before mealtimes). The usual duration of action of a dose is two to four hours.

The total daily dose is usually in the range of 5-20 tablets but doses higher than these may be needed by some patients.

Newborn infants: Neostigmine bromide ampoules are recommended.

Older children: Children under 6 years old should receive an initial dose of half a tablet (7.5 mg) of Neostigmine Bromide; children 6-12 years old should receive one tablet (15 mg). Dosage requirements should be adjusted according to the response but are usually in the range of 15-90 mg orally per day.

The requirement for Neostigmine Bromide is usually markedly decreased after thymectomy, or when additional therapy (steroids, immunosuppressant drugs) is given.

When relatively large doses of Neostigmine Bromide are taken by myasthenic patients, it may be necessary to give atropine or other anticholinergic drugs to counteract the muscarinic effects. It should be noted that the slower gastro-intestinal motility caused by these drugs may affect the absorption of oral Neostigmine Bromide.

In all patients the possibility of 'cholinergic crisis', due to overdosage of Neostigmine Bromide, and its differentiation from 'myasthenic crisis', due to increased severity of disease, must be borne in mind. Both types of crisis are manifested by increased muscle weakness, but whereas myasthenic crisis may require more intensive anticholinesterase treatment, cholinergic crisis calls for immediate discontinuation of this treatment and institution of appropriate supportive measures, including respiratory assistance.

Other indications

Adults: The usual dose is 1 to 2 tablets orally.

Children: 2.5-15 mg orally.

The frequency of these doses may be varied according to the needs of the patient.

The elderly: There are no specific dosage recommendations for Neostigmine Bromide in elderly patients.

4.3 Contraindications

Neostigmine Bromide should not be given to patients with mechanical gastro-intestinal or urinary obstruction.

Neostigmine Bromide is contra-indicated in patients with known hypersensitivity to the drug and to bromides.

Neostigmine Bromide should not be used in conjunction with depolarising muscle relaxants such as suxamethonium as neuromuscular blockade may be potentiated and prolonged apnoea may result.

4.4 Special warnings and precautions for use

Extreme caution is required when administering Neostigmine Bromide to patients with bronchial asthma.

Care should also be taken in patients with bradycardia, recent coronary occlusion, hypotension, peptic ulcer, vagotonia, epilepsy or Parkinsonism.

4.5 Interaction with other medicinal products and other forms of interaction

Neostigmine Bromide should not be given during cyclopropane or halothane anaesthesia; however, it may be used after withdrawal of these agents.

4.6 Pregnancy and lactation

The safety of Neostigmine Bromide during pregnancy or lactation has not been established. Although the possible hazards to mother and child must therefore be weighed against the potential benefits in every case, experience with Neostigmine Bromide in pregnant patients with myasthenia gravis has revealed no untoward effect of the drug on the course of pregnancy.

As the severity of myasthenia gravis often fluctuates considerably, particular care is required to avoid cholinergic crisis, due to overdosage of the drug, but otherwise management is no different from that in non-pregnant patients.

Observations indicate that only negligible amounts of Neostigmine Bromide are excreted in breast milk; nevertheless due regard should be paid to possible effects on the breast-feeding infant.

4.7 Effects on ability to drive and use machines

Not known.

4.8 Undesirable effects

There is no evidence to suggest that Neostigmine Bromide has any special effects in the elderly, however, elderly patients may be more susceptible to dysrhythmias than the younger adult.

Side-effects and adverse reactions may include nausea and vomiting, increased salivation, diarrhoea and abdominal cramps.

4.9 Overdose

Signs of overdose due to muscarinic effects may include abdominal cramps, increased peristalsis, diarrhoea, nausea and vomiting, increased bronchial secretions, salivation, diaphoresis and miosis. Nicotinic effects consist of muscular cramps, fasciculations and general weakness. Bradycardia and hypotension may also occur.

Artificial ventilation should be instituted if respiration is severely depressed. Atropine sulphate 1 to 2 mg intravenously is an antidote to the muscarinic effects.

5. PHARMACOLOGICAL PROPERTIES

5.1 Pharmacodynamic properties

Neostigmine Bromide is an antagonist to cholinesterase, the enzyme which normally destroys acetylcholine. The action of Neostigmine Bromide can briefly be described, therefore, as the potentiation of naturally occurring acetylcholine.

5.2 Pharmacokinetic properties

Neostigmine Bromide is a quaternary ammonium compound and is poorly absorbed from the gastro-intestinal tract. Following parenteral administration as the methylsulphate, neostigmine is rapidly eliminated with a plasma half-life of 50-90 minutes and is excreted in the urine both as unchanged drug and metabolites. It is metabolised partly by hydrolysis of the ester linkage.

5.3 Preclinical safety data
Neostigmine has not been reported to have mutagenic or carcinogenic potential. In rats, acute and chronic exposure causes changes in the fine structure at the end-plate region of muscle.

6. PHARMACEUTICAL PARTICULARS

6.1 List of excipients
Lactose

Maize starch

Talc

Magnesium stearate

6.2 Incompatibilities
None known.

6.3 Shelf life
Five years

6.4 Special precautions for storage
The recommended maximum storage temperature is 30°C. The tablets should be protected from light.

6.5 Nature and contents of container
White pigmented HDPE bottles with plastic snap-on caps, each containing 140 tablets.

6.6 Special precautions for disposal and other handling
None.

7. MARKETING AUTHORISATION HOLDER
Lifehealth Limited

23 Winkfield Road

Windsor

Berkshire

SL4 4BA.

8. MARKETING AUTHORISATION NUMBER(S)
PL 14576/0004

9. DATE OF FIRST AUTHORISATION/RENEWAL OF THE AUTHORISATION
23rd October 1995

10. DATE OF REVISION OF THE TEXT
January 2001

Neotigason 10mg Capsules

(Actavis UK Ltd)

1. NAME OF THE MEDICINAL PRODUCT
Neotigason 10mg capsules

2. QUALITATIVE AND QUANTITATIVE COMPOSITION
Capsules with brown cap and white body with actavis printed in black on the cap and "10" printed in black on the body, containing 10mg acitretin.

Excipients include glucose (see section *4.3 Contraindications*).

For a full list of excipients, see section *6.1*.

3. PHARMACEUTICAL FORM
Capsules for oral administration.

4. CLINICAL PARTICULARS

4.1 Therapeutic indications
Severe extensive psoriasis which is resistant to other forms of therapy.

Palmo-plantar pustular psoriasis.

Severe congenital ichthyosis.

Severe Darier's disease (keratosis follicularis).

4.2 Posology and method of administration
It is recommended that Neotigason be given only by, or under supervision of, a dermatological specialist.

Neotigason capsules are for oral administration.

The capsules should be taken once daily with meals or with milk.

There is a wide variation in the absorption and rate of metabolism of Neotigason. This necessitates individual adjustment of dosage. For this reason the following dosage recommendations can serve only as a guide.

Adults

Initial daily dose should be 25mg or 30mg for 2 to 4 weeks. After this initial treatment period the involved areas of the skin should show a marked response and/or side-effects should be apparent. Following assessment of the initial treatment period, titration of the dose upwards or downwards may be necessary to achieve the desired therapeutic response with the minimum of side-effects. In general, a daily dosage of 25 - 50mg taken for a further 6 to 8 weeks achieves optimal therapeutic results. However, it may be necessary in some cases to increase the dose up to a maximum of 75mg/day.

In patients with Darier's disease a starting dose of 10mg may be appropriate. The dose should be increased cautiously as isomorphic reactions may occur.

Therapy can be discontinued in patients with psoriasis whose lesions have improved sufficiently. Relapses should be treated as described above.

Patients with severe congenital ichthyosis and severe Darier's disease may require therapy beyond 3 months. The lowest effective dosage, not exceeding 50mg/day, should be given.

Continuous use beyond 6 months is contra-indicated as only limited clinical data are available on patients treated beyond this length of time.

Elderly

Dosage recommendations are the same as for other adults.

Children

In view of possible severe side-effects associated with long-term treatment, Neotigason is contra-indicated in children unless, in the opinion of the physician, the benefits significantly outweigh the risks.

The dosage should be established according to bodyweight. The daily dosage is about 0.5mg/kg. Higher doses (up to 1mg/kg daily) may be necessary in some cases for limited periods, but only up to a maximum of 35mg/day. The maintenance dose should be kept as low as possible in view of possible long-term side-effects.

Combination therapy

Other dermatological therapy, particularly with keratolytics, should normally be stopped before administration of Neotigason. However, the use of topical corticosteroids or bland emollient ointment may be continued if indicated.

When Neotigason is used in combination with other types of therapy, it may be possible, depending on the individual patient's response, to reduce the dosage of Neotigason.

4.3 Contraindications
Neotigason is highly teratogenic. Its use is contra-indicated in pregnant women and women who might become pregnant during or within 2 years of the cessation of treatment (see section *4.4 Special warnings and special precautions for use*).

The use of Neotigason is contra-indicated in women who are breast feeding.

Neotigason is contra-indicated in patients with hepatic or renal impairment and in patients with chronic abnormally elevated blood lipid values.

Rare cases of benign intracranial hypertension have been reported after Neotigason and after tetracyclines. Supplementary treatment with antibiotics such as tetracyclines is therefore contra-indicated.

An increased risk of hepatitis has been reported following the concomitant use of methotrexate and etretinate. Consequently, the concomitant use of methotrexate and Neotigason should be avoided.

Concomitant administration of Neotigason with other retinoids or preparations containing high doses of Vitamin A, (i.e. more than the recommended dietary allowance of 4,000 - 5,000 i.u. per day) is contra-indicated due to the risk of hypervitaminosis A.

Neotigason is contra-indicated in cases of hypersensitivity to the preparation (acitretin or excipients) or to other retinoids.

Owing to the presence of glucose, patients with rare glucose-galactose malabsorption should not take this medicine.

4.4 Special warnings and precautions for use
Neotigason should only be prescribed by physicians who are experienced in the use of systemic retinoids and understand the risk of teratogenicity associated with acitretin therapy.

Neotigason is highly teratogenic. The risk of giving birth to a deformed child is exceptionally high if Neotigason is taken before or during pregnancy, no matter for how long or at what dosage. Foetal exposure to Neotigason always involves a risk of congenital malformation.

Neotigason is contra-indicated in women of childbearing potential unless the following criteria are met:

1. Pregnancy has been excluded before instituting therapy with Neotigason (negative pregnancy test within 2 weeks prior to therapy). Whenever practicable a monthly repetition of the pregnancy test is recommended during therapy.

2. She starts Neotigason therapy only on the second or third day of the next menstrual cycle.

3. Having excluded pregnancy, any woman of childbearing potential who is receiving Neotigason must practice effective contraception for at least one month before treatment, during the treatment period and for at least 2 years following its cessation.

Even female patients who normally do not practice contraception because of a history of infertility should be advised to do so, while taking Neotigason.

4. The same effective and uninterrupted contraceptive measures must also be taken every time therapy is repeated, however long the intervening period may have been, and must be continued for 2 years afterwards.

5. Any pregnancy occurring during treatment with Neotigason, or in the 2 years following its cessation, carries a high risk of severe foetal malformation. Therefore, before instituting Neotigason the treating physician must explain clearly and in detail what precautions must be taken. This should include the risks involved and the possible consequences of pregnancy occurring during Neotigason treatment or in the 2 years following its cessation.

6. She is reliable and capable of understanding the risk and complying with effective contraception, and confirms that she has understood the warnings.

In view of the importance of the above precautions, Neotigason Patient Information Leaflets are available to doctors and it is strongly recommended that these be given to all patients.

If oral contraception is chosen as the most appropriate contraceptive method for women undergoing retinoid treatment, then a combined oestrogen-progestogen formulation is recommended.

Patients should not donate blood either during or for at least one year following discontinuation of therapy with Neotigason. Theoretically there would be a small risk to a woman in the first trimester of pregnancy who received blood donated by a patient on Neotigason therapy.

Acitretin has been shown to affect diaphyseal and spongy bone adversely in animals at high doses in excess of those recommended for use in man. Since skeletal hyperostosis and extraosseous calcification have been reported following long-term treatment with etretinate in man, this effect should be expected with acitretin therapy.

Since there have been occasional reports of bone changes in children, including premature epiphyseal closure, skeletal hyperostosis and extraosseous calcification after long-term treatment with etretinate, these effects may be expected with acitretin. Neotigason therapy in children is not, therefore, recommended. If, in exceptional circumstances, such therapy is undertaken the child should be carefully monitored for any abnormalities of musculo-skeletal development.

In adults receiving long-term treatment with Neotigason, appropriate examinations should be periodically performed in view of possible ossification abnormalities (see section *4.8 Undesirable effects*). Any patients complaining of atypical musculo-skeletal symptoms on treatment with Neotigason should be promptly and fully investigated to exclude possible acitretin-induced bone changes. If clinically significant bone or joint changes are found, Neotigason therapy should be discontinued.

The effects of UV light are enhanced by retinoid therapy, therefore patients should avoid excessive exposure to sunlight and the unsupervised use of sun lamps.

Hepatic function should be checked before starting treatment with Neotigason, every 1 - 2 weeks for the first 2 months after commencement and then every 3 months during treatment. If abnormal results are obtained, weekly checks should be instituted. If hepatic function fails to return to normal or deteriorates further, Neotigason must be withdrawn. In such cases it is advisable to continue monitoring hepatic function for at least 3 months.

Serum cholesterol and serum triglycerides (fasting values) must be monitored, especially in high-risk patients (disturbances of lipid metabolism, diabetes mellitus, obesity, alcoholism) and during long-term treatment.

In diabetic patients, retinoids can alter glucose tolerance. Blood sugar levels should therefore be checked more frequently than usual at the beginning of the treatment period.

Patients should be warned of the possibility of alopecia occurring (see section *4.8 Undesirable effects*).

4.5 Interaction with other medicinal products and other forms of interaction
Existing data suggests that concurrent intake of acitretin with ethanol led to the formation of etretinate. However, etretinate formation without concurrent alcohol intake cannot be excluded. Therefore, since the elimination half-life of etretinate is 120 days the post-therapy contraception period in women of childbearing potential must be 2 years (see section *4.4 Special warnings and precautions for use).*

An increased risk of hepatitis has been reported following the concomitant use of methotrexate and etretinate. Consequently, the concomitant use of methotrexate and Neotigason should be avoided (see section *4.3 Contra-indications).*

In concurrent treatment with phenytoin, it must be remembered that Neotigason partially reduces the protein binding of phenytoin. The clinical significance of this is as yet unknown.

Interaction studies show acitretin does not interfere with the anti-ovulatory action of the combined oral contraceptives.

Interactions between Neotigason and other substances (e.g. digoxin, cimetidine) have not been observed to date.

4.6 Pregnancy and lactation
Neotigason is contra-indicated during pregnancy as it is a known human teratogen.

The use of Neotigason is contra-indicated in women who are breast feeding. It is also contra-indicated in women of childbearing potential unless specific criteria are met, (see section *4.4 Special warnings and special precautions for use*).

4.7 Effects on ability to drive and use machines

Decreased night vision has been reported with Neotigason therapy. Patients should be advised of this potential problem and warned to be cautious when driving or operating any vehicle at night. Visual problems should be carefully monitored (see section *4.8 Undesirable effects*).

4.8 Undesirable effects

Most of the clinical side-effects of Neotigason are dose-related and are usually well-tolerated at the recommended dosages. However, the toxic dose of Neotigason is close to the therapeutic dose and most patients experience some side-effects during the initial period whilst dosage is being adjusted. They are usually reversible with reduction of dosage or discontinuation of therapy.

The skin and mucous membranes are most commonly affected, and it is recommended that patients should be so advised before treatment is commenced.

Skin: Dryness of the skin may be associated with scaling, thinning, erythema (especially of the face) and pruritus. Palmar and plantar exfoliation may occur. Sticky skin and dermatitis occur frequently. Epidermal fragility, nail fragility and paronychia have been observed.

Occasionally bullous eruptions and abnormal hair texture have been reported. Hair thinning and frank alopecia may occur, usually noted 4 to 8 weeks after starting therapy, and are reversible following discontinuation of Neotigason. Full recovery usually occurs within 6 months of stopping treatment in the majority of patients.

Granulomatous lesions have occasionally been observed.

Sweating has been reported infrequently.

Rarely, patients may experience photosensitivity reactions.

Mucous membranes: Dryness of mucous membranes, sometimes with erosion, involving the lips, mouth, conjunctivae and nasal mucosa have been reported. Corneal ulcerations have been observed rarely.

Dryness of the conjunctivae may lead to mild-to-moderate conjunctivitis or xerophthalmia and result in intolerance of contact lenses; it may be alleviated by lubrication with artificial tears or topical antibiotics.

Cheilitis, rhagades of the corner of the mouth, dry mouth and thirst have occurred. Occasionally stomatitis, gingivitis and taste disturbance have been reported.

Rhinitis and epistaxis have been observed.

Central nervous system: Headache has occurred infrequently. Benign intracranial hypertension has been reported. Patients with severe headache, nausea, vomiting and visual disturbance should discontinue Neotigason immediately and be referred for neurological evaluation and care.

Neuro-sensory system: Blurred or decreased night vision has been reported occasionally.

Musculo-skeletal system: Myalgia and arthralgia may occur and be associated with reduced tolerance to exercise. Bone pain has also been reported.

Maintenance treatment may result in hyperostosis and extraskeletal calcification, as observed in long-term systemic treatment with other retinoids.

Gastrointestinal tract: Nausea has been reported infrequently. Vomiting, diarrhoea and abdominal pain have been observed rarely.

Liver and biliary system disorders: Transient, usually reversible elevation of serum levels of liver enzymes may occur. When significant, dosage reduction or discontinuation of therapy may be necessary. Jaundice and hepatitis have occurred rarely.

Metabolic: Elevation of serum triglycerides above the normal range has been observed, especially where predisposing factors such as a family history of lipid disorders, obesity, alcohol abuse, diabetes mellitus or smoking are present. The changes are dose-related and may be controlled by dietary means (including restriction of alcohol intake) and/or by reduction of dosage of Neotigason. Increases in serum cholesterol have occurred.

Cardiovascular system: Occasionally peripheral oedema and flushing have been reported.

Miscellaneous reactions: Increased incidence of vulvovaginitis due to Candida albicans has been noted during treatment with acitretin. Malaise and drowsiness have been infrequently reported.

4.9 Overdose

Manifestations of acute Vitamin A toxicity include severe headache, nausea or vomiting, drowsiness, irritability and pruritus. Signs and symptoms of accidental or deliberate overdosage with Neotigason would probably be similar. They would be expected to subside without need for treatment.

Because of the variable absorption of the drug, gastric lavage may be worthwhile within the first few hours after ingestion.

5. PHARMACOLOGICAL PROPERTIES

5.1 Pharmacodynamic properties

Retinol (Vitamin A) is known to be essential for normal epithelial growth and differentiation, though the mode of this effect is not yet established. Both retinol and retinoic acid are capable of reversing hyperkeratotic and metaplastic skin changes. However, these effects are generally only obtained at dosages associated with considerable local or systemic toxicity. Acitretin, a synthetic aromatic derivative of retinoic acid, has a favourable therapeutic ratio, with a greater and more specific inhibitory effect on psoriasis and disorders of epithelial keratinisation. The usual therapeutic response to acitretin consists of desquamation (with or without erythema) followed by more normal re-epithelialisation.

Acitretin is the main active metabolite of etretinate.

5.2 Pharmacokinetic properties

Absorption

Acitretin reaches peak plasma concentration 1 - 4 hours after ingestion of the drug. Bioavailability of orally administered acitretin is enhanced by food. Bioavailability of a single dose is approximately 60%, but inter-patient variability is considerable (36 - 95%).

Distribution

Acitretin is highly lipophilic and penetrates readily into body tissues. Protein binding of acitretin exceeds 99%. In animal studies, acitretin passed the placental barrier in quantities sufficient to produce foetal malformations. Due to its lipophilic nature, it can be assumed that acitretin passes into breast milk in considerable quantities.

Metabolism

Acitretin is metabolised by isomerisation into its 13-cis isomer (cis acitretin), by glucuronidation and cleavage of the side chain.

Elimination

Multiple-dose studies in patients aged 21 - 70 years showed an elimination half-life of approximately 50 hours for acitretin and 60 hours for its main metabolite in plasma, *cis* acitretin, which is also a teratogen. From the longest elimination half-life observed in these patients for acitretin (96 hours) and *cis* acitretin (123 hours), and assuming linear kinetics, it can be predicted that more than 99% of the drug is eliminated within 36 days after cessation of long-term therapy. Furthermore, plasma concentrations of acitretin and *cis* acitretin dropped below the sensitivity limit of the assay (< 6ng/ml) within 36 days following cessation of treatment. Acitretin is excreted entirely in the form of its metabolites, in approximately equal parts via the kidneys and the bile.

5.3 Preclinical safety data

None stated.

6. PHARMACEUTICAL PARTICULARS

6.1 List of excipients

Capsule content:

Glucose, liquid, spray-dried

Sodium ascorbate

Gelatin

Purified water

Microcrystalline cellulose

Capsule shell:

Gelatin

Iron oxide black (E172)

Iron oxide yellow (E172)

Iron oxide red (E172)

Titanium dioxide (E171)

Printing ink:

Shellac

N-Butyl alcohol

Isopropyl alcohol

Propylene glycol

Ammonium hydroxide

Iron oxide black (E172)

6.2 Incompatibilities

None.

6.3 Shelf life

Neotigason capsules have a shelf-life of 3 years.

6.4 Special precautions for storage

Store in the original package. Do not store above 25°C.

6.5 Nature and contents of container

All aluminium blisters containing 56 capsules.

PVC/PVDC (Duplex) or PVC/PE/PVDC (Triplex) blisters with aluminium cover foil containing 56 or 60 capsules.

Amber glass bottles with metal screw caps containing 30 or 100 capsules.

6.6 Special precautions for disposal and other handling

None.

7. MARKETING AUTHORISATION HOLDER

Actavis Group PTC ehf

Reykjavíkurvegi 76-78

220 Hafnarfjordur

Iceland.

8. MARKETING AUTHORISATION NUMBER(S)

PL 30306/0096

9. DATE OF FIRST AUTHORISATION/RENEWAL OF THE AUTHORISATION

22nd April 2008

10. DATE OF REVISION OF THE TEXT

October 2008

Neotigason 25mg Capsules

(Actavis UK Ltd)

1. NAME OF THE MEDICINAL PRODUCT

Neotigason 25mg capsules

2. QUALITATIVE AND QUANTITATIVE COMPOSITION

Capsules with brown cap and yellow body with actavis printed in black on the cap and "25" printed in black on the body, containing 25mg acitretin.

Excipients include glucose (see section *4.3 Contraindications*).

For a full list of excipients, see section *6.1*.

3. PHARMACEUTICAL FORM

Capsules for oral administration.

4. CLINICAL PARTICULARS

4.1 Therapeutic indications

Severe extensive psoriasis which is resistant to other forms of therapy.

Palmo-plantar pustular psoriasis.

Severe congenital ichthyosis.

Severe Darier's disease (keratosis follicularis).

4.2 Posology and method of administration

It is recommended that Neotigason be given only by, or under supervision of, a dermatological specialist.

Neotigason capsules are for oral administration.

The capsules should be taken once daily with meals or with milk.

There is a wide variation in the absorption and rate of metabolism of Neotigason. This necessitates individual adjustment of dosage. For this reason the following dosage recommendations can serve only as a guide.

Adults

Initial daily dose should be 25mg or 30mg for 2 to 4 weeks. After this initial treatment period the involved areas of the skin should show a marked response and/or side-effects should be apparent. Following assessment of the initial treatment period, titration of the dose upwards or downwards may be necessary to achieve the desired therapeutic response with the minimum of side-effects. In general, a daily dosage of 25 - 50mg taken for a further 6 to 8 weeks achieves optimal therapeutic results. However, it may be necessary in some cases to increase the dose up to a maximum of 75mg/day.

In patients with Darier's disease a starting dose of 10mg may be appropriate. The dose should be increased cautiously as isomorphic reactions may occur.

Therapy can be discontinued in patients with psoriasis whose lesions have improved sufficiently. Relapses should be treated as described above.

Patients with severe congenital ichthyosis and severe Darier's disease may require therapy beyond 3 months. The lowest effective dosage, not exceeding 50mg/day, should be given.

Continuous use beyond 6 months is contra-indicated as only limited clinical data are available on patients treated beyond this length of time.

Elderly

Dosage recommendations are the same as for other adults.

Children

In view of possible severe side-effects associated with long-term treatment, Neotigason is contra-indicated in children unless, in the opinion of the physician, the benefits significantly outweigh the risks.

The dosage should be established according to body-weight. The daily dosage is about 0.5mg/kg. Higher doses (up to 1mg/kg daily) may be necessary in some cases for limited periods, but only up to a maximum of 35mg/day. The maintenance dose should be kept as low as possible in view of possible long-term side-effects.

Combination therapy

Other dermatological therapy, particularly with keratolytics, should normally be stopped before administration of Neotigason. However, the use of topical corticosteroids or bland emollient ointment may be continued if indicated.

When Neotigason is used in combination with other types of therapy, it may be possible, depending on the individual patient's response, to reduce the dosage of Neotigason.

4.3 Contraindications

Neotigason is highly teratogenic. Its use is contra-indicated in pregnant women and women who might become pregnant during or within 2 years of the cessation of treatment (see section *4.4 Special warnings and special precautions for use*).

The use of Neotigason is contra-indicated in women who are breast feeding.

Neotigason is contra-indicated in patients with hepatic or renal impairment and in patients with chronic abnormally elevated blood lipid values.

Rare cases of benign intracranial hypertension have been reported after Neotigason and after tetracyclines. Supplementary treatment with antibiotics such as tetracyclines is therefore contra-indicated.

An increased risk of hepatitis has been reported following the concomitant use of methotrexate and etretinate. Consequently, the concomitant use of methotrexate and Neotigason should be avoided.

Concomitant administration of Neotigason with other retinoids or preparations containing high doses of Vitamin A, (i.e. more than the recommended dietary allowance of 4,000 - 5,000 i.u. per day) is contra-indicated due to the risk of hypervitaminosis A.

Neotigason is contra-indicated in cases of hypersensitivity to the preparation (acitretin or excipients) or to other retinoids.

Owing to the presence of glucose, patients with rare glucose-galactose malabsorption should not take this medicine.

4.4 Special warnings and precautions for use

Neotigason should only be prescribed by physicians who are experienced in the use of systemic retinoids and understand the risk of teratogenicity associated with acitretin therapy.

Neotigason is highly teratogenic. The risk of giving birth to a deformed child is exceptionally high if Neotigason is taken before or during pregnancy, no matter for how long or at what dosage. Foetal exposure to Neotigason always involves a risk of congenital malformation.

Neotigason is contra-indicated in women of childbearing potential unless the following criteria are met:

1. Pregnancy has been excluded before instituting therapy with Neotigason (negative pregnancy test within 2 weeks prior to therapy). Whenever practicable a monthly repetition of the pregnancy test is recommended during therapy.

2. She starts Neotigason therapy only on the second or third day of the next menstrual cycle.

3. Having excluded pregnancy, any woman of childbearing potential who is receiving Neotigason must practice effective contraception for at least one month before treatment, during the treatment period and for at least 2 years following its cessation.

Even female patients who normally do not practice contraception because of a history of infertility should be advised to do so, while taking Neotigason.

4. The same effective and uninterrupted contraceptive measures must also be taken every time therapy is repeated, however long the intervening period may have been, and must be continued for 2 years afterwards.

5. Any pregnancy occurring during treatment with Neotigason, or in the 2 years following its cessation, carries a high risk of severe foetal malformation. Therefore, before instituting Neotigason the treating physician must explain clearly and in detail what precautions must be taken. This should include the risks involved and the possible consequences of pregnancy occurring during Neotigason treatment or in the 2 years following its cessation.

6. She is reliable and capable of understanding the risk and complying with effective contraception, and confirms that she has understood the warnings.

In view of the importance of the above precautions, Neotigason Patient Information Leaflets are available to doctors and it is strongly recommended that these be given to all patients.

If oral contraception is chosen as the most appropriate contraceptive method for women undergoing retinoid treatment, then a combined oestrogen-progestogen formulation is recommended.

Patients should not donate blood either during or for at least one year following discontinuation of therapy with Neotigason. Theoretically there would be a small risk to a woman in the first trimester of pregnancy who received blood donated by a patient on Neotigason therapy.

Acitretin has been shown to affect diaphyseal and spongy bone adversely in animals at high doses in excess of those recommended for use in man. Since skeletal hyperostosis and extraosseous calcification have been reported following long-term treatment with etretinate in man, this effect should be expected with acitretin therapy.

Since there have been occasional reports of bone changes in children, including premature epiphyseal closure, skeletal hyperostosis and extraosseous calcification after long-term treatment with etretinate, these effects may be expected with acitretin. Neotigason therapy in children is not, therefore, recommended. If, in exceptional circumstances, such therapy is undertaken the child should be carefully monitored for any abnormalities of musculo-skeletal development.

In adults receiving long-term treatment with Neotigason, appropriate examinations should be periodically performed in view of possible ossification abnormalities (see section *4.8 Undesirable effects*). Any patients complaining of atypical musculo-skeletal symptoms on treatment with Neotigason should be promptly and fully investigated to exclude possible acitretin-induced bone changes. If clinically significant bone or joint changes are found, Neotigason therapy should be discontinued.

The effects of UV light are enhanced by retinoid therapy, therefore patients should avoid excessive exposure to sunlight and the unsupervised use of sun lamps.

Hepatic function should be checked before starting treatment with Neotigason, every 1 - 2 weeks for the first 2 months after commencement and then every 3 months during treatment. If abnormal results are obtained, weekly checks should be instituted. If hepatic function fails to return to normal or deteriorates further, Neotigason must be withdrawn. In such cases it is advisable to continue monitoring hepatic function for at least 3 months.

Serum cholesterol and serum triglycerides (fasting values) must be monitored, especially in high-risk patients (disturbances of lipid metabolism, diabetes mellitus, obesity, alcoholism) and during long-term treatment.

In diabetic patients, retinoids can alter glucose tolerance. Blood sugar levels should therefore be checked more frequently than usual at the beginning of the treatment period.

Patients should be warned of the possibility of alopecia occurring (see section *4.8 Undesirable effects*).

4.5 Interaction with other medicinal products and other forms of interaction

Existing data suggests that concurrent intake of acitretin with ethanol led to the formation of etretinate. However, etretinate formation without concurrent alcohol intake cannot be excluded. Therefore, since the elimination half-life of etretinate is 120 days the post-therapy contraception period in women of childbearing potential must be 2 years (see section *4.4 Special warnings and precautions for use)*.

An increased risk of hepatitis has been reported following the concomitant use of methotrexate and etretinate. Consequently, the concomitant use of methotrexate and Neotigason should be avoided (see section *4.3 Contra-indications)*.

In concurrent treatment with phenytoin, it must be remembered that Neotigason partially reduces the protein binding of phenytoin. The clinical significance of this is as yet unknown.

Interaction studies show acitretin does not interfere with the anti-ovulatory action of the combined oral contraceptives.

Interactions between Neotigason and other substances (e.g. digoxin, cimetidine) have not been observed to date.

4.6 Pregnancy and lactation

Neotigason is contra-indicated during pregnancy as it is a known human teratogen.

The use of Neotigason is contra-indicated in women who are breast feeding. It is also contra-indicated in women of childbearing potential unless specific criteria are met, (see section *4.4 Special warnings and special precautions for use*).

4.7 Effects on ability to drive and use machines

Decreased night vision has been reported with Neotigason therapy. Patients should be advised of this potential problem and warned to be cautious when driving or operating any vehicle at night. Visual problems should be carefully monitored (see section *4.8 Undesirable effects*).

4.8 Undesirable effects

Most of the clinical side-effects of Neotigason are dose-related and are usually well-tolerated at the recommended dosages. However, the toxic dose of Neotigason is close to the therapeutic dose and most patients experience some side-effects during the initial period whilst dosage is being adjusted. They are usually reversible with reduction of dosage or discontinuation of therapy.

The skin and mucous membranes are most commonly affected, and it is recommended that patients should be so advised before treatment is commenced.

Skin: Dryness of the skin may be associated with scaling, thinning, erythema (especially of the face) and pruritus. Palmar and plantar exfoliation may occur. Sticky skin and dermatitis occur frequently. Epidermal fragility, nail fragility and paronychia have been observed.

Occasionally bullous eruptions and abnormal hair texture have been reported. Hair thinning and frank alopecia may occur, usually noted 4 to 8 weeks after starting therapy, and are reversible following discontinuation of Neotigason. Full recovery usually occurs within 6 months of stopping treatment in the majority of patients.

Granulomatous lesions have occasionally been observed.

Sweating has been reported infrequently.

Rarely, patients may experience photosensitivity reactions.

Mucous membranes: Dryness of mucous membranes, sometimes with erosion, involving the lips, mouth, conjunctivae and nasal mucosa have been reported. Corneal ulcerations have been observed rarely.

Dryness of the conjunctivae may lead to mild-to-moderate conjunctivitis or xerophthalmia and result in intolerance of contact lenses; it may be alleviated by lubrication with artificial tears or topical antibiotics.

Cheilitis, rhagades of the corner of the mouth, dry mouth and thirst have occurred. Occasionally stomatitis, gingivitis and taste disturbance have been reported.

Rhinitis and epistaxis have been observed.

Central nervous system: Headache has occurred infrequently. Benign intracranial hypertension has been reported. Patients with severe headache, nausea, vomiting and visual disturbance should discontinue Neotigason immediately and be referred for neurological evaluation and care.

Neuro-sensory system: Blurred or decreased night vision has been reported occasionally.

Musculo-skeletal system: Myalgia and arthralgia may occur and be associated with reduced tolerance to exercise. Bone pain has also been reported.

Maintenance treatment may result in hyperostosis and extraskeletal calcification, as observed in long-term systemic treatment with other retinoids.

Gastrointestinal tract: Nausea has been reported infrequently. Vomiting, diarrhoea and abdominal pain have been observed rarely.

Liver and biliary system disorders: Transient, usually reversible elevation of serum levels of liver enzymes may occur. When significant, dosage reduction or discontinuation of therapy may be necessary. Jaundice and hepatitis have occurred rarely.

Metabolic: Elevation of serum triglycerides above the normal range has been observed, especially where predisposing factors such as a family history of lipid disorders, obesity, alcohol abuse, diabetes mellitus or smoking are present. The changes are dose-related and may be controlled by dietary means (including restriction of alcohol intake) and/or by reduction of dosage of Neotigason. Increases in serum cholesterol have occurred.

Cardiovascular system: Occasionally peripheral oedema and flushing have been reported.

Miscellaneous reactions: Increased incidence of vulvovaginitis due to Candida albicans has been noted during treatment with acitretin. Malaise and drowsiness have been infrequently reported.

4.9 Overdose

Manifestations of acute Vitamin A toxicity include severe headache, nausea or vomiting, drowsiness, irritability and pruritus. Signs and symptoms of accidental or deliberate overdosage with Neotigason would probably be similar. They would be expected to subside without need for treatment.

Because of the variable absorption of the drug, gastric lavage may be worthwhile within the first few hours after ingestion.

5. PHARMACOLOGICAL PROPERTIES

5.1 Pharmacodynamic properties

Retinol (Vitamin A) is known to be essential for normal epithelial growth and differentiation, though the mode of this effect is not yet established. Both retinol and retinoic acid are capable of reversing hyperkeratotic and metaplastic skin changes. However, these effects are generally only obtained at dosages associated with considerable local or systemic toxicity. Acitretin, a synthetic aromatic derivative of retinoic acid, has a favourable therapeutic ratio, with a greater and more specific inhibitory effect on psoriasis and disorders of epithelial keratinisation. The usual therapeutic response to acitretin consists of desquamation (with or without erythema) followed by more normal re-epithelialisation.

Acitretin is the main active metabolite of etretinate.

5.2 Pharmacokinetic properties

Absorption

Acitretin reaches peak plasma concentration 1 - 4 hours after ingestion of the drug. Bioavailability of orally administered acitretin is enhanced by food. Bioavailability of a single dose is approximately 60%, but inter-patient variability is considerable (36 - 95%).

Distribution

Acitretin is highly lipophilic and penetrates readily into body tissues. Protein binding of acitretin exceeds 99%. In animal studies, acitretin passed the placental barrier in quantities sufficient to produce foetal malformations. Due to its lipophilic nature, it can be assumed that acitretin passes into breast milk in considerable quantities.

Metabolism

Acitretin is metabolised by isomerisation into its 13-cis isomer (*cis* acitretin), by glucuronidation and cleavage of the side chain.

Elimination

Multiple-dose studies in patients aged 21 - 70 years showed an elimination half-life of approximately 50 hours for acitretin and 60 hours for its main metabolite in plasma, *cis* acitretin, which is also a teratogen. From the longest elimination half-life observed in these patients for acitretin (96 hours) and *cis* acitretin (123 hours), and assuming linear kinetics, it can be predicted that more than 99% of the drug is eliminated within 36 days after cessation of long-term therapy. Furthermore, plasma concentrations of acitretin and *cis* acitretin dropped below the sensitivity limit of the assay (< 6ng/ml) within 36 days following cessation of treatment. Acitretin is excreted entirely in the form of its metabolites, in approximately equal parts via the kidneys and the bile.

5.3 Preclinical safety data
None stated.

6. PHARMACEUTICAL PARTICULARS

6.1 List of excipients

Capsule content:

Glucose, liquid, spray-dried

Sodium ascorbate

Gelatin

Purified water

Microcrystalline cellulose

Capsule shell:

Gelatin

Iron oxide black (E172)

Iron oxide yellow (E172)

Iron oxide red (E172)

Titanium dioxide (E171)

Printing ink:

Shellac

N-Butyl alcohol

Isopropyl alcohol

Propylene glycol

Ammonium hydroxide

Iron oxide black (E172)

6.2 Incompatibilities
None.

6.3 Shelf life
Neotigason capsules have a shelf-life of 3 years.

6.4 Special precautions for storage
Store in the original package. Do not store above 25°C.

6.5 Nature and contents of container
All aluminium blisters containing 56 capsules.

PVC/PVDC (Duplex) or PVC/PE/PVDC (Triplex) blisters with aluminium cover foil containing 56 or 60 capsules.

Amber glass bottles with metal screw caps containing 30 or 100 capsules.

6.6 Special precautions for disposal and other handling
None.

7. MARKETING AUTHORISATION HOLDER
Actavis Group PTC ehf

Reykjavíkurvegi 76-78

220 Hafnarfjordur

Iceland.

8. MARKETING AUTHORISATION NUMBER(S)
PL 30306/0097

9. DATE OF FIRST AUTHORISATION/RENEWAL OF THE AUTHORISATION
23rd April 2008

10. DATE OF REVISION OF THE TEXT
October 2008

Neupro 1 mg/24 h, 2 mg/24 h, 3 mg/24 h, 4 mg/24 h, 6 mg/24 h, 8 mg/24 h Transdermal Patch & Parkinson's disease Treatment Initiation Pack

(UCB Pharma Limited)

1. NAME OF THE MEDICINAL PRODUCT
Neupro 1 mg/24 h transdermal patch ▼

Neupro 2 mg/24 h transdermal patch ▼

Neupro 3 mg/24 h transdermal patch ▼

Neupro 4 mg/24 h transdermal patch ▼

Neupro 6 mg/24 h transdermal patch ▼

Neupro 8 mg/24 h transdermal patch ▼

2. QUALITATIVE AND QUANTITATIVE COMPOSITION
Neupro 1 mg/24 h transdermal patch

Each patch releases 1 mg of rotigotine per 24 hours. Each patch of 5 cm^2 contains 2.25 mg of rotigotine.

Neupro 2 mg/24 h transdermal patch

Each patch releases 2 mg of rotigotine per 24 hours. Each patch of 10 cm^2 contains 4.5 mg of rotigotine.

Neupro 3 mg/24 h transdermal patch

Each patch releases 3 mg of rotigotine per 24 hours. Each patch of 15 cm^2 contains 6.75 mg of rotigotine.

Neupro 4 mg/24 h transdermal patch

Each patch releases 4 mg of rotigotine per 24 hours. Each patch of 20 cm^2 contains 9.0 mg of rotigotine.

Neupro 6 mg/24 h transdermal patch

Each patch releases 6 mg of rotigotine per 24 hours. Each patch of 30 cm^2 contains 13.5 mg of rotigotine.

Neupro 8 mg/24 h transdermal patch

Each patch releases 8 mg of rotigotine per 24 hours. Each patch of 40 cm^2 contains 18.0 mg of rotigotine.

For a full list of excipients, see section 6.1.

3. PHARMACEUTICAL FORM
Transdermal patch.

Thin, matrix-type, square-shaped with rounded edges, consisting of three layers. The outside of the backing layer is tan-coloured and imprinted with Neupro 1 mg/24 h, 2 mg/24 h, 3 mg/24 h, 4 mg/24 h, 6 mg/24 h or 8 mg/24 h.

4. CLINICAL PARTICULARS

4.1 Therapeutic indications

Restless Legs Syndrome

Neupro is indicated for the symptomatic treatment of moderate to severe idiopathic Restless Legs Syndrome in adults.

Parkinson's disease

Neupro is indicated for the treatment of the signs and symptoms of early-stage idiopathic Parkinson's disease as monotherapy (i.e. without levodopa) or in combination with levodopa, i.e. over the course of the disease, through to late stages when the effect of levodopa wears off or becomes inconsistent and fluctuations of the therapeutic effect occur (end of dose or 'on-off' fluctuations).

4.2 Posology and method of administration
Neupro is applied once a day. The patch should be applied at approximately the same time every day. The patch remains on the skin for 24 hours and will then be replaced by a new one at a different site of application.

If the patient forgets to apply the patch at the usual time of the day or if the patch becomes detached, another patch should be applied for the remainder of the day.

Dosage

The dose recommendations made are in nominal dose.

Restless Legs Syndrome

A single daily dose should be initiated at 1 mg/24 h. Depending on the individual patient response, the dose may be increased in weekly increments of 1 mg/24 h to a maximal dose of 3 mg/24 h. The need for treatment continuation should be reconsidered every 6 months.

Parkinson's disease

Dosing in patients with early-stage Parkinson's disease:

A single daily dose should be initiated at 2 mg/24 h and then increased in weekly increments of 2 mg/24 h to an effective dose up to a maximal dose of 8 mg/24 h.

4 mg/24 h may be an effective dose in some patients. For most patients an effective dose is reached within 3 or 4 weeks at doses of 6 mg/24 h or 8 mg/24 h, respectively.

The maximal dose is 8 mg/24 h.

Dosing in patients with advanced stage Parkinson's disease with fluctuations:

A single daily dose should be initiated at 4 mg/24 h and then increased in weekly increments of 2 mg/24 h to an effective dose up to a maximal dose of 16 mg/24 h.

4 mg/24 h or 6 mg/24 h may be effective doses in some patients. For most patients an effective dose is reached within 3 to 7 weeks at doses of 8 mg/24 h up to a maximum dose of 16 mg/24 h.

For doses higher than 8 mg/24 h multiple patches may be used to achieve the final dose e.g. 10 mg/24 h may be reached by combination of a 6 mg/24 h and a 4 mg/24 h patch.

Parkinson's disease Treatment Initiation Pack:

Neupro treatment initiation pack contains 4 different packages (one for each strength) with 7 patches each, for the first four weeks of therapy.

Depending on the patient's response, not all of the following dose steps may be required or additional higher doses may be needed after week 4, which are not covered by this package.

On the first day of treatment the patient starts with Neupro 2 mg/24 h. During the second week, the patient takes Neupro 4 mg/24 h. During the third week, he or she takes Neupro 6 mg/24 h and during the fourth week Neupro 8 mg/24 h. The packages are marked with "Week 1 (2, 3 or 4)".

Treatment discontinuation

Restless Legs Syndrome

Neupro should be discontinued gradually. The daily dose should be reduced in steps of 1 mg/24 h with a dose reduction preferably every other day, until complete withdrawal of Neupro (see section 4.4). Following this procedure, rebound (worsening of symptoms beyond initial intensity after discontinuation of treatment) was not observed.

Parkinson's disease

Neupro should be discontinued gradually. The daily dose should be reduced in steps of 2 mg/24 h with a dose reduction preferably every other day, until complete withdrawal of Neupro (see section 4.4).

Hepatic and renal impairment: Adjustment of the dose is not necessary in patients with mild to moderate hepatic impairment or in patients with mild to severe renal impairment including those requiring dialysis. Caution is advised when treating patients with severe hepatic impairment, which may result in lower rotigotine clearance. Neupro has not been investigated in this patient group. A dose reduction might be needed in case of worsening of the hepatic impairment. Unexpected accumulation of rotigotine levels may also occur at acute worsening of renal function (see section 5.2).

Children and adolescents: Neupro is not recommended for use in children and adolescents due to a lack of data on safety and efficacy.

Method of administration

The patch should be applied to clean, dry, intact healthy skin on the abdomen, thigh, hip, flank, shoulder, or upper arm. Reapplication to the same site within 14 days should be avoided. Neupro should not be placed on skin that is red, irritated or damaged. (see section 4.4)

Use and handling:

Each patch is packed in a sachet and should be applied directly after the sachet has been opened. One half of the protective liner should be removed and the sticky side should be applied and pressed firmly to the skin. Then, the patch is folded back and the second part of the release liner is removed. The sticky side of the patch should not be touched. The patch should be pressed down firmly with the palm of the hand for about 20 to 30 seconds, so that it sticks well.

In the event that a patch should fall off, a new patch should be applied for the remainder of the 24 hour dosing interval.

The patch should not be cut into pieces.

4.3 Contraindications
Hypersensitivity to the active substance or to any of the excipients.

Magnetic resonance imaging or cardioversion (see section 4.4).

4.4 Special warnings and precautions for use
If a Parkinson's disease patient is insufficiently controlled while on treatment with rotigotine switching to another dopamine agonist might provide additional benefit (see section 5.1)

The backing layer of Neupro contains aluminium. To avoid skin burns, Neupro should be removed if the patient has to undergo magnetic resonance imaging (MRI) or cardioversion.

Dopamine agonists are known to impair the systemic regulation of the blood pressure resulting in postural/orthostatic hypotension. These events were also observed during treatment with Neupro, however the incidence was similar to that in placebo-treated patients.

Syncope was observed in association with Neupro, but also at a similar rate in patients treated with placebo.

It is recommended to monitor blood pressure, especially at the beginning of treatment, due to the general risk of orthostatic hypotension associated with dopaminergic therapy.

Neupro has been associated with somnolence and episodes of sudden sleep onset. Sudden onset of sleep during daily activities, in some cases without awareness of any warning signs, has been reported. Prescribers should continually reassess patients for drowsiness or sleepiness, as patients may not acknowledge drowsiness or sleepiness until directly questioned. A reduction of dosage or termination of therapy should be carefully considered.

Pathologic gambling, increased libido and hypersexuality have been reported in patients treated with dopamine agonists, including rotigotine.

Although not reported with Neupro, symptoms suggestive of neuroleptic malignant syndrome have been reported with abrupt withdrawal of dopaminergic therapy. Therefore it is recommended to taper treatment (see section 4.2).

Hallucinations have been reported and patients should be informed that hallucinations can occur.

Fibrotic complications: Cases of retroperitoneal fibrosis, pulmonary infiltrates, pleural effusion, pleural thickening, pericarditis and cardiac valvulopathy have been reported in some patients treated with ergot-derived dopaminergic agents. While these complications may resolve when treatment is discontinued, complete resolution does not always occur.

Although these adverse reactions are believed to be related to the ergoline structure of these compounds, whether other, nonergot derived dopamine agonists can cause them is unknown.

Neuroleptics given as antiemetic should not be given to patients taking dopamine agonists (see also section 4.5).

Ophthalmologic monitoring is recommended at regular intervals or if vision abnormalities occur.

Augmentation may occur. Augmentation refers to the earlier onset of symptoms in the evening (or even the afternoon), increase in severity of symptoms, and spread of symptoms to involve other body parts. Based on two open-label follow-up studies with one year duration, symptoms reflecting clinically relevant and not relevant augmentation may be as high as 9.4%. However, based on two 6-month, double-blind, placebo-controlled studies, clinically relevant augmentation was observed in 1.5% of rotigotine-treated patients versus 0.5% of placebo treated patients. In two open-label, follow-up studies over a subsequent 12 months, the rate of clinically relevant augmentation was

2.9%. None of these patients discontinued therapy because of augmentation.

External heat (excessive sunlight, heating pads and other sources of heat such as sauna, hot bath) should not be applied to the area of the patch.

Application site skin reactions may occur and are usually mild or moderate in intensity. It is recommended that the application site should be rotated on a daily basis (e.g. from the right side to the left side and from the upper body to the lower body). The same site should not be used within 14 days. If application site reactions occur which last for more than a few days or are persistent, if there is an increase in severity, or if the skin reaction spreads outside the application site, an assessment of the risk/benefit balance for the individual patient should be conducted.

If there is a skin rash or irritation from the transdermal system, direct sunlight on the area should be avoided until the skin heals. Exposure could lead to changes in the skin color.

If a generalised skin reaction (e.g. allergic rash, including erythematous, macular, papular rash or pruritus) associated with the use of Neupro is observed, Neupro should be discontinued.

The incidence of some dopaminergic adverse events, such as hallucinations, dyskinesia, and peripheral oedema generally is higher when given in combination with L-dopa in Parkinson's patients. This should be considered when prescribing rotigotine.

In clinical studies in Parkinson's patients, the 6 month-specific rates of peripheral edema remained at about 4% through the entire observation period up to 36 months.

4.5 Interaction with other medicinal products and other forms of interaction

Because rotigotine is a dopamine agonist, it is assumed that dopamine antagonists, such as neuroleptics (e.g. phenothiazines, butyrophenones, thioxanthenes) or metoclopramide, may diminish the effectiveness of Neupro, and co-administration should be avoided. Because of possible additive effects, caution should be advised when patients are taking sedating medicinal products or other CNS (central nervous system) depressants (e.g. benzodiazepines, antipsychotics, antidepressants) or alcohol in combination with rotigotine.

Co-administration of L-dopa and carbidopa with rotigotine had no effect on the pharmacokinetics of rotigotine, and rotigotine had no effect on the pharmacokinetics of L-dopa and carbidopa.

Co-administration of domperidone with rotigotine had no effect on the pharmacokinetics of rotigotine.

Co-administration of omeprazole (inhibitor of CYP2C19), in doses of 40 mg/day, had no effect on the pharmacokinetics and metabolism of rotigotine in healthy volunteers.

Neupro may potentiate the dopaminergic adverse reaction of L-dopa and may cause and/or exacerbate pre-existing dyskinesia, as described with other dopamine agonists.

Co-administration of rotigotine (3 mg/24 h) did not affect the pharmacodynamics and pharmacokinetics of oral contraceptives (0.03 mg ethinylestradiol, 0.15 mg levonorgestrel).

Interactions with other forms of hormonal contraception have not been investigated.

4.6 Pregnancy and lactation

There are no adequate data from the use of Neupro in pregnant women. Animal studies do not indicate any teratogenic effects in rats and rabbits, but embryo-toxicity was observed in rats and mice at materno-toxic doses (see section 5.3). The potential risk for humans is unknown. Rotigotine should not be used during pregnancy.

Because rotigotine decreases prolactin secretion in humans, inhibition of lactation is expected. Studies in rats have shown that rotigotine and/or its metabolite(s) is excreted in breast milk. In the absence of human data, breast-feeding should be discontinued.

4.7 Effects on ability to drive and use machines

Rotigotine may have major influence on the ability to drive and use machines.

Patients being treated with rotigotine and presenting with somnolence and/or sudden sleep episodes must be informed not to drive or engage in activities (e.g. operating machines) where impaired alertness may put themselves or others at risk of serious injury or death until such recurrent episodes and somnolence have resolved (see also sections 4.4 and 4.5).

4.8 Undesirable effects

Restless Legs Syndrome

Based on the analysis of pooled placebo-controlled clinical trials comprising a total of 748 Neupro- and 214 placebo-treated patients, 65.0% of the patients on Neupro and 32.7% of patients on placebo reported at least one adverse reaction.

At the beginning of therapy dopaminergic adverse reactions such as nausea and vomiting may occur. These are usually mild or moderate in intensity and transient even if treatment is continued.

Adverse drug reactions (ADRs) reported in more than 10% of patients treated with Neupro are nausea, application site reactions, fatigue and headache.

In trials where the application sites were rotated as reflected in the instructions provided in the SPC and package leaflet, 34.2% of 748 patients using Neupro, experienced application site reactions. The majority of these reactions were mild or moderate in intensity, limited to the application areas and resulted in discontinuation of Neupro in 7.2% of subjects.

The following table covers adverse drug reactions from all studies in patients with Restless Legs Syndrome. Within each frequency grouping, undesirable effects are presented in order of decreasing seriousness.

(see Table 1 below)

The discontinuation rate was studied in 3 clinical trials ranging up to 3 years in duration. The percentage of subjects discontinuing was 25-38% over the first year, 10% in the second year, and 11% in the third year. Periodic assessment of efficacy should be performed, along with evaluation of safety, including augmentation.

Parkinson's disease

Based on the analysis of pooled placebo-controlled clinical trials comprising a total of 1,083 Neupro- and 508 placebo-treated patients, 73.0% of the patients on Neupro and 56.3% of patients on placebo reported at least one adverse reaction.

At the beginning of therapy dopaminergic adverse reactions such as nausea and vomiting may occur. These are usually mild or moderate in intensity and transient even if treatment is continued.

Adverse drug reactions (ADRs) reported in more than 10% of patients treated with Neupro transdermal patch are nausea, dizziness, somnolence and application site reactions.

In trials where the application sites were rotated as reflected in the instructions provided in SPC and package leaflet, 35.7% of 830 patients using the Neupro transdermal patch, experienced application site reactions. The majority of these reactions were mild or moderate in intensity, limited to the application areas and resulted in discontinuation of treatment with Neupro in only 4.3% of all subjects receiving Neupro.

Within each frequency grouping, undesirable effects are presented in order of decreasing seriousness.

The following table covers adverse drug reactions from all studies in patients with Parkinson's disease.

(see Table 2 on next page)

Both indications

Neupro has been associated with somnolence including excessive daytime somnolence and sudden sleep onset episodes. In isolated cases "sudden onset of sleep" occurred while driving and resulted in motor vehicle accidents. See also section 4.4 and 4.7.

Patients treated with dopamine agonists including Neupro, have been reported as exhibiting signs of pathological gambling, increased libido and hypersexuality, generally reversible upon reduction of the dose or treatment discontinuation.

4.9 Overdose

The most likely adverse reactions would be those related to the pharmacodynamic profile of a dopamine agonist, including nausea, vomiting, hypotension, involuntary movements, hallucinations, confusion, convulsions and other signs of central dopaminergic stimulation.

There is no known antidote for overdose of dopamine agonists. In case of suspected overdose, the patch(es) should immediately be removed from the patient. Levels of rotigotine decrease after patch removal. Before stopping use of rotigotine completely see section 4.2.

The patient should be monitored closely, including heart rate, heart rhythm and blood pressure. Because rotigotine is over 90% protein bound, dialysis would not be expected to be beneficial.

Treatment of overdose may require general supportive measures to maintain the vital signs.

5. PHARMACOLOGICAL PROPERTIES

5.1 Pharmacodynamic properties

Pharmacotherapeutic group: Dopamine agonists; ATC code: N04BC09

Rotigotine is a non-ergolinic $D_3/D_2/D_1$ dopamine agonist for the treatment of Parkinson's disease. It is believed to elicit its beneficial effect by activation of the D_3, D_2 and D_1 receptors of the caudate-putamen in the brain.

Rotigotine alleviates signs and symptoms of idiopathic Parkinson's disease.

Clinical studies:

The efficacy of Neupro was evaluated in 5 placebo-controlled trials with more than 1,400 patients with idiopathic Restless Legs Syndrome (RLS). Efficacy was demonstrated in controlled trials in patients treated for up to 29 weeks. The effect was maintained over a 6 months period.

The changes from baseline in the International RLS Rating Scale (IRLS) and CGI-item 1 (severity of illness) were primary efficacy parameters. For both primary endpoints statistically significant differences have been observed for the doses 1 mg/24 h, 2 mg/24 h and 3 mg/24 h in comparison to placebo. After 6 months of maintenance treatment in patients with moderate to severe RLS, the baseline IRLS score improved from 30.7 to 20.7 for placebo and from 30.2 to 13.8 for Neupro. The adjusted mean difference was -6.5 points ($CI_{95\%}$ -8.7; -4.4, $p < 0.0001$). CGI-I responder rates (much improved, very much improved) were 43.0% and 67.5% for placebo and Neupro respectively (difference 24.5% $CI_{95\%}$: 14.2%; 34.8%, $p < 0.0001$).

In a placebo-controlled, 7-week trial polysomnographic parameters were investigated. Neupro significantly reduced the periodic limb movement index (PLMI) from 50.9 to 7.7 *versus* 37.4 to 32.7 for placebo ($p < 0.0001$).

Clinical studies in Parkinson's disease

The effectiveness of Neupro in the treatment of the signs and symptoms of idiopathic Parkinson's disease was evaluated in a multinational drug development program consisting of four pivotal, parallel, randomized, double-blind placebo controlled studies.

Table 1

System/organ classes acc. to MedDRA	Very common ≥ 1/10	Common ≥ 1/100, < 1/10	Uncommon ≥ 1/1,000, < 1/100	Rare ≥ 1/10,000, ≤ 1/1,000
Gastrointestinal disorders	Nausea	Vomiting, Dyspepsia		
General disorders and administration site conditions	Application and instillation site reactions[a] (incl. erythema, pruritus, irritation, rash, dermatitis, vesicles, pain, eczema, inflammation, swelling, discolouration, papules, excoriation, urticaria, hypersensitivity) Fatigue	Irritability		
Immune system disorders		Hypersensitivity		
Nervous system disorders	Headache	Somnolence		
Psychiatric disorders		Sleep attacks, Sexual desire disorder[a] (incl. hypersexuality, libido increased), Insomnia, Sleep disorder, Abnormal dreams	Impulse control disorder[a] (incl. pathological gambling, punding)	Obsessive compulsive disorder
Skin and subcutaneous tissue disorders		Pruritus		
Vascular disorders		Hypertension	Orthostatic hypotension	

a) High Level Term

Table 2

System/organ classes acc. to MedDRA	Very common > 1/10	Common >1/100, ≤1/10	Uncommon >1/1,000, ≤1/100	Rare ≤1/1,000
Immune system disorder			Hypersensitivity	
Metabolism and nutrition disorders			Anorexia, Decreased appetite	
Psychiatric disorders		Perception disturbances[b] (hallucination[a], visual hallucination[a], auditory hallucination, illusion), Confusion state, Abnormal dreams[a], Insomnia[a]	Sleep attacks[a], Psychotic disorder (including paranoid psychosis), Compulsive disorders (including pathologic gambling, punding), Increased libido (including hypersexuality), Anxiety, Sleep disorder[a], Nightmares, Disorientation	
Nervous system disorders	Somnolence[a], Dizziness[a]	Dyskinesia[a], Dizziness postural, Headache[a]	Syncope, Vasovagal syncope, Dystonia, Hypersomnia, Lethargia, Disturbance in attention, Memory impaired, Paraesthesia, Dysgeusia, Balance disorder, Tremor	Convulsion, Loss of consciousness
Eye disorders (see section 4.4)			Visual disturbance, Photopsia, Blurred vision	
Ear and labyrinth disorders			Vertigo (incl. positional)	
Cardiac disorders			Atrial fibrillation, Heart rate increased, Palpitations	Supraventricular Tachycardia
Vascular disorders		Orthostatic hypotension (see section 4.4)	Hypertension[a], Hypotension	
Respiratory, thoracic and mediastinal disorders			Cough, Hiccup[a], Dyspnoea	
Gastrointestinal disorders	Nausea[a]	Vomiting[a], Diarrhoea[a], Constipation[a], Dyspepsia[a], Dry mouth[a]	Abdominal pain (incl. upper abdominal pain), Stomach discomfort	
Hepato-biliary disorder		Hepatic enzyme increased (including GGT, ALAT, ASAT)		
Skin and subcutaneous tissue disorders		Rash (incl. rash, allergic; macular, exanthema)(see section 4.4), Erythema[a]; Pruritus, Hyperhydrosis[a],	Generalized pruritus, Dermatitis contact, Skin irritation	
Musculoskeletal and connective tissue disorder			Joint swelling	
Reproductive system and breast disorder			Erectile dysfunction	
General disorders and administration site conditions	Application site reactions[b] (including erythema[a], pruritus[a], irritation[a], burning[a], dermatitis[a], inflammation, papulae, vesicle, blister, pain, hypersensitivity) (see section 4.4)	Oedema peripheral[a], Asthenic conditions[b] (incl. fatigue[a], asthenia, malaise), Weight decreased	Gait disturbance[a], Feeling abnormal, Weight increased[a],	
Injury, poisoning and procedural complications		Fall		

[a] These adverse drug reactions have been reported in the pooled placebo-controlled trials 1% more frequent than in the placebo-treated patients

[b] High Level Term

Two trials investigating the effectiveness of Neupro in the treatment of the signs and symptoms of idiopathic Parkinson's disease were conducted in patients who were not receiving concomitant dopamine agonist therapy and were either L-dopa naïve or previous L-dopa treatment was ≤ 6 months. The primary outcome assessment was the score for the Activities of Daily Living (ADL) component (Part II) plus the Motor Examination component (Part III) of the Unified Parkinson's Disease Rating Scale (UPDRS).

Efficacy was determined by the subject's response to therapy in terms of responder and absolute points improvement in the scores of ADL and Motor Examination combined (UPDRS part II+III).

In one double blind study, 177 patients received rotigotine and 96 patients received placebo. The patients were titrated to their optimal dose of rotigotine or placebo in weekly increments of 2 mg/24 h starting at 2 mg/24 h to a maximum dose of 6 mg/24 h. Patients in each treatment group were maintained at their optimal dose for 6 months.

At the end of the maintenance treatment in 91% of the subjects in the rotigotine arm, the optimal dose was the maximal dose allowed i.e. 6 mg/24 h. An improvement of 20% was seen in 48% of the subjects receiving rotigotine and in 19% of the subjects receiving placebo (Difference 29% $CI_{95\%}$ 18%; 39%, $p<0.0001$). With rotigotine, the mean improvement in the UPDRS score (Parts II + III) was -3.98 points (baseline 29.9 point) whereas in the placebo-treated arm a worsening of 1.31 points was observed (baseline 30.0 points) The difference was 5.28 points and statistically significant ($p<0.0001$).

In a second double-blind study, 213 patients received rotigotine, 227 received ropinirole and 117 patients received placebo. The patients were titrated to their optimal dose of rotigotine in weekly increments of 2 mg/24 h starting at 2 mg/24 h to a maximum dose of 8 mg/24 h over 4 weeks. In the ropinirole group, patients were titrated to their optimal dose up to a maximum of 24 mg/day over 13 weeks. Patients in each treatment group were maintained for 6 months.

At the end of the maintenance treatment in 92% of the subjects in the rotigotine arm, the optimal dose was the maximal dose allowed i.e. 8 mg/24 h. An improvement of 20% was seen in 52% of the subjects receiving rotigotine, 68% of the subjects receiving ropinirole and 30% of the subjects receiving placebo (Difference rotigotine *versus* placebo 21.7%; $CI_{95\%}$ 11.1%; 32.4%, difference ropinirole *versus* placebo 38.4% $CI_{95\%}$ 28.1%; 48.6%, difference ropinirole *versus* rotigotine 16.6%; $CI_{95\%}$ .7.6%; 25.7%). The mean improvement in the UPDRS score (Parts II + III) was 6.83 points (baseline 33.2 points) in the rotigotine arm, 10.78 point in the ropinirole arm (baseline 32.2 points) and 2.33 points in the placebo arm (baseline 31.3 points). All differences between the active treatments and placebo were statistically significant. The difference in effect between ropinirole and rotigotine was also statistically significant in favour of ropinirole.

Two additional trials were conducted in patients who were receiving concomitant levodopa therapy. The primary outcome assessment was the reduction in "off" time (hours). Efficacy was determined by the subject's response to therapy in terms of responder and absolute improvement in the time spent "off".

In one double blind study, 113 patients received rotigotine up to a maximum dose of 8 mg/24 h, 109 patients received rotigotine up to a maximum dose of 12 mg/24 h and 119 patients received placebo. The patients were titrated to their optimal doses of rotigotine or placebo in weekly increments of 2 mg/24 h starting at 4 mg/24 h. Patients in each treatment group were maintained at their optimal dose for 6 months. At the end of the maintenance treatment an improvement of at least 30% was seen in 57% and 55% of the subjects receiving rotigotine 8 mg/24 h and 12 mg/24 h, respectively and in 34% of the subjects receiving placebo (Differences 22% and 21%, respectively $CI_{95\%}$ 10%; 35% and 8%; 33%, respectively, $p<0.001$ for both rotigotine groups). With rotigotine, the mean reductions in "off" time were 2.7 and 2.1 hours, respectively whereas in the placebo-treated arm a reduction of 0.9 hours was observed. The differences were statistically significant ($p<0.001$ and $p=0.003$, respectively).

In a second double-blind study, 201 patients received rotigotine, 200 received pramipexole and 100 patients received placebo. The patients were titrated to their optimal dose of rotigotine in weekly increments of 2 mg/24 h starting at 4 mg/24 h to a maximum dose of 16 mg/24 h. In the pramipexole group, patients received 0,375 mg in the first week, 0.75 mg in the second week and were titrated further in weekly increments of 0.75 mg to their optimal dose up to a maximum of 4.5 mg/day. Patients in each treatment group were maintained for 4 months.

At the end of the maintenance treatment an improvement of at least 30% was seen in 60% of the subjects receiving rotigotine, 67% of the subjects receiving pramipexole and 35% of the subjects receiving placebo (Difference rotigotine *versus* placebo 25%; $CI_{95\%}$ 13%; 36%, difference pramipexole *versus* placebo 32% $CI_{95\%}$ 21%; 43%, difference pramipexole *versus* rotigotine 7%; $CI_{95\%}$ -2%; 17%). The mean reduction in the "off" time was 2.5 hours in the rotigotine arm, 2.8 hours in the pramipexole arm and 0.9 hours in the placebo arm. All differences between the active treatments and placebo were statistically significant.

5.2 Pharmacokinetic properties

Absorption

Following application, rotigotine is continuously released from the transdermal patch and absorbed through the skin. Steady-state concentrations are reached after one to two days of patch application and are maintained at a stable level by once daily application in which the patch is worn for 24 hours. Rotigotine plasma concentrations increase dose-proportionally over a dose range of 1 mg/24 h to 24 mg/24 h.

Approximately 45% of the active substance within the patch is released to the skin in 24 hours. The absolute bioavailability after transdermal application is approximately 37%.

Rotating the site of patch application may result in day-to-day differences in plasma levels. Differences in bioavailability of rotigotine ranged from 2% (upper arm *versus* flank) to 46% (shoulder *versus* thigh). However, there is no indication of a relevant impact on the clinical outcome.

Distribution

The *in vitro* binding of rotigotine to plasma proteins is approximately 92%.

The apparent volume of distribution in humans is approximately 84 l/kg.

Metabolism

Rotigotine is metabolised to a great extent. Rotigotine is metabolised by N-dealkylation as well as direct and secondary conjugation. *In vitro* results indicate that different CYP isoforms are able to catalyse the N-dealkylation of rotigotine. Main metabolites are sulfates and glucuronide conjugates of the parent compound as well as N-desalkyl-metabolites, which are biologically inactive.

The infomation on metabolites is incomplete.

Elimination

Approximately 71% of the rotigotine dose is excreted in urine and a smaller part of about 23% is excreted in faeces.

The clearance of rotigotine after transdermal administration is approximately 10 l/min and its elimination half-life is 5 to 7 hours.

Because the patch is administered transdermally, no effect of food and gastrointestinal conditions is expected.

Special patient groups

Because therapy with Neupro is initiated at a low dose and gradually titrated according to clinical tolerability to obtain the optimum therapeutic effect, adjustment of the dose based on gender, weight, or age is not necessary.

In subjects with moderate hepatic impairment or mild to severe renal impairment, no relevant increases of rotigotine plasma levels were observed. Neupro was not investigated in patients with severe hepatic impairment.

Plasma levels of conjugates of rotigotine and its desalkyl metabolites increase with impaired renal function. However, a contribution of these metabolites to clinical effects is unlikely.

5.3 Preclinical safety data

In repeated dose and long-term toxicity studies, the major effects were associated with the dopamine agonist related pharmacodynamic effects and the consequent decrease of prolactin secretion.

After a single dose of rotigotine, binding to melanin-containing tissues (i.e., eyes) in the pigmented rat and monkey was evident, but was slowly cleared over the 14-day observation period.

Retinal degeneration was observed by transmission microscopy at a dose equivalent to 2.8 times the maximum recommended human dose on a mg/m^2 basis in a 3-month study in albino rats. The effects were more pronounced in female rats. Additional studies to further evaluate the specific pathology have not been performed. Retinal degeneration was not observed during the routine histopathological evaluation of the eyes in any of the toxicology studies in any species used. The relevance of these findings to humans is not known.

In a carcinogenicity study, male rats developed Leydig cell tumours and hyperplasia. Malignant tumours were noted predominantly in the uterus of mid- and high-dose females. These changes are well-known effects of dopamine agonists in rats after life-long therapy and assessed as not relevant to man.

The effects of rotigotine on reproduction have been investigated in rats, rabbits and mice. Rotigotine was not teratogenic in all three species, but was embryotoxic in rats and mice at materno-toxic doses. Rotigotine did not influence male fertility in rats, but clearly reduced female fertility in rats and mice, because of the effects on prolactin levels which are particularly significant in rodents.

Rotigotine did not induce gene mutations in the Ames test, but did show effects in the *in vitro* Mouse Lymphoma Assay with metabolic activation and weaker effects without metabolic activation. This mutagenic effect could be attributed to a clastogenic effect of rotigotine. This effect was not confirmed *in vivo* in the Mouse Micronucleus Test in the rat Unscheduled DNA Synthesis (UDS) test. Since it ran more or less parallel with a decreased relative total growth of the cells, it may be related to a cytotoxic effect of the compound. Therefore, the relevance of the one positive *in vitro* mutagenicity test is not known.

6. PHARMACEUTICAL PARTICULARS

6.1 List of excipients

Backing layer:

Polyester film, siliconized, aluminized,

colour coated with a pigment (titanium dioxide (E171), pigment yellow 95, pigment red 166) layer and imprinted (pigment red 144, pigment yellow 95, pigment black 7).

Self adhesive matrix layer:

Poly(dimethylsiloxane, trimethylsilyl silicate)-copolymerisate,

Povidone K90,

sodium metabisulphite (E223),

ascorbyl palmitate (E304) and

DL-α-tocopherol (E307).

Protective liner:

Transparent fluoropolymer coated polyester film.

6.2 Incompatibilities

Not applicable.

6.3 Shelf life

12 months.

6.4 Special precautions for storage

Store in a refrigerator (2°C – 8°C).

Store in the original package.

6.5 Nature and contents of container

Peel off sachet in a cardboard carton: One side is composed of an ethylene copolymer (innermost layer), an aluminium foil, low density polyethylene film and paper; the other side is composed of polyethylene (innermost layer), aluminium, ethylene copolymer and paper.

The carton contains 7, 20, 28, 30, 56, 60, 84, 90 or 100 transdermal patches, individually sealed in sachets.

The treatment initiation pack contains 28 transdermal patches in 4 cartons with 7 patches of 2 mg, 4 mg, 6 mg, and 8 mg each, individually sealed in sachets.

Not all pack sizes may be marketed.

6.6 Special precautions for disposal and other handling

After use the patch still contains active substance. After removal, the used patch should be folded in half, adhesive side inwards so that the matrix layer is not exposed, placed in the original sachet and then discarded out of the reach of children. Any used or unused patches should be disposed of in accordance with local requirements or returned to the pharmacy.

7. MARKETING AUTHORISATION HOLDER

SCHWARZ PHARMA Ltd.

Shannon, Industrial Estate,

Co. Clare, Ireland

8. MARKETING AUTHORISATION NUMBER(S)

Neupro 1 mg/24 h: EU/1/05/331/038 - 046

Neupro 2 mg/24 h: EU/1/05/331/001 - 003, EU/1/05/331/014 - 019

Neupro 3 mg/24 h: EU/1/05/331/047 - 055

Neupro 4 mg/24 h: EU/1/05/331/004 - 006, EU/1/05/331/020 - 025

Neupro 6 mg/24 h: EU/1/05/331/007 - 009, EU/1/05/331/026 - 031

Neupro 8 mg/24 h: EU/1/05/331/010 - 012, EU/1/05/331/032 - 037

Parkinson's disease Treatment Initiation Pack: EU/1/05/331/013

9. DATE OF FIRST AUTHORISATION/RENEWAL OF THE AUTHORISATION

15/02/2006

10. DATE OF REVISION OF THE TEXT

08/2009

NeuroBloc 5000 U/ml solution for injection

(Eisai Ltd)

1. NAME OF THE MEDICINAL PRODUCT

NeuroBloc 5000 U/ml solution for injection.

2. QUALITATIVE AND QUANTITATIVE COMPOSITION

One ml contains 5000 U Botulinum Toxin Type B.

NeuroBloc 5000U/ml contains less than 1 mmol sodium per ml.

For a full list of excipients, see section 6.1.

3. PHARMACEUTICAL FORM

Solution for injection.

Clear and colourless to light yellow solution.

4. CLINICAL PARTICULARS

4.1 Therapeutic indications

NeuroBloc is indicated for the treatment of cervical dystonia (torticollis).

See Section 5.1 for data on efficacy in patients responsive / resistant to Botulinum Toxin Type A.

4.2 Posology and method of administration

NeuroBloc should only be administered by intramuscular injection by a medical specialist with experience in the treatment of cervical dystonia and in the use of botulinum toxins.

The dosage units are specific to NeuroBloc and are not interchangeable with those used to quantify the dose of other botulinum toxin products.

The dose and frequency of administration should be adjusted for each patient depending on the clinical response. The initial dose is 10,000 U and should be divided between the two to four most affected muscles. Data from clinical trials suggest that efficacy is dose dependent but these trials, because they were not powered for a comparison, do not show a significant difference between 5000 U and 10,000 U. Therefore an initial dose of 5000 U may also be considered but a dose of 10,000 U may increase the likelihood of clinical benefit.

Care should be taken to ensure that NeuroBloc is not injected into a blood vessel.

NeuroBloc may be diluted with sodium chloride 9 mg/ml (0.9%) solution for injection.

Injections should be repeated as required to maintain good function and minimise pain. In long term clinical studies, the average dosing frequency was approximately every 12 weeks, however this may vary between subjects and a proportion of patients maintained a significant improvement relative to baseline for 16 weeks or longer. The dosing frequency should therefore be adapted based on the clinical assessment of an individual patient.

Adults (including the elderly ≥65 years old)

The dose recommended for cervical dystonia is applicable to adults of all ages, including the elderly.

For patients with reduced muscle mass the dose should be adjusted according to individual patient need.

Children and Adolescents

The safety and efficacy of NeuroBloc have not been demonstrated in children.

NeuroBloc is not recommended in children and adolescents until further data become available.

Hepatic and renal impairment

Studies have not been carried out in patients with hepatic or renal impairment. However, the pharmacological characteristics do not indicate any need to adjust the dose.

4.3 Contraindications

Hypersensitivity to the active substance or to any of the excipients.

Individuals with other known neuromuscular diseases (e.g. ALS or peripheral neuropathy) or known neuromuscular junctional disorders (e.g. myasthenia gravis or Lambert-Eaton syndrome) should not be given NeuroBloc.

4.4 Special warnings and precautions for use

NeuroBloc is recommended for intramuscular administration only. Particular caution should be paid to ensure that it is not injected into a blood vessel.

As with many biological/biotechnology proteins used as therapeutic agents, repeated administration of NeuroBloc may be associated with development of antibodies to Botulinum Toxin Type B in some patients. Immunogenicity data from three long term clinical studies indicate that approximately one third of patients develop antibodies, as determined by the mouse neutralisation / mouse protection assay dependent on duration of exposure (See Section 5.1).

An investigation into the consequence of seroconversion showed that the presence of antibodies was not synonymous with a loss of clinical response, and did not have an impact on the overall safety profile. However, the clinical relevance of the presence of antibodies as determined by the mouse neutralisation / mouse protection assay is uncertain.

As with all injected medicines, caution should be used in patients with bleeding disorders or receiving anticoagulant therapy.

Neuromuscular effects related to spread of toxin, distant from the site of administration have been reported (see section 4.8).

Patients treated with therapeutic doses may experience exaggerated muscle weakness.

There have been spontaneous reports of dysphagia, aspiration pneumonia and/or potentially fatal respiratory disease, after treatment with botulinum toxin type A/B.

Patients with underlying neuromuscular disorders including swallowing disorders are at increased risk of these undesirable effects. In patients with neuromuscular disorders or history of dysphagia and aspiration, botulinum toxins should be used under close medical supervision and only if the benefit clearly outweighs the risk.

Following NeuroBloc treatment, all patients and caregivers should be advised to seek medical attention for respiratory difficulties, choking or any new or worsening dysphagia.

Dysphagia has been reported following injection to sites other than the cervical musculature.

The initial starting dose of 10,000 U (or 5000 U) is relevant only to NeuroBloc (Botulinum Toxin Type B). These dosage units are specific to NeuroBloc only and are not relevant to preparations of Botulinum Toxin Type A. The unit dose recommendations for Botulinum Toxin Type A are significantly lower than those for NeuroBloc and administration of Botulinum Toxin Type A at the unit dose recommended for NeuroBloc may result in systemic toxicity and life-threatening clinical sequelae.

4.5 Interaction with other medicinal products and other forms of interaction

The effect of administering different botulinum neurotoxin serotypes concurrently is unknown. However, in clinical trials, NeuroBloc was administered 16 weeks after the injection of Botulinum Toxin Type A.

Co-administration of NeuroBloc and aminoglycosides or agents interfering with neuromuscular transmission (e.g. curare-like compounds) should be considered with caution.

4.6 Pregnancy and lactation

Animal studies are insufficient with respect to effects on pregnancy and embryonal/foetal development. The potential risk for humans is unknown. NeuroBloc should not be used during pregnancy unless clearly necessary.

It is unknown whether Botulinum Toxin Type B is excreted in human breast milk. The excretion of Botulinum Toxin Type B in milk has not been studied in animals. A decision on whether to continue/discontinue breast-feeding or to continue/discontinue therapy with NeuroBloc should be made taking into account the benefit of breast-feeding to the child and the benefit of NeuroBloc therapy to the women.

4.7 Effects on ability to drive and use machines

No studies on the effects on the ability to drive and use machines have been performed. However, the pharmacological characteristics do not indicate that they would be affected.

4.8 Undesirable effects

Undesirable effects, typically dry mouth, dysphagia and blurred vision, may occur following NeuroBloc injection. The two most commonly reported undesirable effects in clinical studies among patients with prior Botulinum Toxin Type A exposure were dry mouth and dysphagia, which were reported at a frequency of 41% and 29%, respectively. Data from clinical studies indicate that there is a tendency for the proportion of treatments associated with dysphagia to increase with higher doses injected into the sternocleidomastoid muscle. Injection site pain was also reported.

The two most commonly reported undesirable effects in a Phase IV comparative clinical study among toxin naïve patients treated with NeuroBloc 10,000 U to 15,000 U were dry mouth and dysphagia, which were reported at a frequency of 44% and 35%, respectively.

Adverse reactions seen in all trials are listed below according to MedDRA system organ class and in decreasing frequency which is defined as follows: Very Common (≥1/10); Common (≥1/100 to <1/10); Uncommon (≥1/1000 to <1/100).

Patients with Prior Botulinum Toxin Type A Exposure

System Organ Class	Very Common	Common
Nervous system disorders	dry mouth	torticollis (worsening from baseline), taste perversion
Respiratory thoracic and mediastinal disorders		voice alteration
Gastrointestinal disorders	dysphagia	dyspepsia
Musculoskeletal connective tissue and bone disorders		myasthenia
General disorders and administration site conditions	injection site pain	neck pain

Patients Naïve to Botulinum Toxins

System Organ Class	Very Common	Common
Nervous system disorders	dry mouth, headache	torticollis
Eye disorders:		blurred vision
Respiratory thoracic and mediastinal disorders		dysphonia
Gastrointestinal disorders	dysphagia	dyspepsia
General disorders and administration site conditions		injection site pain

In common with Botulinum Toxin Type A, electrophysiological jitter, which is not associated with clinical weakness or other electrophysiological abnormalities, may be experienced in some distant muscles.

Post marketing experience

Side effects related to spread of toxin distant from the site of administration have been reported (exaggerated muscle weakness, dysphagia, dyspnoea, aspiration pneumonia with fatal outcome in some cases) (see section 4.4).

The following effects have also been reported during post marketing use: abnormal accommodation, ptosis, vomiting, constipation, flu-like symptoms, and asthenia.

4.9 Overdose

Cases of overdose (some with signs of systemic toxicity) have been reported. In the event of an overdose, general medical supportive measures should be instituted. Doses of up to 15,000 U have infrequently resulted in clinically significant systemic toxicity in adults. However, in children (non-approved use) clinically significant systemic toxicity has occurred at doses approved for the treatment of adult patients. If botulism is clinically suspected, hospitalisation for the monitoring of respiratory function (incipient respiratory failure) may be required.

In the event of an overdose or injection into a muscle that normally compensates for the cervical dystonia, it is conceivable that the dystonia may worsen. As with other botulinum toxins spontaneous recovery will occur over a period of time.

5. PHARMACOLOGICAL PROPERTIES

5.1 Pharmacodynamic properties

Pharmacotherapeutic group: muscle relaxant, peripherally acting agent, ATC code: M03A X 01

NeuroBloc is a neuromuscular blocking agent. The mechanism of action of NeuroBloc in blocking neuromuscular conduction occurs by a three-step process:

1. Extracellular binding of the toxin to specific acceptors on motor nerve terminals

2. Internalisation and release of the toxin into the cytosol of the nerve terminals

3. Inhibition of acetylcholine release from nerve terminals at the neuromuscular junction

When injected directly into a muscle, NeuroBloc causes a localised paralysis that gradually reverses over time. The mechanism by which muscle paralysis is reversed over time remains unknown, but may be associated with the intraneuronal turnover of the affected protein and/or sprouting of the nerve ending.

A series of clinical studies have been conducted to evaluate the efficacy and safety of NeuroBloc in the treatment of cervical dystonia. These studies have demonstrated the activity of NeuroBloc in both treatment-naïve patients, and patients who have previously received treatment with Botulinum Toxin Type A, including those that were considered clinically resistant to Botulinum Toxin Type A.

Two Phase III randomised, multicentre, double-blind, placebo-controlled studies were conducted in patients with cervical dystonia. Both studies enrolled adult patients (≥ 18 years) who had a history of receiving Botulinum Toxin Type A. The first study enrolled patients who were clinically resistant to type A toxin **(A-non responders)**, confirmed by a Frontalis Type A test. The second study enrolled patients who continued to respond to type A toxin **(A-responders)**. In the first study, type A resistant patients **(A-non responders)** were randomised to receive placebo or 10,000 U of NeuroBloc and in the second, type A toxin responsive patients **(A-responders)** were randomised to receive placebo, 5000 U or 10,000 U of toxin. Study drug was injected on a single occasion into 2 to 4 of the following muscles: splenius capitus, sternocleidomastoid, levator scapulae, trapezius, semispinalis capitus and scalene. The total dose was divided between the selected muscles and 1 to 5 injections per muscle were administered. There were 77 subjects enrolled into the first study and 109 into the second. Patient evaluations continued for 16 weeks post injection.

The primary efficacy outcome variable for both studies was the Toronto Western Spasmodic Torticollis Rating Scale TWSTRS-Total score (range of possible scores is 0-87) at Week 4. The secondary endpoints included Visual Analogue Scales (VAS) to quantify the Patient Global Assessment of change and the Physician Global Assessment of change, both from baseline to Week 4. On these scales, scores of 50 indicate no change, 0 much worse, and 100 much better. Results of comparisons of the primary and secondary efficacy variables are summarised in Table 1. Analysis of the TWSTRS sub scales revealed significant effects on the severity of cervical dystonia and its associated pain and disability.

(see Table 1 below)

A further randomised, multicentre, double-blind study was conducted to compare the efficacy of NeuroBloc (10,000 U) to Botulinum Toxin Type A (150 U) in patients with cervical dystonia who have never previously received a botulinum toxin product. The primary efficacy assessment was the TWSTRS Total score, and secondary efficacy assessments included VAS assessment of change evaluated by patient and investigator, conducted at 4, 8 and 12 weeks after treatment. The study met the pre-defined criteria for non-inferiority of NeuroBloc compared to Botulinum Toxin Type A, both in terms of mean TWSTRS total score at week 4 after first and second treatment sessions, and in terms of duration of effect.

The non-inferiority of NeuroBloc compared to Botulinum Toxin Type A was further supported by a responder analysis where similar percentages of subjects showed improvement in the TWSTRS score at Week 4 of Session 1 (86% NeuroBloc and 85% Botox), and a similar proportion of subjects experienced at least a 20% decrease from baseline in the TWSTRS score at Week 4 of Session 1 (51% NeuroBloc, 47% Botox).

Further clinical studies and open label follow-up have shown that subjects can continue to respond to NeuroBloc for prolonged periods of time, with some subjects receiving more than 14 treatment sessions over a period of more than 3.5 years. In addition to improved function as demonstrated by a reduction in TWSTRS-total score, treatment with NeuroBloc was associated with a significant reduction in TWSTRS-Pain and pain VAS scores at each treatment session at weeks 4, 8 and 12 relative to baseline. In these studies, the average dosing frequency was approximately every 12 weeks.

The immunogenicity of NeuroBloc has been evaluated in two clinical studies and an open-label extension study. The presence of antibodies in these studies was assessed using the mouse protection assay (also known as the Mouse Neutralization Assay, MNA).

Immunogenicity data from three long term clinical studies indicate that approximately one third of patients develop antibodies, as determined by the mouse neutralisation / mouse protection assay dependent on duration of exposure. Specifically, these studies showed approximately 19-25% seroconverted within 18 months of initiation of treatment, increasing to approximately 33-44% with up to 45 months of treatment. An investigation into the consequence of seroconversion showed that the presence of antibodies was not synonymous with a loss of clinical response, and did not have an impact on the overall safety profile. However, the clinical relevance of the presence of antibodies as determined by the mouse neutralisation / mouse protection assay is uncertain.

The extent and time course of seroconversion were similar in patients with prior toxin A exposure and those who were toxin A naïve, and between toxin A resistant and toxin A responsive patients.

5.2 Pharmacokinetic properties

NeuroBloc injected intramuscularly produces localised muscle weakness by chemical denervation. Following local intramuscular injection of NeuroBloc serious adverse events that may have been due to systemic effects of Botulinum Toxin Type B, were observed in 12% of adverse drug reaction cases reported during the post-marketing experience (including the following adverse events: dry mouth, dysphagia and blurred vision). However, no pharmacokinetic or Absorption, Distribution, Metabolism and Excretion (ADME) studies have been performed.

5.3 Preclinical safety data

Single dose pharmacology studies in cynomolgus monkeys have shown no effects other than the anticipated dose-dependent paralysis of injected muscles, together with some diffusion of toxin at high doses producing similar effects in neighbouring non-injected muscles.

Table 1: Efficacy Results from Phase III NeuroBloc Studies

	STUDY 1 (A-Resistant Patients)		STUDY 2 (A-Responsive Patients)		
Assessments	**Placebo**	**10,000 U**	**Placebo**	**5000 U**	**10,000 U**
	n = 38	n = 39	n = 36	n = 36	n = 37
TWSTRS-TOTAL					
Mean At Baseline	51.2	52.8	43.6	46.4	46.9
Mean at Week 4	49.2	41.8	39.3	37.1	35.2
Change from Baseline	-2.0	-11.1	-4.3	-9.3	-11.7
P-Value*		0.0001		0.0115	0.0004
Patient Global					
Mean at Week 4	39.5	60.2	43.6	60.6	64.6
P-Value*		0.0001		0.0010	0.0001
Physician Global					
Mean at Week 4	47.9	60.6	52.0	65.3	64.2
P-Value*		0.0001		0.0011	0.0038

* Analysis of covariance, two-tailed tests, $\alpha = 0.05$

Single dose intramuscular toxicology studies have been performed in cynomolgus monkeys. The systemic No Observed Effect Level (NOEL) was shown to be approximately 960 U/kg. The dose resulting in death was 2400 U/kg.

Because of the nature of the product, no animal studies have been carried out to establish the carcinogenic effects of NeuroBloc. Standard tests to investigate the mutagenicity of NeuroBloc have not been performed.

Development studies in rats and rabbits have shown no evidence of foetal malformations or changes to fertility. In the development studies, the No Observed Adverse Effect Dose Level (NOAEL) in rats was 1000 U/kg/day for maternal effects and 3000 U/kg/day for foetal effects. In rabbits, the NOAEL was 0.1 U/kg/day for maternal effects and 0.3 U/kg/day for foetal effects. In the fertility studies the NOAEL was 300 U/kg/day for general toxicity in both males and females and 1000 U/kg/day for fertility and reproductive performance.

6. PHARMACEUTICAL PARTICULARS

6.1 List of excipients

Disodium succinate

Sodium chloride

Human serum albumin (containing sodium caprylate andsodium acetyltryptophanate as excipients)

Hydrochloric acid for pH adjustment

Water for injections

6.2 Incompatibilities

In the absence of incompatibility studies, NeuroBloc must not be mixed with other medicinal products.

6.3 Shelf life

3 years.

From a microbiological point of view, unless the method of opening/dilution precludes the risk of microbial contamination the product should be used immediately.

6.4 Special precautions for storage

Store in a refrigerator (2°C - 8°C). Do not freeze.

Keep the container in the outer carton in order to protect from light.

Within its shelf-life, the product may be stored below 25°C for up to 3 months, without being refrigerated again during this period, and must be withdrawn if not used after this.

6.5 Nature and contents of container

NeuroBloc is supplied in 3.5 ml Type I glass vials, with siliconised grey butyl rubber stoppers oversealed by aluminium crimped caps.

Carton containing a single vial containing 0.5 ml, 1.0 ml or 2.0 ml of solution.

6.6 Special precautions for disposal and other handling

NeuroBloc is provided as a clear and colourless to light yellow sterile injectable solution in vials for single use only. Any unused solution should be discarded (see instructions below). Vials should be visually inspected prior to use. If the NeuroBloc solution is not clear and colourless/light yellow or if the vial appears damaged the product should be discarded as Medical Biohazardous Waste in accordance with local requirements.

The solution in the vials is ready for use.

NeuroBloc may be diluted with sodium chloride 9 mg/ml (0.9%) solution for injection.

Do not shake.

Decontaminate any spill with 10% caustic solution, or sodium hypochlorite (household chlorine bleach – 2 ml (0.5%): 1 litre water) solution. Wear waterproof gloves and soak up the liquid with an appropriate absorbent. Place the absorbed toxin in an autoclave bag, seal it and process as Medical Biohazardous Waste in accordance with local requirements.

7. MARKETING AUTHORISATION HOLDER

Eisai Limited

European Knowledge Centre

Mosquito Way

Hatfield

Hertfordshire

AL10 9SN

United Kingdom

8. MARKETING AUTHORISATION NUMBER(S)

EU/1/00/166/001 – 2500 U

EU/1/00/166/002 – 5000 U

EU/1/00/166/003 – 10,000 U

9. DATE OF FIRST AUTHORISATION/RENEWAL OF THE AUTHORISATION

Date of first authorisation: 22 January 2001

Date of latest renewal: 22 January 2006

10. DATE OF REVISION OF THE TEXT

27 July 2009

Detailed information on this medicinal product is available on the website of the European Medicines Agency (EMEA) http://www.emea.europa.eu/

11. LEGAL CATEGORY

POM – medicinal product subject to medical prescription

Neurontin Capsules and Tablets

(Pfizer Limited)

1. NAME OF THE MEDICINAL PRODUCT

Neurontin 100mg Hard Capsules

Neurontin 300mg Hard Capsules

Neurontin 400mg Hard Capsules

Neurontin 600mg Film-coated Tablets

Neurontin 800mg Film-coated Tablets

2. QUALITATIVE AND QUANTITATIVE COMPOSITION

Each 100 mg hard capsule contains 100 mg gabapentin.

Each 300mg hard capsule contains 300 mg gabapentin.

Each 400mg hard capsule contains 400 mg gabapentin.

Each 600 mg film-coated tablet contains 600 mg gabapentin.

Each 800 mg film-coated tablet contains 800 mg gabapentin.

Excipients:

Each 100 mg hard capsule contains 13 mg lactose (as monohydrate).

Each 300 mg hard capsule contains 41 mg lactose (as monohydrate).

Each 400 mg hard capsule contains 54 mg lactose (as monohydrate).

For a full list of excipients, see section 6.1.

3. PHARMACEUTICAL FORM

Neurontin Hard Capsules

Capsule, hard

Neurontin 100 mg Hard Capsules: A two-piece, white opaque hard capsule, imprinted with 'Neurontin 100 mg' and 'PD' and containing a white to off-white powder.

Neurontin 300 mg Hard Capsules: A two-piece, yellow opaque hard capsule, imprinted with 'Neurontin 300 mg' and 'PD' and containing a white to off-white powder.

Neurontin 400 mg Hard Capsules: A two-piece, orange opaque hard gelatin capsule, imprinted with 'Neurontin 400 mg' and 'PD' and containing a white to off-white powder.

Neurontin Film-Coated Tablets

Neurontin 600 mg Film-coated Tablets: White, elliptical film-coated tablets with a bisecting score on both sides and debossed with "NT" and "16" on one side.

Neurontin 800 mg Film-coated Tablets: White, elliptical film-coated tablets with a bisecting score on both sides and debossed with "NT" and "26" on one side.

The tablet can be divided into equal halves.

4. CLINICAL PARTICULARS

4.1 Therapeutic indications

Epilepsy

Gabapentin is indicated as adjunctive therapy in the treatment of partial seizures with and without secondary generalization in adults and children aged 6 years and above (see section 5.1).

Gabapentin is indicated as monotherapy in the treatment of partial seizures with and without secondary generalization in adults and adolescents aged 12 years and above.

Treatment of peripheral neuropathic pain

Gabapentin is indicated for the treatment of peripheral neuropathic pain such as painful diabetic neuropathy and post-herpetic neuralgia in adults.

4.2 Posology and method of administration

For oral use.

Gabapentin can be given with or without food and should be swallowed whole with sufficient fluid-intake (e.g. a glass of water).

For all indications a titration scheme for the initiation of therapy is described in Table 1, which is recommended for adults and adolescents aged 12 years and above. Dosing instructions for children under 12 years of age are provided under a separate sub-heading later in this section.

Table 1

DOSING CHART – INITIAL TITRATION		
Day 1	Day 2	Day 3
300 mg once a day	300 mg two times a day	300 mg three times a day

Discontinuation of gabapentin

In accordance with current clinical practice, if gabapentin has to be discontinued it is recommended this should be done gradually over a minimum of 1 week independent of the indication.

Epilepsy

Epilepsy typically requires long-term therapy. Dosage is determined by the treating physician according to individual tolerance and efficacy.

Adults and adolescents:

In clinical trials, the effective dosing range was 900 to 3600 mg/day. Therapy may be initiated by titrating the dose as described in Table 1 or by administering 300 mg three times a day (TID) on Day 1. Thereafter, based on individual patient response and tolerability, the dose can be further increased in 300 mg/day increments every 2-3 days up to a maximum dose of 3600 mg/day. Slower titration of gabapentin dosage may be appropriate for individual patients. The minimum time to reach a dose of 1800 mg/day is one week, to reach 2400 mg/day is a total of 2 weeks, and to reach 3600 mg/day is a total of 3 weeks. Dosages up to 4800 mg/day have been well tolerated in long-term open-label clinical studies. The total daily dose should be divided in three single doses, the maximum time interval between the doses should not exceed 12 hours to prevent breakthrough convulsions.

Children aged 6 years and above:

The starting dose should range from 10 to 15 mg/kg/day and the effective dose is reached by upward titration over a period of approximately three days. The effective dose of gabapentin in children aged 6 years and older is 25 to 35 mg/kg/day. Dosages up to 50 mg/kg/day have been well tolerated in a long-term clinical study. The total daily dose should be divided in three single doses, the maximum time interval between doses should not exceed 12 hours.

It is not necessary to monitor gabapentin plasma concentrations to optimize gabapentin therapy. Further, gabapentin may be used in combination with other antiepileptic medicinal products without concern for alteration of the plasma concentrations of gabapentin or serum concentrations of other antiepileptic medicinal products.

Peripheral neuropathic pain

Adults

The therapy may be initiated by titrating the dose as described in Table 1. Alternatively, the starting dose is 900 mg/day given as three equally divided doses. Thereafter, based on individual patient response and tolerability, the dose can be further increased in 300 mg/day increments every 2-3 days up to a maximum dose of 3600 mg/day. Slower titration of gabapentin dosage may be appropriate for individual patients. The minimum time to reach a dose of 1800 mg/day is one week, to reach 2400 mg/day is a total of 2 weeks, and to reach 3600 mg/day is a total of 3 weeks.

In the treatment of peripheral neuropathic pain such as painful diabetic neuropathy and post-herpetic neuralgia, efficacy and safety have not been examined in clinical studies for treatment periods longer than 5 months. If a patient requires dosing longer than 5 months for the treatment of peripheral neuropathic pain, the treating physician should assess the patient's clinical status and determine the need for additional therapy.

Instruction for all areas of indication

In patients with poor general health, i.e., low body weight, after organ transplantation etc., the dose should be titrated more slowly, either by using smaller dosage strengths or longer intervals between dosage increases.

Use in elderly patients (over 65 years of age)

Elderly patients may require dosage adjustment because of declining renal function with age (see Table 2). Somnolence, peripheral oedema and asthenia may be more frequent in elderly patients.

Use in patients with renal impairment

Dosage adjustment is recommended in patients with compromised renal function as described in Table 2 and/or those undergoing haemodialysis. Gabapentin 100 mg capsules can be used to follow dosing recommendations for patients with renal insufficiency.

Table 2

DOSAGE OF GABAPENTIN IN ADULTS BASED ON RENAL FUNCTION	
Creatinine Clearance (ml/min)	Total Daily Dose[a] (mg/day)
≥80	900-3600
50-79	600-1800
30-49	300-900
15-29	150[b]-600
<15[c]	150[b]-300

a Total daily dose should be administered as three divided doses. Reduced dosages are for patients with renal impairment (creatinine clearance < 79 ml/min).

b To be administered as 300 mg every other day.

c For patients with creatinine clearance <15 ml/min, the daily dose should be reduced in proportion to creatinine clearance (e.g., patients with a creatinine clearance of 7.5 ml/min should receive one-half the daily dose that patients with a creatinine clearance of 15 ml/min receive).

Use in patients undergoing haemodialysis

For anuric patients undergoing haemodialysis who have never received gabapentin, a loading dose of 300 to 400 mg, then 200 to 300 mg of gabapentin following each 4 hours of haemodialysis, is recommended. On dialysis-free days, there should be no treatment with gabapentin.

For renally impaired patients undergoing haemodialysis, the maintenance dose of gabapentin should be based on the dosing recommendations found in Table 2. In addition to the maintenance dose, an additional 200 to 300 mg dose following each 4-hour haemodialysis treatment is recommended.

4.3 Contraindications

Hypersensitivity to the active substance or to any of the excipients.

4.4 Special warnings and precautions for use

Suicidal ideation and behaviour have been reported in patients treated with anti-epileptic agents in several indications. A meta-analysis of randomised placebo controlled trials of anti-epileptic drugs has also shown a small increased risk of suicidal ideation and behaviour. The mechanism of this risk is not known and the available data do not exclude the possibility of an increased risk for gabapentin.

Therefore patients should be monitored for signs of suicidal ideation and behaviours and appropriate treatment should be considered. Patients (and caregivers of patients) should be advised to seek medical advice should signs of suicidal ideation or behaviour emerge.

If a patient develops acute pancreatitis under treatment with gabapentin, discontinuation of gabapentin should be considered (see section 4.8).

Although there is no evidence of rebound seizures with gabapentin, abrupt withdrawal of anticonvulsant agents in epileptic patients may precipitate status epilepticus (see section 4.2).

As with other antiepileptic medicinal products, some patients may experience an increase in seizure frequency or the onset of new types of seizures with gabapentin.

As with other anti-epileptics, attempts to withdraw concomitant anti-epileptics in treatment refractive patients on more than one anti-epileptic, in order to reach gabapentin monotherapy have a low success rate.

Gabapentin is not considered effective against primary generalized seizures such as absences and may aggravate these seizures in some patients. Therefore, gabapentin should be used with caution in patients with mixed seizures including absences.

No systematic studies in patients 65 years or older have been conducted with gabapentin. In one double blind study in patients with neuropathic pain, somnolence, peripheral oedema and asthenia occurred in a somewhat higher percentage in patients aged 65 years or above, than in younger patients. Apart from these findings, clinical investigations in this age group do not indicate an adverse event profile different from that observed in younger patients.

The effects of long-term (greater than 36 weeks) gabapentin therapy on learning, intelligence, and development in children and adolescents have not been adequately studied. The benefits of prolonged therapy must therefore be weighed against the potential risks of such therapy.

Laboratory tests

False positive readings may be obtained in the semi-quantitative determination of total urine protein by dipstick tests. It is therefore recommended to verify such a positive dipstick test result by methods based on a different analytical principle such as the Biuret method, turbidimetric or dye-binding methods, or to use these alternative methods from the beginning.

Neurontin hard capsules contain lactose. Patients with rare hereditary problems of galactose intolerance, the Lapp lactase deficiency or glucose-galactose malabsorption should not take Neurontin Capsules.

4.5 Interaction with other medicinal products and other forms of interaction

In a study involving healthy volunteers (N=12), when a 60-mg controlled-release morphine capsule was administered 2 hours prior to a 600-mg gabapentin capsule, mean gabapentin AUC increased by 44% compared to gabapentin administered without morphine. Therefore, patients should be carefully observed for signs of CNS depression, such as somnolence, and the dose of gabapentin or morphine should be reduced appropriately.

No interaction between gabapentin and phenobarbital, phenytoin, valproic acid, or carbamazepine has been observed.

Gabapentin steady-state pharmacokinetics are similar for healthy subjects and patients with epilepsy receiving these anti-epileptic agents.

Coadministration of gabapentin with oral contraceptives containing norethindrone and/or ethinyl estradiol, does not influence the steady-state pharmacokinetics of either component.

Coadministration of gabapentin with antacids containing aluminium and magnesium, reduces gabapentin bioavailability up to 24%. It is recommended that gabapentin be taken at the earliest two hours following antacid administration.

Renal excretion of gabapentin is unaltered by probenecid.

A slight decrease in renal excretion of gabapentin that is observed when it is coadministered with cimetidine is not expected to be of clinical importance.

4.6 Pregnancy and lactation

Risk related to epilepsy and antiepileptic medicinal products in general

The risk of birth defects is increased by a factor of 2 – 3 in the offspring of mothers treated with an antiepileptic medicinal product. Most frequently reported are cleft lip, cardiovascular malformations and neural tube defects. Multiple antiepileptic drug therapy may be associated with a higher risk of congenital malformations than monotherapy, therefore it is important that monotherapy is practised whenever possible. Specialist advice should be given to women who are likely to become pregnant or who are of childbearing potential and the need for antiepileptic treatment should be reviewed when a woman is planning to become pregnant. No sudden discontinuation of antiepileptic therapy should be undertaken as this may lead to breakthrough seizures, which could have serious consequences for both mother and child. Developmental delay in children of mothers with epilepsy has been observed rarely. It is not possible to differentiate if the developmental delay is caused by genetic, social factors, maternal epilepsy or the antiepileptic therapy.

Risk related to gabapentin

There are no adequate data from the use of gabapentin in pregnant women.

Studies in animals have shown reproductive toxicity (see section 5.3). The potential risk for humans is unknown. Gabapentin should not be used during pregnancy unless the potential benefit to the mother clearly outweighs the potential risk to the foetus.

No definite conclusion can be made as to whether gabapentin is associated with an increased risk of congenital malformations when taken during pregnancy, because of epilepsy itself and the presence of concomitant antiepileptic medicinal products during each reported pregnancy.

Gabapentin is excreted in human milk. Because the effect on the breast-fed infant is unknown, caution should be exercised when gabapentin is administered to a breast-feeding mother. Gabapentin should be used in breast-feeding mothers only if the benefits clearly outweigh the risks.

4.7 Effects on ability to drive and use machines

Gabapentin may have minor or moderate influence on the ability to drive and use machines. Gabapentin acts on the central nervous system and may cause drowsiness, dizziness or other related symptoms. Even, if they were only of mild or moderate degree, these undesirable effects could be potentially dangerous in patients driving or operating machinery. This is especially true at the beginning of the treatment and after increase in dose.

4.8 Undesirable effects

The adverse reactions observed during clinical studies conducted in epilepsy (adjunctive and monotherapy) and neuropathic pain have been provided in a single list below by class and frequency (very common ($\geq$ 1/10); common ($\geq$ 1/100 to $<$ 1/10); uncommon ($\geq$ 1/1000 to $<$ 1/100); rare ($\geq$ 1/10000 to $<$ 1/1000); very rare ($<$ 1/10000). Where an adverse reaction was seen at different frequencies in clinical studies, it was assigned to the highest frequency reported.

Additional reactions reported from post-marketing experience are included as frequency Not known (cannot be estimated from the available data) in italics in the list below.

Within each frequency grouping, undesirable effects are presented in order of decreasing seriousness.

Body System	**Adverse drug reactions**
Infections and infestations	
Very Common	Viral infection
Common	Pneumonia, respiratory infection, urinary tract infection, infection, otitis media
Blood and the lymphatic system disorders	
Common	leucopenia
Not known	*thrombocytopenia*
Immune system disorders	
Uncommon	allergic reactions (e.g. urticaria)
Metabolism and Nutrition Disorders	
Common	anorexia, increased appetite
Psychiatric disorders	
Common	hostility, confusion and emotional lability, depression, anxiety, nervousness, thinking abnormal
Not known	*hallucinations*
Nervous system disorders	
Very Common	somnolence, dizziness, ataxia
Common	convulsions, hyperkinesias, dysarthria, amnesia, tremor, insomnia, headache, sensations such as paresthesia, hypaesthesia, coordination abnormal, nystagmus, increased, decreased, or absent reflexes
Uncommon	hypokinesia
Not known	*other movement disorders (e.g. choreoathetosis, dyskinesia, dystonia)*
Eye disorders	
Common	visual disturbances such as amblyopia, diplopia
Ear and Labyrinth disorders	
Common	vertigo
Not known	*tinnitus*
Cardiac disorders	
Uncommon	palpitations
Vascular disorders	
Common	hypertension, vasodilatation
Respiratory, thoracic and mediastinal disorders	
Common	dyspnoea, bronchitis, pharyngitis, cough, rhinitis
Gastrointestinal disorders	
Common	vomiting, nausea, dental abnormalities, gingivitis, diarrhea, abdominal pain, dyspepsia, constipation, dry mouth or throat, flatulence
Not known	*pancreatitis*
Hepatobiliary disorders	
Not known	*hepatitis, jaundice*
Skin and subcutaneous tissue disorders	
Common	facial oedema, purpura most often described as bruises resulting from physical trauma, rash, pruritus, acne
Not known	*Stevens-Johnson syndrome, angioedema, erythema multiforme, alopecia*
Musculoskeletal, connective tissue and bone disorders	
Common	arthralgia, myalgia, back pain, twitching
Not known	*myoclonus*
Renal and urinary disorder	
Not known	*acute renal failure, incontinence*
Reproductive system and breast disorders	
Common	impotence
Not known	*breast hypertrophy, gynaecomastia*
General disorders and administration site conditions	
Very Common	fatigue, fever
Common	peripheral oedema, abnormal gait, asthenia, pain, malaise, flu syndrome
Uncommon Not known	generalized oedema *withdrawal reactions (mostly anxiety, insomnia, nausea, pains, sweating), chest pain. Sudden unexplained deaths have been reported where a causal relationship to treatment with gabapentin has not been established.*
Investigations	
Common Uncommon	WBC (white blood cell count) decreased, weight gain elevated liver function tests SGOT (AST), SGPT (ALT) and bilirubin
Not known	*blood glucose fluctuations in patients with diabetes*
Injury and poisoning	
Common	accidental injury, fracture, abrasion

Under treatment with gabapentin cases of acute pancreatitis were reported. Causality with gabapentin is unclear (see section 4.4).

In patients on haemodialysis due to end-stage renal failure, myopathy with elevated creatine kinase levels has been reported.

Respiratory tract infections, otitis media, convulsions and bronchitis were reported only in clinical studies in children. Additionally, in clinical studies in children, aggressive behaviour and hyperkinesias were reported commonly.

4.9 Overdose

Acute, life-threatening toxicity has not been observed with gabapentin overdoses of up to 49 grams. Symptoms of the overdoses included dizziness, double vision, slurred speech, drowsiness, lethargy and mild diarrhoea. All patients recovered fully with supportive care. Reduced absorption of gabapentin at higher doses may limit drug absorption at the time of overdosing and, hence, minimise toxicity from overdoses.

Overdoses of gabapentin, particularly in combination with other CNS depressant medications, may result in coma.

Although gabapentin can be removed by haemodialysis, based on prior experience it is not usually required. However, in patients with severe renal impairment, haemodialysis may be indicated.

An oral lethal dose of gabapentin was not identified in mice and rats given doses as high as 8000 mg/kg. Signs of acute toxicity in animals included ataxia, laboured breathing, ptosis, hypoactivity, or excitation.

5. PHARMACOLOGICAL PROPERTIES

5.1 Pharmacodynamic properties

Pharmacotherapeutic groups: Other antiepileptics ATC code: N03AX12

The precise mechanism of action of gabapentin is not known.

Gabapentin is structurally related to the neurotransmitter GABA (gamma-aminobutyric acid) but its mechanism of action is different from that of several other active substances that interact with GABA synapses including valproate, barbiturates, benzodiazepines, GABA transaminase inhibitors, GABA uptake inhibitors, GABA agonists, and GABA prodrugs. *In vitro* studies with radiolabeled gabapentin have characterized a novel peptide binding site in rat brain tissues including neocortex and hippocampus that may relate to anticonvulsant and analgesic activity of gabapentin and its structural derivatives.

The binding site for gabapentin has been identified as the $alpha_2$-delta subunit of voltage-gated calcium channels.

Gabapentin at relevant clinical concentrations does not bind to other common drug or neurotransmitter receptors of the brain including $GABA_A$, $GABA_B$, benzodiazepine, glutamate, glycine or N-methyl-d-aspartate receptors.

Gabapentin does not interact with sodium channels *in vitro* and so differs from phenytoin and carbamazepine. Gabapentin partially reduces responses to the glutamate agonist N-methyl-D-aspartate (NMDA) in some test systems *in vitro*, but only at concentrations greater than 100 µM, which are not achieved *in vivo*. Gabapentin slightly reduces the release of monoamine neurotransmitters in vitro. Gabapentin administration to rats increases GABA turnover in several brain regions in a manner similar to valproate sodium, although in different regions of brain. The relevance of these various actions of gabapentin to the anticonvulsant effects remains to be established. In animals, gabapentin readily enters the brain and prevents seizures from maximal electroshock, from chemical convulsants including inhibitors of GABA synthesis, and in genetic models of seizures.

A clinical trial of adjunctive treatment of partial seizures in paediatric subjects ranging in age from 3 to 12 years, showed a numerical but not statistically significant difference in the 50% responder rate in favour of the gabapentin group compared to placebo. Additional post-hoc analyses of the responder rates by age did not reveal a statistically significant effect of age, either as a continuous or dichotomous variable (age groups 3-5 and 6-12 years).

The data from this additional post-hoc analysis are summarised in the table below:

(see Table 2a below)

5.2 Pharmacokinetic properties

Absorption

Following oral administration, peak plasma gabapentin concentrations are observed within 2 to 3 hours. Gabapentin bioavailability (fraction of dose absorbed) tends to decrease with increasing dose. Absolute bioavailability of a 300 mg capsule is approximately 60%. Food, including a high-fat diet, has no clinically significant effect on gabapentin pharmacokinetics.

Gabapentin pharmacokinetics are not affected by repeated administration. Although plasma gabapentin concentrations were generally between 2 µg/ml and

Table 3 Summary of gabapentin mean (%CV) steady-state pharmacokinetic parameters following every eight hours administration

Pharmacokinetic parameter	300 mg (N = 7)		400 mg (N = 14)		800 mg (N=14)	
	Mean	%CV	Mean	%CV	Mean	%CV
C_{max} (µg/ml)	4.02	(24)	5.74	(38)	8.71	(29)
t_{max} (hr)	2.7	(18)	2.1	(54)	1.6	(76)
T1/2 (hr)	5.2	(12)	10.8	(89)	10.6	(41)
AUC (0-8) µg•hr/ml)	24.8	(24)	34.5	(34)	51.4	(27)
Ae% (%)	NA	NA	47.2	(25)	34.4	(37)

C_{max} = Maximum steady state plasma concentration

t_{max} = Time for C_{max}

T1/2 = Elimination half-life

AUC(0-8) = Steady state area under plasma concentration-time curve from time 0 to 8 hours postdose

Ae% = Percent of dose excreted unchanged into the urine from time 0 to 8 hours postdose

NA = Not available

20 µg/ml in clinical studies, such concentrations were not predictive of safety or efficacy. Pharmacokinetic parameters are given in Table 3.

Table 3

Summary of gabapentin mean (%CV) steady-state pharmacokinetic parameters following every eight hours administration

(see Table 3 above)

Distribution

Gabapentin is not bound to plasma proteins and has a volume of distribution equal to 57.7 litres. In patients with epilepsy, gabapentin concentrations in cerebrospinal fluid (CSF) are approximately 20% of corresponding steady-state trough plasma concentrations. Gabapentin is present in the breast milk of breast-feeding women.

Metabolism

There is no evidence of gabapentin metabolism in humans. Gabapentin does not induce hepatic mixed function oxidase enzymes responsible for drug metabolism.

Elimination

Gabapentin is eliminated unchanged solely by renal excretion. The elimination half-life of gabapentin is independent of dose and averages 5 to 7 hours.

In elderly patients, and in patients with impaired renal function, gabapentin plasma clearance is reduced. Gabapentin elimination-rate constant, plasma clearance, and renal clearance are directly proportional to creatinine clearance.

Gabapentin is removed from plasma by haemodialysis. Dosage adjustment in patients with compromised renal function or undergoing haemodialysis is recommended (see section 4.2).

Gabapentin pharmacokinetics in children were determined in 50 healthy subjects between the ages of 1 month and 12 years. In general, plasma gabapentin concentrations in children > 5 years of age are similar to those in adults when dosed on a mg/kg basis.

Linearity/Non-linearity

Gabapentin bioavailability (fraction of dose absorbed) decreases with increasing dose which imparts non-linearity to pharmacokinetic parameters which include the bioavailability parameter (F) e.g. Ae%, CL/F, Vd/F. Elimination pharmacokinetics (pharmacokinetic parameters which do not include F such as CLr and T1/2), are best described by linear pharmacokinetics. Steady state plasma gabapentin concentrations are predictable from single-dose data.

5.3 Preclinical safety data

Carcinogenesis

Gabapentin was given in the diet to mice at 200, 600, and 2000 mg/kg/day and to rats at 250, 1000, and 2000 mg/kg/day for two years. A statistically significant increase in the incidence of pancreatic acinar cell tumours was found only in male rats at the highest dose. Peak plasma drug concentrations in rats at 2000 mg/kg are 10 times higher than plasma concentrations in humans given 3600 mg/day. The pancreatic acinar cell tumours in male rats are low-grade malignancies, did not affect survival, did not metastasize or invade surrounding tissue, and were similar to those seen

Table 2a

Response (≥ 50% Improved) by Treatment and Age MITT* Population			
Age Category	Placebo	Gabapentin	P-Value
< 6 Years Old	4/21 (19.0%)	4/17 (23.5%)	0.7362
6 to 12 Years Old	17/99 (17.2%)	20/96 (20.8%)	0.5144

*The modified intent to treat population was defined as all patients randomised to study medication who also had evaluable seizure diaries available for 28 days during both the baseline and double-blind phases.

in concurrent controls. The relevance of these pancreatic acinar cell tumours in male rats to carcinogenic risk in humans is unclear.

Mutagenesis

Gabapentin demonstrated no genotoxic potential. It was not mutagenic *in vitro* in standard assays using bacterial or mammalian cells. Gabapentin did not induce structural chromosome aberrations in mammalian cells *in vitro* or *in vivo*, and did not induce micronucleus formation in the bone marrow of hamsters.

Impairment of Fertility

No adverse effects on fertility or reproduction were observed in rats at doses up to 2000 mg/kg (approximately five times the maximum daily human dose on a mg/m2 of body surface area basis).

Teratogenesis

Gabapentin did not increase the incidence of malformations, compared to controls, in the offspring of mice, rats, or rabbits at doses up to 50, 30 and 25 times respectively, the daily human dose of 3600 mg, (four, five or eight times, respectively, the human daily dose on a mg/m2 basis).

Gabapentin induced delayed ossification in the skull, vertebrae, forelimbs, and hindlimbs in rodents, indicative of fetal growth retardation. These effects occurred when pregnant mice received oral doses of 1000 or 3000 mg/kg/day during organogenesis and in rats given 500, 1000, or 2000 mg/kg prior to and during mating and throughout gestation. These doses are approximately 1 to 5 times the human dose of 3600 mg on a mg/m2 basis.

No effects were observed in pregnant mice given 500 mg/kg/day (approximately 1/2 of the daily human dose on a mg/m2 basis).

An increased incidence of hydroureter and/or hydronephrosis was observed in rats given 2000 mg/kg/day in a fertility and general reproduction study, 1500 mg/kg/day in a teratology study, and 500, 1000, and 2000 mg/kg/day in a perinatal and postnatal study. The significance of these findings is unknown, but they have been associated with delayed development. These doses are also approximately 1 to 5 times the human dose of 3600 mg on a mg/m2 basis.

In a teratology study in rabbits, an increased incidence of post-implantation fetal loss, occurred in doses given 60, 300, and 1500 mg/kg/day during organogenesis. These doses are approximately 1/4 to 8 times the daily human dose of 3600 mg on a mg/m2 basis.

6. PHARMACEUTICAL PARTICULARS

6.1 List of excipients

Neurontin Hard Capsules

Each hard capsule contains the following excipients: lactose monohydrate, maize starch and talc.

Capsule shell: gelatin, purified water and sodium lauryl sulphate.

The 100 mg hard capsules contain the colouring E171 (titanium dioxide), the 300 mg hard capsules contain the colourings E171 (titanium dioxide) and E172 (yellow iron oxide) and the 400 mg hard capsules contain the colourings E171 (titanium dioxide) and E172 (red and yellow iron oxide).

The printing ink used on all hard capsules contains shellac, E171 (titanium dioxide) and E132 (indigocarmine).

Neurontin Film-coated Tablets

Each film-coated tablet contains the following excipients: Poloxamer 407 (ethylene oxide and propylene oxide), copovidone, maize starch, magnesium stearate

Film-coating: Opadry white YS-1-18111 (hydroxypropylcellulose, talc)

Polishing agent: candelilla wax

6.2 Incompatibilities

Not applicable

6.3 Shelf life

Neurontin Capsules: Three years

Neurontin Tablets: Two years

6.4 Special precautions for storage

Neurontin Capsules: Do not store above 30°C.

Neurontin Tablets: Do not store above 25°C.

6.5 Nature and contents of container

Neurontin Hard Capsules, hard: PVC/PVDC/aluminium foil blister packs

Supplied in packs of 20, 30, 50, 84, 90, 98, 100, 200, 500, 1000 capsules.

Neurontin Film-coated Tablets: PVC/ PE /PVDC/aluminium foil blister packs

Supplied in packs of: 20, 30, 45, 50, 84, 90, 100, 200, 500 tablets

Not all pack sizes may be marketed.

6.6 Special precautions for disposal and other handling

No special requirements.

7. MARKETING AUTHORISATION HOLDER

Pfizer Limited,

Sandwich,

Kent,

CT13 9NJ,

United Kingdom.

8. MARKETING AUTHORISATION NUMBER(S)

Neurontin 100mg hard capsules PL 00057/0853

Neurontin 300mg hard capsules PL 00057/0536

Neurontin 400mg hard capsules PL 00057/0537

Neurontin 600mg film-coated tablets PL 00057/0538

Neurontin 800mg film-coated tablets PL 00057/0539

9. DATE OF FIRST AUTHORISATION/RENEWAL OF THE AUTHORISATION

Neurontin Hard Capsules: 28th May 2008

Neurontin Film-coated Tablets: 28th May 2008

10. DATE OF REVISION OF THE TEXT

01 December 2008

11. LEGAL CATEGORY

POM

Neurontin is a registered trademark

Company reference NN 16_0

Nexium 20mg & 40mg Tablets

(AstraZeneca UK Limited)

1. NAME OF THE MEDICINAL PRODUCT

Nexium 20 mg Tablets

Nexium 40 mg Tablets

2. QUALITATIVE AND QUANTITATIVE COMPOSITION

Each tablet contains: 20 mg esomeprazole (as magnesium trihydrate).

Each tablet contains: 40 mg esomeprazole (as magnesium trihydrate).

For excipients see 6.1.

3. PHARMACEUTICAL FORM

Gastro-resistant tablet

20 mg: A light pink, oblong, biconvex, film-coated tablet engraved 20 mg on one side and A/EH on the other side.

40 mg: A pink, oblong, biconvex, film-coated tablet engraved 40 mg on one side and A/EI on the other side.

4. CLINICAL PARTICULARS

4.1 Therapeutic indications

Nexium tablets are indicated for:

Gastro-Oesophageal Reflux Disease (GORD)

- treatment of erosive reflux oesophagitis

- long-term management of patients with healed oesophagitis to prevent relapse

- symptomatic treatment of gastro-oesophageal reflux disease (GORD)

In combination with an appropriate antibacterial therapeutic regimen for the eradication of *Helicobacter pylori* and

- healing of *Helicobacter pylori* associated duodenal ulcer and

- prevention of relapse of peptic ulcers in patients with *Helicobacter pylori* associated ulcers.

Patients requiring continued NSAID therapy

Healing of gastric ulcers associated with NSAID therapy.

Prevention of gastric and duodenal ulcers associated with NSAID therapy, in patients at risk.

Prolonged treatment after IV induced prevention of rebleeding of peptic ulcers.

Treatment of Zollinger Ellison Syndrome

4.2 Posology and method of administration

The tablets should be swallowed whole with liquid. The tablets should not be chewed or crushed. For patients who have difficulty in swallowing, the tablets can also be dispersed in half a glass of non-carbonated water. No other liquids should be used as the enteric coat may be dissolved. Stir until the tablets disintegrate and drink the liquid with the pellets immediately or within 30 minutes. Rinse the glass with half a glass of water and drink. The pellets must not be chewed or crushed.

For patients who cannot swallow, the tablets can be dispersed in non-carbonated water and administered through a gastric tube. It is important that the appropriateness of the selected syringe and tube is carefully tested.

For preparation and administration instructions see section 6.6.

Adults and adolescents from the age of 12 years.

Gastro-Oesophageal Reflux Disease (GORD)

- treatment of erosive reflux oesophagitis

40 mg once daily for 4 weeks.

An additional 4 weeks treatment is recommended for patients in whom oesophagitis has not healed or who have persistent symptoms.

- long-term management of patients with healed oesophagitis to prevent relapse

20 mg once daily.

- symptomatic treatment of gastro-oesophageal reflux disease (GORD)

20 mg once daily in patients without oesophagitis. If symptom control has not been achieved after four weeks, the patient should be further investigated. Once symptoms have resolved, subsequent symptom control can be achieved using 20 mg once daily. In adults, an on demand regimen taking 20 mg once daily, when needed, can be used. In NSAID treated patients at risk of developing gastric and duodenal ulcers, subsequent symptom control using an on demand regimen is not recommended.

Adults

In combination with an appropriate antibacterial therapeutic regimen for the eradication of *Helicobacter pylori* and

- healing of *Helicobacter pylori* associated duodenal ulcer and

- prevention of relapse of peptic ulcers in patients with *Helicobacter pylori* associated ulcers.

20 mg Nexium with 1 g amoxicillin and 500 mg clarithromycin, all twice daily for 7 days.

Patients requiring continued NSAID therapy

Healing of gastric ulcers associated with NSAID therapy:

The usual dose is 20 mg once daily. The treatment duration is 4-8 weeks.

Prevention of gastric and duodenal ulcers associated with NSAID therapy in patients at risk:

20 mg once daily.

Prolonged treatment after IV induced prevention of rebleeding of peptic ulcers.

40 mg once daily for 4 weeks after IV induced prevention of rebleeding of peptic ulcers.

Treatment of Zollinger Ellison Syndrome

The recommended initial dosage is Nexium 40 mg twice daily. The dosage should then be individually adjusted and treatment continues as long as clinically indicated. Based on the clinical data available, the majority of patients can be controlled on doses between 80 and 160 mg esomeprazole daily. With doses above 80 mg daily, the dose should be divided and given twice-daily.

Children below the age of 12 years

Nexium should not be used in children younger than 12 years since no data is available.

Impaired renal function

Dose adjustment is not required in patients with impaired renal function. Due to limited experience in patients with severe renal insufficiency, such patients should be treated with caution, (see section 5.2).

Impaired hepatic function

Dose adjustment is not required in patients with mild to moderate liver impairment. For patients with severe liver impairment, a maximum dose of 20 mg Nexium should not be exceeded, (see section 5.2).

Elderly

Dose adjustment is not required in the elderly.

4.3 Contraindications

Known hypersensitivity to esomeprazole, substituted benzimidazoles or any other constituents of the formulation.

Esomeprazole, like other PPIs, should not be administered with atazanavir (see section 4.5).

4.4 Special warnings and precautions for use

In the presence of any alarm symptom (e.g. significant unintentional weight loss, recurrent vomiting, dysphagia, haematemesis or melaena) and when gastric ulcer is suspected or present, malignancy should be excluded, as treatment with Nexium may alleviate symptoms and delay diagnosis.

Patients on long-term treatment (particularly those treated for more than a year) should be kept under regular surveillance.

Patients on on-demand treatment should be instructed to contact their physician if their symptoms change in character. When prescribing esomeprazole for on-demand therapy, the implications for interactions with other pharmaceuticals, due to fluctuating plasma concentrations of esomeprazole should be considered, see section 4.5.

When prescribing esomeprazole for eradication of *Helicobacter pylori* possible drug interactions for all components in the triple therapy should be considered. Clarithromycin is a potent inhibitor of CYP3A4 and hence contraindications and interactions for clarithromycin should be considered when the triple therapy is used in patients concurrently taking other drugs metabolised via CYP3A4 such as cisapride.

This medicinal product contains sucrose. Patients with rare hereditary problems of fructose intolerance, glucose-galactose malabsorption or sucrase-isomaltase insufficiency should not take this medicine.

Treatment with proton pump inhibitors may lead to slightly increased risk of gastrointestinal infections such as Salmonella and Campylobacter (see section 5.1).

4.5 Interaction with other medicinal products and other forms of interaction

Effects of esomeprazole on the pharmacokinetics of other drugs

Medicinal products with pH dependent absorption

The decreased intragastric acidity during treatment with esomeprazole, might increase or decrease the absorption of drugs if the mechanism of absorption is influenced by gastric acidity. In common with the use of other inhibitors of acid secretion or antacids, the absorption of ketoconazole and itraconazole can decrease during treatment with esomeprazole.

Co-administration of omeprazole (40 mg once daily) with atazanavir 300 mg/ritonavir 100 mg to healthy volunteers resulted in a substantial reduction in atazanavir exposure (approximately 75% decrease in AUC, C_{max} and C_{min}). Increasing the atazanavir dose to 400 mg did not compensate for the impact of omeprazole on atazanavir exposure. PPIs including esomeprazole should not be co-administered with atazanavir (see section 4.3).

Drugs metabolised by CYP2C19

Esomeprazole inhibits CYP2C19, the major esomeprazole metabolising enzyme. Thus, when esomeprazole is combined with drugs metabolised by CYP2C19, such as diazepam, citalopram, imipramine, clomipramine, phenytoin etc., the plasma concentrations of these drugs may be increased and a dose reduction could be needed. This should be considered especially when prescribing esomeprazole for on-demand therapy. Concomitant administration of 30 mg esomeprazole resulted in a 45% decrease in clearance of the CYP2C19 substrate diazepam. Concomitant administration of 40 mg esomeprazole resulted in a 13% increase in trough plasma levels of phenytoin in epileptic patients. It is recommended to monitor the plasma concentrations of phenytoin when treatment with esomeprazole is introduced or withdrawn. Omeprazole (40 mg once daily) increased voriconazole (a CYP2C19 substrate) C_{max} and AUC_{τ} by 15% and 41%, respectively.

Concomitant administration of 40 mg esomeprazole to warfarin-treated patients in a clinical trial showed that coagulation times were within the accepted range. However, post-marketing, a few isolated cases of elevated INR of clinical significance have been reported during concomitant treatment. Monitoring is recommended when initiating and ending concomitant esomeprazole treatment during treatment with warfarin or other coumarine derivatives.

In healthy volunteers, concomitant administration of 40 mg esomeprazole resulted in a 32% increase in area under the plasma concentration-time curve (AUC) and a 31% prolongation of elimination half-life($t_{1/2}$) but no significant increase in peak plasma levels of cisapride. The slightly prolonged QTc interval observed after administration of cisapride alone, was not further prolonged when cisapride was given in combination with esomeprazole (see also section 4.4).

Esomeprazole has been shown to have no clinically relevant effects on the pharmacokinetics of amoxicillin or quinidine.

Studies evaluating concomitant administration of esomeprazole and either naproxen or rofecoxib did not identify any clinically relevant pharmacokinetic interactions during short-term studies.

Effects of other drugs on the pharmacokinetics of esomeprazole

Esomeprazole is metabolised by CYP2C19 and CYP3A4. Concomitant administration of esomeprazole and a CYP3A4 inhibitor, clarithromycin (500 mg b.i.d.), resulted in a doubling of the exposure (AUC) to esomeprazole. Concomitant administration of esomeprazole and a combined inhibitor of CYP2C19 and CYP 3A4 may result in more than doubling of the esomeprazole exposure. The CYP2C19 and CYP3A4 inhibitor voriconazole increased omeprazole AUC_{τ} by 280%. A dose adjustment of esomeprazole is not regularly required in either of these situations. However, dose adjustment should be considered in patients with severe hepatic impairment and if long-term treatment is indicated.

4.6 Pregnancy and lactation

For Nexium, clinical data on exposed pregnancies are insufficient. With the racemic mixture omeprazole data on a larger number of exposed pregnancies stemmed from epidemiological studies indicate no malformative nor foetotoxic effects. Animal studies with esomeprazole do not indicate direct or indirect harmful effects with respect to embryonal/fetal development. Animal studies with the racemic mixture do not indicate direct or indirect harmful effects with respect to pregnancy, parturition or postnatal development. Caution should be exercised when prescribing to pregnant women.

It is not known whether esomeprazole is excreted in human breast milk. No studies in lactating women have been performed. Therefore Nexium should not be used during breast-feeding.

4.7 Effects on ability to drive and use machines

No effects have been observed.

4.8 Undesirable effects

The following adverse drug reactions have been identified or suspected in the clinical trials programme for esomeprazole and post-marketing. None was found to be dose-related. The reactions are classified according to frequency (common >1/100, <1/10; uncommon >1/1000, <1/100; rare >1/10000, <1/1000; very rare <1/10000).

Blood and lymphatic system disorders

Rare: Leukopenia, thrombocytopenia

Very rare: Agranulocytosis, pancytopenia

Immune system disorders

Rare: Hypersensitivity reactions e.g. fever, angioedema and anaphylactic reaction/shock

Metabolism and nutrition disorders

Uncommon: Peripheral oedema

Rare: Hyponatraemia

Psychiatric disorders

Uncommon: Insomnia

Rare: Agitation, confusion, depression

Very rare: Aggression, hallucinations

Nervous system disorders

Common: Headache

Uncommon: Dizziness, paraesthesia, somnolence

Rare: Taste disturbance

Eye disorders

Rare: Blurred vision

Ear and labyrinth disorders

Uncommon: Vertigo

Respiratory, thoracic and mediastinal disorders

Rare: Bronchospasm

Gastrointestinal disorders

Common: Abdominal pain, constipation, diarrhoea, flatulence, nausea/vomiting

Uncommon: Dry mouth

Rare: Stomatitis, gastrointestinal candidiasis

Hepatobiliary disorders

Uncommon: Increased liver enzymes

Rare: Hepatitis with or without jaundice

Very rare: Hepatic failure, encephalopathy in patients with pre-existing liver disease

Skin and subcutaneous tissue disorders

Uncommon: Dermatitis, pruritus, rash, urticaria

Rare: Alopecia, photosensitivity

Very rare: Erythema multiforme, Stevens-Johnson syndrome, toxic epidermal necrolysis (TEN)

Musculoskeletal, connective tissue and bone disorders

Rare: Arthralgia, myalgia

Very rare: Muscular weakness

Renal and urinary disorders

Very rare: Interstitial nephritis

Reproductive system and breast disorders

Very rare: Gynaecomastia

General disorders and administration site conditions

Rare: Malaise, increased sweating

4.9 Overdose

There is very limited experience to date with deliberate overdose. The symptoms described in connection with 280mg were gastrointestinal symptoms and weakness. Single doses of 80 mg esomeprazole were uneventful. No specific antidote is known. Esomeprazole is extensively plasma protein bound and is therefore not readily dialyzable. As in any case of overdose, treatment should be symptomatic and general supportive measures should be utilised.

5. PHARMACOLOGICAL PROPERTIES

5.1 Pharmacodynamic properties

Pharmacotherapeutic group: Proton Pump Inhibitor

ATC Code: A02B C05.

Esomeprazole is the *S*-isomer of omeprazole and reduces gastric acid secretion through a specific targeted mechanism of action. It is a specific inhibitor of the acid pump in the parietal cell. Both the R- and S-isomer of omeprazole have similar pharmacodynamic activity.

Site and mechanism of action

Esomeprazole is a weak base and is concentrated and converted to the active form in the highly acidic environment of the secretory canaliculi of the parietal cell, where it inhibits the enzyme H^+K^+-ATPase – the acid pump and inhibits both basal and stimulated acid secretion.

Effect on gastric acid secretion

After oral dosing with esomeprazole 20 mg and 40 mg the onset of effect occurs within one hour. After repeated administration with 20 mg esomeprazole once daily for five days, mean peak acid output after pentagastrin stimulation is decreased 90% when measured 6 – 7 hours after dosing on day five.

After five days of oral dosing with 20 mg and 40 mg of esomeprazole, intragastric pH above 4 was maintained for a mean time of 13 hours and 17 hours, respectively over 24 hours in symptomatic GORD patients. The proportion of patients maintaining an intragastric pH above 4 for at least 8, 12 and 16 hours respectively were for esomeprazole 20 mg 76%, 54% and 24%. Corresponding proportions for esomeprazole 40 mg were 97%, 92% and 56%.

Using AUC as a surrogate parameter for plasma concentration, a relationship between inhibition of acid secretion and exposure has been shown.

Therapeutic effects of acid inhibition

Healing of reflux oesophagitis with esomeprazole 40 mg occurs in approximately 78% of patients after four weeks, and in 93% after eight weeks.

One week treatment with esomeprazole 20 mg b.i.d. and appropriate antibiotics, results in successful eradication of *H. pylori* in approximately 90% of patients.

After eradication treatment for one week there is no need for subsequent monotherapy with antisecretory drugs for effective ulcer healing and symptom resolution in uncomplicated duodenal ulcers.

In a randomised, double blind, placebo-controlled clinical study, patients with endoscopically confirmed peptic ulcer bleeding characterised as Forrest Ia, Ib, IIa or IIb (9%, 43%, 38% and 10% respectively) were randomised to receive Nexium solution for infusion (n=375) or placebo (n=389). Following endoscopic hemostasis, patients received either 80 mg esomeprazole as an intravenous infusion over 30 minutes followed by a continuous infusion of 8 mg per hour or placebo for 72 hours. After the initial 72 hour period, all patients received open label 40 mg oral Nexium for 27 days for acid suppression. The occurrence of rebleeding within 3 days was 5.9% in the Nexium treated group compared to 10.3% for the placebo group. At 30 days post-treatment, the occurrence of rebleeding in the Nexium treated versus the placebo treated group was 7.7% vs 13.6%.

Other effects related to acid inhibition

During treatment with antisecretory drugs serum gastrin increases in response to the decreased acid secretion.

An increased number of ECL cells possibly related to the increased serum gastrin levels, have been observed in some patients during long-term treatment with esomeprazole.

During long-term treatment with antisecretory drugs gastric glandular cysts have been reported to occur at a somewhat increased frequency. These changes are a physiological consequence of pronounced inhibition of acid secretion, are benign and appear to be reversible.

Decreased gastric acidity due to any means including proton pump inhibitors, increases gastric counts of bacteria normally present in the gastrointestinal tract. Treatment with proton pump inhibitors may lead to slightly increased risk of gastrointestinal infections such as *Salmonella* and *Campylobacter*.

In two studies with ranitidine as an active comparator, Nexium showed better effect in healing of gastric ulcers in patients using NSAIDs, including COX-2 selective NSAIDs.

In two studies with placebo as comparator, Nexium showed better effect in the prevention of gastric and duodenal ulcers in patients using NSAIDs (aged >60 and/or with previous ulcer), including COX-2 selective NSAIDs.

5.2 Pharmacokinetic properties

Absorption and distribution

Esomeprazole is acid labile and is administered orally as enteric-coated granules. *In vivo* conversion to the R-isomer is negligible. Absorption of esomeprazole is rapid, with peak plasma levels occurring approximately 1-2 hours after dose. The absolute bioavailability is 64% after a single dose of 40 mg and increases to 89% after repeated once-daily administration. For 20 mg esomeprazole the corresponding values are 50% and 68%, respectively. The apparent volume of distribution at steady state in healthy subjects is approximately 0.22 L/kg body weight. Esomeprazole is 97% plasma protein bound.

Food intake both delays and decreases the absorption of esomeprazole although this has no significant influence on the effect of esomeprazole on intragastric acidity.

Metabolism and excretion

Esomeprazole is completely metabolised by the cytochrome P450 system (CYP). The major part of the metabolism of esomeprazole is dependent on the polymorphic CYP2C19, responsible for the formation of the hydroxy- and desmethyl metabolites of esomeprazole. The remaining part is dependent on another specific isoform, CYP3A4, responsible for the formation of esomeprazole sulphone, the main metabolite in plasma.

The parameters below reflect mainly the pharmacokinetics in individuals with a functional CYP2C19 enzyme, extensive metabolisers.

Total plasma clearance is about 17 L/h after a single dose and about 9 L/h after repeated administration. The plasma elimination half-life is about 1.3 hours after repeated once-daily dosing. The pharmacokinetics of esomeprazole has been studied in doses up to 40 mg b.i.d. The area under the plasma concentration-time curve increases with repeated administration of esomeprazole. This increase is dose-dependent and results in a more than dose proportional increase in AUC after repeated administration. This time - and dose-dependency is due to a decrease of first pass metabolism and systemic clearance probably caused by an inhibition of the CYP2C19 enzyme by esomeprazole and/or its sulphone metabolite. Esomeprazole is completely eliminated from plasma between doses with no tendency for accumulation during once-daily administration.

The major metabolites of esomeprazole have no effect on gastric acid secretion. Almost 80% of an oral dose of esomeprazole is excreted as metabolites in the urine, the remainder in the faeces. Less than 1% of the parent drug is found in urine.

Special patient populations

Approximately 2.9 ±1.5% of the population lack a functional CYP2C19 enzyme and are called poor metabolisers. In these individuals the metabolism of esomeprazole is probably mainly catalysed by CYP3A4. After repeated once-daily administration of 40 mg esomeprazole, the mean area under the plasma concentration-time curve was approximately 100% higher in poor metabolisers than in subjects having a functional CYP2C19 enzyme (extensive metabolisers). Mean peak plasma concentrations were increased by about 60%. These findings have no implications for the posology of esomeprazole.

The metabolism of esomeprazole is not significantly changed in elderly subjects (71-80 years of age).

Following a single dose of 40 mg esomeprazole the mean area under the plasma concentration-time curve is approximately 30% higher in females than in males. No gender difference is seen after repeated once-daily administration. These findings have no implications for the posology of esomeprazole.

Impaired organ function

The metabolism of esomeprazole in patients with mild to moderate liver dysfunction may be impaired. The metabolic rate is decreased in patients with severe liver dysfunction resulting in a doubling of the area under the plasma concentration-time curve of esomeprazole. Therefore, a maximum of 20 mg should not be exceeded in patients with severe dysfunction. Esomeprazole or its major metabolites do not show any tendency to accumulate with once-daily dosing.

No studies have been performed in patients with decreased renal function. Since the kidney is responsible for the excretion of the metabolites of esomeprazole but not for the elimination of the parent compound, the metabolism of esomeprazole is not expected to be changed in patients with impaired renal function.

Paediatric

Adolescents 12-18 years:

Following repeated dose administration of 20 mg and 40 mg esomeprazole, the total exposure (AUC) and the time to reach maximum plasma drug concentration (t_{max}) in 12 to 18 year-olds was similar to that in adults for both esomeprazole doses.

5.3 Preclinical safety data

Preclinical bridging studies reveal no particular hazard for humans based on conventional studies of repeated dose toxicity, genotoxicity, and toxicity to reproduction. Carcinogenicity studies in the rat with the racemic mixture have shown gastric ECL-cell hyperplasia and carcinoids. These gastric effects in the rat are the result of sustained, pronounced hypergastrinaemia secondary to reduced production of gastric acid and are observed after long-term treatment in the rat with inhibitors of gastric acid secretion.

6. PHARMACEUTICAL PARTICULARS

6.1 List of excipients

Glycerol monostearate 40-55

hyprolose

hypromellose

iron oxide (20 mg & 40 mg tablets: reddish-brown; 20 mg tablets: yellow) (E 172)

magnesium stearate

methacrylic acid ethyl acrylate copolymer (1:1) dispersion 30 per cent

cellulose microcrystalline

synthetic paraffin

macrogol

polysorbate 80

crospovidone

sodium stearyl fumarate

sugar spheres (sucrose and maize starch)

talc

titanium dioxide (E 171)

triethyl citrate.

6.2 Incompatibilities
Not applicable

6.3 Shelf life
3 years

2 years in climate zones III-IV

6.4 Special precautions for storage
Do not store above 30°C

Keep the container tightly closed (bottle). Store in the original package (blister).

6.5 Nature and contents of container
In the UK it is aluminium blister packages.

Pack sizes for Nexium 20 and 40 mg Tablets are 7 and 28 as hospital packs, and 28 as standard sales packs.

6.6 Special precautions for disposal and other handling
Administration through gastric tube

1. Put the tablet into an appropriate syringe and fill the syringe with approximately 25 mL water and approximately 5 mL air. For some tubes, dispersion in 50 mL water is needed to prevent the pellets from clogging the tube.

2. Immediately shake the syringe for approximately 2 minutes to disperse the tablet.

3. Hold the syringe with the tip up and check that the tip has not clogged.

4. Attach the syringe to the tube whilst maintaining the above position.

5. Shake the syringe and position it with the tip pointing down. Immediately inject 5-10 mL into the tube. Invert the syringe after injection and shake (the syringe must be held with the tip pointing up to avoid clogging of the tip).

6. Turn the syringe with the tip down and immediately inject another 5-10 mL into the tube. Repeat this procedure until the syringe is empty.

7. Fill the syringe with 25 mL of water and 5 mL of air and repeat step 5 if necessary to wash down any sediment left in the syringe. For some tubes, 50 mL water is needed.

7. MARKETING AUTHORISATION HOLDER
AstraZeneca UK Limited

600 Capability Green

Luton, LU1 3LU, UK

8. MARKETING AUTHORISATION NUMBER(S)
PL 17901/0068

PL 17901/0069

9. DATE OF FIRST AUTHORISATION/RENEWAL OF THE AUTHORISATION
10th March 2005

10. DATE OF REVISION OF THE TEXT
21st May 2009

Nexium I.V. 40mg Powder for solution for injection/infusion

(AstraZeneca UK Limited)

1. NAME OF THE MEDICINAL PRODUCT
Nexium I.V. 40 mg Powder for solution for injection/infusion

2. QUALITATIVE AND QUANTITATIVE COMPOSITION
Each vial contains esomeprazole 40 mg (as sodium salt).

For excipients see 6.1.

3. PHARMACEUTICAL FORM
Powder for solution for injection/infusion.

White to off-white porous cake or powder.

4. CLINICAL PARTICULARS

4.1 Therapeutic indications
Nexium for injection and infusion is indicated for:

• gastric antisecretory treatment when the oral route is not possible, such as:

• gastroesophageal reflux disease in patients with oesophagitis and/or severe symptoms of reflux

• healing of gastric ulcers associated with NSAID therapy

• prevention of gastric and duodenal ulcers associated with NSAID therapy, in patients at risk.

• prevention of rebleeding following therapeutic endoscopy for acute bleeding gastric or duodenal ulcers.

4.2 Posology and method of administration
Gastric antisecretory treatment when the oral route is not possible

Patients who cannot take oral medication may be treated parenterally with 20–40 mg once daily. Patients with reflux oesophagitis should be treated with 40 mg once daily. Patients treated symptomatically for reflux disease should be treated with 20 mg once daily. For healing of gastric ulcers associated with NSAID therapy the usual dose is 20 mg once daily. For prevention of gastric and duodenal ulcers associated with NSAID therapy, patients at risk should be treated with 20 mg once daily. Usually the i.v. treatment duration is short and transfer to oral treatment should be made as soon as possible.

Prevention of rebleeding of gastric and duodenal ulcers

Following therapeutic endoscopy for acute bleeding gastric or duodenal ulcers, 80 mg should be administered as a bolus infusion over 30 minutes, followed by a continuous intravenous infusion of 8 mg/h given over 3 days (72 hours).

The parenteral treatment period should be followed by oral acid-suppression therapy.

Method of administration

Injection

40 mg dose

The reconstituted solution should be given as an intravenous injection over a period of at least 3 minutes.

20 mg dose

Half of the reconstituted solution should be given as an intravenous injection over a period of approximately 3 minutes. Any unused solution should be discarded.

Infusion

40 mg dose

The reconstituted solution should be given as an intravenous infusion over a period of 10 to 30 minutes.

20 mg dose

Half of the reconstituted solution should be given as an intravenous infusion over a period of 10 to 30 minutes. Any unused solution should be discarded.

80 mg bolus dose

The reconstituted solution should be given as a continuous intravenous infusion over 30 minutes.

8 mg/h dose

The reconstituted solution should be given as a continuous intravenous infusion over a period of 71.5 hours (calculated rate of infusion of 8 mg/h. See section 6.3 for shelf-life of the reconstituted solution).

Children and adolescents

Nexium I.V. should not be used in children since no data is available.

Impaired renal function

Dose adjustment is not required in patients with impaired renal function. Due to limited experience in patients with severe renal insufficiency, such patients should be treated with caution. (See section 5.2.)

Impaired hepatic function

GORD: Dose adjustment is not required in patients with mild to moderate liver impairment. For patients with severe liver impairment, a maximum daily dose of 20 mg Nexium I.V. should not be exceeded. (See section 5.2.)

Bleeding ulcers: Dose adjustment is not required in patients with mild to moderate liver impairment. For patients with severe liver impairment, following an initial bolus dose of 80 mg Nexium for infusion, a continuous intravenous infusion dose of 4 mg/h for 71.5 hours may be sufficient (see section 5.2).

Elderly

Dose adjustment is not required in the elderly.

4.3 Contraindications
Hypersensitivity to the active substance esomeprazole or to other substituted benzimidazoles or to any of the excipients of this medicinal product.

Esomeprazole, like other PPIs, should not be administered with atazanavir (see section 4.5).

4.4 Special warnings and precautions for use
In the presence of any alarm symptom (e.g. significant unintentional weight loss, recurrent vomiting, dysphagia, haematemesis or melaena) and when gastric ulcer is suspected or present, malignancy should be excluded, as treatment with Nexium I.V. may alleviate symptoms and delay diagnosis.

Treatment with proton pump inhibitors may lead to slightly increased risk of gastrointestinal infections such as Salmonella and Campylobacter (see section 5.1).

4.5 Interaction with other medicinal products and other forms of interaction
Effects of esomeprazole on the pharmacokinetics of other drugs

Medicinal products with pH dependent absorption

The decreased intragastric acidity during treatment with esomeprazole might increase or decrease the absorption of drugs if the mechanism of absorption is influenced by gastric acidity. In common with the use of other inhibitors of acid secretion or antacids, the absorption of ketoconazole and itraconazole can decrease during treatment with esomeprazole.

Co-administration of omeprazole (40 mg once daily) with atazanavir 300 mg/ritonavir 100 mg to healthy volunteers resulted in a substantial reduction in atazanavir exposure (approximately 75% decrease in AUC, C_{max} and C_{min}). Increasing the atazanavir dose to 400 mg did not compensate for the impact of omeprazole on atazanavir exposure. PPIs including esomeprazole should not be co-administered with atazanavir (see section 4.3).

Drugs metabolised by CYP2C19

Esomeprazole inhibits CYP2C19, the major esomeprazole-metabolising enzyme. Thus, when esomeprazole is combined with drugs metabolised by CYP2C19, such as diazepam, citalopram, imipramine, clomipramine, phenytoin etc., the plasma concentrations of these drugs may be increased and a dose reduction could be needed. Concomitant oral administration of 30 mg esomeprazole resulted in a 45% decrease in clearance of the CYP2C19 substrate diazepam. Concomitant oral administration of 40 mg esomeprazole and phenytoin resulted in a 13% increase in trough plasma levels of phenytoin in epileptic patients. It is recommended to monitor the plasma concentrations of phenytoin when treatment with esomeprazole is introduced or withdrawn. Omeprazole (40 mg once daily) increased voriconazole (a CYP2C19 substrate) C_{max} and AUC $_{\tau}$ by 15% and 41%, respectively.

Concomitant oral administration of 40 mg esomeprazole to warfarin-treated patients in a clinical trial showed that coagulation times were within the accepted range. However, post-marketing of oral esomeprazole, a few isolated cases of elevated INR of clinical significance have been reported during concomitant treatment. Monitoring is recommended when initiating and ending concomitant esomeprazole treatment during treatment with warfarin or other coumarine derivatives.

In healthy volunteers, concomitant oral administration of 40 mg esomeprazole and cisapride resulted in a 32% increase in area under the plasma concentration-time curve (AUC) and a 31% prolongation of elimination half-life($t_{1/2}$) but no significant increase in peak plasma levels of cisapride. The slightly prolonged QTc interval observed after administration of cisapride alone, was not further prolonged when cisapride was given in combination with esomeprazole.

Esomeprazole has been shown to have no clinically relevant effects on the pharmacokinetics of amoxicillin or quinidine.

No in vivo interaction studies have been performed with the high dose IV regimen (80 mg + 8 mg/h). The effect of esomeprazole on drugs metabolised by CYP2C19 may be more pronounced during this regimen, and patients should be monitored closely for adverse effects during the 3-day IV treatment period.

Effects of other drugs on the pharmacokinetics of esomeprazole

Esomeprazole is metabolised by CYP2C19 and CYP3A4. Concomitant oral administration of esomeprazole and a CYP3A4 inhibitor, clarithromycin (500 mg b.i.d.), resulted in a doubling of the exposure (AUC) to esomeprazole. Concomitant administration of esomeprazole and a combined inhibitor of CYP2C19 and CYP 3A4 may result in more than doubling of the esomeprazole exposure. The CYP2C19 and CYP3A4 inhibitor voriconazole increased omeprazole AUC $_{\tau}$ by 280%. A dose adjustment of esomeprazole is not regularly required in either of these situations. However, dose adjustment should be considered in patients with severe hepatic impairment and if long-term treatment is indicated.

4.6 Pregnancy and lactation
For esomeprazole, limited data on exposed pregnancies are available. Animal studies with esomeprazole do not indicate direct or indirect harmful effects with respect to embryonal/foetal development. Animal studies with the racemic mixture do not indicate direct or indirect harmful effects with respect to pregnancy, parturition or postnatal development. Caution should be exercised when prescribing Nexium I.V. to pregnant women.

It is not known whether esomeprazole is excreted in human breast milk. No studies in lactating women have been performed. Therefore Nexium I.V. should not be used during breast-feeding.

4.7 Effects on ability to drive and use machines
Nexium I.V. is not likely to affect the ability to drive or use machines.

4.8 Undesirable effects
The following adverse drug reactions have been identified or suspected in the clinical trials programme for esomeprazole administered orally or intravenously and post-marketing when administered orally. The reactions are classified according to frequency (common >1/100, <1/10; uncommon >1/1000, <1/100; rare >1/10000, <1/1000; very rare <1/10000).

Blood and lymphatic system disorders

Rare: Leukopenia, thrombocytopenia

Very rare: Agranulocytosis, pancytopenia

Immune system disorders

Rare: Hypersensitivity reactions e.g. fever, angioedema and anaphylactic reaction/shock

Metabolism and nutrition disorders

Uncommon: Peripheral oedema

Rare: Hyponatraemia

Psychiatric disorders

Uncommon: Insomnia

Rare: Agitation, confusion, depression

Very rare: Aggression, hallucinations

Nervous system disorders

Common: Headache

Uncommon: Dizziness, paraesthesia, somnolence

Rare: Taste disturbance

Eye disorders

Uncommon: Blurred vision

Ear and labyrinth disorders

Uncommon: Vertigo

Respiratory, thoracic and mediastinal disorders

Rare: Bronchospasm

Gastrointestinal disorders

Common: Abdominal pain, constipation, diarrhoea, flatulence, nausea/vomiting

Uncommon: Dry mouth

Rare: Stomatitis, gastrointestinal candidiasis

Hepatobiliary disorders

Uncommon: Increased liver enzymes

Rare: Hepatitis with or without jaundice

Very rare: Hepatic failure, encephalopathy in patients with pre-existing liver disease

Skin and subcutaneous tissue disorders

Common: Administration site reactions*

Uncommon: Dermatitis, pruritus, rash, urticaria

Rare: Alopecia, photosensitivity

Very rare: Erythema multiforme, Stevens-Johnson syndrome, toxic epidermal necrolysis (TEN)

Musculoskeletal, connective tissue and bone disorders

Rare: Arthralgia, myalgia

Very rare: Muscular weakness

Renal and urinary disorders

Very rare: Interstitial nephritis

Reproductive system and breast disorders

Very rare: Gynaecomastia

General disorders and administration site conditions

Rare: Malaise, increased sweating

*Administration site reactions have mainly been observed in a study with high-dose exposure over 3 days (72 hours). See section 5.3.

Irreversible visual impairment has been reported in isolated cases of critically ill patients who have received omeprazole (the racemate) intravenous injection, especially at high doses, but no causal relationship has been established.

4.9 Overdose

There is very limited experience to date with deliberate overdose. The symptoms described in connection with an oral dose of 280 mg were gastrointestinal symptoms and weakness. Single oral doses of 80 mg esomeprazole and intravenous doses of 308 mg esomeprazole over 24 hours were uneventful. No specific antidote is known. Esomeprazole is extensively plasmaprotein bound and is therefore not readily dialyzable. As in any case of overdose, treatment should be symptomatic and general supportive measures should be utilised.

5. PHARMACOLOGICAL PROPERTIES

5.1 Pharmacodynamic properties

Pharmacotherapeutic group: Proton pump inhibitor

ATC Code: A02B C05

Esomeprazole is the S-isomer of omeprazole and reduces gastric acid secretion through a specific targeted mechanism of action. It is a specific inhibitor of the acid pump in the parietal cell. Both the R- and S-isomer of omeprazole have similar pharmacodynamic activity.

Site and mechanism of action

Esomeprazole is a weak base and is concentrated and converted to the active form in the highly acidic environment of the secretory canaliculi of the parietal cell, where it inhibits the enzyme H^+K^+-ATPase – the acid pump and inhibits both basal and stimulated acid secretion.

Effect on gastric acid secretion

After 5 days of oral dosing with 20 mg and 40 mg of esomeprazole, intragastric pH above 4 was maintained for a mean time of 13 hours and 17 hours respectively, over 24 hours in symptomatic GORD patients. The effect is similar irrespective of whether esomeprazole is administered orally or intravenously.

Using AUC as a surrogate parameter for plasma concentration, a relationship between inhibition of acid secretion and exposure has been shown after oral administration of esomeprazole.

During intravenous administration of 80 mg esomeprazole as a bolus infusion over 30 minutes followed by a continuous intravenous infusion of 8 mg/h for 23.5 hours, intragastric pH above 4, and pH above 6 was maintained for a mean time of 21 hours and 11-13 hours, respectively, over 24 hours in healthy subjects.

Therapeutic effects of acid inhibition

Healing of reflux oesophagitis with esomeprazole 40 mg occurs in approximately 78% of patients after 4 weeks, and in 93% after 8 weeks of oral treatment.

In a randomised, double blind, placebo-controlled clinical study, patients with endoscopically confirmed peptic ulcer bleeding characterised as Forrest Ia, Ib, IIa or IIb (9%, 43%, 38% and 10% respectively) were randomised to receive Nexium solution for infusion (n=375) or placebo (n=389). Following endoscopic haemostasis, patients received either 80 mg esomeprazole as an intravenous infusion over 30 minutes followed by a continuous infusion of 8 mg per hour or placebo for 72 hours. After the initial 72 hour period, all patients received open-label 40 mg oral Nexium for 27 days for acid suppression. The occurrence of rebleeding within 3 days was 5.9% in the Nexium treated group compared to 10.3% for the placebo group. At 30 days post-treatment, the occurrence of rebleeding in the Nexium treated versus the placebo treated group was 7.7% vs 13.6%.

Other effects related to acid inhibition

During treatment with antisecretory drugs, serum gastrin increases in response to the decreased acid secretion.

An increased number of ECL cells possibly related to the increased serum gastrin levels, have been observed in some patients during long-term treatment with orally administered esomeprazole.

During long-term oral treatment with antisecretory drugs, gastric glandular cysts have been reported to occur at a somewhat increased frequency. These changes are a physiological consequence of pronounced inhibition of acid secretion, are benign and appear to be reversible.

Decreased gastric acidity due to any means including proton pump inhibitors, increases gastric counts of bacteria normally present in the gastrointestinal tract. Treatment with proton pump inhibitors may lead to slightly increased risk of gastrointestinal infections such as *Salmonella* and *Campylobacter*.

5.2 Pharmacokinetic properties

Distribution

The apparent volume of distribution at steady state in healthy subjects is approximately 0.22 L/kg body weight. Esomeprazole is 97% plasma protein bound.

Metabolism and excretion

Esomeprazole is completely metabolised by the cytochrome P450 system (CYP). The major part of the metabolism of esomeprazole is dependent on the polymorphic CYP2C19, responsible for the formation of the hydroxy- and desmethyl metabolites of esomeprazole. The remaining part is dependent on another specific isoform, CYP3A4, responsible for the formation of esomeprazole sulphone, the main metabolite in plasma.

The parameters below reflect mainly the pharmacokinetics in individuals with a functional CYP2C19 enzyme, extensive metabolisers.

Total plasma clearance is about 17 L/h after a single dose and about 9 L/h after repeated administration. The plasma elimination half-life is about 1.3 hours after repeated once daily dosing. Total exposure (AUC) increases with repeated administration of esomeprazole. This increase is dose-dependent and results in a non-linear dose-AUC relationship after repeated administration. This time-and dose-dependency is due to a decrease of first pass metabolism and systemic clearance, probably caused by inhibition of the CYP2C19 enzyme by esomeprazole and/or its sulphone metabolite. Esomeprazole is completely eliminated from plasma between doses with no tendency for accumulation during once daily administration. There is a dose-linear increase in total exposure following intravenous administration of esomeprazole as a 30-minute infusion (40 mg, 80 mg or 120 mg) followed by a continuous infusion (4 mg/h or 8 mg/h) over 23.5 hours.

Following repeated doses of 40 mg administered as intravenous injections, the mean peak plasma concentration is approx. 13.6 micromol/L. The mean peak plasma concentration after corresponding oral doses is approx. 4.6 micromol/L. A smaller increase (of approx 30%) can be seen in total exposure after intravenous administration compared to oral administration.

The major metabolites of esomeprazole have no effect on gastric acid secretion. Almost 80% of an oral dose of esomeprazole is excreted as metabolites in the urine, the remainder in the faeces. Less than 1% of the parent drug is found in urine.

Special patient populations

Approximately 2.9 ±1.5% of the population lack a functional CYP2C19 enzyme and are called poor metabolisers. In these individuals, the metabolism of esomeprazole is probably mainly catalysed by CYP3A4. After repeated once daily administration of 40 mg oral esomeprazole, the mean total exposure was approximately 100% higher in poor metabolisers than in subjects with a functional CYP2C19 enzyme (extensive metabolisers). Mean peak plasma concentrations were increased by about 60%. Similar differences have been seen for intravenous administration of esomeprazole. These findings have no implications for the posology of esomeprazole.

The metabolism of esomeprazole is not significantly changed in elderly subjects (71–80 years of age).

Following a single oral dose of 40 mg esomeprazole the mean total exposure is approximately 30% higher in females than in males. No gender difference is seen after repeated once daily administration. Similar differences have been observed for intravenous administration of esomeprazole. These findings have no implications for the posology of esomeprazole.

The metabolism of esomeprazole in patients with mild to moderate liver dysfunction may be impaired. The metabolic rate is decreased in patients with severe liver dysfunction resulting in a doubling of the total exposure of esomeprazole. Therefore, a maximum dose of 20 mg should not be exceeded in GORD patients with severe dysfunction. For patients with bleeding ulcers and severe liver impairment, following an initial bolus dose of 80 mg, a maximum continuous intravenous infusion dose of 4 mg/h for 71.5 hours may be sufficient. Esomeprazole or its major metabolites do not show any tendency to accumulate with once daily dosing.

No studies have been performed in patients with decreased renal function. Since the kidney is responsible for the excretion of the metabolites of esomeprazole but not for the elimination of the parent compound, the metabolism of esomeprazole is not expected to be changed in patients with impaired renal function.

5.3 Preclinical safety data

Preclinical studies reveal no particular hazard for humans, based on conventional studies of single and repeated dose toxicity, embryo-foetal toxicity and mutagenicity. Oral carcinogenicity studies in the rat with the racemic mixture have shown gastric ECL-cell hyperplasia and carcinoids. These gastric effects are the result of sustained, pronounced hypergastrinaemia secondary to reduced production of gastric acid, and are observed after long-term treatment in the rat with inhibitors of gastric acid secretion. In the non-clinical program for esomeprazole intravenous formulation there was no evidence of vaso-irritation but a slight tissue inflammatory reaction at the injection site after subcutaneous (paravenous) injection was noted. See section 4.8.

6. PHARMACEUTICAL PARTICULARS

6.1 List of excipients

Disodium edetate

Sodium hydroxide

6.2 Incompatibilities

This medicinal product should not be used with other medicinal products except those mentioned in section 6.6.

6.3 Shelf life

2 years in all climate zones.

Shelf-life after reconstitution

Chemical and physical in-use stability has been demonstrated for 12 hours at 30°C. From a microbiological point of view, the product should be used immediately.

6.4 Special precautions for storage

Store in the original package, in order to protect from light. Vials can however, be stored exposed to normal indoor light outside the box for up to 24 hours. Do not store above 30°C.

6.5 Nature and contents of container

5 mL vial made of colourless borosilicate glass, type I. Stopper made of bromobutyl latex-free rubber. Cap made of aluminium and a plastic flip-off seal.

Pack sizes: 1 vial, 1x10 vials.

Not all pack sizes may be marketed.

6.6 Special precautions for disposal and other handling

The reconstituted solution should be inspected visually for particulate matter and discoloration prior to administration. Only clear solution should be used. For single use only.

When administering a 20 mg dose, only half of the reconstituted solution should be used. Any unused solution should be discarded.

Injection

A solution for injection is prepared by adding 5 mL of 0.9% sodium chloride for intravenous use to the vial with esomeprazole.

The reconstituted solution for injection is clear and colourless to very slightly yellow.

Infusion

A solution for infusion is prepared by dissolving the content of one vial with esomeprazole in up to 100 mL 0.9% sodium chloride for intravenous use.

The reconstituted solution for infusion is clear and colourless to very slightly yellow.

Infusion 80 mg

A solution for infusion is prepared by dissolving the content of two vials of esomeprazole 40 mg in up to 100 ml of 0.9% sodium chloride for intravenous use.

7. MARKETING AUTHORISATION HOLDER

AstraZeneca UK Limited,

600 Capability Green,

Luton, LU1 3LU,

United Kingdom.

8. MARKETING AUTHORISATION NUMBER(S)

PL 17901/0221

9. DATE OF FIRST AUTHORISATION/RENEWAL OF THE AUTHORISATION

10th March 2005

10. DATE OF REVISION OF THE TEXT

21st May 2009

Niaspan 375 mg, 500mg, 750mg and 1000mg Prolonged-Release Tablets

(Abbott Laboratories Limited)

1. NAME OF THE MEDICINAL PRODUCT

Niaspan 375 mg Prolonged-Release Tablets

Niaspan 500 mg Prolonged-Release Tablets

Niaspan 750 mg Prolonged-Release Tablets

Niaspan 1000 mg Prolonged-Release Tablets

2. QUALITATIVE AND QUANTITATIVE COMPOSITION

Each Niaspan 375 mg prolonged-release tablet contains 375 mg nicotinic acid.

Each Niaspan 500 mg prolonged-release tablet contains 500 mg nicotinic acid.

Each Niaspan 750 mg prolonged-release tablet contains 750 mg nicotinic acid.

Each Niaspan 1000 mg prolonged-release tablet contains 1000 mg nicotinic acid.

For a full list of excipients, see section 6.1.

3. PHARMACEUTICAL FORM

Prolonged-release tablet

White to off-white capsule-shaped tablet. Each tablet is embossed with the tablet strength on one side.

4. CLINICAL PARTICULARS

4.1 Therapeutic indications

Treatment of dyslipidaemia, particularly in patients with combined mixed dyslipidaemia, characterised by elevated levels of LDL-cholesterol and triglycerides and low HDL-cholesterol, and in patients with primary hypercholesterolaemia. Niaspan should be used in patients in combination with HMG-CoA reductase inhibitors (statins), when the cholesterol lowering effect of HMG-CoA reductase inhibitor monotherapy is inadequate. Niaspan can be used as monotherapy only in patients who do not tolerate HMG-CoA reductase inhibitors. Diet and other non-pharmacological treatments (e.g. exercise, weight reduction) should be continued during therapy with Niaspan.

4.2 Posology and method of administration

Niaspan should be taken at bedtime, after a low-fat snack (e.g. an apple, low fat yoghurt, slice of bread) and doses should be individualised according to the patient's response.

Initial dose

Therapy with Niaspan must be initiated with a low dose and increased gradually. The recommended dose escalation schedule is shown below in Table 1:

Table 1: Dose escalation schedule

(see Table 1 below)

Maintenance dose

The recommended maintenance dose is 1000 mg (two 500 mg tablets) to 2000 mg (two 1000 mg tablets) once daily at bedtime depending on the patient's response and tolerance. If the response to 1000 mg daily is inadequate, the dose may be increased to 1500 mg daily and subsequently to 2000 mg daily.

The daily dosage of Niaspan should not be increased by more than 500 mg in any four-week period after the initial titration to 1000 mg. The maximum dose is 2000 mg per day.

The different Niaspan tablet strengths have different bioavailability and are therefore not interchangeable.

Niaspan must not be replaced with other nicotinic acid preparations, see section 4.4.

In patients previously treated with other nicotinic acid products, Niaspan treatment must be initiated with the recommended Niaspan dose escalation schedule. The maintenance dose should subsequently be individualised according to the patient's response.

If Niaspan therapy is discontinued for an extended period, re-institution of therapy must include a dose escalation.

Niaspan tablets must not be broken, crushed or chewed before swallowing.

Renal impairment

No studies have been performed in patients with impaired renal function, Niaspan must be used with caution in patients with renal disease.

Hepatic impairment

No studies have been performed in patients with impaired hepatic function. Niaspan must be used with caution in patients with a history of liver disease and who consume substantial quantities of alcohol, see section 4.4. Niaspan is contraindicated in patients with significant hepatic dysfunction, see section 4.3.

Elderly

No dose adjustment is necessary.

Children

The safety and efficacy of nicotinic acid therapy in children and adolescents has not been established. Use in children and adolescents is not recommended.

4.3 Contraindications

Niaspan is contraindicated in patients with

- hypersensitivity to nicotinic acid or to any of the excipients, see section 6.1,
- significant hepatic dysfunction,
- active peptic ulcer disease,
- arterial bleeding.

4.4 Special warnings and precautions for use

Niaspan must not be replaced with other nicotinic acid preparations. When switching from other nicotinic acid preparations to Niaspan, therapy with Niaspan must be initiated with the recommended dose escalation schedule, see section 4.2.

Liver

Nicotinic acid preparations have been associated with abnormal liver tests. Severe hepatic toxicity, including fulminant hepatic necrosis, has occurred in patients who have taken long-acting nicotinic acid products in place of immediate-release nicotinic acid. Since the pharmacokinetics of Niaspan are different to other nicotinic acid preparations, Niaspan must not be replaced with other preparations. The prescribing information of the HMG-CoA reductase inhibitor should also be consulted for warnings and precautions for use.

Caution is advised when Niaspan is used in patients who consume substantial quantities of alcohol and/or have a past history of liver disease.

Elevated liver transaminases have been observed with Niaspan therapy. However, transaminase elevations were reversible upon discontinuation of Niaspan.

Liver tests including AST and ALT must be performed periodically in all patients during therapy with Niaspan and prior to treatment in case of history and/or symptoms of hepatic dysfunction (e.g. jaundice, nausea, fever, and/or malaise). If the transaminase levels show evidence of progression, particularly if they rise to three times the upper limit of normal, the drug must be discontinued.

Skeletal muscle

Single reports on rhabdomyolysis in patients on combined therapy with Niaspan and HMG-CoA reductase inhibitors have been received from spontaneous reporting. Physicians contemplating combined therapy with HMG-CoA reductase inhibitors and Niaspan should carefully weigh the potential benefits and risks and should carefully monitor patients for any symptoms of rhabdomyolysis e.g. muscle pain, tenderness or weakness, particularly during the initial months of therapy and during any periods of upward dosage titration of either drug. Periodic serum creatine phosphokinase (CPK) and potassium determinations should be considered in such situations.

A CPK level should be measured before starting such a combination in patients with pre-disposing factors for rhabdomyolysis, as follows:

- renal impairment
- hypothyroidism
- alcohol abuse
- age > 70 years
- personal or family history of hereditary muscular disorders
- previous history of muscular toxicity with fibrate or HMG-CoA reductase inhibitor

Muscle damage must be considered in any patient presenting with diffuse myalgia, muscle tenderness and/or marked increase in muscle CK levels (> 5 × ULN); under these conditions treatment must be discontinued.

The prescribing information of the HMG-CoA reductase inhibitors should be consulted.

Glucose Intolerance

Diabetic or potentially diabetic patients should be observed closely since there may be a dose-related increase in glucose intolerance. Adjustment of diet and/or oral antidiabetics and/or insulin therapy may become necessary.

Unstable angina and acute myocardial infarction

Caution is advised when Niaspan is used in patients with unstable angina or in the acute phase of myocardial infarction, particularly when such patients are also receiving vasoactive drugs such as nitrates, calcium channel blockers, or adrenergic blocking agents.

Uric acid

Elevated uric acid levels have occurred with Niaspan therapy. Monitoring of patients predisposed to gout is recommended.

Coagulation

Niaspan may affect platelet count and prothrombin time, see section 4.5. Patients undergoing surgery should be carefully evaluated. Caution is also advised when Niaspan is administered concomitantly with anti-coagulants; patients receiving anti-coagulants must be monitored closely for prothrombin time and platelet count.

Hypophosphataemia

Niaspan has been associated with reductions in phosphorous levels. Although these reductions were transient, monitoring of phosphorous levels is recommended in patients at risk of hypophosphataemia.

Other

Patients with a history of jaundice, hepatobiliary disease, or peptic ulcer should be observed closely during Niaspan therapy.

4.5 Interaction with other medicinal products and other forms of interaction

Concomitant alcohol or hot drinks may increase undesirable flushing and pruritus and should be avoided around the time of Niaspan ingestion.

Niaspan has been associated with small but statistically significant dose-related reductions in platelet count (mean of -11% with 2000 mg). In addition, Niaspan has been associated with small but statistically significant increases in prothrombin time (mean of approximately +4%). When Niaspan is administered concomitantly with anti-coagulants, prothrombin time and platelet counts must be monitored closely.

Nicotinic acid may potentiate the blood-pressure lowering effect of ganglionic blocking agents e.g. transdermal nicotine or vasoactive drugs such as nitrates, calcium channel blockers or adrenergic blocking agents.

Bile acid sequestrants bind to other orally administered medicinal products and should be taken separately, see also prescribing information of the concerned product.

Nicotinic acid may produce false elevations in some fluorometric determinations of plasma or urinary catecholamines. Nicotinic acid may also give false-positive reactions with cupric sulphate solution (Benedict's reagent) in urine glucose tests.

Combination of nicotinic acid with HMG-CoA reductase inhibitors may increase the risk for myopathy and rhabdomyolysis, see also section 4.4. The prescribing information of the HMG-CoA reductase inhibitor should also be consulted.

4.6 Pregnancy and lactation

Pregnancy

It is not known whether nicotinic acid at doses typically used for lipid disorders can cause foetal harm when administered to pregnant women or whether it can affect reproductive capacity. Animal studies are incomplete, see section 5.3.

Niaspan should not be prescribed to pregnant women unless strictly necessary.

Lactation

Nicotinic acid has been reported to appear in breast milk. Because of the potential for serious adverse reactions in nursing infants from lipid-altering doses of nicotinic acid, a decision should be made whether to discontinue nursing or to discontinue the drug, taking into account the importance of the drug to the mother. No studies have been conducted with Niaspan in nursing mothers.

4.7 Effects on ability to drive and use machines

Niaspan has no or negligible influence on the ability to drive and use machines.

4.8 Undesirable effects

Flush

In the placebo-controlled clinical trials, flushing episodes (i.e. warmth, redness, itching and/or tingling) were the most common treatment-emergent adverse events for Niaspan (reported by 88% of patients). In these studies fewer than 6% of Niaspan patients discontinued due to flushing.

In comparisons of immediate-release (IR) nicotinic acid and Niaspan, although the number of patients who flushed was similar, fewer flushing episodes were reported by patients who received Niaspan. Following four weeks of maintenance therapy with Niaspan at daily doses of

Table 1: Dose escalation schedule

	Week(s)	Dosage		Daily nicotinic acid dose
↑	1	Niaspan 375 mg	1 tablet at bedtime	375 mg
INITIAL TITRATION SCHEDULE	2	Niaspan 500 mg	1 tablet at bedtime	500 mg
	3	Niaspan 750 mg	1 tablet at bedtime	750 mg
↓	4-7	Niaspan 500 mg	2 tablets at bedtime	1000 mg
		Niaspan 750 mg	2 tablets at bedtime	1500 mg
		Niaspan 1000 mg	2 tablets at bedtime	2000 mg

1500mg, the frequency of flushing over the four week period averaged 1.88 events per patient.

Flushing reactions generally occur during early treatment and the dose titration phase. They are thought to be mediated by the release of prostaglandin D2 and tolerance to flushing usually develops over the course of several weeks.

Spontaneous reports suggest that in rare cases, flushing may be more severe and accompanied by symptoms of dizziness, tachycardia, palpitations, dyspnoea, sweating, chills and/or oedema, which in rare cases may lead to syncope. Medical treatment should be administered as necessary.

Hypersensitivity reactions

Hypersensitivity reactions have been reported very rarely. These may be characterised by symptoms such as generalised exanthema, flush, urticaria, vesiculobullous rash, angioedema, laryngospasm, dyspnoea, hypotension, and circulatory collapse. Medical treatment should be administered as necessary.

The following adverse reactions have been observed in clinical studies or in routine patient management, in patients receiving the recommended daily maintenance doses (1000, 1500, and 2000mg) of Niaspan. They are presented by system organ class and frequency grouping (very common >1/10; common >1/100, <1/10; uncommon >1/1,000, <1/100; rare >1/10,000, <1/1,000; very rare <1/10,000, including isolated reports). In general, the incidence of adverse reactions was higher in women compared to men. (Please refer to Table 2 below).

Table 2: Adverse reactions

(see Table 2 below)

4.9 Overdose

Information on acute overdose with Niaspan in humans is limited. The signs and symptoms of an acute overdose are anticipated to be those of excessive pharmacological effect: severe flushing, nausea/vomiting, diarrhoea, dyspepsia, dizziness, syncope, hypotension, potential cardiac arrhythmias and clinical laboratory abnormalities including elevations in liver function tests. The patient should be carefully observed and given supportive treatment. Insufficient information is available on the dialysis potential of nicotinic acid.

5. PHARMACOLOGICAL PROPERTIES

5.1 Pharmacodynamic properties

Pharmacotherapeutic group: nicotinic acid, ATC code: C10AD02

Nicotinic acid is a water-soluble B-complex vitamin which is a naturally occurring constituent of foods. The human body is not entirely dependent on dietary sources of nicotinic acid, since it may also be synthesised from tryptophan.

The mechanism of action by which nicotinic acid modify lipid profiles is not fully elucidated. However, it is recognised that nicotinic acid inhibits the release of free fatty acids from adipose tissue resulting in less free fatty acids being presented to the liver. Since fewer fatty acids are being transported to the liver, fewer are esterified to triglycerides and then incorporated into VLDL. This may lead to a decrease in LDL generation. By increasing lipoprotein lipase activity, nicotinic acid may increase the rate of chylomicron triglycerides removal from plasma. Thus, nicotinic acid decreases the rate of hepatic synthesis of VLDL and subsequently LDL. It does not appear to affect faecal excretion of fats, sterols, or bile acids.

At the recommended maintenance dose, Niaspan (but not nicotinamide) resulted in a clinical reduction in total cholesterol to HDL ratio [-17, to -27%], LDL [-8 to -16%], triglycerides [-14 to -35%] with an increase in HDL [16% to 26%]. In addition to the above mentioned reduction in LDL levels, nicotinic acid causes a shift in LDL composition from the small dense LDL particles (major atherogenic lipoprotein) to the larger, more buoyant LDL particles (less atherogenic). The increase in HDL is also associated with a shift in the distribution of HDL sub-fractions including an increase in the HDL2 to HDL3 ratio, the protective effect of HDL being mainly due to HDL2. Moreover, nicotinic acid increases serum levels of apolipoprotein A1 (Apo 1), one of the two major lipoproteins of HDL, while decreases concentrations of apolipoprotein B-100 (Apo B), the major protein component of the very low-density lipoprotein (VLDL) and LDL fractions known to play important roles in atherogenesis. The serum levels of lipoprotein a, [Lp (a)], which present great homology with LDL but considered as an independent risk factor for coronary heart disease, are also significantly reduced by Niaspan.

Data from clinical trials suggest that women have a greater hypolipidaemic response than men at equivalent doses of Niaspan.

There are no specific studies of the combination of Niaspan with statins.

The beneficial effect of Niaspan on morbidity and mortality has not been directly assessed. However, relevant clinical data are available with immediate release (IR) nicotinic acid.

5.2 Pharmacokinetic properties

Absorption

Nicotinic acid is rapidly and extensively absorbed when administered orally (at least 60-76% of dose).

Peak steady-state nicotinic acid concentrations were 0.6, 4.9, and 15.5 microgram/ml after doses of 1000, 1500, and 2000 mg Niaspan once daily (given as two 500 mg, two 750 mg, and two 1000 mg tablets, respectively).

Single-dose bioavailability studies have demonstrated that Niaspan tablet strengths are not interchangeable.

Distribution

Studies using radiolabelled nicotinic acid in mice show that nicotinic acid and its metabolites concentrate in the liver, kidney and adipose tissue.

Metabolism

The pharmacokinetic profile of nicotinic acid is complicated due to rapid and extensive first-pass metabolism which is species and dose-rate specific. In humans, one pathway (Pathway 1) is through a simple conjugation step with glycine to form nicotinuric acid (NUA). NUA is then excreted in the urine, although there may be a small amount of reversible metabolism back to nicotinic acid. There is evidence to suggest that nicotinic acid metabolism along this pathway leads to flush. The other pathway (Pathway 2) results in the formation of nicotinamide adenine dinucleotide (NAD). A predominance of metabolism down Pathway 2 may lead to hepatotoxicity. It is unclear whether nicotinamide is formed as a precursor to, or following the synthesis of, NAD. Nicotinamide is further metabolised to at least N-methylnicotinamide (MNA) and nicotinamide N-oxide (NNO). MNA is further metabolised to two other compounds, N-methyl-2-pyridone-5-carboxamide (2PY) and N-methyl-4-pyridone-5-carboxamide (4PY). The formation of 2PY appears to predominate over 4PY in humans. At the doses used to treat hyperlipidaemia, these metabolic pathways are saturable, which explains the non-linear relationship between nicotinic acid dose and plasma concentrations following multiple dose Niaspan administration.

Nicotinamide does not have hypolipidaemic activity; the activity of the other metabolites is unknown.

Elimination

Nicotinic acid and its metabolites are rapidly eliminated in the urine. Following single and multiple doses, approximately 60-76% of the dose administered as Niaspan was recovered in the urine as nicotinic acid and metabolites; up to 12% was recovered as unchanged nicotinic acid after multiple dosing. The ratio of metabolites recovered in the urine was dependent on the dose administered.

Gender differences

Steady state plasma concentrations of nicotinic acid and metabolites after administration of Niaspan are generally higher in women than in men, with the magnitude of difference varying with dose and metabolite. Recovery of

Table 2: Adverse reactions

Organ Class	Very common >1/10	Common >1/100, <1/10	Uncommon >1/1,000, <1/100	Rare >1/10,000, <1/1,000	Very rare <1/10,000, including isolated reports
Immune system disorders					Hypersensitivity reaction
Metabolism and nutrition disorders				Decreased glucose tolerance	Anorexia, gout
Psychiatric disorders				Insomnia, nervousness	
Nervous system disorders			Headache, dizziness	Syncope, paraesthesia	Migraine
Eye disorders				Visual disturbance	Toxic amblyopia, cystoid macular oedema
Cardiac disorders			Tachycardia, palpitations		Atrial fibrillation, other cardiac dysrhythmias
Vascular disorders	Flushing episodes (warmth, redness, itching, tingling)			Hypotension, postural hypotension	Collapse
Respiratory, thoracic and mediastinal disorders			Dyspnoea	Rhinitis	
Gastrointestinal disorders		Diarrhoea, nausea, vomiting, abdominal pain, dyspepsia		Flatulence, eructation	Activation of peptic ulcers, peptic ulceration
Hepatobiliary disorders					Jaundice
Skin and subcutaneous tissue disorders		Pruritus, rash	Sweating, generalised exanthema, urticaria, dry skin	Face oedema, vesiculobullous rash, maculopapular rash	Hyperpigmentation, acanthosis nigricans
Musculoskeletal, connective tissue and bone disorders				Leg cramps, myalgia, myopathy, myasthenia	
General disorders and administration site conditions			Pain, asthenia, chills, peripheral oedema	Chest pain	
Investigations			Elevations in serum transaminases (AST, ALT), alkaline phosphatase, total bilirubin, LDH, amylase, fasting glucose, uric acid; slight reduction in platelet counts, prolongation of prothrombin time, reduction in phosphorus, CK increase		

nicotinic acid and metabolites in urine, however, is generally similar for men and women, indicating the absorption is similar for both genders. The gender differences observed in plasma levels of nicotinic acid and its metabolites may be due to gender-specific differences in metabolic rate or volume of distribution.

5.3 Preclinical safety data

Nicotinic acid has been shown to be of low toxicity in customary animal studies.

Female rabbits have been dosed with 0.3g nicotinic acid per day from pre-conception to lactation, and gave birth to offspring without teratogenic effects. Further specific animal reproduction studies have not been conducted with nicotinic acid or with Niaspan.

In a life-time study in mice, high dose levels of nicotinic acid showed no treatment-related carcinogenic effects and no effects on survival rates.

6. PHARMACEUTICAL PARTICULARS

6.1 List of excipients

Hypromellose

Povidone

Stearic acid

6.2 Incompatibilities

Not applicable

6.3 Shelf life

3 years

6.4 Special precautions for storage

Do not store above 25°C

Blisters: Store in the original package to protect from moisture.

Bottles: Keep the bottle tightly closed to protect from moisture.

6.5 Nature and contents of container

Blisters

Niaspan 375 mg, 500 mg, 750 mg and 1000 mg prolonged-release tablets are packed in individually sealed strips (PVC/Chlortrifluoroethylene/PE/Aluminium).

Blisters of 7, 10, 14, 20, 21, 28, 30, 50, 56, 60, 84, 90, 91, 98, 100 and 105 tablets are available.

Bottles

The Niaspan 500 mg, 750 mg or 1000 mg prolonged-release tablet strengths are packaged in tablet containers (white, round, HDPE bottles). Each container is provided with a silica gel dessicant, a purified cotton wool plug, and a 38 mm child-resistant, PP screw closure. Each container holds 100 tablets.

Not all containers or pack sizes may be marketed.

6.6 Special precautions for disposal and other handling

No special requirements

7. MARKETING AUTHORISATION HOLDER

Abbott Laboratories Ltd

Queenborough

Kent

ME11 5EL

United Kingdom

8. MARKETING AUTHORISATION NUMBER(S)

PL 00037/0636-0639

9. DATE OF FIRST AUTHORISATION/RENEWAL OF THE AUTHORISATION

15 January 2009

10. DATE OF REVISION OF THE TEXT

15 January 2009

Niaspan Prolonged-Release Tablets Starter Pack

(Abbott Laboratories Limited)

1. NAME OF THE MEDICINAL PRODUCT

Niaspan Prolonged-Release Tablets- Starter Pack

2. QUALITATIVE AND QUANTITATIVE COMPOSITION

Starter Pack contains 7 tablets each:

Prolonged-Release Tablets containing 375 mg nicotinic acid

Prolonged-Release Tablets containing 500 mg nicotinic acid

Prolonged-Release Tablets containing 750 mg nicotinic acid

For excipients, see section 6.1.

3. PHARMACEUTICAL FORM

Prolonged-release tablets

White to off-white capsule-shaped tablets. Each tablet is embossed with the tablet strength on one side.

4. CLINICAL PARTICULARS

4.1 Therapeutic indications

Treatment of dyslipidaemia, particularly in patients with combined mixed dyslipidaemia, characterised by elevated levels of LDL-cholesterol and triglycerides and low HDL-cholesterol, and in patients with primary hypercholesterolaemia. Niaspan should be used in patients in combination with HMG-CoA reductase inhibitors (statins), when the cholesterol lowering effect of HMG-CoA reductase inhibitor monotherapy is inadequate. Niaspan can be used as monotherapy only in patients who do not tolerate HMG-CoA reductase inhibitors. Diet and other non-pharmacological treatments (e.g. exercise, weight reduction) should be continued during therapy with Niaspan.

4.2 Posology and method of administration

Niaspan Prolonged-Release Tablets Starter Pack is only a starter pack presentation for initial dose titration.

Niaspan should be taken at bedtime, after a low-fat snack (e.g. an apple, low fat yoghurt, slice of bread) and doses should be individualised according to the patient's response.

Initial dose

Therapy with Niaspan must be initiated with a low dose and increased gradually. The recommended dose escalation schedule is shown below in Table 1:

Table 1: Dose escalation schedule

(see Table 1 below)

Maintenance dose

The recommended maintenance dose is 1000mg (two 500mg tablets) to 2000mg (two 1000mg tablets) once daily at bedtime depending on the patient's response and tolerance. If the response to 1000mg daily is inadequate, the dose may be increased to 1500mg daily and subsequently to 2000mg daily.

The daily dosage of Niaspan should not be increased by more than 500mg in any four-week period after the initial titration to 1000mg. The maximum dose is 2000mg per day.

The different Niaspan tablet strengths have different bioavailability and are therefore not interchangeable.

Niaspan must not be replaced with other nicotinic acid preparations, see section 4.4.

In patients previously treated with other nicotinic acid products, Niaspan treatment must be initiated with the recommended Niaspan dose escalation schedule. The maintenance dose should subsequently be individualised according to the patient's response.

If Niaspan therapy is discontinued for an extended period, re-institution of therapy must include a dose escalation.

Niaspan tablets must not be broken, crushed or chewed before swallowing.

Renal impairment

No studies have been performed in patients with impaired renal function, Niaspan must be used with caution in patients with renal disease.

Hepatic impairment

No studies have been performed in patients with impaired hepatic function. Niaspan must be used with caution in patients with a history of liver disease and who consume substantial quantities of alcohol, see section 4.4. Niaspan is contraindicated in patients with significant hepatic dysfunction, see section 4.3.

Elderly

No dose adjustment is necessary.

Children

The safety and efficacy of nicotinic acid therapy in children and adolescents has not been established. Use in children and adolescents is not recommended.

4.3 Contraindications

Niaspan is contraindicated in patients with

- hypersensitivity to nicotinic acid or to any of the excipients, see section 6.1,
- significant hepatic dysfunction,
- active peptic ulcer disease,
- arterial bleeding.

4.4 Special warnings and precautions for use

Niaspan must not be replaced with other nicotinic acid preparations. When switching from other nicotinic acid preparations to Niaspan, therapy with Niaspan must be initiated with the recommended dose escalation schedule, see section 4.2.

Liver

Nicotinic acid preparations have been associated with abnormal liver tests. Severe hepatic toxicity, including fulminant hepatic necrosis, has occurred in patients who have taken long-acting nicotinic acid products in place of immediate-release nicotinic acid. Since the pharmacokinetics of Niaspan are different to other nicotinic acid preparations, Niaspan must not be replaced with other preparations. The prescribing information of the HMG-CoA reductase inhibitor should also be consulted for warnings and precautions for use.

Caution is advised when Niaspan is used in patients who consume substantial quantities of alcohol and/or have a past history of liver disease.

Elevated liver transaminases have been observed with Niaspan therapy. However, transaminase elevations were reversible upon discontinuation of Niaspan.

Liver tests including AST and ALT must be performed periodically in all patients during therapy with Niaspan and prior to treatment in case of history and/or symptoms of hepatic dysfunction (e.g. jaundice, nausea, fever, and/or malaise). If the transaminase levels show evidence of progression, particularly if they rise to three times the upper limit of normal, the drug must be discontinued.

Skeletal muscle

Single reports on rhabdomyolysis in patients on combined therapy with Niaspan and HMG-CoA reductase inhibitors have been received from spontaneous reporting. Physicians contemplating combined therapy with HMG-CoA reductase inhibitors and Niaspan should carefully weigh the potential benefits and risks and should carefully monitor patients for any symptoms of rhabdomyolysis e.g. muscle pain, tenderness or weakness, particularly during the initial months of therapy and during any periods of upward dosage titration of either drug. Periodic serum creatine phosphokinase (CPK) and potassium determinations should be considered in such situations.

A CPK level should be measured before starting such a combination in patients with pre-disposing factors for rhabdomyolysis, as follows:

- renal impairment
- hypothyroidism
- alcohol abuse
- age > 70 years
- personal or family history of hereditary muscular disorders
- previous history of muscular toxicity with fibrate or HMG-CoA reductase inhibitor

Muscle damage must be considered in any patient presenting with diffuse myalgia, muscle tenderness and/or marked increase in muscle CK levels (>5 × ULN); under these conditions treatment must be discontinued.

The prescribing information of the HMG-CoA reductase inhibitors should be consulted.

Glucose Intolerance

Diabetic or potentially diabetic patients should be observed closely since there may be a dose-related increase in glucose intolerance. Adjustment of diet and/or oral antidiabetics and/or insulin therapy may become necessary.

Unstable angina and acute myocardial infarction

Caution is advised when Niaspan is used in patients with unstable angina or in the acute phase of myocardial infarction, particularly when such patients are also receiving vasoactive drugs such as nitrates, calcium channel blockers, or adrenergic blocking agents.

Uric acid

Elevated uric acid levels have occurred with Niaspan therapy. Monitoring of patients predisposed to gout is recommended.

Coagulation

Niaspan may affect platelet count and prothrombin time, see section 4.5. Patients undergoing surgery should be carefully evaluated. Caution is also advised when Niaspan is administered concomitantly with anti-coagulants; patients receiving anti-coagulants must be monitored closely for prothrombin time and platelet count.

Table 1: Dose escalation schedule

	Week(s)	Dosage		Daily nicotinic acid dose	
↑	1	Niaspan 375mg	1 tablet at bedtime	375mg	↑
INITIAL TITRATION SCHEDULE	2	Niaspan 500mg	1 tablet at bedtime	500mg	TITRATION STARTER PACK
	3	Niaspan 750mg	1 tablet at bedtime	750mg	↓
↓	4-7	Niaspan 500mg	2 tablets at bedtime	1000mg	
		Niaspan 750mg	2 tablets at bedtime	1500mg	
		Niaspan 1000mg	2 tablets at bedtime	2000mg	

Hypophosphataemia

Niaspan has been associated with reductions in phosphorous levels. Although these reductions were transient, monitoring of phosphorous levels is recommended in patients at risk of hypophosphataemia.

Other

Patients with a history of jaundice, hepatobiliary disease, or peptic ulcer should be observed closely during Niaspan therapy.

4.5 Interaction with other medicinal products and other forms of interaction

Concomitant alcohol or hot drinks may increase undesirable flushing and pruritus and should be avoided around the time of Niaspan ingestion.

Niaspan has been associated with small but statistically significant dose-related reductions in platelet count (mean of -11% with 2000mg). In addition, Niaspan has been associated with small but statistically significant increases in prothrombin time (mean of approximately +4%). When Niaspan is administered concomitantly with anti-coagulants, prothrombin time and platelet counts must be monitored closely.

Nicotinic acid may potentiate the blood-pressure lowering effect of ganglionic blocking agents e.g. transdermal nicotine or vasoactive drugs such as nitrates, calcium channel blockers or adrenergic blocking agents.

Bile acid sequestrants bind to other orally administered medicinal products and should be taken separately, see also prescribing information of the concerned product.

Nicotinic acid may produce false elevations in some fluorometric determinations of plasma or urinary catecholamines. Nicotinic acid may also give false-positive reactions with cupric sulphate solution (Benedict's reagent) in urine glucose tests.

Combination of nicotinic acid with HMG-CoA reductase inhibitors may increase the risk for myopathy and rhabdomyolysis, see also section 4.4. The prescribing information of the HMG-CoA reductase inhibitor should also be consulted.

4.6 Pregnancy and lactation

Pregnancy

It is not known whether nicotinic acid at doses typically used for lipid disorders can cause foetal harm when administered to pregnant women or whether it can affect reproductive capacity. Animal studies are incomplete, see section 5.3.

Niaspan should not be prescribed to pregnant women unless strictly necessary.

Lactation

Nicotinic acid has been reported to appear in breast milk. Because of the potential for serious adverse reactions in nursing infants from lipid-altering doses of nicotinic acid, a decision should be made whether to discontinue nursing or to discontinue the drug, taking into account the importance of the drug to the mother. No studies have been conducted with Niaspan in nursing mothers.

4.7 Effects on ability to drive and use machines

Niaspan has no or negligible influence on the ability to drive and use machines.

4.8 Undesirable effects

Flush

In the placebo-controlled clinical trials, flushing episodes (i.e. warmth, redness, itching and/or tingling) were the most common treatment-emergent adverse events for Niaspan (reported by 88% of patients). In these studies fewer than 6% of Niaspan patients discontinued due to flushing.

In comparisons of immediate-release (IR) nicotinic acid and Niaspan, although the number of patients who flushed was similar, fewer flushing episodes were reported by patients who received Niaspan. Following four weeks of maintenance therapy with Niaspan at daily doses of 1500mg, the frequency of flushing over the four week period averaged 1.88 events per patient.

Flushing reactions generally occur during early treatment and the dose titration phase. They are thought to be mediated by the release of prostaglandin D2 and tolerance to flushing usually develops over the course of several weeks.

Spontaneous reports suggest that in rare cases, flushing may be more severe and accompanied by symptoms of dizziness, tachycardia, palpitations, dyspnoea, sweating, chills and/or oedema which in rare cases may lead to syncope. Medical treatment should be administered as necessary.

Hypersensitivity reactions

Hypersensitivity reactions have been reported very rarely. These may be characterised by symptoms such as generalised exanthema, flush, urticaria, vesiculobullous rash, angioedema, laryngospasm, dyspnoea, hypotension, and circulatory collapse. Medical treatment should be administered as necessary.

The following adverse reactions have been observed in clinical studies or in routine patient management, in patients receiving the recommended daily maintenance doses (1000, 1500, and 2000mg) of Niaspan. They are presented by system organ class and frequency grouping (very common >1/10; common >1/100, <1/10; uncommon >1/1,000, <1/100; rare >1/10,000, <1/1,000; very rare <1/10,000, including isolated reports). In general, the incidence of adverse reactions was higher in women compared to men. (Please refer to Table 2 below).

Table 2: Adverse reactions

(see Table 2 below)

4.9 Overdose

Information on acute overdose with Niaspan in humans is limited. The signs and symptoms of an acute overdose are anticipated to be those of excessive pharmacological effect: severe flushing, nausea/vomiting, diarrhoea, dyspepsia, dizziness, syncope, hypotension, potential cardiac arrhythmias and clinical laboratory abnormalities including elevations in liver function tests. The patient should be carefully observed and given supportive treatment. Insufficient information is available on the dialysis potential of nicotinic acid.

5. PHARMACOLOGICAL PROPERTIES

5.1 Pharmacodynamic properties

Pharmacotherapeutic group: nicotinic acid, ATC code: C10AD02

Nicotinic acid is a water-soluble B-complex vitamin which is a naturally occurring constituent of foods. The human body is not entirely dependent on dietary sources of nicotinic acid, since it may also be synthesised from tryptophan.

The mechanism of action by which nicotinic acid modify lipid profiles is not fully elucidated. However, it is recognised that nicotinic acid inhibits the release of free fatty acids from adipose tissue resulting in less free fatty acids being presented to the liver. Since fewer fatty acids are being transported to the liver, fewer are esterified to triglycerides and then incorporated into VLDL. This may lead to a decrease in LDL generation. By increasing lipoprotein lipase activity, nicotinic acid may increase the rate of chylomicron triglycerides removal from plasma. Thus, nicotinic acid decreases the rate of hepatic synthesis of VLDL and subsequently LDL. It does not appear to affect faecal excretion of fats, sterols, or bile acids.

At the recommended maintenance dose, Niaspan (but not nicotinamide) resulted in a clinical reduction in total cholesterol to HDL ratio [-17, to -27%], LDL [-8 to -16%], triglycerides [-14 to -35%] with an increase in HDL [16% to 26%]. In addition to the above mentioned reduction in LDL levels, nicotinic acid causes a shift in LDL composition from the small dense LDL particles (major atherogenic lipoprotein) to the larger, more buoyant LDL particles (less atherogenic). The increase in HDL is also associated with a shift in the distribution of HDL sub-fractions including an

Table 2: Adverse reactions

Organ Class	Very common >1/10	Common >1/100, <1/10	Uncommon >1/1,000, <1/100	Rare >1/10,000, <1/1,000	Very rare <1/10,000, including isolated reports
Immune system disorders					Hypersensitivity reaction
Metabolism and nutrition disorders				Decreased glucose tolerance	Anorexia, gout
Psychiatric disorders				Insomnia, nervousness	
Nervous system disorders			Headache, dizziness	Syncope, paraesthesia	Migraine
Eye disorders				Visual disturbance	Toxic amblyopia, cystoid macular oedema
Cardiac disorders			Tachycardia, palpitations		Atrial fibrillation, other cardiac dysrhythmias
Vascular disorders	Flushing episodes (warmth, redness, itching, tingling)			Hypotension, postural hypotension	Collapse
Respiratory, thoracic and mediastinal disorders			Dyspnoea	Rhinitis	
Gastrointestinal disorders		Diarrhoea, nausea, vomiting, abdominal pain, dyspepsia		Flatulence, eructation	Activation of peptic ulcers, peptic ulceration
Hepatobiliary disorders					Jaundice
Skin and subcutaneous tissue disorders		Pruritus, rash	Sweating, generalised exanthema, urticaria, dry skin	Face oedema, vesiculobullous rash, maculopapular rash	Hyperpigmentation, acanthosis nigricans
Musculoskeletal, connective tissue and bone disorders				Leg cramps, myalgia, myopathy, myasthenia	
General disorders and administration site conditions			Pain, asthenia, chills, peripheral oedema	Chest pain	
Investigations			Elevations in serum transaminases (AST, ALT), alkaline phosphatase, total bilirubin, LDH, amylase, fasting glucose, uric acid; slight reduction in platelet counts, prolongation of prothrombin time, reduction in phosphorus, CK increase		

increase in the HDL2 to HDL3 ratio, the protective effect of HDL being mainly due to HDL2. Moreover, nicotinic acid increases serum levels of apolipoprotein A1 (Apo 1), one of the two major lipoproteins of HDL, while decreases concentrations of apolipoprotein B-100 (Apo B), the major protein component of the very low-density lipoprotein (VLDL) and LDL fractions known to play important roles in atherogenesis. The serum levels of lipoprotein a, [Lp (a)], which present great homology with LDL but considered as an independent risk factor for coronary heart disease, are also significantly reduced by Niaspan.

Data from clinical trials suggest that women have a greater hypolipidaemic response than men at equivalent doses of Niaspan.

There are no specific studies of the combination of Niaspan with statins.

The beneficial effect of Niaspan on morbidity and mortality has not been directly assessed. However, relevant clinical data are available with immediate release (IR) nicotinic acid.

5.2 Pharmacokinetic properties

Absorption

Nicotinic acid is rapidly and extensively absorbed when administered orally (at least 60-76% of dose).

Peak steady-state nicotinic acid concentrations were 0.6, 4.9, and 15.5 microgram/ml after doses of 1000, 1500, and 2000mg Niaspan once daily (given as two 500mg, two 750mg, and two 1000mg tablets, respectively).

Single-dose bioavailability studies have demonstrated that Niaspan tablet strengths are not interchangeable.

Distribution

Studies using radio-labelled nicotinic acid in mice show that nicotinic acid and its metabolites concentrate in the liver, kidney and adipose tissue.

Metabolism

The pharmacokinetic profile of nicotinic acid is complicated due to rapid and extensive first-pass metabolism which is species and dose-rate specific. In humans, one pathway (Pathway 1) is through a simple conjugation step with glycine to form nicotinuric acid (NUA). NUA is then excreted in the urine, although there may be a small amount of reversible metabolism back to nicotinic acid. There is evidence to suggest that nicotinic acid metabolism along this pathway leads to flush. The other pathway (Pathway 2) results in the formation of nicotinamide adenine dinucleotide (NAD). A predominance of metabolism down Pathway 2 may lead to hepatotoxicity. It is unclear whether nicotinamide is formed as a precursor to, or following the synthesis of, NAD. Nicotinamide is further metabolised to at least N-methylnicotinamide (MNA) and nicotinamide N-oxide (NNO). MNA is further metabolised to two other compounds, N-methyl-2-pyridone-5-carboxamide (2PY) and N-methyl-4-pyridone-5-carboxamide (4PY). The formation of 2PY appears to predominate over 4PY in humans. At the doses used to treat hyperlipidaemia, these metabolic pathways are saturable, which explains the non-linear relationship between nicotinic acid dose and plasma concentrations following multiple dose Niaspan administration.

Nicotinamide does not have hypolipidaemic activity; the activity of the other metabolites is unknown.

Elimination

Nicotinic acid and its metabolites are rapidly eliminated in the urine. Following single and multiple doses, approximately 60-76% of the dose administered as Niaspan was recovered in the urine as nicotinic acid and metabolites; up to 12% was recovered as unchanged nicotinic acid after multiple dosing. The ratio of metabolites recovered in the urine was dependent on the dose administered.

Gender differences

Steady state plasma concentrations of nicotinic acid and metabolites after administration of Niaspan are generally higher in women than in men, with the magnitude of difference varying with dose and metabolite. Recovery of nicotinic acid and metabolites in urine, however, is generally similar for men and women, indicating the absorption is similar for both genders. The gender differences observed in plasma levels of nicotinic acid and its metabolites may be due to gender-specific differences in metabolic rate or volume of distribution.

5.3 Preclinical safety data

Nicotinic acid has been shown to be of low toxicity in customary animal studies.

Female rabbits have been dosed with 0.3g nicotinic acid per day from pre-conception to lactation, and gave birth to offspring without teratogenic effects. Further specific animal reproduction studies have not been conducted with nicotinic acid or with Niaspan.

In a life-time study in mice, high dose levels of nicotinic acid showed no treatment-related carcinogenic effects and no effects on survival rates.

6. PHARMACEUTICAL PARTICULARS

6.1 List of excipients

Povidone

Hypromellose

Stearic acid

6.2 Incompatibilities

Not applicable

6.3 Shelf life

3 years

6.4 Special precautions for storage

Do not store above 25°C

Blister: Store in the original package to protect from moisture

6.5 Nature and contents of container

Starter Pack: Niaspan Prolonged Release Tablets Starter Pack are presented in a 21 tablet starter pack containing three weeks supply of medication packed in three individually sealed strips (PVC/Chlortrifluoroethylene/PE/aluminium) as follows:

Week 1: seven Niaspan 375mg Prolonged Release Tablets

Week 2: seven Niaspan 500mg Prolonged Release Tablets

Week 3: seven Niaspan 750mg Prolonged Release Tablets

6.6 Special precautions for disposal and other handling

No special requirements

7. MARKETING AUTHORISATION HOLDER

Abbott Laboratories Ltd

Queenborough

Kent

ME11 5EL

United Kingdom

8. MARKETING AUTHORISATION NUMBER(S)

PL 00037/0635

9. DATE OF FIRST AUTHORISATION/RENEWAL OF THE AUTHORISATION

04th June 2009

10. DATE OF REVISION OF THE TEXT

04th June 2009

Nicam 4% w/w Gel

(Dermal Laboratories Limited)

1. NAME OF THE MEDICINAL PRODUCT

NICAM™ 4% w/w GEL

2. QUALITATIVE AND QUANTITATIVE COMPOSITION

Nicotinamide 4% w/w.

3. PHARMACEUTICAL FORM

Topical gel.

4. CLINICAL PARTICULARS

4.1 Therapeutic indications

For the topical treatment of mild to moderate inflammatory acne vulgaris.

4.2 Posology and method of administration

Apply to the affected area twice daily after the skin has been thoroughly washed with warm water and soap. Enough gel should be used to cover the affected area.

No difference in dose or dose schedule is recommended for adults, children or the elderly.

For topical administration only.

4.3 Contraindications

Contraindicated in persons who have shown hypersensitivity to any of its components.

4.4 Special warnings and precautions for use

For external use only and to be kept away from the eyes and mucous membranes, including those of the nose and mouth. If excessive dryness, irritation or peeling occurs reduce the dosage to one application per day or every other day.

4.5 Interaction with other medicinal products and other forms of interaction

None known.

4.6 Pregnancy and lactation

Vitamin B derivative requirements such as nicotinamide, are increased during pregnancy and infancy. Nicotinamide is excreted in breast milk. As with all medicines, care should be exercised during the first trimester of pregnancy.

4.7 Effects on ability to drive and use machines

None known.

4.8 Undesirable effects

The most frequently encountered adverse effect reported is dryness of the skin. Other less frequent adverse effects include pruritus, erythema, burning sensation and irritation.

4.9 Overdose

Not applicable.

5. PHARMACOLOGICAL PROPERTIES

5.1 Pharmacodynamic properties

Niacin (nicotinic acid) is an essential B complex Vitamin (B_3), whose deficiency results in the clinical syndrome known as pellagra. Nicotinic acid is converted in the body to nicotinamide adenine dinucleotide (NAD) or nicotinamide adenine dinucleotide phosphate (NADP), which function as coenzymes for a wide variety of vital oxidation-reduction reactions. Nicotinamide (niacinamide), the active ingredient, is the physiologically active form of niacin and is the chemical form of Vitamin B_3 found in virtually all multivitamin products. Though nicotinic acid and nicotinamide are so closely related chemically, they differ somewhat in pharmacological properties. Nicotinic acid products exhibit moderately intense cutaneous vasodilation, resulting frequently in mild headaches and flushing or tingling of the skin, but such reactions have not been observed with nicotinamide. Nicotinic acid has also been used for its effect to lower plasma cholesterol, again a property not shared by nicotinamide.

Nicotinamide has demonstrated beneficial effects on inflammatory acne. It is considered that these effects are related to its significant anti-inflammatory activity.

5.2 Pharmacokinetic properties

Following oral administration, nicotinamide is readily absorbed from the gastro-intestinal tract and widely distributed in the body tissues. The main route of metabolism is the conversion to N-methylnicotinamide and the 2-pyridone and 4-pyridone derivatives; nicotinuric acid is also formed. Small amounts of nicotinamide are excreted unchanged in the urine; this amount increases with larger doses.

5.3 Preclinical safety data

Nicotinic acid amide (nicotinamide) has been recognised since 1937 as an essential B complex vitamin whose deficiency results in the clinical syndrome known as pellagra. It is widely available, in tablets and in sterile solution in water for intravenous administration, for the prophylaxis and treatment of pellagra and nutritional deficiency.

In the United States, nicotinamide is included in the Food and Drug Administration's listing of nutritional agents which are Generally Recognised As Safe (GRAS).

6. PHARMACEUTICAL PARTICULARS

6.1 List of excipients

Aluminium Magnesium Silicate; Hypromellose; Citric Acid Anhydrous; Macrogol Lauryl Ether; Ethanol Anhydrous; Purified Water.

6.2 Incompatibilities

None known.

6.3 Shelf life

36 months.

6.4 Special precautions for storage

Do not store above 25°C.

6.5 Nature and contents of container

60g LDPE or co-extruded low density polyethylene laminate tube with white polypropylene cap.

6.6 Special precautions for disposal and other handling

None stated.

7. MARKETING AUTHORISATION HOLDER

Dermal Laboratories

Tatmore Place, Gosmore

Hitchin, Herts SG4 7QR, UK.

8. MARKETING AUTHORISATION NUMBER(S)

00173/0166.

9. DATE OF FIRST AUTHORISATION/RENEWAL OF THE AUTHORISATION

10 September 2002.

10. DATE OF REVISION OF THE TEXT

October 2008.

Nicotinell liquorice 4mg medicated chewing gum

(Novartis Consumer Health)

1. NAME OF THE MEDICINAL PRODUCT

Nicotinell® liquorice 4mg medicated chewing gum

2. QUALITATIVE AND QUANTITATIVE COMPOSITION

One piece of medicated chewing gum contains 4mg nicotine (as 20 mg nicotine – polacrilin (1:4)).

For excipients, see section 6.1

3. PHARMACEUTICAL FORM

Medicated chewing gum.

Each piece of coated chewing gum is off-white in colour and rectangular in shape.

4. CLINICAL PARTICULARS

4.1 Therapeutic indications

Nicotinell gum is indicated for the relief of nicotine withdrawal symptoms, as an aid to smoking cessation.

Concurrent counselling/behavioural support is recommended as it is likely to increase the chances of a successful quit.

4.2 Posology and method of administration

Adults and elderly

Users should stop smoking completely during treatment with Nicotinell gum.

One piece of Nicotinell gum to be chewed when the user feels the urge to smoke. Normally, 8-12 pieces per day can be used, up to a maximum of 15 pieces per day.

The 4 mg chewing gum is intended to be used by smokers with a strong or very strong nicotine dependency and those who have previously failed to stop smoking with the aid of nicotine replacement therapy.

The optimal dosage form is selected according to the following table:

(see Table 1 below)

If an adverse event is noted when high dose forms are initiated, this should be replaced by the lower dosage form.

The characteristics of chewing-gum as a pharmaceutical form are such that individually different nicotine levels can result in the blood. Therefore, dosage frequency should be adjusted according to individual requirements within the stated maximum limit.

Directions for use:

1. One piece of gum should be chewed until the taste becomes strong.
2. The chewing gum should be rested between the gum and cheek.
3. When the taste fades, chewing should commence again.
4. The chewing routine should be repeated for 30 minutes.

The treatment time is individual. Normally, treatment should continue for at least 3 months.

After three months, the user should gradually cut down the number of pieces chewed each day until they have stopped using the product.

Treatment should be discontinued when the dose has been reduced to 1-2 pieces of gum per day. Use of nicotine products like Nicotinell gum beyond 6 months is generally not recommended. Some ex-smokers may need treatment with the gum for longer to avoid returning to smoking. Patients who have been using oral nicotine replacement therapy beyond 9 months are advised to seek additional help and information from health care professionals.

Nicotinell gum is sugar free.

Adolescents (aged 12-18 years of age)

The above recommendation can be used for adolescents aged between 12 and 18 years of age. As data are limited in this age group, medical advice should be obtained should it be found necessary to use the gum beyond 12 weeks.

Concomitant use of acidic beverages such as coffee or soda may decrease the buccal absorption of nicotine. Acidic beverages should be avoided for 15 minutes prior to chewing the gum.

4.3 Contraindications

Hypersensitivity to nicotine or any components of the gum.

Nicotinell gum should not be used by non-smokers.

Due to the presence of liquorice (glycyrrhizin), these gums are contraindicated in pregnancy and lactation (see section 4.6).

4.4 Special warnings and precautions for use

Any risks that may be associated with nicotine replacement therapy are substantially outweighed by the well established dangers of continued smoking.

Precautions: Users should stop smoking completely during therapy with Nicotinell gum. They should be informed that if they continue to smoke while using the gums they may experience increased adverse effects due to the hazards of smoking, including cardiovascular effects.

Cardiovascular disease

In stable cardiovascular disease Nicotinell gum presents a lesser hazard than continuing to smoke. However dependant smokers currently hospitalised as a result of a recent myocardial infarction, severe disrythmia, or recent cerebrovascular accident who are considered to be haemodynamically unstable should be encouraged to stop smoking with non-pharmacological interventions. If this fails, Nicotinell gum may be considered but as data on safety in this patient group are limited, initiation should only be under medical supervision.

Diabetes mellitus

Patients with diabetes mellitus should be advised to monitor their blood sugar levels more closely than usual when nicotine replacement therapy is initiated as catecholamines released by nicotine can affect carbohydrate metabolism.

Allergic reactions

Angioedema and urticaria have been reported.

Gastro-intestinal disease

Swallowed nicotine may exacerbate symptoms in patients suffering from oesophagitis, gastritis, or peptic ulcers and oral nicotine replacement therapy preparations should be used with caution in these conditions. Ulcerative stomatitis have been reported.

Renal and or hepatic impairment

Should be used with caution in patients with moderate to severe hepatic impairment and/or severe renal impairment as the clearance of nicotine or its metabolites may be decreased with the potential for increased adverse effects.

Danger in small children

Doses of nicotine tolerated by adult and adolescent smokers can produce severe toxicity in small children that may be fatal. Products containing nicotine should not be left where they may be misused, handled or ingested by children. Nicotinell gum should be disposed of with care.

Pheochromocytoma and uncontrolled hyperthyroidism

Nicotinell gum should be used with caution in patients with uncontrolled hyperthyroidism or pheochromocytoma as nicotine causes the release of catecholamines.

Transferred dependence

Transferred dependence is rare and is both less harmful and easier to break than smoking dependence.

Stopping smoking

Polycyclic aromatic hydrocarbons in tobacco smoke induce the metabolism of drugs catalysed by CYP 1A2 (and possibly CYP 1A1). When a smoker stops, this may result in slower metabolism and a consequential rise in blood levels of drugs such as theophylline, tacrine, olanzapine and clozapine.

Other warnings

If denture wearers experience difficulty in chewing the gum, it is recommended that they use a different pharmaceutical form of nicotine replacement therapy.

Patients with rare hereditary problems of fructose intolerance should not take this medicine.

Nicotinell 4mg gum contains sorbitol (E420) 0.17g per gum, a source of 0.03g fructose. Calorific value 0.9 kcal/piece of gum.

Nicotinell 4mg gum contains sodium 11.52 mg per piece of gum.

4.5 Interaction with other medicinal products and other forms of interaction

No information is available on interactions between Nicotinell gum and other drugs. No clinically relevant interactions between nicotine replacement therapy and other drugs has definitely been established, however nicotine may possibly enhance the haemodynamic effects of adenosine.

4.6 Pregnancy and lactation

There are no adequate data from the use of preparations containing glycyrrhizin in pregnant and lactating women. Nicotinell Liquorice gum should therefore not be used during pregnancy and lactation. Where use of nicotine replacement therapy is recommended the use other flavoured nicotine gums (e.g. fruit or mint) may be considered.

4.7 Effects on ability to drive and use machines

Not applicable.

4.8 Undesirable effects

Some symptoms such as dizziness, headache and sleep disturbances may be related to the withdrawal of nicotine associated with stopping smoking.

In principle, Nicotinell gums can cause adverse reactions similar to those associated with nicotine administered by other means (including smoking) and these are mainly dose dependant. At recommended doses Nicotinell gum has not been found to cause any serious adverse effects. Excessive consumption of Nicotinell gum by those who have not been in the habit of inhaling tobacco smoke could possibly lead to nausea, faintness or headaches.

Most of the side effects which are reported by patients occur generally during the first 3-4 weeks after initiation of therapy.

Nicotine from gums may sometimes cause a slight irritation of the throat and increase salivation at the start of the treatment.

The gum may stick to and in rare cases damage dentures and dental appliances.

Common ($\geq$ 1/100).

Nervous system disorders: headache, dizziness

Gastrointestinal disorders: hiccups, gastric symptoms e.g. nausea, vomiting, indigestion, heartburn, increased salivation, irritation or sore mouth or throat

Musculoskeletal, connective and bone disorders: jaw muscle ache.

Uncommon (>1/1,000, <1/100)

Cardiac disorders: palpitations

Skin and subcutaneous tissue disorders: erythema, urticaria

Rare (<1/1,000)

Cardiac disorders: cardiac arrhythmias (e.g. atrial fibrillation)

Immune system disorders: hypersensitivity, angioneurotic oedema and anaphylactic reactions.

4.9 Overdose

In overdose, symptoms corresponding to heavy smoking may be seen, however the toxicity of nicotine cannot be directly compared with that of smoking, because tobacco smoke contains additional toxic substances (eg. carbon monoxide and tar).

Overdose with Nicotinell gum may only occur if many pieces are chewed simultaneously. Nicotine toxicity after ingestion will most likely be minimized as a result of early nausea and vomiting that occur following excessive nicotine exposure. Risk of poisoning by swallowing the gum is small. Since the release of nicotine from the gum is slow, very little nicotine is absorbed from the stomach and intestine, and if any is, it will be inactivated in the liver.

Chronic smokers can tolerate doses of nicotine that, in a non-smoker, would be more toxic, because of the development of tolerance.

Symptoms

The minimum lethal dose of nicotine in a non-tolerant man has been estimated to be 40-60mg. Symptoms of acute nicotine poisoning include nausea, salivation, abdominal pain, diarrhoea, sweating, headache, dizziness, disturbed hearing and marked weakness. In extreme cases, these symptoms may be followed by hypotension, rapid or weak or irregular pulse, breathing difficulties, prostration, circulatory collapse and terminal convulsions.

Management of overdose

Following overdose, symptoms may be rapid particularly in children. All nicotine intake should stop immediately and the patient should be treated symptomatically. Artificial respiration with oxygen should be instituted if necessary. Activated charcoal reduces the gastro-intestinal absorption of nicotine.

5. PHARMACOLOGICAL PROPERTIES

5.1 Pharmacodynamic properties

ATC Code: N07B A01

Pharmacotherapeutic group: Drugs used in nicotine dependence

Nicotine, the primary alkaloid in tobacco products and a naturally occurring autonomous substance, is a nicotine receptor agonist in the peripheral and central nervous systems and has pronounced CNS and cardiovascular effects. On consumption of tobacco products, nicotine has proven to be addictive, resulting in craving and other withdrawal symptoms when administration is stopped. This craving and these withdrawal symptoms include a strong urge to smoke, dysphoria, insomnia, irritability, frustration or anger, anxiety, concentration difficulties agitation and increased appetite or weight gain. The gum replaces part of the nicotine that would have been administrated via tobacco and reduces the intensity of the withdrawal symptoms and smoking urge.

5.2 Pharmacokinetic properties

When the gum is chewed, nicotine is steadily released into the mouth and is rapidly absorbed through the buccal mucosa. A proportion, by the swallowing of nicotine containing saliva, reaches the stomach and intestine where it is inactivated.

The nicotine peak plasma mean concentration after a single dose of the 4 mg coated gum is approximately 9.3 nanograms per ml (after 60 minutes) (average plasma concentration of nicotine when smoking a cigarette is 15-30 nanograms per ml).

Nicotine is eliminated mainly via hepatic metabolism; small amounts of nicotine are eliminated in unchanged form via the kidneys. The plasma half-life is approximately three

Table 1

Low to moderate dependency	Moderate to strong dependency	Strong to very strong dependency
Less than 20 cigarettes / day	From 20 to 30 cigarettes / day	Over 30 cigarettes / day
Low dose forms are preferable (2 mg gum)	Low (2 mg gum) or high (4 mg gum) dose forms are acceptable depending on patient characteristics and preference.	High dose forms are preferable (4 mg gum)

Low dosage forms acceptable →

← High dosage forms acceptable

hours. Nicotine crosses the blood-brain barrier, the placenta and is detectable in breast milk.

5.3 Preclinical safety data

No definite conclusion can be drawn on the genotoxic activity of nicotine in vitro. Nicotine was negative in in-vivo tests.

Animal experiments have shown that nicotine induces post-implantation loss and reduces the growth of foetuses.

The results of carcinogenicity assays did not provide any clear evidence of a tumorigenic effect of nicotine.

6. PHARMACEUTICAL PARTICULARS

6.1 List of excipients

Gum base (containing butylhydroxytoluene)
Calcium carbonate
Sorbitol (E420)
Sodium carbonate anhydrous
Sodium hydrogen carbonate
Polacrilin
Glycerol
Purified water
Anise oil
Exctractum Glycyrrhizae soluble
Levomenthol
Eucalyptus oil
Saccharin
Sodium saccharin
Acesulfame potassium
Xylitol
Mannitol (E421)
Gelatin
Titanium dioxide (E171)
Carnauba wax
Talc.

6.2 Incompatibilities

Not applicable.

6.3 Shelf life

2 years

6.4 Special precautions for storage

Do not store above 25°C.

6.5 Nature and contents of container

The chewing-gum is packed in PVC/PVdC/aluminium blisters each containing either 2 or 12 pieces of gum. The blisters are packed in boxes containing 2, 12, 24, 36, 48, 60, 72, 96, 108, 120 & 204 pieces of gum.

Not all pack sizes may be marketed.

6.6 Special precautions for disposal and other handling

No special requirements.

7. MARKETING AUTHORISATION HOLDER

Novartis Consumer Health UK Ltd
Trading as Novartis Consumer Health
Wimblehurst Road,
Horsham,
West Sussex RH12 5AB

8. MARKETING AUTHORISATION NUMBER(S)

PL 00030/0434

9. DATE OF FIRST AUTHORISATION/RENEWAL OF THE AUTHORISATION

14/11/2008

10. DATE OF REVISION OF THE TEXT

14/11/2008

Legal category: GSL

Nicotinell Mint 2mg Lozenge

(Novartis Consumer Health)

1. NAME OF THE MEDICINAL PRODUCT

Nicotinell® Mint 2 mg lozenge

2. QUALITATIVE AND QUANTITATIVE COMPOSITION

Each lozenge contains:

Active substance: 2 mg nicotine (corresponding to 6.144 mg nicotine bitartrate dihydrate).

Excipient(s): aspartame (0.01 g), maltitol (0.9 g).

For a full list of excipients, see section 6.1.

3. PHARMACEUTICAL FORM

Compressed lozenge

White, mint flavoured, round biconvex lozenge.

4. CLINICAL PARTICULARS

4.1 Therapeutic indications

Nicotinell treatment is indicated for the relief of nicotine withdrawal symptoms, in nicotine dependency as an aid to smoking cessation.

Advice and support normally improve the success rate.

4.2 Posology and method of administration

Adults and elderly

Users should stop smoking completely during treatment with Nicotinell lozenge.

Nicotinell Mint 2 mg lozenge is intended to be used by smokers with a strong or very strong nicotine dependency and those who have previously failed to stop smoking with the aid of nicotine replacement therapy.

The optimal dosage form is selected according to the following table:

(see Table 1 below)

If an adverse event is noted when high dose forms are initiated, this should be replaced by the lower dosage form.

The initial dosage should be individualised on the basis of the patients nicotine dependence. One piece of lozenge to suck when the user feels the urge to smoke.

Initially, 1 lozenge should be taken every 1-2 hours. The usual dosage is 8-12 lozenges per day. The maximum daily dose is 15 lozenges.

Directions for use:

1. One lozenge to be sucked until the taste becomes strong.
2. The lozenge should then be lodged between the gum and cheek.
3. When the taste fades, sucking of the lozenge should commence again
4. The sucking routine will be adapted individually and should be repeated until the lozenge dissolves completely (about 30 minutes)

The treatment duration is individual. Normally, treatment should continue for at least 3 months. After 3 months, the user should gradually reduce the number of lozenges or alternatively the user should switch to nicotine 1 mg lozenges and then gradually reduce the number of lozenges per day.

Treatment should be discontinued when the dose has been reduced to 1-2 lozenges per day. Use of nicotine medicinal products like Nicotinell Mint 2 mg lozenge beyond 6 months is generally not recommended. Some ex-smokers may need treatment with the lozenge for longer to avoid returning to smoking. Patients who have been using oral nicotine replacement therapy beyond 9 months are advised to seek additional help and information from health care professionals.

Counselling may help smokers to quit.

Concomitant use of acidic beverages such as coffee or soda may decrease the buccal absorption of nicotine. Acidic beverages should be avoided for 15 minutes prior to sucking the lozenge.

Children and adolescents (≤ 18 years)

Nicotinell lozenge should not be used by people under 18 years of age without recommendation from a physician. There is no experience in treating adolescents under the age of 18 with Nicotinell lozenge.

4.3 Contraindications

Hypersensitivity to any excipients of the lozenge.

Nicotinell lozenge should not be used by non-smokers.

4.4 Special warnings and precautions for use

Dependent smokers with a recent myocardial infarction, unstable or worsening angina including Prinzmetal's angina, severe cardiac arrhythmias, uncontrolled hypertensions or recent cerebrovascular accident should be encouraged to stop smoking with non-pharmacological interventions (such as counselling). If this fails, Nicotinell lozenges may be considered but as data on safety in this patient group are limited, initiation should only be under close medical supervision.

Nicotinell lozenges should be used with caution in patients with hypertension, stable angina pectoris, cerebrovascular disease, occlusive peripheral arterial disease, heart failure, diabetes mellitus, hyperthyroidism or pheochromocytoma and severe hepatic and/or renal impairment.

Patients should initially be encouraged to stop smoking with non-pharmacological interventions (such as counselling).

Swallowed nicotine may exacerbate symptoms in patients suffering from active oesophagitis, oral and pharyngeal inflammation, gastritis or peptic ulcer.

Doses of nicotine that are tolerated by adult smokers during treatment may produce severe symptoms of poisoning in small children and may prove fatal (please see Section 4.9).

Special warnings about excipients

Nicotinell Mint 2 mg lozenges contain sweeteners, including aspartame and maltitol.

Each Nicotinell Mint 2 mg lozenge contains aspartame, a source of phenylalanine equivalent to 5 mg/dose and may be harmful for people with phenylketonuria.

Because Nicotinell Mint 2 mg lozenge contains maltitol (E965):

- patients with rare hereditary problems of fructose intolerance should not take this medicine.
- patients may have a mild laxative effect.

Calorific value 2.3 kcal/g maltitol.

Nicotinell Mint 2 mg lozenge contains 9.8 mg of sodium per piece.

4.5 Interaction with other medicinal products and other forms of interaction

Drug Interactions: No information is available on interactions between Nicotinell lozenge and other medicinal products.

Smoking Cessation: Smoking but not nicotine is associated with increased CYP1A2 activity. After stopping smoking there may be reduced clearance of substrates for this enzyme and increased plasma levels of some medicinal products of potential clinical importance because of their narrow therapeutic window e.g. theophylline, tacrine and clozapine.

The plasma concentrations of other drugs metabolized by CYP1A2 e.g. olanzapine, caffeine, paracetamol, phenazone, phenylbutazone, pentazocine, lidocaine, benzodiazepines, warfarin, oestrogen and vitamin B12 may also increase. However the clinical significance of this effect for these drugs is unknown.

Smoking may lead to reduced analgesic effects of propoxyphene, reduced diuretic response to furosemide (furosemide), reduced effect of propranolol on blood pressure and heart rate reduction and reduced responder rates in ulcer healing with H2-antagonists.

Smoking and nicotine may raise the blood levels of cortisol and catecholamines, i.e. may lead to a reduced effect of nifedipine or adrenergic antagonists and to an increased effect of adrenergic agonists.

Increased subcutaneous absorption of insulin which occurs upon smoking cessation may necessitate a reduction in insulin dose.

4.6 Pregnancy and lactation

Pregnancy

In pregnant women complete cessation of tobacco smoking should always be recommended without nicotine replacement therapy.

Nevertheless, in the case of failure in highly dependent pregnant smokers, tobacco withdrawal via nicotine replacement therapy may be recommended. Indeed, fetal risk is probably lower than that expected with tobacco smoking, due to:

- lower maximal plasma nicotine concentration than with inhaled nicotine
- no additional exposure to polycyclic hydrocarbons and carbon monoxide
- improved chances of quitting smoking by the third trimester.

Smoking continued during the third trimester may lead to intra-uterine growth retardation or even premature birth or stillbirth, depending on the daily amount of tobacco.

Tobacco withdrawal with or without nicotine replacement therapy should not be undertaken alone but as part of a medically supervised smoking cessation program.

In the third trimester nicotine has haemodynamic effects (e.g. changes in fetal heart rate) which could affect the fetus close to delivery. Therefore, after the sixth month of

Table 1

Low to moderate dependency	Moderate to strong dependency	Strong to very strong dependency
Less than 20 cigarettes / day	From 20 to 30 cigarettes / day	Over 30 cigarettes / day
Low dose forms are preferable (1mg lozenge)	Low (1mg lozenge) or high (2mg lozenge) dose forms are acceptable depending on patient characteristics and preference.	High dose forms are preferable (2mg lozenge)

Low dosage forms acceptable

High dosage forms acceptable

pregnancy, the lozenge should only be used under medical supervision in pregnant smokers who have failed to stop smoking by the third trimester.

Lactation

Nicotine is excreted in breast milk in quantities that may affect the child even in therapeutic doses. The lozenge, like smoking itself, should therefore be avoided during breast-feeding. Should smoking withdrawal not be achieved, use of the lozenge by breast feeding smokers should only be initiated after advice from a physician. Where nicotine replacement therapy is used whilst breast-feeding, the lozenge should be taken just after breast-feeding and not during the two hours before breast-feeding.

4.7 Effects on ability to drive and use machines

There is no evidence of any risks associated with driving or operating machinery when the lozenge is used following the recommended dose. Nevertheless smoking cessation can cause behavioural changes.

4.8 Undesirable effects

Nicotinell lozenge can cause adverse reactions similar to those associated with nicotine administered by smoking. These can be attributed to the pharmacological effects of nicotine, which are dose-dependent.

Most of the side effects which are reported by patients occur generally during the first 3-4 weeks after initiation of therapy.

Nicotine from lozenges may sometimes cause a slight irritation of the throat and increase salivation at the start of the treatment. Excessive swallowing of nicotine which is released in the saliva may, at first, cause hiccups. Those with a tendency to indigestion may suffer initially from slight dyspepsia or heartburn.

Slower sucking will usually overcome this problem.

Excessive consumption of lozenges by subjects who have not been in the habit of inhaling tobacco smoke, could possibly lead to nausea, faintness and headache.

Common ($\geqslant$1/100)

Nervous system disorders: Dizziness, headache

Gastrointestinal disorders: Nausea, flatulence, hiccups, gastritis, dry mouth, stomatitis and oesophagitis.

Uncommon ($\geqslant$1/1,000, $<$1/100)

Cardiac disorders: Palpitations

Rare ($\geqslant$ 1/10,000 to $<$1/1,000)

Cardiac disorders: Atrial arrhythmia.

Immune system disorders: hypersensitivity, angioneurotic oedema and anaphylactic reactions.

Certain symptoms which have been reported such as dizziness, headache and insomnia may be ascribed to withdrawal symptoms in connection with smoking cessation and may be due to insufficient administration of nicotine.

Cold sores may develop in connection with smoking cessation, but any relation with the nicotine treatment is unclear.

The patient may still experience nicotine dependence after smoking cessation.

4.9 Overdose

In overdose, symptoms corresponding to heavy smoking may be seen.

The acute lethal oral dose of nicotine is about 0.5 – 0.75 mg per kg body weight, corresponding in an adult to 40 – 60 mg. Even small quantities of nicotine are dangerous in children, and may result in severe symptoms of poisoning which may prove fatal. If poisoning is suspected in a child, a doctor must be consulted immediately.

Overdose with Nicotinell Mint 2 mg lozenge may only occur if many pieces are sucked simultaneously. Nicotine toxicity after ingestion will most likely be minimized as a result of early nausea and vomiting that occur following excessive nicotine exposure.

General symptoms of nicotine poisoning include: weakness, perspiration, salivation, throat burn, nausea, vomiting, diarrhoea, abdominal pain, hearing and visual disturbances, headache, tachycardia and cardiac arrhythmia, dyspnoea, prostration, circulatory collapse, coma and terminal convulsions.

Treatment of overdosage:

Following overdose, symptoms may be rapid particularly in children. Emesis is usually spontaneous. Administration of oral activated charcoal and gastric lavage should be considered as soon as possible and within 1 hour of ingestion. Monitor vital signs and treat symptomatically.

5. PHARMACOLOGICAL PROPERTIES

5.1 Pharmacodynamic properties

ATC Code: N07B A01

Pharmacotherapeutic group: Drugs used in nicotine dependence

Nicotine, the primary alkaloid in tobacco products and a naturally occurring autonomous substance, is a nicotine receptor agonist in the peripheral and central nervous systems and has pronounced CNS and cardiovascular effects. On consumption of tobacco products, nicotine has proven to be addictive, resulting in craving and other withdrawal symptoms when administration is stopped. This craving and these withdrawal symptoms include a strong urge to smoke, dysphoria, insomnia, irritability, frustration or anger, anxiety, concentration difficulties agitation and increased appetite or weight gain. The lozenge replaces part of the nicotine that would have been administrated via tobacco and reduces the intensity of the withdrawal symptoms and smoking urge.

5.2 Pharmacokinetic properties

The absorbed amount of nicotine depends on the amount released into the mouth and absorbed through the buccal mucosa.

The main part of nicotine in Nicotinell Mint 2 mg lozenge is absorbed through the buccal mucosa. A proportion, by the swallowing of nicotine containing saliva, reaches the stomach and intestine where it is inactivated. Due to the first-pass effect in the liver, the systemic bioavailability of nicotine is low. Consequently, in the treatment with Nicotinell Mint 2 mg lozenge the high and quick systemic nicotine concentration, as seen when smoking, is rarely obtained.

Distribution volume after i.v. administration of nicotine is approximately (2-)3 1/kg and the half-life is 2 hours. Nicotine is metabolised principally in the liver and the plasma clearance is approximately 1.2 l/min; nicotine also metabolises in the kidney and lungs. Nicotine crosses the blood-brain barrier.

More than 20 metabolites have been identified, all believed to be less active than nicotine. The main metabolite is cotinine which has a half-life of 15-20 hours and with approximately 10 times higher plasma concentration than nicotine. Nicotine's plasma-protein binding is less than 5%. Changes in nicotine binding from the use of concomitant medicinal products or due to altered disease state are not expected to have significant effect on nicotine kinetics. The main metabolite in urine is cotinine (15% of the dose) and trans-3-hydroxy cotinine (45% of the dose).

About 10% of the nicotine is excreted unchanged. Up to 30% may be excreted with urine in increased diuresis and the acidity under pH 5.

The peak value for the plasma concentration of 2 mg lozenge after a single dose is approximately 7.0 nanogram per ml and the maximal concentration at steady state (one 2 mg lozenge/hour for 12 hours) is approximately 22.5 nanogram per ml (average plasma concentration of nicotine after smoking one cigarette is 15-30 nanogram per ml). Peak plasma concentration is reached after about 48 minutes following sucking of a single lozenge and after about 30 minutes at steady state.

Studies have demonstrated that there is a linear dose-concentration proportionality between the 1 mg and 2 mg Nicotinell lozenges for both C_{max} and AUC. The T_{max} are similar for both strengths.

5.3 Preclinical safety data

Nicotine was positive in some *in-vitro* genotoxicity tests but there are also negative results with the same test systems. Nicotine was negative in standard *in-vivo* tests.

Animal experiments have shown that nicotine induces post-implantation loss and reduces the growth of fetuses.

The results of carcinogenicity assays did not provide any clear evidence of a tumorigenic effect of nicotine.

6. PHARMACEUTICAL PARTICULARS

6.1 List of excipients

Maltitol (E965)

Sodium carbonate anhydrous

Sodium hydrogen carbonate

Polyacrylate dispersion 30 per cent

Xanthan gum

Colloidal anhydrous silica

Levomenthol

Peppermint oil

Aspartame (E951)

Magnesium stearate

6.2 Incompatibilities

Not applicable.

6.3 Shelf life

3 years

6.4 Special precautions for storage

Do not store above 25°C. Store in the original package.

6.5 Nature and contents of container

12, 36, 72, 96, 144 or 204 lozenges in opaque blister packs consisting of aluminium foil and PVC/PE/PVDC/PE/PVC-film. Not all pack sizes may be marketed.

6.6 Special precautions for disposal and other handling

No special requirements.

7. MARKETING AUTHORISATION HOLDER

Novartis Consumer Health UK Ltd

Trading as Novartis Consumer Health

Wimblehurst Road

Horsham

West Sussex

RH12 5AB

8. MARKETING AUTHORISATION NUMBER(S)

PL 00030/0202

9. DATE OF FIRST AUTHORISATION/RENEWAL OF THE AUTHORISATION

31 July 2002 / 2 April 2004

10. DATE OF REVISION OF THE TEXT

10 January 2008

Legal Category:

GSL

Nicotinell mint 4mg medicated chewing gum

(Novartis Consumer Health)

1. NAME OF THE MEDICINAL PRODUCT

Nicotinell® Mint 4mg Medicated Chewing Gum

2. QUALITATIVE AND QUANTITATIVE COMPOSITION

One piece of medicated chewing gum contains 4 mg nicotine (as 20 mg nicotine – polacrilin (1:4)).

For excipients, see section 6.1.

3. PHARMACEUTICAL FORM

Medicated chewing gum.

Each piece of coated chewing gum is off-white in colour and rectangular in shape.

4. CLINICAL PARTICULARS

4.1 Therapeutic indications

Nicotinell gum is indicated for the relief of nicotine withdrawal symptoms, as an aid to smoking cessation. Nicotinell Mint 4mg gum is for use when severe withdrawal symptoms are experienced.

Concurrent counselling/behavioural support is recommended as it is likely to increase the chances of a successful quit.

4.2 Posology and method of administration

Adults and elderly

Users should stop smoking completely during treatment with Nicotinell gum.

One piece of Nicotinell gum to be chewed when the user feels the urge to smoke. Normally, 8-12 pieces per day can be used, up to a maximum of 15 pieces per day.

The 4 mg chewing gum is intended to be used by smokers with a strong or very strong nicotine dependency and those who have previously failed to stop smoking with the aid of nicotine replacement therapy.

The optimal dosage form is selected according to the following table:

(see Table 1 on next page)

If an adverse event is noted when high dose forms are initiated, this should be replaced by the lower dosage form.

The characteristics of chewing-gum as a pharmaceutical form are such that individually different nicotine levels can result in the blood. Therefore, dosage frequency should be adjusted according to individual requirements within the stated maximum limit.

Directions for use:

1. One piece of gum should be chewed until the taste becomes strong.
2. The chewing gum should be rested between the gum and cheek.
3. When the taste fades, chewing should commence again.
4. The chewing routine should be repeated for 30 minutes.

The treatment time is individual. Normally, treatment should continue for at least 3 months.

After three months, the user should gradually cut down the number of pieces chewed each day until they have stopped using the product.

Treatment should be discontinued when the dose has been reduced to 1-2 pieces of gum per day. Use of nicotine products like Nicotinell gum beyond 6 months is generally not recommended. Some ex-smokers may need treatment with the gum for longer to avoid returning to smoking. Patients who have been using oral nicotine replacement therapy beyond 9 months are advised to seek additional help and information from health care professionals.

Nicotinell gum is sugar free.

Adolescents (aged 12-18 years of age)

The above recommendation can be used for adolescents aged between 12 and 18 years of age. As data are limited in this age group, medical advice should be obtained should it be found necessary to use the gum beyond 12 weeks.

Concomitant use of acidic beverages such as coffee or soda may decrease the buccal absorption of nicotine. Acidic beverages should be avoided for 15 minutes prior to chewing the gum.

4.3 Contraindications

Hypersensitivity to nicotine or any components of the gum.

Nicotinell gum should not be used by non-smokers.

4.4 Special warnings and precautions for use

Any risks that may be associated with nicotine replacement therapy are substantially outweighed by the well established dangers of continued smoking.

Table 1

Low to moderate dependency	Moderate to strong dependency	Strong to very strong dependency
Less than 20 cigarettes / day	From 20 to 30 cigarettes / day	Over 30 cigarettes / day
Low dose forms are preferable (2 mg gum)	Low (2 mg gum) or high (4 mg gum) dose forms are acceptable depending on patient characteristics and preference.	High dose forms are preferable (4 mg gum)

Low dosage forms acceptable

High dosage forms acceptable

Precautions: Users should stop smoking completely during therapy with Nicotinell gum. They should be informed that if they continue to smoke while using the gums they may experience increased adverse effects due to the hazards of smoking, including cardiovascular effects.

Cardiovascular disease

In stable cardiovascular disease Nicotinell gum presents a lesser hazard than continuing to smoke. However dependant smokers currently hospitalised as a result of a recent myocardial infarction, severe disrythmia, or recent cerebrovascular accident who are considered to be haemodynamically unstable should be encouraged to stop smoking with non-pharmacological interventions. If this fails, Nicotinell gum may be considered but as data on safety in this patient group are limited, initiation should only be under medical supervision.

Diabetes mellitus

Patients with diabetes mellitus should be advised to monitor their blood sugar levels more closely than usual when nicotine replacement therapy is initiated as catecholamines released by nicotine can affect carbohydrate metabolism.

Allergic reactions

Angioedema and urticaria have been reported.

Gastro-intestinal disease

Swallowed nicotine may exacerbate symptoms in patients suffering from oesophagitis, gastritis, or peptic ulcers and oral nicotine replacement therapy preparations should be used with caution in these conditions. Ulcerative stomatitis have been reported.

Renal and or hepatic impairment

Should be used with caution in patients with moderate to severe hepatic impairment and/or severe renal impairment as the clearance of nicotine or its metabolites may be decreased with the potential for increased adverse effects.

Danger in small children

Doses of nicotine tolerated by adult and adolescent smokers can produce severe toxicity in small children that may be fatal. Products containing nicotine should not be left where they may be misused, handled or ingested by children. Nicotinell gum should be disposed of with care.

Pheochromocytoma and uncontrolled hyperthyroidism

Nicotinell gum should be used with caution in patients with uncontrolled hyperthyroidism or pheochromocytoma as nicotine causes the release of catecholamines.

Transferred dependence

Transferred dependence is rare and is both less harmful and easier to break than smoking dependence.

Stopping smoking

Polycyclic aromatic hydrocarbons in tobacco smoke induce the metabolism of drugs catalysed by CYP 1A2 (and possibly CYP 1A1). When a smoker stops, this may result in slower metabolism and a consequential rise in blood levels of drugs such as theophylline, tacrine, olanzaprine and clozaprine.

Other warnings

If denture wearers experience difficulty in chewing the gum, it is recommended that they use a different pharmaceutical form of nicotine replacement therapy.

Patients with rare hereditary problems of fructose intolerance should not take this medicine.

Nicotinell 4mg gum contains sorbital (E420) 0.2g per gum, a source of 0.04g fructose. Calorific value 0.9 kcal/piece of gum.

Nicotinell 4mg gum contains sodium 11.52 mg per piece of gum.

4.5 Interaction with other medicinal products and other forms of interaction

No information is available on interactions between Nicotinell gum and other drugs. No clinically relevant interactions between nicotine replacement therapy and other drugs has definitely been established, however nicotine may possibly enhance the haemodynamic effects of adenosine.

4.6 Pregnancy and lactation

Pregnancy

Smoking during pregnancy is associated with risks such as intra-uterine growth retardation, premature birth or still birth. Stopping smoking is the single most effective intervention for improving the health of the pregnant smoker and her baby. The earlier abstinence is achieved the better.

Ideally smoking cessation during pregnancy should be achieved without nicotine replacement therapy. For women unable to quit on their own nicotine replacement therapy may be recommended to assist a quit attempt. The risk of using nicotine replacement therapy to the foetus is lower than that expected with tobacco smoking, due to lower maximal plasma concentrations and no additional exposure to polycyclic hydrocarbons and carbon monoxide.

However as nicotine passes to the foetus affecting breathing movements and has a dose-dependant effect on placental/foetal circulation, the decision to use nicotine replacement therapy should be made on a risk-benefit assessment as early on in pregnancy as possible with the aim of discontinuing use after 2-3 months.

Intermittent dose products may be preferable as these usually provide a lower daily dose of nicotine than patches. However, patches may be preferred if the woman is suffering from nausea during pregnancy. If patches are used they should be removed before going to bed to avoid exposure overnight when the foetus would not normally be subjected to smoke derived nicotine.

Lactation

Nicotine from smoking and nicotine replacement therapy is found in breast milk. However the amounts of nicotine the infant is exposed to is relatively small and less hazardous than the second-hand smoke they would otherwise be exposed to.

Using intermittent dose products, compared to patches, may minimize the amount of nicotine in the breast milk as the time between administrations of nicotine replacement therapy and feeding can be more easily prolonged.

4.7 Effects on ability to drive and use machines

Not applicable.

4.8 Undesirable effects

Some symptoms such as dizziness, headache and sleep disturbances may be related to the withdrawal of nicotine associated with stopping smoking.

In principle, Nicotinell gums can cause adverse reactions similar to those associated with nicotine administered by other means (including smoking) and these are mainly dose dependant. At recommended doses Nicotinell gum has not been found to cause any serious adverse effects. Excessive consumption of Nicotinell gum by those who have not been in the habit of inhaling tobacco smoke could possibly lead to nausea, faintness or headaches.

Most of the side effects which are reported by patients occur generally during the first 3-4 weeks after initiation of therapy.

Nicotine from gums may sometimes cause a slight irritation of the throat and increase salivation at the start of the treatment.

The gum may stick to and in rare cases damage dentures and dental appliances.

Common (> 1/100).

Nervous system disorders: headache, dizziness

Gastrointestinal disorders: hiccups, gastric symptoms e.g. nausea, vomiting, indigestion, heartburn, increased salivation, irritation or sore mouth or throat.

Musculoskeletal, connective and bone disorders: jaw muscle ache.

Uncommon (>1/1,000, <1/100)

Cardiac disorders: palpitations

Skin and subcutaneous tissue disorders: erythema, urticaria

Rare (<1/1,000)

Cardiac disorders: cardiac arrhythmias (e.g. atrial fibrillation)

Immune system disorders: hypersensitivity, angioneurotic oedema and anaphylactic reactions.

4.9 Overdose

In overdose, symptoms corresponding to heavy smoking may be seen, however the toxicity of nicotine cannot be directly compared with that of smoking, because tobacco smoke contains additional toxic substances (eg. carbon monoxide and tar).

Overdose with Nicotinell gum may only occur if many pieces are chewed simultaneously. Nicotine toxicity after ingestion will most likely be minimized as a result of early nausea and vomiting that occur following excessive nicotine exposure. Risk of poisoning by swallowing the gum is small. Since the release of nicotine from the gum is slow, very little nicotine is absorbed from the stomach and intestine, and if any is, it will be inactivated in the liver.

Chronic smokers can tolerate doses of nicotine that, in a non-smoker, would be more toxic, because of the development of tolerance.

Symptoms

The minimum lethal dose of nicotine in a non-tolerant man has been estimated to be 40-60mg. Symptoms of acute nicotine poisoning include nausea, salivation, abdominal pain, diarrhoea, sweating, headache, dizziness, disturbed hearing and marked weakness. In extreme cases, these symptoms may be followed by hypotension, rapid or weak or irregular pulse, breathing difficulties, prostration, circulatory collapse and terminal convulsions.

Management of overdose

Following overdose, symptoms may be rapid particularly in children. All nicotine intake should stop immediately and the patient should be treated symptomatically. Artificial respiration with oxygen should be instituted if necessary. Activated charcoal reduces the gastro-intestinal absorption of nicotine.

5. PHARMACOLOGICAL PROPERTIES

5.1 Pharmacodynamic properties

ATC Code: N07B A01

Pharmacotherapeutic group: Drugs used in nicotine dependence

Nicotine, the primary alkaloid in tobacco products and a naturally occurring autonomous substance, is a nicotine receptor agonist in the peripheral and central nervous systems and has pronounced CNS and cardiovascular effects. On consumption of tobacco products, nicotine has proven to be addictive, resulting in craving and other withdrawal symptoms when administration is stopped. This craving and these withdrawal symptoms include a strong urge to smoke, dysphoria, insomnia, irritability, frustration or anger, anxiety, concentration difficulties agitation and increased appetite or weight gain. The gum replaces part of the nicotine that would have been administrated via tobacco and reduces the intensity of the withdrawal symptoms and smoking urge.

5.2 Pharmacokinetic properties

When the gum is chewed, nicotine is steadily released into the mouth and is rapidly absorbed through the buccal mucosa. A proportion, by the swallowing of nicotine containing saliva, reaches the stomach and intestine where it is inactivated.

The nicotine peak plasma mean concentration after a single dose of the 4 mg coated gum is approximately 9.3 nanograms per ml (after approximately 60 minutes) (average plasma concentration of nicotine when smoking a cigarette is 15-30 nanograms per ml).

Nicotine is eliminated mainly via hepatic metabolism; small amounts of nicotine are eliminated in unchanged form via the kidneys. The plasma half-life is approximately three hours. Nicotine crosses the blood-brain barrier, the placenta and is detectable in breast milk.

5.3 Preclinical safety data

No definite conclusion can be drawn on the genotoxic activity of nicotine in vitro. Nicotine was negative in in-vivo tests.

Animal experiments have shown that nicotine induces post-implantation loss and reduces the growth of foetuses.

The results of carcinogenicity assays did not provide any clear evidence of a tumorigenic effect of nicotine.

6. PHARMACEUTICAL PARTICULARS

6.1 List of excipients

Gum base (containing butylhydroxytoluene)
Calcium carbonate
Sorbitol (E420)
Sodium carbonate anhydrous
Sodium hydrogen carbonate
Polacrilin
Glycerol
Purified water
Levomenthol
Peppermint oil
Eucalyptus oil
Saccharin
Sodium saccharin
Acesulfame potassium
Xylitol
Mannitol (E421)
Gelatin
Titanium dioxide (E171)
Carnauba wax
Talc.

6.2 Incompatibilities
Not applicable.

6.3 Shelf life
2 years.

6.4 Special precautions for storage
Do not store above 25°C.

6.5 Nature and contents of container
The chewing-gum is packed in PVC/PVdC/aluminium blisters each containing either 2 or 12 pieces of gum. The blisters are packed in boxes containing 2, 12, 24, 36, 48, 60, 72, 96 108, 120 and 204 pieces of gum.

Not all pack sizes may be marketed.

6.6 Special precautions for disposal and other handling
No special requirements.

7. MARKETING AUTHORISATION HOLDER
Novartis Consumer Health UK Ltd

Trading as Novartis Consumer Health

Wimblehurst Road,

Horsham,

West Sussex RH12 5AB

8. MARKETING AUTHORISATION NUMBER(S)
PL 00030/0428

9. DATE OF FIRST AUTHORISATION/RENEWAL OF THE AUTHORISATION
8 December 2006

10. DATE OF REVISION OF THE TEXT
12 June 2008

Legal category: GSL

Nicotinell TTS 30

(Novartis Consumer Health)

1. NAME OF THE MEDICINAL PRODUCT
Nicotinell® TTS 30

2. QUALITATIVE AND QUANTITATIVE COMPOSITION
Each Nicotinell TTS 30 patch contains 52.5 mg S(-)-nicotine which provides an average absorption rate of 21 mg nicotine in 24 hours.

3. PHARMACEUTICAL FORM
Transdermal patch.

The Nicotinell TTS patch is a transdermal therapeutic system, consisting of a round, flat, matrix-type self-adhesive, yellowish-ochre coloured patch. It is protected by a rectangular metallic release liner backing to be discarded before application.

Nicotinell TTS 30 patch 21mg/24 Hour has a drug releasing area of 30 cm^2 and is printed CG EME on the patch surface.

4. CLINICAL PARTICULARS

4.1 Therapeutic indications
Relief of nicotine withdrawal symptoms as an aid to smoking cessation.

Concurrent counselling/behavioural support is recommended as it is likely to increase the chances of a successful quit attempt

Route of administration: transdermal.

4.2 Posology and method of administration
Adults:

Users should stop smoking completely during treatment with Nicotinell TTS patch.

For individuals smoking 20 cigarettes or more a day, it is recommended that treatment be started with Nicotinell TTS 30 (Step 1) once daily, applied to a dry non-hairy area of the skin on the trunk or upper arm. Those smoking less than this are recommended to start with Nicotinell TTS 20 (Step 2). Sizes of 30cm^2, 20cm^2 and 10cm^2 are available to permit gradual withdrawal of nicotine replacement, using treatment periods of 3-4 weeks (for each size). The size of patch may be adjusted according to individual response, maintaining or increasing the dose if abstinence is not achieved or if withdrawal symptoms are experienced. Total treatment periods of more than 3 months and daily doses above 30cm^2 have not been evaluated. The treatment is designed to be used continuously for 3 months but not beyond. However, if abstinence is not achieved at the end of the 3 month treatment period, further treatments may be recommended.

Those who use nicotine replacement therapy beyond 9 months are recommended to seek additional help and advice from a healthcare professional.

The dosage must not be adjusted by cutting a patch.

The patch should be used as soon as it has been removed from the child-resistant pouch. Following removal of the metallic backing, the patch should be applied to the skin and held in position for 10-20 seconds with the palm of the hand. Each patch should be removed after 24 hours and disposed of safely (see "Warnings"). A different site of application should be chosen each day and several days should be allowed to elapse before a new patch is applied to the same area of skin.

Use for 24 hours optimizes the effect against morning cravings but in pregnant patients, it is recommended that the patch is removed before going to bed (see section 4.6)

Children and young adults:

The above recommendation can be used for adolescences between 12 and 18 years of age. As data are limited in this age group, medical advice should be obtained should it be found necessary to use the patch beyond 12 weeks.

Elderly:

Experience in the use of these patches in smokers over the age of 65 years is limited. Nicotinell TTS does not appear to pose safety problems in this age group.

Potential for abuse and dependence:

Transdermal nicotine is likely to have a very low abuse potential (see also section 4.4 *Transferred Dependence*) because of its slow onset of action, low fluctuations in blood concentrations, inability to produce high blood concentrations of nicotine, and the infrequent (once daily) use. Moreover, gradual weaning from the patches is instituted within the treatment schedule, and the risk of dependence after therapy is minimal. The effects of abrupt withdrawal from Nicotinell TTS are likely to be similar to those observed with tobacco withdrawal from comparable nicotine concentrations.

4.3 Contraindications
Nicotinell TTS should not be administered to non-smokers or occasional smokers. The system is contraindicated in diseases of the skin which may complicate patch therapy, and known hypersensitivity to nicotine or any of the components of the patch.

4.4 Special warnings and precautions for use
Any risks that may be associated with nicotine replacement therapy are substantially outweighed by the well established dangers of continued smoking.

Precautions: Users should stop smoking completely during therapy with Nicotinell TTS. They should be informed that if they continue to smoke while using the patches, they may experience increased adverse effects due to the hazards of smoking, including cardiovascular effects.

Underlying cardiovascular disease

In stable cardiovascular disease Nicotinell TTS presents a lesser hazard than continuing to smoke. However dependent smokers currently hospitalized as a result of a recent myocardial infarction, severe dysrhythmia or recent cerebrovascular accident and who are considered to be haemodynamically unstable should be encouraged to stop smoking with non-pharmacological interventions. If this fails, Nicotinell TTS may be considered but as data on safety in this patient group are limited, initiation should only be under medical supervision.

Diabetes mellitus

Patients with diabetes mellitus should be advised to monitor their blood sugar levels more closely than usual when nicotine replacement therapy is initiated as catecholamines released by nicotine can affect carbohydrate metabolism.

Allergic reactions

Discontinuation of treatment may be advisable in cases of severe or persistent allergic reactions.

Angioedema and urticaria have been reported. Contact sensitisation was reported in a few patients using transdermal nicotine in clinical trials. Patients who develop contact sensitisation to nicotine should be cautioned that a severe reaction could occur from smoking or exposure to other nicotine containing products.

Renal and or hepatic impairment

Should be used in caution in patients with moderate to severe hepatic impairment and/or severe impairment as the clearance of nicotine or its metabolites may be decreased with the potential for increased adverse effects.

Gastro-Intestinal disease

Nicotinell TTS should be used with caution in patients with peptic ulcers.

Pheochromocytoma and uncontrolled hyperthyroidism

Nicotinell TTS should be used with caution in patients with uncontrolled hyperthyroidism or pheochromocytoma as nicotine causes release of catecholamines.

Transferred dependence

Transferred dependence is rare and is both less harmful and easier to break than smoking dependence.

Danger in small children

Doses of nicotine that are tolerated by adult and adolescent smokers can produce severe toxicity in small children that may be fatal. Both before and after use, the patch contains a significant amount of nicotine. Subjects must be cautioned that the patches must not be handled casually or left where they might be inadvertently misused or consumed by children. Used patches must be disposed of with care by folding them in half with the adhesive sides inwards, and ensuring that they do not fall into the hands of children under any circumstances.

Stopping smoking

Polycyclic aromatic hydrocarbons in tobacco smoke induce the metabolism of drugs catalysed by CYP 1A2 (and possibly by CYP 1A1). When a smoker stops, this may result in slower metabolism and a consequent rise in blood levels of such drugs.

4.5 Interaction with other medicinal products and other forms of interaction
No information is available on interactions between Nicotinell TTS and other drugs. No clinically relevant interactions between nicotine replacement therapy and other drugs has definitely been established, however nicotine may possibly enhance the haemodynamic effects of adenosine.

4.6 Pregnancy and lactation
Pregnancy

Smoking during pregnancy is associated with risks such as intra-uterine growth retardation, premature birth or still birth. Stopping smoking is the single most effective intervention for improving the health of both pregnant smoker and her baby. The earlier abstinence is achieved the better.

Ideally smoking cessation during pregnancy should be achieved without nicotine replacement therapy. For women unable to quit on their own, nicotine replacement therapy may be recommended to assist a quit attempt. The risk of using nicotine replacement therapy to the foetus is lower than that expected with tobacco smoking, due to lower maximal plasma nicotine concentrations and no additional exposure to polycyclic hydrocarbons and carbon monoxide.

As nicotine passes to the foetus affecting breathing movements and has a dose-dependent effect on the placental/foetal circulation, the decision to use nicotine replacement therapy should be made on a risk-benefit assessment as early on in pregnancy as possible with the aim of discontinuing use after 2-3 months.

Intermittent dose products may be preferable as these usually provide a lower daily dose of nicotine than patches. However, patches may be preferred if the woman is suffering from nausea during pregnancy. If patches are used they should be removed before going to bed to avoid exposure overnight, when the foetus would not normally be subjected to smoke-derived nicotine).

Lactation

Nicotine from smoke and nicotine replacement therapy is found in breast milk. However the amounts of nicotine the infant is exposed to is relatively small and less hazardous than the second-hand smoke they would otherwise be exposed to.

Using intermittent dose products, compared to patches, may minimize the amount of nicotine in the breast milk as the time between administrations of nicotine replacement therapy and feeding can be more easily prolonged.

4.7 Effects on ability to drive and use machines
Not applicable.

4.8 Undesirable effects
In principle, the Nicotinell TTS can cause adverse reactions similar to those associated with nicotine administered by other means (including smoking) and these are mainly dose dependent. Some symptoms such as dizziness, headache, and sleep disturbance may be related to the withdrawal of nicotine associated with stopping smoking. Since the maximum plasma concentrations of nicotine that are produced by the patch are lower than those produced by smoking and fluctuate less, nicotine-related adverse reactions occurring during treatment with the patch can be expected to be less marked than during smoking.

At recommended doses Nicotinell TTS has not been found to cause any serious adverse effects. Excessive consumption of Nicotinell TTS by those who have not been in the habit of inhaling tobacco smoke could possibly lead to nausea, faintness or headaches.

Some of the symptoms listed below are hard to differentiate from recognised tobacco withdrawal symptoms when comparison with placebo is made. The placebo used contained about 13% of the nicotine of a matching Nicotinell TTS (to match colour and odour for blinding purposes).

The main unwanted effect of Nicotinell TTS is application site reaction. This led to premature discontinuation of patches in about 6% of clinical trial participants. Skin reactions consisted of erythema or pruritus at the patch site. Oedema, burning sensation, blisters, rash, or pinching sensation at the application site was also noted. The majority of these reactions were mild. Most of the skin reactions resolved within 48 hours, but in more severe cases the erythema and infiltration lasted from 1 to 3 weeks. The time of onset of important skin reactions was between 3 and 8 weeks from the start of therapy. In isolated cases the skin reactions extended beyond the application sites. Isolated cases of urticaria, angioneurotic oedema and dyspnoea were reported.

The following are the adverse events/withdrawal symptoms most commonly reported in three double-blind clinical trials irrespective of causal association to study drug.

	Nicotinell TTS (N=401)	Placebo (N=391)
Application site reaction	34.9%	17.6%
Headache	29.7%	29.2%
Cold and flu-like symptoms	12.0%	8.4%

Dysmenorrhoea (% of female subjects)	6.6%	8.8%
Insomnia	6.5%	5.4%
Nausea	6.2%	4.6%
Myalgia	6.0%	4.1%
Dizziness	6.0%	5.9%

Other unwanted experiences reported (irrespective of causal association with Nicotinell TTS) with an incidence of 1% - 5.9% and more frequently than placebo, included: abdominal pain, vomiting, dyspepsia, allergy, motor dysfunction, chest pain, vivid dreams, blood pressure changes, generalised rash, somnolence, impaired concentration and fatigue.

4.9 Overdose

The toxicity of nicotine cannot be directly compared with that of smoking, because tobacco smoke contains additional toxic substances (eg carbon monoxide, and tar).

Chronic smokers can tolerate doses of nicotine that, in a non-smoker, would be more toxic, because of the development of tolerance.

Symptoms

The minimum lethal dose of nicotine in a non-tolerant man has been estimated to be 40 to 60 mg. Symptoms of acute nicotine poisoning include nausea, salivation, abdominal pain, diarrhoea, sweating, headache, dizziness, disturbed hearing and marked weakness. In extreme cases, these symptoms may be followed by hypotension, rapid or weak or irregular pulse, breathing difficulties, prostration, circulatory collapse and terminal convulsions.

Management of overdose

If the patient shows signs of overdose, the patch should be removed immediately. The skin surface may be washed with water and dried (no soap should be used). The skin will continue to deliver nicotine into the blood stream for several hours after removal of the system, possibly because of a depot of nicotine in the skin. Tthe patient should then be treated symptomatically. Artificial respiration with oxygen should be instituted if necessary.

5. PHARMACOLOGICAL PROPERTIES

5.1 Pharmacodynamic properties

S(-)-nicotine is the most pharmacologically active form of nicotine, the major alkaloid of tobacco. S(-)-nicotine acts primarily on cholinergic receptors of the nicotinic type in the peripheral and central nervous system. For many effects, low doses of S(-)-nicotine have a stimulant action, and high doses a depressant effect. Intermittent administration of S(-)-nicotine affects neurohormonal pathways, and results in the release of acetylcholine, noradrenaline, dopamine, serotinin, vasopressin, beta-endorphin, growth hormone, cortisol and ACTH. These neuroregulators may be involved in the reported behavioral and subjective effects of smoking.

Nicotine replacement therapy is an established therapy as an aid to smoking cessation. Nicotinell TTS provides for a convenient once daily administration by exploiting the fact that S(-)-nicotine is readily absorbed through the skin into the systemic circulation. Placebo-controlled, double-blind studies have shown that nicotine replacement therapy with the patch produces smoking abstinence rates statistically significantly better than placebo, with or without group support. There was also a strong trend towards reduction of withdrawal symptoms.

Application of Nicotinell TTS to smokers abstinent overnight resulted in small increases in mean heart rate and systolic blood pressure and a decrease in stroke volume. The effects were smaller in magnitude than those produced by cigarette smoking.

5.2 Pharmacokinetic properties

Following a single application of the Nicotinell TTS to the skin of healthy abstinent smokers there is an initial 1-2 hours delay followed by a progressive rise in nicotine plasma concentrations, with a plateau attained at about 8-10 hours after application.

In the majority of subjects the area under the plasma concentration curve (AUC 0-24 hours) varies approximately in proportion to the drug releasing area of the patch. The patch is designed to deliver approximately 0.7mg/cm^2/24 hours. In comparison with an i.v. infusion, 76.8% of the nicotine released from the Nicotinell TTS is systemically available. Steady state plasma concentrations after repeated daily administration are within the range observed during moderate cigarette smoking.

Absorption of nicotine over 24 hours varies by a factor of two between different individuals; however within-individual variability is small indicating consistent performance of the transdermal system.

S(-)-nicotine is distributed widely in the body with a volume of distribution of approximately 180 litres. It crosses the blood-brain barrier, placenta and is detectable in breast milk. Plasma protein binding is only 5%. Total plasma clearance of nicotine ranges from 0.92 to 2.43 litres/min. It is eliminated mainly via hepatic metabolism. Only small amounts of nicotine are eliminated in unchanged form via the kidneys, a process which is pH dependent, being negligible under alkaline conditions.

5.3 Preclinical safety data

No additional data.

6. PHARMACEUTICAL PARTICULARS

6.1 List of excipients

Pad

Polyester film

Acrylate esters vinylacetate co-polymers

Fractionated coconut oil

Methacrylic acid esters co-polymers

Aluminised polyester backing film

Aluminised and siliconised polyester film release liner.

6.2 Incompatibilities

None known.

6.3 Shelf life

36 months.

6.4 Special precautions for storage

Do not store above 25°C

6.5 Nature and contents of container

Heat-seal paper/aluminium/polyamide/polyacrylnitrile pouches (child-resistant) enclosed in a cardboard carton.

or

Heat-sealed paper/ aluminium polyacrylnitrile pouches. Each pouch is enclosed within a child-resistant sachet. Sachets are packed in a cardboard container.

Nicotinell TTS 30 are available in pack sizes of: 2, 3, 7, 14, 21 & 28 patches.

Not all pack sizes may be marketed.

6.6 Special precautions for disposal and other handling

Keep all medicines out of the reach of children.

7. MARKETING AUTHORISATION HOLDER

Novartis Consumer Health UK Limited

Wimblehurst Road

Horsham

West Sussex

RH12 5AB

Trading as: Novartis Consumer Health.

8. MARKETING AUTHORISATION NUMBER(S)

PL 00030/0109

9. DATE OF FIRST AUTHORISATION/RENEWAL OF THE AUTHORISATION

Date of first authorisation: 1 August 1997

Date of last renewal: 11 February 1998

10. DATE OF REVISION OF THE TEXT

8 September 2008

Legal category

GSL

Nimbex Forte Injection 5mg/ml

(GlaxoSmithKline UK)

1. NAME OF THE MEDICINAL PRODUCT

Nimbex Forte 5mg/ml, solution for injection.

2. QUALITATIVE AND QUANTITATIVE COMPOSITION

AND QUANTITATIVE COMPOSITION

Cisatracurium 5mg as cisatracurium besilate 6.70mg per 1ml

One vial of 30ml contains 150mg of cisatracurium

For excipients, see Section 6.1.

3. PHARMACEUTICAL FORM

Solution for Injection.

Colourless to pale yellow or greenish yellow solution. Practically free from visible particulate matter.

4. CLINICAL PARTICULARS

Nimbex is an intermediate-duration, non-depolarising neuromuscular blocking agent for intravenous administration.

4.1 Therapeutic indications

Nimbex is indicated for use during surgical and other procedures and in intensive care. Nimbex can be used as an adjunct to general anaesthesia, or sedation in the Intensive Care Unit (ICU) to relax skeletal muscles, and to facilitate tracheal intubation and mechanical ventilation.

4.2 Posology and method of administration

Please note that Nimbex should not be mixed in the same syringe or administered simultaneously through the same needle as propofol injectable emulsion or with alkaline solutions such as sodium thiopentone. (see section 6.2).

Nimbex contains no antimicrobial preservative and is intended for single patient use.

4.2.1 Monitoring advice

As with other neuromuscular blocking agents, monitoring of neuromuscular function is recommended during the use of Nimbex in order to individualise dosage requirements.

4.2.2 Use by intravenous bolus injection

4.2.2.1 Dosage in adults

Tracheal Intubation. The recommended intubation dose of Nimbex for adults is 0.15mg/kg (body weight). This dose produced good to excellent conditions for tracheal intubation 120 seconds after administration of Nimbex, following induction of anaesthesia with propofol.

Higher doses will shorten the time to onset of neuromuscular block.

The following table summarises mean pharmacodynamic data when Nimbex was administered at doses of 0.1 to 0.4mg/kg (body weight) to healthy adult patients during opioid (thiopentone/fentanyl/midazolam) or propofol anaesthesia.

(see Table 1 on next page)

Enflurane or isoflurane anaesthesia may extend the clinically effective duration of an initial dose of Nimbex by as much as 15%.

Maintenance. Neuromuscular block can be extended with maintenance doses of Nimbex. A dose of 0.03 mg/kg (body weight) provides approximately 20 minutes of additional clinically effective neuromuscular block during opioid or propofol anaesthesia.

Consecutive maintenance doses do not result in progressive prolongation of effect.

Spontaneous Recovery. Once spontaneous recovery from neuromuscular block is underway, the rate is independent of the Nimbex dose administered. During opioid or propofol anaesthesia, the median times from 25 to 75% and from 5 to 95% recovery are approximately 13 and 30 minutes, respectively.

Reversal. Neuromuscular block following Nimbex administration is readily reversible with standard doses of anticholinesterase agents. The mean times from 25 to 75% recovery and to full clinical recovery (T_4:T_1 ratio $\geq$ 0.7) are approximately 4 and 9 minutes respectively, following administration of the reversal agent at an average of 10% T_1 recovery.

4.2.2.2 Dosage in paediatric patients

Tracheal Intubation (paediatric patients aged 1 month to 12 years): As in adults, the recommended intubation dose of Nimbex is 0.15 mg/kg (body weight) administered rapidly over 5 to 10 seconds. This dose produces good to excellent conditions for tracheal intubation 120 seconds following injection of Nimbex. Pharmacodynamic data for this dose are presented in the tables below.

Nimbex has not been studied for intubation in ASA Class III-IV paediatric patients. There are limited data on the use of Nimbex in paediatric patients under 2 years of age undergoing prolonged or major surgery.

In paediatric patients aged 1 month to 12 years, Nimbex has a shorter clinically effective duration and a faster spontaneous recovery profile than those observed in adults under similar anaesthetic conditions. Small differences in the pharmacodynamic profile were observed between the age ranges 1 to 11 months and 1 to 12 years which are summarised in the tables below:

Paediatric Patients aged 1 to 11 months

(see Table 2 on next page)

Paediatric Patients aged 1 to 12 years

(see Table 3 on next page)

When Nimbex is not required for intubation: A dose of less than 0.15mg/kg can be used. Pharmacodynamic data for doses of 0.08 and 0.1 mg/kg for paediatric patients aged 2 to 12 years are presented in the table below:

(see Table 4 on next page)

Administration of Nimbex following suxamethonium has not been studied in paediatric patients (see section 4.5).

Halothane may be expected to extend the clinically effective duration of a dose of Nimbex by up to 20%. No information is available on the use of Nimbex in children during anaesthesia with other halogenated fluorocarbon anaesthetic agents, but these agents may also be expected to extend the clinically effective duration of a dose of Nimbex.

Maintenance (paediatric patients aged 2-12 years). Neuromuscular block can be extended with maintenance doses of Nimbex. In paediatric patients aged 2 to 12 years, a dose of 0.02 mg/kg (body weight) provides approximately 9 minutes of additional clinically effective neuromuscular block during halothane anaesthesia. Consecutive maintenance doses do not result in progressive prolongation of effect.

There are insufficient data to make a specific recommendation for maintenance dosing in paediatric patients under 2 years of age. However, very limited data from clinical studies in paediatric patients under 2 years of age suggest that a maintenance dose of 0.03mg/kg may extend clinically effective neuromuscular block for a period of up to 25 minutes during opioid anaesthesia.

Spontaneous Recovery. Once recovery from neuromuscular block is underway, the rate is independent of the Nimbex dose administered. During opioid or halothane anaesthesia, the median times from 25 to 75% and from 5 to 95% recovery are approximately 11 and 28 minutes, respectively.

Reversal. Neuromuscular block following Nimbex administration is readily reversible with standard doses of anticholinesterase agents. The mean times from 25 to 75% recovery and to full clinical recovery (T_4:T_1 ratio $\geq$ 0.7) are approximately 2 and 5 minutes respectively, following

Table 1

Initial Nimbex Dose mg/kg (body weight)	Anaesthetic Background	Time to 90% T1* Suppression (min)	Time to Maximum T1* Suppression (min)	Time to 25% Spontaneous T1* Recovery (min)
0.1	Opioid	3.4	4.8	45
0.15	Propofol	2.6	3.5	55
0.2	Opioid	2.4	2.9	65
0.4	Opioid	1.5	1.9	91

* T_1 Single twitch response as well as the first component of the Train-of-four response of the adductor pollicis muscle following supramaximal electrical stimulation of the ulnar nerve.

Table 2 Paediatric Patients aged 1 to 11 months

Nimbex Dose mg/kg (body weight)	Anaesthetic Background	Time to 90% Suppression (min)	Time to Maximum Suppression (min)	Time to 25% Spontaneous T1 Recovery (min)
0.15	Halothane	1.4	2.0	52
0.15	Opioid	1.4	1.9	47

Table 3 Paediatric Patients aged 1 to 12 years

Nimbex Dose mg/kg (body weight)	Anaesthetic Background	Time to 90% Suppression (min)	Time to Maximum Suppression (min)	Time to 25% Spontaneous T1 Recovery (min)
0.15	Halothane	2.3	3.0	43
0.15	Opioid	2.6	3.6	38

Table 4

Nimbex Dose mg/kg (body weight)	Anaesthetic Background	Time to 90% Suppression (min)	Time to Maximum Suppression (min)	Time to 25% Spontaneous T1 Recovery (min)
0.08	Halothane	1.7	2.5	31
0.1	Opioid	1.7	2.8	28

administration of the reversal agent at an average of 13% T_1 recovery.

4.2.3 Use by intravenous infusion

4.2.3.1 Dosage in adults and children aged 2 to 12 years

Maintenance of neuromuscular block may be achieved by infusion of Nimbex. An initial infusion rate of 3 μg/kg (body weight)/min (0.18 mg/kg/hr) is recommended to restore 89 to 99% T_1 suppression following evidence of spontaneous recovery. After an initial period of stabilisation of neuromuscular block, a rate of 1 to 2 μg/kg (body weight)/min (0.06 to 0.12 mg/kg/hr) should be adequate to maintain block in this range in most patients.

Reduction of the infusion rate by up to 40% may be required when Nimbex is administered during isoflurane or enflurane anaesthesia.(see section 4.5).

The infusion rate will depend upon the concentration of cisatracurium in the infusion solution, the desired degree of neuromuscular block, and the patient's weight. The following table provides guidelines for delivery of undiluted Nimbex.

Infusion Delivery Rate of Nimbex injection 2mg/ml

(see Table 5 opposite)

Steady rate continuous infusion of Nimbex is not associated with a progressive increase or decrease in neuromuscular blocking effect.

Following discontinuation of infusion of Nimbex, spontaneous recovery from neuromuscular block proceeds at a rate comparable to that following administration of a single bolus.

4.2.4 Dosage in neonates (aged less than 1 month)

The use of Nimbex in neonates is not recommended as it has not been studied in this patient population.

4.2.5 Dosage in elderly patients

No dosing alterations are required in elderly patients. In these patients Nimbex has a similar pharmacodynamic profile to that observed in young adult patients but, as with other neuromuscular blocking agents, it may have a slightly slower onset.

4.2.6 Dosage in patients with renal impairment

No dosing alterations are required in patients with renal failure.

In these patients Nimbex has a similar pharmacodynamic profile to that observed in patients with normal renal function but it may have a slightly slower onset.

4.2.7 Dosage in patients with hepatic impairment

No dosing alterations are required in patients with end-stage liver disease. In these patients Nimbex has a similar pharmacodynamic profile to that observed in patients with normal hepatic function but it may have a slightly faster onset.

4.2.8 Dosage in patients with cardiovascular disease

When administered by rapid bolus injection (over 5 to 10 seconds) to adult patients with serious cardiovascular disease (New York Heart Association Class I-III) undergoing coronary artery bypass graft (CABG) surgery, Nimbex has not been associated with clinically significant cardiovascular effects at any dose studied (up to and including 0.4 mg/kg (8x ED_{95}). However, there are limited data for doses above 0.3 mg/kg in this patient population).

Nimbex has not been studied in children undergoing cardiac surgery.

4.2.9 Dosage in Intensive Care Unit (ICU) patients

Nimbex may be administered by bolus dose and/or infusion to adult patients in the ICU.

An initial infusion rate of Nimbex of 3 μg/kg (body weight)/min (0.18 mg/kg/hr) is recommended for adult ICU patients. There may be wide interpatient variation in dosage requirements and these may increase or decrease with time. In clinical studies the average infusion rate was 3 μg/kg/min [range 0.5 to 10.2 μg/kg (body weight)/min (0.03 to 0.6mg/kg/hr)]

Table 5 Infusion Delivery Rate of Nimbex injection 2mg/ml

Patient (body weight)	Dose (μg/kg/min)				Infusion Rate
(kg)	1.0	1.5	2.0	3.0	
20	0.6	0.9	1.2	1.8	mL/hr
70	2.1	3.2	4.2	6.3	mL/hr
100	3.0	4.5	6.0	9.0	mL/hr

Table 6 Infusion Delivery Rate of Nimbex Forte injection 5mg/ml

Patient (body weight)	Dose (μg/kg/min)				Infusion Rate
(kg)	1.0	1.5	2.0	3.0	
70	0.8	1.2	1.7	2.5	mL/hr
100	1.2	1.8	2.4	3.6	mL/hr

The median time to full spontaneous recovery following long-term (up to 6 days) infusion of Nimbex in ICU patients was approximately 50 minutes.

Infusion Delivery Rate of Nimbex Forte injection 5mg/ml

(see Table 6 below)

The recovery profile after infusions of Nimbex to ICU patients is independent of duration of infusion.

4.3 Contraindications

Nimbex is contra-indicated in patients known to be hypersensitive to cisatracurium, atracurium, or benzenesulfonic acid.

4.4 Special warnings and precautions for use

4.4.1 Product specific topics

Cisatracurium paralyses the respiratory muscles as well as other skeletal muscles but has no known effect on consciousness or pain threshold. Nimbex should be only administered by or under the supervision of anaesthetists or other clinicians who are familiar with the use and action of neuromuscular blocking agents. Facilities for tracheal intubation, and maintenance of pulmonary ventilation and adequate arterial oxygenation have to be available.

Caution should be exercised when administering Nimbex to patients who have shown hypersensitivity to other neuromuscular blocking agents since a high rate of cross-sensitivity (greater than 50%) between neuromuscular blocking agents has been reported (see section 4.3).

Cisatracurium does not have significant vagolytic or ganglion- blocking properties. Consequently, Nimbex has no clinically significant effect on heart rate and will not counteract the bradycardia produced by many anaesthetic agents or by vagal stimulation during surgery.

Patients with myasthenia gravis and other forms of neuromuscular disease have shown greatly increased sensitivity to non-depolarising blocking agents. An initial dose of not more than 0.02 mg/kg Nimbex is recommended in these patients.

Severe acid-base and/or serum electrolyte abnormalities may increase or decrease the sensitivity of patients to neuromuscular blocking agents.

There is no information on the use of Nimbex in neonates aged less than one month since it has not been studied in this patient population.

Cisatracurium has not been studied in patients with a history of malignant hyperthermia. Studies in malignant hyperthermia- susceptible pigs indicated that cisatracurium does not trigger this syndrome.

There have been no studies of cisatracurium in patients undergoing surgery with induced hypothermia (25 to 28°C). As with other neuromuscular blocking agents the rate of infusion required to maintain adequate surgical relaxation under these conditions may be expected to be significantly reduced.

Cisatracurium has not been studied in patients with burns; however, as with other non-depolarising neuromuscular blocking agents, the possibility of increased dosing requirements and shortened duration of action must be considered if Nimbex injection is administered to these patients.

Nimbex is hypotonic and must not be applied into the infusion line of a blood transfusion.

Intensive Care Unit (ICU) Patients: -

When administered to laboratory animals in high doses, laudanosine, a metabolite of cisatracurium and atracurium, has been associated with transient hypotension and in some species, cerebral excitatory effects. In the most sensitive animal species, these effects occurred at laudanosine plasma concentrations similar to those that have been observed in some ICU patients following prolonged infusion of atracurium.

Consistent with the decreased infusion rate requirements of cisatracurium, plasma laudanosine concentrations are approximately one third those following atracurium infusion.

There have been rare reports of seizures in ICU patients who have received atracurium and other agents. These patients usually had one or more medical conditions predisposing to seizures (eg. cranial trauma, hypoxic encephalopathy, cerebral oedema, viral encephalitis, uraemia). A causal relationship to laudanosine has not been established.

4.5 Interaction with other medicinal products and other forms of interaction

Many drugs have been shown to influence the magnitude and/or duration of action of non-depolarising neuromuscular blocking agents, including the following:-

Increased Effect:

By anaesthetic agents such as enflurane, isoflurane, halothane (see section 4.2) and ketamine, by other non-depolarising neuromuscular blocking agents or by other drugs such as antibiotics (including the aminoglycosides, polymyxins, spectinomycin, tetracyclines, lincomycin and clindamycin), anti- arrhythmic drugs (including propranolol, calcium channel blockers, lignocaine, procainamide and quinidine), diuretics, (including frusemide and possibly thiazides, mannitol and acetazolamide), magnesium and lithium salts and ganglion blocking drugs (trimetaphan, hexamethonium).

A decreased effect is seen after prior chronic administration of phenytoin or carbamazepine.

Prior administration of suxamethonium has no effect on the duration of neuromuscular block following bolus doses of Nimbex or on infusion rate requirements.

Administration of suxamethonium to prolong the effects of non- depolarising neuromuscular blocking agents may result in a prolonged and complex block which can be difficult to reverse with anticholinesterases.

Rarely, certain drugs may aggravate or unmask latent myasthenia gravis or actually induce a myasthenic syndrome; increased sensitivity to non-depolarising neuromuscular blocking agents might result. Such drugs include various antibiotics, β-blockers (propranolol, oxprenolol), anti-arrhythmic drugs (procainamide, quinidine), anti-rheumatic drugs (chloroquine, D-penicillamine), trimetaphan, chlorpromazine, steroids, phenytoin and lithium.

Treatment with anticholinesterases, commonly used in the treatment of Alzheimer's disease e.g. donepezil, may shorten the duration and diminish the magnitude of neuromuscular blockade with cisatracurium.

4.6 Pregnancy and lactation

There are no adequate data from the use of Nimbex in pregnant women. Animal studies are insufficient with respect to effects on pregnancy, embryonal/foetal development, parturition and postnatal development (see section 5.3). The potential risk for humans is unknown.

Nimbex should not be used during pregnancy.

It is not known whether cisatracurium or its metabolites are excreted in human milk.

4.7 Effects on ability to drive and use machines

This precaution is not relevant to the use of Nimbex. Nimbex will always be used in combination with a general anaesthetic and therefore the usual precautions relating to performance of tasks following general anaesthesia apply.

4.8 Undesirable effects

Data from pooled internal clinical trials were used to determine the frequency of very common to uncommon adverse reactions.

The following convention has been used for the classification of frequency:- very common $\geqslant 1/10$, common $\geqslant 1/100$ and $< 1/10$, uncommon $\geqslant 1/1000$ and $< 1/100$, rare $\geqslant 1/10{,}000$ and $< 1/1000$, very rare $< 1/10{,}000$.

Clinical Trial Data

Cardiac disorders

Common	Bradycardia

Vascular disorders

Common	Hypotension
Uncommon	Cutaneous flushing

Respiratory, thoracic and mediastinal disorders

Uncommon	Bronchospasm

Skin and subcutaneous tissue disorders

Uncommon	Rash

Postmarketing Data

Immune system disorders

Very rare	Anaphylactic reaction

Anaphylactic reactions of varying degrees of severity have been observed after the administration of neuromuscular blocking agents. Very rarely, severe anaphylactic reactions have been reported in patients receiving Nimbex in conjunction with one or more anaesthetic agents.

Musculoskeletal and connective tissue disorders

Very rare	Myopathy, muscle weakness

There have been some reports of muscle/weakness and/or myopathy following prolonged use of muscle relaxants in severely ill patients in the ICU. Most patients were receiving concomitant corticosteroids. These events have been reported infrequently in association with Nimbex and a causal relationship has not been established.

4.9 Overdose

4.9.1 Symptoms and signs

Prolonged muscle paralysis and its consequences are expected to be the main signs of overdosage with Nimbex.

4.9.2 Management

It is essential to maintain pulmonary ventilation and arterial oxygenation until adequate spontaneous respiration returns. Full sedation will be required since consciousness is not impaired by Nimbex. Recovery may be accelerated by the administration of anti- cholinesterase agents once evidence of spontaneous recovery is present.

5. PHARMACOLOGICAL PROPERTIES

5.1 Pharmacodynamic properties

Cisatracurium is a neuromuscular blocking agent, ATC code: M03A C11.

Cisatracurium is an intermediate-duration, non-depolarising benzylisoquinolinium skeletal muscle relaxant.

Clinical studies in man indicated that Nimbex is not associated with dose dependent histamine release even at doses up to and including 8 × ED_{95}.

5.1.1 Mode of action

Cisatracurium binds to cholinergic receptors on the motor end-plate to antagonise the action of acetylcholine, resulting in a competitive block of neuromuscular transmission. This action is readily reversed by anti-cholinesterase agents such as neostigmine or edrophonium.

The ED_{95} (dose required to produce 95% depression of the twitch response of the adductor pollicis muscle to stimulation of the ulnar nerve) of cisatracurium is estimated to be 0.05 mg/kg bodyweight during opioid anaesthesia (thiopentone/fentanyl/midazolam).

The ED_{95} of cisatracurium in children during halothane anaesthesia is 0.04 mg/kg.

5.2 Pharmacokinetic properties

Cisatracurium undergoes degradation in the body at physiological pH and temperature by Hofmann elimination (a chemical process) to form laudanosine and the monoquaternary acrylate metabolite. The monoquaternary acrylate undergoes hydrolysis by non-specific plasma esterases to form the monoquaternary alcohol metabolite. Elimination of cisatracurium is largely organ independent but the liver and kidneys are primary pathways for the clearance of its metabolites.

These metabolites do not possess neuromuscular blocking activity.

5.2.1 Pharmacokinetics in adult patients

Non-compartmental pharmacokinetics of cisatracurium are independent of dose in the range studied (0.1 to 0.2 mg/kg, i.e. 2 to 4 × ED_{95}).

Population pharmacokinetic modelling confirms and extends these findings up to 0.4 mg/kg (8 × ED_{95}). Pharmacokinetic parameters after doses of 0.1 and 0.2 mg/kg Nimbex administered to healthy adult surgical patients are summarised in the table below:

Parameter	Range of Mean Values
Clearance	4.7 to 5.7 mL/min/kg
Volume of distribution at steady state	121 to 161 mL/kg
Elimination half-life	22 to 29 min

5.2.2 Pharmacokinetics in elderly patients

There are no clinically important differences in the pharmacokinetics of cisatracurium in elderly and young adult patients. The recovery profile is also unchanged.

5.2.3 Pharmacokinetics in patients with renal/hepatic impairment

There are no clinically important differences in the pharmacokinetics of cisatracurium in patients with end-stage renal failure or end stage liver disease and in healthy adult patients. Their recovery profiles are also unchanged.

5.2.4 Pharmacokinetics during infusions

The pharmacokinetics of cisatracurium after infusions of Nimbex are similar to those after single bolus injection. The recovery profile after infusion of Nimbex is independent of duration of infusion and is similar to that after single bolus injection.

5.2.5 Pharmacokinetics in Intensive Care Unit (ICU) patients

The pharmacokinetics of cisatracurium in ICU patients receiving prolonged infusions are similar to those in healthy surgical adults receiving infusions or single bolus injections. The recovery profile after infusions of Nimbex in ICU patients is independent of duration of infusion.

Concentrations of metabolites are higher in ICU patients with abnormal renal and/or hepatic function (see section 4.4). These metabolites do not contribute to neuromuscular block.

5.3 Preclinical safety data

5.3.1 Acute toxicity

Meaningful acute studies with cisatracurium could not be performed.

For symptoms of toxicity see "Overdosage"

Subacute Toxicity:

Studies with repeated administration for three weeks in dogs and monkeys showed no compound specific toxic signs.

5.3.2 Mutagenicity

Cisatracurium was not mutagenic in an in vitro microbial mutagenicity test at concentrations up to 5000μg/plate.

In an in vivo cytogenetic study in rats, no significant chromosomal abnormalities were seen at s.c doses up to 4mg/kg.

Cisatracurium was mutagenic in an in vitro mouse lymphoma cell mutagenicity assay, at concentrations of 40μg/ml and higher.

A single positive mutagenic response for a drug used infrequently and/or briefly is of questionable clinical relevance.

5.3.3 Carcinogenicity

Carcinogenicity studies have not been performed.

5.3.4 Reproductive toxicology

Fertility studies have not been performed. Reproductive studies in rats have not revealed any adverse effects of cisatracurium on foetal development.

5.3.5 Local tolerance

The result of an intra-arterial study in rabbits showed that Nimbex injection is well tolerated and no drug related changes were seen.

6. PHARMACEUTICAL PARTICULARS

6.1 List of excipients

Benzene sulfonic acid solution 32% w/v, water for injections.

6.2 Incompatibilities

Degradation of cisatracurium besilate has been demonstrated to occur more rapidly in lactated Ringer's Injection and 5% Dextrose and lactated Ringer's Injection than in the infusion fluids listed under Section 6.6.

Therefore it is recommended that lactated Ringer's Injection and 5% Dextrose and lactated Ringer's Injection are not used as the diluent in preparing solutions of Nimbex for infusion.

Since Nimbex is stable only in acidic solutions it should not be mixed in the same syringe or administered simultaneously through the same needle with alkaline solutions, e.g., sodium thiopentone. It is not compatible with ketorolac trometamol or propofol injectable emulsion.

6.3 Shelf life

Shelf-life before dilution: 2 years.

Chemical and physical in-use stability has been demonstrated for at least 24 hours at 5°C and 25°C (see section 6.6).

From a microbiological point of view, the product should be used immediately. If not used immediately, in-use storage times and conditions prior to use are the responsibility of the user and would normally not be longer than 24 hours at 2 to 8°C, unless reconstitution has taken place in controlled and validated aseptic conditions.

6.4 Special precautions for storage

Store in a refrigerator (2- to 8°C). Do not freeze. Keep vial in the outer carton.

Protect from light.

6.5 Nature and contents of container

Nimbex 5mg/ml, solution for injection

30ml in vial (glass): box of 1

Type I, clear, neutral glass vial with a polymeric coated synthetic bromobutyl rubber stopper and aluminium collar with plastic flip-top cover.

NOT ALL PACK SIZES MAY BE MARKETED

6.6 Special precautions for disposal and other handling

This product is for single use only. Use only clear and almost colourless up to slightly yellow/greenish yellow coloured solutions. The product should be visually inspected before use, and if the visual appearance has changed or if the container is damaged, the product must be discarded.

Diluted Nimbex is physically and chemically stable for at least 24 hours at 5°C and 25°C at concentrations between 0.1 and 2 mg/mL in the following infusion fluids, in either polyvinyl chloride or polypropylene containers.

Sodium Chloride (0.9% w/v) Intravenous Infusion.

Glucose (5% w/v) Intravenous Infusion.

Sodium Chloride (0.18% w/v) and Glucose (4% w/v) Intravenous Infusion.

Sodium Chloride (0.45% w/v) and Glucose (2.5% w/v) Intravenous Infusion.

However, since the product contains no antimicrobial preservative, dilution should be carried out immediately prior to use, or failing this be stored as directed under section 6.3.

Nimbex has been shown to be compatible with the following commonly used peri-operative drugs, when mixed in conditions simulating administration into a running intravenous infusion via a Y-site injection port: alfentanil hydrochloride, droperidol, fentanyl citrate, midazolam hydrochloride and sufentanil citrate. Where other drugs are administered through the same indwelling needle or cannula as Nimbex, it is recommended that each drug be flushed through with an adequate volume of a suitable intravenous fluid, e.g., Sodium Chloride Intravenous Infusion (0.9% w/v).

As with other drugs administered intravenously, when a small vein is selected as the injection site, Nimbex should be flushed through the vein with a suitable intravenous fluid, e.g., sodium chloride intravenous infusion (0.9% w/v).

7. MARKETING AUTHORISATION HOLDER
The Wellcome Foundation Limited

Trading as GlaxoSmithKline UK, Stockley Park West, Uxbridge, Middlesex, UB11 1BT

8. MARKETING AUTHORISATION NUMBER(S)
PL 00003/0365

9. DATE OF FIRST AUTHORISATION/RENEWAL OF THE AUTHORISATION
Date of first authorisation: 07 August 1995

Date of last renewal: 06 August 2005

10. DATE OF REVISION OF THE TEXT
13 March 2009

11. LEGAL STATUS
POM

Nimbex Injection 2mg/ml

(GlaxoSmithKline UK)

1. NAME OF THE MEDICINAL PRODUCT
Nimbex 2mg/ml, solution for injection.

2. QUALITATIVE AND QUANTITATIVE COMPOSITION
Cisatracurium 2mg as cisatracurium besilate 2.68mg per 1ml

One ampoule of 2.5ml contains 5mg of cisatracurium

One ampoule of 5ml contains 10mg of cisatracurium

One ampoule of 10ml contains 20mg of cisatracurium

One ampoule of 25ml contains 50mg of cisatracurium

For excipients, see Section 6.1.

3. PHARMACEUTICAL FORM
Solution for Injection.

Colourless to pale yellow or greenish yellow solution. Practically free from visible particulate matter.

4. CLINICAL PARTICULARS
Nimbex is an intermediate-duration, non-depolarising neuromuscular blocking agent for intravenous administration.

4.1 Therapeutic indications
Nimbex is indicated for use during surgical and other procedures and in intensive care. Nimbex can be used as an adjunct to general anaesthesia, or sedation in the Intensive Care Unit (ICU) to relax skeletal muscles, and to facilitate tracheal intubation and mechanical ventilation.

4.2 Posology and method of administration
Please note that Nimbex should not be mixed in the same syringe or administered simultaneously through the same needle as propofol injectable emulsion or with alkaline solutions such as sodium thiopentone. (see section 6.2).

Nimbex contains no antimicrobial preservative and is intended for single patient use.

Monitoring advice

As with other neuromuscular blocking agents, monitoring of neuromuscular function is recommended during the use of Nimbex in order to individualise dosage requirements.

Use by intravenous bolus injection

Dosage in adults

Tracheal Intubation. The recommended intubation dose of Nimbex for adults is 0.15mg/kg (body weight). This dose produced good to excellent conditions for tracheal intubation 120 seconds after administration of Nimbex, following induction of anaesthesia with propofol.

Higher doses will shorten the time to onset of neuromuscular block.

The following table summarises mean pharmacodynamic data when Nimbex was administered at doses of 0.1 to 0.4mg/kg (body weight) to healthy adult patients during opioid (thiopentone/fentanyl/midazolam) or propofol anaesthesia.

(see Table 1 above)

Enflurane or isoflurane anaesthesia may extend the clinically effective duration of an initial dose of Nimbex by as much as 15%.

Maintenance. Neuromuscular block can be extended with maintenance doses of Nimbex. A dose of 0.03 mg/kg (body weight) provides approximately 20 minutes of additional clinically effective neuromuscular block during opioid or propofol anaesthesia.

Consecutive maintenance doses do not result in progressive prolongation of effect.

Spontaneous Recovery. Once spontaneous recovery from neuromuscular block is underway, the rate is independent of the Nimbex dose administered. During opioid or propofol anaesthesia, the median times from 25 to 75% and from 5 to 95% recovery are approximately 13 and 30 minutes, respectively.

Reversal. Neuromuscular block following Nimbex administration is readily reversible with standard doses of anticholinesterase agents. The mean times from 25 to 75% recovery and to full clinical recovery (T_4:T_1 ratio $\geq$ 0.7) are approximately 4 and 9 minutes respectively, following administration of the reversal agent at an average of 10% T_1 recovery.

Dosage in paediatric patients

Tracheal Intubation (paediatric patients aged 1 month to 12 years): As in adults, the recommended intubation dose of Nimbex is 0.15 mg/kg (body weight) administered rapidly over 5 to 10 seconds. This dose produces good to excellent conditions for tracheal intubation 120 seconds following injection of Nimbex. Pharmacodynamic data for this dose are presented in the tables below.

Nimbex has not been studied for intubation in ASA Class III-IV paediatric patients. There are limited data on the use of Nimbex in paediatric patients under 2 years of age undergoing prolonged or major surgery.

In paediatric patients aged 1 month to 12 years, Nimbex has a shorter clinically effective duration and a faster spontaneous recovery profile than those observed in adults under similar anaesthetic conditions. Small differences in the pharmacodynamic profile were observed between the age ranges 1 to 11 months and 1 to 12 years which are summarised in the tables below.

Paediatric Patients aged 1 to 11 months

(see Table 2 below)

Paediatric Patients aged 1 to 12 years

(see Table 3 below)

When Nimbex is not required for intubation: A dose of less than 0.15mg/kg can be used. Pharmacodynamic data for doses of 0.08 and 0.1 mg/kg for paediatric patients aged 2 to 12 years are presented in the table below:

(see Table 4 below)

Administration of Nimbex following suxamethonium has not been studied in paediatric patients (see section 4.5).

Halothane may be expected to extend the clinically effective duration of a dose of Nimbex by up to 20%. No information is available on the use of Nimbex in children during anaesthesia with other halogenated fluorocarbon anaesthetic agents, but these agents may also be expected to extend the clinically effective duration of a dose of Nimbex.

Maintenance (paediatric patients aged 2-12 years). Neuromuscular block can be extended with maintenance doses of Nimbex. In paediatric patients aged 2 to 12 years, a dose of 0.02 mg/kg (body weight) provides approximately 9 minutes of additional clinically effective neuromuscular block during halothane anaesthesia. Consecutive maintenance doses do not result in progressive prolongation of effect.

There are insufficient data to make a specific recommendation for maintenance dosing in paediatric patients under 2 years of age. However, very limited data from clinical studies in paediatric patients under 2 years of age suggest that a maintenance dose of 0.03mg/kg may extend clinically effective neuromuscular block for a period of up to 25 minutes during opioid anaesthesia.

Spontaneous Recovery. Once recovery from neuromuscular block is underway, the rate is independent of the Nimbex dose administered. During opioid or halothane anaesthesia, the median times from 25 to 75% and from 5 to 95% recovery are approximately 11 and 28 minutes, respectively.

Reversal. Neuromuscular block following Nimbex administration is readily reversible with standard doses of anticholinesterase agents. The mean times from 25 to 75% recovery and to full clinical recovery (T_4:T_1 ratio $\geq$ 0.7) are approximately 2 and 5 minutes respectively, following administration of the reversal agent at an average of 13% T_1 recovery.

Use by intravenous infusion

Dosage in adults and children aged 2 to 12 years

Maintenance of neuromuscular block may be achieved by infusion of Nimbex. An initial infusion rate of 3 µg/kg (body weight)/min (0.18 mg/kg/hr) is recommended to restore 89 to 99% T_1 suppression following evidence of spontaneous recovery. After an initial period of stabilisation of neuromuscular block, a rate of 1 to 2 µg/kg (body weight)/min (0.06 to 0.12 mg/kg/hr) should be adequate to maintain block in this range in most patients.

Reduction of the infusion rate by up to 40% may be required when Nimbex is administered during isoflurane or enflurane anaesthesia.(see section 4.5).

The infusion rate will depend upon the concentration of cisatracurium in the infusion solution, the desired degree of neuromuscular block, and the patient's weight. The following table provides guidelines for delivery of undiluted Nimbex.

Infusion Delivery Rate of Nimbex injection 2mg/ml

(see Table 5 on next page)

Table 1

Initial Nimbex Dose mg/kg (body weight)	Anaesthetic Background	Time to 90% T1* Suppression (min)	Time to Maximum T1* Suppression (min)	Time to 25% Spontaneous T1* Recovery (min)
0.1	Opioid	3.4	4.8	45
0.15	Propofol	2.6	3.5	55
0.2	Opioid	2.4	2.9	65
0.4	Opioid	1.5	1.9	91

* T_1 Single twitch response as well as the first component of the Train-of-four response of the adductor pollicis muscle following supramaximal electrical stimulation of the ulnar nerve.

Table 2 Paediatric Patients aged 1 to 11 months

Nimbex Dose mg/kg (body weight)	Anaesthetic Background	Time to 90% Suppression (min)	Time to Maximum Suppression (min)	Time to 25% Spontaneous T1 Recovery (min)
0.15	Halothane	1.4	2.0	52
0.15	Opioid	1.4	1.9	47

Table 3 Paediatric Patients aged 1 to 12 years

Nimbex Dose mg/kg (body weight)	Anaesthetic Background	Time to 90% Suppression (min)	Time to Maximum Suppression (min)	Time to 25% Spontaneous T1 Recovery (min)
0.15	Halothane	2.3	3.0	43
0.15	Opioid	2.6	3.6	38

Table 4

Nimbex Dose mg/kg (body weight)	Anaesthetic Background	Time to 90% Suppression (min)	Time to Maximum Suppression (min)	Time to 25% Spontaneous T1 Recovery (min)
0.08	Halothane	1.7	2.5	31
0.1	Opioid	1.7	2.8	28

Table 5 Infusion Delivery Rate of Nimbex injection 2mg/ml

Patient (body weight) (kg)	Dose (μg/kg/min)				Infusion Rate
	1.0	1.5	2.0	3.0	
20	0.6	0.9	1.2	1.8	mL/hr
70	2.1	3.2	4.2	6.3	mL/hr
100	3.0	4.5	6.0	9.0	mL/hr

Steady rate continuous infusion of Nimbex is not associated with a progressive increase or decrease in neuromuscular blocking effect.

Following discontinuation of infusion of Nimbex, spontaneous recovery from neuromuscular block proceeds at a rate comparable to that following administration of a single bolus.

Dosage in neonates (aged less than 1 month)

The use of Nimbex in neonates is not recommended as it has not been studied in this patient population.

Dosage in elderly patients

No dosing alterations are required in elderly patients. In these patients Nimbex has a similar pharmacodynamic profile to that observed in young adult patients but, as with other neuromuscular blocking agents, it may have a slightly slower onset.

Dosage in patients with renal impairment

No dosing alterations are required in patients with renal failure.

In these patients Nimbex has a similar pharmacodynamic profile to that observed in patients with normal renal function but it may have a slightly slower onset.

Dosage in patients with hepatic impairment

No dosing alterations are required in patients with end-stage liver disease. In these patients Nimbex has a similar pharmacodynamic profile to that observed in patients with normal hepatic function but it may have a slightly faster onset.

Dosage in patients with cardiovascular disease

When administered by rapid bolus injection (over 5 to 10 seconds) to adult patients with serious cardiovascular disease (New York Heart Association Class I-III) undergoing coronary artery bypass graft (CABG) surgery, Nimbex has not been associated with clinically significant cardiovascular effects at any dose studied (up to and including 0.4 mg/kg (8x ED_{95}). However, there are limited data for doses above 0.3 mg/kg in this patient population).

Nimbex has not been studied in children undergoing cardiac surgery.

Dosage in Intensive Care Unit (ICU) patients

Nimbex may be administered by bolus dose and/or infusion to adult patients in the ICU.

An initial infusion rate of Nimbex of 3 μg/kg (body weight)/min (0.18 mg/kg/hr) is recommended for adult ICU patients. There may be wide interpatient variation in dosage requirements and these may increase or decrease with time. In clinical studies the average infusion rate was 3 μg/kg/min [range 0.5 to 10.2 μg/kg (body weight)/min (0.03 to 0.6mg/kg/hr)]

The median time to full spontaneous recovery following long-term (up to 6 days) infusion of Nimbex in ICU patients was approximately 50 minutes.

Infusion Delivery Rate of Nimbex Forte injection 5mg/ml

(see Table 6 below)

The recovery profile after infusions of Nimbex to ICU patients is independent of duration of infusion.

4.3 Contraindications

Nimbex is contra-indicated in patients known to be hypersensitive to cisatracurium, atracurium, or benzenesulfonic acid.

4.4 Special warnings and precautions for use

Product specific topics

Cisatracurium paralyses the respiratory muscles as well as other skeletal muscles but has no known effect on consciousness or pain threshold. Nimbex should be only administered by or under the supervision of anaesthetists or other clinicians who are familiar with the use and action of neuromuscular blocking agents. Facilities for tracheal intubation, and maintenance of pulmonary ventilation and adequate arterial oxygenation have to be available.

Caution should be exercised when administering Nimbex to patients who have shown hypersensitivity to other neuromuscular blocking agents since a high rate of cross-sensitivity (greater than 50%) between neuromuscular blocking agents has been reported (see section 4.3).

Cisatracurium does not have significant vagolytic or ganglion- blocking properties. Consequently, Nimbex has no clinically significant effect on heart rate and will not counteract the bradycardia produced by many anaesthetic agents or by vagal stimulation during surgery.

Patients with myasthenia gravis and other forms of neuromuscular disease have shown greatly increased sensitivity to non-depolarising blocking agents. An initial dose of not more than 0.02 mg/kg Nimbex is recommended in these patients.

Severe acid-base and/or serum electrolyte abnormalities may increase or decrease the sensitivity of patients to neuromuscular blocking agents.

There is no information on the use of Nimbex in neonates aged less than one month since it has not been studied in this patient population.

Cisatracurium has not been studied in patients with a history of malignant hyperthermia. Studies in malignant hyperthermia- susceptible pigs indicated that cisatracurium does not trigger this syndrome.

There have been no studies of cisatracurium in patients undergoing surgery with induced hypothermia (25 to 28°C). As with other neuromuscular blocking agents the rate of infusion required to maintain adequate surgical relaxation under these conditions may be expected to be significantly reduced.

Cisatracurium has not been studied in patients with burns; however, as with other non-depolarising neuromuscular blocking agents, the possibility of increased dosing requirements and shortened duration of action must be considered if Nimbex injection is administered to these patients.

Nimbex is hypotonic and must not be applied into the infusion line of a blood transfusion.

Intensive Care Unit (ICU) Patients: -

When administered to laboratory animals in high doses, laudanosine, a metabolite of cisatracurium and atracurium, has been associated with transient hypotension and in some species, cerebral excitatory effects. In the most sensitive animal species, these effects occurred at laudanosine plasma concentrations similar to those that have been observed in some ICU patients following prolonged infusion of atracurium.

Consistent with the decreased infusion rate requirements of cisatracurium, plasma laudanosine concentrations are approximately one third those following atracurium infusion.

There have been rare reports of seizures in ICU patients who have received atracurium and other agents. These patients usually had one or more medical conditions predisposing to seizures (eg. cranial trauma, hypoxic encephalopathy, cerebral oedema, viral encephalitis, uraemia). A causal relationship to laudanosine has not been established.

4.5 Interaction with other medicinal products and other forms of interaction

Many drugs have been shown to influence the magnitude and/or duration of action of non-depolarising neuromuscular blocking agents, including the following:-

Increased Effect:

By anaesthetic agents such as enflurane, isoflurane, halothane (see section 4.2) and ketamine, by other non-depolarising neuromuscular blocking agents or by other drugs such as antibiotics (including the aminoglycosides, polymyxins, spectinomycin, tetracyclines, lincomycin and clindamycin), anti- arrhythmic drugs (including propranolol, calcium channel blockers, lignocaine, procainamide and quinidine), diuretics, (including frusemide and possibly thiazides, mannitol and acetazolamide), magnesium and lithium salts and ganglion blocking drugs (trimetaphan, hexamethonium).

Table 6 Infusion Delivery Rate of Nimbex Forte injection 5mg/ml

Patient (body weight) (kg)	Dose (μg/kg/min)				Infusion Rate
	1.0	1.5	2.0	3.0	
70	0.8	1.2	1.7	2.5	mL/hr
100	1.2	1.8	2.4	3.6	mL/hr

A decreased effect is seen after prior chronic administration of phenytoin or carbamazepine.

Prior administration of suxamethonium has no effect on the duration of neuromuscular block following bolus doses of Nimbex or on infusion rate requirements.

Administration of suxamethonium to prolong the effects of non- depolarising neuromuscular blocking agents may result in a prolonged and complex block which can be difficult to reverse with anticholinesterases.

Rarely, certain drugs may aggravate or unmask latent myasthenia gravis or actually induce a myasthenic syndrome; increased sensitivity to non-depolarising neuromuscular blocking agents might result. Such drugs include various antibiotics, b-blockers (propranolol, oxprenolol), anti-arrhythmic drugs (procainamide, quinidine), anti-rheumatic drugs (chloroquine, D-penicillamine), trimetaphan, chlorpromazine, steroids, phenytoin and lithium.

Treatment with anticholinesterases, commonly used in the treatment of Alzheimer's disease e.g. donepezil, may shorten the duration and diminish the magnitude of neuromuscular blockade with cisatracurium.

4.6 Pregnancy and lactation

There are no adequate data from the use of Nimbex in pregnant women. Animal studies are insufficient with respect to effects on pregnancy, embryonal/foetal development, parturition and postnatal development (see section 5.3). The potential risk for humans is unknown.

Nimbex should not be used during pregnancy.

It is not known whether cisatracurium or its metabolites are excreted in human milk.

4.7 Effects on ability to drive and use machines

This precaution is not relevant to the use of Nimbex. Nimbex will always be used in combination with a general anaesthetic and therefore the usual precautions relating to performance of tasks following general anaesthesia apply.

4.8 Undesirable effects

Data from pooled internal clinical trials were used to determine the frequency of very common to uncommon adverse reactions.

The following convention has been used for the classification of frequency:- very common $\geqslant$ 1/10, common $\geqslant$ 1/100 and $<$1/10, uncommon $\geqslant$ 1/1000 and $<$1/100, rare $\geqslant$ 1/10,000 and $<$1/1000, very rare $<$ 1/10,000.

Clinical Trial Data

Cardiac disorders

Common	Bradycardia

Vascular disorders

Common	Hypotension
Uncommon	Cutaneous flushing

Respiratory, thoracic and mediastinal disorders

Uncommon	Bronchospasm

Skin and subcutaneous tissue disorders

Uncommon	Rash

Postmarketing Data

Immune system disorders

Very rare	Anaphylactic reaction

Anaphylactic reactions of varying degrees of severity have been observed after the administration of neuromuscular blocking agents. Very rarely, severe anaphylactic reactions have been reported in patients receiving Nimbex in conjunction with one or more anaesthetic agents.

Musculoskeletal and connective tissue disorders

Very rare	Myopathy, muscle weakness

There have been some reports of muscle/weakness and/or myopathy following prolonged use of muscle relaxants in severely ill patients in the ICU. Most patients were receiving concomitant corticosteroids. These events have been reported infrequently in association with Nimbex and a causal relationship has not been established.

4.9 Overdose

4.9.1 Symptoms and signs

Prolonged muscle paralysis and its consequences are expected to be the main signs of overdosage with Nimbex.

Management

It is essential to maintain pulmonary ventilation and arterial oxygenation until adequate spontaneous respiration returns. Full sedation will be required since consciousness is not impaired by Nimbex. Recovery may be accelerated by the administration of anti- cholinesterase agents once evidence of spontaneous recovery is present.

5. PHARMACOLOGICAL PROPERTIES

5.1 Pharmacodynamic properties

Cisatracurium is a neuromuscular blocking agent, ATC code: M03A C11.

Cisatracurium is an intermediate-duration, non-depolarising benzylisoquinolinium skeletal muscle relaxant.

Clinical studies in man indicated that Nimbex is not associated with dose dependent histamine release even at doses up to and including 8 × ED_{95}.

Mode of action

Cisatracurium binds to cholinergic receptors on the motor end-plate to antagonise the action of acetylcholine, resulting in a competitive block of neuromuscular transmission. This action is readily reversed by anti-cholinesterase agents such as neostigmine or edrophonium.

The ED_{95} (dose required to produce 95% depression of the twitch response of the adductor pollicis muscle to stimulation of the ulnar nerve) of cisatracurium is estimated to be 0.05 mg/kg bodyweight during opioid anaesthesia (thiopentone/fentanyl/midazolam).

The ED_{95} of cisatracurium in children during halothane anaesthesia is 0.04 mg/kg.

5.2 Pharmacokinetic properties

Cisatracurium undergoes degradation in the body at physiological pH and temperature by Hofmann elimination (a chemical process) to form laudanosine and the monoquaternary acrylate metabolite. The monoquaternary acrylate undergoes hydrolysis by non-specific plasma esterases to form the monoquaternary alcohol metabolite. Elimination of cisatracurium is largely organ independent but the liver and kidneys are primary pathways for the clearance of its metabolites.

These metabolites do not possess neuromuscular blocking activity.

Pharmacokinetics in adult patients

Non-compartmental pharmacokinetics of cisatracurium are independent of dose in the range studied (0.1 to 0.2 mg/kg, i.e. 2 to 4 × ED_{95}).

Population pharmacokinetic modelling confirms and extends these findings up to 0.4 mg/kg (8 × ED_{95}). Pharmacokinetic parameters after doses of 0.1 and 0.2 mg/kg Nimbex administered to healthy adult surgical patients are summarised in the table below:

Parameter	Range of Mean Values
Clearance	4.7 to 5.7 mL/min/kg
Volume of distribution at steady state	121 to 161 mL/kg
Elimination half-life	22 to 29 min

Pharmacokinetics in elderly patients

There are no clinically important differences in the pharmacokinetics of cisatracurium in elderly and young adult patients. The recovery profile is also unchanged.

Pharmacokinetics in patients with renal/hepatic impairment

There are no clinically important differences in the pharmacokinetics of cisatracurium in patients with end-stage renal failure or end stage liver disease and in healthy adult patients. Their recovery profiles are also unchanged.

Pharmacokinetics during infusions

The pharmacokinetics of cisatracurium after infusions of Nimbex are similar to those after single bolus injection. The recovery profile after infusion of Nimbex is independent of duration of infusion and is similar to that after single bolus injection.

Pharmacokinetics in Intensive Care Unit (ICU) patients

The pharmacokinetics of cisatracurium in ICU patients receiving prolonged infusions are similar to those in healthy surgical adults receiving infusions or single bolus injections. The recovery profile after infusions of Nimbex in ICU patients is independent of duration of infusion.

Concentrations of metabolites are higher in ICU patients with abnormal renal and/or hepatic function (see section 4.4). These metabolites do not contribute to neuromuscular block.

5.3 Preclinical safety data

Acute toxicity

Meaningful acute studies with cisatracurium could not be performed.

For symptoms of toxicity see "Overdosage"

Subacute Toxicity:

Studies with repeated administration for three weeks in dogs and monkeys showed no compound specific toxic signs.

Mutagenicity

Cisatracurium was not mutagenic in an in vitro microbial mutagenicity test at concentrations up to 5000µg/plate.

In an in vivo cytogenetic study in rats, no significant chromosomal abnormalities were seen at s.c doses up to 4mg/kg.

Cisatracurium was mutagenic in an in vitro mouse lymphoma cell mutagenicity assay, at concentrations of 40µg/ml and higher.

A single positive mutagenic response for a drug used infrequently and/or briefly is of questionable clinical relevance.

Carcinogenicity

Carcinogenicity studies have not been performed.

Reproductive toxicology

Fertility studies have not been performed. Reproductive studies in rats have not revealed any adverse effects of cisatracurium on foetal development.

Local tolerance

The result of an intra-arterial study in rabbits showed that Nimbex injection is well tolerated and no drug related changes were seen.

6. PHARMACEUTICAL PARTICULARS

6.1 List of excipients

Benzene sulfonic acid solution 32% w/v, water for injections.

6.2 Incompatibilities

Degradation of cisatracurium besilate has been demonstrated to occur more rapidly in lactated Ringer's Injection and 5% Dextrose and lactated Ringer's Injection than in the infusion fluids listed under Section 6.6.

Therefore it is recommended that lactated Ringer's Injection and 5% Dextrose and lactated Ringer's Injection are not used as the diluent in preparing solutions of Nimbex for infusion.

Since Nimbex is stable only in acidic solutions it should not be mixed in the same syringe or administered simultaneously through the same needle with alkaline solutions, e.g., sodium thiopentone. It is not compatible with ketorolac trometamol or propofol injectable emulsion.

6.3 Shelf life

Shelf life before dilution: 2 years.

Chemical and physical in-use stability has been demonstrated for at least 24 hours at 5°C and 25°C (see section 6.6).

From a microbiological point of view, the product should be used immediately. If not used immediately, in-use storage times and conditions prior to use are the responsibility of the user and would normally not be longer than 24 hours at 2 to 8°C, unless reconstitution has taken place in controlled and validated aseptic conditions.

6.4 Special precautions for storage

Store in a refrigerator (2- to 8°C). Do not freeze. Keep ampoules in the outer carton.

Protect from light.

6.5 Nature and contents of container

Nimbex 2mg/ml, solution for injection

2.5ml in ampoule (glass): box of 5

5ml in ampoule (glass): box of 5

10ml in ampoule (glass): box of 5

25ml in ampoule (glass): box of 2

Type I, clear, neutral glass ampoules.

NOT ALL PACK SIZES MAY BE MARKETED

6.6 Special precautions for disposal and other handling

This product is for single use only. Use only clear and almost colourless up to slightly yellow/greenish yellow coloured solutions. The product should be visually inspected before use, and if the visual appearance has changed or if the container is damaged, the product must be discarded.

Diluted Nimbex is physically and chemically stable for at least 24 hours at 5°C and 25°C at concentrations between 0.1 and 2 mg/mL in the following infusion fluids, in either polyvinyl chloride or polypropylene containers.

Sodium Chloride (0.9% w/v) Intravenous Infusion.

Glucose (5% w/v) Intravenous Infusion.

Sodium Chloride (0.18% w/v) and Glucose (4% w/v) Intravenous Infusion.

Sodium Chloride (0.45% w/v) and Glucose (2.5% w/v) Intravenous Infusion.

However, since the product contains no antimicrobial preservative, dilution should be carried out immediately prior to use, or failing this be stored as directed under section 6.3.

Nimbex has been shown to be compatible with the following commonly used peri-operative drugs, when mixed in conditions simulating administration into a running intravenous infusion via a Y-site injection port: alfentanil hydrochloride, droperidol, fentanyl citrate, midazolam hydrochloride and sufentanil citrate. Where other drugs are administered through the same indwelling needle or cannula as Nimbex, it is recommended that each drug be flushed through with an adequate volume of a suitable intravenous fluid, e.g., Sodium Chloride Intravenous Infusion (0.9% w/v).

As with other drugs administered intravenously, when a small vein is selected as the injection site, Nimbex should be flushed through the vein with a suitable intravenous fluid, e.g., sodium chloride intravenous infusion (0.9% w/v).

Instructions to open the ampoule (only applicable to 2mg/ml ampoule)

Ampoules are equipped with the OPC (One Point Cut) opening system and must be opened following the below instructions:

- Hold with the hand the bottom part of the ampoule as indicated in picture 1
- Put the other hand on the top of the ampoule positioning the thumb above the coloured point and press as indicated in picture 2

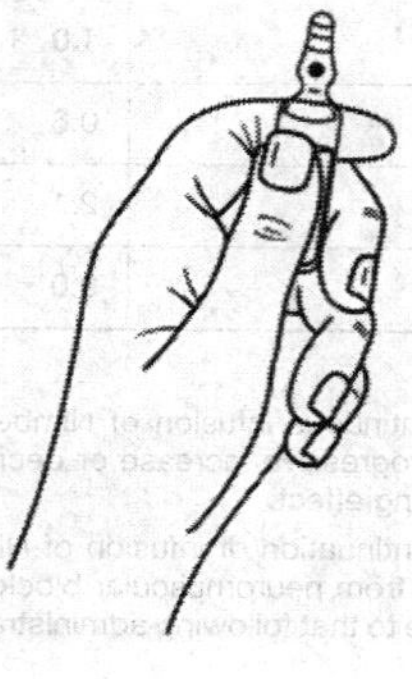

Picture 1

Picture 2

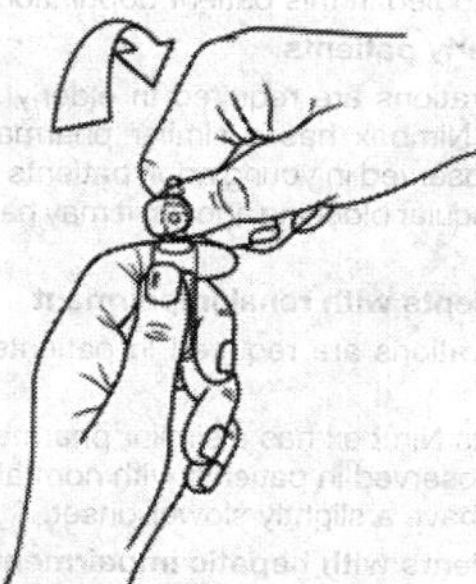

Administrative Data

7. MARKETING AUTHORISATION HOLDER

The Wellcome Foundation Limited

Trading as GlaxoSmithKline UK, Stockley Park West, Uxbridge, Middlesex, UB11 1BT

8. MARKETING AUTHORISATION NUMBER(S)

PL 00003/0364

9. DATE OF FIRST AUTHORISATION/RENEWAL OF THE AUTHORISATION

Date of first authorisation: 07 August 1995

Date of last renewal: 06 August 2005

10. DATE OF REVISION OF THE TEXT

13 March 2009

11. LEGAL STATUS

POM

NIOPAM 150

(Bracco UK Limited)

1. NAME OF THE MEDICINAL PRODUCT

NIOPAM 150

2. QUALITATIVE AND QUANTITATIVE COMPOSITION

30.62 w/v Iopamidol equivalent to 150mg iodine/ml.

Each ml contains 306.2 mg Iopamidol.

For excipients, see 6.1.

3. PHARMACEUTICAL FORM

Solution for injection.

Clear aqueous solution filled into colourless glass ampoules or bottles.

4. CLINICAL PARTICULARS

4.1 Therapeutic indications

X-ray contrast medium for injection, particularly in digital subtraction angiography.

4.2 Posology and method of administration

Route of administration

In digital subtraction angiography:

- Intra-ventricular
- Intra-arterial

Dosage

NIOPAM 150: DOSAGE SCHEDULE

Procedure	Dosage
Intra arterial procedures	Adults: 1-40 ml Children: 0.5 - 0.75 ml/kg
Ventricular angiography	Children: 1-1.5 ml/kg

Elderly: Dosage as for adults. The lowest effective dose should be used.

Method of administration

No other drugs should be mixed with the contrast medium.

Digital subtraction angiography

For cardiac imaging the contrast medium may be administered intra-arterially by selective catheterisation to provide subtracted images. Niopam 340 and 370 injected intravenously either centrally or peripherally is also recommended for use in this modality.

4.3 Contraindications

Use in patients with proven or suspected hypersensitivity to iodine containing preparations of this type.

4.4 Special warnings and precautions for use

A positive history of allergy, asthma or untoward reaction during previous similar investigations indicates a need for extra caution; the benefit should clearly outweigh the risk in such patients. Appropriate resuscitative measures should be immediately available.

X-ray examination of women should if possible be conducted during the pre-ovulation phase of the menstrual cycle and should be avoided during pregnancy.

When examining small children or babies, do not limit fluid intake before administering a hypertonic contrast solution. Also, correct any existing water and electrolyte imbalance.

Care should be exercised in carrying out radiographic procedures with contrast media in patients with severe functional impairment of the liver or myocardium, severe systemic disease and in myelomatosis (including Waldenströms macroglobulinemia, multiple myeloma).

In the latter condition patients should not be exposed to dehydration; similarly abnormalities of fluid or electrolyte balance should be corrected prior to use.

Particular care should also be exercised in patients with moderate to severe impairment of renal function (as reflected by a raised blood urea) or in diabetes. Substantial deterioration in renal function is minimised if the patient is well hydrated. Renal function parameters should be monitored after the procedure in these patients.

Patients with severe hepato-renal insufficiency should not be examined unless absolutely indicated. Re-examination should be delayed for 5-7 days.

Special care should be exercised when this product is injected into the right heart or pulmonary artery in patients with pulmonary hypertension. Right heart angiography should be carried out only when absolutely indicated.

Niopam should be administered with caution in elderly patients and patients with increased intracranial pressure or suspicion of intracranial tumour, abscess or haematoma, and in those with a history of a previous reaction to contrast media, asthma, allergy, epilepsy, severe cardiovascular disease, renal impairment, chronic alcoholism or multiple sclerosis. Patients with these conditions have an increased risk of neurological complications.

General anaesthesia may be indicated in selected patients. However, a higher incidence of adverse reactions has been reported in these patients, probably due to the hypotensive effect of the anaesthetic.

Contrast media may promote sickling in individuals who are homozygous for sickle cell disease when injected intravenously.

Patients with phaeochromocytoma may develop severe hypertensive crisis following intravascular Iopamidol. Pre-medication with α-receptor blockers is recommended.

The administration of iodinated contrast media may aggravate the symptoms of myasthenia gravis.

Patients with congestive heart failure should be observed for several hours following the procedure to detect delayed haemodynamic disturbances, which may be associated with a transitory increase in the circulating osmotic load. All other patients should be observed for at least one hour after the procedure, as most of the adverse events occur in this period. The patient should also be informed that allergic reactions may develop up to several days after the procedure; in such case, a physician should be consulted immediately.

In patients who are known epileptics or have a history of epilepsy, anticonvulsant therapy should be maintained before and following myelographic procedures. In some instances, anticonvulsant therapy may be increased for 48 hours before the examination.

Neuroleptics must be absolutely avoided because they lower the seizure threshold. The same applies to analgesics, anti-emetics, antihistamines and sedatives of the phenothiazine group. Whenever possible, treatment with such drugs should be discontinued at least 48 hours before administration of the contrast medium and not be resumed less than 12 hours after completion of the procedure.

Non-ionic contrast media have less anti-coagulant activity in-vitro than ionic media. Meticulous attention should therefore be paid to angiographic technique. Non-ionic media should not be allowed to remain in contact with blood in the syringe and intravascular catheters should be flushed frequently, to minimise the risk of clotting, which rarely has led to serious thromboembolic complications after procedures.

The presence of renal damage in diabetic patients is one of the factors predisposing to renal impairment following contrast media administration. This may precipitate lactic acidosis in patients who are taking metformin. As a precaution, metformin should be discontinued at the time of, or prior to, the procedure and withheld for 48 hours subsequent to the procedure and re-instituted only after renal function has been re-evaluated and found to be normal.

Niopam should be used with caution in patients with hyperthyroidism. It is possible that hyperthyroidism may recur in patients previously treated for Graves' disease.

4.5 Interaction with other medicinal products and other forms of interaction

Thyroid function tests: use of iodinated contrast media may interfere with tests for thyroid function which depend on iodine estimations, such as Protein Binding Iodine and radioactive iodine uptake. As a consequence they will not accurately reflect thyroid function for up to 16 days following administration of iodinated contrast media. Thyroid function tests not depending on iodine estimations, e.g. T3 resin uptake and total or free thyroxine (T4) assays are not affected.

No other specific interference with physiological functions has been noted.

The administration of an X-ray contrast medium in diabetic patients with nephropathy who are taking biguanides may precipitate lactic acidosis.

Arterial thrombosis has been reported when Iopamidol was given following papaverine.

The administration of vasopressors strongly potentiates the neurological effect of the intra-arterial contrast media.

Contrast media may interfere with laboratory tests for bilirubin, proteins or inorganic substances (e.g. iron, copper, calcium, phosphate). These substances should not be assayed during the same day following the administration of contrast media.

4.6 Pregnancy and lactation

X-ray examination of women should if possible be conducted during the pre-ovulation phase of the menstrual cycle and should be avoided during pregnancy; also, since it has not been demonstrated that Niopam is safe for use in pregnant women, it should be administered only if the procedure is considered essential by the physician.

Niopam is poorly excreted in human milk. From animal experience, Niopam is non toxic in animals after oral administration. Although, no serious adverse reactions have been reported in nursing infants, Niopam should be administered to lactating women only if considered essential by the physician.

4.7 Effects on ability to drive and use machines

There is no known effect on the ability to drive and operate machines. However, because of the risk of early reactions, driving or operating machinery is not advisable for one hour following the last injection.

4.8 Undesirable effects

The use of iodinated compounds may cause untoward side effects and manifestations of anaphylaxis. The symptoms include nausea, vomiting, diffuse erythema, feeling hot, headache, rhinitis or laryngeal oedema, fever, sweating, asthenia, dizziness, pallor, dyspnoea, moderate hypotension. Skin reactions may occur in the form of various types of rash or diffuse blisters. More severe reactions involving the cardiovascular system such as vasodilatation with pronounced hypotension, tachycardia, dyspnoea, agitation, cyanosis, loss of consciousness and cardiac arrest, may require emergency treatment.

The occurrence of delayed intolerance reactions, most commonly pruritus and urticaria, has been reported up to several days post administration.

During intra-cardiac and/or coronary arteriography, ventricular arrhythmias may infrequently occur.

Also cases of myocardial ischemia or infarction and/or cardiac failure/cardiac arrest have been reported rarely.

Other undesirable effects are:

- renal impairment,
- thrombocytopaenia,
- asthma/bronchospasm, and
- pulmonary oedema.

Hyperthyroidism may recur in patients previously treated for Graves' disease.

After cerebral angiography, confusion; stupor; coma; paresis; cortical blindness (usually transient); and convulsions may occur.

Rarely, Steven-Johnson syndrome has been reported.

Local pain and swelling at the injection site may occur.

4.9 Overdose

Treatment of overdosage is directed toward the support of all vital functions and the elimination of the contrast medium while maintaining the patient well hydrated.

If needed, haemodialysis can be used to eliminate Iopamidol from the body.

5. PHARMACOLOGICAL PROPERTIES

Pharmacotherapeutic group; ATC code: V08A B04

5.1 Pharmacodynamic properties

Iopamidol is contrast medium belonging to the new generation of non-ionic compound whose solubility is due to the presence of hydrophilic substitutes in the molecule. This results in a solution of low osmolality when compared with ionic media.

Iopamidol has been shown to be effective as an X-ray contrast medium in neuroradiology, angiography, venography, arthrography, urography, cerebral angiography and left ventriculography and coronary arteriography. Its toxicity particularly cardiac and CNS toxicity are less than those of ionic contrast media.

5.2 Pharmacokinetic properties

The pharmacokinetics of Iopamidol conform to an open two compartment pharmacokinetic model with first order elimination.

Distribution volume is equivalent to extracellular fluid.

Elimination is almost completely through the kidneys. Less that 1% of the administered dose has been recovered in the faeces up to 72 hours after dosing. Elimination is rapid; up to half the administered dose may be recovered in the urine in the first two hours of dosing.

There is no evidence of biotransformation.

Serum protein binding is negligible.

5.3 Preclinical safety data

No adverse effects can be predicted from animal toxicology studies other than those documented from human use of Iopamidol.

6. PHARMACEUTICAL PARTICULARS

6.1 List of excipients

Excipients are: are trometamol, hydrochloric acid and edetate calcium disodium.

6.2 Incompatibilities

No other drug should be mixed with the contrast medium.

6.3 Shelf life

5 years.

6.4 Special precautions for storage

Protect from light.

6.5 Nature and contents of container

5ml, 10ml and 20ml clear, colourless Type I glass ampoules.

30ml, 50ml, 100ml, 250ml and 200ml clear, colourless Type I or Type II glass bottles with rubber closures and aluminium caps.

6.6 Special precautions for disposal and other handling

Discard if the solution is not clear of particulate matter.

Exceptionally, the event of crystallisation of Niopam could occur. It has been shown that such a phenomenon is caused by a damaged or defective container and therefore the product should not be used in this case.

The bottle, once opened, must be used immediately.

Any residue of contrast medium must be discarded.

Niopam, as other iodinated contrast media, can react with metallic surfaces containing copper (e.g. brass), therefore the use of equipment, in which the product comes into direct contact with such surfaces, should be avoided.

7. MARKETING AUTHORISATION HOLDER

Bracco U.K. Ltd,

Bracco House, Mercury Park,

Wycombe Lane, Wooburn Green,

Buckinghamshire HP10 OHH

8. MARKETING AUTHORISATION NUMBER(S)

PL 18920/0007

9. DATE OF FIRST AUTHORISATION/RENEWAL OF THE AUTHORISATION

6th October 1986 / 9th January 2002

10. DATE OF REVISION OF THE TEXT

29th July 2005

NIOPAM 200

(Bracco UK Limited)

1. NAME OF THE MEDICINAL PRODUCT

NIOPAM 200

2. QUALITATIVE AND QUANTITATIVE COMPOSITION

40.8% w/v Iopamidol equivalent to 200mg iodine/ml.

Each ml contains 408.2 mg Iopamidol.

For excipients, see 6.1.

3. PHARMACEUTICAL FORM

Solution for injection.

Clear aqueous solution filled into colourless glass ampoules or bottles.

4. CLINICAL PARTICULARS

4.1 Therapeutic indications

X-ray contrast medium for use in lumbar and thoraco-cervical myelography, computer tomography enhancement.

4.2 Posology and method of administration

Route of administration

Intra-ventricular

Intra-venous

Intra-thecal

Intra-cisternal

Dosage

NIOPAM 200: DOSAGE SCHEDULE

Procedure	Dosage
Lumbar Myelography	Adults 10 - 15 ml
Thoraco-Cervical Myelography	Adults 5 - 15 ml
Computer Tomography Enhancement	Adults: Brain scanning 50 - 100ml Whole body scanning 40-100ml

Elderly: dosage as for adults. The lowest effective dose should be used.

Method of administration

No other drugs should be mixed with the contrast medium.

Lumbar myelography

A slow sub-arachnoid injection is made through a fine lumbar puncture needle into one of the lower lumbar interspinous spaces (L3-L4 or L4-L5) Optimum contrast appears immediately after injections and films should be obtained promptly.

Thoraco-cervical myelography

Following a slow sub-arachnoid injection the patient should be turned on his side and tilted 10°-20° head down under fluoroscopic control. In this manner it is possible to control movement of the contrast medium column into the dorsal region.

If the cervical region is to be examined, the contrast medium should be run into the cervical region first, before the examination of the dorsal areas where it is progressively diluted.

Niopam may also be injected sub-occipitally or by lateral cervical puncture technique. Care should be taken to ensure that the contrast medium does not move intracranially.

Following intra-thecal use, the patient should rest with the head and chest elevated for one hour and be kept well hydrated. Thereafter, he/she may ambulate carefully but bending down be avoided. If remaining in bed, the head and chest should be kept elevated for 6 hours. Patients suspected of having a low seizure threshold should be observed during this period.

Computer tomography enhancement

Contrast enhancement for brain scans can be achieved between one and three minutes after i.v. injection. Niopam 200 is also used for total body scanning examinations after i.v. administration as a bolus, as a drip infusion or by a combination of the two methods.

4.3 Contraindications

Use in patients with proven or suspected hypersensitivity to iodine containing preparations of this type.

Because of overdosage considerations, immediate repeat myelography in the event of technical failure is contraindicated.

4.4 Special warnings and precautions for use

A positive history of allergy, asthma or untoward reaction during previous similar investigations indicates a need for extra caution; the benefit should clearly outweigh the risk in such patients. Appropriate resuscitative measures should be immediately available.

X-ray examination of women should if possible be conducted during the pre-ovulation phase of the menstrual cycle and should be avoided during pregnancy.

Care should be exercised in carrying out radiographic procedures with contrast media in patients with severe functional impairment of the liver or myocardium, severe systemic disease and in myelomatosis (including Waldenströms macroglobulinemia, multiple myeloma). In the latter condition patients should not be exposed to dehydration; similarly abnormalities of fluid or electrolyte balance should be corrected prior to use.

Particular care should also be exercised in patients with moderate to severe impairment of renal function (as reflected by a raised blood urea) or in diabetes. Substantial deterioration in renal function is minimised if the patient is well hydrated. Renal function parameters should be monitored after the procedure in these patients.

Patients with severe hepato-renal insufficiency should not be examined unless absolutely indicated. Re-examination should be delayed for 5-7 days.

Special care should be exercised when this product is injected into the right heart or pulmonary artery in patients with pulmonary hypertension. Right heart angiography should be carried out only when absolutely indicated.

Niopam should be administered with caution in elderly patients and patients with increased intracranial pressure or suspicion of intracranial tumour, abscess or haematoma, and in those with a history of epilepsy, severe cardiovascular disease, renal impairment, chronic alcoholism or multiple sclerosis. Patients with these conditions have an increased risk of neurological complications.

General anaesthesia may be indicated in selected patients. However, a higher incidence of adverse reactions has been reported in these patients, probably due to the hypotensive effect of the anaesthetic.

Contrast media may promote sickling in individuals who are homozygous for sickle cell disease when injected intravenously.

Patients with phaeochromocytoma may develop severe hypertensive crisis following intravascular Iopamidol. Pre-medication with α-receptor blockers is recommended.

The administration of iodinated contrast media may aggravate the symptoms of myasthenia gravis.

Patients with congestive heart failure should be observed for several hours following the procedure to detect delayed haemodynamic disturbances, which may be associated with a transitory increase in the circulating osmotic load. All other patients should be observed for at least one hour after the procedure, as most of the adverse events occur in this period. The patient should also be informed that allergic reactions may develop up to several days after the procedure; in such case, a physician should be consulted immediately.

In neonates, and particularly in premature neonates, it is recommended that tests of thyroid function (typically TSH and T4), should be checked 7-10 days and 1 month after the administration of iodinated contrast media because of the risk of hypothyroidism due to iodine overload. In patients scheduled for thyroid examination with a radioactive iodine tracer, one must take into consideration that iodine uptake in the thyroid gland will be reduced for several days (up to two weeks) after dosing with an iodinized contrast medium that is eliminated through the kidneys.

Local tissue irritation can occur as an event of perivascular infiltration.

In patients who are known epileptics or have a history of epilepsy, anticonvulsant therapy should be maintained before and following myelographic procedures. In some instances, anticonvulsant therapy may be increased for 48 hours before the examination.

Neuroleptics must be absolutely avoided because they lower the seizure threshold. The same applies to analgesics, anti-emetics, antihistamines and sedatives of the phenothiazine group. Whenever possible, treatment with such drugs should be discontinued at least 48 hours before administration of the contrast medium and not be resumed less than 12 hours after completion of the procedure.

Serious neurological events have been observed following direct injection of contrast media into cerebral arteries or vessels supplying the spinal cord or in angiocardiography due to inadvertent filling of the carotids.

Non-ionic contrast media have less anti-coagulant activity *in-vitro* than ionic media. Meticulous attention should therefore be paid to angiographic technique. Non-ionic media should not be allowed to remain in contact with blood in the syringe and intravascular catheters should be flushed frequently, to minimise the risk of clotting, which rarely has led to serious thromboembolic complications after procedures.

Niopam should be used with caution in patients with hyperthyroidism. It is possible that hyperthyroidism may recur in patients previously treated for Graves' disease.

The presence of renal damage in diabetic patients is one of the factors predisposing to renal impairment following contrast media administration. This may precipitate lactic acidosis in patients who are taking metformin. As a precaution, metformin should be discontinued at the time of, or prior to, the procedure and withheld for 48 hours subsequent to the procedure and re-instituted only after renal function has been re-evaluated and found to be normal.

4.5 Interaction with other medicinal products and other forms of interaction

Thyroid function tests: use of iodinated contrast media may interfere with tests for thyroid function which depend on iodine estimations, such as Protein Binding Iodine and radioactive iodine uptake. As a consequence they will not accurately reflect thyroid function for up to 16 days following administration of iodinated contrast media. Thyroid function tests not depending on iodine estimations, e.g. T3 resin uptake and total or free thyroxine (T4) assays are not affected.

No other specific interference with physiological functions have been noted.

The administration of an X-ray contrast medium in diabetic patients with nephropathy who are taking biguanides may precipitate lactic acidosis.

Arterial thrombosis has been reported when Iopamidol was given following papaverine. The administration of vasopressors strongly potentiates the neurological effect of the intra-arterial contrast media.

Contrast media may interfere with laboratory tests for bilirubin, proteins or inorganic substances (eg iron, copper, calcium, phosphate). These substances should not be assayed during the same day following the administration of contrast media.

4.6 Pregnancy and lactation

X-ray examination of women should if possible be conducted during the pre-ovulation phase of the menstrual cycle and should be avoided during pregnancy; also, since it has not been demonstrated that Niopam is safe for use in pregnant women, it should be administered only if the procedure is considered essential by the physician.

Niopam is poorly excreted in human milk. From animal experience, Niopam is non toxic in animals after oral administration. Although, no serious adverse reactions have been reported in nursing infants, Niopam should be administered to lactating women only if considered essential by the physician.

4.7 Effects on ability to drive and use machines

There is no known effect on the ability to drive and operate machines. However, because of the risk of early reactions, driving or operating machinery is not advisable for one hour following the last injection.

4.8 Undesirable effects

The use of iodinated compounds may cause untoward side effects and manifestations of anaphylaxis. The symptoms include nausea, vomiting, diffuse erythema, feeling hot, headache, rhinitis or laryngeal oedema, fever, sweating, asthenia, dizziness, pallor, dyspnoea, moderate hypotension. Skin reactions may occur in the form of various types of rash or diffuse blisters. More severe reactions involving the cardiovascular system such as vasodilatation with pronounced hypotension, tachycardia, dyspnoea, agitation, cyanosis, loss of consciousness and cardiac arrest, may require emergency treatment.

The occurrence of delayed intolerance reactions, most commonly pruritus and urticaria, has been reported up to several days post administration.

During intra-cardiac and/or coronary arteriography, ventricular arrhythmias may infrequently occur.

Also cases of myocardial ischemia or infarction and/or cardiac failure/cardiac arrest have been reported rarely.

Other undesirable effects are:

- renal impairment,
- thrombocytopaenia,
- asthma/bronchospasm, and
- pulmonary oedema.

Hyperthyroidism may recur in patients previously treated for Graves' disease.

After cerebral angiography, confusion; stupor; coma, paresis, cortical blindness (usually transient), and convulsions may occur.

Rarely, Steven-Johnson syndrome has been reported.

Local pain and swelling at the injection site may occur.

Following use in myelography, water soluble non-ionic contrast media have been reported to cause neurological side effects. These include rare cases of seizures, transient confusion or transient motor or sensory dysfunction. Meningism and meningitis have also been reported. The possibility of an infective meningitis should be considered. Headaches, dizziness, nausea and vomiting, pain in limbs, back, or neck pain may also occur.

4.9 Overdose

Treatment of overdosage is directed toward the support of all vital functions and the elimination of the contrast medium while maintaining the patient well hydrated.

If needed, hemodyalisis can be used to eliminate Iopamidol from the body.

5. PHARMACOLOGICAL PROPERTIES

Pharmacotherapeutic group; ATC code: V08A B04

5.1 Pharmacodynamic properties

Iopamidol is contrast medium belonging to the new generation of non-ionic compound whose solubility is due to the presence of hydrophilic substitutes in the molecule. This results in a solution of low osmolality when compared with ionic media.

Iopamidol has been shown to be effective as an X-ray contrast medium in neuroradiology, angiography, venography, arthrography, urography, cerebral angiography and left ventriculography and coronary arteriography. Its toxicity particularly cardiac and CNS toxicity are less than those of ionic contrast media.

5.2 Pharmacokinetic properties

The pharmacokinetics of Iopamidol conform to an open two compartment pharmacokinetic model with first order elimination.

Distribution volume is equivalent to extra-cellular fluid.

Elimination is almost completely through the kidneys. Less that 1% of the administered dose has been recovered in the faeces up to 72 hours after dosing. Elimination is rapid; up to half the administered dose may be recovered in the urine in the first two hours of dosing.

There is no evidence of biotransformation.

Serum protein binding is negligible.

5.3 Preclinical safety data

No adverse effects can be predicted from animal toxicology studies other than those documented from human use of Iopamidol.

6. PHARMACEUTICAL PARTICULARS

6.1 List of excipients

Excipients are: trometamol, hydrochloric acid and edetate calcium disodium.

6.2 Incompatibilities

No other drug should be mixed with the contrast medium.

6.3 Shelf life

5 years.

6.4 Special precautions for storage
Protect from light.

6.5 Nature and contents of container
10ml clear, colourless Type I glass ampoules.

20 and 30ml clear, colourless Type I or Type II glass vials with rubber closures and aluminium caps.

20, 50, 70, 100, 200 and 250ml clear, colourless Type I or Type II glass bottles with rubber closures and aluminium caps.

6.6 Special precautions for disposal and other handling
Discard if the solution is not clear of particulate matter.

Exceptionally, the event of crystallisation of Niopam could occur. It has been shown that such a phenomenon is caused by a damaged or defective container and therefore the product should not be used in this case. The bottle, once opened, must be used immediately.

Any residue of contrast medium must be discarded.

Niopam, as other iodinated contrast media, can react with metallic surfaces containing copper (e.g. brass), therefore the use of equipment, in which the product comes into direct contact with such surfaces, should be avoided.

7. MARKETING AUTHORISATION HOLDER
Bracco U.K. Ltd,
Bracco House, Mercury Park,
Wycombe Lane, Wooburn Green,
Buckinghamshire HP10 OHH

8. MARKETING AUTHORISATION NUMBER(S)
PL 18920/0008

9. DATE OF FIRST AUTHORISATION/RENEWAL OF THE AUTHORISATION
22nd March 1982 / 9th January 2002

10. DATE OF REVISION OF THE TEXT
29th July 2005

NIOPAM 300
(Bracco UK Limited)

1. NAME OF THE MEDICINAL PRODUCT
NIOPAM 300, solution for injection

2. QUALITATIVE AND QUANTITATIVE COMPOSITION
61.2% w/v Iopamidol equivalent to 300mg iodine/ml.

Each ml contains 612 mg iopamidol.

For excipients, see 6.1.

3. PHARMACEUTICAL FORM
Solution for injection.

Clear aqueous solution filled into colourless glass ampoules or bottles.

4. CLINICAL PARTICULARS
4.1 Therapeutic indications
X-ray contrast medium for use in lumbar and thoraco-cervical myelography, cerebral angiography, peripheral angiography, venography, computer tomography enhancement, urography and arthrography.

4.2 Posology and method of administration
Route of administration:
Intra-ventricular
Intra-arterial
Intra-venous
Intra-articular
Intra-thecal
Intra-cisternal

Dosage

NIOPAM 300: DOSAGE SCHEDULE

Procedure	Dosage
Lumbar Myelography	Adults 5 - 10 ml
Thoraco-Cervical Myelography	Adults 5 - 10 ml
Cerebral Angiography	Adults 5 - 10 ml * Children **
Peripheral Arteriography	Adults 20 - 50 ml * Children **
Venography	Adults 20 - 50 ml * Children ** **Do not exceed 250 ml**
Computer Tomography Enhancement	Adults: Brain scanning 50 - 100ml Whole body scanning 40-100ml
Intravenous Urography	Adults 40 - 80 ml In severe renal failure the usual high dose methods should be employed. (up to 1.5 mg/kg) Children 1 - 2.5 mg/kg or **
Arthrography	Adults 1 - 10 ml according to the joint being examined.

* repeat as necessary; ** according to body size and age; Single injection volume depends on the vascular area to be examined.

Elderly: dosage as for adults. The lowest effective dose should be used.

Method of administration

No other drugs should be mixed with the contrast medium.

Lumbar myelography

A slow sub-arachnoid injection is made through a fine lumbar puncture needle into one of the lower lumbar interspinous spaces (L3-L4 or L4-L5). Optimum contrast appears immediately after injections and films should be obtained promptly.

Thoraco-cervical myelography

Following a slow sub-arachnoid injection the patient should be turned on his side and tilted 10°-20° head down under fluoroscopic control. In this manner it is possible to control movement of the contrast medium column into the dorsal region.

If the cervical region is to be examined, the contrast medium should be run into the cervical region first, before the examination of the dorsal areas where it is progressively diluted.

Niopam may also be injected sub-occipitally or by lateral cervical puncture technique. Care should be taken to ensure that the contrast medium does not move intracranially.

Following intrathecal use, the patient should rest with the head and chest elevated for one hour and be kept well hydrated. Thereafter, he/she may ambulate carefully but bending down be avoided. If remaining in bed, the head and chest should be kept elevated for 6 hours. Patients suspected of having a low seizure threshold should be observed during this period.

Cerebral angiography

Any of the current techniques is suitable for radiological visualisation of the cerebral vasculature with Niopam 300. Carotid and vertebral angiography, performed by catheterisation or percutaneous injection techniques, require rapid injection, which, if necessary may be repeated.

Peripheral arteriography and phlebography (venography)

Percutaneous injection into the appropriate blood vessel is used for visualisation of peripheral arteries and veins.

Computer tomography enhancement

Contrast enhancement for brain scans can be achieved between one and three minutes after i.v. injection. Niopam 200, 300 and 340 are also used for total body scanning examinations after i.v. administration as a bolus, as a drip infusion or by a combination of the two methods.

Urography

The contrast medium is injected intravenously and rapidly eliminated through the kidneys. In patients with severe renal failure, high dose urography should be used.

Arthrography

Visualisation of joint cavities and articular surfaces can be achieved by either single or double contrast examination.

4.3 Contraindications
Use in patients with proven or suspected hypersensitivity to iodine containing preparations of this type.

Because of overdosage considerations, immediate repeat myelography in the event of technical failure is contra-indicated.

4.4 Special warnings and precautions for use
A positive history of allergy, asthma or untoward reaction during previous similar investigations indicates a need for extra caution; the benefit should clearly outweigh the risk in such patients. Appropriate resuscitative measures should be immediately available.

X-ray examination of women should if possible be conducted during the pre-ovulation phase of the menstrual cycle and should be avoided during pregnancy.

When examining small children or babies, do not limit fluid intake before administering a hypertonic contrast solution. Also, correct any existing water and electrolyte imbalance.

Care should be exercised in carrying out radiographic procedures with contrast media in patients with severe functional impairment of the liver or myocardium, severe systemic disease and in myelomatosis (including Waldenströms macroglobulinemia, multiple myeloma). In the latter condition patients should not be exposed to dehydration; similarly abnormalities of fluid or electrolyte balance should be corrected prior to use.

Particular care should also be exercised in patients with moderate to severe impairment of renal function (as reflected by a raised blood urea) or in diabetes. Substantial deterioration in renal function is minimised if the patient is well hydrated. Renal function parameters should be monitored after the procedure in these patients.

Patients with severe hepato-renal insufficiency should not be examined unless absolutely indicated. Re-examination should be delayed for 5-7 days.

Niopam should be administered with caution in elderly patients and patients with increased intracranial pressure or suspicion of intracranial tumour, abscess or haematoma, and in those with a history of epilepsy, severe cardiovascular disease, renal impairment, chronic alcoholism or multiple sclerosis.

Patients with these conditions have an increased risk of neurological complications.

General anaesthesia may be indicated in selected patients. However, a higher incidence of adverse reactions has been reported in these patients, probably due to the hypotensive effect of the anaesthetic.

Contrast media may promote sickling in individuals who are homozygous for sickle cell disease when injected intravenously and intra-arterially.

Patients with phaeochromocytoma may develop severe hypertensive crisis following intravascular Niopam. Premedication with α-receptor blockers is recommended.

The administration of iodinated contrast media may aggravate the symptoms of myasthenia gravis.

Patients with congestive heart failure should be observed for several hours following the procedure to detect delayed haemodynamic disturbances, which may be associated with a transitory increase in the circulating osmotic load. All other patients should be observed for at least one hour after the procedure, as most of the adverse events occur in this period. The patient should also be informed that allergic reactions may develop up to several days after the procedure; in such case, a physician should be consulted immediately.

In neonates, and particularly in premature neonates, it is recommended that tests of thyroid function (typically TSH and T4), should be checked 7-10 days and 1 month after the administration of iodinated contrast media because of the risk of hypothyroidism due to iodine overload.

In patients scheduled for thyroid examination with a radioactive iodine tracer, one must take into consideration that iodine uptake in the thyroid gland will be reduced for several days (up to two weeks) after dosing with an iodinized contrast medium that is eliminated through the kidneys.

Local tissue irritation can occur as an event of perivascular infiltration.

Neuroradiology

In patients who are known epileptics or have a history of epilepsy, anticonvulsant therapy should be maintained before and following myelographic procedures. In some instances anticonvulsant therapy may be increased for 48 hours before the examination.

Neuroleptics must be absolutely avoided because they lower the seizure threshold. The same applies to analgesics, antiemetics, antihistamines and sedatives of the phenothiazine group. Whenever possible, treatment with such drugs should be discontinued at least 48 hours before administration of the contrast medium and not be resumed less than 12 hours after completion of the procedure.

Angiography

In patients undergoing angiocardiographic procedures special attention should be paid to the status of the right heart and pulmonary circulation. Right heart insufficiency and pulmonary hypertension may precipitate bradycardia and systemic hypotension, when the organic iodine solution is injected. Right heart angiography should be carried out only when absolutely indicated.

In angiographic procedures, the possibility of dislodging plaque or damaging or perforating the vessel wall should be considered during catheter manipulation and contrast medium injection. Test injections to ensure proper catheter placements are recommended.

Angiography should be avoided whenever possible in patients with homocystinuria due to an increased risk of thrombosis and embolism.

In patients undergoing peripheral angiography, there should be pulsation in the artery into which the X-ray contrast medium will be injected. In patients with thromboangiitis obliterans or ascending infections in combination with serious ischemia the angiography should be performed, if at all, with special caution.

In patients undergoing venography, special caution should be exercised in patients with suspected phlebitis, serious ischaemia, local infections, or a complete venous occlusion. Serious neurological events have been observed following direct injection of contrast media into cerebral arteries or vessels supplying the spinal cord or in angiocardiography due to inadvertent filling of the carotids.

In paediatric roentgenology, one should proceed with great caution when injecting the contrast medium into the right heart chambers of cyanotic neonates with pulmonary hypertension and impaired cardiac function.

In examinations of the aortic arch the tip of the catheter should be positioned carefully to avoid hypotension, bradycardia and CNS injury due to excess pressure transmitted from the injector pump to the brachiocephalic branches of the aorta.

Urography

Care should be exercised in patients with moderate to severe impairment of renal function (as reflected by a raised blood urea). Substantial deterioration in renal function is minimized if the patient is well hydrated. Renal function parameters, especially urinary output should be monitored after the examination in these patients.

Re-examination should be delayed 5-7 days.

Non-ionic contrast media have less anti-coagulant activity *in-vitro* than ionic media. Meticulous attention should therefore be paid to angiographic technique. Non-ionic media should not be allowed to remain in contact with blood in the syringe and intravascular catheters should be flushed frequently, to minimise the risk of clotting, which rarely has led to serious thromboembolic complications after procedures.

Niopam should be used with caution in patients with hyperthyroidism. It is possible that hyperthyroidism may recur in patients previously treated for Graves' disease.

The presence of renal damage in diabetic patients is one of the factors predisposing to renal impairment following contrast media administration. This may precipitate lactic acidosis in patients who are taking metformin. As a precaution, metformin should be discontinued at the time of, or prior to, the procedure and withheld for 48 hours subsequent to the procedure and re-instituted only after renal function has been re-evaluated and found to be normal.

4.5 Interaction with other medicinal products and other forms of interaction

Thyroid function tests: use of iodinated contrast media may interfere with tests for thyroid function which depend on iodine estimations, such as Protein Binding Iodine and radioactive iodine uptake. As a consequence they will not accurately reflect thyroid function for up to 16 days following administration of iodinated contrast media. Thyroid function tests not depending on iodine estimations, e.g. T3 resin uptake and total or free thyroxine (T4) assays are not affected.

No other specific interference with physiological functions have been noted.

The administration of an X-ray contrast medium in diabetic patients with nephropathy who are taking biguanides may precipitate lactic acidosis.

Arterial thrombosis has been reported when iopamidol was given following papaverine.

The administration of vasopressors strongly potentiate the neurological effect of the intra-arterial contrast media.

Contrast media may interfere with laboratory tests for bilirubin, proteins or inorganic substances (eg iron, copper, calcium, phosphate). These substances should not be assayed during the same day following the administration of contrast media.

4.6 Pregnancy and lactation

X-ray examination of women should if possible be conducted during the pre-ovulation phase of the menstrual cycle and should be avoided during pregnancy; also, since it has not been demonstrated that Niopam is safe for use in pregnant women, it should be administered only if the procedure is considered essential by the physician.

Niopam is poorly excreted in human milk. From animal experience, Niopam is non toxic in animals after oral administration. Although, no serious adverse reactions have been reported in nursing infants, Niopam should be administered to lactating women only if considered essential by the physician.

4.7 Effects on ability to drive and use machines

There is no known effect on the ability to drive and operate machines. However, because of the risk of early reactions, driving or operating machinery is not advisable for one hour following the last injection.

4.8 Undesirable effects

As with all other contrast media, this product may provoke anaphylaxis or other manifestations of arrhythmias may infrequently occur.

The use of iodinated compounds may cause untoward side effects and manifestations of anaphylaxis. The symptoms include nausea, vomiting, diffuse erythema, feeling hot, headache, rhinitis or laryngeal oedema, fever, sweating, asthenia, dizziness, pallor, dyspnoea, moderate hypotension. Skin reactions may occur in the form of various types of rash or diffuse blisters. More severe reactions involving the cardiovascular system such as vasodilatation with pronounced hypotension, tachycardia, dyspnea, agitation, cyanosis, loss of consciousness and cardiac arrest may require emergency treatment.

The occurrence of delayed intolerance reactions, most commonly pruritus and urticaria, has been reported up to several days post administration.

During intra-cardiac and/or coronary arteriography, ventricular arrhythmias may infrequently occur.

Also cases of myocardial ischemia or infarction and/or cardiac failure/cardiac arrest have been reported rarely.

Other undesirable effects are:

- renal impairment,
- thrombocytopaenia,
- asthma/bronchospasm, and
- pulmonary oedema.

Hyperthyroidism may recur in patients previously treated for Graves' disease.

After cerebral angiography, confusion, stupor, coma, paresis, cortical blindness (usually transient), and convulsions may occur.

Rarely, Steven-Johnson syndrome has been reported.

Local pain and swelling at the injection site may occur.

Following use in myelography, water soluble non-ionic contrast media have been reported to cause neurological side effects. These include rare cases of seizures, transient confusion or transient motor or sensory dysfunction. Meningism and meningitis have also been reported. The possibility of an infective meningitis should be considered. Headaches, dizziness, nausea and vomiting, pain in limbs, back, or neck pain may also occasionally occur.

4.9 Overdose

Treatment of overdosage is directed toward the support of all vital functions and the elimination of the contrast medium while maintaining the patient well hydrated.

If needed, hemodyalisis can be used to eliminate iopamidol from the body.

5. PHARMACOLOGICAL PROPERTIES

Pharmacotherapeutic group; ATC code: V08A B04

5.1 Pharmacodynamic properties

Iopamidol is contrast medium belonging to the new generation of non-ionic compound whose solubility is due to the presence of hydrophilic substitutes in the molecule. This results in a solution of low osmolality when compared with ionic media.

Iopamidol has been shown to be effective as an X-ray contrast medium in neuroradiology, angiography, venography, arthrography, urography, cerebral angiography and left ventriculography and coronary arteriography. Its toxicity particularly cardiac and CNS toxicity are less than those of ionic contrast media.

5.2 Pharmacokinetic properties

The pharmacokinetics of iopamidol conform to an open two compartment pharmacokinetic model with first order elimination.

Distribution volume is equivalent to extracellular fluid.

Elimination is almost completely through the kidneys. Less that 1% of the administered dose has been recovered in the faeces up to 72 hours after dosing. Elimination is rapid; up to half the administered dose may be recovered in the urine in the first two hours of dosing.

There is no evidence of biotransformation.

Serum protein binding is negligible.

5.3 Preclinical safety data

No adverse effects can be predicted from animal toxicology studies other than those documented from human use of iopamidol.

6. PHARMACEUTICAL PARTICULARS

6.1 List of excipients

Excipients are trometamol, hydrochloric acid and edetate calcium disodium.

6.2 Incompatibilities

No other drug should be mixed with the contrast medium.

6.3 Shelf life

5 years.

6.4 Special precautions for storage

Protect from light.

6.5 Nature and contents of container

10ml clear, colourless Type I glass ampoules.

20 and 30ml clear, colourless Type I or Type II glass vials with rubber closures and aluminium caps.

20, 50, 70, 100, 200 and 250ml clear, colourless Type I or Type II glass bottles with rubber closures and aluminium caps.

6.6 Special precautions for disposal and other handling

Discard if the solution is not clear of particulate matter.

Exceptionally, the event of crystallisation of Niopam could occur. It has been shown that such a phenomenon is caused by a damaged or defective container and therefore the product should not be used in this case.

The bottle, once opened, must be used immediately.

Any residue of contrast medium must be discarded.

Niopam, as other iodinated contrast media, can react with metallic surfaces containing copper (e.g. brass), therefore the use of equipment, in which the product comes into direct contact with such surfaces, should be avoided.

7. MARKETING AUTHORISATION HOLDER

Bracco U.K. Ltd,

Bracco House, Mercury Park,

Wycombe Lane, Wooburn Green,

Buckinghamshire HP10 OHH

8. MARKETING AUTHORISATION NUMBER(S)

PL 18920/0009

9. DATE OF FIRST AUTHORISATION/RENEWAL OF THE AUTHORISATION

22nd March 1982/ 9th January 2002

10. DATE OF REVISION OF THE TEXT

29th July 2005

NIOPAM 340

(Bracco UK Limited)

1. NAME OF THE MEDICINAL PRODUCT

NIOPAM 340, solution for injection

2. QUALITATIVE AND QUANTITATIVE COMPOSITION

69.4% w/v Iopamidol equivalent to 340mg iodine/ml.

Each ml contains 694 mg Iopamidol.

For excipients, see 6.1.

3. PHARMACEUTICAL FORM

Solution for injection.

Clear aqueous solution filled into colourless glass bottles.

4. CLINICAL PARTICULARS

4.1 Therapeutic indications

X-ray contrast medium for use in peripheral arteriography, angiocardiography and left ventriculography, coronary arteriography, aortography - retrograde, selective renal arteriography, selective visceral angiography, digital subtraction angiography, computer tomography enhancement, urography and arthrography.

4.2 Posology and method of administration

Route of administration

Intra-ventricular

Intra-arterial

Intravenous

Intra-articular

Dosage

NIOPAM 340: DOSAGE SCHEDULE

Procedure	Dosage
Peripheral arteriography and venography	Adults 10 - 50 ml Children: **
Angiocardiography and left ventriculography	Adults 30 - 80 ml Children **
Coronary arteriography	Adults: 4 - 8 ml * per artery
Aortography - retrograde	Adults: 30 - 80 ml *
Selective renal arteriography	Adults: 5 - 10ml Children: **
Selective visceral angiography	
Hepatic	Adults: 30 - 70 ml
Coeliac	Adults: 40 - 70ml
Superior Mesenteric	Adults: 25 - 70ml
Inferior Mesenteric	Adults: 5 - 30ml
Digital subtraction angiography (DSA)	
Intravenous injection	Adults 30 - 50 ml Children: **
Coronary arteriography - by intra-arterial DSA,	Adults: 2-5ml
Ventriculography	Adults: 25ml* Children: 1.0-1.5ml/kg
Computer tomography enhancement	Adults: 50 - 100ml
Intravenous urography	Adults: up to 1.5ml/kg Children: 1-2.5ml/kg or **
Arthrography	Adults: 1 - 10ml according to the joint being examined

* repeat as necessary; ** according to body size and age; Do not exceed 250 ml. Single injection volume depends on the vascular area to be examined.

Elderly: dosage as for adults. The lowest effective dose should be used.

Method of administration

No other drugs should be mixed with the contrast medium.

Peripheral arteriography and phlebography (venography)

Percutaneous injection into the appropriate blood vessel is used for visualisation of peripheral arteries and veins.

Angiocardiography, left ventriculography, selective coronary arteriography

Niopam may be administered by rapid injection through a catheter into a suitable peripheral artery or vein. It can also be introduced under pressure through a cardiac catheter into any of the heart chambers, or injected into large vessels for immediate visualisation. The contrast medium may also be administered during selective catheterisation of the coronary arteries.

Aortography

The contrast medium may be introduced directly by intra-arterial injection (retro-grade method) for visualisation of the aorta and its main branches.

Arthrography

Visualisation of joint cavities and articular surfaces can be achieved by either single or double contrast examination.

Selective visceral angiography

Visualisation can be achieved by selective catheterisation and injection into the hepatic, coeliac or mesenteric arteries.

Digital subtraction angiography

For cardiac imaging the contrast medium may be administered intra-arterially by selective catheterisation to provide subtracted images. Niopam 340 and 370 injected intravenously either centrally or peripherally is also recommended for use in this modality.

Urography

The contrast medium is injected intravenously and rapidly eliminated through the kidneys. In patients with severe renal failure, high dose urography should be used.

Computer tomography enhancement

Contrast enhancement for brain scans can be achieved between one and three minutes after i.v. injection. Niopam

200 and 300 are also used for total body scanning examinations after i.v. administration as a bolus, as a drip infusion or by a combination of the two methods.

4.3 Contraindications

Use in patients with proven or suspected hypersensitivity to iodine containing preparations of this type.

4.4 Special warnings and precautions for use

A positive history of allergy, asthma or untoward reaction during previous similar investigations indicates a need for extra caution; the benefit should clearly outweigh the risk in such patients. Appropriate resuscitative measures should be immediately available.

X-ray examination of women should if possible be conducted during the pre-ovulation phase of the menstrual cycle and should be avoided during pregnancy.

When examining small children or babies, do not limit fluid intake before administering a hypertonic contrast solution. Also, correct any existing water and electrolyte imbalance.

Care should be exercised in carrying out radiographic procedures with contrast media in patients with severe functional impairment of the liver or myocardium, severe systemic disease and in myelomatosis (including Waldenströms macroglobulinemia, multiple myeloma).

In the latter condition patients should not be exposed to dehydration; similarly abnormalities of fluid or electrolyte balance should be corrected prior to use.

Particular care should also be exercised in patients with moderate to severe impairment of renal function (as reflected by a raised blood urea) or in diabetes. Substantial deterioration in renal function is minimised if the patient is well hydrated. Renal function parameters should be monitored after the procedure in these patients.

Patients with severe hepato-renal insufficiency should not be examined unless absolutely indicated. Re-examination should be delayed for 5-7 days.

Special care should be exercised when this product is injected into the right heart or pulmonary artery in patients with pulmonary hypertension. Right heart angiography should be carried out only when absolutely indicated.

Niopam should be administered with caution in elderly patients and patients with increased intracranial pressure or suspicion of intracranial tumour, abscess or haematoma, and in those with a history of a previous reaction to contrast media, asthma, allergy, epilepsy, severe cardiovascular disease, renal impairment, chronic alcoholism or multiple sclerosis.

Patients with these conditions have an increased risk of neurological complications.

General anaesthesia may be indicated in selected patients. However, a higher incidence of adverse reactions has been reported in these patients, probably due to the hypotensive effect of the anaesthetic.

Contrast media may promote sickling in individuals who are homozygous for sickle cell disease when injected intravenously and intra-arterially.

Patients with phaeochromocytoma may develop severe hypertensive crisis following intravascular Iopamidol. Pre-medication with α-receptor blockers is recommended.

The administration of iodinated contrast media may aggravate the symptoms of myasthenia gravis.

Patients with congestive heart failure should be observed for several hours following the procedure to detect delayed haemodynamic disturbances, which may be associated with a transitory increase in the circulating osmotic load. All other patients should be observed for at least one hour after the procedure, as most of the adverse events occur in this period. The patient should also be informed that allergic reactions may develop up to several days after the procedure; in such case, a physician should be consulted immediately.

In neonates, and particularly in premature neonates, it is recommended that tests of thyroid function (typically TSH and T4), should be checked 7-10 days and 1 month after the administration of iodinated contrast media because of the risk of hypothyroidism due to iodine overload.

In patients scheduled for thyroid examination with a radioactive iodine tracer, one must take into consideration that iodine uptake in the thyroid gland will be reduced for several days (up to two weeks) after dosing with an iodinized contrast medium that is eliminated through the kidneys.

Local tissue irritation can occur as an event of perivascular infiltration.

Neuroradiology

In patients who are known epileptics or have a history of epilepsy, anticonvulsant therapy should be maintained before and following myelographic procedures. In some instances, anticonvulsant therapy may be increased for 48 hours before the examination.

Neuroleptics must be absolutely avoided because they lower the seizure threshold. The same applies to analgesics, anti-emetics, antihistamines and sedatives of the phenothiazine group. Whenever possible, treatment with such drugs should be discontinued at least 48 hours before administration of the contrast medium and not be resumed less than 12 hours after completion of the procedure.

Angiography

In patients undergoing angiocardiographic procedures special attention should be paid to the status of the right heart and pulmonary circulation. Right heart insufficiency and pulmonary hypertension may precipitate bradycardia and systemic hypotension, when the organic iodine solution is injected. Right heart angiography should be carried out only when absolutely indicated.

In angiographic procedures, the possibility of dislodging plaque or damaging or perforating the vessel wall should be considered during catheter manipulation and contrast medium injection. Test injections to ensure proper catheter placements are recommended.

Angiography should be avoided whenever possible in patients with homocystinuria due to an increased risk of thrombosis and embolism.

In patients undergoing peripheral angiography, there should be pulsation in the artery into which the X-ray contrast medium will be injected. In patients with thromboangiitis obliterans or ascending infections in combination with serious ischemia the angiography should be performed, if at all, with special caution.

In patients undergoing venography, special caution should be exercised in patients with suspected phlebitis, serious ischaemia, local infections, or a complete venous occlusion.

Serious neurological events have been observed following direct injection of contrast media into cerebral arteries or vessels supplying the spinal cord or in angiocardiography due to inadvertent filling of the carotids.

In paediatric roentgenology, one should proceed with great caution when injecting the contrast medium into the right heart chambers of cyanotic neonates with pulmonary hypertension and impaired cardiac function.

In examinations of the aortic arch the tip of the catheter should be positioned carefully to avoid hypotension, bradycardia and CNS injury due to excess pressure transmitted from the injector pump to the brachiocephalic branches of the aorta.

Urography

Care should be exercised in patients with moderate to severe impairment of renal function (as reflected by a raised blood urea). Substantial deterioration in renal function is minimized if the patient is well hydrated. Renal function parameters, especially urinary output should be monitored after the examination in these patients.

Re-examination should be delayed 5-7 days.

Non-ionic contrast media have less anti-coagulant activity *in-vitro* than ionic media. Meticulous attention should therefore be paid to angiographic technique. Non-ionic media should not be allowed to remain in contact with blood in the syringe and intravascular catheters should be flushed frequently, to minimise the risk of clotting, which rarely has led to serious thromboembolic complications after procedures.

Niopam should be used with caution in patients with hyperthyroidism. It is possible that hyperthyroidism may recur in patients previously treated for Graves' disease.

The presence of renal damage in diabetic patients is one of the factors predisposing to renal impairment following contrast media administration. This may precipitate lactic acidosis in patients who are taking metformin. As a precaution, metformin should be discontinued at the time of, or prior to, the procedure and withheld for 48 hours subsequent to the procedure and re-instituted only after renal function has been re-evaluated and found to be normal.

4.5 Interaction with other medicinal products and other forms of interaction

Thyroid function tests: use of iodinated contrast media may interfere with tests for thyroid function which depend on iodine estimations, such as Protein Binding Iodine and radioactive iodine uptake. As a consequence they will not accurately reflect thyroid function for up to 16 days following administration of iodinated contrast media. Thyroid function tests not depending on iodine estimations, e.g. T3 resin uptake and total or free thyroxine (T4) assays are not affected.

No other specific interference with physiological functions has been noted.

The administration of an X-ray contrast medium in diabetic patients with nephropathy who are taking biguanides may precipitate lactic acidosis.

Arterial thrombosis has been reported when Iopamidol was given following papaverine.

The administration of vasopressors strongly potentiates the neurological effect of the intra-arterial contrast media.

Contrast media may interfere with laboratory tests for bilirubin, proteins or inorganic substances (eg iron, copper, calcium, phosphate). These substances should not be assayed during the same day following the administration of contrast media.

4.6 Pregnancy and lactation

X-ray examination of women should if possible be conducted during the pre-ovulation phase of the menstrual cycle and should be avoided during pregnancy; also, since it has not been demonstrated that Niopam is safe for use in pregnant women, it should be administered only if the procedure is considered essential by the physician.

Niopam is poorly excreted in human milk. From animal experience, Niopam is non toxic in animals after oral administration. Although, no serious adverse reactions have been reported in nursing infants, Niopam should be administered to lactating women only if considered essential by the physician.

4.7 Effects on ability to drive and use machines

There is no known effect on the ability to drive and operate machines. However, because of the risk of early reactions, driving or operating machinery is not advisable for one hour following the last injection.

4.8 Undesirable effects

The use of iodinated compounds may cause untoward side effects and manifestations of anaphylaxis. The symptoms include nausea, vomiting, diffuse erythema, feeling hot, headache, rhinitis or laryngeal oedema, fever, sweating, asthenia, dizziness, pallor, dyspnoea, moderate hypotension. Skin reactions may occur in the form of various types of rash or diffuse blisters. More severe reactions involving the cardiovascular system such as vasodilatation with pronounced hypotension, tachycardia, dyspnoea, agitation, cyanosis, loss of consciousness and cardiac arrest may require emergency treatment.

The occurrence of delayed intolerance reactions, most commonly pruritus and urticaria, has been reported up to several days post administration.

During intracardiac and/or coronary arteriography, ventricular arrhythmias may infrequently occur.

Also cases of myocardial ischemia or infarction and/or cardiac failure/cardiac arrest have been reported rarely.

Other undesirable effects are:

- renal impairment,
- thrombocytopaenia,
- asthma/bronchospasm, and
- pulmonary oedema.

Hyperthyroidism may recur in patients previously treated for Graves' disease.

After cerebral angiography, confusion, stupor, coma, paresis, cortical blindness (usually transient), and convulsions may occur.

Rarely, Steven-Johnson syndrome has been reported.

Local pain and swelling at the injection site may occur.

Following use in myelography, water soluble non-ionic contrast media have been reported to cause neurological side effects. These include rare cases of seizures, transient confusion or transient motor or sensory dysfunction. Meningism and meningitis have also been reported. The possibility of an infective meningitis should be considered. Headaches, dizziness, nausea and vomiting, pain in limbs, back, or neck pain may also occur.

4.9 Overdose

Treatment of overdosage is directed toward the support of all vital functions and the elimination of the contrast medium while maintaining the patient well hydrated.

If needed, hemodyalisis can be used to eliminate Iopamidol from the body.

5. PHARMACOLOGICAL PROPERTIES

Pharmacotherapeutic group; ATC code: V08A B04

5.1 Pharmacodynamic properties

Iopamidol is contrast medium belonging to the new generation of non-ionic compound whose solubility is due to the presence of hydrophilic substitutes in the molecule. This results in a solution of low osmolality when compared with ionic media.

Iopamidol has been shown to be effective as an X-ray contrast medium in neuroradiology, angiography, venography, arthrography, urography, cerebral angiography and left ventriculography and coronary arteriography. Its toxicity particularly cardiac and CNS toxicity are less than those of ionic contrast media.

5.2 Pharmacokinetic properties

The pharmacokinetics of Iopamidol conform to an open two compartment pharmacokinetic model with first order elimination.

Distribution volume is equivalent to extracellular fluid.

Elimination is almost completely through the kidneys. Less that 1% of the administered dose has been recovered in the faeces up to 72 hours after dosing. Elimination is rapid; up to half the administered dose may be recovered in the urine in the first two hours of dosing.

There is no evidence of biotransformation.

Serum protein binding is negligible.

5.3 Preclinical safety data

No adverse effects can be predicted from animal toxicology studies other than those documented from human use of Iopamidol.

6. PHARMACEUTICAL PARTICULARS

6.1 List of excipients

Excipients are: trometamol, hydrochloric acid and edetate calcium disodium.

6.2 Incompatibilities

No other drug should be mixed with the contrast medium.

6.3 Shelf life
5 years.

6.4 Special precautions for storage
Protect from light.

6.5 Nature and contents of container
50, 70, 100 and 200ml clear, colourless Type I or Type II glass bottles with rubber closures and aluminium caps.

6.6 Special precautions for disposal and other handling
Discard if the solution is not clear of particulate matter.

Exceptionally, the event of crystallisation of Niopam could occur. It has been shown that such a phenomenon is caused by a damaged or defective container and therefore the product should not be used in this case.

The bottle, once opened, must be used immediately.

Any residue of contrast medium must be discarded.

Niopam, as other iodinated contrast media, can react with metallic surfaces containing copper (e.g. brass), therefore the use of equipment, in which the product comes into direct contact with such surfaces, should be avoided.

7. MARKETING AUTHORISATION HOLDER
Bracco U.K. Ltd,

Bracco House, Mercury Park,

Wycombe Lane, Wooburn Green,

Buckinghamshire HP10 OHH

8. MARKETING AUTHORISATION NUMBER(S)
PL 18920/0010

9. DATE OF FIRST AUTHORISATION/RENEWAL OF THE AUTHORISATION
13th January 1989 / 9th January 2002

10. DATE OF REVISION OF THE TEXT
29th July 2005

NIOPAM 370

(Bracco UK Limited)

1. NAME OF THE MEDICINAL PRODUCT
NIOPAM 370, solution for injection.

2. QUALITATIVE AND QUANTITATIVE COMPOSITION
75.5% w/v Iopamidol equivalent to 370mg iodine/ml.

Each ml contains 755.3 mg Iopamidol.

For excipients, see 6.1.

3. PHARMACEUTICAL FORM
Solution for injection.

Clear aqueous solution filled into colourless glass ampoules or bottles.

4. CLINICAL PARTICULARS
4.1 Therapeutic indications
X-ray contrast medium for use in:

Peripheral arteriography

Angiocardiography and left ventriculography

Coronary arteriography

Aortography - retrograde

Selective renal arteriography

Selective visceral angiography

Digital subtraction angiography

Urography

4.2 Posology and method of administration
<u>Route of administration</u>

Intra-arterial

Intra-venous

Intra-ventricular

<u>Dosage</u>

NIOPAM 370: DOSAGE SCHEDULE

Procedure	Dosage
Peripheral Arteriography	Adults 20 - 50 ml * Children **
Venography	Adults 20 - 50 ml * Children **
Angiocardiography and Left Ventriculography	Adults 30 - 80 ml Children **
Coronary Arteriography	Adults 4 - 8 ml per artery *
Aortography - Retrograde	Adults 30 - 80 ml Children **
Selective Renal Arteriography	Adults 5 - 10 ml Children **
Selective Visceral Angiography:	
Hepatic	Adults 30 - 70 ml
Coeliac	40 - 70 ml
Superior mesenteric, inferior mesenteric	5 - 30 ml
	Children **
Digital Subtraction Angiography:	
Intravenous injection	Adults 50 ml Children 0.5 - 0.75 ml/kg
Left ventriculography	Adults 25 ml Children 1 - 1.5 ml/kg
Selective coronary arteriography by intra-arterial DSA	Adults 2 - 5 ml
Intravenous Urography	Adults 40 - 80 ml In severe renal failure the usual high dose methods should be employed. (up to 1.5 mg/kg or**) Children 1- 2.5 ml/Kg**

*repeat as necessary; ** according to body size and age;

Do not exceed 250 ml. Single injection volume depends on the vascular area to be examined

Elderly: dosage as for adults. The lowest effective dose should be used.

<u>Method of administration</u>

No other drugs should be mixed with the contrast medium.

Peripheral arteriography and phlebography (venography)

Percutaneous injection into the appropriate blood vessel is used for visualisation of peripheral arteries and veins.

Angiocardiography, left ventriculography, selective coronary arteriography

Niopam may be administered by rapid injection through a catheter into a suitable peripheral artery or vein. It can also be introduced under pressure through a cardiac catheter into any of the heart chambers, or injected into large vessels for immediate visualisation. The contrast medium may also be administered during selective catheterisation of the coronary arteries.

Aortography

The contrast medium may be introduced directly by intra-arterial injection (retro-grade method) for visualisation of the aorta and its main branches.

Selective visceral angiography

Visualisation can be achieved by selective catheterisation and injection into the hepatic, coeliac or mesenteric arteries.

Digital subtraction angiography

For cardiac imaging the contrast medium may be administered intra-arterially by selectivecatheterisation to provide subtracted images. Niopam 340 and 370 injected intravenously either centrally or peripherally is also recommended for use in this modality.

Urography

The contrast medium is injected intravenously and rapidly eliminated through the kidneys. In patients with severe renal failure, high dose urography should be used.

4.3 Contraindications
Use in patients with proven or suspected hypersensitivity to iodine containing preparations of this type.

4.4 Special warnings and precautions for use
A positive history of allergy, asthma or untoward reaction during previous similar investigations indicates a need for extra caution; the benefit should clearly outweigh the risk in such patients. Appropriate resuscitative measures should be immediately available.

X-ray examination of women should if possible be conducted during the pre-ovulation phase of the menstrual cycle and should be avoided during pregnancy.

When examining small children or babies, do not limit fluid intake before administering a hypertonic contrast solution. Also, correct any existing water and electrolyte imbalance.

Care should be exercised in carrying out radiographic procedures with contrast media in patients with severe functional impairment of the liver or myocardium, severe systemic disease and in myelomatosis (including Waldenströms macroglobulinemia, multiple myeloma).

In the latter condition patients should not be exposed to dehydration; similarly abnormalities of fluid or electrolyte balance should be corrected prior to use.

Particular care should also be exercised in patients with moderate to severe impairment of renal function (as reflected by a raised blood urea) or in diabetes. Substantial deterioration in renal function is minimised if the patient is well hydrated. Renal function parameters should be monitored after the procedure in these patients.

Patients with severe hepato-renal insufficiency should not be examined unless absolutely indicated. Re-examination should be delayed for 5-7 days.

Special care should be exercised when this product is injected into the right heart or pulmonary artery in patients with pulmonary hypertension. Right heart angiography should be carried out only when absolutely indicated.

Niopam should be administered with caution in elderly patients and patients with increased intracranial pressure or suspicion of intracranial tumour, abscess or haematoma, and in those with a history of a previous reaction to contrast media, asthma, allergy, epilepsy, severe cardiovascular disease, renal impairment, chronic alcoholism or multiple sclerosis.

Patients with these conditions have an increased risk of neurological complications.

General anaesthesia may be indicated in selected patients. However, a higher incidence of adverse reactions has been reported in these patients, probably due to the hypotensive effect of the anaesthetic.

Contrast media may promote sickling in individuals who are homozygous for sickle cell disease when injected intravenously and intra-arterially.

Patients with phaeochromocytoma may develop severe hypertensive crisis following intravascular iopamidol. Pre-medication with α-receptor blockers is recommended. The administration of iodinated contrast media may aggravate the symptoms of myasthenia gravis.

Patients with congestive heart failure should be observed for several hours following the procedure to detect delayed haemodynamic disturbances, which may be associated with a transitory increase in the circulating osmotic load. All other patients should be observed for at least one hour after the procedure, as most of the adverse events occur in this period. The patient should also be informed that allergic reactions may develop up to several days after the procedure; in such case, a physician should be consulted immediately.

In neonates, and particularly in premature neonates, it is recommended that tests of thyroid function (typically TSH and T4), should be checked 7-10 days and 1 month after the administration of iodinated contrast media because of the risk of hypothyroidism due to iodine overload.

In patients scheduled for thyroid examination with a radioactive iodine tracer, one must take into consideration that iodine uptake in the thyroid gland will be reduced for several days (up to two weeks) after dosing with an iodinized contrast medium that is eliminated through the kidneys.

Local tissue irritation can occur as an event of perivascular infiltration.

Neuroradiology

In patients who are known epileptics or have a history of epilepsy, anticonvulsant therapy should be maintained before and following myelographic procedures. In some instances anticonvulsant therapy may be increased for 48 hours before the examination.

Neuroleptics must be absolutely avoided because they lower the seizure threshold. The same applies to analgesics, anti-emetics, antihistamines and sedatives of the phenothiazine group. Whenever possible, treatment with such drugs should be discontinued at least 48 hours before administration of the contrast medium and not be resumed less than 12 hours after completion of the procedure.

Angiography

In patients undergoing angiocardiographic procedures special attention should be paid to the status of the right heart and pulmonary circulation. Right heart insufficiency and pulmonary hypertension may precipitate bradycardia and systemic hypotension, when the organic iodine solution is injected. Right heart angiography should be carried out only when absolutely indicated.

In angiographic procedures, the possibility of dislodging plaque or damaging or perforating the vessel wall should be considered during catheter manipulation and contrast medium injection. Test injections to ensure proper catheter placements are recommended.

Angiography should be avoided whenever possible in patients with homocystinuria due to an increased risk of thrombosis and embolism.

In patients undergoing peripheral angiography, there should be pulsation in the artery into which the X-ray contrast medium will be injected. In patients with thromboangiitis obliterans or ascending infections in combination with serious ischemia the angiography should be performed, if at all, with special caution.

In patients undergoing venography, special caution should be exercised in patients with suspected phlebitis, serious ischaemia, local infections, or a complete venous occlusion.

Serious neurological events have been observed following direct injection of contrast media into cerebral arteries or vessels supplying the spinal cord or in angiocardiography due to inadvertent filling of the carotids.

In paediatric roentgenology, one should proceed with great caution when injecting the contrast medium into the right heart chambers of cyanotic neonates with pulmonary hypertension and impaired cardiac function.

In examinations of the aortic arch the tip of the catheter should be positioned carefully to avoid hypotension, bradycardia and CNS injury due to excess pressure transmitted from the injector pump to the brachiocephalic branches of the aorta.

Urography

Care should be exercised in patients with moderate to severe impairment of renal function (as reflected by a raised blood urea). Substantial deterioration in renal function is minimized if the patient is well hydrated. Renal function parameters, especially urinary output should be monitored after the examination in these patients.

Re-examination should be delayed 5-7 days.

Non-ionic contrast media have less anti-coagulant activity in-vitro than ionic media. Meticulous attention should therefore be paid to angiographic technique. Non-ionic media should not be allowed to remain in contact with blood in the syringe and intravascular catheters should be flushed frequently, to minimise the risk of clotting, which rarely has led to serious thromboembolic complications after procedures.

Niopam should be used with caution in patients with hyperthyroidism. It is possible that hyperthyroidism may recur in patients previously treated for Graves' disease.

The presence of renal damage in diabetic patients is one of the factors predisposing to renal impairment following contrast media administration. This may precipitate lactic acidosis in patients who are taking metformin. As a precaution, metformin should be discontinued at the time of, or prior to, the procedure and withheld for 48 hours subsequent to the procedure and re-instituted only after renal function has been re-evaluated and found to be normal.

4.5 Interaction with other medicinal products and other forms of interaction

Thyroid function tests: use of iodinated contrast media may interfere with tests for thyroid function which depend on iodine estimations, such as Protein Binding Iodine and radioactive iodine uptake. As a consequence they will not accurately reflect thyroid function for up to 16 days following administration of iodinated contrast media. Thyroid function tests not depending on iodine estimations, e.g. T3 resin uptake and total or free thyroxine (T4) assays are not affected.

No other specific interference with physiological functions have been noted.

The administration of an X-ray contrast medium in diabetic patients with nephropathy who are taking biguanides may precipitate lactic acidosis.

Arterial thrombosis has been reported when iopamidol was given following papaverine. The administration of vasopressors strongly potentiate the neurological effect of the intra-arterial contrast media.

Contrast media may interfere with laboratory tests for bilirubin, proteins or inorganic substances (eg iron, copper, calcium, phosphate). These substances should not be assayed during the same day following the administration of contrast media

4.6 Pregnancy and lactation

X-ray examination of women should if possible be conducted during the pre-ovulation phase of the menstrual cycle and should be avoided during pregnancy; also, since it has not been demonstrated that Niopam is safe for use in pregnant women, it should be administered only if the procedure is considered essential by the physician.

Niopam is poorly excreted in human milk. From animal experience, Niopam is non toxic in animals after oral administration. Although, no serious adverse reactions have been reported in nursing infants, Niopam should be administered to lactating women only if considered essential by the physician

4.7 Effects on ability to drive and use machines

There is no known effect on the ability to drive and operate machines. However, because of the risk of early reactions, driving or operating machinery is not advisable for one hour following the last injection.

4.8 Undesirable effects

The use of iodinated compounds may cause untoward side effects and manifestations of anaphylaxis. The symptoms include nausea, vomiting, diffuse erythema, feeling hot, headache, rhinitis or laryngeal oedema, fever, sweating, asthenia, dizziness, pallor, dyspnoea, moderate hypotension. Skin reactions may occur in the form of various types of rash or diffuse blisters. More severe reactions involving the cardiovascular system such as vasodilatation with pronounced hypotension, tachycardia, dyspnoea, agitation, cyanosis, loss of consciousness and cardiac arrest may require emergency treatment.

The occurrence of delayed intolerance reactions, most commonly pruritus and urticaria, has been reported up to several days post administration.

During intracardiac and/or coronary arteriography, ventricular arrhythmias may infrequently occur.

Also cases of myocardial ischemia or infarction and/or cardiac failure/cardiac arrest have been reported rarely.

Other undesirable effects are:

- renal impairment,
- thrombocytopaenia,
- asthma/bronchospasm, and
- pulmonary oedema.

Hyperthyroidism may recur in patients previously treated for Graves' disease.

After cerebral angiography, confusion; stupor; coma; paresis; cortical blindness (usually transient); and convulsions may occur.

Rarely, Steven-Johnson syndrome has been reported.

Local pain and swelling at the injection site may occur.

4.9 Overdose

Treatment of overdosage is directed toward the support of all vital functions and the elimination of the contrast medium while maintaining the patient well hydrated.

If needed, hemodyalisis can be used to eliminate iopamidol from the body.

5. PHARMACOLOGICAL PROPERTIES

Pharmacotherapeutic group; ATC code: V08A B04

5.1 Pharmacodynamic properties

Iopamidol is contrast medium belonging to the new generation of non-ionic compound whose solubility is due to the presence of hydrophilic substitutes in the molecule. This results in a solution of low osmolality when compared with ionic media.

Iopamidol has been shown to be effective as an X-ray contrast medium in neuroradiology, angiography, venography, arthrography, urography, cerebral angiography and left ventriculography and coronary arteriography. Its toxicity particularly cardiac and CNS toxicity are less than those of ionic contrast media.

5.2 Pharmacokinetic properties

The pharmacokinetics of iopamidol conform to an open two compartment pharmacokinetic model with first order elimination.

Distribution volume is equivalent to extra-cellular fluid.

Elimination is almost completely through the kidneys. Less that 1% of the administered dose has been recovered in the faeces up to 72 hours after dosing. Elimination is rapid; up to half the administered dose may be recovered in the urine in the first two hours of dosing.

There is no evidence of biotransformation.

Serum protein binding is negligible.

5.3 Preclinical safety data

No adverse effects can be predicted from animal toxicology studies other than those documented from human use of iopamidol.

6. PHARMACEUTICAL PARTICULARS

6.1 List of excipients

Excipients are: trometamol, hydrochloric acid and edetate calcium disodium.

6.2 Incompatibilities

No other drug should be mixed with the contrast medium.

6.3 Shelf life

5 years.

6.4 Special precautions for storage

Protect from light.

6.5 Nature and contents of container

10, 20 ml clear, colourless Type I glass ampoules.

30ml clear, colourless Type I or Type II glass vials with rubber closures and aluminium caps.

50, 70, 100, 200 and 250ml clear, colourless Type I or Type II glass bottles with rubber closures and aluminium caps.

6.6 Special precautions for disposal and other handling

Discard if the solution is not clear of particulate matter.

Exceptionally, the event of crystallisation of Niopam could occur. It has been shown that such a phenomenon is caused by a damaged or defective container and therefore the product should not be used in this case.

The bottle, once opened, must be used immediately.

Any residue of contrast medium must be discarded.

Niopam, as other iodinated contrast media, can react with metallic surfaces containing copper (e.g. brass), therefore the use of equipment, in which the product comes into direct contact with such surfaces, should be avoided.

7. MARKETING AUTHORISATION HOLDER

Bracco U.K. Ltd,

Bracco House, Mercury Park,

Wycombe Lane, Wooburn Green,

Buckinghamshire HP10 OHH

8. MARKETING AUTHORISATION NUMBER(S)

PL 18920/0011

9. DATE OF FIRST AUTHORISATION/RENEWAL OF THE AUTHORISATION

22nd March 1982 / 9th January 2002

10. DATE OF REVISION OF THE TEXT

29th July 2005

Nitrazepam Mixture BP (SOMNITE Suspension)

(Norgine Limited)

1. NAME OF THE MEDICINAL PRODUCT

Nitrazepam Mixture BP (SOMNITE Suspension).

2. QUALITATIVE AND QUANTITATIVE COMPOSITION

Each 5 ml spoonful contains 2.5 mg Nitrazepam BP.

3. PHARMACEUTICAL FORM

Oral suspension.

4. CLINICAL PARTICULARS

4.1 Therapeutic indications

For the short term treatment of insomnia where daytime sedation is acceptable.

Benzodiazepines should be used to treat insomnia only when it is severe, disabling, or subjecting the individual to extreme distress.

4.2 Posology and method of administration

Nitrazepam is a long acting benzodiazepine, and the lowest dose which can control the symptoms should be used. If possible, treatment should be intermittent. The maximum dose should not be exceeded.

Adults: 5 mg (two 5 ml spoonfuls) before retiring to bed. This dose may, if necessary, be increased to 10 mg (four 5 ml spoonfuls).

Elderly and patients with impaired liver and/or renal function: 2.5 mg (one 5 ml spoonful) before retiring to bed. This dose may, if necessary, be increased to 5 mg (two 5 ml spoonfuls)

Children: Not recommended.

Generally the duration of treatment varies from a few days to two weeks with a maximum, including the tapering off process, of four weeks.

Patients who have taken benzodiazepines chronically may require a longer tapering off period. In certain cases extension beyond the maximum treatment period may be necessary; if so, it should not take place without re-evaluation of the patient's status.

4.3 Contraindications

Chronic psychosis

Myasthenia gravis

Severe hepatic insufficiency

Severe respiratory insufficiency

Sleep apnoea syndrome

Acute Porphyria.

Hypersensitivity to benzodiazepines and other ingredients

4.4 Special warnings and precautions for use

Tolerance: Some loss of efficacy to the hypnotic effects of benzodiazepines may develop after repeated use for a few weeks.

Dependence: Use of benzodiazepines may lead to the development of physical and psychic dependence upon these products. The risk of dependence increases with dose and duration of treatment; it is also greater in patients with a history of alcohol or drug abuse.

Once physical dependence has developed, abrupt termination of treatment will be accompanied by withdrawal symptoms. These may consist of headaches, muscle pain, extreme anxiety, tension, restlessness, confusion and irritability. In severe cases the following symptoms may occur: derealization, depersonalisation, hyperacusis, numbness and tingling of the extremities, hypersensitivity to light, noise and physical contact, hallucinations or epileptic seizures.

Rebound insomnia and anxiety: a transient syndrome whereby the symptoms that led to treatment with a benzodiazepine recur in an enhanced form, may occur on withdrawal of treatment. It may be accompanied by other reactions including mood changes, anxiety or sleep disturbances and restlessness. Since the risk of withdrawal phenomena/rebound phenomena is greater after abrupt discontinuation of treatment, it is recommended that the dosage is decreased gradually.

Duration of treatment: The duration of treatment should be as short as possible (see Posology) depending on the indication, but should not exceed 4 weeks including any dose-tapering period for insomnia. Extension beyond this period should not take place without re-evaluation of the situation.

It may be useful to inform the patient when treatment is started that it will be of limited duration and to explain precisely how the dosage will be progressively decreased. Moreover it is important that the patient should be aware of the possibility of rebound phenomena, thereby minimising anxiety over such symptoms should they occur while SOMNITE is being discontinued.

If a change is made to a benzodiazepine with a short duration of action, the patient should be warned that withdrawal symptoms may develop.

Amnesia: Benzodiazepines may induce anterograde amnesia. The condition occurs most often several hours after ingesting the product and therefore to reduce the risk patients should ensure that they will be able to have an uninterrupted sleep of 7-8 hours (see also Undesirable Effects).

Psychiatric and paradoxical reactions: Reactions like restlessness, agitation, confusion, irritability, aggressiveness, delusion, rages, nightmares, hallucinations, psychoses, inappropriate behaviour and other adverse behavioural effects are known to occur when using benzodiazepines. They may be quite severe and are more likely in children and the elderly. Should they occur, use of the medicinal product should be discontinued.

Specific patient groups: Benzodiazepines should not be given to children without careful assessment of the need to do so; the duration of treatment must be kept to a minimum. Elderly should be given a reduced dose (see Posology). A lower dose is also recommended for patients with chronic respiratory insufficiency due to the risk of respiratory depression (cross refer to section 4.3 -

contraindicated in severe respiratory insufficiency). Benzodiazepines are not indicated to treat patients with severe hepatic insufficiency as they may precipitate encephalopathy.

Benzodiazepines are not recommended for the primary treatment of psychotic illness.

Benzodiazepines should not be used alone to treat depression or anxiety associated with depression (suicide may be precipitated in such patients).

Benzodiazepines should be used with extreme caution in patients with a history of alcohol or drug abuse.

4.5 Interaction with other medicinal products and other forms of interaction

Not recommended: Concomitant intake with alcohol. The sedative effect may be enhanced when the product is used in combination with alcohol. This affects the ability to drive or use machines.

Take into account: Combination with CNS depressants.

Enhancement of the central depressive effect may occur in cases of concomitant use with antipsychotics (neuroleptics), hypnotics, anxiolytics/sedatives, antidepressant agents, narcotic analgesics, anti-epileptic products, anaesthetics and sedative antihistamines.

In the case of narcotic analgesics enhancement of the euphoria may also occur leading to an increase in psychic dependence.

In the case of anti-epileptics, the following

Barbiturates

Carbamazepine

Hydantoins

are inducers of hepatic metabolism and may enhance the metabolism of benzodiazepines.

Phenytoin concentration may be increased or decreased.

Compounds which inhibit certain hepatic enzymes (particularly cytochrome P450) may enhance the activity of benzodiazepines. To a lesser degree this also applies to benzodiazepines that are metabolised only by conjugation.

Cimetidine inhibits the metabolism of nitrazepam.

Benzodiazepines possibly antagonise the effects of levodopa.

Rifampicin, by enzyme induction, reduces the half-life of nitrazepam and increases the clearance.

Probenecid may increase the sedative effects, possibly excessively.

4.6 Pregnancy and lactation

If the product is prescribed to a woman of childbearing potential, she should be warned to contact her physician regarding discontinuance of the product if she intends to become or suspects that she is pregnant.

If, for compelling medical reasons, the product is administered during the late phase of pregnancy, or during labour at high doses, effects on the neonate, such as hypothermia, hypotonia and moderate respiratory depression, can be expected, due to the pharmacological action of the compound.

Moreover, infants born to mothers who took benzodiazepines chronically during the latter stages of pregnancy may have developed physical dependence and may be at some risk for developing withdrawal symptoms in the postnatal period.

Since benzodiazepines are found in the breast milk, benzodiazepines should not be given to breast feeding mothers.

4.7 Effects on ability to drive and use machines

Sedation, amnesia, impaired concentration and impaired muscular function may adversely affect the ability to drive or to use machines. If insufficient sleep duration occurs, the likelihood of impaired alertness may be increased (See also Interactions).

4.8 Undesirable effects

The following occur predominantly at the start of therapy and usually disappear with repeated administration:

ataxia or double vision, confusion, dizziness, drowsiness, fatigue, headache, muscle weakness, numbed emotions, reduced alertness.

Undesirable effects may persist into the following day due to the long half-life.

Other side effects like gastrointestinal disturbances, changes in libido, skin reactions, have been reported occasionally.

Blood dyscrasias, jaundice, hypotension and urinary retention have been reported rarely.

Amnesia: Anterograde amnesia may occur using therapeutic dosages, the risk increasing at higher dosages. Amnestic effect may be associated with inappropriate behaviour. (See Special Warnings and Special Precautions for Use).

Depression: Pre-existing depression may be unmasked during benzodiazepine use.

Psychiatric and Paradoxical Reactions: Psychiatric and paradoxical reactions are known to occur. (See Special Warnings and Special Precautions for Use).

Dependence: Use (even at therapeutic doses) may lead to the development of physical dependence: discontinuation of the therapy may result in withdrawal or rebound phenomena. (See Special Warnings and Special Precautions for Use). Psychic dependence may occur.

Abuse:

Abuse of benzodiazepines has been reported.

4.9 Overdose

Benzodiazepines commonly cause drowsiness, ataxia, dysarthria and nystagmus. Coma, hypotension and respiratory depression occasionally occur but are seldom serious if these drugs are taken alone. Coma usually lasts only a few hours but in elderly people it may be more protracted and cyclical. Benzodiazepine respiratory depressant effects are more serious in patients with severe chronic respiratory disease.

Benzodiazepines potentiate the effects of other central nervous system depressants, including alcohol.

Management

Consider activated charcoal in adults or children who have taken more than 1mg/kg within 1 hour, provided they are not too drowsy. Gastric lavage is unnecessary if these drugs have been taken alone. Patients who are asymptomatic at four hours are unlikely to develop symptoms. Institute supportive measures as indicated by the patient's clinical state.

If CNS depression is severe consider the use of flumazenil (Anexate) a benzodiazepine antagonist. This should rarely be required. It has a short half-life (about an hour) and should NOT BE USED IN MIXED OVERDOSE OR AS A "DIAGNOSTIC" TEST. It is contraindicated in the presence of drugs that reduce seizure threshold (e.g. tricyclic antidepressants).

5. PHARMACOLOGICAL PROPERTIES

5.1 Pharmacodynamic properties

Nitrazepam is a long acting benzodiazepine with anxiolytic, sedative and hypnotic characteristics

5.2 Pharmacokinetic properties

SOMNITE is well absorbed from the GI tract with peak blood levels of nitrazepam being achieved within 2-3 hours of administration.

Half life is approximately 24 hours and plasma steady state levels are achieved after 5 days.

5.3 Preclinical safety data

Preclinical studies provide only limited evidence of safety. Nitrazepam has no significant systemic toxicity potential at the doses in clinical use with the exception of use in pregnancy and lactation for which evidence of safety is lacking.

6. PHARMACEUTICAL PARTICULARS

6.1 List of excipients

Sucrose

Microcrystalline cellulose

Carboxymethyl cellulose sodium

Mixed esters of p-hydroxybenzoic acid

Cherry flavour

Water

6.2 Incompatibilities

None known.

6.3 Shelf life

2 years.

6.4 Special precautions for storage

Do not store above 25°C. Protect from light. Do not freeze.

6.5 Nature and contents of container

Amber glass bottles containing 150 ml of suspension.

6.6 Special precautions for disposal and other handling

The bottle should be shaken before use.

7. MARKETING AUTHORISATION HOLDER

Norgine Limited

Chaplin House

Widewater Place

Moorhall Road

Harefield

UXBRIDGE

Middlesex, UB9 6NS

United Kingdom

8. MARKETING AUTHORISATION NUMBER(S)

PL 00322/0039

9. DATE OF FIRST AUTHORISATION/RENEWAL OF THE AUTHORISATION

26 February 1982/ 01 April 2005

10. DATE OF REVISION OF THE TEXT

January 2009

Legal Category

Prescription Only Medicine

Nitrocine

(UCB Pharma Limited)

1. NAME OF THE MEDICINAL PRODUCT

Nitrocine 1mg/ml, solution for infusion

2. QUALITATIVE AND QUANTITATIVE COMPOSITION

Ampoules containing 10 mg glyceryl trinitrate in 10 ml, or as glass bottles containing 50 mg glyceryl trinitrate in 50 ml.

For excipients see 6.1.

3. PHARMACEUTICAL FORM

Isotonic sterile solution for infusion

4. CLINICAL PARTICULARS

4.1 Therapeutic indications

Surgery:

Nitrocine is indicated for:

1. the rapid control of hypertension during cardiac surgery.

2. reducing blood pressure and maintaining controlled hypotension during surgical procedures.

3. controlling myocardial ischaemia during and after cardiovascular surgery.

Unresponsive congestive heart failure:

Nitrocine may be used to treat unresponsive congestive heart failure secondary to acute myocardial infarction.

Unstable angina:

Nitrocine may be used to treat unstable angina, which is refractory to treatment with beta blockers and sublingual nitrates.

4.2 Posology and method of administration

Adults and Elderly

The dose of Nitrocine should be adjusted to meet the individual needs of the patient.

The recommended dosage range is 10 - 200 mcg/min but up to 400 mcg/min may be necessary during some surgical procedures.

Children:

The safety and efficacy of Nitrocine has not yet been established in children.

Surgery:

A starting dose of 25 mcg/min is recommended for the control of hypertension, or to produce hypotension during surgery. This may be increased by increments of 25 mcg/min at 5 minute intervals until the blood pressure is stabilized. Doses between 10 - 200 mcg/min are usually sufficient during surgery, although doses of up to 400 mcg/min have been required in some cases.

The treatment of perioperative myocardial ischaemia may be started with a dose of 15 - 20 mcg/min, with subsequent increments of 10 - 15 mcg/min until the required effect is obtained.

Unresponsive congestive heart failure:

The recommended starting dose is 20 - 25 mcg/min. This may be decreased to 10 mcg/min, or increased in steps of 20-25 mcg/min every 15 - 30 minutes until the desired effect is obtained.

Unstable angina:

An initial dose of 10 mcg/min is recommended with increments of 10mcg/min being made at approximately 30 minute intervals according to the needs of the patient.

Administration

Nitrocine can be administered undiluted by slow intravenous infusion using a syringe pump incorporating a glass or rigid plastic syringe.

Alternatively, Nitrocine may be administered intravenously as an admixture using a suitable vehicle such as Sodium Chloride Injection B.P. or Dextrose Injection B.P.

Prepared admixtures should be given by intravenous infusion or with the aid of a syringe pump to ensure a constant rate of infusion.

During Nitrocine administration there should be close haemodynamic monitoring of the patient.

Example of admixture preparation

To obtain an admixture of GTN at a concentration of 100 mcg/ml, add 50 ml Nitrocine solution (containing 50 mg glyceryl trinitrate) to 450 ml of infusion vehicle to give a final volume of 500 ml.

A dosage of 100 mcg/min. can be obtained by giving 60 ml of the admixture per hour. This is equivalent to a drip rate of 60 paediatric microdrops per minute or 20 standard drops per minute. At this drip rate the admixture provides enough solution for an infusion time of 8 hours 20 minutes.

For full details it is advisable to consult the dosage chart on the package insert.

Bottles of Nitrocine are for single use only and should not be regarded as multi-dose containers.

4.3 Contraindications

Nitrocine should not be used in the following cases:

Known hypersensitivity to nitrates, marked anaemia, severe cerebral haemorrhage, head trauma, uncorrected hypovolaemia or severe hypotension.

As the safety of Nitrocine during pregnancy and lactation has not yet been established, it should not be used unless considered absolutely essential.

Sildenafil has been shown to potentiate the hypotensive effects of nitrates, and its co-administration with nitrates or nitric oxide donors is therefore contraindicated.

4.4 Special warnings and precautions for use

Close attention to pulse and blood pressure is necessary during the administration of Nitrocine infusions.

Nitrocine should be used with caution in patients suffering from hypothyroidism, severe liver or renal disease, hypothermia and malnutrition.

4.5 Interaction with other medicinal products and other forms of interaction

Concurrent intake of drugs with blood pressure lowering properties e.g. beta blockers, calcium antagonists, vasodilators etc. and/or alcohol may potentiate the hypotensive effect of Nitrocine. The hypotensive effect of nitrates are potentiated by concurrent administration of sildenafil (Viagra®). This might also occur with neuroleptics and tricyclic antidepressants.

4.6 Pregnancy and lactation

There is no, or inadequate, evidence of safety of the drug in human pregnancy or lactation, but it has been in widespread use for many years without apparent ill consequence, animal studies having shown no hazard. If drug therapy is needed in pregnancy, this product can be used if there is no safer alternative.

4.7 Effects on ability to drive and use machines

None stated.

4.8 Undesirable effects

In common with other nitrates, headaches and nausea may occur during administration. Other possible adverse reactions include hypotension, tachycardia, retching, diaphoresis, apprehension, restlessness, muscle twitching, retrosternal discomfort, palpitations, dizziness and abdominal pain. Paradoxical bradycardia has also been observed.

4.9 Overdose

Mild overdose usually results in hypotension and tachycardia. If arterial systolic blood pressure drops below 90 mmHg and if heart rate increases 10% above its initial value, the infusion should be discontinued to allow a return to pre-treatment levels. If hypotension persists, or in more severe cases, this may be reversed by elevating the legs and/or treatment with hypertensive agents.

5. PHARMACOLOGICAL PROPERTIES

5.1 Pharmacodynamic properties

ATC Code: C01DA 02 – Organic Nitrates

Glyceryl trinitrate reduces the tone of vascular smooth muscle. This action is more marked on the venous capacitance vessels than the arterial vessels. There is a reduction in venous return to the heart and a lowering of elevated filling pressure. This lowering of filling pressure reduces the left ventricular end diastolic volume and preload. The net effect is a lowering of myocardial oxygen consumption.

Systemic vascular resistance, pulmonary vascular pressure and arterial pressure are also reduced by glyceryl trinitrate and there is a net reduction in the afterload.

By reducing the preload and afterload, glyceryl trinitrate reduces the workload on the heart.

Glyceryl trinitrate affects oxygen supply by redistributing blood flow along collateral channels from the epicardial to endocardial regions.

5.2 Pharmacokinetic properties

As with all commonly used organic nitrates the metabolic degradation of glyceryl trinitrate occurs via denitration and glucuronidation. The less active metabolites resulting from this biotransformation can be recovered from the urine within 24 hours.

Glyceryl trinitrate is eliminated from plasma with a short half-life of about 2-3 minutes. This rapid disappearance from plasma is consistent with the high systemic clearance values for this drug (up to 3270 L/hour)

5.3 Preclinical safety data

None stated

6. PHARMACEUTICAL PARTICULARS

6.1 List of excipients

Glucose

Propylene glycol

Water for injection.

Hydrochloric acid (for pH adjustment)

6.2 Incompatibilities

Nitrocine contains glyceryl trinitrate in isotonic sterile solution and is compatible with commonly employed infusion solutions. No incompatibilities have so far been demonstrated.

Nitrocine is compatible with glass infusion bottles and with rigid infusion packs made of polyethylene. Nitrocine may also be infused slowly using a syringe pump with a glass or plastic syringe.

Nitrocine is incompatible with polyvinylchloride (PVC) and severe losses of glyceryl trinitrate (over 40%) may occur if this material is used. Contact with polyvinylchloride bags should be avoided. Polyurethane also induces a loss of the active ingredient.

6.3 Shelf life

Glass ampoules 5 years

Glass vials 5 years

For admixture shelf life, refer to section 6.4.

6.4 Special precautions for storage

Chemical and physical in-use stability of the admixture has been demonstrated for 24 hours at 25°C in suitable containers.

From a microbiological point of view, in-use storage times and conditions prior to use are the responsibility of the user and would normally not be longer than 24 hours at 2 to 8°C, unless dilution has taken place in controlled and validated aseptic conditions.

6.5 Nature and contents of container

Glass ampoules 10 ml (Type I glass)

Glass, rubber stoppered vials 50 ml (Type II glass)

6.6 Special precautions for disposal and other handling

Bottles of Nitrocine are for single use only and should not be regarded as multi-dose containers.

Admixtures are prepared by replacing a given volume of infusion vehicle with an equal volume of the product to produce the final infusion solution. For admixture storage, refer to section 6.4.

7. MARKETING AUTHORISATION HOLDER

UCB Pharma Limited

208 Bath Road

Slough

Berkshire

SL1 3WE

United Kingdom

8. MARKETING AUTHORISATION NUMBER(S)

PL 00039/0747

9. DATE OF FIRST AUTHORISATION/RENEWAL OF THE AUTHORISATION

21 January 2009

10. DATE OF REVISION OF THE TEXT

Nitrolingual Pump Spray

(Merck Serono)

1. NAME OF THE MEDICINAL PRODUCT

Nitrolingual Pumpspray

2. QUALITATIVE AND QUANTITATIVE COMPOSITION

Each metered dose contains 400 micrograms glyceryl trinitrate.

3. PHARMACEUTICAL FORM

Sublingual spray.

4. CLINICAL PARTICULARS

4.1 Therapeutic indications

For the treatment and prophylaxis of angina pectoris and the treatment of variant angina.

4.2 Posology and method of administration

Adults and the Elderly:

At the onset of an attack or prior to a precipitating event: one or two 400 microgram metered doses sprayed under the tongue. It is recommended that no more than three metered-doses are taken at any one time and that there should be a minimum interval of 15 minutes between consecutive treatments.

For the prevention of exercise induced angina or in other precipitating conditions: one or two 400 microgram metered doses sprayed under the tongue immediately prior to the event.

Children:

Nitrolingual Pumpspray is not recommended for use.

Administration:

The bottle should be held vertically with the valve head uppermost. If the pump is new, or has not been used for a week or more, the first actuation should be released into the air. The spray orifice should then be placed as close to the mouth as possible. The dose should be sprayed under the tongue and the mouth should be closed immediately after each dose. The spray should not be inhaled. Patients should be instructed to familiarise themselves with the position of the spray orifice, which can be identified by the finger rest on the top of the valve, in order to facilitate orientation for administration at night. During application the patient should rest, ideally in the sitting position.

4.3 Contraindications

Hypersensitivity to nitrates or any constituent of the formulation. Hypotension, hypovolaemia, severe anaemia, cerebral haemorrhage and brain trauma, mitral stenosis and angina caused by hypertrophic obstructive cardiomyopathy. Concomitant administration of phosphodiesterase inhibitors used for the treatment of erectile dysfunction (section 4.5).

4.4 Special warnings and precautions for use

Any lack of effect may be an indicator of early myocardial infarction.

As with all glyceryl trinitrate preparations, use in patients with incipient glaucoma should be avoided.

4.5 Interaction with other medicinal products and other forms of interaction

Tolerance to this drug and cross tolerance to other nitrates may occur. Alcohol may potentiate any hypotensive effect.

The hypotensive effects of nitrates are potentiated by concurrent administration of phosphodiesterase inhibitors used for the treatment of erectile dysfunction. A severe and possibly dangerous fall in blood pressure may occur. This can result in collapse, unconsciousness and may be fatal. Such use is therefore contra-indicated (section 4.3)

If a patient treated with these drugs for erectile dysfunction needs a rapidly effective nitrate, he/she should be closely monitored.

4.6 Pregnancy and lactation

Nitrolingual Pump spray is not generally recommended and should be used only if its potential benefit justifies any potential risk to the foetus or neonate.

4.7 Effects on ability to drive and use machines

Only as a result of hypotension.

4.8 Undesirable effects

Headache, dizziness, postural hypotension, flushing, tachycardia and paradoxical bradycardia have been reported.

4.9 Overdose

Signs and symptoms:

Flushing, severe headache, a feeling of suffocation, hypotension, fainting, restlessness, blurred vision, impairment of respiration, bradycardia and rarely, cyanosis and methaemoglobinaemia may occur. In a few patients there may be a reaction comparable to shock with nausea, vomiting, weakness, sweating and syncope.

Treatment:

Recovery often occurs without special treatment. Hypotension may be corrected by elevation of the legs to promote venous return. Methaemoglobinaemia should be treated by intravenous methylene blue.

Symptomatic treatment should be given for respiratory and circulatory defects in more serious cases.

5. PHARMACOLOGICAL PROPERTIES

5.1 Pharmacodynamic properties

Glyceryl trinitrate relieves angina pectoris by reduction of cardiac work and dilation of the coronary arteries. In this way, not only is there a lessening in arterial oxygen requirement but the amount of oxygenated blood reaching the ischaemic heart is increased.

5.2 Pharmacokinetic properties

The pharmacokinetics of glyceryl trinitrate are complex; venous plasma levels of the drug show wide and variable fluctuations and are not predictive of clinical effect. In a human pharmacodynamic study, pharmacological activity had commenced one minute after dosing and was obvious by two minutes.

5.3 Preclinical safety data

None stated.

6. PHARMACEUTICAL PARTICULARS

6.1 List of excipients

Fractionated coconut oil, ethanol (absolute), medium chain partial glycerides, peppermint oil.

6.2 Incompatibilities

None known.

6.3 Shelf life

3 years.

6.4 Special precautions for storage

Do not store above 25°C.

6.5 Nature and contents of container

Red plastic coated glass bottle fitted with metering pump. Each bottle contains 4.9 or 11.2g solution (equivalent to about 75 or 200 doses).

6.6 Special precautions for disposal and other handling

See 'Administration' section.

7. MARKETING AUTHORISATION HOLDER

Lipha Pharmaceuticals Limited

Harrier House

High Street

West Drayton

Middlesex

UB7 7QG

United Kingdom

8. MARKETING AUTHORISATION NUMBER(S)

PL 03759/0042

9. DATE OF FIRST AUTHORISATION/RENEWAL OF THE AUTHORISATION

28 November 2005

10. DATE OF REVISION OF THE TEXT

28 November 2005

LEGAL CATEGORY Pharmacy

Nitronal

(Merck Serono)

1. NAME OF THE MEDICINAL PRODUCT

Nitronal®

2. QUALITATIVE AND QUANTITATIVE COMPOSITION
Glyceryl trinitrate 1 mg/ml.

3. PHARMACEUTICAL FORM
Solution for infusion.

4. CLINICAL PARTICULARS

4.1 Therapeutic indications

(1) Unresponsive congestive heart failure, including that secondary to acute myocardial infarction.

(2) Refractory unstable angina pectoris and coronary insufficiency, including Prinzmetal's angina.

(3) Control of hypertensive episodes and / or myocardial ischaemia during and after cardiac surgery. For the induction of controlled hypotension for surgery.

4.2 Posology and method of administration

For intravenous use. Nitronal® should be administered by means of a micro-drip set infusion pump or similar device which permits maintenance of constant infusion rate.

Adults and the elderly - the dose should be titrated against the individual clinical response.

(1) Unresponsive congestive heart failure. The normal dose range is 10-100 micrograms / minute administered as a continuous intravenous infusion with frequent monitoring of blood pressure and heart rate. The infusion should be started at the lower rate and increased cautiously until the desired clinical response is achieved. Other haemodynamic measurements are extremely important in monitoring response to the drug: These may include pulmonary capillary wedge pressure, cardiac output and precordial electrocardiogram depending on the clinical picture.

(2) Refractory unstable angina pectoris. An initial infusion rate of 10-15 micrograms / minute is recommended; this may be increased cautiously in increments of 5-10 micrograms until either relief of angina is achieved, headache prevents further increase in dose, or the mean arterial pressure falls by more than 20 mm Hg.

(3) Use in surgery. An initial infusion rate of 25 micrograms / minute is recommended; this should be increased gradually until the desired systolic arterial pressure is attained. The usual dose is 25-200 micrograms / minute.

Children - Not recommended for use in children.

4.3 Contraindications

Hypersensitivity to nitrates. Hypotensive shock, severe anaemia, cerebral haemorrhage, arterial hypoxaemia, uncorrected hypovolaemia and angina caused by hypertrophic obstructive cardiomyopathy. Concomitant administration of sildenafil (section 4.5).

4.4 Special warnings and precautions for use

Caution should be exercised in patients with severe liver or renal disease, hypothermia, hypothyroidism.

Nitronal® should not be given by bolus injection.

4.5 Interaction with other medicinal products and other forms of interaction

Glyceryl trinitrate may potentiate the action of other hypotensive drugs, and the hypotensive and anticholinergic effects of tricyclic anti-depressants; it may also slow the metabolism of morphine-like analgesics.

The hypotensive effects of nitrates are potentiated by concurrent administration of sildenafil. A severe and possibly dangerous fall in blood pressure may occur. This can result in collapse, unconsciousness and may be fatal. Such use is therefore contra-indicated (section 4.3).

4.6 Pregnancy and lactation

This product should not be used in pregnancy or in women who are breast feeding infants unless considered essential by the physician.

4.7 Effects on ability to drive and use machines

No information available.

4.8 Undesirable effects

Nitronal® is generally well tolerated because a minimum dose is administered in unit time. Headache, dizziness, flushing, hypotension and tachycardia may be encountered, particularly if the infusion is administered too rapidly. Nausea, diaphoresis, restlessness, retrosternal discomfort, abdominal pain and paradoxical bradycardia have been reported. These symptoms should be readily reversible on reducing the rate of infusion or, if necessary, discontinuing treatment.

4.9 Overdose

Signs and symptoms: Vomiting, restlessness, hypotension, syncope, cyanosis, coldness of the skin, impairment of respiration, bradycardia, psychosis and methaemoglobinaemia may occur.

Treatment: The symptoms may be readily reversed by discontinuing treatment; if hypotension persists, raising the foot of the bed and the use of vasoconstrictors such as intravenous methoxamine or phenylephrine are recommended. Methaemoglobinaemia should be treated by intravenous methylene blue. Oxygen and assisted respiration may be required.

5. PHARMACOLOGICAL PROPERTIES

5.1 Pharmacodynamic properties

Glyceryl trinitrate exerts a spasmolytic action on smooth muscle, particularly in the vascular system. The predominant effect is an increase in venous capacitance resulting in marked diminution of both the left ventricular filling pressure and volume (preload). There is also a reduction in afterload due to moderate dilation of the arteriolar resistance vessels. These haemodynamic changes lower the myocardial oxygen demand. By direct action and through the reduction of myocardial wall tension glyceryl trinitrate also lowers the resistance to flow in the coronary collateral channels and allows re-distribution of blood flow to ischaemic areas of the myocardium.

Administration of Nitronal® by intravenous infusion to patients with congestive heart failure results in a marked improvement in haemodynamics, reduction of elevated left ventricular filling pressure and systolic wall tension, and an increase in the depressed cardiac output. It reduces the imbalance that exists between myocardial oxygen demand and delivery, thereby diminishing myocardial ischaemia and controlling ischaemia-induced ventricular arrhythmias.

5.2 Pharmacokinetic properties

It is important that the dose of Nitronal® be titrated against the individual clinical response.

After intravenous administration, glyceryl trinitrate is widely distributed in the body with an estimated apparent volume of distribution of approximately 200 litres, and is rapidly metabolised to dinitrate and mononitrate with an estimated half life of 1 to 4 minutes, resulting in plasma levels of less than 1 microgram / ml.

5.3 Preclinical safety data

None, of relevance to the prescriber, which are not given elsewhere in this document.

6. PHARMACEUTICAL PARTICULARS

6.1 List of excipients

Glucose, water for injections, hydrochloric acid.

6.2 Incompatibilities

Glyceryl trinitrate is adsorbed onto administration systems composed of polyvinyl chloride, - see 6.6.

6.3 Shelf life

Ampoules: 4 years

Vial: 2 years

The diluted solution should be administered as soon as possible; it is stable for up to 24 hours in the recommended infusion system.

6.4 Special precautions for storage

Do not store above 25°C. Store in the original container.

6.5 Nature and contents of container

Cartons of 10 ampoules or single vials.

Amber glass ampoule (containing 5ml or 25ml).

Clear glass vial (containing 50ml).

6.6 Special precautions for disposal and other handling

Nitronal® need not be diluted before use but can be diluted with Dextrose Injection BP, Sodium Chloride and Dextrose Injection BP, 0.9% Sodium Chloride Injection BP or other protein-free infusion solution, if required.

The solution, whether or not diluted, should be infused slowly (see dosage section) and not given by bolus injection.

To ensure a constant infusion rate of glyceryl trinitrate it is recommended that Nitronal® be administered by means of a syringe pump or polyethylene infusion bag with a counter, or with a glass or rigid polyethylene syringe and polyethylene tubing. Systems made of polyvinyl chloride may absorb up to 50% of the glyceryl trinitrate from the solution, thus reducing the efficacy of the infusion. If the recommended type of system is unavailable, a 1:10 dilution of Nitronal® should be used and the infusion rate modified according to the haemodynamic response of the patient, until the required parameters are attained.

7. MARKETING AUTHORISATION HOLDER

Lipha Pharmaceuticals Limited
Harrier House
High Street
West Drayton
Middlesex
UB7 7QG

8. MARKETING AUTHORISATION NUMBER(S)

PL 03759 / 0025

9. DATE OF FIRST AUTHORISATION/RENEWAL OF THE AUTHORISATION

30 January 2000

10. DATE OF REVISION OF THE TEXT

18 December 2003

Legal Category POM

Nivaquine Syrup

(sanofi-aventis)

1. NAME OF THE MEDICINAL PRODUCT

Nivaquine Syrup

2. QUALITATIVE AND QUANTITATIVE COMPOSITION

Chloroquine Sulphate BP 68 mg/5 ml.

3. PHARMACEUTICAL FORM

Syrup.

4. CLINICAL PARTICULARS

4.1 Therapeutic indications

Nivaquine is a 4-aminoquinoline compound which has a high degree of activity against the asexual erythrocytic forms of all species of malaria parasites. It is indicated for the suppression and clinical cure of all forms of malaria and, in addition, produces radical cure of falciparum malaria.

Nivaquine also exerts a beneficial effect in certain collagen diseases and protects against the effects of solar radiation. It is employed in the treatment of rheumatoid arthritis, juvenile arthritis, discoid and systemic lupus erythematosus and skin conditions aggravated by sunlight.

Nivaquine is also active against *Entamoeba histolytica* and *Giardia lamblia* and when Flagyl (metronidazole) is not available it may be used in hepatic amoebiasis and giardiasis.

Packs for supply directly to the public: For the prevention of malaria.

Route of administration: oral.

4.2 Posology and method of administration

Rheumatoid arthritis

Adults:	3 × 5 ml Nivaquine Syrup (150 mg chloroquine base) daily.
Children:	3 mg/kg bodyweight daily. Treatment should be discontinued if no improvement has occurred after 6 months.

Systemic lupus erythematosus

Adults:	3 × 5 ml Nivaquine Syrup (150 mg chloroquine base) daily until maximum improvement is obtained followed by smaller maintenance dosage.
Children:	3 mg/kg bodyweight daily. Treatment should be discontinued if no improvement has occurred after 6 months.

Light sensitive skin eruptions

Adults:	3 to 6 × 5 ml Nivaquine Syrup (150 mg to 300 mg chloroquine base) daily during the period of maximum light exposure.
Children:	3 mg/kg body weight daily. Treatment should be discontinued if no improvement has occurred after 6 months.

Suppression of malaria

Adults:	6 × 5 ml Nivaquine Syrup (300 mg chloroquine base) to be taken once a week on the same day each week.
Infants and children up To 12 years:	5 mg chloroquine base per kg bodyweight to be taken once a week on the same day each week.

It is advisable to start taking Nivaquine 1 week before entering an endemic area and to continue for 4 weeks after leaving.

Treatment of malaria

1. Partially immune adults

A single dose of 12 × 5 ml Nivaquine Syrup (600 mg chloroquine base) will provide a safe and effective course of treatment.

2. Non-immune adults

Day 1:	12 × 5 ml Nivaquine Syrup (600 mg chloroquine base) in one dose followed by a further 6 × 5 ml syrup (300 mg chloroquine base) six hours later.
Day 2:	6 × 5 ml Nivaquine Syrup (300 mg chloroquine base).
Day 3:	6 × 5 ml Nivaquine Syrup (300 mg chloroquine base).

The above dosage is intended as a guide in the treatment of *Plasmodium falciparum* malaria. However, due to a variation in the strain sensitivity, it may sometimes be necessary to increase the duration of treatment by administering 6 × 5 ml Nivaquine Syrup (300 mg chloroquine base) daily on days 4 to 7.

3. Non-immune or partially immune infants and children

Nivaquine Syrup can be conveniently used in patients in this age group to permit flexibility of dosage.

Day 1:	10 mg chloroquine base/kg bodyweight (maximum 600 mg base) followed by 5 mg chloroquine base/kg bodyweight (maximum 300 mg base) six hours later.
Day 2:	5 mg chloroquine base/kg bodyweight (maximum 300 mg base).
Day 3:	5 mg chloroquine base/kg bodyweight (maximum 300 mg base).

4.3 Contraindications

The use of chloroquine is contraindicated in patients with known hypersensitivity to 4-aminoquinoline compounds.

Nivaquine is generally contraindicated in pregnancy. However, clinicians may decide to administer Nivaquine to pregnant women for the prevention or treatment of malaria. Ocular or inner ear damage may occur in infants born of mothers who receive high doses of chloroquine throughout pregnancy.

4.4 Special warnings and precautions for use

Nivaquine should be used with care in patients with a history of epilepsy as it has been reported to provoke seizures. Caution is advised in cases of porphyria (precipitated disease may be especially apparent in patients with a high alcohol intake), hepatic disease (particularly cirrhosis) or renal disease, severe gastrointestinal, neurological and blood disorders and in patients receiving anticoagulant therapy.

Nivaquine should be used with care in patients with psoriasis as the condition may be exacerbated.

Although Nivaquine may have a temporary effect on visual accommodation during short term treatment, irreversible retinal damage may occur with prolonged treatment (see sections 4.7 and 4.8, below). Therefore, patients should be advised to discontinue the medication and seek immediate medical advice if they notice any deterioration in their vision which persists for more than 48 hours. Ophthalmological examination should always be carried out before and regularly (3-6 monthly intervals) during prolonged treatment. Retinal damage is particularly likely to occur if treatment has been given for longer than one year, or if the total dosage has exceeded 1.6 g/kg bodyweight. These precautions also apply to patients receiving chloroquine continuously at weekly intervals as a prophylactic against malarial attack for more than three years.

Bone marrow depression, including aplastic anaemia occurs rarely. Full blood counts should therefore be carried out regularly during extended treatment. Caution is required if drugs known to induce blood disorders are used concurrently.

Resistance of Plasmodium falciparum to chloroquine is well documented. When used as malaria prophylaxis official guidelines and local information on prevalence of resistance to anti-malarial drugs should be taken into consideration.

4.5 Interaction with other medicinal products and other forms of interaction

Concomitant administration of chloroquine with magnesium-containing antacids or kaolin may result in reduced absorption of chloroquine. Chloroquine should, therefore, be administered at least two hours apart from antacids or kaolin.

Concomitant use of cimetidine and chloroquine may result in an increased half-life and a decreased clearance of chloroquine.

Chloroquine and mefloquine can lower the convulsive threshold. Co-administration of chloroquine and mefloquine may increase the risk of convulsions. Also, the activity of antiepileptic drugs might be impaired if co-administered with chloroquine.

There have been isolated case reports of an increased plasma ciclosporin level when ciclosporin and chloroquine were co-administered.

Chloroquine may affect the antibody response to rabies vaccine (HDCV).

Caution is advised in patients receiving anticoagulant therapy.

Co-administration of chloroquine and other drugs that have arrhythmogenic potential (e.g. amiodarone) may increase the risk of cardiac arrhythmias.

Concomitant administration of chloroquine and digoxin may increase plasma concentrations of digoxin.

Concomitant use of chloroquine with neostigmine or pyridostigmine has the potential to increase the symptoms of myasthenia gravis and thus diminish the effects of neostigmine and pyridostigmine.

4.6 Pregnancy and lactation

Nivaquine is generally contraindicated in pregnancy. However, clinicians may decide to administer Nivaquine to pregnant women for the prevention or treatment of malaria. Ocular or inner ear damage may occur in infants born of mothers who receive high doses of chloroquine throughout pregnancy.

Although chloroquine is excreted in breast milk, the amount is insufficient to confer any benefit on the infant. Separate chemoprophylaxis for the infant is required. When used for rheumatoid disease breast feeding is not recommended.

4.7 Effects on ability to drive and use machines

Nivaquine has a temporary effect on visual accommodation and patients should be warned that they should not drive or operate machinery if they are affected.

4.8 Undesirable effects

Cardiovascular

- cardiomyopathy has been reported during long term therapy at high doses,

- cardiac dysrhythmias at high doses can occur,

- hypotension.

Central Nervous System (See Section 4.4)

- seizures,

- convulsions have been reported rarely (these may result from cerebral malaria. Such patients should receive an injections of phenobarbital to prevent seizures, in a dose of 3.5mg/kg in addition to intravenous administration of Nivaquine),

- psychiatric disorders such as anxiety, confusion, hallucinations, delirium.

Eye disorders (See Sections 4.4 and 4.7)

- transient blurred vision and reversible corneal opacity,

- cases of retinopathy as well as cases of irreversible retinal damage have been reported during long term, high dose therapy.

- macular defects of colour vision, optic atrophy, scotomas, field defects, blindness and pigmented deposits, difficult in focusing, diplopia.

Gastro-intestinal

- gastrointestinal disturbances such as nausea, vomiting, diarrhoea, abdominal cramps.

General

- headache.

Haematological (See Section 4.4)

- bone marrow depression, including aplastic anaemia, agranulocytosis, thrombocytopenia, neutropenia occurs rarely.

Hepatic

- changes in liver function, including hepatitis and abnormal liver function tests, have been reported rarely.

Hypersensitivity

- allergic and anaphylactic reactions, urticaria and angiodema have occurred rarely.

Hearing disorders

- ototoxicity such as tinnitus, reduced hearing, nerve deafness.

Muscular

- neuropathy, myopathy.

Skin (See Section 4.4)

- skin eruptions, pruritis, depigmentation, loss of hair, exacerbation of psoriasis, photosensitivity, pigmentation of the nails and mucosae (long term use).

- Rare reports of erythema multiforme, Stevens-Johnson syndrome, toxic epidermal necrolysis, exfoliative dermatitis and similar desquamation-type events.

4.9 Overdose

Chloroquine is highly toxic in overdosage; children are particularly susceptible to toxic doses of chloroquine. The chief symptoms of overdose include circulatory collapse due to a potent cardiotoxic effect, respiratory arrest and coma. Symptoms may progress rapidly after initial headache, drowsiness, visual disturbancesnausea and vomiting. Death may result from circulatory or respiratory failure or cardiac dysrhythmia.

Gastric lavage should be carried out urgently, first protecting the airways and instituting artificial ventilation where necessary. There is a risk of cardiac arrest following aspiration of gastric contents in more serious cases. Activated charcoal left in the stomach may reduce absorption of any remaining chloroquine from the gut. Circulatory status (with central venous pressure measurement), respiration, plasma electrolytes and blood gases should be monitored, with correction of hypokalaemia and acidosis if indicated. Cardiac arrhythmias should not be treated unless life threatening; drugs with quinidine-like effects should be avoided.

Early administration of the following has been shown to improve survival in cases of serious poisoning:

1) Adrenaline infusion (0.25 micrograms/kg/min initially, with increments of 0.25 micrograms/kg/min until adequate systolic blood pressure (more than 100 mm mercury) is restored; adrenaline reduces the effects of chloroquine on the heart through its inotropic and vasoconstrictor effects.

2) Diazepam infusion (2 mg/kg over 30 minutes as a loading dose, followed by 1-2 mg/kg/day for up to 2-4 days). Diazepam may minimise cardiotoxicity.

Acidification of the urine, haemodialysis, peritoneal dialysis or exchange transfusions have not been shown to be of value in treating chloroquine -poisoning. Chloroquine is excreted very slowly, therefore symptomatic cases merit observation for several days.

5. PHARMACOLOGICAL PROPERTIES

5.1 Pharmacodynamic properties

Chloroquine is used for the suppression and treatment of malaria. It has rapid schizonticidal effect and appears to affect cell growth by interfering with DNA; its activity also seems to depend on preferential accumulation in the infected erythrocyte. Chloroquine kills the erythrocytic forms of malaria parasites at all stages of development. In addition to its antimalarial properties, it possesses other pharmacological properties. Its anti-inflammatory properties enable Nivaquine to be used in certain collagen diseases and it protects against the effects of solar radiation. Nivaquine is also active against *Entamoeba histolytica* and *Giardia lamblia*. It may be used in hepatic amoebiasis and giardiasis.

5.2 Pharmacokinetic properties

Chloroquine is readily absorbed from the gastro-intestinal tract and about 55% in the circulation is bound to plasma proteins. It accumulates in high concentrations in some tissues, such as kidneys, liver, lungs and spleen and is strongly bound in melanin containing cells such as those in the eyes and the skin; it is also bound to double stranded DNA, present in red blood cells containing schizonts. Chloroquine is eliminated very slowly from the body and it may persist in tissues for a long period. Up to 70% of a dose may be excreted unchanged in urine and up to 25% may be excreted also in the urine as the desethyl metabolite. The rate of urinary excretion of chloroquine is increased at low pH values.

5.3 Preclinical safety data

No additional preclinical data of relevance to the prescriber.

6. PHARMACEUTICAL PARTICULARS

6.1 List of excipients

Sucrose,

Monosodium glutamate,

Saccharin sodium,

Propylene glycol,

Methyl parahydroxybenzoate,

Propyl parahydroxybenzoate,

Peppermint Oil,

Pineapple flavour,

Caramel,

Purified water

6.2 Incompatibilities

None known.

6.3 Shelf life

3 years.

6.4 Special precautions for storage

Nivaquine should be stored below 25°C, protected from light.

6.5 Nature and contents of container

Amber glass bottle containing 100 ml. Either with rolled on pilfer proof aluminium cap and PVDC emulsion coated wad, or HDPE/polypropylene child resistant cap with a tamper evident band.

6.6 Special precautions for disposal and other handling

None stated.

7. MARKETING AUTHORISATION HOLDER

Sanofi-aventis

One Onslow Street

Guildford

Surrey, GU1 4YS, UK

8. MARKETING AUTHORISATION NUMBER(S)

PL 04425/0329

9. DATE OF FIRST AUTHORISATION/RENEWAL OF THE AUTHORISATION

06 March 2003

10. DATE OF REVISION OF THE TEXT

8 September 2008

Legal category

POM

When used solely for the prevention of malaria: Pharmacy Medicine.

Nizoral 2% Cream/Daktarin Gold

(Janssen-Cilag Ltd)

1. NAME OF THE MEDICINAL PRODUCT

POM: Nizoral 2% Cream

P: Daktarin Gold

2. QUALITATIVE AND QUANTITATIVE COMPOSITION

Ketoconazole 2% w/w (each gram of cream contains 20mg).

For a full list of excipients, see 6.1.

3. PHARMACEUTICAL FORM

Cream

4. CLINICAL PARTICULARS

4.1 Therapeutic indications

POM

For topical application in the treatment of dermatophyte infections of the skin such as tinea corporis, tinea cruris, tinea manus and tinea pedis infections due to Trichophyton spp, Microsporon spp and Epidermophyton spp. Nizoral cream is also indicated for the treatment of cutaneous candidosis (including vulvitis), tinea (pityriasis) versicolor and seborrhoeic dermatitis caused by Malassezia (previously called Pityrosporum) spp.

P

For the treatment of the following mycotic infections of the skin: tinea pedis, tinea cruris and candidal intertrigo.

4.2 Posology and method of administration

POM

Tinea pedis:

Nizoral cream should be applied to the affected areas twice daily. The usual duration of treatment for mild infections is 1 week. For more severe or extensive infections (e.g.

Table 1

System Organ Class	Adverse Drug Reactions Frequency Category Very Common ≥1/10	Common ≥1/100 to <1/10	Uncommon ≥1/1,000 to <1/100	Rare ≥1/10,000 to <1/1,000	Very Rare <1/10,000	Not Known
General disorders and administration site conditions		Application site erythema Application site pruritus	Application site bleeding; Application site discomfort; Application site dryness; Application site inflammation; Application site irritation; Application site paraesthesia; Application site reaction.			Urticaria
Skin and subcutaneous tissue disorders		Skin burning sensation	Bullous eruption; Dermatitis contact; Rash; Skin exfoliation; Sticky skin.			
Immune system disorders			Hypersensitivity.			

involving the sole or sides of the feet) treatment should be continued until a few days after all signs and symptoms have disappeared in order to prevent relapse.

For other infections:

Nizoral cream should be applied to the affected areas once or twice daily, depending on the severity of the infection.

The treatment should be continued until a few days after the disappearance of all signs and symptoms. The usual duration of treatment is: tinea versicolor 2-3 weeks, tinea corporis 3-4 weeks.

The diagnosis should be reconsidered if no clinical improvement is noted after 4 weeks. General measures in regard to hygiene should be observed to control sources of infection or reinfection.

Seborrhoeic dermatitis is a chronic condition and relapse is highly likely.

P

For the treatment of tinea pedis (athlete's foot) and tinea cruris (dhobie itch) and candidal intertrigo (sweat rash).

For tinea pedis, Daktarin Gold cream should be applied to the affected areas twice daily. The usual duration of treatment for mild infections is 1 week. For more severe or extensive infections (e.g. involving the sole or sides of the feet) treatment should be continued for 2-3 days after all signs of infection have disappeared to prevent relapse.

For tinea cruris and candidal intertrigo, apply cream to the affected areas once or twice daily until 2-3 days after all signs of infection have disappeared to prevent relapse. Treatment for up to 6 weeks may be necessary. If no improvement in symptoms is experienced after 4 weeks treatment, a doctor should be consulted.

Method of administration: Topical administration.

4.3 Contraindications

Ketoconazole cream is contra-indicated in patients with a known hypersensitivity to any of the ingredients or to ketoconazole itself.

4.4 Special warnings and precautions for use

Not for ophthalmic use.

If a potent topical corticosteroid has been used previously in the treatment of seborrhoeic dermatitis, a recovery period of 2 weeks should be allowed before using Nizoral cream, as an increased incidence of steroid induced skin sensitisation has been reported when no recovery period is allowed.

4.5 Interaction with other medicinal products and other forms of interaction

None known

4.6 Pregnancy and lactation

There are no adequate and well-controlled studies in pregnant or lactating women. To date, no other relevant epidemiological data are available. Data on a limited number of exposed pregnancies indicate no adverse effects of topical ketoconazole on pregnancy or on the health of the foetus/newborn child. Animal studies have shown reproductive toxicity following oral administration of ketoconazole. (see Preclinical safety data, section 5.3). No effects on the breastfed newborn/infant are anticipated. See Pharmacokinetic properties, section 5.2

4.7 Effects on ability to drive and use machines

None.

4.8 Undesirable effects

The safety of ketoconazole cream was evaluated in 1117 subjects who participated in 31 clinical trials. Each subject received at least one topical administration of ketoconazole cream.

Commonly observed adverse reactions to Ketoconazole cream in clinical trials were burning sensation, application site erythema and pruritus.

Including the above-mentioned adverse drug reactions (ADRs), the following table displays ADRs that have been reported with the use of ketoconazole cream from either clinical trial or postmarketing experiences. The displayed frequency categories use the following convention:

Very Common (≥1/10)

Common (≥1/100 to <1/10)

Uncommon (≥1/1,000 to <1/100)

Rare (≥1/10,000 to <1/1,000)

Very rare (<1/10,000)

Not Known (cannot be estimated from the clinical trial data).

(see Table 1 above)

4.9 Overdose

Exaggerated topical application may lead to erythema, oedema and a burning sensation, which will disappear upon discontinuation of the treatment.

If accidental ingestion of ketoconazole cream occurs, No special measures have to be taken.

5. PHARMACOLOGICAL PROPERTIES

5.1 Pharmacodynamic properties

Pharmacotherapeutic group: ATC Code: D01AC08

Ketoconazole has a potent antimycotic action against dermatophytes and yeasts. Ketoconazole cream acts rapidly on the pruritus, which is commonly seen in dermatophyte and yeast infections. This symptomatic improvement often occurs before the first signs of healing are observed.

A study in 250 patients has shown that application twice daily for 7 days of ketoconazole 2% cream vs clotrimazole 1% cream for 4 weeks on both feet demonstrated efficacy in patients with tinea pedis (athlete's foot) presenting lesions between the toes. The primary efficacy endpoint was negative microscopic KOH examination at 4 weeks. Ketoconazole 2% treatment showed equivalent efficacy to 4 weeks clotrimazole 1% treatment. There was no evidence of relapse following treatment with ketoconazole cream at 8 weeks.

5.2 Pharmacokinetic properties

Plasma concentrations of ketoconazole were not detectable after topical administration of Nizoral Cream in adults on the skin. In one study in infants with seborrhoeic dermatitis (n = 19), where approximately 40 g of Nizoral Cream was applied daily on 40% of the body surface area, plasma levels of ketoconazole were detected in 5 infants, ranging from 32 to 133 ng/mL.

5.3 Preclinical safety data

Since ketoconazole administered topically as a cream is not systemically absorbed and does not produce detectable plasma concentrations, there is no specific relevant information.

6. PHARMACEUTICAL PARTICULARS

6.1 List of excipients

Propylene Glycol

Stearyl Alcohol

Cetyl Alcohol

Sorbitan Stearate

Polysorbate 60

Isopropyl Myristate

Sodium Sulphite Anhydrous (E221)

Polysorbate 80

Purified Water

6.2 Incompatibilities

Not applicable.

6.3 Shelf life

60 months.

6.4 Special precautions for storage

Do not store above 25°C.

6.5 Nature and contents of container

Tube made of 99.7% aluminum, lined on inner side with heat polymerised epoxyphenol resin with a latex coldseal ring at the end of the tube. The cap is made of 60% polypropylene, 30% calcium carbonate and 10% glyceryl monostearate.

Tubes of 5g, 15g and 30g.

Not all pack sizes may be marketed

6.6 Special precautions for disposal and other handling

Not applicable.

7. MARKETING AUTHORISATION HOLDER

Janssen-Cilag Ltd

50-100 Holmers Farm Way

High Wycombe

Bucks

HP12 4EG

UK

8. MARKETING AUTHORISATION NUMBER(S)

PL 00242/0107

9. DATE OF FIRST AUTHORISATION/RENEWAL OF THE AUTHORISATION

Renewed 3 December 2002

10. DATE OF REVISION OF THE TEXT

22 April 2009

Legal Category

POM: Nizoral Cream

P: Daktarin Gold

Nizoral 2% Shampoo

(Janssen-Cilag Ltd)

1. NAME OF THE MEDICINAL PRODUCT

Nizoral 2% Shampoo

2. QUALITATIVE AND QUANTITATIVE COMPOSITION

Ketoconazole 2% w/w. (each gram contains 20 mg)

For a full list of excipients, see 6.1

3. PHARMACEUTICAL FORM

Pink viscous shampoo.

4. CLINICAL PARTICULARS

4.1 Therapeutic indications

Prevention and treatment of infections in which the yeast Malassezia (previously called Pityrosporum) is likely to be involved, such as dandruff, seborrhoeic dermatitis and tinea (pityriasis) versicolor.

4.2 Posology and method of administration

For topical administration.

Adults, Elderly and Children:

Wash affected areas and leave for 3-5 minutes before rinsing.

Treatment:

Dandruff and seborrhoeic dermatitis: Wash hair twice weekly for 2-4 weeks.

Tinea versicolor: Once daily for a maximum of 5 days.

Prophylaxis:

Dandruff and seborrhoeic dermatitis: Use once every 1-2 weeks.

Tinea versicolor: Once daily for a maximum of 3 days before exposure to sunshine.

4.3 Contraindications

Known hypersensitivity to ketoconazole or any of the excipients.

4.4 Special warnings and precautions for use

Seborrhoeic dermatitis and dandruff are often associated with increased hair shedding and this has also been reported, although rarely, with the use of Nizoral Shampoo.

In patients who have been on prolonged treatment with topical corticosteroids, it is recommended that the steroid therapy be gradually withdrawn over a period of 2 to 3 weeks, while using Nizoral Shampoo, to prevent any potential rebound effect.

Keep out of the eyes. If the shampoo should get into the eyes, they should be bathed with water.

4.5 Interaction with other medicinal products and other forms of interaction
None Known.

4.6 Pregnancy and lactation
There are no adequate and well-controlled studies in pregnant or lactating women. To date, no other relevant epidemiological data are available. Data on a limited number of exposed pregnancies indicate no adverse effects of topical ketoconazole on pregnancy or on the health of the foetus/newborn child. Animal studies have shown reproductive toxicity following oral administration of ketoconazole. (see Preclinical safety data, section 5.3). No effects on the breastfed newborn/infant are anticipated. See Pharmacokinetic properties, section 5.2

4.7 Effects on ability to drive and use machines
None likely.

4.8 Undesirable effects
As with other shampoos, a local burning sensation, itching, or contact dermatitis (due to irritation or allergy) may occur on exposed areas. Oily and dry hair have been reported rarely with the use of Nizoral shampoo.

In rare instances, mainly in patients with chemically damaged hair or grey hair, a discolouration of the hair has been observed with the use of Nizoral Shampoo.

Additional adverse drug reactions reported in postmarketing reports with Nizoral® Shampoo are included in Table 1. The frequencies are based on spontaneous reporting rates, according to the following convention:

Very common ⩾1/10

Common ⩾1/100 and < 1/10

Uncommon ⩾1/1,000 and <1/100

Rare ⩾1/10,000, <1/1,000

Very rare <1/10,000, including isolated reports

Table 1. Adverse Drug Reactions Identified During Postmarketing Experience with NIZORAL® SHAMPOO by Frequency Category Estimated from Spontaneous Reporting Rates

Immune System Disorders

Very rare Hypersensitivity

Skin and Subcutaneous Tissue Disorder

Very rare Alopecia (Also see Section 4.4 under Special Warnings and Special Precautions For Use), Rash, Urticaria, Skin irritation, Dry skin

General Disorders and Administration Site Conditions

Very rare Application site reaction

4.9 Overdose
In the event of accidental ingestion, only supportive measures should be carried out. In order to avoid aspiration, neither emesis nor gastric lavage should be instigated.

5. PHARMACOLOGICAL PROPERTIES

5.1 Pharmacodynamic properties
Ketoconazole is an imidazole-dioxolane antimycotic, active against yeasts, including Malassezia and dermatophytes. Its broad spectrum of activity is already well known.

5.2 Pharmacokinetic properties
Plasma concentrations of ketoconazole were not detectable after topical administration of Nizoral Shampoo on the scalp. Plasma levels were detected after topical administration of Nizoral Shampoo on the whole body.

5.3 Preclinical safety data
No relevant information additional to that contained elsewhere in the Summary of Product Characteristics.

6. PHARMACEUTICAL PARTICULARS

6.1 List of excipients
Sodium lauryl ether sulphate
Disodium monolauryl ether sulphosuccinate
Coconut fatty acid diethanolamide
Laurdimonium hydrolysed animal collagen
Macrogol 120 methyl glucose dioleate
Sodium chloride
Concentrated hydrochloric acid
Imidurea
Sodium hydroxide
Erythrosine sodium
Purified water

6.2 Incompatibilities
None known.

6.3 Shelf life
36 months.

6.4 Special precautions for storage
Store below 25°C.

6.5 Nature and contents of container
Aluminium sachet lined with polyethylene, containing 7.5 ml* shampoo.

Boxes of 2, 6 and 12 sachets.

High density polyethylene bottles, containing 60ml*, 100ml* or 120 ml shampoo.

*Not all pack sizes are marketed.

6.6 Special precautions for disposal and other handling
Not applicable.

7. MARKETING AUTHORISATION HOLDER
Janssen-Cilag Ltd
50-100 Holmers Farm Way
High Wycombe
Bucks
HP12 4EG
UK

8. MARKETING AUTHORISATION NUMBER(S)
00242/0139

9. DATE OF FIRST AUTHORISATION/RENEWAL OF THE AUTHORISATION
Date of First Authorisation: 18 April 1988

Date of Renewal of Authorisation: 24 June 2008

10. DATE OF REVISION OF THE TEXT
22 April 2009

Legal category POM

Nizoral 200 mg Tablets

(Janssen-Cilag Ltd)

1. NAME OF THE MEDICINAL PRODUCT
Nizoral® 200 mg Tablets.

2. QUALITATIVE AND QUANTITATIVE COMPOSITION
Each tablet contains 200 mg ketoconazole.

For excipients, see section 6.1.

3. PHARMACEUTICAL FORM
Tablet.

White, circular, flat bevelled-edge, half scored tablet marked 'JANSSEN' on one side and 'K/200' on the other side.

4. CLINICAL PARTICULARS

4.1 Therapeutic indications
Because of the risk for serious hepatic toxicity, Nizoral tablets should be used only when the potential benefits are considered to outweigh the potential risks, taking into consideration the availability of other effective antifungal therapy.

Indications are:

Treatment of dermatophytosis and Malassezia (previously called Pityrosporum) folliculitis that cannot be treated topically because of the site, extent of the lesion or deep infection of the skin, in patients resistant to, or intolerant of, fluconazole, terbinafine and itraconazole.

Treatment of chronic mucocutaneous candidosis, cutaneous candidosis, and oropharyngeal candidosis that cannot be treated topically because of the site, extent of the lesion or deep infection of the skin, in patients resistant to or intolerant of both fluconazole and itraconazole.

4.2 Posology and method of administration
Method of administration:

Oral.

Nizoral should be taken during meals for maximal absorption.

Dosage:

Adults

One tablet (= 200 mg) once daily with a meal. If no adequate response is obtained with this dose, the dose should be increased to 2 tablets (= 400 mg) once daily.

Children

- Children weighing from 15 to 30 kg: half a tablet (=100 mg) once daily with a meal.

- Children weighing more than 30 kg: same as for adults.

Duration of Treatment

For all indications, treatment should be continued without interruption until clinical parameters or laboratory tests indicate that the fungal infection has resolved. An inadequate treatment period may lead to recurrence of the active infection. However, the risk of serious hepatic toxicity increases with longer duration of treatment; courses of greater than 10 days should only be given after full consideration of the extent of treatment response and the risk benefit of continuing treatment, and liver function should be closely monitored (see section 4.4 Special warnings and precautions for use)

For the treatment of Malassezia infections, treatment should not normally exceed 4 weeks.

Special Patient Population: Hepatic Impairment (see 4.3 Contraindications)

4.3 Contraindications
Nizoral tablets are contraindicated in the following situations:

- in patients with a known hypersensitivity to ketoconazole, to any of the other ingredients, or to any other imidazole antifungal.

- In patients with acute or chronic liver disease.

- Co-administration of the CYP3A4 substrates astemizole, bepridil, halofantrine, disopyramide, cisapride, dofetilide, levacetylmethadol (levomethadyl), mizolastine, pimozide, quinidine, sertindole or terfenadine with Nizoral Tablets is contraindicated since increased plasma concentrations of these medicinal products can lead to QT prolongation and rare occurrences of torsades de pointes.

- Co-administration of triazolam and oral midazolam.

- Co-administration of CYP3A4 metabolised HMG-CoA reductase inhibitors such as simvastatin and lovastatin.

- Co-administration of ergot alkaloids such as dihydroergotamine, ergometrine (ergonovine), ergotamine and methylergometrine (methylergonovine).

- Co-administration of nisoldipine

- Co-administration of eplerenone

- Co-administration of irinotecan

- Co-administration of everolimus and sirolimus (= rapamycin)

See also 4.5 Interaction with other medicinal products and other forms of interaction.

4.4 Special warnings and precautions for use
Because of the risk for serious hepatic toxicity, Nizoral tablets should be used only when the potential benefits are considered to outweigh the potential risks, taking into consideration the availability of other effective antifungal therapy.

Hepatic toxicity

Very rare cases of serious hepatic toxicity, including cases with a fatal outcome or requiring liver transplantation, have occurred with the use of oral ketoconazole (see 4.8 Undesirable effects). Some patients had no obvious risk factors for liver disease. Cases have been reported that occurred within the first month of treatment, including some within the first week.

The risk of serious hepatic toxicity increases with longer duration of treatment; courses of greater than 10 days should only be given after full consideration of the extent of treatment response and the risk benefit of continuing treatment

All patients should be counselled at the start of treatment with basic knowledge of the signs and symptoms suggestive of liver toxicity. The patient should be informed to discontinue treatment if they feel unwell or in the event of symptoms such as anorexia, nausea, vomiting, fatigue, jaundice, abdominal pain or dark urine. If these occur, treatment should be stopped immediately and liver function testing should be conducted.

Monitoring of hepatic function

Liver function must be monitored in all patients receiving treatment with Nizoral tablets.

Monitor liver function prior to treatment to rule out acute or chronic liver disease (see 4.3 Contraindication).

Liver function must be monitored at weeks 2 and 4 of treatment, then continued monthly, with discontinuation of treatment if any liver parameters are elevated above 3 times the normal limit.

In patients with raised liver enzymes, or those who have experienced liver toxicity with other drugs, treatment should only be started in exceptional cases, where the expected benefit exceeds the risk of hepatic injury, and consideration should be given to monitoring liver function tests (LFTs) more frequently.

Decreased gastric acidity

Absorption is impaired when gastric acidity is decreased. Acid neutralising medicines (e.g. aluminium hydroxide), should not be administered for at least 2 hours after the intake of Nizoral Tablets. In patients with achlorhydria, such as certain AIDS patients and patients on acid secretion suppressors (e.g. H_2-antagonists, proton pump inhibitors), it is advisable to administer Nizoral Tablets with a cola beverage.

Monitoring of adrenal function

In volunteers on daily doses of 400 mg and more, ketoconazole has been shown to reduce the cortisol response to ACTH stimulation. Therefore, adrenal function should be monitored in patients with Addison's Disease, adrenal insufficiency or borderline adrenal function and in patients under prolonged periods of stress (major surgery, intensive care, etc.), and in patients on prolonged therapy presenting signs and symptoms suggestive of adrenal insufficiency.

Documented use of Nizoral tablets in children weighing less than 15 kg is very limited. Therefore it is not recommended to administer Nizoral tablets to small children.

A risk/benefit evaluation should be made before ketoconazole is used in cases of non-life threatening diseases requiring long treatment periods.

Table 1: Adverse Experiences With an Incidence ⩾ 0.5% During Ketoconazole Treatment in 1361 Cases With Various Superficial and Deep Mycoses

System Organ Class AE Preferred term	Superficial Mycosis	Deep Mycosis	Total
	% (N=1,026)	% (N=335)	% (N=1361)
Nervous system disorder			
Headache	0.7	0.9	0.7
Dizziness	0.5	1.2	0.7
Somnolence	0.5	1.2	0.7
Gastrointestinal disorders			
Nausea/Vomiting	1.8	6.9	3.0
Abdominal pain	1.2	1.2	1.2
Diarrhoea	0.7	0.6	0.7
Skin and subcutaneous tissue disorders			
Pruritus	0.8	3.3	1.4

Drug interaction potential

Nizoral has a potential for clinically important drug interactions (see 4.5 Interaction with other medicinal products and other forms of interaction).

Use with domperidone

A slight increase of QT interval (mean less than 10msec) was reported in a drug-drug interaction study with oral domperidone. Even if the significance of this study is not fully clear, alternative therapeutic options should be considered if oral ketoconazole treatment is required (see also sections 4.5).

Lactose

Patients with rare hereditary problems of galactose intolerance, the Lapp lactase deficiency or glucose-galactose malabsorption should not take this medicine.

4.5 Interaction with other medicinal products and other forms of interaction

1. Drugs affecting the absorption of ketoconazole

Drugs affecting gastric acidity impair the absorption of ketoconazole: see 4.4 Special warnings and special precautions for use.

2. Drugs affecting the metabolism of ketoconazole

Ketoconazole is mainly metabolised through the cytochrome CYP3A4.

Enzyme-inducing drugs such as rifampicin, rifabutin, carbamazepine, isoniazid, nevirapine and phenytoin significantly reduce the bioavailability of ketoconazole. As plasma levels are lower than those expected if ketoconazole is used alone (no co-medication), it is not really necessary to monitor plasma levels. The combination of ketoconazole with potent enzyme inducers is not recommended.

Ritonavir increases the bioavailability of ketoconazole. Therefore, when it is given concomitantly, a dose reduction of ketoconazole should be considered.

3. Effect of ketoconazole on the metabolism of other drugs

Ketoconazole can inhibit the metabolism of drugs metabolised by certain hepatic P450 enzymes, especially of the CYP3A family. This can result in an increase and/or prolongation of their effects including adverse effects.

Co-administration of ketoconazole and domperidone is not recommended since the combination can lead to increased plasma concentrations of domperidone and QT prolongation.

Drugs that are contraindicated during treatment with ketoconazole (see 4.3 Contraindications):

Co-administration of the CYP3A4 substrates astemizole, bepridil, halofantrine, disopyramide, cisapride, dofetilide, levacetylmethadol (levomethadyl), mizolastine, pimozide, quinidine, sertindole or terfenadine with NIZORAL Tablets is contraindicated since increased plasma concentrations of these medicinal products can lead to QT prolongation and rare occurrences of torsades de pointes.

Co-administration of triazolam and oral midazolam is contraindicated because of an exaggerated and prolonged pharmacodynamic response.

Co-administration of CYP3A4 metabolised HMG-CoA reductase inhibitors such as simvastatin and lovastatin.

Co-administration of ergot alkaloids such as dihydroergotamine, ergometrine (ergonovine), ergotamine and methylergometrine (methylergonovine))

Co-administration of nisoldipine.

Co-administration of eplerenone.

Co-administration of irinotecan

Co-administration of everolimus and sirolimus (= rapamycin)

When co-administered with oral ketoconazole the following drugs should be used with caution and their plasma concentrations, effects or adverse effects should be monitored. Their dosage, if coadministered with ketoconazole, should be reduced if necessary. This should be considered when prescribing concomitant medication.

Examples include:

- Oral anticoagulants.
- HIV Protease Inhibitors such as indinavir, saquinavir.
- Certain antineoplastic agents such as vinca alkaloids, busulphan, docetaxel, erlotinib and imatinib;
- CYP3A4 metabolised calcium channel blockers such as the dihydropyridines and probably verapamil.
- Certain immunosuppressive agents: ciclosporin and tacrolimus
- Certain CYP3A4 metabolised HMG-CoA reductase inhibitors such as atorvastatin
- Certain glucocorticoids such as budesonide, fluticasone, dexamethasone and methylprednisolone
- Digoxin (via inhibition of P-glycoprotein)
- Others: cilostazol, buspirone, alfentanil, fentanyl, sildenafil, solifenacin, alprazolam, brotizolam, intravenous midazolam, quetiapine, repaglinide, tolterodine, trimetrexate, ebastine, eletriptan and reboxetine

Exceptional cases of a disulfiram-like reaction to alcohol, characterised by flushing, rash, peripheral oedema, nausea and headache, have been reported. All symptoms resolved completely within a few hours.

4.6 Pregnancy and lactation

Pregnancy

There is limited information on the use of Nizoral tablets during pregnancy. Animal studies have shown reproductive toxicity (see 5.3 Preclinical safety data). The potential risk to humans is unknown. Therefore, Nizoral tablets should not be used during pregnancy unless the potential benefit to the mother outweighs the possible risk to the foetus.

Lactation

Since ketoconazole is excreted in the milk, mothers who are under treatment should not breast-feed whilst being treated with Nizoral tablets.

4.7 Effects on ability to drive and use machines

None known.

4.8 Undesirable effects

Clinical trials

In a multinational multi-centre, open label study in patients with various superficial and deep mycoses, adverse events during ketoconazole treatment were evaluable in 1361 cases, 149 (11%) reported adverse events. The adverse events were summarised regardless of the causality assessment of the investigator. The most frequently reported adverse events were of gastrointestinal origin, i.e. nausea and vomiting. Adverse events that were reported with an incidence of ⩾0.5% are presented in Table 1.

(see Table 1 above)

Postmarketing Experience

Including the above mentioned Adverse Drug Reactions (ADRs), the following ADR's have been observed from post-markleting experiences reported with the use of Nizoral tablets. Unlike for clinical trials, precise frequencies cannot be provided for spontaneous reports. The frequency for these reports is therefore classified as 'not known'.

Table 2. Postmarketing reports of adverse drug reactions

Blood and the lymphatic system disorders	
Not Known	thrombocytopenia;
Immune system disorders	
Not Known	allergic conditions including anaphylactic shock anaphylactoid and anaphylactic reactions and angioneurotic oedema
Endocrine disorders	
Not Known	adrenocortical insufficiency
Nervous system disorders	
Not Known	Reversible increased intracranial pressure (e.g. papilloedema, fontanelle bulging in infants), paraesthesia
Eye disorders	
Not Known	photophobia
Gastrointestinal disorders	
Not Known	dyspepsia,
Hepato-biliary disorders	
Not Known	serious hepatotoxicity, including jaundice, hepatitis, biopsy-confirmed hepatic necrosis, cirrhosis, hepatic failure including cases resulting in transplantation or death. (see 4.4 Special warnings and special precautions for use), liver function test abnormal
Skin & and subcutaneous tissue disorders	
Not Known	urticaria, alopecia, photosensitivity
Reproductive system and breast disorders	
Not Known	erectile dysfunction, gynaecomastia, menstrual disorder; with doses higher than the recommended therapeutic dose of 200 or 400mg daily azoospermia

4.9 Overdose

There is no known antidote to ketoconazole.

In the event of accidental overdose, treatment consists of supportive measures. Within the first hour after ingestion gastric lavage may be performed. Activated charcoal may be given if considered appropriate.

5. PHARMACOLOGICAL PROPERTIES

5.1 Pharmacodynamic properties

Pharmacotherapeutic classification: Antimycotics for systemic use, imidazole derivatives

ATC code: J02A B02

Ketoconazole is an imidazole-dioxolane anti-mycotic, which is effective after oral administration and has a broad spectrum of activity against dermatophytes, yeasts and other pathogenic fungi.

In vitro studies have demonstrated that ketoconazole impairs the synthesis of ergosterol in fungal cells. Ergosterol is a vital cell membrane component in fungi. Impairment of its synthesis ultimately results in an antifungal effect.

Data from some clinical PK/PD studies and drug interaction studies suggest that oral dosing with ketoconazole at 200 mg twice daily for 3-7 days can result in a small increase of the QTc interval: a mean maximum increase of about 6 to 12 msec was seen at ketoconazole peak plasma levels, about 1-4 hours after ketoconazole administration. This small prolongation of the QTc interval, however, is not considered to be clinically relevant.

At the therapeutic dosage of 200 mg once daily, a transient decrease in the plasma concentrations of testosterone can be observed. Testosterone concentrations return to predose concentrations within 24 hours after administration of ketoconazole has stopped. During long-term therapy at this dosage, testosterone concentrations are usually not significantly different from controls.

In volunteers on daily doses of 400 mg and more, ketoconazole has been shown to reduce the cortisol response to ACTH stimulation (see 4.4 Special warnings and special precautions for use).

5.2 Pharmacokinetic properties

Absorption

Ketoconazole is a weak dibasic agent and thus requires acidity for dissolution and absorption. Mean peak plasma concentrations of approximately 3.5 µg/ml are reached within 1 to 2 hours, following oral administration of a single 200 mg dose taken with a meal.

Distribution

In vitro, the plasma protein binding is about 99% mainly to the albumin fraction. Ketoconazole is widely distributed into tissues; however, only a negligible proportion of ketoconazole reaches the cerebral-spinal fluid.

Metabolism

Following absorption from the gastro-intestinal tract, ketoconazole is converted into several inactive metabolites. The major identified metabolic pathways are oxidation and degradation of the imidazole and piperazine rings, oxidative O-dealkylation and aromatic hydroxylation.

Excretion

Plasma elimination is biphasic with a half-life of 2 hours during the first 10 hours and 8 hours thereafter. About 13%

of the dose is excreted in the urine, of which 2 to 4% is unchanged drug. The major route of excretion is through the bile into the intestinal tract.

Conditions in special populations

In patients with hepatic or renal insufficiency the overall pharmacokinetics of ketoconazole were not significantly different when compared with healthy subjects. See 4.3 Contraindications and 4.4 Special warnings and precautions for use.

5.3 Preclinical safety data

Slight pathological changes in the kidney, adrenals and ovaries were noted in an 18-month repeated dose rat study. In addition, female rats showed an increase in bone fragility. The No Observed Adverse Effect Level (NOAEL) in both these studies was 10 mg/kg/day.

In reproduction studies, at very high, maternally toxic doses (80 mg/kg/day and higher), ketoconazole impaired female fertility in the rat, and produced embryotoxic and teratogenic (oligodactylia and syndactylia) effects in pups. At 40 mg/kg in rats and rabbits, ketoconazole was devoid of embryotoxicity, teratogenicity and effects on fertility. No teratogenic effects were observed in mice at any dose level tested up to a maximum of 160 mg/kg. In pre-clinical studies, ketoconazole was not carcinogenic or genotoxic.

Electrophysiological studies have shown that ketoconazole inhibits the rapidly activating component of the cardiac delayed rectifier potassium current, prolongs the action potential duration, and may prolong the QT interval.

6. PHARMACEUTICAL PARTICULARS

6.1 List of excipients

Maize starch

Lactose

Polyvidone K90

Microcrystalline cellulose

Colloidal anhydrous silica

Magnesium stearate

6.2 Incompatibilities

None known.

6.3 Shelf life

Five years.

6.4 Special precautions for storage

Store in a dry place between 15°C and 30°C.

6.5 Nature and contents of container

PVC/aluminium blister packs containing 30 tablets

6.6 Special precautions for disposal and other handling

Not applicable.

7. MARKETING AUTHORISATION HOLDER

Janssen-Cilag Ltd

50-100 Holmers Farm Way

High Wycombe

Bucks

HP12 4EG

UK

8. MARKETING AUTHORISATION NUMBER(S)

PL 00242/0083

9. DATE OF FIRST AUTHORISATION/RENEWAL OF THE AUTHORISATION

Date of First Authorisation: 22 December 1980

10. DATE OF REVISION OF THE TEXT

October 2008

Nolvadex D

(AstraZeneca UK Limited)

1. NAME OF THE MEDICINAL PRODUCT

Nolvadex D

2. QUALITATIVE AND QUANTITATIVE COMPOSITION

Tamoxifen Citrate Ph. Eur. 30.4 mg (equivalent to 20 mg tamoxifen).

3. PHARMACEUTICAL FORM

Tablet.

4. CLINICAL PARTICULARS

4.1 Therapeutic indications

Nolvadex is indicated for:

1. The treatment of breast cancer.

2. The treatment of anovulatory infertility.

4.2 Posology and method of administration

Route of administration: Oral

1. Breast Cancer

Adults

The recommended daily dose of tamoxifen is normally 20 mg. No additional benefit, in terms of delayed recurrence or improved survival in patients, has been demonstrated with higher doses. Substantive evidence supporting the use of treatment with 30–40 mg per day is not available, although these doses have been used in some patients with advanced disease.

Elderly patients

Similar dosing regimens of Nolvadex have been used in elderly patients with breast cancer and in some of these patients it has been used as sole therapy.

2. Anovulatory Infertility

Before commencing any course of treatment, whether initial or subsequent, the possibility of pregnancy must be excluded. In women who are menstruating regularly, but with anovular cycles, the initial course of treatment consists of 20 mg given daily on the second, third, fourth and fifth days of the menstrual cycle. If unsatisfactory basal temperature records or poor pre-ovulatory cervical mucus indicate that this initial course of treatment has been unsuccessful, further courses may be given during subsequent menstrual periods, increasing the dosage to 40 mg and then to 80 mg daily.

In women who are not menstruating regularly, the initial course may begin on any day. If no signs of ovulation are demonstrable, then a subsequent course of treatment may start 45 days later, with dosage increased as above. If a patient responds with menstruation, then the next course of treatment is commenced on the second day of the cycle.

Use in children

The use of Nolvadex is not recommended in children, as safety and efficacy have not been established (see sections 5.1 and 5.2).

4.3 Contraindications

Nolvadex must not be given during pregnancy. Premenopausal patients must be carefully examined before treatment for breast cancer or infertility to exclude the possibility of pregnancy (see also section 4.6).

'Nolvadex' should not be given to patients who have experienced hypersensitivity to the product or any of its ingredients.

Concurrent anastrozole therapy (see section 4.5).

Treatment for infertility: Patients with a personal or family history of confirmed idiopathic venous thromboembolic events or a known genetic defect.

4.4 Special warnings and precautions for use

Menstruation is suppressed in a proportion of premenopausal women receiving Nolvadex for the treatment of breast cancer.

An increased incidence of endometrial changes including hyperplasia, polyps, cancer and uterine sarcoma (mostly malignant mixed Mullerian tumours), has been reported in association with Nolvadex treatment. The underlying mechanism is unknown but may be related to the oestrogen-like effect of Nolvadex. Any patient receiving or having previously received Nolvadex who report abnormal gynaecological symptoms, especially vaginal bleeding, or who presents with menstrual irregularities, vaginal discharge and symptoms such as pelvic pain or pressure should be promptly investigated.

A number of second primary tumours, occurring at sites other than the endometrium and the opposite breast, have been reported in clinical trials, following the treatment of breast cancer patients with tamoxifen. No causal link has been established and the clinical significance of these observations remains unclear.

Venous thromboembolism

- A 2–3-fold increase in the risk for VTE has been demonstrated in healthy tamoxifen-treated women (see section 4.8).
- In patients with *breast cancer*, prescribers should obtain careful histories with respect to the patient's personal and family history of VTE. If suggestive of a prothrombotic risk, patients should be screened for thrombophilic factors. Patients who test positive should be counselled regarding their thrombotic risk. The decision to use tamoxifen in these patients should be based on the overall risk to the patient. In selected patients, the use of tamoxifen with prophylactic anticoagulation may be justified (cross-reference section 4.5).
- The risk of VTE is further increased by severe obesity, increasing age and all other risk factors for VTE. The risks and benefits should be carefully considered for *all* patients before treatment with tamoxifen. In patients with *breast cancer*, this risk is also increased by concomitant chemotherapy (see section 4.5). Long-term anticoagulant prophylaxis may be justified for some patients with *breast cancer* who have multiple risk factors for VTE.
- Surgery and immobility: For patients being treated for *infertility*, tamoxifen should be stopped at least 6 weeks before surgery or long-term immobility (when possible) and re-started only when the patient is fully mobile. For patients with *breast cancer*, tamoxifen treatment should only be stopped if the risk of tamoxifen-induced thrombosis clearly outweighs the risks associated with interrupting treatment. All patients should receive appropriate thrombosis prophylactic measures and should include graduated compression stockings for the period of hospitalisation, early ambulation, if possible, and anticoagulant treatment.
- If *any* patient presents with VTE, tamoxifen should be stopped immediately and appropriate anti-thrombosis measures initiated. In patients being treated for *infertility*, tamoxifen should not be re-started unless there is a compelling alternative explanation for their thrombotic event. In patients receiving tamoxifen for *breast cancer*, the decision to re-start tamoxifen should be made with respect to the overall risk for the patient. In selected patients with *breast cancer*, the continued use of tamoxifen with prophylactic anticoagulation may be justified.
- *All* patients should be advised to contact their doctors immediately if they become aware of any symptoms of VTE.

In an uncontrolled trial in 28 girls aged 2–10 years with McCune Albright Syndrome (MAS), who received 20 mg once a day for up to 12 months duration, mean uterine volume increased after 6 months of treatment and doubled at the end of the one-year study. While this finding is in line with the pharmacodynamic properties of tamoxifen, a causal relationship has not been established (see section 5.1).

4.5 Interaction with other medicinal products and other forms of interaction

When Nolvadex is used in combination with coumarin-type anticoagulants, a significant increase in anticoagulant effect may occur. Where such co-administration is initiated, careful monitoring of the patient is recommended.

When Nolvadex is used in combination with cytotoxic agents for the treatment of breast cancer, there is increased risk of thromboembolic events occurring. (See also sections 4.4 and 4.8). Because of this increase in risk of VTE, thrombosis prophylaxis should be considered for these patients for the period of concomitant chemotherapy.

The use of tamoxifen in combination with anastrozole as adjuvant therapy has not shown improved efficacy compared with tamoxifen alone.

As Nolvadex is metabolised by cytochrome P450 3A4, care is required when co-administering with drugs, such as rifampicin, known to induce this enzyme as tamoxifen levels may be reduced. The clinical relevance of this reduction is unknown.

Pharmacokinetic interaction with CYP2D6 inhibitors, showing a reduction in plasma level of an active tamoxifen metabolite, 4-hydroxy-N-desmethyltamoxifen (endoxifen), has been reported in the literature. The relevance of this to clinical practice is not known.

4.6 Pregnancy and lactation

Pregnancy

Nolvadex must not be administered during pregnancy. There have been a small number of reports of spontaneous abortions, birth defects and foetal deaths after women have taken Nolvadex, although no causal relationship has been established.

Reproductive toxicology studies in rats, rabbits and monkeys have shown no teratogenic potential.

In rodent models of foetal reproductive tract development, tamoxifen was associated with changes similar to those caused by estradiol, ethinylestradiol, clomiphene and diethylstilboestrol (DES). Although the clinical relevance of these changes is unknown, some of them, especially vaginal adenosis, are similar to those seen in young women who were exposed to DES *in utero* and who have a 1 in 1000 risk of developing clear-cell carcinoma of the vagina or cervix. Only a small number of pregnant women have been exposed to tamoxifen. Such exposure has not been reported to cause subsequent vaginal adenosis or clear-cell carcinoma of the vagina or cervix in young women exposed *in utero* to tamoxifen.

Women should be advised not to become pregnant whilst taking Nolvadex and should use barrier or other non-hormonal contraceptive methods if sexually active. Premenopausal patients must be carefully examined before treatment to exclude pregnancy. Women should be informed of the potential risks to the foetus, should they become pregnant whilst taking Nolvadex or within two months of cessation of therapy.

Lactation

It is not known if Nolvadex is excreted in human milk and therefore the drug is not recommended during lactation. The decision either to discontinue nursing or discontinue Nolvadex should take into account the importance of the drug to the mother.

4.7 Effects on ability to drive and use machines

There is no evidence that Nolvadex results in impairment of these activities.

4.8 Undesirable effects

Side effects can be classified as either due to the pharmacological action of the drug, e.g. hot flushes, vaginal bleeding, vaginal discharge, pruritus vulvae and tumour flare, or as more general side effects, e.g. gastrointestinal intolerance, headache, light-headedness and occasionally, fluid retention and alopecia.

When side effects are severe, it may be possible to control them by a simple reduction of dosage (to not less than 20 mg/day) without loss of control of the disease. If side effects do not respond to this measure, it may be necessary to stop the treatment.

Skin rashes (including isolated reports of erythema multiforme, Stevens-Johnson syndrome and bullous pemphigoid) and rare hypersensitivity reactions including angioedema have been reported.

A small number of patients with bony metastases have developed hypercalcaemia on initiation of therapy.

Falls in platelet count, usually to 80,000 to 90,000 per cu mm but occasionally lower, have been reported in patients taking tamoxifen for breast cancer.

A number of cases of visual disturbance including reports of corneal changes and retinopathy have been described in patients receiving Nolvadex. An increased incidence of cataracts has been reported in association with the administration of Nolvadex.

Cases of optic neuropathy and optic neuritis have been reported in patients receiving tamoxifen and, in a small number of cases, blindness has occurred.

Uterine fibroids, endometriosis and other endometrial changes including hyperplasia and polyps have been reported.

Cystic ovarian swellings have occasionally been observed in premenopausal women receiving Nolvadex.

Leucopenia has been observed following the administration of Nolvadex, sometimes in association with anaemia and/or thrombocytopenia. Neutropenia has been reported on rare occasions; this can sometimes be severe.

There is evidence of an increased incidence of ischaemic cerebrovascular events and thromboembolic events, including deep vein thrombosis and pulmonary embolism, during tamoxifen therapy (see sections 4.3, 4.4 and 4.5). When Nolvadex is used in combination with cytotoxic agents, there is an increased risk of thromboembolic events occurring.

Leg cramps have been reported commonly in patients receiving Nolvadex.

Very rarely, cases of interstitial pneumonitis have been reported.

Nolvadex has been associated with changes in liver enzyme levels and on rare occasions with a spectrum of more severe liver abnormalities including fatty liver, cholestasis and hepatitis.

Rarely, elevation of serum triglyceride levels, in some cases with pancreatitis, may be associated with the use of Nolvadex.

An increased incidence of endometrial cancer and uterine sarcoma (mostly malignant mixed Mullerian tumours) has been reported in association with Nolvadex treatment.

4.9 Overdose

On theoretical grounds, an overdosage would be expected to cause enhancement of the pharmacological side effects mentioned above. Observations in animals show that extreme overdosage (100–200 times recommended daily dose) may produce oestrogenic effects.

There have been reports in the literature that Nolvadex given at several times the standard dose may be associated with prolongation of the QT interval of the ECG.

There is no specific antidote to overdosage, and treatment must be symptomatic.

5. PHARMACOLOGICAL PROPERTIES

5.1 Pharmacodynamic properties

Nolvadex (tamoxifen) is a non-steroidal, triphenylethylene-based drug which displays a complex spectrum of oestrogen antagonist and oestrogen agonist-like pharmacological effects in different tissues. In breast cancer patients, at the tumour level, tamoxifen acts primarily as an antioestrogen, preventing oestrogen binding to the oestrogen receptor. In the clinical situation, it is recognised that tamoxifen leads to reductions in levels of blood total cholesterol and low density lipoproteins in postmenopausal women of the order of 10–20%. Tamoxifen does not adversely affect bone mineral density.

An uncontrolled trial was undertaken in a heterogenous group of 28 girls aged 2 to 10 years with McCune Albright Syndrome (MAS), who received 20 mg once a day for up to 12 months duration. Among the patients who reported vaginal bleeding during the pre-study period, 62% (13 out of 21 patients) reported no bleeding for a 6-month period and 33% (7 out of 21 patients) reported no vaginal bleeding for the duration of the trial. Mean uterine volume increased after 6 months of treatment and doubled at the end of the one-year study. While this finding is in line with the pharmacodynamic properties of tamoxifen, a causal relationship has not been established (see section 4.4). There are no long-term safety data in children. In particular, the long-term effects of tamoxifen on growth, puberty and general development have not been studied.

5.2 Pharmacokinetic properties

After oral administration, tamoxifen is absorbed rapidly with maximum serum concentrations attained within 4–7 hours. Steady state concentrations (about 300 ng/ml) are achieved after four weeks treatment with 40 mg daily. The drug is highly protein bound to serum albumin (>99%). Metabolism is by hydroxylation, demethylation and conjugation, giving rise to several metabolites which have a similar pharmacological profile to the parent compound and thus contribute to the therapeutic effect. Excretion occurs primarily via the faeces and an elimination half-life of approximately seven days has been calculated for the drug itself, whereas that for N-desmethyltamoxifen, the principal circulating metabolite, is 14 days.

In a clinical study where girls between 2 and 10 years with McCune Albright Syndrome (MAS) received 20 mg tamoxifen once a day for up to 12 months duration, there was an age-dependent decrease in clearance and an increase in exposure (AUC), (with values up to 50% higher in the youngest patients) compared with adults.

5.3 Preclinical safety data

Tamoxifen was not mutagenic in a range of *in vitro* and *in vivo* mutagenicity tests. Tamoxifen was genotoxic in some *in vitro* and *in vivo* genotoxicity tests in rodents. Gonadal tumours in mice and liver tumours in rats receiving tamoxifen have been reported in long-term studies. The clinical relevance of these findings has not been established.

Tamoxifen is a drug on which extensive clinical experience has been obtained. Relevant information for the prescriber is provided elsewhere in the Summary of Product Characteristics.

6. PHARMACEUTICAL PARTICULARS

6.1 List of excipients

Croscarmellose Sodium USNF

Gelatin BP

Lactose Ph. Eur.

Macrogol 300 B.P.

Magnesium Stearate Ph. Eur.

Maize Starch Ph. Eur.

Hydroxypropylmethylcellulose USP

Titanium Dioxide Ph. Eur. (E171)

6.2 Incompatibilities

None known.

6.3 Shelf life

5 years.

6.4 Special precautions for storage

Do not store above 30°C. Store in the original container.

6.5 Nature and contents of container

Aluminium blister pack containing 30 or 250 tablets.

HDPE bottles containing 30 or 250 tablets.

6.6 Special precautions for disposal and other handling

Use as directed by the prescriber.

7. MARKETING AUTHORISATION HOLDER

AstraZeneca UK Limited,

600 Capability Green,

Luton, LU1 3LU, UK.

8. MARKETING AUTHORISATION NUMBER(S)

PL 17901/0034

9. DATE OF FIRST AUTHORISATION/RENEWAL OF THE AUTHORISATION

11th June 2000

10. DATE OF REVISION OF THE TEXT

19th June 2008

Nootropil 800mg & 1200mgTablets and Solution

(UCB Pharma Limited)

1. NAME OF THE MEDICINAL PRODUCT

Nootropil Tablets 1200 mg

Nootropil Tablets 800 mg

Nootropil Solution 33%

2. QUALITATIVE AND QUANTITATIVE COMPOSITION

Piracetam - 1200 mg per tablet

Piracetam - 800 mg per tablet

Piracetam – 33% w/v

3. PHARMACEUTICAL FORM

Tablet for oral administration.

Solution for oral administration.

4. CLINICAL PARTICULARS

4.1 Therapeutic indications

NOOTROPIL is indicated for patients suffering from myoclonus of cortical origin, irrespective of aetiology, and should be used in combination with other anti-myoclonic therapies.

4.2 Posology and method of administration

Adults:

The dosage regime shows important interindividual variability, requiring an individualised dose finding approach. A reasonable protocol would be to introduce piracetam at a dosage of 7.2 g/day, increasing by 4.8 g/day every 3 to 4 days up to a maximum of 20g/day, given in either 2 or 3 divided doses while keeping other antimyoclonic drugs unchanged at their optimal dosage. If possible, depending on clinical benefit, an attempt should be made to subsequently reduce the dosage of other antimyoclonic drugs.

4.3 Contraindications

Piracetam is contra-indicated in patients with severe renal impairment (renal creatinine clearance of less than 20 ml per minute), hepatic impairment and to those under 16 years of age. It is also contraindicated in patients with cerebral haemorrhage and in those with hypersensitivity to piracetam, other pyrrolidone derivatives or any of the excipients.

4.4 Special warnings and precautions for use

Due to the effect of piracetam on platelet aggregation (see section 5.1. Pharmacodynamic Properties), caution is recommended in patients with underlying disorders of haemostasis, major surgery or severe haemorrhage.

Abrupt discontinuation of treatment should be avoided as this may induce myoclonic or generalised seizures in some myoclonic patients.

As piracetam is almost exclusively excreted by the kidneys caution should be exercised in treating patients with known renal impairment. In renally impaired and elderly patients an increase in terminal half-life is directly related to renal function as measured by creatinine clearance.

The daily dose must be individualized according to renal function. Refer to the following table and adjust the dose as indicated. To use this dosing table, an estimate of the patient's creatinine clearance (CLcr) in ml/min is needed. The CLcr in ml/min may be estimated from serum creatinine (mg/dl) determination using the following formula:

$$CLcr = \frac{[140 - \text{age } (years)] \times \text{weight } (kg)}{72 \times \text{serum creatinine } (mg/dl)} (\times 0.85 \text{ for women})$$

Group	Creatinine clearance (ml/min)	Posology and frequency
Normal	> 80	usual daily dose, 2 to 4 sub-doses
Mild	50-79	2/3 usual daily dose, 2 or 3 sub-doses
Moderate	30-49	1/3 usual daily dose, 2 sub-doses
Severe	< 30	1/6 usual daily dose, 1 single intake
	< 20	contraindicated

4.5 Interaction with other medicinal products and other forms of interaction

In a single case, confusion, irritability and sleep disorders were reported in concomitant use with thyroid extract (T3 + T4). At present although based on a small number of patients, no interaction has been found with the following anti-epileptic medications: clonazepam, carbamazepine, phenytoin, phenobarbitone and sodium valproate.

In a published single-blind study on patients with severe recurrent venous thrombosis, piracetam 9.6 g/d did not modify the doses of acenocoumarol necessary to reach INR 2.5 to 3.5, but compared with the effects of acenocoumarol alone, the addition of piracetam 9.6 g/d significantly decreased platelet aggregation, β-thromboglobulin release, levels of fibrinogen and von Willebrand's factors (VIII: C; VIII: vW: Ag; VIII: vW: RCo) and whole blood and plasma viscosity.

To date, there are no known interactions with other drugs.

4.6 Pregnancy and lactation

In animal studies piracetam was not teratogenic and had no effect on fertility at the maximal tested dose of 2.7 /g/kg/day for the rabbit and 4.8 g/kg/day for rats and mice.

Piracetam readily crosses the placental barrier. Since the safety of use in human pregnancy is not established, piracetam is to be avoided during pregnancy.

Piracetam is excreted in human breast milk. Therefore, piracetam should be avoided during breastfeeding or breastfeeding should be discontinued, while receiving treatment with piracetam.

Young women using the product should be taking adequate contraceptive precautions.

4.7 Effects on ability to drive and use machines

In clinical studies, at dosages between 1.6 - 15 grams per day, hyperkinesia, somnolence, nervousness and depression were reported more frequently in patients on piracetam than on placebo. There is no experience on driving ability in dosages between 15 and 20 grams daily. Caution should therefore be exercised by patients intending to drive or use machinery whilst taking piracetam.

4.8 Undesirable effects

A. Clinical studies

Double-blind placebo-controlled clinical or pharmacoclinical trials, of which quantified safety data are available (extracted from the UCB Documentation Data Bank on June 1997), included more than 3000 subjects receiving piracetam, regardless of indication, dosage form, daily dosage or population characteristics.

When adverse events are grouped together according to WHO System Organ Classes, the following classes were found to be related to a statistically significantly higher occurrence under treatment with piracetam: psychiatric disorders, central and peripheral nervous system disorders, metabolic and nutritional disorders, body as a whole - general disorders.

Following adverse experiences were reported for piracetam with a statistically significantly higher incidence than placebo. Incidences are given for piracetam versus placebo treated patients.

WHO System Organ Class	Common (> 1 %, ≤ 10 %)	Uncommon (> 0.1 %, ≤ 1 %)
Central and peripheral nervous system disorders	Hyperkinesia (1.72 versus 0.42 %)	
Metabolic and nutritional disorders	Weight increase (1.29 versus 0.39 %)	
Psychiatric disorders	Nervousness (1.13 versus 0.25 %)	Somnolence (0.96 versus 0.25 %) Depression (0.83 versus 0.21 %)
Body as a whole - general disorders		Asthenia (0.23 versus 0.00 %)

B. Post-marketing experience

From the post-marketing experience, the following adverse drug reactions have been reported (sorted according to MedDRA System Organ Classes). Data are insufficient to support an estimate of their incidence in the population to be treated.

- Ear and labyrinth disorders:

vertigo

- Gastrointestinal disorders:

abdominal pain, abdominal pain upper, diarrhoea, nausea, vomiting

- Immune system disorders:

anaphylactoid reaction, hypersensitivity

- Nervous system disorders:

ataxia, balance impaired, epilepsy aggravated, headache, insomnia, somnolence

- Psychiatric disorders:

agitation, anxiety, confusion, hallucination

- Skin and subcutaneous tissue disorders:

angioneurotic oedema, dermatitis, pruritus, urticaria, rash

4.9 Overdose

Acute toxicological studies in animals showed lethal doses were obtained in mice (18.2 g/kg and higher) but not in rats and dogs dosed respectively at 21 g/kg or 10 g/kg.

No specific measure is indicated. The patient's general condition should be closely monitored. Close attention should be given to keeping the patient well hydrated and monitoring the urine flow.

5. PHARMACOLOGICAL PROPERTIES

5.1 Pharmacodynamic properties

Piracetam's mode of action in cortical myoclonus is as yet unknown.

Piracetam exerts its haemorrheological effects on the platelets, red blood cells, and vessel walls by increasing erythrocyte deformability and by decreasing platelet aggregation, erythrocyte adhesion to vessel walls and capillary vasospasm.

- Effects on the red blood cells:

In patients with sickle cell anemia, piracetam improves the deformability of the erythrocyte membrane, decreases blood viscosity, and prevents rouleaux formation.

- Effects on platelets:

In open studies in healthy volunteers and in patients with Raynaud's phenomenon, increasing doses of piracetam up to 12 g was associated with a dose-dependent reduction in platelet functions compared with pre-treatment values (tests of aggregation induced by ADP, collagen, epinephrine and βTG release), without significant change in platelet count. In these studies, piracetam prolonged bleeding time.

- Effects on blood vessels:

In animal studies, piracetam inhibited vasospasm and counteracted the effects of various spasmogenic agents. It lacked any vasodilatory action and did not induce "steal"phenomenon, nor low or no reflow, nor hypotensive effects.

In healthy volunteers, piracetam reduced the adhesion of RBCs to vascular endothelium and possessed also a direct stimulant effect on prostacycline synthesis in healthy endothelium.

-Effects on coagulation factors:

In healthy volunteers, compared with pre-treatment values, piracetam up to 9.6 g reduced plasma levels of fibrinogen and von Willebrand's factors (VIII: C; VIII R: AG; VIII R: vW) by 30 to 40 %, and increased bleeding time.

In patients with both primary and secondary Raynaud phenomenon, compared with pre-treatment values, piracetam 8 g/d during 6 months reduced plasma levels of fibrinogen and von Willebrand's factors (VIII: C; VIII R: AG; VIII R: vW (RCF)) by 30 to 40 %, reduced plasma viscosity, and increased bleeding time.

5.2 Pharmacokinetic properties

Piracetam is rapidly and almost completely absorbed. Peak plasma levels are reached within 1.5 hours after administration. The extent of oral bioavailability, assessed from the Area Under Curve (AUC), is close to 100% for capsules, tablets and solution. Peak levels and AUC are proportional to the dose given. The volume of distribution of piracetam is 0.7 L/kg, and the plasma half-life is 5.0 hours, in young adult men. Piracetam crosses the blood-brain and the placental barrier and diffuses across membranes used in renal dialysis. Up to now, no metabolite of piracetam has been found. Piracetam is excreted almost completely in urine and the fraction of the dose excreted in urine is independent of the dose given. Excretion half-life values are consistent with those calculated from plasma / blood data. Clearance of the compound is dependent on the renal creatinine clearance and would be expected to diminish with renal insufficiency.

5.3 Preclinical safety data

Single doses of piracetam yielded LD 50 values at 26 g/kg in mice but LD 50 values were not reached in rats. In dogs, clinical signs after acute oral dosing were mild and lethality was not observed at the maximum tested dose of 10 g/kg.

Repeated oral treatment for up to 1 year in dogs (10 g/kg) and 6 months in rats (2 g/kg) was very well tolerated: no target organ toxicity or signs of (irreversible) toxicity were clearly demonstrated. Safe dose levels represent a multiple of the maximum intended human daily dose of 0.4 g/kg.

In terms of exposure (C max) safe levels obtained in the rat and the dog represent respectively 8 fold and 50 fold of the maximum human therapeutic level. AUC levels obtained in the same animals were a multiple of the human AUC level at the maximum intended daily dose.

The only change which might eventually be attributed to chronic treatment in male, but not in female, rats was an increase of the incidence over control animals of progressive glomerulonephrosis at the dose of 2.4 g/kg/day given for 112 weeks.

Although piracetam crosses the placenta into the foetal circulation, no teratogenic effects were observed at dose levels up to 4.8 g/kg/day (mice, rats) and 2.7 g/kg/day (rabbits). Furthermore, the compound affects neither fertility nor the peri- or postnatal development of the pregnancy at doses up to 2.7 g/kg/day.

Piracetam was found to be devoid of any mutagenic or clastogenic activity and does not represent any genotoxic or carcinogenic risk to man.

6. PHARMACEUTICAL PARTICULARS

6.1 List of excipients

Nootropil 800 and 1200 mg Tablets:

Polyethylene glycol 6000

Colloidal anhydrous silica

Magnesium stearate

Methocel

Titanium dioxide (E171)

Polyethylene glycol 400

Nootropil Solution 33%:

Glycerol

Methy parahydroxybenzoate

Propyl parahydroxybenzoate

Sodium acetate

Acetic acid

Purified water

6.2 Incompatibilities

None known.

6.3 Shelf life

Nootropil 800 and 1200 mg Tablets:

Four (4) years.

Nootropil Solution 33%:

Five (5) years.

6.4 Special precautions for storage

Nootropil 800 and 1200 mg Tablets:

None.

Nootropil Solution 33%:

Do not store above 25°C.

6.5 Nature and contents of container

Nootropil 800 mg Tablets - Blister pack in an outer cardboard carton (90 tablets per carton).

Nootropil 1200 mg Tablets – Blister pack in an outer cardboard carton (60 tablets per carton).

Nootropil Solution 33% - Glass bottle containing 125 ml or 300 ml solution.

6.6 Special precautions for disposal and other handling

Tablets – None.

Solution – Do not store above 25°C.

It is advisable to follow each dose with a drink of water or a soft drink to reduce the bitter taste of the solution.

7. MARKETING AUTHORISATION HOLDER

UCB Pharma Ltd.,

208 Bath Road

Slough

Berkshire

SL1 3WE

8. MARKETING AUTHORISATION NUMBER(S)

Nootropil Tablets 800 mg: PL 00039/0535

Nootropil Tablets 1200 mg: PL 00039/0536

Nootropil Solution 33%: PL 00039/0534

9. DATE OF FIRST AUTHORISATION/RENEWAL OF THE AUTHORISATION

14 December 1992/03 December 1998/18 November 2004

10. DATE OF REVISION OF THE TEXT

06 December 2006

Norditropin SimpleXx 5 mg/1.5 ml, Norditropin SimpleXx 10 mg/1.5 ml, Norditropin SimpleXx 15 mg/1.5 ml

(Novo Nordisk Limited)

1. NAME OF THE MEDICINAL PRODUCT

Norditropin® SimpleXx® 5 mg/1.5 ml, solution for injection.

Norditropin® SimpleXx® 10 mg/1.5 ml, solution for injection.

Norditropin® SimpleXx® 15 mg/1.5 ml, solution for injection.

2. QUALITATIVE AND QUANTITATIVE COMPOSITION

Norditropin SimpleXx:

Somatropin 5 mg/1.5 ml (3.3 mg/ml), 10 mg/1.5 ml (6.7 mg/ml) and 15 mg/1.5 ml (10 mg/ml).

Somatropin (epr).

1 mg of somatropin corresponds to 3 IU (International Unit) of somatropin.

3. PHARMACEUTICAL FORM

Solution for injection.

4. CLINICAL PARTICULARS

4.1 Therapeutic indications

Children:

Growth failure due to growth hormone insufficiency.

Growth failure in girls due to gonadal dysgenesis (Turner's Syndrome).

Growth retardation in prepubertal children due to chronic renal disease.

Growth disturbance (current height SDS < -2.5 and parental adjusted height SDS < -1) in short children born small for gestational age (SGA), with a birth weight and/or length below -2 SD, who failed to show catch-up growth (HV SDS <0 during the last year) by 4 years of age or later.

Adults:

Pronounced growth hormone deficiency in known hypothalamic-pituitary disease (one other deficient axis, other than prolactin), demonstrated by one provocative test after institution of adequate replacement therapy for any other deficient axis.

Childhood onset growth hormone insufficiency, reconfirmed by two provocative tests.

In adults, the insulin tolerance test is the provocative test of choice. When the insulin tolerance test is contraindicated, alternative provocative tests must be used. The combined arginine-growth hormone releasing hormone is recommended. An arginine or glucagon test may also be considered; however these tests have less established diagnostic value than the insulin tolerance test.

4.2 Posology and method of administration

The dosage is individual and must always be adjusted in accordance with the individual's response to therapy.

Prescription only.

Norditropin should only be prescribed by doctors with special knowledge of the therapeutic indication of use.

Generally, daily subcutaneous administration in the evening is recommended. The injection site should be varied to prevent lipoatrophy.

Generally recommended dosages:

Children:

Growth hormone insufficiency

25-35 μg/kg/day or 0.7-1.0 mg/m²/day

Equal to: 0.07-0.1 IU/kg/day (2-3 IU/m²/day)

Turner's syndrome

45-67 μg/kg/day or 1.3-2.0 mg/m²/day

Equal to: 0.13-0.2 IU/kg/day (3.9-6 IU/m²/day)

Chronic Renal Disease

50 μg/kg/day or 1.4 mg/m²/day

Equal to: 0.14 IU/kg/day (4.3 IU/m²/day)

Small for Gestational Age

35 μg/kg/day or 1 mg/m²/day

Equal to: 0.1 IU/kg/day (3 IU/m²/day)

A dose of 0.035 mg/kg/day is usually recommended until final height is reached. (See section 5.1).

Treatment should be discontinued after the first year of treatment, if the height velocity SDS is below +1.

Treatment should be discontinued if height velocity is < 2 cm/year and, if confirmation is required, bone age is

> 14 years (girls) or > 16 years (boys), corresponding to closure of the epiphyseal growth plates.

Adults:

Replacement therapy in adults

The dosage must be adjusted to the need of the individual patient. It is recommended to start treatment with a low dose 0.15-0.3 mg/day (equal to 0.45-0.9 IU/day). It is recommended to increase the dosage gradually at monthly intervals based on the clinical response and the patient's experience of adverse events. Serum insulin-like growth factor I (IGF-I) can be used as guidance for the dose titration.

Dose requirements decline with age. Maintenance dosage varies considerably from person to person, but seldom exceeds 1.0 mg/day (equal to 3 IU/day).

4.3 Contraindications

Any evidence of active malignant tumours.

Intracranial neoplasm must be inactive and anti-tumour therapy should be completed prior to institution of therapy.

Pregnancy and lactation. Please refer to Section 4.6.

Patients with acute critical illness suffering complications following open heart surgery, abdominal surgery, multiple accidental trauma, acute respiratory failure or similar conditions should not be treated with Norditropin.

Hypersensitivity to somatropin or to any of the excipients.

In the children with chronic renal disease treatment with Norditropin SimpleXx should be discontinued at renal transplantation.

4.4 Special warnings and precautions for use

Children treated with Norditropin SimpleXx should be regularly assessed by a specialist in child growth. Norditropin SimpleXx treatment should always be instigated by a physician with special knowledge of growth hormone insufficiency and its treatment. This is true also for the management of Turner's syndrome and chronic renal disease and SGA. Data of final adult height following the use of Norditropin for children with chronic renal disease are not available.

The stimulation of skeletal growth in children can only be expected until the epiphyseal discs are closed.

The dosage in children with chronic renal disease is individual and must be adjusted according to the individual response to therapy. The growth disturbance should be clearly established before Norditropin SimpleXx treatment by following growth on optimal treatment for renal disease over one year. Conservative management of uraemia with customary medication and if needed dialysis should be maintained during Norditropin SimpleXx therapy.

Patients with chronic renal disease normally experience a decline in renal function as part of the natural course of their illness. However, as a precautionary measure during Norditropin SimpleXx treatment renal function should be monitored for an excessive decline, or increase in the glomerular filtration rate (which could imply hyperfiltration).

In short children born SGA other medical reasons or treatments that could explain growth disturbance should be ruled out before starting treatment.

In SGA children it is recommended to measure fasting insulin and blood glucose before start of treatment and annually thereafter. In patients with increased risk for diabetes mellitus (e.g. familial history of diabetes, obesity, severe insulin resistance, acanthosis nigricans) oral glucose tolerance testing (OGTT) should be performed. If overt diabetes occurs, growth hormone should not be administered.

In SGA children it is recommended to measure the IGF-I level before start of treatment and twice a year thereafter. If on repeated measurements IGF-I levels exceed +2 SD compared to references for age and pubertal status, the IGF-I / IGFBP-3 ratio could be taken into account to consider dose adjustment.

Experience in initiating treatment in SGA patients near onset of puberty is limited. It is therefore not recommended to initiate treatment near onset of puberty.

Experience with patients with Silver-Russell syndrome is limited.

Some of the height gain obtained with treating short children born SGA with growth hormone may be lost if treatment is stopped before final height is reached.

Somatropin has been found to influence carbohydrate metabolism, therefore, patients should be observed for evidence of glucose intolerance.

Serum thyroxine levels may fall during treatment with Norditropin SimpleXx due to the increased peripheral deiodination of T4 to T3.

In patients with a pituitary disease in progression, hypothyroidism may develop.

Patients with Turner's syndrome have an increased risk of developing primary hypothyroidism associated with anti-thyroid antibodies.

As hypothyroidism interferes with the response to Norditropin SimpleXx therapy patients should have their thyroid function tested regularly, and should receive replacement therapy with thyroid hormone when indicated.

In insulin treated patients adjustment of insulin dose may be needed after initiation of Norditropin SimpleXx treatment.

Patients with growth hormone deficiency secondary to an intracranial lesion should be examined frequently for progression or recurrence of the underlying disease process.

Leukaemia has been reported in a small number of growth hormone deficient patients some of whom have been treated with somatropin. Based on 10 years global assessment there is no increased risk of development of leukaemia during somatropin treatment. In patients in complete remission from tumours or malignant disease, growth hormone therapy has not been associated with an increased relapse rate. Nevertheless, patients who have achieved complete remission of malignant disease should be followed closely for relapse after commencement of Norditropin SimpleXx therapy.

Slipped capital femoral epiphysis may occur more frequently in patients with endocrine disorders and Legg-Calvé-Perthes disease may occur more frequently in patients with short stature. These diseases may present as the development of a limp or complaints of hip or knee pain and physicians and parents should be alerted to this possibility.

Scoliosis may progress in any child during rapid growth. Signs of scoliosis should be monitored during treatment. However, growth hormone treatment has not been shown to increase the incidence or severity of scoliosis.

In the event of severe or recurrent headache, visual problems, nausea, and/or vomiting, a funduscopy for papilloedema is recommended. If papilloedema is confirmed, a diagnosis of benign intracranial hypertension should be considered and if appropriate the growth hormone treatment should be discontinued.

At present there is insufficient evidence to guide clinical decision making in patients with resolved intracranial hypertension. If growth hormone treatment is restarted, careful monitoring for symptoms of intracranial hypertension is necessary.

Growth hormone deficiency in adults is a lifelong disease and needs to be treated accordingly, however, experience in patients older than 60 years and in patients with more than five years of treatment in adult growth hormone deficiency is still limited.

Two placebo-controlled clinical trials of patients in intensive care units have demonstrated an increased mortality among patients suffering from acute critical illness due to complications following open heart or abdominal surgery, multiple accidental trauma or acute respiratory failure, who were treated with somatropin in high doses (5.3 – 8 mg/day). The safety of continuing growth hormone treatment in patients receiving replacement doses for approved indications who concurrently develop these illnesses has not been established. Therefore, the potential benefit of treatment continuation with growth hormone in patients having acute critical illness should be weighed against the potential risk.

4.5 Interaction with other medicinal products and other forms of interaction

Concomitant glucocorticoid therapy may inhibit growth and thereby oppose the growth promoting effect of Norditropin SimpleXx. The effect of growth hormone on final height can also be influenced by additional therapy with other hormones, e.g. gonadotrophin, anabolic steroids, estrogen and thyroid hormone.

4.6 Pregnancy and lactation

Currently there is insufficient evidence of safety of somatropin therapy during pregnancy. The possibility that somatropin is secreted in breast milk cannot be discounted.

4.7 Effects on ability to drive and use machines

No effects.

4.8 Undesirable effects

Growth hormone deficient patients are characterised by extracellular volume deficit. When treatment with somatropin is initiated, this deficit is corrected. Fluid retention with peripheral oedema may occur especially in adults. Carpal tunnel syndrome is uncommon, but may be seen in adults. The symptoms are usually transient dose dependent and may require dose reduction. Mild arthralgia, muscle pain and paresthesia may also occur, but is usually self-limiting.

Adverse reactions in children are uncommon or rare.

Clinical trial experience:

Nervous system disorders

Common (>1/100, <1/10): In adults headache and paraesthesia.

Uncommon (>1/1000, <1/100): In adults carpal tunnel syndrome. In children headache.

Musculoskeletal, connective tissue and bone disorders

Common (>1/100, <1/10): In adults arthralgia, joint stiffness and myalgia.

Uncommon (>1/1000, <1/100): In adults muscle stiffness.

Rare (>1/10000, <1/1000): In children arthralgia and myalgia.

General disorders and administration site conditions

Very common (>1/10): In adults peripheral oedema

Uncommon (>1/1000, <1/100): In adults and children injection site pain. In children injection site reaction NOS.

Rare (>1/10000, <1/1000): In children peripheral oedema.

Skin and subcutaneous tissue disorders

Uncommon (>1/1000, <1/100): In adults pruritus.

Rare (>1/10000, <1/1000): In children rash NOS.

Metabolism and nutrition disorders

Uncommon (>1/1000, <1/100): In adults Diabetes mellitus type 2 (See Post marketing experience)

Post marketing experience:

Very rare cases of hypersensitivity reactions have been reported (please refer to section 4.3).

Formation of antibodies directed against somatropin has rarely been observed during Norditropin therapy. The titres and binding capacities of these antibodies have been very low and have not interfered with the growth response to Norditropin administration.

Very rare cases of decrease in serum thyroxin levels have been reported during treatment with Norditropin (see under 4.4.). Increase in blood alkaline phosphatase level may be seen during the treatment with Norditropin.

Very rare cases of benign intracranial hypertension have been reported.

Very rare cases of diabetes mellitus type 2 have been reported, but most of the available literature does not demonstrate an increased incidence of diabetes associated with somatropin treatment.

4.9 Overdose

Information on overdose and poisoning is lacking.

Acute overdosage can lead to low blood glucose levels initially, followed by high blood glucose levels. These decreased glucose levels have been detected biochemically, but without clinical signs of hypoglycaemia. Long-term overdosage could result in signs and symptoms consistent with the known effects of human growth hormone excess.

5. PHARMACOLOGICAL PROPERTIES

5.1 Pharmacodynamic properties

ATC:H 01 AC 01.

Norditropin SimpleXx contains somatropin, which is human growth hormone produced by recombinant DNA-technology. It is an anabolic peptide of 191 amino acids stabilised by two disulphide bridges with a molecular weight of approximately 22,000 Daltons.

The major effects of Norditropin SimpleXx are stimulation of skeletal and somatic growth and pronounced influence on the body's metabolic processes.

When growth hormone deficiency is treated a normalisation of body composition takes place resulting in an increase in lean body mass and a decrease in fat mass. Somatropin exerts most of its actions through insulin-like growth factor I (IGF-I), which are produced in tissues throughout the body, but predominantly by the liver.

More than 90% of IGF-I is bound to binding proteins (IGFBPs) of which IGFBP-3 is the most important.

A lipolytic and protein sparing effect of the hormone becomes of particular importance during stress.

Somatropin also increases bone turnover indicated by an increase in plasma levels of biochemical bone markers. In adults bone mass is slightly decreased during the initial months of treatment due to more pronounced bone resorption, however, bone mass increases with prolonged treatment.

In clinical trials in short children born SGA doses of 0.033 and 0.067 mg/kg/day have been used for treatment until final height. In 56 patients who were continuously treated and have reached (near) final height, the mean change from height at start of treatment was +1.90 SDS (0.033 mg/kg/day) and +2.19 SDS (0.067 mg/kg/day). Literature data from untreated SGA children without early spontaneous catch-up suggest a late growth of 0.5 SDS. Long-term safety data are still limited.

5.2 Pharmacokinetic properties

I.v. infusion of Norditropin (33 ng/kg/min for 3 hours) to nine growth hormone deficient patients, gave the following results: serum half-time of 21.1 ± 1.7 min., metabolic clearance rate of 2.33 ± 0.58 ml/kg/min. and a distribution space of 67.6 ± 14.6 ml/kg.

S.c. injection of Norditropin SimpleXx (2.5 mg/m^2) to 31 healthy subjects (with endogenous somatropin suppressed by continuous infusion of somatostatin) gave the following results:

Maximal concentration of human growth hormone (42-46 ng/ml) after approximately 4 hours. Thereafter human growth hormone declined with a half life of approximately 2.6 hours.

In addition the different strengths of Norditropin SimpleXx were demonstrated to be bioequivalent to each other and to conventional Norditropin after subcutaneous injection to healthy subjects.

5.3 Preclinical safety data

The general pharmacological effects on the CNS, cardiovascular and respiratory systems following administration of Norditropin SimpleXx with and without forced degradation were investigated in mice and rats; renal function was also evaluated. The degraded product showed no difference in effect when compared with Norditropin SimpleXx and Norditropin. All three preparations showed the expected dose dependent decrease in urine volume and retention of sodium and chloride ions.

In rats, similar pharmacokinetics has been demonstrated between Norditropin SimpleXx and Norditropin. Degraded Norditropin SimpleXx has also been demonstrated to be bioequivalent with Norditropin SimpleXx.

Single and repeated dose toxicity and local tolerance studies of Norditropin SimpleXx or the degraded product did not reveal any toxic effect or damage to the muscle tissue.

The toxicity of Poloxamer 188 has been tested in mice, rats, rabbits and dogs and no findings of toxicological relevance were revealed.

Poloxamer 188 was rapidly absorbed from the injection site with no significant retention of the dose at the site of injection. Poloxamer 188 was excreted primarily via the urine.

6. PHARMACEUTICAL PARTICULARS

6.1 List of excipients

Mannitol, Histidine, Poloxamer 188, Phenol, Water for Injections.

6.2 Incompatibilities

In the absence of compatibility studies, the medicinal product must not be mixed with other medicinal products.

6.3 Shelf life

Norditropin SimpleXx 5 mg/1.5 ml and 10 mg/1.5 ml:

The shelf life is 2 years.

After first opening: store for a maximum of 28 days at + 2°C - + 8°C.

Alternatively, the medicinal product may be stored for a maximum of 21 days not above +25°C.

Norditropin SimpleXx 15 mg/1.5 ml

The shelf life is 2 years.

After first opening: store for a maximum of 28 days at + 2°C - + 8°C.

6.4 Special precautions for storage

Norditropin SimpleXx 5 mg/1.5 ml and 10 mg/1.5 ml:

Before use: Store at + 2°C - + 8°C in the outer carton. Do not freeze.

Once opened, the product may be stored for a maximum of 28 days at + 2°C - + 8°C, *alternatively* stored not above + 25°C for a maximum of 21 days. Store in the pen (NordiPen®) during use. Do not freeze.

Norditropin SimpleXx 15 mg/1.5 ml

Before use: Store at + 2°C - + 8°C in the outer carton. Do not freeze.

Once opened, the product may be stored for a maximum of 28 days at + 2°C - + 8°C. Store in the pen (NordiPen®) during use. Do not freeze.

6.5 Nature and contents of container

Norditropin SimpleXx is contained in a colourless cartridge made of type I glass. The cartridge is closed at the bottom with a rubber stopper shaped as a plunger and at the top with a laminated rubber stopper shaped as a disc and sealed with an aluminium cap. The aluminium cap is finally sealed with a coloured cap (5 mg/1.5 ml (yellow), 10 mg/ 1.5 ml (blue), 15 mg/1.5 ml (green)).

The cartridge is contained in a blister packed in a carton.

Pack sizes: Norditropin SimpleXx 1 × 5mg/1.5ml

Norditropin SimpleXx 1 × 10mg/1.5ml

Norditropin SimpleXx 1 × 15 mg/1.5ml

6.6 Special precautions for disposal and other handling

Patients should be reminded to wash their hands thoroughly with soap and water and/or disinfectant prior to any contact with Norditropin. Norditropin should not be shaken vigorously at any time.

Norditropin SimpleXx 5 mg/1.5 ml, 10 mg/1.5 ml and 15 mg/1.5 ml should only be prescribed for use with the matching NordiPen® (NordiPen® 5, 10 and 15 respectively). Instructions for use of Norditropin SimpleXx in NordiPen® are provided within the respective packs. Patients should be advised to read these instructions very carefully.

Do not use Norditropin SimpleXx if it does not appear water clear and colourless.

7. MARKETING AUTHORISATION HOLDER

Novo Nordisk Limited

BroadfieldPark, Brighton Road

Crawley, West Sussex

RH11 9RT

8. MARKETING AUTHORISATION NUMBER(S)

Norditropin® SimpleXx® 5 mg/1.5 ml - PL 03132/0131

Norditropin® SimpleXx® 10 mg/1.5 ml - PL 03132/0132

Norditropin® SimpleXx® 15 mg/1.5 ml - PL 03132/0133

9. DATE OF FIRST AUTHORISATION/RENEWAL OF THE AUTHORISATION

October 1999/31 December 2003

10. DATE OF REVISION OF THE TEXT

January 2009

Legal Status

POM (Prescription Only Medicine), CD (Sch. 4).

Norgalax

(Norgine Limited)

1. NAME OF THE MEDICINAL PRODUCT

NORGALAX

2. QUALITATIVE AND QUANTITATIVE COMPOSITION

Norgalax contains the active ingredient Docusate Sodium 0.12 g in each 10 g micro-enema:

3. PHARMACEUTICAL FORM

Rectal gel.

4. CLINICAL PARTICULARS

4.1 Therapeutic indications

For the symptomatic treatment of constipation whenever an enema is required and for the preparation of the colon and rectum for endoscopic examination.

4.2 Posology and method of administration

Adults: use one micro-enema. If required, a second micro-enema may be used on the same or the next day.

Children: not recommended for children under 12 years old.

Norgalax is to be administered rectally. Remove the protective cap and insert the applicator into the rectum, squeezing gently until the tube is empty. A drop of the gel may be used as a lubricant if required.

4.3 Contraindications

Haemorrhoids, anal fissures, rectocolitis, anal bleeding, abdominal pain, intestinal obstruction, nausea, vomiting, inflammatory bowel disease, ileus and known hypersensitivity to any of the ingredients.

4.4 Special warnings and precautions for use

As with all laxatives, Norgalax should not be administered chronically. Prolonged use can precipitate the onset of an atonic non-functioning colon and hypokalaemia.

4.5 Interaction with other medicinal products and other forms of interaction

Norgalax may increase the resorption of medicines and is not to be used in combination with hepatotoxic agents.

4.6 Pregnancy and lactation

Norgalax may be used during pregnancy and lactation.

4.7 Effects on ability to drive and use machines

None known.

4.8 Undesirable effects

Anal or rectal burning and pain, usually short lasting diarrhoea, congestion of the rectal mucosa and rectal bleeding may occur occasionally. Hepatotoxicity has been reported especially when used in association with other laxatives.

4.9 Overdose

Overdose will lead to excessive purgation which should be treated symptomatically.

5. PHARMACOLOGICAL PROPERTIES

5.1 Pharmacodynamic properties

Docusate sodium is an anionic surfactant and used as a faecal softening agent. It is considered to ease constipation by increasing the penetration of fluid into the faeces thereby causing them to soften. Norgalax is usually effective in 5 to 20 minutes

5.2 Pharmacokinetic properties

Norgalax has a local effect in the rectum. Minimal absorption cannot be ruled out even with a rectal application.

6. PHARMACEUTICAL PARTICULARS

6.1 List of excipients

Glycerol

Sodium carboxymethyl cellulose

Purified Water

6.2 Incompatibilities

None known

6.3 Shelf life

The shelf life is 4 years.

6.4 Special precautions for storage

Do not store above 25°C.

6.5 Nature and contents of container

A polyethylene tube with fixed applicator and a cap closure, containing 10g of gel in pack sizes of 6 and 100 tubes.

6.6 Special precautions for disposal and other handling

None.

7. MARKETING AUTHORISATION HOLDER

Norgine Limited

Chaplin House

Widewater Place

Moorhall Road

Harefield

UXBRIDGE

Middlesex UB9 6NS

United Kingdom

8. MARKETING AUTHORISATION NUMBER(S)

PL 0322/0065.

9. DATE OF FIRST AUTHORISATION/RENEWAL OF THE AUTHORISATION

February 1999

10. DATE OF REVISION OF THE TEXT

January 2009

Noriday Tablets

(Pharmacia Limited)

1. NAME OF THE MEDICINAL PRODUCT

Noriday®

2. QUALITATIVE AND QUANTITATIVE COMPOSITION

Each tablet contains 350 micrograms norethisterone.

3. PHARMACEUTICAL FORM

White, flat, circular, bevel-edged tablet inscribed 'SEARLE' on one side and 'NY' on the other side.

4. CLINICAL PARTICULARS

4.1 Therapeutic indications

Noriday is a progestogen-only oral contraceptive. It is particularly useful for women for whom oestrogens may not be appropriate.

4.2 Posology and method of administration

Oral Administration

Starting on the first day of menstruation, one pill every day without a break in medication for as long as contraception is required. Additional contraceptive precautions (such as a condom) should be taken for the first 7 days of the first pack. Pills should be taken at the same time each day.

Missed Pills

If a pill is missed within 3 hours of the correct dosage time then the missed pill should be taken as soon as possible; this will ensure that contraceptive protection is maintained. If a pill is taken 3 or more hours late it is recommended that the woman takes the last missed pill as soon as possible and then continues to take the rest of the pills in the normal manner. However, to provide continued contraceptive protection it is recommended that an alternative method of contraception, such as a condom, is used for the next 7 days.

Changing from another oral contraceptive

In order to ensure that contraception is maintained it is advised that the first pill is taken on the day immediately after the patient has finished the previous pack.

Use after childbirth, miscarriage or abortion

The first pill should be taken on the 21st day after childbirth. This will ensure the patient is protected immediately. If there is any delay in taking the first pill, contraception may not be established until 7 days after the first pill has been taken. In these circumstances women should be advised that extra contraceptive methods will be necessary.

After a miscarriage or abortion patients can take the first pill on the next day; in this way they will be protected immediately.

Vomiting and diarrhoea

Gastrointestinal upsets, such as vomiting and diarrhoea, may interfere with the absorption of the pill leading to a reduction in contraceptive efficacy. Women should continue to take Noriday, but they should also be advised to use another contraceptive method during the period of gastrointestinal upset and for the next 7 days.

4.3 Contraindications

The contraindications for progestogen-only oral contraceptives are:

(i) known, suspected, or a past history of breast, genital or hormone dependent cancer;

(ii) acute or severe chronic liver diseases including past or present liver tumours, Dubin-Johnson or Rotor syndrome;

(iii) active liver disease;

(iv) history during pregnancy of idiopathic jaundice or severe pruritus;

(v) disorders of lipid metabolism;

(vi) undiagnosed abnormal vaginal bleeding;

(vii) known or suspected pregnancy;

(viii) hypersensitivity to any component.

Combined oestrogen/progestogen preparations have been associated with an increase in the risk of thromboembolic and thrombotic disease. Risk has been reported to be related to both oestrogenic and progestogenic activity. In the absence of long term epidemiological studies with progestogen-only oral contraceptives, it is required that the existence, or history of thrombophlebitis, thromboembolic disorders, cerebral vascular disease, myocardial infarction, angina, or coronary artery disease be described as a contraindication to Noriday as it is to oestrogen containing oral contraceptives.

4.4 Special warnings and precautions for use

Assessment of women prior to starting oral contraceptives (and at regular intervals thereafter) should include a personal and family medical history of each woman. Physical examination should be guided by this and by the contraindications (section 4.3) and warnings (section 4.4) for this product. The frequency and nature of these assessments should be adapted to the individual woman, but should include measurement of blood pressure and, if judged appropriate by the clinician, breast, abdominal and pelvic examination including cervical cytology.

Malignant hepatic tumours have been reported on rare occasions in long-term users of contraceptives. Benign hepatic tumours have also been associated with oral contraceptive usage. A hepatic tumour should be considered in the differential diagnosis when upper abdominal pain, enlarged liver or signs of intra-abdominal haemorrhage occur.

A statistical association between the use of oral contraceptives and the occurrence of thrombosis, embolism or haemorrhage has been reported. Patients receiving oral contraceptives should be kept under regular surveillance, in view of the possibility of development of conditions such as thrombo-embolism.

The risk of coronary artery disease in women taking oral contraceptives is increased by the presence ofother predisposing factors such as cigarette smoking, hypercholesterolaemia, obesity, diabetes, history of pre-eclamptic toxaemia and increasing age. After the age of thirty-five years, the patient and physician should carefully re-assess the risk/benefit ratio of using oral contraceptives as opposed to alternative methods of contraception.

Noriday should be discontinued at least 4 weeks before elective surgery or during periods of prolonged immobilisation. It would be reasonable to resume Noriday 2 weeks after surgery provided the woman is ambulant. However, every woman should be considered individually with regard to the nature of the operation, the extent of immobilisation, the presence of additional risk factors and the chance of unwanted conception.

Noriday should be discontinued if there is a gradual or sudden, partial or complete loss of vision or any evidence of ocular changes, onset or aggravation of migraine or development of headache of a new kind which is recurrent, persistent or severe, suspicion of thrombosis or infarction, significant rise in blood pressure or if jaundice occurs.

Caution should be exercised where there is the possibility of an interaction between a pre-existing disorder and a known or suspected side effect. The use of Noriday in women suffering from epilepsy, or with a history of migraine or cardiac or renal dysfunction may result in exacerbation of these disorders because of fluid retention. Caution should also be observed in women who wear contact lenses, women with impaired carbohydrate tolerance, depression, gallstones, a past history of liver disease, varicose veins, hypertension, asthma or any disease that is prone to worsen during pregnancy (e.g. multiple sclerosis, porphyria, tetany and otosclerosis).

An increased risk of congenital abnormalities, including heart defects and limb defects, has been reported following the use of sex hormones, including oral contraceptives, in pregnancy. If the patient does not adhere to the prescribed schedule, the possibility of pregnancy should be considered at the time of the first missed period and further use of oral contraceptives should be withheld until pregnancy has been ruled out. It is recommended that for any patient who has missed two consecutive periods, pregnancy should be ruled out before continuing the contraceptive regimen. If pregnancy is confirmed the patient should be advised of the potential risks to the foetus and the advisability of continuing the pregnancy should be discussed in the light of these risks. It is advisable to discontinue Noriday three months before a planned pregnancy.

Progestogen-only oral contraceptives may offer less protection against ectopic pregnancy, than against intrauterine pregnancy.

A meta-analysis from 54 epidemiological studies reported that there is a slightly increased relative risk of having breast cancer diagnosed in women who are currently using oral contraceptives (OC). The observed pattern of increased risk may be due to an earlier diagnosis of breast cancer in OC users, the biological effects of OCs or a combination of both. The additional breast cancers diagnosed in current users of OCs or in women who have used OCs in the last ten years are more likely to be localised to the breast than those in women who never used OCs.

Breast cancer is rare among women under 40 years of age whether or not they take OCs. Whilst the background risk increases with age, the excess number of breast cancer diagnoses in current and recent progesterone-only pill (POP) users is small in relation to the overall risk of breast cancer, possibly of similar magnitude to that associated with combined OCs. However, for POPs, the evidence is based on much smaller populations of users and so is less conclusive than that for combined OCs.

The most important risk factor for breast cancer in POP users is the age women discontinue the POP; the older the age at stopping, the more breast cancers are diagnosed. Duration of use is less important and the excess risk gradually disappears during the course of the 10 years after stopping POP use, such that by 10 years there appears to be no excess.

The evidence suggests that compared with never-users, among 10,000 women who use POPs for up to 5 years but stop by age 20, there would be much less than 1 extra case of breast cancer diagnosed up to 10 years afterwards. For those stopping by age 30 after 5 years use of the POP, there would be an estimated 2-3 extra cases (additional to the 44 cases of breast cancer per 10,000 women in this age group never exposed to oral contraceptives). For those stopping by age 40 after 5 years use, there would be an estimated 10 extra cases diagnosed up to 10 years afterwards (additional to the 160 cases of breast cancer per 10,000 never-exposed women in this age group).

It is important to inform patients that users of all contraceptive pills appear to have a small increase in the risk of being diagnosed with breast cancer, compared with non-users of oral contraceptives, but this has to be weighed against the known benefits.

4.5 Interaction with other medicinal products and other forms of interaction

The herbal remedy St John's wort (*Hypericum perforatum*) should not be taken concomitantly with this medicine as this could potentially lead to a loss of contraceptive effect.

Some drugs may modify the metabolism of Noriday reducing its effectiveness; these include certain sedatives, antibiotics, and antiepileptics. During the time such agents are used concurrently, it is advised that an alternative method of contraception, such as a condom, is also used.

The serum levels of prednisone, prednisolone, cloprednol and possibly other corticosteroids are considerably increased in those taking oral contraceptives. Both the therapeutic and toxic effects may be expected to increase accordingly.

4.6 Pregnancy and lactation

Noriday is contraindicated in women with suspected pregnancy. Several reports suggest an association between foetal exposure to female sex hormones, including oral contraceptives, and congenital anomalies.

There is no evidence that Noriday tablets diminish the yield of breast milk. Small amounts of steroid materials appear in the milk; their effect on the breast-fed child has not been determined.

4.7 Effects on ability to drive and use machines

None known.

4.8 Undesirable effects

The incidence of side effects in clinical trials was lower than that experienced with oestrogen-containing oral contraceptives. Side effects which did occur included some cycle irregularity during the first few months of therapy, spotting or breakthrough bleeding, amenorrhoea, breast discomfort, gastrointestinal symptoms, rash, headaches, migraine, depression, fatigue, nervousness, disturbance of appetite and changes in weight and libido.

Hypertension, which is usually reversible on discontinuing treatment, has occurred in a small percentage of women taking oral contraceptives.

Menstrual pattern: Women taking Noriday for the first time should be informed that they may initially experience menstrual irregularity. This may include amenorrhoea, prolonged bleeding and/or spotting but such irregularity tends to decrease with time. If a woman misses two consecutive periods, pregnancy should be ruled out before continuing the contraceptive regimen.

4.9 Overdose

Serious ill effects have not been reported following acute ingestion of large doses of oral contraceptives by young children. Overdosage may be manifested by nausea, vomiting, breast enlargement and vaginal bleeding. There is no specific antidote and treatment should be symptomatic. Gastric lavage may be employed if the overdose is large and the patient is seen sufficiently early (within four hours).

5. PHARMACOLOGICAL PROPERTIES

5.1 Pharmacodynamic properties

Norethisterone administration increases the protein and sialic acid content of cervical mucus which prevents penetration of the mucus by spermatozoa. It causes changes in the structure of the endometrium such that implantation of blastocysts is impaired. It also reduces numbers and height of cilia on cells lining the fallopian tube, which could delay tubal transport of ova.

5.2 Pharmacokinetic properties

Norethisterone is rapidly and completely absorbed after oral administration, peak plasma concentrations occurring in the majority of subjects between 1 and 3 hours. Due to first-pass metabolism, blood levels after oral administration are 60% of those after i.v. administration. The half life of elimination varies from 5 to 12 hours, with a mean of 7.6 hours. Norethisterone is metabolised mainly in the liver. Approximately 60% of the administered dose is excreted as metabolites in urine and faeces.

5.3 Preclinical safety data

The toxicity of norethisterone is very low. Reports of teratogenic effects in animals are uncommon. No carcinogenic effects have been found even in long-term studies. In subacute and chronic studies only minimal differences between treated and control animals are observed.

6. PHARMACEUTICAL PARTICULARS

6.1 List of excipients

Noriday tablets contain:

Maize starch, polyvidone, magnesium stearate and lactose.

6.2 Incompatibilities

None known.

6.3 Shelf life

The shelf life of Noriday tablets is 5 years.

6.4 Special precautions for storage

Store in a cool, dry place away from direct sunlight.

6.5 Nature and contents of container

Noriday tablets are supplied in pvc/foil blister packs of 28 and 84 tablets.

Blister packaging consists of 250 micron PVC and 20 micron aluminium foil.

6.6 Special precautions for disposal and other handling

None

7. MARKETING AUTHORISATION HOLDER

Pharmacia Limited

Ramsgate Road

Sandwich

Kent, CT13 9NJ

United Kingdom

8. MARKETING AUTHORISATION NUMBER(S)

PL. 00032/0410

9. DATE OF FIRST AUTHORISATION/RENEWAL OF THE AUTHORISATION

26th July 2002

10. DATE OF REVISION OF THE TEXT

March 2004

11. LEGAL CATEGORY

POM

Ref: NO1_0 UK

Norimin Tablets

(Pharmacia Limited)

1. NAME OF THE MEDICINAL PRODUCT

Norimin.

2. QUALITATIVE AND QUANTITATIVE COMPOSITION

Each tablet contains 1 milligram norethisterone and 35 micrograms ethinylestradiol.

3. PHARMACEUTICAL FORM

White round flat tablets with bevel-edged tablet inscribed 'SEARLE' on one side and 'BX' on the other.

4. CLINICAL PARTICULARS

4.1 Therapeutic indications

Norimin is indicated for oral contraception, with the benefit of a low intake of oestrogen.

4.2 Posology and method of administration

Oral Administration: The dosage of Norimin for the initial cycle of therapy is 1 tablet taken at the same time each day from the first day of the menstrual cycle. For subsequent cycles, no tablets are taken for 7 days, then a new course is started of 1 tablet daily for the next 21 days. This sequence of 21 days on treatment, seven days off treatment is repeated for as long as contraception is required.

Patients unable to start taking Norimin tablets on the first day of the menstrual cycle may start treatment on any day up to and including the 5th day of the menstrual cycle.

Patients starting on day 1 of their period will be protected at once. Those patients delaying therapy up to day 5 may not be protected immediately and it is recommended that another method of contraception is used for the first 7 days of tablet-taking. Suitable methods are condoms, caps plus spermicides and intra-uterine devices. The rhythm, temperature and cervical-mucus methods should not be relied upon.

Tablet omissions

Tablets must be taken daily in order to maintain adequate hormone levels and contraceptive efficacy.

If a tablet is missed within 12 hours of the correct dosage time then the missed tablet should be taken as soon as possible, even if this means taking 2 tablets on the same day, this will ensure that contraceptive protection is maintained. If one or more tablets are missed for more than 12 hours from the correct dosage time it is recommended that the patient takes the last missed tablet as soon as possible and then continues to take the rest of the tablets in the normal manner. In addition, it is recommended that extra contraceptive protection, such as a condom, is used for the next 7 days.

Patients who have missed one or more of the last 7 tablets in a pack should be advised to start the next pack of tablets as soon as the present one has finished (i.e. without the normal seven day gap between treatments). This reduces the risk of contraceptive failure resulting from tablets being missed close to a 7 day tablet free period.

Changing from another oral contraceptive

In order to ensure that contraception is maintained it is advised that the first dose of Norimin tablets is taken on the day immediately after the patient has finished the previous pack of tablets.

Use after childbirth, miscarriage or abortion

Providing the patient is not breast feeding the first dose of Norimin tablets should be taken on the 21st day after childbirth. This will ensure the patient is protected immediately. If there is any delay in taking the first dose, contraception may not be established until 7 days after the first tablet has been taken. In these circumstances patients should be advised that extra contraceptive methods will be necessary.

After a miscarriage or abortion patients can take the first dose of Norimin tablets on the next day; in this way they will be protected immediately.

4.3 Contraindications

As with all combined progestogen/oestrogen oral contraceptives, the following conditions should be regarded as contra-indications:

i. History of confirmed venous thromboembolic disease (VTE), family history of idiopathic VTE and other known risk factors of VTE

ii. Thrombophlebitis, cerebrovascular disorders, coronary artery disease, myocardial infarction, angina, hyperlipidaemia or a history of these conditions.

iii. Acute or severe chronic liver disease, including liver tumours, Dubin-Johnson or Rotor syndrome.

iv. History during pregnancy of idiopathic jaundice, severe pruritus or pemphigoid gestationis.

v. Known or suspected breast or genital cancer.

vi. Known or suspected oestrogen-dependent neoplasia.

vii. Undiagnosed abnormal vaginal bleeding.

viii. A history of migraines classified as classical focal or crescendo.

ix. Pregnancy.

4.4 Special warnings and precautions for use

Assessment of women prior to starting oral contraceptives (and at regular intervals thereafter) should include a personal and family medical history of each woman. Physical examination should be guided by this and by the contra-indications (section 4.3) and warnings (section 4.4) for this product. The frequency and nature of these assessments should be based upon relevant guidelines and should be adapted to the individual woman, but should include measurement of blood pressure and, if judged appropriate by the clinician, breast, abdominal and pelvic examination including cervical cytology.

Women taking oral contraceptives require careful observation if they have or have had any of the following conditions: breast nodules; fibrocystic disease of the breast or an abnormal mammogram; uterine fibroids; a history of severe depressive states; varicose veins; sickle-cell anaemia; diabetes; hypertension; cardiovascular disease; migraine; epilepsy; asthma; otosclerosis; multiple sclerosis; porphyria; tetany; disturbed liver functions; gallstones; kidney disease; chloasma; any condition that is likely to worsen during pregnancy. The worsening or first appearance of any of these conditions may indicate that the oral contraceptive should be stopped. Discontinue treatment if there is a gradual or sudden, partial or complete loss of vision or any evidence of ocular changes, onset or aggravation of migraine or development of headache of a new kind which is recurrent, persistent or severe.

Gastro-intestinal upsets, such as vomiting and diarrhoea, may interfere with the absorption of the tablets leading to a reduction in contraceptive efficacy. Patients should continue to take Norimin, but they should also be encouraged to use another contraceptive method during the period of gastro-intestinal upset and for the next 7 days.

Progestogen oestrogen preparations should be used with caution in patients with a history of hepatic dysfunction or hypertension.

An increased risk of venous thromboembolic disease (VTE) associated with the use of oral contraceptives is well established but is smaller than that associated with pregnancy, which has been estimated at 60 cases per 100,000 pregnancies. Some epidemiological studies have reported a greater risk of VTE for women using combined oral contraceptives containing desogestrel or gestodene (the so-called 'third generation' pills) than for women using pills containing levonorgestrel or norethisterone (the so-called 'second generation' pills

The spontaneous incidence of VTE in healthy non-pregnant women (not taking any oral contraceptive) is about 5 cases per 100,000 per year. The incidence in users of second generation pills is about 15 per 100,000 women per year of use. The incidence in users of third generation pills is about 25 cases per 100,000 women per year of use; this excess incidence has not been satisfactorily explained by bias or confounding. The level of all of these risks of VTE increases with age and is likely to be further increased in women with other known risk factors for VTE such as obesity. The excess risk of VTE is highest during the first year a woman ever uses a combined oral contraceptive.

Figure 1

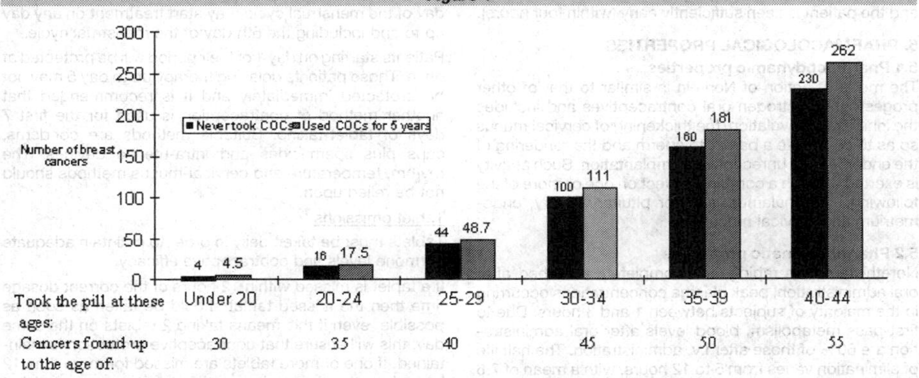

Patients receiving oral contraceptives should be kept under regular surveillance, in view of the possibility of developments such as thromboembolism.

The risk of coronary artery disease in women taking oral contraceptives is increased by the presence of other predisposing factors such as cigarette smoking, hypercholesterolaemia, obesity, diabetes, history of pre-eclamptic toxaemia and increasing age. After the age of thirty-five years, the patient and physician should carefully re-assess the risk/benefit ratio of using combined oral contraceptives as opposed to alternative methods of contraception.

Norimin should be discontinued at least four weeks before, and for two weeks following, elective operations and during immobilisation. Patients undergoing injection treatment for varicose veins should not resume taking Norimin until 3 months after the last injection.

Benign and malignant liver tumours have been associated with oral contraceptive use. The relationship between occurrence of liver tumours and use of female sex hormones is not known at present. These tumours may rupture causing intra-abdominal bleeding. If the patient presents with a mass or tenderness in the right upper quadrant or an acute abdomen, the possible presence of a tumour should be considered.

An increased risk of congenital abnormalities, including heart defects and limb defects, has been reported following the use of sex hormones, including oral contraceptives, in pregnancy. If the patient does not adhere to the prescribed schedule, the possibility of pregnancy should be considered at the time of the first missed period and further use of oral contraceptives should be withheld until pregnancy has been ruled out. It is recommended that for any patient who has missed two consecutive periods, pregnancy should be ruled out before continuing the contraceptive regimen. If pregnancy is confirmed the patient should be advised of the potential risks to the foetus and the advisability of continuing the pregnancy should be discussed in the light of these risks. It is advisable to discontinue Norimin three months before a planned pregnancy.

The risk of arterial thrombosis associated with combined oral contraceptives increases with age, and this risk is aggravated by cigarette smoking. The use of combined oral contraceptives by women in the older age group, especially those who are cigarette smokers, should therefore be discouraged and alternative methods advised.

The use of this product in patients suffering from epilepsy, migraine, asthma or cardiac dysfunction may result in exacerbation of these disorders because of fluid retention. Caution should also be observed in patients who wear contact lenses.

Decreased glucose tolerance may occur in diabetic patients on this treatment, and their control must be carefully supervised.

The use of oral contraceptives has also been associated with a possible increased incidence of gall bladder disease.

Women with a history of oligomenorrhoea or secondary amenorrhoea or young women without regular cycles may have a tendency to remain anovulatory or to become amenorrhoeic after discontinuation of oral contraceptives. Women with these pre-existing problems should be advised of this possibility and encouraged to use other contraceptive methods.

Numerous epidemiological studies have been reported on the risks of ovarian, endometrial, cervical and breast cancer in women using combined oral contraceptives. The evidence is clear that combined oral contraceptives offer substantial protection against both ovarian and endometrial cancer.

An increased risk of cervical cancer in long-term users of combined oral contraceptives has been reported in some studies, but there continues to be controversy about the extent to which this is attributable to the confounding effects of sexual behaviour and other factors.

A meta-analysis from 54 epidemiological studies reported that there is a slightly increased relative risk (RR = 1.24) of having breast cancer diagnosed in women who are currently using combined oral contraceptives (COCs). The observed pattern of increased risk may be due to an earlier diagnosis of breast cancer in COC users, the biological effects of COCs or a combination of both. The additional breast cancers diagnosed in current users of COCs or in women who have used COCs in the last ten years are more likely to be localised to the breast than those in women who never used COCs.

Breast cancer is rare among women under 40 years of age whether or not they take COCs. Whilst this background risk increases with age, the excess number of breast cancer diagnoses in current and recent COC users is small in relation to the overall risk of breast cancer (see bar chart).

The most important risk factor for breast cancer in COC users is the age women discontinue the COC; the older the age at stopping, the more breast cancers are diagnosed. Duration of use is less important and the excess risk gradually disappears during the course of the 10 years after stopping COC use such that by 10 years there appears to be no excess.

The possible increase in risk of breast cancer should be discussed with the user and weighed against the benefits of COCs taking into account the evidence that they offer substantial protection against the risk of developing certain other cancers (e.g. ovarian and endometrial cancer).

Estimated cumulative numbers of breast cancers per 10,000 women diagnosed in 5 years of use and up to 10 years after stopping COCs, compared with numbers of breast cancers diagnosed in 10,000 women who had never used COCs.

(see Figure 1 above)

4.5 Interaction with other medicinal products and other forms of interaction

The herbal remedy St John's wort (*Hypericum perforatum*) should not be taken concomitantly with this medicine as this could potentially lead to a loss of contraceptive effect.

Some drugs may modify the metabolism of Norimin reducing its effectiveness; these include certain sedatives, antibiotics, anti-epileptic and anti-arthritic drugs. During the time such agents are used concurrently, it is advised that mechanical contraceptives also be used.

The results of a large number of laboratory tests have been shown to be influenced by the use of oestrogen containing oral contraceptives, which may limit their diagnostic value. Among these are: biochemical markers of thyroid and liver function; plasma levels of carrier proteins, triglycerides, coagulation and fibrinolysis factors.

4.6 Pregnancy and lactation

Contra-indicated in pregnancy.

Patients who are fully breast-feeding should not take Norimin tablets since, in common with other combined oral contraceptives, the oestrogen component may reduce the amount of milk produced. In addition, active ingredients or their metabolites have been detected in the milk of mothers taking oral contraceptives. The effect of Norimin on breast-fed infants has not been determined.

4.7 Effects on ability to drive and use machines

Not applicable.

4.8 Undesirable effects

As with all oral contraceptives, there may be slight nausea at first, weight gain or breast discomfort, which soon disappear.

Other side-effects known or suspected to occur with oral contraceptives include gastro-intestinal symptoms, changes in libido and appetite, headache, exacerbation of existing uterine fibroid disease, depression, and changes in carbohydrate, lipid and vitamin metabolism.

Spotting or bleeding may occur during the first few cycles. Usually menstrual bleeding becomes light and occasionally there may be no bleeding during the tablet-free days.

Hypertension, which is usually reversible on discontinuing treatment, has occurred in a small percentage of women taking oral contraceptives.

4.9 Overdose

Overdosage may be manifested by nausea, vomiting, breast enlargement and vaginal bleeding. There is no specific antidote and treatment should be symptomatic.

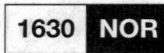

Gastric lavage may be employed if the overdose is large and the patient is seen sufficiently early (within four hours).

5. PHARMACOLOGICAL PROPERTIES

5.1 Pharmacodynamic properties

The mode of action of Norimin is similar to that of other progestogen/oestrogen oral contraceptives and includes the inhibition of ovulation, the thickening of cervical mucus so as to constitute a barrier to sperm and the rendering of the endometrium unreceptive to implantation. Such activity is exerted through a combined effect on one or more of the following: hypothalamus, anterior pituitary, ovary, endometrium and cervical mucus.

5.2 Pharmacokinetic properties

Norethisterone is rapidly and completely absorbed after oral administration, peak plasma concentrations occurring in the majority of subjects between 1 and 3 hours. Due to first-pass metabolism, blood levels after oral administration are 60% of those after i.v. administration. The half life of elimination varies from 5 to 12 hours, with a mean of 7.6 hours. Norethisterone is metabolised mainly in the liver. Approximately 60% of the administered dose is excreted as metabolites in urine and faeces.

Ethinylestradiol is rapidly and well absorbed from the gastro-intestinal tract but is subject to some first-pass metabolism in the gut-wall. Compared to many other oestrogens it is only slowly metabolised in the liver. Excretion is via the kidneys with some appearing also in the faeces.

5.3 Preclinical safety data

The toxicity of norethisterone is very low. Reports of teratogenic effects in animals are uncommon. No carcinogenic effects have been found even in long-term studies.

Long-term continuous administration of oestrogens in some animals increases the frequency of carcinoma of the breast, cervix, vagina and liver.

6. PHARMACEUTICAL PARTICULARS

6.1 List of excipients

Norimin tablets contain:

Maize starch, polyvidone, magnesium stearate and lactose.

6.2 Incompatibilities

None stated.

6.3 Shelf life

The shelf life of Norimin tablets is 5 years.

6.4 Special precautions for storage

Store in a dry place, below 25°C, away from direct sunlight.

6.5 Nature and contents of container

Norimin tablets are supplied in pvc/foil blister packs of 21 and 63 tablets.

6.6 Special precautions for disposal and other handling

None.

7. MARKETING AUTHORISATION HOLDER

Pharmacia Limited
Ramsgate Road
Sandwich
Kent CT13 9NJ, UK

8. MARKETING AUTHORISATION NUMBER(S)

PL 00032/0411.

9. DATE OF FIRST AUTHORISATION/RENEWAL OF THE AUTHORISATION

8 July 2002

10. DATE OF REVISION OF THE TEXT

June 2007

NM 2_0

Norinyl-1 Tablets

(Pharmacia Limited)

1. NAME OF THE MEDICINAL PRODUCT

Norinyl-1.

2. QUALITATIVE AND QUANTITATIVE COMPOSITION

Each tablet contains 1 milligram norethisterone and 50 micrograms mestranol.

3. PHARMACEUTICAL FORM

White, flat, circular, bevel-edged tablet inscribed 'SEARLE' on one side and '1' on the other side.

4. CLINICAL PARTICULARS

4.1 Therapeutic indications

Norinyl-1 is indicated for oral contraception.

4.2 Posology and method of administration

Oral Administration: The dosage of Norinyl-1 for the initial cycle of therapy is 1 tablet taken at the same time each day from the first day of the menstrual cycle. For subsequent cycles, no tablets are taken for 7 days, then a new course is started of 1 tablet daily for the next 21 days. This sequence of 21 days on treatment, seven days off treatment is repeated for as long as contraception is required.

Patients unable to start taking Norinyl-1 tablets on the first day of the menstrual cycle may start treatment on any day up to and including the 5th day of the menstrual cycle.

Patients starting on day 1 of their period will be protected at once. Those patients delaying therapy up to day 5 may not be protected immediately and it is recommended that another method of contraception is used for the first 7 days of tablet-taking. Suitable methods are condoms, caps plus spermicides and intra-uterine devices. The rhythm, temperature and cervical-mucus methods should not be relied upon.

Tablet omissions

Tablets must be taken daily in order to maintain adequate hormone levels and contraceptive efficacy.

If a tablet is missed within 12 hours of the correct dosage time then the missed tablet should be taken as soon as possible, even if this means taking 2 tablets on the same day, this will ensure that contraceptive protection is maintained. If one or more tablets are missed for more than 12 hours from the correct dosage time it is recommended that the patient takes the last missed tablet as soon as possible and then continues to take the rest of the tablets in the normal manner. In addition, it is recommended that extra contraceptive protection, such as a condom, is used for the next 7 days.

Patients who have missed one or more of the last 7 tablets in a pack should be advised to start the next pack of tablets as soon as the present one has finished (i.e. without the normal seven day gap between treatments). This reduces the risk of contraceptive failure resulting from tablets being missed close to a 7 day tablet free period.

Changing from another oral contraceptive

In order to ensure that contraception is maintained it is advised that the first dose of Norinyl-1 tablets is taken on the day immediately after the patient has finished the previous pack of tablets.

Use after childbirth, miscarriage or abortion

Providing the patient is not breast feeding the first dose of Norinyl-1 tablets should be taken on the 21st day after childbirth. This will ensure the patient is protected immediately. If there is any delay in taking the first dose, contraception may not be established until 7 days after the first tablet has been taken. In these circumstances patients should be advised that extra contraceptive methods will be necessary.

After a miscarriage or abortion patients can take the first dose of Norinyl-1 tablets on the next day; in this way they will be protected immediately.

4.3 Contraindications

As with all combined progestogen/oestrogen oral contraceptives, the following conditions should be regarded as contra-indications:

i. History of confirmed venous thromboembolic disease (VTE), family history of idiopathic VTE and other known risk factors of VTE

ii. Thrombophlebitis, cerebrovascular disorders, coronary artery disease, myocardial infarction, angina, hyperlipidaemia or a history of these conditions.

iii. Acute or severe chronic liver disease, including liver tumours, Dubin-Johnson or Rotor syndrome.

iv. History during pregnancy of idiopathic jaundice, severe pruritus or pemphigoid gestationis.

v. Known or suspected breast or genital cancer

vi. Known or suspected oestrogen-dependent neoplasia.

vii. Undiagnosed abnormal vaginal bleeding.

viii. A history of migraines classified as classical focal or crescendo.

ix. Pregnancy.

4.4 Special warnings and precautions for use

Assessment of women prior to starting oral contraceptives (and at regular intervals thereafter) should include a personal and family medical history of each woman. Physical examination should be guided by this and by the contra-indications (section 4.3) and warnings (section 4.4) for this product. The frequency and nature of these assessments should be based upon relevant guidelines and should be adapted to the individual woman, but should include measurement of blood pressure and, if judged appropriate by the clinician, breast, abdominal and pelvic examination including cervical cytology.

Women taking oral contraceptives require careful observation if they have or have had any of the following conditions: breast nodules; fibrocystic disease of the breast or an abnormal mammogram; uterine fibroids; a history of severe depressive states; varicose veins; sickle-cell anaemia; diabetes; hypertension; cardiovascular disease; migraine; epilepsy; asthma; otosclerosis; multiple sclerosis; porphyria; tetany; disturbed liver functions; gallstones; kidney disease; chloasma; any condition that is likely to worsen during pregnancy. The worsening or first appearance of any of these conditions may indicate that the oral contraceptive should be stopped. Discontinue treatment if there is a gradual or sudden, partial or complete loss of vision or any evidence of ocular changes, onset or aggravation of migraine or development of headache of a new kind which is recurrent, persistent or severe.

Gastro-intestinal upsets, such as vomiting and diarrhoea, may interfere with the absorption of the tablets leading to a reduction in contraceptive efficacy. Patients should continue to take Norinyl-1, but they should also be encouraged to use another contraceptive method during the period of gastro-intestinal upset and for the next 7 days.

Progestogen oestrogen preparations should be used with caution in patients with a history of hepatic dysfunction or hypertension.

An increased risk of venous thromboembolic disease (VTE) associated with the use of oral contraceptives is well established but is smaller than that associated with pregnancy, which has been estimated at 60 cases per 100,000 pregnancies. Some epidemiological studies have reported a greater risk of VTE for women using combined oral contraceptives containing desogestrel or gestodene (the so-called 'third generation' pills) than for women using pills containing levonorgestrel or norethisterone (the so-called 'second generation' pills).

The spontaneous incidence of VTE in healthy non-pregnant women (not taking any oral contraceptive) is about 5 cases per 100,000 per year. The incidence in users of second generation pills is about 15 per 100,000 women per year of use. The incidence in users of third generation pills is about 25 cases per 100,000 women per year of use; this excess incidence has not been satisfactorily explained by bias or confounding. The level of all of these risks of VTE increases with age and is likely to be further increased in women with other known risk factors for VTE such as obesity). The excess risk of VTE is highest during the first year a woman ever uses a combined oral contraceptive.

Patients receiving oral contraceptives should be kept under regular surveillance, in view of the possibility of development of such conditions as thromboembolism.

The risk of coronary artery disease in women taking oral contraceptives is increased by the presence of other predisposing factors such as cigarette smoking, hypercholesterolaemia, obesity, diabetes, history of pre-eclamptic toxaemia and increasing age. After the age of thirty-five years, the patient and physician should carefully re-assess the risk/benefit ratio of using combined oral contraceptives as opposed to alternative methods of contraception.

Norinyl-1 should be discontinued at least four weeks before, and for two weeks following, elective operations and during immobilisation. Patients undergoing injection treatment for varicose veins should not resume taking Norinyl-1 until 3 months after the last injection.

Benign and malignant liver tumours have been associated with oral contraceptive use. The relationship between occurrence of liver tumours and use of female sex hormones is not known at present. These tumours may rupture causing intra-abdominal bleeding. If the patient presents with a mass or tenderness in the right upper quadrant or an acute abdomen, the possible presence of a tumour should be considered.

An increased risk of congenital abnormalities, including heart defects and limb defects, has been reported following the use of sex hormones, including oral contraceptives, in pregnancy. If the patient does not adhere to the prescribed schedule, the possibility of pregnancy should be considered at the time of the first missed period and further use of oral contraceptives should be withheld until pregnancy has been ruled out. It is recommended that for any patient who has missed two consecutive periods, pregnancy should be ruled out before continuing the contraceptive regimen. If pregnancy is confirmed the patient should be advised of the potential risks to the foetus and the advisability of continuing the pregnancy should be discussed in the light of these risks. It is advisable to discontinue Norinyl-1 three months before a planned pregnancy.

The risk of arterial thrombosis associated with combined oral contraceptives increases with age, and this risk is aggravated by cigarette smoking. The use of combined oral contraceptives by women in the older age group, especially those who are cigarette smokers, should therefore be discouraged and alternative methods advised.

The use of this product in patients suffering from epilepsy, migraine, asthma or cardiac dysfunction may result in exacerbation of these disorders because of fluid retention. Caution should also be observed in patients who wear contact lenses.

Decreased glucose tolerance may occur in diabetic patients on this treatment, and their control must be carefully supervised.

The use of oral contraceptives has also been associated with a possible increased incidence of gall bladder disease.

Women with a history of oligomenorrhoea or secondary amenorrhoea or young women without regular cycles may have a tendency to remain anovulatory or to become amenorrhoeic after discontinuation of oral contraceptives. Women with these pre-existing problems should be advised of this possibility and encouraged to use other contraceptive methods.

Numerous epidemiological studies have been reported on the risks of ovarian, endometrial, cervical and breast cancer in women using combined oral contraceptives. The evidence is clear that combined oral contraceptives offer

Figure 1

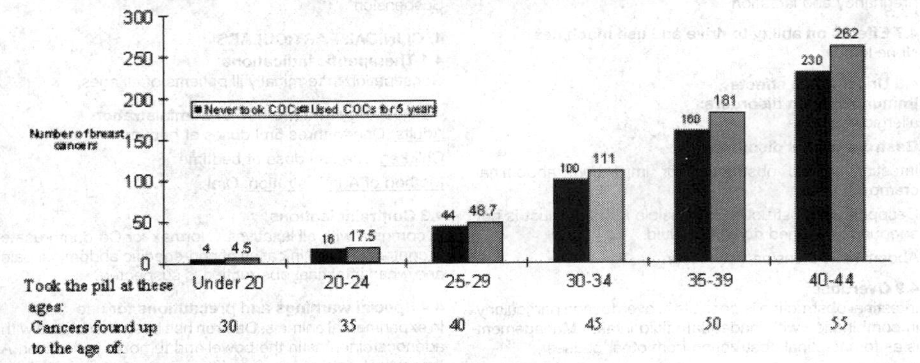

substantial protection against both ovarian and endometrial cancer.

An increased risk of cervical cancer in long-term users of combined oral contraceptives has been reported in some studies, but there continues to be controversy about the extent to which this is attributable to the confounding effects of sexual behaviour and other factors.

A meta-analysis from 54 epidemiological studies reported that there is a slightly increased relative risk (RR = 1.24) of having breast cancer diagnosed in women who are currently using combined oral contraceptives (COCs). The observed pattern of increased risk may be due to an earlier diagnosis of breast cancer in COC users, the biological effects of COCs or a combination of both. The additional breast cancers diagnosed in current users of COCs or in women who have used COCs in the last ten years are more likely to be localised to the breast than those in women who never used COCs.

Breast cancer is rare among women under 40 years of age whether or not they take COCs. Whilst this background risk increases with age, the excess number of breast cancer diagnoses in current and recent COC users is small in relation to the overall risk of breast cancer (see bar chart).

The most important risk factor for breast cancer in COC users is the age women discontinue the COC; the older the age at stopping, the more breast cancers are diagnosed. Duration of use is less important and the excess risk gradually disappears during the course of the 10 years after stopping COC use such that by 10 years there appears to be no excess.

The possible increase in risk of breast cancer should be discussed with the user and weighed against the benefits of COCs taking into account the evidence that they offer substantial protection against the risk of developing certain other cancers (e.g. ovarian and endometrial cancer).

Estimated cumulative numbers of breast cancers per 10,000 women diagnosed in 5 years of use and up to 10 years after stopping COCs, compared with numbers of breast cancers diagnosed in 10,000 women who had never used COCs.

(see Figure 1 above)

4.5 Interaction with other medicinal products and other forms of interaction

The herbal remedy St John's wort (*Hypericum perforatum*) should not be taken concomitantly with this medicine as this could potentially lead to a loss of contraceptive effect.

Some drugs may modify the metabolism of Norinyl-1 reducing its effectiveness; these include certain sedatives, antibiotics, anti-epileptic and anti-arthritic drugs. During the time such agents are used concurrently, it is advised that mechanical contraceptives also be used.

The results of a large number of laboratory tests have been shown to be influenced by the use of oestrogen containing oral contraceptives, which may limit their diagnostic value. Among these are: biochemical markers of thyroid and liver function; plasma levels of carrier proteins, triglycerides, coagulation and fibrinolysis factors.

4.6 Pregnancy and lactation

Contra-indicated in pregnancy.

Patients who are fully breast-feeding should not take Norinyl-1 tablets since, in common with other combined oral contraceptives, the oestrogen component may reduce the amount of milk produced. In addition, active ingredients or their metabolites have been detected in the milk of mothers taking oral contraceptives. The effect of Norinyl-1 on breast-fed infants has not been determined.

4.7 Effects on ability to drive and use machines

Not applicable.

4.8 Undesirable effects

As with all oral contraceptives, there may be slight nausea at first, weight gain or breast discomfort, which soon disappear.

Other side-effects known or suspected to occur with oral contraceptives include gastro-intestinal symptoms, changes in libido and appetite, headache, exacerbation of existing uterine fibroid disease, depression, and changes in carbohydrate, lipid and vitamin metabolism.

Spotting or bleeding may occur during the first few cycles. Usually menstrual bleeding becomes light and occasionally there may be no bleeding during the tablet-free days.

Hypertension, which is usually reversible on discontinuing treatment, has occurred in a small percentage of women taking oral contraceptives.

4.9 Overdose

Overdosage may be manifested by nausea, vomiting, breast enlargement and vaginal bleeding. There is no specific antidote and treatment should be symptomatic. Gastric lavage may be employed if the overdose is large and the patient is seen sufficiently early (within four hours).

5. PHARMACOLOGICAL PROPERTIES

5.1 Pharmacodynamic properties

The mode of action of Norinyl-1 is similar to that of other progestogen/oestrogen oral contraceptives and includes the inhibition of ovulation, the thickening of cervical mucus so as to constitute a barrier to sperm and the rendering of the endometrium unreceptive to implantation. Such activity is exerted through a combined effect on one or more of the following: hypothalamus, anterior pituitary, ovary, endometrium and cervical mucus.

5.2 Pharmacokinetic properties

Norethisterone is rapidly and completely absorbed after oral administration, peak plasma concentrations occurring in the majority of subjects between 1 and 3 hours. Due to first-pass metabolism, blood levels after oral administration are 60% of those after i.v. administration. The half life of elimination varies from 5 to 12 hours, with a mean of 7.6 hours. Norethisterone is metabolised mainly in the liver. Approximately 60% of the administered dose is excreted as metabolites in urine and faeces.

Mestranol is rapidly absorbed and extensively metabolised to ethinyloestradiol. Ethinyloestradiol is rapidly and well absorbed from the gastro-intestinal tract but is subject to some first-pass metabolism in the gut-wall. Compared to many other oestrogens it is only slowly metabolised in the liver. Excretion is via the kidneys with some appearing also in the faeces.

5.3 Preclinical safety data

The toxicity of norethisterone is very low. Reports of teratogenic effects in animals are uncommon. No carcinogenic effects have been found even in long-term studies.

Long-term continuous administration of oestrogens in some animals increases the frequency of carcinoma of the breast, cervix, vagina and liver.

6. PHARMACEUTICAL PARTICULARS

6.1 List of excipients

Norinyl-1 tablets contain:

Maize starch, polyvidone, magnesium stearate and lactose.

6.2 Incompatibilities

None stated.

6.3 Shelf life

The shelf life of Norinyl-1 tablets is 5 years.

6.4 Special precautions for storage

Store in a dry place below 25°C away from direct sunlight.

6.5 Nature and contents of container

Norinyl-1 tablets are supplied in pvc/foil blister packs of 21 and 63 tablets.

6.6 Special precautions for disposal and other handling

None.

7. MARKETING AUTHORISATION HOLDER

Pharmacia Limited
Ramsgate Road
Sandwich
Kent CT13 9NJ
UK

8. MARKETING AUTHORISATION NUMBER(S)

PL 00032/0412

9. DATE OF FIRST AUTHORISATION/RENEWAL OF THE AUTHORISATION

May 16th 1996

10. DATE OF REVISION OF THE TEXT

May 2007

NR2_0

Normacol

(Norgine Limited)

1. NAME OF THE MEDICINAL PRODUCT

NORMACOL.

2. QUALITATIVE AND QUANTITATIVE COMPOSITION

The active ingredient is Sterculia 62% w/w.

3. PHARMACEUTICAL FORM

Oral granules.

4. CLINICAL PARTICULARS

4.1 Therapeutic indications

The treatment of constipation, particularly simple or idiopathic constipation and constipation during pregnancy.

Management of colostomies and ileostomies.

The 'High Residue Diet' management of diverticular disease of the colon and other conditions requiring a high fibre regimen.

The initiation and maintenance of bowel action after rectal and anal surgery.

Administration after ingestion of sharp foreign bodies to provide a coating and reduce the possibility of intestinal damage during transit.

4.2 Posology and method of administration

Adults: 1 or 2 sachets or 1-2 heaped 5ml spoonfuls, once or twice daily after meals.

Elderly: As adult dose.

Children: (6-12 years): one half the above amount.

The granules should be placed dry on the tongue and without chewing or crushing, swallowed immediately with plenty of water or a cool drink. Prior to drinking they may also be sprinkled onto and taken with soft food such as yoghurt.

4.3 Contraindications

Intestinal obstruction, faecal impaction, and total atony of the colon.

Known hypersensitivity to any of the ingredients.

4.4 Special warnings and precautions for use

Caution should be exercised in cases of ulcerative colitis.

Patients with rare hereditary problems of fructose intolerance, glucose –galactose malabsorption or sucrase-isomaltase insufficiency should not take this medicine.

Not to be taken immediately before going to bed or in a recumbent position especially in the elderly. Adequate fluid should be maintained.

Not to be taken for more than 4 days if there has been no movement of the bowels.

It is not unusual for stool to appear paler in colour than normal as a result of local contact with sterculia. This does not indicate anything untoward.

4.5 Interaction with other medicinal products and other forms of interaction

None known.

4.6 Pregnancy and lactation

NORMACOL may be recommended during pregnancy or lactation.

4.7 Effects on ability to drive and use machines

None known.

4.8 Undesirable effects

Immune system disorders:

allergic reactions

Gastrointestinal disorders:

Intestinal/colonic obstruction or impaction, flatulence.

Occasionally mild abdominal distension may occur.

Oesophageal obstruction is possible if the product is taken in overdosage or if it is not adequately washed down with fluid.

4.9 Overdose

Intestinal obstruction is possible in overdosage particularly in combination with inadequate fluid intake. Management is as for intestinal obstruction from other causes.

5. PHARMACOLOGICAL PROPERTIES

5.1 Pharmacodynamic properties

Sterculia acts in the colon by forming a soft bulky stool and inducing a laxative effect.

5.2 Pharmacokinetic properties

Sterculia is not absorbed or digested in the gastrointestinal tract and its laxative action is normally effective within 12 hours of oral administration.

5.3 Preclinical safety data

There is no evidence that Sterculia has a significant systemic toxicity potential.

6. PHARMACEUTICAL PARTICULARS

6.1 List of excipients

Sodium bicarbonate

Sucrose

Talc

Paraffin wax

Titanium dioxide

Vanillin

6.2 Incompatibilities

None known.

6.3 Shelf life

Sachet and lined carton: 2 years

6.4 Special precautions for storage

Store in a dry place below 25°C.

6.5 Nature and contents of container

Sachet containing 7 g of white granules in boxes of 2, 7, 30 or 60 sachets.

Lined box of 100 g or 500 g of white granules.

6.6 Special precautions for disposal and other handling

None.

7. MARKETING AUTHORISATION HOLDER

Norgine Limited

Chaplin House

Widewater Place

Moorhall Road

Harefield

UXBRIDGE

Middlesex UB9 6NS

United Kingdom

8. MARKETING AUTHORISATION NUMBER(S)

PL 0322/5010R

9. DATE OF FIRST AUTHORISATION/RENEWAL OF THE AUTHORISATION

January 1991

10. DATE OF REVISION OF THE TEXT

June 2009

Normacol Plus

(Norgine Limited)

1. NAME OF THE MEDICINAL PRODUCT

NORMACOL Plus

2. QUALITATIVE AND QUANTITATIVE COMPOSITION

The active ingredients are 62% Sterculia and 8.0% Frangula.

3. PHARMACEUTICAL FORM

Brown granules.

4. CLINICAL PARTICULARS

4.1 Therapeutic indications

The treatment of constipation, particularly hypertonic or slow transit constipation, resistant to bulk alone.

The initiation and maintenance of bowel action after rectal surgery and after haemorrhoidectomy.

4.2 Posology and method of administration

Adults (including the elderly): 1 or 2 sachets or 1-2 heaped 5ml spoonfuls, once or twice daily after meals.

Children (6 – 12 years): A reduced amount may be given at the discretion of the physician.

The granules should be placed on the tongue and, without chewing or crushing, swallowed immediately with plenty of water or a cool drink. Prior to drinking they may also be sprinkled on and taken with soft food such as yoghurt.

4.3 Contraindications

Intestinal obstruction, faecal impaction and total atony of the colon.

Known hypersensitivity to the ingredients.

4.4 Special warnings and precautions for use

Caution should be exercised in the use of NORMACOL Plus in cases of ulcerative colitis. Patients should be advised to maintain an adequate fluid intake, to avoid NORMACOL Plus immediately before going to bed or in a recumbent position (especially if they are elderly) and to suspend treatment if bowel movements do not occur within four days.

Prolonged and excessive use of stimulant laxatives can cause dependence and loss of normal bowel function

Patients with rare hereditary problems of fructose intolerance, glucose-galactose malabsorption or sucrase-isomaltase insufficiency should not take this medicine.

4.5 Interaction with other medicinal products and other forms of interaction

None known.

4.6 Pregnancy and lactation

Not recommended.

NORMACOL (Sterculia alone) is available if required in pregnancy and lactation

4.7 Effects on ability to drive and use machines

None known.

4.8 Undesirable effects

Immune system disorders:

allergic reactions

Gastrointestinal disorders:

Intestinal/colonic obstruction or impaction, abdominal cramp

Oesophageal obstruction is possible if the product is not adequately washed down with fluid.

Abdominal distension may occur.

4.9 Overdose

Intestinal obstruction is possible in overdosage particularly in combination with inadequate fluid intake. Management is as for intestinal obstruction from other causes.

If there is profound diarrhoea, dehydration and electrolyte depletion may occur.

5. PHARMACOLOGICAL PROPERTIES

5.1 Pharmacodynamic properties

Sterculia acts in the colon by forming a soft bulky stool and inducing a laxative effect. Frangula acts as a mild peristaltic stimulant and aids the evacuation of the softened faecal mass.

5.2 Pharmacokinetic properties

Sterculia is not absorbed in the gastrointestinal tract; Frangula acts locally on the wall of the intestinal tract. The laxative action of NORMACOL Plus is normally effective within 12 hours of oral administration.

5.3 Preclinical safety data

There are no preclinical data of relevance to the prescriber except as already included in the SPC.

6. PHARMACEUTICAL PARTICULARS

6.1 List of excipients

Sucrose

Talc

Sodium bicarbonate

Paraffin wax

Peppermint flavouring

Colourings: E110, E127 and E132

The sugar provides 7 – 14 calories per dose (1.7 to 3.4g carbohydrate per dose). The sodium content is 1.25 to 2.5 mmol per does. NORMACOL Plus is gluten free.

6.2 Incompatibilities

None known.

6.3 Shelf life

Sachet and lined carton: 2 years.

6.4 Special precautions for storage

Store in a dry place below 25°C.

6.5 Nature and contents of container

Sachets containing 7g of granules in cartons of 2, 7, 10, 30 or 60 sachets.

Lined carton of 200g or 500g of granules.

6.6 Special precautions for disposal and other handling

None.

7. MARKETING AUTHORISATION HOLDER

Norgine Limited

Chaplin House

Widewater Place

Moorhall Road

Harefield

Uxbridge

Middlesex UB9 6NS

United Kingdom

8. MARKETING AUTHORISATION NUMBER(S)

PL 00322/5011R

9. DATE OF FIRST AUTHORISATION/RENEWAL OF THE AUTHORISATION

January 1991

10. DATE OF REVISION OF THE TEXT

December 2008

Legal category: GSL

Normax Suspension or Co-danthrusate Suspension

(UCB Pharma Limited)

1. NAME OF THE MEDICINAL PRODUCT

'Normax' Suspension or Co-danthrusate Suspension

2. QUALITATIVE AND QUANTITATIVE COMPOSITION

Each 5 ml containing 60 mg Sodium Docusate BP and 50 mg Dantron BP

For excipients, see 6.1

3. PHARMACEUTICAL FORM

Suspension

4. CLINICAL PARTICULARS

4.1 Therapeutic indications

Constipation in terminally ill patients of all ages.

4.2 Posology and method of administration

Adults: One to three 5ml doses at bedtime

Children One 5ml dose at bedtime

Method of Administration: Oral

4.3 Contraindications

In common with all laxatives, 'Normax' or Co-danthrusate is contraindicated in cases of non-specific abdominal pain and when intestinal obstruction is suspected.

4.4 Special warnings and precautions for use

In experimental animals, Dantron has been associated with adenocarcinomas in the bowel and tumours in the liver. A theoretical risk of similar effects in humans cannot be excluded.

Dantron is excreted in the urine and metabolised dantron in the faeces. There is evidence that these may cause perineal erythema in patients with urinary and or faecal incontinence. It is recommended therefore that co-danthrusate should be used with caution in all incontinent patients.

Prolonged use is not recommended.

4.5 Interaction with other medicinal products and other forms of interaction

Docusate may enhance the gastrointestinal or hepatic cell uptake of other drugs potentiating their activity and possibly increasing their toxicity.

4.6 Pregnancy and lactation

Co-danthrusate should not be used in pregnancy or lactation.

4.7 Effects on ability to drive and use machines

None known.

4.8 Undesirable effects

Occasionally an orange tint in the urine may be observed due to the Dantron component.

Skin rash may occur and reports of skin irritation, skin discolouration and superficial sloughing of the perianal skin have been reported after prolonged use of co-danthrusate.

Melanosis coli (discolouration of the colonic mucosa) after prolonged use or high doses of Co-Danthrusate

4.9 Overdose

The patient should be encouraged to drink fluids. An anticholinergic preparation may be used to ease excessive intestinal motility if necessary.

5. PHARMACOLOGICAL PROPERTIES

5.1 Pharmacodynamic properties

ATC Code: A06A G10

Dantron is a mild peristaltic stimulant acting on the lower bowel to encourage normal bowel movement without causing irritation. Docusate sodium is a softening agent which prevents excessive colonic dehydration and hardening of stools.

5.2 Pharmacokinetic properties

Not available

5.3 Preclinical safety data

No further information

6. PHARMACEUTICAL PARTICULARS

6.1 List of excipients

Methylcellulose

Xanthan Gum

Glycerol

Propyl Parahydroxybenzoate

Methyl Parahydroxybenzoate

Sorbitol Powder (E200)

Saccharin Sodium

Disodium Hydrogen Orthophosphate (Anhydrous)

Sodium Dihydrogen Orthophosphate

Peppermint Oil

Purified Water

6.2 Incompatibilities

Not known

6.3 Shelf life

36 month (200 ml)

24 month (30 ml)

6.4 Special precautions for storage

Do not store above 25°C. Store in the original package.

6.5 Nature and contents of container

Amber glass bottle with either roll-on pilfer proof aluminium cap with 'steran' faced wad or plastic cap with 'saranex' faced wad. The 30ml volume is for promotional purposes only. The 200ml volume is for prescription.

6.6 Special precautions for disposal and other handling

None

7. MARKETING AUTHORISATION HOLDER
UCB Pharma Limited
208 Bath Road
Slough
Berkshire
SL1 3WE
UK

8. MARKETING AUTHORISATION NUMBER(S)
PL 00039/0381

9. DATE OF FIRST AUTHORISATION/RENEWAL OF THE AUTHORISATION
8 June 1994 / 8 June 1999 / January 2005

10. DATE OF REVISION OF THE TEXT
November 2008

POM

Norprolac Tablets 25, 50 and 75 micrograms

(Ferring Pharmaceuticals Ltd)

1. NAME OF THE MEDICINAL PRODUCT
NORPROLAC®Tablets 25 micrograms
NORPROLAC®Tablets 50 micrograms
NORPROLAC®Tablets 75 micrograms

2. QUALITATIVE AND QUANTITATIVE COMPOSITION
Quinagolide, as the hydrochloride, 25, 50 and 75 micrograms

3. PHARMACEUTICAL FORM
Tablet for oral administration

4. CLINICAL PARTICULARS

4.1 Therapeutic indications
Hyperprolactinaemia (idiopathic or originating from a prolactin-secreting pituitary microadenoma or macroadenoma).

4.2 Posology and method of administration
Since dopaminergic stimulation may lead to symptoms of orthostatic hypotension, the dosage of NORPROLAC should be initiated gradually with the aid of the 'starter pack', and given only at bedtime.

Adults
The optimal dose must be titrated individually on the basis of the prolactin-lowering effect and tolerability.

With the 'starter pack' treatment begins with 25 micrograms/day for the first 3 days, followed by 50 micrograms/day for a further 3 days. From day 7 onwards, the recommended dose is 75 micrograms/day.

If necessary, the daily dose may then be increased stepwise until the optimal individual response is attained. The usual maintenance dosage is 75 to 150 micrograms/day.

Daily doses of 300 micrograms or higher doses are required in less than one-third of the patients.

In such cases, the daily dosage may be increased in steps of 75 to 150 micrograms at intervals not shorter than 4 weeks until satisfactory therapeutic effectiveness is achieved or reduced tolerability, requiring the discontinuation of treatment, occurs.

Elderly
Experience with the use of NORPROLAC in elderly patients is not available.

Children
Experience with the use of NORPROLAC in children is not available.

Method of Administration
NORPROLAC should be taken once a day with some food at bedtime.

4.3 Contraindications
Hypersensitivity to the drug
Impaired hepatic or renal function
For procedure during pregnancy, (see 'Section 4.6 Pregnancy and lactation').

4.4 Special warnings and precautions for use
Fertility may be restored by treatment with NORPROLAC. Women of child-bearing age who do not wish to conceive should therefore be advised to practice a reliable method of contraception.

Since orthostatic hypotension may result in syncope, it is recommended to check blood pressure both lying and standing during the first days of therapy and following dosage increases.

In a few cases, including patients with no previous history of mental illness, treatment with NORPROLAC has been associated with the occurrence of acute psychosis, usually reversible upon discontinuation. Particular caution is required in patients who have had psychotic episodes in their previous history.

To date no data is available with the use of NORPROLAC in patients with impaired renal or hepatic function (see Section 4.3 Contraindications).

NORPROLAC has been associated with somnolence. Other dopamine agonists can be associated with sudden sleep onset episodes, particularly in patients with Parkinson's disease. Patients must be informed of this and advised to exercise caution whilst driving or operating machines during treatment with NORPROLAC.

Patients who have experienced somnolence must not drive or operate machines. Furthermore, a reduction of dosage or termination of therapy may be considered (see Section 4.7 Effects on the ability to drive and use machines).

Pathological gambling, increased libido and hypersexuality have been reported in patients treated with dopamine agonists for Parkinson's disease, including quinagolide.

NORPROLAC should be kept out of the reach and sight of children.

4.5 Interaction with other medicinal products and other forms of interaction
No interactions between NORPROLAC and other drugs have so far been reported. On theoretical grounds, a reduction of the prolactin-lowering effect could be expected when drugs (e.g. neuroleptic agents) with strong dopamine antagonistic properties are used concomitantly. As the potency of NORPROLAC for 5-HT_1 and 5-HT_2 receptors is some 100 times lower than that for D_2 receptors, an interaction between NORPROLAC and 5-HT_{1a} receptors is unlikely. However, care should be taken when using these medicaments concomitantly.

The tolerability of NORPROLAC may be reduced by alcohol.

4.6 Pregnancy and lactation
Pregnancy
Animal data provide no evidence that NORPROLAC has any embryotoxic or teratogenic potential, but experience in pregnant women is still limited. In patients wishing to conceive, NORPROLAC should be discontinued when pregnancy is confirmed, unless there is a medical reason for continuing therapy. No increased incidence of abortion has been observed following withdrawal of the drug at this point.

If pregnancy occurs in the presence of a pituitary adenoma and NORPROLAC treatment has been stopped, close supervision throughout pregnancy is essential.

Lactation
Breast-feeding is usually not possible since NORPROLAC suppresses lactation. If lactation should continue during treatment, breast-feeding cannot be recommended because it is not known whether quinagolide passes into human breast milk.

4.7 Effects on ability to drive and use machines
Since, especially during the first days of treatment, hypotensive reactions may occasionally occur and result in reduced alertness, patients should be cautious when driving a vehicle or operating machinery.

Patients being treated with NORPROLAC and presenting with somnolence must be advised not to drive or engage in activities where impaired alertness may put themselves or others at risk of serious injury or death (eg. operating machines) unless patients have overcome such experiences of somnolence (see Section 4.4 Special warnings and precautions for use).

4.8 Undesirable effects
Frequency estimate: very common ≥10%, common ≥1% to <10%, uncommon ≥0.1% to <1%, rare ≥0.01% to <0.1%, very rare <0.01%.

The adverse reactions reported with the use of NORPROLAC are characteristic for dopamine receptor agonist therapy. They are usually not sufficiently serious to require discontinuation of treatment and tend to disappear when treatment is continued.

Very common undesirable effects are nausea, vomiting, headache, dizziness and fatigue. They occur predominantly during the first few days of the initial treatment or, as a mostly transient event, following dosage increase. If necessary, nausea and vomiting may be prevented by the intake of a peripheral dopaminergic antagonist, such as domperidone, for a few days, at least 1 hour before ingestion of NORPROLAC.

Common undesirable effects include anorexia, abdominal pain, constipation or diarrhoea, insomnia, oedema, flushing, nasal congestion and hypotension. Orthostatic hypotension may result in faintness or syncope (see 4.4 Special warnings and precautions for use).

Rarely NORPROLAC has been associated with somnolence.

In very rare cases, treatment with NORPROLAC has been associated with the occurrence of acute psychosis, reversible upon discontinuation.

Patients treated with dopamine agonists for the treatment of Parkinson's disease including quinagolide, especially at high doses, have been reported as exhibiting signs of pathological gambling, increased libido and hypersexuality, generally reversible upon reduction of the dose or treatment discontinuation.

4.9 Overdose
Symptoms
Acute overdosage with NORPROLAC tablets has not been reported. It would be expected to cause severe nausea, vomiting, headache, dizziness, drowsiness, hypotension and possibly collapse. Hallucinations could also occur.

Treatment
Should be symptomatic.

5. PHARMACOLOGICAL PROPERTIES

5.1 Pharmacodynamic properties
Pharmacotherapeutic group: prolactin inhibitors (ATC code G02C B04).

Quinagolide, the active ingredient of NORPROLAC, is a selective dopamine D_2-receptor agonist not belonging to the chemical classes of ergot or ergoline compounds. Owing to its dopaminergic action, the drug exerts a strong inhibitory effect on the secretion of the anterior pituitary hormone prolactin, but does not reduce normal levels of other pituitary hormones. In some patients the reduction of prolactin secretion may be accompanied by short-lasting, small increases in plasma growth hormone levels, the clinical significance of which is unknown.

As a specific inhibitor of prolactin secretion with a prolonged duration of action, NORPROLAC has been shown to be effective and suitable for once-a-day oral treatment of patients presenting with hyperprolactinaemia and its clinical manifestations such as galactorrhoea, oligomenorrhoea, amenorrhoea, infertility and reduced libido.

5.2 Pharmacokinetic properties
After oral administration of radiolabelled drug, quinagolide is rapidly and well absorbed. Plasma concentration values obtained by a non-selective radio-immunoassay (RIA), measuring quinagolide together with some of its metabolites, were close to the limit of quantification and gave no reliable information.

The apparent volume of distribution of quinagolide after single oral administration of radiolabelled compound was calculated to be approx. 100L. For the parent drug, a terminal half-life of 11.5 hours has been calculated under single dose conditions, and of 17 hours at steady state.

Quinagolide is extensively metabolised during its first pass. Studies performed with ^{3}H-labelled quinagolide revealed that more than 95% of the drug is excreted as metabolites. About equal amounts of total radioactivity are found in faeces and urine.

In blood, quinagolide and its N-desethyl analogue are the biologically active but minor components. Their inactive sulphate or glucuronide conjugates represent the major circulating metabolites. In urine, the main metabolites are the glucuronide and sulphate conjugates of quinagolide and the N-desethyl, N,N-didesethyl analogues. In the faeces the unconjugated forms of the three components were found.

The protein binding of quinagolide is approximately 90% and is non-specific.

The results, obtained in pharmacodynamic studies, indicate that with the recommended therapeutic dosage a clinically significant prolactin-lowering effect occurs within 2 hours after ingestion, reaches a maximum of 4 to 6 hours and is maintained for about 24 hours.

A definite dose-response relationship could be established for the duration, but not for the magnitude, of the prolactin-lowering effect which, with a single oral dose of 50 micrograms was close to maximum. Higher doses did not result in a considerably greater effect but prolonged its duration.

5.3 Preclinical safety data
Acute toxicity
The LD_{50} of quinagolide was determined for several species after single oral administration: mice 357 to > 500 mg/kg; rats > 500 mg/kg; rabbits > 150 mg/kg.

Chronic toxicity
Decreased cholesterol levels of treated female rats suggest that quinagolide influences lipid metabolism. Since similar observations have been made with other dopaminergic drugs, a causal relationship with low prolactin levels is assumed. In several chronic studies with rats, enlarged ovaries resulting from an increased number of corpora lutea and, additionally, hydrometra and endometritis were observed. These changes were reversible and reflect the pharmacodynamic effect of quinagolide: suppression of prolactin secretion inhibits luteolysis in rats and thus influences the normal sexual cycle. In humans, however, prolactin is not involved in luteolysis.

Carcinogenic and mutagenic potential
In comprehensive in vitro and in vivo mutagenic studies there was no evidence of a mutagenic effect.

The changes which were observed in carcinogenicity studies reflect the pharmacodynamic activity of quinagolide. The drug modulates the prolactin level as well as, especially in male rats, the level of luteinizing hormone and, in female rodents, and the ratio of progesterone to oestrogen.

Long-term studies with high doses of quinagolide revealed Leydig cell tumours in rats and mesenchymal uterine tumours in mice. The incidence of Leydig cell tumours in a carcinogenicity study in rats was increased even at low doses (0.01 mg/kg). These results were without relevance for the therapeutic application in humans since there are fundamental differences between humans and rodents in the regulation of the endocrine system.

Reproductive toxicity

Animal studies in rats and rabbits showed no evidence for embryotoxic or teratogenic effects. The prolactin inhibiting effect led to a decrease of milk production in rats, which was associated with an increased loss of rat pups. Possible post-natal effects of exposure during fetal development (2nd and 3rd trimester) and effects on female fertility are not sufficiently investigated.

6. PHARMACEUTICAL PARTICULARS

6.1 List of excipients

Silica, colloidal anhydrous; magnesium stearate; methylhydroxypropylcellulose; maize starch; cellulose, microcrystalline; lactose.

Colourings

25 micrograms: Iron oxide, red

50 micrograms: Indigotin lake

6.2 Incompatibilities

Not applicable

6.3 Shelf life

The shelf life is 5 years. The expiry date is printed on the box. On the blister the expiry date is marked with the letters EXP.

6.4 Special precautions for storage

The expiry date refers to original unopened boxes, which were stored below 25°C. No special warning with respect to light sensitivity or humidity is necessary because the tablets are protected by the packaging.

6.5 Nature and contents of container

The 'starter pack' (NORPROLAC 25/50) consists of 3 tablets of 25 micrograms and 3 tablets of 50 micrograms. These tablets are packed in an aluminium PVC/PVDC blister which is sealed in a moisture-proof aluminium bag.

The 75 microgram tablets are in packs of 30 tablets (3 times 10 tablets) in aluminium blisters.

6.6 Special precautions for disposal and other handling

None

7. MARKETING AUTHORISATION HOLDER

Ferring Pharmaceuticals Ltd

The Courtyard

Waterside Drive

Langley

Berkshire

SL3 6EZ.

8. MARKETING AUTHORISATION NUMBER(S)

NORPROLAC®Tablets 25 micrograms – PL 03194/0096

NORPROLAC®Tablets 50 micrograms – PL 03194/0097

NORPROLAC®Tablets 75 micrograms – PL 03194/0098

9. DATE OF FIRST AUTHORISATION/RENEWAL OF THE AUTHORISATION

15th December 2004

10. DATE OF REVISION OF THE TEXT

January 2007

11. LEGAL CATEGORY

POM

Norprolac is a registered trademark

Norvir Oral Solution

(Abbott Laboratories Limited)

1. NAME OF THE MEDICINAL PRODUCT

Norvir 80 mg/ml oral solution

2. QUALITATIVE AND QUANTITATIVE COMPOSITION

Each ml of oral solution contains 80 mg of ritonavir.

Excipients:

Alcohol (43% v/v)

Polyoxyl 35 Castor Oil

Sunset Yellow (E110)

For a full list of excipients, see section 6.1.

3. PHARMACEUTICAL FORM

Oral solution

The solution is a practically clear, orange solution for oral administration.

4. CLINICAL PARTICULARS

4.1 Therapeutic indications

Ritonavir is indicated in combination with other antiretroviral agents for the treatment of HIV-1 infected patients (adults and children of 2 years of age and older).

4.2 Posology and method of administration

Ritonavir should be administered by physicians who are experienced in the treatment of HIV infection.

Norvir solution is administered orally and should preferably be ingested with food.

Ritonavir dosed as a pharmacokinetic enhancer

The following HIV-1 protease inhibitors have been approved for use with ritonavir as a pharmacokinetic enhancer at the noted doses.

Adult use:

Amprenavir 600 mg twice daily with ritonavir 100 mg twice daily

Atazanavir 300 mg daily with ritonavir 100 mg daily

Fosamprenavir 700 mg twice daily with ritonavir 100 mg twice daily

Lopinavir 400 mg co-formulated with ritonavir 100 mg twice daily

Saquinavir 1000 mg twice daily with ritonavir 100 mg twice daily

Tipranavir 500 mg twice daily with ritonavir 200 mg twice daily

Darunavir 600 mg twice daily with ritonavir 100 mg twice daily

Paediatric use: Lopinavir co-formulated with ritonavir is recommended for children 2 years of age and older. For further dosage recommendations, refer to the product information of other Protease Inhibitors approved for co-administered with ritonavir.

Renal impairment: As ritonavir is primarily metabolised by the liver, ritonavir may be appropriate for use with caution as a pharmacokinetic enhancer in patients with renal insufficiency depending on the specific protease inhibitor with which it is co-administered. However, since the renal clearance of ritonavir is negligible, the decrease in the total body clearance is not expected in patients with renal impairment. For specific dosing information in patients with renal impairment, refer to the Summary of Product Characteristics (SPC) of the co-administered protease inhibitor.

Hepatic impairment: Ritonavir should not be given as a pharmacokinetic enhancer to patients with decompensated liver disease. In the absence of pharmacokinetic studies in patients with stable severe hepatic impairment (Child Pugh Grade C) without decompensation, caution should be exercised when ritonavir is used as a pharmacokinetic enhancer as increased levels of the co-administered PI may occur. Specific recommendations for use of ritonavir as a pharmacokinetic enhancer in patients with hepatic impairment are dependent on the protease inhibitor with which it is co-administered. The SPC of the co-administered PI should be reviewed for specific dosing information in this patient population.

Ritonavir dosed as an antiretroviral agent

Adult use: The recommended dosage of Norvir solution is 600 mg (7.5 ml) twice daily by mouth.

Gradually increasing the dose of ritonavir when initiating therapy may help to improve tolerance. Treatment should be initiated at 300 mg (3.75 ml) twice daily for a period of three days and increased by 100 mg (1.25 ml) twice daily increments up to 600 mg twice daily over a period of no longer than 14 days. Patients should not remain on 300 mg twice daily for more than 3 days.

Paediatric use (2 years of age and above): the recommended dosage of Norvir solution in children is 350 mg/m^2 by mouth twice daily and should not exceed 600 mg twice daily. Norvir should be started at 250 mg/m^2 and increased at 2 to 3 day intervals by 50 mg/m^2 twice daily. When possible, dose should be administered using a calibrated dosing syringe.

Paediatric Dosage Guidelines

(see Table 1 below)

Table 1 Paediatric Dosage Guidelines

Body Surface area* (m^2)	Twice daily dose 250 mg/m^2	Twice daily dose 300 mg/m^2	Twice daily dose 350 mg/m^2
0.25	0.8 ml (62.5 mg)	0.9 ml (75 mg)	1.1 ml (87.5 mg)
0.50	1.6 ml (125 mg)	1.9 ml (150 mg)	2.2 ml (175 mg)
1.00	3.1 ml (250 mg)	3.8 ml (300 mg)	4.4 ml (350 mg)
1.25	3.9 ml (312.5 mg)	4.7 ml (375 mg)	5.5 ml (437.5 mg)
1.50	4.7 ml (375 mg)	5.6 ml (450 mg)	6.6 ml (525 mg)

* Body surface area can be calculated with the following equation

BSA (m^2) = $\sqrt{}$Height (cm) X Weight (kg)/ 3600)

Doses for intermediate body surface areas not included in the above table can be calculated using the following equations:

To calculate the volume to be administered (in ml) the body surface area should be multiplied by a factor of: 3.1 for a dose of 250 mg/m^2; 3.8 for one of 300 mg/m^2; and by 4.4 for 350 mg/m^2.

Renal impairment: Currently, there are no data specific to this patient population and therefore specific dosage recommendations cannot be made. The renal clearance of ritonavir is negligible; therefore, a decrease in the total body clearance is not expected in patients with renal impairment. Because ritonavir is highly protein bound it is unlikely that it will be significantly removed by haemodialysis or peritoneal dialysis.

Hepatic impairment: Ritonaviris principally metabolised and eliminated by the liver. Pharmacokinetic data indicate that no dose adjustment is necessary in patients with mild to moderate hepatic impairment (see section 5.2). Ritonavir should not be given to patients with severe hepatic impairment (see section 4.3).

Special Populations: Pharmacokinetic data indicated that no dose adjustment is necessary for elderly patients (see section 5.2).

The bitter taste of Norvir solution may be lessened if mixed with chocolate milk.

4.3 Contraindications

Hypersensitivity to the active substance or to any of the excipients.

When ritonavir is used as a pharmacokinetic enhancer of other PIs, consult the Summary of Product Characteristics of the co-administered protease inhibitor for contraindications.

Ritonavir should not be given as a pharmacokinetic enhancer or as an antiretroviral agent to patients with decompensated liver disease.

In vitro and *in vivo* studies have demonstrated that ritonavir is a potent inhibitor of CYP3A- and CYP2D6- mediated biotransformations. The following medicines are contraindicated when used with ritonavir and unless otherwise noted, the contraindication is based on the potential for ritonavir to inhibit metabolism of the co-administered drug, resulting in increased exposure to the co-administered drug and risk of clinically significant adverse effects.

The enzyme-modulating effect of ritonavir may be dose dependent. For some products, contraindications may be more relevant when ritonavir is used as an antiretroviral agent than when ritonavir is used as a pharmacokinetic enhancer (eg rifabutin and voriconazole):

(see Table 2 on next page)

4.4 Special warnings and precautions for use

Ritonavir is not a cure for HIV-1 infection or AIDS. Patients receiving ritonavir or any other antiretroviral therapy may continue to develop opportunistic infections and other complications of HIV-1 infection.

Patients should be advised that current antiretroviral therapy has not been proven to prevent the risk of transmission of HIV to others through blood or sexual contact. Appropriate precautions should continue to be used.

When ritonavir is used as a pharmacokinetic enhancer with other PIs, full details on the warnings and precautions relevant to that particular PI should be considered, therefore the Summary of Product Characteristics for the particular PI must be consulted.

Ritonavir dosed as an antiretroviral agent or as a pharmacokinetic enhancer

Patients with chronic diarrhoea or malabsorption: Extra monitoring is recommended when diarrhoea occurs. The relatively high frequency of diarrhoea during treatment with ritonavir may compromise the absorption and efficacy (due to decreased compliance) of ritonavir or other concurrent medications. Serious persistent vomiting and/or diarrhoea associated with ritonavir use might also compromise renal function. It is advisable to monitor renal function in patients with renal function impairment.

Haemophilia: there have been reports of increased bleeding, including spontaneous skin haematomas and haemarthroses, in haemophiliac patients type A and B treated with protease inhibitors. In some patients additional factor VIII was given. In more than a half of the reported cases, treatment with protease inhibitors was continued or reintroduced if treatment had been discontinued. A causal relationship has been evoked, although the mechanism of action has not been elucidated. Haemophiliac patients should therefore be made aware of the possibility of increased bleeding.

Diabetes mellitus and hyperglycaemia: New onset diabetes mellitus, hyperglycaemia or exacerbation of existing diabetes mellitus has been reported in patients receiving protease inhibitors. In some of these the hyperglycaemia was severe and in some cases also associated with ketoacidosis. Many patients had confounding medical conditions, some of which required therapy with agents that have been associated with the development of diabetes mellitus or hyperglycaemia.

Lipodystrophy: Combination antiretroviral therapy has been associated with redistribution of body fat (lipodystrophy) in HIV patients. The long-term consequences of these

Table 2

Drug Class	Drugs within Class	Rationale
Concomitant Drug Levels Increased		
α_1-Adrenoreceptor Antagonist	Alfuzosin	Increased plasma concentrations of alfuzosin which may lead to severe hypotension (see section 4.5).
Analgesics	Pethidine, piroxicam, propoxyphne	Increased plasma concentrations of norpethidine, piroxicam and propoxyphene. Thereby, increasing the risk of serious respiratory depression or haematologic abnormalities, or other serious adverse effects from these agents.
Antiarrthymics	Amiodarone, bepridil, encainide, flecanide, propafenone, quinidine	Increased plasma concentrations of amiodarone, bepridil, encainide, flecanide, propafenone, quinidine. Thereby, increasing the risk of arrhythmias or other serious adverse effects from these agents.
Antibiotic	Fusidic Acid	Increased plasma concentrations of fusidic acid and ritonavir.
Antifungal	Voriconazole	Concomitant use of ritonavir (400 mg twice daily and more) and voriconazole is contraindicated due to a reduction in voriconazole plasma concentrations and possible loss of effect (see section 4.5)
Antihistamines	Astemizole, terfenadine	Increased plasma concentrations of astemizole and terfenadine. Thereby, increasing the risk of serious arrhythmias from these agents.
Antimycobacterial	Rifabutin	Concomitant use of ritonavir dosed as an antiretroviral agent (600 mg twice daily) and rifabutin due to an increase of rifabutin serum concentrations and risk of adverse events including uveitis (see section 4.4). Recommendations regarding use of ritonavir dosed as a pharmacokinetic enhancer with rifabutin are noted in section 4.5
Antipsychotics/ Neuroleptics	Clozapine, pimozide	Increased plasma concentrations of clozapine and pimozide. Thereby, increasing the risk of serious haematologic abnormalities, or other serious adverse effects from these agents.
Ergot Derivatives	Dihydroergotamine, ergonovine, ergotamine, methylergonovine	Increased plasma concentrations of ergot derivatives leading to acute ergot toxicity, including vasospasm and ischaemia.
GI motility agent	Cisapride	Increased plasma concentrations of cisapride. Thereby, increasing the risk of serious arrhythmias from this agent.
HMG Co-A Reductase Inhibitor	Lovastatin, simvastatin	Increased plasma concentrations of lovastatin and simvastatin; thereby, increasing the risk of myopathy including rhabdomyolysis (see section 4.5).
Sedatives/hypnotics	Clorazepate, diazepam, estazolam, flurazepam, oral midazolam and triazolam	Increased plasma concentrations of clorazepate, diazepam, estazolam, flurazepam, oral midazolam and triazolam. Thereby, increasing the risk of extreme sedation and respiratory depression from these agents. (For caution on parenterally administered midazolam, see section 4.5).
Ritonavir Drug Level Decreased		
Herbal Preparation	St. John's Wort	Herbal preparations containing St John's wort (*Hypericum perforatum*) due to the risk of decreased plasma concentrations and reduced clinical effects of ritonavir (see section 4.5).

events are currently unknown. Knowledge about the mechanism is incomplete. A connection between visceral lipomatosis and PIs and lipoatrophy and nucleoside reverse transcriptase inhibitors (NRTIs) has been hypothesised. A higher risk of lipodystrophy has been associated with individual factors such as older age, and with drug related factors such as longer duration of antiretroviral treatment and associated metabolic disturbances. Clinical examination should include evaluation for physical signs of fat redistribution. Consideration should be given to measurement of fasting serum lipids and blood glucose. Lipid disorders should be managed as clinically appropriate (see section 4.8).

Pancreatitis: Pancreatitis should be considered if clinical symptoms (nausea, vomiting, abdominal pain) or abnormalities in laboratory values (such as increased serum lipase or amylase values) suggestive of pancreatitis should occur. Patients who exhibit these signs or symptoms should be evaluated and Norvir therapy should be discontinued if a diagnosis of pancreatitis is made (see section 4.8).

Immune Reactivation Syndrome: in HIV-infected patients with severe immune deficiency at the time of institution of combination antiretroviral therapy (CART), an inflammatory reaction to asymtomatic or residual opportunistic pathogens may arise and cause serious clinical conditions, or aggravation of symptoms. Typically, such reactions have been observed within the first few weeks or months of initiation of CART. Relevant examples are cytomegalovirus retinitis, generalised and/or focal mycobacterial infections, and Pneumocystis carinii pneumonia. Any inflammatory symptoms should be evaluated and treatment instituted when necessary.

Liver disease: Ritonavir should not be given to patients with decompensated liver disease. For patients with stable severe hepatic impairment (Child Pugh Grade C) without decompensation see section 4.2. Patients with chronic hepatitis B or C and treated with combination antiretroviral therapy are at an increased risk for severe and potentially fatal hepatic adverse events. In case of concomitant antiviral therapy for hepatitis B or C, please refer to the relevant product information for these medicinal products.

Patients with pre-existing liver dysfunction including chronic active hepatitis have an increased frequency of liver function abnormalities during combination antiretroviral therapy and should be monitored according to standard practice. If there is evidence of worsening liver disease in such patients, interruption or discontinuation of treatment must be considered.

Renal disease: Since the renal clearance of ritonavir is negligible, the decrease in the total body clearance is not expected in patients with renal impairment. For specific dosing information in patients with renal impairment, refer to the Summary of Product Characteristics (SPC) of the co-administered protease inhibitor. See also section 4.2.

Ritonavir oral solution contains castor oil polyoxyl which may cause stomach upset and diarrhoea. Ritonavir oral solution also contains the azo-colouring agent sunset yellow (E110) which may cause allergic reactions.

Ritonavir oral solution contains alcohol (43% v/v), ie up to 258 mg per maximum dose of 600 mg, equivalent to 65 ml beer, 27 ml wine per dose. Each 100 mg dose contains up to 43 mg alcohol and each 200 mg dose contains 86 mg alcohol. Therefore concomitant administration of Norvir with disulfiram or medicines with disulfiram-like reactions (eg metronidazole) should be avoided. Also to be taken into account in pregnant or breast-feeding women, children and high-risk groups such as patients with liver disease or epilepsy.

Osteonecrosis: Although the etiology is considered to be multifactorial (including corticosteroid use, alcohol consumption, severe immunosuppression, higher body mass index), cases of osteonecrosis have been reported in patients with advanced HIV-disease and/or long-term exposure to combination antiretroviral therapy (CART). Patients should be advised to seek medical advice if they experience joint aches and pain, joint stiffness or difficulty in movement.

PR interval prolongation: ritonavir has been shown to cause modest asymptomatic prolongation of the PR interval in some healthy adult subjects. Rare reports of 2nd or 3rd degree atrioventricular block in patients with underlying structural heart disease and pre-existing conduction system abnormalities or in patients receiving drugs known to prolong the PR interval (such as verapamil or atazanavir) have been reported in patients receiving ritonavir. Norvir should be used with caution in such patients (see section 5.1).

Interactions with other medicinal products

Ritonavir dosed as an antiretroviral agent

The following Warnings and Precautions should be considered when ritonavir is used as an antiretroviral agent. When ritonavir is used as a pharmacokinetic enhancer at the 100 mg and 200 mg level it cannot be assumed that the following warnings and precautions will also apply. When ritonavir is used as a pharmacokinetic enhancer, full details on the warnings and precautions relevant to that particular PI must be considered, therefore the Summary of Product Characteristics, section 4.4, for the particular PI must be consulted to determine if the information below is applicable.

PDE5 inhibitors: Particular caution should be used when prescribing sildenafil, tadalafil or vardenafil in patients receiving ritonavir. Co-administration of ritonavir with these medicinal products is expected to substantially increase their concentrations and may result in associated adverse events such as hypotension and prolonged erection (see section 4.5).

HMG-CoA reductase inhibitors: The HMG-CoA reductase inhibitors simvastatin and lovastatin are highly dependent on CYP3A for metabolism, thus concomitant use of ritonavir with simvastatin or lovastatin is not recommended due to an increased risk of myopathy including rhabdomyolysis. Caution must also be exercised and reduced doses should be considered if ritonavir is used concurrently with atorvastatin, which is metabolised to a lesser extent by CYP3A. While rosuvastatin elimination is not dependent on CYP3A, an elevation of rosuvastatin exposure has been reported with ritonavir co-administration. The mechanism of this interaction is not clear, but may be the result of transporter inhibition. When used with ritonavir dosed as a pharmacokinetic enhancer or as an antiretroviral agent, the lowest doses of atorvastatin or rosuvastatin should be administered. The metabolism of pravastatin and fluvastatin is not dependent of CYP3A, and interactions are not expected with ritonavir. If treatment with an HMG-CoA reductase inhibitor is indicated, pravastatin or fluvastatin is recommended (see section 4.5).

Digoxin: Particular caution should be used when prescribing ritonavir in patients taking digoxin since co-administration of ritonavir with digoxin is expected to increase digoxin levels. The increased digoxin levels may lessen over time (see section 4.5).

In patients who are already taking digoxin when ritonavir is introduced, the digoxin dose should be reduced to one-half of the patients' normal dose and patient need to be followed more closely than usual for several weeks after initiating co-administration of ritonavir and digoxin.

In patients who are already taking ritonavir when digoxin is introduced, digoxin should be introduced more gradually than usual. Digoxin levels should be monitored more intensively than usual during this period, with dose adjustments made, as necessary, based on clinical, electrocardiographic and digoxin level findings.

Ethinyl estradiol: Barrier or other non-hormonal methods of contraception should be considered when administering ritonavir at therapeutic or low doses as ritonavir is likely to reduce the effect and change the uterine bleeding profile when co-administered with estradiol-containing contraceptives.

Glucocorticoids: Concomitant use of ritonavir and fluticasone or other glucocorticoids that are metabolised by CYP3A4 is not recommended unless the potential benefit of treatment outweighs the risk of systemic corticosteroid effects, including Cushing's syndrome and adrenal suppression (see section 4.5).

Trazodone: Particular caution should be used when prescribing ritonavir in patients using trazodone. Trazodone is a CYP3A4 substrate and co-administration of ritonavir is expected to increase trazodone levels. Adverse events of nausea, dizziness, hypotension and syncope have been observed in single dose interaction studies in healthy volunteers (see section 4.5)

Ritonavir dosed as a pharmacokinetic enhancer

The interaction profiles of HIV-protease inhibitors, co-administered with low dose ritonavir, are dependant on the specific co-administered protease inhibitor.

For a description of the mechanisms and potential mechanisms contributing to the interaction profile of the PIs, see section 4.5. Please also review the Summary of Product Characteristics for the particular boosted PI.

Saquinavir: Doses of ritonavir higher than 100 mg twice daily should not be used. Higher doses of ritonavir have been shown to be associated with an increased incidence of adverse events. Co-administration of saquinavir and ritonavir has led to severe adverse events, mainly diabetic ketoacidosis and liver disorders, especially in patients with pre-existing liver disease.

Saquinavir/ritonavir should not be given together with rifampicin, due to the risk of severe hepatotoxicity (presenting as increased hepatic transaminases) if the three medicines are given together (see section 4.5).

Tipranavir: co-administered with 200 mg of ritonavir has been associated with reports of clinical hepatitis and hepatic decompensation including some fatalities. Extra vigilance is warranted in patients with chronic hepatitis B or hepatitis C co-infection, as these patients have an increased risk of hepatotoxicity.

Doses of ritonavir lower than 200 mg twice daily should not be used as they might alter the efficacy profile of the combination.

Fosamprenavir: Co-administration of fosamprenavir with ritonavir in doses greater than 100 mg twice daily has not been clinically evaluated. The use of higher ritonavir doses might alter the safety profile of the combination and therefore is not recommended.

Atazanavir: Co-administration of atazanavir with ritonavir at doses greater than 100 mg once daily has not been clinically evaluated. The use of higher ritonavir doses may alter the safety profile of atazanavir (cardiac effects, hyperbilirubinemia) and therefore is not recommended. Only when atazanavir with ritonavir is co-administered with efavirenz, a dose increase of ritonavir to 200mg once daily could be considered. In this instance, close clinical monitoring is warranted. Refer to the Reyataz Summary of Product Characteristics for further details.

4.5 Interaction with other medicinal products and other forms of interaction

Ritonavir dosed as a pharmacokinetic enhancer or as an antiretroviral agent

Ritonavir has a high affinity for several cytochrome P450 (CYP) isoforms and may inhibit oxidation with the following ranked order: CYP3A4> CYP2D6. Co-administration of Norvir and medicinal products primarily metabolised by CYP3A may result in increased plasma concentrations of the other medicinal product, which could increase or prolong its therapeutic and adverse effects. For select medicinal products (eg alprazolam) the inhibitory effects of ritonavir on CYP3A4 may decrease over time. Ritonavir also has a high affinity for P-glycoprotein and may inhibit this transporter. The inhibitory effect of ritonavir (with or without other protease inhibitors) on P-gp activity may decrease over time (eg digoxin and fexofenadine-see table "Ritonavir effects on non-antiretroviral drugs" below). Ritonavir may induce glucuronidation and oxidation by CYP1A2, CYP2C8, CYP2C9 and CYP2C19 thereby increasing the biotransformation of some medicinal products metabolised by these pathways, and may result in decreased systemic exposure to such medicinal products, which could decease or shorten their therapeutic effect.

Important information regarding drug interactions when ritonavir is used as a pharmacokinetic enhancer is also contained in the Summary of Product Characteristics of the co-administered protease inhibitor.

Drugs that affect ritonavir levels

Serum levels of ritonavir can be reduced by concomitant use of herbal preparations containing St John's wort (*Hypericum perforatum*). This is due to the induction of drug metabolising enzymes by St John's wort. Herbal preparations containing St John's wort must not be used in combination with ritonavir. If a patient is already taking St John's wort, stop St John's wort and if possible check viral levels. Ritonavir levels may increase on stopping St John's wort. The dose of ritonavir may need adjusting. The inducing effect may persist for at least 2 weeks after cessation of treatment with St John's wort (see section 4.3).

Serum levels of ritonavir may be affected by select co-administered medicinal products (eg delavirdine, efavirenz, phenytoin and rifampicin). These interactions are noted in the drug interaction tables below.

Drugs that are affected by the use of ritonavir

Interactions between ritonavir and protease inhibitors, antiretroviral agents other than protease inhibitors and other non-antiretroviral drugs are listed in the tables below.

(see Table 3 on next page)

Cardiac and neurologic events have been reported when ritonavir has been co-administered with disopyramide, mexiletine or nefazadone. The possibility of drug interaction cannot be excluded.

In addition to the interactions listed above, as ritonavir is highly protein bound, the possibility of increased therapeutic and toxic effects due to protein binding displacement of concomitant medications should be considered.

Ritonavir dosed as a pharmacokinetic enhancer

Important information regarding drug interactions when ritonavir is used a pharmacokinetic enhancer is also contained in the Summary of Product Characteristics of the co-administered protease inhibitor.

Proton pump inhibitors and H_2-receptor antagonists: proton pump inhibitors and H_2-receptor antagonists (e.g. omeprazole or ranitidine) may reduce concentrations for co-administered protease inhibitors. For specific information regarding the impact of co-administration of acid reducing agents, refer to the SmPC of the co-administered protease inhibitor. Based on interaction studies with the ritonavir boosted protease inhibitors (lopinavir/ritonavir, atazanavir), concurrent administration of omeprazole or ranitidine does not significantly modify ritonavir efficacy as a pharmacokinetic enhancer despite a slight change of exposure (about 6 - 18%).

4.6 Pregnancy and lactation

A limited number (> 800) of pregnant women were exposed to ritonavir during pregnancy; a very limited number (< 300) were exposed during the first trimester. These data largely refer to exposures where ritonavir was used in combination therapy and not at therapeutic ritonavir doses but at lower doses as a pharmacokinetic enhancer for other PIs. These limited data indicate no increase in the rate of birth defects compared to rates observed in population-based birth defect surveillance systems. Animal data have shown reproductive toxicity (see 5.3). The use of Norvir may be considered in pregnancy only when the benefits outweigh the risk to the foetus.

Ritonavir adversely interacts with oral contraceptives (OCs). Therefore, an alternative, effective and safe method of contraception should be used during treatment.

It is not known whether this medicine is excreted in human milk. Milk excretion has not been measured in the animal studies, however a study in rats showed some effects on offspring development during lactation which are compatible with excretion of ritonavir in milk in that species. HIV infected women should not breast-feed their infants under any circumstances to avoid transmission of HIV.

4.7 Effects on ability to drive and use machines

No studies on the effects on the ability to drive and use machines have been performed. As somnolence and dizziness are known undesirable effects, this should be taken into account when driving or using machinery.

Norvir oral solution contains alcohol (43%).

4.8 Undesirable effects

Ritonavir dosed as a pharmacokinetic enhancer

Adverse events associated with the use of ritonavir as a pharmacokinetic enhancer are dependent on the specific co-administered PI. For information on adverse events refer to the SPC of the specific co-administered PI.

Ritonavir dosed as an antiretroviral agent

In the original clinical studies (Phase II/III), adverse events with possible, probable or unknown relationship to ritonavir were reported in ⩾ 2% of 1033 patients.

The following adverse reactions of moderate to severe intensity with possible or probable relationship to ritonavir have been reported. Within each frequency grouping, undesirable effects are presented in order of decreasing seriousness: very common (> 1/10); common (> 1/100 to < 1/10); uncommon (> 1/1000 to < 1/100); rare(> 1/10,000 to < 1/1,000).

(see Table 4 on page 4931642)

Events noted as having Unknown frequency were identified via post-marketing surveillance.

Hepatic transaminase elevations exceeding five times the upper limit or normal, clinical hepatitis, and jaundice have occurred in patients receiving ritonavir alone or in combination with other antiretrovirals.

Combination antiretroviral therapy has been associated with redistribution of body fat (lipodystrophy) in HIV patients including the loss of peripheral and facial subcutaneous fat, increased intra-abdominal and visceral fat, breast hypertrophy and dorsocervical fat accumulation (buffalo hump).

Combination antiretroviral therapy has been associated with metabolic abnormalities such as hypertriglyceridaemia, hypercholesterolaemia, insulin resistance, hyperglycaemia and hyperlactataemia (see section 4.4).

In HIV-infected patients with severe immune deficiency at the time of initiation of combination antiretroviral therapy (CART), an inflammatory reaction to asymptomatic or residual opportunistic infections may arise (see section 4.4).

Pancreatitis has been observed in patients receiving ritonavir therapy, including those who developed hypertriglyceridemia. In some cases fatalities have been observed. Patients with advanced HIV disease may be at risk of elevated triglycerides and pancreatitis (see section 4.4).

Cases of osteonecrosis have been reported, particularly in patients with generally acknowledged risk factors, advanced HIV disease or long-term exposure to combination antiretroviral therapy (CART). The frequency of this is unknown (see section 4.4).

4.9 Overdose

Human experience of acute overdose with ritonavir is limited. One patient in clinical trials took ritonavir 1500 mg/day for two days and reported paraesthesia, which resolved after the dose was decreased. A case of renal failure with eosinophilia has been reported.

The signs of toxicity observed in animals (mice and rats) included decreased activity, ataxia, dyspnoea and tremors.

There is no specific antidote for overdose with ritonavir. Treatment of overdose with ritonavir should consist of general supportive measures including monitoring of vital signs and observation of the clinical status of the patient. Due to the solubility characteristics and possibility of transintestinal elimination, it is proposed that management of overdose could entail gastric lavage and administration of activated charcoal. Since ritonavir is extensively metabolised by the liver and is highly protein bound, dialysis is unlikely to be beneficial in significant removal of the medicine.

5. PHARMACOLOGICAL PROPERTIES

5.1 Pharmacodynamic properties

Pharmaco-therapeutic group: antiviral for systemic use, ATC code: J05A E03

Ritonavir dosed as a pharmacokinetic enhancer

Pharmacokinetic enhancement by ritonavir is based on ritonavir's activity as a potent inhibitor of CYP3A- mediated metabolism. The degree of enhancement is related to the metabolic pathway of the co-administered protease inhibitor and the impact of the co-administered protease inhibitor on the metabolism of ritonavir. Maximal inhibition of metabolism of the co-administered protease inhibitor is generally achieved with ritonavir doses of 100 mg daily to 200 mg twice daily, and is dependent on the co-administered protease inhibitor. For additional information on the effect of ritonavir on co-administered protease inhibitor metabolism, see section 4.5 and refer to the Summary of Product Characteristics of the particular co-administered PIs.

Ritonavir dosed as an antiretroviral agent

Ritonavir is an orally active peptidomimetic inhibitor of the HIV-1 and HIV-2 aspartyl proteases. Inhibition of HIV protease renders the enzyme incapable of processing the *gag-pol* polyprotein precursor which leads to the production of HIV particles with immature morphology that are unable to initiate new rounds of infection. Ritonavir has selective affinity for the HIV protease and has little inhibitory activity against human aspartyl proteases.

Ritonavir was the first protease inhibitor (approved in 1996) for which efficacy was proven in a study with clinical end-points. However, due to ritonavir's metabolic inhibitory properties its use as a pharmacokinetic enhancer of other protease inhibitors is the prevalent use of ritonavir in clinical practice (see section 4.2).

Effects on the Electrocardiogram

QTcF interval was evaluated in a randomised, placebo and active (moxifloxacin 400 mg once daily) controlled cross-over study in 45 healthy adults, with 10 measurements over 12 hours on Day 3. The maximum mean (95% upper confidence bound) difference in QTcF from placebo was 5.5 (7.6) for 400 mg twice daily ritonavir. The Day 3 ritonavir exposure was approximately 1.5 fold higher than that observed with the 600 mg twice daily dose at steady state. No subject experienced an increase in QTcF of ⩾ 60 msec from baseline or a QTcF interval exceeding the potentially clinically relevant threshold of 500 msec.

Modest prolongation of the PR interval was also noted in subjects receiving ritonavir in the same study on Day 3. The mean changes from baseline in PR interval ranged from 11.0 to 24.0 msec in the 12 hour interval post dose. Maximum PR interval was 252 msec and no second or third degree heart block was observed (see section 4.4).

Resistance

Ritonavir-resistant isolates of HIV-1 have been selected *in vitro* and isolated from patients treated with therapeutic doses of ritonavir.

Reduction in the antiretroviral activity of ritonavir is primarily associated with the protease mutations V82A/F/T/S and I84V. Accumulation of other mutations in the protease gene (including at positions 20, 33, 36, 46, 54, 71, and 90) can also contribute to ritonavir resistance. In general, as mutations associated with ritonavir resistance accumulate, susceptibility to select other PIs may decrease due to cross-resistance. The Summary of Product Characteristics of

Table 3

Drug Interactions – Ritonavir with Protease Inhibitors					
Co-administered Drug	**Dose of Co-administered Drug (mg)**	**Dose of NORVIR (mg)**	**Drug Assessed**	**AUC**	**C_{min}**
Amprenavir	600 q12h	100 q12h	Amprenavir[2]	↑ 64%	↑ 5 fold
	Ritonavir increases the serum levels of amprenavir as a result of CYP3A4 inhibition. Clinical trials confirmed the safety and efficacy of 600 mg amprenavir twice daily with ritonavir 100 mg twice daily. Norvir oral solution should not be co-administered with amprenavir oral solution to children due to the risk of toxicity from excipients in the two formulations. For further information, physicians should refer to the Agenerase Summary of Product Characteristics.				
Atazanavir	300 q24h	100 q24h	Atazanavir	↑ 86%	↑ 11 fold
			Atazanavir[1]	↑ 2 fold	↑ 3-7 fold
	Ritonavir increases the serum levels of atazanavir as a result of CYP3A4 inhibition. Clinical trials confirmed the safety and efficacy of 300 mg atazanavir once daily with ritonavir 100 mg once daily in treatment experienced patients. For further information, physicians should refer to the Reyataz Summary of Product Characteristics.				
Darunavir	600, single	100 q12h	Darunavir	↑ 14 fold	
	Ritonavir increases the serum levels of darunavir as a result of CYP3A inhibition. Darunavir must be given with ritonavir to ensure its therapeutic effect. Ritonavir doses higher than 100 mg twice daily have not been studied with darunavir. For further information, refer to the Summary of Product Characteristics for Prezista.				
Fosamprenavir	700 q12h	100 q12h	Amprenavir	↑ 2.4 fold	↑ 11 fold
	Ritonavir increases the serum levels of amprenavir (from fosamprenavir) as a result of CYP3A4 inhibition. Fosamprenavir must be given with ritonavir to ensure its therapeutic effect. Clinical trials confirmed the safety and efficacy of fosamprenavir 700 mg twice daily with ritonavir 100 mg twice daily. Ritonavir doses higher than 100 mg twice daily have not been studied with fosamprenavir. For further information, physicians should refer to the Telzir Summary of Product Characteristics.				
Indinavir	800 q12h	100 q12h	Indinavir[3]	↑ 178%	ND
			Ritonavir	↑ 72%	ND
	400 q12h	400 q12h	Indinavir[3]	↔	↑ 4 fold
			Ritonavir	↔	↔
	Ritonavir increases the serum levels of indinavir as a result of CYP3A inhibition. Appropriate doses for this combination, with respect to efficacy and safety, have not been established. Minimal benefit of ritonavir-mediated pharmacokinetic enhancement is achieved with doses higher than 100 mg twice daily. In cases of co-administration of ritonavir (100 mg twice daily) and indinavir (800 mg twice daily) caution is warranted as the risk of nephrolithiasis may be increased.				
Nelfinavir	1250 q12h	100 q12h	Nelfinavir	↑ 20to39%	ND
	750, single	500 q12h	Nelfinavir	↑ 152%	ND
			Ritonavir		↔
	Ritonavir increases the serum levels of nelfinavir as a result of CYP3A4 inhibition. Appropriate doses for this combination, with respect to efficacy and safety, have not been established. Minimal benefit of ritonavir-mediated pharmacokinetic enhancement is achieved with doses higher than 100 mg twice daily.				
Saquinavir	1000 q12h	100 q12h	Saquinavir[4]	↑ 15-fold	↑ 5-fold
			Ritonavir	↔	↔
	400 q12h	400 q12h	Saquinavir[4]	↑ 17-fold	ND
			Ritonavir	↔	↔
	Ritonavir increases the serum levels of saquinavir as a result of CYP3A4 inhibition. Saquinavir should only be given in combination with ritonavir. Ritonavir 100 mg twice daily with saquinavir 1000 mg twice daily provides saquinavir systemic exposure over 24 hours similar to or greater than those achieved with saquinavir 1200 mg three times daily without ritonavir. In a clinical study investigating the interaction of rifampicin 600 mg once daily and saquinavir 1000 mg with ritonavir 100 mg twice daily in healthy volunteers, severe hepatocellular toxicity with transaminase elevations up to > 20-fold the upper limit of normal after 1 to 5 days of co-administration was noted. Due to the risk of severe hepatoxicity, saquinavir/ritonavir should not be given together with rifampicin. For further information, physicians should refer to the Invirase or Fortovase Summary of Product Characteristics.				
Tipranavir	500 q12h	200 q12h	Tipranavir	↑ 11 fold	↑ 29 fold
			Ritonavir	↓ 40%	ND
	Ritonavir increases the serum levels of tipranavir as a result of CYP3A inhibition. Tipranavir must be given with low dose ritonavir to ensure its therapeutic effect. Doses of ritonavir less than 200 mg twice daily should not be used with tipranavir as they might alter the efficacy of the combination. For further information, physicians should refer to the Aptivus Summary of Product Characteristics.				
	ND: Not determined. 1. Based on cross-study comparison to 400 mg atazanavir once daily alone. 2. Based on cross-study comparison to 1200 mg amprenavir twice daily alone. 3. Based on cross-study comparison to 800 mg indinavir three times daily alone. 4. Based on cross-stud y comparison to 600 mg saquinavir three times daily alone.				
Drug Interactions – Ritonavir with Antiretroviral Agents Other Than Protease Inhibitors					
Didanosine	200 q12h	600 q12h 2 h later	Didanosine	↓ 13%	↔
	As ritonavir is recommended to be taken with food and didanosine should be taken on an empty stomach, dosing should be separated by 2.5 h. Dose alterations should not be necessary.				
Delavirdine	400 q8h	600 q12h	Delavirdine[1]	↔	↔
			Ritonavir	↑ 50%	↑ 75%
	Based on comparison to historical data, the pharmacokinetics of delavirdine did not appear to be affected by ritonavir. When used in combination with delavirdine, dose reduction of ritonavir may be considered.				
Efavirenz	600 q24h	500 q12h	Efavirenz	↑ 21%	
			Ritonavir	↑ 17%	
	A higher frequency of adverse events (eg, dizziness, nausea, paraesthesia) and laboratory abnormalities (elevated liver enzymes) have been observed when efavirenz is co-administered with ritonavir dosed as an antiretroviral agent.				

Drug Interactions – Ritonavir with Protease Inhibitors

Co-administered Drug	Dose of Co-administered Drug (mg)	Dose of NORVIR (mg)	Drug Assessed	AUC	C_{min}
Maraviroc	100 q12h	100 q12h	Maraviroc	↑ 161%	↑ 28%
	Ritonavir increases the serum levels of maraviroc as a result of CYP3A inhibition. Maraviroc may be given with ritonavir to increase the maraviroc exposure. For further information, refer to the Summary of Product Characteristics for Celsentri.				
Nevirapine	200 q12h	600 q12h	Nevirapine	↔	↔
			Ritonavir	↔	↔
	Co-administration of ritonavir with nevirapine does not lead to clinically relevant changes in the pharmacokinetics of either nevirapine or ritonavir.				
Zidovudine	200 q8h	300 q6h	Zidovudine	↓ 25%	ND
	Ritonavir may induce the glucuronidation of zidovudine, resulting in slightly decreased levels of zidovudine. Dose alterations should not be necessary.				
	ND: Not determined 1. Based on parallel group comparison.				

Ritonavir effects on Non-antiretroviral Co-administered Drugs

Co-administered Drug	Dose of Co-administered Drug (mg)	Dose of NORVIR (mg)	Effect on Co-administered Drug AUC	Effect on Co-administered Drug C_{max}
Alpha $_1$ -Adrenoreceptor Antagonist				
Alfuzosin	Ritonavir co-administration is likely to result in increased plasma concentrations of alfuzosin and is therefore **contraindicated** (see section 4.3).			
Amphetamine Derivatives				
Amphetamine	Ritonavir dosed as an antiretroviral agent is likely to inhibit CYP2D6 and as a result is expected to increase concentrations of amphetamine and its derivatives. Careful monitoring of therapeutic and adverse effects is recommended when these medicines are concomitantly administered with antiretroviral doses of ritonavir (see section 4.4).			
Analgesics				
Buprenorphine	16 q24h	100 q12h	↑ 57%	↑ 77%
Norbuprenorphine			↑ 33%	↑ 108%
Glucuronide metabolites			↔	↔
	The increases of plasma levels of buprenorphine and its active metabolite did not lead to clinically significant pharmacodynamic changes in a population of opioid tolerant patients. Adjustment to the dose of buprenorphine or ritonavir may therefore not be necessary when the two are dosed together. When ritonavir is used in combination with another protease inhibitor and buprenorphine, the SPC of the co-administered protease inhibitor should be reviewed for specific dosing information.			
Pethidine, piroxicam, propoxyphene	Ritonavir co-administration is likely to result in increased plasma concentrations of pethidine, piroxicam, and propoxyphene and is therefore **contraindicated** (see section 4.3).			
Fentanyl	Ritonavir dosed as a pharmacokinetic enhancer or as an antiretroviral agent inhibits CYP3A4 and as a result is expected to increase the plasma concentrations of fentanyl. Careful monitoring of therapeutic and adverse effects is recommended when fentanyl is concomitantly administered with ritonavir.			
Methadone[1]	5, single dose	500 q12h,	↓ 36%	↓ 38%
	Increased methadone dose may be necessary when concomitantly administered with ritonavir dosed as an antiretroviral agent or as a pharmacokinetic enhancer due to induction of glucuronidation. Dose adjustment should be considered based on the patient's clinical response to methadone therapy.			
Morphine	Morphine levels may be decreased due to induction of glucuronidation by co-administered ritonavir dosed as an antiretroviral agent or as a pharmacokinetic enhancer.			
Antiarrhythmics				
Amiodarone, bepridil, encainide, flecanide, propafenone, quinidine	Ritonavir co-administration is likely to result in increased plasma concentrations of amiodarone, bepridil, encainide, flecanide, propafenone, and quinidine and is therefore **contraindicated** (see section 4.3).			
Digoxin	0.5 single IV dose	300 q12h, 3 days	↑ 86%	ND
	0.4 single oral dose	200 q12h, 13 days	↑ 22%	↔
	This interaction may be due to modification of P-glycoprotein mediated digoxin efflux by ritonavir dosed as an antiretroviral agent or as a pharmacokinetic enhancer. Increased digoxin levels observed in patients receiving ritonavir may lessen over time as induction develops (see section 4.4).			
Antiasthmatic				
Theophylline[1]	3 mg/kg q8h	500 q12h	↓ 43%	↓ 32%
	An increased dose of theophyline may be required when co-administered with ritonavir, due to induction of CYP1A2.			
Anticancer agents				
Vincristine, vinblastine	Serum concentrations may be increased when co-administered with ritonavir resulting in the potential for increased incidence of adverse events.			
Anticoagulant				
Warfarin S-Warfarin R-Warfarin	5, single dose	400 q12h	↑ 9% ↓ 33%	↓ 9% ↔
	Induction of CYP1A2 and CYP2C9 lead to decreased levels of R-warfarin while little pharmacokinetic effect is noted on S- warfarin when co-administered with ritonavir. Decreased R-warfarin levels may lead to reduced anticoagulation, therefore it is recommended that anticoagulation parameters are monitored when warfarin is co-administered with ritonavir dosed as an antiretroviral agent or as a pharmacokinetic enhancer.			
Anticonvulsants				
Carbamazepine	Ritonavir dosed as a pharmacokinetic enhancer or as an antiretroviral agent inhibits CYP3A4 and as a result is expected to increase the plasma concentrations of carbamazepine. Careful monitoring of therapeutic and adverse effects is recommended when carbamazepine is concomitantly administered with ritonavir.			

Ritonavir effects on Non-antiretroviral Co-administered Drugs

Co-administered Drug	Dose of Co-administered Drug (mg)	Dose of NORVIR (mg)	Effect on Co-administered Drug AUC	Effect on Co-administered Drug C_{max}
Divalproex, lamotrigine, phenytoin	Ritonavir dosed as a pharmacokinetic enhancer or as an antiretroviral agent induces oxidation by CYP2C9 and glucuronidation and as a result is expected to decrease the plasma concentrations of anticonvulsants. Careful monitoring of serum levels or therapeutic effects is recommended when these medicines are concomitantly administered with ritonavir. Phenytoin may decrease serum levels of ritonavir.			
Antidepressants				
Amitriptyline, fluoxetine, imipramine, nortriptyline, paroxetine, sertraline	Ritonavir dosed as an antiretroviral agent is likely to inhibit CYP2D6 and as a result is expected to increase concentrations of desipramine, imipramine, amitriptyline, nortriptyline, fluoxetine, paroxetine or sertraline. Careful monitoring of therapeutic and adverse effects is recommended when these medicines are concomitantly administered with antiretroviral doses of ritonavir (see section 4.4).			
Desipramine	100 single oral dose	500 q12h	↑ 145%	↑ 22%
	The AUC and Cmax of the 2-hydroxy metabolite were decreased 15 and 67%, respectively. Dosage reduction of desipramine is recommended when co-administered with ritonavir dosed as an antiretroviral agent.			
Trazodone	50, single dose	200 q12h	↑ 2.4-fold	↑ 34%
	An increase in the incidence in trazodone-related adverse events was noted when co-administered with ritonavir dosed as an antiretroviral agent or as a pharmacokinetic enhancer. If trazodone is co-administered with ritonavir, the combination should be used with caution, initiating trazodone at the lowest dosage and monitoring for clinical response and tolerability.			
Antihistamines				
Astemizole, terfenadine	Ritonavir co-administration is likely to result in increased plasma concentrations of astemizole and terfenadine and is therefore **contraindicated** (see section 4.3).			
Fexofenadine	Ritonavir may modify P-glycoprotein mediated fexofenadine efflux when dosed as an antriretroviral agent or as a pharmacokinetic enhancer resulting in increased concentrations of fexofenadine. Increased fexofenadine levels may lessen over time as induction develops.			
Loratadine	Ritonavir dosed as a pharmacokinetic enhancer or as an antiretroviral agent inhibits CYP3A and as a result is expected to increase the plasma concentrations of loratadine. Careful monitoring of therapeutic and adverse effects is recommended when loratidine is concomitantly administered with ritonavir.			
Anti-infectives				
Fusidic Acid	Ritonavir co-administration is likely to result in increased plasma concentrations of both fusidic acid and ritonavir and is therefore **contraindicated** (see section 4.3).			
Rifabutin[1] 25-*O*-desacetyl rifabutin metabolite	150 daily	500 q12h,	↑ 4-fold ↑ 38-fold	↑ 2.5-fold ↑ 16-fold
	Due to the large increase in rifabutin AUC, the concomitant use of rifabutin with ritonavir dosed as an antiretroviral agent is **contraindicated** (see section 4.3). The reduction of the rifabutin dose to 150 mg 3 times per week may be indicated for select PIs when co-administered with ritonavir as a pharmacokinetic enhancer. The Summary of Product Characteristics of the co-administered protease inhibitor should be consulted for specific recommendations. Consideration should be given to official guidance on the appropriate treatment of tuberculosis in HIV-infected patients.			
Rifampicin	Although rifampicin may induce metabolism of ritonavir, limited data indicate that when high doses of ritonavir (600 mg twice daily) is co-administered with rifampicin, the additional inducing effect of rifampicin (next to that of ritonavir itself) is small and may have no clinical relevant effect on ritonavir levels in high-dose ritonavir therapy. The effect of ritonavir on rifampicin is not known.			
Voriconazole	200 q12h	400 q12h	↓ 82%	↓ 66%
	200 q12h	100 q12h	↓ 39%	↓ 24%
	Concomitant use of ritonavir dosed as an antiretroviral agent and voriconazole is **contraindicated** due to reduction in voriconazole concentrations (see section 4.3). Co-administration of voriconazole and ritonavir dosed as a pharmacokinetic enhancer should be avoided, unless an assessment of the benefit/risk to the patient justifies the use of voriconazole.			
Atovaquone	Ritonavir dosed as a pharmacokinetic enhancer or as an antiretroviral agent induces glucuronidation and as a result is expected to decrease the plasma concentrations of atovaquone. Careful monitoring of serum levels or therapeutic effects is recommended when atovaquone is concomitantly administered with ritonavir.			
Clarithromycin 14-OH clarithromycin metabolite	500 q12h,	200 q8h	↑ 77% ↓ 100%	↑ 31% ↓ 99%
	Due to the large therapeutic window of clarithromycin no dose reduction should be necessary in patients with normal renal function. Clarithromycin doses greater than 1 g per day should not be co-administered with ritonavir dosed as an antiretroviral agent or as a pharmacokinetic enhancer. For patients with renal impairment, a clarithromycin dose reduction should be considered: for patients with creatinine clearance of 30 to 60 ml/min the dose should be reduced by 50%, for patients with creatinine clearance less than 30 ml/min the dose should be reduced by 75%.			
Erythromycin, itraconazole	Ritonavir dosed as a pharmacokinetic enhancer or as an antiretroviral agent inhibits CYP3A4 and as a result is expected to increase the plasma concentrations of erythromycin and itraconazole. Careful monitoring of therapeutic and adverse effects is recommended when erythromycin or itraconazole is used concomitantly administered with ritonavir.			
Ketoconazole	200 daily	500 q12h	↑ 3.4-fold	↑ 55%
	Ritonavir inhibits CYP3A-mediated metabolism of ketoconazole. Due to an increased incidence of gastrointestinal and hepatic adverse events, a dose reduction of ketoconazole should be considered when co-administered with ritonavir dosed as an antiretroviral agent or as a pharmacokinetic enhancer.			
Sulfamethoxazole/ Trimethoprim[2]	800/160, single dose	500 q12h	↓ 20% / ↑ 20%	↔
	Dose alteration of sulfamethoxazole/trimethoprim during concomitant ritonavir therapy should not be necessary.			
Antipsychotics/ Neuroleptics				
Clozapine, pimozide	Ritonavir co-administration is likely to result in increased plasma concentrations of clozapine or pimozide and is therefore **contraindicated** (see section 4.3).			
Haloperidol, risperidone, thioridazine	Ritonavir dosed as an antiretroviral agent is likely to inhibit CYP2D6 and as a result is expected to increase concentrations of haloperidol, risperidone and thioridazine. Careful monitoring of therapeutic and adverse effects is recommended when these medicines are concomitantly administered with antiretroviral doses of ritonavir (see section 4.3).			
Calcium channel antagonists				
Amlodipine, diltiazem, nifedipine	Ritonavir dosed as a pharmacokinetic enhancer or as an antiretroviral agent inhibits CYP3A4 and as a result is expected to increase the plasma concentrations of calcium channel antagonists. Careful monitoring of therapeutic and adverse effects is recommended when these medicines are concomitantly administered with ritonavir.			

Ritonavir effects on Non-antiretroviral Co-administered Drugs

Co-administered Drug	Dose of Co-administered Drug (mg)	Dose of NORVIR (mg)	Effect on Co-administered Drug AUC	Effect on Co-administered Drug C_{max}
Ergot Derivatives				
Dihydroergotamine, ergonovine, ergotamine, methylergonovine	Ritonavir co-administration is likely to result in increased plasma concentrations of ergot derivatives and is therefore **contraindicated** (see section 4.3).			
GI motility agent				
Cisapride	Ritonavir co-administration is likely to result in increased plasma concentrations of cisapride and is therefore **contraindicated** (see section 4.3).			
HMG Co-A Reductase Inhibitors				
Atorvastatin, Fluvastatin, Lovastatin, Pravstatin, Rosuvastatin, Simvastatin	HMG-CoA reductase inhibitors which are highly dependent on CYP3A metabolism, such as lovastatin and simvastatin, are expected to have markedly increased plasma concentrations when co-administered with ritonavir dosed as an antiretroviral agent or as a pharmacokinetic enhancer. Since increased concentrations of lovastatin and simvastatin may predispose patients to myopathies, including rhabdomyolysis, the combination of these medicinal products with ritonavir is **contraindicated** (see section 4.3). Atorvastatin is less dependent on CYP3A for metabolism. While rosuvastatin elimination is not dependent on CYP3A, an elevation of rosuvastatin exposure has been reported with ritonavir co-administration. The mechanism of this interaction is not clear, but may be the result of transporter inhibition. When used with ritonavir dosed as a pharmacokinetic enhancer or as an antiretroviral agent, the lowest possible doses of atorvastatin or rosuvastatin should be administered. The metabolism of pravastatin and fluvastatin is not dependent on CYP3A, and interactions are not expected with ritonavir. If treatment with an HMG-CoA reductase inhibitor is indicated, pravastatin or fluvastatin is recommended.			
Hormonal contraceptive				
Ethinyl estradiol	50 µg single dose	500 q12h	↓ 40%	↓ 32%
	Due to reductions in ethinyl estradiol concentrations, barrier or other non-hormonal methods of contraception should be considered with concomitant ritonavir use when dosed as an antiretroviral agent or as a pharmacokinetic enhancer. Ritonavir is likely to change the uterine bleeding profile and reduce the effectiveness of estradiol-containing contraceptives (see section 4.4).			
Immunosupressants				
Cyclosporine, tacrolimus, everolimus	Ritonavir dosed as a pharmacokinetic enhancer or as an antiretroviral agent inhibits CYP3A4 and as a result is expected to increase the plasma concentrations of cyclosporine, tacrolimus or everolimus. Careful monitoring of therapeutic and adverse effects is recommended when these medicines are concomitantly administered with ritonavir.			
Phosphodiesterase inhibitors				
Sildenafil	100, single dose	500 q12h	↑ 11-fold	↑ 4-fold
	Concomitant use of sildenafil with ritonavir dosed as an antiretroviral agent or as a pharmacokinetic enhancer is not recommended and in no instance should sildenafil doses exceed 25 mg in 48 hours (see also section 4.4). Concomitant use of sildenafil with ritonavir is **contraindicated** in pulmonary arterial hypertension patients.			
Tadalafil	20, single dose	200 q12h	↑ 124%	↔
	The concomitant use of tadalafil with ritonavir dosed as an antiretroviral agent or as a pharmacokinetic enhancer should be with caution at reduced doses of no more than 10 mg tadalafil every 72 hours with increased monitoring for adverse events (see section 4.4).			
Vardenafil	5, single dose	600 q12h	↑ 49-fold	↑ 13-fold
	The concomitant use of vardenafil and ritonavir dosed as an antiretroviral agent or as a pharmacokinetic enhancer should be with caution at reduced doses of no more than 2.5 mg every 72 hours with increased monitoring for adverse events (see section 4.4).			
Sedatives/hynoptics				
Clorazepate, diazepam, estazolam, flurazepam, oral and parenteral midazolam and triazolam	Ritonavir co-administration is likely to result in increased plasma concentrations of clorazepate, diazepam, estazolam and flurazepam and is therefore **contraindicated** (see section 4.3). Midazolam is extensively metabolised by CYP3A4. Co-administration with Norvir may cause a large increase in the concentration of this benzodiazepine. No drug interaction study has been performed for the co-administration of Norvir with benzodiazepines. Based on data for other CYP3A4 inhibitors, plasma concentrations of midazolam are expected to be significantly higher when midazolam is given orally. Therefore, Norvir should not be co-administered with orally administered midazolam (see section 4.3), whereas caution should be used with co-administration of Norvir and parenteral midazolam. Data from concomitant use of parenteral midazolam with other protease inhibitors suggest a possible 3 – 4 fold increase in midazolam plasma levels. If Norvir is co-administered with parenteral midazolam, it should be done in an intensive care unit (ICU) or similar setting which ensures close clinical monitoring and appropriate medical management in case of respiratory depression and/or prolonged sedation. Dosage adjustment for midazolam should be considered, especially if more than a single dose of midazolam is administered.			
Triazolam	0.125 single dose	200, 4 doses	↑ > 20 fold	↑ 87%
	Ritonavir co-administration is likely to result in increased plasma concentrations of triazolam and is therefore **contraindicated** (see section 4.3).			
Pethidine Norpethidine metabolite	50 oral single dose	500 q12h	↓ 62% ↑ 47%	↓ 59% ↑ 87%
	The use of pethidine and ritonavir is **contraindicated** due to the increased concentrations of the metabolite, norpethidine, which has both analgesic and CNS stimulant activity. Elevated norpethidine concentrations may increase the risk of CNS effects (eg, seizures), see section 4.3.			
Alprazolam	1, single dose	200 q12h, 2 days	↑ 2.5 fold	↔
		500 q12h, 10 days	↓ 12%	↓ 16%
	Alprazolam metabolism was inhibited following the introduction of ritonavir. After ritonavir use for 10 days, no inhibitory effect of ritonavir was observed. Caution is warranted during the first several days when alprazolam is co-administered with ritonavir dosed as an antiretroviral agent or as a pharmacokinetic enhancer, before induction of alprazolam metabolism develops.			
Buspirone	Ritonavir dosed as a pharmacokinetic enhancer or as an antiretroviral agent inhibits CYP3A and as a result is expected to increase the plasma concentrations of buspirone. Careful monitoring of therapeutic and adverse effects is recommended when buspirone concomitantly administered with ritonavir.			
Sleeping agent				
Zolpidem	5	200, 4 doses	↑ 28%	↑ 22%
	Zolpidem and ritonavir may be co-administered with careful monitoring for excessive sedative effects.			

Ritonavir effects on Non-antiretroviral Co-administered Drugs				
Co-administered Drug	**Dose of Co-administered Drug (mg)**	**Dose of NORVIR (mg)**	**Effect on Co-administered Drug AUC**	**Effect on Co-administered Drug C_{max}**
Smoke cessation				
Bupropion	150 mg	100 mg q12h	↓ 22%	↓ 21%
	150 mg	600 mg q12h	↓ 66%	↓ 62%
	Bupropion is primarily metabolised by CYP2B6. Concurrent administration of bupropion with repeated doses of ritonavir is expected to decrease bupropion levels. These effects are thought to represent induction of bupropion metabolism. However, because ritonavir has also been shown to inhibit CYP2B6 in vitro, the recommended dose of bupropion should not be exceeded. In contrast to long-term administration of ritonavir, there was no significant interaction with bupropion after short-term administration of low doses of ritonavir (200 mg twice daily for 2 days), suggesting reductions in bupropion concentrations may have onset several days after initiation of ritonavir co-administration.			
Steroids				
Fluticasone propionate aqueous nasal spray	200 µg qd	100 q12h	↑ ~350-fold	↑ ~ 25-fold
	Systemic corticosteroid effects including Cushing's syndrome and adrenal suppression (plasma cortisol levels were noted to be decreased 86% in the above study) have been reported in patients receiving ritonavir and inhaled or intranasal fluticasone propionate; similar effects could also occur with other corticosteroids metabolised by CYP3A eg, budesonide. Consequently, concomitant administration of ritonavir dosed as an antiretroviral agent or as a pharmacokinetic enhancer and these glucocorticoids is not recommended unless the potential benefit of treatment outweighs the risk of systemic corticosteroid effects (see section 4.4). A dose reduction of the glucocorticoid should be considered with close monitoring of local and systemic effects or a switch to a glucocorticoid, which is not a substrate for CYP3A4 (eg, beclomethasone). Moreover, in case of withdrawal of glucocorticoids progressive dose reduction may be required over a longer period.			
Dexamethasone	Ritonavir dosed as a pharmacokinetic enhancer or as an antiretroviral agent inhibits CYP3A and as a result is expected to increase the plasma concentrations of dexamethasone. Careful monitoring of therapeutic and adverse effects is recommended when dexamethasone is concomitantly administered with ritonavir.			
Prednisolone	20	200 q12h	↑ 28%	↑ 9%
	Careful monitoring of therapeutic and adverse effects is recommended when prednisolone is concomitantly administered with ritonavir. The AUC of the metabolite prednisolone increased by 37 and 28% after 4 and 14 days ritonavir, respectively.			
	ND: Not determined 1. Based on a parallel group comparison 2. Sulfamethoxazole was co-administered with trimethoprim.			

other protease inhibitors or official continuous updates should be consulted for specific information regarding protease mutations associated with reduced response to these agents.

Clinical pharmacodynamic data

The effects of ritonavir (alone or combined with other antiretroviral agents) on biological markers of disease activity such as CD4 cell count and viral RNA were evaluated in several studies involving HIV-1 infected patients. The following studies are the most important.

Adult Use

A controlled study completed in 1996 with ritonavir as add-on therapy in HIV-1 infected patients extensively pre-treated with nucleoside analogues and baseline CD4 cell counts ⩽ 100 cells/µl showed a reduction in mortality and AIDS defining events. The mean average change from baseline over 16 weeks for HIV RNA levels was -0.79 $\log_{10}$ (maximum mean decrease: 1.29 $\log_{10}$) in the ritonavir group versus -0.01 $\log_{10}$ in the control group. The most frequently used nucleosides in this study were zidovudine, stavudine, didanosine and zalcitabine.

In a study completed in 1996 recruiting less advanced HIV-1 infected patients (CD4 200-500 cells/µl) without previous antiretroviral therapy, ritonavir in combination with zidovudine or alone reduced viral load in plasma and increased CD4 count. The mean average change from baseline over 48 weeks for HIV RNA levels was -0.88 $\log_{10}$ in the ritonavir group versus -0.66 $\log_{10}$ in the ritonavir + zidovudine group versus -0.42 $\log_{10}$ in the zidovudine group.

The continuation of ritonavir therapy should be evaluated by viral load because of the possibility of the emergence of resistance as described under section 4.1 Therapeutic indications.

Paediatric Use

In an open label trial completed in 1998 in HIV infected, clinically stable children there was a significant difference (p = 0.03) in the detectable RNA levels in favour of a triple regimen (ritonavir, zidovudine and lamivudine) following 48 weeks treatment.

In a study completed in 2003, 50 HIV-1 infected, protease inhibitor and lamivudine naïve children age 4 weeks to 2 years received ritonavir 350 or 450 mg/m^2 every 12 hours co-administered with zidovudine 160 mg/m^2 every 8 hours and lamivudine 4 mg/kg every 12 hours. In intent to treat analyses, 72% and 36% of patients achieved reduction in plasma HIV-1 RNA of ⩽ 400 copies/ml at Week 16 and 104, respectively. Response was similar in both dosing regimens and across patient age.

In a study completed in 2000, 76 HIV-1 infected children aged 6 months to 12 years who were protease inhibitor naive and naive to lamivudine and/or stavudine received ritonavir 350 or 450 mg/m^2 every 12 hours co-administered with lamivudine and stavudine. In intent to treat analyses, 50% and 57% of patients in the 350 and 450 mg/m^2 dose groups, respectively, achieved reduction in plasma HIV-1 RNA to ⩽ 400 copies/ml at Week 48.

5.2 Pharmacokinetic properties

Absorption:

There is no parenteral formulation of ritonavir, therefore the extent of absorption and absolute bioavailability have not been determined. The pharmacokinetics of ritonavir during multiple dose regimens were studied in non-fasting HIV-infected adult volunteers. Upon multiple dosing, ritonavir accumulation is slightly less than predicted from a single dose due to a time and dose-related increase in apparent clearance (Cl/F). Trough concentrations of ritonavir decrease over time, possibly due to enzyme induction, but appeared to stabilise by the end of 2 weeks. The time to maximum concentration (T_{max}) remained constant at approximately 4 hours with increasing dose. Renal clearance averaged less than 0.1 l/h and was relatively constant throughout the dosage range.

The pharmacokinetic parameters observed with various dosing schemes of ritonavir alone are shown in the table below.

(see Table 5 on next page)

Effects of food on oral absorption:

Ingestion of ritonavir with food results in higher ritonavir exposure than ingestion in the fasted state.

Distribution:

The apparent volume of distribution (V_B/F) of ritonavir is approximately 20 - 40 l after a single 600 mg dose. The protein binding of ritonavir in human plasma is approximately 98 - 99% and is constant over the concentration range of 1.0 – 100 µg /ml. Ritonavir binds to both human alpha 1-acid glycoprotein (AAG) and human serum albumin (HSA) with comparable affinities.

Tissue distribution studies with ^{14}C-labelled ritonavir in rats showed the liver, adrenals, pancreas, kidneys and thyroid to have the highest concentrations of ritonavir. Tissue to plasma ratios of approximately 1 measured in rat lymph nodes suggests that ritonavir distributes into lymphatic tissues. Ritonavir penetrates minimally into the brain.

Metabolism:

Ritonavir was noted to be extensively metabolised by the hepatic cytochrome P450 system, primarily by the CYP3A isozyme family and to a lesser extent by the CYP2D6 isoform. Animal studies as well as *in vitro* experiments with human hepatic microsomes indicated that ritonavir primarily underwent oxidative metabolism. Four ritonavir metabolites have been identified in man. The isopropylthiazole oxidation metabolite (M-2) is the major metabolite and has antiviral activity similar to that of parent drug. However, the AUC of the M-2 metabolite was approximately 3% of the AUC of parent drug.

Low doses of ritonavir have shown profound effects on the pharmacokinetics of other protease inhibitors (and other products metabolised by CYP3A4) and other protease inhibitors may influence the pharmacokinetics of ritonavir (see section 4.5).

Elimination:

Human studies with radiolabelled ritonavir demonstrated that the elimination of ritonavir was primarily via the hepatobiliary system; approximately 86% of radiolabel was recovered from stool, part of which is expected to be unabsorbed ritonavir. In these studies renal elimination was not found to be a major route of elimination of ritonavir. This was consistent with the observations in animal studies.

Special Populations: No clinically significant differences in AUC or C_{max} were noted between males and females. Ritonavir pharmacokinetic parameters were not statistically significantly associated with body weight or lean body mass. Ritonavir plasma exposures in patients 50 – 70 years of age when dosed 100 mg in combination with lopinavir or at higher doses in the absence of other protease inhibitors is similar to that observed in younger adults.

Patients with impaired liver function: after multiple dosing of ritonavir to healthy volunteers (500 mg twice daily) and subjects with mild to moderate hepatic impairment (Child Pugh Class A and B, 400 mg twice daily) exposure to ritonavir after dose normalisation was not significantly different between the two groups.

Patients with impaired renal function: Ritonavir pharmacokinetic parameters have not been studied in patients with renal impairment. However, since the renal clearance of ritonavir is negligible, no changes in the total body clearance are expected in patients with renal impairment.

Paediatric Patients: Ritonavir steady-state pharmacokinetic parameters were evaluated in HIV infected children above 2 years of age receiving doses ranging from 250 mg/m^2 twice daily to 400 mg/m^2 twice daily. Ritonavir concentrations obtained after 350 to 400 mg/m^2 twice daily in paediatric patients were comparable to those obtained in adults receiving 600 mg (approximately 330 mg/m^2) twice daily. Across dose groups, ritonavir oral clearance (CL/F/m^2) was approximately 1.5 to 1.7 times faster in paediatric patients above 2 years of age than in adult subjects.

Ritonavir steady-state pharmacokinetic parameters were evaluated in HIV infected children less than 2 years of age receiving doses ranging from 350 to 450 mg/m^2 twice daily. Ritonavir concentrations in this study were highly variable and somewhat lower than those obtained in adults receiving 600 mg (approximately 330 mg/m^2) twice daily. Across dose groups, ritonavir oral clearance (CL/F/m^2) declined with age with median values of 9.0 L/h/m^2 in children less than 3 months of age, 7.8 L/h/m^2 in children between 3 and 6 months of age and 4.4 L/h/m^2 in children between 6 and 24 months of age.

5.3 Preclinical safety data

Repeated dose toxicity studies in animals identified major target organs as the liver, retina, thyroid gland and kidney. Hepatic changes involved hepatocellular, biliary and phagocytic elements and were accompanied by increases in hepatic enzymes. Hyperplasia of the retinal pigment epithelium (RPE) and retinal degeneration have been seen in all of the rodent studies conducted with ritonavir, but

Table 4

Undesirable Effects in Clinical Studies and Post-marketing in Adult Patients		
Immune system disorders	Common	Allergic reactions including urticaria, mild skin eruptions, bronchospasm and angioedema
	Rare	Anaphylaxis and Stevens Johnson syndrome
Blood and lymphatic system disorders	Common	Decreased WBC, decreased haemoglobin, decreased neutrophils, increased eosinophils
	Uncommon	Increased WBC, increased neutrophils and increased prothrombin time
	Unknown frequency	Thrombocytopenia
Metabolic and nutritional disorders	Uncommon	Dehydration, diabetes mellitus
	Rare	Hyperglycaemia
	Unknown frequency	Hypertriglyceridaemia, hypercholesterolaemia, hyperuricaemia
Nervous system disorders	Very common	Taste perversion, circumoral and peripheral paresthesia, headache
	Common	Dizziness, paraesthesia, hyperaesthesia, somnolence, insomnia, anxiety
	Unknown frequency	Seizure, syncope
Vascular disorders	Common	Vasodilation
	Unknown frequency	Orthostatic hypotension
Respiratory, thoracic and mediastinal disorders	Common	Pharyngitis, cough increased
Gastrointestinal disorders	Very common	Abdominal pain, nausea, diarrhoea, vomiting
	Common	Dyspepsia, anorexia, local throat irritation, flatulence, dry mouth, eructation, mouth ulcer
Hepatobiliary disorders	Uncommon	Hepatitis and jaundice
Skin and subcutaneous tissue disorders	Common	Rash, pruritus, sweating, lipodystrophy
Musculoskeletal and connective tissue disorders	Common	Increased CPK, myalgia
	Uncommon	Myositis, rhabdomyolysis
Renal and urinary disorders	Unknown frequency	Acute renal failure
Reproductive system and breast disorders	Unknown frequency	Menorrhagia
General disorders and administration site conditions	Very common	Asthenia
	Common	Fever, pain weight loss
Investigations	Common	Increased GGT, increased CPK, increased triglycerides, increased SGPT, increased SGOT, increased amylase, increased uric acid, decreased potassium, decreased free and total thyroxin
	Uncommon	Increased glucose, decreased total calcium, increased magnesium, increased bilirubin, increased alkaline phosphatase

have not been seen in dogs. Ultrastructural evidence suggests that these retinal changes may be secondary to phospholipidosis. However, clinical trials revealed no evidence of drug-induced ocular changes in humans. All thyroid changes were reversible upon discontinuation of ritonavir. Clinical investigation in humans has revealed no clinically significant alteration in thyroid function tests. Renal changes including tubular degeneration, chronic inflammation and proteinurea were noted in rats and are felt to be attributable to species-specific spontaneous disease. Furthermore, no clinically significant renal abnormalities were noted in clinical trials.

Developmental toxicity observed in rats (embryolethality, decreased foetal body weight and ossification delays and visceral changes, including delayed testicular descent) occurred mainly at a maternally toxic dosage. Developmental toxicity in rabbits (embryolethality, decreased litter size and decreased foetal weights) occurred at a maternally toxic dosage.

Ritonavir was not found to be mutagenic or clastogenic in a battery of *in vitro* and *in vivo* assays including the Ames bacterial reverse mutation assay using *S. typhimurium* and *E. coli*, the mouse lymphoma assay, the mouse micronucleus test and chromosomal aberration assays in human lymphocytes.

Long term carcinogenicity studies of ritonavir in mice and rats revealed tumourigenic potential specific for these species, but are regarded as of no relevance for humans.

Table 5

Ritonavir Dosing Regimen	100 mg once daily	100 mg twice daily[1]	200 mg once daily	200 mg twice daily	600 mg twice daily
C_{max} (μg/ml)	0.84 ± 0.39	0.89	3.4 ± 1.3	4.5 ± 1.3	11.2 ± 3.6
C_{trough} (μg/ml)	0.08 ± 0.04	0.22	0.16 ± 0.10	0.6 ± 0.2	3.7 ± 2.6
$AUC_{12\ or\ 24}$ (μg•h/ml)	6.6 ± 2.4	6.2	20.0 ± 5.6	21.92 ± 6.48	77.5 ± 31.5
$t_{½}$ (h)	~5	~5	~4	~8	~3 to 5
Cl/F (L/h)	17.2 ± 6.6	16.1	10.8 ± 3.1	10.0 ± 3.2	8.8 ± 3.2

[1] Values expressed as geometric means. Note: ritonavir was dosed after a meal for all listed regimens.

6. PHARMACEUTICAL PARTICULARS

6.1 List of excipients

Norvir oral solution contains:

alcohol,

purified water,

polyoxyl 35 castor oil,

propylene glycol,

anhydrous citric acid,

saccharin sodium,

peppermint oil,

creamy caramel flavour,

sunset yellow E110

6.2 Incompatibilities

Norvir should not be diluted with water.

6.3 Shelf life

6 months

6.4 Special precautions for storage

Store below 25°C and use within the expiry date shown on the bottle. Do not refrigerate or freeze.

Avoid exposure to excessive heat. Keep the bottle tightly closed.

6.5 Nature and contents of container

Norvir oral solution is supplied in amber coloured multiple-dose polyethylene terephthalate (PET) bottles in a 90 ml size. Each pack contains 5 bottles of 90 ml (450 ml). A dosage cup containing graduations at 3.75 ml (300 mg dose), 5 ml (400 mg dose), 6.25 ml (500 mg dose) and 7.5 ml (600 mg dose) is provided.

6.6 Special precautions for disposal and other handling

Shake well before each use. If, after shaking, particles or precipitate can be seen in the solution, the patient should take the next dose and see their doctor about a fresh supply.

The dosage cup or oral syringe should be cleaned immediately with hot water and dish soap after use. When cleaned immediately, drug residue is removed. The device **must** be dry prior to use

7. MARKETING AUTHORISATION HOLDER

Abbott Laboratories Limited

Queenborough

Kent ME11 5EL

United Kingdom

8. MARKETING AUTHORISATION NUMBER(S)

EU/1/96/016/001

9. DATE OF FIRST AUTHORISATION/RENEWAL OF THE AUTHORISATION

Date of first authorisation: 26 August 1996

Date of last renewal: 27 August 2006

10. DATE OF REVISION OF THE TEXT

2nd September 2009

Norvir Soft Capsules

(Abbott Laboratories Limited)

1. NAME OF THE MEDICINAL PRODUCT

Norvir 100 mg soft capsules

2. QUALITATIVE AND QUANTITATIVE COMPOSITION

Each soft capsule contains 100 mg ritonavir.

Excipients (per soft capsule):

Alcohol (12%w/w)

Castor Oil Polyoxyl 35

For a full list of excipients, see section 6.1.

3. PHARMACEUTICAL FORM

Soft capsule.

The capsule is white with "Abbott A" and the code "DS100" imprinted on the shell in black ink.

4. CLINICAL PARTICULARS

4.1 Therapeutic indications

Ritonavir is indicated in combination with other antiretroviral agents for the treatment of HIV-1 infected patients (adults and children of 2 years of age and older).

4.2 Posology and method of administration

Ritonavir should be administered by physicians who are experienced in the treatment of HIV infection.

Ritonavir soft capsules are administered orally and should preferably be ingested with food.

Ritonavir dosed as a pharmacokinetic enhancer

The following HIV-1 protease inhibitors have been approved for use with ritonavir as a pharmacokinetic enhancer at the noted doses.

Adult use:

Amprenavir 600 mg twice daily with ritonavir 100 mg twice daily

Atazanavir 300 mg daily with ritonavir 100 mg daily

Fosamprenavir 700 mg twice daily with ritonavir 100 mg twice daily

Lopinavir 400 mg co-formulated with ritonavir 100 mg twice daily

Saquinavir 1000 mg twice daily with ritonavir 100 mg twice daily

Tipranavir 500 mg twice daily with ritonavir 200 mg twice daily

Darunavir 600 mg twice daily with ritonavir 100 mg twice daily

Paediatric use: Lopinavir co-formulated with ritonavir is recommended for children 2 years of age and older. For further dosage recommendations, refer to the product information of other Protease Inhibitors approved for co-administered with ritonavir.

Renal impairment: As ritonavir is primarily metabolised by the liver, ritonavir may be appropriate for use with caution as a pharmacokinetic enhancer in patients with renal insufficiency depending on the specific protease inhibitor with which it is co-administered. However, since the renal clearance of ritonavir is negligible, the decrease in the total body clearance is not expected in patients with renal impairment. For specific dosing information in patients with renal impairment, refer to the Summary of Product Characteristics (SPC) of the co-administered protease inhibitor.

Hepatic impairment: Ritonavir should not be given as a pharmacokinetic enhancer to patients with decompensated liver disease. In the absence of pharmacokinetic studies in patients with stable severe hepatic impairment (Child Pugh Grade C) without decompensation, caution should be exercised when ritonavir is used as a pharmacokinetic enhancer as increased levels of the co-administered PI may occur. Specific recommendations for use of ritonavir as a pharmacokinetic enhancer in patients with hepatic impairment are dependent on the protease inhibitor with which it is co-administered. The SPC of the co-administered PI should be reviewed for specific dosing information in this patient population.

Ritonavir dosed as an antiretroviral agent

Adult use: The recommended dosage of Norvir soft capsules is 600 mg (6 capsules) twice daily by mouth.

Gradually increasing the dose of ritonavir when initiating therapy may help to improve tolerance. Treatment should be initiated at 300 mg (3 capsules) twice daily for a period of three days and increased by 100 mg (1 capsule) twice daily increments up to 600 mg twice daily over a period of no longer than 14 days. Patients should not remain on 300 mg twice daily for more than 3 days.

Paediatric use (2 years of age and above): the recommended dosage of Norvir in children is 350 mg/m^2 by mouth twice daily and should not exceed 600 mg twice daily. Norvir should be started at 250 mg/m^2 and increased at 2 to 3 day intervals by 50 mg/m^2 twice daily (please refer to the Norvir 80 mg/ml oral solution Summary of Product Characteristics)

For older children it may be feasible to substitute soft capsules for the maintenance dose of the oral solution.

Dosage conversion from oral solution to soft capsules for children

Oral solution dose	Capsule dose
175 mg (2.2 ml) twice daily	200 mg in the morning and 200 mg in the evening
350 mg (4.4 ml) twice daily	400 mg in the morning and 300 mg in the evening
437.5 mg (5.5 ml) twice daily	500 mg in the morning and 400 mg in the evening
525 mg (6.6 ml) twice daily	500 mg in the morning and 500 mg in the evening

The safety and efficacy of ritonavir in children under the age of 2 have not been established.

Renal impairment: Currently, there are no data specific to this patient population and therefore specific dosage recommendations cannot be made. The renal clearance of ritonavir is negligible, therefore, a decrease in the total body clearance is not expected in patients with renal impairment. Because ritonavir is highly protein bound it is unlikely that it will be significantly removed by haemodialysis or peritoneal dialysis.

Hepatic impairment: Ritonaviris principally metabolised and eliminated by the liver. Pharmacokinetic data indicate that no dose adjustment is necessary in patients with mild to moderate hepatic impairment (see section 5.2). Ritonavir should not be given to patients with severe hepatic impairment (see section 4.3).

Special Populations: Pharmacokinetic data indicated that no dose adjustment is necessary for elderly patients (see section 5.2).

4.3 Contraindications

Hypersensitivity to the active substance or to any of the excipients.

When ritonavir is used as a pharmacokinetic enhancer of other PIs, consult the Summary of Product Characteristics of the co-administered protease inhibitor for contraindications.

Ritonavir should not be given as a pharmacokinetic enhancer or as an antiretroviral agent to patients with decompensated liver disease.

In vitro and *in vivo* studies have demonstrated that ritonavir is a potent inhibitor of CYP3A- and CYP2D6- mediated biotransformations. The following medicines are contraindicated when used with ritonavir and unless otherwise noted, the contraindication is based on the potential for ritonavir to inhibit metabolism of the co-administered drug, resulting in increased exposure to the co-administered drug and risk of clinically significant adverse effects.

The enzyme-modulating effect of ritonavir may be dose dependent. For some products, contraindications may be more relevant when ritonavir is used as an antiretroviral agent than when ritonavir is used as a pharmacokinetic enhancer (eg rifabutin and voriconazole):

(see Table 1 below)

4.4 Special warnings and precautions for use

Ritonavir is not a cure for HIV-1 infection or AIDS. Patients receiving Ritonavir or any other antiretroviral therapy may continue to develop opportunistic infections and other complications of HIV-1 infection.

Patients should be advised that current antiretroviral therapy has not been proven to prevent the risk of transmission of HIV to others through blood or sexual contact. Appropriate precautions should continue to be used.

When ritonavir is used as a pharmacokinetic enhancer with other PIs, full details on the warnings and precautions relevant to that particular PI should be considered, therefore the Summary of Product Characteristics for the particular PI must be consulted.

Ritonavir dosed as an antiretroviral agent or as a pharmacokinetic enhancer

Patients with chronic diarrhoea or malabsorption: Extra monitoring is recommended when diarrhoea occurs. The relatively high frequency of diarrhoea during treatment with ritonavir may compromise the absorption and efficacy (due to decreased compliance) of ritonavir or other concurrent medications. Serious persistent vomiting and/or diarrhoea associated with ritonavir use might also compromise renal function. It is advisable to monitor renal function in patients with renal function impairment.

Haemophilia: there have been reports of increased bleeding, including spontaneous skin haematomas and haemarthroses, in haemophiliac patients type A and B treated with protease inhibitors. In some patients additional factor VIII was given. In more than a half of the reported cases, treatment with protease inhibitors was continued or reintroduced if treatment had been discontinued. A causal relationship has been evoked, although the mechanism of action has not been elucidated. Haemophiliac patients should therefore be made aware of the possibility of increased bleeding.

Diabetes mellitus and hyperglycaemia: New onset diabetes mellitus, hyperglycaemia or exacerbation of existing diabetes mellitus has been reported in patients receiving protease inhibitors. In some of these the hyperglycaemia was severe and in some cases also associated with ketoacidosis. Many patients had confounding medical conditions, some of which required therapy with agents that have been associated with the development of diabetes mellitus or hyperglycaemia.

Lipodystrophy: Combination antiretroviral therapy has been associated with redistribution of body fat (lipodystrophy) in HIV patients. The long-term consequences of these events are currently unknown. Knowledge about the mechanism is incomplete. A connection between visceral lipomatosis and PIs and lipoatrophy and nucleoside reverse transcriptase inhibitors (NRTIs) has been hypothesised. A higher risk of lipodystrophy has been associated with individual factors such as older age, and with drug related factors such as longer duration of antiretroviral treatment and associated metabolic disturbances. Clinical examination should include evaluation for physical signs of fat redistribution. Consideration should be given to measurement of fasting serum lipids and blood glucose. Lipid disorders should be managed as clinically appropriate (see section 4.8).

Pancreatitis: Pancreatitis should be considered if clinical symptoms (nausea, vomiting, abdominal pain) or

Table 1

Drug Class	Drugs within Class	Rationale
Concomitant Drug Levels Increased		
α_1-Adrenoreceptor Antagonist	Alfuzosin	Increased plasma concentrations of alfuzosin which may lead to severe hypotension (see section 4.5).
Analgesics	Pethidine, piroxicam, propoxyphne	Increased plasma concentrations of norpethidine, piroxicam and propoxyphene. Thereby, increasing the risk of serious respiratory depression or haematologic abnormalities, or other serious adverse effects from these agents.
Antiarrhythmics	Amiodarone, bepridil, encainide, flecanide, propafenone, quinidine	Increased plasma concentrations of amiodarone, bepridil, encainide, flecanide, propafenone, quinidine. Thereby, increasing the risk of arrhythmias or other serious adverse effects from these agents.
Antibiotic	Fusidic Acid	Increased plasma concentrations of fusidic acid and ritonavir.
Antifungal	Voriconazole	Concomitant use of ritonavir (400 mg twice daily and more) and voriconazole is contraindicated due to a reduction in voriconazole plasma concentrations and possible loss of effect (see section 4.5)
Antihistamines	Astemizole, terfenadine	Increased plasma concentrations of astemizole and terfenadine. Thereby, increasing the risk of serious arrhythmias from these agents.
Antimycobacterial	Rifabutin	Concomitant use of ritonavir dosed as an antiretroviral agent (600 mg twice daily) and rifabutin due to an increase of rifabutin serum concentrations and risk of adverse events including uveitis (see section 4.4). Recommendations regarding use of ritonavir dosed as a pharmacokinetic enhancer with rifabutin are noted in section 4.5
Antipsychotics/ Neuroleptics	Clozapine, pimozide	Increased plasma concentrations of clozapine and pimozide. Thereby, increasing the risk of serious haematologic abnormalities, or other serious adverse effects from these agents.
Ergot Derivatives	Dihydroergotamine, ergonovine, ergotamine, methylergonovine	Increased plasma concentrations of ergot derivatives leading to acute ergot toxicity, including vasospasm and ischaemia.
GI motility agent	Cisapride	Increased plasma concentrations of cisapride. Thereby, increasing the risk of serious arrhythmias from this agent.
HMG Co-A Reductase Inhibitor	Lovastatin, simvastatin	Increased plasma concentrations of lovastatin and simvastatin; thereby, increasing the risk of myopathy including rhabdomyolysis (see section 4.5).
Sedatives/hypnotics	Clorazepate, diazepam, estazolam, flurazepam, oral midazolam and triazolam	Increased plasma concentrations of clorazepate, diazepam, estazolam, flurazepam, oral midazolam and triazolam. Thereby, increasing the risk of extreme sedation and respiratory depression from these agents. (For caution on parenterally administered midazolam, see section 4.5.)
Ritonavir Drug Level Decreased		
Herbal Preparation	St. John's Wort	Herbal preparations containing St John's wort (*Hypericum perforatum*) due to the risk of decreased plasma concentrations and reduced clinical effects of ritonavir (see section 4.5).

abnormalities in laboratory values (such as increased serum lipase or amylase values) suggestive of pancreatitis should occur. Patients who exhibit these signs or symptoms should be evaluated and Norvir therapy should be discontinued if a diagnosis of pancreatitis is made (see section 4.8).

Immune Reactivation Syndrome: in HIV-infected patients with severe immune deficiency at the time of institution of combination antiretroviral therapy (CART), an inflammatory reaction to asymtomatic or residual opportunistic pathogens may arise and cause serious clinical conditions, or aggravation of symptoms. Typically, such reactions have been observed within the first few weeks or months of initiation of CART. Relevant examples are cytomegalovirus retinitis, generalised and/or focal mycobacterial infections, and Pneumocystis carinii pneumonia. Any inflammatory symptoms should be evaluated and treatment instituted when necessary.

Liver disease: Ritonavir should not be given to patients with decompensated liver disease. For patients with stable severe hepatic impairment (Child Pugh Grade C) without decompensation see section 4.2. Patients with chronic hepatitis B or C and treated with combination antiretroviral therapy are at an increased risk for severe and potentially fatal hepatic adverse events. In case of concomitant antiviral therapy for hepatitis B or C, please refer to the relevant product information for these medicinal products.

Patients with pre-existing liver dysfunction including chronic active hepatitis have an increased frequency of liver function abnormalities during combination antiretroviral therapy and should be monitored according to standard practice. If there is evidence of worsening liver disease in such patients, interruption or discontinuation of treatment must be considered.

Renal disease: Since the renal clearance of ritonavir is negligible, the decrease in the total body clearance is not expected in patients with renal impairment. For specific dosing information in patients with renal impairment, refer to the Summary of Product Characteristics (SPC) of the co-administered protease inhibitor. See also section 4.2.

Osteonecrosis: Although the etiology is considered to be multifactorial (including corticosteroid use, alcohol consumption, severe immunosuppression, higher body mass index), cases of osteonecrosis have been reported in patients with advanced HIV-disease and/or long-term exposure to combination antiretroviral therapy (CART). Patients should be advised to seek medical advice if they experience joint aches and pain, joint stiffness or difficulty in movement.

This medicinal product contains small amounts of ethanol (alcohol), less than 100 mg per maximum dose of 600 mg.

PR interval prolongation: ritonavir has been shown to cause modest asymptomatic prolongation of the PR interval in some healthy adult subjects. Rare reports of 2nd or 3rd degree atrioventricular block in patients with underlying structural heart disease and pre-existing conduction system abnormalities or in patients receiving drugs known to prolong the PR interval (such as verapamil or atazanavir) have been reported in patients receiving ritonavir. Norvir should be used with caution in such patients (see section 5.1).

Interactions with other medicinal products

Ritonavir dosed as an antiretroviral agent

The following Warnings and Precautions should be considered when ritonavir is used as a antiretroviral agent. When ritonavir is used as a pharmacokinetic enhancer at the 100 mg and 200 mg level it cannot be assumed that the following warnings and precautions will also apply. When ritonavir is used as a pharmacokinetic enhancer, full details on the warnings and precautions relevant to that particular PI must be considered, therefore the Summary of Product Characteristics, section 4.4, for the particular PI must be consulted to determine if the information below is applicable.

PDE5 inhibitors: Particular caution should be used when prescribing sildenafil, tadalafil or vardenafil in patients receiving ritonavir. Co-administration of ritonavir with these medicinal products is expected to substantially increase their concentrations and may result in associated adverse events such as hypotension and prolonged erection (see section 4.5).

HMG-CoA reductase inhibitors: The HMG-CoA reductase inhibitors simvastatin and lovastatin are highly dependent on CYP3A for metabolism, thus concomitant use of ritonavir with simvastatin or lovastatin is not recommended due to an increased risk of myopathy including rhabdomyolysis. Caution must also be exercised and reduced doses should be considered if ritonavir is used concurrently with atorvastatin, which is metabolised to a lesser extent by CYP3A. While rosuvastatin elimination is not dependent on CYP3A, an elevation of rosuvastatin exposure has been reported with ritonavir co-administration. The mechanism of this interaction is not clear, but may be the result of transporter inhibition. When used with ritonavir dosed as a pharmacokinetic enhancer or as an antiretroviral agent, the lowest doses of atorvastatin or rosuvastatin should be administered. The metabolism of pravastatin and fluvastatin is not dependent of CYP3A, and interactions are not expected with ritonavir. If treatment with an HMG-CoA reductase inhibitor is indicated, pravastatin or fluvastatin is recommended (see section 4.5).

Digoxin: Particular caution should be used when prescribing ritonavir in patients taking digoxin since co-administration of ritonavir with digoxin is expected to increase digoxin levels. The increased digoxin levels may lessen over time (see section 4.5).

In patients who are already taking digoxin when ritonavir is introduced, the digoxin dose should be reduced to one-half of the patients' normal dose and patients need to be followed more closely than usual for several weeks after initiating co-administration of ritonavir and digoxin.

In patients who are already taking ritonavir when digoxin is introduced, digoxin should be introduced more gradually than usual. Digoxin levels should be monitored more intensively than usual during this period, with dose adjustments made, as necessary, based on clinical, electrocardiographic and digoxin level findings.

Ethinyl estradiol: Barrier or other non-hormonal methods of contraception should be considered when administering ritonavir at therapeutic or low doses as ritonavir is likely to reduce the effect and change the uterine bleeding profile when co-administered with estradiol-containing contraceptives.

Glucocorticoids: Concomitant use of ritonavir and fluticasone or other glucocorticoids that are metabolised by CYP3A4 is not recommended unless the potential benefit of treatment outweighs the risk of systemic corticosteroid effects, including Cushing's syndrome and adrenal suppression (see section 4.5).

Trazodone: Particular caution should be used when prescribing ritonavir in patients using trazodone. Trazodone is a CYP3A4 substrate and co-administration of ritonavir is expected to increase trazodone levels. Adverse events of nausea, dizziness, hypotension and syncope have been observed in single dose interaction studies in healthy volunteers (see section 4.5)

Ritonavir dosed as a pharmacokinetic enhancer

The interaction profiles of HIV-protease inhibitors, co-administered with low dose ritonavir, are dependant on the specific co-administered protease inhibitor.

For a description of the mechanisms and potential mechanisms contributing to the interaction profile of the PIs, see section 4.5. Please also review the Summary of Product Characteristics for the particular boosted PI.

Saquinavir: Doses of ritonavir higher than 100 mg twice daily should not be used. Higher doses of ritonavir have been shown to be associated with an increased incidence of adverse events. Co-administration of saquinavir and ritonavir has led to severe adverse events, mainly diabetic ketoacidosis and liver disorders, especially in patients with pre-existing liver disease.

Saquinavir/ritonavir should not be given together with rifampicin, due to the risk of severe hepatotoxicity (presenting as increased hepatic transaminases) if the three medicines are given together (see section 4.5).

Tipranavir: co-administered with 200 mg of ritonavir has been associated with reports of clinical hepatitis and hepatic decompensation including some fatalities. Extra vigilance is warranted in patients with chronic hepatitis B or hepatitis C co-infection, as these patients have an increased risk of hepatotoxicity.

Doses of ritonavir lower than 200 mg twice daily should not be used as they might alter the efficacy profile of the combination.

Fosamprenavir: Co-administration of fosamprenavir with ritonavir in doses greater than 100 mg twice daily has not been clinically evaluated. The use of higher ritonavir doses might alter the safety profile of the combination and therefore is not recommended.

Atazanavir: Co-administration of atazanavir with ritonavir at doses greater than 100 mg once daily has not been clinically evaluated. The use of higher ritonavir doses may alter the safety profile of atazanavir (cardiac effects, hyperbilirubinemia) and therefore is not recommended. Only when atazanavir with ritonavir is co-administered with efavirenz, a dose increase of ritonavir to 200mg once daily could be considered. In this instance, close clinical monitoring is warranted. Refer to the Reyataz Summary of Product Characteristics for further details.

4.5 Interaction with other medicinal products and other forms of interaction

Ritonavir dosed as a pharmacokinetic enhancer or as an antiretroviral agent

Ritonavir has a high affinity for several cytochrome P450 (CYP) isoforms and may inhibit oxidation with the following ranked order: CYP3A4 > CYP2D6. Co-administration of Norvir and medicinal products primarily metabolised by CYP3A may result in increased plasma concentrations of the other medicinal product, which could increase or prolong its therapeutic and adverse effects. For select medicinal products (eg alprazolam) the inhibitory effects of ritonavir on CYP3A4 may decrease over time. Ritonavir also has a high affinity for P-glycoprotein and may inhibit this transporter. The inhibitory effect of ritonavir (with or without other protease inhibitors) on P-gp activity may decrease over time (eg digoxin and fexofenadine-see table "Ritonavir effects on non-antiretroviral drugs" below). Ritonavir may induce glucuronidation and oxidation by CYP1A2, CYP2C8, CYP2C9 and CYP2C19 thereby increasing the biotransformation of some medicinal products metabolised by these pathways, and may result in decreased systemic exposure to such medicinal products, which could decease or shorten their therapeutic effect.

Important information regarding drug interactions when ritonavir is used as a pharmacokinetic enhancer is also contained in the Summary of Product Characteristics of the co-administered protease inhibitor.

Drugs that affect ritonavir levels

Serum levels of ritonavir can be reduced by concomitant use of herbal preparations containing St John's wort (*Hypericum perforatum*). This is due to the induction of drug metabolising enzymes by St John's wort. Herbal preparations containing St John's wort must not be used in combination with ritonavir. If a patient is already taking St John's wort, stop St John's wort and if possible check viral levels. Ritonavir levels may increase on stopping St John's wort. The dose of ritonavir may need adjusting. The inducing effect may persist for at least 2 weeks after cessation of treatment with St John's wort (see section 4.3).

Serum levels of ritonavir may be affected by select co-administered medicinal products (eg delavirdine, efavirenz, phenytoin and rifampicin). These interactions are noted in the drug interaction tables below.

Drugs that are affected by the use of ritonavir

Interactions between ritonavir and protease inhibitors, antiretroviral agents other than protease inhibitors and other non-antiretroviral drugs are listed in the tables below.

(see Table 2 on next page)

Cardiac and neurologic events have been reported when ritonavir has been co-administered with disopyramide, mexiletine or nefazadone. The possibility of drug interaction cannot be excluded.

In addition to the interactions listed above, as ritonavir is highly protein bound, the possibility of increased therapeutic and toxic effects due to protein binding displacement of concomitant medications should be considered.

Ritonavir dosed as a pharmacokinetic enhancer

Important information regarding drug interactions when ritonavir is used a pharmacokinetic enhancer is also contained in the Summary of Product Characteristics of the co-administered protease inhibitor.

Proton pump inhibitors and H_2-receptor antagonists: proton pump inhibitors and H_2-receptor antagonists (e.g. omeprazole or ranitidine) may reduce concentrations for co-administered protease inhibitors. For specific information regarding the impact of co-administration of acid reducing agents, refer to the SmPC of the co-administered protease inhibitor. Based on interaction studies with the ritonavir boosted protease inhibitors (lopinavir/ritonavir, atazanavir), concurrent administration of omeprazole or ranitidine does not significantly modify ritonavir efficacy as a pharmacokinetic enhancer despite a slight change of exposure (about 6 - 18%).

4.6 Pregnancy and lactation

A limited number (> 800) of pregnant women were exposed to ritonavir during pregnancy; a very limited number (< 300) were exposed during the first trimester. These data largely refer to exposures where ritonavir was used in combination therapy and not at therapeutic ritonavir doses but at lower doses as a pharmacokinetic enhancer for other PIs. These limited data indicate no increase in the rate of birth defects compared to rates observed in population-based birth defect surveillance systems. Animal data have shown reproductive toxicity (see 5.3). The use of Norvir may be considered in pregnancy only when the benefits outweigh the risk to the foetus.

Ritonavir adversely interacts with oral contraceptives (OCs). Therefore, an alternative, effective and safe method of contraception should be used during treatment.

It is not known whether this medicine is excreted in human milk. Milk excretion has not been measured in the animal studies, however a study in rats showed some effects on offspring development during lactation which are compatible with excretion of ritonavir in milk in that species. HIV infected women should not breast-feed their infants under any circumstances to avoid transmission of HIV.

4.7 Effects on ability to drive and use machines

No studies on the effects on the ability to drive and use machines have been performed. As somnolence and dizziness are known undesirable effects, this should be taken into account when driving or using machinery.

4.8 Undesirable effects

Ritonavir dosed as a pharmacokinetic enhancer

Adverse events associated with the use of ritonavir as a pharmacokinetic enhancer are dependent on the specific co-administered PI. For information on adverse events refer to the SPC of the specific co-administered PI.

Ritonavir dosed as an antiretroviral agent

In the original clinical studies (Phase II/III), adverse events with possible, probable or unknown relationship to ritonavir were reported in ⩾ 2% of 1033 patients.

The following adverse reactions of moderate to severe intensity with possible or probable relationship to Ritonavir have been reported. Within each frequency grouping, undesirable effects are presented in order of decreasing

Table 2

Drug Interactions – Ritonavir with Protease Inhibitors

Co-administered Drug	Dose of Co-administered Drug (mg)	Dose of NORVIR (mg)	Drug Assessed	AUC	Cmin
Amprenavir	600 q12h	100 q12h	Amprenavir[2]	↑ 64%	↑ 5 fold
	Ritonavir increases the serum levels of amprenavir as a result of CYP3A4 inhibition. Clinical trials confirmed the safety and efficacy of 600 mg amprenavir twice daily with ritonavir 100 mg twice daily. Norvir oral solution should not be co-administered with amprenavir oral solution to children due to the risk of toxicity from excipients in the two formulations. For further information, physicians should refer to the Agenerase Summary of Product Characteristics.				
Atazanavir	300 q24h	100 q24h	Atazanavir	↑ 86%	↑ 11 fold
			Atazanavir[1]	↑ 2 fold	↑ 3-7 fold
	Ritonavir increases the serum levels of atazanavir as a result of CYP3A4 inhibition. Clinical trials confirmed the safety and efficacy of 300 mg atazanavir once daily with ritonavir 100 mg once daily in treatment experienced patients. For further information, physicians should refer to the Reyataz Summary of Product Characteristics.				
Darunavir	600, single	100 q12h	Darunavir	↑ 14 fold	
	Ritonavir increases the serum levels of darunavir as a result of CYP3A inhibition. Darunavir must be given with ritonavir to ensure its therapeutic effect. Ritonavir doses higher than 100 mg twice daily have not been studied with darunavir. For further information, refer to the Summary of Product Characteristics for Prezista.				
Fosamprenavir	700 q12h	100 q12h	Amprenavir	↑ 2.4 fold	↑ 11 fold
	Ritonavir increases the serum levels of amprenavir (from fosamprenavir) as a result of CYP3A4 inhibition. Fosamprenavir must be given with ritonavir to ensure its therapeutic effect. Clinical trials confirmed the safety and efficacy of fosamprenavir 700 mg twice daily with ritonavir 100 mg twice daily. Ritonavir doses higher than 100 mg twice daily have not been studied with fosamprenavir. For further information, physicians should refer to the Telzir Summary of Product Characteristics.				
Indinavir	800 q12h	100 q12h	Indinavir[3]	↑ 178%	ND
			Ritonavir	↑ 72%	ND
	400 q12h	400 q12h	Indinavir[3]	↔	↑ 4 fold
			Ritonavir	↔	↔
	Ritonavir increases the serum levels of indinavir as a result of CYP3A4 inhibition. Appropriate doses for this combination, with respect to efficacy and safety, have not been established. Minimal benefit of ritonavir-mediated pharmacokinetic enhancement is achieved with doses higher than 100 mg twice daily. In cases of co-administration of ritonavir (100 mg twice daily) and indinavir (800 mg twice daily) caution is warranted as the risk of nephrolithiasis may be increased.				
Nelfinavir	1250 q12h	100 q12h	Nelfinavir	↑ 20to39%	ND
	750, single	500 q12h	Nelfinavir	↑ 152%	ND
			Ritonavir	↔	↔
	Ritonavir increases the serum levels of nelfinavir as a result of CYP3A4 inhibition. Appropriate doses for this combination, with respect to efficacy and safety, have not been established. Minimal benefit of ritonavir-mediated pharmacokinetic enhancement is achieved with doses higher than 100 mg twice daily.				
Saquinavir	1000 q12h	100 q12h	Saquinavir[4]	↑ 15-fold	↑ 5-fold
			Ritonavir	↔	↔
	400 q12h	400 q12h	Saquinavir[4]	↑ 17-fold	ND
			Ritonavir	↔	↔
	Ritonavir increases the serum levels of saquinavir as a result of CYP3A4 inhibition. Saquinavir should only be given in combination with ritonavir. Ritonavir100 mg twice daily with saquinavir 1000 mg twice daily provides saquinavir systemic exposure over 24 hours similar to or greater than those achieved with saquinavir 1200 mg three times daily without ritonavir. In a clinical study investigating the interaction of rifampicin 600 mg once daily and saquinavir 1000 mg with ritonavir 100 mg twice daily in healthy volunteers, severe hepatocellular toxicity with transaminase elevations up to > 20-fold the upper limit of normal after 1 to 5 days of co-administration was noted. Due to the risk of severe hepatoxicity, saquinavir/ritonavir should not be given together with rifampicin. For further information, physicians should refer to the Invirase or Fortovase Summary of Product Characteristics.				
Tipranavir	500 q12h	200 q12h	Tipranavir	↑ 11 fold	↑ 29 fold
			Ritonavir	↓ 40%	ND
	Ritonavir increases the serum levels of tipranavir as a result of CYP3A inhibition. Tipranavir must be given with low dose ritonavir to ensure its therapeutic effect. Doses of ritonavir less than 200 mg twice daily should not be used with tipranavir as they might alter the efficacy of the combination. For further information, physicians should refer to the Aptivus Summary of Product Characteristics.				
	ND: Not determined. 1. Based on cross-study comparison to 400 mg atazanavir once daily alone. 2. Based on cross-study comparison to 1200 mg amprenavir twice daily alone. 3. Based on cross-study comparison to 800 mg indinavir three times daily alone. 4. Based on cross-stud y comparison to 600 mg saquinavir three times daily alone.				

Drug Interactions – Ritonavir with Antiretroviral Agents Other Than Protease Inhibitors

Co-administered Drug	Dose of Co-administered Drug (mg)	Dose of NORVIR (mg)	Drug Assessed	AUC	Cmin
Didanosine	200 q12h	600 q12h 2 h later	Didanosine	↓ 13%	↔
	As ritonavir is recommended to be taken with food and didanosine should be taken on an empty stomach, dosing should be separated by 2.5 h. Dose alterations should not be necessary.				
Delavirdine	400 q8h	600 q12h	Delavirdine[1]	↔	↔
			Ritonavir	↑ 50%	↑ 75%
	Based on comparison to historical data, the pharmacokinetics of delavirdine did not appear to be affected by ritonavir. When used in combination with delavirdine, dose reduction of ritonavir may be considered.				
Efavirenz	600 q24h	500 q12h	Efavirenz	↑ 21%	
			Ritonavir	↑ 17%	
	A higher frequency of adverse events (eg, dizziness, nausea, paraesthesia) and laboratory abnormalities (elevated liver enzymes) have been observed when efavirenz is co-administered with ritonavir dosed as an antiretroviral agent.				

Drug Interactions – Ritonavir with Protease Inhibitors

Co-administered Drug	Dose of Co-administered Drug (mg)	Dose of NORVIR (mg)	Drug Assessed	AUC	Cmin
Maraviroc	100 q12h	100 q12h	Maraviroc	↑ 161%	↑ 28%
	Ritonavir increases the serum levels of maraviroc as a result of CYP3A inhibition. Maraviroc may be given with ritonavir to increase the maraviroc exposure. For further information, refer to the Summary of Product Characteristics for Celsentri.				
Nevirapine	200 q12h	600 q12h	Nevirapine	↔	↔
			Ritonavir	↔	↔
	Co-administration of ritonavir with nevirapine does not lead to clinically relevant changes in the pharmacokinetics of either nevirapine or ritonavir.				
Zidovudine	200 q8h	300 q6h	Zidovudine	↓ 25%	ND
	Ritonavir may induce the glucuronidation of zidovudine, resulting in slightly decreased levels of zidovudine. Dose alterations should not be necessary.				
	ND: Not determined 1. Based on parallel group comparison.				

Ritonavir effects on Non-antiretroviral Co-administered Drugs

Co-administered Drug	Dose of Co-administered Drug (mg)	Dose of NORVIR (mg)	Effect on Co-administered Drug AUC	Effect on Co-administered Drug Cmax
Alpha $_1$ - Adrenoreceptor Antagonist				
Alfuzosin	Ritonavir co-administration is likely to result in increased plasma concentrations of alfuzosin and is therefore **contraindicated** (see section 4.3).			
Amphetamine Derivatives				
Amphetamine	Ritonavir dosed as an antiretroviral agent is likely to inhibit CYP2D6 and as a result is expected to increase concentrations of amphetamine and its derivatives. Careful monitoring of therapeutic and adverse effects is recommended when these medicines are concomitantly administered with antiretroviral doses of ritonavir (see section 4.4).			
Analgesics				
Buprenorphine	16 q24h	100 q12h	↑ 57%	↑ 77%
Norbuprenorphine			↑ 33%	↑ 108%
Glucuronide metabolites			↔	↔
	The increases of plasma levels of buprenorphine and its active metabolite did not lead to clinically significant pharmacodynamic changes in a population of opioid tolerant patients. Adjustment to the dose of buprenorphine or ritonavir may therefore not be necessary when the two are dosed together. When ritonavir is used in combination with another protease inhibitor and buprenorphine, the SPC of the co-administered protease inhibitor should be reviewed for specific dosing information.			
Pethidine, piroxicam, propoxyphene	Ritonavir co-administration is likely to result in increased plasma concentrations of pethidine, piroxicam, and propoxyphene and is therefore **contraindicated** (see section 4.3).			
Fentanyl	Ritonavir dosed as a pharmacokinetic enhancer or as an antiretroviral agent inhibits CYP3A4 and as a result is expected to increase the plasma concentrations of fentanyl. Careful monitoring of therapeutic and adverse effects is recommended when fentanyl is concomitantly administered with ritonavir.			
Methadone[1]	5, single dose	500 q12h,	↓ 36%	↓ 38%
	Increased methadone dose may be necessary when concomitantly administered with ritonavir dosed as an antiretroviral agent or as a pharmacokinetic enhancer due to induction of glucuronidation. Dose adjustment should be considered based on the patient's clinical response to methadone therapy.			
Morphine	Morphine levels may be decreased due to induction of glucuronidation by co-administered ritonavir dosed as an antiretroviral agent or as a pharmacokinetic enhancer.			
Antiarrthymics				
Amiodarone, bepridil, encainide, flecanide, propafenone, quinidine	Ritonavir co-administration is likely to result in increased plasma concentrations of amiodarone, bepridil, encainide, flecanide, propafenone, and quinidine and is therefore **contraindicated** (see section 4.3).			
Digoxin	0.5 single IV dose	300 q12h, 3 days	↑ 86%	ND
	0.4 single oral dose	200 q12h, 13 days	↑ 22%	↔
	This interaction may be due to modification of P-glycoprotein mediated digoxin efflux by ritonavir dosed as an antriretroviral agent or as a pharmacokinetic enhancer. Increased digoxin levels observed in patients receiving ritonavir may lessen over time as induction develops (see section 4.4).			
Antiasthmatic				
Theophylline[1]	3 mg/kg q8h	500 q12h	↓ 43%	↓ 32%
	An increased dose of theophyline may be required when co-administered with ritonavir, due to induction of CYP1A2.			
Anticancer agents				
Vincristine, vinblastine	Serum concentrations may be increased when co-administered with ritonavir resulting in the potential for increased incidence of adverse events.			
Anticoagulant				
Warfarin S-Warfarin R-Warfarin	5, single dose	400 q12h	↑ 9% ↓ 33%	↓ 9% ↔
	Induction of CYP1A2 and CYP2C9 lead to decreased levels of R-warfarin while little pharmacokinetic effect is noted on S- warfarin when co-administered with ritonavir. Decreased R-warfarin levels may lead to reduced anticoagulation, therefore it is recommended that anticoagulation parameters are monitored when warfarin is co-administered with ritonavir dosed as an antiretroviral agent or as a pharmacokinetic enhancer.;			
Anticonvulsants				
Carbamazepine	Ritonavir dosed as a pharmacokinetic enhancer or as an antiretroviral agent inhibits CYP3A4 and as a result is expected to increase the plasma concentrations of carbamazepine. Careful monitoring of therapeutic and adverse effects is recommended when carbamazepine is concomitantly administered with ritonavir.			

Ritonavir effects on Non-antiretroviral Co-administered Drugs				
Co-administered Drug	**Dose of Co-administered Drug (mg)**	**Dose of NORVIR (mg)**	**Effect on Co-administered Drug AUC**	**Effect on Co-administered Drug Cmax**
Divalproex, lamotrigine, phenytoin	Ritonavir dosed as a pharmacokinetic enhancer or as an antiretroviral agent induces oxidation by CYP2C9 and glucuronidation and as a result is expected to decrease the plasma concentrations of anticonvulsants. Careful monitoring of serum levels or therapeutic effects is recommended when these medicines are concomitantly administered with ritonavir. Phenytoin may decrease serum levels of ritonavir.			
Antidepressants				
Amitriptyline, fluoxetine, imipramine, nortriptyline, paroxetine, sertraline	Ritonavir dosed as an antiretroviral agent is likely to inhibit CYP2D6 and as a result is expected to increase concentrations of desipramine, imipramine, amitriptyline, nortriptyline, fluoxetine, paroxetine or sertraline. Careful monitoring of therapeutic and adverse effects is recommended when these medicines are concomitantly administered with antiretroviral doses of ritonavir (see section 4.4).			
Desipramine	100 single oral dose	500 q12h	↑ 145%	↑ 22%
	The AUC and Cmax of the 2-hydroxy metabolite were decreased 15 and 67%, respectively. Dosage reduction of desipramine is recommended when co-administered with ritonavir dosed as an antiretroviral agent.			
Trazodone	50, single dose	200 q12h	↑ 2.4-fold	↑ 34%
	An increase in the incidence in trazodone-related adverse events was noted when co-administered with ritonavir dosed as an antiretroviral agent or as a pharmacokinetic enhancer. If trazodone is co-administered with ritonavir, the combination should be used with caution, initiating trazodone at the lowest dosage and monitoring for clinical response and tolerability.			
Antihistamines				
Astemizole, terfenadine	Ritonavir co-administration is likely to result in increased plasma concentrations of astemizole and terfenadine and is therefore **contraindicated** (see section 4.3).			
Fexofenadine	Ritonavir may modify P-glycoprotein mediated fexofenadine efflux when dosed as an antriretroviral agent or as a pharmacokinetic enhancer resulting in increased concentrations of fexofenadine. Increased fexofenadine levels may lessen over time as induction develops.			
Loratadine	Ritonavir dosed as a pharmacokinetic enhancer or as an antiretroviral agent inhibits CYP3A and as a result is expected to increase the plasma concentrations of loratadine. Careful monitoring of therapeutic and adverse effects is recommended when loratidine is concomitantly administered with ritonavir.			
Anti-infectives				
Fusidic Acid	Ritonavir co-administration is likely to result in increased plasma concentrations of both fusidic acid and ritonavir and is therefore **contraindicated** (see section 4.3).			
Rifabutin[1] 25-*O*-desacetyl rifabutin metabolite	150 daily	500 q12h,	↑ 4-fold ↑ 38-fold	↑ 2.5-fold ↑ 16-fold
	Due to the large increase in rifabutin AUC, the concomitant use of rifabutin with ritonavir dosed as an antiretroviral agent is **contraindicated** (see section 4.3). The reduction of the rifabutin dose to 150 mg 3 times per week may be indicated for select PIs when co-administered with ritonavir as a pharmacokinetic enhancer. The Summary of Product Characteristics of the co-administered protease inhibitor should be consulted for specific recommendations. Consideration should be given to official guidance on the appropriate treatment of tuberculosis in HIV-infected patients.			
Rifampicin	Although rifampicin may induce metabolism of ritonavir, limited data indicate that when high doses of ritonavir (600 mg twice daily) is co-administered with rifampicin, the additional inducing effect of rifampicin (next to that of ritonavir itself) is small and may have no clinical relevant effect on ritonavir levels in high-dose ritonavir therapy. The effect of ritonavir on rifampicin is not known.			
Voriconazole	200 q12h	400 q12h	↓ 82%	↓ 66%
	200 q12h	100 q12h	↓ 39%	↓ 24%
	Concomitant use of ritonavir dosed as an antiretroviral agent and voriconazole is **contraindicated** due to reduction in voriconazole concentrations (see section 4.3). Co-administration of voriconazole and ritonavir dosed as a pharmacokinetic enhancer should be avoided, unless an assessment of the benefit/risk to the patient justifies the use of voriconazole.			
Atovaquone	Ritonavir dosed as a pharmacokinetic enhancer or as an antiretroviral agent induces glucuronidation and as a result is expected to decrease the plasma concentrations of atovaquone. Careful monitoring of serum levels or therapeutic effects is recommended when atovaquone is concomitantly administered with ritonavir.			
Clarithromycin 14-OH clarithromycin metabolite	500 q12h,	200 q8h	↑ 77% ↓ 100%	↑ 31% ↓ 99%
	Due to the large therapeutic window of clarithromycin no dose reduction should be necessary in patients with normal renal function. Clarithromycin doses greater than 1 g per day should not be co-administered with ritonavir dosed as an antiretroviral agent or as a pharmacokinetic enhancer. For patients with renal impairment, a clarithromycin dose reduction should be considered: for patients with creatinine clearance of 30 to 60 ml/min the dose should be reduced by 50%, for patients with creatinine clearance less than 30 ml/min the dose should be reduced by 75%.			
Erythromycin, itraconazole	Ritonavir dosed as a pharmacokinetic enhancer or as an antiretroviral agent inhibits CYP3A4 and as a result is expected to increase the plasma concentrations of erythromycin and itraconazole. Careful monitoring of therapeutic and adverse effects is recommended when erythromycin or itraconazole is used concomitantly administered with ritonavir.			
Ketoconazole	200 daily	500 q12h	↑ 3.4-fold	↑ 55%
	Ritonavir inhibits CYP3A-mediated metabolism of ketoconazole. Due to an increased incidence of gastrointestinal and hepatic adverse events, a dose reduction of ketoconazole should be considered when co-administered with ritonavir dosed as an antiretroviral agent or as a pharmacokinetic enhancer.			
Sulfamethoxazole/ Trimethoprim[2]	800/160, single dose	500 q12h	↓ 20% / ↑ 20%	↔
	Dose alteration of sulfamethoxazole/trimethoprim during concomitant ritonavir therapy should not be necessary.			
Antipsychotics/ Neuroleptics				
Clozapine, pimozide	Ritonavir co-administration is likely to result in increased plasma concentrations of clozapine or pimozide and is therefore **contraindicated** (see section 4.3).			
Haloperidol, risperidone, thioridazine	Ritonavir dosed as an antiretroviral agent is likely to inhibit CYP2D6 and as a result is expected to increase concentrations of haloperidol, risperidone and thioridazine. Careful monitoring of therapeutic and adverse effects is recommended when these medicines are concomitantly administered with antiretroviral doses of ritonavir (see section 4.3).			
Calcium channel antagonists				
Amlodipine, diltiazem, nifedipine	Ritonavir dosed as a pharmacokinetic enhancer or as an antiretroviral agent inhibits CYP3A4 and as a result is expected to increase the plasma concentrations of calcium channel antagonists. Careful monitoring of therapeutic and adverse effects is recommended when these medicines are concomitantly administered with ritonavir.			

Ritonavir effects on Non-antiretroviral Co-administered Drugs				
Co-administered Drug	**Dose of Co-administered Drug (mg)**	**Dose of NORVIR (mg)**	**Effect on Co-administered Drug AUC**	**Effect on Co-administered Drug Cmax**
Ergot Derivatives				
Dihydroergotamine, ergonovine, ergotamine, methylergonovine	Ritonavir co-administration is likely to result in increased plasma concentrations of ergot derivatives and is therefore **contraindicated** (see section 4.3).			
GI motility agent				
Cisapride	Ritonavir co-administration is likely to result in increased plasma concentrations of cisapride and is therefore **contraindicated** (see section 4.3).			
HMG Co-A Reductase Inhibitors				
Atorvastatin, Fluvastatin, Lovastatin, Pravstatin, Rosuvastatin, Simvastatin	HMG-CoA reductase inhibitors which are highly dependent on CYP3A metabolism, such as lovastatin and simvastatin, are expected to have markedly increased plasma concentrations when co-administered with ritonavir dosed as an antiretroviral agent or as a pharmacokinetic enhancer. Since increased concentrations of lovastatin and simvastatin may predispose patients to myopathies, including rhabdomyolysis, the combination of these medicinal products with ritonavir is **contraindicated** (see section 4.3). Atorvastatin is less dependent on CYP3A for metabolism. While rosuvastatin elimination is not dependent on CYP3A, an elevation of rosuvastatin exposure has been reported with ritonavir co-administration. The mechanism of this interaction is not clear, but may be the result of transporter inhibition. When used with ritonavir dosed as a pharmacokinetic enhancer or as an antiretroviral agent, the lowest possible doses of atorvastatin or rosuvastatin should be administered. The metabolism of pravastatin and fluvastatin is not dependent on CYP3A, and interactions are not expected with ritonavir. If treatment with an HMG-CoA reductase inhibitor is indicated, pravastatin or fluvastatin is recommended.			
Hormonal contraceptive				
Ethinyl estradiol	50 µg single dose	500 q12h	↓ 40%	↓ 32%
	Due to reductions in ethinyl estradiol concentrations, barrier or other non-hormonal methods of contraception should be considered with concomitant ritonavir use when dosed as an antiretroviral agent or as a pharmacokinetic enhancer. Ritonavir is likely to change the uterine bleeding profile and reduce the effectiveness of estradiol-containing contraceptives (see section 4.4).			
Immunosupressants				
Cyclosporine, tacrolimus, everolimus	Ritonavir dosed as a pharmacokinetic enhancer or as an antiretroviral agent inhibits CYP3A4 and as a result is expected to increase the plasma concentrations of cyclosporine, tacrolimus or everolimus. Careful monitoring of therapeutic and adverse effects is recommended when these medicines are concomitantly administered with ritonavir.			
Phosphodiesterase inhibitors				
Sildenafil	100, single dose	500 q12h	↑ 11-fold	↑ 4-fold
	Concomitant use of sildenafil with ritonavir dosed as an antiretroviral agent or as a pharmacokinetic enhancer is not recommended and in no instance should sildenafil doses exceed 25 mg in 48 hours (see also section 4.4). Concomitant use of sildenafil with ritonavir is **contraindicated** in pulmonary arterial hypertension patients.			
Tadalafil	20, single dose	200 q12h	↑ 124%	↔
	The concomitant use of tadalafil with ritonavir dosed as an antiretroviral agent or as a pharmacokinetic enhancer should be with caution at reduced doses of no more than 10 mg tadalafil every 72 hours with increased monitoring for adverse events (see section 4.4).			
Vardenafil	5, single dose	600 q12h	↑ 49-fold	↑ 13-fold
	The concomitant use of vardenafil and ritonavir dosed as an antiretroviral agent or as a pharmacokinetic enhancer should be with caution at reduced doses of no more than 2.5 mg every 72 hours with increased monitoring for adverse events (see section 4.4).			
Sedatives/hynoptics				
Clorazepate, diazepam, estazolam, flurazepam, oral and parenteral midazolam and triazolam	Ritonavir co-administration is likely to result in increased plasma concentrations of clorazepate, diazepam, estazolam and flurazepam and is therefore **contraindicated** (see section 4.3). Midazolam is extensively metabolised by CYP3A4. Co-administration with Norvir may cause a large increase in the concentration of this benzodiazepine. No drug interaction study has been performed for the co-administration of Norvir with benzodiazepines. Based on data for other CYP3A4 inhibitors, plasma concentrations of midazolam are expected to be significantly higher when midazolam is given orally. Therefore, Norvir should not be co-administered with orally administered midazolam (see section 4.3), whereas caution should be used with co-administration of Norvir and parenteral midazolam. Data from concomitant use of parenteral midazolam with other protease inhibitors suggest a possible 3 – 4 fold increase in midazolam plasma levels. If Norvir is co-administered with parenteral midazolam, it should be done in an intensive care unit (ICU) or similar setting which ensures close clinical monitoring and appropriate medical management in case of respiratory depression and/or prolonged sedation. Dosage adjustment for midazolam should be considered, especially if more than a single dose of midazolam is administered.			
Triazolam	0.125 single dose	200, 4 doses	↑ > 20 fold	↑ 87%
	Ritonavir co-administration is likely to result in increased plasma concentrations of triazolam and is therefore **contraindicated** (see section 4.3).			
Pethidine	50 oral single dose	500 q12h	↓ 62%	↓ 59%
Norpethidine metabolite			↑ 47%	↑ 87%
	The use of pethidine and ritonavir is **contraindicated** due to the increased concentrations of the metabolite, norpethidine, which has both analgesic and CNS stimulant activity. Elevated norpethidine concentrations may increase the risk of CNS effects (eg, seizures), see section 4.3.			
Alprazolam	1, single dose	200 q12h, 2 days	↑ 2.5 fold	↔
		500 q12h, 10 days	↓ 12%	↓ 16%
	Alprazolam metabolism was inhibited following the introduction of ritonavir. After ritonavir use for 10 days, no inhibitory effect of ritonavir was observed. Caution is warranted during the first several days when alprazolam is co-administered with ritonavir dosed as an antiretroviral agent or as a pharmacokinetic enhancer, before induction of alprazolam metabolism develops.			
Buspirone	Ritonavir dosed as a pharmacokinetic enhancer or as an antiretroviral agent inhibits CYP3A and as a result is expected to increase the plasma concentrations of buspirone. Careful monitoring of therapeutic and adverse effects is recommended when buspirone concomitantly administered with ritonavir.			
Sleeping agent				
Zolpidem	5	200, 4 doses	↑ 28%	↑ 22%
	Zolpidem and ritonavir may be co-administered with careful monitoring for excessive sedative effects.			
Smoke cessation				
Bupropion	150 mg	100 mg q12h	↓ 22%	↓ 21%
	150 mg	600 mg q12h	↓ 66%	↓ 62%

Ritonavir effects on Non-antiretroviral Co-administered Drugs				
Co-administered Drug	**Dose of Co-administered Drug (mg)**	**Dose of NORVIR (mg)**	**Effect on Co-administered Drug AUC**	**Effect on Co-administered Drug Cmax**
	Bupropion is primarily metabolised by CYP2B6. Concurrent administration of bupropion with repeated doses of ritonavir is expected to decrease bupropion levels. These effects are thought to represent induction of bupropion metabolism. However, because ritonavir has also been shown to inhibit CYP2B6 in vitro, the recommended dose of bupropion should not be exceeded. In contrast to long-term administration of ritonavir, there was no significant interaction with bupropion after short-term administration of low doses of ritonavir (200 mg twice daily for 2 days), suggesting reductions in bupropion concentrations may have onset several days after initiation of ritonavir co-administration.			
Steroids				
Fluticasone propionate aqueous nasal spray	200 µg qd	100 q12h	↑ ~350-fold	↑ ~ 25-fold
	Systemic corticosteroid effects including Cushing's syndrome and adrenal suppression (plasma cortisol levels were noted to be decreased 86% in the above study) have been reported in patients receiving ritonavir and inhaled or intranasal fluticasone propionate; similar effects could also occur with other corticosteroids metabolised by CYP3A eg, budesonide. Consequently, concomitant administration of ritonavir dosed as an antiretroviral agent or as a pharmacokinetic enhancer and these glucocorticoids is not recommended unless the potential benefit of treatment outweighs the risk of systemic corticosteroid effects (see section 4.4). A dose reduction of the glucocorticoid should be considered with close monitoring of local and systemic effects or a switch to a glucocorticoid, which is not a substrate for CYP3A4 (eg, beclomethasone). Moreover, in case of withdrawal of glucocorticoids progressive dose reduction may be required over a longer period.			
Dexamethasone	Ritonavir dosed as a pharmacokinetic enhancer or as an antiretroviral agent inhibits CYP3A and as a result is expected to increase the plasma concentrations of dexamethasone. Careful monitoring of therapeutic and adverse effects is recommended when dexamethasone is concomitantly administered with ritonavir.			
Prednisolone	20	200 q12h	↑ 28%	↑ 9%
	Careful monitoring of therapeutic and adverse effects is recommended when prednisolone is concomitantly administered with ritonavir. The AUC of the metabolite prednisolone increased by 37 and 28% after 4 and 14 days ritonavir, respectively.			
	ND: Not determined 1. Based on a parallel group comparison 2. Sulfamethoxazole was co-administered with trimethoprim.			

seriousness: very common (> 1/10); common (> 1/100 to < 1/10); uncommon (> 1/1000 to < 1/100); rare (> 1/10,000 to < 1/1,000).

(see Table 3 on next page)

Events noted as having Unknown frequency were identified via post-marketing surveillance.

Hepatic transaminase elevations exceeding five times the upper limit or normal, clinical hepatitis, and jaundice have occurred in patients receiving ritonavir alone or in combination with other antiretrovirals.

Combination antiretroviral therapy has been associated with redistribution of body fat (lipodystrophy) in HIV patients including the loss of peripheral and facial subcutaneous fat, increased intra-abdominal and visceral fat, breast hypertrophy and dorsocervical fat accumulation (buffalo hump).

Combination antiretroviral therapy has been associated with metabolic abnormalities such as hypertriglyceridaemia, hypercholesterolaemia, insulin resistance, hyperglycaemia and hyperlactataemia (see section 4.4).

In HIV-infected patients with severe immune deficiency at the time of initiation of combination antiretroviral therapy (CART), an inflammatory reaction to asymptomatic or residual opportunistic infections may arise (see section 4.4).

Pancreatitis has been observed in patients receiving ritonavir therapy, including those who developed hypertriglyceridemia. In some cases fatalities have been observed. Patients with advanced HIV disease may be at risk of elevated triglycerides and pancreatitis (see section 4.4).

Cases of osteonecrosis have been reported, particularly in patients with generally acknowledged risk factors, advanced HIV disease or long-term exposure to combination antiretroviral therapy (CART). The frequency of this is unknown (see section 4.4).

4.9 Overdose

Human experience of acute overdose with ritonavir is limited. One patient in clinical trials took ritonavir 1500 mg/day for two days and reported paraesthesia, which resolved after the dose was decreased. A case of renal failure with eosinophilia has been reported.

The signs of toxicity observed in animals (mice and rats) included decreased activity, ataxia, dyspnoea and tremors.

There is no specific antidote for overdose with ritonavir. Treatment of overdose with ritonavir should consist of general supportive measures including monitoring of vital signs and observation of the clinical status of the patient. Due to the solubility characteristics and possibility of transintestinal elimination, it is proposed that management of overdose could entail gastric lavage and administration of activated charcoal. Since ritonavir is extensively metabolised by the liver and is highly protein bound, dialysis is unlikely to be beneficial in significant removal of the medicine.

5. PHARMACOLOGICAL PROPERTIES

5.1 Pharmacodynamic properties

Pharmacotherapeutic group: antiviral for systemic use, ATC code: J05A E03

Ritonavir dosed as a pharmacokinetic enhancer

Pharmacokinetic enhancement by ritonavir is based on ritonavir's activity as a potent inhibitor of CYP3A- mediated metabolism. The degree of enhancement is related to the metabolic pathway of the co-administered protease inhibitor and the impact of the co-administered protease inhibitor on the metabolism of ritonavir. Maximal inhibition of metabolism of the co-administered protease inhibitor is generally achieved with ritonavir doses of 100 mg daily to 200 mg twice daily, and is dependent on the co-administered protease inhibitor. For additional information on the effect of ritonavir on co-administered protease inhibitor metabolism, see Section 4.5 and refer to the Summary of Product Characteristics of the particular co-administered PIs.

Ritonavir dosed as an antiretroviral agent

Ritonavir is an orally active peptidomimetic inhibitor of the HIV-1 and HIV-2 aspartyl proteases. Inhibition of HIV protease renders the enzyme incapable of processing the *gag-pol* polyprotein precursor which leads to the production of HIV particles with immature morphology that are unable to initiate new rounds of infection. Ritonavir has selective affinity for the HIV protease and has little inhibitory activity against human aspartyl proteases.

Ritonavir was the first protease inhibitor (approved in 1996) for which efficacy was proven in a study with clinical endpoints. However, due to ritonavir's metabolic inhibitory properties its use as a pharmacokinetic enhancer of other protease inhibitors is the prevalent use of ritonavir in clinical practice (see section 4.2).

Effects on the Electrocardiogram

QTcF interval was evaluated in a randomised, placebo and active (moxifloxacin 400 mg once daily) controlled crossover study in 45 healthy adults, with 10 measurements over 12 hours on Day 3. The maximum mean (95% upper confidence bound) difference in QTcF from placebo was 5.5 (7.6) for 400 mg twice daily ritonavir. The Day 3 ritonavir exposure was approximately 1.5 fold higher than that observed with the 600 mg twice daily dose at steady state. No subject experienced an increase in QTcF of ⩾ 60 msec from baseline or a QTcF interval exceeding the potentially clinically relevant threshold of 500 msec.

Modest prolongation of the PR interval was also noted in subjects receiving ritonavir in the same study on Day 3. The mean changes from baseline in PR interval ranged from 11.0 to 24.0 msec in the 12 hour interval post dose. Maximum PR interval was 252 msec and no second or third degree heart block was observed (see section 4.4).

Resistance

Ritonavir-resistant isolates of HIV-1 have been selected *in vitro and* isolated from patients treated with therapeutic doses of ritonavir.

Reduction in the antiretroviral activity of ritonavir is primarily associated with the protease mutations V82A/F/T/S and I84V. Accumulation of other mutations in the protease gene (including at positions 20, 33, 36, 46, 54, 71, and 90) can also contribute to ritonavir resistance. In general, as mutations associated with ritonavir resistance accumulate, susceptibility to select other PIs may decrease due to cross-resistance. The Summary of Product Characteristics of other protease inhibitors or official continuous updates should be consulted for specific information regarding protease mutations associated with reduced response to these agents.

Clinical pharmacodynamic data

The effects of ritonavir (alone or combined with other antiretroviral agents) on biological markers of disease activity such as CD4 cell count and viral RNA were evaluated in several studies involving HIV-1 infected patients. The following studies are the most important.

Adult Use

A controlled study completed in 1996 with ritonavir as add-on therapy in HIV-1 infected patients extensively pre-treated with nucleoside analogues and baseline CD4 cell counts ⩽ 100 cells/µl showed a reduction in mortality and AIDS defining events. The mean average change from baseline over 16 weeks for HIV RNA levels was -0.79 $\log_{10}$ (maximum mean decrease: 1.29 $\log_{10}$) in the ritonavir group versus -0.01 $\log_{10}$ in the control group. The most frequently used nucleosides in this study were zidovudine, stavudine, didanosine and zalcitabine.

In a study completed in 1996 recruiting less advanced HIV-1 infected patients (CD4 200-500 cells/µl) without previous antiretroviral therapy, ritonavir in combination with zidovudine or alone reduced viral load in plasma and increased CD4 count. The mean average change from baseline over 48 weeks for HIV RNA levels was -0.88 $\log_{10}$ in the ritonavir group versus -0.66 $\log_{10}$ in the ritonavir + zidovudine group versus -0.42 $\log_{10}$ in the zidovudine group.

The continuation of ritonavir therapy should be evaluated by viral load because of the possibility of the emergence of resistance as described under section 4.1 Therapeutic indications.

Paediatric Use

In an open label trial completed in 1998 in HIV infected, clinically stable children there was a significant difference (p = 0.03) in the detectable RNA levels in favour of a triple regimen (ritonavir, zidovudine and lamivudine) following 48 weeks treatment.

In a study completed in 2003, 50 HIV-1 infected, protease inhibitor and lamivudine naïve children age 4 weeks to 2 years received ritonavir 350 or 450 mg/m^2 every 12 hours co-administered with zidovudine 160 mg/m^2 every 8 hours and lamivudine 4 mg/kg every 12 hours. In intent to treat analyses, 72% and 36% of patients achieved reduction in plasma HIV-1 RNA of ⩽ 400 copies/ml at Week 16 and 104, respectively. Response was similar in both dosing regimens and across patient age.

In a study completed in 2000, 76 HIV-1 infected children aged 6 months to 12 years who were protease inhibitor naive and naive to lamivudine and/or stavudine received ritonavir 350 or 450 mg/m^2 every 12 hours co-administered with lamivudine and stavudine. In intent to treat analyses, 50% and 57% of patients in the 350 and 450 mg/m^2 dose groups, respectively, achieved reduction in plasma HIV-1 RNA to ⩽ 400 copies/ml at Week 48.

5.2 Pharmacokinetic properties

Absorption:

There is no parenteral formulation of ritonavir, therefore the extent of absorption and absolute bioavailability have not been determined. The pharmacokinetics of ritonavir during multiple dose regimens were studied in non-fasting HIV-infected adult volunteers. Upon multiple dosing, ritonavir accumulation is slightly less than predicted from a single dose due to a time and dose-related increase in apparent clearance (Cl/F). Trough concentrations of ritonavir decrease over time, possibly due to enzyme induction, but appeared to stabilise by the end of 2 weeks. The time to maximum concentration (T_{max}) remained constant at approximately 4 hours with increasing dose. Renal clearance averaged less than 0.1 l/h and was relatively constant throughout the dosage range.

Table 3

Undesirable Effects in Clinical Studies and Post-marketing in Adult Patients		
Immune system disorders	Common	Allergic reactions including urticaria, mild skin eruptions, bronchospasm and angioedema
	Rare	Anaphylaxis and Stevens Johnson syndrome
Blood and lymphatic system disorders	Common	Decreased WBC, decreased haemoglobin, decreased neutrophils, increased eosinophils
	Uncommon	Increased WBC, increased neutrophils and increased prothrombin time
	Unknown frequency	Thrombocytopenia
Metabolic and nutritional disorders	Uncommon	Dehydration, diabetes mellitus
	Rare	Hyperglycaemia
	Unknown frequency	Hypertriglyceridaemia, hypercholesterolaemia, hyperuricaemia
Nervous system disorders	Very common	Taste perversion, circumoral and peripheral paresthesia, headache
	Common	Dizziness, paraesthesia, hyperaesthesia, somnolence, insomnia, anxiety
	Unknown frequency	Seizure, syncope
Vascular disorders	Common	Vasodilation
	Unknown frequency	Orthostatic hypotension
Respiratory, thoracic and mediastinal disorders	Common	Pharyngitis, cough increased
Gastrointestinal disorders	Very common	Abdominal pain, nausea, diarrhoea, vomiting
	Common	Dyspepsia, anorexia, local throat irritation, flatulence, dry mouth, eructation, mouth ulcer
Hepatobiliary disorders	Uncommon	Hepatitis and jaundice
Skin and subcutaneous tissue disorders	Common	Rash, pruritus, sweating, lipodystrophy
Musculoskeletal and connective tissue disorders	Common	Increased CPK, myalgia
	Uncommon	Myositis, rhabdomyolysis
Renal and urinary disorders	Unknown frequency	Acute renal failure
Reproductive system and breast disorders	Unknown frequency	Menorrhagia
General disorders and administration site conditions	Very common	Asthenia
	Common	Fever, pain weight loss
Investigations	Common	Increased GGT, increased CPK, increased triglycerides, increased SGPT, increased SGOT, increased amylase, increased uric acid, decreased potassium, decreased free and total thyroxin
	Uncommon	Increased glucose, decreased total calcium, increased magnesium, increased bilirubin, increased alkaline phosphatase

The pharmacokinetic parameters observed with various dosing schemes of ritonavir alone are shown in the table below.

(see Table 4 below)

Effects of food on oral absorption:

Ingestion of ritonavir with food results in higher ritonavir exposure than ingestion in the fasted state.

Distribution:

The apparent volume of distribution (V_B/F) of ritonavir is approximately 20 - 40 l after a single 600 mg dose. The protein binding of ritonavir in human plasma is approximately 98 - 99% and is constant over the concentration range of 1.0 – 100 µg /ml. Ritonavir binds to both human alpha 1-acid glycoprotein (AAG) and human serum albumin (HSA) with comparable affinities.

Tissue distribution studies with ^{14}C-labelled ritonavir in rats showed the liver, adrenals, pancreas, kidneys and thyroid to have the highest concentrations of ritonavir. Tissue to plasma ratios of approximately 1 measured in rat lymph nodes suggests that ritonavir distributes into lymphatic tissues. Ritonavir penetrates minimally into the brain.

Metabolism:

Ritonavir was noted to be extensively metabolised by the hepatic cytochrome P450 system, primarily by the CYP3A isozyme family and to a lesser extent by the CYP2D6 isoform. Animal studies as well as *in vitro* experiments with human hepatic microsomes indicated that ritonavir primarily underwent oxidative metabolism. Four ritonavir metabolites have been identified in man. The isopropylthiazole oxidation metabolite (M-2) is the major metabolite and has antiviral activity similar to that of parent drug. However, the AUC of the M-2 metabolite was approximately 3% of the AUC of parent drug.

Low doses of ritonavir have shown profound effects on the pharmacokinetics of other protease inhibitors (and other products metabolised by CYP3A4) and other protease inhibitors may influence the pharmacokinetics of ritonavir (see section 4.5).

Elimination:

Human studies with radiolabelled ritonavir demonstrated that the elimination of ritonavir was primarily via the hepatobiliary system; approximately 86% of radiolabel was recovered from stool, part of which is expected to be unabsorbed ritonavir. In these studies renal elimination was not found to be a major route of elimination of ritonavir. This was consistent with the observations in animal studies.

Special Populations: No clinically significant differences in AUC or C_{max} were noted between males and females. Ritonavir pharmacokinetic parameters were not statistically significantly associated with body weight or lean body mass. Ritonavir plasma exposures in patients 50 – 70 years of age when dosed 100 mg in combination with lopinavir or at higher doses in the absence of other protease inhibitors is similar to that observed in younger adults.

Patients with impaired liver function: after multiple dosing of ritonavir to healthy volunteers (500 mg twice daily) and subjects with mild to moderate hepatic impairment (Child Pugh Class A and B, 400 mg twice daily) exposure to ritonavir after dose normalisation was not significantly different between the two groups.

Patients with impaired renal function: Ritonavir pharmacokinetic parameters have not been studied in patients with renal impairment. However, since the renal clearance of ritonavir is negligible, no changes in the total body clearance are expected in patients with renal impairment.

Paediatric patients: Ritonavir steady-state pharmacokinetic parameters were evaluated in HIV infected children above 2 years of age receiving doses ranging from 250 mg/m^2 twice daily to 400 mg/m^2 twice daily. Ritonavir concentrations obtained after 350 to 400 mg/m^2 twice daily in paediatric patients were comparable to those obtained in adults receiving 600 mg (approximately 330 mg/m^2) twice daily. Across dose groups, ritonavir oral clearance (CL/F/m^2) was approximately 1.5 to 1.7 times faster in paediatric patients above 2 years of age than in adult subjects.

Ritonavir steady-state pharmacokinetic parameters were evaluated in HIV infected children less than 2 years of age receiving doses ranging from 350 to 450 mg/m^2 twice daily. Ritonavir concentrations in this study were highly variable and somewhat lower than those obtained in adults receiving 600 mg (approximately 330 mg/m^2) twice daily. Across dose groups, ritonavir oral clearance (CL/F/m^2) declined with age with median values of 9.0 L/h/m^2 in children less than 3 months of age, 7.8 L/h/m^2 in children between 3 and 6 months of age and 4.4 L/h/m^2 in children between 6 and 24 months of age.

5.3 Preclinical safety data

Repeated dose toxicity studies in animals identified major target organs as the liver, retina, thyroid gland and kidney. Hepatic changes involved hepatocellular, biliary and phagocytic elements and were accompanied by increases in hepatic enzymes. Hyperplasia of the retinal pigment epithelium (RPE) and retinal degeneration have been seen in all of the rodent studies conducted with ritonavir, but have not been seen in dogs. Ultrastructural evidence suggests that these retinal changes may be secondary to phospholipidosis. However, clinical trials revealed no evidence of drug-induced ocular changes in humans. All thyroid changes were reversible upon discontinuation of ritonavir. Clinical investigation in humans has revealed no clinically significant alteration in thyroid function tests. Renal changes including tubular degeneration, chronic inflammation and proteinurea were noted in rats and are felt to be attributable to species-specific spontaneous disease. Furthermore, no clinically significant renal abnormalities were noted in clinical trials.

Developmental toxicity observed in rats (embryolethality, decreased foetal body weight and ossification delays and visceral changes, including delayed testicular descent) occurred mainly at a maternally toxic dosage. Developmental toxicity in rabbits (embryolethality, decreased litter size and decreased foetal weights) occurred at a maternally toxic dosage.

Ritonavir was not found to be mutagenic or clastogenic in a battery of *in vitro* and *in vivo* assays including the Ames bacterial reverse mutation assay using *S. typhimurium* and *E. coli*, the mouse lymphoma assay, the mouse micronucleus test and chromosomal aberration assays in human lymphocytes.

Long term carcinogenicity studies of ritonavir in mice and rats revealed tumourigenic potential specific for these species, but are regarded as of no relevance for humans.

6. PHARMACEUTICAL PARTICULARS

6.1 List of excipients

Capsule contents:

alcohol,

butylated hydroxytoluene (E321),

oleic acid,

polyoxyl 35 castor oil.

Table 4

Ritonavir Dosing Regimen	100 mg once daily	100 mg twice daily[1]	200 mg once daily	200 mg twice daily	600 mg twice daily
C_{max} (µg/ml)	0.84 ± 0.39	0.89	3.4 ± 1.3	4.5 ± 1.3	11.2 ± 3.6
C_{trough} (µg/ml)	0.08 ± 0.04	0.22	0.16 ± 0.10	0.6 ± 0.2	3.7 ± 2.6
$AUC_{12 \text{ or } 24}$ (µg•h/ml)	6.6 ± 2.4	6.2	20.0 ± 5.6	21.92 ± 6.48	77.5 ± 31.5
$t_{½}$ (h)	~5	~5	~4	~8	~3 to 5
Cl/F (L/h)	17.2 ± 6.6	16.1	10.8 ± 3.1	10.0 ± 3.2	8.8 ± 3.2

[1] Values expressed as geometric means. Note: ritonavir was dosed after a meal for all listed regimens.

Capsule shell:

gelatine,

"sorbitol special" (ie sorbitol sorbitolanhydrides and mannitol),

glycerine,

titanium dioxide (white colour),

medium chain triglycerides,

lecithin,

black ink containing: propylene glycol, black iron oxide, polyvinyl acetate phthalate, polyethylene glycol 400 and ammonium hydroxide.

6.2 Incompatibilities

Not applicable

6.3 Shelf life

2 years

6.4 Special precautions for storage

Store in a refrigerator (2°C - 8°C) until they are dispensed to the patient. Refrigeration by the patient is not required if used within 30 days and stored below 25°C.

Avoid exposure to freezing and excessive heat. Keep the bottle tightly closed.

6.5 Nature and contents of container

Norvir soft capsules are supplied in white high density polyethylene (HDPE) bottles closed with polypropylene caps containing 84 capsules.

Two pack sizes are available for Norvir soft capsules:

– 1 bottle of 84 capsules (84 capsules)

– 4 bottles of 84 capsules (336 capsules)

Not all pack sizes may be marketed.

6.6 Special precautions for disposal and other handling

No special requirements.

7. MARKETING AUTHORISATION HOLDER

Abbott Laboratories Limited

Queenborough

Kent ME11 5EL

United Kingdom

8. MARKETING AUTHORISATION NUMBER(S)

EU/1/96/016/003-004

9. DATE OF FIRST AUTHORISATION/RENEWAL OF THE AUTHORISATION

Date of first authorisation: 26 August 1996

Date of last renewal: 27 August 2006

10. DATE OF REVISION OF THE TEXT

2nd September 2009

Novgos 3.6mg Implant

(Genus Pharmaceuticals)

1. NAME OF THE MEDICINAL PRODUCT

Novgos 3.6 mg Implant

2. QUALITATIVE AND QUANTITATIVE COMPOSITION

One implant contains 3.6 mg goserelin (as goserelin acetate)

Excipients:

For a full list of excipients, see section 6.1.

3. PHARMACEUTICAL FORM

Implant, pre-filled syringe.

The sterile, cylindrical, white to cream coloured implant is placed in a sterile injection needle.

4. CLINICAL PARTICULARS

4.1 Therapeutic indications

Novgos is a luteinization hormone releasing hormone (LHRH)- Agonist (analogue of the natural LHRH).

Novgos is used for treatment of patients with advanced prostate cancer where endocrine treatment is indicated.

4.2 Posology and method of administration

1 implant every month.

Novgos is injected subcutaneously into the anterior abdominal wall.

Generally treatment of prostate cancer with Goserelin is a long-term treatment. Regular control examinations as performed usually in prostate cancer patients are recommended to assess the therapeutic effect.

Remarks for injection technique:

1. The implant consists of two bags, the sterile injection needle and the sterile applicator. Note that the implant is visibly fixed in the injection needle. Open both bags and connect the injection needle to the applicator via the Luer lock. Make sure that the connection is tight and that the plunger remains unchanged in its position.

2. Check that the implant is visible in the control window in the needle.

3. Remove the locking device from the plunger. Insert the cannula into the anterior abdominal wall and insert the implant by depressing the plunger completely.

Paediatric Patients

Novgos is contraindicated in children and adolescents (see section 4.3).

Special Patient Groups

No dosage or interval adjustment is necessary for patients with renal or hepatic impairment or in the elderly.

4.3 Contraindications

Hypersensitivity to the active substance or to any of the excipients.

Novgos is not indicated for use in children and adolescents, as efficacy and tolerability for this group of patients has not been investigated.

4.4 Special warnings and precautions for use

Special caution should be given to patients at particular risk of developing ureteric obstruction or spinal cord compression. Administration of Novgos should be carefully judged and closely monitored during the first months of therapy.

If spinal cord compression or renal impairment due to ureteric obstruction are present or develop, specific standard treatment of these complications should be instituted.

Consideration should be given to the initial use of an anti-androgen at the start of Novgos therapy since this has been reported to prevent the possible sequelae.

Continuous suppression of sexual hormone production leads to infertility in men.

4.5 Interaction with other medicinal products and other forms of interaction

No interaction studies have been performed.

4.6 Pregnancy and lactation

Not applicable as Novgos is intended for male patients only.

4.7 Effects on ability to drive and use machines

No studies on the effects on the ability to drive and use machines have been performed.

4.8 Undesirable effects

The adverse events are listed by system organ class and frequency using the following convention:

very common (≥1/10)

common (≥1/100 to <1/10)

uncommon (≥1/1,000 to <1/100)

rare (≥1/10,000 to <1/1,000)

very rare (<1/10,000), not known (cannot be estimated from the available data).

Within each frequency grouping, undesirable effects are presented in order of decreasing seriousness.

General

Cardiac disorders:

uncommon: changes in blood pressure (hypotension or hypertension)

Nervous system disorders:

very common: non-specific paraesthesias

very rare: pituitary apoplexy following initial administration

Skin and subcutaneous tissue disorders:

common: mild skin rash

Musculoskeletal and connective tissue disorders:

very rare: arthralgia/bone pain

General disorders and administration site conditions:

rare: local reactions at the injection site

Immune system disorders:

rare: hypersensitivity reactions, including symptoms of anaphylaxia

At the beginning of the therapy

Initially, there is a short-term increase in serum testosterone inducing a temporary increase of specific symptoms:

Nervous system disorders:

very rare: spinal cord compression

Renal and urinary disorders:

very rare: ureteric obstruction (due to obstruction of the urinary tract passage)

Musculoskeletal and connective tissue disorders:

common: bone pain

In these cases, the patients must be closely monitored and treated symptomatically during the first month of treatment.

During the therapy

Due to the decrease in serum testosterone during the treatment the use of LHRH-agonists causes loss in bone mineral density. For this reason, during long-term therapy with Novgos an increased fracture risk cannot be excluded, although no increased fracture rates have been observed so far.

Nervous system disorders:

very rare: pituitary adenomas

Endocrine disorders:

very common: hot flushes and sweating

Reproductive system and breast disorders:

very common: decrease in libido and potency, testicular atrophy

common: breast swelling

very rare: breast tenderness

Pituitary adenomas occur more often in prostate cancer patients. However, as no medical reports on the initial state of the pituitary gland were available for these few cases monitored under treatment, it cannot be excluded with certainty that their development was favoured by the use of Novgos.

4.9 Overdose

There is only limited experience of overdosage in humans. In cases where goserelin has unintentionally been re-administered early or given at a higher dose, no clinically relevant adverse reactions have been seen.

Animal tests suggest that no effect other than the intended therapeutic effects on sex hormone concentrations and on the reproductive tract will be evident with higher doses.

In case of toxication symptomatic treatment is required.

5. PHARMACOLOGICAL PROPERTIES

5.1 Pharmacodynamic properties

Pharmacotherapeutic group: LHRH-agonist

ATC code: L02A E03

The treatment with Novgos in men leads to fall of serum testosterone to the castration range.

Treatment with Novgos causes inhibition of growth or regression of hormone dependent cancer of the prostatic gland (oestradiol and/or progesterone receptor positive tumours).

Biosynthesis and secretion of the male and female sexual hormones (testosterone and oestradiol, respectively) are controlled by the hypothalamic LHRH and by luteinization hormone (LH) and follicle stimulating hormone (FSH) which are produced in the pituitary gland. The pulsating release of the natural LHRH from the hypothalamus triggers synthesis and excretion of LH and FSH from the anterior lobe of the pituitary gland.

Goserelin acetate, the active substance of Novgos, is a LHRH analogue with higher activity and longer half life as the natural hormone.

Long-term treatment with goserelin acetate leads to a receptor-down-regulation of the pituitary gland. The number of LHRH- receptors decreases. Thereby LH and FSH secretion and biosynthesis of oestradiol and testosterone in the gonads is suppressed.

After an initial increase during the first 3-5 days in men testosterone levels decrease. Castration range is normally achieved between the second and third week after the beginning of treatment with Novgos. Suppression of serum testosterone with Novgos is equal to the results of orchiectomy.

5.2 Pharmacokinetic properties

The active substance is spread in a completely biodegradable matrix of Poly(D,L-lactide-co-glycolide). An average of 120 μg goserelin per day is released from Novgos. Seven to14 days after administration of Novgos, the maximum serum levels of goserelin are achieved. Subsequently they slowly fall during the third and fourth week of therapy. No accumulation occurs.

Goserelin slightly binds to serum protein (25 %). After subcutaneous administration of a single dose (aqueous solution of 250 μg) of goserelin in patients with normal renal function, elimination half time of 4.2 h in men was observed.

The influence of impaired renal function on goserelin serum levels and total body clearance has been investigated in male patients suffering from prostate cancer. With increasing renal impairment elimination of the substance was delayed. In this case, a close correlation between creatinine clearance and total body clearance could be shown.

However, goserelin was eliminated relatively fast (half-life 12.1h) in patients with severe renal impairment (creatinine-clearance <20ml/min), leading to the conclusion of an additional non-renal elimination pathway possibly located in the liver. Accumulation of goserelin associated with chronic application can therefore not be expected in patients with limited renal impairment.

There is no significant change in pharmacokinetics in patients with hepatic failure.

5.3 Preclinical safety data

Preclinical studies with LHRH agonists revealed in both sexes effects on the reproductive system, which were expected from the known pharmacological properties. These effects were shown to be reversible after discontinuation of the treatment and a due period of regeneration.

Goserelin acetate did not show teratogenicity in rats and rabbits. Based on the pharmacological effects of LHRH agonists on the reproductive system, embryotoxicity and - lethality was observed in rabbits.

Goserelin acetate was not mutagenic in a set of *in vitro* and *in vivo* assays.

Carcinogenicity studies were performed with other LHRH analogues in rats and mice over 24 months. In rats, a dose-related increase in pituitary adenomas was observed after subcutaneous administration at doses of 0.6 to 4 mg/kg/day. No such effect was observed in mice, allowing to regard the effect in rats as species-specific, having no relevance for humans.

6. PHARMACEUTICAL PARTICULARS

6.1 List of excipients

Poly(D,L-lactide-co-glycolide) (1:1).

6.2 Incompatibilities

Not applicable.

6.3 Shelf life

2 years.

From a microbiological point of view, the product should be used immediately. If not used immediately, in-use storage times and conditions are the responsibility of the user.

6.4 Special precautions for storage

Do not store above 25°C.

Store in the original package.

6.5 Nature and contents of container

Each implant is placed in a sterile, siliconised stainless steel injection needle closed with a Luer-Lock screw cap and a needle cover. The needle unit is packaged together with a desiccant in a polyester/aluminium/polyethylene pouch. A sterilised applicator is provided packed in a separate pouch.

Novgos is available in packs of 1, 3 and 6 implants.

Not all pack sizes may be marketed.

6.6 Special precautions for disposal and other handling

No special requirements.

7. MARKETING AUTHORISATION HOLDER

Genus Pharmaceuticals Limited

T/A Genus Pharmaceuticals

Park View House

65 London Road

Newbury

Berkshire, RG14 1JN, UK

8. MARKETING AUTHORISATION NUMBER(S)

PL 06831/0233

9. DATE OF FIRST AUTHORISATION/RENEWAL OF THE AUTHORISATION

02/04/09

10. DATE OF REVISION OF THE TEXT

02/04/09

Novofem film-coated tablets.

(Novo Nordisk Limited)

1. NAME OF THE MEDICINAL PRODUCT

Novofem® film-coated tablet

2. QUALITATIVE AND QUANTITATIVE COMPOSITION

One red film-coated tablet contains:

Estradiol 1 mg (as estradiol hemihydrate)

One white film-coated tablet contains:

Estradiol 1 mg (as estradiol hemihydrate) and norethisterone acetate 1 mg

Excipient: Lactose monohydrate 38.4 mg (red film-coated tablet) and 37.9 mg (white film-coated tablet)

For a full list of excipients, see section 6.1.

3. PHARMACEUTICAL FORM

Film-coated tablet

Red film-coated, biconvex tablets engraved with NOVO 282. Diameter: 6mm.

White film-coated, biconvex tablets engraved with NOVO 283. Diameter: 6mm.

4. CLINICAL PARTICULARS

4.1 Therapeutic indications

Hormone Replacement Therapy (HRT) for oestrogen deficiency symptoms in postmenopausal women with an intact uterus.

Prevention of osteoporosis in postmenopausal women at high risk of future fractures who are intolerant of, or contraindicated for, other medicinal products approved for the prevention of osteoporosis.

The experience of treating women older than 65 years is limited.

4.2 Posology and method of administration

Novofem is a continuous sequential preparation for hormone replacement therapy. The oestrogen is dosed continuously. The progestogen is added for 12 days of every 28 day cycle in a sequential manner.

One tablet is taken daily in the following order: oestrogen therapy (red film-coated tablet) over 16 days, followed by 12 days of oestrogen/progestogen therapy (white film-coated tablet).

After intake of the last white tablet, treatment is continued with the first red tablet of a new pack on the next day. A menstruation-like bleeding usually occurs at the beginning of a new treatment cycle.

In women who are not taking HRT or women transferring from a continuous combined HRT product, treatment may be started on any convenient day. In women transferring from a sequential HRT regimen, treatment should begin the day following completion of the prior regimen.

For initiation and continuation of treatment of postmenopausal symptoms, the lowest effective dose for the shortest duration (see also section 4.4) should be used.

A switch to a higher dose combination product could be indicated if the response after three months is insufficient for satisfactory symptom relief.

If the patient has forgotten to take one tablet, the forgotten tablet is to be discarded. Forgetting a dose may increase the likelihood of breakthrough bleeding and spotting.

4.3 Contraindications

- Known, past or suspected breast cancer
- Known or suspected oestrogen-dependent malignant tumours (e.g. endometrial cancer)
- Undiagnosed genital bleeding
- Untreated endometrial hyperplasia
- Previous idiopathic or current venous thromboembolism (deep venous thrombosis, pulmonary embolism)
- Active or recent arterial thromboembolic disease (e.g. angina, myocardial infarction)
- Acute liver disease or a history of liver disease, as long as liver function tests have failed to return to normal
- Known hypersensitivity to the active substances or to any of the excipients
- Porphyria

4.4 Special warnings and precautions for use

For the treatment of postmenopausal symptoms, HRT should only be initiated for symptoms that adversely affect quality of life. In all cases, a careful appraisal of the risks and benefits should be undertaken at least annually and HRT should only be continued as long as the benefit outweighs the risk.

Medical examination/follow-up

Before initiating or reinstituting HRT, a complete personal and family medical history should be taken. Physical (including pelvic and breast) examination should be guided by this and by the contraindications and warnings for use. During treatment, periodic check-ups are recommended of a frequency and nature adapted to the individual woman. Women should be advised what changes in their breasts should be reported to their doctor or nurse (please see the 'Breast cancer' section below). Investigations, including mammography, should be carried out in accordance with currently accepted screening practices, modified to the clinical needs of the individual.

Conditions which need supervision:

If any of the following conditions are present, have occurred previously and/or have been aggravated during pregnancy or previous hormone treatment, the patient should be closely supervised. It should be taken into account that these conditions may recur or be aggravated during treatment with Novofem, in particular:

- Leiomyoma (uterine fibroids) or endometriosis
- A history of or risk factors for thromboembolic disorders (see below)
- Risk factors for oestrogen dependent tumours, e.g. 1st degree heredity for breast cancer
- Hypertension
- Liver disorders (e.g. liver adenoma)
- Diabetes mellitus with or without vascular involvement
- Cholelithiasis
- Migraine or (severe) headache
- Systemic lupus erythematosus
- A history of endometrial hyperplasia (see below)
- Epilepsy
- Asthma
- Otosclerosis

Reasons for immediate withdrawal of therapy:

Therapy should be discontinued in case a contraindication is discovered and in the following situations:

- Jaundice or deterioration in liver function
- Significant increase in blood pressure
- New onset of migraine-type headache
- Pregnancy

Endometrial hyperplasia

The risk of endometrial hyperplasia and carcinoma is increased when oestrogens are administered alone for prolonged periods (see section 4.8). The addition of a progestogen, for at least 12 days per cycle in non-hysterectomised women greatly reduces this risk.

Breakthrough bleeding and spotting may occur during the first months of treatment. If breakthrough bleeding or spotting appears after some time on therapy, or continues after treatment has been discontinued, the reason should be investigated, which may include endometrial biopsy to exclude endometrial malignancy.

Breast Cancer

A randomised placebo-controlled trial, the Women's Health Initiative study (WHI), and epidemiological studies, including the Million Women Study (MWS), have reported an increased risk of breast cancer in women taking oestrogens, oestrogen-progestogen combinations or tibolone for HRT for several years (see section 4.8).

For all HRT, an excess risk becomes apparent within a few years of use and increases with duration of intake but returns to baseline within a few (at most five) years after stopping treatment.

In the MWS, the relative risk of breast cancer with conjugated equine oestrogens (CEE) or estradiol (E2) was greater when a progestogen was added, either sequentially or continuously, and regardless of type of progestogen. There was no evidence of a difference in risk between the different routes of administration.

In the WHI study, the continuous combined conjugated equine oestrogen and medroxyprogesterone acetate (CEE + MPA) product used was associated with breast cancers that were slightly larger in size and more frequently had local lymph node metastases compared to placebo.

HRT, especially oestrogen-progestogen combined treatment, increases the density of mammographic images which may adversely affect the radiological detection of breast cancer.

Venous thromboembolism

HRT is associated with a higher relative risk of developing venous thromboembolism (VTE), i.e. deep vein thrombosis or pulmonary embolism. One randomised controlled trial and epidemiological studies found a two- to three-fold higher risk for users compared with non-users. For non-users it is estimated that the number of cases of VTE that will occur over a 5 year period is about 3 per 1000 women aged 50-59 years and 8 per 1000 women aged between 60-69 years. It is estimated that in healthy women who use HRT for 5 years, the number of additional cases of VTE over a 5 year period will be between 2 and 6 (best estimate =4) per 1000 women aged 50-59 years and between 5 and 15 (best estimate =9) per 1000 women aged 60-69 years. The occurrence of such an event is more likely in the first year of HRT than later.

Generally recognised risk factors for VTE include a personal history or family history, severe obesity (BMI > 30 kg/m^2) and systemic lupus erythematosus (SLE). There is no consensus about the possible role of varicose veins in VTE.

Patients with a history of VTE or known thrombophilic states have an increased risk of VTE. HRT may add to this risk. Personal or strong family history of thromboembolism, or recurrent spontaneous abortion, should be investigated in order to exclude a thrombophilic predisposition. Until a thorough evaluation of thrombophilic factors has been made or anticoagulant treatment initiated, use of HRT in such patients should be viewed as contraindicated. Those women already on anticoagulant treatment require careful consideration of the benefit-risk of use of HRT.

The risk of VTE may be temporarily increased with prolonged immobilisation, major trauma or major surgery. As in all postoperative patients, scrupulous attention should be given to prophylactic measures to prevent VTE following surgery. Where prolonged immobilisation is liable to follow elective surgery, particularly abdominal or orthopaedic surgery to the lower limbs, consideration should be given to temporarily stopping HRT four to six weeks earlier, if possible. Treatment should not be restarted until the woman is completely mobilised.

If VTE develops after initiating therapy, the drug should be discontinued. Patients should be told to contact their doctors immediately when they are aware of a potential thromboembolic symptom (e.g., painful swelling of a leg, sudden pain in the chest, dyspnea).

Coronary artery disease (CAD)

There is no evidence from randomised controlled trials of cardiovascular benefit with continuous combined conjugated oestrogens and medroxyprogesterone acetate (MPA). Two large clinical trials (WHI and HERS i.e. Heart and Estrogen/progestin Replacement Study) showed a possible increased risk of cardiovascular morbidity in the first year of use and no overall benefit. For other HRT products there are only limited data from randomised controlled trials examining effects in cardiovascular morbidity or mortality. Therefore, it is uncertain whether these findings also extend to other HRT products.

Stroke

One large randomised clinical trial (WHI-trial) found, as a secondary outcome, an increased risk of ischaemic stroke in healthy women during treatment with continuous combined conjugated oestrogens and MPA. For women who do not use HRT, it is estimated that the number of cases of stroke that will occur over a 5 year period is about 3 per 1000 women aged 50-59 years and 11 per 1000 women aged 60-69 years. It is estimated that for women who use conjugated oestrogens and MPA for 5 years, the number of additional cases will be between 0 and 3 (best estimate = 1) per 1000 users aged 50-59 years and between 1 and 9 (best estimate = 4) per 1000 users aged 60-69 years. It is unknown whether the increased risk also extends to other HRT products.

Ovarian cancer

Long-term (at least 5-10 years) use of oestrogen-only HRT products in hysterectomised women has been associated with an increased risk of ovarian cancer in some epidemiological studies. It is uncertain whether long-term use of combined HRT confers a different risk than oestrogen-only products.

Other conditions

Oestrogens may cause fluid retention and, therefore patients with cardiac or renal dysfunction should be carefully observed. Patients with terminal renal insufficiency should be closely observed since it is expected that the level of circulating active ingredients in Novofem will increase.

Women with pre-existing hypertriglyceridemia should be followed closely during oestrogen replacement or hormone replacement therapy, since rare cases of large increases of plasma triglycerides leading to pancreatitis have been reported with oestrogen therapy in this condition.

Oestrogens increase thyroid binding globulin (TBG), leading to increased circulating total thyroid hormone, as measured by protein-bound iodine (PBI), T4 levels (by column or by radio-immunoassay) or T3 levels (by radio-immunoassay). T3 resin uptake is decreased, reflecting the elevated TBG. Free T4 and free T3 concentrations are unaltered. Other binding proteins may be elevated in serum, i.e. corticoid binding globulin (CBG), sex-hormone-binding globulin (SHBG) leading to increased circulating corticosteroids and sex steroids, respectively. Free or biological active hormone concentrations are unchanged. Other plasma proteins may be increased (angiotensinogen/renin substrate, alpha-I-antitrypsin, ceruloplasmin).

There is no conclusive evidence for improvement of cognitive function. There is some evidence from the WHI trial of increased risk of probable dementia in women who start using continuous combined CEE and MPA after the age of 65. It is unknown whether the findings apply to younger post-menopausal women or other HRT products.

Novofem tablets contain lactose. Patients with rare hereditary problems of galactose intolerance, the Lapp lactase deficiency or glucose-galactose malabsorption should not take this medicine.

4.5 Interaction with other medicinal products and other forms of interaction

The metabolism of oestrogens and protestogens may be increased at concomitant use of substances known to induce drug-metabolising enzymes, specifically cytochrome P450 enzymes such as anticonvulsants (e.g. phenobarbital, phenytoin, carbamezapin) and anti-infectives (e.g. rifampicin, rifabutin, nevirapine, efavirenz). Ritonavir and nelfinavir, although known as strong inhibitors, by contrast exhibit inducing properties when used concomitantly with steroid hormones. Herbal preparations containing St John's Wort (*Hypericum perforatum*) may induce the metabolism of oestrogens and progestogens.

Clinically, an increased metabolism of oestrogens and progestogens may lead to decreased effect and changes in the uterine bleeding profile.

Reduced estradiol levels have been observed under the simultaneous use of antibiotics e.g. penicillins and tetracycline.

Oestrogens can enhance the effects and side effects of imipramine.

If cyclosporin is given concomitantly, there may be increased blood levels of cyclosporin, creatinine and transaminases due to the decreased hepatic excretion of cyclosporin.

The requirement of treatment with oral antidiabetic drugs or with insulin may change due to the oestrogen effect on glucose tolerance (will be decreased) and the response to insulin, i.e. the requirement of insulin or oral antidiabetics can be increased as a consequence of a reduced glucose tolerance.

4.6 Pregnancy and lactation

Novofem is not indicated during pregnancy.

If pregnancy occurs during medication with Novofem, treatment should be withdrawn immediately.

Data on a limited number of exposed pregnancies indicate adverse effects of norethisterone on the foetus. At doses higher than normally used in OC and HRT formulations masculinisation of female foetuses was observed.

The results of most epidemiological studies to date relevant to inadvertent foetal exposure to combinations of oestrogens and progestogens indicate no teratogenic or foetotoxic effect.

Lactation

Novofem is not indicated during lactation.

4.7 Effects on ability to drive and use machines

No effects known.

4.8 Undesirable effects

Clinical experience:

The most frequently reported adverse event during treatment in clinical trials conducted with an HRT product similar to Novofem is breast tenderness and headache (>1/10).

The adverse events listed below may occur during oestrogen-progestogen treatment. The frequencies are derived from clinical trials conducted with an HRT product similar to Novofem and from a Post Marketing Surveillance study on Novofem.

(see Table 1 below)

Breast cancer

According to evidence from a large number of epidemiological studies and one randomised placebo-controlled trial, the Women's Health Initiative (WHI), the overall risk of breast cancer increases with increasing duration of HRT use in current or recent HRT users.

For *oestrogen-only* HRT, estimates of relative risk (RR) from a reanalysis of original data from 51 epidemiological studies (in which >80% of HRT use was oestrogen-only HRT) and from the epidemiological Million Women Study (MWS) are similar at 1.35 (95% CI: 1.21-1.49) and 1.30 (95% CI: 1.21-1.40), respectively.

For *oestrogen plus progestogen* combined HRT, several epidemiological studies have reported an overall higher risk for breast cancer than with oestrogens alone.

The MWS reported that, compared to never users, the use of various types of oestrogen-progestogen combined HRT was associated with a higher risk of breast cancer (RR = 2.00, 95% CI: 1.88-2.12) than use of oestrogens alone (RR = 1.30, 95% CI: 1.21-1.40) or use of tibolone (RR = 1.45, 95% CI: 1.25-1.68).

The WHI trial reported a risk estimate of 1.24 (95% CI: 1.01-1.54) after 5.6 years of use of oestrogen-progestogen combined HRT (CEE + MPA) in all users compared with placebo.

The absolute risks calculated from the MWS and the WHI trials are presented below:

The MWS has estimated, from the known average incidence of breast cancer in developed countries, that:

• For women not using HRT, about 32 in every 1000 are expected to have breast cancer diagnosed between the ages of 50 and 64 years.

• For 1000 current or recent users of HRT, the number of *additional* cases during the corresponding period will be

• For users of *oestrogen-only* replacement therapy,

- between 0 and 3 (best estimate = 1.5) for 5 years' use

- between 3 and 7 (best estimate = 5) for 10 years' use.

• For users of *oestrogen plus progestogen* combined HRT,

- between 5 and 7 (best estimate = 6) for 5 years' use

- between 18 and 20 (best estimate = 19 for 10 years use.

The WHI trial estimated that after 5.6 years of follow-up of women between the ages of 50 and 79 years, an *additional* 8 cases of invasive breast cancer would be due to *oestrogen-progestogen combined* HRT (CEE + MPA) per 10,000 women years. According to calculations from the trial data, it is estimated that:

• For 1000 women in the placebo group,

- about 16 cases of invasive breast cancer would be diagnosed in 5 years.

• For 1000 women who used oestrogen + progestogen combined HRT (CEE + MPA), the number of additional cases would be

- between 0 an 9 (best estimate = 4) for 5 years' use.

The number of additional cases of breast cancer in women who use HRT is broadly similar for women who start HRT irrespective of age at start of use (between the ages of 45-65) (see section 4.4).

Endometrial cancer

In women with an intact uterus, the risk of endometrial hyperplasia and endometrial cancer increases with increasing duration of use of unopposed oestrogens. According to data from epidemiological studies, the best estimate of the risk is that for women not using HRT, about 5 in every 1000 are expected to have endometrial cancer diagnosed between the ages of 50 and 65. Depending on the duration of treatment and oestrogen dose, the reported increase in endometrial cancer risk among unopposed oestrogen users varies from 2- to 12-fold greater compared with non-users. Adding a progestogen to oestrogen-only therapy greatly reduces this increased risk.

Post-marketing experience:

In addition to the above mentioned adverse drug reactions, those presented below have been spontaneously reported, and are by an overall judgment considered possibly related to Novofem treatment. The reporting rate of these spontaneous adverse drug reactions is very rare: (<1/10,000 patient years). Post-marketing experience is subject to underreporting especially with regard to trivial and well known adverse drug reactions. The presented frequencies should be interpreted in that light:

Reproductive system and breast disorders: Hyperplasia of endometrium (for further information see section 4.4)

Skin and subcutaneous tissue disorders: Hirsutism.

Other adverse reactions have been reported in association with oestrogen/progestogen treatment:

- Oestrogen-dependent neoplasms benign and malignant, e.g. endometrial cancer.

- Venous thromboembolism, i.e. deep leg or pelvic venous thrombosis and pulmonary embolism, is more frequent among hormone replacement therapy users than among non-users. For further information, see sections 4.3 Contraindications and 4.4 Special warnings and precautions for use.

- Myocardial infarction and stroke

- Skin and subcutaneous disorders: chloasma, erythema multiforme, erythema nodosum, haemorrhagic eruption, vascular purpura.

- Probable dementia (see section 4.4)

- Gallbladder disease.

Table 1

System organ class	Very common >1/10	Common >1/100; <1/10	Uncommon >1/1,000; <1/100	Rare >1/10,000; <1/1,000
Infections and infestations		Vaginal candidiasis		
Immune system disorders				Allergic reaction
Psychiatric disorders				Nervousness
Nervous system disorders	Headache	Dizziness Insomnia Depression	Migraine Libido disorder NOS (not otherwise specified	Vertigo
Vascular disorders		Increased blood pressure Aggravated hypertension	Peripheral embolism and thrombosis	
Gastrointestinal disorders		Dyspepsia Abdominal pain Flatulence Nausea	Vomiting	Diarrhoea Bloating
Hepatobiliary disorders			Gallbladder disease Gallstones	
Skin and subcutaneous tissue disorders		Rash Pruritus	Alopecia	Acne
Musculoskeletal and connective tissue disorders			Muscle cramps	
Reproductive system and breast disorders	Breast tenderness	Vaginal haemorrhage Uterine fibroids aggravated		Uterine fibroid
General disorders and administration site conditions		Oedema		
Investigations		Weight increased		

4.9 Overdose

Overdose may be manifested by nausea and vomiting. Treatment should be symptomatic.

5. PHARMACOLOGICAL PROPERTIES

5.1 Pharmacodynamic properties

ATC Code G03F B05

Oestrogen and progestogen, sequential combination for continuous treatment.

Estradiol: The active ingredient, synthetic 17β-estradiol, is chemically and biologically identical to endogenous human estradiol. It substitutes for the loss of oestrogen production in menopausal women, and alleviates menopausal symptoms.

Oestrogens prevent bone loss following menopause or ovariectomy.

Norethisterone acetate: As oestrogens promote the growth of the endometrium, unopposed oestrogens increase the risk of endometrial hyperplasia and cancer. The addition of a progestogen greatly reduces the oestrogen-induced risk of endometrial hyperplasia in non-hysterectomised women.

Relief of menopausal symptoms is achieved during the first few weeks of treatment.

In a PMS study regular withdrawal bleeding with a mean duration of 3-4 days occurred in 91% of women, who took Novofem over 6 month. Withdrawal bleeding usually started a few days after the last tablet of the progestogen phase.

Oestrogen deficiency at menopause is associated with an increasing bone turnover and decline in bone mass. The effect of oestrogens on the bone mineral density is dose-dependent. Protection appears to be effective for as long as treatment is continued. After discontinuation of HRT, bone mass is lost at a rate similar to that in untreated women.

Evidence from the WHI trial and meta-analysed trials shows that current use of HRT, alone or in combination with a progestogen – given to predominantly healthy women – reduces the risk of hip, vertebral, and other osteoporotic fractures. HRT may also prevent fractures in women with low bone density and/or established osteoporosis, but the evidence for that is limited.

Randomised, double-blind, placebo-controlled studies showed that 1 mg estradiol prevents the postmenopausal loss of bone minerals and increases the bone mineral density. The responses in the spine, femoral neck and trochanter were 2.8%, 1.6% and 2.5%, respectively, over 2 years with 1mg 17β-estradiol unopposed.

5.2 Pharmacokinetic properties

Following oral administration of 17β-estradiol in micronised form, rapid absorption from the gastrointestinal tract occurs. It undergoes extensive first-pass metabolism in the liver and other enteric organs, and a peak plasma concentration of approximately 27 pg/ml (range 13-40 pg/ml) occurs within 6 hours after intake of 1 mg. The area under the curve (AUC_{0-tz}) = 629 h × pg/ml. The half-life of 17β-estradiol is about 25 hours. It circulates bound to SHBG (37%) and to albumin (61%), while only approximately 1-2% is unbound. Metabolism of 17β-estradiol occurs mainly in the liver and gut but also in target organs, and involves the formation of less active or inactive metabolites, including oestrone, catecholoestrogens and several oestrogen sulphates and glucuronides. Oestrogens are partly excreted with the bile, hydrolysed and reabsorbed (enterohepatic circulation), and mainly eliminated in urine in biologically inactive form.

After oral administration, norethisterone acetate is rapidly absorbed and transformed to norethisterone (NET). It undergoes first-pass metabolism in the liver and other enteric organs, and a peak plasma concentration of approximately 9 ng/ml (range 6-11 ng/ml) occurs within 1 hour after intake of 1 mg. The area under the curve (AUC_{0-tz}) = 29 h × pg/ml. The terminal half-life of NET is about 10 hours. NET binds to SHBG (36%) and to albumin (61%). The most important metabolites are isomers of 5α-dihydro-NET and of tetrahydro-NET, which are excreted mainly in the urine as sulphate or glucuronide conjugates. The pharmacokinetics in the elderly have not been studied.

5.3 Preclinical safety data

Animal studies with estradiol and norethisterone acetate have shown expected oestrogenic and progestogenic effects. Both compounds induced adverse effects in preclinical reproductive toxicity studies, in particular embryotoxic effects and anomalies in urogenital tract development. Concerning other preclinic effects, the toxicity profiles of estradiol and norethisterone acetate are well known and reveal no particular human risks beyond those discussed in other sections of the SPC and which generally apply to hormone substitution therapy.

6. PHARMACEUTICAL PARTICULARS

6.1 List of excipients

Both the white and the red tablets contain:

Lactose monohydrate

Maize starch

Gelatin

Talc

Magnesium stearate

Film-coating

White film-coated tablet:

Hypromellose, triacetin, talc

Red film-coated tablet:

Hypromellose, red iron oxide (E 172), titanium dioxide (E 171), propylene glycol and talc

6.2 Incompatibilities

Not applicable.

6.3 Shelf life

3 years.

6.4 Special precautions for storage

Do not store above 25°C. Do not refrigerate. Keep the container in the outer carton.

6.5 Nature and contents of container

1 × 28 tablets or 3 × 28 tablets in calendar dial packs.

The calendar dial pack with 28 tablets consists of the following 3 parts:

- The base made of coloured non-transparent polypropylene,

- The ring-shaped lid made of transparent polystyrene,

- The centre-dial made of coloured non-transparent polystyrene.

Not all pack sizes may be marketed.

6.6 Special precautions for disposal and other handling

No special requirements.

7. MARKETING AUTHORISATION HOLDER

Novo Nordisk Limited

Broadfield Park, Brighton Road,

Crawley, West Sussex, RH11 9RT

8. MARKETING AUTHORISATION NUMBER(S)

PL 03132/0141

9. DATE OF FIRST AUTHORISATION/RENEWAL OF THE AUTHORISATION

May 2002

10. DATE OF REVISION OF THE TEXT

August 2006

LEGAL STATUS

POM (Prescription only medicine)

NovoMix 30 Penfill 100 U/ml, NovoMix 30 FlexPen 100 U/ml

(Novo Nordisk Limited)

1. NAME OF THE MEDICINAL PRODUCT

NovoMix 30 Penfill 100 U/ml, suspension for injection in a cartridge.

NovoMix 30 FlexPen 100 U/ml, suspension for injection in a pre-filled pen.

2. QUALITATIVE AND QUANTITATIVE COMPOSITION

Soluble insulin aspart*/protamine-crystallised insulin aspart* .... 100 U/ml in the ratio of 30/70

* produced by recombinant DNA technology in *Saccharomyces cerevisiae*.

One unit of insulin aspart corresponds to 6 nmol, 0.035 mg salt-free anhydrous insulin aspart.

1 cartridge contains 3 ml equivalent to 300 U.

1 pre-filled pen contains 3 ml equivalent to 300 U.

For a full list of excipients, see section 6.1.

3. PHARMACEUTICAL FORM

Suspension for injection in a cartridge.

Suspension for injection in a pre-filled pen.

NovoMix 30 is a white suspension.

4. CLINICAL PARTICULARS

4.1 Therapeutic indications

Treatment of diabetes mellitus.

4.2 Posology and method of administration

NovoMix 30 has a faster onset of action than biphasic human insulin and should generally be given immediately before a meal. When necessary, NovoMix 30 can be given soon after a meal.

NovoMix 30 is administered subcutaneously in the thigh or in the abdominal wall. If convenient, the gluteal or deltoid region may be used. Injection sites should be rotated within the same region. As with all insulins the duration of action will vary according to the dose, injection site, blood flow, temperature and level of physical activity. The influence of different injection sites on the absorption of NovoMix 30 has not been investigated. NovoMix 30 should never be administered intravenously.

Renal or hepatic impairment may reduce the patient's insulin requirements.

NovoMix 30 can be used in children and adolescents aged 10 years and above when premixed insulin is preferred. For children 6-9 years limited clinical data exists (see section 5.1)

No studies have been performed in children under the age of 6 years.

Dose recommendation

Dosage of NovoMix 30 is individual and determined in accordance with the needs of the patient.

In patients with type 2 diabetes, NovoMix 30 can be given in monotherapy or in combination with oral antidiabetic drugs for which the combination with insulin is approved, when the blood glucose is inadequately controlled with those oral antidiabetic drugs alone. For patients with type 2 diabetes, the recommended starting dose of NovoMix 30 is 6 U at breakfast and 6 U at dinner (evening meal). NovoMix 30 can also be initiated once daily with 12 U at dinner (evening meal). When using NovoMix 30 once daily, it is generally recommended to move to twice-daily when reaching 30 units by splitting the dose into equal breakfast and dinner doses. If twice daily dosing with NovoMix 30 results in recurrent daytime hypoglycaemic episodes, the morning dose can be split into morning and lunchtime doses (thrice daily dosing).

The following titration guideline is recommended for dose adjustments:

Pre-meal blood glucose level		NovoMix 30 dose adjustment
< 4.4 mmol/l	< 80 mg/dL	- 2 U
4.4 – 6.1 mmol/l	80 – 110 mg/dL	0
6.2 – 7.8 mmol/l	111 – 140 mg/dL	+ 2 U
7.9 – 10 mmol/l	141 – 180 mg/dL	+ 4 U
> 10 mmol/l	> 180 mg/dL	+ 6 U

The lowest of three previous days' pre-meal levels should be used. The dose should not be increased if hypoglycaemia occurred within these days. Dose adjustments can be made once a week until target HbA_{1c} is reached. Pre-meal blood glucose levels should be used to evaluate the adequacy of the preceding dose.

The combination of NovoMix 30 with pioglitazone should only be considered following clinical evaluation of the patient's risk of developing signs or symptoms of fluid-related adverse events. The initiation of NovoMix 30 should be undertaken cautiously titrating to the lowest dose required to achieve glycaemic control. (see section 4.4)

In patients with type 1 diabetes the individual insulin requirement is usually between 0.5 and 1.0 Units/kg/day. NovoMix 30 may fully or partially meet this requirement.

The daily insulin requirement may be higher in patients with insulin resistance (e.g. due to obesity), and lower in patients with residual endogenous insulin production.

When transferring a patient from biphasic human insulin to NovoMix 30, start with the same dose and regimen. Then titrate according to individual needs (See titration guidelines in table above).

NovoMix 30 can be used in elderly patients; however there is limited experience with the use of NovoMix 30 in combination with OADs in patients older than 75 years.

4.3 Contraindications

o Hypersensitivity to the active substance or to any of the excipients.

o Hypoglycaemia.

4.4 Special warnings and precautions for use

The use of dosages which are inadequate or discontinuation of treatment, especially in insulin-dependent diabetics, may lead to hyperglycaemia and diabetic ketoacidosis; conditions which are potentially lethal.

Omission of a meal or unplanned, strenuous physical exercise may lead to hypoglycaemia (see section 4.8 and section 4.9). Compared with biphasic human insulin, NovoMix 30 may have a more pronounced glucose lowering effect up to 6 hours after injection. This may have to be compensated for in the individual patient, through adjustment of insulin dose and/or food intake.

Patients, whose blood glucose control is greatly improved, e.g. by intensified insulin therapy, may experience a change in their usual warning symptoms of hypoglycaemia, and should be advised accordingly.

Tighter control of glucose levels can increase the potential for hypoglycaemic episodes and therefore require special attention during dose intensification as outlined in section 4.2.

NovoMix 30 should be administered in immediate relation to a meal. The rapid onset of action should therefore be considered in patients with concomitant diseases or treatment with other medicinal products where a delayed absorption of food might be expected.

Concomitant illness, especially infections, usually increases the patient's insulin requirements.

When patients are transferred between different types of insulin products, the early warning symptoms of hypoglycaemia may change or become less pronounced than those experienced with their previous insulin.

Transferring a patient to a new type or brand of insulin should be done under strict medical supervision. Changes in strength, brand (manufacturer), type, origin (animal, human, human insulin analogue), and/or method of manufacture (recombinant DNA versus animal source insulin) may result in the need for a change in dosage. Patients taking NovoMix 30 may need a change in dosage from that used with their usual insulin. If a dosage adjustment is needed, it may be done with the first dose or during the first few weeks or months.

Adjustment of dosage may also be necessary if patients undertake increased physical activity or change their usual diet. Exercise taken immediately after a meal may increase the risk of hypoglycaemia.

Insulin suspensions are not to be used in insulin infusion pumps.

As with any insulin therapy, injection site reactions may occur and include pain, itching, hives, swelling and inflammation. Continuous rotation of the injection site within a given area may help to reduce or prevent these reactions. Reactions usually resolve in a few days to a few weeks. On rare occasions, injection site reactions may require discontinuation of NovoMix 30.

Combination of NovoMix 30 with pioglitazone:

There have been cases of cardiac failure reported from the market when pioglitazone was used in combination with insulin, especially in patients with risk factors for development of cardiac heart failure. Patients should be observed for signs and symptoms of heart failure, weight gain and oedema when NovoMix 30 is used in combination with pioglitazone. As a consequence of increased insulin sensitivity, patients receiving pioglitazone in dual therapy with insulin may be at risk for dose-related hypoglycaemia, and a reduction in the dose of insulin may be necessary.

4.5 Interaction with other medicinal products and other forms of interaction

A number of medicinal products are known to interact with the glucose metabolism.

The following substances may reduce the patient's insulin requirements:

Oral antidiabetic drugs (OAD), octreotide, monoamine oxidase inhibitors (MAOIs), non-selective beta-adrenergic blocking agents, angiotensin converting enzyme (ACE) inhibitors, salicylates, alcohol, anabolic steroids and sulphonamides.

The following substances may increase the patient's insulin requirements:

Oral contraceptives, thiazides, glucocorticoids, thyroid hormones, sympathomimetics and danazol.

Beta-blocking agents may mask the symptoms of hypoglycaemia.

Alcohol may intensify and prolong the glucose-lowering effect of insulin.

4.6 Pregnancy and lactation

There is limited clinical experience with NovoMix 30 in pregnancy.

Animal reproduction studies have not revealed any differences between insulin aspart and human insulin regarding embryotoxicity or teratogenicity.

In general, intensified blood glucose control and monitoring of pregnant women with diabetes are recommended throughout pregnancy and when contemplating pregnancy. Insulin requirements usually fall in the first trimester and increase subsequently during the second and third trimesters. After delivery, insulin requirements return rapidly to pre-pregnancy levels.

There are no restrictions on treatment with NovoMix 30 during lactation. Insulin treatment of the breast-feeding mother presents no risk to the baby. However, the NovoMix 30 dosage may need to be adjusted.

4.7 Effects on ability to drive and use machines

No studies on the effects on the ability to drive and use machines have been performed.

The patient's ability to concentrate and react may be impaired as a result of hypoglycaemia. This may constitute a risk in situations where these abilities are of special importance (e.g. driving a car or operating machinery).

Patients should be advised to take precautions in order to avoid hypoglycaemia whilst driving. This is particularly important in those who have reduced or absent awareness of the warning signs of hypoglycaemia or have frequent episodes of hypoglycaemia. The advisability of driving should be considered in these circumstances.

4.8 Undesirable effects

Adverse drug reactions observed in patients using NovoMix products are mainly dose-dependent and due to the pharmacologic effect of insulin. As for other insulin products, hypoglycaemia, in general is the most frequently occurring undesirable effect. It may occur if the insulin dose is too high in relation to the insulin requirement and therefore require special attention during dose intensification as outlined in section 4.2. Severe hypoglycaemia may lead to unconsciousness and/or convulsions and may result in temporary or permanent impairment of brain function or even death.

In clinical trials and during marketed use the frequency varies with patient population and dose regimens therefore no specific frequency can be presented. During clinical trials the overall rates of hypoglycaemia did not differ between patients treated with insulin aspart compared to human insulin.

Figure 1 Glucose infusion rate

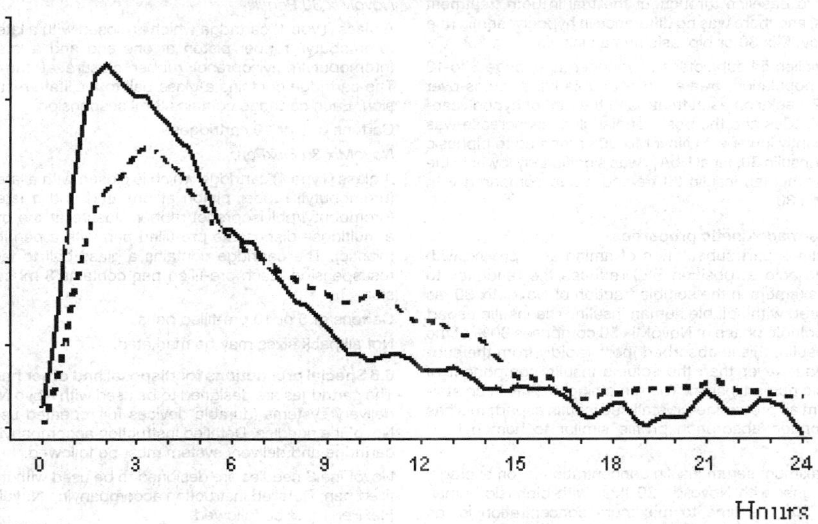

Figure 1: Activity profile of NovoMix 30 (—) and biphasic human insulin 30 (—) in healthy subjects.

Frequencies of adverse drug reactions from clinical trials, which by an overall judgement are considered related to insulin aspart are listed below. The frequencies are defined as: Uncommon (>1/1,000, <1/100) and rare (>1/10,000, <1/1,000). Isolated spontaneous cases are presented as very rare defined as (<1/10,000), including isolated reports.

Within each frequency grouping, undesirable effects are presented in order of decreasing seriousness.

Immune system disorders

Uncommon – Urticaria, rash, eruptions

Very rare – Anaphylactic reactions

Symptoms of generalised hypersensitivity may include generalised skin rash, itching, sweating, gastrointestinal upset, angioneurotic oedema, difficulties in breathing, palpitation and reduction in blood pressure. Generalised hypersensitivity reactions are potentially life threatening.

Nervous system disorders

Rare – Peripheral neuropathy

Fast improvement in blood glucose control may be associated with a condition termed acute painful neuropathy, which is usually reversible.

Eye disorders

Uncommon – Refraction disorder

Refraction anomalies may occur upon initiation of insulin therapy. These symptoms are usually of transitory nature.

Uncommon – Diabetic retinopathy

Long-term improved glycaemic control decreases the risk of progression of diabetic retinopathy. However, intensification of insulin therapy with abrupt improvement in glycaemic control may be associated with worsening of diabetic retinopathy.

Skin and subcutaneous tissue disorders

Uncommon – Lipodystrophy

Lipodystrophy may occur at the injection site as a consequence of failure to rotate injection sites within an area.

Uncommon – Local hypersensitivity

Local hypersensitivity reactions (redness, swelling and itching at the injection site) may occur during treatment with insulin. These reactions are usually transitory and normally they disappear during continued treatment.

General disorders and administration site conditions

Uncommon – Oedema

Oedema may occur upon initiation of insulin therapy. These symptoms are usually of transitory nature. Oedema and weight increase may occur when NovoMix 30 is used in combination with OADs.

4.9 Overdose

A specific overdose for insulin cannot be defined, however, hypoglycaemia may develop over sequential stages if too high doses relative to the patient's requirement are administered:

• Mild hypoglycaemic episodes can be treated by oral administration of glucose or sugary products. It is therefore recommended that the diabetic patient always carry sugar-containing products

• Severe hypoglycaemic episodes, where the patient has become unconscious, can be treated by glucagon (0.5 to 1 mg) given intramuscularly or subcutaneously by a trained person or glucose given intravenously by a medical professional. Glucose must also be given intravenously if the patient does not respond to glucagon within 10 to 15 minutes. Upon regaining consciousness administration of oral carbohydrate is recommended for the patient in order to prevent relapse.

5. PHARMACOLOGICAL PROPERTIES

5.1 Pharmacodynamic properties

Pharmacotherapeutic group: Drugs used in diabetes. Insulins and analogues for injection, intermediate-acting combined with fast-acting. ATC code: A10AD05.

NovoMix 30 is a biphasic suspension of insulin aspart (rapid-acting human insulin analogue) and protamine-crystallised insulin aspart (intermediate-acting human insulin analogue).

The blood glucose lowering effect of insulin occurs when the molecules facilitate the uptake of glucose by binding to insulin receptors on muscle and fat cells - and simultaneously inhibit the output of glucose from the liver.

NovoMix 30 is a biphasic insulin, which contains 30% soluble insulin aspart. This has a rapid onset of action, thus allowing it to be given closer to a meal (within zero to 10 minutes of the meal) when compared to soluble human insulin. The crystalline phase (70%) consists of protamine-crystallised insulin aspart, which has an activity profile that is similar to that of human NPH insulin (Figure 1).

When NovoMix 30 is injected subcutaneously, the onset of action will occur within 10 to 20 minutes of injection. The maximum effect is exerted between 1 and 4 hours after injection. The duration of action is up to 24 hours.

(see Figure 1 above)

In a 3 month trial in patients with type 1 and type 2 diabetes NovoMix 30 showed equal control of glycosylated haemoglobin compared to treatment with biphasic human insulin 30. Insulin aspart is equipotent to human insulin on a molar basis. Compared to biphasic human insulin 30, administration of NovoMix 30 before breakfast and dinner resulted in lower postprandial blood glucose after both meals (breakfast and dinner).

A meta-analysis including nine trials in patients with type 1 and type 2 diabetes showed **that** fasting blood glucose was higher in patients treated with NovoMix 30, than inpatients treated with biphasic human insulin 30.

In one study, 341 patients with type 2 diabetes were randomised to treatment with NovoMix 30 either alone or in combination with metformin, or to metformin together with sulfonylurea. The primary efficacy variable – HbA_{1c} after 16 weeks of treatment – did not differ between patients with NovoMix 30 combined with metformin and patients with metformin plus sulfonylurea. In this trial 57% of the patients had baseline HbA_{1c} above 9%; in these patients treatment with NovoMix 30 in combination with metformin resulted in significantly lower HbA_{1c} than metformin in combination with sulfonylurea.

In one study, patients with type 2 diabetes, insufficiently controlled on oral hypoglycaemic agents alone, were randomised to treatment with twice daily NovoMix 30 (117 patients) or once daily insulin glargine (116 patients). After 28 weeks treatment following the dosing guideline outlined in section 4.2, the mean reduction in HbA_{1c} was 2.8% with NovoMix 30 (mean at baseline = 9.7%). With NovoMix 30, 66% and 42% of the patients reached HbA_{1c} levels below 7% and 6.5%, respectively, and mean FPG was reduced by about 7 mmol/L (from 14.0 mmol/L at baseline to 7.1 mmol/L).

In patients with type 2 diabetes a meta-analysis showed a reduced risk of overall nocturnal hypoglycaemic episodes and major hypoglycaemia with NovoMix 30 compared to biphasic human insulin 30. The risk of overall daytime hypoglycaemic episodes was increased in patients treated with NovoMix 30.

Children and adolescents: A 16 week clinical trial comparing postprandial glycaemic control of meal-related NovoMix 30 with meal-related human insulin/biphasic human insulin 30 and bedtime NPH insulin was performed in 167 subjects aged 10 to 18 years. Mean HbA1c remained similar to baseline throughout the trial in both treatment groups, and there was no difference in hypoglycaemia rate with NovoMix 30 or biphasic human insulin 30.

In a smaller (54 subjects) and younger (age range 6 to 12 years) population, treated in a double-blind, cross-over trial (12 weeks on each treatment) the rate of hypoglycaemic episodes and the postprandial glucose increase was significantly lower with NovoMix 30 compared to biphasic human insulin 30. Final HbA_{1c} was significantly lower in the biphasic human insulin 30 treated group compared with NovoMix 30.

5.2 Pharmacokinetic properties

In insulin aspart substitution of amino acid proline with aspartic acid at position B28 reduces the tendency to form hexamers in the soluble fraction of NovoMix 30, as compared with soluble human insulin. The insulin aspart in the soluble phase of NovoMix 30 comprises 30% of the total insulin: this is absorbed more rapidly from the subcutaneous layer than the soluble insulin component of biphasic human insulin. The remaining 70% is in crystalline form as protamine-crystallised insulin aspart; this has a prolonged absorption profile similar to human NPH insulin.

The maximum serum insulin concentration is, on average, 50% higher with NovoMix 30 than with biphasic human insulin 30. The time to maximum concentration is, on average, half of that for biphasic human insulin 30. In healthy volunteers a mean maximum serum concentration of 140 ± 32 pmol/l was reached about 60 minutes after a subcutaneous dose of 0.20 U/kg body weight. The mean half life ($t_{½}$) of NovoMix 30, reflecting the absorption rate of the protamine bound fraction, was about 8-9 hours. Serum insulin levels returned to baseline 15-18 hours after a subcutaneous dose. In type 2 diabetic patients, the maximum concentration was reached about 95 minutes after dosing, and concentrations well above zero for not less than 14 hours post-dosing were measured.

Children and adolescents: The pharmacokinetics of NovoMix 30 has not been investigated in children or adolescents. However, the pharmacokinetic and pharmacodynamic properties of soluble insulin aspart have been investigated in children (6-12 years) and adolescents (13-17 years) with type 1 diabetes. Insulin aspart was rapidly absorbed in both age groups, with similar t_{max} as in adults. However C_{max} differed between the age groups, stressing the importance of the individual titration of insulin aspart.

The pharmacokinetics of NovoMix 30 has not been investigated in elderly, or patients with impaired renal or liver function.

5.3 Preclinical safety data

Non-clinical data with insulin aspart reveal no special hazard for humans based on conventional studies of safety pharmacology, repeated dose toxicity, genotoxicity and toxicity to reproduction.

In *in vitro* tests, including binding to insulin and IGF-1 receptor sites and effects on cell growth, insulin aspart behaved in a manner that closely resembled human insulin. Studies also demonstrate that the dissociation of binding to the insulin receptor of insulin aspart is equivalent to human insulin.

6. PHARMACEUTICAL PARTICULARS

6.1 List of excipients

Glycerol

Phenol

Metacresol

Zinc (as chloride)

Sodium chloride

Disodium phosphate dihydrate

Protamine sulphate

Sodium hydroxide (for pH adjustment)

Hydrochloric acid (for pH adjustment)

Water for injections

6.2 Incompatibilities

In absence of compatibility studies, this medicinal product must not be mixed with other medicinal products.

6.3 Shelf life

2 years

The in-use shelf life is 4 weeks (not above 30°C).

6.4 Special precautions for storage

Store in a refrigerator (2°C – 8°C) away from the freezing compartment. Do not freeze.

NovoMix 30 Penfill cartridges and NovoMix 30 FlexPen in use or carried as a spare: can be kept at ambient temperature (below 30°C) for up to 4 weeks, but any remainder must then be discarded. Do not refrigerate. Do not store above 30°C. Keep the cartridges in the outer carton or keep the cap on the pen when NovoMix 30 FlexPen is not in use in order to protect from light.

After removing NovoMix 30 Penfill and NovoMix 30 FlexPen from the refrigerator it is recommended to allow them to reach room temperature before resuspending the insulin as instructed for the first time use.

6.5 Nature and contents of container

NovoMix 30 Penfill:

A glass (Type 1) cartridge which is closed with a latex-free (bromobutyl) rubber piston at one end and a latex-free (bromobutyl/polyisoprene) rubber closure at the other. The cartridge contains a glass ball to facilitate resuspension. Each cartridge contains 3 ml suspension.

Cartons of 5 or 10 cartridges.

NovoMix 30 FlexPen:

A glass (Type 1) cartridge which is closed with a latex-free (bromobutyl) rubber piston at one end and a latex-free (bromobutyl/polyisoprene) rubber closure at the other in a multidose disposable pre-filled pen with a pen injector (plastic). The cartridge contains a glass ball to facilitate resuspension. Each pre-filled pen contains 3 ml suspension.

Cartons of 5 or 10 pre-filled pens.

Not all pack sizes may be marketed.

6.6 Special precautions for disposal and other handling

The cartridges are designed to be used with Novo Nordisk delivery systems (durable devices for repeated use) and NovoFine needles. Detailed instruction accompanying the cartridge and delivery system must be followed.

NovoFine **S** needles are designed to be used with the pre-filled pen. Detailed instruction accompanying NovoMix 30 FlexPen must be followed.

NovoMix 30 Penfill and NovoMix 30 FlexPen are for use by one person only. The cartridge and NovoMix 30 FlexPen must not be refilled.

The necessity of resuspending the NovoMix 30 suspension immediately before use is to be stressed to the patient. The resuspended liquid must appear uniformly white and cloudy.

NovoMix 30 which has been frozen must not be used.

The patient should be advised to discard the needle after each injection.

Any unused product or waste material should be disposed of in accordance with local requirements.

7. MARKETING AUTHORISATION HOLDER

Novo Nordisk A/S

Novo Allé

DK-2880 Bagsværd

Denmark

8. MARKETING AUTHORISATION NUMBER(S)

NovoMix 30 Penfill	EU/1/00/142/004-005
NovoMix 30 FlexPen	EU/1/00/142/009-010

9. DATE OF FIRST AUTHORISATION/RENEWAL OF THE AUTHORISATION

Date of first authorisation: 1 August 2000

Date of last renewal: 1 August 2005

10. DATE OF REVISION OF THE TEXT

07/2008

LEGAL CATEGORY

POM (Prescription Only Medicine)

NovoRapid 100 U/ml, NovoRapid Penfill 100 U/ml, NovoRapid FlexPen 100 U/ml

(Novo Nordisk Limited)

1. NAME OF THE MEDICINAL PRODUCT

NovoRapid 100 U/ml solution for injection in vial.

NovoRapid Penfill 100 U/ml solution for injection in cartridge.

NovoRapid FlexPen 100 U/ml solution for injection in pre-filled pen.

2. QUALITATIVE AND QUANTITATIVE COMPOSITION

1 ml of the solution contains 100 U of insulin aspart* (equivialent to 3.5mg). 1 vial contains 10 ml equivalent to 1,000 U.

1 ml of the solution contains 100 U of insulin aspart* (equivialent to 3.5mg). 1 cartridge contains 3 ml equivalent to 300 U.

1 ml of the solution contains 100 U of insulin aspart* (equivialent to 3.5mg). 1 pre-filled pen contains 3 ml equivalent to 300 U.

*Insulin aspart is produced by recombinant DNA technology in *Saccharomyces cerevisiae*.

For a full list of excipients, see section 6.1.

3. PHARMACEUTICAL FORM

Solution for injection in vial.

Solution for injection in cartridge. Penfill.

Solution for injection in pre-filled pen. FlexPen.

Clear, colourless, aqueous solution.

4. CLINICAL PARTICULARS

4.1 Therapeutic indications

Treatment of diabetes mellitus in adults and adolescents and children aged 2 to 17 years.

4.2 Posology and method of administration

NovoRapid is a rapid-acting insulin analogue.

Posology

NovoRapid dosing is individual and determined in accordance with the needs of the patient. It should normally be used in combination with intermediate-acting or long-acting insulin given at least once a day. Blood glucose monitoring and insulin dose adjustments are recommended to achieve optimal glycaemic control.

The individual insulin requirement in adults and children is usually between 0.5 and 1.0 U/kg/day. In a basal-bolus treatment regimen 50-70% of this requirement may be provided by NovoRapid and the remainder by intermediate-acting or long-acting insulin. Adjustment of dosage may be necessary if patients undertake increased physical activity, change their usual diet or during concomitant illness.

Special population

As with all insulin products, in elderly patients and patients with renal or hepatic impairment, glucose monitoring should be intensified and insulin aspart dosage adjusted on an individual basis.

Paediatric use

No studies have been performed in children below the age of 2 years. NovoRapid should only be used in this age group under careful medical supervision.

NovoRapid can be used in children in preference to soluble human insulin when a rapid onset of action might be beneficial (see section 5.1 and 5.2). For example, in the timing of the injections in relation to meals.

Transfer from other insulin products

NovoRapid has a faster onset and a shorter duration of action than soluble human insulin. When injected subcutaneously into the abdominal wall, the onset of action will occur within 10-20 minutes of injection. The maximum effect is exerted between 1 and 3 hours after the injection. The duration of action is 3 to 5 hours.

Due to the faster onset of action, NovoRapid should generally be given immediately before a meal. When necessary NovoRapid can be given soon after a meal. The faster onset of action compared to soluble human insulin is maintained regardless of injection site. When transferring from other insulin products, adjustment of the NovoRapid dose and the dose of the basal insulin may be necessary.

Method of administration

Administration with a syringe:

NovoRapid is administered subcutaneously by injection in the abdominal wall, the thigh, the upper arm, the deltoid region or the gluteal region. Injection sites should therefore always be rotated within the same region. As with all insulin products, subcutaneous injection in the abdominal wall ensures a faster absorption than other injection sites. The duration of action will vary according to the dose, injection site, blood flow, temperature and level of physical activity.

Administration with an insulin delivery system:

NovoRapid Penfill is designed to be used with Novo Nordisk insulin delivery systems and NovoFine needles.

NovoRapid Penfill is accompanied by a package leaflet with detailed instruction for use to be followed.

Administration with FlexPen:

NovoRapid FlexPen are pre-filled pens designed to be used with NovoFine or NovoTwist needles. FlexPen delivers 1-60 units in increments of 1 unit.

NovoRapid FlexPen is colour coded and accompanied by a package leaflet with detailed instruction for use to be followed.

Continuous Subcutaneous Insulin Infusion (CSII):

NovoRapid may be used for Continuous Subcutaneous Insulin Infusion (CSII) in pump systems suitable for insulin infusion. CSII should be administered in the abdominal wall. Infusion sites should be rotated.

When used with an insulin infusion pump, NovoRapid should not be mixed with any other insulin products.

Patients using CSII should be comprehensively instructed in the use of the pump system and use the correct reservoir and tubing for the pump (see section 6.6). The infusion set (tubing and cannula) should be changed in accordance with the instructions in the product information supplied with the infusion set.

Patients administering NovoRapid by CSII must have alternative insulin available in case of pump system failure.

Intravenous use:

If necessary, NovoRapid can be administered intravenously which should be carried out by health care professionals.

For intravenous use, infusion systems with NovoRapid 100 U/ml at concentrations from 0.05 U/ml to 1.0 U/ml insulin aspart in the infusion fluids 0.9% sodium chloride, 5% dextrose or 10% dextrose inclusive 40 mmol/l potassium chloride using polypropylene infusion bags are stable at room temperature for 24 hours.

Although stable over time, a certain amount of insulin will be initially adsorbed to the material of the infusion bag. Monitoring of blood glucose is necessary during insulin infusion.

4.3 Contraindications

Hypersensitivity to the active substance or to any of the excipients.

4.4 Special warnings and precautions for use

Inadequate dosing or discontinuation of treatment, especially in type 1 diabetes, may lead to hyperglycaemia and diabetic ketoacidosis.

Usually the first symptoms of hyperglycaemia develop gradually over a period of hours or days. They include thirst, increased frequency of urination, nausea, vomiting, drowsiness, flushed dry skin, dry mouth, loss of appetite as well as acetone odour of breath. In type 1 diabetes, untreated hyperglycaemic events eventually lead to diabetic ketoacidosis, which is potentially lethal.

Before travelling between different time zones the patient should seek the doctor's advice since this may mean that the patient has to take the insulin and meals at different times.

Hypoglycaemia

Omission of a meal or unplanned strenuous physical exercise may lead to hypoglycaemia.

Hypoglycaemia may occur if the insulin dose is too high in relation to the insulin requirement (see sections 4.8 and 4.9).

Patients whose blood glucose control is greatly improved, e.g. by intensified insulin therapy, may experience a change in their usual warning symptoms of hypoglycaemia, and should be advised accordingly. Usual warning symptoms may disappear in patients with longstanding diabetes.

A consequence of the pharmacodynamics of rapid-acting insulin analogues is that if hypoglycaemia occurs, it may occur earlier after an injection when compared with soluble human insulin.

Since NovoRapid should be administered in immediate relation to a meal the rapid onset of action should be considered in patients with concomitant diseases or medication where a delayed absorption of food might be expected.

Concomitant illness, especially infections and feverish conditions, usually increases the patient's insulin requirements.

When patients are transferred between different types of insulin products, the early warning symptoms of hypoglycaemia may change or become less pronounced than those experienced with their previous insulin.

Transfer from other insulin products

Transferring a patient to another type or brand of insulin should be done under strict medical supervision. Changes in strength, brand (manufacturer), type, origin (animal, human, human insulin analogue) and/or method of manufacture (recombinant DNA versus animal source insulin) may result in the need for a change in dosage. Patients transferred to NovoRapid from another type of insulin may require an increased number of daily injections or a change in dosage from that used with their usual insulins. If an adjustment is needed, it may occur with the first dose or during the first few weeks or months.

Injection site reactions

As with any insulin therapy, injection site reactions may occur and include pain, redness, hives, inflammation, swelling and itching. Continuous rotation of the injection site within a given area may help to reduce or prevent these reactions. Reactions usually resolve in a few days to a few weeks. On rare occasions, injection site reactions may require discontinuation of NovoRapid.

4.5 Interaction with other medicinal products and other forms of interaction

A number of medicinal products are known to interact with the glucose metabolism.

The following substances may reduce the patient's insulin requirements:

Oral antidiabetic medicinal products, monoamine oxidase inhibitors (MAOI), beta-blockers, angiotensin converting enzyme (ACE) inhibitors, salicylates, anabolic steroids and sulphonamides.

The following substances may increase the patient's insulin requirements:

Oral contraceptives, thiazides, glucocorticoids, thyroid hormones, sympathomimetics, growth hormone and danazol.

Beta-blocking agents may mask the symptoms of hypoglycaemia.

Octreotide/lanreotide may both increase or decrease insulin requirement.

Alcohol may intensify or reduce the hypoglycaemic effect of insulin.

4.6 Pregnancy and lactation

Pregnancy

NovoRapid (insulin aspart) can be used in pregnancy. Data from two randomised controlled clinical trials (322 and 27 exposed pregnancies) do not indicate any adverse effect of insulin aspart on pregnancy or on the health of the foetus/newborn when compared to human insulin (see section 5.1).

Table 1

Nervous system disorders	Rare - Peripheral neuropathy Fast improvement in blood glucose control may be associated with a condition termed "acute painful neuropathy", which is usually reversible.
Eye disorders	Uncommon - Refraction disorders Refraction anomalies may occur upon initiation of insulin therapy. These symptoms are usually of transitory nature.
	Uncommon - Diabetic retinopathy Long-term improved glycaemic control decreases the risk of progression of diabetic retinopathy. However, intensification of insulin therapy with abrupt improvement in glycaemic control may be associated with temporary worsening of diabetic retinopathy.
Skin and subcutaneous tissue disorders	Uncommon – Lipodystrophy Lipodystrophy may occur at the injection site as a consequence of failure to rotate injection sites within an area.
	Uncommon - Local hypersensitivity Local hypersensitivity reactions (pain, redness, hives, inflammation, swelling and itching at the injection site) may occur during treatment with insulin. These reactions are usually transitory and normally they disappear during continued treatment.
General disorders and administration site conditions	Uncommon – Oedema Oedema may occur upon initiation of insulin therapy. These symptoms are usually of transitory nature.
Immune system disorders	Uncommon - Urticaria, rash, eruptions
	Very rare - Anaphylactic reactions Symptoms of generalised hypersensitivity may include generalised skin rash, itching, sweating, gastrointestinal upset, angioneurotic oedema, difficulties in breathing, palpitation and reduction in blood pressure. Generalised hypersensitivity reactions are potentially life threatening.

Intensified blood glucose control and monitoring of pregnant women with diabetes (type 1 diabetes, type 2 diabetes or gestational diabetes) are recommended throughout pregnancy and when contemplating pregnancy. Insulin requirements usually fall in the first trimester and increase subsequently during the second and third trimester. After delivery, insulin requirements normally return rapidly to pre-pregnancy values.

Breast-feeding

There are no restrictions on treatment with NovoRapid during breast-feeding. Insulin treatment of the nursing mother presents no risk to the baby. However, the NovoRapid dosage may need to be adjusted.

4.7 Effects on ability to drive and use machines

The patient's ability to concentrate and react may be impaired as a result of hypoglycaemia. This may constitute a risk in situations where these abilities are of special importance (e.g. driving a car or operating machinery).

Patients should be advised to take precautions to avoid hypoglycaemia while driving. This is particularly important in those who have reduced or absent awareness of the warning signs of hypoglycaemia or have frequent episodes of hypoglycaemia. The advisability of driving should be considered in these circumstances.

4.8 Undesirable effects

Adverse reactions observed in patients using NovoRapid are mainly dose-dependent and due to the pharmacologic effect of insulin.

Hypoglycaemia is a common undesirable effect. It may occur if the insulin dose is too high in relation to the insulin requirement. Severe hypoglycaemia may lead to unconsciousness and/or convulsions and may result in temporary or permanent impairment of brain function or even death.

In clinical trials and during marketed use the frequency varies with patient population and dose regimens therefore no specific frequency can be presented. During clinical trials the overall rates of hypoglycaemia did not differ between patients treated with insulin aspart compared to human insulin.

Adverse reactions listed below are classified according to frequency and System Organ Class. Frequency categories are defined according to the following convention: Very common ($\geq 1/10$); common ($\geq 1/100$ to $< 1/10$); uncommon ($\geq 1/1,000$ to $\leq 1/100$); rare ($\geq 1/10,000$ to $\leq 1/1,000$); very rare ($\leq 1/10,000$), not known (cannot be estimated fromthe available data).

(see Table 1 above)

4.9 Overdose

A specific overdose for insulin cannot be defined, however, hypoglycaemia may develop over sequential stages if too high doses relative to the patient's requirement are administered:

- Mild hypoglycaemic episodes can be treated by oral administration of glucose or sugary products. It is therefore recommended that the diabetic patient always carries sugar containing products
- Severe hypoglycaemic episodes, where the patient has become unconscious, can be treated by glucagon (0.5 to 1 mg) given intramuscularly or subcutaneously by a trained person, or by glucose given intravenously by a health care professional. Glucose must also be given intravenously, if the patient does not respond to glucagon within 10 to 15 minutes. Upon regaining consciousness, administration of oral carbohydrates is recommended for the patient in order to prevent a relapse.

5. PHARMACOLOGICAL PROPERTIES

5.1 Pharmacodynamic properties

Pharmacotherapeutic group: Insulins and analogues for injection, fast-acting: ATC code A10AB05.

Mechanism of action

The blood glucose lowering effect of insulin aspart is due to the facilitated uptake of glucose following binding of insulin to receptors on muscle and fat cells and to the simultaneous inhibition of glucose output from the liver.

NovoRapid produces a more rapid onset of action compared to soluble human insulin, together with a lower glucose concentration, as assessed within the first four hours after a meal. NovoRapid has a shorter duration of action compared to soluble human insulin after subcutaneous injection.

(see Figure 1 on next page)

When NovoRapid is injected subcutaneously, the onset of action will occur within 10 to 20 minutes of injection. The maximum effect is exerted between 1 and 3 hours after injection. The duration of action is 3 to 5 hours.

Adults

Clinical trials in patients with type 1 diabetes have demonstrated a lower postprandial blood glucose with NovoRapid compared to soluble human insulin (Fig. I). In two long-term open label trials in patients with type 1 diabetes comprising 1070 and 884 patients, respectively, NovoRapid reduced glycosylated haemoglobin by 0.12 [95% C.I. 0.03; 0.22] percentage points and by 0.15 [95% C.I. 0.05; 0.26] percentage points compared to human insulin; a difference of doubtful clinical significance.

Elderly

A randomised, double-blind cross-over PK/PD trial comparing insulin aspart with soluble human insulin was performed in elderly patients with type 2 diabetes (19 patients aged 65-83 years, mean age 70 years). The relative differences in the pharmacodynamic properties (GIR_{max}, $AUC_{GIR,\ 0\text{-}120\ min}$) between insulin aspart and human insulin in elderly were similar to those seen in healthy subjects and in younger subjects with diabetes.

Children and adolescent

A clinical trial comparing preprandial soluble human insulin with postprandial insulin aspart was performed in small children (20 patients aged 2 to less than 6 years, studied for 12 weeks, among those four were younger than 4 years old) and a single dose PK/PD trial was performed in children (6-12 years) and adolescents (13-17 years). The pharmacodynamic profile of insulin aspart in children was similar to that seen in adults.

Figure 1

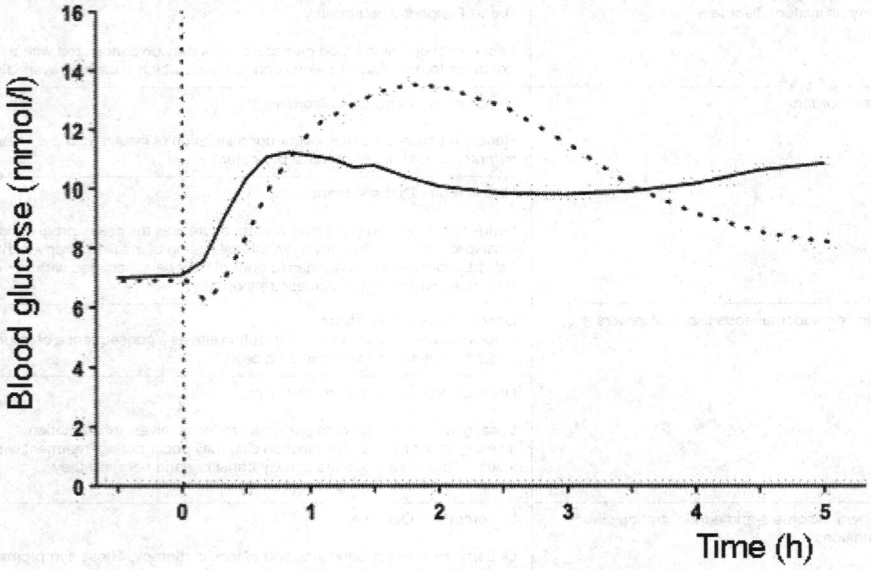

Fig. I. Blood glucose concentrations following a single pre-meal dose of NovoRapid injected immediately before a meal (solid curve) or soluble human insulin administered 30 minutes before a meal (hatched curve) in patients with type 1 diabetes mellitus.

Clinical trials in patients with type 1 diabetes have demonstrated a reduced risk of nocturnal hypoglycaemia with insulin aspart compared with soluble human insulin. The risk of daytime hypoglycaemia was not significantly increased.

Pregnancy

A clinical trial comparing safety and efficacy of insulin aspart vs. human insulin in the treatment of pregnant women with type 1 diabetes (322 exposed pregnancies (insulin aspart: 157; human insulin: 165)) did not indicate any adverse effect of insulin aspart on pregnancy or on the health of the foetus/newborn.

In addition the data from a clinical trial including 27 women with gestational diabetes randomised to treatment with insulin aspart vs. human insulin (insulin aspart: 14; human insulin: 13) showed similar safety profiles between treatments.

Insulin aspart is equipotent to soluble human insulin on a molar basis.

5.2 Pharmacokinetic properties

In NovoRapid substitution of amino acid proline with aspartic acid at position B28 reduces the tendency to form hexamers as observed with soluble human insulin. NovoRapid is therefore more rapidly absorbed from the subcutaneous layer compared to soluble human insulin.

The time to maximum concentration is, on average, half of that for soluble human insulin. A mean maximum plasma concentration of 492±256 pmol/l was reached 40 (interquartile range: 30–40) minutes after a subcutaneous dose of 0.15 U/kg bodyweight in type 1 diabetic patients. The insulin concentrations returned to baseline about 4 to 6 hours after dose. The absorption rate was somewhat slower in type 2 diabetic patients, resulting in a lower C_{max} (352±240 pmol/l) and later t_{max} (60 (interquartile range: 50–90) minutes). The intra-individual variability in time to maximum concentration is significantly less for NovoRapid than for soluble human insulin, whereas the intra-individual variability in C_{max} for NovoRapid is larger.

Children and adolescent

The pharmacokinetic and pharmacodynamic properties of NovoRapid were investigated in children (6–12 years) and adolescents (13–17 years) with type 1 diabetes. Insulin aspart was rapidly absorbed in both age groups, with similar t_{max} as in adults. However, C_{max} differed between the age groups, stressing the importance of the individual titration of NovoRapid.

Elderly

The relative differences in pharmacokinetic properties between insulin aspart and soluble human insulin in elderly subjects (65-83 years, mean age 70 years) with type 2 diabetes were similar to those observed in healthy subjects and in younger subjects with diabetes. A decreased absorption rate was observed in elderly subjects, resulting in a later t_{max} (82 (interquartile range: 60-120) minutes), whereas C_{max} was similar to that observed in younger subjects with type 2 diabetes and slightly lower than in subjects with type 1 diabetes.

Hepatic impairment

A single dose pharmacokinetic study of insulin aspart was performed in 24 subjects with hepatic function ranging from normal to severely impaired. In subjects with hepatic impairment absorption rate was decreased and more variable, resulting in delayed t_{max} from about 50 min in subjects with normal hepatic function to about 85 min in subjects with moderate and severe hepatic impairment. AUC, C_{max} and CL/F were similar in subjects with reduced hepatic function compared with subjects with normal hepatic function.

Renal impairment

A single dose pharmacokinetic study of insulin aspart in 18 subjects with renal function ranging from normal to severely impaired was performed. No apparent effect of creatinine clearance values on AUC, C_{max}, CL/F and t_{max} of insulin aspart was found. Data were limited in subjects with moderate and severe renal impairment. Subjects with renal failure necessitating dialysis treatment were not investigated.

5.3 Preclinical safety data

Non-clinical data reveal no special hazard for humans based on conventional studies of safety pharmacology, repeated dose toxicity, genotoxicity and toxicity to reproduction.

In *in vitro* tests, including binding to insulin and IGF-1 receptor sites and effects on cell growth, insulin aspart behaved in a manner that closely resembled human insulin. Studies also demonstrate that the dissociation of binding to the insulin receptor of insulin aspart is equivalent to human insulin.

6. PHARMACEUTICAL PARTICULARS

6.1 List of excipients

Glycerol

Phenol

Metacresol

Zinc chloride

Disodium phosphate dihydrate

Sodium chloride

Hydrochloric acid (for pH adjustment)

Sodium hydroxide (for pH adjustment)

Water for injections

6.2 Incompatibilities

Substances added to NovoRapid may cause degradation of insulin aspart, e.g. if the medicinal product contains thiols or sulphites.

This medicinal product must not be mixed with other medicinal products. Exceptions are NPH (Neutral Protamine Hagedorn) insulin and infusion fluids as described in section 4.2.

6.3 Shelf life

30 months.

After first opening: A maximum of 4 weeks when stored below 30°C.

6.4 Special precautions for storage

Store in a refrigerator (2°C - 8°C). Keep away from the cooling element. Do not freeze.

Keep the vial in the outer carton in order to protect from light.

Keep the cartridge in the outer carton in order to protect from light.

Keep the cap on FlexPen in order to protect from light.

After first opening or carried as a spare: Do not refrigerate. Store below 30°C.

NovoRapid must be protected from excessive heat and light.

6.5 Nature and contents of container

10 ml solution in vial (type 1 glass) closed with a disc (bromobutyl/polyisoprene rubber) and a protective tamper-proof plastic cap.

Pack sizes of 1 and 5 vials and a multipack with 5 × (1 × 10 ml) vials. Not all pack sizes may be marketed.

3 ml solution in cartridge (type 1 glass) with a plunger (bromobutyl) and a stopper (bromobutyl/polyisoprene) in a carton.

Pack sizes of 5 and 10 cartridges. Not all pack sizes may be marketed.

3 ml solution in cartridge (type 1 glass) with a plunger (bromobutyl) and a stopper (bromobutyl/polyisoprene) contained in a pre-filled multidose disposable pen made of polypropylene.

Pack sizes of 1, 5 and 10 pre-filled pens. Not all pack sizes may be marketed.

6.6 Special precautions for disposal and other handling

NovoRapid vials are for use with insulin syringes with the corresponding unit scale.

NovoRapid Penfill is for use by one person only. The cartridge must not be refilled.

NovoRapid FlexPen is for use by one person only. The cartridge must not be refilled.

The patient should be advised to discard the needle after each injection.

NovoRapid must not be used if it does not appear clear and colourless.

NovoRapid which has been frozen must not be used.

NovoRapid may be used in an infusion pump system (CSII) as described in section 4.2. Tubings in which the inner surface materials are made of polyethylene or polyolefin have been evaluated and found compatible with pump use.

In case of emergency in current NovoRapid users (hospitalisation or insulin pen malfunction), NovoRapid can be withdrawn with an U100 insulin syringe from the cartridge.

7. MARKETING AUTHORISATION HOLDER

Novo Nordisk A/S

Novo Allé

DK-2880 Bagsværd

Denmark

8. MARKETING AUTHORISATION NUMBER(S)

NovoRapid 10 ml EU/1/99/119/001, 008

NovoRapid Penfill 3 ml EU/1/99/119/003, 006

NovoRapid FlexPen 3ml EU/1/99/119/009, 010, 011

9. DATE OF FIRST AUTHORISATION/RENEWAL OF THE AUTHORISATION

Date of first authorisation: 7 September 1999

Date of last renewal: 30 April 2009

10. DATE OF REVISION OF THE TEXT

07/2009

LEGAL CATEGORY

Prescription only medicine (POM)

NovoSeven 1 mg (50KIU) powder and solvent for solution for injection. NovoSeven 2 mg (100 KIU) powder and solvent for solution for injection. NovoSeven 5 mg (250 KIU) powder and solvent for solution for injection.

(Novo Nordisk Limited)

1. NAME OF THE MEDICINAL PRODUCT

NovoSeven ▼ 1 mg (50 KIU) powder and solvent for solution for injection

NovoSeven ▼ 2 mg (100 KIU) powder and solvent for solution for injection

NovoSeven ▼ 5 mg (250 KIU) powder and solvent for solution for injection

2. QUALITATIVE AND QUANTITATIVE COMPOSITION

NovoSeven is presented as powder and solvent for solution for injection containing

1 mg eptacog alfa (activated) per vial (corresponds to 50 KIU/vial).

2 mg eptacog alfa (activated) per vial (corresponds to 100 KIU/vial).

5 mg eptacog alfa (activated) per vial (corresponds to 250 KIU/vial).

1 KIU equals 1000 IU (International Units).

eptacog alfa (activated) is recombinant coagulation factor VIIa (rFVIIa) with a molecular mass of approximately 50,000 Dalton produced in baby hamster kidney cells (BHK Cells) by recombinant DNA technology.

After reconstitution, the product contains 1 mg/ml eptacog alfa (activated) and 10 mg/ml sucrose when reconstituted with solvent.

For a full list of excipients, see Section 6.1.

3. PHARMACEUTICAL FORM

Powder and solvent for solution for injection.

White lyophilized powder. Solvent: clear colourless solution. The reconstituted solution has a pH of approximately 6.0.

4. CLINICAL PARTICULARS

4.1 Therapeutic indications

NovoSeven is indicated for the treatment of bleeding episodes and for the prevention of bleeding in those undergoing surgery or invasive procedures in the following patient groups:

- in patients with congenital haemophilia with inhibitors to coagulation factors VIII or IX> 5 Bethesda Units (BU)
- in patients with congenital haemophilia who are expected to have a high anamnestic response to factor VIII or factor IX administration
- in patients with acquired haemophilia
- in patients with congenital FVII deficiency
- in patients with Glanzmann's thrombasthenia with antibodies to GP IIb - IIIa and/or HLA, and with past or present refractoriness to platelet transfusions.

4.2 Posology and method of administration

Treatment should be initiated under the supervision of a physician experienced in the treatment of haemophilia and/or bleeding disorders.

Posology

Haemophilia A or B with inhibitors or expected to have a high anamnestic response

Dose

NovoSeven should be given as early as possible after the start of a bleeding episode. The recommended initial dose, administered by intravenous bolus injection, is 90 µg per kg body weight.

Following the initial dose of NovoSeven further injections may be repeated. The duration of treatment and the interval between injections will vary with the severity of the haemorrhage, the invasive procedures or surgery being performed.

Dosing in children

Current clinical experience does not warrant a general differentiation in dosing between children and adults, although children have faster clearance than adults. Therefore, higher doses of rFVIIa may be needed in paediatric patients to achieve similar plasma concentrations as in adult patients (see Section 5.2).

Dose interval

Initially 2 - 3 hours to obtain haemostasis.

If continued therapy is needed, the dose interval can be increased successively once effective haemostasis is achieved to every 4, 6, 8 or 12 hours for as long as treatment is judged as being indicated.

Mild to moderate bleeding episodes (including home therapy)

Early intervention has been shown to be efficacious in the treatment of mild to moderate joint, muscle and mucocutaneous bleeds. Two dosing regimens can be recommended:

1) Two to three injections of 90 µg per kg body weight administered at three-hour intervals

If further treatment is required, one additional dose of 90 µg per kg body weight can be administered

2) One single injection of 270 µg per kg body weight

The duration of the home therapy should not exceed 24 hours.

There is no clinical experience with administration of a single dose of 270 µg per kg body weight in elderly patients.

Serious bleeding episodes

An initial dose of 90 µg per kg body weight is recommended and could be administered on the way to the hospital where the patient is usually treated. The following dose varies according to the type and severity of the haemorrhage. Dosing frequency should initially be every second hour until clinical improvement is observed. If continued therapy is indicated, the dose interval can then be increased to 3 hours for 1 - 2 days. Thereafter, the dose interval can be increased successively to every 4, 6, 8 or 12 hours for as long as treatment is judged as being indicated. A major bleeding episode may be treated for 2 - 3 weeks but can be extended beyond this if clinically warranted.

Invasive procedure/surgery

An initial dose of 90 µg per kg body weight should be given immediately before the intervention. The dose should be repeated after 2 hours and then at 2 - 3 hour intervals for the first 24 - 48 hours depending on the intervention performed and the clinical status of the patient. In major surgery, the dose should be continued at 2 - 4 hour intervals for 6 - 7 days. The dose interval may then be increased to 6 - 8 hours for another 2 weeks of treatment. Patients undergoing major surgery may be treated for up to 2 - 3 weeks until healing has occurred.

Acquired Haemophilia

Dose and dose interval

NovoSeven should be given as early as possible after the start of a bleeding episode. The recommended initial dose, administered by intravenous bolus injection, is 90 µg per kg body weight. Following the initial dose of NovoSeven further injections may be given if required. The duration of treatment and the interval between injections will vary with the severity of the haemorrhage, the invasive procedures or the surgery being performed.

The initial dose interval should be 2 - 3 hours. Once haemostasis has been achieved, the dose interval can be increased successively to every 4, 6, 8 or 12 hours for as long as treatment is judged to be indicated.

Factor VII deficiency

Dose, dose range and dose interval

The recommended dose range for treatment of bleeding episodes and for the prevention of bleeding in patients undergoing surgery or invasive procedures is 15 - 30 µg per kg body weight every 4 - 6 hours until haemostasis is achieved. Dose and frequency of injections should be adapted to each individual.

Glanzmann's thrombasthenia

Dose, dose range and dose interval

The recommended dose for treatment of bleeding episodes and for the prevention of bleeding in patients undergoing surgery or invasive procedures is 90 µg (range 80 - 120 µg) per kg body weight at intervals of two hours (1.5 - 2.5 hours). At least three doses should be administered to secure effective haemostasis. The recommended route of administration is bolus injection as lack of efficacy may appear in connection with continuous infusion.

For those patients who are not refractory, platelets are the first line treatment for Glanzmann's thrombasthenia.

Method of administration

Reconstitute the solution as described under section 6.6 and administer as an intravenous bolus injection over 2 - 5 minutes.

Monitoring of treatment – laboratory tests

There is no requirement for monitoring of NovoSeven therapy. Severity of bleeding condition and clinical response to NovoSeven administration must guide dosing requirements.

After administration of rFVIIa, prothrombin time (PT) and activated partial thromboplastin time (aPTT) have been shown to shorten, however no correlation has been demonstrated between PT and aPTT and clinical efficacy of rFVIIa.

4.3 Contraindications

Hypersensitivity to the active substance, or to any of the excipients, or to mouse, hamster or bovine protein.

4.4 Special warnings and precautions for use

In pathological conditions in which tissue factor may be expressed more extensively than considered normal, there may be a potential risk of development of thrombotic events or induction of Disseminated Intravascular Coagulation (DIC) in association with NovoSeven treatment.

Such situations may include patients with advanced atherosclerotic disease, crush injury, septicaemia or DIC. Because of the risk of thromboembolic complications, caution should be excercised when administering NovoSeven to patients with a history of coronary heart disease, to patients with liver disease, to patients post-operatively, to neonates, or to patients at risk of thromboembolic phenomena or disseminated intravascular coagulation. In each of these situations, the potential benefit of treatment with NovoSeven should be weighed against the risk of these complications.

As recombinant coagulation factor VIIa NovoSeven may contain trace amounts of mouse IgG, bovine IgG and other residual culture proteins (hamster and bovine serum proteins), the remote possibility exists that patients treated with the product may develop hypersensitivity to these proteins. In such cases treatment with antihistamines i.v. should be considered.

If allergic or anaphylactic-type reactions occur, the administration should be discontinued immediately. In case of shock, standard medical treatment for shock should be implemented. Patients should be informed of the early signs of hypersensitivity reactions. If such symptoms occur, the patient should be advised to discontinue use of the product immediately and contact their physician.

In case of severe bleeds the product should be administered in hospitals preferably specialized in treatment of haemophilia patients with coagulation factor VIII or IX inhibitors, or if not possible in close collaboration with a physician specialized in haemophilia treatment.

If bleeding is not kept under control hospital care is mandatory. Patients/carers should inform the physician/supervising hospital at the earliest possible opportunity about all usages of NovoSeven.

Factor VII deficient patients should be monitored for prothrombin time and factor VII coagulant activity before and after administration of NovoSeven. In case the factor VIIa activity fails to reach the expected level or bleeding is not controlled after treatment with the recommended doses, antibody formation may be suspected and analysis for antibodies should be performed. The risk of thrombosis in factor VII deficient patients treated with NovoSeven is unknown.

Patients with rare hereditary problems of fructose intolerance, glucose malabsorption or sucrose-isomaltase insufficiency should not take this medicine

4.5 Interaction with other medicinal products and other forms of interaction

The risk of a potential interaction between NovoSeven and coagulation factor concentrates is unknown. Simultaneous use of prothrombin complex concentrates, activated or not, should be avoided.

Anti-fibrinolytics have been reported to reduce blood loss in association with surgery in haemophilia patients, especially in orthopaedic surgery and surgery in regions rich in fibrinolytic activity, such as the oral cavity. Experience with concomitant administration of anti-fibrinolytics and rFVIIa treatment is however limited.

4.6 Pregnancy and lactation

Pregnancy

As a precautionary measure, it is preferable to avoid use of NovoSeven during pregnancy. Data on a limited number of exposed pregnancies within approved indications indicate no adverse effects of rFVIIa on pregnancy or on the health of the foetus/new-born child. To date, no other relevant epidemiological data are available. Animal studies do not indicate direct or indirect harmful effects with respect to pregnancy, embryonal/foetal development, parturition or postnatal development (see Section 5.3).

Lactation

It is unknown whether rFVIIa is excreted in human breast milk. The excretion of rFVIIa in milk has not been studied in animals. A decision on whether to continue/discontinue breast-feeding or to continue/discontinue therapy with NovoSeven should be made taking into account the benefit of breast-feeding to the child and the benefit of NovoSeven therapy to the woman.

4.7 Effects on ability to drive and use machines

No studies on the effect on the ability to drive and use machines have been performed.

4.8 Undesirable effects

The frequencies of both serious and non-serious adverse drug reactions are listed by system organ classes in the table below.

(see Table 1 on next page)

Patients with acquired haemophilia

Clinical trials conducted in 61 patients with acquired haemophilia with a total of 100 treatment episodes, showed that certain adverse drug reactions were reported more frequent (1% based on treatment episodes): Arterial thromboembolic events (cerebral artery occlusion, cerebrovascular accident), venous thromboembolic events (pulmonary embolism and deep vein thrombosis), angina pectoris, nausea, pyrexia, erythematous rash and investigation of increased levels of fibrin degradation products.

Inhibitory antibody formation

In post-marketing experience, there have been no reports of antibodies against NovoSeven or FVII in patients with haemophilia A or B.

In clinical trials of patients with factor VII deficiency, formation of antibodies against NovoSeven and FVII is the only adverse drug reaction reported (frequency: common ($\geqslant$ 1/100 to < 1/10)). In some cases, the antibodies showed inhibitory effect *in vitro*. Risk factors that may have contributed to antibody development including previous treatment with human plasma and/or plasma-derived factor VII, severe mutation of FVII gene, and overdose of NovoSeven, were present. Patients with factor VII deficiency treated with NovoSeven should be monitored for factor VII antibodies, (see Section 4.4).

Thromboembolic events

When NovoSeven is administered to patients outside approved indications, arterial thromboembolic events are common ($\geqslant$ 1/100 to < 1/10). A higher risk of arterial thromboembolic adverse events (5.6% in patients treated with NovoSeven versus 3.0% in placebo-treated patients) has been shown in a meta-analysis of pooled data from placebo-controlled trials conducted outside current approved indications in various clinical settings, each of these having distinct patient characteristics and hence different underlying risk profiles.

Safety and efficacy of NovoSeven have not been established outside the approved indications and therefore NovoSeven should not be used.

Thromboembolic events may lead to cardiac arrest.

4.9 Overdose

Dose limiting toxicities of NovoSeven have not been investigated in clinical trials.

Three cases of overdose have been reported in patients with haemophilia in 13 years. The only complication reported in connection with an overdose was a slight transient increase in blood pressure in a 16 year-old patient receiving 24 mg rFVIIa instead of 5.5 mg.

No cases of overdose have been reported in patients with acquired haemophilia or Glanzmann's thrombasthenia.

In patients with factor VII deficiency, where the recommended dose is 15 – 30 µg/kg rFVIIa, one episode of overdose has been associated with a thrombotic event (occipital stroke) in an elderly (> 80 year) male patient

Table 1

Blood and the lymphatic system disorders	
Rare (> 1/10,000, < 1/1,000)	– Disseminated intravascular coagulation and related laboratory findings including elevated levels of D-dimer and AT-III, (see Section 4.4) – Coagulopathy.
Immune system disorders	
Rare (> 1/10,000, < 1/1,000)	– Hypersensitivity, (see Sections 4.3 and 4.4)
Not known	– Anaphylactic reaction.
Nervous system disorders	
Rare (> 1/10,000, < 1/1,000)	– Headache.
Vascular disorders	
Rare (> 1/10,000, < 1/1,000)	– Arterial thromboembolic events (myocardial infarction, cerebral infarction, cerebral ischaemia, cerebral artery occlusion, cerebrovascular accident, renal artery thrombosis, peripheral ischaemia, peripheral arterial thrombosis and intestinal ischaemia)
Uncommon (> 1/1,000, < 1/100)	– Venous thromboembolic events (deep vein thrombosis, thrombosis at i.v. site, pulmonary embolism, thromboembolic events of the liver including portal vein thrombosis, renal vein thrombosis, thrombophlebitis, superficial thrombophlebitis and intestinal ischaemia)
Rare (> 1/10,000, < 1/1,000)	– Angina pectoris.
Gastrointestinal disorders	
Rare (> 1/10,000, < 1/1,000)	– Nausea.
Skin and subcutaneous disorders	
Uncommon (> 1/1,000, < 1/100)	– Rash (including allergic dermatitis and rash erythematous) – Pruritus and urticaria
Not known	– Flushing – Angioedema.
General disorders and administration site conditions	
Uncommon (> 1/1,000, < 1/100)	– Therapeutic response decreased* – Pyrexia
Rare (> 1/10,000, < 1/1,000)	– Injection site reaction including injection site pain.
Investigations	
Rare (> 1/10,000, < 1/1,000)	– Increased fibrin degradation products – Increase in alanine aminotransferase, alkaline phosphatase, lactate dehydrogenase and prothrombin.

Within each frequency grouping, undesirable effects are presented in order of decreasing seriousness.

Adverse drug reaction reported post-marketing only (i.e. not in clinical trials) are presented with a frequency of not known.

* Lack of efficacy (therapeutic response decreased) has been reported. It is important that the dosage regimen of NovoSeven is compliant with the recommended dosage as stated in Section 4.2.

treated with 10 – 20 times the recommended dose. In addition, the development of antibodies against NovoSeven and FVII has been associated with overdose in one patient with factor VII deficiency.

The dose schedule should not be intentionally increased above the recommended doses due to the absence of information on the additional risk that may be incurred.

5. PHARMACOLOGICAL PROPERTIES

5.1 Pharmacodynamic properties

Pharmacotherapeutic group: Blood coagulation factors, ATC code: B02BD08

NovoSeven contains activated recombinant coagulation factor VII. The mechanism of action includes the binding of factor VIIa to exposed tissue factor. This complex activates factor IX into factor IXa and factor X into factor Xa, leading to the initial conversion of small amounts of prothrombin into thrombin. Thrombin leads to the activation of platelets and factors V and VIII at the site of injury and to the formation of the haemostatic plug by converting fibrinogen into fibrin. Pharmacological doses of NovoSeven activate factor X directly on the surface of activated platelets, localized to the site of injury, independently of tissue factor. This results in the conversion of prothrombin into large amounts of thrombin independently of tissue factor. Accordingly, the pharmacodynamic effect of factor VIIa gives rise to an increased local formation of factor Xa, thrombin and fibrin.

A theoretical risk for the development of systemic activation of the coagulation system in patients suffering from underlying diseases predisposing them to DIC cannot be totally excluded.

5.2 Pharmacokinetic properties

Healthy subjects

Using the FVII clotting assay, the pharmacokinetics of rFVIIa were investigated in 35 healthy Caucasian and Japanese subjects in a dose-escalation study. Subjects were stratified according to sex and ethnic group and dosed with 40, 80 and 160 µg rFVIIa per kg body weight and/or placebo (3 doses each). The pharmacokinetic profiles indicated dose proportionality. The pharmacokinetics were similar across sex and ethnic groups. The mean steady state volume of distribution ranged from 130 to 165 ml/kg, the mean values of clearance ranged from 33.3 to 37.2 ml/h × kg, and the mean terminal half-life ranged from 3.9 to 6.0 hours.

Haemophilia A and B with inhibitors

Using the FVIIa assay, the pharmacokinetic properties of rFVIIa were studied in 12 paediatric (2 - 12 years) and 5 adult patients in non bleeding state. Dose proportionality was established in children for the investigated doses of 90 and 180 µg per kg body weight, which is in accordance with previous findings at lower doses (17.5 - 70 µg/kg rFVIIa). Mean clearance was approximately 50% higher in paediatric patients relative to adults (78 versus 53 ml/h × kg), whereas the mean terminal half life was determined to 2.3 hours in both groups. Mean volume of distribution at steady state was 196 ml/kg in paediatric patients versus 159 ml/kg in adults. Clearance appears related with age, therefore in younger patients clearance may be increased by more than 50%.

Factor VII deficiency

Single dose pharmacokinetics of rFVIIa, 15 and 30 µg per kg body weight, showed no significant difference between the two doses used with regard to dose-independent parameters: total body clearance (70.8 - 79.1 ml/h × kg), volume of distribution at steady state (280 - 290 ml/kg), mean residence time (3.75 - 3.80 h), and half-life (2.82 - 3.11 h). The mean *in vivo* plasma recovery was approximately 20%.

Glanzmann's thrombasthenia

Pharmacokinetics of NovoSeven in patients with Glanzmann's thrombasthenia have not been investigated, but are expected to be similar to the pharmacokinetics in haemophilia A and B patients.

5.3 Preclinical safety data

All findings in the preclinical safety programme were related to the pharmacological effect of rFVIIa.

6. PHARMACEUTICAL PARTICULARS

6.1 List of excipients

Powder

Sodium chloride

Calcium chloride dihydrate

Glycylglycine

Polysorbate 80

Mannitol

Sucrose

Methionine

Hydrochloric acid (for pH-adjustment)

Sodium hydroxide (for pH-adjustment)

Solvent

Histidine

Hydrochloric acid (for pH-adjustment)

Sodium hydroxide (for pH-adjustment)

Water for injections

6.2 Incompatibilities

NovoSeven must not be mixed with infusion solutions or be given in a drip.

6.3 Shelf life

The shelf life is 2 years for the product packed for sale.

After reconstitution, chemical and physical stability have been demonstrated for 6 hours at 25°C and 24 hours at 5°C.

From a microbiological point of view, the product should be used immediately. If not used immediately, storage time and storage conditions prior to use are the responsibility of the user, and should not be longer than 24 hours at 2°C - 8°C, unless reconstitution has taken place in controlled and validated aseptic conditions.

6.4 Special precautions for storage

– Store powder and solvent below 25°C.

– Store powder and solvent protected from light.

– Do not freeze to prevent damage to the solvent vial.

– For storage conditions of the reconstituted medicinal product, see Section 6.3.

6.5 Nature and contents of container

The NovoSeven package contains Type I glass vials closed with a chlorobutyl rubber stopper, covered with an aluminium cap. The closed vials are equipped with a tamper-evident snap-off cap which is made of polypropylene.

Each NovoSeven package contains:

1 mg & 2 mg

– 1 vial (2 ml) with white powder for solution for injection

– 1 vial (2 ml) with solvent for reconstitution

5 mg

– 1 vial (12 ml) with white powder for solution for injection

– 1 vial (12 ml) with solvent for reconstitution

6.6 Special precautions for disposal and other handling

Always use an aseptic technique

Reconstitution

• NovoSeven powder and solvent vials should be at room temperature at reconstitution. Remove the plastic caps from the two vials. If the caps are loose or missing, do not use the vials. Clean the rubber stoppers on the vials with alcohol swabs and allow them to dry before use. Use a disposable syringe of an appropriate size and a vial adapter, transfer needle (20 - 26G) or other suitable device.

• Attach the vial adapter to the solvent vial. If using a transfer needle, screw the transfer needle tightly onto the syringe.

• Pull the plunger to draw in a volume of air that is equal to the amount of solvent in the solvent vial (ml equals cc on the syringe).

• Screw the syringe tightly onto the vial adapter on the solvent vial. If using a transfer needle, insert the transfer needle into the rubber stopper of the solvent vial. Inject air into the vial by pushing the plunger until you feel a clear resistance.

• Hold the syringe with the solvent vial upside down. If using a transfer needle, make sure the transfer needle tip is in the solvent. Pull the plunger to draw the solvent into the syringe.

• Remove the empty solvent vial. If using a vial adapter, tip the syringe to remove it from the vial.

• Attach the syringe with the vial adapter or transfer needle to the powder vial. If using a transfer needle, make sure to penetrate the centre of the rubber stopper. Hold the syringe slightly tilted with the vial facing downwards. Push the plunger slowly to inject the solvent into the powder vial. Make sure not to aim the stream of solvent directly at the NovoSeven powder as this will cause foaming.

• Gently swirl the vial until all the powder is dissolved. Do not shake the vial as this will cause foaming.

NovoSeven reconstituted solution is colourless and should be inspected visually for particulate matter and discolouration prior to administration.

Do not store reconstituted NovoSeven in plastic syringes.

It is recommended to use NovoSeven immediately after reconstitution.

Administration

• Ensure that the plunger is pushed all the way in before turning the syringe upside down (it may have been pushed out by the pressure in the syringe). If using a transfer needle, make sure the transfer needle tip is in the solution. Hold the syringe with the vial upside down and pull the plunger to draw all the solution into the syringe.

• If using a vial adapter, unscrew the vial adapter with the empty vial. If using a transfer needle, remove the transfer needle from the vial, replace the transfer needle cap, and twist the transfer needle off the syringe.

• NovoSeven is now ready for injection. Locate a suitable site, and slowly inject NovoSeven into a vein over a period of 2 - 5 minutes without removing the needle from the injection site.

Safely dispose of the syringe, vials and any unused product. Any unused product or waste material should be disposed of in accordance with local requirements.

7. MARKETING AUTHORISATION HOLDER

Novo Nordisk A/S

Novo Allé

DK-2880 Bagsværd

Denmark

8. MARKETING AUTHORISATION NUMBER(S)

NovoSeven® 1 mg	EU/1/96/006/004
NovoSeven® 2 mg	EU/1/96/006/005
NovoSeven® 5 mg	EU/1/96/006/006

9. DATE OF FIRST AUTHORISATION/RENEWAL OF THE AUTHORISATION

Date of first authorisation: 23 February 1996

Date of latest renewal: 23 February 2006

10. DATE OF REVISION OF THE TEXT

05/2009

Detailed information on this product is available on the website of the European Medicines Agency (EMEA) http://www.emea.europa.eu/

Nozinan injection

(sanofi-aventis)

1. NAME OF THE MEDICINAL PRODUCT

Nozinan injection.

2. QUALITATIVE AND QUANTITATIVE COMPOSITION

Levomepromazine INN (methotrimeprazine BAN) hydrochloride 25mg per ml.

3. PHARMACEUTICAL FORM

Solution for injection.

4. CLINICAL PARTICULARS

4.1 Therapeutic indications

Management of the terminally ill patient. Levomepromazine resembles chlorpromazine and promethazine in the pattern of its pharmacology. It possesses anti-emetic, antihistamine and anti-adrenaline activity and exhibits a strong sedative effect.

Nozinan potentiates the action of other central nervous system depressants but may be given in conjunction with appropriately modified doses of narcotic analgesics in the management of severe pain. Nozinan does not significantly depress respiration and is particularly useful where pulmonary reserve is low.

Nozinan is indicated in the management of pain and accompanying restlessness or distress in the terminally ill patient.

4.2 Posology and method of administration

Intramuscular and intravenous injection

Dosage varies with the condition and individual response of the patient. Nozinan injection may be administered by intramuscular injection or intravenous injection after dilution with an equal volume of normal saline.

The usual dose for adults and the elderly is 12.5mg to 25mg (0.5ml to 1ml) by intramuscular injection, or by the intravenous route after dilution with an equal volume of normal saline immediately before use. In cases of severe agitation, up to 50mg (2ml) may be used, repeated every 6 to 8 hours.

Continuous subcutaneous infusion

Nozinan injection may be administered over a 24 hour period via a syringe driver. The required dose of Nozinan injection (25mg to 200mg per day) should be diluted with the calculated volume of normal saline. Diamorphine hydrochloride is compatible with this solution and may be added if greater analgesia is required.

Nozinan tablets 25mg may be substituted for the injection if oral therapy is more convenient.

Children

Clinical experience with parenteral levomepromazine in children is limited. Where indicated, doses of 0.35mg/kg/day to 3.0mg/kg/day are recommended.

4.3 Contraindications

Safety in pregnancy has not been established. There are no absolute contraindications to the use of Nozinan in terminal care.

4.4 Special warnings and precautions for use

The drug should be avoided, or used with caution, in patients with liver dysfunction or cardiac disease.

The hypotensive effects of Nozinan should be taken into account when it is administered to patients with cardiac disease and the elderly or debilitated. Patients receiving large initial doses should be kept in bed.

As with other neuroleptics, cases of QT interval prolongation have been reported with levomepromazine very rarely. Consequently, and if the clinical situation permits, absence of the following risk factors for onset of this type of arrhythmia should be verified prior to administration:

- Bradycardia or 2nd or 3rd degree heart block.
- Metabolic abnormalities such as hypokalaemia, hypocalcaemia or hypomagnesaemia.
- Starvation or alcohol abuse.
- A history of QT interval prolongation, ventricular arrhythmias or Torsades de Pointes.
- A family history of QT interval prolongation.
- Ongoing treatment with another drug liable to induce marked bradycardia, hypokalaemia, slowed intracardiac conduction or prolonged QT interval.

It is recommended, as part of the initial evaluation in patients to be treated with levomepromazine, that an ECG is performed with measurement of serum calcium, magnesium and potassium levels. Periodic serum electrolyte levels should be monitored and corrected especially when long-term chronic usage is anticipated. An ECG should be repeated to assess the QT interval whenever dose escalation is proposed and when the maximum therapeutic dose is reached.

4.5 Interaction with other medicinal products and other forms of interaction

Cytochrome P450 2D6 Metabolism: Levomepromazine and its non-hydroxylated metabolites are reported to be potent inhibitors of cytochrome P450 2D6. Co-administration of levomepromazine and drugs primarily metabolised by the cytochrome P450 2D6 enzyme system may result in increased plasma concentrations of the drugs that could increase or prolong both therapeutic or adverse effects of those drugs.

There is an increased risk of arrhythmias when neuroleptics are used with drugs that prolong the QT interval such as certain anti-arrhythmics, antidepressants and other antipsychotics. If these drugs are co-administered this should be done with ECG monitoring.

The anticholinergic effect of neuroleptics may be enhanced by other anticholinergic drugs.

Simultaneous administration of desferrioxamine and prochlorperazine has been observed to induce a transient metabolic encephalopathy, characterised by loss of consciousness for 48 to 72 hours. It is possible that this may occur with Nozinan, since it shares many of the pharmacological activities of prochlorperazine. Adrenaline (epinephrine) must not be used in patients overdosed with neuroleptics. Alcohol should be avoided.

4.6 Pregnancy and lactation

Safety in pregnancy has not been established.

4.7 Effects on ability to drive and use machines

Nozinan can cause drowsiness, disorientation, confusion or excessive hypotension, which may affect the patient's ability to drive or operate machinery.

4.8 Undesirable effects

Somnolence and asthenia are frequent side effects. Dry mouth is encountered occasionally. Hypotension may occur, especially in elderly patients. A raised ESR may occasionally be encountered. Agranulocytosis has been reported, as have photosensitivity and allergic skin reactions.

Parkinsonian-like reactions may occur in patients receiving prolonged high dosage. Jaundice is a rare side effect. Other adverse effects common to phenothiazine neuroleptics may be seen, such as heat stroke in hot and humid conditions, constipation that may become severe leading to paralytic ileus, neuroleptic malignant syndrome and rare cases of cardiac rhythm disturbances and prolongation of the QT interval.

Very rarely cases of Torsades de Pointes have been reported, treatment of which should include discontinuation of levomepromazine and correction of hypoxia, electrolyte abnormalities and acid base disturbances.

Necrotizing enterocolitis which can be fatal, has been very rarely reported in patients treated with levomepromazine. Priapism has also been very rarely reported.

4.9 Overdose

Symptoms of levomepromazine overdosage include drowsiness or loss of consciousness, hypotension, tachycardia, ECG changes, ventricular arrhythmias and hypothermia. Severe extrapyramidal dyskinesias may occur.

General vasodilatation may result in circulatory collapse; raising the patient's legs may suffice but, in severe cases, volume expansion by intravenous fluids may be needed; infusion fluids should be warmed before administration in order not to aggravate hypothermia.

Positive inotropic agents such as dopamine may be tried if fluid replacement is insufficient to correct the circulatory collapse. Peripheral vasoconstrictor agents are not generally recommended; avoid use of adrenaline (epinephrine).

Ventricular or supraventricular tachy-arrhythmias usually respond to restoration of normal body temperature and correction of circulatory or metabolic disturbances. If persistent or life-threatening, appropriate anti-arrhythmic therapy may be considered. Avoid lidocaine (lignocaine) and, as far as possible, long acting anti-arrhythmic drugs.

Pronounced central nervous system depression requires airway maintenance or, in extreme circumstances, assisted respiration. Severe dystonic reactions usually respond to procyclidine (5mg to 10mg) or orphenadrine (20mg to 40mg) administered intramuscularly or intravenously. Convulsions should be treated with intravenous diazepam. Neuroleptic malignant syndrome should be treated with cooling. Dantrolene sodium may be tried.

5. PHARMACOLOGICAL PROPERTIES

5.1 Pharmacodynamic properties

Levomepromazine resembles chlorpromazine and promethazine in the pattern of its pharmacology. It possesses anti-emetic, antihistamine and anti-adrenaline activity and exhibits a strong sedative effect.

5.2 Pharmacokinetic properties

Maximum serum concentrations are achieved in 2 to 3 hours depending on the route of administration. Excretion is slow, with a half-life of about 30 hours. It is eliminated via urine and faeces.

5.3 Preclinical safety data

There are no pre-clinical safety data of relevance to the prescriber which are additional to those already included in other sections of the Summary of Product Characteristics.

6. PHARMACEUTICAL PARTICULARS

6.1 List of excipients

Ascorbic acid, sodium sulphite, sodium chloride, Water for Injections, nitrogen.

6.2 Incompatibilities

Incompatible with alkaline solutions.

6.3 Shelf life

60 months.

6.4 Special precautions for storage

Protect from light.

6.5 Nature and contents of container

Colourless type I glass ampoule. Each pack contains 10 ampoules.

6.6 Special precautions for disposal and other handling

Nozinan may be administered by intramuscular injection or intravenous injection after dilution with an equal volume of normal saline, or by continuous subcutaneous infusion with an appropriate volume of normal saline.

Diamorphine hydrochloride is compatible with this solution.

7. MARKETING AUTHORISATION HOLDER

Archimedes Pharma UK Limited

250 South Oak Way

Green Park

Reading

Berkshire

RG2 6UG

United Kingdom

8. MARKETING AUTHORISATION NUMBER(S)

PL 12406/0006

9. DATE OF FIRST AUTHORISATION/RENEWAL OF THE AUTHORISATION

12th May 1999 / 11 May 2004

10. DATE OF REVISION OF THE TEXT

13 November 2007

® Nozinan is a registered trade mark

NOZI010-SPC05A

Nozinan tablets

(sanofi-aventis)

1. NAME OF THE MEDICINAL PRODUCT

Nozinan tablets.

2. QUALITATIVE AND QUANTITATIVE COMPOSITION

Levomepromazine maleate INN (methotrimeprazine maleate BAN) 25mg per tablet.

3. PHARMACEUTICAL FORM

Tablets.

4. CLINICAL PARTICULARS

4.1 Therapeutic indications

Nozinan is a neuroleptic with indications in psychiatry and general medicine, particularly in terminal illness. Clinically it is more sedative and more potent than chlorpromazine in the management of psychotic conditions and in the relief of severe chronic pain.

Psychiatry

As an alternative to chlorpromazine in schizophrenia especially when it is desirable to reduce psychomotor activity.

General medicine

Alone, or together with appropriately modified doses of analgesics and narcotics, in the relief of severe pain and accompanying anxiety and distress.

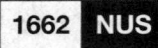

4.2 Posology and method of administration
Dosage varies with the condition under treatment and the individual response of the patient.

1. Terminal illness
Nozinan tablets 25mg may be substituted for the injection if oral therapy is more convenient, the dosage being 12.5mg to 50mg every 4 to 8 hours.

Elderly
No specific dosage recommendations.

2. Psychiatric conditions
Adults
Ambulant patients: initially the total daily oral dose should not exceed 25mg to 50mg usually divided into 3 doses; a larger portion of the dosage may be taken at bedtime to minimise diurnal sedation. The dosage is then gradually increased to the most effective level compatible with sedation and other side effects.

Bed patients: initially the total daily oral dosage may be 100mg to 200mg, usually divided into 3 doses, gradually increased to 1g daily if necessary. When the patient is stable attempts should be made to reduce the dosage to an adequate maintenance level.

Children
Children are very susceptible to the hypotensive and soporific effects of levomepromazine. It is advised that a total daily oral dosage of 1½ tablets should not be exceeded. The average effective daily intake for a ten year old is ½ to 1 tablet.

Elderly patients
It is not advised to give levomepromazine to ambulant patients over 50 years of age unless the risk of a hypotensive reaction has been assessed.

4.3 Contraindications
Safety in pregnancy has not been established.

There are no absolute contraindications to the use of Nozinan in terminal care.

4.4 Special warnings and precautions for use
The drug should be avoided, or used with caution, in patients with liver dysfunction or cardiac disease.

The hypotensive effects of Nozinan should be taken into account when it is administered to patients with cardiac disease and the elderly or debilitated. Patients receiving large initial doses should be kept in bed.

As with other neuroleptics, cases of QT interval prolongation have been reported with levomepromazine very rarely. Consequently, and if the clinical situation permits, absence of the following risk factors for onset of this type of arrhythmia should be verified prior to administration:

- Bradycardia or 2nd or 3rd degree heart block.
- Metabolic abnormalities such as hypokalaemia, hypocalcaemia or hypomagnesaemia.
- Starvation or alcohol abuse.
- A history of QT interval prolongation, ventricular arrhythmias or Torsades de Pointes.
- A family history of QT interval prolongation.
- Ongoing treatment with another drug liable to induce marked bradycardia, hypokalaemia, slowed intracardiac conduction or prolonged QT interval.

It is recommended, as part of the initial evaluation in patients to be treated with levomepromazine, that an ECG is performed with measurement of serum calcium, magnesium and potassium levels. Periodic serum electrolyte levels should be monitored and corrected especially when long-term chronic usage is anticipated. An ECG should be repeated to assess the QT interval whenever dose escalation is proposed and when the maximum therapeutic dose is reached.

4.5 Interaction with other medicinal products and other forms of interaction
Cytochrome P450 2D6 Metabolism: Levomepromazine and its non-hydroxylated metabolites are reported to be potent inhibitors of cytochrome P450 2D6. Co-administration of levomepromazine and drugs primarily metabolised by the cytochrome P450 2D6 enzyme system may result in increased plasma concentrations of the drugs that could increase or prolong both therapeutic or adverse effects of those drugs.

There is an increased risk of arrhythmias when neuroleptics are used with drugs that prolong the QT interval such as certain antiarrhythmics, antidepressants and other antipsychotics. If these drugs are co-administered this should be done with ECG monitoring.

The anticholinergic effect of neuroleptics may be enhanced by other anticholinergic drugs.

Simultaneous administration of desferrioxamine and prochlorperazine has been observed to induce a transient metabolic encephalopathy, characterised by loss of consciousness for 48 to 72 hours. It is possible that this may occur with Nozinan since it shares many of the pharmacological activities of prochlorperazine. Adrenaline (epinephrine) must not be used in patients overdosed with neuroleptics. Alcohol should be avoided.

4.6 Pregnancy and lactation
Safety in pregnancy has not been established.

4.7 Effects on ability to drive and use machines
Nozinan can cause drowsiness, disorientation, confusion or excessive hypotension, which may affect the patient's ability to drive or operate machinery.

4.8 Undesirable effects
Somnolence and asthenia are frequent side effects. Dry mouth is encountered occasionally. Hypotension may occur, especially in elderly patients. A raised ESR may occasionally be encountered. Agranulocytosis has been reported, as have photosensitivity and allergic skin reactions.

Parkinsonian-like reactions may occur in patients receiving prolonged high dosage. Jaundice is a rare side effect. Other adverse effects common to phenothiazine neuroleptics may be seen, such as heat stroke in hot and humid conditions, constipation that may become severe leading to paralytic ileus, neuroleptic malignant syndrome and rare cases of cardiac rhythm disturbances and prolongation of the QT interval.

Very rarely cases of Torsades de Pointes have been reported, treatment of which should include discontinuation of levomepromazine and correction of hypoxia, electrolyte abnormalities and acid base disturbances.

Necrotizing enterocolitis which can be fatal, has been very rarely reported in patients treated with levomepromazine. Priapism has also been very rarely reported.

4.9 Overdose
Symptoms of levomepromazine overdosage include drowsiness or loss of consciousness, hypotension, tachycardia, ECG changes, ventricular arrhythmias and hypothermia. Severe extrapyramidal dyskinesias may occur.

If the patient is seen sufficiently soon (up to 6 hours) after ingestion of a toxic dose, gastric lavage may be attempted. Pharmacological induction of emesis is unlikely to be of any use. Activated charcoal should be given. There is no specific antidote. Treatment is supportive.

Generalised vasodilatation may result in circulatory collapse; raising the patient's legs may suffice but, in severe cases, volume expansion by intravenous fluids may be needed; infusion fluids should be warmed before administration in order not to aggravate hypothermia.

Positive inotropic agents such as dopamine may be tried if fluid replacement is insufficient to correct the circulatory collapse. Peripheral vasoconstrictor agents are not generally recommended; avoid use of adrenaline (epinephrine).

Ventricular or supraventricular tachy-arrhythmias usually respond to restoration of normal body temperature and correction of circulatory or metabolic disturbances. If persistent or life-threatening, appropriate anti-arrhythmic therapy may be considered. Avoid lidocaine (lignocaine) and, as far as possible, long acting anti-arrhythmic drugs.

Pronounced central nervous system depression requires airway maintenance or, in extreme circumstances, assisted respiration. Severe dystonic reactions usually respond to procyclidine (5mg to 10mg) or orphenadrine (20mg to 40mg) administered intramuscularly or intravenously. Convulsions should be treated with intravenous diazepam.

Neuroleptic malignant syndrome should be treated with cooling. Dantrolene sodium may be tried.

5. PHARMACOLOGICAL PROPERTIES
5.1 Pharmacodynamic properties
Levomepromazine resembles chlorpromazine and promethazine in the pattern of its pharmacology. It possesses anti-emetic, antihistamine and anti-adrenaline activity and exhibits a strong sedative effect.

5.2 Pharmacokinetic properties
Maximum serum concentrations are achieved in 2 to 3 hours depending on the route of administration. Excretion is slow, with a half-life of about 30 hours. It is eliminated via urine and faeces.

5.3 Preclinical safety data
There are no pre-clinical safety data of relevance to the prescriber which are additional to those already included in other sections of the Summary of Product Characteristics.

6. PHARMACEUTICAL PARTICULARS
6.1 List of excipients
Potato starch, calcium hydrogen phosphate, magnesium stearate, sodium lauryl sulphate.

6.2 Incompatibilities
Not applicable.

6.3 Shelf life
36 months for blister pack.

60 months for polyethylene or polypropylene containers.

Not all pack sizes may be marketed

6.4 Special precautions for storage
Store below 25°C. Store in original container and protect from light.

6.5 Nature and contents of container
PVC/PVdC/aluminium foil blister pack containing 84 tablets.

OR

High density polyethylene bottle with flip cap or polypropylene tablet container. Each pack contains 500 tablets.

Not all pack sizes may be marketed

6.6 Special precautions for disposal and other handling
None.

7. MARKETING AUTHORISATION HOLDER
Link Pharmaceuticals Limited, Bishops Weald House, Albion Way, Horsham, West Sussex, RH12 1AH, United Kingdom

8. MARKETING AUTHORISATION NUMBER(S)
PL 12406/0007

9. DATE OF FIRST AUTHORISATION/RENEWAL OF THE AUTHORISATION
12th May 1999 / 11 May 2004

10. DATE OF REVISION OF THE TEXT
August 2005

NOZT084-eMC05

Nu-Seals 300

(Alliance Pharmaceuticals)

1. NAME OF THE MEDICINAL PRODUCT
Nu-Seals 300

Aspirin 300mg Enteric Coated

2. QUALITATIVE AND QUANTITATIVE COMPOSITION
Acetylsalicylic Acid 300mg

3. PHARMACEUTICAL FORM
White, enteric coated tablets, coded "300" in red or "GP" in black

4. CLINICAL PARTICULARS
4.1 Therapeutic indications
Aspirin has analgesic, antipyretic and anti-inflammatory actions. It can also be used for the secondary prevention of thrombotic cerebrovascular or cardiovascular disease and following by-pass surgery (see below).

Aspirin has an anti-thrombotic action, mediated through inhibition of platelet activation, which has been shown to be useful in secondary prophylaxis following myocardial infarction, and in patients with unstable angina or ischaemic stroke including cerebral transient attacks.

Nu-Seals 300 is indicated wherever high and prolonged dosage of aspirin is required. The special coating resists dissolution in gastric juice, but will dissolve readily in the relatively less acid environment of the duo-denum. Owing to the delay that the coating imposes on the release of the active ingredient, Nu-Seals 300 is unsuitable for the short-term relief of pain.

4.2 Posology and method of administration
Nu-Seals 300 is for oral administration to adults only.

Analgesic, antipyretic and anti-inflammatory actions: The usual dose of aspirin is 300-900mg repeated three to four times daily according to clinical needs. In acute rheumatic disorders the dose is in the range of 4-8 g daily, taken in divided doses.

Antithrombotic action: Patients should seek the advice of a doctor before commencing therapy for the first time. The usual dosage, for long-term use following myocardial infarction, transient ischaemic attack, or in patients with unstable angina, is 75-150mg once daily. In some circumstances a higher dose may be appropriate, especially in the short term, and up to 300mg a day may be used on the advice of a doctor.

The elderly: *Analgesic, antipyretic and anti-inflammatory actions*: As for adults. The elderly are more likely to experience gastric side-effects and tinnitus. *Antithrombotic action:* The risk-benefit ratio has not been fully established.

Children: Do not give to children aged under 16 years, unless specifically indicated (e.g. for Kawasaki's disease). See 'Special Warnings and Special Precautions for Use'.

4.3 Contraindications
Hypersensitivity to aspirin. Hypoprothrombinaemia, haemophilia and active peptic ulceration or a history of peptic ulceration.

4.4 Special warnings and precautions for use
There is a possible association between aspirin and Reye's syndrome when given to children. Reye's syndrome is a very rare disease, which affects the brain and liver, and can be fatal. For this reason aspirin should not be given to children aged under 16 years unless specifically indicated (e.g. for Kawasaki's disease).

Before commencing long-term aspirin therapy for the management of cerebrovascular or cardiovascular disease patients should consult their doctor who can advise on the relative benefits versus the risks for the individual patient.

Aspirin decreases platelet adhesiveness and increases bleeding time. Haematological and haemorrhagic effects can occur, and may be severe. Patients should report any unusual bleeding symptoms to their physician.

Salicylates should be used with caution in patients with a history of peptic ulceration or coagulation abnormalities. They may also induce gastro-intestinal haemorrhage, occasionally major.

They may also precipitate bronchospasm or induce attacks of asthma in susceptible subjects.

Aspirin should be used with caution in patients with impaired renal or hepatic function (avoid if severe), or in patients who are dehydrated.

Patients with hypertension should be carefully monitored.

4.5 Interaction with other medicinal products and other forms of interaction

Salicylates may enhance the effect of oral hypoglycaemic agents, phenytoin and sodium valproate. They inhibit the uricosuric effect of probenecid and may increase the toxicity of sulphonamides.

Aspirin may potentiate the effect of heparin and increases the risk of bleeding with oral anticoagulants, antiplatelet agents and fibrinolytics.

Plasma salicylate concentrations may be reduced by concurrent use of corticosteroids, and salicylate toxicity may occur following withdrawal of the corticosteroids. The risk of gastrointestinal ulceration and bleeding may be increased when aspirin and corticosteroids are co-administered.

Concurrent use of aspirin and other NSAIDs should be avoided. Use of two or more NSAID preparations increases the risk of serious gastrointestinal haemorrhage.

Concurrent administration of carbonic anhydrase inhibitors such as acetazolamide and salicylates may result in severe acidosis and increased central nervous system toxicity.

In large doses, salicylates may also decrease insulin requirements.

Patients using enteric coated aspirin should be advised against ingesting antacids simultaneously to avoid premature drug release.

Experimental data suggest that ibuprofen may inhibit the effect of low dose aspirin on platelet aggregation when they are dosed concomitantly. However, the limitations of these data and the uncertainties regarding extrapolation of *ex-vivo* data to the clinical situation imply that no firm conclusions can be made for regular ibuprofen use, and no clinically relevant effect is considered to be likely for occasional ibuprofen use (see section 5.1).

4.6 Pregnancy and lactation

Pregnancy: Although clinical and epidemiological evidence suggests the safety of aspirin for use in pregnancy, caution should be exercised when considering use in pregnant patients. Aspirin has the ability to alter platelet function and there may be a risk of haemorrhage in infants whose mothers have consumed aspirin during pregnancy. Prolonged pregnancy and labour, with increased bleeding before and after delivery, decreased birth weight and increased rate of stillbirth have been reported with high blood salicylate levels. With high doses there may be premature closure of the ductus arteriosus and possible persistent pulmonary hypertension in the newborn. Analgesic doses of aspirin should be avoided during the last trimester of pregnancy.

Lactation: As aspirin is excreted in breast milk, Nu-Seals should not be taken by patients who are breast-feeding, as there is a risk of Reye's syndrome in the infant. High maternal doses may impair platelet function in the infant.

4.7 Effects on ability to drive and use machines

None known.

4.8 Undesirable effects

Gastrointestinal irritation is common in patients taking aspirin preparations, and nausea, vomiting, dyspepsia, gastritis, gastrointestinal erosions and ulceration have been reported. Anaemia may occur following chronic gastrointestinal blood loss or acute haemorrhage.

Aspirin prolongs bleeding time, and bleeding disorders, such as epistaxis, haematuria, purpura, ecchymoses, haemoptysis, gastrointestinal bleeding, haematoma and cerebral haemorrhage have occasionally been reported. Fatalities have occurred.

Hypersensitivity reactions include skin rashes, urticaria, angioedema, asthma, bronchospasm and rarely, anaphylaxis.

Other side effects: urate kidney stones and tinnitus.

4.9 Overdose

Salicylate poisoning is usually associated with plasma concentrations >350 mg/L (2.5 mmol/L). Most adult deaths occur in patients whose concentrations exceed 700 mg/L (5.1 mmol/L). Single doses less than 100 mg/kg are unlikely to cause serious poisoning.

Symptoms

Common features include vomiting, dehydration, tinnitus, vertigo, deafness, sweating, warm extremities with bounding pulses, increased respiratory rate and hyperventilation. Some degree of acid-base disturbance is present in most cases.

A mixed respiratory alkalosis and metabolic acidosis with normal or high arterial pH (normal or reduced hydrogen ion concentration) is usual in adults and children over the age of 4 years. In children aged 4 years or less, a dominant metabolic acidosis with low arterial pH (raised hydrogen ion concentration) is common. Acidosis may increase salicylate transfer across the blood brain barrier.

Uncommon features include haematemesis, hyperpyrexia, hypoglycaemia, hypokalaemia, thrombocytopenia, increased INR/PTR, intravascular coagulation, renal failure and non-cardiogenic pulmonary oedema.

Central nervous system features including confusion, disorientation, coma and convulsions are less common in adults than in children.

Management

Give activated charcoal if an adult presents within one hour of ingestion of more than 250 mg/kg. The plasma salicylate concentration should be measured, although the severity of poisoning cannot be determined from this alone and the clinical and biochemical features must be taken into account. Elimination is increased by urinary alkalisation, which is achieved by the administration of 1.26% sodium bicarbonate. The urine pH should be monitored. Correct metabolic acidosis with intravenous 8.4% sodium bicarbonate (first check serum potassium). Forced diuresis should not be used since it does not enhance salicylate excretion and may cause pulmonary oedema.

Haemodialysis is the treatment of choice for severe poisoning and should be considered in patients with plasma salicylate concentrations >700 mg/L (5.1 mmol/L), or lower concentrations associated with severe clinical or metabolic features. Patients under 10 years and over 70 have increased risk of salicylate toxicity, and may require dialysis at an earlier stage.

5. PHARMACOLOGICAL PROPERTIES

5.1 Pharmacodynamic properties

Aspirin has analgesic, antipyretic and anti-inflammatory actions.

It also has antithrombotic action, which is mediated through inhibition of platelet activation.

Nu-Seals 300 tablets have an enteric coat sandwiched between a sealing coat and a top coat. The enteric coat is intended to resist gastric fluid whilst allowing disintegration in the intestinal fluid.

Owing to the delay that the coating imposes on the release of the active ingredient, Nu-Seals 300 is unsuitable for the short-term relief of pain.

Experimental data suggest that ibuprofen may inhibit the effect of low dose aspirin on platelet aggregation when they are dosed concomitantly. In one study, when a single dose of ibuprofen 400mg was taken within 8 hours before or within 30 minutes after immediate release aspirin (81mg), a decreased effect of aspirin on the formation of thromboxane or platelet aggregation occurred. However, the limitations of these data and the uncertainties regarding extrapolation of *ex vivo* data to the clinical situation imply that no firm conclusions can be made for regular ibuprofen use, and no clinically relevant effect is considered to be likely for occasional ibuprofen use.

5.2 Pharmacokinetic properties

In a bioequivalence study comparing the pharmacokinetics of the 300mg product with 4 × 75mg presentation in human volunteers, measures such as terminal phase half-life, area-under-the curve and peak plasma concentrations were recorded on days 1 and 4. On day 1 salicylate reached a peak plasma concentration of between 10.34 and 31.57 mcg/ml and between 11.76 and 27.47mcg/ml for the 300mg and 75mg tablets respectively. Time to peak concentration ranged from 4 to 8 hours and from 3 to 6 hours respectively. AUC ranged from 54.0 to 131.2 and from 64.3 to 137.6 h.mcg/ml respectively. The terminal phase half-life ranged from 1.33 to 2.63 hours and from 1.47 to 2.59 hours respectively. On day 4 C_{max} varied from 15.01 to 48.97 mcg/ml for the 300mg tablet and from 11.26 to 60.21 mcg/ml for 4 × 75mg tablets. T_{max} ranged from 4 to 8 hours and from 3 to 8 hours, whilst AUC ranged from 89.8 to 297.4 h.mcg/ml and from 61.5 to 293.4 h.mcg/ml respectively.

5.3 Preclinical safety data

There are no pre-clinical data of relevance to the prescriber in addition to that summarised in other sections of the Summary of Product Characteristics.

6. PHARMACEUTICAL PARTICULARS

6.1 List of excipients

Maize Starch

Hypromellose

Talc

Methacrylic acid – ethyl acrylate (1:1) copolymer dispersion 30 per cent

Polyethylene Glycol 3350

Propylene Glycol

Benzyl Alcohol

Emulsion silicone

Edible Printing Ink – containing either: E124 Red and Shellac or: E172 Black, Shellac and E322 Lecithin

6.2 Incompatibilities

None

6.3 Shelf life

2 years

6.4 Special precautions for storage

Do not store above 25°C. Keep containers tightly closed.

6.5 Nature and contents of container

HDPE bottles with screw caps containing 14, 56, 100 or 500 tablets.

6.6 Special precautions for disposal and other handling

None

7. MARKETING AUTHORISATION HOLDER

Alliance Pharmaceuticals Ltd

Avonbridge House

Bath Road

Chippenham

Wiltshire

SN15 2BB

8. MARKETING AUTHORISATION NUMBER(S)

PL 16853/0063

9. DATE OF FIRST AUTHORISATION/RENEWAL OF THE AUTHORISATION

Date of first authorisation: 22 May 1973

Date of last renewal of authorisation: 12 May 2006

10. DATE OF REVISION OF THE TEXT

19th June 2009

Nu-Seals 75

(Alliance Pharmaceuticals)

1. NAME OF THE MEDICINAL PRODUCT

Nu-Seals 75, Aspirin 75mg Enteric Coated Tablets, PostMI 75EC, Nu-Seals Cardio 75

2. QUALITATIVE AND QUANTITATIVE COMPOSITION

Acetylsalicylic Acid 75mg

3. PHARMACEUTICAL FORM

White, enteric coated tablets, coded "75" or "GP".

4. CLINICAL PARTICULARS

4.1 Therapeutic indications

For the secondary prevention of thrombotic cerebrovascular or cardiovascular disease and following by-pass surgery (see below).

Aspirin has an antithrombotic action, mediated through inhibition of platelet activation, which has been shown to be useful in secondary prophylaxis following myocardial infarction and in patients with unstable angina or ischaemic stroke including cerebral transient attacks.

Nu-Seals 75 is indicated when prolonged dosage of aspirin is required. The special coating resists dissolution in gastric juice, but will dissolve readily in the relatively less acid environment of the duodenum. Owing to the delay that the coating imposes on the release of the active ingredient, Nu-Seals 75 is unsuitable for the short-term relief of pain.

4.2 Posology and method of administration

Nu-Seals 75 is for oral administration to adults only.

Patients should seek the advice of a doctor before commencing therapy for the first time.

The usual dosage, for long-term use, is 75-150mg once daily. In some circumstances a higher dose may be appropriate, especially in the short term, and up to 300mg a day may be used on the advice of a doctor.

Antithrombotic action: 150mg at diagnosis and 75mg daily thereafter. Tablets taken at diagnosis should be chewed in order to gain rapid absorption.

The elderly: The risk-benefit ratio of the antithrombotic action of aspirin has not been fully established.

Children:

Do not give to children aged under 16 years, unless specifically indicated (e.g. for Kawasaki's disease). See 'Special warnings and precautions for use'.

4.3 Contraindications

Hypersensitivity to aspirin. Hypoprothrombinaemia, haemophilia and active peptic ulceration or a history of peptic ulceration.

4.4 Special warnings and precautions for use

There is a possible association between aspirin and Reye's syndrome when given to children. Reye's syndrome is a very rare disease, which affects the brain and liver, and can be fatal. For this reason aspirin should not be given to children aged under 16 years unless specifically indicated (e.g. for Kawasaki's disease).

Before commencing long-term aspirin therapy for the management of cerebrovascular or cardiovascular disease patients should consult their doctor who can advise on the relative benefits versus the risks for the individual patient.

Aspirin decreases platelet adhesiveness and increases bleeding time. Haematological and haemorrhagic effects can occur, and may be severe. Patients should report any unusual bleeding symptoms to their physician.

Salicylates should be used with caution in patients with a history of peptic ulceration or coagulation abnormalities.

They may also induce gastro-intestinal haemorrhage, occasionally major.

They may also precipitate bronchospasm or induce attacks of asthma in susceptible subjects.

Aspirin should be used with caution in patients with impaired renal or hepatic function (avoid if severe), or in patients who are dehydrated.

Patients with hypertension should be carefully monitored.

4.5 Interaction with other medicinal products and other forms of interaction

Salicylates may enhance the effect of oral hypoglycaemic agents, phenytoin and sodium valproate. They inhibit the uricosuric effect of probenecid and may increase the toxicity of sulphonamides.

Aspirin may potentiate the effect of heparin and increases the risk of bleeding with oral anticoagulants, antiplatelet agents and fibrinolytics.

Plasma salicylate concentrations may be reduced by concurrent use of corticosteroids, and salicylate toxicity may occur following withdrawal of the corticosteroids. The risk of gastrointestinal ulceration and bleeding may be increased when aspirin and corticosteroids are co-administered.

Concurrent use of aspirin and other NSAIDs should be avoided. Use of two or more NSAID preparations increases the risk of serious gastrointestinal haemorrhage.

Concurrent administration of carbonic anhydrase inhibitors such as acetazolamide and salicylates may result in severe acidosis and increased central nervous system toxicity.

In large doses, salicylates may also decrease insulin requirements.

Patients using enteric coated aspirin should be advised against ingesting antacids simultaneously to avoid premature drug release.

Experimental data suggest that ibuprofen may inhibit the effect of low dose aspirin on platelet aggregation when they are dosed concomitantly. However, the limitations of these data and the uncertainties regarding extrapolation of *ex-vivo* data to the clinical situation imply that no firm conclusions can be made for regular ibuprofen use, and no clinically relevant effect is considered to be likely for occasional ibuprofen use (see section 5.1).

4.6 Pregnancy and lactation

Pregnancy: Although clinical and epidemiological evidence suggests the safety of aspirin for use in pregnancy, caution should be exercised when considering use in pregnant patients. Aspirin has the ability to alter platelet function and there may be a risk of haemorrhage in infants whose mothers have consumed aspirin during pregnancy. Prolonged pregnancy and labour, with increased bleeding before and after delivery, decreased birth weight and increased rate of stillbirth have been reported with high blood salicylate levels. With high doses there may be premature closure of the ductus arteriosus and possible persistent pulmonary hypertension in the newborn. Analgesic doses of aspirin should be avoided during the last trimester of pregnancy.

Lactation: As aspirin is excreted in breast milk, Nu-Seals should not be taken by patients who are breast-feeding, as there is a risk of Reye's syndrome in the infant. High maternal doses may impair platelet function in the infant.

4.7 Effects on ability to drive and use machines

None known.

4.8 Undesirable effects

Gastrointestinal irritation is common in patients taking aspirin preparations, and nausea, vomiting, dyspepsia, gastritis, gastrointestinal erosions and ulceration have been reported. Anaemia may occur following chronic gastrointestinal blood loss or acute haemorrhage.

Aspirin prolongs bleeding time, and bleeding disorders, such as epistaxis, haematuria, purpura, ecchymoses, haemoptysis, gastrointestinal bleeding, haematoma and cerebral haemorrhage have occasionally been reported. Fatalities have occurred.

Hypersensitivity reactions include skin rashes, urticaria, angioedema, asthma, bronchospasm and rarely, anaphylaxis.

Other side effects: urate kidney stones and tinnitus.

4.9 Overdose

Salicylate poisoning is usually associated with plasma concentrations >350 mg/L (2.5 mmol/L). Most adult deaths occur in patients whose concentrations exceed 700 mg/L (5.1 mmol/L). Single doses less than 100 mg/kg are unlikely to cause serious poisoning.

Symptoms

Common features include vomiting, dehydration, tinnitus, vertigo, deafness, sweating, warm extremities with bounding pulses, increased respiratory rate and hyperventilation. Some degree of acid-base disturbance is present in most cases.

A mixed respiratory alkalosis and metabolic acidosis with normal or high arterial pH (normal or reduced hydrogen ion concentration) is usual in adults and children over the age of 4 years. In children aged 4 years or less, a dominant metabolic acidosis with low arterial pH (raised hydrogen ion concentration) is common. Acidosis may increase salicylate transfer across the blood brain barrier.

Uncommon features include haematemesis, hyperpyrexia, hypoglycaemia, hypokalaemia, thrombocytopenia, increased INR/PTR, intravascular coagulation, renal failure and non-cardiogenic pulmonary oedema.

Central nervous system features including confusion, disorientation, coma and convulsions are less common in adults than in children.

Management

Give activated charcoal if an adult presents within one hour of ingestion of more than 250 mg/kg. The plasma salicylate concentration should be measured, although the severity of poisoning cannot be determined from this alone and the clinical and biochemical features must be taken into account. Elimination is increased by urinary alkalisation, which is achieved by the administration of 1.26% sodium bicarbonate. The urine pH should be monitored. Correct metabolic acidosis with intravenous 8.4% sodium bicarbonate (first check serum potassium). Forced diuresis should not be used since it does not enhance salicylate excretion and may cause pulmonary oedema.

Haemodialysis is the treatment of choice for severe poisoning and should be considered in patients with plasma salicylate concentrations >700 mg/L (5.1 mmol/L), or lower concentrations associated with severe clinical or metabolic features. Patients under 10 years and over 70 have increased risk of salicylate toxicity, and may require dialysis at an earlier stage.

5. PHARMACOLOGICAL PROPERTIES

5.1 Pharmacodynamic properties

Aspirin has analgesic, antipyretic and anti-inflammatory actions.

It also has antithrombotic action which is mediated through inhibition of platelet activation.

Nu-Seals 75 tablets have an enteric coat sandwiched between a sealing coat and a top coat. The enteric coat is intended to resist gastric fluid whilst allowing disintegration in the intestinal fluid.

Owing to the delay that the coating imposes on the release of the active ingredient, Nu-Seals 75 is unsuitable for the short-term relief of pain.

Experimental data suggest that ibuprofen may inhibit the effect of low dose aspirin on platelet aggregation when they are dosed concomitantly. In one study, when a single dose of ibuprofen 400mg was taken within 8 hours before or within 30 minutes after immediate release aspirin (81mg), a decreased effect of aspirin on the formation of thromboxane or platelet aggregation occurred. However, the limitations of these data and the uncertainties regarding extrapolation of *ex vivo* data to the clinical situation imply that no firm conclusions can be made for regular ibuprofen use, and no clinically relevant effect is considered to be likely for occasional ibuprofen use.

5.2 Pharmacokinetic properties

In a bioequivalence study comparing the pharmacokinetics of the 300mg product with 4 × 75mg presentation in human volunteers, measures such as terminal phase half-life, area-under-the curve and peak plasma concentrations were recorded on days 1 and 4. On day 1 salicylate reached a peak plasma concentration of between 10.34 and 31.57 mcg/ml and between 11.76 and 27.47mcg/ml for the 300mg and 75mg tablets respectively. Time to peak concentration ranged from 4 to 8 hours and from 3 to 6 hours respectively. AUC ranged from 54.0 to 131.2 and from 64.3 to 137.6 h.mcg/ml respectively. The terminal phase half-life ranged from 1.33 to 2.63 hours and from 1.47 to 2.59 hours respectively. On day 4 C_{max} varied from 15.01 to 48.97 mcg/ml for the 300mg tablet and from 11.26 to 60.21 mcg/ml for 4 × 75mg tablets. T_{max} ranged from 4 to 8 hours and from 3 to 8 hours, whilst AUC ranged from 89.8 to 297.4 h.mcg/ml and from 61.5 to 293.4 h.mcg/ml respectively.

5.3 Preclinical safety data

There are no pre-clinical data of relevance to the prescriber in addition to that summarised in other sections of the Summary of Product Characteristics.

6. PHARMACEUTICAL PARTICULARS

6.1 List of excipients

Maize Starch

Hypromellose

Talc

Methacrylic acid – ethyl acrylate (1:1) copolymer dispersion 30 per cent

Polyethylene Glycol 3350

Propylene Glycol

Benzyl Alcohol

Emulsion silicone

Edible Printing Ink - containing either: E124 Red and Shellac or: E172 Black, Shellac and E322 Lecithin

6.2 Incompatibilities

None known.

6.3 Shelf life

2 years.

6.4 Special precautions for storage

Do not store above 25°C. Keep containers tightly closed.

6.5 Nature and contents of container

Blisters comprising of UPVC on one side and aluminium foil on the other containing 14, 28, 56 or 84 tablets. HDPE bottles with screw caps containing 500 tablets.

6.6 Special precautions for disposal and other handling

None.

7. MARKETING AUTHORISATION HOLDER

Alliance Pharmaceuticals Ltd

Avonbridge House

Bath Road

Chippenham

Wiltshire

SN15 2BB

8. MARKETING AUTHORISATION NUMBER(S)

PL 16853/0062

9. DATE OF FIRST AUTHORISATION/RENEWAL OF THE AUTHORISATION

Date of first authorisation: 21 April 1994

Date of last renewal of authorisation: 12 May 2006

10. DATE OF REVISION OF THE TEXT

19th June 2009

Nutraplus Cream

(Galderma (U.K) Ltd)

1. NAME OF THE MEDICINAL PRODUCT

Nutraplus Cream

2. QUALITATIVE AND QUANTITATIVE COMPOSITION

Urea 10% w/w

For excipients see section 6.1

3. PHARMACEUTICAL FORM

Cream

Smooth white, almost odourless cream (water in oil emulsion).

4. CLINICAL PARTICULARS

4.1 Therapeutic indications

An emollient, moisturising and protective cream for the treatment of dry or damaged skin.

4.2 Posology and method of administration

Adults, elderly and children

Apply evenly to the dry skin areas two to three times daily, or as directed by the physician or pharmacist.

4.3 Contraindications

None

4.4 Special warnings and precautions for use

Avoid contact with the eyes. If irritation occurs, discontinue use temporarily.

4.5 Interaction with other medicinal products and other forms of interaction

None known

4.6 Pregnancy and lactation

No known effects. Use at the discretion of the physician or pharmacist.

4.7 Effects on ability to drive and use machines

Not applicable.

4.8 Undesirable effects

None known.

4.9 Overdose

Not applicable

5. PHARMACOLOGICAL PROPERTIES

5.1 Pharmacodynamic properties

Urea is a recognised hydrating agent that has been widely used topically to treat dry or damaged skin.

5.2 Pharmacokinetic properties

Not applicable. Nutraplus is a topical (cutaneous) preparation.

5.3 Preclinical safety data

No specific information is presented given the widespread use of topically applied urea on humans over many years.

6. PHARMACEUTICAL PARTICULARS

6.1 List of excipients

Glycerol monostearate

Octyl palmitate

Myristyl lactate

Mineral oil

Promulgen D (contains Cetearyl alcohol and ceteareth-20)

Propylene glycol

Propyl parahydroxybenzoate (E216)

Methyl parahydroxybenzoate (E218)

Purified water

6.2 Incompatibilities

None known.

6.3 Shelf life
Thirty six months.

6.4 Special precautions for storage
Do not store above 25°C.

As with all medicines, Nutraplus Cream should be stored out of the sight and reach of children.

6.5 Nature and contents of container
White, polyethylene tube with a white polypropylene screw cap as the closure.

Pack sizes: 60g and 100g

6.6 Special precautions for disposal and other handling
No special instructions.

7. MARKETING AUTHORISATION HOLDER
Galderma (UK) Limited

Meridien House

69-71 Clarendon Road

Watford

Herts.

WD17 1DS

UK

8. MARKETING AUTHORISATION NUMBER(S)
PL 10590/0002

9. DATE OF FIRST AUTHORISATION/RENEWAL OF THE AUTHORISATION
4 June 1991

10. DATE OF REVISION OF THE TEXT
February 2006

Nutrizym 10

(Merck Serono)

1. NAME OF THE MEDICINAL PRODUCT
Nutrizym 10

2. QUALITATIVE AND QUANTITATIVE COMPOSITION
Each capsule contains Pancreatin BP 155mg with not less than the following activities. Lipase 10,000 BP Units, Protease 500 BP Units and Amylase 9000 BP Units.

3. PHARMACEUTICAL FORM
Hard gelatin capsule containing enteric coated pancreatin minitablets for oral administration.

4. CLINICAL PARTICULARS

4.1 Therapeutic indications
For the symptomatic relief of pancreatic exocrine insufficiency such as in fibrocystic disease of the pancreas and chronic pancreatitis.

4.2 Posology and method of administration
Adults (including the elderly) and children:

1-2 capsules with meals and 1 capsule with snacks.

Since the individual response to pancreatin supplements is variable, the number of capsules taken may need to be titrated to the individual according to symptoms and at the discretion of the physician. Dose increase, if required should be added slowly with careful monitoring of response and symptomatology.

Colonic damage has been reported in patients with cystic fibrosis taking in excess of 10,000 units of lipase/kg/day. The dose of Nutrizym 10 should usually not exceed this dose.

Capsules should be swallowed whole with water. Where swallowing of capsules proves to be difficult, the minitablets may be removed and taken with water or mixed with a small amount of soft food and swallowed immediately without chewing.

Adequate patient hydration should be ensured at all times whilst treating with Nutrizym 10.

4.3 Contraindications
Known hypersensitivity to the active ingredient (porcine pancreatin) or any of the excipients.

4.4 Special warnings and precautions for use
Hyperuricaemia and hyperuricosuria have been reported to occur in cystic fibrosis patients; pancreatin extracts contain a small amount of purine which might, in high doses, contribute to this condition.

4.5 Interaction with other medicinal products and other forms of interaction
None known.

4.6 Pregnancy and lactation
Safety has not been established and animal toxicological studies are lacking, therefore Nutrizym 10 should not be used in pregnancy and lactation unless clearly necessary, but if required should be used in doses sufficient to provide adequate nutritional status.

4.7 Effects on ability to drive and use machines
Not known.

4.8 Undesirable effects
Hypersensitivity reactions may occur. As with any pancreatin extract, high doses may cause buccal and perianal irritation, in some cases resulting in inflammation.

Stricture of the ileo-caecum and large bowel, and colitis have been reported in children with cystic fibrosis taking pancreatic enzymes. Abdominal symptoms (those not usually experienced by the patient) or changes in abdominal symptoms should be reviewed to exclude the possibility of colonic damage - especially if the patient is taking in excess of 10,000 units of lipase/kg/day.

4.9 Overdose
Inappropriately large doses could result in abdominal discomfort, nausea, vomiting and perianal irritation or inflammation.

5. PHARMACOLOGICAL PROPERTIES

5.1 Pharmacodynamic properties
The active ingredient is a preparation of porcine pancreas with lipase, amylase and protease activity. Lipase enzymes hydrolyse fats to glycerol and fatty acids. Amylase converts starch into dextrins and sugars and protease enzymes change proteins into proteoses and derived substances.

5.2 Pharmacokinetic properties
The active ingredient of Nutrizym 10 is pancreatin which is a substance involved in the digestive process. During the enzymatic degradation of food substances the enzymes themselves are degraded. Any breakdown products are those that would be expected to appear following normal digestion.

5.3 Preclinical safety data
Preclinical data are not available.

6. PHARMACEUTICAL PARTICULARS

6.1 List of excipients
Uncoated minitablets:

Castor Oil (hydrogenated)

Silicon dioxide, colloidal

Magnesium stearate

Sodium carboxymethylcellulose

Microcrystalline cellulose

Minitablet coating:

Simethicone emulsion

Methacrylic acid copolymer, type C (Eudragit L30D)

Talc

Triethyl citrate

Gelatin capsules:

Titanium dioxide

Iron oxide, red

Iron oxide, yellow

Gelatin

6.2 Incompatibilities
Not known.

6.3 Shelf life
Two years.

6.4 Special precautions for storage
Store below 25°C in tightly closed containers.

6.5 Nature and contents of container
Polyethylene or polypropylene containers with polyethylene tamper evident closures containing 50, 100, 200 or 500 capsules.

6.6 Special precautions for disposal and other handling
Not relevant.

7. MARKETING AUTHORISATION HOLDER
E. Merck Ltd

Bedfont Cross, Stanwell Road

Feltham, Middlesex,

TW14 8NX, UK

8. MARKETING AUTHORISATION NUMBER(S)
PL 00493/0157

9. DATE OF FIRST AUTHORISATION/RENEWAL OF THE AUTHORISATION
17 August 1992

10. DATE OF REVISION OF THE TEXT
22 October 2007

Legal Category
P

Nutrizym 22

(Merck Serono)

1. NAME OF THE MEDICINAL PRODUCT
Nutrizym 22

2. QUALITATIVE AND QUANTITATIVE COMPOSITION
Each capsule contains Pancreatin BP 340mg with not less than the following activities. Lipase 22,000 BP Units, Protease 1,100 BP Units and Amylase 19,800 BP Units.

3. PHARMACEUTICAL FORM
Hard gelatin capsule containing enteric coated pancreatin minitablets for oral administration.

4. CLINICAL PARTICULARS

4.1 Therapeutic indications
For the symptomatic relief of pancreatic exocrine insufficiency such as in fibrocystic disease of the pancreas and chronic pancreatitis.

4.2 Posology and method of administration
Adults (including the elderly) and children:

1-2 capsules with meals and 1 capsule with snacks.

Since the individual response to pancreatin supplements is variable, the number of capsules taken may need to be titrated to the individual according to symptoms and at the discretion of the physician. Dose increase, if required should be added slowly with careful monitoring of response and symptomatology.

Colonic damage has been reported in patients with cystic fibrosis taking in excess of 10,000 units of lipase/kg/day. The dose of Nutrizym 22 should usually not exceed this dose.

Where a patient is already receiving a lower unit dose enteric coated pancreatic supplement, then Nutrizym 22 may be substituted at 1/2 of the number of capsules normally consumed with the previous preparation.

Capsules should be swallowed whole with water. Where swallowing of capsules proves to be difficult, the minitablets may be removed and taken with water or mixed with a small amount of soft food and swallowed immediately without chewing.

Adequate patient hydration should be ensured at all times whilst treating with Nutrizym 22.

4.3 Contraindications
In children aged 15 years and under with cystic fibrosis. Known hypersensitivity to the active ingredient (porcine pancreatin) or any of the excipients.

4.4 Special warnings and precautions for use
Hyperuricaemia and hyperuricosuria have been reported to occur in cystic fibrosis patients; pancreatin extracts contain a small amount of purine which might, in high doses, contribute to this condition.

4.5 Interaction with other medicinal products and other forms of interaction
None known.

4.6 Pregnancy and lactation
Safety has not been established and animal toxicological studies are lacking, therefore Nutrizym 22 should not be used in pregnancy and lactation unless clearly necessary, but if required should be used in doses sufficient to provide adequate nutritional status.

Refer to section 4.8 for the potential side - effects of high doses of pancreatic enzymes in patients with cystic fibrosis.

4.7 Effects on ability to drive and use machines
Not known.

4.8 Undesirable effects
Hypersensitivity reactions may occur. As with any pancreatin extract, high doses may cause buccal and perianal irritation, in some cases resulting in inflammation.

Stricture of the ileo-caecum and large bowel, and colitis have been reported in children with cystic fibrosis taking Nutrizym 22. Abdominal symptoms (those not usually experienced by the patient) or changes in abdominal symptoms should be reviewed to exclude the possibility of colonic damage - especially if the patient is taking in excess of 10,000 units of lipase/kg/day.

4.9 Overdose
Inappropriately large doses could result in abdominal discomfort, nausea, vomiting and perianal irritation or inflammation.

5. PHARMACOLOGICAL PROPERTIES

5.1 Pharmacodynamic properties
The active ingredient is a preparation of porcine pancreas with lipase, amylase and protease activity. Lipase enzymes hydrolyse fats to glycerol and fatty acids. Amylase converts starch into dextrins and sugars and protease enzymes change proteins into proteoses and derived substances.

5.2 Pharmacokinetic properties
The active ingredient of Nutrizym 22 is pancreatin which is a substance involved in the digestive process. During the enzymatic degradation of food substances the enzymes themselves are degraded. Any breakdown products are those that would be expected to appear following normal digestion.

5.3 Preclinical safety data
Preclinical data are not available.

6. PHARMACEUTICAL PARTICULARS

6.1 List of excipients
Uncoated minitablets:

Castor Oil (hydrogenated)

Silicon dioxide, colloidal

Magnesium stearate

Sodium carboxymethylcellulose

Microcrystalline cellulose

Minitablet coating:

Simethicone emulsion

Methacrylic acid copolymer, type C (Eudragit L30D)

Talc

Triethyl citrate

Gelatin capsules:

Titanium dioxide

Iron oxide, red

Iron oxide, yellow

Gelatin

6.2 Incompatibilities
Not known.

6.3 Shelf life
Two years.

6.4 Special precautions for storage
Store below 25 degree C in tightly closed containers.

6.5 Nature and contents of container
Polyethylene or polypropylene containers with polyethylene tamper evident closures containing 50, 100, 200 or 500 capsules.

6.6 Special precautions for disposal and other handling
Not relevant.

7. MARKETING AUTHORISATION HOLDER
E. Merck Ltd

Bedfont Cross, Stanwell Road

Feltham, Middlesex,

TW14 8NX, UK

8. MARKETING AUTHORISATION NUMBER(S)
PL 00493/0158

9. DATE OF FIRST AUTHORISATION/RENEWAL OF THE AUTHORISATION
14 October 2002

10. DATE OF REVISION OF THE TEXT
22 October 2008

LEGAL CATEGORY
POM

NutropinAq 10mg/2ml

(Ipsen Ltd)

1. NAME OF THE MEDICINAL PRODUCT
NutropinAq 10 mg/2 ml (30 IU) solution for injection

2. QUALITATIVE AND QUANTITATIVE COMPOSITION
One cartridge contains 10 mg (30 IU) of somatropin*

* human growth hormone produced in *Escherichia coli* cells by recombinant DNA technology.

For a full list of excipients, see section 6.1.

3. PHARMACEUTICAL FORM
Solution for injection.

NutropinAq is a solution for subcutaneous use. The clear, colourless, sterile solution for multidose use is contained in a glass cartridge, closed with a rubber stopper and a rubber seal.

4. CLINICAL PARTICULARS

4.1 Therapeutic indications
- Long-term treatment of children with growth failure due to inadequate endogenous growth hormone secretion.

- Long-term treatment of growth failure associated with Turner syndrome.

- Treatment of prepubertal children with growth failure associated with chronic renal insufficiency up to the time of renal transplantation.

- Replacement of endogenous growth hormone in adults with growth hormone deficiency of either childhood or adult-onset etiology. Growth hormone deficiency should be confirmed appropriately prior to treatment (see section 4.4).

4.2 Posology and method of administration
Diagnosis and therapy with somatropin should be initiated and monitored by physicians who are appropriately qualified and experienced in the diagnosis and management of patients with the therapeutic indication of use.

The NutropinAq dosage and administration schedule should be individualised for each patient.

Dosage

Growth failure in children due to inadequate growth hormone secretion:

0.025 - 0.035 mg/kg bodyweight given as a daily subcutaneous injection.

Somatropin therapy should be continued in children and adolescents until their epiphysis are closed.

Growth failure associated with Turner syndrome:

Up to 0.05 mg/kg bodyweight given as a daily subcutaneous injection.

Somatropin therapy should be continued in children and adolescents until their epiphysis are closed.

Growth failure associated with chronic renal insufficiency:

Up to 0.05 mg/kg bodyweight given as a daily subcutaneous injection.

Somatropin therapy should be continued in children and adolescents until their epiphysis are closed, or up to the time of renal transplantation.

Growth hormone deficiency in adults:

At the start of somatropin therapy, low initial doses of 0.15 - 0.3 mg are recommended, given as a daily subcutaneous injection. The dose should be adjusted stepwise, controlled by serum Insulin-like Growth Factor-1 (IGF-1) values. The recommended final dose seldom exceeds 1.0 mg/day. In general, the lowest efficacious dose should be administered. In older or overweight patients, lower doses may be necessary.

Administration

The solution for injection should be administered subcutaneously each day. The site of injection should be changed.

For instructions for use and handling, see section 6.6.

4.3 Contraindications
Hypersensitivity to the active substance or to any of the excipients.

Somatropin should not be used for growth promotion in patients with closed epiphyses.

Growth hormone should not be used in patients with active neoplasm. NutropinAq therapy should be discontinued if evidence of tumour growth develops.

Growth hormone should not be initiated to treat patients with acute critical illness due to complications following open-heart or abdominal surgery, multiple accidental traumas or to treat patients having acute respiratory failure.

4.4 Special warnings and precautions for use
In adults with growth hormone deficiency the diagnosis should be established depending on the etiology:

Adult-onset: The patient must have growth hormone deficiency as a result of hypothalamic or pituitary disease, and at least one other hormone deficiency diagnosed (except for prolactin). Test for growth hormone deficiency should not be performed until adequate replacement therapy for other hormone deficiencies have been instituted.

Childhood-onset: Patients who have had growth hormone deficiency as a child should be retested to confirm growth hormone deficiency in adulthood before replacement therapy with NutropinAq is started.

In patients with previous malignant disease, special attention should be given to signs and symptoms of relapse.

Patients with a history of an intracranial lesion should be examined frequently for progression or recurrence of the lesion.

NutropinAq is not indicated for the long-term treatment of paediatric patients who have growth failure due to genetically confirmed Prader-Willi syndrome, unless they also have a diagnosis of growth hormone deficiency. There have been reports of sleep apnoea and sudden death after initiating therapy with growth hormone in paediatric patients with Prader-Willi syndrome who had one or more of the following risk factors: severe obesity, history of upper airway obstruction or sleep apnoea, or unidentified respiratory infection.

The effects of growth hormone on recovery were studied in two placebo-controlled clinical trials involving 522 adult patients who were critically ill due to complications following open-heart or abdominal surgery, multiple accidental traumas, or who were having acute respiratory failure. Mortality was higher (41.9 % vs. 19.3 %) among growth hormone treated patients (doses 5.3 - 8 mg/day) compared to those receiving placebo.

The safety of continuing somatropin treatment in patients with acute critical illness in intensive care units due to complications following open-heart or abdominal surgery, multiple accidental trauma or acute respiratory failure receiving replacement doses for approved indications has not been established. Therefore, the benefit-risk assessment for continuing treatment should be performed carefully.

Patients with growth hormone failure secondary to CRI should be examined periodically for evidence of progression of renal osteodystrophy. Slipped capital femoral epiphyses and aseptic necrosis of the femoral head may be seen in children with advanced renal osteodystrophy and in growth hormone deficiency, and it is uncertain whether these problems are affected by GH therapy. Physicians and parents should be alert to the development of a limp or complaints of hip or knee pain in patients treated with NutropinAq.

Scoliosis may progress in any child during rapid growth. Signs of scoliosis should be monitored during treatment. However, growth hormone treatment has not been shown to increase the incidence or severity of scoliosis.

Because somatropin may reduce insulin sensitivity, patients should be monitored for evidence of glucose intolerance. For patients with diabetes mellitus, the insulin dose may require adjustment after NutropinAq therapy is instituted. Patients with diabetes or glucose intolerance should be monitored closely during somatropin therapy.

Intracranial hypertension with papilloedema, visual changes, headache, nausea and/or vomiting has been reported in a small number of patients treated with somatropin. Symptoms usually occur within the first eight weeks of the initiation of NutropinAq therapy. In all reported cases, intracranial hypertension-associated signs and symptoms resolved after reduction of the somatropin dose or termination of the therapy. Funduscopic examination is recommended at the initiation and periodically during the course of treatment.

Hypothyroidism may develop during treatment with somatropin, and untreated hypothyroidism may prevent optimal response to NutropinAq. Therefore, patients should have periodic thyroid function tests and should be treated with thyroid hormone when indicated. Patients with severe hypothyroidism should be treated accordingly prior to the start of NutropinAq therapy.

Since somatropin therapy following renal transplantation has not been adequately tested, NutropinAq treatment should be terminated after that surgery.

Concomitant treatment with glucocorticoids inhibits the growth-promoting effects of NutropinAq. Patients with ACTH deficiency should have their glucocorticoid replacement therapy carefully adjusted to avoid any inhibitory effect on growth. The use of NutropinAq in patients with chronic renal insufficiency receiving glucocorticoid therapy has not been evaluated.

4.5 Interaction with other medicinal products and other forms of interaction
Limited published data indicate that growth hormone treatment increases cytochrome P450 mediated antipyrine clearance in man. Monitoring is advisable when NutropinAq is administered in combination with medicinal products known to be metabolised by CYP450 liver enzymes, such as corticosteroids, sex steroids, anticonvulsants, and cyclosporin.

4.6 Pregnancy and lactation
For NutropinAq, no clinical data on exposed pregnancies are available. Thus, the risk for humans is unknown. Although animal studies do not point to a potential risk during pregnancy, NutropinAq should be discontinued if pregnancy occurs. During pregnancy, maternal somatropin will largely be replaced by placental growth hormone.

It is not known whether somatropin is excreted in human milk, however, absorption of intact protein from the gastrointestinal tract of the infant is unlikely.

4.7 Effects on ability to drive and use machines
No studies on the effects of NutropinAq on the ability to drive and use machines have been performed.

Somatropin has no known effect on the ability to drive or to use machines.

4.8 Undesirable effects
Safety data from 9829 patients treated with Nutropin or NutropinAq - derived from a post-marketing surveillance survey in the United States - demonstrate that approximately 2% of patients have been shown to experience drug-related adverse reactions. Most of these adverse drug reactions were reported in the "general disorders and administration site conditions" system organ class.

The adverse reactions are listed in the table below, based on experience from clinical trials and a post-marketing surveillance survey. Within the system organ classes, adverse reactions are listed under headings of frequency using the following categories: very common (≥ 1/10), common (≥ 1/100, < 1/10); uncommon (≥ 1/1000, < 1/100); rare (≥ 1/10,000, < 1/1,000).

Neoplasms benign, malignant and unspecified (including cysts and polyps)	Uncommon: neoplasm malignant, neoplasm
Blood and lymphatic system disorders	Uncommon: anaemia
Immune system disorders	Common: antibody building
Endocrine disorders	Common: hypothyroidism
Metabolism and nutrition disorders	Common: glucose tolerance impaired Uncommon: hypoglycaemia, hyperphosphatemia Rare: diabetes mellitus
Psychiatric disorders	Uncommon: personality disorder
Nervous system disorders	Common: headache, hypertonia Uncommon: somnolence, nystagmus Rare: neuropathy, intracranial pressure increased
Eye disorders	Uncommon: papilloedema, diplopia
Ear and labyrinth disorders	Uncommon: vertigo

Cardiac disorders	Uncommon: tachycardia, hypertension
Gastrointestinal disorders	Uncommon: vomiting, abdominal pain, flatulence, nausea Rare: diarrhoea
Skin and subcutaneous tissue disorders	Uncommon: lipodystrophy, skin atrophy, dermatitis exfoliative, urticaria, hirsutism, skin hypertrophy
Musculoskeletal and connective tissue disorders	Very common in adults, common in children: arthralgia, myalgia Uncommon: muscle atrophy, bone pain, carpal tunnel syndrome
Renal and urinary disorders	Uncommon: urinary incontinence, haematuria, polyuria, urine frequency/ pollakiuria, urine abnormality
Reproductive system and breast disorders	Uncommon: genital discharge
General disorders and administration site conditions	Very common in adults, common in children: oedema, peripheral oedema Common: injection site reactions, asthenia Uncommon: injection site atrophy, injection site haemorrhage, injection site mass, hypertrophy
Investigations	Rare: renal function test abnormal

As with all medicinal products, a small percentage of patients may develop antibodies to the protein somatropin. The binding capacity of growth hormone antibodies was lower than 2 mg/l in NutropinAq subjects tested, which has not been associated with adversely affected growth rate.

Leukaemia has been reported in a small number of growth hormone deficient patients treated with growth hormone. A causal relationship to somatropin therapy is unlikely.

Patients with endocrinological disorders are more prone to develop an epiphysiolysis.

Indication-specific adverse drug reactions from clinical trials

Paediatric patients:

Patients with growth failure due to inadequate growth hormone secretion

Common: central nervous system neoplasm.

Patients with growth failure associated with Turner syndrome

Common: menorrhagia.

Patients with growth failure associated with chronic renal insufficiency

Common: renal failure, peritonitis, osteonecrosis, blood creatinine increase.

Children with chronic renal insufficiency receiving NutropinAq are more likely to develop intracranial hypertension. The greatest risk is at the beginning of treatment.

Adult patients:

Adults with growth hormone deficiency

Very common: paraesthesia.

Common: hyperglycaemia, hyperlipidaemia, insomnia, synovial disorder, arthrosis, muscular weakness, back pain, breast pain, gynaecomastia.

4.9 Overdose

Acute overdose could lead to hyperglycaemia. Long-term overdose could result in signs and symptoms of gigantism and/or acromegaly consistent with the known effects of excess growth hormone.

5. PHARMACOLOGICAL PROPERTIES

5.1 Pharmacodynamic properties

Pharmacotherapeutic group: Somatropin and analogues, ATC Code: H01 AC 01

Somatropin stimulates growth rate and increases adult height in children who lack endogenous growth hormone. Treatment of growth hormone deficient adults with somatropin results in reduced fat mass, increased lean body mass and increased spine bone mineral density. Metabolic alterations in these patients include normalisation of IGF-1 serum levels.

In vitro and *in vivo* preclinical and clinical tests have demonstrated that somatropin is therapeutically equivalent to human growth hormone of pituitary origin.

Actions that have been demonstrated for human growth hormone include:

Tissue Growth

1. Skeletal growth: growth hormone and its mediator IGF-1 stimulate skeletal growth in growth hormone deficient children by an effect on the epiphyseal plates of long bones. This results in a measurable increase in body length until these growth plates fuse at the end of puberty.

2. Cell growth: Treatment with somatropin results in an increase in both the number and size of skeletal muscle cells.

3. Organ growth: Growth hormone increases the size of internal organs, including kidneys, and increases red blood cell mass.

Protein metabolism

Linear growth is facilitated in part by growth hormone-stimulated protein synthesis. This is reflected by nitrogen retention as demonstrated by a decline in urinary nitrogen excretion and blood urea nitrogen during growth hormone therapy.

Carbohydrate metabolism

Patients with inadequate growth hormone secretion sometimes experience fasting hypoglycaemia that is improved by treatment with somatropin. Growth hormone therapy may decrease insulin sensitivity and impair glucose tolerance.

Mineral metabolism

Somatropin induces retention of sodium, potassium and phosphorus. Serum concentration of inorganic phosphorus are increased in patients with growth hormone deficiency after NutropinAq therapy due to metabolic activity associated with bone growth and increased tubular reabsorption in the kidney. Serum calcium is not significantly altered by somatropin. Adults with growth hormone deficiency show low bone mineral density and in the childhood-onset patient, NutropinAq has been shown to increase spine bone mineral density in a dose-dependent manner.

Connective tissue metabolism

Somatropin stimulates the synthesis of chondroitin sulphate and collagen as well as the urinary excretion of hydroxyproline.

Body composition

Adult growth hormone deficient patients treated with somatropin at a mean dosage of 0.014 mg/kg bodyweight daily demonstrate a decrease in fat mass and increase in lean body mass. When these alterations are coupled with the increase in total body water and bone mass, the overall effect of somatropin therapy is to modify body composition, an effect that is maintained with continued treatment.

5.2 Pharmacokinetic properties

General characteristics

The pharmacokinetic properties of NutropinAq have only been investigated in healthy adult males.

Absorption*:* The absolute bioavailability of recombinant human growth hormone after subcutaneous administration is about 80%.

Distribution*:* Animal studies with somatropin showed that growth hormone localises to highly perfused organs, particularly the liver and kidney. The volume of distribution at steady state for somatropin in healthy adult males is about 50 ml/kg bodyweight, approximating the serum volume.

Metabolism*:* Both the liver and the kidney have been shown to be important protein catabolising organs for growth hormone. Animal studies suggest that the kidney is the dominant organ of clearance. Growth hormone is filtered at the glomerulus and reabsorbed in the proximal tubules. It is then cleaved within renal cells into its constituent amino acids, which return to the systemic circulation.

Elimination*:* After subcutaneous bolus administration, the mean terminal half-life $t_{1/2}$ of somatropin is about 2.3 hours. After intravenous bolus administration of somatropin, the mean terminal half-life $t_{1/2}\beta$ or $t_{1/2}\gamma$ is about 20 minutes and the mean clearance is reported to be in the range of 116 - 174 ml/h/kg.

Available literature data suggest that somatropin clearance is similar in adults and children.

Characteristics in patients

Clearance and mean terminal half-life $t_{1/2}$ of somatropin in adult and paediatric growth hormone deficient patients are similar to those observed in healthy subjects.

Children and adults with chronic renal failure and end-stage renal disease tend to have decreased clearance compared to normal subjects. Endogenous growth hormone production may also increase in some individuals with end-stage renal disease. However, no somatropin accumulation has been reported in children with chronic renal failure or end-stage renal disease dosed with current regimens.

Limited published data for exogenously-administered somatropin suggest absorption and elimination half-lives and time of maximum concentration t_{max} in Turner patients are similar to those observed in both normal and growth hormone deficient populations.

In patients with severe liver dysfunction a reduction in somatropin clearance has been noted. The clinical significance of this decrease is unknown.

5.3 Preclinical safety data

The toxicity of NutropinAq has been tested in rats and monkeys and no findings of toxicological relevance were revealed.

Due to its hormonal activity, somatropin may exert a promotional effect on tumour growth in tumour-bearing subjects. To date, this has not been confirmed in patients.

Local tolerance studies with NutropinAq showed no substantial adverse local reactions.

Studies in transgenic mice suggest a low antibody provoking potential of (aged) liquid Nutropin.

No common reproduction studies were performed. However, long-term treatment of monkeys during pregnancy and lactation and of newborn animals until adolescence, sexual maturity and reproduction did not indicate substantial disturbances of fertility, pregnancy, delivery, nursing or development of progeny.

6. PHARMACEUTICAL PARTICULARS

6.1 List of excipients

Sodium chloride

Phenol

Polysorbate 20

Sodium citrate and citric acid anhydrous

Water for injections

6.2 Incompatibilities

In the absence of compatibility studies, this medicinal productmust not be mixed with other medicinal products.

6.3 Shelf life

2 years

Chemical and physical in-use stability has been demonstrated for 28 days at 2°C - 8°C.

From a microbiological point of view, once opened, the product may be stored for a maximum of 28 days at 2°C - 8°C. NutropinAq is designed to withstand a nominal (one hour maximum) period of time outside of the refrigerator on a daily basis.

6.4 Special precautions for storage

Store in a refrigerator (2°C - 8°C).

Do not freeze.

Keep the blister in the outer carton

For in-use storage conditions of the medicinal product, see section 6.3.

6.5 Nature and contents of container

2 ml of solution in a cartridge (Type I glass) closed with a stopper (butyl rubber) and a seal (rubber).

Pack sizes of 1, 3 and 6 cartridges.

Not all pack sizes may be marketed.

6.6 Special precautions for disposal and other handling

No special requirements.

Instructions for use and handling

NutropinAq is supplied as a sterile solution with preservative for multiple use. The solution should be clear immediately after removal from the refrigerator. If the solution is cloudy, the content must not be injected. Gently swirl. Do not shake vigorously in order not to denature the protein.

NutropinAq is intended for use only with the NutropinAq Pen. Wipe the rubber seal of the NutropinAq with rubbing alcohol or an antiseptic solution to prevent contamination of the contents by microorganisms that may be introduced by repeated needle insertions. It is recommended that NutropinAq be administered using sterile, disposable needles.

The NutropinAq Pen allows for administration of a minimum dose of 0.1 mg to a maximum dose of 4.0 mg, in 0.1 mg increments.

A cartridge that is in the pen should not be removed during injections.

7. MARKETING AUTHORISATION HOLDER

IPSEN Ltd.

190 Bath Road

Slough, Berkshire

SL1 3XE, United Kingdom

8. MARKETING AUTHORISATION NUMBER(S)

EU/1/00/164/003

EU/1/00/164/004

EU/1/00/164/005

9. DATE OF FIRST AUTHORISATION/RENEWAL OF THE AUTHORISATION

Date of first authorisation:16 February 2001

Date of last renewal: 16 February 2006

10. DATE OF REVISION OF THE TEXT

30th October 2006

Occlusal

(Alliance Pharmaceuticals)

1. NAME OF THE MEDICINAL PRODUCT
Occlusal.

26% w/w cutaneous solution

2. QUALITATIVE AND QUANTITATIVE COMPOSITION
Salicylic Acid 26% w/w.

For excipients, see 6.1

3. PHARMACEUTICAL FORM
Cutaneous solution

A colourless to pale yellow solution with a characteristic smell of nail varnish

4. CLINICAL PARTICULARS
4.1 Therapeutic indications
Occlusal is indicated for the treatment and removal of common and plantar warts (verrucae).

4.2 Posology and method of administration
For topical application.

Prior to application soak wart in warm water for five minutes. Remove loose tissue with a brush, emery board, pumice or abrasive sponge, being careful to avoid causing pin-point bleeding or abrading the surrounding healthy skin. Dry thoroughly with a towel not used by others to avoid contagion. Carefully apply Occlusal twice to the wart using the brush applicator allowing the first application to dry before applying the second. Thereafter repeat treatment once daily or as directed by physician. Do not apply to surrounding healthy skin. Clinically visible improvement should occur in one to two weeks but maximum effect may be expected after four to six weeks.

There are no differences in dosage for children, adults or the elderly.

4.3 Contraindications
Occlusal should not be used by diabetics or patients with impaired blood circulation. Do not use on moles, birthmarks, unusual warts with hair growth, on facial warts, or in the anal or perineal region.

4.4 Special warnings and precautions for use
Occlusal is for external use only. Do not permit contact with eyes or mucous membranes. If contact occurs flush with water for 15 minutes. Do not allow contact with normal skin around wart. Avoid using on areas of broken or damaged skin. Discontinue treatment if excessive irritation occurs.

4.5 Interaction with other medicinal products and other forms of interaction
None known.

4.6 Pregnancy and lactation
The chronic use of this product during pregnancy and lactation, particularly when large areas of skin are involved, should be avoided.

4.7 Effects on ability to drive and use machines
None known.

4.8 Undesirable effects
A localised irritant reaction may occur if Occlusal is applied to normal skin surrounding the wart. This may normally be controlled by temporarily discontinuing the use of Occlusal and by being careful to apply the solution only to the wart itself when treatment is resumed.

4.9 Overdose
Salicylism can occur following large doses of salicylic acid or prolonged use of topical salicylic preparations, or in the unlikely event of accidental consumption.

5. PHARMACOLOGICAL PROPERTIES
5.1 Pharmacodynamic properties
Salicylic acid has bacteriostatic and fungicidal actions, but it is its keratolytic properties which are important for this medicinal product. When applied externally it produces slow and painless destruction of the epithelium. Salicylic acid is usually applied in the form of a paint in a collodian base (10 to 17%) or as a plaster (20 to 50%) to destroy warts or corns.

5.2 Pharmacokinetic properties
Not applicable.

5.3 Preclinical safety data
None presented.

6. PHARMACEUTICAL PARTICULARS
6.1 List of excipients
Polyvinyl butyral

Dibutyl phthalate

Isopropyl alcohol

Butyl acetate

Acrylates copolymer

6.2 Incompatibilities
Not applicable

6.3 Shelf life
2 years.

6.4 Special precautions for storage
Do not store above 25°C

6.5 Nature and contents of container
The product is presented in a 10ml amber glass bottle with cap brush assembly. The cap brush assembly comprises of a black cap and a white polythene wand nylon brush with stainless steel staple.

6.6 Special precautions for disposal and other handling
Occlusal is flammable and should be kept away from flame or fire. Keep the bottle tightly capped when not in use. Do not allow the solution to drip from the brush onto the bottle neck thread, otherwise subsequent opening of the bottle may be difficult.

7. MARKETING AUTHORISATION HOLDER
Alliance Pharmaceuticals Limited

Avonbridge House

2 Bath Road

Chippenham

Wiltshire, SN15 2BB

UK

8. MARKETING AUTHORISATION NUMBER(S)
PL 16853/0071

9. DATE OF FIRST AUTHORISATION/RENEWAL OF THE AUTHORISATION
7th September 1998/18th May 2005

10. DATE OF REVISION OF THE TEXT
May 2005

Octim Injection

(Ferring Pharmaceuticals Ltd)

1. NAME OF THE MEDICINAL PRODUCT
OCTIM® Injection

2. QUALITATIVE AND QUANTITATIVE COMPOSITION
Desmopressin acetate 15 micrograms per ml

3. PHARMACEUTICAL FORM
Solution for injection.

4. CLINICAL PARTICULARS
4.1 Therapeutic indications
OCTIM Injection is indicated as follows:

1. To increase Factor VIII:C and Factor VIII:Ag in patients with mild to moderate haemophilia or von Willebrand's disease undergoing surgery or following trauma.

2. To test for fibrinolytic response

4.2 Posology and method of administration
Mild to Moderate Haemophilia and von Willebrand's Disease:

By subcutaneous or intravenous administration.

The dose for adults, children and infants is 0.3 micrograms per kilogram body weight, administered by subcutaneous injection or intravenous infusion. Further doses may be administered at 12 hourly intervals so long as cover is required. As some patients have shown a diminishing response to successive doses, it is recommended that monitoring of Factor VIII levels should continue.

For intravenous infusion, the dose should be diluted in 50ml of 0.9% sodium chloride for injection and given over 20 minutes. This dose should be given immediately prior to surgery or following trauma. During administration of intravenous desmopressin, vasodilation may occur resulting in decreased blood pressure and tachycardia with facial flushing in some patients.

Increase of Factor VIII levels are dependent on basal levels and are normally between 2 and 5 times the pre-treatment levels. If results from a previous administration of desmopressin are not available then blood should be taken predose and 20 minutes post-dose for assay of Factor VIII levels in order to monitor response.

Unless contraindicated, when surgery is undertaken tranexamic acid may be given orally at the recommended dose from 24 hours beforehand until healing is complete.

Fibrinolytic Response Testing:

By subcutaneous or intravenous administration.

The dose for adults and children is 0.3 micrograms per kilogram body weight, administered by subcutaneous injection or intravenous infusion.

For intravenous infusion, the dose should be diluted in 50ml of 0.9% sodium chloride for injection and given over 20 minutes.

A sample of venous blood should be taken 20 minutes after the administration. In patients with a normal response the sample should show fibrinolytic activity of euglobulin clot precipitate on fibrin plates of at least 240mm^2.

4.3 Contraindications
OCTIM Injection is contraindicated in cases of:

- habitual and psychogenic polydipsia
- unstable angina pectoris
- decompensated cardiac insufficiency
- von Willebrand's Disease Type IIB where the administration of desmopressin may result in pseudothrombocytopenia due to the release of abnormal clotting factors which cause platelet aggregation.

Fibrinolytic Response Testing should not be carried out in patients with hypertension, heart disease, cardiac insufficiency and other conditions requiring treatment with diuretic agents.

4.4 Special warnings and precautions for use
Precautions to prevent fluid overload must be taken in:

- conditions characterised by fluid and/or electrolyte imbalance
- patients at risk for increased intracranial pressure

Care should be taken with patients who have reduced renal function and/or cardiovascular disease.

When repeated doses are used to control bleeding in haemophilia or von Willebrand's disease, care should be taken to prevent fluid overload. Fluid should not be forced, orally or parenterally, and patients should only take as much fluid as they require to satisfy thirst. Intravenous infusions should not be left up as a routine after surgery. Fluid accumulation can be readily monitored by weighing the patient or by determining plasma sodium or osmolality.

Measures to prevent fluid overload must be taken in patients with conditions requiring treatment with diuretic agents.

Special attention must be paid to the risk of water retention. The fluid intake should be restricted to the least possible and the body weight should be checked regularly.

If there is a gradual increase of the body weight, decrease of serum sodium to below 130mmol/l or plasma osmolality to below 270mOsm/kg, the fluid intake must be reduced drastically and the administration of OCTIM Injection interrupted.

During administration of OCTIM Injection, it is recommended that the patient's blood pressure is monitored continuously.

OCTIM Injection does not reduce prolonged bleeding time in thrombocytopenia.

4.5 Interaction with other medicinal products and other forms of interaction
Substances which are known to induce SIADH e.g. tricyclic antidepressants, selective serotonin re-uptake inhibitors, chlorpromazine and carbamazepine, may cause an additive antidiuretic effect leading to an increased risk of water retention and/or hyponatraemia.

NSAIDs may induce water retention and/or hyponatraemia.

4.6 Pregnancy and lactation
Pregnancy:

Data on a limited number (n=53) of exposed pregnancies in women with diabetes insipidus indicate rare cases of malformations in children treated during pregnancy. To date, no other relevant epidemiological data are available. Animal studies do not indicate direct or indirect harmful effects with respect to pregnancy, embryonal/fetal development, parturition or postnatal development.

Caution should be exercised when prescribing to pregnant women. Blood pressure monitoring is recommended due to the increased risk of pre-eclampsia.

Lactation:

Results from analyses of milk from nursing mothers receiving 300 micrograms desmopressin intranasally indicate that the amounts of desmopressin that may be transferred to the child are considerably less than the amounts required to influence diuresis or haemostasis.

4.7 Effects on ability to drive and use machines
None

4.8 Undesirable effects
Side-effects include headache, stomach pain and nausea. Isolated cases of allergic skin reactions and more severe general allergic reactions have been reported. Very rare cases of emotional disorders including aggression in children have been reported. Treatment with desmopressin without concomitant reduction of fluid intake may lead to water retention/hyponatraemia with accompanying

symptoms of headache, nausea, vomiting, weight gain, decreased serum sodium and in serious cases, convulsions.

During intravenous infusion of OCTIM Injection, vasodilation may occur, resulting in decreased blood pressure and tachycardia with facial flushing. This side effect is normally avoided by infusing the product over 20 minutes.

4.9 Overdose
An overdose of OCTIM Injection leads to a prolonged duration of action with an increased risk of water retention and/or hyponatraemia.

Treatment:

Although the treatment of hyponatraemia should be individualised, the following general recommendations can be given. Hyponatraemia is treated by discontinuing the desmopressin treatment, fluid restriction and symptomatic treatment if needed.

5. PHARMACOLOGICAL PROPERTIES

5.1 Pharmacodynamic properties
Desmopressin is a structural analogue of vasopressin, with two chemical changes namely desamination of the N-terminal and replacement of the 8-L-Arginine by 8-D-Arginine. These changes have increased the antidiuretic activity and prolonged the duration of action. The pressor activity is reduced to less than 0.01% of the natural peptide as a result of which side-effects are rarely seen.

Like vasopressin, desmopressin also increases concentrations of Factor VIII:C, Factor VIII:Ag (vWF) and Plasminogen Activator (t-PA).

5.2 Pharmacokinetic properties
Following intravenous injection, plasma concentrations of desmopressin follow a biexponential curve. The initial fast phase of a few minutes duration and with a half life of less than 10 minutes is thought mainly to represent the diffusion of desmopressin from plasma to its volume of distribution. The second phase with a half life of 51-158 minutes represents the elimination rate of desmopressin from the body.

As a comparison, the half life of vasopressin is less than 10 minutes.

Subcutaneous administration of desmopressin results in a later T_{max} and lower C_{max} values but comparable bioavailability.

In vitro, in human liver microsome preparations, it has been shown that no significant amount of desmopressin is metabolised in the liver and thus human liver metabolism *in vivo* is not likely to occur.

It is unlikely that desmopressin will interact with drugs affecting hepatic metabolism, since desmopressin has been shown not to undergo significant liver metabolism in *in vitro* studies with human microsomes. However, formal *in vivo* interaction studies have not been performed.

5.3 Preclinical safety data
There are no pre-clinical data of relevance to the prescriber which are additional to those already included in other sections of the SPC.

6. PHARMACEUTICAL PARTICULARS

6.1 List of excipients
Sodium chloride Ph. Eur.

Hydrochloric acid Ph. Eur.

Water for injection Ph. Eur.

6.2 Incompatibilities
None

6.3 Shelf life
48 months.

6.4 Special precautions for storage
Store in a refrigerator at 2°C- 8°C and protect from light.

6.5 Nature and contents of container
Clear glass ampoules.

6.6 Special precautions for disposal and other handling
The injection is administered by subcutaneous injection or intravenous infusion.

For intravenous infusion, the dose should be diluted in 50ml of 0.9% sodium chloride for injection and given over 20 minutes.

7. MARKETING AUTHORISATION HOLDER
Ferring Pharmaceuticals Ltd.

The Courtyard

Waterside Drive

Langley

Berkshire SL3 6EZ.

8. MARKETING AUTHORISATION NUMBER(S)
PL 03194/0055

9. DATE OF FIRST AUTHORISATION/RENEWAL OF THE AUTHORISATION
11th February 2002

10. DATE OF REVISION OF THE TEXT
October 2008

Octim Nasal Spray

(Ferring Pharmaceuticals Ltd)

1. NAME OF THE MEDICINAL PRODUCT
OCTIM® Nasal Spray

2. QUALITATIVE AND QUANTITATIVE COMPOSITION
Desmopressin acetate 150 micrograms per actuation

For excipients, see 6.1

3. PHARMACEUTICAL FORM
Nasal Spray, Solution

Clear, colourless solution

4. CLINICAL PARTICULARS

4.1 Therapeutic indications
OCTIM Nasal Spray is indicated as follows:

1) To increase Factor VIIIC and Factor VIII:Ag (vWf) in patients with mild to moderate haemophilia or von Willebrand's disease undergoing surgery, following trauma or with other bleeding episodes such as menorrhagia and epistaxis.

2) To test for fibrinolytic response.

4.2 Posology and method of administration

Mild to moderate haemophilia and von Willebrand's disease:

Adults (including the elderly) should take 300 micrograms (one spray into each nostril) half an hour before surgery or at bleeding.

Under direct medical supervision, further doses may be administered at 12 hourly intervals so long as cover is required. As some patients have shown a diminishing response to successive doses, Factor VIII levels should continue to be monitored.

Unless specifically directed by the doctor, when OCTIM Nasal Spray is self-administered by the patient, there should be an interval of at least three days between doses.

Increase of Factor VIII levels are dependent on basal levels and are normally between 2 and 5 times the pre-treatment levels. If results from a previous administration of desmopressin are not available then blood should be taken predose and 60 minutes post-dose for assay of Factor VIII levels in order to monitor response.

Fibrinolytic response testing:

Adults (including the elderly) should take 300 micrograms (one spray in each nostril). A sample of venous blood should be taken 60 minutes later.

In patients with a normal response, the sample should show fibrinolytic activity of euglobulin clot precipitate on fibrin plates of at least $240mm^2$.

4.3 Contraindications
OCTIM Nasal Spray is contraindicated in cases of:

- habitual and psychogenic polydipsia
- unstable angina pectoris
- decompensated cardiac insufficiency
- von Willebrand's Disease Type IIB where the administration of desmopressin may result in pseudothrombocytopenia due to the release of abnormal clotting factors which cause platelet aggregation.

Fibrinolytic response testing should not be carried out in patients with hypertension, heart disease, cardiac insufficiency and other conditions requiring treatment with diuretic agents.

4.4 Special warnings and precautions for use
Precautions to prevent fluid overload must be taken in:

- conditions characterised by fluid and/or electrolyte imbalance
- patients at risk for increased intracranial pressure.

Care should be taken with patients who have reduced renal function and or cardiovascular disease or cystic fibrosis.

When repeated doses are used to control bleeding in haemophilia or von Willebrand's disease, care should be taken to prevent fluid overload. Patients should only take as much fluid as they require to satisfy thirst. Intravenous infusions should not be left up as a routine after surgery. Fluid accumulation can be readily monitored by weighing the patient or by determining plasma sodium or osmolality.

Measures to prevent fluid overload must be taken in patients with conditions requiring treatment with diuretic agents.

Special attention must be paid to the risk of water retention. The fluid intake should be restricted to the least possible and the body weight should be checked regularly.

If there is a gradual increase of the body weight, decrease of serum sodium to 130mmol/l or plasma osmolality to below 270mOsm/kg, the fluid intake must be reduced drastically and the administration of OCTIM Nasal Spray interrupted.

OCTIM Nasal Spray does not reduce prolonged bleeding time in thrombocytopenia.

4.5 Interaction with other medicinal products and other forms of interaction
Indomethacin may augment the magnitude but not the duration of response to desmopressin.

Substances which are known to release antidiuretic hormone e.g. tricyclic antidepressants, chlorpromazine and carbamazepine, may cause an additive antidiuretic effect and increase the risk of water retention.

4.6 Pregnancy and lactation
Pregnancy:

OCTIM Nasal Spray should be given with caution to pregnant patients, although the oxytocic effect of desmopressin is very low.

Reproduction studies performed in rats and rabbits with doses of more than 100 times the human dose have revealed no evidence of a harmful action of desmopressin on the fetus. There have been rare reports of malformations in children born to mothers treated for diabetes insipidus during pregnancy. However, a review of available data suggests no increase in the rate of malformations in children exposed to desmopressin throughout pregnancy.

Lactation:

Results from analyses of milk from nursing mothers receiving 300 micrograms desmopressin intranasally indicate that the amounts of desmopressin that may be transferred to the child are considerably less than the amounts required to influence diuresis or haemostasis.

4.7 Effects on ability to drive and use machines
None

4.8 Undesirable effects
Side-effects include headache, stomach pain, nausea, nasal congestion, rhinitis and epistaxis. Isolated cases of allergic skin reactions and more severe general allergic reactions have been reported. Very rare cases of emotional disorders including aggression in children have been reported. Treatment with desmopressin without concomitant reduction of fluid intake may lead to water retention/hyponatraemia with accompanying symptoms of headache, nausea, vomiting, weight gain, decreased serum sodium and in serious cases, convulsions.

4.9 Overdose
Overdose of OCTIM Nasal Spray can lead to hyponatraemia and convulsions.

Treatment:

Overdosage increases the risk of fluid retention and hyponatraemia. If hyponatraemia occurs, desmopressin treatment should immediately be discontinued and fluid intake restricted until serum sodium is normalised.

5. PHARMACOLOGICAL PROPERTIES

5.1 Pharmacodynamic properties
Desmopressin is an analogue of the hormone vasopressin in which the antidiuretic activity has been enhanced by the order of 10, whilst the vasopressor effect has been reduced by the order of 1500. The duration of activity has also been extended.

Like vasopressin, desmopressin also increases concentrations of Factor VIII:C, Factor VIII:Ag (vWf) and plasminogen activator (t-PA)

5.2 Pharmacokinetic properties
ATC code H01B A02

Following intranasal administration, the bioavailability of desmopressin is of the order of 6-10%. Peak plasma levels are achieved in approximately 50 minutes and the mean plasma half-life is about three hours.

5.3 Preclinical safety data
There are no pre-clinical data of relevance to the prescriber which are additional to that already included in other sections of the SPC

6. PHARMACEUTICAL PARTICULARS

6.1 List of excipients
Sodium chloride

Citric acid monohydrate

Disodium phosphate dihydrate

Benzalkonium chloride soln 50%

Purified water

6.2 Incompatibilities
Not applicable

6.3 Shelf life
36 months

6.4 Special precautions for storage
Do not store above 25°C. Keep vial in the outer carton.

Do not freeze.

6.5 Nature and contents of container
Multidose container, Type I glass vial with a pre-compression pump set comprising of a spray pump with a metering valve, nasal applicator and protection cap.

Pack size: 2.5ml (25 sprays)

6.6 Special precautions for disposal and other handling
None

7. MARKETING AUTHORISATION HOLDER
Ferring Pharmaceuticals Ltd.

The Courtyard

Waterside Drive

Langley

Berkshire SL3 6EZ.

8. MARKETING AUTHORISATION NUMBER(S)
PL 03194/0056

9. DATE OF FIRST AUTHORISATION/RENEWAL OF THE AUTHORISATION
25th October 2002

10. DATE OF REVISION OF THE TEXT
MAY 2008

Ocufen

(Allergan Ltd)

1. NAME OF THE MEDICINAL PRODUCT
Ocufen®

2. QUALITATIVE AND QUANTITATIVE COMPOSITION
Flurbiprofen sodium 0.03% w/v

3. PHARMACEUTICAL FORM
Eye drops.

4. CLINICAL PARTICULARS

4.1 Therapeutic indications
Ocufen is indicated for

1) the inhibition of intraoperative miosis. Ocufen does not have intrinsic mydriatic properties and does not replace mydriatic agents.

2) the management of post-operative and post-laser trabeculoplasty inflammation in the anterior segment of the eye in patients in whom steroid therapy is not recommended.

4.2 Posology and method of administration
Adult dosage: For the inhibition of intraoperative miosis, 1 drop is instilled every half hour starting 2 hours before surgery. The final drop should be given not less than 30 minutes before surgery.

To control post-operative and post-laser trabeculoplasty inflammation the dosing regimen above should be followed. Beginning twenty-four hours after surgery, one drop is administered four times daily for at least one week after laser trabeculoplasty or for two to three weeks after other surgery.

In accordance with standard practice, other topical medication should not be co-administered with Ocufen. When administering other topical medications, a minimum interval of 5 minutes between instillations is recommended.

Use in children: Safety and effectiveness in children have not been established.

Administration: Topical by instillation into the conjunctival sac.

4.3 Contraindications
Ocufen is contra-indicated in epithelial herpes simplex keratitis (dendritic keratitis) and in individuals hypersensitive to any component of the medication.

The potential exists for cross-sensitivity to acetylsalicylic acid and other non-steroidal anti-inflammatory drugs. Ocufen is contra-indicated in individuals who have previously exhibited sensitivities to these drugs.

Use of Ocufen is contra-indicated in patients with known haemostatic defects or who are receiving other medications which may prolong bleeding time. Ocufen is contra-indicated for intraocular use during surgical procedures.

4.4 Special warnings and precautions for use
Wound healing may be delayed with the use of Ocufen.

There have been reports that Ocufen may cause an increased bleeding tendency of ocular tissues in conjunction with surgery.

Patients with a history of herpes simplex keratitis should be monitored closely.

4.5 Interaction with other medicinal products and other forms of interaction
Although clinical studies with acetylcholine chloride and animal studies with acetylcholine chloride or carbachol revealed no interference, and there is no known pharmacological basis for an interaction, there have been reports that acetylcholine chloride and carbachol have been ineffective when used in some surgical patients treated with Ocufen.

4.6 Pregnancy and lactation
Use in pregnancy: Safety of use in pregnant women has not been established. Ocufen should be used during pregnancy only if the potential benefit justifies the potential risk to the foetus.

4.7 Effects on ability to drive and use machines
None known.

4.8 Undesirable effects
The most frequent adverse reactions reported with the use of Ocufen are transient burning and stinging on instillation, and other minor signs of ocular irritation.

4.9 Overdose
No adverse effects are likely to be experienced following overdosage.

5. PHARMACOLOGICAL PROPERTIES

5.1 Pharmacodynamic properties
Flurbiprofen sodium is a non steroidal anti inflammatory agent which inhibits prostaglandin synthesis by inhibition of the cyclo-oxygenase enzyme.

Ophthalmic surgery causes prostaglandin release, with the effect that prostaglandin- mediated miosis may occur.

Treatment with Ocufen prior to surgery has been shown to inhibit intra-operative miosis and it is believed that this is brought about by inhibition of ocular prostaglandin release.

The sympathetic nervous system is not affected by this mechanism and acetylcholine- induced miosis has not been found to be inhibited in clinical trials.

Prostaglandins have also been shown to be mediators of certain kinds of intraocular inflammatory processes. In studies performed on animal eyes, prostaglandins have been shown to produce disruption of the blood-aqueous humour barrier, vasodilation, increased vascular permeability, leukocytosis and increased intraocular pressure.

5.2 Pharmacokinetic properties
Flurbiprofen concentrations of 213 ng/ml in aqueous humour have been reported following half hourly treatment for two hours preceding surgery.

5.3 Preclinical safety data
There are no preclinical data of relevance to the prescriber which are additional to that already included in the Summary of Product Characteristics.

6. PHARMACEUTICAL PARTICULARS

6.1 List of excipients
Liquifilm® (polyvinyl alcohol)
Potassium chloride
Sodium chloride
Sodium citrate dihydrate
Citric acid monohydrate
Sodium hydroxide or
Hydrochloric acid (to adjust pH)
Purified water

6.2 Incompatibilities
None known.

6.3 Shelf life
The shelf life is 24 months for the unopened vial. The vial should be discarded after a single dose.

6.4 Special precautions for storage
Store at or below 25°C.

6.5 Nature and contents of container
Clear, plastic unit dose vial, each containing 0.4 ml of solution.

6.6 Special precautions for disposal and other handling
Each vial of Ocufen should be used for a single dose and discarded after use.

7. MARKETING AUTHORISATION HOLDER
Allergan Limited
Marlow International
The Parkway
Marlow
Buckinghamshire SL7 1YL
United Kingdom

8. MARKETING AUTHORISATION NUMBER(S)
PL 00426/0069

9. DATE OF FIRST AUTHORISATION/RENEWAL OF THE AUTHORISATION
28th June 1991/17th May 2005

10. DATE OF REVISION OF THE TEXT
24th November 2006

Oestrogel Pump-Pack Gel

(Ferring Pharmaceuticals Ltd)

1. NAME OF THE MEDICINAL PRODUCT
Oestrogel Pump-Pack

2. QUALITATIVE AND QUANTITATIVE COMPOSITION
Oestrogel contains estradiol as active ingredient, 0.06% w/w.

3. PHARMACEUTICAL FORM
Transdermal gel.

4. CLINICAL PARTICULARS

4.1 Therapeutic indications
Hormone replacement therapy (HRT) for oestrogen deficiency symptoms in postmenopausal women.

Prevention of osteoporosis in postmenopausal women at high risk of future fractures who are intolerant of, or contra-indicated for, other medicinal products approved for the prevention of osteoporosis.

(See also Section 4.4)

4.2 Posology and method of administration
Oestrogel is an oestrogen-only product. Oestrogel should be administered daily on a continuous basis.

Adults and the Elderly:

For initiation and continuation of treatment of postmenopausal symptoms, the lowest effective dose for the shortest duration (see also Section 4.4) should be used.

Menopausal symptoms:

The usual starting dose is two measures (2.5g) of Oestrogel once daily (1.5mg estradiol). In the majority of women this dose will provide effective relief of menopausal symptoms. If after one month's treatment effective relief is not obtained, the dosage may be increased accordingly to a maximum of four measures (5g) of Oestrogel daily (3.0mg estradiol).

Prevention of osteoporosis:

The minimum effective dose is 2.5g of Oestrogel once daily for most patients.

Use with progestagen:

In women with an intact uterus the recommended dose of a progestagen should be administered for at least 12 days of each month, in accordance with the manufacturers recommendations. Unless there is a previous diagnosis of endometriosis, it is not recommended to add a progestagen in hysterectomised women.

Initiation of treatment:

Women who have never taken HRT and have regular menstrual cycles: treatment with Oestrogel can be started within 5 days of start of bleed.

Women who have never taken HRT and are post-menopausal or have very infrequent menstrual cycles: treatment with Oestrogel can be started on any day.

Switching from a continuous oestrogen-progestagen combined HRT: treatment with Oestrogel can be started on any day of the cycle.

Switching from a cyclic or continuous sequential HRT treatment: finish the therapeutic sequence before beginning treatment with Oestrogel.

How to apply Oestrogel:

Each measure from the dispenser is 1.25g of Oestrogel.

The correct dose of gel should be dispensed and applied to clean, dry, intact areas of skin e.g. on the arms and shoulders, or inner thighs. The area of application should be at least 750cm^2, twice the area of the template provided. One measure from the dispenser, or half the prescribed dose, should be applied to each arm/shoulder (or thigh). Oestrogel should NOT be applied on or near the breasts or on the vulval region.

Oestrogel should be allowed to dry for 5 minutes before covering the skin with clothing.

The gel should be applied by the patient herself, not by anyone else, and skin contact, particularly with a male partner, should be avoided for one hour after application.

Washing the skin or contact with other skin products should be avoided until at least one hour after application of Oestrogel.

Missed dose advice:

If the patient forgets to apply a dose, and it is more than 12 hours until the next dose, the missed dose should be applied and normal dosing resumed the next day. If the next dose is less than 12 hours away, it is best just to wait and apply the next dose normally.

Patients should be advised not to apply two doses at the same time.

Forgetting a dose may increase the likelihood of breakthrough bleeding and spotting.

4.3 Contraindications
- Known, past or suspected breast cancer;
- Known or suspected oestrogen-dependent malignant tumours (e.g. endometrial cancer);
- Undiagnosed genital bleeding;
- Untreated endometrial hyperplasia;
- Previous idiopathic or current venous thromboembolism (deep venous thrombosis, pulmonary embolism);
- Active or recent arterial thromboembolic disease (e.g. angina, myocardial infarction);
- Acute liver disease, or a history of liver disease as long as liver function tests have failed to return to normal;
- Known hypersensitivity to the active substances or to any of the excipients;
- Porphyria

4.4 Special warnings and precautions for use
For the treatment of postmenopausal symptoms, HRT should only be initiated for symptoms that adversely affect quality of life. In all cases, a careful appraisal of the risks and benefits should be undertaken at least annually and HRT should only be continued as long as the benefit outweighs the risk.

Assessment of each women prior to taking hormone replacement therapy (and at regular intervals thereafter) should include a personal and family medical history. Physical examination should be guided by this and by the contra-indications (section 4.3) and warnings (section 4.4) for this product. During assessment of each individual woman, clinical examination of the breasts and pelvic examination should be performed where clinically indicated rather than as a routine procedure. Women should be encouraged to participate in the national breast cancer screening programme (mammography) and the national cervical cancer screening programme (cervical cytology) as appropriate for their age. Breast awareness should also be encouraged and women advised to report any changes in their breasts to their doctor or nurse.

If any of the following conditions are present, have occurred previously, and/or have been aggravated during pregnancy or previous hormone treatment, the patient should be closely supervised. It should be taken into account that these conditions may recur or be aggravated during treatment with Oestrogel, in particular:

- Leiomyoma (uterine fibroids) or endometriosis
- A history of, or risk factors for thromboembolic disorders (see below)
- Risk factors for oestrogen dependent tumours, e.g. 1st degree heredity for breast cancer

Hypertension

- Liver disorders (e.g. liver adenoma)
- Diabetes mellitus with or without vascular involvement
- Cholelithiasis
- Migraine or (severe) headache
- Systemic lupus erythematosus
- A history of endometrial hyperplasia (see below)
- Epilepsy
- Asthma
- Otosclerosis

Reasons for immediate withdrawal of therapy:

Therapy should be discontinued in case of a contraindication is discovered and in the following situations:

- Jaundice or deterioration in liver function
- Significant increase in blood pressure
- New onset of migraine-type headache
- Pregnancy

Endometrial hyperplasia:

Prolonged use of unopposed oestrogens may increase the risk of endometrial hyperplasia and carcinoma (see Section 4.8). In women with an intact uterus the addition of a progestagen for at least 12 days per cycle greatly reduces this risk.

Break-through bleeding and spotting may occur during the first months of treatment. If break-through bleeding or spotting appears after some time on therapy, or continues after treatment has been discontinued, the reason should be investigated, which may include endometrial biopsy to exclude endometrial malignancy.

Unopposed oestrogen stimulation may lead to premalignant or malignant transformation in the residual foci of endometriosis. Therefore, the addition of progestagens to oestrogen replacement therapy should be considered in women who have undergone hysterectomy because of endometriosis if they are known to have residual endometriosis.

Breast cancer:

A randomised placebo-controlled trial, the Women's Health Initiative study (WHI), and epidemiological studies, including the Million Women Study (MWS), have reported an increased risk of breast cancer in women taking oestrogens, oestrogen-progestagen combinations or tibolone for HRT for several years (see Section 4.8).

For all HRT, an excess risk becomes apparent within a few years of use and increases with duration of intake but returns to baseline within a few (at most five) years after stopping treatment.

In the MWS, the relative risk of breast cancer with conjugated equine oestrogens (CEE) or estradiol (E2) was greater when a progestagen was added, either sequentially or continuously, and regardless of type of progestagen. There was no evidence of a difference in risk between the different routes of administration.

In the WHI study, the continuous combined conjugated equine oestrogen and medroxyprogesterone acetate (CEE + MPA) product used was associated with breast cancers that were slightly larger in size and more frequently had local lymph node metastases compared to placebo.

HRT, especially oestrogen-progestagen combined treatment, increases the density of mammographic images which may adversely affect the radiological detection of breast cancer.

Venous thromboembolism:

HRT is associated with a higher relative risk of developing venous thromboembolism (VTE), i.e. deep vein thrombosis or pulmonary embolism. One randomised controlled trial and epidemiological studies found a two to threefold higher risk for users compared with non-users. For non-users it is estimated that the number of cases of VTE that will occur over a 5-year period is about 3 per 1000 women aged 50-59 years and 8 per 1000 women aged between 60-69 years. It is estimated that in healthy women who use HRT for 5 years, the number of additional cases of VTE over a 5-year period will be between 2 and 6 (best estimate=4) per 1000 women aged 50-59 years and between 5 and 15 (best estimate=9) per 1000 women aged 60-69 years. he occurrence of such an event is more likely in the first year of HRT than later.

Generally recognised risk factors for VTE include a personal history or family history, severe obesity (BMI > 30kg/m^2) and systemic lupus erythaematosus (SLE). There is no consensus about the possible role of varicose veins in VTE.

Patients with a history of VTE or known thrombophilic states have an increased risk of VTE. HRT may add to this risk. Personal or strong family history of thromboembolism or recurrent spontaneous abortion should be investigated in order to exclude thrombophilic predisposition. Until a thorough evaluation of thrombophilic factors has been made or anticoagulant treatment initiated, use of HRT in such patients should be viewed as contraindicated. Those women already on anticoagulant treatment require careful consideration of the benefit-risk of use of HRT.

The risk of VTE may be temporarily increased with prolonged immobilisation, major trauma or major surgery. As in all postoperative patients, scrupulous attention should be given to prophylactic measures to prevent VTE following surgery. Where prolonged immobilisation is liable to follow elective surgery, particularly abdominal or orthopaedic surgery to the lower limbs, consideration should be given to temporarily stopping HRT 4 to 6 weeks earlier, if possible. Treatment should not be restarted until the woman is completely mobilised.

If VTE develops after initiating therapy, the drug should be discontinued. Patients should be told to contact their doctors immediately when they are aware of a potential thromboembolic symptom (e.g. painful swelling of a leg, sudden pain in the chest, dyspnea).

Coronary Artery Disease (CAD):

There is no evidence from randomised controlled trials of cardiovascular benefit with continuous combined conjugated and oestrogens and medroxyprogesterone acetate (MPA). Two large clinical trials (WHI and HERS i.e. Heart and Estrogen/progestin Replacement Study) showed a possible increased risk of cardiovascular morbidity in the first year of use and no overall benefit. For other HRT products there are only limited data from randomised controlled trials to date examining effects in cardiovascular morbidity or mortality. Therefore, it is uncertain whether these findings also extend to other HRT products.

Stroke:

One large randomised clinical trial (WHI-trial) found, as a secondary outcome, an increased risk of ischaemic stroke in healthy women during treatment with continuous combined conjugated oestrogens and MPA. For women who do not use HRT, it is estimated that the number of cases of stroke that will occur over a 5 year period is about 3 per 1000 women aged 50-59 years and 11 per 1000 women 60-69 years. It is estimated that for women who use conjugated oestrogens and MPA for 5 years, the number of additional cases will be between 0 and 3 (best estimate =1) per 1000 users aged 50-59 and between 1 and 9 (best estimate = 4) per 1000 users aged 60-69. It is unknown whether the increased risk also extends to other HRT products.

Ovarian cancer:

Long-term (at least 5-10 years) use of oestrogen only HRT products in hysterectomised women has been associated with an increased risk of ovarian cancer in some epidemiological studies. It is uncertain whether long-term use of combined HRTs confers to a different risk than oestrogen-only products.

Other conditions:

Oestrogens may cause fluid retention, and therefore patients with cardiac or renal dysfunction should be closely observed. Patients with terminal renal insufficiency should also be closely observed, since it is expected that the level of circulating active ingredients in Oestrogel is increased.

Women with pre-existing hypertriglyceridaemia should be followed closely during oestrogen replacement or hormone replacement therapy, since rare cases of large increases of plasma triglycerides leading to pancreatitis have been reported with oestrogen therapy in this condition.

Oestrogens increase thyroid binding globulin (TBG), leading to increased circulating total thyroid hormone, as measured by protein-bound iodine (PBI)), T4 levels (by column or by radio-immunoassay) or T3 levels (by radio-immunoassay). T3 resin uptake is decreased, reflecting the elevated TBG. Free T4 and free T3 concentrations are unaltered. Other binding proteins may be elevated in serum, i.e. corticoid binding globulin (CBG), sex-hormone-binding globulin (SHBG) leading to increased circulating corticosteroids and sex steroids respectively. Free or biological active hormone concentrations are unchanged. Other plasma proteins may be increased (angiotensinogen/renin substrate, alpha-I-antitrypsin, ceruloplasmin).

There is no conclusive evidence for improvement of cognitive function. There is some evidence from the WHI trial of increased risk of probable dementia in women who start using continuous combined CEE and MPA after the age of 65. It is unknown whether the findings apply to younger post-menopausal women or other HRT products.

4.5 Interaction with other medicinal products and other forms of interaction

Treatment with surface active agents (e.g. sodium lauryl sulphate), or other drugs which alter barrier structure or function, could remove drug bound to the skin, altering transdermal flux. Therefore patients should avoid the use of strong skin cleansers and detergents (e.g. benzalkonium or benzothonium chloride products), skin care products of high alcoholic content (astringents, sunscreens) and keratolytics (e.g. salicylic acid, lactic acid).

The use of any concomitant skin medication which alters skin production (e.g. cytotoxic drugs) should be avoided.

The metabolism of oestrogens may be increased by concomitant use of substances known to induce drug-metabolising enzymes, specifically cytochrome P450 enzymes, such as anticonvulsants (e.g. phenobarbital, phenytoin, carbamezapin) and anti-infectives (e.g. rifampicin, rifabutin, nevirapine, efavirenz).

Ritonavir and nelfinavir, although known as strong inhibitors, by contrast exhibit inducing properties when used concomitantly with steroid hormones. Herbal preparations containing St John's wort (Hypericum Perforatum) may induce the metabolism of oestrogens.

At transdermal administration, the first-pass effect in the liver is avoided and thus, transdermally applied oestrogens might be less affected than oral hormones by enzyme inducers.

Clinically, an increased metabolism of oestrogens and progestagens may lead to decreased effect and changes in the uterine bleeding profile.

4.6 Pregnancy and lactation

Oestrogel is not indicated during pregnancy and lactation. If pregnancy occurs during medication with Oestrogel, treatments should be withdrawn immediately.

The results of most epidemiological studies to date, relevant to inadvertent foetal exposure to oestrogens indicate no teratogenic of foetotoxic effects.

4.7 Effects on ability to drive and use machines

None known.

4.8 Undesirable effects

Skin: Irritation, reddening of the skin or mild and transient erythema at the site of application have been occasionally reported. In this instance a different site of application should be used, but if the topical side-effects continue, consideration should be given to discontinuation of treatment.

CNS: headache, migraine and mood changes.

Gastrointestinal tract: nausea

Genito-urinary tract: increase in the size of uterine fibromyomata, excessive production of cervical mucus.

Breast: pain, enlargement and secretion.

Breast cancer:

According to evidence from a large number of epidemiological studies and one randomised placebo-controlled trial, the Women's Health Initiative (WHI), the overall risk of breast cancer increases with increasing duration of HRT use in current or recent HRT users.

For *oestrogen-only* HRT, estimates of relative risk (RR) from a reanalysis of original data from 51 epidemiological studies (in which >80% of HRT use was oestrogen-only HRT) and from the epidemiological Million Women Study (MWS) are similar at 1.35 (95%CI 1.21 – 1.49) and 1.30 (95%CI 1.21 – 1.40), respectively.

For *oestrogen plus progestagen* combined HRT, several epidemiological studies have reported an overall higher risk for breast cancer than with oestrogens alone.

The MWS reported that, compared to never users, the use of various types of oestrogen-progestagen combined HRT was associated with a higher risk of breast cancer (RR = 2.00, 95%CI: 1.88 – 2.12) than use of oestrogens alone (RR = 1.30, 95%CI: 1.21 – 1.40) or use of tibolone (RR=1.45; 95%CI 1.25-1.68).

The WHI trial reported a risk estimate of 1.24 (95%CI 1.01 – 1.54) after 5.6 years of use of oestrogen-progestagen combined HRT (CEE + MPA) in all users compared with placebo.

The absolute risks calculated from the MWS and the WHI trial are presented below:

The MWS has estimated, from the known average incidence of breast cancer in developed countries, that:

- *For women not using HRT, about 32 in every 1000 are expected to have breast cancer diagnosed between the ages of 50 and 64 years.*
- For 1000 current or recent users of HRT, the number of *additional* cases during the corresponding period will be
  - For users of *oestrogen-only* replacement therapy
    - o between 0 and 3 (best estimate = 1.5) for 5 years' use
    - o between 3 and 7 (best estimate = 5) for 10 years' use.
  - For users of *oestrogen plus progestagen* combined HRT,
    - o between 5 and 7 (best estimate = 6) for 5 years' use
    - o between 18 and 20 (best estimate = 19) for 10 years' use.

The WHI trial estimated that after 5.6 years of follow-up of women between the ages of 50 and 79 years, an *additional*

8 cases of invasive breast cancer would be due to *oestrogen-progestagen combined* HRT (CEE + MPA) per 10,000 women years.

According to calculations from the trial data, it is estimated that:

- For 1000 women in the placebo group,
  - about 16 cases of invasive breast cancer would be diagnosed in 5 years.
- For 1000 women who used oestrogen + progestagen combined HRT (CEE + MPA), the number of *additional* cases would be
  - between 0 and 9 (best estimate = 4) for 5 years' use.

The number of additional cases of breast cancer in women who use HRT is broadly similar for women who start HRT irrespective of age at start of use (between the ages of 45-65) (see section 4.4).

Endometrial cancer:

In women with an intact uterus, the risk of endometrial hyperplasia and endometrial cancer increases with increasing duration of use of unopposed oestrogens. According to data from epidemiological studies, the best estimate of the risk is that for women not using HRT, about 5 in every 1000 are expected to have endometrial cancer diagnosed between the ages of 50 and 65. Depending on the duration of treatment and oestrogen dose, the reported increase in endometrial cancer risk among unopposed oestrogen users varies from 2-to 12-fold greater compared with non-users. Adding a progestagen to oestrogen-only therapy greatly reduces this increased risk.

Other adverse reactions have been reported in association with oestrogen/progestagen treatment:

- Oestrogen-dependent neoplasms benign and malignant, e.g. endometrial cancer.
- Venous thromboembolism, i.e. deep leg or pelvic venous thrombosis and pulmonary embolism, is more frequent among hormone replacement therapy users than among non-users. For further information, see section 4.3 -Contra-indications and 4.4 Special warnings and precautions for use.
- Myocardial infarction and stroke
- Gall bladder disease.
- Skin and subcutaneous disorders: chloasma, erythema multiforme, erythema nodosum, vascular purpura.
- Probable dementia (see section 4.4)

4.9 Overdose

Pain in the breasts or excessive production of cervical mucus may be indicative of too high a dosage, but acute overdosage has not been reported and is unlikely to be a problem. Overdosages of oestrogen may cause nausea, and withdrawal bleeding may occur. There are no specific antidotes and treatment should be symptomatic.

5. PHARMACOLOGICAL PROPERTIES

5.1 Pharmacodynamic properties

The active ingredient, estradiol, is chemically and biologically identical to endogenous human estradiol. It substitutes for the loss of oestrogen in menopausal women, and alleviates menopausal symptoms.

Oestrogel prevents bone loss following menopause or ovariectomy.

Relief of menopausal symptoms

Relief of menopausal symptoms was achieved during the first few weeks of treatment. The rate of regular withdrawal bleeding or amenorrhoea depends on the individual posology and may vary on the individual patient.

Prevention of osteoporosis

Oestrogen deficiency at menopause is associated with an increasing bone turnover and decline in bone mass. The effect of oestrogens on the bone mineral density is dose-dependent. Protection appears to be effective for as long as treatment is continued. After discontinuation of HRT, bone mass is lost at a similar rate to that in untreated women.

Evidence from the WHI trial and meta-analysed trials shows that current use of HRT, alone or in combination with a progestagen – given to predominantly healthy women- reduces the risk of hip, vertebral, and other osteoporotic fractures. HRT may also prevent fractures in women with low bone density and/or established osteoporosis, but the evidence for this is limited.

5.2 Pharmacokinetic properties

Pharmacokinetic studies indicate that, when applied topically to a large area of skin in a volatile solvent, approximately 10% of the estradiol is percutaneously absorbed into the vascular system, regardless of the age of the patient. Daily application of 2.5g or 5g Oestrogel over a surface area of 400-750cm^2 results in a gradual increase in oestrogen blood levels to steady state after approximately 3-5 days and provides circulating levels of both estradiol and estrone equivalent in absolute concentrations and in their respective ratio to those obtained during the early-mid follicular phase of the menstrual cycle.

Oestrogel was administered to 17 postmenopausal women once daily on the posterior surface of one arm from wrist to shoulder for 14 consecutive days.

Maximum serum concentrations (C_{max}) of estradiol and estrone on Day 12 were 117pg/ml and 128pg/ml, respectively.

The time-averaged serum estradiol and estrone concentrations ($C_{average}$) over the 24 hour dose interval after administration of 2.5g of Oestrogel on Day 12 were 76.8pg/ml and 95.7pg/ml, respectively.

Metabolism of estradiol takes place mainly in the liver under oestriol, estrone and their conjugated metabolites (glucuronides, sulphates). These metabolites also undergo enterohepatic recirculation.

When treatment is stopped, estradiol and urinary conjugated estradiol concentrations return to baseline in about 76 hours.

5.3 Preclinical safety data

No relevant information additional to that already contained in the SPC.

6. PHARMACEUTICAL PARTICULARS

6.1 List of excipients

Ethanol

Carbomer

Triethanolamine

Purified water

6.2 Incompatibilities

None known.

6.3 Shelf life

24 months

6.4 Special precautions for storage

Do not store above 25°C.

6.5 Nature and contents of container

Rigid plastic container enclosing a LDPE bag fitted with a metering valve and closed with a polypropylene cap, containing 80g.

6.6 Special precautions for disposal and other handling

Not applicable.

7. MARKETING AUTHORISATION HOLDER

Besins International Healthcare S.A.

Rue Vilain XIIII

1000 Brussels

Belgium

8. MARKETING AUTHORISATION NUMBER(S)

PL 28397/0001

9. DATE OF FIRST AUTHORISATION/RENEWAL OF THE AUTHORISATION

1 November 1997

10. DATE OF REVISION OF THE TEXT

March 2006

Legal category

POM

Oilatum Cream

(Stiefel Laboratories (UK) Limited)

1. NAME OF THE MEDICINAL PRODUCT

Oilatum Cream

2. QUALITATIVE AND QUANTITATIVE COMPOSITION

Contains Light Liquid Paraffin 6.0% w/w and White Soft Paraffin 15.0% w/w in a cream base.

3. PHARMACEUTICAL FORM

Cream for topical application.

4. CLINICAL PARTICULARS

4.1 Therapeutic indications

Oilatum Cream is indicated in the treatment of contact dermatitis, atopic eczema, senile pruritus, ichthyosis and related dry skin conditions.

4.2 Posology and method of administration

Oilatum Cream may be used as often as required. Apply to the affected area and rub in well. It is especially effective after washing when the sebum content of the stratum corneum may be depleted resulting in excessive moisture loss.

Oilatum Cream is suitable for adults, children and the elderly.

4.3 Contraindications

Should not be used in patients with known hypersensitivity to any of the ingredients.

4.4 Special warnings and precautions for use

Pack sizes 40g and 150g: None.

Pack sizes 500ml and 1050ml: Hospital users should follow local procedures and policies for using topical products on in-patients.

4.5 Interaction with other medicinal products and other forms of interaction

None.

4.6 Pregnancy and lactation

There are no restrictions on the use of Oilatum Cream during pregnancy or lactation.

4.7 Effects on ability to drive and use machines

None.

4.8 Undesirable effects

May cause irritation in patients hypersensitive to any of the ingredients.

4.9 Overdose

Accidental ingestion may cause nausea and vomiting. Administer copious quantities of water as required. Excessive topical application should cause no untoward effects other than greasy skin.

5. PHARMACOLOGICAL PROPERTIES

5.1 Pharmacodynamic properties

Light Liquid Paraffin and White Soft Paraffin exert an emollient effect by forming an occlusive film which reduces trans-epidermal water loss, thus helping to maintain normal skin humidity levels. Polyvinyl pyrrolidone enhances the strength and longevity of the occlusive film formed by the oil on the skin.

5.2 Pharmacokinetic properties

Not applicable.

5.3 Preclinical safety data

White Soft Paraffin and Light Liquid Paraffin have been used in pharmaceutical and cosmetic preparations for many years. The formulation contains excipients that are commonly used in such preparations. The safety of these substances is well established by common use over long periods in man.

6. PHARMACEUTICAL PARTICULARS

6.1 List of excipients

PEG 1000 Monostearate

Cetostearyl alcohol

Glycerol

Potassium sorbate

Benzyl alcohol

Citric acid monohydrate

Povidone K29/32

Purified water

6.2 Incompatibilities

None.

6.3 Shelf life

Pack sizes 40g and 150g: Three years.

Pack sizes 500ml and 1050ml: 30 months.

6.4 Special precautions for storage

Pack sizes 40g and 150g: None.

Pack sizes 500ml and 1050ml: Do not store above 25°C.

6.5 Nature and contents of container

Pack size 40g: Internally lacquered, membrane sealed aluminium tube fitted with a polypropylene screw cap and packed into a carton.

Pack size 150g: High density polyethylene tube.

Pack Size 500ml: High density polyethylene bottle fitted with a mechanical pump dispenser.

Pack Size 1050ml: Polypropylene container and lid, fitted with a mechanical pump dispenser (polypropylene components), utilising a follower plate (HDPE)

6.6 Special precautions for disposal and other handling

None.

7. MARKETING AUTHORISATION HOLDER

Stiefel Laboratories (UK) Ltd

Holtspur Lane

Wooburn Green

High Wycombe

Bucks

HP10 0AU

UK

8. MARKETING AUTHORISATION NUMBER(S)

40g and 150g: PL 0174/0207

500ml and 1050ml: PL 0174/0219

9. DATE OF FIRST AUTHORISATION/RENEWAL OF THE AUTHORISATION

Date of first authorisation PL 0174/0207: 24th January 2001

Date of first authorisation PL 0174/0219: 28th October 2005

10. DATE OF REVISION OF THE TEXT

PL 0174/0207: 14th November 2001

PL 0174/0219: 1st June 2006

Oilatum Emollient

(Stiefel Laboratories (UK) Limited)

1. NAME OF THE MEDICINAL PRODUCT

Oilatum Emollient

2. QUALITATIVE AND QUANTITATIVE COMPOSITION
Light Liquid Paraffin 63.4% w/w

3. PHARMACEUTICAL FORM
Liquid Bath Additive

4. CLINICAL PARTICULARS

4.1 Therapeutic indications
Oilatum Emollient is indicated in the treatment of contact dermatitis, atopic dermatitis, senile pruritus, ichthyosis and related dry skin conditions. Oilatum Emollient replaces oil and water and hydrates the keratin. Oilatum Emollient is particularly suitable for infant bathing. The preparation also overcomes the problem of cleansing the skin in conditions where the use of soaps, soap substitutes and colloid or oatmeal baths proves irritating.

4.2 Posology and method of administration
Oilatum Emollient should always be used with water, either added to the water or applied to wet skin.

Adult bath:

Add 1-3 capfuls to an 8-inch bath of water, soak for 10-20 minutes. Pat dry.

Infant bath:

Add ½-2 capfuls to a basin of water, Apply gently over entire body with a sponge. Pat dry.

Skin cleansing:

Rub a small amount of oil into wet skin. Rinse and pat dry.

Where conditions permit, and particularly in cases of extensive areas of dry skin, Oilatum Emollient should be used as a bath oil, ensuring complete coverage by immersion. In addition to the therapeutic benefits, this method of use provides a means of sedating tense patients, particularly relevant in cases of acute pruritic dermatoses where relaxation of tension appears to relieve symptoms.

The product is suitable for use in adults, children and the elderly.

4.3 Contraindications
None

4.4 Special warnings and precautions for use
The patient should be advised to use care to avoid slipping in the bath. If a rash or skin irritation occurs, stop using the product and consult your doctor.

4.5 Interaction with other medicinal products and other forms of interaction
None known

4.6 Pregnancy and lactation
There is no, or inadequate, evidence of the safety of Oilatum Emollient in human pregnancy or lactation, but it has been in wide use for many years without ill consequence.

4.7 Effects on ability to drive and use machines
None

4.8 Undesirable effects
None

4.9 Overdose
Not applicable

5. PHARMACOLOGICAL PROPERTIES

5.1 Pharmacodynamic properties
Light liquid paraffin exerts an emollient effect by forming an occlusive oil film on the stratum corneum. This prevents excessive evaporation of water from the skin surface and aids in the prevention of dryness.

5.2 Pharmacokinetic properties
Not applicable

5.3 Preclinical safety data
Not applicable

6. PHARMACEUTICAL PARTICULARS

6.1 List of excipients
Acetylated Lanolin Alcohols

Isopropyl Palmitate

Polyethylene Glycol 400 dilaurate

Polyoxyethylene 40 sorbital septaoleate

Floral Spice

6.2 Incompatibilities
None

6.3 Shelf life
5 years

6.4 Special precautions for storage
None

6.5 Nature and contents of container
High density polyethylene bottles with a screw cap. Capacity: 25ml, 150ml, 200ml, 250ml, 300ml, 350ml, 400ml, 500ml, 600ml, 1000ml.

6.6 Special precautions for disposal and other handling
There are no special instructions for use or handling

7. MARKETING AUTHORISATION HOLDER
Stiefel Laboratories (UK) Ltd

Eurasia Headquarters

Concorde Road

Maidenhead

SL6 4BY

UK

8. MARKETING AUTHORISATION NUMBER(S)
PL0174/5010R

9. DATE OF FIRST AUTHORISATION/RENEWAL OF THE AUTHORISATION
8th December 1989 / 8th July 2008

10. DATE OF REVISION OF THE TEXT
August 2009

Oilatum Gel
(Stiefel Laboratories (UK) Limited)

1. NAME OF THE MEDICINAL PRODUCT
Oilatum Gel

2. QUALITATIVE AND QUANTITATIVE COMPOSITION
Light liquid paraffin 70% w/w

3. PHARMACEUTICAL FORM
Shower gel.

4. CLINICAL PARTICULARS

4.1 Therapeutic indications
For the treatment of contact dermatitis, atopic dermatitis, senile pruritus ichthyosis and related dry skin conditions.

4.2 Posology and method of administration
Topical

Adults, children and the elderly:

Oilatum Gel may be used as frequently as necessary. Oilatum Gel should always be applied to wet skin, normally as a shower gel.

Shower as usual. Apply Oilatum Gel liberally to wet skin and massage gently. Rinse briefly and lightly pat the skin dry.

4.3 Contraindications
None.

4.4 Special warnings and precautions for use
Take care to avoid slipping in the shower.

Oilatum Gel should not be used on greasy skin.

4.5 Interaction with other medicinal products and other forms of interaction
None.

4.6 Pregnancy and lactation
There is no or inadequate evidence of the safety of Oilatum Gel in human pregnancy and lactation. Topical preparations containing light liquid paraffin have been in wide use for many years without apparent ill consequence.

4.7 Effects on ability to drive and use machines
None.

4.8 Undesirable effects
None

4.9 Overdose
Not applicable.

5. PHARMACOLOGICAL PROPERTIES

5.1 Pharmacodynamic properties
Light liquid paraffin exerts an emollient effect by forming an occlusive oil film on the stratum corneum. This prevents excessive evaporation of water from the skin surface and aids in the prevention of dryness.

5.2 Pharmacokinetic properties
Not applicable.

5.3 Preclinical safety data
There are no pre-clinical data of relevance to the prescriber which are additional to those already stated in other sections of the SPC.

6. PHARMACEUTICAL PARTICULARS

6.1 List of excipients
Polyethylene 617A

2-octadodecanol

Polyethylene glycol 400 dilaurate.

Polyoxyethylene 40 sorbital septaoleate

Polyethylene glycol-2-myristyl ether propionate

Polyphenylmethyl siloxane copolymer

Floral spice

6.2 Incompatibilities
None.

6.3 Shelf life

a) For the product as packaged for sale

3 years

b) After first opening the container

Comply with expiry date

6.4 Special precautions for storage
Store below 25°C.

6.5 Nature and contents of container
High density polyethylene tubes of 15g, 25g, 50g, 60g, 65g, 70g, 75g, 125g and 150g

6.6 Special precautions for disposal and other handling
There are no special instructions for use or handling of Oilatum Gel.

7. MARKETING AUTHORISATION HOLDER
Stiefel Laboratories (UK) Ltd

Eurasia Headquarters

Concorde Road

Maidenhead

SL6 4BY

UK

8. MARKETING AUTHORISATION NUMBER(S)
PL 0174/0072

9. DATE OF FIRST AUTHORISATION/RENEWAL OF THE AUTHORISATION
7th November 1991 / 6th August 2004

10. DATE OF REVISION OF THE TEXT
August 2009

Oilatum Junior
(Stiefel Laboratories (UK) Limited)

1. NAME OF THE MEDICINAL PRODUCT
Oilatum Junior

2. QUALITATIVE AND QUANTITATIVE COMPOSITION
Light Liquid Paraffin 63.4% w/w

3. PHARMACEUTICAL FORM
Liquid bath Additive

4. CLINICAL PARTICULARS

4.1 Therapeutic indications
Oilatum Junior is indicated in the treatment of contact dermatitis, atopic dermatitis, senile pruritus, ichthyosis and related dry skin conditions.

Route of administration: Topical

4.2 Posology and method of administration
Oilatum Junior may be used as frequently as necessary. Oilatum Junior should always be used with water, either added to the water or applied to wet skin.

For adults add 1-3 capfuls to an 8 inch bath of water. Soak for 10-20 minutes. Pat dry.

For infants, add ½-2 capfuls to a basin of water. Apply gently over entire body with a sponge. Pat dry.

4.3 Contraindications
None.

4.4 Special warnings and precautions for use
Patients should be advised to use care to avoid slipping in the bath. If a rash or skin irritation should occur, stop using the product and consult your doctor.

4.5 Interaction with other medicinal products and other forms of interaction
None known

4.6 Pregnancy and lactation
There is no or inadequate evidence of the safety of Oilatum Junior in human pregnancy or lactation, but it has been in wide use for many years without ill consequence.

4.7 Effects on ability to drive and use machines
None.

4.8 Undesirable effects
None.

4.9 Overdose
Not applicable.

5. PHARMACOLOGICAL PROPERTIES

5.1 Pharmacodynamic properties
Light liquid paraffin exerts an emollient effect by forming an occlusive oil film on the stratum corneum. This prevents excessive evaporation of water from the skin surface and aids in the prevention of dryness.

5.2 Pharmacokinetic properties
Not applicable.

5.3 Preclinical safety data
None.

6. PHARMACEUTICAL PARTICULARS

6.1 List of excipients
Acetylated Lanolin Alcohols

Isopropyl Palmitate

Polyethylene Glycol 400 dilaurate

Macrogol ester.

6.2 Incompatibilities
Not applicable.

6.3 Shelf life
For the product as packaged for sale: 5 years

6.4 Special precautions for storage
None.

6.5 Nature and contents of container
High density polyethylene bottles with a screw cap. Capacity: 25ml, 150ml, 200ml, 250ml, 300ml, 350ml, 400ml, 500ml, 600ml, 1000ml.

6.6 Special precautions for disposal and other handling
There are no special instructions for use or handling of Oilatum Junior.

7. MARKETING AUTHORISATION HOLDER
Stiefel Laboratories (UK) Ltd
Eurasia Headquarters
Concorde Road
Maidenhead
SL6 4BY
UK

8. MARKETING AUTHORISATION NUMBER(S)
PL0174/0182

9. DATE OF FIRST AUTHORISATION/RENEWAL OF THE AUTHORISATION
Date of first authorisation: 24th June 1993
Date of latest renewal: 2nd July 2004

10. DATE OF REVISION OF THE TEXT
August 2009

Oilatum Junior Cream
(Stiefel Laboratories (UK) Limited)

1. NAME OF THE MEDICINAL PRODUCT
Oilatum Junior Cream

2. QUALITATIVE AND QUANTITATIVE COMPOSITION
Contains Light Liquid Paraffin 6.0% w/w and White Soft Paraffin 15.0% w/w in a cream base.

3. PHARMACEUTICAL FORM
Cream for topical application.

4. CLINICAL PARTICULARS
4.1 Therapeutic indications
Oilatum Junior Cream is indicated in the treatment of contact dermatitis, atopic eczema, senile pruritus, ichthyosis and related dry skin conditions.

4.2 Posology and method of administration
Oilatum Junior Cream may be used as often as required. Apply to the affected area and rub in well. It is especially effective after washing when the sebum content of the stratum corneum may be depleted resulting in excessive moisture loss.

Oilatum Junior Cream is suitable for adults, children and the elderly.

4.3 Contraindications
Should not be used in patients with known hypersensitivity to any of the ingredients.

4.4 Special warnings and precautions for use
Hospital users should follow local procedures and policies for using topical products on in-patients.

4.5 Interaction with other medicinal products and other forms of interaction
None.

4.6 Pregnancy and lactation
There are no restrictions on the use of Oilatum Junior Cream during pregnancy or lactation.

4.7 Effects on ability to drive and use machines
None.

4.8 Undesirable effects
May cause irritation in patients hypersensitive to any of the ingredients.

4.9 Overdose
Accidental ingestion may cause nausea and vomiting. Administer copious quantities of water as required. Excessive topical application should cause no untoward effects other than greasy skin.

5. PHARMACOLOGICAL PROPERTIES
5.1 Pharmacodynamic properties
Light Liquid Paraffin and White Soft Paraffin exert an emollient effect by forming an occlusive film which reduces trans-epidermal water loss, thus helping to maintain normal skin humidity levels. Polyvinyl pyrrolidone enhances the strength and longevity of the occlusive film formed by the oil on the skin.

5.2 Pharmacokinetic properties
Not applicable.

5.3 Preclinical safety data
White Soft Paraffin and Light Liquid Paraffin have been used in pharmaceutical and cosmetic preparations for many years. The formulation contains excipients that are commonly used in such preparations. The safety of these substances is well established by common use over long periods in man.

6. PHARMACEUTICAL PARTICULARS
6.1 List of excipients
PEG 1000 Monostearate
Cetostearyl alcohol
Glycerol
Potassium sorbate
Benzyl alcohol
Citric acid monohydrate
Povidone K29/32
Purified water

6.2 Incompatibilities
None.

6.3 Shelf life
30 months.

6.4 Special precautions for storage
Do not store above 25 Degrees C.

6.5 Nature and contents of container
High density polyethylene bottle fitted with a mechanical pump dispenser. Pack size 500ml and 1050ml.

6.6 Special precautions for disposal and other handling
None.

7. MARKETING AUTHORISATION HOLDER
Stiefel Laboratories (UK) Ltd
Holtspur Lane
Wooburn Green
High Wycombe
Bucks HP10 0AU

8. MARKETING AUTHORISATION NUMBER(S)
PL 0174/0219

9. DATE OF FIRST AUTHORISATION/RENEWAL OF THE AUTHORISATION
28th October 2005

10. DATE OF REVISION OF THE TEXT
28th September 2006

Oilatum Plus
(Stiefel Laboratories (UK) Limited)

1. NAME OF THE MEDICINAL PRODUCT
Oilatum Plus

2. QUALITATIVE AND QUANTITATIVE COMPOSITION
Light liquid paraffin 52.5% w/w, benzalkonium chloride solution 12.0% w/w, triclosan 2% w/w

3. PHARMACEUTICAL FORM
Solution

4. CLINICAL PARTICULARS
4.1 Therapeutic indications
Topical as a bath additive.

For the prophylactic treatment of eczemas at risk from infection.

4.2 Posology and method of administration
Oilatum Plus should always be diluted with water. It is an effective cleanser and should not be used with soap.

Adults and children: In an eight inch bath add 2 capfuls, in a four inch bath add 1 capful

Infants: Add 1 ml (just sufficient to cover the bottom of the cap) and mix well with water

Do not use for babies younger than 6 months

4.3 Contraindications
Patients with a known hypersensitivity to any of the ingredients should not use the product.

4.4 Special warnings and precautions for use
Avoid contact of the undiluted product with the eyes. If the undiluted product comes into contact with the eye, reddening may occur. Eye irrigation should be performed for 15 minutes and then the eye examined under fluorescein stain. If there is persistent irritation or any uptake of fluorescein, the patient should be referred for ophthalmological opinion.

The product should not be used with soap.

4.5 Interaction with other medicinal products and other forms of interaction
None known.

4.6 Pregnancy and lactation
No restrictions on the use of the product in pregnancy and lactation are proposed.

4.7 Effects on ability to drive and use machines
None known.

4.8 Undesirable effects
None known.

4.9 Overdose
The product is intended for topical use only. Accidental ingestion may cause gastro intestinal irritation with vomiting and diarrhoea. Vomiting may result in foam aspiration. In the case of accidental ingestion, give 1 to 2 glasses of milk or water to drink. If a large quantity of the product is ingested, the patient should be observed in hospital and the use of activated charcoal may be considered.

5. PHARMACOLOGICAL PROPERTIES
5.1 Pharmacodynamic properties
Benzalkonium chloride and triclosan are anti-bacterial agents with proven efficacy against *Staphylococcus aureus*, the principal causative organism in infected eczemas.

Light liquid paraffin is an emollient widely used in the treatment of eczema.

5.2 Pharmacokinetic properties
Not applicable.

5.3 Preclinical safety data
Not applicable.

6. PHARMACEUTICAL PARTICULARS
6.1 List of excipients
Acetylated lanolin alcohols
Isopropyl palmitate
Oleyl alcohol
Polyoxyethylene lauryl ether

6.2 Incompatibilities
None known.

6.3 Shelf life
a) For the product as packaged for sale
3 years
b) After first opening the container
Comply with expiry date

6.4 Special precautions for storage
None.

6.5 Nature and contents of container
White polyvinyl chloride or high density polyethylene bottles containing 20ml, 25ml, 150ml, 250ml, 350ml, 500ml, 600ml, 1000ml with white urea cap.

6.6 Special precautions for disposal and other handling
There are no special instructions for use or handling of Oilatum Plus/Oilatum Junior Flare-Up.

7. MARKETING AUTHORISATION HOLDER
Stiefel Laboratories (UK) Ltd
Eurasia Headquarters
Concorde Road
Maidenhead
SL6 4BY
UK

8. MARKETING AUTHORISATION NUMBER(S)
PL 0174/0070

9. DATE OF FIRST AUTHORISATION/RENEWAL OF THE AUTHORISATION
Date of first authorisation: 16th February 1990
Date of latest renewal: 25th February 2009

10. DATE OF REVISION OF THE TEXT
August 2009

Oily Phenol Injection BP (UCB Pharma Ltd)
(UCB Pharma Limited)

1. NAME OF THE MEDICINAL PRODUCT
Oily Phenol Injection BP 5% w/v

2. QUALITATIVE AND QUANTITATIVE COMPOSITION
Phenol BP 5.00 % w/v

3. PHARMACEUTICAL FORM
Sterile solution intended for parenteral use

4. CLINICAL PARTICULARS
4.1 Therapeutic indications
Scleropathy of haemorrhoids

4.2 Posology and method of administration
Injected into sub-mucosal layer at the base of the haemorrhoid

ADULTS

2-3 ml of oily phenol injection into the sub-mucosal layer at the base of the pile; Several injections may be given at different sites but not more than a total volume of 10 ml should be used at any one time.

CHILDREN

Use of this product is not advised

ELDERLY

No alternative dosage schedules have been suggested.

4.3 Contraindications
Oily Phenol Injection, BP is contraindicated in patients who are hypersensitive to phenol, nuts and in particular almond oil or any component of the product. It should not be used

over large areas, since sufficient amounts may be absorbed to give rise to toxic symptoms. Oily Phenol Injection, BP is also contraindicated in neonates and children.

4.4 Special warnings and precautions for use
For submucosal injection only. Not for intrathecal use. Complications of therapy can include local ulceration and sterile abscess formation. These complications may be serious following a misplaced injection (eg prostatic abscess). Care in choosing the correct site of injection is mandatory.

4.5 Interaction with other medicinal products and other forms of interaction
None stated

4.6 Pregnancy and lactation
Safety in pregnancy has not been established. The effects on the foetus are unknown, therefore Oily Phenol is not recommended for use during pregnancy.

It is not known whether Oily Phenol is excreted in breast milk. Since safety in infants has not been established, Oily Phenol injection is not recommended for use whilst breast-feeding.

4.7 Effects on ability to drive and use machines
Effects of phenol oily injection are not likely to affect the patient's ability to drive and use machinery.

4.8 Undesirable effects
General disorders and administration site conditions:
Pyrexia
Pain
Discomfort
Ulcer
Immune system disorders:
Hypersensitivity
Nervous system disorders:
Dizziness
Hepatobiliary disorders:
Hepatitis
Infections and infestations:
Abscess
Prostatic abscess
Necrotizing fasciitis
Retroperitoneal sepsis
Renal and urinary disorders:
Dysuria
Urinary incontinence
Reproductive system and breast disorders:
Impotence

4.9 Overdose
Symptoms:

The symptoms of overdosage after submucosal injection of Oily Phenol are not known, but are likely to be similar to symptoms observed after excessive exposure to phenol in other preparations. Absorption of phenol after application of dilute phenol solutions to extensive wounds has resulted in abdominal pains, dizziness, methaemoglobinaemia, haemoglobinurea, cyanosis, cardiac arrhythmias, ECG abnormalities, and may result in respiratory failure, circulatory failure, coma and death.

Treatment:

There is no specific antidote for acute phenol overdose. Treatment of overdose is symptomatic and supportive.

5. PHARMACOLOGICAL PROPERTIES

5.1 Pharmacodynamic properties
Oily phenol injection acts as an analgesic and thrombotic agent by numbimg the sensory nerve endings and precipitating proteins.

5.2 Pharmacokinetic properties
Phenol is absorbed from the gastro-intestinal tract and through skin and mucous membranes. It is metabolised to phenylglucoronide and phenylsulphate and small amounts are oxidised to catechol and quinol which are mainly conjugated. The metabolites are excreted in the urine; on oxidation to quinones they may tint the urine green.

5.3 Preclinical safety data
No data available

6. PHARMACEUTICAL PARTICULARS

6.1 List of excipients
Almond oil

6.2 Incompatibilities
Incompatible with alkaline salts, acetanilide, phenazone, piperazine, quinine salts, phenacetin and iron salts. Phenol coagulates albumin and gelatinises collodion.

6.3 Shelf life
3 years

6.4 Special precautions for storage
Store below 25°C

6.5 Nature and contents of container
5 ml neutral glass (type 1) ampoules supplied in cartons of 10

6.6 Special precautions for disposal and other handling
None stated

7. MARKETING AUTHORISATION HOLDER
UCB Pharma Limited
208 Bath Road
Slough
Berkshire
SL1 3WE
UK

8. MARKETING AUTHORISATION NUMBER(S)
PL 0039/5690R

9. DATE OF FIRST AUTHORISATION/RENEWAL OF THE AUTHORISATION
20 March 1987 / 15 October 1997

10. DATE OF REVISION OF THE TEXT
23rd September 2008

Olbetam Capsules 250

(Pharmacia Limited)

1. NAME OF THE MEDICINAL PRODUCT
Olbetam Capsules 250

2. QUALITATIVE AND QUANTITATIVE COMPOSITION
Acipimox INN 250.00 mg

3. PHARMACEUTICAL FORM
Red-brown/dark pink hard gelatin capsules, size no. 1, containing a white to cream powder.

4. CLINICAL PARTICULARS

4.1 Therapeutic indications
Olbetam is indicated for the treatment of lipid disorders characterised, according to Fredrickson, by elevated plasma levels of triglycerides (type IV hyperlipo-proteinaemia), or cholesterol (type IIA hyperlipoproteinaemia) and triglycerides and cholesterol (type IIB hyperlipoproteinaemia).

4.2 Posology and method of administration
To be given orally.

The daily dosage should be adjusted individually depending on plasma triglyceride and cholesterol levels.

The recommended dosage is one 250 mg capsule 2 or 3 times daily to be taken with or after meals. The lower dose is advised in type IV and the higher dose in types IIA and IIB hyperlipoproteinaemias.

Daily dosages of up to 1200 mg have been safely administered for long periods. Improvement in the plasma lipid's picture is usually seen within the first month of therapy.

In patients with slight renal impairment (creatinine clearance values > 60 ml/min) no dose reduction is required. For patients with moderate to severe renal impairment (creatinine clearance values between 60 and 30 ml/min) the dose needs to be reduced accordingly. Acipimox is eliminated entirely through the kidneys, therefore, accumulation can be expected and is related to the degree of renal impairment. It is advised that longer intervals are left between doses of the drug in patients with renal impairment.

4.3 Contraindications
Olbetam is contra-indicated in patients who are hypersensitive to the drug and those with peptic ulceration.

Olbetam should not be given to patients with severe renal impairment (creatinine clearance < 30 ml/min)

4.4 Special warnings and precautions for use
Modification of hyperlipidaemia is recommended only for patients with hyperlipoproteinaemia of a degree and type considered appropriate for treatment.

Low cholesterol and low-fat diets, together with cessation of alcohol consumption, are preferable therapeutic approaches to be tried before starting treatment with Olbetam.

The absorption of Olbetam is not affected by the concomitant administration of colestyramine

Evidence of clinical efficacy in the prevention of heart disease has not been established.

The possible beneficial and adverse, long-term consequences of some drugs used in the hyperlipidaemias are still the subject of scientific discussion.

4.5 Interaction with other medicinal products and other forms of interaction
No interaction has been shown with other lipid lowering agents. However, the combination with statins or fibrates should be used with caution due to reports of an increased risk of musculoskeletal events with nicotinic acid, as strict analogue of acipimox, is used in combination with such lipid-lowering agents.

4.6 Pregnancy and lactation
There is no evidence from the animal studies that acipimox is teratogenic. However, a higher incidence of immature and underweight foetuses was seen in pregnant animals given higher doses of acipimox. This effect may be due to maternal toxicity.

There is only limited experience to date of administration of acipimox to humans therefore epidemiological data is not available. Taking into account the present experience of administration to humans of acipimox and that the safety of acipimox in human pregnancy has not yet been ascertained, it is recommended, therefore, that acipimox not be administered to women who are, or may be pregnant.

In the absence of animal data on the levels of acipimox excreted in milk, Olbetam should not be administered to women who are breast-feeding.

4.7 Effects on ability to drive and use machines
None stated.

4.8 Undesirable effects
The drug may induce skin vasodilatation giving rise to a sensation of heat, flushing or itching, especially at the beginning of therapy and also rash and erythema. These reactions usually disappear rapidly during the first day of treatment. Moderate gastric disturbances (heartburn, epigastric pain, nausea and diarrhoea) have been reported occasionally, as well as headache, malaise, eye symptoms (dry or gritty eye), myositis, myalgia, weakness, arthralgiaand urticaria. On rare occasions patients have developed angioedema and bronchospasm; and anaphylactoid reactions have also been reported.

4.9 Overdose
If toxic effects are observed, supportive care and symptomatic treatment should be administered.

5. PHARMACOLOGICAL PROPERTIES

5.1 Pharmacodynamic properties
Acipimox inhibits the release of fatty acids from adipose tissue and reduces the blood concentrations of very low density lipoproteins (VLDL or Pre-beta) and low density lipoproteins (LDL or beta) with a subsequent overall reduction in triglyceride and cholesterol levels.

Acipimox also has a favourable effect on high density lipoproteins (HDL or alpha) which increase during treatment.

5.2 Pharmacokinetic properties
Acipimox is rapidly and completely absorbed orally, reaching peak plasma levels within two hours. The half-life is about two hours. It does not bind to plasma proteins; it is not significantly metabolised and is eliminated almost completely intact by the urinary route.

5.3 Preclinical safety data
There is no evidence from the animal studies that acipimox is teratogenic. However, a higher incidence of immature and underweight foetuses was seen in pregnant animals given higher doses of acipimox. This effect may be due to maternal toxicity.

6. PHARMACEUTICAL PARTICULARS

6.1 List of excipients
Physically modified corn starch (STA-RX 1500)
Silica gel (Syloid 244) USP
Magnesium stearate Ph. Eur
Sodium lauryl sulphate Ph. Eur
Hard gelatin capsules shell:
Gelatin USP
Titanium dioxide (E171)
Iron oxide red (E172)
Iron oxide yellow (E172)

6.2 Incompatibilities
None stated.

6.3 Shelf life
48 months

6.4 Special precautions for storage
Store at a temperature below 30°C in a dry place.

6.5 Nature and contents of container
Packed in blisters of 10 capsules per strip, inside cartons. Each carton contains 90 capsules.

6.6 Special precautions for disposal and other handling
None given.

Administrative Data

7. MARKETING AUTHORISATION HOLDER
Pharmacia Limited
Ramsgate Road
Sandwich
Kent CT13 9NJ
United Kingdom

8. MARKETING AUTHORISATION NUMBER(S)
PL 00032/0322

9. DATE OF FIRST AUTHORISATION/RENEWAL OF THE AUTHORISATION
2 May 2003

10. DATE OF REVISION OF THE TEXT
31 May 2007

Company Ref: OB2_0

OLMETEC film-coated tablets

(Daiichi Sankyo UK Limited)

1. NAME OF THE MEDICINAL PRODUCT

Olmetec 10 mg film-coated tablet

Olmetec 20 mg film-coated tablet

Olmetec 40 mg film-coated tablet

2. QUALITATIVE AND QUANTITATIVE COMPOSITION

Olmesartan medoxomil

Each 10 mg tablet contains 10 mg of olmesartan medoxomil

Each 20 mg tablet contains 20 mg of olmesartan medoxomil

Each 40 mg tablet contains 40 mg of olmesartan medoxomil

Excipients: lactose monohydrate (see section 4.4)

For a full list of excipients, see section 6.1

3. PHARMACEUTICAL FORM

Film-coated tablet.

Olmetec 10 and 20 mg tablets: White, circular, film-coated tablets with C13 and C14 embossed on one side.

Olmetec 40 mg tablets: White, oval, film-coated tablets with C15 embossed on one side.

4. CLINICAL PARTICULARS

4.1 Therapeutic indications

Treatment of essential hypertension.

4.2 Posology and method of administration

Adults

The recommended starting dose of olmesartan medoxomil is 10 mg once daily. In patients whose blood pressure is not adequately controlled at this dose, the dose of olmesartan medoxomil may be increased to 20 mg once daily as the optimal dose. If additional blood pressure reduction is required, olmesartan medoxomil dose may be increased to a maximum of 40 mg daily or hydrochlorothiazide therapy may be added.

The antihypertensive effect of olmesartan medoxomil is substantially present within 2 weeks of initiating therapy and is maximal by about 8 weeks after initiating therapy. This should be borne in mind when considering changing the dose regimen for any patient.

In order to assist compliance, it is recommended that Olmetec tablets be taken at about the same time each day, with or without food, for example at breakfast time.

Elderly

No adjustment of dosage is generally required in elderly patients (see below for dose recommendations in patients with renal impairment). If up-titration to the maximum dose of 40 mg daily is required, blood pressure should be closely monitored.

Renal impairment

The maximum dose in patients with mild to moderate renal impairment (creatinine clearance of 20 – 60 mL/min) is 20 mg olmesartan medoxomil once daily, owing to limited experience of higher dosages in this patient group. The use of olmesartan medoxomil in patients with severe renal impairment (creatinine clearance < 20 mL/min) is not recommended, since there is only limited experience in this patient group (see sections 4.4, 5.2).

Hepatic impairment

No adjustment of dosage recommendations is required for patients with mild hepatic impairment. In patients with moderate hepatic impairment, an initial dose of 10 mg olmesartan medoxomil once daily is recommended and the maximum dose should not exceed 20 mg once daily. Close monitoring of blood pressure and renal function is advised in hepatically-impaired patients who are already receiving diuretics and/or other antihypertensive agents. There is no experience of olmesartan medoxomil in patients with severe hepatic impairment, therefore use is not recommended in this patient group (see sections 4.4 and 5.2). Olmesartan medoxomil should not be used in patients with biliary obstruction (see 4.3).

Children and adolescents

Olmetec is not recommended for use in children below 18 years due to a lack of data on safety and efficacy.

4.3 Contraindications

Hypersensitivity to the active substance or to any of the excipients (see section 6.1).

Second and third trimesters of pregnancy (see sections 4.4 and 4.6).

Lactation (see section 4.6).

Biliary obstruction (see section 5.2).

4.4 Special warnings and precautions for use

Intravascular volume depletion:

Symptomatic hypotension, especially after the first dose, may occur in patients who are volume and/or sodium depleted by vigorous diuretic therapy, dietary salt restriction, diarrhoea or vomiting. Such conditions should be corrected before the administration of olmesartan medoxomil.

Other conditions with stimulation of the renin-angiotensin-aldosterone system:

In patients whose vascular tone and renal function depend predominantly on the activity of the renin-angiotensin-aldosterone system (e.g. patients with severe congestive heart failure or underlying renal disease, including renal artery stenosis), treatment with other drugs that affect this system has been associated with acute hypotension, azotaemia, oliguria or, rarely, acute renal failure. The possibility of similar effects cannot be excluded with angiotensin II receptor antagonists.

Renovascular hypertension:

There is an increased risk of severe hypotension and renal insufficiency when patients with bilateral renal artery stenosis or stenosis of the artery to a single functioning kidney are treated with medicinal products that affect the renin-angiotensin-aldosterone system.

Renal impairment and kidney transplantation:

When olmesartan medoxomil is used in patients with impaired renal function, periodic monitoring of serum potassium and creatinine levels is recommended. Use of olmesartan medoxomil is not recommended in patients with severe renal impairment (creatinine clearance < 20 mL/min) (see sections 4.2, 5.2). There is no experience of the administration of olmesartan medoxomil in patients with a recent kidney transplant or in patients with end-stage renal impairment (i.e. creatinine clearance <12 mL/min).

Hepatic impairment:

There is no experience in patients with severe hepatic impairment and therefore use of olmesartan medoxomil in this patient group is not recommended (see section 4.2 for dosage recommendations in patients with mild or moderate hepatic impairment).

Hyperkalaemia:

The use of medicinal products that affect the renin-angiotensin-aldosterone system may cause hyperkalaemia.

The risk, that may be fatal, is increased in elderly, in patients with renal insufficiency and in diabetic patients, in patients concomitantly treated with other medicinal products that may increase potassium levels, and/or in patients with intercurrent events.

Before considering the concomitant use of medicinal products that affect the renin-angiotensin-aldosterone system, the benefit risk ratio should be evaluated and other alternatives considered.

The main risk factors for hyperkalaemia to be considered are:

- Diabetes, renal impairment, age (> 70 years)

- Combination with one or more other medicinal products that affect the renin-angiotensin-aldosterone system and/or potassium supplements. Some medicinal products or therapeutic class of medicinal products may provoke a hyperkalaemia: salt substitutes containing potassium, potassium-sparing diuretics, ACE inhibitors, angiotensin II receptors antagonists, non steroidal anti-inflammatory drugs (including selective COX-2 inhibitors), heparin, immunosuppressor as ciclosporin or tacrolimus, trimethoprim

- Intercurrent events, in particular dehydration, acute cardiac decompensation, metabolic acidosis, worsening of renal function, sudden worsening of the renal condition (e.g. infectious diseases), cellular lysis (e.g. acute limb ischemia, rhabdomyolysis, extended trauma).

Close-monitoring of serum potassium in at risk patients is recommended (see section 4.5).

Lithium:

As with other angiotensin-II receptor antagonists, the combination of lithium and olmesartan medoxomil is not recommended (see section 4.5).

Aortic or mitral valve stenosis; obstructive hypertrophic cardiomyopathy:

As with other vasodilators, special caution is indicated in patients suffering from aortic or mitral valve stenosis, or obstructive hypertrophic cardiomyopathy.

Primary aldosteronism:

Patients with primary aldosteronism generally will not respond to antihypertensive drugs acting through inhibition of the renin-angiotensin system. Therefore, the use of olmesartan medoxomil is not recommended in such patients.

Ethnic differences:

As with all other angiotensin II antagonists, the blood pressure lowering effect of olmesartan medoxomil is somewhat less in black patients than in non-black patients, possibly because of a higher prevalence of low-renin status in the black hypertensive population.

Pregnancy:

Angiotensin II antagonists should not be initiated during pregnancy. Unless continued angiotensin II antagonists therapy is considered essential, patients planning pregnancy should be changed to alternative anti-hypertensive treatments which have an established safety profile for use in pregnancy. When pregnancy is diagnosed, treatment with angiotensin II antagonists should be stopped immediately and, if appropriate, alternative therapy should be started (see sections 4.3 and 4.6).

Other:

As with any antihypertensive agent, excessive blood pressure decrease in patients with ischaemic heart disease or ischaemic cerebrovascular disease could result in a myocardial infarction or stroke.

This medicinal product contains lactose. Patients with rare hereditary problems of galactose intolerance, the Lapp-lactase deficiency or glucose-galactose malabsorption should not take this medicinal product.

4.5 Interaction with other medicinal products and other forms of interaction

Interaction studies have only been performed in adults.

Effects of other medicinal products on olmesartan medoxomil:

Potassium supplements and potassium sparing diuretics:

Based on experience with the use of other drugs that affect the renin-angiotensin system, concomitant use of potassium-sparing diuretics, potassium supplements, salt substitutes containing potassium or other drugs that may increase serum potassium levels (e.g. heparin) may lead to increases in serum potassium (see section 4.4). Such concomitant use is therefore not recommended.

Other antihypertensive medications:

The blood pressure lowering effect of olmesartan medoxomil can be increased by concomitant use of other antihypertensive medications.

Non-steroidal anti-inflammatory drugs (NSAIDs):

NSAIDs (including acetylsalicylic acid at doses (> 3 g/day and also COX-2 inhibitors) and angiotensin-II receptor antagonists may act synergistically by decreasing glomerular filtration. The risk of the concomitant use of NSAIDs and angiotensin II antagonists is the occurrence of acute renal failure. Monitoring of renal function at the beginning of treatment should be recommended as well as regular hydration of the patient.

Additionally, concomitant treatment can reduce the antihypertensive effect of angiotensin II receptor antagonists, leading to their partial loss of efficacy.

Other compounds:

After treatment with antacid (aluminium magnesium hydroxide), a modest reduction in bioavailability of olmesartan was observed. Coadministration of warfarin and digoxin had no effect on the pharmacokinetics of olmesartan.

Effects of olmesartan medoxomil on other medicinal products:

Lithium:

Reversible increases in serum lithium concentrations and toxicity have been reported during concomitant administration of lithium with angiotensin converting enzyme inhibitors and angiotensin II antagonists. Therefore use of olmesartan medoxomil and lithium in combination is not recommended (see section 4.4). If use of the combination proves necessary, careful monitoring of serum lithium levels is recommended.

Other compounds:

Compounds which have been investigated in specific clinical studies in healthy volunteers include warfarin, digoxin, an antacid (magnesium aluminium hydroxide), hydrochlorothiazide and pravastatin. No clinically relevant interactions were observed and in particular olmesartan medoxomil had no significant effect on the pharmacokinetics or pharmacodynamics of warfarin or the pharmacokinetics of digoxin.

Olmesartan had no clinically relevant inhibitory effects on *in vitro* human cytochrome P450 enzymes 1A1/2, 2A6, 2C8/9, 2C19, 2D6, 2E1 and 3A4, and had no or minimal inducing effects on rat cytochrome P450 activities. Therefore *in vivo* interaction studies with known cytochrome P450 enzyme inhibitors and inducers were not conducted, and no clinically relevant interactions between olmesartan and drugs metabolised by the above cytochrome P450 enzymes are expected.

4.6 Pregnancy and lactation

Use in pregnancy (see section 4.3):

The use of angiotensin II antagonists is not recommended during the first trimester of pregnancy (see section 4.4). The use of angiotensin II antagonists is contraindicated during the second and third trimester of pregnancy (see sections 4.3 and 4.4).

Epidemiological evidence regarding the risk of teratogenicity following exposure to angiotensin receptor blockers during the first trimester of pregnancy has not been conclusive; however a small increase in risk cannot be excluded. Whilst there is no controlled epidemiological data on the risk with angiotensin II antagonists, similar risks may exist for this class of drugs. Unless continued angiotensin receptor blocker therapy is considered essential, patients planning pregnancy should be changed to alternative anti-hypertensive treatments which have an established safety profile for use in pregnancy. When pregnancy is diagnosed, treatment with angiotensin II antagonists should be stopped immediately, and, if appropriate, alternative therapy should be started.

Angiotensin II antagonists therapy exposure during the second and third trimesters is known to induce human fetotoxicity (decreased renal function, oligohydramnios, skull ossification retardation) and neonatal toxicity (renal failure, hypotension, hyperkalaemia).

Should exposure to angiotensin II antagonists have occurred from the second trimester of pregnancy, ultrasound check of renal function and skull is recommended.

Infants whose mothers have taken angiotensin II antagonists should be closely observed for hypotension (see also sections 4.3 and 4.4).

Use during lactation (see section 4.3):

Olmesartan is excreted in the milk of lactating rats but it is not known whether olmesartan is excreted in human milk. Mothers must not breast-feed if they are taking olmesartan medoxomil.

4.7 Effects on ability to drive and use machines

No studies on the effect on the ability to drive and use machines have been performed. With respect to driving vehicles or operating machines, it should be taken into account that occasionally dizziness or fatigue may occur in patients taking antihypertensive therapy.

4.8 Undesirable effects

Market experience

The following adverse reactions have been reported in post-marketing experience.

They are listed by System Organ Class and ranked under headings of frequency using the following convention: very common (≥1/10); common (≥1/100, <1/10); uncommon (≥1/1,000, <1/100); rare (≥1/10,000, <1/1,000); very rare (<1/10,000) including isolated reports.

System Organ Class	*Very rare*
Blood and lymphatic system disorders	Thrombocytopenia
Metabolism and nutrition disorders	Hyperkalaemia
Nervous system disorders	Dizziness, headache
Respiratory, thoracic and mediastinal disorders	Cough
Gastrointestinal disorders	Abdominal pain, nausea, vomiting
Skin and subcutaneous tissue disorders	Pruritus, exanthem, rash Allergic conditions such as angioneurotic oedema, dermatitis allergic, face oedema and urticaria
Musculoskeletal and connective tissue disorders	Muscle cramp, myalgia
Renal and urinary disorders	Acute renal failure and renal insufficiency (See also under Investigations)
General disorders and administration site conditions	Asthenic conditions such as asthenia, fatigue, lethargy, malaise
Investigations	Abnormal renal function tests such as blood creatinine increased and blood urea increased Increased hepatic enzymes

Single cases of rhabdomyolysis have been reported in temporal association with the intake of angiotensin II receptor blockers. A causal relationship, however, has not been established.

Clinical trials

In double-blind, placebo-controlled monotherapy studies, the overall incidence of treatment-emergent adverse events was 42.4% on olmesartan medoxomil and 40.9% on placebo.

In placebo-controlled monotherapy studies, the only adverse drug reaction that was unequivocally related to treatment was dizziness (2.5% incidence on olmesartan medoxomil and 0.9% on placebo).

In long-term (2-year) treatment, the incidence of withdrawals due to adverse events on olmesartan medoxomil 10 – 20 mg once daily was 3.7%. The following adverse events have been reported across all clinical trials with olmesartan medoxomil (including trials with active as well as placebo control), irrespective of causality or incidence relative to placebo. They are listed by body system and ranked under headings of frequency using the conventions described above:

Central nervous system disorders:

Common: Dizziness

Uncommon: Vertigo

Cardiovascular disorders:

Rare: Hypotension

Uncommon: Angina pectoris

Respiratory system disorders:

Common: Bronchitis, cough, pharyngitis, rhinitis

Gastro-intestinal disorders:

Common: Abdominal pain, diarrhoea, dyspepsia, gastroenteritis, nausea

Skin and appendages disorders:

Uncommon: Rash

Musculoskeletal disorders:

Common: Arthritis, back pain, skeletal pain

Urinary system disorders:

Common: Haematuria, urinary tract infection

General disorders:

Common: Chest pain, fatigue, influenza-like symptoms, peripheral oedema, pain

Laboratory parameters

In placebo-controlled monotherapy studies, the incidence was somewhat higher on olmesartan medoxomil compared with placebo for hypertriglyceridaemia (2.0% versus 1.1%) and for raised creatine phosphokinase (1.3% versus 0.7%).

Laboratory adverse events reported across all clinical trials with olmesartan medoxomil (including trials without a placebo control), irrespective of causality or incidence relative to placebo, included:

Metabolic and nutritional disorders:

Common: Increased creatine phosphokinase, hypertriglyceridaemia, hyperuricaemia

Rare: Hyperkalaemia

Liver and biliary disorders:

Common: Liver enzyme elevations.

Additional information on special populations

In elderly patients the frequency of hypotension is slightly increased from rare to uncommon.

4.9 Overdose

Only limited information is available regarding overdosage in humans. The most likely effect of overdosage is hypotension. In the event of overdosage, the patient should be carefully monitored and treatment should be symptomatic and supportive.

No information is available regarding the dialysability of olmesartan.

5. PHARMACOLOGICAL PROPERTIES

5.1 Pharmacodynamic properties

Pharmaco-therapeutic group:

Angiotensin II antagonists, ATC code: C09C A 08.

Olmesartan medoxomil is a potent, orally active, selective angiotensin II receptor (type AT_1) antagonist. It is expected to block all actions of angiotensin II mediated by the AT_1 receptor, regardless of the source or route of synthesis of angiotensin II. The selective antagonism of the angiotensin II (AT_1) receptors results in increases in plasma renin levels and angiotensin I and II concentrations, and some decrease in plasma aldosterone concentrations.

Angiotensin II is the primary vasoactive hormone of the renin-angiotensin-aldosterone system and plays a significant role in the pathophysiology of hypertension via the type 1 (AT_1) receptor.

In hypertension, olmesartan medoxomil causes a dose-dependent, long-lasting reduction in arterial blood pressure. There has been no evidence of first-dose hypotension, of tachyphylaxis during long-term treatment, or of rebound hypertension after cessation of therapy.

Once daily dosing with olmesartan medoxomil provides an effective and smooth reduction in blood pressure over the 24 hour dose interval. Once daily dosing produced similar decreases in blood pressure as twice daily dosing at the same total daily dose.

With continuous treatment, maximum reductions in blood pressure are achieved by 8 weeks after the initiation of therapy, although a substantial proportion of the blood pressure lowering effect is already observed after 2 weeks of treatment. When used together with hydrochlorothiazide, the reduction in blood pressure is additive and coadministration is well tolerated.

The effect of olmesartan on mortality and morbidity is not yet known.

5.2 Pharmacokinetic properties

Absorption and distribution

Olmesartan medoxomil is a prodrug. It is rapidly converted to the pharmacologically active metabolite, olmesartan, by esterases in the gut mucosa and in portal blood during absorption from the gastrointestinal tract.

No intact olmesartan medoxomil or intact side chain medoxomil moiety have been detected in plasma or excreta. The mean absolute bioavailability of olmesartan from a tablet formulation was 25.6%.

The mean peak plasma concentration (C_{max}) of olmesartan is reached within about 2 hours after oral dosing with olmesartan medoxomil, and olmesartan plasma concentrations increase approximately linearly with increasing single oral doses up to about 80 mg.

Food had minimal effect on the bioavailability of olmesartan and therefore olmesartan medoxomil may be administered with or without food.

No clinically relevant gender-related differences in the pharmacokinetics of olmesartan have been observed.

Olmesartan is highly bound to plasma protein (99.7%), but the potential for clinically significant protein binding displacement interactions between olmesartan and other highly bound coadministered drugs is low (as confirmed by the lack of a clinically significant interaction between olmesartan medoxomil and warfarin). The binding of olmesartan to blood cells is negligible. The mean volume of distribution after intravenous dosing is low (16 – 29 L).

Metabolism and elimination

Total plasma clearance was typically 1.3 L/h (CV, 19%) and was relatively slow compared to hepatic blood flow (ca 90 L/h). Following a single oral dose of ^{14}C-labelled olmesartan medoxomil, 10 - 16% of the administered radioactivity was excreted in the urine (the vast majority within 24 hours of dose administration) and the remainder of the recovered radioactivity was excreted in the faeces. Based on the systemic availability of 25.6%, it can be calculated that absorbed olmesartan is cleared by both renal excretion (ca 40%) and hepato-biliary excretion (ca 60%). All recovered radioactivity was identified as olmesartan. No other significant metabolite was detected. Enterohepatic recycling of olmesartan is minimal. Since a large proportion of olmesartan is excreted via the biliary route, use in patients with biliary obstruction is contraindicated (see section 4.3).

The terminal elimination half life of olmesartan varied between 10 and 15 hours after multiple oral dosing. Steady state was reached after the first few doses and no further accumulation was evident after 14 days of repeated dosing. Renal clearance was approximately 0.5 – 0.7 L/h and was independent of dose.

Pharmacokinetics in special populations

Elderly:

In hypertensive patients, the AUC at steady state was increased by ca 35% in elderly patients (65 – 75 years old) and by ca 44% in very elderly patients (≥ 75 years old) compared with the younger age group. This may be at least in part related to a mean decrease in renal function in this group of patients.

Renal impairment:

In renally impaired patients, the AUC at steady state increased by 62%, 82% and 179% in patients with mild, moderate and severe renal impairment, respectively, compared to healthy controls (see sections 4.2, 4.4).

Hepatic impairment:

After single oral administration, olmesartan AUC values were 6% and 65% higher in mildly and moderately hepatically impaired patients, respectively, than in their corresponding matched healthy controls. The unbound fraction of olmesartan at 2 hours post-dose in healthy subjects, in patients with mild hepatic impairment and in patients with moderate hepatic impairment was 0.26%, 0.34% and 0.41%, respectively. Following repeated dosing in patients with moderate hepatic impairment, olmesartan mean AUC was again about 65% higher than in matched healthy controls. Olmesartan mean C_{max} values were similar in hepatically-impaired and healthy subjects. Olmesartan medoxomil has not been evaluated in patients with severe hepatic impairment (see sections 4.2, 4.4).

5.3 Preclinical safety data

In chronic toxicity studies in rats and dogs, olmesartan medoxomil showed similar effects to other AT_1 receptor antagonists and ACE inhibitors: raised blood urea (BUN) and creatinine (through functional changes to the kidneys caused by blocking AT_1 receptors); reduction in heart weight; a reduction of red cell parameters (erythrocytes, haemoglobin, haematocrit); histological indications of renal damage (regenerative lesions of the renal epithelium, thickening of the basal membrane, dilatation of the tubules). These adverse effects caused by the pharmacological action of olmesartan medoxomil have also occurred in preclinical trials on other AT_1 receptor antagonists and ACE inhibitors and can be reduced by simultaneous oral administration of sodium chloride.

In both species, increased plasma renin activity and hypertrophy/hyperplasia of the juxtaglomerular cells of the kidney were observed. These changes, which are a typical effect of the class of ACE inhibitors and other AT_1 receptor antagonists, would appear to have no clinical relevance.

Like other AT_1 receptor antagonists olmesartan medoxomil was found to increase the incidence of chromosome breaks in cell cultures *in vitro*. No relevant effects were observed in several *in vivo* studies using olmesartan medoxomil at very high oral doses of up to 2000 mg/kg. The overall data of a comprehensive genotoxicity testing suggest that olmesartan is very unlikely to exert genotoxic effects under conditions of clinical use.

Olmesartan medoxomil was not carcinogenic, neither in rats in a 2 year study nor in mice when tested in two 6 month carcinogenicity studies using transgenic models.

In reproductive studies in rats, olmesartan medoxomil did not affect fertility and there was no evidence of a teratogenic effect. In common with other angiotensin II antagonists, survival of offspring was reduced following exposure to olmesartan medoxomil and pelvic dilatation of the kidney was seen after exposure of the dams in late pregnancy and lactation. In common with other antihypertensive agents, olmesartan medoxomil was shown to be more toxic to pregnant rabbits than to pregnant rats, however, there was no indication of a fetotoxic effect.

6. PHARMACEUTICAL PARTICULARS

6.1 List of excipients

Tablet core

Cellulose, microcrystalline

Lactose monohydrate

Hydroxypropylcellulose

Low substituted hydroxypropylcellulose

Magnesium stearate

Tablet coat

Titanium dioxide (E 171)

Talc

Hypromellose

6.2 Incompatibilities

Not applicable.

6.3 Shelf life

3 years.

6.4 Special precautions for storage

This medicinal product does not require any special storage conditions.

6.5 Nature and contents of container

Laminated polyamide/ aluminium/polyvinyl chloride / aluminium blister pack.

Packs of 28 film-coated tablets.

6.6 Special precautions for disposal and other handling

No special requirements.

7. MARKETING AUTHORISATION HOLDER

Daiichi Sankyo UK Limited

Chiltern Place

Chalfont Park

Gerrards Cross

Buckinghamshire

SL9 0BG

UK

8. MARKETING AUTHORISATION NUMBER(S)

Olmetec 10 mg: PL 08265/0015

Olmetec 20 mg: PL 08265/0016

Olmetec 40 mg: PL 08265/0017

9. DATE OF FIRST AUTHORISATION/RENEWAL OF THE AUTHORISATION

22 May 2003/12 August 2007

10. DATE OF REVISION OF THE TEXT

12 August 2007

OLMETEC Plus film-coated tablets

(Daiichi Sankyo UK Limited)

1. NAME OF THE MEDICINAL PRODUCT

Olmetec Plus 20 mg/12.5 mg film-coated tablets ▼

Olmetec Plus 20 mg/25 mg film-coated tablets ▼

2. QUALITATIVE AND QUANTITATIVE COMPOSITION

Olmetec Plus 20 mg/12.5 mg film-coated tablets: Each film-coated tablet contains 20 mg olmesartan medoxomil and 12.5 mg hydrochlorothiazide

Olmetec Plus 20 mg/25 mg film-coated tablets: Each film-coated tablet contains 20 mg olmesartan medoxomil and 25 mg hydrochlorothiazide

For excipients, see section 6.1.

3. PHARMACEUTICAL FORM

Film-coated tablet.

Olmetec Plus 20 mg/12.5 mg film-coated tablets: Reddish-yellow, round, film-coated tablet with C22 debossed on one side.

Olmetec Plus 20 mg/25 mg film-coated tablets: Pinkish, round, film-coated tablet with C24 debossed on one side.

4. CLINICAL PARTICULARS

4.1 Therapeutic indications

Treatment of essential hypertension.

Olmetec Plus fixed dose combination is indicated in patients whose blood pressure is not adequately controlled on olmesartan medoxomil alone.

4.2 Posology and method of administration

Adults

Olmetec Plus is not for use as initial therapy, but in patients whose blood pressure is not adequately controlled by 20 mg olmesartan medoxomil alone. Olmetec Plus is administered once daily, with or without food.

When clinically appropriate, direct change from monotherapy with 20 mg olmesartan medoxomil to the fixed combination may be considered, taking into account that theantihypertensive effect of olmesartan medoxomil is maximal by about 8 weeks after initiating therapy (see section 5.1). Dose titration of the individual components is recommended:

20 mg olmesartan medoxomil/12.5 mg hydrochlorothiazide may be administered in patients whose blood pressure is not adequately controlled by the optimal monotherapy olmesartan medoxomil 20 mg alone.

20 mg olmesartan medoxomil/25 mg hydrochlorothiazide may be administered in patients whose blood pressure is not adequately controlled by 20 mg olmesartan medoxomil/ 12.5 mg hydrochlorothiazide.

A maximum daily dose of 20 mg olmesartan medoxomil and 25 mg hydrochlorothiazide in combination should not be exceeded.

Elderly

In elderly patients the same dosage of the combination is recommended as for adults.

Renal impairment

When Olmetec Plus is used in patients with mild to moderate renal impairment (creatinine clearance of 30 – 60 ml/min) periodic monitoring of renal function is advised (see section 4.4). Olmetec Plus is contraindicated in patients with severe renal impairment (creatinine clearance < 30 mL/min) (see section 4.3).

Hepatic impairment

The use of Olmetec Plus in patients with hepatic impairment is not recommended since there is currently only limited experience of olmesartan medoxomil in this patient group (see sections 4.4, 5.2).

Children and adolescents

As the safety and efficacy of administration of Olmetec Plus to children have not been established, treatment of children up to 18 years is not recommended.

4.3 Contraindications

Hypersensitivity to the active substances, to any of the excipients (see section 6.1) or to other sulfonamide-derived substances (since hydrochlorothiazide is a sulfonamide-derived medicinal product).

Severe renal impairment (creatinine clearance < 30 mL/min).

Refractory hypokalaemia, hypercalcaemia, hyponatraemia and symptomatic hyperuricaemia.

Severe hepatic impairment, cholestasis and biliary obstructive disorders.

Second and third trimesters of pregnancy (see section 4.6).

Lactation (see section 4.6).

4.4 Special warnings and precautions for use

Intravascular volume depletion:

Symptomatic hypotension, especially after the first dose, may occur in patients who are volume and/or sodium depleted by vigorous diuretic therapy, dietary salt restriction, diarrhoea or vomiting. Such conditions should be corrected before the administration of Olmetec Plus.

Other conditions with stimulation of the renin-angiotensin-aldosterone system:

In patients whose vascular tone and renal function depend predominantly on the activity of the renin-angiotensin-aldosterone system (eg patients with severe congestive heart failure or underlying renal disease, including renal artery stenosis), treatment with medicinal products that affect this system has been associated with acute hypotension, azotaemia, oliguria or, rarely, acute renal failure.

Renovascular hypertension:

There is an increased risk of severe hypotension and renal insufficiency when patients with bilateral renal artery stenosis or stenosis of the artery to a single functioning kidney are treated with medicinal products that affect the renin-angiotensin-aldosterone system.

Renal impairment and kidney transplantation:

Olmetec Plus should not be used in patients with severe renal impairment (creatinine clearance < 30 ml/min) (see section 4.3). No dosage adjustment is necessary in patients with mild to moderate renal impairment (creatinine clearance is ≥ 30 ml/min, < 60 mL/min). However, in such patients Olmetec Plus should be administered with caution and periodic monitoring of serum potassium, creatinine and uric acid levels is recommended. Thiazide diuretic-associated azotaemia may occur in patients with impaired renal function. If progressive renal impairment becomes evident, careful reappraisal of therapy is necessary, with consideration given to discontinuing diuretic therapy. There is no experience of the administration of Olmetec Plus in patients with a recent kidney transplantation.

Hepatic impairment:

There is currently limited experience of olmesartan medoxomil in patients with mild to moderate hepatic impairment and no experience in patients with severe hepatic impairment. Furthermore, minor alterations of fluid and electrolyte balance during thiazide therapy may precipitate hepatic coma in patients with impaired hepatic function or progressive liver disease. Therefore use of Olmetec Plus in patients with hepatic impairment is not recommended (see section 4.2). Use of Olmetec Plus in patients with severe hepatic impairment, cholestasis and biliary obstruction is contraindicated (see sections 4.3, 5.2).

Aortic and mitral valve stenosis, obstructive hypertrophic cardiomyopathy:

As with other vasodilators, special caution is indicated in patients suffering from aortic or mitral stenosis, or obstructive hypertrophic cardiomyopathy.

Primary aldosteronism:

Patients with primary aldosteronism generally will not respond to anti-hypertensive medicinal products acting through inhibition of the renin-angiotensin system. Therefore, the use of Olmetec Plus is not recommended in such patients.

Metabolic and endocrine effects:

Thiazide therapy may impair glucose tolerance. In diabetic patients dosage adjustments of insulin or oral hypoglycaemic agents may be required (see section 4.5). Latent diabetes mellitus may become manifest during thiazide therapy.

Increases in cholesterol and triglyceride levels are undesirable effects known to be associated with thiazide diuretic therapy.

Hyperuricaemia may occur or frank gout may be precipitated in some patients receiving thiazide therapy.

Electrolyte imbalance:

As for any patient receiving diuretic therapy, periodic determination of serum electrolytes should be performed at appropriate intervals.

Thiazides, including hydrochlorothiazide, can cause fluid or electrolyte imbalance (including hypokalaemia, hyponatraemia and hypochloraemic alkalosis). Warning signs of fluid or electrolyte imbalance are dryness of the mouth, thirst, weakness, lethargy, drowsiness, restlessness, muscle pain or cramps, muscular fatigue, hypotension, oliguria, tachycardia, and gastrointestinal disturbances such as nausea or vomiting (see section 4.8).

The risk of hypokalaemia is greatest in patients with cirrhosis of the liver, in patients experiencing brisk diuresis, in patients who are receiving inadequate oral intake of electrolytes and in patients receiving concomitant therapy with corticosteroids or ACTH (see section 4.5). Conversely, due to antagonism at the angiotensin-II receptors (AT_1) through the olmesartan medoxomil component of Olmetec Plus hyperkalaemia may occur, especially in the presence of renal impairment and/or heart failure, and diabetes mellitus. Adequate monitoring of serum potassium in patients at risk is recommended. Potassium-sparing diuretics, potassium supplements or potassium-containing salt substitutes and other medicinal products that may increase serum potassium levels (e.g. heparin) should be co-administered cautiously with Olmetec Plus (see section 4.5).

There is no evidence that olmesartan medoxomil would reduce or prevent diuretic-induced hyponatraemia. Chloride deficit is generally mild and usually does not require treatment.

Thiazides may decrease urinary calcium excretion and cause an intermittent and slight elevation of serum calcium in the absence of known disorders of calcium metabolism. Hypercalcaemia may be evidence of hidden hyperparathyroidism. Thiazides should be discontinued before carrying out tests for parathyroid function.

Thiazides have been shown to increase the urinary excretion of magnesium, which may result in hypomagnesaemia.

Dilutional hyponatraemia may occur in oedematous patients in hot weather.

Lithium:

As with other medicinal products containing angiotensin II receptor antagonists and thiazide in combination, the coadministration of Olmetec Plus and lithium is not recommended (see section 4.5).

Ethnic differences:

As with all other angiotensin II antagonists, the blood pressure lowering effect of olmesartan medoxomil is somewhat less in black patients than in non-black patients, possibly because of a higher prevalence of low-renin status in the black hypertensive population.

Anti-doping test:

Hydrochlorothiazide contained in this medicinal product could produce a positive analytic result in an anti-doping test.

Other:

In general arteriosclerosis, in patients with ischaemic heart disease or ischaemic cerebrovascular disease, there is always a risk that excessive blood pressure decrease could result in a myocardial infarction or stroke.

Hypersensitivity reactions to hydrochlorothiazide may occur in patients with or without a history of allergy or bronchial asthma, but are more likely in patients with such a history.

Exacerbation or activation of systemic lupus erythematosus has been reported with the use of thiazide diuretics.

This medicinal product contains lactose. Patients with rare hereditary problems of galactose intolerance, the Lapp lactase deficiency or glucose-galactose malapsorption should not take this medicinal product.

4.5 Interaction with other medicinal products and other forms of interaction

Potential interactions related to both olmesartan medoxomil and hydrochloro-thiazide:

Concomitant use not recommended

Lithium:

Reversible increases in serum lithium concentrations and toxicity have been reported during concomitant administration of lithium with angiotensin converting enzyme inhibitors and, rarely, with angiotensin II antagonists. In addition, renal clearance of lithium is reduced by thiazides and consequently the risk of lithium toxicity may be increased. Therefore use of Olmetec Plus and lithium in combination is not recommended (see section 4.4). If use of the combination proves necessary, careful monitoring of serum lithium levels is recommended.

Concomitant use requiring caution

Baclofen:

Potentiation of antihypertensive effect may occur.

Non-steroidal anti-inflammatory medicinal products:

NSAIDs (ie acetylsalicylic acid > 3 g/day), COX-2 inhibitors and non-selective NSAIDs) may reduce the antihypertensive effect of thiazide diuretics and angiotensin II antagonists.

In some patients with compromised renal function (eg dehydrated patients or elderly patients with compromised renal function) the co-administration of angiotensin II antagonists and agents that inhibit cyclo-oxygenase may result in further deterioration of renal function, including possible acute renal failure, which is usually reversible. Therefore, the combination should be administered with caution, especially in the elderly. Patients should be adequately hydrated and consideration should be given to monitoring of renal function after initiation of concomitant therapy and periodically thereafter.

Concomitant use to be taken into account

Amifostine:

Potentiation of antihypertensive effect may occur.

Other antihypertensive agents:

The blood pressure lowering effect of Olmetec Plus can be increased by concomitant use of other antihypertensive medicinal products.

Alcohol, barbiturates, narcotics or antidepressants:

Potentiation of orthostatic hypotension may occur.

Potential interactions related to olmesartan medoxomil:

Concomitant use not recommended

Medicinal products affecting potassium levels:

Based on experience with the use of other medicinal products that affect the renin-angiotensin system, concomitant use of potassium-sparing diuretics, potassium supplements, salt substitutes containing potassium or other medicinal products that may increase serum potassium levels (eg heparin, ACE inhibitors) may lead to increases in serum potassium (see section 4.4). If medicinal product which affect potassium levels are to be prescribed in combination with Olmetec Plus, monitoring of potassium plasma levels is advised.

Additional information

After treatment with antacid (aluminium magnesium hydroxide), a modest reduction in bioavailability of olmesartan was observed.

Olmesartan medoxomil had no significant effect on the pharmacokinetics or pharmacodynamics of warfarin or the pharmacokinetics of digoxin.

Coadministration of olmesartan medoxomil with pravastatin had no clinically relevant effects on the pharmacokinetics of either component in healthy subjects.

Olmesartan had no clinically relevant inhibitory effects on human cytochrome P450 enzymes 1A1/2, 2A6, 2C8/9, 2C19, 2D6, 2E1 and 3A4 *in vitro*, and had no or minimal inducing effects on rat cytochrome P450 activities. No clinically relevant interactions between olmesartan and medicinal products metabolised by the above cytochrome P450 enzymes are expected.

Potential interactions related to hydrochlorothiazide:

Concomitant use not recommended

Medicinal products affecting potassium levels:

The potassium-depleting effect of hydrochlorothiazide (see section 4.4) may be potentiated by the coadministration of other medicinal products associated with potassium loss and hypokalaemia (eg other kaliuretic diuretics, laxatives, corticosteroids, ACTH, amphotericin, carbenoxolone, penicillin G sodium or salicylic acid derivatives). Such concomitant use is therefore not recommended.

Concomitant use requiring caution

Calcium salts:

Thiazide diuretics may increase serum calcium levels due to decreased excretion. If calcium supplements must be prescribed, serum calcium levels should be monitored and calcium dosage adjusted accordingly.

Cholestyramine and colestipol resins:

Absorption of hydrochlorothiazide is impaired in the presence of anionic exchange resins.

Digitalis glycosides:

Thiazide-induced hypokalaemia or hypomagnesaemia may favour the onset of digitalis-induced cardiac arrhythmias.

Medicinal products affected by serum potassium disturbances:

Periodic monitoring of serum potassium and ECG is recommended when Olmetec Plus is administered with medicinal products affected by serum potassium disturbances (eg digitalis glycosides and antiarrhythmics) and with the following torsades de pointes (ventricular tachycardia)-inducing medicinal products (including some antiarrhythmics), hypokalaemia being a predisposing factor to torsades de pointes (ventricular tachycardia):

- Class Ia antiarrythmics (eg quinidine, hydroquinidine, disopyramide).
- Class III antiarrythmics (eg amiodarone, sotalol, dofetilide, ibutilide).
- Some antipsychotics (eg thioridazine, chlorpromazine, levomepromazine, trifluoperazine, cyamemazine, sulpiride, sultopride, amisulpride, tiapride, pimozide, haloperidol, droperidol).
- Others (eg bepridil, cisapride, diphemanil, erythromycin IV, halofantrin, mizolastin, pentamidine, sparfloxacin, terfenadine, vincamine IV).

Non-depolarizing skeletal muscle relaxants (eg tubocurarine):

The effect of nondepolarizing skeletal muscle relaxants may be potentiated by hydrochlorothiazide.

Anticholinergic agents (eg atropine, biperiden):

Increase of the bioavailability of thiazide-type diuretics by decreasing gastrointestinal motility and stomach emptying rate.

Antidiabetic medicinal products (oral agents and insulin):

The treatment with a thiazide may influence the glucose tolerance. Dosage adjustment of the antidiabetic medicinal product may be required (see section 4.4).

Metformin:

Metformin should be used with caution because of the risk of lactic acidosis induced by possible functional renal failure linked to hydrochlorothiazide.

Beta-blockers and diazoxide:

The hyperglycaemic effect of beta-blockers and diazoxide may be enhanced by thiazides.

Pressor amines (eg noradrenaline):

The effect of pressor amines may be decreased.

Medicinal products used in the treatment of gout (probenecid, sulfinpyrazone and allopurinol):

Dosage adjustment of uricosuric medicinal products may be necessary since hydrochlorothiazide may raise the level of serum uric acid. Increase in dosage of probenecid or sulfinpyrazone may be necessary. Coadministration of a thiazide may increase the incidence of hypersensitivity reactions to allopurinol.

Amantadine:

Thiazides may increase the risk of adverse effects caused by amantadine.

Cytotoxic agents (eg cyclophosphamide, methotrexate):

Thiazides may reduce the renal excretion of cytotoxic medicinal products and potentiate their myelosuppressive effects.

Salicylates:

In case of high dosages of salicylates hydrochlorothiazide may enhance the toxic effect of the salicylates on the central nervous system.

Methyldopa:

There have been isolated reports of haemolytic anaemia occurring with concomitant use of hydrochlorothiazide and methyldopa.

Ciclosporin:

Concomitant treatment with cyclosporine may increase the risk of hyperuricaemia and gout-type complications.

Tetracyclines:

Concomitant administration of tetracyclines and thiazides increases the risk of tetracycline-induced increase in urea. This interaction is probably not applicable to doxycycline.

4.6 Pregnancy and lactation

Pregnancy (see section 4.3):

As a precaution Olmetec Plus should not be used during the first trimester of pregnancy. A change to a suitable alternative treatment should occur before a planned pregnancy. If pregnancy is determined, Olmetec Plus must be discontinued as soon as possible.

The use of Olmetec Plus is thus contraindicated during the second and third trimesters of pregnancy (see section 4.3).

There is no experience on the use of Olmetec Plus in pregnant women. Animal studies of the combination olmesartan medoxomil/hydrochlorothiazide did not indicate a teratogenic effect; however, they did show fetotoxicity (see section 5.3).

During the second and third trimester of pregnancy, substances that act on the renin-angiotensin system may cause damage (hypotension, impairment of renal function, oliguria and/or anuria, oligohydramnia, cranial hypoplasia, intrauterine growth retardation) and death in fetuses and neonates. Cases of pulmonary hypoplasia, facial anomalies and contractions of limbs were also reported. Animal experimental studies with olmesartan medoxomil have shown furthermore that renal damage may occur in the late fetal and neonatal phase. The mechanism is probably a result of pharmacological actions on the renin-angiotensin-aldosterone system.

Hydrochlorothiazide may reduce both plasma volume and uteroplacental blood flow. Thiazides pass the placental barrier and are found in cord blood. They may cause fetal electrolyte disturbances and possibly other reactions that have been observed in adults. Cases of thrombocytopenia in neonates and fetal or neonatal jaundice were reported after treating the mother with thiazides. Should exposure to Olmetec Plus have occurred from the second trimester of pregnancy, skull and fetal renal function should be checked with echography.

Lactation (see section 4.3):

Olmesartan is excreted into the milk of lactating rats. However, it is not known whether olmesartan passes into human milk. Thiazides pass into human milk and may inhibit lactation. The use of Olmetec Plus during lactation is therefore contraindicated (see section 4.3). A decision should be made whether to discontinue breast-feeding or discontinue the drug, taking into account the importance of the drug to the mother.

4.7 Effects on ability to drive and use machines

No studies on the ability to drive and use machines have been performed. However, it should be borne in mind that dizziness or fatigue may occasionally occur in patients taking antihypertensive therapy.

4.8 Undesirable effects

Fixed dose combination:

In clinical trials involving 1155 patients treated with olmesartan medoxomil/hydrochlorothiazide combinations at dosages of 20/12.5 mg or 20/25 mg and 466 patients treated with placebo for periods of up to 21 months, the overall frequency of adverse events on olmesartan medoxomil/hydrochlorothiazide combination therapy was similar to that on placebo. Discontinuations due to adverse events were also similar for olmesartan medoxomil/hydrochlorothiazide 20/12.5 mg - 20/25 mg (2%) and placebo (3%). The frequency of adverse events on olmesartan medoxomil/hydrochlorothiazide overall relative to placebo appeared to be unrelated to age (<65 years versus ≥ 65 years), gender or race although the frequency of dizziness was somewhat increased in patients aged ≥ 75 years.

The most frequent adverse event on olmesartan medoxomil/hydrochlorothiazide 20/12.5 mg – 20/25 mg, and the only adverse event for which the frequency exceeded that on placebo by at least 1%, was dizziness (2.6% on olmesartan medoxomil/hydrochlorothiazide 20/12.5 mg - 20/25 mg and 1.3% on placebo).

Adverse events of potential clinical relevance are listed below by system organ class. Frequencies are defined as: common (≥1/100, <1/10); uncommon (≥1/1000, <1/100); rare (≥1/10000, <1/1000); very rare (<1/10000).

Metabolism and nutrition disorders:

Uncommon: Hyperuricaemia, hypertriglyceridaemia

Nervous system disorders:

Common: Dizziness

Uncommon: Syncope

Cardiac disorders:

Uncommon: Palpitations

Vascular disorders:

Uncommon: Hypotension, orthostatic hypotension

Skin and subcutaneous tissue disorders:

Uncommon: Rash, eczema

General disorders and administration site conditions:

Common: Fatigue

Uncommon: Weakness

Investigations:

Uncommon: Blood potassium decreased, blood potassium increased, blood calcium increased, blood urea increased, blood lipids increased

Laboratory findings

In clinical trials, clinically important changes in standard laboratory parameters were rarely associated with olmesartan medoxomil/hydrochlorothiazide.

Minor increases in mean uric acid, blood urea nitrogen and creatinine values and minor decreases in mean haemoglobin and haematocrit values were observed during treatment with olmesartan medoxomil/hydrochlorothiazide.

Additional information on individual components:

Undesirable effects previously reported with either of the individual components may be potential undesirable effects with Olmetec Plus, even if not observed in clinical trials with this product.

Olmesartan medoxomil:

Market experience

The following adverse reactions have been reported in post-marketing experience.

They are listed by System Organ Class and ranked under headings of frequency using the following convention: very common (≥1/10); common (≥1/100, <1/10); uncommon (≥1/1,000, <1/100); rare (≥1/10,000, <1/1,000); very rare (<1/10,000) including isolated reports.

System Organ Class	Very rare
Blood and lymphatic system disorders	Thrombocytopenia
Nervous system disorders	Dizziness, headache
Respiratory, thoracic and mediastinal disorders	Cough
Gastrointestinal disorders	Abdominal pain, nausea, vomiting
Skin and subcutaneous tissue disorders	Pruritus, exanthem, rash Allergic conditions such as angioneurotic oedema, dermatitis allergic, face oedema and urticaria
Musculoskeletal and connective tissue disorders	Muscle cramp, myalgia
Renal and urinary disorders	Acute renal failure and renal insufficiency (See also under Investigations)
General disorders and administration site conditions	Asthenic conditions such as asthenia, fatigue, lethargy, malaise
Investigations	Abnormal renal function tests such as blood creatinine increased and blood urea increased Increased hepatic enzymes

Clinical trials

In double-blind, placebo-controlled monotherapy studies, the overall incidence of treatment-emergent adverse events was similar on olmesartan medoxomil and on placebo.

In placebo-controlled monotherapy studies, the only adverse drug reaction that was unequivocally related to treatment was dizziness (2.5% incidence on olmesartan medoxomil and 0.9% on placebo).

In long-term (2-year) treatment, the incidence of withdrawals due to adverse events on olmesartan medoxomil 10-20 mg once daily was 3.7%.

The following adverse events have been reported across all clinical trials with olmesartan medoxomil (including trials with active as well as placebo control), irrespective of causality or incidence relative to placebo. They are listed by body system and ranked under headings of frequency using the conventions described above:

Central nervous system disorders:

Common: Dizziness

Uncommon: Vertigo

Cardiovascular disorders:

Rare: Hypotension

Uncommon: Angina pectoris

Respiratory system disorders:

Common: Bronchitis, cough, pharyngitis, rhinitis

Gastrointestinal disorders:

Common: Abdominal pain, diarrhoea, dyspepsia, gastro-enteritis, nausea

Skin and appendages disorders:

Uncommon: Rash

Musculoskeletal disorders:

Common: Arthritis, back pain, skeletal pain

Urinary system disorders:

Common: Haematuria, urinary tract infection

General disorders:

Common: Chest pain, fatigue, influenza-like symptoms, peripheral oedema, pain

Laboratory findings

In placebo-controlled monotherapy studies the incidence was somewhat higher on olmesartan medoxomil compared with placebo for hypertriglyceridaemia (2.0% versus 1.1%) and for raised creatine phosphokinase (1.3% versus 0.7%).

Laboratory adverse events reported across all clinical trials with olmesartan medoxomil (including trials without a placebo control), irrespective of causality or incidence relative to placebo, included:

Metabolic and nutritional disorders:

Common: Increased creatine phosphokinase, hypertriglyceridaemia, hyperuricaemia.

Rare: Hyperkalaemia

Liver and biliary disorders:

Common: Liver enzyme elevations.

Hydrochlorothiazide:

Hydrochlorothiazide may cause or exacerbate volume depletion which may lead to electrolyte imbalance (see section 4.4).

Adverse events reported with the use of hydrochlorothiazide alone include:

Infections and infestations:

Rare: Sialadenitis

Blood and lymphatic system disorders:

Rare: Leukopenia, neutropenia/agranulocytosis, thrombocytopenia, aplastic anaemia, haemolytic anaemia, bone marrow depression

Metabolism and nutrition disorders:

Common: Hyperglycaemia, glycosuria, hyperuricaemia, electrolyte imbalance (including hyponatraemia, hypomagnesaemia, hypochloraemia, hypokalaemia and hypercalcaemia), increases in cholesterol and triglycerides

Uncommon: Anorexia

Psychiatric disorders:

Rare: Restlessness, depression, sleep disturbances, apathy

Nervous system disorders:

Common: Light-headedness, confusional state

Uncommon: Loss of appetite

Rare: Paraesthesia, convulsions

Eye disorders:

Rare: Xanthopsia, transient blurred vision, lacrimation decreased

Ear and labyrinth disorders:

Common: Vertigo

Cardiovascular disorders:

Uncommon: Orthostatic hypotension

Rare: Cardiac arrhythmias, necrotising angiitis (vasculitis, cutaneous vasculitis), thrombosis, embolism

Respiratory, thoracic and mediastinal disorders:

Rare: Dispnoea (including interstitial pneumonia and pulmonary oedema)

Gastrointestinal disorders:

Common: Gastric irritation, nausea, vomiting, diarrhoea, constipation, meteorism and abdominal pain

Rare: Pancreatitis

Very rare: Paralytic ileus

Hepatobiliary disorders:

Rare: Jaundice (intrahepatic cholestatic icterus), acute cholecystitis

Skin and subcutaneous tissue disorders:

Uncommon: Photosensitivity reactions, rash, urticaria

Rare: Cutaneous lupus erythematosus-like reactions, reactivation of cutaneous lupus erythematosus, anaphylactic reactions, toxic epidermal necrolysis

Musculoskeletal and connective tissue disorders:

Rare: Muscle spasm, muscle weakness, paresis

Renal and urinary disorders:

Rare: Renal dysfunction, increase of substances in the serum that are obligatory excreted by urine (creatinine, urea), interstitial nephritis, acute renal failure

Reproductive Symptoms and Breast disorders

Rare: Erectile dysfunction

General disorders and administration site conditions:

Common: Weakness, headache and fatigue

Rare: Fever

4.9 Overdose

No specific information is available on the effects or treatment of Olmetec Plus overdosage. The patient should be closely monitored, and the treatment should be symptomatic and supportive. Management depends upon the time since ingestion and the severity of the symptoms. Suggested measures include induction of emesis and/or gastric lavage. Activated charcoal may be useful in the treatment of overdosage. Serum electrolytes and creatinine should be monitored frequently. If hypotension occurs, the patient should be placed in a supine position, with salt and volume replacements given quickly.

The most likely manifestations of olmesartan overdosage are expected to be hypotension and tachycardia; bradycardia might also occur. Overdosage with hydrochlorothiazide is associated with electrolyte depletion (hypokalaemia, hypochloraemia) and dehydration resulting from excessive diuresis. The most common signs and symptoms of overdosage are nausea and somnolence. Hypokalaemia may result in muscle spasm and/or accentuate cardiac arrhythmias associated with the concomitant use of digitalis glycosides or certain anti-arrhythmic medicinal products.

No information is available regarding the dialysability of olmesartan or hydrochlorothiazide.

5. PHARMACOLOGICAL PROPERTIES

5.1 Pharmacodynamic properties

Pharmaco-therapeutic group: Angiotensin II antagonists and diuretics, ATC code C09D A 08.

Olmetec Plus is a combination of an angiotensin II receptor antagonist, olmesartan medoxomil, and a thiazide diuretic, hydrochlorothiazide. The combination of these ingredients has an additive antihypertensive effect, reducing blood pressure to a greater degree than either component alone.

Once daily dosing with Olmetec Plus provides an effective and smooth reduction in blood pressure over the 24 hour dose interval.

Olmesartan medoxomil is an orally active, selective angiotensin II receptor (type AT_1) antagonist. Angiotensin II is the primary vasoactive hormone of the renin-angiotensin-aldosterone system and plays a significant role in the pathophysiology of hypertension. The effects of angiotensin II include vasoconstriction, stimulation of the synthesis and release of aldosterone, cardiac stimulation and renal reabsorption of sodium. Olmesartan blocks the vasoconstrictor and aldosterone-secreting effects of angiotensin II by blocking its binding to the AT_1 receptor in tissues including vascular smooth muscle and the adrenal gland. The action of olmesartan is independent of the source or route of synthesis of angiotensin II. The selective antagonism of the angiotensin II (AT_1) receptors by olmesartan results in increases in plasma renin levels and angiotensin I and II concentrations, and some decrease in plasma aldosterone concentrations.

In hypertension, olmesartan medoxomil causes a dose-dependent, long-lasting reduction in arterial blood pressure. There has been no evidence of first-dose hypotension, of tachyphylaxis during long-term treatment, or of rebound hypertension after abrupt cessation of therapy.

Once daily dosing with olmesartan medoxomil provides an effective and smooth reduction in blood pressure over the 24 hour dose interval. Once daily dosing produced similar decreases in blood pressure as twice daily dosing at the same total daily dose.

With continuous treatment, maximum reductions in blood pressure are achieved by 8 weeks after the initiation of therapy, although a substantial proportion of the blood pressure lowering effect is already observed after 2 weeks of treatment.

The effect of olmesartan medoxomil on mortality and morbidity is not yet known.

Hydrochlorothiazide is a thiazide diuretic. The mechanism of the antihypertensive effect of thiazide diuretics is not fully known. Thiazides affect the renal tubular mechanisms of electrolyte reabsorption, directly increasing excretion of sodium and chloride in approximately equivalent amounts. The diuretic action of hydrochlorothiazide reduces plasma volume, increases plasma renin activity and increases aldosterone secretion, with consequent increases in urinary potassium and bicarbonate loss, and decreases in serum potassium. The renin-aldosterone link is mediated by angiotensin II and therefore coadministration of an angiotensin II receptor antagonist tends to reverse the potassium loss associated with thiazide diuretics. With hydrochlorothiazide, onset of diuresis occurs at about 2 hours and peak effect occurs at about 4 hours post-dose, whilst the action persists for approximately 6-12 hours.

Epidemiological studies have shown that long-term treatment with hydrochlorothiazide monotherapy reduces the risk of cardiovascular mortality and morbidity.

The combination of olmesartan medoxomil and hydrochlorothiazide produces additive reductions in blood pressure which generally increase with the dose of each component. In pooled placebo-controlled studies, administration of the 20/12.5 mg and 20/25 mg combinations of olmesartan medoxomil/hydrochlorothiazide resulted in mean placebo-subtracted systolic/diastolic blood pressure reductions at trough of 12/7 mm Hg and 16/9 mm Hg, respectively. Age and gender had no clinically relevant effect on response to treatment with olmesartan medoxomil /hydrochlorothiazide combination therapy.

Administration of 12.5 mg and 25 mg hydrochlorothiazide in patients insufficiently controlled by olmesartan medoxomil 20 mg monotherapy gave additional reductions in 24-hour systolic/diastolic blood pressures measured by ambulatory blood pressure monitoring of 7/5 mm Hg and 12/7 mm Hg, respectively, compared with olmesartan medoxomil monotherapy baseline. The additional mean systolic/diastolic blood pressure reductions at trough compared with baseline, measured conventionally, were 11/10 mm Hg and 16/11 mm Hg, respectively.

The effectiveness of olmesartan medoxomil/hydrochlorothiazide combination therapy was maintained over long-term (one-year) treatment. Withdrawal of olmesartan medoxomil therapy, with or without concomitant hydrochlorothiazide therapy, did not result in rebound hypertension.

The effects of fixed dose combination of olmesartan medoxomil/hydrochlorothiazide on mortality and cardiovascular morbidity are currently unknown.

5.2 Pharmacokinetic properties

Absorption and distribution

Olmesartan medoxomil:

Olmesartan medoxomil is a prodrug. It is rapidly converted to the pharmacologically active metabolite, olmesartan, by esterases in the gut mucosa and in portal blood during absorption from the gastrointestinal tract. No intact olmesartan medoxomil or intact side chain medoxomil moiety have been detected in plasma or excreta. The mean absolute bioavailability of olmesartan from a tablet formulation was 25.6%.

The mean peak plasma concentration (C_{max}) of olmesartan is reached within about 2 hours after oral dosing with olmesartan medoxomil, and olmesartan plasma concentrations increase approximately linearly with increasing single oral doses up to about 80 mg.

Food had minimal effect on the bioavailability of olmesartan and therefore olmesartan medoxomil may be administered with or without food.

No clinically relevant gender-related differences in the pharmacokinetics of olmesartan have been observed.

Olmesartan is highly bound to plasma protein (99.7%), but the potential for clinically significant protein binding displacement interactions between olmesartan and other highly bound coadministered active substances is low (as confirmed by the lack of a clinically significant interaction between olmesartan medoxomil and warfarin). The binding of olmesartan to blood cells is negligible. The mean volume of distribution after intravenous dosing is low (16 – 29 L).

Hydrochlorothiazide:

Following oral administration of olmesartan medoxomil and hydrochlorothiazide in combination, the median time to peak concentrations of hydrochlorothiazide was 1.5 to 2 hours after dosing. Hydrochlorothiazide is 68 % protein bound in the plasma and its apparent volume of distribution is 0.83 – 1.14 L/kg.

Metabolism and elimination

Olmesartan medoxomil:

Total plasma clearance of olmesartan was typically 1.3 L/h (CV, 19%) and was relatively slow compared to hepatic blood flow (ca 90 L/h). Following a single oral dose of ^{14}C-labelled olmesartan medoxomil, 10 - 16% of the administered radioactivity was excreted in the urine (the vast majority within 24 hours of dose administration) and the remainder of the recovered radioactivity was excreted in the faeces. Based on the systemic availability of 25.6%, it can be calculated that absorbed olmesartan is cleared by both renal excretion (ca 40%) and hepato-biliary excretion (ca 60%). All recovered radioactivity was identified as olmesartan. No other significant metabolite was detected. Enterohepatic recycling of olmesartan is minimal. Since a large proportion of olmesartan is excreted via the biliary route, use in patients with biliary obstruction is contraindicated (see section 4.3).

The terminal elimination half life of olmesartan varied between 10 and 15 hours after multiple oral dosing. Steady state was reached after the first few doses and no further accumulation was evident after 14 days of repeated dosing. Renal clearance was approximately 0.5 – 0.7 L/h and was independent of dose.

Hydrochlorothiazide:

Hydrochlorothiazide is not metabolised in man and is excreted almost entirely as unchanged active substance in urine. About 60 % of the oral dose is eliminated as unchanged active substance within 48 hours. Renal clearance is about 250-300 mL/min. The terminal elimination half-life of hydrochlorothiazide is 10-15 hours.

Olmetec Plus

The systemic availability of hydrochlorothiazide is reduced by about 20% when co-administered with olmesartan medoxomil, but this modest decrease is not of any clinical relevance. The kinetics of olmesartan are unaffected by the co-administration of hydrochlorothiazide.

Pharmacokinetics in special populations

Elderly:

In hypertensive patients, the olmesartan AUC at steady state was increased by ca 35% in elderly patients (65 – 75 years old) and by ca 44% in very elderly patients (≥ 75 years old) compared with the younger age group (see section 4.2).

Limited data suggest that the systemic clearance of hydrochlorothiazide is reduced in both healthy and hypertensive elderly patients subjects compared to young healthy volunteers.

Renal impairment:

In renally impaired patients, the olmesartan AUC at steady state increased by 62%, 82% and 179% in patients with mild, moderate and severe renal impairment, respectively, compared to healthy controls (see sections 4.2, 4.4).

The half-life of hydrochlorothiazide is prolonged in patients with impaired renal function.

Hepatic impairment:

After single oral administration, olmesartan AUC values were 6% and 65% higher in mildly and moderately hepatically impaired patients, respectively, than in their corresponding matched healthy controls. The unbound fraction of olmesartan at 2 hours post-dose in healthy subjects, in patients with mild hepatic impairment and in patients with moderate hepatic impairment was 0.26%, 0.34% and 0.41%, respectively. Olmesartan medoxomil has not been evaluated in patients with severe hepatic impairment (see sections 4.2, 4.4).

Hepatic impairment does not significantly influence the pharmacokinetics of hydrochlorothiazide.

5.3 Preclinical safety data

The toxic potential of olmesartan medoxomil/hydrochlorothiazide combinationswas evaluated in repeated dose oral toxicity studies for up to six months in rats and dogs. As for each of the individual substances and other medicinal products in this class, the main toxicological target organ of the combination was the kidney. The combination of olmesartan medoxomil/hydrochlorothiazide induced functional renal changes (increases in serum urea nitrogen and in serum creatinine). High dosages caused tubular degeneration and regeneration in the kidneys of rats and dogs, probably via a change in renal haemodynamics (reduced renal perfusion resulting from hypotension with tubular hypoxia and tubular cell degeneration). In addition the olmesartan medoxomil/ hydrochlorothiazide combination caused a decrease in red blood cell parameters (erythrocytes, haemoglobin and haematocrit) and a reduction in heart weight in rats.

These effects have also been observed for other AT_1 receptor antagonists and for ACE inhibitors and they seem to have been induced by the pharmacological action of high dosages of olmesartan medoxomil and seem to be not relevant to humans at the recommended therapeutic doses.

Genotoxicity studies using combined olmesartan medoxomil and hydrochlorothiazide as well as the individual components have not shown any signs of a clinically relevant genotoxic activity.

The carcinogenic potential of a combination of olmesartan medoxomil and hydrochlorothiazide was not investigated as there was no evidence of relevant carcinogenic effects for the two individual components under conditions of clinical use.

There was no evidence of teratogenicity in mice or rats treated with olmesartan medoxomil/hydrochlorothiazide combinations. As expected from this class of medicinal product, fetal toxicity was observed in rats, as evidenced by significantly reduced fetal body weights, when treated with olmesartan medoxomil /hydrochlorothiazide combinations during gestation (see sections 4.3 and 4.6).

6. PHARMACEUTICAL PARTICULARS

6.1 List of excipients

Tablet core

Microcrystalline cellulose

Lactose monohydrate

Low substituted hydroxypropylcellulose

Hydroxypropylcellulose

Magnesium stearate

Tablet coat

Talc

Hypromellose

Titanium dioxide (E 171)

Iron (III) oxide yellow (E172)

Iron (III) oxide red (E172)

6.2 Incompatibilities

Not applicable.

6.3 Shelf life

3 years.

6.4 Special precautions for storage

This medicinal product does not require any special storage conditions.

6.5 Nature and contents of container

Laminated polyamide/aluminium/polyvinyl chloride/aluminium blister.

Packs of 28 film-coated tablets.

6.6 Special precautions for disposal and other handling

No special requirements.

7. MARKETING AUTHORISATION HOLDER

Daiichi Sankyo UK Limited

Chiltern Place

Chalfont Park

Gerrards Cross

Buckinghamshire

SL9 0BG

UK

8. MARKETING AUTHORISATION NUMBER(S)

Olmetec Plus 20 mg/12.5 mg film-coated tablets: PL 08265/0022

Olmetec Plus 20 mg/25 mg film-coated tablets: PL 08265/0023

9. DATE OF FIRST AUTHORISATION/RENEWAL OF THE AUTHORISATION

14th February 2006

10. DATE OF REVISION OF THE TEXT

August 2006

Omacor

(Solvay Healthcare Limited)

1. NAME OF THE MEDICINAL PRODUCT

Omacor, capsule, soft

2. QUALITATIVE AND QUANTITATIVE COMPOSITION

Omega-3-acid ethyl esters 90 —1000 mg

comprising 840 mg eicosapentaenoic acid (EPA) ethyl ester (460mg) and docosahexaenoic acid (DHA) ethyl ester (380mg).

For one capsule.

For a full list of excipients see section 6.1.

3. PHARMACEUTICAL FORM

Capsule, soft.

Soft, oblong, transparent gelatin capsules containing pale yellow oil.

4. CLINICAL PARTICULARS

4.1 Therapeutic indications

Post Myocardial Infarction

Adjuvant treatment in secondary prevention after myocardial infarction, in addition to other standard therapy (e.g. statins, anti-platelet medicinal products, beta-blockers, ACE inhibitors).

Hypertriglyceridaemia

Endogenous hypertriglyceridaemia as a supplement to diet when dietary measures alone are insufficient to produce an adequate response:

- type IV in monotherapy,

- type IIb/III in combination with statins, when control of triglycerides is insufficient.

4.2 Posology and method of administration

Post Myocardial Infarction

One capsule daily.

Hypertriglyceridaemia

Initial treatment two capsules daily. If adequate response is not obtained, the dose may be increased to four capsules daily.

The capsules may be taken with food to avoid gastrointestinal disturbances.

There is no information regarding the use of Omacor in children, in elderly patients over 70 years of age, or in patients with hepatic impairment (see section 4.4), and only limited information regarding the use in patients with renal impairment.

4.3 Contraindications

Hypersensitivity to the active substance, to soya or to any of the excipients.

4.4 Special warnings and precautions for use

Warnings

Because of the moderate increase in bleeding time (with the high dosage, i.e. 4 capsules), patients receiving anticoagulant therapy must be monitored and the dosage of anticoagulant adjusted if necessary (see section 4.5 Interaction with other Medicinal Products and other forms of Interaction). Use of this medication does not eliminate the need for the surveillance usually required for patients of this type.

Make allowance for the increased bleeding time in patients at high risk of haemorrhage (because of severe trauma, surgery, etc).

In the absence of efficacy and safety data, use of this medication in children is not recommended.

Omacor is not indicated in exogenous hypertriglyceridaemia (type 1 hyperchylomicronaemia). There is only limited experience in secondary endogenous hypertriglyceridaemia (especially uncontrolled diabetes).

There is no experience regarding hypertriglyceridaemia in combination with fibrates.

Special precaution

Regular monitoring of hepatic function (ASAT and ALAT) is required in patients with hepatic impairment (in particular with the high dosage, i.e. 4 capsules).

4.5 Interaction with other medicinal products and other forms of interaction

Oral anticoagulants: See Section 4.4 Special warnings and precautions for use.

Omacor has been given in conjunction with warfarin without haemorrhagic complications. However, the prothrombin time must be checked when Omacor is combined with warfarin or when treatment with Omacor is stopped.

4.6 Pregnancy and lactation

Pregnancy

There are no adequate data from the use of Omacor in pregnant women.

Studies in animals have not shown reproductive toxicity. The potential risk for humans is unknown and therefore Omacor should not be used during pregnancy unless clearly necessary.

Lactation

There are no data on the excretion of Omacor in animal and human milk. Omacor should not be used during lactation.

4.7 Effects on ability to drive and use machines

Not relevant.

4.8 Undesirable effects

The frequencies of adverse reactions are ranked according to the following: common (> 1/100, < 1/10); uncommon

(>1/1000 < 1/100); rare (>1/10000, < 1/1000); very rare (< 1/10000), including isolated reports.

Infection and infestations

Uncommon: gastroenteritis

Immune system disorders:

Uncommon: hypersensitivity

Metabolism and nutrition disorders:

Rare: hyperglycaemia

Nervous system disorders:

Uncommon: dizziness, dysgeusia

Rare: headache

Vascular disorders:

Very rare: hypotension

Respiratory thoracic and mediastinal disorders:

Very rare: nasal dryness

Gastrointestinal disorders:

Common: dyspepsia, nausea

Uncommon: abdominal pain, gastrointestinal disorders, gastritis, abdominal pain upper

Rare: gastrointestinal pain

Very rare: lower gastrointestinal haemorrhage

Hepatobiliary disorders:

Rare: hepatic disorders

Skin and subcutaneous tissue disorders:

Rare: acne, rash pruritic

Very rare: urticaria

General disorders and administration site conditions:

Rare: Ill-defined disorders

Investigations:

Very rare: white blood count increased, blood lactate dehydrogenase increased

Moderate elevation of transaminases has been reported in patients with hypertriglyceridaemia.

4.9 Overdose

There are no special recommendations.

Administer symptomatic treatment.

5. PHARMACOLOGICAL PROPERTIES

5.1 Pharmacodynamic properties

Other cholesterol and triglycerides reducers, ATC code: C10AX06.

The omega-3 series polyunsaturated fatty acids, eicosapentaenoic acid (EPA) and docosahexaenoic acid (DHA), are essential fatty acids.

Omacor is active on the plasma lipids by lowering triglyceride levels as a result of a fall in VLDL (very low density lipoprotein), and the substance is also active on haemostasis and blood pressure.

Omacor reduces the synthesis of triglycerides in the liver because EPA and DHA are poor substrates for the enzymes responsible for triglyceride synthesis and they inhibit esterification of other fatty acids.

The increase in peroxisomes of β-oxidation of fatty acids in the liver also contributes to the fall in triglycerides, by reducing the quantity of free fatty acids available for their synthesis. The inhibition of this synthesis lowers VLDL.

Omacor increases LDL-cholesterol in some patients with hypertriglyceridaemia. A rise in HDL-cholesterol is only small, significantly smaller than seen after administration of fibrates, and not consistent.

The long-term lipid-lowering effect (after more than one year) is not known. Otherwise there is no strong evidence that lowering triglycerides reduces the risk of ischaemic heart disease.

During treatment with Omacor, there is a fall in thromboxane A2 production and a slight increase in bleeding time. No significant effect has been observed on the other coagulation factors.

11324 patients, with recent MI (<3 months) and receiving a recommended preventative treatment associated with a Mediterranean diet, were randomised in the GISSI-Prevenzione study in order to receive Omacor (n=2836), vitamin E (n=2830), Omacor + vitamin E (n=2830) or no treatment (n=2828). GISSI-P was a multicentre, randomised, open-label study performed in Italy.

The results observed over 3.5 years, with Omacor 1g/day, have shown a significant reduction of a combined endpoint including all-cause death, non fatal MI and non fatal stroke (decrease in relative risk of 15% [2-26] p=0.0226 in patients taking Omacor alone compared to control, and of 10% [1-18] p=0.0482 in patients taking Omacor with or without vitamin E). A reduction of the second pre-specified endpoint criteria including cardiovascular deaths, non fatal MI and non-fatal stroke has been shown (decrease in relative risk of 20% [5-32] p=0.0082 in patients taking Omacor alone compared to control, decrease in relative risk of 11% [1-20] p= 0.0526 in patients taking Omacor with or without vitamin E). The secondary analysis for each component of the primary endpoints has shown a significant reduction of all cause deaths and cardiovascular deaths, but no reduction of non fatal cardiovascular events or fatal and non fatal strokes.

5.2 Pharmacokinetic properties

During and after absorption, there are three main pathways for the metabolism of the omega-3 fatty acids:

- the fatty acids are first transported to the liver where they are incorporated into various categories of lipoproteins and then channelled to the peripheral lipid stores;
- the cell membrane phospholipids are replaced by lipoprotein phospholipids and the fatty acids can then act as precursors for various eicosanoids;
- the majority is oxidised to meet energy requirements.

The concentration of omega-3 fatty acids, EPA and DHA, in the plasma phospholipids corresponds to the EPA and DHA incorporated into the cell membranes.

Animal pharmacokinetic studies have shown that there is a complete hydrolysis of the ethyl ester accompanied by satisfactory absorption and incorporation of EPA and DHA into the plasma phospholipids and cholesterol esters.

5.3 Preclinical safety data

No safety issues have been identified relevant to human use at the recommended daily intake.

6. PHARMACEUTICAL PARTICULARS

6.1 List of excipients

Capsule core:

Alpha-tocopherol

Capsule shell:

Gelatin

Glycerol

purified water

Medium-chain triglycerides

Lecithin (soya)

6.2 Incompatibilities

Not applicable.

6.3 Shelf life

3 years.

6.4 Special precautions for storage

Do not store above 25°C. Do not freeze.

6.5 Nature and contents of container

White (HDPE) bottle

- 1 × 20 capsules
- 1 × 28 capsules
- 1 × 60 capsules
- 1 × 100 capsules
- 10 × 28 capsules

Not all pack sizes may be marketed.

6.6 Special precautions for disposal and other handling

No special requirements.

7. MARKETING AUTHORISATION HOLDER

Pronova BioPharma Norge AS

P.0 Box 420

1327 Lysaker

Norway

8. MARKETING AUTHORISATION NUMBER(S)

PL 15905/0001

9. DATE OF FIRST AUTHORISATION/RENEWAL OF THE AUTHORISATION

22 July 2001

10. DATE OF REVISION OF THE TEXT

March 2008

LEGAL STATUS

P

Omnitrope 3.3 mg/ml solution for Injection

(Sandoz Limited)

1. NAME OF THE MEDICINAL PRODUCT

Omnitrope ▼ 3.3 mg/ml solution for injection

2. QUALITATIVE AND QUANTITATIVE COMPOSITION

Somatropin* 3.3 mg (corresponding to 10 IU)/ ml.

One cartridge contains 1.5 ml corresponding to 5 mg Somatropin* (15 IU).

* produced in *Escherichia coli* by recombinant DNA technology.

Excipients:

One ml contains 9 mg benzyl alcohol.

For a full list of excipients, see section 6.1.

3. PHARMACEUTICAL FORM

Solution for injection

The solution is clear and colourless.

4. CLINICAL PARTICULARS

4.1 Therapeutic indications

Infants, children and adolescents

- Growth disturbance due to insufficient secretion of growth hormone (GH).
- Growth disturbance associated with Turner syndrome.
- Growth disturbance associated with chronic renal insufficiency.
- Growth disturbance (current height standard deviation score (SDS) < -2.5 and parental adjusted SDS < -1) in short children/adolescents born small for gestational age (SGA), with a birth weight and/or length below -2 standard deviation (SD), who failed to show catch-up growth (height velocity (HV) SDS < 0 during the last year) by 4 years of age or later.
- Prader-Willi syndrome (PWS), for improvement of growth and body composition. The diagnosis of PWS should be confirmed by appropriate genetic testing.

Adults

- Replacement therapy in adults with pronounced growth hormone deficiency. Patients with severe growth hormone deficiency in adulthood are defined as patients with known hypothalamic pituitary pathology and at least one known deficiency of a pituitary hormone not being prolactin. These patients should undergo a single dynamic test in order to diagnose or exclude a growth hormone deficiency. In patients with childhood onset isolated GH deficiency (no evidence of hypothalamic-pituitary disease or cranial irradiation), two dynamic tests should be recommended, except for those having low IGF-I concentrations (SDS < -2) who may be considered for one test. The cut-off point of the dynamic test should be strict.

4.2 Posology and method of administration

Diagnosis and therapy with somatropin should be initiated and monitored by physicians who are appropriately qualified and experienced in the diagnosis and management of patients with growth disorders.

The posology and administration schedule should be individualised.

Growth disturbance due to insufficient secretion of growth hormone in paediatric patients:

Generally a dose of 0.025 - 0.035 mg/kg body weight per day or 0.7 - 1.0 mg/m^2 body surface area per day is recommended. Even higher doses have been used.

Prader-Willi syndrome, for improvement of growth and body composition in paediatric patients:

Generally a dose of 0.035 mg/kg body weight per day or 1.0 mg/m^2 body surface area per day is recommended. Daily doses of 2.7 mg should not be exceeded. Treatment should not be used in paediatric patients with a growth velocity less than 1 cm per year and near closure of epiphyses.

Growth disturbance due to Turner syndrome:

A dose of 0.045 - 0.050 mg/kg body weight per day or 1.4 mg/m^2 body surface area per day is recommended.

Growth disturbance in chronic renal insufficiency:

A dose of 1.4 mg/m^2 body surface area per day (0.045 - 0.050 mg/kg body weight per day) is recommended. Higher doses may be needed if growth velocity is too low. A dose correction may be needed after six months of treatment (see section 4.4).

Growth disturbance in short children/adolescents born small for gestational age (SGA):

A dose of 0.035 mg/kg body weight per day (1 mg/m^2 body surface area per day) is usually recommended until final height is reached (see section 5.1). Treatment should be discontinued after the first year of treatment if the height velocity SDS is below + 1. Treatment should be discontinued if height velocity is < 2 cm/year and, if confirmation is required, bone age is > 14 years (girls) or > 16 years (boys), corresponding to epiphyseal closure.

Dose recommendations for paediatric patients

Indication	mg/kg body weight dose per day	mg/m^2 body surface area dose per day
Growth hormone deficiency	0.025 - 0.035	0.7 - 1.0
Prader-Willi syndrome	0.035	1.0
Turner syndrome	0.045 - 0.050	1.4
Chronic renal insufficiency	0.045 - 0.050	1.4
Children/adolescents born small for gestational age (SGA)	0.035	1.0

Growth hormone deficient adult patients:

Therapy should start with a low dose, 0.15 - 0.3 mg per day. The dose should be gradually increased according to individual patient requirements as determined by the IGF-I concentration. Treatment goal should be insulin-like growth factor (IGF-I) concentrations within 2 SDS from the age corrected mean of healthy adults. Patients with normal IGF-I concentrations at the start of the treatment should be administered growth hormone up to an IGF-I level into the upper range of normal, not exceeding the 2 SDS. Clinical response and undesirable effects may also be used as guidance for dose titration. The daily maintenance dose rarely exceeds 1.0 mg per day. Women may require higher doses than men, while men show an increasing IGF-I sensitivity over time. This means that there is a risk that women, especially those on oral oestrogen replacement are under-treated while men are over-treated. The accuracy of the growth hormone dose should therefore be controlled every 6 months. As normal physiological growth hormone production decreases with age, dose requirements may be reduced. The minimum effective dose should be used.

The injection should be given subcutaneously and the site varied to prevent lipoatrophy.

For instructions for use and handling see section 6.6.

4.3 Contraindications

- Hypersensitivity to somatropin or to any of the excipients.

- Somatropin must not be used when there is any evidence of tumour activity and anti-tumour therapy must be completed prior to starting therapy.

- Somatropin must not be used for growth promotion in patients with closed epiphyses.

- Patients with acute critical illness suffering complications following open heart surgery, abdominal surgery, multiple accidental trauma, acute respiratory failure or similar conditions must not be treated with somatropin. With regard to patients undergoing substitution therapy, see section 4.4.

4.4 Special warnings and precautions for use

Somatropin may induce a state of insulin resistance and in some patients hyperglycaemia. Therefore patients should be observed for evidence of glucose intolerance. In rare cases the diagnostic criteria for diabetes mellitus type II may be fulfilled as a result of the somatropin therapy, but risk factors such as obesity (including obese PWS patients), family history, steroid treatment, or pre-existing impaired glucose tolerance have been present in most cases where this occurred. In patients with already manifested diabetes mellitus, the anti-diabetic therapy might require adjustment when somatropin is instituted.

During treatment with somatropin, an enhanced T4 to T3 conversion has been found which may result in a reduction in serum T4 and an increase in serum T3 concentrations. In general, the peripheral thyroid hormone levels have remained within the reference ranges for healthy subjects. The effects of somatropin on thyroid hormone levels may be of clinical relevance in patients with central subclinical hypothyroidism in whom hypothyroidism theoretically may develop. Conversely, in patients receiving replacement therapy with thyroxin mild hyperthyroidism may occur. It is therefore particularly advisable to test thyroid function after starting treatment with somatropin and after dose adjustments.

Somatropin has been reported to reduce serum cortisol levels, possibly by affecting carrier proteins or by increasing hepatic clearance. The clinical relevance of these findings may be limited. Nevertheless, corticosteroid replacement therapy should be optimised before initiation of Omnitrope therapy.

In growth hormone deficiency, secondary to treatment of malignant disease, it is recommended to pay attention to signs of relapse of the malignancy.

In patients with endocrine disorders, including growth hormone deficiency, slipped epiphyses of the hip may occur more frequently than in the general population. Patients limping during treatment with somatropin, should be examined clinically.

In case of severe or recurrent headache, visual problems, nausea and/or vomiting, a fundoscopy for papilloedema is recommended. If papilloedema is confirmed, a diagnosis of benign intracranial hypertension should be considered and, if appropriate, the growth hormone treatment should be discontinued. At present there is insufficient evidence to give specific advice on the continuation of growth hormone treatment in patients with resolved intracranial hypertension. However, clinical experience has shown that reinstitution of the therapy is often possible without recurrence of the intracranial hypertension. If growth hormone treatment is restarted, careful monitoring for symptoms of intracranial hypertension is necessary.

Experience in patients above 60 years is limited.

In patients with PWS, treatment should always be in combination with a calorie-restricted diet.

There have been reports of fatalities associated with the use of growth hormone in paediatric patients with PWS who had one or more of the following risk factors: severe obesity, history of respiratory impairment, sleep apnoea or unidentified respiratory infection. Patients with PWS and one or more of these risk factors may be at greater risk.

Patients with PWS should be evaluated for upper airway obstruction, sleep apnoea or respiratory infections before initiation of treatment with somatropin.

In case of signs of upper airway obstruction, the problem should be solved by a specialist before starting treatment with somatropin.

Sleep apnoea should be assessed before onset of growth hormone treatment by recognised methods such as polysomnography or overnight oxymetry, and monitored if sleep apnoea is suspected.

If during treatment with somatropin patients show signs of upper airway obstruction (including onset of or increased snoring), treatment should be interrupted, and a new ENT assessment performed.

All patients with PWS should be evaluated for sleep apnoea and monitored if sleep apnoea is suspected.

All patients with PWS should be monitored for signs of respiratory infections which should be diagnosed as early as possible and treated aggressively.

All patients with PWS should have effective weight control before and during treatment with somatropin.

Scoliosis is common in patients with PWS. Scoliosis may progress in any child during rapid growth. Signs of scoliosis should be monitored during treatment. However, growth hormone treatment has not been shown to increase the incidence or severity of scoliosis.

Experience with long term treatment in adults and in patients with PWS is limited.

In short children/adolescents born SGA, other medical reasons or treatments that could explain growth disturbance should be ruled out before starting treatment.

In SGA children/adolescents it is recommended to measure fasting insulin and blood glucose before start of treatment and annually thereafter. In patients with increased risk for diabetes mellitus (e.g. familial history of diabetes, obesity, severe insulin resistance, acanthosis nigricans) oral glucose tolerance testing (OGTT) should be performed. If overt diabetes occurs, growth hormone should not be administered.

In SGA children/adolescents it is recommended to measure the IGF-I level before start of treatment and twice a year thereafter. If on repeated measurements IGF-I levels exceed +2 SD compared to references for age and pubertal status, the IGF-I / IGFBP-3 ratio could be taken into account to consider dose adjustment.

Experience in initiating treatment in SGA patients near onset of puberty is limited. It is therefore not recommended to initiate treatment near onset of puberty. Experience in patients with Silver-Russell syndrome is limited.

Some of the height gain obtained with treating short children/adolescents born SGA with growth hormone may be lost if treatment is stopped before final height is reached.

In chronic renal insufficiency, renal function should be below 50 percent of normal before institution of therapy. To verify growth disturbance, growth should be followed for a year preceding institution of therapy. During this period, conservative treatment for renal insufficiency (which includes control of acidosis, hyperparathyroidism and nutritional status) should have been established and should be maintained during treatment.

The treatment should be discontinued at renal transplantation.

To date, no data on final height in patients with chronic renal insufficiency treated with Omnitrope are available.

The effects of somatropin on recovery were studied in two placebo controlled trials involving 522 critically ill adult patients suffering complications following open heart surgery, abdominal surgery, multiple accidental trauma or acute respiratory failure. Mortality was higher in patients treated with 5.3 or 8 mg somatropin daily compared to patients receiving placebo, 42% vs. 19%. Based on this information, these types of patients should not be treated with somatropin. As there is no information available on the safety of growth hormone substitution therapy in acutely critically ill patients, the benefits of continued treatment in this situation should be weighed against the potential risks involved.

In all patients developing other or similar acute critical illness, the possible benefit of treatment with somatropin must be weighed against the potential risk involved.

This medicinal product contains less than 1 mmol sodium (23 mg) per ml, i.e. essentially 'sodium- free'.

Because of the presence of benzyl alcohol the medicinal product must not be given to premature babies or neonates. It may cause toxic reactions and anaphylactoid reactions in infants and children up to 3 years old.

4.5 Interaction with other medicinal products and other forms of interaction

Data from an interaction study performed in growth hormone deficient adults suggests that somatropin administration may increase the clearance of compounds known to be metabolised by cytochrome P450 isoenzymes. The clearance of compounds metabolised by cytochrome P 450 3A4 (e.g. sex steroids, corticosteroids, anticonvulsants and ciclosporin) may be especially increased resulting in lower plasma levels of these compounds. The clinical significance of this is unknown.

Also see section 4.4 for statements regarding diabetes mellitus and thyroid disorder and section 4.2 for statement on oral oestrogen replacement therapy.

4.6 Pregnancy and lactation

For Omnitrope no clinical data on exposed pregnancies are available. Animal experimental data on reproductive toxicity of Omnitrope are not available. Treatment with Omnitrope should be interrupted if pregnancy occurs.

During normal pregnancy levels of pituitary growth hormone fall markedly after 20 gestation weeks, being replaced almost entirely by placental growth hormone by 30 weeks. In view of this, it is unlikely that continued replacement therapy with somatropin would be necessary in growth hormone deficient women in the third trimester of pregnancy.

It is not known if somatropin is excreted into breast milk, but absorption of intact protein from the gastrointestinal tract of the infant is extremely unlikely.

Caution should be exercised when Omnitrope is administered to breast-feeding women.

4.7 Effects on ability to drive and use machines

No studies on the effects on the ability to drive and use machines have been performed.

4.8 Undesirable effects

Within the organ system classes, adverse reactions are listed under headings of frequency (number of patients expected to experience the reaction), using the following categories: very common (⩾ 1/10); common (⩾ 1/100, < 1/10); uncommon (⩾ 1/1,000, < 1/100); rare (⩾ 1/10,000, < 1/1,000); very rare (< 1/10,000).

Patients with growth hormone deficiency are characterised by extracellular volume deficit. When treatment with somatropin is started this deficit is rapidly corrected. In adult patients, adverse reactions related to fluid retention, such as peripheral oedema, stiffness in the extremities, arthralgia, myalgia and paraesthesia are common. In general these adverse reactions are mild to moderate, arise within the first months of treatment and subside spontaneously or with dose-reduction. The incidence of these undesirable effects is related to the administered dose, the age of patients, and possibly inversely related to the age of patients at the onset of growth hormone deficiency. In paediatric patients such undesirable effects are uncommon.

Neoplasms benign, malignant and unspecified (incl cysts and polyps)

Very rare:	Leukemia. Very rare cases of leukaemia have been reported in growth hormone deficient paediatric patients treated with somatropin, but the incidence appears to be similar to that in the paediatric subjects without growth hormone deficiency.

Immune system disorders

Common:	Formation of antibodies. Somatropin has given rise to the formation of antibodies in approximately 1% of the patients. The binding capacity of these antibodies has been low and no clinical changes have been associated with their formation.

Endocrine disorders

Rare:	Diabetes mellitus type II

Nervous system disorders

Common:	In adults: paraesthesia
Uncommon:	In adults: carpal tunnel syndrome; In paediatric patients: paraesthesia
Rare:	Benign intracranial hypertension

Musculoskeletal and connective tissue disorders

Common:	In adults: stiffness in the extremities, arthralgia, myalgia
Uncommon:	In paediatric patients: stiffness in the extremities, arthralgia, myalgia

General disorders and administration site conditions

Common:	In adults: peripheral oedema; In paediatric patients: transient local skin reactions at the injection site
Uncommon:	In paediatric patients: peripheral oedema

4.9 Overdose

No case of overdose has been reported.

Acute overdose could lead initially to hypoglycaemia and subsequently to hyperglycaemia.

Long-term overdose could result in signs and symptoms consistent with the known effects of human growth hormone excess.

5. PHARMACOLOGICAL PROPERTIES

5.1 Pharmacodynamic properties

Pharmacotherapeutic group: anterior pituitary lobe hormones and analogues.

ATC code: H01AC01.

Somatropin is a potent metabolic hormone of importance for the metabolism of lipids, carbohydrates and proteins. In children with inadequate endogenous growth hormone, somatropin stimulates linear growth and increases growth rate. In adults as well as in children, somatropin maintains a normal body composition by increasing nitrogen retention and stimulation of skeletal muscle growth, and by mobilisation of body fat. Visceral adipose tissue is particularly responsive to somatropin. In addition to enhanced lipolysis, somatropin decreases the uptake of triglycerides into body fat stores. Serum concentrations of IGF-I (Insulin-like Growth Factor-I) and IGFBP3 (Insulin-like Growth Factor Binding Protein 3) are increased by somatropin. In addition, the following actions have been demonstrated.

Lipid metabolism:

Somatropin induces hepatic LDL cholesterol receptors, and affects the profile of serum lipids and lipoproteins. In general, administration of somatropin to growth hormone deficient patients results in reduction in serum LDL and apolipoprotein B. A reduction in serum total cholesterol may also be observed.

Carbohydrate metabolism:

Somatropin increases insulin but fasting blood glucose is commonly unchanged. Children with hypopituitarism may experience fasting hypoglycaemia. This condition is reversed by somatropin.

Water and mineral metabolism:

Growth hormone deficiency is associated with decreased plasma and extracellular volumes. Both are rapidly increased after treatment with somatropin. Somatropin induces the retention of sodium, potassium and phosphorus.

Bone metabolism:

Somatropin stimulates the turnover of skeletal bone. Long-term administration of somatropin to growth hormone deficient patients with osteopenia results in an increase in bone mineral content and density at weight-bearing sites.

Physical capacity:

Muscle strength and physical exercise capacity are improved after long-term treatment with somatropin. Somatropin also increases cardiac output, but the mechanism has yet to be clarified. A decrease in peripheral vascular resistance may contribute to this effect.

In clinical trials in short children/adolescents born SGA doses of 0.033 and 0.067 mg somatropin/kg body weight per day have been used for treatment until final height is reached. In 56 patients who are continuously treated and have reached (near) final height, the mean change from height at start of treatment was +1.90 SDS (0.033 mg/kg body weight per day) and +2.19 SDS (0.067 mg/kg body weight per day). Literature data from untreated SGA children/adolescents without early spontaneous catch-up suggest a late growth of 0.5 SDS. Long-term safety data are still limited.

5.2 Pharmacokinetic properties

Absorption

The bioavailability of subcutaneously administered somatropin is approximately 80% in both healthy subjects and growth hormone deficient patients. A subcutaneous dose of 5 mg of Omnitrope 3.3 mg/ml solution for injection in healthy adults results in plasma Cmax and tmax values of 72 ± 28 μg/l and 4.0 ± 2.0 hours, respectively.

Elimination

The mean terminal half-life of somatropin after intravenous administration in growth hormone deficient adults is about 0.4 hours. However, after subcutaneous administration of Omnitrope 3.3 mg/ml solution for injection, a half-life of 3 hours is achieved. The observed difference is likely due to slow absorption from the injection site following subcutaneous administration.

Sub-populations

The absolute bioavailability of somatropin seems to be similar in males and females following subcutaneous administration.

Information about the pharmacokinetics of somatropin in geriatric and paediatric populations, in different races and in patients with renal, hepatic or cardiac insufficiency is either lacking or incomplete.

5.3 Preclinical safety data

In studies with Omnitrope regarding subacute toxicity and local tolerance, no clinically relevant effects have been observed.

In other studies with somatropin regarding general toxicity, local tolerance and reproduction toxicity no clinically relevant effects have been observed.

With somatropins, in vitro and in vivo genotoxicity studies on gene mutations and induction of chromosome aberrations have been negative.

An increased chromosome fragility has been observed in one *in vitro* study on lymphocytes taken from patients after long term treatment with somatropin and following the addition of the radiomimetic medicinal product bleomycin. The clinical significance of this finding is unclear.

In another study with somatropin, no increase in chromosomal abnormalities was found in the lymphocytes of patients who had received long-term somatropin therapy.

6. PHARMACEUTICAL PARTICULARS

6.1 List of excipients

disodium hydrogen phosphate heptahydrate

sodium dihydrogen phosphate dihydrate

mannitol

poloxamer 188

benzyl alcohol

water for injections

6.2 Incompatibilities

In the absence of compatibility studies, this medicinal product must not be mixed with other medicinal products.

6.3 Shelf life

2 years.

Shelf life after first use:

After first use the cartridge should remain in the pen and has to be kept in a refrigerator (2°C - 8°C) for a maximum of 28 days. Store and transport refrigerated (2°C - 8°C). Do not freeze. Store in the original pen in order to protect from light.

6.4 Special precautions for storage

Unopened cartridge: Store and transport refrigerated (2°C - 8°C). Do not freeze. Store in the original package in order to protect from light.

For storage conditions of the in-use medicinal product, see section 6.3.

6.5 Nature and contents of container

1.5 ml of solution in a cartridge (colourless type I glass) with plunger on one side (siliconised bromobutyl), a disc (bromobutyl) and a cap (aluminium) on the other side.

Pack sizes of 1, 5 and 10.

Not all pack sizes may be marketed.

6.6 Special precautions for disposal and other handling

Omnitrope 3.3 mg/ml solution for injection is a sterile, ready-to-use solution for subcutaneous injection filled in a glass cartridge.

This presentation is intended for multiple use. It should only be administered with the Omnitrope Pen 5, an injection device specifically developed for use with Omnitrope 3.3 mg/ml solution for injection. It has to be administered using sterile, disposable pen needles. Patients and caregivers have to receive appropriate training and instruction on the proper use of the Omnitrope cartridges and the pen from the physician or other suitable qualified health professionals.

The following is a general description of the administration process. The manufacturer's instructions with each pen must be followed for loading the cartridge, attaching the injection needle and for the administration.

1. Hands should be washed.
2. If the solution is cloudy or contains particulate matter, it should not be used. The content must be clear and colourless.
3. Disinfect the rubber membrane of the cartridge with a cleansing swab
4. Insert the cartridge into the Omnitrope Pen 5 following the instructions for use provided with the pen.
5. Clean the site of injection with an alcohol swab.
6. Administer the appropriate dose by subcutaneous injection using a sterile pen needle. Remove the pen needle and dispose of it in accordance with local requirements.

7. MARKETING AUTHORISATION HOLDER

Sandoz GmbH

Biochemiestrasse 10

A-6250 Kundl

Austria

8. MARKETING AUTHORISATION NUMBER(S)

EU/1/06/332/004

EU/1/06/332/005

EU/1/06/332/006

9. DATE OF FIRST AUTHORISATION/RENEWAL OF THE AUTHORISATION

12 April 2006

10. DATE OF REVISION OF THE TEXT

18 March 2008

Omnitrope 6.7 mg/ml solution for Injection

(Sandoz Limited)

1. NAME OF THE MEDICINAL PRODUCT

Omnitrope ▼6.7 mg/ml solution for injection

2. QUALITATIVE AND QUANTITATIVE COMPOSITION

Somatropin* 6.7 mg (corresponding to 20 IU)/ ml.

One cartridge contains 1.5 ml corresponding to 10 mg Somatropin* (30 IU).

* produced in *Escherichia coli* by recombinant DNA technology.

For a full list of excipients, see section 6.1.

3. PHARMACEUTICAL FORM

Solution for injection

The solution is clear and colourless.

4. CLINICAL PARTICULARS

4.1 Therapeutic indications

Infants, children and adolescents

- Growth disturbance due to insufficient secretion of growth hormone (GH).
- Growth disturbance associated with Turner syndrome.
- Growth disturbance associated with chronic renal insufficiency.
- Growth disturbance (current height standard deviation score (SDS) < -2.5 and parental adjusted SDS < -1) in short children/adolescents born small for gestational age (SGA), with a birth weight and/or length below -2 standard deviation (SD), who failed to show catch-up growth (height velocity (HV) SDS < 0 during the last year) by 4 years of age or later.
- Prader-Willi syndrome (PWS), for improvement of growth and body composition. The diagnosis of PWS should be confirmed by appropriate genetic testing.

Adults

- Replacement therapy in adults with pronounced growth hormone deficiency. Patients with severe growth hormone deficiency in adulthood are defined as patients with known hypothalamic pituitary pathology and at least one known deficiency of a pituitary hormone not being prolactin. These patients should undergo a single dynamic test in order to diagnose or exclude a growth hormone deficiency. In patients with childhood onset isolated GH deficiency (no evidence of hypothalamic-pituitary disease or cranial irradiation), two dynamic tests should be recommended, except for those having low IGF-I concentrations (SDS < -2) who may be considered for one test. The cut-off point of the dynamic test should be strict.

4.2 Posology and method of administration

Diagnosis and therapy with somatropin should be initiated and monitored by physicians who are appropriately qualified and experienced in the diagnosis and management of patients with growth disorders.

The posology and administration schedule should be individualised.

Growth disturbance due to insufficient secretion of growth hormone in paediatric patients:

Generally a dose of 0.025 - 0.035 mg/kg body weight per day or 0.7 - 1.0 mg/m^2 body surface area per day is recommended. Even higher doses have been used.

Prader-Willi syndrome, for improvement of growth and body composition in paediatric patients:

Generally a dose of 0.035 mg/kg body weight per day or 1.0 mg/m^2 body surface area per day is recommended. Daily doses of 2.7 mg should not be exceeded. Treatment should not be used in paediatric patients with a growth velocity less than 1 cm per year and near closure of epiphyses.

Growth disturbance due to Turner syndrome:

A dose of 0.045 - 0.050 mg/kg body weight per day or 1.4 mg/m^2 body surface area per day is recommended.

Growth disturbance in chronic renal insufficiency:

A dose of 1.4 mg/m^2 body surface area per day (0.045 - 0.050 mg/kg body weight per day) is recommended. Higher doses may be needed if growth velocity is too low. A dose correction may be needed after six months of treatment (see section 4.4).

Growth disturbance in short children/adolescents born small for gestational age (SGA):

A dose of 0.035 mg/kg body weight per day (1 mg/m^2 body surface area per day) is usually recommended until final height is reached (see section 5.1). Treatment should be discontinued after the first year of treatment if the height velocity SDS is below + 1. Treatment should be discontinued if height velocity is < 2 cm/year and, if confirmation is required, bone age is > 14 years (girls) or > 16 years (boys), corresponding to epiphyseal closure.

Dose recommendations for paediatric patients

Indication	mg/kg body weight dose per day	mg/m^2 body surface area dose per day
Growth hormone deficiency	0.025 - 0.035	0.7 - 1.0
Prader-Willi syndrome	0.035	1.0
Turner syndrome	0.045 - 0.050	1.4
Chronic renal insufficiency	0.045 - 0.050	1.4
Children/adolescents born small for gestational age (SGA)	0.035	1.0

Growth hormone deficient adult patients:

Therapy should start with a low dose, 0.15 - 0.3 mg per day. The dose should be gradually increased according to individual patient requirements as determined by the IGF-I concentration. Treatment goal should be insulin-like growth factor (IGF-I) concentrations within 2 SDS from the age corrected mean of healthy adults. Patients with normal IGF-I concentrations at the start of the treatment should be administered growth hormone up to an IGF-I level into the upper range of normal, not exceeding the 2 SDS. Clinical response and undesirable effects may also be used as guidance for dose titration. The daily maintenance dose rarely exceeds 1.0 mg per day. Women may require higher doses than men, while men show an increasing IGF-I sensitivity over time. This means that there is a risk that women, especially those on oral oestrogen replacement are under-treated while men are over-treated. The accuracy of the growth hormone dose should therefore be controlled every 6 months. As normal physiological growth hormone production decreases with age, dose requirements may be reduced. The minimum effective dose should be used.

The injection should be given subcutaneously and the site varied to prevent lipoatrophy.

For instructions for use and handling see section 6.6.

4.3 Contraindications

- Hypersensitivity to somatropin or to any of the excipients.

- Somatropin must not be used when there is any evidence of tumour activity and anti-tumour therapy must be completed prior to starting therapy.

- Somatropin must not be used for growth promotion in patients with closed epiphyses.

- Patients with acute critical illness suffering complications following open heart surgery, abdominal surgery, multiple accidental trauma, acute respiratory failure or similar conditions must not be treated with somatropin. With regard to patients undergoing substitution therapy, see section 4.4.

4.4 Special warnings and precautions for use

Somatropin may induce a state of insulin resistance and in some patients hyperglycaemia. Therefore patients should be observed for evidence of glucose intolerance. In rare cases the diagnostic criteria for diabetes mellitus type II may be fulfilled as a result of the somatropin therapy, but risk factors such as obesity (including obese PWS patients), family history, steroid treatment, or pre-existing impaired glucose tolerance have been present in most cases where this occurred. In patients with already manifested diabetes mellitus, the anti-diabetic therapy might require adjustment when somatropin is instituted.

During treatment with somatropin, an enhanced T4 to T3 conversion has been found which may result in a reduction in serum T4 and an increase in serum T3 concentrations. In general, the peripheral thyroid hormone levels have remained within the reference ranges for healthy subjects. The effects of somatropin on thyroid hormone levels may be of clinical relevance in patients with central subclinical hypothyroidism in whom hypothyroidism theoretically may develop. Conversely, in patients receiving replacement therapy with thyroxin mild hyperthyroidism may occur. It is therefore particularly advisable to test thyroid function after starting treatment with somatropin and after dose adjustments.

Somatropin has been reported to reduce serum cortisol levels, possibly by affecting carrier proteins or by increasing hepatic clearance. The clinical relevance of these findings may be limited. Nevertheless, corticosteroid replacement therapy should be optimised before initiation of Omnitrope therapy.

In growth hormone deficiency, secondary to treatment of malignant disease, it is recommended to pay attention to signs of relapse of the malignancy.

In patients with endocrine disorders, including growth hormone deficiency, slipped epiphyses of the hip may occur more frequently than in the general population. Patients limping during treatment with somatropin, should be examined clinically.

In case of severe or recurrent headache, visual problems, nausea and/or vomiting, a fundoscopy for papilloedema is recommended. If papilloedema is confirmed, a diagnosis of benign intracranial hypertension should be considered and, if appropriate, the growth hormone treatment should be discontinued. At present there is insufficient evidence to give specific advice on the continuation of growth hormone treatment in patients with resolved intracranial hypertension. However, clinical experience has shown that reinstitution of the therapy is often possible without recurrence of the intracranial hypertension. If growth hormone treatment is restarted, careful monitoring for symptoms of intracranial hypertension is necessary.

Experience in patients above 60 years is limited.

In patients with PWS, treatment should always be in combination with a calorie-restricted diet.

There have been reports of fatalities associated with the use of growth hormone in paediatric patients with PWS who had one or more of the following risk factors: severe obesity, history of respiratory impairment, sleep apnoea or unidentified respiratory infection. Patients with PWS and one or more of these risk factors may be at greater risk.

Patients with PWS should be evaluated for upper airway obstruction, sleep apnoea or respiratory infections before initiation of treatment with somatropin.

In case of signs of upper airway obstruction, the problem should be solved by a specialist before starting treatment with somatropin.

Sleep apnoea should be assessed before onset of growth hormone treatment by recognised methods such as polysomnography or overnight oxymetry, and monitored if sleep apnoea is suspected.

If during treatment with somatropin patients show signs of upper airway obstruction (including onset of or increased snoring), treatment should be interrupted, and a new ENT assessment performed.

All patients with PWS should be evaluated for sleep apnoea and monitored if sleep apnoea is suspected.

All patients with PWS should be monitored for signs of respiratory infections which should be diagnosed as early as possible and treated aggressively.

All patients with PWS should have effective weight control before and during treatment with somatropin.

Scoliosis is common in patients with PWS. Scoliosis may progress in any child during rapid growth. Signs of scoliosis should be monitored during treatment. However, growth hormone treatment has not been shown to increase the incidence or severity of scoliosis.

Experience with long term treatment in adults and in patients with PWS is limited.

In short children/adolescents born SGA, other medical reasons or treatments that could explain growth disturbance should be ruled out before starting treatment.

In SGA children/adolescents it is recommended to measure fasting insulin and blood glucose before start of treatment and annually thereafter. In patients with increased risk for diabetes mellitus (e.g. familial history of diabetes, obesity, severe insulin resistance, acanthosis nigricans) oral glucose tolerance testing (OGTT) should be performed. If overt diabetes occurs, growth hormone should not be administered.

In SGA children/adolescents it is recommended to measure the IGF-I level before start of treatment and twice a year thereafter. If on repeated measurements IGF-I levels exceed +2 SD compared to references for age and pubertal status, the IGF-I / IGFBP-3 ratio could be taken into account to consider dose adjustment.

Experience in initiating treatment in SGA patients near onset of puberty is limited. It is therefore not recommended to initiate treatment near onset of puberty. Experience in patients with Silver-Russell syndrome is limited.

Some of the height gain obtained with treating short children/adolescents born SGA with growth hormone may be lost if treatment is stopped before final height is reached.

In chronic renal insufficiency, renal function should be below 50 percent of normal before institution of therapy. To verify growth disturbance, growth should be followed for a year preceding institution of therapy. During this period, conservative treatment for renal insufficiency (which includes control of acidosis, hyperparathyroidism and nutritional status) should have been established and should be maintained during treatment.

The treatment should be discontinued at renal transplantation.

To date, no data on final height in patients with chronic renal insufficiency treated with Omnitrope are available.

The effects of somatropin on recovery were studied in two placebo controlled trials involving 522 critically ill adult patients suffering complications following open heart surgery, abdominal surgery, multiple accidental trauma or acute respiratory failure. Mortality was higher in patients treated with 5.3 or 8 mg somatropin daily compared to patients receiving placebo, 42% vs. 19%. Based on this information, these types of patients should not be treated with somatropin. As there is no information available on the safety of growth hormone substitution therapy in acutely critically ill patients, the benefits of continued treatment in this situation should be weighed against the potential risks involved.

In all patients developing other or similar acute critical illness, the possible benefit of treatment with somatropin must be weighed against the potential risk involved.

This medicinal product contains less than 1 mmol sodium (23 mg) per ml, i.e. essentially 'sodium- free'.

4.5 Interaction with other medicinal products and other forms of interaction

Data from an interaction study performed in growth hormone deficient adults suggests that somatropin administration may increase the clearance of compounds known to be metabolised by cytochrome P450 isoenzymes. The clearance of compounds metabolised by cytochrome P 450 3A4 (e.g. sex steroids, corticosteroids, anticonvulsants and ciclosporin) may be especially increased resulting in lower plasma levels of these compounds. The clinical significance of this is unknown.

Also see section 4.4 for statements regarding diabetes mellitus and thyroid disorder and section 4.2 for statement on oral oestrogen replacement therapy.

4.6 Pregnancy and lactation

For Omnitrope no clinical data on exposed pregnancies are available. Animal experimental data on reproductive toxicity of Omnitrope are not available. Treatment with Omnitrope should be interrupted if pregnancy occurs.

During normal pregnancy levels of pituitary growth hormone fall markedly after 20 gestation weeks, being replaced almost entirely by placental growth hormone by 30 weeks. In view of this, it is unlikely that continued replacement therapy with somatropin would be necessary in growth hormone deficient women in the third trimester of pregnancy.

It is not known if somatropin is excreted into breast milk, but absorption of intact protein from the gastrointestinal tract of the infant is extremely unlikely.

Caution should be exercised when Omnitrope is administered to breast-feeding women.

4.7 Effects on ability to drive and use machines

No studies on the effects on the ability to drive and use machines have been performed.

4.8 Undesirable effects

Within the organ system classes, adverse reactions are listed under headings of frequency (number of patients expected to experience the reaction), using the following categories: very common (⩾ 1/10); common (⩾ 1/100, < 1/10); uncommon (⩾ 1/1,000, < 1/100); rare (⩾ 1/10,000, < 1/1,000); very rare (< 1/10,000).

Patients with growth hormone deficiency are characterised by extracellular volume deficit. When treatment with somatropin is started this deficit is rapidly corrected. In adult patients, adverse reactions related to fluid retention, such as peripheral oedema, stiffness in the extremities, arthralgia, myalgia and paraesthesia are common. In general these adverse reactions are mild to moderate, arise within the first months of treatment and subside spontaneously or with dose-reduction. The incidence of these undesirable effects is related to the administered dose, the age of patients, and possibly inversely related to the age of patients at the onset of growth hormone deficiency. In paediatric patients such undesirable effects are uncommon.

Neoplasms benign, malignant and unspecified (incl cysts and polyps)

Very rare:	Leukemia. Very rare cases of leukaemia have been reported in growth hormone deficient paediatric patients treated with somatropin, but the incidence appears to be similar to that in the paediatric subjects without growth hormone deficiency.

Immune system disorders

Common:	Formation of antibodies. Somatropin has given rise to the formation of antibodies in approximately 1% of the patients. The binding capacity of these antibodies has been low and no clinical changes have been associated with their formation.

Endocrine disorders

Rare:	Diabetes mellitus type II

Nervous system disorders

Common:	In adults: paraesthesia
Uncommon:	In adults: carpal tunnel syndrome; In paediatric patients: paraesthesia
Rare:	Benign intracranial hypertension

Musculoskeletal and connective tissue disorders

Common:	In adults: stiffness in the extremities, arthralgia, myalgia
Uncommon:	In paediatric patients: stiffness in the extremities, arthralgia, myalgia

General disorders and administration site conditions

Common:	In adults: peripheral oedema; In paediatric patients: transient local skin reactions at the injection site
Uncommon:	In paediatric patients: peripheral oedema

4.9 Overdose

No case of overdose has been reported.

Acute overdose could lead initially to hypoglycaemia and subsequently to hyperglycaemia.

Long-term overdose could result in signs and symptoms consistent with the known effects of human growth hormone excess.

5. PHARMACOLOGICAL PROPERTIES

5.1 Pharmacodynamic properties

Pharmacotherapeutic group: anterior pituitary lobe hormones and analogues.

ATC code: H01AC01.

Somatropin is a potent metabolic hormone of importance for the metabolism of lipids, carbohydrates and proteins. In children with inadequate endogenous growth hormone, somatropin stimulates linear growth and increases growth rate. In adults as well as in children, somatropin maintains a normal body composition by increasing nitrogen retention and stimulation of skeletal muscle growth, and by mobilisation of body fat. Visceral adipose tissue is particularly responsive to somatropin. In addition to enhanced lipolysis, somatropin decreases the uptake of triglycerides into body fat stores. Serum concentrations of IGF-I (Insulin-like Growth Factor-I) and IGFBP3 (Insulin-like Growth Factor Binding Protein 3) are increased by somatropin. In addition, the following actions have been demonstrated.

Lipid metabolism:

Somatropin induces hepatic LDL cholesterol receptors, and affects the profile of serum lipids and lipoproteins. In general, administration of somatropin to growth hormone deficient patients results in reduction in serum LDL and apolipoprotein B. A reduction in serum total cholesterol may also be observed.

Carbohydrate metabolism:

Somatropin increases insulin but fasting blood glucose is commonly unchanged. Children with hypopituitarism may experience fasting hypoglycaemia. This condition is reversed by somatropin.

Water and mineral metabolism:

Growth hormone deficiency is associated with decreased plasma and extracellular volumes. Both are rapidly increased after treatment with somatropin. Somatropin induces the retention of sodium, potassium and phosphorus.

Bone metabolism:

Somatropin stimulates the turnover of skeletal bone. Long-term administration of somatropin to growth hormone deficient patients with osteopoenia results in an increase in bone mineral content and density at weight-bearing sites.

Physical capacity:

Muscle strength and physical exercise capacity are improved after long-term treatment with somatropin. Somatropin also increases cardiac output, but the mechanism has yet to be clarified. A decrease in peripheral vascular resistance may contribute to this effect.

In clinical trials in short children/adolescents born SGA doses of 0.033 and 0.067 mg somatropin/kg body weight per day have been used for treatment until final height is reached. In 56 patients who are continuously treated and have reached (near) final height, the mean change from height at start of treatment was +1.90 SDS (0.033 mg/kg body weight per day) and +2.19 SDS (0.067 mg/kg body weight per day). Literature data from untreated SGA children/adolescents without early spontaneous catch-up suggest a late growth of 0.5 SDS. Long-term safety data are still limited.

5.2 Pharmacokinetic properties

Absorption

The bioavailability of subcutaneously administered somatropin is approximately 80% in both healthy subjects and growth hormone deficient patients. A subcutaneous dose of 5 mg of Omnitrope 6.7 mg/ml solution for injection in healthy adults results in plasma Cmax and tmax values of 74 ± 22 μg/l and 3.9 ± 1.2 hours, respectively.

Elimination

The mean terminal half-life of somatropin after intravenous administration in growth hormone deficient adults is about 0.4 hours. However, after subcutaneous administration of Omnitrope 6.7 mg/ml solution for injection, a half-life of 3 hours is achieved. The observed difference is likely due to slow absorption from the injection site following subcutaneous administration.

Sub-populations

The absolute bioavailability of somatropin seems to be similar in males and females following subcutaneous administration.

Information about the pharmacokinetics of somatropin in geriatric and paediatric populations, in different races and in patients with renal, hepatic or cardiac insufficiency is either lacking or incomplete.

5.3 Preclinical safety data

In studies with Omnitrope regarding subacute toxicity and local tolerance, no clinically relevant effects have been observed.

In other studies with somatropin regarding general toxicity, local tolerance and reproduction toxicity no clinically relevant effects have been observed.

With somatropins, in vitro and in vivo genotoxicity studies on gene mutations and induction of chromosome aberrations have been negative.

An increased chromosome fragility has been observed in one *in vitro* study on lymphocytes taken from patients after long term treatment with somatropin and following the addition of the radiomimetic medicinal product bleomycin. The clinical significance of this finding is unclear.

In another study with somatropin, no increase in chromosomal abnormalities was found in the lymphocytes of patients who had received long-term somatropin therapy.

6. PHARMACEUTICAL PARTICULARS

6.1 List of excipients

disodium hydrogen phosphate heptahydrate

sodium dihydrogen phosphate dihydrate

glycine

poloxamer 188

phenol

water for injections

6.2 Incompatibilities

In the absence of compatibility studies, this medicinal product must not be mixed with other medicinal products.

6.3 Shelf life

18 months.

Shelf life after first use:

After first use the cartridge should remain in the pen and has to be kept in a refrigerator (2°C - 8°C) for a maximum of 28 days. Store and transport refrigerated (2°C - 8°C). Do not freeze. Store in the original pen in order to protect from light.

6.4 Special precautions for storage

Unopened cartridge: Store and transport refrigerated (2°C - 8°C). Do not freeze. Store in the original package in order to protect from light.

For storage conditions of the in-use medicinal product, see section 6.3.

6.5 Nature and contents of container

1.5 ml of solution in a cartridge (colourless type I glass) with plunger on one side (siliconised bromobutyl), a disc (bromobutyl) and a cap (aluminium) on the other side.

Pack sizes of 1, 5 and 10.

Not all pack sizes may be marketed.

6.6 Special precautions for disposal and other handling

Omnitrope 6.7 mg/ml solution for injection is a sterile, ready-to-use solution for subcutaneous injection filled in a glass cartridge.

This presentation is intended for multiple use. It should only be administered with the Omnitrope Pen 10, an injection device specifically developed for use with Omnitrope 6.7 mg/ml solution for injection. It has to be administered using sterile, disposable pen needles. Patients and caregivers have to receive appropriate training and instruction on the proper use of the Omnitrope cartridges and the pen from the physician or other suitable qualified health professionals.

The following is a general description of the administration process. The manufacturer's instructions with each pen must be followed for loading the cartridge, attaching the injection needle and for the administration.

1. Hands should be washed.

2. If the solution is cloudy or contains particulate matter, it should not be used. The content must be clear and colourless.

3. Disinfect the rubber membrane of the cartridge with a cleansing swab

4. Insert the cartridge into the Omnitrope Pen 10 following the instructions for use provided with the pen.

5. Clean the site of injection with an alcohol swab.

6. Administer the appropriate dose by subcutaneous injection using a sterile pen needle. Remove the pen needle and dispose of it in accordance with local requirements.

7. MARKETING AUTHORISATION HOLDER

Sandoz GmbH

Biochemiestrasse 10

A-6250 Kundl

Austria

8. MARKETING AUTHORISATION NUMBER(S)

EU/1/06/332/007

EU/1/06/332/008

EU/1/06/332/009

9. DATE OF FIRST AUTHORISATION/RENEWAL OF THE AUTHORISATION

12 April 2006

10. DATE OF REVISION OF THE TEXT

18 March 2008

Ondemet 2mg/ml Injection

(Beacon Pharmaceuticals)

1. NAME OF THE MEDICINAL PRODUCT

Ondemet 2mg/ml Injection

2. QUALITATIVE AND QUANTITATIVE COMPOSITION

1 ml solution for injection and infusion contains 2mg ondansetron as ondansetron hydrochloride dihydrate.

Each 2 ml ampoule contains 4 mg of ondansetron

Each 4 ml ampoule contains 8 mg of ondansetron.

For excipients, see section 6.1.

3. PHARMACEUTICAL FORM

Solution for injection and infusion, ampoule.

Clear solution.

4. CLINICAL PARTICULARS

4.1 Therapeutic indications

Ondemet 2mg/ml Injection is indicated for the management of nausea and vomiting induced by cytotoxic chemotherapy and radiotherapy, and for the prevention of post-operative nausea and vomiting (PONV).

4.2 Posology and method of administration

For intravenous injection or after dilution for intravenous infusion.

Chemotherapy and radiotherapy induced nausea and vomiting

Adults

The emetogenic potential of cancer treatment varies according to the doses and combinations of chemotherapy and radiotherapy regimens used. The route of administration and dose of ondansetron should be flexible and selected as shown below.

Emetogenic chemotherapy and radiotherapy

For patients receiving emetogenic chemotherapy or radiotherapy ondansetron can be given either by oral or intravenous administration.

For most patients receiving emetogenic chemotherapy or radiotherapy, ondansetron should initially be administered intravenously immediately before treatment, followed by 8 mg orally twelve hourly.

For oral administration: 8 mg 1-2 hours before treatment, followed by 8 mg 12 hours later.

To protect against delayed or prolonged emesis after the first 24 hours, oral treatment with ondansetron should be continued for up to 5 days after a course of treatment. The recommended dose for oral administration is 8 mg twice daily.

Highly emetogenic chemotherapy

Adults: Either 8 mg as a slow intravenous bolus injection or as a short-term infusion lasting 15 minutes immediately before chemotherapy. If this initial dose has insufficient effect it can be supplemented by either 8 mg (intravenous bolus or 15 minutes infusion) every 4th hour, at most twice, or continuous infusion of 1 mg/hour for 24 hours. In some cases the initial dose can be increased to 32 mg diluted with a compatible infusion fluid as an infusion lasting at least 15 minutes immediately before chemotherapy.

After 24 hours treatment is changed to the oral route.

The effect of ondansetron may be enhanced by the simultaneous administration of 20 mg dexamethasone intravenously or an equally potent dose of another glucocorticoid for intravenous use.

Children (aged 2 years and over) and adolescents (< 18 years)

Experience in paediatric patients is limited. In children older than two years, ondansetron may be administered as a single intravenous dose of 5 mg/m^2 over 15 minutes immediately before chemotherapy, followed by 4 mg orally twelve hours later. Oral treatment with a dose according to the body area should be continued for up to 5 days after a course of treatment. Children with a total body area between 0.6 and 1.2 m^2 should receive a dosage schedule of 4 mg 3 times a day, while children with a body area above 1.2 m^2 should receive 8 mg 3 times a day.

There is no experience in children younger than 2 years old.

Ondemet 2mg/ml Injection cannot be used in children with a total body surface below 0.6 m^2.

Elderly

Ondansetron is well tolerated by patients over 65 years and no alteration of dosage, dosing frequency or route of administration are required.

Please refer also to "Special populations".

Post-operative nausea and vomiting (PONV)

Prevention of PONV

For the prevention of PONV ondansetron can be administered orally or by intravenous injection.

Adults: 8 mg as a slow intravenous bolus injection at induction of anaesthesia.

Children aged 2 years and over: 0.1 mg/kg up to a maximum of 4 mg as a slow intravenous bolus injection either before, at or after induction of anaesthesia.

Treatment of established PONV

For the treatment of established PONV intravenous administration is recommended.

Up to 8 mg as a slow bolus injection intravenously or intramuscularly.

Children (aged 2 years and over) and adolescents (< 18 years)

For the prevention and treatment of PONV slow intravenous injection is recommended.

0.1 mg/kg up to a maximum of 4 mg as a slow intravenous bolus injection

Elderly

There is limited experience in the use of ondansetron in the prevention and treatment of post-operative nausea and vomiting (PONV) in the elderly, however ondansetron is well tolerated in patients over 65 years receiving chemotherapy.

Please refer also to "Special populations".

Special populations

Patients with renal impairment

No alteration of daily dosage or frequency of dosing, or route of administration are required.

Patients with hepatic impairment

Clearance of ondansetron is significantly reduced and serum half life significantly prolonged in subjects with moderate or severe impairment of hepatic function. In such patients a total daily dose of 8 mg should not be exceeded.

Patients with poor sparteine/debrisoquine metabolism

The elimination half-life of ondansetron is not altered in subjects classified as poor metabolisers of sparteine and debrisoquine. Consequently in such patients, repeat dosing will give medicinal product exposure levels no different from those of the general population. No alteration of daily dosage or frequency of dosing are required.

4.3 Contraindications
Hypersensitivity to ondansetron or to other selective 5-HT3-receptor antagonists (e.g. granisetron, dolasetron) or to any of the excipients.

4.4 Special warnings and precautions for use
Hypersensitivity reactions have been reported in patients who have exhibited hypersensitivity to other selective 5-HT3 receptor antagonists.

As ondansetron is known to increase large bowel transit time, patients with signs of subacute intestinal obstruction should be monitored following administration.

In patients with adenotonsillar surgery prevention of nausea and vomiting with ondansetron may mask occult bleeding. Therefore, such patients should be followed carefully after ondansetron.

Since there is little experience to date of the use of ondansetron in cardiac patients, caution should be exercised if ondansetron is coadministered with anaesthetics to patients with arrhythmias or cardiac conduction disorders or to patients who are being treated with antiarrhythmic agents or beta-blockers.

The solution for injection contains less than 1 mmol sodium (23 mg) per ampoule, i.e. essentially 'sodium- free'.

Ondemet 2mg/ml Injection should not be used in children with a total body surface below 0.6 m^2.

The medicinal product should not be used for children younger than two years, as for these patients the experience is limited.

4.5 Interaction with other medicinal products and other forms of interaction
There is no evidence that ondansetron either induces or inhibits the metabolism of other medicinal products commonly coadministered with it. Specific studies have shown that ondansetron does not interact with alcohol, temazepam, furosemide, alfentanil, propofol and thiopental.

Ondansetron is metabolised by multiple hepatic cytochrome P-450 enzymes: CYP3A4, CYP2D6 and CYP1A2. Due to the multiplicity of metabolic enzymes capable of metabolising ondansetron, enzyme inhibition or reduced activity of one enzyme (e.g. CYP2D6 genetic deficiency) is normally compensated by other enzymes and should result in little or no significant change in overall ondansetron clearance or dose requirement.

Phenytoin, Carbamazepine and Rifampicin: In patients treated with potent inducers of CYP3A4 (i.e. phenytoin, carbamazepine, and rifampicin), the clearance of ondansetron was increased and ondansetron blood concentrations were decreased.

Tramadol: Data from small studies indicate that ondansetron may reduce the analgesic effect of tramadol.

4.6 Pregnancy and lactation
Pregnancy
Data on a limited number of exposed pregnancies indicate no adverse effects of ondansetron on pregnancy or on the health of the foetus/newborn child. To date, no other relevant epidemiological data are available. Animal studies do not indicate direct or indirect harmful effects with respect to pregnancy, embryonal/foetal development, parturition or postnatal development. Use in human pregnancy has not been established and is not recommended. If it is absolutely necessary that ondansetron be given caution should be exercised when prescribing to pregnant women especially in the first trimester. A careful risk/benefit assessment should be performed.

Lactation
Tests have shown that ondansetron passes into the milk of lactating animals (see section 5.3). It is therefore recommended that mothers receiving ondansetron should not breast-feed their babies.

4.7 Effects on ability to drive and use machines
Ondansetron has no or negligible influence on the ability to drive and use machines.

4.8 Undesirable effects
Adverse events are listed below by system organ class and frequency. Frequencies are defined as: very common (≥ 1/10), common (≥ 1/100 and < 1/10), uncommon (≥ 1/1000 and < 1/100), rare (≥ 1/10,000 and < 1/1000) and very rare (< 1/10,000) including isolated reports. Very common, common and uncommon events were generally determined from clinical trial data. The incidence in placebo was taken into account. Rare and very rare events were generally determined from post-marketing spontaneous data.

The following frequencies are estimated at the standard recommended doses of ondansetron according to indication and formulation.

Immune system disorders
Rare: Immediate hypersensitivity reactions sometimes severe, including anaphylaxis.

Nervous system disorders
Very common: Headache.

Uncommon: Extrapyramidal reactions (such as oculogyric crisis/dystonic reactions) have been observed without definitive evidence of persistent clinical sequelae; seizures.

Rare: Dizziness during rapid intravenous administration.

Eye disorders
Rare: Transient visual disturbances (eg. blurred vision) predominantly during rapid intravenous administration.

Very rare: transient blindness predominantly during intravenous administration.

The majority of the blindness cases reported resolved within 20 minutes. Most patients had received chemotherapeutic agents, which included cisplatin. Some cases of transient blindness were reported as cortical in origin.

Cardiac disorders
Uncommon: Arrhythmias, chest pain with or without ST segment depression, bradycardia.

Vascular disorders
Common: Sensation of warmth or flushing.

Uncommon: Hypotension.

Respiratory, thoracic and mediastinal disorders
Uncommon: Hiccups.

Gastrointestinal disorders
Common: Constipation. Local burning sensation following insertion of suppositories.

Hepatobiliary disorders
Uncommon: Asymptomatic increases in liver function tests.

These events were observed commonly in patients receiving chemotherapy with cisplatin.

General disorders and administration site conditions
Common: Local intravenous injection site reactions

4.9 Overdose
Little is known at present about overdosage with ondansetron, however, a limited number of patients received overdoses. Manifestations that have been reported include visual disturbances, severe constipation, hypotension and a vasovagal episode with transient second degree AV block. In all instances, the events resolved completely. There is no specific antidote for ondansetron, therefore in all cases of suspected overdose, symptomatic and supportive therapy should be given as appropriate.

5. PHARMACOLOGICAL PROPERTIES

5.1 Pharmacodynamic properties
Pharmacotherapeutic group: Antiemetics and antinauseants, Serotonin (5-HT3) antagonists

ATC Code: A04AA01

Ondansetron is a potent, highly selective 5-HT3 receptor-antagonist.

Its precise antiemetic and antinauseant mechanism of action is not known. Chemotherapeutic agents and radiotherapy may cause release of 5-HT in the small intestine initiating a vomiting reflex by activating vagal afferents via 5-HT3 receptors. Ondansetron blocks the initiation of this reflex. Activation of vagal afferents may also cause a release of 5-HT in the area postrema, located on the floor of the fourth ventricle, and this may also promote emesis through a central mechanism. Thus, the effect of ondansetron in the management of the nausea and vomiting induced by cytotoxic chemotherapy and radiotherapy is probably due to antagonism of 5-HT3 receptors on neurons located both in the peripheral and central nervous system. The mechanisms of action in post-operative nausea and vomiting are not known but there may be common pathways with cytotoxic induced nausea and vomiting.

In a pharmaco-psychological study in volunteers ondansetron has not shown a sedative effect.

Ondansetron does not alter plasma prolactin concentrations.

The role of ondansetron in opiate-induced emesis is not yet established.

5.2 Pharmacokinetic properties
Following oral administration, ondansetron is passively and completely absorbed from the gastrointestinal tract and undergoes first pass metabolism (bioavailability is about 60%). Peak plasma concentrations of about 30 ng/ml are attained approximately 1.5 hours after an 8 mg dose. For doses above 8 mg the increase in ondansetron systemic exposure with dose is greater than proportional; this may reflect some reduction in first pass metabolism at higher oral doses. Bioavailability, following oral administration, is slightly enhanced by the presence of food but unaffected by antacids. Studies in healthy elderly volunteers have shown slight, but clinically insignificant, age-related increases in both oral bioavailability (65%) and half-life (5 hours) of ondansetron. Gender differences were shown in the disposition of ondansetron, with females having a greater rate and extent of absorption following an oral dose and reduced systemic clearance and volume of distribution (adjusted for weight).

The disposition of ondansetron following oral, intramuscular(IM) and intravenous(IV) dosing is similar with a terminal half life of about 3 hours and steady state volume of distribution of about 140 L. Equivalent systemic exposure is achieved after IM and IV administration of ondansetron.

The protein binding of ondansetron is 70-76%. A direct effect of plasma concentration and anti-emetic effect has not been established. Ondansetron is cleared from the systemic circulation predominantly by hepatic metabolism through multiple enzymatic pathways. Less than 5% of the absorbed dose is excreted unchanged in the urine. The absence of the enzyme CYP2D6 has no effect on ondansetron's pharmacokinetics. The pharmacokinetic properties of ondansetron are unchanged on repeat dosing.

Following oral, intravenous or intramuscular dosing in patients with severe hepatic impairment, ondansetron's systemic clearance is markedly reduced with prolonged elimination half-lives (15-32 h) and an oral bioavailability approaching 100% due to reduced pre-systemic metabolism.

5.3 Preclinical safety data
Preclinical data revealed no special hazard for humans based on conventional studies of safety pharmacology, repeated dose toxicity, genotoxicity and carcinogenic potential.

Ondansetron and its metabolites accumulate in the milk of rats, milk/plasma-ratio was 5.2.

A study in cloned human cardiac ion channels has shown ondansetron has the potential to affect cardiac repolarisation via blockade of HERG potassium channels. The clinical relevance of this finding is uncertain.

6. PHARMACEUTICAL PARTICULARS

6.1 List of excipients
Sodium chloride.

Citric acid monohydrate.

Sodium citrate.

Water for injections.

6.2 Incompatibilities
This medicinal product must not be mixed with other medicinal products except those mentioned in section 6.6.

6.3 Shelf life
Unopened 3 years.

After opening: 24 hours stored in a refrigerator (2-8°C).

6.4 Special precautions for storage
This medicinal product does not require any special storage precautions.

Chemical and physical in-use stability has been demonstrated for 24 hours at 2-8°C.

From a microbiological point of view, unless the method of opening/reconstitution/dilution precludes the risk of microbial contamination, the product should be used immediately.

If not used immediately, in-use storage times and conditions are the responsibility of the user

6.5 Nature and contents of container
Amber glass ampoules, type 1, containing 2 ml or 4 ml solution

Packs of 5 and 5 × 5 ampoules.

Not all pack sizes may be marketed.

6.6 Special precautions for disposal and other handling
For single use only. Any unused solution should be discarded.

The solution is to be visually inspected prior to use (also after dilution). Only clear solutions practically free from particles should be used.

May be diluted with solution for infusion containing: sodium chloride 9 mg/ml (0.9%), glucose 50 mg/ml (5 %), mannitol 100 mg/ml (10 %) potassium chloride 3 mg/ml (0.3%)+ sodium chloride 9 mg/ml (0.9 %) and potassium chloride 3 mg/ml (0.3%) + glucose 50 mg/ml (5 %) as well as Ringer solution for infusion.

Should not be mixed with other pharmaceutical products.

7. MARKETING AUTHORISATION HOLDER
Beacon Pharmaceuticals Ltd

The Regent

The Broadway

Crowborough

East Sussex,

TN6 1DA

UK.

8. MARKETING AUTHORISATION NUMBER(S)
PL 18157/0018

9. DATE OF FIRST AUTHORISATION/RENEWAL OF THE AUTHORISATION
24/03/2006

10. DATE OF REVISION OF THE TEXT
24/03/2006

Ondemet 4mg Tablets

(Beacon Pharmaceuticals)

1. NAME OF THE MEDICINAL PRODUCT
Ondemet 4mg Tablets

2. QUALITATIVE AND QUANTITATIVE COMPOSITION
Each film-coated tablet contains 4 mg ondansetron (as hydrochloride dihydrate).

For excipients, see section 6.1.

3. PHARMACEUTICAL FORM

Film coated tablet

Pale yellow, round biconvex, film-coated tablet embossed with 41 on one side, diameter 7.2 mm.

4. CLINICAL PARTICULARS

4.1 Therapeutic indications

Ondemet 4mg tablets is indicated for the management of nausea and vomiting induced by cytotoxic chemotherapy and radiotherapy, and for the prevention of post-operative nausea and vomiting (PONV).

4.2 Posology and method of administration

Oral use

For the different dosage regimens appropriate strengths and formulations are available.

Chemotherapy and radiotherapy induced nausea and vomiting

Adults

The emetogenic potential of cancer treatment varies according to the doses and combinations of chemotherapy and radiotherapy regimens used. The route of administration and dose of ondansetron should be flexible and selected as shown below.

Emetogenic chemotherapy and radiotherapy

For patients receiving emetogenic chemotherapy or radiotherapy ondansetron can be given either by oral or intravenous administration.

For most patients receiving emetogenic chemotherapy or radiotherapy, ondansetron should initially be administered intravenously immediately before treatment, followed by 8 mg orally twelve hourly.

For oral administration: 8 mg 1-2 hours before treatment, followed by 8 mg 12 hours later.

To protect against delayed or prolonged emesis after the first 24 hours, oral treatment with ondansetron should be continued for up to 5 days after a course of treatment. The recommended dose for oral administration is 8 mg twice daily.

Highly emetogenic chemotherapy

For patients receiving highly emetogenic chemotherapy, e.g. high-dose cisplatin, ondansetron can be given by intravenous administration.

To protect against delayed or prolonged emesis after the first 24 hours, oral treatment with ondansetron should be continued for up to 5 days after a course of treatment. The recommended dose for oral administration is 8 mg twice daily.

Children (aged 2 years and over) and adolescents (< 18 years)

Experience in paediatric patients is limited. In children older than two years, ondansetron may be administered as a single intravenous dose of 5 mg/m^2 over 15 minutes immediately before chemotherapy, followed by 4 mg orally twelve hours later. Oral treatment with a dose according to the body area should be continued for up to 5 days after a course of treatment. Children with a total body area between 0.6 and 1.2 m^2 should receive a dosage schedule of 4 mg 3 times a day, while children with a body area above 1.2 m^2 should receive 8 mg 3 times a day.

There is no experience in children younger than 2 years old.

Ondemet Tablets cannot be used in children with a total body surface below 0.6 m^2.

Elderly

Ondansetron is well tolerated by patients over 65 years and no alteration of dosage, dosing frequency or route of administration are required.

Please refer also to "Special populations".

Post-operative nausea and vomiting (PONV)

Adults

Prevention of PONV

For the prevention of PONV ondansetron can be administered orally or by intravenous injection.

For oral administration:

16 mg one hour prior to anaesthesia.

Alternatively, 8 mg one hour prior to anaesthesia followed by two further doses of 8 mg at eight hourly intervals.

Treatment of established PONV

For the treatment of established PONV intravenous administration is recommended.

Children (aged 2 years and over) and adolescents (< 18 years)

For the prevention and treatment of PONV slow intravenous injection is recommended.

Elderly

There is limited experience in the use of ondansetron in the prevention and treatment of post-operative nausea and vomiting (PONV) in the elderly, however ondansetron is well tolerated in patients over 65 years receiving chemotherapy.

Please refer also to "Special populations".

Special populations

Patients with renal impairment

No alteration of daily dosage or frequency of dosing, or route of administration are required.

Patients with hepatic impairment

Clearance of Ondansetron is significantly reduced and serum half life significantly prolonged in subjects with moderate or severe impairment of hepatic function. In such patients a total daily dose of 8 mg should not be exceeded.

Patients with poor sparteine/debrisoquine metabolism

The elimination half-life of ondansetron is not altered in subjects classified as poor metabolisers of sparteine and debrisoquine. Consequently in such patients, repeat dosing will give medicinal product exposure levels no different from those of the general population. No alteration of daily dosage or frequency of dosing are required.

4.3 Contraindications

Hypersensitivity to ondansetron or to other selective 5-HT3-receptor antagonists (e.g. granisetron, dolasetron) or to any of the excipients.

4.4 Special warnings and precautions for use

Hypersensitivity reactions have been reported in patients who have exhibited hypersensitivity to other selective 5-HT3 receptor antagonists.

As ondansetron is known to increase large bowel transit time, patients with signs of subacute intestinal obstruction should be monitored following administration.

In patients with adenotonsillar surgery prevention of nausea and vomiting with ondansetron may mask occult bleeding. Therefore, such patients should be followed carefully after ondansetron.

Since there is little experience to date of the use of ondansetron in cardiac patients, caution should be exercised if ondansetron is coadministered with anaesthetics to patients with arrhythmias or cardiac conduction disorders or to patients who are being treated with antiarrhythmic agents or beta-blockers.

Patients with rare hereditary problems of galactose intolerance, Lapp lactase deficiency or glucose-galactose malabsorption should not take this medicine.

Ondemet Tablets should not be used in children with a total body surface below 0.6 m^2.

The medicinal product should not be used for children younger than two years, as for these patients the experience is limited.

4.5 Interaction with other medicinal products and other forms of interaction

There is no evidence that ondansetron either induces or inhibits the metabolism of other medicinal products commonly coadministered with it. Specific studies have shown that ondansetron does not interact with alcohol, temazepam, furosemide, alfentanil, propofol and thiopental.

Ondansetron is metabolised by multiple hepatic cytochrome P-450 enzymes: CYP3A4, CYP2D6 and CYP1A2. Due to the multiplicity of metabolic enzymes capable of metabolising ondansetron, enzyme inhibition or reduced activity of one enzyme (e.g. CYP2D6 genetic deficiency) is normally compensated by other enzymes and should result in little or no significant change in overall ondansetron clearance or dose requirement.

Phenytoin, Carbamazepine and Rifampicin: In patients treated with potent inducers of CYP3A4 (i.e. phenytoin, carbamazepine, and rifampicin), the clearance of ondansetron was increased and ondansetron blood concentrations were decreased.

Tramadol: Data from small studies indicate that ondansetron may reduce the analgesic effect of tramadol.

4.6 Pregnancy and lactation

Pregnancy

Use in pregnancy has not been established and is not recommended.

Data on a limited number of exposed pregnancies indicate no adverse effects of ondansetron on pregnancy or on the health of the foetus/newborn child. To date, no other relevant epidemiological data are available. Animal studies do not indicate direct or indirect harmful effects with respect to pregnancy, embryonal/foetal development, parturition or postnatal development. Use in human pregnancy has not been established and is not recommended. If it is absolutely necessary that Ondansetron be given caution should be exercised when prescribing to pregnant women especially in the first trimester. A careful risk/benefit assessment should be performed.

Lactation

Tests have shown that ondansetron passes into the milk of lactating animals (see section 5.3). It is therefore recommended that mothers receiving ondansetron should not breast-feed their babies.

4.7 Effects on ability to drive and use machines

Ondansetron has no or negligible influence on the ability to drive and use machines.

4.8 Undesirable effects

Adverse events are listed below by system organ class and frequency. Frequencies are defined as: very common (≥ 1/10), common (≥ 1/100 and < 1/10), uncommon (≥ 1/1000 and < 1/100), rare (≥ 1/10,000 and < 1/1000) and very rare (< 1/10,000) including isolated reports. Very common, common and uncommon events were generally determined from clinical trial data. The incidence in placebo was taken into account. Rare and very rare events were generally determined from post-marketing spontaneous data.

The following frequencies are estimated at the standard recommended doses of ondansetron according to indication and formulation.

Immune system disorders

Rare: Immediate hypersensitivity reactions sometimes severe, including anaphylaxis.

Nervous system disorders

Very common: Headache.

Uncommon: Extrapyramidal reactions (such as oculogyric crisis/dystonic reactions) have been observed without definitive evidence of persistent clinical sequelae; seizures.

Rare: Dizziness during rapid intravenous administration.

Eye disorders

Rare: Transient visual disturbances (eg. blurred vision) predominantly during rapid intravenous administration.

Very rare: transient blindness predominantly during intravenous administration.

The majority of the blindness cases reported resolved within 20 minutes. Most patients had received chemotherapeutic agents, which included cisplatin. Some cases of transient blindness were reported as cortical in origin.

Cardiac disorders

Uncommon: Arrhythmias, chest pain with or without ST segment depression, bradycardia.

Vascular disorders

Common: Sensation of warmth or flushing.

Uncommon: Hypotension.

Respiratory, thoracic and mediastinal disorders

Uncommon: Hiccups.

Gastrointestinal disorders

Common: Constipation. Local burning sensation following insertion of suppositories.

Hepatobiliary disorders

Uncommon: Asymptomatic increases in liver function tests.

These events were observed commonly in patients receiving chemotherapy with cisplatin.

General disorders and administration site conditions

Common: Local intravenous injection site reactions.

4.9 Overdose

Little is known at present about overdosage with ondansetron, however, a limited number of patients received overdoses. Manifestations that have been reported include visual disturbances, severe constipation, hypotension and a vasovagal episode with transient second degree AV block. In all instances, the events resolved completely. There is no specific antidote for ondansetron, therefore in all cases of suspected overdose, symptomatic and supportive therapy should be given as appropriate.

5. PHARMACOLOGICAL PROPERTIES

5.1 Pharmacodynamic properties

Pharmacotherapeutic group: Antiemetics and antinauseants, Serotonin (5-HT3) antagonists

ATC Code: A04AA01

Ondansetron is a potent, highly selective 5-HT3 receptor-antagonist.

Its precise antiemetic and antinauseal mechanism of action is not known. Chemotherapeutic agents and radiotherapy may cause release of 5-HT in the small intestine initiating a vomiting reflex by activating vagal afferents via 5-HT3 receptors. Ondansetron blocks the initiation of this reflex. Activation of vagal afferents may also cause a release of 5-HT in the area postrema, located on the floor of the fourth ventricle, and this may also promote emesis through a central mechanism. Thus, the effect of ondansetron in the management of the nausea and vomiting induced by cytotoxic chemotherapy and radiotherapy is probably due to antagonism of 5-HT3 receptors on neurons located both in the peripheral and central nervous system. The mechanisms of action in post-operative nausea and vomiting are not known but there may be common pathways with cytotoxic induced nausea and vomiting.

In a pharmaco-psychological study in volunteers ondansetron has not shown a sedative effect.

Ondansetron does not alter plasma prolactin concentrations.

The role of ondansetron in opiate-induced emesis is not yet established.

5.2 Pharmacokinetic properties

Following oral administration, ondansetron is passively and completely absorbed from the gastrointestinal tract and undergoes first pass metabolism (bioavailability is about 60%). Peak plasma concentrations of about 30 ng/ml are attained approximately 1.5 hours after an 8 mg dose. For doses above 8 mg the increase in ondansetron systemic exposure with dose is greater than proportional; this may reflect some reduction in first pass metabolism at higher oral doses. Bioavailability, following oral administration, is slightly enhanced by the presence of food but unaffected by antacids. Studies in healthy elderly volunteers have shown slight, but clinically insignificant, age-related increases in both oral bioavailability (65%) and half-life (5 hours) of ondansetron. Gender differences were shown in the disposition of ondansetron, with females having a greater rate and extent of absorption following an oral dose and reduced systemic clearance and volume of distribution (adjusted for weight).

The disposition of ondansetron following oral, intramuscular(IM) and intravenous(IV) dosing is similar with a terminal half life of about 3 hours and steady state volume of distribution of about 140 L. Equivalent systemic exposure is achieved after IM and IV administration of ondansetron.

The protein binding of ondansetron is 70-76%. A direct effect of plasma concentration and anti-emetic effect has not been established. Ondansetron is cleared from the systemic circulation predominantly by hepatic metabolism through multiple enzymatic pathways. Less than 5% of the absorbed dose is excreted unchanged in the urine. The absence of the enzyme CYP2D6 has no effect on ondansetron's pharmacokinetics. The pharmacokinetic properties of ondansetron are unchanged on repeat dosing.

Following oral, intravenous or intramuscular dosing in patients with severe hepatic impairment, ondansetron's systemic clearance is markedly reduced with prolonged elimination half-lives (15-32 h) and an oral bioavailability approaching 100% due to reduced pre-systemic metabolism.

5.3 Preclinical safety data

Preclinical data revealed no special hazard for humans based on conventional studies of safety pharmacology, repeated dose toxicity, genotoxicity and carcinogenic potential.

Ondansetron and its metabolites accumulate in the milk of rats, milk/plasma-ratio was 5.2.

A study in cloned human cardiac ion channels has shown ondansetron has the potential to affect cardiac repolarisation via blockade of HERG potassium channels. The clinical relevance of this finding is uncertain.

6. PHARMACEUTICAL PARTICULARS

6.1 List of excipients

Tablet core:

Cellulose, microcrystalline

Lactose monohydrate

Starch, pregelatinised (maize)

Magnesium stearate

Film coating:

Hypromellose

Hydroxypropylcellulose

Propylene glycol

Sorbitan oleate

Sorbic acid

Vanillin

Titanium dioxide (E171)

Quinoline yellow (E 104).

6.2 Incompatibilities

Not applicable.

6.3 Shelf life

3 years.

6.4 Special precautions for storage

This medicinal product does not require any special storage precautions.

6.5 Nature and contents of container

Blister (PVC/Al)

4 mg: 10, 50 and 100 film coated tablets.

Not all pack sizes may be marketed.

6.6 Special precautions for disposal and other handling

No special requirements.

7. MARKETING AUTHORISATION HOLDER

Beacon Pharmaceuticals Ltd

The Regent

The Broadway

Crowborough

East Sussex

TN6 1DA

UK

8. MARKETING AUTHORISATION NUMBER(S)

PL 18157/0016

9. DATE OF FIRST AUTHORISATION/RENEWAL OF THE AUTHORISATION

24/03/2006

10. DATE OF REVISION OF THE TEXT

24/03/2006

Ondemet 8 mg Tablets

(Beacon Pharmaceuticals)

1. NAME OF THE MEDICINAL PRODUCT

Ondemet 8mg Tablets

2. QUALITATIVE AND QUANTITATIVE COMPOSITION

Each film-coated tablet contains 8 mg ondansetron (as hydrochloride dihydrate).

For excipients, see section 6.1.

3. PHARMACEUTICAL FORM

Film coated tablet

Pale yellow, round biconvex, film-coated tablet embossed 42 on one side, diameter 9.2 mm

4. CLINICAL PARTICULARS

4.1 Therapeutic indications

Ondemet 8mg Tablets is indicated for the management of nausea and vomiting induced by cytotoxic chemotherapy and radiotherapy, and for the prevention of post-operative nausea and vomiting (PONV).

4.2 Posology and method of administration

Oral use

For the different dosage regimens appropriate strengths and formulations are available.

Chemotherapy and radiotherapy induced nausea and vomiting

Adults

The emetogenic potential of cancer treatment varies according to the doses and combinations of chemotherapy and radiotherapy regimens used. The route of administration and dose of Ondansetron should be flexible and selected as shown below.

Emetogenic chemotherapy and radiotherapy

For patients receiving emetogenic chemotherapy or radiotherapy ondansetron can be given either by oral or intravenous administration.

For most patients receiving emetogenic chemotherapy or radiotherapy, ondansetron should initially be administered intravenously immediately before treatment, followed by 8 mg orally twelve hourly.

For oral administration: 8 mg 1-2 hours before treatment, followed by 8 mg 12 hours later.

To protect against delayed or prolonged emesis after the first 24 hours, oral treatment with ondansetron should be continued for up to 5 days after a course of treatment. The recommended dose for oral administration is 8 mg twice daily.

Highly emetogenic chemotherapy

For patients receiving highly emetogenic chemotherapy, e.g. high-dose cisplatin, ondansetron can be given by intravenous administration.

To protect against delayed or prolonged emesis after the first 24 hours, oral treatment with ondansetron should be continued for up to 5 days after a course of treatment. The recommended dose for oral administration is 8 mg twice daily.

Children (aged 2 years and over) and adolescents (< 18 years)

Experience in paediatric patients is limited. In children older than two years, ondansetron may be administered as a single intravenous dose of 5 mg/m^2 over 15 minutes immediately before chemotherapy, followed by 4 mg orally twelve hours later. Oral treatment with a dose according to the body area should be continued for up to 5 days after a course of treatment. Children with a total body area between 0.6 and 1.2 m^2 should receive a dosage schedule of 4 mg 3 times a day, while children with a body area above 1.2 m^2 should receive 8 mg 3 times a day.

There is no experience in children younger than 2 years old.

Ondemet Tablets cannot be used in children with a total body surface below 0.6 m^2.

Elderly

Ondansetron is well tolerated by patients over 65 years and no alteration of dosage, dosing frequency or route of administration are required.

Please refer also to "Special populations".

Post-operative nausea and vomiting (PONV)

Adults

Prevention of PONV

For the prevention of PONV ondansetron can be administered orally or by intravenous injection.

For oral administration:

16 mg one hour prior to anaesthesia.

Alternatively, 8 mg one hour prior to anaesthesia followed by two further doses of 8 mg at eight hourly intervals.

Treatment of established PONV

For the treatment of established PONV intravenous administration is recommended.

Children (aged 2 years and over) and adolescents (< 18 years)

For the prevention and treatment of PONV slow intravenous injection is recommended.

Elderly

There is limited experience in the use of ondansetron in the prevention and treatment of post-operative nausea and vomiting (PONV) in the elderly, however ondansetron is well tolerated in patients over 65 years receiving chemotherapy.

Please refer also to "Special populations".

Special populations

Patients with renal impairment

No alteration of daily dosage or frequency of dosing, or route of administration are required.

Patients with hepatic impairment

Clearance of Ondansetron is significantly reduced and serum half life significantly prolonged in subjects with moderate or severe impairment of hepatic function. In such patients a total daily dose of 8 mg should not be exceeded.

Patients with poor sparteine/debrisoquine metabolism

The elimination half-life of ondansetron is not altered in subjects classified as poor metabolisers of sparteine and debrisoquine. Consequently in such patients, repeat dosing will give medicinal product exposure levels no different from those of the general population. No alteration of daily dosage or frequency of dosing are required.

4.3 Contraindications

Hypersensitivity to ondansetron or to other selective 5-HT3-receptor antagonists (e.g. granisetron, dolasetron) or to any of the excipients.

4.4 Special warnings and precautions for use

Hypersensitivity reactions have been reported in patients who have exhibited hypersensitivity to other selective 5-HT3 receptor antagonists.

As ondansetron is known to increase large bowel transit time, patients with signs of subacute intestinal obstruction should be monitored following administration.

In patients with adenotonsillar surgery prevention of nausea and vomiting with ondansetron may mask occult bleeding. Therefore, such patients should be followed carefully after ondansetron.

Since there is little experience to date of the use of ondansetron in cardiac patients, caution should be exercised if ondansetron is coadministered with anaesthetics to patients with arrhythmias or cardiac conduction disorders or to patients who are being treated with antiarrhythmic agents or beta-blockers.

Patients with rare hereditary problems of galactose intolerance, Lapp lactase deficiency or glucose-galactose malabsorption should not take this medicine.

Ondemet Tablets should not be used in children with a total body surface below 0.6 m^2.

The medicinal product should not be used for children younger than two years, as for these patients the experience is limited.

4.5 Interaction with other medicinal products and other forms of interaction

There is no evidence that ondansetron either induces or inhibits the metabolism of other medicinal products commonly coadministered with it. Specific studies have shown that ondansetron does not interact with alcohol, temazepam, furosemide, alfentanil, propofol and thiopental.

Ondansetron is metabolised by multiple hepatic cytochrome P-450 enzymes: CYP3A4, CYP2D6 and CYP1A2. Due to the multiplicity of metabolic enzymes capable of metabolising ondansetron, enzyme inhibition or reduced activity of one enzyme (e.g. CYP2D6 genetic deficiency) is normally compensated by other enzymes and should result in little or no significant change in overall ondansetron clearance or dose requirement.

Phenytoin, Carbamazepine and Rifampicin: In patients treated with potent inducers of CYP3A4 (i.e. phenytoin, carbamazepine, and rifampicin), the clearance of ondansetron was increased and ondansetron blood concentrations were decreased.

Tramadol: Data from small studies indicate that ondansetron may reduce the analgesic effect of tramadol.

4.6 Pregnancy and lactation

Pregnancy

Use in pregnancy has not been established and is not recommended.

Data on a limited number of exposed pregnancies indicate no adverse effects of ondansetron on pregnancy or on the health of the foetus/newborn child. To date, no other relevant epidemiological data are available. Animal studies do not indicate direct or indirect harmful effects with respect to pregnancy, embryonal/foetal development, parturition or postnatal development. Use in human pregnancy has not been established and is not recommended. If it is absolutely necessary that Ondansetron be given caution should be exercised when prescribing to pregnant women especially in the first trimester. A careful risk/benefit assessment should be performed.

Lactation

Tests have shown that ondansetron passes into the milk of lactating animals (see section 5.3). It is therefore recommended that mothers receiving ondansetron should not breast-feed their babies.

4.7 Effects on ability to drive and use machines

Ondansetron has no or negligible influence on the ability to drive and use machines.

4.8 Undesirable effects

Adverse events are listed below by system organ class and frequency. Frequencies are defined as: very common

(≥ 1/10), common (≥ 1/100 and < 1/10), uncommon (≥ 1/1000 and < 1/100), rare (≥ 1/10,000 and < 1/1000) and very rare (< 1/10,000) including isolated reports. Very common, common and uncommon events were generally determined from clinical trial data. The incidence in placebo was taken into account. Rare and very rare events were generally determined from post-marketing spontaneous data.

The following frequencies are estimated at the standard recommended doses of ondansetron according to indication and formulation.

Immune system disorders

Rare: Immediate hypersensitivity reactions sometimes severe, including anaphylaxis.

Nervous system disorders

Very common: Headache.

Uncommon: Extrapyramidal reactions (such as oculogyric crisis/dystonic reactions) have been observed without definitive evidence of persistent clinical sequelae; seizures.

Rare: Dizziness during rapid intravenous administration.

Eye disorders

Rare: Transient visual disturbances (eg. blurred vision) predominantly during rapid intravenous administration.

Very rare: transient blindness predominantly during intravenous administration.

The majority of the blindness cases reported resolved within 20 minutes. Most patients had received chemotherapeutic agents, which included cisplatin. Some cases of transient blindness were reported as cortical in origin.

Cardiac disorders

Uncommon: Arrhythmias, chest pain with or without ST segment depression, bradycardia.

Vascular disorders

Common: Sensation of warmth or flushing.

Uncommon: Hypotension.

Respiratory, thoracic and mediastinal disorders

Uncommon: Hiccups.

Gastrointestinal disorders

Common: Constipation. Local burning sensation following insertion of suppositories.

Hepatobiliary disorders

Uncommon: Asymptomatic increases in liver function tests.

These events were observed commonly in patients receiving chemotherapy with cisplatin.

General disorders and administration site conditions

Common: Local intravenous injection site reactions.

4.9 Overdose

Little is known at present about overdosage with ondansetron, however, a limited number of patients received overdoses. Manifestations that have been reported include visual disturbances, severe constipation, hypotension and a vasovagal episode with transient second degree AV block. In all instances, the events resolved completely. There is no specific antidote for ondansetron, therefore in all cases of suspected overdose, symptomatic and supportive therapy should be given as appropriate.

5. PHARMACOLOGICAL PROPERTIES

5.1 Pharmacodynamic properties

Pharmacotherapeutic group: Antiemetics and antinauseants, Serotonin (5-HT3) antagonists

ATC Code: A04AA01

Ondansetron is a potent, highly selective 5-HT3 receptor-antagonist.

Its precise antiemetic and antinauseal mechanism of action is not known. Chemotherapeutic agents and radiotherapy may cause release of 5-HT in the small intestine initiating a vomiting reflex by activating vagal afferents via 5-HT3 receptors. Ondansetron blocks the initiation of this reflex. Activation of vagal afferents may also cause a release of 5-HT in the area postrema, located on the floor of the fourth ventricle, and this may also promote emesis through a central mechanism. Thus, the effect of ondansetron in the management of the nausea and vomiting induced by cytotoxic chemotherapy and radiotherapy is probably due to antagonism of 5-HT3 receptors on neurons located both in the peripheral and central nervous system. The mechanisms of action in post-operative nausea and vomiting are not known but there may be common pathways with cytotoxic induced nausea and vomiting.

In a pharmaco-psychological study in volunteers ondansetron has not shown a sedative effect.

Ondansetron does not alter plasma prolactin concentrations.

The role of ondansetron in opiate-induced emesis is not yet established.

5.2 Pharmacokinetic properties

Following oral administration, ondansetron is passively and completely absorbed from the gastrointestinal tract and undergoes first pass metabolism (bioavailability is about 60%). Peak plasma concentrations of about 30 ng/ml are attained approximately 1.5 hours after an 8 mg dose. For doses above 8 mg the increase in ondansetron systemic exposure with dose is greater than proportional; this may reflect some reduction in first pass metabolism at higher oral doses. Bioavailability, following oral administration, is slightly enhanced by the presence of food but unaffected by antacids. Studies in healthy elderly volunteers have shown slight, but clinically insignificant, age-related increases in both oral bioavailability (65%) and half-life (5 hours) of ondansetron. Gender differences were shown in the disposition of ondansetron, with females having a greater rate and extent of absorption following an oral dose and reduced systemic clearance and volume of distribution (adjusted for weight).

The disposition of ondansetron following oral, intramuscular(IM) and intravenous(IV) dosing is similar with a terminal half life of about 3 hours and steady state volume of distribution of about 140 L. Equivalent systemic exposure is achieved after IM and IV administration of ondansetron.

The protein binding of ondansetron is 70-76%. A direct effect of plasma concentration and anti-emetic effect has not been established. Ondansetron is cleared from the systemic circulation predominantly by hepatic metabolism through multiple enzymatic pathways. Less than 5% of the absorbed dose is excreted unchanged in the urine. The absence of the enzyme CYP2D6 has no effect on ondansetron's pharmacokinetics. The pharmacokinetic properties of ondansetron are unchanged on repeat dosing.

Following oral, intravenous or intramuscular dosing in patients with severe hepatic impairment, ondansetron's systemic clearance is markedly reduced with prolonged elimination half-lives (15-32 h) and an oral bioavailability approaching 100% due to reduced pre-systemic metabolism.

5.3 Preclinical safety data

Preclinical data revealed no special hazard for humans based on conventional studies of safety pharmacology, repeated dose toxicity, genotoxicity and carcinogenic potential.

Ondansetron and its metabolites accumulate in the milk of rats, milk/plasma-ratio was 5.2.

A study in cloned human cardiac ion channels has shown ondansetron has the potential to affect cardiac repolarisation via blockade of HERG potassium channels. The clinical relevance of this finding is uncertain.

6. PHARMACEUTICAL PARTICULARS

6.1 List of excipients

Tablet core:

Cellulose, microcrystalline

Lactose monohydrate

Starch, pregelatinised (maize)

Magnesium stearate

Film coating:

Hypromellose

Hydroxypropylcellulose

Propylene glycol

Sorbitan oleate

Sorbic acid

Vanillin

Titanium dioxide (E171)

Quinoline yellow (E 104).

6.2 Incompatibilities

Not applicable.

6.3 Shelf life

3 years.

6.4 Special precautions for storage

This medicinal product does not require any special storage precautions.

6.5 Nature and contents of container

Blister (PVC/Al)

8 mg: 10, 15, 30, 50 and 100 film coated tablets.

Not all pack sizes may be marketed.

6.6 Special precautions for disposal and other handling

No special requirements.

7. MARKETING AUTHORISATION HOLDER

Beacon Pharmaceuticals Ltd

The Regent

The Broadway

Crowborough

East Sussex

TN6 1DA

UK

8. MARKETING AUTHORISATION NUMBER(S)

PL 18157/0017

9. DATE OF FIRST AUTHORISATION/RENEWAL OF THE AUTHORISATION

24/03/2006

10. DATE OF REVISION OF THE TEXT

24/03/2006

One-Alpha Capsules

(Leo Laboratories Limited)

1. NAME OF THE MEDICINAL PRODUCT

One-Alpha® Capsules 1 microgram.

One-Alpha® Capsules 0.25 microgram.

One-Alpha® Capsules 0.5 microgram.

2. QUALITATIVE AND QUANTITATIVE COMPOSITION

One-Alpha® Capsules 1 microgram: alfacalcidol (1-α hydroxyvitamin D3) 1 μg.

One-Alpha® Capsules 0.25 microgram: alfacalcidol (1-α hydroxyvitamin D3) 0.25 μg.

One-Alpha® Capsules 0.5 microgram: alfacalcidol 0.5 μg.

3. PHARMACEUTICAL FORM

One-Alpha® Capsules 1 microgram: brown soft gelatin capsules.

One-Alpha® Capsules 0.25 microgram: white soft gelatin capsules.

One-Alpha® Capsules 0.5 microgram: red soft gelatin capsules.

4. CLINICAL PARTICULARS

4.1 Therapeutic indications

One-Alpha® is indicated in all conditions where there is a disturbance of calcium metabolism due to impaired 1-α hydroxylation such as when there is reduced renal function. The main indications are:

a) Renal osteodystrophy

b) Hyperparathyroidism (with bone disease)

c) Hypoparathyroidism

d) Neonatal hypocalcaemia

e) Nutritional and malabsorptive rickets and osteomalacia

f) Pseudo-deficiency (D-dependent) rickets and osteomalacia

g) Hypophosphataemic vitamin D resistant rickets and osteomalacia

4.2 Posology and method of administration

Route of administration: oral

Initial dose for all indications:

Adults	1 microgram/day
Dosage in the elderly	0.5 microgram/day
Neonates and premature infants	0.05 - 0.1 microgram/kg/day
Children under 20 kg bodyweight	0.05 microgram/kg/day
Children over 20 kg bodyweight	1 microgram/day

The dose of One-Alpha® should be adjusted thereafter to avoid hypercalcaemia according to the biochemical response. Indices of response include plasma levels of calcium (ideally corrected for protein binding), alkaline phosphatase, parathyroid hormone, as well as radiographic and histological investigations.

Plasma levels should initially be measured at weekly intervals. The daily dose of One-Alpha® may be increased by increments of 0.25 - 0.5 microgram. When the dose is stabilised, measurements may be taken every 2 - 4 weeks.

Most adult patients respond to doses between 1 and 3 micrograms per day. When there is biochemical or radiographic evidence of bone healing, (and in hypoparathyroid patients when normal plasma calcium levels have been attained), the dose generally decreases. Maintenance doses are generally in the range of 0.25 to 1 microgram per day. If hypercalcaemia occurs, One-Alpha® should be stopped until plasma calcium returns to normal (approximately 1 week) then restarted at half the previous dose.

(a) Renal bone disease:

Patients with relatively high initial plasma calcium levels may have autonomous hyperparathyroidism, often unresponsive to One-Alpha®. Other therapeutic measures may be indicated.

Before and during treatment with One-Alpha®, phosphate binding agents should be considered to prevent hyperphosphataemia. It is particularly important to make frequent plasma calcium measurements in patients with chronic renal failure because prolonged hypercalcaemia may aggravate the decline of renal function.

(b) Hyperparathyroidism:

In patients with primary or tertiary hyperparathyroidism about to undergo parathyroidectomy, pre-operative treatment with One-Alpha® for 2-3 weeks alleviates bone pain and myopathy without aggravating pre-operative hypercalcaemia. In order to decrease post-operative hypocalcaemia, One-Alpha® should be continued until plasma alkaline phosphatase levels fall to normal or hypercalcaemia occurs.

(c) Hypoparathyroidism:

In contrast to the response to parent vitamin D, low plasma calcium levels are restored to normal relatively quickly with One-Alpha®. Severe hypocalcaemia is corrected more rapidly with higher doses of One-Alpha® (e.g. 3-5 micrograms) together with calcium supplements.

(d) Neonatal hypocalcaemia:

Although the normal starting dose of One-Alpha® is 0.05-0.1 microgram/kg/day (followed by careful titration) in severe cases doses of up to 2 microgram/kg/day may be required. Whilst ionised serum calcium levels may provide a guide to response, measurement of plasma alkaline phosphatase activity may be more useful. Levels of alkaline phosphatase approximately 7.5 times above the adult range indicates active disease.

A dose of 0.1 microgram/kg/day of One-Alpha® has proven effective as prophylaxis against early neonatal hypocalcaemia in premature infants.

(e) Nutritional and malabsorptive rickets and osteomalacia:

Nutritional rickets and osteomalacia can be cured rapidly with One-Alpha®. Malabsorptive osteomalacia (responding to large doses of IM or IV parent vitamin D) will respond to small doses of One-Alpha®.

(f) Pseudo-deficiency (D-dependent) rickets and osteomalacia:

Although large doses of parent vitamin D would be required, effective doses of One-Alpha® are similar to those required to heal nutritional vitamin D deficiency rickets and osteomalacia.

(g) Hypophosphataemic vitamin D-resistant rickets and osteomalacia:

Neither large doses of parent vitamin D nor phosphate supplements are entirely satisfactory. Treatment with One-Alpha® at normal dosage rapidly relieves myopathy when present and increases calcium and phosphate retention. Phosphate supplements may also be required in some patients.

4.3 Contraindications

Hypercalcaemia, metastatic calcification.

Hypersensitivity to alfacalcidol or any of the other ingredients.

4.4 Special warnings and precautions for use

One-Alpha® should be used with caution for:

- patients being treated with cardioactive glycosides or digitalis as hypercalcaemia may lead to arrhythmia in such patients
- patients with nephrolithiasis

During treatment with One-Alpha® serum calcium and serum phosphate should be monitored regularly especially in children, patients with renal impairment and patients receiving high doses. To maintain serum phosphate at an acceptable level in patients with renal bone disease a phosphate binding agent may be used.

Hypercalcaemia may appear in patients treated with One-Alpha®, the early symptoms are as follows:

- polyuria
- polydipsia
- weakness, headache, nausea, constipation
- dry mouth
- muscle and bone pain
- metallic taste

Hypercalcaemia can be rapidly corrected by stopping treatment until plasma calcium levels return to normal (in about one week). One-Alpha® treatment may then be restarted at a reduced dose (half the previous dose).

4.5 Interaction with other medicinal products and other forms of interaction

Patients taking barbiturates or anticonvulsants may require larger doses of One-Alpha® to produce the desired effect due to the induction of hepatic detoxification enzymes.

Concomitant administration of colestyramine may interfere with the intestinal absorption of alfacalcidol.

Use with caution in patients being treated with thiazide diuretics as they may have an increased risk of developing hypercalcaemia.

4.6 Pregnancy and lactation

There are no adequate data from the use of alfacalcidol in pregnant women. Animal studies are insufficient with respect to effects on pregnancy. The potential risks for humans are unknown. Caution should be taken when prescribing to pregnant women as hypercalcaemia during pregnancy may produce congenital disorders in the offspring.

Although it has not been established, it is likely that increased amounts of 1,25-dihydroxyvitamin D will be found in the milk of lactating mothers treated with One-Alpha®. This may influence calcium metabolism in the infant.

4.7 Effects on ability to drive and use machines

One-Alpha® has no or negligible influence on the ability to drive or use machines.

4.8 Undesirable effects

The most frequently reported undesirable effects are hypercalcaemia and various skin reactions. Hypercalcaemia can be rapidly corrected by stopping treatment until plasma calcium levels return to normal (about 1 week). One-Alpha® treatment may then be re-started at half the previous dose.

Based on data from post-market use the total undesirable effect "reporting rate" is rare or very rare being approximately 1:10,000 patients treated.

• Metabolism and Nutrition Disorders

Hypercalcaemia

Hyperphosphataemia

• Skin and Subcutaneous Tissue Disorders

Pruritis

Rash

Urticaria

• Renal and Urinary Disorders

Nephrocalcinosis

Renal impairment

4.9 Overdose

Hypercalcaemia is treated by suspending the administration of One-Alpha®.

In severe cases of hypercalcaemia general supportive measures should be undertaken. Keep the patient well hydrated by i.v. infusion of saline (force diuresis), measure electrolytes, calcium and renal function indices; assess electrocardiographic abnormalities, especially in patients on digitalis. More specifically, treatment with glucocorticosteroids, loop diuretics, biphosphonates, calcitonin and eventually haemodialysis with low calcium content should be considered.

5. PHARMACOLOGICAL PROPERTIES

5.1 Pharmacodynamic properties

Alfacalcidol is converted rapidly in the liver to 1,25-dihydroxyvitamin D. This is the metabolite of vitamin D which acts as a regulator of calcium and phosphate metabolism. Since this conversion is rapid, the clinical effects of One-Alpha® and 1,25-dihydroxyvitamin D are very similar.

Impaired 1-α hydroxylation by the kidneys reduces endogenous 1,25-dihydroxyvitamin D production. This contributes to the disturbances in mineral metabolism found in several disorders, including renal bone disease, hypoparathyroidism, neonatal hypocalcaemia and vitamin D dependent rickets. These disorders, which require high doses of parent vitamin D for their correction, will respond to small doses of One-Alpha®.

The delay in response and high dosage required in treating these disorders with parent vitamin D makes dosage adjustment difficult. This can result in unpredictable hypercalcaemia which may take weeks or months to reverse. The major advantage of One-Alpha® is the more rapid onset of response, which allows a more accurate titration of dosage. Should inadvertent hypercalcaemia occur it can be reversed within days of stopping treatment.

5.2 Pharmacokinetic properties

In patients with renal failure, 1-5 μg/day of 1α-hydroxyvitamin D (1α-OHD3) increased intestinal calcium and phosphorus absorption in a dose-related manner. This effect was observed within 3 days of starting the drug and conversely, it was reversed within 3 days of its discontinuation.

In patients with nutritional osteomalacia, increases in calcium absorption were noted within 6 hours of giving 1 μg 1α-OHD3 orally and usually peaked at 24 hours. 1α-OHD3 also produced increases in plasma inorganic phosphorus due to increased intestinal absorption and renal tubular re-absorption. This latter effect is a result of PTH suppression by 1α-OHD3. The effect of the drug on calcium was about double its effect on phosphorus absorption.

Patients with chronic renal failure have shown increased serum calcium levels within 5 days of receiving 1α-OHD3 in a dose of 0.5 - 1.0 μg/day. As serum calcium rose, PTH levels and alkaline phosphatase decreased toward normal.

5.3 Preclinical safety data

There are no pre-clinical data of relevance to the prescriber which are additional to that already included in other sections of the SPC.

6. PHARMACEUTICAL PARTICULARS

6.1 List of excipients

One-Alpha® Capsules 1 microgram: sesame oil, dl-α-tocopherol, gelatin, glycerol, potassium sorbate, black iron oxide, red iron oxide.

One-Alpha® Capsules 0.25 microgram: sesame oil, dl-α-tocopherol, gelatin, glycerol, potassium sorbate, titanium dioxide.

One-Alpha® Capsules 0.5 microgram: sesame oil, dl-α-tocopherol, gelatin, glycerol, potassium sorbate, red iron oxide, titanium dioxide.

6.2 Incompatibilities

Not applicable.

6.3 Shelf life

2 years.

6.4 Special precautions for storage

Do not store above 25°C.

6.5 Nature and contents of container

PVC/AL blister of 30 (OP), with polyamide-coated aluminium cover.

6.6 Special precautions for disposal and other handling

None.

7. MARKETING AUTHORISATION HOLDER

LEO Laboratories Limited

Longwick Road

Princes Risborough

Bucks HP27 9RR

UK

8. MARKETING AUTHORISATION NUMBER(S)

One-Alpha® Capsules 1 microgram: PL 0043/0050.

One-Alpha® Capsules 0.25 microgram: PL 0043/0052.

One-Alpha® Capsules 0.5 microgram: PL 0043/0206.

9. DATE OF FIRST AUTHORISATION/RENEWAL OF THE AUTHORISATION

One-Alpha® Capsules 1 microgram: 26 January 1978/13 January 1994.

One-Alpha® Capsules 0.25 microgram: 8 November 2006.

One-Alpha® Capsules 0.5 microgram: 22 September 1999.

10. DATE OF REVISION OF THE TEXT

One-Alpha® Capsules 1 microgram: March 2007

One-Alpha® Capsules 0.25 microgram: March 2007

One-Alpha® Capsules 0.5 microgram: March 2007

One-Alpha Drops

(Leo Laboratories Limited)

1. NAME OF THE MEDICINAL PRODUCT

One-Alpha® Drops.

2. QUALITATIVE AND QUANTITATIVE COMPOSITION

Alfacalcidol 2 micrograms/ml

3. PHARMACEUTICAL FORM

Oral drops, solution.

4. CLINICAL PARTICULARS

4.1 Therapeutic indications

One-Alpha® is indicated in all conditions where there is a disturbance of calcium metabolism due to impaired 1-α hydroxylation such as when there is reduced renal function. The main indications are:

a) Renal osteodystrophy

b) Hyperparathyroidism (with bone disease)

c) Hypoparathyroidism

d) Neonatal hypocalcaemia

e) Nutritional and malabsorptive rickets and osteomalacia

f) Pseudo-deficiency (D-dependent) rickets and osteomalacia

g) Hypophosphataemic vitamin D resistant rickets and osteomalacia

4.2 Posology and method of administration

One-Alpha® Drops should be administered orally, using the integral dropper. One drop = 0.1 microgram.

Initial dose for all indications:

Adults	1 microgram/day
Dosage in the elderly	0.5 microgram/day
Neonates and premature infants	0.05 - 0.1 microgram/kg/day
Children under 20 kg bodyweight	0.05 microgram/kg/day
Children over 20 kg bodyweight	1 microgram/day

Half-drop doses should be rounded up to the next whole number of drops.

The dose of One-Alpha® should be adjusted thereafter to avoid hypercalcaemia according to the biochemical response. Indices of response include plasma levels of calcium (ideally corrected for protein binding), alkaline phosphatase, parathyroid hormone, as well as radiographic and histological investigations.

Plasma levels should initially be measured at weekly intervals. The daily dose of One-Alpha® may be increased by increments of 0.25 - 0.5 microgram. When the dose is stabilised, measurements may be taken every 2 - 4 weeks.

Most adult patients respond to doses between 1 and 3 micrograms per day. When there is biochemical or radiographic evidence of bone healing, (and in hypoparathyroid patients when normal plasma calcium levels have been attained), the dose generally decreases. Maintenance doses are generally in the range of 0.25 to 1 microgram per day. If hypercalcaemia occurs, One-Alpha® should be stopped until plasma calcium returns to normal (approximately 1 week) then restarted at half the previous dose.

(a) Renal bone disease:

Patients with relatively high initial plasma calcium levels may have autonomous hyperparathyroidism, often unresponsive to One-Alpha®. Other therapeutic measures may be indicated.

Before and during treatment with One-Alpha®, phosphate binding agents should be considered to prevent hyperphosphataemia. It is particularly important to make frequent plasma calcium measurements in patients with chronic renal failure because prolonged hypercalcaemia may aggravate the decline of renal function.

(b) Hyperparathyroidism:

In patients with primary or tertiary hyperparathyroidism about to undergo parathyroidectomy, pre-operative treatment with One-Alpha® for 2-3 weeks alleviates bone pain and myopathy without aggravating pre-operative hypercalcaemia. In order to decrease post-operative hypocalcaemia, One-Alpha® should be continued until plasma alkaline phosphatase levels fall to normal or hypercalcaemia occurs.

(c) Hypoparathyroidism:

In contrast to the response to parent vitamin D, low plasma calcium levels are restored to normal relatively quickly with One-Alpha®. Severe hypocalcaemia is corrected more rapidly with higher doses of One-Alpha® (eg 3-5 micrograms) together with calcium supplements.

(d) Neonatal hypocalcaemia:

Although the normal starting dose of One-Alpha® is 0.05-0.1 microgram/kg/day (followed by careful titration) in severe cases doses of up to 2 microgram/kg/day may be required. Whilst ionised serum calcium levels may provide a guide to response, measurement of plasma alkaline phosphatase activity may be more useful. Levels of alkaline phosphatase approximately 7.5 times above the adult range indicates active disease.

A dose of 0.1 microgram/kg/day of One-Alpha® has proven effective as prophylaxis against early neonatal hypocalcaemia in premature infants.

(e) Nutritional and malabsorptive rickets and osteomalacia:

Nutritional rickets and osteomalacia can be cured rapidly with One-Alpha®. Malabsorptive osteomalacia (responding to large doses of IM or IV parent vitamin D) will respond to small doses of One-Alpha®.

(f) Pseudo-deficiency (D-dependent) rickets and osteomalacia:

Although large doses of parent vitamin D would be required, effective doses of One-Alpha® are similar to those required to heal nutritional vitamin D deficiency rickets and osteomalacia.

(g) Hypophosphataemic vitamin D-resistant rickets and osteomalacia:

Neither large doses of parent vitamin D nor phosphate supplements are entirely satisfactory. Treatment with One-Alpha® at normal dosage rapidly relieves myopathy when present and increases calcium and phosphate retention. Phosphate supplements may also be required in some patients.

4.3 Contraindications

Hypercalcaemia, metastatic calcification.

Hypersensitivity to alfacalcidol or any of the other ingredients.

Patients with rare hereditary problems of fructose intolerance should not take this medicine.

4.4 Special warnings and precautions for use

One-Alpha® should be used with caution for:

- patients being treated with cardioactive glycosides or digitalis as hypercalcaemia may lead to arrhythmia in such patients
- patients with nephrolithiasis

During treatment with One-Alpha® serum calcium and serum phosphate should be monitored regularly especially in children, patients with renal impairment and patients receiving high doses. To maintain serum phosphate at an acceptable level in patients with renal bone disease a phosphate binding agent may be used.

Hypercalcaemia may appear in patients treated with One-Alpha®, the early symptoms are as follows:

- polyuria
- polydipsia
- weakness, headache, nausea, constipation
- dry mouth
- muscle and bone pain
- metallic taste

Hypercalcaemia can be rapidly corrected by stopping treatment until plasma calcium levels return to normal (in about one week). One-Alpha® treatment may then be restarted at a reduced dose (half the previous dose).

4.5 Interaction with other medicinal products and other forms of interaction

Patients taking barbiturates or anticonvulsants may require larger doses of One-Alpha® to produce the desired effect due to the induction of hepatic detoxification enzymes.

Concomitant administration of colestyramine may interfere with the intestinal absorption of alfacalcidol.

Use with caution in patients being treated with thiazide diuretics as they may have an increased risk of developing hypercalcaemia.

4.6 Pregnancy and lactation

There are no adequate data from the use of alfacalcidol in pregnant women. Animal studies are insufficient with respect to effects on pregnancy. The potential risks for humans are unknown. Caution should be taken when prescribing to pregnant women as hypercalcaemia during pregnancy may produce congenital disorders in the offspring.

Although it has not been established, it is likely that increased amounts of 1,25-dihydroxyvitamin D will be found in the milk of lactating mothers treated with One-Alpha®. This may influence calcium metabolism in the infant.

4.7 Effects on ability to drive and use machines

One-Alpha® has no or negligible influence on the ability to drive or use machines.

4.8 Undesirable effects

The most frequently reported undesirable effects are hypercalcaemia and various skin reactions. Hypercalcaemia can be rapidly corrected by stopping treatment until plasma calcium levels return to normal (about 1 week). One-Alpha® treatment may then be re-started at half the previous dose.

Based on data from post-market use the total undesirable effect 'reporting rate' is rare or very rare being approximately 1:10,000 patients treated.

- **Metabolism and Nutrition Disorders**

Hypercalcaemia

Hyperphosphataemia

- **Skin and Subcutaneous Tissue Disorders**

Pruritus

Rash

Urticaria

- **Renal and Urinary Disorders**

Nephrocalcinosis

Renal impairment

4.9 Overdose

Hypercalcaemia is treated by suspending the administration of One-Alpha®.

In severe cases of hypercalcaemia general supportive measures should be undertaken. Keep the patient well hydrated by i.v. infusion of saline (force diuresis), measure electrolytes, calcium and renal function indices; assess electrocardiographic abnormalities, especially in patients on digitalis. More specifically, treatment with glucocorticosteroids, loop diuretics, bisphosphonates, calcitonin and eventually haemodialysis with low calcium content should be considered.

5. PHARMACOLOGICAL PROPERTIES

5.1 Pharmacodynamic properties

Alfacalcidol is converted rapidly in the liver to 1,25-dihydroxyvitamin D. This is the metabolite of vitamin D which acts as a regulator of calcium and phosphate metabolism. Since this conversion is rapid, the clinical effects of One-Alpha® and 1,25-dihydroxyvitamin D are very similar.

Impaired 1-α hydroxylation by the kidneys reduces endogenous 1,25- dihydroxyvitamin D production. This contributes to the disturbances in mineral metabolism found in several disorders, including renal bone disease, hypoparathyroidism, neonatal hypocalcaemia and vitamin D dependent rickets. These disorders, which require high doses of parent vitamin D for their correction, will respond to small doses of One-Alpha®.

The delay in response and high dosage required in treating these disorders with parent vitamin D makes dosage adjustment difficult. This can result in unpredictable hypercalcaemia which may take weeks or months to reverse. The major advantage of One-Alpha® is the more rapid onset of response, which allows a more accurate titration of dosage. Should inadvertent hypercalcaemia occur it can be reversed within days of stopping treatment.

5.2 Pharmacokinetic properties

In patients with renal failure, 1-5 μg/day of 1α-hydroxyvitamin D (1α-OHD3) increased intestinal calcium and phosphorus absorption in a dose-related manner. This effect was observed within 3 days of starting the drug and, conversely, it was reversed within 3 days of its discontinuation.

In patients with nutritional osteomalacia, increases in calcium absorption were noted within 6 hours of giving 1 μg 1α-OHD3 orally and usually peaked at 24 hours. 1α-OHD3 also produced increases in plasma inorganic phosphorus due to increased intestinal absorption and renal tubular reabsorption. This latter effect is a result of PTH suppression by 1α-OHD3. The effect of the drug on calcium was about double its effect on phosphorus absorption.

Patients with chronic renal failure have shown increased serum calcium levels within 5 days of receiving 1α-OHD3 in a dose of 0.5 - 1.0 μg/day. As serum calcium rose, PTH levels and alkaline phosphatase decreased toward normal.

5.3 Preclinical safety data

There are no pre-clinical data of relevance to the prescriber which are additional to that already included in other sections of the SPC.

6. PHARMACEUTICAL PARTICULARS

6.1 List of excipients

Ethanol, polyoxyl 40 hydrogenated castor oil, methylparahydroxybenzoate, citric acid monohydrate, sodium citrate, sorbitol, dl-α-tocopherol and purified water.

6.2 Incompatibilities

None known.

6.3 Shelf life

3 years.

6.4 Special precautions for storage

Store at 2 - 8°C (in a refrigerator). Keep the container in the outer carton.

6.5 Nature and contents of container

Amber glass bottles of 10 ml with a polyethylene dropping device and a polypropylene screw cap.

6.6 Special precautions for disposal and other handling

None.

7. MARKETING AUTHORISATION HOLDER

LEO Laboratories Limited

Longwick Road

Princes Risborough

Bucks HP27 9RR

UK

8. MARKETING AUTHORISATION NUMBER(S)

PL 0043/0207

9. DATE OF FIRST AUTHORISATION/RENEWAL OF THE AUTHORISATION

3 March 2000

10. DATE OF REVISION OF THE TEXT

October 2006

One-Alpha Injection

(Leo Laboratories Limited)

1. NAME OF THE MEDICINAL PRODUCT

One-Alpha® Injection

2. QUALITATIVE AND QUANTITATIVE COMPOSITION

Alfacalcidol (1α-hydroxyvitamin D_3) 2 micrograms/ml.

3. PHARMACEUTICAL FORM

Injection

4. CLINICAL PARTICULARS

4.1 Therapeutic indications

One-Alpha® is indicated in all conditions where there is a disturbance of calcium metabolism due to impaired 1 α-hydroxylation such as when there is reduced renal function.

The main indications are:

a) Renal osteodystrophy

b) Hyperparathyroidism (with bone disease)

c) Hypoparathyroidism

d) Neonatal hypocalcaemia

e) Nutritional and malabsorptive rickets and osteomalacia

f) Pseudo - deficiency (D - dependent) rickets and osteomalacia

g) Hypophosphataemic vitamin D resistant rickets and osteomalacia

4.2 Posology and method of administration

One-Alpha® Injection should be administered intravenously as a bolus over approximately 30 seconds. Shake the ampoule for a minimum of 5 seconds before use.

The dosage of One-Alpha® Injection is the same as for One-Alpha® in its oral presentations.

Initial dosage for all indications is:

Adults	1 microgram/day
Dosage in the elderly	0.5 microgram/day
Neonates and premature infants	0.05 - 0.1 microgram/kg/day
Children under 20 kg bodyweight	0.05 microgram/kg/day
Children over 20 kg bodyweight	1 microgram/day

The dose of One-Alpha® should be adjusted thereafter to avoid hypercalcaemia according to the biochemical response.

Indices of response include plasma levels of calcium (ideally corrected for protein binding), alkaline phosphatase, parathyroid hormone, as well as radiographic and histological investigations.

Maintenance doses are generally in the range of 0.25 - 1 microgram per day.

When administered as intravenous injection to patients undergoing haemodialysis the initial dosage for adults is 1 microgram per dialysis. The maximum dose recommended is 6 micrograms per dialysis and not more than 12 micrograms per week. The injection should be administered into the return line from the haemodialysis machine at the end of each dialysis.

(a) Renal bone disease:

Patients with relatively high initial plasma calcium levels may have autonomous hyperparathyroidism, often unresponsive to One-Alpha®. Other therapeutic measures may be indicated.

Before and during treatment with One-Alpha®, phosphate binding agents should be considered to prevent hyperphosphataemia. It is particularly important to make frequent plasma calcium measurements in patients with chronic renal failure because prolonged hypercalcaemia may aggravate the decline of renal function.

(b) Hyperparathyroidism:

In patients with primary or tertiary hyperparathyroidism about to undergo parathyroidectomy, pre-operative treatment with One-Alpha® for 2-3 weeks alleviates bone pain and myopathy without aggravating pre-operative hypercalcaemia. In order to decrease post-operative hypocalcaemia, One-Alpha® should be continued until plasma alkaline phosphatase levels fall to normal or hypercalcaemia occurs.

(c) Hypoparathyroidism:

In contrast to the response to parent vitamin D, low plasma calcium levels are restored to normal relatively quickly with One-Alpha®. Severe hypocalcaemia is corrected more rapidly with higher doses of One-Alpha® (eg 3-5 micrograms) together with calcium supplements.

(d) Neonatal hypocalcaemia:

Although the normal starting dose of One-Alpha® is 0.05-0.1 microgram/kg/day (followed by careful titration), in severe cases, doses of up to 2 microgram/kg/day may be required. Whilst ionised serum calcium levels may provide a guide to response, measurement of plasma alkaline phosphatase activity may be more useful. Levels of alkaline phosphatase approximately 7.5 times above the adult range indicates active disease.

(e) Nutritional and malabsorptive rickets and osteomalacia:

Nutritional rickets and osteomalacia can be cured rapidly with One-Alpha®. Malabsorptive osteomalacia (responding to large doses of IM or IV parent vitamin D) will respond to small doses of One-Alpha®.

(f) Pseudo-deficiency (D-dependent) rickets and osteomalacia:

Although large doses of parent vitamin D would be required, effective doses of One-Alpha® are similar to those required to heal nutritional Vitamin D deficiency rickets and osteomalacia.

(g) Hypophosphataemic vitamin D-resistant rickets and osteomalacia:

Neither large doses of parent vitamin D nor phosphate supplements are entirely satisfactory. Treatment with One-Alpha® at normal dosage rapidly relieves myopathy when present and increases calcium and phosphate retention. Phosphate supplements may also be required in some patients.

4.3 Contraindications

Hypercalcaemia, metastatic calcification.

Hypersensitivity to alfacalcidol or any of the other ingredients.

4.4 Special warnings and precautions for use

One-Alpha® Injection should be avoided in patients with known sensitivity to injections containing propylene glycol.

One-Alpha® should be used with caution for:

- small premature infants
- patients being treated with cardioactive glycosides or digitalis as hypercalcaemia may lead to arrhythmia in such patients
- patients with nephrolithiasis

During treatment with One-Alpha® serum calcium and serum phosphate should be monitored regularly especially in children, patients with renal impairment and patients receiving high doses. To maintain serum phosphate at an acceptable level in patients with renal bone disease a phosphate binding agent may be used.

Hypercalcaemia may appear in patients treated with One-Alpha®, the early symptoms are as follows:

- polyurina
- polydipsia
- weakness, headache, nausea, constipation
- dry mouth
- muscle and bone pain
- metallic taste

Hypercalcaemia can be rapidly corrected by stopping treatment until plasma calcium levels return to normal (in about one week). One-Alpha® treatment may then be restarted at a reduced dose (half the previous dose).

4.5 Interaction with other medicinal products and other forms of interaction

Patients taking barbiturates or anticonvulsants may require larger doses of One-Alpha® to produce the desired effect due to the induction of hepatic detoxification enzymes.

Use with caution in patients being treated with thiazide diuretics as they may have an increased risk of developing hypercalcaemia.

4.6 Pregnancy and lactation

There are no adequate data from the use of alfacalcidol in pregnant women. Animal studies are insufficient with respect to effects on pregnancy. The potential risks for humans are unknown. Caution should be taken when prescribing to pregnant women as hypercalcaemia during pregnancy may produce congenital disorders in the offspring.

Although it has not been established, it is likely that increased amounts of 1,25 dihydroxyvitamin D will be found in the milk of lactating mothers treated with One-Alpha®. This may influence calcium metabolism in the infant.

4.7 Effects on ability to drive and use machines

One-Alpha® has no or negligible influence on the ability to drive or use machines.

4.8 Undesirable effects

The most frequently reported undesirable effects are hypercalcaemia and various skin reactions. Hypercalcaemia can be rapidly corrected by stopping treatment until plasma calcium levels return to normal (about 1 week). One-Alpha® treatment may then be restarted at half the previous dose.

Based on data from post-market use the total undesirable effect 'reporting rate' is rare or very rare being approximately 1:10,000 patients treated.

- **Metabolism and Nutrition Disorders**

Hypercalcaemia

Hyperphosphataemia

- **Skin and Subcutaneous Tissue Disorders**

Pruritus

Rash

Urticaria

- **Renal and Urinary Disorders**

Nephrocalcinosis

Renal impairment

4.9 Overdose

Hypercalcaemia is treated by suspending the administration of One-Alpha®.

In severe cases of hypercalcaemia general supportive measures should be undertaken. Keep the patient well hydrated by i.v. infusion of saline (force diuresis), measure electrolytes, calcium and renal function indices; assess electrocardiographic abnormalities, especially in patients on digitalis. More specifically, treatment with glucocorticosteroids, loop diuretics, bisphosphonates, calcitonin and eventually haemodialysis with low calcium content should be considered.

5. PHARMACOLOGICAL PROPERTIES

5.1 Pharmacodynamic properties

Alfacalcidol is converted rapidly in the liver to 1,25 dihydroxyvitamin D. This is the metabolite of vitamin D which acts as a regulator of calcium and phosphate metabolism. Since this conversion is rapid, the clinical effects of One-Alpha® and 1,25 dihydroxyvitamin D are very similar.

Impaired 1 α-hydroxylation reduces 1,25 dihydroxyvitamin D production. This contributes to the disturbances in mineral metabolism found in several disorders, including renal bone disease, hypoparathyroidism, neonatal hypocalcaemia and vitamin D dependent rickets. These disorders, which require high doses of parent vitamin D for their correction, will respond to small doses of One-Alpha®.

The delay in response and high dosage required in treating these disorders with parent vitamin D makes dosage adjustment difficult. This can result in unpredictable hypercalcaemia which may take weeks or months to reverse. The major advantage of One-Alpha® is the more rapid onset of response, which allows a more accurate titration of dosage. Should inadvertent hypercalcaemia occur it can be reversed within days of stopping treatment.

5.2 Pharmacokinetic properties

In patients on regular haemodialysis administration of doses between 1 - 4 micrograms of intravenous 1 α-hydroxyvitamin D_3 resulted in increased levels of 1,25 dihydroxyvitamin D. Formation of 1,25 dihydroxyvitamin D_3 occurred within 1 hour after intravenous 1 α-hydroxyvitamin D_3 and peak concentrations were reached between 2 and 5 hours. Elimination half life of the formed 1,25 dihydroxyvitamin D was between 14 and 30 hours.

5.3 Preclinical safety data

There are no pre-clinical data of relevance to the prescriber which are additional to that already included in other sections of the SPC.

6. PHARMACEUTICAL PARTICULARS

6.1 List of excipients

Citric acid, ethanol, sodium citrate, propylene glycol and water for injection.

6.2 Incompatibilities

None known.

6.3 Shelf life

3 years.

6.4 Special precautions for storage

Store at 2-8°C.

6.5 Nature and contents of container

10 × 0.5ml amber glass ampoules.

10 × 1.0ml amber glass ampoules.

6.6 Special precautions for disposal and other handling

None.

7. MARKETING AUTHORISATION HOLDER

LEO Laboratories Limited

Longwick Road

Princes Risborough

Bucks

HP27 9RR

8. MARKETING AUTHORISATION NUMBER(S)

PL 0043/0183

9. DATE OF FIRST AUTHORISATION/RENEWAL OF THE AUTHORISATION

11/11/2005

10. DATE OF REVISION OF THE TEXT

February 2009

Opizone 50mg film-coated Tablets

(Britannia Pharmaceuticals)

1. NAME OF THE MEDICINAL PRODUCT

Opizone 50 mg film-coated tablets

2. QUALITATIVE AND QUANTITATIVE COMPOSITION

Each film-coated tablet contains 50 mg naltrexone hydrochloride.

For a full list of excipients, see section 6.1.

3. PHARMACEUTICAL FORM

Film-coated tablet.

Capsule shaped, beige film-coated tablets with a breakscore on each side.

The tablet can be divided into equal halves.

4. CLINICAL PARTICULARS

4.1 Therapeutic indications

For use as an additional therapy within a comprehensive treatment program including psychological guidance for detoxified patients who have been opioid-dependent. (see 4.2 and 4.4)

4.2 Posology and method of administration

Opizone treatment should be initiated and supervised by suitable qualified physicians.

Use in adults

The recommended initial dose of naltrexone hydrochloride is 25 mg (half a tablet) followed by 50 mg per day (one tablet).

The dosage-regimen can be modified in order to improve compliance to a three-times-a-week dosing schedule as follows: administration of 2 tablets (= 100 mg naltrexone hydrochloride) on Monday and on Wednesday and 3 tablets (= 150 mg naltrexone hydrochloride) on Friday.

A missed dose can be managed by providing 1 tablet per day till the next regular dosage-administration.

Opizone administered to opioid-dependent persons can cause life-threatening withdrawal symptoms. Patients suspected of using or being addicted to opioids must undergo a naloxone provocation test (see 4.4), unless it can be verified that the patient has not taken any opioids for 7-10 days (urine test) prior to the initiation of treatment with naltrexone.

As Opizone is an adjunctive therapy and the full recovery process in opioid-dependent patients is individually variable, no standard duration of treatment can be stated; an initial period of three months should be considered. However, prolonged administration may be necessary.

Use in children and adolescents

Opizone is not recommended for use in children and adolescents below 18 due to a lack of data on safety and efficacy.

Use in elderly

The experience in elderly patients is limited.

4.3 Contraindications

- Hypersensitivity to naltrexone hydrochloride or to any of the excipients

- Acute hepatitis

- Severe hepatic impairment

- Severe renal impairment

- Opioid addicted patients with a current abuse of opioids since an acute withdrawal syndrome may ensue.

- Positive screening result for opioids or after failure of the naloxone provocation test.

4.4 Special warnings and precautions for use

In accordance to national guidance the therapy should be initiated and supervised by a physician experienced in treatment of opioid-addicted patients.

High dose opioid intake, concomitant with Opizone treatment, can lead to life-threatening opioid poisoning from respiratory and circulatory impairment.

Should Opizone be used in opioid-dependent patients a withdrawal syndrome may occur rapidly: the first symptoms can occur within 5 minutes, the last after 48 hours. The treatment of withdrawal symptoms is symptomatic.

Patients must be warned against the concomitant use of opioids (e.g. opioids in cough medication, opioids in symptomatic medication for the treatment of common colds, or opioids contained in anti diarrhoeal agents, etc.) during Opizone treatment (see section 4.3).

During treatment with Opizone, painful conditions should be treated with non-opioid analgesia only.

If a patient needs opioid treatment, e.g. opioid analgesia or anaesthesia in emergency situations, the opioid dose needed to achieve the desired therapeutic effect may be larger than normal. In these cases, respiratory depression and circulatory effects will be more profound and longer lasting. Symptoms related to release of histamine (diaphoresis, itching and other skin and subcutaneous manifestations) can also be manifested more easily. The patient requires specific attention and care in these situations.

Patients suspected of using or being addicted to opioids must undergo a naloxone provocation test, unless it can be verified that the patient has not taken any opioids for 7-10 days (urine test) prior to the initiation of treatment with naltrexone.

A withdrawal syndrome precipitated by naloxone will be of shorter duration than withdrawal precipitated by naltrexone.

The recommended procedure is as follows:

Intravenous provocation

- Intravenous injection of 0.2 mg naloxone
- If after 30 seconds no adverse reactions occur, a further i.v. injection of 0.6 mg naloxone may be administered.

The patient should be observed continuously for 30 minutes for any detectable sign of withdrawal symptoms.

If any symptoms of withdrawal occur Opizone-therapy must not be undertaken. If the test-result is negative the treatment can be initiated. If any doubt exists that the patient is opioid-free, the challenge may be repeated with the dosage of 1.6 mg. If no reaction occurs after this, 25 mg of naltrexone hydrochloride can be administered to the patient.

A naloxone hydrochloride provocation test should not be made in patients with clinically prominent withdrawal symptoms nor in any case of a positive urine test for opioids.

Patients should be warned that large doses of opioids to overcome the blockade may after the cessation of the Opizone result in an acute opioid overdose, with possible fatal outcome.

Patients might be more sensitive to opioid containing medicines after treatment with Opizone.

Naltrexone hydrochloride is extensively metabolised by the liver and excreted predominantly in the urine. Therefore, caution should be observed in administering the medicinal product to patients with impaired hepatic or renal function. Liver function tests should be carried out both before and during treatment.

Patients with rare hereditary problems of galactose intolerance, the Lapp lactase deficiency or glucose-galactose malabsorption should not take this medicine.

4.5 Interaction with other medicinal products and other forms of interaction

Presently, clinical experience and experimental data on the effect of naltrexone on the pharmacokinetics of other substances are limited. Concomitant treatment with naltrexone and other medicinal products should be conducted with caution and should be followed carefully.

No interaction studies have been performed.

In vitro studies have shown that neither naltrexone nor its main metabolite 6-β-naltrexol is metabolised via human CYP450 enzymes. Therefore it is unlikely that the pharmacokinetics of naltrexone is affected by cytochrome P450 enzyme inhibiting drugs.

One case of lethargy and somnolence has been reported after concomitant use of naltrexone and thioridazine.

Until now no interaction between cocaine and naltrexone hydrochloride has been described.

There are no known interactions between naltrexone and alcohol.

For interactions with opioid containing drugs please see 4.4.

4.6 Pregnancy and lactation

Pregnancy:

There are no clinical data on naltrexone hydrochloride use in pregnancy. Data from animal studies have shown reproductive toxicity (see section 5.3.). The data are insufficient to establish clinical relevance. The potential risk for humans is unknown. Naltrexone should only be given to pregnant women when, in the judgement of the attending physician the potential benefits outweigh and the possible risk.

Lactation:

There are no clinical data on naltrexone hydrochloride use in lactation. It is unknown whether naltrexone or 6-beta-naltrexol is excreted in human breast milk. During treatment breast feeding is not recommended.

4.7 Effects on ability to drive and use machines

Opizone has minor or moderate influence on the ability to drive and use machines.

4.8 Undesirable effects

The following undesirable effects are ranked according to system organ class and to their frequency:

Very common (⩾ 1/10)

Common (⩾1/100 to < 1/10)

Uncommon (⩾1/1.000 to < 1/100)

Rare (⩾ 1/10.000 to < 1/1.000)

Very rare (< 1/10.000)

MedDRA system organ class	Symptom
Very common	
Nervous system disorder	Headache
	Sleep disorders
	Restlessness
	Nervousness
Gastrointestinal disorder	Abdominal pain
	Abdominal cramps
	Nausea
	Inclination to vomit
Musculoskeletal and connective tissue disorders	Joint and muscle pain
General disorder and administration site conditions	Feebleness
Common	
Nervous system disorders	Thirst
	Dizziness
	Shivering
	Increased transpiration
	Vertigo
Eye disorders	Increased lacrimation
Respiratory, thoracic and mediastinal disorder	Pain in the chest
Gastrointestinal disorders	Diarrhoea
	Constipation
Renal and urinary disorders	Urine retention
Skin and subcutaneous tissue disorder	Rash
General disorders and administration site conditions	Lack of appetite
Reproductive system and breast disorders	Delayed ejaculation
	Decreased potency
Psychiatric disorders	Anxiety
	Increased energy
	Despondency
	Irritability
	Mood swings
Rare	
Nervous system disorders	Speech disorder
Gastrointestinal disorders	Hepatic disorders
Psychiatric disorders	Depression
	Suicidal ideation
	Attempted suicide
Very rare	
Blood and lymphatic system disorders	Idiopathic thrombocytopenic purpurea
Nervous system disorders	Tremor
Skin and subcutaneous tissue disorders	Exanthema
Psychiatric disorders	Agitation
	Euphoria
	Hallucination

4.9 Overdose

Symptoms

There is limited clinical experience with naltrexone overdose in patients. There was no evidence of toxicity in volunteers receiving 800 mg/day for seven days.

Treatment

In case of overdose, patients should be monitored and treated symptomatically in a closely supervised environment.

5. PHARMACOLOGICAL PROPERTIES

5.1 Pharmacodynamic properties

Pharmacotherapeutic group: Opioid antagonist

ATC code: V03A B30

Naltrexone is a specific opioid antagonist with only minimal agonistic activity. It acts by stereospecific competition with receptors which are mainly located in the central and peripheral nervous system. Naltrexone competitively binds to these receptors and blocks the access for exogenously administered opioids.

Naltrexone treatment does not lead to physical or mental dependence. No tolerance for the opioid antagonising effect is seen.

Opizone 50 mg film-coated tablet reduces the risk of relapse and supports abstinence from opioids.

Opizone 50 mg film-coated tablet is a non-aversive therapy and does not cause reactions after opioid intake. Therefore it does not cause a disulfiram-type reaction.

5.2 Pharmacokinetic properties

Naltrexone is rapidly and almost completely absorbed from the gastrointestinal tract after oral administration.

It undergoes a liver first-pass effect and peak plasma concentration is reached within approximately one hour.

Naltrexone is hydroxylated in the liver basically to the main active metabolite 6-beta-naltrexol and, to a lesser extent, to 2-hydroxy-3-methoxy-6-beta-naltrexol.

The plasma-half-life of naltrexone is approximately 4 hours, the average blood level is 8.55 mg/ml, and plasma-protein-binding is 21%. The plasma-half-life of 6-beta-naltrexol is 13 hours.

The medicinal product is excreted primarily renal. About 60% of the peroral dose is excreted within 48 hours as glucuronidised 6-beta-naltrexol and naltrexone.

5.3 Preclinical safety data

Preclinical data reveal no special hazard for humans based on conventional studies of safety, pharmacology, repeated dose toxicity, genotoxicity, carcinogenic potential, toxicity to reproduction. However, there is some evidence on hepatotoxicity with increasing dose, since reversible increases of liver enzymes have been found in humans with therapeutic and higher doses (see section 4.4 and 4.8).

Naltrexone (100 mg/kg, approximately 140 times the human therapeutic dose) caused a significant increase in pseudo-pregnancy in the rat. A decrease in the pregnancy rate of mated female rats also occurred. The relevance of these observations to human fertility is not known.

Naltrexone has been shown to have an embryocidal effect in the rat and rabbit when given in doses approximately 140 times the human therapeutic dose. This effect was demonstrated in rats dosed with 100 mg/kg of naltrexone prior to and throughout gestation, and rabbits treated with 60 mg/kg of naltrexone during the period of organogenesis.

6. PHARMACEUTICAL PARTICULARS

6.1 List of excipients

Tablet core

Lactose monohydrate

Powdered cellulose

Microcrystalline cellulose

Silica, colloidal anhydrous

Crospovidone

Magnesium stearate

Film-coat: Opadry 31 F 27245 Beige

Lactose monohydrate

Hypromellose

Titanium dioxide (E171)

Macrogol 4000

Black ferric oxide (E172)

Red ferric oxide (E172)

Yellow ferric oxide (E172)

6.2 Incompatibilities

Not applicable.

6.3 Shelf life

2 years.

6.4 Special precautions for storage

Do not store above 25°C

Store in the original package in order to protect from moisture.

6.5 Nature and contents of container

Pack size: 7, 14, 28 and 56 tablets in PCV/PVDC Aluminium blister.

Not all pack sizes may be marketed.

6.6 Special precautions for disposal and other handling

No special requirements.

7. MARKETING AUTHORISATION HOLDER

AOP Orphan Pharmaceuticals AG

Wilhelminenstrasse 91/II f

1160 Vienna

Austria

8. MARKETING AUTHORISATION NUMBER(S)
PL Number: 21344/0002

9. DATE OF FIRST AUTHORISATION/RENEWAL OF THE AUTHORISATION
14.08.2006

10. DATE OF REVISION OF THE TEXT
14.11.2008

Opticrom Aqueous Eye Drops

(sanofi-aventis)

1. NAME OF THE MEDICINAL PRODUCT
Opticrom™ Aqueous Eye Drops

2. QUALITATIVE AND QUANTITATIVE COMPOSITION
Sodium cromoglicate 2.0% w/v.

3. PHARMACEUTICAL FORM
A clear colourless to pale yellow solution for administration to the eye.

4. CLINICAL PARTICULARS

4.1 Therapeutic indications
For the prophylaxis and symptomatic treatment of acute allergic conjunctivitis, chronic allergic conjunctivitis and vernal kerato conjunctivitis.

4.2 Posology and method of administration
Adults and children: one or two drops into each eye four times daily or as indicated by the doctor.

Elderly: no current evidence for alteration of the dose.

Route of administration: topical ophthalmic.

4.3 Contraindications
The product is contraindicated in patients who have shown hypersensitivity to Sodium cromoglicate, Benzalkonium chloride or Disodium edetate.

4.4 Special warnings and precautions for use
Discard any remaining contents four weeks after opening the bottle.

As with other ophthalmic solutions containing Benzalkonium chloride, soft contact lenses should not be worn during treatment period.

4.5 Interaction with other medicinal products and other forms of interaction
None known.

4.6 Pregnancy and lactation
As with all medication, caution should be exercised especially during the first trimester of pregnancy. Cumulative experience with Sodium cromoglicate suggests that it has no adverse effects on foetal development. It should be used in pregnancy only where there is a clear clinical need.

It is not known whether Sodium cromoglicate is excreted in human breast milk but, on the basis of its physicochemical properties, this is considered unlikely. There is no information to suggest the use of Sodium cromoglicate has any undesirable effects on the baby.

4.7 Effects on ability to drive and use machines
As with all eye drops, instillation of Opticrom may cause a transient blurring of vision.

4.8 Undesirable effects
Transient stinging and burning may occur after instillation. Other symptoms of local irritation have been reported rarely.

4.9 Overdose
No action other than medical observation should be necessary.

5. PHARMACOLOGICAL PROPERTIES

5.1 Pharmacodynamic properties
In vitro and *in vivo* animal studies have shown that Sodium cromoglicate inhibits the degranulation of sensitised mast cells which occurs after exposure to specific antigens. Sodium cromoglicate acts by inhibiting the release of histamine and various membrane derived mediators from the mast cell.

Sodium cromoglicate has demonstrated the activity *in vitro* to inhibit the degranulation of non-sensitised rat mast cells by phospholipase A and subsequent release of chemical mediators. Sodium cromoglicate did not inhibit the enzymatic activity of released phospholipase A on its specific substrate.

Sodium cromoglicate has no intrinsic vasoconstrictor or antihistamine activity.

5.2 Pharmacokinetic properties
Sodium cromoglicate is poorly absorbed. When multiple doses of Sodium cromoglicate ophthalmic solution are instilled into normal rabbit eyes, less than 0.07% of the administered dose of Sodium cromoglicate is absorbed into the systemic circulation (presumably by way of the eye, nasal passages, buccal cavity and gastrointestinal tract). Trace amounts (less than 0.01%) of the sodium cromoglicate does penetrate into the aqueous humour and clearance from this chamber is virtually complete within 24 hours after treatment is stopped.

In normal volunteers, analysis of drug excretion indicates that approximately 0.03% of Sodium cromoglicate is absorbed following administration to the eye.

5.3 Preclinical safety data
None stated.

6. PHARMACEUTICAL PARTICULARS

6.1 List of excipients
Benzalkonium chloride, Disodium edetate, Purified water.

6.2 Incompatibilities
None known.

6.3 Shelf life
3 years.

The eye drops should be used within 4 weeks of opening the container. Any remaining after this time should be discarded.

6.4 Special precautions for storage
Store below 30°C.

Protect from direct sunlight.

6.5 Nature and contents of container
Low density polyethylene bottle and plug with a polypropylene cap with a shrink type security seat containing 13.5 ml.

6.6 Special precautions for disposal and other handling
None.

7. MARKETING AUTHORISATION HOLDER
Sanofi-aventis
One Onslow Street
Guildford
Surrey
GU1 4YS
UK

8. MARKETING AUTHORISATION NUMBER(S)
PL 04425/0324

9. DATE OF FIRST AUTHORISATION/RENEWAL OF THE AUTHORISATION
28 February 2003

10. DATE OF REVISION OF THE TEXT
December 2006

11 LEGAL CLASSIFICATION
POM

Optimax

(Merck Serono)

1. NAME OF THE MEDICINAL PRODUCT
Optimax Tablets 500 mg

2. QUALITATIVE AND QUANTITATIVE COMPOSITION
Each tablet contains 500 mg L-tryptophan.

For excipients, see section 6.1.

3. PHARMACEUTICAL FORM
Tablet

White, capsule-shaped, engraved with 'OPT' on one side, break line on the reverse

4. CLINICAL PARTICULARS

4.1 Therapeutic indications
In treatment-resistant depression after trials of standard antidepressant drug treatments, and as an adjunct to other anti-depressant medication.

Treatment with Optimax should only be initiated by hospital specialists. Patients may subsequently be prescribed Optimax in the community by their general practitioner.

4.2 Posology and method of administration
For oral use

Adults: The usual dose is two tablets, three times daily; for some patients, up to 6g L-tryptophan may be required.

Elderly: A lower dose may be appropriate, especially where there is evidence of renal or hepatic impairment.

Children: Not recommended. Safety has not been established.

4.3 Contraindications
Patients with a previous history of eosinophilia myalgia syndrome (EMS) following the use of L-tryptophan. This syndrome, which is a multisystem disorder, is characterised by raised eosinophils ($>1.0 \times 10^9$/L), and severe myalgia in the absence of either an infectious or neoplastic cause.

Patients with a known hypersensitivity to the active substance or any of the excipients.

4.4 Special warnings and precautions for use
Suicide/suicidal thoughts or clinical worsening
Depression is associated with an increased risk of suicidal thoughts, self harm and suicide (suicide-related events). This risk persists until significant remission occurs. As improvement may not occur during the first few weeks or more of treatment, patients should be closely monitored until such improvement occurs. It is general clinical experience that the risk of suicide may increase in the early stages of recovery.

Patients with a history of suicide-related events, or those exhibiting a significant degree of suicidal ideation prior to commencement of treatment are known to be at greater risk of suicidal thoughts or suicide attempts, and should receive careful monitoring during treatment. A meta-analysis of placebo-controlled clinical trials of antidepressant drugs in adult patients with psychiatric disorders showed an increased risk of suicidal behaviour with antidepressants compared to placebo in patients less than 25 years old.

Close supervision of patients and in particular those at high risk should accompany drug therapy especially in early treatment and following dose changes. Patients (and caregivers of patients) should be alerted about the need to monitor for any clinical worsening, suicidal behaviour or thoughts and unusual changes in behaviour and to seek medical advice immediately if these symptoms present.

Eosinophilia Myalgia Syndrome
Eosinophilia Myalgia Syndrome (EMS) has been reported in association with the use of oral L-tryptophan-containing products. It is a multisystem disorder which is usually reversible but, rarely, fatal. Various investigations have not as yet identified the aetiological factors precisely.

The symptoms of EMS have been reported to include eosinophilia, arthralgia or myalgia, fever, dyspnoea, neuropathy, peripheral oedema and skin lesions which can include sclerosis or papular and urticarial lesions.

Caution should be exercised with patients who experience some but not all of the symptoms of EMS after taking L-tryptophan. Treatment should be withheld and the symptoms investigated until the possibility of EMS can be excluded.

Serotonin syndrome
The possible interaction between L-tryptophan and 5HT reuptake inhibitors could lead to the "serotonin syndrome" characterised by a combination of agitation, restlessness and gastro-intestinal symptoms including diarrhoea. Combinations with 5HT reuptake inhibitors should only be used with care (see Section 4.5).

4.5 Interaction with other medicinal products and other forms of interaction
Where L-tryptophan is combined with an MAO Inhibitor the side effects of the latter may be enhanced. Use of L-tryptophan in combination with a 5HT reuptake inhibitor has the potential for increasing the severity of the adverse effects of the latter and could lead to serotonin syndrome (see Section 4.4).

In patients taking L-tryptophan in conjunction with phenothiazines or benzodiazepines there have been isolated reports of sexual disinhibition.

4.6 Pregnancy and lactation
Safety in pregnancy or lactation has not been established

4.7 Effects on ability to drive and use machines
L-tryptophan may produce drowsiness. Patients who drive and operate machinery should be warned of the possible hazard.

4.8 Undesirable effects
In some patients, L-tryptophan may cause a slight feeling of nausea which usually disappears within 2 or 3 days. Such nausea can be minimised by giving L-tryptophan after food. Other adverse reactions include headache and light-headedness.

Cases of suicidal ideation and suicidal behaviours (frequency not known) have been reported during L-tryptophan therapy or early after treatment discontinuation (see section 4.4).

4.9 Overdose
Drowsiness and vomiting may occur; supportive measures should be employed.

5. PHARMACOLOGICAL PROPERTIES

5.1 Pharmacodynamic properties
Pharmacotherapeutic group: Antidepressants

ATC Code: NO6A X 02

L-tryptophan is an essential dietary amino acid and, following hydroxylation and decarboxylation, is the major source of 5-hydroxytryptamine (5-HT). L-tryptophan, 5-HT and 5-HT metabolite levels are lower than normal in patients with depression. Administration of L-tryptophan re-establishes the inhibitory action of 5-HT on the amygdaloid nuclei, thereby reducing feelings of anxiety and depression.

5.2 Pharmacokinetic properties
L-tryptophan is readily absorbed after oral administration. The elimination half-life when administered orally or intravenously to healthy humans is in the range of 1-3 hours. L-tryptophan is bound to plasma proteins to a large extent and is eliminated primarily by metabolism.

5.3 Preclinical safety data
None reported

6. PHARMACEUTICAL PARTICULARS

6.1 List of excipients

Sta-RX Starch,

maize starch,

Explotab,

saccharin sodium,

magnesium stearate,

Aerosil

6.2 Incompatibilities

None known

6.3 Shelf life

3 years

6.4 Special precautions for storage

None

6.5 Nature and contents of container

Polypropylene bottle containing 84 tablets

6.6 Special precautions for disposal and other handling

Not applicable

7. MARKETING AUTHORISATION HOLDER

E Merck Ltd.

Bedfont Cross, Stanwell Road

Feltham, Middlesex,

TW14 8NX, UK

8. MARKETING AUTHORISATION NUMBER(S)

PL 0493/5900

9. DATE OF FIRST AUTHORISATION/RENEWAL OF THE AUTHORISATION

11/01/82 / 08/07/02

10. DATE OF REVISION OF THE TEXT

22 October 2008

Oramorph Oral Solution

(Boehringer Ingelheim Limited)

1. NAME OF THE MEDICINAL PRODUCT

Oramorph Oral Solution 10 mg/5 ml

2. QUALITATIVE AND QUANTITATIVE COMPOSITION

Each 5 ml contains 10 mg of Morphine Sulphate BP.

Excipients: 30 % w/v sucrose, 10.5 % w/v Ethanol (96%), methyl parahydroxybenzoate (E218) and propyl parahydroxybenzoate (E216).

For full list of excipients, see Section 6.1.

3. PHARMACEUTICAL FORM

A clear, colourless solution for oral administration.

4. CLINICAL PARTICULARS

4.1 Therapeutic indications

For the relief of severe pain.

4.2 Posology and method of administration

Adults: Usual dose 10-20 mg (5-10 ml) every 4 hours.

Children 6-12 years: Maximum dose 5-10 mg (2.5-5 ml) every 4 hours.

Children 1-5 years: Maximum dose 5 mg (2.5 ml) every 4 hours.

Children under 1 year: Not recommended.

Dosage can be increased under medical supervision according to the severity of the pain and the patient's previous history of analgesic requirements. Reductions in dosage may be appropriate in the elderly, patients with moderate-severe renal or hepatic impairment, or where sedation is undesirable.

Morphine Sulphate BP is readily absorbed from the gastro-intestinal tract following oral administration. However, when Oramorph Oral Solution is used in place of parenteral morphine, a 50% to 100% increase in dosage is usually required in order to achieve the same level of analgesia.

4.3 Contraindications

Respiratory depression, obstructive airways disease, known morphine sensitivity, acute hepatic disease, acute alcoholism, head injuries, coma, convulsive disorders and where the intracranial pressure is raised, paralytic ileus. Concurrent administration of monoamine oxidase inhibitors or within two weeks of discontinuation of their use.

Oramorph is contraindicated in patients known to be hypersensitive to morphine sulphate or to any other component of the product.

Morphine and some other opioids can induce the release of endogenous histamine and thereby stimulate catecholamine release making them unsuitable for use in patients with phaeochromocytoma.

Opioids are contraindicated in acute asthma exacerbations, see section 4.4 for information relating to use in controlled asthma.

4.4 Special warnings and precautions for use

Care should be exercised if morphine sulphate is given in the first 24 hours post-operatively, in hypothyroidism, and where there is reduced respiratory reserve, such as kyphoscoliosis, emphysema and severe obesity. Opioids are contra-indicated in acute asthma exacerbations. However, it has been suggested that they can be used with caution in controlled asthma.

Morphine sulphate should not be given if paralytic ileus is likely to occur (see section 4.3) or where there is an obstructive bowel disorder or prostatic hyperplasia. If constipation occurs, this may be treated with appropriate laxatives.

It is wise to reduce dosage in chronic hepatic and renal disease, myxoedema, adrenocortical insufficiency, prostatic hypertrophy or shock.

The administration of morphine may result in severe hypotension in individuals whose ability to maintain homeostatic blood pressure has already been compromised by depleted blood volume or the concurrent administration of drugs such as phenothiazine or certain anaesthetics.

Tolerance and dependence may occur. Withdrawal symptoms may occur on abrupt discontinuation or on the administration of a narcotic antagonist e.g. naloxone.

Hypersensitivity and anaphylactic reaction have both occurred with the use of Oramorph. Care should be taken to elicit any history of allergic reactions to opiates.

4.5 Interaction with other medicinal products and other forms of interaction

Phenothiazine antiemetics may be given with morphine, but it should be noted that morphine potentiates the effects of tranquillisers, anaesthetics, hypnotics, sedatives, antipsychotics, tricyclic antidepressants and alcohol. Morphine may possibly increase plasma concentrations of esmolol.

Cimetidine inhibits the metabolism of morphine. Opioid analgesics including morphine may antagonise the actions of domperidone and metoclopramide on gastro-intestinal activity. Concomitant use of ritonavir should be avoided as the plasma concentration of morphine may be increased. The absorption of mexiletine may be delayed by concurrent use of morphine.

Monoamine oxidase inhibitors are known to interact with narcotic analgesics producing CNS excitation or depression with hyper- or hypotensive crisis, please see section 4.3.

Interactions have been reported in those subjects taking oramorph and voriconazole. Interactions have been reported in those taking oramorph and gabapentin. Both interactions suggest an increase in opioid adverse events when co-prescribed, the mechanism of which is not known. Caution should be taken where these medicines are co-prescribed.

In a study involving healthy volunteers (N=12), when a 60 mg controlled-release morphine capsule was administered 2 hours prior to a 600 mg gabapentin capsule, mean gabapentin AUC increased by 44% compared to gabapentin administered without morphine. Therefore, patients should be carefully observed for signs of CNS depression, such as somnolence, and the dose of gabapentin or morphine should be reduced appropriately.

4.6 Pregnancy and lactation

Although morphine sulphate has been in general use for many years, there is inadequate evidence of safety in human pregnancy and lactation.

Morphine is known to cross the placenta, and is excreted in breast milk, and may thus cause respiratory depression in the newborn infant. Infants born from mothers who have been taking morphine on a chronic basis may exhibit withdrawal symptoms.

Gastric stasis and risk of inhalation pneumonia in mother during labour.

Medicines should not be used in pregnancy, especially the first trimester unless the expected benefit is thought to outweigh any possible risk to the foetus.

4.7 Effects on ability to drive and use machines

Morphine sulphate is likely to impair ability to drive and to use machinery. This effect is even more enhanced, when used in combination with alcohol or CNS depressants. Patients should be warned not to drive or operate dangerous machinery after taking Oramorph.

4.8 Undesirable effects

In routine clinical practice, the commonest side effects of morphine sulphate are nausea, vomiting, constipation, drowsiness and confusion If constipation occurs, this may be treated with appropriate laxatives.

Other adverse reactions include:

Cardiovascular: bradycardia, tachycardia, palpitations, orthostatic hypotension and hypothermia. Raised intracranial pressure occurs in some patients.

Central Nervous system: headache, restlessness, vertigo, mood changes, hallucinations, dependence, muscle rigidity.

Gastrointestinal: dry mouth, biliary spasm.

Genitourinary: decreased libido/potency, micturation may be difficult and there may be ureteric spasm. There is also an antidiuretic effect.

General: sweating, facial flushing and miosis.

These effects are more common in ambulant patients than in those who are bedridden.

Immune system disorders: hypersensitivity reactions including anaphylaxis. Urticaria, pruritis.

4.9 Overdose

Symptoms: Signs of morphine toxicity and overdosage are likely to consist of pin-point pupils, respiratory depression and hypotension. Circulatory failure and deepening coma may occur in more severe cases. Convulsions may occur in infants and children. Death may occur from respiratory failure.

Treatment of morphine overdose: Administer 0.4-2 mg of naloxone intravenously. Repeat at 2-3 minute intervals as necessary to a maximum of 10mg, or by an infusion of 2mg in 500 ml of normal saline or 5 % dextrose (4 microgram/ml). Empty the stomach. A 0.02% aqueous solution of potassium permanganate may be used for lavage. Care should always be taken that the airway is maintained. Assist respiration if necessary. Maintain fluid and electrolyte levels, oxygen, i.v. fluids, vasopressors and other supportive measures should be employed as indicated.

Caution: the duration of the effect of naloxone (2-3 hours) may be shorter than the duration of the effect of the morphine overdose. It is recommended that a patient who has regained consciousness after naloxone treatment should be observed for at least 6 hours after the last dose of naloxone.

5. PHARMACOLOGICAL PROPERTIES

5.1 Pharmacodynamic properties

Morphine binds to opiate receptors, which are located on the cell surfaces of the brain and nervous tissue. This action results in alteration of neurotransmitter release and calcium uptake. It has been postulated that this is the basis of the modulation of sensory input from afferent nerves sensitive to pain.

5.2 Pharmacokinetic properties

Morphine N-methyl ^{14}C sulphate administered orally to humans reaches a peak plasma level after around 15 minutes: levels of plasma-conjugated morphine peak at about 3 hours, and slowly decrease over the following 24 hours. After the first hour no significant differences in total plasma levels of radioactivity are seen whether administration is by intravenous, intramuscular, subcutaneous or oral route.

Morphine is a basic amine, and rapidly leaves the plasma and concentrates in the tissues. In animals it has been shown that a relatively small amount of free morphine crosses the blood-brain barrier. Morphine is metabolised in the liver and probably also in the mucosal cells of the small intestine. The metabolites recovered in the urine, in addition to free morphine, are morphine-3-glucuronide and morphine ethereal sulphate. These account for over 65 % of administered radioactivity; further radioactivity can be recovered as exhaled $^{14}CO_2$.

5.3 Preclinical safety data

No further relevant preclinical data are available.

6. PHARMACEUTICAL PARTICULARS

6.1 List of excipients

Ethanol (96%), corn syrup, sucrose, methyl parahydroxybenzoate (E218), propyl parahydroxybenzoate (E216) and purified water.

6.2 Incompatibilities

None stated.

6.3 Shelf life

3 years.

Discard Oramorph Oral Solution 3 months after first opening.

6.4 Special precautions for storage

Do not store above 25°C. Store in the original container to protect from light.

6.5 Nature and contents of container

Amber glass bottles with a tamper–evident, child resistant polypropylene closure with expanded PE liner are available in packs of 100 ml, 250 ml, 300 ml or 500 ml.

Not all pack sizes may be marketed.

6.6 Special precautions for disposal and other handling

None stated.

7. MARKETING AUTHORISATION HOLDER

Boehringer Ingelheim Limited

Ellesfield Avenue

Bracknell

Berkshire

RG12 8YS

United Kingdom

8. MARKETING AUTHORISATION NUMBER(S)

PL 0015/0122

9. DATE OF FIRST AUTHORISATION/RENEWAL OF THE AUTHORISATION

Date of first authorisation: 8th March 1988 /

Date of last renewal: 8th March 1993

10. DATE OF REVISION OF THE TEXT

August 2009

Legal category

POM

Orap 4 mg tablets.

(Janssen-Cilag Ltd)

1. NAME OF THE MEDICINAL PRODUCT
Orap™ 4 mg tablets.

2. QUALITATIVE AND QUANTITATIVE COMPOSITION
Each tablet contains pimozide 4 mg.

3. PHARMACEUTICAL FORM
Tablet

Green, circular, biconvex, normally arched tablets, cross-scored on one side and 'JANSSEN' on the other side.

4. CLINICAL PARTICULARS

4.1 Therapeutic indications
Orap is an antipsychotic of the diphenylbutyl-piperidine series and is indicated in:

- Chronic schizophrenia, for the treatment of symptoms and prevention of relapse.

- Other psychoses, especially paranoid and monosymptomatic hypochondriacal psychoses (eg delusional parasitosis).

4.2 Posology and method of administration
Orap is intended for once daily oral administration in adults and children over 12 years of age.

Since individual response to antipsychotic drugs is variable, dosage should be individually determined and is best initiated and titrated under close clinical supervision. In determining the initial dose, consideration should be given to the patient's age, severity of symptoms and previous response to other neuroleptic drugs. Dose increases should be made at weekly intervals or longer, and by increments of 2-4 mg in the daily dose.

The patient should be reviewed regularly to ensure the minimum effective dose is being used.

Chronic schizophrenia:

The dose ranges between 2 and 20 mg daily, with 2 mg as a starting dose. This may be increased according to response and tolerance to achieve an optimum response.

Other psychoses, paranoid states and monosymptomatic hypochondriacal psychoses (MHP):

An initial dose of 4 mg daily which may then be gradually increased, if necessary, according to response, to a maximum of 16 mg daily.

Use in elderly:

Elderly patients require half the normal starting dose of pimozide.

Method of Administration

Oral use.

4.3 Contraindications
In common with several other neuroleptics, pimozide has been reported to prolong the QT interval. It is, therefore, contra-indicated in patients with a pre-existing congenital prolongation of QT, or with a history of this syndrome, and in patients with a history of cardiac arrhythmias and a history of Torsades de pointes. Orap should not be used in the case of acquired long QT interval, such as that associated with the concomitant use of drugs known to prolong the QT interval (see section 4.5 Interactions), known uncorrected hypokalaemia or hypomagnesaemia, or clinically significant cardiac disorders (eg recent acute myocardial infarction, uncompensated heart failure, arrhythmias treated with class IA and III antiarrhythmic medicinal products) or clinically significant bradycardia.

Orap is also contra-indicated in patients with severe central nervous system depression and in patients with a known hypersensitivity to pimozide or other diphenylbutyl-piperidine derivatives. It should not be used in patients with depression or Parkinson's syndrome.

The concomitant use of orally or parenterally administered cytochrome P450 CYP 3A4 inhibiting drugs such as azole antimycotics, antiviral protease inhibitors, macrolide antibiotics and nefazodone is contra-indicated. The concomitant use of CYP 2D6 inhibiting drugs such as quinidine is also contra-indicated. The inhibition of either or both cytochrome P450 systems may result in the elevation of pimozide blood concentration and increase the possibility of QT-prolongation.

Orap is contraindicated with concomitant use of serotonin uptake inhibitors such as sertraline, paroxetine, citalopram and escitalopram (see Section 4.5).

4.4 Special warnings and precautions for use
Please also refer to Drug Interactions section.

Cardiac monitoring

There have been very rare reports of QT prolongation, ventricular arrhythmias, and Torsade de Pointes in patients without risk factors for QT prolongation administered therapeutic doses of pimozide, and in the setting of overdose. Ventricular tachycardia and ventricular fibrillation (in some cases with fatal outcomes) have also been reported, in addition to very rare reports of sudden death and cardiac arrest.

As with other neuroleptics, cases of sudden unexpected death have been reported with pimozide at recommended doses and in the setting of overdose. An ECG should be

Table 1

System Organ Class	Adverse Drug Reactions Frequency Category Very Common (≥ 1/10)	Common (≥ 1/100 to < 1/10)	Uncommon (≥ 1/1,000 to < 1/100)	Not Known
Endocrine Disorders				Hyperglycaemia (in patients with pre-existing diabetes); Blood Prolactin Increased
Metabolism and Nutrition Disorders		Anorexia		
Psychiatric Disorders		Depression; Insomnia; Agitation; Restlessness		Libido Decreased
Nervous System Disorders	Dizziness; Somnolence;	Extrapyramidal Disorder; Akathisia; Headache; Tremor; Lethargy; Muscle Rigidity	Bradykinesia; Cogwheel Rigidity; Dyskinesia; Dystonia; Dysarthria	Neuroleptic Malignant Syndrome; Grand Mal Convulsion; Tardive Dyskinesia; Neck Rigidity
Eye Disorders		Vision Blurred	Oculogyric crisis	
Cardiac Disorders				Torsade de Pointes; Ventricular Tachycardia; Ventricular Fibrillation
Gastrointestinal Disorders		Constipation; Dry Mouth; Vomiting; Salivary Hypersecretion		
Skin and subcutaneous tissue disorders	Hyperhidrosis	Sebaceous Gland Overactivity		Rash, Urticaria; Pruritus
Musculoskeletal and Connective Tissue Disorders			Muscle Spasms	
Renal and urinary disorders	Nocturia	Urinary frequency		Glycosuria
Reproductive System and Breast Disorders		Erectile Dysfunction	Amenorrhoea	Galactorrhoea; Gynaecomastia
General Disorders and Administration Site Conditions		Extreme exhaustion	Face oedema	Body Temperature Dysregulation; Hypothermia
Investigations				Electrocardiogram QT Interval Prolonged; Electroencephalogram Abnormal

performed prior to initiation of treatment with pimozide, as well as periodically during treatment. If repolarization changes (prolongation of QT interval, T-wave changes or U-wave development) appear or arrhythmias develop, the need for treatment with pimozide in these patients should be reviewed. They should be closely monitored and their dose of pimozide should be reduced or the drug discontinued. If QT or QTc exceeds 500 msec, pimozide should be discontinued.

As with other neuroleptics, caution is advised in patients with cardiovascular diseases, patients with a family history of QT prolongation. Hypotension may very rarely occur.

Electrolyte disturbances should also be considered a risk factor (see Section 4.3 Contraindications and Section 4.5 Interaction with other medicinal products and other forms of interaction) and periodic electrolyte monitoring is recommended.

Drugs which may cause electrolyte disturbances are not recommended in patients receiving long-term pimozide (please also refer to the Drug Interactions section.)

Liver disease

Caution is advised in patients with liver disease because pimozide is metabolized in the liver.

Kinetics of response/withdrawal

In schizophrenia, the response to antipsychotic drug treatment may be delayed. If drugs are withdrawn, recurrence of symptoms may not become apparent for several weeks or months.

Acute withdrawal symptoms, including nausea, vomiting, sweating and insomnia, have been described after abrupt cessation of antipsychotic drugs. Recurrence of psychotic symptoms may also occur, and the emergence of involuntary movement disorders (such as akathisia, dystonia and dyskinesia) has been reported. Therefore, gradual withdrawal is advisable.

Extrapyramidal symptoms

In common with all neuroleptics, extrapyramidal symptoms may occur (see Section 4.8). Antiparkinson drugs of the anticholinergic type may be prescribed as required, but should not be prescribed routinely as a preventive measure (see tardive dyskinesia below).

Tardive dyskinesia

As with all antipsychotic agents, tardive dyskinesia may appear in some patients on long-term therapy or after drug discontinuation. The syndrome is mainly characterized by rhythmical involuntary movements of the tongue, face, mouth or jaw. The manifestations may be permanent in some patients.

The syndrome may be masked when treatment is reinstituted, when the dosage is increased or when a switch is made to a different antipsychotic drug. Treatment should be discontinued as soon as possible.

There is no known treatment for tardive dyskinesia. The antipsychotic drug may mask it, as may anticholinergic agents. Although the latter do not predispose to tardive dyskinesia, they should not be used routinely to mask the Parkinsonian effects of antipsychotic drugs as they may mask the early signs of tardive dyskinesia.

Neuroleptic malignant syndrome

In common with other antipsychotic drugs, pimozide has been associated with neuroleptic malignant syndrome: an idiosyncratic response characterized by hyperthermia, generalised muscle rigidity, autonomic instability, altered consciousness. Hyperthermia is often an early sign of this syndrome.

Antipsychotic treatment should be withdrawn immediately and appropriate supportive therapy and careful monitoring instituted.

Seizures

As with other antipsychotic drugs, pimozide should be used cautiously in patients with a history of seizures or other conditions that potentially lower the seizure threshold (e.g. alcohol withdrawal or brain damage). In addition, grand mal convulsions have been reported in association with pimozide.

Body Temperature Regulation

Disruption of the body's ability to reduce core body temperature has been attributed to antipsychotic agents.

Appropriate care is advised when prescribing pimozide to patients who will be experiencing conditions which may contribute to an elevation in core body temperature, e.g., exercising strenuously, exposure to extreme heat, receiving concomitant medication with anticholinergic activity or being subject to dehydration.

Endocrine Effects

Hormonal effects of antipsychotic neuroleptic drugs include hyperprolactinaemia, which may cause galactorrhoea, gynaecomastia, oligomenorrhoea or amenorrhoea, and erectile dysfunction.

Pimozide should only be used with great caution in patients with thyrotoxicosis.

Other

Caution is also advised in patients with renal failure, Parkinson's disease and phaeochromocytoma.

Concomitant use of pimozide with other neuroleptics should be avoided.

4.5 Interaction with other medicinal products and other forms of interaction

Please also refer to the Precautions and Warnings and Contra-indications sections.

As with other neuroleptics, Orap may increase the central nervous system depression produced by other CNS depressant drugs, including alcohol, hypnotics, sedatives or strong analgesics.

Orap may impair the anti-Parkinson effect of levodopa. The dosage of anticonvulsants may need to be increased to take account of lowered seizure threshold.

Concomitant use of pimozide with drugs known to prolong the QT interval are contra-indicated (see section 4.3). Examples include certain antiarrhythmics, such as those of Class 1A (such as quinidine, disopyramide and procainamide) and Class III (such as amiodarone and sotalol), tricyclic antidepressants (such as amitriptyline), certain tetracyclic antidepressants (such as maprotiline), certain other antipsychotic medications (such as phenothiazines and sertindole), certain antihistamines (such as terfenadine), cisapride, bretylium and certain antimalarials such as quinine and mefloquine. This list is not comprehensive.

There is an increased risk of extrapyramidal effects with anti-emetics such as metoclopramide.

Avoid concomitant use with sibutramine due to an increased risk of CNS toxicity.

Concomitant use with calcium channel blockers may result in an enhanced hypotensive effect.

Concurrent treatment with neuroleptics should be kept to a minimum as they may predispose to the cardiotoxic effects of pimozide. Particular care should be exercised in patients who are using depot neuroleptics. Low potency neuroleptics such as chlorpromazine and thioridazine should not be used concomitantly with pimozide.

Pimozide is metabolised mainly via the cytochrome P450 subtype 3A4 (CYP 3A4) enzyme system and, to a lesser extent, via the CYP 2D6 subtype.

In vitro data indicate that highly potent inhibitors of the CYP 3A4 enzyme system, such as azole antimycotics, antiviral protease inhibitors, macrolide antibiotics and nefazodone will inhibit the metabolism of pimozide, resulting in markedly elevated plasma levels of pimozide.

In vitro data also indicated that quinidine diminishes the CYP 2D6 dependent metabolism of pimozide.

Elevated pimozide levels may enhance the risk of QT-prolongation.

As grapefruit juice is known to inhibit the metabolism of CYP3A4 metabolised drugs, concomitant use of grapefruit juice with pimozide should be avoided.

An *in vivo* study of pimozide added to steady state sertraline revealed a 40% increase in the pimozide AUC and Cmax (see Section 4.3).

An *in vivo* study of co-administered pimozide and citalopram resulted in a mean increase of QTc values of approximately 10 milliseconds. Citalopram did not alter the AUC and Cmax of pimozide (see Section 4.3).

An *in vivo* study of co-administered pimozide (a single 2 mg dose) and paroxetine (60 mg daily) was associated with mean increases of 151% in pimozide AUC and 62% in pimozide Cmax (see Section 4.3).

As CYP1A2 may also contribute to the metabolism of pimozide, prescribers should be aware of the theoretical potential for drug interactions with inhibitors of this enzymatic system.

Concurrent use of drugs causing electrolyte imbalance is not recommended. Diuretics, in particular those causing hypokalemia, should be avoided but, if necessary, potassium-sparing diuretics are preferred.

4.6 Pregnancy and lactation

The safety of Orap in human pregnancy has not been established. Studies in animals have not demonstrated teratogenic effects. As with other drugs, it is not advisable to administer Orap in pregnancy.

Orap may be excreted in breast milk. If the use of Orap is considered essential, breast feeding should be discontinued.

4.7 Effects on ability to drive and use machines

Orap may impair alertness, especially at the start of treatment. These effects may be potentiated by alcohol. Patients should be warned of the risks of sedation and advised not to drive or operate machinery during treatment until their susceptibility is known.

4.8 Undesirable effects

The safety of ORAP was evaluated in 165 pimozide-treated subjects who participated in seven placebo-controlled trials of patients with schizophrenia, or patients with anxiety or behavioural disorders, and in 303 pimozide-treated subjects who participated in eleven active-comparator controlled clinical trials in patients with schizophrenia (10 trials, including chronic schizophrenia) or psychic fatigability (1 trial). Based on pooled safety data from these clinical trials, the most commonly reported (≥ 9% incidence) Adverse Drug Reactions (ADRs) were (with % incidence): Nervous System Disorders: Dizziness (11) and Somnolence (11), Extrapyramidal Disorder (9); Muscle Rigidity (9); Hyperhidrosis (13); Nocturia (12).

Including the above-mentioned ADRs, the following table (next page) displays ADRs that have been reported with the use of ORAP from either clinical-trial or post-marketing experiences. The displayed frequency categories use the following convention:

Very common (≥ 1/10); common (≥ 1/100 to < 1/10); uncommon (≥ 1/1,000 to < 1/100); rare (≥ 1/10,000 to <1/1,000); very rare (<1/10,000), not known (cannot be estimated form the available data)

(see Table 1 on previous page)

In addition to the above, cardiac arrest and sudden unexplained death have been reported with the use of pimozide. These events should be considered ADRs associated with the class of medicinal products, the D2, dopamine-antagonist neuroleptics.

4.9 Overdose

In general, the signs and symptoms of overdose with Orap would be an exaggeration of known pharmacological effects, the most prominent of which would be severe extrapyramidal symptoms, hypotension or sedation. The risk of cardiac arrhythmias, possibly associated with QT-prolongation and ventricular arrhythmias including Torsade de Pointes, should be considered. The patient may appear comatose with respiratory depression and hypotension which could be severe enough to produce a shock-like state.

Treatment:

There is no specific antidote to pimozide. Gastric lavage, establishment of a patent airway and, if necessary, mechanically assisted respiration are advised. Continuous electrocardiographic monitoring should be performed due to the risk of QT interval prolongation and ventricular arrhythmias including Torsade de Pointes and continued until the ECG returns to normal. Hypotension and circulatory collapse may be counteracted by the use of intravenous fluids, plasma or concentrated albumin, and vasopressor agents such as noradrenaline.

Adrenaline should not be used.

In cases of severe extrapyramidal symptoms, anti-Parkinson medication should be administered.

Because of the long half-life of pimozide, patients who have taken an overdose should be observed for at least 4 days.

5. PHARMACOLOGICAL PROPERTIES

5.1 Pharmacodynamic properties

Pimozide is an orally active neuroleptic drug which blocks central dopaminergic receptors. Pimozide antagonises many of the actions of amphetamine and apomorphine.

5.2 Pharmacokinetic properties

The mean serum elimination half-life in schizophrenic patients is approximately 55 hours. This is highly variable and may be as long as 150 hours in some individuals. There is a 13-fold interindividual difference in the area under the serum pimozide concentration-time curve and an equivalent degree of variation in peak serum levels among patients studied. The significance of this is unclear since there are few correlations between plasma levels and clinical findings.

5.3 Preclinical safety data

No relevant information additional to that contained elsewhere in the Summary of Product Characteristics.

6. PHARMACEUTICAL PARTICULARS

6.1 List of excipients

Calcium hydrogen phosphate dihydrate

Maize starch

Microcrystalline cellulose

Polyvidone K30

Talc

Cottonseed Oil Hydrogenated

Ferric oxide (E172)

Indigotindisulphonate (E132) - aluminium lake

Purified water*

* not in final product

6.2 Incompatibilities

None known.

6.3 Shelf life

36 months.

6.4 Special precautions for storage

Do not store above 25°C.

6.5 Nature and contents of container

PVC/aluminium foil blister packs, containing 28*, 100 or 250* tablets.

* *not marketed*

6.6 Special precautions for disposal and other handling

Not applicable.

7. MARKETING AUTHORISATION HOLDER

Janssen-Cilag Ltd

50-100 Holmers Farm Way

High Wycombe

Buckinghamshire

HP12 4EG

UK

8. MARKETING AUTHORISATION NUMBER(S)

PL 0242/0038R

9. DATE OF FIRST AUTHORISATION/RENEWAL OF THE AUTHORISATION

Renewal of Authorisation: 7 April 2002

10. DATE OF REVISION OF THE TEXT

11 February 2009

Orelox Paediatric Granules for Oral Suspension

(sanofi-aventis)

1. NAME OF THE MEDICINAL PRODUCT

Orelox™ Paediatric Granules for Oral Suspension.

2. QUALITATIVE AND QUANTITATIVE COMPOSITION

When reconstituted each 5ml volume contains 52mg of cefpodoxime proxetil (equivalent to 40mg cefpodoxime).

3. PHARMACEUTICAL FORM

Granules for the preparation of an oral suspension.

4. CLINICAL PARTICULARS

4.1 Therapeutic indications

Orelox is a bactericidal cephalosporin antibiotic active against a wide range of Gram-negative and Gram-positive organisms. It is indicated for the treatment of the following infections either before the infecting organism has been identified or when caused by bacteria of established sensitivity.

Indications include:

Upper respiratory tract infections caused by organisms sensitive to cefpodoxime, including acute otitis media, sinusitis, tonsillitis and pharyngitis.

Orelox should be reserved for recurrent or chronic infections, or for infections where the causative organism is known or suspected to be resistant to commonly used antibiotics.

Lower respiratory tract infections caused by organisms sensitive to cefpodoxime. Including pneumonia, acute bronchitis and when bacterial super-infection complicates bronchiolitis.

Upper and lower urinary tract infections caused by organisms sensitive to cefpodoxime including cystitis and acute pyelonephritis.

Skin and soft tissue infections caused by organisms sensitive to cefpodoxime such as abscesses, cellulitis, infected wounds, furuncles, folliculitis, paronychia, carbuncles and ulcers.

4.2 Posology and method of administration

Route of administration: oral.

Adults and Elderly:

Not applicable for this product.

Children:

The recommended mean dosage for children is 8mg/kg/day administered in two divided doses at 12 hour intervals.

The following dosage regimen is proposed as a guide to prescribing:-

Below 6 months: 8mg/kg/day in 2 divided doses

6 months-2 years: 5.0 ml twice daily

3-8 years: 10.0 ml twice daily

Above 9 years: 12.5ml twice daily or 100mg tablet twice daily

Orelox should not be used in infants less than 15 days old, as no experience yet exists in this age group.

A measuring spoon (5ml) is provided with the bottle to aid correct dosing. One measuring spoon (5ml) contains the equivalent of 40 mg cefpodoxime.

The product should be taken during meals for optimal absorption.

Renal Impairment:

The dosage of Orelox does not require modification if creatinine clearance exceeds 40 $ml.min^{-1}/1.73m^2$.

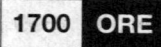

Below this value, pharmacokinetic studies indicate an increase in plasma elimination half-life and the maximum plasma concentrations, and hence the dosage should be adjusted appropriately.

CREATININE CLEARANCE (ML/MIN)	
39 – 10	Unit dose[1] administered as a single dose every 24 hours (i.e half of the usual adult dose).
< 10	Unit dose[1] administered as a single dose every 48 hours (i.e quarter of the usual adult dose).
Haemodialysis Patients	Unit dose[1] administered after each dialysis session.

NOTE:

[1]The unit dose is either 100mg or 200mg, depending on the type of infection.

Hepatic Impairment:

The dosage does not require modification in cases of hepatic impairment.

Instructions for Reconstitution:

Before preparing the suspension the silica gel desiccant contained in a capsule inside the cap must be removed and disposed of. The suspension is prepared by adding water to the bottle up to the calibrated mark and shaking thoroughly to obtain an evenly dispersed suspension

4.3 Contraindications

Patients with hypersensitivity to cephalosporin antibiotics.

Patients with phenylketonuria since the product contains aspartame.

Patients with rare hereditary problems of galactose intolerance, fructose intolerance, the Lapp lactase deficiency, glucose-galactose malabsorption or sucrase-isomaltase insufficiency should not take this medicine.

4.4 Special warnings and precautions for use

Preliminary enquiry about allergy to penicillin is necessary before prescribing cephalosporins since cross allergy to penicillins occurs in 5-10% of cases.

Particular care will be needed in patients sensitive to penicillin: strict medical surveillance is necessary from the very first administration. Where there is doubt, medical assistance should be available at the initial administration, in order to treat any anaphylactic episode.

In patients who are allergic to other cephalosporins, the possibility of cross allergy to Orelox should be borne in mind. Orelox should not be given to those patients with a previous history of immediate type hypersensitivity to cephalosporins.

Hypersensitivity reactions (anaphylaxis) observed with beta-lactam antibiotics can be serious and occasionally fatal.

The onset of any manifestation of hypersensitivity indicates that treatment should be stopped.

Orelox is not the preferred antibiotic for the treatment of staphylococcal pneumonia and should not be used in the treatment of atypical pneumonia caused by organisms such as *Legionella*, *Mycoplasma* and *Chlamydia*.

In cases of severe renal insufficiency it may be necessary to reduce the dosage regimen dependent on the creatinine clearance.

Antibiotics should always be prescribed with caution in patients with a history of gastrointestinal disease, particularly colitis. Orelox may induce diarrhoea, antibiotic associated colitis and pseudomembranous colitis. These side-effects, which may occur more frequently in patients receiving higher doses for prolonged periods, should be considered as potentially serious. The presence of *C. difficile* should be investigated. In all potential cases of colitis, the treatment should be stopped immediately. The diagnosis should be confirmed by sigmoidoscopy and specific antibiotic therapy (vancomycin) substituted if considered clinically necessary. The administration of products which cause faecal stasis must be avoided. Although any antibiotic may cause pseudomembranous colitis, the risk may be higher with broad-spectrum drugs, such as the cephalosporins.

As with all beta-lactam antibiotics, neutropenia, and more rarely agranulocytosis may develop, particularly during extended treatment. For cases of treatment lasting longer than 10 days, blood count should therefore be monitored, and treatment discontinued if neutropenia is found.

Cephalosporins may be absorbed onto the surface of red cell membranes and react with antibiotics directed against the drug. This can produce a positive Coombs' test and very rarely, haemolytic anaemia. Cross-reactivity may occur with penicillin for this reaction.

The product should not be used in infants less than 15 days old as no clinical trial data in this age group yet exists.

Changes in renal function have been observed with antibiotics of the same class, particularly when given concurrently with potentially nephrotoxic drugs such as aminoglycosides and/or potent diuretics. In such cases, renal function should be monitored.

As with other antibiotics, the prolonged use of cefpodoxime proxetil may result in the overgrowth of non-susceptible organisms. With oral antibiotics the normal colonic flora may be altered, allowing overgrowth by clostridia with consequent pseudomembranous colitis. Repeated evaluation of the patient is essential and if superinfection occurs during therapy, appropriate measures should be taken.

4.5 Interaction with other medicinal products and other forms of interaction

No clinically significant drug interactions have been reported during the course of clinical studies.

Histamine H2-antagonists and antacids reduce the bioavailibility of cefpodoxime. Probenecid reduces the excretion of cephalosporins. Cephlasporins potentially enhance the anticoagulant effect of coumarins and reduce the contraceptive effect of oestrogens.

As with other cephalosporins, isolated cases showing development of a positive Coombs' test have been reported (see Precautions).

Studies have shown that bioavailability is decreased by approximately 30% when Orelox is administered with drugs which neutralise gastric pH or inhibit acid secretions. Therefore, such drugs as antacids of the mineral type and H_2 blockers such as ranitidine, which cause an increase in gastric pH, should be taken 2 or 3 hours after Orelox administration.

In contrast, drugs which decrease gastric pH such as pentagastrine will increase bioavailability. The clinical consequences remain to be established.

The bioavailability increases if the product is administered during meals.

A false positive reaction for glucose in the urine may occur with Benedict's or Fehling's solutions or with copper sulphate test tablets, but not with tests based on enzymatic glucose oxidase reactions.

4.6 Pregnancy and lactation

Not applicable.

4.7 Effects on ability to drive and use machines

Not applicable.

4.8 Undesirable effects

Possible side effects include gastrointestinal disorders such as diarrhoea and rarely antibiotic-associated colitis (see Section 4.4: Special Warnings and Precautions for Use), nausea, vomiting and abdominal pain and rash, urticaria and itching. Changes in renal function have been observed with antibiotics from the same group as cefpodoxime, particularly when co-prescribed with aminoglycosides and/or potent diuretics.

Occasional cases have been reported of headaches, dizziness, tinnitus, parethesia, asthenia and malaise. Rare cases of allergic reactions including hypersensitivity mucocutaneous reactions, skin rashes and pruritus. Occasional cases of bullous reactions including Stevens-Johnson syndrome, toxic epidermal necrolysis and erythema multiforme have also been received. Transient moderate elevations of ASAT, ALAT and alkaline phosphatases and/or bilirubin have been reported. These laboratory abnormalities which may also be explained by the infection, may rarely exceed twice the upper limit of the named range and elicit a pattern of liver injury, usually cholestatic and most often asymptomatic. Slight increases in blood urea and creatinine have also been reported. Exceptionally rare are the occurrence of liver damage and of haematological disorders such as reduction in haemoglobin, thrombocytosis, thrombocytopenia, leucopenia and eosinophilia. Haemolytic anaemia has extremely rarely been reported.

As with other β-lactam antibiotics, neutropenia and, more rarely, agranulocytosis may develop during treatment with cefpodoxime, particularly if given over long periods.

As with other cephalosporins there have been rare reports of anaphylactic reactions, bronchospasm, purpura and angiodema, serum sickness-like reactions with rashes, fever and arthralgia.

4.9 Overdose

In the event of overdosage with Orelox, supportive and symptomatic therapy is indicated.

In cases of overdosage, particularly in patients with renal insufficiency, encephalopathy may occur. The encephalopathy is usually reversible once cefpodoxime plasma levels have fallen.

5. PHARMACOLOGICAL PROPERTIES

5.1 Pharmacodynamic properties

Orelox (Cefpodoxime proxetil) is a beta-lactam antibiotic, a 3rd generation oral cephalosporin. It is the prodrug of cefpodoxime.

Following oral administration, Orelox is taken up by the gastro-intestinal wall where it is rapidly hydrolysed to cefpodoxime, a bactericidal antibiotic, which is then absorbed systemically.

BACTERIOLOGY:

The mechanism of action of cefpodoxime is based on inhibition of bacterial cell wall synthesis. It is stable to numerous beta-lactamases.

Cefpodoxime has been shown to possess *in vitro* bactericidal activity against numerous Gram-positive and Gram-negative bacteria.

ANTIBACTERIAL ACTIVITY:

It is highly active against the Gram-positive organisms:

- *Streptococcus pneumoniae*
- Streptococci of Groups A (*S. pyogenes*), B (*S. agalactiae*), C, F and G
- Other streptococci (*S. mitis*, *S. sanguis* and *S. salivarius*)
- *Propionibacterium acnes*
- *Corynebacterium diphtheriae*

It is highly active against the Gram-negative organisms:

- *Haemophilus influenzae* (beta-lactamase and non beta-lactamase producing strains)
- *Haemophilus para-influenzae* (beta-lactamase and non beta-lactamase producing strains)
- *Moraxella catarrhalis* (beta-lactamase and non beta-lactamase producing strains)
- *Escherichia coli*
- *Klebsiella* Spp. (*K. pneumoniae*)
- *Proteus mirabilis*

It is moderately active against:

- Meticillin-sensitive staphylococci, penicillinase and non-penicillinase producing strains (*S. aureus* and *S. epidermidis*)

In addition, as with many cephalosporins, the following are resistant to cefpodoxime.

- Enterococci
- Meticillin-resistant staphylococci (*S. aureus* and *S. coagulase* (negative))
- *Staphylococcus saprophyticus*
- *Pseudomonas aeruginosa* and *Pseudomonas* Spp.
- *Clostridium difficile*
- *Bacteroides fragilis* and related species

As with all antibiotics, whenever possible, sensitivity should be confirmed by *in vitro* testing.

5.2 Pharmacokinetic properties

Orelox is taken up in the intestine and is hydrolysed to the active metabolite cefpodoxime. When cefpodoxime proxetil is administered orally to fasting subjects as a tablet corresponding to 100mg of cefpodoxime, 51.5% is absorbed and absorption is increased by food intake. The volume of distribution is 32.3 l and peak levels of cefpodoxime occur 2 to 3 hrs after dosing. The maximum plasma concentration is 1.2mg/l and 2.5mg/l after doses of 100mg and 200mg respectively. Following administration of 100mg and 200mg twice daily over 14.5 days, the plasma pharmacokinetic parameters of cefpodoxime remain unchanged.

Serum protein binding of cefpodoxime, 40% principally to albumin. This binding is non saturable in type.

Concentrations of cefpodoxime in excess of the minimum inhibitory levels (MIC) for common pathogens can be achieved in lung parenchyma, bronchial mucosa, pleural fluid, tonsils, interstitial fluid and prostate tissue.

As the majority of cefpodoxime is eliminated in the urine, the concentration is high. (Concentrations in 0-4, 4-8, 8-12 hr fractions after a single dose exceed MIC_{90} of common urinary pathogens). Good diffusion of cefpodoxime is also seen into renal tissue, with concentrations above MIC_{90} of the common urinary pathogens, 3-12hrs after an administration of a single 200mg dose (1.6-3.1μG/G). Concentrations of cefpodoxime in the medullary and cortical tissues is similar.

Studies in healthy volunteers show median concentrations of cefpodoxime in the total ejaculate 6-12hrs following administration of a single 200mg dose to be above the MIC_{90} of *N. gonorrhoeae*.

The main route of excretion is renal, 80% is excreted unchanged in the urine, with an elimination half life of approx 2.4 hours.

CHILDREN

In children, studies have shown the maximum plasma concentration occurs approximately 2-4 hours after dosing. A single 5mg/kg dose in 4-12 year olds produced a maximum concentration similar to that in adults given a 200mg dose.

In patients below 2 years receiving repeated doses of 5mg/kg 12 hourly, the average plasma concentrations, 2hrs post dose, are between 2.7mg/l (1-6 months) and 2.0mg/l (7 months-2 years).

In patients between 1 month and 12 years receiving repeated doses of 5mg/kg 12 hourly, the residual plasma concentrations at steady state are between 0.2-0.3mg/l (1 month-2 years) and 0.1mg/l (2-12 years).

5.3 Preclinical safety data

Not applicable.

6. PHARMACEUTICAL PARTICULARS

6.1 List of excipients

The product contains anhydrous colloidal silica, aspartame, banana flavour, carboxymethylcellulose calcium, carboxymethylcellulose sodium, citric acid monohydrate, hydroxypropylcellulose, yellow iron oxide, lactose monohydrate, monosodium glutamate, potassium sorbate, sodium chloride, sorbitan trioleate, sucrose and talc.

6.2 Incompatibilities
None reported during clinical studies.

6.3 Shelf life
24 months.

Reconstituted suspension: can be stored for up to 10 days refrigerated (2-8°C).

6.4 Special precautions for storage
Bottles: unreconstituted product should be stored below 30°C.

6.5 Nature and contents of container
Amber glass bottle with a calibration marking. This is fitted with a polyethylene dehydrating capsule containing silica gel, closed by a cardboard disc make up part of closure. There is a polyethylene pilfer and childproof screw cap fitted with tight triseal joint.

Pack sizes of 100ml of suspension.

A 5ml plastic spoon is supplied with the pack.

6.6 Special precautions for disposal and other handling
Before preparing the suspension the silica gel desiccant contained in a capsule inside the cap must be removed and disposed of. The suspension is prepared by adding water to the bottle up to the calibrated mark and shaking thoroughly to obtain an evenly dispersed suspension.

7. MARKETING AUTHORISATION HOLDER
Sanofi-aventis
One Onslow Street
Guildford
Surrey
GU1 4YS
UK

8. MARKETING AUTHORISATION NUMBER(S)
PL 04425/0251

9. DATE OF FIRST AUTHORISATION/RENEWAL OF THE AUTHORISATION
23rd July 2004

10. DATE OF REVISION OF THE TEXT
December 2006

LEGAL CATEGORY
POM

Orelox Tablets 100mg

(sanofi-aventis)

1. NAME OF THE MEDICINAL PRODUCT
Orelox™ Tablets 100mg.

2. QUALITATIVE AND QUANTITATIVE COMPOSITION
Each Orelox tablet contains 130mg of cefpodoxime proxetil (equivalent to 100mg cefpodoxime).

3. PHARMACEUTICAL FORM
Tablet for oral use.

4. CLINICAL PARTICULARS

4.1 Therapeutic indications
Orelox is a bactericidal cephalosporin antibiotic active against a wide range of Gram-negative and Gram-positive organisms. It is indicated for the treatment of the following infections either before the infecting organism has been identified or when caused by bacteria of established sensitivity.

Upper respiratory tract infections caused by organisms sensitive to cefpodoxime, including sinusitis.

In tonsillitis and pharyngitis, Orelox should be reserved for recurrent or chronic infections, or for infections where the causative organism is known or suspected to be resistant to commonly used antibiotics.

Lower respiratory tract infections caused by organisms sensitive to cefpodoxime, including acute bronchitis, relapses or exacerbations of chronic bronchitis and bacterial pneumonia.

Upper and lower urinary tract infections caused by organisms sensitive to cefpodoxime including cystitis and acute pyelonephritis.

Skin and soft tissue infections caused by organisms sensitive to cefpodoxime such as abscesses, cellulitis, infected wounds, furuncles, folliculitis, paronychia, carbuncles and ulcers.

Gonorrhoea - uncomplicated gonococcal urethritis.

4.2 Posology and method of administration
Route of administration: oral.

<u>Adults</u>:

Adults with normal renal function:

Upper respiratory tract infections: For upper respiratory tract infections caused by organisms sensitive to cefpodoxime, including sinusitis. In tonsillitis and pharyngitis, Orelox should be reserved for recurrent or chronic infections, or for infections where the causative organism is known or suspected to be resistant to commonly used antibiotics. Sinusitis: 200mg twice daily. Other upper respiratory tract infections: 100mg twice daily.

Lower respiratory tract infections: For lower respiratory tract infections caused by organisms sensitive to cefpodoxime, including acute bronchitis, relapses or exacerbations of chronic bronchitis and bacterial pneumonia: 100-200 mg twice daily, dependent on the severity of the infection.

Urinary tract infections:

Uncomplicated lower urinary tract infections: 100mg should be taken twice daily.

Uncomplicated upper urinary tract infections: 200mg should be taken twice daily.

Uncomplicated gonococcal urethritis: 200mg should be taken as a single dose.

Skin and soft tissue infections: 200mg should be taken twice daily.

Tablets should be taken during meals for optimum absorption.

<u>Elderly</u>:

It is not necessary to modify the dose in elderly patients with normal renal function.

<u>Children</u>:

Orelox Paediatric is available to treat infants (over 15 days old) and children. Please refer to the separate Summary of Product Characteristics for details.

<u>**Hepatic Impairment:**</u>

The dosage does not require modification in cases of hepatic impairment.

<u>**Renal Impairment:**</u>

The dosage of Orelox does not require modification if creatinine clearance exceeds 40 ml/min.

Below this value, pharmacokinetic studies indicate an increase in plasma elimination half-life and the maximum plasma concentrations, and hence the dosage should be adjusted appropriately.

CREATININE CLEARANCE (ML/MIN)	
39 – 10	Unit dose[1] administered as a single dose every 24 hours (i.e half of the usual adult dose).
< 10	Unit dose[1] administered as a single dose every 48 hours (i.e quarter of the usual adult dose).
Haemodialysis Patients	Unit dose[1] administered after each dialysis session.

NOTE:
[1]The unit dose is either 100mg or 200mg, depending on the type of infection.

4.3 Contraindications
Hypersensitivity to cephalosporin antibiotics.

Patients with rare hereditary problems of galactose intolerance, the Lapp lactase deficiency or glucose-galactose malabsorption should not take this medicine.

4.4 Special warnings and precautions for use
Preliminary enquiry about allergy to penicillin is necessary before prescribing cephalosporins since cross allergy to penicillins occurs in 5-10% of cases.

Particular care will be needed in patients sensitive to penicillin: strict medical surveillance is necessary from the very first administration. Where there is doubt, medical assistance should be available at the initial administration, in order to treat any anaphylactic episode.

In patients who are allergic to other cephalosporins, the possibility of cross allergy to Orelox should be borne in mind. Orelox should not be given to those patients with a previous history of immediate type hypersensitivity to cephalosporins.

Hypersensitivity reactions (anaphylaxis) observed with beta-lactam antibiotics can be serious and occasionally fatal.

The onset of any manifestation of hypersensitivity indicates that treatment should be stopped.

Orelox is not the preferred antibiotic for the treatment of staphylococcal pneumonia and should not be used in the treatment of atypical pneumonia caused by organisms such as *Legionella*, *Mycoplasma* and *Chlamydia*.

In cases of severe renal insufficiency it may be necessary to reduce the dosage regimen dependent on the creatinine clearance.

Possible side effects include gastrointestinal disorders such as nausea, vomiting and abdominal pain. Antibiotics should always be prescribed with caution in patients with a history of gastrointestinal disease, particularly colitis. Orelox may induce diarrhoea, antibiotic associated colitis and pseudomembranous colitis. These side-effects, which may occur more frequently in patients receiving higher doses for prolonged periods, should be considered as potentially serious. The presence of *C. difficile* should be investigated. In all potential cases of colitis, the treatment should be stopped immediately. The diagnosis should be confirmed by sigmoidoscopy and specific antibiotic therapy (vancomycin) substituted if considered clinically necessary. The administration of products which cause faecal stasis must be avoided. Although any antibiotic may cause pseudomembranous colitis, the risk may be higher with broad-spectrum drugs, such as the cephalosporins.

As with all beta-lactam antibiotics, neutropenia, and more rarely agranulocytosis may develop, particularly during extended treatment. For cases of treatment lasting longer than 10 days, blood count should therefore be monitored, and treatment discontinued if neutropenia is found.

Cephalosporins may be absorbed onto the surface of red cell membranes and react with antibodies directed against the drug. This can produce a positive Coombs' test and very rarely, haemolytic anaemia. Cross-reactivity may occur with penicillin for this reaction.

Changes in renal function have been observed with antibiotics of the same class, particularly when given concurrently with potentially nephrotoxic drugs such as aminoglycosides and/or potent diuretics. In such cases, renal function should be monitored.

As with other antibiotics, the prolonged use of cefpodoxime proxetil may result in the overgrowth of non-susceptible organisms. With oral antibiotics the normal colonic flora may be altered, allowing overgrowth by clostridia with consequent pseudomembranous colitis. Repeated evaluation of the patient is essential and if superinfection occurs during therapy, appropriate measures should be taken.

4.5 Interaction with other medicinal products and other forms of interaction
No clinically significant drug interactions have been reported during the course of clinical studies.

Histamine H2-antagonists and antacids reduce the bioavailibility of cefpodoxime. Probenecid reduces the excretion of cephalosporins. Cephlasporins potentially enhance the anticoagulant effect of coumarins and reduce the contraceptive effect of oestrogens.

As with other cephalosporins, isolated cases showing development of a positive Coombs' test have been reported (see Precautions).

Studies have shown that bioavailability is decreased by approximately 30% when Orelox is administered with drugs which neutralise gastric pH or inhibit acid secretions. Therefore, such drugs as antacids of the mineral type and H_2 blockers such as ranitidine, which can cause an increase in gastric pH, should be taken 2 to 3 hours after Orelox administration.

The bioavailability increases if the product is administered during meals.

A false positive reaction for glucose in the urine may occur with Benedict's or Fehling's solutions or with copper sulphate test tablets, but not with tests based on enzymatic glucose oxidase reactions.

4.6 Pregnancy and lactation
Studies carried out in several animal species have not shown any teratogenic or foetotoxic effects. However, the safety of cefpodoxime proxetil in pregnancy has not been established and, as with all drugs, it should be administered with caution during the early months of pregnancy.

Cefpodoxime is excreted in human milk. Either breastfeeding or treatment of the mother should be stopped.

4.7 Effects on ability to drive and use machines
Attention should be drawn to the risk of dizzy sensations.

4.8 Undesirable effects
Possible side effects include gastrointestinal disorders such as diarrhoea and rarely antibiotic-associated colitis, (see Section 4.4: Special Warnings and Precautions for Use), nausea, vomiting and abdominal pain and rash, urticaria and itching. Changes in renal function have been observed with antibiotics from the same group as cefpodoxime, particularly when co-prescribed with aminoglycosides and/or potent diuretics.

Occasional cases have been reported of headaches, dizziness, tinnitus, parethesia, asthenia and malaise. Rare cases of allergic reactions include hypersensitivity mucocutaneous reactions, skin rashes and pruritus. Occasional cases of bullous reactions such as Stevens-Johnson syndrome, toxic epidermal necrolysis and erythema multiforme have also been received. Transient moderate elevations of ASAT, ALAT and alkaline phosphatases and/or bilirubin have been reported. These laboratory abnormalities which may be explained by the infection, may rarely exceed twice the upper limit of the named range and elicit a pattern of liver injury, usually cholestatic and most often asymptomatic. Slight increases in blood urea and creatinine have also been reported. Exceptionally rare are the occurrence of liver damage and of haematological disorders such as reduction in haemoglobin, thrombocytosis, thrombocytopenia, leucopenia and eosinophilia. Haemolytic anaemia has extremely rarely been reported.

As with other β-lactam antibiotics, neutropenia and, more rarely, agranulocytosis may develop during treatment with cefpodoxime, particularly if given over long periods.

As with other cephalosporins, there have been rare reports of anaphylactic reactions, bronchospasm, purpura and angioema, serum-sickness-like reactions with rashes, fever and arthralgia.

4.9 Overdose

In the event of overdosage with Orelox, supportive and symptomatic therapy is indicated.

In cases of overdosage, particularly in patients with renal insufficiency, encephalopathy may occur. The encephalopathy is usually reversible once cefpodoxime plasma levels have fallen.

5. PHARMACOLOGICAL PROPERTIES

5.1 Pharmacodynamic properties

Orelox (Cefpodoxime proxetil) is a beta-lactam antibiotic, a 3rd generation oral cephalosporin. It is the prodrug of cefpodoxime.

Following oral administration, Orelox is taken up by the gastro-intestinal wall where it is rapidly hydrolysed to cefpodoxime, a bactericidal antibiotic, which is then absorbed systemically.

BACTERIOLOGY:

The mechanism of action of cefpodoxime is based on inhibition of bacterial cell wall synthesis. It is stable to numerous beta-lactamases.

Cefpodoxime has been shown to possess *in vitro* bactericidal activity against numerous Gram-positive and Gram-negative bacteria.

It is highly active against the Gram-positive organisms:

- *Streptococcus pneumoniae*
- Streptococci of Groups A (*S. pyogenes*), B (*S. agalactiae*), C, F and G
- Other streptococci (*S. mitis, S. sanguis* and *S. salivarius*)
- *Corynebacterium diphtheriae*

It is highly active against the Gram-negative organisms:

- *Haemophilus influenzae* (beta-lactamase and non beta-lactamase producing strains)
- *Haemophilus para-influenzae* (beta-lactamase and non beta-lactamase producing strains)
- *Branhamella catarrhalis* (beta-lactamase and non beta-lactamase producing strains)
- *Neisseria meningitidis*
- *Neisseria gonorrhoeae*
- *Escherichia coli*
- *Klebsiella* Spp. (*K. pneumoniae*; *K. oxytoca*)
- *Proteus mirabilis*

It is moderately active against meticillin-sensitive staphylococci, penicillinase and non-penicillinase producing strains (*S. aureus* and *S. epidermidis*).

In addition, as with many cephalosporins, the following are resistant to cefpodoxime: enterococci, meticillin-resistant staphylococci (*S. aureus* and *S. epidermidis*), *Staphylococcus saprophyticus, Pseudomonas aeruginosa and Pseudomonas* Spp., *Clostridium difficile, Bacteroides fragilis* and related species.

As with all antibiotics, whenever possible, sensitivity should be confirmed by *in vitro* testing.

5.2 Pharmacokinetic properties

Orelox is taken up in the intestine and is hydrolysed to the active metabolite cefpodoxime. When cefpodoxime proxetil is administered orally to fasting subjects as a tablet corresponding to 100mg of cefpodoxime, 51.5% is absorbed and absorption is increased by food intake. The volume of distribution is 32.3 l and peak levels of cefpodoxime occur 2 to 3 hrs after dosing. The maximum plasma concentration is 1.2mg/l and 2.5mg/l after doses of 100mg and 200mg respectively. Following administration of 100mg and 200mg twice daily over 14.5 days, the plasma pharmacokinetic parameters of cefpodoxime remain unchanged.

Serum protein binding of cefpodoxime, 40% principally to albumin. This binding is non saturable in type.

Concentrations of cefpodoxime in excess of the minimum inhibitory levels (MIC) for common pathogens can be achieved in lung parenchyma, bronchial mucosa, pleural fluid, tonsils, interstitial fluid and prostate tissue.

As the majority of cefpodoxime is eliminated in the urine, the concentration is high. (Concentrations in 0-4, 4-8, 8-12 hr fractions after a single dose exceed MIC_{90} of common urinary pathogens). Good diffusion of cefpodoxime is also seen into renal tissue, with concentrations above MIC_{90} of the common urinary pathogens, 3-12hrs after an administration of a single 200mg dose (1.6-3.1μG/G). Concentrations of cefpodoxime in the medullary and cortical tissues is similar.

Studies in healthy volunteers show median concentrations of cefpodoxime in the total ejaculate 6-12hrs following administration of a single 200mg dose to be above the MIC_{90} of *N. gonorrhoeae*.

The main route of excretion is renal, 80% is excreted unchanged in the urine, with an elimination half life of approx 2.4 hours.

5.3 Preclinical safety data

Not applicable.

6. PHARMACEUTICAL PARTICULARS

6.1 List of excipients

The product contains magnesium stearate, carboxymethylcellulose calcium, hydroxypropylcellulose, sodium lauryl sulphate, lactose, ethyl alcohol and purified water. The coating contains titanium dioxide, talc and hydroxypropylmethylcellulose 6CP.

6.2 Incompatibilities

None reported during clinical studies.

6.3 Shelf life

36 months.

6.4 Special precautions for storage

Store below 25°C.

6.5 Nature and contents of container

Orelox tablets are supplied in blister packs of 10 tablets.

6.6 Special precautions for disposal and other handling

None.

7. MARKETING AUTHORISATION HOLDER

Sanofi-aventis

One Onslow Street

Guildford

Surrey

GU1 4YS

UK

8. MARKETING AUTHORISATION NUMBER(S)

PL 04425/0252

9. DATE OF FIRST AUTHORISATION/RENEWAL OF THE AUTHORISATION

12 February 2004

10. DATE OF REVISION OF THE TEXT

December 2006

LEGAL CATEGORY

POM

Ortho-Gynest Pessaries

(Janssen-Cilag Ltd)

1. NAME OF THE MEDICINAL PRODUCT

Ortho-Gynest 0.5mg Pessaries

2. QUALITATIVE AND QUANTITATIVE COMPOSITION

Estriol 0.5mg

Excipients: Benzoic acid, Butylated hydroxytoluene

For a full list of excipients, see section 6.1

3. PHARMACEUTICAL FORM

Pessary

Description of the product:

Ortho-Gynest Pessaries are yellowish-white, egg-shaped vaginal pessaries. Their consistency is that of soft paraffin. They will liquefy at body temperature within 30 minutes.

4. CLINICAL PARTICULARS

4.1 Therapeutic indications

1. Hormonal replacement for the treatment of atrophic vaginitis and kraurosis vulvae (due to estrogen deficiency) in post-menopausal women.

2. Treatment of pruritus vulvae and dyspareunia associated with atrophic vaginal epithelium.

4.2 Posology and method of administration

Ortho-Gynest Pessaries are an estrogen-only product for intravaginal use.

No progestogen needs to be added (but please refer to section 4.4).

Guidance on how to start therapy and maintenance

Ortho-Gynest Pessaries can be started any time after the manifestation of atrophic vaginitis or associated symptoms (eg dyspareunia, pruritus). The recommended initial dose is one pessary per day.

A maintenance dose of one pessary every three or four days (twice a week) may be used after restoration of the vaginal mucosa has been achieved.

For initiation and continuation of treatment of postmenopausal symptoms, the lowest effective dose for the shortest (see also Section 4.4) should be used. Attempts to taper and discontinue medication should be made at three to six month intervals following physical examination.

Administration

Insert the pessary high into the vagina, preferably in the evening

Advice when a dose is forgotten

If a dose is forgotten, a pessary should be inserted as soon as possible.

There is no relevant indication for use of Ortho-Gynest in children.

4.3 Contraindications

Hypersensitivity to estriol or to any of the excipients.

- Known, past or suspected breast cancer
- Known or suspected estrogen-dependent malignant tumuours (eg endometrial cancer)
- Undiagnosed genital bleeding
- Untreated endometrial hyperplasia
- Previous idiopathic or current venous thrombo-embolism (deep venous thrombosis, pulmonary embolism)
- Active or recent arterial thrombo-embolic disease (eg angina, myocardial infarction)
- Acute liver disease, or a history of liver disease as long as liver function tests have failed to return to normal
- Porphyria

4.4 Special warnings and precautions for use

For the treatment of postmenopausal symptoms, HRT should only be initiated for symptoms that adversely affect quality of life. In all cases, a careful appraisal of the risks and benefits should be undertaken at least annually and HRT should only be continued as long as the benefit outweighs the risk

Medical examination/follow-up

Before initiating or re-instituting HRT, a complete personal and family medical history should be taken. Physical (including pelvic and breast) examination should be guided by this and by the contra-indications and warnings for use. During treatment, periodic check-ups are recommended of a frequency and nature adapted to the individual woman. Women should be advised what changes in their breasts should be reported to their doctor or nurse (see 'Breast cancer' below). Investigations, including mammography, should be carried out in accordance with currently accepted screening practices, modified to the clinical needs of the individual.

Conditions which need supervision

If any of the following conditions are present, have occurred previously, and/or have been aggravated during pregnancy or previous hormone treatment, the patient should be closely supervised. It should be taken into account that these conditions may recur or be aggravated during treatment with Ortho-Gynest Pessaries, in particular:

- Leiomyoma (uterine fibroids) or endometriosis
- A history of, or risk factors for, thrombo-embolic disorders (see below)
- Risk factors for estrogen dependent tumours, eg 1st degree heredity for breast cancer
- Hypertension
- Liver disorders (eg liver adenoma)
- Diabetes mellitus with or without vascular involvement
- Cholelithiasis
- Migraine or (severe) headache
- Systemic lupus erythematosus
- A history of endometrial hyperplasia (see below)
- Epilepsy
- Asthma
- Otosclerosis

Reasons for immediate withdrawal of therapy:

Therapy should be discontinued if a contra-indication is discovered and in the following situations:

- Jaundice or deterioration in liver function
- Significant increase in blood pressure
- New onset of migraine-type headache
- Pregnancy

Endometrial hyperplasia

The risk of endometrial hyperplasia and carcinoma is increased when systemic estrogens are administered alone for prolonged periods of time. The endometrial safety of long-term or repeated use of topical vaginal estrogens is uncertain. Therefore, if repeated, treatment should be reviewed at least annually, with special consideration given to any symptoms of endometrial hyperplasia or carcinoma.

If break-through bleeding or spotting appears at any time on therapy, the reason should be investigated, which may include endometrial biopsy to exclude endometrial malignancy.

Unopposed estrogen stimulation may lead to premalignant or malignant transformation in the residual foci of endometriosis. Therefore, caution is advised when using this product in women who have undergone hysterectomy because of endometriosis, if they are known to have residual endometriosis.

Breast cancer

A randomised placebo-controlled trial, the Women's Health Initiative (WHI) and epidemiological studies, including the Million Women Study (MWS) have reported an increased risk of breast cancer in women taking estrogens or estrogen-progestogen combinations or tibolone for HRT for several years (see Section 4.8).

For all HRT, an excess risk becomes apparent within a few years of use and increases with duration of intake but returns to baseline within a few (at most five) years after stopping treatment.

In the MWS, the relative risk of breast cancer with conjugated equine estrogens (CEE) or estradiol (E2) was greater when a progestogen was added, either sequentially or continuously, and regardless of type of progestogen. There was no evidence of a difference in risk between the different routes of administration.

In the WHI study, the continuous combined conjugated equine estrogen and medroxyprogesterone acetate (CEE + MPA) product used was associated with breast cancers that were slightly larger in size and more frequently had local lymph node metastases compared to placebo.

HRT, especially estrogen-progestogen combined treatment, increases the density of mammographic images which may adversely affect the radiological detection of breast cancer.

Venous thrombo-embolism

HRT is associated with a higher relative risk of developing venous thrombo-embolism (VTE), i.e. deep vein thrombosis or pulmonary embolism. One randomised controlled trial and epidemiological studies found a two- to threefold higher risk for users compared with non-users. For non-users it is estimated that the number of cases of VTE that will occur over a 5 year period is about 3 per 1000 women aged 50-59 years and 8 per 1000 women aged 60-69 years. It is estimated that in healthy women who use HRT for 5 years, the number of additional cases of VTE over a 5 year period will be between 2 and 6 (best estimate =4) per 1000 women aged 50-59 years and between 5 and 15 (best estimate =9) per 1000 women aged 60-69 years. The occurrence of such an event is more likely in the first year of HRT than later.

Generally recognised risk factors for VTE include a personal history or family history, severe obesity (BMI > 30 kg/m^2) and systemic lupus erythematosus (SLE). There is no consensus about the possible role of varicose veins in VTE.

Patients with a history of VTE or known thrombophilic states have an increased risk of VTE. HRT may add to this risk. Personal or strong family history of thrombo-embolism or recurrent spontaneous abortion should be investigated in order to exclude a thrombophilic predisposition. Until a thorough evaluation of thrombophilic factors has been made or anticoagulant treatment initiated, use of HRT in such patients should be viewed as contra-indicated. The women already on anticoagulant treatment require careful consideration of the benefit-risk of use of HRT.

The risk of VTE may be temporarily increased with prolonged immobilisation, major trauma or major surgery. As in all postoperative patients, scrupulous attention should be given to prophylactic measures to prevent VTE following surgery. Where prolonged immobilisation is liable to follow elective surgery, particularly abdominal or orthopaedic surgery to the lower limbs, consideration should be given to temporarily stopping HRT 4 weeks earlier, if this is possible. Treatment should not be restarted until the woman is completely mobilised.

If VTE develops after initiating therapy, the drug should be discontinued. Patients should be told to contact their doctors immediately when they are aware of a potential thrombo-embolic symptom (eg, painful swelling of a leg, sudden pain in the chest, dyspnoea).

Coronary artery disease (CAD)

There is no evidence from randomised controlled trials of cardiovascular benefit with continuous combined conjugated estrogens and medroxyprogesterone acetate MPA. Two large clinical trials (WHI and HERS i.e. Heart and Estrogen/progestin Replacement Study) showed a possible increased risk of cardiovascular morbidity in the first year of use and no overall benefit. For other HRT products there are only limited data from randomised controlled trials examining effects in cardiovascular morbidity or mortality. Therefore, it is uncertain whether these findings also extend to other HRT products.

Stroke

One large randomised clinical trial (WHI-trial) found, as a secondary outcome, an increased risk of ischaemic stroke in healthy women during treatment with continuous combined conjugated estrogens and MPA. For women who do not use HRT, it is estimated that the number of cases of stroke that will occur over a 5 year period is about 3 per 1000 women aged 50-59 years and 11 per 1000 women aged 60-69 years. It is estimated that for women who use conjugated estrogens and MPA for 5 years, the number of additional cases will be between 0 and 3 (best estimate = 1) per 1000 users aged 50-59 years and between 1 and 9 (best estimate = 4) per 1000 users aged 60-69 years. It is unknown whether the increased risk also extends to other HRT products.

Ovarian cancer

Long-term (at least 5-10 years) use of estrogen-only HRT products in hysterectomised women has been associated with an increased risk of ovarian cancer in some epidemiological studies. It is uncertain whether long-term use of combined HRT confers a different risk than estrogen-only products.

Other conditions

Estrogens may cause fluid retention, and therefore patients with cardiac or renal dysfunction should be carefully observed. Patients with terminal renal insufficiency should be closely observed, since it is expected that the level of circulating active ingredients in Ortho-Gynest Pessaries is increased.

Women with pre-existing hypertriglyceridaemia should be followed closely during estrogen replacement or hormone replacement therapy, since rare cases of large increases of plasma triglycerides leading to pancreatitis have been reported with estrogen therapy in this condition.

Oral estrogens increase thyroid binding globulin (TBG), leading to increased circulating total thyroid hormone, as measured by protein-bound iodine (PBI), T4 levels (by column or radio-immunoassay) or T3 levels (by radio-immunoassay). T3 resin uptake is decreased, reflecting the elevated TBG. Free T4 and free T3 concentrations are unaltered. Other binding proteins may be elevated in serum, i.e. corticoid binding globulin (CBG), sex-hormone-binding globulin (SHBG) leading to increased circulating corticosteroids and sex steroids, respectively. Free or biological active hormone concentrations are unchanged. Other plasma proteins may be increased (angiotensinogen/renin substrate, alpha-I-antitrypsin, ceruloplasmin). With vaginal administration, stimulation of the liver by the first-pass effect is avoided and thus, transvaginal estrogens might affect hormone binding proteins and other serum proteins produced by the liver less than oral hormones.

There is no conclusive evidence for improvement of cognitive function. There is some evidence from the WHI trial of increased risk of probable dementia in women who start using continuous combined CEE and MPA after the age of 65. It is unknown whether the findings apply to younger post-menopausal women or other HRT products.

4.5 Interaction with other medicinal products and other forms of interaction

The serum concentration and efficacy of estrogens could be reduced and its metabolism increased by concomitant administration of drugs known to induce drug metabolising enzymes, specifically CYP 450 enzymes, such as anticonvulsants (eg phenobarbital, phenytoin, carbamazepine) and anti-infectives (eg rifampicin, rifabutin, nevirapine, efavirenz) and also bosentan.

Ritonavir and nelfinavir, although known as strong inhibitors, by contrast exhibit inducing properties when used concomitantly with steroid hormones. Herbal preparations containing St. John's Wort (*Hypericum perforatum*) may raise the metabolism of estrogens. With intravaginal administration, the first-pass effect in the liver is avoided and thus, estriol given intravaginally might be less affected by enzyme inducers than oral hormones.

Clinically, an increased metabolism of estrogens may lead to decreased effect.

Contact between contraceptive diaphragm or condoms and Ortho-Gynest Pessaries must be avoided since the rubber may be damaged by this preparation.

Estrogen-containing oral contraceptives have been shown to significantly decrease plasma concentrations of lamotrigine when co-administered due to induction of lamotrigine glucuronidation. This may reduce seizure control. Although the potential interaction between estrogen-containing hormone replacement therapy and lamotrigine has not been studied, it is expected that a similar interaction exists, which may lead to a reduction in seizure control among women taking both drugs together. Therefore, dose adjustment of lamotrigine may be necessary.

4.6 Pregnancy and lactation

Pregnancy

Ortho-Gynest Pessaries are not indicated during pregnancy. If pregnancy occurs during use of Ortho-Gynest Pessaries, treatment should be withdrawn immediately.

There are no clinical data on exposed pregnancies.

The results of most epidemiological studies to date relevant to inadvertent foetal exposure to estrogens indicate no teratogenic or foetotoxic effect.

Lactation

Ortho-Gynest Pessaries are not indicated during lactation.

4.7 Effects on ability to drive and use machines

No studies on the effects on the ability to drive and use machines have been performed.

4.8 Undesirable effects

In a double-blind, placebo controlled clinical trial of 30 women treated with Ortho-Gynest, the following undesirable effects were reported in the estriol pessary treatment group more frequently than in the placebo group:

Breast pain, micturition frequency increased, vaginal discharge, cystitis, leg pain, pre-menstrual tension, lower abdominal pain, palpitations and depression.

The following adverse reactions, associated with estrogen treatment, may occur during estriol overdose: breast pain or tenderness nausea, break-through bleeding, abdominal cramps and/or bloating.

Breast cancer

According to evidence from a large number of epidemiological studies and one randomised placebo-controlled trial, the Women's Health Initiative(WHI), the overall risk of breast cancer increases with increasing duration of HRT use in current or recent HRT users.

For *estrogen-only* HRT, estimates of relative risk (RR) from a re-analysis of original data from 51 epidemiological studies (in which >80% of HRT use was estrogen-only HRT) and from the epidemiological Million Women Study (MWS) are similar at 1.35 (95%CI 1.21 – 1.49) and 1.30 (95%CI 1.21 – 1.40), respectively.

For *estrogen plus progestogen* combined HRT, several epidemiological studies have reported an overall higher risk for breast cancer than with estrogens alone.

The MWS reported that, compared to never users, the use of various types of estrogen-progestogen combined HRT was associated with a higher risk of breast cancer (RR = 2.00, 95%CI: 1.88 – 2.12) than use of estrogens alone (RR = 1.30, 95%CI: 1.21 – 1.40) or use of tibolone (RR=1.45; 95%CI 1.25-1.68).

The WHI trial reported a risk estimate of 1.24 (95%CI 1.01 – 1.54) after 5.6 years of use of estrogen-progestogen combined HRT (CEE + MPA) in all users compared with placebo.

The absolute risks calculated from the MWS and the WHI trial are presented below:

The MWS has estimated, from the known average incidence of breast cancer in developed countries, that:

- For women not using HRT, about 32 in every 1000 are expected to have breast cancer diagnosed between the ages of 50 and 64 years.
- For 1000 current or recent users of HRT, the number of *additional* cases during the corresponding period will be
- For users of *estrogen-only* replacement therapy

between 0 and 3 (best estimate = 1.5) for 5 years' use

between 3 and 7 (best estimate = 5) for 10 years' use.

- For users of *estrogen plus progestogen* combined HRT,

between 5 and 7 (best estimate = 6) for 5 years' use

between 18 and 20 (best estimate = 19) for 10 years' use.

The WHI trial estimated that after 5.6 years of follow-up of women between the ages of 50 and 79 years, an *additional* 8 cases of invasive breast cancer would be due to *estrogen-progestogen combined* HRT (CEE + MPA) per 10,000 women years.

According to calculations from the trial data, it is estimated that:

- For 1000 women in the placebo group, about 16 cases of invasive breast cancer would be diagnosed in 5 years.
- For 1000 women who used estrogen + progestogen combined HRT (CEE+ MPA), the number of *additional* cases would be between 0 and 9 (best estimate = 4) for 5 years' use.

The number of additional cases of breast cancer in women who use HRT is broadly similar for women who start HRT irrespective of age at start of use (between the ages of 45-65) (see section 4.4).

Other adverse events which have been reported in association with estrogen/progestogen treatment are:

- Estrogen-dependent neoplasms benign and malignant; eg endometrial cancer; breast cancer.
- Venous thrombo-embolism. Deep leg or pelvic venous thrombosis and pulmonary embolism are more frequent among HRT users than among non-users. For further information, see section 4.3 Contra-indications and 4.4 Special Warnings and Precautions for Use.
- Myocardial infarction and stroke.
- Gall bladder disease.
- Skin and subcutaneous tissue disorders: chloasma; erythema multiforme; erythema nodosum; vascular purpura, urticaria, angioedema.
- Probable dementia (see section 4.4).

4.9 Overdose

Symptoms of overdose of estrogen therapy may include breast pain or tenderness, nausea, break-through bleeding, abdominal cramps and/or bloating. Vaginal lavage should be considered. If accidental ingestion of large quantities of the product occurs, an appropriate method of gastric emptying may be considered.

5. PHARMACOLOGICAL PROPERTIES

5.1 Pharmacodynamic properties

Pharmacotherapeutic group: Natural and semisynthetic estrogens, plain; ATC code: G03CA04

The active ingredient, synthetic estriol, is chemically and biologically identical to endogenous human estriol. Estriol, a weak estrogen, is a natural metabolite of estradiol, the predominant estrogen. Estriol exerts estrogenicity by binding to estrogen receptors present in the female genital tract.

Oral or vaginal estriol, similar to estradiol, corrects lowered proliferation and abnormal physiology in the atrophic vaginal epithelium seen in estrogen deficient states, such as after natural or surgical menopause. Studies of the endometrium after using Ortho-Gynest Pessaries rarely show minor signs of proliferation in previously atrophic endometria.

Clinical trial information

Improvement of vaginal epithelial cytology was noted in 50 subjects with vaginal atrophy already after 7 days of daily treatment with Ortho-Gynest Pessaries. Improvement was sustained over 7 or more weeks in a total of 70 patients studied in two clinical trials. Alleviation of associated symptoms (eg dyspareunia, urethral symptoms) was first observed after 4 weeks of daily treatment with Ortho-Gynest Pessaries in a total of 110 women in four clinical trials and further improvement was seen over subsequent months.

5.2 Pharmacokinetic properties
Estriol is readily absorbed following intravaginal application. Peak serum estriol concentrations are generally observed within 2 hours following intravaginal application and remain elevated for 6 hours. Systemic bioavailability on vaginal administration is better than after oral administration. Intravaginal application of 1 mg estriol in women with senile atrophy of the vaginal epithelium results in serum levels similar to those seen after oral administration of 10 mg estriol.

Upon first use of an Ortho-Gynest Pessary, plasma levels of estriol rise within 2 hours to 450 +/- 113 pmol/L (156+/- 39 pg/mL) (mean+/- SD), and remain elevated for at least 6 hours in supine subjects, while levels decline to baseline within 4 hours in active subjects. Upon continuous use, little if any accumulation occurs, as plasma estriol levels 8-10 hours after last administration were detectable only in one third of subjects.

Estriol circulates with the blood, about 14% free, 8% bound to SHBG and the rest bound to albumin. Primary metabolites of estriol include the 16-alpha-glucuronide, 3-glucuronide, 3-sulfate and 3-sulfate 16-alpha-glucuronide. More than 95% of estriol is excreted in the urine, predominantly in the form of glucuronides.

5.3 Preclinical safety data
No relevant information additional to that contained elsewhere in the Summary of Product Characteristics.

6. PHARMACEUTICAL PARTICULARS

6.1 List of excipients
Benzoic acid
Butylated hydroxytoluene
Polyethylene glycol 400
Polyethylene glycol 1000
Sorbitan monostearate
Witepsol S 55

6.2 Incompatibilities
Not applicable

6.3 Shelf life
2 years

6.4 Special precautions for storage
Do not store above 30°C

6.5 Nature and contents of container
PVC or PVC/PE moulds, containing 5* or 15 pessaries.

* Not currently marketed

6.6 Special precautions for disposal and other handling
Please refer to Section 4.2 Posology and Method of Administration.

Empty blisters may be disposed of in household waste. Return unused drug to your pharmacy for destruction. Do not dispose of unused drug in household waste or flush it down the toilet

7. MARKETING AUTHORISATION HOLDER
Janssen-Cilag Ltd
50 -100 Holmers Farm Way
High Wycombe
Buckinghamshire
HP12 4EG
UK

8. MARKETING AUTHORISATION NUMBER(S)
PL 00242/0250

9. DATE OF FIRST AUTHORISATION/RENEWAL OF THE AUTHORISATION
Date of first authorisation: 1 December 1995

Date of latest renewal: 19 May 2006

10. DATE OF REVISION OF THE TEXT
8th June 2009

Orudis 100

(sanofi-aventis)

1. NAME OF THE MEDICINAL PRODUCT
Orudis 100

2. QUALITATIVE AND QUANTITATIVE COMPOSITION
In terms of the active ingredient

Ketoprofen 100mg

3. PHARMACEUTICAL FORM
Capsules

4. CLINICAL PARTICULARS

4.1 Therapeutic indications
Recommended in the management of rheumatoid arthritis, osteoarthritis, ankylosing spondylitis, acute articular and periarticular disorders, (bursitis, capsulitis, synovitis, tendinitis), cervical spondylitis, low back pain (strain, lumbago, sciatica, fibrositis), painful musculoskeletal conditions, acute gout, dysmenorrhoea and control of pain and inflammation following orthopaedic surgery.

Orudis reduces joint pain and inflammation and facilitates increase in mobility and functional independence.

It does not cure the underlying disease.

4.2 Posology and method of administration
Oral dosage 50 - 100mg twice daily, morning and evening, depending on patient's weight and on the severity of symptoms.

The maximum daily dose is 200mg. The balance of risks and benefits should be carefully considered before commencing treatment with 200mg daily, and higher doses are not recommended (see also section 4.4).

Best results are obtained by titrating dosage to suit each patient: start with a low dosage in mild chronic disease and a high dosage in acute or severe disease. Some patients derive greater benefit by treatment with capsules only, some with a combined capsule/suppository regimen and others with a higher dosage at night time than at early morning. Where patients require a maximum oral dosage initially, an attempt should be made to reduce this dosage for maintenance since lower dosage might be better tolerated for purposes of long-term treatment.

Elderly: The elderly are at increased risk of the serious consequences of adverse reactions. If an NSAID is considered necessary, the lowest effective dose should be used and for the shortest possible duration. The patient should be monitored regularly for GI bleeding during NSAID therapy.

Paediatric dosage: Not established.

To limit occurrence of gastrointestinal disturbance, capsules should always be taken with food (milk, meals).

Undesirable effects may be minimised by using the lowest effective dose for the shortest duration necessary to control symptoms (see section 4.4).

4.3 Contraindications
Ketoprofen is contraindicated in patients who have a history of hypersensitivity reactions such as asthmatic attacks, rhinitis, angioedema, urticaria or other allergic-type reactions to ketoprofen, any other ingredients in this medicine, ASA or other NSAIDs. Severe, rarely fatal, anaphylactic reactions have been reported in such patients (see section 4.8 – Undesirable effects).

Ketoprofen is also contraindicated in the following cases:

– Severe heart failure

– active peptic ulcer or any history of gastrointestinal haemorrhage, ulceration or perforation

– History of gastrointestinal bleeding or perforation, related to previous NSAIDs therapy

– severe hepatic insufficiency

– severe renal insufficiency

– third trimester of pregnancy

Disease in children (safety/dosage during long-term treatment has not been established).

4.4 Special warnings and precautions for use
Undesirable effects may be minimised by using the lowest effective dose for the shortest duration necessary to control symptoms (see section 4.2, and GI and cardiovascular risks below).

The use of Orudis with concomitant NSAIDs including cyclooxygenase-2 selective inhibitors should be avoided (see section 4.5).

Elderly:
The elderly have an increased risk of adverse reactions to NSAIDs, especially gastro-intestinal bleeding and perforation which may be fatal (see Section 4.2 – Posology and method of administration).

Cardiovascular, Renal and Hepatic impairment:
At the start of treatment, renal function must be carefully monitored in patients with heart impairment, heart failure, liver dysfunction, cirrhosis and nephrosis, in patients receiving diuretic therapy, in patients with chronic renal impairment, particularly if the patient is elderly. In these patients, administration of ketoprofen may induce a reduction in renal blood flow caused by prostaglandin inhibition and lead to renal decomposition. (see also Section 4.3 – Contra-indications).

NSAIDs have also been reported to cause nephrotoxicity in various forms and this can lead to interstitial nephritis, nephrotic syndrome and renal failure.

In patients with abnormal liver function tests or with a history of liver disease, transaminase levels should be evaluated periodically, particularly during longterm therapy. Rare cases of jaundice and hepatitis have been described with ketoprofen.

Cardiovascular and cerebrovascular effects
Appropriate monitoring and advice are required for patients with a history of hypertension and/or mild to moderate congestive heart failure as fluid retention and oedema have been reported in association with NSAID therapy.

Clinical trial and epidemiological data suggest that use of some NSAIDs (particularly at high doses and in long term treatment) may be associated with a small increased risk of arterial thrombotic events (for example myocardial infarction or stroke). There are insufficient data to exclude such a risk for ketoprofen.

Patients with uncontrolled hypertension, congestive heart failure, established ischaemic heart disease, peripheral arterial disease, and/or cerebrovascular disease should only be treated with ketoprofen after careful consideration. Similar consideration should be made before initiating longer-term treatment of patients with risk factors for cardiovascular disease (e.g. hypertension, hyperlipidaemia, diabetes mellitus, smoking).

Respiratory disorders:
Caution is required if NSAIDs are administered to patients suffering from, or with a previous history of, bronchial asthma, since NSAIDs have been reported to cause bronchospasm in such patients.

Gastro-intestinal bleeding, ulceration and perforation:
GI bleeding, ulceration or perforation, which can be fatal, has been reported with all NSAIDs at any time during treatment, with or without warning symptoms or a previous history of serious GI events.

Some epidemiological evidence suggests that ketoprofen may be associated with a high risk of serious gastrointestinal toxicity, relative to some other NSAIDs, especially at high doses (see also section 4.2 and 4.3).

The risk of GI bleeding, ulceration or perforation is higher with increasing NSAID doses, in patients with a history of ulcer, particularly if complicated with haemorrhage or perforation (see section 4.3), and in the elderly. These patients should commence treatment on the lowest dose available. Combination therapy with protective agents (e.g. misoprostol or proton pump inhibitors) should be considered for these patients, and also for patients requiring concomitant low dose aspirin, or other drugs likely to increase gastrointestinal risk (see below and section 4.5).

NSAIDs should only be given with care to patients with a history of gastro-intestinal disease (e.g. ulcerative colitis, Crohn's disease) as these conditions may be exacerbated (see Section 4.8 – Undesirable effects). Patients with a history of GI toxicity, particularly when elderly, should report any unusual abdominal symptoms (especially GI bleeding), particularly in the initial stages of treatment.

Caution should be advised in patients receiving concomitant medications which could increase the risk of ulceration or bleeding, such as corticosteroids, or anti-coagulants such as warfarin, selective serotonin-reuptake inhibitors or anti-platelet agents such as aspirin (see Section 4.5).

When GI bleeding or ulceration occurs in patients receiving ketoprofen, the treatment should be withdrawn.

SLE and mixed connective tissue disease:
In patients with systemic lupus erythematosus (SLE) and mixed connective tissue disorders, there may be an increased risk of aseptic meningitis (see Section 4.8 - Undesirable effects).

Female fertility:
The use of ketoprofen, as with other NSAIDs, may impair female fertility and is not recommended in women attempting to conceive. In women who have difficulty conceiving or who are undergoing investigation of infertility, withdrawal of ketoprofen should be considered.

Skin reactions:
Serious skin reactions, some of them fatal, including exfoliative dermatitis, Stevens-Johnson syndrome, and toxic epidermal necrolysis, have been reported very rarely in association with the use of NSAIDs. Patients appear to be at highest risk of these reactions early in the course of therapy, the onset of the reaction occurring in the majority of cases within the first month of treatment. Treatment should be discontinued at the first appearance of skin rash, mucosal lesions, or any other sign of hypersensitivity.

Infectious disease:
As with other NSAIDs, in the presence of an infectious disease, it should be noted that the anti-inflammatory, analgesic and the antipyretic properties of ketoprofen may mask the usual signs of infection progression such as fever.

Visual disturbances:
If visual disturbances such a blurred vision occur, treatment should be discontinued.

4.5 Interaction with other medicinal products and other forms of interaction
Anticoagulants (heparin and warfarin) and platelet aggregation inhibitors (i.e.ticlopidine, clopidogrel):

Increased risk of bleeding. If coadministration is unavoidable, patient should be closely monitored. (see section 4.4 – Special warnings and precautions for use)

Lithium: Ketoprofen can increase lithium blood levels to possibly toxic levels due to decreased elimination of lithium. If administered together, plasma concentrations of lithium should be monitored in order to adjust the lithium dose.

Other analgesics/NSAIDs (including cyclooxygenase-2 selective inhibitors) and high dose salicylates:
Avoid concomitant use of two or more NSAIDs (including aspirin) as this may increase the risk of adverse effects, particularly gastrointestinal ulceration and bleeding. (see Section 4.4 – Special warnings and precautions for use).

Methotrexate: Serious interactions have been recorded after the use of high dose methotrexate with NSAIDs, including ketoprofen, due to decreased elimination of methotrexate. At doses greater than 15mg/week:

Increased risk of haematologic toxicity of methotrexate, particularly if administered at high doses (> 15 mg/week), possibly related to displacement of protein-bound methotrexate and to its decreased renal clearance. At doses lower than 15mg/week: During the first weeks of combination treatment, full blood count should be monitored weekly. If there is any alteration of the renal function or if the patient is elderly, monitoring should be done more frequently.

Mifepristone: NSAIDs should not be used for 8-12 days after mifepristone administration as NSAIDs can reduce the effect of mifepristone.

Pentoxifylline: There is an increased risk of bleeding. More frequent clinical monitoring and monitoring of bleeding time is required.

Antihypertensives: Reduced antihypertensive effect.

Diuretics: Risk of reduced diuretic effect. Patients and particularly dehydrated patients taking diuretics are at a greater risk of developing renal failure secondary to a decrease in renal blood flow caused by prostaglandin inhibition. Such patients should be rehydrated before initiating coadministration therapy and renal function monitored when the treatment is started (see section 4.4 – Special warnings and precautions for use).

Cardiac glycosides: NSAIDs may exacerbate cardiac failure, reduce GFR and increase plasma glycoside levels.

Cyclosporin: Increased risk of nephrotoxicity.

Corticosteroids: Increased risk of GI ulceration or bleeding. (see Section 4.4 Special warnings and precautions for use).

Quinolone antibiotics: Animal data indicate that NSAIDs can increase the risk of convulsions associated with quinolone antibiotics. Patients taking NSAIDs and quinolones may have an increased risk of developing convulsions.

Tacrolimus: Possible increased risk of nephrotoxicity when NSAIDs are given with tacrolimus.

Thrombolytics: Increased risk of bleeding.

Probenecid: Concomitant administration of probenecid may markedly reduce the plasma clearance of ketoprofen.

Anti-platelet agents and Selective serotonin reuptake inhibitors (SSRIs): increased risk of gastrointestinal bleeding (section 4.4 – Special warnings and precautions for use).

ACE inhibitors and Angiotensin II Antagonists:

In patients with compromised renal function (e.g. dehydrated patients or elderly patients the co-administration of an ACE inhibitor or Angiotensin II antagonist and agents that inhibit cyclo-oxygenase may result in further deterioration of renal function, including possible acute renal failure.

Zidovudine: increased risk of haematological toxicity when NSAIDs are given with zidovudine. There is evidence of an increased risk of haemarthroses and haematoma in HIV(+) haemophiliacs receiving concurrent treatment with zidovudine and ibuprofen.

4.6 Pregnancy and lactation

Pregnancy

No embryopathic effects have been demonstrated in animals. Congenital abnormalities have been reported in association with NSAID administration in man; however, these are low in frequency and do not appear to follow any discernable pattern.

It is recommended to avoid ketoprofen during the first two trimesters of pregnancy or labour unless the potential benefit to the patient outweighs the potential risk to the foetus.

In view of the known effects of NSAIDs on the foetal cardiovascular system (risk of premature closure of the ductus arteriosus), use in the last trimester of pregnancy is contra-indicated (see Section 4.3 - Contra-indications). The onset of labour may be delayed and the duration increased with an increased bleeding tendency in both mother and child.

Lactation

In limited studies so far available, NSAIDs can appear in breast milk in very low concentrations. Avoid use of ketoprofen unless considered essential.

See Section 4.4 – Special warnings and precautions for use, regarding female fertility.

4.7 Effects on ability to drive and use machines

Undesirable effects such as dizziness, drowsiness, fatigue and visual disturbances are possible after taking NSAIDs. If affected patients should not drive or operate machinery.

4.8 Undesirable effects

Blood and the lymphatic system disorder:

– thrombocytopenia, anemia due to bleeding, neutropenia, agranulocytosis, bone marrow aplasia and haemolytic anaemia

Immune system disorders:

– dermatological reactions: rash, pruritus, urticaria, angioedema

– respiratory reactions: aggravated asthma, asthmatic attack, dyspnoea, bronchospasm (particularly in patients with known hypersensitivity to ASA and other NSAIDs)

– anaphylactic reactions (including shock)

- non-specific allergic reactions

Psychiatric disorders:

– somnolence, mood disorders

Nervous system disorders:

– Depression, confusion, hallucinations, vertigo, dizziness, paraesthesia, convulsions

- malaise, fatigue and drowsiness

- reports of aseptic meningitis (especially in patients with existing auto-immune disorders such as systemic lupus erythematosis, mixed connective tissue disease) with symptoms such as stiff neck, headache, nausea, vomiting, fever or disorientation (See section 4.4).

Eye disorders:

– visual disturbances such as blurred vision (see section 6)

- optic neuritis

Ear and labyrinth disorders:

– tinnitus

Cardiac disorders:

– oedema, hypertension, vasodilatation, cardiac failure

Clinical trial and epidemiological data suggest that use of some NSAIDs (particularly at high doses and in long term treatment) may be associated with an increased risk of arterial thrombotic events (for example myocardial infarction or stroke) (see section 4.4).

Gastrointestinal disorders:

– gastralgia, dyspepsia, abdominal pain, nausea, vomiting, diarrhoea, constipation, flatulence

– gastritis, stomatitis, exacerbation of colitis and Crohn's disease

– peptic ulcer, gastrointestinal bleeding and perforation

- melaena, haematemesis

- pancreatitis; very rare reports of pancreatitis have been noted with NSAIDs

Gastro-intestinal bleeding may sometimes be fatal, particularly in the elderly (see Section 4.4 Special warnings and precautions for use).

Hepato-biliary disorders:

– elevation of transaminase levels, abnormal liver function, jaundice and rare cases of hepatitis

Skin and subcutaneous tissue disorders:

- Photosensitivity reactions, alopecia, purpura, exfoliative and bullous dermatoses (including epidermal necrolysis, erythema multiforme, Stevens Johnson Syndrome and Toxic Epidermal Necrolysis).

Renal and urinary disorders:

– abnormal renal function tests, acute renal failure, interstitial nephritis, nephriticsyndrome

General disorders and administration site conditions:

– headache, oedema, weight gain, taste perversion

In all cases of major adverse effects Orudis should be withdrawn at once.

4.9 Overdose

Symptoms

Like other propionic acid derivatives, ketoprofen is of low toxicity in overdosage; symptoms after acute ketoprofen intoxication are largely limited to drowsiness, abdominal pain and vomiting. Headache, nausea, rarely diarrhoea, disorientation, excitation, coma, dizziness, tinnitus, fainting, occasionally convulsions may also occur. Adverse effects seen after overdosage with propionic acid derivatives such as hypotension, bronchospasm and gastrointestinal haemorrhage should be anticipated.

In cases of significant poisoning, acute renal failure and liver damage are possible.

Therapeutic measures:

Treatment is supportive and symptomatic.

Within one hour of ingestion, consideration should be given to administering activated charcoal. Alternatively, in adults, gastric lavage should be considered if the patient presents within 1 hour of ingesting a potentially toxic amount.

Good urine output should be ensured.

Renal and liver function should be closely monitored.

Patients should be observed for at least four hours after ingestion of potentially toxic amounts.

Frequent or prolonged convulsions should be treated with intravenous diazepam.

The benefit of gastric decontamination is uncertain.

Other measures may be indicated by the patient's clinical condition.

5. PHARMACOLOGICAL PROPERTIES

5.1 Pharmacodynamic properties

Ketoprofen overall has the properties of a potent non-steroidal anti-inflammatory agent. It has the following pharmacological effects.

Anti-inflammatory

It inhibits the development of carageenan-induced abscesses in rats at 1mg/kg and UV-radiation induced erythema in guinea pigs at 6mg/kg. It is also a potent inhibitor of PGE_2 and $PGF_{2\alpha}$ synthesis in guinea pigs and human chopped lung preparations.

Analgesic

Ketoprofen effectively reduced visceral pain in mice caused by phenyl benzoquinone or by bradykinin following P.O. administration at about 6mg/kg.

Antipyretic

Ketoprofen (2 and 6mg/kg) inhibited hyperthermia caused by s.c. injection of brewer's yeast in rats and, at 1mg/kg, hyperthermia caused by i.v. administration of antigonococcal vaccine to rabbits.

Ketoprofen at 10mg/kg i.v. did not affect the cardiovascular, respiratory, central nervous system or autonomic nervous systems.

5.2 Pharmacokinetic properties

Ketoprofen is completely absorbed from Orudis capsules and maximum plasma concentrations occur after ½ - 1 hour. It declines thereafter with a elimination half-life of about 2 - 3 hours. There is no accumulation on continued daily dosing.

5.3 Preclinical safety data

No additional data of relevance to the prescriber

6. PHARMACEUTICAL PARTICULARS

6.1 List of excipients

Lactose
Magnesium Stearate
Capsule shells
Red Iron Oxide
Titanium Dioxide (E171)
Gelatin

6.2 Incompatibilities

None stated.

6.3 Shelf life

60 months

6.4 Special precautions for storage

Store in a dry place below 25°C. Protect from light.

6.5 Nature and contents of container

Cardboard carton containing blister packs of 56 capsules

6.6 Special precautions for disposal and other handling

None stated

7. MARKETING AUTHORISATION HOLDER

Sanofi-aventis

One Onslow Street

Guildford

Surrey

GU1 4YS

UK

8. MARKETING AUTHORISATION NUMBER(S)

PL 04425/0577

9. DATE OF FIRST AUTHORISATION/RENEWAL OF THE AUTHORISATION

09/10/2006

10. DATE OF REVISION OF THE TEXT

8 July 2009

11. LEGAL CLASSIFICATION

POM

Orudis 50

(sanofi-aventis)

1. NAME OF THE MEDICINAL PRODUCT

Orudis 50

2. QUALITATIVE AND QUANTITATIVE COMPOSITION

In terms of the active ingredient

Ketoprofen 50mg

3. PHARMACEUTICAL FORM

Capsules

4. CLINICAL PARTICULARS

4.1 Therapeutic indications

Recommended in the management of rheumatoid arthritis, osteoarthritis, ankylosing spondylitis, acute articular and periarticular disorders, (bursitis, capsulitis, synovitis, tendinitis), cervical spondylitis, low back pain (strain, lumbago, sciatica, fibrositis), painful musculoskeletal conditions, acute gout, dysmenorrhoea and control of pain and inflammation following orthopaedic surgery.

Orudis reduces joint pain and inflammation and facilitates increase in mobility and functional independence.

It does not cure the underlying disease.

4.2 Posology and method of administration

Oral dosage 50 - 100mg twice daily, morning and evening, depending on patient's weight and on the severity of symptoms.

The maximum daily dose is 200mg. The balance of risks and benefits should be carefully considered before commencing treatment with 200mg daily, and higher doses are not recommended (see also section 4.4).

Best results are obtained by titrating dosage to suit each patient: start with a low dosage in mild chronic disease and a high dosage in acute or severe disease. Some patients derive greater benefit by treatment with capsules only, some with a combined capsule/suppository regimen and others with a higher dosage at night time than at early morning. Where patients require a maximum oral dosage initially, an attempt should be made to reduce this dosage for maintenance since lower dosage might be better tolerated for purposes of long-term treatment.

Elderly: The elderly are at increased risk of the serious consequences of adverse reactions. If an NSAID is considered necessary, the lowest effective dose should be used and for the shortest possible duration. The patient should be monitored regularly for GI bleeding during NSAID therapy.

Paediatric dosage: Not established.

To limit occurrence of gastrointestinal disturbance, capsules should always be taken with food (milk, meals).

Undesirable effects may be minimised by using the lowest effective dose for the shortest duration necessary to control symptoms (see section 4.4).

4.3 Contraindications

Ketoprofen is contraindicated in patients who have a history of hypersensitivity reactions such as asthmatic attacks, rhinitis, angioedema, urticaria or other allergic-type reactions to ketoprofen, any other ingredients in this medicine, ASA or other NSAIDs. Severe, rarely fatal, anaphylactic reactions have been reported in such patients (see section 4.8 – Undesirable effects).

Ketoprofen is also contraindicated in the following cases:

– Severe heart failure

– active peptic ulcer or any history of gastrointestinal haemorrhage, ulceration or perforation

– History of gastrointestinal bleeding or perforation, related to previous NSAIDs therapy

– severe hepatic insufficiency

– severe renal insufficiency

– third trimester of pregnancy

Disease in children (safety/dosage during long-term treatment has not been established).

4.4 Special warnings and precautions for use

Undesirable effects may be minimised by using the lowest effective dose for the shortest duration necessary to control symptoms (see section 4.2, and GI and cardiovascular risks below).

The use of Orudis with concomitant NSAIDs including cyclooxygenase-2 selective inhibitors should be avoided (see section 4.5.

Elderly:

The elderly have an increased risk of adverse reactions to NSAIDs, especially gastro-intestinal bleeding and perforation which may be fatal (see Section 4.2 – Posology and method of administration).

Cardiovascular, Renal and Hepatic impairment:

At the start of treatment, renal function must be carefully monitored in patients with heart impairment, heart failure, liver dysfunction, cirrhosis and nephrosis, in patients receiving diuretic therapy, in patients with chronic renal impairment, particularly if the patient is elderly. In these patients, administration of ketoprofen may induce a reduction in renal blood flow caused by prostaglandin inhibition and lead to renal decomposition. (see also Section 4.3 – Contra-indications).

NSAIDs have also been reported to cause nephrotoxicity in various forms and this can lead to interstitial nephritis, nephrotic syndrome and renal failure.

In patients with abnormal liver function tests or with a history of liver disease, transaminase levels should be evaluated periodically, particularly during longterm therapy. Rare cases of jaundice and hepatitis have been described with ketoprofen.

Cardiovascular and cerebrovascular effects

Appropriate monitoring and advice are required for patients with a history of hypertension and/or mild to moderate congestive heart failure as fluid retention and oedema have been reported in association with NSAID therapy.

Clinical trial and epidemiological data suggest that use of some NSAIDs (particularly at high doses and in long term treatment) may be associated with a small increased risk of arterial thrombotic events (for example myocardial infarction or stroke). There are insufficient data to exclude such a risk for ketoprofen.

Patients with uncontrolled hypertension, congestive heart failure, established ischaemic heart disease, peripheral arterial disease, and/or cerebrovascular disease should only be treated with ketoprofen after careful consideration. Similar consideration should be made before initiating longer-term treatment of patients with risk factors for cardiovascular disease (e.g. hypertension, hyperlipidaemia, diabetes mellitus, smoking).

Respiratory disorders:

Caution is required if NSAIDs are administered to patients suffering from, or with a previous history of, bronchial asthma, since NSAIDs have been reported to cause bronchospasm in such patients.

Gastro-intestinal bleeding, ulceration and perforation:

GI bleeding, ulceration or perforation, which can be fatal, has been reported with all NSAIDs at any time during treatment, with or without warning symptoms or a previous history of serious GI events.

Some epidemiological evidence suggests that ketoprofen may be associated with a high risk of serious gastrointestinal toxicity, relative to some other NSAIDs, especially at high doses (see also section 4.2 and 4.3).

The risk of GI bleeding, ulceration or perforation is higher with increasing NSAID doses, in patients with a history of ulcer, particularly if complicated with haemorrhage or perforation (see section 4.3), and in the elderly. These patients should commence treatment on the lowest dose available. Combination therapy with protective agents (e.g. misoprostol or proton pump inhibitors) should be considered for these patients, and also for patients requiring concomitant low dose aspirin, or other drugs likely to increase gastrointestinal risk (see below and section 4.5).

NSAIDs should only be given with care to patients with a history of gastro-intestinal disease (e.g. ulcerative colitis, Crohn's disease) as these conditions may be exacerbated (see Section 4.8 – Undesirable effects). Patients with a history of GI toxicity, particularly when elderly, should report any unusual abdominal symptoms (especially GI bleeding), particularly in the initial stages of treatment.

Caution should be advised in patients receiving concomitant medications which could increase the risk of ulceration or bleeding, such as corticosteroids, or anti-coagulants such as warfarin, selective serotonin-reuptake inhibitors or anti-platelet agents such as aspirin (see Section 4.5).

When GI bleeding or ulceration occurs in patients receiving ketoprofen, the treatment should be withdrawn.

SLE and mixed connective tissue disease:

In patients with systemic lupus erythematosus (SLE) and mixed connective tissue disorders, there may be an increased risk of aseptic meningitis (see Section 4.8 - Undesirable effects).

Female fertility:

The use of ketoprofen, as with other NSAIDs, may impair female fertility and is not recommended in women attempting to conceive. In women who have difficulty conceiving or who are undergoing investigation of infertility, withdrawal of ketoprofen should be considered.

Skin reactions:

Serious skin reactions, some of them fatal, including exfoliative dermatitis, Stevens-Johnson syndrome, and toxic epidermal necrolysis, have been reported very rarely in association with the use of NSAIDs. Patients appear to be at highest risk of these reactions early in the course of therapy, the onset of the reaction occurring in the majority of cases within the first month of treatment. Treatment should be discontinued at the first appearance of skin rash, mucosal lesions, or any other sign of hypersensitivity.

Infectious disease:

As with other NSAIDs, in the presence of an infectious disease, it should be noted that the anti-inflammatory, analgesic and the antipyretic properties of ketoprofen may mask the usual signs of infection progression such as fever.

Visual disturbances:

If visual disturbances such a blurred vision occur, treatment should be discontinued.

4.5 Interaction with other medicinal products and other forms of interaction

Anticoagulants (heparin and warfarin) and platelet aggregation inhibitors (i.e.ticlopidine, clopidogrel):

Increased risk of bleeding. If coadministration is unavoidable, patient should be closely monitored. (see section 4.4 – Special warnings and precautions for use)

Lithium: Ketoprofen can increase lithium blood levels to possibly toxic levels due to decreased elimination of lithium. If administered together, plasma concentrations of lithium should be monitored in order to adjust the lithium dose.

Other analgesics/NSAIDs (including cyclooxygenase-2 selective inhibitors) and high dose salicylates:

Avoid concomitant use of two or more NSAIDs (including aspirin) as this may increase the risk of adverse effects, particularly gastrointestinal ulceration and bleeding. (see Section 4.4 – Special warnings and precaurtions for use).

Methotrexate: Serious interactions have been recorded after the use of high dose methotrexate with NSAIDs, including ketoprofen, due to decreased elimination of methotrexate. At doses greater than 15mg/week:

Increased risk of haematologic toxicity of methotrexate, particularly if administered at high doses (> 15 mg/week), possibly related to displacement of protein-bound methotrexate and to its decreased renal clearance. At doses lower than 15mg/week: During the first weeks of combination treatment, full blood count should be monitored weekly. If there is any alteration of the renal function or if the patient is elderly, monitoring should be done more frequently.

Mifepristone: NSAIDs should not be used for 8-12 days after mifepristone administration as NSAIDs can reduce the effect of mifepristone.

Pentoxifylline: There is an increased risk of bleeding. More frequent clinical monitoring and monitoring of bleeding time is required.

Antihipertensives: Reduced antihypertensive effect.

Diuretics: Risk of reduced diuretic effect. Patients and particularly dehydrated patients taking diuretics are at a greater risk of developing renal failure secondary to a decrease in renal blood flow caused by prostaglandin inhibition. Such patients should be rehydrated before initiating coadministration therapy and renal function monitored when the treatment is started (see section 4.4 – Special warnings and precautions for use).

Cardiac glycosides: NSAIDs may exacerbate cardiac failure, reduce GFR and increase plasma glycoside levels.

Cyclosporin: Increased risk of nephrotoxicity.

Corticosteroids: Increased risk of GI ulceration or bleeding. (see Section 4.4 Special warnings and precautions for use).

Quinolone antibiotics: Animal data indicate that NSAIDs can increase the risk of convulsions associated with quinolone antibiotics. Patients taking NSAIDs and quinolones may have an increased risk of developing convulsions.

Tacrolimus: Possible increased risk of nephrotoxicity when NSAIDs are given with tacrolimus.

Thrombolytics: Increased risk of bleeding.

Probenecid: Concomitant administration of probenecid may markedly reduce the plasma clearance of ketoprofen.

Anti-platelet agents and Selective serotonin reuptake inhibitors (SSRIs): increased risk of gastrointestinal bleeding (section 4.4 – Special warnings and precautions for use).

ACE inhibitors and Angiotensin II Antagonists:

In patients with compromised renal function (e.g. dehydrated patients or elderly patients the co-administration of an ACE inhibitor or Angiotensin II antagonist and agents that inhibit cyclo-oxygenase may result in further deterioration of renal function, including possible acute renal failure.

Zidovudine: increased risk of haematological toxicity when NSAIDs are given with zidovudine. There is evidence of an increased risk of haemarthroses and haematoma in HIV(+) haemophiliacs receiving concurrent treatment with zidovudine and ibuprofen.

4.6 Pregnancy and lactation

Pregnancy

No embryopathic effects have been demonstrated in animals. Congenital abnormalities have been reported in association with NSAID administration in man; however, these are low in frequency and do not appear to follow any discernable pattern.

It is recommended to avoid ketoprofen during the first two trimesters of pregnancy or labour unless the potential benefit to the patient outweighs the potential risk to the foetus.

In view of the known effects of NSAIDs on the foetal cardiovascular system (risk of premature closure of the ductus arteriosus), use in the last trimester of pregnancy is contra-indicated (see Section 4.3 - Contra-indications). The onset of labour may be delayed and the duration increased with an increased bleeding tendency in both mother and child.

Lactation

In limited studies so far available, NSAIDs can appear in breast milk in very low concentrations. Avoid use of ketoprofen unless considered essential.

See Section 4.4 – Special warnings and precautions for use, regarding female fertility.

4.7 Effects on ability to drive and use machines

Undesirable effects such as dizziness, drowsiness, fatigue and visual disturbances are possible after taking NSAIDs. If affected patients should not drive or operate machinery.

4.8 Undesirable effects

Blood and the lymphatic system disorder:

– thrombocytopenia, anemia due to bleeding, neutropenia, agranulocytosis, bone marrow aplasia and haemolytic anaemia

Immune system disorders:

– dermatological reactions: rash, pruritus, urticaria, angioedema

– respiratory reactions: aggravated asthma, asthmatic attack, dyspnoea, bronchospasm (particularly in patients with known hypersensitivity to ASA and other NSAIDs)

– anaphylactic reactions (including shock)

- non-specific allergic reactions

Psychiatric disorders:

– somnolence, mood disorders

Nervous system disorders:

– Depression, confusion, hallucinations, vertigo, dizziness, paraesthesia, convulsions

- malaise, fatigue and drowsiness

- reports of aseptic meningitis (especially in patients with existing auto-immune disorders such as systemic lupus erythematosis, mixed connective tissue disease) with symptoms such as stiff neck, headache, nausea, vomiting, fever or disorientation (See section 4.4).

Eye disorders:

– visual disturbances such as blurred vision (see section 6)

- optic neuritis

Ear and labyrinth disorders:

–tinnitus

Cardiac disorders:

– oedema, hypertension, vasodilatation, cardiac failure

Clinical trial and epidemiological data suggest that use of some NSAIDs (particularly at high doses and in long term treatment) may be associated with an increased risk of arterial thrombotic events (for example myocardial infarction or stroke) (see section 4.4).

Gastrointestinal disorders:

– gastralgia, dyspepsia, abdominal pain, nausea, vomiting, diarrhoea, constipation, flatulence

– gastritis, stomatitis, exacerbation of colitis and Crohn's disease

– peptic ulcer, gastrointestinal bleeding and perforation

- melaena, haematemesis

- pancreatitis; very rare reports of pancreatitis have been noted with NSAIDs

Gastro-intestinal bleeding may sometimes be fatal, particularly in the elderly (see Section 4.4 Special warnings and precautions for use).

Hepato-biliary disorders:

– elevation of transaminase levels, abnormal liver function, jaundice and rare cases of hepatitis

Skin and subcutaneous tissue disorders:

- Photosensitivity reactions, alopecia, purpura, exfoliative and bullous dermatoses (including epidermal necrolysis, erythema multiforme, Stevens Johnson Syndrome and Toxic Epidermal Necrolysis).

Renal and urinary disorders:

– abnormal renal function tests, acute renal failure, interstitial nephritis, nephriticsyndrome

General disorders and administration site conditions:

– headache, oedema, weight gain, taste perversion

In all cases of major adverse effects Orudis should be withdrawn at once.

4.9 Overdose

Symptoms

Like other propionic acid derivatives, ketoprofen is of low toxicity in overdosage; symptoms after acute ketoprofen intoxication are largely limited to drowsiness, abdominal pain and vomiting. Headache, nausea, rarely diarrhoea, disorientation, excitation, coma, dizziness, tinnitus, fainting, occasionally convulsions may also occur. Adverse effects seen after overdosage with propionic acid derivatives such as hypotension, bronchospasm and gastro-intestinal haemorrhage should be anticipated.

In cases of significant poisoning, acute renal failure and liver damage are possible.

Therapeutic measures:

Treatment is supportive and symptomatic.

Within one hour of ingestion, consideration should be given to administering activated charcoal. Alternatively, in adults, gastric lavage should be considered if the patient presents within 1 hour of ingesting a potentially toxic amount.

Good urine output should be ensured.

Renal and liver function should be closely monitored.

Patients should be observed for at least four hours after ingestion of potentially toxic amounts.

Frequent or prolonged convulsions should be treated with intravenous diazepam.

The benefit of gastric decontamination is uncertain.

Other measures may be indicated by the patient's clinical condition.

5. PHARMACOLOGICAL PROPERTIES

5.1 Pharmacodynamic properties

Ketoprofen overall has the properties of a potent non-steroidal anti-inflammatory agent. It has the following pharmacological effects.

Anti-inflammatory

It inhibits the development of carageenan-induced abscesses in rats at 1mg/kg and UV-radiation induced erythema in guinea pigs at 6mg/kg. It is also a potent inhibitor of PGE_2 and $PGF_{2\alpha}$ synthesis in guinea pigs and human chopped lung preparations.

Analgesic

Ketoprofen effectively reduced visceral pain in mice caused by phenyl benzoquinone or by bradykinin following P.O. administration at about 6mg/kg.

Antipyretic

Ketoprofen (2 and 6mg/kg) inhibited hyperthermia caused by s.c. injection of brewer's yeast in rats and, at 1mg/kg, hyperthermia caused by i.v. administration of antigonococcal vaccine to rabbits.

Ketoprofen at 10mg/kg i.v. did not affect the cardiovascular, respiratory, central nervous system or autonomic nervous systems.

5.2 Pharmacokinetic properties

Ketoprofen is completely absorbed from Orudis capsules and maximum plasma concentrations occur after ½ - 1 hour. It declines thereafter with a elimination half-life of about 2 - 3 hours. There is no accumulation on continued daily dosing.

5.3 Preclinical safety data

No additional data of relevance to the prescriber

6. PHARMACEUTICAL PARTICULARS

6.1 List of excipients

Lactose, magnesium stearate

Capsule shells (Elanco & Scherer)

Opaque purple cap: Brilliant Blue FCF (E133), Erythrosine (E127), Titanium Dioxide (E171), Gelatin. Opaque green base: Brilliant Blue FCF (E133), Yellow iron Oxide (E172), Titanium Dioxide (E171), Gelatin

Capsule shells (Capsulgel)

Opaque purple cap: Patent Blue V (E131), Erythrosine (E127), Titanium Dioxide (E171), Gelatin. Opaque green base: Yellow iron Oxide (E172), Patent Blue V (E131), Titanium Dioxide (E171), Gelatin

6.2 Incompatibilities

None stated

6.3 Shelf life

60 months

6.4 Special precautions for storage

Store in a dry place below 25°C. Protect from light.

6.5 Nature and contents of container

Cardboard carton containing blister packs of 112 capsules

6.6 Special precautions for disposal and other handling

None stated.

7. MARKETING AUTHORISATION HOLDER

Sanofi-aventis

One Onslow Street

Guildford

Surrey

GU1 4YS

UK

8. MARKETING AUTHORISATION NUMBER(S)

PL 04425/0576

9. DATE OF FIRST AUTHORISATION/RENEWAL OF THE AUTHORISATION

13/09/2006

10. DATE OF REVISION OF THE TEXT

8 July 2009

11. LEGAL CLASSIFICATION

POM

Orudis Suppositories 100mg

(sanofi-aventis)

1. NAME OF THE MEDICINAL PRODUCT

Orudis Suppositories 100mg

2. QUALITATIVE AND QUANTITATIVE COMPOSITION

In terms of the active ingredient

Ketoprofen 100 mg

For a full list of excipients, see section 6.1.

3. PHARMACEUTICAL FORM

Suppository

4. CLINICAL PARTICULARS

4.1 Therapeutic indications

Orudis is a potent non steroidal anti-inflammatory analgesic agent and strong inhibitor of prostaglandin synthetase.

Orudis is recommended in the management of rheumatoid arthritis, osteoarthritis, ankylosing spondilitis, acute articular and peri-articular disorders (bursitis, capsulitis, synovitis, tendinitis), cervical spondylitis, low back pain (strain, lumbago, sciatica, fibrositis), painful musculo-skeletal conditions, acute gout and control of pain and inflammation following orthopaedic surgery.

Orudis reduces joint pain and inflammation and facilitates increase in mobility and functional independence. As with other non-steroidal anti-inflammatory agents, it does not cure the underlying disease.

4.2 Posology and method of administration

Rectal dosage is one suppository (100 mg) late at night supplemented as required with Orudis capsules during daytime.

Elderly: The elderly are at increased risk of serious adverse reactions from NSAIDs. If an NSAID is considered necessary, it is generally advisable to begin ketoprofen therapy at the lower end of the dose range and to maintain such patients on the lowest effective dosage, for the shortest possible duration. The patient should be monitored regularly for GI bleeding during NSAID therapy.

Paediatric dosage is not established.

Route of administration is rectal.

Undesirable effects may be minimised by using the lowest effective dose for the shortest duration necessary to control symptoms (see section 4.4).

4.3 Contraindications

Ketoprofen is contraindicated in patients who have a history of hypersensitivity reactions such as asthmatic attacks, rhinitis, angioedema, urticaria or other allergic-type reactions to ketoprofen, any other ingredients in this medicine, ASA or other NSAIDs. Severe, rarely fatal, anaphylactic reactions have been reported in such patients (see section 4.8 – Undesireable effects).

Ketoprofen is also contraindicated in the following cases:

– Severe heart failure

– active peptic ulcer or any history of gastrointestinal hemorrhage, ulceration or perforation

– History of gastrointestinal bleeding or perforation, related to previous NSAIDs therapy

– severe hepatic insufficiency

– severe renal insufficiency

– third trimester of pregnancy

– rectitis or history of proctorrhagia (rectal administration) (see section 4.4 – Special warnings and precautions for use).

Disease in children (safety/dosage during long term treatment has not been established).

4.4 Special warnings and precautions for use

Undesirable effects may be minimised by using the lowest effective dose for the shortest duration necessary to control symptoms (see section 4.2, and GI and cardiovascular risks below).

The use of Orudis with concomitant NSAIDs including cyclooxygenase-2 selective inhibitors should be avoided (see section 4.5).

Elderly:

The elderly have an increased risk of adverse reactions to NSAIDs, especially gastro-intestinal bleeding and perforation which may be fatal (see Section 4.2 – Posology and method of administration).

Cardiovascular, Renal and Hepatic impairment:

At the start of treatment, renal function must be carefully monitored in patients with heart impairment, heart failure, liver dysfunction, cirrhosis and nephrosis, in patients receiving diuretic therapy, in patients with chronic renal impairment, particularly if the patient is elderly. In these patients, administration of ketoprofen may induce a reduction in renal blood flow caused by prostaglandin inhibition and lead to renal decompensation. (see also Section 4.3 – Contra-indications).

NSAIDs have also been reported to cause nephrotoxicity in various forms and this can lead to interstitial nephritis, nephrotic syndrome and renal failure.

In patients with abnormal liver function tests or with a history of liver disease, transaminase levels should be evaluated periodically, particularly during longterm therapy. Rare cases of jaundice and hepatitis have been described with ketoprofen.

Cardiovascular and cerebrovascular effects

Appropriate monitoring and advice are required for patients with a history of hypertension and/or mild to moderate congestive heart failure as fluid retention and oedema have been reported in association with NSAID therapy.

Clinical trial and epidemiological data suggest that use of some NSAIDs (particularly at high doses and in long term treatment) may be associated with a small increased risk of arterial thrombotic events (for example myocardial infarction or stroke). There are insufficient data to exclude such a risk for ketoprofen.

Patients with uncontrolled hypertension, congestive heart failure, established ischaemic heart disease, peripheral arterial disease, and/or cerebrovascular disease should only be treated with ketoprofen after careful consideration. Similar consideration should be made before initiating longer-term treatment of patients with risk factors for cardiovascular disease (e.g. hypertension, hyperlipidaemia, diabetes mellitus, smoking).

Respiratory disorders:

Caution is required if NSAIDs are administered to patients suffering from, or with a previous history of, bronchial asthma since NSAIDs have been reported to cause bronchospasm in such patients.

Gastro-intestinal bleeding, ulceration and perforation:

GI bleeding, ulceration or perforation, which can be fatal, has been reported with all NSAIDs at any time during treatment, with or without warning symptoms or a previous history of serious GI events.

Some epidemiological evidence suggests that ketoprofen may be associated with a high risk of serious gastrointestinal toxicity, relative to some other NSAIDs, especially at high doses (see also section 4.2 and 4.3).

The risk of GI bleeding, ulceration or perforation is higher with increasing NSAID doses, in patients with a history of ulcer, particularly if complicated with haemorrhage or perforation (see section 4.3), and in the elderly. These patients should commence treatment on the lowest dose available. Combination therapy with protective agents (e.g. misoprostol or proton pump inhibitors) should be considered for these patients, and also for patients requiring concomitant low dose aspirin, or other drugs likely to increase gastrointestinal risk (see below and section 4.5).

NSAIDs should only be given with care to patients with a history of gastro-intestinal disease (e.g. ulcerative colitis, Crohn's disease) as these conditions may be exacerbated (see Section 4.8 – Undesirable effects). Patients with a history of GI toxicity, particularly when elderly, should report any unusual abdominal symptoms (especially GI bleeding), particularly in the initial stages of treatment.

Caution should be advised in patients receiving concomitant medications which could increase the risk of ulceration or bleeding, such as corticosteroids, or anti-coagulants such as warfarin, selective serotonin-reuptake inhibitors or anti-platelet agents such as aspirin (see Section 4.5).

When GI bleeding or ulceration occurs in patients receiving ketoprofen, the treatment should be withdrawn.

SLE and mixed connective tissue disease:

In patients with systemic lupus erythematosus (SLE) and mixed connective tissue disorders, there may be an increased risk of aseptic meningitis (see Section 4.8 - Undesirable effects).

Female fertility:

The use of ketoprofen, as with other NSAIDs, may impair female fertility and is not recommended in women attempting to conceive. In women who have difficulty conceiving or who are undergoing investigation of infertility, withdrawal of ketoprofen should be considered.

Skin reactions:

Serious skin reactions, some of them fatal, including exfoliative dermatitis, Stevens-Johnson syndrome, and toxic epidermal necrolysis, have been reported very rarely in association with the use of NSAIDs. Patients appear to be at highest risk of these reactions early in the course of therapy, the onset of the reaction occurring in the majority of cases within the first month of treatment. Treatment should be discontinued at the first appearance of skin rash, mucaosal lesions, or any other sign of hypersensitivity.

Infectious disease:

As with other NSAIDs, in the presence of an infectious disease, it should be noted that the anti-inflammatory, analgesic and the antipyretic properties of ketoprofen may mask the usual signs of infection progression such as fever.

Visual disturbances:

If visual disturbances such a blurred vision occur, treatment should be discontinued.

4.5 Interaction with other medicinal products and other forms of interaction

Anticoagulants (heparin and warfarin) and platelet aggregation inhibitors (i.e.ticlopidine, clopidogrel):

Increased risk of bleeding. If coadministration is unavoidable, patient should be closely monitored. (see section 4.4 – Special warnings and precautions for use)

Lithium: Ketoprofen can increase lithium blood levels to possibly toxic levels due to decreased elimination of lithium. If administered together, plasma concentrations of lithium should be monitored in order to adjust the lithium dose.

Other analgesics/NSAIDs (including cyclooxygenase-2 selective inhibitors) and high dose salicylates:

Avoid concomitant use of two or more NSAIDs (including aspirin) as this may increase the risk of adverse effect, particularly gastrointestinal ulceration and bleeding. (see Section 4.4 – Special warnings and precautions for use).

Methotrexate: Serious interactions have been recorded after the use of high dose methotrexate with NSAIDs, including ketoprofen, due to decreased elimination of methotrexate. At doses greater than 15mg/week:

Increased risk of haematologic toxicity of methotrexate, particularly if administered at high doses (> 15 mg/week), possibly related to displacement of protein-bound methotrexate and to its decreased renal clearance. At doses lower than 15mg/week: During the first weeks of combination treatment, full blood count should be monitored weekly. If there is any alteration of the renal function or if the patient is elderly, monitoring should be done more frequently.

Mifepristone: NSAIDs should not be used for 8-12 days after mifepristone administration as NSAIDs can reduce the effect of mifepristone.

Pentoxifylline: There is an increased risk of bleeding. More frequent clinical monitoring and monitoring of bleeding time is required.

Anti-hypertensives: Risk of reduced anti-hypertensive effect.

Diuretics: Risk of reduced diuretic effect. Patients and particularly dehydrated patients taking diuretics are at a greater risk of developing renal failure secondary to a decrease in renal blood flow caused by prostaglandin inhibition. Such patients should be rehydrated before initiating coadministration therapy and renal function monitored when the treatment is started (see section 4.4 – Special warnings and precautions for use).

Cardiac glycosides: NSAIDs may exacerbate cardiac failure, reduce GFR and increase plasma glycoside levels.

Ciclosporin: Increased risk of nephrotoxicity of NSAIDs.

Corticosteroids: Increased risk of GI ulceration or bleeding (see Section 4.4 Special warnings and precautions for use).

Quinolone antibiotics: Animal data indicate that NSAIDs can increase the risk of convulsions associated with quinolone antibiotics. Patients taking NSAIDs and quinolones may have an increased risk of developing convulsions.

Tacrolimus: Possible increased risk of nephrotoxicity when NSAIDs are given with tacrolimus.

Thrombolytics: Increased risk of bleeding.

Probenecid: Concomitant administration of probenecid may markedly reduce the plasma clearance of ketoprofen.

Anti-platelet agents and Selective serotonin reuptake inhibitors (SSRIs): increased risk of gastrointestinal bleeding (section 4.4 – Special warnings and precautions for use).

ACE inhibitors and Angiotensin II Antagonists:

In patients with compromised renal function (e.g. dehydrated patients or elderly patients the co-administration of an ACE inhibitor or Angiotensin II antagonist and agents that inhibit cyclo-oxygenase may result in further deterioration of renal function, including possible acute renal failure.

Zidovudine: increased risk of haematological toxicity when NSAIDs are given with zidovudine. There is evidence of an increased risk of haemarthroses and haematoma in HIV(+) haemophiliacs receiving concurrent treatment with zidovudine and ibuprofen.

4.6 Pregnancy and lactation

Pregnancy

No embryopathic effects have been demonstrated in animals. Congenital abnormalities have been reported in association with NSAID administration in man; however, these are low in frequency and do not appear to follow any discernable pattern.

It is recommended to avoid ketoprofen during the first two trimesters of pregnancy or labour unless the potential benefit to the patient outweighs the potential risk to the foetus.

In view of the known effects of NSAIDs on the foetal cardiovascular system (risk of premature closure of the ductus arteriosus), use in the last trimester of pregnancy is contra-indicated (see Section 4.3 - Contra-indications). The onset of labour may be delayed and the duration increased with an increased bleeding tendency in both mother and child.

Lactation

Trace amounts of ketoprofen are excreted in breast milk. Avoid use of ketoprofen unless it is considered essential.

See Section 4.4 – Special warnings and precautions for use, regarding female fertility.

4.7 Effects on ability to drive and use machines

Undesirable effects such as dizziness, drowsiness, fatigue and visual disturbances are possible after taking NSAIDs. If affected, patients should not drive or operate machinery.

4.8 Undesirable effects

Blood and the lymphatic system disorders:

– thrombocytopenia, anemia due to bleeding, neutropenia, agranulocytosis, bone marrow aplasia and haemolytic anaemia

Immune system disorders:

– dermatological reactions: rash, pruritus, urticaria, angioedema

– respiratory reactions: aggravated asthma, asthmatic attack, dyspnoea, bronchospasm (particularly in patients with known hypersensitivity to ASA and other NSAIDs)

– anaphylactic reactions (including shock)

– non-specific allergic reactions

Psychiatric disorders

– somnolence, mood disorders

Nervous system disorders

– depression, confusion, hallucinations, vertigo, dizziness, paresthesia, convulsions

– malaise, fatigue and drowsiness

– reports of aseptic meningitis (especially in patients with existing autoimmune disorders, such as systemic lupus erythematosus, mixed connective tissue disease), with symptoms such as stiff neck, headache, nausea, vomiting, fever or disorientation (See section 4.4)

Eye disorders

– visual disturbances such as blurred vision (see section 4.6)

– optic neuritis

Ear and labyrinth disorders:

– tinnitus

Cardiac disorders:

– oedema, hypertension, vasodilatation, cardiac failure

Clinical trial and epidemiological data suggest that use of some NSAIDs (particularly at high doses and in long term treatment) may be associated with an increased risk of arterial thrombotic events (for example myocardial infarction or stroke) (see section 4.4).

Gastro-intestinal disorders:

– gastralgia, dyspepsia, abdominal pain, nausea, vomiting, diarrhoea, constipation, flatulence

– gastritis, stomatitis, exacerbation of colitis and Crohn's disease

– peptic ulcer, gastrointestinal bleeding and perforation

– melaena, haematemesis, proctitis

– pancreatitis; very rare reports of pancreatitis have been noted with NSAIDs

Gastro-intestinal bleeding may sometimes be fatal, particularly in the elderly (see Section 4.4 Special warnings and precautions for use).

Hepato-biliary disorders:

– elevation of transaminase levels, abnormal liver function, jaundice and rare cases of hepatitis

Skin and subcutaneous tissue disorders:

– Photosensitivity, alopecia purpura, exfoliative and bullous dermatoses including epidermal necrolysis, erythema multiforme, Stevens Johnson Syndrome and Toxic Epidermal Necrolysis).

Renal and urinary disorders:

– abnormal renal function tests, acute renal failure, interstitial nephritis, nephritic syndrome

General disorders and administration site conditions

– headache, oedema, weight gain, taste perversion

In all cases of major adverse effects Orudis should be withdrawn at once.

4.9 Overdose

Symptoms

Like other propionic acid derivatives, ketoprofen is of low toxicity in overdosage; symptoms after acute ketoprofen intoxication are largely limited to drowsiness, abdominal pain and vomiting. Headache, nausea, rarely diarrhoea, disorientation, excitation, coma, dizziness, tinnitus, fainting, occasionally convulsions may also occur. Adverse effects seen after overdosage with propionic acid derivatives such as hypotension, bronchospasm and gastro-intestinal haemorrhage should be anticipated.

In cases of significant poisoning, acute renal failure and liver damage are possible.

Therapeutic measures:

Treatment is supportive and symptomatic.

Within one hour of ingestion, consideration should be given to administering activated charcoal. Alternatively, in adults, gastric lavage should be considered if the patient presents within 1 hour of ingesting a potentially toxic amount.

Good urine output should be ensured.

Renal and liver function should be closely monitored.

Patients should be observed for at least four hours after ingestion of potentially toxic amounts.

Frequent or prolonged convulsions should be treated with intravenous diazepam.

The benefit of gastric decontamination is uncertain.

Other measures may be indicated by the patient's clinical condition.

5. PHARMACOLOGICAL PROPERTIES

5.1 Pharmacodynamic properties

Ketoprofen overall has the properties of a potent non-steroidal anti-inflammatory agent. It has the following pharmacological effects:

Anti-inflammatory

It inhibits the development of carageenan-induced abscesses in rats at 1mg/kg and UV-radiation induced erythema in guinea pigs at 6mg/kg. It is also a potent inhibitor of PGE_2 and $PGF_{2\alpha}$ synthesis in guinea pig and human chopped lung preparations.

Analgesic

Ketoprofen effectively reduced visceral pain in mice caused by phenyl benzoquinone or by bradykinin following p.o. administration at about 6mg/kg.

Antipyretic

Ketoprofen (2 and 6mg/kg) inhibited hyperthermia caused by s.c. injection of brewer's yeast in rats and, at 1mg/kg hyperthermia caused by i.v. administration of antigonococcal vaccine to rabbits.

Ketoprofen at 10mg/kg i.v. did not affect the cardiovascular, respiratory, central nervous system or autonomic nervous systems.

5.2 Pharmacokinetic properties

The bioavailability of ketoprofen from the suppository formulation (1 × 100 mg suppositories) has been compared with that from the capsule formulation (2 × 50 mg capsules). The results indicated that there was no significant difference between the bioavailability of the two dosage forms. It is for this reason that toxicological studies by the oral route are considered relevant to the present application for Orudis suppositories.

Ketoprofen is completely absorbed from Orudis capsules and maximum plasma concentrations occur after ½ - 1 hour. It declines thereafter with an elimination half life of about 2-3 hours. There is no accumulation on daily dosing.

5.3 Preclinical safety data

No additional pre-clinical data of relevance to the prescriber.

6. PHARMACEUTICAL PARTICULARS

6.1 List of excipients

Hydrophobic silica

Hard fat

6.2 Incompatibilities

None stated

6.3 Shelf life

36 months

6.4 Special precautions for storage

Store in a dry place below 25°C

6.5 Nature and contents of container

Cardboard carton containing sealed PVC/polyethylene laminate, 2 × 5 suppositories

6.6 Special precautions for disposal and other handling

None stated

7. MARKETING AUTHORISATION HOLDER

Sanofi-aventis,

One Onslow Street,

Guildford,

Surrey,

GU1 4YS

8. MARKETING AUTHORISATION NUMBER(S)

PL 04425/0596

9. DATE OF FIRST AUTHORISATION/RENEWAL OF THE AUTHORISATION

16 October 2006

10. DATE OF REVISION OF THE TEXT

February 2009

Legal category

POM

Oruvail

(sanofi-aventis)

1. NAME OF THE MEDICINAL PRODUCT

Oruvail 100

Oruvail 150

Oruvail 200

2. QUALITATIVE AND QUANTITATIVE COMPOSITION

Ketoprofen 100mg

Ketoprofen 150mg

Ketoprofen 200mg

3. PHARMACEUTICAL FORM

Controlled release capsules

4. CLINICAL PARTICULARS

4.1 Therapeutic indications

Oruvail is recommended in the management of rheumatoid arthritis, osteoarthritis, ankylosing spondylitis, acute articular and peri-articular disorders, (bursitis, capsulitis, synovitis, tendinitis), cervical spondylitis, low back pain (strain, lumbago, sciatica, fibrositis), painful musculo-skeletal conditions, acute gout, dysmenorrhoea and control of pain and inflammation following orthopaedic surgery.

Oruvail reduces joint pain and inflammation and facilitates increase in mobility and functional independence. As with other non-steroidal anti-inflammatory agents, it does not cure the underlying disease.

4.2 Posology and method of administration

Oral dosage 50 - 100mg twice daily, morning and evening, depending on patient's weight and on the severity of symptoms.

The maximum daily dose is 200mg. The balance of risks and benefits should be carefully considered before commencing treatment with 200mg daily, and higher doses are not recommended (see also section 4.4).

Best results are obtained by titrating dosage to suit each patient: start with a low dosage in mild chronic disease and a high dosage in acute or severe disease. Some patients derive greater benefit by treatment with capsules only, some with a combined capsule/suppository regimen and others with a higher dosage at night time than at early morning. Where patients require a maximum oral dosage initially, an attempt should be made to reduce this dosage for maintenance since lower dosage might be better tolerated for purposes of long-term treatment.

Elderly: The elderly are at increased risk of the serious consequences of adverse reactions. If an NSAID is considered necessary, the lowest effective dose should be used and for the shortest possible duration. The patient should be monitored regularly for GI bleeding during NSAID therapy.

Paediatric dosage: Not established.

To limit occurrence of gastrointestinal disturbance, capsules should always be taken with food (milk, meals).

Undesirable effects may be minimised by using the lowest effective dose for the shortest duration necessary to control symptoms (see section 4.4).

4.3 Contraindications

Active peptic ulceration, a history of recurrent peptic ulceration or chronic dyspepsia, severe renal dysfunction.

Oruvail should not be given to patients who have previously shown hypersensitivity reactions (e.g. asthma, rhinitis or urticaria) in response to ketoprofen, any of the other ingredients contained, or to aspirin, ibuprofen or other non-steroidal anti-inflammatory agents. As with other non-steroidal anti-inflammatory agents, severe bronchospasm might be precipitated in these subjects, and in patients suffering from or with a history of, bronchial asthma or allergic disease.

Severe heart failure

4.4 Special warnings and precautions for use

Ketoprofen should be used with caution in patients with renal, hepatic or cardiac impairment. Inhibition of renal prostaglandin synthesis by non- steroidal anti-inflammatory agents may interfere with renal function especially in the presence of existing renal disease. The dose should be kept as low as possible and renal function should be monitored in these patients. NSAIDs should be given with care to patients with a history of heart failure or hypertension since oedema has been reported in association with NSAID administration.

Caution is required if NSAIDs are administered to patients suffering from, or with a previous history of, bronchial asthma, since NSAIDs have been reported to cause bronchospasm in such patients.

NSAIDs should only be given with care to patients with a history of gastrointestinal disease. Oruvail capsules should always be prescribed, "to be taken with food" to minimise gastric intolerance

Undesirable effects may be minimised by using the minimum effective dose for the shortest possible duration.

Undesirable effects may be minimised by using the lowest effective dose for the shortest duration necessary to control symptoms (see section 4.2, and GI and cardiovascular risks below).

Cardiovascular and cerebrovascular effects

Appropriate monitoring and advice are required for patients with a history of hypertension and/or mild to moderate congestive heart failure as fluid retention and oedema have been reported in association with NSAID therapy.

Clinical trial and epidemiological data suggest that use of some NSAIDs (particularly at high doses and in long term treatment) may be associated with a small increased risk of arterial thrombotic events (for example myocardial infarction or stroke). There are insufficient data to exclude such a risk for ketoprofen.

Patients with uncontrolled hypertension, congestive heart failure, established ischaemic heart disease, peripheral arterial disease, and/or cerebrovascular disease should only be treated with ketoprofen after careful consideration. Similar consideration should be made before initiating longer-term treatment of patients with risk factors for cardiovascular disease (e.g. hypertension, hyperlipidaemia, diabetes mellitus, smoking).

4.5 Interaction with other medicinal products and other forms of interaction

Ketoprofen is highly protein bound, concomitant use of other protein-binding drugs e.g. anticoagulants, sulphonamides, hydantoins, might necessitate modification of dosage in order to avoid increased levels of such drugs resulting from competition for plasma protein-binding sites.

Similar acting drugs such as aspirin or other NSAIDS should not be administered concomitantly with ketoprofen as the potential for adverse reactions is increased.

Serious interactions have been recorded after the use of high dose methotrexate with non-steroidal anti-inflammatory agents, including ketoprofen. Decreased elimination of methotrexate has been reported.

NSAIDs should not be used for 8-12 days after mifepristone administration as NSAIDs can reduce the effect of mifepristone.

Care should be taken in patients treated with any of the following drugs, as interactions with NSAIDs have been reported in some patients:

Antihypertensives: Reduced anti-hypertensive effect.

Diuretics: Reduced diuretic effect. Diuretics can increase the risk of nephrotoxicity of NSAIDs.

Cardiac glycosides: NSAIDs may exacerbate cardiac failure, reduce GFR and increase plasma glycoside levels.

Lithium: Decreased elimination of lithium.

Cyclosporin: Increased risk of nephrotoxicity.

Corticosteroids: Increased risk of GI bleeding.

Anticoagulants: Enhanced anticoagulant effect.

Quinolone antibiotics: Animal data indicate that NSAIDs can increase the risk of convulsions associated with quinolone antibiotics. Patients taking NSAIDs and quinolones may have an increased risk of developing convulsions.

4.6 Pregnancy and lactation

Pregnancy

No embryopathic effects have been demonstrated in animals. Congenital abnormalities have been reported in association with NSAID administration in man; however, these are low in frequency and do not appear to follow any discernable pattern.

It is recommended to avoid ketoprofen during the first two trimesters of pregnancy or labour unless the potential benefit to the patient outweighs the potential risk to the foetus.

In view of the known effects of NSAIDs on the foetal cardiovascular system (risk of premature closure of the ductus arteriosus), use in the last trimester of pregnancy is contraindicated. The onset of labour may be delayed and the duration increased with an increased bleeding tendency in both mother and child (see Section 4.3 - Contra-indications).

Lactation

In limited studies so far available, NSAIDs can appear in breast milk in very low concentrations. Avoid use of ketoprofen unless considered essential.

See Section 4.4 – Special warnings and precautions for use, regarding female fertility.

4.7 Effects on ability to drive and use machines

Undesirable effects such as dizziness, drowsiness, fatigue and visual disturbances are possible after taking NSAIDs. If affected patients should not drive or operate machinery

4.8 Undesirable effects

Blood and the lymphatic system disorders:

– thrombocytopenia, anemia due to bleeding, neutropenia, agranulocytosis, bone marrow aplasia and haemolytic anaemia

Immune system disorders:

– dermatological reactions: rash, pruritus, urticaria, angioedema

– respiratory reactions: aggravated asthma, asthmatic attack, dyspnoea, bronchospasm (particularly in patients with known hypersensitivity to ASA and other NSAIDs)

– anaphylactic reactions (including shock)

- non-specific allergic reactions

Psychiatric disorders:

– somnolence, mood disorders

Nervous system disorders:

– Depression, confusion, hallucinations, vertigo, dizziness, paraesthesia, convulsions

- malaise, fatigue and drowsiness

- reports of aseptic meningitis (especially in patients with existing auto-immune disorders such as systemic lupus erythematosis, mixed connective tissue disease) with symptoms such as stiff neck, headache, nausea, vomiting, fever or disorientation (See section 4.4).

Eye disorders

– visual disturbances such as blurred vision (see section 6)

- optic neuritis

Ear and labyrinth disorders

– tinnitus

Cardiac disorders:

– oedema, hypertension, vasodilatation, cardiac failure

Clinical trial and epidemiological data suggest that use of some NSAIDs (particularly at high doses and in long term treatment) may be associated with an increased risk of arterial thrombotic events (for example myocardial infarction or stroke) (see section 4.4).

Gastrointestinal disorders:

– gastralgia, dyspepsia, abdominal pain, nausea, vomiting, diarrhoea, constipation, flatulence

– gastritis, stomatitis, exacerbation of colitis and Crohn's disease

– peptic ulcer, gastrointestinal bleeding and perforation

- melaena, haematemesis

- pancreatitis; very rare reports of pancreatitis have been noted with NSAIDs

Gastro-intestinal bleeding may sometimes be fatal, particularly in the elderly (see Section 4.4 Special warnings and precautions for use).

Hepato-biliary disorders:

– elevation of transaminase levels, abnormal liver function, jaundice and rare cases of hepatitis

- Skin and subcutaneous tissue disorders:

- Photosensitivity reactions, alopecia, purpura, exfoliative and bullous dermatoses (including epidermal necrolysis, erythema multiforme, Stevens Johnson Syndrome and Toxic Epidermal Necrolysis).

Renal and urinary disorders:

– abnormal renal function tests, acute renal failure, interstitial nephritis, nephriticsyndrome

General disorders and administration site conditions:

– headache, oedema, weight gain, taste perversion

In all cases of major adverse effects Orudis should be withdrawn at once.

4.9 Overdose
Symptoms

Like other propionic acid derivatives, ketoprofen is of low toxicity in overdosage; symptoms after acute ketoprofen intoxication are largely limited to drowsiness, abdominal pain and vomiting. Headache, nausea, rarely diarrhoea, disorientation, excitation, coma, dizziness, tinnitus, fainting, occasionally convulsions may also occur. Adverse effects seen after overdosage with propionic acid derivatives such as hypotension, bronchospasm and gastro-intestinal haemorrhage should be anticipated.

In cases of significant poisoning, acute renal failure and liver damage are possible.

Therapeutic measures:

Treatment is supportive and symptomatic.

Within one hour of ingestion, consideration should be given to administering activated charcoal. Alternatively, in adults, gastric lavage should be considered if the patient presents within 1 hour of ingesting a potentially toxic amount.

Good urine output should be ensured.

Renal and liver function should be closely monitored.

Patients should be observed for at least four hours after ingestion of potentially toxic amounts.

Frequent or prolonged convulsions should be treated with intravenous diazepam.

The benefit of gastric decontamination is uncertain.

Other measures may be indicated by the patient's clinical condition.

5. PHARMACOLOGICAL PROPERTIES

5.1 Pharmacodynamic properties

Ketoprofen overall has the properties of a potent non-steroidal anti- inflammatory agent. It has the following pharmacological effects:

Anti-inflammatory

It inhibits the development of carageenan-induced abscesses in rats at 1mg/kg, UV-radiation induced erythema in guinea pigs at 6mg/kg. It is also a potent inhibitor of $PGE_{2\ \infty}$ and $PFG_{2\ \infty}$ synthesis in guinea pig and human chopped lung preparations.

Analgesic

Ketoprofen effectively reduced visceral pain in mice caused by phenyl benzoquinone or by bradykinin following p.o. Administration at about 6mg/kg.

Antipyretic

Ketoprofen (2 and 6mg/kg) inhibited hyperthermia caused by s.c injection of brewer's yeast in rats and, at 1mg/kg hyperthermia caused by i.v. administration of anticoagulant vaccine to rabbits.

Ketoprofen at 10mg/kg i.v. did not affect the cardiovascular, respiratory, central nervous system or autonomic nervous systems.

5.2 Pharmacokinetic properties

Ketoprofen is slowly but completely absorbed from Oruvail capsules. Maximum plasma concentration occurs after 6 - 8 hours. It declines thereafter with a half-life of about 8 hours. There is no accumulation on continued daily dosing. Ketoprofen is very highly bound to plasma protein

5.3 Preclinical safety data

No additional data of relevance to the prescriber

6. PHARMACEUTICAL PARTICULARS

6.1 List of excipients

Pellets

Sugar spheres

Colloidal anhydrous silica

Shellac

Ethylcellulose

Talc

Capsule shell-body

Gelatin

Erythrosine (E127)

Capsule shell – cap

Gelatin

Titanium dioxide (E171)

Erythrosine (E127) – 100mg and 150mg only

Patent blue V (E131) – 100mg only

6.2 Incompatibilities

None stated

6.3 Shelf life

36 months

6.4 Special precautions for storage

Store below 25°C in a dry place and protect from light.

6.5 Nature and contents of container

UPVC/Aluminium foil blister or UPVC coated with PVDC aluminium foil blister containing 28 capsules

6.6 Special precautions for disposal and other handling

None stated

7. MARKETING AUTHORISATION HOLDER

Sanofi-aventis

One Onslow Street

Guildford

Surrey

GU1 4YS

UK

8. MARKETING AUTHORISATION NUMBER(S)

100mg capsules: PL 04425/0597

150mg capsules: PL04425/0598

200mg capsules: PL 04425/0599

9. DATE OF FIRST AUTHORISATION/RENEWAL OF THE AUTHORISATION

100mg capsules: 04 September 2006

150mg capsules: 09 January 2007

200mg capsules: 21 September 2006

10. DATE OF REVISION OF THE TEXT

8 July 2009

11. LEGAL CLASSIFICATION

POM

Oruvail Gel 2.5%

(sanofi-aventis)

1. NAME OF THE MEDICINAL PRODUCT

Oruvail Gel 2.5%

2. QUALITATIVE AND QUANTITATIVE COMPOSITION

Ketoprofen 2.5% w/w

3. PHARMACEUTICAL FORM

Gel

4. CLINICAL PARTICULARS

4.1 Therapeutic indications

Ketoprofen is a non-steroidal anti-inflammatory drug. It has anti-inflammatory and analgesic actions.

Indications recommended for packs supplied within pharmacy only legal status

Relief of backache, muscular pain and rheumatic pain, sprains and strains.

Relief of musculoskeletal pain and swelling caused by sports injuries.

Pain of non serious arthritis.

Indications recommended when prescribed by a physician as a prescription only medicine

Relief of acute painful musculoskeletal conditions caused by trauma, such as sports injuries, sprains, strains and contusions.

Pain of non serious arthritis.

4.2 Posology and method of administration

Recommended dose and dosage schedule for packs supplied with pharmacy only legal status

Adults: Apply a thin layer of gel to the affected area three times a day for up to 7 days. After the gel is applied it should be rubbed in well.

Elderly: As above.

Children: Not to be applied to children under 12 year of age.

Recommended dose and dosage schedule when prescribed by a physician as a prescription only medicine

Adults: To be applied two to four times daily to the skin in the painful or inflamed region for up to 7 days. Apply gently but massage well to ensure gel penetration. The usual recommended dose is 15g per day (7.5 grams correspond to approximately 14cm of gel).

Elderly: There are no specific dosage recommendations for the elderly.

Children: Not recommended as safety in children has not been established.

4.3 Contraindications

Patients with a known hypersensitivity to ketoprofen or any of the excipients, aspirin or other non-steroidal anti-inflammatory agents; patients suffering from or with a history of bronchial asthma or allergic disease. Oruvail gel should be avoided in patients with exudative dermatoses, eczema, sores and infected skin lesions or broken skin. Oruvail gel should not be applied to mucous membranes, anal or genital areas, eyes or used with occlusive dressings.

4.4 Special warnings and precautions for use

Although systemic effects are minimal, the gel should be used with caution in patients with severe renal impairment. Should a skin rash occur after gel application, treatment must be stopped. Do not apply Oruvail gel beneath occlusive dressings. Areas of skin treated with Oruvail gel should not be exposed directly sunlight, or solarium ultraviolet light, either during treatment or for two weeks following treatment discontinuation. Keep the gel away from naked flames. Do not incinerate.

4.5 Interaction with other medicinal products and other forms of interaction

Interactions are unlikely as serum concentrations following topical administration are low.

Serious interactions have been recorded after the use of high dose methotrexate with non-steroidal anti-inflammatory agents, including ketoprofen, when administered by the systemic route.

4.6 Pregnancy and lactation

No embryopathic effects have been demonstrated in animals and there is epidemiological evidence of the safety of ketoprofen in human pregnancy. Nevertheless, it is recommended that ketoprofen should be avoided during pregnancy. Non-steroidal anti-inflammatory drugs may also delay labour.

Trace amounts of ketoprofen are excreted in breast milk, therefore Oruvail Gel should not be used during breast feeding.

4.7 Effects on ability to drive and use machines

None known.

4.8 Undesirable effects

Adverse reactions: Skin reactions, including photosensitivity reactions, pruritus, localised erythema. These are usually mild and resolve after cessation of the gel. Cases of more severe reactions such as bullous or phylcytenar eczema which may spread or become generalised have occurred rarely.

4.9 Overdose

Overdose is unlikely by topical administration.

If accidentally ingested, the gel may cause systemic adverse effects depending on the amount ingested. However, if they occur, treatment should be supportive and symptomatic.

5. PHARMACOLOGICAL PROPERTIES

5.1 Pharmacodynamic properties

Ketoprofen is a non-steroidal anti-inflammatory drug. It has anti-inflammatory and analgesic actions.

5.2 Pharmacokinetic properties

Plasma and tissue levels of ketoprofen have been measured in 24 patients undergoing knee surgery. After repeated percutaneous administration of Oruvail gel the plasma levels were about 60 fold less (9 - 39 ng/g) than those obtained after a single oral dose of ketoprofen (490 - 3300 ng/g). Tissue levels at the area of application were within the same concentration range for the gel as for the oral treatment, although the gel was associated with a considerably higher inter-individual variability.

The bioavailability of ketoprofen after topical administration has been estimated to be approximately 5% of the level obtained after an orally administered dose, based on urinary excretion data.

The protein binding in plasma is approximately 99%. Ketoprofen is excreted through the kidneys mainly as glucuronide conjugate.

5.3 Preclinical safety data

No additional pre-clinical data of relevance to the prescriber.

6. PHARMACEUTICAL PARTICULARS

6.1 List of excipients

Carbopol

Triethanolamine

Lavender Oil

Ethanol

Purified water

6.2 Incompatibilities

The gel should not be diluted.

6.3 Shelf life

36 months.

6.4 Special precautions for storage

Do not store above 25°C

6.5 Nature and contents of container

Cardboard carton containing aluminium tube internally coated with polycondensed epoxyphenol varnish with the tip sealed with the same material containing either 30 or 100g of gel.

6.6 Special precautions for disposal and other handling

Wash your hands following application

Keep gel away from naked flames.

Do not incinerate.

The tube should be closed after use.

7. MARKETING AUTHORISATION HOLDER

Sanofi-aventis

One Onslow Street

Guildford

Surrey

GU1 4YS

UK

8. MARKETING AUTHORISATION NUMBER(S)

PL 00012/0243

9. DATE OF FIRST AUTHORISATION/RENEWAL OF THE AUTHORISATION

28.07.97

10. DATE OF REVISION OF THE TEXT

November 2006

Legal Category

POM for pack sizes larger than 30g

PHARMACY for pack sizes up to and including 30g

Oruvail I.M. Injection

(sanofi-aventis)

1. NAME OF THE MEDICINAL PRODUCT

Oruvail IM Injection

2. QUALITATIVE AND QUANTITATIVE COMPOSITION

In terms of the active ingredient

Ketoprofen BP 100mg in 2 ml.

3. PHARMACEUTICAL FORM

Solution for IM injection

4. CLINICAL PARTICULARS

4.1 Therapeutic indications

Oruvail injection is recommended in the management of acute exacerbations of:

- Rheumatoid arthritis, osteoarthritis, ankylosing spondylitis.
- Periarticular conditions such as fibrositis, bursitis, capsulitis, tendinitis and tenosynovitis.
- Low back pain of musculoskeletal origin and sciatica.
- Other painful musculoskeletal conditions.
- Acute gout.
- Control of pain and inflammation following orthopaedic surgery.

4.2 Posology and method of administration

Adults: 50 to 100 mg every four hours, repeated up to a maximum of 200 mg in twenty-four hours. Following a satisfactory response, oral therapy should be instituted with ketoprofen capsules. It is recommended that the injection should not normally be continued for longer than three days.

Elderly: The elderly are at increased risk of the serious consequences of adverse reactions. If an NSAID is considered necessary, the lowest effective dose should be used and for the shortest possible duration. The patient should be monitored regularly for GI bleeding during NSAID therapy.

Paediatric dosage: not established.

Oruvail IM Injection is for intramuscular injection only.

Undesirable effects may be minimised by using the lowest effective dose for the shortest duration necessary to control symptoms (see section 4

4.3 Contraindications

Hypersensitivity to ketoprofen or to any of the excipients.

NSAIDs are contraindicated in patients who have previously shown hypersensitivity reactions (e.g. asthma, rhinitis, angioedema or urticaria) in response to ibuprofen, Aspirin, or other non-steroidal anti-inflammatory drugs.

Active peptic ulcer, or any history of gastrointestinal bleeding, ulceration or perforation

History of gastrointestinal bleeding or perforation, related to previous NSAIDs therapy.

Severe heart failure, hepatic failure and renal failure (see section 4.4).

During the last trimester of pregnancy (see section 4.6)

4.4 Special warnings and precautions for use

Oruvail injection is for intramuscular use only.

Undesirable effects may be minimised by using the lowest effective dose for the shortest duration necessary to control symptoms (see section 4.2, and GI and cardiovascular risks below).

Use with concomitant NSAIDs including cyclooxygenase-2 selective inhibitors should be avoided (see section 4.5 – Interaction with other medicinal products and other forms of interactions).

Elderly:

The elderly have an increased risk of adverse reactions to NSAIDs, especially gastro-intestinal bleeding and perforation which may be fatal (see Section 4.2).

Cardiovascular, Renal and Hepatic impairment:

The administration of an NSAID may cause a dose dependent reduction in prostaglandin formation and precipitate renal failure. Patients at greatest risk of this reaction are those with impaired renal function, cardiac impairment, liver dysfunction, those taking diuretics and the elderly. Renal function should be monitored in these patients (see also section 4.3).

Cardiovascular and cerebrovascular effects

Appropriate monitoring and advice are required for patients with a history of hypertension and/or mild to moderate congestive heart failure as fluid retention and oedema have been reported in association with NSAID therapy.

Clinical trial and epidemiological data suggest that use of some NSAIDs (particularly at high doses and in long term treatment) may be associated with a small increased risk of arterial thrombotic events (for example myocardial infarction or stroke). There are insufficient data to exclude such a risk for ketoprofen.

Patients with uncontrolled hypertension, congestive heart failure, established ischaemic heart disease, peripheral arterial disease, and/or cerebrovascular disease should only be treated with ketoprofen after careful consideration. Similar consideration should be made before initiating longer-term treatment of patients with risk factors for cardiovascular disease (e.g. hypertension, hyperlipidaemia, diabetes mellitus, smoking).

Respiratory disorders:

Caution is required if NSAIDs are administered to patients suffering from, or with a previous history of, bronchial asthma, since NSAIDs have been reported to cause bronchospasm in such patients.

Gastro-intestinal bleeding, ulceration and perforation:

GI bleeding, ulceration or perforation, which can be fatal, has been reported with all NSAIDs at any time during treatment, with or without warning symptoms or a previous history of serious GI events.

Some epidemiological evidence suggests that ketoprofen may be associated with a high risk of serious gastrointestinal toxicity, relative to some other NSAIDs, especially at high doses (see also section 4.2 and 4.3).

The risk of GI bleeding, ulceration or perforation is higher with increasing NSAID doses, in patients with a history of ulcer, particularly if complicated with haemorrhage or perforation (see section 4.3), and in the elderly. These patients should commence treatment on the lowest dose available. Combination therapy with protective agents (e.g. misoprostol or proton pump inhibitors) should be considered for these patients, and also for patients requiring concomitant low dose aspirin, or other drugs likely to increase gastrointestinal risk (see below and section 4.5).

NSAIDs should only be given with care to patients with a history of gastro-intestinal disease (e.g. ulcerative colitis, Crohn's disease) as these conditions may be exacerbated (see Section 4.8 – Undesirable effects). Patients with a history of GI toxicity, particularly when elderly, should report any unusual abdominal symptoms (especially GI bleeding), particularly in the initial stages of treatment.

Caution should be advised in patients receiving concomitant medications which could increase the risk of ulceration or bleeding, such as oral corticosteroids, anticoagulants such as warfarin, selective serotonin-reuptake inhibitors or anti-platelet agents such as aspirin (see section 4.5).

When GI bleeding or ulceration occurs in patients receiving ketoprofen, the treatment should be withdrawn.

SLE and mixed connective tissue disease:

In patients with systemic lupus erythematosus (SLE) and mixed connective tissue disorders there may be an increased risk of aseptic meningitis (see section 4.8).

Impaired female fertility:

The use of ketoprofen, as with other NSAIDs, may impair female fertility and is not recommended in women attempting to conceive. In women who have difficulties conceiving or who are undergoing investigation of infertility, withdrawal of ketoprofen should be considered.

Skin reactions:

Serious skin reactions, some of them fatal, including exfoliative dermatitis, Stevens-Johnson syndrome, and toxic epidermal necrolysis, have been reported very rarely in association with the use of NSAIDs (see section 4.8). Patients appear to be at highest risk for these reactions early in the course of therapy: the onset of the reaction occurring in the majority of cases within the first month of treatment. Treatment should be discontinued at the first appearance of skin rash, mucosal lesions, or any other sign of hypersensitivity.

4.5 Interaction with other medicinal products and other forms of interaction

Other analgesics including cyclooxygenase-2 selective inhibitors: Avoid concomitant use of two or more NSAIDs (including aspirin) as this may increase the risk of adverse effects (see section 4.4).

Anti-coagulants: NSAIDs may enhance the effects of anti-coagulants, such as Warfarin.

Anti-platelet agents and selective serotonin reuptake inhibitors (SSRIs): Increased risk of gastrointestinal bleeding.

Lithium: Decreased elimination of lithium

Methotrexate: Decreased elimination of methotrexate.

Mifepristone: NSAIDs should not be used for 8-12 days after mifepristone administration as NSAIDs can reduce the effect of mifepristone.

Anti-hypertensives: Reduced anti-hypertensive effect.

Diuretics: Reduced diuretic effect. Diuretics can increase the risk of nephrotoxicity of NSAIDs.

Cardiac glycosides: NSAIDs may exacerbate cardiac failure, reduce GFR and increase plasma glycoside levels.

Ciclosporin: Increased risk of nephrotoxicity

Corticosteroids: Increased risk of gastrointestinal ulceration or bleeding

Quinolone antibiotics: Animal data indicate that NSAIDs can increase the risk of convulsions associated with quinolone antibiotics. Patients taking NSAIDs and quinolones may have an increased risk of developing convulsions.

Tacrolimus: Possible increased risk of nephrotoxicity when NSAIDs are given with tacrolimus.

Zidovudine: increased risk of haematological toxicity when NSAIDs are given with zidovudine. There is evidence of an increased risk of haemarthroses and haematoma in HIV(+) haemophiliacs receiving concurrent treatment with zidovudine and ibuprofen.

4.6 Pregnancy and lactation

Pregnancy

No embryopathic effects have been demonstrated in animals. Congenital abnormalities have been reported in association with NSAID administration in man; however, these are low in frequency and do not appear to follow any discernable pattern.

It is recommended to avoid ketoprofen during the first two trimesters of pregnancy or labour unless the potential benefit to the patient outweighs the potential risk to the foetus.

In view of the known effects of NSAIDs on the foetal cardiovascular system (risk of premature closure of the ductus arteriosus), use in the last trimester of pregnancy is contra-indicated (see Section 4.3 - Contra-indications). The onset of labour may be delayed and the duration increased with an increased bleeding tendency in both mother and child.

Lactation

Trace amounts of ketoprofen are excreted in breast milk. Avoid use of ketoprofen unless it is considered essential.

See Section 4.4 – Special warnings and precautions for use, regarding female fertility.

4.7 Effects on ability to drive and use machines

CNS side effects have been observed in some patients (see section 4.8). If affected patients should not drive or operate machinery.

4.8 Undesirable effects

Gastrointestinal: The most commonly observed adverse events are gastrointestinal in nature. Peptic ulcers, perforation or GI bleeding, sometimes fatal, particularly in the elderly, may occur (see section 4.4). Nausea, vomiting, diarrhoea, flatulence, constipation, dyspepsia, abdominal pain, melaena, haematemesis, ulcerative stomatitis, exacerbation of colitis and Crohn's disease (see section 4.4) have been r3eported following administration. Less frequently, gastritis has been observed. Pancreatitis has been reported very rarely.

Hypersensitivity: Hypersensitivity reactions have been reported following treatment with NSAIDs. These may consist of (a) non-specific allergic reactions and anaphylaxis (b) respiratory tract reactivity comprising asthma, aggravated asthma, bronchospasm or dyspnoea, or (c) assorted skin disorders, including rashes of various types, pruritus, urticaria, purpura, angiodema and, more rarely exfoliative and bullous dermatoses (including epidermal necrolysis and erythema multiforme).

Local reactions can occur and may include pain or a burning sensation. In all cases of major adverse effects Oruvail should be withdrawn at once.

Cardiovascular and cerebrovascular:

Oedema, hypertension, and cardiac failure, have been reported in association with NSAID treatment.

Clinical trial and epidemiological data suggest that use of some NSAIDs (particularly at high doses and in long term treatment) may be associated with an increased risk of arterial thrombotic events (for example myocardial infarction or stroke) (see section 4.4).

Other adverse reactions reported less commonly include:

Renal: Nephrotoxicity in various forms, including interstitial nephritis, nephritic syndrome and renal failure.

Hepatic: abnormal liver function, hepatitis and jaundice.

Neurological and special senses: Visual disturbances, optic neuritis, headaches, paraesthesia, reports of aseptic meningitis (especially in patients with existing autoimmune disorders, such as systemic lupus erythematosus, mixed connective tissue disease), with symptoms such as stiff neck, headache, nausea, vomiting, fever or disorientation (See section 4.4), depression, confusion, hallucinations, tinnitus, vertigo, dizziness, malaise, fatigue and drowsiness.

Haematological: Thrombocytopenia, neutropenia, agranulocytosis, aplastic anaemia and haemolytic anaemia.

Dermatological: Bullous reactions including Stevens Johnson Syndrome and Toxic Epidermal Necrolysis (very rare). Photosensitivity.

4.9 Overdose

Symptoms

Like other propionic acid derivatives, ketoprofen is of low toxicity in overdosage. Symptoms after acute ketoprofen intoxication are largely limited to drowsiness, abdominal pain and vomiting. Headache, nausea, rarely diarrhoea, disorientation, excitation, coma, dizziness, tinnitus, fainting, occasionally convulsions may also occur. A dverse effects seen after overdosage with propionic acid derivatives such as hypotension, bronchospasm and gastro-intestinal haemorrhage should be anticipated.

In cases of significant poisoning, acute renal failure and liver damage are possible.

Therapeutic measures:

Treatment is otherwise supportive and symptomatic.

Good urine output should be ensured.

Renal and liver function should be closely monitored.

Frequent or prolonged convulsions should be treated with intravenous diazepam.

Other measures may be indicated by the patient's clinical condition.

5. PHARMACOLOGICAL PROPERTIES

5.1 Pharmacodynamic properties

Ketoprofen is a pharmacopoeial non-steroidal anti-inflammatory drug (NSAID). It is a strong inhibitor of prostaglandin synthetase and potent analgesic agent. Studies in vitro and in vivo show that ketoprofen possesses powerful anti-inflammatory, antipyretic, antibradykinin and lysosomal membrane stabilising properties.

5.2 Pharmacokinetic properties

Peak concentrations of approximately 10 mg/L are reached at about 0.5-0.75 H after a 100 mg dose. The elimination half life is approximately 1.88 H. Apart from earlier Tmax values, there are no significant differences between the pharmacokinetics of Oruvail IM injection and conventional release capsules (Orudis).

5.3 Preclinical safety data

No additional data of relevance to the prescriber.

6. PHARMACEUTICAL PARTICULARS

6.1 List of excipients

Arginine	BP
Benzyl Alcohol	BP
Citric Acid anhydrous (E330)	BP
Water For Injections	BP

6.2 Incompatibilities

None stated

6.3 Shelf life

36 months

6.4 Special precautions for storage

Store below 30°C. Protect from light.

6.5 Nature and contents of container

Cartons containing 10 ampoules each having 2 ml. of injection.

6.6 Special precautions for disposal and other handling

None stated

7. MARKETING AUTHORISATION HOLDER

Sanofi-aventis

One Onslow Street

Guildford

Surrey, GU1 4YS, UK

8. MARKETING AUTHORISATION NUMBER(S)

PL 04425/0377

9. DATE OF FIRST AUTHORISATION/RENEWAL OF THE AUTHORISATION

15 November 2005

10. DATE OF REVISION OF THE TEXT

06 July 2009

LEGAL CATEGORY; POM

Otosporin Ear Drops

(GlaxoSmithKline UK)

1. NAME OF THE MEDICINAL PRODUCT

Otosporin Ear Drops

2. QUALITATIVE AND QUANTITATIVE COMPOSITION

Polymyxin B Sulphate EP 10,000 units per ml

Neomycin Sulphate EP 3,400 units per ml

Hydrocortisone EP 1.0% w/v

3. PHARMACEUTICAL FORM

Liquid for topical application to humans

4. CLINICAL PARTICULARS

4.1 Therapeutic indications

Otosporin Ear Drops are indicated for the treatment of otitis externa due to, or complicated by, bacterial infection.

Route of Administration

Topical

In Vitro Activity

Otosporin Ear Drops are active against a wide range of bacterial pathogens. The range of activity includes:-

Gram-Positive Organisms:

Staphylococcus Epidermis and *Staphylococcus Aureus:*

Gram-Negative Organisms:

Enterobacter Spp.

Escherichia Spp.

Haemophilus Spp.

Klebsiella Spp.

Proteus Spp.

Pseudomonas Aeruginosa

Otosporin Ear Drops are not expected to be active against streptococci, including *Streptococcus Pyogenes*

Hydrocortisone possesses anti-inflammatory, anti-allergic and antipruritic activity.

4.2 Posology and method of administration

Adults

Following cleansing and drying of the external auditory meatus and canal as appropriate, three drops should be instilled into the affected ear three or four times daily. Alternatively, a gauze wick may be introduced into the external auditory canal and kept saturated with the solution; the wick may be left in place for 24 to 48 hours.

Treatment should not be continued for more than 7 days without medical supervision.

Soap should not be used for cleansing of the external auditory meatus and canal as it may inactivate the antibiotics.

Children

Otosporin Ear Drops are suitable for use in children (3 years and over) at the same dose as adults. A possibility of increased absorption exists in very young children, thus Otosporin Ear Drops are not recommended in neonates and infants (<3 years). (See 4.3 Contra-indications, 4.4 Special Warnings and Precautions for Use).

Use in the Elderly

As for adults. Caution should be exercised in cases where a decrease in renal function exists and significant systemic absorption of neomycin sulphate may occur (see 4.4 Special Warnings and Precautions for Use).

Use in Renal Impairment

Dosage should be reduced in patients with reduced renal function (see 4.4 Special Warnings and Precautions for Use).

4.3 Contraindications

The use of Otosporin Ear Drops is contra-indicated in patients in whom perforation of the tympanic membrane is known or suspected.

Due to the known ototoxic and nephrotoxic potential of neomycin sulphate, the use of Otosporin Ear Drops in large quantities or on large areas for prolonged periods of time is not recommended in circumstances where significant systemic absorption may occur.

The use of Otosporin Ear Drops is contra-indicated in patients who have demonstrated allergic hypersensitivity to any of the components of the preparation or to cross-sensitising substances such as framycetin, kanamycin, gentamicin and other related antibiotics.

The use of Otosporin Ear Drops is contra-indicated in the presence of untreated viral, fungal and tubercular infections.

A possibility of increased absorption exists in very young children, thus Otosporin Ear Drops are not recommended for use in neonates and infants (up to 3years). In neonates and infants, absorption by immature skin may be enhanced and renal function may be immature.

4.4 Special warnings and precautions for use

Occasionally, delayed hypersensitivity to corticosteroids may occur. Treatment with topical steroid antibiotic combinations should not be continued for more than seven days in the absence of any clinical improvement, since prolonged use may lead to occult extension of infection due to the masking effect of the steroid. Prolonged use may also lead to skin sensitisation and the emergence of resistant organisms.

Following significant systemic absorption, aminoglycosides such as neomycin can cause irreversible ototoxicity; neomycin and polymyxin B sulphate have nephrotoxic potential and polymyxin B sulphate has neurotoxic potential.

All topically active corticosteroids possess the potential to suppress the pituitary-adrenal axis following systemic absorption. Development of adverse systemic effects due to the hydrocortisone component of Otosporin Ear Drops is considered to be unlikely, although the recommended dosage should not be exceeded, particularly in infants.

Prolonged, unsupervised, use should be avoided as it may lead to irreversible partial or total deafness, especially in the elderly and in patients with impaired renal function. In renal impairment the plasma clearance of neomycin is reduced (see Dosage in Renal Impairment).

Use in the immediate pre- and post- operative period is not advised as neomycin may rarely cause neuro-muscular block; because it potentiates skeletal muscle relaxant drugs, it may cause respiratory depression and arrest.

4.5 Interaction with other medicinal products and other forms of interaction

Following significant systemic absorption, both neomycin sulphate and polymyxin b sulphate can intensify and prolong the respiratory depressant effects of neuromuscular blocking agents.

4.6 Pregnancy and lactation

There is little information to demonstrate the possible effect of topically applied neomycin in pregnancy and lactation. However, neomycin present in maternal blood can cross the placenta and may give rise to a theoretical risk of foetal toxicity thus use of Otosporin Ear Drops is not recommended in pregnancy or lactation.

4.7 Effects on ability to drive and use machines

None known.

4.8 Undesirable effects

The incidence of allergic hypersensitivity reactions to neomycin sulphate in the general population is low. There is, however, an increased incidence of hypersensitivity to neomycin in certain selected groups of patients in dermatological practice, particularly those with venous stasis eczema and ulceration, and chronic otitis externa.

Allergic hypersensitivity reactions following topical application of polymyxin B sulphate and hydrocortisone are rare.

Allergic hypersensitivity to neomycin following topical use may manifest itself as an eczematous exacerbation with reddening, scaling, swelling and itching or as a failure of the lesion to heal.

Stinging and burning have occasionally been reported when Otosporin Ear Drops gained access to the middle ear.

Otosporin Ear Drops should only be used in the ear and are not suitable for use in the eye.

4.9 Overdose

Symptoms and signs:-

Possible symptoms or signs associated with excessive use of Otosporin Ear Drops are those due to significant systemic absorption (see Special Warnings and Precautions for Use).

Management:-

Use of the product should be stopped and the patient's general status, hearing acuity, renal and neuromuscular functions should be monitored.

In overdose, blood concentrations of neomycin sulphate, and polymyxin B sulphate should be determined. Haemodialysis may reduce the serum level of neomycin sulphate.

5. PHARMACOLOGICAL PROPERTIES

5.1 Pharmacodynamic properties

Otosporin solution is a bactericidal preparation active against all the pathogens commonly found in bacterial infections of the ear. Polymyxin B is bactericidal against a wide range of gram negative bacilli including *Pseudomonas* Spp., *Escherichea coli*, *Enterobacter* Spp., *Klebsiella* Spp., and *Haemophilus influenzae*. It exerts a bactericidal effect by binding to acid phospholipids in the cell wall and membranes of the bacterium, thereby rendering ineffective the osmotic barrier normally provided by the cell membrane. This leads to escape of the cell contents and the death of the organism.

Neomycin sulphate is bactericidal against a wide range of gram positive and negative bacterial pathogens including *staphylococci, streptococci, Escherichia, Enterobacter, Klebsiella, Haemophilus, Proteus, Salmonella* and *Shigella* species. It is also active against some strains of the *pseudomonas aeruginosa* and against *mycobacterium tuberculosis* and *Neisseria gonorrhoea*. Neomycin exerts its bactericidal effect by interfering with the protein synthesis of susceptible organisms.

5.2 Pharmacokinetic properties

No data are available regarding the pharmacokinetics of this product. However since this is a topical preparation and significant systemic absorption is unlikely to occur, the data are irrelevant.

Systemically absorbed neomycin is predominantly excreted by the kidney and the total amount excreted in the urine varies between 30% and 50%. The pharmacokinetics of systemically absorbed polymyxin B has been described.

5.3 Preclinical safety data

None stated.

6. PHARMACEUTICAL PARTICULARS

6.1 List of excipients

Cetostearyl Alcohol EP

Sorbitan Laurate BP

Polysorbate 20 EP

Methyl Hydroxybenzoate EP

Dilute Sulphuric Acid BP

Purified Water EP

6.2 Incompatibilities

None known

6.3 Shelf life
36 months

6.4 Special precautions for storage
Do not store above 25°C

Protect from light

6.5 Nature and contents of container
Polypropylene bottles with integral nozzles and pilfer proof caps

5ml or 10ml pack sizes

Not all pack sizes may be marketed

6.6 Special precautions for disposal and other handling
None stated.

Administrative Data

7. MARKETING AUTHORISATION HOLDER
The Wellcome Foundation Ltd

Glaxo Wellcome House

Berkeley Avenue

Greenford

Middlesex

Trading as

GlaxoSmithKline UK

Stockley Park West

Uxbridge

Middlesex UB11 1BT

8. MARKETING AUTHORISATION NUMBER(S)
PL0003/5106R

9. DATE OF FIRST AUTHORISATION/RENEWAL OF THE AUTHORISATION
21 May 2008

10. DATE OF REVISION OF THE TEXT
21 May 2008

Otrivine Adult Nasal Spray

(Novartis Consumer Health)

1. NAME OF THE MEDICINAL PRODUCT
Otrivine Adult Nasal Spray

2. QUALITATIVE AND QUANTITATIVE COMPOSITION
Xylometazoline Hydrochloride 0.1% w/v

For excipients see section 6.1

3. PHARMACEUTICAL FORM
Nasal spray, solution

The spray is a clear, colourless solution

4. CLINICAL PARTICULARS

4.1 Therapeutic indications
For the treatment of nasal congestion, perennial and allergic rhinitis (including hay fever), sinusitis.

4.2 Posology and method of administration
Adults, children over 12 years and the elderly: One application in each nostril 2 or 3 times daily

Route of administration: Nasal use

4.3 Contraindications
Known hypersensitivity to Otrivine.

Patients with trans-sphenoidal hypophysectomy or surgery exposing the dura mater.

4.4 Special warnings and precautions for use
Patients are advised not to take decongestants for more than seven consecutive days. Otrivine, like other preparations belonging to the same class of active substances, should be used only with caution in patients showing a strong reaction to sympathomimetic agents as evidenced by signs of insomnia, dizziness etc.

- Do not exceed the recommended dosage
- Decongestants should not be used for more than seven consecutive days. If symptoms persist consult your doctor
- If you are pregnant or taking other medicines or are under a doctor's care consult him before using Otrivine
- The adult spray should not be used for infants or children under 12 years
- Each Otrivine pack should be used by one person only to prevent any cross infection
- Some patients who have sensitive nasal passages may feel some local discomfort when applying nasal drops. Other side effects are very rare
- Keep medicines out of reach of children

4.5 Interaction with other medicinal products and other forms of interaction
None

4.6 Pregnancy and lactation
No foetal toxicity or fertility studies have been carried out in animals. In view of its potential systemic vasoconstrictor effect, it is advisable to take the precaution of not using Otrivine during pregnancy.

Label warning: If you are pregnant or taking any other medicines or are under a doctor's care, consult him before using Otrivine.

4.7 Effects on ability to drive and use machines
None

4.8 Undesirable effects
The following side effects have occasionally been encountered: A burning sensation in the nose and throat, local irritation, nausea, headache, and dryness of the nasal mucosa.
Systemic cardiovascular effects have occurred, and this should be kept in mind when giving Otrivine to people with cardiovascular disease.

4.9 Overdose
No cases of overdosage in adults have yet been reported. In rare instances of accidental poisoning in children, the clinical picture has been marked chiefly by signs such as acceleration and irregularity of the pulse, elevated blood pressure, drowsiness, respiratory depression or irregularity. There is no specific treatment and appropriate supportive treatment should be initiated.

5. PHARMACOLOGICAL PROPERTIES

5.1 Pharmacodynamic properties
Otrivine is a sympathomimetic agent with marked alpha-adrenergic activity, and is intended for use in the nose. It constricts the nasal blood vessels, thereby decongesting the mucosa of the nose and neighbouring regions of the pharynx. This enables patients suffering from colds to breathe more easily through the nose. The effect of Otrivine begins within a few minutes and lasts for up to 10 hours. Otrivine is generally well tolerated and does not impair the function of ciliated epithelium.

5.2 Pharmacokinetic properties
Systemic absorption may occur following nasal application of xylometazoline hydrochloride solutions. It is not used systemically.

5.3 Preclinical safety data
There are no findings in the preclinical testing which are of relevance to the prescriber.

6. PHARMACEUTICAL PARTICULARS

6.1 List of excipients
Benzalkonium chloride

Disodium phosphate dodecahydrate (Sodium phosphate)

Disodium edetate

Sodium dihydrogen phosphate dihydrate (Sodium acid phosphate)

Sodium chloride

Purified water

6.2 Incompatibilities
None

6.3 Shelf life
Unopened: 36 months

After the container is opened for the first time: 28 days

6.4 Special precautions for storage
Do not store above 25°C.

6.5 Nature and contents of container

Bottle:	Low density polyethylene
Cap:	High density polyethylene
Spray valve and capillary:	Low density polyethylene
Carton:	Cardboard
Pack size:	10 ml

6.6 Special precautions for disposal and other handling
Keep all medicines out of the reach of children

Administrative Data

7. MARKETING AUTHORISATION HOLDER
Novartis Consumer Health UK Limited

Wimblehurst Road

Horsham

West Sussex

RH12 5AB

Trading as: Novartis Consumer Health

8. MARKETING AUTHORISATION NUMBER(S)
PL 00030/0116

9. DATE OF FIRST AUTHORISATION/RENEWAL OF THE AUTHORISATION
Date of first authorisation: 1 October 1997

10. DATE OF REVISION OF THE TEXT
16 December 2003

Legal category:
GSL

Otrivine Child Nasal Drops

(Novartis Consumer Health)

1. NAME OF THE MEDICINAL PRODUCT
Otrivine® Child Nasal Drops

2. QUALITATIVE AND QUANTITATIVE COMPOSITION
Xylometazoline Hydrochloride 0.05% w/v

For excipients see 6.1

3. PHARMACEUTICAL FORM
Nasal drops, solution

The product is a clear, colourless solution

4. CLINICAL PARTICULARS

4.1 Therapeutic indications
For the treatment of nasal congestion, perennial and allergic rhinitis (including hay fever), sinusitis.

4.2 Posology and method of administration
Adults and elderly: Not applicable.

Otrivine Child Nasal Drops are contra-indicated in children under 6 years of age.

Children between 6 and 12 years (all indications):

1 or 2 drops, in each nostril 1 or 2 times daily.

Not to be used for more than 5 days without the advice of a doctor. Parents or carers should seek medical attention if the child's condition deteriorates during treatment.

Not more than 2 doses should be given in any 24 hours.

Route of administration: Nasal use

Do not exceed the stated dose

Keep out of the reach and sight of children.

4.3 Contraindications

- Known hypersensitivity to Otrivine or any of the excipients
- Concomitant use of other sympathomimetic decongestants
- Cardiovascular disease including hypertension
- Diabetes mellitus
- Phaeochromocytoma
- Hyperthyroidism
- Closed angle glaucoma
- Monoamine oxidase inhibitors (MAOIs, or within 14 days of stopping treatment, see section 4.5)
- Beta-blockers – (see section 4.5)
- Inflammation of the skin and/or mucosa of the nasal vestibule
- Trans-sphenoidal hypophysectomy or nasal surgery exposing the dura mater
- Not to be used in children under the age of 6 years

4.4 Special warnings and precautions for use
Patients are advised not to take decongestants for more than five consecutive days, without the advice of a doctor. Otrivine Child Nasal Drops like other preparations belonging to the same class of active substances, should be used only with caution in patients showing a strong reaction to sympathomimetic agents as evidenced by signs of insomnia, dizziness etc.

- Do not exceed the recommended dosage
- Do not take with any other cough and cold medicine.
- Decongestants should not be used for more than five consecutive days. If symptoms persist consult your doctor
- If your child is receiving medication or is under a doctor's care, consult him before giving Otrivine Child Nasal Drops
- Each Otrivine Child Nasal Drops pack should be used by one person only to prevent any cross infection
- Some patients who have sensitive nasal passages may feel some local discomfort when applying nasal drops. Other side effects are very rare
- Occasionally small children may show restlessness or sleep disturbance or experience hallucinations when Otrivine Child Nasal Drops is used. If this occurs Otrivine Child Nasal Drops should be stopped
- Keep medicines out of reach and sight of children
- Expectant mothers should consult their doctors before using Otrivine Child Nasal Drops for themselves
- Use with caution in occlusive vascular disease
- Keep away from the eyes

4.5 Interaction with other medicinal products and other forms of interaction
MAOIs and /or RIMAs: should not be given to patients treated with MAOIs or within 14 days of stopping treatment: increased risk of hypertensive crisis

- **Moclobemide:** risk of hypertensive crisis
- **Antihypertensives** (including adrenergic neurone blockers & beta-blockers): Otrivine Child Nasal Drops may block the hypotensive effects
- **Cardiac glycosides:** increased risk of dysrhythmias
- **Ergot alkaloids** (ergotamine & methysergide): increased risk of ergotism
- **Appetite suppressants and amphetamine-like psychostimulants:** risk of hypertension
- **Oxytocin**– risk of hypertension

4.6 Pregnancy and lactation
No foetal toxicity or fertility studies have been carried out in animals. In view of its potential systemic vasoconstrictor effect, it is advisable to take the precaution of not using Otrivine Child Nasal Drops during pregnancy.

Label warning: Expectant mothers should consult their doctor before using Otrivine Child Nasal Drops for themselves

4.7 Effects on ability to drive and use machines
None

4.8 Undesirable effects
The following side effects have occasionally been encountered: A burning sensation in the nose and throat, local irritation, nausea, headache, and dryness of the nasal mucosa.

Systemic cardiovascular effects have occurred, and this should be kept in mind when giving Otrivine Child Nasal Drops to people with cardiovascular disease.

Oral agents

Cardiovascular effects

- Tachycardia/palpitations
- Other cardiac dysrhythmias and hypertension
- CNS effects
- Irritability
- Anxiety
- Restlessness
- Excitability
- Insomnia
- Hallucinations and paranoid delusions

Skin reactions including rash

Hypersensitivity reactions – including that cross-sensitivity may occur with other sympathomimetics

Other reactions

- Nausea and/or vomiting
- Headache
- Urinary retention

Topical agents

- Local effects – irritation and dryness
- Nausea
- Headache
- Rebound congestion (rhinitis medicamentosa) – especially with prolonged and/or heavy use
- Tolerance with diminished effect – especially with prolonged and/or heavy use
- Cardiovascular effects (as with oral agents) particularly with prolonged and/or excessive use
- CNS effects (as with oral agents) particularly with prolonged and/or excessive use

4.9 Overdose
No cases of overdosage in adults have yet been reported. In rare instances of accidental poisoning in children, the clinical picture has been marked chiefly by signs such as acceleration and irregularity of the pulse, elevated blood pressure, drowsiness, respiratory depression or irregularity. There is no specific treatment and appropriate supportive treatment should be initiated.

5. PHARMACOLOGICAL PROPERTIES

5.1 Pharmacodynamic properties
Otrivine Child Nasal Drops is a sympathomimetic agent with marked alpha-adrenergic activity, and is intended for use in the nose. It constricts the nasal blood vessels, thereby decongesting the mucosa of the nose and neighbouring regions of the pharynx. This enables patients suffering from colds to breathe more easily through the nose. The effect of Otrivine Child Nasal Drops begins within a few minutes and lasts for up to 10 hours. Otrivine Child Nasal Drops is generally well tolerated and does not impair the function of ciliated epithelium.

5.2 Pharmacokinetic properties
Systemic absorption may occur following nasal application of xylometazoline hydrochloride solutions. It is not used systemically.

5.3 Preclinical safety data
There are no findings in the preclinical testing which are of relevance to the prescriber.

6. PHARMACEUTICAL PARTICULARS

6.1 List of excipients
Benzalkonium chloride

Disodium phosphate dodecahydrate (Sodium phosphate)

Disodium edetate

Sodium dihydrogen phosphate dihydrate (Sodium acid phosphate)

Sodium chloride

Sorbitol

Hypromellose

Purified water

6.2 Incompatibilities
None

6.3 Shelf life
Unopened: 36 months

After the container is opened for the first time: 28 days

6.4 Special precautions for storage
Protect from heat

6.5 Nature and contents of container

Bottle:	High density polyethylene
Cap:	Polypropylene
Pipette rod:	Low density polythene
Pipette bulb:	Halogenated butyl elastomer
Carton:	Cardboard

The pipette forms an integral part of the cap.

Pack size: 10 ml

6.6 Special precautions for disposal and other handling
Keep all medicines out of the reach of children

7. MARKETING AUTHORISATION HOLDER
Novartis Consumer Health UK Limited

Wimblehurst Road

Horsham

West Sussex

RH12 5AB

Trading as: Novartis Consumer Health

8. MARKETING AUTHORISATION NUMBER(S)
PL 00030/0114

9. DATE OF FIRST AUTHORISATION/RENEWAL OF THE AUTHORISATION
15 November 2003

10. DATE OF REVISION OF THE TEXT
21 May 2009

Legal category: P

Ovitrelle 250 micrograms/0.5 ml prefilled syringe

(Merck Serono)

1. NAME OF THE MEDICINAL PRODUCT
Ovitrelle® 250 micrograms/0.5ml, solution for injection in a pre-filled syringe

2. QUALITATIVE AND QUANTITATIVE COMPOSITION
Choriogonadotropin alfa* 250 micrograms in 0.5 ml. (equivalent to approximately 6500 IU)

Excipients: 27.3 mg mannitol, 0.05 mg poloxamer 188, 0.1 mg L-methionine

* Produced by recombinant DNA technology in CHO

For a full list of excipients, see section 6.1.

3. PHARMACEUTICAL FORM
Solution for injection

Clear, colourless solution.

The pH of the solution is 7.0 ± 0.3, its osmolarity 250-400 mOsm/L

4. CLINICAL PARTICULARS

4.1 Therapeutic indications
Ovitrelle is indicated in the treatment of

Women undergoing superovulation prior to assisted reproductive techniques such as in vitro fertilisation (IVF): Ovitrelle is administered to trigger final follicular maturation and luteinisation after stimulation of follicular growth,

Anovulatory or oligo-ovulatory women: Ovitrelle is administered to trigger ovulation and luteinisation in anovulatory or oligo-ovulatory patients after stimulation of follicular growth.

4.2 Posology and method of administration
Ovitrelle is intended for subcutaneous administration.

Treatment with Ovitrelle should be performed under the supervision of a physician experienced in the treatment of fertility problems.

The following dosing regimen should be used:

Women undergoing superovulation prior to assisted reproductive techniques such as in vitro fertilisation (IVF):

One pre-filled syringe of Ovitrelle (250 micrograms) is administered 24 to 48 hours after the last administration of an FSH- or hMG preparation, i.e. when optimal stimulation of follicular growth is achieved.

Anovulatory or oligo-ovulatory women:

One pre-filled syringe of Ovitrelle (250 micrograms) is administered 24 to 48 hours after optimal stimulation of follicular growth is achieved. The patient is recommended to have coitus on the day of, and the day after, Ovitrelle injection.

4.3 Contraindications
Ovitrelle is contraindicated for safety reasons in case of:

- Tumours of the hypothalamus and pituitary gland
- Hypersensitivity to the active substance or to any of the excipients
- Ovarian enlargement or cyst due to reasons other than polycystic ovarian disease
- Gynaecological haemorrhages of unknown aetiology
- Ovarian, uterine or mammary carcinoma
- Extrauterine pregnancy in the previous 3 months
- Active thrombo-embolic disorders

Ovitrelle must not be used when an effective response cannot be obtained, for example:

- Primary ovarian failure
- Malformations of sexual organs incompatible with pregnancy
- Fibroid tumours of the uterus incompatible with pregnancy
- Postmenopausal women

4.4 Special warnings and precautions for use
To date, there is no clinical experience with Ovitrelle in other indications commonly treated with urine derived human chorionic gonadotropin.

Before starting treatment, the couple's infertility should be assessed as appropriate and putative contraindications for pregnancy evaluated. In particular, patients should be evaluated for hypothyroidism, adrenocortical deficiency, hyperprolactinemia and pituitary or hypothalamic tumours, and appropriate specific treatment given.

Special precautions should be taken before administering Ovitrelle to patients with clinically significant systemic disease where pregnancy could lead to a worsening of the condition.

Patients undergoing ovarian stimulation are at an increased risk of developing ovarian hyperstimulation syndrome (OHSS) due to multiple follicular development.

Ovarian hyperstimulation syndrome may become a serious medical event characterised by large ovarian cysts, which are prone to rupture and the presence of ascites within a clinical picture of circulatory dysfunction. Ovarian hyperstimulation syndrome due to excessive ovarian response can be avoided by withholding hCG administration. Patients should be advised to refrain from coitus or use barrier methods for at least 4 days.

Careful monitoring of estradiol levels and ovarian response, based on ultrasound is recommended prior to and during stimulation therapy, for all patients.

The risk of multiple pregnancy following assisted reproductive technologies is related to the number of embryos replaced. In patients undergoing induction of ovulation, the incidence of multiple pregnancies and births (mostly twins) is increased compared with natural conception.

To minimise the risk of OHSS and of multiple pregnancy, ultrasound scans as well as estradiol measurements are recommended. In anovulation, the risk of OHSS is increased by a serum estradiol level > 1500 pg/ml (5400 pmol/l) and more than 3 follicles of 14 mm or more in diameter. In assisted reproductive techniques, there is an increased risk of OHSS with a serum estradiol > 3000 pg/ml (11000 pmol/l) and 20 or more follicles of 12 mm or more in diameter. When the estradiol level is > 5500 pg/ml (20000 pmol/l) and when there are 40 or more follicles in total, it may be necessary to withhold hCG administration.

Severe ovarian hyperstimulation syndrome could be complicated in rare cases by haemoperitoneum, acute pulmonary distress, ovarian torsion, and thromboembolism.

Adherence to recommended Ovitrelle dosage, regimen of administration and careful monitoring of therapy will minimise the incidence of ovarian hyperstimulation and multiple pregnancy.

The rate of miscarriage, in both anovulatory patients and women undergoing assisted reproductive techniques, is higher than that found in the normal population but comparable with the rates observed in women with other fertility problems.

During Ovitrelle therapy, a minor thyroid stimulation is possible, of which the clinical relevance is unknown.

Self-administration of Ovitrelle should only be performed by patients who are adequately trained and have access to expert advice.

4.5 Interaction with other medicinal products and other forms of interaction
No specific interaction studies with Ovitrelle and other medicines have been performed however no clinically significant drug interactions have been reported during hCG therapy. Following administration, Ovitrelle may interfere for up to ten days with the immunological determination of serum / urinary hCG, leading to a false positive pregnancy test.

4.6 Pregnancy and lactation
Considering the indication, Ovitrelle should not be used during pregnancy and lactation. No clinical data on exposed pregnancies are available. No reproduction studies with choriogonadotropin alfa in animals were performed (see section 5.3). The potential risk for humans is unknown.

There are no data on the excretion of choriogonadotropin alfa in milk.

4.7 Effects on ability to drive and use machines
No studies on the effects on the ability to drive and use machines have been performed.

4.8 Undesirable effects
In comparative trials with different doses of Ovitrelle, the following undesirable effects were found to be associated with Ovitrelle in a dose-related fashion: ovarian hyperstimulation syndrome, and vomiting and nausea. Ovarian hyperstimulation syndrome was observed in approximately 4% of patients treated with Ovitrelle. Severe ovarian hyperstimulation syndrome was reported in less than 0.5% patients (see section 4.4).

In rare instances, thromboembolisms have been associated with menotrophin/hCG therapy. Although this adverse event was not observed, there is the possibility that this may also occur with Ovitrelle.

Ectopic pregnancy, ovarian torsion and other complications have been reported in patients after hCG administration. These are considered concomitant effects related to Assisted Reproductive Technologies (ART).

After best evidence assessment, the following undesirable effects may be observed after administration of Ovitrelle. Within each frequency grouping, undesirable effects are presented in order of decreasing seriousness.

Common (>1/100, <1/10)

Gastrointestinal disorders: Vomiting/nausea, abdominal pain

Reproductive system and breast disorders: Mild or moderate ovarian hyperstimulation syndrome

General disorders and administration site conditions: Headache, tiredness, local reaction/pain at injection site.

Uncommon (>1/1000, <1/100)

Psychiatric disorders: Depression, irritability, restlessness,

Gastrointestinal disorders: Diarrhoea,

Reproductive system and breast disorders: Severe ovarian hyperstimulation syndrome, breast pain

Very rare (<1/10,000)

Immune system disorders: allergic reactions

Skin and subcutaneous tissue disorders: Mild reversible skin reactions manifesting as rash.

4.9 Overdose

No case of overdose has been reported.

Nevertheless, there is a possibility that ovarian hyperstimulation syndrome (OHSS) may result from an overdosage of Ovitrelle (see section 4.4).

5. PHARMACOLOGICAL PROPERTIES

5.1 Pharmacodynamic properties

Pharmacotherapeutic group: gonadotropins, ATC code: G03G A08

Ovitrelle is a medicinal product of chorionic gonadotropin produced by recombinant DNA techniques. It shares the amino acid sequence with urinary hCG. Chorionic gonadotropin binds on the ovarian theca (and granulosa) cells to a transmembrane receptor shared with the luteinising hormone, the LH/CG receptor.

The principal pharmacodynamic activity in women is oocyte meiosis resumption, follicular rupture (ovulation), corpus luteum formation and production of progesterone and estradiol by the corpus luteum.

In women, chorionic gonadotropin acts as a surrogate LH-surge that triggers ovulation.

Ovitrelle is used to trigger final follicular maturation and early luteinisation after use of medicinal products for stimulation of follicular growth.

In comparative clinical trials, administration of a dose of 250 micrograms of Ovitrelle was as effective as 5000 IU and 10000 IU of urinary hCG in inducing final follicular maturation and early luteinisation in assisted reproductive techniques, and as effective as 5000 IU of urinary hCG in ovulation induction.

So far, there are no signs of antibody development in humans to Ovitrelle. Repeated exposure to Ovitrelle was investigated in male patients only. Clinical investigation in women for the indication of ART and anovulation was limited to one treatment cycle.

5.2 Pharmacokinetic properties

Following intravenous administration, choriogonadotropin alfa is distributed to the extracellular fluid space with a distribution half-life of around 4.5 hours. The steady-state volume of distribution and the total clearance are 6 l and 0.2 l/h, respectively. There are no indications that choriogonadotropin alfa is metabolised and excreted differently than endogenous hCG.

Following subcutaneous administration, choriogonadotropin alfa is eliminated from the body with a terminal half-life of about 30 hours, and the absolute bioavailability is about 40 %.

A comparative study between the currently registered freeze-dried formulation and the liquid formulation showed bioequivalence between the two formulations.

5.3 Preclinical safety data

Non-clinical data reveal no special hazard for humans based on conventional studies of safety pharmacology, repeated dose toxicity and genotoxicity. Studies on carcinogenic potential were not performed. This is justified, given the proteinous nature of the drug substance and the negative outcome of the genotoxicity testing.

Studies on reproduction were not performed in animals.

6. PHARMACEUTICAL PARTICULARS

6.1 List of excipients

Mannitol

Methionine

Poloxamer 188

Diluted phosphoric acid

Sodium hydroxide

Water for injections

6.2 Incompatibilities

In the absence of compatibility studies, this medicinal product must not be mixed with other medicinal products.

6.3 Shelf life

2 years.

After opening, the product should be used immediately. However, the in-use stability has been demonstrated for 24 hours at +2° to 8°C.

6.4 Special precautions for storage

Store in a refrigerator (2°C – 8°C). Store in the original package. Within its shelf-life, the solution may be stored at or below 25°C for up to 30 days without being refrigerated again during this period. It must be discarded if not used after these 30 days.

6.5 Nature and contents of container

0.5 ml of solution in a pre-filled syringe (type I glass) with a plunger stopper (halobutyl rubber) and plunger (plastic), and with a needle for injection (stainless) – pack of 1.

6.6 Special precautions for disposal and other handling

Only clear solution without particles should be used. Any unused product or waste material should be disposed of in accordance with local requirements.

For single use only.

7. MARKETING AUTHORISATION HOLDER

Merck Serono Europe Limited

56, Marsh Wall

London E14 9TP

United Kingdom

8. MARKETING AUTHORISATION NUMBER(S)

Authorisation number	Presentations
EU/1/00/165/007	Ovitrelle – 250 micrograms/0.5 ml – Solution for injection – 1 pre-filled syringe

9. DATE OF FIRST AUTHORISATION/RENEWAL OF THE AUTHORISATION

2 February 2001 / 31 January 2006

10. DATE OF REVISION OF THE TEXT

July 2009

LEGAL STATUS

POM

NAME AND ADDRESS OF DISTRIBUTOR IN UK

Merck Serono Ltd

Bedfont Cross

Stanwell Road

Feltham

Middlesex

TW14 8NX

NAME AND ADDRESS OF DISTRIBUTOR IN IRELAND

Allphar Services Limited

Pharmaceutical Agents and Distributors

Belgard Road

Tallaght

Dublin 24

Ovranette

(Wyeth Pharmaceuticals)

1. NAME OF THE MEDICINAL PRODUCT

Ovranette Tablets.

2. QUALITATIVE AND QUANTITATIVE COMPOSITION

Each tablet contains 0.15mg levonorgestrel and 0.03mg ethinylestradiol.

For excipients see 6.1

3. PHARMACEUTICAL FORM

Sugar-coated tablets.

4. CLINICAL PARTICULARS

4.1 Therapeutic indications

Oral contraception.

Treatment of endometriosis.

Treatment of spasmodic dysmenorrhoea and premenstrual tension.

Treatment of functional uterine bleeding (menorrhagia, metrorrhagia, metropathia haemorrhatica).

Emergency treatment of acute uterine bleeding.

4.2 Posology and method of administration

For oral administration

Dosage and Administration

First treatment cycle: 1 tablet daily for 21 days, starting with the tablet marked number 1, on the first day of the menstrual cycle. Additional contraception (barriers and spermicides) is not required.

Subsequent cycles: Each subsequent course is started when seven tablet-free days have followed the preceding course. A withdrawal bleed should occur during the 7 tablet-free days.

Changing from another 21 day combined oral contraceptive: The first tablet of Ovranette should be taken on the first day immediately after the end of the previous oral contraceptive course. Additional precautions are not required. A withdrawal bleed should not be expected until the end of the first pack.

Changing from an Every Day (ED) 28 day combined oral contraceptive: The first tablet of Ovranette should be taken on the day immediately after the day on which the last active pill in the ED pack has been taken. The remaining tablets in the ED pack should be discarded. Additional precautions are not required. A withdrawal bleed should not be expected until the end of the first pack.

Changing from a Progestogen-only-Pill (POP): The first tablet of Ovranette should be taken on the first day of menstruation even if the POP for that day has already been taken. The remaining tablets in the POP pack should be discarded. Additional precautions are not required.

Post-partum and post-abortum use: After pregnancy, combined oral contraception can be started in non-lactating women 21 days after a vaginal delivery, provided that the patient is fully ambulant and there are no puerperal complications. If the pill is started later than 21 days after delivery, then alternative contraception (barriers and spermicides) should be used until oral contraception is started and for the first 7 days of pill-taking. If unprotected intercourse has taken place after 21 days post partum, then oral contraception should not be started until the first menstrual bleed after childbirth. After miscarriage or abortion oral contraception may be started immediately.

Other indications

Endometriosis: Continuous treatment with two tablets daily.

Spasmodic dysmenorrhoea, premenstrual tension: Dosage as for oral contraception.

Functional uterine bleeding: Two tablets are taken daily on a cyclic basis as for oral contraception. In the first one or two cycles it may be necessary to give four tablets, or in exceptional cases, five.

Emergency treatment of acute uterine bleeding: Four tablets are given initially and, if necessary, 4-8 tablets daily.

Elderly: Not applicable

Children: Not applicable

Special Circumstances Requiring Additional Contraception

Missed Pills: If a tablet is delayed, it should be taken as soon as possible, and if it is taken within 12 hours of the correct time, additional contraception is not needed. Further tablets should then be taken at the usual time. If the delay exceeds 12 hours, the last missed pill should be taken when remembered, the earlier missed pills left in the pack and normal pill-taking resumed. If one or more tablets are omitted from the 21 days of pill-taking, addition contraception (barriers and spermicides) should be used for the next 7 days of pill-taking. In addition, if one or more pills are missed during the last 7 days of pill-taking, the subsequent pill-free interval should be disregarded and the next pack started the day after taking the last tablet from the previous pack. In this case, a period should not be expected until the end of the second pack. If the patient does not have a period at the end of the second pack, she must return to her doctor to exclude the possibility of pregnancy.

Gastro-intestinal upset: Vomiting or diarrhoea may reduce the efficacy by preventing full absorption. Additional contraception (barriers and spermicides) should be used during the stomach upset and for the 7 days following the upset. If these 7 days overrun the end of a pack, the next pack should be started without a break. In this case, a period should not be expected until the end of the second pack. If the patient does not have a period at the end of the second pack, she must return to her doctor to exclude the possibility of pregnancy.

Mild laxatives do not impair contraceptive action.

Interaction with other drugs:

Some drugs may reduce the efficacy of oral contraceptives (refer to "4.5. Interaction with other medicaments and other forms of interaction."). It is, therefore, advisable to use non-hormonal methods of contraception (barriers and spermicides) in addition to the oral contraceptive as long as an extremely high degree of protection is required during treatment with such drugs. The additional contraception should be used while the concurrent medication continues and for 7 days afterwards. If these extra precautions overrun the end of the pack, the next pack should be started without a break. In this case a withdrawal bleed should not be expected until the end of the second pack. If the patient does not have a withdrawal bleed at the end of the second pack, she must return to her doctor to exclude the possibility of pregnancy.

4.3 Contraindications

1. Suspected pregnancy

2. History of confirmed venous thromboembolism (VTE). Family history of idiopathic VTE. Other known risk factors for VTE.

3. Arterial thrombotic disorders and a history of these conditions, disorders of lipid metabolism and other

conditions in which, in individual cases, there is known or suspected to be a much increased risk of thrombosis.

4. Sickle-cell anaemia

5. Acute or severe chronic liver diseases. Dubin-Johnson syndrome. Rotor syndrome. History, during pregnancy, of idiopathic jaundice or severe pruritis.

6. History of herpes gestationis.

7. Mammary or endometrial carcinoma, or a history of these conditions.

8. Abnormal vaginal bleeding of unknown cause.

9. Deterioration of otosclerosis during pregnancy.

4.4 Special warnings and precautions for use

Warnings:

1. Venous and Arterial Thrombosis and Thromboembolism

Use of COCs is associated with an increased risk of venous and arterial thrombotic and thromboembolic events.

Minimising exposure to oestrogens and progestogens is in keeping with good principles of therapeutics. For any particular oestrogen/progestogen combination, the dosage regimen prescribed should be one that contains the least amount of oestrogen and progestogen that is compatible with a low failure rate and the needs of the patient.

Unless clinically indicated otherwise, new users of COCs should be started on preparations containing less than 50μg of oestrogen.

Venous Thrombosis and Thromboembolism

Use of COCs increases the risk of venous thrombotic and thromboembolic events. Reported events include deep venous thrombosis and pulmonary embolism.

The use of any COC carries an increased risk of venous thrombotic and thromboembolic events compared with no use. The excess risk is highest during the first year a woman ever uses a combined oral contraceptive. This increased risk is less than the risk of venous thrombotic and thromboembolic events associated with pregnancy which is estimated as 60 cases per 100,000 woman-years. Venous thromboembolism is fatal in 1-2% of cases.

Some epidemiological studies have reported a greater risk of VTE for women using combined oral contraceptives containing desogestrel or gestodene (the so-called third generation pills) than for women using pills containing levonorgestrel (the so-called second generation pills).

The spontaneous incidence of VTE in healthy non-pregnant women (not taking any oral contraceptive) is about 5 cases per 100,000 women per year. The incidence in users of the second generation pills (such as Ovranette) is about 15 per 100,000 women per year of use. The incidence in users of third generation pills is about 25 cases per 100,000 women per year of use; this excess incidence has not been satisfactorily explained by bias or confounding. The level of all these risks of VTE increases with age and is likely to be further increased in women with other known risk factors of VTE.

All this information should be taken into account when prescribing this COC. When counselling on the choice of contraceptive method(s) all of the above information should be considered.

The risk of venous thrombotic and thromboembolic events is further increased in women with conditions predisposing for venous thrombosis and thromboembolism. Caution must be exercised when prescribing COCs for such women.

Examples of predisposing conditions for venous thrombosis are:

- Certain inherited or acquired thrombophilias (the presence of an inherited thrombophilia may be indicated by a family history of venous thrombotic/thromboembolic events
- Obesity (body mass index of 30kg/m^2 or over)
- Surgery or trauma with increased risk of thrombosis (see reasons for discontinuation)
- Recent delivery or second-trimester abortion
- Prolonged immobilisation
- Increasing age
- Systemic Lupus Erythematosus (SLE)

The relative risk of post-operative thromboembolic complications has been reported to be increased two- or fourfold with the use of COCs (see reasons for discontinuation).

Since the immediate post-partum period is associated with an increased risk of thromboembolism, COCs should be started no earlier than day 28 after delivery or second-trimester abortion.

Arterial Thrombosis and Thromboembolism

The use of COCs increases the risk or arterial thrombotic and thromboembolic events. Reported events include myocardial infarction and cerebrovascular events (ischaemic and haemorrhagic stroke).

The risk of arterial thrombotic and thromboembolic events is further increased in women with underlying risk factors.

Caution must be exercised when prescribing COCs for women with risk factors for arterial thrombotic and thromboembolic events.

Figure 1

Estimated cumulative numbers of breast cancers per 10,000 women diagnosed in 5 years of use and up to 10 years after stopping COCs, compared with numbers of breast cancers diagnosed in 10,000 women who had never used COCs

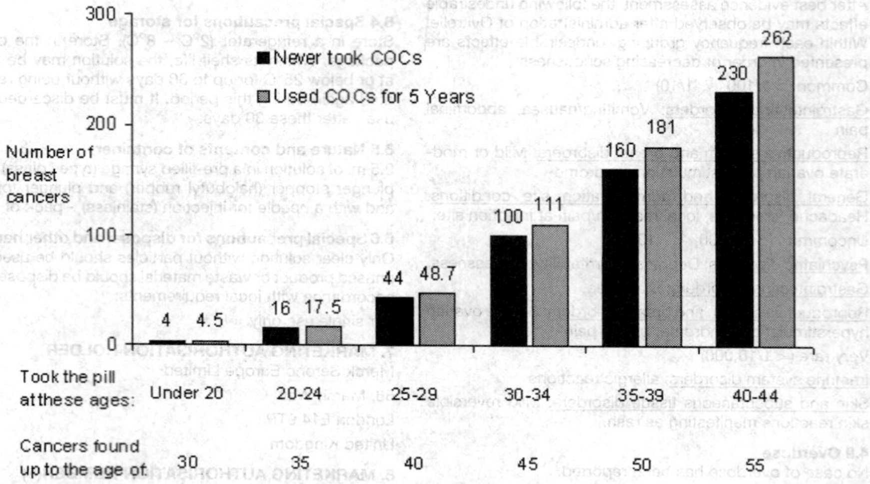

Examples of risk factors for arterial thrombotic and thromboembolic event are:

- Smoking, especially over the age of 35
- Certain inherited and acquired thrombophilias
- Hypertension
- Dyslipoproteinaemias
- Thrombogenic valvular heart disease, atrial fibillation
- Obesity (body mass index of 30kg/m^2)
- Increasing age
- Diabetes
- Systemic Lupus Erythematosus (SLE)

COC users with migraine (particularly migraine with aura) may be at increased risk of stroke.

There is no consensus about the possible role of varicose veins and superficial thrombophlebitis in venous thromboembolism

The suitability of a combined oral contraceptive should be judged according to the severity of such conditions in the individual case, and should be discussed with the patient before she decides to take it.

2. The risk of arterial thrombosis associated with combined oral contraceptives increases with age, and this risk is aggravated by cigarette smoking. The use of combined oral contraceptives by women in the older age group, especially those who are cigarette smokers, should therefore be discouraged and alternative methods used.

3. The possibility cannot be ruled out that certain chronic diseases may occasionally deteriorate during the use of combined oral contraceptives. (See 'Precautions').

4. Malignant liver tumours have been reported on rare occasions in long-term users of oral contraceptives. Benign hepatic tumours have also been associated with oral contraceptive usage. A hepatic tumour should be considered in the differential diagnosis when upper abdominal pain, enlarged liver or signs of intra-abdominal haemorrhage occur.

5. Numerous epidemiological studies have been reported on the risks of ovarian, endometrial, cervical and breast cancer in women using combined oral contraceptives. The evidence is clear that combined oral contraceptives offer substantial protection against both ovarian and endometrial cancer.

An increased risk of cervical cancer in long term users of combined oral contraceptives has been reported in some studies, but there continues to be controversy about the extent to which this is attributable to the confounding effects of sexual behaviour and other factors.

A meta-analysis from 54 epidemiological studies reported that there is a slightly increased relative risk (RR = 1.24) of having breast cancer diagnosed in women who are currently using combined oral contraceptives (COCs). The observed pattern of increased risk may be due to an earlier diagnosis of breast cancer in COC users, the biological effects of COCs or a combination of both. The additional breast cancers diagnosed in current users of COCs or in women who have used COCs in the last ten years are more likely to be localised to the breast than those in women who never used COCs.

Breast cancer is rare among women under 40 years of age whether or not they take COCs. Whilst this background risk increases with age, the excess number of breast cancer diagnoses in current and recent COC users is small in relation to the overall risk of breast cancer (see bar chart).

(see Figure 1 above)

The most important risk factor for breast cancer in COC users is the age women discontinue the COC; the older the age at stopping, the more breast cancers are diagnosed. Duration of use is less important and the excess risk gradually disappears during the course of the 10 years after stopping COC use such that by 10 years there appears to be no excess.

The possible increase in risk of breast cancer should be discussed with the user and weighed against the benefits of COCs taking into account the evidence that they offer substantial protection against the risk of developing certain other cancers (e.g. ovarian and endometrial cancer).

Reasons for stopping oral contraception immediately:

1. Occurrence of migraine in patients who have never previously suffered from it. Exacerbation of pre-existing migraine. Any unusually frequent or unusually severe headaches.

2. Any kind of acute disturbance of vision.

3. Suspicion of thrombosis or infarction including symptoms such as unusual pains in or swelling of the legs, stabbing pains on breathing, persistent cough or coughing blood, pain or tightness in the chest.

4. Six weeks before elective operations, or treatment of varicose veins by sclerotherapy and during immobilisation, e.g. after accidents, etc.

5. Significant rise in blood-pressure.

6. Jaundice.

7. Clear exacerbation of conditions known to be capable of deteriorating during oral contraception or pregnancy.

8. Pregnancy is a reason for stopping immediately because it has been suggested by some investigations that oral contraceptives taken in early pregnancy may slightly increase the risk of foetal malformations. Other investigations have failed to support these findings. The possibility therefore cannot be excluded, but it is certain that if a risk exists at all, it is very small.

If oral contraception is stopped for any reason and pregnancy is not desired, it is recommended that alternative non-hormonal methods of contraception (such as barriers or spermicides) are used to ensure contraceptive protection is maintained.

Precautions:

1. Assessment of women prior to starting oral contraceptives (and at regular intervals thereafter) should include a personal and family medical history of each woman. Physical examination should be guided by this and by the contraindications (section 4.3) and warnings (section 4.4) for this product. The frequency and nature of these assessments should be based upon relevant guidelines and should be adapted to the individual woman, but should include measurement of blood pressure and, if judged appropriate by the clinician, breast, abdominal and pelvic examination including cervical cytology.

2. Before starting treatment, pregnancy must be excluded.

3. The following conditions require careful observation during medication: a history of severe depressive states, varicose veins, diabetes, hypertension, epilepsy, otosclerosis, multiple sclerosis, porphyria, tetany, disturbed liver function, gall-stones, cardiovascular diseases, renal diseases, chloasma, uterine fibroids, asthma, the wearing of contact lenses, or any disease that is prone to worsen during pregnancy. The first appearance or deterioration of

any of these conditions may indicate that the oral contraceptive should be stopped.

4. The risk of the deterioration of chloasma, which is often not fully reversible, is reduced by the avoidance of excessive exposure to sunlight.

Menstrual changes:

1. Reduction of menstrual flow: This is not abnormal and it is to be expected in some patients.

2. Missed menstruation: Occasionally withdrawal bleeding may not occur at all. If the tablets have been taken correctly, pregnancy is very unlikely but should be ruled out before a new course of tablets is started.

Intermenstrual bleeding:

Very light "spotting" or heavier "break through bleeding" may occur during tablet-taking, especially in the first few cycles. It appears to be generally of no significance, except where it indicates errors of tablet-taking, or where the possibility of interaction with other drugs exists. However, if irregular bleeding is persistent an organic cause should be considered.

4.5 Interaction with other medicinal products and other forms of interaction

Some drugs accelerate the metabolism of oral contraceptives when taken concurrently and these include barbiturates, phenytoin, phenylbutazone and rifampicin. Other drugs suspected of having the capacity to reduce the efficacy of oral contraceptives include ampicillin and other antibiotics. It is therefore, advisable to use non-hormonal methods of contraception (barriers and spermicides). Please refer to "4.2 Posology and Method of Administration, Interaction with other drugs".

The response to metyrapone is less pronounced in women taking oral contraceptives.

ACTH function test remains unchanged. Reduction in corticosteriod excretion and elevation or plasma corticosteriods are due to increased cortisol binding capacity of plasma proteins.

Serum protein-bound iodine levels should not be used for evaluation of thyroid function as levels may rise due to increased thyroid hormone binding capacity of plasma proteins.

Erythrocyte sedimentation may be accelerated in absence of any disease due to change in proportion of plasma protein fractions. Increases in plasma copper, iron and alkaline phosphatase have been recorded.

The herbal remedy, St John's Wort (*Hypericum perforatum*) should not be taken concomitantly with this medicine as it could potentially lead to a loss of contraceptive effect.

4.6 Pregnancy and lactation

Pregnancy is a reason for stopping administration immediately because it has been suggested by some investigations that oral contraceptives taken in early pregnancy may slightly increase the risk of foetal malformations. Other investigations have failed to support these findings. The possibility therefore cannot be excluded, but it is certain that if a risk exists at all, it is very small. After pregnancy, combined oral contraception can be started in non-lactating women 21 days after vaginal delivery, provided that the patient is fully ambulant and there are no puerperal complications.

Please refer to recommended dosage schedule: Post-partum and post-abortum use.

Administration of oestrogens to lactating women may decrease the quantity or quality of the milk.

4.7 Effects on ability to drive and use machines

None known.

4.8 Undesirable effects

See 'Special Warnings and Special Precautions for Use'.

There is an increased risk of venous thromboembolism for all women using a combined oral contraceptive. For information on differences in risk between oral contraceptives, see Section 4.4.

Occasional side-effect may include nausea, vomiting, headaches, breast tenderness, irregular bleeding or missed bleeds, changed body weight or libido, depressive moods, chloasma and altered serum lipid profile.

4.9 Overdose

There have been no reports of serious ill-effects from overdosage, even when a considerable number of tablets have been taken by a small child. In general, it is, therefore, unnecessary to treat overdosage. However, if overdosage is discovered within two or three hours and is so large that treatment seems desirable, gastric lavage can be safely used.

There are no specific antidotes and further treatment should be symptomatic.

5. PHARMACOLOGICAL PROPERTIES

5.1 Pharmacodynamic properties

Ethinylestradiol is a synthetic oestrogen which has actions and uses similar to those of oestradiol, but is much more potent.

Norgestrel is a progestational agent with actions similar to those of progesterone. It is more potent as an inhibitor of ovulation than norethisterone and has androgenic activity.

5.2 Pharmacokinetic properties

Ethinylestradiol is absorbed by the gastro-intestinal tract. It is only slowly metabolised and excreted in the urine.

Norgestrel is absorbed from the gastrointestinal tract. Metabolites are excreted in the urine and faeces as glucuronide and sulphate conjugates.

5.3 Preclinical safety data

Nothing of relevance to the prescriber.

6. PHARMACEUTICAL PARTICULARS

6.1 List of excipients

Core: lactose, maize starch, povidone 25, magnesium stearate, talc, purified water.

Coating: sucrose, polyethylene glycol 6000, calcium carbonate, talc, povidone 90, purified water, white wax and wax carnauba.

6.2 Incompatibilities

None known.

6.3 Shelf life

36 months.

6.4 Special precautions for storage

Store at or below room temperature.

6.5 Nature and contents of container

Aluminium foil and PVC blister packs of 21 tablets.

Cartons containing 1, 3 and 50 blisters.

6.6 Special precautions for disposal and other handling

Not applicable.

7. MARKETING AUTHORISATION HOLDER

John Wyeth & Brother Limited

t/a Wyeth Laboratories

Huntercombe Lane South

Taplow, Maidenhead

Berkshire SL6 0PH

8. MARKETING AUTHORISATION NUMBER(S)

PL 0011/0041

9. DATE OF FIRST AUTHORISATION/RENEWAL OF THE AUTHORISATION

26 February 1996 / 05 December 2008

10. DATE OF REVISION OF THE TEXT

05 December 2008

Ovysmen Oral Contraceptive Tablets

(Janssen-Cilag Ltd)

1. NAME OF THE MEDICINAL PRODUCT

OVYSMEN® Oral Contraceptive Tablets

2. QUALITATIVE AND QUANTITATIVE COMPOSITION

OVYSMEN are tablets for oral administration.

Each tablet contains norethisterone PhEur 0.5 mg and ethinylestradiol PhEur 0.035 mg.

3. PHARMACEUTICAL FORM

Tablet.

4. CLINICAL PARTICULARS

4.1 Therapeutic indications

Contraception and the recognised indications for such oestrogen/progestogen combinations.

4.2 Posology and method of administration

For Oral Administration

Adults

It is preferable that tablet intake from the first pack is started on the first day of menstruation in which case no extra contraceptive precautions are necessary.

If menstruation has already begun (that is 2, 3 or 4 days previously), tablet taking should commence on day 5 of the menstrual period. In this case, additional contraceptive precautions must be taken for the first 7 days of tablet taking.

If menstruation began more than 5 days previously then the patient should be advised to wait until her next menstrual period before starting to take OVYSMEN.

How to take OVYSMEN:

One tablet is taken daily at the same time (preferably in the evening) without interruption for 21 days, followed by a break of 7 tablet-free days. Each subsequent pack is started after the 7 tablet-free days have elapsed. Additional contraceptive precautions are not then required.

Elderly:

Not applicable

Children:

Not recommended

4.3 Contraindications

Absolute contra-indications

– Pregnancy or suspected pregnancy (that cannot yet be excluded).

– Circulatory disorders (cardiovascular or cerebrovascular) such as thrombophlebitis and thrombo-embolic processes, or a history of these conditions (including history of confirmed venous thrombo-embolism (VTE), family history of idiopathic VTE and other known risk factors for VTE), moderate to severe hypertension, hyperlipoproteinaemia. In addition the presence of more than one of the risk factors for arterial disease.

– Severe liver disease, cholestatic jaundice or hepatitis (viral or non-viral) or a history of these conditions if the results of liver function tests have failed to return to normal, and for 3 months after liver function tests have been found to be normal; a history of jaundice of pregnancy or jaundice due to the use of steroids, Rotor syndrome and Dubin-Johnson syndrome, hepatic cell tumours and porphyria.

– Cholelithiasis.

– Known or suspected oestrogen-dependent tumours; endometrial hyperplasia; undiagnosed vaginal bleeding.

– Systemic lupus erythematosus or a history of this condition.

– A history during pregnancy or previous use of steroids of:

- severe pruritus
- herpes gestationis
- a manifestation or deterioration of otosclerosis

Relative contra-indications:

If any relative contra-indication listed below is present, the benefits of oestrogen/progestogen-containing preparations must be weighed against the possible risk for each individual case and the patient kept under close supervision. In case of aggravation or appearance of any of these conditions whilst the patient is taking the pill, its use should be discontinued.

– Conditions implicating an increasing risk of developing venous thrombo-embolic complications, e.g. severe varicose veins or prolonged immobilisation or major surgery. Disorders of coagulation.

– Presence of any risk factor for arterial disease e.g. smoking, hyperlipidaemia or hypertension.

– Other conditions associated with an increased risk of circulatory disease such as latent or overt cardiac failure, renal dysfunction, or a history of these conditions.

– Epilepsy or a history of this condition.

– Migraine or a history of this condition.

– A history of cholelithiasis.

– Presence of any risk factor for oestrogen-dependent tumours; oestrogen-sensitive gynaecological disorders such as uterine fibromyomata and endometriosis.

– Diabetes mellitus.

– Severe depression or a history of this condition. If this is accompanied by a disturbance in tryptophan metabolism, administration of vitamin B6 might be of therapeutic value.

– Sickle cell haemoglobinopathy, since under certain circumstances, e.g. during infections or anoxia, oestrogen-containing preparations may induce thrombo-embolic process in patients with this condition.

– If the results of liver function tests become abnormal, use should be discontinued.

4.4 Special warnings and precautions for use

Post partum administration

Following a vaginal delivery, oral contraceptive administration to non-breast-feeding mothers can be started 21 days post-partum provided the patient is fully ambulant and there are no puerperal complications. No additional contraceptive precautions are required. If post-partum administration begins more than 21 days after delivery, additional contraceptive precautions are required for the first 7 days of pill-taking.

If intercourse has taken place post-partum, oral contraceptive use should be delayed until the first day of the first menstrual period.

After miscarriage or abortion, administration should start immediately, in which case no additional contraceptive precautions are required.

Changing from a 21 day pill or 22 day pill to OVYSMEN

All tablets in the old pack should be finished. The first OVYSMEN tablet is taken the next day ie no gap is left between taking tablets nor does the patient need to wait for her period to begin. Tablets should be taken as instructed in 'How to take OVYSMEN' (see 4.2). Additional contraceptive precautions are not required. The patient will not have a period until the end of the first OVYSMEN pack, but this is not harmful, nor does it matter if she experiences some bleeding on tablet-taking days.

Changing from a combined every day pill (28 day tablets) to OVYSMEN

OVYSMEN should be started after taking the last active tablet from the 'Every day Pill' pack (ie after taking 21 or 22 tablets). The first OVYSMEN tablet is taken the next day ie no gap is left between taking tablets nor does the patient need to wait for her period to begin. Tablets should be taken as instructed in 'How to take OVYSMEN' (see 4.2). Additional contraceptive precautions are not required. Remaining tablets from the every day (ED) pack should be discarded.

The patient will not have a period until the end of the first OVYSMEN pack, but this is not harmful, nor does it matter if she experiences some bleeding on tablet-taking days.

Changing from a progestogen-only pill (POP or mini pill) to OVYSMEN

The first OVYSMEN tablet should be taken on the first day of the period, even if the patient has already taken a mini pill on that day. Tablets should be taken as instructed in 'How to take OVYSMEN' (see 4.2). Additional contraceptive precautions are not required. All the remaining progestogen-only pills in the mini pill pack should be discarded.

If the patient is taking a mini pill, then she may not always have a period, especially when she is breast-feeding. The first OVYSMEN tablet should be taken on the day after stopping the mini pill. All remaining pills in the mini pill packet must be discarded. Additional contraceptive precautions must be taken for the first 7 days.

To skip a period

To skip a period, a new pack of OVYSMEN should be started on the day after finishing the current pack (the patient skips the tablet-free days). Tablet-taking should be continued in the usual way.

During the use of the second pack she may experience slight spotting or break- through bleeding but contraceptive protection will not be diminished provided there are no tablet omissions.

The next pack of OVYSMEN is started after the usual 7 tablet-free days, regardless of whether the period has completely finished or not.

Reduced reliability

When OVYSMEN is taken according to the directions for use the occurrence of pregnancy is highly unlikely. However, the reliability of oral contraceptives may be reduced under the following circumstances:

(i) Forgotten tablets

If the patient forgets to take a tablet, she should take it as soon as she remembers and take the next one at the normal time. This may mean that two tablets are taken in one day. Provided she is less than 12 hours late in taking her tablet, OVYSMEN will still give contraceptive protection during this cycle and the rest of the pack should be taken as usual.

If she is more than 12 hours late in taking one or more tablets then she should take the last missed pill as soon as she remembers but leave the other missed pills in the pack. She should continue to take the rest of the pack as usual but must use extra precautions (eg sheath, diaphragm, plus spermicide) and follow the '7-day rule' (see Further Information for the '7-day rule').

If there are 7 or more pills left in the pack after the missed and delayed pills then the usual 7-day break can be left before starting the next pack. If there are less than 7 pills left in the pack after the missed and delayed pills then when the pack is finished the next pack should be started the next day. If withdrawal bleeding does not occur at the end of the second pack then a pregnancy test should be performed.

(ii) Vomiting or diarrhoea

If after tablet intake, vomiting or diarrhoea occurs, a tablet may not be absorbed properly by the body. If the symptoms disappear within 12 hours of tablet-taking, the patient should take an extra tablet from a spare pack and continue with the rest of the pack as usual.

However, if the symptoms continue beyond those 12 hours, additional contraceptive precautions are necessary for any sexual intercourse during the stomach or bowel upset and for the following 7 days (the patient must be advised to follow the '7-day rule').

(iii) Change in bleeding pattern

If after taking OVYSMEN for several months, there is a sudden occurrence of spotting or breakthrough bleeding (not observed in previous cycles) or the absence of withdrawal bleeding, contraceptive effectiveness may be reduced. If withdrawal bleeding fails to occur and none of the above mentioned events has taken place, pregnancy is highly unlikely and oral contraceptive use can be continued until the end of the next pack. (If withdrawal bleeding fails to occur at the end of the second cycle, tablet intake should be discontinued and pregnancy excluded before oral contraceptive use can be resumed.) However, if withdrawal bleeding is absent and any of the above mentioned events has occurred, tablet intake should be discontinued and pregnancy excluded before oral contraceptive use can be resumed.

Medical examination/consultation

Assessment of women prior to starting oral contraceptives (and at regular intervals thereafter) should include a personal and family medical history of each woman. Physical examination should be guided by this and by the contra-indications (Section 4.3) and warnings (Section 4.4) for this product. The frequency and nature of these assessments should be based upon relevant guidelines and should be adapted to the individual woman, but should include measurement of blood pressure and, if judged appropriate by the clinician, breast, abdominal and pelvic examination including cervical cytology.

Caution should be observed when prescribing oral contraceptives to young women whose cycles are not yet stabilised.

Venous thrombo-embolic disease

An increased risk of venous thrombo-embolic disease (VTE) associated with the use of oral contraceptives is well established but is smaller than that associated with pregnancy, which has been estimated at 60 cases per 100,000 pregnancies. Some epidemiological studies have reported a greater risk of VTE for women using combined oral contraceptives containing desogestrel or gestodene (the so-called 'third generation' pills) than for women using pills containing levonorgestrel or norethisterone (the so-called 'second generation' pills).

The spontaneous incidence of VTE in healthy non-pregnant women (not taking any oral contraceptive) is about 5 cases per 100,000 per year. The incidence in users of second generation pills is about 15 per 100,000 women per year of use. The incidence in users of third generation pills is about 25 cases per 100,000 women per year of use; this excess incidence has not been satisfactorily explained by bias or confounding. The level of all of these risks of VTE increases with age and is likely to be further increased in women with other known risk factors for VTE such as obesity. The excess risk of VTE is highest during the first year a woman ever uses a combined oral contraceptive.

Surgery, varicose veins or immobilisation

In patients using oestrogen-containing preparations, the risk of deep vein thrombosis may be temporarily increased when undergoing a major operation (eg abdominal, orthopaedic), and surgery to the legs, medical treatment for varicose veins or prolonged immobilisation. Therefore, it is advisable to discontinue oral contraceptive use at least 4 to 6 weeks prior to these procedures if performed electively and to (re)start not less than 2 weeks after full ambulation. The latter is also valid with regard to immobilisation after an accident or emergency surgery. In case of emergency surgery, thrombotic prophylaxis is usually indicated e.g. with subcutaneous heparin.

Chloasma

Chloasma may occasionally occur, especially in women with a history of chloasma gravidarum. Women with a tendency to chloasma should avoid exposure to the sun or ultraviolet radiation whilst taking this preparation. Chloasma is often not fully reversible.

Laboratory tests

The use of steroids may influence the results of certain laboratory tests. In the literature, at least a hundred different parameters have been reported to possibly be influenced by oral contraceptive use, predominantly by the oestrogenic component. Among these are: biochemical parameters of the liver, thyroid, adrenal and renal function, plasma levels of (carrier) proteins and lipid/lipoprotein fractions and parameters of coagulation and fibrinolysis.

Further information

Additional contraceptive precautions

When additional contraceptive precautions are required, the patient should be advised either not to have sex, or to use a cap plus spermicide or for her partner to use a condom. Rhythm methods should not be advised as the pill disrupts the usual cyclical changes associated with the natural menstrual cycle e.g. changes in temperature and cervical mucus.

The 7-day rule

If any one tablet is forgotten for more than 12 hours.

If the patient has vomiting or diarrhoea for more than 12 hours.

If the patient is taking any of the drugs listed under 'Interactions':

The patient should continue to take her tablets as usual and:

- Additional contraceptive precautions must be taken for the next 7 days.

But - if these 7 days run beyond the end of the current pack, the next pack must be started as soon as the current one is finished, i.e. no gap should be left between packs. (This prevents an extended break in tablet taking which may increase the risk of the ovaries releasing an egg and thus reducing contraceptive protection.) The patient will not have a period until the end of 2 packs but this is not harmful nor does it matter if she experiences some bleeding on tablet taking days.

4.5 Interaction with other medicinal products and other forms of interaction

Irregular cycles and reduced reliability of oral contraceptives may occur when these preparations are used concomitantly with drugs such as anticonvulsants, barbiturates, antibiotics, (eg tetracyclines, ampicillin, rifampicin, etc.), griseofulvin, activated charcoal and certain laxatives. Special consideration should be given to patients being treated with antibiotics for acne. They should be advised to use a non-hormonal method of contraception, or to use an oral contraceptive containing a progestogen showing minimal androgenicity, which have been reported as helping to improve acne without using an antibiotic. Oral contraceptives may diminish glucose tolerance and increase the need for insulin or other antidiabetic drugs in diabetics.

The herbal remedy St John's Wort *(Hypericum perforatum)* should not be taken concomitantly with this medicine as this could potentially lead to a loss of contraceptive effect.

4.6 Pregnancy and lactation

OVYSMEN is contra-indicated for use during pregnancy or suspected pregnancy, since it has been suggested that combined oral contraceptives, in common with many other substances, might be capable of affecting the normal development of the child in the early stages of pregnancy. It can be definitely concluded, however, that, if a risk of abnormality exists at all, it must be very small.

Mothers who are breast-feeding should be advised not to use the combined pill since this may reduce the amount of breast-milk, but may be advised instead to use a progestogen-only pill (POP).

4.7 Effects on ability to drive and use machines

Not applicable.

4.8 Undesirable effects

Various adverse reactions have been associated with oral contraceptive use. The first appearance of symptoms indicative of any one of these reactions necessitates immediate cessation of oral contraceptive use while appropriate diagnostic and therapeutic measures are undertaken.

Serious Adverse Reactions

There is a general opinion, based on statistical evidence, that users of combined oral contraceptives experience more often than non-users various disorders of the coagulation. How often these disorders occur in users of modern low-oestrogen oral contraceptives is unknown, but there are reasons for suggesting that they may occur less often than with the older types of pill which contain more oestrogen.

Various reports have associated oral contraceptive use with the occurrence of deep venous thrombosis, pulmonary embolism and other embolisms. Other investigations of these oral contraceptives have suggested an increased risk of oestrogen and/or progestogen dose-dependent coronary and cerebrovascular accidents, predominantly in heavy smokers. Thrombosis has very rarely been reported to occur in other veins or arteries, e.g. hepatic, mesenteric, renal or retinal.

It should be noted that there is no consensus about often contradictory findings obtained in early studies. The physician should bear in mind the possibility of vascular accidents occurring and that there may not be full recovery from such disorders and they may be fatal. The physician should take into account the presence of risk factors for arterial disease and deep venous thrombosis when prescribing oral contraceptives. Risk factors for arterial disease include smoking, the presence of hyperlipidaemia, hypertension or diabetes.

Signs and symptoms of a thrombotic event may include: sudden severe pain in the chest, whether or not reaching to the left arm; sudden breathlessness; and unusual severe, prolonged headache, especially if it occurs for the first time or gets progressively worse, or is associated with any of the following symptoms: sudden partial or complete loss of vision or diplopia, aphasia, vertigo, a bad fainting attack or collapse with or without focal epilepsy, weakness or very marked numbness suddenly affecting one side or one part of the body, motor disturbances; severe pain in the calf of one leg; acute abdomen.

Cigarette smoking increases the risk of serious cardiovascular adverse reactions to oral contraceptive use. The risk increases with age and with heavy smoking and is more marked in women over 35 years of age. Women who use oral contraceptives should be strongly advised not to smoke.

The use of oestrogen-containing oral contraceptives may promote growth of existing sex steroid dependent tumours. For this reason, the use of these oral contraceptives in patients with such tumours is contra-indicated. Numerous epidemiological studies have been reported on the risk of ovarian, endometrial, cervical and breast cancer in women using combined oral contraceptives. The evidence is clear that combined oral contraceptives offer substantial protection against both ovarian and endometrial cancer. An increased risk of cervical cancer in long term users of combined oral contraceptives has been reported in some studies, but there continues to be controversy about the extent to which this is attributable to the confounding effects of sexual behaviour and other factors.

A meta-analysis from 54 epidemiological studies reported that there is a slightly increased relative risk (RR = 1.24) of having breast cancer diagnosed in women who are currently using combined oral contraceptives (COCs). The observed pattern of increased risk may be due to an earlier diagnosis of breast cancer in COC users, the biological effects of COCs or a combination of both. The additional breast cancers diagnosed in current users of COCs or in women who have used COCs in the last 10 years are more likely to be localised to the breast than those in women who never used COCs.

Breast cancer is rare among women under 40 years of age whether or not they take COCs. Whilst this background risk increases with age, the excess number of breast cancer diagnoses in current and recent COC users is small in relation to the overall risk of breast cancer (see bar chart).

The most important risk factor for breast cancer in COC users is the age women discontinue the COC; the older the age at stopping, the more breast cancers are diagnosed. Duration of use is less important and the excess risk gradually disappears during the course of the 10 years after stopping COC use such that by 10 years there appears to be no excess.

The possible increase in risk of breast cancer should be discussed with the user and weighed against the benefits of COCs taking into account the evidence that they offer

Figure 1

Estimated number of breast cancers found in 10,000 women who took the Pill for 5 years then stopped, or who never took the Pill

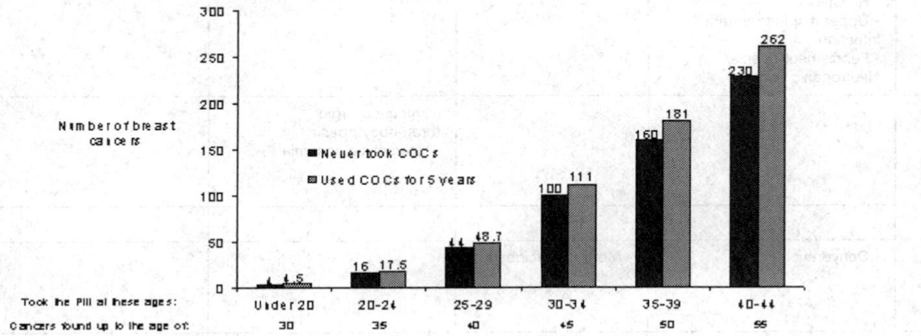

substantial protection against the risk of developing certain other cancers (e.g. ovarian and endometrial cancer).

(see Figure 1 above)

Malignant hepatic tumours have been reported on rare occasions in long-term users of oral contraceptives. Benign hepatic tumours have also been associated with oral contraceptive usage. A hepatic tumour should be considered in the differential diagnosis when upper abdominal pain, enlarged liver or signs of intra-abdominal haemorrhage occur.

The use of oral contraceptives may sometimes lead to the development of cholestatic jaundice or cholelithiasis.

On rare occasions the use of oral contraceptives may trigger or reactivate systemic lupus erythematosus.

A further rare complication of oral contraceptive use is the occurrence of chorea which can be reversed by discontinuing the pill. The majority of cases of oral contraceptive-induced chorea show a pre-existing predisposition which often relates to acute rheumatism.

Other Adverse Reactions

Cardiovascular System

Rise of blood pressure. If hypertension develops, treatment should be discontinued.

Genital Tract

Intermenstrual bleeding, post-medication amenorrhoea, changes in cervical secretion, increase in size of uterine fibromyomata, aggravation of endometriosis, certain vaginal infections, eg candidiasis.

Breast

Tenderness, pain, enlargement, secretion.

Gastro-intestinal Tract

Nausea, vomiting, cholelithiasis, cholestatic jaundice.

Skin

Erythema nodosum, rash, chloasma, erythema multiforme, hirsutism, loss of scalp hair.

Eyes

Discomfort of the cornea if contact lenses are used.

CNS

Headache, migraine, mood changes, depression.

Metabolic

Fluid retention, change in body weight, reduced glucose tolerance.

Other

Changes in libido, leg cramps.

4.9 Overdose

There have been no reports of serious ill-health from overdosage even when a considerable number of tablets have been taken by a small child. In general, it is therefore unnecessary to treat overdosage. However, if overdosage is discovered within two or three hours and is large, then gastric lavage can be safely used. There are no antidotes and further treatment should be symptomatic.

5. PHARMACOLOGICAL PROPERTIES

5.1 Pharmacodynamic properties

OVYSMEN acts through the mechanism of gonadotrophin suppression by the oestrogenic and progestational actions of ethinylestradiol and norethisterone. The primary mechanism of action is inhibition of ovulation, but alterations to the cervical mucus and to the endometrium may also contribute to the efficacy of the product.

5.2 Pharmacokinetic properties

Norethisterone and ethinylestradiol are absorbed from the gastro-intestinal tract and metabolised in the liver. To obtain maximal contraceptive effectiveness the tablets should be taken as directed and at approximately the same time each day.

Because the active ingredients are metabolised in the liver, reduced contraceptive efficacy has been associated with concomitant use of oral contraceptives and rifampicin. A similar association has been suggested with oral contraceptives and barbiturates, phenytoin sodium, phenylbutazone, griseofulvin and ampicillin.

5.3 Preclinical safety data

The toxicology of norethisterone and ethinylestradiol has been extensively investigated in animal studies and through long term clinical experience with widespread use in contraceptives.

6. PHARMACEUTICAL PARTICULARS

6.1 List of excipients

Lactose (anhydrous)

Magnesium stearate

Pregelatinised starch

Methanol (does not appear in final product)

6.2 Incompatibilities

Not applicable.

6.3 Shelf life

Two years.

6.4 Special precautions for storage

Do not store above 30°C.

Protect from light.

6.5 Nature and contents of container

Carton containing 3 PVC/foil blister strips of 21 tablets each.

6.6 Special precautions for disposal and other handling

Not applicable.

7. MARKETING AUTHORISATION HOLDER

Janssen-Cilag Limited

50-100 Holmers Farm Way

High Wycombe

Bucks

HP12 4EG

UK

8. MARKETING AUTHORISATION NUMBER(S)

PL 00242/0253

9. DATE OF FIRST AUTHORISATION/RENEWAL OF THE AUTHORISATION

24 February 2009

10. DATE OF REVISION OF THE TEXT

24 February 2009

Legal category POM

Oxaliplatin 5 mg/ml, powder for solution for infusion (medac UK)

(medac GmbH)

1. NAME OF THE MEDICINAL PRODUCT

Oxaliplatin 5 mg/ml, powder for solution for infusion

2. QUALITATIVE AND QUANTITATIVE COMPOSITION

One ml of reconstituted solution contains 5 mg oxaliplatin.

50mg vial:

each vial contains 50mg of Oxaliplatin for reconstitution in 10ml of solvent.

100mg vial:

each vial contains 100mg of Oxaliplatin for reconstitution in 20ml of solvent.

150mg vial:

each vial contains 150mg of Oxaliplatin for reconstitution in 30ml of solvent.

For a full list of excipients, see section 6.1.

3. PHARMACEUTICAL FORM

Powder for solution for infusion

White powder for solution for infusion.

4. CLINICAL PARTICULARS

4.1 Therapeutic indications

Oxaliplatin in combination with 5-fluorouracil (5-FU) and folinic acid (FA) is indicated for:

- Adjuvant treatment of stage III (Duke's C) colon cancer after complete resection of primary tumor
- Treatment of metastatic colorectal cancer.

4.2 Posology and method of administration

Posology

FOR ADULTS ONLY

The recommended dose for oxaliplatin in adjuvant setting is 85 mg/m^2 intravenously repeated every two weeks for 12 cycles (6 months).

The recommended dose for oxaliplatin in treatment of metastatic colorectal cancer is 85 mg/m^2 intravenously repeated every 2 weeks.

Dosage given should be adjusted according to tolerability (see section 4.4).

Oxaliplatin should always be administered before fluoropyrimidines.

Oxaliplatin is administered as a 2- to 6-hour intravenous infusion in 250 to 500 ml of 5% glucose solution to give a concentration between 0.2 mg/ml and 0.70 mg/ml; 0.70 mg/ml is the highest concentration in clinical practice for an oxaliplatin dose of 85 mg/m^2.

Oxaliplatin was mainly used in combination with continuous infusion 5-fluorouracil based regimens. For the two-weekly treatment schedule 5-fluorouracil regimens combining bolus and continuous infusion were used.

- Special Populations

- Renal impairment:

Oxaliplatin has not been studied in patients with severe renal impairment (see section 4.3).

In patients with moderate renal impairment, treatment may be initiated at the normally recommended dose (see section 4.4). There is no need for dose adjustment in patients with mild renal dysfunction.

- Hepatic impairment:

In a phase I study including patients with several levels of hepatic impairment, frequency and severity of hepato-biliary disorders appeared to be related to progressive disease and impaired liver function tests at baseline. During clinical development no specific dose adjustment for patients with abnormal liver function tests were performed.

- Elderly patients:

No increase in severe toxicities was observed when oxaliplatin was used as a single agent or in combination with 5-fluorouracil in patients over the age of 65. In consequence no specific dose adaptation is required for elderly patients.

Method of administration

Oxaliplatin is administered by intravenous infusion.

The administration of oxaliplatin does not require hyperhydration.

Oxaliplatin diluted in 250 to 500 ml of 5% glucose solution to give a concentration not less than 0.2 mg/ml must be infused via a central venous line or peripheral vein over 2 to 6 hours. Oxaliplatin infusion should always precede that of 5-fluorouracil.

In the event of extravasation, administration must be discontinued immediately.

Instructions for use:

Oxaliplatin must be reconstituted and further diluted before use. Only the recommended diluents should be used to reconstitute and then dilute the freeze-dried product. (See section 6.6).

4.3 Contraindications

Oxaliplatin is contra-indicated in patients who

- have a known history of hypersensitivity to oxaliplatin or to the excipient.
- are breast feeding.
- have myelosuppression prior to starting first course, as evidenced by baseline neutrophils $< 2 \times 10^9$/l and/or platelet count of $< 100 \times 10^9$/l.
- have a peripheral sensory neuropathy with functional impairment prior to first course.
- have a severely impaired renal function (creatinine clearance less than 30 ml/min).

4.4 Special warnings and precautions for use

Oxaliplatin should only be used in specialised departments of oncology and should be administered under the supervision of an experienced oncologist.

For use in pregnant women see section 4.6.

Genotoxic effects were observed with oxaliplatin in the preclinical studies. Therefore male patients treated with oxaliplatin are advised not to father a child during and up to 6 months after treatment and to seek advice on conservation of sperm prior to treatment because oxaliplatin may have an anti-fertility effect which could be irreversible. Women should not become pregnant during treatment with oxaliplatin and should use an effective method of contraception (see section 4.6)

Appropriate contraceptive measures must be taken during and after cessation of therapy during 4 months for women and 6 months for men.

Table 1

MedDRA Organ system classes	Very common	Common	Uncommon	Rare	Very rare
Infections and infestations *	- Infection	- Rhinitis - Upper respiratory tract infection - Febrile neutropenia/ Neutropenic sepsis			
Blood and the lymphatic system disorders*	- Anaemia - Neutropenia - Thrombocytopenia - Leucopenia - Lymphopenia			- Immunoallergic thrombocytopenia - Haemolytic anaemia	
Immune system disorders*	- Allergy/ allergic reaction+				
Metabolism and nutrition disorders	- Anorexia - Glycaemia abnormalities - Hypokalaemia - Natraemia abnormalities	- Dehydration	- Metabolic acidosis		
Psychiatric disorders		- Depression - Insomnia	- Nervousness		
Nervous system disorders*	- Peripheral sensory neuropathy - Sensory disturbance - Dysgeusia - Headache	- Dizziness - Motor neuritis - Meningism		- Dysarthria	
Eye disorders		- Conjunctivitis - Visual disturbance		- Visual acuity reduced transiently - Visual field disturbances	- Optic neuritis
Ear and labyrinth disorders			- Ototoxicity	- Deafness	
Vascular disorders	- Epistaxis	- Haemorrhage - Flushing - Deep vein thrombosis - Pulmonary embolism			
Respiratory, thoracic and mediastinal disorders	- Dyspnoea - Cough	- Hiccups - Chest pain		- Interstitial lung disease - Pulmonary fibrosis**	
Gastrointestinal disorders*	- Nausea - Diarrhoea - Vomiting - Stomatitis/ Mucositis - Abdominal pain - Constipation	- Dyspepsia - Gastroesophageal reflux - Rectal haemorrhage	- Ileus - Intestinal obstruction	- Colitis including clostridium difficile diarrhoea	
Hepatobiliary disorders					Liver sinusoidal obstruction syndrome
Skin and subcutaneous tissue disorders	- Skin disorder - Alopecia	- Skin exfoliation (i.e. Hand & Foot syndrome) - Rash erythematous - Rash - Hyperhidrosis - Nail disorder			
Musculoskeletal, connective tissue and bone disorders	- Back pain	- Arthralgia - Bone pain			
Renal and urinary disorders		- Dysuria - Haematuria - Micturition frequency abnormal			Acute tubulo-interstitial nephropathy leading to acute renal failure
General disorders and administration site conditions	- Fatigue - Fever++ - Asthenia - Pain - Injection site reaction+++				
Investigations	- Hepatic enzyme increase - Blood alkaline phosphatase increase - Blood bilirubin increase - Blood lactate dehydrogenase increase - Weight increase (adjuvant setting)	- Blood creatinine increase - Weight decrease (metastatic setting)			

* See detailed section below

** See section 4.4.

+ Common allergic reactions such as skin rash (particularly urticaria), conjunctivitis, rhinitis.

Common anaphylactic reactions, including bronchospasm, sensation of chest pain, angioedema, hypotension and anaphylactic shock.

++ Very common fever, rigors (tremors), either from infection (with or without febrile neutropenia) or possibly from immunological mechanism.

+++ Injection site reactions including local pain, redness, swelling and thrombosis have been reported. Extravasation may also result in local pain and inflammation which may be severe and lead to complications including necrosis, especially when oxaliplatin is infused through a peripheral vein (see section 4.4).

Due to limited information on safety in patients with moderately impaired renal function, administration should only be considered after suitable appraisal of the benefit/risk for the patient.

In this situation, renal function should be closely monitored and dose adjusted according to toxicity.

Patients with a history of allergic reaction to platinum compounds should be monitored for allergic symptoms. In case of an anaphylactic-like reaction to oxaliplatin, the infusion should be immediately discontinued and appropriate symptomatic treatment initiated. Oxaliplatin rechallenge is contra-indicated.

In case of oxaliplatin extravasation, the infusion must be stopped immediately and usual local symptomatic treatment initiated.

Neurological toxicity of oxaliplatin should be carefully monitored, especially if co-administered with other medications with specific neurological toxicity. A neurological examination should be performed before each administration and periodically thereafter.

For patients who develop acute laryngopharyngeal dysaesthesia (see section 4.8), during or within the hours following the 2-hour infusion, the next oxaliplatin infusion should be administered over 6 hours.

If neurological symptoms (paraesthesia, dysaesthesia) occur, the following recommended oxaliplatin dosage adjustment should be based on the duration and severity of these symptoms:

- If symptoms last longer than seven days and are troublesome, the subsequent oxaliplatin dose should be reduced from 85 to 65 mg/m^2 (metastatic setting) or 75 mg/m^2 (adjuvant setting).

- If paraesthesia without functional impairment persists until the next cycle, the subsequent oxaliplatin dose should be reduced from 85 to 65 mg/m^2 (metastatic setting) or 75 mg/m^2 (adjuvant setting).

- If paraesthesia with functional impairment persists until the next cycle, oxaliplatin should be discontinued.

- If these symptoms improve following discontinuation of oxaliplatin therapy, resumption of therapy may be considered.

Patients should be informed of the possibility of persistent symptoms of peripheral sensory neuropathy after the end of the treatment. Localised moderate paraesthesias or paraesthesias that may interfere with functional activities can persist after up to 3 years following treatment cessation in the adjuvant setting.

Gastrointestinal toxicity, which manifests as nausea and vomiting, warrants prophylactic and/or therapeutic anti-emetic therapy (see section 4.8).

Dehydration, paralytic ileus, intestinal obstruction, hypokalemia, metabolic acidosis and renal impairment may be caused by severe diarrhoea/emesis particularly when combining oxaliplatin with 5-fluorouracil.

If haematological toxicity occurs (neutrophils $< 1.5 \times 10^9$/l or platelets $< 50 \times 10^9$/l), administration of the next course of therapy should be postponed until haematological values return to acceptable levels. A full blood count with white cell differential should be performed prior to start of therapy and before each subsequent course.

Patients must be adequately informed of the risk of diarrhoea/emesis, mucositis/stomatitis and neutropenia after oxaliplatin and 5-fluorouracil administration so that they can urgently contact their treating physician for appropriate management.

If mucositis/stomatitis occurs with or without neutropenia, the next treatment should be delayed until recovery from mucositis/stomatitis to grade 1 or less and/or until the neutrophil count is $\geqslant 1.5 \times 10^9$/l.

For oxaliplatin combined with 5-fluorouracil (with or without folinic acid), the usual dose adjustments for 5-fluorouracil associated toxicities should apply.

If grade 4 diarrhoea (WHO), grade 3-4 neutropenia (neutrophils $< 1.0 \times 10^9$/l), grade 3-4 thrombo-cytopenia (platelets $< 50 \times 10^9$/l) occur, the dose of oxaliplatin should be reduced from 85 mg/m^2 to 65 mg/m^2 (metastatic setting) or 75 mg/m^2 (adjuvant setting), in addition to any 5-fluorouracil dose reductions required.

In case of abnormal liver function test results or portal hypertension which does not obviously result from liver metastases, very rare cases of drug-induced hepatic vascular disorders should be considered.

In the case of unexplained respiratory symptoms such as non-productive cough, dyspnoea, crackles or radiological pulmonary infiltrates, oxaliplatin should be discontinued until further pulmonary investigations exclude an interstitial lung disease or pulmonary fibrosis (see section 4.8).

4.5 Interaction with other medicinal products and other forms of interaction

In patients who have received a single dose of 85 mg/m^2 of oxaliplatin, immediately before administration of 5-fluorouracil, no change in the level of exposure to 5-fluorouracil has been observed.

In vitro, no significant displacement of oxaliplatin binding to plasma proteins has been observed with the following agents: erythromycin, salicylates, granisetron, paclitaxel, and sodium valproate.

4.6 Pregnancy and lactation

To date there is no available information on safety of use in pregnant women. In animal studies, reproductive toxicity was observed. Consequently, oxaliplatin is not recommended during pregnancy and in women of childbearing potential not using contraceptive measures. The use of oxaliplatin should only be considered after suitably appraising the patient of the risk to the foetus and with the patient's consent.

Appropriate contraceptive measures must be taken during and after cessation of therapy during 4 months for women and 6 months for men.

Excretion in breast milk has not been studied. Breast-feeding is contra-indicated during oxaliplatin therapy.

Oxaliplatin may have an anti-fertility effect (see section 4.4).

4.7 Effects on ability to drive and use machines

No studies on the effects on the ability to drive and use machines have been performed. However oxaliplatin treatment resulting in an increase risk of dizziness, nausea and vomiting, and other neurologic symptoms that affect gait and balance may lead to a minor or moderate influence on the ability to drive and use machines.

4.8 Undesirable effects

The most frequent adverse events of oxaliplatin in combination with 5-fluorouracil/folinic acid (5-FU/FA) were gastrointestinal (diarrhea, nausea, vomiting and mucositis), haematological (neutropenia, thrombocytopenia) and neurological (acute and dose cumulative peripheral sensory neurophathy). Overall, these adverse events were more frequent and severe with oxaliplatin and 5-FU/FA combination than with 5-FU/FA alone.

The frequencies reported in the table below are derived from clinical trials in the metastatic and adjuvant settings (having included 416 and 1108 patients respectively in the FOLFOX arm) and from post marketing experience.

Frequencies in this table are defined using the following convention: very common ($\geqslant$ 1/10) common ($\geqslant$ 1/100 to $<$ 1/10), uncommon ($\geqslant$ 1/1,000 to $<$ 1/100), rare ($\geqslant$ 1/10,000 to $<$ 1/1,000), very rare ($<$ 1/10,000), not known (cannot be estimated from the available data).

(see Table 1 on previous page)

<u>*Haematological toxicity*</u>

Table 2: Incidence by patient (%), by grade

(see Table 2 below)

<u>*Digestive toxicity*</u>

Table 3: Incidence by patient (%), by grade

(see Table 3 below)

Prophylaxis and/or treatment with potent antiemetic agents is indicated.

Dehydration, paralytic ileus, intestinal obstruction, hypokalemia, metabolic acidosis and renal impairment may be caused by severe diarrhoea/emesis particularly when combining oxaliplatin with 5-fluorouracil (see section 4.4).

In single cases pancreatitis is reported.

<u>*Nervous system:*</u>

The dose limiting toxicity of oxaliplatin is neurological. It involves a sensory peripheral neuropathy characterised by dysaesthesia and/or paraesthesia of the extremities with or without cramps, often triggered by the cold. These symptoms occur in up to 95 % of patients treated. The duration of these symptoms, which usually regress between courses of treatment, increases with the number of treatment cycles.

The onset of pain and/or a functional disorder are indications, depending on the duration of the symptoms, for dose adjustment, or even treatment discontinuation (see section 4.4).

This functional disorder includes difficulties in executing delicate movements and is a possible consequence of sensory impairment. The risk of occurrence of persistent symptoms for a cumulative dose of 850 mg/m^2 (10 cycles) is approximately 10 % and 20 % for a cumulative dose of 1020 mg/m^2 (12 cycles).

In the majority of the cases, the neurological signs and symptoms improve or totally recover when treatment is discontinued. In the adjuvant setting of colon cancer, 6 months after treatment cessation, 87 % of patients had no or mild symptoms. After up to 3 years of follow up, about 3 % of patients presented either with persisting localised paresthesias of moderate intensity (2.3 %) or with paraesthesias that may interfere with functional activities (0.5 %).

Acute neurosensory manifestations (see section 5.3) have been reported. They start within hours of administration and often occur on exposure to cold. They usually present as transient paraesthesia, dysaesthesia and hypoesthesia. An acute syndrome of pharyngolaryngeal dysaesthesia occurs in 1% - 2% of patients and is characterised by subjective sensations of dysphagia or dyspnoea/feeling of suffocation, without any objective evidence of respiratory distress (no cyanosis or hypoxia) or of laryngospasm or bronchospasm (no stridor or wheezing). Although antihistamines and bronchodilators have been administered in such cases, the symptoms are rapidly reversible even in the absence of treatment. Prolongation of the infusion helps to reduce the incidence of this syndrome (see section 4.4).

Occasionally other symptoms that have been observed include jaw spasm/muscle spasms/muscle contractions-involuntary/muscle twitching/myoclonus, coordination abnormal/gait abnormal/ ataxia/ balance disorders, throat or chest tightness/ pressure/ discomfort/pain. In addition, cranial nerve dysfunctions may be associated, or also occur as an isolated event such as ptosis, diplopia, aphonia/ dysphonia/ hoarseness, sometimes described as vocal cord paralysis, abnormal tongue sensation or dysarthria, sometimes described as aphasia, trigeminal neuralgia/ facial pain/ eye pain, decrease in visual acuity, visual field disorders.

Other neurological symptoms such as dysarthria, loss of deep tendon reflex and Lhermitte's sign were reported during treatment with oxaliplatin. Isolated cases of optic neuritis have been reported.

<u>*Allergic reactions:*</u>

Table 4: Incidence by patient (%), by grade

(see Table 4 on next page)

<u>*Hepatobiliary disorders*</u>

Liver sinusoidal obstruction syndrome, also known as veno-occlusive disease of liver, or pathological manifestations related to such liver disorder, including peliosis hepatis, nodular regenerative hyperplasia, perisinusoidal fibrosis. Clinical manifestations may be portal hypertension and/or increased transaminases.

4.9 Overdose

There is no known antidote to oxaliplatin. In cases of overdose, exacerbation of adverse events can be expected. Monitoring of haematological parameters should be initiated and symptomatic treatment given.

5. PHARMACOLOGICAL PROPERTIES

5.1 Pharmacodynamic properties

CYTOSTATIC AGENT

Pharmacotherapeutic group: other antineoplastic agents, platinum compounds ATC code: L01XA 03

Oxaliplatin is an antineoplastic drug belonging to a new class of platinum-based compounds in which the platinum atom is complexed with 1,2-diaminocyclohexane ("DACH") and an oxalate group.

Oxaliplatin is a single enantiomer, the Cis-[oxalato(trans-l-1,2- DACH)platinum].

Oxaliplatin exhibits a wide spectrum of both *in vitro* cytotoxicity and *in vivo* antitumour activity in a variety of tumour model systems including human colorectal cancer models. Oxaliplatin also demonstrates *in vitro* and *in vivo* activity in various cisplatin resistant models.

A synergistic cytotoxic action has been observed in combination with 5-fluorouracil both *in vitro* and *in vivo*.

Studies on the mechanism of action of oxaliplatin, although not completely elucidated, show that the aqua-derivatives resulting from the biotransformation of oxaliplatin, interact with DNA to form both inter and intra-strand cross-links, resulting in the disruption of DNA synthesis leading to cytotoxic and antitumour effects.

In patients with metastatic colorectal cancer, the efficacy of oxaliplatin (85mg/m^2 repeated every two weeks) combined with 5-fluorouracil/folinic acid (5-FU/FA) is reported in three clinical studies:

- In front-line treatment, the 2-arm comparative phase III EFC2962 study randomised 420 patients either to 5-FU/FA alone (LV5FU2, N=210) or the combination of oxaliplatin with 5-FU/FA (FOLFOX4, N=210).

- In pretreated patients, the comparative three arms phase III study EFC4584 randomised 821 patients refractory to an irinotecan (CPT-11) + 5-FU/FA combination either to 5-FU/

Table 2 Incidence by patient (%), by grade

Oxaliplatin and 5-FU/FA 85 mg/m^2 every 2 weeks	Metastatic Setting			Adjuvant Setting		
	All grades	Gr 3	Gr 4	All grades	Gr 3	Gr 4
Anemia	82.2	3	< 1	75.6	0.7	0.1
Neutropenia	71.4	28	14	78.9	28.8	12.3
Thrombocytopenia	71.6	4	< 1	77.4	1.5	0.2
Febrile neutropenia	5.0	3.6	1.4	0.7	0.7	0.0
Neutropenic sepsis	1.1	0.7	0.4	1.1	0.6	0.4

Table 3 Incidence by patient (%), by grade

Oxaliplatin and 5-FU/FA 85 mg/m^2 every 2 weeks	Metastatic Setting			Adjuvant Setting		
	All grades	Gr 3	Gr 4	All grades	Gr 3	Gr 4
Nausea	69.9	8	< 1	73.7	4.8	0.3
Diarrhoea	60.8	9	2	56.3	8.3	2.5
Vomiting	49.0	6	1	47.2	5.3	0.5
Mucositis / Stomatitis	39.9	4	< 1	42.1	2.8	0.1

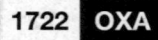

Table 4 Incidence by patient (%), by grade

Oxaliplatin and 5-FU/FA 85 mg/m² every 2 weeks	Metastatic Setting			Adjuvant Setting		
	All grades	Gr 3	Gr 4	All grades	Gr 3	Gr 4
Allergic reactions / Allergy	9.1	1	< 1	10.3	2.3	0.6

Table 5 Response rate under FOLFOX4 versus LV5FU2

Response rate, % (95% CI) independent radiological review ITT analysis	LV5FU2	FOLFOX4	Oxaliplatin Single agent
Front-line treatment EFC2962	22 (16-27)	49 (42-46)	NA*
Response assessment every 8 weeks	P value = 0.0001		
Pretreated patients EFC4584	0.7 (0.0-2.7)	11.1 (7.6-15.5)	1.1 (0.2-3.2)
(refractory to CPT-11 + 5-FU/FA) *Response assessment every 6 weeks*	P value < 0.0001		
Pretreated patients EFC2964 (refractory to 5-FU/FA) *Response assessment every 12 weeks*	NA*	23 (13-36)	NA*

* NA: Not applicable.

Table 6 Median Progression Free Survival (PFS) / Median Time to Progression (TTP) FOLFOX4 versus LV5FU2

Median PFS/TTP, Months (95% CI) independent radiological review ITT analysis	LV5FU2	FOLFOX4	Oxaliplatin Single agent
Front-line treatment EFC2962 (PFS)	6.0 (5.5-6.5)	8.2 (7.2-8.8)	NA*
	Log-rank P value = 0.0003		
Pretreated patients EFC4584 (TTP) (refractory to CPT-11 + 5-FU/FA)	2.6 (1.8-2.9)	5.3 (4.7-6.1)	2.1 (1.6-2.7)
	Log-rank P value < 0.0001		
Pretreated patients EFC2964 (refractory to 5-FU/FA)	NA*	5.1 (3.1-5.7)	NA*

NA: Not applicable.

Table 7 Median Overall Survival (OS) under FOLFOX4 versus LV5FU2

Median OS, months (95% CI) ITT analysis	LV5FU2	FOLFOX4	Oxaliplatin Single agent
Front-line treatment EFC2962	14.7 (13.0-18.2)	16.2 (14.7-18.2)	NA*
	Log-rank P value = 0.12		
Pretreated patients EFC4584 (TTP) (refractory to CPT-11 + 5-FU/FA)	8.8 (7.3-9.3)	9.9 (9.1-10.5)	8.1 (7.2-8.7)
	Log-rank P value = 0.09		
Pretreated patients EFC2964 (refractory to 5-FU/FA)	NA*	10.8 (9.3-12.8)	NA*

* NA: Not applicable.

FA alone (LV5FU2, N=275), oxaliplatin single agent (N=275), or combination of oxaliplatin with 5-FU/FA (FOLFOX4, N=271).

- Finally, the uncontrolled phase II EFC2964 study included patients refractory to 5-FU/FA alone, that were treated with the oxaliplatin and 5-FU/FA combination (FOLFOX4, N=57)

The two randomised clinical trials, EFC2962 in front-line therapy and EFC4584 in pretreated patients, demonstrated a significantly higher response rate and a prolonged progression free survival (PFS)/time to progression (TTP) as compared to treatment with 5-FU/FA alone. In EFC4584 performed in refractory pretreated patients, the difference in median overall survival (OS) between the combination of oxaliplatin and 5-FU/FA did not reach statistical significance.

Table 5: Response rate under FOLFOX4 versus LV5FU2

(see Table 5 above)

Table 6: Median Progression Free Survival (PFS) / Median Time to Progression (TTP) FOLFOX4 versus LV5FU2

(see Table 6 above)

Table 7: Median Overall Survival (OS) under FOLFOX4 versus LV5FU2

(see Table 7 above)

In pretreated patients (EFC4584), who were symptomatic at baseline, a higher proportion of those treated with oxaliplatin and 5-FU/FA experienced a significant improvement of their disease-related symptoms compared to those treated with 5-FU/FA alone (27.7 % vs 14.6 % p = 0.0033).

In non-pretreated patients (EFC2962), no statistically significant difference between the two treatment groups was found for any of the quality of life dimensions. However, the quality of life scores were generally better in the control arm for measurement of global health status and pain and worse in the oxaliplatin arm for nausea and vomiting.

In the adjuvant setting, the MOSAÏC comparative phase III study (EFC3313) randomised 2246 patients (899 stage II/Duke's B2 and 1347 stage III/Duke's C) further to complete resection of the primary tumour of colon cancer either to 5-FU/FA alone (LV5FU2, N=1123 (B2/C=448/675)) or to combination of oxaliplatin and 5-FU/FA (FOLFOX4, N=1123 (B2/C=451/672)).

Table 8: EFC 3313 3-year disease free survival (ITT analysis)*

Treatment arm	LV5FU2	FOLFOX4
Percent 3-year disease free survival (95% CI)	73.3 (70.6-75.6)	78.7 (76.2-81.1)
Hazard ratio (95% CI)	0.76 (0.64-0.89)	
Stratified log rank test	P = 0.0008	

* median follow up 44.2 months (all patients followed for at least 3 years)

The study demonstrated an overall significant advantage in 3-year disease free survival for the oxaliplatin and 5-FU/FA combination (FOLFOX4) over 5-FU/FA alone (LV5FU2).

Table 9: EFC 3313 3-year Disease Free Survival (ITT analysis)* according to Stage of Disease

(see Table 9 on next page)

Overall Survival (ITT analysis):

At time of the analysis of the 3-year disease free survival, which was the primary endpoint of the MOSAIC trial, 85.1 % of the patients were still alive in the FOLFOX4 arm versus 83.8 % in the LV5FU2 arm. This translated into an overall reduction in mortality risk of 10 % in favour of FOLFOX4 not reaching statistical significance (hazard ratio = 0.90). The figures were 92.2 % versus 92.4 % in the stage II (Duke's B2) sub-population (hazard ratio = 1.01) and 80.4 % versus 78.1 % in the stage III (Duke's C) sub-population (hazard ratio = 0.87), for FOLFOX4 and LV5FU2, respectively.

5.2 Pharmacokinetic properties

The pharmacokinetics of individual active compounds have not been determined. The pharmacokinetics of ultrafiltrable platinum, representing a mixture of all unbound, active and inactive platinum species, following a two-hour infusion of oxaliplatin at 130 mg/m² every three weeks for 1 to 5 cycles and oxaliplatin at 85 mg/m² every two weeks for 1 to 3 cycles are as follows:

Table 10: Summary of Platinum Pharmacokinetic Parameter Estimates in Ultrafiltrate Following Multiple Doses of Oxaliplatin at 85 mg/m² Every Two Weeks or at 130 mg/m² Every Three Weeks

(see Table 10 on next page)

At the end of a 2-hour infusion, 15 % of the administered platinum is present in the systemic circulation, the remaining 85 % being rapidly distributed into tissues or eliminated in the urine. Irreversible binding to red blood cells and plasma, results in half-lives in these matrices that are close to the natural turnover of red blood cells and serum albumin. No accumulation was observed in plasma ultrafiltrate following 85 mg/m² every two weeks or 130 mg/m² every three weeks and steady state was attained by cycle one in this matrix. Inter- and intra-subject variability is generally low.

Biotransformation *in vitro* is considered to be the result of non-enzymatic degradation and there is no evidence of cytochrome P450-mediated metabolism of the diaminocyclohexane (DACH) ring.

Oxaliplatin undergoes extensive biotransformation in patients, and no intact drug was detectable in plasma ultrafiltrate at the end of a 2h-infusion. Several cytotoxic biotransformation products including the monochloro-, dichloro- and diaquo-DACH platinum species have been identified in the systemic circulation together with a number of inactive conjugates at later time points.

Platinum is predominantly excreted in urine, with clearance mainly in the 48 hours following administration.

By day 5, approximately 54 % of the total dose was recovered in the urine and < 3 % in the faeces.

A significant decrease in clearance from 17.6 ± 2.18 l/h to 9.95 ± 1.91 l/h in renal impairment was observed together with a statistically significant decrease in distribution volume from 330 ± 40.9 to 241 ± 36.1 l. The effect of severe renal impairment on platinum clearance has not been evaluated.

5.3 Preclinical safety data

The target organs identified in preclinical species (mice, rats, dogs, and/or monkeys) in single- and multiple-dose studies included the bone marrow, the gastrointestinal system, the kidney, the testes, the nervous system, and the heart. The target organ toxicities observed in animals are consistent with those produced by other platinum-containing drugs and DNA-damaging, cytotoxic drugs used in the treatment of human cancers with the exception of the effects produced on the heart. Effects on the heart were observed only in the dog and included electrophysiological disturbances with lethal ventricular fibrillation.

Table 9 EFC 3313 3-year Disease Free Survival (ITT analysis)* according to Stage of Disease

Patient stage	Stage II (Duke's B2)		Stage III (Duke's C)	
Treatment arm	LV5FU2	FOLFOX4	LV5FU2	FOLFOX4
Percent 3-year disease free survival (95% CI)	84.3 (80.9-87.7)	87.4 (84.3-90.5)	65.8 (62.1-69.5)	72.8 (69.4-76.2)
Hazard ratio (95% CI)	0.79 (0.57-1.09)		0.75 (0.62-0.90)	
Stratified log rank test	P = 0.151		P = 0.002	

* median follow up 44.2 months (all patients followed for at least 3 years)

Table 10 Summary of Platinum Pharmacokinetic Parameter Estimates in Ultrafiltrate Following Multiple Doses of Oxaliplatin at 85 mg/m² Every Two Weeks or at 130 mg/m² Every Three Weeks

Dose	C_{max}	AUC_{0-48}	AUC	$t_{1/2\alpha}$	$t_{1/2\beta}$	$t_{1/2\gamma}$	V_{ss}	CL
	μg/ml	μg * h /ml	μg * h /ml	h	h	h	l	l / h
85 mg/m² Mean	0.814	4.19	4.68	0.43	16.8	391	440	17.4
SD	0.193	0.647	1.40	0.35	5.74	406	199	6.35
130 mg/m² Mean	1.21	8.20	11.9	0.28	16.3	273	582	10.1
SD	0.10	2.40	4.60	0.06	2.90	19.0	261	3.07

Mean AUC_{0-48} and C_{max} values were determined on Cycle 3 (85 mg/m²) or cycle 5 (130 mg/m²).
Mean AUC, Vss, CL, and CL_{R0-48} values were determined on Cycle 1.
C_{end}, C_{max}, AUC, AUC_{0-48}, V_{ss} and CL values were determined by non-compartmental analysis.
$t_{1/2\alpha}$, $t_{1/2\beta}$, $t_{1/2\gamma}$ were determined by compartmental analysis (Cycles 1-3 combined).

Cardiotoxicity is considered specific to the dog not only because it was observed in the dog alone but also because doses similar to those producing lethal cardiotoxicity in dogs (150 mg/m²) were well-tolerated by humans. Preclinical studies using rat sensory neurons suggest that the acute neurosensory symptoms related to Oxaliplatin may involve an interaction with voltage-gated Na+ channels.

Oxaliplatin was mutagenic and clastogenic in mammalian test systems and produced embryo-fetal toxicity in rats. Oxaliplatin is considered a probable carcinogen, although carcinogenic studies have not been conducted.

6. PHARMACEUTICAL PARTICULARS

6.1 List of excipients

Lactose monohydrate.

6.2 Incompatibilities

The diluted medicinal product should not be mixed with other medications in the same infusion bag or infusion line. Under instructions for use described in section 6.6, oxaliplatin can be co-administered with folinic acid via a Y-line.

- DO NOT use in association with alkaline drugs or solutions, in particular 5-fluorouracil, basic solutions, trometamol and folinic acid products containing trometamol as an excipient and trometamol salts of other drugs. Alkaline drugs or solutions will adversely affect the stability of oxaliplatin (see section 6.6).

- DO NOT reconstitute or dilute oxaliplatin with saline or other solutions containing chloride ions (including calcium, potassium or sodium chlorides).

- DO NOT mix with other drugs in the same infusion bag or infusion line (see section 6.6 for instructions concerning simultaneous administration with folinic acid).

- DO NOT use injection equipment containing aluminium.

6.3 Shelf life

Medicinal product as packaged for sale:

2 years

Reconstituted concentrate solution in the original vial:

From a microbiological and chemical point of view, the reconstituted concentrate solution should be diluted immediately.

Solution for infusion after dilution:

Chemical and physical in-use stability has been demonstrated for 24 hours at 2°C to 8°C.

From a microbiological point of view, the infusion preparation should be used immediately.

If not used immediately, in-use storage times and conditions prior to use are the responsibility of the user and would normally not be longer than 24 hours at 2°C to 8°C.

6.4 Special precautions for storage

Medicinal product as packaged for sale: This medicinal product does not require any special storage conditions. Do not freeze.

For storage conditions of the reconstituted medicinal product, see section 6.3.

Reconstituted concentrate solution: should be diluted immediately.

Solution for infusion after dilution: store at 2°C to 8°C for not longer than 24 hours.

Inspect visually prior to use. Only clear solutions without particles should be used.

The medicinal product is for single use only. Any unused solution should be discarded.

6.5 Nature and contents of container

Clear glass vial (type I) with chlorobutyl rubber stopper.

Pack sizes: 1 vial containing 50 mg, 100 mg and 150 mg of oxaliplatin.

Not all pack sizes may be marketed.

6.6 Special precautions for disposal and other handling

As with other potentially toxic compounds, caution should be exercised when handling and preparing oxaliplatin solutions.

Instructions for Handling

The handling of this cytotoxic agent by nursing or medical personnel requires every precaution to guarantee the protection of the handler and his surroundings.

The preparation of injectable solutions of cytotoxic agents must be carried out by trained specialist personnel with knowledge of the medicines used, in conditions that guarantee the integrity of the product, the protection of the environment and in particular the protection of the personnel handling the medicines, in accordance with the hospital policy. It requires a preparation area reserved for this purpose. It is forbidden to smoke, eat or drink in this area.

Personnel must be provided with appropriate handling materials, notably long sleeved gowns, protection masks, caps, protective goggles, sterile single-use gloves, protective covers for the work area, containers and collection bags for waste.

Excreta and vomit must be handled with care.

Pregnant women must be warned to avoid handling cytotoxic agents.

Any broken container must be treated with the same precautions and considered as contaminated waste. Contaminated waste should be incinerated in suitably labelled rigid containers. See below section "Disposal".

If oxaliplatin powder, reconstituted solution or infusion solution, should come into contact with skin, wash immediately and thoroughly with water.

If oxaliplatin powder, reconstituted solution or infusion solution, should come into contact with mucous membranes, wash immediately and thoroughly with water.

Special precautions for administration

- DO NOT use injection material containing aluminium.
- DO NOT administer undiluted.
- Only glucose 5% infusion solution (50 mg/ml) is to be used as a diluent.
- DO NOT reconstitute or dilute for infusion with sodium chloride or chloride containing solutions.
- DO NOT mix with any other medication in the same infusion bag or administer simultaneously by the same infusion line.
- DO NOT mix with alkaline drugs or solutions, in particular 5-fluorouracil, folinic acid preparations containing trometamol as an excipient and trometamol salts of other drugs. Alkaline drugs or solutions will adversely affect the stability of oxaliplatin.

Instruction for use with folinic acid (as calcium folinate or disodium folinate)

Oxaliplatin 85mg/m² IV infusion in 250 to 500 ml of 5% glucose solution (50 mg/ml) is given at the same time as folinic acid IV infusion in 5% glucose solution, over 2 to 6 hours, using a Y-line placed immediately before the site of infusion.

These two drugs should **not** be combined in the same infusion bag. Folinic acid must not contain trometamol as an excipient and must only be diluted using isotonic 5% glucose solution, never in alkaline solutions or sodium chloride or chloride containing solutions.

Instruction for use with 5-fluorouracil

Oxaliplatin should always be administered before fluoropyrimidines – i.e. 5-fluorouracil.

After oxaliplatin administration, flush the line and then administer 5-fluorouracil.

For additional information on drugs combined with oxaliplatin, see the corresponding manufacturer's summary of product characteristics.

Reconstitution of the powder

- Water for injections or 5 % glucose solution should be used to reconstitute the solution.
- For a vial of 50 mg: add 10 ml of solvent to obtain a concentration of 5 mg oxaliplatin/ml.
- For a vial of 100 mg: add 20 ml of solvent to obtain a concentration of 5 mg oxaliplatin/ml.
- For a vial of 150 mg: add 30 ml of solvent to obtain a concentration of 5 mg oxaliplatin/ml.

Inspect visually prior to use. Only clear solutions without particles should be used.

The medicinal product is for single use only. Any unused solution should be discarded.

Dilution before infusion

Withdraw the required amount of reconstituted concentrate solution from the vial(s) and then dilute with 250 ml to 500 ml of a 5 % glucose solution to give an oxaliplatin concentration not less than 0.2 mg/ml and 0.7 mg/ml, concentration range for which the physico-chemical stability of oxaliplatin has been demonstrated.

Administer by IV infusion.

After dilution in 5% glucose, chemical and physical in-use stability has been demonstrated for 24 hours at 2°C to 8°C.

From a microbiological point of view, this infusion preparation should be used immediately.

If not used immediately, in-use storage times and conditions prior to use are the responsibility of the user and would normally not be longer than 24 hours at 2°C to 8°C unless dilution has taken place in controlled and validated aseptic conditions.

Inspect visually prior to use. Only clear solutions without particles should be used.

The medicinal product is for single use only. Any unused solution should be discarded.

NEVER use sodium chloride solution for either reconstitution or dilution.

The compatibility of oxaliplatin solution for infusion has been tested with representative, PVC-based, administration sets.

Infusion

The administration of oxaliplatin does not require prehydration. Oxaliplatin diluted in 250 to 500 ml of a 5 % glucose solution to give a concentration not less than 0.2 mg/ml must be infused either by peripheral vein or central venous line over 2 to 6 hours. When oxaliplatin is administered with 5-fluorouracil, the oxaliplatin infusion should precede that of 5-fluorouracil.

Disposal

Remnants of the medicinal product as well as all materials that have been used for reconstitution, for dilution and administration must be destroyed according to hospital standard procedures applicable to cytotoxic agents with due regard to current laws related to the disposal of hazardous waste.

7. MARKETING AUTHORISATION HOLDER

medac
Gesellschaft für klinische
Spezialpräparate mbH
Fehlandtstr. 3
D-20354 Hamburg, Germany

8. MARKETING AUTHORISATION NUMBER(S)

PL 11587/0048

9. DATE OF FIRST AUTHORISATION/RENEWAL OF THE AUTHORISATION

02/08/2007

10. DATE OF REVISION OF THE TEXT

06/01/2009

Oxis Turbohaler 12, inhalation powder

(AstraZeneca UK Limited)

1. NAME OF THE MEDICINAL PRODUCT

Oxis Turbohaler 12, inhalation powder.

2. QUALITATIVE AND QUANTITATIVE COMPOSITION

Each delivered dose (i.e. the dose leaving the mouthpiece) from Oxis Turbohaler 12 contains 9 micrograms formoterol fumarate dihydrate which is derived from a metered dose of 12 micrograms.

Excipient: Lactose monohydrate 450 micrograms per delivered dose (corresponding to 600 micrograms per metered dose).

For a full list of excipients, see section 6.1.

3. PHARMACEUTICAL FORM

Inhalation powder.

White powder.

4. CLINICAL PARTICULARS

4.1 Therapeutic indications

Oxis Turbohaler is indicated as add on therapy to maintenance treatment with inhaled corticosteroids, for the relief of broncho-obstructive symptoms and prevention of exercise-induced symptoms, in patients with asthma when adequate treatment with corticosteroids is not sufficient. Oxis Turbohaler is also indicated for the relief of broncho-obstructive symptoms in patients with chronic obstructive pulmonary disease (COPD).

4.2 Posology and method of administration

Use of doses above those normally required by the individual patient on more than 2 days per week, is a sign of suboptimal disease control and maintenance treatment should be reassessed.

Oxis Turbohaler is not recommended for use in children below 6 years due to insufficient data on safety and efficacy.

Asthma:

In asthma, Oxis Turbohaler can be used once or twice daily ('regular dosage') and as 'relief medication' to relieve acute broncho-obstructive symptoms.

Adults aged > 18 years:

Relief medication: 1 inhalation for the relief of acute broncho-obstructive symptoms.

Regular dosage: 1 inhalation once or twice daily. Some patients may need 2 inhalations once or twice daily.

Prevention of exercise-induced bronchoconstriction: 1 inhalation before exercise.

The daily dose for regular use should not exceed 4 inhalations, however occasionally up to a maximum of 6 inhalations may be allowed within a 24-hour period.

No more than 3 inhalations should be taken on any single occasion.

Children and adolescents 6 years and older:

Relief medication: 1 inhalation for the relief of acute broncho-obstructive symptoms.

Regular dosage: 1 inhalation once or twice daily.

Prevention of exercise-induced bronchoconstriction: 1 inhalation before exercise.

The regular daily dose should not exceed 2 inhalations, however, occasionally up to a maximum of 4 inhalations may be allowed within a 24-hour period. No more than 1 inhalation should be taken on any single occasion.

COPD:

Regular dosage: 1 inhalation once or twice daily.

The daily dose for regular use should not exceed 2 inhalations.

If required, additional inhalations above those prescribed for regular therapy may be used for relief of symptoms, up to a maximum total daily dose of 4 inhalations (regular plus as required). More than 2 inhalations should not be taken on any single occasion.

Special patient groups: There are no special dosing requirements for elderly patients. There are no data available for use of Oxis Turbohaler in patients with hepatic or renal impairment (see also section 5.2).

NB! A lower strength is also available.

Oxis Turbohaler is inspiratory flow driven which means that, when the patient inhales through the mouthpiece, the substance will follow the inspired air into the airways.

Note! It is important to instruct the patient to breathe in forcefully and deeply through the mouthpiece to ensure that an optimal dose is obtained.

It is important to instruct the patient never to chew or bite on the mouthpiece and never to use the inhaler if it has been damaged or if the mouthpiece has become detached.

The patient may not taste or feel any medication when using Oxis Turbohaler due to the small amount of drug dispensed.

Detailed instructions for use are packed together with each inhaler.

4.3 Contraindications

Hypersensitivity to formoterol or to lactose (which contains small amounts of milk proteins).

4.4 Special warnings and precautions for use

Oxis Turbohaler should not be used (and is not sufficient) as the first treatment for asthma.

Asthmatic patients who require therapy with long acting β_2-agonists, should also receive optimal maintenance anti-inflammatory therapy with corticosteroids. Patients must be advised to continue taking their anti-inflammatory therapy after the introduction of Oxis Turbohaler even when symptoms decrease. Should symptoms persist, or treatment with β_2-agonists need to be increased, this indicates a worsening of the underlying condition and warrants a reassessment of the maintenance therapy.

Although Oxis Turbohaler may be introduced as add-on therapy when inhaled corticosteroids do not provide adequate control of asthma symptoms, patients should not be initiated on Oxis Turbohaler during an acute severe asthma exacerbation, or if they have significantly worsening or acutely deteriorating asthma. Serious asthma-related adverse events and exacerbations may occur during treatment with Oxis Turbohaler. Patients should be asked to continue treatment but to seek medical advice if asthma symptoms remain uncontrolled or worsen after initiation on Oxis Turbohaler. Once asthma symptoms are controlled, consideration may be given to gradually reducing the dose of Oxis Turbohaler. Regular review of patients as treatment is stepped down is important. The lowest effective dose of Oxis Turbohaler should be used.

The maximum daily dose should not be exceeded. The long-term safety of regular treatment at higher doses than 36 micrograms per day in adults with asthma, 18 micrograms per day in children with asthma and 18 micrograms per day in patients with COPD, has not been established.

Frequent need of medication (i.e. prophylactic treatment e.g. corticosteroids and long-acting β_2-agonists) for the prevention of exercise-induced bronchoconstriction several times every week, despite an adequate maintenance treatment, can be a sign of suboptimal asthma control, and warrants a reassessment of the asthma therapy and an evaluation of the compliance.

Caution should be observed when treating patients with thyrotoxicosis, phaeochromocytoma, hypertrophic obstructive cardiomyopathy, idiopathic subvalvular aortic stenosis, severe hypertension, aneurysm or other severe cardiovascular disorders, such as ischaemic heart disease, tachyarrhythmias or severe heart failure.

Formoterol may induce prolongation of the QTc-interval. Caution should be observed when treating patients with prolongation of the QTc-interval and in patients treated with drugs affecting the QTc-interval (see 4.5).

Due to the hyperglycaemic effects of β_2-agonists, additional blood glucose monitoring is recommended initially in diabetic patients.

Potentially serious hypokalaemia may result from β_2-agonist therapy. Particular caution is recommended in acute severe asthma as the associated risk may be augmented by hypoxia. The hypokalaemic effect may be potentiated by concomitant treatment with xanthine-derivatives, steroids and diuretics. The serum potassium levels should therefore be monitored.

As with other inhalation therapy, the potential for paradoxical bronchospasm should be considered.

Oxis Turbohaler contains lactose, 450 micrograms per delivered dose (corresponding to 600 micrograms per metered dose). This amount does not normally cause problems in lactose intolerant people. Patients with rare hereditary problems of galactose intolerance, the Lapp lactase deficiency or glucose-galactose malabsorption should not take this medicine.

Children up to the age of 6 years should not be treated with Oxis Turbohaler, as no sufficient experience is available for this group.

4.5 Interaction with other medicinal products and other forms of interaction

No specific interaction studies have been carried out with Oxis Turbohaler.

Concomitant treatment with other sympathomimetic substances such as other β_2-agonists or ephedrine may potentiate the undesirable effects of Oxis Turbohaler and may require titration of the dose.

Concomitant treatment with xanthine derivatives, steroids or diuretics such as thiazides and loop diuretics may potentiate a rare hypokalaemic adverse effect of β_2-agonists. Hypokalaemia may increase the disposition towards arrhythmias in patients who are treated with digitalis glycosides.

There is a theoretical risk that concomitant treatment with other drugs known to prolong the QTc-interval may give rise to a pharmacodynamic interaction with formoterol and increase the possible risk of ventricular arrhythmias. Examples of such drugs include certain antihistamines (e.g. terfenadine, astemizole, mizolastine), certain antiarrhythmics (e.g. quinidine, disopyramide, procainamide), erythromycin and tricyclic antidepressants.

There is an elevated risk of arrhythmias in patients receiving concomitant anaesthesia with halogenated hydrocarbons.

Beta-adrenergic blockers can weaken or inhibit the effect of Oxis Turbohaler. Oxis Turbohaler should therefore not be given together with beta-adrenergic blockers (including eye drops) unless there are compelling reasons.

4.6 Pregnancy and lactation

There are no adequate data from the use of formoterol in pregnant women. In animal studies formoterol has caused implantation losses as well as decreased early postnatal survival and birth weight. The effects appeared at considerably higher systemic exposures than those reached during clinical use of Oxis Turbohaler. Treatment with Oxis Turbohaler may be considered at all stages of pregnancy if needed to obtain asthma control and if the expected benefit to the mother is greater than any possible risk to the foetus. The potential risk for human is unknown.

It is not known whether formoterol passes into human breast milk. In rats, small amounts of formoterol have been detected in maternal milk. Administration of Oxis Turbohaler to women who are breastfeeding should only be considered if the expected benefit to the mother is greater than any possible risk to the child.

4.7 Effects on ability to drive and use machines

Oxis Turbohaler has no influence on the ability to drive and use machines.

4.8 Undesirable effects

The most commonly reported adverse events of β_2-agonist therapy, such as tremor and palpitations, tend to be mild and disappear within a few days of treatment.

Adverse reactions, which have been associated with formoterol are given below, listed by system organ class and frequency. Frequency are defined as: very common ($\geq$1/10), common ($\geq$1/100 and $<$1/10), uncommon ($\geq$1/1 000 and $<$1/100), rare ($\geq$1/10 000 and $<$1/1000) and very rare $<$1/10 000).

Cardiac disorders	Common	Palpitations
	Uncommon	Tachycardia
	Rare	Cardiac arrhythmias, e.g. atrial fibrillation, supraventricular tachycardia, extrasystoles.
	Very rare	Angina pectoris
Gastrointestinal disorders	Rare	Nausea
Immune system disorders	Rare	Hypersensitivity reactions, e.g. bronchospasm, exanthema, urticaria, pruritus
Investigations	Very rare	Prolongation of QTc-interval
Metabolic and nutrition disorders	Rare	Hypokalemia/ Hyperkalemia
	Very rare	Hyperglycemia
Musculoskeletal, connective tissue and bone disorders	Uncommon	Muscle cramps
Nervous system disorders	Common	Headache, tremor
	Very rare	Taste disturbances, dizziness
Psychiatric disorders	Uncommon	Agitation, restlessness, sleep disturbances
Vascular disorders	Very rare	Variations in blood pressure

As with all inhalation therapy, paradoxical bronchospasm may occur in very rare cases.

Treatment with β_2-agonists may result in an increase in blood levels of insulin, free fatty acids, glycerol and ketone bodies.

The excipient lactose contains small amounts of milk proteins. These may cause allergic reactions.

4.9 Overdose

There is limited clinical experience on the management of overdose. An overdose would likely lead to effects that are typical of β_2-agonists: tremor, headache, palpitations. Symptoms reported from isolated cases are tachycardia, hyperglycaemia, hypokalaemia, prolonged QTc-interval, arrhythmia, nausea and vomiting. Supportive and symptomatic treatment is indicated.

Use of cardioselective beta-blockers may be considered, but only subject to extreme caution since the use of β-adrenergic blocker medication may provoke bronchospasm. Serum potassium should be monitored.

5. PHARMACOLOGICAL PROPERTIES

5.1 Pharmacodynamic properties

Pharmacotherapeutic group: selective β_2-agonist, formoterol, ATC code: R03A C13.

Formoterol is a selective β_2-adrenoceptor agonist that produces relaxation of bronchial smooth muscle. Formoterol thus has a bronchodilating effect in patients with reversible airways obstruction. The bronchodilating effect sets in rapidly, within 1-3 minutes after inhalation and has a mean duration of 12 hours after a single dose.

5.2 Pharmacokinetic properties

Absorption

Inhaled formoterol is rapidly absorbed. Peak plasma concentration is reached about 10 minutes after inhalation.

In studies the mean lung deposition of formoterol after inhalation via Turbohaler ranged from 28-49% of the delivered dose (corresponding to 21-37% of the metered dose). The total systemic availability for the higher lung deposition was around 61% of the delivered dose (corresponding to 46% of the metered dose).

Distribution and metabolism

Plasma protein binding is approximately 50%.

Formoterol is metabolised via direct glucuronidation and O-demethylation. The enzyme responsible for O-demethylation has not been identified. Total plasma clearance and volume of distribution has not been determined.

Elimination

The major part of the dose of formoterol is eliminated via metabolism. After inhalation 8-13% of the delivered dose (corresponding to 6-10% of the metered dose) of formoterol is excreted unmetabolised in the urine. About 20% of an intravenous dose is excreted unchanged in the urine. The terminal half-life after inhalation is estimated to be 17 hours.

Special populations:

The effect of decreased liver or kidney function on the pharmacokinetics of formoterol and the pharmacokinetics in the elderly is not known. As formoterol is primarily eliminated via liver metabolism an increased exposure can be expected in patients with severe liver cirrhosis.

5.3 Preclinical safety data

The effects of formoterol seen in toxicity studies in rats and dogs were mainly on the cardiovascular system and consisted of hyperaemia, tachycardia, arrhythmias and myocardial lesions. These effects are known pharmacological manifestations seen after the administration of high doses of β_2-agonists.

A somewhat reduced fertility in male rats was observed at high systemic exposure to formoterol.

No genotoxic effects of formoterol have been observed in in-vitro or in vivo tests. In rats and mice a slight increase in the incidence of benign uterine leiomyomas has been observed. This effect is looked upon as a class-effect observed in rodents after long exposure to high doses of β_2-agonists.

6. PHARMACEUTICAL PARTICULARS

6.1 List of excipients

Lactose monohydrate (which contains milk proteins).

6.2 Incompatibilities

Not applicable.

6.3 Shelf life

2 years.

6.4 Special precautions for storage

Do not store above 30°C. Keep the container/cap tightly closed.

6.5 Nature and contents of container

Oxis Turbohaler is a multidose, inspiratory flow driven, dry powder inhaler. The inhaler is made of plastic parts (PP, PC, HDPE, LDPE, LLDPE, PBT).

Each inhaler contains 60 doses.

Each pack contains either 60 doses (1 inhaler), 3x60 doses (3 inhalers), 10x60 doses (10 inhalers), 18x60 doses (18 inhalers) or 20x60 doses (20 inhalers).

Not all pack-sizes may be marketed.

6.6 Special precautions for disposal and other handling

No special requirements.

Any unused product or waste material should be disposed of in accordance with the local requirements.

7. MARKETING AUTHORISATION HOLDER

AstraZeneca UK Ltd.

600 Capability Green

Luton

Bedfordshire

LU1 3LU

UK

8. MARKETING AUTHORISATION NUMBER(S)

PL17901/0153

9. DATE OF FIRST AUTHORISATION/RENEWAL OF THE AUTHORISATION

10 March 2007

10. DATE OF REVISION OF THE TEXT

10th November 2008

Oxis Turbohaler 6, inhalation powder

(AstraZeneca UK Limited)

1. NAME OF THE MEDICINAL PRODUCT

Oxis Turbohaler 6, inhalation powder.

2. QUALITATIVE AND QUANTITATIVE COMPOSITION

Each delivered dose (i.e. the dose leaving the mouthpiece) from Oxis Turbohaler 6 contains 4.5 micrograms formoterol fumarate dihydrate, which is derived from a metered dose of 6 micrograms.

Excipient: Lactose monohydrate 450 micrograms per delivered dose (corresponding to 600 micrograms per metered dose).

For a full list of excipients, see section 6.1.

3. PHARMACEUTICAL FORM

Inhalation powder.

White powder.

4. CLINICAL PARTICULARS

4.1 Therapeutic indications

Oxis Turbohaler is indicated as add on therapy to maintenance treatment with inhaled corticosteroids, for the relief of broncho-obstructive symptoms and prevention of exercise-induced symptoms, in patients with asthma when adequate treatment with corticosteroids is not sufficient. Oxis Turbohaler is also indicated for the relief of broncho-obstructive symptoms in patients with chronic obstructive pulmonary disease (COPD).

4.2 Posology and method of administration

Use of doses above those normally required by the individual patient on more than 2 days per week, is a sign of suboptimal disease control and maintenance treatment should be reassessed.

Oxis Turbohaler is not recommended for use in children below 6 years due to insufficient data on safety and efficacy.

Asthma:

In asthma, Oxis Turbohaler can be used once or twice daily ('regular dosage') and as 'relief medication' to relieve acute broncho-obstructive symptoms.

Adults aged > 18 years:

Relief medication: 1 or 2 inhalations for the relief of acute broncho-obstructive symptoms.

Regular dosage: 1 or 2 inhalations once or twice daily. Some patients may need 4 inhalations once or twice daily.

Prevention of exercise-induced bronchoconstriction: 2 inhalations before exercise.

The daily dose for regular use should not exceed 8 inhalations, however occasionally up to a maximum of 12 inhalations may be allowed within a 24-hour period.

No more than 6 inhalations should be taken on any single occasion.

Children and adolescents 6 years and older:

Relief medication: 1 or 2 inhalations for the relief of acute broncho-obstructive symptoms.

Regular dosage: 2 inhalations once or twice daily.

Prevention of exercise-induced bronchoconstriction: 1 or 2 inhalations before exercise.

The regular daily dose should not exceed 4 inhalations, however occasionally up to 8 inhalations may be allowed within a 24-hour period. No more than 2 inhalations should be taken on any single occasion.

COPD:

Regular dosage: 2 inhalations once or twice daily.

The daily dose for regular use should not exceed 4 inhalations.

If required, additional inhalations above those prescribed for regular therapy may be used for relief of symptoms, up to a maximum total daily dose of 8 inhalations (regular plus as required). More than 4 inhalations should not be taken on any single occasion.

Special patient groups: There are no special dosing requirements for elderly patients. There are no data available for use of Oxis Turbohaler in patients with hepatic or renal impairment (see also section 5.2).

NB! A higher strength is available as an alternative for patients requiring 2 or more inhalations.

Oxis Turbohaler is inspiratory flow driven which means that, when the patient inhales through the mouthpiece, the substance will follow the inspired air into the airways.

Note! It is important to instruct the patient to breathe in forcefully and deeply through the mouthpiece to ensure that an optimal dose is obtained.

It is important to instruct the patient never to chew or bite on the mouthpiece and never to use the inhaler if it has been damaged or if the mouthpiece has become detached.

The patient may not taste or feel any medication when using Oxis Turbohaler due to the small amount of drug dispensed.

Detailed instructions for use are packed together with each inhaler.

4.3 Contraindications

Hypersensitivity to formoterol or to lactose (which contains small amounts of milk proteins).

4.4 Special warnings and precautions for use

Oxis Turbohaler should not be used (and is not sufficient) as the first treatment for asthma.

Asthmatic patients who require therapy with long acting β_2-agonists, should also receive optimal maintenance anti-inflammatory therapy with corticosteroids. Patients must be advised to continue taking their anti-inflammatory therapy after the introduction of Oxis Turbohaler even when symptoms decrease. Should symptoms persist, or treatment with β_2-agonists need to be increased, this indicates a worsening of the underlying condition and warrants a reassessment of the maintenance therapy.

Although Oxis Turbohaler may be introduced as add-on therapy when inhaled corticosteroids do not provide adequate control of asthma symptoms, patients should not be initiated on Oxis Turbohaler during an acute severe asthma exacerbation, or if they have significantly worsening or acutely deteriorating asthma. Serious asthma-related adverse events and exacerbations may occur during treatment with Oxis Turbohaler. Patients should be asked to continue treatment but to seek medical advice if asthma symptoms remain uncontrolled or worsen after initiation on Oxis Turbohaler. Once asthma symptoms are controlled, consideration may be given to gradually reducing the dose of Oxis Turbohaler. Regular review of patients as treatment is stepped down is important. The lowest effective dose of Oxis Turbohaler should be used.

The maximum daily dose should not be exceeded. The long-term safety of regular treatment at higher doses than 36 micrograms per day in adults with asthma, 18 micrograms per day in children with asthma and 18 micrograms per day in patients with COPD, has not been established.

Frequent need of medication (i.e. prophylactic treatment e.g. corticosteroids and long-acting β_2-agonists) for the prevention of exercise-induced bronchoconstriction several times every week, despite an adequate maintenance treatment, can be a sign of suboptimal asthma control, and warrants a reassessment of the asthma therapy and an evaluation of the compliance.

Caution should be observed when treating patients with thyrotoxicosis, phaeochromocytoma, hypertrophic obstructive cardiomyopathy, idiopathic subvalvular aortic stenosis, severe hypertension, aneurysm or other severe cardiovascular disorders, such as ischaemic heart disease, tachyarrhythmias or severe heart failure.

Formoterol may induce prolongation of the QTc-interval. Caution should be observed when treating patients with prolongation of the QTc-interval and in patients treated with drugs affecting the QTc-interval (see 4.5).

Due to the hyperglycaemic effects of β_2-agonists, additional blood glucose monitoring is recommended initially in diabetic patients.

Potentially serious hypokalaemia may result from β_2-agonist therapy. Particular caution is recommended in acute severe asthma as the associated risk may be augmented by hypoxia. The hypokalaemic effect may be potentiated by concomitant treatment with xanthine-derivatives, steroids and diuretics. The serum potassium levels should therefore be monitored.

As with other inhalation therapy, the potential for paradoxical bronchospasm should be considered.

Oxis Turbohaler contains lactose 450 micrograms per delivered dose (corresponding to 600 micrograms per metered dose). This amount does not normally cause problems in lactose intolerant people. Patients with rare hereditary problems of galactose intolerance, the Lapp lactase deficiency or glucose-galactose malabsorption should not take this medicine.

Children up to the age of 6 years should not be treated with Oxis Turbohaler, as no sufficient experience is available for this group.

4.5 Interaction with other medicinal products and other forms of interaction

No specific interaction studies have been carried out with Oxis Turbohaler.

Concomitant treatment with other sympathomimetic substances such as other β_2-agonists or ephedrine may potentiate the undesirable effects of Oxis Turbohaler and may require titration of the dose.

Concomitant treatment with xanthine derivatives, steroids or diuretics such as thiazides and loop diuretics may potentiate a rare hypokalaemic adverse effect of β_2-agonists. Hypokalaemia may increase the disposition towards arrhythmias in patients who are treated with digitalis glycosides.

There is a theoretical risk that concomitant treatment with other drugs known to prolong the QTc-interval may give rise to a pharmacodynamic interaction with formoterol and increase the possible risk of ventricular arrhythmias. Examples of such drugs include certain antihistamines (e.g. terfenadine, astemizole, mizolastine), certain antiarrhythmics (e.g. quinidine, disopyramide, procainamide), erythromycin and tricyclic antidepressants.

There is an elevated risk of arrhythmias in patients receiving concomitant anaesthesia with halogenated hydrocarbons.

Beta-adrenergic blockers can weaken or inhibit the effect of Oxis Turbohaler. Oxis Turbohaler should therefore not be given together with beta-adrenergic blockers (including eye drops) unless there are compelling reasons.

4.6 Pregnancy and lactation

There are no adequate data from the use of formoterol in pregnant women. In animal studies formoterol has caused implantation losses as well as decreased early postnatal survival and birth weight. The effects appeared at considerably higher systemic exposures than those reached during clinical use of Oxis Turbohaler. Treatment with Oxis Turbohaler may be considered at all stages of pregnancy if needed to obtain asthma control and if the expected benefit to the mother is greater than any possible risk to the foetus. The potential risk for human is unknown.

It is not known whether formoterol passes into human breast milk. In rats, small amounts of formoterol have been detected in maternal milk. Administration of Oxis Turbohaler to women who are breastfeeding should only be considered if the expected benefit to the mother is greater than any possible risk to the child.

4.7 Effects on ability to drive and use machines

Oxis Turbohaler has no influence on the ability to drive and use machines.

4.8 Undesirable effects

The most commonly reported adverse events of β_2-agonist therapy, such as tremor and palpitations, tend to be mild and disappear within a few days of treatment.

Adverse reactions, which have been associated with formoterol are given below, listed by system organ class and frequency. Frequency are defined as: very common ($\geq$1/10), common ($\geq$1/100 and <1/10), uncommon ($\geq$1/1 000 and <1/100), rare ($\geq$1/10 000 and <1/1000) and very rare (<1/10 000).

Cardiac disorders	Common	Palpitations
	Uncommon	Tachycardia
	Rare	Cardiac arrhythmias, e.g. atrial fibrillation, supraventricular tachycardia, extrasystoles.
	Very rare	Angina pectoris
Gastrointestinal disorders	Rare	Nausea
Immune system disorders	Rare	Hypersensitivity reactions, e.g. bronchospasm, exanthema, urticaria, pruritus
Investigations	Very rare	Prolongation of QTc-interval
Metabolic and nutrition disorders	Rare	Hypokalemia/ Hyperkalemia
	Very rare	Hyperglycemia
Musculoskeletal, connective tissue and bone disorders	Uncommon	Muscle cramps
Nervous system disorders	Common	Headache, tremor
	Very rare	Taste disturbances, dizziness
Psychiatric disorders	Uncommon	Agitation, restlessness, sleep disturbances
Vascular disorders	Very rare	Variations in blood pressure

As with all inhalation therapy, paradoxical bronchospasm may occur in very rare cases.

Treatment with β_2-agonists may result in an increase in blood levels of insulin, free fatty acids, glycerol and ketone bodies.

The excipient lactose contains small amounts of milk proteins. These may cause allergic reactions.

4.9 Overdose

There is limited clinical experience on the management of overdose. An overdose would likely lead to effects that are typical of β_2-agonists: tremor, headache, palpitations. Symptoms reported from isolated cases are tachycardia, hyperglycaemia, hypokalaemia, prolonged QTc-interval, arrhythmia, nausea and vomiting. Supportive and symptomatic treatment is indicated.

Use of cardioselective beta-blockers may be considered, but only subject to extreme caution since the use of β-adrenergic blocker medication may provoke bronchospasm. Serum potassium should be monitored.

5. PHARMACOLOGICAL PROPERTIES

5.1 Pharmacodynamic properties

Pharmacotherapeutic group: selective β_2-agonist, formoterol, ATC code: R03A C13.

Formoterol is a selective β_2-adrenoceptor agonist that produces relaxation of bronchial smooth muscle. Formoterol thus has a bronchodilating effect in patients with reversible airways obstruction. The bronchodilating effect sets in rapidly, within 1-3 minutes after inhalation and has a mean duration of 12 hours after a single dose.

5.2 Pharmacokinetic properties

Absorption

Inhaled formoterol is rapidly absorbed. Peak plasma concentration is reached about 10 minutes after inhalation.

In studies the mean lung deposition of formoterol after inhalation via Turbohaler ranged from 28-49% of the delivered dose (corresponding to 21-37% of the metered dose). The total systemic availability for the higher lung deposition was around 61% of the delivered dose (corresponding to 46% of the metered dose).

Distribution and metabolism

Plasma protein binding is approximately 50%.

Formoterol is metabolised via direct glucuronidation and O-demethylation. The enzyme responsible for O-demethylation has not been identified. Total plasma clearance and volume of distribution has not been determined.

Elimination

The major part of the dose of formoterol is eliminated via metabolism. After inhalation 8-13% of the delivered dose (corresponding to 6-10% of the metered dose) of formoterol is excreted unmetabolised in the urine. About 20% of an intravenous dose is excreted unchanged in the urine. The terminal half-life after inhalation is estimated to be 17 hours.

Special populations:

The effect of decreased liver or kidney function on the pharmacokinetics of formoterol and the pharmacokinetics in the elderly is not known. As formoterol is primarily eliminated via liver metabolism an increased exposure can be expected in patients with severe liver cirrhosis.

5.3 Preclinical safety data

The effects of formoterol seen in toxicity studies in rats and dogs were mainly on the cardiovascular system and consisted of hyperaemia, tachycardia, arrhythmias and myocardial lesions. These effects are known pharmacological manifestations seen after the administration of high doses of β_2-agonists.

A somewhat reduced fertility in male rats was observed at high systemic exposure to formoterol.

No genotoxic effects of formoterol have been observed in in-vitro or in vivo tests. In rats and mice a slight increase in the incidence of benign uterine leiomyomas has been observed. This effect is looked upon as a class-effect observed in rodents after long exposure to high doses of β_2-agonists.

6. PHARMACEUTICAL PARTICULARS

6.1 List of excipients

Lactose monohydrate(which contains milk proteins).

6.2 Incompatibilities

Not applicable.

6.3 Shelf life

2 years.

6.4 Special precautions for storage

Do not store above 30°C. Keep the container/cap tightly closed.

6.5 Nature and contents of container

Oxis Turbohaler is a multidose, inspiratory flow driven, dry powder inhaler.

The inhaler is made of plastic parts (PP, PC, HDPE, LDPE, LLDPE, PBT).

Each inhaler contains 60 doses.

Each pack contains either 60 doses (1 inhaler), 3x60doses (3 inhalers), 10x60 doses (10 inhalers), 18x60 doses (18 inhalers), 20x60 doses (20 inhalers).

Not all pack-sizes may be marketed.

6.6 Special precautions for disposal and other handling

No special requirements.

Any unused product or waste material should be disposed of in accordance with the local requirements.

7. MARKETING AUTHORISATION HOLDER

AstraZeneca UK Ltd.

600 Capability Green

Luton

Bedfordshire

LU1 3LU

UK

8. MARKETING AUTHORISATION NUMBER(S)

PL 17901/0154

9. DATE OF FIRST AUTHORISATION/RENEWAL OF THE AUTHORISATION

10 March 2007

10. DATE OF REVISION OF THE TEXT

10th November 2008

OxyContin tablets

(Napp Pharmaceuticals Limited)

1. NAME OF THE MEDICINAL PRODUCT

OxyContin®5 mg, 10 mg, 20 mg, 40 mg, 80 mg film-coated, prolonged release tablets

2. QUALITATIVE AND QUANTITATIVE COMPOSITION

5 mg tablet contains 4.5 mg of oxycodone as 5 mg of oxycodone hydrochloride.

10 mg tablet contains 9.0 mg of oxycodone as 10 mg of oxycodone hydrochloride.

20 mg tablet contains 18.0 mg of oxycodone as 20 mg of oxycodone hydrochloride.

40 mg tablet contains 36.0 mg of oxycodone as 40 mg of oxycodone hydrochloride.

80 mg tablet contains 72.0 mg of oxycodone as 80 mg of oxycodone hydrochloride.

For excipients see section 6.1.

3. PHARMACEUTICAL FORM

Film coated, prolonged release, round, convex tablet.

The 5 mg tablets are light blue, marked OC on one side and 5 on the other.

The 10 mg tablets are white, marked OC on one side and 10 on the other.

The 20 mg tablets are pink, marked OC on one side and 20 on the other.

The 40 mg tablets are yellow, marked OC on one side and 40 on the other.

The 80 mg tablets are green, marked OC on one side and 80 on the other.

4. CLINICAL PARTICULARS

4.1 Therapeutic indications

For the treatment of moderate to severe pain in patients with cancer and post-operative pain.

For the treatment of severe pain requiring the use of a strong opioid.

4.2 Posology and method of administration

OxyContin tablets must be swallowed whole, and not chewed.

Elderly and adults over 18 years:

OxyContin tablets should be taken at 12-hourly intervals. The dosage is dependent on the severity of the pain, and the patient's previous history of analgesic requirements.

OxyContin is not intended for use as a prn analgesic.

Increasing severity of pain will require an increased dosage of ***OxyContin*** tablets using the 5 mg, 10 mg, 20 mg, 40 mg or 80 mg tablet strengths, either alone or in combination, to achieve pain relief. The correct dosage for any individual patient is that which controls the pain and is well tolerated for a full 12 hours. Patients should be titrated to pain relief unless unmanageable adverse drug reactions prevent this. If higher doses are necessary increases should be made, where possible, in 25% - 50% increments. The need for escape medication more than twice a day indicates that the dosage of ***OxyContin*** tablets should be increased.

The usual starting dose for opioid naïve patients or patients presenting with severe pain uncontrolled by weaker opioids is 10 mg, 12-hourly. Some patients may benefit from a starting dose of 5 mg to minimise the incidence of side effects. The dose should then be carefully titrated, as frequently as once a day if necessary, to achieve pain relief. For the majority of patients, the maximum dose is 200 mg 12-hourly. However, a few patients may require higher doses. Doses in excess of 1000 mg have been recorded.

Patients receiving oral morphine before ***OxyContin*** therapy should have their daily dose based on the following ratio: 10 mg of oral oxycodone is equivalent to 20 mg of oral morphine. It must be emphasised that this is a guide to the dose of ***OxyContin*** tablets required. Inter-patient variability requires that each patient is carefully titrated to the appropriate dose.

Controlled pharmacokinetic studies in elderly patients (aged over 65 years) have shown that, compared with younger adults, the clearance of oxycodone is only slightly reduced. No untoward adverse drug reactions were seen based on age, therefore adult doses and dosage intervals are appropriate.

Children under 18 years:

There were no studies in patients below 18 years of age, therefore ***OxyContin*** should not be used in patients under 18 years.

Adults with mild to moderate renal impairment and mild hepatic impairment:

The plasma concentration in this population may be increased. Therefore dose initiation should follow a conservative approach. Patients should be started on ***OxyContin*** 5 mg 12-hourly or ***OxyNorm*** liquid 2.5 mg 6-hourly and titrated to pain relief as described above.

Use in non-malignant pain:

Opioids are not first line therapy for chronic non-malignant pain, nor are they recommended as the only treatment. Types of chronic pain which have been shown to be alleviated by strong opioids include chronic osteoarthritic pain and intervertebral disc disease. The need for continued treatment in non-malignant pain should be assessed at regular intervals.

Cessation of therapy:

When a patient no longer requires therapy with oxycodone, it may be advisable to taper the dose gradually to prevent symptoms of withdrawal.

4.3 Contraindications

Hypersensitivity to any of the constituents, respiratory depression, head injury, paralytic ileus, acute abdomen, delayed gastric emptying, chronic obstructive airways disease, cor pulmonale, chronic bronchial asthma, hypercarbia, known oxycodone sensitivity or in any situation where opioids are contra-indicated, moderate to severe hepatic impairment, severe renal impairment (creatinine clearance <10 ml/min), chronic constipation, concurrent administration of monoamine oxidase inhibitors or within 2 weeks of discontinuation of their use. Not recommended for pre-operative use or for the first 24 hours post-operatively. Patients with rare hereditary problems of galactose intolerance, the Lapp lactase deficiency or glucose-galactose malabsorption should not take this medicine. Pregnancy.

4.4 Special warnings and precautions for use

The major risk of opioid excess is respiratory depression. As with all narcotics, a reduction in dosage may be advisable in hypothyroidism. Use with caution in patients with raised intracranial pressure, hypotension, hypovolaemia, toxic psychosis, diseases of the biliary tract, pancreatitis, inflammatory bowel disorders, prostatic hypertrophy, adrenocortical insufficiency, acute alcoholism, delirium tremens, chronic renal and hepatic disease or severe pulmonary disease, and debilitated, elderly and infirm patients. ***OxyContin*** tablets should not be used where there is a possibility of paralytic ileus occurring. Should paralytic ileus be suspected or occur during use, ***OxyContin*** tablets should be discontinued immediately. As with all opioid preparations, patients about to undergo additional pain relieving procedures (e.g. surgery, plexus blockade) should not receive ***OxyContin*** tablets for 12 hours prior to the intervention. If further treatment with ***OxyContin*** tablets is indicated then the dosage should be adjusted to the new post-operative requirement.

OxyContin 80 mg should not be used in patients not previously exposed to opioids. This tablet strength may cause fatal respiratory depression when administered to opioid naïve patients.

As with all opioid preparations, ***OxyContin*** tablets should be used with caution following abdominal surgery as opioids are known to impair intestinal motility and should not be used until the physician is assured of normal bowel function.

For appropriate patients who suffer with chronic non-malignant pain, opioids should be used as part of a comprehensive treatment programme involving other medications and treatment modalities. A crucial part of the assessment of a patient with chronic non-malignant pain is the patient's addiction and substance abuse history. There is potential for development of psychological dependence (addiction) to opioid analgesics, including oxycodone. ***OxyContin*** tablets, like all opioids, should be used with particular care in patients with a history of alcohol and drug abuse.

If opioid treatment is considered appropriate for the patient, then the main aim of treatment is not to minimise the dose of opioid but rather to achieve a dose which provides adequate pain relief with a minimum of side effects. There must be frequent contact between physician and patient so that dosage adjustments can be made. It is strongly recommended that the physician defines treatment outcomes in accordance with pain management guidelines. The physician and patient can then agree to discontinue treatment if these objectives are not met.

OxyContin has an abuse profile similar to other strong opioids. Oxycodone may be sought and abused by people with latent or manifest addiction disorders.

In-vitro data have demonstrated that the release rate of oxycodone from the ***OxyContin*** formulation is maintained in varying concentrations of ethanol. Therefore, patients already established on an alcohol-resistant prolonged release formulation of oxycodone should not be switched to an alternative alcohol-susceptible formulation of oxycodone. As with all opioids, concomitant administration of alcohol is not recommended due to the increased CNS depressant effects (see also section 4.5 and 5.3).

As with other opioids, infants who are born to dependent mothers may exhibit withdrawal symptoms and may have respiratory depression at birth.

OxyContin tablets must be swallowed whole, and not broken, chewed or crushed. The administration of broken, chewed or crushed ***OxyContin*** tablets leads to a rapid release and absorption of a potentially fatal dose of oxycodone (see Section 4.9). Abuse of the tablets by parenteral administration can be expected to result in other serious adverse events, such as local tissue necrosis, infection, pulmonary granulomas, increased risk of endocarditis, and valvular heart injury, which may be fatal.

4.5 Interaction with other medicinal products and other forms of interaction

OxyContin, like other opioids, potentiates the effects of tranquillisers, anaesthetics, hypnotics, anti-depressants, sedatives, phenothiazines, neuroleptic drugs, alcohol, other opioids, muscle relaxants and antihypertensives. Monoamine oxidase inhibitors are known to interact with narcotic analgesics, producing CNS excitation or depression with hypertensive or hypotensive crisis. Concurrent administration of quinidine, an inhibitor of cytochrome P450-2D6, resulted in an increase in oxycodone C_{max} by 11%, AUC by 13%, and $t_{½}$elim. by 14%. Also an increase in noroxycodone level was observed, (C_{max} by 50%; AUC by 85%, and $t_{½}$elim. by 42%). The pharmacodynamic effects of oxycodone were not altered. This interaction may be observed for other potent inhibitors of cytochrome P450-2D6 enzyme. Cimetidine and inhibitors of cytochrome P450-3A such as ketoconazole and erythromycin may inhibit the metabolism of oxycodone.

4.6 Pregnancy and lactation

OxyContin tablets are not recommended for use in pregnancy nor during labour. Infants born to mothers who have received opioids during pregnancy should be monitored for respiratory depression.

Oxycodone may be secreted in breast milk and may cause respiratory depression in the newborn. ***OxyContin*** tablets should, therefore, not be used in breast-feeding mothers.

4.7 Effects on ability to drive and use machines

Oxycodone may modify patients' reactions to a varying extent depending on the dosage and individual susceptibility. Therefore patients should not drive or operate machinery if affected.

4.8 Undesirable effects

Adverse drug reactions are typical of full opioid agonists. Tolerance and dependence may occur (see *Tolerance and Dependence*, below). Constipation may be prevented with an appropriate laxative. If nausea and vomiting are troublesome, oxycodone may be combined with an anti-emetic.

Common (incidence of ⩾1%) and uncommon (incidence of ⩽1%) adverse drug reactions are listed in the table below.

Body System	Common	Uncommon
Immune system disorders		Anaphylactic reaction
		Anaphylactoid reaction
		Hypersensitivity
Metabolism and nutritional disorders	Anorexia	Dehydration
Psychiatric disorders	Anxiety	Affect lability
	Confusional state	Agitation
	Insomnia	Depression
	Nervousness	Drug dependence
	Thinking disturbances	Euphoria
	Abnormal dreams	Hallucinations
		Disorientation
		Mood altered
		Restlessness
		Dysphoria
Nervous system disorders	Headache	Amnesia
	Dizziness	Hypertonia
	Sedation	Tremor
	Somnolence	Hypoaesthesia
		Hypotonia
		Paraesthesia
		Speech disorder
		Convulsions
		Muscle contractions involuntary
		Taste perversion
		Syncope
Eye disorders		Miosis
		Visual disturbance
Ear and labyrinth disorders		Vertigo
Cardiac disorders		Supraventricular tachycardia
Vascular disorders		Hypotension
		Orthostatic hypotension
		Vasodilatation
		Facial flushing
Respiratory, thoracic and mediastinal disorders	Bronchospasm	Respiratory depression
	Dyspnoea	Hiccups
	Cough decreased	
Gastrointestinal disorders	Constipation	Dysphagia
	Nausea	Eructation
	Vomiting	Flatulence
	Dry mouth	Gastrointestinal disorders
		Ileus
	Dyspepsia	Gastritis
	Abdominal pain	
	Diarrhoea	
Hepato-biliary disorders		Biliary colic
		Increased hepatic enzymes
Skin and subcutaneous tissue disorders	Hyperhidrosis	Dry skin
	Pruritus	Exfoliative dermatitis
	Rash	Urticaria
Musculoskeletal and connective tissue disorders		Muscular rigidity
Renal and urinary disorders		Urinary retention
		Ureteral spasm
Reproductive system and breast disorders		Amenorrhoea
		Libido decreased
		Erectile dysfunction
General disorders and administration site conditions	Asthenia	Drug tolerance
	Chills	Oedema
		Oedema peripheral
		Malaise
		Thirst
		Pyrexia
		Drug withdrawal syndrome

Tolerance and Dependence:

The patient may develop tolerance to the drug with chronic use and require progressively higher doses to maintain pain control. Prolonged use of ***OxyContin*** tablets may lead to physical dependence and a withdrawal syndrome may occur upon abrupt cessation of therapy. When a patient no longer requires therapy with oxycodone, it may be advisable to taper the dose gradually to prevent symptoms of withdrawal. The opioid abstinence or withdrawal syndrome is characterised by some or all of the following: restlessness, lacrimation, rhinorrhea, yawning, perspiration, chills, myalgia, mydriasis and palpitations. Other symptoms also may develop, including: irritability, anxiety, backache, joint pain, weakness, abdominal cramps, insomnia, nausea, anorexia, vomiting, diarrhoea, or increased blood pressure, respiratory rate or heart rate.

4.9 Overdose

Signs of oxycodone toxicity and overdosage are pin-point pupils, respiratory depression and hypotension. Circulatory failure and somnolence progressing to stupor or deepening coma, skeletal muscle flaccidity, bradycardia and death may occur in more severe cases.

Treatment of oxycodone overdosage: Primary attention should be given to the establishment of a patent airway and institution of assisted or controlled ventilation.

In the case of massive overdosage, administer naloxone intravenously (0.4 to 2 mg for an adult and 0.01 mg/kg body weight for children), if the patient is in a coma or respiratory depression is present. Repeat the dose at 2 minute intervals if there is no response. If repeated doses are required then an infusion of 60% of the initial dose per hour is a useful starting point. A solution of 10 mg made up in 50 ml dextrose will produce 200 micrograms/ml for infusion using an IV pump (dose adjusted to the clinical response). Infusions are not a substitute for frequent review of the patient's clinical state. Intramuscular naloxone is an alternative in the event IV access is not possible. As the duration of action of naloxone is relatively short, the patient must be carefully monitored until spontaneous respiration is reliably re-established. Naloxone is a competitive antagonist and large doses (4 mg) may be required in seriously poisoned patients.

For less severe overdosage, administer naloxone 0.2 mg intravenously followed by increments of 0.1 mg every 2 minutes if required.

Naloxone should not be administered in the absence of clinically significant respiratory or circulatory depression secondary to oxycodone overdosage. Naloxone should be administered cautiously to persons who are known, or suspected, to be physically dependent on oxycodone. In such cases, an abrupt or complete reversal of opioid effects may precipitate pain and an acute withdrawal syndrome.

Additional/other considerations:

- Consider activated charcoal (50 g for adults, 10 -15 g for children), if a substantial amount has been ingested within 1 hour, provided the airway can be protected. It may be reasonable to assume that late administration of activated charcoal may be beneficial for prolonged release preparations; however there is no evidence to support this.
- ***OxyContin*** tablets will continue to release and add to the oxycodone load for up to 12 hours after administration and management of oxycodone overdosage should be modified accordingly. Gastric contents may need to be emptied as this can be useful in removing unabsorbed drug, particularly when a prolonged release formulation has been taken.

5. PHARMACOLOGICAL PROPERTIES

5.1 Pharmacodynamic properties

Pharmacotherapeutic group: Natural opium alkaloids

ATC code: NO2A AO5

Oxycodone is a full opioid agonist with no antagonist properties. It has an affinity for kappa, mu and delta opiate receptors in the brain and spinal cord. Oxycodone is similar to morphine in its action. The therapeutic effect is mainly analgesic, anxiolytic and sedative.

Clinical studies

The efficacy of ***OxyContin*** tablets has been demonstrated in cancer pain, post-operative pain and severe non-malignant pain such as diabetic neuropathy, postherpetic neuralgia, low back pain and osteoarthritis. In the latter indication, treatment was continued for up to 18 months and proved effective in many patients for whom NSAIDs alone provided inadequate relief. The efficacy of ***OxyContin*** tablets in neuropathic pain was confirmed by three placebo-controlled studies.

In patients with chronic non-malignant pain, maintenance of analgesia with stable dosing was demonstrated for up to three years.

5.2 Pharmacokinetic properties

Compared with morphine, which has an absolute bioavailability of approximately 30%, oxycodone has a high absolute bioavailability of up to 87% following oral administration. Oxycodone has an elimination half-life of approximately 3 hours and is metabolised principally to noroxycodone and oxymorphone. Oxymorphone has some analgesic activity but is present in the plasma in low concentrations and is not considered to contribute to oxycodone's pharmacological effect.

The release of oxycodone from ***OxyContin*** tablets is biphasic with an initial relatively fast release providing an early onset of analgesia followed by a more controlled release which determines the 12 hour duration of action. The mean apparent elimination half-life of ***OxyContin*** is 4.5 hours which leads to steady-state being achieved in about one day.

Release of oxycodone from ***OxyContin*** tablets is independent of pH.

OxyContin tablets have an oral bioavailability comparable with conventional oral oxycodone, but the former achieve maximal plasma concentrations at about 3 hours rather than about 1 to 1.5 hours. Peak and trough concentrations of oxycodone from ***OxyContin*** tablets 10 mg administered 12-hourly are equivalent to those achieved from conventional oxycodone 5 mg administered 6-hourly.

OxyContin tablets 5 mg, 10 mg, 20 mg, 40 mg and 80 mg are bioequivalent in terms of both rate and extent of absorption. Ingestion of a standard high-fat meal does not alter the peak oxycodone concentration or the extent of oxycodone absorption from ***OxyContin*** tablets.

Elderly

The AUC in elderly subjects is 15% greater when compared with young subjects.

Gender

Female subjects have, on average, plasma oxycodone concentrations up to 25% higher than males on a body weight adjusted basis. The reason for this difference is unknown.

Patients with renal impairment

Preliminary data from a study of patients with mild to moderate renal dysfunction show peak plasma oxycodone and noroxycodone concentrations approximately 50% and 20% higher, respectively and AUC values for oxycodone, noroxycodone and oxymorphone approximately 60%, 60% and 40% higher than normal subjects, respectively. There was an increase in $t_{½}$ of elimination for oxycodone of only 1 hour.

Patients with mild to moderate hepatic impairment

Patients with mild to moderate hepatic dysfunction showed peak plasma oxycodone and noroxycodone concentrations approximately 50% and 20% higher, respectively, than normal subjects. AUC values were approximately 95% and 75% higher, respectively. Oxymorphone peak plasma concentrations and AUC values were lower by 15% to 50%. The $t_{½}$ elimination for oxycodone increased by 2.3 hours.

5.3 Preclinical safety data

Oxycodone was not mutagenic in the following assays: Ames Salmonella and E. Coli test with and without metabolic activation at doses of up to 5000 μg, chromosomal aberration test in human lymphocytes (in the absence of metabolic activation and with activation after 48 hours of exposure) at doses of up to 1500 μg/ml, and in the *in vivo* bone marrow micronucleus assay in mice (at plasma levels of up to 48 μg/ml). Mutagenic results occurred in the presence of metabolic activation in the human chromosomal aberration test (at greater than or equal to 1250 μg/ml) at 24 but not 48 hours of exposure and in the mouse lymphoma assay at doses of 50 μg/ml or greater with metabolic activation and at 400 μg/ml or greater without metabolic activation. The data from these tests indicate that the genotoxic risk to humans may be considered low.

Studies of oxycodone in animals to evaluate its carcinogenic potential have not been conducted owing to the length of clinical experience with the drug substance.

In vitro dissolution data generated using the standard dissolution method, show that in the presence of ethanol, at concentrations up to 40%, the prolonged release characteristics of the ***OxyContin*** formulation were maintained and no breakdown of the prolonged release mechanism was observed.

6. PHARMACEUTICAL PARTICULARS

6.1 List of excipients

Lactose monohydrate

Povidone

Ammoniomethacrylate co-polymer

Sorbic acid

Glyceryl triacetate

Stearyl alcohol

Talc

Magnesium stearate

Hypromellose (E464)

Titanium dioxide (E171)

Macrogol

In addition the tablets contain the following:

5 mg	Brilliant blue (E133)
10 mg	Hydroxypropylcellulose
20 mg and 40 mg	Polysorbate 80, iron oxide (E172).
80 mg	Hydroxypropylcellulose, iron oxide (E172), indigo carmine (E132)

6.2 Incompatibilities

Not applicable

6.3 Shelf life

Three years.

6.4 Special precautions for storage

Do not store above 25°C.

6.5 Nature and contents of container

PVC blister packs with aluminium foil backing containing 28 tablets (5 mg) or 56 tablets (10, 20, 40, 80 mg).

6.6 Special precautions for disposal and other handling

None.

7. MARKETING AUTHORISATION HOLDER

Napp Pharmaceuticals Ltd
Cambridge Science Park
Milton Road
Cambridge CB4 0GW

8. MARKETING AUTHORISATION NUMBER(S)

PL 16950/0097-0100, 0123

9. DATE OF FIRST AUTHORISATION/RENEWAL OF THE AUTHORISATION

10, 20, 40, 80 mg tablets: 5 March 1999/ 30 June 2005

5 mg tablets: 21 May 2002/ 30 June 2005

10. DATE OF REVISION OF THE TEXT

November 2008

11. LEGAL CATEGORY

CD (Sch 2) POM

® OxyContin and the Napp Device are Registered Trade Marks.

OxyNorm 10 mg/ml solution for injection or infusion

(Napp Pharmaceuticals Limited)

1. NAME OF THE MEDICINAL PRODUCT

OxyNorm® 10 mg/ml, solution for injection or infusion

2. QUALITATIVE AND QUANTITATIVE COMPOSITION

Oxycodone hydrochloride 10 mg/ml (equivalent to 9 mg/ml oxycodone)

For excipients, see Section 6.1

3. PHARMACEUTICAL FORM

Solution for injection or infusion.

4. CLINICAL PARTICULARS

4.1 Therapeutic indications

For the treatment of moderate to severe pain in patients with cancer and post-operative pain. For the treatment of severe pain requiring the use of a strong opioid.

4.2 Posology and method of administration

Route of administration:

Subcutaneous injection or infusion

Intravenous injection or infusion.

Posology:

The dose should be adjusted according to the severity of pain, the total condition of the patient and previous or concurrent medication.

Adults over 18 years:

The following starting doses are recommended. A gradual increase in dose may be required if analgesia is inadequate or if pain severity increases.

i.v. (Bolus): Dilute to 1 mg/ml in 0.9% saline, 5% dextrose or water for injections. Administer a bolus dose of 1 to 10 mg slowly over 1-2 minutes.

Doses should not be administered more frequently than every 4 hours.

i.v. (Infusion): Dilute to 1 mg/ml in 0.9% saline, 5% dextrose or water for injections. A starting dose of 2 mg/hour is recommended.

i.v. (PCA): Dilute to 1 mg/ml in 0.9% saline, 5% dextrose or water for injections. Bolus doses of 0.03 mg/kg should be administered with a minimum lock-out time of 5 minutes.

s.c. (Bolus): Use as 10 mg/ml concentration. A starting dose of 5 mg is recommended, repeated at 4-hourly intervals as required.

s.c. (Infusion): Dilute in 0.9% saline, 5% dextrose or water for injections if required. A starting dose of 7.5 mg/day is recommended in opioid naïve patients, titrating gradually according to symptom control. Cancer patients transferring from oral oxycodone may require much higher doses (see below).

Transferring patients between oral and parenteral oxycodone:

The dose should be based on the following ratio: 2 mg of oral oxycodone is equivalent to 1 mg of parenteral oxycodone. It must be emphasised that this is a guide to the dose required. Inter-patient variability requires that each patient is carefully titrated to the appropriate dose.

Elderly:

Elderly patients should be treated with caution. The lowest dose should be administered with careful titration to pain control.

Patients with renal and hepatic impairment:

Patients with mild to moderate renal impairment and/or mild hepatic impairment should be treated with caution. The lowest dose should be given with careful titration to pain control.

Children under 18 years:

There are no data on the use of ***OxyNorm*** injection in patients under 18 years of age.

Use in non-malignant pain:

Opioids are not first-line therapy for chronic non-malignant pain, nor are they recommended as the only treatment. Types of chronic pain which have been shown to be alleviated by strong opioids include chronic osteoarthritic pain and intervertebral disc disease. The need for continued treatment in non-malignant pain should be assessed at regular intervals.

Cessation of therapy:

When a patient no longer requires therapy with oxycodone, it may be advisable to taper the dose gradually to prevent symptoms of withdrawal.

4.3 Contraindications

OxyNorm injection is contraindicated in patients with known hypersensitivity to oxycodone or any of the other constituents, or in any situation where opioids are contra-indicated; respiratory depression; head injury; paralytic ileus; acute abdomen; chronic obstructive airways disease; cor pulmonale; chronic bronchial asthma; hypercarbia; moderate to severe hepatic impairment; severe renal impairment (creatinine clearance <10 ml/min); chronic constipation; concurrent administration of monoamine oxidase inhibitors or within 2 weeks of discontinuation of their use; pregnancy.

4.4 Special warnings and precautions for use

The major risk of opioid excess is respiratory depression. As with all opioids, a reduction in dosage may be advisable in hypothyroidism. Use with caution in patients with raised intracranial pressure, hypotension, hypovolaemia, toxic psychoses, diseases of the biliary tract, inflammatory bowel disorders, prostatic hypertrophy, adrenocortical insufficiency, acute alcoholism, delirium tremens, pancreatitis, chronic renal and hepatic disease or severe pulmonary disease and debilitated, elderly and infirm patients. ***OxyNorm*** injection should not be used where there is a possibility of paralytic ileus occurring. Should paralytic ileus be suspected or occur during use, ***OxyNorm*** injection should be discontinued immediately.

The patient may develop tolerance to oxycodone with chronic use and require progressively higher doses to maintain pain control. The patient may develop physical dependence, in which case an abstinence syndrome may be seen following abrupt cessation.

For appropriate patients who suffer with chronic non-malignant pain, opioids should be used as part of a comprehensive treatment programme involving other medications and treatment modalities. A crucial part of the assessment of a patient with chronic non-malignant pain is the patient's addiction and substance abuse history. There is potential for development of psychological dependence (addiction) to opioid analgesics, including oxycodone. ***OxyNorm*** injection, like all opioids, should be used with particular care in patients with a history of alcohol and drug abuse.

If opioid treatment is considered appropriate for the patient, then the main aim of treatment is not to minimise the dose of opioid but rather to achieve a dose which provides adequate pain relief with a minimum of side effects. There must be frequent contact between physician and patient so that dosage adjustments can be made. It is strongly recommended that the physician defines treatment outcomes in accordance with pain management guidelines. The physician and patient can then agree to discontinue treatment if these objectives are not met.

Oxycodone has an abuse profile similar to other strong opioids and should be used with caution in opioid-dependent patients. Oxycodone may be sought and abused by people with latent or manifest addiction disorders.

As with other opioids, infants who are born to dependent mothers may exhibit withdrawal symptoms and may have respiratory depression at birth.

4.5 Interaction with other medicinal products and other forms of interaction

There is an enhanced CNS depressant effect with drugs such as tranquillisers, anaesthetics, hypnotics, anti-depressants, sedatives, phenothiazines, neuroleptic drugs, alcohol, other opioids, muscle relaxants and anti-hypertensives. Monoamine oxidase inhibitors are known to interact with narcotic analgesics, producing CNS excitation or depression with hypertensive or hypotensive crisis.

Oxycodone is metabolised in part via the CYP2D6 and CYP3A4 pathways. While these pathways may be blocked by a variety of drugs, such blockade has not yet been shown to be of clinical significance with this agent.

4.6 Pregnancy and lactation

The effect of oxycodone in human reproduction has not been adequately studied. No studies on fertility or the post-natal effects of intrauterine exposure have been carried out. However, studies in rats and rabbits with oral doses of oxycodone equivalent to 3 and 47 times an adult dose of 160 mg/day, respectively, did not reveal evidence of harm to the foetus due to oxycodone. ***OxyNorm*** injection is not recommended for use in pregnancy nor during labour. Infants born to mothers who have received opioids during pregnancy should be monitored for respiratory depression.

Oxycodone may be secreted in breast milk and may cause respiratory depression in the newborn. Oxycodone should therefore not be used in breast-feeding mothers.

4.7 Effects on ability to drive and use machines

Oxycodone may modify patients' reactions to a varying extent depending on the dosage and individual susceptibility. Therefore patients should not drive or operate machinery, if affected.

4.8 Undesirable effects

Adverse drug reactions are typical of full opioid agonists. Tolerance and dependence may occur (see Tolerance and Dependence, below). Constipation may be prevented with an appropriate laxative. If nausea or vomiting are troublesome, oxycodone may be combined with an antiemetic.

Common (incidence of $\geqslant$ 1%) and uncommon (incidence of $\leqslant$ 1%) adverse drug reactions to oxycodone are listed in the table below.

Body System	Common	Uncommon
Immune system disorders		Anaphylactic reaction
		Anaphylactoid reaction
		Hypersensitivity
Metabolism and nutritional disorders	Anorexia	Dehydration
Psychiatric disorders	Anxiety	Affect lability
	Confusional state	Agitation
	Insomnia	Depression
	Nervousness	Drug dependence
	Thinking disturbances	Euphoria
	Abnormal dreams	Hallucinations
		Disorientation
		Mood altered
		Restlessness
		Dysphoria
Nervous system disorders	Headache	Amnesia
	Dizziness	Hypertonia
	Sedation	Tremor
	Somnolence	Hypoaesthesia
		Hypotonia
		Paraesthesia
		Speech disorder
		Convulsions
		Muscle contractions involuntary
		Taste perversion
		Syncope
Eye disorders		Miosis
		Visual disturbance
Ear and labyrinth disorders		Vertigo
Cardiac disorders		Supraventricular tachycardia
Vascular disorders		Hypotension
		Orthostatic hypotension
		Vasodilatation
		Facial flushing
Respiratory, thoracic and mediastinal disorders	Bronchospasm	Respiratory depression
	Dyspnoea	Hiccups
	Cough decreased	
Gastrointestinal disorders	Constipation	Dysphagia
	Nausea	Eructation
	Vomiting	Flatulence
	Dry mouth	Gastrointestinal disorders
	Dyspepsia	Ileus
	Abdominal pain	Gastritis
	Diarrhoea	
Hepato-biliary disorders		Biliary colic
		Increased hepatic enzymes
Skin and subcutaneous tissue disorders	Hyperhidrosis	Dry skin
	Pruritus	Exfoliative dermatitis
	Rash	Urticaria
Musculoskeletal and connective tissue disorders		Muscular rigidity
Renal and urinary disorders		Urinary retention
		Ureteral spasm
Reproductive system and breast disorders		Amenorrhoea
		Libido decreased
		Erectile dysfunction
General disorders and administration site conditions	Asthenia	Drug tolerance
	Chills	Oedema
		Oedema peripheral
		Malaise
		Thirst
		Pyrexia
		Drug withdrawal syndrome

Tolerance and Dependence:

The patient may develop tolerance to the drug with chronic use and require progressively higher doses to maintain pain control. Prolonged use of ***OxyNorm*** injection may lead to physical dependence and a withdrawal syndrome may occur upon abrupt cessation of therapy. When a patient no longer requires therapy with oxycodone, it may be advisable to taper the dose gradually to prevent symptoms of withdrawal. The opioid abstinence or withdrawal syndrome is characterised by some or all of the following: restlessness, lacrimation, rhinorrhoea, yawning, perspiration, chills, myalgia, mydriasis and palpitations. Other symptoms also may develop, including: irritability, anxiety, backache, joint pain, weakness, abdominal cramps, insomnia, nausea, anorexia, vomiting, diarrhoea, or increased blood pressure, respiratory rate or heart rate.

4.9 Overdose

Symptoms of overdosage

Signs of oxycodone toxicity and overdosage are pin-point pupils, respiratory depression, hypotension and hallucinations. Nausea and vomiting are common in less severe cases. Non-cardiac pulmonary oedema and rhabdomyolysis are particularly common after intravenous injection of opioid analgesics. Circulatory failure and somnolence progressing to stupor or coma, skeletal muscle flaccidity, bradycardia and death may occur in more severe cases.

The effects of overdosage will be potentiated by the simultaneous ingestion of alcohol or other psychotropic drugs.

Treatment of overdosage

Primary attention should be given to the establishment of a patent airway and institution of assisted or controlled ventilation.

In the case of massive overdosage, administer naloxone intravenously (0.4 to 2mg for an adult and 0.01mg/kg body weight for children) if the patient is in a coma or respiratory depression is present. Repeat the dose at 2 minute intervals if there is no response. If repeated doses are required then an infusion of 60% of the initial dose per hour is a useful starting point. A solution of 10 mg made up in 50 ml dextrose will produce 200 micrograms/ml for infusion using an IV pump (dose adjusted to the clinical response). Infusions are not a substitute for frequent review of the patient's clinical state.

Intramuscular naloxone is an alternative in the event that IV access is not possible. As the duration of action of naloxone is relatively short, the patient must be carefully monitored until spontaneous respiration is reliably re-established. Naloxone is a competitive antagonist and large doses (4 mg) may be required in seriously poisoned patients.

For less severe overdosage, administer naloxone 0.2 mg intravenously followed by increments of 0.1 mg every 2 minutes if required.

The patient should be observed for at least 6 hours after the last dose of naloxone.

Naloxone should not be administered in the absence of clinically significant respiratory or circulatory depression secondary to oxycodone overdosage. Naloxone should be administered cautiously to persons who are known, or suspected, to be physically dependent on oxycodone. In such cases, an abrupt or complete reversal of opioid effects may precipitate pain and an acute withdrawal syndrome.

5. PHARMACOLOGICAL PROPERTIES

5.1 Pharmacodynamic properties

Pharmacotherapeutic group: Natural opium alkaloids

ATC code: N02A A05

Oxycodone is a full opioid agonist with no antagonist properties. It has an affinity for kappa, mu and delta opioid receptors in the brain and spinal cord. Oxycodone is similar to morphine in its action. The therapeutic effect is mainly analgesic, anxiolytic, antitussive and sedative.

Opioids may influence the hypothalamic-pituitary-adrenal or gonadal axes. Some changes that can be seen include an increase in serum prolactin and decreases in plasma cortisol and testosterone. Clinical symptoms may be manifest from these hormonal changes.

In vitro and animal studies indicate various effects of natural opioids, such as morphine, on components of the immune system; the clinical significance of these findings is unknown. Whether oxycodone, a semisynthetic opioid, has immunological effects similar to morphine is unknown.

5.2 Pharmacokinetic properties

Pharmacokinetic studies in healthy subjects demonstrated an equivalent availability of oxycodone from ***OxyNorm*** injection when administered by the intravenous and subcutaneous routes, as a single bolus dose or a continuous infusion over 8 hours.

Following absorption, oxycodone is distributed throughout the entire body. Approximately 45% is bound to plasma protein. It is metabolised in the liver to produce noroxycodone, oxymorphone and various conjugated glucuronides. The analgesic effects of the metabolites are clinically insignificant.

The active drug and its metabolites are excreted in both urine and faeces.

The plasma concentrations of oxycodone are only minimally affected by age, being 15% greater in elderly as compared to young subjects.

Female subjects have, on average, plasma oxycodone concentrations up to 25% higher than males on a body weight adjusted basis.

The drug penetrates the placenta and can be found in breast milk.

When compared to normal subjects, patients with mild to severe hepatic dysfunction may have higher plasma concentrations of oxycodone and noroxycodone, and lower plasma concentrations of oxymorphone. There may be an increase in the elimination half-life of oxycodone and this may be accompanied by an increase in drug effects.

When compared to normal subjects, patients with mild to severe renal dysfunction may have higher plasma concentrations of oxycodone and its metabolites. There may be an increase in the elimination half-life of oxycodone and this may be accompanied by an increase in drug effects.

5.3 Preclinical safety data

Oxycodone was not mutagenic in the following assays: Ames Salmonella and E. Coli test with and without metabolic activation at doses of up to 5000 mg, chromosomal aberration test in human lymphocytes (in the absence of metabolic activation and with activation after 48 hours of exposure) at doses of up to 1500 mg/ml, and in the in vivo bone marrow micronucleus assay in mice (at plasma levels of up to 48 mg/ml). Mutagenic results occurred in the presence of metabolic activation in the human chromosomal aberration test (at greater than or equal to 1250 mg/ml) at 24 but not 48 hours of exposure and in the mouse lymphoma assay at doses of 50 mg/ml or greater with metabolic activation and at 400 mg/ml or greater without metabolic activation. The data from these tests indicate that the genotoxic risk to humans may be considered low.

Studies of oxycodone in animals to evaluate its carcinogenic potential have not been conducted owing to the length of clinical experience with the drug substance.

6. PHARMACEUTICAL PARTICULARS

6.1 List of excipients

Citric acid monohydrate

Sodium citrate

Sodium chloride

Hydrochloric acid, dilute

Sodium hydroxide

Water for injections

6.2 Incompatibilities

This medicinal product must not be mixed with other medicinal products except those mentioned in section 6.6.

Cyclizine at concentrations of 3 mg/ml or less, when mixed with ***OxyNorm*** injection, either undiluted or diluted with water for injections, shows no sign of precipitation over a period of 24 hours storage at room temperature. Precipitation has been shown to occur in mixtures with ***OxyNorm*** injection at cyclizine concentrations greater than 3 mg/ml or when diluted with 0.9% saline. It is recommended that water for injections be used as a diluent when cyclizine and oxycodone hydrochloride are co-administered either intravenously or subcutaneously as an infusion.

Prochlorperazine is chemically incompatible with ***OxyNorm*** injection.

6.3 Shelf life

3 years unopened.

After opening use immediately.

For further information see Section 6.6.

6.4 Special precautions for storage

No special precautions for storage prior to opening.

For further information on use after opening see Section 6.6.

6.5 Nature and contents of container

Clear glass ampoules: 1 ml and 2 ml.

Pack size: 5 ampoules.

Not all pack sizes may be marketed.

6.6 Special precautions for disposal and other handling

Each ampoule is for single use in a single patient. The injection should be given immediately after opening the ampoule, and any unused portion be discarded. Chemical and physical in-use stability has been demonstrated for 24 hours at room temperature.

From a microbiological point of view, the product should be used immediately. If not used immediately, in-use storage times and conditions prior to use are the responsibility of the user and would normally not be longer than 24 hours at 2 to 8°C, unless reconstitution, dilution, etc has taken place in controlled and validated aseptic conditions.

OxyNorm injection has been shown to be **compatible** with the following drugs:

Hyoscine butylbromide

Hyoscine hydrobromide

Dexamethasone sodium phosphate

Haloperidol

Midazolam hydrochloride

Metoclopramide hydrochloride

Levomepromazine hydrochloride

OxyNorm injection, undiluted or diluted to 1 mg/ml with 0.9% w/v saline, 5% w/v dextrose or water for injections, is physically and chemically stable when in contact with representative brands of polypropylene or polycarbonate syringes, polyethylene or PVC tubing, and PVC or EVA infusion bags, over a 24 hour period at room temperature.

The injection, whether undiluted or diluted to 1 mg/ml in the infusion fluids used in these studies and contained in the various assemblies, does not need to be protected from light.

Inappropriate handling of the undiluted solution after opening of the original ampoule, or of the diluted solutions may compromise the sterility of the product.

7. MARKETING AUTHORISATION HOLDER

Napp Pharmaceuticals Ltd

Cambridge Science Park

Milton Road

Cambridge CB4 0GW

8. MARKETING AUTHORISATION NUMBER(S)

PL 16950/0128

9. DATE OF FIRST AUTHORISATION/RENEWAL OF THE AUTHORISATION

14 April 2003

10. DATE OF REVISION OF THE TEXT

September 2008

11. LEGAL CATEGORY

CD (Sch 2) POM

®***OxyNorm*** and the NAPP device are Registered Trade Marks.

OxyNorm 5, 10, 20 mg

(Napp Pharmaceuticals Limited)

1. NAME OF THE MEDICINAL PRODUCT

OxyNorm® 5, 10, 20 mg

2. QUALITATIVE AND QUANTITATIVE COMPOSITION

Each capsule contains 4.5, 9, or 18 mg of oxycodone as 5, 10, or 20 mg of oxycodone hydrochloride.

For excipients, see section 6.1.

3. PHARMACEUTICAL FORM

Capsule, hard.

OxyNorm capsules 5 mg are orange/beige, printed ONR 5.

OxyNorm capsules 10 mg are white/beige, printed ONR 10.

OxyNorm capsules 20 mg are pink/beige, printed ONR 20.

4. CLINICAL PARTICULARS

4.1 Therapeutic indications

For the treatment of moderate to severe pain in patients with cancer and post-operative pain.

For the treatment of severe pain requiring the use of a strong opioid.

4.2 Posology and method of administration

Route of administration:

Oral

In common with other strong opioids, the need for continued treatment should be assessed at regular intervals.

Elderly and adults over 18 years:

OxyNorm capsules should be taken at 4-6 hourly intervals. The dosage is dependent on the severity of the pain, and the patient's previous history of analgesic requirements.

Increasing severity of pain will require an increased dosage of ***OxyNorm*** capsules. The correct dosage for any individual patient is that which controls the pain and is well tolerated throughout the dosing period. Patients should be titrated to pain relief unless unmanageable adverse drug reactions prevent this.

The usual starting dose for opioid naive patients or patients presenting with severe pain uncontrolled by weaker opioids is 5 mg, 4-6 hourly. The dose should then be carefully titrated, as frequently as once a day if necessary, to achieve pain relief. The majority of patients will not require a daily dose greater than 400 mg. However, a few patients may require higher doses.

Patients receiving oral morphine before oxycodone therapy should have their daily dose based on the following ratio: 10 mg of oral oxycodone is equivalent to 20 mg of oral morphine. It must be emphasised that this is a guide to the dose of ***OxyNorm*** capsules required. Inter-patient variability requires that each patient is carefully titrated to the appropriate dose.

Controlled pharmacokinetic studies in elderly patients (aged over 65 years) have shown that, compared with younger adults, the clearance of oxycodone is only slightly reduced. No untoward adverse drug reactions were seen based on age, therefore adult doses and dosage intervals are appropriate.

Adults with mild to moderate renal impairment and mild hepatic impairment. The plasma concentration in this patient population may be increased. Therefore, dose initiation should follow a conservative approach. The starting dose for opioid naive patients is 2.5 mg oxycodone 6-hourly, given as ***OxyNorm*** liquid.

Children under 18 years:

OxyNorm capsules should not be used in patients under 18 years.

Use in non-malignant pain:

Opioids are not first line therapy for chronic non-malignant pain, nor are they recommended as the only treatment. Types of chronic pain which have been shown to be alleviated by strong opioids include chronic osteoarthritic pain and intervertebral disc disease. The need for continued treatment in non-malignant pain should be assessed at regular intervals.

Cessation of Therapy:

When a patient no longer requires therapy with oxycodone, it may be advisable to taper the dose gradually to prevent symptoms of withdrawal.

4.3 Contraindications

Hypersensitivity to any of the constituents, respiratory depression, head injury, paralytic ileus, acute abdomen, delayed gastric emptying, chronic obstructive airways disease, cor pulmonale, chronic bronchial asthma, hypercarbia, known oxycodone sensitivity or in any situation where opioids are contra-indicated, moderate to severe hepatic impairment, severe renal impairment (creatinine clearance < 10 ml/min), chronic constipation, concurrent administration of monoamine oxidase inhibitors or within 2 weeks of discontinuation of their use. Pregnancy.

4.4 Special warnings and precautions for use

The major risk of opioid excess is respiratory depression. As with all narcotics, a reduction in dosage may be advisable in hypothyroidism. Use with caution in opioid dependent patients and in patients with raised intracranial pressure, hypotension, hypovolaemia, toxic psychosis, diseases of the biliary tract, pancreatitis, inflammatory bowel disorders, prostatic hypertrophy, adrenocortical insufficiency, acute alcoholism, delirium tremens, chronic renal and hepatic disease, or severe pulmonary disease and debilitated, elderly and infirm patients. ***OxyNorm*** capsules should not be used where there is a possibility of paralytic ileus occurring. Should paralytic ileus be suspected or occur during use, ***OxyNorm*** capsules should be discontinued immediately. As with all opioid preparations, patients about to undergo additional pain relieving procedures (e.g. surgery, plexus blockade) should not receive ***OxyNorm*** capsules for 6 hours prior to the intervention. If further treatment with oxycodone is indicated then the dosage should be adjusted to the new post-operative requirement.

Oxycodone should be used with caution following abdominal surgery as opioids are known to impair intestinal motility and should not be used until the physician is assured of normal bowel function.

For appropriate patients who suffer with chronic non-malignant pain, opioids should be used as part of a comprehensive treatment programme involving other medications and treatment modalities. A crucial part of the assessment of a patient with chronic non-malignant pain is the patient's addiction and substance abuse history. There is potential for development of psychological dependence (addiction) to opioid analgesics, including oxycodone. ***OxyNorm*** capsules, like all opioids, should be used with particular care in patients with a history of alcohol and drug abuse.

If opioid treatment is considered appropriate for the patient, then the main aim of treatment is not to minimise the dose of opioid but rather to achieve a dose which provides adequate pain relief with a minimum of side effects. There must be frequent contact between physician and patient so that dosage adjustments can be made. It is strongly recommended that the physician defines treatment outcomes in accordance with pain management guidelines. The physician and patient can then agree to discontinue treatment if these objectives are not met.

Sunset yellow, a constituent of the 5 mg capsule, can cause allergic type reactions such as asthma. This is more common in people who are allergic to aspirin.

Oxycodone has an abuse profile similar to other strong opioids. Oxycodone may be sought and abused by people with latent or manifest addiction disorders.

As with other opioids, infants who are born to dependent mothers may exhibit withdrawal symptoms and may have respiratory depression at birth.

The capsules should be swallowed whole, and not chewed or crushed. Abuse of oral dosage forms by parenteral administration can be expected to result in serious adverse events, which may be fatal.

4.5 Interaction with other medicinal products and other forms of interaction

Oxycodone, like other opioids, potentiates the effects of tranquillisers, anaesthetics, hypnotics, anti-depressants, sedatives, phenothiazines, neuroleptic drugs, alcohol, other opioids muscle relaxants and antihypertensives. Monoamine oxidase inhibitors are known to interact with narcotic analgesics, producing CNS excitation or depression with hypertensive or hypotensive crisis. Concurrent administration of quinidine, an inhibitor of cytochrome P450-2D6, resulted in an increase in oxycodone C_{max} by 11%, AUC by 13%, and $t_{½}$ elim. by 14%. Also an increase in noroxycodone level was observed, (C_{max} by 50%, AUC by 85%, and $t_{½}$ elim. by 42%). The pharmacodynamic effects of oxycodone were not altered. This interaction may be observed for other potent inhibitors of cytochrome P450-2D6 enzyme. Cimetidine and inhibitors of cytochrome P450-3A such as ketoconazole and erythromycin may inhibit the metabolism of oxycodone.

4.6 Pregnancy and lactation

OxyNorm capsules are not recommended for use in pregnancy nor during labour. Infants born to mothers who have received opioids during pregnancy should be monitored for respiratory depression.

Oxycodone may be secreted in breast milk and may cause respiratory depression in the newborn. ***OxyNorm*** capsules should, therefore, not be used in breast-feeding mothers.

4.7 Effects on ability to drive and use machines

Oxycodone may modify patients' reactions to a varying extent depending on the dosage and individual susceptibility. Therefore patients should not drive or operate machinery if affected.

4.8 Undesirable effects

Adverse drug reactions are typical of full opioid agonists. Tolerance and dependence may occur (see *Tolerance and Dependence*, below). Constipation may be prevented with an appropriate laxative. If nausea and vomiting are troublesome, oxycodone may be combined with an anti-emetic.

Common (incidence of ≥ 1%) and uncommon (incidence of ≤ 1%) adverse drug reactions are listed in the table below.

Body System	Common	Uncommon
Immune system disorders		Anaphylactic reaction
		Anaphylactoid reaction
		Hypersensitivity
Metabolism and nutritional disorders	Anorexia	Dehydration
Psychiatric disorders	Anxiety	Affect lability
	Confusional state	Agitation
	Insomnia	Depression
	Nervousness	Drug dependence
	Thinking disturbances	Euphoria
	Abnormal dreams	Hallucinations
		Disorientation
		Mood altered
		Restlessness
		Dysphoria
Nervous system disorders	Headache	Amnesia
	Dizziness	Hypertonia
	Sedation	Tremor
	Somnolence	Hypoaesthesia
		Hypotonia
		Paraesthesia
		Speech disorder
		Convulsions
		Muscle contractions involuntary
		Taste perversion
		Syncope
Eye disorders		Miosis
		Visual disturbance
Ear and labyrinth disorders		Vertigo
Cardiac disorders		Supraventricular tachycardia
Vascular disorders		Hypotension
		Orthostatic hypotension
		Vasodilatation
		Facial flushing
Respiratory, thoracic and mediastinal disorders	Bronchospasm	Respiratory depression
	Dyspnoea	Hiccups
	Cough decreased	
Gastrointestinal disorders	Constipation	Dysphagia
	Nausea	Eructation
	Vomiting	Flatulence
	Dry mouth	Gastrointestinal disorders
	Dyspepsia	Ileus
	Abdominal pain	Gastritis
	Diarrhoea	
Hepato-biliary disorders		Biliary colic
		Increased hepatic enzymes
Skin and subcutaneous tissue disorders	Hyperhidrosis	Dry skin
	Pruritus	Exfoliative dermatitis
	Rash	Urticaria
Musculoskeletal and connective tissue disorders		Muscular rigidity
Renal and urinary disorders		Urinary retention
		Ureteral spasm
Reproductive system and breast disorders		Amenorrhoea
		Libido decreased
		Erectile dysfunction
General disorders and administration site conditions	Asthenia	Drug tolerance
	Chills	Oedema
		Oedema peripheral
		Malaise
		Thirst
		Pyrexia
		Drug withdrawal syndrome

Tolerance and Dependence:

The patient may develop tolerance to the drug with chronic use and require progressively higher doses to maintain pain control. Prolonged use of ***OxyNorm*** capsules may lead to physical dependence and a withdrawal syndrome may occur upon abrupt cessation of therapy. When a patient no longer requires therapy with oxycodone, it may be advisable to taper the dose gradually to prevent symptoms of withdrawal. The opioid abstinence or withdrawal syndrome is characterised by some or all of the following: restlessness, lacrimation, rhinorrhoea, yawning, perspiration, chills, myalgia, mydriasis and palpitations. Other symptoms also may develop, including: irritability, anxiety, backache, joint pain, weakness, abdominal cramps, insomnia, nausea, anorexia, vomiting, diarrhoea, or increased blood pressure, respiratory rate or heart rate.

OxyNorm capsules should be used with particular care in patients with a history of alcohol and drug abuse.

4.9 Overdose

Signs of oxycodone toxicity and overdosage are pin-point pupils, respiratory depression and hypotension. Circulatory failure and somnolence progressing to stupor or deepening coma, skeletal muscle flaccidity, bradycardia and death may occur in more severe cases.

Treatment of oxycodone overdosage: Primary attention should be given to the establishment of a patent airway and institution of assisted or controlled ventilation.

In the case of massive overdosage, administer naloxone intravenously (0.4 to 2 mg for an adult and 0.01 mg/kg body weight for children), if the patient is in a coma or respiratory depression is present. Repeat the dose at 2 minute intervals if there is no response. If repeated doses are required then an infusion of 60% of the initial dose per hour is a useful starting point. A solution of 10 mg made up in 50 ml dextrose will produce 200 micrograms/ml for infusion using an IV pump (dose adjusted to the clinical response). Infusions are not a substitute for frequent review of the patient's clinical state. Intramuscular naloxone is an alternative in the event IV access is not possible. As the duration of action of naloxone is relatively short, the patient must be carefully monitored until spontaneous respiration is reliably established. Naloxone is a competitive antagonist and large doses (4 mg) may be required in seriously poisoned patients.

For less severe overdosage, administer naloxone 0.2 mg intravenously followed by increments of 0.1 mg every 2 minutes if required.

Naloxone should not be administered in the absence of clinically significant respiratory or circulatory depression secondary to oxycodone overdosage. Naloxone should be administered cautiously to persons who are known, or suspected, to be physically dependent on oxycodone. In such cases, an abrupt or complete reversal of opioid effects may precipitate pain and an acute withdrawal syndrome.

Additional/other considerations:

- Consider activated charcoal (50 g for adults, 10 -15 g for children), if a substantial amount has been ingested within 1 hour, provided the airway can be protected.
- Gastric contents may need to be emptied as this can be useful in removing unabsorbed drug.

5. PHARMACOLOGICAL PROPERTIES

5.1 Pharmacodynamic properties

Pharmacotherapeutic group: Natural opium alkaloids

ATC code: N02A A05

Oxycodone is a full opioid agonist with no antagonist properties. It has an affinity for kappa, mu and delta opiate receptors in the brain and spinal cord. The therapeutic effect is mainly analgesic, anxiolytic and sedative.

5.2 Pharmacokinetic properties

Compared with morphine, which has an absolute bioavailability of approximately 30%, oxycodone has a high absolute bioavailability of up to 87% following oral administration. Oxycodone has an elimination half-life of approximately 3 hours and is metabolised principally to noroxycodone via CYP450-3A and oxymorphone via CYP450-2D6. Oxymorphone has some analgesic activity but is present in the plasma in low concentrations and is not considered to contribute to oxycodone's pharmacological effect.

5.3 Preclinical safety data

Oxycodone was not mutagenic in the following assays: Ames Salmonella and E. Coli test with and without metabolic activation at doses of up to 5000 μg, chromosomal aberration test in human lymphocytes (in the absence of metabolic activation and with activation after 48 hours of exposure) at doses of up to 1500 μg/ml, and in the *in vivo* bone marrow micronucleus assay in mice (at plasma levels of up to 48 μg/ml). Mutagenic results occurred in the presence of metabolic activation in the human chromosomal aberration test (at greater than or equal to 1250 μg/ml) at 24 but not 48 hours of exposure and in the mouse lymphoma assay at doses of 50 μg/ml or greater with metabolic activation and at 400 μg/ml or greater without metabolic activation. The data from these tests indicate that the genotoxic risk to humans may be considered low.

Studies of oxycodone in animals to evaluate its carcinogenic potential have not been conducted owing to the length of clinical experience with the drug substance.

6. PHARMACEUTICAL PARTICULARS

6.1 List of excipients

Cellulose, microcrystalline

Magnesium stearate

Titanium dioxide (E171)

Iron oxide (E172)

Indigo carmine (E132)

Sodium laurylsulphate

Gelatin

In addition, the 5 mg capsule contains Sunset Yellow (E110).

The capsules are printed with ink containing shellac, iron oxide (E172) and propylene glycol.

6.2 Incompatibilities

Not applicable

6.3 Shelf life

Four years

6.4 Special precautions for storage

Do not store above 30°C.

6.5 Nature and contents of container

PVdC coated PVC blister packs with aluminium backing foil.

Pack size: 56 capsules.

6.6 Special precautions for disposal and other handling

None stated.

7. MARKETING AUTHORISATION HOLDER

Napp Pharmaceuticals Ltd

Cambridge Science Park

Milton Road

Cambridge CB4 0GW

8. MARKETING AUTHORISATION NUMBER(S)

PL 16950/0106-0108

9. DATE OF FIRST AUTHORISATION/RENEWAL OF THE AUTHORISATION

26th October 1999/25 June 2005

10. DATE OF REVISION OF THE TEXT

July 2008

11 LEGAL CATEGORY

CD (Sch 2) POM

OxyNorm 50 mg/ml, solution for injection or infusion

(Napp Pharmaceuticals Limited)

1. NAME OF THE MEDICINAL PRODUCT

OxyNorm® 50 mg/ml, solution for injection or infusion

2. QUALITATIVE AND QUANTITATIVE COMPOSITION

Oxycodone hydrochloride 50 mg/ml (equivalent to 45 mg/ml oxycodone)

For excipients, see Section 6.1

3. PHARMACEUTICAL FORM

Solution for injection or infusion.

4. CLINICAL PARTICULARS

4.1 Therapeutic indications

For the treatment of moderate to severe pain in patients with cancer and post-operative pain. For the treatment of severe pain requiring the use of a strong opioid.

4.2 Posology and method of administration

Route of administration:

Subcutaneous injection or infusion

Intravenous injection or infusion.

Posology:

The dose should be adjusted according to the severity of pain, the total condition of the patient and previous or concurrent medication.

Adults over 18 years:

The following starting doses are recommended. A gradual increase in dose may be required if analgesia is inadequate or if pain severity increases.

i.v. (Bolus): Dilute in 0.9% saline, 5% dextrose or water for injections. Administer a bolus dose of 1 to 10 mg slowly over 1-2 minutes in opioid naïve patients.

Doses should not be administered more frequently than every 4 hours.

i.v. (Infusion): Dilute in 0.9% saline, 5% dextrose or water for injections. A starting dose of 2 mg/hour is recommended for opioid naïve patients.

i.v. (PCA): Dilute in 0.9% saline, 5% dextrose or water for injections. Bolus doses of 0.03 mg/kg should be administered with a minimum lock-out time of 5 minutes for opioid naïve patients.

s.c. (Bolus): Dilute in 0.9% saline, 5% dextrose or water for injections. A starting dose of 5 mg is recommended, repeated at 4-hourly intervals as required for opioid naïve patients.

s.c. (Infusion): Dilute in 0.9% saline, 5% dextrose or water for injections if required. A starting dose of 7.5 mg/day is recommended in opioid naïve patients, titrating gradually according to symptom control.

Cancer patients transferring from oral oxycodone may require much higher doses (see below).

Transferring patients between oral and parenteral oxycodone:

The dose should be based on the following ratio: 2 mg of oral oxycodone is equivalent to 1 mg of parenteral oxycodone. It must be emphasised that this is a guide to the dose required. Inter-patient variability requires that each patient is carefully titrated to the appropriate dose.

Elderly:

Elderly patients should be treated with caution. The lowest dose should be administered with careful titration to pain control.

Patients with renal and hepatic impairment:

Patients with mild to moderate renal impairment and/or mild hepatic impairment should be treated with caution. The lowest dose should be given with careful titration to pain control.

Children under 18 years:

There are no data on the use of ***OxyNorm*** injection in patients under 18 years of age.

Use in non-malignant pain:

Opioids are not first-line therapy for chronic non-malignant pain, nor are they recommended as the only treatment. Types of chronic pain which have been shown to be alleviated by strong opioids include chronic osteoarthritic pain and intervertebral disc disease. The need for continued treatment in non-malignant pain should be assessed at regular intervals

Cessation of therapy:

When a patient no longer requires therapy with oxycodone, it may be advisable to taper the dose gradually to prevent symptoms of withdrawal.

4.3 Contraindications

OxyNorm injection is contraindicated in patients with known hypersensitivity to oxycodone or any of the other constituents, or in any situation where opioids are contraindicated; respiratory depression; head injury; paralytic ileus; acute abdomen; chronic obstructive airways disease; cor pulmonale; chronic bronchial asthma; hypercarbia; moderate to severe hepatic impairment; severe renal impairment (creatinine clearance <10 ml/min); chronic constipation; concurrent administration of monoamine oxidase inhibitors or within 2 weeks of discontinuation of their use; pregnancy.

4.4 Special warnings and precautions for use

The major risk of opioid excess is respiratory depression. As with all opioids, a reduction in dosage may be advisable in hypothyroidism. Use with caution in patients with raised intracranial pressure, hypotension, hypovolaemia, toxic psychoses, diseases of the biliary tract, inflammatory bowel disorders, prostatic hypertrophy, adrenocortical insufficiency, acute alcoholism, delirium tremens, pancreatitis, chronic renal and hepatic disease or severe pulmonary disease and debilitated, elderly and infirm patients. ***OxyNorm*** injection should not be used where there is a possibility of paralytic ileus occurring. Should paralytic ileus be suspected or occur during use, ***OxyNorm*** injection should be discontinued immediately.

The patient may develop tolerance to oxycodone with chronic use and require progressively higher doses to maintain pain control. The patient may develop physical dependence, in which case an abstinence syndrome may be seen following abrupt cessation.

For appropriate patients who suffer with chronic non-malignant pain, opioids should be used as part of a comprehensive treatment programme involving other medications and treatment modalities. A crucial part of the assessment of a patient with chronic non-malignant pain is the patient's addiction and substance abuse history. ***OxyNorm*** injection should be used with particular care in patients with a history of alcohol and drug abuse.

If opioid treatment is considered appropriate for the patient, then the main aim of treatment is not to minimise the dose of opioid but rather to achieve a dose which provides adequate pain relief with a minimum of side effects. There must be frequent contact between physician and patient so that dosage adjustments can be made. It is strongly recommended that the physician defines treatment outcomes in accordance with pain management guidelines. The physician and patient can then agree to discontinue treatment if these objectives are not met.

Oxycodone has an abuse liability similar to other strong opioids and should be used with caution in opioid-dependent patients. Oxycodone may be sought and abused by people with latent or manifest addiction disorders.

As with other opioids, infants who are born to dependent mothers may exhibit withdrawal symptoms and may have respiratory depression at birth.

4.5 Interaction with other medicinal products and other forms of interaction

There is an enhanced CNS depressant effect with drugs such as tranquillisers, anaesthetics, hypnotics, anti-depressants, sedatives, phenothiazines, neuroleptic drugs, alcohol, other opioids, muscle relaxants and antihypertensives. Monoamine oxidase inhibitors are known to interact with narcotic analgesics, producing CNS excitation or depression with hypertensive or hypotensive crisis.

Oxycodone is metabolised in part via the CYP2D6 and CYP3A4 pathways. While these pathways may be blocked by a variety of drugs, such blockade has not yet been shown to be of clinical significance with this agent.

4.6 Pregnancy and lactation

The effect of oxycodone in human reproduction has not been adequately studied. No studies on fertility or the postnatal effects of intrauterine exposure have been carried out. However, studies in rats and rabbits with oral doses of oxycodone equivalent to 3 and 47 times an adult dose of 160 mg/day, respectively, did not reveal evidence of harm to the foetus due to oxycodone. ***OxyNorm*** injection is not recommended for use in pregnancy nor during labour. Infants born to mothers who have received opioids during pregnancy should be monitored for respiratory depression.

Oxycodone may be secreted in breast milk and may cause respiratory depression in the newborn. Oxycodone should therefore not be used in breast-feeding mothers.

4.7 Effects on ability to drive and use machines

Oxycodone may modify patients' reactions to a varying extent depending on the dosage and individual susceptibility. Therefore patients should not drive or operate machinery, if affected.

4.8 Undesirable effects

Adverse drug reactions are typical of full opioid agonists. Tolerance and dependence may occur (see Tolerance and Dependence, below). Constipation may be prevented with an appropriate laxative. If nausea or vomiting are troublesome, oxycodone may be combined with an antiemetic.

Common (incidence of ≥ 1%) and uncommon (incidence of ≤ 1%) adverse drug reactions to oxycodone are listed in the table below.

Body System	Common	Uncommon
Gastrointestinal	Constipation	Biliary spasm
	Nausea	Hepatic enzyme increased.
	Vomiting	Dysphagia
	Dry mouth	Eructation
	Anorexia	Flatulence
	Dyspepsia	Gastrointestinal disorders
	Abdominal pain	Ileus
	Diarrhoea	Taste perversion
		Gastritis
		Hiccups
Central Nervous System	Headache	Vertigo
	Confusion	Hallucinations
	Asthenia	Disorientation
	Faintness	Mood changes
	Dizziness	Restlessness
	Sedation	Agitation

	Anxiety	Depression
	Abnormal dreams	Tremor
	Nervousness	Withdrawal syndrome
	Insomnia	Amnesia
	Thought abnormalities	Hypoaesthesia
	Drowsiness	Hypertonia
	Twitching	Hypotonia
		Malaise
		Paraesthesia
		Speech disorder
		Euphoria
		Dysphoria
		Seizure
		Vision abnormalities
Genitourinary		Urinary retention
		Ureteric spasm
		Impotence
		Amenorrhoea
		Decreased libido
Cardiovascular	Orthostatic hypotension	Palpitations
		Supraventricular tachycardia
		Hypotension
		Syncope
		Vasodilation
Metabolic and Nutritional		Dehydration
		Oedema
		Peripheral oedema
		Thirst
Respiratory	Bronchospasm	Overdose may produce respiratory depression
	Dyspnoea	
	Decreased cough reflex	
Dermatological	Rash	Dry skin
	Pruritus	Exfoliative dermatitis
		Urticaria
General	Sweating	Facial flushing
	Chills	Miosis
		Allergic reaction
		Fever
		Anaphylaxis

Tolerance and Dependence:

The patient may develop tolerance to the drug with chronic use and require progressively higher doses to maintain pain control. Prolonged use of ***OxyNorm*** injection may lead to physical dependence and a withdrawal syndrome may occur upon abrupt cessation of therapy. When a patient no longer requires therapy with oxycodone, it may be advisable to taper the dose gradually to prevent symptoms of withdrawal. The opioid abstinence or withdrawal syndrome is characterised by some or all of the following: restlessness, lacrimation, rhinorrhoea, yawning, perspiration, chills, myalgia and mydriasis. Other symptoms also may develop, including: irritability, anxiety, backache, joint pain, weakness, abdominal cramps, insomnia, nausea, anorexia, vomiting, diarrhoea, or increased blood pressure, respiratory rate or heart rate.

OxyNorm injection should be used with particular care in patients with a history of alcohol and drug abuse.

4.9 Overdose

Symptoms of overdosage

Signs of oxycodone toxicity and overdosage are pin-point pupils, respiratory depression, hypotension and hallucinations. Nausea and vomiting are common in less severe cases. Non-cardiac pulmonary oedema and rhabdomyolysis are particularly common after intravenous injection of opioid analgesics. Circulatory failure and somnolence progressing to stupor or coma, skeletal muscle flaccidity, bradycardia and death may occur in more severe cases.

The effects of overdosage will be potentiated by the simultaneous ingestion of alcohol or other psychotropic drugs.

Treatment of overdosage

Primary attention should be given to the establishment of a patent airway and institution of assisted or controlled ventilation.

In the case of massive overdosage, administer naloxone intravenously (0.4 to 2mg for an adult and 0.01mg/kg body weight for children) if the patient is in a coma or respiratory depression is present. Repeat the dose at 2 minute intervals if there is no response. If repeated doses are required then an infusion of 60% of the initial dose per hour is a useful starting point. A solution of 10 mg made up in 50 ml dextrose will produce 200 micrograms/ml for infusion using an IV pump (dose adjusted to the clinical response). Infusions are not a substitute for frequent review of the patient's clinical state.

Intramuscular naloxone is an alternative in the event that IV access is not possible. As the duration of action of naloxone is relatively short, the patient must be carefully monitored until spontaneous respiration is reliably re-established. Naloxone is a competitive antagonist and large doses (4 mg) may be required in seriously poisoned patients.

For less severe overdosage, administer naloxone 0.2 mg intravenously followed by increments of 0.1 mg every 2 minutes if required.

The patient should be observed for at least 6 hours after the last dose of naloxone.

Naloxone should not be administered in the absence of clinically significant respiratory or circulatory depression secondary to oxycodone overdosage. Naloxone should be administered cautiously to persons who are known, or suspected, to be physically dependent on oxycodone. In such cases, an abrupt or complete reversal of opioid effects may precipitate pain and an acute withdrawal syndrome.

5. PHARMACOLOGICAL PROPERTIES

5.1 Pharmacodynamic properties

Pharmacotherapeutic group: Natural opium alkaloids

ATC code: N02A A05

Oxycodone is a full opioid agonist with no antagonist properties. It has an affinity for kappa, mu and delta opioid receptors in the brain and spinal cord. Oxycodone is similar to morphine in its action. The therapeutic effect is mainly analgesic, anxiolytic, antitussive and sedative.

Opioids may influence the hypothalamic-pituitary-adrenal or gonadal axes. Some changes that can be seen include an increase in serum prolactin and decreases in plasma cortisol and testosterone. Clinical symptoms may be manifest from these hormonal changes.

In vitro and animal studies indicate various effects of natural opioids, such as morphine, on components of the immune system; the clinical significance of these findings is unknown. Whether oxycodone, a semisynthetic opioid, has immunological effects similar to morphine is unknown.

5.2 Pharmacokinetic properties

Pharmacokinetic studies in healthy subjects demonstrated an equivalent availability of oxycodone from ***OxyNorm*** injection when administered as a 5 mg dose by the intravenous and subcutaneous routes, as a single bolus dose or a continuous infusion over 8 hours.

Following absorption, oxycodone is distributed throughout the entire body. Approximately 45% is bound to plasma protein. It is metabolised in the liver to produce noroxycodone, oxymorphone and various conjugated glucuronides. The analgesic effects of the metabolites are clinically insignificant. The active drug and its metabolites are excreted in both urine and faeces.

The plasma concentrations of oxycodone are only minimally affected by age, being 15% greater in elderly as compared to young subjects.

Female subjects have, on average, plasma oxycodone concentrations up to 25% higher than males on a body weight adjusted basis.

The drug penetrates the placenta and can be found in breast milk.

When compared to normal subjects, patients with mild to severe hepatic dysfunction may have higher plasma concentrations of oxycodone and noroxycodone, and lower plasma concentrations of oxymorphone. There may be an increase in the elimination half-life of oxycodone and this may be accompanied by an increase in drug effects.

When compared to normal subjects, patients with mild to severe renal dysfunction may have higher plasma concentrations of oxycodone and its metabolites. There may be an increase in the elimination half-life of oxycodone and this may be accompanied by an increase in drug effects.

5.3 Preclinical safety data

Non-clinical data reveal no special hazard for humans based on conventional studies of safety pharmacology, repeated dose toxicity, and genotoxicity.

Teratogenicity

Oxycodone had no effect on fertility or early embryonic development in male and female rats at doses as high as 8 mg/kg/d. Also, oxycodone did not induce any deformities in rats at doses as high as 8 mg/kg/d or in rabbits at doses as high as 125 mg/kg/d. Dose-related increases in developmental variations (increased incidences of extra (27) presacral vertebrae and extra pairs of ribs) were observed in rabbits when the data for individual fetuses were analyzed. However, when the same data were analyzed using litters as opposed to individual fetuses, there was no dose-related increase in developmental variations although the incidence of extra presacral vertebrae remained significantly higher in the 125 mg/kg/d group compared to the control group. Since this dose level was associated with severe pharmacotoxic effects in the pregnant animals, the fetal findings may have been a secondary consequence of severe maternal toxicity.

In a study of peri- and postnatal development in rats, maternal body weight and food intake parameters were reduced for doses ⩾ 2 mg/kg/d compared to the control group. Body weights were lower in the F1 generation from maternal rats in the 6 mg/kg/d dosing group. There were no effects on physical, reflexological, or sensory developmental parameters or on behavioural and reproductive indices in the F1 pups (the NOEL for F1 pups was 2 mg/kg/d based on body weight effects seen at 6 mg/kg/d). There were no effects on the F2 generation at any dose in the study.

Mutagenicity

The results of *in vitro* and *in vivo* studies indicate that the genotoxic risk of OxyNorm to humans is minimal or absent at the systemic oxycodone concentrations that are achieved therapeutically.

Oxycodone was not genotoxic in a bacterial mutagenicity assay or in an in vivo micronucleus assay in the mouse. Oxycodone produced a positive response in the in vitro mouse lymphoma assay in the presence of rat liver S9 metabolic activation at dose levels greater than 25 µg/mL. Two in vitro chromosomal aberrations assays with human lymphocytes were conducted. In the first assay, oxycodone was negative without metabolic activation but was positive with S9 metabolic activation at the 24 hour time point but not at other time points or at 48 hour after exposure. In the second assay, oxycodone did not show any clastogenicity either with or without metabolic activation at any concentration or time point.

No animal studies to evaluate the carcinogenic potential of oxycodone have been conducted.

6. PHARMACEUTICAL PARTICULARS

6.1 List of excipients

Citric acid monohydrate

Sodium citrate

Sodium chloride

Hydrochloric acid, dilute

Sodium hydroxide

Water for injections

6.2 Incompatibilities

This medicinal product must not be mixed with other medicinal products except those mentioned in section 6.6.

Cyclizine at concentrations of 3 mg/ml or less, when mixed with ***OxyNorm*** injection, either undiluted or diluted with water for injections, shows no sign of precipitation over a period of 24 hours storage at room temperature. Precipitation has been shown to occur in mixtures with ***OxyNorm*** injection at cyclizine concentrations greater than 3 mg/ml or when diluted with 0.9% saline. However, if the dose of OxyNorm injection is reduced and the solution is sufficiently diluted with Water for Injections, concentrations greater than 3 mg/ml are possible. It is recommended that Water for Injections be used as a diluent when cyclizine and oxycodone hydrochloride are co-administered either intravenously or subcutaneously as an infusion.

Prochlorperazine is chemically incompatible with ***OxyNorm*** injection.

6.3 Shelf life

3 years unopened.

After opening use immediately.

For further information see Section 6.6.

6.4 Special precautions for storage

No special precautions for storage prior to opening.

For further information on use after opening see Section 6.6.

6.5 Nature and contents of container

Clear glass ampoules: 1 ml

Pack size: 5 ampoules.

6.6 Special precautions for disposal and other handling

The injection should be given immediately after opening the ampoule. Once opened, any unused portion should be discarded. Chemical and physical in-use stability has been demonstrated for 24 hours at room temperature.

From a microbiological point of view, the product should be used immediately. If not used immediately, in-use storage times and conditions prior to use are the responsibility of the user and would normally not be longer than 24 hours at 2 to 8°C, unless reconstitution, dilution, etc has taken place in controlled and validated aseptic conditions.

No evidence of incompatibility was observed between ***OxyNorm*** injection and representative bands of injectable forms of the following drugs, when stored in high and low dose combinations in polypropylene syringes over a 24 hour period at ambient temperature.

Hyoscine butylbromide

Hyoscine hydrobromide

Dexamethasone sodium phosphate

Haloperidol

Midazolam hydrochloride

Metoclopramide hydrochloride

Levomepromazine hydrochloride

Glycopyrronium bromide

Ketamine hydrochloride

OxyNorm 50 mg/ml injection, undiluted or diluted to 3 mg/ml with 0.9% w/v saline, 5% w/v dextrose or water for injections, is physically and chemically stable when in contact with representative brands of polypropylene or polycarbonate syringes, polyethylene or PVC tubing, and PVC or EVA infusion bags, over a 24 hour period at room temperature (25°C).

The 50 mg/ml injection, whether undiluted or diluted to 3 mg/ml in the infusion fluids used in these studies and contained in the various assemblies, does not need to be protected from light.

Inappropriate handling of the undiluted solution after opening of the original ampoule, or of the diluted solutions may compromise the sterility of the product.

7. MARKETING AUTHORISATION HOLDER

Napp Pharmaceuticals Ltd

Cambridge Science Park

Milton Road

Cambridge CB4 0GW

8. MARKETING AUTHORISATION NUMBER(S)

PL 16950/0155

9. DATE OF FIRST AUTHORISATION/RENEWAL OF THE AUTHORISATION

14/01/2009

10. DATE OF REVISION OF THE TEXT

14/01/2009

OxyNorm liquid and OxyNorm concentrate

(Napp Pharmaceuticals Limited)

1. NAME OF THE MEDICINAL PRODUCT

OxyNorm® liquid 5 mg/5 ml

OxyNorm® concentrate 10 mg/ml

2. QUALITATIVE AND QUANTITATIVE COMPOSITION

Each 5 ml ***OxyNorm*** liquid contains oxycodone base 4.5 mg as oxycodone hydrochloride 5 mg.

Each 1 ml ***OxyNorm*** concentrate contains oxycodone base 9 mg as oxycodone hydrochloride 10 mg.

For excipients, see section 6.1.

3. PHARMACEUTICAL FORM

OxyNorm liquid is a clear colourless/straw-coloured solution.

OxyNorm concentrate is a clear orange solution.

4. CLINICAL PARTICULARS

4.1 Therapeutic indications

For the treatment of moderate to severe pain in patients with cancer and post-operative pain.

For the treatment of severe pain requiring the use of a strong opioid.

4.2 Posology and method of administration

Route of administration:

Oral

Post-operative pain:

In common with other strong opioids, the need for continued treatment should be assessed at regular intervals.

Elderly and adults over 18 years:

OxyNorm liquids should be taken at 4-6 hourly intervals. The dosage is dependent on the severity of the pain, and the patient's previous history of analgesic requirements.

Increasing severity of pain will require an increased dosage of ***OxyNorm*** liquids. The correct dosage for any individual patient is that which controls the pain and is well tolerated throughout the dosing period. Patients should be titrated to pain relief unless unmanageable adverse drug reactions prevent this.

The usual starting dose for opioid naïve patients or patients presenting with severe pain uncontrolled by weaker opioids is 5 mg, 4-6 hourly. The dose should then be carefully titrated, as frequently as once a day if necessary, to achieve pain relief. The majority of patients will not require a daily dose greater than 400 mg. However, a few patients may require higher doses.

Patients receiving oral morphine before oxycodone therapy should have their daily dose based on the following ratio: 10 mg of oral oxycodone is equivalent to 20 mg of oral morphine. It must be emphasised that this is a guide to the dose of ***OxyNorm*** liquids required. Inter-patient variability requires that each patient is carefully titrated to the appropriate dose.

Controlled pharmacokinetic studies in elderly patients (aged over 65 years) have shown that, compared with younger adults, the clearance of oxycodone is only slightly reduced. No untoward adverse drug reactions were seen based on age, therefore adult doses and dosage intervals are appropriate.

Adults with mild to moderate renal impairment and mild hepatic impairment: The plasma concentration in this patient population may be increased. Therefore, dose initiation should follow a conservative approach. The starting dose for opioid naïve patients is 2.5 mg, 6-hourly.

Children under 18 years:

OxyNorm liquids should not be used in patients under 18 years.

Use in non-malignant pain:

Opioids are not first line therapy for chronic non-malignant pain, nor are they recommended as the only treatment. Types of chronic pain which have been shown to be alleviated by strong opioids include chronic osteoarthritic pain and intervertebral disc disease. The need for continued treatment in non-malignant pain should be assessed at regular intervals.

Cessation of therapy:

When a patient no longer requires therapy with oxycodone, it may be advisable to taper the dose gradually to prevent symptoms of withdrawal.

4.3 Contraindications

Respiratory depression, head injury, paralytic ileus, acute abdomen, delayed gastric emptying, chronic obstructive airways disease, cor pulmonale, chronic bronchial asthma, hypercarbia, known oxycodone sensitivity or in any situation where opioids are contra-indicated, moderate to severe hepatic impairment, severe renal impairment (creatinine clearance $<$ 10 ml/min), chronic constipation, concurrent administration of monoamine oxidase inhibitors or within 2 weeks of discontinuation of their use, pregnancy and lactation, hypersensitivity to any of the constituents of the product.

4.4 Special warnings and precautions for use

The major risk of opioid excess is respiratory depression. As with all narcotics, a reduction in dosage may be advisable in hypothyroidism. Use with caution in opioid dependent patients and in patients with raised intracranial pressure, hypotension, hypovolaemia, toxic psychosis, diseases of the biliary tract, pancreatitis, inflammatory bowel disorders, prostatic hypertrophy, adrenocortical insufficiency, acute alcoholism, delirium tremens, chronic renal and hepatic disease, or severe pulmonary disease and debilitated, elderly and infirm patients. ***OxyNorm*** liquids should not be used where there is a possibility of paralytic ileus occurring. Should paralytic ileus be suspected or occur during use, ***OxyNorm*** liquids should be discontinued immediately. As with all opioid preparations, patients about to undergo additional pain relieving procedures (e.g. surgery, plexus blockade) should not receive ***OxyNorm*** liquids for 6 hours prior to the intervention. If further treatment with oxycodone is indicated then the dosage should be adjusted to the new post-operative requirement.

Oxycodone should be used with caution following abdominal surgery as opioids are known to impair intestinal motility and should not be used until the physician is assured of normal bowel function.

For appropriate patients who suffer with chronic non-malignant pain, opioids should be used as part of a comprehensive treatment programme involving other medications and treatment modalities. A crucial part of the assessment of a patient with chronic non-malignant pain is the patient's addiction and substance abuse history. There is potential for development of psychological dependence (addiction) to opioid analgesics, including oxycodone. ***OxyNorm*** liquids, like all opioids, should be used with particular care in patients with a history of alcohol and drug abuse.

If opioid treatment is considered appropriate for the patient, then the main aim of treatment is not to minimise the dose of opioid but rather to achieve a dose which provides adequate pain relief with a minimum of side effects. There must be frequent contact between physician and patient so that dosage adjustments can be made. It is strongly recommended that the physician defines treatment outcomes in accordance with pain management guidelines. The physician and patient can then agree to discontinue treatment if these objectives are not met.

Sunset yellow, a constituent of ***OxyNorm*** concentrate, can cause allergic-type reactions such as asthma. This is more common in people who are allergic to aspirin.

Both ***OxyNorm*** liquid and ***OxyNorm*** concentrate contain the preservative sodium benzoate. This is a mild irritant to the skin, eyes and mucous membrane.

Oxycodone has an abuse profile similar to other strong opioids. Oxycodone may be sought and abused by people with latent or manifest addiction disorders.

As with other opioids, infants who are born to dependent mothers may exhibit withdrawal symptoms and may have respiratory depression at birth.

Abuse of oral dosage forms by parenteral administration can be expected to result in serious adverse events, which may be fatal.

4.5 Interaction with other medicinal products and other forms of interaction

Oxycodone, like other opioids, potentiates the effects of tranquillisers, anaesthetics, hypnotics, anti-depressants, sedatives, phenothiazines, neuroleptic drugs, alcohol, other opioids, muscle relaxants and antihypertensives. Monoamine oxidase inhibitors are known to interact with narcotic analgesics, producing CNS excitation or depression with hypertensive or hypotensive crisis. Concurrent administration of quinidine, an inhibitor of cytochrome P450-2D6 with a modified release oxycodone tablet, resulted in an increase in oxycodone C_{max} by 11%, AUC by 13%, and $t_{½}$ elim. by 14%. Also an increase in noroxycodone level was observed, (C_{max} by 50%, AUC by 85%, and $t_{½}$ elim. by 42%). The pharmacodynamic effects of oxycodone were not altered. This interaction may be observed for other potent inhibitors of cytochrome P450-2D6 enzyme. Cimetidine and inhibitors of cytochrome P450-3A4 such as ketoconazole and erythromycin may inhibit the metabolism of oxycodone.

4.6 Pregnancy and lactation

OxyNorm liquids are not recommended for use in pregnancy nor during labour. Infants born to mothers who have received opioids during pregnancy should be monitored for respiratory depression.

Oxycodone may be secreted in breast milk and may cause respiratory depression in the newborn. ***OxyNorm*** liquids should, therefore, not be used in breast-feeding mothers.

4.7 Effects on ability to drive and use machines

Oxycodone may modify patients' reactions to a varying extent depending on the dosage and individual susceptibility. Therefore patients should not drive or operate machinery if affected.

4.8 Undesirable effects

Adverse drug reactions are typical of full opioid agonists. Tolerance and dependence may occur (see *Tolerance and Dependence*, below). Constipation may be prevented with an appropriate laxative. If nausea and vomiting are troublesome, oxycodone may be combined with an anti-emetic.

Common (incidence of $\geqslant$ 1%) and uncommon (incidence of $\leqslant$ 1%) adverse drug reactions are listed in the table below.

Body System	Common	Uncommon
Immune system disorders		Anaphylactic reaction
		Anaphylactoid reaction
		Hypersensitivity
Metabolism and nutritional disorders	Anorexia	Dehydration
Psychiatric disorders	Anxiety	Affect lability
	Confusional state	Agitation
	Insomnia	Depression
	Nervousness	Drug dependence
	Thinking disturbances	Euphoria
	Abnormal dreams	Hallucinations
		Disorientation
		Mood altered
		Restlessness
		Dysphoria
Nervous system disorders	Headache	Amnesia
	Dizziness	Hypertonia
	Sedation	Tremor
	Somnolence	Hypoaesthesia
		Hypotonia
		Paraesthesia
		Speech disorder
		Convulsions

		Muscle contractions involuntary
		Taste perversion
		Syncope
Eye disorders		Miosis
		Visual disturbance
Ear and labyrinth disorders		Vertigo
Cardiac disorders		Supraventricular tachycardia
Vascular disorders		Hypotension
		Orthostatic hypotension
		Vasodilatation
		Facial flushing
Respiratory, thoracic and mediastinal disorders	Bronchospasm	Respiratory depression
	Dyspnoea	Hiccups
	Cough decreased	
Gastrointestinal disorders	Constipation	Dysphagia
	Nausea	Eructation
	Vomiting	Flatulence
	Dry mouth	Gastrointestinal disorders
	Dyspepsia	Ileus
	Abdominal pain	Gastritis
	Diarrhoea	
Hepato-biliary disorders		Biliary colic
		Increased hepatic enzymes
Skin and subcutaneous tissue disorders	Hyperhidrosis	Dry skin
	Pruritus	Exfoliative dermatitis
	Rash	Urticaria
Musculoskeletal and connective tissue disorders		Muscular rigidity
Renal and urinary disorders		Urinary retention
		Ureteral spasm
Reproductive system and breast disorders		Amenorrhoea
		Libido decreased
		Erectile dysfunction
General disorders and administration site conditions	Asthenia	Drug tolerance
	Chills	Oedema
		Oedema peripheral
		Malaise
		Thirst
		Pyrexia
		Drug withdrawal syndrome

Tolerance and Dependence:

The patient may develop tolerance to the drug with chronic use and require progressively higher doses to maintain pain control. Prolonged use of ***OxyNorm*** liquids may lead to physical dependence and a withdrawal syndrome may occur upon abrupt cessation of therapy. When a patient no longer requires therapy with oxycodone, it may be advisable to taper the dose gradually to prevent symptoms of withdrawal. The opioid abstinence or withdrawal syndrome is characterised by some or all of the following: restlessness, lacrimation, rhinorrhoea, yawning, perspiration, chills, myalgia, mydriasis and palpitations. Other symptoms also may develop, including: irritability, anxiety, backache, joint pain, weakness, abdominal cramps, insomnia, nausea, anorexia, vomiting, diarrhoea, or increased blood pressure, respiratory rate or heart rate.

4.9 Overdose

Signs of oxycodone toxicity and overdosage are pin-point pupils, respiratory depression and hypotension. Circulatory failure and somnolence progressing to stupor or deepening coma, skeletal muscle flaccidity, bradycardia and death may occur in more severe cases.

Treatment of oxycodone overdosage: Primary attention should be given to the establishment of a patent airway and institution of assisted or controlled ventilation.

In the case of massive overdosage, administer naloxone intravenously (0.4 to 2 mg for an adult and 0.01 mg/kg body weight for children), if the patient is in a coma or respiratory depression is present. Repeat the dose at 2 minute intervals if there is no response. If repeated doses are required then an infusion of 60% of the initial dose per hour is a useful starting point. A solution of 10 mg made up in 50 ml dextrose will produce 200 micrograms/ml for infusion using an IV pump (dose adjusted to the clinical response). Infusions are not a substitute for frequent review of the patient's clinical state. Intramuscular naloxone is an alternative in the event IV access is not possible. As the duration of action of naloxone is relatively short, the patient must be carefully monitored until spontaneous respiration is reliably established. Naloxone is a competitive antagonist and large doses (4 mg) may be required in seriously poisoned patients.

For less severe overdosage, administer naloxone 0.2 mg intravenously followed by increments of 0.1 mg every 2 minutes if required.

Naloxone should not be administered in the absence of clinically significant respiratory or circulatory depression secondary to oxycodone overdosage. Naloxone should be administered cautiously to persons who are known, or suspected, to be physically dependent on oxycodone. In such cases, an abrupt or complete reversal of opioid effects may precipitate pain and an acute withdrawal syndrome.

Additional/other considerations:

- Consider activated charcoal (50 g for adults, 10 -15 g for children), if a substantial amount has been ingested within 1 hour, provided the airway can be protected.
- Gastric contents may need to be emptied as this can be useful in removing unabsorbed drug.

5. PHARMACOLOGICAL PROPERTIES

5.1 Pharmacodynamic properties

Pharmacotherapeutic group: Natural opium alkaloids

ATC code: N02A A05

Oxycodone is a full opioid agonist with no antagonist properties. It has an affinity for kappa, mu and delta opiate receptors in the brain and spinal cord. Oxycodone is similar to morphine in its action. The therapeutic effect is mainly analgesic, anxiolytic and sedative.

5.2 Pharmacokinetic properties

Compared with morphine, which has an absolute bioavailability of approximately 30%, oxycodone has a high absolute bioavailability of up to 87% following oral administration. Oxycodone has an elimination half life of approximately 3-4 hours and is metabolised principally to noroxycodone and oxymorphone. Oxymorphone has some analgesic activity but is present in the plasma at low concentrations and is not considered to contribute to oxycodone's pharmacological effect.

A pharmacokinetic study in healthy volunteers has demonstrated that, following administration of a single 10 mg dose, ***OxyNorm*** liquid 5 mg/5 ml and ***OxyNorm*** concentrate 10 mg/ml provided an equivalent rate and extent of absorption of oxycodone. Mean peak plasma concentrations of approximately 20 ng/ml were achieved within 1.5 hours of administration, median t_{max} values from both strengths of liquid being less than one hour.

Studies involving controlled release oxycodone have demonstrated that the oral bioavailability of oxycodone is only slightly increased (16%) in the elderly. In patients with renal and hepatic impairment, the bioavailability of oxycodone was increased by 60% and 90% respectively, and a reduced initial dose is recommended in these groups.

5.3 Preclinical safety data

Oxycodone was not mutagenic in the following assays: Ames Salmonella and E. Coli test with and without metabolic activation at doses of up to 5000 μg, chromosomal aberration test in human lymphocytes (in the absence of metabolic activation and with activation after 48 hours of exposure) at doses of up to 1500 μg/ml, and in the *in vivo* bone marrow micronucleus assay in mice (at plasma levels of up to 48 μg/ml). Mutagenic results occurred in the presence of metabolic activation in the human chromosomal aberration test (at greater than or equal to 1250 μg/ml) at 24 but not 48 hours of exposure and in the mouse lymphoma assay at doses of 50 μg/ml or greater with metabolic activation and at 400 μg/ml or greater without metabolic activation. The data from these tests indicate that the genotoxic risk to humans may be considered low. Studies of oxycodone in animals to evaluate its carcinogenic potential have not been conducted owing to the length of clinical experience with the drug substance.

6. PHARMACEUTICAL PARTICULARS

6.1 List of excipients

Saccharin sodium

Sodium benzoate

Citric acid monohydrate

Sodium citrate

Hydrochloric acid

Sodium hydroxide

Purified water

In addition, ***OxyNorm*** liquid contains hypromellose and ***OxyNorm*** concentrate contains Sunset Yellow (E110).

6.2 Incompatibilities

Not applicable.

6.3 Shelf life

Four years

6.4 Special precautions for storage

Do not store above 30°C

6.5 Nature and contents of container

OxyNorm liquid is supplied in 250 ml amber glass bottles with polyethylene/polypropylene screw caps. ***OxyNorm*** concentrate is supplied in 120 ml amber glass bottles with polyethylene/polypropylene caps. A graduated dropper or an oral syringe is also supplied with ***OxyNorm*** concentrate.

6.6 Special precautions for disposal and other handling

OxyNorm concentrate may be mixed with a soft drink for ease of administration and to improve palatability.

7. MARKETING AUTHORISATION HOLDER

Napp Pharmaceuticals Ltd

Cambridge Science Park

Milton Road

Cambridge CB4 0GW

8. MARKETING AUTHORISATION NUMBER(S)

PL 16950/0003, 4

9. DATE OF FIRST AUTHORISATION/RENEWAL OF THE AUTHORISATION

9th December 1999/ 25 June 2005

10. DATE OF REVISION OF THE TEXT

July 2008

11 LEGAL CATEGORY

CD (Sch 2) POM

Pabal 100 micrograms in 1ml solution for injection

(Ferring Pharmaceuticals Ltd)

1. NAME OF THE MEDICINAL PRODUCT

PABAL ▼ 100 micrograms/ml solution for injection

2. QUALITATIVE AND QUANTITATIVE COMPOSITION

Carbetocin 100 micrograms/ml.

Oxytocic activity: approximately 50 IU of oxytocin/ ampoule

For a full list of excipients, see section 6.1.

3. PHARMACEUTICAL FORM

Solution for injection.

A clear colourless solution.

4. CLINICAL PARTICULARS

4.1 Therapeutic indications

PABAL is indicated for the prevention of uterine atony following delivery of the infant by Caesarean section under epidural or spinal anaesthesia.

4.2 Posology and method of administration

Withdraw 1 ml of PABAL containing 100 micrograms carbetocin and administer only by intravenous injection, under adequate medical supervision in a hospital.

PABAL must be administered only after delivery of the infant by Caesarean section. It should be given as soon as possible after delivery, preferably before removal of the placenta. PABAL is intended for single use only. No further doses of carbetocin should be administered.

4.3 Contraindications

- During pregnancy and labour before delivery of the infant.
- Carbetocin must not be used for the induction of labour.
- Hypersensitivity to carbetocin, oxytocin or to any of the excipients.
- Hepatic or renal disease.
- Cases of pre-eclampsia and eclampsia.
- Serious cardiovascular disorders.
- Epilepsy.

4.4 Special warnings and precautions for use

Carbetocin is intended for use only at well equipped specialist obstetrics units with experienced and qualified staff available at all times.

The use of carbetocin at any stage before delivery of the infant is not appropriate because its uterotonic activity persists for several hours after a single bolus injection. This is in marked contrast to the rapid reduction of effect observed after discontinuation of an oxytocin infusion.

In case of persistent uterine bleeding after administration of carbetocin the cause must be determined. Consideration should be given to causes such as retained placental fragments, inadequate emptying or repair of the uterus, or disorders of blood coagulation.

Carbetocin is intended for single administration only. In case of persisting uterine hypotonia or atonia and the consequent excessive bleeding, additional therapy with oxytocin and/or ergometrine should be considered. There are no data on additional doses of carbetocin or on the use of carbetocin following persisting uterine atony after oxytocin.

Animal studies have shown carbetocin to possess some antidiuretic activity (vasopressin activity: <0,025 IU/ampoule) and therefore the possibility of hyponatraemia cannot be excluded, particularly in patients also receiving large volumes of intravenous fluids. The early signs of drowsiness, listlessness and headache should be recognised to prevent convulsions and coma.

In general, carbetocin should be used cautiously in the presence of migraine, asthma and cardiovascular disease or any state in which a rapid addition to extracellular water may produce hazard for an already overburdened system. The decision of administering carbetocin can be made by the physician after carefully weighing the potential benefit carbetocin may provide in these particular cases.

Specific studies have not been undertaken in gestational diabetes mellitus.

The efficacy of carbetocin has not been assessed following vaginal delivery.

4.5 Interaction with other medicinal products and other forms of interaction

During clinical trials, carbetocin has been administered in association with a number of analgesics, spasmolytics and agents used for epidural or spinal anaesthesia, and no drug interactions have been identified. Specific interaction studies have not been undertaken.

Since carbetocin is closely related in structure to oxytocin, the occurrence of interactions known to be associated with oxytocin cannot be excluded:

Severe hypertension has been reported when oxytocin was given 3 to 4 hours following prophylactic administration of a vasoconstrictor in conjunction with caudal-block anaesthesia.

During combination with ergot-alkaloids, such as methylergometrine, oxytocin and carbetocin may enhance the blood pressure enhancing effect of these agents. If oxytocin or methylergometrine are administered after carbetocin there may be a risk of cumulative exposure.

Since it has been found that prostaglandins potentiate the effect of oxytocin, it is expected that this can also occur with carbetocin. Therefore, it is not recommended that prostaglandins and carbetocin be used together. If they are concomitantly administered, the patient should be carefully monitored.

Some inhalation-anesthetics, such as halothane and cyclopropane may enhance the hypotensive effect and weaken the effect of carbetocin on the uterus. Arrhythmias have been reported for oxytocin during concomitant use.

4.6 Pregnancy and lactation

Carbetocin is contraindicated during pregnancy and must not be used for the induction of labour (see section 4.3).

No significant effects on milk let-down have been reported during clinical trials. Small amounts of carbetocin have been shown to pass from plasma into breast milk of nursing women (see section 5.2). The small amounts transferred into colostrum or breast milk after a single injection of carbetocin, and subsequently ingested by the infant are assumed to be degraded by enzymes in the gut.

4.7 Effects on ability to drive and use machines

Not relevant.

4.8 Undesirable effects

The adverse events observed with carbetocin during the clinical trials were of the same type and frequency as the adverse events observed with oxytocin when administered after Caesarean section under spinal or epidural anaesthesia.

System Organ Class	Very common ≥ 1/10	Common ≥ 1/100 and < 1/10
Blood and lymphatic system disorders		Anaemia
Nervous system disorders	Headache, tremor	Dizziness
Vascular disorders	Hypotension, flushing	
Respiratory, thoracic and mediastinal disorders		Chest pain, dyspnoea
Gastrointestinal disorders	Nausea, abdominal pain	Metallic taste, vomiting
Skin and subcutaneous tissue disorders	Pruritus	
Musculosceletal and connective tissue disorders		Back pain
General disorders and administration site conditions	Feeling of warmth	Chills, pain

In the clinical trials sweating and tachycardia were reported as sporadic cases.

4.9 Overdose

Overdosage of carbetocin may produce uterine hyperactivity whether or not due to hypersensitivity to this agent.

Hyperstimulation with strong (hypertonic) or prolonged (tetanic) contractions resulting from oxytocin overdose can lead to uterine rupture or postpartum haemorrhage.

Overdosage of oxytocin may lead to hyponatraemia and water intoxication in severe cases, especially when associated with excessive concomitant fluid intake. As carbetocin is an analogue of oxytocin, the possibility of a similar event cannot be excluded.

Treatment of overdosage of carbetocin consists of symptomatic and supportive therapy. When signs or symptoms of overdosage occur oxygen should be given to the mother. In cases of water intoxication it is essential to restrict fluid intake, promote diuresis, correct electrolyte imbalance, and control convulsions that may eventually occur.

5. PHARMACOLOGICAL PROPERTIES

5.1 Pharmacodynamic properties

Pharmacotherapeutic group: Oxytocin and analogues

ATC code: H01BB03

The pharmacological and clinical properties of carbetocin are those of a long acting oxytocin agonist.

Like oxytocin, carbetocin selectively binds to oxytocin receptors in the smooth muscle of the uterus, stimulates rhythmic contractions of the uterus, increases the frequency of existing contractions, and raises the tone of the uterus musculature.

On the postpartum uterus, carbetocin is capable of increasing the rate and force of spontaneous uterine contractions. The onset of uterine contraction following carbetocin is rapid, with a firm contraction being obtained within 2 minutes.

A single 100 micrograms intravenous dose of carbetocin administered after the delivery of the infant is sufficient to maintain adequate uterine contraction that prevents uterine atony and excessive bleeding comparable with an oxytocin infusion lasting for several hours.

5.2 Pharmacokinetic properties

Carbetocin shows a biphasic elimination after intravenous administration with linear pharmacokinetics in the dose range of 400 to 800 micrograms. The terminal elimination half-life is approximately 40 minutes. Renal clearance of the unchanged form is low, with <1% of the injected dose excreted unchanged by the kidney.

In 5 healthy nursing mothers, plasma carbetocin concentrations were detectable by 15 min and peaked at a maximum of 1035 ± 218 pg/ml within 60 min. Peak concentrations in milk were approximately 56 times lower than in plasma at 120 min.

5.3 Preclinical safety data

Non-clinical data reveal no special hazard for humans based on conventional studies of safety pharmacology, repeated dose toxicology and genotoxicity. A reproductive toxicity study in rats, with daily drug administration from parturition to day 21 of lactation, showed a reduction in offspring body weight gain. No other toxic effects were observed. The indication did not warrant studies on fertility or embryotoxicity.

Carcinogenicity studies have not been performed with carbetocin due to the single dose nature of the indication

6. PHARMACEUTICAL PARTICULARS

6.1 List of excipients

Sodium chloride

Glacial acetic acid for pH adjustment

Water for injections.

6.2 Incompatibilities

In the absence of compatibility studies, this medicinal product must not be mixed with other medicinal products.

6.3 Shelf life

2 years.

Shelf life after first opening the container:

After first opening the ampoule: the solution should be used immediately.

6.4 Special precautions for storage

Keep ampoules in the outer carton, in order to protect from light. Store in a refrigerator (2°C to 8°C). Do not freeze.

6.5 Nature and contents of container

Type I glass ampoule with a white identification ring and a blue dot indicating the pre-cut area containing 1 ml of solution for injection.

Packs of 5 ampoules

6.6 Special precautions for disposal and other handling

PABAL is for intravenous use only.

Only clear solutions practically free from particles should be used.

Any unused product or waste material should be disposed of in accordance with local requirements.

7. MARKETING AUTHORISATION HOLDER

Ferring Pharmaceuticals Ltd

The Courtyard

Waterside Drive

Langley

Berkshire

SL3 6EZ

8. MARKETING AUTHORISATION NUMBER(S)

PL 03194/0058

9. DATE OF FIRST AUTHORISATION/RENEWAL OF THE AUTHORISATION

6th October 2002.

10. DATE OF REVISION OF THE TEXT
Feburary 2007

Paclitaxel medac 6 mg/ml concentrate for solution for infusion (medac UK)

(medac GmbH)

1. NAME OF THE MEDICINAL PRODUCT
Paclitaxel medac 6 mg/ml concentrate for solution for infusion

2. QUALITATIVE AND QUANTITATIVE COMPOSITION
1 ml concentrate for solution for infusion contains 6 mg paclitaxel.

One vial of 5 ml contains 30 mg paclitaxel.

One vial of 16.7 ml contains 100 mg paclitaxel.

One vial of 50 ml contains 300 mg paclitaxel.

Excipients:

Macrogolglycerol ricinoleate 527 mg/ml

Ethanol, anhydrous 395 mg/ml

For a full list of excipients, see section 6.1.

3. PHARMACEUTICAL FORM
Concentrate for solution for infusion

Paclitaxel medac is a clear, colourless to light yellowish viscous solution.

4. CLINICAL PARTICULARS

4.1 Therapeutic indications

***Ovarian carcinoma:* For first-line treatment of carcinoma of the ovary,** paclitaxel is indicated in combination with cisplatin in patients with advanced disease or a residual tumour (> 1 cm) following laparotomy.

For second-line treatment of carcinoma of the ovary, paclitaxel is indicated for treatment of metastatic carcinoma of the ovary after failure of standard therapy with platinum-containing preparations.

Breast carcinoma: As adjuvant treatment paclitaxel is indicated in treatment of node-positive breast carcinoma after anthracycline and cyclophosphamide (AC) treatment. Adjuvant treatment with paclitaxel should be considered as an alternative to prolonged AC treatment.

Paclitaxel is indicated as initial treatment of locally advanced or metastatic breast carcinoma either in combination with anthracycline in patients in whom anthracycline treatment is suitable or in combination with trastuzumab, in patients who over-express HER-2 at a level of 3+ as determined by immunohistochemistry methods and to patients to whom anthracycline treatment is not suitable (see sections 4.4 and 5.1).

Paclitaxel is indicated as a single agent for treatment of metastatic breast carcinoma in patients in whom standard anthracycline therapy has failed or in whom anthracycline therapy is not suitable.

Advanced non-small-cell lung carcinoma: Paclitaxel, in combination with cisplatin, is indicated for treatment of non-small-cell lung carcinoma (NSCLC) in patients who are not candidates for potentially curative surgery and/or radiotherapy.

AIDS-related Kaposi's sarcoma: paclitaxel is indicated for the treatment of patients with advanced AIDS-related Kaposi's sarcoma (KS) who have failed prior liposomal anthracycline therapy.

Limited efficacy data supports this indication, a summary of the relevant studies is shown in section 5.1.

4.2 Posology and method of administration
All patients must be premedicated with corticosteroids, antihistamines, and H_2 antagonists prior to paclitaxel therapy, e.g.

Drug	Dose	Administration prior to paclitaxel
dexamethasone	20 mg oral* or i.v.	For oral administration: approximately 12 and 6 hours or for i.v. administration: 30 to 60 minutes
diphenhydramine**	50 mg i.v.	30 - 60 minutes
cimetidine	300 mg i.v.	30 - 60 minutes
or		
ranitidine	50 mg i.v.	30 - 60 minutes

* 8-20 mg for KS patients

** equivalent antihistamine (e.g. chlorpheniramine)

Paclitaxel should be administered through an in-line filter with a microporous membrane ⩽ 0.22 μm (see section 6.6).

First-line treatment of ovarian carcinoma:

Although other dosage regimens are being investigated, a combination regimen of paclitaxel and cisplatin is recommended. Depending on the duration of the infusion, two doses of paclitaxel are recommended: paclitaxel 175 mg/m² administered intravenously over three hours, followed by cisplatin at a dose of 75 mg/m² in three week intervals, or paclitaxel 135 mg/m², as a 24-hour infusion, followed by cisplatin 75 mg/m², with a three-week interval between treatment cycles (see section 5.1).

Second-line treatment of ovarian carcinoma:

The recommended dose for paclitaxel is 175 mg/m² administered over a period of three hours, with a three-week interval between treatment cycles.

Adjuvant chemotherapy of breast carcinoma:

The recommended dose for paclitaxel is 175 mg/m² administered over a period of three hours, with a three-week interval during 4 treatment cycles, after AC treatment.

First-line treatment of breast carcinoma:

When paclitaxel is used in combination with doxorubicin (50 mg/m²), paclitaxel should be administered 24 hours after doxorubicin. The recommended dose for paclitaxel is 220 mg/m² administered intravenously over a period of three hours, with a three-week interval between treatment cycles (see sections 4.5 and 5.1). In combination with trastuzumab, the recommended dose of paclitaxel is 175 mg/m² administered intravenously over a period of three hours, with a three-week interval between treatment cycles (see section 5.1). In combination with trastuzumab the paclitaxel infusion can begin on the day after the first trastuzumab dose or directly after a follow-up dose of trastuzumab if the preceding trastuzumab dose was well tolerated (see the Summary of Product Characteristics of trastuzumab for detailed information on dosing).

Second-line treatment of breast carcinoma:

The recommended dose for paclitaxel is 175 mg/m² administered over a period of three hours, with a three-week interval between treatment cycles.

Treatment of advanced NSCLC:

The recommended dose for paclitaxel is 175 mg/m² administered over a period of three hours, followed by cisplatin 80 mg/m², with a three-week interval between treatment cycles.

Treatment of AIDS-related KS:

The recommended dose of paclitaxel is 100 mg/m² administered as a 3-hour intravenous infusion every two weeks.

The following doses of paclitaxel should be administered according to individual patient tolerance.

Administration of paclitaxel should not be repeated until the neutrophil count is ⩾ 1.5 × 10^9/l (⩾ 1 × 10^9/l for KS patients) and the platelet count is ⩾ 100 × 10^9/l (⩾ 75 × 10^9/l for KS patients). If patients develop severe neutropenia (neutrophils < 0.5 × 10^9/l for seven days or more) or severe peripheral neuropathy, the dosage in subsequent treatment cycles should be reduced by 20 % (25 % for KS patients) (see section 4.4).

Patients with hepatic impairment: Inadequate data are available to recommend dosage alterations in patients with mild to moderate hepatic impairments (see sections 4.4 and 5.2).

Patients with severe hepatic impairment should not be treated with paclitaxel.

4.3 Contraindications
Paclitaxel is contraindicated in patients with severe hypersensitivity to paclitaxel or to any excipient, particularly macrogolglycerol ricinoleate (see section 4.4).

Paclitaxel is contraindicated during pregnancy and lactation (see section 4.6), and should not be used in patients with baseline neutrophils < 1.5 × 10^9/l (< 1 × 10^9/l for KS patients).

In KS, paclitaxel is also contraindicated in patients with concurrent, serious, uncontrolled infections.

4.4 Special warnings and precautions for use
Paclitaxel should be given under the supervision of a physician with experience in using cancer chemotherapeutic agents. Appropriate equipment for emergency treatment should be available, since severe hypersensitivity reactions may occur.

The patient should be premedicated with corticosteroids, antihistamines and H_2 antagonists before treatment with paclitaxel (see section 4.2).

Paclitaxel should be given *before* cisplatin when used in combination (see section 4.5).

Severe hypersensitivity reactions, characterised by dyspnoea and hypotension requiring treatment, angioedema and generalised urticaria have occurred in < 1 % of the patients treated with paclitaxel after adequate premedication. These reactions are probably histamine-mediated. At the first sign of severe hypersensitivity reactions, the paclitaxel infusion should be discontinued immediately. Symptomatic treatment should be initiated and the patient should not be treated with paclitaxel again.

Myelosuppression (primarily neutropenia) is the dose-limiting toxicity. The blood count should be monitored frequently during the paclitaxel treatment. The patient should not be treated until the neutrophil count is ⩾ 1.5 × 10^9/l (⩾ 1 × 10^9/l for KS patients) and the platelets are ⩾ 100 × 10^9/l (⩾ 75 × 10^9/l for KS patients). In the KS clinical study, most of patients received Granulocyte-Colony Stimulating Factor (G-CSF).

Severe cardiac conduction disorders have seldom been reported after treatment with paclitaxel as a single agent. If patients develop clear cardiac conduction disorders during treatment with paclitaxel, suitable treatment should be initiated and the cardiac function monitored continuously during subsequent treatment with paclitaxel. Hypotension, hypertension, and bradycardia have been seen during administration of paclitaxel; the patients are normally asymptomatic and in general they do not require any treatment. Frequent monitoring of vital signs is recommended, especially during the first hour of the paclitaxel infusion. Severe cardiovascular events were seen more often in patients with NSCLC than in patients with breast or ovarian carcinoma. A single case of heart failure related to paclitaxel was seen in the AIDS-KS clinical study.

When paclitaxel is used in combination with doxorubicin or trastuzumab for initial treatment of metastatic breast carcinoma, special attention to monitoring of the cardiac function should be given. Patients, who are candidates for treatment with paclitaxel in these combinations should undergo baseline cardiac examinations, including medical history, clinical examination, ECG, echocardiogram, and/or MUGA scan. Cardiac function should be monitored during the entire treatment period (e.g. every three months). Monitoring may help to identify patients who develop cardiac dysfunction and the treating physician should carefully evaluate the cumulative dose (mg/m²) of anthracycline when making decisions regarding the frequency of examination of the ventricular function. If the examination indicates aggravation of the cardiac function, even if it is asymptomatic, the treating physician should carefully assess the clinical benefits of further treatment in relation to the potential to induce cardiac impairment, including potentially irreversible injury. If further treatment is administered, the cardiac function should be monitored more frequent (e.g every second treatment cycle). For further information see Summary of Products Characteristics for trastuzumab or doxorubicin.

Although **peripheral neuropathy** can often occur, the development of serious symptoms is rare. In severe cases, a dose reduction of 20 % (25 % for KS patients) is recommended for all subsequent treatment cycles with paclitaxel. Severe neurotoxicity occurred more often in patients with NSCLC and ovarian carcinoma having undergone first-line chemotherapy with paclitaxel given as a three-hour infusion in combination with cisplatin, than in patients who received either paclitaxel alone or cyclophosphamide followed by cisplatin.

Patients with hepatic impairment may be at increased risk of toxicity, particularly grade III-IV myelosuppression. There is no evidence that the toxicity of paclitaxel is increased when given as a 3-hour infusion to patients with mildly abnormal liver function. When paclitaxel is given as a longer infusion, increased myelosuppression may be seen in patients with moderate to severe hepatic impairment. Patients should be monitored closely for the development of profound myelosuppression (see section 4.2). Inadequate data are available to recommend dosage alterations in patients with mild to moderate hepatic impairments (see section 5.2).

No data are available for patients with severe baseline cholestasis. Patients with severe hepatic impairment should not be treated with paclitaxel.

Since Paclitaxel medac contains ethanol (395 mg/ml), possible CNS and other influences should be considered.

Cautions should be observed to avoid intra-arterial administration of paclitaxel, since severe tissue reactions have been seen after intra-arterial administration in animal local tolerance studies.

Pseudomembranous colitis has been rarely reported. Pseudomembranous colitis has been seen even in patients who were not given concomitant antibiotic treatment. This reaction should be considered in the differential diagnosis of cases of severe or persistent diarrhoea occurring during or shortly after treatment with paclitaxel.

Paclitaxel may in combination with radiotherapy of the lung and irrespective of the chronological order contribute to the development of interstitial pneumonitis.

In KS patients, severe mucositis is rare. If severe reactions occur, the paclitaxel dose should be reduced by 25 %.

This medicinal product contains macrogolglycerol ricinoleate, which may cause severe allergic reactions.

4.5 Interaction with other medicinal products and other forms of interaction
Paclitaxel clearance is not influenced by premedication with cimetidine.

It is recommended to administer paclitaxel *before* cisplatin in first-line paclitaxel treatment of ovarian carcinoma. If paclitaxel is given *before* cisplatin, the safety profile of paclitaxel is consistent with that reported for single-agent use. When paclitaxel is given *after* cisplatin, patients showed a more profound myelosuppression and an approximately 20 % decrease in paclitaxel clearance. Patient who are treated with paclitaxel and cisplatin may have increased risk of renal impairment as seen in treatment with cisplatin alone in gynecological carcinoma.

The elimination of doxorubicin and its active metabolites may be reduced when paclitaxel and doxorubicin are administered too close in time and therefore paclitaxel as initial treatment of metastatic breast carcinoma should be administered 24 hours after doxorubicin (see section 5.2).

Metabolism of paclitaxel is partly catalysed by cytochrome P450 isoenzymes CYP2C8 and 3A4 (see section 5.2). Clinical studies have demonstrated that CYP2C8-mediated metabolism of paclitaxel to 6α-hydroxypaclitaxel is the major metabolic pathway in humans. Based on current knowledge no clinically relevant interactions between paclitaxel and other CYP2C8 substances are to be expected. Concomitant administration of ketoconazole, a known potent inhibitor of CYP3A4, does not inhibit the elimination of paclitaxel in patients; subsequently the two medicinal products can be administered concomitantly without dosage adjustment. Further data concerning potential of drug interactions between paclitaxel and other CYP3A4 substrates/inhibitors are limited. Caution is therefore required when concurrently administering paclitaxel with medicinal products known to inhibit (e.g erythromycin, fluoxetine, gemfibrozil) or induce (e.g. rifampicin, carbamazepine, phenytoin, phenobarbital, efavirenz, nevirapine) either CYP2C8 or 3A4.

Studies in KS patients, who were taking multiple concomitant medications, suggest that the systemic clearance of paclitaxel was significantly lower in the presence of nelfinavir and ritonavir, but not with indinavir. Insufficient information is available on interactions with other protease inhibitors. Consequently, paclitaxel should be administered with caution in patients receiving protease inhibitors as concomitant therapy.

4.6 Pregnancy and lactation

Pregnancy:

Paclitaxel has been shown to be embryotoxic and foetotoxic in rabbits, and to reduce the fertility in rats.

There is no information on the use of paclitaxel in pregnant women. As with other cytotoxic drugs, paclitaxel may cause foetal harm in treatment of pregnant women. Paclitaxel is contraindicated during pregnancy. Women should be advised to avoid becoming pregnant during treatment with paclitaxel, and to inform the treating physician immediately if pregnancy occurs.

Lactation:

It is not known whether paclitaxel is excreted into human breast milk. Paclitaxel is contraindicated in lactating women. Breast-feeding should be interrupted during paclitaxel treatment.

4.7 Effects on ability to drive and use machines

It has not been shown that paclitaxel affect this ability. However, paclitaxel contains alcohol (see sections 4.4 and 6.1). The ability to drive or to use machines may be decreased due to the alcohol content of the medicinal product.

4.8 Undesirable effects

Unless otherwise mentioned, the following description refers to the collected database of 812 patients with solid tumours treated with monotherapy of paclitaxel in clinical studies.

As the KS population is very specific, a special chapter based on a clinical study with 107 patients, is presented at the end of this section,

Unless otherwise mentioned, the incidence and severity of the reported adverse events was generally similar in patients receiving paclitaxel for treatment of ovarian or breast carcinoma, or NSCLC. None of the observed toxicities were clearly affected by age.

The most frequent adverse reaction was **myelosuppression.** Severe neutropenia ($< 0.5 \times 10^9$/l) was observed in 28 % of the patients, but had no association to episodes of fever. Only 1 % of the patients had severe neutropenia for $\geqslant$ 7 days. Thrombocytopenia was observed in 11 % of the patients. 3 % of the patients had a platelet count nadir of $< 50 \times 10^9$/l at least once during the study. Anaemia was seen in 64 % of the patients, but was only severe (Hb < 5 mmol/l) in 6 % of the patients. The incidence and severity of the anaemia is related to the baseline haemoglobin values.

Neurotoxicity, primarily peripheral neuropathy, appeared to be more frequent and more severe from a 3-hour infusion of 175 mg/m^2 (85 % neurotoxicity, 15 % severe) than from 24-hour infusion of 135 mg/m^2 (25 % peripheral neuropathy, 3 % severe) when paclitaxel was combined with cisplatin. There is an apparent increase in the incidence of severe neurotoxicity in patients with NSCLC and ovarian carcinoma given a 3-hour infusion of paclitaxel followed by cisplatin. Peripheral neuropathy may occur during the first treatment cycle and can deteriorate with increasing exposure to paclitaxel. Peripheral neuropathy caused discontinuation of paclitaxel in a few cases. Sensory symptoms improved or abated within a few months after the discontinuation of paclitaxel. Pre-existing neuropathy resulting from prior treatment is not a contraindication for treatment with paclitaxel.

Arthralgia or myalgia were seen in 60 % of the patients and was severe in 13 % of the patients.

Serious hypersensitivity reactions with possibly fatal outcome (defined as hypotension requiring treatment, angioedema, respiratory distress requiring bronchodilator treatment, or generalised urticaria) were seen in 2 patients (< 1 % of the patients). 34 % of the patients (17 % of all treatment cycles) experienced mild hypersensitivity reactions. These mild reactions, mainly flush and rash, did not require any treatment or discontinuation of paclitaxel.

Injection site reactions during intravenous administration may lead to local oedema, pain, erythema, and induration. Extravasations may result in cellulitis. Skin sloughing and/or peeling has been reported, sometimes related to extravasation. Skin discoloration may also occur. There are single reports about skin reactions so called "recall", at sites of previous extravasations following administration of paclitaxel at a different site. A specific treatment of extravasation reactions is unknown at this time.

The table below shows undesirable effects independent of their intensity associated with single treatment with paclitaxel given as 3-hour infusion in metastatic disease (812 patients treated in clinical trials) and undesirable effects reported in post-marketing surveillance* of paclitaxel.

The occurrence of undesirable effects is described below and defined according to the following rules: Very common ($\geq$ 1/10), common ($\geq$ 1/100, < 1/10), uncommon ($\geq$ 1/1,000, <1 /100), rare ($\geq$ 1/10,000, < 1/1,000), very rare (< 1/10,000).

Infections and infestations	*Very common*: infection (mainly urinary tract infections and infections in the upper respiratory tract) with reported cases of fatal outcome. *Uncommon:* septic shock *Rare**: pneumonia, peritonitis, sepsis
Blood and lymphatic system disorders	*Very common*: myelosuppression, neutropenia, anaemia, thrombocytopenia, leukopenia, bleeding *Rare**: febrile neutropenia *Very rare**: acute myeloid leukaemia, myelodysplastic syndrome
Immune system disorders	*Very common*: mild hypersensitivity reactions (mainly flush and rash) *Uncommon*: significant hypersensitivity reactions requiring treatment (e.g. hypotension, angioneurotic oedema, respiratory distress, generalised urticaria, chills, back pain, chest pain, tachycardia, abdominal pain, pain in the limbs, diaphoresis and hypertension) *Rare**: anaphylactic reactions *Very rare**: anaphylactic shock
Metabolism and nutrition disorders	*Very rare**: anorexia
Psychiatric disorders	*Very rare**: confusional state
Nervous system disorders	*Very common*: neurotoxicity (mainly peripheral neuropathy) *Rare**: motor neuropathy (with resultant minor distal weakness) *Very rare**: autonomic neuropathy (resulting in paralytic ileus and orthostatic hypotension), grand mal seizures, convulsions, encephalopathy, dizziness, headache, ataxia
Eye disorders	*Very rare**: optic nerve and/or visual disturbances (scintillating scotomata), particularly in patients who have received higher doses than recommended
Ear and labyrinth disorders	*Very rare**: ototoxicity, loss of hearing, tinnitus, vertigo
Cardiac disorders	*Common*: bradycardia *Uncommon*: cardiomyopathy, asymptomatic ventricular tachycardia, tachycardia with extrasystole, AV-block and syncope, myocardial infarction *Very rare**: atrial fibrillation, supraventricular tachycardia
Vascular disorders	*Very common*: hypotension *Uncommon*: hypertension, thrombosis, thrombophlebitis *Very rare**: shock
Respiratory, thoracic and mediastinal disorders	*Rare**: dyspnoea, pleural effusion, interstitial pneumonia, lung fibrosis, pulmonary embolism, respiratory failure *Very rare**: cough
Gastrointestinal disorders	*Very common*: nausea, vomiting, diarrhoea, mucositis *Uncommon**: bowel obstruction, bowel perforation, ischemic colitis, pancreatitis *Very rare**: mesenteric thrombosis, pseudomembranous colitis, oesophagitis, constipation, ascites, neutropenic colitis
Hepatobiliary disorders	*Very rare**: hepatic necrosis, hepatic encephalopathy (both with reported cases of fatal outcome)
Skin and subcutaneous tissue disorders	*Very common*: alopecia *Common*: transient, mild nail and skin changes *Rare**: pruritus, rash, erythema *Very rare**: Stevens-Johnson syndrome, epidermal necrolysis, erythema multiforme, exfoliative dermatitis, urticaria, onycholysis (patients on therapy should use sun protection on hands and feet)
Musculoskeletal and connective tissue disorders	*Very common:* arthralgia, myalgia
General disorders and administration site conditions	*Common*: injection site reactions (including localised oedema, pain, erythema, induration, occasionally extravasation can result in cellulites, skin fibrosis and skin necrosis) *Rare**: asthenia, pyrexia, dehydration, oedema, malaise
Investigations	*Common*: severe elevation of AST (SGOT), severe elevation of alkaline phosphatase *Uncommon*: severe elevation of bilirubin *Rare**: increase in blood creatinine

Patients with breast carcinoma, who received paclitaxel as an adjuvant treatment after AC, experienced neurotoxicity, allergic reactions, arthralgia/myalgia, anemia, infection, fever, nausea/vomiting and diarrhoea more often compared to patients, who received AC alone. The frequency of these adverse reactions was consistent with the use of paclitaxel alone, as reported above.

Combination treatment

The following description refers to two large studies of first-line chemotherapy in ovarian carcinoma (paclitaxel + cisplatin: more than 1050 patients), two phase III studies in first-line treatment of metastatic breast carcinoma, one which investigated the combination with doxorubicin (paclitaxel + doxorubicin: 267 patients), and another which investigated the combination with trastuzumab (planned subgroup analysis paclitaxel + trastuzumab: 188 patients) and two phase III studies in treatment of advanced NSCLC (paclitaxel + cisplatin: more than 360 patients) (see section 5.1).

Neurotoxicity, arthralgia/myalgia and hypersensitivity were reported more often and were more severe in patients given paclitaxel as a 3-hour infusion followed by cisplatin for first-line chemotherapy of ovarian carcinoma than in those treated with cyclophosphamide followed by cisplatin. Myelosuppression appeared less often and to a lesser degree with 3-hour paclitaxel infusion followed by cisplatin compared to cyclophosphamide followed by cisplatin.

In first-line chemotherapy in metastatic breast carcinoma, neutropenia, anaemia, peripheral neuropathy, arthralgia/myalgia, asthenia, fever and diarrhoea were more severe and frequently reported when paclitaxel (220 mg/m^2) was administered as 3-hour infusion 24 hours after doxorubicin (50 mg/m^2) compared to standard FAC treatment (5-FU 500 mg/m^2, doxorubicin 50 mg/m^2, cyclophosphamide 500 mg/m^2). Nausea and vomiting seemed to occur more seldom and were less severe with paclitaxel (220 mg/m^2) / doxorubicin (50 mg/m^2) regimen compared to standard FAC regimen. The use of corticosteroids may have contributed to lower occurrence and less severity of the nausea and vomiting in the paclitaxel/doxorubicin group.

When paclitaxel was administered with trastuzumab as a 3-hour infusion for first-line treatment of patients with metastatic breast carcinoma, the following events were reported more often than with paclitaxel given as monotherapy (regardless of a relationship to paclitaxel or trastuzumab): heart failure (8 % vs 1 %), infection (46 % vs 27 %), chills (42 % vs 4 %), fever (47 % vs 23 %), cough (42 % vs 22 %), rash (39 % vs 18 %), arthralgia (37 % vs 21 %), tachycardia (12 % vs 4 %), diarrhoea (45 % vs 30 %), hypertension (11 % vs 3 %), epistaxis (18 % vs 4 %), acne (11 % vs 3 %), herpes simplex (12 % vs 3 %), accidental injury (13 % vs 3 %), insomnia (25 % vs 13 %), rhinitis (22 % vs 5 %), sinusitis (21 % vs 7 %) and injection site reactions (7 % vs 1 %). Some of these frequency differences can be attributed to a greater number and duration of treatment cycles with the paclitaxel / trastuzumab combination compared to paclitaxel as monotherapy. Severe adverse events were reported at a similar rate for paclitaxel / trastuzumab and paclitaxel monotherapy.

When doxorubicin was administered in combination with paclitaxel in metastatic breast carcinoma, **abnormal heart contraction** ($\geqslant$ 20 % reduction of the left ventricular output fraction) were observed in 15 % of the patients compared with 10 % treated with standard FAC regimen. **Congestive heart failure** was observed in < 1 % in both paclitaxel/doxorubicin and standard FAC treatment. Administration of trastuzumab in combination with paclitaxel in patients previously treated with anthracyclines showed an increase of the number and severity of **cardiac dysfunction** as compared with paclitaxel monotherapy (NYHA class I/II: 10 % vs 0 %; NYHA class III/IV: 2 % vs 1 %) and is seldom associated with death (see Summary of Product Characteristics for trastuzumab). Aside from these rare cases, all patients responded to appropriate medical treatment.

Radiation pneumonitis has been reported in patients concurrently receiving radiotherapy.

AIDS-related Kaposi's sarcoma:

Except for haematologic and hepatic undesirable effects (see below), the frequency and severity of undesirable effects are generally similar between KS patients and patients treated with paclitaxel monotherapy for other solitd tumours, based on a clinical study including 107 patients.

Blood and lymphatic system disorders:

Myelosuppression was the major dose limiting toxicity. Neutropenia is the most important haematological toxicity. During the initial treatment severe neutropenia occurred ($< 0.5 \times 10^9$/l) in 20 % of the patients. Through the entire treatment period severe neutropenia was observed in 39 % of the patients. Neutropenia was seen for > 7 days in 41 % of the patients and for 30-35 days in 8 % of the patients. Within 35 days the neutropenia had disappeared in all patients who were examined. The occurrence of grade 4 neutropenia, which lasted ≥ 7 days was 22 %.

Neutropenic fever related to paclitaxel was reported in 14 % of the patients and in 1.3 % of the treatment cycles. There were 3 fatal septic episodes (2.8 %) during the paclitaxel administration, which were related to the medicinal product.

Thrombocytopenia was observed in 50 % of the patients, and was severe ($< 50 \times 10^9$/l) in 9 % of the cases. Only 14 % experienced fall in the number of platelets $< 75 \times 10^9$/l, at least once during the treatment. Bleeding episodes related to paclitaxel was reported in < 3 % of the patients, but the bleedings were found.

Anaemia (Hb < 11 g/dL) was observed in 61 % of the patients and was severe (Hb < 8 g/dL) in 10 % of the cases. Red cell transfusions were needed in 21 % of the patients.

Hepatobiliary disorders: In the patients (> 50 % used protease inhibitor) with normal baseline liver function, 28 % had enhanced bilirubin, 43 % enhanced alkaline phosphatase and 44 % enhanced AST (SGOT). For each of these parameters the increase was severe in 1 % of the cases.

4.9 Overdose

No antidote is known for paclitaxel overdose. The commonly expected complications of over-dose will be myelosuppression, peripheral neuropathy and mucositis.

5. PHARMACOLOGICAL PROPERTIES

5.1 Pharmacodynamic properties

Pharmacotherapeutic group: Plant alkaloids and other natural products, taxanes,

ATC-Code: L01C D01

Paclitaxel is a novel antimicrotubuler agent that promotes the assembly of microtubules from tubulin dimers and stabilises microtubules by preventing depolymerization. This stability results in the inhibition of the normal dynamic re-organisation of the microtubule network that is essential for vital interphase and mitotic cellular functions. In addition, paclitaxel induces abnormal arrays or bundles of microtubules throughout the cell cycle and multiple asters of microtubules during mitosis.

In the first-line chemotherapy of ovarian carcinoma, the safety and efficacy of paclitaxel were evaluated in two major, randomised, controlled (vs. cyclophosphamide 750 mg/m²/cisplatin 75 mg/m²) trials. In the Intergroup trial (B-MS CA 139-209), over 650 patients with stage II_{b-c}, III or IV primary ovarian cancer received a maximum of 9 treatment courses of paclitaxel (175 mg/m² over 3 hours) followed by cisplatin (75 mg/m²) or control. The second major trial (GOG-111/B-MS CA 139-022) evaluated a maximum of 6 courses of either paclitaxel (135 mg/m² over 24 hours) followed by cisplatin (75 mg/m²) or control in over 400 patients with stage III/IV primary ovarian cancer, with a > 1 cm residual disease after staging laparotomy, or with distant metastases. While the two different paclitaxel posologies were not compared with each other directly, in both trials patients treated with paclitaxel in combination with cisplatin had a significantly higher response rate, longer time to progression, and longer survival time when compared with standard therapy. Increased neurotoxicity, arthralgia/myalgia but reduced myelosuppression were observed in advanced ovarian cancer patients administered three-hour infusion paclitaxel/cisplatin as compared to patients who received cyclophosphamide/cisplatin.

In the adjuvant treatment of breast carcinoma, 3121 patients with node-positive breast carcinoma were treated with adjuvant paclitaxel therapy or no chemotherapy following 4 courses of doxorubicin and cyclophosphamide (CALGB 9344, BMS CA 139-223). Median follow-up was 69 months. Overall, paclitaxel patients had a significant reduction of 18 % in the risk of disease recurrence to patients receiving AC alone (p=0.0014), and a significant reduction of 19 % in the risk of death (p=0.0044) relative to patients receiving AC alone. Retrospective analyses show benefit in all patient subsets. In patients with hormone receptor negative/unknown tumours, reduction in risk of disease recurrence was 28 % (95 % CI: 0.59-0.86). In the patient subgroup with hormone receptor positive tumours, the risk reduction of disease recurrence was 9 % (95 % CI: 0.78-1.07). However, the design of the study did not investigate the effect of extended AC therapy beyond 4 cycles. It cannot be excluded on the basis of this study alone that the observed effects could be partly due to the difference in duration of chemotherapy between the two arms (AC 4 cycles; AC + paclitaxel 8 cycles). Therefore, adjuvant treatment with paclitaxel should be regarded as an alternative to extended AC therapy.

In a second large clinical study in adjuvant node-positive breast cancer with a similar design, 3060 patients were randomised to receive or not 4 courses of paclitaxel at a higher dose of 225 mg/m² following 4 courses of AC (NSABP B-28, BMS CA139-270). At a median follow-up of 64 months, paclitaxel patients had a significant reduction of 17 % in the risk of disease recurrence relative to the patients who received AC alone (p=0.006); paclitaxel treatment was associated with a reduction in the risk of death of 7 % (95 % CI: 0.78-1.12). All subset analyses favoured the paclitaxel arm. In this study patients with hormone receptor positive tumours had a reduction in the risk of disease recurrence of 23 % (95 % CI: 0.6-0.92); in the patient subgroup with hormone receptor negative tumours the risk reduction of disease recurrence was 10 % (95 % CI: 0.7-1.11).

In the first-line treatment of metastatic breast cancer, the efficacy and safety of paclitaxel were evaluated in two pivotal, phase III, randomised, controlled open-label trials.

In the first study (BMS CA139-278), the combination of bolus doxorubicin (50 mg/m²) followed after 24 hours by paclitaxel (220 mg/m² by 3-hour infusion) (AT), was compared versus standard FAC regimen (5-FU 500 mg/m², doxorubicin 50 mg/m², cyclophosphamide 500 mg/m²), both administered every three weeks for 8 courses. In this randomised study, 267 patients with metastatic breast cancer, who had either received no prior chemotherapy or only non-anthracycline chemotherapy in the adjuvant setting, were enrolled. Results showed a significant difference in time to progression for patients receiving AT compared to those receiving FAC (8.2 vs 6.2 months; p=0.029). The median survival was in favour of paclitaxel/doxorubicin vs. FAC (23.0 vs. 18.3 months; p=0.004). In the AT and FAC treatment arm 44 % and 48 % respectively received follow-up chemotherapy which included taxanes in 7 % and 50 % respectively. The overall response rate was also significantly higher in the AT arm compared to the FAC arm (68 % vs. 55 %).

Complete responses were seen in 19 % of the paclitaxel/doxorubicin arm patients vs. 8 % of the FAC arm patients. All efficacy results have been subsequently confirmed by a blinded independent review.

In the second pivotal study, the efficacy and safety of paclitaxel and trastuzumab was evaluated in a planned subgroup analysis (metastatic breast cancer patients who formerly received adjuvant anthracyclines) of the study HO648g. The efficacy of trastuzumab in combination with paclitaxel in patients who did not received prior adjuvant anthracyclines has not been proven. The combination of trastuzumab (4 mg/kg loading dose then 2 mg/kg weekly) and paclitaxel (175 mg/m²) 3-hour infusion, every three weeks was compared to single-agent paclitaxel (175 mg/m²) 3-hour infusion, every three weeks in 188 patients with metastatic breast cancer over-expressing HER-2 (2+ or 3+ measured by immunohistochemistry), who had previously been treated with anthracyclines. Paclitaxel was administered every three weeks for at least six courses while trastuzumab was given weekly until disease progression. The study showed a significant benefit for the paclitaxel/trastuzumab combination in terms of time to progression (6.9 vs. 3.0 months), response rate (41 % vs. 17 %), and duration of response (10.5 vs. 4.5 months) when compared to paclitaxel alone. The most significant toxicity observed with the paclitaxel/trastuzumab combination was cardiac dysfunction (see section 4.8).

In the treatment of advanced NSCLC, paclitaxel 175 mg/m² followed by cisplatin 80 mg/m² has been evaluated in two phase III trials (367 patients on paclitaxel containing regimens). Both were randomised trials, one compared to treatment with cisplatin 100 mg/m², the other used teniposide 100 mg/m² teniposide followed by cisplatin 80 mg/m² as comparator (367 patients on comparator). Results in each trial were similar. For the primary outcome of mortality, there was no significant difference between the paclitaxel containing regimen and the comparator (median survival times 8.1 and 9.5 months on paclitaxel containing regimens, 8.6 and 9.9 months on comparators). Similarly, for progression-free survival there was no significant difference between treatments. There was a significant benefit in terms of clinical response rate. Quality of life results are suggestive of a benefit on paclitaxel containing regimens in terms of appetite loss and provide clear evidence of the inferiority of paclitaxel containing regimens in terms of peripheral neuropathy (p < 0.008).

In the treatment of AIDS-related KS, the efficacy and safety of paclitaxel were investigated in a non-comparative study in patients with advanced KS, previously treated with systemic chemotherapy. The primary end-point was best tumour response. Of the 107 patients, 63 were considered resistant to liposomal anthracyclines. This subgroup is considered to constitute the core efficacy population. The overall success rate (complete/partial response) after 15 cycles of treatment was 57 % (CI 44 – 70 %) in liposomal anthracycline-resistant patients. Over 50 % of the responses were apparent after the first 3 cycles. In liposomal anthracycline-resistant patiens, the response rates were comparable for patients who had never received protease inhibitor (55.6 %) and those who received one at least 2 months prior to treatment with paclitaxel (60.9 %). The median time to progression in the core population was 468 days (95 % CI 257-NE). Median survival could not be computed, but the lower 95 % bound was 617 days in core patients.

5.2 Pharmacokinetic properties

Following intravenous administration, paclitaxel exhibits a biphasic decline in plasma concentrations.

The pharmacokinetics of paclitaxel were determined following 3- and 24-hour infusions at doses of 135 mg/m² and 175 mg/m². Mean terminal half-life estimates ranged from 3.0 to 52.7 hours, and mean, non-compartmentally derived, values for total body clearance ranged from 11.6 to 24.0 l/hour/m²; total body clearance appeared to decrease with higher plasma concentrations of paclitaxel. Mean steady-state volume of distribution ranged from 198 to 688 l/m², indicating extensive extravascular distribution and/or tissue binding. With the 3-hour infusion, increasing doses result in non-linear pharmacokinetics. For a 30 % increase in dose from 135 mg/m² to 175 mg/m² the C_{max} and $AUC_{>\infty}$ values increased 75 % and 81 %, respectively.

Following an intravenous dose of 100 mg/m² given as a 3-hour infusion to 19 KS patients, the mean C_{max} was 1,530 ng/ml (range 761-2,860 ng/mL) and the mean AUC 5,619 ng hr/mL (range 2,609-9,428 ng hr/mL). Clearance was 20.6 l/h/m² (range 11-38 l/h/m²) and the volume of distribution was 291 l/m² (range 121-638 l/m²). The terminal elimination half-time averaged 23.7 hours (range 12-33 hours).

Intra-patient variability in systemic paclitaxel exposure was minimal. There was no evidence for accumulation of paclitaxel with multiple treatment courses.

In vitro studies of binding to human serum proteins indicate that 89-98 % of drug is bound. The presence of cimetidine, ranitidine, dexamethasone or diphenhydramine did not affect protein binding of paclitaxel.

The metabolic disposition of paclitaxel has not been fully elucidated in humans. Mean values for cumulative urinary recovery of unchanged drug have ranged from 1.3 to 12.6 % of the dose, indicating extensive non-renal clearance. Hepatic metabolism and biliary clearance may be the principal mechanisms for disposition of paclitaxel. Paclitaxel appears to be metabolised primarily by cytochrome P450 enzymes. Following administration of a radiolabelled paclitaxel, an average of 26 %, 2 % and 6 % of the radioactivity was excreted in the faeces as 6α-hydroxypaclitaxel, 3'-p-hydroxy-paclitaxel, and 6α-3'-p-dihydroxy-paclitaxel, respectively. The formation of these hydroxylated metabolites is catalysed by CYP2C8, -3A4 and both - 2C8 and -3A4 respectively. The effect of renal or hepatic dysfunction on the disposition of paclitaxel following a 3-hour infusion has not been investigated formally. Pharmacokinetic parameters obtained from one patient undergoing haemodialysis who receive a 3-hour infusion of paclitaxel 135 mg/m² were within the range of those defined in non-dialysis patients.

In clinical trials where paclitaxel and doxorubicin were administered concomitantly, the distribution and elimination of doxorubicin and its metabolites were prolonged. Total plasma exposure to doxorubicin was 30 % higher when paclitaxel immediately followed doxorubicin than when there was a 24-hour interval between drugs.

For use of paclitaxel in combination with other therapies, please consult the Summary of Product Characteristics of cisplatin, doxorubicin or trastuzumab for information on the use of these medicinal products.

5.3 Preclinical safety data

The carcinogenic potential of paclitaxel has not been studied. However, paclitaxel may be carcinogenic and genotoxic due to its mechanism of action. Paclitaxel has been shown to be mutagenic in both *in vitro* and *in vivo* mammalian test systems.

6. PHARMACEUTICAL PARTICULARS

6.1 List of excipients

Macrogolglycerol ricinoleate

Ethanol, anhydrous

Citric acid, anhydrous

6.2 Incompatibilities

Polyethoxylated castor oil can result in DEHP (di-(2-ethylhexyl)phthalate) leaching from polyvinyl chloride (PVC) containers at levels which increases with time and concentration. Consequently the preparation, storage and administration of diluted Paclitaxel medac should be carried out using equipment not containing PVC.

6.3 Shelf life

Unopened vial: 3 years

After opening:

From a microbiological, chemical and physical point of view the product may be stored for maximum 28 days at 25 °C. Other storage periods and storage conditions are the responsibility of the user.

After dilution:

Diluted solution for infusion has been shown to be chemically and physically stable for up to 72 hours at 25°C.

Diluted solutions should not be stored in a refrigerator (see section 6.6).

From a microbiological point of view, diluted solution should be used immediately.

6.4 Special precautions for storage
Do not store above 25°C.

Store in the original package in order to protect from light.

6.5 Nature and contents of container
Type I glass vials (with a PTFE coated bromobutyl rubber closure) containing 30 mg, 100 mg, or 300 mg paclitaxel in 5 ml, 16.7 ml or 50 ml solution respectively.

Each vial is packed separately in a box. Multi-pack with 10 boxes is also available.

Not all pack sizes may be marketed.

6.6 Special precautions for disposal and other handling
The current national guidelines for handling of chemotherapeutic agents should be followed.

Handling: As with all chemotherapeutic agents, caution should be exercised when handling paclitaxel. The dilution should be done by trained personnel in specially designated areas under aseptic conditions. Adequate protective gloves should be used. Precautions should be taken in order to avoid contact with the skin and mucous membrane. In case of contact with the skin the area must be rinsed with soap and water. After topic exposure tingling and burning sensation and redness have been observed. In the event of contact with mucous membranes, they should be rinsed immediately with water. Dyspnoea, chest pain, burning throat and nausea have been reported after inhalation.

Refrigerated storage of unopened vials can lead to precipitates, which re-dissolve with little or no agitation when the preparation has reached room temperature. The quality of the product is not affected. The vial should be discarded if the solution remains cloudy or if an insoluble precipitate is found.

Following multiple needle entries and product withdrawals, the vial maintain microbial, chemical and physical stability for up to 28 days at 25°C. Other storage times and conditions are the responsibility of the user.

Use of the Chemo-Dispensing Pin or Spike is not recommended since it can damage the stopper, resulting in loss of sterility.

Preparation of the solution for infusion: Prior to infusion the paclitaxel should be diluted under aseptic conditions. Paclitaxel is diluted with 0.9% NaCl solution or 5% glucose solution or 5% glucose/0.9% NaCl solution or Ringer's solution plus 5% glucose to a concentration of 0.3 – 1.2 mg/ml.

Chemical and physical stability of diluted infusion at 25°C is 72 hours.

From a microbiological point of view, the product should be used immediately. If the product is not used immediately the storage time and condition are the responsibility of the user.

After dilution the solution may be cloudy. This is attributed to the formulation vehicle and is not removed by filtration. Paclitaxel should be infused through an in-line filter with a microporous membrane with a pore diameter not larger than 0.22 μm. Testing of an infusion system using an in-line filter revealed no significant losses in potency.

There have been rare reports of precipitates during the infusion of paclitaxel, usually at the end of a 24-hour infusion. Even though the cause of the precipitation is not known it may be due to possible supersaturating of the solution. In order to reduce the risk of precipitation paclitaxel should be used as quickly as possible after dilution and excessive vibration or shaking should be avoided. The infusion sets should be flushed thoroughly before use. The appearance of the solution should be checked frequently during the infusion, and the infusion stopped if precipitates appear.

In order to minimise the exposure of the patients to DEHP (di-(2-ethylhexyl)phthalate), which may leach from PVC infusion bags, sets, and other medical equipments, diluted paclitaxel solution for infusion should be stored in non-PVC bottles (glass, polypropylene) or plastic containers (polypropylene, polyolefin) and administered through polyethylene-lined infusion sets. Filters (e.g. Ivex-2®) with short PVC inlets and outlets have not resulted in significant leaching of DEHP.

Disposal: All items used in the preparation, administration or otherwise coming into contact with paclitaxel must be disposed in accordance with local guidelines for disposal of chemotherapeutic agents.

7. MARKETING AUTHORISATION HOLDER
medac Gesellschaft für klinische Spezialpräparate mbH

Fehlandtstraβe 3

20354 Hamburg

Germany

8. MARKETING AUTHORISATION NUMBER(S)
PL 11587/0044

9. DATE OF FIRST AUTHORISATION/RENEWAL OF THE AUTHORISATION
10/09/2007

10. DATE OF REVISION OF THE TEXT
10/09/2007

Palladone capsules

(Napp Pharmaceuticals Limited)

1. NAME OF THE MEDICINAL PRODUCT
PALLADONE® capsules 1.3 mg and 2.6 mg.

2. QUALITATIVE AND QUANTITATIVE COMPOSITION
PALLADONE capsules contain Hydromorphone Hydrochloride USP 1.3 mg or 2.6 mg.

For excipients, see 6.1

3. PHARMACEUTICAL FORM
PALLADONE capsules 1.3 mg are orange/clear capsules marked HNR 1.3.

PALLADONE capsules 2.6 mg are red/clear capsules marked HNR 2.6.

4. CLINICAL PARTICULARS

4.1 Therapeutic indications
For the relief of severe pain in cancer.

4.2 Posology and method of administration
Route of administration

The capsules can be swallowed whole or opened and their contents sprinkled on to cold soft food.

Dosage and administration

Adults and children over 12 years

PALLADONE capsules should be used at 4-hourly intervals. The dosage is dependent upon the severity of the pain and the patient's previous history of analgesic requirements. 1.3 mg of hydromorphone has an efficacy approximately equivalent to 10 mg of morphine given orally. A patient presenting with severe pain should normally be started on a dosage of one PALLADONE capsule 4-hourly. Increasing severity of pain will require increased dosage of hydromorphone to achieve the desired relief.

Elderly and patients with renal impairment

The elderly and patients with renal impairment should be dose titrated with PALLADONE capsules in order to achieve adequate analgesia. It should be noted, however, that these patients may require a lower dosage to achieve adequate analgesia.

Patients with hepatic impairment

Contra-indicated.

Children under 12 years

Not recommended.

4.3 Contraindications
Hydromorphone is contra-indicated in patients with known hypersensitivity to hydromorphone or other ingredients in the formulation.

It is also contra-indicated in respiratory depression with hypoxia or elevated carbon dioxide levels in the blood, pregnancy, coma, acute abdomen, hepatic impairment, paralytic ileus, concurrent administration of monoamine oxidase inhibitors or within 2 weeks of discontinuation of their use. Hydromorphone should be avoided in patients with raised intracranial pressure or head injury, and also in patients with convulsive disorders or acute alcoholism.

4.4 Special warnings and precautions for use
The major risk of opioid excess is respiratory depression. As with all narcotics, a reduction in dosage may be advised in the elderly or infirm patients with severely impaired pulmonary function, toxic psychosis, delirium tremens, pancreatitis, hypothyroidism, hypotension with hypovolaemia, chronic obstructive airways disease, renal or adrenocortical insufficiency, prostatic hypertrophy, shock or reduced respiratory reserve. PALLADONE capsules are not recommended in the first 24 hours post-operatively. After this time they should be used with caution, particularly following abdominal surgery.

PALLADONE capsules should not be used where there is the possibility of paralytic ileus occurring. Should paralytic ileus be suspected or occur during use, PALLADONE capsules should be discontinued immediately.

Patients about to undergo cordotomy or other pain-relieving surgical procedures should not receive PALLADONE capsules for 4 hours prior to surgery. If further treatment with PALLADONE capsules is indicated, the dosage should be adjusted to the new post-operative requirement.

The patient may develop tolerance to the drug with chronic use and require progressively higher doses to maintain pain control. The patient may develop physical dependence; an abstinence syndrome may be seen following abrupt cessation. When a patient no longer requires therapy with hydromorphone, it may be advisable to taper the dose gradually to prevent symptoms of withdrawal.

Hydromorphone has a morphine-like abuse profile and may be sought and abused by people with latent or manifest addiction disorders. Hydromorphone should be used with particular care in patients with a history of alcohol and drug abuse.

Abuse of oral dosage forms by parenteral administration can be expected to result in serious adverse events, which may be fatal.

4.5 Interaction with other medicinal products and other forms of interaction
Centrally acting drugs such as major and minor tranquillisers, anaesthetics, barbiturates, antiemetics, antidepressants, alcohol, neuroleptics, hypnotics, other opioids, monoamine oxidase inhibitors (see section 4.3) and sedatives may interact with hydromorphone and potentiate the effects of either drug, e.g. sedation, respiratory depression, etc.

4.6 Pregnancy and lactation
PALLADONE capsules are not recommended in pregnancy or in the breast-feeding mother as there are insufficient animal or human data to justify such use.

4.7 Effects on ability to drive and use machines
Hydromorphone may cause drowsiness and patients should not drive or operate machinery if affected.

4.8 Undesirable effects
Hydromorphone may cause constipation, nausea and vomiting. Constipation may be treated with appropriate laxatives. When nausea and vomiting are troublesome, PALLADONE capsules can be readily combined with anti-emetics.

Common (incidence of ⩾ 1%) and uncommon (⩽ 1%) adverse drug reactions are listed in the table below.

	Common	Uncommon
Cardiac and vascular disorders	Hypotension	
Eye disorders		Blurred vision Miosis
Gastrointestinal and hepatobiliary disorders	Constipation Dry mouth Nausea Vomiting	Biliary colic Paralytic ileus
General disorders	Asthenic conditions	Drug withdrawal syndrome Drug tolerance Peripheral oedema
Immune system disorders		Hypersensitivity reactions (including oropharyngeal swelling)
Nervous system disorders	Dizziness Somnolence	Convulsions Dyskinesia Headache Sedation Tremor In particular in high doses hyperalgesia that will not respond to a further dose of hydromorphone (possibly dose reduction or change in opioid required).
Psychiatric disorders	Confusion	Drug addiction Agitation Dysphoria Euphoria Hallucination
Renal and urinary disorders	Urinary retention	
Respiratory, thoracic and mediastinal disorders		Respiratory depression
Skin and subcutaneous tissue disorders	Pruritus Rash Sweating	Urticaria

4.9 Overdose
Signs of hydromorphone toxicity and overdosage are pinpoint pupils, respiratory depression and hypotension. Circulatory failure and somnolence progressing to stupor or deepening coma, skeletal muscle flaccidity, bradycardia and death may occur in more severe cases. Rhabdomyolosis progressing to renal failure has been reported in opioid overdosage.

Treatment of overdosage:

Primary attention should be given to the establishment of a patent airway and institution of assisted or controlled ventilation.

In the case of massive overdosage, administer naloxone intravenously (0.4 to 2 mg for an adult and 0.01 mg/kg bodyweight for children), if the patient is in a coma or respiratory depression is present. Repeat the dose at 2 minute intervals if there is no response. If repeated doses are required then an infusion of 60% of the initial dose per hour is a useful starting point. A solution of 10 mg made up in 50 ml dextrose will produce 200 micrograms/ml for infusion using an IV pump (dose adjusted to the clinical response). Infusions are not a substitute for frequent review of the patient's clinical state.

Intramuscular naloxone is an alternative in the event IV access is not possible. As the duration of action of naloxone is relatively short, the patient must be carefully monitored until spontaneous respiration is reliably re-established. Naloxone is a competitive antagonist and large doses (4 mg) may be required in seriously poisoned patients. For less severe overdosage, administer naloxone 0.2 mg intravenously followed by increments of 0.1 mg every 2 minutes if required.

Naloxone should not be administered in the absence of clinically significant respiratory or circulatory depression secondary to hydromorphone overdosage. Naloxone should be administered cautiously to persons who are known, or suspected, to be physically dependent on hydromorphone. In such cases, an abrupt or complete reversal of opioid effects may precipitate an acute withdrawal syndrome.

Other supportive measures as indicated by the patient's progress and clinical condition should be considered.

Additional /other considerations:

Consider activated charcoal (50 g for adult, 1g/kg for children), if a substantial amount has been ingested within 1 hour, provided the airway can be protected.

Gastric contents may need to be emptied as this can be useful in removing unabsorbed drug.

5. PHARMACOLOGICAL PROPERTIES

5.1 Pharmacodynamic properties

Pharmacotherapeutic group: Natural opium alkaloid ATC code: NO2A A03

Like morphine, hydromorphone is an agonist of mu receptors. The pharmacological actions of hydromorphone and morphine do not differ significantly. The oral analgesic potency ratio of hydromorphone to morphine is approximately 5-10:1. Hydromorphone and related opioids produce their major effects on the central nervous system and bowel. The effects are diverse and include analgesia, drowsiness, changes in mood, respiratory depression, decreased gastrointestinal motility, nausea, vomiting, and alteration of the endocrine and autonomic nervous system.

5.2 Pharmacokinetic properties

Hydromorphone is absorbed from the gastrointestinal tract and undergoes pre-systemic elimination resulting in an oral bioavailability of about 50%. It is metabolised and excreted in the urine mainly as conjugated hydromorphone, dihydroisomorphine and dihydromorphine.

5.3 Preclinical safety data

There are no pre-clinical data of relevance to the prescriber which are additional to that already included in other sections of the SPC.

6. PHARMACEUTICAL PARTICULARS

6.1 List of excipients

Microcrystalline cellulose

Lactose (anhydrous)

Capsule shells

Gelatin

Erythrosine (E127)

Iron oxide (E172)

Titanium dioxide (E171)

Sodium dodecylsulphate

Black Printing Ink

Shellac

Propylene glycol

Iron oxide (E172)

6.2 Incompatibilities

None known.

6.3 Shelf life

Two years.

6.4 Special precautions for storage

Do not store above 25°C. Store in the original package.

6.5 Nature and contents of container

PVdC coated PVC blisters with aluminium backing foil containing 56 capsules.

6.6 Special precautions for disposal and other handling

None stated

7. MARKETING AUTHORISATION HOLDER

Napp Pharmaceuticals Limited

Cambridge Science Park

Milton Road

Cambridge

CB4 0GW

8. MARKETING AUTHORISATION NUMBER(S)

PL 16950/0049, 0050

9. DATE OF FIRST AUTHORISATION/RENEWAL OF THE AUTHORISATION

12 February 1997

10. DATE OF REVISION OF THE TEXT

September 2008

Palladone SR capsules

(Napp Pharmaceuticals Limited)

1. NAME OF THE MEDICINAL PRODUCT

PALLADONE®SR capsules 2 mg, 4 mg, 8 mg, 16 mg, 24 mg.

2. QUALITATIVE AND QUANTITATIVE COMPOSITION

The capsules contain Hydromorphone Hydrochloride USP 2 mg, 4 mg, 8 mg, 16 mg, 24 mg.

For excipients, see 6.1.

3. PHARMACEUTICAL FORM

Prolonged release capsule.

Hard gelatin capsule containing spherical prolonged release pellets.

PALLADONE SR capsules 2 mg are yellow/white capsules marked HCR 2.

PALLADONE SR capsules 4 mg are pale blue/clear capsules marked HCR 4.

PALLADONE SR capsules 8 mg are pink/clear capsules marked HCR 8.

PALLADONE SR capsules 16 mg are brown/clear capsules marked HCR 16.

PALLADONE SR capsules 24 mg are dark blue/clear capsules marked HCR 24.

4. CLINICAL PARTICULARS

4.1 Therapeutic indications

For the relief of severe pain in cancer.

4.2 Posology and method of administration

Route of administration

The capsules can be swallowed whole or opened and their contents sprinkled on to cold soft food.

Dosage and administration

Adults and children over 12 years

PALLADONE SR capsules should be used at 12-hourly intervals. The dosage is dependent upon the severity of the pain and the patient's previous history of analgesic requirements. 4 mg of hydromorphone has an efficacy approximately equivalent to 30 mg of morphine sulphate given orally. A patient presenting with severe pain should normally be started on a dosage of 4 mg PALLADONE SR capsules 12-hourly. Increasing severity of pain will require increased dosage of hydromorphone to achieve the desired relief.

Elderly and patients with renal impairment

The elderly and patients with renal impairment should be dose titrated with PALLADONE SR capsules in order to achieve adequate analgesia. It should be noted, however, that these patients may require a lower dosage to achieve adequate analgesia.

Patients with hepatic impairment

Contra-indicated.

Children under 12 years

Not recommended.

4.3 Contraindications

Hydromorphone is contra-indicated in patients with known hypersensitivity to hydromorphone or other ingredients in the formulation.

It is also contra-indicated in respiratory depression with hypoxia or elevated carbon dioxide levels in the blood, pregnancy, coma, acute abdomen, hepatic impairment, paralytic ileus, concurrent administration of monoamine oxidase inhibitors or within 2 weeks of discontinuation of their use. Use of PALLADONE SR capsules should be avoided in patients with raised intracranial pressure or head injury, and also in patients with convulsive disorders or acute alcoholism.

Pre-operative administration of PALLADONE SR capsules is not recommended and is not an approved indication.

4.4 Special warnings and precautions for use

The major risk of opioid excess is respiratory depression. As with all narcotics, a reduction in dosage may be advised in the elderly or infirm patients with severely impaired pulmonary function, toxic psychosis, delirium tremens, pancreatitis, hypothyroidism, hypotension with hypovolaemia, chronic obstructive airways disease, renal or adrenocortical insufficiency, prostatic hypertrophy, shock or reduced respiratory reserve. PALLADONE SR capsules are not recommended in the first 24 hours post-operatively. After this time they should be used with caution, particularly following abdominal surgery.

PALLADONE SR capsules should not be used where there is the possibility of paralytic ileus occurring. Should paralytic ileus be suspected or occur during use, PALLADONE SR capsules should be discontinued.

Patients about to undergo cordotomy or other pain relieving surgical procedures should not receive PALLADONE SR capsules for 24 hours prior to surgery. If further treatment with PALLADONE SR capsules is indicated, then the dosage should be adjusted to the new post-operative requirement.

The patient may develop tolerance to the drug with chronic use and require progressively higher doses to maintain pain control. The patient may develop physical dependence; an abstinence syndrome may be seen following abrupt cessation.

When a patient no longer requires therapy with hydromorphone, it may be advisable to taper the dose gradually to prevent symptoms of withdrawal.

Hydromorphone has a morphine-like abuse profile and may be sought and abused by people with latent or manifest addiction disorders. Hydromorphone should be used with particular care in patients with a history of alcohol and drug abuse.

The prolonged release capsules may be opened and their contents sprinkled on to soft cold food. However the capsule contents should not be chewed or crushed. The administration of chewed or crushed hydromorphone pellets may lead to a rapid release and absorption of a potentially fatal dose of hydromorphone (see section 4.9).

Abuse of oral dosage forms by parenteral administration can be expected to result in serious adverse events, which may be fatal.

4.5 Interaction with other medicinal products and other forms of interaction

Centrally acting drugs such as major and minor tranquillisers, anaesthetics, barbiturates, antiemetics, antidepressants, alcohol, neuroleptics, hypnotics, other opioids, monoamine oxidase inhibitors (see section 4.3) and sedatives may interact with hydromorphone, and the effects of either drug, e.g. sedation, respiratory depression, etc.

4.6 Pregnancy and lactation

PALLADONE SR capsules are not recommended in pregnancy or in the breast-feeding mother as there are insufficient animal or human data to justify such use.

4.7 Effects on ability to drive and use machines

Hydromorphone may cause drowsiness and patients should not drive or operate machinery if affected.

4.8 Undesirable effects

Hydromorphone may cause constipation, nausea and vomiting. Constipation may be treated with appropriate laxatives. When nausea and vomiting are troublesome, PALLADONE SR capsules can be readily combined with anti-emetics

Common (incidence of ⩾ 1%) and uncommon (⩽ 1%) adverse drug reactions are listed in the table below:

	Common	Uncommon
Cardiac and vascular disorders	Hypotension	
Eye disorders		Blurred vision Miosis
Gastrointestinal and hepatobiliary disorders	Constipation Dry mouth Nausea Vomiting	Biliary colic Paralytic ileus
General disorders	Asthenic conditions	Drug withdrawal syndrome Drug tolerance Peripheral oedema
Immune system disorders		Hypersensitivity reactions (including oropharyngeal swelling)
Nervous system disorders	Dizziness Somnolence	Convulsions Dyskinesia Headache Sedation Tremor In particular in high doses hyperalgesia that will not respond to a further dose of hydromorphone (possibly dose reduction or change in opioid required).
Psychiatric disorders	Confusion	Drug addiction Agitation Dysphoria Euphoria Hallucination
Renal and urinary disorders	Urinary retention	
Respiratory, thoracic and mediastinal disorders		Respiratory depression
Skin and subcutaneous tissue disorders	Pruritus Rash Sweating	Urticaria

4.9 Overdose

Signs of hydromorphone toxicity and overdosage are pin-point pupils, respiratory depression and hypotension. Circulatory failure and somnolence progressing to stupor or deepening coma, skeletal muscle flaccidity, bradycardia and death may occur in more severe cases. Rhabdomyolosis progressing to renal failure has been reported in opioid overdosage.

Treatment of overdosage:

Primary attention should be given to the establishment of a patent airway and institution of assisted or controlled ventilation.

In the case of massive overdosage, administer naloxone intravenously (0.4 to 2 mg for an adult and 0.01mg/kg body weight for children), if the patient is in a coma or respiratory depression is present. Repeat the dose at 2 minute intervals if there is no response. If repeated doses are required then an infusion of 60% of the initial dose per hour is a useful starting point. A solution of 10 mg made up in 50 ml dextrose will produce 200 micrograms/ml for infusion using an IV pump (dose adjusted to the clinical response). Infusions are not a substitute for frequent review of the patient's clinical state.

Intramuscular naloxone is an alternative in the event IV access is not possible. As the duration of action of naloxone is relatively short, the patient must be carefully monitored until spontaneous respiration is reliably re-established. Naloxone is a competitive antagonist and large doses (4 mg) may be required in seriously poisoned patients. For less severe overdosage, administer naloxone 0.2 mg intravenously followed by increments of 0.1 mg every 2 minutes if required.

Naloxone should not be administered in the absence of clinically significant respiratory or circulatory depression secondary to hydromorphone overdosage. Naloxone should be administered cautiously to persons who are known, or suspected, to be physically dependent on hydromorphone. In such cases, an abrupt or complete reversal of opioid effects may precipitate an acute withdrawal syndrome.

Other supportive measures as indicated by the patient's progress and clinical condition should be considered.

Additional/other considerations:

Consider activated charcoal (50 g for adults, 1g/kg for children), if a substantial amount has been ingested within 1 hour, provided the airway can be protected. It may be reasonable to assume that late administration of activated charcoal may be beneficial for prolonged release preparations; however there is no evidence to support this.

PALLADONE SR capsules will continue to release and add to the hydromorphone load for up to 12 hours after administration and management of hydromorphone overdosage should be monitored accordingly. Gastric contents may need to be emptied as this can be useful in removing unabsorbed drug, particularly when a prolonged release formulation has been taken.

5. PHARMACOLOGICAL PROPERTIES

5.1 Pharmacodynamic properties

Pharmacotherapeutic group: Natural opium alkaloid

ATC code: NO2A A03

Like morphine, hydromorphone is an agonist of mu receptors. The pharmacological actions of hydromorphone and morphine do not differ significantly. The oral analgesic potency ratio of hydromorphone to morphine is approximately 5-10:1. Hydromorphone and related opioids produce their major effects on the central nervous system and bowel. The effects are diverse and include analgesia, drowsiness, changes in mood, respiratory depression, decreased gastrointestinal motility, nausea, vomiting and alteration of the endocrine and autonomic nervous system.

5.2 Pharmacokinetic properties

Hydromorphone is absorbed from the gastrointestinal tract and undergoes pre-systemic elimination resulting in an oral bioavailability of about 50%. It is metabolised and excreted in the urine mainly as conjugated hydromorphone and with smaller amounts of unchanged hydromorphone, dihydroisomorphine and dihydromorphine. PALLADONE SR capsules have been formulated to produce therapeutic plasma levels following 12-hourly dosing.

5.3 Preclinical safety data

There are no pre-clinical data of relevance to the prescriber which are additional to that already included in other sections of the SPC.

6. PHARMACEUTICAL PARTICULARS

6.1 List of excipients

Microcrystalline cellulose

Hypromellose

Ethylcellulose (N10)

Colloidal anhydrous silica

Dibutyl sebacate

Capsule shells

Gelatin

Sodium dodecylsulphate

Titanium dioxide (E171)

Black Printing ink

Shellac

Propylene glycol

Iron oxide (E172)

The following colours are included in the capsule shells:

2 mg Quinoline yellow (E104);

4 mg Erythrosine (E127), indigo carmine (E132);

8 mg Erythrosine (E127);

16 mg Iron oxide (E172);

24 mg Indigo carmine (E132).

6.2 Incompatibilities

None known.

6.3 Shelf life

Eighteen months.

6.4 Special precautions for storage

Do not store above 25°C. Store in the original package.

6.5 Nature and contents of container

PVdC/PVC blister packs with aluminium backing foil containing 56 capsules.

6.6 Special precautions for disposal and other handling

None stated.

7. MARKETING AUTHORISATION HOLDER

Napp Pharmaceuticals Limited

Cambridge Science Park

Milton Road

Cambridge

CB4 0GW

8. MARKETING AUTHORISATION NUMBER(S)

PL 16950/0051-0055

9. DATE OF FIRST AUTHORISATION/RENEWAL OF THE AUTHORISATION

12 February 1997 / 17 January 2006

10. DATE OF REVISION OF THE TEXT

September 2008

Paludrine Tablets

(AstraZeneca UK Limited)

1. NAME OF THE MEDICINAL PRODUCT

Paludrine Tablets

2. QUALITATIVE AND QUANTITATIVE COMPOSITION

Proguanil hydrochloride 100 mg

3. PHARMACEUTICAL FORM

Tablets for oral administration.

4. CLINICAL PARTICULARS

4.1 Therapeutic indications

Paludrine is an effective antimalarial agent. It is recommended for the prevention and suppression of malaria.

4.2 Posology and method of administration

Non-immune subjects entering a malarious area are advised to begin treatment with Paludrine 1 week before, or if this is not possible, then at least 2 days before entering the malarious area. The daily dose of Paludrine should be continued throughout exposure to risk and for 4 weeks after leaving the area.

Adults:	Two tablets (200 mg) daily.	
Children:	Under 1 year:	1/4 tablet (25 mg) daily
	1 to 4 years:	1/2 tablet (50 mg) daily
	5 to 8 years:	1 tablet (100 mg) daily
	9 to 14 years:	1 1/2 tablets (150 mg) daily
	Over 14 years:	Adult dose daily

The daily dose is best taken with water, after food, at the same time each day.

Provided the tablet fragment gives the minimum amount specified, precise accuracy in children's dosage is not essential since the drug possesses a wide safety margin.

For a young child, the dose may be administered crushed and mixed with milk, honey or jam. The treatment should be started at least two days before entering the malarious area and continued for the whole period of stay and 4 weeks after leaving the area.

Elderly patients: There are no special dosage recommendations for the elderly, but it may be advisable to monitor elderly patients so that optimum dosage can be individually determined.

Renal Impairment: Based on a theoretical model derived from a single dose pharmacokinetic study, the following guidance is given for adults with renal impairment. (See also Sections 4.3 and 4.4)

Creatinine clearance (ml/min 1.73 m²)	Dosage
⩾ 60	200 mg once daily (standard dose)
20 to 59	100 mg once daily
10 to 19	50 mg every second day
< 10	50 mg once weekly

The grade of renal impairment and/or the serum creatinine concentration may be approximately equated to creatinine clearance levels as indicated below.

Creatinine Clearance (ml/min/1.73 m²)	Approx* serum Creatinine (micromol/1)	Renal Impairment Grade (arbitrarily divided for dosage purposes)
⩾ 60	-	-
20 to 59	150 to 300	Mild
10 to 19	300 to 700	Moderate
< 10	> 700	Severe

*Serum creatinine concentration is only an approximate guide to renal function unless corrected for age, weight and sex.

4.3 Contraindications

Paludrine should be used with caution in patients with severe renal impairment. (See also Sections 4.2 and 4.4)

4.4 Special warnings and precautions for use

Paludrine should be used with caution in patients with severe renal impairment. (See also Section 4.2) There have been rare reports of haematological changes in such patients.

In any locality where drug-resistant malaria is known or suspected, it is essential to take local medical advice on what prophylactic regimen is appropriate. Prophylactic use of Paludrine alone may not be sufficient.

4.5 Interaction with other medicinal products and other forms of interaction

Antacids may reduce the absorption of proguanil, so should be taken at least 2-3 hours apart.

Proguanil can potentiate the anticoagulant effect of warfarin and related anticoagulants through a possible interference with their metabolic pathways. Caution is advised when initiating or withdrawing malaria prophylaxis with Paludrine in patients on continuous treatment with anticoagulants.

4.6 Pregnancy and lactation

Pregnancy: Paludrine has been widely used for over 40 years and a causal connection between its use and any adverse effect on mother or foetus has not been established.

However, Paludrine should not be used during pregnancy unless, in the judgement of the physician, potential benefit outweighs the risk.

Malaria in pregnant women increases the risk of maternal death, miscarriage, still-birth and low birth weight with the associated risk of neonatal death. Although travel to malarious areas should be avoided during pregnancy, if this is unavoidable effective prophylaxis is therefore strongly advised in pregnant women.

Lactation: Although Paludrine is excreted in breast milk, the amount is insufficient to confer any benefit on the infant. Separate chemoprophylaxis for the infant is required.

4.7 Effects on ability to drive and use machines

There is no evidence to suggest that Paludrine causes sedation or is likely to affect concentration.

4.8 Undesirable effects

At normal dosage levels the side effect most commonly encountered is mild gastric intolerance, including diarrhoea and constipation. This usually subsides as treatment is continued.

Mouth ulceration and stomatitis have on occasion been reported. Isolated cases of skin reactions and reversible hair loss have been reported in association with the use of proguanil.

Rarely, allergic reactions, which manifest as urticaria or angioedema and very rarely vasculitis, have been reported.

Drug fever and cholestasis may very rarely occur in patients receiving Paludrine.

Haematological changes in patients with severe renal impairment have been reported.

4.9 Overdose

The following effects have been reported in cases of overdosage:

Haematuria, renal irritation, epigastric discomfort and vomiting. There is no specific antidote and symptoms should be treated as they arise.

5. PHARMACOLOGICAL PROPERTIES

5.1 Pharmacodynamic properties

Proguanil is an antimalarial drug and dihydrofolate reductase inhibitor. It acts like the other antifolate antimalarials by interfering with the folic-folinic acid systems and thus exerts its effect mainly at the time the nucleus is dividing. Since its activity is dependent on its metabolism, proguanil has a slow schizonticidal effect in the blood. It also has some schizonticidal activity in the tissues.

Proguanil is effective against the exoerythrocytic forms of some strains of plasmodium falciparum but it has little or no activity against the exoerythrocytic forms of p. Vivax. It has a marked sporonticidal effect against some strains of p falciparum; it does not kill the gametocytes, but renders them non-infective for the mosquito while the drug is present in the blood. Malaria parasites in the red blood cells are killed more rapidly by chloroquine or quinine than by proguanil, which is therefore not the best drug to use for the treatment of acute malaria.

Soon after proguanil was introduced, it was observed that the drug was inactive as an inhibitor of the in vitro growth of p. Gallinaceum and p. Cynomolgi, but that sera from dosed monkeys were active against p. Cynomolgi in vitro. These findings suggested that proguanil was activated in vivo.

Since that time it has been accepted by most investigators in this field that cycloguanil is the active metabolite of proguanil and that parent compound is inactive per se.

Cycloguanil acts by binding to the enzyme dihydrofolate reductase in the malaria parasite. The effect of this action is to prevent the completion of schizogony. This is seen in the asexual blood stages as an arrest of maturation of the developing schizonts and an accumulation of large, abnormal looking trophozoites.

Proguanil is highly active against the primary exoerythocytic forms of p. Falciparum and it has a fleeting inhibiting action on those of p. Vivax. Proguanil is therefore a valuable drug for causal prophylaxis in falciparum malaria.

5.2 Pharmacokinetic properties

Absorption: Rapid, reaching a peak at 3 to 4 hours. The active metabolite (cycloguanil) peaks somewhat later (4 to 9 hours).

Half-life: The half-life of proguanil is 14 to 20 hours, whilst cycloguanil has a half-life of the order of 20 hours. Accumulation during repeated dosing is therefore limited, steady-state being reached within approximately 3 days.

Metabolism: Transformation of proguanil into cycloguanil is associated with cytochrome P450, CYP 2C19, activity. A smaller part of the transformation of proguanil into cycloguanil is probably catalysed by CYP 3A4.

Elimination: Elimination occurs both in the faeces and, principally, in the urine.

In the event of a daily dose being missed, the blood levels fall rapidly but total disappearance of the drug only occurs 3 to 5 days after stopping treatment.

5.3 Preclinical safety data

Proguanil is a drug on which extensive clinical experience has been obtained. All relevant information for the prescriber is provided elsewhere in the Summary of Product Characteristics.

6. PHARMACEUTICAL PARTICULARS

6.1 List of excipients

Calcium carbonate

Gelatin

Magnesium stearate

Maize starch

6.2 Incompatibilities

None known.

6.3 Shelf life

5 years.

6.4 Special precautions for storage

Store below 30°C.

6.5 Nature and contents of container

HDPE bottles (100) and blister packs (98).

6.6 Special precautions for disposal and other handling

Use as directed by the prescriber.

7. MARKETING AUTHORISATION HOLDER

AstraZeneca UK Limited,
600 Capability Green,
Luton, LU1 3LU, UK.

8. MARKETING AUTHORISATION NUMBER(S)

PL 17901/0036

9. DATE OF FIRST AUTHORISATION/RENEWAL OF THE AUTHORISATION

18th June 2000

10. DATE OF REVISION OF THE TEXT

18th April 2005

Paludrine/Avloclor Anti-Malarial Travel Pack Chloroquine & Proguanil Anti-Malarial Tablets

(AstraZeneca UK Limited)

1. NAME OF THE MEDICINAL PRODUCT

Paludrine/Avloclor Anti-malarial Travel Pack.

Chloroquine and Proguanil Anti-malarial Tablets.

2. QUALITATIVE AND QUANTITATIVE COMPOSITION

Paludrine tablets containing 100 mg proguanil hydrochloride

Avloclor tablets containing 250 mg chloroquine phosphate, which is equivalent to 155 mg chloroquine base.

3. PHARMACEUTICAL FORM

Tablets.

4. CLINICAL PARTICULARS

4.1 Therapeutic indications

Prophylaxis and suppression of malaria.

4.2 Posology and method of administration

Non-immune subjects entering a malarious area are advised to begin daily treatment with Paludrine 1 week before, or if this is not possible, then at least 2 days before entering the malarious area. The daily dose of Paludrine should be continued throughout exposure to risk and for 4 weeks after leaving the area.

A single dose of Avloclor should be taken each week on the same day each week. Start one week before exposure to risk and continue until 4 weeks after leaving the malarious area.

Each dose should be taken with water after food.

Adults and children over 14 years: Take two Paludrine tablets daily as directed above. Take two Avloclor tablets once a week as directed above.

Children: Do not give to children under 1 year. The following single dose of Paludrine should be taken at the same time each day and the following single dose of Avloclor should be taken once a week on the same day each week.

	Paludrine (at the same time each day)	**Avloclor (on the same day each week)**
1 to 4 years	Half of a tablet	Half of a tablet
5 to 8 years	One tablet	One tablet
9 to 14 years	One and a half tablets	One and a half tablets

For a young child the dose may be administered crushed and mixed with milk, honey or jam.

Provided the Paludrine tablet fragment gives the minimum amount specified, precise accuracy in children's dosage is not essential since the drug possesses a wide safety margin.

The Avloclor dose given to children should be calculated on their body weight (5 mg chloroquine base/kg/week) and must not exceed the adult dose regardless of weight.

Elderly Patients: There are no special dosage recommendations for the elderly, but it may be advisable to monitor elderly patients so that optimum dosage can be individually determined.

Paludrine and Renal Impairment: Based on a theoretical model derived from a single dose pharmacokinetic study, the following guidance is given for adults with renal impairment. (See also Sections 4.3 and 4.4).

Creatinine clearance (ml/min/1.73 m²)	**Dosage**
⩾ 60	200 mg once daily (standard dose)
20 to 59	100 mg once daily
10 to 19	50 mg every second day
< 10	50 mg once weekly

The grade of renal impairment and/or the serum creatinine concentration may be approximately equated to creatinine clearance levels as indicated below.

Creatinine clearance (ml/min/1.73 m²)	**Approx* serum creatinine (micromol/1)**	**Renal Impairment Grade (arbitrarily divided for dosage purposes)**
⩾ 60	-	
20 to 59	150 to 300	Mild
10 to 19	300 to 700	Moderate
< 10	> 700	Severe

*Serum creatinine concentration is only an approximate guide to renal function unless corrected for age, weight and sex.

Avloclor and Hepatic or Renally Impaired Patients: Caution is necessary when giving Avloclor to patients with renal disease or hepatic disease.

4.3 Contraindications

Known hypersensitivity to chloroquine or any other ingredients of the formulation.

4.4 Special warnings and precautions for use

When used as malaria prophylaxis official guidelines and local information on prevalence of resistance to anti-malarial drugs should be taken into consideration.

Paludrine should be used with caution in patients with severe renal impairment. (See also Section 4.2). There have been rare reports of haematological changes in such patients. Caution is necessary when giving Avloclor to patients with renal disease.

Caution is necessary when giving Avloclor to patients with impaired hepatic function, particularly when associated with cirrhosis.

Caution is also necessary in patients with porphyria. Avloclor may precipitate severe constitutional symptoms and an increase in the amount of porphyrins excreted in the urine. This reaction is especially apparent in patients with high alcohol intake.

Avloclor should be used with care in patients with a history of epilepsy. Potential risks and benefits should be carefully evaluated before use in subjects taking anti-convulsant therapy or with a history of epilepsy as, rarely, cases of convulsions have been reported in association with chloroquine.

The use of Avloclor in patients with psoriasis may precipitate a severe attack.

Caution is advised in patients with glucose-6-phosphate dehydrogenase deficiency, as there may be a risk of haemolysis.

Prolonged or high dose Avloclor therapy:

Considerable caution is needed in the use of Avloclor for long-term high dosage therapy and such use should only be considered when no other drug is available.

Irreversible retinal damage and corneal changes may develop during long term therapy and after the drug has been discontinued. Ophthalmic examination prior to and at 3 – 6 monthly intervals during use is required if patients are receiving chloroquine

- At continuous high doses for longer than 12 months
- As weekly treatment for longer than 3 years
- When total consumption exceeds 1.6g/kg (cumulative dose 100g).

Full blood counts should be carried out regularly during extended treatment as bone marrow suppression may occur rarely.

4.5 Interaction with other medicinal products and other forms of interaction

Antacids (aluminium, calcium and magnesium salts) may reduce the absorption of proguanil and chloroquine, so antacids should be taken well separated from Paludrine and Avloclor (at least two hours before or after).

If the patient is taking cyclosporin then chloroquine may cause an increase in cyclosporin levels.

Pre-exposure intradermal human diploid-cell rabies vaccine should not be administered to patients taking chloroquine as this may suppress antibody response. When vaccinated against rabies, that vaccine should precede the start of antimalarial dosing, otherwise the effectiveness of the vaccine might be reduced.

Chloroquine significantly reduces levels of praziquantel. Caution is therefore advised during co-administration. Prescribers may consider increasing the dose of praziquantel if the patient does not respond to the initial dose.

Amiodarone:	chloroquine and hydroxychloroquine increase the risk of cardiac arrhythmias including ventricular arrhythmias, bradycardias and cardiac conduction defect. Concurrent use is contra-indicated.
Anticoagulants:	proguanil can potentiate the anticoagulant effect of warfarin and related anticoagulants through a possible interference with their metabolic pathways. Caution is advised when initiating or withdrawing malaria prophylaxis with Paludrine in patients on continuous treatment with anticoagulants.
Other antimalarials:	increased risk of convulsion with mefloquine.
Cardiac glycosides:	hydroxychloroquine and possibly chloroquine increase plasma concentration of digoxin.
Parasympathomimetics:	chloroquine and hydroxychloroquine have potential to increase symptoms of myasthenia gravis and thus diminish effect of neostigmine and pyridostigmine.
Ulcer healing drugs:	cimetidine inhibits metabolism of chloroquine (increased plasma concentration).

4.6 Pregnancy and lactation

Pregnancy

Avloclor and Paludrine should not be used during pregnancy unless, in the judgement of the physician, potential benefit outweighs the risk.

Short-term malaria prophylaxis:

Malaria in pregnant women increases the risk of maternal death, miscarriage, still-birth and low birth weight with the associated risk of neonatal death. Travel to malarious areas should be avoided during pregnancy but, if this is not possible, women should receive effective prophylaxis.

Long-term high dose Avloclor therapy:

There is evidence to suggest that Avloclor given to women in high doses throughout pregnancy can give rise to foetal abnormalities including visual loss, ototoxicity and cochlear-vestibular dysfunction. Paludrine has been widely used for over 40 years and a causal connection between its use and any adverse effect on mother or foetus has not been established.

Lactation

Although both Paludrine and Avloclor are excreted in breast milk, the amount is too small to be harmful when used for malaria prophylaxis but as a consequence is insufficient to confer any benefit on the infant. Separate chemoprophylaxis for the infant is required. However, when long-term high doses of chloroquine are used for rheumatoid disease, breast feeding is not recommended.

4.7 Effects on ability to drive and use machines

Defects in visual accommodation may occur on first taking Avloclor and patients should be warned regarding driving or operating machinery.

There is no evidence to suggest that Paludrine causes sedation or is likely to affect concentration.

4.8 Undesirable effects

The adverse reactions which may occur at doses used in the prophylaxis of malaria are generally not of a serious nature. Where prolonged high dosage of chloroquine is required, i.e. in the treatment of rheumatoid arthritis, adverse reactions can be of a more serious nature.

Paludrine

At normal dosage levels the side effect most commonly encountered is mild gastric intolerance, including diarrhoea and constipation. This usually subsides as treatment is continued.

Mouth ulceration and stomatitis have on occasion been reported. Isolated cases of skin reactions and reversible hair loss have been reported in association with the use of proguanil.

Rarely, allergic reactions which manifest as urticaria or angioedema and very rarely vasculitis, have been reported.

Drug fever and cholestasis may very rarely occur in patients receiving Paludrine.

Haematological changes in patients with severe renal impairment have been reported.

Avloclor

Adverse reactions reported after Avloclor use are:

Cardiovascular:	hypotension and ECG changes (at high doses), cardiomyopathy.
Central nervous system:	convulsions and psychotic reactions including hallucinations (rare), anxiety, personality changes.
Eye disorders:	retinal degeneration, macular defects of colour vision, pigmentation, optic atrophy scotomas, field defects, blindness, corneal opacities and pigmented deposits, blurring of vision, difficulty in accommodation, diplopia.
Gastro-intestinal:	gastro-intestinal disturbances, nausea, vomiting, diarrhoea, abdominal cramps.
General:	headache.
Haematological:	bone marrow depression, aplastic anaemia, agranulocytosis, thrombocytopenia, neutropenia.
Hepatic:	changes in liver function, including hepatitis and abnormal liver function tests, have been reported rarely.
Hypersensitivity:	allergic and anaphylactic reactions, including urticaria, angioedema and vasculitis.
Hearing disorders:	tinnitus, reduced hearing, nerve deafness.
Muscular:	neuromyopathy and myopathy.
Skin:	macular, urticarial and purpuric skin eruptions, occasional depigmentation or loss of hair, erythema multiforme, Stevens-Johnson syndrome, toxic epidermal necrolysis, precipitation of psoriasis, pruritus, photosensitivity, lichen-planus type reaction, pigmentation of the skin and mucous membranes (long term use).

4.9 Overdose

Paludrine

The following effects have been reported in cases of overdosage:

Haematuria, renal irritation, epigastric discomfort and vomiting. There is no specific antidote and symptoms should be treated as they arise.

Avloclor

Chloroquine is highly toxic in overdose and children are particularly susceptible. The chief symptoms of overdosage include circulatory collapse due to a potent cardiotoxic effect, respiratory arrest and coma. Symptoms may progress rapidly after initial nausea and vomiting. Cardiac complications may occur without progressively deepening coma.

Death may result from circulatory or respiratory failure or cardiac arrhythmia. If there is no demonstrable cardiac output due to arrhythmias, asystole or electromechanical dissociation, external chest compression should be persisted with for as long as necessary, or until adrenaline and diazepam can be given (see below).

Gastric lavage should be carried out urgently, first protecting the airway and instituting artificial ventilation where necessary. There is a risk of cardiac arrest following aspiration of gastric contents in more serious cases. Activated charcoal left in the stomach may reduce absorption of any remaining chloroquine from the gut. Circulatory status (with central venous pressure measurement), respiration, plasma electrolytes and blood gases should be monitored, with correction of hypokalaemia and acidosis if indicated. Cardiac arrhythmias should not be treated unless life threatening; drugs with quinidine-like effects should be avoided. Intravenous sodium bicarbonate 1-2mmol/kg over 15 minutes may be effective in conduction disturbances, and DC shock is indicated for ventricular tachycardia and ventricular fibrillation.

Early administration of the following has been shown to improve survival in cases of serious poisoning:

1. Adrenaline infusion 0.25 micrograms/kg/min initially, with increments of 0.25 micrograms/kg/min until adequate systolic blood pressure (more than 100mm/Hg) is restored; adrenaline reduces the effects of chloroquine on the heart through its inotropic and vasoconstrictor effects.

2. Diazepam infusion (2mg/kg over 30 minutes as a loading dose, followed by 1-2mg/kg/day for up to 2-4 days). Diazepam may minimise cardiotoxicity.

Acidification of the urine, haemodialysis, peritoneal dialysis or exchange transfusion have not been shown to be of value in treating chloroquine poisoning. Chloroquine is excreted very slowly, therefore cases of overdosage require observation for several days.

5. PHARMACOLOGICAL PROPERTIES

5.1 Pharmacodynamic properties

Paludrine

Proguanil is an antimalarial drug and dihydrofolate reductase inhibitor. It acts like the other antifolate antimalarials by interfering with the folic-folinic acid systems and thus exerts its effect mainly at the time the nucleus is dividing. Since its activity is dependent on its metabolism, proguanil has a slow schizonticidal effect in the blood. It also has some schizonticidal activity in the tissues.

Proguanil is effective against the exoerythrocytic forms of some strains of *plasmodium falciparum* but it has little or no activity against the exoerythrocytic forms of *p. Vivax*. It has a marked sporonticidal effect against some strains of *p falciparum*; it does not kill the gametocytes, but renders them non-infective for the mosquito while the drug is present in the blood. Malaria parasites in the red blood cells are killed more rapidly by chloroquine or quinine than by proguanil, which is therefore not the best drug to use for the treatment of acute malaria.

Soon after proguanil was introduced, it was observed that the drug was inactive as an inhibitor of the in vitro growth of *p. Gallinaceum* and *p. Cynomolgi*, but that sera from dosed monkeys were active against *p. Cynomolgi* in vitro. These findings suggested that proguanil was activated in vivo.

Since that time it has been accepted by most investigators in this field that cycloguanil is the active metabolite of proguanil and that parent compound is inactive per se.

Cycloguanil acts by binding to the enzyme dihydrofolate reductase in the malaria parasite. The effect of this action is to prevent the completion of schizogony. This is seen in the asexual blood stages as an arrest of maturation of the developing schizonts and an accumulation of large, abnormal looking trophozoites.

Proguanil is highly active against the primary exoerythocytic forms of *p. Falciparum* and it has a fleeting inhibiting action on those of *p. Vivax*. Proguanil is therefore a valuable drug for causal prophylaxis in falciparum malaria.

Avloclor

The mode of action of chloroquine on plasmodia has not been fully elucidated. Chloroquine binds to and alters the properties of DNA. Chloroquine also binds to ferriprotoporphyrin IX and this leads to lysis of the plasmodial membrane.

In suppressive treatment, chloroquine inhibits the erythrocytic stage of development of plasmodia. In acute attacks of malaria, it interrupts erythrocytic schizogony of the parasite. Its ability to concentrate in parasitised erythrocytes may account for the selective toxicity against the erythrocytic stages of plasmodial infection.

5.2 Pharmacokinetic properties

Paludrine

Absorption: Rapid, reaching a peak at 3 to 4 hours. The active metabolite (cycloguanil) peaks somewhat later (4 to 9 hours).

Half-life: The half-life of proguanil is 14 to 20 hours, whilst cycloguanil has a half-life of the order of 20 hours. Accumulation during repeated dosing is therefore limited, steady-state being reached within approximately 3 days.

Metabolism: Transformation of proguanil into cycloguanil is associated with cytochrome P450, CYP 2C19, activity. A smaller part of the transformation of proguanil into cycloguanil is probably catalysed by CYP 3A4.

Elimination: Elimination occurs both in the faeces and, principally, in the urine.

In the event of a daily dose being missed, the blood levels fall rapidly but total disappearance of the drug only occurs 3 to 5 days after stopping treatment.

Avloclor

Studies in volunteers using single doses of chloroquine phosphate equivalent to 300mg base have found peak plasma levels to be achieved within one to six hours. These levels are in the region of 54-102 microgram/litre, the concentration in whole blood being some 4 to 10 times higher. Following a single dose, chloroquine may be detected in plasma for more than four weeks. Mean bioavailability from tablets of chloroquine phosphate is 89%. Chloroquine is widely distributed in body tissues such as the eyes, kidneys, liver, and lungs where retention is prolonged. The elimination of chloroquine is slow, with a multi exponential decline in plasma concentration. The initial distribution phase has a half-life of 2-6 days while the terminal elimination phase is 10-60 days. Approximately 50-70% of chloroquine in plasma is bound to the plasma proteins.

The principal metabolite is monodesethylchloroquine, which reaches a peak concentration of 10-20 microgram/litre within a few hours. Mean urinary recovery, within 3-13 weeks, is approximately 50% of the administered dose, most being unchanged drug and the remainder as metabolite. Chloroquine may be detected in urine for several months.

5.3 Preclinical safety data

Both Paludrine and Avloclor have been extensively used for many years in clinical practice. All relevant information for the prescriber is provided elsewhere in this document.

6. PHARMACEUTICAL PARTICULARS

6.1 List of excipients

Paludrine	Avloclor
Calcium carbonate	Magnesium stearate
Gelatin	Maize starch
Magnesium stearate	
Maize starch	

6.2 Incompatibilities

None known.

6.3 Shelf life

5 years.

6.4 Special precautions for storage

Do not store above 30°C. Store in the original package.

6.5 Nature and contents of container

PVC/PVDC Aluminium Foil Blister Pack of 112's containing 98 Paludrine and 14 Avloclor tablets.

6.6 Special precautions for disposal and other handling

No special instructions.

7. MARKETING AUTHORISATION HOLDER

AstraZeneca UK Limited,

600 Capability Green,

Luton, LU1 3LU, UK.

8. MARKETING AUTHORISATION NUMBER(S)

PL 17901/0037

9. DATE OF FIRST AUTHORISATION/RENEWAL OF THE AUTHORISATION

18th June 2000/5th November 2002

10. DATE OF REVISION OF THE TEXT

23rd June 2005

Pancrease HL Capsules

(Janssen-Cilag Ltd)

1. NAME OF THE MEDICINAL PRODUCT

Pancrease™ HL Capsules

2. QUALITATIVE AND QUANTITATIVE COMPOSITION

Each capsule contains pancreatin, equivalent to 25000 units of lipase, 22500 units of amylase and 1250 units of protease.

3. PHARMACEUTICAL FORM

Size 0, elongated hard gelatin capsule, with a white opaque body and a white opaque cap, each ringed with a red band and the letters HL in red, containing enterically coated minitablets.

4. CLINICAL PARTICULARS

4.1 Therapeutic indications

Exocrine pancreatic enzyme deficiency as in cystic fibrosis, chronic pancreatitis, post pancreatectomy, post gastro-intestinal bypass surgery (eg Billroth II gastroenterostomy), and ductal obstruction from neoplasm (eg of the pancreas or common bile duct).

4.2 Posology and method of administration

For oral administration.

Patients with pancreatic insufficiency should undergo regular nutritional assessments as a component of routine care and additionally, when dosing of pancreatic enzyme replacement is altered.

Dosage should be individualised to each patient, with therapy being initiated at the lowest possible dose and gradually increase until the desired control of steatorrhoea is obtained.

Adults and children

One or two capsules during each meal and one capsule with snacks. The interindividual response to pancreatin supplements is variable and the number of capsules may need to be titrated to the individual based upon parameters of steatorrhoea and symptomatology. Further dose increases, if required, should be added slowly, with careful monitoring of response and symptomatology.

Where patients are already in receipt of lower unit dose enteric coated pancreatin supplements, then Pancrease

HL Capsules may be substituted at one-third of the number of capsules of the previous preparation.

Where swallowing of capsules is difficult, then they may be opened and the minitablets taken with liquid or soft foods which do not require chewing. To protect the enteric coating, the minitablets should not be crushed or chewed.

Contact of the minitablets with food having a pH higher than 5.0 can dissolve the protective coating and will reduce the efficacy of the product.

It is important to ensure adequate hydration of patients at all times whilst dosing Pancrease HL Capsules.

Patients who are taking or have been given in excess of 10,000 units of lipase/kg/day are at risk of developing colon damage. The dose of Pancrease HL should usually not exceed this dose.

4.3 Contraindications
Pancrease HL Capsules are contra-indicated in patients known to be hypersensitive to pork protein or any other component of this product.

Children aged 15 or under with cystic fibrosis.

4.4 Special warnings and precautions for use
Contact of the minitablets with food or liquid having a pH higher than 5.0 can dissolve the protective coating and will reduce efficacy of the product.

Cases of fibrotic strictures in the colon have been reported primarily in cystic fibrosis patients with the use of enzyme supplements, generally at dosages above the recommended range. If symptoms suggestive of gastrointestinal obstruction occur, the possibility of bowel strictures should be considered. In some cases surgery including resection of the bowel is required and the need for this should also be considered.

Any change in pancreatic enzyme replacement therapy (e.g., dose or brand of medication) should be made cautiously and only under medical supervision.

4.5 Interaction with other medicinal products and other forms of interaction
None stated.

4.6 Pregnancy and lactation
No adequate, well-controlled studies have been conducted in pregnant women. Pancrease HL capsules should be used during pregnancy only if the potential benefit justifies the potential risk to the foetus. Pancrease HL should not be used in pregnancy and lactation unless clearly necessary but if required should be used in doses sufficient to provide adequate nutritional status (see warnings about high dose sections 4.2 & 4.8)

The possibility of protein constituents appearing in the breast milk cannot be excluded; therefore caution should be exercised when prescribing Pancrease HL capsules to lactating women.

4.7 Effects on ability to drive and use machines
None stated.

4.8 Undesirable effects
Postmarketing Experience
Adverse drug reactions from spontaneous reports during the worldwide postmarketing experience with Pancrelipase Capsules that meet threshold criteria are included in Table 1. The adverse drug reactions are ranked by frequency, using the following convention:

Very common $\geq$1/10
Common $\geq$1/100 and < 1/10
Uncommon $\geq$1/1,000 and <1/100
Rare $\geq$1/10,000 and <1/1,000
Very rare <1/10,000, including isolated reports

The frequencies provided below reflect reporting rates for adverse drug reactions from spontaneous reports, and do not represent more precise estimates that might be obtained in clinical trials or epidemiological studies.

The most frequently reported adverse events were of gastrointestinal origin i.e. nausea, vomiting and diarrhoea.

Table 1. Postmarketing reports of adverse drug reactions

Metabolism and Nutrition Disorders	
Very rare	weight decrease
Investigations	
Very rare	hyperuricosuria, hyperuricaemia
Gastrointestinal disorders	
Very rare	abdominal distention, abdominal pain, abnormal faeces, colonic stenosis, diarrhoea, intestinal bleeding, perianal irritation, dyspepsia, fibrosing colonopathy, flatulence, ileal stenosis, intestinal obstruction, melaena, nausea, constipation, vomiting.
General disorders and administration site conditions	
Very rare	oedema, pain,
Skin and subcutaneous tissue disorders	
Very rare	pruritus, rash

4.9 Overdose
Overdosage is unlikely and has not been experienced to date with Pancrease HL. Inappropriately large doses could result in symptoms such as abdominal discomfort, nausea, vomiting, perianal irritation or inflammation.

5. PHARMACOLOGICAL PROPERTIES
5.1 Pharmacodynamic properties
The enzymes catalyse the hydrolysis of fats into glycerol and fatty acids, protein into proteoses and derived substances, and starch into dextrins and sugars.

5.2 Pharmacokinetic properties
Pancreatin is not systemically absorbed from the gastro-intestinal tract.

5.3 Preclinical safety data
No relevant information additional to that contained elsewhere in the Summary of Product Characteristics.

6. PHARMACEUTICAL PARTICULARS
6.1 List of excipients
Castor oil, hydrogenated
Silica Colloidal Anhydrous
Magnesium stearate
Croscarmellose Sodium
Cellulose microcrystalline
Coat composition:
Simethicone emulsion
Methacryllic acid-ethyl acrylate copolymer (1:1)
Talc
Triethyl citrate
Purified water
Capsule composition (body and cap):
Titanium dioxide
Gelatin
Ink composition:
Shellac
Red iron oxide (E172)
Industrial methylated spirits
Purified Water
Propylene Glycol
Isopropyl Alcohol
n-Butyl Alcohol
OR
Shellac
Red Iron Oxide (E172)
Dehydrated Alcohol
Propylene Glycol
Isopropyl Alcohol
Butyl Alcohol
Strong Ammonia Solution
Potassium Hydroxide
Purified Water.

6.2 Incompatibilities
None stated.

6.3 Shelf life
2 years.

6.4 Special precautions for storage
Do not store above 25°C. Keep bottle tightly closed. Do not refrigerate or freeze.

6.5 Nature and contents of container
High density polyethylene bottles with a low density polyethylene snap top lid, containing 100 or 500 capsules.

6.6 Special precautions for disposal and other handling
Not applicable.

7. MARKETING AUTHORISATION HOLDER
Janssen-Cilag Ltd
50-100 Holmers Farm Way
High Wycombe
Bucks
HP12 4EG
UK

8. MARKETING AUTHORISATION NUMBER(S)
0242/0255

9. DATE OF FIRST AUTHORISATION/RENEWAL OF THE AUTHORISATION
1 October 1995

10. DATE OF REVISION OF THE TEXT
August 2009

Legal category POM

Pancrex Granules

(Paines & Byrne Limited)

1. NAME OF THE MEDICINAL PRODUCT
Pancrex Granules.

2. QUALITATIVE AND QUANTITATIVE COMPOSITION
Pancreatin BP to provide enzymatic activity per gram not less than:

Free protease	300 BP units
Lipase	5000 BP units
Amylase	4000 BP units

3. PHARMACEUTICAL FORM
Granules.

4. CLINICAL PARTICULARS
4.1 Therapeutic indications
Pancrex is used to compensate for reduced intestinal enzyme activity in pancreatic deficiency states.

It is indicated for the treatment of fibrocystic disease of the pancreas (cystic fibrosis), chronic pancreatitis and pancreatic steatorrhoea following pancreatectomy. It may also be indicated following gastrectomy as an aid to digestion.

4.2 Posology and method of administration
Dosage should be adjusted according to the needs of the individual patient and the amount and type of food consumed.

The following dosage ranges provide a suitable basis for adjustment.

Adults, the Elderly, and Children

5 g - 10 g swallowed dry or mixed with a little water or milk just before meals

4.3 Contraindications
Hypersensitivity to the active ingredient (porcine pancreatin) or any of the excipients.

4.4 Special warnings and precautions for use
Unsuitable for people with lactase insufficiency, galactosaemia or glucose/galactose malabsorption syndrome.

It is possible that some irritation of the skin of the mouth may occur if the granules are chewed or retained in the mouth. Irritation of the anus may also occur. A barrier cream may prevent this local irritation.

If the granules are mixed with liquids the resulting mixture should not be allowed to stand for more than one hour prior to use.

4.5 Interaction with other medicinal products and other forms of interaction
None known.

4.6 Pregnancy and lactation
Pancrex should not be used in pregnancy and lactation unless clearly necessary but if required should be used in doses sufficient to provide adequate nutritional status.

4.7 Effects on ability to drive and use machines
None.

4.8 Undesirable effects
Rare cases of hyperuricosuria and hyperuricaemia have been reported when extremely high doses of pancreatin have been taken.

Strictures of the ileo-caecum and large bowel, and colitis, have been reported in children with cystic fibrosis taking high doses of pancreatic enzyme supplements. To date Pancrex and Pancrex V presentations have not been implicated in the development of colonic damage. However unusual abdominal symptoms or changes in abdominal symptoms should be reviewed to exclude the possibility of colonic damage especially if the patient is taking in excess of 10,000 units/kg/day of lipase.

4.9 Overdose
None stated.

5. PHARMACOLOGICAL PROPERTIES
5.1 Pharmacodynamic properties
Pancreatin is derived from porcine pancreas and contains the enzymes, amylase, protease and lipase. The enzymes have the same actions as pancreatic juice and when administered to patients with pancreatic insufficiency improve the ability to metabolise starches, proteins and fats.

5.2 Pharmacokinetic properties
Pancreatin hydrolyses fats to glycerol and fatty acids, changes proteins into proteases and derived substances, and converts starch into dextrins and sugars.

5.3 Preclinical safety data
No relevant pre-clinical safety data has been generated.

6. PHARMACEUTICAL PARTICULARS
6.1 List of excipients
Lactose, acacia (E414), Opaseal P17-0200 containing IMS, polyvinyl acetate phthalate and stearic acid (E570).

This medicinal product contains approximately 70g of lactose per 100g. When taken according to the dosage recommendations each dose supplies up to 7g of lactose.

6.2 Incompatibilities
None known.

6.3 Shelf life
2 years.

6.4 Special precautions for storage
Store at a temperature not exceeding 15°C.

6.5 Nature and contents of container
Securitainer; 100, 300 and 500 g.

6.6 Special precautions for disposal and other handling
Not applicable.

7. MARKETING AUTHORISATION HOLDER
Paines and Byrne Limited
Lovett House
Lovett Road
Staines
TW18 3AZ
United Kingdom

8. MARKETING AUTHORISATION NUMBER(S)
PL0051/5003R

9. DATE OF FIRST AUTHORISATION/RENEWAL OF THE AUTHORISATION
First authorisation granted 1 May 1987 / October 2003

10. DATE OF REVISION OF THE TEXT
25 October 2007

11. Legal category
P

Pancrex V Capsules

(Paines & Byrne Limited)

1. NAME OF THE MEDICINAL PRODUCT
Pancrex V Capsules.

2. QUALITATIVE AND QUANTITATIVE COMPOSITION
Pancreatin BP to provide enzymatic activity per capsule not less than:

Free protease	430 BP units
Lipase	8000 BP units
Amylase	9000 BP units

3. PHARMACEUTICAL FORM
Capsule.

4. CLINICAL PARTICULARS
4.1 Therapeutic indications
Pancrex is used to compensate for reduced intestinal enzyme activity in pancreatic deficiency states.

It is indicated for the treatment of fibrocystic disease of the pancreas (cystic fibrosis), chronic pancreatitis and pancreatic steatorrhoea following pancreatectomy. It may also be indicated following gastrectomy as an aid to digestion.

4.2 Posology and method of administration
Dosage should be adjusted according to the needs of the individual patient and the amount and type of food consumed.

The following dosage ranges provide a suitable basis for adjustment.

Infants: the contents of 1 - 2 capsules mixed with feeds.

Older Children and Adults: the contents of 2 - 6 capsules with each snack or meal. The capsules may be swallowed.

The capsules may provide a suitable alternative to the enteric coated presentations in cases where the pH of the duodenum is not sufficiently alkaline to dissolve the enteric coat.

Capsules provide a simple and convenient method of dose measurement of pancreatin for administration to younger children requiring a low dose.

4.3 Contraindications
Hypersensitivity to the active ingredient (porcine pancreatin) or any of the excipients.

4.4 Special warnings and precautions for use
It is possible that some irritation of the skin of the mouth may occur if capsules are chewed or the contents retained in the mouth. Irritation of the anus may also occur. A barrier cream may prevent this local irritation.

Allergic/asthmatic reactions have occasionally occurred on handling the capsule contents.

If the capsule contents are mixed with liquids or feeds the resulting mixture should not be allowed to stand for more than one hour prior to use.

4.5 Interaction with other medicinal products and other forms of interaction
None known.

4.6 Pregnancy and lactation
Pancrex should not be used in pregnancy and lactation unless clearly necessary but if required should be used in doses sufficient to provide adequate nutritional status.

4.7 Effects on ability to drive and use machines
None.

4.8 Undesirable effects
Rare cases of hyperuricosuria and hyperuricaemia have been reported when extremely high doses of pancreatin have been taken.

Strictures of the ileo-caecum and large bowel, and colitis, have been reported in children with cystic fibrosis taking high doses of pancreatic enzyme supplements. To date Pancrex and Pancrex V presentations have not been implicated in the development of colonic damage. However unusual abdominal symptoms or changes in abdominal symptoms should be reviewed to exclude the possibility of colonic damage especially if the patient is taking in excess of 10,000 units/kg/day of lipase.

4.9 Overdose
None stated.

5. PHARMACOLOGICAL PROPERTIES
5.1 Pharmacodynamic properties
Pancreatin is derived from porcine pancreas and contains the enzymes, amylase, protease and lipase. The enzymes have the same actions as pancreatic juice and when administered to patients with pancreatic insufficiency improve the ability to metabolise starches, proteins and fats.

5.2 Pharmacokinetic properties
Pancreatin hydrolyses fats to glycerol and fatty acids, changes proteins into proteases and derived substances, and converts starch into dextrins and sugars.

5.3 Preclinical safety data
No relevant pre-clinical safety data has been generated.

6. PHARMACEUTICAL PARTICULARS
6.1 List of excipients
Aluminium oxide, magnesium stearate, microcrystalline cellulose gelatin, titanium dioxide, yellow iron oxide (E172), quinoline yellow (E104).

6.2 Incompatibilities
None known.

6.3 Shelf life
2 years.

6.4 Special precautions for storage
Store at a temperature not exceeding 15°C.

6.5 Nature and contents of container
Securitainer; 100, 300 and 500 capsules.

6.6 Special precautions for disposal and other handling
Not applicable.

Administrative Data
7. MARKETING AUTHORISATION HOLDER
Paines and Byrne Limited
Lovett House
Lovett Road
Staines
TW18 3AZ
United Kingdom

8. MARKETING AUTHORISATION NUMBER(S)
PL0051/5043R

9. DATE OF FIRST AUTHORISATION/RENEWAL OF THE AUTHORISATION
First authorisation granted 13 November 1985
Renewal granted 31st May 2001

10. DATE OF REVISION OF THE TEXT
25 October 2007

11. LEGAL CATEGORY
P

Pancrex V Capsules 125mg

(Paines & Byrne Limited)

1. NAME OF THE MEDICINAL PRODUCT
Pancrex V Capsules 125 mg.

2. QUALITATIVE AND QUANTITATIVE COMPOSITION
Pancreatin BP to provide enzymatic activity per capsule not less than:

Free protease	160 BP units
Lipase	2950 BP units
Amylase	3300 BP units

3. PHARMACEUTICAL FORM
Capsule.

4. CLINICAL PARTICULARS
4.1 Therapeutic indications
Pancrex is used to compensate for reduced intestinal enzyme activity in pancreatic deficiency states.

It is indicated for the treatment of fibrocystic disease of the pancreas (cystic fibrosis), chronic pancreatitis and pancreatic steatorrhoea following pancreatectomy. It may also be indicated following gastrectomy as an aid to digestion.

4.2 Posology and method of administration
These low dose capsules may be used when small amounts of Pancrex are required, for example for neonates.

Dosage should be adjusted according to the needs of the individual patient and the amount of food consumed.

The following dosage scale provides a suitable basis for adjustment.

Neonates: the contents of 1 - 2 capsules mixed with feeds.

4.3 Contraindications
Hypersensitivity to the active ingredient (porcine pancreatin) or any of the excipients.

4.4 Special warnings and precautions for use
It is possible that some irritation of the skin of the mouth may occur if capsules 125 mg are chewed or the contents retained in the mouth. Irritation of the anus may also occur. A barrier cream may prevent this local irritation.

Allergic/asthmatic reactions have occasionally occurred on handling the capsule contents.

If the capsule contents are mixed with liquids or feeds the resulting mixture should not be allowed to stand for more than one hour prior to use.

4.5 Interaction with other medicinal products and other forms of interaction
None known.

4.6 Pregnancy and lactation
Pancrex should not be used in pregnancy and lactation unless clearly necessary but if required should be used in doses sufficient to provide adequate nutritional status.

4.7 Effects on ability to drive and use machines
None.

4.8 Undesirable effects
Rare cases of hyperuricosuria and hyperuricaemia have been reported when extremely high doses of pancreatin have been taken.

Strictures of the ileo-caecum and large bowel, and colitis, have been reported in children with cystic fibrosis taking high doses of pancreatic enzyme supplements. To date Pancrex and Pancrex V presentations have not been implicated in the development of colonic damage. However unusual abdominal symptoms or changes in abdominal symptoms should be reviewed to exclude the possibility of colonic damage especially if the patient is taking in excess of 10,000 units/kg/day of lipase.

4.9 Overdose
None stated.

5. PHARMACOLOGICAL PROPERTIES
5.1 Pharmacodynamic properties
Pancreatin is derived from porcine pancreas and contains the enzymes, amylase, protease and lipase. The enzymes have the same actions as pancreatic juice and when administered to patients with pancreatic insufficiency improve the ability to metabolise starches, proteins and fats.

5.2 Pharmacokinetic properties
Pancreatin hydrolyses fats to glycerol and fatty acids, changes proteins into proteases and derived substances, and converts starch into dextrins and sugars.

5.3 Preclinical safety data
No relevant pre-clinical safety data has been generated.

6. PHARMACEUTICAL PARTICULARS
6.1 List of excipients
Aluminium oxide, magnesium stearate, microcrystalline cellulose.

6.2 Incompatibilities
None known.

6.3 Shelf life
2 years.

6.4 Special precautions for storage
Store at a temperature not exceeding 15°C.

6.5 Nature and contents of container
Securitainer; 300 and 500 capsules.

6.6 Special precautions for disposal and other handling
Not applicable.

Administrative Data
7. MARKETING AUTHORISATION HOLDER
Paines and Byrne Limited
Lovett House
Lovett Road
Staines
TW18 3AZ
United Kingdom

8. MARKETING AUTHORISATION NUMBER(S)
PL0051/5104R

9. DATE OF FIRST AUTHORISATION/RENEWAL OF THE AUTHORISATION
First authorisation granted 13 November 1985
Renewal granted 4 November 2003

10. DATE OF REVISION OF THE TEXT
25 October 2007

11. Legal category
P

Pancrex V Forte Tablets

(Paines & Byrne Limited)

1. NAME OF THE MEDICINAL PRODUCT
Pancrex V Forte Tablets

2. QUALITATIVE AND QUANTITATIVE COMPOSITION
Pancreatin BP to provide enzymatic activity per tablet not less than:

Free protease	330 BP units
Lipase	5600 BP units
Amylase	5000 BP units

3. PHARMACEUTICAL FORM
Tablet.

4. CLINICAL PARTICULARS
4.1 Therapeutic indications
Pancrex is used to compensate for reduced intestinal enzyme activity in pancreatic deficiency states.

It is indicated for the treatment of fibrocystic disease of the pancreas (cystic fibrosis), chronic pancreatitis and pancreatic steatorrhoea following pancreatectomy. It may also be indicated following gastrectomy as an aid to digestion.

4.2 Posology and method of administration
Dosage should be adjusted according to the needs of the individual patient and the amount and type of food consumed.

The following dosage ranges provide a suitable basis for adjustment.

Adults, the Elderly, and Children

6 - 10 tablets before each snack or meal, swallowed whole

4.3 Contraindications
Hypersensitivity to the active ingredient (porcine pancreatin) or any of the excipients.

4.4 Special warnings and precautions for use
Unsuitable for people with lactase insufficiency, galactosaemia or glucose/galactose malabsorption syndrome.

Variations in response to treatment may be due to enteric coating. It is possible that some irritation of the skin of the mouth may occur if tablets are chewed or preparations retained in the mouth. Irritation of the anus may also occur. A barrier cream may prevent this local irritation.

4.5 Interaction with other medicinal products and other forms of interaction
None known.

4.6 Pregnancy and lactation
Pancrex should not be used in pregnancy and lactation unless clearly necessary but if required should be used in doses sufficient to provide adequate nutritional status.

4.7 Effects on ability to drive and use machines
None.

4.8 Undesirable effects
Rare cases of hyperuricosuria and hyperuricaemia have been reported when extremely high doses of pancreatin have been taken.

Strictures of the ileo-caecum and large bowel, and colitis, have been reported in children with cystic fibrosis taking high doses of pancreatic enzyme supplements. To date Pancrex and Pancrex V presentations have not been implicated in the development of colonic damage. However unusual abdominal symptoms or changes in abdominal symptoms should be reviewed to exclude the possibility of colonic damage especially if the patient is taking in excess of 10,000 units/kg/day of lipase.

4.9 Overdose
None stated.

5. PHARMACOLOGICAL PROPERTIES
5.1 Pharmacodynamic properties
Pancreatin is derived from porcine pancreas and contains the enzymes, amylase, protease and lipase. The enzymes have the same actions as pancreatic juice and when administered to patients with pancreatic insufficiency improve the ability to metabolise starches, proteins and fats.

5.2 Pharmacokinetic properties
Pancreatin hydrolyses fats to glycerol and fatty acids, changes proteins into proteases and derived substances, and converts starch into dextrins and sugars.

5.3 Preclinical safety data
No relevant pre-clinical safety data has been generated.

6. PHARMACEUTICAL PARTICULARS
6.1 List of excipients
Lactose, povidone, stearic acid, Opaseal P17-28901 (containing IMS, titanium dioxide (E171), polyvinyl acetate phthalate, and stearic acid (E570)) talc, sucrose, acacia, calcium carbonate, titanium dioxide, Opalux AS 7000B (containing sucrose, sodium benzoate (E211), titanium dioxide (E171), and indigo carmine aluminium lake (E132)), syrup, Opagloss 6000P (containing ethanol, shellac (E904), white beeswax (E901), yellow carnuba wax (E903)).

This medicinal product contains approximately 0.13g of lactose. When taken according to the dosage recommendations each dose supplies up to 1.3g of lactose.

6.2 Incompatibilities
None known.

6.3 Shelf life
2 years.

6.4 Special precautions for storage
Store at a temperature not exceeding 15°C.

6.5 Nature and contents of container
Securitainer: 100, 250, 300 and 500 tablets.

6.6 Special precautions for disposal and other handling
Not applicable.

Administrative Data
7. MARKETING AUTHORISATION HOLDER
Paines and Byrne Limited
Lovett House
Lovett Road
Staines
TW18 3AZ
United Kingdom

8. MARKETING AUTHORISATION NUMBER(S)
PL0051/5000R

9. DATE OF FIRST AUTHORISATION/RENEWAL OF THE AUTHORISATION
First authorisation granted 22 November 1985 / October 2003

10. DATE OF REVISION OF THE TEXT
25 October 2007.

11. Legal Category
P

Pancrex V Powder

(Paines & Byrne Limited)

1. NAME OF THE MEDICINAL PRODUCT
Pancrex V Powder

2. QUALITATIVE AND QUANTITATIVE COMPOSITION
Pancreatin BP to provide enzymatic activity per gram not less than:

Free protease	1400 BP units
Lipase	25000 BP units
Amylase	30000 BP units

3. PHARMACEUTICAL FORM
Powder.

4. CLINICAL PARTICULARS
4.1 Therapeutic indications
Pancrex is used to compensate for reduced intestinal enzyme activity in pancreatic deficiency states.

It is indicated for the treatment of fibrocystic disease of the pancreas (cystic fibrosis), chronic pancreatitis and pancreatic steatorrhoea following pancreatectomy. It may also be indicated following gastrectomy as an aid to digestion.

4.2 Posology and method of administration
Dosage should be adjusted according to the needs of the individual patient and the amount and type of food consumed.

The following dosage ranges provide a suitable basis for adjustment.

Adults, the Elderly, and Children

0.5 g - 2 g swallowed dry or mixed with a little water or milk before each snack or meal

New-born infants

0.25 g - 0.5 g with each feed

4.3 Contraindications
Hypersensitivity to the active ingredient (porcine pancreatin) or any of the excipients.

4.4 Special warnings and precautions for use
It is possible that some irritation of the skin of the mouth may occur if the powder is retained in the mouth. Irritation of the anus may also occur. A barrier cream may prevent this local irritation.

Allergic/asthmatic reactions have occasionally occurred on handling the powder.

If the powder is mixed with liquids or feeds the resulting mixture should not be allowed to stand for more than one hour prior to use.

4.5 Interaction with other medicinal products and other forms of interaction
None known.

4.6 Pregnancy and lactation
Pancrex should not be used in pregnancy and lactation unless clearly necessary but if required should be used in doses sufficient to provide adequate nutritional status.

4.7 Effects on ability to drive and use machines
None.

4.8 Undesirable effects
Rare cases of hyperuricosuria and hyperuricaemia have been reported when extremely high doses of pancreatin have been taken.

Strictures of the ileo-caecum and large bowel, and colitis, have been reported in children with cystic fibrosis taking high doses of pancreatic enzyme supplements. To date Pancrex and Pancrex V presentations have not been implicated in the development of colonic damage. However unusual abdominal symptoms or changes in abdominal symptoms should be reviewed to exclude the possibility of colonic damage especially if the patient is taking in excess of 10,000 units/kg/day of lipase.

4.9 Overdose
None stated.

5. PHARMACOLOGICAL PROPERTIES
5.1 Pharmacodynamic properties
Pancreatin is derived from porcine pancreas and contains the enzymes, amylase, protease and lipase. The enzymes have the same actions as pancreatic juice and when administered to patients with pancreatic insufficiency improve the ability to metabolise starches, proteins and fats.

5.2 Pharmacokinetic properties
Pancreatin hydrolyses fats to glycerol and fatty acids, changes proteins into proteases and derived substances, and converts starch into dextrins and sugars.

5.3 Preclinical safety data
No relevant pre-clinical safety data has been generated.

6. PHARMACEUTICAL PARTICULARS
6.1 List of excipients
None.

6.2 Incompatibilities
None known.

6.3 Shelf life
2 years.

6.4 Special precautions for storage
Store at a temperature not exceeding 15°C.

6.5 Nature and contents of container
Securitainer; 100 g, 250 g and 300 g.

6.6 Special precautions for disposal and other handling
Not applicable.

Administrative Data
7. MARKETING AUTHORISATION HOLDER
Paines & Byrne Limited
Lovett House
Lovett Road
Staines
TW18 3AZ
United Kingdom

8. MARKETING AUTHORISATION NUMBER(S)
PL0051/5004R

9. DATE OF FIRST AUTHORISATION/RENEWAL OF THE AUTHORISATION
First authorisation granted 13 November 1985 / October 2003

10. DATE OF REVISION OF THE TEXT
25 October 2007

11. Legal Category
P

Pancrex V Tablets

(Paines & Byrne Limited)

1. NAME OF THE MEDICINAL PRODUCT
Pancrex V Tablets.

2. QUALITATIVE AND QUANTITATIVE COMPOSITION
Pancreatin BP to provide enzymatic activity per tablet not less than:

Free protease	110 BP units
Lipase	1900 BP units
Amylase	1700 BP units

3. PHARMACEUTICAL FORM
Tablet.

4. CLINICAL PARTICULARS
4.1 Therapeutic indications
Pancrex is used to compensate for reduced intestinal enzyme activity in pancreatic deficiency states.

It is indicated for the treatment of fibrocystic disease of the pancreas (cystic fibrosis), chronic pancreatitis and pancreatic steatorrhoea following pancreatectomy. It may also be indicated following gastrectomy as an aid to digestion.

4.2 Posology and method of administration
Dosage should be adjusted according to the needs of the individual patient and the amount and type of food consumed.

The following dosage ranges provide a suitable basis for adjustment.

Adults, the Elderly, and Children

5 - 15 tablets before each snack or meal, swallowed whole

4.3 Contraindications
Hypersensitivity to the active ingredient (porcine pancreatin) or any of the excipients.

4.4 Special warnings and precautions for use
Unsuitable for people with lactase insufficiency, galactosaemia or glucose/galactose malabsorption syndrome.

Variations in response to treatment may be due to enteric coating. It is possible that some irritation of the skin of the mouth may occur if tablets are chewed or preparations retained in the mouth. Irritation of the anus may also occur. A barrier cream may prevent this local irritation.

4.5 Interaction with other medicinal products and other forms of interaction
None known.

4.6 Pregnancy and lactation
Pancrex should not be used in pregnancy and lactation unless clearly necessary but if required should be used in doses sufficient to provide adequate nutritional status.

4.7 Effects on ability to drive and use machines
None.

4.8 Undesirable effects
Rare cases of hyperuricosuria and hyperuricaemia have been reported when extremely high doses of pancreatin have been taken.

Strictures of the ileo-caecum and large bowel, and colitis, have been reported in children with cystic fibrosis taking high doses of pancreatic enzyme supplements. To date Pancrex and Pancrex V presentations have not been implicated in the development of colonic damage. However unusual abdominal symptoms or changes in abdominal symptoms should be reviewed to exclude the possibility of colonic damage especially if the patient is taking in excess of 10,000 units/kg/day of lipase.

4.9 Overdose
None stated.

5. PHARMACOLOGICAL PROPERTIES

5.1 Pharmacodynamic properties
Pancreatin is derived from porcine pancreas and contains the enzymes, amylase, protease and lipase. The enzymes have the same actions as pancreatic juice and when administered to patients with pancreatic insufficiency improve the ability to metabolise starches, proteins and fats.

5.2 Pharmacokinetic properties
Pancreatin hydrolyses fats to glycerol and fatty acids, changes proteins into proteases and derived substances, and converts starch into dextrins and sugars.

5.3 Preclinical safety data
No relevant pre-clinical safety data has been generated.

6. PHARMACEUTICAL PARTICULARS

6.1 List of excipients
Lactose, povidone, stearic acid, Opaseal P17-28901 (containing IMS, titanium dioxide (E171), polyvinyl acetate phthalate, and stearic acid (E570)), talc, sucrose, acacia, calcium carbonate, titanium dioxide, Opalux AS 7000B (containing sucrose, sodium benzoate (E211), titanium dioxide (E171), and indigo carmine aluminium lake (E132)), syrup, Opagloss 6000P (containing ethanol, shellac (E904), white beeswax (E901), yellow carnuba wax (E903)).

This medicinal product contains approximately 0.055g of lactose. When taken according to the dosage recommendations each dose supplies up to 0.83g of lactose.

6.2 Incompatibilities
None known.

6.3 Shelf life
2 years.

6.4 Special precautions for storage
Store at a temperature not exceeding 15°C.

6.5 Nature and contents of container
Securitainer; 100, 300 and 500 tablets.

6.6 Special precautions for disposal and other handling
Not applicable.

Administrative Data

7. MARKETING AUTHORISATION HOLDER
Paines & Byrne Limited

Lovett House

Lovett Road

Staines

TW18 3AZ

United Kingdom

8. MARKETING AUTHORISATION NUMBER(S)
PL0051/5002R

9. DATE OF FIRST AUTHORISATION/RENEWAL OF THE AUTHORISATION
First authorisation granted 30 October 1985 / October 2003

10. DATE OF REVISION OF THE TEXT
25 October 2007

11. LEGAL CATEGORY
P

PanOxyl 5 Cream

(Stiefel Laboratories (UK) Limited)

1. NAME OF THE MEDICINAL PRODUCT
PanOxyl 5 Cream

2. QUALITATIVE AND QUANTITATIVE COMPOSITION
Benzoyl peroxide 5.0% w/w

3. PHARMACEUTICAL FORM
Cream for cutaneous use

4. CLINICAL PARTICULARS

4.1 Therapeutic indications
PanOxyl 5 Cream is indicated for the treatment of acne vulgaris.

4.2 Posology and method of administration
Adults

Apply to the whole of the affected area once daily. Washing with soap and water prior to application greatly enhances the efficacy of the preparation.

Elderly patients

There are no specific recommendations. Acne vulgaris does not present in the elderly.

Paediatric use

The product is not intended for use in pre-pubescent children since acne vulgaris rarely presents in this age group.

4.3 Contraindications
Patients with a known hypersensitivity to any of the ingredients should not use the product.

4.4 Special warnings and precautions for use
Avoid contact with the eyes, mouth and other mucous membranes. Care should be taken when applying the product to the neck and other sensitive areas.

The product may bleach dyed fabrics.

4.5 Interaction with other medicinal products and other forms of interaction
None.

4.6 Pregnancy and lactation
There are no restrictions on the use of the product during pregnancy or lactation.

4.7 Effects on ability to drive and use machines
None

4.8 Undesirable effects
In normal use, a mild burning sensation will probably be felt on first application and a moderate reddening and peeling of the skin will occur within a few days. During the first few weeks of treatment a sudden increase in peeling will occur in most patients; this is not harmful and will normally subside in a day or two if treatment is temporarily discontinued.

4.9 Overdose
Not applicable.

5. PHARMACOLOGICAL PROPERTIES

5.1 Pharmacodynamic properties
Benzoyl peroxide has antibacterial activity against *Propionibacterium acnes*, the organism implicated in acne vulgaris. It has kerolytic activity and is sebostatic, counteracting the hyperkeratinisation and excessive sebum production associated with acne.

5.2 Pharmacokinetic properties
Not applicable.

5.3 Preclinical safety data
Not applicable. Benzoyl peroxide has been in widespread use for many years.

6. PHARMACEUTICAL PARTICULARS

6.1 List of excipients
Macrogol 1000 monostearate

Stearic acid

Glyceryl monostearate

Isopropyl palmitate

Propylene glycol

Zinc stearate

Purified water

6.2 Incompatibilities
None

6.3 Shelf life

a) For the product as packaged for sale
3 years

b) After first opening the container
Comply with expiry date

6.4 Special precautions for storage
Store below 25°C.

6.5 Nature and contents of container
Internally lacquered aluminium tubes of 40g. High density polyethylene tubes of 25g.

6.6 Special precautions for disposal and other handling
There are no special instructions for use or handling of PanOxyl 5 Cream.

7. MARKETING AUTHORISATION HOLDER
Stiefel Laboratories (UK) Ltd

Eurasia Headquarters

Concorde Road

Maidenhead

SL6 4BY

UK

8. MARKETING AUTHORISATION NUMBER(S)
PL 0174/5007R

9. DATE OF FIRST AUTHORISATION/RENEWAL OF THE AUTHORISATION
26th February 1990

10. DATE OF REVISION OF THE TEXT
August 2009

Panoxyl Acne Gel 5, 10

(Stiefel Laboratories (UK) Limited)

1. NAME OF THE MEDICINAL PRODUCT
Panoxyl Acnegel 5

Panoxyl Acnegel 10

2. QUALITATIVE AND QUANTITATIVE COMPOSITION
Panoxyl Acnegel 5: Benzoyl peroxide 5.0% w/w

Panoxyl Acnegel 10: Benzoyl peroxide 10.0% w/w

3. PHARMACEUTICAL FORM
Gel for cutaneous use

4. CLINICAL PARTICULARS

4.1 Therapeutic indications
Indicated for the treatment of acne vulgaris

4.2 Posology and method of administration
Adults

Apply to the whole of the affected area once daily. Washing with soap and water prior to application greatly enhances the efficacy of the preparation.

Elderly Patients

There are no specific recommendations. Acne vulgaris does not present in the elderly.

Paediatric Use

The product is not intended for use in pre-pubescent children since acne vulgaris rarely presents in this age group.

4.3 Contraindications
Patients with a known hypersensitivity to any of the ingredients should not use the product.

4.4 Special warnings and precautions for use
Avoid contact with the eyes, mouth and other mucous membranes. Care should be taken when applying the product to the neck and other sensitive areas.

The product may bleach dyed fabrics.

4.5 Interaction with other medicinal products and other forms of interaction
None

4.6 Pregnancy and lactation
There are no restrictions on the use of the product during pregnancy or lactation.

4.7 Effects on ability to drive and use machines
None

4.8 Undesirable effects
In normal use, a mild burning sensation will probably be felt on first application and a moderate reddening and peeling of the skin will occur within a few days. During the first few weeks of treatment a sudden increase in peeling will occur in most patients; this is not harmful and will normally subside in a day or two if treatment is temporarily discontinued.

4.9 Overdose
Not applicable

5. PHARMACOLOGICAL PROPERTIES

5.1 Pharmacodynamic properties
Benzoyl peroxide has anti-bacterial activity against Propionibacterium acnes, the organism implicated in acne vulgaris. It has keratolytic activity and is sebostatic, counteracting the hyperkeratinisation and excessive sebum production associated with acne.

5.2 Pharmacokinetic properties
Not applicable

5.3 Preclinical safety data
Not applicable. Benzoyl peroxide has been in widespread use for many years.

6. PHARMACEUTICAL PARTICULARS

6.1 List of excipients

Colloidal Magnesium Aluminium Silicate

Hydroxypropylmethylcellulose

Polyoxyethylene lauryl ether

Denatured alcohol

Citric acid monohydrate

Alpine Essence 6565A

Purified water.

6.2 Incompatibilities

None

6.3 Shelf life

36 months

Panoxyl Acnegel 10: Comply with expiry date

6.4 Special precautions for storage

Store in a cool place

6.5 Nature and contents of container

Internally lacquered aluminium tubes of 40g

6.6 Special precautions for disposal and other handling

There are no special instructions for use or handling the product.

7. MARKETING AUTHORISATION HOLDER

Stiefel Laboratories (UK) Ltd

Holtspur Lane

Wooburn Green

High Wycombe

Bucks HPIO OAU

8. MARKETING AUTHORISATION NUMBER(S)

Panoxyl Acnegel 5: PL0174/0019R

Panoxyl Acnegel 10: PL0174/0020R

9. DATE OF FIRST AUTHORISATION/RENEWAL OF THE AUTHORISATION

23.04.90

10. DATE OF REVISION OF THE TEXT

Panoxyl Acnegel 5: 08.08.94

Panoxyl Acnegel 10: 30.03.95

Panoxyl Aquagel 2.5, 5, 10

(Stiefel Laboratories (UK) Limited)

1. NAME OF THE MEDICINAL PRODUCT

PanOxyl Aquagel 2.5

PanOxyl Aquagel 5

PanOxyl Aquagel 10

2. QUALITATIVE AND QUANTITATIVE COMPOSITION

PanOxyl Aquagel 2.5: Benzoyl peroxide 2.5% w/w

PanOxyl Aquagel 5: Benzoyl peroxide 5% w/w

PanOxyl Aquagel 10: Benzoyl peroxide 10% w/w

3. PHARMACEUTICAL FORM

Gel

4. CLINICAL PARTICULARS

4.1 Therapeutic indications

The product is indicated for use in the topical treatment of acne vulgaris.

4.2 Posology and method of administration

Treatment should normally begin with PanOxyl Aquagel 2.5. Apply to the affected areas once daily. Washing prior to application enhances the efficacy of the preparation.

The reaction of the skin to benzoyl peroxide differs in individual patients. The higher concentration in PanOxyl Aquagel 5 or 10 may be required to produce a satisfactory response.

4.3 Contraindications

PanOxyl Aquagel should not be prescribed for patients with a known hypersensitivity to benzoyl peroxide.

4.4 Special warnings and precautions for use

Avoid contact with the eyes, mouth and mucous membranes. Care should be taken when applying the product to the neck and other sensitive areas.

During the first few days of treatment a moderate reddening and peeling will occur. During the first few weeks of treatment a sudden increase in peeling will occur in most patients. This is not harmful and will normally subside within a day or two if treatment is discontinued. If excessive irritation, redness or peeling occurs, discontinue use.

The product may bleach dyed fabrics.

4.5 Interaction with other medicinal products and other forms of interaction

None

4.6 Pregnancy and lactation

There are no restriction on the use of PanOxyl Aquagel in pregnancy and lactation.

4.7 Effects on ability to drive and use machines

None

4.8 Undesirable effects

None

4.9 Overdose

Not applicable.

5. PHARMACOLOGICAL PROPERTIES

5.1 Pharmacodynamic properties

Benzoyl peroxide has sebostatic and keratolytic activity coupled with antibacterial activity against *Propionibacterium acnes*, the organism implicated in acne vulgaris. Its use in the treatment of acne is well established.

5.2 Pharmacokinetic properties

Not applicable.

5.3 Preclinical safety data

Not applicable. Benzoyl peroxide has been in widespread use for many years.

6. PHARMACEUTICAL PARTICULARS

6.1 List of excipients

Carbomer 940

Di-isopropanolamine

Propylene glycol

Polyoxyethylene lauryl ether

Sodium lauryl sulphate

Purified water

6.2 Incompatibilities

None

6.3 Shelf life

2 years

6.4 Special precautions for storage

Store below 25°C.

6.5 Nature and contents of container

Internally lacquered aluminium tubes with screw caps. Licensed pack sizes: 40g

6.6 Special precautions for disposal and other handling

There are no special instructions for use or handling of PanOxyl Aquagel.

7. MARKETING AUTHORISATION HOLDER

Stiefel Laboratories (UK) Ltd

Eurasia Headquarters

Concorde Road

Maidenhead

SL6 4BY

UK

8. MARKETING AUTHORISATION NUMBER(S)

PanOxyl Aquagel 2.5: PL 0174/0049

PanOxyl Aquagel 5: PL 0174/0050

PanOxyl Aquagel 10: PL 0174/0051

9. DATE OF FIRST AUTHORISATION/RENEWAL OF THE AUTHORISATION

21st August 1984

10. DATE OF REVISION OF THE TEXT

August 2009

PanOxyl Wash 10%

(Stiefel Laboratories (UK) Limited)

1. NAME OF THE MEDICINAL PRODUCT

PanOxyl Wash 10%

2. QUALITATIVE AND QUANTITATIVE COMPOSITION

Benzoyl peroxide10.0% w/w

3. PHARMACEUTICAL FORM

Lotion for cutaneous use

4. CLINICAL PARTICULARS

4.1 Therapeutic indications

PanOxyl Wash 10% is indicated for the treatment of acne vulgaris.

4.2 Posology and method of administration

Adults

Wet the affected area with water and wash thoroughly with PanOxyl Wash. Rinse well with warm water, then rinse with cold water. Pat dry with a clean towel. Use once a day.

Elderly patients

There are no specific recommendations. Acne vulgaris does not present in the elderly.

Paediatric use

The product is not intended for use in pre-pubescent children since acne vulgaris rarely presents in this age group.

4.3 Contraindications

Patients with a known hypersensitivity to any of the ingredients should not use the product.

4.4 Special warnings and precautions for use

Avoid contact with the eyes, mouth and other mucous membranes. Care should be taken when applying the product to the neck and other sensitive areas.

The product may bleach dyed fabrics.

4.5 Interaction with other medicinal products and other forms of interaction

None

4.6 Pregnancy and lactation

There are no restrictions on the use of the product during pregnancy or lactation.

4.7 Effects on ability to drive and use machines

None

4.8 Undesirable effects

In normal use, a mild burning sensation will probably be felt on first application and a moderate reddening and peeling of the skin will occur within a few days. During the first few weeks of treatment a sudden increase in peeling will occur in most patients; this is not harmful and will normally subside in a day or two if treatment is temporarily discontinued.

4.9 Overdose

Not applicable.

5. PHARMACOLOGICAL PROPERTIES

5.1 Pharmacodynamic properties

Benzoyl peroxide has antibacterial activity against *Propionibacterium acnes*, the organism implicated in acne vulgaris. It has keratolytic activity and is sebostatic, counteracting the hyperkeratinisation and excessive sebum production associated with acne.

5.2 Pharmacokinetic properties

Not applicable.

5.3 Preclinical safety data

Not applicable. Benzoyl peroxide has been in widespread use for many years.

6. PHARMACEUTICAL PARTICULARS

6.1 List of excipients

Magnesium aluminium silicate

Citric acid monohydrate

Sodium alkyl aryl polyether sulphonate

Sodium dihexyl sulphosuccinate

Sodium lauryl sulphoacetate

Hydroxypropylmethylcellulose

Polyoxyethylene lauryl ether

Imidurea

Purified water

6.2 Incompatibilities

None

6.3 Shelf life

a) For the product as packaged for sale

2 years

b) After first opening the container

Comply with expiry date

6.4 Special precautions for storage

Store below 25°C.

6.5 Nature and contents of container

Flip top polyethylene bottle containing 150 ml.

6.6 Special precautions for disposal and other handling

There are no special instructions for use or handling of PanOxyl Wash 10%.

7. MARKETING AUTHORISATION HOLDER

Stiefel Laboratories (UK) Ltd

Eurasia Headquarters

Concorde Road

Maidenhead

SL6 4BY

UK

8. MARKETING AUTHORISATION NUMBER(S)

PL 0174/0048

9. DATE OF FIRST AUTHORISATION/RENEWAL OF THE AUTHORISATION

25th June 1985 / 20th October 2005

10. DATE OF REVISION OF THE TEXT

August 2009

Paramax 500mg/5mg Tablets, Paramax 500mg/5mg Effervescent Powder

(sanofi-aventis)

1. NAME OF THE MEDICINAL PRODUCT

Paramax 500mg/5mg Tablets

Paramax 500mg/5mg Effervescent Powder

2. QUALITATIVE AND QUANTITATIVE COMPOSITION

500mg paracetamol with 5mg metoclopramide hydrochloride (calculated with reference to anhydrous substance).

3. PHARMACEUTICAL FORM

Tablets

Effervescent powder

4. CLINICAL PARTICULARS

4.1 Therapeutic indications

Paramax is indicated for the symptomatic treatment of migraine

4.2 Posology and method of administration

Paramax should be taken at the first warning of an attack. If symptoms persist, further doses may be taken at four-hourly intervals. Total dosage in any 24-hour period should not exceed the quantity stated.

The dosage recommendations given below should be strictly adhered to if side-effects of the dystonic type are to be avoided. It should be noted that at total daily dosage of metoclopramide, especially for adolescents and young adults, should not normally exceed 0.5mg/kg body weight.

Usual Recommended Dosage (number of tablets/sachets)

	Initial dose at first warning of attack	Maximum dosage in any 24-hour period
Adults (including elderly patients)	2	6
Young adults (12-19 years)	1	3

Young adults and adolescents: Paramax should only be used after careful examination to avoid masking an underlying disorder, e.g. cerebral irritation. In the treatment of this group attention should be given primarily to bodyweight.

Children: A presentation of Paramax suitable for the treatment of children under 12 years of age is not available.

Paramax sachets are emptied into about $^{1}/_{4}$ of a glass of water and stirred before taking.

For oral administration only.

4.3 Contraindications

Hypersensitivity to paracetamol, metoclopramide or any other constituents.

Gastrointestinal haemorrhage, obstruction or perforation, since stimulation of gastrointestinal motility constitutes a risk in these situations.

History of neuroleptic or metoclopramide-induced tardive dyskinesia.

Confirmed epilepsy, since the frequency and severity of seizures may be increased.

Confirmed or suspected phaeochromocytoma, because of the risk of hypertensive crisis.

Combination with levodopa because of a mutual antagonism.

Metoclopramide should be not be used in the immediate post-operative period (up to 3-4 days) following pyloroplasty or gut anastomosis, as vigorous gastro-intestinal contractions may adversely affect healing.

4.4 Special warnings and precautions for use

Patients should not take Paramax with any other paracetamol-containing products.

Care is advised in the administration of paracetamol to patients with severe renal or severe hepatic impairment. The hazards of overdose are greater in those with (non-cirrhotic) alcoholic liver disease.

Care should be exercised in the event of Paramax being prescribed concurrently with a phenothiazine since extrapyramidal symptoms may occur with both products (see section 4.5).

Extrapyramidal disorders, drowsiness, decreased level of consciousness, confusion and hallucination occur more frequently when high doses of metoclopramide are used (see adverse reactions).

Children, young patients and the elderly should be treated with care as they are at increased risk of extrapyramidal reactions (see section 4.8).

Symptomatic treatment of extrapyramidal reactions may be necessary (benzodiazepines in children and/or anticholinergic anti-parkinsonian drugs in adults).

If vomiting persists the patient should be re-assessed to exclude the possibility of an underlying disorder, e.g. cerebral irritation.

Care should be exercised in patients being treated with other centrally active drugs (see section 4.5).

Neuroleptic Malignant Syndrome (NMS), a potentially fatal symptom complex with hyperthermia, muscle rigidity, extrapyramidal symptoms, altered mental status and autonomic dysfunction, may occur. The management of NMS should include

1) immediate discontinuation of the product,

2) intensive symptomatic treatment and medical monitoring, and

3) treatment of any concomitant serious medical problems for which specific treatments are available.

Methemoglobinemia which could be related to NADH cytochrome b5 reductase deficiency has been reported. In such cases, metoclopramide should be immediately and permanently discontinued and appropriate measures initiated.

Care should be exercised when using Paramax in patients with a history of atopy (including asthma) or porphyria.

4.5 Interaction with other medicinal products and other forms of interaction

Contraindicated combination:

Levodopa: Levodopa and metoclopramide have a mutual antagonism (see section 4.3)

Combination to be avoided:

Alcohol: Alcohol potentiates the sedative effect of metoclopramide.

Paracetamol may potentiate the effects of alcohol. Therefore, the risk of sedation and the effects of alcohol may be increased when Paramax is taken with alcohol.

Chloramphenicol: Paracetamol may increase the elimination half-life of chloramphenicol.

Oral contraceptives: Oral contraceptives may increase the rate of paracetamol clearance.

Metoclopramide or domperidone: The speed of absorption of paracetamol may be increased by metoclopramide or domperidone.

Colestyramine: The speed of absorption of paracetamol may be reduced by colestyramine.

Warfarin and other coumarins: The anticoagulant effect of warfarin and other coumarins may be enhanced by prolonged regular use of paracetamol with increased risk of bleeding; occasional doses have no significant effect.

Combination to be taken into account:

Anticholinergics and morphine derivatives: Anticholinergics and morphine derivatives antagonise the effects of metoclopramide on the gastrointestinal motility.

CNS depressants (morphine derivatives, hypnotics, anxiolytics, sedative H1 antihistamines, sedative antidepressants, barbiturates, clonidine and related): Combination of CNS depressants with metoclopramide may result in potentiation of sedative effects.

Antipsychotics: Combination of antipsychotics with metoclopramide may result in potentiation of extrapyramidal effects.

Due to the promotion of gastric emptying and normal peristalsis (see section 5.1) caused by metoclopramide, the absorption of certain drugs may be modified:

Digoxin: Metoclopramide decreases the gastric absorption of digoxin. Therefore, dose adjustment may be required.

Ciclosporin: Metoclopramide increases ciclosporin bioavailability. Dose adjustment may be required. In one study, dosing requirements for ciclosporin were reduced by 20% when metoclopramide was administered concomitantly. To avoid toxicity, careful monitoring of ciclosporin plasma concentration in therefore required.

4.6 Pregnancy and lactation

Animal studies, carried out on the individual active components, have not demonstrated any teratogenic effect. These studies have not been carried out on the combination product. In the absence of a teratogenic effect in animals, a malformative effect in humans is not anticipated.

Metoclopramide: data on pregnant patients (> 1000) indicate no malformative nor foeto/ neonatal toxicity during 1rst trimester of pregnancy. A limited amount of data on pregnant patients (> 300) indicate no neonatal toxicity in other trimesters. Animal studies do not indicate reproductive toxicity.

Exposure of pregnant women to the individual active components indicates no adverse effect on pregnancy or on the health of the foetus/new born child. To date, no epidemiological data are available for the combination product. Paramax should only be used during pregnancy when there are compelling reasons and like all drugs avoid use in the first and second trimester unless the physician believes the benefits outweigh the risk. Thereafter, patients should follow the advice of their doctor regarding its use.

During lactation, metoclopramide and paracetamol are excreted in breast milk and adverse reactions in the breast-fed baby cannot be excluded. A decision should be made whether to discontinue breast-feeding or to abstain from Paramax treatment.

4.7 Effects on ability to drive and use machines

Paramax may cause drowsiness. The ability to drive vehicles or operate machinery can be impaired, particularly if Paramax is administered with CNS depressants or alcohol.

4.8 Undesirable effects

Nervous system and psychiatric disorders

The following reactions, sometimes associated, occur more frequently when high doses are used:

- Extrapyramidal symptoms: acute dystonia and dyskinesia, parkinsonian syndrome, akathisia may increase following administration of a single dose particularly in children, young adults and the elderly (see section 4.4 Special warnings and precautions for use). Although, rarely, tardive dyskinesia may be irreversible.

The incidence of extrapyramidal symptoms in children and young adults may increase if the metoclopramide dosage exceeds 0.5mg/kg body weight/day.

Reactions include spasm of the facial muscles, trismus, rhythmic protrusion of the tongue, a bulbar type of speech, spasm of extra-ocular muscles including oculogyric crises, unnatural positioning of the head and shoulders and opisthotonos. There may be a generalised increase in muscle tone. The majority of reactions occur within 36 hours of starting treatment and the effects usually disappear within 24 hours of withdrawal of the drug. Should treatment of a dystonic reaction be required, a benzodiazepine or an anticholinergic anti-Parkinsonian drug may be used.

- Drowsiness, decreased level of consciousness, confusion, hallucination.

Other reactions may occur:

- Tardive dyskinesia, particularly in elderly patients and following or after prolonged treatment.

- Restlessness, anxiety

- Depression

- Seizures

- Neuroleptic malignant syndrome.

Gastrointestinal disorders

- Diarrhoea

Blood and Lymphatic system disorders

Metoclopramide may cause:

- Methaemoglobinaemia which could be related to NADH cytochrome b5 reductase deficiency have been reported, particularly in neonates.

- Sulfhaemoglobinaemia, mainly with concomitant administration of high doses of sulfur-releasing drugs.

- Blood dyscrasias including thrombocytopenia and agranulocytosis,

Endocrine disorders

- Hyperprolactinaemia with (amenorrhea, galactorrhea, gynaecomastia).

General disorders and administration site conditions

- Very rarely hypersensitivity, including anaphylaxis has been reported.

- Asthenia.

- Skin rash

- Cardiac and vascular disorders

- Hypotension.

- Bradycardia, heart block have been reported with metoclopramide, particularly the intravenous formulation.

Since extrapyramidal symptoms may occur with both metoclopramide and phenothiazines, care should be exercised in the event of both drugs being prescribed concurrently.

4.9 Overdose

Paracetamol overdose

Liver damage is possible in adults who have taken 10g or more of paracetamol. Ingestion of 5g or more of paracetamol may lead to liver damage if the patient has risk factors (see below).

Risk factors

If the patient:

- Is on long term treatment with carbamazepine, phenobarbital, phenytoin, primidone, rifampicin, St John's Wort or other drugs that induce liver enzymes.
- Regularly consumes ethanol in excess of recommended amounts.
- Is likely to be glutathione deplete e.g. eating disorders, cystic fibrosis, HIV infection, starvation, cachexia.

Symptoms

Symptoms of paracetamol overdosage in the first 24 hours are pallor, nausea, vomiting, anorexia and abdominal pain. Liver damage may become apparent 12 to 48 hours after ingestion. Abnormalities of glucose metabolism and metabolic acidosis may occur. In severe poisoning, hepatic failure may progress to encephalopathy, haemorrhage, hypoglycaemia, cerebral oedema, and death. Acute renal failure with acute tubular necrosis, strongly suggested by loin pain, haematuria and proteinuria, may develop even in the absence of severe liver damage. Cardiac arrhythmias and pancreatitis have been reported.

Management

Immediate treatment is essential in the management of paracetamol overdose. Despite a lack of significant early symptoms, patients should be referred to hospital urgently for immediate medical attention. Symptoms may be limited to nausea or vomiting and may not reflect the severity of overdose or the risk of organ damage. Management should be in accordance with established treatment guidelines, see BNF overdose section.

Treatment with activated charcoal should be considered if the overdose has been taken within 1 hour. Plasma paracetamol concentration should be measured at 4 hours or later after ingestion (earlier concentrations are unreliable). Treatment with N-acetylcysteine may be used up to 24 hours after ingestion of paracetamol, however, the maximum protective effect is obtained up to 8 hours post-ingestion. The effectiveness of the antidote declines sharply after this time. If required the patient should be given intravenous N-acetylcysteine, in line with the established dosage schedule. If vomiting is not a problem, oral methionine may be a suitable alternative for remote areas, outside hospital. Management of patients who present with serious hepatic dysfunction beyond 24h from ingestion should be discussed with the NPIS or a liver unit.

Metoclopramide overdose

Metoclopramide overdose may cause extrapyramidal disorders and drowsiness, decreased level of consciousness, confusion, hallucinations and convulsions.

Decreased level of consciousness, confusion, hallucinations resolve after metoclopramide withdrawal.

Treatment for extrapyramidal disorders caused by metoclopramide overdose is symptomatic (benzodiazepines in children and/or anticholinergic anti-parkinsonian drugs in adults).

5. PHARMACOLOGICAL PROPERTIES

5.1 Pharmacodynamic properties

The mechanism of action of metoclopramide in the gastrointestinal tract remains unclear and current hypotheses have been reviewed by Harrington et al (1983). It appears that metoclopramide has both central and local mechanisms of action; at the local level metoclopramide may have a direct effect on gastric muscle, stimulating contractility (Hay, 1975).

The addition of metoclopramide to paracetamol therapy for migraine has the additional benefit of combating the nausea and vomiting which are often experienced by migraine sufferers. The antiemetic activity of metoclopramide is probably mediated, at least in part, by blockade of dopamine receptors in the chemoreceptor trigger zone for vomiting (Harrington et al 1983).

5.2 Pharmacokinetic properties

Published data concerning the pharmacokinetics of Paramax is limited. In a study involving four healthy volunteers in which plasma paracetamol concentrations were compared following administration of Paramax tablets (1g paracetamol + 10mg metoclopramide), Panadol tablets (1g paracetamol) and Solpadeine effervescent tablets (1g paracetamol + 16mg codeine phosphate + 16mg caffeine), absorption of paracetamol from Paramax tablets was found not to differ significantly from absorption from Panadol or Solpadeine (Dougall et al, 1983).

Oral paracetamol is largely absorbed from the small intestine, the rate of absorption depending on the rate of gastric emptying (Heading et al, 1973; Clements et al, 1978).

Gastric emptying is often severely delayed during migraine attacks (Kreel, 1969); absorption of oral paracetamol has been shown to be delayed and impaired in patients during a migraine attack compared to when the same patients are headache free (Tokala and Neuvonen, 1984). Metoclopramide stimulates gastric emptying and has been shown to accelerate absorption of paracetamol (Nimmo *et al.* 1973 and Crome *et al.* 1981).

5.3 Preclinical safety data

Paracetamol and metoclopramide hydrochloride are well established drug substances and results of preclinical testing are well documented.

6. PHARMACEUTICAL PARTICULARS

6.1 List of excipients

Tablets: Colloidal silica dioxide, Magnesium stearate, Microcrystalline cellulose

Effervescent powder: Sodium carbonate, Saccharin sodium, Lemon flavour, Sodium dihydrogen, citrate, anhydrous, Sodium bicarbonate, Gelatin

6.2 Incompatibilities

None stated

6.3 Shelf life

Shelf life allocation: 5 years

Do not use after expiry date given on the label

6.4 Special precautions for storage

Tablets: Store in the original container. Do not store above 30°C.

Effervescent powder: Store in original package. Do not store above 25°C.

6.5 Nature and contents of container

PVC aluminium blister packs containing 42 tablets.

Packs of 42 sachets packed into cartons.

6.6 Special precautions for disposal and other handling

No special instructions for use

7. MARKETING AUTHORISATION HOLDER

Sanofi-aventis

One Onslow Street

Guildford

Surrey

GU1 4YS

UK

8. MARKETING AUTHORISATION NUMBER(S)

Tablets: PL 04425/0614

Sachets: PL 04425/0196

9. DATE OF FIRST AUTHORISATION/RENEWAL OF THE AUTHORISATION

03 March 2009

10. DATE OF REVISION OF THE TEXT

July 2009

Legal Status

POM

Paramol Soluble Tablets

(SSL International plc)

1. NAME OF THE MEDICINAL PRODUCT

Paramol Soluble Tablets.

2. QUALITATIVE AND QUANTITATIVE COMPOSITION

Paracetamol 500 mg

Dihydrocodeine tartrate 7.46 mg

3. PHARMACEUTICAL FORM

Effervescent tablet

4. CLINICAL PARTICULARS

4.1 Therapeutic indications

For the treatment of mild to moderate pain; including headache, migraine, feverish conditions, period pain, toothache and other dental pain, back pain, muscular and joint pains, neuralgia, the aches and pains of cold and flu, and as an antipyretic.

4.2 Posology and method of administration

For oral administration.

Dosage and administration

Paramol Soluble Tablets should be taken during or after meals. The tablets should be dissolved in water.

Adults and children over 12 years:

1 or 2 tablets every four to six hours. Do not exceed eight tablets in any 24-hour period. Do not take for more than 3 days continuously without medical review.

Children under 12 years:

Not recommended.

Elderly:

Caution should be observed in increasing the dose in the elderly.

4.3 Contraindications

Known hypersensitivity to paracetamol, dihydrocodeine, other opioids or other constituents of the tablets.

Respiratory depression, obstructive airways disease, convulsive disorders.

Diarrhoea caused by poisoning until the toxic material has been eliminated, or diarrhoea associated with pseudomembranous colitis.

4.4 Special warnings and precautions for use

Paramol Soluble Tablets should be used with caution in patients with:

- Hepatic function impairment (avoid if severe) and those with non-cirrhotic alcoholic liver disease. The hazards of overdose are greater in those with alcoholic liver disease.
- Prolonged use of Paramol Soluble Tablets may cause hepatic necrosis.
- Renal function impairment.
- Hypothyroidism (risk of depression and prolonged CNS depression is increased)
- Inflammatory bowel disease – risk of toxic megacolon
- Opioids should not be administered during an asthma attack
- Convulsions - may be induced or exacerbated
- Drug abuse, dependence (including alcoholism), enhanced instability, suicidal ideation or attempts – predisposed to drug abuse
- Head injuries or conditions where intracranial pressure is raised
- Gall bladder disease or gall stones - opioids may cause biliary contraction
- Gastro-intestinal surgery - use with caution after recent GI surgery as opioids may alter GI motility
- Prostatic hypertrophy or recent urinary tract surgery
- Adrenocortical insufficiency, e.g. Addison's Disease
- Hypotension and shock
- Myasthenia gravis
- Phaeochromocytoma - opioids may stimulate catecholamine release by inducing the release of endogenous histamine

The label will state:

Do not exceed the recommended dose.

Do not take with any other paracetamol-containing products. Immediate medical attention should be sought in the event of an overdose, even if you feel well.

May cause dizziness, if affected do not drive or operate machinery.

If symptoms persist, consult your doctor.

Keep out of the reach and sight of children.

The label will state (to be displayed prominently on outer pack, not boxed):

If you need to use this medicine for more than three days at a time, see your doctor or pharmacist. Taking dihydrocodeine regularly for a long time can lead to addiction. Taking a painkiller for headaches too often or for too long can make them worse.

The leaflet will state:

Immediate medical advice should be sought in the event of an overdose, even if you feel well, because of the risk of delayed, serious liver damage.

The leaflet will state in a prominent position in the before taking section:

If you need to use this medicine for more than three days at a time, see your doctor, pharmacist or healthcare professional. Taking codeine regularly for a long time can lead to addiction, which might cause you to feel restless and irritable when you stop taking the tablets. Taking a painkiller for headaches too often or for too long can make them worse.

4.5 Interaction with other medicinal products and other forms of interaction

The speed of absorption of paracetamol may be increased by metoclopramide or domperidone and absorption reduced by cholestyramine.

The anticoagulant effect of warfarin and other coumarins may be enhanced by prolonged regular daily use of paracetamol with increased risk of bleeding. Occasional doses have no significant effect.

The depressant effects of opioid analgesics are enhanced by other CNS depressants such as alcohol, anaesthetics, anxiolytics, hypnotics, tricyclic antidepressants and antipsychotics.

Dihydrocodeine tartrate may interact with monoamine oxidase inhibitors (MAOI's), such that opioids should not be used in patients taking MAOI's or within 14 days of stopping such treatment. If opioid analgesics are required they should be given with extreme caution.

The effects of dihydrocodeine tartrate in reducing gastrointestinal motility may interfere with the absorption of such as mexiletine, and may counteract the stimulatory effect of metoclopramide and domperidone.

Cimetidine inhibits the metabolism of some opioids

4.6 Pregnancy and lactation

Epidemiological studies in human pregnancy have shown no effects due to paracetamol used in the recommended dosage. However, paracetamol should be avoided in pregnancy unless considered essential by the physician.

Risk benefit must be considered because opioid analgesics cross the placenta. Studies in animals have shown opioids to cause delayed ossification in mice and increased resorption in rats.

Regular use during pregnancy may cause physical dependence in the fetus, leading to withdrawal symptoms in the neonate. During labour opioids enter the fetal circulation and may cause respiratory depression in the neonate.

Administration should be avoided during the late stages of labour and during the delivery of a premature infant.

Paracetamol is excreted in breast milk but not in a clinically significant amount.

Available published data do not contraindicate breast feeding; however some opioids are distributed in breast milk in small amounts and it is advisable to avoid administration of opioids in a breastfeeding woman.

4.7 Effects on ability to drive and use machines

Opioid analgesics can impair mental function and can cause blurred vision and dizziness. Patients should make sure they are not affected before driving or operating machinery.

4.8 Undesirable effects

Adverse effects of paracetamol are rare but hypersensitivity, including skin rash, may occur. There have been rare reports of blood dyscrasias including thrombocytopenia and agranulocytosis, but these were not necessarily causally related to paracetamol. Constipation if it occurs, is readily treated with a mild laxative. Nausea, headache, vertigo, dizziness and urinary retention may occur in a few patients.

Regular prolonged use of dihydrocodeine is known to lead to addiction and symptoms of restlessness and irritability may result when treatment is stopped. Prolonged use of a painkiller for headaches can make them worse.

4.9 Overdose

Paracetamol:

Symptoms: Pallor, nausea, vomiting, anorexia and abdominal pain in the first 24 hours. Liver damage may become apparent 12 to 48 hours after ingestion.

Abnormalities of glucose metabolism and metabolic acidosis may occur. In severe poisoning, hepatic failure may progress to encephalopathy, coma and death.

Acute renal failure with acute tubular necrosis may develop even in the absence of severe liver damage. Cardiac arrhythmias have been reported.

Liver damage is likely in adults who have taken 10g or more of paracetamol. It is considered that excess quantities of a toxic metabolite (usually adequately detoxified by glutathione when normal doses of paracetamol are ingested), become irreversibly bound to liver tissue.

Treatment: Immediate treatment is essential in the management of paracetamol overdose. Despite a lack of significant early symptoms, patients should be referred to hospital urgently for immediate medical attention and any patient who had ingested around 7.5g or more of paracetamol in the preceding 4 hours should undergo gastric lavage. Administration of oral methionine or intravenous N-acetylcysteine, which may have a beneficial effect up to at least 48 hours after the overdose, may be required.

General supportive measures must be available.

Opioids:

Symptoms: cold clammy skin, confusion, convulsions, severe drowsiness, tiredness, low blood pressure, pinpoint pupils of eyes, slow heart beat and respiratory rate coma.

Treatment: Treat respiratory depression or other life-threatening adverse effects first.

Empty the stomach via gastric lavage or induction of emesis.

The opioid antagonist naloxone (0.4-2mg subcutaneous) can be given and repeated at 2-3 minute intervals to a maximum of 10mg. Naloxone may also be given by intramuscular injection or intravenous infusion. The patient should be monitored as the duration of opioid analgesic may exceed that of the antagonist.

5. PHARMACOLOGICAL PROPERTIES

5.1 Pharmacodynamic properties

Paracetamol is an effective analgesic possessing a remarkably low level of side effects. Its broad clinical utility has been extensively reported, and it now largely replaces aspirin for routine use. Paracetamol is well tolerated, having a bland effect on gastric mucosa, unlike aspirin, it neither exacerbates symptoms of peptic ulcer nor precipitates bleeding. Dihydrocodeine tartrate has been widely used for a number of years as a powerful analgesic; 30 mg of dihydrocodeine has been reported to have analgesic potency equal to 60 or 120 mg codeine.

In addition the compound exhibits well-defined anti-tussive activity.

Fortifying paracetamol with 7.46 mg dihydrocodeine tartrate provides an effective combination of drugs for the treatment of severe pain.

5.2 Pharmacokinetic properties

Dihydrocodeine is well absorbed from the gastrointestinal tract. Like other phenanthrene derivatives, dihydrocodeine is mainly metabolised in the liver with the resultant metabolites being excreted mainly in the urine. Metabolism of dihydrocodeine includes o-demethylation, n-demethylation and 6-keto reduction.

Paracetamol is readily absorbed from the gastrointestinal tract with peak plasma concentrations occurring 30 minutes to 2 hours after ingestion. It is metabolised in the liver and excreted in the urine mainly as the glucuronide and sulphate conjugates.

5.3 Preclinical safety data

Not applicable.

6. PHARMACEUTICAL PARTICULARS

6.1 List of excipients

Citric acid (anhydrous, added as citric acid monohydrate)

Sodium hydrogen carbonate

Sodium carbonate (anhydrous)

Sodium benzoate

Saccharin sodium

Povidone

6.2 Incompatibilities

None known.

6.3 Shelf life

24 months.

6.4 Special precautions for storage

Store at or below 25°C.

6.5 Nature and contents of container

1. Blister packs: 43 μm soft tempered aluminium foil coated with 25 μm polyethylene on the inside.

2. Aluminium foil strip packs: 25 μm aluminium foil coated with 40g/m^2 paper and 12g/m^2 polyethylene on the outside and 18g/m^2 surlyn on the inside.

Pack sizes: 2, 12, 24 tablets

6.6 Special precautions for disposal and other handling

None stated.

7. MARKETING AUTHORISATION HOLDER

Seton Products Ltd.

Tubiton House

Oldham

OL1 3HS

8. MARKETING AUTHORISATION NUMBER(S)

PL 11314/0058.

9. DATE OF FIRST AUTHORISATION/RENEWAL OF THE AUTHORISATION

20th December 1995.

10. DATE OF REVISION OF THE TEXT

June 2007

Paramol Tablets (New Capsule Shape)

(SSL International plc)

1. NAME OF THE MEDICINAL PRODUCT

Paramol Tablets.

2. QUALITATIVE AND QUANTITATIVE COMPOSITION

Paracetamol 500mg

Dihydrocodeine Tartrate 7.46mg

3. PHARMACEUTICAL FORM

Film coated tablets

4. CLINICAL PARTICULARS

4.1 Therapeutic indications

For the treatment of mild to moderate pain and as antipyretic in conditions such as: headache; migraine; feverish conditions; period pain; toothache and other dental pain; back pain; muscular and joint pains; neuralgia and the aches and pains of colds and flu.

4.2 Posology and method of administration

Route of Administration: Oral

Recommended doses and dosage schedules:

Paramol Tablets should, if possible, be taken during or after meals.

Adults and children over 12 years:

One or two tablets every four to six hours.

Do not exceed 8 tablets in any 24 hour period.

Do not take for more than 3 days continuously without medical review.

Children under 12 years:

Not recommended

The Elderly:

Caution should be exercised when increasing the dose in the elderly.

4.3 Contraindications

Hypersensitivity to paracetamol or any other constituents, respiratory depression, obstructive airways disease.

4.4 Special warnings and precautions for use

Paramol Tablets should be given with caution to patients with allergic disorders and should not be given during an attack of asthma.

Dosage should be reduced in the elderly, in hyperthyroidism and in chronic hepatic disease. An overdose can cause hepatic necrosis.

Care is advised in the administration of paracetamol to patients with severe renal or severe hepatic impairment. The hazard of overdose is greater in those with non-cirrhotic alcoholic liver disease.

The label will state:

Do not exceed the recommended dose.

Do not take with any other paracetamol-containing products.

Immediate medical attention should be sought in the event of an overdose, even if you feel well because of the risk of delayed, serious liver damage.

If symptoms persist, consult your doctor.

Keep out of reach of children.

The label will state (to be displayed prominently on outer pack, not boxed):

If you need to use this medicine for more than three days at a time, see your doctor or pharmacist. Taking dihydrocodeine regularly, for a long time, can lead to addiction. Taking a painkiller for headaches too often or for too long can make them worse.

The leaflet will state in a prominent position in the before taking section:

If you need to use this medicine for more than three days at a time, see your doctor, pharmacist or healthcare professional. Taking dihydrocodeine regularly, for a long time, can lead to addiction, which might cause you to feel restless and irritable when you stop taking the tablets. Taking a painkiller for headaches too often or for too long can make them worse.

4.5 Interaction with other medicinal products and other forms of interaction

The speed of absorption of paracetamol may be increased by metoclopramide or domperidone and absorption reduced by cholyestyramine. The anticoagulant effect of warfarin and other coumarins may be enhanced by prolonged regular daily use of paracetamol with increased risk of bleeding; occasional doses have no significant effect. Additive central nervous system depression may occur with alcohol.

4.6 Pregnancy and lactation

Epidemiological studies in human pregnancy have shown no ill effects due to paracetamol used in the recommended dosage, but patients should follow the advice of their doctor regarding its use. Paracetamol is excreted in breast milk but not in a clinically significant amount. Available published data do not contraindicate breast-feeding.

4.7 Effects on ability to drive and use machines

None stated.

4.8 Undesirable effects

Adverse effects of paracetamol are rare but hypersensitivity, including skin rash, may occur. There have been rare reports of blood dyscrasias including thrombocytopenia and agranulocytosis, but these were not necessarily causally related to paracetamol. Constipation if it occurs, is readily treated with a mild laxative. Nausea, vertigo, headache and giddiness may occur in a few patients.

Regular prolonged use of dihydrocodeine is known to lead to addiction and symptoms of restlessness and irritability may result when treatment is stopped. Prolonged use of a painkiller for headaches can make them worse.

4.9 Overdose

Symptoms of paracetamol overdose in the first 24 hours are pallor, nausea, vomiting, anorexia and abdominal pain. Liver damage may become apparent 12 to 48 hours after ingestion. Abnormalities of glucose metabolism and metabolic acidosis may occur. In severe poisoning, hepatic failure may progress to encephalopathy, coma and death. Acute renal failure with acute tubular necrosis may develop even in the absence of severe liver damage. Cardiac arrhythmias and pancreatitis have been reported. Liver damage is possible in adults who have taken 10g or more of paracetamol. It is considered that excess quantities of a toxic metabolite (usually adequately detoxified by glutathione when normal doses of paracetamol are ingested) become irreversibly bound to liver tissue.

Treatment:

Immediate treatment is essential in the management of paracetamol overdose. Despite a lack of significant early symptoms, patients should be referred to hospital urgently for immediate medical attention and any patient who has ingested around 7.5g or more of paracetamol in the preceding 4 hours should undergo gastric lavage. Administration of oral methionine or intravenous N-acetylcysteine, which may have a beneficial effect up to at least 48 hours after the overdose, may be required. General supportive measures must be available.

5. PHARMACOLOGICAL PROPERTIES

5.1 Pharmacodynamic properties

Paracetamol is an effective analgesic possessing a remarkably low level of side effects. Its broad clinical utility has been extensively reported and now largely replaces aspirin for routine use. Paracetamol is well tolerated, having a bland effect on the gastric mucosa, unlike aspirin, it neither exacerbates symptoms of peptic ulcer nor precipitates bleeding. Dihydrocodeine tartrate has been widely used for a number of years as a powerful analgesic. 30mg of dihydrocodeine has the analgesic potency of 60 to 120mg of codeine. In addition the product exhibits well-defined anti-tussive activity. Fortifying paracetamol with dihydrocodeine tartrate provides an effective combination of drugs for the treatment of mild to moderate pain and acts as an anti-pyretic.

5.2 Pharmacokinetic properties

Dihydrocodeine is well absorbed from the gastrointestinal tract. Like other Phenanthrene derivatives, dihydrocodeine is largely metabolised in the liver with the resultant metabolites being excreted mainly in the urine. Metabolism of dihyrocodeine includes O-Demethylation, N-Demethylation and 6-Ketoreduction. Paracetamol is readily absorbed from the gastro-intestinal tract with peak plasma concentrations occurring 30 minutes to 2 hours after ingestion. It is metabolised in the liver, and excreted in the urine mainly as glucuronide and sulphate conjugates.

5.3 Preclinical safety data

There are no pre-clinical tests performed on the product.

6. PHARMACEUTICAL PARTICULARS

6.1 List of excipients

Magnesium Stearate

Maize Starch

Povidone

Opadry White (Hypromellose, Titanium Dioxide and Macrogol 400)

6.2 Incompatibilities

None stated.

6.3 Shelf life

24 months.

6.4 Special precautions for storage

Do not store above 25°C.

6.5 Nature and contents of container

Blister Strips: 250μ PVC base material with an aluminium foil 20μ coated with a 15μ PVC layer. Pack Sizes are 12, 24, or 32 tablets.

6.6 Special precautions for disposal and other handling

None stated.

7. MARKETING AUTHORISATION HOLDER

Seton Products Ltd., Tubiton House, Oldham OL1 3HS.

8. MARKETING AUTHORISATION NUMBER(S)

PL 11314/0128.

9. DATE OF FIRST AUTHORISATION/RENEWAL OF THE AUTHORISATION
16/09/1999

10. DATE OF REVISION OF THE TEXT
October 2006

Pardelprin MR Capsules 75mg
(Actavis UK Ltd)

1. NAME OF THE MEDICINAL PRODUCT
PARDELPRIN MR CAPSULES 75mg
INDOMETACIN MODIFIED RELEASE CAPSULES

2. QUALITATIVE AND QUANTITATIVE COMPOSITION
Each capsule contains 75mg of Indometacin.

3. PHARMACEUTICAL FORM
Dark blue (head) and clear (body) hard gelatin Size 2 capsules printed "C" and "IR" in grey.

4. CLINICAL PARTICULARS
4.1 Therapeutic indications
Indometacin has non-steroidal analgesic and anti-inflammatory properties.
It is indicated for the following conditions:

• active stages of rheumatoid arthritis, osteoarthritis, ankylosing spondylitis, degenerative joint disease of the hip, acute musculoskeletal disorders and low back pain.

• periarticular disorders such as bursitis, tendinitis, synovitis, tenosynovitis and capsulitis.

• inflammation, pain and oedema following orthopaedic procedures

• treatment of pain and associated symptoms of primary dysmenorrhoea.

4.2 Posology and method of administration
Pardelprin is for oral administration and should always be given with food or milk to reduce the chance of gastro-intestinal disturbance. To minimise the evolution of unwanted reactions it is helpful in chronic conditions to start the therapy with a low dosage, increasing as required.

Adults: One capsule once or twice daily, depending on patient needs and response.

Dysmenorrhoea: One capsule a day, starting with onset of cramps or bleeding, and continuing for as long as symptoms usually last.

Elderly: The elderly are at increased risk of the serious consequences of adverse reactions. If an NSAID is considered necessary, the lowest effective dose should be used and for the shortest possible duration. The patient should be monitored regularly for GI bleeding during NSAID therapy

Children: Safety for use in children has not been established.

Undesirable effects may be minimised by using the lowest effective dose for the shortest duration necessary to control symptoms (see section 4.4).

Method of Administration
Oral use.

4.3 Contraindications
• Known hypersensitivity to NSAIDs, other ingredients in the product or other non-steroidal anti-inflammatory drugs.
• NSAIDs are contraindicated in patients with angioneurotic oedema or who have, with aspirin or other non-steroidal anti-inflammatory drugs experienced acute asthmatic attacks, urticaria or rhinitis in response to aspirin or other NSAIDs.
• Use with concomitant NSAIDs including cyclooxygenase 2 specific inhibitors (see section 4.5).
• Active peptic ulcer, a history of gastro-intestinal lesions.
• Severe hepatic, renal and cardiac failure (see section 4.4).
• Severe heart failure.
• Not to be used in patients with nasal polyps.
• During the last trimester of pregnancy (see section 4.6).
• Safety in children has not been established.

4.4 Special warnings and precautions for use
• Undesirable effects may be minimised by using the lowest effective dose for the shortest duration necessary to control symptoms (see section 4.2, and GI and cardiovascular risks below).

•*Cardiovascular and cerebrovascular effects*
Appropriate monitoring and advice are required for patients with a history of hypertension and/or mild to moderate congestive heart failure as fluid retention and oedema have been reported in association with NSAID therapy.

Clinical trial and epidemiological data suggest that use of some NSAIDs (particularly at high doses and in long term treatment) may be associated with a small increased risk of arterial thrombotic events (for example myocardial infartion or stroke). There are insufficient data to exclude such a risk for indometacin.

Patients with uncontrolled hypertension, congestive heart failure, established ischaemic heart disease, peripheral arterial disease, and/or cerebrovascular disease should only be treated with indometacin after careful consideration. Similar consideration should be made before initiating longer-term treatment of patients with risk factors for cardiovascular disease (e.g. hypertension, hyperlipidaemia, diabetes mellitus, smoking).

• Patients with rare hereditary problems of fructose or galactose intolerance, the Lapp lactase deficiency or glucose-galactose malabsorption or sucrase-isomaltase insufficiency should not take this medicine.

• Gastro-intestinal disorders which occur can be reduced by giving indometacin with food, milk or antacids.

• Patients should be carefully observed to detect any unusual manifestations of drug sensitivity.

• Indometacin should be used cautiously in patients with impaired renal function, bleeding disorders, psychiatric disorders, epilepsy or parkinsonism, as it may tend to aggravate these.

• Indometacin may mask the signs and symptoms of infectious disease and this should be borne in mind in order to avoid delay in starting treatment for infections. Indometacin should be used with caution in patients with an existing, albeit controlled infection. Caution is advised with concomitant use of live vaccines.

• In patients with renal, cardiac, hepatic impairment, hypertension, heart failure or conditions predisposing to fluid retention caution is required since the use of NSAIDs may result in deterioration of renal function (see section 4.8). The dose should be kept as low as possible and renal function should be monitored. NSAIDs may also cause fluid retention which may further aggravate these conditions.

• In patients with reduced renal blood flow where renal prostaglandins play a major role in maintaining renal perfusion, administration of a NSAID may precipitate overt renal decompensation. Patients at greatest risk of this reaction are those with renal or hepatic dysfunction, diabetes mellitus, advanced age, extracellular volume depletion, congestive heart failure, sepsis or concomitant use of any nephrotoxic drug. Indometacin should be given with caution and renal function should be monitored in any patient who may have reduced renal reserve. Discontinuation of NSAID therapy is usually followed by recovery to the pre-treatment state.

• Particular care should be taken with older patients who are more susceptible to side-effects from indometacin (see section 4.2).

• Caution is required if administered to patients suffering from or with a previous history of bronchial asthma since NSAIDs have been reported to precipitate bronchospasm in such patients.

• Caution is advised in patients with pre-existing sigmoid lesions (such as diverticulum or carcinoma) or ulcerative colitis or Crohns disease(or the development of these conditions) as indometacin can aggravate these conditions.

• Patients with a history of GI toxicity, particularly the elderly, should report any unusual abdominal symptoms (especially GI bleeding) particularly in the initial stages of treatment.

• GI bleeding, ulceration or perforation, which can be fatal, has been reported with all NSAIDs at any time during treatment, with or without warning symptoms or previous history of serious GI events. When GI bleeding or ulceration occurs in patients receiving indometacin, the treatment should be withdrawn.

• In patients with systemic lupus erythematosus (SLE) and mixed connective tissue disorders there may be an increased risk of aseptic meningitis (see section 4.8).

• The use of indometacin may impair female fertility and is not recommended in women attempting to conceive. In women who have difficulties conceiving or who are undergoing investigation of infertility, withdrawal of indometacin should be considered.

• Indometacin should be used with caution in patients with coagulation defects as indometacin can inhibit platelet aggregation. This effect may be exaggerated in patients with underlying haemostatic defects. Inhibition of platelet aggregation usually disappears within 24 hours of discontinuing indometacin.

• Caution is required in post-operative patients as bleeding time is prolonged (but within normal range) in normal adults.

• During prolonged therapy, periodic ophthalmic examinations are recommended, as corneal deposits and retinal disturbances have been reported. In patients with rheumatoid arthritis, eye changes may occur which may be related to the underlying disease or to the therapy. Therefore, in chronic rheumatoid disease, ophthalmological examinations are periodic intervals are recommended. Therapy should be discontinued if eye changes are observed.

• Patients should be periodically observed to allow early detection of any unwanted effects on peripheral blood (anaemia), liver function (also see section 4.8 Undesirable effects), or gastrointestinal tract especially during prolonged therapy.

• Caution should be advised in patients receiving concomitant medications which could increase the risk of gastro-toxicity or bleeding, such as corticoseroids, anticoagulants such as warfarin or anti-platelet agents such as aspirin (see section 4.5).

• Avoid concomitant use of two or more NSAIDs.

4.5 Interaction with other medicinal products and other forms of interaction
• Analgesics – avoid concomitant use of two or more NSAIDs (including aspirin) as this may increase the risk of adverse effects.

• Antibacterials - NSAIDs possibly increase the risk of convulsions with 4-quinolones. Also skin reactions and neurotoxicity have been reported with ciprofloxacin.

• Anticoagulants- NSAIDs may enhance the effects of anti-coagulants, such as warfarin (see section 4.4).

• Antidepressants (SSRI) – increased risk of bleeding.

• Antidiabetics – the effect of sulphonylureas may be increased by NSAIDs. Isolated case of metabolic acidosis with metformin.

• Antiepileptics – effect of phenytoin possibly increased by NSAIDs.

• Antihypertensives - indometacin may acutely reduce the antihypertensive effect of beta-blockers due partly to indometacin's inhibition of prostaglandin synthesis. Patients receiving dual therapy should have the antihypertensive effect of their therapy reassessed. Therefore, caution should be exercised when considering the addition of indometacin to the regimen of a patient taking any of the following antihypertensive agents: alpha-adrenergic blocking agents, ACE inhibitors, beta-adrenergic blocking agents, angiotensin-2-receptor antagonists, hydralazine or nifedipine. Hyperkalaemia has also been reported with ACE inhibitors.

• Antiplatelet drugs – increased risk of bleeding with clopidogrel. Indometacin can inhibit platelet aggregation an effect which disappears within 24 hours of discontinuation; the bleeding time may be prolonged and this effect may be exaggerated in patients with an underlying haemostatic defect.

• Antipsychotics – increased drowsiness with indometacin and haloperidol.

• Antivirals – pharmacokinetic changes have been recorded with zalcitabine/indometacin. Also increased risk of haematological toxicity with zidovudine. Risk of indometacin toxicity with ritonavir, avoid concomitant use.

• Benzodiazepines – increased risk of dizziness with diazepam and indometacin.

• Cardiac Glycosides - NSAIDs may exacerbate heart failure, reduce GFR, and increase plasma-cardiac glycoside concentration.

• Ciclosporin - administration of NSAIDs concomitantly with ciclosporin has been associated with an increase in ciclosporin-induced toxicity, possibly due to decreased synthesis of renal prostacyclin. NSAIDs should be used with caution in patients taking ciclosporin, and renal function should be monitored carefully.

• Corticosteroids – increased risk of gastrointestinal bleeding and ulceration (see section 4.4). If the patient is receiving corticosteroids concomitantly, a reduction in dosage of these may be possible but should only be effected slowly under supervision.

• Cytotoxics – caution should be employed in use with cyclophosphamide as acute water intoxication has been reported. Indometacin may decrease the tubular secretion of methotrexate thus potentiating toxicity; simultaneous use should be undertaken with caution.

• Desmopressin – effect potentiated by indometacin.

• Diflunisal- avoid concomitant use. Increased plasma levels of indometacin by about a third with a concomitant decrease in renal clearance occurs. Fatal gastro-intestinal haemorrhage has occurred.

• Diuretics – NSAIDS may reduce the effectiveness of all types of diuretics. Indometacin may reduce the diuretic and antihypertensive effect of thiazides and furosemide in some patients. Indometacin may cause blocking of the furosemide -induced increase in plasma renin activity. Diuretics can increase the risk of nephrotoxicity of NSAIDs.

• Lithium - indometacin is an inhibitor of prostaglandin synthesis and therefore the following drug interactions may occur; indometacin may raise plasma lithium levels and reduce lithium clearance in subjects with steady state plasma lithium concentrations. At the onset of such combined therapy, plasma lithium concentration should be monitored more frequently.

• Mifepristone - manufacturer recommends avoid NSAIDs until 8-12 days after mifepristone administration.

• Muscle Relaxants – increased risk of baclofen toxicity due to reduced rate of excretion.

• Muromonab-CD3 - significant rise in incidence of psychosis and encephalopathy in patients receiving both these drugs.

• Probenecid - co-administration of probenecid may increase plasma levels of indometacin. When increases in the dose of indometacin are made under these circumstances, they should be made cautiously and in small increments.

• Salicylates-use of indometacin with aspirin or other salicylates is not recommended because there is no enhancement of therapeutic effect while the incidence of gastro-intestinal side-effects is increased. Moreover, co-administration of aspirin may decrease the blood concentration of indometacin.

• Tacrolimus – increased risk of nephrotoxicity

• Tiludronic acid – bisphosphonates bioavailability increased by indometacin.

• Triamterene - indometacin and triamterene should not be administered together since reversible renal failure may be induced.

• Vasodilators – possible increased risk of bleeding with NSAIDs.

• Laboratory tests: borderline elevations of one or more liver tests may occur, and significant elevations of ALT (SGPT) or AST (SGOT) have been seen in less than 1% of patients receiving therapy with NSAIDs in controlled clinical trials. If abnormal liver tests persist or worsen, if clinical signs and symptoms consistent with liver disease develop, or if systemic manifestations such as rash or eosinophilia occur, indometacin should be stopped. False-negative results in the dexamethasone suppression test (DST) in patients being treated with indometacin have been reported. Thus, results of this test should be used with caution in these patients.

4.6 Pregnancy and lactation

Pregnancy: Congenital abnormalities have been reported in association with NSAID administration in man; however, these are low in frequency and do not appear to follow any discernible pattern. In view of the known effects of NSAIDs on the foetal cardiovascular system (risk of closure of the ductus arteriosus), use in the last trimester of pregnancy is contraindicated. The onset of labour may be delayed and the duration increased with an increased bleeding tendency in both mother and child (see section 4.3). NSAIDs should not be used during the first two trimesters of pregnancy or labour unless the potential benefit to the patients outweighs the potential risk to the foetus.

Lactation: In limited studies so far available, NSAIDs can appear in breast milk in very low concentrations. NSAIDs should, if possible, be avoided when breastfeeding.

See section 4.4 for information on female fertility.

4.7 Effects on ability to drive and use machines

Patients should be warned not to drive as they may experience dizziness, drowsiness, fatigue or visual disturbances. They should make sure they are not affected before driving or operating machinery.

4.8 Undesirable effects

• *Blood and lymphatic system disorders:* blood dyscrasias (thrombocytopenia, neutropenia, leukopenia, agranulocytosis, petechiae, ecchymosis, purpura, aplastic or haemolytic anaemia), bone marrow depression, petechiae, elevation of blood urea, epistaxis, ecchymosis, purpura, and disseminated intravascular coagulation) may occur infrequently. Some patients manifest anaemia secondary to obvious or occult gastro-intestinal bleeding.

• *Hypersensitivity:* hypersensitivity reactions have been reported following treatment with NSAIDs. These may consist of (a) non-specific allergic reactions and anaphylaxis, (b) respiratory tract reactivity comprising asthma, aggravated asthma, bronchospasm or dyspnoea, or (c) assorted skin disorders, including rashes of various types, pruritus, urticaria, purpura, angiodema and, more rarely exfoliative and bullous dermatoses (including epidermal necrolysis and erythema multiforme).

• *Metabolism and nutrition disorders:* hyperglycaemia, hyperkalaemia and glycosuria have been reported rarely.

• *Nervous system disorders:* headache, dizziness and light-headedness are common side effects. Starting therapy with a low dose and increasing gradually minimises the incidence of headache. These symptoms frequently disappear on continued therapy or reducing the dosage, but if headache persists despite dosage reduction, indometacin should be withdrawn. Other CNS effects include reports of aseptic meningitis (especially in patients with existing auto-immune disorders, such as systemic lupus erythematosus or mixed connective tissue disease) with symptoms such as stiff neck, headache, nausea, vomiting, fever or disorientation (see section 4.4), depression, vertigo, fatigue, malaise, dysarthria, syncope, coma, cerebral oedema, nervousness, confusion, anxiety and other psychiatric disturbances, depersonalisation, hallucinations, drowsiness, convulsions and aggravation of epilepsy, peripheral neuropathy, paraesthesia, involuntary movements, insomnia and parkinsonism. These effects are often transient and abate or disappear on reduced or stopping treatment. However, the severity of these may, on occasion, require cessation of therapy.

• *Eye disorders:* blurred vision, optic neuritis, diplopia and orbital and peri-orbital pain are seen infrequently. Corneal deposits and retinal or macular disturbances disturbances have been reported in some patients with rheumatoid arthritis on prolonged therapy with indometacin, and ophthalmic examinations are desirable in patients given prolonged treatment.

• *Ear disorders:* tinnitus or hearing disturbances (rarely deafness) have been reported.

• *Cardiac disorders:* there have been reports of oedema, hypertension, hypotension, tachycardia, chest pain, arrhythmia, palpitations and cardiac failure.

• *Vascular disorders:* flushing has been reported.

• *Respiratory, thoracic and mediastinal disorders*: pulmonary eosinophilia. There may be bronchospasm in patients with a history of bronchial asthma or other allergic disease.

• *Gastrointestinal disorders:* nausea, anorexia, vomiting, gastritis, epigastric discomfort or abdominal pain, constipation or diarrhoea all have been reported; more rarely, stomatitis, flatulence, ulceration at any point in the gastro-intestinal tract (even with resultant stenosis and obstruction), bleeding (even without obvious ulceration or from a diverticulum) and perforation of pre-existing sigmoid lesions (such as diverticulum or carcinoma) have occurred; and increased abdominal pain or exacerbation of the condition in patients with ulcerative colitis or Crohns disease (or the development of this condition) and regional ileitis have been rarely reported. Peptic ulcers, perforation or GI bleeding, sometimes fatal, particularly in the elderly, may occur (see section 4.4). If gastro-intestinal bleeding does occur treatment with indometacin should be discontinued. Gastro-intestinal disorders which occur can be reduced by giving indometacin with food, milk or antacids.

• *Hepato-biliary disorders:* cholestasis, elevation of LFTs (see section 4.5). Rarely hepatitis and jaundice (associated with some fatalities).

• *Skin and subcutaneous tissue disorders:* itching, urticaria, angioneurotic oedema, angiitis, photosensitivity, erythema nodosum, rash and exfoliative dermatitis all have been reported infrequently - as have Stevens Johnson syndrome, erythema multiforme, toxic epidermal necrolysis, hair loss, sweating and exacerbation of psoriasis.

• *Musculo-skeletal, connective tissue and bone disorders:* muscle weakness and acceleration of cartilage degeneration.

• *Renal and urinary disorders:* haematuria, nephrotic syndrome, proteinuria, interstitial nephritis, renal insufficiency or failure have all been reported. In patients with renal, cardiac or hepatic impairment, caution is required since the use of non-steroidal anti-inflammatory drugs may result in deterioration of renal function. The dose should be kept as low as possible and renal function should be monitored.

• *Reproductive system and breast disorders:* vaginal bleeding, interstitial nephritis, breast changes (enlargement, tenderness, gynaecomastia).

• Clinical trial and epidemiological data suggest that the use of some NSAIDs (particularly at high doses and in long term treatment) may be associated with an increased risk of arterial thrombotic events (for example myocardial infarction or stroke) (see section 4.4).

4.9 Overdose

Symptoms: headache, nausea, vomiting, epigastric pain, gastrointestinal bleeding, rarely diarrhoea, disorientation, excitation, coma, drowsiness, dizziness, tinnitus, fainting, occasionally convulsions. In cases of significant poisoning acute renal failure and liver damage are possible.

Treatment: patients should be treated symptomatically as required. Within one hour of ingestion of a potentially toxic amount, activated charcoal should be considered. Alternatively, in adults, gastric lavage should be considered. Good urine output should be ensured. Renal and liver function should be closely monitored. Patients should be observed for at least four hours after ingestion of potentially toxic amounts. Frequent or prolonged convulsions should be treated with intravenous diazepam.

5. PHARMACOLOGICAL PROPERTIES

5.1 Pharmacodynamic properties

ATC CODE: M01A B01

Indometacin is a non-steroidal anti-inflammatory agent with analgesic and antipyretic properties.

The analgesic properties have been attributed to both central and peripheral effect, which are distinct from its anti-inflammatory activity.

5.2 Pharmacokinetic properties

Absorption: The formulation has a gradual in vitro release profile over 8 hours.

Distribution: More than 90% is bound to plasma proteins. It is distributed into synovial fluid, CNS and placenta. Low concentrations have been found in breast milk.

Metabolism: It is metabolised in the liver primarily by demethylation and deacetylation, it also undergoes glucuronidation and enterohepatic circulation. Half-life is between 3 – 11 hours.

Elimination: Mainly excreted in the urine, approximately 60%, the pH of the urine can affect this amount. Lesser amounts in the faeces. Indometacin is also excreted in milk in small amounts.

The following pharmacokinetic particulars were obtained with indometacin MR 75mg Capsules; (n=8)

$t_{½\infty}$	3.999 hours
$t_{½\beta}$	3.853 hours
Tmax	6.182 hours
Cmax	2.192 μg/ml
AUC0-24	31.190 μg/ml/hours

5.3 Preclinical safety data

None stated.

6. PHARMACEUTICAL PARTICULARS

6.1 List of excipients

Also contains: sucrose, corn starch, lactose, povidone, talc, magnesium stearate, polymers of methacrylic acid, acrylic acid esters and methacrylic acid esters. Capsule shell: titanium dioxide (E171), erythrosine (E127), indigotine (E132), yellow iron oxide (E172) and gelatin.

Printing ink: shellac glaze, titanium dioxide (E171) and iron oxide black (E172).

6.2 Incompatibilities

See under interactions with other medicaments and other forms of interaction section.

6.3 Shelf life

Shelf-life

In the medicinal product as packaged for sale: 36 months.

Shelf-life after dilution/reconstitution

Not applicable.

Shelf-life after first opening

Not applicable.

6.4 Special precautions for storage

Store in a dry place below 25°C.

Protect from light.

6.5 Nature and contents of container

Capsule container: ie polypropylene securitainer with polyethylene closure.

Number of capsules per container: 28 or 100.

6.6 Special precautions for disposal and other handling

Not applicable.

Administrative Data

7. MARKETING AUTHORISATION HOLDER

Name or style and permanent address of registered place of business of the holder of the Marketing Authorisation:

Actavis UK Limited

(Trading style: Actavis)

Whiddon Valley

BARNSTAPLE

N Devon EX32 8NS

8. MARKETING AUTHORISATION NUMBER(S)

PL 0142/0436

9. DATE OF FIRST AUTHORISATION/RENEWAL OF THE AUTHORISATION

12.8.97

Renewed – 18.03.09

10. DATE OF REVISION OF THE TEXT

11.05.09

Pariet 10mg & 20mg

(Eisai Ltd)

1. NAME OF THE MEDICINAL PRODUCT

PARIET® 10mg gastro-resistant tablet

PARIET® 20mg gastro-resistant tablet

2. QUALITATIVE AND QUANTITATIVE COMPOSITION

10mg rabeprazole sodium, equivalent to 9.42mg rabeprazole

20mg rabeprazole sodium, equivalent to 18.85mg rabeprazole

For a full list of excipients, see section 6.1.

3. PHARMACEUTICAL FORM

Gastro-resistant tablet.

10mg: Pink, film coated biconvex tablet with 'E 241' printed on one side.

20mg: Yellow, film coated biconvex tablet with 'E 243' printed on one side.

4. CLINICAL PARTICULARS

4.1 Therapeutic indications

PARIET tablets are indicated for the treatment of:

• Active duodenal ulcer

• Active benign gastric ulcer

• Symptomatic erosive or ulcerative gastro-oesophageal reflux disease (GORD).

• Gastro-Oesophageal Reflux Disease Long-term Management (GORD Maintenance)

• Symptomatic treatment of moderate to very severe gastro-oesophageal reflux disease (symptomatic GORD)

• Zollinger-Ellison Syndrome

• In combination with appropriate antibacterial therapeutic regimens for the eradication of *Helicobacter pylori* in patients with peptic ulcer disease. See section 4.2

4.2 Posology and method of administration

Adults/elderly:

Active Duodenal Ulcer and Active Benign Gastric Ulcer: The recommended oral dose for both active duodenal ulcer and active benign gastric ulcer is 20mg to be taken once daily in the morning.

Most patients with active duodenal ulcer heal within four weeks. However a few patients may require an additional four weeks of therapy to achieve healing. Most patients with active benign gastric ulcer heal within six weeks. However again a few patients may require an additional six weeks of therapy to achieve healing.

Erosive or Ulcerative Gastro-Oesophageal Reflux Disease (GORD): The recommended oral dose for this condition is 20mg to be taken once daily for four to eight weeks.

Gastro-Oesophageal Reflux Disease Long-term Management (GORD Maintenance): For long-term management, a maintenance dose of PARIET 20mg or 10mg once daily can be used depending upon patient response.

Symptomatic treatment of moderate to very severe gastro-oesophageal reflux disease (symptomatic GORD): 10mg once daily in patients without oesophagitis. If symptom control has not been achieved during four weeks, the patient should be further investigated. Once symptoms have resolved, subsequent symptom control can be achieved using an on-demand regimen taking 10mg once daily when needed.

Zollinger-Ellison Syndrome: The recommended adult starting dose is 60 mg once a day. The dose may be titrated upwards to 120mg/day based on individual patient needs. Single daily doses up to 100mg/day may be given. 120mg dose may require divided doses, 60mg twice daily. Treatment should continue for as long as clinically indicated.

Eradication of H. pylori: Patients with *H. pylori* infection should be treated with eradication therapy. The following combination given for 7 days is recommended.

PARIET 20mg twice daily + clarithromycin 500mg twice daily and amoxicillin 1g twice daily.

For indications requiring once daily treatment PARIET tablets should be taken in the morning, before eating; and although neither the time of day nor food intake was shown to have any effect on rabeprazole sodium activity, this regimen will facilitate treatment compliance.

Patients should be cautioned that the PARIET tablets should not be chewed or crushed, but should be swallowed whole.

Renal and hepatic impairment: No dosage adjustment is necessary for patients with renal or hepatic impairment.

See section 4.4 Special Warnings and Precautions for Use of PARIET in the treatment of patients with severe hepatic impairment.

Children:

PARIET is not recommended for use in children, as there is no experience of its use in this group.

4.3 Contraindications

PARIET is contra-indicated in patients with known hypersensitivity to rabeprazole sodium, or to any excipient used in the formulation. PARIET is contra-indicated in pregnancy and during breast feeding.

4.4 Special warnings and precautions for use

Symptomatic response to therapy with rabeprazole sodium does not preclude the presence of gastric or oesophageal malignancy, therefore the possibility of malignancy should be excluded prior to commencing treatment with PARIET.

Patients on long-term treatment (particularly those treated for more than a year) should be kept under regular surveillance.

A risk of cross-hypersensitivity reactions with other proton pump inhibitor or substituted benzimidazoles cannot be excluded.

Patients should be cautioned that PARIET tablets should not be chewed or crushed, but should be swallowed whole.

PARIET is not recommended for use in children, as there is no experience of its use in this group.

There have been post marketing reports of blood dyscrasias (thrombocytopenia and neutropenia). In the majority of cases where an alternative aetiology cannot be identified, the events were uncomplicated and resolved on discontinuation of rabeprazole.

Hepatic enzyme abnormalities have been seen in clinical trials and have also been reported since market authorisation. In the majority of cases where an alternative aetiology cannot be identified, the events were uncomplicated and resolved on discontinuation of rabeprazole.

No evidence of significant drug related safety problems was seen in a study of patients with mild to moderate hepatic impairment versus normal age and sex matched controls. However because there are no clinical data on the use of PARIET in the treatment of patients with severe hepatic dysfunction the prescriber is advised to exercise caution when treatment with PARIET is first initiated in such patients.

Co-administration of atazanavir with PARIET is not recommended (see section 4.5).

4.5 Interaction with other medicinal products and other forms of interaction

Rabeprazole sodium produces a profound and long lasting inhibition of gastric acid secretion. An interaction with compounds whose absorption is pH dependent may occur. Co-administration of rabeprazole sodium with ketoconazole or itraconazole may result in a significant decrease in antifungal plasma levels. Therefore individual patients may need to be monitored to determine if a dosage adjustment is necessary when ketoconazole or itraconazole are taken concomitantly with PARIET.

In clinical trials, antacids were used concomitantly with the administration of PARIET and, in a specific drug-drug interaction study, no interaction with liquid antacids was observed.

Co-administration of atazanavir 300mg/ritonavir 10mg with omeprazole (40 mg once daily) or atazanavir 400mg with lansoprazole (60mg once daily) to healthy volunteers resulted in a substantial reduction in atazanavir exposure. The absorption of atazanavir is pH dependent. Although not studied, similar results are expected with other proton pump inhibitors. Therefore PPIs, including rabeprazole, should not be co-administered with atazanavir (see Section 4.4).

4.6 Pregnancy and lactation

Pregnancy:

There are no data on the safety of rabeprazole in human pregnancy. Reproduction studies performed in rats and rabbits have revealed no evidence of impaired fertility or harm to the foetus due to rabeprazole sodium, although low foeto-placental transfer occurs in rats. PARIET is contraindicated during pregnancy.

Lactation:

It is not known whether rabeprazole sodium is excreted in human breast milk. No studies in lactating women have been performed. Rabeprazole sodium is however excreted in rat mammary secretions. Therefore PARIET should not be used during breast feeding.

4.7 Effects on ability to drive and use machines

Based on the pharmacodynamic properties and the adverse events profile, it is unlikely that PARIET would cause an impairment of driving performance or compromise the ability to use machinery. If however, alertness is impaired due to somnolence, it is recommended that driving and operating complex machinery be avoided.

4.8 Undesirable effects

The most commonly reported adverse drug reactions, during controlled clinical trials with rabeprazole were headache, diarrhoea, abdominal pain, asthenia, flatulence, rash and dry mouth. The majority of adverse events experienced during clinical studies were mild or moderate in severity, and transient in nature.

The following adverse events have been reported from clinical trial and post-marketed experience.

Frequencies are defined as: common (>1/100, <1/10), uncommon (> 1/1,000, <1/100), rare (>1/10,000, <1/1000) and very rare (<1/10,000).

(see Table 1 on next page)

4.9 Overdose

Experience to date with deliberate or accidental overdose is limited. The maximum established exposure has not exceeded 60mg twice daily, or 160mg once daily. Effects are generally minimal, representative of the known adverse event profile and reversible without further medical intervention. No specific antidote is known. Rabeprazole sodium is extensively protein bound and is, therefore, not dialysable. As in any case of overdose, treatment should be symptomatic and general supportive measures should be utilised.

5. PHARMACOLOGICAL PROPERTIES

5.1 Pharmacodynamic properties

Pharmacotherapeutic group: Alimentary tract and metabolism, Drugs for peptic ulcer and gastro-oesophageal reflux disease (GORD), proton pump inhibitors,

ATC code: A02B C04

Mechanism of Action: Rabeprazole sodium belongs to the class of anti-secretory compounds, the substituted benzimidazoles, that do not exhibit anticholinergic or H_2 histamine antagonist properties, but suppress gastric acid secretion by the specific inhibition of the H^+/K^+-ATPase enzyme (the acid or proton pump) The effect is dose-related and leads to inhibition of both basal and stimulated acid secretion irrespective of the stimulus. Animal studies indicate that after administration, rabeprazole sodium rapidly disappears from both the plasma and gastric mucosa. As a weak base, rabeprazole is rapidly absorbed following all doses and is concentrated in the acid environment of the parietal cells. Rabeprazole is converted to the active sulphenamide form through protonation and it subsequently reacts with the available cysteines on the proton pump.

Anti-secretory Activity: After oral administration of a 20mg dose of rabeprazole sodium the onset of the anti-secretory effect occurs within one hour, with the maximum effect occurring within two to four hours. Inhibition of basal and food stimulated acid secretion 23 hours after the first dose of rabeprazole sodium are 69% and 82% respectively and the duration of inhibition lasts up to 48 hours. The inhibitory effect of rabeprazole sodium on acid secretion increases slightly with repeated once-daily dosing, achieving steady state inhibition after three days. When the drug is discontinued, secretory activity normalises over 2 to 3 days.

Serum Gastrin Effects: In clinical studies patients were treated once daily with 10 or 20mg rabeprazole sodium, for up to 43 months duration. Serum gastrin levels increased during the first 2 to 8 weeks reflecting the inhibitory effects on acid secretion and remained stable while treatment was continued. Gastrin values returned to pre-treatment levels, usually within 1 to 2 weeks after discontinuation of therapy.

Human gastric biopsy specimens from the antrum and the fundus from over 500 patients receiving rabeprazole or comparator treatment for up to 8 weeks have not detected changes in ECL cell histology, degree of gastritis, incidence of atrophic gastritis, intestinal metaplasia or distribution of *H. pylori* infection. In over 250 patients followed for 36 months of continuous therapy, no significant change in findings present at baseline was observed.

Other Effects: Systemic effects of rabeprazole sodium in the CNS, cardiovascular and respiratory systems have not been found to date. Rabeprazole sodium, given in oral doses of 20mg for 2 weeks, had no effect on thyroid function, carbohydrate metabolism, or circulating levels of parathyroid hormone, cortisol, oestrogen, testosterone, prolactin, cholecystokinin, secretin, glucagon, follicle stimulating hormone (FSH), luteinising hormone (LH), renin, aldosterone or somatotrophic hormone.

Studies in healthy subjects have shown that rabeprazole sodium does not have clinically significant interactions with amoxicillin. Rabeprazole does not adversely influence plasma concentrations of amoxicillin or clarithromycin when co-administered for the purpose of eradicating upper gastrointestinal *H. pylori* infection.

5.2 Pharmacokinetic properties

Absorption: PARIET is an enteric-coated (gastro-resistant) tablet formulation of rabeprazole sodium. This presentation is necessary because rabeprazole is acid-labile. Absorption of rabeprazole therefore begins only after the tablet leaves the stomach. Absorption is rapid, with peak plasma levels of rabeprazole occurring approximately 3.5 hours after a 20mg dose. Peak plasma concentrations (C_{max}) of rabeprazole and AUC are linear over the dose range of 10mg to 40mg. Absolute bioavailability of an oral 20mg dose (compared to intravenous administration) is about 52% due in large part to pre-systemic metabolism. Additionally the bioavailability does not appear to increase with repeat administration. In healthy subjects the plasma half-life is approximately one hour (range 0.7 to 1.5 hours), and the total body clearance is estimated to be 283 ± 98 ml/min. There was no clinically relevant interaction with food. Neither food nor the time of day of administration of the treatment affect the absorption of rabeprazole sodium.

Distribution: Rabeprazole is approximately 97% bound to human plasma proteins.

Metabolism and excretion: Rabeprazole sodium, as is the case with other members of the proton pump inhibitor (PPI) class of compounds, is metabolised through the cytochrome P450 (CYP450) hepatic drug metabolising system. *In vitro* studies with human liver microsomes indicated that rabeprazole sodium is metabolised by isoenzymes of CYP450 (CYP2C19 and CYP3A4). In these studies, at expected human plasma concentrations rabeprazole neither induces nor inhibits CYP3A4; and although *in vitro* studies may not always be predictive of *in vivo* status these findings indicate that no interaction is expected between rabeprazole and cyclosporin. In humans the thioether (M1) and carboxylic acid (M6) are the main plasma metabolites with the sulphone (M2), desmethyl-thioether (M4) and mercapturic acid conjugate (M5) minor metabolites observed at lower levels. Only the desmethyl metabolite (M3) has a small amount of anti-secretory activity, but it is not present in plasma.

Following a single 20mg ^{14}C labelled oral dose of rabeprazole sodium, no unchanged drug was excreted in the urine. Approximately 90% of the dose was eliminated in urine mainly as the two metabolites: a mercapturic acid conjugate (M5) and a carboxylic acid (M6), plus two unknown metabolites. The remainder of the dose was recovered in faeces.

Gender: Adjusted for body mass and height, there are no significant gender differences in pharmacokinetic parameters following a single 20mg dose of rabeprazole.

Renal dysfunction: In patients with stable, end-stage, renal failure requiring maintenance haemodialysis (creatinine clearance $\leqslant 5ml/min/1.73m^2$), the disposition of rabeprazole was very similar to that in healthy volunteers. The AUC and the C_{max} in these patients was about 35% lower than the corresponding parameters in healthy volunteers. The mean half-life of rabeprazole was 0.82 hours in healthy volunteers, 0.95 hours in patients during haemodialysis and 3.6 hours post dialysis. The clearance of the drug in patients with renal disease requiring maintenance haemodialysis was approximately twice that in healthy volunteers.

Hepatic dysfunction: Following a single 20mg dose of rabeprazole to patients with chronic mild to moderate hepatic impairment the AUC doubled and there was a 2-3 fold increase in half-life of rabeprazole compared to the healthy volunteers. However, following a 20mg dose daily for 7 days the AUC had increased to only 1.5-fold and the C_{max} to only 1.2-fold. The half-life of rabeprazole in patients with hepatic impairment was 12.3 hours compared to 2.1 hours in healthy volunteers. The pharmacodynamic

Table 1

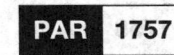

System Organ Class	Common	Uncommon	Rare	Very Rare	Not Known
Infections and infestations	Infection				
Blood and the lymphatic system disorders			Neutropenia Leucopenia Thrombocytopenia Leucocytosis		
Immune system disorders			Hypersensitivity[1,2]		
Metabolism and nutrition disorders			Anorexia		Hyponatremia
Psychiatric disorders	Insomnia	Nervousness	Depression		Confusion
Nervous system disorders	Headache Dizziness	Somnolence			
Eye disorders			Visual disturbance		
Vascular disorders					Peripheral oedema
Respiratory, thoracic and mediastinal disorders	Cough Pharyngitis Rhinitis	Bronchitis Sinusitis			
Gastrointestinal disorders	Diarrhoea Vomiting Nausea Abdominal pain Constipation Flatulence	Dyspepsia Dry mouth Eructation	Gastritis Stomatitis Taste disturbance		
Hepato-biliary disorders			Hepatitis Jaundice Hepatic encephalopathy[3]		
Skin and subcutaneous tissue disorders		Rash Erythema[2]	Pruritus Sweating Bullous reactions[2]	Erythema multiforme, toxic epidermal necrolysis (TEN), Stevens-Johnson syndrome (SJS)	
Musculoskeletal, connective tissue and bone disorders	Non-specific pain Back pain	Myalgia Leg cramps Arthralgia			
Renal and urinary disorders		Urinary tract infection	Interstitial nephritis		
Reproductive system and breast disorders					Gynaecomastia
General disorders and administration site conditions	Asthenia Influenza like illness	Chest pain Chills Pyrexia			
Investigations		Increased hepatic enzymes[3]	Weight increased		

[1] Includes facial swelling, hypotension and dyspnoea

[2] Erythema, bullous reactions and hypersensitivity reactions have usually resolved after discontinuation of therapy.

[3] Rare reports of hepatic encephalopathy have been received in patients with underlying cirrhosis. In treatment of patients with severe hepatic dysfunction the prescriber is advised to exercise caution when treatment with PARIET is first initiated in such patients (see section 4.4).

response (gastric pH control) in the two groups was clinically comparable.

Elderly: Elimination of rabeprazole was somewhat decreased in the elderly. Following 7 days of daily dosing with 20mg of rabeprazole sodium, the AUC approximately doubled, the C_{max} increased by 60% and t½ increased by approximately 30% as compared to young healthy volunteers. However there was no evidence of rabeprazole accumulation.

CYP2C19 Polymorphism: Following a 20mg daily dose of rabeprazole for 7 days, CYP2C19 slow metabolisers, had AUC and t½ which were approximately 1.9 and 1.6 times the corresponding parameters in extensive metabolisers whilst C_{max} had increased by only 40%.

5.3 Preclinical safety data

Non-clinical effects were observed only at exposures sufficiently in excess of the maximum human exposure that make concerns for human safety negligible in respect of animal data.

Studies on mutagenicity gave equivocal results. Tests in mouse lymphoma cell line were positive, but *in vivo* micronucleus and *in vivo* and *in vitro* DNA repair tests were negative. Carcinogenicity studies revealed no special hazard for humans.

6. PHARMACEUTICAL PARTICULARS

6.1 List of excipients

Core tablet: Mannitol, magnesium oxide, low-substituted hyprolose, hyprolose, magnesium stearate

Undercoating: ethylcellulose, magnesium oxide

Enteric coating: hypromellose phthalate, diacetylated monoglycerides, talc, titanium dioxide (E171), red iron oxide (E172) – 10mg only, yellow iron oxide (E172) – 20mg only, carnauba wax

Printing ink – Pariet 10mg: White Shellac, black iron oxide (E172), Dehydrated Ethyl Alcohol, 1-Butanol.

Printing ink – Pariet 20mg: White Shellac, Red Iron Oxide (E172), Carnauba wax, Glycerine fatty acid ester, Dehydrated Ethyl Alcohol, 1-Butanol.

6.2 Incompatibilities

Not applicable.

6.3 Shelf life

2 years.

6.4 Special precautions for storage

Do not store above 25°C. Do not refrigerate

6.5 Nature and contents of container

Blister strips (aluminium/aluminium)

Pack sizes: 1,5, 7, 14, 15, 25, 28, 30, 50, 56, 75, 98, 112, or 120 tablets

Not all pack sizes may be marketed.

6.6 Special precautions for disposal and other handling

No special requirements.

7. MARKETING AUTHORISATION HOLDER

Eisai Limited, European Knowledge Centre, Mosquito Way, Hatfield, Hertfordshire, AL10 9SN, United Kingdom

8. MARKETING AUTHORISATION NUMBER(S)

Pariet 10mg: PL 10555/0010 (10mg tablets)

Pariet 20mg: PL10555/0008 (20mg tablets)

9. DATE OF FIRST AUTHORISATION/RENEWAL OF THE AUTHORISATION

8 May 1998/May 2008

10. DATE OF REVISION OF THE TEXT

May 2009

11. LEGAL CATEGORY

POM – Medicinal product subject to medical prescription

Parvolex Injection

(UCB Pharma Limited)

1. NAME OF THE MEDICINAL PRODUCT

Parvolex Solution for Infusion.

2. QUALITATIVE AND QUANTITATIVE COMPOSITION

Acetylcysteine 200mg/ml.

For excipients, see 6.1.

3. PHARMACEUTICAL FORM

Solution for infusion.

4. CLINICAL PARTICULARS

4.1 Therapeutic indications

For the treatment of paracetamol overdosage.

4.2 Posology and method of administration

The injection is administered by intravenous infusion. The following infusion fluids may be used: 5% dextrose, 0.9% sodium chloride, 0.3% potassium chloride with 5% glucose, or 0.3% potassium chloride with 0.9% sodium chloride.

Adults:

An initial dose of 150mg/kg body weight of acetylcysteine is infused in 200ml of the recommended infusion fluid over 15 minutes, followed by 50mg/kg in 500ml infusion fluid over the next 4 hours, then 100mg/kg in 1 litre infusion fluid over the next 16 hours. (This gives a total dose of 300mg/kg in 20 hours.)

Children:

Children should be treated with the same doses and regimen as adults; however, the quantity of intravenous fluid used should be modified to take into account age and weight, as fluid overload is a potential danger. The National Poisons Centres in the UK have provided the following guidance:

Children weighing 20kg or more:

150mg/kg intravenous infusion in 100ml infusion fluid over 15 minutes; then 50mg/kg in 250ml infusion fluid over 4 hours; then 100mg/kg in 500ml infusion fluid over 16 hours.

Children under 20kg:

Volumes for infusion of the above doses are the responsibility of the prescriber and should be based on the daily maintenance requirements of the child by weight.

Critical times:

Acetylcysteine (Parvolex®) is very effective in preventing paracetamol-induced hepatotoxicity when administered during the first 8 hours after a paracetamol overdose. When administered after the first 8 hours, the protective effect diminishes progressively as the overdose-treatment interval increases. However, clinical experience indicates that acetylcysteine can still be of benefit when administered up to 24 hours after paracetamol overdose, without any change in its safety profile. It may also be administered after 24 hours in patients at risk of severe liver damage. In general, for patients presenting later than 24 hours after a paracetamol overdose, guidance should be sought from a National Poisons Centre.

Treatment 'nomogram':

Plasma paracetamol concentration in relation to time after the overdose is commonly used to determine whether a patient is at risk of hepatotoxicity and should, therefore, receive treatment with an antidote such as acetylcysteine. For the majority of otherwise healthy patients, a line joining points of 200mg/l at 4 hours and 30mg/l at 15 hours on a semilogarithmic plot is used. (Treatment line A - see graph.) This line can be extended to 24 hours after overdose, based on a paracetamol half-life of 4 hours. It is recommended that patients whose plasma paracetamol concentrations fall on or above this line receive acetylcysteine. If there is doubt about the timing of the overdose, consideration should be given to treatment with acetylcysteine.

Patients with induced hepatic microsomal oxidase enzymes (such as chronic alcoholics and patients taking anticonvulsant drugs) are susceptible to paracetamol-induced hepatotoxicity at lower plasma paracetamol concentrations (see section 4.4 - Special Warnings and Precautions for Use) and should be assessed against treatment line B (see graph).

In patients who have taken staggered overdoses, blood levels are meaningless in relation to the treatment graph. These patients should all be considered for treatment with acetylcysteine.

NB: Blood samples taken less than 4 hours after a paracetamol overdose give unreliable estimates of the serum paracetamol concentration.

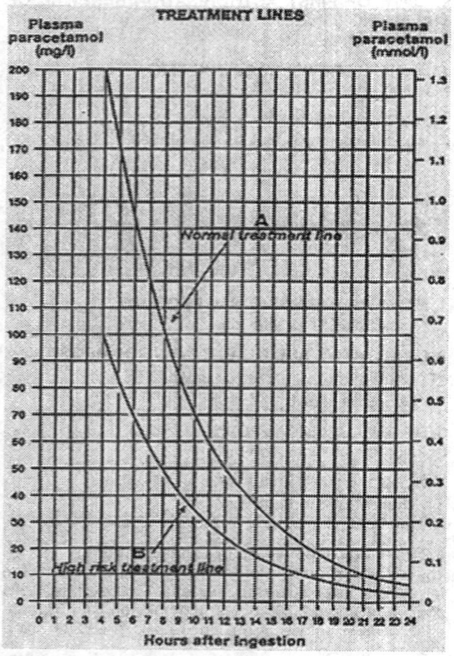

Plasma paracetamol concentrations in relation to time after overdosage as a guide to prognosis.

From guidelines agreed by National Poisons Centres - June 1995.

Parvolex is indicated in patients with values on or above the appropriate treatment line.

4.3 Contraindications
Hypersensitivity to any ingredient in the preparation.

4.4 Special warnings and precautions for use
Precautions:

Administer with caution in patients with asthma or a history of bronchospasm.

Liver enzyme-inducing drugs; chronic alcohol abuse:

Patients taking drugs that induce liver enzymes, such as some anticonvulsant drugs (e.g. phenytoin, phenobarbitone, primidone and carbamazepam) and rifampicin, and patients who routinely consume alcohol above recommended levels are believed to be at risk of hepatotoxicity from paracetamol poisoning at lower plasma paracetamol concentrations than other patients. It is recommended that such patients whose plasma paracetamol concentrations fall on or above a treatment line joining 100mg/l at 4 hours after overdose and 15mg/l at 15 hours after overdose on a semilogarithmic plot (i.e. treatment line B - see graph), be given acetylcysteine.

Other patients predisposed to toxicity:

Patients suffering from malnutrition, for example, patients with anorexia or AIDS, may have depleted glutathione reserves. It has been recommended that paracetamol overdose in such patients be treated as for chronic alcohol consumers or patients taking anticonvulsant drugs (treatment line B - see graph).

4.5 Interaction with other medicinal products and other forms of interaction
There are no known interactions.

4.6 Pregnancy and lactation
The safety of acetylcysteine in pregnancy has not been investigated in formal prospective clinical trials. However, clinical experience indicates that use of acetylcysteine in pregnancy for the treatment of paracetamol overdose is effective. Prior to use in pregnancy, the potential risks should be balanced against the potential benefits.

4.7 Effects on ability to drive and use machines
There are no known effects on ability to drive and use machines.

4.8 Undesirable effects
'Anaphylactoid' or 'hypersensitivity-like' reactions have been reported. They include nausea/vomiting, injection-site reactions, flushing, itching, rashes/urticaria, angioedema, bronchospasm/respiratory distress, hypotension, and rarely, tachycardia or hypertension. These have usually occurred between 15 and 60 minutes after the start of infusion. In many cases, symptoms have been relieved by stopping the infusion. Occasionally, an antihistamine drug may be necessary. Corticosteroids may occasionally be required. Once an anaphylactoid reaction is under control, the infusion can normally be restarted at the lowest infusion rate (100mg/kg in 1 litre over 16 hours).

In rare instances, the following side-effects have occurred: coughing, chest tightness or pain, puffy eyes, sweating, malaise, raised temperature, vasodilation, blurred vision, bradycardia, facial or eye pain, syncope, acidosis, thrombocytopenia, respiratory or cardiac arrest, stridor, anxiety, extravasation, arthropathy, arthralgia, deterioration of liver function, generalised seizure, cyanosis, lowered blood urea. Rare instances of fatality have also occurred.

Hypokalaemia and ECG changes have been noted in patients with paracetamol poisoning irrespective of the treatment given. Monitoring of plasma potassium concentration is, therefore, recommended.

If any side-effects to Parvolex® (acetylcysteine) develop, advice should be sought from a National Poisons Centre to ensure that the patients receives adequate treatment of the paracetamol overdose.

4.9 Overdose
There is a theoretical risk of hepatic encephalopathy. Overdosage of acetylcysteine has been reported to be associated with effects similar to the 'anaphylactoid' reactions noted in section 4.8 (Undesirable Effects), but they may be more severe. General supportive measures should be carried out. Such reactions are managed with antihistamines and steroids in the usual way. There is no specific antidote.

5. PHARMACOLOGICAL PROPERTIES

5.1 Pharmacodynamic properties
Acetylcysteine is considered to reduce the hepatic toxicity of NAPQI (n-acetyl-p-benzo-quinoneimine), the highly reactive intermediate metabolite following ingestion of a high dose of paracetamol, by at least two mechanisms. First, acetylcysteine acts as a precursor for the synthesis of glutathione and, therefore, maintains cellular glutathione at a level sufficient to inactivate NAPQI. This is thought to be the main mechanism by which acetylcysteine acts in the early stages of paracetamol toxicity.

Acetylcysteine has been shown to still be effective when infusion is started at up to 12 hours after paracetamol ingestion, when most of the analgesic will have been metabolised to its reactive metabolite. At this stage, acetylcysteine is thought to act by reducing oxidised thiol groups in key enzymes.

When acetylcysteine treatment is begun more than 8 to 10 hours after paracetamol overdose, its efficacy in preventing hepatotoxicity (based on serum indicators) declines progressively with further lengthening of the overdose-treatment interval (the time between paracetamol overdose and start of treatment). However, there is now evidence that it can still be beneficial when given up to 24 hours after overdose. At this late stage of paracetamol hepatotoxicity, acetylcysteine's beneficial effects may be due to its ability to improve systematic haemodynamics and oxygen transport, although the mechanism by which this may occur has yet to be determined.

5.2 Pharmacokinetic properties
Following intravenous administration of acetylcysteine using the standard 20-hour intravenous regimen, plasma levels of 300 to 900mg/l have been reported to occur shortly after the start of the infusion, falling to 11 to 90mg/l at the end of the infusion period. Elimination half-lives of 2 to 6 hours have been reported after intravenous dosing, with 20 to 30% of the administered dose being recovered unchanged in the urine.

Metabolism appears to be rapid and extensive. There is no information on whether acetylcysteine crosses the blood-brain barrier or the placenta, or whether it is excreted in breast milk.

5.3 Preclinical safety data
None stated.

6. PHARMACEUTICAL PARTICULARS

6.1 List of excipients
Disodium Edetate

Sodium Hydroxide

Water for Injections

6.2 Incompatibilities
Acetylcysteine is not compatible with rubber or metals, particularly iron, copper and nickel. Silicone rubber and plastic are satisfactory for use with Parvolex®.

A change in the colour of the solution to light purple has sometimes been noted and is not thought to indicate significant impairment of safety or efficacy.

6.3 Shelf life
3 years.

6.4 Special precautions for storage
Store below 25°C.

6.5 Nature and contents of container
Clear, Type I glass, 10ml snap ring ampoules. 10 × 10ml ampoules are packed in cartons.

6.6 Special precautions for disposal and other handling
Acetylcysteine to be diluted for intravenous infusion using either 5% dextrose, 0.9% sodium chloride, 0.3% potassium chloride with 5% glucose, or 0.3% potassium chloride with 0.9% sodium chloride. The volumes to be used are as directed in section 4.2.

7. MARKETING AUTHORISATION HOLDER
UCB Pharma Limited

208 Bath Road

Slough

Berkshire

SL1 3WE

UK

8. MARKETING AUTHORISATION NUMBER(S)
PL 00039/0410

9. DATE OF FIRST AUTHORISATION/RENEWAL OF THE AUTHORISATION
14 October 1992, 31 October 1997, June 2002

10. DATE OF REVISION OF THE TEXT
June 2005

11. Legal Category

POM

Pavacol-D

(Alliance Pharmaceuticals)

1. NAME OF THE MEDICINAL PRODUCT
Pavacol-D®

2. QUALITATIVE AND QUANTITATIVE COMPOSITION
Dark brown liquid containing 5 mg of Pholcodine BP in each 5 ml

3. PHARMACEUTICAL FORM
Liquid for oral administration

4. CLINICAL PARTICULARS

4.1 Therapeutic indications
Cough suppressant for relief of acute non-productive cough associated with upper respiratory tract infection.

4.2 Posology and method of administration
Adults

One or two 5 ml spoonfuls as required. The dose may be increased to three 5 ml spoonfuls if necessary. No more than 60 ml should be taken in 24 hours.

Children

Do not give to children under 6 years of age (See Section 4.3, "Contraindications").

From 6 to 12 years: one 5 ml spoon four to five times daily. No more than 25ml should be taken in 24 hours. Not to be used for more than 5 days.

Parents or carers should seek medical attention if the child's condition deteriorates during treatment.

Pavacol-D may be diluted with sorbitol solution BPC.

No specific information on the use of this product in the elderly is available. Clinical trials have included patients over 65 years and no adverse reactions specific to this age group have been reported.

4.3 Contraindications
Hypersensitivity to any of the ingredients, liver disease or ventilatory failure.

Not to be used in children under the age of 6 years.

Pholcodine should not be given to subjects in or at risk of developing respiratory failure.

Patients with chronic bronchitis, COPD, bronchiolitis or bronchiectasis due to sputum retention.

Patients taking monoamine oxidase inhibitors (MAOIs) or within 14 days of stopping such treatment (See Section 4.5, "Interactions with other medicinal products and other forms of interaction").

4.4 Special warnings and precautions for use
As pholcodine is a sedative, caution is needed in those patients who have airway disease e.g. asthma, as respiratory depression may occur.

Ask a doctor before use if you suffer from a chronic or persistent cough, if you have asthma, suffering from an acute asthma attack or where the cough is accompanied by excessive secretions.

Caution is also needed in patients with kidney disease or a history of drug abuse.

Pholcodine should not be taken with any other cough or cold medicine (See Section 4.5, "Interactions with other medicinal products and other forms of interaction").

Use of pholcodine with alcohol or other CNS depressants may increase the effects on the CNS and cause toxicity in relatively smaller doses.

4.5 Interaction with other medicinal products and other forms of interaction

Alcohol or other CNS depressants may lead to greater drowsiness and sedation.

Pholcodine should not be taken with any other cough or cold medicine.

Not to be used in patients taking MAOIs or within 14 days of stopping treatment.

Interaction with neuromuscular blocking agents (anaphylaxis) has been reported.

Pholcodine may accentuate the hypotensive effects of antihypertensives. The same effect may be seen when administered with diuretics.

Pholcodine may enhance the sedative effects of central nervous system depressants including alcohol, barbiturates, hypnotics, narcotic analgesics, sedatives and tranquillisers (phenothiazines and tricyclic antidepressants).

4.6 Pregnancy and lactation

Although Pavacol-D has been in general use for many years, there is no evidence of ill consequences during human pregnancy.

Medicines should not be used in pregnancy, especially the first trimester, unless the expected benefit is thought to outweigh any possible risk to the foetus.

4.7 Effects on ability to drive and use machines

Drowsiness occurs occasionally after taking pholcodine.

4.8 Undesirable effects

The following side effects may be associated with the use of pholcodine:

Occasional drowsiness, dizziness, excitation, confusion, sputum retention, vomiting, gastrointestinal disturbances (nausea and constipation) and skin reactions including rash.

Immune system disorders have been noted including hypersensitivity reactions and anaphylaxis.

4.9 Overdose

Pholcodine is thought to be of low toxicity but the effects in overdosage will be potentiated by simultaneous ingestion of alcohol and psychotropic drugs.

Symptoms: These include nausea, drowsiness, restlessness, excitement, ataxia and respiratory depression.

Management: Treatment of overdose should be symptomatic and supportive. Gastric lavage may be of use. Naloxone has been used successfully to reverse central or peripheral opioid effects in children (0.01 mg/kg body weight). Activated charcoal may also be used (1 g/kg body weight) if more than 4 mg/kg has been ingested within 1 hour, provided the airway can be protected.

5. PHARMACOLOGICAL PROPERTIES

5.1 Pharmacodynamic properties

Pholcodine is a specific anti-tussive lacking the unwanted side-effects of opium and its derivatives. The specificity of action suggests that pholcodine acts via a distinct subset of opioid receptors.

5.2 Pharmacokinetic properties

In a study in male volunteers receiving 15, 30, and 60 mg doses of pholcodine at 7 day intervals, pharmacokinetics were found to be independent of dose. The elimination of pholcodine is described by a two-compartment model with elimination half-life of 37± 4.2 hours. Pholcodine undergoes little conjugation and is not transformed to morphine.

5.3 Preclinical safety data

None stated.

6. PHARMACEUTICAL PARTICULARS

6.1 List of excipients

Tolu balsam

Ethanol 96%

Anise Oil

Clove Oil

Peppermint Oil

Capsicum Tincture

Strong Ginger tincture

Sorbitol solution

Saccharin Sodium

Hydroxyethylcellulose

Treacle Flavour

Caramel

L-menthol

Methyl Paraben

Propyl Paraben

Purified Water

6.2 Incompatibilities

None.

6.3 Shelf life

The shelf life expiry date for Pavacol-D is 3 years from the date of its manufacture.

When Pavacol-D is diluted an in-use shelf life of 14 days is recommended.

6.4 Special precautions for storage

Store below 25°C. Protect from light.

6.5 Nature and contents of container

50 ml, 100 ml, 150 ml, 250 ml, 300 ml, and 1000 ml round amber glass bottle (type III glass) with an aluminium roll-on pilfer proof cap.

Not all pack sizes may be marketed.

6.6 Special precautions for disposal and other handling

None stated.

7. MARKETING AUTHORISATION HOLDER

Alliance Pharmaceuticals Limited

Avonbridge House

Chippenham

Wiltshire

SN15 2BB

United Kingdom

8. MARKETING AUTHORISATION NUMBER(S)

PL 16853/0100

9. DATE OF FIRST AUTHORISATION/RENEWAL OF THE AUTHORISATION

14th November 2003

10. DATE OF REVISION OF THE TEXT

19th May 2009

Pegasys 135mcg and 180mcg solution for injection in Pre-filled Syringe

(Roche Products Limited)

1. NAME OF THE MEDICINAL PRODUCT

Pegasys 135 micrograms solution for injection in pre-filled syringe

Pegasys 180 micrograms solution for injection in pre-filled syringe

2. QUALITATIVE AND QUANTITATIVE COMPOSITION

One pre-filled syringe contains

peginterferon alfa-2a* .... 135 micrograms

One pre-filled syringe contains

peginterferon alfa-2a* .... 180 micrograms

Each syringe of 0.5ml solution contains 135 micrograms peginterferon alfa-2a*. The strength indicates the quantity of the interferon alfa-2a moiety of peginterferon alfa-2a without consideration of the pegylation.

Each syringe of 0.5 ml solution contains 180 micrograms peginterferon alfa-2a*. The strength indicates the quantity of the interferon alfa-2a moiety of peginterferon alfa-2a without consideration of the pegylation.

*The active substance, peginterferon alfa-2a, is a covalent conjugate of the protein interferon alfa-2a produced by recombinant DNA technology in *Escherichia coli* with bis-[monomethoxy polyethylene glycol].

The potency of this product should not be compared to the one of another pegylated or non-pegylated protein of the same therapeutic class. For more information, see section 5.1.

For a full list of excipients, see section 6.1.

Excipient:

Benzyl alcohol (10 mg/ 1 ml)

3. PHARMACEUTICAL FORM

Solution for injection in pre-filled syringe.

The solution is clear and colourless to light yellow.

4. CLINICAL PARTICULARS

4.1 Therapeutic indications

Chronic hepatitis B:

Pegasys is indicated for the treatment of HBeAg-positive or HBeAg-negative chronic hepatitis B in adult patients with compensated liver disease and evidence of viral replication, increased ALT and histologically verified liver inflammation and/or fibrosis (see sections 4.4 and 5.1).

Chronic hepatitis C:

Pegasys is indicated for the treatment of chronic hepatitis C in adult patients who are positive for serum HCV-RNA, including patients with compensated cirrhosis and/or co-infected with clinically stable HIV (see section 4.4).

The optimal way to use Pegasys in patients with chronic hepatitis C is in combination with ribavirin. The combination of Pegasys and ribavirin is indicated in naive patients and patients who have failed previous treatment with interferon alpha (pegylated or non-pegylated) alone or in combination therapy with ribavirin.

Monotherapy is indicated mainly in case of intolerance or contraindication to ribavirin.

4.2 Posology and method of administration

Treatment should be initiated only by a physician experienced in the treatment of patients with hepatitis B or C.

Please refer also to the ribavirin Summary of Product Characteristics (SPC) when Pegasys is to be used in combination with ribavirin.

Dose to be administered and duration of treatment

Chronic hepatitis B:

The recommended dosage and duration of Pegasys for both HBeAg-positive and HBeAg-negative chronic hepatitis B is 180 micrograms once weekly for 48 weeks by subcutaneous administration in the abdomen or thigh.

Chronic hepatitis C – treatment-naïve patients:

The recommended dose for Pegasys is 180 micrograms once weekly by subcutaneous administration in the abdomen or thigh given in combination with oral ribavirin or as monotherapy.

The dose of ribavirin to be used in combination with Pegasys is given in Table 1.

The ribavirin dose should be administered with food.

Duration of treatment

The duration of combination therapy with ribavirin for chronic hepatitis C depends on viral genotype. Patients infected with HCV genotype 1 who have detectable HCV RNA at week 4 regardless of pre-treatment viral load should receive 48 weeks of therapy.

Treatment for 24 weeks may be considered in patients infected with

- genotype 1 with low viral load (LVL) (⩽ 800,000 IU/mL) at baseline or

- genotype 4

who become HCV RNA negative at week 4 and remain HCV RNA negative at week 24. However, an overall 24 weeks treatment duration may be associated with a higher risk of relapse than a 48 weeks treatment duration (see section 5.1). In these patients, tolerability to combination therapy and additional prognostic factors such as degree of fibrosis should be taken into account when deciding on treatment duration. Shortening the treatment duration in patients with genotype 1 and high viral load (HVL) (>800, 000 IU/ml) at baseline who become HCV RNA negative at week 4 and remain HCV RNA negative at week 24 should be considered with even more caution since the limited data available suggest that this may significantly negatively impact the sustained virologic response.

Patients infected with HCV genotype 2 or 3 who have detectable HCV RNA at week 4, regardless of pre-treatment viral load should receive 24 weeks of therapy. Treatment for only 16 weeks may be considered in selected patients infected with genotype 2 or 3 with LVL (⩽ 800,000 IU/mL) at baseline who become HCV negative by week 4 of treatment and remain HCV negative by week 16. Overall 16 weeks of treatment may be associated with a lower chance of response and is associated with a higher risk of relapse than a 24 week treatment duration (see section 5.1). In these patients, tolerability to combination therapy and the presence of additional clinical or prognostic factors such as degree of fibrosis should be taken into account when considering deviations from standard 24 weeks treatment duration. Shortening the treatment duration in patients infected with genotype 2 or 3 with HVL (> 800,000 IU/mL) at baseline who become HCV negative by week 4 should be considered with more caution as this may significantly negatively impact the sustained virological response (see Table 1).

Available data for patients infected with genotype 5 or 6 are limited; therefore combination treatment with 1000/1200 mg of ribavirin for 48 weeks is recommended.

Table 1: Dosing Recommendations for Combination therapy for HCV Patients

(see Table 1 on next page)

The ultimate clinical impact of a shortened initial treatment of 16 weeks instead of 24 weeks is unknown, taking into account the need for retreating non-responding and relapsing patients.

The recommended duration of Pegasys monotherapy is 48 weeks.

Chronic hepatitis C – treatment-experienced patients:

The recommended dose of Pegasys in combination with ribavirin is 180 mcg once weekly by subcutaneous administration. For patients <75 kg and ⩾75 kg, 1000 mg daily and 1200 mg daily of ribavirin, respectively, should be administered.

Patients who have detectable virus at week 12 should stop therapy. The recommended total duration of therapy is 48 weeks. If patients infected with virus genotype 1, not responding to prior treatment with PEG-IFN and ribavirin are considered for treatment, the recommended total duration of therapy is 72 weeks (see section 5.1).

HIV-HCV co-infection

The recommended dosage for Pegasys, alone or in combination with 800 milligrams of ribavirin, is 180 micrograms once weekly subcutaneously for 48 weeks, regardless of genotype. The safety and efficacy of combination therapy with ribavirin doses greater than 800 milligrams daily is currently being studied. A duration of therapy less than 48 weeks has not been adequately studied.

Predictability of response and non-response – treatment-naïve patients

Early virological response by week 12, defined as a 2 log viral load decrease or undetectable levels of HCV RNA has been shown to be predictive for sustained response (see Tables 2 and 6).

Table 1 Dosing Recommendations for Combination therapy for HCV Patients

Genotype	Pegasys Dose	Ribavirin Dose	Duration
Genotype 1 LVL with RVR*	180 micrograms	<75 kg = 1000 mg ≥75 kg = 1200 mg	24 weeks or 48 weeks
Genotype 1 HVL with RVR*	180 micrograms	<75 kg = 1000 mg ≥75 kg = 1200 mg	48 weeks
Genotype 4 with RVR*	180 micrograms	<75 kg = 1000 mg ≥75 kg = 1200 mg	24 weeks or 48 weeks
Genotype 1 or 4 without RVR*	180 micrograms	<75 kg = 1000 mg ≥75 kg = 1200 mg	48 weeks
Genotype 2 or 3 without RVR**	180 micrograms	800 mg	24 weeks
Genotype 2 or 3 LVL with RVR**	180 micrograms	800 mg[(a)]	16 weeks[(a)] or 24 weeks
Genotype 2 or 3 HVL with RVR**	180 micrograms	800 mg	24 weeks

*RVR = rapid viral response (HCV RNA undetectable) at week 4 and HCV RNA undetectable at week 24;

**RVR = rapid viral response (HCV RNA negative) by week 4

LVL= ≤800,000 IU/mL; HVL=> 800,000 IU/mL

[(a)] It is presently not clear whether a higher dose of ribavirin (e.g. 1000/1200 mg/day based on body weight) results in higher SVR rates than does the 800 mg/day, when treatment is shortened to 16 weeks.

Table 2: Predictive Value of Week 12 Virological Response at the Recommended Dosing Regimen while on Pegasys Combination Therapy

(see Table 2 below)

The negative predictive value for sustained response in patients treated with Pegasys in monotherapy was 98%.

A similar negative predictive value has been observed in HIV-HCV co-infected patients treated with Pegasys monotherapy or in combination with ribavirin (100% (130/130) or 98% (83/85), respectively). Positive predictive values of 45% (50/110) and 70% (59/84) were observed for genotype 1 and genotype 2/3 HIV-HCV co-infected patients receiving combination therapy.

Predictability of response and non-response – treatment-experienced patients

In non-responder patients re-treated for 48 or 72 weeks, viral suppression at week 12 (undetectable HCV RNA defined as <50 IU/mL) has been shown to be predictive for sustained virological response. The probabilities of not achieving a sustained virological response with 48 or 72 weeks of treatment if viral suppression was not achieved at week 12 were 96% (363 of 380) and 96% (324 of 339), respectively. The probabilities of achieving a sustained virological response with 48 or 72 weeks of treatment if viral suppression was achieved at week 12 were 35% (20 of 57) and 57% (57 of 100), respectively.

Dose adjustment for adverse reactions

General

Where dose adjustment is required for moderate to severe adverse reactions (clinical and/or laboratory) initial dose reduction to 135 micrograms is generally adequate. However, in some cases, dose reduction to 90 micrograms or 45 micrograms is necessary. Dose increases to or towards the original dose may be considered when the adverse reaction abates (see section 4.4 for use and section 4.8).

Haematological (see also Table 3)

Dose reduction is recommended if the neutrophil count is < 750/mm³. For patients with Absolute Neutrophil Count (ANC) < 500/mm³ treatment should be suspended until ANC values return to > 1000/mm³. Therapy should initially be re-instituted at 90 micrograms Pegasys and the neutrophil count monitored.

Dose reduction to 90 micrograms is recommended if the platelet count is < 50,000/mm³. Cessation of therapy is recommended when platelet count decreases to levels < 25,000/mm³.

Specific recommendations for management of treatment-emergent anaemia are as follows: ribavirin should be reduced to 600 milligrams/day (200 milligrams in the morning and 400 milligrams in the evening) if either of the following apply: (1) a patient without significant cardiovascular disease experiences a fall in haemoglobin to < 10 g/dl and ≥ 8.5 g/dl, or (2) a patient with stable cardiovascular disease experiences a fall in haemoglobin by ≥ 2 g/dl during any 4 weeks of treatment. A return to original dosing is not recommended. Ribavirin should be discontinued if either of the following apply: (1) A patient without significant cardiovascular disease experiences a fall in haemoglobin confirmed to < 8.5 g/dl; (2) A patient with stable cardiovascular disease maintains a haemoglobin value < 12 g/dl despite 4 weeks on a reduced dose. If the abnormality is reversed, ribavirin may be restarted at 600 milligrams daily, and further increased to 800 milligrams daily at the discretion of the treating physician. A return to original dosing is not recommended.

(see Table 3 below)

In case of intolerance to ribavirin, Pegasys monotherapy should be continued.

Liver function

Fluctuations in abnormalities of liver function tests are common in patients with chronic hepatitis C. As with other alpha interferons, increases in ALT levels above baseline (BL) have been observed in patients treated with Pegasys, including patients with a virological response.

In chronic hepatitis C clinical trials, isolated increases in ALT (≥ 10x ULN, or ≥ 2x BL for patients with a BL ALT ≥ 10x ULN) which resolved without dose-modification were observed in 8 of 451 patients treated with combination therapy. If ALT increase is progressive or persistent, the dose should be reduced initially to 135 micrograms. When increase in ALT levels is progressive despite dose reduction, or is accompanied by increased bilirubin or evidence of hepatic decompensation, therapy should be discontinued (see section 4.4).

For chronic hepatitis B patients, transient flares of ALT levels sometimes exceeding 10 times the upper limit of normal are not uncommon, and may reflect immune clearance. Treatment should normally not be initiated if ALT is > 10 times the upper limit of normal. Consideration should be given to continuing treatment with more frequent monitoring of liver function during ALT flares. If the Pegasys dose is reduced or withheld, therapy can be restored once the flare is subsiding (see section 4.4).

Special populations

Elderly

Adjustments in the recommended dosage of 180 micrograms once weekly are not necessary when instituting Pegasys therapy in elderly patients (see section 5.2).

Children and adolescents

Only limited safety and efficacy data are available in children and adolescents (6-18 years) (see section 5.1). Pegasys is contraindicated in neonates and young children up to 3 years old because of the excipient benzyl alcohol (see sections 4.3 and 4.4).

Patients with renal impairment

In patients with end stage renal disease, a starting dose of 135 micrograms should be used (see section 5.2). Regardless of the starting dose or degree of renal impairment, patients should be monitored and appropriate dose reductions of Pegasys during the course of therapy should be made in the event of adverse reactions.

Patients with hepatic impairment

In patients with compensated cirrhosis (eg, Child-Pugh A), Pegasys has been shown to be effective and safe. Pegasys has not been evaluated in patients with decompensated cirrhosis (eg, Child-Pugh B or C or bleeding oesophageal varices) (see section 4.3).

The Child-Pugh classification divides patients into groups A, B, and C, or "Mild", "Moderate" and "Severe" corresponding to scores of 5-6, 7-9 and 10-15, respectively.

Modified Assessment

Assessment	Degree of abnormality	Score
Encephalopathy	None Grade 1-2 Grade 3-4*	1 2 3
Ascites	Absent Slight Moderate	1 2 3
S-Bilirubin (mg/dl)	<2 2.0-3 >3	1 2 3
SI unit = μmol/l)	<34 34-51 >51	1 2 3
S-Albumin (g/dl)	>3.5 3.5-2.8 <2.8	1 2 3
INR	<1.7 1.7-2.3 >2.3	1 2 3

*Grading according to Trey, Burns and Saunders (1966)

4.3 Contraindications

• Hypersensitivity to the active substance, to alpha interferons, or to any of the excipients

• Autoimmune hepatitis

• Severe hepatic dysfunction or decompensated cirrhosis of the liver

• Neonates and young children up to 3 years old, because of the excipient benzyl alcohol (see section 4.4 for benzyl alcohol)

• A history of severe pre-existing cardiac disease, including unstable or uncontrolled cardiac disease in the previous six months (see section 4.4)

• Initiation of Pegasys is contraindicated in HIV-HCV patients with cirrhosis and a Child-Pugh score ≥ 6

For contraindications to ribavirin, please refer also to the ribavirin Summary of Product Characteristics (SPC) when Pegasys is to be used in combination with ribavirin.

Table 2 Predictive Value of Week 12 Virological Response at the Recommended Dosing Regimen while on Pegasys Combination Therapy

Genotype	Negative			Positive		
	No response by week 12	No sustained response	Predictive Value	Response by week 12	Sustained response	Predictive Value
Genotype 1 (N= 569)	102	97	**95%** (97/102)	467	271	**58%** (271/467)
Genotype 2 and 3 (N=96)	3	3	**100%** (3/3)	93	81	**87%** (81/93)

Table 3 Dose Adjustment for Adverse Reaction (For further guidance see also text above)

	Reduce ribavirin to 600 mg	Withhold ribavirin	Reduce Pegasys to 135/90/45 micrograms	Withhold Pegasys	Discontinue Combination
Absolute Neutrophil Count			< 750/mm³	< 500/mm³	
Platelet Count			< 50,000/mm³ > 25,000/mm³		< 25,000/mm³
Haemoglobin - no cardiac disease	< 10 g/dl, and ≥ 8.5 g/dl	< 8.5 g/dl			
Haemoglobin - stable cardiac disease	decrease ≥ 2 g/dl during any 4 weeks	< 12 g/dl despite 4 weeks at reduced dose			

4.4 Special warnings and precautions for use

Psychiatric and Central Nervous System (CNS):
Severe CNS effects, particularly depression, suicidal ideation and attempted suicide have been observed in some patients during Pegasys therapy, and even after treatment discontinuation mainly during the 6-month follow-up period. Other CNS effects including aggressive behaviour (sometimes directed against others), bipolar disorders, mania, confusion and alterations of mental status have been observed with alpha interferons. Patients should be closely monitored for any signs or symptoms of psychiatric disorders. If such symptoms appear, the potential seriousness of these undesirable effects must be borne in mind by the prescribing physician and the need for adequate therapeutic management should be considered. If psychiatric symptoms persist or worsen, or suicidal ideation is identified, it is recommended that treatment with Pegasys be discontinued, and the patient followed, with psychiatric intervention as appropriate.

Patients with existence of, or history of severe psychiatric conditions:
If treatment with Pegasys is judged necessary in patients with existence or history of severe psychiatric conditions, this should only be initiated after having ensured appropriate individualised diagnostic and therapeutic management of the psychiatric condition.

Please refer also to the ribavirin Summary of Product Characteristics (SPC) when Pegasys is to be used in combination with ribavirin.

All patients in the chronic hepatitis C studies had a liver biopsy before inclusion, but in certain cases (ie, patients with genotype 2 or 3), treatment may be possible without histological confirmation. Current treatment guidelines should be consulted as to whether a liver biopsy is needed prior to commencing treatment.

In patients with normal ALT, progression of fibrosis occurs on average at a slower rate than in patients with elevated ALT. This should be considered in conjunction with other factors, such as HCV genotype, age, extrahepatic manifestations, risk of transmission, etc. which influence the decision to treat or not.

Excipient: Benzyl alcohol. Pegasys is contraindicated in infants or young children up to 3 years old because of the excipient benzyl alcohol.

Laboratory tests prior to and during therapy

Prior to beginning Pegasys therapy, standard haematological and biochemical laboratory tests are recommended for all patients.

The following may be considered as baseline values for initiation of treatment:

- Platelet count $\geq$ 90,000/mm^3
- Absolute neutrophil counts $\geq$ 1500/mm^3
- Adequately controlled thyroid function (TSH and T4)

Haematological tests should be repeated after 2 and 4 weeks and biochemical tests should be performed at 4 weeks. Additional testing should be performed periodically during therapy.

In clinical trials, Pegasys treatment was associated with decreases in both total white blood cell (WBC) count and absolute neutrophil count (ANC), usually starting within the first 2 weeks of treatment (see section 4.8). Progressive decreases after 8 weeks of therapy were infrequent. The decrease in ANC was reversible upon dose reduction or cessation of therapy (see section 4.2), reached normal values by 8 weeks in the majority of patients and returned to baseline in all patients after about 16 weeks.

Pegasys treatment has been associated with decreases in platelet count, which returned to pre-treatment levels during the post-treatment observation period (see section 4.8). In some cases, dose modification may be necessary (see section 4.2).

The occurrence of anaemia (haemoglobin $<$10 g/dl) has been observed in up to 15% of chronic hepatitis C patients in clinical trials on the combined treatment of Pegasys with ribavirin. The frequency depends on the treatment duration and the dose of ribavirin (see section 4.8,). The risk of developing anaemia is higher in the female population.

As with other interferons, caution should be exercised when administering Pegasys in combination with other potentially myelosuppressive agents.

The use of Pegasys and ribavirin combination therapy in chronic hepatitis C patients who failed prior treatment has not been adequately studied in patients who discontinued prior therapy for haematological adverse events. Physicians considering treatment in these patients should carefully weigh the risks versus the benefits of re-treatment.

Endocrine system

Thyroid function abnormalities or worsening of pre-existing thyroid disorders have been reported with the use of alpha interferons, including Pegasys. Prior to initiation of Pegasys therapy, TSH and T4 levels should be evaluated. Pegasys treatment may be initiated or continued if TSH levels can be maintained in the normal range by medication. TSH levels should be determined during the course of therapy if a patient develops clinical symptoms consistent with possible thyroid dysfunction (see section 4.8). As with other interferons, hypoglycaemia, hyperglycaemia and diabetes mellitus have been observed with Pegasys (see section 4.8). Patients with these conditions who cannot be effectively controlled by medication should not begin Pegasys monotherapy nor Pegasys/ribavirin combination therapy. Patients who develop these conditions during treatment and cannot be controlled with medication should discontinue Pegasys or Pegasys/ribavirin therapy.

Cardiovascular system

Hypertension, supraventricular arrhythmias, congestive heart failure, chest pain and myocardial infarction have been associated with alpha interferon therapies, including Pegasys. It is recommended that patients who have pre-existing cardiac abnormalities have an electrocardiogram prior to initiation of Pegasys therapy. If there is any deterioration of cardiovascular status, therapy should be suspended or discontinued. In patients with cardiovascular disease, anaemia may necessitate dose reduction or discontinuation of ribavirin (see section 4.2).

Liver function

In patients who develop evidence of hepatic decompensation during treatment, Pegasys should be discontinued. As with other alpha interferons, increases in ALT levels above baseline have been observed in patients treated with Pegasys, including patients with a viral response. When the increase in ALT levels is progressive and clinically significant, despite dose reduction, or is accompanied by increased direct bilirubin, therapy should be discontinued (see sections 4.2 and 4.8).

In chronic hepatitis B, unlike chronic hepatitis C, disease exacerbations during therapy are not uncommon and are characterised by transient and potentially significant increases in serum ALT. In clinical trials with Pegasys in HBV, marked transaminase flares have been accompanied by mild changes in other measures of hepatic function and without evidence of hepatic decompensation. In approximately half the cases of flares exceeding 10 times the upper limit of normal, Pegasys dosing was reduced or withheld until the transaminase elevations subsided, while in the rest therapy was continued unchanged. More frequent monitoring of hepatic function was recommended in all instances.

Hypersensitivity

Serious, acute hypersensitivity reaction (eg, urticaria, angioedema, bronchoconstriction, anaphylaxis) have been rarely observed during alpha interferon therapy. If this occurs, therapy must be discontinued and appropriate medical therapy instituted immediately. Transient rashes do not necessitate interruption of treatment.

Autoimmune disease

The development of auto-antibodies and autoimmune disorders has been reported during treatment with alpha interferons. Patients predisposed to the development of autoimmune disorders may be at increased risk. Patients with signs or symptoms compatible with autoimmune disorders should be evaluated carefully, and the benefit-risk of continued interferon therapy should be reassessed (see also *Endocrine System* in sections 4.4 and 4.8).

Cases of Vogt-Koyanagi-Harada (VKH) syndrome have been reported in patients with chronic hepatitis C treated with interferon. This syndrome is a granulomatous inflammatory disorder affecting the eyes, auditory system, meninges, and skin. If VKH syndrome is suspected, antiviral treatment should be withdrawn and corticosteroid therapy discussed (see section 4.8).

Fever/infections

While fever may be associated with the flu-like syndrome reported commonly during interferon therapy, other causes of persistent fever, particularly serious infections (bacterial, viral, fungal) must be ruled out, especially in patients with neutropenia. Serious infections (bacterial, viral, fungal) and sepsis have been reported during treatment with alpha interferons including Pegasys. Appropriate anti-infective therapy should be started immediately and discontinuation of therapy should be considered.

Ocular changes

As with other interferons retinopathy including retinal haemorrhages, cotton wool spots, papilloedema, optic neuropathy and retinal artery or vein obstruction which may result in loss of vision have been reported in rare instances with Pegasys. All patients should have a baseline eye examination. Any patient complaining of decrease or loss of vision must have a prompt and complete eye examination. Patients with preexisting ophthalmologic disorders (eg, diabetic or hypertensive retinopathy) should receive periodic ophthalmologic exams during Pegasys therapy. Pegasys treatment should be discontinued in patients who develop new or worsening ophthalmologic disorders.

Pulmonary changes

As with other alpha interferons, pulmonary symptoms, including dyspnoea, pulmonary infiltrates, pneumonia, and pneumonitis have been reported during therapy with Pegasys. In case of persistent or unexplained pulmonary infiltrates or pulmonary function impairment, treatment should be discontinued.

Skin disorder

Use of alpha interferons has been associated with exacerbation or provocation of psoriasis and sarcoidosis. Pegasys must be used with caution in patients with psoriasis, and in cases of onset or worsening of psoriatic lesions, discontinuation of therapy should be considered.

Transplantation

The safety and efficacy of Pegasys treatment have not been established in patients with liver transplantation.

HIV-HCV coinfection

Please refer to the respective Summary of Product Characteristics of the antiretroviral medicinal products that are to be taken concurrently with HCV therapy for awareness and management of toxicities specific for each product and the potential for overlapping toxicities with Pegasys with or without ribavirin. In study NR15961, patients concurrently treated with stavudine and interferon therapy with or without ribavirin, the incidence of pancreatitis and/or lactic acidosis was 3% (12/398).

Patients co-infected with HIV and receiving Highly Active Anti-Retroviral Therapy (HAART) may be at increased risk of developing lactic acidosis. Caution should therefore be exercised when adding Pegasys and ribavirin to HAART therapy (see ribavirin SPC).

Co-infected patients with advanced cirrhosis receiving HAART may also be at increased risk of hepatic decompensation and possibly death if treated with ribavirin in combination with interferons, including Pegasys. Baseline variables in co-infected cirrhotic patients that may be associated with hepatic decompensation include: increased serum bilirubin, decreased haemoglobin, increased alkaline phosphatase or decreased platelet count, and treatment with didanosine (ddI).

The concomitant use of ribavirin with zidovudine is not recommended due to an increased risk of anaemia (see section 4.5).

Co-infected patients should be closely monitored, assessing their Child-Pugh score during treatment, and should be immediately discontinued if they progress to a Child-Pugh score of 7 or greater.

In patients co-infected with HIV-HCV, limited efficacy and safety data (N = 51) are available in subjects with CD4 counts less than 200 cells/uL. Caution is therefore warranted in the treatment of patients with low CD4 counts.

Dental and periodontal disorders

Dental and periodontal disorders, which may lead to loss of teeth, have been reported in patients receiving Pegasys and ribavirin combination therapy. In addition, dry mouth could have a damaging effect on teeth and mucous membranes of the mouth during long-term treatment with the combination of Pegasys and ribavirin. Patients should brush their teeth thoroughly twice daily and have regular dental examinations. In addition some patients may experience vomiting. If this reaction occurs, they should be advised to rinse out their mouth thoroughly afterwards.

Use of peginterferon as long term maintenance monotherapy (unapproved use)

In a randomised, controlled US study (HALT-C) of HCV non-responder patients with varied degrees of fibrosis where 3.5 years of treatment with 90 micrograms/week of Pegasys monotherapy was studied, no significant reductions were observed in the rate of fibrosis progression or related clinical events.

4.5 Interaction with other medicinal products and other forms of interaction

Interaction studies have only been performed in adults.

Administration of Pegasys 180 micrograms once weekly for 4 weeks in healthy male subjects did not show any effect on mephenytoin, dapsone, debrisoquine and tolbutamide pharmacokinetics profiles, suggesting that Pegasys has no effect on in vivo metabolic activity of cytochrome P450 3A4, 2C9, 2C19 and 2D6 isozymes.

In the same study, a 25% increase in the AUC of theophylline (marker of cytochrome P450 1A2 activity) was observed, demonstrating that Pegasys is an inhibitor of cytochrome P450 1A2 activity. Serum concentrations of theophylline should be monitored and appropriate dose adjustments of theophylline made for patients taking theophylline and Pegasys concomitantly. The interaction between theophylline and Pegasys is likely to be maximal after more than 4 weeks of Pegasys therapy.

HCV monoinfected patients and HBV monoinfected patients

In a pharmacokinetic study of 24 HCV patients concomitantly receiving methadone maintenance therapy (median dose 95 mg; range 30 mg to 150 mg), treatment with Pegasys 180 micrograms sc once weekly for 4 weeks was associated with mean methadone levels that were 10% to 15% higher than at baseline. The clinical significance of this finding is unknown; nonetheless, patients should be monitored for the signs and symptoms of methadone toxicity. Especially in patients on a high dose of methadone, the risk for QTc prolongation should be considered.

Results from pharmacokinetic substudies of pivotal phase III trials demonstrated no pharmacokinetic interaction of lamivudine on Pegasys in HBV patients or between Pegasys and ribavirin in HCV patients.

A clinical trial investigating the combination of telbivudine 600 mg daily, with pegylated interferon alfa-2a, 180 micrograms once weekly by subcutaneous administration for the treatment of HBV, indicates that the combination is associated with an increased risk for developing peripheral neuropathy. The mechanism behind these events is not known; thus, co-treatment with telbivudine and other interferons (pegylated or standard) may also entail an excess risk. Moreover, the benefit of the combination of telbivudine with interferon alfa (pegylated or standard) is not currently established.

HIV-HCV co-infected patients

No apparent evidence of drug interaction was observed in 47 HIV-HCV co-infected patients who completed a 12 week pharmacokinetic substudy to examine the effect of ribavirin on the intracellular phosphorylation of some nucleoside reverse transcriptase inhibitors (lamivudine and zidovudine or stavudine). However, due to high variability, the confidence intervals were quite wide. Plasma exposure of ribavirin did not appear to be affected by concomitant administration of nucleoside reverse transcriptase inhibitors (NRTIs).

Co-administration of ribavirin and didanosine is not recommended. Exposure to didanosine or its active metabolite (dideoxyadenosine 5'-triphosphate) is increased *in vitro* when didanosine is co-administered with ribavirin. Reports of fatal hepatic failure as well as peripheral neuropathy, pancreatitis, and symptomatic hyperlactataemia/lactic acidosis have been reported with use of ribavirin.

Exacerbation of anaemia due to ribavirin has been reported when zidovudine is part of the regimen used to treat HIV although the exact mechanism remains to be elucidated. The concomitant use of ribavirin with zidovudine is not recommended due to an increased risk of anaemia (see section 4.4). Consideration should be given to replacing zidovudine in a combination ART regimen if this is already established. This would be particularly important in patients with a known history of zidovudine induced anaemia.

4.6 Pregnancy and lactation

There are no adequate data on the use of peginterferon alfa-2a in pregnant women. Studies in animals with interferon alfa-2a have shown reproductive toxicity (see section 5.3) and the potential risk for humans is unknown. Pegasys is to be used during pregnancy only if the potential benefit justifies the potential risk to the foetus.

It is not known whether the components of this medicinal product are excreted in human milk. Because of the potential for adverse reactions in nursing infants, nursing should be discontinued prior to initiation of treatment.

Use with ribavirin

Significant teratogenic and/or embryocidal effects have been demonstrated in all animal species exposed to ribavirin. Ribavirin therapy is contraindicated in women who are pregnant. Extreme care must be taken to avoid pregnancy in female patients or in partners of male patients taking Pegasys in combination with ribavirin. Female patients of childbearing potential and their partners must each use an effective contraceptive during treatment and for 4 months after treatment has been concluded. Male patients and their female partners must each use an effective contraceptive during treatment and for 7 months after treatment has been concluded. Please refer to the ribavirin SPC.

4.7 Effects on ability to drive and use machines

Pegasys has a minor or moderate influence on the ability to drive and use machines. Patients who develop dizziness, confusion, somnolence or fatigue should be cautioned to avoid driving or operating machinery.

4.8 Undesirable effects

Experience from clinical trials

Chronic hepatitis C

The frequency and severity of the most commonly reported adverse reactions with Pegasys are similar to those reported with interferon alfa-2a (see Table 4). The most frequently reported adverse reactions with Pegasys 180 micrograms were mostly mild to moderate in severity and were manageable without the need for modification of doses or discontinuation of therapy.

Chronic hepatitis B

In clinical trials of 48 week treatment and 24 weeks follow-up, the safety profile for Pegasys in chronic hepatitis B was similar to that seen in chronic hepatitis C. With the exception of pyrexia the frequency of the majority of the reported adverse reactions was notably less in CHB patients treated with Pegasys monotherapy compared with HCV patients treated with Pegasys monotherapy (see Table 4). Adverse events were experienced by 88% of Pegasys-treated patients as compared with 53% of patients in the lamivudine comparator group, while 6% of the Pegasys-treated and 4% of the lamivudine-treated patients experienced serious adverse events during the studies. Adverse events or laboratory abnormalities led to 5% of patients withdrawing from Pegasys treatment, while less than 1% of patients withdrew from lamivudine treatment for these reasons. The percentage of patients with cirrhosis who withdrew from treatment was similar to that of the overall population in each treatment group.

Chronic hepatitis C in prior non-responder patients

Overall, the safety profile for Pegasys in combination with ribavirin in prior non-responder patients was similar to that in naïve patients. In a clinical trial of non-responder patients to prior pegylated interferon alfa-2b/ribavirin, which exposed patients to either 48 or 72 weeks of treatment, the frequency of withdrawal for adverse events or laboratory abnormalities from Pegasys treatment and ribavirin treatment was 6% and 7%, respectively, in the 48 week arms and 12% and 13%, respectively, in the 72 week arms. Similarly for patients with cirrhosis or transition to cirrhosis, the frequencies of withdrawal from Pegasys treatment and ribavirin treatment were higher in the 72-week treatment arms (13% and 15%) than in the 48-week arms (6% and 6%). Patients who withdrew from previous therapy with pegylated interferon alfa-2b/ribavirin because of haematological toxicity were excluded from enrolling in this trial.

In another clinical trial, non-responder patients with advanced fibrosis or cirrhosis (Ishak score of 3 to 6) and baseline platelet counts as low as 50,000/mm^3 were treated for 48 weeks. Haematologic laboratory abnormalities observed during the first 20 weeks of the trial included anaemia (26% of patients experienced a haemoglobin level of <10 g/dL), neutropenia (30% experienced an ANC <750/mm^3), and thrombocytopenia (13% experienced a platelet count <50,000/ mm^3) (see section 4.4).

Chronic hepatitis C and HIV co-infection

In HIV-HCV co-infected patients, the clinical adverse event profiles reported for Pegasys, alone or in combination with ribavirin, were similar to those observed in HCV mono-infected patients For HIV-HCV patients receiving Pegasys and ribavirin combination therapy other undesirable effects have been reported in ≥ 1% to ≤ 2% of patients: hyperlactacidaemia/lactic acidosis, influenza, pneumonia, affect lability, apathy, tinnitus, pharyngolaryngeal pain, cheilitis, acquired lipodystrophy and chromaturia. Pegasys treatment was associated with decreases in absolute CD4+ cell counts within the first 4 weeks without a reduction in CD4+ cell percentage. The decrease in CD4+ cell counts was reversible upon dose reduction or cessation of therapy. The use of Pegasys had no observable negative impact on the control of HIV viraemia during therapy or follow-up. Limited safety data (N= 51) are available in co-infected patients with CD4+ cell counts <200/μl.

Table 4 summarises the undesirable effects reported with Pegasys monotherapy in CHB or CHC patients and with Pegasys in combination with ribavirin in CHC patients.

Table 4: Undesirable Effects Reported with Pegasys Monotherapy for HBV or HCV or In Combination with Ribavirin for HCV Patients

(see Table 4 on next page)

Post marketing adverse events

Infections and infestations:

Sepsis: frequency unknown.

As with other alpha interferons, sepsis has been reported with Pegasys.

Blood and lymphatic system disorders:

Pure red cell aplasia: frequency unknown.

As with other alpha interferons, pure red cell aplasia has been reported with Pegasys.

Immune system disorders:

A wide variety of autoimmune and immune-mediated disorders have been reported with alpha interferons including thyroid disorders, systemic lupus erythematosus, rheumatoid arthritis (new or aggravated), idiopathic and thrombotic thrombocytopenic purpura, vasculitis, neuropathies including mononeuropathies and Vogt-Koyanagi-Harada disease (see also section 4.4. Autoimmune disease).

Psychiatric disorders:

Mania, bipolar disorders: frequency unknown.

As with other alpha interferons, mania and bipolar disorders have been reported with Pegasys.

Nervous System Disorders:

Cerebral ischaemia: frequency unknown.

Eye Disorders:

Serous retinal detachment: frequency unknown.

As with other alpha interferons, serous retinal detachment has been reported with Pegasys.

Vascular disorders:

Peripheral ischaemia: frequency unknown.

As with other alpha interferons, peripheral ischaemia has been reported with Pegasys.

Gastrointestinal disorders:

Ischaemic colitis: frequency unknown.

As with other alpha interferons, ischaemic colitis has been reported with Pegasys.

Musculoskeletal connective tissue and bone disorders:

Rhabdomyolysis: frequency unknown.

Laboratory values

Pegasys treatment was associated with abnormal laboratory values: ALT increase, bilirubin increase, electrolyte disturbance (hypokalaemia, hypocalcaemia, hypophosphataemia), hyperglycaemia, hypoglycaemia and elevated triglycerides (see section 4.4.). With both Pegasys monotherapy, and also the combined treatment with ribavirin, up to 2% of patients experienced increased ALT levels that led to dose modification or discontinuation of the treatment.

Treatment with Pegasys was associated with decreases in haematological values (leucopenia, neutropenia, lymphopenia, thrombocytopenia and haemoglobin), which generally improved with dose modification, and returned to pretreatment levels within 4-8 weeks upon cessation of therapy (see sections 4.2 and 4.4).

Moderate (ANC: 0.749 - 0.5 × 10^9/l) and severe (ANC: < 0.5 × 10^9/l) neutropenia was observed respectively in 24% (216/887) and 5% (41/887) of patients receiving Pegasys 180 micrograms and ribavirin 1000/1200 milligrams for 48 weeks.

Anti-interferon antibodies

1-5% of patients treated with Pegasys developed neutralising anti-interferon antibodies. As with other interferons, a higher incidence of neutralising antibodies was seen in chronic hepatitis B. However in neither disease was this correlated with lack of therapeutic response.

Thyroid function

Pegasys treatment was associated with clinically significant abnormalities in thyroid laboratory values requiring clinical intervention (see section 4.4). The frequencies observed (4.9%) in patients receiving Pegasys/ribavirin (NV15801) are similar to those observed with other interferons.

Laboratory values for HIV-HCV co-infected patients

Although haematological toxicities of neutropenia, thrombocytopenia and anaemia occurred more frequently in HIV-HCV patients, the majority could be managed by dose modification and the use of growth factors and infrequently required premature discontinuation of treatment. Decrease in ANC levels below 500 cells/mm^3 was observed in 13% and 11% of patients receiving Pegasys monotherapy and combination therapy, respectively. Decrease in platelets below 50,000/mm^3 was observed in 10% and 8% of patients receiving Pegasys monotherapy and combination therapy, respectively. Anaemia (haemoglobin < 10g/dL) was reported in 7% and 14% of patients treated with Pegasys monotherapy or in combination therapy, respectively.

4.9 Overdose

Overdoses involving between two injections on consecutive days (instead of weekly interval) up to daily injections for 1 week (ie, 1260 micrograms/week) have been reported. None of these patients experienced unusual, serious or treatment-limiting events. Weekly doses of up to 540 and 630 micrograms have been administered in renal cell carcinoma and chronic myelogenous leukaemia clinical trials, respectively. Dose limiting toxicities were fatigue, elevated liver enzymes, neutropenia and thrombocytopenia, consistent with interferon therapy.

5. PHARMACOLOGICAL PROPERTIES

5.1 Pharmacodynamic properties

Pharmacotherapeutic group: Immunostimulating Agent/ Cytokine, ATC code: L03A B11

The conjugation of PEG reagent (bis-monomethoxypolyethylene glycol) to interferon alfa-2a forms a pegylated interferon alfa-2a (Pegasys). Pegasys possesses the *in vitro* antiviral and antiproliferative activities that are characteristic of interferon alfa-2a.

Interferon alfa-2a is conjugated with bis-[monomethoxy polyethylene glycol] at a degree of substitution of one mole of polymer/mole of protein. The average molecular mass is approximately 60,000 of which the protein moiety constitutes approximately 20,000.

HCV RNA levels decline in a biphasic manner in responding patients with hepatitis C who have received treatment with 180 micrograms Pegasys. The first phase of decline occurs 24 to 36 hours after the first dose of Pegasys is followed by and the second phase of decline which continues over the next 4 to 16 weeks in patients who achieve a sustained response. Ribavirin had no significant effect on the initial viral kinetics over the first 4 to 6 weeks in patients treated with the combination of ribavirin and pegylated interferon alfa-2a or interferon alfa.

Chronic hepatitis B:

Clinical trial results

All clinical trials recruited patients with chronic hepatitis B who had active viral replication measured by HBV DNA, elevated levels of ALT and a liver biopsy consistent with chronic hepatitis. Study WV16240 recruited patients who were positive for HBeAg, while study WV16241 recruited patients who were negative for HBeAg and positive for anti-HBe. In both studies the treatment duration was 48 weeks, with 24 weeks of treatment-free follow-up. Both studies compared Pegasys plus placebo vs Pegasys plus lamivudine vs lamivudine alone. No HBV-HIV co-infected patients were included in these clinical trials.

Response rates at the end of follow-up for the two studies are presented in Table 5. In study WV16240, the primary efficacy endpoints were HBeAg seroconversion and HBV-DNA below 10^5 copies/ml. In study WV16241, the primary efficacy endpoints were ALT normalisation and HBV-DNA below 2 × 10^4 copies/ml. HBV-DNA was measured by the COBAS AMPLICOR® HBV MONITOR Assay (limit of detection 200 copies/ml).

A total of 283/1351 (21%) of patients had advanced fibrosis or cirrhosis, 85/1351 (6%) had cirrhosis. There was no

Table 4 Undesirable Effects Reported with Pegasys Monotherapy for HBV or HCV or In Combination with Ribavirin for HCV Patients

Body system	Very Common ≥1 /10	Common ≥1 /100 to < 1 /10	Uncommon ≥1 /1000 to < 1 /100	Rare ≥1 /10,000 to < 1 /1000	Very rare <1/10,000
Infections and infestations		Upper respiratory infection, bronchitis, oral candidiasis, herpes simplex, fungal, viral and bacterial infections	Pneumonia, skin infection	Endocarditis, otitis externa	
Neoplasms benign and malignant			Hepatic neoplasm		
Blood and lymphatic system disorders		Thrombocytopenia, anaemia, lymphadenopathy		Pancytopenia	Aplastic anaemia
Immune system disorders			Sarcoidosis, thyroiditis	Anaphylaxis, systemic lupus erythematosus rheumatoid arthritis	Idiopathic or thrombotic thrombocytopenic purpura
Endocrine disorders		Hypothyroidism, hyperthyroidism	Diabetes	Diabetic ketoacidosis	
Metabolism and Nutrition Disorders	Anorexia		Dehydration		
Psychiatric disorders	Depression*, anxiety, insomnia*	Emotional disorders, mood alteration Aggression, nervousness, libido decreased	Suicidal ideation, hallucinations	Suicide, psychotic disorder	
Nervous system disorders	Headache, dizziness*, concentration impaired	Memory impairment, syncope, weakness, migraine, hypoaesthesia, hyperaesthesia, paraesthesia, tremor, taste disturbance, nightmares, somnolence	Peripheral neuropathy	Coma, convulsions, facial palsy	
Eye disorders		Vision blurred, eye pain, eye inflammation, xerophthalmia	Retinal haemorrhage	Optic neuropathy, Papilloedema, retinal vascular disorder, retinopathy, corneal ulcer	Vision loss,
Ear and labyrinth disorders		Vertigo, earache	Hearing loss		
Cardiac disorders		Tachycardia, palpitations, oedema peripheral		Myocardial infarction, congestive heart failure, angina, supraventricular tachycardia, arrhythmia, atrial fibrillation, pericarditis, cardiomyopathy	
Vascular disorders		Flushing	Hypertension	Cerebral haemorrhage, vasculitis	
Respiratory, thoracic and mediastinal disorders	Dyspnoea, cough	Dyspnoea exertional, epistaxis, nasopharyngitis, sinus congestion, nasal congestion, rhinitis, sore throat	Wheezing	Interstitial pneumonitis including fatal outcome, pulmonary embolism	
Gastrointestinal disorders	Diarrhoea*, nausea*, abdominal pain*	Vomiting, dyspepsia, dysphagia, mouth ulceration, gingival bleeding, glossitis, stomatitis, flatulence, dry mouth	Gastrointestinal bleeding	Peptic ulcer, pancreatitis	
Hepato-biliary disorders			Hepatic dysfunction	Hepatic failure, cholangitis, fatty liver	
Skin and subcutaneous tissue disorders	Alopecia, dermatitis, pruritus, dry skin	Rash, sweating increased, psoriasis, urticaria, eczema, skin disorder, photosensitivity reaction, night sweats			Toxic epidermal necrolysis, Stevens-Johnson syndrome, angioedema, erythema multiforme
Musculoskeletal connective tissue and bone disorders	Myalgia, arthralgia	Back pain, arthritis, muscle weakness, bone pain, neck pain, musculoskeletal pain, muscle cramps		Myositis	
Renal and urinary disorders				Renal insufficiency	
Reproductive system and breast disorders		Impotence			
General disorders and administration site conditions	Pyrexia, rigors*, pain*, asthenia, fatigue, injection site reaction*, irritability*	Chest pain, influenza like illness, malaise, lethargy, hot flushes, thirst			
Investigations		Weight decreased			
Injury and poisoning				Substance overdose	

*These adverse reactions were common (≥1/100 to < 1/10) in CHB patients treated with Pegasys monotherapy

difference in response rate between these patients and those without advanced fibrosis or cirrhosis.

Table 5: Serological, Virological and Biochemical Responses in Chronic Hepatitis B

(see Table 5 on next page)

Histological response was similar across the three treatment groups in each study; however, patients showing a sustained response 24 weeks after the end of treatment were significantly more likely to also show histological improvement.

All patients who completed the phase III studies were eligible for entry into a long-term follow-up study (WV16866). Among patients from study WV16240, who received Pegasys monotherapy and entered the long-term follow-up study, the rate of sustained HBeAg seroconversion 12 months after the end of therapy was 48% (73/153). In patients receiving Pegasys monotherapy in study WV16241, the rate of HBV DNA response and ALT normalisation 12 months after end of treatment were 42% (41/97) and 59% (58/99), respectively.

<u>Chronic hepatitis C</u>

Predictability of response

Please refer to section 4.2, in Table 2.

Dose-response in monotherapy

In a direct comparison with 90 micrograms, the 180 micrograms-dose was associated with superior sustained virological response in patients with cirrhosis, but in a study in non-cirrhotic patients very similar results were obtained with doses of 135 micrograms and 180 micrograms.

Confirmatory clinical trials in treatment-naïve patients

All clinical trials recruited interferon-naïve patients with chronic hepatitis C confirmed by detectable levels of serum HCV RNA, elevated levels of ALT (with the exception of study NR16071) and a liver biopsy consistent with chronic hepatitis. Study NV15495 specifically recruited patients with a histological diagnosis of cirrhosis (about 80%) or transition to cirrhosis (about 20%). Only HIV-HCV co-infected patients were included in the study NR15961 (see Table 14). These patients had stable HIV disease and mean CD4 T-cell count was about 500 cells/μL.

For HCV monoinfected patients and HIV-HCV co-infected patients, for treatment regimens, duration of therapy and study outcome see Tables 6, 7, 8 and Table 14, respectively. Virological response was defined as undetectable HCV RNA as measured by the COBAS AMPLICOR® HCV Test, version 2.0 (limit of detection 100 copies/ml equivalent to 50 International Units/ml) and sustained response as one negative sample approximately 6 months after end of therapy.

(see Table 6 on next page)

The virological responses of HCV monoinfected patients treated with Pegasys monotherapy and with Pegasys and ribavirin combination therapy in relation to genotype and pre-treatment viral load and in relation to genotype, pre-treatment viral load and rapid virological response at week 4 are summarised in Table 7 and Table 8, respectively. The results of study NV15942 provide the rationale for recommending treatment regimens based on genotype, baseline viral load and virological response at week 4 (see Tables 1, 7 and 8).

The difference between treatment regimens was in general not influenced by presence/absence of cirrhosis; therefore treatment recommendations for genotype 1, 2 or 3 are independent of this baseline characteristic.

Table 7: Sustained Virological Response Based on Genotype and Pre-treatment Viral Load after Pegasys Combination Therapy with Ribavirin in HCV Patients

(see Table 7 on next page)

The possibility to consider shortening treatment duration to 24 weeks in genotype 1 and 4 patients was examined based on a sustained rapid virological response observed in patients with rapid virological response at week 4 in studies NV15942 and ML17131 (see Table 8).

Table 8: Sustained Virological Response Based on Rapid Viral Response at week 4 for Genotype 1 and 4 after Pegasys Combination Therapy with Ribavirin in HCV Patients

(see Table 8 on page 4931765)

Although limited, data indicated that shortening treatment to 24 weeks might be associated with a higher risk of relapse (see Table 9).

Table 9: Relapse of Virological Response at the End of Treatment for Rapid Virological Response Population

(see Table 9 on page 4931765)

The possibility of shortening treatment duration to 16 weeks in genotype 2 or 3 patients was examined based on a sustained virological response observed in patients with rapid virological response by week 4 in study NV17317 (see Table 10).

In study NV17317 in patients infected with viral genotype 2 or 3, all patients received Pegasys 180 μg sc qw and a ribavirin dose of 800 mg and were randomised to treatment for either 16 or 24 weeks. Overall treatment for 16 weeks resulted in lower sustained viral response (65%) than treatment for 24 weeks (76%) ($p < 0.0001$).

The sustained viral response achieved with 16 weeks of treatment and with 24 weeks of treatment was also

Table 5 Serological, Virological and Biochemical Responses in Chronic Hepatitis B

	HBeAg positive Study WV16240			HBeAg negative / anti-HBe positive Study WV16241		
Response Parameter	**Pegasys** 180 mcg & **Placebo** (N=271)	**Pegasys** 180 mcg & **Lamivudine** 100 mg (N=271)	**Lamivudine** 100 mg (N=272)	**Pegasys** 180 mcg & **Placebo** (N=177)	**Pegasys** 180 mcg & **Lamivudine** 100 mg (N=179)	**Lamivudine** 100 mg (N=181)
HBeAg Sero-conversion	32% #	27%	19%	N/A	N/A	N/A
HBV DNA response *	32% #	34%	22%	43% #	44%	29%
ALT Normal-isation	41% #	39%	28%	59% #	60%	44%
HBsAg Sero-conversion	3% #	3%	0%	3%	2%	0%

*** For HBeAg-positive patients: HBV DNA < 10^5 copies/ml**
For HBeAg-negative /anti-HBe-positive patients: HBV DNA < 2 × 10^4 copies/ml
 # p-value (vs. lamivudine) ≤ 0.01 (stratified Cochran-Mantel-Haenszel test)

Table 6 Virological Response in HCV Patients

	Pegasys Monotherapy				Pegasys Combination Therapy		
	non-cirrhotic and cirrhotic		cirrhotic		non-cirrhotic and cirrhotic		
	Study NV15496 + NV15497 + NV15801		Study NV15495		Study NV15942	Study NV15801	
	Pegasys 180 mcg (N=701) 48 weeks	**Interferon alfa-2a** 6 MIU/3 MIU & 3 MIU (N=478) 48 weeks	**Pegasys** 180 mcg (N=87) 48 weeks	**Interferon alfa-2a** 3 MIU (N=88) 48 weeks	**Pegasys** 180 mcg & **Ribavirin** 1000/1200 mg (N=436) 48 weeks	**Pegasys** 180 mcg & **Ribavirin** 1000/1200 mg (N=453) 48 weeks	**Interferon Alfa-2b** 3 MIU & **Ribavirin** 1000/1200 mg (N=444) 48 weeks
Response at End of Treatment	55 - 69%	22 - 28%	44%	14%	68%	69%	52%
Overall Sustained Response	28 - 39%	11 - 19%	30%*	8%*	63%	54%**	45%**

*** 95% CI for difference: 11% to 33% p-value (stratified Cochran-Mantel-Haenszel test) = 0.001**
**** 95% CI for difference: 3% to 16% p-value (stratified Cochran-Mantel-Haenszel test)=0.003**

Table 7 Sustained Virological Response Based on Genotype and Pre-treatment Viral Load after Pegasys Combination Therapy with Ribavirin in HCV Patients

	Study NV15942				Study NV15801	
	Pegasys 180 mcg & **Ribavirin** 800 mg 24 weeks	**Pegasys** 180 mcg & **Ribavirin** 1000/1200 mg 24 weeks	**Pegasys** 180 mcg & **Ribavirin** 800 mg 48 weeks	**Pegasys** 180 mcg & **Ribavirin** 1000/1200 mg 48 weeks	**Pegasys** 180 mcg & **Ribavirin** 1000/1200 mg 48 weeks	**Interferon alfa-2b** 3 MIU & **Ribavirin** 1000/1200 mg 48 weeks
Genotype 1	29% (29/101)	42% (49/118)*	41% (102/250)*	**52%** (142/271)*	45% (134/298)	36% (103/285)
Low viral load	41% (21/51)	52% (37/71)	55% (33/60)	**65%** (55/85)	53% (61/115)	44% (41/94)
High viral load	16% (8/50)	26% (12/47)	36% (69/190)	**47%** (87/186)	40% (73/182)	33% (62/189)
Genotype 2/3	**84%** (81/96)	81% (117/144)	79% (78/99)	80% (123/153)	71% (100/140)	61% (88/145)
Low viral load	**85%** (29/34)	83% (39/47)	88% (29/33)	77% (37/48)	76% (28/37)	65% (34/52)
High viral load	**84%** (52/62)	80% (78/97)	74% (49/66)	82% (86/105)	70% (72/103)	58% (54/93)
Genotype 4	(0/5)	(8/12)	(5/8)	(9/11)	(10/13)	(5/11)

Low viral load= ≤ 800,000 IU/mL; High viral load= > 800,000 IU/mL

*Pegasys 180 mcg ribavirin 1000/1200 mg, 48 w *vs.* Pegasys 180 mcg ribavirin 800 mg, 48 w: Odds Ratio (95% CI) = 1.52 (1.07 to 2.17) P-value (stratified Cochran-Mantel-Haenszel test) = 0.020

*Pegasys 180 mcg ribavirin 1000/1200 mg, 48 w *vs.* Pegasys 180 mcg ribavirin 1000/1200 mg, 24 w: Odds Ratio (95% CI) = 2.12 (1.30 to 3.46) P-value (stratified Cochran-Mantel-Haenszel test) = 0.002.

examined in a retrospective subgroup analysis of patients who were HCV RNA negative by week 4 and had a LVL at baseline (see Table 10)

Table 10: Sustained Virological Response Overall and Based on Rapid Viral Response by Week 4 for Genotype 2 or 3 after Pegasys Combination Therapy with Ribavirin in HCV Patients

(see Table 10 on next page)

It is presently not clear whether a higher does of ribavirin (e.g. 1000/1200 mg/day based on body weight) results in higher SVR rates than does the 800 mg/day, when treatment is shortened to 16 weeks.

The data indicated that shortening treatment to 16 weeks is associated with a higher risk of relapse (see Table 11).

Table 11: Relapse of Virological Response after the End of Treatment in Genotype 2 or 3 Patients with a Rapid Viral Response

(see Table 11 on next page)

Superior efficacy of Pegasys compared to interferon alfa-2a was demonstrated also in terms of histological response, including patients with cirrhosis and/or HIV-HCV co-infection.

Chronic hepatitis C prior treatment non-responder patients

In study MV17150, patients who were non-responders to previous therapy with pegylated interferon alfa-2b plus ribavirin were randomised to four different treatments:

- Pegasys 360 mcg/week for 12 weeks, followed by 180 mcg/week for a further 60 weeks
- Pegasys 360 mcg/week for 12 weeks, followed by 180 mcg/week for a further 36 weeks
- Pegasys 180 mcg/week for 72 weeks
- Pegasys 180 mcg/week for 48 weeks

All patients received ribavirin (1000 or 1200 mg/day) in combination with Pegasys. All treatment arms had 24 week treatment-free follow-up.

Multiple regression and pooled group analyses evaluating the influence of treatment duration and use of induction dosing clearly identified treatment duration for 72 weeks as the primary driver for achieving a sustained virological response. Differences in sustained virological response (SVR) based on treatment duration, demographics and best responses to previous treatment are displayed in Table 12.

Table 12: Week 12 Virological Response (VR) and Sustained Virological Response (SVR) in Patients with Virological Response at Week 12 after Treatment with Pegasys and Ribavirin Combination Therapy in Non-responders to Peginterferon alfa-2b plus Ribavirin.

(see Table 12 on page 4931766)

In the HALT-C study, patients with chronic hepatitis C and advanced fibrosis or cirrhosis who were non-responders to previous treatment with interferon alfa or pegylated interferon alfa monotherapy or in combination therapy with ribavirin were treated with Pegasys 180 mcg/week and ribavirin 1000/1200 mg daily. Patients who achieved undetectable levels of HCV RNA after 20 weeks of treatment remained on Pegasys plus ribavirin combination therapy for a total of 48 weeks and were then followed for 24 weeks after the end of treatment. The probability for sustained virological response varied depending upon the previous treatment regimen; see Table 13.

Table 13 Sustained Virological Response in HALT-C by Previous Treatment

Regimen in Non-responder Population

Previous Treatment	**Pegasys** 180 mcg & **Ribavirin** 1000/1200 mg 48 weeks
Interferon	27% (70/255)
Pegylated interferon	34% (13/38)
Interferon plus ribavirin	13% (90/692)
Pegylated interferon plus ribavirin	11% (7/61)

HIV-HCV co-infected patients

The virological responses of patients treated with Pegasys monotherapy and with Pegasys and ribavirin combination therapy in relation to genotype and pre-treatment viral load for HIV-HCV co-infected patients are summarised below in Table 14.

Table 14: Sustained Virological Response based on Genotype and Pre-treatment Viral Load after Pegasys Combination Therapy with Ribavirin in HIV-HCV Co-infected Patients

(see Table 14 on page 4931766)

HCV patients with normal ALT

In study NR16071, HCV patients with normal ALT values were randomised to receive Pegasys 180 micrograms/week and ribavirin 800 milligrams/day for either 24 or 48 weeks followed by a 24 week treatment free follow-up period or no treatment for 72 weeks. The SVRs reported in the treatment arms of this study were similar to the corresponding treatment arms from study NV15942.

Children and adolescents

In the investigator sponsored CHIPS study (Chronic Hepatitis C International Paediatric Study), 65 children and adolescents (6-18 years) with chronic HCV infection were treated with PEG-IFN alfa 2a 100 mcg/m^2 sc once weekly and ribavirin 15 mg/kg/day for 24 weeks (genotypes 2 and 3) or 48 weeks (all other genotypes). Preliminary and limited safety data demonstrated no obvious departure from the known safety profile of the combination in adults with chronic HCV infection, but, importantly, the potential impact on growth has not been reported. Efficacy results were similar to those reported in adults.

5.2 Pharmacokinetic properties

Following a single subcutaneous injection of Pegasys 180 micrograms in healthy subjects, serum concentrations of peginterferon alfa-2a are measurable within 3 to 6 hours. Within 24 hours, about 80% of the peak serum concentration is reached. The absorption of Pegasys is sustained with peak serum concentrations reached 72 to 96 hours after dosing. The absolute bioavailability of Pegasys is 84% and is similar to that seen with interferon alfa-2a.

Peginterferon alfa-2a is found predominantly in the bloodstream and extracellular fluid as seen by the volume of distribution at steady-state (V_d) of 6 to 14 litres in humans after intravenous administration. From mass balance, tissue distribution and whole body autoradioluminography studies performed in rats, peginterferon alfa-2a is distributed to the liver, kidney and bone marrow in addition to being highly concentrated in the blood.

The metabolism of Pegasys is not fully characterised; however studies in rats indicate that the kidney is a major organ for excretion of radiolabelled material. In humans, the systemic clearance of peginterferon alfa-2a is about 100-fold lower than that of the native interferon alfa-2a. After intravenous administration, the terminal half-life of

Table 8 Sustained Virological Response Based on Rapid Viral Response at week 4 for Genotype 1 and 4 after Pegasys Combination Therapy with Ribavirin in HCV Patients

	Study NV15942		Study ML17131
	Pegasys 180 mcg & **Ribavirin** 1000/1200 mg 24 weeks	**Pegasys** 180 mcg & **Ribavirin** 1000/1200 mg 48 weeks	**Pegasys** 180 mcg & **Ribavirin** 1000/1200 mg 24 weeks
Genotype 1 RVR Low viral load High viral load	90% (28/31) 93% (25/27) 75% (3/4)	92% (47/51) 96% (26/27) 88% (21/24)	77% (59/77) 80% (52/65) 58% (7/12)
Genotype 1 non RVR Low viral load High viral load	24% (21/87) 27% (12/44) 21% (9/43)	43% (95/220) 50% (31/62) 41% (64/158)	- - -
Genotype 4 RVR	(5/6)	(5/5)	92% (22/24)
Genotype 4 non RVR	(3/6)	(4/6)	-

Low viral load= ⩽ 800,000 IU/mL; High viral load=> 800,000 IU/mL

RVR = rapid viral response (HCV RNA undetectable) at week 4 and HCV RNA undetectable at week 24

Table 9 Relapse of Virological Response at the End of Treatment for Rapid Virological Response Population

	Study NV15942		Study NV15801
	Pegasys 180 mcg & **Ribavirin** 1000/1200 mg 24 weeks	**Pegasys** 180 mcg & **Ribavirin** 1000/1200 mg 48 weeks	**Pegasys** 180 mcg & **Ribavirin** 1000/1200 mg 48 weeks
Genotype 1 RVR Low viral load High viral load	6.7% (2/30) 3.8% (1/26) 25% (1/4)	4.3% (2/47) 0% (0/25) 9.1% (2/22)	0% (0/24) 0% (0/17) 0% (0/7)
Genotype 4 RVR	(0/5)	(0/5)	0% (0/4)

Table 10 Sustained Virological Response Overall and Based on Rapid Viral Response by Week 4 for Genotype 2 or 3 after Pegasys Combination Therapy with Ribavirin in HCV Patients

Study NV17317				
	Pegasys 180 mcg & **Ribavirin** 800 mg 16 weeks	**Pegasys** 180 mcg & **Ribavirin** 800 mg 24 weeks	Treatment difference 95%CI	p value
Genotype 2 or 3	65% (443/679)	76% (478/630)	-10.6% [-15.5%; -0.06%]	P<0.0001
Genotype 2 or 3 RVR Low viral load High viral load	82% (378/461) 89% (147/166) 78% (231/295)	90% (370/410) 94% (141/150) 88% (229/260)	-8.2% [-12.8%; -3.7%] -5.4% [-12%; 0.9%] -9.7% [-15.9%;-3.6%]	P=0.0006 P=0.11 P=0.002

Low viral load= ⩽ 800,000 IU/mL; High viral load=> 800,000 IU/mL

RVR = rapid viral response (HCV RNA undetectable) at week 4

Table 11 Relapse of Virological Response after the End of Treatment in Genotype 2 or 3 Patients with a Rapid Viral Response

Study NV17317				
	Pegasys 180 mcg & **Ribavirin** 800 mg 16 weeks	**Pegasys** 180 mcg & **Ribavirin** 800 mg 24 weeks	Treatment difference 95%CI	p value
Genotype 2 or 3 RVR Low viral load High viral load	15% (67/439) 6% (10/155) 20% (57/284)	6% (23/386) 1% (2/141) 9% (21/245)	9.3% [5.2%; 13.6%] 5% [0.6%; 10.3%] 11.5% [5.6%; 17.4%]	P<0.0001 P=0.04 P=0.0002

Low viral load= ⩽ 800,000 IU/mL; High viral load=> 800,000 IU/mL

RVR = rapid viral response (HCV RNA undetectable) at week 4

peginterferon alfa-2a in healthy subjects is approximately 60 to 80 hours compared to values of 3-4 hours for standard interferon. The terminal half-life after subcutaneous administration in patients is longer with a mean value of 160 hours (84 to 353 hours). The terminal half-life may not only reflect the elimination phase of the compound, but may also reflect the sustained absorption of Pegasys.

Dose-proportional increases in exposure of Pegasys are seen in healthy subjects and in patients with chronic hepatitis B or C after once-weekly dosing.

In chronic hepatitis B or C patients, peginterferon alfa-2a serum concentrations accumulate 2 to 3 fold after 6 to 8 weeks of once weekly dosing compared to single dose values. There is no further accumulation after 8 weeks of once weekly dosing. The peak to trough ratio after 48 weeks of treatment is about 1.5 to 2. Peginterferon alfa-2a serum concentrations are sustained throughout one full week (168 hours).

Patients with renal impairment

Renal impairment is associated with slightly decreased CL/F and prolonged half-life. In patients (n=3) with CL_{crea} between 20 and 40 ml/min, the average CL/F is reduced by 25% compared with patients with normal renal function. In patients with end stage renal disease undergoing haemodialysis, there is a 25% to 45% reduction in the clearance, and doses of 135 micrograms result in similar exposure as 180 micrograms doses in patients with normal renal function (see section 4.2).

Please refer also to the ribavirin Summary of Product Characteristics (SPC) when Pegasys is to be used in combination with ribavirin.

Gender

The pharmacokinetics of Pegasys after single subcutaneous injections were comparable between male and female healthy subjects.

Elderly

In subjects older than 62 years, the absorption of Pegasys after a single subcutaneous injection of 180 micrograms was delayed but still sustained compared to young healthy subjects (t_{max} of 115 hours vs. 82 hours, older than 62 years vs. younger, respectively). The AUC was slightly increased (1663 vs. 1295 ng·h/ml) but peak concentrations (9.1 vs. 10.3 ng/ml) were similar in subjects older than 62 years. Based on drug exposure, pharmacodynamic response and tolerability, a lower dose of Pegasys is not needed in the geriatric patient (see section 4.2).

Hepatic impairment

The pharmacokinetics of Pegasys were similar between healthy subjects and patients with hepatitis B or C. Comparable exposure and pharmacokinetic profiles were seen in cirrhotic (Child-Pugh Grade A) and non-cirrhotic patients.

Site of administration

Subcutaneous administration of Pegasys should be limited to the abdomen and thigh, as the extent of absorption based on AUC was about 20% to 30% higher upon injection in the abdomen and thigh. Exposure to Pegasys was decreased in studies following administration of Pegasys in the arm compared to administration in the abdomen and thigh.

5.3 Preclinical safety data

The Non-clinical toxicity studies conducted with Pegasys were limited due to species specificity of interferons. Acute and chronic toxicity studies have been carried out in cynomolgus monkeys, and the findings observed in peginterferon dosed animals were similar in nature to those produced by interferon alfa-2a.

Reproductive toxicity studies have not been performed with Pegasys. As with other alpha interferons, prolongation of the menstrual cycle was observed following administration of peginterferon alfa-2a to female monkeys. Treatment with interferon alfa-2a resulted in a statistically significant increase in abortifacient activity in rhesus monkeys. Although no teratogenic effects were seen in the offspring delivered at term, adverse effects in humans cannot be excluded.

Pegasys plus ribavirin

When used in combination with ribavirin, Pegasys did not cause any effects in monkeys not previously seen with either active substance alone. The major treatment-related change was reversible mild to moderate anaemia, the severity of which was greater than that produced by either active substance alone.

6. PHARMACEUTICAL PARTICULARS

6.1 List of excipients

sodium chloride

polysorbate 80

benzyl alcohol (10 mg/ 1 ml)

sodium acetate

acetic acid

water for injections

6.2 Incompatibilities

In the absence of compatibility studies, this medicinal product must not be mixed with other medicinal products.

6.3 Shelf life

3 years

6.4 Special precautions for storage

Store in a refrigerator (2°C-8°C). Do not freeze.

Keep the pre-filled syringe in the outer carton in order to protect from light.

6.5 Nature and contents of container

0.5 ml of solution for injection in pre-filled syringe (siliconised Type I glass) with a plunger stopper and tip cap (butyl rubber laminated on the product facing side with fluororesin) with a needle. Available in packs of 1, 4 or 12. Not all pack-sizes may be marketed.

6.6 Special precautions for disposal and other handling

The solution for injection is for single use only. It should be inspected visually for particulate matter and discoloration before administration.

Any unused product or waste material should be disposed of in accordance with local requirements.

Table 12 Week 12 Virological Response (VR) and Sustained Virological Response (SVR) in Patients with Virological Response at Week 12 after Treatment with Pegasys and Ribavirin Combination Therapy in Non-responders to Peginterferon alfa-2b plus Ribavirin.

	Pegasys 360/180 or 180 µg & **Ribavirin** 1000/1200 mg 72 or 48 Weeks (N = 942) **Pts with VR at Wk 12 [a] (N = 876)**	**Pegasys** 360/180 or 180 µg & **Ribavirin** 1000/1200 mg 72 Weeks (N = 473) **SVR in Pts with VR at Wk 12 [b] (N = 100)**	**Pegasys** 360/180 or 180 µg & **Ribavirin** 1000/1200 mg 48 Weeks (N = 469) **SVR in Pts with VR at Wk 12 [b] (N = 57)**
Overall	18% (157/876)	57% (57/100)	35% (20/57)
Low viral load	35% (56/159)	63% (22/35)	38% (8/21)
High viral load	14% (97/686)	54% (34/63)	32% (11/34)
Genotype 1/4	17% (140/846)	55% (52/94)	35% (16/46)
Low viral load	35% (54/154)	63% (22/35)	37% (7/19)
High viral load	13% (84/663)	52% (30/58)	35% (9/26)
Genotype 2/3	58% (15/26)	(4/5)	(3/10)
Low viral load	(2/5)	—	(1/2)
High viral load	(11/19)	(3/4)	(1/7)
Cirrhosis Status			
Cirrhosis	8% (19/239)	(6/13)	(3/6)
Noncirrhosis	22% (137/633)	59% (51/87)	34% (17/50)
Best Response during Previous Treatment			
≥2log$_{10}$ decline in HCV RNA	28% (34/121)	68% (15/22)	(6/12)
<2log$_{10}$ decline in HCV RNA	12% (39/323)	64% (16/25)	(5/14)
Missing best previous response	19% (84/432)	49% (26/53)	29% (9/31)

High viral load =>800,000 IU/mL, low viral load = ≤ 800,000 IU/mL.

a Patients who achieved viral suppression (undetectable HCV RNA, <50 IU/mL) at week 12 were considered to have a virological response at week 12. Patients missing HCV RNA results at week 12 have been excluded from the analysis.

b Patients who achieved viral suppression at week 12 but were missing HCV RNA results at the end of follow-up were considered to be non-responders

Table 14 Sustained Virological Response based on Genotype and Pre-treatment Viral Load after Pegasys Combination Therapy with Ribavirin in HIV-HCV Co-infected Patients

Study NR15961			
	Interferon alfa-2a 3 MIU & **Ribavirin 800 mg** 48 weeks	**Pegasys** 180 mcg & **Placebo** 48 weeks	**Pegasys** 180 mcg & **Ribavirin 800 mg** 48 weeks
All patients	12% (33/285)*	20% (58/286)*	40% (116/289)*
Genotype 1	7% (12/171)	14% (24/175)	29% (51/176)
Low viral load	19% (8/42)	38% (17/45)	61% (28/46)
High viral load	3% (4/129)	5% (7/130)	18% (23/130)
Genotype 2-3	20% (18/89)	36% (32/90)	62% (59/95)
Low viral load	27% (8/30)	38% (9/24)	61% (17/28)
High viral load	17% (10/59)	35% (23/66)	63% (42/67)

Low viral load= ≤ 800,000 IU/mL; High viral load=> 800,000 IU/mL

* Pegasys 180 mcg ribavirin 800 mg vs. Interferon alfa-2a 3MIU ribavirin 800 mg: Odds Ratio (95% CI) = 5.40 (3.42 to 8.54), ...P-value (stratified Cochran-Mantel-Haenszel test) = < 0.0001

* Pegasys 180 mcg ribavirin 800 mg vs. Pegasys 180µg: Odds Ratio (95% CI) = 2.89 (1.93 to 4.32), ...P-value (stratified Cochran-Mantel-Haenszel test) = < 0.0001

* Interferon alfa-2a 3MIU ribavirin 800 mg vs. Pegasys 180 mcg: Odds Ratio (95% CI) = 0.53 (0.33 to 0.85), ...P-value (stratified Cochran-Mantel-Haenszel test) = < 0.0084

7. MARKETING AUTHORISATION HOLDER

Roche Registration Limited
6 Falcon Way
Shire Park
Welwyn Garden City
AL7 1TW
United Kingdom

8. MARKETING AUTHORISATION NUMBER(S)

EU/1/02/221/005
EU/1/02/221/006
EU/1/02/221/007
EU/1/02/221/008
EU/1/02/221/009
EU/1/02/221/010

9. DATE OF FIRST AUTHORISATION/RENEWAL OF THE AUTHORISATION

20 June 2002/ 20 June 2007

10. DATE OF REVISION OF THE TEXT

21 August 2009

LEGAL STATUS

POM

Pentacarinat 300mg

(sanofi-aventis)

1. NAME OF THE MEDICINAL PRODUCT

Pentacarinat 300mg

2. QUALITATIVE AND QUANTITATIVE COMPOSITION

in terms of the active ingredient

Pentamidine Isetionate BP 300 mg (Equivalent to 172.4 mg pentamidine base)

3. PHARMACEUTICAL FORM

Sterile powder for use after reconstitution

4. CLINICAL PARTICULARS

4.1 Therapeutic indications

Pentamidine is indicated in the treatment of:

Pneumonia due to Pneumocystis carinii (PCP)

Leishmaniasis including visceral and cutaneous

Early phase African sleeping sickness caused by Trypanosoma gambiense.

All indications can be treated by deep intramuscular injection or intravenous injection.

Pneumocystis carinii pneumonia can also be treated by the inhalation route.

Pentacarinat is also indicated in the prevention of Pneumocystis carinii pneumonia in patients infected by the human immunodeficiency virus (HIV) who have experienced a previous episode of PCP. Administration is by the inhalation route.

4.2 Posology and method of administration

Pentamidine powder is reconstituted before use with Water for Injections BP. For intravenous use the required dose of pentamidine isetionate is diluted further in 50-250ml of glucose intravenous infusion BP or 0.9% (normal) Sodium Chloride Injection BP.

The following dosage regimens are recommended for adults, children and infants.

Treatment:

Pneumocystis carinii pneumonia:

By slow iv infusion, 4 mg/kg bodyweight of pentamidine isetionate once daily for at least 14 days.

If administered by inhalation, two 300 mg vials are dissolved in 6 ml of water for injection and the resultant solution administered by a suitable nebuliser once daily for three weeks.

Leishmaniasis

Visceral: 3-4 mg/kg bodyweight of pentamidine isetionate on alternate days to a maximum of 10 injections, preferably by im injection. A repeat course may be necessary.

Cutaneous: 3-4 mg/kg bodyweight, once or twice weekly by im injection until the condition resolves.

Trypanosomiasis:

4mg/kg bodyweight of pentamidine isetionate once daily or on alternate days to a total of 7-10 injections. The im or iv infusion route may be used.

There are no specific dosage recommendations for the elderly.

In renal failure the following recommendations are made for a creatinine clearance of less than 10ml/min.:

P. carinii pneumonia: in life threatening cases, 4 mg/kg bodyweight once daily for 7 to 10 days, then 4 mg/kg bodyweight on alternate days, to complete the course of at least 14 doses. In less severe cases, 4 mg/kg bodyweight on alternate days, to complete the course of at least 14 doses.

No dosage reductions are necessary in renally impaired patients with leishmaniasis or trypanosomiasis.

Hepatic failure: no specific dosage recommendations.

Prevention

Dissolve the contents of one pentacarinat vial (300 mg pentamidine isetionate) in 4-6 ml water for injections BP.

In the prophylaxis of P. carinii pneumonia, the adult dosage is 300 mg every 4 weeks or 150mg every 2 weeks.

4.3 Contraindications

The drug should not be administered to patients with a known hypersensitivity to pentamidine.

4.4 Special warnings and precautions for use

Pentamidine isetionate should be used with particular caution in patients with hepatic and/or renal dysfunction, hypertension or hypotension, hyperglycaemia or hypoglycaemia, leucopenia, thrombocytopenia or anaemia.

Fatalities due to severe hypotension, hypoglycaemia, acute pancreatitis and cardiac arrhythmias have been reported in patients treated with pentamidine isetionate, by both the intramuscular and intravenous routes. Baseline blood pressure should be established and patients should receive the drug lying down. Blood pressure should be closely monitored during administration and at regular intervals until treatment is concluded.

Therefore patients receiving pentamidine by inhalation should be closely monitored for the development of severe adverse reactions.

Pentamidine isetionate may prolong the QT interval. Cardiac arrhythmias indicative of QT prolongation, such as Torsades de Pointes, have been reported in isolated cases with administration of pentamidine isetionate. Therefore, pentamidine isetionate should be used with care in patients with coronary heart disease, a history of ventricular arrhythmias, uncorrected hypokalaemia and or hypomagnesaemia, bradycardia (<50 bpm), or during concomitant administration of pentamidine isetionate with QT prolonging agents.

Particular caution is necessary if the QTc exceeds 500 msec whilst receiving pentamidine isetionate therapy, continuous cardiac monitoring should be considered in this case.

Should the QTc interval exceed 550 msec then an alternative regimen should be considered

Laboratory monitoring: The following tests should be carried out before, during and after therapy by the parenteral route:

I) Blood urea, nitrogen and serum creatinine daily during therapy.

II) Complete blood and platelet counts daily during therapy.

III) Fasting blood glucose measurements daily during therapy, and at regular intervals after completion of therapy. Hyperglycaemia and diabetes mellitus, with or without preceding hypoglycaemia have occurred up to several months after cessation of therapy.

IV) Liver function tests (LFTS) including bilirubin, alkaline phosphatase, aspartate aminotransferase (AST/GOT), and alkaline aminotransferase (ALT/GPT). If baseline measurements are normal and remain so during therapy, test weekly. When there is baseline elevation in LFTS and/or LFTS increase during therapy, continue monitoring weekly unless the patient is on other hepatotoxic agents, when monitoring every 3-5 days is appropriate.

V) Serum calcium, test weekly. Serum magnesium, test twice weekly.

VI) Electrocardiograms at regular intervals.

VII) Urine analysis and serum electrolytes daily during therapy.

The benefit of aerosolised pentamidine therapy in patients at high risk of a pneumothorax should be weighed against the clinical consequences of such a manifestation.

4.5 Interaction with other medicinal products and other forms of interaction

Caution is advised when pentamidine isetionate is concomitantly used with drugs that are known to prolong the QT interval such as phenothiazines, tricyclic antidepressants, terfenadine and astemizole, IV erythromycin, halofantrine and quinolone antibiotics (see Warnings section).

4.6 Pregnancy and lactation

There is no evidence of the safety of pentamidine isetionate in human pregnancy. A miscarriage within the first trimester of pregnancy has been reported following aerosolised prophylactic administration. Pentamidine isetionate should not be administered to pregnant patients unless considered essential.

Lactation: The use of pentamidine isetionate is contra-indicated in breast feeding mothers unless considered essential by the physician.

4.7 Effects on ability to drive and use machines

Pentamidine has no known effect on the ability to drive and use machines.

4.8 Undesirable effects

Pentamidine isetionate may prolong the QT interval. Isolated cases of Torsades de Pointes have been reported with the administration of pentamidine isetionate.

Parenteral Route

Severe reactions which may be life threatening include hypotension, hypoglycaemia, pancreatitis, cardiac arrythmias, leucopenia, thrombocytopenia, acute renal failure, hypocalcaemia. A possible case of Stevens-Johnson syndrome has been reported.

Less severe reactions include azotemia, abnormal liver function tests, leucopenia, anaemia, thrombocytopenia, macroscopic haematuria, hypomagnesaemia, hyperkalaemia, nausea and vomiting, hypotension, dizziness, syncope, flushing, hypoglycaemia, hyperglycaemia, rash, taste disturbances.

Rhabdomyolysis has been rarely reported following intramuscular administration of pentamidine isetionate.

Local reactions can occur ranging in severity from discomfort and pain to induration, abscess formation and muscle necrosis.

Reversible renal side effects occur with the highest frequency (over 20% of patients) with a slightly lower frequency of local reactions.

Side effects including metabolic disturbances, hepatic, haematological, or hypotensive episodes occur much less frequently (5-10% patients).

Inhalation Route:

Bronchospasm has been reported to occur following use of the nebuliser. This has been particularly noted in patients who have a history of smoking or asthma. This can usually be controlled by prior use of bronchodilators.

The occurrence of cases of pneumothorax has been reported in patients presenting a history of PCP. Although the aetiology of the pneumothorax was not linked primarily to the aerosolised administration of pentamidine in the majority of cases, a causal relationship to pentamidine cannot be ruled out.

Local reactions involving the upper respiratory tract can occur ranging in severity from cough, shortness of breath and wheezing, bronchospasms to eosinophilic pneumonia.

Other side effects reported were hypotention, hypoglycaemia, acute pancreatitis, renal insufficiency rash, fever, decrease in appetite, taste disturbances, fatigue, lightheadedness and nausea.

4.9 Overdose

Treatment is symptomatic. Cardiac rhythm disorders, including Torsades de Pointes, have been reported following overdose of pentamidine isetionate.

5. PHARMACOLOGICAL PROPERTIES

5.1 Pharmacodynamic properties

Pentamidine isetionate is an aromatic diamine. It is an antiprotozoal agent which acts by interfering with DNA and folate transformation, and by the inhibition of RNA and protein synthesis.

5.2 Pharmacokinetic properties

After intravenous infusion, plasma levels of pentamidine fall rapidly during the first two hours to one twentieth of peak levels, followed by a much slower decline thereafter. After intramuscular administration, the apparent volume of distribution of pentamidine is significantly greater (>3 times) than that observed following intravenous administration.

Elimination of half-lives after parenteral administration were estimated to be about 6 hours after intravenous infusion in patients with a normal renal function. The elimination of half-life following intramuscular injection was found to be about 9 hours.

Following parenteral administration, pentamidine appears to be widely distributed in the body and probably accumulates in tissue, particularly the liver and kidney. Only a small amount is excreted unchanged in the urine.

When administered by the use of a nebuliser, human kinetic studies revealed significant differences when compared to parenteral administration. Aerosol administration resulted in a 10-fold increase in bronchial alveolar lavage (BAL) supernatant fluid and an 80-fold increase in BAL sediment concentrations in comparison with those seen with equivalent intravenous doses.

Limited data suggests that the half-life of pentamidine in BAL fluid is greater than 10 to 14 days. Peak plasma concentrations after inhalation therapy were found to be approximately 10% of those observed with equivalent intramuscular doses and less than 5% of those observed following intravenous administration. This suggests that systemic effects by the inhalation route are less likely.

Long term pulmonary parenchymal effects of aerosolised pentamidine are not known. Lung volume and alveolar capillary diffusion, however, have not been shown to be affected by high doses of pentamidine administered by inhalation to AIDS patients.

5.3 Preclinical safety data

No additional data of relevance to the prescriber

6. PHARMACEUTICAL PARTICULARS

6.1 List of excipients

Not applicable

6.2 Incompatibilities

Pentamidine isetionate solution should not be mixed with any injection solutions other than Water for Injections BP, Glucose Intravenous Infusion BP and 0.9% (normal) Sodium Chloride Injection BP.

6.3 Shelf life

60 months when unopened. After reconstitution 24 hours.

6.4 Special precautions for storage

Store the dry product below 30°C.

Store the reconstituted product (for intravenous infusion) at 2-8°C. Use within 24 hours.

6.5 Nature and contents of container

Cardboard carton containing 5 × 10 ml glass vials each with rubber bung and aluminium ring. Each vial contains 300 mg Pentamidine Isetionate BP.

6.6 Special precautions for disposal and other handling

This product should be reconstituted in a fume cupboard. Store the dry product below 30°C. Store dilute reconstituted drug solutions between 2-8C, and discard all unused portions within 24 hours of preparation. Concentrated solutions for administration by the inhalation or intramuscular routes should be used immediately.

After reconstitution with Water for Injections BP, pentacarinat should not be mixed with any injection solutions other than Glucose Intravenous Infusion 5% BP and 0.9% (normal) Sodium Chloride Injection BP.

The optimal particle size for alveolar deposition is between 1 and 2 microns.

The freshly prepared solution should be administered by inhalation using a suitable nebuliser such as a Respirgard II (trade mark of Marquest Medical Products Inc.), Modified Acorn system 22 (trade mark of Medic-Aid) or an equivalent device with either a compressor or piped oxygen at a flow rate of 6 to 10 Litres/Minute.

The nebuliser should be used in a vacated, well ventilated room. Only staff wearing adequate protective clothing (mask, goggles, gloves) should be in the room when nebulisers are being used.

A suitable well fitted one-way system should be employed such that the nebuliser stores the aerosolised drug during exhalations and disperses exhaled pentamidine into a reservoir. A filter should be fitted to the exhaust line to reduce atmospheric pollution. It is advisable to use a suitable exhaust tube which vents directly through a window to the external atmosphere. Care should be taken to ensure that passers-by will not be exposed to the exhaust.

All bystanders including medical personnel, women of child bearing potential, pregnant women, children, and people with a history of asthma, should avoid exposure to atmospheric pentamidine resulting from nebuliser usage.

Dosage equivalence: 4 mG of pentamidine isetionate contains 2.3 mG pentamidine base; 1 mg of pentamidine base is equivalent to 1.74 mG pentamidine isetionate.

Displacement value: 300 mG of pentamidine isetionate displace approximately 0.15 ml of water.

7. MARKETING AUTHORISATION HOLDER

Sanofi-aventis
One Onslow Street
Guildford
Surrey
GU1 4YS
UK

8. MARKETING AUTHORISATION NUMBER(S)

PL 04425/0572

9. DATE OF FIRST AUTHORISATION/RENEWAL OF THE AUTHORISATION

18th September 2006

10. DATE OF REVISION OF THE TEXT

21st December 2006

Legal category

POM

Pentacarinat Ready-to-Use Solution

(sanofi-aventis)

1. NAME OF THE MEDICINAL PRODUCT

Pentacarinat Ready-to-Use solution

2. QUALITATIVE AND QUANTITATIVE COMPOSITION

In terms of the active ingredient

Pentamidine Isetionate 300mg

(Equivalent to 172.4mg Pentamidine base)

3. PHARMACEUTICAL FORM

Nebuliser Solution

4. CLINICAL PARTICULARS

4.1 Therapeutic indications

Pentacarinat Ready-to-Use Solution is indicated in the treatment of Pneumocystis carinii pneumonia (PCP) in patients infected by the human immunodeficiency virus (HIV).

Pentacarinat Ready-to-Use Solution is also indicated for the prevention of Pneumocystis carinii pneumonia in patients infected by the human immunodeficiency virus who have experienced a previous episode of PCP.

4.2 Posology and method of administration

Adults

Treatment of Pneumocystis carinii pneumonia

600mg, (two bottles) given once daily for 3 weeks, administered by a suitable nebuliser.

Prevention of Pneumocystis carinii pneumonia

300mg given once a month or 150mg given every two weeks, administered using a suitable nebuliser.

There are no specific dosage recommendations for the elderly.

Hepatic failure

No information is available.

4.3 Contraindications

The drug should not be administered to patients with a known hypersensitivity to pentamidine.

4.4 Special warnings and precautions for use

Fatalities due to severe hypotension, hypoglycaemia, acute pancreatitis and cardiac arrhythmias have been reported in patients treated with pentamidine isetionate, by both the intramuscular and intravenous routes. Therefore patients receiving pentamidine by inhalation should be closely monitored for the development of severe adverse reactions.

Pentamidine isetionate should be used with particular caution in patients with hepatic and/or renal dysfunction, hypertension, hyperglycaemia, hypoglycaemia, leucopenia, thrombocytopenia or anaemia. Bronchospasm has been reported to occur following the use of the nebuliser. This has been particularly noted in patients who have a history of smoking or asthma. This can be controlled by prior use of bronchodilators.

The benefit of aerosolised pentamidine therapy in patients at high risk of a pneumothorax should be weighed against the clinical consequences of such a manifestation.

Pentamidine isetionate may prolong the QT interval. Cardiac arrhythmias indicative of QT prolongation, such as Torsades de Pointes, have been reported in isolated cases with administration of pentamidine isetionate. Therefore, pentamidine isetionate should be used with care in patients with coronary heart disease, a history of ventricular arrhythmias, uncorrected hypokalaemia and or hypomagnesaemia, bradycardia (<50 bpm), or during concomitant administration of pentamidine isetionate with QT prolonging agents.

Particular caution is necessary if the QTc exceeds 500 msec whilst receiving pentamidine isetionate therapy, continuous cardiac monitoring should be considered in this case.

Should the QTc-interval exceed 550 msec then an alternative regimen should be considered.

4.5 Interaction with other medicinal products and other forms of interaction

Caution is advised when pentamidine isetionate is concomitantly used with drugs that are known to prolong the QT interval such as phenothiazines, tricyclic antidepressants, terfenadine and astemizole, IV erythromycin, halofantrine, and quinolene antibiotics (see Warnings section).

4.6 Pregnancy and lactation

There is no evidence on the safety of aerosolised pentamidine in human pregnancy. A miscarriage within the first trimester of pregnancy has been reported following aerosolised prophylactic administration. Pentamidine isetionate should not be administered to pregnant patients unless considered essential. The use of pentamidine isetionate is contraindicated in breast feeding mothers unless considered essential by the physician.

4.7 Effects on ability to drive and use machines

Pentamidine has no known effect on the ability to drive and use machines.

4.8 Undesirable effects

Cases of pneumothorax have been reported in patients with a history of PCP. Although the aetiology of the pneumothorax was not linked primarily to the aerosolised administration of pentamidine in the majority of cases, a causal relationship cannot be ruled out. Local reactions involving the respiratory tract can occur, ranging in severity from cough, shortness of breath and wheezing, bronchospasms to eosinophilic pneumonia. Other adverse effects reported with the use of aerosolised pentamidine are rash, hypotension, hypoglycaemia, acute pancreatitis, renal insufficiency, fever, decrease in appetite, taste disturbances, fatigue, lightheadedness and nausea.

Pentamidine isetionate may prolong the QT interval. Isolated cases of Torsades de Pointes have been reported with the administration of pentamidine isetionate.

4.9 Overdose

Should overdosage occur, treatment is symptomatic.

Cardiac rhythm disorders, including Torsades de Pointes, have been reported following overdose of pentamidine isetionate.

5. PHARMACOLOGICAL PROPERTIES

5.1 Pharmacodynamic properties

Pentamidine isetionate is an aromatic diamine. It is an antiprotozoal agent which acts by interfering with DNA and folate transformation, and by the inhibition of RNA and protein synthesis.

5.2 Pharmacokinetic properties

When administered by the use of a nebuliser, human kinetic studies revealed significant differences when compared to parenteral administration. Aerosol administration resulted in a 10-fold increase in bronchial alveolar lavage (BAL) supernatant fluid and an 80-fold increase in BAL sediment concentrations in comparison with those seen with equivalent parenteral doses.

Limited data suggests that the half life of pentamidine in BAL fluid is greater than 10-14 days.

Long term pulmonary parenchymal effects of aerosolised pentamidine are not known. Lung volume and alveolar capillary diffusion, however, have not been shown to be affected by high doses of pentamidine administered by inhalation to AIDS patients.

5.3 Preclinical safety data

No additional data of relevance to the prescriber.

6. PHARMACEUTICAL PARTICULARS

6.1 List of excipients

Glucose

Sodium acetate

Glacial acetic acid

Water for Injections

6.2 Incompatibilities

Pentamidine nebuliser solution should not be mixed with any other solution.

6.3 Shelf life

12 months.

6.4 Special precautions for storage

Store below 25°C. Do not refrigerate. See 6.6 (Instructions for Use/Handling)

6.5 Nature and contents of container

Low density polyethylene bottles and plug with yellow high density polyethylene tamper evident caps

6.6 Special precautions for disposal and other handling

Any solid material evident in the polyethylene bottle should be re-dissolved by gentle warming in the hand before use. The solution placed in the nebuliser reservoir should be visually inspected prior to use. Any solution containing particulate matter should be discarded and the nebuliser reservoir rinsed with sterile water prior to re-use.

The optimal particle size for alveolar deposition is between 1 and 2 microns.

The solution containing the required dosage should be administered by inhalation using a suitable nebuliser such as a Respirgard II (trade mark of Marquest Medical Products inc.), modified Acorn system 22 (trade mark of Medic-Aid) or an equivalent device with either a compressor or piped oxygen at a flow rate of 6 to 10 litres/minute.

The nebuliser should be used in a vacated well ventilated room. Only staff wearing adequate protective clothing (mask, goggles, gloves) should be in the room when nebulisers are being used.

A suitable well fitted one way system should be employed such that the nebuliser stores the aerosolised drug during exhalations and disperses exhaled pentamidine into a reservoir. A filter should be fitted to the exhaust line to reduce atmospheric pollution. It is advisable to use a suitable exhaust tube which vents directly through a window to the external atmosphere. Care should be taken to ensure that passers-by will not be exposed to the exhaust. All bystanders including medical personnel, women of child bearing potential, pregnant women, children and people with a history of asthma should avoid exposure to atmospheric pentamidine resulting from nebuliser usage.

Dosage equivalence: 4 mg pentamidine isetionate contain 2.3 mg pentamidine base. 1 mg pentamidine base is equivalent to 1.74 mg pentamidine isetionate.

7. MARKETING AUTHORISATION HOLDER

Sanofi-aventis

One Onslow Street

Guildford

Surrey

GU1 4YS

UK

8. MARKETING AUTHORISATION NUMBER(S)

PL 04425/0571

9. DATE OF FIRST AUTHORISATION/RENEWAL OF THE AUTHORISATION

1st September 1997

10. DATE OF REVISION OF THE TEXT

21st December 2006

Legal Category: POM

Pentagastrin Injection BP (Cambridge Laboratories)

(Cambridge Laboratories)

1. NAME OF THE MEDICINAL PRODUCT

Pentagastrin Injection BP

2. QUALITATIVE AND QUANTITATIVE COMPOSITION

Pentagastrin BP 0.025% w/v

3. PHARMACEUTICAL FORM

Solution for Injection.

4. CLINICAL PARTICULARS

4.1 Therapeutic indications

Pentagastrin Injection BP is used for the diagnostic testing of gastric secretion.

4.2 Posology and method of administration

For administration either subcutaneously or by continuous intravenous infusion.

Adults (including the elderly) and Children

The following procedure is adopted for testing gastric secretion with Pentagastrin Injection BP:

The patient receives no medication (eg. antacids, etc.) that might affect the results of the test for 24 hours and no food for 12 hours before the test. On the morning of the test a radio-opaque tube (Leven no. 7 or Ryles's 12 – 16Fr.) is passed into the patients by the way of the nose. Radiological observation is used to ensure that the tube is correctly positioned in the lower part of the body of the stomach.

The tube is securely fastened to the patient's nose and forehead with adhesive tape to ensure that it is not displaced. The patient lies on his left side.

The gastric juices are then collected by applying continuous suction (at 30-50 mm Hg below atmospheric pressure) to this tube, supplemented by manual suction. The patient takes occasional deep breaths to improve collection. The basal secretion is obtained by collecting samples at 15 minute intervals over an hour.

Pentagastrin Injection BP is then given, either at a dose of:

(a) 6 micrograms/kg bodyweight subcutaneously, or

(b) 0.6 micrograms/kg/hour as a continuous intravenous infusion. A tuberculin syringe is used to give a dose correct to 0.01 ml.

If dilution is required normal saline may be used.

Specimens of the gastric juices are again collected over periods of 10 or 15 minutes. The volume of the sample is measured and it is immediately filtered through gauze into a bottle. The acidity of each sample is determined by titration.

4.3 Contraindications

When the patient has previously shown a severe idiosyncratic response to the drug, Pentagastrin Injection BP should not be administered.

4.4 Special warnings and precautions for use

As pentagastrin stimulates gastric acid secretion it should be used with caution in patients with acute or bleeding peptic ulcer disease, though there is no clinical evidence to contraindicate use.

4.5 Interaction with other medicinal products and other forms of interaction

None known.

4.6 Pregnancy and lactation

Pregnancy: Pentagastrin Injection BP should not be administered during pregnancy.

Lactation: no special precautions are required.

4.7 Effects on ability to drive and use machines

No precautions are required.

4.8 Undesirable effects

At the recommended dosage the incidence of side effects is extremely small, although very occasionally an individual may respond with hypotension and associated dizziness and faintness. Other unwanted effects reported are mild abdominal discomfort, abdominal cramps, nausea, vomiting, flushing, sweating, headaches, drowsiness or exhaustion, heaviness or weakness of the legs, allergic reactions, bradycardia, tachycardia, anxiety and panic attacks. These effects disappear once administration of 'Pentagastrin Injection BP' has ceased.

4.9 Overdose

The form of presentation makes it unlikely that overdosage will occur, and no such occurrence has been reported. As maximal secretory response is produced by the normal dosage, increased dosage would be expected to have no sequel other than an accentuation of the known side effects.

5. PHARMACOLOGICAL PROPERTIES

5.1 Pharmacodynamic properties

Pentagastrin is a synthetic pentapeptide containing the carboxyl terminal tetrapeptide responsible for the actions of natural gastrins. The most prominent action of pentagastrin is to stimulate the secretion of gastric acid, pepsin and intrinsic factor. Additonally, it stimulates pancreatic secretion, inhibits absorption of water and electrolytes from the ileum, contracts the smooth muscle of the lower oesophageal sphincter and stomach (but delays gastric emptying time), relaxes the sphincter of Oddi and increases blood flow in the gastric mucosa.

5.2 Pharmacokinetic properties

Pentagastrin stimulates gastric acid secretion approximately ten minutes after subcutaneous injection, with peak response occurring in most cases twenty to thirty minutes after administration. Duration of activity is usually between sixty and eighty minutes.

Pentagastrin is rapidly absorbed after administration. Pentagastrin has a short half-live (10 minutes or less) in the circulation. It is metabolised primarily in the liver and excretion is mainly by the kidneys.

5.3 Preclinical safety data

Pentagastrin is a drug on which extensive clinical experience has been obtained. All relevant information for the prescriber is provided elsewhere in the Summary of Product Characteristics.

6. PHARMACEUTICAL PARTICULARS

6.1 List of excipients

Sodium chloride Ph.Eur

Water for Injections Ph.Eur

Ammonium bicarbonate BP

N. Ammonia solution } pH Adjustment

N. Hydrochloric acid }

Final Excipient Composition in Solution

Sodium chloride

Water

Ammonium chloride

6.2 Incompatibilities

None known.

6.3 Shelf life

24 months

6.4 Special precautions for storage

Store in a refrigerator. Do not freeze. Keep container in the outer carton.

6.5 Nature and contents of container

2 ml glass ampoules in boxes of 5.

6.6 Special precautions for disposal and other handling

If dilution is required Sodium Chloride Injection BP may be used. This solution should be prepared immediately before it is required for use.

Administrative Data

7. MARKETING AUTHORISATION HOLDER

Cambridge Laboratories Limited

Deltic House

Kingfisher Way

Silverlink Business Park

Wallsend

Tyne & Wear

NE28 9NX

8. MARKETING AUTHORISATION NUMBER(S)
PL 12070/0020

9. DATE OF FIRST AUTHORISATION/RENEWAL OF THE AUTHORISATION
First authorisation 9/2/73

Renewed 15/10/95

10. DATE OF REVISION OF THE TEXT
March 2005

Pentasa Mesalazine Enema

(Ferring Pharmaceuticals Ltd)

1. NAME OF THE MEDICINAL PRODUCT
PENTASA® Mesalazine Enema.

2. QUALITATIVE AND QUANTITATIVE COMPOSITION
Each enema bottle contains mesalazine 1g in 100ml.

3. PHARMACEUTICAL FORM
Rectal suspension.

Each bottle contains 100ml of a colourless to faint yellow suspension containing 1g mesalazine

4. CLINICAL PARTICULARS

4.1 Therapeutic indications
PENTASA Mesalazine Enema is indicated for the treatment of ulcerative colitis affecting the distal colon and rectum.

4.2 Posology and method of administration
Adults: The recommended dosage is one enema at bedtime.

Children: Not recommended.

PENTASA Mesalazine Enemas are for rectal administration

4.3 Contraindications
PENTASA is contraindicated in:
- patients with known sensitivity to salicylates
- patients with severe liver and/or renal impairment
- patients allergic to any of the ingredients

4.4 Special warnings and precautions for use
Serious blood dyscrasias have been reported rarely with mesalazine. Haematological investigations should be performed if the patient develops unexplained bleeding, bruising, purpura, anaemia, fever or sore throat. Treatment should be stopped if there is suspicion or evidence of blood dyscrasia.

Most patients who are intolerant or hypersensitive to sulphasalazine are able to use PENTASA without risk of similar reactions. However, caution is recommended when treating patients allergic to sulphasalazine (risk of allergy to salicylates). Caution is recommended in patients with impaired liver function.

It is recommended that mesalazine is used with extreme caution in patients with mild to moderate renal impairment (see section 4.3).

If a patient develops dehydration while on treatment with mesalazine, normal electrolyte levels and fluid balance should be restored as soon as possible.

Mesalazine induced cardiac hypersensitivity reactions (myocarditis and pericarditis) have been reported rarely. Treatment should be discontinued on suspicion or evidence of these reactions.

4.5 Interaction with other medicinal products and other forms of interaction
The concurrent use of mesalazine with other known nephrotoxic agents, such as NSAIDs and azathioprine, may increase the risk of renal reactions (see section 4.4).

Concomitant treatment with mesalazine can increase the risk of blood dyscrasia in patients receiving azathioprine or 6-mercaptopurine.

4.6 Pregnancy and lactation
PENTASA should be used with caution during pregnancy and lactation and only if the potential benefit outweighs the possible hazards in the opinion of the physician.

Mesalazine is known to cross the placental barrier, but the limited data available on its use in pregnant women do not allow assessment of possible adverse effects. No teratogenic effects have been observed in animal studies.

Blood disorders (leucopenia, thrombocytopenia, anaemia) have been reported in new-borns of mothers being treated with PENTASA.

Mesalazine is excreted in breast milk. The mesalazine concentration in breast milk is lower than in maternal blood, whereas the metabolite, acetyl mesalazine appears in similar or increased concentrations. There is limited experience of the use of oral mesalazine in lactating women. No controlled studies with PENTASA during breast-feeding have been carried out. Hypersensitivity reactions like diarrhoea in the infant cannot be excluded.

4.7 Effects on ability to drive and use machines
No adverse effects.

4.8 Undesirable effects
Mesalazine may be associated with an exacerbation of the symptoms of colitis in those patients who have previously had such problems with sulphasalazine.

Undesirable effects are as follows:

Common	*Gastrointestinal disorders:*
(≥1% and <10%)	Nausea, vomiting, diarrhoea, abdominal pain
	Skin disorders:
	Rash (including urticaria and erythematous rash)
	General:
	Headache
Rare	*Blood disorders:*
(≥0.01% and < 0.1%)	Leucopenia (including granulocytopenia), neutropenia, agranulocytosis, aplastic anaemia, thrombocytopenia
	Nervous system disorders:
	Peripheral neuropathy
	Cardiac disorders:
	Myocarditis, pericarditis
	Respiratory disorders:
	Allergic lung reactions (including dyspnoea, coughing, allergic alveolitis, pulmonary eosinophilia, pulmonary infiltration, pneumonitis)
	Gastrointestinal disorders:
	Pancreatitis, increased amylase
	Liver:
	Abnormalities of hepatic function and hepatotoxicity (including, hepatitis, cirrhosis, hepatic failure)
	Urogenital:
	Abnormal renal function (including interstitial nephritis, nephrotic syndrome), urine discolouration (*see additional text)
	Collagen disorders:
	Lupus erythematosus-like reactions
Very rare	*Blood disorders:*
(<0.01%)	Anaemia, eosinophilia (as part of an allergic reaction) and pancytopenia
	Liver:
	Increased liver enzymes and bilirubin
	Skin disorders:
	Reversible alopecia, bullous skin reactions including erythema multiforme and Stevens-Johnson syndrome
	Musculo-skeletal disorders:
	Myalgia, arthralgia
	Allergic reactions:
	Hypersensitivity reactions, drug fever

*Renal failure has been reported. Mesalazine-induced nephrotoxicity should be suspected in patients developing renal dysfunction during treatment.

The mechanism of mesalazine induced myocarditis, pericarditis, pancreatitis, nephritis and hepatitis is unknown, but it might be of allergic origin.

Following rectal administration local reactions such as pruritus, rectal discomfort and urge may occur.

4.9 Overdose
Acute experience in animals:

Single oral doses of mesalazine of up to 5g/kg in pigs or a single intravenous dose of mesalazine at 920mg/kg in rats were not lethal.

Human experience:

No cases of overdose have been reported.

Management of overdose in man:

Symptomatic treatment at hospital. Close monitoring of renal function. Intravenous infusion of electrolytes may be used to promote diuresis.

5. PHARMACOLOGICAL PROPERTIES

5.1 Pharmacodynamic properties
Pharmacotherapeutic group: Intestinal anti-inflammatory agents.

Mechanism of action and pharmacodynamic effects:

Mesalazine is recognised as the active moiety of sulphasalazine in the treatment of ulcerative colitis. It is thought to act locally on the gut wall in inflammatory bowel disease, although its precise mechanism of action has not been fully elucidated.

Increased leucocyte migration, abnormal cytokine production, increased production of arachidonic acid metabolites, particularly leukotriene B4 and increased free radical formation in the inflamed intestinal tissue are all present in patients with inflammatory bowel disease. Mesalazine has in-vitro and in-vivo pharmacological effects that inhibit leucocyte chemotaxis, decrease cytokine and leukotriene production and scavenge for free radicals. It is currently unknown which, if any of these mechanisms play a predominant role in the clinical efficacy of mesalazine.

5.2 Pharmacokinetic properties
General characteristics of the active substance

Disposition and local availability:

PENTASA enemas are designed to provide the distal part of the intestinal tract with high concentrations of mesalazine and a low systemic absorption. The enemas have been shown to reach and cover the descending colon.

Biotransformation:

Mesalazine is metabolised both pre-systemically by the intestinal mucosa and systemically in the liver to N-acetyl mesalazine (acetyl mesalazine). The acetylation seems to be independent of the acetylator phenotype of the patient. Some acetylation also occurs through the action of colonic bacteria.

Acetyl mesalazine is thought to be clinically as well as toxicologically inactive, although this remains to be confirmed.

Absorption:

The absorption following rectal administration is low, but depends on the dose, the formulation and the extent of spread. Based on urine recoveries in healthy volunteers under steady-state conditions given a daily dose of 2g (1g × 2), about 15-20% of the dose is absorbed after administration of enemas.

Distribution:

Mesalazine and acetyl mesalazine do not cross the blood brain barrier. Protein binding of mesalazine is approximately 50% and of acetyl mesalazine about 80%.

Elimination:

The plasma half-life of pure mesalazine is approximately 40 minutes and for acetyl mesalazine approximately 70 minutes. Both substances are excreted in urine and faeces. The urinary excretion consists mainly of acetyl mesalazine.

Characteristics in patients:

The systematic absorption following administration of PENTASA enemas has been shown to be significantly decreased in patients with active ulcerative colitis compared to those in remission.

In patients with impaired liver and kidney functions, the resultant decrease in the rate of elimination and increased systemic concentration of mesalazine may constitute an increased risk of nephrotoxic adverse reactions.

5.3 Preclinical safety data
There are no pre-clinical data of relevance to the prescriber which are additional to that already included in other sections of the SPC.

6. PHARMACEUTICAL PARTICULARS

6.1 List of excipients
Disodium edetate

Sodium metabisulphite

Sodium acetate

Hydrochloric acid, concentrated

Purified water

6.2 Incompatibilities
None known.

6.3 Shelf life
24 months.

6.4 Special precautions for storage
Do not store above 25°C. Keep bottle in the outer carton.

6.5 Nature and contents of container
Polyethylene enema bottles fitted with a tip and valve for rectal application, supplied in nitrogen-filled aluminium-foil bags. Presented in cartons containing 7 × 100ml bottles individually foil-wrapped.

6.6 Special precautions for disposal and other handling
None.

7. MARKETING AUTHORISATION HOLDER
Ferring Pharmaceuticals Ltd.,

The Courtyard

Waterside Drive

Langley

Berkshire SL3 6EZ.

8. MARKETING AUTHORISATION NUMBER(S)
PL 3194/0027

9. DATE OF FIRST AUTHORISATION/RENEWAL OF THE AUTHORISATION
4th February 2004

10. DATE OF REVISION OF THE TEXT
February 2005

11. LEGAL CATEGORY
POM

Pentasa Sachet 1g

(Ferring Pharmaceuticals Ltd)

1. NAME OF THE MEDICINAL PRODUCT
PENTASA Sachet 1g prolonged release granules

Table 1 Frequency of adverse effects, based on clinical trials and reports from post-marketing surveillance

System Organ Classes	Common ≥1/100 to <1/10	Rare ≥1/10,000 to <1/1,000	Very rare <1/10,000	Not Known
Blood and the lymphatic system disorders			Eosinophilia (as part of an allergic reaction) Anaemia Aplastic anaemia Leukopenia (incl. Granulocytopenia) Thrombocytopenia Agranulocytosis Pancytopenia	
Immune system disorders				Hypersensitivity reaction
Nervous system disorders	Headache		Peripheral neuropathy Benign intracranial hypertension in adolescents	
Cardiac disorders		Myocarditis* Pericarditis*		
Respiratory, thoracic and mediastinal disorders			Allergic lung reactions (incl. dyspnoea, cough, allergic alveolitis, pulmonary eosinophilia, lung infiltration, pneumonitis)	
Gastrointestinal disorders	Diarrhoea Abdominal pain Nausea Vomiting	Pancreatitis* Increased amylase (blood and/or urine)		
Hepato-biliary disorders			Increased liver enzymes and bilirubin, hepatotoxicity (incl. hepatitis*, cirrhosis, hepatic failure)	
Skin and subcutaneous tissue disorders	Rash, (incl. urticaria, erythematous rash		Reversible alopecia Quincke's oedema	
Musculoskeletal, connective tissue and bone disorders			Myalgia Arthralgia Single cases of lupus erythematosus-like reactions	
Renal and urinary disorders			Renal impairment, interstitial nephritis*, nephritic syndrome, urine discolouration	
General disorders and administration site conditions				Drug fever

(*) The mechanism of mesalazine-induced myo- and pericarditis, pancreatitis, nephritis and hepatitis in unknown, but it might be of allergic origin.

2. QUALITATIVE AND QUANTITATIVE COMPOSITION

Each sachet contains mesalazine 1 g

For a full list of excipients, see section 6.1.

3. PHARMACEUTICAL FORM

Prolonged release granules

Whitish to pale brown granules

4. CLINICAL PARTICULARS

4.1 Therapeutic indications

Mild to moderate ulcerative colitis

4.2 Posology and method of administration

Ulcerative colitis

Active disease

Individual dosage, up to 4 g mesalazine daily divided into 2-4 doses.

Maintenance treatment

Individual dosage. Recommended dosage, 2 g mesalazine once daily.

There is no dosage recommendation in children due to limited clinical data.

The granules must not be chewed.

The contents of the sachet should be emptied onto the tongue and washed down with some water or orange juice.

4.3 Contraindications

Hypersensitivity to mesalazine, any other component of the product, or salicylates.

Severe liver and/or renal impairment.

Children under 12 years of age.

4.4 Special warnings and precautions for use

Caution is recommended when treating patients allergic to sulphasalazine (risk of allergy to salicylates). In case of acute symptoms of intolerance, i.e. cramps, abdominal pain, fever, severe headache and rash, the treatment should be discontinued immediately.

Caution is recommended in patients with impaired liver or renal function and in patients with haemorrhagic diathesis. The drug is not recommended for use in patients with renal impairment. The renal function should be regularly monitored (e.g. serum creatinine), especially during the initial phase of treatment. Mesalazine induced nephrotoxicity should be suspected in patients developing renal dysfunction during treatment.

Blood tests (differential blood count; liver function parameters like ALT or AST) should be assessed prior to and during treatment, at the discretion of the treating physician.

The concurrent use of other known nephrotoxic agents, such as NSAIDs and azathioprine, may increase the risk of renal reactions (see section 4.5).

Caution is recommended in patients with active peptic ulcer.

Mesalazine-induced cardiac hypersensitivity reactions (myo- and pericarditis) have been reported rarely. Serious blood dyscrasias have been reported very rarely with mesalazine. Treatment should be discontinued on suspicion or evidence of these adverse reactions.

4.5 Interaction with other medicinal products and other forms of interaction

No specific interaction studies have been performed. Concomitant treatment with mesalazine can increase the risk of blood dyscrasia in patients receiving azathioprine or 6-mercaptopurine.

4.6 Pregnancy and lactation

PENTASA Sachet should not be used during pregnancy and lactation except when the potential benefits of the treatment outweigh the possible hazards in the opinion of the physician.

Pregnancy:

Mesalazine is known to cross the placental barrier. The limited data available on the use of this compound in pregnant women do not allow assessment of possible adverse effects. No teratogenic effects have been observed in animal studies and in a controlled human study.

Blood disorders (leucopenia, thrombocytopenia, anaemia) have been reported in new-borns of mothers being treated with PENTASA.

Lactation:

Mesalazine is excreted in breast milk. The mesalazine concentration in breast milk is lower than in maternal blood, whereas the metabolite-acetyl mesalazine-appears in similar or increased concentrations. No controlled studies with PENTASA during breast-feeding have been carried out. Only limited experience during lactation in women after oral application is available to date. Hypersensitivity reactions like diarrhoea can not be excluded.

4.7 Effects on ability to drive and use machines

None known.

4.8 Undesirable effects

The most frequent adverse reactions seen in clinical trials are diarrhoea (3%), nausea (3%), abdominal pain (3%), headache (3%), vomiting (1%) and rash (1%). Hypersensitivity reactions and drug fever may occasionally occur

Frequency of adverse effects, based on clinical trials and reports from post-marketing surveillance

(see Table 1 opposite)

It is important to note that several of these disorders can also be attributed to the inflammatory bowel disease itself.

4.9 Overdose

Experience in animals:

A single intravenous dose of mesalazine in rats of 920 mg/kg and single oral doses of mesalazine in pigs up to 5g/kg were not lethal.

Human experience:

No experience

Management of overdose in man:

Symptomatic treatment at hospital. Close monitoring of renal function.

5. PHARMACOLOGICAL PROPERTIES

5.1 Pharmacodynamic properties

Pharmacotherapeutic group: Intestinal anti-inflammatory agents

ATC-Code: A 07E C02

Mesalazine is the active component of sulphasalazine, which has been used for a long time in the treatment of ulcerative colitis and Crohn's disease.

The therapeutic value of mesalazine appears to be due to local effect on the inflamed intestinal tissue, rather than to systemic effect.

Increased leucocyte migration, abnormal cytokine production, increased production of arachidonic acid metabolites particularly leukotriene B4, and increased free radical formation in the inflamed intestinal tissue are all present in patients with inflammatory bowel disease. Mesalazine has in-vitro and in-vivo pharmacological effects that inhibit leucocyte chemotaxis, decrease cytokine and leukotriene production and scavenge for free radicals. The mechanism of action of mesalazine is, however, still not understood.

5.2 Pharmacokinetic properties

General characteristics of the active substance

PENTASA Sachet prolonged release granules consist of ethylcellulose coated microgranules of mesalazine. Following administration mesalazine is released continuously throughout the gastrointestinal tract in any enteral pH conditions. The microgranules enter the duodenum within an hour of administration, independent of food co-administration. The average small intestinal transit time is approximately 3 – 4 hrs in healthy volunteers.

Biotransformation:

Mesalazine is metabolised into N-acetyl-mesalazine (acetyl mesalazine) both pre-systematically by the intestinal mucosa and systemically in the liver. Some acetylation also occurs through the action of colonic bacteria. The acetylation seems to be independent of the acetylator phenotype of the patient. Acetyl mesalazine is believed to be clinically as well as toxicologically inactive.

Absorption:

30-50% of an oral dose is absorbed, predominantly from the small intestine. Maximum plasma concentrations are seen 1-4 hours post-dose. The plasma concentration of mesalazine decreases gradually and is no longer detectable 12 hours post-dose. The plasma concentration curve for acetyl-mesalazine follows the same pattern, but the concentration is generally higher and the elimination is slower.

The metabolic ratio of acetyl-mesalazine to mesalazine in plasma after oral administration ranges from 3.5 to 1.3 after daily doses of 500mg × 3 and 2g × 3, respectively, implying a dose-dependent acetylation which may be subject to saturation.

Mean steady-state plasma concentrations of mesalazine are approximately 2μmol/l, 8μmol/l and 12μmol/l after 1.5g, 4g and 6g daily dosages, respectively. For acetyl mesalazine the corresponding concentrations are 6μmol/1, 13μmol/1 and 16μmol/1.

The transit and release of mesalazine after oral administration are independent of food co-administration, whereas the systemic absorption will be reduced.

Distribution:

Mesalazine and acetyl-mesalazine do not cross the blood-brain barrier. Protein binding of mesalazine is approximately 50% and of acetyl-mesalazine about 80%.

Elimination:

The plasma half-life following i.v. administration of mesalazine is approximately 40 minutes and for acetyl-mesalazine approximately 70 minutes. Due to the continuous release of mesalazine throughout the gastrointestinal tract, the elimination half-life cannot be determined after oral administration. Tests have shown that steady-state is reached after a treatment period of 5 days following oral administration.

Both mesalazine and acetyl-mesalazine are excreted with the urine and faeces. The urinary excretion consists mainly of acetyl-mesalazine.

Characteristics in patients

The delivery of mesalazine to the intestinal mucosa after oral administration is only slightly affected by pathophysiologic changes such as diarrhoea and increased bowel acidity observed during active inflammatory bowel disease. A reduction in systemic absorption to 20-25% of the daily dose has been observed in patients with accelerated intestinal transit. Likewise, a corresponding increase in faecal excretion has been seen.

In patients with impaired liver and kidney functions, the resultant decrease in the rate of elimination may constitute an increased risk of nephrotoxic adverse reactions.

5.3 Preclinical safety data

Definitive nephrotoxicity and possible gastrointestinal toxicity is demonstrated in all species examined, and nephrotoxicity is evident with doses 5 – 10 times those used in humans.

In vitro test systems and in-vivo studies showed no evidence of mutagenic effects. Studies on the tumourigenic potential carried out in rats showed no evidence of any substance-related increase in the incidence of tumours.

6. PHARMACEUTICAL PARTICULARS

6.1 List of excipients

Ethylcellulose, microcrystalline cellulose

6.2 Incompatibilities

Not applicable

6.3 Shelf life

2 years

The granules should be used immediately after first opening of the sachet.

6.4 Special precautions for storage

This medicinal product does not require any special storage conditions.

6.5 Nature and contents of container

Aluminium foil single dose container

Pack sizes:

1 $\times$ 50 sachets

2 $\times$ 50 or 100 sachets

3 $\times$ 50 or 150 sachets

Not all pack sizes may be marketed

6.6 Special precautions for disposal and other handling

Any unused product or waste material should be disposed of in accordance with local requirements.

7. MARKETING AUTHORISATION HOLDER

Ferring Pharmaceuticals Ltd

The Courtyard

Waterside Drive

Langley

Berkshire SL3 6EZ.

United Kingdom

8. MARKETING AUTHORISATION NUMBER(S)

PL 03194/0075

9. DATE OF FIRST AUTHORISATION/RENEWAL OF THE AUTHORISATION

5th December 2007

10. DATE OF REVISION OF THE TEXT

December 2008.

Pentasa Sachet 2g

(Ferring Pharmaceuticals Ltd)

1. NAME OF THE MEDICINAL PRODUCT

Pentasa Sachet 2g prolonged release granules

2. QUALITATIVE AND QUANTITATIVE COMPOSITION

Each sachet contains mesalazine 2g.

For a full list of excipients, see section 6.1.

3. PHARMACEUTICAL FORM

Prolonged release granules

Whitish to pale brown granules

4. CLINICAL PARTICULARS

4.1 Therapeutic indications

Mild to moderate Ulcerative colitis

4.2 Posology and method of administration

Ulcerative colitis

Active disease

Individual dosage, up to 4 g mesalazine daily divided into 2-4 doses.

Maintenance treatment

Individual dosage. Recommended dosage, 2 g mesalazine once daily.

There is no dosage recommendation in children due to limited clinical data.

The granules must not be chewed.

The contents of the sachet should be emptied onto the tongue and washed down with some water or orange juice.

4.3 Contraindications

Hypersensitivity to mesalazine, any other component of the product, or salicylates.

Severe liver and/or renal impairment.

Children under 12 years of age.

4.4 Special warnings and precautions for use

Caution is recommended when treating patients allergic to sulphasalazine (risk of allergy to salicylates). In case of acute symptoms of intolerance, i.e. cramps, abdominal pain, fever, severe headache and rash, the treatment should be discontinued immediately.

Caution is recommended in patients with impaired liver or renal function and in patients with haemorrhagic diathesis. The drug is not recommended for use in patients with renal impairment. The renal function should be regularly monitored (e.g. serum creatinine), especially during the initial phase of treatment. Mesalazine induced nephrotoxicity should be suspected in patients developing renal dysfunction during treatment.

Blood tests (differential blood count; liver function parameters like ALT or AST) should be assessed prior to and during treatment, at the discretion of the treating physician.

The concurrent use of other known nephrotoxic agents, such as NSAIDs and azathioprine, may increase the risk of renal reactions.

Caution is recommended in patients with active peptic ulcer.

Mesalazine-induced cardiac hypersensitivity reactions (myo- and pericarditis) have been reported rarely. Serious blood dyscrasias have been reported very rarely with mesalazine (see section 4.5). Treatment should be discontinued on suspicion or evidence of these adverse reactions.

4.5 Interaction with other medicinal products and other forms of interaction

No specific interaction studies have been performed. Concomitant treatment with mesalazine can increase the risk of blood dyscrasia in patients receiving azathioprine or 6-mercaptopurine.

4.6 Pregnancy and lactation

Pentasa Sachet should not be used during pregnancy and lactation except when the potential benefits of the treatment outweigh the possible hazards in the opinion of the physician.

Pregnancy: Mesalazine is known to cross the placental barrier. The limited data available on the use of this compound in pregnant women do not allow assessment of possible adverse effects. No teratogenic effects have been observed in animal studies and in a controlled human study.

Blood disorders (leucopenia, thrombocytopenia, anaemia) have been reported in new-borns of mothers being treated with Pentasa Sachet.

Lactation: Mesalazine is excreted into breast milk. The mesalazine concentration in breast milk is lower than that in maternal blood, whereas the metabolite - acetyl-mesalazine - appears in similar or increased concentrations. No controlled studies have been carried out with Pentasa Sachet during breast-feeding. To date, only limited experience is available for oral use in women during lactation. Hypersensitivity reactions like diarrhoea can not be excluded.

4.7 Effects on ability to drive and use machines

None known.

4.8 Undesirable effects

The most frequent adverse reactions seen in clinical trials are diarrhoea (3%), nausea (3%), abdominal pain (3%), headache (3%), vomiting (1%) and rash (1%). Hypersensitivity reactions and drug fever may occasionally occur

Frequency of adverse effects, based on clinical trials and reports from post-marketing surveillance

(see Table 1 on next page)

It is important to note that several of these disorders can also be attributed to the inflammatory bowel disease itself.

4.9 Overdose

Experience in animals: A single intravenous dose of mesalazine in rats of 920 mg/kg and single oral doses of mesalazine in pigs up to 5g/kg were not lethal.

Human experience: No experience.

Management of overdose in man: Symptomatic treatment at hospital. Close monitoring of renal function.

5. PHARMACOLOGICAL PROPERTIES

5.1 Pharmacodynamic properties

Pharmacotherapeutic group: Intestinal anti-inflammatory agents

ATC code: A07E C02

Mesalazine is the active component of sulfasalazine, which has been used for a long time in the treatment of ulcerative colitis and Crohn's disease.

The therapeutic value of mesalazine appears to be due to local effect on the inflamed intestinal tissue, rather than to systemic effect.

Increased leukocyte migration, abnormal cytokine production, increased production of arachidonic acid metabolites, particularly leukotriene B4, and increased free radical formation in the inflamed intestinal tissue are all present in patients with inflammatory bowel disease. Mesalazine has *in vitro* and *in vivo* pharmacological effects that inhibit leukocyte chemotaxis, decrease cytokine and leukotriene production and scavenge for free radicals. The mechanism of action of mesalazine is, however, still not understood.

5.2 Pharmacokinetic properties

General Characteristics of the Active Substance

Pentasa Sachet prolonged release granules consist of ethylcellulose coated microgranules of mesalazine. Following administration mesalazine is released continuously throughout the gastroentestinal tract in any enteral pH conditions. The microgranules enter the duodenum within an hour of administration, independent of food co-administration. The average small intestinal transit time is approximately 3-4 hours in healthy volunteers.

Biotransformation: Mesalazine is metabolised into N-acetyl-mesalazine (acetyl-mesalazine) both pre-systemically by the intestinal mucosa and systemically in the liver. Some acetylation also occurs through the action of colonic bacteria. The acetylation seems to be independent of the acetylator phenotype of the patient.

Acetyl-mesalazine is believed to be clinically as well as toxicologically inactive.

Absorption: 30-50% of an oral dose is absorbed, predominantly from the small intestine. Maximum plasma concentrations are seen 1-4 hours post-dose. The plasma concentration of mesalazine decreases gradually and is no longer detectable 12 hours post-dose. The plasma concentration curve for acetyl-mesalazine follows the same pattern, but the concentration is generally higher and the elimination is slower.

The metabolic ratio of acetyl-mesalazine to mesalazine in plasma after oral administration ranges from 3.5 to 1.3 after daily doses of 500mg $\times$ 3 and 2g $\times$ 3, respectively, implying a dose-dependent acetylation which may be subject to saturation.

Mean steady-state plasma concentrations of mesalazine are approximately 2 μmol/l, 8μmol/l and 12μmol/l after 1.5g, 4g and 6g daily dosages, respectively. For acetyl-mesalazine the corresponding concentrations are 6 μmol/l, 13μmol/l and 16μmol/l.

The transit and release of mesalazine after oral administration are independent of food co-administration, whereas the systemic absorption will be reduced.

Distribution: Mesalazine and acetyl-mesalazine do not cross the blood-brain barrier. Protein binding of mesalazine is approximately 50% and of acetyl-mesalazine about 80%.

Elimination: The plasma half-life following i.v. administration of mesalazine is approximately 40 minutes and for acetyl-mesalazine approximately 70 minutes. Due to the continuous release of mesalazine throughout the gastrointestinal tract, the elimination half-life cannot be determined after oral administration. Tests have shown that steady-state is reached after a treatment period of 5 days following oral administration.

Both mesalazine and acetyl-mesalazine are excreted with the urine and faeces. The urinary excretion consists mainly of acetyl-mesalazine.

Characteristics in Patients

The delivery of mesalazine to the intestinal mucosa after oral administration is only slightly affected by pathophysiologic changes such as diarrhoea and increased bowel acidity observed during active inflammatory bowel disease. A reduction in systemic absorption to 20-25% of the daily dose has been observed in patients with accelerated intestinal transit. Likewise, a corresponding increase in faecal excretion has been seen.

In patients with impaired liver and kidney functions, the resultant decrease in the rate of elimination may constitute an increased risk of nephrotoxic adverse reactions.

5.3 Preclinical safety data

Definitive nephrotoxicity and possible gastrointestinal toxicity is demonstrated in all species examined, and nephrotoxicity is evident with doses 5 – 10 times those used in humans.

In vitro test systems and *in vivo* studies showed no evidence of mutagenic effects. Studies on the tumourigenic potential carried out in rats showed no evidence of any substance-related increase in the incidence of tumours.

Table 1 Frequency of adverse effects, based on clinical trials and reports from post-marketing surveillance

System Organ Classes	Common ≥1/100 to <1/10	Rare ≥1/10,000 to <1/1,000	Very rare <1/10,000	Not Known
Blood and the lymphatic system disorders			Eosinophilia (as part of an allergic reaction) Anaemia Aplastic anaemia Leukopenia (incl. Granulocytopenia) Thrombocytopenia Agranulocytosis Pancytopenia	
Immune system disorders				Hypersensitivity reaction
Nervous system disorders	Headache		Peripheral neuropathy Benign intracranial hypertension in adolescents	
Cardiac disorders		Myocarditis* Pericarditis*		
Respiratory, thoracic and mediastinal disorders			Allergic lung reactions (incl. dyspnoea, cough, allergic alveolitis, pulmonary eosinophilia, lung infiltration, pneumonitis)	
Gastrointestinal disorders	Diarrhoea Abdominal pain Nausea Vomiting	Pancreatitis* Increased amylase (blood and/or urine)		
Hepato-biliary disorders			Increased liver enzymes and bilirubin, hepatotoxicity (incl. hepatitis*, cirrhosis, hepatic failure)	
Skin and subcutaneous tissue disorders	Rash, (incl. urticaria, erythematous rash		Reversible alopecia Quincke's oedema	
Musculoskeletal, connective tissue and bone disorders			Myalgia Arthralgia Single cases of lupus erythematosus-like reactions	
Renal and urinary disorders			Renal impairment, interstitial nephritis*, nephritic syndrome, urine discolouration	
General disorders and administration site conditions				Drug fever

(*) The mechanism of mesalazine-induced myo- and pericarditis, pancreatitis, nephritis and hepatitis in unknown, but it might be of allergic origin.

6. PHARMACEUTICAL PARTICULARS

6.1 List of excipients

Ethylcellulose

Microcrystalline cellulose

6.2 Incompatibilities

Not applicable.

6.3 Shelf life

2 years.

The granules should be used immediately after first opening of the sachet.

6.4 Special precautions for storage

This medicinal product does not require any special conditions.

6.5 Nature and contents of container

Aluminium foil single dose container.

Pack sizes:

1 × 60 sachets

1 × 10 sachets

Not all pack sizes may be marketed.

6.6 Special precautions for disposal and other handling

Any unused product or waste material should be disposed of in accordance with local requirements.

7. MARKETING AUTHORISATION HOLDER

Ferring Pharmaceuticals Ltd

The Courtyard

Waterside Drive

Langley

Berkshire

SL3 6EZ.

United Kingdom

8. MARKETING AUTHORISATION NUMBER(S)

PL 03194/0102

9. DATE OF FIRST AUTHORISATION/RENEWAL OF THE AUTHORISATION

12th December 2007

10. DATE OF REVISION OF THE TEXT

December 2008

Pentasa Slow Release Tablets 500mg

(Ferring Pharmaceuticals Ltd)

1. NAME OF THE MEDICINAL PRODUCT

PENTASA® Slow Release Tablets 500mg

2. QUALITATIVE AND QUANTITATIVE COMPOSITION

Each tablet contains mesalazine 500mg

3. PHARMACEUTICAL FORM

Tablet

White-grey to pale-brown, specked round tablets, scored and marked 500mg on one side and 'PENTASA' on the reverse side.

4. CLINICAL PARTICULARS

4.1 Therapeutic indications

PENTASA Slow Release Tablets 500mg are indicated for the treatment of mild to moderate exacerbations of ulcerative colitis. For the maintenance of remission of ulcerative colitis.

4.2 Posology and method of administration

Ulcerative Colitis

The tablets must not be crushed or chewed. They may be swallowed whole or broken up. To facilitate swallowing they may be dispersed in 50ml of cold water. Stir and drink immediately.

Adults: Acute treatment: Individual dosage of up to 4g mesalazine daily in two or three divided doses.

Maintenance treatment: Individual dosage. Recommended starting dose is 1.5g mesalazine daily in two or three divided doses.

Children: Not recommended.

Elderly Patients: The usual adult dose applies.

Route of administration: oral.

4.3 Contraindications

PENTASA is contraindicated in:

- patients with known sensitivity to salicylates
- children under the age of 15 years
- patients with severe liver and/or renal impairment
- patients allergic to any of the ingredients

4.4 Special warnings and precautions for use

Serious blood dyscrasias have been reported rarely with mesalazine. Haematological investigations should be performed if the patient develops unexplained bleeding, bruising, purpura, anaemia, fever or sore throat. Treatment should be stopped if there is suspicion or evidence of blood dyscrasia.

Most patients who are intolerant or hypersensitive to sulphasalazine are able to take PENTASA without risk of similar reactions. However, caution is recommended when treating patients allergic to sulphasalazine (risk of allergy to salicylates). Caution is recommended in patients with impaired liver function.

It is recommended that mesalazine is used with extreme caution in patients with mild to moderate renal impairment (see section 4.3).

Patients on any oral formulation of mesalazine should have renal function monitored, with serum creatinine levels measured prior to treatment start, every 3 months for the first year, then 6 monthly for the next 4 years and annually thereafter. Treatment with mesalazine should be discontinued if renal function deteriorates.

If a patient develops dehydration while on treatment with mesalazine, normal electrolyte levels and fluid balance should be restored as soon as possible.

Mesalazine induced cardiac hypersensitivity reactions (myocarditis and pericarditis) have been reported rarely. Treatment should be discontinued on suspicion or evidence of these reactions.

4.5 Interaction with other medicinal products and other forms of interaction

The concurrent use of mesalazine with other known nephrotoxic agents, such as NSAIDs and azathioprine, may increase the risk of renal reactions (see section 4.4).

Concomitant treatment with mesalazine can increase the risk of blood dyscrasia in patients receiving azathioprine or 6-mercaptopurine.

4.6 Pregnancy and lactation

PENTASA should be used with caution during pregnancy and lactation and only if the potential benefit outweighs the possible hazards in the opinion of the physician.

Mesalazine is known to cross the placental barrier, but the limited data available on its use in pregnant women do not allow assessment of possible adverse effects. No teratogenic effects have been observed in animal studies.

Blood disorders (leucopenia, thrombocytopenia, anaemia) have been reported in new-borns of mothers being treated with PENTASA.

Mesalazine is excreted in breast milk. The mesalazine concentration in breast milk is lower than in maternal blood, whereas the metabolite, acetyl mesalazine appears in similar or increased concentrations. There is limited experience of the use of oral mesalazine in lactating women. No controlled studies with PENTASA during breast-feeding have been carried out. Hypersensitivity reactions like diarrhoea in the infant cannot be excluded.

4.7 Effects on ability to drive and use machines

No adverse effects.

4.8 Undesirable effects

Mesalazine may be associated with an exacerbation of the symptoms of colitis in those patients who have previously had such problems with sulphasalazine.

Undesirable effects are as follows:

Common (≥1% and <10%)	*Gastrointestinal disorders:* Nausea, vomiting, diarrhoea, abdominal pain *Skin disorders:* Rash (including urticaria and erythematous rash) *General:* Headache
Rare (≥0.01% and < 0.1%)	*Blood disorders:* Leucopenia (including granulocytopenia), neutropenia, agranulocytosis, aplastic anaemia, thrombocytopenia *Nervous system disorders* Peripheral neuropathy *Cardiac disorders:* Myocarditis, pericarditis *Respiratory disorders:* Allergic lung reactions (including dyspnoea, coughing, allergic alveolitis, pulmonary eosinophilia, pulmonary infiltration, pneumonitis) *Gastrointestinal disorders:* Pancreatitis, increased amylase

	Liver:
	Abnormalities of hepatic function and hepatotoxicity (including, hepatitis, cirrhosis, hepatic failure)
	Urogenital:
	Abnormal renal function (including interstitial nephritis, nephrotic syndrome), urine discolouration (*see additional text)
	Collagen disorders:
	Lupus erythematosus-like reactions
Very rare (<0.01%)	*Blood disorders:*
	Anaemia, eosinophilia (as part of an allergic reaction) and pancytopenia
	Liver:
	Increased liver enzymes and bilirubin
	Skin disorders:
	Reversible alopecia, bullous skin reactions including erythema multiforme and Stevens-Johnson syndrome
	Musculo-skeletal disorders:
	Myalgia, arthralgia
	Allergic reactions:
	Hypersensitivity reactions, drug fever

*Renal failure has been reported. Mesalazine-induced nephrotoxicity should be suspected in patients developing renal dysfunction during treatment.

The mechanism of mesalazine induced myocarditis, pericarditis, pancreatitis, nephritis and hepatitis is unknown, but it might be of allergic origin.

4.9 Overdose

Acute experience in animals:

Single oral doses of mesalazine of up to 5g/kg in pigs or a single intravenous dose of mesalazine at 920mg/kg in rats were not lethal.

Human experience:

No cases of overdose have been reported.

Management of overdose in man:

Symptomatic treatment at hospital. Close monitoring of renal function. Intravenous infusion of electrolytes may be used to promote diuresis.

5. PHARMACOLOGICAL PROPERTIES

5.1 Pharmacodynamic properties

Pharmacotherapeutic group: Intestinal anti-inflammatory agents.

Mechanism of action and pharmacodynamic effects:

Mesalazine is recognised as the active moiety of sulphasalazine in the treatment of ulcerative colitis. It is thought to act locally on the gut wall in inflammatory bowel disease, although its precise mechanism of action has not been fully elucidated.

Increased leucocyte migration, abnormal cytokine production, increased production of arachidonic acid metabolites, particularly leukotriene B4 and increased free radical formation in the inflamed intestinal tissue are all present in patients with inflammatory bowel disease. Mesalazine has in-vitro and in-vivo pharmacological effects that inhibit leucocyte chemotaxis, decrease cytokine and leukotriene production and scavenge for free radicals. It is currently unknown which, if any of these mechanisms play a predominant role in the clinical efficacy of mesalazine.

5.2 Pharmacokinetic properties

General characteristics of the active substance

Disposition and local availability:

PENTASA tablets consist of ethylcellulose-coated microgranules of mesalazine. Following administration and tablet disintegration the microgranules act as discrete slow-release formulations which allow a continuous release of drug from duodenum to rectum at all enteral pH conditions. The microgranules enter the duodenum within an hour of administration, independent of food co-administration. In healthy volunteers the average small intestinal transit time is approximately 3-4 hours.

Biotransformation:

Mesalazine is metabolised both pre-systemically by the intestinal mucosa and systemically in the liver to N-acetyl mesalazine (acetyl mesalazine). The acetylation seems to be independent of the acetylator phenotype of the patient. Some acetylation also occurs through the action of colonic bacteria.

Acetyl mesalazine is thought to be clinically as well as toxicologically inactive, although this remains to be confirmed.

Absorption:

Based on urine recovery data in healthy volunteers, 30-50% of the ingested dose is absorbed following oral administration, predominantly from the small intestine. Mesalazine is detectable in plasma approximately 15 minutes following administration. Maximum plasma concentrations are seen 1 - 4 hours post-dose. After a gradual decrease, mesalazine will no longer be detectable 12 hours post-dose. The plasma concentration curve for acetyl mesalazine follows the same pattern, but the concentrations are generally higher and the elimination is slower.

The metabolic ratio of acetyl mesalazine to mesalazine in plasma after oral administration ranges from 3.5 to 1.3 after daily doses of 500mg × 3 and 2g × 3 respectively, implying a dose-dependent acetylation which may be subject to saturation.

Mean steady-state plasma concentrations of mesalazine are approximately 2 micromoles/l, 8 micromoles/l and 12 micromoles/l after daily doses of 1.5g, 4g and 6g respectively. For acetyl mesalazine the corresponding concentrations are 6 micromoles/l, 13 micromoles/l and 16 micromoles/l respectively.

The transit and release of mesalazine after oral administration are independent of food co-administration, whereas the systemic absorption is reduced.

Distribution:

Mesalazine and acetyl mesalazine do not cross the blood-brain barrier. Protein binding of mesalazine is approximately 50% and of acetyl mesalazine about 80%.

Elimination:

The plasma half-life of pure mesalazine is approximately 40 minutes and for acetyl mesalazine approximately 70 minutes. Due to continuous release of mesalazine from PENTASA throughout the gastrointestinal tract, the elimination half-life cannot be determined after oral administration. However, steady-state is reached after a treatment period of 5 days following oral administration. Both substances are excreted in urine and faeces. The urinary excretion consists mainly of acetyl mesalazine.

Characteristics in patients:

The delivery of mesalazine to its site of action after oral administration is only slightly affected by pathophysiological changes such as diarrhoea and increased bowel activity observed during active inflammatory bowel disease. A reduction in systemic absorption to 20 – 25% of the daily dose has been observed in patients with accelerated intestinal transit. A corresponding increase in faecal excretion has been seen.

In patients with impaired liver and kidney functions, the resultant decrease in the rate of elimination and increased systemic concentration of mesalazine may constitute an increased risk of nephrotoxic adverse reactions.

5.3 Preclinical safety data

There are no pre-clinical data of relevance to the prescriber which are additional to that already included in other sections of the SPC.

6. PHARMACEUTICAL PARTICULARS

6.1 List of excipients

Povidone

Ethylcellulose

Magnesium stearate

Talc

Microcrystalline cellulose

6.2 Incompatibilities

None known

6.3 Shelf life

36 months

6.4 Special precautions for storage

Do not store above 25°C.

Store in the original package.

6.5 Nature and contents of container

Blister: Double aluminium foil. Pack size: 100 Tablets

6.6 Special precautions for disposal and other handling

None

7. MARKETING AUTHORISATION HOLDER

Ferring Pharmaceuticals Ltd.,

The Courtyard

Waterside Drive

Langley

Berkshire SL3 6EZ

8. MARKETING AUTHORISATION NUMBER(S)

PL 3194/0044

9. DATE OF FIRST AUTHORISATION/RENEWAL OF THE AUTHORISATION

30th March 2004

10. DATE OF REVISION OF THE TEXT

February 2005

11 LEGAL CATEGORY

POM

Pentasa Suppositories 1g

(Ferring Pharmaceuticals Ltd)

1. NAME OF THE MEDICINAL PRODUCT

PENTASA® Suppositories 1g

2. QUALITATIVE AND QUANTITATIVE COMPOSITION

Each suppository contains mesalazine 1g

3. PHARMACEUTICAL FORM

Suppositories

Oblong, compressed white to light tan, speckled suppositories

4. CLINICAL PARTICULARS

4.1 Therapeutic indications

PENTASA Suppositories are indicated for the treatment of ulcerative proctitis.

4.2 Posology and method of administration

Ulcerative Proctitis:

Usual adult dose: Acute treatment: 1 suppository daily for 2 to 4 weeks.

Maintenance treatment: 1 suppository daily.

Children: Not recommended.

Elderly Patients: The usual adult dose applies.

4.3 Contraindications

PENTASA is contraindicated in:

- patients with known sensitivity to salicylates
- children under the age of 15 years
- patients with severe liver and/or renal impairment
- patients allergic to any of the ingredients

4.4 Special warnings and precautions for use

Serious blood dyscrasias have been reported rarely with mesalazine. Haematological investigations should be performed if the patient develops unexplained bleeding, bruising, purpura, anaemia, fever or sore throat. Treatment should be stopped if there is suspicion or evidence of blood dyscrasia.

Most patients who are intolerant or hypersensitive to sulphasalazine are able to use PENTASA without risk of similar reactions. However, caution is recommended when treating patients allergic to sulphasalazine (risk of allergy to salicylates). Caution is recommended in patients with impaired liver function.

It is recommended that mesalazine is used with extreme caution in patients with mild to moderate renal impairment (see section 4.3).

If a patient develops dehydration while on treatment with mesalazine, normal electrolyte levels and fluid balance should be restored as soon as possible.

Mesalazine induced cardiac hypersensitivity reactions (myocarditis and pericarditis) have been reported rarely. Treatment should be discontinued on suspicion or evidence of these reactions.

4.5 Interaction with other medicinal products and other forms of interaction

The concurrent use of mesalazine with other known nephrotoxic agents, such as NSAIDs and azathioprine, may increase the risk of renal reactions (see section 4.4).

Concomitant treatment with mesalazine can increase the risk of blood dyscrasia in patients receiving azathioprine or 6-mercaptopurine.

4.6 Pregnancy and lactation

PENTASA should be used with caution during pregnancy and lactation and only if the potential benefit outweighs the possible hazards in the opinion of the physician.

Mesalazine is known to cross the placental barrier, but the limited data available on its use in pregnant women do not allow assessment of possible adverse effects. No teratogenic effects have been observed in animal studies.

Blood disorders (leucopenia, thrombocytopenia, anaemia) have been reported in new-borns of mothers being treated with PENTASA.

Mesalazine is excreted in breast milk. The mesalazine concentration in breast milk is lower than in maternal blood, whereas the metabolite, acetyl mesalazine appears in similar or increased concentrations. There is limited experience of the use of oral mesalazine in lactating women. No controlled studies with PENTASA during breast-feeding have been carried out. Hypersensitivity reactions like diarrhoea in the infant cannot be excluded.

4.7 Effects on ability to drive and use machines

No adverse effects.

4.8 Undesirable effects

Mesalazine may be associated with an exacerbation of the symptoms of colitis in those patients who have previously had such problems with sulphasalazine.

Undesirable effects are as follows:

Common (≥1% and <10%)	*Gastrointestinal disorders:*
	Nausea, vomiting, diarrhoea, abdominal pain
	Skin disorders:
	Rash (including urticaria and erythematous rash)
	General:
	Headache
Rare (≥0.01% and < 0.1%)	*Blood disorders:*
	Leucopenia (including granulocytopenia), neutropenia, agranulocytosis, aplastic anaemia, thrombocytopenia

	Nervous system disorders:	Peripheral neuropathy
	Cardiac disorders:	Myocarditis, pericarditis
	Respiratory disorders:	Allergic lung reactions (including dyspnoea, coughing, allergic alveolitis, pulmonary eosinophilia, pulmonary infiltration, pneumonitis)
	Gastrointestinal disorders:	Pancreatitis, increased amylase
	Liver:	Abnormalities of hepatic function and hepatotoxicity (including hepatitis, cirrhosis, hepatic failure)
	Urogenital:	Abnormal renal function (including interstitial nephritis, nephrotic syndrome), urine discolouration (*see additional text)
	Collagen disorders:	Lupus erythematosus-like reactions
Very rare (<0.01%)	*Blood disorders:*	Anaemia, eosinophilia (as part of an allergic reaction) and pancytopenia
	Liver:	Increased liver enzymes and bilirubin
	Skin disorders:	Reversible alopecia, bullous skin reactions including erythema multiforme and Stevens-Johnson syndrome
	Musculo-skeletal disorders:	Myalgia, arthralgia
	Allergic reactions:	Hypersensitivity reactions, drug fever

*Renal failure has been reported. Mesalazine-induced nephrotoxicity should be suspected in patients developing renal dysfunction during treatment.

The mechanism of mesalazine induced myocarditis, pericarditis, pancreatitis, nephritis and hepatitis is unknown, but it might be of allergic origin.

Following rectal administration local reactions such as pruritus, rectal discomfort and urge may occur.

4.9 Overdose

Acute experience in animals:

Single oral doses of mesalazine of up to 5g/kg in pigs or a single intravenous dose of mesalazine at 920mg/kg in rats were not lethal.

Human experience:

No cases of overdose have been reported.

Management of overdose in man:

Symptomatic treatment at hospital. Close monitoring of renal function. Intravenous infusion of electrolytes may be used to promote diuresis.

5. PHARMACOLOGICAL PROPERTIES

5.1 Pharmacodynamic properties

Pharmacotherapeutic group: Intestinal anti-inflammatory agents.

Mechanism of action and pharmacodynamic effects:

Mesalazine is recognised as the active moiety of sulphasalazine in the treatment of ulcerative colitis. It is thought to act locally on the gut wall in inflammatory bowel disease, although its precise mechanism of action has not been fully elucidated.

Increased leucocyte migration, abnormal cytokine production, increased production of arachidonic acid metabolites, particularly leukotriene B4 and increased free radical formation in the inflamed intestinal tissue are all present in patients with inflammatory bowel disease. Mesalazine has in-vitro and in-vivo pharmacological effects that inhibit leucocyte chemotaxis, decrease cytokine and leukotriene production and scavenge for free radicals. It is currently unknown which, if any of these mechanisms play a predominant role in the clinical efficacy of mesalazine.

5.2 Pharmacokinetic properties

General characteristics of the active substance:

Disposition and local availability:

PENTASA suppositories are designed to provide the distal part of the intestinal tract with high concentrations of mesalazine and a low systemic absorption. They are used to treat the rectum.

Biotransformation:

Mesalazine is metabolised both pre-systemically by the intestinal mucosa and systemically in the liver to N-acetyl mesalazine (acetyl mesalazine). The acetylation seems to be independent of the acetylator phenotype of the patient. Some acetylation also occurs through the action of colonic bacteria.

Acetyl mesalazine is thought to be clinically as well as toxicologically inactive, although this remains to be confirmed.

Absorption:

The absorption following rectal administration is low, but depends on the dose, the formulation and the extent of spread. Based on urine recoveries in healthy volunteers under steady-state conditions given a daily dose of 2g (1g × 2), approximately 10% of the dose is absorbed after administration of suppositories.

Distribution:

Mesalazine and acetyl mesalazine do not cross the blood brain barrier. Protein binding of mesalazine is approximately 50% and of acetyl mesalazine about 80%.

Elimination:

The plasma half-life of pure mesalazine is approximately 40 minutes and for acetyl mesalazine approximately 70 minutes. Both substances are excreted in urine and faeces. The urinary excretion consists mainly of acetyl mesalazine.

Characteristics in patients:

In patients with impaired liver and kidney functions, the resultant decrease in the rate of elimination and increased systemic concentration of mesalazine may constitute an increased risk of nephrotoxic adverse reactions.

5.3 Preclinical safety data

There are no pre-clinical data of relevance to the prescriber which are additional to that already included in other sections of the SPC.

6. PHARMACEUTICAL PARTICULARS

6.1 List of excipients

Povidone Ph. Eur.

Macrogol 6000 Ph. Eur.

Magnesium stearate Ph. Eur.

Talc Ph. Eur.

6.2 Incompatibilities

None known

6.3 Shelf life

36 months

6.4 Special precautions for storage

Do not store above 25°C. Store in the original package.

6.5 Nature and contents of container

Double aluminium foil blister strips of 7 suppositories each.

Pack size: 28

6.6 Special precautions for disposal and other handling

None

7. MARKETING AUTHORISATION HOLDER

Ferring Pharmaceuticals Ltd.

The Courtyard

Waterside Drive

Langley

Berkshire SL3 6EZ

8. MARKETING AUTHORISATION NUMBER(S)

PL 3194/0045

9. DATE OF FIRST AUTHORISATION/RENEWAL OF THE AUTHORISATION

5th December 2002

10. DATE OF REVISION OF THE TEXT

February 2005

11. LEGAL CATEGORY

POM

Pentostam Injection

(GlaxoSmithKline UK)

1. NAME OF THE MEDICINAL PRODUCT

Pentostam Injection.

2. QUALITATIVE AND QUANTITATIVE COMPOSITION

Sodium Stibogluconate equivalent to 100 mg pentavalent antimony in each ml.

3. PHARMACEUTICAL FORM

Injection.

4. CLINICAL PARTICULARS

4.1 Therapeutic indications

Pentostam is indicated for the following diseases:

Visceral leishmaniasis (kala azar).

Cutaneous leishmaniasis.

South American mucocutaneous leishmaniasis.

Pentostam may also be of value in the treatment of leishmaniasis recidivans and diffuse cutaneous leishmaniasis in the New World.

Note: Cutaneous and diffuse cutaneous leishmaniasis caused by *Leishmania aethiopica* infections are unresponsive to treatment with pentavalent antimony compounds, including Pentostam, at conventional dosage, but may respond slowly at higher dosage.

4.2 Posology and method of administration

Route of administration

Except where otherwise stated, all doses should be given by the intravenous or intramuscular route (see Warnings and Precautions).

Due to the presence of particulates (size range 20 to 300 microns) Pentostam solution should be drawn up through a filter immediately prior to administration. These particulates are insoluble complexes formed by an interaction between product preservative and the antioxidant in the rubber stopper. Filters of pore size 5 micron or less and membrane types polyvinylidene difluoride, polyethersulphone, polysulphone, nylon, surfactant-free cellulose acetate and mixed cellulose esters have been shown to be suitable. Where sterile filters are not available the risks and benefits of administering unfiltered Pentostam therapy should be assessed by the clinician on an individual basis.

All dosage recommendations are based on the findings of the WHO Expert Committee on leishmaniasis which met in 1984. There are no special recommendations for different age groups.

Visceral leishmaniasis: 10 to 20 mg Sb^{5+} (0.1 to 0.2 ml Pentostam)/kg bodyweight to a maximum of 850 mg (8.5 ml Pentostam) daily for a minimum period of 20 days. Patients should be examined for evidence of relapse after 2 and 6 months, and in Africa after 12 months.

Cutaneous leishmaniasis NOT caused by L. aethiopica: The dosage regimen outlined for visceral leishmaniasis is recommended. Alternatively, single, non-inflamed nodular lesions known not to be due to *L. braziliensis* may be treated with intralesional injections of 100 to 300 mg Sb^{5+} (1 to 3 ml Pentostam) repeated once or twice if necessary at intervals of 1 to 2 days. Infiltration must be thorough and produce complete blanching of the base of the lesion.

Individuals with cutaneous leishmaniasis due to *L. braziliensis* should be treated systematically for several days after the lesion is healed.

Note: After successful treatment of *L. braziliensis*, anti-leishmania antibody titres decline steadily over 4 to 24 months.

Muco-cutaneous leishmaniasis: Patients with parasitologically confirmed leishmaniasis should be treated with 20 mg Sb^{5+} (0.2 ml Pentostam)/kg bodyweight to a maximum of 850 mg (8.5 ml Pentostam) daily, continuing this dosage for several days longer than it takes to achieve parasitological and clinical cure.

In the event of relapse, a further course should be given for at least twice the previous duration.

Diffuse cutaneous leishmaniasis in the New World and leishmaniasis recidivans: Owing to the rarity of these conditions, precise data on dosage are not available. A dose of 10 to 20 mg Sb^{5+} (0.1 to 0.2 ml Pentostam)/kg bodyweight to a maximum of 850 mg (8.5 ml Pentostam) may be given daily for 2 to 3 weeks. If there is a response, then treatment should be maintained until several days after clinical cure of leishmaniasis recidivans and for several months after clinical and parasitological cure of diffuse cutaneous leishmaniasis.

Use in the elderly: There is little information on the effects of Pentostam on elderly individuals. If treatment of cutaneous leishmaniasis is necessary then local infiltration is preferred. The normal precautions should be strictly adhered to when treating older patients for visceral leishmaniasis.

4.3 Contraindications

Pentostam should not be given to any patient with significantly impaired renal function.

Pentostam should not be given to any patient who has experienced a serious adverse reaction to a previous dose.

4.4 Special warnings and precautions for use

Intravenous injection should be filtered immediately before use (see Posology and Method of Administration). Administer very slowly over 5 minutes to reduce the risk of local thrombosis. In the unlikely event of coughing, vomiting or substernal pain occurring, administration should be discontinued immediately. In such cases, extreme care should be taken if Pentostam is re-administered by this route.

Successful treatment of mucocutaneous leishmaniasis may induce severe inflammation around the lesion. In cases of pharyngeal or tracheal involvement, this may be life-threatening. Under such circumstances, corticosteroids may be used.

Very rarely, anaphylactic shock may develop during treatment for which adrenaline injection and appropriate supportive measures should be given immediately.

Prolongation of the QTc interval has been observed in some patients taking sodium stibogluconate and appears to be dose-related. There have also been reports of fatal cardiac arrhythmias in patients receiving higher dose antimonial therapy for visceral leishmaniasis. Therefore, ECG monitoring is recommended before and during therapy with sodium stibogluconate. Where ECG monitoring is not available, the risks and benefits of sodium stibogluconate therapy should be assessed on an individual basis.

If clinically significant prolongation of QTc interval occurs, sodium stibogluconate should be discontinued. Electrocardiographic changes, notably alterations in T wave amplitude may be expected in the majority of patients given sodium stibogluconate, these appear to be reversible on cessation of therapy and are not of serious significance.

Sodium stibogluconate should be used with caution in patients with cardiovascular disease, a history of ventricular arrhythmias or other risk factors known to predispose towards QT prolongation: for example, those with congenital QTc prolongation or taking concomitant drugs known to significantly prolong the QT interval (e.g. class III antiarrhythmics such as sotalol and amiodarone).

As there appears to be a dose relationship in the development of ECG abnormalities, prior exposure to antimonial therapy should be considered when assessing a patient's suitability for initiating or continuing therapy with sodium stibogluconate.

Patients who have recently received other antimonial drugs should be monitored closely for signs of antimony intoxication such as bradycardia and cardiac arrhythmias during administration of sodium stibogluconate.

Intercurrent infections, such as pneumonia, should be sought and treated concomitantly.

High concentrations of antimony are found in the livers of animals after repeated dosage with pentavalent antimony. Pentostam should therefore be used with caution in patients with hepatic disease. However, some abnormalities of liver function may be expected in cases of visceral leishmaniasis. In such patients the benefit of pentavalent antimony treatment outweighs the risk. Pentostam may induce mild elevation of hepatic enzymes in serum which later return to normal.

The Pack for this product carries the following statements:

Keep out of the reach and sight of children

Do not store above 25°C. Do not freeze.

Protect from light

Poison

In addition the 100 ml pack will have the following statement:

The contents should not be used more than 1 month after removing the first dose.

4.5 Interaction with other medicinal products and other forms of interaction
No interactions with Pentostam have been reported.

4.6 Pregnancy and lactation
Although no effects on the foetus have been reported, Pentostam should be withheld during pregnancy unless the potential benefits to the patient outweigh the possible risk to the foetus.

Children should not be breast-fed by mothers receiving Pentostam.

4.7 Effects on ability to drive and use machines
None known.

4.8 Undesirable effects
Approximately 1 to 2% of patients complain of nausea, vomiting and/or diarrhoea and a slightly higher number of abdominal pain.

Other common side-effects include anorexia, malaise, myalgia, arthralgia headache and lethargy.

ECG changes, including reduction in T-wave amplitude, T-wave inversion and QT prolongation have been observed (see Section 4.4 Special Warnings and Precautions for Use).

Transient coughing immediately following injection was reported with varying frequency during several trials.

Intravenous injection of Pentostam may cause transient pain along the course of the vein and eventually thrombosis of that vein.

Transient rises in serum lipase and amylase usually occur during treatment with sodium stibogluconate. Symptomatic pancreatitis has also been reported.

During some early trials of sodium stibogluconate, pneumonia occurred in a small number of patients treated for visceral leishmaniasis and this occasionally proved fatal. Pneumonia is a feature of the visceral leishmaniasis disease process; however, it has been associated with the toxicity profile of trivalent antimony. It is, therefore, not possible to determine whether these cases were due to the disease or to Pentostam.

Other (rarely reported) side-effects include fever, rigor, sweating, vertigo, facial flushing, worsening of lesions on the cheek, bleeding from the nose or gum, substernal pain, jaundice and rash.

Transient reductions in platelets, white blood cells and haemoglobin.

4.9 Overdose
The main symptoms of antimony overdosage are gastrointestinal disturbances (nausea, vomiting and severe diarrhoea). Haemorrhagic nephritis and hepatitis may also occur.

There is only limited information on the use of chelating agents in the treatment of intoxication with antimony compounds. Dimercaprol has been reported to be effective: a dose of 200 mg by intramuscular injection, every six hours until recovery is complete, is suggested.

2,3-dimercaptosuccinic acid (DMSA) may also be effective treatment.

5. PHARMACOLOGICAL PROPERTIES

5.1 Pharmacodynamic properties
The mode of action of Pentostam is unknown. *In vitro* exposure of amastigotes to 500 mg Sb^{5+}/ml results in a greater than 50% decrease in parasite DNA, RNA protein and purine nucleoside triphosphate levels. It has been postulated that the reduction in ATP (adenosine triphosphate) and GTP (guanosine triphosphate) synthesis contributes to decreased macromolecular synthesis.

5.2 Pharmacokinetic properties
Following intravenous or intramuscular administration of sodium stibogluconate, antimony is excreted rapidly via the kidneys, the majority of the dose being detected in the first 12-hour urine collection. This rapid excretion is reflected by a marked fall in serum or whole blood antimony levels to approximately 1 to 4% of the peak level by 8 hours after an intravenous dose. During daily administration, there is a slow accumulation of sodium stibogluconate into the central compartment so that tissue concentrations reach a theoretical maximum level after at least 7 days.

5.3 Preclinical safety data
There are no preclinical data of relevance to the prescriber which are additional to that in other sections of the SPC.

6. PHARMACEUTICAL PARTICULARS

6.1 List of excipients
Chlorocresol BP

Glucono-delta-lactone HSE

Water for Injections EP

6.2 Incompatibilities
None known.

6.3 Shelf life
36 months.

6.4 Special precautions for storage
Do not store above 25°C. Do not freeze.

Protect from light.

6.5 Nature and contents of container
Amber glass vials sealed with synthetic butyl rubber closures and aluminium collars.

Pack sizes: 6 and 100ml.

6.6 Special precautions for disposal and other handling
Pentostam solution should be filtered immediately prior to use (see Posology and Method of Administration).

7. MARKETING AUTHORISATION HOLDER
The Wellcome Foundation Ltd

Glaxo Wellcome House

Berkeley Avenue

Greenford

Middlesex

UB6 ONN

Trading as:

GlaxoSmithKline UK

Stockley Park West

Uxbridge

Middlesex UB11 1BT.

8. MARKETING AUTHORISATION NUMBER(S)
PL 0003/5105R

9. DATE OF FIRST AUTHORISATION/RENEWAL OF THE AUTHORISATION
Renewal of the Authorisation: 12/01/2007

10. DATE OF REVISION OF THE TEXT
12/01/2007

Pentrax Shampoo (Alliance Pharmaceuticals)

(Alliance Pharmaceuticals)

1. NAME OF THE MEDICINAL PRODUCT
Pentrax 4.3% w/v Shampoo

2. QUALITATIVE AND QUANTITATIVE COMPOSITION
Fractar 5 7.71%

(equivalent to coal tar 4.3% w/v)

For excipients, see Section 6.1

3. PHARMACEUTICAL FORM
Shampoo

A burgundy-brown liquid of medium viscosity and a coal-tar odour.

4. CLINICAL PARTICULARS

4.1 Therapeutic indications
For the relief of itching, irritation, redness, flaking and/or scaling due to dandruff, seborrhoeic dermatitis, or psoriasis of the scalp.

4.2 Posology and method of administration
For topical administration.

Adults:
Pentrax Shampoo should be massaged into wet hair and scalp to produce a lather. The hair should be rinsed and the procedure repeated applying a liberal amount of Pentrax and allowing the lather to remain on the hair for up to 10 minutes. Hair should be rinsed thoroughly.

Use at least twice weekly or as directed by a physician.

Children:
As for adults.

Elderly:
As for adults.

4.3 Contraindications
Pentrax Shampoo is contra-indicated in persons with a sensitivity to any of the ingredients.

4.4 Special warnings and precautions for use
Avoid contact with the eyes. If shampoo gets into the eyes rinse thoroughly with water.

If the condition worsens or does not improve after regular use of the product as directed, consult a physician.

4.5 Interaction with other medicinal products and other forms of interaction
None known.

4.6 Pregnancy and lactation
The safety of Pentrax has not been established.

4.7 Effects on ability to drive and use machines
None known.

4.8 Undesirable effects
There have been no reports of adverse effects following the use of Pentrax Shampoo. However, coal tar may cause irritation to the skin. Erythema and hypersensitivity to coal tar has been reported. Although carcinogenicity of coal tar has been demonstrated in animal studies, no studies demonstrating an increased risk to skin cancer with normal therapeutic use in humans have been reported. There is no unequivocal evidence to link the use of topically applied coal tar products, with skin cancer.

4.9 Overdose
There is no evidence of systemic absorption following the use of this shampoo. There are no reports available of its ingestion.

5. PHARMACOLOGICAL PROPERTIES

5.1 Pharmacodynamic properties
Coal tar is an antipruritic, keratolytic and a weak antiseptic.

5.2 Pharmacokinetic properties
There is no evidence of systemic absorption following the use of Pentrax Shampoo.

5.3 Preclinical safety data
Tar preparations have been in wide use for many years. Although tar preparations containing polycyclic aromatic hydrocarbons (PAHs) have been demonstrated to be carcinogenic in the skin of experimental animals, present evidence, based on epidemiology studies and follow up trials, reveals no evidence of increased risk of skin or internal cancer, particularly when the product is used as directed.

6. PHARMACEUTICAL PARTICULARS

6.1 List of excipients
Dioctyl sodium sulphosuccinate

Laureth 23

Polyethylene glycol 8

Sodium lauryl sulphate

Cocamide DEA

Lauramine oxide

6.2 Incompatibilities
None known.

6.3 Shelf life
48 months.

6.4 Special precautions for storage
Do not store above 30°C.

6.5 Nature and contents of container
Pentrax Shampoo is supplied in a polyvinylchloride bottle with a polypropylene screw cap with triseal. Each bottle contains either 30ml, 120ml or 240ml of Pentrax Shampoo.

6.6 Special precautions for disposal and other handling
No special requirements.

7. MARKETING AUTHORISATION HOLDER
Alliance Pharmaceuticals Ltd

Avonbridge House

Bath Road

Chippenham

Wiltshire

SN15 2BB

8. MARKETING AUTHORISATION NUMBER(S)
PL 16853/0075

9. DATE OF FIRST AUTHORISATION/RENEWAL OF THE AUTHORISATION
1st July 1999

10. DATE OF REVISION OF THE TEXT
December 2005

Pepcid 20 and 40 mg Tablets

(Merck Sharp & Dohme Limited)

1. NAME OF THE MEDICINAL PRODUCT
PEPCID® 20 mg Tablets

PEPCID® 40 mg Tablets

2. QUALITATIVE AND QUANTITATIVE COMPOSITION
'Pepcid' 20 mg, each tablet contains 20 mg of famotidine.

'Pepcid' 40 mg, each tablet contains 40 mg of famotidine.

3. PHARMACEUTICAL FORM
Film-coated tablets.

Beige, round-cornered square tablets, marked 'MSD 963' on one side and plain on the other.

Brown, round-cornered square tablets, marked 'MSD 964' on one side and plain on the other.

4. CLINICAL PARTICULARS

4.1 Therapeutic indications
Duodenal ulcer.

Prevention of relapses of duodenal ulceration.

Benign gastric ulcer.

Hypersecretory conditions such as Zollinger-Ellison syndrome.

Treatment of gastro-oesophageal reflux disease.

Prevention of relapse of symptoms and erosions or ulcerations associated with gastro-oesophageal reflux disease.

4.2 Posology and method of administration
In benign gastric and duodenal ulceration, the dose of 'Pepcid' is one 40 mg tablet at night.

Duodenal ulcer

The recommended initial dose is one 40 mg tablet of 'Pepcid' at night. Treatment should continue for four to eight weeks. In most patients, healing occurs on this regimen within four weeks. In those patients whose ulcers have not healed completely after four weeks, a further four-week period of treatment is recommended.

Maintenance therapy: For preventing the recurrence of duodenal ulceration, the reduced dose of 20 mg of 'Pepcid' at night is recommended.

Benign gastric ulcer

The recommended dose is one 40 mg tablet of 'Pepcid' at night. Treatment should continue for four to eight weeks unless endoscopy reveals earlier healing.

Zollinger-Ellison syndrome

Patients without prior antisecretory therapy should be started on 20 mg of 'Pepcid' every six hours. Dosage should then be adjusted to individual response: doses up to 800 mg daily have been used up to one year without the development of significant adverse effects or tachyphylaxis. Patients who have been receiving another H_2 antagonist may be switched directly to 'Pepcid' at a dose higher than that recommended for new cases. This starting dose will depend on the severity of the condition and the last dose of H_2 antagonist previously used.

Gastro-oesophageal reflux disease

The recommended dosage for the symptomatic relief of gastro-oesophageal reflux disease is 20 mg of famotidine twice daily, which may be given for six to twelve weeks. Most patients experience improvement after two weeks.

Where gastro-oesophageal reflux disease is associated with the presence of oesophageal erosion or ulceration, the recommended dosage is 40 mg of famotidine twice daily, which may be given for six to twelve weeks.

Maintenance therapy: For the prevention of recurrence of symptoms and erosions or ulcerations associated with gastro-oesophageal reflux disease, the recommended dosage is 20 mg of famotidine twice daily.

Use in the elderly: The recommended dosage in most elderly patients is the same as in younger patients for all indications (see above).

Use in impaired renal function: To avoid excess accumulation of the drug in patients with moderate or severe renal insufficiency, the dose of PEPCID may be reduced to half the dose or the dosing interval may be prolonged to 36-48 hours as indicated by the patient's clinical response.

Paediatric use

The efficacy and safety of 'Pepcid' in children have not been established.

4.3 Contraindications
Hypersensitivity to any component of this product. Cross sensitivity in this class of compounds has been observed. Therefore 'Pepcid' should not be administered to patients with a history of hypersensitivity to other H_2-receptor antagonists.

4.4 Special warnings and precautions for use
Gastric carcinoma

Gastric malignancy should be excluded prior to initiation of therapy of gastric ulcer with 'Pepcid'. Symptomatic response of gastric ulcer to therapy with 'Pepcid' does not preclude the presence of gastric malignancy.

Impaired renal function

Since 'Pepcid' is primarily excreted via the kidney, caution should be exercised when treating patients with impaired renal function. The dose should be reduced to 20 mg *nocte* when creatinine clearance falls below 10 ml/min.

4.5 Interaction with other medicinal products and other forms of interaction
'Pepcid' does not inhibit the hepatic cytochrome P450 enzyme system. Furthermore, clinical studies have shown that famotidine does not potentiate the actions of warfarin, theophylline, phenytoin, diazepam, propranolol, aminopyrine and antipyrine, which are inactivated by this system.

Probenecid

The administration of probenecid can delay the elimination of famotidine. Concomitant use of probenecid and famotidine tablets should be used with caution.

Antacids

Bioavailability may be slightly increased by food, or slightly decreased by antacids; however, these effects are of no clinical consequence.

Ketonconazole / Itraconazole

During concomitant use of substances whose absorption is affected by gastric acid levels, a possible change in the absorption of these substances should be considered. The absorption of ketonconazole or itraconazole can be reduced; ketonconazole should be administered two hours before administering famotidine.

4.6 Pregnancy and lactation
Pregnancy: 'Pepcid' is not recommended for use in pregnancy, and should be prescribed only if clearly needed. Before a decision is made to use 'Pepcid' during pregnancy, the physician should weigh the potential benefits from the drug against the possible risks involved.

Breast-feeding mothers: 'Pepcid' is secreted in human milk, therefore breast-feeding mothers should either stop breast-feeding or stop taking the drug.

4.7 Effects on ability to drive and use machines
None known.

4.8 Undesirable effects
General disorders and administration site conditions:

Very rare: fatigue

Nervous system disorders:

Rare: headache, dizziness,

Very rare: epileptic seizures/convulsions (in patients with impaired renal function), paraesthesia

Gastrointestinal disorders:

Rare: constipation, diarrhoea

Very rare: dry mouth, dysgeusia, nausea and/or vomiting, abdominal discomfort of distension, anorexia

Hepatobiliary disorders:

Very rare: liver enzyme abnormalities, cholestatic jaundice

Isolated cases: worsening of hepatic disease however a causal relationship to therapy with 'Pepcid' has not been established.

Skin and subcutaneous tissue disorders:

Very rare: rash, pruritus, Stevens Johnson Syndrome/toxic epidermal necrolysis

Immune system disorders:

Very rare: urticaria, anaphylaxis, angioedema

Musculoskeletal and connective tissue disorders:

Very rare: arthralgia, muscle cramps

Psychiatric disorders:

Very rare: reversible psychic disturbances including depression, anxiety disorders, agitation, confusion and hallucinations, reduced libido, insomnia

Hematologic:

Very rare: pancytopenia, leucopenia; thrombocytopenia, agranulocytosis, neutropenia.

Reproductive system and breast disorders:

Rare: impotence, reversible gynaecomastia

Cardic disorders:

Very rare: A-V block, interstitial pneumonia.

4.9 Overdose
The adverse reactions in overdose cases are similar to the adverse reactions encountered in normal clinical experience (see section 4.8).

Patients with Zollinger-Ellison syndrome have tolerated doses up to 800 mg daily for more than a year without the development of significant adverse effects.

The usual measures to remove unabsorbed material from the gastro-intestinal tract, clinical monitoring, and supportive therapy should be employed.

5. PHARMACOLOGICAL PROPERTIES

5.1 Pharmacodynamic properties
'Pepcid', in single oral doses of 5 mg to 40 mg, produced dose-related inhibition of basal and pentagastrin, betazole, or insulin-stimulated gastric secretion in healthy volunteers. The inhibition affected volume, acid, and pepsin content of the gastric juice. In patients with benign gastric or duodenal ulceration, similar inhibitory effects on gastric secretion were noted.

In volunteers given a second pentagastrin challenge 5-7 hours after the dose of 'Pepcid' the inhibition of gastric secretion persisted, in contrast to control subjects on cimetidine 300 mg or on placebo.

A single oral dose of 40 mg of 'Pepcid' given at 9 pm was effective for more than 12 hours after administration. The 40 mg dose also had some continuing effect through the breakfast meal. The 80 mg dose of 'Pepcid' administered at 9 pm had no longer duration of action than the 40 mg dose.

Basal serum gastrin levels were increased by 20 mg and 10 mg doses of 'Pepcid' in some studies but unchanged in others. Gastric emptying was not affected by 'Pepcid', nor were hepatic and portal blood flows altered. 'Pepcid' did not cause changes in endocrine function.

5.2 Pharmacokinetic properties
'Pepcid' obeys linear kinetics. 'Pepcid' is rapidly absorbed, with dose-related peak plasma concentrations reached in one to three hours. Bioavailability is not affected by the presence of food in the stomach. Repeated doses do not lead to accumulation of the drug.

Protein binding in the plasma is relatively low (15-20%). The plasma half-life after a single oral dose or multiple repeated doses (for 5 days) was approximately 3 hours.

Metabolism of the drug occurs in the liver, with formation of the inactive sulphoxide metabolite.

Approximately 25-60% of the oral dosage is excreted in the urine, mainly as unchanged drug. A small amount may be excreted as the sulphoxide.

5.3 Preclinical safety data
No relevant information.

6. PHARMACEUTICAL PARTICULARS

6.1 List of excipients
Magnesium Stearate (E572)

Microcrystalline Cellulose (E460)

Pregelatinised Starch

Talc

Hydroxypropyl Cellulose (E463)

Hypromellose (E464)

Red Iron Oxide (E172)

Titanium Dioxide (E171)

Yellow Iron Oxide (E172)

Carnauba Wax (E903)

6.2 Incompatibilities
None.

6.3 Shelf life
24 months.

6.4 Special precautions for storage
Do not store above 25°C.

6.5 Nature and contents of container
Opacified PVC-aluminium blister packs of 2 and 4 tablets and calendar packs of 28 tablets.

Amber glass, high density polyethylene or polypropylene bottles of 50 tablets.

6.6 Special precautions for disposal and other handling
None.

7. MARKETING AUTHORISATION HOLDER
Merck Sharp & Dohme Limited

Hertford Road, Hoddesdon, Hertfordshire EN11 9BU, UK.

8. MARKETING AUTHORISATION NUMBER(S)
20 mg tablet: PL 0025/0215

40 mg tablet: PL 0025/0216

9. DATE OF FIRST AUTHORISATION/RENEWAL OF THE AUTHORISATION
Date granted: 8 September 1987

Last Renewed: 5 June 2008

10. DATE OF REVISION OF THE TEXT
01 May 2009

11. LEGAL CATEGORY
POM

® denotes registered trademark of Merck & Co., Inc., Whitehouse Station, NJ, USA

SPC.PCD.08.UK.3001

Perdix 15mg

(UCB Pharma Limited)

1. NAME OF THE MEDICINAL PRODUCT
Perdix 15 mg film-coated tablets

2. QUALITATIVE AND QUANTITATIVE COMPOSITION
Each Perdix 15 mg tablet contains moexipril hydrochloride 15 mg.

3. PHARMACEUTICAL FORM
Film-coated tablet.

4. CLINICAL PARTICULARS

4.1 Therapeutic indications
For the treatment of hypertension as monotherapy.

As second line therapy for the treatment of hypertension in combination with diuretics or calcium antagonists e.g. hydrochlorothiazide or nifedipine.

4.2 Posology and method of administration

Initial therapy:

In patients with uncomplicated essential hypertension not on diuretic therapy, the recommended initial dose is 7.5 mg once a day. Dosage should be adjusted according to blood pressure response. The usual dosage is 7.5 to 15 mg moexipril daily, administered in a single dose. Some patients may benefit from a further increase to 30 mg per day.

Doses over 30 mg have been used, but do not appear to give a greater effect.

If blood pressure is not controlled with Perdix alone, a low dose of a diuretic may be added. Hydrochlorothiazide 12.5 mg has been shown to provide an additive effect.

With concomitant diuretic therapy, it may be possible to reduce the dose of Perdix.

Diuretic treated patients:

In hypertensive patients who are currently being treated with a diuretic, symptomatic hypotension may occur occasionally following the initial dose of Perdix. The diuretic should be discontinued, if possible, for two to three days before beginning therapy with Perdix to reduce the likelihood of hypotension (see "Warnings"). The dosage of Perdix should be adjusted according to blood pressure response. If the patient's blood pressure is not controlled with Perdix alone, diuretic therapy may be resumed as described above.

If the diuretic cannot be discontinued or the diuretic has recently been withdrawn, an initial dose of 3.75 mg (half 7.5 mg tablet) should be used under medical supervision for at least two hours and until blood pressure has stabilised for at least an additional hour (see "Warnings and Precautions").

Concomitant administration of Perdix with potassium supplements, potassium salt substitutes, or potassium-sparing diuretics may lead to increases of serum potassium (see "Precautions").

Nifedipine treated patients:

As add-on therapy, Perdix has been investigated in combination with nifedipine. If Perdix is used as add-on therapy to nifedipine, the starting dose of Perdix should be 3.75 mg (half 7.5 mg tablet).

Elderly patients:

In elderly patients, an initial dosage of 3.75 mg (half 7.5 mg tablet) once daily is recommended followed by titration to the optimal response.

Children:

Not recommended. Safety and efficacy in children has not been established.

Renal failure:

In patients with creatinine clearance ⩽ 40 ml/min, an initial dose of 3.75 mg of moexipril (half 7.5 mg tablet) is recommended.

Hepatic cirrhosis:

In patients with hepatic cirrhosis, an initial dose of 3.75 mg of moexipril (half 7.5 mg tablet) is recommended.

Afro-Caribbean patients:

Where Perdix is used as a single agent in hypertension, Afro-Caribbean patients may show a reduced therapeutic response.

4.3 Contraindications

Perdix is contra-indicated in patients who are hypersensitive to this product and in patients with a history of angioedema related to previous treatment with an angiotensin converting enzyme inhibitor.

Second and third trimesters of pregnancy (see sections 4.4 and 4.6).

4.4 Special warnings and precautions for use

Warnings:

Angioedema:

Angioedema involving the extremities, face, lips, mucous membranes, tongue, glottis or larynx has been reported in patients treated with ACE inhibitors. If angioedema involves the tongue, glottis or larynx, airway obstruction may occur and be fatal. If laryngeal stridor or angioedema of the face, lips, mucous membranes, tongue, glottis or extremities occur, treatment with Perdix should be discontinued and appropriate therapy instituted immediately. Where there is involvement of the tongue, glottis, or larynx, likely to cause airway obstruction, appropriate therapy, e.g. subcutaneous epinephrine solution 1:1000 (0.3 ml to 0.5 ml) should be promptly administered (see "Precautions").

Intestinal angioedema has been reported in patients treated with ACE inhibitors. These patients presented with abdominal pain (with or without nausea and vomiting); in some cases there was no prior history of facial angioedema and C1-esterase levels were normal. The angioedema was diagnosed by procedures including abdominal CT scan or ultrasound, or at surgery, and symptoms resolved after stopping the ACE inhibitor. Intestinal angioedema should be included in the differential diagnosis of patients on ACE inhibitors presenting with abdominal pain.

Cough:

During treatment with an ACE inhibitor a dry and non-productive cough may occur which disappears after discontinuation.

Hypotension:

Perdix can cause symptomatic hypotension. Like other ACE inhibitors, Perdix has been only rarely associated with hypotension in hypertensive patients receiving monotherapy. Symptomatic hypotension is most likely to occur in patients who have been volume – and/or salt – depleted as a result of prolonged diuretic therapy, dietary salt restriction, dialysis, diarrhoea, or vomiting. Volume and/or salt depletion should be corrected before initiating therapy with Perdix.

If hypotension occurs, the patient should be placed in a supine position and, if necessary, treated with intravenous infusion of physiological saline. Perdix treatment usually can be continued following restoration of blood pressure and volume.

Neutropenia/agranulocytosis:

ACE inhibitors have been shown to cause agranulocytosis and bone marrow depression, rarely in uncomplicated patients, but more frequently in patients with renal impairment, especially if they also have a collagen-vascular disease such as systemic lupus erythematosus or scleroderma. Available data from clinical trials of Perdix are insufficient to show that Perdix does not cause agranulocytosis at similar rates. Monitoring of white blood cell counts should be considered in patients with collagen-vascular disease, especially if the disease is associated with impaired renal function.

Proteinuria:

Proteinuria may occur, particularly in patients with existing renal function impairment or on higher doses of Perdix.

Dialysis:

Patients who are dialysed using high-flux polyacrylonitrile membranes and treated with ACE inhibitors may experience anaphylactoid reactions such as facial swelling, flushing, hypotension and dyspnoea within a few minutes of commencing haemodialysis. It is recommended that an alternative membrane or an alternative antihypertensive drug be used.

LDL apheresis/Desensibilisation:

During LDL (low-density lipoprotein) apheresis (in patients with severe hypercholesterinemia) life-threatening hypersensitivity reactions may occur in patients under ACE inhibitor therapy.

During desensibilisation therapy against insect poisons (e.g. bee or wasp stings) and concomitant treatment with an ACE inhibitor, life-threatening hypersensitivity reactions (e.g. blood pressure fall, dyspnoea, vomiting, allergic skin reactions) may occur.

If LDL apheresis or desensibilisation therapy against insect poisons is required, the ACE inhibitor should be substituted by a different antihypertensive drug temporarily.

Pregnancy

ACE inhibitors should not be initiated during pregnancy. Unless continued ACE inhibitor therapy is considered essential, patients planning pregnancy should be changed to alternative antihypertensive treatments which have an established safety profile for use in pregnancy. When pregnancy is diagnosed, treatment with ACE inhibitors should be stopped immediately, and, if appropriate, alternative therapy should be started (see sections 4.3 and 4.6).

Precautions:

Impaired renal function:

As a consequence of inhibiting the renin-angiotensin-aldosterone system, changes in renal function may be anticipated in susceptible individuals.

Oliguria and/or progressive azotemia and rarely acute renal failure and/or death have been reported in association with ACE inhibitors in patients with severe congestive heart failure whose renal function may depend on the activity of the renin-angiotensin-aldosterone system.

In hypertensive patients with renal artery stenosis in a solitary kidney or bilateral renal artery stenosis, increases in blood urea nitrogen and serum creatinine may occur. Experience with other angiotensin converting enzyme inhibitors suggests that these increases are usually reversible upon discontinuation of ACE inhibitor and/or diuretic therapy. In such patients, renal function should be monitored during the first few weeks of therapy.

Some hypertensive patients with no apparent pre-existing renal vascular disease have developed increases in blood urea nitrogen and serum creatinine, usually minor and transient, especially when Perdix has been given concomitantly with a diuretic. This is more likely to occur in patients with pre-existing renal impairment. Dosage reduction of Perdix and/or discontinuation of the diuretic may be required.

Evaluation of the hypertensive patient should always include assessment of renal function.

Impaired renal function decreases total clearance of moexiprilat and approximately doubles AUC.

Hyperkalaemia:

In clinical trials, hyperkalaemia (serum potassium greater than 10% above the upper limit of normal) has occurred in approximately 2.6% of hypertensive patients receiving Perdix. In most cases, these were isolated values, which resolved despite continued therapy. In clinical trials, 0.1% of patients (two patients) were discontinued from therapy due to an elevated serum potassium. Risk factors for the development of hyperkalaemia include renal insufficiency, diabetes mellitus and the concomitant use of potassium-sparing diuretics, potassium supplements and/or potassium-containing salt substitutes, which should be used cautiously, if at all, with Perdix (see "Precautions").

Hepatic cirrhosis:

Since Perdix is primarily metabolised by hepatic and gut wall esterases to its active moiety, moexiprilat, patients with impaired liver function could develop elevated plasma levels of unchanged Perdix. In a study in patients with alcoholic or biliary cirrhosis, the extent of hydrolysis was unaffected, although the rate was slowed. In these patients, the apparent total body clearance of moexiprilat was decreased and the plasma AUC approximately doubled.

Surgery/anaesthesia:

In patients undergoing surgery or during anaesthesia with agents that produce hypotension, Perdix will block the angiotensin II formation that could otherwise occur secondary to compensatory renin release. Hypotension that occurs as a result of this mechanism can be corrected by volume expansion.

Aortic stenosis/hypertrophic cardiomyopathy:

Perdix should be used with caution in patients with an obstruction in the outflow tract of the left ventricle.

4.5 Interaction with other medicinal products and other forms of interaction

Diuretics:

Excessive reductions in blood pressure, especially in patients in whom diuretic therapy was recently instituted, have been reported with ACE inhibitors. The possibility of hypotensive effects with Perdix can be minimised by discontinuing diuretic therapy or increasing salt intake for several days before initiation of treatment with Perdix. If this is not possible, the starting dose should be reduced (see also 4.2 and 4.4).

Nifedipine:

The co-administration of nifedipine with Perdix gives rise to an enhanced antihypertensive effect.

Potassium supplements and potassium-sparing diuretics:

Perdix can attenuate potassium loss caused by thiazide diuretics. Potassium-sparing diuretics (spironolactone, triamterene, amiloride, and others) or potassium supplements have been shown to increase the risk of hyperkalaemia when used concomitantly with ACE inhibitors. Therefore, if concomitant use of such agents is indicated, they should be given with caution and the patient's serum potassium should be monitored frequently.

Oral anticoagulants:

Interaction studies with warfarin failed to identify any clinically important effects on the serum concentrations of the anticoagulants or on their anticoagulant effects.

Lithium:

Increased serum lithium levels and symptoms of lithium toxicity have been reported in patients receiving ACE inhibitors during therapy with lithium. These drugs should be co-administered with caution, and frequent monitoring of serum lithium levels is recommended. If a diuretic is also used, the risk of lithium toxicity may be increased.

Anaesthetic drugs:

Perdix may enhance the hypotensive effects of certain anaesthetic drugs.

Narcotic drugs/Antipsychotics:

Postural hypotension may occur.

Allopurinol, cytostatic or immunosuppressive agents, systemic corticosteroids or procainamide:

Concomitant administration with Perdix may lead to an increased risk for leucopenia.

Non-Steroidal anti-inflammatory drugs:

The administration of NSAIDs may reduce the antihypertensive effect of Perdix. Furthermore, it has been reported that NSAIDs and ACE inhibitors exert an additive effect on increase in serum potassium, whereas renal function may decrease. These effects are in principle reversible, and occur especially in patients with compromised renal function.

Alcohol enhances the hypotensive effect of Perdix.

Other agents:

No clinically important pharmacokinetic interactions occurred when Perdix was administered concomitantly with hydrochlorothiazide, digoxin, cimetidine, or nifedipine in healthy volunteers. However, in hypertensive patients, the antihypertensive effect of Perdix was enhanced when given in combination with diuretics, or calcium antagonists.

4.6 Pregnancy and lactation

The use of ACE inhibitors is not recommended during the first trimester of pregnancy (see section 4.4). The use of ACE inhibitors is contraindicated during the second and third trimester of pregnancy (see sections 4.3 and 4.4).

Epidemiological evidence regarding the risk of teratogenicity following exposure to ACE inhibitors during the first trimester of pregnancy has not been conclusive; however a small increase in risk cannot be excluded. Unless continued ACE inhibitor therapy is considered essential, patients planning pregnancy should be changed to alternative antihypertensive treatments which have an established safety profile for use in pregnancy. When pregnancy is diagnosed, treatment with ACE inhibitors should be stopped immediately, and, if appropriate, alternative therapy should be started.

Exposure to ACE inhibitor therapy during the second and third trimesters is known to induce human foetotoxicity (decreased renal function, oligohydramnios, skull ossification retardation) and neonatal toxicity (renal failure, hypotension, hyperkalaemia). (See section 5.3). Should exposure to ACE inhibitor have occurred from the second trimester of pregnancy, ultrasound check of renal function and skull is recommended. Infants whose mothers have taken ACE inhibitors should be closely observed for hypotension (see sections 4.3 and 4.4).

Lactation

Because no information is available regarding the use of Perdix during breast-feeding, Perdix is not recommended and alternative treatments with better established safety profiles during breast-feeding are preferable, especially while nursing a newborn or preterm infant.

4.7 Effects on ability to drive and use machines

The intake of ACE inhibitors may – as any antihypertensive therapy – induce hypotension with subsequent impairment of reactivity. Alcohol intake may enhance this effect.

4.8 Undesirable effects

The most commonly reported undesirable effects (more than 1% of patients treated with Perdix in controlled trials) were cough (4.0%), headache (3.6%), dizziness (3.3%), fatigue (1.2%), flushing (1.2%), and rash (1.0%).

Other adverse experiences possibly or probably related, or of uncertain relationship to therapy, reported in controlled or uncontrolled clinical trials occurring in less than 1% of Perdix patients and less frequent clinically significant events which have been attributed to ACE inhibitors include the following:

Cardiovascular:

Symptomatic hypotension, postural hypotension, or syncope was seen in < 1% of patients; these reactions led to discontinuation of therapy in controlled trials in 2 patients (0.1%) who had received Perdix monotherapy and in 1 patient (0.05%) who had received Perdix with hydrochlorothiazide. Other reports included chest pain, angina/myocardial infarction, tachycardia, palpitations, rhythm disturbances, transient ischaemic attacks, cerebrovascular accident.

Renal:

Of hypertensive patients with no apparent pre-existing renal disease, 0.8% of patients receiving Perdix alone and 1.5% of patients receiving Perdix with hydrochlorothiazide have experienced increases in serum creatinine to at least 140% of their baseline values.

Acute renal failure has been reported for ACE inhibitors including Perdix (see section 4.4 Special Warnings and Precautions for use).

Gastrointestinal:

Abdominal pain, dyspepsia, constipation, nausea, vomiting, diarrhoea, appetite/weight change, dry mouth, pancreatitis, hepatitis.

Intestinal Angioedema:

Intestinal Angioedema has been reported in patients treated with ACE inhibitors (see section 4.4 Special Warnings and Precautions for use).

Respiratory:

Upper respiratory infection, pharyngitis, sinusitis/rhinitis, bronchospasm, dyspnoea.

Urogenital:

Renal insufficiency.

Dermatologic:

Occasionally allergic and hypersensitivity reactions can occur like rash, pruritus, urticaria, erythema multiforme, Stevens-Johnson syndrome, toxic epidermic necrolysis, psoriasis-like efflorescence, pemphigus and alopecia. This can be accompanied by fever, myalgia, arthralgia, eosinophilia and/or increased ANA-titres. ACE inhibitors have been associated with the onset of angioneurotic oedema in a small subset of patients involving the face and oropharyngeal tissues.

Neurological and psychiatric:

Headache or tiredness may occasionally occur; rarely there may be drowsiness, depression, sleep disturbances, impotence, tingling sensations, numbness or paraesthesia, disturbances of balance, confusion, tinnitus, blurred vision, and alterations of taste or a transient loss of taste.

Other

Sweating, flu syndrome, malaise.

Clinical Laboratory Test Findings:

Decreases in haemoglobin, haematocrit, platelets and white cell count and individual cases of agranulocytosis or pancytopenia, as well as elevation of liver enzymes and serum bilirubin have been reported in a few patients. In patients with congenital deficiency concerning G-6-PDH individual cases of haemolytic anaemia have been reported.

In rare cases, especially in patients with impaired kidney function or collagen disease, or those simultaneously receiving treatment will allopurinol, procainamide or certain drugs which suppress the defence reactions, there may be anaemia, thrombocytopenia, neutropenia, eosinophilia and in isolated cases, even agranulocytosis or pancytopenia.

Creatinine and blood urea nitrogen:

As with other ACE inhibitors, minor increases in blood urea nitrogen or serum creatinine, reversible upon discontinuation of therapy, were observed in approximately 1% of patients with essential hypertension who were treated with Perdix. Increases are more likely to occur in patients receiving concomitant diuretics or in patients with compromised renal function.

Potassium:

Since moexipril decreases aldosterone secretion, elevation of serum potassium can occur. Potassium supplements and potassium-sparing diuretics should be given with caution and the patient's serum potassium should be monitored frequently.

Other:

Clinically important changes in standard laboratory tests were rarely associated with Perdix administration. Elevations of liver enzymes and uric acid have been reported. In trials, less than 1% of moexipril-treated patients discontinued Perdix treatment because of laboratory abnormalities.

4.9 Overdose

Symptoms and treatment:

To date, no case of overdosage has been reported. Signs and symptoms expected in cases of overdosage would be related to hypotension and should be relieved by intravenous infusion of isotonic saline solution.

5. PHARMACOLOGICAL PROPERTIES

5.1 Pharmacodynamic properties

In animals as well as in humans, interactions between the renin-angiotensin-aldosterone system and the kallikrein-kinin system provide an important biochemical basis for blood pressure homeostasis. In hypertension the normal feedback mechanism formed by the renin-angiotensin system (RAS) may be dysfunctional, resulting in a self-perpetuating hypertensive condition.

Angiotensin converting enzyme (ACE) inhibitors were developed to interrupt this system and thereby to lower blood pressure. Perdix potently inhibits ACE and by this the formation of angiotensin II, the active agent of the RAS, thus blocking its vasoconstrictor and sodium-retaining effects with a consequent reduction in blood pressure.

Since ACE is identical to kininase II, an enzyme that degrades the potent vasodilator bradykinin, inhibition of ACE leads to an additional, non renin-mediated reduction in systemic blood pressure. The antihypertensive effects of ACE inhibitors are accompanied by a reduction in peripheral vascular resistance.

5.2 Pharmacokinetic properties

The prodrug moexipril is rapidly absorbed and de-esterified to the active metabolite moexiprilate. The pharmacokinetic parameters for moexipril and moexiprilate were similar after both, single and multiple does of moexipril and appear to be dose-proportional.

Moexipril and moexiprilate are moderately bound to plasma proteins, predominately albumin. Therefore, concurrently administered drugs are unlikely to interfere with the binding of moexipril and moexiprilate in any clinically significant way. Metabolites of moexipril present in the diketopiperazine derivatives of moexipril and moexiprilate. Both, moexipril and moexiprilate are eliminated in the urine, and moexiprilate is eliminated in the faeces.

The pharmacokinetic profile of moexipril and moexiprilate should allow the same dosage recommendation in patients with mild to moderate renal dysfunction ($Cl_{cr} > 40$ ml/min) as in patients with normal renal function. With severe renal dysfunction, dosage reduction is recommended. In patients with liver cirrhosis, the pharmacokinetics of moexipril and moexiprilate were significantly altered as compared with normal subjects. In such patients, therapy with Perdix should be started with 3.75 mg (half 7.5 mg tablet).

There were no apparent pharmacokinetic drug interactions with HCTZ, digoxin, cimetidine, warfarin or nifedipine.

5.3 Preclinical safety data

Acute toxicity:

Findings of the acute toxicity studies in animals do not raise questions as to the safety of moexipril HCl as well as the main metabolite moexiprilate under the conditions of proposed clinical usage.

Subacute/chronic toxicity:

Subacute and chronic toxicity studies in rats and dogs with repeated oral administration of moexipril HCl up to 12 months, revealed mainly heart and kidney as target organs. The effects are completely comparable with those of other ACE inhibitors and can be interpreted as results of highly exaggerated pharmacological activity.

First unspecific drug-related side-effects after long-term administration were seen at 75 mg/kg, i.e. a dose which corresponds 150 times the maximum recommended total daily dose in humans when compared on the basis of body weight.

Reproduction studies:

Studies in rats and rabbits including all segments of reproduction revealed no direct effects of moexipril HCl on fertility, reproduction and abnormalities in F_1– or F_2– pups.

Regarding precautions in women of child bearing potential and use during pregnancy and lactation see 4.3 and 4.6.

Mutagenicity:

As conclusion of different 'in vitro' and one 'in vivo' mutagenicity studies, the mutagenic potential of moexipril HCl for human beings should be extremely low.

Carcinogenicity:

Neither the long-term toxicity studies in rats and dogs nor special carcinogenicity studies in mice and rats over 78 and 104 weeks respectively, indicated neoplastigenic properties of moexipril HCl. Therefore, it can be concluded that the carcinogenic risk for human beings will be extremely low.

6. PHARMACEUTICAL PARTICULARS

6.1 List of excipients

Lactose

Crospovidone

Light magnesium oxide

Gelatine

Magnesium stearate

Methylhydroxypropylcellulose

Hydroxypropylcellulose

Polyethyleneglycol 6000

Titanium dioxide

Ferric oxide

Purified water (not present in the finished product)

6.2 Incompatibilities

No incompatibilities have so far been demonstrated.

6.3 Shelf life

5 years.

6.4 Special precautions for storage

Store in the original package.

6.5 Nature and contents of container

Calendar packs containing 28 tablets, 14 per Al/Al blister pack.

6.6 Special precautions for disposal and other handling

No special instruction necessary

7. MARKETING AUTHORISATION HOLDER

UCB Pharma Limited

208 Bath Road

Slough

Berkshire

SL1 3WE

United Kingdom

8. MARKETING AUTHORISATION NUMBER(S)

PL 00039/0755

9. DATE OF FIRST AUTHORISATION/RENEWAL OF THE AUTHORISATION

01 April 2009

10. DATE OF REVISION OF THE TEXT

Perdix 7.5mg

(UCB Pharma Limited)

1. NAME OF THE MEDICINAL PRODUCT

Perdix 7.5 mg film-coated tablets

2. QUALITATIVE AND QUANTITATIVE COMPOSITION

Each Perdix 7.5 mg tablet contains moexipril hydrochloride 7.5 mg.

3. PHARMACEUTICAL FORM

Film-coated tablet.

4. CLINICAL PARTICULARS

4.1 Therapeutic indications

For the treatment of hypertension as monotherapy.

As second line therapy for the treatment of hypertension in combination with diuretics or calcium antagonists e.g. hydrochlorothiazide or nifedipine.

4.2 Posology and method of administration

Initial therapy:

In patients with uncomplicated essential hypertension not on diuretic therapy, the recommended initial dose is 7.5 mg once a day. Dosage should be adjusted according to blood pressure response. The usual dosage is 7.5 to 15 mg moexipril daily, administered in a single dose. Some patients may benefit from a further increase to 30 mg per day.

Doses over 30 mg have been used, but do not appear to give a greater effect.

If blood pressure is not controlled with Perdix alone, a low dose of a diuretic may be added. Hydrochlorothiazide 12.5 mg has been shown to provide an additive effect.

With concomitant diuretic therapy, it may be possible to reduce the dose of Perdix.

Diuretic treated patients:

In hypertensive patients who are currently being treated with a diuretic, symptomatic hypotension may occur occasionally following the initial dose of Perdix. The diuretic should be discontinued, if possible, for two to three days before beginning therapy with Perdix to reduce the likelihood of hypotension (see "Warnings"). The dosage of Perdix should be adjusted according to blood pressure response. If the patient's blood pressure is not controlled with Perdix alone, diuretic therapy may be resumed as described above.

If the diuretic cannot be discontinued or the diuretic has recently been withdrawn, an initial dose of 3.75 mg (half 7.5 mg tablet) should be used under medical supervision for at least two hours and until blood pressure has stabilised for at least an additional hour (see "Warnings and Precautions").

Concomitant administration of Perdix with potassium supplements, potassium salt substitutes, or potassium-sparing diuretics may lead to increases of serum potassium (see "Precautions").

Nifedipine treated patients:

As add-on therapy, Perdix has been investigated in combination with nifedipine. If Perdix is used as add-on therapy to nifedipine, the starting dose of Perdix should be 3.75 mg (half 7.5 mg tablet).

Elderly patients:

In elderly patients, an initial dosage of 3.75 mg (half 7.5 mg tablet) once daily is recommended followed by titration to the optimal response.

Children:

Not recommended. Safety and efficacy in children has not been established.

Renal failure:

In patients with creatinine clearance ⩽ 40 ml/min, an initial dose of 3.75 mg of moexipril (half 7.5 mg tablet) is recommended.

Hepatic cirrhosis:

In patients with hepatic cirrhosis, an initial dose of 3.75 mg of moexipril (half 7.5 mg tablet) is recommended.

Afro-Caribbean patients:

Where Perdix is used as a single agent in hypertension, Afro-Caribbean patients may show a reduced therapeutic response.

4.3 Contraindications

Perdix is contra-indicated in patients who are hypersensitive to this product and in patients with a history of angioedema related to previous treatment with an angiotensin converting enzyme inhibitor.

Second and third trimesters of pregnancy (see sections 4.4 and 4.6).

4.4 Special warnings and precautions for use

Warnings:

Angioedema:

Angioedema involving the extremities, face, lips, mucous membranes, tongue, glottis or larynx has been reported in patients treated with ACE inhibitors. If angioedema involves the tongue, glottis or larynx, airway obstruction may occur and be fatal. If laryngeal stridor or angioedema of the face, lips, mucous membranes, tongue, glottis or extremities occur, treatment with Perdix should be discontinued and appropriate therapy instituted immediately. Where there is involvement of the tongue, glottis, or larynx, likely to cause airway obstruction, appropriate therapy, e.g. subcutaneous epinephrine solution 1:1000 (0.3 ml to 0.5 ml) should be promptly administered (see "Precautions").

Intestinal angioedema has been reported in patients treated with ACE inhibitors. These patients presented with abdominal pain (with or without nausea and vomiting); in some cases there was no prior history of facial angioedema and C1-esterase levels were normal. The angioedema was diagnosed by procedures including abdominal CT scan or ultrasound, or at surgery, and symptoms resolved after stopping the ACE inhibitor. Intestinal angioedema should be included in the differential diagnosis of patients on ACE inhibitors presenting with abdominal pain.

Cough:

During treatment with an ACE inhibitor a dry and non-productive cough may occur which disappears after discontinuation.

Hypotension:

Perdix can cause symptomatic hypotension. Like other ACE inhibitors, Perdix has been only rarely associated with hypotension in hypertensive patients receiving monotherapy. Symptomatic hypotension is most likely to occur in patients who have been volume – and/or salt – depleted as a result of prolonged diuretic therapy, dietary salt restriction, dialysis, diarrhoea, or vomiting. Volume and/or salt depletion should be corrected before initiating therapy with Perdix.

If hypotension occurs, the patient should be placed in a supine position and, if necessary, treated with intravenous infusion of physiological saline. Perdix treatment usually can be continued following restoration of blood pressure and volume.

Neutropenia/agranulocytosis:

ACE inhibitors have been shown to cause agranulocytosis and bone marrow depression, rarely in uncomplicated patients, but more frequently in patients with renal impairment, especially if they also have a collagen-vascular disease such as systemic lupus erythematosus or scleroderma. Available data from clinical trials of Perdix are insufficient to show that Perdix does not cause agranulocytosis at similar rates. Monitoring of white blood cell counts should be considered in patients with collagen-vascular disease, especially if the disease is associated with impaired renal function.

Proteinuria:

Proteinuria may occur, particularly in patients with existing renal function impairment or on higher doses of Perdix.

Dialysis:

Patients who are dialysed using high-flux polyacrylonitrile membranes and treated with ACE inhibitors may experience anaphylactoid reactions such as facial swelling, flushing, hypotension and dyspnoea within a few minutes of commencing haemodialysis. It is recommended that an alternative membrane or an alternative antihypertensive drug be used.

LDL apheresis/Desensibilisation:

During LDL (low-density lipoprotein) apheresis (in patients with severe hypercholesterinemia) life-threatening hypersensitivity reactions may occur in patients under ACE inhibitor therapy.

During desensibilisation therapy against insect poisons (e.g. bee or wasp stings) and concomitant treatment with an ACE inhibitor, life-threatening hypersensitivity reactions (e.g. blood pressure fall, dyspnoea, vomiting, allergic skin reactions) may occur.

If LDL apheresis or desensibilisation therapy against insect poisons is required, the ACE inhibitor should be substituted by a different antihypertensive drug temporarily.

Pregnancy

ACE inhibitors should not be initiated during pregnancy. Unless continued ACE inhibitor therapy is considered essential, patients planning pregnancy should be changed to alternative antihypertensive treatments which have an established safety profile for use in pregnancy. When pregnancy is diagnosed, treatment with ACE inhibitors should be stopped immediately, and, if appropriate, alternative therapy should be started (see sections 4.3 and 4.6).

Precautions:

Impaired renal function:

As a consequence of inhibiting the renin-angiotensin-aldosterone system, changes in renal function may be anticipated in susceptible individuals.

Oliguria and/or progressive azotemia and rarely acute renal failure and/or death have been reported in association with ACE inhibitors in patients with severe congestive heart failure whose renal function may depend on the activity of the renin-angiotensin-aldosterone system.

In hypertensive patients with renal artery stenosis in a solitary kidney or bilateral renal artery stenosis, increases in blood urea nitrogen and serum creatinine may occur. Experience with other angiotensin converting enzyme inhibitors suggests that these increases are usually reversible upon discontinuation of ACE inhibitor and/or diuretic therapy. In such patients, renal function should be monitored during the first few weeks of therapy.

Some hypertensive patients with no apparent pre-existing renal vascular disease have developed increases in blood urea nitrogen and serum creatinine, usually minor and transient, especially when Perdix has been given concomitantly with a diuretic. This is more likely to occur in patients with pre-existing renal impairment. Dosage reduction of Perdix and/or discontinuation of the diuretic may be required.

Evaluation of the hypertensive patient should always include assessment of renal function.

Impaired renal function decreases total clearance of moexiprilat and approximately doubles AUC.

Hyperkalaemia:

In clinical trials, hyperkalaemia (serum potassium greater than 10% above the upper limit of normal) has occurred in approximately 2.6% of hypertensive patients receiving Perdix. In most cases, these were isolated values, which resolved despite continued therapy. In clinical trials, 0.1% of patients (two patients) were discontinued from therapy due to an elevated serum potassium. Risk factors for the development of hyperkalaemia include renal insufficiency, diabetes mellitus and the concomitant use of potassium-sparing diuretics, potassium supplements and/or potassium-containing salt substitutes, which should be used cautiously, if at all, with Perdix (see "Precautions").

Hepatic cirrhosis:

Since Perdix is primarily metabolised by hepatic and gut wall esterases to its active moiety, moexiprilat, patients with impaired liver function could develop elevated plasma levels of unchanged Perdix. In a study in patients with alcoholic or biliary cirrhosis, the extent of hydrolysis was unaffected, although the rate was slowed. In these patients, the apparent total body clearance of moexiprilat was decreased and the plasma AUC approximately doubled.

Surgery/anaesthesia:

In patients undergoing surgery or during anaesthesia with agents that produce hypotension, Perdix will block the angiotensin II formation that could otherwise occur secondary to compensatory renin release. Hypotension that occurs as a result of this mechanism can be corrected by volume expansion.

Aortic stenosis/hypertrophic cardiomyopathy:

Perdix should be used with caution in patients with an obstruction in the outflow tract of the left ventricle.

4.5 Interaction with other medicinal products and other forms of interaction

Diuretics:

Excessive reductions in blood pressure, especially in patients in whom diuretic therapy was recently instituted, have been reported with ACE inhibitors. The possibility of hypotensive effects with Perdix can be minimised by discontinuing diuretic therapy or increasing salt intake for several days before initiation of treatment with Perdix. If this is not possible, the starting dose should be reduced (see also 4.2 and 4.4).

Nifedipine:

The co-administration of nifedipine with Perdix gives rise to an enhanced antihypertensive effect.

Potassium supplements and potassium-sparing diuretics:

Perdix can attenuate potassium loss caused by thiazide diuretics. Potassium-sparing diuretics (spironolactone, triamterene, amiloride, and others) or potassium supplements have been shown to increase the risk of hyperkalaemia when used concomitantly with ACE inhibitors. Therefore, if concomitant use of such agents is indicated, they should be given with caution and the patient's serum potassium should be monitored frequently.

Oral anticoagulants:

Interaction studies with warfarin failed to identify any clinically important effects on the serum concentrations of the anticoagulants or on their anticoagulant effects.

Lithium:

Increased serum lithium levels and symptoms of lithium toxicity have been reported in patients receiving ACE inhibitors during therapy with lithium. These drugs should be co-administered with caution, and frequent monitoring of serum lithium levels is recommended. If a diuretic is also used, the risk of lithium toxicity may be increased.

Anaesthetic drugs:

Perdix may enhance the hypotensive effects of certain anaesthetic drugs.

Narcotic drugs/Antipsychotics:

Postural hypotension may occur.

Allopurinol, cytostatic or immunosuppressive agents, systemic corticosteroids or procainamide:

Concomitant administration with Perdix may lead to an increased risk for leucopenia.

Non-Steroidal anti-inflammatory drugs:

The administration of NSAIDs may reduce the antihypertensive effect of Perdix. Furthermore, it has been reported that NSAIDs and ACE inhibitors exert an additive effect on increase in serum potassium, whereas renal function may decrease. These effects are in principle reversible, and occur especially in patients with compromised renal function.

Alcohol enhances the hypotensive effect of Perdix.

Other agents:

No clinically important pharmacokinetic interactions occurred when Perdix was administered concomitantly with hydrochlorothiazide, digoxin, cimetidine, or nifedipine in healthy volunteers. However, in hypertensive patients, the antihypertensive effect of Perdix was enhanced when given in combination with diuretics, or calcium antagonists.

4.6 Pregnancy and lactation

> The use of ACE inhibitors is not recommended during the first trimester of pregnancy (see section 4.4). The use of ACE inhibitors is contraindicated during the second and third trimester of pregnancy (see sections 4.3 and 4.4).

Epidemiological evidence regarding the risk of teratogenicity following exposure to ACE inhibitors during the first trimester of pregnancy has not been conclusive; however a small increase in risk cannot be excluded. Unless continued ACE inhibitor therapy is considered essential, patients planning pregnancy should be changed to alternative antihypertensive treatments which have an established safety profile for use in pregnancy. When pregnancy is diagnosed, treatment with ACE inhibitors should be stopped immediately, and, if appropriate, alternative therapy should be started.

Exposure to ACE inhibitor therapy during the second and third trimesters is known to induce human foetotoxicity (decreased renal function, oligohydramnios, skull ossification retardation) and neonatal toxicity (renal failure, hypotension, hyperkalaemia). (See section 5.3). Should exposure to ACE inhibitor have occurred from the second trimester of pregnancy, ultrasound check of renal function and skull is recommended. Infants whose mothers have taken ACE inhibitors should be closely observed for hypotension (see sections 4.3 and 4.4).

Lactation

Because no information is available regarding the use of Perdix during breast-feeding, Perdix is not recommended and alternative treatments with better established safety profiles during breast-feeding are preferable, especially while nursing a newborn or preterm infant.

4.7 Effects on ability to drive and use machines

The intake of ACE inhibitors may – as any antihypertensive therapy – induce hypotension with subsequent impairment of reactivity. Alcohol intake may enhance this effect.

4.8 Undesirable effects

The most commonly reported undesirable effects (more than 1% of patients treated with Perdix in controlled trials) were cough (4.0%), headache (3.6%), dizziness (3.3%), fatigue (1.2%), flushing (1.2%), and rash (1.0%).

Other adverse experiences possibly or probably related, or of uncertain relationship to therapy, reported in controlled or uncontrolled clinical trials occurring in less than 1% of Perdix patients and less frequent clinically significant events which have been attributed to ACE inhibitors include the following:

Cardiovascular:

Symptomatic hypotension, postural hypotension, or syncope was seen in < 1% of patients; these reactions led to discontinuation of therapy in controlled trials in 2 patients (0.1%) who had received Perdix monotherapy and in 1 patient (0.05%) who had received Perdix with hydrochlorothiazide. Other reports included chest pain, angina/myocardial infarction, tachycardia, palpitations, rhythm disturbances, transient ischaemic attacks, cerebrovascular accident.

Renal:

Of hypertensive patients with no apparent pre-existing renal disease, 0.8% of patients receiving Perdix alone and 1.5% of patients receiving Perdix with hydrochlorothiazide have experienced increases in serum creatinine to at least 140% of their baseline values.

Acute renal failure has been reported for ACE inhibitors including Perdix (see section 4.4 Special Warnings and Precautions for use).

Gastrointestinal:

Abdominal pain, dyspepsia, constipation, nausea, vomiting, diarrhoea, appetite/weight change, dry mouth, pancreatitis, hepatitis.

Intestinal Angioedema:

Intestinal Angioedema has been reported in patients treated with ACE inhibitors (see section 4.4 Special Warnings and Precautions for use).

Respiratory:

Upper respiratory infection, pharyngitis, sinusitis/rhinitis, bronchospasm, dyspnoea.

Urogenital:

Renal insufficiency.

Dermatologic:

Occasionally allergic and hypersensitivity reactions can occur like rash, pruritus, urticaria, erythema multiforme, Stevens-Johnson syndrome, toxic epidermic necrolysis, psoriasis-like efflorescence, pemphigus and alopecia. This can be accompanied by fever, myalgia, arthralgia, eosinophilia and/or increased ANA-titres. ACE inhibitors have been associated with the onset of angioneurotic oedema in a small subset of patients involving the face and oropharyngeal tissues.

Neurological and psychiatric:

Headache or tiredness may occasionally occur; rarely there may be drowsiness, depression, sleep disturbances, impotence, tingling sensations, numbness or paraesthesia, disturbances of balance, confusion, tinnitus, blurred vision, and alterations of taste or a transient loss of taste.

Other

Sweating, flu syndrome, malaise.

Clinical Laboratory Test Findings:

Decreases in haemoglobin, haematocrit, platelets and white cell count and individual cases of agranulocytosis or pancytopenia, as well as elevation of liver enzymes and serum bilirubin have been reported in a few patients. In patients with congenital deficiency concerning G-6-PDH individual cases of haemolytic anaemia have been reported.

In rare cases, especially in patients with impaired kidney function or collagen disease, or those simultaneously receiving treatment will allopurinol, procainamide or certain drugs which suppress the defence reactions, there may be anaemia, thrombocytopenia, neutropenia, eosinophilia and in isolated cases, even agranulocytosis or pancytopenia.

Creatinine and blood urea nitrogen:

As with other ACE inhibitors, minor increases in blood urea nitrogen or serum creatinine, reversible upon discontinuation of therapy, were observed in approximately 1% of patients with essential hypertension who were treated with Perdix. Increases are more likely to occur in patients receiving concomitant diuretics or in patients with compromised renal function.

Potassium:

Since moexipril decreases aldosterone secretion, elevation of serum potassium can occur. Potassium supplements and potassium-sparing diuretics should be given with caution and the patient's serum potassium should be monitored frequently.

Other:

Clinically important changes in standard laboratory tests were rarely associated with Perdix administration. Elevations of liver enzymes and uric acid have been reported. In trials, less than 1% of moexipril-treated patients discontinued Perdix treatment because of laboratory abnormalities.

4.9 Overdose

Symptoms and treatment:

To date, no case of overdosage has been reported. Signs and symptoms expected in cases of overdosage would be related to hypotension and should be relieved by intravenous infusion of isotonic saline solution.

5. PHARMACOLOGICAL PROPERTIES

5.1 Pharmacodynamic properties

In animals as well as in humans, interactions between the renin-angiotensin-aldosterone system and the kallikrein-kinin system provide an important biochemical basis for blood pressure homeostasis. In hypertension the normal feedback mechanism formed by the renin-angiotensin system (RAS) may be dysfunctional, resulting in a self-perpetuating hypertensive condition.

Angiotensin converting enzyme (ACE) inhibitors were developed to interrupt this system and thereby to lower blood pressure. Perdix potently inhibits ACE and by this the formation of angiotensin II, the active agent of the RAS, thus blocking its vasoconstrictor and sodium-retaining effects with a consequent reduction in blood pressure.

Since ACE is identical to kininase II, an enzyme that degrades the potent vasodilator bradykinin, inhibition of ACE leads to an additional, non renin-mediated reduction in systemic blood pressure. The antihypertensive effects of ACE inhibitors are accompanied by a reduction in peripheral vascular resistance.

5.2 Pharmacokinetic properties

The prodrug moexipril is rapidly absorbed and de-esterified to the active metabolite moexiprilate. The pharmacokinetic parameters for moexipril and moexiprilate were similar after both, single and multiple does of moexipril and appear to be dose-proportional.

Moexipril and moexiprilate are moderately bound to plasma proteins, predominately albumin. Therefore, concurrently administered drugs are unlikely to interfere with the binding of moexipril and moexiprilate in any clinically significant way. Metabolites of moexipril present in the diketopiperazine derivatives of moexipril and moexiprilate. Both, moexipril and moexiprilate are eliminated in the urine, and moexiprilate is eliminated in the faeces.

The pharmacokinetic profile of moexipril and moexiprilate should allow the same dosage recommendation in patients with mild to moderate renal dysfunction (Cl_{cr} > 40 ml/min) as in patients with normal renal function. With severe renal dysfunction, dosage reduction is recommended. In patients with liver cirrhosis, the pharmacokinetics of moexipril and moexiprilate were significantly altered as compared with normal subjects. In such patients, therapy with Perdix should be started with 3.75 mg (half 7.5 mg tablet).

There were no apparent pharmacokinetic drug interactions with HCTZ, digoxin, cimetidine, warfarin or nifedipine.

5.3 Preclinical safety data

Acute toxicity:

Findings of the acute toxicity studies in animals do not raise questions as to the safety of moexipril HCl as well as the main metabolite moexiprilate under the conditions of proposed clinical usage.

Subacute/chronic toxicity:

Subacute and chronic toxicity studies in rats and dogs with repeated oral administration of moexipril HCl up to 12 months, revealed mainly heart and kidney as target organs. The effects are completely comparable with those of other ACE inhibitors and can be interpreted as results of highly exaggerated pharmacological activity.

First unspecific drug-related side-effects after long-term administration were seen at 75 mg/kg, i.e. a dose which corresponds 150 times the maximum recommended total daily dose in humans when compared on the basis of body weight.

Reproduction studies:

Studies in rats and rabbits including all segments of reproduction revealed no direct effects of moexipril HCl on fertility, reproduction and abnormalities in F_1– or F_2– pups. Regarding precautions in women of child bearing potential and use during pregnancy and lactation see 4.3 and 4.6.

Mutagenicity:

As conclusion of different 'in vitro' and one 'in vivo' mutagenicity studies, the mutagenic potential of moexipril HCl for human beings should be extremely low.

Carcinogenicity:

Neither the long-term toxicity studies in rats and dogs nor special carcinogenicity studies in mice and rats over 78 and 104 weeks respectively, indicated neoplastigenic properties of moexipril HCl. Therefore, it can be concluded that the carcinogenic risk for human beings will be extremely low.

6. PHARMACEUTICAL PARTICULARS

6.1 List of excipients

Lactose

Crospovidone

Light magnesium oxide

Gelatine

Magnesium stearate

Methylhydroxypropylcellulose

Hydroxypropylcellulose

Polyethyleneglycol 6000

Titanium dioxide

Ferric oxide

Purified water (not present in the finished product)

6.2 Incompatibilities

No incompatibilities have so far been demonstrated.

6.3 Shelf life

5 years.

6.4 Special precautions for storage

Store in the original package.

6.5 Nature and contents of container

Calendar packs containing 28 tablets, 14 per Al/Al blister pack.

6.6 Special precautions for disposal and other handling

No special instruction necessary

7. MARKETING AUTHORISATION HOLDER

UCB Pharma Limited

208 Bath Road

Slough

Berkshire

SL1 3WE

United Kingdom

8. MARKETING AUTHORISATION NUMBER(S)

PL 00039/0754

9. DATE OF FIRST AUTHORISATION/RENEWAL OF THE AUTHORISATION

01 April 2009

10. DATE OF REVISION OF THE TEXT

Pergoveris 150 IU/75 IU powder and solvent for solution for injection

(Merck Serono)

1. NAME OF THE MEDICINAL PRODUCT

Pergoveris 150 IU/75 IU powder and solvent for solution for injection.

2. QUALITATIVE AND QUANTITATIVE COMPOSITION

One vial contains 150 IU (equivalent to 11 micrograms) of follitropin alfa (r-hFSH) and 75 IU (equivalent to 3.0 micrograms) of lutropin alfa (r-hLH).

The reconstituted solution contains 150 IU r-hFSH and 75 IU r-hLH per milliliter. Follitropin alfa and lutropin alfa are produced in genetically engineered Chinese Hamster Ovary (CHO) cells.

Excipients: sucrose, disodium phosphate dihydrate, sodium dihydrogen phosphate monohydrate.

For a full list of excipients, see section 6.1.

3. PHARMACEUTICAL FORM

Powder and solvent for solution for injection.

Powder: white lyophilised pellet.

Solvent: clear colourless solution.

The pH of the reconstituted solution is 6.5 - 7.5.

4. CLINICAL PARTICULARS

4.1 Therapeutic indications

Pergoveris is indicated for the stimulation of follicular development in women with severe LH and FSH deficiency.

In clinical trials, these patients were defined by an endogenous serum LH level < 1.2 IU/l.

4.2 Posology and method of administration

Treatment with Pergoveris should be initiated under the supervision of a physician experienced in the treatment of fertility problems.

Pergoveris is intended for subcutaneous administration. The powder should be reconstituted immediately prior to use with the solvent provided.

In LH and FSH deficient women (hypogonadotrophic hypogonadism), the objective of Pergoveris therapy is to develop a single mature Graafian follicle from which the oocyte will be liberated after the administration of human chorionic gonadotrophin (hCG). Pergoveris should be given as a course of daily injections. Since these patients are amenorrhoeic and have low endogenous oestrogen secretion, treatment can commence at any time.

Treatment should be tailored to the individual patient's response as assessed by measuring follicle size by ultrasound and oestrogen response. A recommended regimen commences with one vial of Pergoveris daily. If less than one vial of Pergoveris daily is used, the follicular response may be unsatisfactory because the amount of lutropin alfa may be insufficient (see section 5.1).

If an FSH dose increase is deemed appropriate, dose adaptation should preferably be after 7-14 day intervals and preferably by 37.5-75 IU increments using a licensed follitropin alfa preparation. It may be acceptable to extend the duration of stimulation in any one cycle to up to 5 weeks.

When an optimal response is obtained, a single injection of 5,000 IU to 10,000 IU hCG should be administered 24-48 hours after the last Pergoveris injection. The patient is recommended to have coitus on the day of, and on the day following, hCG administration. Alternatively, intrauterine insemination (IUI) may be performed.

Luteal phase support may be considered since lack of substances with luteotrophic activity (LH/hCG) after ovulation may lead to premature failure of the corpus luteum.

If an excessive response is obtained, treatment should be stopped and hCG withheld. Treatment should recommence in the next cycle at a dose of FSH lower than that of the previous cycle.

In clinical trials, patients with severe FSH and LH deficiency were defined by an endogenous serum LH level <1.2 IU/l as measured in a central laboratory. However, it should be taken into account that there are variations between LH measurements performed in different laboratories. In these trials the ovulation rate per cycle was 70-75%.

4.3 Contraindications

Pergoveris is contraindicated in patients with:

- hypersensitivity to the active substances follitropin alfa and lutropin alfa or to any of the excipients
- case of tumours of the hypothalamus and pituitary gland
- ovarian enlargement or cyst not due to polycystic ovarian disease
- gynaecological haemorrhages of unknown aetiology
- ovarian, uterine or mammary carcinoma

Pergoveris must not be used when an effective response cannot be obtained, such as:

- primary ovarian failure
- malformations of sexual organs incompatible with pregnancy
- fibroid tumours of the uterus incompatible with pregnancy

4.4 Special warnings and precautions for use

Pergoveris contains potent gonadotrophic substances capable of causing mild to severe adverse reactions, and should only be used by physicians who are thoroughly familiar with infertility problems and their management.

Gonadotrophin therapy requires a certain time commitment by physicians and supportive health professionals, as well as the availability of appropriate monitoring facilities. In women, safe and effective use of Pergoveris calls for monitoring of ovarian response with ultrasound, alone or preferably in combination with measurement of serum oestradiol levels, on a regular basis. There may be a degree of interpatient variability in response to FSH/LH administration, with a poor response to FSH/LH in some patients. The lowest effective dose in relation to the treatment objective should be used in women.

Self-administration of Pergoveris should only be performed by patients who are well motivated, adequately trained and with access to expert advice.

The first injection of Pergoveris should be performed under direct medical supervision.

Patients with porphyria or a family history of porphyria should be closely monitored during treatment with Pergoveris. Deterioration or a first appearance of this condition may require cessation of treatment.

Pergoveris contains less than 1 mmol sodium (23 mg) per dose, i.e. essentially "sodium-free".

Pergoveris contains 30 mg of sucrose per dose. This should be taken into account in patients with diabetes mellitus.

Before starting treatment, the couple's infertility should be assessed as appropriate and putative contraindications for pregnancy evaluated. In particular, patients should be evaluated for the following:

- hypothyroidism
- adrenocortical deficiency
- hyperprolactinemia and pituitary or hypothalamic tumours

Appropriate specific treatment should be given.

Patients undergoing stimulation of follicular growth are at an increased risk of developing hyperstimulation in view of possible excessive oestrogen response and multiple follicular development.

In clinical trials, lutropin alfa in combination with follitropin alfa has been shown to increase the ovarian sensitivity to gonadotropins. If an FSH dose increase is deemed appropriate, dose adaptation should preferably be at 7-14 day intervals and preferably with 37.5-75 IU increments using a licensed follitropin alfa preparation.

Ovarian Hyperstimulation Syndrome (OHSS) is a medical event distinct from uncomplicated ovarian enlargement. OHSS is a syndrome that can manifest itself with increasing degrees of severity. It comprises marked ovarian enlargement, high serum sex steroids, and an increase in vascular permeability which can result in an accumulation of fluid in the peritoneal, pleural and, rarely, in the pericardial cavities.

The following symptomatology may be observed in severe cases of OHSS:

- abdominal pain
- abdominal distension
- severe ovarian enlargement
- weight gain
- dyspnoea
- oliguria and gastrointestinal symptoms including nausea, vomiting and diarrhoea.

Clinical evaluation may reveal:

- hypovolaemia
- haemoconcentration
- electrolyte imbalances
- ascites
- haemoperitoneum
- pleural effusions
- hydrothorax
- acute pulmonary distress, and thromboembolic events.

Very rarely, severe OHSS may be complicated by pulmonary embolism, ischemic stroke and myocardial infarction.

Excessive ovarian response seldom gives rise to significant hyperstimulation unless hCG is administered to induce ovulation. Therefore in cases of ovarian hyperstimulation it is prudent to withhold hCG in such cases and advise the patient to refrain from coitus or use barrier methods for at least 4 days. OHSS may progress rapidly (within 24 hours to several days) to become a serious medical event, therefore patients should be followed for at least two weeks after hCG administration.

To minimise the risk of OHSS or of multiple pregnancy (see below), ultrasound scans as well as oestradiol measurements are recommended. In anovulation the risk of OHSS is increased by a serum oestradiol level > 900 pg/ml (3,300 pmol/l) and by the presence of more than 3 follicles of 14 mm or more in diameter.

Adherence to recommended Pergoveris and FSH dosage and regimen of administration and careful monitoring of therapy will minimise the incidence of ovarian hyperstimulation and multiple pregnancy (see below).

OHSS may be more severe and more protracted if pregnancy occurs. Most often, OHSS occurs after hormonal treatment has been discontinued and reaches its maximum at about seven to ten days following treatment. Usually, OHSS resolves spontaneously with the onset of menses.

If severe OHSS occurs, gonadotrophin treatment should be stopped if still ongoing. The patient should be hospitalised and specific therapy for OHSS started.

This syndrome occurs with higher incidence in patients with polycystic ovarian disease.

In patients undergoing induction of ovulation, the incidence of multiple pregnancies and births is increased compared with natural conception. The majority of multiple conceptions are twins. To minimise the risk of multiple pregnancy, careful monitoring of ovarian response is recommended.

The patients should be advised of the potential risk of multiple births before starting treatment.

The incidence of pregnancy wastage by miscarriage or abortion is higher in patients undergoing stimulation of follicular growth for ovulation induction than in the normal population.

When risk of OHSS or multiple pregnancies is assumed, treatment discontinuation should be considered.

Women with a history of tubal disease are at risk of ectopic pregnancy, whether the pregnancy is obtained by spontaneous conception or with fertility treatments. The prevalence of ectopic pregnancy after IVF was reported to be 2 to 5%, as compared to 1 to 1.5% in the general population.

There have been reports of ovarian and other reproductive system neoplasms, both benign and malignant, in women who have undergone multiple drug regimens for infertility treatment. It is not yet established whether or not treatment with gonadotrophins increases the baseline risk of these tumours in infertile women.

The prevalence of congenital malformations after ART may be slightly higher than after spontaneous conceptions. This is thought to be due to differences in parental characteristics (e.g. maternal age, sperm characteristics) and multiple pregnancies.

In women with generally recognised risk factors for thrombo-embolic events, such as personal or family history, treatment with gonadotrophins may further increase the risk. In these women, the benefits of gonadotrophin administration need to be weighed against the risks. It should be noted however, that pregnancy itself also carries an increased risk of thrombo-embolic events.

4.5 Interaction with other medicinal products and other forms of interaction

Pergoveris should not be administered as a mixture with other medicinal products, in the same injection, except follitropin alfa.

4.6 Pregnancy and lactation

Pergoveris should not be used during pregnancy or lactation.

4.7 Effects on ability to drive and use machines

No studies on the effects on the ability to drive and use machines have been performed.

4.8 Undesirable effects

Within each frequency grouping, undesirable effects are presented in order of decreasing seriousness.

Nervous system disorders	Very Common (≥1/10)	Headache
	Common (≥1/100 to <1/10)	Somnolence
Respiratory, thoracic and mediastinal disorders	Very rare (<1/10,000)	Exacerbation or worsening of asthma
Gastrointestinal disorders	Common (≥1/100 to <1/10)	Abdominal pain and gastrointestinal symptoms such as nausea, vomiting, diarrhoea, abdominal cramps and bloating
Vascular disorders	Very rare (<1/10,000)	Thromboembolism, usually associated with severe ovarian hyperstimulation syndrome (OHSS)
General disorders and administration site conditions	Very Common (≥1/10)	Mild to severe injection site reaction (pain, redness, bruising, swelling and/or irritation at the site of injection)
Immune system disorders	Very rare (<1/10,000)	Mild systemic allergic reactions (e.g. mild forms of erythema, rash, facial swelling, urticaria, oedema, difficulty breathing). Serious cases of allergic reactions, including anaphylactic reactions, have also been reported.
Reproductive system and breast disorders	Very Common (≥1/10)	Ovarian cysts
	Common (≥1/100 to <1/10)	Breast pain, pelvic pain, mild to moderate OHSS
	Uncommon (≥1/1,000 to <1/100)	Severe OHSS
	Rare (≥1/10,000 to <1/1,000)	Ovarian torsion, a complication of OHSS

4.9 Overdose

The effects of an overdose of Pergoveris are unknown. Nevertheless one could expect ovarian hyperstimulation syndrome to occur, which is further described in section 4.4.

5. PHARMACOLOGICAL PROPERTIES

5.1 Pharmacodynamic properties

Pharmacotherapeutic group: Gonadotrophins, ATC code: G03GA05 / G03GA07.

Pergoveris is a preparation of follicle stimulating hormone and luteinising hormone produced by genetically engineered Chinese Hamster Ovary (CHO) cells.

In clinical trials the efficacy of the combination of follitropin alfa and lutropin alfa has been demonstrated in women with hypogonadotropic hypogonadism.

In the stimulation of follicular development in anovulatory women deficient in LH and FSH, the primary effect resulting from administration of lutropin alfa is an increase in oestradiol secretion by the follicles, the growth of which is stimulated by FSH.

In one clinical study of women with hypogonadotrophic hypogonadism and an endogenous serum LH concentration below 1.2 IU/L the appropriate dose of r-hLH (lutropin alfa) was investigated. A dose of 75 IU r-hLH daily (in combination with 150 IU follitropin alfa (r-hFSH)) resulted in adequate follicular development and oestrogen production. A dose of 25 IU r-hLH daily (in combination with 150 IU follitropin alfa) resulted in insufficient follicular development. Therefore, administration of less than one vial of Pergoveris daily may provide too little LH-activity to ensure adequate follicular development.

5.2 Pharmacokinetic properties

Follitropin alfa and lutropin alfa have shown the same pharmacokinetic profile as follitropin alfa and lutropin alfa separately.

Follitropin alfa

Following intravenous administration, follitropin alfa is distributed to the extracellular fluid space with an initial half-life of around 2 hours and eliminated from the body with a terminal half-life of about one day. The steady state volume of distribution and total clearance are 10 l and 0.6 l/h, respectively. One-eighth of the follitropin alfa dose is excreted in the urine.

Following subcutaneous administration, the absolute bioavailability is about 70%. Following repeated administration, follitropin alfa accumulates 3-fold achieving asteady-state within 3-4 days. In women whose endogenous gonadotrophin secretion is suppressed, follitropin alfa has nevertheless been shown to effectively stimulate follicular development and steroidogenesis, despite unmeasurable LH levels.

Lutropin alfa

Following intravenous administration, lutropin alfa is rapidly distributed with an initial half-life of approximately one hour and eliminated from the body with a terminal half-life of about 10-12 hours. The steady state volume of distribution is around 10-14 l. Lutropin alfa shows linear pharmacokinetics, as assessed by AUC which is directly proportional to the dose administered. Total clearance is around 2 l/h, and less than 5% of the dose is excreted in the urine. The mean residence time is approximately 5 hours.

Following subcutaneous administration, the absolute bioavailability is approximately 60%; the terminal half-life is slightly prolonged. The lutropin alfa pharmacokinetics following single and repeated administration of lutropin alfa are comparable and the accumulation ratio of lutropin alfa is minimal. There is no pharmacokinetic interaction with follitropin alfa when administered simultaneously.

5.3 Preclinical safety data

Non-clinical data reveal no special hazard for humans based on conventional studies of safety pharmacology, repeated dose toxicity and genotoxicity.

6. PHARMACEUTICAL PARTICULARS

6.1 List of excipients

Powder:

Sucrose

Polysorbate 20

Methionine

Disodium phosphate dihydrate

Sodium dihydrogen phosphate monohydrate

Phosphoric acid, concentrated for pH adjustment

Sodium hydroxide for pH adjustment

Solvent:

Water for Injections

6.2 Incompatibilities

This medicinal product must not be mixed with other medicinal products except those mentioned in section 6.6.

6.3 Shelf life

3 years.

For immediate and single use following first opening and reconstitution.

6.4 Special precautions for storage

Do not store above 25°C.

Store in the original package in order to protect from light.

6.5 Nature and contents of container

Powder: 3 ml vials (Type I glass) with a stopper (bromobutyl rubber) and aluminium flip-off cap.

1 vial contains 11 micrograms r-hFSH and 3 micrograms r-hLH.

Solvent: 3 ml vials (Type I glass) with a Teflon coated rubber stopper and aluminium flip-off cap.

1 vial of solvent contains 1 ml of water for injections.

The medicinal product is supplied in pack sizes of 1, 3 and 10 vials with the corresponding number of 1, 3 and 10 vials of solvent.

Not all pack sizes may be marketed.

6.6 Special precautions for disposal and other handling

For single use only.

Pergoveris must be reconstituted with the solvent before use.

The reconstituted solution should not be administered if it contains particles or is not clear.

Pergoveris may be mixed with follitropin alfa and co-administered as a single injection.

Any unused medicinal product or waste material should be disposed of in accordance with local requirements.

7. MARKETING AUTHORISATION HOLDER

Merck Serono Europe Limited

56 Marsh Wall

London E14 9TP

United Kingdom

8. MARKETING AUTHORISATION NUMBER(S)

EU/1/07/396/001

EU/1/07/396/002

EU/1/07/396/003

9. DATE OF FIRST AUTHORISATION/RENEWAL OF THE AUTHORISATION

25 June 2007

10. DATE OF REVISION OF THE TEXT

July 2009

Periactin

(Merck Sharp & Dohme Limited)

1. NAME OF THE MEDICINAL PRODUCT

PERIACTIN® 4 mg Tablets

2. QUALITATIVE AND QUANTITATIVE COMPOSITION

Each 'Periactin' tablet contains cyproheptadine hydrochloride equivalent to 4 mg anhydrous cyproheptadine hydrochloride.

3. PHARMACEUTICAL FORM

White round bevelled edged tablet with a scoreline on one side and marked 'MSD 62' on the other.

4. CLINICAL PARTICULARS

4.1 Therapeutic indications

'Periactin' is a serotonin and histamine antagonist with anticholinergic and sedative properties.

In allergy and pruritus: 'Periactin' has a wide range of antiallergic and antipruritic activity, and can be used successfully in the treatment of acute and chronic allergic and pruritic conditions, such as dermatitis, including neurodermatitis and neurodermatitis circumscripta; eczema; eczematoid dermatitis; dermatographism; mild, local allergic reactions to insect bites; hay fever and other seasonal rhinitis; perennial allergic and vasomotor rhinitis; allergic conjunctivitis due to inhalant allergens and foods; urticaria; angioneurotic oedema; drug and serum reactions; anogenital pruritus; pruritus of chicken-pox.

'Periactin' is indicated as adjunctive therapy to adrenaline and other standard measures for the relief of anaphylactic reactions after the acute manifestations have been controlled.

In migraine and vascular headache: 'Periactin' has been reported to have beneficial effects in a significant number of patients having vascular types of headache. Many patients who have responded inadequately to all other agents have reported amelioration of symptoms with 'Periactin'. The characteristic headache and feeling of malaise may disappear within an hour or two of the first dose.

4.2 Posology and method of administration

Route of administration: oral.

There is no recommended dosage for children under 2 years old. 'Periactin' is not recommended for elderly, debilitated patients.

For the treatment of allergy and pruritus:

Dosage must be determined on an individual basis. The effect of a single dose usually lasts for four to six hours. For continuous effective relief, the daily requirement should be given in divided doses, usually three times a day, or as often as necessary, to provide continuous relief.

Adults: The therapeutic range is 4-20 mg (1 to 5 tablets) a day, most patients requiring 12-16 mg a day. It is recommended that dosage be initiated with 4 mg three times a day and then adjusted according to the weight and response of the patient up to a maximum of 32 mg a day.

Children aged 7-14 years: Usually 4 mg two or three times a day, according to the patient's weight and response. If an additional dose is required, it should be given at bedtime. Maximum 16 mg a day.

Children aged 2-6 years: Initially 2 mg two or three times a day, adjusted according to the patient's weight and response. If an additional dose is required, it should be given at bedtime. Maximum 12 mg a day.

For treatment of vascular headache and migraine

For both prophylactic and therapeutic use, an initial dose of 4 mg, repeated if necessary after half an hour. Patients who respond usually obtain relief with 8 mg, and this dose should not be exceeded within a 4- to 6-hour period.

Maintenance: 4 mg every four to six hours.

Use in the elderly: 'Periactin' should not be used in elderly, debilitated patients. Elderly patients are more likely to experience dizziness, sedation, and hypotension.

4.3 Contraindications

'Periactin' is contraindicated in:

- patients undergoing therapy for an acute asthmatic attack;
- newborn or premature infants; use in infants has been associated with apnoea, cyanosis and respiratory difficulty
- breast-feeding mothers;
- patients with known sensitivity to cyproheptadine hydrochloride or drugs with similar chemical structure;
- concurrent use with monoamine oxidase inhibitors;
- glaucoma;
- patients with pyloroduodenal obstruction, stenosing peptic ulcer, symptomatic prostatic hypertrophy, predisposition to urinary retention or bladder neck obstruction;
- elderly, debilitated patients.

4.4 Special warnings and precautions for use

Antihistamines should not be used to treat lower respiratory tract symptoms, including those of acute asthma.

The safety and efficacy of 'Periactin' is not established in children under 2 years old.

Overdosage of antihistamines, particularly in infants and children, may produce hallucinations, central nervous system depression, convulsions, respiratory and cardiac arrest, and death.

Antihistamines may diminish mental alertness; conversely, particularly in the young child, they may occasionally produce excitation.

Patients should be warned against engaging in activities requiring motor co-ordination and mental alertness, such as driving a car or operating machinery (see section 4.7 'Effects on ability to drive and use machines').

Rarely, prolonged therapy with antihistamines may cause blood dyscrasias.

Because 'Periactin' has an atropine-like action, it should be used cautiously in patients with a history of bronchial asthma, increased intra-ocular pressure, hyperthyroidism, cardiovascular disease, or hypertension.

Excipients

Patients with rare hereditary problems of galactose intolerance, the Lapp lactase deficiency or glucose-galactose malabsorption should not take this medicine.

4.5 Interaction with other medicinal products and other forms of interaction

MAO inhibitors prolong and intensify the anticholinergic effects of antihistamines.

Antihistamines may have additive effects with alcohol and other CNS depressants, e.g. hypnotics, sedatives, tranquillisers and anti-anxiety agents.

Drugs with anti-serotonin activity, such as cyproheptadine, may interfere with serotonin-enhancing anti-depressants including selective serotonin re-uptake inhibitors (SSRI's). This may result in possible recurrence of depression and related symptoms.

Cyproheptadine may cause a false positive test result for tricyclic antidepressant drugs (TCA) when evaluating a drug screen (e.g. urine, serum). Because cyproheptadine and TCAs may produce similar overdose symptoms, physicians should carefully monitor patients for TCA toxicity in the event of combined overdose.

4.6 Pregnancy and lactation

The use of any drug in pregnancy or in women of child-bearing age requires that the potential benefit of the drug should be weighed against possible hazards to the embryo and foetus. It is not known whether 'Periactin' is excreted in human milk, and because of the potential for serious adverse reactions in breast-feeding infants from 'Periactin', a decision should be made whether to discontinue breast-feeding or to discontinue the drug, taking into account the importance of the drug to the mother (see section 4.3 'Contraindications').

4.7 Effects on ability to drive and use machines

This product may cause drowsiness and somnolence. Patients receiving it should not drive or operate machinery unless it has been shown that their physical and mental capacity remains unaffected.

4.8 Undesirable effects

The side effects that appear frequently are drowsiness and somnolence. Many patients who initially complain of drowsiness may no longer do so after the first three to four days of continuous administration.

Side effects reported with antihistamines are:

Central nervous system: Sedation, sleepiness (often transient), dizziness, disturbed co-ordination, confusion, restlessness, excitation, nervousness, tremor, irritability, aggressive behaviour, insomnia, paraesthesiae, neuritis, convulsions, euphoria, hallucinations, hysteria, faintness.

Integumentary: Allergic manifestations of rash and oedema, excessive perspiration, urticaria, photosensitivity.

Special senses: Acute labyrinthitis, blurred vision, diplopia, vertigo, tinnitus.

Cardiovascular: Hypotension, palpitation, tachycardia, extrasystoles, anaphylactic shock.

Haematological: Haemolytic anaemia, leucopenia, agranulocytosis, thrombocytopenia.

Digestive system: Cholestasis, hepatic failure, hepatitis, hepatic function abnormality, dryness of mouth, epigastric distress, anorexia, nausea, vomiting, diarrhoea, constipation, jaundice.

Genito-urinary: Frequency and difficulty of micturition, urinary retention, early menses.

Respiratory: Dryness of the nose and throat, thickening of bronchial secretions, tightness of chest and wheezing, nasal stuffiness, epistaxis.

Miscellaneous: Fatigue, rigors, headache, increased appetite/weight gain.

4.9 Overdose

Antihistamine overdosage reactions may vary from CNS depression or stimulation to convulsions, respiratory and cardiac arrest and death, especially in infants and children. Atropine-like and gastro-intestinal symptoms may occur.

If vomiting has not occurred spontaneously, it should be induced in the conscious patient with syrup of ipecac. If the patient cannot vomit, gastric lavage with isotonic or half isotonic saline is indicated, followed by activated charcoal. Precautions against aspiration must be taken, especially in infants and children.

Life-threatening CNS signs and symptoms should be treated appropriately.

Saline cathartics usefully draw water into the bowel by osmosis to dilute bowel content rapidly.

Central stimulants must not be used, but vasopressors may be used to counteract hypotension.

5. PHARMACOLOGICAL PROPERTIES

5.1 Pharmacodynamic properties

Cyproheptadine hydrochloride is a serotonin and histamine antagonist with anticholinergic and sedative effects. Antiserotonin and antihistamine drugs appear to compete with serotonin and histamine, respectively, for receptor sites.

Cyproheptadine hydrochloride antagonises the following effects of serotonin, in laboratory animals:

Bronchoconstrictor (guinea-pig)

Vasopressor (dog)

Spasmogenic (isolated rat uterus)

Oedema (rat)

Lethal (haemophilus pertussis-treated mouse)

In these effects it equals or surpasses the activity of many of the activities of specific serotonin antagonists, such as 1-Benzyl-2-methyl-5-methoxy-tryptame (BAS) and 1 Benzyl-2methyl-5-hydroxy-tryptamine (BMS), in contrast, specific antihistamines, even the most potent, show little or no serotonin antagonism.

Cyproheptadine hydrochloride antagonises or blocks the following effects of histamine in laboratory animals:

Bronchoconstrictor (guinea-pig)

Vasopressor (dog)

Spasmogenic (isolated rat uterus)

Anaphylactic shock, active and passive (guinea-pig and mouse)

Increased gastric secretion (Heidenhain pouch dog.)

It is unusual that cyproheptadine hydrochloride protects both the guinea-pig and mice against anaphylactic shock. In guinea-pigs, the pulmonary aspects of anaphylactic shock are attributable to the release of endogenous histamine and can be controlled by substances with specific antihistamine activity. In mice however, where histamine release seems to be less important and serotonin release may be involved, specific antihistamines are of little value in protecting against anaphylaxis. Thus the protective effect of cyproheptadine hydrochloride in mice may be an anti-serotonin effect.

The inhibitory effect of cyproheptadine in histamine-induced gastric secretion is also unusual as specific antihistamines do not influence this effect.

Cyproheptadine has appetite stimulation properties in laboratory animals.

5.2 Pharmacokinetic properties

After a single 4 mg oral dose of ^{14}C-labelled cyproheptadine hydrochloride in normal subjects given as tablets or syrup, 2 to 20% of the radioactivity was excreted in the stools. Only about 34% of the stool radioactivity was unchanged drug, corresponding to less than 5.7% of the dose. At least 40% of the administered radioactivity was excreted in the urine.

No significant difference in the mean urinary excretion exists between the tablet and syrup formulations. No detectable amounts of unchanged drug were present in the urine of patients on chronic 12-20 mg daily doses of 'Periactin' syrup. The principle metabolite found in human urine has been identified as a quaternary ammonium glucuronide conjugate of cyproheptadine. Elimination is diminished in renal insufficiency.

5.3 Preclinical safety data

No relevant information.

6. PHARMACEUTICAL PARTICULARS

6.1 List of excipients

'Periactin' tablets contain the following inactive ingredients: calcium hydrogen phosphate E341, lactose, magnesium stearate E572, potato starch and pregelatinised maize starch.

6.2 Incompatibilities

None known.

6.3 Shelf life

3 years.

6.4 Special precautions for storage

Do not store above 25°C. Store in the original package.

6.5 Nature and contents of container

30 tablets in opaque PVC blisters with hard-temper aluminium lidding.

6.6 Special precautions for disposal and other handling

None.

7. MARKETING AUTHORISATION HOLDER

Merck Sharp & Dohme Limited

Hertford Road, Hoddesdon, Hertfordshire EN11 9BU, UK.

8. MARKETING AUTHORISATION NUMBER(S)

Tablets PL 0025/5017R

9. DATE OF FIRST AUTHORISATION/RENEWAL OF THE AUTHORISATION

Licence granted: 3 October 1990

Last renewed: 14 August 2001

10. DATE OF REVISION OF THE TEXT

14 November 2008

LEGAL CATEGORY

P.

® denotes registered trademark of Merck & Co., Inc., Whitehouse Station, NJ, USA.

SPC.PCTT.07.UK.2804

Perinal Cutaneous Spray

(Dermal Laboratories Limited)

1. NAME OF THE MEDICINAL PRODUCT

PERINAL™ CUTANEOUS SPRAY

2. QUALITATIVE AND QUANTITATIVE COMPOSITION

Hydrocortisone 0.2 % w/w; Lidocaine Hydrochloride 1.0% w/w.

3. PHARMACEUTICAL FORM

Colourless to pale yellow aqueous cutaneous spray solution.

4. CLINICAL PARTICULARS

4.1 Therapeutic indications

For the symptomatic relief of anal and perianal itch, irritation and pain, such as associated with haemorrhoids.

4.2 Posology and method of administration

The same dosage schedule applies to all age groups, although the spray is not normally recommended for children under 14 years unless on medical advice:-

Spray once over the affected area up to three times daily, depending on the severity of the condition.

4.3 Contraindications

Not to be used if sensitive to lidocaine or any of the other ingredients. Not to be used on broken or infected skin. Not to be used internally (inside the anus), or anywhere other than the anal area.

4.4 Special warnings and precautions for use

Perinal Spray is intended for use for limited periods and so should not be used continuously for longer than 7 days without medical advice. Patients should be instructed to seek medical advice if they experience persistent pain or bleeding from the anus, especially where associated with a change in bowel habit, if the stomach is distended or if they are losing weight. Prompt medical treatment may be very important under such circumstances. Perinal Spray should be kept away from the eyes, nose and mouth.

The label will state:-

Perinal Spray should not be used during pregnancy, while breast feeding or by children under the age of 14 without medical advice. Keep spray away from the eyes, nose and mouth, and do not apply to broken or infected skin, or to any part of the body except the anal area. Prime pump before initial use by depressing its top once or twice. Wash hands, and replace cap after use. Consult your doctor if the condition does not improve, or if rectal bleeding occurs. Do not use continuously for more than 7 days, unless recommended by your doctor. Do not use if sensitive to any of the ingredients. Keep out of the reach of children. For external use only.

4.5 Interaction with other medicinal products and other forms of interaction

No known interactions. Medical supervision is required if used in conjunction with other medicines containing steroids, owing to possible additive effects.

4.6 Pregnancy and lactation

There is inadequate evidence of safety in human pregnancy. Topical administration of corticosteroids to pregnant animals can cause abnormalities of foetal development including cleft palate and intra-uterine growth retardation. There may therefore be a very small risk of such effects in the human foetus. The risk/benefit needs to be carefully assessed, therefore, before prescribing this medicine.

4.7 Effects on ability to drive and use machines

None known.

4.8 Undesirable effects

A temporary tingling sensation may be experienced locally after initial application. Hypersensitivity to lidocaine has rarely been reported.

4.9 Overdose

Under exceptional circumstances, if Perinal Spray is used excessively, particularly in young children, it is theoretically possible that adrenal suppression and skin thinning may occur. The symptoms are normally reversible on cessation of treatment.

5. PHARMACOLOGICAL PROPERTIES

5.1 Pharmacodynamic properties

The preparation combines the well-known local anti-inflammatory and anti-pruritic properties of hydrocortisone and the analgesic effect of lidocaine in an aqueous spray formulation. On application, finger contact with the affected area can be avoided which makes for improved hygiene, and lessens the risk of infection.

5.2 Pharmacokinetic properties

The active ingredients of the formulation are readily available for intimate contact with the skin and mucous membranes, as the preparation is sprayed in small droplets which dry after application to leave the active ingredients in close contact with the affected area.

Because the preparation is a clear solution, it is entirely homogeneous, and the availability of the active ingredient is optimal.

5.3 Preclinical safety data

No special information.

6. PHARMACEUTICAL PARTICULARS

6.1 List of excipients

Cetomacrogol 1000; Citric Acid Monohydrate; Sodium Citrate; Propyl Gallate; Phenoxyethanol; Purified Water.

6.2 Incompatibilities

None known.

6.3 Shelf life

30 months.

6.4 Special precautions for storage

Do not store above 25°C.

6.5 Nature and contents of container

30 ml collapsible laminate tube with metering-dose spray pump and cap, which is ozone-friendly.

The spray operates when held in any direction. It is *not* an aerosol and does *not* contain any potentially irritant propellants.

6.6 Special precautions for disposal and other handling

Not applicable.

7. MARKETING AUTHORISATION HOLDER

Dermal Laboratories

Tatmore Place, Gosmore

Hitchin, Herts SG4 7QR, UK.

8. MARKETING AUTHORISATION NUMBER(S)

00173/0049.

9. DATE OF FIRST AUTHORISATION/RENEWAL OF THE AUTHORISATION

5 June 2002.

10. DATE OF REVISION OF THE TEXT

August 2008.

Periostat 20mg film-coated tablets

(Alliance Pharmaceuticals)

1. NAME OF THE MEDICINAL PRODUCT

PERIOSTAT® 20 mg film-coated tablets

2. QUALITATIVE AND QUANTITATIVE COMPOSITION

Each film-coated tablet contains 23.08 mg doxycycline hyclate equivalent to 20 mg doxycycline.

For excipients, see 6.1

3. PHARMACEUTICAL FORM

Film-coated tablet

White to off-white round tablets imprinted on one side with PS-20

4. CLINICAL PARTICULARS

4.1 Therapeutic indications

For patients with adult periodontitis. PERIOSTAT is indicated as an adjunct to supra-gingival and sub-gingival scaling and root planing, with oral hygiene instruction, carried out by a dental practitioner or hygienist as appropriate.

4.2 Posology and method of administration

Adults and the elderly:

PERIOSTAT 20 mg should be administered twice daily, at least one hour before meals or before bedtime. Tablets should be swallowed whole with adequate fluids (at least 100ml of water) and should be taken in an upright sitting or standing position (see 4.4: Special warnings and Precautions for Use).

PERIOSTAT is indicated for treatment periods of 3 months. PERIOSTAT should not be administered for more than 3 consecutive three month periods.

No dosage modification is necessary in elderly patients.

Renal Impairment:

No dosage adjustment is necessary in the presence of renal impairment.

Children:

For use in children, see 'Contraindications'.

4.3 Contraindications

In common with other drugs of the tetracycline class, PERIOSTAT is contra-indicated in infants and children up to 12 years of age.

Doxycycline should not be administered to patients who have shown hypersensitivity to doxycycline hyclate, other tetracyclines or to any of the excipients.

Patients known to have, or suspected to have, achlorhydria should not be prescribed doxycycline.

Use of doxycycline is contra-indicated during pregnancy and lactation (See 4.6 Pregnancy and lactation).

4.4 Special warnings and precautions for use

Tablet forms of the tetracycline class of drugs may cause oesophageal irritation and ulceration. To avoid oesophageal irritation and ulceration, adequate fluids should be taken with this medication. PERIOSTAT should be swallowed whilst in an upright sitting or standing posture. Tablets taken in the evening should be taken well in advance of retiring (see 4.2: Posology and Method of Administration).

Whilst no overgrowth by opportunistic microorganisms such as yeast were noted during clinical studies, PERIOSTAT therapy may result in overgrowth of nonsusceptible microorganisms including fungi (with clinical symptoms of persistent bad breath, reddening of the gums, etc.). Periodic observation of the patient is essential. PERIOSTAT therapy has been associated with diarrhoea, colitis and vaginal moniliasis which may suggest overgrowth of non-susceptible micro-organisms. If overgrowth by resistant organisms appears, PERIOSTAT therapy should be discontinued and an appropriate treatment instituted.

PERIOSTAT should be used with caution in patients with a history of or predisposition to oral candidosis. The safety and effectiveness of PERIOSTAT has not been established for the treatment of periodontitis in patients with coexistent oral candidosis. Whilst not observed during clinical trials with PERIOSTAT, the use of tetracyclines may increase the incidence of vaginal candidosis.

The blood doxycycline levels in patients treated with PERIOSTAT are lower than in those treated with conventional antimicrobial formulations of doxycycline. As, however, there are no data to support safety in hepatic impairment at this lower dose, PERIOSTAT should be administered with caution to patients with hepatic impairment or to those receiving potentially hepatotoxic drugs.

Caution should be observed in the treatment of patients with myasthenia gravis who may be at risk of worsening of the condition.

All patients receiving doxycycline including PERIOSTAT should be advised to avoid excessive sunlight or artificial ultraviolet light while receiving doxycycline and to discontinue therapy if phototoxicity (e.g., skin eruption etc) occurs. Sunscreen or sunblock should be considered. Treatment should cease at the first sign of skin erythema.

In common with the use of antimicrobial drugs in general, there is a risk of the development of pseudomembranous colitis with doxycycline treatment. In the event of the development of diarrhoea during treatment with PERIOSTAT, the possibility of pseudomembranous colitis should be considered and appropriate therapy instituted. This may include the discontinuation of doxycycline and the institution of specific antibiotic therapy (e.g vancomycin). Agents inhibiting peristalsis should not be employed in this situation.

In the event of a severe acute hypersensitivity reaction (e.g. anaphylaxis), treatment with PERIOSTAT must be stopped at once and the usual emergency measures taken (e.g. administration of antihistamines, corticosteroids, sympathomimetics and if necessary artificial respiration instituted).

Patients with rare hereditary problems of galactose intolerance, the Lapp lactase deficiency or glucose-galactose malabsorption should not take this medicine.

4.5 Interaction with other medicinal products and other forms of interaction

These recommendations regarding the potential interactions between doxycycline and other medications are based upon the larger doses generally used in antimicrobial formulations of doxycycline rather than with PERIOSTAT. However at the present time, insufficient data exist for reassurance that the interactions described with higher doses of doxycycline will not occur with PERIOSTAT.

The absorption of doxycycline from the gastro-intestinal tract may be inhibited by bi- or tri- valent ions such as aluminium, zinc, calcium (found for example in milk, dairy products and calcium-containing fruit juices), by magnesium (found for example in antacids) or by iron preparations, activated charcoal, cholestyramine, bismuth chelates and sucralfate. Therefore such medicines or foodstuffs should be taken after a period of 2 to 3 hours following ingestion of PERIOSTAT. Didanosine tablets may decrease the absorption of doxycycline due to the gastric pH increase as a consequence of the antacid content of the didanosine tablets. Didanosine should therefore be taken at least 2 hours after doxycycline. Quinapril may reduce the absorption of doxycycline due to the high magnesium content in quinapril tablets.

Doxycycline has been shown to potentiate the hypoglycaemic effect of sulfonylurea oral antidiabetic agents. If administered in combination with these drugs, blood sugar levels should be monitored and if necessary, the doses of the above drugs reduced.

Doxycycline has been shown to depress plasma prothrombin activity thereby potentiating the effect of anticoagulants of the dicoumarol type. If administered in combination with these agents, coagulation parameters, including INR, should be monitored and if necessary, the doses of the above drugs reduced. The possibility of an increased risk of bleeding events should be borne in mind.

When doxycycline is administered shortly before, during or after courses of isotretinoin, there is the possibility of potentiation between the drugs to cause reversible pressure increase in the intracranial cavity (pseudotumour cerebri). Concomitant administration should therefore be avoided.

Bacteriostatic drugs including doxycycline may interfere with the bacteriocidal action of penicillin and betalactam antibiotics. It is advisable that PERIOSTAT and betalactam antibiotics should not therefore be used in combination.

Rifampicin, barbiturates, carbamazepine, diphenylhydantoin, primidone, phenytoin, and chronic alcohol abuse, may accelerate the decomposition of doxycycline due to enzyme induction in the liver thereby decreasing its half-life. Sub-therapeutic doxycycline concentrations may result. Doxycycline used concurrently with cyclosporin has been reported to decrease the half-life of doxycycline.

Tetracyclines and methoxyflurane used in combination have been reported to result in fatal renal toxicity.

Tetracyclines used concurrently with oral contraceptives have in a few cases resulted in either breakthrough bleeding or pregnancy.

4.6 Pregnancy and lactation

Use in Pregnancy:

Studies in animals have not demonstrated a teratogenic effect. In humans, the use of tetracyclines during a limited number of pregnancies has not revealed any specific malformation to date. The administration of tetracyclines during the second and the third trimesters results in permanent discolouration of the deciduous teeth in the offspring.

As a consequence, PERIOSTAT is contraindicated during pregnancy (see 4.3: Contraindications).

Use in Lactation:

Tetracyclines are secreted into the milk of lactating women. PERIOSTAT should therefore not be used in breast-feeding mothers.

4.7 Effects on ability to drive and use machines

PERIOSTAT therapy has been associated with nausea and dizziness. Those affected should not drive or operate machinery.

4.8 Undesirable effects

The most commonly reported adverse reactions in Phase III trials were headache (26%) and common cold (22%). The following table lists those adverse reactions occurring in four Phase III trials conducted in 213 patients.

(see Table 1 below)

The following adverse reactions have been observed in patients receiving tetracyclines, including doxycycline:-

Gastrointestinal: Anorexia, nausea, vomiting, diarrhoea, glossitis, dysphagia, enterocolitis and inflammatory lesions with monilial overgrowth in the anogenital region.

Table 1

Organ System	Undesirable Effect	Very Common (>1/10)	Common (>1/100, <1/10)	Uncommon (>1/1000, <1/100)	Rare (>1/10000, <1/1000)
Infections & Infestations	Infection Periodontal Abscess		4 8		
Respiratory	Common Cold	47			
	Flu Symptoms	24			
	Sinusitis		18		
	Coughing		9		
	Bronchitis		7		
Gastrointestinal	Dyspepsia		13		
	Diarrhoea		12		
	Acid Indigestion		8		
Skin Disorders	Rash		8		
Musculoskeletal	Toothache		14		
	Joint Pain		12		
	Back Pain		11		
	Pain		8		
	Muscle Pain			2	
	Gum Pain			1	
Reproductive	Menstrual Cramps		9		
General	Headache	55			
	Nausea		17		
	Tooth Disorder		13		
	Sore Throat		11		
	Sinus Headache		8		
Injury	Accidental Injury		11		

Hepatotoxicity has been reported rarely. These reactions have been caused by both the oral and parenteral administration of tetracyclines. Oesophagitis and oesophageal ulceration have been reported, most often in patients administered the hyclate salt in capsule form. Most of these patients took medication just prior to going to bed.

Skin: Maculo papular, erythematous rashes and Stevens-Johnson syndrome. Skin photosensitivity can occur. Exfoliative dermatitis has been reported but is uncommon.

Renal: An apparently dose related increase in blood urea has been reported with tetracyclines.

Blood: Thrombocytopenia, neutropenia, haemolytic anaemia, eosinophilia and porphyriahave been reported with tetracyclines.

Hypersensitivity reactions: Exacerbation of systemic lupus erythematosus, anaphylaxis, anaphylactoid purpura, pericarditis, urticaria and angioneurotic oedema.

Musculoskeletal: Arthralgia

Other: Bulging fontanelles in infants and benign intracranial hypertension in adults has been reported with the use of tetracyclines. Treatment should cease if evidence of raised intracranial pressure develops. These conditions disappeared rapidly when the drug was discontinued. Brown-black microscopic discolouration of thyroid tissue has been reported with long-term use of tetracyclines. Thyroid function is normal.

Adverse reactions typical of the tetracycline class of drugs are less likely to occur during medication with PERIOSTAT, due to the reduced dosage and the relatively low serum levels involved. This assertion is supported by several clinical trials which suggest that no significant differences exist with regard to frequency of adverse events between active and placebo groupings. However, the clinician should always be aware of the possibility of adverse events occurring and should monitor patients accordingly.

The following adverse events have been reported during post-marketing:

(Frequency estimate: very common > 1 in 10; common >1 in 100 to <1 in 10; uncommon >1 in 1000 to <1 in 100; rare >1 in 10,000 to <1 in 1000; very rare <1 in 10,000)

<u>Infections</u>

Rare: Vaginal moniliasis, Anogenital moniliasis

<u>Immune system disorders</u>

Rare: Mild allergic reactions

<u>Nervous system disorders</u>

Rare: Headache

Very rare: Dizziness

<u>Gastrointestinal disorders</u>

Rare: Nausea, diarrhoea, dyspepsia

Very rare: Abdominal pain, constipation, dry mouth, superficial tooth discolouration

There have been isolated case reports of bloody diarrhoea, colitis and pseudomembranous colitis.

<u>Skin and subcutaneous tissue disorders</u>

Rare: Rash

Very rare: Urticaria, pruritus, skin photosensitivity

<u>Musculoskeletal disorders</u>

Very rare: Arthralgia

<u>General disorders</u>

Very rare: Asthenia

4.9 Overdose

To date no significant acute toxicity has been described in the case of a single oral intake of a multiple of therapeutic doses of doxycycline. In case of overdosage there is, however, a risk of parenchymatous hepatic and renal damage and of pancreatitis.

The usual dose of PERIOSTAT is low when compared with the usual doses for doxycycline when used for antimicrobial therapy. Therefore clinicians should bear in mind that a significant proportion of overdoses are likely to produce blood concentrations of doxycycline within the therapeutic range of antimicrobial treatment, for which there is a large quantity of data supporting the safety of the drug. In these cases observation is recommended. In cases of significant overdosage, doxycycline therapy should be stopped immediately; and symptomatic measures undertaken as required. Intestinal absorption of unabsorbed doxycycline should be minimised by producing non-absorbable chelate complexes by the administration of magnesium or calcium salt containing antacids. Gastric lavage should be considered.

Dialysis does not alter serum half-life and thus would not be of benefit in treating cases of overdosage.

5. PHARMACOLOGICAL PROPERTIES

5.1 Pharmacodynamic properties

Pharmacotherapeutic group: Tetracyclines

ATC code: J01A A02

The active ingredient of PERIOSTAT, doxycycline, is synthetically derived from oxytetracycline, with a molecular formula of $C_{22}H_{24}N_2O_8 \bullet HCl \bullet \frac{1}{2} C_2H_5OH \bullet \frac{1}{2} H_2O$.

PERIOSTAT is an inhibitor of collagenase activity. Studies have shown that at the proposed 20 mg b.i.d. dose level, PERIOSTAT reduces the elevated collagenase activity in the gingival crevicular fluid of patients with chronic adult periodontitis, whilst not demonstrating any clinical evidence of anti-microbial activity.

Susceptibility

The dosage achieved with this product during administration is well below the concentration required to inhibit microorganisms commonly associated with adult periodontitis. Clinical studies with this product demonstrated no effect on total anaerobic and facultative bacteria in plaque samples from patients administered this dose regimen for 9 to 18 months. This product **SHOULD NOT** be used for reducing the numbers of, or eliminating, those microorganisms associated with periodontitis.

5.2 Pharmacokinetic properties

Absorption:

Doxycycline is almost completely absorbed after oral administration. Following ingestion of 20 mg doxycycline twice daily, mean maximum plasma concentrations were 0.79 μg/ml. Peak levels were generally achieved 2 hours after administration. Food intake reduced the extent of absorption by 10% and decreased and delayed the peak plasma levels.

Distribution:

Doxycycline is greater than 90% bound to plasma proteins and has an apparent volume of distribution of 50L.

Metabolism:

Major metabolic pathways of doxycycline have not been identified, however, enzyme inducers decrease the half-life of doxycycline.

Elimination:

Doxycycline is excreted in the urine and faeces as unchanged drug. Between 40% and 60% of an administered dose can be accounted for in the urine by 92 hours, and approximately 30% in the faeces. The terminal half-life after a single 20 mg doxycycline dose averaged 18h.

Special populations:

The half-life is not significantly altered in patients with severely impaired renal function. Doxycycline is not eliminated to any great extent during haemodialysis.

5.3 Preclinical safety data

The carcinogenic potential of doxycycline has been investigated and no changes indicative of a direct carcinogenic effect were seen. Increases in benign tumours of the mammary gland (fibroadenoma), uterus (polyp) and thyroid (C-cell adenoma), which are consistent with a hormonal effect, were observed in treated females. Doxycycline has shown no mutagenic activity and no convincing evidence of clastogenic activity.

Effects on fertility and reproductive performance and on pre- and post-natal toxicity have been assessed in rats over the dose range 50 to 500 mg/kg/day. At 50 mg/kg/day (88 times the human dose) there was a decrease in the straight-line velocity of sperm, but there was no apparent effect on male or female fertility or on sperm morphology. Maternal toxicity at 500 mg/kg/day was shown by noisy breathing, loose faeces, and transient reductions in both body weight gain and food consumption after parturition with a slight increase in the duration of gestation. No maternal toxicity was apparent at or below 100 mg/kg/day and there was no effect on the F1 generation at 50 mg/kg/day during parturition, lactation or post-weaning. Developmental toxicity studies have not been conducted, but doxycycline is known to cross the placenta.

Hyperpigmentation of the thyroid following administration of members of the tetracycline class has been observed in rats, minipigs, dogs and monkeys and thyroid hyperplasia has occurred in rats, dogs, chickens and mice.

The anticipated human dose for doxycycline, 20 mg b.i.d. is equivalent to ~0.5 mg/kg/day for a 70 kg man. At this dose plasma C_{max} and AUC_{0-24} were 780 ng/ml and 10954 ng*h/ml respectively.

Toxicity following repeated oral administration has been evaluated in rats and cynomolgus monkeys. Discolouration of the thyroid was a finding common to rats exposed at 25 mg/kg/day for 13 weeks or 20 mg/kg/day for 26 weeks, and to cynomolgus monkeys at 30 mg/kg/day for 1 year. C_{max} and AUC_{0-24} following a single oral dose of 25 mg/kg were 2.2 and 1.6 times respectively the values recorded in man. Dose-related increases in both the incidence and severity of tubular degeneration/regeneration in the kidney were seen following administration to cynomolgus monkeys for 28 days or 52 weeks. At 5 mg/kg/day, focal lesions were present after 28 days, but no lesions were present in monkeys treated for 52 weeks. Mean plasma C_{max} and AUC_{0-24} values at 28 days in monkeys receiving 5 mg/kg/day were 1235 ng/ml and 11600 ng*h/ml respectively and there was no evidence of accumulation.

In humans the use of tetracyclines during tooth development may cause permanent discolouration of the teeth (yellow-grey-brown). This reaction is more common during long-term use of the drug but has been observed following repeated short-term courses. Enamel hypoplasia has also been reported. As for other tetracyclines, doxycycline forms a stable calcium complex in any bone-forming tissue. A decrease in the fibula growth has been observed in premature infants given oral tetracycline in doses of 25 mg/kg every 6 hours. This reaction was shown to be reversible when the drug was discontinued.

6. PHARMACEUTICAL PARTICULARS

6.1 List of excipients

Tablet core:

Magnesium stearate

Microcrystalline cellulose

Film coating:

Lactose monohydrate

Hypromellose (E464)

Titanium dioxide (E171)

Triacetin

6.2 Incompatibilities

Not applicable.

6.3 Shelf life

Three years

6.4 Special precautions for storage

Do not store above 25°C.

6.5 Nature and contents of container

PVC Aclar/aluminium foil blisters containing 14 tablets. Carton pack sizes: 28 and 56 tablets.

A 120ml white high density polyethylene tablet container with child resistant polypropylene closure. Each HDPE container contains 60 tablets.

Not all pack sizes may be marketed.

6.6 Special precautions for disposal and other handling

No special requirements.

7. MARKETING AUTHORISATION HOLDER

Alliance Pharmaceuticals Limited

Avonbridge House

Bath Road

Chippenham

Wiltshire SN15 2BB

United Kingdom

8. MARKETING AUTHORISATION NUMBER(S)

PL 16853/0078

9. DATE OF FIRST AUTHORISATION/RENEWAL OF THE AUTHORISATION

20/12/2005

10. DATE OF REVISION OF THE TEXT

May 2006

LEGAL CATEGORY

POM

Persantin Retard 200mg

(Boehringer Ingelheim Limited)

1. NAME OF THE MEDICINAL PRODUCT

Persantin Retard 200 mg Modified Release Capsules, Hard

2. QUALITATIVE AND QUANTITATIVE COMPOSITION

Each modified release capsule contains dipyridamole 200 mg.

For excipients, see 6.1

3. PHARMACEUTICAL FORM

Modified release capsules, hard.

Hard gelatin capsules consisting of a red cap and an orange body.

4. CLINICAL PARTICULARS

4.1 Therapeutic indications

- Secondary prevention of ischaemic stroke and transient ischaemic attacks either alone or in conjunction with aspirin.

- An adjunct to oral anti-coagulation for prophylaxis of thromboembolism associated with prosthetic heart valves.

4.2 Posology and method of administration

For oral administration.

<u>Adults, including the elderly</u>

The recommended dose is one capsule twice daily, usually one in the morning and one in the evening preferably with meals.

The capsules should be swallowed whole without chewing.

<u>Children</u>

PERSANTIN Retard 200 mg is not recommended for children.

4.3 Contraindications

Hypersensitivity to any component of the product.

4.4 Special warnings and precautions for use

Among other properties, dipyridamole acts as a potent vasodilator. It should therefore be used with caution in patients with severe coronary artery disease including unstable angina and/or recent myocardial infarction, left ventricular outflow obstruction or haemodynamic instability (e.g. decompensated heart failure).

Patients being treated with regular oral doses of PERSANTIN Retard should not receive additional intravenous dipyridamole. Clinical experience suggests that patients being treated with oral dipyridamole who also require pharmacological stress testing with intravenous dipyridamole, should discontinue drugs containing oral dipyridamole for twenty-four hours prior to stress testing.

In patients with myasthenia gravis readjustment of therapy may be necessary after changes in dipyridamole dosage. (See Interactions).

PERSANTIN should be used with caution in patients with coagulation disorders.

4.5 Interaction with other medicinal products and other forms of interaction

Dipyridamole increases the plasma levels and cardiovascular effects of adenosine. Adjustment of adenosine dosage should therefore be considered if use with dipyridamole is unavoidable.

There is evidence that the effects of acetylsalicylic acid and dipyridamole on platelet behaviour are additive.

When dipyridamole is used in combination with anticoagulants or acetylsalicylic acid, the statements on intolerance and risks for these preparations must be observed. Addition of dipyridamole to acetylsalicylic acid does not increase the incidence of bleeding events. When dipyridamole was administered concomitantly with warfarin, bleeding was no greater in frequency or severity than that observed when warfarin was administered alone.

Dipyridamole may increase the hypotensive effect of blood pressure lowering drugs and may counteract the anticholinesterase effect of cholinesterase inhibitors thereby potentially aggravating myasthenia gravis.

4.6 Pregnancy and lactation

There is inadequate evidence of safety in human pregnancy, but dipyridamole has been used for many years without apparent ill-consequence. Animal studies have shown no hazard. Nevertheless, medicines should not be used in pregnancy, especially the first trimester unless the expected benefit is thought to outweigh the possible risk to the foetus.

PERSANTIN Retard 200 mg should only be used during lactation if considered essential by the physician.

4.7 Effects on ability to drive and use machines

None stated.

4.8 Undesirable effects

Adverse reactions at therapeutic doses are usually mild. Vomiting, diarrhoea and symptoms such as dizziness, nausea, dyspepsia, headache and myalgia have been observed. These tend to occur early after initiating treatment and may disappear with continued treatment.

As a result of its vasodilating properties, PERSANTIN Retard 200 mg may cause hypotension, hot flushes and tachycardia. Worsening of the symptoms of coronary heart disease such as angina and arrhythmias.

Hypersensitivity reactions such as rash, urticaria, severe bronchospasm and angio-odema have been reported. In very rare cases, increased bleeding during or after surgery has been observed.

Isolated cases of thrombocytopenia have been reported in conjunction with treatment with PERSANTIN.

Dipyridamole has been shown to be incorporated into gallstones.

4.9 Overdose

Symptoms

Due to the low number of observations, experience with dipyridamole overdose is limited. Symptoms such as feeling warm, flushes, sweating, accelerated pulse, restlessness, feeling of weakness, dizziness, drop in blood pressure and anginal complaints can be expected.

Therapy

Symptomatic therapy is recommended. Administration of xanthine derivatives (e.g. aminophylline) may reverse the haemodynamic effects of dipyridamole overdose. ECG monitoring is advised in such a situation. Due to its wide distribution to tissues and its predominantly hepatic elimination, dipyridamole is not likely to be accessible to enhanced removal procedures.

5. PHARMACOLOGICAL PROPERTIES

5.1 Pharmacodynamic properties

The antithrombotic action of dipyridamole is based on its ability to modify various aspects of platelet function such as inhibition of platelet adhesion and aggregation, which have been shown to be factors associated with the initiation of thrombus formation, as well as lengthening shortened platelet survival time.

5.2 Pharmacokinetic properties

PERSANTIN Retard 200 mg given twice daily has been shown to be bioequivalent to the same total daily dose of PERSANTIN Tablets given in four divided doses.

Peak plasma concentrations are reached 2 - 3 hours after administration. Steady state conditions are reached within 3 days.

Metabolism of dipyridamole occurs in the liver predominantly by conjugation with glucuronic acid to form a monoglucuronide. In plasma about 70 - 80% of the total amount is present as parent compound and 20 - 30% as the monoglucuronide.

Renal excretion is very low (1 - 5%).

5.3 Preclinical safety data

Dipyridamole has been extensively investigated in animal models and no clinically significant findings have been observed at doses equivalent to therapeutic doses in humans.

6. PHARMACEUTICAL PARTICULARS

6.1 List of excipients

Tartaric acid

Povidone

Methacrylic acid - methyl methacrylate copolymer (1:2)

Talc

Acacia

Hypromellose

Hypromellose phthalate

Triacetin

Dimethicone 350

Stearic acid

and in the capsule shells

Gelatin

Titanium dioxide; E171

Red and yellow iron oxides; E172

6.2 Incompatibilities

Not applicable.

6.3 Shelf life

3 years.

Discard any capsules remaining 6 weeks after first opening.

6.4 Special precautions for storage

Do not store above 25°C.

6.5 Nature and contents of container

White polypropylene tubes with low-density polyethylene Air-sec stoppers filled with desiccating agent (90% white silicon gel/10% molecular sieves).

Packs contain 30, 60 or 100 capsules. Not all pack sizes may be marketed.

6.6 Special precautions for disposal and other handling

No special requirements

7. MARKETING AUTHORISATION HOLDER

Boehringer Ingelheim Limited

Ellesfield Avenue

Bracknell

Berkshire

RG12 8YS

United Kingdom

8. MARKETING AUTHORISATION NUMBER(S)

PL 00015/0206

9. DATE OF FIRST AUTHORISATION/RENEWAL OF THE AUTHORISATION

3 February 1997

10. DATE OF REVISION OF THE TEXT

19/04/2007

11. Legal category

Prescription Only Medicine

P2b/UK/SPC/10

Pevaryl 1% Topical Cream

(Janssen-Cilag Ltd)

1. NAME OF THE MEDICINAL PRODUCT

Pevaryl 1% Topical Cream.

2. QUALITATIVE AND QUANTITATIVE COMPOSITION

Econazole nitrate. 1.0% w/w.

Each gram of cream contains 10 mg econazole nitrate

Excipients: each gram of cream contains 2 mg benzoic acid and

52 micrograms butylated hydroxyanisole

For a full list of excipients, see section 6.1

3. PHARMACEUTICAL FORM

Cream.

4. CLINICAL PARTICULARS

4.1 Therapeutic indications

For the treatment of fungal infections of the skin.

4.2 Posology and method of administration

For cutaneous administration.

Dosage

The dosage regimen is the same for all patients.

Apply twice daily to the affected part and rub into the skin gently with the finger. Continue the application until all skin lesions are healed.

In the treatment of fungal infections of the nail, the cream should be applied once a day and covered with an occlusive dressing.

4.3 Contraindications

Pevaryl Topical Cream is contraindicated in individuals who have shown hypersensitivity to any of its ingredients.

4.4 Special warnings and precautions for use

Hypersensitivity has rarely been recorded, if it should occur, administration of the product should be discontinued.

4.5 Interaction with other medicinal products and other forms of interaction

Econazole administered systemically is known to inhibit CYP3A4/2C9. Due to the limited systemic availability after topical application, clinically relevant interactions are rare. However, in patients on oral anticoagulants, such as warfarin, caution should be exercised and anticoagulant effect should be monitored.

4.6 Pregnancy and lactation

Only small amounts of the drug are absorbed through the skin and no teratogenic effects have been observed in animals. Hence the product may be used with caution during pregnancy.

4.7 Effects on ability to drive and use machines

None known.

4.8 Undesirable effects

Rarely, transient local irritation may occur after immediate application. If this persists please contact your doctor for advice.

4.9 Overdose

This product is for topical application only.

If large amounts have been taken by mouth or swallowed, gastric emptying may be considered desirable.

5. PHARMACOLOGICAL PROPERTIES

5.1 Pharmacodynamic properties

Econazole nitrate is a broad spectrum antimycotic with activity against dermatophytes, yeasts and moulds. A clinically relevant action against Gram positive bacteria has also been found.

5.2 Pharmacokinetic properties

Econazole nitrate is only slightly absorbed from the skin. No active drug has been detected in the serum. Radio labelling shows that less than 0.1% of an oral dose is absorbed. Peak serum levels are achieved after 2 hours and 90% binds to plasma proteins. Metabolism is limited but occurs primarily in the liver with excretion of metabolites in the urine.

5.3 Preclinical safety data

No relevant information additional to that contained elsewhere in the Summary of Product Characteristics.

6. PHARMACEUTICAL PARTICULARS

6.1 List of excipients

Pegoxyl-7-stearate

Peglicol-5-oleate

Liquid paraffin

Butylated hydroxyanisole (E320)

Benzoic acid (E210)

Flower Perfume 4074

Purified water

6.2 Incompatibilities

None stated.

6.3 Shelf life

24 months.

6.4 Special precautions for storage

Do not store above 25°C.

6.5 Nature and contents of container

Resin lined, aluminium tubes containing 15 g or 30 g of cream.

6.6 Special precautions for disposal and other handling

No special requirements.

Any unused product or waste material should be disposed of in accordance with local requirements

7. MARKETING AUTHORISATION HOLDER

Janssen-Cilag Limited

50-100 Holmers Farm Way

High Wycombe

Buckinghamshire

HP12 4EG

UK

8. MARKETING AUTHORISATION NUMBER(S)

PL 00242/0259

9. DATE OF FIRST AUTHORISATION/RENEWAL OF THE AUTHORISATION

Date of first authorisation: 01/07/95

Renewal of authorisation 18th March 2009

10. DATE OF REVISION OF THE TEXT

11th September 2009

PHARMORUBICIN

(Pharmacia Limited)

1. NAME OF THE MEDICINAL PRODUCT

Pharmorubicin Rapid Dissolution 10 mg, 20 mg, 50 mg & 150 mg

Pharmorubicin Solution for Injection 2 mg/ml

2. QUALITATIVE AND QUANTITATIVE COMPOSITION

Pharmorubicin Rapid Dissolution 10 mg, 20 mg, 50 mg and 150 mg

After reconstitution, each vial contains 2 mg/ml epirubicin hydrochloride

5 ml vials contain 10 mg of epirubicin hydrochloride

10 ml vials contain 20 mg of epirubicin hydrochloride

25 ml vials contain 50 mg of epirubicin hydrochloride

75 ml vials contain 150 mg epirubicin hydrochloride.

Pharmorubicin Solution for Injection 2 mg/ml

Each vial contains 2 mg/ml epirubicin hydrochloride

5 ml vials contain 10 mg of epirubicin hydrochloride

10 ml vials contain 20 mg of epirubicin hydrochloride

25 ml vials contain 50 mg of epirubicin hydrochloride

100 ml vials contain 200 mg epirubicin hydrochloride.

For excipients, see section 6.1.

3. PHARMACEUTICAL FORM

Powder for solution for injection or infusion.

Solution for injection or infusion.

Red, freeze-dried, sterile, powder for injection containing 10 mg, 20 mg, 50 mg and 150 mg epirubicin hydrochloride.

Red, sterile, preservative-free, aqueous solution.

4. CLINICAL PARTICULARS

4.1 Therapeutic indications

Pharmorubicin has produced responses in a wide range of neoplastic conditions, including breast, ovarian, gastric, lung and colorectal carcinomas, malignant lymphomas, leukaemias and multiple myeloma.

Intravesical administration of Pharmorubicin has been found to be beneficial in the treatment of superficial bladder cancer, carcinoma-in-situ and in the prophylaxis of recurrences after transurethral resection.

4.2 Posology and method of administration

Intravenous administration: Pharmorubicin is not active when given orally and should not be injected intramuscularly or intrathecally.

It is advisable to give the drug via the tubing of a freely running IV saline infusion after checking that the needle is well placed in the vein. This method minimises the risk of drug extravasation and makes sure that the vein is flushed with saline after the administration of the drug. Extravasation of Pharmorubicin from the vein during injection may give rise to severe tissue lesions, even necrosis. Venous sclerosis may result from injection into small vessels or repeated injections into the same vein.

Conventional doses:

When Pharmorubicin is used as a single agent, the recommended dosage in adults is 60-90 mg/m^2 body area; the drug should be injected IV over 3-5 minutes and, depending on the patients' haematomedullary status, the dose should be repeated at 21 day intervals.

High doses:

Pharmorubicin as a single agent for the treatment of lung cancer at high doses should be administered according to the following regimens:

Lung cancer

Small cell lung cancer (previously untreated): 120 mg/m^2 day 1, every 3 weeks.

Non-small cell lung cancer (squamous, large cell, and adenocarcinoma previously untreated): 135 mg/m^2 day 1 or 45 mg/m^2 days 1, 2, 3, every 3 weeks.

Breast cancer

In the adjuvant treatment of early breast cancer patients with positive lymph nodes, intravenous doses of epirubicin ranging from 100 mg/m^2 (as a single dose on day 1) to 120 mg/m^2 (in two divided doses on days 1 and 8) every 3-4 weeks, in combination with intravenous cyclophosphamide and 5-fluorouracil and oral tamoxifen, are recommended.

The drug should be given as an I.V. bolus over 3-5 minutes or as an infusion up to 30 minutes. Lower doses (60-75 mg/m^2 for conventional treatment and 105-120 mg/ m^2 for high dose schedules) are recommended for patients whose bone marrow function has already been impaired by previous chemotherapy or radiotherapy, by age, or neoplastic bone-marrow infiltration. The total dose per cycle may be divided over 2-3 successive days.

When the drug is used in combination with other antitumour agents, the doses need to be adequately reduced. Since the major route of elimination of Pharmorubicin is the hepatobiliary system, the dosage should be reduced in patients with impaired liver function, in order to avoid an increase of overall toxicity. Moderate liver impairment (bilirubin: 1.4-3 mg/100ml) requires a 50% reduction of dose, while severe impairment (bilirubin > 3 mg/100 ml) necessitates a dose reduction of 75%.

Moderate renal impairment does not appear to require a dose reduction in view of the limited amount of Pharmorubicin excreted by this route.

Intravesical administration:

Pharmorubicin may be given by intravesical administration for the treatment of superficial bladder cancer and carcinoma-in-situ. It should not be used in this way for the treatment of invasive tumours which have penetrated the bladder wall where systemic therapy or surgery is more appropriate. Epirubicin has also been successfully used intravesically as a prophylactic agent after transurethral resection of superficial tumours in order to prevent recurrences.

While many regimens have been used, the following may be helpful as a guide: for therapy 8 × weekly instillations of 50 mg/50 ml (diluted with saline or distilled sterile water). In the case of local toxicity (chemical cystitis), a dose reduction to 30 mg per 50 ml is advised. For carcinoma-in-situ, depending on the individual tolerability of the patient, the dose may be increased up to 80 mg/50 ml. For prophylaxis, 4 × weekly administrations of 50 mg/50 ml followed by 11 × monthly instillations at the same dosage, is the schedule most commonly used

The solution should be retained intravesically for 1 hour. To avoid undue dilution with urine, the patient should be instructed not to drink any fluid in the 12 hours prior to instillation. During the instillation, the patient should be rotated occasionally and should be instructed to void at the end of the instillation time.

4.3 Contraindications

Pharmorubicin is contraindicated in patients with marked myelosuppression induced by previous treatment with other antitumour agents or by radiotherapy and in patients already treated with maximal cumulative doses of other anthracyclines such as Doxorubicin or Daunorubicin.

The drug is contraindicated in patients with current or previous history of cardiac impairment.

4.4 Special warnings and precautions for use

Pharmorubicin should be administered only under the supervision of qualified physicians experienced in antiblastic and cytotoxic therapy. Treatment with high dose Pharmorubicin in particular requires the availability of facilities for the care of possible clinical complications due to myelosuppression.

Initial treatment calls for a careful baseline monitoring of various laboratory parameters and cardiac function.

During each cycle of treatment with Pharmorubicin, patients must be carefully and frequently monitored. Red and white blood cells, neutrophils and platelet counts should be carefully assessed both before and during each cycle of therapy. Leukopenia and neutropenia are usually transient with conventional and high-dose schedules, reaching a nadir between the 10th and 14th day and returning to normal values by the 21st day; they are more severe with high dose schedules. Very few patients, even receiving high doses, experience thrombocytopenia (< 100,000 platelets/mm^3).

Before starting therapy and if possible during treatment, liver function should be evaluated (SGOT, SGPT, alkaline phosphatase, bilirubin). A cumulative dose of 900-1000 mg/m^2 should only be exceeded with extreme caution with both conventional and high doses.

Above this level the risk of irreversible congestive cardiac failure increases greatly. There is objective evidence that the cardiac toxicity may occur rarely below this range. However, cardiac function must be carefully monitored during treatment to minimise the risk of cardiac failure of the type described for other anthracyclines.

Heart failure can appear even several weeks after discontinuing treatment, and may prove unresponsive to specific medical treatment. The potential risk of cardiotoxicity may increase in patients who have received concomitant, or prior, radiotherapy to the mediastinal pericardial area.

In establishing the maximal cumulative doses of Pharmorubicin, any concomitant therapy with potentially cardiotoxic drugs should be taken intoaccount.

It is recommended that an ECG before and after each treatment cycle should be carried out. Alterations in the ECG tracing, such as flattening or inversion of the T-wave, depression of the S-T segment, or the onset of arrhythmias, generally transient and reversible, need not necessarily be taken as indications to discontinue treatment.

Cardiomyopathy induced by anthracyclines, is associated with a persistent reduction of the QRS voltage, prolongation beyond normal limits of the systolic interval (PEP/LVET) and a reduction of the ejection fraction. Cardiac monitoring of patients receiving Pharmorubicin treatment is highly important and it is advisable to assess cardiac function by non-invasive techniques such as ECG, echocardiography and, if necessary, measurement of ejection fraction by radionuclide angiography.

Like other cytotoxic agents, Pharmorubicin may induce hyperuricaemia as a result of rapid lysis of neoplastic cells. Blood uric acid levels should therefore be carefully checked so that this phenomenon may be controlled pharmacologically.

Pharmorubicin may impart a red colour to the urine for 1-2 days after administration.

4.5 Interaction with other medicinal products and other forms of interaction

It is not recommended that Pharmorubicin be mixed with other drugs. But Pharmorubicin can be used in combination with other anticancer drugs.

Cimetidine increases the formation of the active metabolite of epirubicin and the exposure of the unchanged epirubicin by pharmacokinetic interaction.

4.6 Pregnancy and lactation

There is no conclusive information as to whether epirubicin may adversely affect human fertility or cause teratogenesis. Experimental data, however, suggest that epirubicin may harm the foetus. This product should not normally be administered to patients who are pregnant or to mothers who are breast-feeding. Like most other anti-cancer agents, epirubicin has shown mutagenic and carcinogenic properties in animals.

4.7 Effects on ability to drive and use machines

There have been no reports of particular adverse events relating to effects on ability to drive and to use machines.

4.8 Undesirable effects

Apart from myelosuppression and cardiotoxicity, the following adverse reactions have been described:

Alopecia, normally reversible, appears in 60-90% of treated cases; it is accompanied by lack of beard growth in males.

Mucositis may appear 5-10 days after the start of treatment, and usually involves stomatitis with areas of painful erosions, mainly along the side of the tongue and the sublingual mucosa.

Gastro-intestinal disturbances, such as nausea, vomiting and diarrhoea.

Hyperpyrexia.

Fever, chills and urticaria have been rarely reported; anaphylaxis may occur.

High doses of pharmorubicin have been safely administered in a large number of untreated patients having various solid tumours and has caused adverse events which are no different from those seen at conventional doses with the exception of reversible severe neutropenia (< 500 neutrophils/mm^3 for < 7 days) which occurred in the majority of patients. Only a few patients required hospitalisation and supportive therapy for severe infectious complications at high doses.

During intravesical administration, as drug absorption is minimal, systemic side effects are rare; more frequently chemical cystitis, sometimes haemorrhagic, has been observed.

Haematological

The occurrence of secondary acute myeloid leukaemia with or without a pre-leukaemic phase has been reported rarely in patients concurrently treated with epirubicin in association with DNA- damaging antineoplastic agents. Such cases could have a short (1-3 year) latency period.

4.9 Overdose

Very high single doses of epirubicin may be expected to cause acute myocardial degeneration within 24 hours and severe myelosuppression within 10-14 days. Treatment should aim to support the patient during this period and should utilise such measures as blood transfusion and reverse barrier nursing. Delayed cardiac failure has been seen with the anthracyclines up to 6 months after the overdose. Patients should be observed carefully and should, if signs of cardiac failure arise, be treated along conventional lines.

5. PHARMACOLOGICAL PROPERTIES

5.1 Pharmacodynamic properties

Pharmacotherapeutic group (ATC code) – L01D B

The mechanism of action of Pharmorubicin is related to its ability to bind to DNA. Cell culture studies have shown rapid cell penetration, localisation in the nucleus and inhibition of nucleic acid synthesis and mitosis. Pharmorubicin has proved to be active on a wide spectrum of experimental tumours including L1210 and P388 leukaemias, sarcomas SA180 (solid and ascitic forms), B16 melanoma, mammary carcinoma, Lewis lung carcinoma and colon carcinoma 38. It has also shown activity against human tumours transplanted into athymic nude mice (melanoma, mammary lung, prostatic and ovarian carcinomas).

5.2 Pharmacokinetic properties

In patients with normal hepatic and renal function, plasma levels after I.V. injection of 60-150mg/m^2 of the drug follow a tri-exponential decreasing pattern with a very fast first phase and a slow terminal phase with a mean half-life of about 40 hours. These doses are within the limits of pharmacokinetic linearity both in terms of plasma clearance values and metabolic pathway. The major metabolites that have been identified are epirubicinol (13-OH-epirubicin) and glucuronides of epirubicin and epirubicinol.

The 4'-O-glucuronidation distinguishes epirubicin from doxorubicin and may account for the faster elimination of epirubicin and its reduced toxicity. Plasma levels of the main metabolite, the 13-OH derivative (epirubicinol) are consistently lower and virtually parallel those of the unchanged drug.

Pharmorubicin is eliminated mainly through the liver; high plasma clearance values (0.9 l/min) indicate that this slow elimination is due to extensive tissue distribution.

Urinary excretion accounts for approximately 9-10% of the administered dose in 48 hours. Biliary excretion represents the major route of elimination, about 40% of the administered dose being recovered in the bile in 72 hours.

The drug does not cross the blood-brain-barrier. When Pharmorubicin is administered intravesically the systemic absorption is minimal.

5.3 Preclinical safety data

The main target organs in rat, rabbit and dog following repeated dosing were the haemolymphopoietic system, GI tract, kidney, liver and reproductive organs. Epirubicin was also cardiotoxic in the species tested.

It was genotoxic, and, like other anthracyclines, carcinogenic in rats.

Epirubicin was embryotoxic in rats. No malformations were seen in rats or rabbits, but like other anthracyclines and cytotoxic drugs, epirubicin must be considered potentially teratogenic.

A local tolerance study in rats and mice showed extravasation of epirubicin causes tissue necrosis.

6. PHARMACEUTICAL PARTICULARS

6.1 List of excipients

Pharmorubicin Rapid Dissolution 10 mg, 20 mg, 50 mg & 150 mg

Methyl hydroxybenzoate
Lactose monohydrate

Pharmorubicin Solution for Injection 2 mg/ml

Hydrochloric acid

Sodium chloride

Water for Injections

6.2 Incompatibilities

Prolonged contact with any solution of an alkaline pH should be avoided as it will result in hydrolysis of the drug. Pharmorubicin should not be mixed with heparin due to chemical incompatibility, which may lead to precipitation when the drugs are in certain proportions.

Pharmorubicin can be used in combination with other antitumour agents, but it is not recommended that it be mixed with other drugs.

6.3 Shelf life

a) Shelf life of the product as package for sale.

Pharmorubicin Rapid Dissolution 10 mg, 20 mg, 50 mg & 150 mg

Four years.

Pharmorubicin Solution for Injection 2 mg/ml

Glass vials: 3 years

Polypropylene Cytosafe™ vials: 3 years

b) Shelf life after first opening the container/reconstitution according to directions:

Pharmorubicin Solution for Injection does not contain a preservative or bacteriostatic agent. Vials are, therefore for single use only and any unused portion must be discarded after use.

From a microbiological point of view, the product should be used immediately after first penetration of the rubber stopper. If not used immediately, in use storage times and conditions are the responsibility of the user.

6.4 Special precautions for storage

Pharmorubicin Rapid Dissolution 10 mg, 20 mg, 50 mg & 150 mg

Keep the container in the outer carton

Pharmorubicin Solution for Injection 2 mg/ml

Store at 2°C - 8°C (in a refrigerator)

Keep the container in outer carton

6.5 Nature and contents of container

Pharmorubicin Rapid Dissolution 10 mg, 20 mg, 50 mg & 150 mg

5 ml, 10 ml, 50 ml and 75 ml colourless glass vial Type I with chlorobutyl rubber bung and aluminium snap cap.

Pharmorubicin Solution for Injection 2 mg/ml

Colourless glass 5ml, 10ml, 25ml, or 100ml vial (type I), with Teflon-faced chlorobutyl rubber bung and aluminium cap with inset grey polypropylene disk.

Colourless polypropylene 5ml, 10ml, 25ml or 100ml vial with Teflon-faced halobutyl rubber stopper and aluminium cap with plastic flip-off top:

6.6 Special precautions for disposal and other handling

Pharmorubicin Rapid Dissolution 10 mg, 20 mg, 50 mg & 150 mg only:

Preparation of the freeze-dried powder for intravenous administration. Dissolve in sodium chloride/water for injection. The vial contents will be under a negative pressure. To minimize aerosol formation during reconstitution, particular care should be taken when the needle is inserted. Inhalation of any aerosol produced during reconstitution must be avoided. After gentle agitation the reconstituted solution will be transparent and red in appearance.

The product should be dissolved in 0.9% sodium chloride or water for injection to get the final concentration of 2 mg/ml according to the following instructions:

Strength (mg)	Solvent volume (ml)
10	5
20	10
50	25
150	75

Pharmorubicin Rapid Dissolution 10 mg, 20 mg, 50 mg & 150 mg

Pharmorubicin Solution for Injection 2 mg/ml

Intravenous administration. Epirubicin should be administered into the tubing of a freely flowing intravenous infusion (0.9% sodium chloride). To minimize the risk of thrombosis or perivenous extravasation, the usual infusion times range between 3 and 20 minutes depending upon dosage and volume of the infusion solution. A direct push injection is not recommended due to the risk of extravasation, which may occur even in the presence of adequate blood return upon needle aspiration (see Warning and Precautions).

Discard any unused solution.

Intravesical administration. Epirubicin should be instilled using a catheter and retained intravesically for 1 hour. During instillation, the patient should be rotated to ensure that the vesical mucosa of the pelvis receives the most extensive contact with the solution. To avoid undue dilution with urine, the patient should be instructed not to drink any fluid in the 12 hours prior to instillation. The patient should be instructed to void at the end of the instillation.

Protective measures: The following protective recommendations are given due to the toxic nature of this substance:

Personnel should be trained in good technique for reconstitution and handling.

• Pregnant staff should be excluded from working with this drug.

• Personnel handling epirubicin should wear protective clothing: goggles, gowns and disposable gloves and masks.

• A designated area should be defined for reconstitution (preferably under a laminar flow system); the work surface should be protected by disposable, plastic-backed, absorbent paper.

• All items used for reconstitution, administration or cleaning, including gloves, should be placed in high-risk, waste disposal bags for high temperature incineration. Spillage or leakage should be treated with dilute sodium hypochlorite (1% available chlorine) solution, preferably by soaking, and then water.

• All cleaning materials should be disposed of as indicated previously.

• In case of skin contact thoroughly wash the affected area with soap and water or sodium bicarbonate solution. However, do not abrade the skin by using a scrub brush. In case of contact with the eye(s), hold back the eyelid of the affected eye(s), and flush with copious amounts of water for at least 15 minutes. Then seek medical evaluation by a physician.

• Always wash hands after removing gloves.

7. MARKETING AUTHORISATION HOLDER

Pharmacia Limited

Ramsgate Road

Sandwich

Kent

CT13 9NJ

United Kingdom

8. MARKETING AUTHORISATION NUMBER(S)

PL 00032/0275 (Pharmorubicin Solution for Injection 2 mg/ml)

PL 00032/0276 (Pharmorubicin Rapid Dissolution)

9. DATE OF FIRST AUTHORISATION/RENEWAL OF THE AUTHORISATION

14 May 2004

10. DATE OF REVISION OF THE TEXT

June 2005

Company Reference: PM 2_0

Phenergan 10mg Tablets

(sanofi-aventis)

1. NAME OF THE MEDICINAL PRODUCT

Phenergan™ 10 mg Tablets.

2. QUALITATIVE AND QUANTITATIVE COMPOSITION

Promethazine hydrochloride 10 mg.

3. PHARMACEUTICAL FORM

Pale blue film coated tablets marked PN 10 on one side.

4. CLINICAL PARTICULARS

4.1 Therapeutic indications

As symptomatic treatment for allergic conditions of the upper respiratory tract and skin including allergic rhinitis, urticaria and anaphylactic reactions to drugs and foreign proteins.

As an adjunct in preoperative sedation in surgery and obstetrics.

As an antiemetic.

For short term use:

Sedation and treatment of insomnia in adults.

As a paediatric sedative.

4.2 Posology and method of administration

Route of administration: Oral.

Not for use in children under the age of 2 years.

As an antihistamine in allergy:

Children 2-5 years	The use of Phenergan Elixir is recommended for this age group.
Children 5-10 years	Either 10 or 20 mg as a single dose*. Or 10 mg bd. Maximum daily dose 20 mg.
Children over 10 years and adults (including elderly)	Initially 10 mg bd. Increasing to a maximum of 20 mg tds as required.

*Single doses are best taken at night.

As an antiemetic:

Children 2-5 years	The use of Phenergan Elixir is recommended for this age group.
Children 5-10 years	10 mg to be taken the night before the journey. To be repeated after 6–8 hours as required.
Children over 10 years and adults (including elderly)	20 mg to be taken the night before the journey. To be repeated after 6–8 hours as required.

Short term sedation:

Children 2-5 years	The use of Phenergan Elixir is recommended for this age group.
Children 5-10 years	20 mg as a single night time dose.
Children over 10 years and adults (including elderly)	20 to 50 mg as a single night time dose.

4.3 Contraindications

Phenergan should not be used in patients in coma or suffering from CNS depression of any cause. Phenergan should not be given to patients with a known hypersensitivity to promethazine or to any of the excipients. Promethazine is contraindicated for use in children less than two years of age because of the potential for fatal respiratory depression. Phenergan should be avoided in patients taking monoamine oxidase inhibitors up to 14 days previously.

4.4 Special warnings and precautions for use

Phenergan may thicken or dry lung secretions and impair expectoration. It should therefore be used with caution in patients with asthma, bronchitis or bronchiectasis.

Use with care in patients with severe coronary artery disease, narrow angle glaucoma, epilepsy or hepatic and renal insufficiency.

Caution should be exercised in patients with bladder neck or pyloro-duodenal obstruction.

The use of promethazine should be avoided in children and adolescents with signs and symptoms suggestive of Reye's Syndrome.

Promethazine may mask the warning signs of ototoxicity caused by ototoxic drugs e.g. salicylates. It may also delay the early diagnosis of intestinal obstruction or raised intracranial pressure through the suppression of vomiting.

Patients with rare hereditary problems of galactose intolerance, the Lapp lactase deficiency or glucose-galactose malabsorption should not take this medicine.

Phenergan should not be used for longer than 7 days without seeking medical advice.

4.5 Interaction with other medicinal products and other forms of interaction

Phenergan will enhance the action of any anticholinergic agent, tricyclic antidepressant, sedative or hypnotic. Alcohol should be avoided during treatment. Phenergan may interfere with immunological urine pregnancy tests to produce false-positive or false-negative results. Phenergan should be discontinued at least 72 hours before the start of skin tests as it may inhibit the cutaneous histamine response thus producing false-negative results.

4.6 Pregnancy and lactation

Phenergan should not be used in pregnancy unless the physician considers it essential. The use of Phenergan is not recommended in the 2 weeks prior to delivery in view of the risk of irritability and excitement in the neonate.

Available evidence suggests that the amount excreted in milk is insignificant. However, there are risks of neonatal irritability and excitement.

4.7 Effects on ability to drive and use machines

Because the duration of action may be up to 12 hours, patients should be advised that if they feel drowsy they should not drive or operate heavy machinery.

4.8 Undesirable effects

Side effects may be seen in a few patients: drowsiness, dizziness, restlessness, headaches, nightmares, tiredness, and disorientation. Anticholinergic side effects such as blurred vision, dry mouth and urinary retention occur occasionally. Infants are susceptible to the anticholinergic effects of promethazine, while other children may display paradoxical hyperexcitability. The elderly are particularly susceptible to the anticholinergic effects and confusion due to promethazine. Other side-effects include urticaria, rash, pruritus, anorexia, gastric irritation, palpitations, hypotension, arrhythmias, extrapyramidal effects, muscle spasms and tic-like movements of the head and face. Anaphylaxis, jaundice and blood dyscrasias including haemolytic anaemia rarely occur. Photosensitive skin reactions have been reported. Strong sunlight should be avoided during treatment.

4.9 Overdose

Symptoms of severe overdosage are variable. They are characterised in children by various combinations of excitation, ataxia, incoordination, athetosis and hallucinations, while adults may become drowsy and lapse into coma. Convulsions may occur in both adults and children: coma or excitement may precede their occurrence. Cardiorespiratory depression is uncommon. If the patient is seen soon enough after ingestion, it should be possible to induce vomiting with ipecacuanha despite the antiemetic effect of promethazine; alternatively, gastric lavage may be used.

Treatment is otherwise supportive with attention to maintenance of adequate respiratory and circulatory status. Convulsions should be treated with diazepam or other suitable anticonvulsant.

5. PHARMACOLOGICAL PROPERTIES

5.1 Pharmacodynamic properties

Pharmacotherapeutic group: Antihistamine for systemic use

ATC code: R06AD02

Potent, long acting, antihistamine with additional anti-emetic central sedative and anti-cholinergic properties.

5.2 Pharmacokinetic properties

Promethazine is distributed widely in the body. It enters the brain and crosses the placenta. Promethazine is slowly excreted via urine and bile. Phenothiazines pass into the milk at low concentrations.

5.3 Preclinical safety data

No additional preclinical data of relevance to the prescriber.

6. PHARMACEUTICAL PARTICULARS

6.1 List of excipients

Lactose

Maize starch

Povidone K30

Magnesium stearate

Polyethylene glycol 200

Opaspray M-1-4210A (contains Titanium dioxide - E 171, Hypromellose - E464 and Indigo carmine aluminium lake FD&C Blue no 2 - E132)

Hypromellose (Pharmacoat 606)

6.2 Incompatibilities

None stated.

6.3 Shelf life

5 years

6.4 Special precautions for storage

Store below 30°C. Store in the original carton in order to protect from light

6.5 Nature and contents of container

Opaque white 250μm uPVC coated with 40gsm PVdC, 20μm hard temper aluminium foil (coated with vinyl heat seal lacquer) backing, of 56 tablets.

6.6 Special precautions for disposal and other handling

None stated.

7. MARKETING AUTHORISATION HOLDER

Sanofi-aventis

One Onslow Street

Guildford

Surrey

GU1 4YS

UK

8. MARKETING AUTHORISATION NUMBER(S)

PL 04425/0631

9. DATE OF FIRST AUTHORISATION/RENEWAL OF THE AUTHORISATION

3rd October 2008

10. DATE OF REVISION OF THE TEXT

October 2008

11 LEGAL CLASSIFICATION

P

Phenergan 25 mg tablets

(sanofi-aventis)

1. NAME OF THE MEDICINAL PRODUCT

Phenergan™ 25 mg Tablets.

2. QUALITATIVE AND QUANTITATIVE COMPOSITION

Promethazine hydrochloride 25 mg.

3. PHARMACEUTICAL FORM

Pale blue film coated tablets marked PN 25 on one side.

4. CLINICAL PARTICULARS

4.1 Therapeutic indications

As symptomatic treatment for allergic conditions of the upper respiratory tract and skin including allergic rhinitis, urticaria and anaphylactic reactions to drugs and foreign proteins.

As an adjunct in preoperative sedation in surgery and obstetrics.

As an antiemetic.

For short term use:

Sedation and treatment of insomnia in adults.

As a paediatric sedative.

4.2 Posology and method of administration

Route of administration: Oral.

Not for use in children under the age of 2 years because the safety of such use has not been established.

As an antihistamine in allergy:

Children 2-5 years	The use of Phenergan Elixir is recommended for this age group.
Children 5-10 years	25 mg as a single dose*. Maximum daily dose 25 mg.
Children over 10 years and adults (including elderly)	25 mg as a single dose*. Increasing to a maximum of 25 mg bd as required.

*Single doses are best taken at night.

As an antiemetic:

Children 2-5 years	The use of Phenergan Elixir is recommended for this age group.
Children 5-10 years	The use of Phenergan Elixir or Phenergan 10 mg Tablets is recommended.
Children over 10 years and adults (including elderly)	25 mg to be taken the night before the journey. To be repeated after 6–8 hours as required.

Short term sedation:

Children 2-5 years	The use of Phenergan Elixir is recommended for this age group.
Children 5-10 years	25 mg as a single night time dose.
Children over 10 years and adults (including elderly)	25 or 50 mg as a single night time dose.

4.3 Contraindications

Phenergan should not be used in patients in coma or suffering from CNS depression of any cause. Phenergan should not be given to patients with a known hypersensitivity to promethazine or to any of the excipients. Promethazine is contraindicated for use in children less than two years of age because of the potential for fatal respiratory depression. Phenergan should be avoided in patients taking monoamine oxidase inhibitors up to 14 days previously.

4.4 Special warnings and precautions for use

Phenergan may thicken or dry lung secretions and impair expectoration. It should therefore be used with caution in patients with asthma, bronchitis or bronchiectasis.

Use with care in patients with severe coronary artery disease, narrow angle glaucoma, epilepsy or hepatic and renal insufficiency.

Caution should be exercised in patients with bladder neck or pyloro-duodenal obstruction.

The use of promethazine should be avoided in children and adolescents with signs and symptoms suggestive of Reye's Syndrome.

Promethazine may mask the warning signs of ototoxicity caused by ototoxic drugs e.g. salicylates. It may also delay the early diagnosis of intestinal obstruction or raised intracranial pressure through the suppression of vomiting.

Patients with rare hereditary problems of galactose intolerance, the Lapp lactase deficiency or glucose-galactose malabsorption should not take this medicine.

Phenergan should not be used for longer than 7 days without seeking medical advice.

4.5 Interaction with other medicinal products and other forms of interaction

Phenergan will enhance the action of any anticholinergic agent, tricyclic antidepressant, sedative or hypnotic. Alcohol should be avoided during treatment. Phenergan may interfere with immunological urine pregnancy tests to produce false-positive or false-negative results. Phenergan should be discontinued at least 72 hours before the start of skin tests as it may inhibit the cutaneous histamine response thus producing false-negative results.

4.6 Pregnancy and lactation

Phenergan should not be used in pregnancy unless the physician considers it essential. The use of Phenergan is not recommended in the 2 weeks prior to delivery in view of the risk of irritability and excitement in the neonate.

Available evidence suggests that the amount excreted in milk is insignificant. However, there are risks of neonatal irritability and excitement.

4.7 Effects on ability to drive and use machines

Because the duration of action may be up to 12 hours, patients should be advised that if they feel drowsy they should not drive or operate heavy machinery.

4.8 Undesirable effects

Side effects may be seen in a few patients: drowsiness, dizziness, restlessness, headaches, nightmares, tiredness, and disorientation. Anticholinergic side effects such as blurred vision, dry mouth and urinary retention occur occasionally. Infants are susceptible to the anticholinergic effects of promethazine, while other children may display paradoxical hyperexcitability. The elderly are particularly susceptible to the anticholinergic effects and confusion due to promethazine. Other side-effects include urticaria, rash, pruritus, anorexia, gastric irritation, palpitations, hypotension, arrhythmias, extrapyramidal effects, muscle spasms and tic-like movements of the head and face. Anaphylaxis, jaundice and blood dyscrasias including haemolytic anaemia rarely occur. Photosensitive skin reactions have been reported. Strong sunlight should be avoided during treatment.

4.9 Overdose

Symptoms of severe overdosage are variable. They are characterised in children by various combinations of excitation, ataxia, incoordination, athetosis and hallucinations, while adults may become drowsy and lapse into coma. Convulsions may occur in both adults and children: coma or excitement may precede their occurrence. Cardiorespiratory depression is uncommon. If the patient is seen soon enough after ingestion, it should be possible to induce vomiting with ipecacuanha despite the antiemetic effect of promethazine; alternatively, gastric lavage may be used.

Treatment is otherwise supportive with attention to maintenance of adequate respiratory and circulatory status. Convulsions should be treated with diazepam or other suitable anticonvulsant.

5. PHARMACOLOGICAL PROPERTIES

5.1 Pharmacodynamic properties

Potent, long acting, antihistamine with additional anti-emetic central sedative and anti-cholinergic properties.

5.2 Pharmacokinetic properties

Promethazine is distributed widely in the body. It enters the brain and crosses the placenta. Promethazine is slowly excreted via urine and bile. Phenothiazines pass into the milk at low concentrations.

5.3 Preclinical safety data

No additional preclinical data of relevance to the prescriber.

6. PHARMACEUTICAL PARTICULARS

6.1 List of excipients

Lactose

Maize starch

Povidone K30

Magnesium stearate

Polyethylene glycol 200

Opaspray M-1-4210A (contains Titanium dioxide- E171, Hypromellose- E464 and Indigo carmine aluminium lake FD&C Blue no 2- E132)

Hypromellose (Pharmacoat 606).

6.2 Incompatibilities

None stated.

6.3 Shelf life
60 months.

6.4 Special precautions for storage
Protect from light. Store below 30°C.

6.5 Nature and contents of container
Opaque white 250μm uPVC coated with 40gsm PVdC. 20μm hard temper aluminium foil (coated with vinyl heat seal lacquer) backing of 56 tablets.

6.6 Special precautions for disposal and other handling
None stated.

7. MARKETING AUTHORISATION HOLDER
Sanofi-aventis
One Onslow Street
Guildford
Surrey
GU1 4YS
UK

8. MARKETING AUTHORISATION NUMBER(S)
PL 04425/0281

9. DATE OF FIRST AUTHORISATION/RENEWAL OF THE AUTHORISATION
17 July 2006

10. DATE OF REVISION OF THE TEXT
1 March 2007

11 LEGAL CLASSIFICATION
P

Phenergan Elixir
(sanofi-aventis)

1. NAME OF THE MEDICINAL PRODUCT
Phenergan Elixir.

2. QUALITATIVE AND QUANTITATIVE COMPOSITION
Promethazine hydrochloride 5 mg / 5 ml.
For excipients see section 6.1

3. PHARMACEUTICAL FORM
Oral solution

4. CLINICAL PARTICULARS
4.1 Therapeutic indications
As symptomatic treatment for allergic conditions of the upper respiratory tract and skin including allergic rhinitis, urticaria and anaphylactic reactions to drugs and foreign proteins.

As an adjunct in preoperative sedation in surgery and obstetrics.

As an antiemetic.

For short term use:

Sedation and treatment of insomnia in adults.

As a paediatric sedative.

4.2 Posology and method of administration
Route of administration: Oral.

Not for use in children under the age of 2 years (see section 4.3)

As an antihistamine in allergy:

Children 2-5 years	Either 5–15 mg as a single dose. Or 5 mg bd. Maximum daily dose 15 mg.
Children 5-10 years	Either 10–25 mg as a single dose. Or 5-10 mg bd. Maximum daily dose 25 mg.
Children over 10 years and adults (including elderly)	Initially 10 mg bd. Increasing to a maximum of 20 mg tds as required.

As an antiemetic:

Children 2-5 years	5 mg to be taken the night before the journey. To be repeated after 6–8 hours as required.
Children 5-10 years	10 mg to be taken the night before the journey. To be repeated after 6–8 hours as required.
Children over 10 years and adults (including elderly)	25 mg to be taken the night before the journey. To be repeated after 6–8 hours as required.

Short term sedation:

Children 2-5 years	15 or 20 mg as a single night time dose.
Children 5-10 years	20 or 25 mg as a single night time dose.
Children over 10 years and adults (including elderly)	25 or 50 mg as a single night time dose. The use of Phenergan tablets to provide these doses is recommended.

4.3 Contraindications
Phenergan should not be used in patients in coma or suffering from CNS depression of any cause. Phenergan should not be given to patients with a known hypersensitivity to promethazine or to any of the excipients. Promethazine is contraindicated for use in children less than two years of age because of the potential for fatal respiratory depression. Phenergan should be avoided in patients taking monoamine oxidase inhibitors up to 14 days previously.

The elixir contains hydrogenated glucose syrup and is not suitable for diabetics.

4.4 Special warnings and precautions for use
Phenergan may thicken or dry lung secretions and impair expectoration. It should therefore be used with caution in patients with asthma, bronchitis or bronchiectasis.

Use with care in patients with severe coronary artery disease, narrow angle glaucoma, epilepsy or hepatic and renal insufficiency.

Caution should be exercised in patients with bladder neck or pyloro-duodenal obstruction.

The use of promethazine should be avoided in children and adolescents with signs and symptoms suggestive of Reye's Syndrome.

Promethazine may mask the warning signs of ototoxicity caused by ototoxic drugs e.g. salicylates. It may also delay the early diagnosis of intestinal obstruction or raised intracranial pressure through the suppression of vomiting.

Patients with rare hereditary problems of fructose intolerance should not take this medicine.

Phenergan Elixir should not be used for longer than 7 days without seeking medical advice.

4.5 Interaction with other medicinal products and other forms of interaction
Phenergan will enhance the action of any anticholinergic agent, tricyclic antidepressant, sedative or hypnotic. Alcohol should be avoided during treatment. Phenergan may interfere with immunological urine pregnancy tests to produce false-positive or false-negative results. Phenergan should be discontinued at least 72 hours before the start of skin tests as it may inhibit the cutaneous histamine response thus producing false-negative results.

4.6 Pregnancy and lactation
Phenergan Elixir should not be used in pregnancy unless the physician considers it essential. The use of Phenergan is not recommended in the 2 weeks prior to delivery in view of the risk of irritability and excitement in the neonate.

Available evidence suggests that the amount excreted in milk is insignificant. However, there are risks of neonatal irritability and excitement.

4.7 Effects on ability to drive and use machines
Because the duration of action may be up to 12 hours, patients should be advised that if they feel drowsy they should not drive or operate heavy machinery.

4.8 Undesirable effects
Side effects may be seen in a few patients: drowsiness, dizziness, restlessness, headaches, nightmares, tiredness, and disorientation. Anticholinergic side effects such as blurred vision, dry mouth and urinary retention occur occasionally. Infants are susceptible to the anticholinergic effects of promethazine, while other children may display paradoxical hyperexcitability. The elderly are particularly susceptible to the anticholinergic effects and confusion due to promethazine. Other side effects include urticaria, rash, pruritus, anorexia, gastric irritation, palpitations, hypotension, arrhythmias, extrapyramidal effects, muscle spasms and tic-like movements of the head and face. Anaphylaxis, jaundice and blood dyscrasias including haemolytic anaemia rarely occur. Photosensitive skin reactions have been reported. Strong sunlight should be avoided during treatment.

The preservatives used in Phenergan Elixir have been reported to cause hypersensitivity reactions, characterised by circulatory collapse with CNS depression in certain susceptible individuals with allergic tendencies.

4.9 Overdose
Symptoms of severe overdosage are variable. They are characterised in children by various combinations of excitation, ataxia, incoordination, athetosis and hallucinations, while adults may become drowsy and lapse into coma. Convulsions may occur in both adults and children: coma or excitement may precede their occurrence. Tachycardia may develop. Cardiorespiratory depression is uncommon. If the patient is seen soon enough after ingestion, it should be possible to induce vomiting with ipecacuanha despite the antiemetic effect of promethazine; alternatively, gastric lavage may be used.

Treatment is otherwise supportive with attention to maintenance of adequate respiratory and circulatory status. Convulsions should be treated with diazepam or other suitable anticonvulsant.

5. PHARMACOLOGICAL PROPERTIES
5.1 Pharmacodynamic properties
Pharmacotherapeutic group: Antihistamine for systemic use ATC code: R06AD02

Potent, long **acting**, antihistamine with additional antiemetic central sedative and anti-cholinergic properties.

5.2 Pharmacokinetic properties
Promethazine is distributed widely in the body. It enters the brain and crosses the placenta. Promethazine is slowly excreted via urine and bile. Phenothiazines pass into the milk at low concentrations.

5.3 Preclinical safety data
No additional preclinical data of relevance to the prescriber.

6. PHARMACEUTICAL PARTICULARS
6.1 List of excipients
Maltitol liquid, Citric acid anhydrous (E330), Sodium citrate (E331), Ascorbic acid (E300), Sodium sulphite anhydrous (E221), Sodium metabisulphite (E223), Sodium benzoate (E211), Orange juice flavour 510844E, Caramel (E150), Acesulfame potassium (E950), Purified water.

6.2 Incompatibilities
None stated.

6.3 Shelf life
2 years when unopened. 1 month when opened.

6.4 Special precautions for storage
Store below 25°C. Keep the bottle in the outer carton in order to protect from light.

6.5 Nature and contents of container
Amber glass type III bottle containing 100 ml. Rolled on pilfer proof aluminium cap and PVDC emulsion coated wad, or HDPE/polypropylene child resistant cap with tamper evident band.

6.6 Special precautions for disposal and other handling
None stated.

7. MARKETING AUTHORISATION HOLDER
Sanofi-aventis
One Onslow Street
Guildford
Surrey, GU1 4YS, UK

8. MARKETING AUTHORISATION NUMBER(S)
PL 04425/0630

9. DATE OF FIRST AUTHORISATION/RENEWAL OF THE AUTHORISATION
October 2008

10. DATE OF REVISION OF THE TEXT
October 2008

Legal category: P

Phenergan Injection
(sanofi-aventis)

1. NAME OF THE MEDICINAL PRODUCT
Phenergan Solution for Injection 2.5% w/v.

2. QUALITATIVE AND QUANTITATIVE COMPOSITION
Promethazine hydrochloride 2.5% w/v.

3. PHARMACEUTICAL FORM
Solution for injection.

4. CLINICAL PARTICULARS
4.1 Therapeutic indications
As symptomatic treatment for allergic conditions of the upper respiratory tract and skin including allergic rhinitis, urticaria and anaphylactic reactions to drugs and foreign proteins.

Sedation and treatment of insomnia in adults.

As an adjunct in preoperative sedation in surgery and obstetrics.

As a paediatric sedative.

Not for use in children under 2 years of age because the safety of such use has not been established.

Route of administration: Intramuscular or intravenous.

4.2 Posology and method of administration
Route of administration: Intramuscular or intravenous (after dilution)

The usual dose is 25 - 50 mg by deep intramuscular injection, or, in emergency, by slow intravenous injection after dilution of the 2.5% solution to 10 times its volume with water for injections immediately before use.

Maximum parenteral dose 100 mg.

Elderly: No specific dosage recommendations.

Children: 6.25 - 12.5 mg for children from 5 - 10 years by deep intramuscular injection. Not for use in children under 2 years of age (see section 4.3).

4.3 Contraindications
Phenergan should not be used in patients in coma or suffering from CNS depression of any cause.

Phenergan should not be given to patients with a known hypersensitivity to promethazine or to any of the excipients.

Promethazine is contraindicated for use in children less than two years of age because of the potential for fatal respiratory depression.

Phenergan should be avoided in patients taking monoamine oxidase inhibitors up to 14 days previously.

4.4 Special warnings and precautions for use

Phenergan may thicken or dry lung secretions and impair expectoration. It should therefore be used with caution in patients with asthma, bronchitis or bronchiectasis.

Use with care in patients with severe coronary artery disease, narrow angle glaucoma, epilepsy or hepatic and renal insufficiency.

Caution should be exercised in patients with bladder neck or pyloro-duodenal obstruction.

The use of promethazine should be avoided in children and adolescents with signs and symptoms suggestive of Reye's Syndrome.

Promethazine may mask the warning signs of ototoxicity caused by ototoxic drugs e.g. salicylates. It may also delay the early diagnosis of intestinal obstruction or raised intracranial pressure through the suppression of vomiting.

Intravenous injection should be performed with extreme care to avoid extravasation or inadvertent intra-arterial injection, which could lead to necrosis and peripheral gangrene. If a patient complains of pain during intravenous injection, stop the injection immediately, as this may be a sign of extravasation or inadvertent intra-arterial injection. Intramuscular injection must also be performed carefully to avoid inadvertent subcutaneous injection, which could lead to local necrosis.

4.5 Interaction with other medicinal products and other forms of interaction

Phenergan will enhance the action of any anticholinergic agent, tricyclic antidepressant, sedative or hypnotic. Alcohol should be avoided during treatment. Phenergan may cause hypotension, and dosage adjustment of antihypertensive therapy may therefore be required. Phenergan may lower the convulsive threshold, and dosage adjustment of anticonvulsant medication may therefore be required. Phenergan may interfere with immunological urine pregnancy tests to produce false-positive or false-negative results. Phenergan should be discontinued at least 72 hours before the start of skin tests as it may inhibit the cutaneous histamine response thus producing false-negative results. Phenergan injection may increase glucose tolerance.

4.6 Pregnancy and lactation

Phenergan Injection should not be used in pregnancy unless the physician considers it essential. The use of Phenergan is not recommended in the 2 weeks prior to delivery in view of the risk of irritability and excitement in the neonate.

Available evidence suggests that the amount excreted in milk is insignificant. However, there are risks of neonatal irritability and excitement.

4.7 Effects on ability to drive and use machines

Ambulant patients receiving Phenergan for the first time should not be in control of vehicles or machinery for the first few days until it is established that they are not hypersensitive to the central nervous effects of the drug and do not suffer from disorientation, confusion or dizziness.

4.8 Undesirable effects

Side effects may be seen in a few patients: drowsiness, dizziness, restlessness, headaches, nightmares, tiredness, and disorientation. Anticholinergic side effects such as blurred vision, dry mouth and urinary retention occur occasionally. Newborn and premature infants are susceptible to the anticholinergic effects of promethazine, while other children may display paradoxical hyperexcitability. The elderly are particularly susceptible to the anticholinergic effects and confusion due to promethazine. Other side-effects include anorexia, gastric irritation, palpitations, hypotension, arrhythmias, extrapyramidal effects, muscle spasms and tic-like movements of the head and face. Jaundice and blood dyscrasias including haemolytic anaemia rarely occur. Very rare cases of allergic reactions, including urticaria, rash, pruritus and anaphylaxis, have been reported.

Photosensitive skin reactions have been reported; strong sunlight should be avoided during treatment.

4.9 Overdose

Symptoms of severe overdosage are variable. They are characterised in children by various combinations of excitation, ataxia, incoordination, athetosis and hallucinations, while adults may become drowsy and lapse into coma. Convulsions may occur in both adults and children: coma or excitement may precede their occurrence. Cardiorespiratory depression is uncommon. If the patient is seen soon enough after ingestion, it should be possible to induce vomiting with ipecacuanha despite the antiemetic effect of promethazine; alternatively, gastric lavage may be used.

Treatment is otherwise supportive with attention to maintenance of adequate respiratory and circulatory status. Convulsions should be treated with diazepam or other suitable anticonvulsant.

5. PHARMACOLOGICAL PROPERTIES

5.1 Pharmacodynamic properties

Potent, long acting, antihistamine with additional anti-emetic central sedative and anti-cholinergic properties.

5.2 Pharmacokinetic properties

Promethazine is slowly excreted via urine and bile. It is distributed widely in the body. It enters the brain and crosses the placenta. Phenothiazines pass into the milk at low concentrations.

5.3 Preclinical safety data

No additional data of relevance to the prescriber.

6. PHARMACEUTICAL PARTICULARS

6.1 List of excipients

Sodium sulphite anhydrous (E221), Sodium metabisulphite (E223), Water for injections.

6.2 Incompatibilities

None stated.

6.3 Shelf life

60 months.

6.4 Special precautions for storage

Protect from light. Keep container in the outer carton.

6.5 Nature and contents of container

Cardboard carton containing 10 × 1 ml ampoules

6.6 Special precautions for disposal and other handling

Discoloured solutions should not be used.

7. MARKETING AUTHORISATION HOLDER

Sanofi-aventis

One Onslow Street

Guildford

Surrey, GU1 4YS, UK

8. MARKETING AUTHORISATION NUMBER(S)

PL 04425/0648

9. DATE OF FIRST AUTHORISATION/RENEWAL OF THE AUTHORISATION

9th February 2009

10. DATE OF REVISION OF THE TEXT

9th February 2009

11 LEGAL CLASSIFICATION

POM

Phenytoin 250mg/5ml Solution for Injection (Beacon Pharmaceuticals)

(Beacon Pharmaceuticals)

1. NAME OF THE MEDICINAL PRODUCT

Phenytoin 250mg/5ml Solution for Injection

2. QUALITATIVE AND QUANTITATIVE COMPOSITION

Each 5 ml ampoule contains 250 mg phenytoin sodium.

For excipients, see 6.1

3. PHARMACEUTICAL FORM

Solution for injection.

Clear, colourless, sterile, solution.

4. CLINICAL PARTICULARS

4.1 Therapeutic indications

Phenytoin Solution for Injection is indicated for

The control of status epilepticus of the tonic-clonic (grand mal type) and the prevention and treatment of seizures occurring during or following neurosurgery and/or severe head injury.

Phenytoin is also used in the treatment of cardiac arrhythmias where first line therapy is not effective. It is of particular value when these are digitalis induced.

4.2 Posology and method of administration

For intravenous administration.

Whenever solution and container permit, parenteral drug products should be inspected visually for particulate matter and discolouration prior to administration. Phenytoin Solution for Injection is suitable for use as long as it remains clear and free of precipitate. Upon refrigeration or freezing a precipitate might form; this will dissolve again after the solution is allowed to stand at room temperature. The product is still suitable for use. Only a clear solution should be used. A faint yellow colouration may develop; however, this has no effect on the potency of this solution.

There is a relatively small margin between full therapeutic effect and minimally toxic doses of this drug. Optimum control without clinical signs of toxicity occurs most often with serum levels between 10 and 20mg/l (40-80 micromoles/l).

Phenytoin Solution for Injection should be injected slowly directly into a large vein through a large-gauge needle or intravenous catheter.

Each injection or infusion of intravenous phenytoin should be preceded and followed by an injection of sterile saline through the same needle or catheter to avoid local venous irritation due to alkalinity of the solution. (See section 4.4.)

For infusion administration the phenytoin solution should be diluted in 50-100ml of normal saline, with the final concentration of phenytoin not exceeding 10mg/ml, the infusion mixture should not be refrigerated. Administration should begin immediately after the infusion mixture has been prepared and must be completed within one hour. An in-line filter (0.22-0.50 microns) should be used.

The diluted form is suitable for use as long as it remains clear and free of precipitate.

It is essential that both electrocardiogram and blood pressure of the patient be continuously monitored. Cardiac resuscitative equipment should be available. The patient should be observed for signs of respiratory depression. If administration of intravenous phenytoin does not terminate seizures, the use of other measures, including general anaesthesia, should be considered.

Use in Status Epilepticus:

In a patient having continuous seizure activity, as compared to the more common rapidly recurring seizures, i.e. serial epilepsy, injection of intravenous diazepam or a short acting barbiturate is recommended because of their rapid onset of action, prior to administration of phenytoin.

Following the use of diazepam in patients having continuous seizures and in the initial management of serial epilepsy a loading dose of phenytoin 10-15mg/kg should be injected slowly intravenously, at a rate not exceeding 50mg per minute in adults (this will require approximately 20 minutes in a 70kg patient). The loading dose should be followed by maintenance doses of 100mg orally or intravenously every 6 to 8 hours.

In neonates, it has been shown that absorption of phenytoin is unreliable after oral administration, but a loading dose of 15-20mg/kg of phenytoin intravenously will usually produce serum concentrations of 10–20 mg/l phenytoin which is within the generally accepted therapeutic range. The drug should be injected slowly intravenously at a rate of 1-3mg/kg/min.

It is advised that the serum levels of phenytoin are determined in the management of status epilepticus and to establish a maintenance dose. The clinically effective level is usually 10-20mg/l although some cases of tonic-clonic seizures may be controlled with lower serum levels of phenytoin.

Intramuscular administration should not be used in the treatment of status epilepticus because the attainment of peak plasma levels may require up to 24 hours.

Use in Cardiac Arrhythmias:

3.5-5mg per kg of bodyweight intravenously initially, repeated once if necessary. The solution should be injected slowly, intravenously and at a uniform rate which should not exceed 1ml (50mg) per minute.

Other clinical conditions:

The intravenous route of administration is preferred. Dosage and dosing interval will, of necessity, be determined by the needs of the individual patient. Factors such as previous antiepileptic therapy, seizure control, age and general medical condition must be considered.

Phenytoin is slowly absorbed when administered intramuscularly; this may be appropriate for the treatment of certain conditions.

When short-term intramuscular administration is necessary for a patient previously stabilised orally, compensating dosage adjustments are essential to maintain therapeutic serum levels. An intramuscular dose 50% greater than the oral dose is necessary to maintain these levels. When returned to oral administration, the dose should be reduced by 50% of the original oral dose, for the same period of time the patient received phenytoin intramuscularly. This is to prevent excessive serum levels due to continued release from intramuscular tissue sites

Neurosurgery:

In a patient who has not previously received the drug, 100-200mg (2-4ml) of phenytoin may be given intramuscularly at approximately 4-hour intervals prophylactically during neurosurgery and continued during the postoperative period for 48-72 hrs. The dosage should then be reduced to a maintenance dose of 300mg and adjusted according to serum level estimations.

If the patient requires more than a week of intramuscular phenytoin, alternative routes should be explored such as gastric intubation. For time periods less than one week, the patient switched from intramuscular administration should receive one half the original oral dose for the same period of time the patient received phenytoin intramuscularly. Measurement of serum levels is of value as a guide to an appropriate adjustment of dosage.

Elderly (over 65 years):

As for adults. However, complications may occur more readily in elderly patients.

Neonates:

In neonates it has been shown that absorption of phenytoin is unreliable after oral administration. Phenytoin should be injected slowly intravenously at a rate of 1-3mg/kg/min at a dose of 15-20mg/kg. This will usually produce serum concentrations of phenytoin within the generally accepted therapeutic range of 10-20mg/l.

Infants and children:

As for adults. Children tend to metabolise phenytoin more rapidly than adults. This should be considered when determining dosage regimens; monitoring serum levels is therefore particularly beneficial in such cases.

4.3 Contraindications

Phenytoin is contra-indicated in patients who are hypersensitive to phenytoin or other hydantoins. Intra-arterial administration must be avoided in view of the high pH of the preparation.

Because of its effect on ventricular automaticity, phenytoin is contra-indicated in sinus bradycardia, sino-atrial block, and second and third degree A-V block, and patients with Adams-Stokes syndrome.

4.4 Special warnings and precautions for use

In adults, intravenous administration should not exceed 50mg per minute. In neonates, the drug should be administered at a rate of 1-3mg/kg/min.

The most notable signs of toxicity associated with the intravenous use of this drug are cardiovascular collapse and/or central nervous system depression. Severe cardiotoxic reactions and fatalities due to depression of atrial and ventricular conduction and ventricular fibrillation, respiratory arrest and tonic seizures have been reported particularly in elderly or gravely ill patients, if the preparation is given too rapidly or in excess.

When the drug is administered rapidly by the intravenous route hypotension usually occurs.

Soft tissue irritation and inflammation has occurred at the site of injection with and without extravasation of intravenous phenytoin. Soft tissue irritation may vary from slight tenderness to extensive necrosis, sloughing and in rare instances has led to amputation. Subcutaneous or perivascular injection should be avoided because of the highly alkaline nature of the solution.

The intramuscular route is not recommended for the treatment of status epilepticus because of slow absorption. Serum levels of phenytoin in the therapeutic range cannot be rapidly achieved by this method.

General:

Intravenous phenytoin should be used with caution in patients with hypotension and severe myocardial insufficiency.

Phenytoin should be discontinued if a skin rash appears. If the rash is exfoliative, purpuric, or bullous or if lupus erythematosus, Stevens-Johnson syndrome, or toxic epidermal necrolysis is suspected, use of this drug should not be resumed and alternative therapy should be considered. If the rash is of a milder type (measles-like or scarlatiniform), therapy may be resumed after the rash has completely disappeared. If the rash recurs upon reinstitution of therapy, further phenytoin medication is contra-indicated.

Phenytoin is not effective for absence (petit mal) seizures. If tonic-clonic (grand mal) and absence (petit mal) seizures are present together, combined drug therapy is needed.

Serum levels of phenytoin sustained above the optimal range may produce confusional states referred to as "delirium", "psychosis", or "encephalopathy", or rarely irreversible cerebellar dysfunction. Accordingly, at the first sign of acute toxicity, serum drug level determinations are recommended. Dose reduction of phenytoin therapy is indicated if serum levels are excessive, if symptoms persist, termination of therapy with phenytoin is recommended.

Herbal preparations containing St John's wort (Hypericum perforatum) should not be used while taking phenytoin due to the risk of decreased plasma concentrations and reduced clinical effects of phenytoin (see Section 4.5).

Phenytoin is highly protein bound and extensively metabolised by the liver. In patients with impaired liver function a reduced maintenance dosage may be required to prevent accumulation and toxicity. Where protein binding is reduced, as in uraemia, total serum phenytoin levels will be reduced accordingly. However, the pharmacologically active free drug concentration is unlikely to be altered. Therefore, under these circumstances therapeutic control may be achieved with total phenytoin levels below the normal range of 10-20mg/l. Dosage should not exceed the minimum necessary to control convulsions.

Biotransformation of phenytoin occurs mainly in the liver. Patients with impaired liver function, elderly patients, or those who are gravely ill may show early signs of toxicity.

Phenytoin may affect glucose metabolism and inhibit insulin release. Hyperglycaemia has been reported. Phenytoin is not indicated for seizures due to hypoglycaemia or other metabolic causes. Therefore it is advised that caution be taken when treating diabetic patients.

It has been rarely reported that the use of phenytoin exacerbates porphyria, therefore caution should be exercised in using this medication in patients suffering from this disease.

Suicidal ideation and behaviour have been reported in patients treated with anti-epileptic agents in several indications. A meta-analysis of randomised placebo controlled trials of anti-epileptic drugs has also shown a small increased risk of suicidal ideation and behaviour. The mechanism of this risk is not known and the available data do not exclude the possibility of an increased risk for phenytoin.

Therefore, patients should be monitored for signs of suicidal ideation and behaviours and appropriate treatment should be considered. Patients and caregivers of patients) should be advised to seek medical advice should signs of suicidal ideation or behaviours emerge.

Laboratory Tests:

Phenytoin serum level determinations may be necessary to achieve optimal dosage adjustments.

4.5 Interaction with other medicinal products and other forms of interaction

Drugs which may increase phenytoin serum levels include: amiodarone, antifungal agents (such as, but not limited to, amphotericin B, fluconazole, ketoconazole, miconazole and itraconazole), chloramphenicol, chlordiazepoxide, diazepam, dicoumarol, diltiazem, disulfiram, oestrogens, fluoxetine, H2-antagonists, halothane, isoniazid, methylphenidate, nifedipine, omeprazole, phenothiazines, phenylbutazone, salicylates, succinimides, sulphonamides, tolbutamide, trazodone, and viloxazine.

Drugs, which may decrease phenytoin serum levels, include folic acid, reserpine, rifampicin, sucralfate, theophylline and vigabatrin.

Serum levels of phenytoin can be reduced by concomitant use of the herbal preparations containing St John's wort (Hypericum perforatum). St John's wort induces enzymes that metabolise phenytoin. Herbal preparations containing St John's wort should therefore not be combined with phenytoin. The inducing effect may persist for at least 2 weeks after cessation of treatment with St John's wort. If a patient is already taking St John's wort check the anticonvulsant levels and stop St John's wort. Anticonvulsant levels may increase on stopping St John's wort. The dose of anticonvulsant may need adjusting.

Drugs, which may either increase or decrease phenytoin serum levels, include carbamazepine, phenobarbital, valproic acid, sodium valproate, antineoplastic agents, certain antacids and ciprofloxacin. Similarly the effect of phenytoin on carbamazepine, phenobarbital, valproic acid and sodium valproate serum levels is unpredictable.

Acute alcoholic intake may increase phenytoin serum levels while chronic alcoholic use may decrease serum levels.

Although not a true pharmacokinetic interaction, tricyclic antidepressants and phenothiazines may precipitate seizures in susceptible patients and phenytoin dosage may need to be adjusted.

Phenytoin impairs the effect of the following drugs: antifungal agents, antineoplastic agents, calcium channel blockers, clozapine, corticosteroids, ciclosporin, dicoumarol, digitoxin, doxycycline, frusemide, lamotrigine, methadone, neuromuscular blockers, oestrogens, oral contraceptives, paroxetine, quinidine, rifampicin, theophylline and vitamin D.

The effect of warfarin is enhanced by phenytoin. The effect of phenytoin on warfarin is variable and prothrombin times should be determined when these agents are combined.

Serum level determinations are especially helpful when possible drug interactions are suspected.

Drug/Laboratory Test Interactions:

Phenytoin may cause a slight decrease in serum levels of total and free thyroxine, possibly as a result of enhanced peripheral metabolism. These changes do not lead to clinical hypothyroidism and do not affect the levels of circulating TSH. The latter can therefore be used for diagnosing hypothyroidism in the patient on phenytoin. Phenytoin does not interfere with uptake and suppression tests used in the diagnosis of hypothyroidism. It may, however, produce lower than normal values for dexamethasone or metapyrone tests. Phenytoin may cause raised serum levels of glucose, alkaline phosphatase, gamma glutamyl transpeptidase and lowered serum levels of calcium and folic acid. It is recommended that serum folate concentrations be measured at least every 6 months, and folic acid supplements given if necessary. Phenytoin may affect blood sugar metabolism tests.

4.6 Pregnancy and lactation

In considering the use of phenytoin intravenously in the management of status epilepticus in pregnancy, the following information should be weighed in assessing the risks and the benefits. The potential adverse effects upon the foetus of status epilepticus, specifically hypoxia, make it imperative to control the condition in the shortest possible time.

There are intrinsic methodologic problems in obtaining adequate data on drug teratogenicity in humans. Genetic factors or the epileptic condition itself may be more important than drug therapy in leading to birth defects. The great majority of mothers on anticonvulsant medication deliver normal infants. It is important to note that anticonvulsant drugs should not be discontinued in patients in whom the drug is administered to prevent major seizures because of the strong possibility of precipitating status epilepticus and attendant hypoxia and threat to life. In individual cases where the severity and frequency of the seizure disorder are such that the removal of medication does not pose a serious threat to the patient, discontinuation of the drug may be considered prior to and during pregnancy although it cannot be said with any confidence that even minor seizures do not pose some hazard to the developing embryo or foetus.

There is some evidence that phenytoin may produce congenital abnormalities in the offspring of a small number of epileptic patients, therefore it should not be used as the first drug during pregnancy, especially early pregnancy, unless in the judgement of the physician the potential benefits outweigh the risk.

In addition to the reports of increased incidence of congenital malformations, such as cleft lip/palate and heart malformations in children of women receiving phenytoin and other antiepileptic drugs, there have been recent reports of a foetal hydantoin syndrome. This consists of prenatal growth deficiency, microencephaly and mental deficiency in children born to mothers who have received phenytoin, barbiturates, alcohol, or trimethadione. However, these features are all interrelated and are frequently associated with intrauterine growth retardation from other causes.

There have been isolated reports of malignancies, including neuroblastoma, in children whose mothers received phenytoin during pregnancy.

An increase in seizure frequency during pregnancy occurs in a proportion of patients, because of altered phenytoin absorption or metabolism. Periodic measurement of serum phenytoin levels is particularly valuable in the management of a pregnant epileptic patient as a guide to an appropriate adjustment of dosage. However, post partum restoration of the original dosage will probably be indicated. Neonatal coagulation defects have been reported within the first 24 hours in babies born to epileptic mothers receiving phenytoin. Vitamin K has been shown to prevent or correct this defect and may be given to the mother before delivery and to the neonate after birth.

Infant breast-feeding is not recommended for women taking this drug because phenytoin appears to be secreted in low concentrations in human milk.

4.7 Effects on ability to drive and use machines

None known.

4.8 Undesirable effects

Signs of toxicity are associated with cardiovascular and central nervous system depression.

Central Nervous System:

The most common adverse reactions with phenytoin therapy occur in the central nervous system and are usually dose-related. These include nystagmus, ataxia, slurred speech, decreased coordination, mental confusion, paraesthesia, drowsiness and vertigo. Dizziness, insomnia, transient nervousness, motor twitching, and headache have also been observed. There have also been rare reports of phenytoin-induced dyskinesia, including chorea, dystonia, tremor, and asterixis, similar to those induced by phenothiazine and other neuroleptic drugs. A predominantly sensory peripheral polyneuropathy has been observed in patients receiving long-term phenytoin therapy. Tonic seizures have also been reported.

Cardiovascular:

Severe cardiotoxic reactions and fatalities have been reported with atrial and ventricular conduction depression and ventricular fibrillation. Severe complications are most commonly encountered in elderly or gravely ill patients.

Respiratory:

Alterations in respiratory function including respiratory arrest may occur.

Injection Site:

Local irritation, inflammation and tenderness. Necrosis and sloughing have been reported after subcutaneous or perivascular injection. Subcutaneous or perivascular injection should be avoided. Soft tissue irritation and inflammation have occurred at the site of injection with and without extravasation of intravenous phenytoin.

Dermatological System:

Dermatological reactions sometimes accompanied by fever have included scarlatiniform or morbilliform rashes. A morbilliform rash (measles-like) is the most common. Other types of dermatitis are seen more rarely. Other more serious forms, which may be fatal, have included bullous, exfoliative or purpuric dermatitis, lupus erythematosus, Stevens-Johnson syndrome, and toxic epidermal necrolysis.

Haemopoietic System:

Haemopoietic complications, some fatal, have occasionally been reported in association with administration of phenytoin. These have included thrombocytopenia, leucopenia, granulocytopenia, agranulocytosis, and pancytopenia with or without bone marrow suppression and aplastic anaemia. While macrocytosis and megaloblastic anaemia have occurred, these conditions usually respond to folic acid therapy. There have been a number of reports suggesting a relationship between phenytoin and the development of lymphadenopathy (local or generalised) including benign lymph node hyperplasia, pseudolymphoma, lymphoma, and Hodgkin's Disease. Although a cause and effect relationship has not been established, the occurrence of lymphadenopathy indicates the need to differentiate such a condition from other types of lymph node pathology. Lymph node involvement may occur with or without symptoms and signs resembling serum sickness, e.g. fever, rash and liver involvement.

In all cases of lymphadenopathy, follow-up observation for an extended period is indicated and every effort should be made to achieve seizure control using alternative antiepileptic drugs.

Gastrointestinal System:

Nausea, vomiting, constipation, toxic hepatitis, and liver damage.

Connective Tissue System:

Coarsening of the facial features, enlargement of the lips, gingival hyperplasia, hirsutism, hypertrichosis, Peyronie's disease and Dupuytren's contracture may occur rarely.

Immune System:

Hypersensitivity syndrome has been reported and may in rare cases be fatal (the syndrome may include, but is not limited to, symptoms such as arthralgias, eosinophilia, fever, liver dysfunction, lymphadenopathy or rash), systemic lupus erythematosus, periarteritis nodosa, and immunoglobulin abnormalities may occur. Several individual case reports have suggested that there may be an increased, although still rare, incidence of hypersensitivity reactions, including skin rash and hepatotoxicity, in black patients.

Other:

Polyarthropathy, interstitial nephritis, pneumonitis.

4.9 Overdose

The lethal dose in children is not known. The mean lethal dose in adults is estimated to be 2 to 5 grams. The initial symptoms are nystagmus, ataxia, and dysarthria. Other signs are tremor, hyperflexia, lethargy, nausea, vomiting. The patient may become comatose and hypotensive. Death is due to respiratory and circulatory depression.

Attempts to relate serum levels of the drug to toxic effects have shown wide interpatient variation. Nystagmus on lateral gaze usually appears at 20mg/l, and ataxia at 30mg/l, dysarthria and lethargy appear when the serum concentration is >40mg/l, but a concentration as high as 50mg/l has been reported without evidence of toxicity.

As much as 25 times the therapeutic dose, which resulted in a serum concentration of 100mg/l, was taken with complete recovery.

Treatment:

Treatment is non-specific since there is no known antidote. The adequacy of the respiratory and circulatory systems should be carefully observed and appropriate supportive measures employed. Haemodialysis can be considered since phenytoin is not completely bound to plasma proteins. Total exchange transfusion has been used in the treatment of severe intoxication in children.

In acute overdosage the possibility of the presence of other CNS depressants, including alcohol, should be borne in mind.

5. PHARMACOLOGICAL PROPERTIES

5.1 Pharmacodynamic properties

Pharmacotherapeutic group: Antiepileptics

ATC code: N03AB 01

Phenytoin is effective in various animal models of generalised convulsive disorders and reasonably effective in models of partial seizures but relatively ineffective in models of myoclonic seizures.

It appears to stabilise rather than raise the seizure threshold and prevents spread of seizure activity rather than abolish the primary focus of seizure discharge.

The mechanism by which phenytoin exerts its anticonvulsant action has not been fully elucidated, however, possible contributory effects include:

1. Non-synaptic effects to reduce sodium conductance, enhance active sodium extrusion, block repetitive firing and reduce post-tetanic potentiation.

2. Post-synaptic action to enhance GABA-mediated inhibition and reduce excitatory synaptic transmission.

3. Pre-synaptic actions to reduce calcium entry and block release of neurotransmitter.

5.2 Pharmacokinetic properties

After injection phenytoin is distributed into body fluids including CSF. Its volume of distribution has been estimated to be between 0.52 and 1.19 litres/kg, and it is highly protein bound (usually 90% in adults).

In serum, phenytoin binds rapidly and reversibly to proteins. About 90% of phenytoin in plasma is bound to albumin. The plasma half-life of phenytoin in man averages 22 hours with a range of 7 to 42 hours.

Phenytoin is hydroxylated in the liver by an enzyme system that is saturable. Small incremental doses may produce very substantial increases in serum levels when these are in the upper range of therapeutic concentrations.

The parameters controlling elimination are also subject to wide interpatient variation. The serum level achieved by a given dose is therefore also subject to wide variation.

5.3 Preclinical safety data

There are no preclinical safety data which could be of relevance to the prescriber and which are not already included in other relevant sections of the SPC.

6. PHARMACEUTICAL PARTICULARS

6.1 List of excipients

Propylene glycol

Ethanol (96%)

Sodium hydroxide

Water for injection.

6.2 Incompatibilities

Phenytoin solution for injection should not be mixed with other drugs because of precipitation of phenytoin acid.

6.3 Shelf life

2 years.

6.4 Special precautions for storage

Do not store above 25°C.

Store in the original package.

Keep out of sight and reach of children.

The product should not be used if a precipitate or haziness is noticed in the ampoule

6.5 Nature and contents of container

Transparent, type I glass ampoules.

Each 5ml ampoule contains 250mg phenytoin sodium.

Packs contain 1 ampoule or 50 ampoules (clinical pack)

6.6 Special precautions for disposal and other handling

Should be used immediately after opening. Discard any unused product once opened.

Refer also to 4.2 above.

7. MARKETING AUTHORISATION HOLDER

Beacon Pharmaceuticals Ltd.

Tunbridge Wells

Kent TN1 1YG

8. MARKETING AUTHORISATION NUMBER(S)

PL 18157/0010

9. DATE OF FIRST AUTHORISATION/RENEWAL OF THE AUTHORISATION

21/08/2006

10. DATE OF REVISION OF THE TEXT

9/9/2008

Phosphate Sandoz

(HK Pharma Limited)

1. NAME OF THE MEDICINAL PRODUCT

PHOSPHATE SANDOZ® Effervescent Tablets

2. QUALITATIVE AND QUANTITATIVE COMPOSITION

PHOSPHATE SANDOZ Effervescent Tablets containing 1.936g of sodium acid phosphate anhydrous.

3. PHARMACEUTICAL FORM

Effervescent Tablets

4. CLINICAL PARTICULARS

4.1 Therapeutic indications

Hypercalcaemia associated with such conditions as hyperparathyroidism, multiple myelomatosis and malignancy.

Hypophosphataemia associated with vitamin D resistant rickets and vitamin D resistant hypophosphataemic osteomalacia.

4.2 Posology and method of administration

PHOSPHATE SANDOZ Effervescent should be dissolved in 1/3 to 1/2 a tumblerful of water and taken orally.

Dosage should be adjusted to suit the requirements of individual patients. Excessive dosage has been reported to produce hypocalcaemia in isolated cases. Particular care should therefore be taken to ensure appropriate dosage in the elderly.

Adults

Hypercalcaemia: up to 6 tablets daily (adjustment being made according to requirements).

Vitamin D resistant hypophosphateaemic osteomalacia: 4-6 tablets daily.

Children under 5 years

Hypercalcaemia: up to 3 tablets daily (adjustment being made according to requirements).

Vitamin D resistant rickets: 2-3 tablets daily.

4.3 Contraindications

None.

4.4 Special warnings and precautions for use

In cases of impaired renal function associated with hypercalcaemia and in cases where restricted sodium intake is required, eg. congestive cardiac failure, hypertension or pre-eclamptic toxaemia, the sodium (20.4mmol per tablet) and potassium (3.1mmol per tablet) content of PHOSPHATE SANDOZ should be taken into consideration. In cases of hypercalcaemia associated with impaired renal function and hyperphosphataemia, the main effect of oral phosphate is to bind calcium in the gut and thus reduce calcium absorption.

The effect of oral phosphate on serum phosphate is likely to be minimal, but close monitoring of serum levels is recommended.

Soft tissue calcification and nephrocalcinosis have been reported in isolated cases following intravenous therapy with phosphate.

This is thought to be a function of dosage and rapidity of phosphate administration. While such effects appear less likely to occur with oral phosphates, careful surveillance of patients is recommended, especially if on long term therapy.

4.5 Interaction with other medicinal products and other forms of interaction

Concurrent administrations of antacids, containing agents such as aluminium hydroxide, may result in displacement of calcium from binding to oral phosphate, thus reducing efficacy.

4.6 Pregnancy and lactation

The safety of PHOSPHATE SANDOZ in human pregnancy has not been formally studied, but the drug has been widely used for many years without ill-consequence.

4.7 Effects on ability to drive and use machines

None.

4.8 Undesirable effects

Apart from gastro-intestinal upsets, nausea and diarrhoea, very few side effects have been reported.

4.9 Overdose

Excessive dosage has been reported to produce hypocalcaemia in isolated cases. This has proved reversible when dosage has been adjusted.

5. PHARMACOLOGICAL PROPERTIES

5.1 Pharmacodynamic properties

Oral administration of inorganic phosphates produces a fall in serum calcium in patients with hypercalcaemia. PHOSPHATE SANDOZ Effervescent Tablets also contain sodium ions which aid the correction of the dehydration and sodium depletion seen in hypercalcaemia.

5.2 Pharmacokinetic properties

Approximately two thirds of ingested phosphate is absorbed from the gastro-intestinal tract; most of the absorbed phosphate is then filtered by the glomeruli and subsequently undergoes reabsorption. Parathyroid hormone and vitamin D stimulate absorption of phosphate from the small intestine and its reabsorption from the proximal tubule. Virtually all absorbed phosphate is eventually excreted in the urine, the remainder being excreted in the faeces.

5.3 Preclinical safety data

PHOSPHATE SANDOZ Effervescent Tablets contain sodium acid phosphate, anhydrous, sodium bicarbonate and potassium bicarbonate (all of which are subject to pharmacopoeial monographs). The physiological, pharmacological and clinical toxicity of potassium salts are well documented and limited animal data are therefore available.

6. PHARMACEUTICAL PARTICULARS

6.1 List of excipients

Potassium bicarbonate, sodium bicarbonate, sodium saccharin, orange flavour 52.570 TP, polyethylene glycol 4000, sugar icing CP, citric acid anhydrous, water.

6.2 Incompatibilities

None.

6.3 Shelf life

36 months.

6.4 Special precautions for storage

Do not store above 25°C. Store in the original container. Keep the container tightly closed

6.5 Nature and contents of container

Polypropylene tubes of 20 effervescent tablets in boxes of 5 tubes (100 tablets).

6.6 Special precautions for disposal and other handling

None.

7. MARKETING AUTHORISATION HOLDER

HK Pharma Ltd

PO Box 105

HITCHIN

SG5 2GG

8. MARKETING AUTHORISATION NUMBER(S)

PL 16784/0001

9. DATE OF FIRST AUTHORISATION/RENEWAL OF THE AUTHORISATION

28th April 1998

10. DATE OF REVISION OF THE TEXT

October 2002

Phyllocontin Continus tablets 225mg, Phyllocontin Forte Continus tablets 350mg

(Napp Pharmaceuticals Limited)

1. NAME OF THE MEDICINAL PRODUCT
PHYLLOCONTIN CONTINUS 225 mg prolonged release tablets.

PHYLLOCONTIN Forte CONTINUS 350 mg prolonged release tablets.

2. QUALITATIVE AND QUANTITATIVE COMPOSITION
Aminophylline hydrate 225 and 350 mg.

For a full list of excipients, see 6.1.

3. PHARMACEUTICAL FORM
Prolonged release tablets

PHYLLOCONTIN CONTINUS tablets 225 mg are pale yellow, film-coated tablets with the Napp logo on one side and SA on the other.

PHYLLOCONTIN Forte CONTINUS tablets 350 mg are pale yellow, film-coated tablets with the Napp logo on one side and SA 350 on the other.

4. CLINICAL PARTICULARS
4.1 Therapeutic indications
For the treatment and prophylaxis of bronchospasm associated with asthma, chronic obstructive pulmonary disease and chronic bronchitis. Also indicated in adults for the treatment of left ventricular and congestive cardiac failure.

4.2 Posology and method of administration
Route of Administration

Oral.

The tablets should be swallowed whole and not chewed.

Children: The maintenance dose (expressed as mg aminophylline) is 12mg/kg twice daily adjusted to the nearest 225mg. It is recommended that half the maintenance dose be given for the first week of therapy if the patient has not previously been receiving xanthine preparations. PHYLLOCONTIN CONTINUS tablets 225mg are, therefore, not suitable as a starting dose for children weighing under 40 kg.

Some children with chronic asthma require and tolerate much higher doses (13-20 mg/kg twice daily). Lower doses (based on the usual adult dose) may be required by adolescents.

Adults: The usual dose is two PHYLLOCONTIN CONTINUS tablets 225 mg, or one or two PHYLLOCONTIN Forte CONTINUS tablets 350mg twice-daily following an initial week of therapy on one tablet twice-daily.

The Elderly: The dose should be adjusted following the response to the initial week of therapy on one tablet twice-daily.

Dose Titration: Patients vary in their response to xanthines and it may be necessary to titrate dosage individually. Steady state theophylline levels are generally attained 3-4 days after dose adjustment. If a satisfactory clinical response is not achieved, serum theophylline should be measured 4-6 hours after the last dose. Based on serum theophylline assay results dosage should be titrated using the following as a guide:

Peak serum theophylline level	Dosage adjustment to nearest 125 mg
< 10 micrograms/ml	Increase total daily dose by half
10-15 micrograms/ml	Increase total daily dose by one quarter if symptoms persist
16-20 micrograms/ml	No adjustment required
21-25 micrograms/ml	Decrease dose by one quarter
26-30 micrograms/ml	Miss next dose and decrease maintenance by one half

4.3 Contraindications
Should not be given concomitantly with ephedrine in children. Hypersensitivity to xanthines or any of the tablet constituents. Porphyria.

4.4 Special warnings and precautions for use
The patient's response to therapy should be carefully monitored – worsening of asthma symptoms requires medical attention.

Use with caution in patients with cardiac arrhythmias, peptic ulcer, hyperthyroidism, severe hypertension, hepatic dysfunction, chronic alcoholism or acute febrile illness.

The half-life of theophylline may be prolonged in the elderly and in patients with heart failure, hepatic impairment or viral infections. Toxic accumulation may occur (see Section 4.9 overdose).

A reduction of dosage may be necessary in the elderly patient.

Avoid concomitant use with other xanthine-containing products.

The hypokalaemia resulting from beta agonist therapy, steroids, diuretics and hypoxia may be potentiated by xanthines. Particular care is advised in patients suffering from severe asthma who require hospitalisation. It is recommended that serum potassium levels are monitored in such situations.

Alternative treatment is advised for patients with a history of seizure activity.

4.5 Interaction with other medicinal products and other forms of interaction
The following increase clearance and it may therefore be necessary to increase dosage to ensure a therapeutic effect: aminoglutethimide, carbamazepine, moracizine, phenytoin, rifampicin, sulphinpyrazone, barbiturates and Hypericum perforatum. Plasma concentrations of theophylline can be reduced by concomitant use of the herbal remedy St John's Wort (Hypericum perforatum). Smoking and alcohol consumption can also increase clearance of theophylline.

The following reduce clearance and a reduced dosage may therefore be necessary to avoid side-effects: allopurinol, carbimazole, cimetidine, ciprofloxacin, clarithromycin, diltiazem, disulfiram, erythromycin, fluconazole, interferon, isoniazid, isoprenaline, methotrexate, mexiletine, nizatidine, norfloxacin, oxpentifylline, propafenone, propranolol, ofloxacin, thiabendazole, verapamil, viloxazine hydrochloride and oral contraceptives. The concomitant use of theophylline and fluvoxamine should usually be avoided. Where this is not possible, patients should have their theophylline dose halved and plasma theophylline should be monitored closely.

Factors such as viral infections, liver disease and heart failure also reduce theophylline clearance. There are conflicting reports concerning the potentiation of theophylline by influenza vaccine and physicians should be aware that interaction may occur. A reduction of dosage may be necessary in elderly patients. Thyroid disease or associated treatment may alter theophylline plasma levels. There is also a pharmacological interaction with adenosine, benzodiazepines, halothane, lomustine and lithium and these drugs should be used with caution.

Theophylline may decrease steady state phenytoin levels.

4.6 Pregnancy and lactation
There are no adequate data from well controlled studies from the use of theophylline in pregnant women. Theophylline has been reported to give rise to teratogenic effects in mice, rats and rabbits (see section 5.3). The potential risk for humans is unknown. Theophylline should not be administered during pregnancy unless clearly necessary. Theophylline is secreted in breast milk, and may be associated with irritability in the infant, therefore it should only be given to breast feeding women when the anticipated benefits outweigh the risk to the child.

4.7 Effects on ability to drive and use machines
No known effects.

4.8 Undesirable effects
The side-effects usually associated with theophylline and xanthine derivatives such are nausea, gastric irritation, headache, CNS stimulation, tachycardia, palpitations, arrhythmias and convulsions.

4.9 Overdose
Over 3 g could be serious in an adult (40 mg/kg in a child). The fatal dose may be as little as 4.5 g in an adult (60 mg/kg in a child), but is generally higher.

Symptoms
Warning: Serious features may develop as long as 12 hours after overdosage with prolonged release formulations.

Alimentary features: Nausea, vomiting (which is often severe), epigastric pain and haematemesis. Consider pancreatitis if abdominal pain persists.

Neurological features: Restlessness, hypertonia, exaggerated limb reflexes and convulsions. Coma may develop in very severe cases.

Cardiovascular features: Sinus tachycardia is common. Ectopic beats and supraventricular and ventricular tachycardia may follow.

Metabolic features: Hypokalaemia due to shift of potassium from plasma into cells is common, can develop rapidly and may be severe. Hyperglycaemia, hypomagnesaemia and metabolic acidosis may also occur. Rhabdomyolysis may also occur.

Management
Activated charcoal or gastric lavage should be considered if a significant overdose has been ingested within 1-2 hours. Repeated doses of activated charcoal given by mouth can enhance theophylline elimination. Measure the plasma potassium concentration urgently, repeat frequently and correct hypokalaemia. BEWARE! If large amounts of potassium have been given, serious hyperkalaemia may develop during recovery. If plasma potassium is low, then the plasma magnesium concentration should be measured as soon as possible.

In the treatment of ventricular arrhythmias, proconvulsant antiarrhythmic agents such as lignocaine (lidocaine) should be avoided because of the risk of causing or exacerbating seizures.

Measure the plasma theophylline concentration regularly when severe poisoning is suspected, until concentrations are falling. Vomiting should be treated with an antiemetic such as metoclopramide or ondansetron.

Tachycardia with an adequate cardiac output is best left untreated. Beta-blockers may be given in extreme cases but not if the patient is asthmatic. Control isolated convulsions with intravenous diazepam. Exclude hypokalaemia as a cause.

5. PHARMACOLOGICAL PROPERTIES
5.1 Pharmacodynamic properties
Pharmacotherapeutic group: Other systemic drugs for obstructive airways diseases.

ATC code: R03D A05

Aminophylline (theophylline) is a bronchodilator. In addition it affects the function of a number of cells involved in the inflammatory processes associated with asthma and chronic obstructive airways disease. Of most importance may be enhanced suppressor T-lymphocyte activity and reduction of eosinophil and neutrophil function. These actions may contribute to an anti-inflammatory prophylactic activity in asthma and chronic obstructive airways disease. Theophylline stimulates the myocardium and produces a diminution of venous pressure in congestive heart failure leading to marked increase in cardiac output.

5.2 Pharmacokinetic properties
Aminophylline (theophylline) is well absorbed from PHYLLOCONTIN CONTINUS tablets and at least 60% may be bound to plasma proteins. The main urinary metabolites are 1,3 dimethyl uric acid and 3-methylxanthine. About 10% is excreted unchanged.

5.3 Preclinical safety data
In studies in which mice, rats and rabbits were dosed during the period of organogenesis, theophylline produced teratogenic effects.

6. PHARMACEUTICAL PARTICULARS
6.1 List of excipients
Hydroxyethylcellulose

Povidone [K25]

Cetostearyl Alcohol

Purified Talc

Magnesium Stearate

Film coat

Hypromellose [E464]

Polyethylene glycol 400

Opaspray M-1-3058 (containing Industrial Methylated Spirit

Hypromellose [E464], Titanium Dioxide [E171], Iron Oxide [E172]).

6.2 Incompatibilities
Not applicable.

6.3 Shelf life
Three years

6.4 Special precautions for storage
Do not store above 25°C.

Store in the original package.

6.5 Nature and contents of container
PHYLLOCONTIN CONTINUS tablets 225 mg are available in PVC blister packs containing 56 tablets.

PHYLLOCONTIN Forte CONTINUS tablets are available in polypropylene containers containing 56 tablets.

6.6 Special precautions for disposal and other handling
No special requirements.

7. MARKETING AUTHORISATION HOLDER
Napp Pharmaceuticals Ltd

Cambridge Science Park

Milton Road

Cambridge CB4 0GW

8. MARKETING AUTHORISATION NUMBER(S)
PL 16950/0057, 0058

9. DATE OF FIRST AUTHORISATION/RENEWAL OF THE AUTHORISATION
PHYLLOCONTIN CONTINUS tablets 225 mg –

7 July 1989 / 28 July 2006

PHYLLOCONTIN Forte CONTINUS tablets 350 mg –

17 August 1983 / 28 July 2006

10. DATE OF REVISION OF THE TEXT
July 2006

® PHYLLOCONTIN, CONTINUS, NAPP and the NAPP device are Registered Trade Marks.

Physiotens Tablets 200 micrograms

(Solvay Healthcare Limited)

1. NAME OF THE MEDICINAL PRODUCT
Physiotens® Tablets 200 micrograms

Cynt Tablets 200 micrograms

Moxonidine 200 micrograms Tablets

2. QUALITATIVE AND QUANTITATIVE COMPOSITION

Each tablet contains 200 micrograms moxonidine.

3. PHARMACEUTICAL FORM

Film coated tablets.

Light pink, round, biconvex, film-coated tablets imprinted '0.2' on one face.

4. CLINICAL PARTICULARS

4.1 Therapeutic indications

Mild to moderate essential or primary hypertension.

4.2 Posology and method of administration

Adults (including the elderly):

Treatment should be started with 200 micrograms of Physiotens/Cynt/Moxonidine in the morning. The dose may be titrated after three weeks to 400 micrograms, given as one dose or as divided doses (morning and evening) until a satisfactory response has been achieved. If the response is still unsatisfactory after a further three weeks' treatment, the dosage can be increased up to a maximum of 600 micrograms in divided doses (morning and evening).

A single dose of 400 micrograms of Physiotens/Cynt/Moxonidine and a daily dose of 600 micrograms in divided doses (morning and evening) should not be exceeded.

In patients with moderate renal dysfunction (GFR above 30 ml/min, but below 60 ml/min), the single dose should not exceed 200 micrograms and the daily dose should not exceed 400 micrograms of moxonidine.

The tablets should be taken with a little liquid. As the intake of food has no influence on the pharmacokinetic properties of moxonidine, the tablets may be taken before, during or after the meal.

Paediatric population

Physiotens/Cynt/Moxonidine is not recommended for use in children and adolescents below 16 years due to lack of data on safety and efficacy.

4.3 Contraindications

Physiotens/Cynt/Moxonidine should not be used in cases of:

- history of angioneurotic oedema
- hypersensitivity to the active substance or to any of the excipients
- sick sinus syndrome or sino-atrial block
- 2nd or 3rd degree atrioventricular block
- bradycardia (below 50 beats/minute at rest)
- malignant arrhythmia
- severe heart failure (see Section 4.4)
- severe coronary artery disease or unstable angina
- severe liver disease
- severe renal dysfunction (GFR $<$30 ml/min, serum creatinine concentration $>$160 μmol/l).

Physiotens/Cynt/Moxonidine should not be used because of lack of therapeutic experience in cases of:

- intermittent claudication
- Raynaud's disease
- Parkinson's disease
- epileptic disorders
- glaucoma
- depression
- pregnancy or lactation
- children and adolescents below 16 years of age.

4.4 Special warnings and precautions for use

If Moxonidine is used in combination with a beta-blocker and both treatments have to be discontinued, the beta-blocker should be discontinued first and Moxonidine only thereafter.

In patients with moderate renal dysfunction (GFR above 30 but below 60 ml/min, serum creatinine above 105 but below 160 μmol), the hypotensive effect of Physiotens/Cynt/Moxonidine should be closely monitored, especially at the start of treatment.

Due to lack of therapeutic experience, the use of Physiotens/Cynt/Moxonidine concomitantly with alcohol or tricyclic antidepressants should be avoided.

Due to a lack of clinical data supporting the safety in patients with co-existing moderate heart failure, Physiotens/Cynt/Moxonidine must be used with caution in such patients.

Treatment with Physiotens/Cynt/Moxonidine should not be discontinued abruptly, but should be withdrawn gradually over a period of two weeks.

Patients with rare hereditary problems of galactose intolerance, the rare Lapp lactase deficiency or glucose-galactose malabsorption should not take this medicine.

4.5 Interaction with other medicinal products and other forms of interaction

Concurrent administration of other antihypertensive agents enhances the hypotensive effect of Physiotens/Cynt/Moxonidine.

The effect of sedatives and hypnotics may be intensified by Physiotens/Cynt/Moxonidine. The sedative effect of benzodiazepines can be enhanced by concurrent administration of Physiotens/Cynt/Moxonidine.

4.6 Pregnancy and lactation

As insufficient data are available, Physiotens/Cynt/Moxonidine should not be used during pregnancy.

Physiotens/Cynt/Moxonidine should not be used during lactation because it is excreted into breast milk.

4.7 Effects on ability to drive and use machines

No data are available to suggest that Physiotens/Cynt/Moxonidine adversely affects the ability to drive or operate machines. However, as somnolence and dizziness have been reported, patients should be cautioned about their ability to undertake potentially hazardous tasks such as driving and operating machinery if so affected.

4.8 Undesirable effects

At the start of treatment dry mouth is frequently observed, while headache, asthenia, dizziness, nausea, sleep disturbances and vasodilatation are observed occasionally. Sedation has been reported in less than 1% of patients. The frequency and intensity of these symptoms often decrease in the course of treatment.

Allergic skin reactions have been reported in very rare cases.

Isolated cases of angioedema have been reported.

4.9 Overdose

Oral dosages up to 2.0 mg/day have been tolerated without the occurrence of serious adverse events. The following case of accidental overdose with Physiotens/Cynt/Moxonidine by a 2 year old child has been reported:

The child ingested an unknown quantity of Physiotens/Cynt/Moxonidine. The maximum dosage possibly ingested was 14 mg. The child had the following symptoms: sedation, coma, hypotension, miosis and dyspnoea. Gastric lavage, glucose infusion, mechanically assisted ventilation and rest resulted in the complete disappearance of the symptoms in 11 hours.

Because of the pharmacodynamic properties of Physiotens/Cynt/Moxonidine, the following symptoms can be expected in adults: sedation, hypotension, orthostatic dysregulation, bradycardia, dry mouth. In rare cases emesis and paradoxical hypertension may occur.

No specific antidote is known. Phentolamine (Rogitine) may, depending on the dose, reverse part of the symptoms of moxonidine overdosage. Measures to support blood circulation are recommended.

5. PHARMACOLOGICAL PROPERTIES

5.1 Pharmacodynamic properties

In different animal models, Physiotens/Cynt/Moxonidine has been shown to be a potent antihypertensive agent. Available experimental data convincingly suggest that the site of the antihypertensive action of Physiotens/Cynt/Moxonidine is the central nervous system (CNS). Within the brainstem, Physiotens/Cynt/Moxonidine has been shown to selectively interact with I_1-imidazoline receptors. These imidazoline-sensitive receptors are concentrated in the rostral ventrolateral medulla, an area critical to the central control of the peripheral sympathetic nervous system. The net effect of this interaction with the I_1-imidazoline receptor appears to result in a reduced activity of sympathetic nerves (demonstrated for cardiac, splanchnic and renal sympathetic nerves).

Physiotens/Cynt/Moxonidine differs from other available centrally acting antihypertensives by exhibiting only low affinity to central α_2-adrenoceptors as compared to I_1-imidazoline receptors; α_2-adrenoceptors are considered the molecular target via which sedation and dry mouth, the most common undesired side effects of centrally acting antihypertensives, are mediated.

In humans, Physiotens/Cynt/Moxonidine leads to a reduction of systemic vascular resistance and consequently in arterial blood pressure.

5.2 Pharmacokinetic properties

Oral moxonidine treatment of rats and dogs resulted in rapid and almost complete absorption and peak plasma levels within $<$0.5 hours. Average plasma concentrations were comparable in both species after p.o. and i.v. administration. The elimination half-lives of radioactivity and unchanged compound were estimated to be 1-3 hours. Moxonidine and its two main metabolites (4,5-dehydromoxonidine and a guanidine derivative) was predominantly excreted in the urine. No indication of moxonidine cumulation was observed in either species during chronic toxicity studies after 52 weeks.

In humans, about 90% of an oral dose of moxonidine is absorbed; it is not subject to first-pass metabolism and its bio-availability is 88%. Food intake does not interfere with moxonidine pharmacokinetics. Moxonidine is 10-20% metabolised, mainly to 4,5-dehydromoxonidine and to a guanidine derivative by opening of the imidazoline ring. The hypotensive effect of 4,5-dehydromoxonidine is only 1/10, and that of the guanidine derivative is less than 1/100 of that of moxonidine. The maximum plasma levels of moxonidine are reached 30-180 minutes after the intake of a film-coated tablet.

Only about 7% of moxonidine is bound to plasma protein (Vd_{ss}=1.8 ± 0.4 l/kg). Moxonidine and its metabolites are eliminated almost entirely via the kidneys. More than 90% of the dose is eliminated via the kidneys in the first 24 hours after administration, while only about 1% is eliminated via the faeces. The cumulative renal excretion of unchanged moxonidine is about 50-75%.

The mean plasma elimination half-life of moxonidine is 2.2-2.3 hours, and the renal elimination half-life is 2.6-2.8 hours.

Pharmacokinetics in the elderly

Small differences between the pharmacokinetic properties of moxonidine in the healthy elderly and younger adults are unlikely to be clinically significant. As there is no accumulation of moxonidine, dosage adjustment is unnecessary provided renal function is normal.

Pharmacokinetics in children

No pharmacokinetic studies have been performed in children.

Pharmacokinetics in renal impairment

In moderately impaired renal function (GFR 30-60 ml/min), AUC increased by 85% and clearance decreased to 52%. In such patients the hypotensive effect of Physiotens/Cynt/Moxonidine should be closely monitored, especially at the start of treatment; additionally, single doses should not exceed 200 micrograms and the daily dose should not exceed 400 micrograms.

5.3 Preclinical safety data

Chronic oral treatment for 52 weeks of rats (with dosages of 0.12-4 mg/kg) and dogs (with dosages of 0.04-0.4 mg/kg) revealed significant effects of moxonidine only at the highest doses. Slight disturbances of electrolyte balance (decrease of blood sodium and increase of potassium, urea and creatinine) were found in the high dose rats and emesis and salivation only for the high dose dogs. In addition slight increases of liver weight were obvious for both high dose species.

Reproductive toxicology did not show moxonidine effects (at oral doses up to 6.4 mg/kg) on fertility of rats and development of the embryo and foetus. Neither was evidence seen of embryotoxic and teratogenic properties in the rat at oral doses up to 27 mg/kg and the rabbit up to 4.9 mg/kg, nor on peri- and post-natal development in the rat after oral dosage up to 9 mg/kg.

Five different studies also did not show any indication of mutagenic or genotoxic effects of moxonidine. In addition, carcinogenicity studies in rats and mice at oral doses of 0.1-7.0 mg/kg did not reveal any evidence of carcinogenic potential.

6. PHARMACEUTICAL PARTICULARS

6.1 List of excipients

Lactose, povidone, crospovidone, magnesium stearate, hypromellose, ethylcellulose, polyethylene glycol 6000, talc, red ferric oxide, titanium dioxide.

6.2 Incompatibilities

No incompatibilities are known.

6.3 Shelf life

2 years.

6.4 Special precautions for storage

Do not store above 25°C.

6.5 Nature and contents of container

The tablets are packed in blister strips of 14. The blister strips are made of PVC/PVdC or PVC film with covering Aluminium foil. Each carton contains 14, 28 or 84 tablets.

6.6 Special precautions for disposal and other handling

None.

7. MARKETING AUTHORISATION HOLDER

Solvay Healthcare Limited

Mansbridge Road

West End

Southampton

SO18 3JD

8. MARKETING AUTHORISATION NUMBER(S)

PL 00512/0152

9. DATE OF FIRST AUTHORISATION/RENEWAL OF THE AUTHORISATION

15 September 1997/ 5 April 2002

10. DATE OF REVISION OF THE TEXT

12 June 2009

Physiotens Tablets 300 micrograms

(Solvay Healthcare Limited)

1. NAME OF THE MEDICINAL PRODUCT

Physiotens® Tablets 300 micrograms

Cynt Tablets 300 micrograms

Moxonidine 300 micrograms Tablets

2. QUALITATIVE AND QUANTITATIVE COMPOSITION

Each tablet contains 300 micrograms moxonidine.

3. PHARMACEUTICAL FORM

Film coated tablets.

Pale red, round, biconvex, film-coated tablets imprinted '0.3' on one face.

4. CLINICAL PARTICULARS

4.1 Therapeutic indications

Mild to moderate essential or primary hypertension.

4.2 Posology and method of administration

Adults (including the elderly):

Treatment should be started with 200 micrograms of Physiotens/Cynt/Moxonidine in the morning. The dose may be titrated after three weeks to 400 micrograms, given as one dose or as divided doses (morning and evening) until a satisfactory response has been achieved. If the response is still unsatisfactory after a further three weeks' treatment, the dosage can be increased up to a maximum of 600 micrograms in divided doses (morning and evening).

A single dose of 400 micrograms of Physiotens/Cynt/Moxonidine and a daily dose of 600 micrograms in divided doses (morning and evening) should not be exceeded.

In patients with moderate renal dysfunction (GFR above 30 ml/min, but below 60 ml/min), the single dose should not exceed 200 micrograms and the daily dose should not exceed 400 micrograms of moxonidine.

The tablets should be taken with a little liquid. As the intake of food has no influence on the pharmacokinetic properties of moxonidine, the tablets may be taken before, during or after the meal.

Paediatric population

Physiotens/Cynt/Moxonidine is not recommended for use in children and adolescents below 16 years due to lack of data on safety and efficacy.

4.3 Contraindications

Physiotens/Cynt/Moxonidine should not be used in cases of:

- history of angioneurotic oedema
- hypersensitivity to the active substance or to any of the excipients
- sick sinus syndrome or sino-atrial block
- 2nd or 3rd degree atrioventricular block
- bradycardia (below 50 beats/minute at rest)
- malignant arrhythmia
- severe heart failure (see Section 4.4)
- severe coronary artery disease or unstable angina
- severe liver disease
- severe renal dysfunction (GFR <30 ml/min, serum creatinine concentration >160 μmol/l).

Physiotens/Cynt/Moxonidine should not be used because of lack of therapeutic experience in cases of:

- intermittent claudication
- Raynaud's disease
- Parkinson's disease
- epileptic disorders
- glaucoma
- depression
- pregnancy or lactation
- children and adolescents below 16 years of age.

4.4 Special warnings and precautions for use

If Moxonidine is used in combination with a beta-blocker and both treatments have to be discontinued, the beta-blocker should be discontinued first and Moxonidine only thereafter.

In patients with moderate renal dysfunction (GFR above 30 but below 60 ml/min, serum creatinine above 105 but below 160 μmol), the hypotensive effect of Physiotens/Cynt/Moxonidine should be closely monitored, especially at the start of treatment.

Due to lack of therapeutic experience, the use of Physiotens/Cynt/Moxonidine concomitantly with alcohol or tricyclic antidepressants should be avoided.

Due to a lack of clinical data supporting the safety in patients with co-existing moderate heart failure, Physiotens/Cynt/Moxonidine must be used with caution in such patients.

Treatment with Physiotens/Cynt/Moxonidine should not be discontinued abruptly, but should be withdrawn gradually over a period of two weeks.

Patients with rare hereditary problems of galactose intolerance, the rare Lapp lactase deficiency or glucose-galactose malabsorption should not take this medicine.

4.5 Interaction with other medicinal products and other forms of interaction

Concurrent administration of other antihypertensive agents enhances the hypotensive effect of Physiotens/Cynt/Moxonidine.

The effect of sedatives and hypnotics may be intensified by Physiotens/Cynt/Moxonidine. The sedative effect of benzodiazepines can be enhanced by concurrent administration of Physiotens/Cynt/Moxonidine.

4.6 Pregnancy and lactation

As insufficient data are available, Physiotens/Cynt/Moxonidine should not be used during pregnancy.

Physiotens/Cynt/Moxonidine should not be used during lactation because it is excreted into breast milk.

4.7 Effects on ability to drive and use machines

No data are available to suggest that Physiotens/Cynt/Moxonidine adversely affects the ability to drive or operate machines. However, as somnolence and dizziness have been reported, patients should be cautioned about their ability to undertake potentially hazardous tasks such as driving and operating machinery if so affected.

4.8 Undesirable effects

At the start of treatment dry mouth is frequently observed, while headache, asthenia, dizziness, nausea, sleep disturbances and vasodilatation are observed occasionally. Sedation has been reported in less than 1% of patients. The frequency and intensity of these symptoms often decrease in the course of treatment.

Allergic skin reactions have been reported in very rare cases.

Isolated cases of angioedema have been reported.

4.9 Overdose

Oral dosages up to 2.0 mg/day have been tolerated without the occurrence of serious adverse events. The following case of accidental overdose with Physiotens/Cynt/Moxonidine by a 2 year old child has been reported:

The child ingested an unknown quantity of Physiotens/Cynt/Moxonidine. The maximum dosage possibly ingested was 14 mg. The child had the following symptoms: sedation, coma, hypotension, miosis and dyspnoea. Gastric lavage, glucose infusion, mechanically assisted ventilation and rest resulted in the complete disappearance of the symptoms in 11 hours.

Because of the pharmacodynamic properties of Physiotens/Cynt/Moxonidine, the following symptoms can be expected in adults: sedation, hypotension, orthostatic dysregulation, bradycardia, dry mouth. In rare cases emesis and paradoxical hypertension may occur.

No specific antidote is known. Phentolamine (Rogitine) may, depending on the dose, reverse part of the symptoms of moxonidine overdosage. Measures to support blood circulation are recommended.

5. PHARMACOLOGICAL PROPERTIES

5.1 Pharmacodynamic properties

In different animal models, Physiotens/Cynt/Moxonidine has been shown to be a potent antihypertensive agent. Available experimental data convincingly suggest that the site of the antihypertensive action of Physiotens/Cynt/Moxonidine is the central nervous system (CNS). Within the brainstem, Physiotens/Cynt/Moxonidine has been shown to selectively interact with I_1-imidazoline receptors. These imidazoline-sensitive receptors are concentrated in the rostral ventrolateral medulla, an area critical to the central control of the peripheral sympathetic nervous system. The net effect of this interaction with the I_1-imidazoline receptor appears to result in a reduced activity of sympathetic nerves (demonstrated for cardiac, splanchnic and renal sympathetic nerves).

Physiotens/Cynt/Moxonidine differs from other available centrally acting antihypertensives by exhibiting only low affinity to central α_2-adrenoceptors as compared to I_1-imidazoline receptors; α_2-adrenoceptors are considered the molecular target via which sedation and dry mouth, the most common undesired side effects of centrally acting antihypertensives, are mediated

In humans, Physiotens/Cynt/Moxonidine leads to a reduction of systemic vascular resistance and consequently in arterial blood pressure.

5.2 Pharmacokinetic properties

Oral moxonidine treatment of rats and dogs resulted in rapid and almost complete absorption and peak plasma levels within <0.5 hours. Average plasma concentrations were comparable in both species after p.o. and i.v. administration. The elimination half-lives of radioactivity and unchanged compound were estimated to be 1-3 hours. Moxonidine and its two main metabolites (4,5-dehydromoxonidine and a guanidine derivative) was predominantly excreted in the urine. No indication of moxonidine cumulation was observed in either species during chronic toxicity studies after 52 weeks.

In humans, about 90% of an oral dose of moxonidine is absorbed; it is not subject to first-pass metabolism and its bio-availability is 88%. Food intake does not interfere with moxonidine pharmacokinetics. Moxonidine is 10-20% metabolised, mainly to 4,5-dehydromoxonidine and to a guanidine derivative by opening of the imidazoline ring. The hypotensive effect of 4,5-dehydromoxonidine is only 1/10, and that of the guanidine derivative is less than 1/100 of that of moxonidine. The maximum plasma levels of moxonidine are reached 30-180 minutes after the intake of a film-coated tablet.

Only about 7% of moxonidine is bound to plasma protein (Vd_{ss}=1.8 ± 0.4 l/kg). Moxonidine and its metabolites are eliminated almost entirely via the kidneys. More than 90% of the dose is eliminated via the kidneys in the first 24 hours after administration, while only about 1% is eliminated via the faeces. The cumulative renal excretion of unchanged moxonidine is about 50-75%.

The mean plasma elimination half-life of moxonidine is 2.2-2.3 hours, and the renal elimination half-life is 2.6-2.8 hours.

Pharmacokinetics in the elderly

Small differences between the pharmacokinetic properties of moxonidine in the healthy elderly and younger adults are unlikely to be clinically significant. As there is no accumulation of moxonidine, dosage adjustment is unnecessary provided renal function is normal.

Pharmacokinetics in children

No pharmacokinetic studies have been performed in children.

Pharmacokinetics in renal impairment

In moderately impaired renal function (GFR 30-60 ml/min), AUC increased by 85% and clearance decreased to 52%. In such patients the hypotensive effect of Physiotens/Cynt/Moxonidine should be closely monitored, especially at the start of treatment; additionally, single doses should not exceed 200 micrograms and the daily dose should not exceed 400 micrograms.

5.3 Preclinical safety data

Chronic oral treatment for 52 weeks of rats (with dosages of 0.12-4 mg/kg) and dogs (with dosages of 0.04-0.4 mg/kg) revealed significant effects of moxonidine only at the highest doses. Slight disturbances of electrolyte balance (decrease of blood sodium and increase of potassium, urea and creatinine) were found in the high dose rats and emesis and salivation only for the high dose dogs. In addition slight increases of liver weight were obvious for both high dose species.

Reproductive toxicology did not show moxonidine effects (at oral doses up to 6.4 mg/kg) on fertility of rats and development of the embryo and foetus. Neither was evidence seen of embryotoxic and teratogenic properties in the rat at oral doses up to 27 mg/kg and the rabbit up to 4.9 mg/kg, nor on peri- and post-natal development in the rat after oral dosage up to 9 mg/kg.

Five different studies also did not show any indication of mutagenic or genotoxic effects of moxonidine. In addition, carcinogenicity studies in rats and mice at oral doses of 0.1-7.0 mg/kg did not reveal any evidence of carcinogenic potential.

6. PHARMACEUTICAL PARTICULARS

6.1 List of excipients

Lactose, povidone, crospovidone, magnesium stearate, hypromellose, ethylcellulose, polyethylene glycol 6000, talc, red ferric oxide, titanium dioxide.

6.2 Incompatibilities

No incompatibilities are known.

6.3 Shelf life

2 years.

6.4 Special precautions for storage

Do not store above 25°C.

6.5 Nature and contents of container

The tablets are packed in blister strips of 14. The blister strips are made of PVC/PVdC or PVC film with covering Aluminium foil. Each carton contains 14, 28 or 84 tablets.

6.6 Special precautions for disposal and other handling

None.

7. MARKETING AUTHORISATION HOLDER

Solvay Healthcare Limited

Mansbridge Road

West End

Southampton

SO18 3JD

8. MARKETING AUTHORISATION NUMBER(S)

PL 00512/0153

9. DATE OF FIRST AUTHORISATION/RENEWAL OF THE AUTHORISATION

15 September 1997/ 5 April 2002

10. DATE OF REVISION OF THE TEXT

12 June 2009

Physiotens Tablets 400 micrograms

(Solvay Healthcare Limited)

1. NAME OF THE MEDICINAL PRODUCT

Physiotens® Tablets 400 micrograms

Cynt Tablets 400 micrograms

Moxonidine 400 micrograms Tablets

2. QUALITATIVE AND QUANTITATIVE COMPOSITION

Each tablet contains 400 micrograms moxonidine.

3. PHARMACEUTICAL FORM

Film coated tablets.

Dull red, round, biconvex, film-coated tablets imprinted '0.4' on one face.

4. CLINICAL PARTICULARS

4.1 Therapeutic indications

Mild to moderate essential or primary hypertension.

4.2 Posology and method of administration

Adults (including the elderly):

Treatment should be started with 200 micrograms of Physiotens/Cynt/Moxonidine in the morning. The dose may be titrated after three weeks to 400 micrograms, given as one dose or as divided doses (morning and evening) until a satisfactory response has been achieved. If the response is still unsatisfactory after a further three weeks' treatment, the dosage can be increased up to a maximum of 600 micrograms in divided doses (morning and evening).

A single dose of 400 micrograms of Physiotens/Cynt/Moxonidine and a daily dose of 600 micrograms in divided doses (morning and evening) should not be exceeded.

In patients with moderate renal dysfunction (GFR above 30 ml/min, but below 60 ml/min), the single dose should not exceed 200 micrograms and the daily dose should not exceed 400 micrograms of moxonidine.

The tablets should be taken with a little liquid. As the intake of food has no influence on the pharmacokinetic properties of moxonidine, the tablets may be taken before, during or after the meal.

Paediatric population

Physiotens/Cynt/Moxonidine is not recommended for use in children and adolescents below 16 years due to lack of data on safety and efficacy.

4.3 Contraindications

Physiotens/Cynt/Moxonidine should not be used in cases of:

- history of angioneurotic oedema
- hypersensitivity to the active substance or to any of the excipients
- sick sinus syndrome or sino-atrial block
- 2nd or 3rd degree atrioventricular block
- bradycardia (below 50 beats/minute at rest)
- malignant arrhythmia
- severe heart failure (see Section 4.4)
- severe coronary artery disease or unstable angina
- severe liver disease
- severe renal dysfunction (GFR <30 ml/min, serum creatinine concentration >160 μmol/l).

Physiotens/Cynt/Moxonidine should not be used because of lack of therapeutic experience in cases of:

- intermittent claudication
- Raynaud's disease
- Parkinson's disease
- epileptic disorders
- glaucoma
- depression
- pregnancy or lactation
- children and adolescents below 16 years of age.

4.4 Special warnings and precautions for use

If Moxonidine is used in combination with a beta-blocker and both treatments have to be discontinued, the beta-blocker should be discontinued first and Moxonidine only thereafter.

In patients with moderate renal dysfunction (GFR above 30 but below 60 ml/min, serum creatinine above 105 but below 160 μmol), the hypotensive effect of Physiotens/Cynt/Moxonidine should be closely monitored, especially at the start of treatment.

Due to lack of therapeutic experience, the use of Physiotens/Cynt/Moxonidine concomitantly with alcohol or tricyclic antidepressants should be avoided.

Due to a lack of clinical data supporting the safety in patients with co-existing moderate heart failure, Physiotens/Cynt/Moxonidine must be used with caution in such patients.

Treatment with Physiotens/Cynt/Moxonidine should not be discontinued abruptly, but should be withdrawn gradually over a period of two weeks.

Patients with rare hereditary problems of galactose intolerance, the rare Lapp lactase deficiency or glucose-galactose malabsorption should not take this medicine.

4.5 Interaction with other medicinal products and other forms of interaction

Concurrent administration of other antihypertensive agents enhances the hypotensive effect of Physiotens/Cynt/Moxonidine.

The effect of sedatives and hypnotics may be intensified by Physiotens/Cynt/Moxonidine. The sedative effect of benzodiazepines can be enhanced by concurrent administration of Physiotens/Cynt/Moxonidine.

4.6 Pregnancy and lactation

As insufficient data are available, Physiotens/Cynt/Moxonidine should not be used during pregnancy.

Physiotens/Cynt/Moxonidine should not be used during lactation because it is excreted into breast milk.

4.7 Effects on ability to drive and use machines

No data are available to suggest that Physiotens/Cynt/Moxonidine adversely affects the ability to drive or operate machines. However, as somnolence and dizziness have been reported, patients should be cautioned about their ability to undertake potentially hazardous tasks such as driving and operating machinery if so affected.

4.8 Undesirable effects

At the start of treatment dry mouth is frequently observed, while headache, asthenia, dizziness, nausea, sleep disturbances and vasodilatation are observed occasionally. Sedation has been reported in less than 1% of patients. The frequency and intensity of these symptoms often decrease in the course of treatment.

Allergic skin reactions have been reported in very rare cases.

Isolated cases of angioedema have been reported.

4.9 Overdose

Oral dosages up to 2.0 mg/day have been tolerated without the occurrence of serious adverse events. The following case of accidental overdose with Physiotens/Cynt/Moxonidine by a 2 year old child has been reported:

The child ingested an unknown quantity of Physiotens/Cynt/Moxonidine. The maximum dosage possibly ingested was 14 mg. The child had the following symptoms: sedation, coma, hypotension, miosis and dyspnoea. Gastric lavage, glucose infusion, mechanically assisted ventilation and rest resulted in the complete disappearance of the symptoms in 11 hours.

Because of the pharmacodynamic properties of Physiotens/Cynt/Moxonidine, the following symptoms can be expected in adults: sedation, hypotension, orthostatic dysregulation, bradycardia, dry mouth. In rare cases emesis and paradoxical hypertension may occur.

No specific antidote is known. Phentolamine (Rogitine) may, depending on the dose, reverse part of the symptoms of moxonidine overdosage. Measures to support blood circulation are recommended.

5. PHARMACOLOGICAL PROPERTIES

5.1 Pharmacodynamic properties

In different animal models, Physiotens/Cynt/Moxonidine has been shown to be a potent antihypertensive agent. Available experimental data convincingly suggest that the site of the antihypertensive action of Physiotens/Cynt/Moxonidine is the central nervous system (CNS). Within the brainstem, Physiotens/Cynt/Moxonidine has been shown to selectively interact with I_1-imidazoline receptors. These imidazoline-sensitive receptors are concentrated in the rostral ventrolateral medulla, an area critical to the central control of the peripheral sympathetic nervous system. The net effect of this interaction with the I_1-imidazoline receptor appears to result in a reduced activity of sympathetic nerves (demonstrated for cardiac, splanchnic and renal sympathetic nerves).

Physiotens/Cynt/Moxonidine differs from other available centrally acting antihypertensives by exhibiting only low affinity to central α_2-adrenoceptors as compared to I_1-imidazoline receptors; α_2-adrenoceptors are considered the molecular target via which sedation and dry mouth, the most common undesired side effects of centrally acting antihypertensives, are mediated.

In humans, Physiotens/Cynt/Moxonidine leads to a reduction of systemic vascular resistance and consequently in arterial blood pressure.

5.2 Pharmacokinetic properties

Oral moxonidine treatment of rats and dogs resulted in rapid and almost complete absorption and peak plasma levels within <0.5 hours. Average plasma concentrations were comparable in both species after p.o. and i.v. administration. The elimination half-lives of radioactivity and unchanged compound were estimated to be 1-3 hours. Moxonidine and its two main metabolites (4,5-dehydromoxonidine and a guanidine derivative) was predominantly excreted in the urine. No indication of moxonidine cumulation was observed in either species during chronic toxicity studies after 52 weeks.

In humans, about 90% of an oral dose of moxonidine is absorbed; it is not subject to first-pass metabolism and its bio-availability is 88%. Food intake does not interfere with moxonidine pharmacokinetics. Moxonidine is 10-20% metabolised, mainly to 4,5-dehydromoxonidine and to a guanidine derivative by opening of the imidazoline ring. The hypotensive effect of 4,5-dehydromoxonidine is only 1/10, and that of the guanidine derivative is less than 1/100 of that of moxonidine. The maximum plasma levels of moxonidine are reached 30-180 minutes after the intake of a film-coated tablet.

Only about 7% of moxonidine is bound to plasma protein (Vd_{ss}=1.8 ± 0.4 l/kg). Moxonidine and its metabolites are eliminated almost entirely via the kidneys. More than 90% of the dose is eliminated via the kidneys in the first 24 hours after administration, while only about 1% is eliminated via the faeces. The cumulative renal excretion of unchanged moxonidine is about 50-75%.

The mean plasma elimination half-life of moxonidine is 2.2-2.3 hours, and the renal elimination half-life is 2.6-2.8 hours.

Pharmacokinetics in the elderly

Small differences between the pharmacokinetic properties of moxonidine in the healthy elderly and younger adults are unlikely to be clinically significant. As there is no accumulation of moxonidine, dosage adjustment is unnecessary provided renal function is normal.

Pharmacokinetics in children

No pharmacokinetic studies have been performed in children.

Pharmacokinetics in renal impairment

In moderately impaired renal function (GFR 30-60 ml/min), AUC increased by 85% and clearance decreased to 52%. In such patients the hypotensive effect of Physiotens/Cynt/Moxonidine should be closely monitored, especially at the start of treatment; additionally, single doses should not exceed 200 micrograms and the daily dose should not exceed 400 micrograms.

5.3 Preclinical safety data

Chronic oral treatment for 52 weeks of rats (with dosages of 0.12-4 mg/kg) and dogs (with dosages of 0.04-0.4 mg/kg) revealed significant effects of moxonidine only at the highest doses. Slight disturbances of electrolyte balance (decrease of blood sodium and increase of potassium, urea and creatinine) were found in the high dose rats and emesis and salivation only for the high dose dogs. In addition slight increases of liver weight were obvious for both high dose species.

Reproductive toxicology did not show moxonidine effects (at oral doses up to 6.4 mg/kg) on fertility of rats and development of the embryo and foetus. Neither was evidence seen of embryotoxic and teratogenic properties in the rat at oral doses up to 27 mg/kg and the rabbit up to 4.9 mg/kg, nor on peri- and post-natal development in the rat after oral dosage up to 9 mg/kg.

Five different studies also did not show any indication of mutagenic or genotoxic effects of moxonidine. In addition, carcinogenicity studies in rats and mice at oral doses of 0.1-7.0 mg/kg did not reveal any evidence of carcinogenic potential.

6. PHARMACEUTICAL PARTICULARS

6.1 List of excipients

Lactose, povidone, crospovidone, magnesium stearate, hypromellose, ethylcellulose, polyethylene glycol 6000, talc, red ferric oxide, titanium dioxide.

6.2 Incompatibilities

No incompatibilities are known.

6.3 Shelf life

2 years.

6.4 Special precautions for storage

Do not store above 25°C.

6.5 Nature and contents of container

The tablets are packed in blister strips of 14. The blister strips are made of PVC/PVdC or PVC film with covering Aluminium foil. Each carton contains 14, 28 or 84 tablets.

6.6 Special precautions for disposal and other handling

None.

7. MARKETING AUTHORISATION HOLDER

Solvay Healthcare Limited

Mansbridge Road

West End

Southampton

SO18 3JD

8. MARKETING AUTHORISATION NUMBER(S)

PL 00512/0154

9. DATE OF FIRST AUTHORISATION/RENEWAL OF THE AUTHORISATION

15 September 1997/ 5 April 2002

10. DATE OF REVISION OF THE TEXT

12 June 2009

Picolax

(Ferring Pharmaceuticals Ltd)

1. NAME OF THE MEDICINAL PRODUCT

PICOLAX

2. QUALITATIVE AND QUANTITATIVE COMPOSITION

Each sachet contains the following active ingredients:

Sodium picosulfate	10.0mg
Magnesium oxide, light	3.5g
Citric acid, anhydrous	12.0g

3. PHARMACEUTICAL FORM

Powder for oral solution.

White crystalline powder.

4. CLINICAL PARTICULARS

4.1 Therapeutic indications

To clean the bowel prior to X-ray examination, endoscopy or surgery.

4.2 Posology and method of administration

Route of administration: Oral

A low residue diet is recommended on the day prior to the hospital procedure. To avoid dehydration during treatment with PICOLAX it is recommended to drink approximately 250ml per hour, of water or other clear fluid while the washout effect persists.

Directions for reconstitution:

Reconstitute the contents of one sachet in a cup of water (approximately 150ml). Stir for 2-3 minutes and drink the solution. If it becomes hot, wait until it cools sufficiently to drink.

Adults (including the elderly):

One sachet reconstituted in water as directed, taken before 8 am on the day before the procedure. Second sachet 6 to 8 hours later.

Children:

1 - 2 years: ¼ sachet morning, ¼ sachet afternoon

2 - 4 years: ½ sachet morning, ½ sachet afternoon

4 - 9 years: 1 sachet morning, ½ sachet afternoon

9 and above: adult dose

4.3 Contraindications

Hypersensitivity to any of the ingredients of the product, congestive cardiac failure, gastric retention, gastro-intestinal ulceration, toxic colitis, toxic megacolon, ileus, nausea and vomiting, acute surgical abdominal conditions such as acute appendicitis and known or suspected gastro-intestinal obstruction or perforation.

In patients with severely reduced renal function, accumulation of magnesium in plasma may occur. Another preparation should be used in such cases.

4.4 Special warnings and precautions for use

Recent gastro-intestinal surgery. Care should also be taken in patients with renal impairment, heart disease or inflammatory bowel disease.

Use with caution in patients on drugs that might affect water and/or electrolyte balance e.g. diuretics, corticosteroids, lithium (see 4.5).

PICOLAX may modify the absorption of regularly prescribed oral medication and should be used with caution e.g. there have been isolated reports of seizures in patients on antiepileptics, with previously controlled epilepsy (see 4.5 and 4.8).

An inadequate oral intake of water and electrolytes could create clinically significant, deficiencies, particularly in less fit patients. In this regard, the elderly, debilitated individuals and patients at risk of hypokalaemia may need particular attention. Prompt corrective action should be taken to restore fluid/electrolyte balance in patients with signs or symptoms of hyponatraemia.

The period of bowel cleansing should not exceed 24 hours because longer preparation may increase the risk of water and electrolyte imbalance.

4.5 Interaction with other medicinal products and other forms of interaction

As a purgative, PICOLAX increases the gastrointestinal transit rate. The absorption of other orally administered medicines (e.g. anti-epileptics, contraceptives, anti-diabetics, antibiotics) may therefore be modified during the treatment period (see 4.4).

The efficacy of PICOLAX is lowered by bulk-forming laxatives.

Care should be taken with patients already receiving drugs which may be associated with hypokalaemia (such as diuretics or corticosteroids, or drugs where hypokalaemia is a particular risk i.e. cardiac glycosides). Caution is also advised when PICOLAX is used in patients on NSAIDs or drugs known to induce SIADH e.g. tricyclic antidepressants, selective serotonin re-uptake inhibitors, antipsychotic drugs and carbamazepine as these drugs may increase the risk of water retention and/or electrolyte imbalance.

4.6 Pregnancy and lactation

Reproduction studies with sodium picosulfate performed in animals have revealed no evidence of a harmful action on the fetus. However, clinical experience of the use of PICOLAX during pregnancy is limited and caution should be observed, particularly during the first trimester.

Neither sodium picosulfate nor magnesium citrate have been shown to be excreted in breast milk.

4.7 Effects on ability to drive and use machines

Not applicable.

4.8 Undesirable effects

Adverse reactions to PICOLAX are very rare (<1 in10,000) and are presented below by System Organ Class and Preferred term.

Immune system disorders

Anaphylactoid reaction, hypersensitivity

Metabolism and nutrition disorders

Hyponatraemia

Nervous system disorders

Epilepsy, grand mal convulsion, convulsions, confusional state, headache

Gastrointestinal disorders

Vomiting, diarrhoea, abdominal pain, nausea, proctalgia

Skin and subcutaneous tissue disorders

Rash (including erythematous and maculo-papular rash), urticaria, pruritus, purpura

General disorders

Drug interaction

Hyponatraemia has been reported with or without associated convulsions (see 4.4). In epileptic patients, there have been isolated reports of seizure/grand mal convulsion without associated hyponatraemia (see 4.4 and 4.5). There have been isolated reports of anaphylactoid reaction (see 4.3). Isolated cases of mild reversible aphthoid ileal ulcers have been reported.

4.9 Overdose

Overdosage would lead to profuse diarrhoea. Treatment is by general supportive measures and maintenance of fluid intake.

5. PHARMACOLOGICAL PROPERTIES

5.1 Pharmacodynamic properties

The active components of PICOLAX are sodium picopsulfate, a stimulant cathartic, active locally in the colon, and magnesium citrate which acts as an osmotic laxative by retaining moisture in the colon. The action is of a powerful 'washing out' effect combined with peristaltic stimulation to clear the bowel prior to radiography, colonoscopy or surgery. The product is not intended for use as a routine laxative.

5.2 Pharmacokinetic properties

Both active components are locally active in the colon, and neither are absorbed in any detectable amounts.

5.3 Preclinical safety data

There are no pre-clinical data of relevance to the prescriber which are additional to that already included in other sections of the SPC.

6. PHARMACEUTICAL PARTICULARS

6.1 List of excipients

Potassium bicarbonate, granular

Sodium saccharin

Natural, spray dried orange flavour which contains acacia gum, lactose, ascorbic acid, butylated hydroxyanisole.

6.2 Incompatibilities

None known

6.3 Shelf life

36 months

6.4 Special precautions for storage

Do not store above 25°C. Store in the original package.

6.5 Nature and contents of container

Sachet:

4 layers: paper-polyethylene-aluminium-surlyn

Each pack contains a pair of sachets that can be separated by tearing apart the perforated strip.

Weight of sachet contents: 16.1g

6.6 Special precautions for disposal and other handling

None

7. MARKETING AUTHORISATION HOLDER

Ferring Pharmaceuticals Limited

The Courtyard

Waterside Drive

Langley

Berkshire

SL3 6EZ

United Kingdom

8. MARKETING AUTHORISATION NUMBER(S)

PL 03194/0014

9. DATE OF FIRST AUTHORISATION/RENEWAL OF THE AUTHORISATION

1st November 2001

10. DATE OF REVISION OF THE TEXT

May 2008

11. DOSIMETRY

(IF APPLICABLE)

12. INSTRUCTIONS FOR PREPARATION OF RADIOPHARMACEUTICALS

(IF APPLICABLE)

Piportil Depot Injection

(sanofi-aventis)

1. NAME OF THE MEDICINAL PRODUCT

Piportil Depot 5% w/v.

2. QUALITATIVE AND QUANTITATIVE COMPOSITION

in terms of the active ingredient

Pipotiazine palmitate 5.0% w/v

3. PHARMACEUTICAL FORM

Depot injection.

4. CLINICAL PARTICULARS

4.1 Therapeutic indications

For the maintenance treatment of schizophrenia and paranoid psychoses and prevention of relapse, especially where compliance with oral medication is a problem

4.2 Posology and method of administration

Patients should be stabilised on Piportil Depot under psychiatric supervision. Administration should be by deep intramuscular injection into the gluteal region. Wide variation of response can be expected. The following dosage recommendations are suitable for either indication.

Adults: Initially 25mg should be given to assess the response of the patient to the drug. Further doses should be administered at appropriate intervals, increasing by increments of 25 or 50 mg until a satisfactory response is obtained. In clinical practice, Piportil Depot has been shown to have a long duration of action, allowing intervals of 4 weeks between injections for maintenance therapy. Dosage should be adjusted under close supervision to suit each individual patient in order to obtain the best therapeutic response compatible with tolerance.

The duration of action depends on the dose administered, allowing dosage intervals to be varied to suit individual circumstances.

Most patients respond favourably to a dose of 50-100 mg every 4 weeks, the maximum recommended dose is 200 mg every four weeks.

Elderly: Neuroleptics should be used cautiously in the elderly: A reduced starting dose is recommended, ie 5-10 mg might be considered.

Children: Not recommended for use in children.

4.3 Contraindications

Piportil Depot should not be administered to patients in a comatose state or with marked cerebral atherosclerosis, phaeochromocytoma, renal or liver failure, severe cardiac insufficiency or hypersensitivity to other phenothiazine derivatives.

4.4 Special warnings and precautions for use

Piportil Depot should be used with caution in patients suffering from or who have a history of, the following conditions: severe respiratory disease, epilepsy, alcohol withdrawal symptoms, brain damage, Parkinson's disease or marked extrapyramidal symptoms with previously used neuroleptics, personal or family history of narrow angle glaucoma, hypothyroidism, myasthenia gravis, prostatic hypertrophy, thyrotoxicosis. Care is required in very hot or very cold weather particularly in elderly frail patients.

Neuroleptic phenothiazines may potentiate QT interval prolongation which increases the risk of onset of serious ventricular arrhythmias of the torsade de pointes type, which is potentially fatal (sudden death). QT prolongation is exacerbated, in particular, in the presence of bradycardia, hypokalaemia, and congenital or acquired (i.e. drug induced) QT prolongation. The risk-benefit should be fully assessed before Piportil treatment is commenced. If the clinical situation permits, medical and laboratory evaluations (e.g. biochemical status and ECG) should be performed to rule out possible risk factors (e.g. cardiac disease; family history of QT prolongation; metabolic abnormalities such as hypokalaemia, hypocalcaemia or hypomagnesaemia; starvation; alcohol abuse; concomitant therapy with other drugs known to prolong the QT interval) before initiating treatment with Piportil and during the initial phase of treatment, or as deemed necessary during the treatment (see also sections 4.5 and 4.8).

Avoid concomitant treatment with other neuroleptics (see section 4.5).

Stroke: In randomised clinical trials versus placebo performed in a population of elderly patients with dementia and treated with certain atypical antipsychotic drugs, a 3-fold increase of the risk of cerebrovascular events has been observed. The mechanism of such risk increase is not known. An increase in the risk with other antipsychotic drugs or other populations of patients cannot be excluded. Piportil should be used with caution in patients with stroke risk factors.

Acute withdrawal symptoms, including nausea, vomiting, sweating, and insomnia have been described after abrupt cessation of antipsychotic drugs. Recurrence of psychotic symptoms may also occur, and the emergence of involuntary movement disorders (such as akathisia, dystonia and dyskinesia) has been reported. Therefore, gradual withdrawal is advisable.

4.5 Interaction with other medicinal products and other forms of interaction

There is an increased risk of arrhythmias when antipsychotics are used with concomitant QT prolonging drugs (including certain antiarrhythmics, antidepressants and other antipsychotics) and drugs causing electrolyte imbalance

The CNS depressant actions of neuroleptic agents may be intensified (additively) by alcohol, barbiturates and other sedatives. Respiratory depression may occur.

The hypotensive effect of most antihypertensive drugs especially alpha adrenoceptor blocking agents may be exaggerated by neuroleptics. This effect may also be observed with anaesthetics and opioid analgesics.

The mild anticholinergic effect of neuroleptics may be enhanced by other anticholinergic drugs possibly leading to constipation, heat stroke, etc.

The action of some drugs may be opposed by phenothiazine neuroleptics; these include amfetamine, levodopa, apomorphine, lisuride, pergolide, bromocriptine, cabergoline, clonidine, guanethidine, adrenaline.

Some drugs may possibly enhance the effects of phenothiazines including cimetidine.

Anticholinergic agents may reduce the antipsychotic effect of neuroleptics.

Some drugs interfere with absorption of neuroleptic agents: antacids, kaolin, anti-Parkinson drugs, lithium. Increases or decreases in the plasma concentrations of a number of drugs, e.g. propranolol, phenobarbital have been observed but were not of clinical significance. Concomitant use with ritonavir may possibly increase the plasma concentration of the antipsychotic.

High doses of neuroleptics reduce the response to hypoglycaemic agents, the dosage of which might have to be raised.

There is an increased risk of extrapyramidal effects with tetrabenazine and lithium, and an increased possibility of neurotoxicity with lithium. Sibutramine can lead to an increased risk of CNS toxicity.

Adrenaline must not be used in patients overdosed with phenothiazine neuroleptics. Most of the above interactions are of a theoretical nature and not dangerous. Simultaneous administration of desferrioxamine and prochlorperazine has been observed to induce a transient metabolic encephalopathy characterised by loss of consciousness for 48–72 hours. It is possible that this may occur with Piportil since it shares many of the pharmacological properties of prochlorperazine.

Avoid concomitant use of Clozapine with depot formulation as it cannot be withdrawn quickly if neutropenia occurs.

4.6 Pregnancy and lactation

There is inadequate evidence of safety of Piportil Depot in human pregnancy, although animal studies have shown no hazard. The drug should not be used during pregnancy or lactation unless the physician considers it essential.

4.7 Effects on ability to drive and use machines

Patients should be warned about drowsiness especially at the start of treatment and advised not to drive or operate machinery.

4.8 Undesirable effects

Minor side effects of neuroleptics are drowsiness, especially at the start of treatment, nasal stuffiness, dry mouth, insomnia, agitation and weight gain. Other possible adverse effects are listed below.

Liver function: jaundice, usually transient, occurs in a very small percentage of patients taking neuroleptics. A premonitory sign may be a sudden onset of fever after one to three weeks of treatment followed by the development of jaundice. Neuroleptic jaundice has the biochemical and other characteristics of obstructive jaundice and is associated with obstructions of the canaliculi by bile thrombi; the frequent presence of an accompanying eosinophilia indicates the allergic nature of this phenomenon. Treatment should be withheld on the development of jaundice.

Cardiorespiratory: Hypotension, usually postural, commonly occurs. Elderly or volume depleted subjects are particularly susceptible; it is more likely to occur after intramuscular administration.

ECG changes include QT prolongation (as with other neuroleptics), ST depression, U-Wave and T-Wave changes. Cardiac arrhythmias, including ventricular arrhythmias and atrial arrhythmias, a-v block, ventricular tachycardia, which may result in ventricular fibrillation or cardiac arrest have been reported during neuroleptic phenothiazine therapy, possibly related to dosage. Pre-existing cardiac disease, old age, hypokalaemia and concurrent tricyclic antidepressants may predispose.

There have been isolated reports of sudden death, with possible causes of cardiac origin (see section 4.4, above), as well as cases of unexplained sudden death, in patients receiving neuroleptic phenothiazines.

Blood picture: A mild leukopenia occurs in up to 30% of patients on prolonged high dosage of neuroleptics. Agranulocytosis may occur rarely; it is not dose-related. The occurrence of unexplained infections or fever requires immediate haematological investigation.

Extrapyramidal: Acute dystonias or dyskinesias, usually transitory, are commoner in children and young adults, and usually occur within the first 4 days of treatment or after dosage increases.

- Akathisia characteristically occurs after large initial doses.

- Parkinsonism is commoner in adults and the elderly. It usually develops after weeks or months of treatment. One or more of the following may be seen: tremor, rigidity, akinesia or other features of Parkinsonism. Commonly just tremor.

- Tardive dyskinesia: If this occurs it is usually, but not necessarily, after prolonged or high dosage. It can even occur after treatment has been stopped. Dosage should therefore be kept low whenever possible.

Skin and eyes: contact skin sensitisation is a serious but rare complication in those frequently handling preparations of phenothiazines; the greatest care must be taken to avoid contact of the drug with the skin. Skin rashes of various kinds may also be seen in patients treated with these drugs. Patients on high dosage should be warned that they may develop photosensitivity in sunny weather and should avoid exposure to direct sunlight.

Ocular changes and the development of a metallic greyish-mauve coloration of exposed skin have been noted in some individuals mainly females, who have received chlorpromazine continuously for long periods (four to eight years). Other neuroleptics have been implicated but less frequently.

Endocrine: hyperprolactinaemia which may result in galactorrhoea, gynaecomastia, amenorrhoea; impotence.

Neuroleptic malignant syndrome (hyperthermia, rigidity, autonomic dysfunction and altered consciousness) may occur with any neuroleptic.

4.9 Overdose

Symptoms of phenothiazine overdosage include drowsiness or loss of consciousness, hypotension, tachycardia, ECG changes, ventricular arrhythmias and hypothermia. Severe extrapyramidal dyskinesias may occur.

Generalised vasodilatation may result in circulatory collapse; raising the patient's legs may suffice, in severe cases, volume expansion by intravenous fluids may be needed; infusion fluids should be warmed before administration in order not to aggravate hypothermia.

Positive inotropic agents such as dopamine may be tried if fluid replacement is insufficient to correct the circulatory collapse. Peripheral vasoconstrictor agents are not generally recommended; avoid the use of adrenaline.

Ventricular or supraventricular tachy-arrhythmias usually respond to restoration of normal body temperature and correction of circulatory or metabolic disturbances. If they are persistent or life threatening, appropriate anti-arrhythmic therapy may be considered. Avoid lidocaine and, as far as possible, long acting anti-arrhythmic drugs.

Pronounced central nervous system depression requires airway maintenance or, in extreme circumstances, assisted respiration. Severe dystonic reactions usually respond to procyclidine (5–10mg) or orphenadrine (20–40mg) administered intramuscularly or intravenously. Convulsions should be treated with intravenous diazepam.

Neuroleptic malignant syndrome should be treated with cooling. Dantrolene sodium may be tried.

5. PHARMACOLOGICAL PROPERTIES

5.1 Pharmacodynamic properties

Slow release phenothiazine neuroleptic

5.2 Pharmacokinetic properties

There is little information about blood levels, distribution and excretion in humans. The rate of metabolism and excretion of phenothiazines decreases in old age

5.3 Preclinical safety data

There are no pre-clinical data of relevance to the prescriber which are additional to that already included in other sections of the SPC.

6. PHARMACEUTICAL PARTICULARS

6.1 List of excipients

Sesame oil, Refined (containing butylhydroxyanisole – E320)

6.2 Incompatibilities

Piportil Depot injection should not be admixed with any other substance.

6.3 Shelf life

60 months

6.4 Special precautions for storage

Protect from light

6.5 Nature and contents of container

1 and 2 ml clear glass ampoules- pack containing 10 ampoules.

6.6 Special precautions for disposal and other handling

None stated

7. MARKETING AUTHORISATION HOLDER

Sanofi-aventis

One Onslow Street

Guildford

Surrey

GU1 4YS

UK

8. MARKETING AUTHORISATION NUMBER(S)

PL04425/0585

9. DATE OF FIRST AUTHORISATION/RENEWAL OF THE AUTHORISATION

8th September 2006

10. DATE OF REVISION OF THE TEXT

15 August 2007

Legal Classification

POM

Plaquenil Tablets

(sanofi-aventis)

1. NAME OF THE MEDICINAL PRODUCT

Plaquenil Tablets

2. QUALITATIVE AND QUANTITATIVE COMPOSITION

Hydroxychloroquine Sulphate BP 200mg

3. PHARMACEUTICAL FORM

Film coated tablet.

4. CLINICAL PARTICULARS

4.1 Therapeutic indications

Treatment of rheumatoid arthritis, juvenile chronic arthritis, discoid and systemic lupus erythematosus, and dermatological conditions caused or aggravated by sunlight.

4.2 Posology and method of administration

Adults (including the elderly)

The minimum effective dose should be employed. This dose should not exceed 6.5mg/kg/day (calculated from ideal body weight and not actual body weight) and will be either 200mg or 400mg per day.

In patients able to receive 400mg daily:

Initially 400mg daily in divided doses. The dose can be reduced to 200mg when no further improvement is evident. The maintenance dose should be increased to 400mg daily if the response lessens.

Children

The minimum effective dose should be employed and should not exceed 6.5mg/kg/day based on ideal body weight. The 200mg tablet is therefore not suitable for use in children with an ideal body weight of less than 31kg.

Each dose should be taken with a meal or glass of milk.

Hydroxychloroquine is cumulative in action and will require several weeks to exert its beneficial effects, whereas minor side effects may occur relatively early. For rheumatic disease treatment should be discontinued if there is no improvement by 6 months. In light-sensitive diseases, treatment should only be given during periods of maximum exposure to light.

The tablets are for oral administration.

4.3 Contraindications

- known hypersensitivity to 4-aminoquinoline compounds
- pre-existing maculopathy of the eye
- pregnancy (see section 4.6 Pregnancy and lactation).

4.4 Special warnings and precautions for use

General

- The occurrence of retinopathy is very uncommon if the recommended daily dose is not exceeded. The administration of doses in excess of the recommended maximum is likely to increase the risk of retinopathy, and accelerate its onset.
- All patients should have an ophthalmological examination before initiating treatment with Plaquenil. Thereafter, ophthalmological examinations must be repeated at least every 12 months.

The examination should include testing visual acuity, careful ophthalmoscopy, fundoscopy, central visual field testing with a red target, and colour vision.

This examination should be more frequent and adapted to the patient in the following situations:

- daily dosage exceeds 6.5mg/kg lean body weight. Absolute body weight used as a guide to dosage could result in an overdosage in the obese.
- renal insufficiency
- visual acuity below 6/8
- age above 65 years
- cumulative dose more than 200 g.

Plaquenil should be discontinued immediately in any patient who develops a pigmentary abnormality, visual field defect, or any other abnormality not explainable by difficulty in accommodation or presence of corneal opacities. Patients should continue to be observed for possible progression of the changes.

Patients should be advised to stop taking the drug immediately and seek the advice of their prescribing doctor if any disturbances of vision are noted, including abnormal colour vision.

Plaquenil should be used with caution in patients taking medicines which may cause adverse ocular or skin reactions. Caution should also be applied when it is used in the following:

- patients with hepatic or renal disease, and in those taking drugs known to affect those organs. Estimation of plasma hydroxychloroquine levels should be undertaken in patients with severely compromised renal or hepatic function and dosage adjusted accordingly.
- patients with severe gastrointestinal, neurological or blood disorders.

Although the risk of bone marrow depression is low, periodic blood counts are advisable as anaemia, aplastic anaemia, agranulocytosis, a decrease in white blood cells, and thrombocytopenia have been reported. Plaquenil should be discontinued if abnormalities develop.

Caution is also advised in patients with a sensitivity to quinine, those with glucose-6-phosphate dehydrogenase deficiency, those with porphyria cutanea tarda which can be exacerbated by hydroxychloroquine and in patients with psoriasis since it appears to increase the risk of skin reactions.

Patients with rare hereditary problems of galactose intolerance, the Lapp lactase deficiency or glucose-galactose malabsorption should not take this medicine.

Small children are particularly sensitive to the toxic effects of 4-aminoquinolines; therefore patients should be warned to keep Plaquenil out of the reach of children.

All patients on long-term therapy should undergo periodic examination of skeletal muscle function and tendon reflexes. If weakness occurs, the drug should be withdrawn.

4.5 Interaction with other medicinal products and other forms of interaction

Hydroxychloroquine sulphate has been reported to increase plasma digoxin levels: serum digoxin levels should be closely monitored in patients receiving combined therapy.

Hydroxychloroquine sulphate may also be subject to several of the known interactions of chloroquine even though specific reports have not appeared. These include: potentiation of its direct blocking action at the neuromuscular junction by aminoglycoside antibiotics; inhibition of its metabolism by cimetidine which may increase plasma concentration of the antimalarial; antagonism of effect of neostigmine and pyridostigmine; reduction of the antibody response to primary immunisation with intradermal human diploid-cell rabies vaccine.

As with chloroquine, antacids may reduce absorption of hydroxychloroquine so it is advised that a 4 hour interval be observed between Plaquenil and antacid dosaging.

As hydroxychloroquine may enhance the effects of a hypoglycaemic treatment, a decrease in doses of insulin or antidiabetic drugs may be required.

4.6 Pregnancy and lactation

Pregnancy:

Hydroxychloroquine crosses the placenta. Data are limited regarding the use of hydroxychloroquine during pregnancy. It should be noted that 4-aminoquinolines in therapeutic doses have been associated with central nervous system damage, including ototoxicity (auditory and vestibular toxicity, congenital deafness), retinal hemorrhages and abnormal retinal pigmentation. Therefore Plaquenil should not be used in pregnancy.

Lactation:

Careful consideration should be given to using hydroxychloroquine during lactation, since it has been shown to be excreted in small amounts in human breast milk, and it is known that infants are extremely sensitive to the toxic effects of 4-aminoquinolines.

4.7 Effects on ability to drive and use machines

Impaired visual accommodation soon after the start of treatment has been reported and patients should be warned regarding driving or operating machinery. If the condition is not self-limiting, it will resolve on reducing the dose or stopping treatment.

4.8 Undesirable effects

• Ocular effects:

Retinopathy with changes in pigmentation and visual field defects can occur, but appears to be uncommon if the recommended daily dose is not exceeded. In its early form it appears reversible on discontinuation of Plaquenil. If allowed to develop, there may be a risk of progression even after treatment withdrawal.

Patients with retinal changes may be asymptomatic initially, or may have scotomatous vision with paracentral, pericentral ring types, temporal scotomas and abnormal colour vision.

Corneal changes including oedema and opacities have been reported. They are either symptomless or may cause disturbances such as haloes, blurring of vision or photophobia. They may be transient and are reversible on stopping treatment.

Blurring of vision due to a disturbance of accommodation which is dose dependent and reversible may also occur.

• Dermatologic effects:

Skin rashes sometimes occur; pruritus, pigmentary changes in skin and mucous membranes, bleaching of hair and alopecia have also been reported. These usually resolve readily on stopping treatment.

Bullous eruptions including very rare cases of erythema multiforme and Stevens-Johnson syndrome, photosensitivity and isolated cases of exfoliative dermatitis have been reported. Very rare cases of acute generalised exanthematous pustulosis (AGEP) has to be distinguished from psoriasis, although hydroxychloroquine may precipitate attacks of psoriasis. It may be associated with fever and hyperleukocytosis. Outcome is usually favourable after drug withdrawal.

• Gastrointestinal effects:

Gastrointestinal disturbances such as nausea, diarrhoea, anorexia, abdominal pain and, rarely, vomiting may occur. These symptoms usually resolve immediately on reducing the dose or on stopping treatment.

• CNS effects:

Less frequently, dizziness, vertigo, tinnitus, hearing loss, headache, nervousness, emotional lability, toxic psychosis and convulsions have been reported with this class of drugs.

• Neuromuscular effects:

Skeletal muscle myopathy or neuromyopathy leading to progressive weakness and atrophy of proximal muscle groups have been noted. Myopathy may be reversible after drug discontinuation, but recovery may take many months.

Associated mild sensory changes, depression of tendon reflexes and abnormal nerve conduction may be observed.

• Cardio-vascular effects:

Cardiomyopathy has been rarely reported.

Chronic toxicity should be suspected when conduction disorders (bundle branch block/atrioventricular heart block) as well as biventricular hypertrophy are found. Drug withdrawal may lead to recovery.

• Hematologic effects:

Rarely, there have been reports of bone-marrow depression. Blood disorders such as anaemia, aplastic anaemia, agranulocytosis, a decrease in white blood cells and thrombocytopenia have been reported.

Hydroxychloroquine may precipitate or exacerbate porphyria.

• Liver effects:

Isolated cases of abnormal liver function tests have been reported; rare cases of fulminant hepatic failure have also been reported.

• Allergic reactions:

Urticaria, angioedema and bronchospasm have been reported.

4.9 Overdose

Overdosage with the 4-aminoquinolines is dangerous particularly in infants, as little as 1-2g having proved fatal.

The symptoms of overdosage may include headache, visual disturbances, cardiovascular collapse, convulsions, hypokalaemia, and rhythm and conduction disorders, followed by sudden and early respiratory and cardiac arrest. Since these effects may appear soon after taking a massive dose, treatment should be prompt and symptomatic. The stomach should be immediately evacuated, either by emesis or by gastric lavage. Activated charcoal in a dose at least five times of the overdose may inhibit further absorption if introduced into the stomach by tube following lavage and within 30 minutes of ingestion of the overdose.

Consideration should be given to administration of parenteral diazepam in cases of overdosage; it has been shown to be beneficial in reversing chloroquine cardiotoxicity.

Respiratory support and shock management should be instituted as necessary.

5. PHARMACOLOGICAL PROPERTIES

5.1 Pharmacodynamic properties

Antimalarial agents like chloroquine and hydroxychloroquine have several pharmacological actions which may be involved in their therapeutic effect in the treatment of rheumatic disease, but the role of each is not known. These include interaction with sulphydryl groups, interference with enzyme activity (including phospholipase, NADH - cytochrome C reductase, cholinesterase, proteases and hydrolases), DNA binding, stabilisation of lysosomal membranes, inhibition of prostaglandin formation, inhibition of polymorphonuclear cell chemotaxis and phagocytosis, possible interference with interleukin 1 production from monocytes and inhibition of neutrophil superoxide release.

5.2 Pharmacokinetic properties

Hydroxychloroquine has actions, pharmacokinetics and metabolism similar to those of chloroquine. Following oral administration, hydroxychloroquine is rapidly and almost completely absorbed. In one study, mean peak plasma hydroxychloroquine concentrations following a single dose of 400mg in healthy subjects ranged from 53-208ng/ml with a mean of 105ng/ml. The mean time to peak plasma concentration was 1.83 hours. The mean plasma elimination half-life varied, depending on the post-administration period, as follows: 5.9 hours (at C_{max}-10 hours), 26.1 hours (at 10-48 hours) and 299 hours (at 48-504 hours). The parent compound and metabolites are widely distributed in the body and elimination is mainly via the urine, where 3% of the administered dose was recovered over 24 hours in one study.

5.3 Preclinical safety data

There are no preclinical safety data of relevance to the prescriber, which are additional to that already included in other sections of the SPC.

6. PHARMACEUTICAL PARTICULARS

6.1 List of excipients

Lactose monohydrate, maize starch, magnesium stearate, polyvidone, Opadry OY-L-28900 (containing hypromellose, macrogol 4000, titanium dioxide (E171), lactose.)

6.2 Incompatibilities

No incompatibilities are known.

6.3 Shelf life

3 years

6.4 Special precautions for storage

Store below 25°C.

6.5 Nature and contents of container

250µm clear PVC/20µm aluminium foil blister pack containing 60 tablets.

6.6 Special precautions for disposal and other handling

None.

7. MARKETING AUTHORISATION HOLDER

Sanofi-aventis

One Onslow Street

Guildford

Surrey GU1 4YS

8. MARKETING AUTHORISATION NUMBER(S)

PL 11723/0150

9. DATE OF FIRST AUTHORISATION/RENEWAL OF THE AUTHORISATION

27 August 1997

10. DATE OF REVISION OF THE TEXT

May 2007

Legal Category

POM

Plavix (sanofi-aventis)

(sanofi-aventis)

1. NAME OF THE MEDICINAL PRODUCT

Plavix 75 mg film-coated tablets

Plavix 300 mg film-coated tablets

2. QUALITATIVE AND QUANTITATIVE COMPOSITION

Plavix 75mg tablets:

Each film-coated tablet contains 75 mg of clopidogrel (as hydrogen sulphate).

Excipients: each tablet contains 3 mg lactose and 3.3 mg hydrogenated castor oil.

Plavix 300mg tablets:

Each film-coated tablet contains 300 mg of clopidogrel (as hydrogen sulphate).

Excipients: each tablet contains 12 mg lactose and 13.2 mg hydrogenated castor oil.

For a full list of excipients, see section 6.1.

3. PHARMACEUTICAL FORM

Film-coated tablets.

Plavix 75mg tablets: Pink, round, biconvex, engraved with «75» on one side and «1171» on the other side.

Plavix 300mg tablets: Pink, oblong, engraved with «300» on one side and «1332» on the other side.

4. CLINICAL PARTICULARS

4.1 Therapeutic indications

Clopidogrel is indicated in adults for the prevention of atherothrombotic events in:

• Patients suffering from myocardial infarction (from a few days until less than 35 days), ischaemic stroke (from 7 days until less than 6 months) or established peripheral arterial disease.

• Patients suffering from acute coronary syndrome:

- Non-ST segment elevation acute coronary syndrome (unstable angina or non-Q-wave myocardial infarction), including patients undergoing a stent placement following percutaneous coronary intervention, in combination with acetylsalicylic acid (ASA).

- ST segment elevation acute myocardial infarction, in combination with ASA in medically treated patients eligible for thrombolytic therapy.

For further information please refer to section 5.1.

4.2 Posology and method of administration

• Adults and elderly

Clopidogrel should be given as a single daily dose of 75 mg with or without food.

The 300 mg tablet of clopidogrel is intended for use as a loading dose in patients suffering from acute coronary syndrome:

– Non-ST segment elevation acute coronary syndrome (unstable angina or non-Q-wave myocardial infarction): clopidogrel treatment should be initiated with a single 300-mg loading dose and then continued at 75 mg once a day (with acetylsalicylic acid (ASA) 75 mg-325 mg daily). Since higher doses of ASA were associated with higher bleeding risk it is recommended that the dose of ASA should not be higher than 100 mg. The optimal duration of treatment has not been formally established. Clinical trial data support use up to 12 months, and the maximum benefit was seen at 3 months (see section 5.1).

- ST segment elevation acute myocardial infarction: clopidogrel should be given as a single daily dose of 75 mg initiated with a 300-mg loading dose in combination with ASA and with or without thrombolytics. For patients over 75 years of age clopidogrel should be initiated without a loading dose. Combined therapy should be started as early as possible after symptoms start and continued for at least four weeks. The benefit of the combination of clopidogrel with ASA beyond four weeks has not been studied in this setting (see section 5.1).

• Pharmacogenetics

CYP2C19 poor metaboliser status is associated with diminished response to clopidogrel. The optimal dose regimen for poor metabolisers has yet to be determined (see Section 5.1).

• Paediatric patients

The safety and efficacy of clopidogrel in children and adolescents have not yet been established.

• Renal impairment

Therapeutic experience is limited in patients with renal impairment (see section 4.4).

• Hepatic impairment

Therapeutic experience is limited in patients with moderate hepatic disease who may have bleeding diatheses (see section 4.4).

4.3 Contraindications

• Hypersensitivity to the active substance or to any of the excipients.

• Severe liver impairment.

• Active pathological bleeding such as peptic ulcer or intracranial haemorrhage.

4.4 Special warnings and precautions for use

Due to the risk of bleeding and haematological undesirable effects, blood cell count determination and/or other appropriate testing should be promptly considered whenever clinical symptoms suggestive of bleeding arise during the course of treatment (see section 4.8). As with other antiplatelet agents, clopidogrel should be used with caution in patients who may be at risk of increased bleeding from trauma, surgery or other pathological conditions and in patients receiving treatment with ASA, heparin, glycoprotein IIb/IIIa inhibitors or non-steroidal anti-inflammatory drugs (NSAIDS) including Cox-2 inhibitors. Patients should be followed carefully for any signs of bleeding including occult bleeding, especially during the first weeks of treatment and/or after invasive cardiac procedures or surgery. The concomitant administration of clopidogrel with oral anticoagulants is not recommended since it may increase the intensity of bleedings (see section 4.5).

If a patient is to undergo elective surgery and antiplatelet effect is temporarily not desirable, clopidogrel should be discontinued 7 days prior to surgery. Patients should inform physicians and dentists that they are taking clopidogrel before any surgery is scheduled and before any new medicinal product is taken. Clopidogrel prolongs bleeding time and should be used with caution in patients who have lesions with a propensity to bleed (particularly gastrointestinal and intraocular).

Patients should be told that it might take longer than usual to stop bleeding when they take clopidogrel (alone or in combination with ASA), and that they should report any unusual bleeding (site or duration) to their physician.

Thrombotic Thrombocytopenic Purpura (TTP) has been reported very rarely following the use of clopidogrel, sometimes after a short exposure. It is characterised by thrombocytopenia and microangiopathic haemolytic anaemia associated with either neurological findings, renal dysfunction or fever. TTP is a potentially fatal condition requiring prompt treatment including plasmapheresis.

In view of the lack of data, clopidogrel cannot be recommended during the first 7 days after acute ischaemic stroke.

Pharmacogenetics: Based on literature data, patients with genetically reduced CYP2C19 function have lower systemic exposure to the active metabolite of clopidogrel and diminished antiplatelet responses, and generally exhibit higher cardiovascular event rates following myocardial infarction than do patients with normal CYP2C19 function (see section 5.2).

Since clopidogrel is metabolised to its active metabolite partly by CYP2C19, use of drugs that inhibit the activity of this enzyme would be expected to result in reduced drug levels of the active metabolite of clopidogrel and a reduction in clinical efficacy. Concomitant use of drugs that inhibit CYP2C19 should be discouraged (see section 4.5 for a list of CYP2C19 inhibitors, see also section 5.2). Although the evidence of CYP2C19 inhibition varies within the class of Proton Pump Inhibitors, clinical studies suggest an interaction between clopidogrel and possibly all members of this class. Therefore, concomitant use of Proton Pump Inhibitors should be avoided unless absolutely necessary. There is no evidence that other drugs that reduce stomach acid such as H2 blockers or antacids interfere with antiplatelet activity of clopidogrel.

Therapeutic experience with clopidogrel is limited in patients with renal impairment. Therefore clopidogrel should be used with caution in these patients (see section 4.2).

Experience is limited in patients with moderate hepatic disease who may have bleeding diatheses. Clopidogrel should therefore be used with caution in this population (see section 4.2).

Plavix contains lactose. Patients with rare hereditary problems of galactose intolerance, the Lapp lactase deficiency or glucose-galactose malabsorption should not take this medicinal product.

This medicinal product contains hydrogenated castor oil which may cause stomach upset and diarrhoea.

4.5 Interaction with other medicinal products and other forms of interaction

Oral anticoagulants: the concomitant administration of clopidogrel with oral anticoagulants is not recommended since it may increase the intensity of bleedings (see section 4.4).

Glycoprotein IIb/IIIa inhibitors: clopidogrel should be used with caution in patients who may be at risk of increased bleeding from trauma, surgery or other pathological conditions that receive concomitant glycoprotein IIb/IIIa inhibitors (see section 4.4).

Acetylsalicylic acid (ASA): ASA did not modify the clopidogrel-mediated inhibition of ADP-induced platelet aggregation, but clopidogrel potentiated the effect of ASA on collagen-induced platelet aggregation. However, concomitant administration of 500 mg of ASA twice a day for one day did not significantly increase the prolongation of bleeding time induced by clopidogrel intake. A pharmacodynamic interaction between clopidogrel and acetylsalicylic acid is possible, leading to increased risk of bleeding. Therefore, concomitant use should be undertaken with caution (see section 4.4). However, clopidogrel and ASA have been administered together for up to one year (see section 5.1).

Heparin: in a clinical study conducted in healthy subjects, clopidogrel did not necessitate modification of the heparin dose or alter the effect of heparin on coagulation. Co-administration of heparin had no effect on the inhibition of platelet aggregation induced by clopidogrel. A pharmacodynamic interaction between clopidogrel and heparin is possible, leading to increased risk of bleeding. Therefore, concomitant use should be undertaken with caution (see section 4.4).

Thrombolytics: the safety of the concomitant administration of clopidogrel, fibrin or non-fibrin specific thrombolytic agents and heparins was assessed in patients with acute myocardial infarction. The incidence of clinically significant bleeding was similar to that observed when thrombolytic agents and heparin are co-administered with ASA (see section 4.8)

NSAIDs: in a clinical study conducted in healthy volunteers, the concomitant administration of clopidogrel and naproxen increased occult gastrointestinal blood loss. However, due to the lack of interaction studies with other NSAIDs it is presently unclear whether there is an increased risk of gastrointestinal bleeding with all NSAIDs. Consequently, NSAIDs including Cox-2 inhibitors and clopidogrel should be co-administered with caution (see section 4.4).

Other concomitant therapy:

Since clopidogrel is metabolised to its active metabolite partly by CYP2C19, use of drugs that inhibit the activity of this enzyme would be expected to result in reduced drug levels of the active metabolite of clopidogrel and a reduction in clinical efficacy. Concomitant use of drugs that inhibit CYP2C19 should be discouraged (see sections 4.4 and 5.2).

Drugs that inhibit CYP2C19 include omeprazole and esomeprazole, fluvoxamine, fluoxetine, moclobemide, voriconazole, fluconazole, ticlopidine, ciprofloxacin, cimetidine, carbamazepine, oxcarbazepine and chloramphenicol.

Proton Pump Inhibitors:

Although the evidence of CYP2C19 inhibition varies within the class of Proton Pump Inhibitors, clinical studies suggest an interaction between clopidogrel and possibly all members of this class. Therefore, concomitant use of Proton Pump Inhibitors should be avoided unless absolutely necessary. There is no evidence that other drugs that reduce stomach acid such as H2 blockers or antacids interfere with antiplatelet activity of clopidogrel.

A number of other clinical studies have been conducted with clopidogrel and other concomitant medicinal products to investigate the potential for pharmacodynamic and pharmacokinetic interactions. No clinically significant pharmacodynamic interactions were observed when clopidogrel was co-administered with atenolol, nifedipine, or both atenolol and nifedipine. Furthermore, the pharmacodynamic activity of clopidogrel was not significantly influenced by the co-administration of phenobarbital, cimetidine, or oestrogen.

The pharmacokinetics of digoxin or theophylline were not modified by the co-administration of clopidogrel. Antacids did not modify the extent of clopidogrel absorption.

Data from studies with human liver microsomes indicated that the carboxylic acid metabolite of clopidogrel could inhibit the activity of Cytochrome P_{450} 2C9. This could potentially lead to increased plasma levels of medicinal products such as phenytoin and tolbutamide and the NSAIDs, which are metabolised by Cytochrome P_{450} 2C9. Data from the CAPRIE study indicate that phenytoin and tolbutamide can be safely co-administered with clopidogrel.

Apart from the specific medicinal product interaction information described above, interaction studies with clopidogrel and some medicinal products commonly administered in patients with atherothrombotic disease have not been performed. However, patients entered into clinical trials with clopidogrel received a variety of concomitant medicinal products including diuretics, beta blockers, ACEI, calcium antagonists, cholesterol lowering agents, coronary vasodilators, antidiabetic agents (including insulin), antiepileptic agents, and GPIIb/IIIa antagonists without evidence of clinically significant adverse interactions.

4.6 Pregnancy and lactation

As no clinical data on exposure to clopidogrel during pregnancy are available, it is preferable not to use clopidogrel during pregnancy as a precautionary measure.

Animal studies do not indicate direct or indirect harmful effects with respect to pregnancy, embryonal/foetal development, parturition or postnatal development (see section 5.3).

It is unknown whether clopidogrel is excreted in human breast milk. Animal studies have shown excretion of clopidogrel in breast milk. As a precautionary measure, breast-feeding should not be continued during treatment with Plavix.

4.7 Effects on ability to drive and use machines

Clopidogrel has no or negligible influence on the ability to drive and use machines.

4.8 Undesirable effects

Clopidogrel has been evaluated for safety in more than 42,000 patients who have participated in clinical studies, including over 9,000 patients treated for 1 year or more. The clinically relevant adverse reactions observed in the CAPRIE, CURE, CLARITY and COMMIT studies are discussed below. Overall, clopidogrel 75 mg/day was comparable to ASA 325 mg/day in CAPRIE regardless of age, gender and race. In addition to clinical studies experience, adverse reactions have been spontaneously reported.

Bleeding is the most common reaction reported both in clinical studies as well as in post-marketing experience where it was mostly reported during the first month of treatment.

In CAPRIE, in patients treated with either clopidogrel or ASA, the overall incidence of any bleeding was 9.3%. The incidence of severe cases was 1.4% for clopidogrel and 1.6% for ASA.

In CURE, the major bleeding event rate for clopidogrel+ASA was dose-dependent on ASA (<100mg: 2.6%; 100-200mg: 3.5%; >200mg: 4.9%) as was the major bleeding event rate for placebo+ASA (<100mg: 2.0%; 100-200mg: 2.3%; >200mg: 4.0%). The risk of bleeding (life-threatening, major, minor, other) decreased during the course of the trial: 0-1 months (clopidogrel: 9.6%; placebo: 6.6%), 1-3 months (clopidogrel: 4.5%; placebo: 2.3%), 3-6 months (clopidogrel: 3.8%; placebo: 1.6%), 6-9 months (clopidogrel: 3.2%; placebo: 1.5%), 9-12 months (clopidogrel: 1.9%; placebo: 1.0%). There was no excess in major bleeds with clopidogrel + ASA within 7 days after coronary bypass graft surgery in patients who stopped therapy more than five days prior to surgery (4.4% clopidogrel+ASA vs. 5.3% placebo+ASA). In patients who remained on therapy within five days of bypass graft surgery, the event rate was 9.6% for clopidogrel+ASA, and 6.3% for placebo+ASA.

In CLARITY, there was an overall increase in bleeding in the clopidogrel + ASA group (17.4%) vs. the placebo + ASA group (12.9%). The incidence of major bleeding was similar between groups (1.3% versus 1.1% for the clopidogrel + ASA and the placebo + ASA groups, respectively). This was consistent across subgroups of patients defined by baseline characteristics, and type of fibrinolytic or heparin therapy.

In COMMIT, the overall rate of noncerebral major bleeding or cerebral bleeding was low and similar in both groups (0.6% versus 0.5% in the clopidogrel + ASA and the placebo + ASA groups, respectively).

Adverse reactions that occurred either during clinical studies or that were spontaneously reported are presented in the table below. Their frequency is defined using the following conventions: common (≥1/100 to <1/10); uncommon (≥1/1,000 to <1/100); rare (≥1/10,000 to <1/1,000); very rare (<1/10,000). Within each system organ class, adverse drug reactions are presented in order of decreasing seriousness.

(see Table 1 on next page)

4.9 Overdose

Overdose following clopidogrel administration may lead to prolonged bleeding time and subsequent bleeding complications. Appropriate therapy should be considered if bleedings are observed.

No antidote to the pharmacological activity of clopidogrel has been found. If prompt correction of prolonged bleeding time is required, platelet transfusion may reverse the effects of clopidogrel.

5. PHARMACOLOGICAL PROPERTIES

5.1 Pharmacodynamic properties

Pharmacotherapeutic group: platelet aggregation inhibitors excl. heparin, ATC Code: B01AC-04.

Clopidogrel is a prodrug, one of whose metabolites is an inhibitor of platelet aggregation. Clopidogrel must be metabolised by CYP450 enzymes to produce the active metabolite that inhibits platelet aggregation. The active metabolite of clopidogrel selectively inhibits the binding of adenosine diphosphate (ADP) to its platelet $P2Y_{12}$ receptor and the subsequent ADP-mediated activation of the glycoprotein GPIIb/IIIa complex, thereby inhibiting platelet aggregation. Due to the irreversible binding, platelets exposed are affected for the remainder of their lifespan (approximately 7-10 days) and recovery of normal platelet function occurs at a rate consistent with platelet turnover. Platelet aggregation induced by agonists other than ADP is

Table 1

System Organ Class	Common	Uncommon	Rare	Very rare
Blood and the lymphatic system disorders		Thrombocytopenia, leucopenia, eosinophilia	Neutropenia, including severe neutropenia	Thrombotic thrombocytopenic purpura (TTP) (see section 4.4), aplastic anaemia, pancytopenia, agranulocytosis, severe thrombocytopenia, granulocytopenia, anaemia
Immune system disorders				Serum sickness, anaphylactoid reactions
Psychiatric disorders				Hallucinations, confusion
Nervous system disorders		Intracranial bleeding (some cases were reported with fatal outcome), headache, paraesthesia, dizziness		Taste disturbances
Eye disorders		Eye bleeding (conjunctival, ocular, retinal)		
Ear and labyrinth disorders			Vertigo	
Vascular disorders	Haematoma			Serious haemorrhage, haemorrhage of operative wound, vasculitis, hypotension
Respiratory, thoracic and mediastinal disorders	Epistaxis			Respiratory tract bleeding (haemoptysis, pulmonary haemorrhage), bronchospasm, interstitial pneumonitis
Gastrointestinal disorders	Gastrointestinal haemorrhage, diarrhoea, abdominal pain, dyspepsia	Gastric ulcer and duodenal ulcer, gastritis, vomiting, nausea, constipation, flatulence	Retroperitoneal haemorrhage	Gastrointestinal and retroperitoneal haemorrhage with fatal outcome, pancreatitis, colitis (including ulcerative or lymphocytic colitis), stomatitis
Hepato-biliary disorders				Acute liver failure, hepatitis, abnormal liver function test
Skin and subcutaneous tissue disorders	Bruising	Rash, pruritus, skin bleeding (purpura)		Bullous dermatitis (toxic epidermal necrolysis, Stevens Johnson Syndrome, erythema multiforme), angioedema, rash erythematous, urticaria, eczema, lichen planus
Musculoskeletal connective tissue and bone disorders				Musculo-skeletal bleeding (haemarthrosis), arthritis, arthralgia, myalgia
Renal and urinary disorders		Haematuria		Glomerulonephritis blood creatinine increased
General disorders and administration site conditions	Bleeding at puncture site			Fever
Investigations		Bleeding time prolonged, neutrophil count decreased, platelet count decreased		

also inhibited by blocking the amplification of platelet activation by released ADP.

Because the active metabolite is formed by CYP450 enzymes, some of which are polymorphic or subject to inhibition by other drugs, not all patients will have adequate platelet inhibition.

Repeated doses of 75 mg per day produced substantial inhibition of ADP-induced platelet aggregation from the first day; this increased progressively and reached steady state between Day 3 and Day 7. At steady state, the average inhibition level observed with a dose of 75 mg per day was between 40% and 60%. Platelet aggregation and bleeding time gradually returned to baseline values, generally within 5 days after treatment was discontinued.

The safety and efficacy of clopidogrel have been evaluated in 4 double-blind studies involving over 80,000 patients: the CAPRIE study, a comparison of clopidogrel to ASA, and the CURE, CLARITY and COMMIT studies comparing clopidogrel to placebo, both medicinal products given in combination with ASA and other standard therapy.

Recent myocardial infarction (MI), recent stroke or established peripheral arterial disease

The CAPRIE study included 19,185 patients with atherothrombosis as manifested by recent myocardial infarction (<35 days), recent ischaemic stroke (between 7 days and 6 months) or established peripheral arterial disease (PAD). Patients were randomised to clopidogrel 75 mg/day or ASA 325 mg/day, and were followed for 1 to 3 years. In the myocardial infarction subgroup, most of the patients received ASA for the first few days following the acute myocardial infarction.

Clopidogrel significantly reduced the incidence of new ischaemic events (combined end point of myocardial infarction, ischaemic stroke and vascular death) when compared to ASA. In the intention to treat analysis, 939 events were observed in the clopidogrel group and 1,020 events with ASA (relative risk reduction (RRR) 8.7%, [95% CI: 0.2 to 16.4]; p = 0.045), which corresponds, for every 1,000 patients treated for 2 years, to 10 [CI: 0 to 20] additional patients being prevented from experiencing a new ischaemic event. Analysis of total mortality as a secondary endpoint did not show any significant difference between clopidogrel (5.8%) and ASA (6.0%).

In a subgroup analysis by qualifying condition (myocardial infarction, ischaemic stroke, and PAD) the benefit appeared to be strongest (achieving statistical significance at p = 0.003) in patients enrolled due to PAD (especially those who also had a history of myocardial infarction) (RRR = 23.7%; CI: 8.9 to 36.2) and weaker (not significantly different from ASA) in stroke patients (RRR = 7.3%; CI: -5.7 to 18.7 [p=0.258]). In patients who were enrolled in the trial on the sole basis of a recent myocardial infarction, clopidogrel was numerically inferior, but not statistically different from ASA (RRR = -4.0%; CI: -22.5 to 11.7 [p=0.639]). In addition, a subgroup analysis by age suggested that the benefit of clopidogrel in patients over 75 years was less than that observed in patients ≤75 years.

Since the CAPRIE trial was not powered to evaluate efficacy of individual subgroups, it is not clear whether the differences in relative risk reduction across qualifying conditions are real, or a result of chance.

Acute coronary syndrome

The CURE study included 12,562 patients with non-ST segment elevation acute coronary syndrome (unstable angina or non-Q-wave myocardial infarction), and presenting within 24 hours of onset of the most recent episode of chest pain or symptoms consistent with ischaemia. Patients were required to have either ECG changes compatible with new ischaemia or elevated cardiac enzymes or troponin I or T to at least twice the upper limit of normal. Patients were randomised to clopidogrel (300 mg loading dose followed by 75 mg/day, N=6,259) or placebo (N=6,303), both given in combination with ASA (75-325 mg once daily) and other standard therapies. Patients were treated for up to one year. In CURE, 823 (6.6%) patients received concomitant GPIIb/IIIa receptor antagonist therapy. Heparins were administered in more than 90% of the patients and the relative rate of bleeding between clopidogrel and placebo was not significantly affected by the concomitant heparin therapy.

The number of patients experiencing the primary endpoint [cardiovascular (CV) death, myocardial infarction (MI), or stroke] was 582 (9.3%) in the clopidogrel-treated group and 719 (11.4%) in the placebo-treated group, a 20% relative risk reduction (95% CI of 10%-28%; p=0.00009) for the clopidogrel-treated group (17% relative risk reduction when patients were treated conservatively, 29% when they underwent percutaneous transluminal coronary angioplasty (PTCA) with or without stent and 10% when they underwent coronary artery bypass graft (CABG)). New cardiovascular events (primary endpoint) were prevented, with relative risk reductions of 22% (CI: 8.6, 33.4), 32% (CI: 12.8, 46.4), 4% (CI: -26.9, 26.7), 6% (CI: -33.5, 34.3) and 14% (CI: -31.6, 44.2), during the 0-1, 1-3, 3-6, 6-9 and 9-12 month study intervals, respectively. Thus, beyond 3 months of treatment, the benefit observed in the clopidogrel + ASA group was not further increased, whereas the risk of haemorrhage persisted (see section 4.4).

The use of clopidogrel in CURE was associated with a decrease in the need of thrombolytic therapy (RRR = 43.3%; CI: 24.3%, 57.5%) and GPIIb/IIIa inhibitors (RRR = 18.2%; CI: 6.5%, 28.3%).

The number of patients experiencing the co-primary endpoint (CV death, MI, stroke or refractory ischaemia) was 1,035 (16.5%) in the clopidogrel-treated group and 1,187 (18.8%) in the placebo-treated group, a 14% relative risk reduction (95% CI of 6%-21%, p=0.0005) for the clopidogrel-treated group. This benefit was mostly driven by the statistically significant reduction in the incidence of MI [287 (4.6%) in the clopidogrel treated group and 363 (5.8%) in the placebo treated group]. There was no observed effect on the rate of rehospitalisation for unstable angina.

The results obtained in populations with different characteristics (e.g. unstable angina or non-Q-wave MI, low to high risk levels, diabetes, need for revascularisation, age, gender, etc.) were consistent with the results of the primary analysis. In particular, in a post-hoc analysis in 2,172 patients (17% of the total CURE population) who underwent stent placement (Stent-CURE), the data showed that clopidogrel compared to placebo, demonstrated a significant RRR of 26.2% favouring clopidogrel for the co-primary endpoint (CV death, MI, stroke) and also a significant RRR of 23.9% for the second co-primary endpoint (CV death, MI, stroke or refractory ischaemia). Moreover, the safety profile of clopidogrel in this subgroup of patients did not raise any particular concern. Thus, the results from this subset are in line with the overall trial results.

The benefits observed with clopidogrel were independent of other acute and long-term cardiovascular therapies (such as heparin/LMWH, GPIIb/IIIa antagonists, lipid lowering medicinal products, beta blockers, and ACE-inhibitors). The efficacy of clopidogrel was observed independently of the dose of ASA (75-325 mg once daily).

In patients with acute ST-segment elevation MI, safety and efficacy of clopidogrel have been evaluated in 2 randomised, placebo-controlled, double-blind studies, CLARITY and COMMIT.

The CLARITY trial included 3,491 patients presenting within 12 hours of the onset of a ST elevation MI and planned for thrombolytic therapy. Patients received clopidogrel (300 mg loading dose, followed by 75 mg/day, n=1,752) or placebo (n=1,739), both in combination with ASA (150 to 325 mg as a loading dose, followed by 75 to 162 mg/day), a fibrinolytic agent and, when appropriate, heparin. The patients were followed for 30 days. The primary endpoint was the occurrence of the composite of an occluded infarct-related artery on the predischarge angiogram, or death or recurrent MI before coronary angiography. For patients who did not undergo angiography, the primary endpoint was death or recurrent myocardial infarction by Day 8 or by hospital discharge. The patient population included 19.7% women and 29.2% patients $\geqslant$ 65 years. A total of 99.7% of patients received fibrinolytics (fibrin specific: 68.7%, non-fibrin specific: 31.1%), 89.5% heparin, 78.7% beta blockers, 54.7% ACE inhibitors and 63% statins.

Fifteen percent (15.0%) of patients in the clopidogrel group and 21.7% in the placebo group reached the primary endpoint, representing an absolute reduction of 6.7% and a 36 % odds reduction in favor of clopidogrel (95% CI: 24, 47%; $p < 0.001$), mainly related to a reduction in occluded infarct-related arteries. This benefit was consistent across all prespecified subgroups including patients' age and gender, infarct location, and type of fibrinolytic or heparin used.

The 2x2 factorial design COMMIT trial included 45,852 patients presenting within 24 hours of the onset of the symptoms of suspected MI with supporting ECG abnormalities (i.e. ST elevation, ST depression or left bundle-branch block). Patients received clopidogrel (75 mg/day, n=22,961) or placebo (n=22,891), in combination with ASA (162 mg/day), for 28 days or until hospital discharge. The co-primary endpoints were death from any cause and the first occurrence of re-infarction, stroke or death. The population included 27.8% women, 58.4% patients $\geqslant$ 60 years (26% $\geqslant$ 70 years) and 54.5% patients who received fibrinolytics.

Clopidogrel significantly reduced the relative risk of death from any cause by 7% (p = 0.029), and the relative risk of the combination of re-infarction, stroke or death by 9% (p = 0.002), representing an absolute reduction of 0.5% and 0.9%, respectively. This benefit was consistent across age, gender and with or without fibrinolytics, and was observed as early as 24 hours.

5.2 Pharmacokinetic properties

Absorption

After single and repeated oral doses of 75 mg per day, clopidogrel is rapidly absorbed. Mean peak plasma levels of unchanged clopidogrel (approximately 2.2-2.5 ng/ml after a single 75 mg oral dose) occurred approximately 45 minutes after dosing. Absorption is at least 50%, based on urinary excretion of clopidogrel metabolites.

Distribution

Clopidogrel and the main circulating (inactive) metabolite bind reversibly *in vitro* to human plasma proteins (98% and 94% respectively). The binding is non-saturable *in vitro* over a wide concentration range.

Metabolism

Clopidogrel is extensively metabolised by the liver. *In vitro* and *in vivo*, clopidogrel is metabolised according to two main metabolic pathways: one mediated by esterases and leading to hydrolysis into its inactive carboxylic acid derivative (85% of circulating metabolites), and one mediated by multiple cytochromes P450. Clopidogrel is first metabolised to a 2-oxo-clopidogrel intermediate metabolite. Subsequent metabolism of the 2-oxo-clopidogrel intermediate metabolite results in formation of the active metabolite, a thiol derivative of clopidogrel. *In vitro*, this metabolic pathway is mediated by CYP3A4, CYP2C19, CYP1A2 and CYP2B6. The active thiol metabolite which has been isolated *in vitro*, binds rapidly and irreversibly to platelet receptors, thus inhibiting platelet aggregation.

Elimination

Following an oral dose of ^{14}C-labelled clopidogrel in man, approximately 50% was excreted in the urine and approximately 46% in the faeces in the 120-hour interval after dosing. After a single oral dose of 75ng, clopidogrel has a half-life of approximately 6 hours. The elimination half-life of the main circulating metabolite was 8 hours after single and repeated administration.

Pharmacogenetics

Several polymorphic CYP450 enzymes activate clopidogrel. CYP2C19 is involved in the formation of both the active metabolite and the 2-oxo-clopidogrel intermediate metabolite. Clopidogrel active metabolite pharmacokinetics and antiplatelet effects, as measured by *ex vivo* platelet aggregation assays, differ according to CYP2C19 genotype. The CYP2C19*1 allele corresponds to fully functional metabolism while the CYP2C19*2 and CYP2C19*3 alleles correspond to reduced metabolism. The CYP2C19*2 and CYP2C19*3 alleles account for 85% of reduced function alleles in whites and 99% in Asians. Other alleles associated with reduced metabolism include CYP2C19*4, *5, *6, *7, and *8, but these are less frequent in the general population. Published frequencies for the common CYP2C19 phenotypes and genotypes are listed in the table below.

CYP2C19 Phenotype and Genotype Frequency

	Frequency (%)		
	White (n=1356)	**Black (n=966)**	**Chinese (n=573)**
Extensive metabolism: CYP2C19*1/*1	74	66	38
Intermediate metabolism: CYP2C19*1/*2 or *1/*3	26	29	50
Poor metabolism: CYP2C19*2/*2, *2/*3 or *3/*3	2	4	14

To date, the impact of CYP2C19 genotype on the pharmacokinetics of the active metabolite of clopidogrel has been evaluated in 227 subjects from 7 reported studies. Reduced CYP2C19 metabolism in intermediate and poor metabolisers decreased the C_{max} and AUC of the active metabolite by 30-50% following 300- or 600-mg loading doses and 75-mg maintenance doses. Lower active metabolite exposure results in less platelet inhibition or higher residual platelet reactivity. To date, diminished antiplatelet responses to clopidogrel have been described for intermediate and poor metabolisers in 21 reported studies involving 4,520 subjects. The relative difference in antiplatelet response between genotype groups varies across studies depending on the method used to evaluate response, but is typically greater than 30%.

The association between CYP2C19 genotype and clopidogrel treatment outcome was evaluated in 2 post hoc clinical trial analyses (substudies of CLARITY [n=465] and TRITON-TIMI 38 [n=1,477]) and 5 cohort studies (total n=6,489). In CLARITY and one of the cohort studies (n=765; Trenk), cardiovascular event rates did not differ significantly by genotype. In TRITON-TIMI 38 and 3 of the cohort studies (n= 3,516; Collet, Sibbing, Giusti), patients with an impaired metaboliser status (intermediate and poor combined) had a higher rate of cardiovascular events (death, myocardial infarction, and stroke) or stent thrombosis compared to extensive metabolisers. In the fifth cohort study (n=2,208; Simon), the increased event rate was observed only in poor metabolisers.

Pharmacogenetic testing can identify genotypes associated with variability in CYP2C19 activity.

There may be genetic variants of other CYP450 enzymes with effects on the ability to form the active metabolite of clopidogrel.

Special populations

The pharmacokinetics of the active metabolite of clopidogrel is not known in these special populations.

Renal impairment

After repeated doses of 75 mg clopidogrel per day in subjects with severe renal disease (creatinine clearance from 5 to 15 ml/min), inhibition of ADP-induced platelet aggregation was lower (25%) than that observed in healthy subjects, however, the prolongation of bleeding time was similar to that seen in healthy subjects receiving 75 mg of clopidogrel per day. In addition, clinical tolerance was good in all patients.

Hepatic impairment

After repeated doses of 75 mg clopidogrel per day for 10 days in patients with severe hepatic impairment, inhibition of ADP-induced platelet aggregation was similar to that observed in healthy subjects. The mean bleeding time prolongation was also similar in the two groups.

Race

The prevalence of CYP2C19 alleles that result in intermediate and poor CYP2C19 metabolism differs according to race/ethnicity (see Pharmacogenetics). From literature, limited data in Asian populations are available to assess the clinical implication of genotyping of this CYP on clinical outcome events.

5.3 Preclinical safety data

During non clinical studies in rat and baboon, the most frequently observed effects were liver changes. These occurred at doses representing at least 25 times the exposure seen in humans receiving the clinical dose of 75 mg/day and were a consequence of an effect on hepatic metabolising enzymes. No effect on hepatic metabolising enzymes was observed in humans receiving clopidogrel at the therapeutic dose.

At very high doses, a poor gastric tolerability (gastritis, gastric erosions and/or vomiting) of clopidogrel was also reported in rat and baboon.

There was no evidence of carcinogenic effect when clopidogrel was administered for 78 weeks to mice and 104 weeks to rats when given at doses up to 77 mg/kg per day (representing at least 25 times the exposure seen in humans receiving the clinical dose of 75 mg/day).

Clopidogrel has been tested in a range of *in vitro* and *in vivo* genotoxicity studies, and showed no genotoxic activity.

Clopidogrel was found to have no effect on the fertility of male and female rats and was not teratogenic in either rats or rabbits. When given to lactating rats, clopidogrel caused a slight delay in the development of the offspring. Specific pharmacokinetic studies performed with radiolabelled clopidogrel have shown that the parent compound or its metabolites are excreted in the milk. Consequently, a direct effect (slight toxicity), or an indirect effect (low palatability) cannot be excluded.

6. PHARMACEUTICAL PARTICULARS

6.1 List of excipients

Core:

Mannitol (E421)

Macrogol 6000

Microcrystalline cellulose

Hydrogenated castor oil

Low substituted hydroxypropylcellulose

Coating:

Hypromellose (E464)

Lactose

Triacetin (E1518)

Titanium dioxide (E171)

Red iron oxide (E172)

Polishing agent:

Carnauba wax

6.2 Incompatibilities

Not applicable

6.3 Shelf life

Plavix 75mg: 3 years

Plavix 300mg: 3 years

6.4 Special precautions for storage

Plavix 75mg tablets: Store below 30°C.

Plavix 300mg tablets: This medicinal product does not require any special storage conditions.

6.5 Nature and contents of container

Plavix 75mg tablets: PVC/PVDC/Aluminium blisters in cardboard cartons containing 30 film-coated tablets.

Plavix 300mg tablets: Aluminium perforated unit-dose blisters in cardboard cartons containing 30x1 film-coated tablets.

6.6 Special precautions for disposal and other handling

Any unused product or waste material should be disposed of in accordance with local requirements.

7. MARKETING AUTHORISATION HOLDER

Sanofi Pharma Bristol-Myers Squibb SNC

174 Avenue de France

F-75013 Paris – France

8. MARKETING AUTHORISATION NUMBER(S)

Plavix 75mg tablets: EU/1/98/069/005a - Cartons of 30 film-coated tablets in PVC/PVDC/Alu blisters

Plavix 300mg tablets: EU/1/98/069/009 - Cartons of 30x1 film-coated tablets in all aluminium perforated unit-dose blisters

9. DATE OF FIRST AUTHORISATION/RENEWAL OF THE AUTHORISATION

Date of first authorisation: 15 July 1998

Date of latest renewal: 15 July 2008

10. DATE OF REVISION OF THE TEXT

75mg tablet: 28 August 2009

300mg tablet: 28 August 2009

Legal Category: POM

Plendil 2.5mg, Plendil 5mg and Plendil 10mg

(AstraZeneca UK Limited)

1. NAME OF THE MEDICINAL PRODUCT

Plendil 2.5mg, Plendil 5mg and Plendil 10mg.

2. QUALITATIVE AND QUANTITATIVE COMPOSITION

Plendil 2.5mg contains Felodipine Ph. Eur. 2.5mg

Plendil 5mg contains Felodipine Ph. Eur. 5mg

Plendil 10mg contains Felodipine Ph. Eur. 10mg

3. PHARMACEUTICAL FORM

Circular biconvex film coated extended-release tablets.

Plendil 2.5mg - yellow tablets coded A/FL and 2.5 on the reverse.

Plendil 5mg - pink tablets coded A/FM and 5 on the reverse.

Plendil 10mg - red-brown tablets coded A/FE and 10 on the reverse.

4. CLINICAL PARTICULARS

4.1 Therapeutic indications

In the management of hypertension and prophylaxis of chronic stable angina pectoris.

4.2 Posology and method of administration

For oral administration.

The tablets should be taken in the morning irrespective of food intake. Plendil tablets must not be chewed or crushed. They should be swallowed whole with half a glass of water.

Hypertension

Adults (including elderly) The dose should be adjusted to the individual requirements of the patient. The recommended starting dose is 5mg once daily. If necessary the dose may be further increased or another antihypertensive agent added. The usual maintenance dose is 5 - 10 mg once daily. Doses higher than 20mg daily are not usually needed. For dose titration purposes a 2.5mg tablet is available. In elderly patients an initial treatment with 2.5mg daily should be considered.

Angina pectoris

Adults The dose should be adjusted individually. Treatment should be started with 5mg once daily and if needed be increased to 10mg once daily.

Children The safety and efficacy of Plendil in children has not been established.

Plendil can be used in combination with β-blockers, ACE inhibitors or diuretics. The effects on blood pressure are likely to be additive and combination therapy will usually enhance the antihypertensive effect. Care should be taken to avoid hypotension.

In patients with severely impaired liver function the dose of felodipine should be low. The pharmacokinetics are not significantly affected in patients with impaired renal function.

4.3 Contraindications

Unstable angina pectoris.

Pregnancy.

Patient with a previous allergic reaction to Plendil or other dihydropyridines because of the theoretical risk of cross-reactivity.

Plendil should not be used in patients with clinically significant aortic stenosis, uncompensated heart failure, and during or within one month of a myocardial infarction.

As with other calcium channel blockers, Plendil should be discontinued in patients who develop cardiogenic shock.

4.4 Special warnings and precautions for use

As with other vasodilators, Plendil may, in rare cases, precipitate significant hypotension with tachycardia which in susceptible individuals may result in myocardial ischaemia.

There is no evidence that Plendil is useful for secondary prevention of myocardial infarction.

The efficacy and safety of Plendil in the treatment of malignant hypertension has not been studied.

Plendil should be used with caution in patients with severe left ventricular dysfunction.

4.5 Interaction with other medicinal products and other forms of interaction

Concomitant administration of substances which interfere with the cytochrome P4503A4 enzyme system may affect plasma concentrations of felodipine. Enzyme inhibitors such as cimetidine, erythromycin, itraconazole and ketoconazole impair the elimination of felodipine, and Plendil dosage may need to be reduced when drugs are given concomitantly. Conversely, powerful enzyme inducing agents such as some anticonvulsants (phenytoin, carbamazepine, phenobarbital) can increase felodipine elimination and higher than normal Plendil doses may be required in patients taking the drugs.

No dosage adjustment is required when Plendil is given concomitantly with digoxin.

Felodipine does not appear to affect the unbound fraction of other extensively plasma protein bound drugs such as warfarin.

Felodipine may increase the concentration of tacrolimus. When used together, the tacrolimus serum concentration should be followed and the tacrolimus dose may need to be adjusted.

Grapefruit juice results in increased peak plasma levels and bioavailability possibly due to an interaction with flavonoids in the fruit juice. This interaction has been seen with other dihydropyridine calcium antagonists and represents a class effect. Therefore grapefruit juice should not be taken together with Plendil tablets.

4.6 Pregnancy and lactation

Felodipine should not be given during pregnancy.

In a study on fertility and general reproductive performance in rats, a prolongation of parturition resulting in difficult labour, increased foetal deaths and early postnatal deaths were observed in the medium-and high-dose groups.

Reproductive studies in rabbits have shown a dose-related reversible enlargement of the mammary glands of the parent animals and dose-related digital abnormalities in the foetuses when felodipine was administered during stages of early foetal development.

Felodipine has been detected in breast milk, but it is unknown whether it has harmful effects on the new-born.

4.7 Effects on ability to drive and use machines

None.

4.8 Undesirable effects

As with other calcium antagonists, flushing, headache, palpitations, dizziness and fatigue may occur. These reactions are usually transient and are most likely to occur at the start of treatment or after an increase in dosage.

As with other calcium antagonists ankle swelling, resulting from precapillary vasodilation, may occur. The degree of ankle swelling is dose related.

In patients with gingivitis/periodontitis, mild gingival enlargement has been reported with Plendil, as with other calcium antagonists. The enlargement can be avoided or reversed by careful dental hygiene.

As with other dihydropyridines, aggravation of angina has been reported in a small number of individuals especially after starting treatment. This is more likely to happen in patients with symptomatic ischaemic heart disease.

The following adverse events have been reported from clinical trials and from Post Marketing Surveillance. In the great majority of cases a causal relationship between these events and treatment with felodipine has not been established.

Skin: very rarely - leucocytoclastic vasculitis, rarely - rash and/or pruritus, and isolated cases of photosensitivity.

Musculoskeletal: in isolated cases arthralgia and myalgia.

Psychiatric: rarely impotence/sexual dysfunction.

Central and peripheral nervous system: headache, dizziness. In isolated cases paraesthesia.

Gastrointestinal: very rarely - gingivitis, in isolated cases abdominal pain, nausea, vomiting, gum hyperplasia.

Hepatic: in isolated cases increased liver enzymes.

Urinary system: very rarely urinary frequency.

Cardiovascular: rarely - tachycardia, palpitations and syncope.

Vascular (extracardiac): peripheral oedema, flush.

Other: very rarely - fever, rarely - fatigue, in isolated cases hypersensitivity reactions e.g. urticaria, angio-oedema.

4.9 Overdose

Symptoms: Overdosage may cause excessive peripheral vasodilatation with marked hypotension which may sometimes be accompanied by bradycardia.

Management: Activated charcoal, induction of vomiting or gastric lavage, if appropriate or indicated. Severe hypotension should be treated symptomatically, with the patient placed supine and the legs elevated. Bradycardia, if present, should be treated with atropine 0.5-1mg i.v. If this is not sufficient, plasma volume should be increased by infusion of e.g. glucose, saline or dextran. Sympathomimetic drugs with predominant effect on the α_1-adrenoceptor may be given e.g. metaraminol or phenylephrine.

5. PHARMACOLOGICAL PROPERTIES

5.1 Pharmacodynamic properties

Felodipine is a vascular selective calcium antagonist, which lowers arterial blood pressure by decreasing peripheral vascular resistance. Due to the high degree of selectivity for smooth muscle in the arterioles, felodipine in therapeutic doses has no direct effect on cardiac contractility or conduction.

It can be used as monotherapy or in combination with other antihypertensive drugs, e.g. β-receptor blockers, diuretics or ACE-inhibitors, in order to achieve an increased antihypertensive effect. Felodipine reduces both systolic and diastolic blood pressure and can be used in isolated systolic hypertension. In a study of 12 patients, felodipine maintained its antihypertensive effect during concomitant therapy with indomethacin.

Because there is no effect on venous smooth muscle or adrenergic vasomotor control, felodipine is not associated with orthostatic hypotension.

Felodipine has anti-anginal and anti-ischaemic effects due to improved myocardial oxygen supply/demand balance. Coronary vascular resistance is decreased and coronary blood flow as well as myocardial oxygen supply are increased by felodipine due to dilation of both epicardial arteries and arterioles. Felodipine effectively counteracts coronary vasospasm. The reduction in systemic blood pressure caused by felodipine leads to decreased left ventricular afterload.

Felodipine improves exercise tolerance and reduces anginal attacks in patients with stable effort induced angina pectoris. Both symptomatic and silent myocardial ischaemia are reduced by felodipine in patients with vasospastic angina. Felodipine can be used as monotherapy or in combination with β-receptor blockers in patients with stable angina pectoris.

Felodipine possesses a mild natriuretic/diuretic effect and generalised fluid retention does not occur.

In a randomised, double-blind, 3-week, parallel group study in children aged 6-16 years with primary hypertension, the antihypertensive effects of once daily felodipine 2.5 mg (n=33), 5 mg (n=33) and 10 mg (n=31) were compared with placebo (n=35). The study failed to demonstrate the efficacy of felodipine in lowering blood pressure in children aged 6-16 years.

The long-term effects of felodipine on growth, puberty and general development have not been studied. The long-term efficacy of felodipine as therapy in childhood to reduce cardiovascular morbidity and mortality in adulthood has also not been established.

Felodipine is well tolerated in patients with concomitant disease such as congestive heart failure well-controlled on appropriate therapy, asthma and other obstructive pulmonary diseases, diabetes, gout, hyperlipidemia impaired renal function, renal transplant recipients and Raynaud's disease. Felodipine has no significant effect on blood glucose levels or lipid profiles.

Haemodynamic effects: The primary haemodynamic effect of felodipine is a reduction of total peripheral vascular resistance which leads to a decrease in blood pressure. These effects are dose-dependent. In patients with mild to moderate essential hypertension, a reduction in blood pressure usually occurs 2 hours after the first oral dose and lasts for at least 24 hours with a trough/peak ratio usually above 50%.

Plasma concentration of felodipine and decrease in total peripheral resistance and blood pressure are positively correlated.

Electrophysiological and other cardiac effects: Felodipine in therapeutic doses has no effect on cardiac contractility or atrioventricular conduction or refractoriness.

Renal effects: Felodipine has a natriuretic and diuretic effect. Studies have shown that the tubular reabsorption of filtered sodium is reduced. This counteracts the salt and water retention observed for other vasodilators. Felodipine does not affect the daily potassium excretion. The renal vascular resistance is decreased by felodipine. Normal glomerular filtration rate is unchanged. In patients with impaired renal function glomerular filtration rate may increase.

Felodipine is well tolerated in renal transplant recipients.

Site and mechanism of action: The predominant pharmacodynamic feature of felodipine is its pronounced vascular versus myocardial selectivity. Myogenically active smooth muscles in arterial resistance vessels are particularly sensitive to felodipine.

Felodipine inhibits electrical and contractile activity of vascular smooth muscle cells via an effect on the calcium channels in the cell membrane.

5.2 Pharmacokinetic properties

Absorption and distribution: Felodipine is completely absorbed from the gastrointestinal tract after administration of felodipine extended release tablets.

The systemic availability of felodipine is approximately 15% in man and is independent of dose in the therapeutic dose range.

With the extended-release tablets the absorption phase is prolonged. This results in even felodipine plasma concentrations within the therapeutic range for 24 hours.

The plasma protein binding of felodipine is approximately 99%. It is bound predominantly to the albumin fraction.

Elimination and metabolism: The average half-life of felodipine in the terminal phase is 25 hours. There is no significant accumulation during long-term treatment. Felodipine is extensively metabolised by the liver and all identified metabolites are inactive. Elderly patients and patients with reduced liver function have an average higher plasma concentration of felodipine than younger patients.

About 70% of a given dose is excreted as metabolites in the urine; the remaining fraction is excreted in the faeces. Less than 0.5% of a dose is recovered unchanged in the urine.

The kinetics of felodipine are not changed in patients with renal impairment.

In a single dose (felodipine extended release 5 mg) pharmacokinetic study in twelve children aged between 6 and 16 years there was no apparent relationship between age and AUC, C_{max} or half-life of felodipine.

5.3 Preclinical safety data

Felodipine is a calcium antagonist and lowers arterial blood pressure by decreasing vascular resistance. In general a reduction in blood pressure is evident 2 hours after the first oral dose and at steady state lasts for at least 24 hours after dose.

Felodipine exhibits a high degree of selectivity for smooth muscles in the arterioles and in therapeutic doses has no direct effect on cardiac contractility. Felodipine does not affect venous smooth muscle and adrenergic vasomotor control.

Electrophysiological studies have shown that felodipine has no direct effect on conduction in the specialised conducting system of the heart and no effect on the AV nodal refractories.

Plendil possesses a mild natriuretic/diuretic effect and does not produce general fluid retention, nor affect daily potassium excretion. Plendil is well tolerated in patients with congestive heart failure.

6. PHARMACEUTICAL PARTICULARS

6.1 List of excipients
Polyoxyl 40 hydrogenated castor oil, Hydroxypropyl cellulose, Propyl gallate, Hydroxypropyl methylcellulose, Sodium aluminium silicate, Microcrystalline cellulose, Lactose anhydrous, Sodium stearyl fumarate, Macrogol, Colour Titanium dioxide (E171), Colour Iron oxide yellow (E172) and Carnauba wax.

6.2 Incompatibilities
None stated.

6.3 Shelf life
Plendil 2.5mg – 24 months
Plendil 5mg – 3 years
Plendil 10mg – 3 years

6.4 Special precautions for storage
Do not store above 25°C.

6.5 Nature and contents of container
1. HDPE Bottles - White, high density polyethylene (PE) bottles with PE screw caps. A break-off ring guarantees the integrity of the unopened package. Each bottle contains 100 tablets.

2. Aclar®Blisters - Press through blister package of aluminium form foil with an aluminium foil as enclosure web. Each blister strip contains 7 tablets. A single pack may contain 7, 14, 28, 56 or 112 tablets as multiplies of blisters of 7.

3. Tristar®Blisters - Press through packages of thermoformed PVC/PVDC with an aluminium foil as enclosure web. Each blister strip contains 7 tablets. A single pack may contain 7, 14, 28, 56 or 112 tablets as multiples of blisters of 7.

4. PVC/PVDC Blisters - Press through blister package of PVC/PVDC form foil with an aluminium foil as enclosure web. Each blister strip contains 7 tablets. A single pack may contain 7, 14, 28, 56 or 112 tablets as multiples of blisters of 7.

6.6 Special precautions for disposal and other handling
None Stated

7. MARKETING AUTHORISATION HOLDER
AstraZeneca UK Ltd.,
600 Capability Green,
Luton, LU1 3LU, UK.

8. MARKETING AUTHORISATION NUMBER(S)

Plendil 2.5mg	PL 17901/0156
Plendil 5mg	PL 17901/0157
Plendil 10mg	PL 17901/0155

9. DATE OF FIRST AUTHORISATION/RENEWAL OF THE AUTHORISATION
3rd February 2002

10. DATE OF REVISION OF THE TEXT
27th September 2007

Pletal 100 mg tablets
(Otsuka Pharmaceuticals (UK) Ltd)

1. NAME OF THE MEDICINAL PRODUCT
Pletal 100 mg tablets

2. QUALITATIVE AND QUANTITATIVE COMPOSITION
One tablet contains 100 mg of cilostazol.
For a full list of excipients, see section 6.1.

3. PHARMACEUTICAL FORM
Tablet
White, round, flat faced tablets debossed with "OG30" on one side.

4. CLINICAL PARTICULARS

4.1 Therapeutic indications
Pletal is indicated for the improvement of the maximal and pain-free walking distances in patients with intermittent claudication, who do not have rest pain and who do not have evidence of peripheral tissue necrosis (peripheral arterial disease Fontaine stage II).

4.2 Posology and method of administration
The recommended dosage of cilostazol is 100 mg twice a day. Cilostazol should be taken 30 minutes before or two hours after breakfast and the evening meal. Taking cilostazol with food has been shown to increase the maximum plasma concentrations (C_{max}) of cilostazol, which may be associated with an increased incidence of adverse effects.

Treatment for 16-24 weeks can result in a significant improvement in walking distance. Some benefit may be observed following treatment for 4-12 weeks.

The physician should consider other treatment options if cilostazol is ineffective after six months.

The elderly
There are no special dosage requirements for the elderly.

Children
Safety and efficacy in children have not been established.

Renal impairment
No dose adjustment is necessary in patients with a creatinine clearance of >25 ml/min. Cilostazol is contraindicated in patients with a creatinine clearance of ≤25 ml/min.

Hepatic impairment
No dosage adjustment is necessary in patients with mild hepatic disease. There are no data in patients with moderate or severe hepatic impairment. Since cilostazol is extensively metabolised by hepatic enzymes, it is contraindicated in patients with moderate or severe hepatic impairment.

4.3 Contraindications
- Known hypersensitivity to cilostazol or to any of the excipients
- Severe renal impairment: creatinine clearance of ≤ 25 ml/min
- Moderate or severe hepatic impairment
- Congestive heart failure
- Pregnancy
- Patients with any known predisposition to bleeding (e.g. active peptic ulceration, recent (within six months) haemorrhagic stroke, proliferative diabetic retinopathy, poorly controlled hypertension)
- Patients with any history of ventricular tachycardia, ventricular fibrillation or multifocal ventricular ectopics, whether or not adequately treated, and in patients with prolongation of the QTc interval

4.4 Special warnings and precautions for use
Patients should be warned to report any episode of bleeding or easy bruising whilst on therapy. In case of retinal bleeding administration of cilostazol should be stopped. Refer to Sections 4.3 *Contraindications* and 4.5 *Interactions with other medicinal products and other forms of interaction* for further advice on bleeding.

Due to cilostazol's platelet aggregation inhibitory effect it is possible that an increased bleeding risk occurs in combination with surgery (including minor invasive measurements like tooth extraction). If a patient is to undergo elective surgery and anti-platelet effect is not necessary, cilostazol should be stopped 5 days prior to surgery.

There have been rare or very rare reports of haematological abnormalities including thrombocytopenia, leucopenia, agranulocytosis, pancytopenia and aplastic anaemia (see section 4.8). Most patients recovered on discontinuation of cilostazol. However, some cases of pancytopenia and aplastic anaemia had a fatal outcome.

In addition to reporting episodes of bleeding and easy bruising, patients should be warned to promptly report any other signs which might also suggest the early development of blood dyscrasia such as pyrexia and sore throat. A full blood count should be performed if infection is suspected or there is any other clinical evidence of blood dyscrasia. Cilostazol should be discontinued promptly if there is clinical or laboratory evidence of haematological abnormalities.

Caution is advised when cilostazol is co-administered with inhibitors or inducers of CYP3A4 and CYP2C19 or with CYP3A4 substrates. See section 4.5 for further information.

Caution should be exercised when prescribing cilostazol for patients with atrial or ventricular ectopy and patients with atrial fibrillation or flutter.

Caution is needed when co-administering cilostazol with any other agent which has the potential to reduce blood pressure due to the possibility that there may be an additive hypotensive effect with a reflex tachycardia. Refer also to Section 4.8.

Caution should be exercised when co-administering cilostazol with any other agents that inhibit platelet aggregation. Refer to section 4.5 *Interactions with other medicinal products and other forms of interaction.*

4.5 Interaction with other medicinal products and other forms of interaction

Inhibitors of platelet aggregation
Cilostazol is a PDE III inhibitor with anti-platelet activity. In a clinical study in healthy subjects, cilostazol given 150mg b.i.d. for five days did not result in prolongation of bleeding time.

Aspirin
Short term (≤4 days) co-administration of aspirin with cilostazol suggested a 23-25% increase in inhibition of ADP-induced *ex vivo* platelet aggregation when compared to aspirin alone.

There were no apparent trends toward a greater incidence of haemorrhagic adverse effects in patients taking cilostazol and aspirin compared to patients taking placebo and equivalent doses of aspirin.

Clopidogrel and other antiplatelet drugs
Concomitant administration of cilostazol and clopidogrel did not have any effect on platelet count, prothrombin time (PT) or activated partial thromboplastin time (aPTT). All healthy subjects in the study had a prolongation of bleeding time on clopidogrel alone and concomitant administration with cilostazol did not result in a significant additional effect on bleeding time. Caution is advised when co-administering cilostazol with any drug that inhibits platelet aggregation. Consideration should be given to monitoring the bleeding time at intervals. Special attention should be paid to patients who are receiving multiple anti-platelet therapies.

Oral Anticoagulants like warfarin
In a single-dose clinical study, no inhibition of the metabolism of warfarin or an effect on the coagulation parameters (PT, aPTT, bleeding time) was observed. However, caution is advised in patients receiving both cilostazol and any anticoagulant agent, and frequent monitoring is required to reduce the possibility of bleeding.

Cytochrome P-450 (CYP) enzyme inhibitors
Cilostazol is extensively metabolised by CYP enzymes, particularly CYP3A4 and CYP2C19 and to a lesser extent CYP1A2. The dehydro metabolite, which has 4-7 times the potency of cilostazol in inhibiting platelet aggregation, appears to be formed primarily via CYP3A4. The 4'-trans-hydroxy metabolite, with potency one-fifth that of cilostazol, appears to be formed primarily via CYP2C19. Therefore, drugs inhibiting CYP3A4 (e.g., some macrolides, azole antifungals, protease inhibitors) or CYP2C19 (like proton pump inhibitors, PPIs) increase the total pharmacological activity by 32 and 42%, respectively and could have the potential to enhance the undesirable effects of cilostazol. A dose reduction to cilostazol 50 mg b.i.d. could be considered based on the individual clinical and tolerance response.

Administration of 100 mg cilostazol on the seventh day of erythromycin (a moderate inhibitor of CYP3A4) 500 mg t.i.d. resulted in an increase in the AUC of cilostazol by 74%, accompanied by a 24% decrease in AUC of the dehydro metabolite but with notable increases in AUC of the 4'-trans-hydroxy metabolite.

Co-administration of single doses of ketoconazole (a strong inhibitor of CYP3A4) 400 mg and cilostazol 100 mg resulted in a 117% increase in the AUC of cilostazol, accompanied by a 15% decrease in the AUC of the dehydro metabolite and a 87% increase in the AUC of the 4'-trans-hydroxymetabolite, which finally increases the total pharmacological activity by 32% as compared to cilostazol alone.

Administration of 100 mg cilostazol b.i.d. with diltiazem (an inhibitor of CYP3A4) 180 mg once daily resulted in an increase in the AUC of cilostazol by 44%. Co-administration did not affect exposure to the dehydro metabolite but increased by 40% the AUC of the 4'-trans-hydroxy metabolite. In patients in clinical trials, concomitant use with diltiazem was shown to increase the AUC of cilostazol by 53%.

Administration of a single dose of 100 mg cilostazol with 240 ml grapefruit juice (an inhibitor of intestinal CYP3A4) did not have a notable effect on the pharmacokinetics of cilostazol.

Administration of a single dose of 100 mg cilostazol on the seventh day of omeprazole (an inhibitor of CYP2C19) 40 mg once daily increased the AUC of cilostazol by 26%, accompanied by a 69% increase in the AUC of the dehydro metabolite and a decrease of 31% in the AUC of the 4'-trans hydroxy metabolite, which finally increases the total pharmacological activity by 42% as compared to cilostazol alone.

Cytochrome P-450 enzyme substrates
Cilostazol has been shown to increase the AUC of lovastatin (sensitive substrate for CYP3A4) and its β-hydroxy acid by 70%. Caution is advised when cilostazol is co-administered with CYP3A4 substrates with a narrow therapeutic index (e.g., cisapride, halofantrine, pimozide, ergot derivates). Caution is advised in case of co-administration with simvastatin.

Cytochrome P-450 enzyme inducers
The effect of CYP3A4 and CYP2C19 inducers (such as carbamazepin, phenytoin, rifampicin and St. John's wort) on cilostazol pharmacokinetics has not been evaluated. The antiplatelet effect may theoretically be altered and should be carefully monitored when cilostazol is co-administered with CYP3A4 and CYP2C19 inducers.

In clinical trials, smoking (which induces CYP1A2) decreased cilostazol plasma concentrations by 18%.

4.6 Pregnancy and lactation

Pregnancy
There are no adequate data in the use of cilostazol in pregnant women. Studies in animals have shown reproductive toxicity (see Section 5.3). The potential risk for humans is unknown. Pletal should not be used during pregnancy.

Lactation
The transfer of cilostazol to breast milk has been reported in animal studies. The excretion of cilostazol in human milk is unknown. Due to the potential harmful effect in the newborn child breast fed by a treated mother, the use of Pletal is not recommended during breast feeding.

4.7 Effects on ability to drive and use machines
Cilostazol may cause dizziness and patients should be warned to exercise caution before they drive or operate machinery.

4.8 Undesirable effects

The most commonly reported adverse reactions in clinical trials were headache (in > 30%), diarrhoea and abnormal stools (in >15% each). These reactions were usually of mild to moderate intensity and were sometimes alleviated by reducing the dose.

Adverse reactions reported in clinical trials and in the post-marketing period are included in the table below.

The frequencies correspond with: Very common (≥1/10)

Common (≥1/100 to <1/10)

Uncommon (≥1/1,000 to <1/100)

Rare (≥1/10,000 to <1/1000)

Very rare (<1/10,000), not known (cannot be estimated from the available data)

The frequencies of reactions observed in the post-marketing period is considered unknown (cannot be estimated from the available data).

(see Table 1 opposite)

An increase in the incidence of palpitation and peripheral oedema was observed when cilostazol was combined with other vasodilators that cause reflex tachycardia e.g. dihydropyridine calcium channel blockers.

The only adverse event resulting in discontinuation of therapy in ≥3% of patients treated with cilostazol was headache. Other frequent causes of discontinuation included palpitation and diarrhoea (both 1.1%).

Cilostazol *per se* may carry an increased risk of bleeding and this risk may be potentiated by co-administration with any other agent with such potential.

The risk of intraocular bleeding may be higher in patients with diabetes.

4.9 Overdose

Information on acute overdose in humans is limited. The signs and symptoms can be anticipated to be severe headache, diarrhoea, tachycardia and possibly cardiac arrhythmias.

Patients should be observed and given supportive treatment. The stomach should be emptied by induced vomiting or gastric lavage, as appropriate.

5. PHARMACOLOGICAL PROPERTIES

5.1 Pharmacodynamic properties

Pharmacotherapeutic group: Antithrombotic agents, platelet aggregation inhibitor excl. heparin.

ATC code: B01A C

From data generated in nine placebo-controlled studies (where 1,634 patients were exposed to cilostazol), it has been demonstrated that cilostazol improves exercise capacity as judged by changes in Absolute Claudication Distance (ACD, or maximal walking distance) and Initial Claudication Distance (ICD, or pain-free walking distance) upon treadmill testing. Following 24 weeks treatment, cilostazol 100 mg b.i.d. increases in mean ACD ranged from 60.4 - 129.1 metres, whilst mean ICD increases ranged from 47.3 - 93.6 metres.

A meta-analysis based on weighted mean differences across the nine studies indicated that there was a significant absolute overall post-baseline improvement of 42 m in maximal walking distance (ACD) for cilostazol 100 mg b.i.d. over the improvement seen under placebo. This corresponds to a relative improvement of 100% over placebo. This effect appeared lower in diabetics than in non-diabetics.

Animal studies have shown cilostazol to have vasodilator effects and this has been demonstrated in small studies in man where ankle blood flow was measured by strain gauge plethysmography. Cilostazol also inhibits smooth muscle cell proliferation in rat and human smooth muscle cells *in vitro*, and inhibits the platelet release reaction of platelet-derived growth factor and PF-4 in human platelets.

Studies in animals and in man (*in vivo* and *ex vivo*) have shown that cilostazol causes reversible inhibition of platelet aggregation. The inhibition is effective against a range of aggregants (including shear stress, arachidonic acid, collagen, ADP and adrenaline); in man the inhibition lasts for up to 12 hours, and on cessation of administration of cilostazol recovery of aggregation occurred within 48-96 hours, without rebound hyperaggregability. Effects on circulating plasma lipids have been examined in patients taking Pletal. After 12 weeks, as compared to placebo, Pletal 100 mg b.i.d. produced a reduction in triglycerides of 0.33 mmol/L (15%) and an increase in HDL-cholesterol of 0.10mmol/L (10%).

A randomized, double-blind, placebo-controlled Phase IV study was conducted to assess the long-term effects of cilostazol, with focus on mortality and safety. In total, 1,439 patients with intermittent claudication and no heart failure have been treated with cilostazol or placebo for up to three years. With respect to mortality, the observed 36-month Kaplan-Meier event rate for deaths on study drug with a median time on study drug of 18 months was 5.6% (95%CI of 2.8 to 8.4%) on cilostazol and 6.8% (95% CI of 1.9 to 11.5%) on placebo. Long-term treatment with cilostazol did not raise safety concerns.

5.2 Pharmacokinetic properties

Following multiple doses of cilostazol 100 mg twice daily in patients with peripheral vascular disease, steady state is achieved within 4 days.

Table 1

Blood and the lymphatic system disorders	Common	Ecchymosis
	Uncommon	Anaemia
	Rare	Bleeding time prolonged, thrombocythaemia
	Unknown	Bleeding tendency, thrombocytopenia, granulocytopenia, agranulocytosis, leukopenia, pancytopenia, aplastic anaemia
Immune system disorders	Uncommon	Allergic reaction
Metabolism and nutrition disorders	Common	Oedema (peripheral, face)
	Uncommon	Hyperglycaemia, Diabetes mellitus
	Unknown	Anorexia
Psychiatric disorders	Uncommon	Anxiety
Nervous system disorders	Very common	Headache
	Common	Dizziness
	Uncommon	Insomnia, abnormal dreams
	Unknown	Paresis, hypoaesthesia
Eye disorders	Unknown	Conjunctivitis
Ear and labyrinth disorders	Unknown	Tinnitus
Cardiac disorders	Common	Palpitation, tachycardia, angina pectoris, arrhythmia, ventricular extrasystoles
	Uncommon	Myocardial infarction, atrial fibrillation, congestive heart failure, supraventricular tachycardia, ventricular tachycardia, syncope
Vascular disorders	Uncommon	Eye haemorrhage, epistaxis, gastrointestinal haemorrhage, haemorrhage unspecified, orthostatic hypotension
	Unknown	Hot flushes, hypertension, hypotension, cerebral haemorrhage, pulmonary haemorrhage, muscle haemorrhage, respiratory tract haemorrhage, subcutaneous haemorrhage
Respiratory, thoracic and mediastinal disorders	Common	Rhinitis, pharyngitis
	Uncommon	Dyspnoea, pneumonia, cough
	Unknown	Interstitial pneumonia
Gastrointestinal disorders	Very common	Diarrhoea, abnormal faeces
	Common	Nausea and vomiting, dyspepsia, flatulence, abdominal pain
	Uncommon	Gastritis
Hepato-biliary disorders	Unknown	Hepatitis, hepatic function abnormal, jaundice
Skin and subcutaneous tissue disorders	Common	Rash, pruritus
	Unknown	Eczema, skin eruptions, Stevens-Johnson syndrome, toxic epidermal necrolysis, urticaria
Musculoskeletal, connective tissue and bone disorders	Uncommon	Myalgia
Renal and urinary disorders	Rare	Renal failure, renal impairment
	Unknown	Haematuria, pollakiuria
General disorders and administration site conditions	Common	Chest pain, asthenia
	Uncommon	Chills
	Unknown	Pyrexia, malaise, pain
Investigations	Unknown	Uric acid level increased, blood urea increased, blood creatinine increased

The C_{max} of cilostazol and its primary circulating metabolites increase less than proportionally with increasing doses. However, the AUC for cilostazol and its metabolites increase approximately proportionately with dose.

The apparent elimination half-life of cilostazol is 10.5 hours. There are two major metabolites, a dehydro-cilostazol and a 4'-trans-hydroxy cilostazol, both of which have similar apparent half-lives. The dehydro metabolite is 4-7 times as active a platelet anti-aggregant as the parent compound and the 4'-trans-hydroxy metabolite is one fifth as active. Plasma concentrations (as measured by AUC) of the dehydro and 4'-trans-hydroxy metabolites are ~41% and ~12% of cilostazol concentrations.

Cilostazol is eliminated predominantly by metabolism and subsequent urinary excretion of metabolites. The primary isoenzymes involved in its metabolism are cytochrome P-450 CYP3A4, to a lesser extent, CYP2C19, and to an even lesser extent CYP1A2.

The primary route of elimination is urinary (74%) with the remainder excreted in the faeces. No measurable amount of unchanged cilostazol is excreted in the urine, and less than 2% of the dose is excreted as the dehydro-cilostazol metabolite. Approximately 30% of the dose is excreted in the urine as the 4'-trans-hydroxy metabolite. The remainder is excreted as metabolites, none of which exceed 5% of the total excreted.

Cilostazol is 95-98% protein bound, predominantly to albumin. The dehydro metabolite and 4'-trans-hydroxy metabolite are 97.4% and 66% protein bound respectively.

There is no evidence that cilostazol induces hepatic microsomal enzymes.

The pharmacokinetics of cilostazol and its metabolites were not significantly affected by age or gender in healthy subjects aged between 50-80 years.

In subjects with severe renal impairment, the free fraction of cilostazol was 27% higher and both C_{max} and AUC were 29% and 39% lower respectively than in subjects with normal renal function. The C_{max} and AUC of the dehydro metabolite were 41% and 47% lower respectively in the severely renally impaired subjects compared to subjects with normal renal function. The C_{max} and AUC of 4'-trans-hydroxy cilostazol were 173% and 209%

greater in subjects with severe renal impairment. The drug should not be administered to patients with a creatinine clearance <25ml/min (see Section 4.3).

There are no data in patients with moderate to severe hepatic impairment and since cilostazol is extensively metabolised by hepatic enzymes, the drug should not be used in such patients (see Section 4.3).

5.3 Preclinical safety data

Cilostazol and several of its metabolites are phosphodiesterase III inhibitors which suppress cyclic AMP degradation, resulting in increased cAMP in a variety of tissues including platelets and blood vessels. As with other positive inotropic and vasodilator agents, cilostazol produced cardiovascular lesions in dogs. Such lesions were not seen in rats or monkeys and are considered species specific. Investigation of QTc in dogs and monkeys showed no prolongation after administration of cilostazol or its metabolites.

Mutagenicity studies were negative in bacterial gene mutation, bacterial DNA repair, mammalian cell gene mutation and mouse *in vivo* bone marrow chromosomal aberrations. In *in vitro* tests on Chinese ovary hamster cells cilostazol produced a weak but significant increase in chromosome aberration frequency. No unusual neoplastic outcomes were observed in two-year carcinogenicity studies in rats at oral (dietary) doses up to 500 mg/kg/day, and in mice at doses up to 1000 mg/kg/day.

In rats dosed during pregnancy, foetal weights were decreased. In addition, an increase in foetuses with external, visceral and skeletal abnormalities was noted at high dose levels. At lower dose levels, retardations of ossification were observed. Exposure in late pregnancy resulted in an increased incidence of stillbirths and lower offspring weights. An increased incidence of retardation of ossification of the sternum was observed in rabbits. As there is no experience of cilostazol use in human pregnancy, it should not be used in women who are pregnant.

6. PHARMACEUTICAL PARTICULARS

6.1 List of excipients

Maize starch, microcrystalline cellulose, carmellose calcium, hypromellose and magnesium stearate.

6.2 Incompatibilities

Not applicable.

6.3 Shelf life

3 years.

6.4 Special precautions for storage

This medicinal product does not require any special storage conditions.

6.5 Nature and contents of container

Cartons containing 14, 20, 28, 30, 50, 56, 98, 100, 112 and 168 tablets as well as hospital packs with 70 (5x14) tablets packed in PVC/Aluminium blisters.

Not all pack sizes may be marketed.

6.6 Special precautions for disposal and other handling

No special requirements.

7. MARKETING AUTHORISATION HOLDER

Otsuka Pharmaceutical Europe Ltd
Hunton House
Highbridge Business Park
Oxford Road
Uxbridge
Middlesex, UB8 1HU
UK

8. MARKETING AUTHORISATION NUMBER(S)

PL 11515/0001

9. DATE OF FIRST AUTHORISATION/RENEWAL OF THE AUTHORISATION

21 March 2000 / 20 March 2005

10. DATE OF REVISION OF THE TEXT

November 2008

Pletal 50 mg tablets

(Otsuka Pharmaceuticals (UK) Ltd)

1. NAME OF THE MEDICINAL PRODUCT

Pletal 50 mg tablets

2. QUALITATIVE AND QUANTITATIVE COMPOSITION

One tablet contains 50 mg of cilostazol.

For a full list of excipients, see section 6.1.

3. PHARMACEUTICAL FORM

Tablet

White, round, flat faced tablets debossed with "OG31" on one side.

4. CLINICAL PARTICULARS

4.1 Therapeutic indications

Pletal is indicated for the improvement of the maximal and pain-free walking distances in patients with intermittent claudication, who do not have rest pain and who do not have evidence of peripheral tissue necrosis (peripheral arterial disease Fontaine stage II).

4.2 Posology and method of administration

The recommended dosage of cilostazol is 100 mg twice a day. Cilostazol should be taken 30 minutes before or two hours after breakfast and the evening meal. Taking cilostazol with food has been shown to increase the maximum plasma concentrations (C_{max}) of cilostazol, which may be associated with an increased incidence of adverse effects.

Treatment for 16-24 weeks can result in a significant improvement in walking distance. Some benefit may be observed following treatment for 4-12 weeks.

The physician should consider other treatment options if cilostazol is ineffective after six months.

<u>The elderly</u>

There are no special dosage requirements for the elderly.

<u>Children</u>

Safety and efficacy in children have not been established.

<u>Renal impairment</u>

No dose adjustment is necessary in patients with a creatinine clearance of >25 ml/min. Cilostazol is contraindicated in patients with a creatinine clearance of ≤25 ml/min.

<u>Hepatic impairment</u>

No dosage adjustment is necessary in patients with mild hepatic disease. There are no data in patients with moderate or severe hepatic impairment. Since cilostazol is extensively metabolised by hepatic enzymes, it is contraindicated in patients with moderate or severe hepatic impairment.

4.3 Contraindications

- Known hypersensitivity to cilostazol or to any of the excipients
- Severe renal impairment: creatinine clearance of ≤ 25 ml/min
- Moderate or severe hepatic impairment
- Congestive heart failure
- Pregnancy
- Patients with any known predisposition to bleeding (e.g. active peptic ulceration, recent (within six months) haemorrhagic stroke, proliferative diabetic retinopathy, poorly controlled hypertension)
- Patients with any history of ventricular tachycardia, ventricular fibrillation or multifocal ventricular ectopics, whether or not adequately treated, and in patients with prolongation of the QTc interval

4.4 Special warnings and precautions for use

Patients should be warned to report any episode of bleeding or easy bruising whilst on therapy. In case of retinal bleeding administration of cilostazol should be stopped. Refer to Sections 4.3 *Contraindications* and 4.5 *Interactions with other medicinal products and other forms of interaction* for further advice on bleeding.

Due to cilostazol's platelet aggregation inhibitory effect it is possible that an increased bleeding risk occurs in combination with surgery (including minor invasive measurements like tooth extraction). If a patient is to undergo elective surgery and anti-platelet effect is not necessary, cilostazol should be stopped 5 days prior to surgery.

There have been rare or very rare reports of haematological abnormalities including thrombocytopenia, leucopenia, agranulocytosis, pancytopenia and aplastic anaemia (see section 4.8). Most patients recovered on discontinuation of cilostazol. However, some cases of pancytopenia and aplastic anaemia had a fatal outcome.

In addition to reporting episodes of bleeding and easy bruising, patients should be warned to promptly report any other signs which might also suggest the early development of blood dyscrasia such as pyrexia and sore throat. A full blood count should be performed if infection is suspected or there is any other clinical evidence of blood dyscrasia. Cilostazol should be discontinued promptly if there is clinical or laboratory evidence of haematological abnormalities.

Caution is advised when cilostazol is co-administered with inhibitors or inducers of CYP3A4 and CYP2C19 or with CYP3A4 substrates. See section 4.5 for further information.

Caution should be exercised when prescribing cilostazol for patients with atrial or ventricular ectopy and patients with atrial fibrillation or flutter.

Caution is needed when co-administering cilostazol with any other agent which has the potential to reduce blood pressure due to the possibility that there may be an additive hypotensive effect with a reflex tachycardia. Refer also to Section 4.8.

Caution should be exercised when co-administering cilostazol with any other agents that inhibit platelet aggregation. Refer to section 4.5 *Interactions with other medicinal products and other forms of interaction.*

4.5 Interaction with other medicinal products and other forms of interaction

<u>Inhibitors of platelet aggregation</u>

Cilostazol is a PDE III inhibitor with anti-platelet activity. In a clinical study in healthy subjects, cilostazol given 150mg b.i.d. for five days did not result in prolongation of bleeding time.

<u>Aspirin</u>

Short term (≤4 days) co-administration of aspirin with cilostazol suggested a 23-25% increase in inhibition of ADP-induced *ex vivo* platelet aggregation when compared to aspirin alone.

There were no apparent trends toward a greater incidence of haemorrhagic adverse effects in patients taking cilostazol and aspirin compared to patients taking placebo and equivalent doses of aspirin.

<u>Clopidogrel and other antiplatelet drugs</u>

Concomitant administration of cilostazol and clopidogrel did not have any effect on platelet count, prothrombin time (PT) or activated partial thromboplastin time (aPTT). All healthy subjects in the study had a prolongation of bleeding time on clopidogrel alone and concomitant administration with cilostazol did not result in a significant additional effect on bleeding time. Caution is advised when co-administering cilostazol with any drug that inhibits platelet aggregation. Consideration should be given to monitoring the bleeding time at intervals. Special attention should be paid to patients who are receiving multiple anti-platelet therapies.

<u>Oral Anticoagulants like warfarin</u>

In a single-dose clinical study, no inhibition of the metabolism of warfarin or an effect on the coagulation parameters (PT, aPTT, bleeding time) was observed. However, caution is advised in patients receiving both cilostazol and any anticoagulant agent, and frequent monitoring is required to reduce the possibility of bleeding.

<u>Cytochrome P-450 (CYP) enzyme inhibitors</u>

Cilostazol is extensively metabolised by CYP enzymes, particularly CYP3A4 and CYP2C19 and to a lesser extent CYP1A2. The dehydro metabolite, which has 4-7 times the potency of cilostazol in inhibiting platelet aggregation, appears to be formed primarily via CYP3A4. The 4'-trans-hydroxy metabolite, with potency one-fifth that of cilostazol, appears to be formed primarily via CYP2C19. Therefore, drugs inhibiting CYP3A4 (e.g., some macrolides, azole antifungals, protease inhibitors) or CYP2C19 (like proton pump inhibitors, PPIs) increase the total pharmacological activity by 32 and 42%, respectively and could have the potential to enhance the undesirable effects of cilostazol. A dose reduction to cilostazol 50 mg b.i.d. could be considered based on the individual clinical and tolerance response.

Administration of 100 mg cilostazol on the seventh day of erythromycin (a moderate inhibitor of CYP3A4) 500 mg t.i.d. resulted in an increase in the AUC of cilostazol by 74%, accompanied by a 24% decrease in AUC of the dehydro metabolite but with notable increases in AUC of the 4'-trans-hydroxy metabolite.

Co-administration of single doses of ketoconazole (a strong inhibitor of CYP3A4) 400 mg and cilostazol 100 mg resulted in a 117% increase in the AUC of cilostazol, accompanied by a 15% decrease in the AUC of the dehydro metabolite and a 87% increase in the AUC of the 4'-trans-hydroxymetabolite, which finally increases the total pharmacological activity by 32% as compared to cilostazol alone.

Administration of 100 mg cilostazol b.i.d. with diltiazem (an inhibitor of CYP3A4) 180 mg once daily resulted in an increase in the AUC of cilostazol by 44%. Co-administration did not affect exposure to the dehydro metabolite but increased by 40% the AUC of the 4'-trans-hydroxy metabolite. In patients in clinical trials, concomitant use with diltiazem was shown to increase the AUC of cilostazol by 53%.

Administration of a single dose of 100 mg cilostazol with 240 ml grapefruit juice (an inhibitor of intestinal CYP3A4) did not have a notable effect on the pharmacokinetics of cilostazol.

Administration of a single dose of 100 mg cilostazol on the seventh day of omeprazole (an inhibitor of CYP2C19) 40 mg once daily increased the AUC of cilostazol by 26%, accompanied by a 69% increase in the AUC of the dehydro metabolite and a decrease of 31% in the AUC of the 4'-trans hydroxy metabolite, which finally increases the total pharmacological activity by 42% as compared to cilostazol alone.

<u>Cytochrome P-450 enzyme substrates</u>

Cilostazol has been shown to increase the AUC of lovastatin (sensitive substrate for CYP3A4) and its β-hydroxy acid by 70%. Caution is advised when cilostazol is co-administered with CYP3A4 substrates with a narrow therapeutic index (e.g., cisapride, halofantrine, pimozide, ergot derivates). Caution is advised in case of co-administration with simvastatin.

<u>Cytochrome P-450 enzyme inducers</u>

The effect of CYP3A4 and CYP2C19 inducers (such as carbamazepin, phenytoin, rifampicin and St. John's wort) on cilostazol pharmacokinetics has not been evaluated. The antiplatelet effect may theoretically be altered and should be carefully monitored when cilostazol is co-administered with CYP3A4 and CYP2C19 inducers.

In clinical trials, smoking (which induces CYP1A2) decreased cilostazol plasma concentrations by 18%.

4.6 Pregnancy and lactation

Pregnancy

There are no adequate data in the use of cilostazol in pregnant women. Studies in animals have shown reproductive toxicity (see Section 5.3). The potential risk for humans is unknown. Pletal should not be used during pregnancy.

Lactation

The transfer of cilostazol to breast milk has been reported in animal studies. The excretion of cilostazol in human milk is unknown. Due to the potential harmful effect in the newborn child breast fed by a treated mother, the use of Pletal is not recommended during breast feeding.

4.7 Effects on ability to drive and use machines

Cilostazol may cause dizziness and patients should be warned to exercise caution before they drive or operate machinery.

4.8 Undesirable effects

The most commonly reported adverse reactions in clinical trials were headache (in > 30%), diarrhoea and abnormal stools (in >15% each). These reactions were usually of mild to moderate intensity and were sometimes alleviated by reducing the dose.

Adverse reactions reported in clinical trials and in the post-marketing period are included in the table below.

The frequencies correspond with: Very common (≥1/10)

Common (≥1/100 to <1/10)

Uncommon (≥1/1,000 to <1/100)

Rare (≥1/10,000 to <1/1000)

Very rare (<1/10,000), not known (cannot be estimated from the ≥available data)

The frequencies of reactions observed in the post-marketing period is considered unknown (cannot be estimated from the available data).

(see Table 1 opposite)

An increase in the incidence of palpitation and peripheral oedema was observed when cilostazol was combined with other vasodilators that cause reflex tachycardia e.g. dihydropyridine calcium channel blockers.

The only adverse event resulting in discontinuation of therapy in ≥3% of patients treated with cilostazol was headache. Other frequent causes of discontinuation included palpitation and diarrhoea (both 1.1%).

Cilostazol *per se* may carry an increased risk of bleeding and this risk may be potentiated by co-administration with any other agent with such potential.

The risk of intraocular bleeding may be higher in patients with diabetes.

4.9 Overdose

Information on acute overdose in humans is limited. The signs and symptoms can be anticipated to be severe headache, diarrhoea, tachycardia and possibly cardiac arrhythmias.

Patients should be observed and given supportive treatment. The stomach should be emptied by induced vomiting or gastric lavage, as appropriate.

5. PHARMACOLOGICAL PROPERTIES

5.1 Pharmacodynamic properties

Pharmacotherapeutic group: Antithrombotic agents, platelet aggregation inhibitor excl. heparin.

ATC code: B01A C

From data generated in nine placebo-controlled studies (where 1,634 patients were exposed to cilostazol), it has been demonstrated that cilostazol improves exercise capacity as judged by changes in Absolute Claudication Distance (ACD, or maximal walking distance) and Initial Claudication Distance (ICD, or pain-free walking distance) upon treadmill testing. Following 24 weeks treatment, cilostazol 100 mg b.i.d. increases in mean ACD ranged from 60.4 - 129.1 metres, whilst mean ICD increases ranged from 47.3 - 93.6 metres.

A meta-analysis based on weighted mean differences across the nine studies indicated that there was a significant absolute overall post-baseline improvement of 42 m in maximal walking distance (ACD) for cilostazol 100 mg b.i.d. over the improvement seen under placebo. This corresponds to a relative improvement of 100% over placebo. This effect appeared lower in diabetics than in non-diabetics.

Animal studies have shown cilostazol to have vasodilator effects and this has been demonstrated in small studies in man where ankle blood flow was measured by strain gauge plethysmography. Cilostazol also inhibits smooth muscle cell proliferation in rat and human smooth muscle cells *in vitro*, and inhibits the platelet release reaction of platelet-derived growth factor and PF-4 in human platelets.

Studies in animals and in man (*in vivo* and *ex vivo*) have shown that cilostazol causes reversible inhibition of platelet aggregation. The inhibition is effective against a range of aggregants (including shear stress, arachidonic acid, collagen, ADP and adrenaline); in man the inhibition lasts for up to 12 hours, and on cessation of administration of cilostazol recovery of aggregation occurred within 48-96 hours, without rebound hyperaggregability. Effects on circulating plasma lipids have been examined in patients taking Pletal. After 12 weeks, as compared to placebo,

Table 1

Blood and the lymphatic system disorders	Common	Ecchymosis
	Uncommon	Anaemia
	Rare	Bleeding time prolonged, thrombocythaemia
	Unknown	Bleeding tendency, thrombocytopenia, granulocytopenia, agranulocytosis, leukopenia, pancytopenia, aplastic anaemia
Immune system disorders	Uncommon	Allergic reaction
Metabolism and nutrition disorders	Common	Oedema (peripheral, face)
	Uncommon	Hyperglycaemia, Diabetes mellitus
	Unknown	Anorexia
Psychiatric disorders	Uncommon	Anxiety
Nervous system disorders	Very common	Headache
	Common	Dizziness
	Uncommon	Insomnia, abnormal dreams
	Unknown	Paresis, hypoaesthesia
Eye disorders	Unknown	Conjunctivitis
Ear and labyrinth disorders	Unknown	Tinnitus
Cardiac disorders	Common	Palpitation, tachycardia, angina pectoris, arrhythmia, ventricular extrasystoles
	Uncommon	Myocardial infarction, atrial fibrillation, congestive heart failure, supraventricular tachycardia, ventricular tachycardia, syncope
Vascular disorders	Uncommon	Eye haemorrhage, epistaxis, gastrointestinal haemorrhage, haemorrhage unspecified, orthostatic hypotension
	Unknown	Hot flushes, hypertension, hypotension, cerebral haemorrhage, pulmonary haemorrhage, muscle haemorrhage, respiratory tract haemorrhage, subcutaneous haemorrhage
Respiratory, thoracic and mediastinal disorders	Common	Rhinitis, pharyngitis
	Uncommon	Dyspnoea, pneumonia, cough
	Unknown	Interstitial pneumonia
Gastrointestinal disorders	Very common	Diarrhoea, abnormal faeces
	Common	Nausea and vomiting, dyspepsia, flatulence, abdominal pain
	Uncommon	Gastritis
Hepato-biliary disorders	Unknown	Hepatitis, hepatic function abnormal, jaundice
Skin and subcutaneous tissue disorders	Common	Rash, pruritus
	Unknown	Eczema, skin eruptions, Stevens-Johnson syndrome, toxic epidermal necrolysis, urticaria
Musculoskeletal, connective tissue and bone disorders	Uncommon	Myalgia
Renal and urinary disorders	Rare	Renal failure, renal impairment
	Unknown	Haematuria, pollakiuria
General disorders and administration site conditions	Common	Chest pain, asthenia
	Uncommon	Chills
	Unknown	Pyrexia, malaise, pain
Investigations	Unknown	Uric acid level increased, blood urea increased, blood creatinine increased

Pletal 100 mg b.i.d. produced a reduction in triglycerides of 0.33 mmol/L (15%) and an increase in HDL-cholesterol of 0.10mmol/L (10%).

A randomized, double-blind, placebo-controlled Phase IV study was conducted to assess the long-term effects of cilostazol, with focus on mortality and safety. In total, 1,439 patients with intermittent claudication and no heart failure have been treated with cilostazol or placebo for up to three years. With respect to mortality, the observed 36-month Kaplan-Meier event rate for deaths on study drug with a median time on study drug of 18 months was 5.6% (95%CI of 2.8 to 8.4%) on cilostazol and 6.8% (95% CI of 1.9 to 11.5%) on placebo. Long-term treatment with cilostazol did not raise safety concerns.

5.2 Pharmacokinetic properties

Following multiple doses of cilostazol 100 mg twice daily in patients with peripheral vascular disease, steady state is achieved within 4 days.

The C_{max} of cilostazol and its primary circulating metabolites increase less than proportionally with increasing doses. However, the AUC for cilostazol and its metabolites increase approximately proportionately with dose.

The apparent elimination half-life of cilostazol is 10.5 hours. There are two major metabolites, a dehydro-cilostazol and a 4'-trans-hydroxy cilostazol, both of which have similar apparent half-lives. The dehydro metabolite is 4-7 times as active a platelet anti-aggregant as the parent compound and the 4'-trans-hydroxy metabolite is one fifth as active. Plasma concentrations (as measured by AUC) of the dehydro and 4'-trans-hydroxy metabolites are ~41% and ~12% of cilostazol concentrations.

Cilostazol is eliminated predominantly by metabolism and subsequent urinary excretion of metabolites. The primary isoenzymes involved in its metabolism are cytochrome P-450 CYP3A4, to a lesser extent, CYP2C19, and to an even lesser extent CYP1A2.

The primary route of elimination is urinary (74%) with the remainder excreted in the faeces. No measurable amount of unchanged cilostazol is excreted in the urine, and less than 2% of the dose is excreted as the dehydro-cilostazol metabolite. Approximately 30% of the dose is excreted in the urine as the 4'-trans-hydroxy metabolite. The remainder is excreted as metabolites, none of which exceed 5% of the total excreted.

Cilostazol is 95-98% protein bound, predominantly to albumin. The dehydro metabolite and 4'-trans-hydroxy metabolite are 97.4% and 66% protein bound respectively.

There is no evidence that cilostazol induces hepatic microsomal enzymes.

The pharmacokinetics of cilostazol and its metabolites were not significantly affected by age or gender in healthy subjects aged between 50-80 years.

In subjects with severe renal impairment, the free fraction of cilostazol was 27% higher and both C_{max} and AUC were 29% and 39% lower respectively than in subjects with normal renal function. The C_{max} and AUC of the dehydro metabolite were 41% and 47% lower respectively in the severely renally impaired subjects compared to subjects with normal renal function. The C_{max} and AUC of 4'-trans-hydroxy cilostazol were 173% and 209% greater in subjects with severe renal impairment. The drug should not be administered to patients with a creatinine clearance <25ml/min (see Section 4.3).

There are no data in patients with moderate to severe hepatic impairment and since cilostazol is extensively metabolised by hepatic enzymes, the drug should not be used in such patients (see Section 4.3).

5.3 Preclinical safety data

Cilostazol and several of its metabolites are phosphodiesterase III inhibitors which suppress cyclic AMP degradation, resulting in increased cAMP in a variety of tissues including platelets and blood vessels. As with other positive inotropic and vasodilator agents, cilostazol produced cardiovascular lesions in dogs. Such lesions were not seen in rats or monkeys and are considered species specific. Investigation of QTc in dogs and monkeys showed no prolongation after administration of cilostazol or its metabolites.

Mutagenicity studies were negative in bacterial gene mutation, bacterial DNA repair, mammalian cell gene mutation and mouse *in vivo* bone marrow chromosomal aberrations. In *in vitro* tests on Chinese ovary hamster cells cilostazol produced a weak but significant increase in chromosome aberration frequency. No unusual neoplastic outcomes were observed in two-year carcinogenicity studies in rats at oral (dietary) doses up to 500 mg/kg/day, and in mice at doses up to 1000 mg/kg/day.

In rats dosed during pregnancy, foetal weights were decreased. In addition, an increase in foetuses with external, visceral and skeletal abnormalities was noted at high dose levels. At lower dose levels, retardations of ossification were observed. Exposure in late pregnancy resulted in an increased incidence of stillbirths and lower offspring weights. An increased incidence of retardation of ossification of the sternum was observed in rabbits. As there is no experience of cilostazol use in human pregnancy, it should not be used in women who are pregnant.

6. PHARMACEUTICAL PARTICULARS

6.1 List of excipients

Maize starch, microcrystalline cellulose, carmellose calcium, hypromellose and magnesium stearate.

6.2 Incompatibilities

Not applicable.

6.3 Shelf life

3 years.

6.4 Special precautions for storage

This medicinal product does not require any special storage conditions.

6.5 Nature and contents of container

Cartons containing 14, 20, 28, 30, 50, 56, 98, 100, 112 and 168 tablets as well as hospital packs with 70 (5x14) tablets packed in PVC/Aluminium blisters.

Not all pack sizes may be marketed.

6.6 Special precautions for disposal and other handling

No special requirements.

7. MARKETING AUTHORISATION HOLDER

Otsuka Pharmaceutical Europe Ltd

Hunton House

Highbridge Business Park

Oxford Road

Uxbridge

Middlesex, UB8 1HU

UK

8. MARKETING AUTHORISATION NUMBER(S)

PL 11515/0002

9. DATE OF FIRST AUTHORISATION/RENEWAL OF THE AUTHORISATION

21 March 2000 / 20 March 2005

10. DATE OF REVISION OF THE TEXT

November 2008

POLLENSHIELD HAYFEVER (P)

(Actavis UK Ltd)

1. NAME OF THE MEDICINAL PRODUCT

Cetirizine Hydrochloride 10mg Tablets

POLLENSHIELD HAYFEVER

2. QUALITATIVE AND QUANTITATIVE COMPOSITION

Each tablet contains 10mg Cetirizine hydrochloride.

For a full list of excipients, see 6.1

3. PHARMACEUTICAL FORM

Film-coated tablet.

Film-coated, white or almost white convex, elliptical, tablets. 5.7 × 11.4mm. The letter "C" on one side and the letters "J" and "E" on either side of a central division line on the reverse.

4. CLINICAL PARTICULARS

4.1 Therapeutic indications

In adults and paediatric patients 6 year and above:

- Cetirizine is indicated for the relief of nasal and ocular symptoms of seasonal and perennial allergic rhinitis.

- Cetirizine is indicated for the relief of symptoms of chronic idiopathic urticaria.

4.2 Posology and method of administration

Children aged from 6 to 12 years: 5mg twice daily (a half tablet twice daily).

Adults and adolescents over 12 years of age: 10mg once daily (1 tablet).

The tablets need to be swallowed with a glass of liquid.

Elderly subjects: data do not suggest that the dose needs to be reduced in elderly subjects provided that the renal function is normal.

Patients with moderate to severe renal impairment: there are no data to document the efficacy/safety ratio in patients with renal impairement. Since cetirizine is mainly excreted via renal route (see section 5.2), in cases no alternative treatment can be used, the dosing intervals must be individualized according to renal function. Refer to the following table and adjust the dose as indicated. To use this dosing table, an estimate of the patient's creatinine clearance (CLcr) in ml/min is needed. The CLcr (ml/min) may be estimated from serum creatinine (mg/dl) determination using the following formula:

$$CL_{cr} = \frac{[140 - age(years)] \times weight(kg)}{72 \times serum\ creatinine\ (mg/dl)} \quad (\times 0.85\ for\ women)$$

Dosing adjustments for adult patients with impaired renal function

Group	Creatinine clearance (ml/min)	Dosage and frequency
Normal	⩾80	10mg once daily
Mild	50 – 79	10mg once daily
Moderate	30 – 49	5mg once daily
Severe	30	5mg once every 2 days
End-stage renal disease	10	Contra-indicated
Patients undergoing dialysis		

In paediatric patients suffering from renal impairment, the dose will have to be adjusted on an individual basis taking into account the renal clearance of the patient, his age and his body weight.

Patients with hepatic impairment: no dose adjustment is needed in patients with solely hepatic impairment.

Patients with hepatic impairment and renal impairment: dose adjustment is recommended (see Patients with moderate to severe renal impairment above).

Method of Administration

For oral use.

4.3 Contraindications

Hypersensitivity to the active substance, to any of the excipients, to hydroxyzine or to any piperazine derivatives.

Patients with severe renal impairment at less than 10ml/min creatinine clearance.

Patients with rare hereditary problems of galactose intolerance, the Lapp lactase deficiency or glucose- galactose malabsorption should not take cetirizine film-coated tablet.

4.4 Special warnings and precautions for use

At therapeutic doses, no clinically significant interactions have been demonstrated with alcohol (for a blood alcohol level of 0.5g/L). Nevertheless, precaution is recommended if alcohol is taken concomitantly.

Caution in epileptic patients and patients at risk of convulsions is recommended.

The use of the film-coated tablet formulation is not recommended in children aged less than 6 years since this formulation does not allow for appropriate dose adaptation.

4.5 Interaction with other medicinal products and other forms of interaction

Due to the pharmacokinetic, pharmacodynamic and tolerance profile of cetirizine, no interactions are expected with this antihistamine. Actually, neither pharmacodynamic nor significant pharmacokinetic interaction was reported in drug-drug interactions studies performed, notably with pseudoephedrine or theophylline (400mg/day).

The extent of absorption of cetirizine is not reduced with food, although the rate of absorption is decreased.

4.6 Pregnancy and lactation

For cetirizine very rare clinical data on exposed pregnancies are available. Animal studies do not indicate direct or indirect harmful effects with respect to pregnancy, embryonal/fetal development, parturition or postnatal development. Caution should be exercised when prescribing to pregnant or breast feeding women because cetirizine passes into breast milk.

4.7 Effects on ability to drive and use machines

Objective measurements of driving ability, sleep latency and assembly line performance have not demonstrated any clinically relevant effects at the recommended dose of 10mg. Patients intending to drive, engaging in potentially hazardous activities or operating machinery should not exceed the recommended dose and should take their response to the medicinal product into account. In these sensitive patients, concurrent use with alcohol or other CNS depressants may cause additional reductions in alertness and impairment of performance.

4.8 Undesirable effects

Clinical studies have shown that cetirizine at the recommended dosage has minor undesirable effects on the CNS, including somnolence, fatigue, dizziness and headache. In some cases, paradoxical CNS stimulation has been reported.

Although cetirizine is a selective antagonist of peripheral H_1-receptors and is relatively free of anticholinergic activity, isolated cases of micturition difficulty, eye accommodation disorders and dry mouth have been reported.

Instances of abnormal hepatic function with elevated hepatic enzymes accompanied by elevated bilirubin have been reported. Mostly this resolves upon discontinuation of the treatment with cetirizine dihydrochloride.

Clinical trials

Double blind controlled clinical or pharmacoclinical trials comparing cetirizine to placebo or other antihistamines at the recommended dosage (10mg daily for cetirizine), of which quantified safety data are available, included more than 3200 subjects exposed to cetirizine. From this pooling, the following adverse events were reported for cetirizine 10mg in the placebo-controlled trials at rates of 1.0% or greater:

Adverse event (WHO-ART)	Cetirizine 10mg (n= 3260)	Placebo (n = 3061)
Body as a whole – general disorders		
Fatigue	1.63%	0.95%
Central and peripheral nervous system disorders		
Dizziness	1.10%	0.98%
Headache	7.42%	8.07%
Gastro-intestinal system disorders		
Abdominal pain	0.98%	1.08%
Dry mouth	2.09%	0.82%
Nausea	1.07%	1.14%
Psychiatric disorders		
Somnolence	9.63%	5.00%
Respiratory system disorders		
Pharyngitis	1.29%	1.34%

Although statistically more common than under placebo, somnolence was mild to moderate in the majority of cases. Objective tests as demonstrated by other studies have demonstrated that usual daily activities are unaffected at the recommended daily dose in healthy young volunteers.

Adverse drug reactions at rates of 1% or greater in children aged from 6 months to 12 years, included in placebo-controlled clinical or pharmacoclinical trials are:

Adverse drug reactions (WHO-ART)	Cetirizine (n=1656)	Placebo (n =1294)
Gastro-intestinal system disorders Diarrhoea	1.0%	0.6%
Psychiatric disorders Somnolence	1.8%	1. 4%
Respiratory system disorders Rhinitis	1.4%	1.1%
Body as a whole – general disorders Fatigue	1.0%	0.3%

Post-marketing experience

In addition to the adverse effects reported during clinical studies and listed above, isolated cases of the following adverse drug reactions have been reported in post-marketing experience. For these less frequently reported undesirable effects, the estimated frequencies (uncommon: $\geq$1/1,000 to 1/100, rare: $\geq$1/10,000 to 1/1,000, very rare: 1/10,000) are made based on post-marketing experience.

Blood and lymphatic disorders:

Very rare: thrombocytopenia

Immune system disorders:

Rare: hypersensitivity

Very rare: anaphylactic shock

Psychiatric disorders:

Uncommon: agitation

Rare: aggression, confusion, depression, hallucination, insomnia

Very rare: tic

Nervous system disorders:

Uncommon: paraesthesia

Rare: convulsions, movements disorders

Very rare: dysgeusia, syncope, tremor, dystonia, dyskinesia

Eye disorders:

Very rare: accommodation disorder, blurred vision, oculogyration

Cardiac disorders:

Rare: tachycardia

Gastro-intestinal disorders:

Uncommon: diarrhoea

Hepatobiliary disorders:

Rare: hepatic function abnormal (increased transaminases, alkaline phosphatase, γ-GT and bilirubin)

Skin and subcutaneous tissue disorders:

Uncommon: pruritus, rash

Rare: urticaria

Very rare: angioneurotic oedema, fixed drug eruption

Renal and urinary disorders:

Very rare: dysuria, enuresis

General disorders and administration site conditions:

Uncommon: asthenia, malaise

Rare: oedema

Investigations:

Rare: weight increased

4.9 Overdose

Symptoms

Symptoms observed after an overdose of cetirizine are mainly associated with CNS effects or with effects that could suggest an anticholinergic effect.

Adverse events reported after an intake of at least 5 times the recommended daily dose are: confusion, diarrhoea, dizziness, fatigue, headache, malaise, mydriasis, pruritus, restlessness, sedation, somnolence, stupor, tachycardia, tremor, and urinary retention.

Management

There is no known specific antidote to cetirizine.

Should overdose occur, symptomatic or supportive treatment is recommended. Gastric lavage should be considered following ingestion of a short occurrence.

Cetirizine is not effectively removed by dialysis.

5. PHARMACOLOGICAL PROPERTIES

5.1 Pharmacodynamic properties

Pharmacotherapeutic group: Piperazine derivatives, ATC code: R06A E07

Cetirizine, a human metabolite of hydroxyzine, is a potent and selective antagonist of peripheral H_1-receptors. *In vitro* receptor binding studies have shown no measurable affinity for other than H_1-receptors.

In addition to its anti-H_1 effect, cetirizine was shown to display anti-allergic activities: at a dose of 10mg once or twice daily, it inhibits the late phase recruitment of eosinophils, in the skin and conjunctiva of atopic subjects submitted to allergen challenge.

Studies in healthy volunteers show that cetirizine, at doses of 5 and 10mg strongly inhibits the wheal and flare reactions induced by very high concentrations of histamine into the skin, but the correlation with efficacy is not established.

In a 35-day study in children aged 5 to 12, no tolerance to the antihistaminic effect (suppression of wheal and flare) of cetirizine was found. When a treatment with cetirizine is stopped after repeated administration, the skin recovers its normal reactivity to histamine within 3 days.

In a six-week, placebo-controlled study of 186 patients with allergic rhinitis and concomitant mild to moderate asthma, cetirizine 10mg once daily improved rhinitis symptoms and did not alter pulmonary function. This study supports the safety of administering cetirizine to allergic patients with mild to moderate asthma.

In a placebo-controlled study, cetirizine given at the high daily dose of 60mg for seven days did not cause statistically significant prolongation of QT interval.

At the recommended dosage, cetirizine has demonstrated that it improves the quality of life of patients with perennial and seasonal allergic rhinitis.

5.2 Pharmacokinetic properties

The steady - state peak plasma concentrations is approximately 300ng/ml and is achieved within 1.0 ± 0.5 h. No accumulation is observed for cetirizine following daily doses of 10mg for 10 days. The distribution of pharmacokinetic parameters such as peak plasma concentration (C_{max}) and area under curve (AUC), is unimodal in human volunteers.

The extent of absorption of cetirizine is not reduced with food, although the rate of absorption is decreased. The extent of bioavailability is similar when cetirizine is given as solutions, capsules or tablets.

The apparent volume of distribution is 0.50l/kg. Plasma protein binding of cetirizine is 93 ± 0.3%. Cetirizine does not modify the protein binding of warfarin.

Cetirizine does not undergo extensive first pass metabolism. About two third of the dose are excreted unchanged in urine. The terminal half-life is approximately 10 hours.

Cetirizine exhibits linear kinetics over the range of 5 to 60mg.

Special populations

Elderly: Following a single 10mg oral dose, half-life increased by about 50% and clearance decreased by 40% in 16 elderly subjects compared to the normal subjects. The decrease in cetirizine clearance in these elderly volunteers appeared to be related to their decreased renal function.

Children, infants and toddlers: The half-life of cetirizine was about 6 hours in children of 6-12 years and 5 hours in children 2-6 years. In infants and toddlers aged 6 to 24 months, it is reduced to 3.1 hours

Renally impaired patients: The pharmacokinetics of the drug were similar in patients with mild impairment (creatinine clearance higher than 40ml/min) and healthy volunteers. Patients with moderate renal impairment had a 3-fold increase in half-life and 70% decrease in clearance compared to healthy volunteers.

Patients on hemodialysis (creatinine clearance less than 7ml/min) given a single oral 10mg dose of cetirizine had a 3-fold increase in half-life and a 70% decrease in clearance compared to normals. Cetirizine was poorly cleared by haemodialysis. Dosing adjustment is necessary in patients with moderate or severe renal impairment (see section 4.2).

Hepatically impaired patients: Patients with chronic liver diseases (hepatocellular, cholestatic, and biliary cirrhosis) given 10 or 20mg of cetirizine as a single dose had a 50% increase in half-life along with a 40% decrease in clearance compared to healthy subjects.

Dosing adjustment is only necessary in hepatically impaired patients if concomitant renal impairment is present.

5.3 Preclinical safety data

Non-clinical data reveal no special hazard for humans based on conventional studies of safety pharmacology, repeated dose toxicity, genotoxicity, carcinogenic potential, toxicity to reproduction.

6. PHARMACEUTICAL PARTICULARS

6.1 List of excipients

Tablet core:

Microcrystalline cellulose (E460), lactose monohydrate, crospovidone, colloidal anhydrous silica, magnesium stearate.

Film coat:

Hypromellose (E464), macrogol stearate, microcrystalline cellulose (E460), propylene glycol, titanium dioxide (E171).

6.2 Incompatibilities

None known.

6.3 Shelf life

24 months.

6.4 Special precautions for storage

Blister pack:

Do not store above 25°C.

Store in the original package

6.5 Nature and contents of container

Blister pack

(i) 60μm PVC/45μm Al/25μm OPA

(ii) 20μm Al

HDPE tablet container with LDPE cap.

HDPE tablet container: 20, 28, 30, 56, 60, 100

Blister pack: 7, 20, 28, 30, 56, 60, 100

6.6 Special precautions for disposal and other handling

Not applicable.

7. MARKETING AUTHORISATION HOLDER

Actavis UK Limited

(Trading style: Actavis)

Whiddon Valley

BARNSTAPLE

N Devon EX32 8NS

8. MARKETING AUTHORISATION NUMBER(S)

PL 0142/0490

9. DATE OF FIRST AUTHORISATION/RENEWAL OF THE AUTHORISATION

27/01/2001

10. DATE OF REVISION OF THE TEXT

24/06/2009

POLLENSHIELD HAYFEVER RELIEF (GSL)

(Actavis UK Ltd)

1. NAME OF THE MEDICINAL PRODUCT

POLLENSHIELD HAYFEVER RELIEF

2. QUALITATIVE AND QUANTITATIVE COMPOSITION

Each tablet contains 10mg Cetirizine hydrochloride.

For a full list of excipients, see 6.1

3. PHARMACEUTICAL FORM

Film-coated tablet.

Film-coated, white or almost white convex, elliptical, tablets. 5.7 × 11.4mm. The letter "C" on one side and the letters "J" and "E" on either side of a central division line on the reverse.

4. CLINICAL PARTICULARS

4.1 Therapeutic indications

In adults and paediatric patients 6 year and above:

- Cetirizine is indicated for the relief of nasal and ocular symptoms of seasonal and perennial allergic rhinitis.
- Cetirizine is indicated for the relief of symptoms of chronic idiopathic urticaria.

4.2 Posology and method of administration

Posology

Children aged from 6 to 12 years: 5mg twice daily (a half tablet twice daily).

Adults and adolescents over 12 years of age: 10mg once daily (1 tablet).

The tablets need to be swallowed with a glass of liquid.

Elderly subjects: data do not suggest that the dose needs to be reduced in elderly subjects provided that the renal function is normal.

Patients with moderate to severe renal impairment: there are no data to document the efficacy/safety ratio in patients with renal impairement. Since cetirizine is mainly excreted via renal route (see section 5.2), in cases no alternative treatment can be used, the dosing intervals must be individualized according to renal function. Refer to the following table and adjust the dose as indicated. To use this dosing table, an estimate of the patient's creatinine clearance (CLcr) in ml/min is needed. The CLcr (ml/min) may be estimated from serum creatinine (mg/dl) determination using the following formula:

$$CL_{cr} = \frac{[140 - age(years)] \times weight(kg)}{(72 \times serum\ creatinine\ (mg/dl)} \quad (\times 0.85 \text{ for women})$$

Dosing adjustments for adult patients with impaired renal function

Group	Creatinine clearance (ml/min)	Dosage and frequency
Normal	≥80	10mg once daily
Mild	50 – 79	10mg once daily
Moderate	30 – 49	5mg once daily
Severe	30	5mg once every 2 days
End-stage renal disease	10	Contra-indicated
Patients undergoing dialysis		

In paediatric patients suffering from renal impairment, the dose will have to be adjusted on an individual basis taking into account the renal clearance of the patient, his age and his body weight.

Patients with hepatic impairment: no dose adjustment is needed in patients with solely hepatic impairment.

Patients with hepatic impairment and renal impairment: dose adjustment is recommended (see Patients with moderate to severe renal impairment above).

Method of Administration

For oral use.

4.3 Contraindications

Hypersensitivity to the active substance, to any of the excipients, to hydroxyzine or to any piperazine derivatives.

Patients with severe renal impairment at less than 10ml/min creatinine clearance.

Patients with rare hereditary problems of galactose intolerance, the Lapp lactase deficiency or glucose- galactose malabsorption should not take cetirizine film-coated tablet.

4.4 Special warnings and precautions for use

At therapeutic doses, no clinically significant interactions have been demonstrated with alcohol (for a blood alcohol level of 0.5g/L). Nevertheless, precaution is recommended if alcohol is taken concomitantly.

Caution in epileptic patients and patients at risk of convulsions is recommended.

The use of the film-coated tablet formulation is not recommended in children aged less than 6 years since this formulation does not allow for appropriate dose adaptation.

4.5 Interaction with other medicinal products and other forms of interaction

Due to the pharmacokinetic, pharmacodynamic and tolerance profile of cetirizine, no interactions are expected with this antihistamine. Actually, neither pharmacodynamic nor significant pharmacokinetic interaction was reported in drug-drug interactions studies performed, notably with pseudoephedrine or theophylline (400mg/day).

The extent of absorption of cetirizine is not reduced with food, although the rate of absorption is decreased.

4.6 Pregnancy and lactation

For cetirizine very rare clinical data on exposed pregnancies are available. Animal studies do not indicate direct or indirect harmful effects with respect to pregnancy, embryonal/fetal development, parturition or postnatal development. Caution should be exercised when prescribing to pregnant or breast feeding women because cetirizine passes into breast milk.

4.7 Effects on ability to drive and use machines

Objective measurements of driving ability, sleep latency and assembly line performance have not demonstrated any clinically relevant effects at the recommended dose of 10mg. Patients intending to drive, engaging in potentially hazardous activities or operating machinery should not exceed the recommended dose and should take their response to the medicinal product into account. In these sensitive patients, concurrent use with alcohol or other CNS depressants may cause additional reductions in alertness and impairment of performance.

4.8 Undesirable effects

Clinical studies have shown that cetirizine at the recommended dosage has minor undesirable effects on the CNS, including somnolence, fatigue, dizziness and headache. In some cases, paradoxical CNS stimulation has been reported.

Although cetirizine is a selective antagonist of peripheral H_1-receptors and is relatively free of anticholinergic activity, isolated cases of micturition difficulty, eye accommodation disorders and dry mouth have been reported.

Instances of abnormal hepatic function with elevated hepatic enzymes accompanied by elevated bilirubin have been reported. Mostly this resolves upon discontinuation of the treatment with cetirizine dihydrochloride.

Clinical trials

Double blind controlled clinical or pharmacoclinical trials comparing cetirizine to placebo or other antihistamines at the recommended dosage (10mg daily for cetirizine), of which quantified safety data are available, included more than 3200 subjects exposed to cetirizine. From this pooling, the following adverse events were reported for cetirizine 10mg in the placebo-controlled trials at rates of 1.0% or greater:

Adverse event (WHO-ART)	Cetirizine 10mg (n= 3260)	Placebo (n = 3061)
Body as a whole – general disorders		
Fatigue	1.63%	0.95%
Central and peripheral nervous system disorders		
Dizziness	1.10%	0.98%
Headache	7.42%	8.07%
Gastro-intestinal system disorders		
Abdominal pain	0.98%	1.08%
Dry mouth	2.09%	0.82%
Nausea	1.07%	1.14%
Psychiatric disorders		
Somnolence	9.63%	5.00%
Respiratory system disorders		
Pharyngitis	1.29%	1.34%

Although statistically more common than under placebo, somnolence was mild to moderate in the majority of cases. Objective tests as demonstrated by other studies have demonstrated that usual daily activities are unaffected at the recommended daily dose in healthy young volunteers.

Adverse drug reactions at rates of 1% or greater in children aged from 6 months to 12 years, included in placebo-controlled clinical or pharmacoclinical trials are:

Adverse drug reactions (WHO-ART)	Cetirizine (n=1656)	Placebo (n =1294)
Gastro-intestinal system disorders Diarrhoea	1.0%	0.6%
Psychiatric disorders Somnolence	1.8%	1. 4%
Respiratory system disorders Rhinitis	1.4%	1.1%
Body as a whole – general disorders Fatigue	1.0%	0.3%

Post-marketing experience

In addition to the adverse effects reported during clinical studies and listed above, isolated cases of the following adverse drug reactions have been reported in post-marketing experience. For these less frequently reported undesirable effects, the estimated frequencies (uncommon: ≥1/1,000 to 1/100, rare: ≥1/10,000 to 1/1,000, very rare: 1/10,000) are made based on post-marketing experience.

Blood and lymphatic disorders:

Very rare: thrombocytopenia

Immune system disorders:

Rare: hypersensitivity

Very rare: anaphylactic shock

Psychiatric disorders:

Uncommon: agitation

Rare: aggression, confusion, depression, hallucination, insomnia

Very rare: tic

Nervous system disorders:

Uncommon: paraesthesia

Rare: convulsions, movements disorders

Very rare: dysgeusia, syncope, tremor, dystonia, dyskinesia

Eye disorders:

Very rare: accommodation disorder, blurred vision, oculogyration

Cardiac disorders:

Rare: tachycardia

Gastro-intestinal disorders:

Uncommon: diarrhoea

Hepatobiliary disorders:

Rare: hepatic function abnormal (increased transaminases, alkaline phosphatase, γ-GT and bilirubin)

Skin and subcutaneous tissue disorders:

Uncommon: pruritus, rash

Rare: urticaria

Very rare: angioneurotic oedema, fixed drug eruption

Renal and urinary disorders:

Very rare: dysuria, enuresis

General disorders and administration site conditions:

Uncommon: asthenia, malaise

Rare: oedema

Investigations:

Rare: weight increased

4.9 Overdose

Symptoms

Symptoms observed after an overdose of cetirizine are mainly associated with CNS effects or with effects that could suggest an anticholinergic effect.

Adverse events reported after an intake of at least 5 times the recommended daily dose are: confusion, diarrhoea, dizziness, fatigue, headache, malaise, mydriasis, pruritus, restlessness, sedation, somnolence, stupor, tachycardia, tremor, and urinary retention.

Management

There is no known specific antidote to cetirizine.

Should overdose occur, symptomatic or supportive treatment is recommended. Gastric lavage should be considered following ingestion of a short occurrence.

Cetirizine is not effectively removed by dialysis.

5. PHARMACOLOGICAL PROPERTIES

5.1 Pharmacodynamic properties

Pharmacotherapeutic group: Piperazine derivatives, ATC code: R06A E07

Cetirizine, a human metabolite of hydroxyzine, is a potent and selective antagonist of peripheral H_1-receptors. *In vitro* receptor binding studies have shown no measurable affinity for other than H_1-receptors.

In addition to its anti-H_1 effect, cetirizine was shown to display anti-allergic activities: at a dose of 10mg once or twice daily, it inhibits the late phase recruitment of eosinophils, in the skin and conjunctiva of atopic subjects submitted to allergen challenge.

Studies in healthy volunteers show that cetirizine, at doses of 5 and 10mg strongly inhibits the wheal and flare reactions induced by very high concentrations of histamine into the skin, but the correlation with efficacy is not established. In a 35-day study in children aged 5 to 12, no tolerance to the antihistaminic effect (suppression of wheal and flare) of cetirizine was found. When a treatment with cetirizine is stopped after repeated administration, the skin recovers its normal reactivity to histamine within 3 days.

In a six-week, placebo-controlled study of 186 patients with allergic rhinitis and concomitant mild to moderate asthma, cetirizine 10mg once daily improved rhinitis symptoms and did not alter pulmonary function. This study supports the safety of administering cetirizine to allergic patients with mild to moderate asthma.

In a placebo-controlled study, cetirizine given at the high daily dose of 60mg for seven days did not cause statistically significant prolongation of QT interval.

At the recommended dosage, cetirizine has demonstrated that it improves the quality of life of patients with perennial and seasonal allergic rhinitis.

5.2 Pharmacokinetic properties

The steady - state peak plasma concentrations is approximately 300ng/ml and is achieved within 1.0 ± 0.5 h. No accumulation is observed for cetirizine following daily doses of 10mg for 10 days. The distribution of pharmacokinetic parameters such as peak plasma concentration (C_{max}) and area under curve (AUC), is unimodal in human volunteers.

The extent of absorption of cetirizine is not reduced with food, although the rate of absorption is decreased. The extent of bioavailability is similar when cetirizine is given as solutions, capsules or tablets.

The apparent volume of distribution is 0.50l/kg. Plasma protein binding of cetirizine is 93 ± 0.3%. Cetirizine does not modify the protein binding of warfarin.

Cetirizine does not undergo extensive first pass metabolism. About two third of the dose are excreted unchanged in urine. The terminal half-life is approximately 10 hours.

Cetirizine exhibits linear kinetics over the range of 5 to 60mg.

Special populations

Elderly: Following a single 10mg oral dose, half-life increased by about 50% and clearance decreased by 40% in 16 elderly subjects compared to the normal subjects. The decrease in cetirizine clearance in these elderly volunteers appeared to be related to their decreased renal function.

Children, infants and toddlers: The half-life of cetirizine was about 6 hours in children of 6-12 years and 5 hours in children 2-6 years. In infants and toddlers aged 6 to 24 months, it is reduced to 3.1 hours

Renally impaired patients: The pharmacokinetics of the drug were similar in patients with mild impairment (creatinine clearance higher than 40ml/min) and healthy volunteers. Patients with moderate renal impairment had a 3-fold increase in half-life and 70% decrease in clearance compared to healthy volunteers.

Patients on hemodialysis (creatinine clearance less than 7ml/min) given a single oral 10mg dose of cetirizine had a 3-fold increase in half-life and a 70% decrease in clearance compared to normals. Cetirizine was poorly cleared by haemodialysis. Dosing adjustment is necessary in patients with moderate or severe renal impairment (see section 4.2).

Hepatically impaired patients: Patients with chronic liver diseases (hepatocellular, cholestatic, and biliary cirrhosis) given 10 or 20mg of cetirizine as a single dose had a 50% increase in half-life along with a 40% decrease in clearance compared to healthy subjects.

Dosing adjustment is only necessary in hepatically impaired patients if concomitant renal impairment is present.

5.3 Preclinical safety data

Non-clinical data reveal no special hazard for humans based on conventional studies of safety pharmacology, repeated dose toxicity, genotoxicity, carcinogenic potential, toxicity to reproduction.

6. PHARMACEUTICAL PARTICULARS

6.1 List of excipients

Tablet core:

Microcrystalline cellulose (E460), lactose monohydrate, crospovidone, colloidal anhydrous silica, magnesium stearate.

Film coat:

Hypromellose (E464), macrogol stearate, microcrystalline cellulose (E460), propylene glycol, titanium dioxide (E171).

6.2 Incompatibilities

None known.

6.3 Shelf life

24 months.

6.4 Special precautions for storage

Blister pack:

Do not store above 25°C.

Store in the original package

6.5 Nature and contents of container
Blister pack

(i) 60μm PVC/45μm Al/25μm OPA

(ii) 20μm Al

Blister pack: 4, 5, 7

6.6 Special precautions for disposal and other handling
Not applicable.

7. MARKETING AUTHORISATION HOLDER
Actavis UK Limited

(Trading style: Actavis)

Whiddon Valley

BARNSTAPLE

N Devon EX32 8NS

8. MARKETING AUTHORISATION NUMBER(S)
PL 0142/0606

9. DATE OF FIRST AUTHORISATION/RENEWAL OF THE AUTHORISATION
June 2004

10. DATE OF REVISION OF THE TEXT
24.06.2009

Legal status
GSL

11. DOSIMETRY

12 INSTRUCTIONS FOR PREPARATION OF RADIOPHARMACEUTICALS (IF APPLICABLE)

Polytar AF

(Stiefel Laboratories (UK) Limited)

1. NAME OF THE MEDICINAL PRODUCT
Polytar AF

2. QUALITATIVE AND QUANTITATIVE COMPOSITION
Tar Blend 1% w/w, Zinc Pyrithione 1% w/w in a shampoo base

Tar Blend comprises:

Pine tar, Cade oil, Coal Tar Solution, Arachis Oil extract of Coal Tar.

3. PHARMACEUTICAL FORM
Medicated Shampoo

4. CLINICAL PARTICULARS

4.1 Therapeutic indications
Polytar AF is indicated in the topical treatment of scalp disorders such as dandruff, seborrhoeic dermatitis and psoriasis.

4.2 Posology and method of administration
Shake the bottle before use. Wet the hair and massage Polytar AF into the hair, scalp and surrounding skin. Leave for 2-3 minutes, then rinse thoroughly.

Polytar AF should be used two or three times weekly for at least 3 weeks or until the condition clears.

4.3 Contraindications
Polytar AF should not be used by patients with known hypersensitivity to any of the ingredients.

4.4 Special warnings and precautions for use
Avoid contact with the eyes. Tar products may cause skin irritation, rashes and, rarely, photosensitivity. Zinc pyrithione may cause dermatitis, should this occur, Polytar AF should be discontinued.

4.5 Interaction with other medicinal products and other forms of interaction
None known.

4.6 Pregnancy and lactation
The safety of Polytar AF in human pregnancy and lactation has not been established.

4.7 Effects on ability to drive and use machines
None.

4.8 Undesirable effects
None.

4.9 Overdose
Not applicable.

5. PHARMACOLOGICAL PROPERTIES

5.1 Pharmacodynamic properties

Tar blend:

Tars suppress DNA synthesis in hyperplastic skin, this inhibits mitotic activity and protein synthesis. By decreasing proliferation and dermal infiltration, they promote a return to normal keratinisation. Tars also have vasoconstricting astringent and antipruritic properties.

Zinc Pyrithione:

Zinc Pyrithione has antibacterial and antifungal properties. It is fungicidal against the pathogenic yeasts of the pityrosporum genus which are implicated in dandruff and seborrhoeic dermatitis.

5.2 Pharmacokinetic properties
Not Applicable.

5.3 Preclinical safety data
Not Applicable.

6. PHARMACEUTICAL PARTICULARS

6.1 List of excipients
Coconut diethanolamide

Triethanolamine Lauryl Sulphate

Carbomer

Sodium Hydroxide

Hypromellose

Octoxinol

Glycerol

Imidurea

Purified Water

6.2 Incompatibilities
None

6.3 Shelf life
24 months

6.4 Special precautions for storage
Store below 25°C

6.5 Nature and contents of container
High density polyethylene bottles of 25ml, 65ml, 150ml, 250ml, 350ml, 400ml, 1000ml

6.6 Special precautions for disposal and other handling
There are no special instructions for use or handling of Polytar AF.

7. MARKETING AUTHORISATION HOLDER
Stiefel Laboratories (UK) Ltd

Eurasia Headquarters

Concorde Road

Maidenhead

SL6 4BY

UK

8. MARKETING AUTHORISATION NUMBER(S)
PL 0174/0071

9. DATE OF FIRST AUTHORISATION/RENEWAL OF THE AUTHORISATION
16th March 1992.

10. DATE OF REVISION OF THE TEXT
August 2009

Polytar Emollient

(Stiefel Laboratories (UK) Limited)

1. NAME OF THE MEDICINAL PRODUCT
Polytar Emollient

2. QUALITATIVE AND QUANTITATIVE COMPOSITION
Tar Blend 25.00% w/w, Light Liquid Paraffin 35.00% w/w

Tar Blend comprises:

Pine tar BP 30% w/w, Cade oil BPC 30% w/w, Coal Tar Solution BP 10% w/w, Arachis Oil extract of Coal Tar BP 30% w/w.

3. PHARMACEUTICAL FORM
Liquid bath additive.

4. CLINICAL PARTICULARS

4.1 Therapeutic indications
Topical.

Polytar Emollient is indicated in the treatment of psoriasis, eczema, atopic and pruritic dermatoses. The use of Polytar Emollient may be combined with ultraviolet radiation and other adjunctive therapy. Polytar Emollient is also of value in removing loose psoriatic scales and paste following dithranol treatment.

4.2 Posology and method of administration
Adults, children and the elderly:

Two to four capfuls of Polytar Emollient should be added to an 8 inch bath and the patient instructed to soak for 20 minutes.

4.3 Contraindications
None.

4.4 Special warnings and precautions for use
Patients should be instructed to guard against slipping when entering or leaving the bath. If skin irritation occurs and persists, discontinue use and consult your doctor. Tar products may stain baths and fabrics.

4.5 Interaction with other medicinal products and other forms of interaction
None known.

4.6 Pregnancy and lactation
There is no, or inadequate evidence of the safety of Polytar Emollient in human pregnancy and lactation but it has been in wide use for many years without apparent ill consequence.

4.7 Effects on ability to drive and use machines
None.

4.8 Undesirable effects
Tar products may cause skin irritation, rashes and rarely, photosensitivity. In the event of such a reaction, discontinue use and consult your doctor.

4.9 Overdose
Not applicable.

5. PHARMACOLOGICAL PROPERTIES

5.1 Pharmacodynamic properties
Tar preparations have keratoplastic and antipruritic activity and are widely used as topical therapy for a range of dermatoses. The use of emollient bath oils in the management of widespread dry and itching skin is well established. Mineral oil exerts its emollient effect by skin absorption. The combination of tar blend with an emollient therefore provides a pharmacological active product with emollient properties.

5.2 Pharmacokinetic properties
Not applicable.

5.3 Preclinical safety data
None stated.

6. PHARMACEUTICAL PARTICULARS

6.1 List of excipients
Octyiphenoxypolythoxy Ethanol

Sorbitan Monooleate

Polyethylene Glycol 400 Dilaurate

Isopropyl Palmitate

6.2 Incompatibilities
None.

6.3 Shelf life
36 months

6.4 Special precautions for storage
None.

6.5 Nature and contents of container
Polyvinyl chloride bottles fitted with a screw cap containing 350ml, 500ml, 600ml, 1000ml.

6.6 Special precautions for disposal and other handling
There are no special instructions for use or handling of Polytar Emollient.

7. MARKETING AUTHORISATION HOLDER
Stiefel Laboratories (UK) Ltd

Eurasia Headquarters

Concorde Road

Maidenhead

SL6 4BY

UK

8. MARKETING AUTHORISATION NUMBER(S)
PL 00174/5011R

9. DATE OF FIRST AUTHORISATION/RENEWAL OF THE AUTHORISATION
31st August 2006

10. DATE OF REVISION OF THE TEXT
August 2009

Polytar Liquid

(Stiefel Laboratories (UK) Limited)

1. NAME OF THE MEDICINAL PRODUCT
Polytar Liquid

2. QUALITATIVE AND QUANTITATIVE COMPOSITION
Tar Blend 1% w/w

Tar Blend comprises:

Pine tar, Cade Oil, Coal Tar Solution, Arachis Oil extract of Coal Tar.

3. PHARMACEUTICAL FORM
Medicated Shampoo

4. CLINICAL PARTICULARS

4.1 Therapeutic indications
Polytar Liquid is indicated in the treatment of scalp disorders including psoriasis, dandruff, seborrhoea, eczema and pruritus. Polytar Liquid is also of value in the removal of ointments and pastes used in the treatment of psoriasis.

4.2 Posology and method of administration
The hair should be wetted and sufficient Polytar Liquid applied to produce an abundant lather. The scalp and adjacent areas should be vigorously massaged with the fingertips. The hair should then be thoroughly rinsed and the procedure repeated.

Polytar Liquid should be used once or twice weekly.

4.3 Contraindications
Patients with a known hypersensitivity to any of the ingredients should not use the product.

4.4 Special warnings and precautions for use
There are no special warnings or precautions.

4.5 Interaction with other medicinal products and other forms of interaction
There are no known interactions with other medicaments or other forms of interaction.

4.6 Pregnancy and lactation
There is no, or inadequate evidence of the safety of Polytar Liquid in human pregnancy and lactation, but it has been in wide use for many years without apparent ill consequence.

4.7 Effects on ability to drive and use machines
The use of this product will not affect the ability to drive and to use machines.

4.8 Undesirable effects
Tar products may cause skin irritation, rashes and rarely, photosensitivity. If irritation occurs and persists, treatment should be discontinued.

4.9 Overdose
The product is intended for external use only. It is applied to the scalp and rinsed off. Use of an excessive quantity is not a cause for concern.

5. PHARMACOLOGICAL PROPERTIES

5.1 Pharmacodynamic properties
Tars suppress DNA synthesis in hyperplastic skin, inhibiting mitotic activity and protein synthesis. They decrease epidermal proliferation and dermal infiltration and thus promote a return to normal keratinisation.

Tars also have vasoconstrictor, antipruritic and antiseptic properties.

5.2 Pharmacokinetic properties
The product is applied topically and acts at the site of application. The potential for systemic absorption from a wash off shampoo is extremely low.

5.3 Preclinical safety data
Tar preparations have been in widespread use for many years and their safety in humans has been established.

6. PHARMACEUTICAL PARTICULARS

6.1 List of excipients
Oleyl alcohol
Coconut diethanolamide
Hexylene glycol
Polysorbate 80
Triethanolamide Lauryl Sulphate
Sodium chloride
Citric acid
Octylphenoxypolyethoxy ethanol
Imidurea
Fragrance 5412
Purified Water

6.2 Incompatibilities
There are no known incompatibilities

6.3 Shelf life
a) For the product as packaged for sale
3 years
b) After first opening the container
Comply with expiry date

6.4 Special precautions for storage
There are no special precautions for storage.

6.5 Nature and contents of container
High density polyethylene bottles of 65ml, 150ml, 200ml, 250ml, 350ml, 400ml, 500ml, 600ml, 1000ml.

6.6 Special precautions for disposal and other handling
There are no special instructions for use or handling of Polytar Liquid.

7. MARKETING AUTHORISATION HOLDER
Stiefel Laboratories (UK) Ltd
Eurasia Headquarters
Concorde Road
Maidenhead
SL6 4BY
UK

8. MARKETING AUTHORISATION NUMBER(S)
PL 0174/5016R

9. DATE OF FIRST AUTHORISATION/RENEWAL OF THE AUTHORISATION
14th March 1990/11th May 2000/11th May 2005/27th February 2009

10. DATE OF REVISION OF THE TEXT
August 2009

Polytar Plus

(Stiefel Laboratories (UK) Limited)

1. NAME OF THE MEDICINAL PRODUCT
Polytar Plus

2. QUALITATIVE AND QUANTITATIVE COMPOSITION
Tar Blend 1% w/w

3. PHARMACEUTICAL FORM
Medicated shampoo for topical use.

4. CLINICAL PARTICULARS

4.1 Therapeutic indications
Polytar Plus is indicated as an aid in the treatment of scalp disorders such as psoriasis, seborrhoea, pruritus and dandruff. Polytar Plus is also of value in the removal of ointments and pastes used in the treatment of psoriasis.

4.2 Posology and method of administration
The following dosages and schedules are applicable for adults, children and the elderly.

The hair should be wetted and sufficient Polytar Plus applied to produce an abundant lather. The scalp and adjacent areas should be vigorously massaged with the fingertips. The hair should then be thoroughly rinsed and the procedure repeated.

Polytar Plus should be used once or twice weekly.

4.3 Contraindications
None stated.

4.4 Special warnings and precautions for use
None stated.

4.5 Interaction with other medicinal products and other forms of interaction
None stated.

4.6 Pregnancy and lactation
There are no restrictions on the use of Polytar Plus during pregnancy or lactation.

4.7 Effects on ability to drive and use machines
None stated.

4.8 Undesirable effects
None stated.

4.9 Overdose
None stated.

5. PHARMACOLOGICAL PROPERTIES

5.1 Pharmacodynamic properties
While the mode of action of tars are not fully established, their therapeutic effect has been observed over many years. It has been postulated that tars work by exerting a cytostatic action following an initial cytoproliferative effect. This slowing of the keratinisation process in the epidermal layer and reduction in the rate of epidermal turnover promoting a return to normal keratinisation.

5.2 Pharmacokinetic properties
Not applicable. The product acts at the site of application.

5.3 Preclinical safety data
Not applicable.

6. PHARMACEUTICAL PARTICULARS

6.1 List of excipients
Coconut diethanolamide, Hexylene glycol, Volpo N10, Oleyl alcohol, Polysorbate 80, Triton X100, Fragrance 5412, Polypeptide SF, Imadozolidinyl Urea, Triethanolamine Lauryl Sulphate, Citric acid, Purified water

6.2 Incompatibilities
None stated.

6.3 Shelf life
a) For the product as packaged for sale
3 years
b) After first opening the container
Comply with expiry date

6.4 Special precautions for storage
None

6.5 Nature and contents of container
Polyethylene screw top bottles of 25ml, 65ml, 125ml, 150ml, 250ml, 350ml, 500ml, 600ml

6.6 Special precautions for disposal and other handling
There are no special instructions for use or handling of Polytar Plus.

7. MARKETING AUTHORISATION HOLDER
Stiefel Laboratories (UK) Ltd
Eurasia Headquarters
Concorde Road
Maidenhead
SL6 4BY
UK

8. MARKETING AUTHORISATION NUMBER(S)
PL 0174/0037

9. DATE OF FIRST AUTHORISATION/RENEWAL OF THE AUTHORISATION
2nd December 1977/2nd December 1982/2nd December 1987/2nd December 1992

10. DATE OF REVISION OF THE TEXT
August 2009

Potassium Iodate Tablets 85mg (Cambridge Laboratories)

(Cambridge Laboratories)

1. NAME OF THE MEDICINAL PRODUCT
Potassium Iodate 85mg Tablets

2. QUALITATIVE AND QUANTITATIVE COMPOSITION
Each tablet contains 85mg Potassium Iodate equivalent to 50mg iodine.

For excipients see Section 6.1.

3. PHARMACEUTICAL FORM
Tablet.
Off white, round tablet with star shaped double break line, engraved 2202.

4. CLINICAL PARTICULARS

4.1 Therapeutic indications
Potassium iodate is indicated as a thyroid-blocking agent to prevent the uptake of radioactive iodine, for example after a nuclear accident.

4.2 Posology and method of administration
For oral administration.

Administration should take place within 3 hours of a nuclear accident, or up to 10 hours after an accident, however, this is less effective.

A single daily dose should be administered. This will protect against exposure lasting up to 24 hours. (see Section 4.4).

Tabletsiodine equivalent

Adults, Elderly 2 tablets 100 mg
and adolescents
(over 12 years)
Children 1 tablet 50 mg
(3-12 years)
Children ½ tablet 25 mg
(1 month – 3 years)
Neonates ¼ tablet 12.5mg
(birth – 1 month) or 12.5mg iodine equivalent as standard solution For neonates living at home a dosage of ¼ tablet is satisfactory. The dosage can be crushed and mixed with milk or water. For neonates in hospital a dosage of 12.5 mg iodine equivalent can be given as a standard solution freshly prepared from KI crystals. It is recommended that maternity wards store KI crystals.

For babies the dose may be crushed and mixed with milk or juice before administration. For children the dose may be crushed and mixed with eg. Jam, honey or yoghurt.

4.3 Contraindications
Potassium iodate is contra-indicated in patients with known iodine sensitivity, renal failure, hypocomplementaemic vasculitis or dermatitis herpetiformis.

4.4 Special warnings and precautions for use
In cases of exposure to radioiodine from nuclear accidents, dosing of potassium iodate should be based on emergency plans and predetermined operational intervention levels. Risk benefit of administration of stable radioiodine should be considered for the different age groups at risk. Pregnant and lactating women, neonates, infants and children should be treated first. A single dose of potassium iodate gives adequate protection for one day. Prolonged exposure may require repeat dosing. Iodine prophylaxis is used against inhaled radioiodine and should not be the main prophylaxis for ingested contamination.

Patients with thyrotoxicosis treated medically, or patients with a past history of thyrotoxicosis treated medically who are now off treatment and apparently in remission, may be at risk.

Iodine induced hyperthyroidism may be precipitated in patients with asymptomatic nodular goitre or latent Graves' disease, who are not under medical care.

Potassium salts should be given cautiously to patients with renal or adrenal insufficiency, acute dehydration or heat cramp.

Care should be exercised if potassium salts are given concomitantly with potassium-sparing diuretics, as hyperkalaemia may result.

The potential benefit of iodine prophylaxis is greatest in the young. The thyroid of the foetus, neonate and young infant has a higher yearly thyroid cancer risk per unit dose of radioactive iodine than the thyroid of an adult.

Potassium iodate prophylaxis is not usually indicated in adults over 40 unless doses to the thyroid from inhalation rise to levels threatening thyroid function, that is of the order of about 5 Gy. The risk of thyroid cancer is extremely low in this group whereas the incidence of thyroid disease is higher in this group therefore the risk of iodine induced thyroid complications are higher.

Neonates in the first days of life are at particular risk from exposure to radioactive iodine and blocking of thyroid function by overload of potassium iodate. The fraction of radioactive uptake is fourfold greater than all other age groups. The neonatal thyroid is especially sensitive to functional blocking caused by overload of potassium iodate. Transient hypothyroidism during this early period of brain development can result in loss of intellectual capacity. If stable iodine is given to neonates close follow up of thyroid function is essential. For neonates who have been administered potassium iodate in the first few weeks of life TSH levels and, if necessary, T4 levels should be monitored and appropriate replacement therapy given.

4.5 Interaction with other medicinal products and other forms of interaction

Several drugs, such as captopril and enalopril can cause hyperkalaemia and this effect may be enhanced if Potassium Iodate is also administered.

The effect of quinidine on the heart is increased by increased plasma concentration of potassium.

Hyperkalaemia results from the interaction between potassium salts and potassium sparing diuretics such as amiloride or triamterene or aldosterone antagonists.

4.6 Pregnancy and lactation

Teratogenic effects such as congenital goitre and hypothyroidism have been reported when iodides, and therefore presumably iodate, are administered to pregnant women.

However, in the event of a nuclear accident, the proper use of potassium iodate in low doses, over a short period of time, as a thyroid blocking agent is not contra-indicated. Prophylactic administration of iodate to the pregnant mother should also be effective for the foetus.

Throughout pregnancy the number of doses of potassium iodate should be kept to a minimum. In areas of iodine deficiency prolonged dosage could lead to maternal or foetal thyroid blockage with possible consequences for foetal development. If potassium iodate is administered late in pregnancy, the thyroid function of the new-born should be monitored. This is generally met by routine screening in the neonatal period. For neonates who have been administered potassium iodate in the first few weeks of life TSH levels and, if necessary, T4 levels should be monitored and appropriate replacement therapy given.

Pregnant women with active hyperthyroidism must not take potassium iodate because of the risk of foetal thyroid blockage.

Iodine is actively transported into breast milk, however those breast feeding should continue to do so (see Section 5.2).

4.7 Effects on ability to drive and use machines

No effect.

4.8 Undesirable effects

Since experience with potassium iodate is limited, presumably the following side effects, which can occur with potassium iodide, can also be associated with potassium iodate.

Hypersensitivity reactions such as skin rashes, swollen salivary glands; headache, bronchospasm and gastro-intestinal disturbances can be mild or severe and may be dose dependent.

Hyperthyroidism, iodine induced autoimmunity (Grave's and Hashimoto type), toxic nodular goitre and iodine-induced hypothyroidism have been reported as side effects of iodine therapy.

An overactive thyroid gland, thyroiditis, and an enlarged thyroid gland with or without development or myxoedema have also been reported.

Continued administration may lead to mental depression, nervousness, sexual impotence and insomnia.

4.9 Overdose

In overdose, symptoms of iodism such as headache, pain and swelling of the salivary glands, fever or laryngitis, swelling or inflammation of the throat, gastrointestinal upset and diarrhoea can occur. Pulmonary oedema can also occur.

Acute ingestion of iodine can result in corrosive injury of the gastrointestinal tract and renal damage. Cardiopulmonary collapse due to circulatory failure should be treated by maintenance of airway and stabilisation of the circulation. Oedema of the glottis resulting in asphyxia or aspiration pneumonia can occur. In acute iodine poisoning large quantities of milk and starch mucilage have been given.

Lavage with starch mucilage or lavage with activated charcoal should be considered if there is no oesophageal damage.

Electrolyte and water losses should be replaced and the circulation should be maintained. Pethidine (100 mg) or morphine sulphate (10 mg) may be given for pain. A tracheostomy may become necessary.

Haemodialysis may reduce excessively elevated serum iodine concentrations.

Retinal toxicity has been associated with potassium iodate overdose.

5. PHARMACOLOGICAL PROPERTIES

5.1 Pharmacodynamic properties

The iodine released from iodide and iodate on absorption from the gut is taken up rapidly and preferentially by the cells of the thyroid gland. Once in the thyroid, it is rapidly incorporated into organic molecules that are synthesised into thyroid hormones and ultimately released into the general circulation.

If excessive amounts of stable iodate are administered to normal adults, the iodine uptake mechanism of the thyroid is saturated and little or no further iodine is taken up. This effectively blocks the uptake of radioactive iodine in the event of accidental exposure to radioiodines.

5.2 Pharmacokinetic properties

Iodine absorbed from the gut is taken up rapidly and preferentially by the cells of the thyroid gland. Renal clearance of iodide/iodate is usually in the range of 30 to 50 ml of serum/minute, is closely related to glomerular filtration, and is little affected by the iodate load. Most radioiodine not taken up by the thyroid gland after a single oral bolus of iodate is excreted in the urine over the subsequent 48-hour period.

As much as a quarter of the iodine taken by the mother may be secreted in the milk within 24 hours. Potassium iodate can partially block transport of radioiodine in the milk. The same criteria should apply when selecting a dose of potassium iodate to protect a lactating mother as that used for other young adults under 40 years of age.

5.3 Preclinical safety data

Preclinical information has not been included because the safety profile of Potassium Iodate has been established after many years of clinical use.

6. PHARMACEUTICAL PARTICULARS

6.1 List of excipients

The tablet contains Calcium Hydrogen Phosphate, Croscarmellose Sodium, Microcrystalline Cellulose and Magnesium Stearate.

6.2 Incompatibilities

None known.

6.3 Shelf life

Polypropylene containers - 30 months

PVC/PVDC/Al Blisters - 30 months

Al/Al blisters - 30 months

Al/Al strips - 30 months

6.4 Special precautions for storage

Do not store above 25°C.

Store in original container.

6.5 Nature and contents of container

In polypropylene containers with caps or child resistant closures in packs of 50, 100, 500 or 1000 tablets.

Blister strips in multiples of 6, 10 or 100 tablets.

6.6 Special precautions for disposal and other handling

Not applicable.

7. MARKETING AUTHORISATION HOLDER

Cambridge Laboratories Ltd, Deltic House, Kingfisher Way, Silverlink Business Park, Wallsend, Tyne and Wear NE28 9NX

8. MARKETING AUTHORISATION NUMBER(S)

PL 12070/0025

9. DATE OF FIRST AUTHORISATION/RENEWAL OF THE AUTHORISATION

19 October 2001

10. DATE OF REVISION OF THE TEXT

November 2004

Powergel 2.5% gel

(A. Menarini Pharma U.K. S.R.L.)

1. NAME OF THE MEDICINAL PRODUCT

POWERGEL 2.5% gel

2. QUALITATIVE AND QUANTITATIVE COMPOSITION

Powergel contains ketoprofen BP 2.5g/100g.

For a full list of excipients, see section 6.1.

3. PHARMACEUTICAL FORM

A colourless, non-greasy, non-staining gel with an aromatic fragrance for topical application.

4. CLINICAL PARTICULARS

4.1 Therapeutic indications

For local relief of pain and inflammation associated with soft tissue injuries and acute strains and sprains.

4.2 Posology and method of administration

Powergel should be applied topically to the affected area two or three times daily. Maximum duration of use should not exceed 7 days if supplied by a pharmacist or 10 days if supplied on prescription. Powergel should be applied with gentle massage only.

Adults and elderly:	**Tube or dispenser:** Apply 5 to 10cm of gel (100-200mg ketoprofen) with each application; for the pump dispenser push the pump 3-6 times.
Children under 12 years of age:	Not recommended as experience in children is limited.

4.3 Contraindications

Hypersensitivity to the active ingredient, to any of the excipients or to other substances which are closely related to these chemically, such as acetyl salicylic acid or other non-steroid anti-inflammatory drugs and fenofibrate. Ketoprofen gel should not be administered to patients in whom acetyl salicylic acid or other NSAIDs have caused asthma, rhinitis or urticaria.

Ketoprofen gel should not be applied to open wounds or lesions of the skin, or near the eyes.

4.4 Special warnings and precautions for use

Discontinue use if skin rash develops.

Hands should be washed immediately after use.

Do not use with occlusive dressing.

Topical application of large amounts may result in systemic effects, including hypersensitivity and asthma.

Ketoprofen gel should be used with caution in patients with serious kidney failure.

The use of topical products, especially if it is prolonged, may give rise to phenomena of sensitisation or local irritation.

To prevent any phenomena of hypersensitivity or photosensitivity, avoid exposure to direct sunlight, including solarium (sunbeds), during the treatment and for 2 weeks afterwards.

Keep out of the reach and sight of children.

"P" warning: If symptoms persist after 7 days, consult your doctor.

4.5 Interaction with other medicinal products and other forms of interaction

No interactions of Powergel with other drugs have been reported. It is, however, advisable to monitor patients under treatment with coumarinic substances.

4.6 Pregnancy and lactation

No embryopathic effects have been demonstrated in animals and there is no epidemiological evidence of the safety of ketoprofen in human pregnancy. Therefore, it is recommended to avoid ketoprofen unless considered essential in which case it should be discontinued within one week of expected confinement when NSAIDs might cause premature closure of the ductus arteriosus or persistent pulmonary hypertension in the neonate. They may also delay labour. Trace amounts of ketoprofen are excreted in breast milk after systemic administration.

4.7 Effects on ability to drive and use machines

No effects on the ability to drive and use machinery have been reported.

4.8 Undesirable effects

The prolonged use of products for topical administration may cause hypersensitivity phenomena. In such cases the treatment should be discontinued and a suitable alternative therapy instituted. Skin photosensitivity has been reported in isolated cases. Although not known for topical use of ketoprofen, the following adverse events are reported for systemic use: Minor adverse events, frequently transient, consist of gastrointestinal effects such as indigestion, dyspepsia, nausea, constipation, diarrhoea, heartburn and various types of abdominal discomfort. Other minor effects such as headache, dizziness, mild confusion, vertigo, drowsiness, oedema, mood change and insomnia may occur less frequently. Major gastrointestinal adverse events such as peptic ulceration, haemorrhage or perforation may rarely occur. Haematological reactions including thrombocytopenia, hepatic or renal damage, dermatological reactions, bronchospasm and anaphylaxis are exceedingly rare.

4.9 Overdose

Considering the low blood levels of ketoprofen by the percutaneous route, no overdosage phenomena have been described yet.

5. PHARMACOLOGICAL PROPERTIES

5.1 Pharmacodynamic properties

Ketoprofen is an inhibitor of both the cyclo-oxygenase and lipoxygenase pathways. Inhibition of prostaglandin synthesis provides for potent anti-inflammatory, analgesic and antipyretic effects. Lipoxygenase inhibitors appear to attenuate cell-mediated inflammation and thus retard the progression of tissue destruction in inflamed joints. In addition, Ketoprofen is a powerful inhibitor of bradykinin (a chemical mediator of pain and inflammation), it stabilises lysosomal membranes against osmotic damage and prevents the release of lysosomal enzymes that mediate tissue destruction in inflammatory reactions.

5.2 Pharmacokinetic properties

Powergel allows the site specific topical delivery of ketoprofen with very low plasma concentrations of drug. Therapeutic levels in the affected tissues provide relief from pain and inflammation, yet will satisfactorily overcome the problem of significant systemic unwanted effects.

5.3 Preclinical safety data

There are no preclinical data of relevance to the prescriber which are additional to that already included in other parts of the SPC.

6. PHARMACEUTICAL PARTICULARS

6.1 List of excipients

Powergel contains the following excipients: carbomer 940, ethanol, neroli essence, lavender essence, trolamine, purified water.

6.2 Incompatibilities
Not applicable.

6.3 Shelf life
Tube and dispenser: 60 months.

6.4 Special precautions for storage
Store below 25°C.

6.5 Nature and contents of container
Soft aluminium tube, treated inside with non-toxic epoxy resin. The tubes are packed in cardboard together with a package insert. The following pack sizes are approved:

P: 30g pack

POM: 30g sample pack, 50g pack, 2x50g twin pack, 100g pack

Dispenser: rigid polypropylene dispenser containing 50g or 100g gel.

Not all pack sizes may be marketed.

6.6 Special precautions for disposal and other handling
Not applicable.

7. MARKETING AUTHORISATION HOLDER
A Menarini Industrie Farmaceutiche Ruinite S.r.l.

Via Sette Santi, 3

50131 Florence

Italy

8. MARKETING AUTHORISATION NUMBER(S)
PL 10649/0001.

9. DATE OF FIRST AUTHORISATION/RENEWAL OF THE AUTHORISATION
28 January 1993/1 May 2008

10. DATE OF REVISION OF THE TEXT
February 2009

Legal Category
P (30g pack, maximum duration of use 7 days).

POM (30g sample pack, 50g pack, 2x50g twinpack, 100g pack, 50 g and 100g dispenser pack).

Pradaxa 110 mg hard capsules

(Boehringer Ingelheim Limited)

1. NAME OF THE MEDICINAL PRODUCT
Pradaxa▼ 110 mg hard capsules

2. QUALITATIVE AND QUANTITATIVE COMPOSITION
Each hard capsule contains 110 mg of dabigatran etexilate (as mesilate)

Excipients: Each hard capsule contains 3 micrograms sunset yellow (E110)

For a full list of excipients, see section 6.1.

3. PHARMACEUTICAL FORM
Hard capsule

Imprinted capsules with light blue, opaque cap and cream-coloured, opaque body of size 1 filled with yellowish pellets. The cap is imprinted with the Boehringer Ingelheim company symbol, the body with "R110".

4. CLINICAL PARTICULARS
4.1 Therapeutic indications
Primary prevention of venous thromboembolic events in adult patients who have undergone elective total hip replacement surgery or total knee replacement surgery.

4.2 Posology and method of administration
Prevention of Venous Thromboembolism (VTE) in patients following elective knee replacement surgery:

The recommended dose of Pradaxa is 220 mg once daily taken as 2 capsules of 110 mg. Treatment should be initiated orally within 1 - 4 hours of completed surgery with a single capsule and continuing with 2 capsules once daily thereafter for a total of 10 days.

Prevention of Venous Thromboembolism (VTE) in patients following elective hip replacement surgery:

The recommended dose of Pradaxa is 220 mg once daily taken as 2 capsules of 110 mg. Treatment should be initiated orally within 1 - 4 hours of completed surgery with a single capsule and continuing with 2 capsules once daily thereafter for a total of 28-35 days.

For both surgeries, if haemostasis is not secured, initiation of treatment should be delayed. If treatment is not started on the day of surgery then treatment should be initiated with 2 capsules once daily.

Special patient populations:

Renal impairment:

Treatment with Pradaxa in patients with severe renal impairment (creatinine clearance < 30 ml/min) is contra-indicated (see section 4.3).

In patients with moderate renal impairment (creatinine clearance 30-50 ml/min), there is limited clinical experience. These patients should be treated with caution. The recommended dose is 150 mg taken once daily as 2 capsules of 75 mg (see section 4.4 and 5.1).

After knee replacement surgery treatment should be initiated orally within 1 - 4 hours of completed surgery with a single capsule and continuing with 2 capsules once daily thereafter for a total of 10 days.

After hip replacement surgery treatment should be initiated orally within 1 - 4 hours of completed surgery with a single capsule and continuing with 2 capsules once daily thereafter for a total of 28-35 days.

Elderly:

In elderly patients (> 75 years) there is limited clinical experience. These patients should be treated with caution. The recommended dose is 150 mg taken once daily as 2 capsules of 75 mg (see section 4.4 and 5.1).

After knee replacement surgery treatment should be initiated orally within 1 - 4 hours of completed surgery with a single capsule and continuing with 2 capsules once daily thereafter for a total of 10 days.

After hip replacement surgery treatment should be initiated orally within 1 - 4 hours of completed surgery with a single capsule and continuing with 2 capsules once daily thereafter for a total of 28-35 days.

Hepatic impairment:

Patients with elevated liver enzymes > 2 upper limit of normal (ULN) were excluded in clinical trials. Therefore the use of Pradaxa is not recommended in this population (see sections 4.4 and 5.2). ALT should be measured as part of the standard pre-operative evaluation (see section 4.4).

Weight:

There is very limited clinical experience in patients with a body weight < 50 kg or > 110 kg at the recommended posology. Given the available clinical and kinetic data no adjustment is necessary (see section 5.2) but close clinical surveillance is recommended (see section 4.4).

Post-surgical patients with an increased risk for bleeding:

Patients at risk for bleeding or patients at risk of overexposure, notably patients with moderate renal impairment (creatinine clearance 30 - 50 ml/min), should be treated with caution (see sections 4.4 and 5.1).

Children and adolescents:

There is no experience in children and adolescents.

Pradaxa is not recommended for use in patients below 18 years due to lack of data on safety and efficacy.

Concomitant use of Pradaxa with Amiodarone:

Dosing should be reduced to 150 mg Pradaxa daily in patients who received concomitantly dabigatran etexilate and amiodarone (see section 4.5).

Switching from Pradaxa treatment to parenteral anticoagulant:

It is recommended to wait 24 hours after the last dose before switching from Pradaxa to a parenteral anticoagulant (see section 4.5).

Switching from parenteral anticoagulants treatment to Pradaxa:

No data are available, therefore it is not recommended to start the administration of Pradaxa before the next scheduled dose of the parenteral anticoagulant would have been due (see section 4.5).

Pradaxa should be swallowed as a whole with water, with or without food.

4.3 Contraindications

- Hypersensitivity to the active substance or to any of the excipients
- Patients with severe renal impairment (CrCl < 30 ml/min)
- Active clinically significant bleeding
- Organic lesion at risk of bleeding
- Spontaneous or pharmacological impairment of haemostasis
- Hepatic impairment or liver disease expected to have any impact on survival
- Concomitant treatment with quinidine (see section 4.5)

4.4 Special warnings and precautions for use
Hepatic impairment:

Patients with elevated liver enzymes > 2 ULN were excluded in controlled clinical trials. Therefore the use of Pradaxa is not recommended in this population. ALT should be measured as part of the standard pre-operative evaluation.

Haemorrhagic risk:

Close clinical surveillance (looking for signs of bleeding or anaemia) is recommended throughout the treatment period, especially in the following situations that may increase the hemorrhagic risk: diseases associated with an increased risk of bleeding, such as congenital or acquired coagulation disorders, thrombocytopenia or functional platelet defects, active ulcerative gastrointestinal disease, recent biopsy or major trauma, recent intracranial haemorrhage or brain, spinal or ophthalmic surgery, bacterial endocarditis.

Patients with moderate renal impairment have an increased exposure to dabigatran. Limited data is available in patients < 50 kg and the elderly (see sections 4.2 and 5.2). In these situations, Pradaxa should be used with caution and a close clinical surveillance (looking for signs of bleeding or anemia) is required throughout the treatment period (see section 4.2).

When severe bleedings occur treatment must be discontinued and the source of bleeding investigated (see section 4.9).

Agents that may enhance the risk of haemorrhage should not be administered concomitantly or should be administered with caution with Pradaxa (see section 4.5).

Patients at high surgical mortality risk and with intrinsic risk factors for thromboembolic events:

There are limited efficacy and safety data for dabigatran available in these patients and therefore they should be treated with caution.

Spinal anaesthesia/epidural anaesthesia/lumbar puncture:

In patients undergoing major orthopaedic surgery, epidural or spinal haematomas that may result in long-term or permanent paralysis cannot be excluded with the concurrent use of dabigatran and spinal/epidural anaesthesia or spinal puncture. The risk of these rare events may be higher with postoperative use of indwelling epidural catheters or the concomitant use of other medicinal products affecting haemostasis.

Therefore the use of Pradaxa is not recommended in patients undergoing anaesthesia with post-operative indwelling epidural catheters.

Administration of the first dose of Pradaxa should occur a minimum of two hours after the catheter is removed. These patients require frequent observation for neurological signs and symptoms.

Hip fracture surgery:

There is no data on the use of Pradaxa in patients undergoing hip fracture surgery. Therefore treatment is not recommended.

Colorants:

Pradaxa hard capsules contain the colorant sunset yellow (E110), which may cause allergic reactions.

4.5 Interaction with other medicinal products and other forms of interaction
Interaction studies have only been performed in adults.

Anticoagulants and platelet aggregation agents:

The following treatments are not recommended concomitantly with Pradaxa: unfractionated heparins and heparin derivatives, low molecular weight heparins (LMWH), fondaparinux, desirudin, thrombolytic agents, GPIIb/IIIa receptor antagonists, clopidogrel, ticlopidine, dextran, sulfinpyrazone and vitamin K antagonists. It should be noted that unfractionated heparin can be administered at doses necessary to maintain a patent central venous or arterial catheter (see sections 4.2 and 4.4).

Interactions linked to dabigatran etexilate and dabigatran metabolic profile:

Dabigatran etexilate and dabigatran are not metabolised by the cytochrome P450 system and have no *in vitro* effects on human cytochrome P450 enzymes. Therefore, related medicinal product interactions are not expected with dabigatran.

NSAIDs: When Pradaxa was coadministered with diclofenac, the plasma exposure of both medicinal products remained unchanged indicating a lack of a pharmacokinetic interaction between dabigatran etexilate and diclofenac. However, due to the risk of haemorrhage, notably with NSAIDs with elimination half-lives > 12 hours, close observation for signs of bleeding is recommended (see section 4.4).

Transporter interactions:

Amiodarone: Amiodarone is an inhibitor of the efflux transporter P-glycoprotein and dabigatran etexilate a substrate of this transporter. When Pradaxa was coadministered with amiodarone, the extent and rate of absorption of amiodarone and its active metabolite DEA were essentially unchanged. The dabigatran AUC and C_{max} were increased by about 60 % and 50 %, respectively. The mechanism of

Table 1 Bleeding events broken down to major and any bleeding in the pivotal hip and knee study

	Dabigatran etexilate 150 mg	Dabigatran etexilate 220 mg	Enoxaparin
	N (%)	N (%)	N (%)
Treated	1866 (100.0)	1825 (100.0)	1848 (100.0)
Major Bleeding	24 (1.3)	33 (1.8)	27 (1.5)
Any bleeding	258 (13.8)	251 (13.8)	247 (13.4)

the interaction has not been completely clarified. In view of the long half-life of amiodarone the potential for drug interaction may exist for weeks after discontinuation of amiodarone.

Dosing should be reduced to 150 mg Pradaxa daily in patients who received concomitantly dabigatran etexilate and amiodarone (see section 4.2).

P- glycoprotein inhibitors:

Caution should be exercised with strong P- glycoprotein inhibitors like verapamil, clarithromycin, and others. The P-glycoprotein inhibitor quinidine is contraindicated (see section 4.3).

P- glycoprotein inducers:

Potent P- glycoprotein inducers such as rifampicin or St John's wort (Hypericum perforatum), may reduce the systemic exposure of dabigatran. Caution is advised when co-administering these medicinal products.

Digoxin: In a study performed with 24 healthy subjects, when Pradaxa was coadministered with digoxin, no changes on digoxin and no clinical relevant changes on dabigatran exposure have been observed.

Gastric pH:

Pantoprazole: When Pradaxa was coadministered with pantoprazole, a decrease in the dabigatran area under the plasma concentration - time curve of approximately 30 % was observed. Pantoprazole and other proton-pump inhibitors were co-administered with Pradaxa in clinical trials and no effects on bleeding or efficacy were observed.

Ranitidine: Ranitidine administration together with Pradaxa had no clinically relevant effect on the extent of absorption of dabigatran.

4.6 Pregnancy and lactation

Pregnancy:

There are no adequate data from the use of Pradaxa in pregnant women.

Studies in animals have shown reproductive toxicity (see section 5.3). The potential risk for humans is unknown.

Women of child-bearing potential should avoid pregnancy during treatment with dabigatran etexilate. Pradaxa should not be used during pregnancy unless clearly necessary.

Lactation:

There are no clinical data of the effect of dabigatran on infants during breast feeding.

Lactation should be discontinued during treatment with Pradaxa.

4.7 Effects on ability to drive and use machines

No studies on the effects on the ability to drive and use machines have been performed.

4.8 Undesirable effects

A total of 10.084 patients were treated in 4 actively controlled VTE prevention trials with at least one dose of the medicinal product. Of these 5419 were treated with 150 mg or 220 mg daily of Pradaxa, while 389 received doses less than 150 mg daily and 1168 received doses in excess of 220 mg daily.

The most commonly reported adverse reactions are bleedings occurring in total in approximately 14 % of patients; the frequency of major bleeds (including wound site bleedings) is less than 2 %.

Although rare in frequency in clinical trials, major or severe bleeding may occur and, regardless of location, may lead to disabling, life-threatening or even fatal outcomes.

The table 1 shows the number (%) of patients experiencing bleeding events during the treatment period in the VTE prevention in the two pivotal clinical trials, according to dose.

Table 1 Bleeding events broken down to major and any bleeding in the pivotal hip and knee study

(see Table 1 on previous page)

Table 2 shows the adverse reactions ranked under headings of SOC and frequency using the following convention: very common (≥ 1/10); common (≥ 1/100, <1/10); uncommon (≥ 1/1,000, <1/100); rare (≥ 1/10,000, <1/1,000); very rare (< 1/10,000).

(see Table 2 opposite)

Beyond the reported ALT findings the following laboratory chemistry data had been measured in phase 3 studies as presented in table 3.

Table 3: ALT findings the following laboratory chemistry

(see Table 3 on next page)

4.9 Overdose

There is no antidote to dabigatran. Doses of dabigatran etexilate beyond those recommended, expose the patient to increased risk of bleeding. In the event of haemorrhagic complications, treatment must be discontinued and the source of bleeding investigated. Since dabigatran is excreted predominantly by the renal route adequate diuresis must be maintained. The initiation of appropriate treatment, e.g. surgical haemostasis or the transfusion of fresh frozen plasma should be considered.

Dabigatran can be dialysed; there is no clinical experience to demonstrate the utility of this approach in clinical studies.

Table 2

SOC / Preferred Term.	Dabigatran etexilate 150 mg	Dabigatran etexilate 220 mg	Enoxaparin
	N (%)	N (%)	N (%)
Number of patients treated	2737 (100)	2682 (100)	3108 (100)
Blood and lymphatic system disorders			
	Common		
Anaemia	110 (4.0)	117 (4.4)	141 (4.5)
	Uncommon		
Thrombocytopenia	5 (0.2)	2 (0.1)	5 (0.2)
Vascular disorders			
	Common		
Haematoma	38 (1.4)	37 (1.4)	55 (1.8)
Traumatic haematoma	37 (1.4)	41 (1.5)	51 (1.6)
Wound haemorrhage	35 (1.3)	28 (1.0)	31 (1.0)
	Uncommon		
Haemorrhage	5 (0.2)	18 (0.7)	21 (0.7)
Respiratory and thoracic system disorders			
	Uncommon		
Epistaxis	19 (0.7)	15 (0.6)	13 (0.4)
Gastrointestinal disorders			
	Common		
Gastrointestinal haemorrhage	33 (1.2)	17 (0.6)	20 (0.6)
	Uncommon		
Rectal haemorrhage	12 (0.4)	15 (0.6)	5 (0.2)
Haemorrhoidal haemorrhage	4 (0.2)	8 (0.3)	2 (0.1)
Hepatobiliary disorders			
	Uncommon		
Alaninine aminotransferase increased	18 (0.7)	7 (0.3)	28 (0.9)
Aspartate aminotransferase increased	9 (0.3)	5 (0.2)	15 (0.5)
Hepatic function abnormal/ Liver function Test abnormal	6 (0.2)	10 (0.4)	7 (0.2)
Hepatic enzyme increased	4 (0.2)	5 (0.2)	11 (0.4)
Hyperbilirubinaemia	4 (0.1)	3 (0.1)	4 (0.1)
Transaminases increased	0 (0.0)	2 (0.1)	1 (0.0)
Skin and subcutaneous tissue disorder			
	Common		
Skin haemorrhage	45 (1.6)	57 (2.1)	61 (2.0)
Musculoskeletal and connective tissue and bone disorders			
	Uncommon		
Haemarthrosis	9 (0.3)	7 (0.3)	17 (0.6)
Renal and urinary disorders			
	Common		
Haematuria	38 (1.4)	33 (1.4)	25 (0.8)
General disorders and administration site conditions			
	Uncommon		
Injection site haemorrhage	21 (0.8)	19 (0.7)	27 (0.9)
Bloody discharge	2 (0.1)	6 (0.2)	6 (0.2)
Catheter site haemorrhage	2 (0.1)	1 (0.0)	7 (0.2)
Investigations			
	Common		
Haemoglobin decreased	45 (1.6)	35 (1.3)	74 (2.4)
	Uncommon		
Haematocrit decreased	0 (0.0)	6 (0.2)	4 (0.1)
Injury, poisoning and procedural complications			
	Common		
Wound secretion	130 (4.8)	130 (4.9)	93 (3.0)
Anaemia postoperative	99 (3.6)	87 (3.2)	120 (3.7)
Post procedural haematoma	66 (2.4)	45 (1.7)	78 (2.5)
Post procedural haemorrhage	37 (1.4)	54 (2.0)	56 (1.8)
Post procedural discharge	31 (1.1)	34 (1.3)	31 (1.0)
Surgical and medial procedures			
	Uncommon		
Post procedural drainage	11 (0.4)	13 (0.5)	16 (0.5)
Wound drainage	1 (0.0)	4 (0.2)	2 (0.1)

Table 3 ALT findings the following laboratory chemistry

	Dabigatran etexilate 150 mg	Dabigatran etexilate 220 mg	Enoxaparin
	N (%)	N (%)	N (%)
Total rates of Alaninine aminotransferase increased 3 × ULN	68 (2.5)	58 (2.2)	95 (3.5)

Table 4 Analysis of major VTE and VTE-related mortality during the treatment period in the RE-MODEL and the RE-NOVATE orthopeadic surgery studies

Trial	Dabigatran etexilate 220 mg	Dabigatran etexilate 150 mg	Enoxaparin 40 mg
RE-NOVATE (hip)			
N	909	888	917
Incidences (%)	28 (3.1)	38 (4.3)	36 (3.9)
Risk ratio over enoxaparin	0.78	1.09	
95% CI	0.48, 1.27	0.70, 1.70	
RE-MODEL (knee)			
N	506	527	511
Incidences (%)	13 (2.6)	20 (3.8)	18 (3.5)
Risk ratio over enoxaparin	0.73	1.08	
95% CI	0.36, 1.47	0.58, 2.01	

Table 5 Analysis of total VTE and all cause mortality during the treatment period in the RE-NOVATE and the RE-MODEL orthopaedic surgery studies

Trial	Dabigatran etexilate 220 mg	Dabigatran etexilate 150 mg	Enoxaparin 40 mg
RE-NOVATE (hip)			
N	880	874	897
Incidences (%)	53 (6.0)	75 (8.6)	60 (6.7)
Risk ratio over enoxaparin	0.9	1.28	
95% CI	(0.63, 1.29)	(0.93, 1.78)	
RE-MODEL (knee)			
N	503	526	512
Incidences (%)	183 (36.4)	213 (40.5)	193 (37.7)
Risk ratio over enoxaparin	0.97	1.07	
95% CI	(0.82, 1.13)	(0.92, 1.25)	

Table 6 Major bleeding events by treatment in the individual RE-MODEL and the RE-NOVATE studies

Trial	Dabigatran etexilate 220 mg	Dabigatran etexilate 150 mg	Enoxaparin 40 mg
RE-NOVATE (hip)			
Treated patients N	1146	1163	1154
Number of MBE N(%)	23 (2.0)	15 (1.3)	18 (1.6)
RE-MODEL (knee)			
Treated patients N	679	703	694
Number of MBE N(%)	10 (1.5)	9 (1.3)	9 (1.3)

5. PHARMACOLOGICAL PROPERTIES

5.1 Pharmacodynamic properties

Pharmacotherapeutic group: direct thrombine inhibitors, ATC code: B01AE07

Dabigatran etexilate is a small molecule prodrug which does not exhibit any pharmacological activity. After oral administration, dabigatran etexilate is rapidly absorbed and converted to dabigatran by esterase-catalysed hydrolysis in plasma and in the liver. Dabigatran is a potent, competitive, reversible direct thrombin inhibitor and is the main active principle in plasma.

Since thrombin (serine protease) enables the conversion of fibrinogen into fibrin during the coagulation cascade, its inhibition prevents the development of thrombus. Dabigatran also inhibits free thrombin, fibrin-bound thrombin and thrombin-induced platelet aggregation.

In-vivo and *ex-vivo* animal studies have demonstrated antithrombotic efficacy and anticoagulant activity of dabigatran after intravenous administration and of dabigatran etexilate after oral administration in various animal models of thrombosis.

There is a clear correlation between plasma dabigatran concentration and degree of anticoagulant effect based on phase II studies.

Steady state (after day 3) dabigatran peak plasma concentration, measured 2 - 4 hours after 220 mg dabigatran etexilate administration, is expected to be around 270 ng/ml, with an expected range of 80 - 460 ng/ml. The dabigatran trough concentration, measured at the end of the dosing interval (24 hours after the last 220 mg dabigatran dose), is expected to be around 40 ng/ml, with expected range of 10-90 ng/ml.

Ethnic origin:

More than 99% of efficacy and safety data were generated in Caucasians.

Clinical trials in Venous Thromboembolism (VTE) prophylaxis following major joint replacement surgery:

In 2 large randomized, parallel group, double-blind, dose-confirmatory trials, patients undergoing elective major orthopaedic surgery (one for knee replacement surgery and one for hip replacement surgery) received Pradaxa 75 mg or 110 mg within 1-4 hours of surgery followed by 150 mg or 220 mg daily thereafter, haemostasis having been secured, or enoxaparin 40 mg on the day prior to surgery and daily thereafter.

In the RE-MODEL trial (knee replacement) treatment was for 6 – 10 days and in the RE-NOVATE trial (hip replacement) for 28 – 35 days. Totals of 2076 patients (knee) and 3494 (hip) were treated respectively.

Composite of total VTE (including PE, proximal and distal DVT, whatever symptomatic or asymptomatic detected by routine venography) and all-cause mortality constituted the primary end-point for both studies. Composite of major VTE (including PE and proximal DVT, whatever symptomatic or asymptomatic detected by routine venography) and VTE-related mortality constituted a secondary end-point and is considered of better clinical relevance.

Results of both studies showed that the antithrombotic effect of Pradaxa 220 mg and 150 mg were statistically non-inferior to that of enoxaparin on total VTE and all-cause mortality. The point estimate for incidence of Major VTE and VTE related mortality for the 150 mg dose was slightly worse than enoxaparin (table 4). Better results were seen with the 220mg dose where the point estimate of Major VTE was slightly better than enoxaparin (table 4)."

The clinical studies have been conducted in a patient population with a mean age > 65 years.

There were no differences in the phase 3 clinical studies for efficacy and safety data between men and women.

In the studied patient population of RE-MODEL and RE-NOVATE (5539 patients treated), 51 % suffered from concomitant hypertension, 9 % from concomitant diabetes, 9 % from concomitant coronary artery disease and 20 % had a history of venous insufficiency. None of these diseases showed an impact on the effects of dabigatran on VTE-prevention or bleeding rates.

Data for the major VTE and VTE-related mortality endpoint were homogeneous with regards to the primary efficacy endpoint and are shown in table 4.

Data for the total VTE and all cause mortality endpoint are shown in table 5.

Data for adjudicated major bleeding endpoints are shown in tables 6 below.

Table 4: Analysis of major VTE and VTE-related mortality during the treatment period in the RE-MODEL and the RE-NOVATE orthopaedic surgery studies

(see Table 4 above)

Table 5: Analysis of total VTE and all cause mortality during the treatment period in the RE-NOVATE and the RE-MODEL orthopaedic surgery studies

(see Table 5 opposite)

Table 6: Major bleeding events by treatment in the individual RE-MODEL and the RE-NOVATE studies

(see Table 6 opposite)

5.2 Pharmacokinetic properties

After oral administration, dabigatran etexilate is rapidly and completely converted to dabigatran, which is the active form in plasma. The cleavage of the prodrug dabigatran etexilate by esterase-catalysed hydrolysis to the active principle dabigatran is the predominant metabolic reaction. The absolute bioavailability of dabigatran following oral administration of Pradaxa was approximately 6.5 %.

After oral administration of Pradaxa in healthy volunteers, the pharmacokinetic profile of dabigatran in plasma is characterized by a rapid increase in plasma concentrations with Cmax attained within 0.5 and 2.0 hours post administration.

Absorption:

A study evaluating post-operative absorption of dabigatran etexilate, 1-3 hours following surgery, demonstrated relatively slow absorption compared with that in healthy volunteers, showing a smooth plasma concentration-time profile without high peak plasma concentrations. Peak plasma concentrations are reached at 6 hours following administration in a postoperative period due to contributing factors such as anesthesia, gastrointestinal paresis, and surgical effects independent of the oral medicinal product formulation. It was demonstrated in a further study that slow and delayed absorption is usually only present on the day of surgery. On subsequent days absorption of dabigatran is rapid with peak plasma concentrations attained 2 hours after medicinal product administration.

Food does not affect the bioavailability of dabigatran etexilate but delays the time to peak plasma concentrations by 2 hours.

Distribution:

Low (34-35 %) concentration independent binding of dabigatran to human plasma proteins was observed. The volume of distribution of dabigatran of 60 – 70 L exceeded the volume of total body water indicating moderate tissue distribution of dabigatran.

Cmax and the area under the plasma concentration-time curve were dose proportional. Plasma concentrations of dabigatran showed a biexponential decline with a mean terminal half-life of 12 - 14 hours in healthy volunteers and 14 – 17 hours in patients undergoing major orthopaedic surgery. The half-life was independent of dose.

Metabolism and elimination:

Metabolism and excretion of dabigatran were studied following a single intravenous dose of radiolabeled dabigatran in healthy male subjects. After an intravenous dose, the dabigatran-derived radioactivity was eliminated primarily in the urine (85 %). Faecal excretion accounted for 6 % of the administered dose. Recovery of the total radioactivity ranged from 88 - 94 % of the administered dose by 168 hours post dose.

Dabigatran is subject to conjugation forming pharmacologically active acylglucuronides. Four positional isomers, 1-O, 2-O, 3-O, 4-O-acylglucuronide exist, each accounts for less than 10 % of total dabigatran in plasma. Traces of other metabolites were only detectable with highly sensitive analytical methods. Dabigatran is eliminated primarily in the unchanged form in the urine, at a rate of approximately 100 ml/min corresponding to the glomerular filtration rate.

Special populations:

Renal insufficiency:

The exposure (AUC) of dabigatran after the oral administration of Pradaxa is approximately 2.7 fold higher in volunteers with moderate renal insufficiency (CrCL between 30 – 50 ml/min) than in those without renal insufficiency.

In a small number of volunteers with severe renal insufficiency (CrCL 10 - 30 ml/min), the exposure (AUC) to dabigatran was approximately 6 times higher and the half-life approximately 2 times longer than that observed in a population without renal insufficiency (see sections 4.2, 4.3 and 4.4).

Elderly patients:

Specific pharmacokinetic studies with elderly subjects showed an increase of 40 to 60 % in the AUC and of more than 25 % in C_{max} compared to young subjects. Population-based pharmacokinetic studies have evaluated the pharmacokinetics of dabigatran after repeated doses in patients (up to 88 years). The observed increase of dabigatran exposure correlated with the age-related reduction in creatinine clearance (see sections 4.2 and 4.4).

Hepatic insufficiency:

No change in dabigatran exposure was seen in 12 subjects with moderate hepatic insufficiency (Child Pugh B) compared to 12 controls (see sections 4.2 and 4.4).

Body weight:

Population pharmacokinetic studies have evaluated the pharmacokinetics of dabigatran in patients of 48 to 120 kg body weight. Body weight had a minor effect on the plasma clearance of dabigatran resulting in higher exposure in patients with low body weight (see section 4.2 and 4.4).

Gender:

Active substance exposure in female patients is about 40 % to 50 % higher than in male patients and no dose adjustment is recommended.

Ethnic origin:

The pharmacokinetics of dabigatran was investigated in Caucasian and Japanese volunteers after single and multiple doses. Ethnic origin does not affect the pharmacokinetics of dabigatran in a clinically relevant manner. No pharmacokinetic data in black patients are available.

Pharmacokinetic interactions:

In vitro interaction studies did not show any inhibition or induction of the principal isoenzymes of cytochrome P450. This has been confirmed by in vivo studies with healthy volunteers, who did not show any interaction between this treatment and the following active substances: atorvastatin (CYP3A4), digoxin (P-glycoprotein transporter interaction) and diclofenac (CYP2C9).

Dabigatran exposure in healthy subjects was increased by 60 % in the presence of amiodarone.

5.3 Preclinical safety data

Non-clinical data reveal no special hazard for humans based on conventional studies of safety pharmacology, repeated dose toxicity and genotoxicity.

Effects observed in the repeat-dose toxicity studies were due to the exaggerated pharmacodynamic effect of dabigatran.

An effect on female fertility was observed in the form of a decrease in implantations and an increase in pre-implantation loss at 70 mg/kg (5-fold the plasma exposure level in patients). At doses that were toxic to the mothers (5 to 10-fold the plasma exposure level in patients), a decrease in foetal body weight and viability along with an increase in foetal variations were observed in rats and rabbits. In the pre- and post-natal study, an increase in foetal mortality was observed at doses that were toxic to the dams (a dose corresponding to a plasma exposure level 4-fold higher than observed in patients).

Carcinogenicity studies have not yet been completed with dabigatran.

6. PHARMACEUTICAL PARTICULARS

6.1 List of excipients

Capsule fill

- Tartaric acid
- Acacia
- Hypromellose
- Dimeticone 350
- Talc
- Hydroxypropylcellulose

Capsule shell

- Carrageenan
- Potassium Chloride
- Titanium Dioxide
- Indigo Carmine (E132)
- Sunset Yellow (E110)
- Hypromellose
- Water purified

Black printing ink

- Shellac
- N-Butyl alcohol
- Isopropyl alcohol
- Industrial methylated spirit
- Iron oxide black (E172)
- Purified water
- Propylene glycol

6.2 Incompatibilities

Not applicable.

6.3 Shelf life

Blister and bottle: 3 years

Once the bottle is opened, the product must be used within 30 days

6.4 Special precautions for storage

Blister:

Store in the original package in order to protect from moisture.

Bottle:

Store in the original package in order to protect from moisture. Keep the bottle tightly closed.

6.5 Nature and contents of container

Cartons containing 1, 3, or 6 blister strips (10 × 1, 30 × 1, 60 × 1) in perforated aluminium unit dose blisters. The blister consists of an aluminium lidding foil coated with polyvinylchloride-polyvinylacetate copolymer-acrylate (PVCAC acrylate) in contact with the product and an aluminium bottom foil with polyvinylchloride (PVC) in contact with the product.

Polypropylene bottle with a screw cap containing 60 hard capsules.

Not all pack sizes may be marketed.

6.6 Special precautions for disposal and other handling

When taking Pradaxa capsules out of the blister pack, the following instructions should be followed:

- The hard capsules should be taken out of the blister card by peeling off the backing foil.
- The hard capsules should not be pushed through the blister foil.
- The blister foil should only be peeled off, when a hard capsule is required.

When taking a hard capsule out of the bottle, please observe the following instructions:

- The cap opens by pushing and turning.

Any unused product or waste material should be disposed of in accordance with local requirements.

7. MARKETING AUTHORISATION HOLDER

Boehringer Ingelheim International GmbH

D-55216 Ingelheim am Rhein

Germany

8. MARKETING AUTHORISATION NUMBER(S)

EU/1/08/442/005 - 10 × 1 capsules - blister (alu/alu)

EU/1/08/442/006 - 30 × 1 capsules - blister (alu/alu)

EU/1/08/442/007 - 60 × 1 capsules - blister (alu/alu)

EU/1/08/442/008 - 60 capsules - bottle (PP)

9. DATE OF FIRST AUTHORISATION/RENEWAL OF THE AUTHORISATION

18th March 2008

10. DATE OF REVISION OF THE TEXT

25th March 2009

LEGAL CATEGORY

POM

Pradaxa 75 mg hard capsules

(Boehringer Ingelheim Limited)

1. NAME OF THE MEDICINAL PRODUCT

Pradaxa▼ 75 mg hard capsules

2. QUALITATIVE AND QUANTITATIVE COMPOSITION

Each hard capsule contains 75 mg of dabigatran etexilate (as mesilate)

Excipients: Each hard capsule contains 2 micrograms sunset yellow (E110)

For a full list of excipients, see section 6.1.

3. PHARMACEUTICAL FORM

Hard capsule

Imprinted capsules with light blue, opaque cap and cream-coloured, opaque body of size 2 filled with yellowish pellets. The cap is imprinted with the Boehringer Ingelheim company symbol, the body with "R75".

4. CLINICAL PARTICULARS

4.1 Therapeutic indications

Primary prevention of venous thromboembolic events in adult patients who have undergone elective total hip replacement surgery or total knee replacement surgery.

4.2 Posology and method of administration

Prevention of Venous Thromboembolism (VTE) in patients following elective knee replacement surgery:

The recommended dose of Pradaxa is 220 mg once daily taken as 2 capsules of 110 mg. Treatment should be initiated orally within 1 – 4 hours of completed surgery with a single capsule and continuing with 2 capsules once daily thereafter for a total of 10 days.

Prevention of Venous Thromboembolism (VTE) in patients following elective hip replacement surgery:

The recommended dose of Pradaxa is 220 mg once daily taken as 2 capsules of 110 mg. Treatment should be initiated orally within 1 – 4 hours of completed surgery with a single capsule and continuing with 2 capsules once daily thereafter for a total of 28-35 days.

For both surgeries, if haemostasis is not secured, initiation of treatment should be delayed. If treatment is not started on the day of surgery then treatment should be initiated with 2 capsules once daily.

Special patient populations:

Renal impairment:

Treatment with Pradaxa in patients with severe renal impairment (creatinine clearance < 30 ml/min) is contra-indicated (see section 4.3).

In patients with moderate renal impairment (creatinine clearance 30-50 ml/min), there is limited clinical experience. These patients should be treated with caution. The recommended dose is 150 mg taken once daily as 2 capsules of 75 mg (see section 4.4 and 5.1).

After knee replacement surgery treatment should be initiated orally within 1 – 4 hours of completed surgery with a single capsule and continuing with 2 capsules once daily thereafter for a total of 10 days.

After hip replacement surgery treatment should be initiated orally within 1 – 4 hours of completed surgery with a single capsule and continuing with 2 capsules once daily thereafter for a total of 28-35 days.

Elderly:

In elderly patients (> 75 years) there is limited clinical experience. These patients should be treated with caution. The recommended dose is 150 mg taken once daily as 2 capsules of 75 mg (see section 4.4 and 5.1).

After knee replacement surgery treatment should be initiated orally within 1 – 4 hours of completed surgery with a single capsule and continuing with 2 capsules once daily thereafter for a total of 10 days.

After hip replacement surgery treatment should be initiated orally within 1 – 4 hours of completed surgery with a single capsule and continuing with 2 capsules once daily thereafter for a total of 28-35 days.

Hepatic impairment:

Patients with elevated liver enzymes > 2 upper limit of normal (ULN) were excluded in clinical trials. Therefore the use of Pradaxa is not recommended in this population (see sections 4.4 and 5.2). ALT should be measured as part of the standard pre-operative evaluation (see section 4.4).

Weight:

There is very limited clinical experience in patients with a body weight < 50 kg or > 110 kg at the recommended posology. Given the available clinical and kinetic data no adjustment is necessary (see section 5.2) but close clinical surveillance is recommended (see section 4.4).

Post-surgical patients with an increased risk for bleeding:

Patients at risk for bleeding or patients at risk of overexposure, notably patients with moderate renal impairment (creatinine clearance 30 – 50 ml/min), should be treated with caution (see sections 4.4 and 5.1).

Children and adolescents:

There is no experience in children and adolescents.

Pradaxa is not recommended for use in patients below 18 years due to lack of data on safety and efficacy.

Concomitant use of Pradaxa with Amiodarone:

Dosing should be reduced to 150 mg Pradaxa daily in patients who received concomitantly dabigatran etexilate and amiodarone (see section 4.5).

Switching from Pradaxa treatment to parenteral anticoagulant:

It is recommended to wait 24 hours after the last dose before switching from Pradaxa to a parenteral anticoagulant (see section 4.5).

Switching from parenteral anticoagulants treatment to Pradaxa:

No data are available, therefore it is not recommended to start the administration of Pradaxa before the next scheduled dose of the parenteral anticoagulant would have been due (see section 4.5).

Pradaxa should be swallowed as a whole with water, with or without food.

4.3 Contraindications

- Hypersensitivity to the active substance or to any of the excipients
- Patients with severe renal impairment (CrCl < 30 ml/min)
- Active clinically significant bleeding
- Organic lesion at risk of bleeding
- Spontaneous or pharmacological impairment of haemostasis
- Hepatic impairment or liver disease expected to have any impact on survival
- Concomitant treatment with quinidine (see section 4.5)

4.4 Special warnings and precautions for use

Hepatic impairment:

Patients with elevated liver enzymes > 2 ULN were excluded in controlled clinical trials. Therefore the use of Pradaxa is not recommended in this population. ALT should be measured as part of the standard pre-operative evaluation.

Haemorrhagic risk:

Close clinical surveillance (looking for signs of bleeding or anaemia) is recommended throughout the treatment period, especially in the following situations that may increase the hemorrhagic risk: diseases associated with an increased risk of bleeding, such as congenital or acquired coagulation disorders, thrombocytopenia or functional platelet defects, active ulcerative gastrointestinal disease, recent biopsy or major trauma, recent intracranial haemorrhage or brain, spinal or ophthalmic surgery, bacterial endocarditis.

Patients with moderate renal impairment have an increased exposure to dabigatran. Limited data is available in patients < 50 kg and the elderly (see sections 4.2 and 5.2). In these situations, Pradaxa should be used with caution and a close clinical surveillance (looking for signs of bleeding or anemia) is required throughout the treatment period (see section 4.2).

When severe bleedings occur treatment must be discontinued and the source of bleeding investigated (see section 4.9).

Agents that may enhance the risk of haemorrhage should not be administered concomitantly or should be administered with caution with Pradaxa (see section 4.5).

Patients at high surgical mortality risk and with intrinsic risk factors for thromboembolic events:

There are limited efficacy and safety data for dabigatran available in these patients and therefore they should be treated with caution.

Spinal anaesthesia/epidural anaesthesia/lumbar puncture:

In patients undergoing major orthopaedic surgery, epidural or spinal haematomas that may result in long-term or permanent paralysis cannot be excluded with the concurrent use of dabigatran and spinal/epidural anaesthesia or spinal puncture. The risk of these rare events may be higher with postoperative use of indwelling epidural catheters or the concomitant use of other medicinal products affecting haemostasis.

Therefore the use of Pradaxa is not recommended in patients undergoing anaesthesia with post-operative indwelling epidural catheters.

Administration of the first dose of Pradaxa should occur a minimum of two hours after the catheter is removed. These patients require frequent observation for neurological signs and symptoms.

Hip fracture surgery:

There is no data on the use of Pradaxa in patients undergoing hip fracture surgery. Therefore treatment is not recommended.

Colorants:

Pradaxa hard capsules contain the colorant sunset yellow (E110), which may cause allergic reactions.

4.5 Interaction with other medicinal products and other forms of interaction

Interaction studies have only been performed in adults.

Anti coagulants and platelet aggregation agents:

The following treatments are not recommended concomitantly with Pradaxa: unfractionated heparins and heparin derivatives, low molecular weight heparins (LMWH), fondaparinux, desirudin, thrombolytic agents, GPIIb/IIIa receptor antagonists, clopidogrel, ticlopidine, dextran, sulfinpyrazone and vitamin K antagonists. It should be noted that unfractionated heparin can be administered at doses necessary to maintain a patent central venous or arterial catheter (see sections 4.2 and 4.4).

Interactions linked to dabigatran etexilate and dabigatran metabolic profile:

Dabigatran etexilate and dabigatran are not metabolised by the cytochrome P450 system and have no *in vitro* effects on human cytochrome P450 enzymes. Therefore, related medicinal product interactions are not expected with dabigatran.

NSAIDs: When Pradaxa was coadministered with diclofenac, the plasma exposure of both medicinal products remained unchanged indicating a lack of a pharmacokinetic interaction between dabigatran etexilate and diclofenac. However, due to the risk of haemorrhage, notably with NSAIDs with elimination half-lives > 12 hours, close observation for signs of bleeding is recommended (see section 4.4).

Transporter interactions:

Amiodarone: Amiodarone is an inhibitor of the efflux transporter P-glycoprotein and dabigatran etexilate a substrate of this transporter. When Pradaxa was coadministered with amiodarone, the extent and rate of absorption of amiodarone and its active metabolite DEA were essentially unchanged. The dabigatran AUC and C_{max} were increased by about 60 % and 50 %, respectively. The mechanism of the interaction has not been completely clarified. In view of the long half-life of amiodarone the potential for drug interaction may exist for weeks after discontinuation of amiodarone.

Dosing should be reduced to 150 mg Pradaxa daily in patients who received concomitantly dabigatran etexilate and amiodarone (see section 4.2).

P- glycoprotein inhibitors:

Caution should be exercised with strong P- glycoprotein inhibitors like verapamil, clarithromycin, and others. The P-glycoprotein inhibitor quinidine is contraindicated (see section 4.3).

P- glycoprotein inducers:

Potent P- glycoprotein inducers such as rifampicin or St John's wort (Hypericum perforatum), may reduce the systemic exposure of dabigatran. Caution is advised when co-administering these medicinal products.

Digoxin: In a study performed with 24 healthy subjects, when Pradaxa was coadministered with digoxin, no changes on digoxin and no clinical relevant changes on dabigatran exposure have been observed.

Gastric pH:

Pantoprazole: When Pradaxa was coadministered with pantoprazole, a decrease in the dabigatran area under the plasma concentration - time curve of approximately 30 % was observed. Pantoprazole and other proton-pump inhibitors were co-administered with Pradaxa in clinical trials and no effects on bleeding or efficacy were observed.

Ranitidine: Ranitidine administration together with Pradaxa had no clinically relevant effect on the extent of absorption of dabigatran.

4.6 Pregnancy and lactation

Pregnancy:

There are no adequate data from the use of Pradaxa in pregnant women.

Studies in animals have shown reproductive toxicity (see section 5.3). The potential risk for humans is unknown.

Women of child-bearing potential should avoid pregnancy during treatment with dabigatran etexilate. Pradaxa should not be used during pregnancy unless clearly necessary.

Lactation:

There are no clinical data of the effect of dabigatran on infants during breast feeding.

Lactation should be discontinued during treatment with Pradaxa.

4.7 Effects on ability to drive and use machines

No studies on the effects on the ability to drive and use machines have been performed.

4.8 Undesirable effects

A total of 10.084 patients were treated in 4 actively controlled VTE prevention trials with at least one dose of the medicinal product. Of these 5419 were treated with 150 mg or 220 mg daily of Pradaxa, while 389 received doses less than 150 mg daily and 1168 received doses in excess of 220 mg daily.

The most commonly reported adverse reactions are bleedings occurring in total in approximately 14 % of patients; the frequency of major bleeds (including wound site bleedings) is less than 2 %.

Although rare in frequency in clinical trials, major or severe bleeding may occur and, regardless of location, may lead to disabling, life-threatening or even fatal outcomes.

The table 1 shows the number (%) of patients experiencing bleeding events during the treatment period in the VTE prevention in the two pivotal clinical trials, according to dose.

Table 1 Bleeding events broken down to major and any bleeding in the pivotal hip and knee study

(see Table 1 below)

Table 2 shows the adverse reactions ranked under headings of SOC and frequency using the following convention: very common (≥ 1/10); common (≥ 1/100, <1/10); uncommon (≥ 1/1,000, <1/100); rare (≥ 1/10,000, <1/1,000); very rare (< 1/10,000).

(see Table 2 on next page)

Beyond the reported ALT findings the following laboratory chemistry data had been measured in phase 3 studies as presented in table 3.

Table 3: ALT findings the following laboratory chemistry

(see Table 3 on page 4931821)

4.9 Overdose

There is no antidote to dabigatran. Doses of dabigatran etexilate beyond those recommended, expose the patient to increased risk of bleeding. In the event of haemorrhagic complications, treatment must be discontinued and the source of bleeding investigated. Since dabigatran is excreted predominantly by the renal route adequate diuresis must be maintained. The initiation of appropriate treatment, e.g. surgical haemostasis or the transfusion of fresh frozen plasma should be considered.

Dabigatran can be dialysed; there is no clinical experience to demonstrate the utility of this approach in clinical studies.

5. PHARMACOLOGICAL PROPERTIES

5.1 Pharmacodynamic properties

Pharmacotherapeutic group: direct thrombine inhibitors, ATC code: B01AE07

Dabigatran etexilate is a small molecule prodrug which does not exhibit any pharmacological activity. After oral administration, dabigatran etexilate is rapidly absorbed and converted to dabigatran by esterase-catalysed hydrolysis in plasma and in the liver. Dabigatran is a potent, competitive, reversible direct thrombin inhibitor and is the main active principle in plasma.

Since thrombin (serine protease) enables the conversion of fibrinogen into fibrin during the coagulation cascade, its inhibition prevents the development of thrombus. Dabigatran also inhibits free thrombin, fibrin-bound thrombin and thrombin-induced platelet aggregation.

In-vivo and *ex-vivo* animal studies have demonstrated antithrombotic efficacy and anticoagulant activity of dabigatran after intravenous administration and of dabigatran etexilate after oral administration in various animal models of thrombosis.

There is a clear correlation between plasma dabigatran concentration and degree of anticoagulant effect based on phase II studies.

Steady state (after day 3) dabigatran peak plasma concentration, measured 2 - 4 hours after 220 mg dabigatran etexilate administration, is expected to be around 270 ng/ml, with an expected range of 80 - 460 ng/ml. The dabigatran trough concentration, measured at the end of the dosing interval (24 hours after the last 220 mg dabigatran dose), is expected to be around 40 ng/ml, with expected range of 10-90 ng/ml.

Ethnic origin:

More than 99% of efficacy and safety data were generated in Caucasians.

Clinical trials in Venous Thromboembolism (VTE) prophylaxis following major joint replacement surgery:

In 2 large randomized, parallel group, double-blind, dose-confirmatory trials, patients undergoing elective major orthopaedic surgery (one for knee replacement surgery and one for hip replacement surgery) received Pradaxa

Table 1 Bleeding events broken down to major and any bleeding in the pivotal hip and knee study

	Dabigatran etexilate 150 mg	Dabigatran etexilate 220 mg	Enoxaparin
	N (%)	N (%)	N (%)
Treated	1866 (100.0)	1825 (100.0)	1848 (100.0)
Major Bleeding	24 (1.3)	33 (1.8)	27 (1.5)
Any bleeding	258 (13.8)	251 (13.8)	247 (13.4)

Table 2

SOC / Preferred Term.	Dabigatran etexilate 150 mg	Dabigatran etexilate 220 mg	Enoxaparin
	N (%)	N (%)	N (%)
Number of patients treated	2737 (100)	2682 (100)	3108 (100)
Blood and lymphatic system disorders			
	Common		
Anaemia	110 (4.0)	117 (4.4)	141 (4.5)
	Uncommon		
Thrombocytopenia	5 (0.2)	2 (0.1)	5 (0.2)
Vascular disorders			
	Common		
Haematoma	38 (1.4)	37 (1.4)	55 (1.8)
Traumatic haematoma	37 (1.4)	41 (1.5)	51 (1.6)
Wound haemorhhage	35 (1.3)	28 (1.0)	31 (1.0)
	Uncommon		
Haemorrhage	5 (0.2)	18 (0.7)	21 (0.7)
Respiratory and thoracic system disorders			
	Uncommon		
Epistaxis	19 (0.7)	15 (0.6)	13 (0.4)
Gastrointestinal disorders			
	Common		
Gastrointestinal haemorrhage	33 (1.2)	17 (0.6)	20 (0.6)
	Uncommon		
Rectal haemorrhage	12 (0.4)	15 (0.6)	5 (0.2)
Haemorrhoidal haemorrhage	4 (0.2)	8 (0.3)	2 (0.1)
Hepatobiliary disorders			
	Uncommon		
Alaninine aminotransferase increased	18 (0.7)	7 (0.3)	28 (0.9)
Aspartate aminotransferase increased	9 (0.3)	5 (0.2)	15 (0.5)
Hepatic function abnormal/ Liver function Test abnormal	6 (0.2)	10 (0.4)	7 (0.2)
Hepatic enzyme increased	4 (0.2)	5 (0.2)	11 (0.4)
Hyperbilirubinaemia	4 (0.1)	3 (0.1)	4 (0.1)
Transaminases increased	0 (0.0)	2 (0.1)	1 (0.0)
Skin and subcutaneous tissue disorder			
	Common		
Skin haemorrhage	45 (1.6)	57 (2.1)	61 (2.0)
Musculoskeletal and connective tissue and bone disorders			
	Uncommon		
Haemarthrosis	9 (0.3)	7 (0.3)	17 (0.6)
Renal and urinary disorders			
	Common		
Haematuria	38 (1.4)	33 (1.4)	25 (0.8)
General disorders and administration site conditions			
	Uncommon		
Injection site haemorrhage	21 (0.8)	19 (0.7)	27 (0.9)
Bloody discharge	2 (0.1)	6 (0.2)	6 (0.2)
Catheter site haemorrhage	2 (0.1)	1 (0.0)	7 (0.2)
Investigations			
	Common		
Haemoglobin decreased	45 (1.6)	35 (1.3)	74 (2.4)
	Uncommon		
Haematocrit decreased	0 (0.0)	6 (0.2)	4 (0.1)
Injury, poisoning and procedural complications			
	Common		
Wound secretion	130 (4.8)	130 (4.9)	93 (3.0)
Anaemia postoperative	99 (3.6)	87 (3.2)	120 (3.7)
Post procedural haematoma	66 (2.4)	45 (1.7)	78 (2.5)
Post procedural haemorrhage	37 (1.4)	54 (2.0)	56 (1.8)
Post procedural discharge	31 (1.1)	34 (1.3)	31 (1.0)
Surgical and medial procedures			
	Uncommon		
Post procedural drainage	11 (0.4)	13 (0.5)	16 (0.5)
Wound drainage	1 (0.0)	4 (0.2)	2 (0.1)

75 mg or 110 mg within 1-4 hours of surgery followed by 150 mg or 220 mg daily thereafter, haemostasis having been secured, or enoxaparin 40 mg on the day prior to surgery and daily thereafter.

In the RE-MODEL trial (knee replacement) treatment was for 6 – 10 days and in the RE-NOVATE trial (hip replacement) for 28 – 35 days. Totals of 2076 patients (knee) and 3494 (hip) were treated respectively.

Composite of total VTE (including PE, proximal and distal DVT, whatever symptomatic or asymptomatic detected by routine venography) and all-cause mortality constituted the primary end-point for both studies. Composite of major VTE (including PE and proximal DVT, whatever symptomatic or asymptomatic detected by routine venography) and VTE-related mortality constituted a secondary end-point and is considered of better clinical relevance.

Results of both studies showed that the antithrombotic effect of Pradaxa 220 mg and 150 mg were statistically non-inferior to that of enoxaparin on total VTE and all-cause mortality. The point estimate for incidence of Major VTE and VTE related mortality for the 150 mg dose was slightly worse than enoxaparin (table 4). Better results were seen with the 220mg dose where the point estimate of Major VTE was slightly better than enoxaparin (table 4)."

The clinical studies have been conducted in a patient population with a mean age > 65 years.

There were no differences in the phase 3 clinical studies for efficacy and safety data between men and women.

In the studied patient population of RE-MODEL and RE-NOVATE (5539 patients treated), 51 % suffered from concomitant hypertension, 9 % from concomitant diabetes, 9 % from concomitant coronary artery disease and 20 % had a history of venous insufficiency. None of these diseases showed an impact on the effects of dabigatran on VTE-prevention or bleeding rates.

Data for the major VTE and VTE-related mortality endpoint were homogeneous with regards to the primary efficacy endpoint and are shown in table 4.

Data for the total VTE and all cause mortality endpoint are shown in table 5.

Data for adjudicated major bleeding endpoints are shown in tables 6 below.

Table 4: Analysis of major VTE and VTE-related mortality during the treatment period in the RE-MODEL and the RE-NOVATE orthopeadic surgery studies

(see Table 4 on next page)

Table 5: Analysis of total VTE and all cause mortality during the treatment period in the RE-NOVATE and the RE-MODEL orthopaedic surgery studies

(see Table 5 on next page)

Table 6: Major bleeding events by treatment in the individual RE-MODEL and the RE-NOVATE studies

(see Table 6 on next page)

5.2 Pharmacokinetic properties

After oral administration, dabigatran etexilate is rapidly and completely converted to dabigatran, which is the active form in plasma. The cleavage of the prodrug dabigatran etexilate by esterase-catalysed hydrolysis to the active principle dabigatran is the predominant metabolic reaction. The absolute bioavailability of dabigatran following oral administration of Pradaxa was approximately 6.5 %.

After oral administration of Pradaxa in healthy volunteers, the pharmacokinetic profile of dabigatran in plasma is characterized by a rapid increase in plasma concentrations with Cmax attained within 0.5 and 2.0 hours post administration.

Absorption:

A study evaluating post-operative absorption of dabigatran etexilate, 1-3 hours following surgery, demonstrated relatively slow absorption compared with that in healthy volunteers, showing a smooth plasma concentration-time profile without high peak plasma concentrations. Peak plasma concentrations are reached at 6 hours following administration in a postoperative period due to contributing factors such as anesthesia, gastrointestinal paresis, and surgical effects independent of the oral medicinal product formulation. It was demonstrated in a further study that slow and delayed absorption is usually only present on the day of surgery. On subsequent days absorption of dabigatran is rapid with peak plasma concentrations attained 2 hours after medicinal product administration.

Food does not affect the bioavailability of dabigatran etexilate but delays the time to peak plasma concentrations by 2 hours.

Distribution:

Low (34-35 %) concentration independent binding of dabigatran to human plasma proteins was observed. The volume of distribution of dabigtran of 60 – 70 L exceeded the volume of total body water indicating moderate tissue distribution of dabigatran.

Cmax and the area under the plasma concentration-time curve were dose proportional. Plasma concentrations of dabigatran showed a biexponential decline with a mean terminal half-life of 12 - 14 hours in healthy volunteers and 14 – 17 hours in patients undergoing major orthopaedic surgery. The half-life was independent of dose.

Table 3 ALT findings the following laboratory chemistry

	Dabigatran etexilate 150 mg	Dabigatran etexilate 220 mg	Enoxaparin
	N (%)	N (%)	N (%)
Total rates of Alaninine aminotransferase increased 3 × ULN	68 (2.5)	58 (2.2)	95 (3.5)

Table 4 Analysis of major VTE and VTE-related mortality during the treatment period in the RE-MODEL and the RE-NOVATE orthopaedic surgery studies

Trial	Dabigatran etexilate 220 mg	Dabigatran etexilate 150 mg	Enoxaparin 40 mg
RE-NOVATE (hip)			
N	909	888	917
Incidences (%)	28 (3.1)	38 (4.3)	36 (3.9)
Risk ratio over enoxaparin	0.78	1.09	
95% CI	0.48, 1.27	0.70, 1.70	
RE-MODEL (knee)			
N	506	527	511
Incidences (%)	13 (2.6)	20 (3.8)	18 (3.5)
Risk ratio over enoxaparin	0.73	1.08	
95% CI	0.36, 1.47	0.58, 2.01	

Table 5 Analysis of total VTE and all cause mortality during the treatment period in the RE-NOVATE and the RE-MODEL orthopaedic surgery studies

Trial	Dabigatran etexilate 220 mg	Dabigatran etexilate 150 mg	Enoxaparin 40 mg
RE-NOVATE (hip)			
N	880	874	897
Incidences (%)	53 (6.0)	75 (8.6)	60 (6.7)
Risk ratio over enoxaparin	0.9	1.28	
95% CI	(0.63, 1.29)	(0.93, 1.78)	
RE-MODEL (knee)			
N	503	526	512
Incidences (%)	183 (36.4)	213 (40.5)	193 (37.7)
Risk ratio over enoxaparin	0.97	1.07	
95% CI	(0.82, 1.13)	(0.92, 1.25)	

Table 6 Major bleeding events by treatment in the individual RE-MODEL and the RE-NOVATE studies

Trial	Dabigatran etexilate 220 mg	Dabigatran etexilate 150 mg	Enoxaparin 40 mg
RE-NOVATE (hip)			
Treated patients N	1146	1163	1154
Number of MBE N(%)	23 (2.0)	15 (1.3)	18 (1.6)
RE-MODEL (knee)			
Treated patients N	679	703	694
Number of MBE N(%)	10 (1.5)	9 (1.3)	9 (1.3)

Metabolism and elimination:

Metabolism and excretion of dabigatran were studied following a single intravenous dose of radiolabeled dabigatran in healthy male subjects. After an intravenous dose, the dabigatran-derived radioactivity was eliminated primarily in the urine (85 %). Faecal excretion accounted for 6 % of the administered dose. Recovery of the total radioactivity ranged from 88 - 94 % of the administered dose by 168 hours post dose.

Dabigatran is subject to conjugation forming pharmacologically active acylglucuronides. Four positional isomers, 1-O, 2-O, 3-O, 4-O-acylglucuronide exist, each accounts for less than 10 % of total dabigatran in plasma. Traces of other metabolites were only detectable with highly sensitive analytical methods. Dabigatran is eliminated primarily in the unchanged form in the urine, at a rate of approximately 100 ml/min corresponding to the glomerular filtration rate.

Special populations:

Renal insufficiency:

The exposure (AUC) of dabigatran after the oral administration of Pradaxa is approximately 2.7 fold higher in volunteers with moderate renal insufficiency (CrCL between 30 – 50 ml/min) than in those without renal insufficiency.

In a small number of volunteers with severe renal insufficiency (CrCL 10 - 30 ml/min), the exposure (AUC) to dabigatran was approximately 6 times higher and the half-life approximately 2 times longer than that observed in a population without renal insufficiency (see sections 4.2, 4.3 and 4.4).

Elderly patients:

Specific pharmacokinetic studies with elderly subjects showed an increase of 40 to 60 % in the AUC and of more than 25 % in C_{max} compared to young subjects. Population-based pharmacokinetic studies have evaluated the pharmacokinetics of dabigatran after repeated doses in patients (up to 88 years). The observed increase of dabigatran exposure correlated with the age-related reduction in creatinine clearance (see sections 4.2 and 4.4).

Hepatic insufficiency:

No change in dabigatran exposure was seen in 12 subjects with moderate hepatic insufficiency (Child Pugh B) compared to 12 controls (see sections 4.2 and 4.4).

Body weight:

Population pharmacokinetic studies have evaluated the pharmacokinetics of dabigatran in patients of 48 to 120 kg body weight. Body weight had a minor effect on the plasma clearance of dabigatran resulting in higher exposure in patients with low body weight (see section 4.2 and 4.4).

Gender:

Active substance exposure in female patients is about 40 % to 50 % higher than in male patients and no dose adjustment is recommended.

Ethnic origin:

The pharmacokinetics of dabigatran was investigated in Caucasian and Japanese volunteers after single and multiple doses. Ethnic origin does not affect the pharmacokinetics of dabigatran in a clinically relevant manner. No pharmacokinetic data in black patients are available.

Pharmacokinetic interactions:

In vitro interaction studies did not show any inhibition or induction of the principal isoenzymes of cytochrome P450. This has been confirmed by in vivo studies with healthy volunteers, who did not show any interaction between this treatment and the following active substances: atorvastatin (CYP3A4), digoxin (P-glycoprotein transporter interaction) and diclofenac (CYP2C9).

Dabigatran exposure in healthy subjects was increased by 60 % in the presence of amiodarone.

5.3 Preclinical safety data

Non-clinical data reveal no special hazard for humans based on conventional studies of safety pharmacology, repeated dose toxicity and genotoxicity.

Effects observed in the repeat-dose toxicity studies were due to the exaggerated pharmacodynamic effect of dabigatran.

An effect on female fertility was observed in the form of a decrease in implantations and an increase in pre-implantation loss at 70 mg/kg (5-fold the plasma exposure level in patients). At doses that were toxic to the mothers (5 to 10-fold the plasma exposure level in patients), a decrease in foetal body weight and viability along with an increase in foetal variations were observed in rats and rabbits. In the pre- and post-natal study, an increase in foetal mortality was observed at doses that were toxic to the dams (a dose corresponding to a plasma exposure level 4-fold higher than observed in patients).

Carcinogenicity studies have not yet been completed with dabigatran.

6. PHARMACEUTICAL PARTICULARS

6.1 List of excipients

Capsule fill

- Tartaric acid
- Acacia
- Hypromellose
- Dimeticone 350
- Talc
- Hydroxypropylcellulose

Capsule shell

- Carrageenan
- Potassium Chloride
- Titanium Dioxide
- Indigo Carmine (E132)
- Sunset Yellow (E110)
- Hypromellose
- Water purified

Black printing ink

- Shellac
- N-Butyl alcohol
- Isopropyl alcohol
- Industrial methylated spirit
- Iron oxide black (E172)
- Purified water
- Propylene glycol

6.2 Incompatibilities

Not applicable.

6.3 Shelf life

Blister and bottle: 3 years

Once the bottle is opened, the product must be used within 30 days

6.4 Special precautions for storage

Blister:

Store in the original package in order to protect from moisture.

Bottle:

Store in the original package in order to protect from moisture. Keep the bottle tightly closed.

6.5 Nature and contents of container

Cartons containing 1, 3, or 6 blister strips (10 × 1, 30 × 1, 60 × 1) in perforated aluminium unit dose blisters. The blister consists of an aluminium lidding foil coated with polyvinylchloride-polyvinylacetate copolymer-acrylate (PVCAC acrylate) in contact with the product and an aluminium bottom foil with polyvinylchloride (PVC) in contact with the product.

Polypropylene bottle with a screw cap containing 60 hard capsules.

Not all pack sizes may be marketed.

6.6 Special precautions for disposal and other handling

When taking Pradaxa capsules out of the blister pack, the following instructions should be followed:

• The hard capsules should be taken out of the blister card by peeling off the backing foil.

• The hard capsules should not be pushed through the blister foil.

• The blister foil should only be peeled off, when a hard capsule is required.

When taking a hard capsule out of the bottle, please observe the following instructions:

• The cap opens by pushing and turning.

Any unused product or waste material should be disposed of in accordance with local requirements.

7. MARKETING AUTHORISATION HOLDER

Boehringer Ingelheim International GmbH

D-55216 Ingelheim am Rhein

Germany

8. MARKETING AUTHORISATION NUMBER(S)

EU/1/08/442/001 - 10 × 1 capsules - blister (alu/alu)

EU/1/08/442/002 - 30 × 1 capsules - blister (alu/alu)

EU/1/08/442/003 - 60 × 1 capsules - blister (alu/alu)

EU/1/08/442/004 - 60 capsules - bottle (PP)

9. DATE OF FIRST AUTHORISATION/RENEWAL OF THE AUTHORISATION

18th March 2008

10. DATE OF REVISION OF THE TEXT

25th March 2009

LEGAL CATEGORY

POM

Prandin 0.5mg, 1mg, 2mg Tablets

(Daiichi Sankyo UK Limited)

1. NAME OF THE MEDICINAL PRODUCT

Prandin 0.5 mg tablets

Prandin 1 mg tablets

Prandin 2 mg tablets

2. QUALITATIVE AND QUANTITATIVE COMPOSITION

Repaglinide 0.5 mg or Repaglinide 1 mg or Repaglinide 2 mg respectively.

For a full list of excipients, see section 6.1.

3. PHARMACEUTICAL FORM

Tablet

Repaglinide tablets are white (0.5 mg), yellow (1 mg), or peach-coloured (2 mg), round and convex and engraved with Novo Nordisk logo (Apis bull).

4. CLINICAL PARTICULARS

4.1 Therapeutic indications

Repaglinide is indicated in patients with type 2 diabetes (Non Insulin-Dependent Diabetes Mellitus (NIDDM)) whose hyperglycaemia can no longer be controlled satisfactorily by diet, weight reduction and exercise. Repaglinide is also indicated in combination with metformin in type 2 diabetes patients who are not satisfactorily controlled on metformin alone.

Treatment should be initiated as an adjunct to diet and exercise to lower the blood glucose in relation to meals.

4.2 Posology and method of administration

Repaglinide is given preprandially and is titrated individually to optimise glycaemic control. In addition to the usual self-monitoring by the patient of blood and/or urinary glucose, the patient's blood glucose must be monitored periodically by the physician to determine the minimum effective dose for the patient. Glycosylated haemoglobin levels are also of value in monitoring the patient's response to therapy. Periodic monitoring is necessary to detect inadequate lowering of blood glucose at the recommended maximum dose level (i.e. primary failure) and to detect loss of adequate blood glucose-lowering response after an initial period of effectiveness (i.e. secondary failure).

Short-term administration of repaglinide may be sufficient during periods of transient loss of control in type 2 diabetic patients usually controlled well on diet.

Repaglinide should be taken before main meals (i.e. preprandially).

Doses are usually taken within 15 minutes of the meal but time may vary from immediately preceding the meal to as long as 30 minutes before the meal (i.e. preprandially 2, 3, or 4 meals a day). Patients who skip a meal (or add an extra meal) should be instructed to skip (or add) a dose for that meal.

In the case of concomitant use with other active substances refer to sections 4.4 and 4.5 to assess the dosage.

Initial dose

The dosage should be determined by the physician, according to the patient's requirements.

The recommended starting dose is 0.5 mg. One to two weeks should elapse between titration steps (as determined by blood glucose response).

If patients are transferred from another oral hypoglycaemic agent the recommended starting dose is 1 mg.

Maintenance

The recommended maximum single dose is 4 mg taken with main meals.

The total maximum daily dose should not exceed 16 mg.

Specific patient groups

Repaglinide is primarily excreted via the bile and excretion is therefore not affected by renal disorders.

Eight percent of one dose of repaglinide is excreted through the kidneys and total plasma clearance of the product is decreased in patients with renal impairment. As insulin sensitivity is increased in diabetic patients with renal impairment, caution is advised when titrating these patients.

No clinical studies have been conducted in patients > 75 years of age or in patients with hepatic insufficiency (see section 4.4).

Repaglinide is not recommended for use in children below age 18 due to a lack of data on safety and/or efficacy.

In debilitated or malnourished patients the initial and maintenance dosage should be conservative and careful dose titration is required to avoid hypoglycaemic reactions.

Patients receiving other oral hypoglycaemic agents (OHAs)

Patients can be transferred directly from other oral hypoglycaemic agents to repaglinide. However, no exact dosage relationship exists between repaglinide and the other oral hypoglycaemic agents. The recommended maximum starting dose of patients transferred to repaglinide is 1 mg given before main meals.

Repaglinide can be given in combination with metformin, when the blood glucose is insufficiently controlled with metformin alone. In this case, the dosage of metformin should be maintained and repaglinide administered concomitantly. The starting dose of repaglinide is 0.5 mg, taken before main meals; titration is according to blood glucose response as for monotherapy.

4.3 Contraindications

• Hypersensitivity to repaglinide or to any of the excipients in Prandin

• Type 1 diabetes (Insulin-Dependent Diabetes Mellitus: IDDM), C-peptide negative

• Diabetic ketoacidosis, with or without coma

• Severe hepatic function disorder

• Concomitant use of gemfibrozil (see section 4.5).

4.4 Special warnings and precautions for use

General

Repaglinide should only be prescribed if poor blood glucose control and symptoms of diabetes persist despite adequate attempts at dieting, exercise and weight reduction.

Repaglinide like other insulin secretagogues, is capable of producing hypoglycaemia.

The blood glucose-lowering effect of oral hypoglycaemic agents decreases in many patients over time. This may be due to progression of the severity of the diabetes or to diminished responsiveness to the product. This phenomenon is known as secondary failure, to distinguish it from primary failure, where the drug is ineffective in an individual patient when first given. Adjustment of dose and adherence to diet and exercise should be assessed before classifying a patient as a secondary failure.

Repaglinide acts through a distinct binding site with a short action on the β-cells. Use of repaglinide in case of secondary failure to insulin secretagogues has not been investigated in clinical trials.

Trials investigating the combination with other insulin secretagogues and acarbose have not been performed.

Trials of combination therapy with Neutral Protamine Hagedorn (NPH) insulin or thiazolidinediones have been performed. However, the benefit risk profile remains to be established when comparing to other combination therapies.

Combination treatment with metformin is associated with an increased risk of hypoglycaemia.

When a patient stabilised on any oral hypoglycaemic agent is exposed to stress such as fever, trauma, infection or surgery, a loss of glycaemic control may occur. At such times, it may be necessary to discontinue repaglinide and treat with insulin on a temporary basis.

The use of repaglinide might be associated with an increased incidence of acute coronary syndrome (e.g. myocardial infarction) (see sections 4.8 and 5.1).

Concomitant use

Repaglinide should be used with caution or be avoided in patients receiving drugs which influence repaglinide metabolism (see section 4.5). If concomitant use is necessary, careful monitoring of blood glucose and close clinical monitoring should be performed.

Specific patient groups

No clinical studies have been conducted in patients with impaired hepatic function. No clinical studies have been performed in children and adolescents < 18 years of age or in patients > 75 years of age. Therefore, treatment is not recommended in these patient groups.

Careful dose titration is recommended in debilitated or malnourished patients. The initial and maintenance dosages should be conservative (see section 4.2).

4.5 Interaction with other medicinal products and other forms of interaction

A number of drugs are known to influence repaglinide metabolism. Possible interactions should therefore be taken into account by the physician:

In vitro data indicate that repaglinide is metabolised predominantly by CYP2C8, but also by CYP3A4. Clinical data in healthy volunteers support CYP2C8 as being the most important enzyme involved in repaglinide metabolism with CYP3A4 playing a minor role, but the relative contribution of CYP3A4 can be increased if CYP2C8 is inhibited. Consequently metabolism, and by that clearance of repaglinide, may be altered by drugs which influence these cytochrome P-450 enzymes via inhibition or induction. Special care should be taken when both inhibitors of CYP2C8 and 3A4 are co-administered simultaneously with repaglinide.

Based on *in vitro* data, repaglinide appears to be a substrate for active hepatic uptake (organic anion transporting protein OATP1B1). Drugs that inhibit OATP1B1 may likewise have the potential to increase plasma concentrations of repaglinide, as has been shown for ciclosporin (see below).

The following substances may enhance and/or prolong the hypoglycaemic effect of repaglinide: Gemfibrozil, clarithromycin, itraconazole, ketoconazole, trimethoprim, ciclosporin, other antidiabetic agents, monoamine oxidase inhibitors (MAOI), non selective beta blocking agents, angiotensin converting enzyme (ACE)-inhibitors, salicylates, NSAIDs, octreotide, alcohol, and anabolic steroids.

Co-administration of gemfibrozil (600 mg twice daily), an inhibitor of CYP2C8, and repaglinide (a single dose of 0.25 mg) increased the repaglinide AUC 8.1-fold and C_{max} 2.4-fold in healthy volunteers. Half-life was prolonged from 1.3 hr to 3.7 hr, resulting in possibly enhanced and prolonged blood glucose-lowering effect of repaglinide, and plasma repaglinide concentration at 7 hr was increased 28.6-fold by gemfibrozil. The concomitant use of gemfibrozil and repaglinide is contraindicated (see section 4.3).

Co-administration of trimethoprim (160 mg twice daily), a moderate CYP2C8 inhibitor, and repaglinide (a single dose of 0.25 mg) increased the repaglinide AUC, C_{max} and $t_{½}$ (1.6-fold, 1.4-fold and 1.2-fold respectively) with no statistically significant effects on the blood glucose levels. This lack of pharmacodynamic effect was observed with a sub-therapeutic dose of repaglinide. Since the safety profile of this combination has not been established with dosages higher than 0.25 mg for repaglinide and 320 mg for trimethoprim, the concomitant use of trimethoprim with repaglinide should be avoided. If concomitant use is necessary, careful monitoring of blood glucose and close clinical monitoring should be performed (see section 4.4).

Rifampicin, a potent inducer of CYP3A4, but also CYP2C8, acts both as an inducer and inhibitor of the metabolism of repaglinide. Seven days pre-treatment with rifampicin (600 mg), followed by co-administration of repaglinide (a single dose of 4 mg) at day seven resulted in a 50% lower AUC (effect of a combined induction and inhibition). When repaglinide was given 24 hours after the last rifampicin dose, an 80% reduction of the repaglinide AUC was observed (effect of induction alone). Concomitant use of rifampicin and repaglinide might therefore induce a need for repaglinide dose adjustment which should be based on carefully monitored blood glucose concentrations at both initiation of rifampicin treatment (acute inhibition), following dosing (mixed inhibition and induction), withdrawal (induction alone) and up to approximately two weeks after withdrawal of rifampicin where the inductive effect of rifampicin is no longer present. It can not be excluded that other inducers, e.g. phenytoin, carbamazepine, phenobarbital, St John's wort, may have a similar effect.

The effect of ketoconazole, a prototype of potent and competitive inhibitors of CYP3A4, on the pharmacokinetics of repaglinide has been studied in healthy subjects.

Co-administration of 200 mg ketoconazole increased the repaglinide (AUC and C_{max}) by 1.2-fold with profiles of blood glucose concentrations altered by less than 8% when administered concomitantly (a single dose of 4 mg repaglinide). Co-administration of 100 mg itraconazole, an inhibitor of CYP3A4, has also been studied in healthy volunteers, and increased the AUC by 1.4-fold. No significant effect on the glucose level in healthy volunteers was observed. In an interaction study in healthy volunteers, co-administration of 250 mg clarithromycin, a potent mechanism-based inhibitor of CYP3A4, slightly increased the repaglinide (AUC) by 1.4-fold and C_{max} by 1.7-fold and increased the mean incremental AUC of serum insulin by 1.5-fold and the maximum concentration by 1.6-fold. The exact mechanism of this interaction is not clear.

In a study conducted in healthy volunteers, the concomitant administration of repaglinide (a single dose of 0.25 mg) and ciclosporin (repeated dose at 100 mg) increased repaglinide AUC and C_{max} about 2.5-fold and 1.8-fold respectively. Since the interaction has not been established with dosages higher than 0.25 mg for repaglinide, the concomitant use of ciclosporin with repaglinide should be avoided. If the combination appears necessary, careful clinical and blood glucose monitoring should be performed (see section 4.4).

β-blocking agents may mask the symptoms of hypoglycaemia.

Co-administration of cimetidine, nifedipine, oestrogen, or simvastatin with repaglinide, all CYP3A4 substrates, did not significantly alter the pharmacokinetic parameters of repaglinide.

Repaglinide had no clinically relevant effect on the pharmacokinetic properties of digoxin, theophylline or warfarin at steady state, when administered to healthy volunteers. Dosage adjustment of these compounds when co-administered with repaglinide is therefore not necessary.

The following substances may reduce the hypoglycaemic effect of repaglinide:

Oral contraceptives, rifampicin, barbiturates, carbamazepine, thiazides, corticosteroids, danazol, thyroid hormones and sympathomimetics.

When these medications are administered to or withdrawn from a patient receiving repaglinide, the patient should be observed closely for changes in glycaemic control.

When repaglinide is used together with other drugs that are mainly secreted by the bile, like repaglinide, any potential interaction should be considered.

4.6 Pregnancy and lactation

There are no studies of repaglinide in pregnant or lactating women. Therefore the safety of repaglinide in pregnant women cannot be assessed. Up to now repaglinide showed not to be teratogenic in animal studies. Embryotoxicity, abnormal limb development in foetuses and new born pups, was observed in rats exposed to high doses in the last stage of pregnancy and during the lactation period. Repaglinide is detected in the milk of experimental animals. For that reason repaglinide should be avoided during pregnancy and should not be used in lactating women.

4.7 Effects on ability to drive and use machines

Patients should be advised to take precautions to avoid hypoglycaemia whilst driving. This is particularly important in those who have reduced or absent awareness of the warning signs of hypoglycaemia or have frequent episodes of hypoglycaemia. The advisability of driving should be considered in these circumstances.

4.8 Undesirable effects

Based on the experience with repaglinide and with other hypoglycaemic agents the following adverse events have been seen: Frequencies are defined as: Common (≥1/100 to <1/10); uncommon (≥1/1,000 to <1/100); rare (≥ 1/10,000 to < 1/1,000); very rare (< 1/10,000); not known (cannot be estimated from the available data).

Immune system disorders

Very rare: Allergy

Generalised hypersensitivity reactions (e.g. anaphylactic reaction), or immunological reactions such as vasculitis.

Metabolism and nutrition disorders

Common: Hypoglycaemia

Not known: Hypoglycaemic coma and hypoglycaemic unconsciousness

As with other hypoglycaemic agents, hypoglycaemic reactions have been observed after administration of repaglinide. These reactions are mostly mild and easily handled through intake of carbohydrates. If severe, requiring third party assistance, infusion of glucose may be necessary. The occurrence of such reactions depends, as for every diabetes therapy, on individual factors, such as dietary habits, dosage, exercise and stress (see section 4.4). Interactions with other medicinal products may increase the risk of hypoglycaemia (see section 4.5). During post marketing experience, cases of hypoglycaemia have been reported in patients treated with repaglinide in combination with metformin or thiazolidinedione.

Gastro-intestinal disorders

Common: Abdominal pain and diarrhoea

Very rare: Vomiting and constipation

Not known: Nausea

Gastro-intestinal complaints such as abdominal pain, diarrhoea, nausea, vomiting and constipation have been reported in clinical trials. The rate and severity of these symptoms did not differ from that seen with other oral insulin secretagogues.

Skin and subcutaneous tissue disorders

Not known: Hypersensitivity

Hypersensitivity reactions of the skin may occur as erythema, itching, rashes and urticaria. There is no reason to suspect cross-allergenicity with sulphonylurea drugs due to the difference of the chemical structure.

Eye disorders

Very rare: Visual disturbances

Changes in blood glucose levels have been known to result in transient visual disturbances, especially at the commencement of treatment. Such disturbances have only been reported in very few cases after initiation of repaglinide treatment. No such cases have led to discontinuation of repaglinide treatment in clinical trials.

Cardiac disorders

Rare: Cardiovascular disease

Type 2 diabetes is associated with an increased risk for cardiovascular disease. In one epidemiological study, a higher incidence of acute coronary syndrome was reported in the repaglinide group. However, the causality of the relationship remains uncertain (see sections 4.4 and 5.1).

Hepato-biliary disorders

Very rare: Hepatic function abnormal

In very rare cases, severe hepatic dysfunction has been reported. However, a causal relationship with repaglinide has not been established.

Very rare: Increased liver enzymes

Isolated cases of increase in liver enzymes have been reported during treatment with repaglinide. Most cases were mild and transient, and very few patients discontinued treatment due to increase in liver enzymes.

4.9 Overdose

Repaglinide has been given with weekly escalating doses from 4 - 20 mg four times daily in a 6 week period. No safety concerns were raised. As hypoglycaemia in this study was avoided through increased calorie intake, a relative overdose may result in an exaggerated glucose-lowering effect with development of hypoglycaemic symptoms (dizziness, sweating, tremor, headache etc.). Should these symptoms occur, adequate action should be taken to correct the low blood glucose (oral carbohydrates). More severe hypoglycaemia with seizure, loss of consciousness or coma should be treated with IV glucose.

5. PHARMACOLOGICAL PROPERTIES

5.1 Pharmacodynamic properties

Pharmaco-therapeutic group: Carbamoylmethyl benzoic acid derivative, ATC code: A10B X02

Repaglinide is a novel short-acting oral secretagogue. Repaglinide lowers the blood glucose levels acutely by stimulating the release of insulin from the pancreas, an effect dependent upon functioning β-cells in the pancreatic islets.

Repaglinide closes ATP-dependent potassium channels in the β-cell membrane via a target protein different from other secretagogues. This depolarises the β-cell and leads to an opening of the calcium channels. The resulting increased calcium influx induces insulin secretion from the β-cell.

In type 2 diabetic patients, the insulinotropic response to a meal occurred within 30 minutes after an oral dose of repaglinide. This resulted in a blood glucose-lowering effect throughout the meal period. The elevated insulin levels did not persist beyond the time of the meal challenge. Plasma repaglinide levels decreased rapidly, and low drug concentrations were seen in the plasma of type 2 diabetic patients 4 hours post-administration.

A dose-dependent decrease in blood glucose was demonstrated in type 2 diabetic patients when administered in doses from 0.5 to 4 mg repaglinide.

Clinical study results have shown that repaglinide is optimally dosed in relation to main meals (preprandial dosing).

Doses are usually taken within 15 minutes of the meal, but the time may vary from immediately preceding the meal to as long as 30 minutes before the meal.

One epidemiological study suggested an increased risk of acute coronary syndrome in repaglinide treated patients as compared to sulfonylurea treated patients (see sections 4.4 and 4.8).

5.2 Pharmacokinetic properties

Repaglinide is rapidly absorbed from the gastrointestinal tract, which leads to a rapid increase in the plasma concentration of the drug. The peak plasma level occurs within one hour post administration. After reaching a maximum, the plasma level decreases rapidly, and repaglinide is eliminated within 4 - 6 hours. The plasma elimination half-life is approximately one hour.

Repaglinide pharmacokinetics are characterised by a mean absolute bioavailability of 63% (CV 11%), low volume of distribution, 30 L (consistent with distribution into intracellular fluid), and rapid elimination from the blood.

A high interindividual variability (60%) in repaglinide plasma concentrations has been detected in the clinical trials. Intraindividual variability is low to moderate (35%) and as repaglinide should be titrated against the clinical response, efficacy is not affected by interindividual variability.

Repaglinide exposure is increased in patients with hepatic insufficiency and in the elderly type 2 diabetic patients. The AUC (SD) after 2 mg single dose exposure (4 mg in patients with hepatic insufficiency) was 31.4 ng/ml × hr (28.3) in healthy volunteers, 304.9 ng/ml × hr (228.0) in patients with hepatic insufficiency, and 117.9 ng/ml × hr (83.8) in the elderly type 2 diabetic patients.

After a 5 day treatment of repaglinide (2 mg × 3/day) in patients with a severe impaired renal function (creatinine clearance: 20-39 ml/min.), the results showed a significant 2-fold increase of the exposure (AUC) and half-life ($t_{1/2}$) as compared to subjects with normal renal function.

Repaglinide is highly bound to plasma proteins in humans (greater than 98%).

No clinically relevant differences were seen in the pharmacokinetics of repaglinide, when repaglinide was administered 0, 15 or 30 minutes before a meal or in fasting state.

Repaglinide is almost completely metabolised, and no metabolites with clinically relevant hypoglycaemic effect have been identified.

Repaglinide and its metabolites are excreted primarily via the bile. A small fraction (less than 8%) of the administered dose appears in the urine, primarily as metabolites. Less than 1% of the parent drug is recovered in faeces.

5.3 Preclinical safety data

Non-clinical data revealed no special hazard for humans based on conventional studies of safety pharmacology, repeated dose toxicity, genotoxicity and carcinogenic potential.

6. PHARMACEUTICAL PARTICULARS

6.1 List of excipients

Microcrystalline cellulose (E460)

Calcium hydrogen phosphate, anhydrous

Maize starch

Amberlite (polacrilin potassium)

Povidone (polyvidone)

Glycerol 85%

Magnesium stearate

Meglumine

Poloxamer

Iron oxide, yellow (1 mg tablets only) (E172)

Iron oxide, red (2 mg tablets only) (E172)

6.2 Incompatibilities

Not applicable.

6.3 Shelf life

5 years.

6.4 Special precautions for storage

Store in the original package.

6.5 Nature and contents of container

The blister pack (aluminium/aluminium) contains 30, 90, 120 or 270 tablets, respectively.

Not all pack sizes may be marketed.

6.6 Special precautions for disposal and other handling

No special requirements.

7. MARKETING AUTHORISATION HOLDER

Novo Nordisk A/S

Novo Allé

DK-2880 Bagsværd

Denmark

8. MARKETING AUTHORISATION NUMBER(S)

Prandin 0.5 mg EU/1/00/162/003-005, EU/1/00/162/021

Prandin 1 mg EU/1/00/162/009-011, EU/1/00/162/020

Prandin 2 mg EU/1/00/162/015-017, EU/1/00/162/019

9. DATE OF FIRST AUTHORISATION/RENEWAL OF THE AUTHORISATION

Date of first authorisation: 29 January 2001

Date of last renewal: 23 July 2008

10. DATE OF REVISION OF THE TEXT

12/2008

Praxilene

(Merck Serono)

1. NAME OF THE MEDICINAL PRODUCT

Praxilene 100mg Capsules

2. QUALITATIVE AND QUANTITATIVE COMPOSITION

100mg naftidrofuryl oxalate equivalent to 81.0 mg naftidrofuryl and 19.0 mg oxalate.

3. PHARMACEUTICAL FORM

Capsule

4. CLINICAL PARTICULARS

4.1 Therapeutic indications

Peripheral vascular disorders - intermittent claudication, night cramps, rest pain, incipient gangrene, trophic ulcers, Raynaud's Syndrome, diabetic arteriopathy and acrocyanosis.

Cerebral vascular disorders - cerebral insufficiency and cerebral atherosclerosis, particularly where these manifest themselves as mental deterioration and confusion in the elderly.

4.2 Posology and method of administration

Peripheral vascular disorders - one or two capsules three times daily for a minimum of three months, or at the discretion of the physician.

Cerebral vascular disorders - one 100mg capsule three times daily for a minimum of three months, or at the discretion of the physician.

There is no recommended use for children.

Administration:

For oral administration. The capsules should be swallowed whole during meals with a sufficient amount of water (minimum) of one glass.

4.3 Contraindications

Hypersensitivity to the drug. Patients with a history of hyperoxaluria or recurrent calcium-containing stones.

4.4 Special warnings and precautions for use

A sufficient amount of liquid should be taken during treatment to maintain an adequate level of diuresis.

4.5 Interaction with other medicinal products and other forms of interaction

None known.

4.6 Pregnancy and lactation

Pregnancy: There is no, or inadequate, evidence of the safety of naftidrofuryl oxalate in human pregnancy, but it has been in wide use for many years without apparent ill consequence, animal studies having shown no hazard. If drug therapy is needed in pregnancy, this drug can be used if there is no safer alternative.

Lactation: No information is available.

4.7 Effects on ability to drive and use machines

None known.

4.8 Undesirable effects

Naftidrofuryl oxalate is normally well tolerated in the dosage recommended. Occasionally nausea, epigastric pain and rashes have been noted.

Rarely, hepatitis has been reported. Very rarely, calcium oxalate kidney stones have been reported.

4.9 Overdose

Signs and symptoms: Depression of cardiac conduction and convulsions may occur.

Treatment: The stomach should be emptied by gastric lavage and emesis. Activated charcoal may be employed if necessary. Cardiovascular function and respiration should be monitored and, in severe cases, electrical pacemaking or the use of isoprenaline should be considered. Convulsions may be managed by diazepam.

5. PHARMACOLOGICAL PROPERTIES

5.1 Pharmacodynamic properties

Naftidrofuryl oxalate has been shown to exert a direct effect on intracellular metabolism. Thus it has been shown in man and animals that it produces an increase of ATP levels and a decrease of lactic acid levels in ischaemic conditions, evidence for an enhancement of cellular oxidative capacity. Furthermore, naftidrofuryl oxalate is a powerful spasmolytic agent.

5.2 Pharmacokinetic properties

Naftidrofuryl oxalate is well absorbed when given orally. Peak plasma levels occur about 30 minutes after dosing and the half life is about an hour, although inter subject variation is relatively high. Accumulation does not occur at a dose level of 200mg three times daily.

The drug becomes extensively bound to plasma proteins and is excreted principally via the urine, all in the form of metabolites.

5.3 Preclinical safety data

No toxic effects were seen in animal studies which provide additional information to that obtained in man. In repeated dose studies the no effect level was 25mg/kg/day or greater. There was no evidence of effects on reproduction below doses which caused maternal toxicity.

6. PHARMACEUTICAL PARTICULARS

6.1 List of excipients

Talc

Magnesium Stearate

Purified Water*

Denatured Ethanol*

Capsule Shells:

Erythrosine (E127)

Titanium Dioxide (E171)

Gelatine

Printing ink:

Black iron oxide (E172)

*Not present in final product

6.2 Incompatibilities

None known.

6.3 Shelf life

36 months.

6.4 Special precautions for storage

Store below 20°C in a dry place away from light.

6.5 Nature and contents of container

Pack size 10 (medical sample), 21 and 84 capsules:-

Cardboard carton containing blister strips comprising heat-sealable PVC (250μm) and aluminium foil (30μm).

Pack size 100 and 500:

Polyethylene securitainers with tamper evident closures.

6.6 Special precautions for disposal and other handling

None.

7. MARKETING AUTHORISATION HOLDER

Merck Serono Ltd

Bedfont Cross

Stanwell Road

Feltham

Middlesex

TW14 8NX, UK

8. MARKETING AUTHORISATION NUMBER(S)

PL 11648/0064

9. DATE OF FIRST AUTHORISATION/RENEWAL OF THE AUTHORISATION

24 March 2009

10. DATE OF REVISION OF THE TEXT

24 March 2009

Pred Forte

(Allergan Ltd)

1. NAME OF THE MEDICINAL PRODUCT

PRED FORTE®

2. QUALITATIVE AND QUANTITATIVE COMPOSITION

1% w/v prednisolone acetate

3. PHARMACEUTICAL FORM

Eye Drops

4. CLINICAL PARTICULARS

4.1 Therapeutic indications

For short-term treatment of steroid-responsive inflammatory conditions of the eye, after excluding the presence of viral, fungal and bacterial pathogens.

4.2 Posology and method of administration

Route of administration is by ocular instillation.

Adults: One to two drops instilled into the conjunctival sac two to four times daily. During the initial 24 to 48 hours the dosing frequency may be safely increased to 2 drops every hour. Care should be taken not to discontinue therapy prematurely.

Children and elderly patients: Pred Forte has not specifically been studied in these patient groups. No adjustment in the adult dosage regimen is recommended.

4.3 Contraindications

Acute untreated purulent ocular infections. Acute superficial herpes simplex (dendritic keratitis); vaccinia, varicella and most other viral diseases of the cornea and conjunctiva. Fungal diseases of the eye. Ocular tuberculosis. Sensitivity to any component of the formulation.

4.4 Special warnings and precautions for use

Acute purulent infections of the eye may be masked or enhanced by the use of topical steroids. Pred Forte contains no antimicrobial agent. If infection is present, appropriate measures must be taken to counteract the infective organisms.

Fungal infections of the cornea have been reported coincidentally with long-term steroid application and fungal invasion may be suspected in any persistent corneal ulceration where a steroid has been used, or is in use.

Various ocular diseases and long-term use of topical corticosteroids have been known to cause corneal or scleral thinning. Use of topical corticosteroids in the presence of thin corneal or scleral tissue may lead to perforation.

Pred Forte contains benzalkonium chloride as a preservative and should not be used in patients continuing to wear soft (hydrophilic) contact lenses.

Patients with a history of herpes simplex keratitis should be treated with caution. Use of steroid medication in the presence of stromal herpes simplex requires caution and should be followed by frequent, mandatory, slit-lamp microscopy.

Use of topical corticosteroids may cause an increase in intraocular pressure in certain individuals. This may result in damage to the optic nerve with resultant defects in visual fields. It is advisable that intraocular pressure be checked frequently during treatment with Pred Forte.

4.5 Interaction with other medicinal products and other forms of interaction

None known

4.6 Pregnancy and lactation

There is inadequate evidence of safety in human pregnancy. Administration of corticosteroids to pregnant animals can cause abnormalities of foetal development including cleft palate and intra-uterine growth retardation. There may therefore be a very small risk of such defects in the human foetus.

4.7 Effects on ability to drive and use machines

Pred Forte may cause short-lasting blurring of vision upon instillation. If affected, the patient should not use machinery/electric tools or drive until vision has returned to normal.

4.8 Undesirable effects

Ocular: irritation, burning or stinging sensations, allergic reaction, blurred vision; increased intraocular pressure; secondary ocular infections from fungi or viruses liberated from ocular tissues; perforation of the globe when used in conditions where there is a thinning of the cornea or sclera. Posterior subcapsular cataract formation has been reported after heavy or protracted use of topical ophthalmic corticosteroids.

Systemic: extensive topical use of corticosteroids may lead to systemic side effects.

4.9 Overdose

There is no clinical experience of overdosage. Acute overdosage is unlikely to occur via the ophthalmic route.

5. PHARMACOLOGICAL PROPERTIES

5.1 Pharmacodynamic properties

Prednisolone acetate is a synthetic adrenocorticoid with the general properties of prednisolone. Adrenocorticoids diffuse across cell membranes to complex with cytoplasmic receptors and subsequently stimulate synthesis of enzymes with anti-inflammatory effects. Glucocorticoids inhibit the oedema, fibrin deposition, capillary dilation and phagocytic migration of the acute inflammatory response as well as capillary proliferation, deposition of collagen and scar formation.

Prednisolone acetate has, on a weight to weight basis, a potency three to five times that of hydrocortisone.

5.2 Pharmacokinetic properties

Prednisolone acetate has been shown to penetrate rapidly the cornea after topical application of a suspension preparation. Aqueous humour T_{max} occurs between 30 and 45 minutes after installation. The half life of prednisolone acetate in human aqueous humour is approximately 30 minutes.

5.3 Preclinical safety data

Not applicable

6. PHARMACEUTICAL PARTICULARS

6.1 List of excipients

Benzalkonium chloride

Hydroxypropylmethylcellulose

Polysorbate 80

Boric acid

Sodium citrate

Sodium chloride

Disodium edetate

Purified water

6.2 Incompatibilities

None known

6.3 Shelf life

24 months unopened.

28 days after first opening.

6.4 Special precautions for storage

Do not store above 25°C. Do not freeze.

6.5 Nature and contents of container

5 ml and 10 ml bottles and dropper tips composed of low density polyethylene. Screw caps are medium impact polystyrene.

6.6 Special precautions for disposal and other handling

Shake the bottle well before use.

7. MARKETING AUTHORISATION HOLDER

Allergan Ltd

Marlow International

The Parkway

Marlow

Bucks

SL7 1YL

UK

8. MARKETING AUTHORISATION NUMBER(S)

PL 00426/0051

9. DATE OF FIRST AUTHORISATION/RENEWAL OF THE AUTHORISATION

18th March 2003

10. DATE OF REVISION OF THE TEXT

20th December 2007

Predfoam

(Forest Laboratories UK Limited)

1. NAME OF THE MEDICINAL PRODUCT
PREDFOAM

2. QUALITATIVE AND QUANTITATIVE COMPOSITION
Each metered dose contains 31.4mg of the active ingredient prednisolone sodium metasulphobenzoate, equivalent to prednisolone 20.0mg.

3. PHARMACEUTICAL FORM
Aerosol foam for rectal administration

4. CLINICAL PARTICULARS

4.1 Therapeutic indications
Treatment of proctitis and ulcerative colitis.

4.2 Posology and method of administration
For adults and elderly patients:

One metered dose rectally once or twice daily for 2 weeks, extending treatment for a further 2 weeks when a good response is obtained. Use should be discontinued at the discretion of the physician once the disease is stable and under control.

For children:

Not recommended.

4.3 Contraindications
Corticosteroids are contra-indicated in local conditions where infection might be masked or healing impaired, e.g. peritonitis fistulae, intestinal obstruction, perforation of the bowel.

4.4 Special warnings and precautions for use
This product should be used with extreme caution in the presence of severe ulcerative colitis. The possibility of masking local or systemic infection should be borne in mind when using this product.

For rectal use only

4.5 Interaction with other medicinal products and other forms of interaction
None stated

4.6 Pregnancy and lactation
There is inadequate evidence of safety in human pregnancy. Topical administration of corticosteroids to pregnant animals can cause abnormalities in foetal development including cleft palate and intrauterine growth retardation. There may therefore be a very small risk of such effects in the human foetus.

4.7 Effects on ability to drive and use machines
None stated

4.8 Undesirable effects
The consequences of systemic absorption should be considered if Predfoam is used extensively over prolonged periods. As with all rectal corticosteroids, prolonged continuous use is undesirable.

4.9 Overdose
Overdosage by this route is unlikely.

5. PHARMACOLOGICAL PROPERTIES

5.1 Pharmacodynamic properties
Prednisolone sodium metasulphobenzoate is a synthetic glucocorticoid with anti-inflammatory action. The product is given rectally to enable local treatment and to reduce side-effects associated with systemic administration of steroids.

5.2 Pharmacokinetic properties
None stated

5.3 Preclinical safety data
There are no preclinical data of relevance to the prescriber which are additional to that already included in other sections of the SPC.

6. PHARMACEUTICAL PARTICULARS

6.1 List of excipients
Non-ionic Emulsifying Wax

Cetostearyl Alcohol

Oleyl Alcohol

Technical White Oils

Phenoxyethanol

Sorbic Acid

Polysorbate 20

Disodium Edetate

Sodium Hydroxide

Purified Water

Butane 48

6.2 Incompatibilities
None stated

6.3 Shelf life
4 years

6.4 Special precautions for storage
Pressurised container containing a flammable propellant. Do not store above 25°C. Protect from sunlight and do not expose to temperatures exceeding 50°C. Do not pierce or burn even after use. Do not spray on naked flame or any incandescent material.

Do not refrigerate

6.5 Nature and contents of container
Each pack contains an aluminium aerosol can fitted with a metering valve containing sufficient for 14 doses plus 14 disposable applicators.

6.6 Special precautions for disposal and other handling
Shake canister before use. When using for the first time remove and discard the small plastic safety tag from under the button. An applicator nozzle is then pushed on to the side arm of the canister. The semi-circular cut-out on the cap is lined up with the nozzle.

The easiest way to administer Predfoam is to stand with one foot raised on a chair and gently insert the nozzle tip into the rectum. Smearing the nozzle with lubricating jelly may help insertion. Holding the canister with the dose button pointing down, press the button on the canister firmly and release. Only press the button once so as not to exceed the recommended dose.

7. MARKETING AUTHORISATION HOLDER
Forest Laboratories UK Limited

Bourne Road

Bexley

Kent DA5 1NX

8. MARKETING AUTHORISATION NUMBER(S)
PL 0108/0101

9. DATE OF FIRST AUTHORISATION/RENEWAL OF THE AUTHORISATION
9 September 1986 / 7 October 1998

10. DATE OF REVISION OF THE TEXT
September 1998

11. Legal Category
POM

Predsol Retention Enema

(UCB Pharma Limited)

1. NAME OF THE MEDICINAL PRODUCT
Predsol Retention Enema

2. QUALITATIVE AND QUANTITATIVE COMPOSITION
20mg prednisolone as the sodium phosphate ester.

For excipients, see 6.1

3. PHARMACEUTICAL FORM
Rectal Solution

100ml disposable plastic bottles, each containing 20mg prednisolone as the sodium phosphate ester in a buffered solution. The product complies with the specification for Prednisolone Enema BP.

4. CLINICAL PARTICULARS

4.1 Therapeutic indications
Predsol Retention Enema provides local corticosteroid treatment for rectal and rectosigmoidal disease in ulcerative colitis and Crohn's disease.

4.2 Posology and method of administration
Adults

1 enema used nightly, for 2 to 4 weeks. Treatment may be continued in patients showing progressive improvement, but it should not be persisted with if the response has been inadequate. Some patients may relapse after an interval but are likely to respond equally well to a repeated course of treatment.

The enema is used each night on retiring. It may be warmed before administration by placing the bottle in a vessel of warm water for a few minutes. Before use lie in bed on the left side with knees drawn up. Hold the bottle upwards. Place hand in the protective plastic cover and remove the cap from the bottle. Attach the nozzle and lubricate with petroleum jelly. Gently insert about half the length of the nozzle into the rectum. The bottle should then be squeezed gently until it is emptied, taking a minute or two to do so. The nozzle should then be removed from the rectum. Invert the plastic protective cover around the bottle and discard the whole unit. The patient should then roll over to lie face down for 3 to 5 minutes but may sleep in any comfortable position.

Although predsol enema is applied locally, it should be born in mind that there is likely to be substantial systemic absorption, especially when the bowel is inflamed.

The volume of the enema is considered to be the optimum to ensure maximum coverage of the affected area. However, undesirable effects may be minimised by using for the minimum period. Frequent patient review is required to monitor therapeutic effect against disease activity.

Children

Predsol retention enema as packed is not suitable for use in children.

Route of Administration:

Rectal

4.3 Contraindications
Systemic or local infection unless specific anti-infective therapy is employed. Hypersensitivity to any ingredient.

4.4 Special warnings and precautions for use
Although Predsol Enema is applied locally, it should be borne in mind that there is likely to be substantial systemic absorption, especially when the bowel is inflamed.

The volume of the enema is considered to be the optimum to ensure maximum coverage of the affected area, however, undesirable effects may be minimised by using for the minimum period. Frequent patient review is required to monitor therapeutic effect against disease activity (see 'Posology and Method of Administration').

Suppression of the inflammatory response and immune system increases the susceptibility to infections and their severity. The clinical presentation may often be atypical and serious infections such as septicaemia and tuberculosis may be masked and may reach an advanced stage before being recognised.

Chickenpox is of particular concern since this normally minor illness may be fatal in immunosuppressed patients. Patients without a definite history of chickenpox should be advised to avoid close contact with chickenpox or herpes zoster and if exposed they should seek medical attention. Passive immunisation with varicella zoster immunoglobulin (VZIG) is needed by exposed non-immune patients who are receiving systemic corticosteroids or who have used them within the previous 3 months; this should be given within 10 days of exposure to chickenpox. If a diagnosis of chickenpox is confirmed, the illness warrants special care and urgent treatment. Corticosteroids should not be stopped and the dose may need to be increased.

Patients should be advised to take particular care to avoid exposure to measles and to seek immediate medical advice if exposure occurs. Prophylaxis with intramuscular normal immunoglobulin may be needed.

Live vaccines should not be given to individuals with impaired immune responsiveness. The antibody response to other vaccines may be diminished.

Corticosteroid treatment may reduce the response of the pituitary adrenal axis to stress, and relative insufficiency can persist for up to a year after withdrawal of prolonged therapy. Withdrawal of corticosteroids after prolonged therapy must therefore always be gradual to avoid acute adrenal insufficiency, being tapered off over weeks or months according to the dose and the duration of treatment. During prolonged therapy any intercurrent illness, trauma or surgical procedure will require a temporary increase in dosage; if corticosteroids have been stopped following prolonged therapy they may need to be temporarily re-introduced.

Use with caution in patients with myasthenia gravis, non-specific ulcerative colitis, diverticulitis and fresh intestinal anastamoses.

Special precautions

Particular care is required when considering the use of systemic corticosteroids in patients with the following conditions and frequent patient monitoring is necessary.

A. Osteoporosis (post-menopausal females are particularly at risk).

B. Hypertension or congestive heart failure.

C. Existing or previous history of severe affective disorders (especially previous steroid psychosis).

D. Diabetes mellitus (or a family history of diabetes).

E. History of tuberculosis.

F. Glaucoma (or a family history of glaucoma).

G. Previous corticosteroid-induced myopathy.

H. Liver failure - blood levels of corticosteroid may be increased, as with other drugs which are metabolised in the liver.

I. Renal insufficiency.

J. Epilepsy.

K. Peptic ulceration.

L. Hypothyroidism

M. Recent myocardial infarction.

Patients should carry "Steroid treatment" cards which give clear guidance on the precautions to be taken to minimise risk and which provide details of the prescriber, drug, dosage and the duration of treatment.

Patients/and or carers should be warned that potentially severe psychiatric adverse reactions may occur with systemic steroids (see section 4.8). Symptoms typically emerge within a few days or weeks of starting treatment. Risks may be higher with high doses/systemic exposure (see also section 4.5 pharmacokinetic interactions that can increase the risk of side effects), although dose levels do not allow prediction of the onset, type, severity or duration of reactions. Most reactions recover after either dose reduction or withdrawal, although specific treatment may be necessary. Patients/carers should be encouraged to seek medical advice if worrying psychological symptoms develop, especially if depressed mood or suicidal ideation is suspected. Patients/carers should also be alert to possible psychiatric disturbances that may occur either during or immediately after dose tapering/withdrawal of systemic steroids, although such reactions have been reported infrequently.

Particular care is required when considering the use of systemic corticosteroids in patients with existing or previous history of severe affective disorders in themselves or in their first degree relatives. These would include depressive or manic-depressive illness and previous steroid psychosis.

Use in the Elderly

The common adverse effects of systemic corticosteroids may be associated with more serious consequences in old age, especially osteoporosis, hypertension, hypokalaemia, diabetes, susceptibility to infection and thinning of the skin. Close clinical supervision is required to avoid life-threatening reactions.

4.5 Interaction with other medicinal products and other forms of interaction

Systemic absorption of prednisolone should be borne in mind, especially when there is local inflammation. Thus the following interactions are possible:

Analgesics:

Increased risk of gastro-intestinal bleeding and ulceration with aspirin and NSAIDs; the renal clearance of salicylates is increased by corticosteroids and steroid withdrawal may result in salicylate intoxication.

Antibacterials:

Rifamycins accelerate metabolism of corticosteroids (reduced effect); erythromycin inhibits metabolism of methylprednisolone and possibly other corticosteroids. *Fluoroquinolones* - Increased risk of tendon rupture.

Anticoagulants:

The efficacy of coumarin anticoagulants may be enhanced by concurrent corticosteroid therapy and close monitoring of the INR or prothrombin time is required to avoid spontaneous bleeding.

Antidiabetics:

Antagonism of hypoglycaemic effect.

Antiepileptics:

Carbamazepine, phenobarbital, phenytoin and primidone accelerate metabolism of corticosteroids (reduced effect).

Antifungals:

Increased risk of hypokalaemia with amphotericin (avoid concomitant use unless corticosteroids are required to control reactions); ketoconazole inhibits metabolism of methylprednisolone and possibly other corticosteroids.

Antihypertensives:

Antagonism of hypotensive effect.

Antimuscarinics:

Decreased effect of antimuscarinics in myasthenia gravis.

Antivirals:

Ritonavir possibly increases plasma concentration of prednisolone.

Cardiac Glycosides:

Increased toxicity if hypokalaemia occurs with corticosteroids.

Ciclosporin:

Increased plasma concentrations of prednisolone.

Cytotoxics:

Increased risk of haematological toxicity with methotrexate.

Diuretics:

Antagonism of diuretic effect; acetazolamide, loop diuretics, and thiazides increased risk of hypokalaemia.

Hormone antagonists:

Aminoglutethimide accelerates metabolism of corticosteroids (reduced effect).

Isoniazid:

Decreased isoniazid concentrations.

Licorice:

Increased corticosteroid levels.

Mifepristone:

Effects of corticosteroids may be reduced for 3-4 days after mifepristone.

Neuromuscular blockers:

Antagonism of the neuromuscular blockade.

Oral Contraceptives:

Alteration in the plasma protein binding and metabolism of prednisolone caused by oestrogens, with or without progesterone, can result in exposure of women to increased levels of unbound prednisolone for prolonged periods of time.

Quetiapine:

Decreased quetiapine concentrations.

Somatropin:

The growth promoting effect of somatropin may be inhibited.

Sympathomimetics:

Increased risk of hypokalaemia if high doses of corticosteroids given with high doses of bambuterol, fenoterol, formoterol, ritodrine, salbutamol, salmeterol, and terbutaline.

Theophylline:

Increased risk of hypokalaemia.

Ulcer-healing drugs:

Carbenoxolone increases the risk of hypokalaemia.

Vaccines:

Live vaccines should not be given to individuals with impaired immune response as a result of treatment with large doses of corticosteroids.

4.6 Pregnancy and lactation

Topical administration of corticosteroids to pregnant animals can cause abnormalities of foetal development including cleft palate and intrauterine growth retardation. There may therefore be a very small risk of such effects in the human foetus. Also, hypoadrenalism may occur in the neonate. When corticosteroids are essential however, patients with normal pregnancies may be treated as though they were in the non-gravid state. Patients with pre-eclampsia or fluid retention require close monitoring.

Corticosteroids are excreted in small amounts in breast milk and infants of mothers taking pharmacological doses of steroids should be monitored carefully for signs of adrenal suppression.

4.7 Effects on ability to drive and use machines

None known.

4.8 Undesirable effects

The incidence of predictable undesirable effects, including hypothalamic - pituitary - adrenal suppression correlates with the relative systemic potency of the drug, dosage, timing of administration and the duration of treatment (see 'Special Warnings and Precautions for Use').

Endocrine/metabolic

Suppression of the hypothalamic - pituitary - adrenal axis, growth suppression in infancy, childhood and adolescence, menstrual irregularity and amenorrhoea. Cushingoid Facies, hirsutism, weight gain, impaired carbohydrate tolerance with increased requirement for antidiabetic therapy. Negative protein and calcium balance. Increased appetite.

Anti-inflammatory and immunosuppressive effects

Increased susceptibility and severity of infections with suppression of clinical symptoms and signs. Opportunistic infections, recurrence of dormant tuberculosis (see 'Special Warnings and Precautions for Use').

Blood and lymphatic system disorders

Alteration in lipid levels (increases in total cholesterol, low density lipoproteins and triglycerides), porphyria, leukemoid reactions.

Musculoskeletal

Osteoporosis, vertebral and long bone fractures, avascular osteonecrosis, tendon rupture, proximal myopathy.

Fluid and electrolyte disturbance

Sodium and water retention, hypertension, potassium loss, hypokalaemic alkalosis.

Neuropsychiatric

Euphoria, psychological dependence, depression, insomnia, and aggravation of schizophrenia. Increased intracranial pressure with papilloedema in children (pseudotumour cerebri), usually after treatment withdrawal. Aggravation of epilepsy.

Ophthalmic

Increased intra-ocular pressure, glaucoma, papilloedema, posterior subcapsular cataracts, corneal or scleral thinning, exacerbation of ophthalmic viral or fungal diseases. Chorioretinopathy.

Cardiac

Myocardial rupture following recent myocardial infarction.

Gastrointestinal

Nausea, hiccups, dyspepsia, peptic ulceration with perforation and haemorrhage, acute pancreatitis, candidiasis.

Dermatological

Impaired healing, skin atrophy, bruising, telangiectasia, striae, acne, dermatitis, increased sweating and toxic epidermal necrolysis.

General

Hypersensitivity including anaphylaxis, has been reported. Leucocytosis. Thrombo-embolism.

Withdrawal symptoms and signs

Too rapid a reduction of corticosteroid dosage following prolonged treatment can lead to acute adrenal insufficiency, hypotension and in severe cases this could be fatal.

A 'withdrawal syndrome' may also occur including fever, myalgia, arthralgia, rhinitis, conjunctivitis, painful itchy skin nodules and loss of weight.

4.9 Overdose

Treatment is unlikely to be needed in cases of acute overdosage.

5. PHARMACOLOGICAL PROPERTIES

5.1 Pharmacodynamic properties

ATC Code: A07E A01

Not applicable

5.2 Pharmacokinetic properties

Not applicable.

5.3 Preclinical safety data

None stated.

6. PHARMACEUTICAL PARTICULARS

6.1 List of excipients

Nipastat GL 75

Disodium edetate

Sodium acid phosphate

Disodium hydrogen phosphate anhydrous

Sodium hydroxide

Purified water

6.2 Incompatibilities

None known.

6.3 Shelf life

24 months.

6.4 Special precautions for storage

Do not store above 25°C. Keep the container in the outer carton.

6.5 Nature and contents of container

Each 100ml single dose is supplied in a low density polythene bottle with a low density polythene cap, with a separate PVC nozzle. Seven bottles, plastic protective covers and instructions for use are supplied in each box.

6.6 Special precautions for disposal and other handling

None stated.

7. MARKETING AUTHORISATION HOLDER

UCB Pharma Limited

208 Bath Road

Slough

Berkshire

SL1 3WE

UK

8. MARKETING AUTHORISATION NUMBER(S)

PL 00039/0396

9. DATE OF FIRST AUTHORISATION/RENEWAL OF THE AUTHORISATION

14 October 1992

10. DATE OF REVISION OF THE TEXT

March 2008

Predsol Suppositories

(UCB Pharma Limited)

1. NAME OF THE MEDICINAL PRODUCT

Predsol Suppositories.

2. QUALITATIVE AND QUANTITATIVE COMPOSITION

5mg prednisolone as the sodium phosphate ester.

For excipients, see 6.1

3. PHARMACEUTICAL FORM

Suppository

4. CLINICAL PARTICULARS

4.1 Therapeutic indications

Prednisolone is a glucocorticosteroid which is about four times as potent as hydrocortisone on a weight for weight basis.

Predsol Suppositories are indicated for the treatment of haemorrhagic and granular proctitis and the anal complications of Crohn's disease.

4.2 Posology and method of administration

Rectal administration in adults and children:

One suppository inserted at night and one in the morning after defaecation. When the response is good, treatment is usually continued for some months. If symptoms recur later, treatment should be resumed.

4.3 Contraindications

Systemic or local infection unless specific anti-infective therapy is employed.

Hypersensitivity to any ingredient.

4.4 Special warnings and precautions for use

Although Predsol Suppositories are applied locally, it should be borne in mind that there is likely to be substantial systemic absorption, especially when the bowel is inflamed.

Undesirable effects may be minimised by using for a minimum period. Frequent patient review is required to monitor therapeutic effect against disease activity.

Suppression of the inflammatory response and immune function increases the susceptibility to infections and their severity. The clinical presentation may often be atypical and serious infections such as septicaemia and tuberculosis may be masked and may reach an advanced stage before being recognised.

Chickenpox is of particular concern since this normally minor illness may be fatal in immunosuppressed patients. Patients without a definite history of chickenpox should be advised to avoid close personal contact with chickenpox or herpes zoster and if exposed they should seek urgent medical attention. Passive immunisation with varicella zoster immunoglobulin (VZIG) is needed by exposed non-immune patients who are receiving systemic corticosteroids or who have used them within the previous 3 months; this should be given within 10 days of exposure to chickenpox. If a diagnosis of chickenpox is confirmed, the illness warrants specialist care and urgent treatment. Corticosteroids should not be stopped and the dose may need to be increased.

Patients should be advised to take particular care to avoid exposure to measles and to seek immediate medical advice if exposure occurs. Prophylaxis with intramuscular normal immunoglobulin may be needed.

Live vaccines should not be given to individuals with impaired immune responsiveness. The antibody response to other vaccines may be diminished.

Corticosteroid treatment may reduce the response of the pituitary adrenal axis to stress, and relative insufficiency can persist for up to a year after withdrawal of prolonged therapy. Withdrawal of corticosteroids after prolonged therapy must therefore always be gradual to avoid acute adrenal insufficiency, being tapered off over weeks or months according to the dose and duration of treatment. During prolonged therapy any intercurrent illness, trauma or surgical procedure will require a temporary increase in dosage. If corticosteroids have been stopped following prolonged therapy they may need to be temporarily re-introduced.

Use with caution in patients with myasthenia gravis, non-specific ulcerative colitis, diverticulitis and fresh intestinal anastamoses.

Special precautions:

Particular care is required when considering the use of systemic corticosteroids in patients with the following conditions and frequent patient monitoring is necessary.

A. Osteoporosis (post-menopausal females are particularly at risk).

B. Hypertension or congestive heart failure.

C. Existing or previous history of severe affective disorders (especially previous steroid psychosis).

D. Diabetes mellitus (or a family history of diabetes).

E. History of tuberculosis.

F. Glaucoma (or a family history of glaucoma).

G. Previous corticosteroid-induced myopathy.

H. Liver failure - blood levels of corticosteroid may be increased, (as with other drugs which are metabolised in the liver).

I. Renal insufficiency.

J. Epilepsy.

K. Peptic ulceration.

L. Hypothyroidism.

M. Recent myocardial infarction.

Patients should carry 'steroid treatment' cards which give clear guidance on the precautions to be taken to minimise risk and which provide details of prescriber, drug, dosage and the duration of treatment.

Patients/and or carers should be warned that potentially severe psychiatric adverse reactions may occur with systemic steroids (see section 4.8). Symptoms typically emerge within a few days or weeks of starting treatment. Risks may be higher with high doses/systemic exposure (see also section 4.5 pharmacokinetic interactions that can increase the risk of side effects), although dose levels do not allow prediction of the onset, type, severity or duration of reactions. Most reactions recover after either dose reduction or withdrawal, although specific treatment may be necessary. Patients/carers should be encouraged to seek medical advice if worrying psychological symptoms develop, especially if depressed mood or suicidal ideation is suspected. Patients/carers should also be alert to possible psychiatric disturbances that may occur either during or immediately after dose tapering/withdrawal of systemic steroids, although such reactions have been reported infrequently.

Use in the elderly:

The common adverse effects of systemic corticosteroids may be associated with more serious consequences in old age, especially osteoporosis, hypertension, hypokalaemia, diabetes, susceptibility to infection and thinning of the skin. Close clinical supervision is required to avoid life-threatening reactions.

4.5 Interaction with other medicinal products and other forms of interaction

Systemic absorption of prednisolone should be borne in mind, especially when there is local inflammation. Thus the following interactions are possible:

Analgesics:

Increased risk of gastro-intestinal bleeding and ulceration with aspirin and NSAIDs; the renal clearance of salicylates is increased by corticosteroids and steroid withdrawal may result in salicylate intoxication.

Antibacterials:

Rifamycins accelerate metabolism of corticosteroids (reduced effect); erythromycin inhibits metabolism of methylprednisolone and possibly other corticosteroids. *Fluoroquinolones* - Increased risk of tendon rupture.

Anticoagulants:

The efficacy of coumarin anticoagulants may be enhanced by concurrent corticosteroid therapy and close monitoring of the INR or prothrombin time is required to avoid spontaneous bleeding.

Antidiabetics:

Antagonism of hypoglycaemic effect.

Antiepileptics:

Carbamazepine, phenobarbital, phenytoin and primidone accelerate metabolism of corticosteroids (reduced effect).

Antifungals:

Increased risk of hypokalaemia with amphotericin (avoid concomitant use unless corticosteroids are required to control reactions); ketoconazole inhibits metabolism of methylprednisolone and possibly other corticosteroids.

Antihypertensives:

Antagonism of hypotensive effect.

Anticholinesterases:

Decreased effect of anticholinesterases in myasthenia gravis.

Antivirals:

Ritonavir possibly increases plasma concentration of prednisolone.

Cardiac Glycosides:

Increased toxicity if hypokalaemia occurs with corticosteroids.

Ciclosporin:

Increased plasma concentrations of prednisolone.

Cytotoxics:

Increased risk of haematological toxicity with methotrexate.

Diuretics:

Antagonism of diuretic effect; acetazolamide, loop diuretics, and thiazides increased risk of hypokalaemia.

Hormone antagonists:

Aminoglutethimide accelerates metabolism of corticosteroids (reduced effect).

Licorice:

Increased corticosteroid levels.

Mifepristone:

Effects of corticosteroids may be reduced for 3-4 days after mifepristone.

Neuromuscular blockers:

Antagonism of the neuromuscular blockade.

Oral Contraceptives:

Alteration in the plasma protein binding and metabolism of prednisolone caused by oestrogens, with or without progesterone, can result in exposure of women to increased levels of unbound prednisolone for prolonged periods of time.

Somatropin:

The growth promoting effect of somatropin may be inhibited.

Sympathomimetics:

Increased risk of hypokalaemia if high doses of corticosteroids given with high doses of bambuterol, fenoterol, formoterol, ritodrine, salbutamol, salmeterol, and terbutaline.

Theophylline:

increased risk of hypokalaemia.

Ulcer-healing drugs:

Carbenoxolone increases the risk of hypokalaemia.

Vaccines:

Live vaccines should not be given to individuals with impaired immune response as a result of treatment with large doses of corticosteroids.

4.6 Pregnancy and lactation

There is inadequate evidence of safety in human pregnancy. Topical administration of corticosteroids to pregnant animals can cause abnormalities of foetal development including cleft palate and intrauterine growth retardation. There may therefore be a very small risk of such effects in the human foetus. Also, hypoadrenalism may occur in the neonate. When corticosteroids are essential however, patients with normal pregnancies may be treated as though they were in the non-gravid state. Patients with pre-eclampsia or fluid retention require close monitoring.

Corticosteroids are excreted in small amounts in breast milk and infants of mothers taking pharmacological doses of steroids should be monitored carefully for signs of adrenal suppression.

4.7 Effects on ability to drive and use machines

None known.

4.8 Undesirable effects

The incidence of predictable undesirable effects, including hypothalamic-pituitary-adrenal (HPA) axis suppression correlates with the relative systemic potency of the drug, dosage, timing of administration and the duration of treatment (see Other Special Warnings and Precautions).

Endocrine/metabolic:

Suppression of the hypothalamic-pituitary-adrenal axis, growth suppression in infancy, childhood and adolescence, menstrual irregularity and amenorrhoea. Cushingoid facies, hirsutism, weight gain, impaired carbohydrate tolerance with increased requirement for antidiabetic therapy. Negative protein and calcium balance. Increased appetite.

Anti-inflammatory and immunosuppressive effects:

Increased susceptibility and severity of infections with suppression of clinical symptoms and signs, opportunistic infections, recurrence of dormant tuberculosis (see Other Special Warnings and Precautions).

Blood and lymphatic system disorders

Alteration in lipid levels (increases in total cholesterol, low density lipoproteins and triglycerides), leukemoid reactions.

Musculoskeletal:

Osteoporosis, vertebral and long bone fractures, avascular osteonecrosis, tendon rupture, proximal myopathy.

Fluid and electrolyte disturbance:

Sodium and water retention, hypertension, potassium loss, hypokalaemic alkalosis.

Neuropsychiatric:

A wide range of psychiatric reactions including affective disorder (such a irritable, euphoric, depressed and labile mood and suicidal thoughts), psychotic reactions (including mania, delusions, hallucinations and aggravation of schizophrenia), behavioural disturbances, irritability, anxiety, sleep disturbances and cognitive dysfunction including confusion and amnesia have been reported. Reactions are common any may occur in both adults and children. In adults, the frequency of severe reactions has been estimated to the 5-6%. Psychological effects have been reported on withdrawal of corticosteroids; the frequency is unknown.

Psychological dependence. Increased intra-cranial pressure with papilloedema in children (pseudotumour cerebri), usually after treatment withdrawal. Aggravation of epilepsy.

Ophthalmic:

Increased intra-ocular pressure, glaucoma, papilloedema, posterior subcapsular cataracts, corneal or scleral thinning, exacerbation of ophthalmic viral or fungal diseases. Chorioretinopathy.

Cardiac

Myocardial rupture following recent myocardial infarction.

Gastrointestinal:

Nausea, hiccups, dyspepsia, peptic ulceration with perforation and haemorrhage, acute pancreatitis, candidiasis.

Dermatological:

Impaired healing, skin atrophy, bruising, telangiectasia, striae, acne, dermatitis and toxic epidermal necrolysis.

General:

Hypersensitivity including anaphylaxis, has been reported. Leucocytosis. Thrombo-embolism.

Withdrawal symptoms and signs:

Too rapid a reduction of corticosteroid dosage following prolonged treatment can lead to acute adrenal insufficiency, hypotension and in severe cases this could be fatal.

A 'withdrawal syndrome' may also occur including; fever, myalgia, arthralgia, rhinitis, conjunctivitis, painful itchy skin nodules and loss of weight.

4.9 Overdose

Treatment is unlikely to be needed in cases of acute overdosage.

5. PHARMACOLOGICAL PROPERTIES

5.1 Pharmacodynamic properties

ATC: A07E A01

Prednisolone sodium phosphate is an active corticosteroid with topical anti-inflammatory activity.

5.2 Pharmacokinetic properties

Corticosteroids are metabolised mainly in the liver but also in the kidney and are excreted in the urine.

Synthetic corticosteroids such as prednisolone have increased potency when compared with the natural corticosteroids, due to their slower metabolism and lower protein-binding affinity.

5.3 Preclinical safety data

None stated.

6. PHARMACEUTICAL PARTICULARS

6.1 List of excipients

Witepsol H15.

6.2 Incompatibilities

None known.

6.3 Shelf life

2 years.

6.4 Special precautions for storage

Store below 25°C.

6.5 Nature and contents of container

Fin sealed plastic cavities moulded from 100 micron non-toxic PVC. Each cartoned plastic mould contains 10 suppositories (2 strips of 5 suppositories).

6.6 Special precautions for disposal and other handling

None stated.

7. MARKETING AUTHORISATION HOLDER
UCB Pharma Limited
208 Bath Road
Slough
Berkshire
SL1 3WE
UK

8. MARKETING AUTHORISATION NUMBER(S)
PL 00039/0395

9. DATE OF FIRST AUTHORISATION/RENEWAL OF THE AUTHORISATION
23 February 1993.

10. DATE OF REVISION OF THE TEXT
March 2008

Pregaday Tablets
(UCB Pharma Limited)

1. NAME OF THE MEDICINAL PRODUCT
Pregaday Tablets

2. QUALITATIVE AND QUANTITATIVE COMPOSITION
Each tablets contains Ferrous Fumarate EP 322.00 mg and Folic Acid EP 0.35 mg.

3. PHARMACEUTICAL FORM
Film-coated tablet

4. CLINICAL PARTICULARS

4.1 Therapeutic indications
There is evidence that a daily intake of 100mg of elemental iron in the ferrous form is adequate to prevent development of iron deficiency in expectant mothers. If a mild iron deficiency is present when Pregaday administration is started, this will be corrected by increased absorption of iron.

The daily folate requirement rises steeply during the final trimester of pregnancy, and evidence of maternal depletion may be found. To ensure normal tissue folate levels in the mother after delivery a daily supplement of about 300 micrograms is required during the second and third trimester of pregnancy. This does not obscure the blood picture of addisonian pernicious anaemia.

Pregaday Tablets are indicated during the second and third trimester of pregnancy for prophylaxis against iron deficiency and megaloblastic anaemia of pregnancy. Pregaday Tablets are not intended as a treatment for established megaloblastic anaemia.

4.2 Posology and method of administration
Adults:
It is usual to begin therapy with Pregaday Tablets about the thirteenth week of pregnancy (see precautions) either as routine prophylaxis or selectively if the haemoglobin concentration is less than 11g/100 ml (less than 75% normal).

One tablet should be taken daily by mouth.

Children: Not applicable

4.3 Contraindications
Known hypersensitivity to the product, Vitamin B_{12} deficiency, paroxysmal nocturnal haemoglobinuria, haemosiderosis, haemochromatosis, active peptic ulcer, repeated blood transfusion, regional enteritis and ulcerative colitis.

Pregaday must not be used in the treatment of anaemias other than those due to iron deficiency.

4.4 Special warnings and precautions for use
The label will state
"Important warning: Contains Iron. Keep out of reach and sight of children, as overdose may be fatal".

This will appear on the front of the pack within a rectangle in which there is no other information.

Some post-gastrectomy patients show poor absorption of iron. Care is needed when treating iron deficiency anaemia in patients with treated or controlled peptic ulceration. Caution should be exercised when administering folic acid to patients who may have folate dependent tumours.

Since anaemia due to combined iron and vitamin B_{12} or folate deficiencies may be microcytic in type, patients with microcytic anaemia resistant to therapy with iron alone should be screened for vitamin B_{12} or folate deficiency.

Pregaday tablets should be kept out of the reach of children.

4.5 Interaction with other medicinal products and other forms of interaction
Iron reduces the absorption of penicillamine. Iron compounds impair the bioavailability of fluoroquinolones, levodopa, carbidopa, thyroxine and bisphosphonates.

Absorption of both iron and antibiotic may be reduced if Pregaday is given with tetracycline.

Absorption of both iron and zinc are reduced if taken concomitantly.

Concurrent administration of antacids may reduce absorption of iron. Co-trimoxazole, chloramphenicol, sulphasalazine, aminopterin, methotrexate, pyrimethamine or sulphonamides may interfere with folate metabolism.

Serum levels of anticonvulsant drugs may be reduced by administration of folate.

Oral chloramphenicol delays plasma iron clearance, incorporation of iron into red blood cells and interferes with erythropoiesis.

Some inhibition of iron absorption may occur if it is taken with cholestyramine, trientine, tea, eggs or milk.

Administration of oral iron may increase blood pressure in patients receiving methyldopa.

Coffee may be a factor in reducing iron bioavailability.

Neomycin may alter the absorption of iron.

4.6 Pregnancy and lactation
Administration of Pregaday Tablets during the first trimester of pregnancy may be undesirable.

A minority of pregnant women are not protected by physiological doses of folic acid. The development of anaemia despite prophylaxis with Pregaday Tablets calls for investigation.

4.7 Effects on ability to drive and use machines
None

4.8 Undesirable effects
Gastro-intestinal disorders have been reported including gastro-intestinal discomfort, anorexia, nausea, vomiting, constipation, diarrhoea. Darkening of the stools may occur.

Rarely allergic reactions may occur.

4.9 Overdose
Acute overdose of oral iron requires emergency treatment. In young children

200-250 mg/kg ferrous fumarate is considered to be extremely dangerous.

Symptoms and signs of abdominal pain, vomiting and diarrhoea appear within 60 minutes. Cardiovascular collapse with coma may follow. Some improvement may occur after this phase which, in some patients, is followed by recovery. In others, after about 16 hours, deterioration may occur involving diffuse vascular congestion, pulmonary oedema, convulsions, anuria, hypothermia, severe shock, metabolic acidosis, coagulation abnormalities and hypoglycaemia.

Vomiting should be induced immediately, followed as soon as possible by parenteral injection of desferrioxamine mesylate, and then gastric lavage. In the meantime, it is helpful to give milk and/or 5% sodium bicarbonate solution by mouth.

Dissolve 2 g desferrioxamine mesylate in 2 to 3 ml of water for injections and give intramuscularly. A solution of 5 g desferrioxamine in 50 to 100 ml of fluid may be left in the stomach. If desferrioxamine is not available, leave 300 ml of 1 % to 5 % sodium bicarbonate in the stomach. Fluid replacement is essential.

Recovery may be complicated by long-term sequelae such as hepatic necrosis, pyloric stenosis or acute toxic encephalitis which may lead to CNS damage.

5. PHARMACOLOGICAL PROPERTIES

5.1 Pharmacodynamic properties
There is evidence that a daily dose of 100mg of elemental iron in the ferrous form is adequate to prevent development of iron deficiency in expectant mothers. If a mild iron deficiency is present when Pregaday administration is started, this will be corrected by increased absorption of iron. The daily folate requirement rises steeply during the final trimester of pregnancy, and evidence of maternal depletion may be found. To ensure normal tissue folate levels in the mother after delivery a daily supplement of about 300 micrograms is required during the second and third trimester of pregnancy. This does not obscure the blood picture of addisonian pernicious anaemia.

5.2 Pharmacokinetic properties
Iron is absorbed chiefly in the duodenum and jejunum, absorption being aided by the acid secretion of the stomach and being more readily effected when the iron is in the ferrous state.

Folic acid is absorbed mainly from the proximal part of the small intestine. Folate polyglutamates are considered to be de-conjugated to monoglutamates during absorption. Folic acid rapidly appears in the blood, where it is extensively bound to plasma proteins. The amounts of folic acid absorbed from normal diets are rapidly distributed in body tissues and about 4 to 5 micrograms is excreted in the urine daily. When larger amounts are absorbed, a high proportion is metabolised in the liver to other active forms of folate and a proportion is stored as reduced and methylated folate. Larger amounts of folate are rapidly excreted in the urine.

5.3 Preclinical safety data
Not stated

6. PHARMACEUTICAL PARTICULARS

6.1 List of excipients
The tablet cores also contain maize starch EP, sodium lauryl sulphate EP, gelatin EP and liquid paraffin EP. The film coat contains **either** hydroxypropylmethyl cellulose EP (E464), acetylated monoglyceride and Opaspray pink **or** hydroxypropylmethyl cellulose EP (E464), propylene glycol EP and Opaspray pink.

Opaspray pink contains hydroxypropyl cellulose (E463), red iron oxide(E172) and titanium dioxide (E171).

6.2 Incompatibilities
None

6.3 Shelf life
36 months

6.4 Special precautions for storage
Protect from light, store below 25°C

6.5 Nature and contents of container
Cartons containing two calendar blister packs of 14 tablets prepared from PVdC coated opaque 250 micron PVC film and 20 micron tempered aluminium foil.

6.6 Special precautions for disposal and other handling
Not applicable

7. MARKETING AUTHORISATION HOLDER
UCB Pharma Limited
208 Bath Road
Slough
Berkshire
SL1 3WE
UK

8. MARKETING AUTHORISATION NUMBER(S)
PL 00039/0398

9. DATE OF FIRST AUTHORISATION/RENEWAL OF THE AUTHORISATION
23 February 1993

10. DATE OF REVISION OF THE TEXT
June 2005

Premarin Tablets
(Wyeth Pharmaceuticals)

1. NAME OF THE MEDICINAL PRODUCT
Premarin 0.3mg
Premarin 0.625mg
Premarin 1.25mg

2. QUALITATIVE AND QUANTITATIVE COMPOSITION
Tablets containing 0.3mg, 0.625mg or 1.25mg Conjugated Estrogens USP.

3. PHARMACEUTICAL FORM
Coated Tablet

Premarin 0.3mg tablets are green oval biconvex, sugar-coated tablets marked with "0.3" in white ink.

Premarin 0.625mg tablets are maroon oval biconvex sugar-coated tablet unmarked or marked with " 0.625" in white ink.

Premarin 1.25mg tablets are yellow oval biconvex sugar coated tablet unmarked or marked with "1.25" in black ink.

4. CLINICAL PARTICULARS

4.1 Therapeutic indications
Premarin 0.3mg, 0.625mg and 1.25mg:

- Hormone replacement therapy for estrogen deficiency symptoms in postmenopausal women.

Premarin 0.625mg and 1.25mg:

- Prevention of osteoporosis in postmenopausal women at high risk of future fractures who are intolerant of, or contra-indicated for, other medicinal products approved for the prevention of osteoporosis.

4.2 Posology and method of administration
Adults:
Premarin is an estrogen only HRT.

Treatment of Postmenopausal Symptoms
Premarin 0.3-1.25mg daily is the usual starting dose for women without a uterus. Continuous administration is recommended.

For initiation and continuation of treatment of postmenopausal symptoms, the lowest effective dose for the shortest duration (see also Section 4.4 Special warnings and precautions for use) should be used. Treatment to control menopausal symptoms should be initiated with Premarin 0.3mg. If symptoms are not adequately controlled, higher doses of Premarin may be prescribed. Once treatment is established the lowest effective dose necessary for the relief of symptoms should be used. Patients should be re-evaluated periodically to determine if treatment for symptoms is still necessary.

Treatment of osteoporosis
The minimum effective dose is 0.625mg daily for most patients. (See section 5.1 Pharmacodynamic properties).

Starting or Changing Treatment
In women who are not taking hormone replacement therapy or women who switch from a continuous combined hormone replacement therapy product, treatment may be started on any convenient day. In women transferring from a sequential hormone replacement therapy regimen,

treatment should begin the day following completion of the prior regimen.

Concomitant progestogen use for women with a uterus

In women with a uterus, where the addition of a progestogen is necessary it should be added for at least 12-14 days every 28 day cycle to reduce the risk to the endometrium.

Unless there is a previous diagnosis of endometriosis, it is not recommended to add a progestogen in hysterectomised women.

The benefits of the lower risk of endometrial hyperplasia and endometrial cancer due to adding progestogen should be weighed against the increased risk of breast cancer (see sections 4.4 Special warnings and precautions for use and 4.8 Undesirable effects).

Forgotten tablet: If a tablet is forgotten, it should be taken as soon as the patient remembers, therapy should then be continued as before. If more than one tablet has been forgotten only the most recent tablet should be taken, the patient should not take double the usual dose to make up for missed tablets.

Missed pills may cause breakthrough bleeding in women with a uterus.

Elderly

There are no special dosage requirements for elderly patients, but as with all medicines, the lowest effective dose should be used.

Children

Not recommended.

4.3 Contraindications

1. Known, past or suspected breast cancer
2. Known or suspected estrogen-dependent malignant tumours (e.g. endometrial cancer)
3. Undiagnosed abnormal genital bleeding
4. Untreated endometrial hyperplasia
5. Active or past history of venous thromboembolism (e.g. deep vein thrombosis, pulmonary embolism)
6. Active or recent arterial thromboembolic disease (e.g. angina, myocardial infarction)
7. Acute liver disease or history of liver disease where the liver function tests have failed to return to normal
8. Known hypersensitivity to the active substances or to any of the excipients of Premarin tablets
9. Porphyria

4.4 Special warnings and precautions for use

For the treatment of postmenopausal symptoms, HRT should only be initiated for symptoms that adversely affect quality of life. In all cases, a careful appraisal of the risks and benefits should be undertaken at least annually and HRT should only be continued as long as the benefit outweighs the risk.

1. Medical examination/Follow up

Before initiating or reinstituting HRT, a complete personal and family medical history should be taken. Physical (including pelvic and breast) examination should be guided by the contraindications and warnings for use. During treatment, periodic check-ups are recommended of a frequency and nature adapted to the individual women. Women should be advised what changes in their breasts should be reported to their doctor or nurse (see 'Breast Cancer' below). Investigations, including mammography, should be carried out in accordance with currently accepted screening practices, modified to the clinical needs of the individual.

2. Conditions that need supervision

If any of the following conditions are present, have occurred previously, and/or have been aggravated during pregnancy or previous hormone treatment, the patient should be closely supervised. It should be taken into account that these conditions may recur or be aggravated during treatment with Premarin, in particular:

- Leiomyoma (uterine fibroids) or endometriosis
- A family history of, or other risk factors for, thromboembolic disorders (see below)
- Risk factors for estrogen dependent tumours (e.g. first degree heredity for breast cancer)
- Hypertension
- Liver disorders (e.g. liver adenoma)
- Diabetes mellitus with or without vascular involvement
- Cholelithiasis
- Migraine or (severe) headaches
- Systemic lupus erythematosus (SLE)
- A history of endometrial hyperplasia (see below)
- Epilepsy
- Asthma
- Otosclerosis

3. Reasons for immediate withdrawal of therapy

Therapy should be discontinued if a contra-indication is discovered and in the following situations:

- Jaundice or deterioration in liver function
- Significant increase in blood pressure
- New onset of migraine-type headache
- Pregnancy

4. Endometrial Hyperplasia

The risk of endometrial hyperplasia and carcinoma is increased when estrogens are administered alone for prolonged periods (see section 4.8 Undesirable effects and section 5.1 Pharmacodynamic Properties). The addition of a progestogen for at least 12 days of the cycle in non-hysterectomised women greatly reduces this risk.

The reduction in risk to the endometrium should be weighed against the increase in the risk of breast cancer of added progestogen (see 'Breast Cancer' below and section 4.8 Undesirable effects).

Break-through bleeding and spotting may occur during the first months of treatment. If break-through bleeding or spotting appears after some time on therapy, or continues after treatment has been discontinued, the reason should be investigated, which may include endometrial biopsy to exclude endometrial malignancy.

Unopposed estrogen stimulation may lead to pre-malignant or malignant transformation in the residual foci of endometriosis. Therefore, the addition of progestogens to estrogen replacement therapy should be considered in women who have undergone hysterectomy because of endometriosis, if they are known to have residual endometriosis (but see above).

5. Breast Cancer

A randomised placebo-controlled trial, the Women's Health Initiative study (WHI), and epidemiological studies, including the Million Women Study (MWS), have reported an increased risk of breast cancer in women taking estrogens, estrogen-progestogen combinations or tibolone for HRT for several years (see Section 4.8 Undesirable effects). For all HRT, an excess risk becomes apparent within a few years of use and increases with the duration of intake but returns to baseline within a few (at most five) years after stopping treatment.

In the MWS, the relative risk of breast cancer with conjugated equine estrogens (CEE) or estradiol (E2) was greater when a progestogen was added, either sequentially or continuously, and regardless of type of progestogen. There was no evidence of a difference in risk between the different routes of administration.

In the WHI study, the continuous combined conjugated equine estrogen and medroxyprogesterone acetate (CEE + MPA) product used was associated with breast cancers that were slightly larger in size and more frequently had local lymph node metastases compared to placebo.

HRT, especially estrogen-progestogen combined treatment, increases the density of mammographic images which may adversely affect the radiological detection of breast cancer.

6. Venous thromboembolism

Hormone replacement therapy (HRT) is associated with a higher relative risk of developing venous thromboembolism (VTE) i.e. deep vein thrombosis or pulmonary embolism. One randomised controlled trial and epidemiological studies found a two to threefold higher risk for users compared with non-users. For non- users it is estimated that the number of cases of VTE that will occur over a 5-year period is about 3 per 1000 women aged 50-59 years and 8 per 1000 women aged between 60-69 years. It is estimated that in healthy women who use HRT for 5 years, the number of additional cases of VTE over a 5-year period will be between 2 and 6 (best estimate = 4) per 1000 women aged 50-59 years and between 5 and 15 (best estimate = 9) per 1000 women aged 60-69 years. The occurrence of such an event is more likely in the first year of HRT than later.

Generally recognised risk factors for VTE include a personal or family history and severe obesity (Body Mass Index $>30kg/m^2$) and systemic lupus erythematosus (SLE). There is no consensus about the possible role of varicose veins in VTE.

Patients with a history of VTE or known thrombophilic states have an increased risk of VTE. HRT may add to this risk. Personal or strong family history of thromboembolism or recurrent spontaneous abortion should be investigated in order to exclude a thrombophilic predisposition. Until a thorough evaluation of thrombophilic factors has been made or anticoagulant treatment initiated, use of HRT in such patients should be viewed as contraindicated. Those women already on anticoagulant treatment require careful consideration of the benefit-risk of use of HRT.

The risk of VTE may be temporarily increased with prolonged immobilisation, major trauma or major surgery. As in all postoperative patients scrupulous attention should be given to prophylactic measures to prevent VTE following surgery. Where prolonged immobilisation is liable to follow elective surgery, particularly abdominal or orthopaedic surgery to the lower limbs, consideration should be given to temporarily stopping HRT 4-6 weeks earlier, if this is possible. Treatment should not be restarted until the woman is completely mobilised.

If VTE develops after initiating therapy, the drug should be discontinued. Patients should be told to contact their doctors immediately when they are aware of potential thromboembolic symptoms (e.g. painful swelling of a leg, sudden pain in the chest, dyspnoea).

7. Coronary Artery Disease (CAD)

There is no evidence from randomised controlled trials of cardiovascular benefit with continuous combined conjugated estrogens and MPA. Two large clinical trials (WHI and HERS i.e. Heart and Estrogen/progestin Replacement Study) showed a possible increased risk of cardiovascular morbidity in the first year of use and no overall benefit. For other HRT products, there are only limited data from randomised controlled trials examining effects in cardiovascular morbidity or mortality. Therefore, it is uncertain whether these findings also extend to other HRT products.

8. Stroke

One large randomised clinical trial (WHI-trial) found, as a secondary outcome, an increased risk of ischaemic stroke in healthy women during treatment with continuous combined conjugated estrogens and MPA. For women who do not use HRT, it is estimated that the number of cases of stroke that will occur over a 5 year period is about 3 per 1000 women aged 50-59 years and 11 per 1000 women aged 60-69 years. It is estimated that for women who use conjugated estrogens and MPA for 5 years, the number of additional cases will be between 0 and 3 (best estimate =1) per 1000 users aged 50-59 years and between 1 and 9 (best estimate = 4) per 1000 users aged 60-69 years. It is unknown whether the increased risk also extends to other HRT products.

9. Ovarian Cancer

Long-term (at least 5-10 years) use of estrogen-only HRT products in hysterectomised women has been associated with an increased risk of ovarian cancer in some epidemiological studies. It is uncertain whether long-term use of combined HRT confers different risk than estrogen-only products.

Other Conditions

10. Estrogens may cause fluid retention and therefore patients with cardiac or renal dysfunction should be carefully observed. Patients with terminal renal insufficiency should be closely observed, since it is expected that the level of circulating active ingredients in Premarin is increased.

11. The use of estrogen may influence the laboratory results of certain endocrine tests and liver enzymes.

Estrogens increase thyroid binding globulin (TBG), leading to increased circulating total thyroid hormone, as measured by protein-bound iodine (PBI), T4 levels (by column or by radio-immunoassay) or T3 levels (by radio-immunoassay). T3 resin uptake is decreased, reflecting the elevated TBG. Free T4 and free T3 concentrations are unaltered.

Other binding proteins may be elevated in serum, i.e. corticoid binding globulin (CBG), sex-hormone-binding globulin (SHBG) leading to increased circulating corticosteroids and sex steroids, respectively. Free or biologically active hormone concentrations are unchanged. Other plasma proteins may be increased (angiotensinogen/renin substrate, alpha-I-antitrypsin, ceruloplasmin).

Some patients dependent on thyroid hormone replacement therapy may require increased doses in order to maintain their free thyroid hormone levels in an acceptable range. Therefore, patients should have their thyroid function monitored more frequently when commencing concurrent treatment in order to maintain their free thyroid hormone levels in an acceptable range.

12. A worsening of glucose tolerance may occur in patients taking estrogens and therefore diabetic patients should be carefully observed while receiving hormone replacement therapy.

This product contains lactose and sucrose. Patients with rare hereditary problems of galactose intolerance, fructose intolerance, the Lapp lactase deficiency, glucose-galactose malabsorption or sucrase-isomaltase insufficiency should not take this medicine.

13. There is an increase in the risk of gallbladder disease in women receiving HRT (see conditions that need supervision).

14. Women with pre-existing hypertriglyceridemia should be followed closely during estrogen replacement or hormone replacement therapy, since rare cases of large increases of plasma triglycerides leading to pancreatitis have been reported with estrogen therapy in this condition.

15. Estrogens should be used with caution in individuals with severe hypocalcaemia.

16. There is no conclusive evidence for improvement of cognitive function. There is some evidence from the WHI trial of increased risk of probable dementia in women who start using continuous combined CEE and MPA after the age of 65. It is unknown whether the findings apply to younger post-menopausal women or other HRT products.

4.5 Interaction with other medicinal products and other forms of interaction

The metabolism of estrogens may be increased by concomitant use of substances known to induce drug-metabolising enzymes, specifically cytochrome P450 enzymes, such as anticonvulsants (e.g. phenobarbital, phenytoin, carbamazepine) and anti-infectives (e.g. rifampicin, rifabutin, nevirapine, efavirenz).

Ritonavir and nelfinavir, although known as strong inhibitors, by contrast exhibit inducing properties when used concomitantly with steroid hormones.

Herbal preparations containing St John's wort *(Hypericum perforatum)* may induce the metabolism of estrogens.

Clinically, an increased metabolism of estrogens and progestogens may lead to decreased effect and changes in the uterine bleeding profile.

The response to metyrapone may be reduced.

4.6 Pregnancy and lactation
Premarin is not indicated during pregnancy.

For women with a uterus

If pregnancy occurs during medication with Premarin treatment should be withdrawn immediately. The results of most epidemiological studies to date relevant to inadvertent foetal exposure to estrogens indicate no teratogenic or foetotoxic effects.

Lactation:

Premarin is not indicated during lactation.

4.7 Effects on ability to drive and use machines
None known.

4.8 Undesirable effects
See also 4.4 Special warnings and precautions for use.

Adverse drug reactions (ADRs)

The adverse reactions listed in the table are based on post-marketing spontaneous (reporting rate), clinical trials and class-effects.

System Organ Class	Adverse Reaction
Reproductive system and breast disorders	Breakthrough bleeding/ spotting; Breast pain, tenderness, enlargement, discharge; Change in menstrual flow; Change in cervical ectropion and secretion; Dysmenorrhoea; Galactorrhoea; Increased size of uterine leiomyomata
Gastrointestinal disorders	Nausea; Bloating; Abdominal pain; Vomiting; Pancreatitis
Nervous	Dizziness; Headache; Migraine; Nervousness; Stroke; Exacerbation of epilepsy
Musculoskeletal, connective tissue and bone disorders	Arthralgias; Leg cramps
Psychiatric disorders	Changes in libido; Mood disturbances; Depression; Irritability
Vascular disorders	Pulmonary embolism; Superficial thrombophlebitis and deep venous thrombophlebitis
Cardiac Disorders	Myocardial Infarction
General disorders and administration site disorders	Oedema
Skin and subcutaneous tissue disorders	Alopecia; Chloasma/ melasma; Hirsutism; Pruritus; Rash
Infections and infestations	Vaginitis, including vaginal candidiasis
Immune system disorders	Urticaria: Angioedeoma: Anaphylactic/anaphylactoid reactions
Metabolism and nutrition disorders	Glucose intolerance
Eye disorders	Intolerance to contact lenses
Respiratory, thoracic and mediastinal disorders	Exacerbation of asthma
Hepatobiliary	Gallbladder disease
Neoplasms benign and malignant	Breast cancer; Fibrocystic breast changes; Ovarian cancer; Endometrial Cancer
Investigations	Changes in weight (increase or decrease); Increased triglycerides

Breast Cancer

According to evidence from a large number of epidemiological studies and one randomised placebo-controlled trial, the Women's Health Initiative (WHI), the overall risk of breast cancer increases with increasing duration of HRT use in current or recent HRT users.

For estrogen-only HRT, estimates of relative risk (RR) from a reanalysis of original data from 51 epidemiological studies (in which >80% of HRT use was estrogen-only HRT) and from the epidemiological Million Women Study (MWS) are similar at 1.35 (95%CI 1.21 – 1.49) and 1.30 (95%CI 1.21 – 1.40), respectively.

For estrogen plus progestogen combined HRT, several epidemiological studies have reported an overall higher risk for breast cancer than with estrogens alone.

The MWS reported that, compared to never users, the use of various types of estrogen-progestogen combined HRT was associated with a higher risk of breast cancer (RR = 2.00, 95%CI: 1.88 – 2.12) than use of estrogens alone (RR = 1.30, 95%CI: 1.21 – 1.40) or use of tibolone (RR=1.45; 95%CI 1.25-1.68).

The WHI trial reported a risk estimate of 1.24 (95%CI 1.01 – 1.54) after 5.6 years of use of estrogen-progestogen combined HRT (CEE + MPA) in all users compared with placebo.

The absolute risks calculated from the MWS and the WHI trial are presented below:

The MWS has estimated, from the known average incidence of breast cancer in developed countries, that:

- For women not using HRT, about 32 in every 1000 are expected to have breast cancer diagnosed between the ages of 50 and 64 years.
- For 1000 current or recent users of HRT, the number of additional cases during the corresponding period will be
  - For users of estrogen-only replacement therapy
    - between 0 and 3 (best estimate = 1.5) for 5 years' use
    - between 3 and 7 (best estimate = 5) for 10 years' use.
  - For users of estrogen plus progestogen combined HRT
    - between 5 and 7 (best estimate = 6) for 5 years' use
    - between 18 and 20 (best estimate = 19) for 10 years' use.

The WHI trial estimated that after 5.6 years of follow-up of women between the ages of 50 and 79 years, an additional 8 cases of invasive breast cancer would be due to estrogen-progestogen combined HRT (CEE + MPA) per 10,000 women years.

According to calculations from the trial data, it is estimated that:

- For 1000 women in the placebo group.
- About 16 cases of invasive breast cancer would be diagnosed in 5 years.
- For 1000 women who used estrogen plus progestogen combined HRT (CEE + MPA), the number of additional cases would be
- Between 0 and 9 (best estimate = 4) for 5 years' use.

The number of additional cases of breast cancer in women who use HRT is broadly similar for women who start HRT irrespective of age at start of use (between the ages of 45-65) (see section 4.4 Special warnings and special precautions for use).

Endometrial Cancer

In women with an intact uterus, the risk of endometrial hyperplasia and endometrial cancer increases with increasing duration of use of unopposed estrogens. According to data from epidemiological studies, the best estimate of the risk is that for women not using HRT, about 5 in every 1000 are expected to have endometrial cancer diagnosed between the ages of 50 and 65. Depending on the duration of treatment and estrogen dose, the reported increase in endometrial cancer risk among unopposed estrogen users varies from 2-to 12-fold greater compared with non-users. Adding a progestogen to estrogen-only therapy greatly reduces this increased risk.

Other adverse reactions reported in association with estrogen/progestogen treatment including Premarin:

- Estrogen-dependent neoplasms benign and malignant, e.g. endometrial hyperplasia, endometrial cancer
- Venous thromboembolism, i.e. deep leg or pelvic venous thrombosis and pulmonary embolism, is more frequent among hormone replacement therapy users than among non-users. For further information, see section 4.3 Contra-indications and 4.4 Special warnings and precautions for use.
- Retinal vascular thrombosis
- Myocardial infarction
- Increases in blood pressure
- Cholestatic jaundice
- Enlargement of hepatic haemangiomas
- Skin and subcutaneous disorders: erythema multiforme, erythema nodosum, vascular purpura
- Probable dementia (see section 4.4 Special warnings and special precautions for use)
- Exacerbation of chorea
- Exacerbation of porphyria,
- Exacerbation of hypocalcaemia
- Exacerbation of otosclerosis

4.9 Overdose
Numerous reports of ingestion of large doses of estrogen-containing oral contraceptives by young children indicate that acute serious ill effects do not occur. Overdosage of estrogen may cause nausea and vomiting, and withdrawal bleeding may occur in females. There is no specific antidote and further treatment should be symptomatic.

5. PHARMACOLOGICAL PROPERTIES

5.1 Pharmacodynamic properties
ATC Code: G03C A57

Conjugated Estrogens

The active ingredients are primarily the sulphate esters of estrone, equilin sulphates, 17α-estradiol and 17β-estradiol. These substitute for the loss of estrogen production in menopausal women, and alleviate menopausal symptoms. Estrogens prevent bone loss following menopause or ovariectomy.

Relief of estrogen-deficiency symptoms

In a 1-year clinical trial (n=2,805), vasomotor symptoms were assessed for efficacy during the first 12 weeks of treatment in a subset of symptomatic women (n=241, 0.625mg n=27, 0.3mg n=30) who had at least 7 moderate or severe hot flushes daily or 50 moderate to severe hot flushes during the week before randomisation. Premarin 0.3mg and 0.625mg tablets were shown to be statistically better than placebo at weeks 4, 8 and 12 for relief of both frequency and severity of moderate to severe vasomotor symptoms.

The incidence of endometrial hyperplasia with Premarin, ie unopposed estrogen, at cycle 13 for 0.625mg (n=249) and 0.3mg (n=269) was assessed. The number of patients with hyperplasia was 20 (8.03%) for 0.625mg and 1 (0.37%) for 0.3mg.

Prevention of osteoporosis

At present there is no established screening programme for determining women at risk of developing osteoporotic fracture. Epidemiological studies suggest a number of individual risk factors which contribute to the development of postmenopausal osteoporosis. These include: early menopause; family history of osteoporosis; thin, small frame; cigarette use; recent prolonged systemic corticosteroid use.

Estrogen deficiency at menopause is associated with an increasing bone turnover and decline in bone mass. The effect of estrogens on the bone mineral density is dose-dependent. Protection appears to be effective for as long as treatment is continued. After discontinuation of HRT, bone mass is lost at a rate similar to that in untreated women.

Evidence from the WHI trial and meta-analysed trials shows that current use of HRT, alone or in combination with a progestogen – given to predominantly healthy women – reduces the risk of hip, vertebral and other osteoporotic fractures. HRT may also help prevent fractures in women with low bone density and/or established osteoporosis, but the evidence for that is limited.

In the HOPE study, prevention of bone loss was assessed by measurement of bone mineral density (BMD), at the final on-therapy evaluation (cycle 26 or the last available evaluation for those who discontinued early), primarily at the anteroposterior lumbar spine (L_2 to L_4 BMD). Secondarily, BMD measurements of the total body, femoral neck and trochanter were analysed.

The mean increase in anteroposterior lumbar spine bone mineral density (L_2 to L_4 BMD) after 2 years treatment was 2.46% ± 0.37 with Premarin 0.625mg.

Premarin also has an effect of the other BMD parameters. The mean increase in total femoral neck BMD was 1.82% ± 0.45 with Premarin 0.625mg. The mean increase in femoral trochanter BMD was 3.82% ± 0.58 with Premarin 0.625mg.

5.2 Pharmacokinetic properties

Absorption

Conjugated estrogens are soluble in water and are well absorbed from the gastrointestinal tract after release from the drug formulation. The Premarin tablets release conjugated estrogens slowly over several hours. The pharmacodynamic profile of unconjugated and conjugated estrogens following doses of 3 × 0.3mg and 2 × 0.625mg are provided in Table 1.

Distribution

The distribution of exogenous estrogen is similar to that of endogenous estrogens. Estrogens are widely distributed in the body and are generally found in higher concentrations in the sex hormone target organs. Estrogens circulate in the blood largely bound to sex hormone binding globulin (SHBG) and albumin.

Metabolism

Exogenous estrogens are metabolised in the same manner as endogenous estrogens. Circulating estrogens exist in dynamic equilibrium of metabolic interconversions. These transformations take place mainly in the liver. Estradiol is converted reversibly to estrone, and both can be converted to estriol, which is the major urinary metabolite. Estrogens also undergo enterohepatic recirculation via sulphate and glucuronide conjugation in the liver, biliary secretion of conjugates into the intestine, and hydrolysis in the gut following reabsorption. In post-menopausal women a significant proportion of the circulating estrogens exists as sulphate conjugates, especially estrone sulphate, which serves as a circulating reservoir for the formation of more active estrogens.

Excretion

Estriol, estrone and estradiol are excreted in the urine along with glucuronide and sulphate conjugates.

Table 1 – Pharmacokinetic parameters for Premarin

Pharmacokinetic profile for unconjugated estrogens following a dose of 3 × 0.3mg or 2 × 0.625mg

(see Table 1 below)

Pharmacokinetic profile for conjugated estrogens following a dose of 3 × 0.3mg or 2 × 0.625mg

(see Table 2 below)

5.3 Preclinical safety data

Long-term continuous administration of natural and synthetic estrogens in certain animal species increases the frequency of carcinomas of the breast, cervix, vagina and liver.

6. PHARMACEUTICAL PARTICULARS

6.1 List of excipients

Premarin 0.3mg:

Calcium sulphate anhydrous
Carnauba wax
Microcrystalline cellulose
Glyceryl mono-oleates
Lactose monohydrate
Magnesium stearate
Methylcellulose
Macrogol
Shellac solution (pharmaceutical glaze)
Sucrose
Titanium dioxide (E171)
Stearic acid
Edible ink (Opacode S-828905)†
Opalux Green AS-R-11501‡

†contains titanium dioxide (E171), purified water, shellac, ethanol, N-butly alcohol, propylene glycol, ammonia solution and ethyl acetate.

‡ contains sucrose, yellow iron oxide (172), indigo carmine aluminium lake(E172), titanium dioxide, polyvinyl pyrrolidone, sodium benzoate, methyl p-hydroxybenzoate, propyl p-hydroxybenzoate and purified water.

Premarin 0.625mg:

Calcium sulphate anhydrous
Carnauba wax
Microcrystalline cellulose
Glyceryl mono-oleate
Lactose monohydrate
Magnesium stearate
Methylcellulose
Macrogol
Shellac solution (pharmaceutical glaze)
Sucrose
Titanium dioxide (E171)
Opalux maroon colour AS-R-3910†
For marked tablets:
Stearic acid
Edible ink (Opacode S-8-28905)††

† Opalux maroon colour contains sucrose, purified water, erythrosine (E127), titanium dioxide (E171), sunset yellow (E110), indigo carmine (E132), polyvinylpyrrolidone and sodium benzoate.

††Edible ink (Opacode S-8-28905) contains titanium dioxide (E171), shellac (E904), purified water, ethanol, N-butyl alcohol, propylene glycol (E1520), ammonia solution and ethyl acetate.

Premarin 1.25mg:

Calcium sulphate
Carnauba wax
Microcrystalline cellulose
Glyceryl mono-oleate
Lactose
Magnesium stearate
Methylcellulose
Macrogol 20000
Shellac solution (Pharmaceutical glaze)
Sucrose
Titanium dioxide (E171)
Colours
Sunset yellow (E110)
Quinoline yellow aluminium lake (E104)
For marked tablets:
Steraric acid
Edible ink (Opacode S-8-27741)††

††Edible ink (Opacode S-8-27741)Iron oxide black, shellac, purified water, ethanol, N-butyl alcohol, propylene glycol, ammonium solution, and ethyl acetate.

6.2 Incompatibilities

Not applicable.

6.3 Shelf life

Three years.

6.4 Special precautions for storage

Do not store above 25°C.

6.5 Nature and contents of container

Polyvinylchloride (PVC)/Aluminium foil blisters containing 28 tablets. One carton pack contains 3 blisters.

Securitainers containing 100 tablets

PVC/Aluminium foil blisters containing 21 tablets

6.6 Special precautions for disposal and other handling

Not applicable.

7. MARKETING AUTHORISATION HOLDER

John Wyeth and Brother Limited
Trading as: Wyeth Pharmaceuticals
Huntercombe Lane South
Taplow, Maidenhead,
Berkshire, SL6 0PH

8. MARKETING AUTHORISATION NUMBER(S)

Premarin tablets 0.3mg PL 0011/0164
Premarin tablets 0.625mg PL 0011/0165
Premarin tablets 1.25mg PL 0011/0166

9. DATE OF FIRST AUTHORISATION/RENEWAL OF THE AUTHORISATION

1972.

10. DATE OF REVISION OF THE TEXT

Approved 30th April 2007

Table 1 Pharmacokinetic parameters for Premarin

	Premarin 0.3mg				Premarin 0.625mg			
Drug PK Parameter Arithmetic Mean (%CV)	C_{max} (pg/mL)	t_{max} (h)	$t_{1/2}$ (h)	AUC (pg.h/mL)	C_{max} (pg/mL)	t_{max} (h)	$t_{1/2}$ (h)	AUC (pg.h/mL)*
estrone	82 (33)	7.8 (27)	54.7 (42)	5390 (50)	139 (37)	8.8 (20)	28.0 (13)	5016 (34)
baseline-adjusted estrone	58 (42)	7.8 (27)	21.1 (45)	1467 (41)	120 (42)	8.8 (20)	17.4 (37)	2956 (39)
equilin	31 (47)	7.2 (28)	18.3 (110)	652 (68)	66 (42)	7.9 (19)	13.6 (52)	1210 (37)

Table 2

	Premarin 0.3mg				Premarin 0.625mg			
Drug PK Parameter Arithmetic Mean (%CV)	C_{max} (ng/mL)	t_{max} (h)	$t_{1/2}$ (h)	AUC (ng.h/mL)	C_{max} (ng/mL)	t_{max} (h)	$t_{1/2}$ (h)	AUC (pg.h/mL)*
total estrone	2.5 (32)	6.5 (29)	25.4 (22)	61.0 (43)	7.3 (41)	7.3 (51)	15.0 (25)	134 (42)
baseline-adjusted total estrone	2.4 (32)	6.5 (29)	16.2 (34)	40.8 (36)	7.1 (41)	7.3 (25)	13.6 (27)	122 (39)
total equilin	1.6 (40)	5.9 (27)	11.8 (21)	22.4 (42)	5.0 (42)	6.2 (26)	10.1 (27)	65 (45)

* $t_{1/2}$ = terminal-phase disposition half-life (0.693/γ)

Premarin Vaginal Cream

(Wyeth Pharmaceuticals)

1. NAME OF THE MEDICINAL PRODUCT

Premarin* Vaginal Cream.

2. QUALITATIVE AND QUANTITATIVE COMPOSITION

Each 1gram of the cream contains 0.625mg conjugated estrogens USP.

3. PHARMACEUTICAL FORM

Cream for intravaginal or topical administration.

4. CLINICAL PARTICULARS

4.1 Therapeutic indications

Short-term treatment of atrophic vaginitis and post-menopausal atrophic urethritis, kraurosis vulvae.

4.2 Posology and method of administration

Adults: The usual recommended dose is 1 to 2g daily administered intravaginally or topically to the vaginal area, depending on the severity of the condition.

The applicator has dosage markings showing how much of the cream is equivalent to 1g or 2g to help you with applying the correct amount of cream.

The following 'Instruction for Use' should be given to the patient and are included in the Patient Information Leaflet:

To apply the cream into the vagina, the applicator should be used as follows:

1. Remove the cap from the aluminium tube of cream and screw the nozzle end of the applicator onto the tube.
2. Gently squeeze the tube to force the cream into the barrel of the applicator. Depending on the dose your doctor advised you to use, fill the applicator with cream up to the appropriate dosage marking.
3. Unscrew the filled applicator from the tube of cream and replace the cap on the tube.
4. To apply the cream, gently insert the applicator into your vagina and then press the plunger back to its original position.
5. After use, remove the empty applicator.

To clean the applicator after use, pull the plunger out from the barrel and wash both parts with mild soap and warm water. Do not boil or use hot water.

Administration should be cyclic (e.g. three weeks on and one week off). It should start on the fifth day of bleeding in the patient who is menstruating and arbitrarily if not.

For initiation and continuation of treatment of postmenopausal symptoms, the lowest effective dose for the shortest duration (see also Section 4.4 Special and special precautions for use) should be used.

The addition of a progestogen is not needed during treatment with Premarin Vaginal Cream (see Section 4.4 Special warnings and special precautions for use)

Missed dose: If the patient forgets to apply a dose, it should be applied as soon as possible. The patient should not use doubled their usual dose to make up for missed applications.

Elderly: There are no special dosage requirements for elderly patients, but as with all medicines, the lowest effective dose should be used.

Children: Not recommended.

4.3 Contraindications

1. Known past or suspected cancer of the breast.
2. Known or suspected estrogen-dependent malignant tumours (e.g. endometrial cancer)
3. Undiagnosed abnormal genital bleeding.
4. Untreated endometrial hyperplasia
5. Active or past history of venous thromboembolism (e.g. deep vein thrombosis, pulmonary embolism)
6. Active or recent arterial thromboembolic disease (e.g. angina, myocardial infarction)
7. Acute liver disease or history of liver disease where the liver function tests have failed to return to normal.
8. Known hypersensitivity to the active substance or to any of the excipients of Premarin Vaginal Cream.
9. Porphyria

4.4 Special warnings and precautions for use

Due to estrogen absorption following the application of Premarin Vaginal Cream, prolonged administration might result in systemic effects. Therefore, the following warnings and precautions should be considered.

For the treatment of postmenopausal symptoms, HRT should only be initiated for symptoms that adversely affect quality of life. In all cases, a careful appraisal of the risks and benefits should be undertaken at least annually and HRT should only be continued as long as the benefit outweighs the risk.

1. Medical Examination/Follow up

Before initiating or reinstituting HRT, a complete personal and family medical history should be taken. Physical (including pelvic and breast) examination should be guided by the contraindications and warnings for use. During treatment, periodic check-ups are recommended of a frequency and nature adapted to the individual women.

Women should be advised what changes in their breasts should be reported to their doctor or nurse (see 'Breast Cancer' below). Investigations, including mammography, should be carried out in accordance with currently accepted screening practices, modified to the clinical needs of the individual.

2. Conditions that need supervision

If any of the following conditions are present, have occurred previously, and/or have been aggravated during pregnancy or previous hormone treatment, the patient should be closely supervised. It should be taken into account that these conditions may recur or be aggravated during treatment with Premarin Vaginal Cream, in particular:

- Leiomyoma (uterine fibroids) or endometriosis
- A family history of, or other risk factors for, thromboembolic disorders (see below)
- Risk factors for estrogen dependent tumours (e.g. first degree heredity for breast cancer)
- Hypertension
- Liver disorders (e.g. liver adenoma)
- Diabetes mellitus with or without vascular involvement
- Cholelithiasis
- Migraine or (severe) headaches
- Systemic lupus erythematosus (SLE)
- A history of endometrial hyperplasia (see below)
- Epilepsy
- Asthma
- Otosclerosis

3. Reasons for immediate withdrawal of therapy

Therapy should be discontinued if a contra-indication is discovered and in the following situations:

- Jaundice or deterioration in liver function
- Significant increase in blood pressure
- New onset of migraine-type headache
- Pregnancy

4. Endometrial Hyperplasia

The risk of endometrial hyperplasia and carcinoma is increased when systemic estrogens are administered alone for prolonged periods of time. The endometrial safety of long-term or repeated use of topical vaginal estrogens is uncertain. Therefore, if repeated, treatment should be reviewed at least annually, with special consideration given to any symptoms of endometrial hyperplasia or carcinoma.

Unopposed Estrogen stimulation may lead to premalignant or malignant transformation in the residual foci of endometriosis. Therefore, caution is advised when using this product in women who have undergone hysterectomy because of endometriosis, especially if they are known to have residual endometriosis.

If break-through bleeding or spotting appears at any time on therapy, the reason should be investigated, which may include endometrial biopsy to exclude endometrial malignancy.

5. Breast Cancer

A randomised placebo-controlled trial, the Women's Health Initiative study (WHI), and epidemiological studies, including the Million Women Study (MWS), have reported an increased risk of breast cancer in women taking estrogens, estrogen-progestogen combinations or tibolone for HRT for several years (see Section 4.8 Undesirable effects). For all HRT, an excess risk becomes apparent within a few years of use and increases with the duration of intake but returns to baseline within a few (at most five) years after stopping treatment.

In the MWS, the relative risk of breast cancer with conjugated equine estrogens (CEE) or estradiol (E2) was greater when a progestogen was added, either sequentially or continuously, and regardless of type of progestogen. There was no evidence of a difference in risk between the different routes of administration.

In the WHI study, the continuous combined conjugated equine estrogen and medroxyprogesterone acetate (CEE + MPA) product used was associated with breast cancers that were slightly larger in size and more frequently had local lymph node metastases compared to placebo.

HRT, especially estrogen-progestogen combined treatment, increases the density of mammographic images which may adversely affect the radiological detection of breast cancer.

6. Venous Thromboembolism

Hormone replacement therapy (HRT) is associated with a higher relative risk of developing venous thromboembolism (VTE) i.e. deep vein thrombosis or pulmonary embolism. One randomised controlled trial and epidemiological studies found a two to threefold higher risk for users compared with non-users. For non- users it is estimated that the number of cases of VTE that will occur over a 5-year period is about 3 per 1000 women aged 50-59 years and 8 per 1000 women aged between 60-69 years. It is estimated that in healthy women who use HRT for 5 years, the number of additional cases of VTE over a 5-year period will be between 2 and 6 (best estimate = 4) per 1000 women aged 50-59 years and between 5 and 15 (best estimate = 9) per 1000 women aged 60-69 years. The occurrence of such an event is more likely in the first year of HRT than later.

Generally recognised risk factors for VTE include a personal or family history and severe obesity (Body Mass Index $>30kg/m^2$) and systemic lupus erythematosus (SLE). There is no consensus about the possible role of varicose veins in VTE.

Patients with a history of VTE or known thrombophilic states have an increased risk of VTE. HRT may add to this risk. Personal or strong family history of thromboembolism or recurrent spontaneous abortion should be investigated in order to exclude a thrombophilic predisposition. Until a thorough evaluation of thrombophilic factors has been made or anticoagulant treatment initiated, use of HRT in such patients should be viewed as contraindicated. Those women already on anticoagulant treatment require careful consideration of the benefit-risk of use of HRT.

The risk of VTE may be temporarily increased with prolonged immobilisation, major trauma or major surgery. As in all postoperative patients scrupulous attention should be given to prophylactic measures to prevent VTE following surgery. Where prolonged immobilisation is liable to follow elective surgery, particularly abdominal or orthopaedic surgery to the lower limbs, consideration should be given to temporarily stopping HRT 4 weeks earlier, if this is possible. Treatment should not be restarted until the woman is completely mobilised.

If venous thromboembolism develops after initiating therapy the drug should be discontinued. Patients should be told to contact their doctors immediately when they are aware of potential thromboembolic symptoms (e.g. painful swelling of leg, sudden pain in the chest, dyspnoea)

7. Coronary Artery Disease (CAD)

There is no evidence from randomised controlled trials of cardiovascular benefit with continuous combined conjugated estrogens and MPA. Two large clinical trials (WHI and HERS i.e. Heart and Estrogen/progestin Replacement Study) showed a possible increased risk of cardiovascular morbidity in the first year of use and no overall benefit. For other HRT products, there are only limited data from randomised controlled trials examining effects in cardiovascular morbidity or mortality. Therefore, it is uncertain whether these findings also extend to other HRT products.

8. Stroke

One large randomised clinical trial (WHI-trial) found, as a secondary outcome, an increased risk of ischaemic stroke in healthy women during treatment with continuous combined conjugated estrogens and MPA. For women who do not use HRT, it is estimated that the number of cases of stroke that will occur over a 5 year period is about 3 per 1000 women aged 50-59 years and 11 per 1000 women aged 60-69 years. It is estimated that for women who use conjugated estrogens and MPA for 5 years, the number of additional cases will be between 0 and 3 (best estimate = 1) per 1000 users aged 50-59 years and between 1 and 9 (best estimate = 4) per 1000 users aged 60-69 years. It is unknown whether the increased risk also extends to other HRT products.

9. Ovarian Cancer

Long term (at least 5 –10 years) use of estrogen-only HRT products in hysterectomised women has been associated with an increased risk of ovarian cancer in some epidemiological studies. It is uncertain whether long-term use of combined HRT confers different risk than estrogen-only products.

Other Conditions

10. Estrogens may cause fluid retention and therefore patients with cardiac or renal dysfunction should be carefully observed. Patients with terminal renal insufficiency should be closely observed, since it is expected that the level of circulating active ingredients in Premarin is increased.

11. Women with an intact uterus of child-bearing potential should be advised to adhere to non-hormonal contraceptive methods.

Premarin Vaginal Cream has been shown to weaken latex condoms. The potential for Premarin Vaginal Cream to weaken and contribute to the failure of condoms, diaphragms or cervical caps made of latex or rubber should be considered. If there is still a possibility that a patient could become pregnant, they should be advised to use an alternative form of non-hormonal contraceptive.

12. The use of estrogen may influence the laboratory results of certain endocrine tests and liver enzymes.

Estrogens increase thyroid binding globulin (TBG), leading to increased circulating total thyroid hormone, as measured by protein-bound iodine (PBI), T4 levels (by column or by radio-immunoassay) or T3 levels (by radio-immunoassay). T3 resin uptake is decreased, reflecting the elevated TBG. Free T4 and free T3 concentrations are unaltered.

Other binding proteins may be elevated in serum, i.e. corticoid binding globulin (CBG), sex-hormone-binding globulin (SHBG) leading to increased circulating corticosteroids and sex steroids, respectively. Free or biologically active hormone concentrations are unchanged. Other plasma proteins may be increased (angiotensinogen/renin substrate, alpha-I-antitrypsin, ceruloplasmin).

Some patients dependent on thyroid hormone replacement therapy may require increased doses in order to maintain their free thyroid hormone levels in an acceptable range. Therefore, these patients should have their thyroid function monitored more frequently when commencing concurrent treatment in order to maintain their free thyroid hormone levels in an acceptable range.

13. There is an increase in the risk of gallbladder disease in women receiving HRT (see conditions that need supervision)

14. A worsening of glucose tolerance may occur in patients taking estrogens and therefore diabetic patients should be carefully observed while receiving hormone replacement therapy.

15. Women with pre-existing hypertriglyceridemia should be followed closely during estrogen replacement or hormone replacement therapy, since rare cases of large increases of plasma triglycerides leading to pancreatitis have been reported with estrogen therapy in this condition.

16. Estrogens should be used with caution in individuals with severe hypocalcaemia

17. There is no conclusive evidence for improvement of cognitive function. There is some evidence from the WHI trial of increased risk of probable dementia in women who start using continuous combined CEE and MPA after the age of 65. It is unknown whether the findings apply to younger post-menopausal women or other HRT products.

4.5 Interaction with other medicinal products and other forms of interaction

The metabolism of estrogens may be increased by concomitant use of substances known to induce drug-metabolising enzymes, specifically cytochrome P450 enzymes, such as anticonvulsants (e.g. phenobarbital, phenytoin, carbamazepine) and anti-infectives (e.g. rifampicin, rifabutin, nevirapine, efavirenz).

Ritonavir and nelfinavir, although known as strong inhibitors, by contrast exhibit inducing properties when used concomitantly with steroid hormones.

Herbal preparations containing St John's wort *(Hypericum perforatum)* may induce the metabolism of estrogens.

Clinically, an increased metabolism of estrogens and progestogens may lead to decreased effect and changes in the uterine bleeding profile.

The response to metyrapone may be reduced.

4.6 Pregnancy and lactation

Premarin is not indicated during pregnancy.

For women with a uterus:

If pregnancy occurs during medication with Premarin, treatment should be withdrawn immediately. The results of most epidemiological studies to date relevant to inadvertent foetal exposure to estrogens indicate no teratogenic or foetotoxic effects.

Lactation:

Premarin is not indicated during lactation.

4.7 Effects on ability to drive and use machines

Not applicable.

4.8 Undesirable effects

See also 4.4 Special warnings and special precautions for use.

Adverse drug reactions (ADRs)

The following adverse reactions have been reported with Premarin Vaginal Cream or are undesirable effects associated with estrogens.

System Organ Class	Adverse Reaction
Reproductive system	Breakthrough bleeding/ spotting Application site reactions of vulvovaginal discomfort including burning, irritation, and genital pruritus Vaginal discharge Increased size of uterine leiomyomata Endometrial hyperplasia
Breast disorders	Breast pain, tenderness, enlargement, discharge
Gastrointestinal disorders	Nausea, vomiting bloating, abdominal pain Pancreatitis
Nervous system disorders	Dizziness, headache, migraine, nervousness, stroke
Musculoskeletal, connective tissue and bone disorders	Arthralgias, leg cramps
Psychiatric disorders	Changes in libido, mood disturbances, irritability, depression
Vascular disorders	Pulmonary embolism. Venous thromboembolism
Cardiac disorders	Myocardial Infarction

General disorders and administration site conditions	Oedema Exacerbation of otosclerosis
Skin and subcutaneous tissue disorders	Alopecia Chloasma, hirsutism, pruritus, rash Erythema multiforme, erythema nodosum
Hepatobiliary disorder	Gallbladder disease Cholestatic jaundice
Infections and Infestations	Vaginitis, including vaginal candidiasis Cystitis
Neoplasms benign and malignant (including cysts and polyps)	Breast cancer*, Fibrocystic breast changes Endometrial cancer, Enlargement of hepatic haemangiomas
Immune system disorders	Urticaria, Angioedema, Anaphylactic/anaphylactoid reactions, Hypersensitivity
Metabolism and nutrition disorders	Glucose intolerance
Eye Disorders	Intolerance to contact lenses
Investigations	Changes in weight (increase or decrease) Increased triglycerides Increases in blood pressure

Breast Cancer

According to evidence from a large number of epidemiological studies and one randomised placebo-controlled trial, the Women's Health Initiative (WHI), the overall risk of breast cancer increases with increasing duration of HRT use in current or recent HRT users.

For estrogen-only HRT, estimates of relative risk (RR) from a reanalysis of original data from 51 epidemiological studies (in which >80% of HRT use was estrogen-only HRT) and from the epidemiological Million Women Study (MWS) are similar at 1.35 (95%CI 1.21 - 1.49) and 1.30 (95%CI 1.21 - 1.40), respectively.

For estrogen plus progestogen combined HRT, several epidemiological studies have reported an overall higher risk for breast cancer than with estrogens alone.

The MWS reported that, compared to never users, the use of various types of estrogen-progestogen combined HRT was associated with a higher risk of breast cancer (RR = 2.00, 95%CI: 1.88 - 2.12) than use of estrogens alone (RR = 1.30, 95%CI: 1.21 - 1.40) or use of tibolone (RR=1.45; 95%CI 1.25-1.68).

The WHI trial reported a risk estimate of 1.24 (95%CI 1.01 - 1.54) after 5.6 years of use of estrogen-progestogen combined HRT (CEE + MPA) in all users compared with placebo.

The absolute risks calculated from the MWS and the WHI trial are presented below:

The MWS has estimated, from the known average incidence of breast cancer in developed countries, that:

- For women not using HRT, about 32 in every 1000 are expected to have breast cancer diagnosed between the ages of 50 and 64 years.
- For 1000 current or recent users of HRT, the number of additional cases during the corresponding period will be
- For users of estrogen-only replacement therapy

- between 0 and 3 (best estimate = 1.5) for 5 years' use
- between 3 and 7 (best estimate = 5) for 10 years' use.

- For users of estrogen plus progestogen combined HRT

- between 5 and 7 (best estimate = 6) for 5 years' use
- between 18 and 20 (best estimate = 19) for 10 years' use.

The WHI trial estimated that after 5.6 years of follow-up of women between the ages of 50 and 79 years, an additional 8 cases of invasive breast cancer would be due to estrogen-progestogen combined HRT (CEE + MPA) per 10,000 women years.

According to calculations from the trial data, it is estimated that:

- For 1000 women in the placebo group.

- About 16 cases of invasive breast cancer would be diagnosed in 5 years.

- For 1000 women who used estrogen plus progestogen combined HRT (CEE + MPA), the number of additional cases would be

- Between 0 and 9 (best estimate = 4) for 5 years' use.

The number of additional cases of breast cancer in women who use HRT is broadly similar for women who start HRT irrespective of age at start of use (between the ages of 45-65) (see section 4.4 Special warnings and special precautions for use).

Other adverse reactions reported in association with estrogen/progestogen treatment including Premarin Vaginal Cream:

- Estrogen-dependent neoplasms benign and malignant, e.g. endometrial hyperplasia, endometrial cancer
- Venous thromboembolism, i.e. deep leg or pelvic venous thrombosis and pulmonary embolism, is more frequent among hormone replacement therapy users than among non-users. For further information, see section 4.3 Contra-indications and 4.4 Special warnings and special precautions for use.
- Retinal vascular thrombosis
- Myocardial infarction
- Increases in blood pressure
- Cholestatic jaundice
- Enlargement of hepatic haemangiomas
- Skin and subcutaneous disorders: erythema multiforme, erythema nodosum, vascular purpura
- Probable dementia (see section 4.4 Special warnings and special precautions for use)
- Exacerbation of chorea
- Exacerbation of porphyria,
- Exacerbation of hypocalcaemia
- Exacerbation of otosclerosis

4.9 Overdose

Numerous reports of ingestion of large doses of estrogen-containing oral contraceptives by young children indicate that acute serious ill effects do not occur. Overdosage of estrogen may cause nausea and vomiting, and withdrawal bleeding may occur in females. There is no specific antidote and further treatment should be symptomatic.

5. PHARMACOLOGICAL PROPERTIES

5.1 Pharmacodynamic properties

ATC Code: G03C A57

Conjugated Estrogens

Conjugated estrogen cream has identical pharmacological actions to endogenous estrogens. The active ingredients are primarily the sulphate esters of estrone, equilin sulphates, 17α-estradiol and 17β-estradiol. These substitute for the loss of estrogen production in menopausal women, and alleviate menopausal symptoms.

5.2 Pharmacokinetic properties

Absorption

The estrogens in Premarin Vaginal Cream are absorbed systemically.

Distribution

The distribution of exogenous estrogen is similar to that of endogenous estrogens. Estrogens are widely distributed in the body and are generally found in higher concentrations in the sex hormone target organs. Estrogens circulate in the blood largely bound to sex hormone binding globulin (SHBG) and albumin.

Metabolism

Exogenous estrogens are metabolised in the same manner as endogenous estrogens. Circulating estrogens exist in dynamic equilibrium of metabolic interconversions. These transformations take place mainly in the liver. Estradiol is converted reversibly to estrone, and both can be converted to estriol, which is the major urinary metabolite. Estrogens also undergo enterohepatic recirculation via sulphate and glucuronide conjugation in the liver, biliary secretion of conjugates into the intestine, and hydrolysis in the gut following reabsorption. In post-menopausal women a significant proportion of the circulating estrogens exists as sulphate conjugates, especially estrone sulphate, which serves as a circulating reservoir for the formation of more active estrogens.

Excretion

Estriol, estrone and estradiol are excreted in the urine along with glucuronide and sulphate conjugates.

5.3 Preclinical safety data

There are no preclinical data of relevance to the prescriber which are additional to that already included in other sections of the SPC.

6. PHARMACEUTICAL PARTICULARS

6.1 List of excipients

Liquid paraffin, glyceryl monostearate, cetyl alcohol, cetyl esters wax, white wax, methyl stearate, sodium lauryl sulphate, phenylethyl alcohol, glycerin, propylene glycol monostearate, purified water.

6.2 Incompatibilities

Not applicable.

6.3 Shelf life

2 years.

6.4 Special precautions for storage

Do not store above 25°C.

6.5 Nature and contents of container

Primary container: Aluminium tube with a white screw-on cap, containing 42.5g of cream.

Secondary container: Cardboard carton.

6.6 Special precautions for disposal and other handling

Not applicable.

7. MARKETING AUTHORISATION HOLDER

John Wyeth and Brother Limited

Trading as Wyeth Pharmaceuticals

Huntercombe Lane South

Taplow, Maidenhead

Berkshire, SL6 0PH

8. MARKETING AUTHORISATION NUMBER(S)

PL 00011/0163.

9. DATE OF FIRST AUTHORISATION/RENEWAL OF THE AUTHORISATION

22 November 1990 / 12 December 1995

10. DATE OF REVISION OF THE TEXT

Approved 6th December 2005

* Trademark

Premique

(Wyeth Pharmaceuticals)

1. NAME OF THE MEDICINAL PRODUCT

Premique*.

2. QUALITATIVE AND QUANTITATIVE COMPOSITION

Premique is a tablet for oral administration containing conjugated estrogens† 0.625mg and medroxyprogesterone acetate (MPA) 5.0mg.

†Conjugated estrogens contain sodium estrone sulphate, sodium equilin sulphate, 17α-dihydroequilin, 17α-estradiol, equilenin, 17α-dihydroequilenin, 17β-dihydroequilenin, 17β-dihydroequilenin, 17β-estradiol and 8,9-dehydro-estrone.

For excipients see 6.1.

3. PHARMACEUTICAL FORM

Coated tablet.

Light blue oval biconvex sugar coated tablet marked with '0.625/5'.

4. CLINICAL PARTICULARS

4.1 Therapeutic indications

Hormone replacement therapy for estrogen deficiency symptoms in postmenopausal women with an intact uterus.

Prevention of osteoporosis in postmenopausal women at high risk of future fractures who are intolerant of, or contra-indicated for, other medicinal products approved for the prevention of osteoporosis.

4.2 Posology and method of administration

Premique is taken orally in a continuous combined 28-day regimen of one tablet daily with no break between packs.

In women who are not taking hormone replacement therapy or women who switch from another continuous combined hormone replacement therapy product, treatment may be started on any convenient day. In women transferring from a sequential hormone replacement therapy regimen, treatment should begin the day following completion of the prior regimen.

For treatment of postmenopausal symptoms: The usual starting dose is one tablet 0.625mg/5.0mg per day.

For prevention and management of osteoporosis associated with estrogen deficiency: The usual starting dose is one tablet 0.625mg/5.0mg per day. (see section 5.1 Pharmacodynamic Properties).

Maintenance/Continuation/Extended treatment

For initiation and continuation of treatment of postmenopausal symptoms, the lowest effective dose for the shortest duration (see also Section 4.4 Special warnings and special precautions for use) should be used. Patients should be re-evaluated periodically to determine if treatment for symptoms is still necessary.

The benefits of the lower risk of endometrial hyperplasia and endometrial cancer due to adding a progestogen should be weighed against the increased risk of breast cancer (see sections 4.4 Special warnings and special precautions for use and 4.8 Undesirable effects).

Forgotten tablet: If a tablet is forgotten, it should be taken as soon as the patient remembers, therapy should then be continued as before. If more than one tablet has been forgotten only the most recent tablet should be taken, the patient should not take double the usual dose to make up for missed tablets.

Missed pills may cause breakthrough bleeding.

Elderly:

There are no special dosage requirements for elderly patients, but, as with all medicines, the lowest effective dose should be used.

Children:

Not recommended.

4.3 Contraindications

1. Known, past or suspected breast cancer
2. Known or suspected estrogen-dependent malignant tumours (e.g. endometrial cancer)
3. Undiagnosed abnormal genital bleeding
4. Untreated endometrial hyperplasia

5. Active or past history of venous thromboembolism (e.g. deep vein thrombosis, pulmonary embolism)

6. Active or recent arterial thromboembolic disease (e.g. angina, myocardial infarction)

7. Acute liver disease or history of liver disease where the liver function tests have failed to return to normal

8. Known hypersensitivity to the active substances or to any of the excipients of Premique tablets

9. Porphyria

4.4 Special warnings and precautions for use

For the treatment of postmenopausal symptoms, HRT should only be initiated for symptoms that adversely affect quality of life. In all cases, a careful appraisal of the risks and benefits should be undertaken at least annually and HRT should only be continued as long as the benefit outweighs the risk.

1. Medical examination/Follow up

Before initiating or reinstituting HRT, a complete personal and family medical history should be taken. Physical (including pelvic and breast) examination should be guided by the contraindications and warnings for use. During treatment, periodic check-ups are recommended of a frequency and nature adapted to the individual women. Women should be advised what changes in their breasts should be reported to their doctor or nurse (see 'Breast Cancer' below). Investigations, including mammography, should be carried out in accordance with currently accepted screening practices, modified to the clinical needs of the individual.

2. Conditions that need supervision

If any of the following conditions are present, have occurred previously, and/or have been aggravated during pregnancy or previous hormone treatment, the patient should be closely supervised. It should be taken into account that these conditions may recur or be aggravated during treatment with Premique, in particular:

– Leiomyoma (uterine fibroids) or endometriosis

– A family history of, or other risk factors for, thromboembolic disorders (see below)

– Risk factors for estrogen dependent tumours (e.g. 1st degree heredity for breast cancer)

– Hypertension

– Liver disorders (e.g. liver adenoma)

– Diabetes mellitus with or without vascular involvement

– Cholelithiasis

– Migraine or (severe) headaches

– Systemic lupus erythematosus (SLE)

– A history of endometrial hyperplasia (see below)

– Epilepsy

– Asthma

– Otosclerosis

3. Reasons for immediate withdrawal of therapy

Therapy should be discontinued if a contra-indication is discovered and in the following situations:

– Jaundice or deterioration in liver function

– Significant increase in blood pressure

– New onset of migraine-type headache

– Pregnancy

4. Endometrial Hyperplasia

The risk of endometrial hyperplasia and carcinoma is increased when estrogens are administered alone for prolonged periods (see section 4.8 Undesirable effects). The addition of a progestogen for at least 12 days of the cycle in non-hysterectomised women greatly reduces this risk. Unless there is a previous diagnosis of endometriosis it is not recommended to add a progestogen in hysterectomised women.

The reduction in risk to the endometrium should be weighed against the increase in the risk of breast cancer of added progestogen (see 'Breast cancer' below and Section 4.8 Undesirable effects).

Break-through bleeding and spotting may occur during the first months of treatment. If break-through bleeding or spotting appears after some time on therapy, or continues after treatment has been discontinued, the reason should be investigated, which may include endometrial biopsy to exclude endometrial malignancy.

5. Breast Cancer

A randomised placebo-controlled trial, the Women's Health Initiative study (WHI), and epidemiological studies, including the Million Women Study (MWS), have reported an increased risk of breast cancer in women taking estrogens, estrogen-progestogen combinations or tibolone for HRT for several years (see Section 4.8 Undesirable effects). For all HRT, an excess risk becomes apparent within a few years of use and increases with the duration of intake but returns to baseline within a few (at most five) years after stopping treatment.

In the MWS, the relative risk of breast cancer with conjugated equine estrogens (CEE) or estradiol (E2) was greater when a progestogen was added, either sequentially or continuously, and regardless of type of progestogen. There was no evidence of a difference in risk between the different routes of administration.

In the WHI study, the continuous combined conjugated equine estrogen and medroxyprogesterone acetate (CEE + MPA) product used was associated with breast cancers that were slightly larger in size and more frequently had local lymph node metastases compared to placebo.

HRT, especially estrogen-progestogen combined treatment, increases the density of mammographic images which may adversely affect the radiological detection of breast cancer.

6. Venous thromboembolism

Hormone replacement therapy (HRT) is associated with a higher relative risk of developing venous thromboembolism (VTE) i.e. deep vein thrombosis or pulmonary embolism. One randomised controlled trial and epidemiological studies found a two to threefold higher risk for users compared with non-users. For non- users it is estimated that the number of cases of VTE that will occur over a 5-year period is about 3 per 1000 women aged 50-59 years and 8 per 1000 women aged between 60-69 years. It is estimated that in healthy women who use HRT for 5 years, the number of additional cases of VTE over a 5-year period will be between 2 and 6 (best estimate 4) per 1000 women aged 50-59 years and between 5 and 15 (best estimate = 9) per 1000 women aged 60-69 years. The occurrence of such an event is more likely in the first year of HRT than later.

Generally recognised risk factors for VTE include a personal or family history and severe obesity (Body Mass Index $>30kg/m^2$) and systemic lupus erythematosus (SLE). There is no consensus about the possible role of varicose veins in VTE.

Patients with a history of VTE or known thrombophilic states have an increased risk of VTE. HRT may add to this risk. Personal or strong family history of thromboembolism or recurrent spontaneous abortion should be investigated in order to exclude a thrombophilic predisposition. Until a thorough evaluation of thrombophilic factors has been made or anticoagulant treatment initiated, use of HRT in such patients should be viewed as contraindicated. Those women already on anticoagulant treatment require careful consideration of the benefit-risk of use of HRT.

The risk of VTE may be temporarily increased with prolonged immobilisation, major trauma or major surgery. As in all postoperative patients scrupulous attention should be given to prophylactic measures to prevent VTE following surgery. Where prolonged immobilisation is liable to follow elective surgery, particularly abdominal or orthopaedic surgery to the lower limbs, consideration should be given to temporarily stopping HRT 4-6 weeks earlier, if this is possible. Treatment should not be restarted until the woman is completely mobilised.

If venous thromboembolism develops after initiating therapy the drug should be discontinued. Patients should be told to contact their doctors immediately when they are aware of potential thromboembolic symptoms (e.g. painful swelling of a leg, sudden pain in the chest, dyspnoea).

7. Coronary Artery Disease (CAD)

There is no evidence from randomised controlled trials of cardiovascular benefit with continuous combined conjugated estrogens and MPA. Two large clinical trials (WHI and HERS i.e. Heart and Estrogen/progestin Replacement Study) showed a possible increased risk of cardiovascular morbidity in the first year of use and no overall benefit. For other HRT products, there are only limited data from randomised controlled trials examining effects in cardiovascular morbidity or mortality. Therefore, it is uncertain whether these findings also extend to other HRT products.

8. Stroke

One large randomised clinical trial (WHI-trial) found, as a secondary outcome, an increased risk of ischaemic stroke in healthy women during treatment with continuous combined conjugated estrogens and MPA. For women who do not use HRT, it is estimated that the number of cases of stroke that will occur over a 5 year period is about 3 per 1000 women aged 50-59 years and 11 per 1000 women aged 60-69 years. It is estimated that for women who use conjugated estrogens and MPA for 5 years, the number of additional cases will be between 0 and 3 (best estimate =1) per 1000 users aged 50-59 years and between 1 and 9 (best estimate = 4) per 1000 users aged 60-69 years. It is unknown whether the increased risk also extends to other HRT products.

9. Ovarian Cancer

Long term (at least 5 –10 years) use of estrogen-only HRT products in hysterectomised women has been associated with an increased risk of ovarian cancer in some epidemiological studies. It is uncertain whether long-term use of combined HRT confers different risk than estrogen-only products.

Other Conditions

10. Estrogens/progestogens may cause fluid retention and therefore patients with cardiac or renal dysfunction should be carefully observed. Patients with terminal renal insufficiency should be closely observed, since it is expected that the level of circulating active ingredients in Premique is increased.

11. The use of estrogen may influence the laboratory results of certain endocrine tests and liver enzymes.

Estrogens increase thyroid binding globulin (TBG), leading to increased circulating total thyroid hormone, as measured by protein-bound iodine (PBI), T4 levels (by column or by radio-immunoassay) or T3 levels (by radio-immunoassay). T3 resin uptake is decreased, reflecting the elevated TBG. Free T4 and free T3 concentrations are usually unaltered.

Other binding proteins may be elevated in serum, i.e. corticoid binding globulin (CBG), sex-hormone-binding globulin (SHBG) leading to increased circulating corticosteroids and sex steroids, respectively. Free or biologically active hormone concentrations are usually unchanged. Other plasma proteins may be increased (angiotensinogen/renin substrate, alpha-I-antitrypsin, ceruloplasmin).

Some patients dependent on thyroid hormone replacement therapy may require increased doses in order to maintain their free thyroid hormone levels in an acceptable range. Therefore, patients should have their thyroid function monitored more frequently when commencing concurrent treatment in order to maintain their free thyroid hormone levels in an acceptable range.

12. There is an increase in the risk of gallbladder disease in women receiving HRT (see conditions that need supervision)

13. A worsening of glucose tolerance may occur in some patients on estrogen/progestogen therapy and therefore diabetic patients should be carefully observed while receiving hormone replacement therapy.

This product contains lactose and sucrose. Patients with rare hereditary problems of galactose intolerance, fructose intolerance, the Lapp lactase deficiency, glucose-galactose malabsorption or sucrase-isomaltase insufficiency should not take this medicine.

14. Women with pre-existing hypertriglyceridemia should be followed closely during estrogen replacement or hormone replacement therapy, since rare cases of large increases of plasma triglycerides leading to pancreatitis have been reported with estrogen therapy in this condition.

15. Estrogens should be used with caution in individuals with severe hypocalcaemia

16. There is no conclusive evidence for improvement of cognitive function. There is some evidence from the WHI trial of increased risk of probable dementia in women who start using continuous combined CEE and MPA after the age of 65. It is unknown whether the findings apply to younger post-menopausal women or other HRT products.

4.5 Interaction with other medicinal products and other forms of interaction

The metabolism of estrogens and progestogens may be increased by concomitant use of substances known to induce drug-metabolising enzymes, specifically cytochrome P450 enzymes, such as anticonvulsants (e.g. phenobarbital, phenytoin, carbamazepine) and anti-infectives (e.g. rifampicin, rifabutin, nevirapine, efavirenz).

Ritonavir and nelfinavir, although known as strong inhibitors, by contrast exhibit inducing properties when used concomitantly with steroid hormones.

Herbal preparations containing St John's wort *(Hypericum perforatum)* may induce the metabolism of estrogens and progestogens.

Clinically, an increased metabolism of estrogens and progestogens may lead to decreased effect and changes in the uterine bleeding profile.

The response to metyrapone may be reduced.

Aminogluthimide administered concomitantly with MPA may significantly depress the bioavailiablity of MPA.

4.6 Pregnancy and lactation

Pregnancy:

Premique is not indicated during pregnancy. If pregnancy occurs during medication with Premique treatment should be withdrawn immediately.

Clinically, data on a limited number of exposed pregnancies indicate no adverse effects of MPA on the foetus.

The results of most epidemiological studies to date relevant to inadvertent foetal exposure to combinations of estrogens and progestogens indicate no teratogenic or foetotoxic effect.

Lactation:

Premique is not indicated during lactation.

4.7 Effects on ability to drive and use machines

Premique should not affect the ability to drive or use machinery.

4.8 Undesirable effects

See also Section 4.4 Special warnings and special precautions for use.

Adverse drug reactions (ADRs)

The adverse reactions listed in the table are based on post-marketing spontaneous (reporting rate), clinical trials and class-effects. Breast pain is a very common adverse event reported in ⩾ 10% of patients.

(see Table 1 on next page)

Breast cancer

According to evidence from a large number of epidemiological studies and one randomised placebo-controlled trial, the Women's Health Initiative (WHI), the overall risk

Table 1

System Organ Class	Very Common ADRs (>1/10)	Common ADRs (>1/100, <1/10)	Uncommon ADRs (>1/1000, <1/100)	Rare ADRs (>1/10000, <1/1000)	Very Rare ADRs (<1/10000), isolated reports
Infections and infestations		Vaginitis,	Vaginal candidiasis		
Neoplasms benign and malignant (including cysts and polyps)				Fibrocystic breast changes Ovarian cancer	Enlargement of hepatic hemangiomas
Immune system disorders				Anaphylactic/ anaphylactoid reactions, including urticaria and angioedema	
Metabolism and nutrition disorders				Glucose intolerance	Exacerbation of porphyria; hypocalcemia
Psychiatric disorders		Depression	Changes in libido; Mood disturbances;	Irritability	
Nervous system disorders			Dizziness; Headache; Migraine; Anxiety	Stroke; Exacerbation of epilepsy;	Exacerbation of chorea
Eye disorders			Intolerance to contact lenses	None	Retinal vascular thrombosis
Cardiac disorders				Myocardial infarction	
Vascular disorders				Pulmonary embolism; Superficial thrombophlebitis	
Respiratory, thoracic and mediastinal disorders				Exacerbation of asthma	
Gastrointestinal disorders			Nausea; Bloating; Abdominal pain	Vomiting; Pancreatitis	
Hepatobiliary disorders			Gallbladder disease	None	Cholestatic jaundice
Skin and subcutaneous tissue disorders			Alopecia; acne; Pruritis	Chloasma/melasma; Hirsutism; Pruritus; Rash	
Musculoskeletal, connective tissue and bone disorders		Arthralgias; Leg cramps			
Reproductive system & breast disorders	Breast pain	Breakthrough bleeding/spotting dysmenorrhea, breast, tenderness, enlargement, discharge	Change in menstrual flow; Change in cervical ectropion and secretion	Galactorrhoea; Increased size of uterine leiomyomata	
General disorders and administration site conditions			Oedema		
Investigations		Changes in weight (increase or decrease) Increased triglycerides			Increase in blood pressure

of breast cancer increases with increasing duration of HRT use in current or recent HRT users.

For estrogen-only HRT, estimates of relative risk (RR) from a reanalysis of original data from 51 epidemiological studies (in which >80% of HRT use was estrogen-only HRT) and from the epidemiological Million Women Study (MWS) are similar at 1.35 (95%CI 1.21 – 1.49) and 1.30 (95%CI 1.21 – 1.40), respectively.

For estrogen plus progestogen combined HRT, several epidemiological studies have reported an overall higher risk for breast cancer than with estrogens alone.

The MWS reported that, compared to never users, the use of various types of estrogen-progestogen combined HRT was associated with a higher risk of breast cancer (RR = 2.00, 95%CI: 1.88 – 2.12) than use of estrogens alone (RR = 1.30, 95%CI: 1.21 – 1.40) or use of tibolone (RR=1.45; 95%CI 1.25-1.68).

The WHI trial reported a risk estimate of 1.24 (95%CI 1.01 – 1.54) after 5.6 years of use of estrogen-progestogen combined HRT (CEE + MPA) in all users compared with placebo.

The absolute risks calculated from the MWS and the WHI trial are presented below:

The MWS has estimated, from the known average incidence of breast cancer in developed countries, that:

- For women not using HRT, about 32 in every 1000 are expected to have breast cancer diagnosed between the ages of 50 and 64 years.
- For 1000 current or recent users of HRT, the number of additional cases during the corresponding period will be
- For users of estrogen-only replacement therapy

o between 0 and 3 (best estimate = 1.5) for 5 years' use

o between 3 and 7 (best estimate = 5) for 10 years' use.

- For users of estrogen plus progestogen combined HRT

o between 5 and 7 (best estimate = 6) for 5 years' use

o between 18 and 20 (best estimate = 19) for 10 years' use.

The WHI trial estimated that after 5.6 years of follow-up of women between the ages of 50 and 79 years, an additional 8 cases of invasive breast cancer would be due to estrogen-progestogen combined HRT (CEE + MPA) per 10,000 women years.

According to calculations from the trial data, it is estimated that:

- For 1000 women in the placebo group.

o About 16 cases of invasive breast cancer would be diagnosed in 5 years.

- For 1000 women who used estrogen plus progestogen combined HRT (CEE + MPA), the number of additional cases would be

o Between 0 and 9 (best estimate = 4) for 5 years' use.

The number of additional cases of breast cancer in women who use HRT is broadly similar for women who start HRT irrespective of age at start of use (between the ages of 45-65) (see section 4.4 Special warnings and special precautions for use).

<u>Endometrial Cancer</u>

In women with an intact uterus, the risk of endometrial hyperplasia and endometrial cancer increases with increasing duration of use of unopposed estrogens. According to data from epidemiological studies, the best estimate of the risk is that for women not using HRT, about 5 in every 1000 are expected to have endometrial cancer diagnosed between the ages of 50 and 65. Depending on the duration of treatment and estrogen dose, the reported increase in endometrial cancer risk among unopposed estrogen users varies from 2-to 12-fold greater compared with non-users. Adding a progestogen to estrogen-only therapy greatly reduces this increased risk.

Other adverse reactions reported in association with estrogen/progestogen treatment including Premique:

- Estrogen-dependent neoplasms benign and malignant, e.g. endometrial hyperplasia, endometrial cancer
- Venous thromboembolism, i.e. deep leg or pelvic venous thrombosis and pulmonary embolism, is more frequent among hormone replacement therapy users than among non-users. For further information, see section 4.3 Contra-indications and 4.4 Special Warnings and Precautions for Use.
- Myocardial infarction
- Stroke
- Skin and subcutaneous disorders: erythema multiforme, erythema nodosum, vascular purpura
- Probable dementia (see section 4.4 Special warnings and special precautions for use)
- Exacerbation of otosclerosis

4.9 Overdose

Symptoms of overdosage of estrogen-containing products in adults and children may include nausea, vomiting, breast tenderness, dizziness, abdominal pain, drowsiness/fatigue and withdrawal bleeding may occur in females. There is no specific antidote, and further treatment should be symptomatic.

5. PHARMACOLOGICAL PROPERTIES

5.1 Pharmacodynamic properties

ATC Code: GO3F A12

<u>Conjugated Estrogens</u>

The active ingredients are primarily the sulphate esters of estrone, equilin sulphates, 17α-estradiol and 17β-estradiol. These substitute for the loss of estrogen production in menopausal women, and alleviate menopausal symptoms. Estrogens prevent bone loss following menopause or ovariectomy.

<u>Progestogen:</u>

As estrogens promote the growth of the endometrium, unopposed estrogens increase the risk of endometrial hyperplasia and cancer. The addition of a progestogen reduces but does not eliminate the estrogen-induced risk of endometrial hyperplasia in non-hysterectomised women.

<u>Relief of estrogen-deficiency symptoms</u>

In a 1-year clinical trial (n=2,808), vasomotor symptoms were assessed for efficacy during the first 12 weeks of treatment in a subset of symptomatic women (n=241) who had at least 7 moderate or severe hot flushes daily or 50 moderate to severe hot flushes during the week before randomisation. Premique 0.625mg/2.5mg (conjugated estrogens/medroxyprogesterone acetate) was shown to be statistically better than placebo at weeks 4, 8 and 12 for relief of both frequency and severity of moderate to severe vasomotor symptoms.

In two clinical trials, the incidence of amenorrhoea (no bleeding or spotting) increased over time in women treated with Premique 0.625mg/2.5mg. Amenorrhoea was seen in 68% of women at cycle 6 and 77% of women at cycle 12. Breakthrough bleeding and/or spotting appeared in 48% during the first 3 months, and in 24% of women during months 10-12 of treatment.

<u>Prevention of osteoporosis</u>

Epidemiological studies suggest a number of individual risk factors which contribute to the development of postmenopausal osteoporosis. These include: early menopause; family history of osteoporosis; thin, small frame; cigarette use; recent prolonged systemic corticosteroid use.

Estrogen deficiency at menopause is associated with an increasing bone turnover and decline in bone mass. The effect of estrogens on the bone mineral density is dose-dependent. Protection appears to be effective for as long as treatment is continued. After discontinuation of HRT, bone mass is lost at a rate similar to that in untreated women.

Evidence from the WHI trial and meta-analysed trials shows that current use of HRT, alone or in combination with a progestogen – given to predominantly healthy women – reduces the risk of hip, vertebral and other osteoporotic fractures. HRT may also help prevent fractures in women with low bone density and/or established osteoporosis, but the evidence for that is limited.

After 3 years of treatment with Premique 0.625mg/2.5mg, the increase in lumbar spine bone mineral density (BMD) was 4.87% ± 0.66. The percentage of women who maintained (less than 1% BMD loss per year) or gained BMD in lumbar zone during treatment was 92%.

Premique 0.625mg/2.5mg also had an effect on hip BMD. The increase after 3 years was 1.94% ± 0.44 at total hip. The percentage of women who maintained (less than 1% BMD loss per year) or gained BMD in hip zone during treatment was 88%.

5.2 Pharmacokinetic properties

Absorption

Conjugated estrogens are soluble in water and are well absorbed from the gastrointestinal tract after release from the drug formulation. However Premique contains a formulation of medroxyprogesterone acetate (MPA) that is immediately released and conjugated estrogens that are slowly released over several hours. MPA is well absorbed from the gastrointestinal tract. Table 1 summarises the mean pharmacokinetic parameters for unconjugated and conjugated estrogens, and medroxyprogesterone acetate following administration of 2 Premique 0.625/2.5mg and 2 Premique 0.625/5mg tablets to healthy postmenopausal women.

Table 2 – Pharmacokinetic parameters for Premique

Pharmacokinetic parameters for unconjugated and conjugated estrogens (CE) and medroxyprogesterone acetate (MPA)

(see Table 2 below)

Distribution

The distribution of exogenous estrogens is similar to that of endogenous estrogens. Estrogens are widely distributed in the body and are generally found in higher concentrations in the sex hormone target organs. Estrogens circulate in the blood largely bound to sex hormone binding globulin (SHBG) and albumin. MPA is approximately 90% bound to plasma proteins but does not bind to SHBG.

Metabolism

Exogenous estrogens are metabolised in the same manner as endogenous estrogens. Circulating estrogens exist in a dynamic equilibrium of metabolic interconversions. These transformations take place mainly in the liver. Estradiol is converted reversibly to estrone, and both can be converted to estriol, which is the major urinary metabolite. Estrogens also undergo enterohepatic recirculation via sulphate and glucuronide conjugation in the liver, biliary secretion of conjugates into the intestine, and hydrolysis in the gut followed by reabsorption. In postmenopausal women a significant proportion of the circulating estrogens exists as sulphate conjugates, especially estrone sulphate, which serves as a circulating reservoir for the formation of more active estrogens. Metabolism and elimination of MPA occur primarily in the liver via hydroxylation, with subsequent conjugation and elimination in the urine.

Excretion

Estradiol, estrone and estriol are excreted in the urine along with glucuronide and sulphate conjugates. Most metabolites of MPA are extracted as glucuronide conjugates with only minor amounts secreted as sulphates.

5.3 Preclinical safety data

Long-term continuous administration of natural and synthetic estrogens in certain animal species increases the frequency of carcinomas of the breast, cervix, vagina and liver.

In a two-year oral study in which female rats were exposed to MPA dosages of up to 5000μg/kg/day in their diets (50 times higher - based on AUC values - than the level observed in women taking 10mg of MPA), a dose-related increase in pancreatic islet cell tumours (adenomas and carcinomas) occurred. Pancreatic tumour incidence was increased at 1000 and 5000μg/kg/day, but not at 200μg/kg/day.

The cortisol activity of MPA at these high doses is thought to increase serum glucose in rats which reactively stimulates the beta cells of the pancreatic islets to produce insulin. This repeated stimulation is thought to cause the tumours in rats. Similar lesions are not likely to occur in humans since the endocrine system of rats is more sensitive to hormones than that of women. When MPA is combined with estrogen, MPA binds to fewer glucocorticosteriod receptors and thus has less effect on plasma glucose. In humans, the diabetogenic response to MPA at therapeutic doses is slight. Moreover, an extensive literature search revealed no evidence that MPA causes pancreatic tumours in humans.

6. PHARMACEUTICAL PARTICULARS

6.1 List of excipients

Tablet core:

Lactose monohydrate

Methylcellulose

Magnesium stearate

Calcium phosphate tribasic

Tablet coating:

Calcium sulphate anhydrous

Macrogol

Glyceryl mono-oleate

Shellac

Microcrystalline cellulose

Sucrose

Titanium dioxide

Povidone

Carnauba wax

Colour (E132)

Stearic acid

Edible Ink (Opacode Black S-8-27741)†

†Opacode black ink contains iron oxide black (E172), shellac, purified water, ethanol, N-butyl alcohol, propylene glycol, ethyl acetate.

6.2 Incompatibilities

None known.

Table 2 Pharmacokinetic parameters for Premique

Drug	2 × 0.625mg CE/2.5mg MPA Combination Tablets (n=54)				2 × 0.625mg CE/5mg MPA Combination Tablets (n=51)			
PK Parameter Arithmetic Mean (%CV)	C_{max} (pg/mL)	t_{max} (h)	$t_{1/2}$ (h)	AUC (pg.h/mL)	C_{max} (pg/mL)	t_{max} (h)	$t_{1/2}$ (h)	AUC (pg.h/mL)
Unconjugated Estrogens								
Estrone	175(23)	7.6(24)	31.6(23)	5358(34)	124(43)	10(35)	62.2(137)	6303(40)
BA*-Estrone	159(26)	7.6(24)	16.9(34)	3313(40)	104(49)	10(35)	26.0(100)	3136(51)
Equilin	71(31)	5.8(34)	9.9(35)	951(43)	54(43)	8.9(34)	15.5(53)	1179(56)
PK Parameter Arithmetic Mean (%CV)	C_{max} (pg/mL)	t_{max} (h)	$t_{1/2}$ (h)	AUC (pg.h/mL)	C_{max} (pg/mL)	t_{max} (h)	$t_{1/2}$ (h)	AUC (pg.h/mL)
Conjugated Estrogens								
Total Estrone	6.6(38)	6.1(28)	20.7(34)	116(59)	6.3(48)	9.1(29)	23.6(36)	151(42)
BA*- Total Estrone	6.4(39)	6.1(28)	15.4(34)	100(57)	6.2(48)	9.1(29)	20.6(35)	139(40)
Total Equilin	5.1(45)	4.6(35)	11.4(25)	50(70)	4.2(52)	7.0(36)	17.2(131)	72(50)
PK Parameter Arithmetic Mean (%CV)	C_{max} (pg/mL)	t_{max} (h)	$t_{1/2}$ (h)	AUC (pg.h/mL)	C_{max} (pg/mL)	t_{max} (h)	$t_{1/2}$ (h)	AUC (pg.h/mL)
Medroxyprogesterone acetate								
MPA	1.5(40)	2.8(54)	37.6(30)	37(30)	4.8(31)	2.4(50)	46.3(39)	102(28)

BA* = Baseline adjusted

$T_{1/2}$ = apparent terminal phase disposition half life ($0.693/\lambda_z$)

6.3 Shelf life

Three years.

6.4 Special precautions for storage

Do not store above 25°C. Keep blister in outer carton to protect from light.

6.5 Nature and contents of container

Primary container

Polyvinylchloride (PVC)/Aluminium foil blister pack.

Secondary container

Cardboard carton.

Presentation

Each carton contains 28 tablets (1 blister pack) or 84 tablets (3 blister packs).

Not all pack sizes may be marketed.

6.6 Special precautions for disposal and other handling

No special instructions.

7. MARKETING AUTHORISATION HOLDER

John Wyeth and Brother Limited

Trading as: Wyeth Pharmaceuticals

Huntercombe Lane South

Taplow, Maidenhead

Berkshire SL6 0PH

8. MARKETING AUTHORISATION NUMBER(S)

PL 00011/0212.

9. DATE OF FIRST AUTHORISATION/RENEWAL OF THE AUTHORISATION

27th September 1995

10. DATE OF REVISION OF THE TEXT

29 July 2008

* Trade Mark

Premique Cycle

(Wyeth Pharmaceuticals)

1. NAME OF THE MEDICINAL PRODUCT

Premique Cycle.

2. QUALITATIVE AND QUANTITATIVE COMPOSITION

Premique Cycle is a combination of conjugated estrogens* USP and medroxyprogesterone acetate (MPA) Ph.Eur.

Premique Cycle is composed of 14 tablets containing 0.625mg conjugated estrogens and 14 combination tablets containing 0.625mg conjugated estrogens and 10mg MPA.

*Conjugated estrogens contain sodium estrone sulphate, sodium equilin sulphate, 17α-dihydroequilin, 17α-estradiol, equilenin, 17α-dihydroequilenin, 17β-dihydroequilin, 17β-dihydroequilenin, 17β-estradiol and 8,9-dehydro-oestrone.

3. PHARMACEUTICAL FORM

Premique Cycle is available for oral administration as conjugated estrogens 0.625mg tablets and conjugated estrogens/MPA (0.625mg/10mg) combination tablets. Conjugated estrogens 0.625mg tablets are white, oval, biconvex sugar-coated tablets marked "0.625". Conjugated estrogens/MPA (0.625mg/10mg) combination tablets are green, oval, biconvex sugar-coated tablets marked "0.625/10".

4. CLINICAL PARTICULARS

4.1 Therapeutic indications

• Hormone replacement therapy for estrogen deficiency symptoms in menopausal and postmenopausal women

• Prevention of osteoporosis in postmenopausal women at high risk of future fractures who are intolerant of, or contra-indicated for, other medicinal products approved for the prevention of osteoporosis.

4.2 Posology and method of administration

Adults:

Premique Cycle is available for oral use in a sequential regimen for treatment of women with a uterus. That is, for the first 14 days of each cycle (days 1-14), one white tablet containing conjugated estrogens 0.625mg is taken daily, and for the last 14 days (days 15-28), one green tablet containing conjugated estrogens 0.625mg and MPA 10mg is taken daily. There should be no break between packs.

For most post-menopausal women, therapy may be commenced at any convenient time, although if the patient is still menstruating, commencement on the first day of bleeding is recommended. In women transferring from another sequential hormone replacement therapy regimen, treatment should begin the day following completion of the prior regimen.

Patients should be advised that a regular withdrawal bleed will usually occur at the end of one cycle of Premique Cycle and the beginning of the next.

For treatment of postmenopausal symptoms: Conjugated estrogens 0.625mg daily for the first 14 days of each cycle, followed by conjugated estrogens/MPA (0.625mg/10mg) combination tablet daily on days 15 to 28.

For prevention and treatment of osteoporosis associated with estrogen deficiency: Conjugated estrogens 0.625mg daily for the first 14 days and conjugated estrogens/MPA (0.625mg/10mg) combination tablet taken daily on days 15 to 28. (See section 5.1 Pharmacological Properties)

Maintenance/Continuation/Extended Treatment:

For initiation and continuation of treatment of postmenopausal symptoms, the lowest effective dose for the shortest duration (see also Section 4.4 Special warnings and special precautions for use) should be used. Patients should be re-evaluated periodically to determine if treatment for symptoms is still necessary.

The benefits of the lower risk of endometrial hyperplasia and endometrial cancer due to adding a progestogen should be weighed against the increased risk of breast cancer (see sections 4.4 Special Warnings and Precautions for Use and 4.8 Undesirable Effects).

Forgotten tablet: If a tablet is forgotten, it should be taken as soon as the patient remembers, therapy should then be continued as before. If more than one tablet has been forgotten only the most recent tablet should be taken. The patient should not take double the usual dose to make up for the missed tablet.

Missed pills may cause breakthrough bleeding.

Elderly:

There are no special dosage requirements for elderly patients, but, as with all medicines, the lowest effective dose should be used.

Children:

Not recommended.

4.3 Contraindications

1. Known, past or suspected cancer of the breast.
2. Known or suspected estrogen-dependent malignant tumours (e.g. endometrial cancer)
3. Undiagnosed abnormal genital bleeding.
4. Untreated endometrial hyperplasia
5. Active or past history of venous thromboembolism (e.g. deep vein thrombosis, pulmonary embolism)
6. Active or recent arterial thromboembolic disease (e.g. angina, myocardial infarction)
7. Acute liver disease or history of liver disease where the liver function tests have failed to return to normal.
8. Known hypersensitivity to the active substances or to any of the excipients of Premique Cycle tablets.
9. Porphyria

4.4 Special warnings and precautions for use

For the treatment of postmenopausal symptoms, HRT should only be initiated for symptoms that adversely affect quality of life. In all cases, a careful appraisal of the risks and benefits should be undertaken at least annually and HRT should only be continued as long as the benefit outweighs the risk.

1. Medical examination/Follow up

Before initiating or reinstituting HRT, a complete personal and family medical history should be taken. Physical (including pelvic and breast) examination should be guided by the contraindications and warnings for use. During treatment, periodic check-ups are recommended of a frequency and nature adapted to the individual women. Women should be advised what changes in their breasts should be reported to their doctor or nurse (see 'Breast Cancer' below). Investigations, including mammography, should be carried out in accordance with currently accepted screening practices, modified to the clinical needs of the individual.

2. Conditions that need supervision

If any of the following conditions are present, have occurred previously, and/or have been aggravated during pregnancy or previous hormone treatment, the patient should be closely supervised. It should be taken into account that these conditions may recur or be aggravated during treatment with Premique Cycle, in particular:

– Leiomyoma (uterine fibroids) or endometriosis

– A family history of, or other risk factors for, thromboembolic disorders (see below)

– Risk factors for estrogen dependent tumours (e.g. 1st degree heredity for breast cancer)

– Hypertension

– Liver disorders (e.g. liver adenoma)

– Diabetes mellitus with or without vascular involvement

– Cholelithiasis

– Migraine or (severe) headaches

– Systemic lupus erythematosus (SLE)

– A history of endometrial hyperplasia (see below)

– Epilepsy

– Asthma

– Otosclerosis

3. Reasons for immediate withdrawal of therapy

Therapy should be discontinued if a contra-indication is discovered and in the following situations:

– Jaundice or deterioration in liver function

– Significant increase in blood pressure

– New onset of migraine-type headache

– Pregnancy

4. Endometrial Hyperplasia

The risk of endometrial hyperplasia and carcinoma is increased when estrogens are administered alone for prolonged periods (see section 4.8 Undesirable effects). The addition of a progestogen for at least 12 days of the cycle in non-hysterectomised women greatly reduces this risk. Unless there is a previous diagnosis of endometriosis it is not recommended to add a progestogen in hysterectomised women.

The reduction in risk to the endometrium should be weighed against the increase in the risk of breast cancer of added progestogen (see 'Breast cancer' below and Section 4.8 Undesirable effects).

Break-through bleeding and spotting may occur during the first months of treatment. If break-through bleeding or spotting appears after some time on therapy, or continues after treatment has been discontinued, the reason should be investigated, which may include endometrial biopsy to exclude endometrial malignancy.

5. Breast Cancer

A randomised placebo-controlled trial, the Women's Health Initiative study (WHI), and epidemiological studies, including the Million Women Study (MWS), have reported an increased risk of breast cancer in women taking estrogens, estrogen-progestogen combinations or tibolone for HRT for several years (see Section 4.8 Undesirable effects). For all HRT, an excess risk becomes apparent within a few years of use and increases with the duration of intake but returns to baseline within a few (at most five) years after stopping treatment.

In the MWS, the relative risk of breast cancer with conjugated equine estrogens (CEE) or estradiol (E2) was greater when a progestogen was added, either sequentially or continuously, and regardless of type of progestogen. There was no evidence of a difference in risk between the different routes of administration.

In the WHI study, the continuous combined conjugated equine estrogen and medroxyprogesterone acetate (CEE + MPA) product used was associated with breast cancers that were slightly larger in size and more frequently had local lymph node metastases compared to placebo.

HRT, especially estrogen-progestogen combined treatment, increases the density of mammographic images which may adversely affect the radiological detection of breast cancer.

6. Venous thromboembolism

Hormone replacement therapy (HRT) is associated with a higher relative risk of developing venous thromboembolism (VTE) i.e. deep vein thrombosis or pulmonary embolism. One randomised controlled trial and epidemiological studies found a two to threefold higher risk for users compared with non-users. For non- users it is estimated that the number of cases of VTE that will occur over a 5-year period is about 3 per 1000 women aged 50-59 years and 8 per 1000 women aged between 60-69 years. It is estimated that in healthy women who use HRT for 5 years, the number of additional cases of VTE over a 5-year period will be between 2 and 6 (best estimate 4) per 1000 women aged 50-59 years and between 5 and 15 (best estimate = 9) per 1000 women aged 60-69 years. The occurrence of such an event is more likely in the first year of HRT than later.

Generally recognised risk factors for VTE include a personal or family history and severe obesity (Body Mass Index $>30kg/m^2$) and systemic lupus erythematosus (SLE). There is no consensus about the possible role of varicose veins in VTE.

Patients with a history of VTE or known thrombophilic states have an increased risk of VTE. HRT may add to this risk. Personal or strong family history of thromboembolism or recurrent spontaneous abortion should be investigated in order to exclude a thrombophilic predisposition. Until a thorough evaluation of thrombophilic factors has been made or anticoagulant treatment initiated, use of HRT in such patients should be viewed as contraindicated. Those women already on anticoagulant treatment require careful consideration of the benefit-risk of use of HRT.

The risk of VTE may be temporarily increased with prolonged immobilisation, major trauma or major surgery. As in all postoperative patients, scrupulous attention should be given to prophylactic measures to prevent VTE following surgery. Where prolonged immobilisation is liable to follow elective surgery, particularly abdominal or orthopaedic surgery to the lower limbs, consideration should be given to temporarily stopping HRT 4-6 weeks earlier, if this is possible. Treatment should not be restarted until the woman is completely mobilised.

If venous thromboembolism develops after initiating therapy, the drug should be discontinued. Patients should be told to contact their doctors immediately when they are aware of potential thromboembolic symptoms (e.g. painful swelling of a leg, sudden pain in the chest, dyspnoea).

7. Coronary Artery Disease (CAD)

There is no evidence from randomised controlled trials of cardiovascular benefit with continuous combined conjugated estrogens and MPA. Two large clinical trials (WHI and HERS i.e. Heart and Estrogen/progestin Replacement Study) showed a possible increased risk of cardiovascular morbidity in the first year of use and no overall benefit. For other HRT products, there are only limited data from randomised controlled trials examining effects in cardiovascular morbidity or mortality. Therefore, it is uncertain whether these findings also extend to other HRT products.

8. Stroke

One large randomised clinical trial (WHI-trial) found, as a secondary outcome, an increased risk of ischaemic stroke in healthy women during treatment with continuous combined conjugated estrogens and MPA. For women who do not use HRT, it is estimated that the number of cases of stroke that will occur over a 5 year period is about 3 per 1000 women aged 50-59 years and 11 per 1000 women aged 60-69 years. It is estimated that for women who use conjugated estrogens and MPA for 5 years, the number of additional cases will be between 0 and 3 (best estimate =1) per 1000 users aged 50-59 years and between 1 and 9 (best estimate = 4) per 1000 users aged 60-69 years. It is unknown whether the increased risk also extends to other HRT products.

9. Ovarian Cancer

Long term (at least 5-10 years) use of estrogen-only HRT products in hysterectomised women has been associated with an increased risk of ovarian cancer in some epidemiological studies. It is uncertain whether long-term use of combined HRT confers different risk than estrogen-only products.

Other Conditions

10. Estrogens/progestogens may cause fluid retention and therefore patients with cardiac or renal dysfunction should be carefully observed. Patients with terminal renal insufficiency should be closely observed, since it is expected that the level of circulating active ingredients in Premique Cycle is increased.

11. The use of estrogen may influence the laboratory results of certain endocrine tests and liver enzymes.

Estrogens increase thyroid binding globulin (TBG), leading to increased circulating total thyroid hormone, as measured by protein-bound iodine (PBI), T4 levels (by column or by radio-immunoassay) or T3 levels (by radio-immunoassay). T3 resin uptake is decreased, reflecting the elevated TBG. Free T4 and free T3 concentrations are unaltered.

Other binding proteins may be elevated in serum, i.e. corticoid binding globulin (CBG), sex-hormone-binding globulin (SHBG) leading to increased circulating corticosteroids and sex steroids, respectively. Free or biologically active hormone concentrations are unchanged. Other plasma proteins may be increased (angiotensinogen/renin substrate, alpha-I-antitrypsin, ceruloplasmin).

Some patients dependent on thyroid hormone replacement therapy may require increased doses in order to maintain their free thyroid hormone levels in an acceptable range. Therefore, patients should have their thyroid function monitored more frequently when commencing concurrent treatment in order to maintain their free thyroid hormone levels in an acceptable range.

12. There is an increase in the risk of gallbladder disease in women receiving HRT (see conditions that need supervision)

13. A worsening of glucose tolerance may occur in some patients on estrogen/progestogen therapy and therefore diabetic patients should be carefully observed while receiving hormone replacement therapy.

This product contains lactose and sucrose. Patients with rare hereditary problems of galactose intolerance, fructose intolerance, the Lapp lactase deficiency, glucose-galactose malabsorption or sucrase-isomaltase insufficiency should not take this medicine.

14. Women with pre-existing hypertriglyceridemia should be followed closely during estrogen replacement or hormone replacement therapy, since rare cases of large increases of plasma triglycerides leading to pancreatitis have been reported with estrogen therapy in this condition.

15. Estrogens should be used with caution in individuals with severe hypocalcaemia.

16. There is no conclusive evidence of improvement of cognitive function. There is some evidence from the WHI trial of increased risk of probable dementia in women who start using continuous combined CEE and MPA after the age of 65. It is unknown whether the findings apply to younger post-menopausal women or other HRT products.

4.5 Interaction with other medicinal products and other forms of interaction

The metabolism of estrogens and progestogens may be increased by concomitant use of substances known to induce drug-metabolising enzymes, specifically cytochrome P450 enzymes, such as anticonvulsants (e.g. phenobarbital, phenytoin, carbamazepine) and anti-infectives (e.g. rifampicin, rifabutin, nevirapine, efavirenz).

Ritonavir and nelfinavir, although known as strong inhibitors, by contrast exhibit inducing properties when used concomitantly with steroid hormones.

Herbal preparations containing St John's wort *(Hypericum perforatum)* may induce the metabolism of estrogens and progestogens.

Clinically, an increased metabolism of estrogens and progestogens may lead to decreased effect and changes in the uterine bleeding profile.

The response to metyrapone may be reduced.

Aminogluthimide administered concomitantly with MPA may significantly depress the bioavailiablity of MPA.

4.6 Pregnancy and lactation

Pregnancy:

Premique Cycle is not indicated during pregnancy. If pregnancy occurs during medication with Premique treatment should be withdrawn immediately.

Clinically, data on a limited number of exposed pregnancies indicate no adverse effects of MPA on the foetus.

The results of most epidemiological studies to date relevant to inadvertent foetal exposure to combinations of estrogens and progestogens indicate no teratogenic or foetotoxic effect.

Lactation:

Premique Cycle is not indicated during lactation.

4.7 Effects on ability to drive and use machines

Premique Cycle should not affect the ability to drive or use machines.

4.8 Undesirable effects

See also 4.4 Special warnings and special precautions for use.

Adverse drug reactions (ADRs)

The adverse reactions listed in the table are based on post-marketing spontaneous (reporting rate), clinical trials and class-effects. Breast pain is a very common adverse event reported in ≥ 10% of patients.

(see Table 1 opposite)

Breast cancer

According to evidence from a large number of epidemiological studies and one randomised placebo-controlled trial, the Women's Health Initiative (WHI), the overall risk of breast cancer increases with increasing duration of HRT use in current or recent HRT users.

For estrogen-only HRT, estimates of relative risk (RR) from a reanalysis of original data from 51 epidemiological studies (in which >80% of HRT use was estrogen-only HRT) and from the epidemiological Million Women Study (MWS) are similar at 1.35 (95%CI 1.21 – 1.49) and 1.30 (95%CI 1.21 – 1.40), respectively.

For estrogen plus progestogen combined HRT, several epidemiological studies have reported an overall higher risk for breast cancer than with estrogens alone.

The MWS reported that, compared to never users, the use of various types of estrogen-progestogen combined HRT was associated with a higher risk of breast cancer (RR = 2.00, 95%CI: 1.88 – 2.12) than use of estrogens alone (RR = 1.30, 95%CI: 1.21 – 1.40) or use of tibolone (RR=1.45; 95%CI 1.25-1.68).

The WHI trial reported a risk estimate of 1.24 (95%CI 1.01 – 1.54) after 5.6 years of use of estrogen-progestogen combined HRT (CEE + MPA) in all users compared with placebo.

The absolute risks calculated from the MWS and the WHI trial are presented below:

The MWS has estimated, from the known average incidence of breast cancer in developed countries, that:

- For women not using HRT, about 32 in every 1000 are expected to have breast cancer diagnosed between the ages of 50 and 64 years.
- For 1000 current or recent users of HRT, the number of additional cases during the corresponding period will be
- For users of estrogen-only replacement therapy
  - o between 0 and 3 (best estimate = 1.5) for 5 years' use
  - o between 3 and 7 (best estimate = 5) for 10 years' use.
- For users of estrogen plus progestogen combined HRT
  - o between 5 and 7 (best estimate = 6) for 5 years' use
  - o between 18 and 20 (best estimate = 19) for 10 years' use.

The WHI trial estimated that after 5.6 years of follow-up of women between the ages of 50 and 79 years, an additional 8 cases of invasive breast cancer would be due to estrogen-progestogen combined HRT (CEE + MPA) per 10,000 women years.

According to calculations from the trial data, it is estimated that:

- For 1000 women in the placebo group.
  - o About 16 cases of invasive breast cancer would be diagnosed in 5 years.
- For 1000 women who used estrogen plus progestogen combined HRT (CEE + MPA), the number of additional cases would be
  - o Between 0 and 9 (best estimate = 4) for 5 years' use.

The number of additional cases of breast cancer in women who use HRT is broadly similar for women who start HRT irrespective of age at start of use (between the ages of 45-65) (see section 4.4 Special warnings and special precautions for use).

Table 1

System Organ Class	Very Common ADRs (>1/10)	Common ADRs (>1/100, <1/10)	Uncommon ADRs (>1/1000, <1/100)	Rare ADRs (>1/10000, <1/1000)	Very Rare ADRs (<1/10000), isolated reports
Infections and infestations		Vaginitis	Vaginal candidiasis		
Neoplasms benign and malignant (including cysts and polyps)				Fibrocystic breast changes Ovarian cancer	Enlargement of hepatic hemangiomas
Immune system disorders				Anaphylactic/anaphylactoid reactions, including urticaria and angioedema	
Metabolism and nutrition disorders				Glucose intolerance	Exacerbation of porphyria; hypocalcemia
Psychiatric disorders		Depression	Changes in libido; Mood disturbances;	Irritability	
Nervous system disorders			Dizziness; Headache; Migraine; Anxiety	Stroke; Exacerbation of epilepsy;	Exacerbation of chorea
Eye disorders			Intolerance to contact lenses	None	Retinal vascular thrombosis
Cardiac disorders				Myocardial infarction	
Vascular disorders				Pulmonary embolism; Superficial thrombophlebitis	
Respiratory, thoracic and mediastinal disorders				Exacerbation of asthma	
Gastrointestinal disorders			Nausea; Bloating; Abdominal pain	Vomiting; Pancreatitis	
Hepatobiliary disorders			Gallbladder disease	None	Cholestatic jaundice
Skin and subcutaneous tissue disorders			Alopecia; acne; Pruritis	Chloasma/melasma; Hirsutism; Pruritus; Rash	
Musculoskeletal, connective tissue and bone disorders		Arthralgias; Leg cramps			
Reproductive system & breast disorders	Breast pain	Breakthrough bleeding/spotting dysmenorrhea, breast, tenderness, enlargement, discharge	Change in menstrual flow; Change in cervical ectropion and secretion	Galactorrhoea; Increased size of uterine leiomyomata	
General disorders and administration site conditions			Oedema		
Investigations		Changes in weight (increase or decrease) Increased triglycerides			Increase in blood pressure

Endometrial Cancer

In women with an intact uterus, the risk of endometrial hyperplasia and endometrial cancer increases with increasing duration of use of unopposed estrogens. According to data from epidemiological studies, the best estimate of the risk is that for women not using HRT, about 5 in every 1000 are expected to have endometrial cancer diagnosed between the ages of 50 and 65. Depending on the duration of treatment and estrogen dose, the reported increase in endometrial cancer risk among unopposed estrogen users varies from 2-to 12-fold greater compared with non-users. Adding a progestogen to estrogen-only therapy greatly reduces this increased risk.

Other adverse reactions reported in association with estrogen/progestogen treatment including Premique:

- Estrogen-dependent neoplasms benign and malignant, e.g. endometrial hyperplasia, endometrial cancer
- Venous thromboembolism, i.e. deep leg or pelvic venous thrombosis and pulmonary embolism, is more frequent among hormone replacement therapy users than among non-users. For further information, see section 4.3 Contra-indications and 4.4 Special Warnings and Precautions for Use.
- Myocardial infarction
- Stroke
- Skin and subcutaneous disorders: erythema multiforme, erythema nodosum, vascular purpura
- Probable dementia (see section 4.4 Special warnings and special precautions for use)
- Exacerbation of otosclerosis

4.9 Overdose

Symptoms of overdosage of estrogen-containing products in adults and children may include nausea, vomiting, breast tenderness, dizziness, abdominal pain, drowsiness/fatigue and withdrawal bleeding may occur in females. There is no specific antidote, and further treatment should be symptomatic.

5. PHARMACOLOGICAL PROPERTIES

5.1 Pharmacodynamic properties

ATC Code: GO3F A12

Conjugated Estrogens

The active ingredients are primarily the sulphate esters of estrone, equilin sulphates, 17α-estradiol and 17β-estradiol. These substitute for the loss of estrogen production in menopausal women, and alleviate menopausal symptoms. Estrogens prevent bone loss following menopause or ovariectomy.

Progestogen:

As estrogens promote the growth of the endometrium, unopposed estrogens increase the risk of endometrial hyperplasia and cancer. The addition of a progestogen reduces but does not eliminate the estrogen-induced risk of endometrial hyperplasia in non-hysterectomised women.

Relief of estrogen-deficiency symptoms

In a 1-year clinical trial (n=2,808), vasomotor symptoms were assessed for efficacy during the first 12 weeks of treatment in a subset of symptomatic women (n=241) who had at least 7 moderate or severe hot flushes daily or 50 moderate to severe hot flushes during the week before randomisation. Premique 0.625mg/2.5mg (conjugated estrogens/medroxyprogesterone acetate) was shown to be statistically better than placebo at weeks 4, 8 and 12 for relief of both frequency and severity of moderate to severe vasomotor symptoms.

In two clinical trials, the incidence of amenorrhoea (no bleeding or spotting) increased over time in women treated with Premique 0.625mg/2.5mg. Amenorrhoea was seen in 68% of women at cycle 6 and 77% of women at cycle 12. Breakthrough bleeding and/or spotting appeared in 48% during the first 3 months, and in 24% of women during months 10-12 of treatment.

Prevention of osteoporosis

Epidemiological studies suggest a number of individual risk factors which contribute to the development of post-menopausal osteoporosis. These include: early menopause; family history of osteoporosis; thin, small frame; cigarette use; recent prolonged systemic corticosteroid use.

Estrogen deficiency at menopause is associated with an increasing bone turnover and decline in bone mass. The effect of estrogens on the bone mineral density is dose-dependent. Protection appears to be effective for as long as treatment is continued. After discontinuation of HRT, bone mass is lost at a rate similar to that in untreated women.

Evidence from the WHI trial and meta-analysed trials shows that current use of HRT, alone or in combination with a progestogen – given to predominantly healthy women – reduces the risk of hip, vertebral and other osteoporotic fractures. HRT may also help prevent fractures in women with low bone density and/or established osteoporosis, but the evidence for that is limited.

After 3 years of treatment with Premique 0.625mg/2.5mg, the increase in lumbar spine bone mineral density (BMD) was 4.87% ± 0.66. The percentage of women who maintained (less than 1% BMD loss per year) or gained BMD in lumbar zone during treatment was 92%.

Premique 0.625mg/2.5mg also had an effect on hip BMD. The increase after 3 years was 1.94% ± 0.44 at total hip. The percentage of women who maintained (less than 1% BMD loss per year) or gained BMD in hip zone during treatment was 88%.

5.2 Pharmacokinetic properties

Absorption

Conjugated estrogens are soluble in water and are well absorbed from the gastrointestinal tract after release from the drug formulation. However Premique contains a formulation of medroxyprogesterone acetate (MPA) that is immediately released and conjugated estrogens that are slowly released over several hours. MPA is well absorbed from the gastrointestinal tract. Table 1 summarises the mean pharmacokinetic parameters for unconjugated and conjugated estrogens, and medroxyprogesterone acetate following administration of 2 Premique 0.625/2.5mg and 2 Premique 0.625/5mg tablets to healthy postmenopausal women.

Distribution

The distribution of exogenous estrogens is similar to that of endogenous estrogens. Estrogens are widely distributed in the body and are generally found in higher concentrations in the sex hormone target organs. Estrogens circulate in the blood largely bound to sex hormone binding globulin (SHBG) and albumin. MPA is approximately 90% bound to plasma proteins but does not bind to SHBG.

Metabolism

Exogenous estrogens are metabolised in the same manner as endogenous estrogens. Circulating estrogens exist in a dynamic equilibrium of metabolic interconversions. These transformations take place mainly in the liver. Estradiol is converted reversibly to estrone, and both can be converted to estriol, which is the major urinary metabolite. Estrogens also undergo enterohepatic recirculation via sulphate and glucuronide conjugation in the liver, biliary secretion of conjugates into the intestine, and hydrolysis in the gut followed by reabsorption. In postmenopausal women a significant proportion of the circulating estrogens exists as sulphate conjugates, especially estrone sulphate, which serves as a circulating reservoir for the formation of more active estrogens. Metabolism and elimination of MPA occur primarily in the liver via hydroxylation, with subsequent conjugation and elimination in the urine.

Excretion

Estradiol, estrone and estriol are excreted in the urine along with glucuronide and sulphate conjugates. Most metabolites of MPA are extracted as glucuronide conjugates with only minor amounts secreted as sulphates.

Table 2 – Pharmacokinetic parameters for Premique

Pharmacokinetic parameters for unconjugated and conjugated estrogens (CE) and medroxyprogesterone acetate (MPA)

(see Table 2 below)

5.3 Preclinical safety data

Long-term continuous administration of natural and synthetic estrogens in certain animal species increases the frequency of carcinomas of the breast, cervix, vagina and liver.

In a two-year oral study in which female rats were exposed to MPA dosages of up to 5000μg/kg/day in their diets (50 times higher – based on AUC values – than the level observed in women taking 10mg of MPA), a dose-related increase in pancreatic islet cell tumours (adenomas and carcinomas) occurred. Pancreatic tumour incidence was increased at 1000 and 5000μg/kg/day, but not at 200μg/kg/day.[†]

The cortisol activity of MPA at these high doses is thought to increase serum glucose in rats which reactively stimulates the beta cells of the pancreatic islets to produce insulin. This repeated stimulation is thought to cause the tumours in rats. Similar lesions are not likely to occur in humans, since the endocrine system of rats is more sensitive to hormones than that of women. When MPA is combined with estrogen, MPA binds to fewer glucocorticosteroid receptors and thus has less effect on plasma glucose. In humans, the diabetogenic response to MPA at therapeutic doses is slight. Moreover, an extensive literature search revealed no evidence that MPA causes pancreatic tumours in humans.

Table 2 Pharmacokinetic parameters for Premique

Drug	2 × 0.625mg CE/2.5mg MPA Combination Tablets (n=54)				2 × 0.625mg CE/5mg MPA Combination Tablets (n=51)			
PK Parameter Arithmetic Mean (%CV)	C_{max} (pg/mL)	t_{max} (h)	$t_{1/2}$ (h)	AUC (pg.h/mL)	C_{max} (pg/mL)	t_{max} (h)	$t_{1/2}$ (h)	AUC (pg.h/mL)
Unconjugated Estrogens								
Estrone	175(23)	7.6(24)	31.6(23)	5358(34)	124(43)	10(35)	62.2(137)	6303(40)
BA*-Estrone	159(26)	7.6(24)	16.9(34)	3313(40)	104(49)	10(35)	26.0(100)	3136(51)
Equilin	71(31)	5.8(34)	9.9(35)	951(43)	54(43)	8.9(34)	15.5(53)	1179(56)
PK Parameter Arithmetic Mean (%CV)	C_{max} (pg/mL)	t_{max} (h)	$t_{1/2}$ (h)	AUC (pg.h/mL)	C_{max} (pg/mL)	t_{max} (h)	$t_{1/2}$ (h)	AUC (pg.h/mL)
Conjugated Estrogens								
Total Estrone	6.6(38)	6.1(28)	20.7(34)	116(59)	6.3(48)	9.1(29)	23.6(36)	151(42)
BA*- Total Estrone	6.4(39)	6.1(28)	15.4(34)	100(57)	6.2(48)	9.1(29)	20.6(35)	139(40)
Total Equilin	5.1(45)	4.6(35)	11.4(25)	50(70)	4.2(52)	7.0(36)	17.2(131)	72(50)
PK Parameter Arithmetic Mean (%CV)	C_{max} (pg/mL)	t_{max} (h)	$t_{1/2}$ (h)	AUC (pg.h/mL)	C_{max} (pg/mL)	t_{max} (h)	$t_{1/2}$ (h)	AUC (pg.h/mL)
Medroxyprogesterone acetate								
MPA	1.5(40)	2.8(54)	37.6(30)	37(30)	4.8(31)	2.4(50)	46.3(39)	102(28)

BA* = Baseline adjusted

$T_{1/2}$ = apparent terminal phase disposition half life ($0.693/\lambda_z$)

6. PHARMACEUTICAL PARTICULARS

6.1 List of excipients

White (conjugated estrogens) tablets: calcium phosphate tribasic, calcium sulphate, carnauba wax, microcrystalline cellulose, glyceryl mono-oleate, lactose, magnesium stearate, methylcellulose, macrogol, shellac, sucrose, titanium dioxide (E171) and edible printing ink (Opacode S-8-27741-Black).[†]

Green (conjugated estrogens/MPA) combination tablets: calcium phosphate tribasic, calcium sulphate, carnauba wax, microcrystalline cellulose, glyceryl mono-oleate, lactose, magnesium stearate, methylcellulose, methyl hydroxybenzoate, macrogol, povidone, propyl hydroxybenzoate, shellac, sodium benzoate, sucrose, indigo carmine (E132), titanium dioxide (E171), iron oxide yellow (E172) and edible printing ink[†].

[†] contains iron oxide black (E172), shellac, propylene glycol, ethanol, ethyl acetate, N-Butyl alcohol, purified water, ammonia solution.

6.2 Incompatibilities

None known.

6.3 Shelf life

Two years.

6.4 Special precautions for storage

Do not store above 25°C. Keep blister in outer carton to protect from light.

6.5 Nature and contents of container

Primary container

Polyvinylchloride (PVC)/Aluminium foil blister pack.

Secondary container

Cardboard carton.

Presentation

Cartons containing 3 blisters (84 tablets). Each blister contains 14 conjugated estrogen tablets 0.625mg and 14 conjugated estrogen 0.625mg/MPA 10mg tablets.

6.6 Special precautions for disposal and other handling

No special instructions.

7. MARKETING AUTHORISATION HOLDER

John Wyeth and Brother Limited

Trading as: Wyeth Pharmaceuticals

Taplow, Maidenhead,

Berkshire SL6 0PH,

England, UK.

8. MARKETING AUTHORISATION NUMBER(S)

PL 0011/0239

9. DATE OF FIRST AUTHORISATION/RENEWAL OF THE AUTHORISATION

30 April 1999

10. DATE OF REVISION OF THE TEXT

22 September 2008

Premique Low Dose 0.3mg/1.5mg Modified Release Tablets

(Wyeth Pharmaceuticals)

1. NAME OF THE MEDICINAL PRODUCT

Premique Low Dose 0.3mg/1.5mg modified release tablets

2. QUALITATIVE AND QUANTITATIVE COMPOSITION

Premique Low Dose 0.3 mg/1.5 mg modified release tablets are for oral administration containing conjugated estrogens[†] 0.3 mg and medroxyprogesterone acetate (MPA) 1.5 mg.

[†]Conjugated estrogens contain the sodium sulphate conjugates of estrone, equilin, 17α-dihydroequilin, 17α-estradiol, 17β-dihydroequilin, 17α-dihydroequilenin, 17β-dihydroequilenin, equilenin, 17β-estradiol and Δ8,9-dehydro-estrone.

For excipients, see section 6.1.

3. PHARMACEUTICAL FORM

Modified release tablet.

Cream oval biconvex sugar coated tablet marked 'W 0.3/ 1.5' in black ink.

4. CLINICAL PARTICULARS

4.1 Therapeutic indications

Hormone replacement therapy for estrogen deficiency symptoms in postmenopausal women with an intact uterus.

4.2 Posology and method of administration

Premique Low Dose is taken orally in a continuous combined 28-day regimen of one tablet daily with no break between packs.

In women who are not taking hormone replacement therapy or women who switch from another continuous combined hormone replacement therapy product, treatment may be started on any convenient day. In women transferring from a sequential hormone replacement therapy regimen, treatment should begin the day following completion of the prior regimen.

For treatment of postmenopausal symptoms: Take one tablet per day.

Breakthrough bleeding and spotting may occur in the early stages of Premique Low Dose therapy. If breakthrough bleeding persists and endometrial abnormality has been ruled out, a higher dose of treatment or cyclic therapy should be considered as an alternative.

The lowest dose and regimen that will control symptoms should be chosen.

Maintenance/Continuation/Extended treatment

For initiation and continuation of treatment of postmenopausal symptoms, the lowest effective dose for the shortest duration (see also Section 4.4 Special warnings and special precautions for use) should be used. Patients should be re-evaluated periodically to determine if treatment for symptoms is still necessary.

The benefits of the lower risk of endometrial hyperplasia and endometrial cancer due to adding a progestogen should be weighed against the increased risk of breast cancer (see section 4.4 Special warnings and special precautions for use and section 4.8 Undesirable effects)

Forgotten tablet: If a tablet is forgotten, it should be taken as soon as the patient remembers, therapy should then be continued as before. If more than one tablet has been forgotten only the most recent tablet should be taken, the patient should not take double the usual dose to make up for missed tablets.

Missed pills may cause breakthrough bleeding.

Elderly:

There are no special dosage requirements for elderly patients, but, as with all medicines, the lowest effective dose should be used.

Children:

Not recommended

4.3 Contraindications

1. Known, past or suspected breast cancer.
2. Known or suspected estrogen-dependent malignant tumours (e.g. endometrial cancer)
3. Undiagnosed abnormal genital bleeding.
4. Untreated endometrial hyperplasia
5. Active or past history of venous thromboembolism (e.g. deep vein thrombosis, pulmonary embolism)
6. Active or recent arterial thromboembolic disease (e.g. angina, myocardial infarction)
7. Acute liver disease or history of liver disease where the liver function tests have failed to return to normal.
8. Known hypersensitivity to the active substances or to any of the excipients of Premique Low Dose tablets.
9. Porphyria

4.4 Special warnings and precautions for use

For the treatment of postmenopausal symptoms, HRT should only be initiated for symptoms that adversely affect the quality of life. In all cases, a careful appraisal of the risks and benefits should be undertaken at least annually and HRT should only be continues as long as the benefit outweighs the risk.

Medical examination/Follow up

Before initiating or reinstituting HRT, a complete personal and family medical history should be taken. Physical (including pelvic and breast) examination should be guided by the contraindications and warnings for use. During treatment, periodic check-ups are recommended of a frequency and nature adapted to the individual woman. Women should be advised what changes in their breasts should be reported to their doctor or nurse (see 'Breast Cancer' below). Investigations, including mammography, should be carried out in accordance with currently accepted screening practices, modified to the clinical needs of the individual.

Conditions that need supervision

If any of the following conditions are present, have occurred previously, and/or have been aggravated during pregnancy or previous hormone treatment, the patient should be closely supervised. It should be taken into account that these conditions may recur or be aggravated during treatment with Premique Low Dose, in particular:

– Leiomyoma (uterine fibroids) or endometriosis
– A family history of, or other risk factors for, thromboembolic disorders (see below)
– Risk factors for estrogen dependent tumours (e.g. 1st degree heredity for breast cancer)
– Hypertension
– Liver disorders (e.g. liver adenoma)
– Diabetes mellitus with or without vascular involvement
– Cholelithiasis
– Migraine or (severe) headaches
– Systemic lupus erythematosus (SLE)
– A history of endometrial hyperplasia (see below)
– Epilepsy
– Asthma
– Otosclerosis

Reasons for immediate withdrawal of therapy

Therapy should be discontinued if a contra-indication is discovered and in the following situations:

– Jaundice or deterioration in liver function
– Significant increase in blood pressure
– New onset of migraine-type headache
– Pregnancy

Endometrial Hyperplasia

The risk of endometrial hyperplasia and carcinoma is increased when estrogens are administered alone for prolonged periods (see section 4.8 Undesirable effects). The addition of a progestogen for at least 12 days of the cycle in non-hysterectomised women greatly reduces this risk. Unless there is a previous diagnosis of endometriosis it is not recommended to add a progestogen in hysterectomised women.

The reduction in risk to the endometrium should be weighed against the increase in the risk of breast cancer of added progestogen (see 'Breast Cancer' below and section 4.8 Undesirable effects).

Break-through bleeding and spotting may occur during the first months of treatment. If break-through bleeding or spotting appears after some time on therapy, or continues after treatment has been discontinued, the reason should be investigated, which may include endometrial biopsy to exclude endometrial malignancy.

Breast Cancer

A randomised controlled trial, the Women's Health Initiative study (WHI), and epidemiological studies, including the Million Women Study (MWS), have reported an increased risk of breast cancer in women taking estrogens, estrogen-progestogen combinations or tibolone for HRT for several years (see Section 4.8 Undesirable effects). For all HRT, an excess risk becomes apparent within a few years of use and increases with the duration of intake but returns to baseline within a few (at most five) years after stopping treatment.

In the MWS, the relative risk of breast cancer with conjugated equine estrogens (CEE) or estradiol (E2) was greater when a progestogen was added, either sequentially or continuously, and regardless of type of progestogen. There was no evidence of a difference in risk between the different routes of administration.

In the WHI study, the continuous combined conjugated equine estrogen and medroxyprogesterone acetate (CEE + MPA) product used was associated with breast cancers that were slightly larger in size and more frequently had local lymph node metastases compared to placebo.

HRT, especially estrogen-progestogen combined treatment, increases the density of mammographic images which may adversely affect the radiological detection of breast cancer.

Venous thromboembolism

Hormone replacement therapy (HRT) is associated with a higher relative risk of developing venous thromboembolism (VTE) i.e. deep vein thrombosis or pulmonary embolism. One randomised controlled trial and epidemiological studies found a two to threefold higher risk for users compared with non-users. For non- users it is estimated that the number of cases of VTE that will occur over a 5-year period is about 3 per 1000 women aged 50-59 years and 8 per 1000 women aged between 60-69 years. It is estimated that in healthy women who use HRT for 5 years, the number of additional cases of VTE over a 5-year period will be between 2 and 6 (best estimate 4) per 1000 women aged 50-59 years and between 5 and 15 (best estimate = 9) per 1000 women aged 60-69 years. The occurrence of such an event is more likely in the first year of HRT than later.

Generally recognised risk factors for VTE include a personal or family history and severe obesity (Body Mass Index >30 kg/m^2) and systemic lupus erythematosus (SLE). There is no consensus about the possible role of varicose veins in VTE.

Patients with a history of VTE or known thrombophilic states have an increased risk of VTE. HRT may add to this risk. Personal or strong family history of thromboembolism or recurrent spontaneous abortion should be investigated in order to exclude a thrombophilic predisposition. Until a thorough evaluation of thrombophilic factors has been made or anticoagulant treatment initiated, use of HRT in such patients should be viewed as contraindicated. Those women already on anticoagulant treatment require careful consideration of the benefit-risk of use of HRT.

The risk of VTE may be temporarily increased with prolonged immobilisation, major trauma or major surgery. As in all postoperative patients scrupulous attention should be given to prophylactic measures to prevent VTE following surgery. Where prolonged immobilisation is liable to follow elective surgery, particularly abdominal or orthopaedic surgery to the lower limbs, consideration should be given to temporarily stopping HRT 4-6 weeks earlier, if this is possible. Treatment should not be restarted until the woman is completely mobilised.

If venous thromboembolism develops after initiating therapy the drug should be discontinued. Patients should be told to contact their doctors immediately when they are aware of potential thromboembolic symptoms (e.g. painful swelling of a leg, sudden pain in the chest, dyspnoea).

Coronary Artery Disease (CAD)

There is no evidence from randomised controlled trials of cardiovascular benefit with continuous combined conjugated estrogens and MPA. Two large clinical trials (WHI and HERS i.e. Heart and Estrogen/progestin Replacement Study) showed a possible increased risk of cardiovascular morbidity in the first year of use and no overall benefit. For other HRT products, there are only limited data randomised controlled trials examining effects in cardiovascular morbidity or mortality. Therefore, it is uncertain whether these findings also extend to other HRT products.

Stroke

One large randomised clinical trial (WHI-trial) found, as a secondary outcome, an increased risk of ischaemic stroke in healthy women during treatment with continuous combined conjugated estrogens and MPA. For women who do not use HRT, it is estimated that the number of cases of stroke that will occur over a 5 year period is about 3 per 1000 women aged 50-59 years and 11 per 1000 women aged 60-69 years. It is estimated that for women who use conjugated estrogens and MPA for 5 years, the number of additional cases will be between 0 and 3 (best estimate =1) per 1000 users aged 50-59 years and between 1 and 9 (best estimate = 4) per 1000 users aged 60-69 years. It is unknown whether the increased risk also extends to other HRT products.

Ovarian Cancer

Long term (at least 5 –10 years) use of estrogen-only HRT products in hysterectomised women has been associated with an increased risk of ovarian cancer in some epidemiological studies. It is uncertain whether long-term use of combined HRT confers different risk than estrogen-only products.

Other Conditions

- Estrogens/progestogens may cause fluid retention and therefore patients with cardiac or renal dysfunction should be carefully observed. Patients with terminal renal insufficiency should be closely observed, since it is expected that the level of circulating active ingredients in Premique Low Dose is increased.
- The use of estrogen may influence the laboratory results of certain endocrine tests and liver enzymes.

Estrogens increase thyroid binding globulin (TBG), leading to increased circulating total thyroid hormone, as measured by protein-bound iodine (PBI), T4 levels (by column or by radio-immunoassay) or T3 levels (by radio-immunoassay). T3 resin uptake is decreased, reflecting the elevated TBG. Free T4 and free T3 concentrations are usually unaltered.

Other binding proteins may be elevated in serum, i.e. corticoid binding globulin (CBG), sex-hormone-binding globulin (SHBG) leading to increased circulating corticosteroids and sex steroids, respectively. Free or biologically active hormone concentrations are usually unchanged. Other plasma proteins may be increased (angiotensinogen/renin substrate, alpha-I-antitrypsin, ceruloplasmin).

Some patients dependent on thyroid hormone replacement therapy may require increased doses in order to maintain their free thyroid hormone levels in an acceptable range. Therefore, patients should have their thyroid function monitored more frequently when commencing concurrent treatment in order to maintain their free thyroid hormone levels in an acceptable range.

- There is an increase in the risk of gallbladder disease in women receiving HRT (see conditions that need supervision)
- A worsening of glucose tolerance may occur in some patients on estrogen/progestogen therapy and therefore diabetic patients should be carefully observed while receiving hormone replacement therapy.

This product contains lactose and sucrose. Patients with rare hereditary problems of galactose intolerance, fructose intolerance, the Lapp lactase deficiency, glucose-galactose malabsorption or sucrase-isomaltase insufficiency should not take this medicine.

- Women with pre-existing hypertriglyceridemia should be followed closely during estrogen replacement or hormone replacement therapy, since rare cases of large increases of plasma triglycerides leading to pancreatitis have been reported with estrogen therapy in this condition.

- Estrogens should be used with caution in individuals with severe hypocalcaemia
- There is no conclusive evidence for improvement of cognitive function. There is some evidence from the WHI trial of increased risk of probable dementia in women who start using continuous combined CEE and MPA after the age of 65. It is unknown whether the findings apply to younger post-menopausal women or other HRT products.

4.5 Interaction with other medicinal products and other forms of interaction

The metabolism of estrogens and progestogens may be increased by concomitant use of substances known to induce drug-metabolising enzymes, specifically cytochrome P450 enzymes, such as anticonvulsants (e.g. phenobarbital, phenytoin, carbamazepine) and anti-infectives (e.g. rifampicin, rifabutin, nevirapine, efavirenz).

Ritonavir and nelfinavir, although known as strong inhibitors, by contrast exhibit inducing properties when used concomitantly with steroid hormones.

Herbal preparations containing St John's wort (Hypericum perforatum) may induce the metabolism of estrogens and progestogens.

Clinically, an increased metabolism of estrogens and progestogens may lead to decreased effect and changes in the uterine bleeding profile.

The response to metyrapone may be reduced.

Aminogluthimide administered concomitantly with MPA may significantly depress the bioavailiablity of MPA.

4.6 Pregnancy and lactation

Pregnancy:

Premique Low Dose is not indicated during pregnancy. If pregnancy occurs during medication with Premique Low Dose treatment should be withdrawn immediately.

Clinically, data on a limited number of exposed pregnancies indicate no adverse effects of MPA on the foetus.

The results of most epidemiological studies to date relevant to inadvertent foetal exposure to combinations of estrogens and progestogens indicate no teratogenic or foetotoxic effect.

Lactation:

Premique Low Dose is not indicated during lactation.

4.7 Effects on ability to drive and use machines

Premique Low Dose should not affect the ability to drive or use machinery.

4.8 Undesirable effects

See also Section 4.4 Special warnings and special precautions for use.

Adverse drug reactions (ADRs)

The adverse reactions listed in the table are based on post-marketing spontaneous (reporting rate), clinical trials and class-effects. Breast pain is a very common adverse event reported in ⩾ 10% of patients.

(see Table 1 opposite)

Table 1

System Organ Class	Very Common ADRs (>1/10)	Common ADRs (>1/100, <1/10)	Uncommon ADRs (>1/1000, <1/100)	Rare ADRs (>1/10000, <1/1000)	Very Rare ADRs (<1/10000), isolated reports
Infections and infestations		Vaginitis	Vaginal candidiasis		
Neoplasms benign and malignant (including cysts and polyps)				Fibrocystic breast changes Ovarian cancer	Enlargement of hepatic hemangiomas
Immune system disorders				Anaphylactic/ anaphylactoid reactions, including urticaria and angioedema	
Metabolism and nutrition disorders				Glucose intolerance	Exacerbation of porphyria; hypocalcemia
Psychiatric disorders		Depression	Changes in libido; Mood disturbances	Irritability	
Nervous system disorders			Dizziness; Headache; Migraine; Anxiety	Stroke; Exacerbation of epilepsy	Exacerbation of chorea
Eye disorders			Intolerance to contact lenses		Retinal vascular thrombosis
Cardiac disorders				Myocardial infarction	
Vascular disorders				Pulmonary embolism; Superficial thrombophlebitis	
Respiratory, thoracic and mediastinal disorders				Exacerbation of asthma	
Gastrointestinal disorders			Nausea; Bloating; Abdominal pain	Vomiting; Pancreatitis	
Hepatobiliary disorders			Gallbladder disease	None	Cholestatic jaundice
Skin and subcutaneous tissue disorders			Alopecia; acne; Pruritis	Chloasma/melasma; Hirsutism; Pruritus; Rash	
Musculoskeletal, connective tissue and bone disorders		Arthralgias; Leg cramps			
Reproductive system & breast disorders	Breast pain	Breakthrough bleeding/spotting dysmenorrhea, breast, tenderness, enlargement, discharge	Change in menstrual flow; Change in cervical ectropion and secretion	Galactorrhoea; Increased size of uterine leiomyomata	
General disorders and administration site conditions			Oedema		
Investigations		Changes in weight (increase or decrease) Increased triglycerides			Increase in blood pressure

Breast cancer

According to evidence from a large number of epidemiological studies and one randomised placebo-controlled trial, the Women's Health Initiative (WHI), the overall risk of breast cancer increases with increasing duration of HRT use in current or recent HRT users.

For estrogen-only HRT, estimates of relative risk (RR) from a reanalysis of original data from 51 epidemiological studies (in which >80% of HRT use was estrogen-only HRT) and from the epidemiological Million Women Study (MWS) are similar at 1.35 (95%CI 1.21 – 1.49) and 1.30 (95%CI 1.21 – 1.40), respectively.

For estrogen plus progestogen combined HRT, several epidemiological studies have reported an overall higher risk for breast cancer than with estrogens alone.

The MWS reported that, compared to never users, the use of various types of estrogen-progestogen combined HRT was associated with a higher risk of breast cancer (RR = 2.00, 95%CI: 1.88 – 2.12) than use of estrogens alone (RR = 1.30, 95%CI: 1.21 – 1.40) or use of tibolone (RR=1.45; 95%CI 1.25-1.68).

The WHI trial reported a risk estimate of 1.24 (95%CI 1.01 – 1.54) after 5.6 years of use of estrogen-progestogen combined HRT (CEE + MPA) in all users compared with placebo.

The absolute risks calculated from the MWS and the WHI trial are presented below:

The MWS has estimated, from the known average incidence of breast cancer in developed countries, that:

- For women not using HRT, about 32 in every 1000 are expected to have breast cancer diagnosed between the ages of 50 and 64 years.
- For 1000 current or recent users of HRT, the number of additional cases during the corresponding period will be
  - For users of estrogen-only replacement therapy
    - o between 0 and 3 (best estimate = 1.5) for 5 years' use
    - o between 3 and 7 (best estimate = 5) for 10 years' use.
  - For users of estrogen plus progestogen combined HRT
    - o between 5 and 7 (best estimate = 6) for 5 years' use
    - o between 18 and 20 (best estimate = 19) for 10 years' use.

The WHI trial estimated that after 5.6 years of follow-up of women between the ages of 50 and 79 years, an additional 8 cases of invasive breast cancer would be due to estrogen-progestogen combined HRT (CEE + MPA) per 10,000 women years.

According to calculations from the trial data, it is estimated that:

- For 1000 women in the placebo group.
  - o About 16 cases of invasive breast cancer would be diagnosed in 5 years.
- For 1000 women who used estrogen plus progestogen combined HRT (CEE + MPA), the number of additional cases would be
  - o Between 0 and 9 (best estimate = 4) for 5 years' use.

The number of additional cases of breast cancer in women who use HRT is broadly similar for women who start HRT irrespective of age at start of use (between the ages of 45-65) (see section 4.4 Special warnings and special precautions for use).

Endometrial Cancer

In women with an intact uterus, the risk of endometrial hyperplasia and endometrial cancer increases with increasing duration of use of unopposed estrogens. According to data from epidemiological studies, the best estimate of the risk is that for women not using HRT, about 5 in every 1000 are expected to have endometrial cancer diagnosed between the ages of 50 and 65. Depending on the duration of treatment and estrogen dose, the reported increase in endometrial cancer risk among unopposed estrogen users varies from 2-to 12-fold greater compared with non-users. Adding a progestogen to estrogen-only therapy greatly reduces this increased risk.

Other adverse reactions reported in association with estrogen/progestogen treatment including Premique:

- Estrogen-dependent neoplasms benign and malignant, e.g. endometrial hyperplasia, endometrial cancer
- Venous thromboembolism, i.e. deep leg or pelvic venous thrombosis and pulmonary embolism, is more frequent among hormone replacement therapy users than among non-users. For further information, see section 4.3 Contra-indications and 4.4 Special Warnings and Precautions for Use.
- Myocardial infarction
- Stroke

• Skin and subcutaneous disorders: erythema multiforme, erythema nodosum, vascular purpura

• Probable dementia (see section 4.4 Special warnings and special precautions for use)

• Exacerbation of otosclerosis

4.9 Overdose

Symptoms of overdosage of estrogen-containing products in adults and children may include nausea, vomiting, breast tenderness, dizziness, abdominal pain, drowsiness/fatigue and withdrawal bleeding may occur in females. There is no specific antidote, and further treatment should be symptomatic.

5. PHARMACOLOGICAL PROPERTIES

5.1 Pharmacodynamic properties

ATC Code: GO3F A12 (Medroxyprogesterone & estrogen)

Conjugated Estrogens

The active ingredients are primarily the sulphate esters of estrone, equilin sulphates, 17α-estradiol and 17β-estradiol. These substitute for the loss of estrogen production in menopausal women, and alleviate menopausal symptoms.

Progestogen:

As estrogens promote the growth of the endometrium, unopposed estrogens increase the risk of endometrial hyperplasia and cancer. The addition of a progestogen reduces but does not eliminate the estrogen-induced risk of endometrial hyperplasia in non-hysterectomised women.

Relief of estrogen-deficiency symptoms

In a 1-year clinical trial (n=2,808), vasomotor symptoms were assessed for efficacy during the first 12 weeks of treatment in a subset of symptomatic women (n=241) who had at least 7 moderate or severe hot flushes daily or 50 moderate to severe hot flushes during the week before randomisation. Premique 0.625mg/2.5mg (conjugated estrogens/medroxyprogesterone acetate) was shown to be statistically better than placebo at weeks 4, 8 and 12 for relief of both frequency and severity of moderate to severe vasomotor symptoms.

In two clinical trials, the incidence of amenorrhoea (no bleeding or spotting) increased over time in women treated with Premique 0.625 mg/2.5 mg. Amenorrhoea was seen in 68% of women at cycle 6 and 77% of women at cycle 12. Breakthrough bleeding and/or spotting appeared in 48% during the first 3 months, and in 24% of women during months 10-12 of treatment.

5.2 Pharmacokinetic properties

Absorption

Conjugated estrogens are soluble in water and are well absorbed from the gastrointestinal tract after release from the drug formulation. However Premique Low Dose contains a formulation of medroxyprogesterone acetate (MPA) that is immediately released and conjugated estrogens that are slowly released over several hours. MPA is well absorbed from the gastrointestinal tract. Table 1 summarises the mean pharmacokinetic parameters for unconjugated and conjugated estrogens, and medroxyprogesterone acetate following administration of 2 Premique Low Dose 0.3 /1.5 mg and 2 Premique Low Dose 0.45/1.5 mg tablets to healthy postmenopausal women.

Distribution

The distribution of exogenous estrogens is similar to that of endogenous estrogens. Estrogens are widely distributed in the body and are generally found in higher concentrations in the sex hormone target organs. Estrogens circulate in the blood largely bound to sex hormone binding globulin (SHBG) and albumin. MPA is approximately 90% bound to plasma proteins but does not bind to SHBG.

Metabolism

Exogenous estrogens are metabolised in the same manner as endogenous estrogens. Circulating estrogens exist in a dynamic equilibrium of metabolic interconversions. These transformations take place mainly in the liver. Estradiol is converted reversibly to estrone, and both can be converted to estriol, which is the major urinary metabolite. Estrogens also undergo enterohepatic recirculation via sulphate and glucuronide conjugation in the liver, biliary secretion of conjugates into the intestine, and hydrolysis in the gut followed by reabsorption. In postmenopausal women a significant proportion of the circulating estrogens exists as sulphate conjugates, especially estrone sulphate, which serves as a circulating reservoir for the formation of more active estrogens. Metabolism and elimination of MPA occur primarily in the liver via hydroxylation, with subsequent conjugation and elimination in the urine.

Excretion

Estradiol, estrone and estriol are excreted in the urine along with glucuronide and sulphate conjugates. Most metabolites of MPA are extracted as glucuronide conjugates with only minor amounts secreted as sulphates.

Table 2 – Pharmacokinetic parameters for Premique Low Dose

(see Table 2 below)

5.3 Preclinical safety data

Long-term continuous administration of natural and synthetic estrogens in certain animal species increases the frequency of carcinomas of the breast, cervix, vagina and liver.

In a two-year oral study in which female rats were exposed to MPA dosages of up to 5000μg/kg/day in their diets (50 times higher - based on AUC values - than the level observed in women taking 10mg of MPA), a dose-related increase in pancreatic islet cell tumours (adenomas and carcinomas) occurred. Pancreatic tumour incidence was increased at 1000 and 5000μg/kg/day, but not at 200μg/kg/day.

The cortisol activity of MPA at these high doses is thought to increase serum glucose in rats which reactively stimulates the beta cells of the pancreatic islets to produce insulin. This repeated stimulation is thought to cause the tumours in rats. Similar lesions are not likely to occur in humans since the endocrine system of rats is more sensitive to hormones than that of women. When MPA is combined with estrogen, MPA binds to fewer glucocorticosteroid receptors and thus has less effect on plasma glucose. In humans, the diabetogenic response to MPA at therapeutic doses is slight. Moreover, an extensive literature search revealed no evidence that MPA causes pancreatic tumours in humans.

Table 2 Pharmacokinetic parameters for Premique Low Dose

Drug	2 × 0.3 mg CE/1.5 mg MPA Combination (n=30)				2 × 0.45 mg CE/1.5 mg MPA Combination (n=61)			
PK Parameter Arithmetic Mean (%CV)	C_{max} (pg/mL)	t_{max} (h)	$t_{1/2}$- (h)	*AUC* (pg.h/mL)	C_{max} (pg/mL)	t_{max} (h)	$t_{1/2}$- (h)	*AUC* (pg.h/mL)
Unconjugated Estrogens								
Estrone	79 (35)	9.4 (86)	51.3 (30)	5029 (45)	91 (30)	9.8 (47)	48.9 (28)	5786 (42)
BA*-Estrone	56 (46)	9.4 (86)	19.8 (39)	1429 (49)	67 (37)	9.8 (47)	21.5 (49)	2042 (52)
Equilin	30 (43)	7.9 (42)	14.0 (75)	590 (42)	35 (40)	8.5 (34)	16.4 (49)	825 (44)
PK Parameter Arithmetic Mean (%CV)	C_{max} (ng/mL)	t_{max} (h)	$t_{1/2}$- (h)	*AUC* (ng.h/mL)	C_{max} (ng/mL)	t_{max} (h)	$t_{1/2}$- (h)	*AUC* (ng.h/mL)
Conjugated Estrogens								
Total Estrone	2.4 (38)	7.1 (27)	26.5 (33)	62 (48)	3.0 (37)	8.2 (39)	25.9 (23)	78 (40)
BA*- Total Estrone	2.2 (36)	7.1 (27)	16.3 (32)	41 (44)	2.8 (36)	8.2 (39)	16.9 (36)	56 (39)
Total Equilin	1.5 (47)	5.5 (29)	11.5 (24)	22 (41)	1.9 (42)	7.2 (33)	12.2 (25)	31 (52)
PK Parameter Arithmetic Mean (%CV)	C_{max} (ng/mL)	t_{max} (h)	$t_{1/2}$- (h)	*AUC* (ng.h/mL)	C_{max} (ng/mL)	t_{max} (h)	$t_{1/2}$- (h)	*AUC* (ng.h/mL)
Medroxyprogesterone acetate								
MPA	1.2 (42)	2.8 (61)	42.3 (34)	29.4 (30)	1.2 (42)	2.7 (52)	47.2 (41)	32.0 (36)

BA* = Baseline adjusted

C_{max} = peak plasma concentration

t_{max} = time peak concentration occurs

$t_{1/2}$ = apparent terminal-phase disposition half life (0.693/λ_z)

AUC = total area under the concentration-time curve

6. PHARMACEUTICAL PARTICULARS

6.1 List of excipients

Tablet core:

Lactose monohydrate

Methylcellulose

Magnesium stearate

Calcium phosphate

Tablet coating:

Macrogol

Glyceryl mono-oleate

Shellac

Calcium sulphate

Microcrystalline cellulose

Sucrose

Titanium dioxide (E171)

Povidone

Carnauba wax

Yellow Ferric Oxide (E172)

Printing on tablet:

Black Tek Print SW-9008 (shellac, propylene glycol, black iron oxide (E172) and potassium hydroxide).

6.2 Incompatibilities

Not applicable.

6.3 Shelf life

24 months.

6.4 Special precautions for storage

Do not store above 25°C. Keep blister in the outer carton to protect from light.

6.5 Nature and contents of container

Polyvinylchloride (PVC)/Aluminium foil blister pack of 28 tablets. Each carton contains 28 tablets (1 blister pack) or 84 tablets (3 blister packs).

Not all pack sizes may be marketed.

6.6 Special precautions for disposal and other handling

Not applicable.

7. MARKETING AUTHORISATION HOLDER

John Wyeth & Brother Limited

Trading as: Wyeth Pharmaceuticals

Huntercombe Lane South

Taplow

Maidenhead

Berkshire SL6 0PH

8. MARKETING AUTHORISATION NUMBER(S)

PL 00011/0256

9. DATE OF FIRST AUTHORISATION/RENEWAL OF THE AUTHORISATION

08 March 2004

10. DATE OF REVISION OF THE TEXT

08 June 2009

Prempak-C

(Wyeth Pharmaceuticals)

1. NAME OF THE MEDICINAL PRODUCT

Prempak-C 0.625mg.

Prempak-C 1.25mg.

2. QUALITATIVE AND QUANTITATIVE COMPOSITION

Prempak-C 0.625mg consists of 28 tablets containing 0.625mg conjugated estrogens USP, and 12 tablets containing 0.15mg norgestrel.

Prempak-C 1.25mg consists of 28 tablets containing 1.25mg conjugated estrogens USP, and 12 tablets containing 0.15mg norgestrel.

For a full list of excipients, see section 6.1.

3. PHARMACEUTICAL FORM

Prempak-C 0.625mg coated tablets

Maroon oval biconvex sugar-coated tablet marked with '0.625' in white ink.

Round light brown sugar coated tablets containing norgestrel 0.15mg.

Prempak-C 1.25mg coated tablets

Yellow oval biconvex sugar coated tablet marked with "1.25" in black ink.

Round light brown sugar coated tablets containing norgestrel 0.15mg.

4. CLINICAL PARTICULARS

4.1 Therapeutic indications

• Hormone replacement therapy for estrogen deficiency symptoms in menopausal and postmenopausal women

• Prevention of osteoporosis in postmenopausal women at high risk of future fractures who are intolerant of, or contra-indicated for, other medicinal products approved for the prevention of osteoporosis.

4.2 Posology and method of administration

Adults:

Prempak-C is available for oral use in a sequential regimen for treatment of women with a uterus. The recommended starting dose is 0.625mg-1.25mg conjugated estrogens daily. One norgestrel tablet should be taken daily from day 17 to day 28 of estrogen therapy. Continuous estrogen administration is recommended. For maintenance, the lowest effective dose should be used.

For treatment of postmenopausal symptoms:

0.625-1.25mg conjugated estrogens daily depending on the response of the individual. One norgestrel tablet should be taken daily from day 17 to day 28 of estrogen therapy.

Prophylaxis of osteoporosis:

The minimum effective dose is 0.625mg daily for most patients. One norgestrel tablet should be taken daily from day 17 to day 28 of estrogen therapy. (See section 5.1 Pharmacological properties)

For most postmenopausal women therapy may be commenced at any convenient time although if the patient is still menstruating, commencement on first day of bleeding is recommended. In women transferring from another sequential hormone replacement therapy regimen, treatment should begin the day following completion of the prior regimen. Withdrawal bleeding usually occurs within three to seven days after the last norgestrel tablet.

Maintenance/Continuation/Extended treatment:

For initiation and continuation of treatment of postmenopausal symptoms, the lowest effective dose for the shortest duration (see also Section 4.4 Special warnings and special precautions for use) should be used. Patients should be re-evaluated periodically to determine if treatment for symptoms is still necessary.

The benefits of the lower risk of endometrial hyperplasia and endometrial cancer due to adding a progestogen should be weighed against the increased risk of breast cancer (see sections 4.4 Special warnings and special precautions for use, and 4.8 Undesirable effects).

Forgotten tablet: If a tablet is forgotten, it should be taken as soon as the patient remembers, therapy should then be continued as before. If more than one tablet has been forgotten only the most recent tablet should be taken. The patient should not take double the usual dose to make up for the missed tablet.

Missed pills may cause breakthrough bleeding.

Elderly:

There are no special dosage requirements for elderly patients, but as with all medicines, the lowest effective dose should be used.

Children:

Not recommended.

4.3 Contraindications

1. Known, past or suspected cancer of the breast
2. Known or suspected estrogen-dependent malignant tumours (e.g. endometrial cancer)
3. Undiagnosed abnormal genital bleeding
4. Untreated endometrial hyperplasia
5. Active or past history of venous thromboembolism (e.g. deep vein thrombosis, pulmonary embolism)
6. Active or recent arterial thromboembolic disease (e.g. angina, myocardial infarction)
7. Acute liver disease or history of liver disease where the liver function tests have failed to return to normal
8. Known hypersensitivity to the active substances or to any of the excipients of Prempak-C tablets
9. Porphyria

4.4 Special warnings and precautions for use

For the treatment of postmenopausal symptoms, HRT should only be initiated for symptoms that adversely affect quality of life. In all cases, a careful appraisal of the risks and benefits should be undertaken at least annually and HRT should only be continued as long as the benefit outweighs the risk.

1. Medical examination/Follow up

Before initiating or reinstituting HRT, a complete personal and family medical history should be taken. Physical (including pelvic and breast) examination should be guided by the contraindications and warnings for use. During treatment, periodic check-ups are recommended of a frequency and nature adapted to the individual women. Women should be advised what changes in their breasts should be reported to their doctor or nurse (see 'Breast Cancer' below). Investigations, including mammography, should be carried out in accordance with currently accepted screening practices, modified to the clinical needs of the individual.

2. Conditions that need supervision

If any of the following conditions are present, have occurred previously, and/or have been aggravated during pregnancy or previous hormone treatment, the patient should be closely supervised. It should be taken into account that these conditions may recur or be aggravated during treatment with Prempak-C, in particular:

– Leiomyoma (uterine fibroids) or endometriosis

– A family history of, or other risk factors for, thromboembolic disorders (see below)

– Risk factors for estrogen dependent tumours (e.g. first degree heredity for breast cancer)

– Hypertension

– Liver disorders (e.g. liver adenoma)

– Diabetes mellitus with or without vascular involvement

– Cholelithiasis

– Migraine or (severe) headaches

– Systemic lupus erythematosus (SLE)

– A history of endometrial hyperplasia (see below)

– Epilepsy

– Asthma

– Otosclerosis

3. Reasons for immediate withdrawal of therapy

Therapy should be discontinued if a contra-indication is discovered and in the following situations:

– Jaundice or deterioration in liver function

– Significant increase in blood pressure

– New onset of migraine-type headache

– Pregnancy

4. Endometrial Hyperplasia

The risk of endometrial hyperplasia and carcinoma is increased when estrogens are administered alone for prolonged periods (see section 4.8 Undesirable effects). The addition of a progestogen for at least 12 days of the cycle in non-hysterectomised women greatly reduces this risk. Unless there is a previous diagnosis of endometriosis it is not recommended to add a progestogen in hysterectomised women.

The reduction in risk to the endometrium should be weighed against the increase in the risk of breast cancer of added progestogen (see 'Breast cancer' below and Section 4.8 Undesirable effects).

Break-through bleeding and spotting may occur during the first months of treatment. If break-through bleeding or spotting appears after some time on therapy, or continues after treatment has been discontinued, the reason should be investigated, which may include endometrial biopsy to exclude endometrial malignancy.

5. Breast Cancer

A randomised placebo-controlled trial, the Women's Health Initiative study (WHI), and epidemiological studies, including the Million Women Study (MWS), have reported an increased risk of breast cancer in women taking estrogens, estrogen-progestogen combinations or tibolone for HRT for several years (see Section 4.8 Undesirable effects). For all HRT, an excess risk becomes apparent within a few years of use and increases with the duration of intake but returns to baseline within a few (at most five) years after stopping treatment.

In the MWS, the relative risk of breast cancer with conjugated equine estrogens (CEE) or estradiol (E2) was greater when a progestogen was added, either sequentially or continuously, and regardless of type of progestogen. There was no evidence of a difference in risk between the different routes of administration.

In the WHI study, the continuous combined conjugated equine estrogen and medroxyprogesterone acetate (CEE + MPA) product used was associated with breast cancers that were slightly larger in size and more frequently had local lymph node metastases compared to placebo.

HRT, especially estrogen-progestogen combined treatment, increases the density of mammographic images which may adversely affect the radiological detection of breast cancer.

6. Venous thromboembolism

Hormone replacement therapy (HRT) is associated with a higher relative risk of developing venous thromboembolism (VTE) i.e. deep vein thrombosis or pulmonary embolism. One randomised controlled trial and epidemiological studies found a two to threefold higher risk for users compared with non-users. For non- users it is estimated that the number of cases of VTE that will occur over a 5-year period is about 3 per 1000 women aged 50-59 years and 8 per 1000 women aged between 60-69 years. It is estimated that in healthy women who use HRT for 5 years, the number of additional cases of VTE over a 5-year period will be between 2 and 6 (best estimate = 4) per 1000 women aged 50-59 years and between 5 and 15 (best estimate = 9) per 1000 women aged 60-69 years. The occurrence of such an event is more likely in the first year of HRT than later.

Generally recognised risk factors for VTE include a personal or family history and severe obesity (Body Mass Index $>30kg/m^2$) and systemic lupus erythematosus (SLE). There is no consensus about the possible role of varicose veins in VTE.

Patients with a history of VTE or known thrombophilic states have an increased risk of VTE. HRT may add to this risk. Personal or strong family history of thromboembolism or recurrent spontaneous abortion should be investigated in order to exclude a thrombophilic predisposition. Until a thorough evaluation of thrombophilic factors has been made or anticoagulant treatment initiated, use of HRT in such patients should be viewed as contraindicated. Those women already on anticoagulant treatment require careful consideration of the benefit-risk of use of HRT.

The risk of VTE may be temporarily increased with prolonged immobilisation, major trauma or major surgery. As in all post-operative patients, scrupulous attention should be given to prophylactic measures to prevent VTE following surgery. Where prolonged immobilisation is liable to follow elective surgery, particularly abdominal or orthopaedic surgery to the lower limbs, consideration should be given to temporarily stopping HRT 4-6 weeks earlier, if this is possible. Treatment should not be restarted until the woman is completely mobilised.

If venous thromboembolism develops after initiating therapy the drug should be discontinued. Patients should be told to contact their doctors immediately when they are aware of potential thromboembolic symptoms (e.g. painful swelling of a leg, sudden pain in the chest, dyspnoea).

7. Coronary Artery Disease (CAD)

There is no evidence from randomised controlled trials of cardiovascular benefit with continuous combined conjugated estrogens and MPA. Two large clinical trials (WHI and HERS i.e. Heart and Estrogen/progestin Replacement Study) showed a possible increased risk of cardiovascular morbidity in the first year of use and no overall benefit. For other HRT products, there are only limited data from randomised controlled trials examining effects in cardiovascular morbidity or mortality. Therefore, it is uncertain whether these findings also extend to other HRT products.

8. Stroke

One large randomised clinical trial (WHI-trial) found, as a secondary outcome, an increased risk of ischaemic stroke in healthy women during treatment with continuous combined conjugated estrogens and MPA. For women who do not use HRT, it is estimated that the number of cases of stroke that will occur over a 5 year period is about 3 per 1000 women aged 50-59 years and 11 per 1000 women aged 60-69 years. It is estimated that for women who use conjugated estrogens and MPA for 5 years, the number of additional cases will be between 0 and 3 (best estimate =1) per 1000 users aged 50-59 years and between 1 and 9 (best estimate = 4) per 1000 users aged 60-69 years. It is unknown whether the increased risk also extends to other HRT products.

9. Ovarian Cancer

Long term (at least 5-10 years) use of estrogen-only HRT products in hysterectomised women has been associated with an increased risk of ovarian cancer in some epidemiological studies. It is uncertain whether long-term use of combined HRT confers different risk than estrogen-only products.

Other Conditions

10. Estrogens/progestogens may cause fluid retention and therefore patients with cardiac or renal dysfunction should be carefully observed. Patients with terminal renal insufficiency should be closely observed, since it is expected that the level of circulating active ingredients in Prempak-C is increased.

11. The use of estrogen may influence the laboratory results of certain endocrine tests and liver enzymes.

Estrogens increase thyroid binding globulin (TBG), leading to increased circulating total thyroid hormone, as measured by protein-bound iodine (PBI), T4 levels (by column or by radio-immunoassay) or T3 levels (by radio-immunoassay). T3 resin uptake is decreased, reflecting the elevated TBG. Free T4 and free T3 concentrations are unaltered.

Other binding proteins may be elevated in serum, i.e. corticoid binding globulin (CBG), sex-hormone-binding globulin (SHBG) leading to increased circulating corticosteroids and sex steroids, respectively. Free or biologically active hormone concentrations are unchanged. Other plasma proteins may be increased (angiotensinogen/renin substrate, alpha-I-antitrypsin, ceruloplasmin).

Some patients dependent on thyroid hormone replacement therapy may require increased doses in order to maintain their free thyroid hormone levels in an acceptable range. Therefore, patients should have their thyroid function monitored more frequently when commencing concurrent treatment in order to maintain their free thyroid hormone levels in an acceptable range.

12. Changed estrogen levels may affect certain endocrine and liver function tests.

13. There is an increase in the risk of gallbladder disease in women receiving HRT (see conditions that need supervision).

14. A worsening of glucose tolerance may occur in patients taking estrogens and therefore diabetic patients should be carefully observed while receiving hormone replacement therapy.

This product contains lactose and sucrose. Patients with rare hereditary problems of galactose intolerance, fructose intolerance, the Lapp lactase deficiency, glucose-galactose malabsorption or sucrase-isomaltase insufficiency should not take this medicine.

15. Women with pre-existing hypertriglyceridemia should be followed closely during estrogen replacement or hormone replacement therapy, since rare cases of large increases of plasma triglycerides leading to pancreatitis have been reported with estrogen therapy in this condition.

16. Estrogens should be used with caution in individuals with severe hypocalcaemia

17. There is no conclusive evidence for improvement of cognitive function. There is some evidence from the WHI trial of increased risk of probable dementia in women who start using continuous combined CEE and MPA after the age of 65. It is unknown whether the findings apply to younger post-menopausal women or other HRT products.

4.5 Interaction with other medicinal products and other forms of interaction

The metabolism of estrogens and progestogens may be increased by concomitant use of substances known to induce drug-metabolising enzymes, specifically cytochrome P450 enzymes, such as anticonvulsants (e.g. phenobarbital, phenytoin, carbamazepine) and anti-infectives (e.g. rifampicin, rifabutin, nevirapine, efavirenz).

Ritonavir and nelfinavir, although known as strong inhibitors, by contrast exhibit inducing properties when used concomitantly with steroid hormones.

Herbal preparations containing St John's wort (*Hypericum perforatum)* may induce the metabolism of estrogens and progestogens.

Clinically, an increased metabolism of estrogens and progestogens may lead to decreased effect and changes in the uterine bleeding profile.

The response to metyrapone may be reduced.

4.6 Pregnancy and lactation

Pregnancy:

Prempak-C is not indicated during pregnancy. If pregnancy occurs during medication with Prempak-C treatment should be withdrawn immediately.

Clinically, data on a limited number of exposed pregnancies indicate no adverse effects of MPA on the foetus.

The results of most epidemiological studies to date relevant to inadvertent foetal exposure to combinations of estrogens and progestogens indicate no teratogenic or foetotoxic effect.

Lactation:

Prempak-C is not indicated during lactation.

4.7 Effects on ability to drive and use machines

None known.

4.8 Undesirable effects

See also 4.4 Special warnings and special precautions for use.

Adverse drug reactions (ADRs)

The adverse reactions listed in the table are based on post-marketing spontaneous (reporting rate), clinical trials and class-effects.

System Organ Class	Adverse Reaction
Infections and infestations	Vaginitis, including vaginal candidiasis
Neoplasms benign and malignant	Fibrocystic breast changes; Ovarian Cancer; Enlargement of hepatic haemangiomas
Immune system disorders	Urticaria; Angioedeoma; Anaphylactic/ anaphylactoid reactions
Metabolism and nutrition disorders	Glucose intolerance; Hypocalcaemia; Exacerbation of porphyria
Psychiatric disorders	Depression; Changes in libido; Mood disturbances; Irritability
Nervous system disorders	Anxiety; Dizziness; Headache (including migraine); Exacerbation of epilepsy; Stroke; Exacerbation of chorea
Eye disorders	Intolerance to contact lenses; Retinal vascular thrombosis
Cardiac disorders	
Vascular disorders	Pulmonary embolism; Deep vein thrombosis, Superficial thrombophlebitis
Respiratory, thoracic and mediastinal disorders	Exacerbation of asthma
Gastrointestinal disorders	Nausea; Bloating; Abdominal pain; Vomiting; Pancreatitis
Hepatobiliary	Gallbladder disease; Cholestatic jaundice
Skin and subcutaneous tissue disorders	Alopecia; Acne; Pruritus; Chloasma/ melasma; Hirsutism; Rash
Musculoskeletal, connective tissue and bone disorders	Arthralgias; Leg cramps
General disorders and administration site disorders	Oedema
Reproductive system & breast disorders	Breakthrough bleeding/spotting; Dysmenorrhoea; Change in menstrual flow; Change in cervical ectropion and secretion; Increased size of uterine leiomyomata (fibroids) Breast pain, tenderness, Enlargement, discharge; Galactorrhoea
Investigations	Changes in weight (increase or decrease), Increased triglycerides; Increased blood pressure

Breast cancer

According to evidence from a large number of epidemiological studies and one randomised placebo-controlled trial, the Women's Health Initiative (WHI), the overall risk of breast cancer increases with increasing duration of HRT use in current or recent HRT users.

For estrogen-only HRT, estimates of relative risk (RR) from a reanalysis of original data from 51 epidemiological studies (in which >80% of HRT use was estrogen-only HRT) and from the epidemiological Million Women Study (MWS) are similar at 1.35 (95%CI 1.21 – 1.49) and 1.30 (95%CI 1.21 – 1.40), respectively.

For estrogen plus progestogen combined HRT, several epidemiological studies have reported an overall higher risk for breast cancer than with estrogens alone.

The MWS reported that, compared to never users, the use of various types of estrogen-progestogen combined HRT was associated with a higher risk of breast cancer (RR = 2.00, 95%CI: 1.88 – 2.12) than use of estrogens alone (RR = 1.30, 95%CI: 1.21 – 1.40) or use of tibolone (RR=1.45; 95%CI 1.25-1.68).

The WHI trial reported a risk estimate of 1.24 (95%CI 1.01 – 1.54) after 5.6 years of use of estrogen-progestogen combined HRT (CEE + MPA) in all users compared with placebo.

The absolute risks calculated from the MWS and the WHI trial are presented below:

The MWS has estimated, from the known average incidence of breast cancer in developed countries, that:

• For women not using HRT, about 32 in every 1000 are expected to have breast cancer diagnosed between the ages of 50 and 64 years.

• For 1000 current or recent users of HRT, the number of additional cases during the corresponding period will be

• For users of estrogen-only replacement therapy

o between 0 and 3 (best estimate = 1.5) for 5 years' use

o between 3 and 7 (best estimate = 5) for 10 years' use.

• For users of estrogen plus progestogen combined HRT

o between 5 and 7 (best estimate = 6) for 5 years' use

o between 18 and 20 (best estimate = 19) for 10 years' use.

The WHI trial estimated that after 5.6 years of follow-up of women between the ages of 50 and 79 years, an additional 8 cases of invasive breast cancer would be due to estrogen-progestogen combined HRT (CEE + MPA) per 10,000 women years.

According to calculations from the trial data, it is estimated that:

• For 1000 women in the placebo group.

o About 16 cases of invasive breast cancer would be diagnosed in 5 years.

• For 1000 women who used estrogen plus progestogen combined HRT (CEE + MPA), the number of additional cases would be

o Between 0 and 9 (best estimate = 4) for 5 years' use.

The number of additional cases of breast cancer in women who use HRT is broadly similar for women who start HRT irrespective of age at start of use (between the ages of 45-65) (see section 4.4 Special warnings and special precautions for use).

Endometrial Cancer

In women with an intact uterus, the risk of endometrial hyperplasia and endometrial cancer increases with increasing duration of use of unopposed estrogens.

According to data from epidemiological studies, the best estimate of the risk is that for women not using HRT about 5 in every 1000 are expected to have endometrial cancer diagnosed between the ages of 50 and 65. Depending on the duration of treatment and estrogen dose, the reported increase in endometrial cancer risk among unopposed estrogen users varies from 2-to 12-fold greater compared with non-users. Adding a progestogen to estrogen-only therapy greatly reduces this increased risk.

Other adverse reactions reported in association with estrogen/progestogen treatment including Prempak-C:

• Estrogen-dependent neoplasms benign and malignant, e.g. endometrial hyperplasia, endometrial cancer

• Venous thromboembolism, i.e. deep leg or pelvic venous thrombosis and pulmonary embolism, is more frequent among hormone replacement therapy users than among non-users. For further information, see section 4.3 Contra-indications and 4.4 Special warnings and special precautions for use.

• Myocardial infarction

• Stroke

• Skin and subcutaneous disorders: erythema multiforme, erythema nodosum, vascular purpura

• Probable dementia (see section 4.4 Special warnings and special precautions for use)

• Exacerbation of otosclerosis

4.9 Overdose

Symptoms of overdosage of estrogen-containing products in adults and children may include nausea, vomiting, breast tenderness, dizziness, abdominal pain, drowsiness/fatigue and withdrawal bleeding may occur in females. There is no specific antidote, and further treatment should be symptomatic.

5. PHARMACOLOGICAL PROPERTIES

5.1 Pharmacodynamic properties

ATC Code: G03F A10

Conjugated Estrogens

The active ingredients are primarily the sulphate esters of estrone, equilin sulphates, 17α-estradiol and 17β-estradiol. These substitute for the loss of estrogen production in menopausal women, and alleviate menopausal symptoms. Estrogens prevent bone loss following menopause or ovariectomy.

Progestogen:

As estrogens promote the growth of the endometrium, unopposed estrogens increase the risk of endometrial hyperplasia and cancer. The addition of a progestogen reduces but does not eliminate the estrogen-induced risk of endometrial hyperplasia in non-hysterectomised women.

The following data are from studies done with a different progestogen to that in Prempak-C. However, since the effect is due to the conjugated estrogens, these results can be extrapolated to other conjugated estrogen plus progestogen combination products.

Relief of estrogen-deficiency symptoms

In a 1-year clinical trial (n=2,808), vasomotor symptoms were assessed for efficacy during the first 12 weeks of treatment in a subset of symptomatic women (n=241) who had at least 7 moderate or severe hot flushes daily or 50 moderate to severe hot flushes during the week before randomisation. Premique 0.625 mg/2.5 mg(conjugated estrogens/medroxyprogesterone acetate) was shown to be statistically better than placebo at weeks 4, 8 and 12 for relief of both frequency and severity of moderate to severe vasomotor symptoms.

Prevention of osteoporosis

Epidemiological studies suggest a number of individual risk factors which contribute to the development of postmenopausal osteoporosis. These include: early menopause; family history of osteoporosis; thin, small frame; cigarette use; recent prolonged systemic corticosteroid use.

Estrogen deficiency at menopause is associated with an increasing bone turnover and decline in bone mass. The effect of estrogens on the bone mineral density is dose-dependent. Protection appears to be effective for as long as treatment is continued. After discontinuation of HRT, bone mass is lost at a rate similar to that in untreated women.

Evidence from the WHI trial and meta-analysed trials shows that current use of HRT, alone or in combination with a progestogen – given to predominantly healthy women – reduces the risk of hip, vertebral and other osteoporotic fractures. HRT may also help prevent fractures in women with low bone density and/or established osteoporosis, but the evidence for that is limited.

After 3 years of treatment with Premique 0.625 mg/2.5 mg, the increase in lumbar spine bone mineral density (BMD) was 4.87% ± 0.66. The percentage of women who maintained (less than 1% BMD loss per year) or gained BMD in lumbar zone during treatment was 92%.

Premique 0.625 mg/2.5 mg also had an effect on hip BMD. The increase after 3 years was 1.94% ± 0.44 at total hip. The percentage of women who maintained (less than 1% BMD loss per year) or gained BMD in hip zone during treatment was 88%.

5.2 Pharmacokinetic properties

Conjugated Estrogens

Absorption

Conjugated estrogens are soluble in water and are well absorbed from the gastrointestinal tract after release from the drug formulation. Premarin tablets (conjugated estrogens only) release conjugated estrogens slowly over several hours. The pharmacodynamic profile of unconjugated and conjugated estrogens following a dose of 2 × 0.625mg is provided in Table 1.

Distribution

The distribution of exogenous estrogen is similar to that of endogenous estrogens. Estrogens are widely distributed in the body and are generally found in higher concentrations in the sex hormone target organs. Estrogens circulate in the blood largely bound to sex hormone binding globulin (SHBG) and albumin.

Metabolism

Exogenous estrogens are metabolised in the same manner as endogenous estrogens. Circulating estrogens exist in dynamic equilibrium of metabolic interconversions. These transformations take place mainly in the liver. Estradiol is converted reversibly to estrone, and both can be converted to estriol, which is the major urinary metabolite. Estrogens also undergo enterohepatic recirculation via sulphate and glucuronide conjugation in the liver, biliary secretion of conjugates into the intestine, and hydrolysis in the gut following reabsorption. In post-menopausal women a significant proportion of the circulating estrogens exists as sulphate conjugates, especially estrone sulphate, which serves as a circulating reservoir for the formation of more active estrogens.

Excretion

Estriol, estrone and estradiol are excreted in the urine along with glucuronide and sulphate conjugates.

Table 1 - Pharmacokinetic parameters for Premarin

Pharmacokinetic profile for unconjugated estrogens following a dose of 2 × 0.625mg

(see Table 1 below)

Pharmacokinetic profile for conjugated estrogens following a dose of 2 × 0.625mg

(see Table 2 below)

Norgestrel

Norgestrel is a racemic mixture consisting of a levo-rotatory isomer, which is biologically inactive, and the biologically active dextro-rotatory isomer, commonly known as levonorgestrel.

The biologically active isomer, levonorgestrel, is rapidly and almost completely absorbed after administration by mouth, and undergoes little first pass hepatic metabolism. It is highly bound to plasma proteins; 42 to 68% to sex hormone binding globulin and 30 to 56% to albumin. Levonorgestrel and norgestrel are metabolised in the liver to sulphate and glucuronide conjugates, which are excreted in the urine and to a lesser extent in the faeces.

The pharmacokinetic profile of levonorgestrel following an oral dose of 150 micrograms and repeat dosing performed until a steady state was achieved is provided in Table 1.

The proportion of levonorgestrel bound to sex hormone binding globulin is higher when it is given with an estrogen. This indicates that the pharmacokinetic parameters for each active substance will differ when used in combination.

Table 3 – Pharmacokinetic parameters for Levonorgestrel following a dose of 150 microgram and repeat dosing until steady state achieved

(see Table 3 below)

5.3 Preclinical safety data

Long-term continuous administration of natural and synthetic estrogens in certain animal species increases the frequency of carcinoma of the breast, cervix, vagina and liver.

6. PHARMACEUTICAL PARTICULARS

6.1 List of excipients

Prempak-C 0.625 Conjugated estrogen tablets:

Calcium sulphate anhydrous
Carnauba wax
Microcrystalline cellulose
Glyceryl mono-oleates
Lactose monohydrate
Magnesium stearate
Methylcellulose
Marcrogol
Shellac solution (pharmaceutical glaze)
Sucrose
Titanium dioxide (E171)
Opalux maroon colour AS-R-3910 †
Stearic acid
Edible ink (Opacode S-8-28905)††

†Opalux maroon colour AS-R-3910 contains sucrose, purified water, erythrosine (E127), titanium dioxide (E171), sunset yellow (E110), indigo carmine (E132), povidone (E1201) and sodium benzoate (E211).

††Edible ink (Opacode S-8-28905) contains titanium dioxide (E171), shellac (E904), purified water, ethanol, N-butyl alcohol, propylene glycol (E1520), ammonia solution and ethyl acetate.

Prempak-C 1.25mg Conjugated estrogen tablets:

Calcium sulphate anhydrous
Carnauba wax
Microcrystalline cellulose
Glyceryl mono-oleates
Lactose
Magnesium stearate
Methylcellulose
Macrogol 20000
Shellac solution (Pharmaceutical glaze)
Sucrose
Titanium dioxide (E171)
Stearic acid

Colours

Sunset yellow (E110)
Quinoline yellow aluminium lake (E104)
Edible ink (Opacode S-8-27741) containing;
Iron oxide black
Shellac
Purified water
Ethanol
N-butyl alcohol
Propylene glycol
Ammonium solution
Ethyl acetate.

Norgestrel tablets:

Bleached wax
Calcium carbonate
Carnauba wax
Lactose
Magnesium stearate
Macrogol
Polyvinyl pyrrolidone
Starch
Sucrose
Talc
Titanium dioxide (E171)
Colour E172.

6.2 Incompatibilities

Not applicable.

6.3 Shelf life

Three years.

6.4 Special precautions for storage

Do not store above 25°C.

6.5 Nature and contents of container

Polyvinylchloride (PVC)/Aluminium foil blisters containing 28 conjugated estrogen and 12 norgestrel tablets. One carton pack contains 3 blisters.

6.6 Special precautions for disposal and other handling

Not applicable.

7. MARKETING AUTHORISATION HOLDER

John Wyeth and Brother Limited
Trading as: Wyeth Pharmaceuticals
Huntercombe Lane South
Taplow, Maidenhead
Berkshire, SL6 0PH

8. MARKETING AUTHORISATION NUMBER(S)

Prempak-C tablets 0.625mg PL 00011/0161
Prempak-C tablets 1.25mg PL00011/0162

9. DATE OF FIRST AUTHORISATION/RENEWAL OF THE AUTHORISATION

1982.

10. DATE OF REVISION OF THE TEXT

29 July 2008

Table 1 Pharmacokinetic parameters for Premarin

Drug PK Parameter Arithmetic Mean (%CV)	C_{max} (pg/mL)	t_{max} (h)	$t_{1/2}$ (h)	AUC (pg.h/mL)*
estrone	139 (37)	8.8 (20)	28.0 (13)	5016 (34)
baseline-adjusted estrone	120 (42)	8.8 (20)	17.4 (37)	2956 (39)
equilin	66 (42)	7.9 (19)	13.6 (52)	1210 (37)

* $t_{1/2}$ = terminal-phase disposition half-life (0.693/γ)

Table 2

Drug PK Parameter Arithmetic Mean (%CV)	C_{max} (ng/mL)	t_{max} (h)	$t_{1/2}$ (h)	AUC (pg.h/mL)*
total estrone	7.3 (41)	7.3 (51)	15.0 (25)	134 (42)
baseline-adjusted total estrone	7.1 (41)	7.3 (25)	13.6 (27)	122 (39)
total equilin	5.0 (42)	6.2 (26)	10.1 (27)	65 (45)

* $t_{1/2}$ = terminal-phase disposition half-life (0.693/γ)

Table 3 Pharmacokinetic parameters for Levonorgestrel following a dose of 150 microgram and repeat dosing until steady state achieved

PK Parameter Mean value (SD provided in square brackets)	C_{max} (µg/L)	t_{max} (h)	$t_{1/2DIST}$ (h)	$t_{1/2\beta}$ (h)	Vd (L)	CL (ml/min/kg)	AUC (µg/L·h)
Single Dose (150µg)	4.3 [1.3]	1.2 [0.5]	0.6 [0.2]	13.9 [3.2]	108 [37]	1.5 [0.6]	30.9 [11.9]
Repeat dose (to steady state)	2.7 [0.3]	1.0 [0.3]	0.5 [0.2]	17.4 [3.6]	226 [61]	2.5 [0.4]	25.0 [5.9]

Preotact

(Nycomed UK Ltd)

1. NAME OF THE MEDICINAL PRODUCT

Preotact▼100 micrograms powder and solvent for solution for injection.

2. QUALITATIVE AND QUANTITATIVE COMPOSITION

Preotact contains parathyroid hormone manufactured using a strain of Escherichia coli modified by recombinant DNA technology.

The medicinal product is supplied in a dual-chamber cartridge.

The first chamber contains 1.61 mg parathyroid hormone. Each dose of 71.4 microliter contains 100 micrograms parathyroid hormone. Each cartridge contains 14 doses.

The second chamber contains a sterile solvent for reconstitution.

For a full list of excipients, see section 6.1.

3. PHARMACEUTICAL FORM

Powder and solvent for solution for injection.

White to off-white powder and clear, colourless solvent.

4. CLINICAL PARTICULARS

4.1 Therapeutic indications

Treatment of osteoporosis in postmenopausal women at high risk of fractures (see section 5.1).

A significant reduction in the incidence of vertebral, but not hip fractures has been demonstrated.

4.2 Posology and method of administration

The recommended dose is 100 micrograms of parathyroid hormone administered once-daily as a subcutaneous injection into the abdomen.

Patients must be trained to use the proper injection techniques (see section 6.6). A user manual is available with the Preotact pen to instruct patients on the correct use of the pen. The pen is not included in the packs with cartridges.

Patients should receive supplemental calcium and vitamin D if dietary intake is inadequate.

Data support continuous treatment with Preotact for up to 24 months (see section 4.4).

Following treatment with Preotact patients can be treated with a bisphosphonate to further increase bone mineral density (see section 5.1).

Specific populations

Renal impairment

No dose adjustment is necessary in patients with mild to moderate renal impairment (creatinine clearance 30 to 80 ml/min). There is no data available in patients with severe renal impairment. Preotact should therefore not be used in patients with severe renal impairment (see section 4.3).

Hepatic impairment

No dose adjustment is needed for patients with mild or moderate hepatic impairment (total score of 7 to 9 on the Child-Pugh scale). There is no data available in patients with severe hepatic impairment. Preotact should therefore not be used in patients with severe hepatic impairment (see section 4.3).

Children and adolescents

The safety and efficacy of Preotact in patients under 18 years have not been studied. Preotact should not be used in paediatric patients or young adults.

Elderly

Dose adjustment based upon age is not required (see section 5.2).

4.3 Contraindications

Preotact is contraindicated in patients

- with hypersensitivity to parathyroid hormone or to any of the excipients (see section 6.1)
- who have previously received radiation therapy to the skeleton
- with pre-existing hypercalcemia and other disturbances in the phosphocalcic metabolism
- with metabolic bone diseases other than primary osteoporosis (including hyperparathyroidism and Paget's disease of the bone)
- with unexplained elevations of bone-specific alkaline phosphatase
- with severe renal impairment
- with severe hepatic impairment

4.4 Special warnings and precautions for use

Patients initiated on Preotact therapy should be monitored at months 1, 3 and 6 for elevated levels of serum and/or urinary calcium. Monitoring beyond 6 months is not recommended for patients whose total serum calcium is within the normal limits at 6 months.

Elevated serum calcium was observed during Preotact treatment. Serum calcium concentrations reach a maximum between 6 and 8 hours post dose and normally return to baseline by 20 to 24 hours after each administration of parathyroid hormone. Therefore if any blood samples are taken from a patient for monitoring of calcium levels, this should be done at least 20 hours after the most recent injection.

Management of elevated serum calcium

Patients with persistent elevated serum calcium (above the upper normal level) should be evaluated for underlying disease (e.g. hyperparathyroidism). If no underlying condition is found, the following management procedures should be followed:

- Calcium and vitamin D supplementation should be withdrawn
- The frequency of Preotact dosing should be changed to 100 micrograms every other day
- If elevated levels continue, Preotact therapy should be stopped and the patient monitored until the abnormal values have reverted to normal

Patients with pre-existing hypercalcemia and/or hypercalciuria

Preotact has been studied in patients with pre-existing hypercalcemia and/or hypercalciuria. In these patients, Preotact treatment was more likely to exacerbate their underlying hypercalcemia and/or hypercalciuria.

Preotact has not been studied in patients with active urolithiasis. Preotact should be used with caution in patients with active or previous urolithiasis.

Caution should be exercised in patients receiving cardiac glucosides (see section 4.5).

Studies in rats indicate an increased incidence of osteosarcoma with long-term administration of Preotact (see section 5.3). The occurrence of osteosarcoma only occurred at doses that produced systemic exposures ≥ 27-times higher than that observed in humans at the 100 micrograms dose. Until further clinical data becomes available the recommended treatment time of 24 months should not be exceeded.

Preotact contains metacresol, which may cause allergic reactions.

This medicinal product contains less than 1 mmol sodium (23 mg) per dose.

4.5 Interaction with other medicinal products and other forms of interaction

Parathyroid hormone is a natural peptide that is not metabolised by, and does not inhibit hepatic microsomal drug-metabolising enzymes (e.g. cytochrome P450 isoenzymes). Furthermore, parathyroid hormone is not protein bound and has a low volume of distribution. Consequently, no interaction with other medicinal products would be anticipated and no specific drug-drug interactions studies were performed. No potential for drug interactions was identified in the clinical program.

Combining parathyroid hormone with alendronate use has not been shown to provide any advantage over either form of treatment alone, when the end point of bone mineral density was evaluated. (see section 5.1).

From the knowledge of the mechanism of action, combined use of Preotact and cardiac glucosides may predispose patients to digitalis toxicity if hypercalcemia develops.

4.6 Pregnancy and lactation

There are no data available from the use of parathyroid hormone during pregnancy and lactation. Animal studies of reproductive toxicity are incomplete (see section 5.3).

Parathyroid hormone should not be used during pregnancy or breast-feeding.

4.7 Effects on ability to drive and use machines

No studies on the effects on the ability to drive and use machines have been performed. As some episodes of dizziness have been described in patients treated with Preotact, patients should refrain from driving or using machines until symptoms have subsided.

4.8 Undesirable effects

The following adverse reaction (ADR) data are based on two placebo-controlled studies involving 2642 postmenopausal osteoporotic women of whom 1341 received parathyroid hormone. Approximately 71.4 % of the patients on parathyroid hormone reported at least one ADR.

Hypercalcemia and/or hypercalciuria reflect the known pharmacodynamic actions of parathyroid hormone in the gastrointestinal tract, the kidney, and the bone. Hypercalcemia was reported in 25.3 % of patients and hypercalciuria in 39.3 % of patients treated with Preotact. Hypercalcemia was transient and was reported most frequently in the first 3 months of treatment. It was managed during the clinical programme by monitoring laboratory values and the use of a pre-specified management algorithm (see sections 4.3, 4.4, and 5.1).

The only other very commonly reported ADR was nausea.

The table below gives an overview of the ADRs where the incidence is at least 0.5 % higher in the parathyroid hormone group compared to placebo. The following categories are used to rank the undesirable effects by frequency of occurrence: very common (> 1/10); common (> 1/100 and < 1/10); uncommon (> 1/1000 and < 1/100); rare (> 1/10,000 and < 1/1000); and very rare (< 1/10,000), including isolated reports.

System organ class	PTH N = 1341 (%)
Infections and Infestations	
Uncommon	
Influenza	0.5
Metabolism and nutrition disorders	
Very common	
Hypercalcemia	25.3
Common	
Blood calcium increased	3.1
Uncommon	
Blood alkaline phosphatase increased	0.8
Anorexia	0.6
Blood uric acid increased	0.6
Nervous system disorders	
Common	
Headache	9.3
Dizziness	3.9
Uncommon	
Dysgeusia	0.8
Parosmia	0.7
Cardiac disorders	
Common	
Palpitations	1.0
Gastrointestinal disorders	
Very common	
Nausea	13.5
Common	
Vomiting	2.5
Constipation	1.8
Dyspepsia	1.3
Diarrhoea	1.0
Uncommon	
Abdominal pain	0.8
Musculoskeletal, connective tissue and bone disorders	
Common	
Muscle cramp	1.1
Pain in extremity	1.1
Back pain	1.0
Renal and urinary disorders	
Very common	
Hypercalciuria	39.3
Common	
Urine calcium/creatinine ratio increased	2.9
Urine calcium increased	2.2
General disorders and administration site conditions	
Common	
Injection site erythema	2.6
Fatigue	1.8
Asthenia	1.2
Uncommon	
Injection site irritation	0.9

Preotact increases serum uric acid concentrations. For all subjects who received parathyroid hormone 100 micrograms blood uric acid increase was reported for 8 subjects (0.6 %) and hyperuricemia was reported for 5 subjects (0.4 %). Although gout, arthralgia and nephrolithiasis were reported as ADRs, the relationship to elevations in uric acid due to Preotact administration has not been fully established.

Antibodies to parathyroid hormone

In a large phase III clinical study, antibodies to parathyroid hormone were detected in 3 % of women receiving Preotact compared to 0.2 % of women receiving placebo. In these women with a positive titer, there was no evidence of hypersensitivity reactions, allergic reactions, effects on bone mineral density response, or effects on serum calcium.

4.9 Overdose

Signs and symptoms

In the Preotact clinical program, accidental overdose was reported for 17 subjects.

Preotact has been administered in single doses up to 5 micrograms/kg and in repeated doses of up to 3 micrograms/kg/day for 3 days and up to 2.5 micrograms/kg/day for 7 days. The effects of overdose that might be expected include delayed hypercalcemia, nausea, vomiting, dizziness and headache.

Overdose management

There is no specific antidote for Preotact. Treatment of suspected overdose should include temporary discontinuation of Preotact, monitoring of serum calcium, and implementation of appropriate, supportive measures, such as hydration. Due to the relatively short duration of the pharmacological activity of Preotact further measures should not be necessary.

5. PHARMACOLOGICAL PROPERTIES

5.1 Pharmacodynamic properties

Pharmacotherapeutic group: parathyroid hormone, ATC code: H05 AA03.

Mechanism of action

Preotact contains recombinant human parathyroid hormone which is identical to the full-length native 84-amino acid polypeptide.

Physiological actions of parathyroid hormone include stimulation of bone formation by direct effects on bone forming cells (osteoblasts) indirectly increasing the intestinal absorption of calcium and increasing the tubular reabsorption of calcium and excretion of phosphate by the kidney.

Pharmacodynamic effects

The skeletal effects of parathyroid hormone depend upon the pattern of systemic exposure. Transient elevations in parathyroid hormone levels after subcutaneous injection of Preotact stimulates new bone formation on trabecular and cortical (periosteal and/or endosteal) bone surfaces by preferential stimulation of osteoblastic activity over osteoclastic activity.

Effects on serum calcium concentrations

Parathyroid hormone is the principal regulator of serum calcium homeostasis. In response to subcutaneous doses of Preotact (100 micrograms parathyroid hormone), serum total calcium levels increase gradually and reach peak concentration (mean increase in 129 patients, 0.15 mmol/l) at approximately 6 to 8 hours after dosing. In general, serum calcium levels return to baseline levels 24 hours after dosing.

Based on two placebo-controlled studies involving 2642 postmenopausal osteoporotic women, hypercalcemia was reported in 25.3 % of patients treated with Preotact compared to 4.3 % of placebo-treated patients. The hypercalcemia was transient and was reported most frequently in the first 3 months of treatment. It was managed during the clinical programme by monitoring laboratory values and the use of a pre-specified management algorithm.(see sections 4.3 and 4.4).

Clinical efficacy

Effect on fracture incidence

The pivotal study was an 18-month double-blind, placebo-controlled, phase III study (TOP) of the effect of Preotact on fracture incidence in women with postmenopausal osteoporosis.

A total of 2532 patients (1286 Preotact and 1246 placebo), aged 45-94 years (8.1 % 45-54 years and 11.4 % ⩾ 75 years), were randomised to receive 100 micrograms/day or placebo with daily calcium (700 mg) and vitamin D (400 IU) supplementation.

Overall, approximately 19 % of the subjects in each treatment group had at least 1 prevalent vertebral fracture at baseline. The mean baseline lumbar T score was approximately -3.0 in each treatment group.

Of the 2532 randomised intention-to-treat (ITT) patients, a total of 59 patients experienced at least one new vertebral fracture, placebo: 42 (3.37 %) – Preotact: 17 (1.32 %), p=0.001. Patients in the Preotact treatment group had a 61 % relative risk reduction of a new vertebral fracture at month 18 compared to the patients in the placebo group.

To prevent one or more new vertebral fractures, 48 women had to be treated for a median of 18 months for the total population. For patients with pre-existing fractures, number needed to treat (NNT) is 21 patients.

There was no significant difference between the treatment groups in the incidence of any non-vertebral clinical fracture: 5.52 % for Preotact vs. 5.86 % for placebo.

The most relevant fracture reduction was observed among patients at high risk of fractures such as patients with previous fractures and in patients with a lumbar spine T-score of ⩽ - 3.

Relatively few patients less than 5 years postmenopausal and 45-54 years of age were enrolled in the phase III study (2-3 %). The results for these subjects were not different from the results in the study as a whole.

Effect on bone mineral density (BMD)

In the pivotal study, Preotact increased BMD in the lumbar spine after 18 months treatment by 6.5 % compared with -0.3 % for placebo ($p<0.001$). Significant increases in hip BMD (total, femoral neck, trochanter) were observed at study endpoint; 1.0, 1.8 and 1.0 %, respectively, for Preotact versus -1.1, -0.7 and -0.6 % for placebo ($p<0.001$).

Continued treatment for up to 24 months in an open-label extension of this study resulted in a continued increase in BMD. The increase from baseline in lumbar spine and femoral neck BMD was 6.8 % and 2.2 %, respectively in patients treated with Preotact.

The effects of Preotact on bone architecture were evaluated using quantitative computed tomography (QCT) and peripheral QCT. Volumetric trabecular BMD at the lumbar spine increased by 38 % over baseline at 18 months. Similarly, volumetric trabecular BMD at the total hip increased by 4.7 %. Similar increases occurred at the femoral neck, trochanter, and intertrochanter. Treatment with Preotact reduced volumetric cortical bone BMD (measured at the distal radius and mid-shaft tibia), while periosteal circumference or indices of cortical bone strength were maintained.

In the 24-month alendronate combination therapy study (PaTH), the effects of Preotact on bone architecture were also evaluated using QCT. Volumetric trabecular BMD at the lumbar spine increased by 26, 13, and 11 % (Preotact, Preotact and alendronate and alendronate, respectively) over baseline at 12 months. Similarly, volumetric trabecular BMD at the total hip increased by 9, 6, and 2 %, respectively, in the 3 groups.

Treatment of osteoporosis with combination and sequential therapy

The PaTH study was a NIH sponsored randomised, placebo-controlled, 2 year, multicenter, double-blind trial of Preotact and alendronate as monotherapy and in combination for the treatment of postmenopausal osteoporosis. Inclusion criterias were; women between 55 and 85 years of age with BMD T-scores below -2.5 or below -2 and at least one additional risk factor for fracture. All women were given calcium (400-500 mg) and vitamin D (400 IU) supplements.

A total of 238 postmenopausal women, were randomly assigned to one of the following treatment groups; Preotact (100 micrograms parathyroid hormone), alendronate (10 mg), or the combination of both, and followed for 12 months. In the second year of the study women in the original Preotact group were randomly assigned to receive either alendronate or matching placebo, and women in the other two groups received alendronate.

At baseline a total of 165 women (69 %) had a T-score below –2.5, and 112 (47 %) reported at least one fracture after menopause.

One year of therapy, showed the following results: The increases in lumbar spine BMD above baseline were similar in the Preotact and combination-therapy groups (6.3 and 6.1 %, respectively), but were somewhat smaller in the alendronate group (4.6 %). Increases in BMD at the total hip were 0.3, 1.9, and 3.0 % for the 3 groups, respectively.

At the end of year 2 (12 months after Preotact was discontinued), there was a 12.1 % mean increase in dual energy X-ray absorptiometry (DXA) spine BMD for patients who received alendronate for the second year. For the patients who received placebo during the second year, the mean percent increase was 4.1 % compared to baseline, but had decreased slightly compared to the end of 12 months of Preotact treatment. For the mean change in hip BMD, there was a 4.5 % increase from baseline with one year of alendronate compared to a 0.1 % decrease after one year of placebo.

Preotact in combination with hormone replacement therapy (HRT) in 180 postmenopausal women has been shown to significantly increase lumbar spine BMD at 12 months compared with HRT alone (7.1 % vs. 1.1 %, $p<0.001$). The combination was effective regardless of age, baseline rate of bone turnover, or baseline BMD.

5.2 Pharmacokinetic properties

Absorption

Subcutaneous administration of 100 micrograms of parathyroid hormone into the abdomen produces a rapid increase in plasma parathyroid hormone levels and achieves a peak at 1 to 2 hours after dosing. The average half-life is of about 1.5 hours. The absolute bioavailability of 100 micrograms of parathyroid hormone after subcutaneous administration in the abdomen is 55 %.

Distribution

The volume of distribution at steady-state following intravenous administration is approximately 5.4 l. Intersubject variability in the volume of distribution of parathyroid hormone is about 40 %.

Biotransformation

Parathyroid hormone is efficiently removed from the blood by a receptor-mediated process in the liver and is broken down into smaller peptide fragments. The fragments derived from the amino-terminus are further degraded within the cell while the fragments derived from the carboxy-terminius are released back into the blood and cleared by the kidney. These carboxy-terminal fragments are thought to play a role in the regulation of parathyroid hormone activity. Under normal physiologic conditions, full-length parathyroid hormone (1-84) constitutes only 5-30 % of the circulating forms of the molecule, while 70-95 % is present as carboxy-terminal fragments. Following a subcutaneous dose of Preotact, C-terminal fragments make up about 60-90% of the circulating forms of the molecule.

Systemic clearance of parathyroid hormone (45.3 l/hour) following an intravenous dose is close to normal liver plasma flow and is consistent with extensive hepatic metabolism of the active substance. Intersubject variability in systemic clearance is about 15 %.

Elimination

Parathyroid hormone is metabolised in the liver and to a lesser degree in the kidney. Parathyroid hormone is not excreted from the body in its intact form. Circulating carboxy-terminal fragments are filtered by the kidney, but are subsequently broken to even smaller fragments during tubular reuptake.

Hepatic impairment

There was a modest increase of about 20 % in the mean baseline corrected exposure (AUC) to parathyroid hormone in a study conducted in 6 men and 6 women with moderate hepatic impairment as compared with a matched group of 12 subjects with normal hepatic function.

No studies have been conducted in patients with severe hepatic impairment.

Renal impairment

The overall exposure and C_{max} of parathyroid hormone were slightly increased (22 % and 56 %, respectively) in a group of 8 male and 8 female subjects with mild-to-moderate renal impairment (creatinine clearances of 30 to 80 ml/min) compared with a matched group of 16 subjects with normal renal function.

The pharmacokinetics of parathyroid hormone in patients with severe renal impairment (creatinine clearance of less than 30 ml/min) has not been investigated.

Elderly

No differences in Preotact pharmacokinetics were detected with regard to age (range 47-88 years). Dosage adjustment based on age is not required.

Gender

The medicinal product has only been studied in postmenopausal women.

5.3 Preclinical safety data

Preclinical data reveal no special hazard for humans based on conventional studies of safety pharmacology, mutagenicity, toxicity to fertility and general reproduction, and local tolerance.

In monkeys receiving daily subcutaneous doses for 6 months, there was an increased occurrence of renal tubular mineralization at exposure levels below clinical exposure levels.

Rats treated with near life-time daily injections had dose-dependent exaggerated bone formation and an increased incidence of bone tumours, including osteosarcoma, most probably due to an epigenetic mechanism. Due to the differences in bone physiology in rats and humans, the clinical relevance of these findings is probably minor. No osteosarcomas have been observed in clinical trials.

There are no studies of foetal, developmental, perinatal or postnatal toxicity. It is unknown whether recombinant human parathyroid hormone is excreted in the milk of lactating animals.

6. PHARMACEUTICAL PARTICULARS

6.1 List of excipients

Powder

Mannitol

Citric acid monohydrate

Sodium chloride

Hydrochloric acid, dilute (for pH adjustment)

Sodium hydroxide 1N (for pH adjustment)

Solvent

Metacresol

Water for injections

6.2 Incompatibilities

Not applicable.

6.3 Shelf life

Powder: 30 months

Mixed solution: chemical and physical in-use stability has been demonstrated for 28 days at 2-8°C. During the 28-day period the mixed solution can be stored for up to 7 days at temperatures below 25°C.

6.4 Special precautions for storage

Do not store above 25°C. Do not freeze.

Keep the cartridge in the outer carton in order to protect from light.

Mixed solution: Store in a refrigerator (2-8°C). Do not freeze. Once the cartridge is mixed it can be stored outside the refrigerator at temperatures below 25°C for up to 7 days during the 28 day use period.(see section 6.3).

6.5 Nature and contents of container

The container closure system is comprised of a dual-chamber cartridge, a center stopper, a crimp cap (containing a rubber seal) sealing the first chamber containing lyophilised powder and an end stopper sealing the second chamber containing the solvent for mixing.

Cartridge: The glass of the dual-chamber cartridge is made of glass Type I.

Stopper (center and end): The stopper is made of bromobutyl rubber, grey.

Crimp cap (containing a rubber seal): The crimp cap is made of aluminium and the rubber seal is made of bromobutyl rubber.

Each dual-chamber cartridge contains 1.61 mg parathyroid hormone and 1.13 ml solvent (14 doses).

Preotact is available in packs of 2 and 6 cartridges. Not all pack sizes may be marketed.

The Preotact pen and needles are not included.

6.6 Special precautions for disposal and other handling

Preotact is injected using the re-usable pen, Preotact pen. The contents of the dual-chamber cartridge is mixed in the Preotact pen. After mixing the liquid should be clear and colourless.

DO NOT SHAKE; shaking may cause denaturation of the active substance.

If the mixed solution is cloudy, coloured or contains particles the cartridge should be removed from the Preotact pen and a new cartridge inserted.

Any unused product or waste material should be disposed of in accordance with local requirements.

7. MARKETING AUTHORISATION HOLDER

Nycomed Danmark ApS

Langebjerg 1

DK-4000 Roskilde

Denmark

8. MARKETING AUTHORISATION NUMBER(S)

EU/1/06/339/001-002

9. DATE OF FIRST AUTHORISATION/RENEWAL OF THE AUTHORISATION
24 April 2006

10. DATE OF REVISION OF THE TEXT

Prevenar Suspension for Injection in Pre-filled Syringe

(Wyeth Pharmaceuticals)

1. NAME OF THE MEDICINAL PRODUCT
Prevenar suspension for injection in pre-filled syringe
Pneumococcal saccharide conjugated vaccine, adsorbed

2. QUALITATIVE AND QUANTITATIVE COMPOSITION
Each 0.5 ml dose contains:

Pneumococcal polysaccharide serotype 4* 2 micrograms

Pneumococcal polysaccharide serotype 6B* 4 micrograms

Pneumococcal polysaccharide serotype 9V* 2 micrograms

Pneumococcal polysaccharide serotype 14* 2 micrograms

Pneumococcal oligosaccharide serotype 18C* 2 micrograms

Pneumococcal polysaccharide serotype 19F* 2 micrograms

Pneumococcal polysaccharide serotype 23F* 2 micrograms

* Conjugated to the CRM_{197} carrier protein and adsorbed on aluminium phosphate (0.5 mg)

For a full list of excipients, see section 6.1.

3. PHARMACEUTICAL FORM
Suspension for injection in pre-filled syringe.

The vaccine is a homogeneous white suspension.

4. CLINICAL PARTICULARS

4.1 Therapeutic indications
Active immunisation against disease caused by *Streptococcus pneumoniae* serotypes 4, 6B, 9V, 14, 18C, 19F and 23F (including sepsis, meningitis, pneumonia, bacteraemia and acute otitis media) in infants and children from 2 months up to 5 years of age (see sections 4.2, 4.4 and 5.1).

For the number of doses to be administered in the different age groups, see section 4.2.

The use of Prevenar should be determined on the basis of official recommendations taking into consideration the impact of invasive disease in different age groups as well as variability of serotype epidemiology in different geographical areas (see sections 4.4, 4.8 and 5.1).

4.2 Posology and method of administration
The vaccine should be given by intramuscular injection. The preferred sites are anterolateral aspect of the thigh (vastus lateralis muscle) in infants or the deltoid muscle of the upper arm in young children.

Immunisation schedules:

The immunisation schedules for Prevenar should be based on official recommendations.

Infants aged 2 - 6 months:

The primary infant series consists of three doses, each of 0.5 ml, the first dose usually given at 2 months of age and with an interval of at least 1 month between doses. A fourth dose is recommended in the second year of life.

Alternatively, when Prevenar is given as part of a routine infant immunisation programme, a two-dose schedule may be considered. The first dose may be given from the age of 2 months with a second dose at least 2 months later and a third (booster) dose at 11-15 months of age (see section 5.1)

Previously unvaccinated older infants and children:

Infants aged 7 - 11 months: two doses, each of 0.5 ml, with an interval of at least 1 month between doses. A third dose is recommended in the second year of life.

Children aged 12 - 23 months: two doses, each of 0.5 ml, with an interval of at least 2 months between doses.

Children aged 24 months – 5 years: one single dose.

The need for a booster dose after these immunisation schedules has not been established.

4.3 Contraindications
Hypersensitivity to the active substances or to any of the excipients, or to diphtheria toxoid.

4.4 Special warnings and precautions for use
As with other vaccines, the administration of Prevenar should be postponed in subjects suffering from acute moderate or severe febrile illness.

As with all injectable vaccines, appropriate medical treatment and supervision should always be readily available in case of a rare anaphylactic event following the administration of the vaccine.

The potential risk of apnoea and the need for respiratory monitoring for 48-72h should be considered when administering the primary immunisation series to very premature infants (born ⩽ 28 weeks of gestation) and particularly for those with a previous history of respiratory immaturity. As the benefit of vaccination is high in this group of infants, vaccination should not be withheld or delayed.

Prevenar will not protect against other *Streptococcus pneumoniae* serotypes than those included in the vaccine nor other micro-organisms that cause invasive disease or otitis media.

This vaccine should not be given to infants or children with thrombocytopenia or any coagulation disorder that would contraindicate intramuscular injection unless the potential benefit clearly outweighs the risk of administration.

Although some antibody response to diphtheria toxoid may occur, immunisation with this vaccine does not substitute for routine diphtheria immunisation.

For children from 2 years through 5 years of age, a single dose immunisation schedule was used. A higher rate of local reactions has been observed in children older than 24 months of age compared with infants (see section 4.8).

Children with impaired immune responsiveness, whether due to the use of immunosuppressive therapy, a genetic defect, HIV infection, or other causes, may have reduced antibody response to active immunisation.

Limited data have demonstrated that Prevenar (three dose primary series) induces an acceptable immune response in infants with sickle cell disease with a safety profile similar to that observed in non-high-risk groups (see section 5.1). Safety and immunogenicity data are not yet available for children in other specific high-risk groups for invasive pneumococcal disease (e.g. children with another congenital or acquired splenic dysfunction, HIV-infected, malignancy, nephrotic syndrome). Vaccination in high-risk groups should be considered on an individual basis.

Children below 2 years old should receive the appropriate-for-age Prevenar vaccination series (see section 4.2). The use of pneumococcal conjugate vaccine does not replace the use of 23-valent pneumococcal polysaccharide vaccines in children ⩾ 24 months of age with conditions (such as sickle cell disease, asplenia, HIV infection, chronic illness or who are immunocompromised) placing them at higher risk for invasive disease due to *Streptococcus pneumoniae*. Whenever recommended, children at risk who are ⩾ 24 months of age and already primed with Prevenar should receive 23-valent pneumococcal polysaccharide vaccine. The interval between the pneumococcal conjugate vaccine (Prevenar) and the 23-valent pneumococcal polysaccharide vaccine should not be less than 8 weeks. There are no data available to indicate whether the administration of 23-valent pneumococcal polysaccharide vaccine to unprimed children or to children primed with Prevenar might result in hyporesponsiveness to further doses of Prevenar.

When Prevenar is co-administered with hexavalent vaccines (DTaP/Hib(PRP-T)/IPV/HepB), the physician should be aware that data from clinical studies indicate that the rate of febrile reactions was higher compared to that occurring following the administration of hexavalent vaccines alone. These reactions were mostly moderate (less than or equal to 39 °C) and transient (see section 4.8).

Antipyretic treatment should be initiated according to local treatment guidelines.

Prophylactic antipyretic medication is recommended:

- for all children receiving Prevenar simultaneously with vaccines containing whole cell pertussis because of higher rate of febrile reactions (see section 4.8).

- for children with seizure disorders or with a prior history of febrile seizures.

Do not administer Prevenar intravenously.

As with any vaccine, Prevenar may not protect all individuals receiving the vaccine from pneumococcal disease. Additionally, for vaccine serotypes, protection against otitis media is expected to be substantially lower than protection against invasive disease. As otitis media is caused by many organisms other than pneumococcal serotypes represented in the vaccine, protection against all otitis media is expected to be low (see section 5.1).

4.5 Interaction with other medicinal products and other forms of interaction
Prevenar can be administered simultaneously with other paediatric vaccines in accordance with the recommended immunisation schedules. Different injectable vaccines should always be given at different injection sites.

The immune response to routine paediatric vaccines co-administered with Prevenar at different injection sites was assessed in 7 controlled clinical studies. The antibody response to Hib tetanus protein conjugate (PRP-T), tetanus and Hepatitis B (HepB) vaccines was similar to controls. For CRM-based Hib conjugate vaccine, enhancement of antibody responses to Hib and diphtheria in the infant series was observed. At the booster, some suppression of Hib antibody level was observed but all children had protective levels. Inconsistent reduction in response to pertussis antigens as well as to inactivated polio vaccine (IPV) were observed. The clinical relevance of these interactions is unknown. Limited results from open label studies showed an acceptable response to MMR and varicella.

Data on concomitant administration of Prevenar with Infanrix hexa (DTaP/Hib(PRP-T)/IPV/HepB vaccine) have shown no clinically relevant interference in the antibody response to each of the individual antigens when given as a 3 dose primary vaccination.

Sufficient data regarding interference on the concomitant administration of other hexavalent vaccines with Prevenar are currently not available.

In a clinical trial that compared separate with concomitant administrations of Prevenar (three doses at 2, 3.5, 6 months and a booster dose at approximately 12 months) and Meningitec (meningococcal C conjugate vaccine; two doses at 2 and 6 months and a booster dose at approximately 12 months) there was no evidence of immune interference between the two conjugate vaccines after the primary series or after the booster doses.

4.6 Pregnancy and lactation
Prevenar is not intended for use in adults. Information on the safety of the vaccine when used during pregnancy and lactation is not available.

4.7 Effects on ability to drive and use machines
Not relevant.

4.8 Undesirable effects
The safety of the vaccine was assessed in different controlled clinical studies in which more than 18,000 healthy infants (6 weeks to 18 months) were included. The majority of the safety experience comes from the efficacy trial in which 17,066 infants received 55,352 doses of Prevenar. Also safety in previously unvaccinated older children has been assessed.

In all studies, Prevenar was administered concurrently with the recommended childhood vaccines.

Amongst the most commonly reported adverse reactions were injection site reactions and fever.

No consistent increased local or systemic reactions within repeated doses were seen throughout the primary series or with the booster dose, the exception being a higher rate of transient tenderness (36.5 %) and tenderness that interfered with limb movement (18.5 %) were seen with the booster dose.

In older children receiving a single dose of vaccine, a higher rate of local reactions has been observed than that previously described in infancy. These reactions were primarily transient in nature. In a post licensure study involving 115 children between 2-5 years of age, tenderness was reported in 39.1 % of children; in 15.7 % of children the tenderness interfered with limb movement. Redness was reported in 40.0 % of children, and induration was reported in 32.2 % of subjects. Redness or induration ≥2cm in diameter was reported in 22.6 % and 13.9% of children respectively.

When Prevenar is co-administered with hexavalent vaccines (DTaP/Hib(PRP-T)/IPV/HepB), fever ⩾ 38 °C per dose was reported in 28.3 % to 48.3 % of infants in the group receiving Prevenar and the hexavalent vaccine at the same time as compared to 15.6 % to 23.4 % in the group receiving the hexavalent vaccine alone. Fever of greater than 39.5 °C per dose was observed in 0.6 to 2.8 % of infants receiving Prevenar and hexavalent vaccines (see section 4.4).

Reactogenicity was higher in children receiving whole cell pertussis vaccines concurrently. In a study, including 1,662 children, fever of ⩾ 38°C was reported in 41.2 % of children who received Prevenar simultaneously with DTP as compared to 27.9 % in the control group. Fever of > 39°C was reported in 3.3 % of children compared to 1.2 % in the control group.

Undesirable effects reported in clinical trials or from the post-marketing experience are listed in the following table per body system and per frequency and this is for all age groups. The frequency is defined as follows: very common: ⩾ 1/10, common: ⩾ 1/100 and < 1/10, uncommon: ⩾ 1/1,000 and < 1/100, rare: ⩾ 1/10,000 and < 1/1,000, very rare: ⩽ 1/10,000.

Within each frequency grouping, undesirable effects are presented in order of decreasing seriousness

Blood and lymphatic system disorders:
Very rare: Lymphadenopathy localised to the region of the injection site

Immune system disorders:
Rare: Hypersensitivity reactions such as, anaphylactic/anaphylactoid reactions including shock, angioneurotic oedema, bronchospasm, dyspnoea, face oedema.

Nervous system disorders:
Rare: Seizures, including febrile seizures.

Gastrointestinal disorders:
Very common: Vomiting, diarrhoea, decreased appetite.

Skin and subcutaneous tissue disorders:
Uncommon: Rash/urticaria.

Very rare: Erythema multiforme.

General disorders and administration site conditions:
Very common: Injection site reactions (e.g. erythema, induration/swelling, pain/tenderness); fever ⩾ 38°C, irritability, crying, drowsiness, restless sleep.

Common: Injection site swelling/induration and erythema >2.4 cm, tenderness interfering with movement, fever > 39°C.

Rare: Hypotonic hyporesponsive episode, injection site hypersensitivity reactions (eg., dermatitis, pruritus, urticaria, flushing).

Apnoea in very premature infants (≤ 28 weeks of gestation) (see section 4.4).

4.9 Overdose

There have been reports of overdose with Prevenar, including cases of administration of a higher than recommended dose and cases of subsequent doses administered closer than recommended to the previous dose. No undesirable effects were reported in the majority of individuals. In general, adverse events reported with overdose have also been reported with recommended single doses of Prevenar.

5. PHARMACOLOGICAL PROPERTIES

5.1 Pharmacodynamic properties

Pharmacotherapeutic group: pneumococcal vaccines, ATC code: J07AL02

Immunogenicity

Significant increases in antibody (measured by ELISA) were seen for all vaccine serotypes following a three-dose primary series of Prevenar in infants and following booster doses although geometric mean concentrations varied between the 7 serotypes. Prevenar has also been shown to elicit functional antibodies (measured by opsonophagocytosis) to all vaccine serotypes following the primary series. Long-term persistence of antibodies has not been investigated after administration of a primary series in infants plus booster or after administration of single priming doses to older children. Administration of unconjugated pneumococcal polysaccharides at 13 months following the primary series with Prevenar elicited an anamnestic antibody response for the 7 serotypes included in the vaccine, indicating that priming had occurred.

The immunogenicity of a two-dose primary series in infants plus a booster at about one year of age has been documented in several studies. Most of the data have indicated that smaller proportions of infants achieved antibody concentrations ≥0.35 μg/mL (the reference antibody concentration recommended by WHO)[1] against serotypes 6B and 23F after two-dose primary series when directly or indirectly compared with three-dose primary series. In addition, GMCs were lower for antibodies to most serotypes after a two-dose infant series than after a three-dose infant series. However, antibody responses to booster doses in toddlers following two-dose or three-dose infant series were comparable for all 7 vaccine serotypes and indicated that both infant regimens had elicited adequate priming.

Significant increases in antibody (measured by ELISA) to all vaccine serotypes were seen after administration of single doses of Prevenar to children aged 2 to 5 years. Antibody concentrations were similar to those achieved following a three-dose infant series and a booster dose at less than 2 years of age. Efficacy trials in the 2- to 5-year-old population have not been conducted.

Clinical trial efficacy of the two-dose infant primary series plus a booster has not been established, and the clinical consequences of lower antibody concentrations against serotypes 6B and 23F after the two-dose infant series are not known.

Efficacy against invasive disease

Estimates of efficacy against invasive disease were obtained in the US population where vaccine serotype coverage ranged from 80 to 89 %. Epidemiological data between 1988 and 2003 indicated that in Europe coverage is lower and varies from country to country. Consequently, Prevenar should cover between 54 % and 84 % of isolates from invasive pneumococcal disease (IPD) in European children less than 2 years of age. In European children between 2 to 5 years of age, Prevenar should cover about 62 % to 83 % of the clinical isolates responsible for invasive pneumococcal disease. It is estimated that more than 80 % of the antimicrobial resistant strains would be covered by the serotypes included in the vaccine. The vaccine serotype coverage in the paediatric population decreases with increasing age. The decrease in the incidence of IPD seen in older children may be partly due to naturally acquired immunity.

Efficacy against invasive disease was assessed in a large-scale randomised, double-blind, clinical trial in a multiethnic population in Northern California (Kaiser Permanente trial). More than 37,816 infants were immunised with either Prevenar or a control vaccine (meningococcal conjugate group C vaccine), at 2, 4, 6 and 12-15 months of age. At the time of the study, the serotypes included in the vaccine accounted for 89 % of IPD.

A total of 52 cases of invasive disease caused by vaccine serotypes had accumulated in a blinded follow-up period through April 20, 1999. The estimate of vaccine serotype specific efficacy was 94 % (95 % CI: 81, 99) in the intent-to-treat population and 97 % (95 % CI: 85, 100) in the per protocol (fully immunised) population (40 cases). In Europe, the estimates of effectiveness in children less than 2 years of age range from 51 % to 79 % when considering vaccine coverage against serotypes causing invasive disease.

Efficacy against pneumonia

In the Kaiser Permanente trial, efficacy was 87.5 % (95 % CI: 7, 99) against bacteraemic pneumonia due to vaccine serotypes of *S. pneumoniae*.

Effectiveness (no microbiological confirmation of diagnosis was performed) against non-bacteraemic pneumonia was also assessed. As many pathogens other than pneumococcal serotypes represented in the vaccine may contribute to the burden of pneumonia in children, protection against all clinical pneumonia is expected to be lower than for invasive pneumococcal disease. In the per-protocol analysis, the estimated risk reduction for the first episode of clinical pneumonia with abnormal chest radiograph (defined as the presence of infiltrates beyond the perihilar area, consolidation, or empyema) was 20.5 % (95 % CI: 4.4, 34.0). Reductions in pneumonia with abnormal chest radiograph were greatest in the first year of life (32.2 %; 95 % CI: 3.3, 52.5) and in the first 2 years of life (23.4 %; 95 % CI: 5.2, 38.1).

Efficacy against otitis media

Acute otitis media (AOM) is a common childhood disease with different aetiologies. Bacteria can be responsible for 60-70% of clinical episodes of AOM. The pneumococcus is responsible for 30-40% of all bacterial AOM and a greater fraction of severe AOM. Theoretically, Prevenar could prevent about 60-80% of serotypes causing pneumococcal AOM. It is estimated that Prevenar could prevent 6-13% of all clinical episodes of AOM.

Efficacy of Prevenar against acute otitis media (AOM) was assessed in a randomised, double blind, clinical trial of 1,662 Finnish infants immunised with either Prevenar or a control vaccine (Hepatitis B vaccine), at 2, 4, 6 and 12-15 months of age. The estimate for vaccine efficacy against vaccine-serotype AOM, the primary endpoint of the trial, was 57 % (95 % CI: 44, 67) in the per-protocol analysis and 54 % (95 % CI: 41, 64) in the intent-to-treat analysis. A 33 % (95 % CI: -1, 80) increase in AOM due to serogroups not included in the vaccine was observed in immunised subjects. However, the overall benefit was a 34 % (95 % CI: 21, 45) reduction in the incidence of all pneumococcal AOM. The impact of the vaccine on total number of episodes of otitis media regardless of etiology was a 6 % (95 % CI: -4, 16) reduction.

A subset of children in this study were followed until they reached 4 to 5 years of age. In this follow-up, vaccine efficacy for frequent OM (defined as at least 3 episodes within 6 months) was 18 % (95 % CI: 1, 32), for chronic otitis media with effusion, 50 % (95 % CI: 15, 71), and for tympanostomy tube placement, 39 % (95 % CI: 4, 61).

Efficacy of Prevenar against AOM was assessed as a secondary endpoint in the Kaiser Permanente trial. Children were followed until 3.5 years of age. The impact of the vaccine on total number of episodes of otitis media regardless of etiology was a 7 % reduction (95 % CI: 4, 10). The effect of the vaccine in the per-protocol analysis was a 9 % reduction (95 % CI: 3, 15) in recurrent AOM (defined as 3 episodes in six months or 4 episodes in one year) or a 23 % (95 % CI: 7,36) reduction for recurrent AOM (5 episodes in six months or 6 episodes in one year). Tympanostomy tube placement was reduced by 24 % (95 % CI: 12, 35) in the per-protocol analysis and by 23 % (95 % CI: 11, 34) in the intent-to-treat analysis.

Effectiveness

The effectiveness of Prevenar against IPD (i.e. comprising the protection afforded by vaccination and from herd immunity due to reduced transmission of vaccine serotypes in the population) has been evaluated in national immunisation programmes that employ three-dose or two-dose infant series, each with booster doses.

In the USA, generalised vaccination with Prevenar using a four-dose series in infants and a catch-up programme for children up to 5 years of age was introduced in 2000. Vaccine effectiveness against IPD caused by vaccine serotypes was evaluated in 3- to 59-month old children within the first four years of the implementation of the programme. When compared with no vaccination, point estimates for the effectiveness of 2-, 3-, or 4-doses given on an infant schedule were similar: 96% (95% CI 88-99); 95% (95% CI 88-99); and 100% (95% CI 94-100), respectively. In the USA in the same time frame, there was a 94% reduction in vaccine type IPD in individuals under 5 years of age, compared to a pre-vaccine baseline (1998/99). In parallel, there was a 62% reduction in vaccine type IPD in individuals over 5 years of age. This indirect or herd effect is due to a reduction in transmission of vaccine serotypes from immunised young children to the rest of the population and coincides with decreased nasopharyngeal carriage of vaccine serotypes.

In Quebec, Canada Prevenar was introduced at 2, 4 and 12 months of age with a single dose catch-up programme in children up to 5 years of age. In the first two years of the programme, with over 90% coverage, the observed effectiveness against IPD caused by vaccine serotypes was 93% (95% CI 75-98) for the 2 dose infant series and 100% (95% CI 91-100) for the completed schedule.

Preliminary data from England and Wales reported less than 1 year following introduction of routine immunisation at 2, 4 and 13 months with a single dose catch-up programme for children 13 to 23 months of age have suggested that effectiveness of this schedule might be lower against serotype 6B than against the other serotypes in the vaccine.

The effectiveness of a two-dose primary series has not been established against pneumonia or acute otitis media.

Additional immunogenicity data

The immunogenicity of Prevenar has been investigated in an open-label, multicenter study in 49 infants with sickle cell disease. Children were vaccinated with Prevenar (3 doses one month apart from the age of 2 months) and 46 of these children also received a 23-valent pneumococcal polysaccharide vaccine at the age of 15-18 months. After primary immunisation, 95.6% of the subjects had antibody levels of at least 0.35 μg/ml for all seven serotypes found in Prevenar. A significant increase was seen in the concentrations of antibodies against the seven serotypes after the polysaccharide vaccination, suggesting that immunological memory was well established.

[1] WHO technical report No 927, 2005; Appendix serological criteria for calculation and licensure of new pneumococcal conjugate vaccine formulations for use in infants.

5.2 Pharmacokinetic properties

Evaluation of pharmacokinetic properties is not available for vaccines.

5.3 Preclinical safety data

A repeated dose intramuscular toxicity study (13 weeks, 5 injections, one every three weeks) of pneumococcal conjugate vaccine in rabbits revealed no evidence of any significant local or systemic toxic effects.

Repeated dose subcutaneous toxicity studies (13 weeks, 7 injections of the clinical dose, one every other week, followed by a 4-week recovery period) of Prevenar in rats and monkeys revealed no evidence of any significant local or systemic toxic effects.

6. PHARMACEUTICAL PARTICULARS

6.1 List of excipients

Sodium chloride

Water for injections

6.2 Incompatibilities

In the absence of compatibility studies, this medicinal product must not be mixed with other medicinal products.

6.3 Shelf life

4 years

6.4 Special precautions for storage

Store in a refrigerator (2°C – 8°C).

Do not freeze.

6.5 Nature and contents of container

0.5 ml suspension for injection in pre-filled syringe (Type I glass) with a plunger rod (polypropylene), a plunger stopper (latex free grey butyl rubber) and a protective-tip cap (latex free grey butyl rubber) - pack size of 1 and 10 with or without needle, and multi pack of 5 packs of 10 pre-filled syringes without needle.

Not all pack sizes may be marketed.

6.6 Special precautions for disposal and other handling

Upon storage, a white deposit and clear supernatant can be observed.

The vaccine should be well shaken to obtain a homogeneous white suspension and be inspected visually for any particulate matter and/or variation of physical aspect prior to administration. Do not use if the content appears otherwise.

Any unused product or waste material should be disposed of in accordance with local requirements.

7. MARKETING AUTHORISATION HOLDER

Wyeth Lederle Vaccines S.A.

Rue du Bosquet, 15

B-1348 Louvain-la-Neuve

Belgium

8. MARKETING AUTHORISATION NUMBER(S)

EU/1/00/167/003 – 1 × pre-filled syringe

EU/1/00/167/004 – 10 × pre-filled syringe

EU/1/00/167/006 – 1 × pre-filled syringe with separate needle

EU/1/00/167/007 – 10 × pre-filled syringe with separate needles

EU/1/00/167/008 – 5 × 10 pre-filled syringes without needle.

9. DATE OF FIRST AUTHORISATION/RENEWAL OF THE AUTHORISATION

Date of first authorisation: 02/02/2001

Date of last renewal: 12/04/2006

10. DATE OF REVISION OF THE TEXT

27 July 2009

PREZISTA 300 mg film-coated tablets

(Janssen-Cilag Ltd)

1. NAME OF THE MEDICINAL PRODUCT

PREZISTA®▼ 300 mg film-coated tablets

2. QUALITATIVE AND QUANTITATIVE COMPOSITION

Each film-coated tablet contains 300 mg of darunavir (as ethanolate).

Excipient: Each tablet contains 1.375 mg sunset yellow FCF (E110). For a full list of excipients, see section 6.1.

3. PHARMACEUTICAL FORM

Film-coated tablet.

Orange oval shaped tablet, debossed with "300MG" on one side and "TMC114" on the other side.

4. CLINICAL PARTICULARS

4.1 Therapeutic indications

PREZISTA, co-administered with low dose ritonavir is indicated in combination with other antiretroviral medicinal products for the treatment of human immunodeficiency virus (HIV-1) infection in antiretroviral treatment (ART) experienced adult patients, including those that have been highly pre-treated and for the treatment of HIV-1 infection in ART-experienced children and adolescents from the age of 6 years and at least 20 kg body weight.

In deciding to initiate treatment with PREZISTA co-administered with low dose ritonavir careful consideration should be given to the treatment history of the individual patient and the patterns of mutations associated with different agents. Genotypic or phenotypic testing (when available) and treatment history should guide the use of PREZISTA.

4.2 Posology and method of administration

Therapy should be initiated by a physician experienced in the management of HIV infection.

PREZISTA must always be given orally with low dose ritonavir as a pharmacokinetic enhancer and in combination with other antiretroviral medicinal products. The Summary of Product Characteristics of ritonavir must therefore be consulted prior to initiation of therapy with PREZISTA.

Adults

ART-experienced patients

The recommended dose of PREZISTA is 600 mg twice daily (b.i.d.) taken with ritonavir 100 mg b.i.d. and with food. The type of food does not affect the exposure to darunavir (see sections 4.4, 4.5 and 5.2).

The use of only 75 mg and 150 mg tablets to achieve the recommended dose of PREZISTA in adults is appropriate when there is a possibility of hypersensitivity to specific colouring agents, or difficulty in swallowing the 300 mg or 600 mg tablets.

ART-naïve patients

PREZISTA 300 mg tablets are not indicated for ART-naïve patients. For dosage recommendations in ART-naïve patients see the Summary of Product Characteristics for PREZISTA 400 mg tablets.

After therapy with PREZISTA has been initiated, patients should be advised not to alter the dosage or discontinue therapy without instruction of their physician.

Children and adolescents

ART-experienced paediatric patients (6 to 17 years of age and weighing at least 20kg)

The recommended dose of PREZISTA with low dose ritonavir for paediatric patients is based on body weight. +of 40 kg or more. For children weighing less than 40 kg, please also refer to the PREZISTA Summary of Product Characteristics of the 75 mg and 150 mg tablets.

Recommended dose for treatment-experienced paediatric patients (6 to 17 years of age) for PREZISTA tablets and ritonavir

Body weight (kg)	Dose
⩾ 20 kg–< 30 kg	375 mg PREZISTA/50 mg ritonavir b.i.d.
⩾ 30 kg–<40 kg	450 mg PREZISTA/60 mg ritonavir b.i.d.
⩾ 40 kg	600 mg PREZISTA/100 mg ritonavir b.i.d.

The recommended dose of PREZISTA with low dose ritonavir should not exceed the recommended adult dose (600/100 mg b.i.d.).

The use of only 75 mg and 150 mg tablets to achieve the recommended dose of PREZISTA could be appropriate when there is a possibility of hypersensitivity to specific colouring agents.

PREZISTA tablets should be taken with ritonavir twice daily and with food. The type of food does not affect the exposure to darunavir.

ART-experienced children less than 6 years of age or less than 20 kg body weight, and ART-naïve paediatric patients

There are insufficient data on the use of PREZISTA with low dose ritonavir in children less than 6 years of age or less than 20 kg body weight. Hence, PREZISTA is not recommended for use in this group (see sections 4.4 and 5.3).

Elderly

Limited information is available in this population and therefore PREZISTA should be used with caution in this age group (see sections 4.4 and 5.2).

Hepatic impairment

Darunavir is metabolised by the hepatic system. No dose adjustment is recommended in patients with mild (Child-Pugh Class A) or moderate (Child-Pugh Class B) hepatic impairment, however, PREZISTA should be used with caution in these patients. No pharmacokinetic data are available in patients with severe hepatic impairment. Severe hepatic impairment could result in an increase of darunavir exposure and a worsening of its safety profile. Therefore, PREZISTA must not be used in patients with severe hepatic impairment (Child-Pugh Class C) (see sections 4.3, 4.4 and 5.2).

Renal impairment

No dose adjustment is required in patients with renal impairment (see sections 4.4 and 5.2).

In case a dose of PREZISTA and/or ritonavir was missed within 6 hours of the time it is usually taken, patients should be instructed to take the prescribed dose of PREZISTA and ritonavir with food as soon as possible. If this was noticed later than 6 hours of the time it is usually taken, the missed dose should not be taken and the patient should resume the usual dosing schedule.

This guidance is based on the 15 hour half-life of darunavir in the presence of ritonavir and the recommended dosing interval of approximately 12 hours.

4.3 Contraindications

Hypersensitivity to the active substance or to any of the excipients.

Patients with severe (Child-Pugh Class C) hepatic impairment.

Combination of rifampicin with PREZISTA with concomitant low dose ritonavir is contraindicated (see section 4.5).

The combination product lopinavir/ritonavir should not be used with PREZISTA because co-administration causes large decreases in darunavir concentrations, which may in turn significantly decrease the darunavir therapeutic effect (see section 4.5).

Herbal preparations containing St John's wort (*Hypericum perforatum*) must not be used while taking PREZISTA due to the risk of decreased plasma concentrations and reduced clinical effects of darunavir (see section 4.5).

Co-administration of PREZISTA with low dose ritonavir, with active substances that are highly dependent on CYP3A for clearance and for which elevated plasma concentrations are associated with serious and/or life-threatening events is contraindicated. These active substances include e.g. antiarrhythmics (amiodarone, bepridil, quinidine, systemic lidocaine), antihistamines (astemizole, terfenadine), ergot derivatives (e.g. dihydroergotamine, ergonovine, ergotamine, methylergonovine), gastrointestinal motility agents (cisapride), neuroleptics (pimozide, sertindole), sedatives/hypnotics [triazolam, midazolam administered orally (for caution on parenterally administered midazolam, see section 4.5)] and HMG-CoA reductase inhibitors (simvastatin and lovastatin) (see section 4.5).

4.4 Special warnings and precautions for use

Patients should be advised that current antiretroviral therapy does not cure HIV and has not been proven to prevent the transmission of HIV to others through blood or sexual contact. Appropriate precautions should continue to be employed.

PREZISTA should only be used in combination with low dose ritonavir as a pharmacokinetic enhancer (see section 5.2).

Increasing the dose of ritonavir from that recommended in section 4.2 did not significantly affect darunavir concentrations and is not recommended.

PREZISTA is not recommended for use in children below 6 years of age or less than 20 kg body weight (see sections 4.2 and 5.3).

Elderly: As limited information is available on the use of PREZISTA in patients aged 65 and over, caution should be exercised in the administration of PREZISTA in elderly patients, reflecting the greater frequency of decreased hepatic function and of concomitant disease or other therapy (see sections 4.2 and 5.2).

Darunavir binds predominantly to α1-acid glycoprotein. This protein binding is concentration dependent indicative for saturation of binding. Therefore, protein displacement of medicinal products highly bound to α1-acid glycoprotein cannot be ruled out.

Severe skin rash, which may be accompanied with fever and/or elevations of transaminases, has occurred in 0.5% of patients treated with PREZISTA. Erythema multiforme and Stevens-Johnson Syndrome have been rarely (< 0.1%) observed. Treatment with PREZISTA should be discontinued if such a condition develops.

Darunavir contains a sulphonamide moiety. PREZISTA should be used with caution in patients with a known sulphonamide allergy.

Patients with coexisting conditions

Hepatic impairment

The safety and efficacy of PREZISTA have not been established in patients with severe underlying liver disorders and PREZISTA is therefore contraindicated in patients with severe hepatic impairment. Due to an increase in the unbound darunavir plasma concentrations, PREZISTA should be used with caution in patients with mild or moderate hepatic impairment (see sections 4.2, 4.3 and 5.2).

Patients with chronic hepatitis B or C and treated with combination antiretroviral therapy are at an increased risk for severe and potentially fatal hepatic adverse events. In case of concomitant antiviral therapy for hepatitis B or C, please refer to the relevant product information for these medicinal products.

Patients with pre-existing liver dysfunction including chronic hepatitis have an increased frequency of liver function abnormalities during combination antiretroviral therapy and should be monitored according to standard practice. If there is evidence of worsening liver disease in such patients, interruption or discontinuation of treatment should be considered.

Renal impairment

No special precautions or dose adjustments are required in patients with renal impairment. As darunavir and ritonavir are highly bound to plasma proteins, it is unlikely that they will be significantly removed by haemodialysis or peritoneal dialysis. Therefore, no special precautions or dose adjustments are required in these patients (see sections 4.2 and 5.2).

Haemophiliac patients

There have been reports of increased bleeding, including spontaneous skin haematomas and haemarthrosis in patients with haemophilia type A and B treated with PIs. In some patients additional factor VIII was given. In more than half of the reported cases, treatment with PIs was continued or reintroduced if treatment had been discontinued. A causal relationship has been suggested, although the mechanism of action has not been elucidated. Haemophiliac patients should therefore be made aware of the possibility of increased bleeding.

Diabetes mellitus/Hyperglycaemia

New onset diabetes mellitus, hyperglycaemia, or exacerbation of existing diabetes mellitus has been reported in patients receiving antiretroviral therapy, including PIs. In some of these patients the hyperglycaemia was severe and in some cases also associated with ketoacidosis. Many patients had confounding medical conditions some of which required therapy with agents that have been associated with the development of diabetes mellitus or hyperglycaemia.

Fat redistribution and metabolic disorders

Combination antiretroviral therapy has been associated with redistribution of body fat (lipodystrophy) in HIV infected patients. The long-term consequences of these events are currently unknown. Knowledge about the mechanism is incomplete. A connection between visceral lipomatosis and PIs and lipoatrophy and NRTIs has been hypothesised. A higher risk of lipodystrophy has been associated with individual factors such as older age and with drug related factors such as longer duration of antiretroviral treatment and associated metabolic disturbances. Clinical examination should include evaluation for physical signs of fat redistribution. Consideration should be given to measurement of fasting serum lipids and blood glucose. Lipid disorders should be managed as clinically appropriate (see section 4.8).

Osteonecrosis

Although the etiology is considered to be multifactorial (including corticosteroid use, alcohol consumption, severe immunosuppression, higher body mass index), cases of osteonecrosis have been reported particularly in patients with advanced HIV disease and/or long-term exposure to combination antiretroviral therapy (CART). Patients should be advised to seek medical advice if they experience joint aches and pain, joint stiffness or difficulty in movement.

Immune reactivation syndrome

In HIV infected patients with severe immune deficiency at the time of institution of combination antiretroviral therapy (CART), an inflammatory reaction to asymptomatic or residual opportunistic pathogens may arise and cause serious clinical conditions, or aggravation of symptoms. Typically, such reactions have been observed within the first weeks or months of initiation of CART. Relevant examples are cytomegalovirus retinitis, generalised and/or focal mycobacterial infections and pneumonia caused by *Pneumocystis jiroveci* (formerly known *as Pneumocystis carinii*). Any inflammatory symptoms should be evaluated and treatment instituted when necessary. In addition, reactivation of herpes simplex and herpes zoster has been observed in clinical studies with PREZISTA co-administered with low dose ritonavir.

Interactions with medicinal products

Several of the interaction studies have been performed at lower than recommended doses of darunavir. The effects on co-administered medicinal products may thus be underestimated and clinical monitoring of safety may be indicated. For full information on interactions with other medicinal products see section 4.5.

PREZISTA tablets contain sunset yellow FCF (E110) which may cause an allergic reaction.

4.5 Interaction with other medicinal products and other forms of interaction

Darunavir and ritonavir are both inhibitors of the CYP3A4 isoform. Co-administration of darunavir and ritonavir and medicinal products primarily metabolised by CYP3A4 may result in increased systemic exposure to such medicinal products, which could increase or prolong their therapeutic effect and adverse reactions.

PREZISTA co-administered with low dose ritonavir must not be combined with medicinal products that are highly dependent on CYP3A4 for clearance and for which increased systemic exposure is associated with serious and/or life-threatening events (narrow therapeutic index). These medicinal products include amiodarone, bepridil, quinidine, systemic lidocaine, astemizole, terfenadine, midazolam administered orally, triazolam, cisapride, pimozide, sertindole, simvastatin, lovastatin and the ergot alkaloids (e.g. ergotamine, dihydroergotamine, ergonovine and methylergonovine) (see section 4.3).

The overall pharmacokinetic enhancement effect by ritonavir was an approximate 14-fold increase in the systemic exposure of darunavir when a single dose of 600 mg darunavir was given orally in combination with ritonavir at 100 mg b.i.d. Therefore, PREZISTA must only be used in combination with low dose ritonavir as a pharmacokinetic enhancer (see sections 4.4 and 5.2).

A clinical study utilising a cocktail of medicinal products that are metabolised by cytochromes CYP2C9, CYP2C19 and CYP2D6 demonstrated an increase in CYP2C9 and CYP2C19 activity and inhibition of CYP2D6 activity in the presence of PREZISTA/rtv, which may be attributed to the presence of low dose ritonavir. Co-administration of darunavir and ritonavir and medicinal products which are primarily metabolised by CYP2D6 (such as flecainide, propafenone, metoprolol) may result in increased plasma concentrations of these medicinal products, which could increase or prolong their therapeutic effect and adverse reactions. Co-administration of darunavir and ritonavir and medicinal products primarily metabolised by CYP2C9 (such as warfarin) and CYP2C19 (such as methadone) may result in decreased systemic exposure to such medicinal products, which could decrease or shorten their therapeutic effect.

Although the effect on CYP2C8 has only been studied *in vitro*, co-administration of darunavir and ritonavir and medicinal products primarily metabolised by CYP2C8 (such as paclitaxel, rosiglitazone, repaglinide) may result in decreased systemic exposure to such medicinal products, which could decrease or shorten their therapeutic effect.

Medicinal products that affect darunavir/ritonavir exposure

Darunavir and ritonavir are metabolised by CYP3A. Medicinal products that induce CYP3A activity would be expected to increase the clearance of darunavir and ritonavir, resulting in lowered plasma concentrations of darunavir and ritonavir (e.g. rifampicin, St John's wort, lopinavir). Co-administration of darunavir and ritonavir and other medicinal products that inhibit CYP3A may decrease the clearance of darunavir and ritonavir and may result in increased plasma concentrations of darunavir and ritonavir (e.g. indinavir, systemic azoles like ketoconazole and clotrimazole). These interactions are described in the interaction tables below.

Interaction table

Interactions between darunavir/ritonavir and protease inhibitors, antiretroviral agents other than protease inhibitors and other non-antiretroviral medicinal products are listed in the tables below (increase is indicated as "↑", decrease as "↓", no change as "↔", not determined as "ND", twice daily as "b.i.d.", once daily as "q.d." and once every other day as "q.o.d.").

Several of the interaction studies (indicated by # in the table below) have been performed at lower than recommended doses of darunavir or with a different dosing regimen (see section 4.2 Posology). The effects on co-administered medicinal products may thus be underestimated and clinical monitoring of safety may be indicated.

Interactions – Darunavir/ritonavir with Protease Inhibitors

The efficacy and safety of the use of PREZISTA with low dose ritonavir and any other PI (e.g. (fos)amprenavir, nelfinavir and tipranavir) has not been established in HIV patients. Generally, dual therapy with protease inhibitors is not recommended.

(see Table 1 on next page)

4.6 Pregnancy and lactation

Pregnancy

There are no adequate and well controlled studies with darunavir in pregnant women. Studies in animals do not indicate direct harmful effects with respect to pregnancy, embryonal/foetal development, parturition or postnatal development (see section 5.3).

PREZISTA co-administered with low dose ritonavir should be used during pregnancy only if the potential benefit justifies the potential risk.

Breast-feeding

It is not known whether darunavir is excreted in human milk. Studies in rats have demonstrated that darunavir is excreted in milk and at high levels (1,000 mg/kg/day) resulted in toxicity. Because of both the potential for HIV transmission and the potential for adverse reactions in breast-fed infants, mothers should be instructed not to breast-feed under any circumstances if they are receiving PREZISTA.

Fertility

No human data on the effect of darunavir on fertility are available. There was no effect on mating or fertility with darunavir treatment in rats (see section 5.3).

4.7 Effects on ability to drive and use machines

No studies on the effects of PREZISTA in combination with ritonavir on the ability to drive and use machines have been performed. However, dizziness has been reported in some patients during treatment with regimens containing PREZISTA co-administered with low dose ritonavir and should be borne in mind when considering a patient's ability to drive or operate machinery (see section 4.8).

4.8 Undesirable effects

Adult patients

The adverse drug reactions are derived from Phase IIb and Phase III trials, in which a total of 1,968 treatment-experienced patients initiated therapy with the recommended dose of PREZISTA 600 mg with ritonavir 100 mg twice daily. Median exposure to PREZISTA/ritonavir in this group was 37.3 weeks. Thirty percent of these patients experienced at least one adverse drug reaction of at least grade 2 severity. The most frequent (⩾ 2%) of those were diarrhoea (3.9%), hypertriglyceridaemia (3.8%), rash (2.8%), nausea (2.6%), hypercholesterolaemia (2.5%) and headache (2.0%).

2.6% of the patients discontinued treatment due to adverse reactions.

Adverse reactions are listed by system organ class (SOC) and frequency. Within each frequency grouping, adverse reactions are presented in order of decreasing seriousness. Frequencies are defined as very common (⩾ 1/10), common (⩾ 1/100 to < 1/10) and uncommon (⩾ 1/1,000 to < 1/100).

(see Table 2 on page 4931854)

In clinical trials (n=1,968), rash (all grades, at least possibly related) occurred in 5.6% of patients treated with PREZISTA. Rash was mostly mild to moderate, often occurring within the first four weeks of treatment and resolving with continued dosing. Grade 2-4 rash was reported in 2.9% of patients. The discontinuation rate due to rash in patients using PREZISTA co-administered with 100 mg ritonavir was 0.5%.

Severe cases of skin rash, including erythema multiforme and Stevens-Johnson Syndrome (both rare) have been reported in ongoing clinical trials with PREZISTA co-administered with 100 mg ritonavir.

The safety assessment in antiretroviral treatment-naïve adult patients (n=343) is based on all safety data from the Phase III trial ARTEMIS comparing PREZISTA/rtv 800/100 mg q.d. versus lopinavir/ritonavir 800/200 mg per day. Median exposure in the PREZISTA/ritonavir group was 56.3 weeks.

0.6% of the patients discontinued treatment due to adverse drug reactions.

In these treatment naïve-patients, the following adverse drug reactions were identified:

ADRs of at least moderate intensity and reported in more than one patient

Common: hypertriglyceridaemia, hypercholesterolaemia, headache, diarrhoea, nausea, increased alanine aminotransferase.

Uncommon: hyperlipidaemia, vomiting, abdominal pain, increased aspartate aminotransferase, rash (including maculopapular rash), allergic dermatitis, pruritus.

ADRs of all severity grades and reported in more than one patient

Very common: diarrhoea, nausea.

Common: hypertriglyceridaemia, hypercholesterolaemia, anorexia, insomnia, headache, dizziness, dysgeusia, vomiting, abdominal pain, abdominal discomfort, abdominal distension, flatulence, increased alanine aminotransferase, rash (including maculopapular, papular rash), alopecia, dry skin, pruritus, fatigue.

Uncommon: upper respiratory tract infection, diabetes mellitus, hyperlipidaemia, abnormal dreams, hypoaesthesia, disturbance in attention, somnolence, dyspepsia, eructation, increased aspartate aminotransferase, allergic dermatitis, urticaria, dermatitis, night sweats, myalgia, muscle spasms, asthenia.

Combination antiretroviral therapy has been associated with redistribution of body fat (lipodystrophy) in HIV patients, including loss of peripheral and facial subcutaneous fat, increased intra-abdominal and visceral fat, breast hypertrophy and dorsocervical fat accumulation (buffalo hump) (see section 4.4).

Combination antiretroviral therapy has also been associated with metabolic abnormalities such as hypertriglyceridaemia, hypercholesterolaemia, insulin resistance, hyperglycaemia and hyperlactataemia (see section 4.4).

Increased CPK, myalgia, myositis and rarely, rhabdomyolysis have been reported with the use of protease inhibitors, particularly in combination with NRTIs.

Cases of osteonecrosis have been reported, particularly in patients with generally acknowledged risk factors, advanced HIV disease or long-term exposure to combination antiretroviral therapy (CART). The frequency of this is unknown (see section 4.4).

In HIV infected patients with severe immune deficiency at the time of initiation of combination antiretroviral therapy, an inflammatory reaction to asymptomatic or residual opportunistic infections may arise (see section 4.4).

There have been reports of increased spontaneous bleeding in haemophiliac patients receiving antiretroviral protease inhibitors (see section 4.4).

Children and adolescents

The safety assessment in children and adolescents is based on the safety data from the Phase II trial DELPHI in which 80 ART-experienced HIV-1 infected paediatric patients aged from 6 to 17 years and weighing at least 20 kg received PREZISTA with low dose ritonavir in combination with other antiretroviral agents (see section 5.1).

Overall, the safety profile in these 80 children and adolescents was similar to that observed in the adult population.

Patients co-infected with hepatitis B and/or hepatitis C virus

Among 1,968 treatment-experienced patients receiving PREZISTA co-administered with ritonavir 600/100 mg b.i.d., 236 patients were co-infected with hepatitis B or C. Co-infected patients were more likely to have baseline and treatment emergent hepatic transaminase elevations than those without chronic viral hepatitis (see section 4.4).

4.9 Overdose

Human experience of acute overdose with PREZISTA co-administered with low dose ritonavir is limited. Single doses up to 3,200 mg of darunavir as oral solution alone and up to 1,600 mg of the tablet formulation of darunavir in combination with ritonavir have been administered to healthy volunteers without untoward symptomatic effects.

There is no specific antidote for overdose with PREZISTA. Treatment of overdose with PREZISTA consists of general supportive measures including monitoring of vital signs and observation of the clinical status of the patient. If indicated, elimination of unabsorbed active substance is to be achieved by emesis or gastric lavage. Administration of activated charcoal may also be used to aid in removal of unabsorbed active substance. Since darunavir is highly protein bound, dialysis is unlikely to be beneficial in significant removal of the active substance.

5. PHARMACOLOGICAL PROPERTIES

5.1 Pharmacodynamic properties

Pharmacotherapeutic group: Antiviral for systemic use, ATC code: J05AE10.

Mechanism of action

Darunavir is an inhibitor of the dimerisation and of the catalytic activity of the HIV-1 protease (K_D of 4.5×10^{-12}M). It selectively inhibits the cleavage of HIV encoded Gag-Pol polyproteins in virus infected cells, thereby preventing the formation of mature infectious virus particles.

Antiviral activity *in vitro*

Darunavir exhibits activity against laboratory strains and clinical isolates of HIV-1 and laboratory strains of HIV-2 in acutely infected T-cell lines, human peripheral blood mononuclear cells and human monocytes/macrophages with median EC_{50} values ranging from 1.2 to 8.5 nM (0.7 to 5.0 ng/ml). Darunavir demonstrates antiviral activity *in vitro* against a broad panel of HIV-1 group M (A, B, C, D, E, F, G) and group O primary isolates with EC_{50} values ranging from < 0.1 to 4.3 nM.

These EC_{50} values are well below the 50% cellular toxicity concentration range of 87 μM to > 100 μM.

The EC_{50} value of darunavir increases by a median factor of 5.4 in the presence of human serum.

Darunavir showed synergistic antiviral activity when studied in combination with the protease inhibitors ritonavir, nelfinavir, or amprenavir and additive antiviral activity when studied in combination with the protease inhibitors indinavir, saquinavir, lopinavir, atazanavir, or tipranavir, the N(t)RTIs zidovudine, lamivudine, zalcitabine, didanosine, stavudine, abacavir, emtricitabine, or tenofovir, the NNRTIs nevirapine, delavirdine, or efavirenz and the fusion inhibitor enfuvirtide. No antagonism was observed between darunavir and any of those antiretrovirals.

Resistance

In vitro selection of darunavir-resistant virus from wild type HIV-1 was lengthy > 3 years). The selected viruses were unable to grow in the presence of darunavir concentrations above 400 nM. Viruses selected in these conditions and showing decreased susceptibility to darunavir (range: 23-50-fold) harboured 2 to 4 amino acid substitutions in the protease gene. Identification of determinants of decreased susceptibility to darunavir in those viruses is under investigation.

In vitro selection of darunavir resistant HIV-1 (range: 53-641-fold change in EC_{50} values [FC]) from 9 HIV-1 strains harbouring multiple PI Resistance-Associated Mutations (RAMs) showed that a minimum of 8 darunavir *in vitro* selected mutations were required in the HIV-1 protease to render a virus resistant (FC> 10) to darunavir.

In a pooled analysis of the POWER 1, 2 and 3 (see Clinical experience subsection) and DUET 1 and 2 (TMC125-C206 and TMC125-C216) trials the amino acid substitutions identified that developed on PREZISTA co-administered with ritonavir (600/100 mg b.i.d.) in ⩾ 20% of the isolates from subjects who experienced virologic failure by rebound were V32I, I54L and L89V. Amino acid

Table 1

Co-administered Medicinal Product	Dose of Co-administered Medicinal Product (mg)	Dose of darunavir/ritonavir (mg)	Medicinal Product Assessed	AUC	C_{min}
Lopinavir/ritonavir	400/100 b.i.d. 533/133.3 b.i.d.	1,200/100 b.i.d. 1,200 b.i.d.	Lopinavir Darunavir Lopinavir Darunavir	↔ ↓ 38%* ↔ ↓ 41%	↔ ↓ 51%* ↔ ↓ 55%
	* based upon not dose normalised values Due to a decrease in the exposure (AUC) of darunavir by 40%, appropriate doses of the combination have not been established. Hence, concomitant use of PREZISTA co-administered with low dose ritonavir and the combination product lopinavir/ritonavir is contraindicated (see section 4.3).				
Saquinavir	1,000 b.i.d.	400/100 b.i.d.#	Darunavir	↓ 26%	↓ 42%
	The study with boosted saquinavir showed no significant effect of darunavir on saquinavir. It is not recommended to combine PREZISTA co-administered with low dose ritonavir with saquinavir.				
Indinavir	800 b.i.d.	400/100 b.i.d. #	Indinavir Darunavir	↑ 23% ↑ 24%	↑ 125% ↑ 44%
	When used in combination with PREZISTA co-administered with low dose ritonavir, dose adjustment of indinavir from 800 mg b.i.d. to 600 mg b.i.d. may be warranted in case of intolerance.				
Atazanavir	300 q.d.	400/100 b.i.d. #	Atazanavir Darunavir	↔ ↔	↔ ↔
	Darunavir/ritonavir did not significantly affect atazanavir exposure, however 90% CI for C_{min} were 99-234%. Atazanavir can be used with PREZISTA co-administered with low dose ritonavir.				
Interactions – Darunavir/ritonavir with Antiretroviral Agents other than Protease Inhibitors					
Co-administered Medicinal Product	**Dose of Co-administered Medicinal Product (mg)**	**Dose of darunavir/ritonavir (mg)**	**Medicinal Product Assessed**	**AUC**	**C_{min}**
Efavirenz	600 q.d.	300/100 b.i.d. #	Efavirenz Darunavir	↑ 21% ↓ 13%	↑ 17% ↓ 31%
	Efavirenz decreases the plasma concentrations of darunavir as a result of CYP3A4 induction. Darunavir/ritonavir increases the plasma concentrations of efavirenz as a result of CYP3A4 inhibition. Clinical monitoring for central nervous system toxicity associated with increased exposure to efavirenz may be indicated when PREZISTA co-administered with low dose ritonavir is given in combination with efavirenz.				
Etravirine	100 b.i.d.*	600/100 b.i.d.	Etravirine Darunavir	↓ 37% ↔	↓ 49% ↔
	* dose used in drug-interaction study. For recommended dose see paragraph below. There was a 37% decrease in etravirine exposure in the presence of darunavir/ritonavir and no relevant change in exposure to darunavir. Therefore, PREZISTA co-administered with low dose ritonavir can be co-administered with etravirine **200 mg b.i.d.** without dose adjustments.				
Nevirapine	200 b.i.d.	400/100 b.i.d. #	Nevirapine Darunavir	↑ 27% ↔	↑ 47% ↔
	Darunavir/ritonavir increases the plasma concentrations of nevirapine as a result of CYP3A4 inhibition. Since this difference is not considered to be clinically relevant, the combination of PREZISTA co-administered with low dose ritonavir and nevirapine can be used without dose adjustments.				
Tenofovir	300 q.d.	300/100 b.i.d. #	Tenofovir Darunavir	↑ 22% ↔	↑ 37% ↔
	Ritonavir effect on MDR-1 transport in renal tubuli has been a proposed mechanism for increased plasma concentrations of tenofovir. Monitoring of renal function may be indicated when PREZISTA co-administered with low dose ritonavir is given in combination with tenofovir, particularly in patients with underlying systemic or renal disease, or in patients taking nephrotoxic agents.				
Zidovudine Zalcitabine Emtricitabine Stavudine Lamivudine Abacavir	Based on the different elimination pathways of the other NRTIs zidovudine, zalcitabine, emtricitabine, stavudine, lamivudine, that are primarily renally excreted, and abacavir for which metabolism is not mediated by CYP450, no interactions are expected for these medicinal compounds and PREZISTA co-administered with low dose ritonavir.				
Didanosine	400 q.d.	600/100 b.i.d.	Didanosine Darunavir	↔ ↔	NA ↔
	Didanosine was administered on an empty stomach 2 hours prior to administration of darunavir/ritonavir. Systemic exposure to darunavir co-administered with low dose ritonavir, with or without didanosine was comparable. The combination of PREZISTA co-administered with low dose ritonavir and didanosine can be used without dose adjustments.				
Maraviroc	150 b.i.d.	600/100 b.i.d.	Maraviroc Darunavir	↑ 305% ↔	ND ND
	The maraviroc dose should be 150 mg twice daily when co-administered with PREZISTA with low dose ritonavir. Darunavir/ritonavir concentrations were consistent with historical data.				
Interactions – Darunavir/ritonavir with Non-antiretroviral co-administered Medicinal Products					
Co-administered Medicinal Product	**Dose of Co-administered Medicinal Product (mg)**	**Dose of darunavir/ritonavir (mg)**	**Medicinal Product Assessed**	**AUC**	**C_{min}**
Antiarrhythmics					
Digoxin	0.4 mg single dose	600/100 b.i.d.	Digoxin	↑ 60%	ND
	Darunavir/ritonavir increases the plasma concentrations of digoxin. Inhibition of Pgp may be a likely explanation. Given that digoxin has as a narrow therapeutic index, it is recommended that the lowest possible dose of digoxin should initially be prescribed in case digoxin is given to patients on darunavir/ritonavir therapy. The digoxin dose should be carefully titrated to obtain the desired clinical effect while assessing the overall clinical state of the subject.				
Antibiotics					
Clarithromycin	500 b.i.d.	400/100 b.i.d. #	Clarithromycin Darunavir	↑ 57% ↔	↑ 174% ↔
	Darunavir/ritonavir increases the plasma concentrations of clarithromycin as a result of CYP3A4 inhibition and possible Pgp inhibition. Concentrations of the metabolite 14-OH-clarithromycin were not detectable. Caution is warranted and clinical monitoring is recommended. For patients with renal impairment, a dose reduction of clarithromycin should be considered.				
Anticoagulant					
Warfarin	Warfarin concentrations may be affected when co-administered with darunavir with ritonavir. The international normalised ratio (INR) should be monitored when warfarin is combined with PREZISTA co-administered with low dose ritonavir.				
Anticonvulsants					
Phenobarbital Phenytoin	Phenobarbital and phenytoin are inducers of CYP450 enzymes. PREZISTA co-administered with low dose ritonavir should not be used in combination with these medicines, as co-administration may cause significant decreases in darunavir plasma concentrations.				
Carbamazepine	200 b.i.d.	600/100 b.i.d.	Carbamazepine Darunavir	↑ 45% ↔	↑ 54% ↔
	Exposure to darunavir, co-administered with ritonavir, was unaffected by carbamazepine. Ritonavir exposure (AUC12h) was decreased by 49%. For carbamazepine, AUC12h was increased by 45%. No dose adjustment for PREZISTA/ritonavir is recommended. If there is a need to combine PREZISTA/ritonavir and carbamazepine, patients should be monitored for potential carbamazepine-related adverse events. Carbamazepine concentrations should be monitored and its dose should be titrated for adequate response. Based upon the findings, the carbamazepine dose may need to be reduced by 25% to 50% in the presence of PREZISTA/ritonavir.				
Antifungals					
Voriconazole	The combined use of voriconazole with darunavir co-administered with low dose ritonavir has not been studied. Voriconazole is metabolised by cytochrome P450 isoenzymes, CYP2C19, CYP2C9 and CYP3A4. Ritonavir, which can induce some of these isoenzymes, may decrease voriconazole plasma concentrations. Voriconazole should not be co-administered with PREZISTA with low dose ritonavir unless an assessment of the benefit/risk ratio justifies the use of voriconazole.				
Ketoconazole	200 b.i.d.	400/100 b.i.d. #	Ketoconazole Darunavir	↑ 212% ↑ 42%	↑ 868% ↑ 73%
	Ketoconazole is a potent inhibitor as well as substrate of CYP3A4. Caution is warranted and clinical monitoring is recommended. When co-administration is required the daily dose of ketoconazole should not exceed 200 mg.				

Co-administered Medicinal Product	Dose of Co-administered Medicinal Product (mg)	Dose of darunavir/ritonavir (mg)	Medicinal Product Assessed	AUC	C_{min}
Itraconazole	Itraconazole, like ketoconazole, is a potent inhibitor as well as substrate of CYP3A4. Concomitant systemic use of itraconazole and darunavir co-administered with low dose ritonavir may increase plasma concentrations of darunavir. Simultaneously, plasma concentrations of itraconazole may be increased by darunavir co-administered with low dose ritonavir. Caution is warranted and clinical monitoring is recommended. When co-administration is required the daily dose of itraconazole should not exceed 200 mg.				
Clotrimazole	Concomitant systemic use of clotrimazole and darunavir co-administered with low dose ritonavir may increase plasma concentrations of darunavir. This was confirmed using a population pharmacokinetic model. The increase in the median darunavir AUC_{24h} value for the patients taking clotrimazole from the overall median was 33%. Caution is warranted and clinical monitoring is recommended, when co-administration of clotrimazole is required.				
Calcium channel blockers					
Felodipine Nifedipine Nicardipine	Darunavir and ritonavir inhibit CYP3A4 and as a result can be expected to increase the plasma concentrations of calcium channel antagonists, which are CYP3A4 substrates. Clinical monitoring of therapeutic and adverse effects is recommended when these medicines are concomitantly administered with PREZISTA with low dose ritonavir.				
HMG Co-A Reductase Inhibitors					
Lovastatin Simvastatin	Lovastatin and simvastatin, which are highly dependent on CYP3A4 metabolism are expected to have markedly increased plasma concentrations when co-administered with darunavir co-administered with low dose ritonavir. This may cause myopathy, including rhabdomyolysis. Concomitant use of PREZISTA co-administered with low dose ritonavir with lovastatin and simvastatin is therefore contraindicated (see section 4.3).				
Atorvastatin	10 q.d.	300/100 b.i.d. #	Atorvastatin Darunavir	3-4 times ↑ ND	3-4 times ↑ ND
	The results of this interaction trial show that atorvastatin (10 mg q.d.) in combination with darunavir/ritonavir (300/100 mg b.i.d.) provides an exposure to atorvastatin, which is only 15% lower than that obtained with (40 mg q.d.) atorvastatin alone. When administration of atorvastatin and PREZISTA co-administered with low dose ritonavir is desired, it is recommended to start with an atorvastatin dose of 10 mg q.d. A gradual dose increase of atorvastatin may be tailored to the clinical response.				
Pravastatin	40 mg single dose	600/100 b.i.d.	Pravastatin	0-5 times ↑	ND
	Darunavir/ritonavir did not increase exposure to a single dose of pravastatin in most subjects but up to 5-fold in a limited subset of subjects. When administration of pravastatin and PREZISTA co-administered with low dose ritonavir is required, it is recommended to start with the lowest possible dose of pravastatin and titrate it up to the desired clinical effect while monitoring for safety.				
Hormonal contraceptive					
Ethinylestradiol Norethindrone	35 µg/1 mg q.d.	600/100 b.i.d.	Ethinylestradiol Norethindrone	↓ 44% ↓ 14%	↓ 62% ↓ 30%
	Alternative or additional contraceptive measures are recommended when oestrogen-based contraceptives are co-administered with PREZISTA and low dose ritonavir. Patients using oestrogens as hormone replacement therapy should be clinically monitored for signs of oestrogen deficiency.				
Immunosupressants					
Cyclosporine Tacrolimus Sirolimus	Exposure to cyclosporine, tacrolimus, or sirolimus will be increased when co-administered with PREZISTA co-administered with low dose ritonavir. Therapeutic drug monitoring of the immunosuppressive agent must be done when co-administration occurs.				
H_2-receptor antagonists and proton pump inhibitors					
Ranitidine	150 b.i.d.	400/100 b.i.d. #	Darunavir	↔	↔
	Based on these results, PREZISTA co-administered with low dose ritonavir can be co-administered with H_2-receptor antagonists without dose adjustments.				
Omeprazole	20 q.d.	400/100 b.i.d. #	Darunavir	↔	↔
	Based on these results, PREZISTA co-administered with low dose ritonavir can be co-administered with proton pump inhibitors without dose adjustments.				
Opiods					
Methadone	55-150 q.d.	600/100 b.i.d. (dosed for 7 days)	R-methadone	↓ 16%	↓ 15%
	Based on pharmacokinetic and clinical findings, no adjustment of methadone dosage is required when initiating co-administration with PREZISTA/ritonavir. However, increased methadone dose may be necessary when concomitantly administered for a longer period of time due to induction of metabolism by ritonavir. Therefore, clinical monitoring is recommended, as maintenance therapy may need to be adjusted in some patients.				
PDE-5 inhibitors					
Sildenafil Vardenafil Tadalafil	In an interaction study a comparable systemic exposure to sildenafil was observed for a single intake of 100 mg sildenafil alone and a single intake of 25 mg sildenafil co-administered with darunavir/ritonavir (400/100 mg b.i.d.). Concomitant use of PDE-5 inhibitors with PREZISTA co-administered with low dose ritonavir should be done with caution. If concomitant use of PREZISTA co-administered with low dose ritonavir with sildenafil, vardenafil, or tadalafil is indicated, sildenafil at a single dose not exceeding 25 mg in 48 hours, vardenafil at a single dose not exceeding 2.5 mg dose in 72 hours or tadalafil at a single dose not exceeding 10 mg dose in 72 hours is recommended.				
Rifamycines					
Rifampicin	Rifampicin is a strong CYP3A4 inducer and has been shown to cause profound decreases in concentrations of other protease inhibitors, which can result in virological failure and resistance development. During attempts to overcome the decreased exposure by increasing the dose of other protease inhibitors with ritonavir, a high frequency of liver reactions was seen. The combination of rifampicin and PREZISTA with concomitant low dose ritonavir is contraindicated (see section 4.3).				
Rifabutin	150 q.o.d.	600/100 b.i.d.	Rifabutin* Darunavir	1.6 times ↑ ↑ 53%	ND ↑ 68%
	* sum of active moieties of rifabutin (parent drug + 25-*O*- desacetyl metabolite) A dose reduction of rifabutin by 75% of the usual dose of 300 mg/day [i.e. rifabutin 150 mg q.o.d. (once every other day)] and increased monitoring for rifabutin related adverse events is warranted in patients receiving the combination. In case of safety issues, a further increase of the dosing interval for rifabutin and/or monitoring of rifabutin levels should be considered. Consideration should be given to official guidance on the appropriate treatment of tuberculosis in HIV infected patients. Rifabutin is an inducer and substrate of CYP3A4. An increase of systemic exposure to darunavir was observed when PREZISTA co-administered with 100 mg ritonavir was co-administered with rifabutin [150 mg q.o.d. (once every other day)]. Based upon the safety profile of PREZISTA/ritonavir, this increase in darunavir exposure in the presence of rifabutin does not warrant a dose adjustment for PREZISTA/ritonavir. The interaction trial showed a comparable daily systemic exposure for rifabutin between treatment at 300 mg q.d. (once daily) alone and 150 mg q.o.d. (once every other day) in combination with PREZISTA/ritonavir (600/100 mg b.i.d.) with an about 10-fold increase in the daily exposure to the active metabolite 25-*O*- desacetylrifabutin. Furthermore, AUC of the sum of active moieties of rifabutin (parent drug + 25-*O*- desacetyl metabolite) was increased 1.6-fold, while C_{max} remained comparable. Data on comparison with a 150 mg q.d. (once daily) reference dose is lacking.				
Sedatives/Hypnotics					
Parenteral midazolam	Midazolam is extensively metabolised by CYP3A4. Co-administration with PREZISTA/ritonavir may cause a large increase in the concentration of this benzodiazepine. No drug interaction study has been performed for the co-administration of PREZISTA/ritonavir with benzodiazepines. Based on data for other CYP3A4 inhibitors, plasma concentrations of midazolam are expected to be significantly higher when midazolam is given orally. Therefore PREZISTA/ritonavir should not be co-administered with orally administered midazolam (see section 4.3), whereas caution should be used with co-administration of PREZISTA/ritonavir and parenteral midazolam. Data from concomitant use of parenteral midazolam with other protease inhibitors suggest a possible 3-4 fold increase in midazolam plasma levels. If PREZISTA/ritonavir is co-administered with parenteral midazolam, it should be done in an intensive care unit (ICU) or similar setting, which ensures close clinical monitoring and appropriate medical management in case of respiratory depression and/or prolonged sedation. Dosage adjustment for midazolam should be considered, especially if more than a single dose of midazolam is administered.				
Selective Serotonin Reuptake Inhibitors (SSRIs)					
Paroxetine	20 q.d.	400/100 b.i.d. #	Paroxetine Darunavir	↓ 39% ↔	↓ 37% ↔
Sertraline	50 q.d.	400/100 b.i.d. #	Sertraline Darunavir	↓ 49% ↔	↓ 49% ↔
	If SSRIs are co-administered with PREZISTA and ritonavir, the recommended approach is a dose titration of the SSRI based on a clinical assessment of antidepressant response. In addition, patients on a stable dose of sertraline or paroxetine who start treatment with PREZISTA co-administered with low dose ritonavir should be monitored for antidepressant response.				
Steroids					
Fluticasone propionate Budesonide	In a clinical study where ritonavir 100 mg capsules b.i.d were co-administered with 50 µg intranasal fluticasone propionate (4 times daily) for 7 days in healthy subjects, fluticasone propionate plasma concentrations increased significantly, whereas the intrinsic cortisol levels decreased by approximately 86% (90% confidence interval 82-89%). Greater effects may be expected when fluticasone propionate is inhaled. Systemic corticosteroid effects including Cushing's syndrome and adrenal suppression have been reported in patients receiving ritonavir and inhaled or intranasally administered fluticasone propionate; this could also occur with other corticosteroids metabolised via the P450 3A pathway e.g. budesonide. Consequently, concomitant administration of PREZISTA, co-administered with low dose ritonavir and these glucocorticoids, is not recommended unless the potential benefit of treatment outweighs the risk of systemic corticosteroid effects. A dose reduction of the glucocorticoid should be considered with close monitoring of local and systemic effects or a switch to a glucocorticoid, which is not a substrate for CYP3A4 (e.g. beclomethasone). Moreover, in case of withdrawal of glucocorticoids progressive dose reduction may have to be performed over a longer period. The effects of high fluticasone systemic exposure on ritonavir plasma levels are as yet unknown.				
Dexamethasone	Systemic dexamethasone induces CYP3A4 and thereby may decrease darunavir exposure. Therefore this combination should be used with caution.				
Others					
St. John's wort	PREZISTA co-administered with low dose ritonavir must not be used concomitantly with products containing St John's wort (*Hypericum perforatum*) because co-administration may cause significant decreases in darunavir plasma concentrations and also in ritonavir concentrations. This is due to the induction of metabolising enzymes by St John's wort. If a patient is already taking St John's wort, stop St John's wort and if possible check viral levels. Darunavir exposure (and also ritonavir exposure) may increase on stopping St John's wort. The inducing effect may persist for at least 2 weeks after cessation of treatment with St John's wort (see section 4.3).				

Table 2

SOC Frequency category	Adverse reaction* All grades	Adverse reaction** Grade 2-4
Infections and infestations		
uncommon	herpes simplex	
Blood and lymphatic system disorders		
uncommon	thrombocytopenia, neutropenia, anaemia, increased eosinophil count, leukopenia	thrombocytopenia, neutropenia, anaemia
Immune system disorders		
uncommon	immune reconstitution syndrome	immune reconstitution syndrome
Endocrine disorders		
uncommon	hypothyroidism, increased blood thyroid stimulating hormone	
Metabolism and nutrition disorders		
common	lipodystrophy (including lipohypertrophy, lipodystrophy, lipoatrophy), hypertriglyceridaemia, hypercholesterolaemia, hyperlipidaemia	hypertriglyceridaemia, hypercholesterolaemia, hyperlipidaemia
uncommon	diabetes mellitus, gout, anorexia, decreased appetite, decreased weight, increased weight, hyperglycaemia, insulin resistance, decreased high density lipoprotein, increased appetite, polydipsia, increased blood lactate dehydrogenase	diabetes mellitus, lipodystrophy (including lipohypertrophy, lipodystrophy, lipoatrophy), gout, anorexia, decreased appetite, decreased weight, increased weight, hyperglycaemia, insulin resistance
Psychiatric disorders		
common	insomnia	
uncommon	depression, confusional state, disorientation, anxiety, altered mood, sleep disorder, abnormal dreams, nightmare, decreased libido, restlessness	depression, confusional state, disorientation, anxiety, altered mood, insomnia, sleep disorder, abnormal dreams
Nervous system disorders		
common	headache, peripheral neuropathy, dizziness	headache
uncommon	syncope, convulsion, lethargy, paraesthesia, hypoaesthesia, ageusia, dysgeusia, disturbance in attention, memory impairment, somnolence, sleep phase rhythm disturbance	peripheral neuropathy, dizziness, lethargy, paraesthesia, hypoaesthesia, somnolence
Eye disorders		
uncommon	visual disturbance, conjunctival hyperaemia, dry eye	conjunctival hyperaemia
Ear and labyrinth disorders		
uncommon	vertigo	vertigo
Cardiac disorders		
uncommon	acute myocardial infarction, myocardial infarction, angina pectoris, prolonged electrocardiogram QT, sinus bradycardia, tachycardia, palpitations	acute myocardial infarction, myocardial infarction, angina pectoris, prolonged electrocardiogram QT
Vascular disorders		
uncommon	hypertension, flushing	hypertension
Respiratory, thoracic and mediastinal disorders		
uncommon	dyspnoea, cough, epistaxis, rhinorrhoea, throat irritation	dyspnoea, cough
Gastrointestinal disorders		
very common	diarrhoea	
common	vomiting, nausea, abdominal pain, increased blood amylase, dyspepsia, abdominal distension, flatulence	vomiting, diarrhoea, nausea, abdominal pain, increased blood amylase
uncommon	pancreatitis, gastritis, gastrooesophageal reflux disease, aphthous stomatitis, stomatitis, retching, haematemesis, dry mouth, abdominal discomfort, constipation, increased lipase, eructation, oral dysaesthesia, cheilitis, dry lip, coated tongue	pancreatitis, gastritis, gastrooesophageal reflux disease, aphthous stomatitis, retching, dry mouth, abdominal distension, abdominal discomfort, flatulence, dyspepsia, constipation, increased lipase
Hepatobiliary disorders		
common	increased alanine aminotransferase, increased aspartate aminotransferase	increased alanine aminotransferase
uncommon	hepatitis, cytolytic hepatitis, hepatic steatosis, hepatomegaly, increased transaminase, increased blood bilirubin, increased blood alkaline phosphatase, increased gamma-glutamyltransferase	hepatitis, cytolytic hepatitis, hepatic steatosis, increased transaminase, increased aspartate aminotransferase, increased blood alkaline phosphatase, increased gamma-glutamyltransferase
Skin and subcutaneous tissue disorders		
common	rash (including macular, maculopapular, papular, erythematous and pruritic rash), pruritus	rash (including macular, maculopapular, papular, erythematous and pruritic rash)
uncommon	generalised rash, allergic dermatitis, face oedema, urticaria, dermatitis, eczema, erythema, hyperhidrosis, night sweats, alopecia, acne, seborrhoeic dermatitis, skin lesion, xeroderma, dry skin, nail pigmentation	generalised rash, allergic dermatitis, urticaria, pruritus, hyperhidrosis, night sweats, alopecia
Musculoskeletal and connective tissue disorders		
uncommon	myalgia, muscle spasms, muscular weakness, musculoskeletal stiffness, arthritis, arthralgia, joint stiffness, pain in extremity, osteoporosis, increased blood creatine phosphokinase	myalgia, arthralgia, pain in extremity, osteoporosis, increased blood creatine phosphokinase
Renal and urinary disorders		
uncommon	acute renal failure, renal failure, nephrolithiasis, increased blood creatinine, decreased creatinine renal clearance, proteinuria, bilirubinuria, dysuria, nocturia, pollakiuria	acute renal failure, renal failure, nephrolithiasis, increased blood creatinine, decreased creatinine renal clearance, proteinuria, bilirubinuria
Reproductive system and breast disorders		
uncommon	erectile dysfunction, gynaecomastia	erectile dysfunction, gynaecomastia
General disorders and administration site conditions		
common	asthenia, fatigue	fatigue
uncommon	pyrexia, chest pain, peripheral oedema, malaise, chills, abnormal feeling, feeling hot, irritability, pain, xerosis	pyrexia, chest pain, asthenia, peripheral oedema, malaise

* Adverse events, considered at least possibly related by the investigator to PREZISTA co-administered with low dose ritonavir, occurring in more than 1 patient.

** Adverse events, at least grade 2 in severity and considered at least possibly related by the investigator to PREZISTA co-administered with low dose ritonavir, occurring in more than 1 patient.

Table 3

	TITAN		
Outcomes	PREZISTA/rtv 600/100 mg b.i.d. + OBR N=298	lopinavir/rtv 400/100 mg b.i.d. + OBR N=297	Treatment difference (95% CI of difference)
HIV-1 RNA < 400 copies/ml[a]	228 (76.5%)	199 (67.0%)	9.5% (2.3; 16.7)[b]
HIV-1 RNA < 50 copies/ml[a]	211 (70.8%)	179 (60.3%)	10.5% (2.9; 18.1)[b]
mean HIV-1 RNA log change from baseline (log_{10} copies/ml)[c]	-1.95	-1.72	-0.23[d] (-0.44; -0.02)[b]
median CD4+ cell count change from baseline (x 10^6/l)[c]	88	81	

[a] Imputations according to the TLOVR algorithm

[b] Based on a normal approximation of the difference in % response

[c] NC=F

[d] Difference in means

Table 4

	POWER 1 and POWER 2 pooled data			POWER 3
Outcomes at 48 weeks				
Baseline characteristics				
Mean plasma HIV-1 RNA	4.61 log_{10} copies/ml (PREZISTA/ritonavir) 4.49 log_{10} copies/ml (control)			4.58 log_{10} copies/ml
Median CD4+ cell count	153 × 10^6 cells/l (PREZISTA/ritonavir) 163 × 10^6 cells/l (control)			120 × 10^6 cells/l
Outcomes	PREZISTA/ritonavir 600/100 mg b.i.d. n=131	Control n=124	Treatment difference	PREZISTA/ritonavir 600/100 mg b.i.d. n=334
HIV-1 RNA log_{10} mean change from baseline (log_{10} copies/ml)[a]	-1.69	-0.37	1.32 (1.58; 1.05)[d]	-1.62
CD4+ cell count mean change from baseline (x 10^6/l)[b]	103	17	86 (57; 114)[d]	105
HIV RNA ≥1 log_{10} below baseline[c]	81 (61.8%)	20 (16.1%)	45.7% (35.0%; 56.4%)[d]	196 (58.7%)
HIV RNA < 400 copies/ml[c]	72 (55.0%)	18 (14.5%)	40.4% (29.8%; 51.1%)[d]	183 (54.8%)
HIV RNA < 50 copies/ml[c]	59 (45.0%)	14 (11.3%)	33.7% (23.4%; 44.1%)[d]	155 (46.4%)

[a] Non-completer is failure imputation: patients who discontinued prematurely are imputed with a change equal to 0

[b] Last Observation Carried Forward imputation

[c] Imputations according to the TLOVR algorithm

[d] 95% confidence intervals.

substitutions that developed in 10 to 20% of the isolates were V11I, I13V, L33F, I50V and F53L. Amino acid substitutions that developed in 5 to 10% of isolates were L10F, I15V, M36L, K43T, M46I, I47V, A71I, G73S, T74P, L76V, V82I and I84V.

Of the viruses isolated from patients experiencing virologic failure by rebound from the PREZISTA/rtv 600/100 mg b.i.d. group of the POWER and DUET trials, 85% of those susceptible to darunavir at baseline developed decreased susceptibility to darunavir during treatment.

In the same group of patients, 71% of viruses that were susceptible to tipranavir at baseline remained susceptible after treatment.

Cross-resistance

Darunavir has a < 10-fold decreased susceptibility against 90% of 3,309 clinical isolates resistant to amprenavir, atazanavir, indinavir, lopinavir, nelfinavir, ritonavir, saquinavir and/or tipranavir showing that viruses resistant to most PIs remain susceptible to darunavir.

Clinical experience

Adult patients

Efficacy of PREZISTA co-administered with 100 mg ritonavir in treatment-naïve patients

There are no data on the efficacy of darunavir co-administered with 100 mg ritonavir in treatment-naïve HIV-1 infected patients.

Efficacy of PREZISTA co-administered with 100 mg ritonavir in treatment-experienced patients

The evidence of efficacy of PREZISTA co-administered with ritonavir (600/100 mg b.i.d.) in treatment-experienced patients is based on the 48 weeks analysis of the Phase III trial TITAN in treatment-experienced lopinavir naïve patients and on the analyses of 96 weeks data from the Phase IIb trials POWER 1, 2 and 3 in patients with high level of PI resistance.

TITAN is an ongoing randomised, controlled, open-label Phase III trial comparing PREZISTA co-administered with ritonavir (600/100 mg b.i.d.) versus lopinavir/ritonavir (400/100 mg b.i.d) in treatment-experienced, lopinavir naïve HIV-1 infected adult patients. Both arms used an Optimised Background Regimen (OBR) consisting of at least 2 antiretrovirals (NRTIs with or without NNRTIs). The mean baseline plasma HIV-1 RNA was 4.33 log_{10} copies/ml and the median baseline CD4+ cell count was 235 × 10^6 cells/l (range 3 – 831 × 10^6 cells/l) in the PREZISTA/ritonavir arm.

The table above shows the efficacy data of the 48 week analysis from the TITAN trial.

(see Table 3 above)

Non-inferiority in virologic response, defined as the percentage of subjects with plasma HIV-1 RNA level < 400 copies/ml, was demonstrated (at the chosen 12% non-inferiority margin) for both Intent-To-Treat and On Protocol populations.

POWER 1 *and* **POWER 2** are randomised, controlled trials consisting of an initial dose-finding part and a second long-term part in which all patients randomised to PREZISTA co-administered with 100 mg ritonavir received the recommended dose of 600/100 mg b.i.d.

HIV-1 infected patients who were eligible for these trials had previously failed more than 1 PI containing regimen. PREZISTA co-administered with 100 mg ritonavir plus an optimised background regimen (OBR) was compared to a control group receiving an investigator-selected PI(s) regimen plus an OBR. The OBR consisted of at least 2 NRTIs with or without enfuvirtide (ENF).

POWER 3: additional data on the efficacy of PREZISTA co-administered with ritonavir 600/100 mg b.i.d. with OBR have been obtained in similar treatment-experienced patients participating in the non-randomised trial TMC114-C215. Entry criteria were the same as and baseline characteristics were comparable to those of POWER 1 and POWER 2.

The table below shows the efficacy data of the 48-week analyses on the recommended 600 mg dose of PREZISTA co-administered with 100 mg ritonavir b.i.d. from the pooled POWER 1 and POWER 2 trials as well as from the POWER 3 trial.

(see Table 4 opposite)

Analyses of data through 96 weeks of treatment in the three POWER trials demonstrated sustained antiretroviral efficacy and immunological benefit. Treatment with PREZISTA co-administered with ritonavir (600/100 mg b.i.d.) resulted in 56.5% (POWER 1 and 2) and 52.2% (POWER 3) of responders with a decrease of at least 1 log10 in HIV RNA from baseline, 38.9% (POWER 1 and 2) and 42.1% (POWER 3) of subjects with an HIV RNA level < 50 copies/ml and 49.6% (POWER 1 and 2) and 50.0% (POWER 3) respectively of subjects with an HIV RNA level less than 400 copies/ml. The mean decrease in HIV RNA level compared to baseline was 1.58 (POWER 1 and 2) and 1.43 (POWER 3) log10 copies/ml and a mean increase in CD4+ cell count of 133 × 10^6 cells/l (POWER 1 and 2) and 103 × 10^6 cells/l (POWER 3) was observed.

Out of the 206 subjects who responded with complete viral suppression (< 50 copies/ml) at week 48, 177 subjects (86% of the responders at week 48) remained responders at week 96.

Baseline genotype or phenotype and virologic outcome

In a pooled analysis of the 600/100 mg b.i.d. groups of the POWER and DUET trials, the presence at baseline of 3 or more of mutations V11I, V32I, L33F, I47V, I50V, I54L or M, T74P, L76V, I84V or L89V was associated with a decreased virologic response to PREZISTA co-administered with 100 mg ritonavir. The presence of these individual mutations was associated with a median of 13 to 15 PI resistance associated mutations of the IAS-USA list of mutations.

In early treatment-experienced patients (TITAN) three or more of these mutations were only found in 4% of the patients at baseline.

Response (HIV-1 RNA < 50 copies/ml at week 24) to PREZISTA co-administered with ritonavir (600/100 mg b.i.d.) by baseline genotype and by use of enfuvirtide (ENF): As treated analysis of the POWER and DUET trials.*

(see Table 5 below)

Baseline darunavir phenotype (shift in susceptibility relative to reference) was shown to be a predictive factor of virologic outcome.

Response (HIV-1 RNA < 50 copies/ml at week 24) to PREZISTA co-administered with ritonavir (600/100 mg b.i.d.) by baseline darunavir phenotype and by use of enfuvirtide: As treated analysis of the POWER and DUET trials.

(see Table 6 on next page)

Children from the age of 6 years and adolescents

DELPHI is an open-label, Phase II trial evaluating the pharmacokinetics, safety, tolerability, and efficacy of PREZISTA with low dose ritonavir in 80 ART-experienced HIV-1 infected paediatric patients aged 6 to 17 years and weighing at least 20 kg. These patients received PREZISTA/ritonavir in combination with other antiretroviral agents (see section 4.2 for dosage recommendations per body weight). Virologic response was defined as a decrease in plasma HIV-1 RNA viral load of at least 1.0 log10 versus baseline.

Table 5

Number of mutations at baseline*	All subjects % n/N	Subjects with no/non-naïve use of ENF % n/N	Subjects with naïve use of ENF % n/N
All ranges	45% 455/1,014	39% 290/741	60% 165/273
0-2	54% 359/660	50% 238/477	66% 121/183
3	39% 67/172	29% 35/120	62% 32/52
≥ 4	12% 20/171	7% 10/135	28% 10/36

* Number of mutations from the list of mutations associated with a diminished response to PREZISTA/ritonavir (V11I, V32I, L33F, I47V, I50V, I54L or M, T74P, L76V, I84V or L89V)

Table 6

Baseline darunavir phenotype	All subjects % n/N	Subjects with no/non-naïve use of ENF % n/N	Subjects with naïve use of ENF % n/N
All ranges	45% 455/1,014	39% 290/741	60% 165/273
⩽ 10	55% 364/659	51% 244/477	66% 120/182
10-40	29% 59/203	17% 25/147	61% 34/56
> 40	8% 9/118	5% 5/94	17% 4/24

In the study, patients who were at risk of discontinuing therapy due to intolerance of ritonavir oral solution (e.g. taste aversion) were allowed to switch to the capsule formulation. Of the 44 patients taking ritonavir oral solution, 27 switched to the 100 mg capsule formulation and exceeded the weight-based ritonavir dose without changes in observed safety.

DELPHI	
Baseline disease characteristics	
Mean plasma HIV-1 RNA	4.64 $\log_{10}$ copies/ml
Median CD4+ cell count	330 × 10^6 cells/l (range: 6 to 1,505 × 10^6 cells/l)
Outcomes at week 48	PREZISTA/ritonavir N=80
HIV-1 RNA ⩾ 1 $\log_{10}$ below baseline[a]	52 (65.0%)
HIV-1 RNA < 50 copies/ml[a]	38 (47.5%)
HIV-1 RNA < 400 copies/ml[a]	47 (58.8%)
HIV-1 RNA $\log_{10}$ mean change from baseline[b]	-1.81
CD4+ cell count mean change from baseline[b]	147

[a] Imputations according to the TLOVR algorithm.

[b] Non-completer is failure imputation: patients who discontinued prematurely are imputed with a change equal to 0.

According to the TLOVR non-virologic failure censored algorithm 24 (30.0%) subjects experienced virological failure, of which 17 (21.3%) subjects were rebounders and 7 (8.8%) subjects were non-responders.

5.2 Pharmacokinetic properties

The pharmacokinetic properties of darunavir, co-administered with ritonavir, have been evaluated in healthy adult volunteers and in HIV-1 infected patients. Exposure to darunavir was higher in HIV-1 infected patients than in healthy subjects. The increased exposure to darunavir in HIV-1 infected patients compared to healthy subjects may be explained by the higher concentrations of alpha-1-acid glycoprotein (AAG) in HIV-1 infected patients, resulting in higher darunavir binding to plasma AAG and, therefore, higher plasma concentrations.

Darunavir is primarily metabolised by CYP3A. Ritonavir inhibits CYP3A, thereby increasing the plasma concentrations of darunavir considerably.

Absorption

Darunavir was rapidly absorbed following oral administration. Maximum plasma concentration of darunavir in the presence of low dose ritonavir is generally achieved within 2.5-4.0 hours.

The absolute oral bioavailability of a single 600 mg dose of darunavir alone was approximately 37% and increased to approximately 82% in the presence of 100 mg b.i.d. ritonavir. The overall pharmacokinetic enhancement effect by ritonavir was an approximate 14-fold increase in the systemic exposure of darunavir when a single dose of 600 mg darunavir was given orally in combination with ritonavir at 100 mg b.i.d. (see section 4.4).

When administered without food, the relative bioavailability of darunavir in the presence of low dose ritonavir is 30% lower as compared to intake with food. Therefore, PREZISTA tablets should be taken with ritonavir and with food. The type of food does not affect exposure to darunavir.

Distribution

Darunavir is approximately 95% bound to plasma protein. Darunavir binds primarily to plasma alpha-1-acid glycoprotein.

Following intravenous administration, the volume of distribution of darunavir alone was 88.1 ± 59.0 l (Mean ± SD) and increased to 131 ± 49.9 l (Mean ± SD) in the presence of 100 mg twice-daily ritonavir.

Metabolism

In vitro experiments with human liver microsomes (HLMs) indicate that darunavir primarily undergoes oxidative metabolism. Darunavir is extensively metabolised by the hepatic CYP system and almost exclusively by isozyme CYP3A4. A ^{14}C-darunavir trial in healthy volunteers showed that a majority of the radioactivity in plasma after a single 400/100 mg darunavir with ritonavir dose was due to the parent active substance. At least 3 oxidative metabolites of darunavir have been identified in humans; all showed activity that was at least 10-fold less than the activity of darunavir against wild type HIV.

Elimination

After a 400/100 mg ^{14}C-darunavir with ritonavir dose, approximately 79.5% and 13.9% of the administered dose of ^{14}C-darunavir could be retrieved in faeces and urine, respectively. Unchanged darunavir accounted for approximately 41.2% and 7.7% of the administered dose in faeces and urine, respectively. The terminal elimination half-life of darunavir was approximately 15 hours when combined with ritonavir.

The intravenous clearance of darunavir alone (150 mg) and in the presence of low dose ritonavir was 32.8 l/h and 5.9 l/h, respectively.

Special Populations

Paediatrics

The pharmacokinetics of darunavir in combination with ritonavir in 74 treatment-experienced paediatric patients, aged 6 to 17 years and weighing at least 20 kg, showed that the administered weight-based doses of PREZISTA/ritonavir resulted in darunavir exposure comparable to that in adults receiving PREZISTA/ritonavir 600/100 mg b.i.d. (see section 4.2).*Elderly*

Population pharmacokinetic analysis in HIV infected patients showed that darunavir pharmacokinetics are not considerably different in the age range (18 to 75 years) evaluated in HIV infected patients (n=12, age ⩾ 65) (see section 4.4). However, only limited data were available in patients above the age of 65 year.

Gender

Population pharmacokinetic analysis showed a slightly higher darunavir exposure (16.8%) in HIV infected females compared to males. This difference is not clinically relevant.

Renal impairment

Results from a mass balance study with ^{14}C-darunavir with ritonavir showed that approximately 7.7% of the administered dose of darunavir is excreted in the urine unchanged.

Although darunavir has not been studied in patients with renal impairment, population pharmacokinetic analysis showed that the pharmacokinetics of darunavir were not significantly affected in HIV infected patients with moderate renal impairment (CrCl between 30-60 ml/min, n=20) (see sections 4.2 and 4.4).

Hepatic impairment

Darunavir is primarily metabolised and eliminated by the liver. In a multiple dose study with PREZISTA co-administered with ritonavir (600/100 mg) twice daily, it was demonstrated that the total plasma concentrations of darunavir in subjects with mild (Child-Pugh Class A, n=8) and moderate (Child-Pugh Class B, n=8) hepatic impairment were comparable with those in healthy subjects. However, unbound darunavir concentrations were approximately 55% (Child-Pugh Class A) and 100% (Child-Pugh Class B) higher, respectively. The clinical relevance of this increase is unknown therefore, PREZISTA should be used with caution. The effect of severe hepatic impairment on the pharmacokinetics of darunavir has not been studied (see sections 4.2, 4.3 and 4.4).

5.3 Preclinical safety data

Animal toxicology studies have been conducted at exposures up to clinical exposure levels with darunavir alone, in mice, rats and dogs and in combination with ritonavir in rats and dogs.

In repeated-dose toxicology studies in mice, rats and dogs, there were only limited effects of treatment with darunavir. In rodents the target organs identified were the haematopoietic system, the blood coagulation system, liver and thyroid. A variable but limited decrease in red blood cell-related parameters was observed, together with increases in activated partial thromboplastin time.

Changes were observed in liver (hepatocyte hypertrophy, vacuolation, increased liver enzymes) and thyroid (follicular hypertrophy). In the rat, the combination of darunavir with ritonavir lead to a small increase in effect on RBC parameters, liver and thyroid and increased incidence of islet fibrosis in the pancreas (in male rats only) compared to treatment with darunavir alone. In the dog, no major toxicity findings or target organs were identified up to exposures equivalent to clinical exposure at the recommended dose.

In a study conducted in rats, the number of corpora lutea and implantations were decreased in the presence of maternal toxicity. Otherwise, there were no effects on mating or fertility with darunavir treatment up to 1,000 mg/kg/day and exposure levels below (AUC-0.5 fold) of that in human at the clinically recommended dose. Up to same dose levels, there was no teratogenicity with darunavir in rats and rabbits when treated alone nor in mice when treated in combination with ritonavir. The exposure levels were lower than those with the recommended clinical dose in humans. In a pre- and postnatal development assessment in rats, darunavir with and without ritonavir, caused a transient reduction in body weight gain of the offspring pre-weaning and there was a slight delay in the opening of eyes and ears. Darunavir in combination with ritonavir caused a reduction in the number of pups that exhibited the startle response on day 15 of lactation and a reduced pup survival during lactation. These effects may be secondary to pup exposure to the active substance via the milk and/or maternal toxicity. No post weaning functions were affected with darunavir alone or in combination with ritonavir. In juvenile rats receiving darunavir up to days 23-26, increased mortality was observed with convulsions in some animals. Exposure in plasma, liver and brain was considerably higher than in adult rats after comparable doses in mg/kg between days 5 and 11 of age. After day 23 of life, the exposure was comparable to that in adult rats. The increased exposure was likely at least partly due to immaturity of the drug-metabolising enzymes in juvenile animals. No treatment related mortalities were noted in juvenile rats dosed at 1,000 mg/kg darunavir (single dose) on day 26 of age or at 500 mg/kg (repeated dose) from day 23 to 50 of age, and the exposures and toxicity profile were comparable to those observed in adult rats.

Due to uncertainties regarding the rate of development of the human blood brain barrier and liver enzymes, PREZISTA with low dose ritonavir should not be used in paediatric patients below 3 years of age.

Darunavir was evaluated for carcinogenic potential by oral gavage administration to mice and rats up to 104 weeks. Daily doses of 150, 450 and 1,000 mg/kg were administered to mice and doses of 50, 150 and 500 mg/kg were administered to rats. Dose-related increases in the incidences of hepatocellular adenomas and carcinomas were observed in males and females of both species. Thyroid follicular cell adenomas were noted in male rats. Administration of darunavir did not cause a statistically significant increase in the incidence of any other benign or malignant neoplasm in mice or rats. The observed hepatocellular and thyroid tumours in rodents are considered to be of limited relevance to humans. Repeated administration of darunavir to rats caused hepatic microsomal enzyme induction and increased thyroid hormone elimination, which predispose rats, but not humans, to thyroid neoplasms. At the highest tested doses, the systemic exposures (based on AUC) to darunavir were between 0.4- and 0.7-fold (mice) and 0.7- and 1-fold (rats), relative to those observed in humans at the recommended therapeutic doses.

After 2 years administration of darunavir at exposures at or below the human exposure, kidney changes were observed in mice (nephrosis) and rats (chronic progressive nephropathy).

Darunavir was not mutagenic or genotoxic in a battery of *in vitro* and *in vivo* assays including bacterial reverse mutation (Ames), chromosomal aberration in human lymphocytes and *in vivo* micronucleus test in mice.

6. PHARMACEUTICAL PARTICULARS

6.1 List of excipients

Tablet core

Microcrystalline cellulose

Colloidal anhydrous silica

Crospovidone

Magnesium stearate

Tablet film-coat

Poly (vinyl alcohol) – partially hydrolyzed

Macrogol 3350

Titanium dioxide (E171)

Talc

Sunset yellow FCF (E110)

6.2 Incompatibilities

Not applicable.

6.3 Shelf life

2 years

6.4 Special precautions for storage

This medicinal product does not require any special storage conditions.

6.5 Nature and contents of container

Opaque, white, high density polyethylene (HDPE) plastic, 160 ml bottle containing 120 tablets, fitted with polypropylene (PP) child resistant closure.

One bottle

6.6 Special precautions for disposal and other handling

No special requirements.

7. MARKETING AUTHORISATION HOLDER

Janssen-Cilag International NV
Turnhoutseweg 30
B-2340 Beerse
Belgium

8. MARKETING AUTHORISATION NUMBER(S)

EU/1/06/380/001

9. DATE OF FIRST AUTHORISATION/RENEWAL OF THE AUTHORISATION

Date of first authorisation: 12 February 2007

Date of latest renewal: 12 February 2009

10. DATE OF REVISION OF THE TEXT

23rd June 2009

Detailed information on this product is available on the website of the European Medicines Agency (EMEA) http://www.emea.europa.eu/.

PREZISTA 400 mg film coated tablets

(Janssen-Cilag Ltd)

1. NAME OF THE MEDICINAL PRODUCT

PREZISTA▼ 400 mg film-coated tablets

2. QUALITATIVE AND QUANTITATIVE COMPOSITION

Each film-coated tablet contains 400 mg of darunavir (as ethanolate).

Excipient: Each tablet contains 0.834 mg sunset yellow FCF (E110).

For a full list of excipients, see section 6.1.

3. PHARMACEUTICAL FORM

Film-coated tablet.

Light orange oval shaped tablet, debossed with "400MG" on one side and "TMC" on the other side.

4. CLINICAL PARTICULARS

4.1 Therapeutic indications

PREZISTA 400 mg, co-administered with low dose ritonavir is indicated in combination with other antiretroviral medicinal products for the treatment of human immunodeficiency virus (HIV-1) infection in antiretroviral therapy (ART) naïve adults.

4.2 Posology and method of administration

Therapy should be initiated by a physician experienced in the management of HIV infection.

PREZISTA must always be given orally with 100 mg ritonavir as a pharmacokinetic enhancer and in combination with other antiretroviral medicinal products. The Summary of Product Characteristics of ritonavir must therefore be consulted prior to initiation of therapy with PREZISTA.

Adults

ART-naïve patients

The recommended dosage of PREZISTA is 800 mg once daily (q.d.) taken with ritonavir 100 mg q.d. and with food. Patients should be instructed to take PREZISTA with low dose ritonavir within 30 minutes after completion of a meal. The type of food does not affect the exposure to darunavir (see sections 4.4, 4.5 and 5.2).

ART-experienced patients

For dosage recommendations in ART-experienced patients see the Summary of Product Characteristics for PREZISTA 300 mg and 600 mg tablets.

After therapy with PREZISTA has been initiated, patients should be advised not to alter the dosage or discontinue therapy without instruction of their physician.

Children and adolescents

PREZISTA is not recommended for use in children and adolescents because due to insufficient data on safety, efficacy and pharmacokinetics.

Elderly

Limited information is available in this population and therefore PREZISTA should be used with caution in this age group (see sections 4.4 and 5.2).

Hepatic impairment

Darunavir is metabolised by the hepatic system. No dose adjustment is recommended in patients with mild (Child-Pugh Class A) or moderate (Child-Pugh Class B) hepatic impairment, however, PREZISTA should be used with caution in these patients. No pharmacokinetic data are available in patients with severe hepatic impairment. Severe hepatic impairment could result in an increase of darunavir exposure and a worsening of its safety profile. Therefore, PREZISTA should not be used in patients with severe hepatic impairment (Child-Pugh Class C) (see sections 4.3, 4.4 and 5.2).

Renal impairment

No dose adjustment is required in patients with renal impairment (see sections 4.4 and 5.2).

If an 800/100 mg once daily dose of PREZISTA/ritonavir is missed within 12 hours of the time it is usually taken, patients should be instructed to take the prescribed dose of PREZISTA and ritonavir with food as soon as possible. If this is noticed later than 12 hours of the time it is usually taken, the missed dose should not be taken and the patient should resume the usual dosing schedule.

This guidance is based on the 15 hour half-life of darunavir in the presence of ritonavir and the recommended dosing interval of approximately 24 hours.

4.3 Contraindications

Hypersensitivity to the active substance or to any of the excipients.

Patients with severe (Child-Pugh Class C) hepatic impairment.

Combination of rifampicin with PREZISTA with concomitant low dose ritonavir is contraindicated (see section 4.5).

The combination product lopinavir/ritonavir should not be used with PREZISTA because co-administration causes large decreases in darunavir concentrations, which may in turn significantly decrease the darunavir therapeutic effect (see section 4.5).

Herbal preparations containing St John's wort (*Hypericum perforatum*) must not be used while taking PREZISTA due to the risk of decreased plasma concentrations and reduced clinical effects of darunavir (see section 4.5).

Co-administration of PREZISTA with 100 mg ritonavir, with active substances that are highly dependent on CYP3A for clearance and for which elevated plasma concentrations are associated with serious and/or life-threatening events is contraindicated. These active substances include e.g. antiarrhythmics (amiodarone, bepridil, quinidine, systemic lidocaine), antihistamines (astemizole, terfenadine), ergot derivatives (e.g. dihydroergotamine, ergonovine, ergotamine, methylergonovine), gastrointestinal motility agents (cisapride), neuroleptics (pimozide, sertindole), sedatives/hypnotics [triazolam, midazolam administered orally (for caution on parenterally administered midazolam, see section 4.5)] and HMG-CoA reductase inhibitors (simvastatin and lovastatin) (see section 4.5).

4.4 Special warnings and precautions for use

Patients should be advised that current antiretroviral therapy does not cure HIV and has not been proven to prevent the transmission of HIV to others through blood or sexual contact. Appropriate precautions should continue to be employed.

PREZISTA should only be used in combination with 100 mg of ritonavir as a pharmacokinetic enhancer (see section 5.2).

Increasing the dose of ritonavir from that recommended in section 4.2 did not significantly affect darunavir concentrations and is not recommended.

Elderly: As limited information is available on the use of PREZISTA in patients aged 65 and over, caution should be exercised in the administration of PREZISTA in elderly patients, reflecting the greater frequency of decreased hepatic function and of concomitant disease or other therapy (see sections 4.2 and 5.2).

Darunavir binds predominantly to α1-acid glycoprotein. This protein binding is concentration dependent indicative for saturation of binding. Therefore, protein displacement of medicinal products highly bound to α1-acid glycoprotein cannot be ruled out.

Severe skin rash, which may be accompanied with fever and/or elevations of transaminases, has occurred in 0.5% of patients treated with PREZISTA. Erythema multiforme and Stevens-Johnson Syndrome have been rarely ($< 0.1\%$) observed. Treatment with PREZISTA should be discontinued if such a condition develops.

Darunavir contains a sulphonamide moiety. PREZISTA should be used with caution in patients with a known sulphonamide allergy.

Patients with coexisting conditions

Hepatic impairment

The safety and efficacy of PREZISTA have not been established in patients with severe underlying liver disorders and PREZISTA is therefore contraindicated in patients with severe hepatic impairment. Due to an increase in the unbound darunavir plasma concentrations, PREZISTA should be used with caution in patients with mild or moderate hepatic impairment (see sections 4.2, 4.3 and 5.2).

Patients with chronic hepatitis B or C and treated with combination antiretroviral therapy are at an increased risk for severe and potentially fatal hepatic adverse events. In case of concomitant antiviral therapy for hepatitis B or C, please refer to the relevant product information for these medicinal products.

Patients with pre-existing liver dysfunction including chronic hepatitis have an increased frequency of liver function abnormalities during combination antiretroviral therapy and should be monitored according to standard practice. If there is evidence of worsening liver disease in such patients, interruption or discontinuation of treatment should be considered.

Renal impairment

No special precautions or dose adjustments are required in patients with renal impairment. As darunavir and ritonavir are highly bound to plasma proteins, it is unlikely that they will be significantly removed by haemodialysis or peritoneal dialysis. Therefore, no special precautions or dose adjustments are required in these patients (see sections 4.2 and 5.2).

Haemophiliac patients

There have been reports of increased bleeding, including spontaneous skin haematomas and haemarthrosis in patients with haemophilia type A and B treated with PIs. In some patients additional factor VIII was given. In more than half of the reported cases, treatment with PIs was continued or reintroduced if treatment had been discontinued. A causal relationship has been suggested, although the mechanism of action has not been elucidated. Haemophiliac patients should therefore be made aware of the possibility of increased bleeding.

Diabetes mellitus/Hyperglycaemia

New onset diabetes mellitus, hyperglycaemia, or exacerbation of existing diabetes mellitus has been reported in patients receiving antiretroviral therapy, including PIs. In some of these patients the hyperglycaemia was severe and in some cases also associated with ketoacidosis. Many patients had confounding medical conditions some of which required therapy with agents that have been associated with the development of diabetes mellitus or hyperglycaemia.

Fat redistribution and metabolic disorders

Combination antiretroviral therapy has been associated with redistribution of body fat (lipodystrophy) in HIV infected patients. The long-term consequences of these events are currently unknown. Knowledge about the mechanism is incomplete. A connection between visceral lipomatosis and PIs and lipoatrophy and NRTIs has been hypothesised. A higher risk of lipodystrophy has been associated with individual factors such as older age and with drug related factors such as longer duration of antiretroviral treatment and associated metabolic disturbances. Clinical examination should include evaluation for physical signs of fat redistribution. Consideration should be given to measurement of fasting serum lipids and blood glucose. Lipid disorders should be managed as clinically appropriate (see section 4.8).

Osteonecrosis

Although the etiology is considered to be multifactorial (including corticosteroid use, alcohol consumption, severe immunosuppression, higher body mass index), cases of osteonecrosis have been reported particularly in patients with advanced HIV disease and/or long-term exposure to combination antiretroviral therapy (CART). Patients should be advised to seek medical advice if they experience joint aches and pain, joint stiffness or difficulty in movement.

Immune reactivation syndrome

In HIV infected patients with severe immune deficiency at the time of institution of combination antiretroviral therapy (CART), an inflammatory reaction to asymptomatic or residual opportunistic pathogens may arise and cause serious clinical conditions, or aggravation of symptoms. Typically, such reactions have been observed within the first weeks or months of initiation of CART. Relevant examples are cytomegalovirus retinitis, generalised and/or focal mycobacterial infections and pneumonia caused by *Pneumocystis jiroveci* (formerly known as *Pneumocystis carinii*). Any inflammatory symptoms should be evaluated and treatment instituted when necessary. In addition, reactivation of herpes simplex and herpes zoster has been observed in clinical studies with PREZISTA co-administered with 100 mg ritonavir.

Interactions with medicinal products

Several of the interaction studies have been performed at lower than recommended doses of darunavir. The effects on co-administered medicinal products may thus be underestimated and clinical monitoring of safety may be indicated. For full information on interactions with other medicinal products see section 4.5.

PREZISTA tablets contain sunset yellow FCF (E110) which may cause an allergic reaction.

4.5 Interaction with other medicinal products and other forms of interaction

Darunavir and ritonavir are both inhibitors of the CYP3A4 isoform. Co-administration of darunavir and ritonavir and medicinal products primarily metabolised by CYP3A4 may result in increased systemic exposure to such medicinal products, which could increase or prolong their therapeutic effect and adverse reactions.

PREZISTA co-administered with 100 mg ritonavir must not be combined with medicinal products that are highly dependent on CYP3A4 for clearance and for which increased systemic exposure is associated with serious and/or life-threatening events (narrow therapeutic index). These medicinal products include amiodarone, bepridil, quinidine, systemic lidocaine, astemizole, terfenadine, midazolam administered orally, triazolam, cisapride, pimozide, sertindole, simvastatin, lovastatin and the ergot alkaloids (e.g. ergotamine, dihydroergotamine, ergonovine and methylergonovine) (see section 4.3).

The overall pharmacokinetic enhancement effect by ritonavir was an approximate 14-fold increase in the systemic exposure of darunavir when a single dose of 600 mg darunavir was given orally in combination with ritonavir at 100 mg b.i.d. Therefore, PREZISTA must only be used in combination with 100 mg of ritonavir as a pharmacokinetic enhancer (see sections 4.4 and 5.2).

A clinical study utilising a cocktail of drugs that are metabolised by cytochromes CYP2C9, CYP2C19 and CYP2D6 demonstrated an increase in CYP2C9 and CYP2C19 activity and inhibition of CYP2D6 activity in the presence of PREZISTA/rtv, which may be attributed to the presence of low dose ritonavir. Co-administration of darunavir and ritonavir and medicinal products which are primarily metabolised by CYP2D6 (such as flecainide, propafenone, metoprolol) may result in increased plasma concentrations of these medicinal products, which could increase or prolong their therapeutic effect and adverse reactions. Co-administration of darunavir and ritonavir and medicinal products primarily metabolised by CYP2C9 (such as warfarin) and CYP2C19 (such as methadone) may result in decreased systemic exposure to such medicinal products, which could decrease or shorten their therapeutic effect.

Although the effect on CYP2C8 has only been studied *in vitro*, co-administration of darunavir and ritonavir and medicinal products primarily metabolised by CYP2C8 (such as paclitaxel, rosiglitazone, repaglinide) may result in decreased systemic exposure to such medicinal products, which could decrease or shorten their therapeutic effect.

Medicinal products that affect darunavir/ritonavir exposure

Darunavir and ritonavir are metabolised by CYP3A. Medicinal products that induce CYP3A activity would be expected to increase the clearance of darunavir and ritonavir, resulting in lowered plasma concentrations of darunavir and ritonavir (e.g. rifampicin, St John's wort, lopinavir). Co-administration of darunavir and ritonavir and other medicinal products that inhibit CYP3A may decrease the clearance of darunavir and ritonavir and may result in increased plasma concentrations of darunavir and ritonavir (e.g. indinavir, systemic azoles like ketoconazole and clotrimazole). These interactions are described in the interaction tables below.

Interaction table

Interactions between darunavir/ritonavir and protease inhibitors, antiretroviral agents other than protease inhibitors and other non-antiretroviral medicinal products are listed in the tables below (increase is indicated as "↑", decrease as "↓", no change as "↔", not determined as "ND", twice daily as "b.i.d.", once daily as "q.d." and once every other day as "q.o.d.").

Several of the interaction studies (indicated by # in the table below) have been performed at lower than recommended doses of darunavir or with a different dosing regimen (see section 4.2 Posology). The effects on co-administered medicinal products may thus be underestimated and clinical monitoring of safety may be indicated.

Interactions – Darunavir/ritonavir with Protease Inhibitors

The efficacy and safety of the use of PREZISTA with 100 mg ritonavir and any other PI (e.g. (fos)amprenavir, nelfinavir and tipranavir) has not been established in HIV patients. Generally, dual therapy with protease inhibitors is not recommended.

(see Table 1 on next page)

4.6 Pregnancy and lactation

Pregnancy

There are no adequate and well controlled studies with darunavir in pregnant women. Studies in animals do not indicate direct harmful effects with respect to pregnancy, embryonal/foetal development, parturition or postnatal development (see section 5.3).

PREZISTA co-administered with 100 mg ritonavir should be used during pregnancy only if the potential benefit justifies the potential risk.

Breast-feeding

It is not known whether darunavir is excreted in human milk. Studies in rats have demonstrated that darunavir is excreted in milk and at high levels (1,000 mg/kg/day) resulted in toxicity. Because of both the potential for HIV transmission and the potential for adverse reactions in breast-fed infants, mothers should be instructed not to breast-feed under any circumstances if they are receiving PREZISTA.

Fertility

No human data on the effect of darunavir on fertility are available. There was no effect on mating or fertility with darunavir treatment in rats (see section 5.3).

4.7 Effects on ability to drive and use machines

No studies on the effects of PREZISTA in combination with ritonavir on the ability to drive and use machines have been performed. However, dizziness has been reported in some patients during treatment with regimens containing PREZISTA co-administered with 100 mg ritonavir and should be borne in mind when considering a patient's ability to drive or operate machinery (see section 4.8).

4.8 Undesirable effects

The adverse drug reactions are derived from Phase IIb and Phase III trials, in which a total of 1,968 treatment-experienced patients initiated therapy with the recommended dose of PREZISTA 600 mg with ritonavir 100 mg twice daily. Median exposure to PREZISTA/ritonavir in this group was 37.3 weeks. Thirty percent of these patients experienced at least one adverse drug reaction of at least grade 2 severity. The most frequent (≥ 2%) of those were diarrhoea (3.9%), hypertriglyceridaemia (3.8%), rash (2.8%), nausea (2.6%), hypercholesterolaemia (2.5%) and headache (2.0%).

2.6% of the patients discontinued treatment due to adverse reactions.

Adverse reactions are listed by system organ class (SOC) and frequency. Within each frequency grouping, adverse reactions are presented in order of decreasing seriousness. Frequencies are defined as very common (≥ 1/10), common (≥ 1/100 to < 1/10) and uncommon (≥ 1/1,000 to < 1/100).

(see Table 2 on page 4931861)

In clinical trials (n=1,968), rash (all grades, at least possibly related) occurred in 5.6% of patients treated with PREZISTA. Rash was mostly mild to moderate, often occurring within the first four weeks of treatment and resolving with continued dosing. Grade 2-4 rash was reported in 2.9% of patients. The discontinuation rate due to rash in patients using PREZISTA co-administered with 100 mg ritonavir was 0.5%.

Severe cases of skin rash, including erythema multiforme and Stevens-Johnson Syndrome (both rare) have been reported in ongoing clinical trials with PREZISTA co-administered with 100 mg ritonavir.

The safety assessment in antiretroviral treatment-naïve adult patients (n=343) is based on all safety data from the Phase III trial ARTEMIS comparing PREZISTA/rtv 800/100 mg q.d. versus lopinavir/ritonavir 800/200 mg per day. Median exposure in the PREZISTA/ritonavir group was 56.3 weeks.

0.6% of the patients discontinued treatment due to adverse drug reactions.

In these treatment naïve-patients, the following adverse drug reactions were identified:

ADRs of at least moderate intensity and reported in more than one patient

Common: hypertriglyceridaemia, hypercholesterolaemia, headache, diarrhoea, nausea, increased alanine aminotransferase.

Uncommon: hyperlipidaemia, vomiting, abdominal pain, increased aspartate aminotransferase, rash (including maculopapular rash), allergic dermatitis, pruritus.

ADRs of all severity grades and reported in more than one patient

Very common: diarrhoea, nausea.

Common: hypertriglyceridaemia, hypercholesterolaemia, anorexia, insomnia, headache, dizziness, dysgeusia, vomiting, abdominal pain, abdominal discomfort, abdominal distension, flatulence, increased alanine aminotransferase, rash (including maculopapular, papular rash), alopecia, dry skin, pruritus, fatigue.

Uncommon: upper respiratory tract infection, diabetes mellitus, hyperlipidaemia, abnormal dreams, hypoaesthesia, disturbance in attention, somnolence, dyspepsia, eructation, increased aspartate aminotransferase, allergic dermatitis, urticaria, dermatitis, night sweats, myalgia, muscle spasms, asthenia.

Combination antiretroviral therapy has been associated with redistribution of body fat (lipodystrophy) in HIV patients, including loss of peripheral and facial subcutaneous fat, increased intra-abdominal and visceral fat, breast hypertrophy and dorsocervical fat accumulation (buffalo hump) (see section 4.4).

Combination antiretroviral therapy has also been associated with metabolic abnormalities such as hypertriglyceridaemia, hypercholesterolaemia, insulin resistance, hyperglycaemia and hyperlactataemia (see section 4.4).

Increased CPK, myalgia, myositis and rarely, rhabdomyolysis have been reported with the use of protease inhibitors, particularly in combination with NRTIs.

Cases of osteonecrosis have been reported, particularly in patients with generally acknowledged risk factors, advanced HIV disease or long-term exposure to combination antiretroviral therapy (CART). The frequency of this is unknown (see section 4.4).

In HIV infected patients with severe immune deficiency at the time of initiation of combination antiretroviral therapy, an inflammatory reaction to asymptomatic or residual opportunistic infections may arise (see section 4.4).

There have been reports of increased spontaneous bleeding in haemophiliac patients receiving antiretroviral protease inhibitors (see section 4.4).

Patients co-infected with hepatitis B and/or hepatitis C virus

Among 1,968 treatment-experienced patients receiving PREZISTA co-administered with ritonavir 600/100 mg b.i.d., 236 patients were co-infected with hepatitis B or C. Co-infected patients were more likely to have baseline and treatment emergent hepatic transaminase elevations than those without chronic viral hepatitis (see section 4.4).

4.9 Overdose

Human experience of acute overdose with PREZISTA co-administered with 100 mg ritonavir is limited. Single doses up to 3,200 mg of darunavir as oral solution alone and up to 1,600 mg of the tablet formulation of darunavir in combination with ritonavir have been administered to healthy volunteers without untoward symptomatic effects.

There is no specific antidote for overdose with PREZISTA. Treatment of overdose with PREZISTA consists of general supportive measures including monitoring of vital signs and observation of the clinical status of the patient. If indicated, elimination of unabsorbed active substance is to be achieved by emesis or gastric lavage. Administration of activated charcoal may also be used to aid in removal of unabsorbed active substance. Since darunavir is highly protein bound, dialysis is unlikely to be beneficial in significant removal of the active substance.

5. PHARMACOLOGICAL PROPERTIES

5.1 Pharmacodynamic properties

Pharmacotherapeutic group: Antiviral for systemic use, ATC code: J05AE10.

Mechanism of action

Darunavir is an inhibitor of the dimerisation and of the catalytic activity of the HIV-1 protease (K_D of 4.5×10^{-12}M). It selectively inhibits the cleavage of HIV encoded Gag-Pol polyproteins in virus infected cells, thereby preventing the formation of mature infectious virus particles.

Antiviral activity *in vitro*

Darunavir exhibits activity against laboratory strains and clinical isolates of HIV-1 and laboratory strains of HIV-2 in acutely infected T-cell lines, human peripheral blood mononuclear cells and human monocytes/macrophages with median EC_{50} values ranging from 1.2 to 8.5 nM (0.7 to 5.0 ng/ml). Darunavir demonstrates antiviral activity *in vitro* against a broad panel of HIV-1 group M (A, B, C, D, E, F, G) and group O primary isolates with EC_{50} values ranging from < 0.1 to 4.3 nM.

These EC_{50} values are well below the 50% cellular toxicity concentration range of 87 μM to > 100 μM.

The EC_{50} value of darunavir increases by a median factor of 5.4 in the presence of human serum.

Darunavir showed synergistic antiviral activity when studied in combination with the protease inhibitors ritonavir, nelfinavir, or amprenavir and additive antiviral activity when studied in combination with the protease inhibitors indinavir, saquinavir, lopinavir, atazanavir, or tipranavir, the N(t)RTIs zidovudine, lamivudine, zalcitabine, didanosine, stavudine, abacavir, emtricitabine, or tenofovir, the NNRTIs nevirapine, delavirdine, or efavirenz and the fusion inhibitor enfuvirtide. No antagonism was observed between darunavir and any of those antiretrovirals.

Resistance

In vitro selection of darunavir-resistant virus from wild type HIV-1 was lengthy (> 3 years). The selected viruses were unable to grow in the presence of darunavir concentrations above 400 nM. Viruses selected in these conditions and showing decreased susceptibility to darunavir (range: 23-50-fold) harboured 2 to 4 amino acid substitutions in the protease gene. Identification of determinants of decreased susceptibility to darunavir in those viruses is under investigation.

In vitro selection of darunavir resistant HIV-1 (range: 53-641-fold change in EC_{50} values [FC]) from 9 HIV-1 strains harbouring multiple PI Resistance-Associated Mutations (RAMs) showed that a minimum of 8 darunavir *in vitro* selected mutations were required in the HIV-1 protease to render a virus resistant (FC > 10) to darunavir.

In the 48 week analysis of the ARTEMIS trial (see Clinical experience subsection ART-naïve patients), 9.9% virologic failures were observed in patients receiving PREZISTA/ritonavir 800/100 mg q.d. In these virologic failures no developing PI RAMs were identified. In 1 virologic failure of the PREZISTA/ritonavir group, 1 developing NRTI RAM at position 184 was identified, which was associated with a decreased susceptibility to emtricitabine included in the background regimen.

In a pooled analysis of the POWER 1, 2 and 3 (see Clinical experience subsection ART-experienced patients) and DUET 1 and 2 (TMC125-C206 and TMC125-C216) trials the amino acid substitutions identified that developed on PREZISTA co-administered with ritonavir (600/100 mg b.i.d.) in ≥ 20% of the isolates from subjects who experienced virologic failure by rebound were V32I, I54L and L89V. Amino acid substitutions that developed in 10 to 20% of the isolates were V11I, I13V, L33F, I50V and F53L. Amino acid substitutions that developed in 5 to 10% of isolates were L10F, I15V, M36L, K43T, M46I, I47V, A71I, G73S, T74P, L76V, V82I and I84V.

Of the viruses isolated from patients experiencing virologic failure by rebound from the PREZISTA/rtv 600/100 mg b.i.d. group of the POWER and DUET trials, 85% of those susceptible to darunavir at baseline developed decreased susceptibility to darunavir during treatment.

In the same group of patients, 71% of viruses that were susceptible to tipranavir at baseline remained susceptible after treatment.

Cross-resistance

Darunavir has a < 10-fold decreased susceptibility against 90% of 3,309 clinical isolates resistant to amprenavir,

Table 1

Co-administered Medicinal Product	Dose of Co-administered Medicinal Product (mg)	Dose of darunavir/ritonavir (mg)	Medicinal Product Assessed	AUC	C_{min}
Lopinavir/ritonavir	400/100 b.i.d.	1,200/100 b.i.d.	Lopinavir	↔	↔
			Darunavir	↓ 38%*	↓ 51%*
	533/133.3 b.i.d.	1,200 b.i.d.	Lopinavir	↔	↔
			Darunavir	↓41%	↓55%
	* based upon not dose normalised values Due to a decrease in the exposure (AUC) of darunavir by 40%, appropriate doses of the combination have not been established. Hence, concomitant use of PREZISTA co-administered with 100 mg ritonavir and the combination product lopinavir/ritonavir is contraindicated (see section 4.3).				
Saquinavir	1,000 b.i.d.	400/100 b.i.d.#	Darunavir	↓26%	↓42%
	The study with boosted saquinavir showed no significant effect of darunavir on saquinavir. It is not recommended to combine PREZISTA co-administered with 100 mg ritonavir with saquinavir.				
Indinavir	800 b.i.d.	400/100 b.i.d.#	Indinavir	↑ 23%	↑ 125%
			Darunavir	↑ 24%	↑ 44%
	When used in combination with PREZISTA co-administered with 100 mg ritonavir, dose adjustment of indinavir from 800 mg b.i.d. to 600 mg b.i.d. may be warranted in case of intolerance.				
Atazanavir	300 q.d.	400/100 b.i.d.#	Atazanavir Darunavir	↔ ↔	↔ ↔
	Darunavir/ritonavir did not significantly affect atazanavir exposure, however 90% CI for C_{min} were 99-234%. Atazanavir can be used with PREZISTA co-administered with 100 mg ritonavir.				
Interactions – Darunavir/ritonavir with Antiretroviral Agents other than Protease Inhibitors					
Co-administered Medicinal Product	**Dose of Co-administered Medicinal Product (mg)**	**Dose of darunavir/ritonavir (mg)**	**Medicinal Product Assessed**	**AUC**	**C_{min}**
Efavirenz	600 q.d.	300/100 b.i.d.#	Efavirenz	↑ 21%	↑ 17%
			Darunavir	↓ 13%	↓ 31%
	Efavirenz decreases the plasma concentrations of darunavir as a result of CYP3A4 induction. Darunavir/ritonavir increases the plasma concentrations of efavirenz as a result of CYP3A4 inhibition. Clinical monitoring for central nervous system toxicity associated with increased exposure to efavirenz may be indicated when PREZISTA co-administered with 100 mg ritonavir is given in combination with efavirenz.				
Etravirine	100 b.i.d.*	600/100 b.i.d.	Etravirine	↓ 37%	↓ 49%
			Darunavir	↔	↔
	* dose used in drug-interaction study. For recommended dose see paragraph below. There was a 37% decrease in etravirine exposure in the presence of darunavir/ritonavir and no relevant change in exposure to darunavir. Therefore, PREZISTA co-administered with low dose ritonavir can be co-administered with etravirine **200 mg b.i.d.** without dose adjustments.				
Nevirapine	200 b.i.d.	400/100 b.i.d.#	Nevirapine	↑ 27%	↑ 47%
			Darunavir	↔	↔
	Darunavir/ritonavir increases the plasma concentrations of nevirapine as a result of CYP3A4 inhibition. Since this difference is not considered to be clinically relevant, the combination of PREZISTA co-administered with 100 mg ritonavir and nevirapine can be used without dose adjustments.				
Tenofovir	300 q.d.	300/100 b.i.d.#	Tenofovir	↑ 22%	↑ 37%
			Darunavir	↔	↔
	Ritonavir effect on MDR-1 transport in renal tubuli has been a proposed mechanism for increased plasma concentrations of tenofovir. Monitoring of renal function may be indicated when PREZISTA co-administered with 100 mg ritonavir is given in combination with tenofovir, particularly in patients with underlying systemic or renal disease, or in patients taking nephrotoxic agents.				
Zidovudine Zalcitabine Emtricitabine Stavudine Lamivudine Abacavir	Based on the different elimination pathways of the other NRTIs zidovudine, zalcitabine, emtricitabine, stavudine, lamivudine, that are primarily renally excreted, and abacavir for which metabolism is not mediated by CYP450, no interactions are expected for these medicinal compounds and PREZISTA co-administered with 100 mg ritonavir.				
Didanosine	400 q.d.	600/100 b.i.d.	Didanosine Darunavir	↔ ↔	NA ↔
	Didanosine was administered on an empty stomach 2 hours prior to administration of darunavir/ritonavir. Systemic exposure to darunavir co-administered with low dose ritonavir, with or without didanosine was comparable. The combination of PREZISTA co-administered with 100 mg ritonavir and didanosine can be used without dose adjustments.				
Maraviroc	150 b.i.d.	600/100 b.i.d.	Maraviroc	↑ 305%	ND
			Darunavir	↔	ND
	The maraviroc dose should be 150 mg twice daily when co-administered with PREZISTA with low dose ritonavir. Darunavir/ritonavir concentrations were consistent with historical data.				
Interactions – Darunavir/ritonavir with Non-antiretroviral co-administered Medicinal Products					
Co-administered Medicinal Product	**Dose of Co-administered Medicinal Product (mg)**	**Dose of darunavir/ritonavir (mg)**	**Medicinal Product Assessed**	**AUC**	**C_{min}**
Antiarrhythmics					
Digoxin	0.4 mg single dose	600/100 b.i.d.	Digoxin	↑ 60%	ND
	Darunavir/ritonavir increases the plasma concentrations of digoxin. Inhibition of Pgp may be a likely explanation. Given that digoxin has as a narrow therapeutic index, it is recommended that the lowest possible dose of digoxin should initially be prescribed in case digoxin is given to patients on darunavir/ritonavir therapy. The digoxin dose should be carefully titrated to obtain the desired clinical effect while assessing the overall clinical state of the subject.				
Antibiotics					
Clarithromycin	500 b.i.d.	400/100 b.i.d.#	Clarithromycin	↑ 57%	↑ 174%
			Darunavir	↔	↔
	Darunavir/ritonavir increases the plasma concentrations of clarithromycin as a result of CYP3A4 inhibition and possible Pgp inhibition. Concentrations of the metabolite 14-OH-clarithromycin were not detectable. Caution is warranted and clinical monitoring is recommended. For patients with renal impairment, a dose reduction of clarithromycin should be considered.				
Anticoagulant					
Warfarin	Warfarin concentrations may be affected when co-administered with darunavir with ritonavir. The international normalised ratio (INR) should be monitored when warfarin is combined with PREZISTA co-administered with 100 mg ritonavir.				
Anticonvulsants					
Phenobarbital Phenytoin	Phenobarbital and phenytoin are inducers of CYP450 enzymes. PREZISTA co-administered with 100 mg ritonavir should not be used in combination with these medicines, as co-administration may cause significant decreases in darunavir plasma concentrations.				
Carbamazepine	200 b.i.d.	600/100 b.i.d.	Carbamazepine	↑ 45%	↑ 54%
			Darunavir	↔	↔
	Exposure to darunavir, co-administered with ritonavir, was unaffected by carbamazepine. Ritonavir exposure (AUC12h) was decreased by 49%. For carbamazepine, AUC12h was increased by 45%. No dose adjustment for PREZISTA/rtv is recommended. If there is a need to combine PREZISTA/rtv and carbamazepine, patients should be monitored for potential carbamazepine-related adverse events. Carbamazepine concentrations should be monitored and its dose should be titrated for adequate response. Based upon the findings, the carbamazepine dose may need to be reduced by 25% to 50% in the presence of PREZISTA/rtv.				
Antifungals					
Voriconazole	The combined use of voriconazole with darunavir co-administered with 100 mg ritonavir has not been studied. Voriconazole is metabolised by cytochrome P450 isoenzymes, CYP2C19, CYP2C9 and CYP3A4. Ritonavir, which can induce some of these isoenzymes, may decrease voriconazole plasma concentrations. Voriconazole should not be co-administered with PREZISTA with 100 mg ritonavir unless an assessment of the benefit/risk ratio justifies the use of voriconazole.				
Ketoconazole	200 b.i.d.	400/100 b.i.d.#	Ketoconazole	↑ 212%	↑ 868%
			Darunavir	↑ 42%	↑ 73%
	Ketoconazole is a potent inhibitor as well as substrate of CYP3A4. Caution is warranted and clinical monitoring is recommended. When co-administration is required the daily dose of ketoconazole should not exceed 200 mg.				

Co-administered Medicinal Product	Dose of Co-administered Medicinal Product (mg)	Dose of darunavir/ritonavir (mg)	Medicinal Product Assessed	AUC	C_{min}
Itraconazole	Itraconazole, like ketoconazole, is a potent inhibitor as well as substrate of CYP3A4. Concomitant systemic use of itraconazole and darunavir co-administered with 100 mg ritonavir may increase plasma concentrations of darunavir. Simultaneously, plasma concentrations of itraconazole may be increased by darunavir co-administered with 100 mg ritonavir. Caution is warranted and clinical monitoring is recommended. When co-administration is required the daily dose of itraconazole should not exceed 200 mg.				
Clotrimazole	Concomitant systemic use of clotrimazole and darunavir co-administered with 100 mg ritonavir may increase plasma concentrations of darunavir. This was confirmed using a population pharmacokinetic model. The increase in the median darunavir AUC_{24h} value for the patients taking clotrimazole from the overall median was 33%. Caution is warranted and clinical monitoring is recommended, when co-administration of clotrimazole is required.				
Calcium channel blockers					
Felodipine Nifedipine Nicardipine	Darunavir and ritonavir inhibit CYP3A4 and as a result can be expected to increase the plasma concentrations of calcium channel antagonists, which are CYP3A4 substrates. Clinical monitoring of therapeutic and adverse effects is recommended when these medicines are concomitantly administered with PREZISTA with 100 mg ritonavir.				
HMG Co-A Reductase Inhibitors					
Lovastatin Simvastatin	Lovastatin and simvastatin, which are highly dependent on CYP3A4 metabolism are expected to have markedly increased plasma concentrations when co-administered with darunavir co-administered with 100 mg ritonavir. This may cause myopathy, including rhabdomyolysis. Concomitant use of PREZISTA co-administered with 100 mg ritonavir with lovastatin and simvastatin is therefore contraindicated (see section 4.3).				
Atorvastatin	10 q.d.	300/100 b.i.d.[#]	Atorvastatin	3-4 times ↑	3-4 times ↑
			Darunavir	ND	ND
	The results of this interaction trial show that atorvastatin (10 mg q.d.) in combination with darunavir/ritonavir (300/100 mg b.i.d.) provides an exposure to atorvastatin, which is only 15% lower than that obtained with (40 mg q.d.) atorvastatin alone. When administration of atorvastatin and PREZISTA co-administered with 100 mg ritonavir is desired, it is recommended to start with an atorvastatin dose of 10 mg q.d. A gradual dose increase of atorvastatin may be tailored to the clinical response.				
Pravastatin	40 mg single dose	600/100 b.i.d.	Pravastatin	0-5 times ↑	ND
	Darunavir/ritonavir did not increase exposure to a single dose of pravastatin in most subjects but up to 5-fold in a limited subset of subjects. When administration of pravastatin and PREZISTA co-administered with 100 mg ritonavir is required, it is recommended to start with the lowest possible dose of pravastatin and titrate it up to the desired clinical effect while monitoring for safety.				
Hormonal contraceptive					
Ethinylestradiol	35 µg/1 mg q.d.	600/100 b.i.d.	Ethinylestradiol	↓ 44%	↓ 62%
Norethindrone			Norethindrone	↓ 14%	↓ 30%
	Alternative or additional contraceptive measures are recommended when oestrogen-based contraceptives are co-administered with PREZISTA and 100 mg ritonavir. Patients using oestrogens as hormone replacement therapy should be clinically monitored for signs of oestrogen deficiency.				
Immunosupressants					
Cyclosporine Tacrolimus Sirolimus	Exposure to cyclosporine, tacrolimus, or sirolimus will be increased when co-administered with PREZISTA co-administered with 100 mg ritonavir. Therapeutic drug monitoring of the immunosuppressive agent must be done when co-administration occurs.				
H_2-receptor antagonists and proton pump inhibitors					
Ranitidine	150 b.i.d.	400/100 b.i.d.[#]	Darunavir	↔	↔
	Based on these results, PREZISTA co-administered with 100 mg ritonavir can be co-administered with H_2-receptor antagonists without dose adjustments.				
Omeprazole	20 q.d.	400/100 b.i.d.[#]	Darunavir	↔	↔
	Based on these results, PREZISTA co-administered with 100 mg ritonavir can be co-administered with proton pump inhibitors without dose adjustments.				
Opiods					
Methadone	55-150 q.d.	600/100 b.i.d. (dosed for 7 days)	R-methadone	↓ 16%	↓ 15%
	Based on pharmacokinetic and clinical findings, no adjustment of methadone dosage is required when initiating co-administration with PREZISTA/ritonavir. However, increased methadone dose may be necessary when concomitantly administered for a longer period of time due to induction of metabolism by ritonavir. Therefore, clinical monitoring is recommended, as maintenance therapy may need to be adjusted in some patients.				
PDE-5 inhibitors					
Sildenafil Vardenafil Tadalafil	In an interaction study a comparable systemic exposure to sildenafil was observed for a single intake of 100 mg sildenafil alone and a single intake of 25 mg sildenafil co-administered with darunavir/ritonavir (400/100 mg b.i.d.). Concomitant use of PDE-5 inhibitors with PREZISTA co-administered with 100 mg ritonavir should be done with caution. If concomitant use of PREZISTA co-administered with 100 mg ritonavir with sildenafil, vardenafil, or tadalafil is indicated, sildenafil at a single dose not exceeding 25 mg in 48 hours, vardenafil at a single dose not exceeding 2.5 mg dose in 72 hours or tadalafil at a single dose not exceeding 10 mg dose in 72 hours is recommended.				
Rifamycines					
Rifampicin	Rifampicin is a strong CYP3A4 inducer and has been shown to cause profound decreases in concentrations of other protease inhibitors, which can result in virological failure and resistance development. During attempts to overcome the decreased exposure by increasing the dose of other protease inhibitors with ritonavir, a high frequency of liver reactions was seen. The combination of rifampicin and PREZISTA with concomitant low dose ritonavir is contraindicated (see section 4.3).				
Rifabutin	150 q.o.d.	600/100 b.i.d.	Rifabutin*	1.6 times ↑	ND
			Darunavir	↑ 53%	↑ 68%
	* sum of active moieties of rifabutin (parent drug + 25-*O*- desacetyl metabolite) A dosage reduction of rifabutin by 75% of the usual dose of 300 mg/day [i.e. rifabutin 150 mg q.o.d. (once every other day)] and increased monitoring for rifabutin related adverse events is warranted in patients receiving the combination. In case of safety issues, a further increase of the dosing interval for rifabutin and/or monitoring of rifabutin levels should be considered. Consideration should be given to official guidance on the appropriate treatment of tuberculosis in HIV infected patients. Rifabutin is an inducer and substrate of CYP3A4. An increase of systemic exposure to darunavir was observed when PREZISTA co-administered with 100 mg ritonavir was co-administered with rifabutin [150 mg q.o.d. (once every other day)]. Based upon the safety profile of PREZISTA/ritonavir, this increase in darunavir exposure in the presence of rifabutin does not warrant a dose adjustment for PREZISTA/ritonavir. The interaction trial showed a comparable daily systemic exposure for rifabutin between treatment at 300 mg q.d. (once daily) alone and 150 mg q.o.d. (once every other day) in combination with PREZISTA/ritonavir (600/100 mg b.i.d.) with an about 10-fold increase in the daily exposure to the active metabolite 25-*O*-desacetylrifabutin. Furthermore, AUC of the sum of active moieties of rifabutin (parent drug + 25-*O*- desacetyl metabolite) was increased 1.6-fold, while C_{max} remained comparable. Data on comparison with a 150 mg q.d. (once daily) reference dose is lacking.				
Sedatives/Hypnotics					
Parenteral midazolam	Midazolam is extensively metabolised by CYP3A4. Co-administration with PREZISTA/ritonavir may cause a large increase in the concentration of this benzodiazepine. No drug interaction study has been performed for the co-administration of PREZISTA/ritonavir with benzodiazepines. Based on data for other CYP3A4 inhibitors, plasma concentrations of midazolam are expected to be significantly higher when midazolam is given orally. Therefore PREZISTA/ritonavir should not be co-administered with orally administered midazolam (see section 4.3), whereas caution should be used with co-administration of PREZISTA/ritonavir and parenteral midazolam. Data from concomitant use of parenteral midazolam with other protease inhibitors suggest a possible 3-4 fold increase in midazolam plasma levels. If PREZISTA/ritonavir is co-administered with parenteral midazolam, it should be done in an intensive care unit (ICU) or similar setting, which ensures close clinical monitoring and appropriate medical management in case of respiratory depression and/or prolonged sedation. Dosage adjustment for midazolam should be considered, especially if more than a single dose of midazolam is administered.				
Selective Serotonin Reuptake Inhibitors (SSRIs)					
Paroxetine	20 q.d.	400/100 b.i.d.[#]	Paroxetine	↓ 39%	↓ 37%
			Darunavir	↔	↔
Sertraline	50 q.d.	400/100 b.i.d.[#]	Sertraline	↓ 49%	↓ 49%
			Darunavir	↔	↔
	If SSRIs are co-administered with PREZISTA and ritonavir, the recommended approach is a dose titration of the SSRI based on a clinical assessment of antidepressant response. In addition, patients on a stable dose of sertraline or paroxetine who start treatment with PREZISTA co-administered with 100 mg ritonavir should be monitored for antidepressant response.				
Steroids					
Fluticasone propionate Budesonide	In a clinical study where ritonavir 100 mg capsules b.i.d were co-administered with 50 µg intranasal fluticasone propionate (4 times daily) for 7 days in healthy subjects, fluticasone propionate plasma concentrations increased significantly, whereas the intrinsic cortisol levels decreased by approximately 86% (90% confidence interval 82-89%). Greater effects may be expected when fluticasone propionate is inhaled. Systemic corticosteroid effects including Cushing's syndrome and adrenal suppression have been reported in patients receiving ritonavir and inhaled or intranasally administered fluticasone propionate; this could also occur with other corticosteroids metabolised via the P450 3A pathway e.g. budesonide. Consequently, concomitant administration of PREZISTA, co-administered with 100 mg ritonavir and these glucocorticoids, is not recommended unless the potential benefit of treatment outweighs the risk of systemic corticosteroid effects. A dose reduction of the glucocorticoid should be considered with close monitoring of local and systemic effects or a switch to a glucocorticoid, which is not a substrate for CYP3A4 (e.g. beclomethasone). Moreover, in case of withdrawal of glucocorticoids progressive dose reduction may have to be performed over a longer period. The effects of high fluticasone systemic exposure on ritonavir plasma levels are as yet unknown.				
Dexamethasone	Systemic dexamethasone induces CYP3A4 and thereby may decrease darunavir exposure. Therefore this combination should be used with caution.				
Others					
St. John's wort	PREZISTA co-administered with 100 mg ritonavir must not be used concomitantly with products containing St John's wort (*Hypericum perforatum*) because co-administration may cause significant decreases in darunavir plasma concentrations and also in ritonavir concentrations. This is due to the induction of metabolising enzymes by St John's wort. If a patient is already taking St John's wort, stop St John's wort and if possible check viral levels. Darunavir exposure (and also ritonavir exposure) may increase on stopping St John's wort. The inducing effect may persist for at least 2 weeks after cessation of treatment with St John's wort (see section 4.3).				

Table 2

SOC Frequency category	Adverse reaction* All grades	Adverse reaction** Grade 2-4
Infections and infestations		
uncommon	herpes simplex	
Blood and lymphatic system disorders		
uncommon	thrombocytopenia, neutropenia, anaemia, increased eosinophil count, leukopenia	thrombocytopenia, neutropenia, anaemia
Immune system disorders		
uncommon	immune reconstitution syndrome	immune reconstitution syndrome
Endocrine disorders		
uncommon	hypothyroidism, increased blood thyroid stimulating hormone	
Metabolism and nutrition disorders		
common	lipodystrophy (including lipohypertrophy, lipodystrophy, lipoatrophy), hypertriglyceridaemia, hypercholesterolaemia, hyperlipidaemia	hypertriglyceridaemia, hypercholesterolaemia, hyperlipidaemia
uncommon	diabetes mellitus, gout, anorexia, decreased appetite, decreased weight, increased weight, hyperglycaemia, insulin resistance, decreased high density lipoprotein, increased appetite, polydipsia, increased blood lactate dehydrogenase	diabetes mellitus, lipodystrophy (including lipohypertrophy, lipodystrophy, lipoatrophy), gout, anorexia, decreased appetite, decreased weight, increased weight, hyperglycaemia, insulin resistance
Psychiatric disorders		
common	insomnia	
uncommon	depression, confusional state, disorientation, anxiety, altered mood, sleep disorder, abnormal dreams, nightmare, decreased libido, restlessness	depression, confusional state, disorientation, anxiety, altered mood, insomnia, sleep disorder, abnormal dreams
Nervous system disorders		
common	headache, peripheral neuropathy, dizziness	headache
uncommon	syncope, convulsion, lethargy, paraesthesia, hypoaesthesia, ageusia, dysgeusia, disturbance in attention, memory impairment, somnolence, sleep phase rhythm disturbance	peripheral neuropathy, dizziness, lethargy, paraesthesia, hypoaesthesia, somnolence
Eye disorders		
uncommon	visual disturbance, conjunctival hyperaemia, dry eye	conjunctival hyperaemia
Ear and labyrinth disorders		
uncommon	vertigo	vertigo
Cardiac disorders		
uncommon	acute myocardial infarction, myocardial infarction, angina pectoris, prolonged electrocardiogram QT, sinus bradycardia, tachycardia, palpitations	acute myocardial infarction, myocardial infarction, angina pectoris, prolonged electrocardiogram QT
Vascular disorders		
uncommon	hypertension, flushing	hypertension
Respiratory, thoracic and mediastinal disorders		
uncommon	dyspnoea, cough, epistaxis, rhinorrhoea, throat irritation	dyspnoea, cough
Gastrointestinal disorders		
very common	diarrhoea	
common	vomiting, nausea, abdominal pain, increased blood amylase, dyspepsia, abdominal distension, flatulence	vomiting, diarrhoea, nausea, abdominal pain, increased blood amylase
uncommon	pancreatitis, gastritis, gastroesophageal reflux disease, aphthous stomatitis, stomatitis, retching, haematemesis, dry mouth, abdominal discomfort, constipation, increased lipase, eructation, oral dysaesthesia, cheilitis, dry lip, coated tongue	pancreatitis, gastritis, gastroesophageal reflux disease, aphthous stomatitis, retching, dry mouth, abdominal distension, abdominal discomfort, flatulence, dyspepsia, constipation, increased lipase
Hepatobiliary disorders		
common	increased alanine aminotransferase, increased aspartate aminotransferase	increased alanine aminotransferase
uncommon	hepatitis, cytolytic hepatitis, hepatic steatosis, hepatomegaly, increased transaminase, increased blood bilirubin, increased blood alkaline phosphatase, increased gamma-glutamyltransferase	hepatitis, cytolytic hepatitis, hepatic steatosis, increased transaminase, increased aspartate aminotransferase, increased blood alkaline phosphatase, increased gamma-glutamyltransferase
Skin and subcutaneous tissue disorders		
common	rash (including macular, maculopapular, papular, erythematous and pruritic rash), pruritus	rash (including macular, maculopapular, papular, erythematous and pruritic rash)
uncommon	generalised rash, allergic dermatitis, face oedema, urticaria, dermatitis, eczema, erythema, hyperhidrosis, night sweats, alopecia, acne, seborrhoeic dermatitis, skin lesion, xeroderma, dry skin, nail pigmentation	generalised rash, allergic dermatitis, urticaria, pruritus, hyperhidrosis, night sweats, alopecia
Musculoskeletal and connective tissue disorders		
uncommon	myalgia, muscle spasms, muscular weakness, musculoskeletal stiffness, arthritis, arthralgia, joint stiffness, pain in extremity, osteoporosis, increased blood creatine phosphokinase	myalgia, arthralgia, pain in extremity, osteoporosis, increased blood creatine phosphokinase
Renal and urinary disorders		
uncommon	acute renal failure, renal failure, nephrolithiasis, increased blood creatinine, decreased creatinine renal clearance, proteinuria, bilirubinuria, dysuria, nocturia, pollakiuria	acute renal failure, renal failure, nephrolithiasis, increased blood creatinine, decreased creatinine renal clearance, proteinuria, bilirubinuria
Reproductive system and breast disorders		
uncommon	erectile dysfunction, gynaecomastia	erectile dysfunction, gynaecomastia
General disorders and administration site conditions		
common	asthenia, fatigue	fatigue
uncommon	pyrexia, chest pain, peripheral oedema, malaise, chills, abnormal feeling, feeling hot, irritability, pain, xerosis	pyrexia, chest pain, asthenia, peripheral oedema, malaise

* Adverse events, considered at least possibly related by the investigator to PREZISTA co-administered with low dose ritonavir, occurring in more than 1 patient.

** Adverse events, at least grade 2 in severity and considered at least possibly related by the investigator to PREZISTA co-administered with low dose ritonavir, occurring in more than 1 patient.

Table 3

	ARTEMIS		
Outcomes	PREZISTA/rtv 800/100 mg q.d. N=343	lopinavir/rtv 800/200 mg per day N=346	treatment difference (95% CI of difference)
HIV-1 RNA < 50 copies/ml[a]	287 (83.7%)	271 (78.3%)	5.3 (-0.5; 11.2)[b]
HIV-1 RNA < 400 copies/ml[a]	301 (87.8%)	295 (85.3%)	2.5 (-2.6; 7.6)[b]
mean HIV-1 RNA log change from baseline (log_{10} copies/ml)[c]	-2.77	-2.65	-0.11[d] (-0.30; 0.07)[b]
median CD4+ cell count change from baseline (x 10^6/l)[c]	137	141	

[a] Imputations according to the TLOVR algorithm
[b] Based on normal approximation to the difference in % response
[c] Non-completer is failure imputation: patients who discontinued prematurely are imputed with a change equal to 0
[d] Difference in means

Table 4

	TITAN		
Outcomes	PREZISTA/rtv 600/100 mg b.i.d. + OBR N=298	lopinavir/rtv 400/100 mg b.i.d. + OBR N=297	Treatment difference (95% CI of difference)
HIV-1 RNA < 400 copies/ml[a]	228 (76.5%)	199 (67.0%)	9.5% (2.3; 16.7)[b]
HIV-1 RNA < 50 copies/ml[a]	211 (70.8%)	179 (60.3%)	10.5% (2.9; 18.1)[b]
mean HIV-1 RNA log change from baseline (log_{10} copies/ml)[c]	-1.95	-1.72	-0.23[d] (-0.44; -0.02)[b]
median CD4+ cell count change from baseline (x 10^6/l)[c]	88	81	

[a] Imputations according to the TLOVR algorithm
[b] Based on a normal approximation of the difference in % response
[c] NC=F
[d] Difference in means

atazanavir, indinavir, lopinavir, nelfinavir, ritonavir, saquinavir and/or tipranavir showing that viruses resistant to most PIs remain susceptible to darunavir.

In the virologic failures of the ARTEMIS trial no cross-resistance with other PIs was observed.

Clinical experience

Efficacy of PREZISTA co-administered with 100 mg ritonavir in ART-naïve patients

The evidence of efficacy of PREZISTA/ritonavir 800/100 mg q.d. is based on the analyses of 48 week data from the ongoing, randomised, controlled, open-label Phase III trial ARTEMIS in antiretroviral treatment-naïve HIV-1 infected patients comparing PREZISTA/ritonavir 800/100 mg q.d. with lopinavir/ritonavir 800/200 mg per day (given as a twice-daily or as a once-daily regimen). Both arms used a fixed background regimen consisting of tenofovir disoproxil fumarate 300 mg q.d. and emtricitabine 200 mg q.d.

HIV-1 infected patients who were eligible for this trial had plasma HIV-1 RNA> 5,000 copies/ml. Randomisation was stratified by screening plasma viral load and screening CD4+ cell count.

The mean baseline plasma HIV-1 RNA was 4.86 log_{10} copies/ml and the median baseline CD4+ cell count was 228 × 10^6 cells/l (range 4–750 × 10^6 cells/l).

The table above shows the efficacy data of the 48 week analyses from the ARTEMIS trial:

(see Table 3 above)

In the 48 week analysis, the virologic response (HIV-1 RNA < 50 copies/ml) for the PREZISTA/ritonavir arm was 83.7% and for the lopinavir/rtv arm 78.3%.

Non-inferiority in virologic response, defined as the percentage of subjects with plasma HIV-1 RNA level < 50 copies/ml, was demonstrated (at the pre-defined 12% non-inferiority margin) for both Intent-To-Treat and On Protocol populations.

Efficacy of PREZISTA co-administered with 100 mg ritonavir in ART-experienced patients

The evidence of efficacy of PREZISTA co-administered with ritonavir (600/100 mg b.i.d.) in treatment-experienced patients is based on the 48 weeks analysis of the Phase III trial TITAN in treatment-experienced lopinavir naïve patients and on the analyses of 96 weeks data from the Phase IIb trials POWER 1, 2 and 3 in patients with high level of PI resistance.

TITAN is an ongoing randomised, controlled, open-label Phase III trial comparing PREZISTA co-administered with ritonavir (600/100 mg b.i.d.) versus lopinavir/ritonavir (400/100 mg b.i.d) in treatment-experienced, lopinavir naïve HIV-1 infected adult patients. Both arms used an Optimised Background Regimen (OBR) consisting of at least 2 antiretrovirals (NRTIs with or without NNRTIs). The mean baseline plasma HIV-1 RNA was 4.33 log_{10} copies/ml and the median baseline CD4+ cell count was 235 × 10^6 cells/l (range 3 – 831 × 10^6 cells/l) in the PREZISTA/ritonavir arm.

The table below shows the efficacy data of the 48 week analysis from the TITAN trial.

(see Table 4 above)

Non-inferiority in virologic response, defined as the percentage of subjects with plasma HIV-1 RNA level < 400 copies/ml, was demonstrated (at the chosen 12% non-inferiority margin) for both Intent-To-Treat and On Protocol populations.

POWER 1 and ***POWER 2*** are randomised, controlled trials consisting of an initial dose-finding part and a second long-term part in which all patients randomised to PREZISTA co-administered with 100 mg ritonavir received the recommended dose of 600/100 mg b.i.d.

HIV-1 infected patients who were eligible for these trials had previously failed more than 1 PI containing regimen. PREZISTA co-administered with 100 mg ritonavir plus an optimised background regimen (OBR) was compared to a control group receiving an investigator-selected PI(s) regimen plus an OBR. The OBR consisted of at least 2 NRTIs with or without enfuvirtide (ENF).

POWER 3*:* additional data on the efficacy of PREZISTA co-administered with ritonavir 600/100 mg b.i.d. with OBR have been obtained in similar treatment-experienced patients participating in the non-randomised trial TMC114-C215. Entry criteria were the same as and baseline characteristics were comparable to those of POWER 1 and POWER 2.

The table below shows the efficacy data of the 48-week analyses on the recommended 600 mg dose of PREZISTA co-administered with 100 mg ritonavir b.i.d. from the pooled POWER 1 and POWER 2 trials as well as from the POWER 3 trial.

(see Table 5 below)

Analyses of data through 96 weeks of treatment in the three POWER trials demonstrated sustained antiretroviral efficacy and immunological benefit. Treatment with PREZISTA co-administered with ritonavir (600/100 mg b.i.d.) resulted in 56.5% (POWER 1 and 2) and 52.2% (POWER 3) of responders with a decrease of at least 1 log_{10} in HIV RNA from baseline, 38.9% (POWER 1 and 2) and 42.1% (POWER 3) of subjects with an HIV RNA level < 50 copies/ml and 49.6% (POWER 1 and 2) and 50.0% (POWER 3) respectively of subjects with an HIV RNA level less than 400 copies/ml. The mean decrease in HIV RNA level compared to baseline was 1.58 (POWER 1 and 2) and 1.43 (POWER 3) log_{10} copies/ml and a mean increase in CD4+ cell count of 133 × 10^6 cells/l (POWER 1 and 2) and 103 × 10^6 cells/l (POWER 3) was observed.

Out of the 206 subjects who responded with complete viral suppression (< 50 copies/ml) at week 48, 177 subjects (86% of the responders at week 48) remained responders at week 96.

Baseline genotype or phenotype and virologic outcome

In a pooled analysis of the 600/100 mg b.i.d. groups of the POWER and DUET trials, the presence at baseline of 3 or more of mutations V11I, V32I, L33F, I47V, I50V, I54L or M, T74P, L76V, I84V or L89V was associated with a decreased virologic response to PREZISTA co-administered with 100 mg ritonavir. The presence of these individual mutations was associated with a median of 13 to 15 PI resistance associated mutations of the IAS-USA list of mutations.

In early treatment-experienced patients (TITAN) three or more of these mutations were only found in 4% of the patients at baseline.

Response (HIV-1 RNA < 50 copies/ml at week 24) to PREZISTA co-administered with ritonavir (600/100 mg b.i.d.) by baseline genotype and by use of enfuvirtide (ENF): As treated analysis of the POWER and DUET trials.*

(see Table 6 on next page)

Baseline darunavir phenotype (shift in susceptibility relative to reference) was shown to be a predictive factor of virologic outcome.

Table 5

	POWER 1 and POWER 2 pooled data			POWER 3
Outcomes at 48 weeks				
Baseline characteristics				
Mean plasma HIV-1 RNA	4.61 log_{10} copies/ml (PREZISTA/ritonavir) 4.49 log_{10} copies/ml (control)			4.58 log_{10} copies/ml
Median CD4+ cell count	153 × 10^6 cells/l (PREZISTA/ritonavir) 163 × 10^6 cells/l (control)			120 × 10^6 cells/l
Outcomes	PREZISTA/ritonavir 600/100 mg b.i.d. n=131	Control n=124	Treatment difference	PREZISTA/ritonavir 600/100 mg b.i.d. n=334
HIV-1 RNA log_{10} mean change from baseline (log_{10} copies/ml)[a]	-1.69	-0.37	1.32 (1.58; 1.05)[d]	-1.62
CD4+ cell count mean change from baseline (x 10^6/l)[b]	103	17	86 (57; 114)[d]	105
HIV RNA ≥1 log_{10} below baseline[c]	81 (61.8%)	20 (16.1%)	45.7% (35.0%; 56.4%)[d]	196 (58.7%)
HIV RNA < 400 copies/ml[c]	72 (55.0%)	18 (14.5%)	40.4% (29.8%; 51.1%)[d]	183 (54.8%)
HIV RNA < 50 copies/ml[c]	59 (45.0%)	14 (11.3%)	33.7% (23.4%; 44.1%)[d]	155 (46.4%)

[a] Non-completer is failure imputation: patients who discontinued prematurely are imputed with a change equal to 0
[b] Last Observation Carried Forward imputation
[c] Imputations according to the TLOVR algorithm
[d] 95% confidence intervals.

Table 6

Number of mutations at baseline*	All subjects % n/N	Subjects with no/non-naïve use of ENF % n/N	Subjects with naïve use of ENF % n/N
All ranges	45% 455/1,014	39% 290/741	60% 165/273
0-2	54% 359/660	50% 238/477	66% 121/183
3	39% 67/172	29% 35/120	62% 32/52
⩾ 4	12% 20/171	7% 10/135	28% 10/36

* Number of mutations from the list of mutations associated with a diminished response to PREZISTA/ritonavir (V11I, V32I, L33F, I47V, I50V, I54L or M, T74P, L76V, I84V or L89V)

Response (HIV-1 RNA < 50 copies/ml at week 24) to PREZISTA co-administered with ritonavir (600/100 mg b.i.d.) by baseline darunavir phenotype and by use of enfuvirtide: As treated analysis of the POWER and DUET trials.

(see Table 7 below)

5.2 Pharmacokinetic properties

The pharmacokinetic properties of darunavir, co-administered with ritonavir, have been evaluated in healthy adult volunteers and in HIV-1 infected patients. Exposure to darunavir was higher in HIV-1 infected patients than in healthy subjects. The increased exposure to darunavir in HIV-1 infected patients compared to healthy subjects may be explained by the higher concentrations of alpha-1-acid glycoprotein (AAG) in HIV-1 infected patients, resulting in higher darunavir binding to plasma AAG and, therefore, higher plasma concentrations.

Darunavir is primarily metabolised by CYP3A. Ritonavir inhibits CYP3A, thereby increasing the plasma concentrations of darunavir considerably.

Absorption

Darunavir was rapidly absorbed following oral administration. Maximum plasma concentration of darunavir in the presence of low dose ritonavir is generally achieved within 2.5-4.0 hours.

The absolute oral bioavailability of a single 600 mg dose of darunavir alone was approximately 37% and increased to approximately 82% in the presence of 100 mg b.i.d. ritonavir. The overall pharmacokinetic enhancement effect by ritonavir was an approximate 14-fold increase in the systemic exposure of darunavir when a single dose of 600 mg darunavir was given orally in combination with ritonavir at 100 mg b.i.d. (see section 4.4).

When administered without food, the relative bioavailability of darunavir in the presence of low dose ritonavir is 30% lower as compared to intake with food. Therefore, PREZISTA tablets should be taken with ritonavir and with food. The type of food does not affect exposure to darunavir.

Distribution

Darunavir is approximately 95% bound to plasma protein. Darunavir binds primarily to plasma alpha-1-acid glycoprotein.

Following intravenous administration, the volume of distribution of darunavir alone was 88.1 ± 59.0 l (Mean ± SD) and increased to 131 ± 49.9 l (Mean ± SD) in the presence of 100 mg twice-daily ritonavir.

Metabolism

In vitro experiments with human liver microsomes (HLMs) indicate that darunavir primarily undergoes oxidative metabolism. Darunavir is extensively metabolised by the hepatic CYP system and almost exclusively by isozyme CYP3A4. A ^{14}C-darunavir trial in healthy volunteers showed that a majority of the radioactivity in plasma after a single 400/100 mg darunavir with ritonavir dose was due to the parent active substance. At least 3 oxidative metabolites of darunavir have been identified in humans; all showed activity that was at least 10-fold less than the activity of darunavir against wild type HIV.

Elimination

After a 400/100 mg ^{14}C-darunavir with ritonavir dose, approximately 79.5% and 13.9% of the administered dose of ^{14}C-darunavir could be retrieved in faeces and urine, respectively. Unchanged darunavir accounted for approximately 41.2% and 7.7% of the administered dose in faeces and urine, respectively. The terminal elimination half-life of darunavir was approximately 15 hours when combined with ritonavir.

The intravenous clearance of darunavir alone (150 mg) and in the presence of low dose ritonavir was 32.8 l/h and 5.9 l/h, respectively.

Special Populations

Paediatrics

There are no pharmacokinetic data available in children and adolescents.

Elderly

Population pharmacokinetic analysis in HIV infected patients showed that darunavir pharmacokinetics are not considerably different in the age range (18 to 75 years) evaluated in HIV infected patients (see section 4.4). However, only limited data were available in patients above the age of 65 year.

Gender

Population pharmacokinetic analysis showed a slightly higher darunavir exposure in HIV infected females compared to males. This difference is not clinically relevant.

Renal impairment

Results from a mass balance study with ^{14}C-darunavir with ritonavir showed that approximately 7.7% of the administered dose of darunavir is excreted in the urine unchanged.

Although darunavir has not been studied in patients with renal impairment, population pharmacokinetic analysis showed that the pharmacokinetics of darunavir were not significantly affected in HIV infected patients with moderate renal impairment (CrCl between 30-60 ml/min, n=20) (see sections 4.2 and 4.4).

Hepatic impairment

Darunavir is primarily metabolised and eliminated by the liver. In a multiple dose study with PREZISTA co-administered with ritonavir (600/100 mg) twice daily, it was demonstrated that the total plasma concentrations of darunavir in subjects with mild (Child-Pugh Class A, n=8) and moderate (Child-Pugh Class B, n=8) hepatic impairment were comparable with those in healthy subjects. However, unbound darunavir concentrations were approximately 55% (Child-Pugh Class A) and 100% (Child-Pugh Class B) higher, respectively. The clinical relevance of this increase is unknown therefore, PREZISTA should be used with caution. The effect of severe hepatic impairment on the pharmacokinetics of darunavir has not been studied (see sections 4.2, 4.3 and 4.4).

5.3 Preclinical safety data

Animal toxicology studies have been conducted at exposures up to clinical exposure levels with darunavir alone, in mice, rats and dogs and in combination with ritonavir in rats and dogs.

In repeated-dose toxicology studies in mice, rats and dogs, there were only limited effects of treatment with darunavir. In rodents the target organs identified were the haematopoietic system, the blood coagulation system, liver and thyroid. A variable but limited decrease in red blood cell-related parameters was observed, together with increases in activated partial thromboplastin time.

Changes were observed in liver (hepatocyte hypertrophy, vacuolation, increased liver enzymes) and thyroid (follicular hypertrophy). In the rat, the combination of darunavir with ritonavir lead to a small increase in effect on RBC parameters, liver and thyroid and increased incidence of islet fibrosis in the pancreas (in male rats only) compared to treatment with darunavir alone. In the dog, no major toxicity findings or target organs were identified up to exposures equivalent to clinical exposure at the recommended dose.

In a study conducted in rats, the number of corpora lutea and implantations were decreased in the presence of maternal toxicity. Otherwise, there were no effects on mating or fertility with darunavir treatment up to 1,000 mg/kg/day and exposure levels below (AUC-0.5 fold) of that in human at the clinically recommended dose. Up to same dose levels, there was no teratogenicity with darunavir in rats and rabbits when treated alone nor in mice when treated in combination with ritonavir. The exposure levels were lower than those with the recommended clinical dose in humans. In a pre- and postnatal development assessment in rats, darunavir with and without ritonavir, caused a transient reduction in body weight gain of the offspring pre-weaning and there was a slight delay in the opening of eyes and ears. Darunavir in combination with ritonavir caused a reduction in the number of pups that exhibited the startle response on day 15 of lactation and a reduced pup survival during lactation. These effects may be secondary to pup exposure to the active substance via the milk and/or maternal toxicity. No post weaning functions were affected with darunavir alone or in combination with ritonavir. In juvenile rats receiving darunavir up to days 23-26, increased mortality was observed with convulsions in some animals. Exposure in plasma, liver and brain was considerably higher than in adult rats after comparable doses in mg/kg between days 5 and 11 of age. After day 23 of life, the exposure was comparable to that in adult rats. The increased exposure was likely at least partly due to immaturity of the drug-metabolising enzymes in juvenile animals. No treatment related mortalities were noted in juvenile rats dosed at 1,000 mg/kg darunavir (single dose) on day 26 of age or at 500 mg/kg (repeated dose) from day 23 to 50 of age, and the exposures and toxicity profile were comparable to those observed in adult rats.

In humans, the activity of drug-metabolising enzymes approaches adult values by 1 to 3 years of age.

Darunavir was evaluated for carcinogenic potential by oral gavage administration to mice and rats up to 104 weeks. Daily doses of 150, 450 and 1,000 mg/kg were administered to mice and doses of 50, 150 and 500 mg/kg were administered to rats. Dose-related increases in the incidences of hepatocellular adenomas and carcinomas were observed in males and females of both species. Thyroid follicular cell adenomas were noted in male rats. Administration of darunavir did not cause a statistically significant increase in the incidence of any other benign or malignant neoplasm in mice or rats. The observed hepatocellular and thyroid tumours in rodents are considered to be of limited relevance to humans. Repeated administration of darunavir to rats caused hepatic microsomal enzyme induction and increased thyroid hormone elimination, which predispose rats, but not humans, to thyroid neoplasms. At the highest tested doses, the systemic exposures (based on AUC) to darunavir were between 0.4- and 0.7-fold (mice) and 0.7- and 1-fold (rats), relative to those observed in humans at the recommended therapeutic doses.

After 2 years administration of darunavir at exposures at or below the human exposure, kidney changes were observed in mice (nephrosis) and rats (chronic progressive nephropathy).

Darunavir was not mutagenic or genotoxic in a battery of *in vitro* and *in vivo* assays including bacterial reverse mutation (Ames), chromosomal aberration in human lymphocytes and *in vivo* micronucleus test in mice.

Table 7

Baseline darunavir phenotype	All subjects % n/N	Subjects with no/non-naïve use of ENF % n/N	Subjects with naïve use of ENF % n/N
All ranges	45% 455/1,014	39% 290/741	60% 165/273
⩽ 10	55% 364/659	51% 244/477	66% 120/182
10-40	29% 59/203	17% 25/147	61% 34/56
> 40	8% 9/118	5% 5/94	17% 4/24

6. PHARMACEUTICAL PARTICULARS

6.1 List of excipients

Tablet core

Microcrystalline cellulose

Colloidal anhydrous silica

Crospovidone

Magnesium stearate

Tablet film-coat

Poly(vinyl alcohol) – partially hydrolyzed

Macrogol 3350

Titanium dioxide (E171)

Talc

Sunset yellow FCF (E110)

6.2 Incompatibilities

Not applicable.

6.3 Shelf life

2 years

6.4 Special precautions for storage
This medicinal product does not require any special storage conditions.

6.5 Nature and contents of container
Opaque, white, high density polyethylene (HDPE) plastic, 160 ml bottle containing 60 tablets, fitted with polypropylene (PP) child resistant closure.

One bottle

6.6 Special precautions for disposal and other handling
No special requirements.

7. MARKETING AUTHORISATION HOLDER
Janssen-Cilag International NV

Turnhoutseweg 30

B-2340 Beerse

Belgium

8. MARKETING AUTHORISATION NUMBER(S)
EU/1/06/380/003

9. DATE OF FIRST AUTHORISATION/RENEWAL OF THE AUTHORISATION
Date of first authorisation: 29 January 2009

10. DATE OF REVISION OF THE TEXT
Detailed information on this product is available on the website of the European Medicines Agency (EMEA) http://www.emea.europa.eu/.

PREZISTA 600 mg film coated tablets

(Janssen-Cilag Ltd)

1. NAME OF THE MEDICINAL PRODUCT
PREZISTA▼ 600 mg film-coated tablets

2. QUALITATIVE AND QUANTITATIVE COMPOSITION
Each film-coated tablet contains 600 mg of darunavir (as ethanolate).

Excipient: Each tablet contains 2.750 mg sunset yellow FCF (E110).

For a full list of excipients, see section 6.1.

3. PHARMACEUTICAL FORM
Film-coated tablet.

Orange oval shaped tablet, debossed with "600MG" on one side and "TMC" on the other side.

4. CLINICAL PARTICULARS

4.1 Therapeutic indications
PREZISTA, co-administered with low dose ritonavir is indicated in combination with other antiretroviral medicinal products for the treatment of human immunodeficiency virus (HIV-1) infection in antiretroviral treatment (ART) experienced adult patients, including those that have been highly pre-treated, and for the treatment of HIV-1 infection in ART-experienced children and adolescents from the age of 6 years and at least 20 kg body weight.

In deciding to initiate treatment with PREZISTA co-administered with low dose ritonavir careful consideration should be given to the treatment history of the individual patient and the patterns of mutations associated with different agents. Genotypic or phenotypic testing (when available) and treatment history should guide the use of PREZISTA.

4.2 Posology and method of administration
Therapy should be initiated by a physician experienced in the management of HIV infection.

PREZISTA must always be given orally with low dose ritonavir as a pharmacokinetic enhancer and in combination with other antiretroviral medicinal products. The Summary of Product Characteristics of ritonavir must therefore be consulted prior to initiation of therapy with PREZISTA.

Adults

ART-experienced patients

The recommended dose of PREZISTA is 600 mg twice daily (b.i.d.) taken with ritonavir 100 mg b.i.d. and with food. The type of food does not affect the exposure to darunavir (see sections 4.4, 4.5 and 5.2).

The use of only 75 mg and 150 mg tablets to achieve the recommended dose of PREZISTA in adults is appropriate when there is a possibility of hypersensitivity to specific colouring agents, or difficulty in swallowing the 300 mg or 600 mg tablets.

ART-naïve patients

PREZISTA 600 mg tablets are not indicated for ART-naïve patients. For dosage recommendations in ART-naïve patients see the Summary of Product Characteristics for PREZISTA 400 mg tablets.

After therapy with PREZISTA has been initiated, patients should be advised not to alter the dosage or discontinue therapy without instruction of their physician.

Children and adolescents

ART-experienced paediatric patients (6 to 17 years of age and weighing at least 20 kg) The recommended dose of PREZISTA with low dose ritonavir for paediatric patients is based on body weight and should not exceed the recommended adult dose (600/100 mg b.i.d.). The adult dose of PREZISTA/ritonavir (600/100 mg b.i.d.) may be used in children of 40 kg or more. For children weighing less than 40 kg, please refer to the PREZISTA Summary of Product Characteristics of the 75 mg and 150 mg tablets.

PREZISTA tablets should be taken with ritonavir twice daily and with food. The type of food does not affect the exposure to darunavir.

ART-experienced children less than 6 years of age or less than 20 kg body weight, and ART-naïve paediatric patients

There are insufficient data on the use of PREZISTA with low dose ritonavir in children less than 6 years of age or less than 20 kg body weight. Hence, PREZISTA is not recommended for use in this group (see sections 4.4 and 5.3).

Elderly

Limited information is available in this population and therefore PREZISTA should be used with caution in this age group (see sections 4.4 and 5.2).

Hepatic impairment

Darunavir is metabolised by the hepatic system. No dose adjustment is recommended in patients with mild (Child-Pugh Class A) or moderate (Child-Pugh Class B) hepatic impairment, however, PREZISTA should be used with caution in these patients. No pharmacokinetic data are available in patients with severe hepatic impairment. Severe hepatic impairment could result in an increase of darunavir exposure and a worsening of its safety profile. Therefore, PREZISTA must not be used in patients with severe hepatic impairment (Child-Pugh Class C) (see sections 4.3, 4.4 and 5.2).

Renal impairment

No dose adjustment is required in patients with renal impairment (see sections 4.4 and 5.2).

In case a dose of PREZISTA and/or ritonavir was missed within 6 hours of the time it is usually taken, patients should be instructed to take the prescribed dose of PREZISTA and ritonavir with food as soon as possible. If this was noticed later than 6 hours of the time it is usually taken, the missed dose should not be taken and the patient should resume the usual dosing schedule.

This guidance is based on the 15 hour half-life of darunavir in the presence of ritonavir and the recommended dosing interval of approximately 12 hours.

4.3 Contraindications
Hypersensitivity to the active substance or to any of the excipients.

Patients with severe (Child-Pugh Class C) hepatic impairment.

Combination of rifampicin with PREZISTA with concomitant low dose ritonavir is contraindicated (see section 4.5).

The combination product lopinavir/ritonavir should not be used with PREZISTA because co-administration causes large decreases in darunavir concentrations, which may in turn significantly decrease the darunavir therapeutic effect (see section 4.5).

Herbal preparations containing St John's wort (*Hypericum perforatum*) must not be used while taking PREZISTA due to the risk of decreased plasma concentrations and reduced clinical effects of darunavir (see section 4.5).

Co-administration of PREZISTA with low dose ritonavir, with active substances that are highly dependent on CYP3A for clearance and for which elevated plasma concentrations are associated with serious and/or life-threatening events is contraindicated. These active substances include e.g. antiarrhythmics (amiodarone, bepridil, quinidine, systemic lidocaine), antihistamines (astemizole, terfenadine), ergot derivatives (e.g. dihydroergotamine, ergonovine, ergotamine, methylergonovine), gastrointestinal motility agents (cisapride), neuroleptics (pimozide, sertindole), sedatives/hypnotics [triazolam, midazolam administered orally (for caution on parenterally administered midazolam, see section 4.5)] and HMG-CoA reductase inhibitors (simvastatin and lovastatin) (see section 4.5).

4.4 Special warnings and precautions for use
Patients should be advised that current antiretroviral therapy does not cure HIV and has not been proven to prevent the transmission of HIV to others through blood or sexual contact. Appropriate precautions should continue to be employed.

PREZISTA should only be used in combination with low dose ritonavir as a pharmacokinetic enhancer (see section 5.2).

Increasing the dose of ritonavir from that recommended in section 4.2 did not significantly affect darunavir concentrations and is not recommended.

PREZISTA is not recommended for use in children below 6 years of age or less than 20 kg body weight (see sections 4.2 and 5.3).

Elderly: As limited information is available on the use of PREZISTA in patients aged 65 and over, caution should be exercised in the administration of PREZISTA in elderly patients, reflecting the greater frequency of decreased hepatic function and of concomitant disease or other therapy (see sections 4.2 and 5.2).

Darunavir binds predominantly to α1-acid glycoprotein. This protein binding is concentration dependent indicative for saturation of binding. Therefore, protein displacement of medicinal products highly bound to α1-acid glycoprotein cannot be ruled out.

Severe skin rash, which may be accompanied with fever and/or elevations of transaminases, has occurred in 0.5% of patients treated with PREZISTA. Erythema multiforme and Stevens-Johnson Syndrome have been rarely (< 0.1%) observed. Treatment with PREZISTA should be discontinued if such a condition develops.

Darunavir contains a sulphonamide moiety. PREZISTA should be used with caution in patients with a known sulphonamide allergy.

Patients with coexisting conditions

Hepatic impairment

The safety and efficacy of PREZISTA have not been established in patients with severe underlying liver disorders and PREZISTA is therefore contraindicated in patients with severe hepatic impairment. Due to an increase in the unbound darunavir plasma concentrations, PREZISTA should be used with caution in patients with mild or moderate hepatic impairment (see sections 4.2, 4.3 and 5.2).

Patients with chronic hepatitis B or C and treated with combination antiretroviral therapy are at an increased risk for severe and potentially fatal hepatic adverse events. In case of concomitant antiviral therapy for hepatitis B or C, please refer to the relevant product information for these medicinal products.

Patients with pre-existing liver dysfunction including chronic hepatitis have an increased frequency of liver function abnormalities during combination antiretroviral therapy and should be monitored according to standard practice. If there is evidence of worsening liver disease in such patients, interruption or discontinuation of treatment should be considered.

Renal impairment

No special precautions or dose adjustments are required in patients with renal impairment. As darunavir and ritonavir are highly bound to plasma proteins, it is unlikely that they will be significantly removed by haemodialysis or peritoneal dialysis. Therefore, no special precautions or dose adjustments are required in these patients (see sections 4.2 and 5.2).

Haemophiliac patients

There have been reports of increased bleeding, including spontaneous skin haematomas and haemarthrosis in patients with haemophilia type A and B treated with PIs. In some patients additional factor VIII was given. In more than half of the reported cases, treatment with PIs was continued or reintroduced if treatment had been discontinued. A causal relationship has been suggested, although the mechanism of action has not been elucidated. Haemophiliac patients should therefore be made aware of the possibility of increased bleeding.

Diabetes mellitus/Hyperglycaemia

New onset diabetes mellitus, hyperglycaemia, or exacerbation of existing diabetes mellitus has been reported in patients receiving antiretroviral therapy, including PIs. In some of these patients the hyperglycaemia was severe and in some cases also associated with ketoacidosis. Many patients had confounding medical conditions some of which required therapy with agents that have been associated with the development of diabetes mellitus or hyperglycaemia.

Fat redistribution and metabolic disorders

Combination antiretroviral therapy has been associated with redistribution of body fat (lipodystrophy) in HIV infected patients. The long-term consequences of these events are currently unknown. Knowledge about the mechanism is incomplete. A connection between visceral lipomatosis and PIs and lipoatrophy and NRTIs has been hypothesised. A higher risk of lipodystrophy has been associated with individual factors such as older age and with drug related factors such as longer duration of antiretroviral treatment and associated metabolic disturbances. Clinical examination should include evaluation for physical signs of fat redistribution. Consideration should be given to measurement of fasting serum lipids and blood glucose. Lipid disorders should be managed as clinically appropriate (see section 4.8).

Osteonecrosis

Although the etiology is considered to be multifactorial (including corticosteroid use, alcohol consumption, severe immunosuppression, higher body mass index), cases of osteonecrosis have been reported particularly in patients with advanced HIV disease and/or long-term exposure to combination antiretroviral therapy (CART). Patients should be advised to seek medical advice if they experience joint aches and pain, joint stiffness or difficulty in movement.

Immune reactivation syndrome

In HIV infected patients with severe immune deficiency at the time of institution of combination antiretroviral therapy (CART), an inflammatory reaction to asymptomatic or residual opportunistic pathogens may arise and cause serious clinical conditions, or aggravation of symptoms. Typically, such reactions have been observed within the first weeks or months of initiation of CART. Relevant examples are cytomegalovirus retinitis, generalised and/or focal mycobacterial infections and pneumonia caused by *Pneumocystis jiroveci* (formerly known as *Pneumocystis carinii*). Any inflammatory symptoms should be evaluated and treatment instituted when necessary. In addition, reactivation of herpes simplex and herpes zoster has been observed in clinical studies with PREZISTA co-administered with low dose ritonavir.

Interactions with medicinal products

Several of the interaction studies have been performed at lower than recommended doses of darunavir. The effects on co-administered medicinal products may thus be underestimated and clinical monitoring of safety may be indicated. For full information on interactions with other medicinal products see section 4.5.

PREZISTA tablets contain sunset yellow FCF (E110) which may cause an allergic reaction.

4.5 Interaction with other medicinal products and other forms of interaction

Darunavir and ritonavir are both inhibitors of the CYP3A4 isoform. Co-administration of darunavir and ritonavir and medicinal products primarily metabolised by CYP3A4 may result in increased systemic exposure to such medicinal products, which could increase or prolong their therapeutic effect and adverse reactions.

PREZISTA co-administered with low dose ritonavir must not be combined with medicinal products that are highly dependent on CYP3A4 for clearance and for which increased systemic exposure is associated with serious and/or life-threatening events (narrow therapeutic index). These medicinal products include amiodarone, bepridil, quinidine, systemic lidocaine, astemizole, terfenadine, midazolam administered orally, triazolam, cisapride, pimozide, sertindole, simvastatin, lovastatin and the ergot alkaloids (e.g. ergotamine, dihydroergotamine, ergonovine and methylergonovine) (see section 4.3).

The overall pharmacokinetic enhancement effect by ritonavir was an approximate 14-fold increase in the systemic exposure of darunavir when a single dose of 600 mg darunavir was given orally in combination with ritonavir at 100 mg b.i.d. Therefore, PREZISTA must only be used in combination with low dose ritonavir as a pharmacokinetic enhancer (see sections 4.4 and 5.2).

A clinical study utilising a cocktail of medicinal products that are metabolised by cytochromes CYP2C9, CYP2C19 and CYP2D6 demonstrated an increase in CYP2C9 and CYP2C19 activity and inhibition of CYP2D6 activity in the presence of PREZISTA/rtv, which may be attributed to the presence of low dose ritonavir. Co-administration of darunavir and ritonavir and medicinal products which are primarily metabolised by CYP2D6 (such as flecainide, propafenone, metoprolol) may result in increased plasma concentrations of these medicinal products, which could increase or prolong their therapeutic effect and adverse reactions. Co-administration of darunavir and ritonavir and medicinal products primarily metabolised by CYP2C9 (such as warfarin) and CYP2C19 (such as methadone) may result in decreased systemic exposure to such medicinal products, which could decrease or shorten their therapeutic effect.

Although the effect on CYP2C8 has only been studied *in vitro*, co-administration of darunavir and ritonavir and medicinal products primarily metabolised by CYP2C8 (such as paclitaxel, rosiglitazone, repaglinide) may result in decreased systemic exposure to such medicinal products, which could decrease or shorten their therapeutic effect.

Medicinal products that affect darunavir/ritonavir exposure

Darunavir and ritonavir are metabolised by CYP3A. Medicinal products that induce CYP3A activity would be expected to increase the clearance of darunavir and ritonavir, resulting in lowered plasma concentrations of darunavir and ritonavir (e.g. rifampicin, St John's wort, lopinavir). Co-administration of darunavir and ritonavir and other medicinal products that inhibit CYP3A may decrease the clearance of darunavir and ritonavir and may result in increased plasma concentrations of darunavir and ritonavir (e.g. indinavir, systemic azoles like ketoconazole and clotrimazole). These interactions are described in the interaction tables below.

Interaction table

Interactions between darunavir/ritonavir and protease inhibitors, antiretroviral agents other than protease inhibitors and other non-antiretroviral medicinal products are listed in the tables below (increase is indicated as "↑", decrease as "↓", no change as "↔", not determined as "ND", twice daily as "b.i.d.", once daily as "q.d." and once every other day as "q.o.d.").

Several of the interaction studies (indicated by # in the table below) have been performed at lower than recommended doses of darunavir or with a different dosing regimen (see section 4.2 Posology). The effects on co-administered medicinal products may thus be underestimated and clinical monitoring of safety may be indicated.

Interactions – Darunavir/ritonavir with Protease Inhibitors

The efficacy and safety of the use of PREZISTA with low dose ritonavir and any other PI (e.g. (fos)amprenavir, nelfinavir and tipranavir) has not been established in HIV patients. Generally, dual therapy with protease inhibitors is not recommended.

(see Table 1 on next page)

4.6 Pregnancy and lactation

Pregnancy

There are no adequate and well controlled studies with darunavir in pregnant women. Studies in animals do not indicate direct harmful effects with respect to pregnancy, embryonal/foetal development, parturition or postnatal development (see section 5.3).

PREZISTA co-administered with low dose ritonavir should be used during pregnancy only if the potential benefit justifies the potential risk.

Breast-feeding

It is not known whether darunavir is excreted in human milk. Studies in rats have demonstrated that darunavir is excreted in milk and at high levels (1,000 mg/kg/day) resulted in toxicity. Because of both the potential for HIV transmission and the potential for adverse reactions in breast-fed infants, mothers should be instructed not to breast-feed under any circumstances if they are receiving PREZISTA.

Fertility

No human data on the effect of darunavir on fertility are available. There was no effect on mating or fertility with darunavir treatment in rats (see section 5.3).

4.7 Effects on ability to drive and use machines

No studies on the effects of PREZISTA in combination with ritonavir on the ability to drive and use machines have been performed. However, dizziness has been reported in some patients during treatment with regimens containing PREZISTA co-administered with low dose ritonavir and should be borne in mind when considering a patient's ability to drive or operate machinery (see section 4.8).

4.8 Undesirable effects

Adult patients

The adverse drug reactions are derived from Phase IIb and Phase III trials, in which a total of 1,968 treatment-experienced patients initiated therapy with the recommended dose of PREZISTA 600 mg with ritonavir 100 mg twice daily. Median exposure to PREZISTA/ritonavir in this group was 37.3 weeks. Thirty percent of these patients experienced at least one adverse drug reaction of at least grade 2 severity. The most frequent (⩾ 2%) of those were diarrhoea (3.9%), hypertriglyceridaemia (3.8%), rash (2.8%), nausea (2.6%), hypercholesterolaemia (2.5%) and headache (2.0%).

2.6% of the patients discontinued treatment due to adverse reactions.

Adverse reactions are listed by system organ class (SOC) and frequency. Within each frequency grouping, adverse reactions are presented in order of decreasing seriousness. Frequencies are defined as very common (⩾ 1/10), common (⩾ 1/100 to < 1/10) and uncommon (⩾ 1/1,000 to < 1/100).

(see Table 2 on page 4931868)

In clinical trials (n=1,968), rash (all grades, at least possibly related) occurred in 5.6% of patients treated with PREZISTA. Rash was mostly mild to moderate, often occurring within the first four weeks of treatment and resolving with continued dosing. Grade 2-4 rash was reported in 2.9% of patients. The discontinuation rate due to rash in patients using PREZISTA co-administered with 100 mg ritonavir was 0.5%.

Severe cases of skin rash, including erythema multiforme and Stevens-Johnson Syndrome (both rare) have been reported in ongoing clinical trials with PREZISTA co-administered with 100 mg ritonavir.

The safety assessment in antiretroviral treatment-naïve adult patients (n=343) is based on all safety data from the Phase III trial ARTEMIS comparing PREZISTA/rtv 800/100 mg q.d. versus lopinavir/ritonavir 800/200 mg per day. Median exposure in the PREZISTA/ritonavir group was 56.3 weeks.

0.6% of the patients discontinued treatment due to adverse drug reactions.

In these treatment naïve-patients, the following adverse drug reactions were identified:

ADRs of at least moderate intensity and reported in more than one patient

Common: hypertriglyceridaemia, hypercholesterolaemia, headache, diarrhoea, nausea, increased alanine aminotransferase.

Uncommon: hyperlipidaemia, vomiting, abdominal pain, increased aspartate aminotransferase, rash (including maculopapular rash), allergic dermatitis, pruritus.

ADRs of all severity grades and reported in more than one patient

Very common: diarrhoea, nausea.

Common: hypertriglyceridaemia, hypercholesterolaemia, anorexia, insomnia, headache, dizziness, dysgeusia, vomiting, abdominal pain, abdominal discomfort, abdominal distension, flatulence, increased alanine aminotransferase, rash (including maculopapular, papular rash), alopecia, dry skin, pruritus, fatigue.

Uncommon: upper respiratory tract infection, diabetes mellitus, hyperlipidaemia, abnormal dreams, hypoaesthesia, disturbance in attention, somnolence, dyspepsia, eructation, increased aspartate aminotransferase, allergic dermatitis, urticaria, dermatitis, night sweats, myalgia, muscle spasms, asthenia.

Combination antiretroviral therapy has been associated with redistribution of body fat (lipodystrophy) in HIV patients, including loss of peripheral and facial subcutaneous fat, increased intra-abdominal and visceral fat, breast hypertrophy and dorsocervical fat accumulation (buffalo hump) (see section 4.4).

Combination antiretroviral therapy has also been associated with metabolic abnormalities such as hypertriglyceridaemia, hypercholesterolaemia, insulin resistance, hyperglycaemia and hyperlactataemia (see section 4.4).

Increased CPK, myalgia, myositis and rarely, rhabdomyolysis have been reported with the use of protease inhibitors, particularly in combination with NRTIs.

Cases of osteonecrosis have been reported, particularly in patients with generally acknowledged risk factors, advanced HIV disease or long-term exposure to combination antiretroviral therapy (CART). The frequency of this is unknown (see section 4.4).

In HIV infected patients with severe immune deficiency at the time of initiation of combination antiretroviral therapy, an inflammatory reaction to asymptomatic or residual opportunistic infections may arise (see section 4.4).

There have been reports of increased spontaneous bleeding in haemophiliac patients receiving antiretroviral protease inhibitors (see section 4.4).

Children and adolescents

The safety assessment in children and adolescents is based on the safety data from the Phase II trial DELPHI in which 80 ART-experienced HIV-1 infected paediatric patients aged from 6 to 17 years and weighing at least 20 kg received PREZISTA with low dose ritonavir in combination with other antiretroviral agents (see section 5.1).

Overall, the safety profile in these 80 children and adolescents was similar to that observed in the adult population.

Patients co-infected with hepatitis B and/or hepatitis C virus

Among 1,968 treatment-experienced patients receiving PREZISTA co-administered with ritonavir 600/100 mg b.i.d., 236 patients were co-infected with hepatitis B or C. Co-infected patients were more likely to have baseline and treatment emergent hepatic transaminase elevations than those without chronic viral hepatitis (see section 4.4).

4.9 Overdose

Human experience of acute overdose with PREZISTA co-administered with low dose ritonavir is limited. Single doses up to 3,200 mg of darunavir as oral solution alone and up to 1,600 mg of the tablet formulation of darunavir in combination with ritonavir have been administered to healthy volunteers without untoward symptomatic effects.

There is no specific antidote for overdose with PREZISTA. Treatment of overdose with PREZISTA consists of general supportive measures including monitoring of vital signs and observation of the clinical status of the patient. If indicated, elimination of unabsorbed active substance is to be achieved by emesis or gastric lavage. Administration of activated charcoal may also be used to aid in removal of unabsorbed active substance. Since darunavir is highly protein bound, dialysis is unlikely to be beneficial in significant removal of the active substance.

5. PHARMACOLOGICAL PROPERTIES

5.1 Pharmacodynamic properties

Pharmacotherapeutic group: Antiviral for systemic use, ATC code: J05AE10.

Mechanism of action

Darunavir is an inhibitor of the dimerisation and of the catalytic activity of the HIV-1 protease (K_D of 4.5×10^{-12}M). It selectively inhibits the cleavage of HIV encoded Gag-Pol polyproteins in virus infected cells, thereby preventing the formation of mature infectious virus particles.

Antiviral activity *in vitro*

Darunavir exhibits activity against laboratory strains and clinical isolates of HIV-1 and laboratory strains of HIV-2 in acutely infected T-cell lines, human peripheral blood mononuclear cells and human monocytes/macrophages with median EC_{50} values ranging from 1.2 to 8.5 nM (0.7 to 5.0 ng/ml). Darunavir demonstrates antiviral activity *in vitro* against a broad panel of HIV-1 group M (A, B, C, D, E, F, G) and group O primary isolates with EC_{50} values ranging from < 0.1 to 4.3 nM.

These EC_{50} values are well below the 50% cellular toxicity concentration range of 87 μM to > 100 μM.

The EC_{50} value of darunavir increases by a median factor of 5.4 in the presence of human serum.

Darunavir showed synergistic antiviral activity when studied in combination with the protease inhibitors ritonavir, nelfinavir, or amprenavir and additive antiviral activity when studied in combination with the protease inhibitors indinavir, saquinavir, lopinavir, atazanavir, or tipranavir, the N(t)RTIs zidovudine, lamivudine, zalcitabine, didanosine, stavudine, abacavir, emtricitabine, or tenofovir, the NNRTIs nevirapine, delavirdine, or efavirenz and the fusion inhibitor enfuvirtide. No antagonism was observed between darunavir and any of those antiretrovirals.

Table 1

Co-administered Medicinal Product	Dose of Co-administered Medicinal Product (mg)	Dose of darunavir/ritonavir (mg)	Medicinal Product Assessed	AUC	C_{min}
Lopinavir/ritonavir	400/100 b.i.d. 533/133.3 b.i.d.	1,200/100 b.i.d. 1,200 b.i.d.	Lopinavir Darunavir Lopinavir Darunavir	↔ ↓ 38%* ↔ ↓ 41%	↔ ↓ 51%* ↔ ↓ 55%
	* based upon not dose normalised values Due to a decrease in the exposure (AUC) of darunavir by 40%, appropriate doses of the combination have not been established. Hence, concomitant use of PREZISTA co-administered with low dose ritonavir and the combination product lopinavir/ritonavir is contraindicated (see section 4.3).				
Saquinavir	1,000 b.i.d.	400/100 b.i.d.#	Darunavir	↓ 26%	↓ 42%
	The study with boosted saquinavir showed no significant effect of darunavir on saquinavir. It is not recommended to combine PREZISTA co-administered with low dose ritonavir with saquinavir.				
Indinavir	800 b.i.d.	400/100 b.i.d.#	Indinavir Darunavir	↑ 23% ↑ 24%	↑ 125% ↑ 44%
	When used in combination with PREZISTA co-administered with low dose ritonavir, dose adjustment of indinavir from 800 mg b.i.d. to 600 mg b.i.d. may be warranted in case of intolerance.				
Atazanavir	300 q.d.	400/100 b.i.d.#	Atazanavir Darunavir	↔ ↔	↔ ↔
	Darunavir/ritonavir did not significantly affect atazanavir exposure, however 90% CI for C_{min} were 99-234%. Atazanavir can be used with PREZISTA co-administered with low dose ritonavir.				
Interactions – Darunavir/ritonavir with Antiretroviral Agents other than Protease Inhibitors					
Co-administered Medicinal Product	**Dose of Co-administered Medicinal Product (mg)**	**Dose of darunavir/ritonavir (mg)**	**Medicinal Product Assessed**	**AUC**	**C_{min}**
Efavirenz	600 q.d.	300/100 b.i.d.	Efavirenz Darunavir	↑ 21% ↓ 13%	↑ 17% ↓ 31%
	Efavirenz decreases the plasma concentrations of darunavir as a result of CYP3A4 induction. Darunavir/ritonavir increases the plasma concentrations of efavirenz as a result of CYP3A4 inhibition. Clinical monitoring for central nervous system toxicity associated with increased exposure to efavirenz may be indicated when PREZISTA co-administered with low dose ritonavir is given in combination with efavirenz.				
Etravirine	100 b.i.d.*	600/100 b.i.d.	Etravirine Darunavir	↓ 37% ↔	↓ 49% ↔
	* dose used in drug-interaction study. For recommended dose see paragraph below. There was a 37% decrease in etravirine exposure in the presence of darunavir/ritonavir and no relevant change in exposure to darunavir. Therefore, PREZISTA co-administered with low dose ritonavir can be co-administered with etravirine **200 mg b.i.d.** without dose adjustments.				
Nevirapine	200 b.i.d.	400/100 b.i.d.#	Nevirapine Darunavir	↑ 27% ↔	↑ 47% ↔
	Darunavir/ritonavir increases the plasma concentrations of nevirapine as a result of CYP3A4 inhibition. Since this difference is not considered to be clinically relevant, the combination of PREZISTA co-administered with low dose ritonavir and nevirapine can be used without dose adjustments.				
Tenofovir	300 q.d.	300/100 b.i.d.#	Tenofovir Darunavir	↑ 22% ↔	↑ 37% ↔
	Ritonavir effect on MDR-1 transport in renal tubuli has been a proposed mechanism for increased plasma concentrations of tenofovir. Monitoring of renal function may be indicated when PREZISTA co-administered with low dose ritonavir is given in combination with tenofovir, particularly in patients with underlying systemic or renal disease, or in patients taking nephrotoxic agents.				
Zidovudine Zalcitabine Emtricitabine Stavudine Lamivudine Abacavir	Based on the different elimination pathways of the other NRTIs zidovudine, zalcitabine, emtricitabine, stavudine, lamivudine, that are primarily renally excreted, and abacavir for which metabolism is not mediated by CYP450, no interactions are expected for these medicinal compounds and PREZISTA co-administered with low dose ritonavir.				
Didanosine	400 q.d.	600/100 b.i.d.	Didanosine Darunavir	↔ ↔	NA ↔
	Didanosine was administered on an empty stomach 2 hours prior to administration of darunavir/ritonavir. Systemic exposure to darunavir co-administered with low dose ritonavir, with or without didanosine was comparable. The combination of PREZISTA co-administered with low dose ritonavir and didanosine can be used without dose adjustments.				
Maraviroc	150 b.i.d.	600/100 b.i.d.	Maraviroc Darunavir	↑ 305% ↔	ND ND
	The maraviroc dose should be 150 mg twice daily when co-administered with PREZISTA with low dose ritonavir. Darunavir/ritonavir concentrations were consistent with historical data.				
Interactions – Darunavir/ritonavir with Non-antiretroviral co-administered Medicinal Products					
Co-administered Medicinal Product	**Dose of Co-administered Medicinal Product (mg)**	**Dose of darunavir/ritonavir (mg)**	**Medicinal Product Assessed**	**AUC**	**C_{min}**
Antiarrhythmics					
Digoxin	0.4 mg single dose	600/100 b.i.d.	Digoxin	↑ 60%	ND
	Darunavir/ritonavir increases the plasma concentrations of digoxin. Inhibition of Pgp may be a likely explanation. Given that digoxin has as a narrow therapeutic index, it is recommended that the lowest possible dose of digoxin should initially be prescribed in case digoxin is given to patients on darunavir/ritonavir therapy. The digoxin dose should be carefully titrated to obtain the desired clinical effect while assessing the overall clinical state of the subject.				
Antibiotics					
Clarithromycin	500 b.i.d.	400/100 b.i.d.#	Clarithromycin Darunavir	↑ 57% ↔	↑ 174% ↔
	Darunavir/ritonavir increases the plasma concentrations of clarithromycin as a result of CYP3A4 inhibition and possible Pgp inhibition. Concentrations of the metabolite 14-OH-clarithromycin were not detectable. Caution is warranted and clinical monitoring is recommended. For patients with renal impairment, a dose reduction of clarithromycin should be considered.				
Anticoagulant					
Warfarin	Warfarin concentrations may be affected when co-administered with darunavir with ritonavir. The international normalised ratio (INR) should be monitored when warfarin is combined with PREZISTA co-administered with low dose ritonavir.				
Anticonvulsants					
Phenobarbital Phenytoin	Phenobarbital and phenytoin are inducers of CYP450 enzymes. PREZISTA co-administered with low dose ritonavir should not be used in combination with these medicines, as co-administration may cause significant decreases in darunavir plasma concentrations.				
Carbamazepine	200 b.i.d.	600/100 b.i.d.	Carbamazepine Darunavir	↑ 45% ↔	↑ 54% ↔
	Exposure to darunavir, co-administered with ritonavir, was unaffected by carbamazepine. Ritonavir exposure (AUC12h) was decreased by 49%. For carbamazepine, AUC12h was increased by 45%. No dose adjustment for PREZISTA/ritonavir is recommended. If there is a need to combine PREZISTA/ritonavir and carbamazepine, patients should be monitored for potential carbamazepine-related adverse events. Carbamazepine concentrations should be monitored and its dose should be titrated for adequate response. Based upon the findings, the carbamazepine dose may need to be reduced by 25% to 50% in the presence of PREZISTA/ritonavir.				
Antifungals					
Voriconazole	The combined use of voriconazole with darunavir co-administered with low dose ritonavir has not been studied. Voriconazole is metabolised by cytochrome P450 isoenzymes, CYP2C19, CYP2C9 and CYP3A4. Ritonavir, which can induce some of these isoenzymes, may decrease voriconazole plasma concentrations. Voriconazole should not be co-administered with PREZISTA with low dose ritonavir unless an assessment of the benefit/risk ratio justifies the use of voriconazole.				
Ketoconazole	200 b.i.d.	400/100 b.i.d.#	Ketoconazole Darunavir	↑ 212% ↑ 42%	↑ 868% ↑ 73%
	Ketoconazole is a potent inhibitor as well as substrate of CYP3A4. Caution is warranted and clinical monitoring is recommended. When co-administration is required the daily dose of ketoconazole should not exceed 200 mg.				
Itraconazole	Itraconazole, like ketoconazole, is a potent inhibitor as well as substrate of CYP3A4. Concomitant systemic use of itraconazole and darunavir co-administered with low dose ritonavir may increase plasma concentrations of darunavir. Simultaneously, plasma concentrations of itraconazole may be increased by darunavir co-administered with low dose ritonavir. Caution is warranted and clinical monitoring is recommended. When co-administration is required the daily dose of itraconazole should not exceed 200 mg.				

Co-administered Medicinal Product	Dose of Co-administered Medicinal Product (mg)	Dose of darunavir/ritonavir (mg)	Medicinal Product Assessed	AUC	C_{min}
Clotrimazole	Concomitant systemic use of clotrimazole and darunavir co-administered with low dose ritonavir may increase plasma concentrations of darunavir. This was confirmed using a population pharmacokinetic model. The increase in the median darunavir AUC_{24h} value for the patients taking clotrimazole from the overall median was 33%. Caution is warranted and clinical monitoring is recommended, when co-administration of clotrimazole is required.				
Calcium channel blockers					
Felodipine Nifedipine Nicardipine	Darunavir and ritonavir inhibit CYP3A4 and as a result can be expected to increase the plasma concentrations of calcium channel antagonists, which are CYP3A4 substrates. Clinical monitoring of therapeutic and adverse effects is recommended when these medicines are concomitantly administered with PREZISTA with low dose ritonavir.				
HMG Co-A Reductase Inhibitors					
Lovastatin Simvastatin	Lovastatin and simvastatin, which are highly dependent on CYP3A4 metabolism are expected to have markedly increased plasma concentrations when co-administered with darunavir co-administered with low dose ritonavir. This may cause myopathy, including rhabdomyolysis. Concomitant use of PREZISTA co-administered with low dose ritonavir with lovastatin and simvastatin is therefore contraindicated (see section 4.3).				
Atorvastatin	10 q.d.	300/100 b.i.d.#	Atorvastatin Darunavir	3-4 times ↑ ND	3-4 times ↑ ND
	The results of this interaction trial show that atorvastatin (10 mg q.d.) in combination with darunavir/ritonavir (300/100 mg b.i.d.) provides an exposure to atorvastatin, which is only 15% lower than that obtained with (40 mg q.d.) atorvastatin alone. When administration of atorvastatin and PREZISTA co-administered with low dose ritonavir is desired, it is recommended to start with an atorvastatin dose of 10 mg q.d. A gradual dose increase of atorvastatin may be tailored to the clinical response.				
Pravastatin	40 mg single dose	600/100 b.i.d.	Pravastatin	0-5 times ↑	ND
	Darunavir/ritonavir did not increase exposure to a single dose of pravastatin in most subjects but up to 5-fold in a limited subset of subjects. When administration of pravastatin and PREZISTA co-administered with low dose ritonavir is required, it is recommended to start with the lowest possible dose of pravastatin and titrate it up to the desired clinical effect while monitoring for safety.				
Hormonal contraceptive					
Ethinylestradiol Norethindrone	35 μg/1 mg q.d.	600/100 b.i.d.	Ethinylestradiol Norethindrone	↓ 44% ↓ 14%	↓ 62% ↓ 30%
	Alternative or additional contraceptive measures are recommended when oestrogen-based contraceptives are co-administered with PREZISTA and low dose ritonavir. Patients using oestrogens as hormone replacement therapy should be clinically monitored for signs of oestrogen deficiency.				
Immunosupressants					
Cyclosporine Tacrolimus Sirolimus	Exposure to cyclosporine, tacrolimus, or sirolimus will be increased when co-administered with PREZISTA co-administered with low dose ritonavir. Therapeutic drug monitoring of the immunosuppressive agent must be done when co-administration occurs.				
H_2-receptor antagonists and proton pump inhibitors					
Ranitidine	150 b.i.d.	400/100 b.i.d.#	Darunavir	↔	↔
	Based on these results, PREZISTA co-administered with low dose ritonavir can be co-administered with H_2-receptor antagonists without dose adjustments.				
Omeprazole	20 q.d.	400/100 b.i.d.#	Darunavir	↔	↔
	Based on these results, PREZISTA co-administered with low dose ritonavir can be co-administered with proton pump inhibitors without dose adjustments.				
Opiods					
Methadone	55-150 q.d.	600/100 b.i.d. (dosed for 7 days)	R-methadone	↓ 16%	↓ 15%
	Based on pharmacokinetic and clinical findings, no adjustment of methadone dosage is required when initiating co-administration with PREZISTA/ritonavir. However, increased methadone dose may be necessary when concomitantly administered for a longer period of time due to induction of metabolism by ritonavir. Therefore, clinical monitoring is recommended, as maintenance therapy may need to be adjusted in some patients.				
PDE-5 inhibitors					
Sildenafil Vardenafil Tadalafil	In an interaction study a comparable systemic exposure to sildenafil was observed for a single intake of 100 mg sildenafil alone and a single intake of 25 mg sildenafil co-administered with darunavir/ritonavir (400/100 mg b.i.d.). Concomitant use of PDE-5 inhibitors with PREZISTA co-administered with low dose ritonavir should be done with caution. If concomitant use of PREZISTA co-administered with low dose ritonavir with sildenafil, vardenafil, or tadalafil is indicated, sildenafil at a single dose not exceeding 25 mg in 48 hours, vardenafil at a single dose not exceeding 2.5 mg dose in 72 hours or tadalafil at a single dose not exceeding 10 mg dose in 72 hours is recommended.				
Rifamycines					
Rifampicin	Rifampicin is a strong CYP3A4 inducer and has been shown to cause profound decreases in concentrations of other protease inhibitors, which can result in virological failure and resistance development. During attempts to overcome the decreased exposure by increasing the dose of other protease inhibitors with ritonavir, a high frequency of liver reactions was seen. The combination of rifampicin and PREZISTA with concomitant low dose ritonavir is contraindicated (see section 4.3).				
Rifabutin	150 q.o.d.	600/100 b.i.d.	Rifabutin* Darunavir	1.6 times ↑ ↑ 53%	ND ↑ 68%
	* sum of active moieties of rifabutin (parent drug + 25-*O*- desacetyl metabolite) A dose reduction of rifabutin by 75% of the usual dose of 300 mg/day [i.e. rifabutin 150 mg q.o.d. (once every other day)] and increased monitoring for rifabutin related adverse events is warranted in patients receiving the combination. In case of safety issues, a further increase of the dosing interval for rifabutin and/or monitoring of rifabutin levels should be considered. Consideration should be given to official guidance on the appropriate treatment of tuberculosis in HIV infected patients. Rifabutin is an inducer and substrate of CYP3A4. An increase of systemic exposure to darunavir was observed when PREZISTA co-administered with 100 mg ritonavir was co-administered with rifabutin [150 mg q.o.d. (once every other day)]. Based upon the safety profile of PREZISTA/ritonavir, this increase in darunavir exposure in the presence of rifabutin does not warrant a dose adjustment for PREZISTA/ritonavir. The interaction trial showed a comparable daily systemic exposure for rifabutin between treatment at 300 mg q.d. (once daily) alone and 150 mg q.o.d. (once every other day) in combination with PREZISTA/ritonavir (600/100 mg b.i.d.) with an about 10-fold increase in the daily exposure to the active metabolite 25-*O*- desacetylrifabutin. Furthermore, AUC of the sum of active moieties of rifabutin (parent drug + 25-*O*- desacetyl metabolite) was increased 1.6-fold, while C_{max} remained comparable. Data on comparison with a 150 mg q.d. (once daily) reference dose is lacking.				
Sedatives/Hypnotics					
Parenteral midazolam	Midazolam is extensively metabolised by CYP3A4. Co-administration with PREZISTA/ritonavir may cause a large increase in the concentration of this benzodiazepine. No drug interaction study has been performed for the co-administration of PREZISTA/ritonavir with benzodiazepines. Based on data for other CYP3A4 inhibitors, plasma concentrations of midazolam are expected to be significantly higher when midazolam is given orally. Therefore PREZISTA/ritonavir should not be co-administered with orally administered midazolam (see section 4.3), whereas caution should be used with co-administration of PREZISTA/ritonavir and parenteral midazolam. Data from concomitant use of parenteral midazolam with other protease inhibitors suggest a possible 3-4 fold increase in midazolam plasma levels. If PREZISTA/ritonavir is co-administered with parenteral midazolam, it should be done in an intensive care unit (ICU) or similar setting, which ensures close clinical monitoring and appropriate medical management in case of respiratory depression and/or prolonged sedation. Dosage adjustment for midazolam should be considered, especially if more than a single dose of midazolam is administered.				
Selective Serotonin Reuptake Inhibitors (SSRIs)					
Paroxetine	20 q.d.	400/100 b.i.d.#	Paroxetine Darunavir	↓ 39% ↔	↓ 37% ↔
Sertraline	50 q.d.	400/100 b.i.d.#	Sertraline Darunavir	↓ 49% ↔	↓ 49% ↔
	If SSRIs are co-administered with PREZISTA and ritonavir, the recommended approach is a dose titration of the SSRI based on a clinical assessment of antidepressant response. In addition, patients on a stable dose of sertraline or paroxetine who start treatment with PREZISTA co-administered with low dose ritonavir should be monitored for antidepressant response.				
Steroids					
Fluticasone propionate Budesonide	In a clinical study where ritonavir 100 mg capsules b.i.d were co-administered with 50 μg intranasal fluticasone propionate (4 times daily) for 7 days in healthy subjects, fluticasone propionate plasma concentrations increased significantly, whereas the intrinsic cortisol levels decreased by approximately 86% (90% confidence interval 82-89%). Greater effects may be expected when fluticasone propionate is inhaled. Systemic corticosteroid effects including Cushing's syndrome and adrenal suppression have been reported in patients receiving ritonavir and inhaled or intranasally administered fluticasone propionate; this could also occur with other corticosteroids metabolised via the P450 3A pathway e.g. budesonide. Consequently, concomitant administration of PREZISTA, co-administered with low dose ritonavir and these glucocorticoids, is not recommended unless the potential benefit of treatment outweighs the risk of systemic corticosteroid effects. A dose reduction of the glucocorticoid should be considered with close monitoring of local and systemic effects or a switch to a glucocorticoid, which is not a substrate for CYP3A4 (e.g. beclomethasone). Moreover, in case of withdrawal of glucocorticoids progressive dose reduction may have to be performed over a longer period. The effects of high fluticasone systemic exposure on ritonavir plasma levels are as yet unknown.				
Dexamethasone	Systemic dexamethasone induces CYP3A4 and thereby may decrease darunavir exposure. Therefore this combination should be used with caution.				
Others					
St. John's wort	PREZISTA co-administered with low dose ritonavir must not be used concomitantly with products containing St John's wort (*Hypericum perforatum*) because co-administration may cause significant decreases in darunavir plasma concentrations and also in ritonavir concentrations. This is due to the induction of metabolising enzymes by St John's wort. If a patient is already taking St John's wort, stop St John's wort and if possible check viral levels. Darunavir exposure (and also ritonavir exposure) may increase on stopping St John's wort. The inducing effect may persist for at least 2 weeks after cessation of treatment with St John's wort (see section 4.3).				

Table 2

SOC Frequency category	Adverse reaction* All grades	Adverse reaction** Grade 2-4
Infections and infestations		
uncommon	herpes simplex	
Blood and lymphatic system disorders		
uncommon	thrombocytopenia, neutropenia, anaemia, increased eosinophil count, leukopenia	thrombocytopenia, neutropenia, anaemia
Immune system disorders		
uncommon	immune reconstitution syndrome	immune reconstitution syndrome
Endocrine disorders		
uncommon	hypothyroidism, increased blood thyroid stimulating hormone	
Metabolism and nutrition disorders		
common	lipodystrophy (including lipohypertrophy, lipodystrophy, lipoatrophy), hypertriglyceridaemia, hypercholesterolaemia, hyperlipidaemia	hypertriglyceridaemia, hypercholesterolaemia, hyperlipidaemia
uncommon	diabetes mellitus, gout, anorexia, decreased appetite, decreased weight, increased weight, hyperglycaemia, insulin resistance, decreased high density lipoprotein, increased appetite, polydipsia, increased blood lactate dehydrogenase	diabetes mellitus, lipodystrophy (including lipohypertrophy, lipodystrophy, lipoatrophy), gout, anorexia, decreased appetite, decreased weight, increased weight, hyperglycaemia, insulin resistance
Psychiatric disorders		
common	insomnia	
uncommon	depression, confusional state, disorientation, anxiety, altered mood, sleep disorder, abnormal dreams, nightmare, decreased libido, restlessness	depression, confusional state, disorientation, anxiety, altered mood, insomnia, sleep disorder, abnormal dreams
Nervous system disorders		
common	headache, peripheral neuropathy, dizziness	headache
uncommon	syncope, convulsion, lethargy, paraesthesia, hypoaesthesia, ageusia, dysgeusia, disturbance in attention, memory impairment, somnolence, sleep phase rhythm disturbance	peripheral neuropathy, dizziness, lethargy, paraesthesia, hypoaesthesia, somnolence
Eye disorders		
uncommon	visual disturbance, conjunctival hyperaemia, dry eye	conjunctival hyperaemia
Ear and labyrinth disorders		
uncommon	vertigo	vertigo
Cardiac disorders		
uncommon	acute myocardial infarction, myocardial infarction, angina pectoris, prolonged electrocardiogram QT, sinus bradycardia, tachycardia, palpitations	acute myocardial infarction, myocardial infarction, angina pectoris, prolonged electrocardiogram QT
Vascular disorders		
uncommon	hypertension, flushing	hypertension
Respiratory, thoracic and mediastinal disorders		
uncommon	dyspnoea, cough, epistaxis, rhinorrhoea, throat irritation	dyspnoea, cough
Gastrointestinal disorders		
very common	diarrhoea	
common	vomiting, nausea, abdominal pain, increased blood amylase, dyspepsia, abdominal distension, flatulence	vomiting, diarrhoea, nausea, abdominal pain, increased blood amylase
uncommon	pancreatitis, gastritis, gastrooesophageal reflux disease, aphthous stomatitis, stomatitis, retching, haematemesis, dry mouth, abdominal discomfort, constipation, increased lipase, eructation, oral dysaesthesia, cheilitis, dry lip, coated tongue	pancreatitis, gastritis, gastrooesophageal reflux disease, aphthous stomatitis, retching, dry mouth, abdominal distension, abdominal discomfort, flatulence, dyspepsia, constipation, increased lipase
Hepatobiliary disorders		
common	increased alanine aminotransferase, increased aspartate aminotransferase	increased alanine aminotransferase
uncommon	hepatitis, cytolytic hepatitis, hepatic steatosis, hepatomegaly, increased transaminase, increased blood bilirubin, increased blood alkaline phosphatase, increased gamma-glutamyltransferase	hepatitis, cytolytic hepatitis, hepatic steatosis, increased transaminase, increased aspartate aminotransferase, increased blood alkaline phosphatase, increased gamma-glutamyltransferase
Skin and subcutaneous tissue disorders		
common	rash (including macular, maculopapular, papular, erythematous and pruritic rash), pruritus	rash (including macular, maculopapular, papular, erythematous and pruritic rash)
uncommon	generalised rash, allergic dermatitis, face oedema, urticaria, dermatitis, eczema, erythema, hyperhidrosis, night sweats, alopecia, acne, seborrhoeic dermatitis, skin lesion, xeroderma, dry skin, nail pigmentation	generalised rash, allergic dermatitis, urticaria, pruritus, hyperhidrosis, night sweats, alopecia
Musculoskeletal and connective tissue disorders		
uncommon	myalgia, muscle spasms, muscular weakness, musculoskeletal stiffness, arthritis, arthralgia, joint stiffness, pain in extremity, osteoporosis, increased blood creatine phosphokinase	myalgia, arthralgia, pain in extremity, osteoporosis, increased blood creatine phosphokinase
Renal and urinary disorders		
uncommon	acute renal failure, renal failure, nephrolithiasis, increased blood creatinine, decreased creatinine renal clearance, proteinuria, bilirubinuria, dysuria, nocturia, pollakiuria	acute renal failure, renal failure, nephrolithiasis, increased blood creatinine, decreased creatinine renal clearance, proteinuria, bilirubinuria
Reproductive system and breast disorders		
uncommon	erectile dysfunction, gynaecomastia	erectile dysfunction, gynaecomastia
General disorders and administration site conditions		
common	asthenia, fatigue	fatigue
uncommon	pyrexia, chest pain, peripheral oedema, malaise, chills, abnormal feeling, feeling hot, irritability, pain, xerosis	pyrexia, chest pain, asthenia, peripheral oedema, malaise

* Adverse events, considered at least possibly related by the investigator to PREZISTA co-administered with low dose ritonavir, occurring in more than 1 patient.

** Adverse events, at least grade 2 in severity and considered at least possibly related by the investigator to PREZISTA co-administered with low dose ritonavir, occurring in more than 1 patient.

Table 3

Outcomes	TITAN PREZISTA/rtv 600/100 mg b.i.d. + OBR N=298	lopinavir/rtv 400/100 mg b.i.d. + OBR N=297	Treatment difference (95% CI of difference)
HIV-1 RNA < 400 copies/ml[a]	228 (76.5%)	199 (67.0%)	9.5% (2.3; 16.7)[b]
HIV-1 RNA < 50 copies/ml[a]	211 (70.8%)	179 (60.3%)	10.5% (2.9; 18.1)[b]
mean HIV-1 RNA log change from baseline (log_{10} copies/ml)[c]	-1.95	-1.72	-0.23[d] (-0.44; -0.02)[b]
median CD4+ cell count change from baseline (x 10^6/l)[c]	88	81	

[a] Imputations according to the TLOVR algorithm

[b] Based on a normal approximation of the difference in % response

[c] NC=F

[d] Difference in means

Table 4

Outcomes at 48 weeks	POWER 1 and POWER 2 pooled data			POWER 3
Baseline characteristics				
Mean plasma HIV-1 RNA	4.61 log_{10} copies/ml (PREZISTA/ritonavir) 4.49 log_{10} copies/ml (control)			4.58 log_{10} copies/ml
Median CD4+ cell count	153 × 10^6 cells/l (PREZISTA/ritonavir) 163 × 10^6 cells/l (control)			120 × 10^6 cells/l
Outcomes	PREZISTA/ritonavir 600/100 mg b.i.d. n=131	Control n=124	Treatment difference	PREZISTA/ritonavir 600/100 mg b.i.d. n=334
HIV-1 RNA log_{10} mean change from baseline (log_{10} copies/ml)[a]	-1.69	-0.37	1.32 (1.58; 1.05)[d]	-1.62
CD4+ cell count mean change from baseline (x 10^6/l)[b]	103	17	86 (57; 114)[d]	105
HIV RNA ≥1 log_{10} below baseline[c]	81 (61.8%)	20 (16.1%)	45.7% (35.0%; 56.4%)[d]	196 (58.7%)
HIV RNA < 400 copies/ml[c]	72 (55.0%)	18 (14.5%)	40.4% (29.8%; 51.1%)[d]	183 (54.8%)
HIV RNA < 50 copies/ml[c]	59 (45.0%)	14 (11.3%)	33.7% (23.4%; 44.1%)[d]	155 (46.4%)

[a] Non-completer is failure imputation: patients who discontinued prematurely are imputed with a change equal to 0

[b] Last Observation Carried Forward imputation

[c] Imputations according to the TLOVR algorithm

[d] 95% confidence intervals.

Resistance

In vitro selection of darunavir-resistant virus from wild type HIV-1 was lengthy (> 3 years). The selected viruses were unable to grow in the presence of darunavir concentrations above 400 nM. Viruses selected in these conditions and showing decreased susceptibility to darunavir (range: 23-50-fold) harboured 2 to 4 amino acid substitutions in the protease gene. Identification of determinants of decreased susceptibility to darunavir in those viruses is under investigation.

In vitro selection of darunavir resistant HIV-1 (range: 53-641-fold change in EC_{50} values [FC]) from 9 HIV-1 strains harbouring multiple PI Resistance-Associated Mutations (RAMs) showed that a minimum of 8 darunavir *in vitro* selected mutations were required in the HIV-1 protease to render a virus resistant (FC > 10) to darunavir.

In a pooled analysis of the POWER 1, 2 and 3 (see Clinical experience subsection) and DUET 1 and 2 (TMC125-C206 and TMC125-C216) trials the amino acid substitutions identified that developed on PREZISTA co-administered with ritonavir (600/100 mg b.i.d.) in ≥ 20% of the isolates from subjects who experienced virologic failure by rebound were V32I, I54L and L89V. Amino acid substitutions that developed in 10 to 20% of the isolates were V11I, I13V, L33F, I50V and F53L. Amino acid substitutions that developed in 5 to 10% of isolates were L10F, I15V, M36L, K43T, M46I, I47V, A71I, G73S, T74P, L76V, V82I and I84V.

Of the viruses isolated from patients experiencing virologic failure by rebound from the PREZISTA/rtv 600/100 mg b.i.d. group of the POWER and DUET trials, 85% of those susceptible to darunavir at baseline developed decreased susceptibility to darunavir during treatment.

In the same group of patients, 71% of viruses that were susceptible to tipranavir at baseline remained susceptible after treatment.

Cross-resistance

Darunavir has a < 10-fold decreased susceptibility against 90% of 3,309 clinical isolates resistant to amprenavir, atazanavir, indinavir, lopinavir, nelfinavir, ritonavir, saquinavir and/or tipranavir showing that viruses resistant to most PIs remain susceptible to darunavir.

Clinical experience

Adult patients

Efficacy of PREZISTA co-administered with 100 mg ritonavir in treatment-naïve patients

There are no data on the efficacy of darunavir co-administered with 100 mg ritonavir in treatment-naïve HIV-1 infected patients.

Efficacy of PREZISTA co-administered with 100 mg ritonavir in treatment-experienced patients

The evidence of efficacy of PREZISTA co-administered with ritonavir (600/100 mg b.i.d.) in treatment-experienced patients is based on the 48 weeks analysis of the Phase III trial TITAN in treatment-experienced lopinavir naïve patients and on the analyses of 96 weeks data from the Phase IIb trials POWER 1, 2 and 3 in patients with high level of PI resistance.

TITAN is an ongoing randomised, controlled, open-label Phase III trial comparing PREZISTA co-administered with ritonavir (600/100 mg b.i.d.) versus lopinavir/ritonavir (400/100 mg b.i.d) in treatment-experienced, lopinavir naïve HIV-1 infected adult patients. Both arms used an Optimised Background Regimen (OBR) consisting of at least 2 antiretrovirals (NRTIs with or without NNRTIs). The mean baseline plasma HIV-1 RNA was 4.33 log_{10} copies/ml and the median baseline CD4+ cell count was 235 × 10^6 cells/l (range 3 – 831 × 10^6 cells/l) in the PREZISTA/ritonavir arm.

The table below shows the efficacy data of the 48 week analysis from the TITAN trial.

(see Table 3 opposite)

Non-inferiority in virologic response, defined as the percentage of subjects with plasma HIV-1 RNA level < 400 copies/ml, was demonstrated (at the chosen 12% non-inferiority margin) for both Intent-To-Treat and On Protocol populations.

POWER 1 and ***POWER 2*** are randomised, controlled trials consisting of an initial dose-finding part and a second long-term part in which all patients randomised to PREZISTA co-administered with 100 mg ritonavir received the recommended dose of 600/100 mg b.i.d.

HIV-1 infected patients who were eligible for these trials had previously failed more than 1 PI containing regimen. PREZISTA co-administered with 100 mg ritonavir plus an optimised background regimen (OBR) was compared to a control group receiving an investigator-selected PI(s) regimen plus an OBR. The OBR consisted of at least 2 NRTIs with or without enfuvirtide (ENF).

POWER 3*:* additional data on the efficacy of PREZISTA co-administered with ritonavir 600/100 mg b.i.d. with OBR have been obtained in similar treatment-experienced patients participating in the non-randomised trial TMC114-C215. Entry criteria were the same as and baseline characteristics were comparable to those of POWER 1 and POWER 2.

The table below shows the efficacy data of the 48-week analyses on the recommended 600 mg dose of PREZISTA co-administered with 100 mg ritonavir b.i.d. from the pooled POWER 1 and POWER 2 trials as well as from the POWER 3 trial.

(see Table 4 opposite)

Analyses of data through 96 weeks of treatment in the three POWER trials demonstrated sustained antiretroviral efficacy and immunological benefit. Treatment with PREZISTA co-administered with ritonavir (600/100 mg b.i.d.) resulted in 56.5% (POWER 1 and 2) and 52.2% (POWER 3) of responders with a decrease of at least 1 log_{10} in HIV RNA from baseline, 38.9% (POWER 1 and 2) and 42.1% (POWER 3) of subjects with an HIV RNA level < 50 copies/ml and 49.6% (POWER 1 and 2) and 50.0% (POWER 3) respectively of subjects with an HIV RNA level less than 400 copies/ml. The mean decrease in HIV RNA level compared to baseline was 1.58 (POWER 1 and 2) and 1.43 (POWER 3) log_{10} copies/ml and a mean increase in CD4+ cell count of 133 × 10^6 cells/l (POWER 1 and 2) and 103 × 10^6 cells/l (POWER 3) was observed.

Out of the 206 subjects who responded with complete viral suppression (< 50 copies/ml) at week 48, 177 subjects (86% of the responders at week 48) remained responders at week 96.

Baseline genotype or phenotype and virologic outcome

In a pooled analysis of the 600/100 mg b.i.d. groups of the POWER and DUET trials, the presence at baseline of 3 or more of mutations V11I, V32I, L33F, I47V, I50V, I54L or M, T74P, L76V, I84V or L89V was associated with a decreased virologic response to PREZISTA co-administered with 100 mg ritonavir. The presence of these individual mutations was associated with a median of 13 to 15 PI resistance associated mutations of the IAS-USA list of mutations.

In early treatment-experienced patients (TITAN) three or more of these mutations were only found in 4% of the patients at baseline.

Response (HIV-1 RNA < 50 copies/ml at week 24) to PREZISTA co-administered with ritonavir (600/100 mg b.i.d.) by baseline genotype and by use of enfuvirtide (ENF): As treated analysis of the POWER and DUET trials.*

(see Table 5 below)

Baseline darunavir phenotype (shift in susceptibility relative to reference) was shown to be a predictive factor of virologic outcome.

Response (HIV-1 RNA < 50 copies/ml at week 24) to PREZISTA co-administered with ritonavir (600/100 mg b.i.d.) by baseline darunavir phenotype and by use of enfuvirtide: As treated analysis of the POWER and DUET trials.

Table 5

Number of mutations at baseline*	All subjects % n/N	Subjects with no/non-naïve use of ENF % n/N	Subjects with naïve use of ENF % n/N
All ranges	45% 455/1,014	39% 290/741	60% 165/273
0-2	54% 359/660	50% 238/477	66% 121/183
3	39% 67/172	29% 35/120	62% 32/52
≥ 4	12% 20/171	7% 10/135	28% 10/36

* Number of mutations from the list of mutations associated with a diminished response to PREZISTA/ritonavir (V11I, V32I, L33F, I47V, I50V, I54L or M, T74P, L76V, I84V or L89V)

Table 6

Baseline darunavir phenotype	All subjects % n/N	Subjects with no/non-naïve use of ENF % n/N	Subjects with naïve use of ENF % n/N
All ranges	45% 455/1,014	39% 290/741	60% 165/273
⩽ 10	55% 364/659	51% 244/477	66% 120/182
10-40	29% 59/203	17% 25/147	61% 34/56
> 40	8% 9/118	5% 5/94	17% 4/24

(see Table 6 above)

Children from the age of 6 years and adolescents

DELPHI is an open-label, Phase II trial evaluating the pharmacokinetics, safety, tolerability, and efficacy of PREZISTA with low dose ritonavir in 80 ART-experienced HIV-1 infected paediatric patients aged 6 to 17 years and weighing at least 20 kg. These patients received PREZISTA/ritonavir in combination with other antiretroviral agents (see section 4.2 for dosage recommendations per body weight). Virologic response was defined as a decrease in plasma HIV-1 RNA viral load of at least 1.0 $\log_{10}$ versus baseline.

In the study, patients who were at risk of discontinuing therapy due to intolerance of ritonavir oral solution (e.g. taste aversion) were allowed to switch to the capsule formulation. Of the 44 patients taking ritonavir oral solution, 27 switched to the 100 mg capsule formulation and exceeded the weight-based ritonavir dose without changes in observed safety.

DELPHI	
Baseline disease characteristics	
Mean plasma HIV-1 RNA	4.64 $\log_{10}$ copies/ml
Median CD4+ cell count	330 × 10^6 cells/l (range: 6 to 1,505 × 10^6 cells/l)
Outcomes at week 48	PREZISTA/ritonavir N=80
HIV-1 RNA ⩾ 1 $\log_{10}$ below baseline[a]	52 (65.0%)
HIV-1 RNA < 50 copies/ml[a]	38 (47.5%)
HIV-1 RNA < 400 copies/ml[a]	47 (58.8%)
HIV-1 RNA $\log_{10}$ mean change from baseline[b]	-1.81
CD4+ cell count mean change from baseline[b]	147

[a] Imputations according to the TLOVR algorithm.

[b] Non-completer is failure imputation: patients who discontinued prematurely are imputed with a change equal to 0.

According to the TLOVR non-virologic failure censored algorithm 24 (30.0%) subjects experienced virological failure, of which 17 (21.3%) subjects were rebounders and 7 (8.8%) subjects were non-responders.

5.2 Pharmacokinetic properties

The pharmacokinetic properties of darunavir, co-administered with ritonavir, have been evaluated in healthy adult volunteers and in HIV-1 infected patients. Exposure to darunavir was higher in HIV-1 infected patients than in healthy subjects. The increased exposure to darunavir in HIV-1 infected patients compared to healthy subjects may be explained by the higher concentrations of alpha-1-acid glycoprotein (AAG) in HIV-1 infected patients, resulting in higher darunavir binding to plasma AAG and, therefore, higher plasma concentrations.

Darunavir is primarily metabolised by CYP3A. Ritonavir inhibits CYP3A, thereby increasing the plasma concentrations of darunavir considerably.

Absorption

Darunavir was rapidly absorbed following oral administration. Maximum plasma concentration of darunavir in the presence of low dose ritonavir is generally achieved within 2.5-4.0 hours.

The absolute oral bioavailability of a single 600 mg dose of darunavir alone was approximately 37% and increased to approximately 82% in the presence of 100 mg b.i.d. ritonavir. The overall pharmacokinetic enhancement effect by ritonavir was an approximate 14-fold increase in the systemic exposure of darunavir when a single dose of 600 mg darunavir was given orally in combination with ritonavir at 100 mg b.i.d. (see section 4.4).

When administered without food, the relative bioavailability of darunavir in the presence of low dose ritonavir is 30% lower as compared to intake with food. Therefore, PREZISTA tablets should be taken with ritonavir and with food. The type of food does not affect exposure to darunavir.

Distribution

Darunavir is approximately 95% bound to plasma protein. Darunavir binds primarily to plasma alpha-1-acid glycoprotein.

Following intravenous administration, the volume of distribution of darunavir alone was 88.1 ± 59.0 l (Mean ± SD) and increased to 131 ± 49.9 l (Mean ± SD) in the presence of 100 mg twice-daily ritonavir.

Metabolism

In vitro experiments with human liver microsomes (HLMs) indicate that darunavir primarily undergoes oxidative metabolism. Darunavir is extensively metabolised by the hepatic CYP system and almost exclusively by isozyme CYP3A4. A ^{14}C-darunavir trial in healthy volunteers showed that a majority of the radioactivity in plasma after a single 400/100 mg darunavir with ritonavir dose was due to the parent active substance. At least 3 oxidative metabolites of darunavir have been identified in humans; all showed activity that was at least 10-fold less than the activity of darunavir against wild type HIV.

Elimination

After a 400/100 mg ^{14}C-darunavir with ritonavir dose, approximately 79.5% and 13.9% of the administered dose of ^{14}C-darunavir could be retrieved in faeces and urine, respectively. Unchanged darunavir accounted for approximately 41.2% and 7.7% of the administered dose in faeces and urine, respectively. The terminal elimination half-life of darunavir was approximately 15 hours when combined with ritonavir.

The intravenous clearance of darunavir alone (150 mg) and in the presence of low dose ritonavir was 32.8 l/h and 5.9 l/h, respectively.

Special Populations

Paediatrics

The pharmacokinetics of darunavir in combination with ritonavir in 74 treatment-experienced paediatric patients, aged 6 to 17 years and weighing at least 20 kg, showed that the administered weight-based doses of PREZISTA/ritonavir resulted in darunavir exposure comparable to that in adults receiving PREZISTA/ritonavir 600/100 mg b.i.d. (see section 4.2).

Elderly

Population pharmacokinetic analysis in HIV infected patients showed that darunavir pharmacokinetics are not considerably different in the age range (18 to 75 years) evaluated in HIV infected patients (n=12, age ⩾ 65) (see section 4.4). However, only limited data were available in patients above the age of 65 year.

Gender

Population pharmacokinetic analysis showed a slightly higher darunavir exposure (16.8%) in HIV infected females compared to males. This difference is not clinically relevant.

Renal impairment

Results from a mass balance study with ^{14}C-darunavir with ritonavir showed that approximately 7.7% of the administered dose of darunavir is excreted in the urine unchanged.

Although darunavir has not been studied in patients with renal impairment, population pharmacokinetic analysis showed that the pharmacokinetics of darunavir were not significantly affected in HIV infected patients with moderate renal impairment (CrCl between 30-60 ml/min, n=20) (see sections 4.2 and 4.4).

Hepatic impairment

Darunavir is primarily metabolised and eliminated by the liver. In a multiple dose study with PREZISTA co-administered with ritonavir (600/100 mg) twice daily, it was demonstrated that the total plasma concentrations of darunavir in subjects with mild (Child-Pugh Class A, n=8) and moderate (Child-Pugh Class B, n=8) hepatic impairment were comparable with those in healthy subjects. However, unbound darunavir concentrations were approximately 55% (Child-Pugh Class A) and 100% (Child-Pugh Class B) higher, respectively. The clinical relevance of this increase is unknown therefore, PREZISTA should be used with caution. The effect of severe hepatic impairment on the pharmacokinetics of darunavir has not been studied (see sections 4.2, 4.3 and 4.4).

5.3 Preclinical safety data

Animal toxicology studies have been conducted at exposures up to clinical exposure levels with darunavir alone, in mice, rats and dogs and in combination with ritonavir in rats and dogs.

In repeated-dose toxicology studies in mice, rats and dogs, there were only limited effects of treatment with darunavir. In rodents the target organs identified were the haematopoietic system, the blood coagulation system, liver and thyroid. A variable but limited decrease in red blood cell-related parameters was observed, together with increases in activated partial thromboplastin time.

Changes were observed in liver (hepatocyte hypertrophy, vacuolation, increased liver enzymes) and thyroid (follicular hypertrophy). In the rat, the combination of darunavir with ritonavir lead to a small increase in effect on RBC parameters, liver and thyroid and increased incidence of islet fibrosis in the pancreas (in male rats only) compared to treatment with darunavir alone. In the dog, no major toxicity findings or target organs were identified up to exposures equivalent to clinical exposure at the recommended dose.

In a study conducted in rats, the number of corpora lutea and implantations were decreased in the presence of maternal toxicity. Otherwise, there were no effects on mating or fertility with darunavir treatment up to 1,000 mg/kg/day and exposure levels below (AUC-0.5 fold) of that in human at the clinically recommended dose. Up to same dose levels, there was no teratogenicity with darunavir in rats and rabbits when treated alone nor in mice when treated in combination with ritonavir. The exposure levels were lower than those with the recommended clinical dose in humans. In a pre- and postnatal development assessment in rats, darunavir with and without ritonavir, caused a transient reduction in body weight gain of the offspring pre-weaning and there was a slight delay in the opening of eyes and ears. Darunavir in combination with ritonavir caused a reduction in the number of pups that exhibited the startle response on day 15 of lactation and a reduced pup survival during lactation. These effects may be secondary to pup exposure to the active substance via the milk and/or maternal toxicity. No post weaning functions were affected with darunavir alone or in combination with ritonavir. In juvenile rats receiving darunavir up to days 23-26, increased mortality was observed with convulsions in some animals. Exposure in plasma, liver and brain was considerably higher than in adult rats after comparable doses in mg/kg between days 5 and 11 of age. After day 23 of life, the exposure was comparable to that in adult rats. The increased exposure was likely at least partly due to immaturity of the drug-metabolising enzymes in juvenile animals. No treatment related mortalities were noted in juvenile rats dosed at 1,000 mg/kg darunavir (single dose) on day 26 of age or at 500 mg/kg (repeated dose) from day 23 to 50 of age, and the exposures and toxicity profile were comparable to those observed in adult rats.

Due to uncertainties regarding the rate of development of the human blood brain barrier and liver enzymes, PREZISTA with low dose ritonavir should not be used in paediatric patients below 3 years of age.

Darunavir was evaluated for carcinogenic potential by oral gavage administration to mice and rats up to 104 weeks. Daily doses of 150, 450 and 1,000 mg/kg were administered to mice and doses of 50, 150 and 500 mg/kg were administered to rats. Dose-related increases in the incidences of hepatocellular adenomas and carcinomas were observed in males and females of both species. Thyroid follicular cell adenomas were noted in male rats. Administration of darunavir did not cause a statistically significant increase in the incidence of any other benign or malignant neoplasm in mice or rats. The observed hepatocellular and thyroid tumours in rodents are considered to be of limited relevance to humans. Repeated administration of darunavir to rats caused hepatic microsomal enzyme induction and increased thyroid hormone elimination, which predispose rats, but not humans, to thyroid neoplasms. At the highest tested doses, the systemic exposures (based on AUC) to darunavir were between 0.4- and 0.7-fold (mice) and 0.7- and 1-fold (rats), relative to those observed in humans at the recommended therapeutic doses.

After 2 years administration of darunavir at exposures at or below the human exposure, kidney changes were observed in mice (nephrosis) and rats (chronic progressive nephropathy).

Darunavir was not mutagenic or genotoxic in a battery of *in vitro* and *in vivo* assays including bacterial reverse mutation (Ames), chromosomal aberration in human lymphocytes and *in vivo* micronucleus test in mice.

6. PHARMACEUTICAL PARTICULARS

6.1 List of excipients

Tablet core

Microcrystalline cellulose

Colloidal anhydrous silica

Crospovidone

Magnesium stearate

Tablet film-coat

Poly(vinyl alcohol) – partially hydrolyzed

Macrogol 3350

Titanium dioxide (E171)

Talc

Sunset yellow FCF (E110)

6.2 Incompatibilities
Not applicable.

6.3 Shelf life
2 years

6.4 Special precautions for storage
This medicinal product does not require any special storage conditions.

6.5 Nature and contents of container
Opaque, white, high density polyethylene (HDPE) plastic, 160 ml bottle containing 60 tablets, fitted with polypropylene (PP) child resistant closure.

One bottle

6.6 Special precautions for disposal and other handling
No special requirements.

7. MARKETING AUTHORISATION HOLDER
Janssen-Cilag International NV

Turnhoutseweg 30

B-2340 Beerse

Belgium

8. MARKETING AUTHORISATION NUMBER(S)
EU/1/06/380/002

9. DATE OF FIRST AUTHORISATION/RENEWAL OF THE AUTHORISATION
Date of first authorisation: 12 February 2007

Date of latest renewal: 12 February 2009

10. DATE OF REVISION OF THE TEXT
23rd June 2009

Detailed information on this product is available on the website of the European Medicines Agency (EMEA) http://www.emea.europa.eu/

PREZISTA 75 mg & 150 mg film-coated tablets

(Janssen-Cilag Ltd)

1. NAME OF THE MEDICINAL PRODUCT
PREZISTA®▼ 75 mg & 150 mg film-coated tablets

2. QUALITATIVE AND QUANTITATIVE COMPOSITION
Each film-coated tablet contains 75 mg or 150 mg of darunavir (as ethanolate).

For a full list of excipients, see section 6.1.

3. PHARMACEUTICAL FORM
Film-coated tablet.

PREZISTA 75 mg: white caplet shaped tablet, debossed with "75" on one side and "TMC" on the other side.

PREZISTA 150 mg: white oval shaped tablet, debossed with "150" on one side and "TMC" on the other side.

4. CLINICAL PARTICULARS

4.1 Therapeutic indications
PREZISTA, co-administered with low dose ritonavir is indicated in combination with other antiretroviral medicinal products for the treatment of human immunodeficiency virus (HIV-1) infection in antiretroviral treatment (ART) experienced adult patients, including those that have been highly pre-treated and for the treatment of HIV-1 infection in ART-experienced children and adolescents from the age of 6 years and at least 20 kg body weight.

In deciding to initiate treatment with PREZISTA co-administered with low dose ritonavir careful consideration should be given to the treatment history of the individual patient and the patterns of mutations associated with different agents. Genotypic or phenotypic testing (when available) and treatment history should guide the use of PREZISTA.

4.2 Posology and method of administration
Therapy should be initiated by a physician experienced in the management of HIV infection.

PREZISTA must always be given orally with low dose ritonavir as a pharmacokinetic enhancer and in combination with other antiretroviral medicinal products. The Summary of Product Characteristics of ritonavir must therefore be consulted prior to initiation of therapy with PREZISTA.

Adults

ART-experienced patients

The recommended dose of PREZISTA is 600 mg twice daily (b.i.d.) taken with ritonavir 100 mg b.i.d. and with food. The type of food does not affect the exposure to darunavir (see sections 4.4, 4.5 and 5.2).

The use of the PREZISTA 75 mg or 150 mg tablets, developed for paediatric use, causes a high pill burden in adults, therefore their use is recommended only when the use of the available PREZISTA 300 mg or 600 mg tablets is deemed not appropriate such as due to difficulty in swallowing or hypersensitivity to specific colouring agents.

ART-naïve patients

PREZISTA 75 mg & 150 mg tablets are not indicated for ART-naïve patients. For dosage recommendations in ART-naïve patients see the Summary of Product Characteristics for PREZISTA 400 mg tablets.

After therapy with PREZISTA has been initiated, patients should be advised not to alter the dosage or discontinue therapy without instruction of their physician.

Children and adolescents

ART-experienced paediatric patients (6 to 17 years of age and weighing at least 20kg)

Recommended dose for treatment-experienced paediatric patients (6 to 17 years of age) for PREZISTA tablets and ritonavir	
Body weight (kg)	**Dose**
⩾ 20 kg–< 30 kg	375 mg PREZISTA/50 mg ritonavir b.i.d.
⩾ 30 kg–<40 kg	450 mg PREZISTA/60 mg ritonavir b.i.d.
⩾ 40 kg	600 mg PREZISTA/100 mg ritonavir b.i.d.

The recommended dose of PREZISTA with low dose ritonavir should not exceed the recommended adult dose (600/100 mg b.i.d.).

The use of only 75 mg and 150 mg tablets to achieve the recommended dose of PREZISTA could be appropriate when there is a possibility of hypersensitivity to specific colouring agents.

PREZISTA tablets should be taken with ritonavir twice daily and with food. The type of food does not affect the exposure to darunavir.

ART-experienced children less than 6 years of age or less than 20 kg body weight, and ART-naïve paediatric patients

There are insufficient data on the use of PREZISTA with low dose ritonavir in children less than 6 years of age or less than 20 kg body weight. Hence, PREZISTA is not recommended for use in this group (see sections 4.4 and 5.3).

Elderly

Limited information is available in this population and therefore PREZISTA should be used with caution in this age group (see sections 4.4 and 5.2).

Hepatic impairment

Darunavir is metabolised by the hepatic system. No dose adjustment is recommended in patients with mild (Child-Pugh Class A) or moderate (Child-Pugh Class B) hepatic impairment, however, PREZISTA should be used with caution in these patients. No pharmacokinetic data are available in patients with severe hepatic impairment. Severe hepatic impairment could result in an increase of darunavir exposure and a worsening of its safety profile. Therefore, PREZISTA must not be used in patients with severe hepatic impairment (Child-Pugh Class C) (see sections 4.3, 4.4 and 5.2).

Renal impairment

No dose adjustment is required in patients with renal impairment (see sections 4.4 and 5.2).

In case a dose of PREZISTA and/or ritonavir was missed within 6 hours of the time it is usually taken, patients should be instructed to take the prescribed dose of PREZISTA and ritonavir with food as soon as possible. If this was noticed later than 6 hours of the time it is usually taken, the missed dose should not be taken and the patient should resume the usual dosing schedule.

This guidance is based on the 15 hour half-life of darunavir in the presence of ritonavir and the recommended dosing interval of approximately 12 hours.

4.3 Contraindications
Hypersensitivity to the active substance or to any of the excipients.

Patients with severe (Child-Pugh Class C) hepatic impairment.

Combination of rifampicin with PREZISTA with concomitant low dose ritonavir is contraindicated (see section 4.5).

The combination product lopinavir/ritonavir should not be used with PREZISTA because co-administration causes large decreases in darunavir concentrations, which may in turn significantly decrease the darunavir therapeutic effect (see section 4.5).

Herbal preparations containing St John's wort (*Hypericum perforatum*) must not be used while taking PREZISTA due to the risk of decreased plasma concentrations and reduced clinical effects of darunavir (see section 4.5).

Co-administration of PREZISTA with low dose ritonavir, with active substances that are highly dependent on CYP3A for clearance and for which elevated plasma concentrations are associated with serious and/or life-threatening events is contraindicated. These active substances include e.g. antiarrhythmics (amiodarone, bepridil, quinidine, systemic lidocaine), antihistamines (astemizole, terfenadine), ergot derivatives (e.g. dihydroergotamine, ergonovine, ergotamine, methylergonovine), gastrointestinal motility agents (cisapride), neuroleptics (pimozide, sertindole), sedatives/hypnotics [triazolam, midazolam administered orally (for caution on parenterally administered midazolam, see section 4.5)] and HMG-CoA reductase inhibitors (simvastatin and lovastatin) (see section 4.5).

4.4 Special warnings and precautions for use
Patients should be advised that current antiretroviral therapy does not cure HIV and has not been proven to prevent the transmission of HIV to others through blood or sexual contact. Appropriate precautions should continue to be employed.

PREZISTA should only be used in combination with low dose ritonavir as a pharmacokinetic enhancer (see section 5.2).

Increasing the dose of ritonavir from that recommended in section 4.2 did not significantly affect darunavir concentrations and is not recommended.

PREZISTA is not recommended for use in children below 6 years of age or less than 20 kg body weight (see sections 4.2 and 5.3).

Elderly: As limited information is available on the use of PREZISTA in patients aged 65 and over, caution should be exercised in the administration of PREZISTA in elderly patients, reflecting the greater frequency of decreased hepatic function and of concomitant disease or other therapy (see sections 4.2 and 5.2).

Darunavir binds predominantly to α1-acid glycoprotein. This protein binding is concentration dependent indicative for saturation of binding. Therefore, protein displacement of medicinal products highly bound to α1-acid glycoprotein cannot be ruled out.

Severe skin rash, which may be accompanied with fever and/or elevations of transaminases, has occurred in 0.5% of patients treated with PREZISTA. Erythema multiforme and Stevens-Johnson Syndrome have been rarely (< 0.1%) observed. Treatment with PREZISTA should be discontinued if such a condition develops.

Darunavir contains a sulphonamide moiety. PREZISTA should be used with caution in patients with a known sulphonamide allergy.

Patients with coexisting conditions

Hepatic impairment

The safety and efficacy of PREZISTA have not been established in patients with severe underlying liver disorders and PREZISTA is therefore contraindicated in patients with severe hepatic impairment. Due to an increase in the unbound darunavir plasma concentrations, PREZISTA should be used with caution in patients with mild or moderate hepatic impairment (see sections 4.2, 4.3 and 5.2).

Patients with chronic hepatitis B or C and treated with combination antiretroviral therapy are at an increased risk for severe and potentially fatal hepatic adverse events. In case of concomitant antiviral therapy for hepatitis B or C, please refer to the relevant product information for these medicinal products.

Patients with pre-existing liver dysfunction including chronic hepatitis have an increased frequency of liver function abnormalities during combination antiretroviral therapy and should be monitored according to standard practice. If there is evidence of worsening liver disease in such patients, interruption or discontinuation of treatment should be considered.

Renal impairment

No special precautions or dose adjustments are required in patients with renal impairment. As darunavir and ritonavir are highly bound to plasma proteins, it is unlikely that they will be significantly removed by haemodialysis or peritoneal dialysis. Therefore, no special precautions or dose adjustments are required in these patients (see sections 4.2 and 5.2).

Haemophiliac patients

There have been reports of increased bleeding, including spontaneous skin haematomas and haemarthrosis in patients with haemophilia type A and B treated with PIs. In some patients additional factor VIII was given. In more than half of the reported cases, treatment with PIs was continued or reintroduced if treatment had been discontinued. A causal relationship has been suggested, although the mechanism of action has not been elucidated. Haemophiliac patients should therefore be made aware of the possibility of increased bleeding.

Diabetes mellitus/Hyperglycaemia

New onset diabetes mellitus, hyperglycaemia, or exacerbation of existing diabetes mellitus has been reported in patients receiving antiretroviral therapy, including PIs. In some of these patients the hyperglycaemia was severe and in some cases also associated with ketoacidosis. Many patients had confounding medical conditions some of which required therapy with agents that have been associated with the development of diabetes mellitus or hyperglycaemia.

Fat redistribution and metabolic disorders

Combination antiretroviral therapy has been associated with redistribution of body fat (lipodystrophy) in HIV infected patients. The long-term consequences of these events are currently unknown. Knowledge about the mechanism is incomplete. A connection between visceral lipomatosis and PIs and lipoatrophy and NRTIs has been hypothesised. A higher risk of lipodystrophy has been associated with individual factors such as older age and with drug related factors such as longer duration of antiretroviral treatment and associated metabolic disturbances. Clinical examination should include evaluation for physical signs of fat redistribution. Consideration should be given to measurement of fasting serum lipids and blood glucose. Lipid disorders should be managed as clinically appropriate (see section 4.8).

Osteonecrosis

Although the etiology is considered to be multifactorial (including corticosteroid use, alcohol consumption, severe immunosuppression, higher body mass index), cases of osteonecrosis have been reported particularly in patients with advanced HIV disease and/or long-term exposure to combination antiretroviral therapy (CART). Patients should be advised to seek medical advice if they experience joint aches and pain, joint stiffness or difficulty in movement.

Immune reactivation syndrome

In HIV infected patients with severe immune deficiency at the time of institution of combination antiretroviral therapy (CART), an inflammatory reaction to asymptomatic or residual opportunistic pathogens may arise and cause serious clinical conditions, or aggravation of symptoms. Typically, such reactions have been observed within the first weeks or months of initiation of CART. Relevant examples are cytomegalovirus retinitis, generalised and/or focal mycobacterial infections and pneumonia caused by *Pneumocystis jiroveci* (formerly known as *Pneumocystis carinii*). Any inflammatory symptoms should be evaluated and treatment instituted when necessary. In addition, reactivation of herpes simplex and herpes zoster has been observed in clinical studies with PREZISTA co-administered with low dose ritonavir.

Interactions with medicinal products

Several of the interaction studies have been performed at lower than recommended doses of darunavir. The effects on co-administered medicinal products may thus be underestimated and clinical monitoring of safety may be indicated. For full information on interactions with other medicinal products see section 4.5.

4.5 Interaction with other medicinal products and other forms of interaction

Darunavir and ritonavir are both inhibitors of the CYP3A4 isoform. Co-administration of darunavir and ritonavir and medicinal products primarily metabolised by CYP3A4 may result in increased systemic exposure to such medicinal products, which could increase or prolong their therapeutic effect and adverse reactions.

PREZISTA co-administered with low dose ritonavir must not be combined with medicinal products that are highly dependent on CYP3A4 for clearance and for which increased systemic exposure is associated with serious and/or life-threatening events (narrow therapeutic index). These medicinal products include amiodarone, bepridil, quinidine, systemic lidocaine, astemizole, terfenadine, midazolam administered orally, triazolam, cisapride, pimozide, sertindole, simvastatin, lovastatin and the ergot alkaloids (e.g. ergotamine, dihydroergotamine, ergonovine and methylergonovine) (see section 4.3).

The overall pharmacokinetic enhancement effect by ritonavir was an approximate 14-fold increase in the systemic exposure of darunavir when a single dose of 600 mg darunavir was given orally in combination with ritonavir at 100 mg b.i.d. Therefore, PREZISTA must only be used in combination with low dose ritonavir as a pharmacokinetic enhancer (see sections 4.4 and 5.2).

A clinical study utilising a cocktail of medicinal products that are metabolised by cytochromes CYP2C9, CYP2C19 and CYP2D6 demonstrated an increase in CYP2C9 and CYP2C19 activity and inhibition of CYP2D6 activity in the presence of PREZISTA/rtv, which may be attributed to the presence of low dose ritonavir. Co-administration of darunavir and ritonavir and medicinal products which are primarily metabolised by CYP2D6 (such as flecainide, propafenone, metoprolol) may result in increased plasma concentrations of these medicinal products, which could increase or prolong their therapeutic effect and adverse reactions. Co-administration of darunavir and ritonavir and medicinal products primarily metabolised by CYP2C9 (such as warfarin) and CYP2C19 (such as methadone) may result in decreased systemic exposure to such medicinal products, which could decrease or shorten their therapeutic effect.

Although the effect on CYP2C8 has only been studied *in vitro*, co-administration of darunavir and ritonavir and medicinal products primarily metabolised by CYP2C8 (such as paclitaxel, rosiglitazone, repaglinide) may result in decreased systemic exposure to such medicinal products, which could decrease or shorten their therapeutic effect.

Medicinal products that affect darunavir/ritonavir exposure

Darunavir and ritonavir are metabolised by CYP3A. Medicinal products that induce CYP3A activity would be expected to increase the clearance of darunavir and ritonavir, resulting in lowered plasma concentrations of darunavir and ritonavir (e.g. rifampicin, St John's wort, lopinavir). Co-administration of darunavir and ritonavir and other medicinal products that inhibit CYP3A may decrease the clearance of darunavir and ritonavir and may result in increased plasma concentrations of darunavir and ritonavir (e.g. indinavir, systemic azoles like ketoconazole and clotrimazole). These interactions are described in the interaction tables below.

Interaction table

Interactions between darunavir/ritonavir and protease inhibitors, antiretroviral agents other than protease inhibitors and other non-antiretroviral medicinal products are listed in the tables below (increase is indicated as "↑", decrease as "↓", no change as "↔", not determined as "ND", twice daily as "b.i.d.", once daily as "q.d." and once every other day as "q.o.d.").

Several of the interaction studies (indicated by # in the table below) have been performed at lower than recommended doses of darunavir or with a different dosing regimen (see section 4.2 Posology). The effects on co-administered medicinal products may thus be underestimated and clinical monitoring of safety may be indicated.

Interactions – Darunavir/ritonavir with Protease Inhibitors

The efficacy and safety of the use of PREZISTA with low dose ritonavir and any other PI (e.g. (fos)amprenavir, nelfinavir and tipranavir) has not been established in HIV patients. Generally, dual therapy with protease inhibitors is not recommended.

(see Table 1 on next page)

4.6 Pregnancy and lactation

Pregnancy

There are no adequate and well controlled studies with darunavir in pregnant women. Studies in animals do not indicate direct harmful effects with respect to pregnancy, embryonal/foetal development, parturition or postnatal development (see section 5.3).

PREZISTA co-administered with low dose ritonavir should be used during pregnancy only if the potential benefit justifies the potential risk.

Breast-feeding

It is not known whether darunavir is excreted in human milk. Studies in rats have demonstrated that darunavir is excreted in milk and at high levels (1,000 mg/kg/day) resulted in toxicity. Because of both the potential for HIV transmission and the potential for adverse reactions in breast-fed infants, mothers should be instructed not to breast-feed under any circumstances if they are receiving PREZISTA.

Fertility

No human data on the effect of darunavir on fertility are available. There was no effect on mating or fertility with darunavir treatment in rats (see section 5.3).

4.7 Effects on ability to drive and use machines

No studies on the effects of PREZISTA in combination with ritonavir on the ability to drive and use machines have been performed. However, dizziness has been reported in some patients during treatment with regimens containing PREZISTA co-administered with low dose ritonavir and should be borne in mind when considering a patient's ability to drive or operate machinery (see section 4.8).

4.8 Undesirable effects

Adult patients

The adverse drug reactions are derived from Phase IIb and Phase III trials, in which a total of 1,968 treatment-experienced patients initiated therapy with the recommended dose of PREZISTA 600 mg with ritonavir 100 mg twice daily. Median exposure to PREZISTA/ritonavir in this group was 37.3 weeks. Thirty percent of these patients experienced at least one adverse drug reaction of at least grade 2 severity. The most frequent (⩾ 2%) of those were diarrhoea (3.9%), hypertriglyceridaemia (3.8%), rash (2.8%), nausea (2.6%), hypercholesterolaemia (2.5%) and headache (2.0%).

2.6% of the patients discontinued treatment due to adverse reactions.

Adverse reactions are listed by system organ class (SOC) and frequency. Within each frequency grouping, adverse reactions are presented in order of decreasing seriousness. Frequencies are defined as very common (⩾ 1/10), common (⩾ 1/100 to < 1/10) and uncommon (⩾ 1/1,000 to < 1/100).

(see Table 2 on page 4931875)

In clinical trials (n=1,968), rash (all grades, at least possibly related) occurred in 5.6% of patients treated with PREZISTA. Rash was mostly mild to moderate, often occurring within the first four weeks of treatment and resolving with continued dosing. Grade 2-4 rash was reported in 2.9% of patients. The discontinuation rate due to rash in patients using PREZISTA co-administered with 100 mg ritonavir was 0.5%.

Severe cases of skin rash, including erythema multiforme and Stevens-Johnson Syndrome (both rare) have been reported in ongoing clinical trials with PREZISTA co-administered with 100 mg ritonavir.

The safety assessment in antiretroviral treatment-naïve adult patients (n=343) is based on all safety data from the Phase III trial ARTEMIS comparing PREZISTA/rtv 800/100 mg q.d. versus lopinavir/ritonavir 800/200 mg per day. Median exposure in the PREZISTA/ritonavir group was 56.3 weeks.

0.6% of the patients discontinued treatment due to adverse drug reactions.

In these treatment naïve-patients, the following adverse drug reactions were identified:

ADRs of at least moderate intensity and reported in more than one patient

Common: hypertriglyceridaemia, hypercholesterolaemia, headache, diarrhoea, nausea, increased alanine aminotransferase.

Uncommon: hyperlipidaemia, vomiting, abdominal pain, increased aspartate aminotransferase, rash (including maculopapular rash), allergic dermatitis, pruritus.

ADRs of all severity grades and reported in more than one patient

Very common: diarrhoea, nausea.

Common: hypertriglyceridaemia, hypercholesterolaemia, anorexia, insomnia, headache, dizziness, dysgeusia, vomiting, abdominal pain, abdominal discomfort, abdominal distension, flatulence, increased alanine aminotransferase, rash (including maculopapular, papular rash), alopecia, dry skin, pruritus, fatigue.

Uncommon: upper respiratory tract infection, diabetes mellitus, hyperlipidaemia, abnormal dreams, hypoaesthesia, disturbance in attention, somnolence, dyspepsia, eructation, increased aspartate aminotransferase, allergic dermatitis, urticaria, dermatitis, night sweats, myalgia, muscle spasms, asthenia.

Combination antiretroviral therapy has been associated with redistribution of body fat (lipodystrophy) in HIV patients, including loss of peripheral and facial subcutaneous fat, increased intra-abdominal and visceral fat, breast hypertrophy and dorsocervical fat accumulation (buffalo hump) (see section 4.4).

Combination antiretroviral therapy has also been associated with metabolic abnormalities such as hypertriglyceridaemia, hypercholesterolaemia, insulin resistance, hyperglycaemia and hyperlactataemia (see section 4.4).

Increased CPK, myalgia, myositis and rarely, rhabdomyolysis have been reported with the use of protease inhibitors, particularly in combination with NRTIs.

Cases of osteonecrosis have been reported, particularly in patients with generally acknowledged risk factors, advanced HIV disease or long-term exposure to combination antiretroviral therapy (CART). The frequency of this is unknown (see section 4.4).

In HIV infected patients with severe immune deficiency at the time of initiation of combination antiretroviral therapy, an inflammatory reaction to asymptomatic or residual opportunistic infections may arise (see section 4.4).

There have been reports of increased spontaneous bleeding in haemophiliac patients receiving antiretroviral protease inhibitors (see section 4.4).

Children and adolescents

The safety assessment in children and adolescents is based on the safety data from the Phase II trial DELPHI in which 80 ART-experienced HIV-1 infected paediatric patients aged from 6 to 17 years and weighing at least 20 kg received PREZISTA with low dose ritonavir in combination with other antiretroviral agents (see section 5.1). Overall, the safety profile in these 80 children and adolescents was similar to that observed in the adult population.

Patients co-infected with hepatitis B and/or hepatitis C virus

Among 1,968 treatment-experienced patients receiving PREZISTA co-administered with ritonavir 600/100 mg b.i.d., 236 patients were co-infected with hepatitis B or C. Co-infected patients were more likely to have baseline and treatment emergent hepatic transaminase elevations than those without chronic viral hepatitis (see section 4.4).

4.9 Overdose

Human experience of acute overdose with PREZISTA co-administered with low dose ritonavir is limited. Single doses up to 3,200 mg of darunavir as oral solution alone and up to 1,600 mg of the tablet formulation of darunavir in combination with ritonavir have been administered to healthy volunteers without untoward symptomatic effects.

There is no specific antidote for overdose with PREZISTA. Treatment of overdose with PREZISTA consists of general supportive measures including monitoring of vital signs and observation of the clinical status of the patient. If indicated, elimination of unabsorbed active substance is to be achieved by emesis or gastric lavage. Administration of activated charcoal may also be used to aid in removal of unabsorbed active substance. Since darunavir is highly protein bound, dialysis is unlikely to be beneficial in significant removal of the active substance.

5. PHARMACOLOGICAL PROPERTIES

5.1 Pharmacodynamic properties

Pharmacotherapeutic group: Antiviral for systemic use, ATC code: J05AE10.

Mechanism of action

Darunavir is an inhibitor of the dimerisation and of the catalytic activity of the HIV-1 protease (K_D of 4.5 × 10^{-12}M). It selectively inhibits the cleavage of HIV encoded

Table 1

Co-administered Medicinal Product	Dose of Co-administered Medicinal Product (mg)	Dose of darunavir/ritonavir (mg)	Medicinal Product Assessed	AUC	C_{min}
Lopinavir/ritonavir	400/100 b.i.d. 533/133.3 b.i.d.	1,200/100 b.i.d. 1,200 b.i.d.	Lopinavir Darunavir Lopinavir Darunavir	↔ ↓38%* ↔ ↓ 41%	↔ ↓51%* ↔ ↓ 55%
	* based upon not dose normalised values Due to a decrease in the exposure (AUC) of darunavir by 40%, appropriate doses of the combination have not been established. Hence, concomitant use of PREZISTA co-administered with low dose ritonavir and the combination product lopinavir/ritonavir is contraindicated (see section 4.3).				
Saquinavir	1,000 b.i.d.	400/100 b.i.d.#	Darunavir	↓ 26%	↓ 42%
	The study with boosted saquinavir showed no significant effect of darunavir on saquinavir. It is not recommended to combine PREZISTA co-administered with low dose ritonavir with saquinavir.				
Indinavir	800 b.i.d.	400/100 b.i.d. #	Indinavir Darunavir	↑ 23% ↑ 24%	↑ 125% ↑ 44%
	When used in combination with PREZISTA co-administered with low dose ritonavir, dose adjustment of indinavir from 800 mg b.i.d. to 600 mg b.i.d. may be warranted in case of intolerance.				
Atazanavir	300 q.d.	400/100 b.i.d. #	Atazanavir Darunavir	↔ ↔	↔ ↔
	Darunavir/ritonavir did not significantly affect atazanavir exposure, however 90% CI for C_{min} were 99-234%. Atazanavir can be used with PREZISTA co-administered with low dose ritonavir.				
Interactions – Darunavir/ritonavir with Antiretroviral Agents other than Protease Inhibitors					
Co-administered Medicinal Product	**Dose of Co-administered Medicinal Product (mg)**	**Dose of darunavir/ritonavir (mg)**	**Medicinal Product Assessed**	**AUC**	**C_{min}**
Efavirenz	600 q.d.	300/100 b.i.d. #	Efavirenz Darunavir	↑ 21% ↓ 13%	↑ 17% ↓ 31%
	Efavirenz decreases the plasma concentrations of darunavir as a result of CYP3A4 induction. Darunavir/ritonavir increases the plasma concentrations of efavirenz as a result of CYP3A4 inhibition. Clinical monitoring for central nervous system toxicity associated with increased exposure to efavirenz may be indicated when PREZISTA co-administered with low dose ritonavir is given in combination with efavirenz.				
Etravirine	100 b.i.d.*	600/100 b.i.d.	Etravirine Darunavir	↓ 37% ↔	↓ 49% ↔
	* dose used in drug-interaction study. For recommended dose see paragraph below. There was a 37% decrease in etravirine exposure in the presence of darunavir/ritonavir and no relevant change in exposure to darunavir. Therefore, PREZISTA co-administered with low dose ritonavir can be co-administered with etravirine **200 mg b.i.d.** without dose adjustments.				
Nevirapine	200 b.i.d.	400/100 b.i.d. #	Nevirapine Darunavir	↑ 27% ↔	↑ 47% ↔
	Darunavir/ritonavir increases the plasma concentrations of nevirapine as a result of CYP3A4 inhibition. Since this difference is not considered to be clinically relevant, the combination of PREZISTA co-administered with low dose ritonavir and nevirapine can be used without dose adjustments.				
Tenofovir	300 q.d.	300/100 b.i.d. #	Tenofovir Darunavir	↑ 22% ↔	↑ 37% ↔
	Ritonavir effect on MDR-1 transport in renal tubuli has been a proposed mechanism for increased plasma concentrations of tenofovir. Monitoring of renal function may be indicated when PREZISTA co-administered with low dose ritonavir is given in combination with tenofovir, particularly in patients with underlying systemic or renal disease, or in patients taking nephrotoxic agents.				
Zidovudine Zalcitabine Emtricitabine Stavudine Lamivudine Abacavir	Based on the different elimination pathways of the other NRTIs zidovudine, zalcitabine, emtricitabine, stavudine, lamivudine, that are primarily renally excreted, and abacavir for which metabolism is not mediated by CYP450, no interactions are expected for these medicinal compounds and PREZISTA co-administered with low dose ritonavir.				
Didanosine	400 q.d.	600/100 b.i.d.	Didanosine Darunavir	↔ ↔	NA ↔
	Didanosine was administered on an empty stomach 2 hours prior to administration of darunavir/ritonavir. Systemic exposure to darunavir co-administered with low dose ritonavir, with or without didanosine was comparable. The combination of PREZISTA co-administered with low dose ritonavir and didanosine can be used without dose adjustments.				
Maraviroc	150 b.i.d.	600/100 b.i.d.	Maraviroc Darunavir	↑ 305% ↔	ND ND
	The maraviroc dose should be 150 mg twice daily when co-administered with PREZISTA with low dose ritonavir. Darunavir/ritonavir concentrations were consistent with historical data.				
Interactions – Darunavir/ritonavir with Non-antiretroviral co-administered Medicinal Products					
Co-administered Medicinal Product	**Dose of Co-administered Medicinal Product (mg)**	**Dose of darunavir/ritonavir (mg)**	**Medicinal Product Assessed**	**AUC**	**C_{min}**
Antiarrhythmics					
Digoxin	0.4 mg single dose	600/100 b.i.d.	Digoxin	↑ 60%	ND
	Darunavir/ritonavir increases the plasma concentrations of digoxin. Inhibition of Pgp may be a likely explanation. Given that digoxin has as a narrow therapeutic index, it is recommended that the lowest possible dose of digoxin should initially be prescribed in case digoxin is given to patients on darunavir/ritonavir therapy. The digoxin dose should be carefully titrated to obtain the desired clinical effect while assessing the overall clinical state of the subject.				
Antibiotics					
Clarithromycin	500 b.i.d.	400/100 b.i.d. #	Clarithromycin Darunavir	↑ 57% ↔	↑ 174% ↔
	Darunavir/ritonavir increases the plasma concentrations of clarithromycin as a result of CYP3A4 inhibition and possible Pgp inhibition. Concentrations of the metabolite 14-OH-clarithromycin were not detectable. Caution is warranted and clinical monitoring is recommended. For patients with renal impairment, a dose reduction of clarithromycin should be considered.				
Anticoagulant					
Warfarin	Warfarin concentrations may be affected when co-administered with darunavir with ritonavir. The international normalised ratio (INR) should be monitored when warfarin is combined with PREZISTA co-administered with low dose ritonavir.				
Anticonvulsants					
Phenobarbital Phenytoin	Phenobarbital and phenytoin are inducers of CYP450 enzymes. PREZISTA co-administered with low dose ritonavir should not be used in combination with these medicines, as co-administration may cause significant decreases in darunavir plasma concentrations.				
Carbamazepine	200 b.i.d.	600/100 b.i.d.	Carbamazepine Darunavir	↑ 45% ↔	↑ 54% ↔
	Exposure to darunavir, co-administered with ritonavir, was unaffected by carbamazepine. Ritonavir exposure (AUC12h) was decreased by 49%. For carbamazepine, AUC12h was increased by 45%. No dose adjustment for PREZISTA/ritonavir is recommended. If there is a need to combine PREZISTA/ritonavir and carbamazepine, patients should be monitored for potential carbamazepine-related adverse events. Carbamazepine concentrations should be monitored and its dose should be titrated for adequate response. Based upon the findings, the carbamazepine dose may need to be reduced by 25% to 50% in the presence of PREZISTA/ritonavir.				
Antifungals					
Voriconazole	The combined use of voriconazole with darunavir co-administered with low dose ritonavir has not been studied. Voriconazole is metabolised by cytochrome P450 isoenzymes, CYP2C19, CYP2C9 and CYP3A4. Ritonavir, which can induce some of these isoenzymes, may decrease voriconazole plasma concentrations. Voriconazole should not be co-administered with PREZISTA with low dose ritonavir unless an assessment of the benefit/risk ratio justifies the use of voriconazole.				
Ketoconazole	200 b.i.d.	400/100 b.i.d. #	Ketoconazole Darunavir	↑ 212% ↑ 42%	↑ 868% ↑ 73%
	Ketoconazole is a potent inhibitor as well as substrate of CYP3A4. Caution is warranted and clinical monitoring is recommended. When co-administration is required the daily dose of ketoconazole should not exceed 200 mg.				
Itraconazole	Itraconazole, like ketoconazole, is a potent inhibitor as well as substrate of CYP3A4. Concomitant systemic use of itraconazole and darunavir co-administered with low dose ritonavir may increase plasma concentrations of darunavir. Simultaneously, plasma concentrations of itraconazole may be increased by darunavir co-administered with low dose ritonavir. Caution is warranted and clinical monitoring is recommended. When co-administration is required the daily dose of itraconazole should not exceed 200 mg.				

Co-administered Medicinal Product	Dose of Co-administered Medicinal Product (mg)	Dose of darunavir/ritonavir (mg)	Medicinal Product Assessed	AUC	C_{min}
Clotrimazole	Concomitant systemic use of clotrimazole and darunavir co-administered with low dose ritonavir may increase plasma concentrations of darunavir. This was confirmed using a population pharmacokinetic model. The increase in the median darunavir AUC_{24h} value for the patients taking clotrimazole from the overall median was 33%. Caution is warranted and clinical monitoring is recommended, when co-administration of clotrimazole is required.				
Calcium channel blockers					
Felodipine Nifedipine Nicardipine	Darunavir and ritonavir inhibit CYP3A4 and as a result can be expected to increase the plasma concentrations of calcium channel antagonists, which are CYP3A4 substrates. Clinical monitoring of therapeutic and adverse effects is recommended when these medicines are concomitantly administered with PREZISTA with low dose ritonavir.				
HMG Co-A Reductase Inhibitors					
Lovastatin Simvastatin	Lovastatin and simvastatin, which are highly dependent on CYP3A4 metabolism are expected to have markedly increased plasma concentrations when co-administered with darunavir co-administered with low dose ritonavir. This may cause myopathy, including rhabdomyolysis. Concomitant use of PREZISTA co-administered with low dose ritonavir with lovastatin and simvastatin is therefore contraindicated (see section 4.3).				
Atorvastatin	10 q.d.	300/100 b.i.d. #	Atorvastatin	3-4 times ↑	3-4 times ↑
			Darunavir	ND	ND
	The results of this interaction trial show that atorvastatin (10 mg q.d.) in combination with darunavir/ritonavir (300/100 mg b.i.d.) provides an exposure to atorvastatin, which is only 15% lower than that obtained with (40 mg q.d.) atorvastatin alone. When administration of atorvastatin and PREZISTA co-administered with low dose ritonavir is desired, it is recommended to start with an atorvastatin dose of 10 mg q.d. A gradual dose increase of atorvastatin may be tailored to the clinical response.				
Pravastatin	40 mg single dose	600/100 b.i.d.	Pravastatin	0-5 times ↑	ND
	Darunavir/ritonavir did not increase exposure to a single dose of pravastatin in most subjects but up to 5-fold in a limited subset of subjects. When administration of pravastatin and PREZISTA co-administered with low dose ritonavir is required, it is recommended to start with the lowest possible dose of pravastatin and titrate it up to the desired clinical effect while monitoring for safety.				
Hormonal contraceptive					
Ethinylestradiol Norethindrone	35 μg/1 mg q.d.	600/100 b.i.d.	Ethinylestradiol Norethindrone	↓ 44% ↓ 14%	↓ 62% ↓ 30%
	Alternative or additional contraceptive measures are recommended when oestrogen-based contraceptives are co-administered with PREZISTA and low dose ritonavir. Patients using oestrogens as hormone replacement therapy should be clinically monitored for signs of oestrogen deficiency.				
Immunosupressants					
Cyclosporine Tacrolimus Sirolimus	Exposure to cyclosporine, tacrolimus, or sirolimus will be increased when co-administered with PREZISTA co-administered with low dose ritonavir. Therapeutic drug monitoring of the immunosuppressive agent must be done when co-administration occurs.				
H_2-receptor antagonists and proton pump inhibitors					
Ranitidine	150 b.i.d.	400/100 b.i.d. #	Darunavir	↔	↔
	Based on these results, PREZISTA co-administered with low dose ritonavir can be co-administered with H_2-receptor antagonists without dose adjustments.				
Omeprazole	20 q.d.	400/100 b.i.d. #	Darunavir	↔	↔
	Based on these results, PREZISTA co-administered with low dose ritonavir can be co-administered with proton pump inhibitors without dose adjustments.				
Opiods					
Methadone	55-150 q.d.	600/100 b.i.d. (dosed for 7 days)	R-methadone	↓ 16%	↓ 15%
	Based on pharmacokinetic and clinical findings, no adjustment of methadone dosage is required when initiating co-administration with PREZISTA/ritonavir. However, increased methadone dose may be necessary when concomitantly administered for a longer period of time due to induction of metabolism by ritonavir. Therefore, clinical monitoring is recommended, as maintenance therapy may need to be adjusted in some patients.				
PDE-5 inhibitors					
Sildenafil Vardenafil Tadalafil	In an interaction study a comparable systemic exposure to sildenafil was observed for a single intake of 100 mg sildenafil alone and a single intake of 25 mg sildenafil co-administered with darunavir/ritonavir (400/100 mg b.i.d.). Concomitant use of PDE-5 inhibitors with PREZISTA co-administered with low dose ritonavir should be done with caution. If concomitant use of PREZISTA co-administered with low dose ritonavir with sildenafil, vardenafil, or tadalafil is indicated, sildenafil at a single dose not exceeding 25 mg in 48 hours, vardenafil at a single dose not exceeding 2.5 mg dose in 72 hours or tadalafil at a single dose not exceeding 10 mg dose in 72 hours is recommended.				
Rifamycines					
Rifampicin	Rifampicin is a strong CYP3A4 inducer and has been shown to cause profound decreases in concentrations of other protease inhibitors, which can result in virological failure and resistance development. During attempts to overcome the decreased exposure by increasing the dose of other protease inhibitors with ritonavir, a high frequency of liver reactions was seen. The combination of rifampicin and PREZISTA with concomitant low dose ritonavir is contraindicated (see section 4.3).				
Rifabutin	150 q.o.d.	600/100 b.i.d.	Rifabutin*	1.6 times ↑	ND
			Darunavir	↑ 53%	↑ 68%
	* sum of active moieties of rifabutin (parent drug + 25-*O*- desacetyl metabolite) A dose reduction of rifabutin by 75% of the usual dose of 300 mg/day [i.e. rifabutin 150 mg q.o.d. (once every other day)] and increased monitoring for rifabutin related adverse events is warranted in patients receiving the combination. In case of safety issues, a further increase of the dosing interval for rifabutin and/or monitoring of rifabutin levels should be considered. Consideration should be given to official guidance on the appropriate treatment of tuberculosis in HIV infected patients. Rifabutin is an inducer and substrate of CYP3A4. An increase of systemic exposure to darunavir was observed when PREZISTA co-administered with 100 mg ritonavir was co-administered with rifabutin [150 mg q.o.d. (once every other day)]. Based upon the safety profile of PREZISTA/ritonavir, this increase in darunavir exposure in the presence of rifabutin does not warrant a dose adjustment for PREZISTA/ritonavir. The interaction trial showed a comparable daily systemic exposure for rifabutin between treatment at 300 mg q.d. (once daily) alone and 150 mg q.o.d. (once every other day) in combination with PREZISTA/ritonavir (600/100 mg b.i.d.) with an about 10-fold increase in the daily exposure to the active metabolite 25-*O*-desacetylrifabutin. Furthermore, AUC of the sum of active moieties of rifabutin (parent drug + 25-*O*- desacetyl metabolite) was increased 1.6-fold, while C_{max} remained comparable. Data on comparison with a 150 mg q.d. (once daily) reference dose is lacking.				
Sedatives/Hypnotics					
Parenteral midazolam	Midazolam is extensively metabolised by CYP3A4. Co-administration with PREZISTA/ritonavir may cause a large increase in the concentration of this benzodiazepine. No drug interaction study has been performed for the co-administration of PREZISTA/ritonavir with benzodiazepines. Based on data for other CYP3A4 inhibitors, plasma concentrations of midazolam are expected to be significantly higher when midazolam is given orally. Therefore PREZISTA/ritonavir should not be co-administered with orally administered midazolam (see section 4.3), whereas caution should be used with co-administration of PREZISTA/ritonavir and parenteral midazolam. Data from concomitant use of parenteral midazolam with other protease inhibitors suggest a possible 3-4 fold increase in midazolam plasma levels. If PREZISTA/ritonavir is co-administered with parenteral midazolam, it should be done in an intensive care unit (ICU) or similar setting, which ensures close clinical monitoring and appropriate medical management in case of respiratory depression and/or prolonged sedation. Dosage adjustment for midazolam should be considered, especially if more than a single dose of midazolam is administered.				
Selective Serotonin Reuptake Inhibitors (SSRIs)					
Paroxetine	20 q.d.	400/100 b.i.d. #	Paroxetine Darunavir	↓ 39% ↔	↓ 37% ↔
Sertraline	50 q.d.	400/100 b.i.d. #	Sertraline Darunavir	↓ 49% ↔	↓ 49% ↔
	If SSRIs are co-administered with PREZISTA and ritonavir, the recommended approach is a dose titration of the SSRI based on a clinical assessment of antidepressant response. In addition, patients on a stable dose of sertraline or paroxetine who start treatment with PREZISTA co-administered with low dose ritonavir should be monitored for antidepressant response.				
Steroids					
Fluticasone propionate Budesonide	In a clinical study where ritonavir 100 mg capsules b.i.d were co-administered with 50 μg intranasal fluticasone propionate (4 times daily) for 7 days in healthy subjects, fluticasone propionate plasma concentrations increased significantly, whereas the intrinsic cortisol levels decreased by approximately 86% (90% confidence interval 82-89%). Greater effects may be expected when fluticasone propionate is inhaled. Systemic corticosteroid effects including Cushing's syndrome and adrenal suppression have been reported in patients receiving ritonavir and inhaled or intranasally administered fluticasone propionate; this could also occur with other corticosteroids metabolised via the P450 3A pathway e.g. budesonide. Consequently, concomitant administration of PREZISTA, co-administered with low dose ritonavir and these glucocorticoids, is not recommended unless the potential benefit of treatment outweighs the risk of systemic corticosteroid effects. A dose reduction of the glucocorticoid should be considered with close monitoring of local and systemic effects or a switch to a glucocorticoid, which is not a substrate for CYP3A4 (e.g. beclomethasone). Moreover, in case of withdrawal of glucocorticoids progressive dose reduction may have to be performed over a longer period. The effects of high fluticasone systemic exposure on ritonavir plasma levels are as yet unknown.				
Dexamethasone	Systemic dexamethasone induces CYP3A4 and thereby may decrease darunavir exposure. Therefore this combination should be used with caution.				
Others					
St. John's wort	PREZISTA co-administered with low dose ritonavir must not be used concomitantly with products containing St John's wort (*Hypericum perforatum)* because co-administration may cause significant decreases in darunavir plasma concentrations and also in ritonavir concentrations. This is due to the induction of metabolising enzymes by St John's wort. If a patient is already taking St John's wort, stop St John's wort and if possible check viral levels. Darunavir exposure (and also ritonavir exposure) may increase on stopping St John's wort. The inducing effect may persist for at least 2 weeks after cessation of treatment with St John's wort (see section 4.3).				

Table 2

SOC Frequency category	Adverse reaction* All grades	Adverse reaction** Grade 2-4
Infections and infestations		
uncommon	herpes simplex	
Blood and lymphatic system disorders		
uncommon	thrombocytopenia, neutropenia, anaemia, increased eosinophil count, leukopenia	thrombocytopenia, neutropenia, anaemia
Immune system disorders		
uncommon	immune reconstitution syndrome	immune reconstitution syndrome
Endocrine disorders		
uncommon	hypothyroidism, increased blood thyroid stimulating hormone	
Metabolism and nutrition disorders		
common	lipodystrophy (including lipohypertrophy, lipodystrophy, lipoatrophy), hypertriglyceridaemia, hypercholesterolaemia, hyperlipidaemia	hypertriglyceridaemia, hypercholesterolaemia, hyperlipidaemia
uncommon	diabetes mellitus, gout, anorexia, decreased appetite, decreased weight, increased weight, hyperglycaemia, insulin resistance, decreased high density lipoprotein, increased appetite, polydipsia, increased blood lactate dehydrogenase	diabetes mellitus, lipodystrophy (including lipohypertrophy, lipodystrophy, lipoatrophy), gout, anorexia, decreased appetite, decreased weight, increased weight, hyperglycaemia, insulin resistance
Psychiatric disorders		
common	insomnia	
uncommon	depression, confusional state, disorientation, anxiety, altered mood, sleep disorder, abnormal dreams, nightmare, decreased libido, restlessness	depression, confusional state, disorientation, anxiety, altered mood, insomnia, sleep disorder, abnormal dreams
Nervous system disorders		
common	headache, peripheral neuropathy, dizziness	headache
uncommon	syncope, convulsion, lethargy, paraesthesia, hypoaesthesia, ageusia, dysgeusia, disturbance in attention, memory impairment, somnolence, sleep phase rhythm disturbance	peripheral neuropathy, dizziness, lethargy, paraesthesia, hypoaesthesia, somnolence
Eye disorders		
uncommon	visual disturbance, conjunctival hyperaemia, dry eye	conjunctival hyperaemia
Ear and labyrinth disorders		
uncommon	vertigo	vertigo
Cardiac disorders		
uncommon	acute myocardial infarction, myocardial infarction, angina pectoris, prolonged electrocardiogram QT, sinus bradycardia, tachycardia, palpitations	acute myocardial infarction, myocardial infarction, angina pectoris, prolonged electrocardiogram QT
Vascular disorders		
uncommon	hypertension, flushing	hypertension
Respiratory, thoracic and mediastinal disorders		
uncommon	dyspnoea, cough, epistaxis, rhinorrhoea, throat irritation	dyspnoea, cough
Gastrointestinal disorders		
very common	diarrhoea	
common	vomiting, nausea, abdominal pain, increased blood amylase, dyspepsia, abdominal distension, flatulence	vomiting, diarrhoea, nausea, abdominal pain, increased blood amylase
uncommon	pancreatitis, gastritis, gastrooesophageal reflux disease, aphthous stomatitis, stomatitis, retching, haematemesis, dry mouth, abdominal discomfort, constipation, increased lipase, eructation, oral dysaesthesia, cheilitis, dry lip, coated tongue	pancreatitis, gastritis, gastrooesophageal reflux disease, aphthous stomatitis, retching, dry mouth, abdominal distension, abdominal discomfort, flatulence, dyspepsia, constipation, increased lipase
Hepatobiliary disorders		
common	increased alanine aminotransferase, increased aspartate aminotransferase	increased alanine aminotransferase
uncommon	hepatitis, cytolytic hepatitis, hepatic steatosis, hepatomegaly, increased transaminase, increased blood bilirubin, increased blood alkaline phosphatase, increased gamma-glutamyltransferase	hepatitis, cytolytic hepatitis, hepatic steatosis, increased transaminase, increased aspartate aminotransferase, increased blood alkaline phosphatase, increased gamma-glutamyltransferase
Skin and subcutaneous tissue disorders		
common	rash (including macular, maculopapular, papular, erythematous and pruritic rash), pruritus	rash (including macular, maculopapular, papular, erythematous and pruritic rash)
uncommon	generalised rash, allergic dermatitis, face oedema, urticaria, dermatitis, eczema, erythema, hyperhidrosis, night sweats, alopecia, acne, seborrhoeic dermatitis, skin lesion, xeroderma, dry skin, nail pigmentation	generalised rash, allergic dermatitis, urticaria, pruritus, hyperhidrosis, night sweats, alopecia
Musculoskeletal and connective tissue disorders		
uncommon	myalgia, muscle spasms, muscular weakness, musculoskeletal stiffness, arthritis, arthralgia, joint stiffness, pain in extremity, osteoporosis, increased blood creatine phosphokinase	myalgia, arthralgia, pain in extremity, osteoporosis, increased blood creatine phosphokinase
Renal and urinary disorders		
uncommon	acute renal failure, renal failure, nephrolithiasis, increased blood creatinine, decreased creatinine renal clearance, proteinuria, bilirubinuria, dysuria, nocturia, pollakiuria	acute renal failure, renal failure, nephrolithiasis, increased blood creatinine, decreased creatinine renal clearance, proteinuria, bilirubinuria
Reproductive system and breast disorders		
uncommon	erectile dysfunction, gynaecomastia	erectile dysfunction, gynaecomastia
General disorders and administration site conditions		
common	asthenia, fatigue	fatigue
uncommon	pyrexia, chest pain, peripheral oedema, malaise, chills, abnormal feeling, feeling hot, irritability, pain, xerosis	pyrexia, chest pain, asthenia, peripheral oedema, malaise

* Adverse events, considered at least possibly related by the investigator to PREZISTA co-administered with low dose ritonavir, occurring in more than 1 patient.

** Adverse events, at least grade 2 in severity and considered at least possibly related by the investigator to PREZISTA co-administered with low dose ritonavir, occurring in more than 1 patient.

Table 3

Outcomes	TITAN PREZISTA/rtv 600/100 mg b.i.d. + OBR N=298	lopinavir/rtv 400/100 mg b.i.d. + OBR N=297	Treatment difference (95% CI of difference)
HIV-1 RNA < 400 copies/ml[a]	228 (76.5%)	199 (67.0%)	9.5% (2.3; 16.7)[b]
HIV-1 RNA < 50 copies/ml[a]	211 (70.8%)	179 (60.3%)	10.5% (2.9; 18.1)[b]
mean HIV-1 RNA log change from baseline ($\log_{10}$ copies/ml)[c]	-1.95	-1.72	-0.23[d] (-0.44; -0.02)[b]
median CD4+ cell count change from baseline (x 10^6/l)[c]	88	81	

[a] Imputations according to the TLOVR algorithm

[b] Based on a normal approximation of the difference in % response

[c] NC=F

[d] Difference in means

Table 4

Outcomes at 48 weeks	POWER 1 and POWER 2 pooled data			POWER 3
Baseline characteristics				
Mean plasma HIV-1 RNA	4.61 $\log_{10}$ copies/ml (PREZISTA/ritonavir) 4.49 $\log_{10}$ copies/ml (control)			4.58 $\log_{10}$ copies/ml
Median CD4+ cell count	153 × 10^6 cells/l (PREZISTA/ritonavir) 163 × 10^6 cells/l (control)			120 × 10^6 cells/l
Outcomes	PREZISTA/ritonavir 600/100 mg b.i.d. n=131	Control n=124	Treatment difference	PREZISTA/ritonavir 600/100 mg b.i.d. n=334
HIV-1 RNA $\log_{10}$ mean change from baseline ($\log_{10}$ copies/ml)[a]	-1.69	-0.37	1.32 (1.58; 1.05)[d]	-1.62
CD4+ cell count mean change from baseline (x 10^6/l)[b]	103	17	86 (57; 114)[d]	105
HIV RNA ≥ 1 $\log_{10}$ below baseline[c]	81 (61.8%)	20 (16.1%)	45.7% (35.0%; 56.4%)[d]	196 (58.7%)
HIV RNA < 400 copies/ml[c]	72 (55.0%)	18 (14.5%)	40.4% (29.8%; 51.1%)[d]	183 (54.8%)
HIV RNA < 50 copies/ml[c]	59 (45.0%)	14 (11.3%)	33.7% (23.4%; 44.1%)[d]	155 (46.4%)

[a] Non-completer is failure imputation: patients who discontinued prematurely are imputed with a change equal to 0

[b] Last Observation Carried Forward imputation

[c] Imputations according to the TLOVR algorithm

[d] 95% confidence intervals.

Gag-Pol polyproteins in virus infected cells, thereby preventing the formation of mature infectious virus particles.

Antiviral activity *in vitro*

Darunavir exhibits activity against laboratory strains and clinical isolates of HIV-1 and laboratory strains of HIV-2 in acutely infected T-cell lines, human peripheral blood mononuclear cells and human monocytes/macrophages with median EC_{50} values ranging from 1.2 to 8.5 nM (0.7 to 5.0 ng/ml). Darunavir demonstrates antiviral activity *in vitro* against a broad panel of HIV-1 group M (A, B, C, D, E, F, G) and group O primary isolates with EC_{50} values ranging from < 0.1 to 4.3 nM.

These EC_{50} values are well below the 50% cellular toxicity concentration range of 87 μM to > 100 μM.

The EC_{50} value of darunavir increases by a median factor of 5.4 in the presence of human serum.

Darunavir showed synergistic antiviral activity when studied in combination with the protease inhibitors ritonavir, nelfinavir, or amprenavir and additive antiviral activity when studied in combination with the protease inhibitors indinavir, saquinavir, lopinavir, atazanavir, or tipranavir, the N(t)RTIs zidovudine, lamivudine, zalcitabine, didanosine, stavudine, abacavir, emtricitabine, or tenofovir, the NNRTIs nevirapine, delavirdine, or efavirenz and the fusion inhibitor enfuvirtide. No antagonism was observed between darunavir and any of those antiretrovirals.

Resistance

In vitro selection of darunavir-resistant virus from wild type HIV-1 was lengthy (> 3 years). The selected viruses were unable to grow in the presence of darunavir concentrations above 400 nM. Viruses selected in these conditions and showing decreased susceptibility to darunavir (range: 23-50-fold) harboured 2 to 4 amino acid substitutions in the protease gene. Identification of determinants of decreased susceptibility to darunavir in those viruses is under investigation.

In vitro selection of darunavir resistant HIV-1 (range: 53-641-fold change in EC_{50} values [FC]) from 9 HIV-1 strains harbouring multiple PI Resistance-Associated Mutations (RAMs) showed that a minimum of 8 darunavir *in vitro* selected mutations were required in the HIV-1 protease to render a virus resistant (FC> 10) to darunavir.

In a pooled analysis of the POWER 1, 2 and 3 (see Clinical experience subsection) and DUET 1 and 2 (TMC125-C206 and TMC125-C216) trials the amino acid substitutions identified that developed on PREZISTA co-administered with ritonavir (600/100 mg b.i.d.) in ≥ 20% of the isolates from subjects who experienced virologic failure by rebound were V32I, I54L and L89V. Amino acid substitutions that developed in 10 to 20% of the isolates were V11I, I13V, L33F, I50V and F53L. Amino acid substitutions that developed in 5 to 10% of isolates were L10F, I15V, M36L, K43T, M46I, I47V, A71I, G73S, T74P, L76V, V82I and I84V.

Of the viruses isolated from patients experiencing virologic failure by rebound from the PREZISTA/rtv 600/100 mg b.i.d. group of the POWER and DUET trials, 85% of those susceptible to darunavir at baseline developed decreased susceptibility to darunavir during treatment.

In the same group of patients, 71% of viruses that were susceptible to tipranavir at baseline remained susceptible after treatment.

Cross-resistance

Darunavir has a < 10-fold decreased susceptibility against 90% of 3,309 clinical isolates resistant to amprenavir, atazanavir, indinavir, lopinavir, nelfinavir, ritonavir, saquinavir and/or tipranavir showing that viruses resistant to most PIs remain susceptible to darunavir.

Clinical experience

Adult patients

Efficacy of PREZISTA co-administered with 100 mg ritonavir in treatment-naïve patients

There are no data on the efficacy of darunavir co-administered with 100 mg ritonavir in treatment-naïve HIV-1 infected patients.

Efficacy of PREZISTA co-administered with 100 mg ritonavir in treatment-experienced patients

The evidence of efficacy of PREZISTA co-administered with ritonavir (600/100 mg b.i.d.) in treatment-experienced patients is based on the 48 weeks analysis of the Phase III trial TITAN in treatment-experienced lopinavir naïve patients and on the analyses of 96 weeks data from the Phase IIb trials POWER 1, 2 and 3 in patients with high level of PI resistance.

TITAN is an ongoing randomised, controlled, open-label Phase III trial comparing PREZISTA co-administered with ritonavir (600/100 mg b.i.d.) versus lopinavir/ritonavir (400/100 mg b.i.d) in treatment-experienced, lopinavir naïve HIV-1 infected adult patients. Both arms used an Optimised Background Regimen (OBR) consisting of at least 2 antiretrovirals (NRTIs with or without NNRTIs). The mean baseline plasma HIV-1 RNA was 4.33 $\log_{10}$ copies/ml and the median baseline CD4+ cell count was 235 × 10^6 cells/l (range 3 – 831 × 10^6 cells/l) in the PREZISTA/ritonavir arm.

The table below shows the efficacy data of the 48 week analysis from the TITAN trial.

(see Table 3 above)

Non-inferiority in virologic response, defined as the percentage of subjects with plasma HIV-1 RNA level < 400 copies/ml, was demonstrated (at the chosen 12% non-inferiority margin) for both Intent-To-Treat and On Protocol populations.

POWER 1 *and* **POWER 2** are randomised, controlled trials consisting of an initial dose-finding part and a second long-term part in which all patients randomised to PREZISTA co-administered with 100 mg ritonavir received the recommended dose of 600/100 mg b.i.d.

HIV-1 infected patients who were eligible for these trials had previously failed more than 1 PI containing regimen. PREZISTA co-administered with 100 mg ritonavir plus an optimised background regimen (OBR) was compared to a control group receiving an investigator-selected PI(s) regimen plus an OBR. The OBR consisted of at least 2 NRTIs with or without enfuvirtide (ENF).

POWER 3: additional data on the efficacy of PREZISTA co-administered with ritonavir 600/100 mg b.i.d. with OBR have been obtained in similar treatment-experienced patients participating in the non-randomised trial TMC114-C215. Entry criteria were the same as and baseline characteristics were comparable to those of POWER 1 and POWER 2.

The table below shows the efficacy data of the 48-week analyses on the recommended 600 mg dose of PREZISTA co-administered with 100 mg ritonavir b.i.d. from the pooled POWER 1 and POWER 2 trials as well as from the POWER 3 trial.

(see Table 4 above)

Analyses of data through 96 weeks of treatment in the three POWER trials demonstrated sustained antiretroviral efficacy and immunological benefit. Treatment with PREZISTA co-administered with ritonavir (600/100 mg b.i.d.) resulted in 56.5% (POWER 1 and 2) and 52.2% (POWER 3) of responders with a decrease of at least 1 log10 in HIV RNA from baseline, 38.9% (POWER 1 and 2) and 42.1% (POWER 3) of subjects with an HIV RNA level < 50 copies/ml and 49.6% (POWER 1 and 2) and 50.0% (POWER 3) respectively of subjects with an HIV RNA level less than 400 copies/ml. The mean decrease in HIV RNA level compared to baseline was 1.58 (POWER 1 and 2) and 1.43 (POWER 3) log10 copies/ml and a mean increase in

Table 5

Number of mutations at baseline*	All subjects % n/N	Subjects with no/non-naïve use of ENF % n/N	Subjects with naïve use of ENF % n/N
All ranges	45% 455/1,014	39% 290/741	60% 165/273
0-2	54% 359/660	50% 238/477	66% 121/183
3	39% 67/172	29% 35/120	62% 32/52
≥ 4	12% 20/171	7% 10/135	28% 10/36

* Number of mutations from the list of mutations associated with a diminished response to PREZISTA/ritonavir (V11I, V32I, L33F, I47V, I50V, I54L or M, T74P, L76V, I84V or L89V)

Table 6

Baseline darunavir phenotype	All subjects % n/N	Subjects with no/non-naïve use of ENF % n/N	Subjects with naïve use of ENF % n/N
All ranges	45% 455/1,014	39% 290/741	60% 165/273
≤ 10	55% 364/659	51% 244/477	66% 120/182
10-40	29% 59/203	17% 25/147	61% 34/56
> 40	8% 9/118	5% 5/94	17% 4/24

CD4+ cell count of 133 × 10^6 cells/l (POWER 1 and 2) and 103 × 10^6 cells/l (POWER 3) was observed.

Out of the 206 subjects who responded with complete viral suppression (< 50 copies/ml) at week 48, 177 subjects (86% of the responders at week 48) remained responders at week 96.

Baseline genotype or phenotype and virologic outcome

In a pooled analysis of the 600/100 mg b.i.d. groups of the POWER and DUET trials, the presence at baseline of 3 or more of mutations V11I, V32I, L33F, I47V, I50V, I54L or M, T74P, L76V, I84V or L89V was associated with a decreased virologic response to PREZISTA co-administered with 100 mg ritonavir. The presence of these individual mutations was associated with a median of 13 to 15 PI resistance associated mutations of the IAS-USA list of mutations.

In early treatment-experienced patients (TITAN) three or more of these mutations were only found in 4% of the patients at baseline.

Response (HIV-1 RNA < 50 copies/ml at week 24) to PREZISTA co-administered with ritonavir (600/100 mg b.i.d.) by baseline genotype and by use of enfuvirtide (ENF): As treated analysis of the POWER and DUET trials.*

(see Table 5 on previous page)

Baseline darunavir phenotype (shift in susceptibility relative to reference) was shown to be a predictive factor of virologic outcome.

Response (HIV-1 RNA < 50 copies/ml at week 24) to PREZISTA co-administered with ritonavir (600/100 mg b.i.d.) by baseline darunavir phenotype and by use of enfuvirtide: As treated analysis of the POWER and DUET trials.

(see Table 6 above)

Children from the age of 6 years and adolescents

DELPHI is an open-label, Phase II trial evaluating the pharmacokinetics, safety, tolerability, and efficacy of PREZISTA with low dose ritonavir in 80 ART-experienced HIV-1 infected paediatric patients aged 6 to 17 years and weighing at least 20 kg. These patients received PREZISTA/ritonavir in combination with other antiretroviral agents (see section 4.2 for dosage recommendations per body weight). Virologic response was defined as a decrease in plasma HIV-1 RNA viral load of at least 1.0 log10 versus baseline.

In the study, patients who were at risk of discontinuing therapy due to intolerance of ritonavir oral solution (e.g. taste aversion) were allowed to switch to the capsule formulation. Of the 44 patients taking ritonavir oral solution, 27 switched to the 100 mg capsule formulation and exceeded the weight-based ritonavir dose without changes in observed safety.

DELPHI	
Baseline disease characteristics	
Mean plasma HIV-1 RNA	4.64 $\log_{10}$ copies/ml
Median CD4+ cell count	330 × 10^6 cells/l (range: 6 to 1,505 × 10^6 cells/l)
Outcomes at week 48	PREZISTA/ritonavir N=80
HIV-1 RNA ≥ 1 $\log_{10}$ below baseline[a]	52 (65.0%)
HIV-1 RNA < 50 copies/ml[a]	38 (47.5%)
HIV-1 RNA < 400 copies/ml[a]	47 (58.8%)
HIV-1 RNA $\log_{10}$ mean change from baseline[b]	-1.81
CD4+ cell count mean change from baseline[b]	147

[a] Imputations according to the TLOVR algorithm.

[b] Non-completer is failure imputation: patients who discontinued prematurely are imputed with a change equal to 0.

According to the TLOVR non-virologic failure censored algorithm 24 (30.0%) subjects experienced virological failure, of which 17 (21.3%) subjects were rebounders and 7 (8.8%) subjects were non-responders.

5.2 Pharmacokinetic properties

The pharmacokinetic properties of darunavir, co-administered with ritonavir, have been evaluated in healthy adult volunteers and in HIV-1 infected patients. Exposure to darunavir was higher in HIV-1 infected patients than in healthy subjects. The increased exposure to darunavir in HIV-1 infected patients compared to healthy subjects may be explained by the higher concentrations of alpha-1-acid glycoprotein (AAG) in HIV-1 infected patients, resulting in higher darunavir binding to plasma AAG and, therefore, higher plasma concentrations.

Darunavir is primarily metabolised by CYP3A. Ritonavir inhibits CYP3A, thereby increasing the plasma concentrations of darunavir considerably.

Absorption

Darunavir was rapidly absorbed following oral administration. Maximum plasma concentration of darunavir in the presence of low dose ritonavir is generally achieved within 2.5-4.0 hours.

The absolute oral bioavailability of a single 600 mg dose of darunavir alone was approximately 37% and increased to approximately 82% in the presence of 100 mg b.i.d. ritonavir. The overall pharmacokinetic enhancement effect by ritonavir was an approximate 14-fold increase in the systemic exposure of darunavir when a single dose of 600 mg darunavir was given orally in combination with ritonavir at 100 mg b.i.d. (see section 4.4).

When administered without food, the relative bioavailability of darunavir in the presence of low dose ritonavir is 30% lower as compared to intake with food. Therefore, PREZISTA tablets should be taken with ritonavir and with food. The type of food does not affect exposure to darunavir.

Distribution

Darunavir is approximately 95% bound to plasma protein. Darunavir binds primarily to plasma alpha-1-acid glycoprotein.

Following intravenous administration, the volume of distribution of darunavir alone was 88.1 ± 59.0 l (Mean ± SD) and increased to 131 ± 49.9 l (Mean ± SD) in the presence of 100 mg twice-daily ritonavir.

Metabolism

In vitro experiments with human liver microsomes (HLMs) indicate that darunavir primarily undergoes oxidative metabolism. Darunavir is extensively metabolised by the hepatic CYP system and almost exclusively by isozyme CYP3A4. A ^{14}C-darunavir trial in healthy volunteers showed that a majority of the radioactivity in plasma after a single 400/100 mg darunavir with ritonavir dose was due to the parent active substance. At least 3 oxidative metabolites of darunavir have been identified in humans; all showed activity that was at least 10-fold less than the activity of darunavir against wild type HIV.

Elimination

After a 400/100 mg ^{14}C-darunavir with ritonavir dose, approximately 79.5% and 13.9% of the administered dose of ^{14}C-darunavir could be retrieved in faeces and urine, respectively. Unchanged darunavir accounted for approximately 41.2% and 7.7% of the administered dose in faeces and urine, respectively. The terminal elimination half-life of darunavir was approximately 15 hours when combined with ritonavir.

The intravenous clearance of darunavir alone (150 mg) and in the presence of low dose ritonavir was 32.8 l/h and 5.9 l/h, respectively.

Special Populations

Paediatrics

The pharmacokinetics of darunavir in combination with ritonavir in 74 treatment-experienced paediatric patients, aged 6 to 17 years and weighing at least 20 kg, showed that the administered weight-based doses of PREZISTA/ritonavir resulted in darunavir exposure comparable to that in adults receiving PREZISTA/ritonavir 600/100 mg b.i.d. (see section 4.2).

Elderly

Population pharmacokinetic analysis in HIV infected patients showed that darunavir pharmacokinetics are not considerably different in the age range (18 to 75 years) evaluated in HIV infected patients (n=12, age ≥ 65) (see section 4.4). However, only limited data were available in patients above the age of 65 year.

Gender

Population pharmacokinetic analysis showed a slightly higher darunavir exposure (16.8%) in HIV infected females compared to males. This difference is not clinically relevant.

Renal impairment

Results from a mass balance study with ^{14}C-darunavir with ritonavir showed that approximately 7.7% of the administered dose of darunavir is excreted in the urine unchanged.

Although darunavir has not been studied in patients with renal impairment, population pharmacokinetic analysis showed that the pharmacokinetics of darunavir were not significantly affected in HIV infected patients with moderate renal impairment (CrCl between 30-60 ml/min, n=20) (see sections 4.2 and 4.4).

Hepatic impairment

Darunavir is primarily metabolised and eliminated by the liver. In a multiple dose study with PREZISTA co-administered with ritonavir (600/100 mg) twice daily, it was demonstrated that the total plasma concentrations of darunavir in subjects with mild (Child-Pugh Class A, n=8) and moderate (Child-Pugh Class B, n=8) hepatic impairment were comparable with those in healthy subjects. However, unbound darunavir concentrations were approximately 55% (Child-Pugh Class A) and 100% (Child-Pugh Class B) higher, respectively. The clinical relevance of this increase is unknown therefore, PREZISTA should be used with caution. The effect of severe hepatic impairment on the pharmacokinetics of darunavir has not been studied (see sections 4.2, 4.3 and 4.4).

5.3 Preclinical safety data

Animal toxicology studies have been conducted at exposures up to clinical exposure levels with darunavir alone, in mice, rats and dogs and in combination with ritonavir in rats and dogs.

In repeated-dose toxicology studies in mice, rats and dogs, there were only limited effects of treatment with darunavir. In rodents the target organs identified were the haematopoietic system, the blood coagulation system, liver and thyroid. A variable but limited decrease in red blood cell-related parameters was observed, together with increases in activated partial thromboplastin time.

Changes were observed in liver (hepatocyte hypertrophy, vacuolation, increased liver enzymes) and thyroid (follicular hypertrophy). In the rat, the combination of darunavir with ritonavir lead to a small increase in effect on RBC parameters, liver and thyroid and increased incidence of islet fibrosis in the pancreas (in male rats only) compared to treatment with darunavir alone. In the dog, no major toxicity findings or target organs were identified up to exposures equivalent to clinical exposure at the recommended dose.

In a study conducted in rats, the number of corpora lutea and implantations were decreased in the presence of maternal toxicity. Otherwise, there were no effects on mating or fertility with darunavir treatment up to 1,000 mg/kg/day and exposure levels below (AUC-0.5 fold) of that in human at the clinically recommended dose. Up to same dose levels, there was no teratogenicity with darunavir in rats and rabbits when treated alone nor in mice when treated in combination with ritonavir. The exposure levels were lower than those with the recommended clinical dose in humans. In a pre- and postnatal development assessment in rats, darunavir with and without ritonavir, caused a transient reduction in body weight gain of the offspring pre-weaning and there was a slight delay in the opening of eyes and ears. Darunavir in combination with ritonavir caused a reduction in the number of pups that exhibited the startle response on day 15 of lactation and a reduced pup survival during lactation. These effects may be secondary to pup exposure to the active substance via the milk and/or maternal toxicity. No post weaning functions were affected with darunavir alone or in combination with ritonavir. In juvenile rats receiving darunavir up to days 23-26, increased mortality was observed with convulsions in some animals. Exposure in plasma, liver and brain was considerably higher than in adult rats after comparable doses in mg/kg between days 5 and 11 of age. After day 23 of life, the exposure was comparable to that in adult rats. The increased exposure was likely at least partly due to immaturity of the drug-metabolising enzymes in juvenile animals. No treatment related mortalities were noted in juvenile rats dosed at 1,000 mg/kg darunavir (single dose) on day 26 of age or at 500 mg/kg (repeated dose) from day 23 to 50 of age, and the exposures and toxicity profile were comparable to those observed in adult rats.

Due to uncertainties regarding the rate of development of the human blood brain barrier and liver enzymes, PREZISTA with low dose ritonavir should not be used in paediatric patients below 3 years of age.

Darunavir was evaluated for carcinogenic potential by oral gavage administration to mice and rats up to 104 weeks. Daily doses of 150, 450 and 1,000 mg/kg were administered to mice and doses of 50, 150 and 500 mg/kg were administered to rats. Dose-related increases in the incidences of hepatocellular adenomas and carcinomas were observed in males and females of both species. Thyroid follicular cell adenomas were noted in male rats.

Administration of darunavir did not cause a statistically significant increase in the incidence of any other benign or malignant neoplasm in mice or rats. The observed hepatocellular and thyroid tumours in rodents are considered to be of limited relevance to humans. Repeated administration of darunavir to rats caused hepatic microsomal enzyme induction and increased thyroid hormone elimination, which predispose rats, but not humans, to thyroid neoplasms. At the highest tested doses, the systemic exposures (based on AUC) to darunavir were between 0.4- and 0.7-fold (mice) and 0.7- and 1-fold (rats), relative to those observed in humans at the recommended therapeutic doses.

After 2 years administration of darunavir at exposures at or below the human exposure, kidney changes were observed in mice (nephrosis) and rats (chronic progressive nephropathy).

Darunavir was not mutagenic or genotoxic in a battery of *in vitro* and *in vivo* assays including bacterial reverse mutation (Ames), chromosomal aberration in human lymphocytes and *in vivo* micronucleus test in mice.

6. PHARMACEUTICAL PARTICULARS

6.1 List of excipients

Tablet core

Microcrystalline cellulose

Colloidal anhydrous silica

Crospovidone

Magnesium stearate

Tablet film-coat

Poly (vinyl alcohol) – partially hydrolyzed

Macrogol 3350

Titanium dioxide (E171)

Talc

6.2 Incompatibilities

Not applicable.

6.3 Shelf life

2 years

6.4 Special precautions for storage

This medicinal product does not require any special storage conditions.

6.5 Nature and contents of container

PREZISTA 75 mg: opaque, white, high density polyethylene (HDPE) plastic, 160 ml bottle containing 480 tablets, fitted with polypropylene (PP) child resistant closure.

PREZISTA 150 mg: opaque, white, high density polyethylene (HDPE) plastic, 160 ml bottle containing 240 tablets, fitted with polypropylene (PP) child resistant closure.

One bottle

6.6 Special precautions for disposal and other handling

No special requirements.

7. MARKETING AUTHORISATION HOLDER

Janssen-Cilag International NV
Turnhoutseweg 30
B-2340 Beerse
Belgium

8. MARKETING AUTHORISATION NUMBER(S)

EU/1/06/380/005

EU/1/06/380/004

9. DATE OF FIRST AUTHORISATION/RENEWAL OF THE AUTHORISATION

Date of first authorisation: 12 February 2007

Date of latest renewal: 12 February 2009

10. DATE OF REVISION OF THE TEXT

Detailed information on this product is available on the website of the European Medicines Agency (EMEA) http://www.emea.europa.eu/.

Priadel 200mg & 400mg prolonged release tablets

(sanofi-aventis)

1. NAME OF THE MEDICINAL PRODUCT

Priadel 400mg prolonged release tablets.

Priadel 200mg prolonged release tablets.

2. QUALITATIVE AND QUANTITATIVE COMPOSITION

Priadel tablets contain 400mg lithium carbonate.

Priadel 200 tablets contain 200mg lithium carbonate.

3. PHARMACEUTICAL FORM

Priadel: White, circular, bi-convex tablets engraved PRIADEL on one side, scored on the other side, in a prolonged release formulation.

Priadel 200: White, scored, capsule-shaped tablets engraved P200 on one side, in a prolonged release formulation.

4. CLINICAL PARTICULARS

4.1 Therapeutic indications

1. In the management of acute manic or hypomanic episodes.

2. In the management of episodes of recurrent depressive disorders where treatment with other antidepressants has been unsuccessful.

3. In the prophylaxis against bipolar affective disorders.

4. Control of aggressive behaviour or intentional self harm.

4.2 Posology and method of administration

A simple treatment schedule has been evolved which except for some minor variations should be followed whether using Priadel therapeutically or prophylactically. The minor variations to this schedule depend on the elements of the illness being treated and these are described later.

1. In patients of average weight (70kg) an initial dose of 400-1,200mg of Priadel may be given as a single daily dose in the morning or on retiring. Alternatively, the dose may be divided and given morning and evening. The tablets should not be crushed or chewed. When changing between lithium preparations serum lithium levels should first be checked, then Priadel therapy commenced at a daily dose as close as possible to the dose of the other form of lithium. As bioavailability varies from product to product (particularly with regard to retard or slow release preparations) a change of product should be regarded as initiation of new treatment.

2. Four to five days after starting treatment (and never longer than one week) a blood sample should be taken for the estimation of serum lithium level.

3. The objective is to adjust the Priadel dose so as to maintain the "Target" serum lithium concentrations at 12 and 24 hours as shown in the table below.

"Target" serum lithium concentration (mmol/l)

	At 12 hours	At 24 hours
Once daily dosage	0.7 – 1.0	0.5 – 0.8
Twice daily dosage	0.5 – 0.8	

Both strengths have break lines, therefore they can be divided accurately to provide dosage requirements as small as 100mg. Serum lithium levels should be monitored weekly until stabilisation is achieved. The serum level should not exceed 1.5 mmol/l.

4. Lithium therapy should not be initiated unless adequate facilities for routine monitoring of serum concentrations are available. Following stabilisation of serum lithium levels, the period between subsequent estimations can be increased gradually but should not normally exceed three months. Additional measurements should be made following alteration of dosage, on development of intercurrent disease, signs of manic or depressive relapse, following significant change in sodium or fluid intake, or if signs of lithium toxicity occur.

5. Whilst a high proportion of acutely ill patients may respond within three to seven days of the commencement of Priadel therapy, Priadel should be continued through any recurrence of the affective disturbance. This is important as the full prophylactic effect may not occur for 6 to 12 months after the initiation of therapy.

6. In patients who show a positive response to Priadel therapy, treatment is likely to be long term. Careful clinical appraisal of the patient should be exercised throughout medication (see precautions).

7. If lithium is to be discontinued, particularly in cases of high doses, the dose should be reduced gradually.

Prophylactic treatment of bipolar affective disorders and control of aggressive behaviour or intentional self harm: It is recommended that the described treatment schedule is followed.

Treatment of acute manic or hypomanic episodes and recurrent depressive disorders: It is likely that a higher than normal Priadel intake may be necessary during an acute phase and divided doses would be required here. The monitoring should maintain serum levels at 0.8-1.5 mmol/l until acute symptoms have been controlled. In all other details the described treatment schedule is recommended.

Elderly:

Elderly patients or those below 50kg in weight, often require lower lithium dosage to achieve therapeutic serum levels. Starting doses of 200mg to 400mg are recommended. Dosage increments of 200 to 400mg every 3 to 5 days are usual. Total daily doses of 800 to 1800mg may be necessary to achieve effective blood lithium levels of 0.8 to 1.0 mmol/l. For prophylaxis, the dosage necessary to reach a blood lithium level of 0.4 to 0.8 mmol/l is generally in the range of 600 to 1200 mg/day.

Children and adolescents:

Not recommended.

4.3 Contraindications

• Hypersensitivity to lithium or to any of the excipients.

• Cardiac disease.

• Clinically significant renal impairment.

• Untreated hypothyroidism.

• Breast-feeding.

• Patients with low body sodium levels, including for example dehydrated patients or those on low sodium diets.

• Addison's disease.

4.4 Special warnings and precautions for use

• When considering Priadel therapy, it is necessary to ascertain whether patients are receiving lithium in any other form. If so, check serum levels before proceeding.

• Before beginning a lithium treatment:

– it is important to ensure that renal function is normal.

– cardiac function should be assessed.

– thyroid function should be evaluated. Patients should be euthyroid before initiation of lithium therapy.

• Renal, cardiac and thyroid functions should be re-assessed periodically.

• The possibility of hypothyroidism and renal dysfunction arising during prolonged treatment should be borne in mind and periodic assessments made.

• Patients receiving long term lithium therapy should be warned by the physician and be given clear instructions regarding the symptoms of impending intoxication (see 4.9 Overdose). They should be warned of the urgency of immediate action should these symptoms appear, and also of the need to maintain a constant and adequate salt and water intake. Treatment should be discontinued immediately on the first signs of toxicity (see 4.9 Overdose).

• Patients should be warned to report if polyuria or polydipsia develop. Episodes of nausea, vomiting, diarrhoea, fluid deprivation (e.g. excessive sweating), and/or other conditions leading to salt/water depletion should also be reported. Drugs likely to upset electrolyte balance such as diuretics (including severe dieting) should also be reported. Indeed, sodium depletion increases the plasma lithium concentration (due to competitive reabsorption at the renal level). In these cases, lithium dosage should be closely monitored and reduction of dosage may be necessary.

• Caution should be exercised to ensure that diet and fluid intake are normal in order to maintain a stable electrolyte balance. This may be of special importance in very hot weather or work environment. Infectious diseases including colds, influenza, gastro-enteritis and urinary infections may alter fluid balance and thus affect serum lithium levels. Treatment should be discontinued during any intercurrent infection and should only be reinstituted after the patient's physical health has returned to normal.

• Elderly patients are particularly liable to lithium toxicity. Use with care as lithium excretion may also be reduced. They may exhibit adverse reactions at serum levels ordinarily tolerated by younger patients.

4.5 Interaction with other medicinal products and other forms of interaction

Interactions which increase lithium concentrations:

If one of the following drugs is initiated, lithium dosage should either be adjusted or concomitant treatment stopped, as appropriate:

• Metronidazole.

• Non-steroidal anti-inflammatory drugs (monitor serum lithium concentrations more frequently if NSAID therapy is initiated or discontinued).

• ACE inhibitors.

• Diuretics (thiazides show a paradoxical antidiuretics effect resulting in possible water retention and lithium intoxication). If a thiazide diuretic has to be prescribed for a lithium-treated patient, lithium dosage should first be reduced and the patient re-stabilised with frequent monitoring. Similar precautions should be exercised on diuretic withdrawal.

• Other drugs affecting electrolyte balance, e.g. steroids, may alter lithium excretion and should therefore be avoided.

• Tetracyclines.

Interactions which decrease serum lithium concentrations:

• Xanthines (theophylline, caffeine).

• Sodium bicarbonate containing products.

• Diuretics (osmotic and carbonic anhydrase inhibitors).

• Urea.

Interactions causing neurotoxicity:

• Neuroleptics (particularly haloperidol at higher dosages), flupentixol, diazepam, thioridazine, fluphenazine, chlorpromazine and clozapine may lead in rare cases to neurotoxicity in the form of confusion, disorientation, lethargy, tremor, extra-pyramidal symptoms and myoclonus.

• Methyldopa.

• Selective Serotonin Re-uptake Inhibitors (e.g. fluvoxamine and fluoxetine) as this combination may precipitate a serotoninergic syndrome, which justifies immediate discontinuation of treatment.

• Calcium channel blockers may lead to a risk of neurotoxicity in the form of ataxia, confusion and somnolence, reversible after discontinuation of the drug. Lithium concentrations may be increased.

• Carbamazepine may lead to dizziness, somnolence, confusion and cerebellar symptoms.

Lithium may prolong the effects of neuromuscular blocking agents. There have been reports of interaction between lithium and phenytoin, indometacin and other prostaglandin-synthetase inhibitors.

4.6 Pregnancy and lactation

4.6.1 Pregnancy

Lithium therapy should not be used during pregnancy, especially during the first trimester, unless considered essential. There is epidemiological evidence that it may be harmful to the foetus in human pregnancy. Lithium crosses the placental barrier. In animal studies lithium has been reported to interfere with fertility, gestation and foetal development. An increase in cardiac and other abnormalities, especially Ebstein anomaly, are reported. Therefore, a pre-natal diagnosis such as ultrasound and electrocardiogram examination is strongly recommended. In certain cases where a severe risk to the patient could exist if treatment were stopped, lithium has been continued during pregnancy.

If it is considered essential to maintain lithium treatment during pregnancy, serum lithium levels should be closely monitored and measured frequently since renal function changes gradually during pregnancy and suddenly at parturition. Dosage adjustments are required. It is recommended that lithium be discontinued shortly before delivery and reinitiated a few days *post-partum*.

Neonates may show signs of lithium toxicity necessitating fluid therapy in the neonatal period. Neonates born with low serum lithium concentrations may have a flaccid appearance that returns to normal without any treatment.

4.6.2 Women of child-bearing potential

It is advisable that women treated with lithium should adopt adequate contraceptive methods. In case of a planned pregnancy, it is strongly recommended to discontinue lithium therapy.

4.6.3 Lactation

Since adequate human data on use during lactation, adequate animal reproduction studies are not available and as lithium is secreted in breast milk, bottle-feeding is recommended (see section 4.3 Contra-indications).

4.7 Effects on ability to drive and use machines

As lithium may cause disturbances of the CNS, patients should be warned of the possible hazards when driving or operating machinery.

4.8 Undesirable effects

Side effects are usually related to serum lithium concentration and are less common in patients with plasma lithium concentrations below 1.0 mmol/l.

Initial therapy: fine tremor of the hands, polyuria and thirst may occur.

Body as a whole: muscle weakness, peripheral oedema.

Cardiovascular: cardiac arrhythmia (NOS), mainly bradycardia, sinus node dysfunction, peripheral circulatory collapse, hypotension, oedema, ECG changes such as reversible flattening or inversion of T-waves and QT prolongation, cardiomyopathy.

CNS: ataxia, hyperactive deep tendon reflexes, extrapyramidal symptoms, seizures, slurred speech, dizziness, nystagmus, stupor, coma, pseudotumor cerebri, myasthenia gravis, vertigo, giddiness, dazed feeling, memory impairment.

Dermatology: alopecia, acne, folliculitis, pruritus, aggravation or occurrence of psoriasis, allergic rashes, acneiform eruptions, papular skin disorders, cutaneous ulcers.

Endocrine: euthyroid goitre, hypothyroidism, hyperthyroidism and thyrotoxicosis. Lithium-induced hypothyroidism may be managed successfully with concurrent levothyroxine. Hypercalcaemia, hypermagnesaemia, hyperparathyroidism have been reported.

Gastrointestinal: anorexia, nausea, vomiting, diarrhoea, excessive salivation, dry mouth, abdominal discomfort, taste disorder, gastritis.

Haematological: leucocytosis.

Metabolic and Nutrional: weight gain, hyperglycaemia.

Renal: polydipsia and/or polyuria, symptoms of nephrogenic diabetes insipidus, histological renal changes with interstitial fibrosis after long term treatment.

High serum concentrations of lithium including episodes of acute lithium toxicity may aggravate these changes. The minimum clinically effective dose of lithium should always be used. In patients who develop polyuria and/or polydipsia, renal function should be monitored, e.g. with measurement of blood urea, serum creatinine and urinary protein levels in addition to the routine serum lithium assessment.

Reproductive: sexual dysfunction.

Senses: dysgeusia, blurred vision, scotomata.

Rare cases of nephrotic syndrome, speech disorder, confusion, impaired consciousness, myoclonus and abnormal reflex have been reported.

If any of the above symptoms appear, treatment should be stopped immediately and arrangements made for serum lithium measurement.

4.9 Overdose

In patients with a raised lithium concentration, the risk of toxicity is greater in those with the following underlying medical conditions: hypertension, diabetes, congestive heart failure, chronic renal failure, schizophrenia, Addison's disease.

Acute

A single acute overdose usually carries low risk and patients tend to show mild symptoms only, irrespective of their serum lithium concentration. However more severe symptoms may occur after a delay if lithium elimination is reduced because of renal impairment, particularly if a slow-release preparation has been taken. The fatal dose, in a single overdose, is probably over 5g.

If an acute overdose has been taken by a patient on chronic lithium therapy, this can lead to serious toxicity occurring even after a modest overdose as the extravascular tissues are already saturated with lithium.

Chronic

Lithium toxicity can also occur in chronic accumulation for the following reasons: Acute or chronic overdosage; dehydration e.g. due to intercurrent illness, deteriorating renal function, drug interactions, most commonly involving a thiazide diuretic or a non-steroidal anti-inflammatory drug (NSAID).

Symptoms

The onset of symptoms may be delayed, with peak effects not occurring for as long as 24 hours, especially in patients who are not receiving chronic lithium therapy or following the use of a sustained release preparation.

Mild: Nausea, diarrhoea, blurred vision, polyuria, light headedness, fine resting tremor, muscular weakness and drowsiness.

Moderate: Increasing confusion, blackouts, fasciculation and increased deep tendon reflexes, myoclonic twitches and jerks, choreoathetoid movements, urinary or faecal incontinence, increasing restlessness followed by stupor. Hypernatraemia.

Severe: Coma, convulsions, cerebellar signs, cardiac dysrythmias including sinoatrial block, sinus and junctional bradycardia and first degree heart block. Hypotension or rarely hypertension, circulatory collapse and renal failure.

Management

There is no specific antidote to lithium poisoning. In the event of accumulation, lithium should be stopped and serum estimation should be carried out every 6 hours. Under no circumstances should a diuretic be used. Osmotic diuresis (mannitol or urea infusion) or alkalinisation of the urine (sodium lactate or sodium bicarbonate infusion) should be initiated. All patients should be observed for a minimum of 24 hours. ECG should be monitored in symptomatic patients. Steps should be taken to correct hypotension.

Consider gastric lavage for non-sustained-release preparations if more than 4 g has been ingested by an adult within 1 hour or definite ingestion of a significant amount by a child. Slow-release tablets do not disintegrate in the stomach and most are too large to pass up a lavage tube. Gut decontamination is not useful for chronic accumulation. Activated charcoal does not adsorb lithium.

Peritoneal or haemodialysis should be instituted promptly if there is deterioration in the patient's condition (e.g. marked neurological or cardiac features), if the serum lithium level is over 4.0 mmol/l, in an acute overdose (not in addition to chronic use), if there is a deterioration in the patient's condition, or if the serum lithium concentration is not falling at a rate corresponding to a half-life of under 30 hours. This should be continued until there is no lithium in the serum or dialysis fluid. Serum lithium levels should be monitored for at least a further week to take account of any possible rebound in serum lithium levels as a result of delayed diffusion from the body tissues.

In cases of acute on chronic overdose or in cases of chronic lithium toxicity if the lithium concentration is >4.0 mmol/l, discuss with your local poisons service.

Clinical improvement generally takes longer than reduction of serum lithium concentrations regardless of the method used.

5. PHARMACOLOGICAL PROPERTIES

5.1 Pharmacodynamic properties

The mode of action of lithium is still not fully understood. However, lithium modifies the production and turnover of certain neurotransmitters, particularly serotonin, and it may also block dopamine receptors.

It modifies concentrations of some electrolytes, particularly calcium and magnesium, and it may reduce thyroid activity.

5.2 Pharmacokinetic properties

Lithium has a half life of about 24-hours although this increases to about 36-hours in the elderly due to a progressive decrease in renal lithium clearance with age. Lithium is 95% eliminated in the urine. Time to peak serum level for prolonged release Priadel tablets is about 2 hours and approximately 90% bioavailability would be expected.

5.3 Preclinical safety data

Nothing of therapeutic relevance.

6. PHARMACEUTICAL PARTICULARS

6.1 List of excipients

Priadel contains Glycerol distearate, mannitol, acacia spray dried, sodium laurilsulfate, magnesium stearate, maize starch and sodium starch glycolate (Type A).

Priadel 200 contains Glycerol monostearate, glycerol distearate, mannitol, acacia spray dried, sodium laurilsulfate, magnesium stearate, maize starch and sodium starch glycolate (Type A).

6.2 Incompatibilities

None stated

6.3 Shelf life

Three years.

6.4 Special precautions for storage

Do not store above 25°C. Store in the original package to protect from moisture.

6.5 Nature and contents of container

Pack sizes:

Priadel: Blister packs 100

Priadel 200: Blister packs 100

6.6 Special precautions for disposal and other handling

Not applicable

7. MARKETING AUTHORISATION HOLDER

sanofi-aventis

One Onslow Street

Guildford

Surrey

GU1 4YS

8. MARKETING AUTHORISATION NUMBER(S)

Priadel: 04425/0325

Priadel 200: 04425/0322

9. DATE OF FIRST AUTHORISATION/RENEWAL OF THE AUTHORISATION

27th January 2009

10. DATE OF REVISION OF THE TEXT

27th January 2009

Legal category

POM

Priadel Liquid

(sanofi-aventis)

1. NAME OF THE MEDICINAL PRODUCT

Priadel Liquid.

2. QUALITATIVE AND QUANTITATIVE COMPOSITION

A clear, colourless, pineapple flavoured, sugar free syrup containing 520mg lithium citrate equivalent to 200mg lithium carbonate per 5ml.

3. PHARMACEUTICAL FORM

Syrup.

4. CLINICAL PARTICULARS

4.1 Therapeutic indications

1. In the management of acute manic or hypomanic episodes.

2. In the management of episodes of recurrent depressive disorders where treatment with other antidepressants has been unsuccessful.

3. In the prophylaxis against bipolar affective disorders.

4. Control of aggressive behaviour or intentional self harm.

4.2 Posology and method of administration

A simple treatment schedule has been evolved which except for some minor variations should be followed whether using Priadel Liquid therapeutically or prophylactically. The minor variations to this schedule depend on the elements of the illness being treated and these are described later.

1. In patients of average weight (70kg) an initial daily dose of 10-30ml Priadel Liquid (equivalent to 400-1200mg lithium carbonate) should be given in divided doses, ideally twice a day. When changing between lithium preparations serum lithium levels should first be checked, then Priadel Liquid therapy commenced at a daily dose as close as possible to the dose of the other form of lithium. As bioavailability varies from product to product (particularly with regard to slow release preparations) a change of product should be regarded as initiation of new treatment.

2. Four to five days after starting treatment (and never longer than one week) a blood sample should be taken for the estimation of serum lithium level.

3. *The objective is to adjust the Priadel dose so as to maintain the "Target" serum lithium concentrations at 12 and 24 hours shown in the table below.*

"Target" serum lithium concentration (mmol/l)

	At 12 hours	At 24 hours
Once daily dosage	0.7 – 1.0	0.5 – 0.8
Twice daily dosage	0.5 – 0.8	

Priadel Liquid is supplied with a 2.5/5ml double ended spoon to provide adjustments equivalent to 100mg and 200mg lithium carbonate respectively. Serum lithium levels should be monitored weekly until stabilisation is achieved. The serum level should not exceed 1.5 mmol/l.

4. Lithium therapy should not be initiated unless adequate facilities for routine monitoring of serum concentrations are available. Following stabilisation of serum lithium levels, the period between subsequent estimations can be increased gradually but should not normally exceed three months. Additional measurements should be made following alteration of dosage, on development of intercurrent disease, signs of manic or depressive relapse, following significant change in sodium or fluid intake, or if signs of lithium toxicity occur.

5. Whilst a high proportion of acutely ill patients may respond within three to seven days of the commencement of therapy with Priadel Liquid it should be continued through any recurrence of the affective disturbance. This is important as the full prophylactic effect may not occur for 6 to 12 months after the initiation of therapy.

6. In patients who show a positive response with Priadel Liquid, treatment is likely to be long term. Careful clinical appraisal of the patient should be exercised throughout medication (see Precautions).

7. If lithium is to be discontinued, particularly in cases of high doses, the dose should be reduced gradually.

Prophylactic treatment of bipolar affective disorders and control of aggressive behaviour or intentional self harm: It is recommended that the described treatment schedule is followed.

Treatment of acute manic or hypomanic episodes and recurrent depressive disorders: It is likely that a higher than normal Priadel Liquid intake may be necessary during an acute phase. The monitoring should maintain serum levels at 0.8 – 1.5 mmol/l until acute symptoms have been controlled. In all other details the described treatment schedule is recommended.

Elderly:

Elderly patients or those below 50kg in weight, often require lower lithium dosage to achieve therapeutic serum levels. Starting doses of 200mg to 400mg are recommended taken twice daily. Dosage increments of 200 to 400mg every 3 to 5 days are usual. Total daily doses of 800 to 1800mg may be necessary to achieve effective blood lithium levels of 0.8 to 1.0 mmol/L. For prophylaxis, the dosage necessary to reach a blood lithium level of 0.4 to 0.8 mmol/L is generally in the range of 600 to 1200 mg/day.

Children and adolescents:

Not recommended.

4.3 Contraindications

• Hypersensitivity to lithium or to any of the excipients.

• Cardiac disease.

• Clinically significant renal impairment.

• Untreated hypothyroidism.

• Breast-feeding.

• Patients with low body sodium levels, including for example dehydrated patients or those on low sodium diets.

• Addison's disease.

4.4 Special warnings and precautions for use

• When considering Priadel therapy, it is necessary to ascertain whether patients are receiving lithium in any other form. If so, check serum levels before proceeding.

• Before beginning a lithium treatment:

– it is important to ensure that renal function is normal.

– cardiac function should be assessed.

– thyroid function should be evaluated. Patients should be euthyroid before initiation of lithium therapy.

• Renal, cardiac and thyroid functions should be re-assessed periodically.

• The possibility of hypothyroidism and renal dysfunction arising during prolonged treatment should be borne in mind and periodic assessments made.

• Patients receiving long term lithium therapy should be warned by the physician and be given clear instructions regarding the symptoms of impending intoxication (see 4.9 Overdosage). They should be warned of the urgency of immediate action should these symptoms appear, and also of the need to maintain a constant and adequate salt and water intake. Treatment should be discontinued immediately on the first signs of toxicity (see 4.9 Overdosage).

• Patients should be warned to report if polyuria or polydipsia develop. Episodes of nausea, vomiting, diarrhoea, fluid deprivation (e.g. excessive sweating), and/or other conditions leading to salt/water depletion should also be reported. Drugs likely to upset electrolyte balance such as diuretics (including severe dieting) should also be reported. Indeed, sodium depletion increases the lithium plasma concentration (due to competitive reabsorption at the renal level). In these cases, lithium dosage should be closely monitored and reduction of dosage may be necessary.

• Caution should be exercised to ensure that diet and fluid intake are normal in order to maintain a stable electrolyte balance. This may be of special importance in very hot weather or work environment. Infectious diseases including colds, influenza, gastro-enteritis and urinary infections may alter fluid balance and thus affect serum lithium levels. Treatment should be discontinued during any intercurrent infection and should only be reinstituted after the patient's physical health has returned to normal.

• Elderly patients are particularly liable to lithium toxicity. Use with care as lithium excretion may also be reduced. They may exhibit adverse reactions at serum levels ordinarily tolerated by younger patients.

4.5 Interaction with other medicinal products and other forms of interaction

<u>Interactions which increase lithium concentrations:</u>

If one of the following drugs is initiated, lithium dosage should either be adjusted or concomitant treatment stopped, as appropriate:

• Metronidazole.

• Non-steroidal anti-inflammatory drugs (monitor serum lithium concentrations more frequently if NSAID therapy is initiated or discontinued).

• ACE inhibitors.

• Diuretics (thiazides show a paradoxical antidiuretics effect resulting in possible water retention and lithium intoxication). If a thiazide diuretic has to be prescribed for a lithium-treated patient, lithium dosage should first be reduced and the patient re-stabilised with frequent monitoring. Similar precautions should be exercised on diuretic withdrawal.

• Other drugs affecting electrolyte balance, e.g. steroids, may alter lithium excretion and should therefore be avoided.

• Tetracyclines.

<u>Interactions which decrease serum lithium concentrations:</u>

• Xanthines (theophylline, caffeine).

• Sodium bicarbonate containing products.

• Diuretics (osmotic and carbonic anhydrase inhibitors).

• Urea.

<u>Interactions causing neurotoxicity:</u>

• Neuroleptics (particularly haloperidol at higher dosages), flupentixol, diazepam, thioridazine, fluphenazine, chlorpromazine and clozapine may lead in rare cases to neurotoxicity in the form of confusion, disorientation, lethargy, tremor, extra-pyramidal symptoms and myoclonus.

• Methyldopa.

• Selective Serotonin Re-uptake Inhibitors (e.g. fluvoxamine and fluoxetine) as this combination may precipitate a serotoninergic syndrome, which justifies immediate discontinuation of treatment.

• Calcium channel blockers may lead to a risk of neurotoxicity in the form of ataxia, confusion and somnolence, reversible after discontinuation of the drug. Lithium concentrations may be increased.

• Carbamazepine may lead to dizziness, somnolence, confusion and cerebellar symptoms.

Lithium may prolong the effects of neuromuscular blocking agents. There have been reports of interaction between lithium and phenytoin, indomethacin and other prostaglandin-synthetase inhibitors.

4.6 Pregnancy and lactation

4.6.1 Pregnancy

Lithium therapy should not be used during pregnancy, especially during the first trimester, unless considered essential. There is epidemiological evidence that it may be harmful to the foetus in human pregnancy. Lithium crosses the placental barrier. In animal studies lithium has been reported to interfere with fertility, gestation and foetal development. An increase in cardiac and other abnormalities, especially Ebstein anomaly, are reported. Therefore, a pre-natal diagnosis such as ultrasound and electrocardiogram examination is strongly recommended. In certain cases where a severe risk to the patient could exist if treatment were stopped, lithium has been continued during pregnancy.

If it is considered essential to maintain lithium treatment during pregnancy, serum lithium levels should be closely monitored and measured frequently since renal function changes gradually during pregnancy and suddenly at parturition. Dosage adjustments are required. It is recommended that lithium be discontinued shortly before delivery and reinitiated a few days *post-partum*.

Neonates may show signs of lithium toxicity necessitating fluid therapy in the neonatal period. Neonates born with low serum lithium concentrations may have a flaccid appearance that returns to normal without any treatment.

4.6.2 Women of child-bearing potential

It is advisable that women treated with lithium should adopt adequate contraceptive methods. In case of a planned pregnancy, it is strongly recommended to discontinue lithium therapy.

4.6.3 Lactation

Since adequate human data on use during lactation, adequate animal reproduction studies are not available and as lithium is secreted in breast milk, bottle-feeding is recommended (see section 4.3 Contraindications).

4.7 Effects on ability to drive and use machines

As lithium may cause disturbances of the CNS, patients should be warned of the possible hazards when driving or operating machinery.

4.8 Undesirable effects

Side effects are usually related to serum lithium concentration and are less common in patients with plasma lithium concentrations below 1.0 mmol/l.

Initial therapy: fine tremor of the hands, polyuria and thirst may occur.

Body as a whole: muscle weakness, peripheral oedema.

Cardiovascular: cardiac arrhythmia (NOS), mainly bradycardia, sinus node dysfunction, peripheral circulatory collapse, hypotension, oedema, ECG changes such as reversible flattening or inversion of T-waves and QT prolongation, cardiomyopathy.

CNS: ataxia, hyperactive deep tendon reflexes, extrapyramidal symptoms, seizures, slurred speech, dizziness, nystagmus, stupor, coma, pseudotumor cerebri, myasthenia gravis, vertigo, giddiness, dazed feeling, memory impairment.

Dermatology: alopecia, acne, folliculitis, pruritus, aggravation or occurrence of psoriasis, allergic rashes, acneiform eruptions, papular skin disorders, cutaneous ulcers.

Endocrine: euthyroid goitre, hypothyroidism, hyperthyroidism and thyrotoxicosis. Lithium-induced hypothyroidism may be managed successfully with concurrent thyroxine. Hypercalcaemia, hypermagnesaemia, hyperparathyroidism have been reported.

Gastrointestinal: anorexia, nausea, vomiting, diarrhoea, excessive salivation, dry mouth, abdominal discomfort, taste disorder, gastritis

Haematological: leucocytosis.

Metabolic and Nutrional: weight gain, hyperglycaemia,

Renal: polydipsia and/or polyuria, symptoms of nephrogenic diabetes insipidus, histological renal changes with interstitial fibrosis after long term treatment.

High serum concentrations of lithium including episodes of acute lithium toxicity may aggravate these changes. The minimum clinically effective dose of lithium should always be used. In patients who develop polyuria and/or polydipsia, renal function should be monitored, e.g. with measurement of blood urea, serum creatinine and urinary protein levels in addition to the routine serum lithium assessment.

Reproductive: sexual dysfunction.

Senses: dysgeusia, blurred vision, scotomata.

Rare cases of nephrotic syndrome, speech disorder, confusion, impaired consciousness, myoclonus and abnormal reflex have been reported.

If any of the above symptoms appear, treatment should be stopped immediately and arrangements made for serum lithium measurement.

4.9 Overdose

In patients with a raised lithium concentration, the risk of toxicity is greater in those with the following underlying medical conditions: hypertension, diabetes, congestive heart failure, chronic renal failure, schizophrenia, Addison's disease.

Acute

A single acute overdose usually carries low risk and patients tend to show mild symptoms only, irrespective of their serum lithium concentration. However more severe symptoms may occur after a delay if lithium elimination is reduced because of renal impairment, particularly if a slow-release preparation has been taken. The fatal dose, in a single overdose, is probably over 5g.

If an acute overdose has been taken by a patient on chronic lithium therapy, this can lead to serious toxicity occurring even after a modest overdose as the extravascular tissues are already saturated with lithium.

Chronic

Lithium toxicity can also occur in chronic accumulation for the following reasons: Acute or chronic overdosage; dehydration e.g. due to intercurrent illness, deteriorating renal function, drug interactions, most commonly involving a thiazide diuretic or a non-steroidal anti-inflammatory drug (NSAID).

Symptoms

The onset of symptoms may be delayed, with peak effects not occurring for as long as 24 hours, especially in patients who are not receiving chronic lithium therapy or following the use of a sustained release preparation.

Mild: Nausea, diarrhoea, blurred vision, polyuria, light headedness, fine resting tremor, muscular weakness and drowsiness.

Moderate: Increasing confusion, blackouts, fasciculation and increased deep tendon reflexes, myoclonic twitches and jerks, choreoathetoid movements, urinary or faecal incontinence, increasing restlessness followed by stupor. Hypernatraemia.

Severe: Coma, convulsions, cerebellar signs, cardiac dysrythmias including sinoatrial block, sinus and junctional bradycardia and first degree heart block. Hypotension or rarely hypertension, circulatory collapse and renal failure.

Management

There is no specific antidote to lithium poisoning. In the event of accumulation, lithium should be stopped and serum estimation should be carried out every 6 hours.

Under no circumstances should a diuretic be used. Osmotic diuresis (mannitol or urea infusion) or alkalinisation of the urine (sodium lactate or sodium bicarbonate infusion) should be initiated. All patients should be observed for a minimum of 24 hours. ECG should be monitored in symptomatic patients. Steps should be taken to correct hypotension.

Consider gastric lavage for non-sustained-release preparations if more than 4 g has been ingested by an adult within 1 hour or definite ingestion of a significant amount by a child. Slow-release tablets do not disintegrate in the stomach and most are too large to pass up a lavage tube. Gut decontamination is not useful for chronic accumulation. Activated charcoal does not adsorb lithium.

Peritoneal or haemodialysis should be instituted promptly if there is deterioration in the patient's condition (e.g. marked neurological or cardiac features), if the serum lithium level is over 4.0 mmol/l, in an acute overdose (not in addition to chronic use), if there is a deterioration in the patient's condition, or if the serum lithium concentration is not falling at a rate corresponding to a half-life of under 30 hours. This should be continued until there is no lithium in the serum or dialysis fluid. Serum lithium levels should be monitored for at least a further week to take account of any possible rebound in serum lithium levels as a result of delayed diffusion from the body tissues.

In cases of acute on chronic overdose or in cases of chronic lithium toxicity if the lithium concentration is >4.0 mmol/l, discuss with your local poisons service.

Clinical improvement generally takes longer than reduction of serum lithium concentrations regardless of the method used.

5. PHARMACOLOGICAL PROPERTIES

5.1 Pharmacodynamic properties

The mode of action of lithium is still not fully understood. However, lithium modifies the production and turnover of certain neurotransmitters, particularly serotonin, and it may also block dopamine receptors.

It modifies concentrations of some electrolytes, particularly calcium and magnesium, and it may reduce thyroid activity.

5.2 Pharmacokinetic properties

Lithium has a half-life of about 24 hours although this increases to about 36 hours in the elderly due to a progressive decrease in renal lithium clearance with age. Lithium is 95% eliminated in the urine. Time to peak serum level for an immediate release product, such as Priadel Liquid, is about 1.5 hours and complete bioavailability would be expected.

5.3 Preclinical safety data

None stated.

6. PHARMACEUTICAL PARTICULARS

6.1 List of excipients

Other ingredients include:

Ethanol, xanthan gum, saccharin sodium, sorbic acid, citric acid, pineapple flavour, purified water.

6.2 Incompatibilities

Dilution of Priadel Liquid is not recommended.

6.3 Shelf life

Two years.

6.4 Special precautions for storage

Store at or below 25°C. Protect from direct sunlight.

6.5 Nature and contents of container

Priadel Liquid is supplied in an amber glass bottle fitted with a one-piece polypropylene screw cap. Packs are available in 150ml and 300ml volumes.

6.6 Special precautions for disposal and other handling

Not applicable.

7. MARKETING AUTHORISATION HOLDER

sanofi-aventis

One Onslow Street

Guildford

Surrey

GU1 4YS

8. MARKETING AUTHORISATION NUMBER(S)

04425/0354

9. DATE OF FIRST AUTHORISATION/RENEWAL OF THE AUTHORISATION

26th March 2009

10. DATE OF REVISION OF THE TEXT

26th March 2009

11 Legal category

POM

Prialt solution for infusion

(Eisai Ltd)

1. NAME OF THE MEDICINAL PRODUCT

Prialt▼ 100 micrograms/ml solution for infusion.

2. QUALITATIVE AND QUANTITATIVE COMPOSITION

One ml solution contains 100 µg ziconotide (as ziconotide acetate).

1 ml vial: Each vial contains 100 µg ziconotide (as ziconotide acetate).

5 ml vial: Each vial contains 500 µg ziconotide (as ziconotide acetate).

For a full list of excipients, see section 6.1.

3. PHARMACEUTICAL FORM

Solution for infusion. Clear, colourless solution, free of visible particles.

4. CLINICAL PARTICULARS

4.1 Therapeutic indications

Ziconotide is indicated for the treatment of severe, chronic pain in patients who require intrathecal (IT) analgesia.

4.2 Posology and method of administration

Treatment with ziconotide should only be undertaken by physicians experienced in intrathecal (IT) administration of medicinal products. Prialt is for intrathecal use only.

For instructions for use and handling, see section 6.6.

Adults (including the elderly ≥ 65 years of age)

Dosing of ziconotide should be initiated at 2.4 µg/day and titrated on an individual patient basis according to the patient's analgesic response and adverse reactions. Patients should be titrated in dose increments of ≤ 2.4 µg/day, up to a maximum dose of 21.6 µg/day. The minimal interval between dose increases is 24 hours; the recommended interval, for safety reasons, is 48 hours or more. If necessary the dose can be decreased by any amount (including stopping the infusion) for the management of adverse reactions. Approximately 75% of patients who respond satisfactorily to treatment require a dose of ≤ 9.6 µg/day.

Ziconotide must be administered as a continuous infusion via an intrathecal catheter, using an external or internally implanted mechanical infusion pump capable of delivering an accurate infusion volume. As the risk of meningitis secondary to prolonged catheterisation of the intrathecal space is greater with an external catheter infusion system, internal systems are recommended to administer ziconotide for prolonged periods. An external catheter system should only be used when an internal system cannot be implanted.

When low doses of ziconotide are required, for example when initiating titration, ziconotide must be diluted before use with preservative-free sodium chloride 9 mg/ml (0.9%) solution for injection. (see section 6.6).

Use in paediatric patients (< 18 years of age)

Prialt is not recommended for use in children below 18 years due to a lack of data on safety and efficacy. There is no experience in children.

Use in patients with impaired hepatic function

Studies have not been conducted in patients with impaired hepatic function. Caution should be exercised when ziconotide is administered to patients with impaired hepatic function.

Use in patients with impaired renal function

Studies have not been conducted in patients with impaired renal function. Caution should be exercised when ziconotide is administered to patients with impaired renal function.

4.3 Contraindications

Hypersensitivity to the active substance or to any of the excipients.

Ziconotide is contraindicated in combination with IT chemotherapy (see section 4.5).

4.4 Special warnings and precautions for use

Although ziconotide has been studied in long-term, open label efficacy and safety clinical trials, controlled studies of longer than 3 weeks duration have not been conducted (see section 5.1). Possible long-term local toxic effects on the spinal cord have not been excluded and preclinical data in this respect are limited (see section 5.3). Therefore, caution is needed during long-term treatment.

The administration of medicinal products by the intrathecal (IT) route carries the risk of potentially serious infections, such as meningitis, which may be life threatening. Meningitis due to the entrance of organisms along the catheter track or inadvertent contamination of the infusion system is a known complication of intrathecal medicinal product administration, especially with external systems.

Patients and physicians must be vigilant for typical symptoms and signs of meningitis.

The optimal intrathecal placement of the catheter tip has not been established. Lower catheter tip placement, e.g. at the lumbar level, may reduce the incidence of ziconotide-related neurological adverse reactions. Therefore, catheter tip placement should be carefully considered to allow adequate access to spinal nociceptive segments whilst minimising medicinal product concentrations at cerebral levels.

Only a small number of patients have received systemic chemotherapy and IT ziconotide. Caution should be exercised when ziconotide is administered to patients who are receiving systemic chemotherapy (see section 4.5).

Elevations in creatine kinase, which are usually asymptomatic, are common amongst patients on intrathecal ziconotide. Progressive elevation of the creatine kinase is uncommon. However monitoring of creatine kinase is recommended. In the event of progressive elevation, or clinically significant elevation in association with clinical features of myopathy or rhabdomyolysis, discontinuation of ziconotide should be considered.

Hypersensitivity reactions including anaphylaxis have not been observed during clinical trials and the immunogenicity of ziconotide administered by the IT route appears to be low. However, the potential for severe allergic reactions cannot be excluded.

Cognitive and neuropsychiatric adverse reactions, particularly confusion, are common in patients treated with ziconotide. Cognitive impairment typically appears after several weeks of treatment. Episodes of acute psychiatric disturbances, such as hallucinations, paranoid reactions, hostility, delirium, psychosis and manic reactions have been reported in patients treated with ziconotide. The ziconotide dose should be reduced or discontinued if signs or symptoms of cognitive impairment or neuropsychiatric adverse reactions develop, but other contributing causes should also be considered. The cognitive effects of ziconotide are typically reversible within 1 - 4 weeks after discontinuation of the medicinal product, but may persist in some cases.

Patients have experienced depressed levels of consciousness while receiving ziconotide. The patient usually remains conscious and breathing is not depressed. The event may be self limited, but ziconotide should be discontinued until the event resolves. The re-introduction of ziconotide is not recommended in these patients. Withdrawal of concomitant CNS depressant medicinal products should also be considered as they may contribute to the reduced level of arousal.

In patients with severe chronic pain there is a higher incidence of suicide and suicide attempts than in the general population. Ziconotide may cause or worsen depression with the risk of suicide in susceptible patients.

4.5 Interaction with other medicinal products and other forms of interaction

Specific clinical medicinal product interaction studies have not been conducted with ziconotide. However, low plasma ziconotide concentrations, metabolism by ubiquitous peptidases and relatively low plasma protein binding (see section 5.2) make metabolic-based interactions or plasma protein displacement type interactions between ziconotide and other medicinal products unlikely.

No clinical data are available on the interaction between IT chemotherapy and IT ziconotide. Ziconotide is contraindicated in combination with IT chemotherapy (see section 4.3).

Only a small number of patients have received systemic chemotherapy and IT ziconotide. Caution should be exercised when ziconotide is administered to patients who are receiving systemic chemotherapy (see section 4.4).

Medicinal products that affect specific peptidases/proteases would not be expected to impact upon ziconotide plasma exposure. Based on very limited clinical investigations, both angiotensin converting enzyme inhibitors (e.g., benazepril, lisinopril and moexipril) and HIV protease inhibitors (e.g., ritonavir, saquinavir, indinavir), have no readily apparent effect on plasma ziconotide exposure.

Ziconotide does not interact with opiate receptors. If discontinuing opiates when initiating ziconotide therapy, opiate withdrawal should be gradual. For patients being withdrawn from IT opiates, the IT opiate infusion dose should be gradually tapered over a few weeks and replaced with a pharmacologically equivalent dose of oral opiates. Adding IT ziconotide to stable doses of IT morphine (see section 5.1), is possible but requires special attention, as a high rate of neuropsychiatric adverse events (confusion/thinking abnormal, paranoid reactions and hallucinations, and abnormal gait), some of them serious, was observed in Study 202 despite a low dose of ziconotide. Vomiting and anorexia, and peripheral edema were also observed when IT ziconotide was added to IT morphine. The addition of IT morphine to stable doses of IT ziconotide is better tolerated (pruritis has been reported). (See section 5.1).

An increased incidence of somnolence has been observed when ziconotide is administered concomitantly with systemic baclofen, clonidine, bupivacaine or propofol.

No data are available regarding the concomitant use of partial opioid agonists (e.g. buprenorphine) with ziconotide.

4.6 Pregnancy and lactation

There are no adequate data from the use of ziconotide in pregnant women. Studies in animals have shown reproductive toxicity (see section 5.3). The potential risk for humans is unknown. Ziconotide should not be used during pregnancy unless clearly necessary.

It is not known whether ziconotide is excreted in breast milk, therefore it should not be administered to breast-feeding women unless clearly necessary.

4.7 Effects on ability to drive and use machines

No studies on the effects on the ability to drive and use machines have been performed.

Ziconotide may cause confusion, somnolence and other neurological adverse reactions, therefore patients must be advised not to drive or operate machines if affected.

4.8 Undesirable effects

The safety of ziconotide administered as a continuous intrathecal infusion has been evaluated in more than 1,400 patients participating in acute and chronic pain clinical trials. The duration of treatment has ranged from one-hour bolus infusion to continuous use for more than 6 years. The median exposure time was 43 days. The infusion dose rate ranged from 0.03 - 912 μg/day, with a median final dose rate of 7.2 μg/day.

In clinical trials, 88% of patients experienced adverse drug reactions (ADRs). The most commonly reported ADRs reported in long-term clinical trials were dizziness (42%), nausea (30%), nystagmus (23%), confusional state (25%), gait abnormal (16%), memory impairment (13%), vision blurred (14%) headache (12%), asthenia (13%), and vomiting (11%) and somnolence (10%). Most ADRs were mild to moderate in severity and resolved over time.

All ADRs reported in the intrathecal clinical trials with ziconotide (short- and long-term exposure) are listed below in order of frequency.

Very Common (> 1/10), Common (> 1/100, < 1/10), Uncommon (> 1/1,000, < 1/100)

Infections and Infestations

Uncommon: sepsis, meningitis

Metabolism and nutrition disorders

Common: appetite decreased, anorexia

Psychiatric disorders

Very common: confusional state

Common: anxiety, auditory hallucination, insomnia, agitation, disorientation, hallucination, visual hallucination, depression, paranoia, irritability, depression aggravated, nervousness, affect lability, mental status changes, anxiety aggravated, confusion aggravated

Uncommon: delirium, psychotic disorder, suicidal ideation, suicide attempt, thought blocking, abnormal dreams

Nervous system disorders

Very Common: dizziness, nystagmus, memory impairment, headache, somnolence

Common: dysarthria, amnesia, dysgeusia, tremor, balance impaired, ataxia, aphasia, burning sensation, sedation, paraesthesia, hypoaesthesia, disturbance in attention, speech disorder, areflexia, coordination abnormal, dizziness postural, cognitive disorder, hyperaesthesia, hyporeflexia, ageusia, depressed level of consciousness, dysaesthesia, parosmia, mental impairment

Uncommon: incoherence, loss of consciousness, coma, stupor, convulsions, cerebrovascular accident, encephalopathy

Eye disorders

Very Common: vision blurred

Common: diplopia, visual disturbance, photophobia

Ear and labyrinth disorders

Common: vertigo, tinnitus

Cardiac disorders

Uncommon: atrial fibrillation

Vascular disorders

Common: orthostatic hypotension, hypotension

Respiratory, thoracic and mediastinal disorders

Common: dyspnoea

Uncommon: respiratory distress

Gastrointestinal disorders

Very Common: nausea, vomiting

Common: diarrhoea, dry mouth, constipation, nausea aggravated, upper abdominal pain

Uncommon: dyspepsia

Skin and subcutaneous tissue disorders

Common: pruritus, sweating increased

Uncommon: rash

Musculoskeletal and connective tissue disorders

Common: pain in limb, myalgia, muscle spasms, muscle cramp, muscle weakness, arthralgia, peripheral swelling

Uncommon: rhabdomyolysis, myositis, back pain, muscle twitching, neck pain

Renal and urinary disorders

Common: urinary retention, urinary hesitation, dysuria, urinary incontinence

Uncommon: acute renal failure

General disorders and administration site conditions

Very Common: gait abnormal, asthenia

Common: fatigue, pyrexia, lethargy, oedema peripheral, rigors, fall, chest pain, feeling cold, pain, feeling jittery, pain exacerbated

Uncommon: difficulty in walking

Investigations

Common: blood creatine phosphokinase increased, weight decreased

Uncommon: electrocardiogram abnormal, aspartate aminotransferase increased, blood creatine phosphokinase MM increased, body temperature increased

Specific comments and particular caution regarding meningitis, elevations of creatine kinase, and CNS adverse events can be found in Section 4.4.

4.9 Overdose

In intravenous infusion studies, healthy male volunteers received ziconotide at doses of up to 70,000 μg/day or 3,200 times the maximum recommended daily intrathecal infusion dose. Postural hypotension was observed in almost all subjects who received high intravenous doses of ziconotide.

The maximum recommended intrathecal dose is 21.6 μg/day. The maximum intended intrathecal dose of ziconotide in clinical trials was 912 μg/day following upward titration over 7 days.

In one clinical study a male cancer patient received an accidental IT ziconotide overdose of 744 μg over a 24-hour period (31 μg/hour) and resumed treatment at the intended dose after experiencing a reduction in Visual Analog Scale of Pain Intensity (VASPI) from 82 to 2.5 mm. In some patients who received intrathecal doses greater than the maximum recommended dose, exaggerated pharmacological effects, e.g., ataxia, nystagmus, dizziness, stupor, depressed level of consciousness, muscle spasms, confusional state, sedation, hypotension, aphasia, speech disorder, nausea and vomiting were observed. There was no indication of respiratory depression. Most patients under observation recovered within 24 hours of withdrawal of the medicinal product.

General medical supportive measures should be administered to patients who receive an overdose until the exaggerated pharmacological effects of the medicinal product have resolved.

5. PHARMACOLOGICAL PROPERTIES

5.1 Pharmacodynamic properties

Pharmacotherapeutic group: Analgesics ATC code: N02BG08

This medicinal product has been authorised under "Exceptional Circumstances". This means that due to the rarity of the disease it has not been possible to obtain complete information on this medicinal product. The European Medicines Agency (EMEA) will review any new information, which may become available every year and this SPC will be updated as necessary.

Ziconotide is a synthetic analogue of a ω-conopeptide, MVIIA, found in the venom of the *Conus magus* marine snail. It is an N-type calcium channel blocker (NCCB). NCCs regulate neurotransmitter release in specific neuronal populations responsible for the spinal processing of pain. In binding to these neuronal NCCs ziconotide inhibits the voltage sensitive calcium current into primary nociceptive afferents terminating in the superficial layers of the dorsal horn of the spinal cord. In turn, this inhibits their release of neurotransmitters (including Substance P) and therefore, the spinal signalling of pain.

Though statistically significant relationships and reasonable correlation between cerebrospinal fluid (CSF) exposure (AUC, C_{max}) and clinical response measures have been observed following 1 hour IT administration, no well-defined dose-concentration-response relationships have yet been identified. Many responsive patients obtain near-maximal analgesia within a few hours of delivery of an appropriate dose. However, maximal effects may be delayed for approximately 24 hours in some patients. Given the occurrence of analgesia and adverse drug reactions at similar doses, the recommended interval between dose increases is 48 hours or more. If necessary the dose can be decreased by any amount (including stopping the infusion) for the management of adverse drug reactions.

Nervous system adverse reactions, particularly dizziness, nausea and abnormal gait appear to be correlated with CSF exposure, though a definitive relationship has not been established.

Low plasma exposure occurs during IT infusion due to the low recommended IT infusion rates and relatively rapid plasma clearance (see section 5.2). Therefore, pharmacological effects related to systemic exposure should be minimal.

The median dose at response is approximately 6.0 μg/day and approximately 75% of responsive patients require ⩽ 9.6 μg/day. To limit the occurrence of serious adverse drug reactions, a maximum dose of 21.6 μg/day is recommended. However, in clinical trials it has been observed that patients who tolerate doses of 21.6 μg/day following slow titration over a 3 to 4-week period, generally tolerate higher doses up to 48.0 μg/day.

There is no evidence of the development of pharmacological tolerance to ziconotide in patients. However, in view of limited data, the development of tolerance cannot be excluded. Examination of the patency of the intrathecal catheter should be considered if the required ziconotide dose continually increases and there is no benefit or increase in drug reactions.

There were three placebo-controlled clinical trials of IT ziconotide.

Two short-term studies, 95-001 (malignant pain) and 96-002 (non malignant pain), involving 366 patients, demonstrated the efficacy of IT ziconotide in severe chronic pain using the percent change in Visual Analog Scale of Pain Intensity (VASPI) as the primary efficacy measure. These studies were of short duration, 5 and 6 days respectively, and used a more rapid dose escalation and higher doses than recommended in Section 4.2.

Efficacy results from study 95-001

(see Table 1 below)

Efficacy results from study 96-002

(see Table 2 on next page)

The aetiologies of pain in studies 95-001 (malignant pain) and 96-002 (non-malignant pain) were varied and included bone pain (n = 38) mostly due to bone metastases (n = 34), myelopathy (n = 38), half of whom had spinal cord injury with paralysis (n = 19), neuropathy (n = 79), radiculopathy (n = 24), spinal pain (n = 91) mostly due to failed back surgery (n = 82), and other aetiologies (n = 82). Some patients had more than one cause of pain. The efficacy of IT ziconotide was apparent in all groups.

Study 301 (n = 220) was of longer duration (21 days), involved more cautious up-titration and lower doses of IT ziconotide, and enrolled the most refractory population of patients studied in the three studies. All patients in the 301 study had failed IT therapy with combinations of analgesics and their physicians considered that 97% of the patients were refractory to currently available treatments. The majority had spinal pain (n = 134), especially failed back surgery (n = 110); a lower proportion had neuropathy (n = 36). Only five had malignant pain. The primary endpoint was the percent change in VASPI score. The efficacy of IT ziconotide in study 301 was lower than in the previous two, short-term studies. The frequency and severity of adverse events were also lower.

Efficacy results from study 301

(see Table 3 on next page)

Combination studies with IT Morphine

Clinical studies 201 and 202 indicate that the combination of IT ziconotide and IT morphine may effectively reduce pain and decrease systemic opioid use over a sustained period of time for patients whose pain was inadequately controlled with their maximum tolerated dose of IT ziconotide (median 8.7 μg/day, mean 25.7 μg/day – study 201) or with IT morphine (study 202) alone. When adding IT

Table 1 Efficacy results from study 95-001

Parameter	Initial Treatment Assignment		
	Ziconotide (n = 71)	Placebo (n = 40)	p-value
Mean VASPI score at baseline in mm (SD)	74.1 (± 13.82)	77.9 (± 13.60)	_
Mean VASPI score at end of initial titration in mm (SD)	35.7 (± 33.27)	61.0 (± 22.91)	
% improvement in VASPI score at end of initial titration (SD)	51.4 (± 43.63)	18.1 (± 28.28)	< 0.001
Responder[a] n (%)	34 (47.9%)	7 (17.5%)	0.001
Dose at end of titration (μg/hr)			
Mean	0.91		
Median	0.60		
Range	0.074 - 9.36		

[a]Responders were defined as those patients who 1) experienced a ⩾ 30% drop in VASPI score compared to baseline; 2) had stable or decreased concomitant opioid analgesics; and 3) had opiate type unchanged from preinfusion if receiving opiates.

SD – Standard Deviation.

Table 2 Efficacy results from study 96-002

Parameter	Initial Treatment Assignment Ziconotide (n = 169)[b]	Placebo (n = 86)	p-value
Mean VASPI score at baseline in mm (SD)	80.1 (± 15.10)	76.9 (± 14.58)	–
Mean VASPI score at end of initial titration in mm (SD)	54.4 (± 29.30)	71.9 (± 30.93)	–
% improvement in VASPI score at end of initial titration (SD)	31.2 (± 38.69)	6.0 (± 42.84)	< 0.001
Responder[a] n (%)	57 (33.7%)	11 (12.8%)	< 0.001
Dose at end of titration (μg/hr)			
Mean	1.02		
Median	0.50		
Range	0.019 - 9.60		

[a]Responders were defined as those patients who 1) experienced a $\geqslant$ 30% drop in VASPI score compared to baseline; 2) had stable or decreased concomitant opioid analgesics; and 3) had opiate type unchanged from preinfusion if receiving opiates.

[b]164 patients provided VASPI scores for ziconotide at the end of titration.

SD – Standard Deviation.

Table 3 Efficacy results from study 301

Parameter	Initial Treatment Assignment Ziconotide (n = 112)	Placebo (n = 108)	p-value
Mean VASPI score at baseline in mm (SD)	80.7 (± 14.98)	80.7 (± 14.91)	-
Mean VASPI score at end of initial titration in mm (SD)	67.9 (± 22.89)	74.1 (± 21.28)	–
% improvement in VASPI score at end of initial titration (SD)	14.7 (± 27.71)	7.2 (± 24.98)	0.0360
Responder[a] n (%)	18 (16.1%)	13 (12.0%)	0.390
Dose at end of titration (μg/hr)			
Mean	0.29		
Median	0.25		
Range	0.0 - 0.80		

[a]Responders were defined as those who experienced a $\geqslant$ 30% drop in VASPI score compared to baseline.

SD – Standard Deviation.

ziconotide to stable doses of IT morphine, as with the initiation of IT ziconotide monotherapy, the appearance of psychotic adverse events (e.g., hallucinations, paranoid reactions) or discontinuation due to increased adverse events may occur. (see section 4.5).

5.2 Pharmacokinetic properties

The CSF pharmacokinetics of ziconotide have been studied following one-hour IT infusions of 1 - 10 μg of ziconotide in patients with chronic pain. The plasma pharmacokinetics following intravenous doses (0.3 – 10 μg/kg/24 hr) were also studied. IT and intravenous pharmacokinetics data are summarised below.

<u>CSF and Plasma Pharmacokinetics of Ziconotide [mean ± SD (median)]</u>

(see Table 4 below)

Absorption: Following one-hour IT administration (1 – 10 μg), both cumulative exposure (AUC; range: 83.6 – 608 ng/hr/ml) and peak exposure (C_{max}; range: 16.4 – 132 ng/ml) values were variable and dose-dependent, but appeared only approximately dose-proportional. Plasma concentrations following continuous ($\geqslant$ 48 h) IT infusion ($\leqslant$ 21.6 μg/day) appear to be relatively low and typically undetectable (i.e., about 80% of plasma samples collected from pain patients contain no quantifiable medicinal product; $<$ 0.04 ng/ml). No accumulation of ziconotide in plasma following long-term IT administration (up to 9 months) has been observed.

Distribution: Median ziconotide CSF volume of distribution (Vd: 99 ml) is between the spinal cord CSF volume (approximately 75 ml) and total CSF volume (approximately 130 ml). Ziconotide appears to distribute mainly within the CSF until transferred to the systemic circulation. Upon reaching the systemic circulation, ziconotide appears to be more extensively distributed, based on a plasma distribution volume of approximately 30 l and is only about 53% bound (non-specifically) to human plasma proteins.

Biotransformation: Ziconotide is a peptide consisting of 25 naturally-occurring amino acids of the L-configuration, and does not appear to be appreciably metabolised in the CSF. Following passage into the systemic circulation, ziconotide is expected to be primarily susceptible to proteolytic cleavage by various ubiquitous peptidases/proteases present in most organs (e.g., kidney, liver, lung, muscle, etc.), and thus degraded to peptide fragments and its individual constituent free amino acids. The generated free amino acids are expected to be taken up by cellular carrier systems and either subjected to normal intermediary metabolism or used as substrates for constitutive biosynthetic processes. Due to the wide distribution of these peptidases it is not expected that hepatic or renal impairment would affect the systemic clearance of ziconotide. The biological activity of the various expected proteolytic degradation products has not been assessed. It is unlikely that the degradation products of ziconotide will have significant biological activity, as peptides consisting of the individual peptide loop structures have been found to have binding affinities for N-type voltage sensitive calcium channels that are several orders of magnitude lower than that of the parent (ziconotide) compound.

Elimination: Mean ziconotide CL (0.38 ml/min) approximates adult human CSF turnover rate (0.3 - 0.4 ml/min). Hence, ziconotide appears to be mainly eliminated from the CSF (mean $t_{1/2}$ = 4.6 hr) by bulk flow of CSF out of the CNS through the arachnoid villi with subsequent transfer into the systemic circulation. Very low circulating plasma concentrations of ziconotide may be observed following IT administration due to both the low IT infusion rate and relatively rapid plasma clearance. The mean plasma elimination half-life ($t_{1/2}$) is 1.3 hr. Ziconotide is a relatively small molecular weight peptide (MW = 2,639) and is filtered by the kidney glomerulus, but only minimal amounts of ziconotide ($<$ 1%) are recovered in human urine following intravenous infusion. This is because almost all of the filtered active substance is rapidly endocytosed and ultimately transported back to the systemic circulation.

Specific populations: Although only limited data are available, there is no obvious effect of race, height, weight, gender or age on CSF ziconotide exposure after IT administration. No formal studies assessing the impact of renal or hepatic dysfunction have been conducted; however, given that peptidases are present in various body organs, it is not anticipated that renal or hepatic dysfunction will significantly impact systemic exposure of ziconotide.

Table 4 CSF and Plasma Pharmacokinetics of Ziconotide [mean ± SD (median)]

Route of administration	Fluid matrix	Number of patients	CL (ml/min)	Vd (ml)	$t_{1/2}$ (hr)
Intrathecal	CSF	23	0.38 ± 0.56 (0.26)	155 ± 263 (99)	4.6 ± 0.9 (4.5)
Intravenous	Plasma	21	270 ± 44 (260)	30,460 ± 6,366 (29,320)	1.3 ± 0.3 (1.3)

CL = clearance; Vd = distribution volume; $t_{1/2}$ = half life

5.3 Preclinical safety data

Preclinical toxic effects related to ziconotide administration were observed only at exposures considered sufficiently in excess of the human exposure to indicate little risk in clinical use.

In subchronic continuous intrathecal infusion studies in rats and dogs, behavioural effects were seen at doses $\geqslant$ 8-fold the maximum recommended clinical intrathecal infusion dose of 21.6 μg/day (on a mg/kg basis). These effects were defined by exaggerated pharmacological actions of ziconotide and not by neurotoxic lesions or target organ toxicity. Observations included transient and reversible neurological effects consisting of tremors, uncoordinated movements and hyper- and hypoactivity.

The long-term consequences to neuronal function of continuous N-type calcium-channel block have not been demonstrated in experimental animals. Changes in neurological signalling have not been studied in experimental animals. Ziconotide did not induce bacterial gene mutation and was not genotoxic. Chronic animal studies have not been performed to assess the carcinogenic potential of ziconotide. However, ziconotide did not induce cell transformation in the *in vitro* Syrian hamster embryo (SHE) assay and did not increase cell proliferation (pre-neoplastic lesion formation) or apoptosis after subchronic intrathecal exposure in dogs.

In rat fertility studies, there were no effects in males while reductions in corpora lutea; implantation sites and number of live embryos were observed in females. No adverse effects on female reproduction and post-natal development in rats were seen at systemic exposures up to 2,300 times human exposures at the maximum recommended intrathecal dose.

Ziconotide was not teratogenic in rats and rabbits at exposures $<$ 100 times human plasma levels.

These results do not indicate a significant risk to humans due to the relatively high systemic exposures needed to elicit these effects in rats and rabbits.

6. PHARMACEUTICAL PARTICULARS

6.1 List of excipients

Methionine

Sodium chloride

Water for injections

Hydrochloric acid (pH adjuster)

Sodium hydroxide (pH adjuster)

6.2 Incompatibilities

This medicinal product must not be mixed with other medicinal products except those mentioned in section 6.6.

6.3 Shelf life

3 years

Chemical and physical in use stability has been demonstrated for 60 days at 37°C.

From a microbiological point of view, if the product is diluted it should be transferred to the infusion pump immediately. If not used immediately, in-use storage times and conditions prior to use are the responsibility of the user and would normally not be longer than 24 hours at 2°C – 8°C, unless dilution has taken place in controlled and validated aseptic conditions.

6.4 Special precautions for storage

Store in a refrigerator (2°C - 8°C). Do not freeze. Keep the vial in the outer carton in order to protect from light.

For storage conditions of the diluted medicinal product, see section 6.3.

6.5 Nature and contents of container

Single-use Type I glass vials with butyl rubber stoppers coated with fluorinated polymer.

Each vial contains 1 or 5 ml solution for infusion.

One vial per carton.

6.6 Special precautions for disposal and other handling

If dilution is required, Prialt must be diluted aseptically with preservative-free sodium chloride 9 mg/ml (0.9%) solution for injection before use. The concentration of the solution used in the infusion pump must be no lower than 5 μg/ml ziconotide in an external pump and 25 μg/ml in an internal pump.

Strict aseptic procedures must be used during the preparation and handling of the solution for infusion and refilling of the pump. The patient and health-care providers must be familiar with the handling of the external or internal infusion system and be aware of the need to guard against infection.

Prialt has been shown to be chemically and physically compatible with the implantable Synchromed pump and the external CADD-Micro pump at the concentration levels indicated above. Chemical and physical in-use stability has been demonstrated for 14 days at 37°C in the Synchromed pump when the pump has not previously been exposed to the medicinal product. The initial fill must therefore be replaced after 14 days.

Prialt was stable for 60 days at 37°C in the Synchromed pump previously exposed to the medicinal product. Stability has been demonstrated for 21 days at room temperature in the CADD-Micro pump.

Specific instructions for using the pumps must be obtained from the manufacturer. CE marked pumps equivalent to the Synchromed and CADD-Micro pump should be used to deliver Prialt. Pumps previously used to deliver other medicinal products must be washed out three times with sodium chloride 9 mg/ml (0.9%) solution for injection (preservative-free) before being filled with Prialt. The introduction of air into the pump reservoir or cartridge should be minimized, as oxygen can degrade ziconotide.

Prior to initiation of therapy, an internal pump must be rinsed three times with 2 ml of Prialt at 25 µg/ml. The concentration of Prialt in a naïve pump may be reduced due to adsorption onto the surfaces of the device, and/or dilution by the residual space of the device. Because of this, after the first use of Prialt, the reservoir should be emptied and refilled after 14 days. Subsequently the pump should be emptied and refilled every 60 days.

Prialt is a clear and colourless solution. It should be inspected visually for particulate matter and discolouration prior to administration. The solution should not be used if discoloured or cloudy or if particulate matter is observed.

For single use only. Any unused solution should be discarded according to local regulations.

7. MARKETING AUTHORISATION HOLDER
Eisai Ltd.,
European Knowledge Centre
Mosquito Way
Hatfield
Herts
AL10 9SN
United Kingdom

8. MARKETING AUTHORISATION NUMBER(S)
EU/1/04/302/001 – 1 ml solution for infusion.
EU/1/04/302/003 – 5 ml solution for infusion.

9. DATE OF FIRST AUTHORISATION/RENEWAL OF THE AUTHORISATION
21 February 2005

10. DATE OF REVISION OF THE TEXT
17th March 2009

Detailed information on this product is available on the website of the European Medicines Agency (EMEA) www.emea.europa.eu

11. LEGAL CATEGORY
POM - Medicinal product subject to medical prescription

Primacor Injection

(sanofi-aventis)

1. NAME OF THE MEDICINAL PRODUCT
Primacor Injection

2. QUALITATIVE AND QUANTITATIVE COMPOSITION
Milrinone 1mg/ml.

(*For full list of excipients see section 6.1*)

3. PHARMACEUTICAL FORM
Solution for Injection.

Clear, colourless to pale yellow liquid.

4. CLINICAL PARTICULARS

4.1 Therapeutic indications
Primacor Injection is indicated for the short-term treatment of severe congestive heart failure unresponsive to conventional maintenance therapy, and for the treatment of patients with acute heart failure, including low output states following cardiac surgery.

4.2 Posology and method of administration
For intravenous administration.

Adults: Primacor Injection should be given as a loading dose of 50µg/kg administered over a period of 10 minutes usually followed by a continuous infusion at a dosage titrated between 0.375µg/kg/min and 0.75µg/kg/min according to haemodynamic and clinical response, but should not exceed 1.13mg/kg/day total dose.

The following provides a guide to maintenance infusion delivery rate based upon a solution containing milrinone 200µg/ml prepared by adding 40ml diluent per 10ml ampoule (400ml diluent per 100ml Primacor Injection). 0.45% saline, 0.9% saline or 5% dextrose may be used as diluents.

Primacor Injection Dose (µg /kg/min)	Infusion Delivery Rate (ml/kg/hr)
0.375	0.11
0.400	0.12
0.500	0.15
0.600	0.18
0.700	0.21
0.750	0.22

Solutions of different concentrations may be used according to patient fluid requirements. The duration of therapy should depend upon the patient's response. In congestive cardiac failure, patients have been maintained on the infusion for up to 5 days, although the usual period is 48 to 72 hours. In acute states following cardiac surgery, it is unlikely that treatment need be maintained for more than 12 hours.

Renal Impairment: Dosage adjustment required. Data obtained from patients with severe renal impairment but without heart failure have demonstrated that the presence of renal impairment significantly increases the terminal elimination half-life of milrinone. For patients with clinical evidence of renal impairment, the following maintenance infusion rates are recommended using the infusion solution described above.

Creatinine Clearance (ml/min/1.73m²)	Primacor Injection Dose (µg/kg/min)	Maintenance Infusion Delivery Rate (ml/kg/hr)
5	0.20	0.06
10	0.23	0.07
20	0.28	0.08
30	0.33	0.10
40	0.38	0.11
50	0.43	0.13

The infusion rate should be adjusted according to haemodynamic response.

Elderly: Experience so far suggests that no special dosage recommendations are necessary.

Children: Safety and effectiveness in children and adolescents under 18 years of age have not been established. Primacor Injection should be used only if the potential benefits outweigh the potential risks.

4.3 Contraindications
Hypersensitivity to milrinone or any of the excipients.

4.4 Special warnings and precautions for use
The use of inotropic agents such as milrinone during the acute phase of a myocardial infarction may lead to an undesirable increase in myocardial oxygen consumption (MVO_2). Primacor Injection is not recommended immediately following acute myocardial infarction until safety and efficacy have been established in this situation.

Careful monitoring should be maintained during Primacor Injection therapy including blood pressure, heart rate, clinical state, electro-cardiogram, fluid balance, electrolytes and renal function (i.e. serum creatinine).

In patients with severe obstructive aortic or pulmonary valvular disease or hypertrophic subaortic stenosis, Primacor Injection should not be used in place of surgical relief of the obstruction. In these conditions it is possible that a drug with inotropic / vasodilator properties might aggravate outflow obstruction.

Supraventricular and ventricular arrhythmias have been observed in the high risk population treated with Primacor Injection. In some patients an increase in ventricular ectopy including non-sustained ventricular tachycardia has been observed which did not affect patient safety or outcome.

As Primacor Injection produces a slight enhancement in A-V node conduction, there is a possibility of an increased ventricular response rate in patients with uncontrolled atrial flutter / fibrillation. Consideration should therefore be given to digitalisation or treatment with other agents to prolong A-V node conduction time prior to starting Primacor Injection therapy, and to discontinuing the therapy if arrhythmias occur.

The potential for arrhythmia, present in heart failure itself, may be increased by many drugs or a combination of drugs. Patients receiving Primacor Injection should be closely monitored during infusion and the infusion should be stopped if arrhythmias develop.

Milrinone may induce hypotension as a consequence of its vasodilatory activity, therefore caution should be exercised when Primacor Injection is administered to patients who are hypotensive prior to treatment. The rate of infusion should be slowed or stopped in patients showing excessive decreases in blood pressure.

If prior vigorous diuretic therapy is suspected of having caused significant decreases in cardiac filling pressure Primacor Injection should be cautiously administered while monitoring blood pressure, heart rate and clinical symptomatology.

Improvement in cardiac output with resultant diuresis may necessitate a reduction in the dose of diuretic. Potassium loss due to excessive diuresis may necessitate a reduction in the dose of diuretic. Potassium loss due to excessive diuresis may predispose digitalised patients to arrhythmias. Therefore, hypokalaemia should be corrected by potassium supplementation in advance of, or during, the use of Primacor Injection.

Cases of infusion site reaction have been reported with Primacor Injection (*see Section 4.8, Undesirable effects*). Consequently, careful monitoring of the infusion site should be maintained so as to avoid possible extravasation

4.5 Interaction with other medicinal products and other forms of interaction
None have been observed during Primacor Injection therapy (*but see Section 6.2, Incompatibilities*).

Whilst there is a theoretical potential interaction with calcium channel blockers, there has been no evidence of a clinically significant interaction to date.

Milrinone has a favourable inotropic effect in fully digitalised patients without causing signs of glycoside toxicity.

4.6 Pregnancy and lactation
Although animal studies have not revealed evidence of drug-induced foetal damage or other deleterious effects on reproductive function, the safety of milrinone in human pregnancy has not yet been established. It should be used during pregnancy only if the potential benefit justifies the potential risk to the foetus.

Caution should be exercised when Primacor Injection is administered to nursing women, since it is not known whether milrinone is excreted in human milk.

4.7 Effects on ability to drive and use machines
Not applicable.

4.8 Undesirable effects
Adverse reactions have been ranked under heading of system-organ class and frequency using the following convention: very common (>= 1/10); common (>= 1/100, <1/10); uncommon (>= 1/1,000, <1/100); rare (>= 1/10,000, <1/1,000); very rare (<1/10,000); not known (cannot be estimated from the available data).

Blood and the lymphatic system disorders:

- Uncommon: Thrombocytopenia

Metabolism and nutrition disorders:

- Uncommon: Hypokalaemia

Nervous system disorders:

- Common: Headaches, usually mild to moderate in severity
- Uncommon: Tremor

Cardiac disorders:

- Common:

- Ventricular ectopic activity
- Non sustained or sustained ventricular tachycardia
- Supraventricular arrhythmias
- Hypotension

- Uncommon:

- Ventricular fibrillation
- Angina/chest pain

- Very rare: Torsades de pointes

The incidence of arrhythmias has not been related to dose or plasma levels of milrinone. These arrhythmias are rarely life threatening. If present, they are often associated with certain underlying factors such as pre-existing arrhythmias, metabolic abnormalities (e.g. hypokalaemia) abnormal digoxin levels and catheter insertion.

Respiratory, thoracic and mediastinal disorders:

- Very rare: Bronchospasm

Hepato-biliary disorders:

- Uncommon: Liver function tests abnormal

Skin and subcutaneous tissue disorders:

- Very rare: Skin reactions such as rash.

General disorders and administration site conditions:

- Very rare: Anaphylactic shock
- Not known: Infusion site reaction

4.9 Overdose
Overdose of intravenous Primacor may produce hypotension (because of its vasodilatory effect) and cardiac arrhythmia. If this occurs, Primacor Injection administration should be reduced or temporarily discontinued until the patient's condition stabilises. No specific antidote is known, but general measures for circulatory support should be taken.

5. PHARMACOLOGICAL PROPERTIES

5.1 Pharmacodynamic properties
Pharmacotherapeutic group; Phosphodiesterase inhibitor, ATC code C01CE02

Milrinone is a positive inotrope and vasodilator, with little chronotropic activity. It also improves left ventricular diastolic relaxation. It differs in structure and mode of action from the digitalis glycosides, catecholamines or angiotensin converting enzyme inhibitors. It is a selective inhibitor of peak III phosphodiesterase isoenzyme in cardiac and vascular muscle. It produces slight enhancement of A-V node conduction, but no other significant electro-physiological effects.

In clinical studies Primacor Injection has been shown to produce prompt improvements in the haemodynamic indices of congestive heart failure, including cardiac output, pulmonary capillary wedge pressure and vascular resistance, without clinically significant effect on heart rate or myocardial oxygen consumption. Haemodynamic improvement during intravenous Primacor therapy is accompanied by clinical symptomatic improvement in congestive cardiac failure, as measured by change in New York Heart Association classification.

5.2 Pharmacokinetic properties
Following intravenous injections of 12.5 to 125mcg/kg to congestive heart failure patients, Primacor Injection had a volume of distribution of 0.38 l/kg/hr, a mean terminal elimination half-life of 2.3 hours, and a clearance of 0.13 l/kg/hr. Following intravenous infusions of 0.2 to 0.7mcg/kg/min to congestive heart failure patients, the drug had a volume of distribution of about 0.45 l/kg, a mean terminal elimination half-life of 2.4 hours, and a clearance of 0.14 l/kg/hr. These pharmacokinetic parameters were not dose-dependent, and the area under the plasma concentration versus time curve following injection was significantly dose-dependent.

The primary route of excretion of milrinone in man is via the urine. Elimination in normal subjects via the urine is rapid, with approximately 60% recovered within the first two hours following dosing, and approximately 90% recovered within the first eight hours following dosing. The mean renal clearance of milrinone is approximately 0.3 l/min, indicative of active secretion.

5.3 Preclinical safety data
There are no preclinical data of relevance to the prescriber which are additional to that already in other sections of the SPC.

6. PHARMACEUTICAL PARTICULARS

6.1 List of excipients
Lactic Acid, Dextrose Anhydrous, Water for Injection, Sodium Hydroxide.

6.2 Incompatibilities
Furosemide or bumetanide should not be administered in intravenous lines containing Primacor Injection since precipitation occurs on admixture. Sodium Bicarbonate Intravenous infusion should not be used for dilution.

Other drugs should not be mixed with Primacor Injection until further compatibility data are available.

6.3 Shelf life
48 months when unopened. A diluted solution of Primacor Injection should be used within 24 hours.

6.4 Special precautions for storage
Do not store above 25°C. Do not freeze.

6.5 Nature and contents of container
Type 1 10ml flint glass ampoules packed in lots of 10.

6.6 Special precautions for disposal and other handling
Infusion solutions diluted as recommended with 0.45% saline, 0.9% saline or 5% dextrose should be freshly prepared before use. Parenteral drug products should be examined visually and should not be used if particulate matter or discolouration are present.

7. MARKETING AUTHORISATION HOLDER
sanofi aventis
One Onslow Street
Guildford
Surrey GU1 4YS

8. MARKETING AUTHORISATION NUMBER(S)
PL 11723/0064

9. DATE OF FIRST AUTHORISATION/RENEWAL OF THE AUTHORISATION
1st June 2003

10. DATE OF REVISION OF THE TEXT
June 2008

Legal category: POM

Primaxin IV Injection

(Merck Sharp & Dohme Limited)

1. NAME OF THE MEDICINAL PRODUCT
'Primaxin' IV 500 mg Injection

2. QUALITATIVE AND QUANTITATIVE COMPOSITION
'Primaxin' IV 500 mg Injection contains 500 mg imipenem (as the monohydrate) with 500 mg cilastatin (as the sodium salt).

3. PHARMACEUTICAL FORM
Powder for concentrate for solution for infusion.

'Primaxin' IV is available as vials containing sterile white to light yellow powder.

4. CLINICAL PARTICULARS

4.1 Therapeutic indications
Broad-spectrum beta-lactam antibiotic.

'Primaxin' contains:

imipenem, a member of a class of beta-lactam antibiotics - the thienamycins cilastatin sodium, a specific enzyme inhibitor, that blocks the metabolism of imipenem in the kidney and substantially increases the concentration of unchanged imipenem in the urinary tract.

'Primaxin' is bactericidal against an unusually wide spectrum of Gram-positive, Gram-negative, aerobic and anaerobic pathogens. 'Primaxin' is useful for treating single and polymicrobic infections, and initiating therapy prior to identification of the causative organisms.

'Primaxin' is indicated for the treatment of the following infections due to susceptible organisms:

'Primaxin' IV

Lower respiratory tract infections

Intra-abdominal infections

Genito-urinary infections

Gynaecological infections

Septicaemia

Bone and joint infections

Skin and soft tissue infections

Note: 'Primaxin' is not indicated against central nervous system infections.

'Primaxin' is indicated against mixed infections caused by susceptible aerobic and anaerobic bacteria. The majority of these infections are associated with contamination by faecal flora, or flora originating from the vagina, skin, and mouth. In these mixed infections, 'Primaxin' is usually effective against *Bacteroides fragilis* sp., the most commonly encountered anaerobic pathogen, which is usually resistant to the aminoglycosides, cephalosporins and penicillins.

Consideration should be given to official local guidance (e.g. national recommendations) on the appropriate use of bacterial agents.

Susceptibility of the causative organism to the treatment should be tested (if possible), although therapy may be initiated before the results are available.

Prophylaxis: 'Primaxin' IV is also indicated for the prevention of certain post-operative infections in patients undergoing contaminated or potentially contaminated surgical procedures or where the occurrence of post-operative infection could be especially serious.

4.2 Posology and method of administration
The total daily dosage and route of administration of 'Primaxin' should be based on the type or severity of infection, consideration of degree of susceptibility of the pathogen(s), renal function and bodyweight. Doses cited are based on a bodyweight of $\geq$70 kg. The total daily requirement should be given in equally divided doses.

The dosage recommendations that follow specify the amounts of imipenem to be given. An equivalent amount of cilastatin is provided with this. One vial of 'Primaxin' IV 500 mg provides the equivalent of 500 mg anhydrous imipenem and 500 mg cilastatin.

Use in the elderly

Age does not usually affect the tolerability and efficacy of 'Primaxin'. The dosage should be determined by the severity of the infection, the susceptibility of the causative organism(s), the patient's clinical condition, and renal function.

INTRAVENOUS ADMINISTRATION

This formulation should not be used intramuscularly. The dosage of 'Primaxin' IV should be determined by the severity of the infection, the antibiotic susceptibility of the causative organism(s) and the condition of the patient.

Note: All recommended doses refer to the imipenem fraction of 'Primaxin'.

Adults (based on 70 kg bodyweight): The usual adult daily dosage is 1-2 g administered in 3-4 equally divided doses (see chart below). In infections due to less sensitive organisms, the daily dose may be increased to a maximum dose of 50 mg/kg/day (not exceeding 4 g daily).

Usual adult intravenous dosage

Each dose of 250 mg or 500 mg should be given by intravenous infusion over 20-30 minutes. Each dose of 1000 mg should be infused over 40-60 minutes. In patients who develop nausea during infusion, the infusion rate may be slowed.

(see Table 1 below)

Primaxin' has been used successfully as monotherapy in immunocompromised cancer patients for confirmed or suspected infections such as sepsis.

Prophylactic use

For prophylaxis against post-surgical infections in adults, 1 g 'Primaxin' IV should be given intravenously on induction of anaesthesia and 1 g three hours later. For high-risk (i.e. colorectal) surgery, two additional 0.5 g doses can be given at 8 and 16 hours after induction.

In patients with renal insufficiency

As in patients with normal renal function, dosing is based on the severity of the infection. The maximum dosage for patients with various degrees of renal functional impairment is shown in the following table. Doses cited are based on a bodyweight of 70 kg. Proportionate reduction in dose administered should be made for patients with lower bodyweight.

Maximum dosage in relation to renal function

(see Table 2 below)

Patients with a creatinine clearance of $\leq$5 ml/min should not receive 'Primaxin' IV unless haemodialysis is started within 48 hours.

'Primaxin' is cleared by haemodialysis. The patient should receive 'Primaxin' IV immediately after haemodialysis and at 12-hourly intervals thereafter. Dialysis patients, especially those with background CNS disease, should be carefully monitored; patients on haemodialysis should receive 'Primaxin' IV only when the benefit outweighs the potential risk of convulsions (see 4.4 'Special warnings and special precautions for use').

There are currently inadequate data to recommend the use of 'Primaxin' IV for patients on peritoneal dialysis.

Paediatric dosage

Age	Dose	Dosage interval	Total daily dose
3 months of age and older (less than 40 kg bodyweight)	15 mg/kg	6 hours	60 mg/kg

The maximum daily dose should not exceed 2 g.

Children over 40 kg bodyweight should receive adult doses.

Clinical data are insufficient to recommend an optimal dose for children under 3 months of age or infants and children with impaired renal function.

Table 1

IV administration			
Severity of infection	Dose	Dosage interval	Total daily dose
Mild	250 mg	6 hours	1.0 g
Moderate	500 mg	8 hours	1.5 g
Severe – fully susceptible	500 mg	6 hours	2.0 g
Severe and/or life-threatening infections due to less sensitive organisms (primarily some strains of *P.aeruginosa*)	1000 mg 1000 mg	8 hours 6 hours	3.0 g 4.0 g

Table 2 Maximum dosage in relation to renal function

Renal function	Creatinine clearance (ml/min)	Dose (mg)	Dosage interval (hrs)	Maximum total daily dose* (g)
Mild impairment	31-70	500	6 - 8	1.5 - 2
Moderate impairment	21-30	500	8 - 12	1 - 1.5
Severe** impairment	0-20	250-500	12	0.5 - 1.0

* The higher dose should be reserved for infections caused by less susceptible organisms.

** Patients with creatinine clearance of 6-20 ml/min should be treated with 250 mg (or 3.5 mg/kg, whichever is lower) every 12 hours for most pathogens. When the 500 mg dose is used in these patients there may be an increased risk of convulsions.

'Primaxin' IV is not recommended for the therapy of meningitis. If meningitis is suspected an appropriate antibiotic should be used.

'Primaxin' IV may be used in children with sepsis as long as they are not suspected of having meningitis.

4.3 Contraindications

Hypersensitivity to this product.

4.4 Special warnings and precautions for use

Warning

There is some clinical and laboratory evidence of partial cross-allergenicity between 'Primaxin' and the other beta-lactam antibiotics, penicillins and cephalosporins. Severe reactions (including anaphylaxis) have been reported with most beta-lactam antibiotics.

Before initiating therapy with 'Primaxin', careful inquiry should be made concerning previous hypersensitivity reactions to beta-lactam antibiotics. If an allergic reaction to 'Primaxin' occurs, the drug should be discontinued and appropriate measures undertaken.

Pseudomembranous colitis, reported with virtually all antibiotics, can range from mild to life-threatening in severity. 'Primaxin' should be prescribed with caution in patients with a history of gastro-intestinal disease, particularly colitis. Treatment-related diarrhoea should always be considered as a pointer to this diagnosis. While studies indicate that a toxin of *Clostridium difficile* is one of the primary causes of antibiotic-associated colitis, other causes should be considered.

Paediatric use

'Primaxin' IV: Efficacy and tolerability in infants under 3 months of age have yet to be established; therefore, 'Primaxin' IV is not recommended for use below this age.

Central nervous system: Patients with CNS disorders and/or compromised renal function (accumulation of 'Primaxin' may occur) have shown CNS side effects, especially when recommended dosages based on bodyweight and renal function were exceeded. Hence it is recommended that the dosage schedules of 'Primaxin' should be strictly adhered to, and established anticonvulsant therapy continued.

If focal tremors, myoclonus or convulsions occur, the patient should be evaluated neurologically and placed on anticonvulsant therapy if not already instituted. If these symptoms continue, the dosage should be reduced, or 'Primaxin' withdrawn completely.

Use in patients with renal insufficiency

Patients with creatinine clearances of $\leq$5 ml/min should not receive 'Primaxin' IV unless haemodialysis is instituted within 48 hours. For patients on haemodialysis, 'Primaxin' IV is recommended only when the benefit outweighs the potential risk of convulsions.

4.5 Interaction with other medicinal products and other forms of interaction

General seizures have been reported in patients who received ganciclovir and 'Primaxin' IV. These drugs should not be used concomitantly unless the potential benefit outweighs the risk.

Decreased serum levels of valproic acid with co-administration of carbapenem antibiotics have been reported during post-marketing and in some cases breakthrough seizures have occurred. Careful monitoring of serum levels of valproic acid should be considered if imipenem is to be co-administered with valproic acid (e.g. sodium valproate).

Concomitant probenecid has been shown to double the plasma level and half-life of cilastatin, but with no effect on its urinary recovery.

Concomitant probenecid showed only minimal increases in plasma level and half-life of imipenem, with urinary recovery of active imipenem decreased to approximately 60% of the administered dose.

4.6 Pregnancy and lactation

Pregnant monkeys showed evidence of maternal and foetal toxicity with bolus injections at doses equivalent to twice the human dose.

The use of 'Primaxin' in pregnant women has not been studied and 'Primaxin' should therefore not be given in pregnancy unless the anticipated benefit to the mother outweighs the possible risk to the foetus.

'Primaxin' has been detected in human milk. If the use of 'Primaxin' is deemed essential, the mother should stop breast-feeding.

4.7 Effects on ability to drive and use machines

There are no specific data; however, some of the CNS side-effects, such as dizziness, psychic disturbances, confusion and seizures, may affect the ability to drive or operate machinery.

4.8 Undesirable effects

Side effects

'Primaxin' is generally well tolerated. Side effects rarely require cessation of therapy and are generally mild and transient; serious side effects are rare.

Local reactions: erythema, local pain and induration, thrombophlebitis.

Allergic: rash, pruritus, urticaria, erythema multiforme, Stevens-Johnson syndrome, angioedema, toxic epidermal necrolysis (rarely), exfoliative dermatitis, (rarely) candidiasis, fever including drug fever, anaphylactic reactions.

Gastro-intestinal: nausea, vomiting, diarrhoea, staining of teeth and/or tongue. Pseudomembranous colitis has been reported.

Blood: eosinophilia, leucopenia, neutropenia including agranulocytosis, thrombocytopenia, thrombocytosis, decreased haemoglobin and prolonged prothrombin time. A positive direct Coombs test may develop.

Liver function: mild increases in serum transaminases, bilirubin and/or serum alkaline phosphatase, hepatitis rarely have been reported.

Renal function: oliguria/anuria, polyuria, acute renal failure (rarely). The role of 'Primaxin' in changes in renal function is difficult to assess, since factors predisposing to pre-renal uraemia or to impaired renal function usually have been present. Elevated serum creatinine and blood urea have been seen. A harmless urine discoloration, not to be confused with haematuria, has been seen in children.

Central nervous system: myoclonic activity, psychic disturbances including hallucinations, paraesthesia, confusional states or convulsions have been reported.

Granulocytopenic patients: drug-related nausea and/or vomiting appear to occur more frequently in granulocytopenic patients than in non-granulocytopenic patients treated with 'Primaxin'.

Special senses: hearing loss, taste perversion.

Other reported reactions with an unknown causal relationship

Gastro-intestinal: haemorrhagic colitis, gastro-enteritis, abdominal pain, glossitis, tongue papillar hypertrophy, heartburn, pharyngeal pain, increased salivation.

Central nervous system: dizziness, somnolence, encephalopathy, vertigo, headache.

Special senses: tinnitus.

Respiratory: chest discomfort, dyspnoea, hyperventilation, thoracic spine pain.

Cardiovascular: hypotension, palpitations, tachycardia.

Skin: flushing, cyanosis, hyperhidrosis, skin texture changes, pruritus vulvae.

Body as a whole: polyarthralgia, asthenia/weakness.

Blood: haemolytic anaemia, pancytopenia, bone marrow depression.

4.9 Overdose

No specific information is available on the treatment of overdosage with 'Primaxin'.

Imipenem-cilastatin sodium is haemodialysable. However, usefulness of this procedure in the overdosage setting is unknown.

5. PHARMACOLOGICAL PROPERTIES

Pharmacotherapeutic group: Antibacterials for systemic use.

ATC code: J01D H51

5.1 Pharmacodynamic properties

Mechanism of Action

Imipenem is a potent inhibitor of bacterial cell wall synthesis and is highly reactive towards penicillin-binding protein. Imipenem is more potent in its bactericidal effect than other antibiotics studied. Imipenem also provides excellent stability to degradative bacterial beta-lactamases. Imipenem is therefore active against a high percentage of organisms resistant to other beta-lactam antibiotics.

Cilastatin sodium is a competitive, reversible, and specific inhibitor of dehydropeptidase-I, the renal enzyme which metabolises and inactivates imipenem. Cilastatin sodium is devoid of intrinsic antibacterial activity itself and does not affect the antibacterial activity of imipenem.

Bacteriology

'Primaxin' has a unique anti-bacterial spectrum. Against Gram-negative species, 'Primaxin' shares the spectrum of the newer cephalosporins and penicillins; against Gram-positive species 'Primaxin' exerts the high bacterial potency previously associated only with narrow-spectrum beta-lactam antibiotics and the first-generation cephalosporins.

The antibiotic spectrum of 'Primaxin' is broader than that of other antibiotics studied and includes virtually all clinically significant pathogenic genera.

In vitro tests show that imipenem acts synergistically with aminoglycoside antibiotics against some isolates of *Pseudomonas aeruginosa*.

Breakpoints (NCCLS)

The general MIC susceptibility test breakpoints to separate sensitive (S) pathogens from resistant (R) pathogens are: S $\leqslant$4 mcg/mL, R $\geqslant$ 16 mcg/mL.

For *Haemophilus spp.* S $\leqslant$ 4 mcg/mL, R MIC breakpoint not defined.

For *Neisseria gonorrhoeae* MIC breakpoints not defined.

For *Streptococcus pneumoniae* S $\leqslant$ 0.12 mcg/mL, R $\geqslant$ 1 mcg/mL

For streptococci other than *S. pneumoniae* MIC breakpoints not defined.

Susceptibility

The prevalence of resistance may vary geographically and with time for selected species and local information on resistance is desirable, particularly when treating severe infections. The information below gives only approximate guidance on the probability as to whether the microorganism will be susceptible to 'Primaxin' or not.

Organism	Prevalence of Resistance (Range) [European Union]
SUSCEPTIBLE	
Gram-positive aerobes:	
Bacillus spp	
Enterococcus faecalis	0 to 7%
Erysipelothrix rhusiopathiae	
Listeria monocytogenes	
Nocardia spp	
Pediococcus spp	
Staphylococcus aureus (methicillin susceptible, including penicillinase-producing strains	0%
Staphylococcus epidermidis (methicillin susceptible, including penicillinase-producing strains)	0 to 7%
Staphylococcus saprophyticus	0%
*Streptococcus agalactiae**	
Streptococcus Group C	
Streptococcus Group G	
Streptococcus pneumoniae	0%
Streptococcus pneumoniae, PRSP	0 to 83%
*Streptococcus pyogenes**	
*Viridans group streptococci** (including alpha and gamma hemolytic strains)	
Gram-negative aerobes:	
Achromobacter spp.	
Acinetobacter baumannii	0 to 67%
Aeromonas hydrophila	0 to 50%
Alcaligenes spp	
Bordetella bronchicanis	
Bordetella bronchiseptica	
Bordetella pertussis	
Brucella melitensis	
Burkholderia pseudomallei (formerly *pseudomonas pseudomallei)*	
Burkholderia stutzeri (formerly *pseudomonas stutzeri)*	
Campylobacter spp.	
Capnocytophaga spp.	
Citrobacter freundii	0%
Citrobacter koseri (formerly *Citrobacter diversus*	0%
Eikenella corrodens	
Enterobacter aerogenes	0%
Enterobacter agglomerans	
Enterobacter cloacae	0 to 13%
Eschericia coli	0%
Gardnerella vaginalis	
Haemophilus ducreyi	
Haemophilus influenzae (including beta-lactamase-producing strains)*	
*Haemophilus parainfluenzae**	
Hafnia alvei	0%
Klebsiella oxytoca	0%
Klebsiella ozaenae	
Klebsiella pneumoniae	0%
Moraxella catarrhalis	0%
Morganella morganii (formerly *Proteus morganii)*	0 to 7%
Neisseria gonorrhoeae (including penicillinase-producing strains)*	
Neisseria meningitidis	
Pasteurella spp	0%
Pasteurella multocida	
Plesiomonas shigelloides	
Proteus mirabilis	0%
Proteus vulgaris	0 to 8%
Providencia alcalifaciens	

Providencia rettgeri (formerly *Proteus rettgeri*)	0 to 20%
Providencia stuartii	0%
Pseudomonas aeruginosa	0 to 20%
Pseudomonas fluorescens	
Pseudomonas putida	
Salmonella spp	0%
Salmonella typhi	
Serratia spp	
Serratia proteamaculans (formerly *Serratia liquefaciens*)	
Serratia marcescens	0%
Shigella spp.	0%
Yersinia spp (formerly *Pasteurella*)	
Yersinia enterocolitica	
Yersinia pseudotuberculosis	
Gram-positive Anaerobes:	
Actinomyces spp	
Bifidobacterium spp.	
Clostridium spp	0%
Clostridium pefringens	
Eubacterium spp.	
Lactobacillus spp.	
Mobiluncus spp.	
Microaerophilic streptococci	
Peptococcus spp.	
Peptostreptococcus spp.	0%
Propionibacterium spp (including *P. acnes*)	
Gram-negative Anaerobes:	
Bacteroides spp.	6%
Bacteroides distasonis	
Bacteroides fragilis	0 to 7%
Bacteroides ovatus	
Bacteroides thetaitaomicron	0%
Bacteroides uniformis	
Bacteroides vulgatus	
Bilophila wadsworthia	
Fusobacterium spp.	
Fusobacterium necrophorum	
Fusobacterium nucleatum	
Porphyromonas asaccharolytica (formerly *Bacteroides asaccharolytica bivius*)	
Prevotella bivia (formerly *Bacteroides bivius*)	
Prevotella disiens (formerly *Bacteroides disiens*)	
Prevotella intermedia (formerly *Bacteroides intermedius*)	
Prevotella melaninogenica (formerly *Bacteroides melaninogenicus*)	
Veillonella spp	
Others:	
Mycobacterium fortuitum	
Myobacterium smegmatis	
RESISTANT	
Gram-positive Aerobes:	
Enterococcus faecium	
methicillin-resistant staphylococci	
Gram-negative Aerobes:	
Stenotrophomonas maltophilia (formerly *Xanthomonas maltophilia*, formerly *Pseudomonas maltophilia*)	
(Some strains of *Burkholderia cepacia* (formerly *Pseudomonas cepacia*)	

*Resistant breakpoint not defined.

Mechanism/s of Resistance

For species considered susceptible to imipenem, resistance was uncommon in surveillance studies in Europe. In resistant isolates, resistance to other antibacterial agents of the carbapenem class was seen in some, but not all isolates. Imipenem is effectively stable to hydrolysis by most classes of beta-lactamases, including penicillinases, cephalosporinases and extended spectrum beta-lactamases, but not metallo-beta-lactamases. Although effectively stable to beta-lactamase activity, resistance, when seen, is generally due to a combination of decreased permeability and low-level beta-lactamase hydrolysis.

The mechanism of action of imipenem differs from that of other classes of antibiotics, such as quinolones, aminoglycosides, macrolides and tetracyclines. There is no target-based cross-resistance between imipenem and these substances. However, micro-organisms may exhibit resistance to more than one class of antibacterial agents when the mechanism is, or includes, impermeability to some compounds.

5.2 Pharmacokinetic properties

'Primaxin' IV

The product is administered intravenously, therefore bioavailability data are not relevant.

Imipenem: Peak plasma levels of 36.4 mcg/ml after 500 mg, half-life 62.0 (±3.9) mins; plasma clearance 225.5 (±15.9) ml/min.

Co-administration of cilastatin sodium increases plasma concentrations of imipenem and increases the AUC by about 20%. There is also a decrease in plasma clearance (194.9 ml/min) and an increase in renal clearance, urinary recovery and urinary concentration.

5.3 Preclinical safety data

No relevant data.

6. PHARMACEUTICAL PARTICULARS

6.1 List of excipients

The only inactive ingredient in 'Primaxin' IV is sodium bicarbonate.

6.2 Incompatibilities

'Primaxin' is chemically incompatible with lactate and should not be reconstituted with diluents containing lactate. 'Primaxin' IV can, however, be administered into an IV tubing through which a lactate solution is being infused. 'Primaxin' should not be mixed or physically added to other antibiotics.

6.3 Shelf life

24 months.

6.4 Special precautions for storage

Vials of dry 'Primaxin' should be stored below 25°C. The container should be kept in the outer carton until immediately before use.

After reconstitution 'Primaxin' IV can be kept at room temperature (below 25°C) for up to three hours or under refrigeration (below 4°C) for up to 24 hours.

6.5 Nature and contents of container

'Primaxin' IV 500 mg strength is available in Type I (20ml) clear glass vials with grey butyl rubber stoppers (West Formula 1816) and aluminium collar seals with plastic flip-off tops. The vial size for 'Primaxin' IV 500 mg strength is 20ml

6.6 Special precautions for disposal and other handling

Preparation of intravenous solution

The following table is provided for convenience in reconstituting 'Primaxin' IV for intravenous infusion.

Strength	Volume of diluent added (ml)	Approximate concentration of imipenem (mg/ml)
'Primaxin' IV 500 mg	100	5

Reconstitution of 20 ml vial

Contents of the vials must be suspended and transferred to 100 mL of an appropriate infusion solution. A suggested procedure is to add approximately 10 mL from the appropriate infusion solution (see 'Compatibility and Stability')) to the vial. Shake well and transfer the resulting suspension to the infusion solution container.

CAUTION: THE SUSPENSION IS NOT FOR DIRECT INFUSION.

Repeat with an additional 10 mL of infusion solution to ensure complete transfer of vial contents to the infusion solution. The resulting mixture should be agitated until clear.

Compatibility and stability

In keeping with good clinical and pharmaceutical practice, 'Primaxin' IV should be administered as a freshly prepared solution. On the few occasions where changing circumstances make this impracticable, reconstituted 'Primaxin' IV retains satisfactory potency for three hours at room temperature (up to 25°C) or 24 hours in a refrigerator (below 4°C) when prepared in any of the following diluents: 0.9% Sodium Chloride Injection; 5% Dextrose and 0.9% Sodium Chloride; 5% Dextrose and 0.225% Sodium Chloride; 5% Mannitol.

'Primaxin' IV is chemically incompatible with lactate and should not be reconstituted with diluents containing lactate. 'Primaxin' IV can, however, be administered into an IV tubing through which a lactate solution is being infused.

'Primaxin' should not be mixed with, or physically added to, other antibiotics.

7. MARKETING AUTHORISATION HOLDER

Merck Sharp & Dohme Limited

Hertford Road, Hoddesdon, Hertfordshire EN11 9BU

8. MARKETING AUTHORISATION NUMBER(S)

PL 0025/0229

9. DATE OF FIRST AUTHORISATION/RENEWAL OF THE AUTHORISATION

Licence first granted 30 June 1988

Licence last renewed 07 October 2005

10. DATE OF REVISION OF THE TEXT

February 2009

LEGAL CATEGORY:

P.O.M.

® denotes registered trademark of Merck & Co., Inc., Whitehouse Station, NJ, USA.

SPC.TENIV.08.UK.2942

Priorix

(GlaxoSmithKline UK)

1. NAME OF THE MEDICINAL PRODUCT

Priorix®

Powder and solvent for solution for injection

Measles, Mumps and Rubella vaccine (live)

2. QUALITATIVE AND QUANTITATIVE COMPOSITION

Each 0.5 ml dose of the reconstituted vaccine contains:

- not less than $10^{3.0}$ $CCID_{50}$* of the Schwarz measles[1]

- not less than $10^{3.7}$ $CCID_{50}$ of the RIT 4385 mumps[1], and

- - not less than $10^{3.0}$ $CCID_{50}$ of the Wistar RA 27/3 rubella[2] virus strains.

*CCID $_{50}$– Cell Culture Infective Dose 50

[1]produced in chick embryo cells

[2]produced in human diploid (MRC-5) cells

For a full list of excipients, see section 6.1

3. PHARMACEUTICAL FORM

Lyophilised vaccine for reconstitution with the sterile diluent provided.

Before reconstitution, the lyophilised vaccine is a white to slightly pink powder and the diluent is a clear colourless liquid.

4. CLINICAL PARTICULARS

4.1 Therapeutic indications

Priorix is indicated for active immunisation against measles, mumps and rubella.

4.2 Posology and method of administration

Posology

0.5 ml of the reconstituted vaccine constitutes one dose.

Priorix may be used for both primary immunisation and revaccination of children over 9 months of age, adolescents and adults. For infants in their first year of life see section 4.4. The vaccine should be given according to the recommended schedule.

Priorix may be given to subjects who have previously been vaccinated with other measles, mumps and rubella vaccines.

Children who suffered idiopathic thrombocytopenic purpura (ITP) within 6 weeks of the first dose of MMR (or its component vaccines) should have their serological status evaluated at the time the second dose is due. If serology testing suggests that a child is not fully immune against measles, mumps and rubella then a second dose of MMR is recommended.

Method of administration

Priorix is for subcutaneous injection.

It may also be given by intramuscular injection. A limited number of subjects received Priorix intramuscularly in clinical trials in which an adequate immune response was obtained for all three components.

PRIORIX SHOULD UNDER NO CIRCUMSTANCES BE ADMINISTERED INTRAVASCULARLY.

Alcohol and other disinfecting agents must be allowed to evaporate from the skin before injection of the vaccine since they can inactivate the attenuated viruses in the vaccine.

For instructions on reconstitution of the product before administration refer to section 6.6.

4.3 Contraindications

Priorix is contraindicated in subjects with known systemic hypersensitivity to any component of the vaccine or to neomycin (see also Section 4.4.) A history of contact dermatitis to neomycin is not a contraindication.

Priorix must not be administered to pregnant women. Furthermore, pregnancy must be avoided for one month after vaccination (see Section 4.6).

Priorix should not be given to subjects with impaired immune function. These include patients with primary or secondary immunodeficiencies.

However, measles, mumps, rubella-combined vaccines can be given to asymptomatic HIV-infected persons without adverse consequences to their illness and may be considered for those who are symptomatic.

As with other vaccines, the administration of Priorix should be postponed in subjects suffering from acute severe febrile illness. The presence of a minor infection, however, is not a contraindication for vaccination.

4.4 Special warnings and precautions for use

As with all injectable vaccines, appropriate medical treatment and supervision should always be readily available in case of a rare anaphylactic event following the administration of the vaccine.

The measles and mumps components of the vaccine are produced in chick embryo cell culture and may therefore contain traces of egg protein. Persons with a history of anaphylactic, anaphylactoid, or other immediate reactions (e.g. generalised urticaria, swelling of the mouth and throat, difficulty breathing, hypotension, or shock) subsequent to egg ingestion may be at an enhanced risk of immediate-type hypersensitivity reactions after vaccination, although these types of reactions have been shown to be very rare. Individuals who have experienced anaphylaxis after egg ingestion should be vaccinated with extreme caution, with adequate treatment for anaphylaxis on hand should such a reaction occur.

Priorix should be given with caution to persons with a history or family history of allergic diseases or those with a history or family history of convulsions.

Limited protection against measles may be obtained by vaccination up to 72 hours after exposure to natural measles.

Infants in their first year of life may not respond sufficiently to the measles component of the vaccine, due to the possible persistence of maternal measles antibodies. This should not preclude the use of the vaccine in infants from the age of 9 months if this is considered necessary (e.g. due to travel to a region with high prevalence of measles or in outbreak situations). In these circumstances further doses of combined measles, mumps and rubella vaccine should be administered in accordance with official recommendations.

Children who suffered idiopathic thrombocytopenic purpura (ITP) within 6 weeks of the first dose of MMR (or its component vaccines) should have their serological status evaluated at the time the second dose is due. If serology testing suggests that a child is not fully immune against measles, mumps and rubella then a second dose of MMR is recommended.

Transmission of measles virus from vaccinees to susceptible contacts has never been documented. Pharyngeal excretion of the rubella virus is known to occur about 7 to 28 days after vaccination with peak excretion around the 11th day. However there is no evidence of transmission of this excreted vaccine virus to susceptible contacts. Studies have shown that recipients of the Jeryl Lynn strain of mumps virus vaccine do not spread this virus to susceptible contacts and that the virus cannot be isolated from blood, urine or saliva.

As with any vaccine, vaccination with Priorix may not result in complete protection of all vaccinees against the infections it is intended to prevent.

4.5 Interaction with other medicinal products and other forms of interaction

It is generally accepted that measles, mumps and rubella-combined vaccine may be given at the same time as the oral polio vaccine (OPV) or inactivated polio vaccine (IPV), the injectable trivalent diphtheria, tetanus and pertussis vaccines (DTPw/DTPa) and *Haemophilus influenzae* type b (Hib). Concomitant vaccines should be given by separate injections into different body sites.

Studies have shown that Priorix can be administered at the same time as the live attenuated varicella vaccine (Varilix) if separate injection sites are used.

If Priorix cannot be given at the same time as other live attenuated vaccines, an interval of 4 weeks should be left between vaccinations.

In subjects who have received human gammaglobulins or a blood transfusion, vaccination should be delayed for at least three months because of the likelihood of vaccine failure due to passively acquired mumps, measles and rubella antibodies. However, if Priorix is being given primarily to achieve protection against rubella, the vaccine may be given within three months of the administration of an immunoglobulin preparation or a blood transfusion. In such instances, serological testing should be performed approximately 8-12 weeks later in order to assess the need for re-immunisation.

If tuberculin testing has to be done it should be carried out before, or simultaneously with, vaccination since it has been reported that live measles (and possibly mumps) vaccine may cause a temporary depression of tuberculin skin sensitivity. This anergy may last for four to six weeks and tuberculin testing should not be performed within that period after vaccination to avoid false negative results.

Priorix may be given as a booster dose in subjects who have previously been vaccinated with another measles mumps and rubella combined vaccine.

4.6 Pregnancy and lactation

Pregnancy

Priorix is contraindicated in pregnant women. Furthermore, pregnancy should be avoided for one month after vaccination.

Lactation

There are no human data regarding use in breast-feeding women. They can be vaccinated where the benefit outweighs the risk.

4.7 Effects on ability to drive and use machines

The vaccine is unlikely to produce an effect on the ability to drive and use machines.

4.8 Undesirable effects

Frequencies are reported as:

Very common: $\geqslant$ 10%

Common: $\geqslant$ 1% and $<$ 10%

Uncommon: $\geqslant$ 0.1% and $<$ 1%

Rare: $\geqslant$ 0.01% and $<$ 0.1%

Very rare: $<$ 0.01%

In controlled clinical studies in children aged from 9 months to 2 years, signs and symptoms were actively monitored during a 42-day follow-up period. Parents/guardians of the vaccinees were also requested to report any adverse events during the study period.

The safety profile presented below is based on a total of approximately 12,000 subjects administered Priorix in clinical trials

Infections and infestations:

Uncommon: otitis media

Common: upper respiratory tract infection

Blood and lymphatic system disorders:

Uncommon: lymphadenopathy

Immune system disorders:

Rare: allergic reactions

Metabolism and nutrition disorders:

Uncommon: anorexia

Psychiatric disorders:

Uncommon: nervousness, abnormal crying, insomnia

Nervous system disorders:

Rare: febrile convulsions

Eye disorders:

Uncommon: conjunctivitis

Respiratory, thoracic and mediastinal disorders:

Uncommon: bronchitis, cough

Gastrointestinal disorders:

Uncommon: parotid gland enlargement, diarrhoea, vomiting

Skin and subcutaneous tissue disorders:

Common: rash

General disorders and administration site conditions:

Very common: redness at the injection site, fever $\geqslant$38°C (rectal) or $\geqslant$37.5°C (axillary/oral)

Common: pain and swelling at the injection site, fever $>$39.5°C (rectal) or $>$39°C (axillary/oral)

In general, the frequency category for adverse reactions was similar for the first and second vaccine doses. The exception to this was pain at the injection site which was "Common" after the first vaccine dose and "Very common" after the second vaccine dose.

During post-marketing surveillance, the following reactions have been reported in temporal association with Priorix vaccination:

Infections and infestations:

Meningitis

Blood and lymphatic system disorders:

Thrombocytopenia, thrombocytopenic purpura

Immune system disorders

Anaphylactic reactions

Nervous system disorders:

Transverse myelitis, Guillain Barré syndrome, peripheral neuritis, encephalitis*

Skin and subcutaneous tissue disorders:

Erythema multiforme

Musculoskeletal and connective tissue disorders:

Arthralgia, arthritis

General disorders and administration site conditions:

Kawasaki syndrome

As in natural rubella infection, arthralgia, or in isolated cases, chronic arthritis as well as myalgia, exanthema and swollen lymph nodes may occur two to four weeks after administration of live rubella vaccines. The incidence of joint reactions increases with the age of the vaccinee. Cases of exudative arthritis are extremely rare.

In rare cases a mumps-like condition with an abbreviated incubation period cannot be ruled out. In isolated cases, a transient, painful swelling of the testicles had been reported after combined mumps, measles, rubella vaccination.

Accidental intravascular administration may give rise to severe reactions or even shock. Immediate measures depend on the severity of the reaction.

In comparative studies with other measles, mumps and rubella vaccines, the incidences of local pain, redness and swelling reported with Priorix were low, while the incidences of other adverse reactions were similar.

* Encephalitis has been reported with a frequency below 1 per 10 million doses. The risk of encephalitis following administration of the vaccine is far below the risk of encephalitis caused by natural diseases (measles: 1 in 1000 to 2000 cases; rubella: approximately 1 in 6000 cases).

In rare cases a measles-like syndrome has been reported following vaccination with Priorix.

4.9 Overdose

Cases of overdose (up to 2 times the recommended dose) have been reported during post-marketing surveillance. No adverse events have been associated to the overdose.

5. PHARMACOLOGICAL PROPERTIES

5.1 Pharmacodynamic properties

Pharmacotherapeutic group: Viral vaccine.

ATC code: J07B D52.

The safety and immunogenicity of Priorix in adolescents and adults has not been specifically studied in clinical trials.

In clinical studies in children aged from 12 months to 2 years Priorix has been demonstrated to be highly immunogenic. Following primary vaccination with a single dose of Priorix in the second year of life antibodies against measles were detected in 98.0%, against mumps in 96.1% and against rubella in 99.3% of previously seronegative vaccinees.

One hundred and fifty five children aged 10 – 22 months at immunisation were followed up for 12 months post vaccination. All remained seropositive for anti-measles and anti-rubella antibodies. 88.4% were still seropositive at month 12 for anti-mumps antibody. This percentage is in line with what was observed for other measles, mumps and rubella-combined vaccines (87%).

5.2 Pharmacokinetic properties

Not applicable.

5.3 Preclinical safety data

Not applicable.

6. PHARMACEUTICAL PARTICULARS

6.1 List of excipients

Vaccine:

Lactose

Mannitol

Sorbitol

The vaccine also contains the following amino acids:

L-alanine,

L-arginine,

glycine,

L-histidine

L-isoleucine

L-leucine

L-lysine HC1

L-methionine

L-phenylalanine

L-proline

L-serine

L-threonine,

L-tryptophan

L-tyrosine

L-valine

L-aspartic acid

L-cysteine

L-cystine,

L-hydroxproline

The vaccine may contain residual amounts of neomycin (25 micrograms maximum).

Diluent: Water for injections.

6.2 Incompatibilities

Priorix should not be mixed with other vaccines in the same syringe.

6.3 Shelf life

The shelf-life of Priorix is two years when the vaccine is stored according to recommendations (see Section 6.4.) The shelf lives of the vaccine and diluent are not identical, therefore their expiry dates are different. The outer carton bears the earlier of the two expiry dates and this date must be respected. The carton and ALL its contents should be discarded on reaching the outer carton expiry date.

6.4 Special precautions for storage

Priorix should be stored in a refrigerator between 2°C and 8°C and protected from light.

Do not freeze.

During transport, recommended conditions of storage should be respected, particularly in hot climates.

6.5 Nature and contents of container

Priorix is presented as a lyophilised pellet in a vial (type I glass) with a stopper (bromobutyl rubber). The sterile diluent is presented in a prefilled syringe (type I glass) with plunger stopper (chlorobutyl rubber) with 2 separate needles or ampoule (type I glass).

Single pack size.

6.6 Special precautions for disposal and other handling

The diluent and reconstituted vaccine should be inspected visually for any foreign particulate matter and/or variation of physical aspects prior to administration. In the event of either being observed, discard the diluent or reconstituted vaccine.

The vaccine must be reconstituted by adding **the entire contents** of the supplied container of diluent to the vial containing the pellet. After the addition of the diluent to the pellet, the mixture should be well shaken until the pellet is completely dissolved in the diluent.

Due to minor variation of its pH, the reconstituted vaccine may vary in colour from clear peach to fuschia pink without deterioration of the vaccine's potency.

Inject the **entire contents** of the vial.

It is normal practice to administer the vaccine immediately after reconstitution with the diluent provided. However, the vaccine may still be used up to 3 hours after reconstitution or to the end of the vaccination session whichever is sooner.

7. MARKETING AUTHORISATION HOLDER

SmithKline Beecham plc

Great West Road, Brentford, Middlesex TW8 9GS

Trading as

GlaxoSmithKline UK

Stockley Park West

Uxbridge

Middlesex

UB11 1BT

8. MARKETING AUTHORISATION NUMBER(S)

PL 10592/0110

9. DATE OF FIRST AUTHORISATION/RENEWAL OF THE AUTHORISATION

4 December 1997 / 3 December 2002

10. DATE OF REVISION OF THE TEXT

4 December 2008

Privigen 100mg/ml solution for infusion

(CSL Behring UK Limited)

1. NAME OF THE MEDICINAL PRODUCT

Privigen®▼ 100 mg/ml solution for infusion

2. QUALITATIVE AND QUANTITATIVE COMPOSITION

Human normal immunoglobulin (IVIg).

One ml contains:

human plasma protein..100 mg

(purity of at least 98% IgG)

One vial of 25 ml contains: 2.5 g

One vial of 50 ml contains: 5 g

One vial of 100 ml contains: 10 g

One vial of 200 ml contains: 20 g

Distribution of the IgG subclasses (average values):

IgG_1	67.8%
IgG_2	28.7%
IgG_3	2.3%
IgG_4	1.2%

The maximum IgA content is 0.025 mg/ml.

For a full list of excipients, see section 6.1.

3. PHARMACEUTICAL FORM

Solution for infusion.

The solution is clear or slightly opalescent and colourless to pale yellow.

Privigen is isotonic, with an osmolality of 320 mOsmol/kg.

4. CLINICAL PARTICULARS

4.1 Therapeutic indications

Replacement therapy in

- Primary immunodeficiency (PID) syndromes such as:
  - congenital agammaglobulinaemia and hypogammaglobulinaemia
  - common variable immunodeficiency
  - severe combined immunodeficiency
  - Wiskott Aldrich syndrome
- Myeloma or chronic lymphocytic leukaemia with severe secondary hypogammaglobulinaemia and recurrent infections.
- Children with congenital AIDS and recurrent infections.

Immunomodulation

- Immune thrombocytopenic purpura (ITP), in children or adults at high risk of bleeding or prior to surgery to correct the platelet count.
- Guillain-Barré syndrome.
- Kawasaki disease.

Allogeneic bone marrow transplantation

4.2 Posology and method of administration

Posology

The dose and dosage regimen is dependent on the indication.

In replacement therapy the dosage may need to be individualised for each patient depending on the pharmacokinetic and clinical response. The following dosage regimens are given as a guideline.

Replacement therapy in primary immunodeficiency syndromes

The dosage regimen should achieve a trough IgG level (measured before the next infusion) of at least 4 to 6 g/l. Three to six months are required after the initiation of therapy for equilibration to occur.

The recommended starting dose is 0.4 to 0.8 g/kg body weight (bw) followed by at least 0.2 g/kg bw every three weeks.

The dose required to achieve a trough level of 6 g/l is of the order of 0.2 to 0.8 g/kg bw/month. The dosage interval when steady state has been reached varies from two to four weeks.

Trough levels should be measured in order to adjust the dose and dosage interval.

Replacement therapy in myeloma or chronic lymphocytic leukaemia with severe secondary hypogammaglobulinaemia and recurrent infections; replacement therapy in children with AIDS and recurrent infections

The recommended dose is 0.2 to 0.4 g/kg bw every three to four weeks.

Immune thrombocytopenic purpura

For the treatment of an acute episode, 0.8 to 1 g/kg bw on day one, which may be repeated once within three days, or 0.4 g/kg bw daily for two to five days. The treatment can be repeated if relapse occurs.

Guillain-Barré syndrome

0.4 g/kg bw/day for three to seven days.

Experience in children is limited.

Kawasaki disease

1.6 to 2.0 g/kg bw should be administered in divided doses over two to five days or 2.0 g/kg bw as a single dose.

Patients should receive concomitant treatment with acetylsalicylic acid.

Allogeneic bone marrow transplantation:

Human normal immunoglobulin treatment can be used as part of the conditioning regimen and after the transplantation.

For the treatment of infections and prophylaxis of graft versus host disease, dosage is individually tailored. The starting dose is normally 0.5 g/kg bw/week, starting seven days before transplantation and continued for up to three months after the transplantation.

In case of persistent lack of antibody production, a dose of 0.5 g/kg bw/month is recommended until antibody levels return to normal.

The dosage recommendations are summarised in the following table:

(see Table 1 below)

Method of administration

Human normal immunoglobulin should be infused intravenously. The initial infusion rate is 0.3 ml/kg bw/hr. If well tolerated, the rate of administration may gradually be increased to 4.8 ml/kg bw/hr.

In PID patients who have tolerated the infusion rate of 4.8ml/kg bw/hr well, the rate may be further increased gradually to 7.2 ml/kg bw/hr.

4.3 Contraindications

Hypersensitivity to the active substance or to any of the excipients.

Hypersensitivity to homologous immunoglobulins, especially in the very rare cases of IgA deficiency when the patient has antibodies against IgA.

Patients with hyperprolinaemia.

4.4 Special warnings and precautions for use

Certain severe adverse drug reactions may be related to the rate of infusion. The recommended infusion rate given under section 4.2 "Method of administration" must be followed closely. Patients must be closely monitored and carefully observed for any symptoms throughout the infusion period.

Certain adverse reactions may occur more frequently:

– in case of high rate of infusion,

– in patients with hypo- or agammaglobulinaemia with or without IgA deficiency,

– in patients who receive human normal immunoglobulin for the first time or, in rare cases, when the human normal immunoglobulin product is switched or when there has been a long interval since the previous infusion.

True hypersensitivity reactions are rare. They can occur in the very rare cases of IgA deficiency with anti-IgA antibodies.

Rarely, human normal immunoglobulin can induce a fall in blood pressure with anaphylactic reaction, even in patients who had tolerated previous treatment with human normal immunoglobulin.

Potential complications can often be avoided by ensuring that patients:

– are not sensitive to human normal immunoglobulin by initially infusing the product slowly (0.3 ml/kg bw/hr);

– are carefully monitored for any symptoms throughout the infusion period. In particular, patients naive to human normal immunoglobulin, patients switched from an alternative IVIg product or when there has been a long interval since the previous infusion should be monitored during the first infusion and for one hour after, in order to detect potential adverse signs. All other patients should be observed for at least twenty minutes after administration.

There is clinical evidence of an association between IVIg administration and thromboembolic events such as myocardial infarction, stroke, pulmonary embolism and deep vein thromboses which is assumed to be related to a relative increase in blood viscosity through the high influx

Table 1

Indication	Dose	Frequency of injections
Replacement therapy		
– in primary immunodeficiency	starting dose: 0.4–0.8 g/kg bw thereafter: 0.2–0.8 g/kg bw	every two to four weeks to obtain IgG trough levels of at least 4–6 g/l
– in secondary immunodeficiency	0.2–0.4 g/kg bw	every three to four weeks to obtain IgG trough levels of at least 4–6 g/l
– Children with AIDS	0.2–0.4 g/kg bw	every three to four weeks
Immunomodulation		
Immune thrombocytopenic purpura	0.8–1 g/kg bw or 0.4 g/kg bw/d	on day one, possibly repeated once within three days for two to five days
– Guillain-Barré syndrome	0.4 g/kg bw/d	for three to seven days
– Kawasaki disease	1.6–2 g/kg bw or 2 g/kg bw	in divided doses over two to five days in association with acetylsalicylic acid in one dose in association with acetylsalicylic acid
Allogeneic bone marrow transplantation		
– treatment of infections and prophylaxis of graft versus host disease	0.5 g/kg bw	every week from seven days before up to three months after transplantation
– persistent lack of antibody production	0.5 g/kg bw	every month until antibody levels return to normal

of immunoglobulin in at-risk patients. Caution should be exercised in prescribing and infusing IVIg in obese patients and in patients with pre-existing risk factors for thrombotic events (such as advanced age, hypertension, diabetes mellitus and a history of vascular disease or thrombotic episodes, patients with acquired or inherited thrombophilic disorders, patients with prolonged periods of immobilisation, severely hypovolaemic patients and patients with diseases which increase blood viscosity).

Cases of acute renal failure have been reported in patients receiving IVIg therapy. In most cases, risk factors have been identified, such as pre-existing renal insufficiency, diabetes mellitus, hypovolaemia, being overweight, concomitant nephrotoxic medicinal products or age over 65.

In case of renal impairment, IVIg discontinuation should be considered.

While these reports of renal dysfunction and acute renal failure have been associated with the use of many of the licensed IVIg products, those containing sucrose as a stabiliser accounted for a disproportionate share of the total number. In patients at risk, the use of IVIg products that do not contain sucrose may be considered. Privigen does not contain sucrose or other sugars.

In patients at risk of acute renal failure or thromboembolic adverse reactions, IVIg products should be administered at the minimum rate of infusion and dose practicable.

In all patients, IVIg administration requires:

– adequate hydration prior to the initiation of the infusion of IVIg

– monitoring of urine output

– monitoring of serum creatinine levels

– avoidance of concomitant use of loop diuretics.

In case of adverse reaction, either the rate of administration must be reduced or the infusion stopped. The treatment required depends on the nature and severity of the side effect.

In case of shock, standard medical treatment for shock should be implemented.

Information on safety with respect to transmissible agents

Standard measures to prevent infections resulting from the use of medicinal products prepared from human blood or plasma include selection of donors, screening of individual donations and plasma pools for specific markers of infection and the inclusion of effective manufacturing steps for the inactivation/removal of viruses. Despite this, when medicinal products prepared from human blood or plasma are administered, the possibility of transmitting infective agents cannot be totally excluded. This also applies to unknown or emerging viruses and other pathogens.

The measures taken are considered effective for enveloped viruses such as HIV, HBV, and HCV, and for the non-enveloped viruses HAV and B19V.

There is reassuring clinical experience regarding the lack of hepatitis A or B19V transmission with immunoglobulins and it is also assumed that the antibody content makes an important contribution to the viral safety.

It is strongly recommended that every time Privigen is administered to a patient, the name and batch number of the product are recorded in order to maintain a link between the patient and the batch of the product.

4.5 Interaction with other medicinal products and other forms of interaction

Live attenuated virus vaccines

Immunoglobulin administration may impair the efficacy of live attenuated virus vaccines such as measles, mumps, rubella and varicella for a period of at least six weeks and up to three months. After administration of this product, an interval of three months should elapse before vaccination with live attenuated virus vaccines. In the case of measles, this impairment may persist for up to one year. Therefore patients receiving measles vaccine should have their antibody status checked.

Interference with serological testing

After injection of immunoglobulin the transitory rise of the various passively transferred antibodies in the patient's blood may result in misleading positive results in serological testing.

Passive transmission of antibodies to erythrocyte antigens, e.g. A, B, D, may interfere with some serological tests for red cell allo-antibodies (e.g. Coombs test).

4.6 Pregnancy and lactation

The safety of this medicinal product for use in human pregnancy has not been established in controlled clinical trials and therefore should only be given with caution to pregnant women and breast-feeding mothers. Clinical experience with immunoglobulins suggests that no harmful effects on the course of pregnancy, or on the foetus and the neonate are to be expected.

Immunoglobulins are excreted into the milk and may contribute to the transfer of protective antibodies to the neonate.

4.7 Effects on ability to drive and use machines

No effects on ability to drive and use machines have been observed.

4.8 Undesirable effects

With human normal immunoglobulin for intravenous administration, adverse reactions such as chills, headache, fever, vomiting, allergic reactions, nausea, arthralgia, low blood pressure and moderate low back pain may occur occasionally.

Table 2 Frequency of Adverse Drug Reactions (ADRs) in clinical studies with Privigen

MedDRA System Organ Class	MedDRA preferred term	ADR frequency category
Investigations	Bilirubin conjugated increased, blood bilirubin unconjugated increased, Coombs direct test positive, Coombs test positive, blood lactate dehydrogenase increased, haematocrit decreased, alanine aminotransferase increased, aspartate aminotransferase increased, blood creatinine increased, blood pressure decreased, blood pressure increased, body temperature increased, haemoglobin decreased	Uncommon
Cardiac disorders	Palpitations	Uncommon
Blood and lymphatic system disorders	Anaemia, anisocytosis	Uncommon
Nervous system disorders	Headache	Very common
	Dizziness, head discomfort, somnolence, tremor, sinus headache	Uncommon
Respiratory, thoracic and mediastinal disorders	Dyspnoea, oropharyngeal blistering, painful respiration, throat tightness	Uncommon
Gastrointestinal disorders	Vomiting, nausea	Common
	Diarrhoea, abdominal pain upper	Uncommon
Renal and urinary disorders	Proteinuria	Uncommon
Skin and subcutaneous tissue disorders	Pruritus, skin disorder, night sweats, urticaria	Uncommon
Musculoskeletal and connective tissue disorders	Back pain	Common
	Neck pain, pain in extremity, musculoskeletal stiffness, muscle spasms, musculoskeletal pain, myalgia	Uncommon
Vascular disorders	Flushing, hypertension, hypotension	Uncommon
General disorders and administration site conditions	Chills, fatigue, pyrexia	Common
	Chest pain, general symptom, asthenia, influenza like illness, hyperthermia, pain, injection site pain	Uncommon
Hepatobiliary disorders	Hyperbilirubinaemia	Uncommon

Rarely human normal immunoglobulins may cause a sudden fall in blood pressure and, in isolated cases, anaphylactic shock, even when the patient has shown no hypersensitivity to previous administration.

Cases of reversible aseptic meningitis, isolated cases of reversible haemolytic anaemia/haemolysis and rare cases of transient cutaneous reactions, have been observed with human normal immunoglobulin.

Increase in serum creatinine level and/or acute renal failure have been observed.

Very rarely: Thromboembolic reactions such as myocardial infarction, stroke, pulmonary embolism and deep vein thromboses.

Three clinical studies with Privigen were performed, two in patients with primary immunodeficiency (PID) and one in patients with immune thrombocytopenic purpura (ITP). In the pivotal PID study 80 subjects were enrolled and treated with Privigen. Of these, 72 completed the twelve months of treatment. In the PID extension study 55 subjects were enrolled and treated with Privigen. The ITP study was performed in 57 patients.

Most adverse drug reactions (ADRs) observed in the three clinical studies were mild to moderate in nature.

The ADRs reported in the three studies are summarised and categorised according to the MedDRA System organ class and frequency below. Frequency per infusion has been evaluated using the following criteria: very common ($\geqslant$1/10), common ($\geqslant$1/100 to $<$1/10), uncommon ($\geqslant$1/1 000 to $<$1/100).

Within each frequency grouping, undesirable effects are presented in order of decreasing severity.

Frequency of Adverse Drug Reactions (ADRs) in clinical studies with Privigen

(see Table 2 below)

For safety with respect to transmissible agents, see section 4.4.

4.9 Overdose

Overdose may lead to fluid overload and hyperviscosity, particularly in patients at risk, including elderly patients or patients with renal impairment.

5. PHARMACOLOGICAL PROPERTIES

5.1 Pharmacodynamic properties

Pharmacotherapeutic group: immune sera and immunoglobulins: immunoglobulins, normal human, for intravascular administration, ATC code: J06BA02.

Human normal immunoglobulin contains mainly immunoglobulin G (IgG) with a broad spectrum of antibodies against infectious agents.

Human normal immunoglobulin contains the IgG antibodies present in the normal population. It is usually prepared from pooled plasma from not fewer than 1,000 donors. It has a distribution of immunoglobulin G subclasses closely proportional to that in native human plasma. Adequate doses of this medicinal product may restore abnormally low immunoglobulin G levels to the normal range.

The mechanism of action in indications other than replacement therapy is not fully elucidated, but includes immunomodulatory effects.

The safety and efficacy of Privigen was evaluated in two prospective, open-label, single-arm, multicenter studies performed in Europe (ITP study) and Europe and USA (PID study).

5.2 Pharmacokinetic properties

Human normal immunoglobulin is immediately and completely bioavailable in the recipient's circulation after intravenous administration. It is distributed relatively rapidly between plasma and extravascular fluid, equilibrium between the intra- and extravascular compartments is reached after approximately three to five days.

The pharmacokinetic parameters for Privigen were determined in a clinical study in PID patients (see section 5.1). Twenty-five patients (aged 13 to 69 years) participated in the pharmacokinetic assessment (see table below). The median half-life of Privigen in primary immunodeficiency patients was 36.6 days. This half-life may vary from patient to patient, particularly in primary immunodeficiency.

Pharmacokinetic parameters of Privigen in 25 PID patients

Parameter	Pivotal Study (N=25) ZLB03_002CR Median (Range)	Extension study (N=13) ZLB05_006CR Median (Range)
C_{max} (peak, g/l)	23.4 (10.4-34.6)	26.3 (20.9-32.9)
C_{min} (trough, g/l)	10.2 (5.8-14.7)	12.3 (10.4-18.8) (3-week schedule) 9.4 (7.3-13.2) (4-week schedule)
$t_{½}$ (days)	36.6 (20.6-96.6)	31.1 (14.6-43.6)

C_{max}, maximum serum concentration; C_{min}, trough (minimum level) serum concentration; $t_{½}$, elimination half-life

IgG and IgG-complexes are broken down in cells of the reticuloendothelial system.

5.3 Preclinical safety data

Immunoglobulins are a normal constituent of the human body. L-proline is a physiological, non-essential amino acid.

The safety of Privigen has been assessed in several preclinical studies, with particular reference to the excipient L-proline. Some published studies pertaining to hyperprolinaemia have shown that long-term, high doses of L-proline have effects on brain development in very young rats. However, in studies where the dosing was designed to reflect the clinical indications for Privigen, no effects on brain development were observed. Non-clinical data reveal no special risk for humans based on safety pharmacology and toxicity studies.

6. PHARMACEUTICAL PARTICULARS

6.1 List of excipients

L-proline

Water for injections

6.2 Incompatibilities

This medicinal product must not be mixed with other medicinal products except those mentioned in section 6.6.

6.3 Shelf life

2 years

6.4 Special precautions for storage

Do not store above 25 °C.

Do not freeze.

Keep the vial in the outer carton in order to protect from light.

6.5 Nature and contents of container

25 ml of solution in a single vial (type I glass), with a stopper (elastomeric), a cap (aluminium crimp), a flip off disc (plastic), label with integrated hanger.

50 or 100 ml of solution in a single vial (type I or II glass), with a stopper (elastomeric), a cap (aluminium crimp), a flip off disc (plastic), label with integrated hanger.

200 ml of solution in a single vial (type II glass), with a stopper (elastomeric), a cap (aluminium crimp), a flip off disc (plastic), label with integrated hanger.

Pack sizes:

1 vial (2.5 g/25 ml, 5 g/50 ml, 10 g/100 ml, 20 g/200 ml),

3 vials (10 g/100 ml, 20 g/200 ml).

Not all pack sizes may be marketed.

6.6 Special precautions for disposal and other handling

Privigen comes as a ready-for-use solution in single-use vials. The product should be at room or body temperature before use. A vented infusion line should be used for the administration of Privigen. Always pierce the stopper at its centre, within the marked area.

The solution should be clear or slightly opalescent. Do not use solutions that are cloudy or have particulate matter.

Once the vial has been entered under aseptic conditions, its contents should be used promptly. Because the solution contains no preservative, Privigen should be infused as soon as possible.

Any unused product or waste material should be disposed of in accordance with local requirements.

7. MARKETING AUTHORISATION HOLDER

CSL Behring GmbH

Emil-von-Behring-Strasse 76

D-35041 Marburg

Germany

8. MARKETING AUTHORISATION NUMBER(S)

2.5 g: EU/1/08/446/004

5 g: EU/1/08/446/001

10 g: EU/1/08/446/002

20 g: EU/1/08/446/003

10g x3: EU/1/08/446/005

20g x3: EU/1/08/446/006

9. DATE OF FIRST AUTHORISATION/RENEWAL OF THE AUTHORISATION

001-003: 25 April 2008

004: 07 May 2009

005-006: 30 June 2009

10. DATE OF REVISION OF THE TEXT

21 August 2009

Detailed information on this product is available on the website of the European Medicines Agency (EMEA): http://www.emea.europa.eu/

Procarbazine Capsules 50mg (Cambridge Laboratories)

(Cambridge Laboratories)

1. NAME OF THE MEDICINAL PRODUCT

Procarbazine Capsules 50mg

2. QUALITATIVE AND QUANTITATIVE COMPOSITION

Each capsule contains 58.3mg Procarbazine hydrochloride (equivalent to 50mg of Procarbazine).

3. PHARMACEUTICAL FORM

Capsules with white opaque cap and body. Marked 'CL 50' on cap.

4. CLINICAL PARTICULARS

4.1 Therapeutic indications

The main indication is Hodgkin's disease (lymphadenoma).

Procarbazine may also be useful in other advanced lymphomata and a variety of solid tumours which have proved resistant to other forms of therapy.

4.2 Posology and method of administration

In combination chemotherapeutic regimens:

Procarbazine is usually administered concomitantly with other appropriate cytostatic drugs in repeated four- to six-weekly cycles. In most such combination chemotherapy regimens currently in use (eg. the so-called MOPP schedule with mustine, Vincristine and Prednisone) Procarbazine is given daily on the first 10 - 14 days of each cycle in a dosage of 100mg per sq. metre of body surface (to nearest 50mg).

As sole therapeutic agent: Adults:

Treatment should begin with small doses which are increased gradually up to a maximum daily dose of 250 or 300mg divided as evenly as possible throughout the day.

Initial dosage scheme

1st day:	50mg	4th day:	200mg
2nd day:	100mg	5th day:	250mg
3rd day:	150mg	6th day et seq:	250-300mg

Further procedure:

Treatment should be continued with 250 or 300mg daily until the greatest possible remission has been obtained, after which a maintenance dose is given.

Maintenance dose:

50 - 150mg daily. Treatment should be continued until a total dose of at least 6g has been given. Otherwise, a negative result is not significant.

Elderly:

Procarbazine should be used with caution in the elderly. Patients in this group should be observed very closely for signs of early failure or intolerance of treatment.

Children:

If, on the recommendation of a physician, a children's dosage is required, 50mg daily should be given for the first week. Daily dosage should then be maintained at 100mg per sq. metre of body surface (to nearest 50mg) until leucopenia or thrombocytopenia occurs or maximum response is obtained.

Procarbazine capsules are for oral administration.

4.3 Contraindications

Pre-existing severe leucopenia or thrombocytopenia from any cause; severe hepatic or renal damage.

Procarbazine should not be used in the management of non-malignant disease.

4.4 Special warnings and precautions for use

Procarbazine should be given only under the supervision of a physician who is experienced in cancer chemotherapy and having facilities for regular monitoring of clinical and haematological effects during and after administration.

Introduction of therapy should only be effected under hospital conditions.

Caution is advisable in patients with hepatic or renal dysfunction, cardiovascular or cerebrovascular disease, phaeochromocytoma, or epilepsy.

Regular blood counts are of great importance. If during the initial treatment the total white cell count falls to 3,000 per mm^3 or the platelet count to 80,000 per mm^3, treatment should be suspended temporarily until the leucocyte and/or platelet levels recover, when therapy with the maintenance dose may be resumed.

Treatment should be interrupted on the appearance of allergic skin reactions.

Procarbazine has been shown to be carcinogenic in animals. The increased risk of carcinogenicity in man should be borne in mind when long-term management of patients is proposed.

4.5 Interaction with other medicinal products and other forms of interaction

Procarbazine is a weak MAO inhibitor and therefore interactions with certain foodstuffs and drugs, although very rare, must be borne in mind. Thus, owing to possible potentiation of the effect of barbiturates, narcotic analgesics (especially Pethidine), drugs with anticholinergic effects (including phenothiazine derivatives and tricyclic antidepressants), other central nervous system depressants (including anaesthetic agents) and anti-hypertensive agents, these drugs should be given concurrently with caution and in low doses. Intolerance to alcohol (Disulfiram-like reaction) may occur.

4.6 Pregnancy and lactation

Procarbazine is teratogenic in animals. Isolated human foetal malformations have been reported following MOPP combination therapy. Therefore Procarbazine should not be administered to patients who are pregnant unless considered absolutely essential by the physician. Procarbazine should not be given to breast feeding mothers.

4.7 Effects on ability to drive and use machines

None known.

4.8 Undesirable effects

Loss of appetite and nausea occur in most cases, sometimes with vomiting. These symptoms are usually confined to the first few days of treatment and then tend to disappear.

Procarbazine causes leucopenia and thrombocytopenia. These haematological changes are almost always reversible and seldom require complete cessation of therapy.

4.9 Overdose

Signs of overdosage include severe nausea and vomiting, dizziness, hallucinations, depression and convulsions; hypotension or tachycardia may occur.

Gastric lavage and general supportive treatment should be performed, with prophylactic treatment against possible infection, and frequent blood counts.

5. PHARMACOLOGICAL PROPERTIES

5.1 Pharmacodynamic properties

Procarbazine, a methylhydrazine derivative, is a cytostatic agent with weak MAO inhibitor properties. Its exact mode of action on tumour cells is unknown. It may be effective in patients who have become resistant to radiation therapy and other cytostatic agents.

5.2 Pharmacokinetic properties

Procarbazine is readily absorbed from the gastrointestinal tract. It is rapidly metabolised, the primary circulating metabolite is the azo derivative while the major urinary metabolite has been shown to be N-isopropyl-terephthalamic acid.

5.3 Preclinical safety data

There are no pre-clinical data of relevance to the prescriber which are additional to that already included in other sections of the SPC.

6. PHARMACEUTICAL PARTICULARS

6.1 List of excipients

Mannitol

Maize starch

Talc

Magnesium stearate

Capsule shell components:

Gelatin

Titanium dioxide E171

Ink components:

Shellac

Soya lethicin

n-Butyl alcohol

Antifoam DC 1510

Black iron oxide E172

6.2 Incompatibilities

None known.

6.3 Shelf life

Three years.

6.4 Special precautions for storage

Store in a dry place. Do not store above 25°C.

6.5 Nature and contents of container

Blister packs of 50 capsules.

6.6 Special precautions for disposal and other handling

Handling guidelines:

Undamaged capsules present minimal risk of contamination, but in accordance with good hygiene requirements, direct handling should be avoided. As with all cytotoxics, precautions should be taken to avoid exposing staff during pregnancy.

Waste material may be disposed of by incineration.

Administrative Data

7. MARKETING AUTHORISATION HOLDER

Cambridge Laboratories Limited

Deltic House

Kingfisher Way

Silverlink Business Park

Wallsend

Tyne & Wear

NE28 9NX

8. MARKETING AUTHORISATION NUMBER(S)

PL 12070/0004

9. DATE OF FIRST AUTHORISATION/RENEWAL OF THE AUTHORISATION

30/08/2006

10. DATE OF REVISION OF THE TEXT

30/08/2006

Procoralan

(Servier Laboratories Limited)

1. NAME OF THE MEDICINAL PRODUCT

▼ Procoralan 5 mg film-coated tablets

▼ Procoralan 7.5 mg film coated tablets

2. QUALITATIVE AND QUANTITATIVE COMPOSITION

Procoralan 5 mg

One film-coated tablet contains 5 mg ivabradine (equivalent to 5.390 mg ivabradine as hydrochloride).

Excipient: 63.91 mg lactose monohydrate

Procoralan 7.5 mg

One film-coated tablet contains 7.5 mg ivabradine (equivalent to 8.085 mg ivabradine as hydrochloride).

Excipient: 61.215 mg lactose monohydrate

For a full list of excipients, see section 6.1.

3. PHARMACEUTICAL FORM

Film-coated tablet.

Procoralan 5 mg: salmon-coloured, oblong, film-coated tablet scored on both sides, engraved with "5" on one face and on the other face.

The tablet can be divided into equal halves.

Procoralan 7.5 mg: salmon-coloured, triangular, film-coated tablet engraved with "7.5" on one face and on the other face.

4. CLINICAL PARTICULARS

4.1 Therapeutic indications

Symptomatic treatment of chronic stable angina pectoris in patients with normal sinus rhythm, who have a contra-indication or intolerance for beta-blockers.

4.2 Posology and method of administration

For the different doses film-coated tablets containing 5 mg and 7.5 mg ivabradine are available.

The usual recommended starting dose of ivabradine is 5 mg twice daily. After three to four weeks of treatment, the dose may be increased to 7.5 mg twice daily depending on the therapeutic response. If, during treatment, heart rate decreases persistently below 50 beats per minute (bpm) at rest or the patient experiences symptoms related to bradycardia such as dizziness, fatigue or hypotension, the dose must be titrated downward including the possible dose of 2.5 mg twice daily (one half 5 mg tablet twice daily). Treatment must be discontinued if heart rate below 50 bpm or symptoms of bradycardia persist (see section 4.4).

Tablets must be taken orally twice daily, i.e. once in the morning and once in the evening during meals (see section 5.2).

Elderly

Since ivabradine has been studied in a limited number of patients aged 75 years or more, a lower starting dose should be considered for these patients (2.5 mg twice daily i.e. one half 5 mg tablet twice daily) before up-titration if necessary.

Renal insufficiency

No dose adjustment is required in patients with renal insufficiency and creatinine clearance above 15 ml/min (see section 5.2).

No data are available in patients with creatinine clearance below 15 ml/min. Ivabradine should therefore be used with precaution in this population.

Hepatic impairment

No dose adjustment is required in patients with mild hepatic impairment. Caution should be exercised when using ivabradine in patients with moderate hepatic impairment. Ivabradine is contra-indicated for use in patients with severe hepatic insufficiency, since it has not been studied in this population and a large increase in systemic exposure is anticipated (see sections 4.3 and 5.2).

Children and adolescents

Procoralan is not recommended for use in children and adolescents due to a lack of data on safety and efficacy.

4.3 Contraindications

- Hypersensitivity to the active substance or to any of the excipients (see section 6.1)
- Resting heart rate below 60 beats per minute prior to treatment
- Cardiogenic shock
- Acute myocardial infarction
- Severe hypotension (< 90/50 mmHg)
- Severe hepatic insufficiency
- Sick sinus syndrome
- Sino-atrial block
- Heart failure patients with NYHA functional classification III-IV due to a lack of data
- Pacemaker dependent
- Unstable angina
- AV-block of 3rd degree
- Combination with strong cytochrome P450 3A4 inhibitors such as azole antifungals (ketoconazole, itraconazole), macrolide antibiotics (clarithromycin, erythromycin *per os*, josamycin, telithromycin), HIV protease inhibitors (nelfinavir, ritonavir) and nefazodone (see sections 4.5 and 5.2)
- Pregnancy, lactation (see section 4.6)

4.4 Special warnings and precautions for use

Special warnings

Cardiac arrhythmias

Ivabradine is not effective in the treatment or prevention of cardiac arrhythmias and likely loses its efficacy when a tachyarrhythmia occurs (eg. ventricular or supraventricular tachycardia). Ivabradine is therefore not recommended in patients with atrial fibrillation or other cardiac arrhythmias that interfere with sinus node function.

It is recommended to regularly clinically monitor ivabradine treated patients for the occurrence of atrial fibrillation (sustained or paroxysmal), which should also include ECG monitoring if clinically indicated (e.g. in case of exacerbated angina, palpitations, irregular pulse).

Use in patients with AV-block of 2nd degree

Ivabradine is not recommended in patients with AV-block of 2nd degree.

Use in patients with a low heart rate

Ivabradine must not be initiated in patients with a pre-treatment resting heart rate below 60 beats per minute (see section 4.3).

If, during treatment, resting heart rate decreases persistently below 50 bpm or the patient experiences symptoms related to bradycardia such as dizziness, fatigue or hypotension, the dose must be titrated downward or treatment discontinued if heart rate below 50 bpm or symptoms of bradycardia persist (see section 4.2).

Combination with other antianginal therapies

Concomitant use of ivabradine with heart rate reducing calcium channel blockers such as verapamil or diltiazem is not recommended (see section 4.5). No safety issue has been raised on the combination of ivabradine with nitrates and dihydropyridine calcium channel blockers such as amlodipine. Additional efficacy of ivabradine in combination with dihydropyridine calcium channel blockers has not been established (see section 5.1).

Chronic heart failure

Heart failure must be appropriately controlled before considering ivabradine treatment. The use of ivabradine is contra-indicated in heart failure patients with NYHA functional classification III-IV, due to a lack of data on clinical efficacy and safety (see section 4.3). Caution is needed in patients with asymptomatic left ventricular dysfunction, as well as in heart failure patients with NYHA functional classification II due to a limited number of patients studied.

Stroke

The use of ivabradine is not recommended immediately after a stroke since no data is available in these situations.

Visual function

Ivabradine influences on retinal function (see section 5.1). To date, there is no evidence of a toxic effect of ivabradine on the retina, but the effects of long-term ivabradine treatment beyond one year on retinal function are currently not known. Cessation of treatment should be considered if any unexpected deterioration in visual function occurs. Caution should be exercised in patients with retinitis pigmentosa.

Precautions for use

Patients with hypotension

Limited data are available in patients with mild to moderate hypotension, and ivabradine should therefore be used with caution in these patients. Ivabradine is contra-indicated in patients with severe hypotension (blood pressure < 90/50 mmHg) (see section 4.3).

Atrial fibrillation - Cardiac arrhythmias

There is no evidence of risk of (excessive) bradycardia on return to sinus rhythm when pharmacological cardioversion is initiated in patients treated with ivabradine. However, in the absence of extensive data, non urgent DC-cardioversion should be considered 24 hours after the last dose of ivabradine.

Use in patients with congenital QT syndrome or treated with QT prolonging medicinal products

The use of ivabradine in patients with congenital QT syndrome or treated with QT prolonging medicinal products should be avoided (see section 4.5). If the combination appears necessary, close cardiac monitoring is needed.

Use in patients with moderate hepatic insufficiency

Caution should be exercised when using ivabradine in patients with moderate hepatic insufficiency (see section 4.2).

Use in patients with severe renal insufficiency

Caution should be exercised when using ivabradine in patients with severe renal insufficiency (creatinine clearance < 15 ml/min) (see section 4.2).

Excipients

Since tablets contain lactose, patients with rare hereditary problems of galactose intolerance, the Lapp lactase deficiency or glucose-galactose malabsorption should not take this medicinal product.

4.5 Interaction with other medicinal products and other forms of interaction

Pharmacodynamic interactions

Concomitant use not recommended

QT prolonging medicinal products

- Cardiovascular QT prolonging medicinal products (e.g. quinidine, disopyramide, bepridil, sotalol, ibutilide, amiodarone).
- Non cardiovascular QT prolonging medicinal products (e.g. pimozide, ziprasidone, sertindole, mefloquine, halofantrine, pentamidine, cisapride, erythromycin IV).

The concomitant use of cardiovascular and non cardiovascular QT prolonging medicinal products with ivabradine should be avoided since QT prolongation may be exacerbated by heart rate reduction. If the combination appears necessary, close cardiac monitoring is needed (see section 4.4).

Pharmacokinetic interactions

Cytochrome P450 3A4 (CYP3A4)

Ivabradine is metabolised by CYP3A4 only and it is a very weak inhibitor of this cytochrome. Ivabradine was shown not to influence the metabolism and plasma concentrations of other CYP3A4 substrates (mild, moderate and strong inhibitors). CYP3A4 inhibitors and inducers are liable to interact with ivabradine and influence its metabolism and pharmacokinetics to a clinically significant extent. Drug-drug interaction studies have established that CYP3A4 inhibitors increase ivabradine plasma concentrations, while inducers decrease them. Increased plasma concentrations of ivabradine may be associated with the risk of excessive bradycardia (see section 4.4).

Contra-indication of concomitant use

The concomitant use of potent CYP3A4 inhibitors such as azole antifungals (ketoconazole, itraconazole), macrolide antibiotics (clarithromycin, erythromycin *per os*, josamycin, telithromycin), HIV protease inhibitors (nelfinavir, ritonavir) and nefazodone is contra-indicated (see section 4.3). The potent CYP3A4 inhibitors ketoconazole (200 mg once daily) and josamycin (1 g twice daily) increased ivabradine mean plasma exposure by 7 to 8 fold.

Concomitant use not recommended

Moderate CYP3A4 inhibitors: specific interaction studies in healthy volunteers and patients have shown that the combination of ivabradine with the heart rate reducing agents diltiazem or verapamil resulted in an increase in ivabradine exposure (2 to 3 fold increase in AUC) and an additional heart rate reduction of 5 bpm. The concomitant use of ivabradine with these medicinal products is not recommended (see section 4.4).

Concomitant use with precautions

- Moderate CYP3A4 inhibitors: the concomitant use of ivabradine with other moderate CYP3A4 inhibitors (e.g. fluconazole) may be considered at the starting dose of 2.5 mg twice daily and if resting heart rate is above 60 bpm, with monitoring of heart rate.
- Grapefruit juice: ivabradine exposure was increased by 2-fold following the co-administration with grapefruit juice. Therefore the intake of grapefruit juice should be restricted during the treatment with ivabradine.
- CYP3A4 inducers: CYP3A4 inducers (e.g. rifampicin, barbiturates, phenytoin, *Hypericum perforatum* [St John's Wort]) may decrease ivabradine exposure and activity. The concomitant use of CYP3A4 inducing medicinal products may require an adjustment of the dose of ivabradine. The combination of ivabradine 10 mg twice daily with St John's Wort was shown to reduce ivabradine AUC by half. The intake of St John's Wort should be restricted during the treatment with ivabradine.

Other concomitant use

Specific drug-drug interaction studies have shown no clinically significant effect of the following medicinal products on pharmacokinetics and pharmacodynamics of ivabradine: proton pump inhibitors (omeprazole, lansoprazole), sildenafil, HMG CoA reductase inhibitors (simvastatin), dihydropyridine calcium channel blockers (amlodipine, lacidipine), digoxin and warfarin. In addition there was no clinically significant effect of ivabradine on the pharmacokinetics of simvastatin, amlodipine, lacidipine, on the pharmacokinetics and pharmacodynamics of digoxin, warfarin and on the pharmacodynamics of aspirin.

In pivotal phase III clinical trials the following medicinal products were not restricted and therefore were routinely combined with ivabradine with no evidence of safety concerns: angiotensin converting enzyme inhibitors, angiotensin II antagonists, diuretics, short and long acting nitrates, HMG CoA reductase inhibitors, fibrates, proton pump inhibitors, oral antidiabetics, aspirin and other anti-platelet agents.

4.6 Pregnancy and lactation

There are no adequate data concerning the use of ivabradine in pregnant women. Animal reproduction studies have shown embryotoxic and teratogenic effects (see section 5.3). The potential risk for humans is unknown. Therefore, ivabradine is contra-indicated during pregnancy.

Animal studies indicate that ivabradine is excreted in milk. Therefore, ivabradine is contra-indicated in breast-feeding women.

4.7 Effects on ability to drive and use machines

A specific study to assess the possible influence of ivabradine on driving performance has been performed in healthy volunteers where no alteration of the driving performance was evidenced. Ivabradine has no influence on the ability to drive and use machines. However, ivabradine may cause transient luminous phenomena consisting mainly of phosphenes (see section 4.8). The possible occurrence of such luminous phenomena should be taken into account when driving or using machines in situations where sudden variations in light intensity may occur, especially when driving at night.

4.8 Undesirable effects

Procoralan has been studied in clinical trials involving nearly 5,000 participants. Approximately 2,900 patients have been treated with ivabradine in phase II-III studies.

The most common undesirable effects with ivabradine are dose dependent and related to the pharmacological effect of the medicinal product.

The following adverse effects or events have been reported during clinical trials and are ranked using the following frequency: very common (>1/10); common (>1/100, <1/10); uncommon (>1/1000, <1/100); rare (>1/10000, <1/1000); very rare (<1/10000); not known (cannot be estimated from the available data).

Investigations:

Uncommon:

- Hyperuricaemia
- Eosinophilia
- Elevated creatinine in blood

Cardiac disorders:

Common:

- Bradycardia: 3.3% of patients particularly within the first 2 to 3 months of treatment initiation. 0.5% of patients experienced a severe bradycardia below or equal to 40 bpm.
- AV 1st degree block (ECG prolonged PQ interval)
- Ventricular extrasystoles

Uncommon:

- Palpitations, supraventricular extrasystoles

The following events reported during clinical trials were of similar incidence than comparators and/or possibly related to the underlying disease: sinus arrhythmia, unstable angina, angina pectoris aggravated, atrial fibrillation, myocardial ischaemia, myocardial infarction and ventricular tachycardia.

Eye disorders:

Very common:

- Luminous phenomena (phosphenes): reported by 14.5% of patients, described as a transient enhanced brightness in a limited area of the visual field. They are usually triggered by sudden variations in light intensity. The onset of phosphenes is generally within the first two months of treatment after which they may occur repeatedly. Phosphenes were generally reported to be of mild to moderate intensity. All phosphenes resolved during or after treatment, of which a majority (77.5%) resolved during treatment. Fewer than 1% of patients changed their daily routine or discontinued the treatment in relation with phosphenes.

Common:

- Blurred vision

Gastrointestinal disorders:

Uncommon:

- Nausea
- Constipation
- Diarrhoea

General disorders and administration site conditions:

Common:

- Headache, generally during the first month of treatment.
- Dizziness, possibly related to bradycardia.

Uncommon:

- Vertigo
- Dyspnoea
- Muscle cramps

4.9 Overdose

Overdose may lead to severe and prolonged bradycardia (see section 4.8).

Severe bradycardia should be treated symptomatically in a specialised environment. In the event of bradycardia with poor haemodynamic tolerance, symptomatic treatment including intravenous beta-stimulating agents such as isoprenaline may be considered. Temporary cardiac electrical pacing may be instituted if required.

5. PHARMACOLOGICAL PROPERTIES

5.1 Pharmacodynamic properties

Pharmacotherapeutic group: other cardiac preparations, ATC code: C01EB17.

Ivabradine is a pure heart rate lowering agent, acting by selective and specific inhibition of the cardiac pacemaker I_f current that controls the spontaneous diastolic depolarisation in the sinus node and regulates heart rate. The cardiac effects are specific to the sinus node with no effect on intra-atrial, atrioventricular or intraventricular conduction times, nor on myocardial contractility or ventricular repolarisation.

Ivabradine can interact also with the retinal current I_h which closely resembles cardiac I_f. It participates in the temporal resolution of the visual system, by curtailing the retinal response to bright light stimuli. Under triggering circumstances (e.g. rapid changes in luminosity), partial inhibition of I_h by ivabradine underlies the luminous phenomena that may be occasionally experienced by patients. Luminous phenomena (phosphenes) are described as a transient enhanced brightness in a limited area of the visual field (see section 4.8).

The main pharmacodynamic property of ivabradine in humans is a specific dose dependent reduction in heart rate. Analysis of heart rate reduction with doses up to 20 mg twice daily indicates a trend towards a plateau effect which is consistent with a reduced risk of severe bradycardia below 40 bpm (see section 4.8).

At usual recommended doses, heart rate reduction is approximately 10 bpm at rest and during exercise. This leads to a reduction in cardiac workload and myocardial oxygen consumption. Ivabradine does not influence intracardiac conduction, contractility (no negative inotropic effect) or ventricular repolarisation:

- in clinical electrophysiology studies, ivabradine had no effect on atrioventricular or intraventricular conduction times or corrected QT intervals;
- in patients with left ventricular dysfunction (left ventricular ejection fraction (LVEF) between 30 and 45%), ivabradine did not have any deleterious influence on LVEF.

The antianginal and anti-ischaemic efficacy of Procoralan was studied in four double-blind randomised trials (two versus placebo, and one each versus atenolol and amlodipine). These trials included a total of 3,222 patients with chronic stable angina pectoris, of whom 2,168 received ivabradine.

Ivabradine 5 mg twice daily was shown to be effective on exercise test parameters within 3 to 4 weeks of treatment. Efficacy was confirmed with 7.5 mg twice daily. In particular, the additional benefit over 5 mg twice daily was established in a reference-controlled study versus atenolol: total exercise duration at trough was increased by about 1 minute after one month of treatment with 5 mg twice daily and further improved by almost 25 seconds after an additional 3-month period with forced titration to 7.5 mg twice daily. In this study, the antianginal and anti-ischaemic benefits of ivabradine were confirmed in patients aged 65 years or more. The efficacy of 5 and 7.5 mg twice daily was consistent across studies on exercise test parameters (total exercise duration, time to limiting angina, time to angina onset and time to 1mm ST segment depression) and was associated with a decrease of about 70% in the rate of angina attacks. The twice-daily dosing regimen of ivabradine gave uniform efficacy over 24 hours.

In a 725-patients randomised placebo-controlled study, ivabradine did not show additional efficacy on top of amlodipine at the trough of drug activity (12 hours after oral intake) while an additional efficacy was shown at peak (3-4 hours after oral intake).

Ivabradine efficacy was fully maintained throughout the 3- or 4-month treatment periods in the efficacy trials. There was no evidence of pharmacological tolerance (loss of efficacy) developing during treatment nor of rebound phenomena after abrupt treatment discontinuation. The antianginal and anti-ischaemic effects of ivabradine were associated with dose-dependent reductions in heart rate and with a significant decrease in rate pressure product (heart rate × systolic blood pressure) at rest and during exercise. The effects on blood pressure and peripheral vascular resistance were minor and not clinically significant.

A sustained reduction of heart rate was demonstrated in patients treated with ivabradine for at least one year (n = 713). No influence on glucose or lipid metabolism was observed.

The antianginal and anti-ischaemic efficacy of ivabradine was preserved in diabetic patients (n = 457) with a similar safety profile as compared to the overall population.

5.2 Pharmacokinetic properties

Under physiological conditions, ivabradine is rapidly released from tablets and is highly water-soluble (>10 mg/ml). Ivabradine is the S-enantiomer with no bioconversion demonstrated *in vivo*. The N-desmethylated derivative of ivabradine has been identified as the main active metabolite in humans.

Absorption and bioavailability

Ivabradine is rapidly and almost completely absorbed after oral administration with a peak plasma level reached in about 1 hour under fasting condition. The absolute bioavailability of the film-coated tablets is around 40%, due to first-pass effect in the gut and liver.

Food delayed absorption by approximately 1 hour, and increased plasma exposure by 20 to 30 %. The intake of the tablet during meals is recommended in order to decrease intra-individual variability in exposure (see section 4.2).

Distribution

Ivabradine is approximately 70% plasma protein bound and the volume of distribution at steady state is close to 100 l in patients. The maximum plasma concentration following chronic administration at the recommended dose of 5 mg twice daily is 22 ng/ml (CV=29%). The average plasma concentration is 10 ng/ml (CV=38%) at steady state.

Biotransformation

Ivabradine is extensively metabolised by the liver and the gut by oxidation through cytochrome P450 3A4 (CYP3A4) only. The major active metabolite is the N-desmethylated derivative (S 18982) with an exposure about 40% of that of the parent compound. The metabolism of this active metabolite also involves CYP3A4. Ivabradine has low affinity for CYP3A4, shows no clinically relevant CYP3A4 induction or inhibition and is therefore unlikely to modify CYP3A4 substrate metabolism or plasma concentrations. Inversely, potent inhibitors and inducers may substantially affect ivabradine plasma concentrations (see section 4.5).

Elimination

Ivabradine is eliminated with a main half-life of 2 hours (70-75% of the AUC) in plasma and an effective half-life of 11 hours. The total clearance is about 400 ml/min and the renal clearance is about 70 ml/min. Excretion of metabolites occurs to a similar extent via faeces and urine. About 4% of an oral dose is excreted unchanged in urine.

Linearity/non linearity

The kinetics of ivabradine is linear over an oral dose range of 0.5 – 24 mg.

Special populations

- Elderly: no pharmacokinetic differences (AUC and Cmax) have been observed between elderly (≥ 65 years) or very elderly patients (≥ 75 years) and the overall population (see section 4.2).
- Renal insufficiency: the impact of renal impairment (creatinine clearance from 15 to 60 ml/min) on ivabradine pharmacokinetic is minimal, in relation with the low contribution of renal clearance (about 20 %) to total elimination for both ivabradine and its main metabolite S 18982 (see section 4.2).
- Hepatic impairment: in patients with mild hepatic impairment (Child Pugh score up to 7) unbound AUC of ivabradine and the main active metabolite were about 20% higher than in subjects with normal hepatic function. Data are insufficient to draw conclusions in patients with moderate hepatic impairment. No data are available in patients with severe hepatic impairment (see sections 4.2 and 4.3).

Pharmacokinetic/pharmacodynamic (PK/PD) relationship

PK/PD relationship analysis has shown that heart rate decreases almost linearly with increasing ivabradine and S 18982 plasma concentrations for doses of up to 15-20 mg twice daily. At higher doses, the decrease in heart rate is no longer proportional to ivabradine plasma concentrations and tends to reach a plateau. High exposures to ivabradine that may occur when ivabradine is given in combination with strong CYP3A4 inhibitors may result in an excessive decrease in heart rate although this risk is reduced with moderate CYP3A4 inhibitors (see sections 4.3, 4.4 and 4.5).

5.3 Preclinical safety data

Reproductive toxicity studies showed no effect of ivabradine on fertility in male and female rats. When pregnant animals were treated during organogenesis at exposures close to therapeutic doses, there was a higher incidence of foetuses with cardiac defects in the rat and a small number of foetuses with ectrodactylia in the rabbit.

In dogs given ivabradine (doses of 2, 7 or 24mg/kg/day) for one year, reversible changes in retinal function were observed but were not associated with any damage to ocular structures. These data are consistent with the pharmacological effect of ivabradine related to its interaction with hyperpolarisation-activated I_h currents in the retina, which share extensive homology with the cardiac pacemaker I_f current.

Other long-term repeat dose and carcinogenicity studies revealed no clinically relevant changes.

6. PHARMACEUTICAL PARTICULARS

6.1 List of excipients

Core

Lactose monohydrate

Magnesium stearate (E 470 B)

Maize starch

Maltodextrin

Silica, colloidal anhydrous (E 551)

Film-coating

Hypromellose (E 464)

Titanium dioxide (E 171)

Macrogol 6000

Glycerol (E 422)

Magnesium stearate (E 470 B)

Yellow iron oxide (E 172)

Red iron oxide (E 172)

6.2 Incompatibilities

Not applicable.

6.3 Shelf life

3 years.

6.4 Special precautions for storage
This medicinal product does not require any special storage conditions.

6.5 Nature and contents of container
Aluminium/PVC blister packed in cardboard boxes.

Pack sizes

Calendar packs containing 14, 28, 56, 84, 98, 100 or 112 film-coated tablets.

Not all pack sizes may be marketed.

6.6 Special precautions for disposal and other handling
No special requirements.

7. MARKETING AUTHORISATION HOLDER
Les Laboratoires Servier

22 rue Garnier

92200 Neuilly sur Seine

France

8. MARKETING AUTHORISATION NUMBER(S)

Procoralan 5 mg	EU/1/05/316/003	(pack of 56 tablets)
Procoralan 7.5 mg	EU/1/05/316/010	(pack of 56 tablets)

9. DATE OF FIRST AUTHORISATION/RENEWAL OF THE AUTHORISATION
25/10/2005

10. DATE OF REVISION OF THE TEXT
05/2009

Proctosedyl Ointment

(sanofi-aventis)

1. NAME OF THE MEDICINAL PRODUCT
Proctosedyl Ointment

2. QUALITATIVE AND QUANTITATIVE COMPOSITION
Cinchocaine Hydrochloride (Micro) BP 0.5 %ww, Hydrocortisone (Micro) EP 0.5 %ww

3. PHARMACEUTICAL FORM
Yellowish-white translucent greasy ointment.

4. CLINICAL PARTICULARS

4.1 Therapeutic indications
The local anaesthetic cinchocaine relieves pain and relaxes sphincteric spasm. Pruritis and inflammation are relieved by hydrocortisone, which also decreases serious discharge.

Proctosedyl is, therefore, useful for the short term relief (not more than 7 days) of pain, irritation and pruritis associated with haemorrhoids and pruritis ani.

4.2 Posology and method of administration
Apply the ointment in small quantities with the finger, on the painful or pruritic area, morning and evening and after each stool. For deep application attach cannula to tube, insert to full extent and squeeze tube gently from lower end whilst withdrawing.

The ointment may be used separately or concurrently with the suppositories.

4.3 Contraindications
Known hypersensitivity to any of the ingredients.

Not for use in the presence of infections.

4.4 Special warnings and precautions for use
Apply only to the region of the rectum and anus and surrounding skin. Hydrocortisone can cause thinning and damage to the skin especially of the face.

As with all preparations containing topical steroids, the possibility of systemic absorption should be considered. In particular, long-term continuous therapy should be avoided in infants. Adrenal suppression can occur even without occlusion.

4.5 Interaction with other medicinal products and other forms of interaction
None known.

4.6 Pregnancy and lactation
In pregnant animals, administration of corticosteroids can cause abnormalities of foetal development. The relevance of this finding to human beings has not been established. However, topical steroids should not be used extensively in pregnancy, i.e. in large amounts or for long periods.

4.7 Effects on ability to drive and use machines
None.

4.8 Undesirable effects
In persons sensitive to any of the ingredients, skin rash may occur. Although less likely to cause adrenal suppression when applied topically, Hydrocortisone, applied to a large enough area, especially of damaged skin for long enough, or if under occlusive dressing, may have this adverse effect.

4.9 Overdose
Not applicable.

5. PHARMACOLOGICAL PROPERTIES

5.1 Pharmacodynamic properties
Cinchocaine is a local anaesthetic of the amide type.

Hydrocortisone is a glucocorticoid with anti-inflammatory and other properties.

5.2 Pharmacokinetic properties
The literature states that absorption of hydrocortisone does occur through the skin, particularly denuded skin. However, this absorption is not of a clinical significance as hydrocortisone topically, has only rarely been associated with side effects resulting from pituitary adrenal suppression.

Cinchocaine is little absorbed through the intact skin, but absorbed through mucous membranes. Like other local anaesthetics of the amide type, cinchocaine is metabolised in the liver.

5.3 Preclinical safety data
None stated.

6. PHARMACEUTICAL PARTICULARS

6.1 List of excipients
Wool fat, liquid paraffin, white soft paraffin.

6.2 Incompatibilities
None stated.

6.3 Shelf life
36 months

6.4 Special precautions for storage
Store below 25°C.

6.5 Nature and contents of container
Aluminium tube with plastic cannula (30g tubes).

6.6 Special precautions for disposal and other handling
None stated.

7. MARKETING AUTHORISATION HOLDER
sanofi-aventis

One Onslow Street

Guildford

Surrey

GU1 4YS

8. MARKETING AUTHORISATION NUMBER(S)
PL 04425/0207

9. DATE OF FIRST AUTHORISATION/RENEWAL OF THE AUTHORISATION
21 July 2005

10. DATE OF REVISION OF THE TEXT
Decemebr 2006

Legal category: POM

Proctosedyl Suppositories

(sanofi-aventis)

1. NAME OF THE MEDICINAL PRODUCT
Proctosedyl Suppositories

2. QUALITATIVE AND QUANTITATIVE COMPOSITION
Cinchocaine Hydrochloride (micro) BP 5mg

Hydrocortisone (micro) EP 5mg

3. PHARMACEUTICAL FORM
Smooth off-white suppositories.

4. CLINICAL PARTICULARS

4.1 Therapeutic indications
The local anaesthetic Cinchocaine relieves pain and relaxes sphincteric spasm. Pruritis and inflammation are relieved by Hydrocortisone which also decreases serous discharge. Proctosedyl is, therefore, useful for the short term relief (not more than 7 days) of pain, irritation and pruritis associated with haemorrhoids, pruritis ani.

4.2 Posology and method of administration
Adults (including the elderly) and children:

A suppository is inserted morning and evening, and after each stool. The ointment may be used concurrently with the suppositories.

4.3 Contraindications
Known hypersensitivity to any of the ingredients. Not for use in the presence of infections.

4.4 Special warnings and precautions for use
As with all preparations containing topical steroids, the possibility of systemic absorption should be considered. In particular, long-term continuous therapy should be avoided in infants. Adrenal suppression can occur even without occlusion.

4.5 Interaction with other medicinal products and other forms of interaction
None known.

4.6 Pregnancy and lactation
In pregnant animals, administration of corticosteroids can cause abnormalities of foetal development. The relevance of this finding to human beings has not been established. However, topical steroids should not be used extensively in pregnancy, i.e. in large amounts or for long periods.

4.7 Effects on ability to drive and use machines
None.

4.8 Undesirable effects
In persons sensitive to any of the ingredients, anal irritation may occur.

4.9 Overdose
Not applicable.

5. PHARMACOLOGICAL PROPERTIES

5.1 Pharmacodynamic properties
Cinchocaine is a local anaesthetic of the amide type.

Hydrocortisone is a glucocorticoid with anti-inflammatory and other properties.

5.2 Pharmacokinetic properties
The literature states that absorption of Hydrocortisone does occur through the skin, particularly denuded skin. However, this absorption is not of a clinical significance as Hydrocortisone topically has only rarely been associated with side effects resulting from pituitary adrenal suppression.

Cinchocaine is little absorbed through the intact skin, but absorbed through mucous membranes. Like other local anaesthetics of the amide type, Cinchocaine is metabolised in the liver.

5.3 Preclinical safety data
None stated.

6. PHARMACEUTICAL PARTICULARS

6.1 List of excipients
Hard Fat

6.2 Incompatibilities
Not applicable.

6.3 Shelf life
18 months.

6.4 Special precautions for storage
Store at 2°C - 8°C

6.5 Nature and contents of container
Each suppository is contained in a pocket formed from white PVC/PE laminate in packs of 12.

6.6 Special precautions for disposal and other handling
None stated.

7. MARKETING AUTHORISATION HOLDER
sanofi-aventis

One Onslow Street

Guildford

Surrey

GU1 4YS

8. MARKETING AUTHORISATION NUMBER(S)
PL 04425/0208

9. DATE OF FIRST AUTHORISATION/RENEWAL OF THE AUTHORISATION
21 July 2005

10. DATE OF REVISION OF THE TEXT
December 2006

Legal category
POM

Pro-Epanutin Concentrate for Infusion / Solution for Injection

(Pfizer Limited)

1. NAME OF THE MEDICINAL PRODUCT
Pro-Epanutin Concentrate for infusion / Solution for injection

2. QUALITATIVE AND QUANTITATIVE COMPOSITION
One ml of Pro-Epanutin contains 75mg of fosphenytoin sodium (equivalent to 50mg of phenytoin sodium) and referred to as 50mg PE (see Section 4.2).

Each 10ml vial contains 750mg of fosphenytoin sodium (equivalent to 500mg of phenytoin sodium) and referred to as 500mg PE.

For excipients, see Section 6.1.

3. PHARMACEUTICAL FORM
Concentrate for infusion / Solution for injection.

Pro-Epanutin is a clear, colourless to pale yellow, sterile solution.

4. CLINICAL PARTICULARS

4.1 Therapeutic indications
Pro-Epanutin is indicated:

• for the control of status epilepticus of the tonic-clonic (grand mal) type **(see Section 4.2 Posology and Method of Administration)**.

• for prevention and treatment of seizures occurring in connection with neurosurgery and/or head trauma.

• as substitute for oral phenytoin if oral administration is not possible and/or contra-indicated.

Table 1

Weight (kg)	Dose (mg PE)	Volume of Pro-Epanutin (50mg PE/ml) No. of 10ml vials to open	Volume (ml) to draw up	Volume (ml) of diluent (5% glucose or 0.9% sodium chloride) for final concentration of 25mg PE/ml	Minimum Infusion Time (mins) to achieve the maximum recommended infusion rate of 150mg PE / minute
100	1500	3	30	30	10
95	1425	3	28.5	28.5	9.5
90	1350	3	27	27	9
85	1275	3	25.5	25.5	8.5
80	1200	3	24	24	8
75	1125	3	22.5	22.5	7.5
70	1050	3	21	21	7
65	975	2	19.5	19.5	6.5
60	900	2	18	18	6
55	825	2	16.5	16.5	5.5
50	750	2	15	15	5
45	675	2	13.5	13.5	4.5

Table 2

Weight (kg)	Dose (mg PE)	Volume of Pro-Epanutin (50mg PE/ml)		Volume (ml) of diluent* (5% glucose or 0.9% sodium chloride)		Minimum Infusion Time (mins) to achieve the maximum recommended infusion rate of 100mg PE / minute
		No. of 10ml vials to open	Volume (ml) to draw up	for final concentration of 25mg PE/ml	for final concentration of 1.5mg PE/ml	
100	500	1	10	10	323	5
90	450	1	9	9	291	4.5
80	400	1	8	8	259	4
70	350	1	7	7	226	3.5
60	300	1	6	6	194	3
50	250	1	5	5	162	2.5

*For IV infusion the final concentration should range between 1.5 and 25mg PE/ml

4.2 Posology and method of administration

IMPORTANT NOTE: Throughout all Pro-Epanutin product labelling, the amount and concentration of fosphenytoin is always expressed in terms of phenytoin sodium equivalents (PE) to avoid the need to perform molecular weight-based adjustments when converting between fosphenytoin and phenytoin sodium doses. Pro-Epanutin should always be prescribed and dispensed in phenytoin sodium equivalent units (PE). Note, however, that fosphenytoin has important differences in administration from parenteral phenytoin sodium (see Section 4.4 Special Warnings and Precautions for Use).

Phenytoin sodium equivalents (PE):

1.5mg of fosphenytoin is equivalent to 1mg PE (phenytoin sodium equivalent)

Administration:

Pro-Epanutin may be administered by IV infusion or by IM injection. The intramuscular route should be considered when there is not an urgent need to control seizures. Pro-Epanutin should not be administered by IM route in emergency situations such as status epilepticus.

Products with particulate matter or discoloration should not be used.

Intravenous infusion:

For IV infusion, Pro-Epanutin should be diluted in 5% glucose or 0.9% sodium chloride solution. The concentration should range from 1.5 to 25mg PE/ml.

Because of the risk of hypotension, the recommended rate of administration by IV infusion in routine clinical settings is 50-100mg PE/minute. Even in an emergency, **it should not exceed 150mg PE/minute.** The use of a device controlling the rate of infusion is recommended.

Please refer to tables 1 to 10 for examples of dosing, dilution and infusion time calculations.

Continuous monitoring of electrocardiogram, blood pressure and respiratory function for the duration of the infusion is essential. The patient should also be observed throughout the period where maximal plasma phenytoin concentrations occur. This is approximately 30 minutes after the end of the Pro-Epanutin infusions.

Cardiac resuscitative equipment should be available **(see Section 4.4 Special Warnings and Precautions for Use).**

DOSAGE IN ADULTS

Status Epilepticus

Loading dose:

In order to obtain rapid seizure control in patients with continuous seizure activity, IV diazepam or lorazepam should be administered prior to administration of Pro-Epanutin.

The loading dose of Pro-Epanutin is 15mg PE/kg administered as a single dose by IV infusion

Recommended IV infusion rate: 100 to 150mg PE/min. **(should not exceed 150mg PE/minute even for emergency use).**

Examples of infusion times are presented in Table 1.

Intramuscular administration of Pro-Epanutin is contraindicated in the treatment of status epilepticus. If administration of Pro-Epanutin does not terminate seizures, the use of alternative anticonvulsants should be considered.

Table 1:

Status Epilepticus: Examples of IV loading doses of 15mg PE/kg, and recommendations for dilution (to 25mg PE/ml) and IV infusion times (at maximum rate of 150mg PE/min by body weight)

(see Table 1 opposite)

Maintenance dose:

The recommended maintenance dose of Pro-Epanutin of 4 to 5mg PE/kg/day may be given by IV infusion or by IM injection. The total daily dose may be given in one or two divided doses.

Recommended IV infusion rate for maintenance dose: 50 to 100mg PE/minute.

Examples of infusion times are provided in Table 2.

Maintenance doses should be adjusted according to patient response and trough plasma phenytoin concentrations **(see Therapeutic Drug Monitoring).**

Transfer to maintenance therapy with oral phenytoin should be made when appropriate.

Table 2:

Status Epilepticus: Examples for maximum IV maintenance doses of 5mg PE/kg, recommendations for dilution* (to 25mg PE/ml or to 1.5mg PE/ml), and IV infusion times (at maximum rate of 100mg PE/minute) by body weight

(see Table 2 opposite)

Treatment or Prophylaxis of Seizures

Loading dose:

The loading dose of Pro-Epanutin is 10 to 15mg PE/kg given as a single dose by IV infusion or by IM injection.

Recommended IV infusion rate for treatment or prophylaxis of seizures:

50 to 100mg PE/minute **(should not exceed 150mg PE/minute).**

Examples of infusion times are presented in Table 3.

Table 3:

Treatment or Prophylaxis of seizures: Examples for IV loading doses of 10mg PE/kg[a], and recommendations for dilution* (to 25mg PE/ml or to 1.5mg PE/ml) and IV infusion times (at maximum rate of 100mg PE/minute) by body weight

(see Table 3 below)

Maintenance dose:

The recommended maintenance dose of Pro-Epanutin of 4 to 5mg PE/kg/day may be given by IV infusion or by IM injection. The total daily dose may be given in one or two divided doses.

*Recommended IV infusion rate for maintenance dose:*50 to 100mg PE/minute.

Examples of infusion times are presented in Table 4.

Maintenance doses should be adjusted according to patient response and trough plasma phenytoin concentrations **(see Therapeutic Drug Monitoring).**

Transfer to maintenance therapy with oral phenytoin should be made when appropriate.

Table 4:

Treatment or Prophylaxis of seizures: Examples for maximum IV maintenance doses of 5mg PE/kg, recommendations for dilution* (to 25mg PE/ml or to 1.5mg PE/ml), and IV infusion times (at maximum infusion rate of 100mg PE/minute) by body weight

(see Table 4 on next page)

Temporary substitution of oral phenytoin therapy with Pro-Epanutin.

The same dose and dosing frequency as for oral phenytoin therapy should be used and can be administered by IV infusion or by IM injection.

Table 3

Weight (kg)	Dose (mg PE)	Volume of Pro-Epanutin (50mg PE/ml)		Volume (ml) of diluent* (5% glucose or 0.9% sodium chloride)		Minimum Infusion Time (mins) to achieve the maximum recommended infusion rate of 100mg PE / minute
		No. of 10ml vials to open	Volume (ml) to draw up	for final concentration of 25mg PE/ml	for final concentration of 1.5mg PE/ml	
100	1000	2	20	20	647	10
90	900	2	18	18	582	9
80	800	2	16	16	517	8
70	700	2	14	14	453	7
60	600	2	12	12	388	6
50	500	1	10	10	323	5

*For IV infusion the final concentration should range between 1.5 and 25mg PE/ml

[a] Please refer to Table 1 for examples of calculations for loading doses of 15mg PE/kg

Table 4

Weight (kg)	Dose (mg PE)	Volume of Pro-Epanutin (50mg PE/ml)		Volume (ml) of diluent* (5% glucose or 0.9% sodium chloride)		Minimum Infusion Time (mins) to achieve the maximum recommended infusion rate of 100mg PE / minute
		No. of 10ml vials to open	Volume (ml) to draw up	for final concentration of 25mg PE/ml	for final concentration of 1.5mg PE/ml	
100	500	1	10	10	323	5
90	450	1	9	9	291	4.5
80	400	1	8	8	259	4
70	350	1	7	7	226	3.5
60	300	1	6	6	194	3
50	250	1	5	5	162	2.5

*For IV infusion the final concentration should range between 1.5 to 25mg PE/ml

Table 5

Dose (mg phenytoin sodium)	Dose (mg PE)	Volume of Pro-Epanutin (50mg PE/ml)		Volume (ml) of diluent* (5% glucose or 0.9% sodium chloride)		Minimum Infusion Time (mins) to achieve the maximum recommended infusion rate of 100mg PE / minute
		No. of 10ml vials to open	Volume (ml) to draw up	for final concentration of 25mg PE/ml	for final concentration of 1.5mg PE/ml	
500	500	1	10	10	323	5
450	450	1	9	9	291	4.5
400	400	1	8	8	259	4
350	350	1	7	7	226	3.5
300	300	1	6	6	194	3
250	250	1	5	5	162	2.5

*For IV infusion the final concentration should range between 1.5 to 25mg PE/ml

Table 6

Weight (kg)	Dose (mg PE)	Volume of Pro-Epanutin (50mg PE/ml)		Volume (ml) of diluent (5% glucose or 0.9% sodium chloride) for final concentration of 25mg PE/ml	Minimum Infusion Time (mins) to achieve the maximum recommended infusion rate of 3mg PE /kg/ minute
		No. of 10ml vials to open	Volume (ml) to draw up		
35	525	2	10.5	10.5	5
32.5	487.5	1	9.75	9.75	5
30	450	1	9	9	5
27.5	412.5	1	8.25	8.25	5
25	375	1	7.5	7.5	5
22.5	337.5	1	6.75	6.75	5
20	300	1	6	6	5
17.5	262.5	1	5.25	5.25	5

Table 7

Weight (kg)	Dose (mg PE)	Volume of Pro-Epanutin (50mg PE/ml)		Volume (ml) of diluent* (5% glucose or >0.9% sodium chloride)		Minimum Infusion Time (mins) to achieve the maximum recommended infusion rate of 2mg PE /kg/ minute
		No. of 10ml vials to open	Volume (ml) to draw up	for final concentration of 25mg PE/ml	for final concentration of 1.5mg PE/ml	
35	175	1	3.5	3.5	113	2.5
32.5	162.5	1	3.25	3.25	105	2.5
30	150	1	3	3	97	2.5
27.5	137.5	1	2.75	2.75	89	2.5
25	125	1	2.5	2.5	81	2.5
22.5	112.5	1	2.25	2.25	73	2.5
20	100	1	2	2	65	2.5
17.5	87.5	1	1.75	1.75	57	2.5

*For IV infusion the final concentration should range between 1.5 and 25mg PE/ml

*Recommended IV infusion rate for temporary substitution dosing:*50 to 100mg PE/minute.

Examples of infusion times are presented in Table 5.

Therapeutic drug monitoring may be useful whenever switching between products and/or routes of administration. Doses should be adjusted according to patient response and trough plasma phenytoin concentrations (see **Therapeutic Drug Monitoring**).

Fosphenytoin has not been evaluated systemically for more than 5 days.

Table 5:

Temporary substitution of oral phenytoin therapy: Examples of equivalent doses and recommendations for dilution* (to 25mg PE/ml or to 1.5mg PE/ml), and IV infusion times (at maximum rate of 100mg PE/minute)

(see Table 5 opposite)

DOSAGE IN CHILDREN

Pro-Epanutin may be administered to children (ages 5 and above) by IV infusion only, at the same mg PE/kg dose used for adults. The doses of Pro-Epanutin for children have been predicted from the known pharmacokinetics of Pro-Epanutin in adults and children aged 5 to 10 years and of parenteral phenytoin in adults and children.

Status Epilepticus

Loading dose

In order to obtain rapid seizure control in patients with continuous seizure activity IV diazepam or lorazepam should be administered prior to administration of Pro-Epanutin.

The loading dose of Pro-Epanutin is 15mg PE/kg administered as a single dose by IV infusion

*Recommended IV infusion rate:*2 to 3mg PE/kg/min. **(should not exceed 3mg PE/kg/minute or 150mg PE/minute).**

The recommended infusion rate is presented in Table 6.

If administration of Pro-Epanutin does not terminate seizures, the use of alternative anticonvulsants should be considered.

Table 6:

Status Epilepticus: Examples of IV loading doses of 15mg PE/kg and recommendations for dilution (to 25mg PE/ml) and IV infusion times (at 3mg PE/kg/minute) by body weight

(see Table 6 opposite)

Maintenance dose:

The recommended maintenance dose of Pro-Epanutin of 4 to 5mg PE/kg/day may be given by IV infusion. The total daily dose may be given in one to four divided doses.

*Recommended IV infusion rate for maintenance dosing:*1 to 2mg PE/kg/minute **(should not exceed 100mg PE/minute).**

The recommended infusion time is presented in Table 7.

Maintenance doses should be adjusted according to patient response and trough plasma phenytoin concentrations **(see Therapeutic Drug Monitoring).**

Transfer to maintenance therapy with oral phenytoin should be made when appropriate.

Table 7:

Status Epilepticus: Examples for maximum IV maintenance doses of 5mg PE/kg, recommendations for dilution* (to 25mg PE/ml or to 1.5mg PE/ml) and IV infusion times (at maximum rate of 2mg PE/kg/minute) by body weight

(see Table 7 opposite)

Treatment or Prophylaxis of Seizures

Loading dose:

The loading dose of Pro-Epanutin is 10 to 15mg PE/kg given as a single dose by IV infusion.

Recommended IV infusion rate fortreatment or prophylaxis of seizures: 1 to 2mg PE/kg/minute **(should not exceed 3mg PE/kg/minute or 150mg PE/minute).**

The recommended infusion time is presented in Table 8.

Table 8:

Treatment or Prophylaxis of seizures: Examples for IV loading doses of 10mg PE/kg[a], and recommendations for dilution* (to 25mg PE/ml or to 1.5mg PE/ml) and IV infusion times (at maximum rate of 2mg PE/kg/minute) by body weight

(see Table 8 on next page)

Maintenance dose:

The recommended maintenance dose of Pro-Epanutin of 4 to 5mg PE/kg/day may be given by IV infusion. The total daily dose may be given in one to four divided doses.

Recommended IV infusion rate for maintenance dosing: 1 to 2mg PE/kg/minute **(should not exceed 100mg PE/minute).**

The recommended infusion time is presented in Table 9.

Maintenance doses should be adjusted according to patient response and trough plasma phenytoin concentrations **(see Therapeutic Drug Monitoring).**

Transfer to maintenance therapy with oral phenytoin should be made when appropriate.

Table 8

Weight (kg)	Dose (mg PE)	Volume of Pro-Epanutin (50mg PE/ml)		Volume (ml) of diluent* (5% glucose or 0.9% sodium chloride)		Minimum Infusion Time (mins) to achieve the maximum recommended infusion rate of 2mg PE /kg/ minute
		No. of 10ml vials to open	Volume (ml) to draw up	for final concentration of 25mg PE/ml	for final concentration of 1.5mg PE/ml	
35	350	1	7	7	226	5
32.5	325	1	6.5	6.5	210	5
30	300	1	6	6	194	5
27.5	275	1	5.5	5.5	178	5
25	250	1	5	5	161	5
22.5	225	1	4.5	4.5	145	5
20	200	1	4	4	129	5
17.5	175	1	3.5	3.5	113	5

***For IV infusion the final concentration should range between 1.5 to 25mg PE/ml**

[a] Please refer to Table 1 for examples of calculations for loading doses of 15mg PE/kg

Table 9

Weight (kg)	Dose (mg PE)	Volume of Pro-Epanutin (50mg PE/ml)		Volume (ml) of diluent* (5% glucose or 0.9% sodium chloride)		Minimum Infusion Time (mins) to achieve the maximum recommended infusion rate of 2mg PE /kg/ minute
		No. of 10ml vials to open	Volume (ml) to draw up	for final concentration of 25mg PE/ml	for final concentration of 1.5mg PE/ml	
35	175	1	3.5	3.5	113	2.5
32.5	162.5	1	3.25	3.25	105	2.5
30	150	1	3	3	97	2.5
27.5	137.5	1	2.75	2.75	89	2.5
25	125	1	2.5	2.5	81	2.5
22.5	112.5	1	2.25	2.25	73	2.5
20	100	1	2	2	65	2.5
17.5	87.5	1	1.75	1.75	57	2.5

***For IV infusion the final concentration should range between 1.5 and 25mg PE/ml**

Table 9:

Treatment or Prophylaxis of seizures: Examples for maximum IV maintenance doses of 5mg PE/kg, recommendations for dilution* (to 25mg PE/ml or to 1.5mg PE/kg), and IV infusion times (at a maximum rate of 2mg PE/kg/minute) by body weight

(see Table 9 above)

Temporary substitution of oral phenytoin therapy with Pro-Epanutin.

The same dose and dosing frequency as for oral phenytoin therapy should be administered by IV infusion.

Recommended IV infusion rate for temporary substitution dosing: 1 to 2 mg PE/kg/minute (**should not exceed 50 to 100 mg PE/minute.)**

The recommended infusion time is presented in Table 10.

Therapeutic drug monitoring may be useful whenever switching between products and/or routes of administration. Doses should be adjusted according to patient response and trough plasma phenytoin concentrations **(see Therapeutic Drug Monitoring).**

Fosphenytoin has not been evaluated systemically for more than 5 days.

Table 10:

Temporary substitution of oral phenytoin therapy: Examples of equivalent doses and recommendations for dilution* (to 25mg PE/ml or to 1.5mg PE/ml), and IV infusion times (at maximum rate of 2mg PE/kg/minute)

(see Table 10 below)

ELDERLY PATIENTS

A lower loading dose and/or infusion rate, and lower or less frequent maintenance dosing of Pro-Epanutin may be required. Phenytoin metabolism is slightly decreased in elderly patients. A 10% to 25% reduction in dose or rate may be considered and careful clinical monitoring is required.

Table 10

Dose (mg phenytoin sodium) 5mg/kg	Dose (mg PE)	Volume of Pro-Epanutin (50mg PE/ml)		Volume (ml) of diluent* (5% glucose or 0.9% sodium chloride)		Minimum Infusion Time (mins) to achieve the maximum recommended infusion rate of 2mg PE /kg/ minute
		No. of 10ml vials to open	Volume (ml) to draw up	for final concentration of 25mg PE/ml	for final concentration of 1.5mg PE/ml	
175	175	1	3.5	3.5	113	2.5
150	150	1	3	3	97	2.5
125	125	1	2.5	2.5	81	2.5
100	100	1	2	2	65	2.5
75	75	1	1.5	1.5	49	2.5
50	50	1	1	1	32	2.5

***For IV infusion the final concentration should range between 1.5 to 25mg PE/ml**

PATIENTS WITH RENAL OR HEPATIC DISEASE

Except in the treatment of status epilepticus, a lower loading dose and/or infusion rate, and lower or less frequent maintenance dosing may be required in patients with renal and/or hepatic disease or in those with hypoalbuminaemia. A 10% to 25% reduction in dose or rate may be considered and careful clinical monitoring is required.

The rate of conversion of IV Pro-Epanutin to phenytoin but not the clearance of phenytoin may be increased in these patients. Plasma unbound phenytoin concentrations may also be elevated. It may therefore, be more appropriate to measure plasma unbound phenytoin concentrations rather than plasma total phenytoin concentrations in these patients.

Therapeutic drug monitoring:

Prior to complete conversion, immunoanalytical techniques may significantly overestimate plasma phenytoin concentrations due to cross-reactivity with fosphenytoin. Chromatographic assay methods (e.g. HPLC) accurately quantitate phenytoin concentrations in biological fluids in the presence of fosphenytoin. It is advised that blood samples to assess phenytoin concentration ***should not*** be obtained for at least 2 hours after IV Pro-Epanutin infusion or 4 hours after IM Pro-Epanutin injection.

Optimal seizure control without clinical signs of toxicity occurs most often with plasma total phenytoin concentrations of between 10 and 20mg/l (40 and 80micromoles/l) or plasma unbound phenytoin concentrations of between 1 and 2mg/l (4 and 8micromoles/l).

Plasma phenytoin concentrations sustained above the optimal range may produce signs of acute toxicity **(see Section 4.4 Special Warnings and Precautions for Use).**

Phenytoin capsules are approximately 90% bioavailable by the oral route. Phenytoin, supplied as Pro-Epanutin, is 100% bioavailable by both the IM and IV routes. For this reason, plasma phenytoin concentrations may increase when IM or IV Pro-Epanutin is substituted for oral phenytoin sodium therapy. However, it is not necessary to adjust the initial doses when substituting oral phenytoin with Pro-Epanutin or vice versa.

Therapeutic drug monitoring may be useful whenever switching between products and/or routes of administration.

4.3 Contraindications

Hypersensitivity to fosphenytoin sodium or the excipients of Pro-Epanutin, or to phenytoin or other hydantoins.

Parenteral phenytoin affects ventricular automaticity. Pro-Epanutin is therefore, contra-indicated in patients with sinus bradycardia, sino-atrial block, second and third degree A-V block and Adams-Stokes syndrome.

Acute intermittent porphyria.

4.4 Special warnings and precautions for use

Doses of Pro-Epanutin are always expressed as their phenytoin sodium equivalents (PE = phenytoin sodium equivalent). Therefore, when Pro-Epanutin is dosed as PE do not make any adjustment in the recommended doses when substituting Pro-Epanutin for phenytoin sodium or vice versa.

Note, however, that Pro-Epanutin has important differences in administration from parenteral phenytoin sodium. Pro-Epanutin should not be administered intravenously at a rate greater than 150mg PE/min while the maximum intravenous infusion rate for phenytoin is 50mg/min (see Section 4.2 Posology and Method of Administration).

Phenytoin is not effective in absence seizures. If tonic-clonic seizures are present simultaneously with absence seizures, combined drug therapy is recommended.

Cardiovascular disease:

Pro-Epanutin should be used with caution in patients with hypotension and severe myocardial insufficiency. Severe cardiovascular reactions including atrial and ventricular conduction depression and ventricular fibrillation, and sometimes, fatalities have been reported following phenytoin and fosphenytoin administration. Hypotension may also occur following IV administration of high doses and/ or high infusion rates of Pro-Epanutin and even within recommended doses and rates. A reduction in the rate of administration or discontinuation of dosing may be necessary **(see Section 4.2 Posology and Method of Administration)**.

Patients with an acute cerebrovascular event may be at increased risk of hypotension and require particularly close monitoring.

Withdrawal Precipitated Seizure/Status Epilepticus:

Abrupt withdrawal of antiepileptic drugs may increase seizure frequency and may lead to status epilepticus.

Suicidal ideation and behaviour:

Suicidal ideation and behaviour have been reported in patients treated with anti-epileptic agents in several indications. A meta-analysis of randomised placebo controlled trials of anti-epileptic drugs has also shown a small increased risk of suicidal ideation and behaviour. The mechanism of this risk is not known and the available data do not exclude the possibility of an increased risk for fosphenytoin.

Therefore patients should be monitored for signs of suicidal ideation and behaviours and appropriate treatment should be considered. Patients (and caregivers of patients) should be advised to seek medical advice should signs of suicidal ideation or behaviour emerge.

Rash:

Pro-Epanutin should be discontinued if a skin rash or signs of an allergic or hypersensitivity reaction or syndrome appear. Rapid substitution with an alternative antiepileptic drug not belonging to the hydantoin chemical class may be necessary.

Hypersensitivity Syndrome and Hepatoxicity:

A hypersensitivity reaction or syndrome has been associated with phenytoin administration. Fever, skin eruptions and lymphadenopathy may occur within the first two months of treatment. Hepatotoxicity is often associated with this hypersensitivity syndrome. Acute hepatotoxicities, including acute hepatic failure, jaundice, hepatomegaly and elevated serum transaminase levels have also been reported. Recovery from acute hepatotoxicity may be prompt, however fatal outcomes have also occurred.

Pro-Epanutin should be discontinued immediately following signs of acute hepatotoxicity and not readministered. Leucocytosis, eosinophilia and arthralgias may also occur. Although still rare, there may be an increased incidence of hypersensitivity reactions in black patients.

Lymphadenopathy:

Lymphadenopathy (local or generalised) including benign lymph node hyperplasia, pseudolymphoma, lymphoma and Hodgkin's Disease have been associated with administration of phenytoin, although a cause and effect relationship has not been established. It is therefore, important to eliminate other types of lymph node pathology before discontinuing therapy with Pro-Epanutin. Lymph node involvement may occur with or without symptoms and signs resembling serum sickness, e.g. fever, rash and liver involvement, as part of the hypersensitivity syndrome described above. In all cases of lymphadenopathy, long term follow-up observations are indicated and every effort should be made to achieve seizure control using alternative antiepileptic drugs.

Acute toxicity:

Confusional states referred to as "delirium", "psychosis" or "encephalopathy" or rarely irreversible cerebellar dysfunction may occur if plasma phenytoin concentrations are sustained above the optimal therapeutic range. Plasma phenytoin concentrations should be determined at the first sign of acute toxicity **(see Section 4.2 Posology and Method of Administration: Therapeutic Drug Monitoring)**. If plasma phenytoin concentrations are excessive, the dose of Pro-Epanutin should be reduced. If symptoms persist, administration of Pro-Epanutin should be discontinued.

Renal or Hepatic Disease:

Pro-Epanutin should be used with caution in patients with renal and/or hepatic disease, or in those with hypoalbuminaemia. Alterations in dosing may be necessary in patients with impaired kidney or liver function, elderly patients or those who are gravely ill **(see Section 4.2 Posology and Method of Administration)**. These patients may show early signs of phenytoin toxicity or an increase in the severity of adverse events due to alterations in Pro-Epanutin and phenytoin pharmacokinetics.

The phosphate load provided by Pro-Epanutin is 0.0037mmol phosphate/mg fosphenytoin sodium. Caution is advised when administering Pro-Epanutin in patients requiring phosphate restriction, such as those with severe renal impairment.

Sensory Disturbances:

Overall these occur in 13% of the patients exposed to Pro-Epanutin. Transient itching, burning, warmth or tingling in the groin during and shortly after intravenous infusion of Pro-Epanutin may occur. The sensations are not consistent with the signs of an allergic reaction and may be avoided or minimised by using a slower rate of IV infusion or by temporarily stopping the infusion.

Diabetes:

Phenytoin may raise blood glucose in diabetic patients.

Alcohol Use:

Acute alcohol intake may increase plasma phenytoin concentrations while chronic alcohol use may decrease plasma phenytoin concentrations.

4.5 Interaction with other medicinal products and other forms of interaction

Drug interactions which may occur following the administration of Pro-Epanutin are those that are expected to occur with drugs known to interact with phenytoin. Phenytoin metabolism is saturable and other drugs that utilise the same metabolic pathways may alter plasma phenytoin concentrations. There are many drugs which may increase or decrease plasma phenytoin concentrations. Equally phenytoin may affect the metabolism of a number of other drugs because of its potent enzyme-inducing potential. Determination of plasma phenytoin concentrations is especially helpful when possible drug interactions are suspected **(see Section 4.2 Posology and Method of Administration: Therapeutic Drug Monitoring)**.

No drugs are known to interfere with the conversion of fosphenytoin to phenytoin.

Phenytoin is extensively bound to plasma proteins and is prone to competitive displacement. Drugs highly bound to albumin could also increase the fosphenytoin unbound fraction with the potential to increase the rate of conversion of fosphenytoin to phenytoin. Phenytoin is metabolised by hepatic cytochrome P450 enzymes. Inhibition of phenytoin metabolism may produce significant increases in plasma phenytoin concentrations and increase the risk of phenytoin toxicity. Phenytoin is also a potent inducer of hepatic drug-metabolising enzymes.

The following drug interactions are the most commonly occurring drug interactions with phenytoin:

Drugs that may ***increase*** plasma phenytoin concentrations include: acute alcohol intake, amiodarone, chloramphenicol, chlordiazepoxide, diazepam, dicoumarol, disulfiram, oestrogens, fluoxetine, H_2-antagonists (e.g. cimetidine), halothane, isoniazid, methylphenidate, phenothiazines, phenylbutazone, salicylates, succinimides (e.g. ethosuximide), sulphonamides, tolbutamide, trazodone, viloxazine, antifungal agents (e.g. amphotericin B, fluconazole, ketoconazole, miconazole and itraconazole) and omeprazole.

Drugs that may ***decrease*** plasma phenytoin concentrations include carbamazepine, chronic alcohol abuse, reserpine, folic acid, sucralfate and vigabatrin.

Drugs that may either ***increase*** or ***decrease*** plasma phenytoin concentrations include: phenobarbitone, valproic acid, sodium valproate, antineoplastic agents, ciprofloxacin and certain antacids. Similarly, the effects of phenytoin on plasma phenobarbitone, valproic acid and sodium valproate concentrations are unpredictable.

Although not a true pharmacokinetic interaction, tricyclic antidepressants and phenothiazines may precipitate seizures in susceptible patients and Pro-Epanutin dosage may need to be adjusted.

Drugs whose efficacy is impaired by phenytoin include: anticoagulants, corticosteroids, dicoumarol, digitoxin, doxycycline, oestrogens, furosemide, oral contraceptives, rifampicin, quinidine, theophylline, vitamin D, antifungal agents, antineoplastic agents and clozapine.

Drugs whose effect is enhanced by phenytoin include: warfarin.

Drug/Laboratory Test Interactions:

Phenytoin may decrease serum concentrations of T_4. It may also produce low results in dexamethasone or metyrapone tests. This may be an artifact. Phenytoin may cause increased blood glucose or serum concentrations of alkaline phosphatase and gamma glutamyl transpeptidase (GGT). Phenytoin may affect blood calcium and blood sugar metabolism tests.

Phenytoin has the potential to lower serum folate levels.

4.6 Pregnancy and lactation

An increase in seizure frequency may occur during pregnancy because of altered phenytoin pharmacokinetics. Periodic measurement of plasma phenytoin concentrations may be valuable in the management of pregnant women as a guide to appropriate adjustment of dosage **(see Section 4.2 Posology and Method of Administration: Therapeutic Drug Monitoring)**. However, postpartum restoration of the original dosage will probably be indicated.

If this drug is used during pregnancy, or if the patient becomes pregnant while taking the drug, the patient should be informed of the potential harm to the foetus.

Prenatal exposure to phenytoin may increase the risks for congenital malformations and other adverse developmental outcomes. Increased frequencies of major malformations (such as orofacial clefts and cardiac defects), minor anomalies (dysmorphic facial features, nail and digit hypoplasia), growth abnormalities (including microcephaly) and mental deficiency have been reported among children born to epileptic women who took phenytoin alone or in combination with other antiepileptic drugs during pregnancy. There have also been several reported cases of malignancies, including neuroblastoma, in children whose mothers received phenytoin during pregnancy. The overall incidence of malformations for children of epileptic women treated with antiepileptic drugs (phenytoin and/or others) during pregnancy is about 10% or two-to-three-fold that in the general population. However, the relative contribution of antiepileptic drugs and other factors associated with epilepsy to this increased risk are uncertain and in most cases it has not been possible to attribute specific developmental abnormalities to particular antiepileptic drugs.

It might be necessary to give vitamin K to the mother during the last gestational month. Neonates of the mother receiving Pro-Epanutin should be monitored for haemorrhagic diathesis and if necessary additional vitamin K should be administered.

Foetal toxicity, developmental toxicity and teratogenicity were observed in offspring of rats given fosphenytoin during pregnancy, similar to those reported with phenytoin. No developmental effects were observed in offspring of pregnant rabbits given fosphenytoin; malformations have been reported in offspring of pregnant rabbits with phenytoin at ⩾75mg/kg.

It is not known whether Pro-Epanutin is excreted in human milk. Following administration of oral phenytoin, phenytoin appears to be excreted in low concentrations in human milk. Therefore, breast-feeding is not recommended for women receiving Pro-Epanutin.

4.7 Effects on ability to drive and use machines

Caution is recommended in patients performing skilled tasks (e.g. driving or operating machinery) as treatment with fosphenytoin may cause central nervous system adverse effects such as dizziness and drowsiness **(see Section 4.8 Undesirable Effects)**.

4.8 Undesirable effects

The following adverse events have been reported in clinical trials in adults receiving Pro-Epanutin. The list also includes adverse effects that have been reported following both the acute and chronic use of phenytoin.

Central Nervous System:

Central nervous system effects are the most common side effects seen following administration of Pro-Epanutin or phenytoin and are usually dose-related. Nystagmus, dizziness, paraesthesia, ataxia, tremor, incoordination, stupor, vertigo, euphoria, drowsiness, motor twitching, transient nervousness, slurred speech, mental confusion and insomnia.

There have also been rare reports of phenytoin-induced dyskinesias, including chorea, dystonia and asterixis, similar to those induced by phenothiazines or other neuroleptic drugs. A predominantly sensory peripheral polyneuropathy has been observed in patients receiving long-term phenytoin therapy. Tonic seizures have also been reported. The incidence and severity of adverse events related to the CNS and sensory disturbances were greater at higher doses and rates.

Cardiovascular and Respiratory systems:

Hypotension, vasodilation, severe cardiotoxic reactions with atrial and ventricular conduction depression (including bradycardia and all degrees of heart block), asystole ventricular fibrillation and cardiovascular collapse. Some of these reactions have been fatal. **(see Section 4.4 Special Warnings and Precautions for Use)**.

Alterations in respiratory function (including respiratory arrest), pneumonitis.

Haemopoietic system:

Ecchymosis, thrombocytopenia, leucopenia, granulocytopenia, agranulocytosis, pancytopenia with or without bone marrow suppression and aplastic anaemia have been occasionally reported with phenytoin administration. Some of these reports have been fatal.

Liver or Kidney:

Toxic hepatitis, liver damage, interstitial nephritis.

Gastrointestinal System:

Nausea, vomiting, dry mouth, taste perversion, constipation.

Skin and Connective Tissue:

Pruritus, rash **(see Section 4.4 Special Warnings and Precautions for Use)**, coarsening of the facial features, enlargement of the lips, gingival hyperplasia, hirsutism, hypertrichosis, Peyronie's disease and Dupuytren's contracture may occur rarely.

Special Senses:

Tinnitus, ear disorder, taste perversion, abnormal vision.

Immune System:

Hypersensitivity syndrome **(see Section 4.4 Special Warnings and Precautions for Use)**, systemic lupus erythematosus, periarteritis nodosa, immunoglobulin abnormalities.

Body as a whole:

Headache, pain, asthenia, chills, injection site reaction, injection site pain, polyarthropathy, hyperglycaemia.

No trends in laboratory changes were observed in Pro-Epanutin treated patients.

4.9 Overdose

Nausea, vomiting, lethargy, tachycardia, bradycardia, asystole, cardiac arrest, hypotension, syncope, hypocalcaemia, metabolic acidosis and death have been reported in cases of overdosage with Pro-Epanutin.

Initial symptoms of Pro-Epanutin toxicity are those associated with acute phenytoin toxicity. These are nystagmus, ataxia and dysarthria. Other signs include tremor, hyperreflexia, lethargy, slurred speech, nausea, vomiting, coma and hypotension. There is a risk of potentially fatal respiratory or circulatory depression. There are marked variations among individuals with respect to plasma phenytoin concentrations where toxicity occurs. Lateral gaze nystagmus usually appears at 20mg/l, ataxia at 30mg/l and dysarthria and lethargy appear when the plasma concentration is over 40mg/l. However, phenytoin concentrations as high as 50mg/l have been reported without evidence of toxicity. As much as 25 times the therapeutic phenytoin dose has been taken, resulting in plasma phenytoin concentrations over 100mg/l, with complete recovery.

Treatment is non-specific since there is no known antidote to Pro-Epanutin or phenytoin overdosage. The adequacy of the respiratory and circulatory systems should be carefully observed and appropriate supportive measures employed. Haemodialysis can be considered since phenytoin is not completely bound to plasma proteins. Total exchange transfusion has been used in the treatment of severe intoxication in children. In acute overdosage the possibility of the use of other CNS depressants, including alcohol, should be borne in mind.

Formate and phosphate are metabolites of fosphenytoin and therefore, may contribute to signs of toxicity following overdosage. Signs of formate toxicity are similar to those of methanol toxicity and are associated with severe anion-gap metabolic acidosis. Large amounts of phosphate, delivered rapidly, could potentially cause hypocalcaemia with paraesthesia, muscle spasms and seizures. Ionised free calcium levels can be measured and, if low, used to guide treatment.

5. PHARMACOLOGICAL PROPERTIES

5.1 Pharmacodynamic properties

ATC-Code: N03AB

Pro-Epanutin is a prodrug of phenytoin and accordingly, its anticonvulsant effects are attributable to phenytoin.

The pharmacological and toxicological effects of fosphenytoin sodium include those of phenytoin.

The cellular mechanisms of phenytoin thought to be responsible for its anticonvulsant actions include modulation of voltage-dependent sodium channels of neurones, inhibition of calcium flux across neuronal membranes, modulation of voltage-dependent calcium channels of neurones and enhancement of the sodium-potassium ATPase activity of neurones and glial cells. The modulation of sodium channels may be a primary anticonvulsant mechanism because this property is shared with several other anticonvulsants in addition to phenytoin.

5.2 Pharmacokinetic properties

Fosphenytoin is a pro-drug of phenytoin and it is rapidly converted into phenytoin mole for mole.

Fosphenytoin Pharmacokinetics

Absorption/Bioavailability:

When Pro-Epanutin is administered by IV infusion, maximum plasma fosphenytoin concentrations are achieved at the end of the infusion. Fosphenytoin is completely bioavailable following IM administration of Pro-Epanutin. Peak concentrations occur at approximately 30 minutes post-dose. Plasma fosphenytoin concentrations following IM administration are lower but more sustained than those following IV administration due to the time required for absorption of fosphenytoin from the injection site.

Distribution:

Fosphenytoin is extensively bound (95% to 99%) to human plasma proteins, primarily albumin. Binding to plasma proteins is saturable with the result that the fraction unbound increases as total fosphenytoin concentrations increase. Fosphenytoin displaces phenytoin from protein binding sites. The volume of distribution of fosphenytoin increases with fosphenytoin sodium dose and rate and ranges from 4.3 to 10.8L.

Metabolism and Excretion:

The hydrolysis of fosphenytoin to phenytoin yields 2 metabolites, phosphate and formaldehyde. Formaldehyde is subsequently converted to formate, which is in turn metabolised via a folate dependent mechanism. Although phosphate and formaldehyde (formate) have potentially important biological effects, these effects typically occur at concentrations considerably in excess of those obtained when Pro-Epanutin is administered under conditions of use recommended in this labelling.

The conversion half-life of fosphenytoin to phenytoin is approximately 15 minutes. The mechanism of fosphenytoin conversion has not been determined but phosphatases probably play a major role. Each mmol of fosphenytoin is metabolised to 1mmol of phenytoin, phosphate and formate.

Fosphenytoin is not excreted in urine.

Phenytoin Pharmacokinetics (after Pro-Epanutin administration):

The pharmacokinetics of phenytoin following IV administration of Pro-Epanutin, are complex and when used in an emergency setting (e.g. status epilepticus), differences in rate of availability of phenytoin could be critical. Studies have, therefore, empirically determined an infusion rate for Pro-Epanutin that gives a rate and extent of phenytoin systemic availability similar to that of a 50mg/min phenytoin sodium infusion. Because Pro-Epanutin is completely absorbed and converted to phenytoin following IM administration, systemic phenytoin concentrations are generated that are similar enough to oral phenytoin to allow essentially interchangeable use and to allow reliable IM loading dose administration.

The following table displays pharmacokinetic parameters of fosphenytoin and phenytoin following IV and IM Pro-Epanutin administration.

Mean Pharmacokinetic Parameter Values by Route of Pro-Epanutin Administration.

(see Table 11 below)

Absorption/Bioavailability:

Fosphenytoin sodium is rapidly and completely converted to phenytoin following IV or IM Pro-Epanutin administration. Therefore, the bioavailability of phenytoin following administration of Pro-Epanutin is the same as that following parenteral administration of phenytoin.

Distribution:

Phenytoin is highly bound to plasma proteins, primarily albumin, although to a lesser extent than fosphenytoin. In the absence of fosphenytoin, approximately 12% of total plasma phenytoin is unbound over the clinically relevant concentration range. However, fosphenytoin displaces phenytoin from plasma protein binding sites. This increases the fraction of phenytoin unbound (up to 30% unbound) during the period required for conversion of fosphenytoin to phenytoin (approximately 0.5 to 1 hour postinfusion).

The volume of distribution for phenytoin ranges from 24.9 to 36.8L.

Metabolism and Excretion:

Phenytoin derived from administration of Pro-Epanutin is extensively metabolised in the liver and excreted in urine primarily as 5-(p-hydroxy-phenyl)-5-phenylhydantoin and its glucuronide; little unchanged phenytoin (1%-5% of the Pro-Epanutin dose) is recovered in urine. Phenytoin hepatic metabolism is saturable and, following administration of single IV Pro-Epanutin doses of 400 to 1200mg PE, total and unbound phenytoin AUC values increase disproportionately with dose. Mean total phenytoin half-life values (12.0 to 28.9 hr) following Pro-Epanutin administration at these doses are similar to those after equal doses of parenteral phenytoin and tend to be longer at higher plasma phenytoin concentrations.

Characteristics in Patients

Patients with Renal or Hepatic Disease:

Fosphenytoin conversion to phenytoin is more rapid in patients with renal or hepatic disease than with other patients because of decreased plasma protein binding, secondary to hypoalbuminaemia, occurring in these disease states. The extent of conversion to phenytoin is not affected. Phenytoin metabolism may be reduced in patients with hepatic impairment resulting in increased plasma phenytoin concentrations **(see Section 4.2 Posology and Method of Administration)**.

Elderly Patients:

Patient age had no significant impact on fosphenytoin pharmacokinetics. Phenytoin clearance tends to decrease with increasing age (20% less in patients over 70 years of age relative to that in patients 20-30 years of age) **(see Section 4.2 Posology and Method of Administration)**.

Gender:

Gender had no significant impact on fosphenytoin or phenytoin pharmacokinetics.

Children:

Limited studies in children (age 5 to 10) receiving Pro-Epanutin have shown similar concentration-time profiles of fosphenytoin and phenytoin to those observed in adult patients receiving comparable mg PE/kg doses.

5.3 Preclinical safety data

The systemic toxicity of fosphenytoin is qualitatively and quantitatively similar to that of phenytoin at comparable exposures.

Carcinogenicity studies with fosphenytoin are not available. Since fosphenytoin is a prodrug of phenytoin, the carcinogenicity results with phenytoin can be extrapolated. An increased incidence of hepatocellular tumors was observed after administration of phenytoin in 1 of 3 studies in rats and 2 of 3 studies in mice. Lymphomas were also observed in susceptible strains of mice. These rodent tumors are of uncertain clinical significance.

Genetic toxicity studies showed that fosphenytoin was not mutagenic in bacteria or in mammalian cells *in vitro*. It was clastogenic in cultured V79 Chinese hamster lung cells in the presence of metabolic activation, but not in an *in vivo* mouse bone marrow micronucleus test. Phenytoin is not genotoxic *in vivo*.

Local irritation following IV or IM dosing or inadvertent perivenous administration was less severe with fosphenytoin than with phenytoin and was generally comparable to that observed with vehicle injections. The potential of fosphenytoin to induce intra-arterial irritation was not assessed.

6. PHARMACEUTICAL PARTICULARS

6.1 List of excipients

Water for injection, trometamol buffer adjusted to pH 8.6 to 9.0 with hydrochloric acid.

6.2 Incompatibilities

This medicinal product must not be mixed with other medicinal products except those mentioned in Section 6.6.

6.3 Shelf life

2 years.

6.4 Special precautions for storage

Store at 2°C to 8°C (under refrigeration). The undiluted product may be stored at room temperature (8°C to 25°C) for up to 24 hours.

6.5 Nature and contents of container

10ml sulphur treated Type I glass vials (10ml solution) with a Teflon coated stopper, an aluminium seal and flip-off cap.

Boxes of 10 vials with 10ml solution for injection.

6.6 Special precautions for disposal and other handling

Pro-Epanutin must be diluted to a concentration ranging from 1.5 to 25mg PE/ml prior to infusion, with 5% glucose or 0.9% saline solution for injection. See Section 4.2 for dilution information. After dilution Pro-Epanutin is suitable only for immediate use.

For single use only. After opening, unused product should be discarded.

Vials that develop particulate matter should not be used.

7. MARKETING AUTHORISATION HOLDER

United Kingdom:

Pfizer Limited,

Sandwich,

Kent,

CT13 9NJ

Ireland:

Pfizer Healthcare Ireland,

9 Riverwalk,

National Digital Park,

Citywest Business Campus,

Dublin 24, Ireland.

Pro-Epanutin is distributed in the UK by Blackstaff Pharmaceuticals Limited.

8. MARKETING AUTHORISATION NUMBER(S)

PL 00057/0551

PA 822/19/1

9. DATE OF FIRST AUTHORISATION/RENEWAL OF THE AUTHORISATION

UK: 28th July 2004

Ireland: 2nd July 2004

10. DATE OF REVISION OF THE TEXT

December 2008

Ref: PJ6_0

Table 11 Mean Pharmacokinetic Parameter Values by Route of Pro-Epanutin Administration

				Fosphenytoin			Total Phenytoin		Free (Unbound) Phenytoin	
Route	**Dose (mg PE)**	**Dose (mg PE/kg)**	**Infusion Rate (mg PE/min)**	**Cmax (µg/ml)**	**tmax (hr)**	**t½ (min)**	**Cmax (µg/ml)**	**tmax (hr)**	**Cmax (µg/ml)**	**tmax (hr)**
Intramuscular	855	12.4	–	18.5	0.61	41.2	14.3	3.23	2.02	4.16
Intravenous	1200	15.6	100	139	0.19	18.9	26.9	1.18	2.78	0.52
Intravenous	1200	15.6	150	156	0.13	20.5	28.2	0.98	3.18	0.58

Dose = Fosphenytoin dose (phenytoin sodium equivalents [mgPE] or phenytoin sodium equivalents/kg [mg PE/kg]).

Infusion Rate = Fosphenytoin infusion rate (mg phenytoin sodium equivalents/min [mg PE/min]).

Cmax = Maximum plasma analyte concentration (µg/ml).

tmax = Time of Cmax (hr).

t½ = Terminal elimination half-life (min).

Proflex Pain Relief Cream

(Novartis Consumer Health)

1. NAME OF THE MEDICINAL PRODUCT

Proflex ®Cream

Proflex® Pain Relief Cream

2. QUALITATIVE AND QUANTITATIVE COMPOSITION

Active ingredient: Ibuprofen BP 5%

For excipients, see Section 6.1.

3. PHARMACEUTICAL FORM

Cream

4. CLINICAL PARTICULARS

4.1 Therapeutic indications

Topical analgesic and anti-inflammatory treatment for the fast relief of the symptoms of rheumatic pain, muscular aches and pains, backache, lumbago, fibrositis, pains or swellings such as strains, sprains, and sports injuries.

Route of Administration

Topical.

4.2 Posology and method of administration

Adults and elderly:

4-10 cm (1½-4 inches) of cream (50-125mg ibuprofen) 3-4 times daily, massaged into the skin over a large area at the affected site. A period of at least 4 hours should be left between each application.

Children:

Not recommended for children under 12 years

Label/Leaflet directionsfor Proflex Pain Relief Cream:

Gently massage a thin layer of cream into the affected area. Repeat 3 or 4 times daily. Do not use under occlusive dressings without consulting your doctor or pharmacist.

4.3 Contraindications

Hypersensitivity to any of the constituents. Hypersensitivity to aspirin or other non-steroidal anti-inflammatory drugs including provocation or exacerbation of asthma, rhinitis, or urticaria.

4.4 Special warnings and precautions for use

Label warnings -

Do not use if you are allergic to ibuprofen or any of the ingredients of Proflex Pain Relief Cream, aspirin or any other painkillers.

Not recommended for children under 12 years. If symptoms persist, consult your doctor or pharmacist. Consult your doctor before use if you are asthmatic, pregnant, are taking aspirin or any other pain relieving or regular medication.

Keep away from inflamed or broken skin, lips and near the eyes. Discontinue if rash develops.

For external use only.

Wash hands after use.

Do not exceed the maximum dose.

Keep out of the reach of children.

4.5 Interaction with other medicinal products and other forms of interaction

Concurrent aspirin or other NSAIDs may result in an increased incidence of adverse reactions.

Experimental data suggest that ibuprofen may inhibit the effect of low dose aspirin on platelet aggregation when they are dosed concomitantly. However, the limitation of these data and the uncertainties regarding extrapolation of ex-vivo data to the clinical situation imply that no firm conclusions can be made for regular ibuprofen use, and no clinically relevant effect is considered to be likely for occasional ibuprofen use (see section 5.1)

4.6 Pregnancy and lactation

Whilst no teratogenic effects have been demonstrated in animal experiments, ibuprofen should be avoided during pregnancy. The onset of labour may be delayed and duration of labour may be increased. Ibuprofen appears in breast milk in very low concentration and is unlikely to affect the breast-fed infant adversely.

4.7 Effects on ability to drive and use machines

Proflex Cream/Proflex Pain Relief Cream will not impair the ability to drive and the ability to use machines.

4.8 Undesirable effects

Skin reactions are most frequently reported.

Skin:

Application site reactions, (see Hypersensitivity for other skin reactions).

Gastro-intestinal:

Abdominal pain, dyspepsia.

Respiratory:

Bronchospasm may be precipitated in patients suffering from or with a previous history of bronchial asthma.

Hypersensitivity:

Hypersensitivity reactions have been reported following treatment with ibuprofen. These may consist of (a) non-specific allergic reaction and anaphylaxis, (b) respiratory tract reactivity comprising of asthma, aggravated asthma, bronchospasm or dyspnoea, or (c) assorted skin disorders, including rashes of various types, pruritus, urticaria, purpura, angiodema and, less commonly, bullous dermatoses (including epidermal necrolysis and erythema multiforme).

4.9 Overdose

Overdosage with a topical presentation of ibuprofen is unlikely. Symptoms of ibuprofen overdose include headache, vomiting, drowsiness and hypotension. Correction of severe electrolyte abnormalities should be considered.

5. PHARMACOLOGICAL PROPERTIES

5.1 Pharmacodynamic properties

Ibuprofen is a phenylpropionic acid derivative which has analgesic anti-inflammatory and anti-pyretic actions.

Experimental data suggest that ibuprofen may inhibit the effect of low dose aspirin on platelet aggregation when they are dosed concomitantly. In one study, when a single dose of ibuprofen 400mg was taken within 8 hours before or within 30 minutes after immediate release aspirin dosing (81mg), a decreased effect of aspirin on the formation of thromboxane or platelet aggregation occurred. However, the limitations of these data and the uncertainties regarding extrapolation of *ex vivo* data to the clinical situation imply that no firm conclusions can be made for regular ibuprofen use and no clinically relevant effect is considered to be likely for occasional ibuprofen use.

5.2 Pharmacokinetic properties

Percutaneous absorption approximately 5% that of oral ibuprofen.

Cmax = 0.64 μg/ml (higher concentrations achieved locally)

Tmax = 2.00h

5.3 Preclinical safety data

Not applicable.

6. PHARMACEUTICAL PARTICULARS

6.1 List of excipients

Fractionated coconut oil

Arlacel 165

Arlatone 983S

Propylene glycol

Sodium methyl hydroxybenzoate

Keltrol F

Purified water

6.2 Incompatibilities

None stated.

6.3 Shelf life

36 months.

6.4 Special precautions for storage

Store in a cool place.

6.5 Nature and contents of container

Internally lacquered aluminium tube.

Pack sizes: 5, 10, 15, 20, 25, 30, 50, 60 and 100.

6.6 Special precautions for disposal and other handling

Keep all medicines out of the reach of children.

For external use only.

Wash hands after use.

7. MARKETING AUTHORISATION HOLDER

Novartis Consumer Health UK Ltd

Wimblehurst Road

Horsham

West Sussex, RH12 5AB.

Trading Style: Novartis Consumer Health

8. MARKETING AUTHORISATION NUMBER(S)

PL 00030/0052

9. DATE OF FIRST AUTHORISATION/RENEWAL OF THE AUTHORISATION

11 September 1990/13 May 2003

10. DATE OF REVISION OF THE TEXT

24th November 2008

Legal category: 30g pack GSL; 100g pack P

Prograf 0.5mg, 1mg, 5mg Hard Capsules

(Astellas Pharma Ltd)

1. NAME OF THE MEDICINAL PRODUCT

Prograf 0.5 mg hard capsules

Prograf 1 mg hard capsules

Prograf 5 mg hard capsules

2. QUALITATIVE AND QUANTITATIVE COMPOSITION

Prograf 0.5 mg hard capsules

Each capsule contains 0.5 mg of tacrolimus (as monohydrate).

Excipient: 62.85 mg of lactose monohydrate

Prograf 1 mg hard capsules

Each capsule contains 1 mg of tacrolimus (as monohydrate).

Excipient: 61.35 mg of lactose monohydrate

Prograf 5 mg hard capsules

Each capsule contains 5 mg of tacrolimus (as monohydrate).

Excipient: 123.60 mg of lactose monohydrate

For a full list of excipients, see section 6.1.

3. PHARMACEUTICAL FORM

Prograf 0.5 mg hard capsules

Capsule, hard

Opaque light yellow hard gelatin capsules imprinted in red with "0.5 mg" and "[f] 607", containing white powder.

Prograf 1 mg hard capsules

Capsule, hard

Opaque white hard gelatin capsules imprinted in red with "1 mg" and "[f] 617", containing white powder.

Prograf 5 mg hard capsules

Capsule, hard

Opaque greyish red hard gelatin capsules imprinted in white with "5 mg" and "[f] 657", containing white powder.

4. CLINICAL PARTICULARS

4.1 Therapeutic indications

Prophylaxis of transplant rejection in liver, kidney or heart allograft recipients.

Treatment of allograft rejection resistant to treatment with other immunosuppressive medicinal products.

4.2 Posology and method of administration

Prograf therapy requires careful monitoring by adequately qualified and equipped personnel. The medicinal product should only be prescribed, and changes in immunosuppressive therapy initiated, by physicians experienced in immunosuppressive therapy and the management of transplant patients.

Inadvertent, unintentional or unsupervised switching of immediate- or prolonged-release formulations of tacrolimus is unsafe. This can lead to graft rejection or increased incidence of side effects, including under- or over immunosuppression, due to clinically relevant differences in systemic exposure to tacrolimus. Patients should be maintained on a single formulation of tacrolimus with the corresponding daily dosing regimen; alterations in formulation or regimen should only take place under the close supervision of a transplant specialist (see sections 4.4 and 4.8). Following conversion to any alternative formulation, therapeutic drug monitoring must be performed and dose adjustments made to ensure that systemic exposure to tacrolimus is maintained.

General considerations

The recommended initial dosages presented below are intended to act solely as a guideline. Prograf dosing should primarily be based on clinical assessments of rejection and tolerability in each patient individually aided by blood level monitoring (see below for recommended target whole blood trough concentrations). If clinical signs of rejection are apparent, alteration of the immunosuppressive regimen should be considered.

Prograf can be administered intravenously or orally. In general, dosing may commence orally; if necessary, by administering the capsule contents suspended in water, via nasogastric tubing.

Prograf is routinely administered in conjunction with other immunosuppressive agents in the initial post-operative period. The Prograf dose may vary depending upon the immunosuppressive regimen chosen.

Method of administration

It is recommended that the oral daily dose be administered in two divided doses (e.g. morning and evening). Capsules should be taken immediately following removal from the blister. Patients should be advised not to swallow the desiccant. The capsules should be swallowed with fluid (preferably water).

Capsules should generally be administered on an empty stomach or at least 1 hour before or 2 to 3 hours after a meal, to achieve maximal absorption (see section 5.2).

Duration of dosing

To suppress graft rejection, immunosuppression must be maintained; consequently, no limit to the duration of oral therapy can be given.

Dosage recommendations – Liver transplantation

Prophylaxis of transplant rejection - adults

Oral Prograf therapy should commence at 0.10 - 0.20 mg/kg/day administered as two divided doses (e.g. morning and evening). Administration should commence approximately 12 hours after the completion of surgery.

If the dose cannot be administered orally as a result of the clinical condition of the patient, intravenous therapy of 0.01 - 0.05 mg/kg/day should be initiated as a continuous 24-hour infusion.

Prophylaxis of transplant rejection - children

An initial oral dose of 0.30 mg/kg/day should be administered in two divided doses (e.g. morning and evening). If the clinical condition of the patient prevents oral dosing, an initial intravenous dose of 0.05 mg/kg/day should be administered as a continuous 24-hour infusion.

Dose adjustment during post-transplant period in adults and children

Prograf doses are usually reduced in the post-transplant period. It is possible in some cases to withdraw concomitant immunosuppressive therapy, leading to Prograf monotherapy. Post-transplant improvement in the condition of the patient may alter the pharmacokinetics of tacrolimus and may necessitate further dose adjustments.

Rejection therapy – adults and children

Increased Prograf doses, supplemental corticosteroid therapy, and introduction of short courses of mono-/polyclonal antibodies have all been used to manage rejection episodes. If signs of toxicity are noted (e.g. pronounced adverse reactions - see section 4.8) the dose of Prograf may need to be reduced.

For conversion to Prograf, treatment should begin with the initial oral dose recommended for primary immunosuppression.

For information on conversion from ciclosporin to Prograf, see below under "Dose adjustments in specific patient populations".

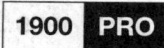

Dosage recommendations - Kidney transplantation

Prophylaxis of transplant rejection – adults

Oral Prograf therapy should commence at 0.20 - 0.30 mg/kg/day administered as two divided doses (e.g. morning and evening). Administration should commence within 24 hours after the completion of surgery.

If the dose cannot be administered orally as a result of the clinical condition of the patient, intravenous therapy of 0.05 - 0.10 mg/kg/day should be initiated as a continuous 24-hour infusion.

Prophylaxis of transplant rejection – children

An initial oral dose of 0.30mg/kg/day should be administered in two divided doses (e.g. morning and evening). If the clinical condition of the patient prevents oral dosing, an initial intravenous dose of 0.075–0.100 mg/kg/day should be administered as a continuous 24-hour infusion.

Dose adjustment during post-transplant period in adults and children

Prograf doses are usually reduced in the post-transplant period. It is possible in some cases to withdraw concomitant immunosuppressive therapy, leading to Prograf-based dual-therapy. Post-transplant improvement in the condition of the patient may alter the pharmacokinetics of tacrolimus and may necessitate further dose adjustments.

Rejection therapy – adults and children

Increased Prograf doses, supplemental corticosteroid therapy, and introduction of short courses of mono-/polyclonal antibodies have all been used to manage rejection episodes. If signs of toxicity are noted (e.g. pronounced adverse reactions - see section 4.8) the dose of Prograf may need to be reduced.

For conversion to Prograf, treatment should begin with the initial oral dose recommended for primary immunosuppression.

For information on conversion from ciclosporin to Prograf, see below under "Dose adjustments in specific patient populations".

Dosage recommendations - Heart transplantation

Prophylaxis of transplant rejection – adults

Prograf can be used with antibody induction (allowing for delayed start of Prograf therapy) or alternatively in clinically stable patients without antibody induction.

Following antibody induction, oral Prograf therapy should commence at a dose of 0.075 mg/kg/day administered as two divided doses (e.g. morning and evening). Administration should commence within 5 days after the completion of surgery as soon as the patient's clinical condition is stabilised. If the dose cannot be administered orally as a result of the clinical condition of the patient, intravenous therapy of 0.01 to 0.02 mg/kg/day should be initiated as a continuous 24-hour infusion.

An alternative strategy was published where oral tacrolimus was administered within 12 hours post transplantation. This approach was reserved for patients without organ dysfunction (e.g. renal dysfunction). In that case, an initial oral tacrolimus dose of 2 to 4 mg per day was used in combination with mycophenolate mofetil and corticosteroids or in combination with sirolimus and corticosteroids.

Prophylaxis of transplant rejection – children

Prograf has been used with or without antibody induction in paediatric heart transplantation.

In patients without antibody induction, if Prograf therapy is initiated intravenously, the recommended starting dose is 0.03 - 0.05 mg/kg/day as a continuous 24-hour infusion targeted to achieve tacrolimus whole blood concentrations of 15 - 25 ng/ml. Patients should be converted to oral therapy as soon as clinically practicable. The first dose of oral therapy should be 0.30 mg/kg/day starting 8 to 12 hours after discontinuing intravenous therapy.

Following antibody induction, if Prograf therapy is initiated orally, the recommended starting dose is 0.10 - 0.30 mg/kg/day administered as two divided doses (e.g. morning and evening).

Dose adjustment during post-transplant period in adults and children

Prograf doses are usually reduced in the post-transplant period. Post-transplant improvement in the condition of the patient may alter the pharmacokinetics of tacrolimus and may necessitate further dose adjustments.

Rejection therapy – adults and children

Increased Prograf doses, supplemental corticosteroid therapy, and introduction of short courses of mono-/polyclonal antibodies have all been used to manage rejection episodes.

In adult patients converted to Prograf, an initial oral dose of 0.15 mg/kg/day should be administered in two divided doses (e.g. morning and evening).

In paediatric patients converted to Prograf, an initial oral dose of 0.20 - 0.30 mg/kg/day should be administered in two divided doses (e.g. morning and evening).

For information on conversion from ciclosporin to Prograf, see below under "Dose adjustments in specific patient populations".

Dosage recommendations - Rejection therapy, other allografts

The dose recommendations for lung, pancreas and intestinal transplantation are based on limited prospective clinical trial data. In lung-transplanted patients Prograf has been used at an initial oral dose of 0.10 - 0.15 mg/kg/day, in pancreas-transplanted patients at an initial oral dose of 0.2 mg/kg/day and in intestinal transplantation at an initial oral dose of 0.3 mg/kg/day.

Dosage adjustments in specific patient populations

Patients with liver impairment

Dose reduction may be necessary in patients with severe liver impairment in order to maintain the blood trough levels within the recommended target range.

Patients with kidney impairment

As the pharmacokinetics of tacrolimus are unaffected by renal function, no dose adjustment should be required. However, owing to the nephrotoxic potential of tacrolimus careful monitoring of renal function is recommended (including serial serum creatinine concentrations, calculation of creatinine clearance and monitoring of urine output).

Paediatric patients

In general, paediatric patients require doses 1½ - 2 times higher than the adult doses to achieve similar blood levels.

Elderly patients

There is no evidence currently available to indicate that dosing should be adjusted in elderly patients.

Conversion from ciclosporin

Care should be taken when converting patients from ciclosporin-based to Prograf-based therapy (see sections 4.4 and 4.5). Prograf therapy should be initiated after considering ciclosporin blood concentrations and the clinical condition of the patient. Dosing should be delayed in the presence of elevated ciclosporin blood levels. In practice, Prograf therapy has been initiated 12 - 24 hours after discontinuation of ciclosporin. Monitoring of ciclosporin blood levels should be continued following conversion as the clearance of ciclosporin might be affected.

Target whole blood trough concentration recommendations

Dosing should primarily be based on clinical assessments of rejection and tolerability in each individual patient.

As an aid to optimise dosing, several immunoassays are available for determining tacrolimus concentrations in whole blood including a semi-automated microparticle enzyme immunoassay (MEIA). Comparisons of concentrations from the published literature to individual values in clinical practice should be assessed with care and knowledge of the assay methods employed. In current clinical practice, whole blood levels are monitored using immunoassay methods.

Blood trough levels of tacrolimus should be monitored during the post-transplantation period. When dosed orally, blood trough levels should be drawn approximately 12 hours post-dosing, just prior to the next dose. The frequency of blood level monitoring should be based on clinical needs. As Prograf is a medicinal product with low clearance, adjustments to the dosage regimen may take several days before changes in blood levels are apparent. Blood trough levels should be monitored approximately twice weekly during the early post-transplant period and then periodically during maintenance therapy. Blood trough levels of tacrolimus should also be monitored following dose adjustment, changes in the immunosuppressive regimen, or following co-administration of substances which may alter tacrolimus whole blood concentrations (see section 4.5).

Clinical study analysis suggests that the majority of patients can be successfully managed if tacrolimus blood trough levels are maintained below 20 ng/ml. It is necessary to consider the clinical condition of the patient when interpreting whole blood levels.

In clinical practice, whole blood trough levels have generally been in the range 5 - 20 ng/ml in liver transplant recipients and 10 - 20 ng/ml in kidney and heart transplant patients in the early post-transplant period. Subsequently, during maintenance therapy, blood concentrations have generally been in the range of 5 - 15 ng/ml in liver, kidney and heart transplant recipients.

4.3 Contraindications

Hypersensitivity to tacrolimus or other macrolides.

Hypersensitivity to any of the excipients.

4.4 Special warnings and precautions for use

During the initial post-transplant period, monitoring of the following parameters should be undertaken on a routine basis: blood pressure, ECG, neurological and visual status, fasting blood glucose levels, electrolytes (particularly potassium), liver and renal function tests, haematology parameters, coagulation values, and plasma protein determinations. If clinically relevant changes are seen, adjustments of the immunosuppressive regimen should be considered.

Medication errors, including inadvertent, unintentional or unsupervised substitution of immediate- or prolonged-release tacrolimus formulations, have been observed. This has led to serious adverse events, including graft rejection, or other side effects which could be a consequence of either under- or over-exposure to tacrolimus. Patients should be maintained on a single formulation of tacrolimus with the corresponding daily dosing regimen; alterations in formulation or regimen should only take place under the close supervision of a transplant specialist (see sections 4.2 and 4.8).

Herbal preparations containing St. John's wort (Hypericum perforatum) or other herbal preparations should be avoided when taking Prograf due to the risk of interactions that lead to decrease in blood concentrations of tacrolimus and reduced clinical effect of tacrolimus (see section 4.5 Interactions with other medicinal products and other forms of interactions).

Since levels of tacrolimus in blood may significantly change during diarrhoea episodes, extra monitoring of tacrolimus concentrations is recommended during episodes of diarrhoea.

The combined administration of ciclosporin and tacrolimus should be avoided and care should be taken when administering tacrolimus to patients who have previously received ciclosporin (see sections 4.2 and 4.5).

Ventricular hypertrophy or hypertrophy of the septum, reported as cardiomyopathies, have been observed on rare occasions. Most cases have been reversible, occurring primarily in children with tacrolimus blood trough concentrations much higher than the recommended maximum levels. Other factors observed to increase the risk of these clinical conditions included pre-existing heart disease, corticosteroid usage, hypertension, renal or hepatic dysfunction, infections, fluid overload, and oedema. Accordingly, high-risk patients, particularly young children and those receiving substantial immunosuppression should be monitored, using such procedures as echocardiography or ECG pre- and post-transplant (e.g. initially at three months and then at 9-12 months). If abnormalities develop, dose reduction of Prograf therapy, or change of treatment to another immunosuppressive agent should be considered. Tacrolimus may prolong the QT interval but at this time lacks substantial evidence for causing Torsades de Pointes. Caution should be exercised in patients with diagnosed or suspected Congenital Long QT Syndrome.

Patients treated with Prograf have been reported to develop EBV-associated lymphoproliferative disorders. Patients switched to Prograf therapy should not receive anti-lymphocyte treatment concomitantly. Very young (< 2 years), EBV-VCA-negative children have been reported to have an increased risk of developing lymphoproliferative disorders. Therefore, in this patient group, EBV-VCA serology should be ascertained before starting treatment with Prograf. During treatment, careful monitoring with EBV-PCR is recommended. Positive EBV-PCR may persist for months and is per se not indicative of lymphoproliferative disease or lymphoma.

Patients treated with tacrolimus have been reported to develop posterior reversible encephalopathy syndrome (PRES). If patients taking tacrolimus present with symptoms indicating PRES such as headache, altered mental status, seizures, and visual disturbances, a radiological procedure (e.g. MRI) should be performed. If PRES is diagnosed, adequate blood pressure control and immediate discontinuation of systemic tacrolimus is advised. Most patients completely recover after appropriate measures are taken.

Patients treated with immunosuppressants, including Prograf are at increased risk of opportunistic infections (bacterial, fungal, viral and protozoal). Among these conditions are BK virus associated nephropathy and JC virus associated progressive multifocal leukoencephalopathy (PML). These infections are often related to a high total immunosuppressive burden and may lead to serious or fatal conditions that physicians should consider in patients with deteriorating renal function or neurological symptoms.

As with other immunosuppressive agents, owing to the potential risk of malignant skin changes, exposure to sunlight and UV light should be limited by wearing protective clothing and using a sunscreen with a high protection factor.

As with other potent immunosuppressive compounds, the risk of secondary cancer is unknown (see section 4.8).

As Prograf contains lactose, special care should be taken in patients with rare hereditary problems of galactose intolerance, the Lapp lactase deficiency or glucose-galactose malabsorption.

4.5 Interaction with other medicinal products and other forms of interaction

Metabolic interactions

Systemically available tacrolimus is metabolised by hepatic CYP3A4. There is also evidence of gastrointestinal metabolism by CYP3A4 in the intestinal wall. Concomitant use of medicinal products or herbal remedies known to inhibit or induce CYP3A4 may affect the metabolism of tacrolimus and thereby increase or decrease tacrolimus blood levels. It is therefore recommended to monitor tacrolimus blood levels whenever substances which have the potential to alter CYP3A metabolism are used concomitantly and to adjust the tacrolimus dose as appropriate in order to maintain similar tacrolimus exposure (see sections 4.2 and 4.4).

Inhibitors of metabolism

Clinically the following substances have been shown to increase tacrolimus blood levels:

Strong interactions have been observed with antifungal agents such as ketoconazole, fluconazole, itraconazole and voriconazole, the macrolide antibiotic erythromycin or HIV protease inhibitors (e.g. ritonavir). Concomitant use of these substances may require decreased tacrolimus doses in nearly all patients.

Weaker interactions have been observed with clotrimazole, clarithromycin, josamycin, nifedipine, nicardipine, diltiazem, verapamil, danazol, ethinylestradiol, omeprazole and nefazodone.

In vitro the following substances have been shown to be potential inhibitors of tacrolimus metabolism: bromocriptine, cortisone, dapsone, ergotamine, gestodene, lidocaine, mephenytoin, miconazole, midazolam, nilvadipine, norethisterone, quinidine, tamoxifen, troleandomycin.

Grapefruit juice has been reported to increase the blood level of tacrolimus and should therefore be avoided.

Inducers of metabolism

Clinically the following substances have been shown to decrease tacrolimus blood levels:

Strong interactions have been observed with rifampicin, phenytoin or St. John's Wort (Hypericum perforatum) which may require increased tacrolimus doses in almost all patients. Clinically significant interactions have also been observed with phenobarbital. Maintenance doses of corticosteroids have been shown to reduce tacrolimus blood levels.

High dose prednisolone or methylprednisolone administered for the treatment of acute rejection have the potential to increase or decrease tacrolimus blood levels.

Carbamazepine, metamizole and isoniazid have the potential to decrease tacrolimus concentrations.

Effect of tacrolimus on the metabolism of other medicinal products

Tacrolimus is a known CYP3A4 inhibitor; thus concomitant use of tacrolimus with medicinal products known to be metabolised by CYP3A4 may affect the metabolism of such medicinal products.

The half-life of ciclosporin is prolonged when tacrolimus is given concomitantly. In addition, synergistic/additive nephrotoxic effects can occur. For these reasons, the combined administration of ciclosporin and tacrolimus is not recommended and care should be taken when administering tacrolimus to patients who have previously received ciclosporin (see sections 4.2 and 4.4).

Tacrolimus has been shown to increase the blood level of phenytoin.

As tacrolimus may reduce the clearance of steroid-based contraceptives leading to increased hormone exposure, particular care should be exercised when deciding upon contraceptive measures.

Limited knowledge of interactions between tacrolimus and statins is available. Available data suggests that the pharmacokinetics of statins are largely unaltered by the co-administration of tacrolimus.

Animal data have shown that tacrolimus could potentially decrease the clearance and increase the half-life of pentobarbital and phenazone.

Other interactions which have led to clinically detrimental effects

Concurrent use of tacrolimus with medicinal products known to have nephrotoxic or neurotoxic effects may increase these effects (e.g., aminoglycosides, gyrase inhibitors, vancomycin, sulfamethoxazole+trimethoprim, NSAIDs, ganciclovir or aciclovir).

Enhanced nephrotoxicity has been observed following the administration of amphotericin B and ibuprofen in conjunction with tacrolimus.

As tacrolimus treatment may be associated with hyperkalaemia, or may increase pre-existing hyperkalaemia, high potassium intake, or potassium-sparing diuretics (e.g., amiloride, triamterene, or spironolactone) should be avoided.

Immunosuppressants may affect the response to vaccination and vaccination during treatment with tacrolimus may be less effective. The use of live attenuated vaccines should be avoided.

Protein binding considerations

Tacrolimus is extensively bound to plasma proteins. Possible interactions with other medicinal products known to have high affinity for plasma proteins should be considered (e.g., NSAIDs, oral anticoagulants, or oral antidiabetics).

4.6 Pregnancy and lactation

Human data show that tacrolimus is able to cross the placenta. Limited data from organ transplant recipients show no evidence of an increased risk of adverse effects on the course and outcome of pregnancy under tacrolimus treatment compared with other immunosuppressive medicinal products. To date, no other relevant epidemiological data are available. Due to the need of treatment, tacrolimus can be considered in pregnant women when there is no safer alternative and when the perceived benefit justifies the potential risk to the foetus. In case of *in utero* exposure, monitoring of the newborn for the potential adverse effects of tacrolimus is recommended (in particular the effects on the kidneys). There is a risk for premature delivery (<37 week) as well as for hyperkalaemia in the newborn, which, however, normalizes spontaneously.

In rats and rabbits, tacrolimus caused embryofoetal toxicity at doses which demonstrated maternal toxicity (see section 5.3). Tacrolimus affected male fertility in rats (see section 5.3).

Lactation

Human data demonstrate that tacrolimus is excreted into breast milk. As detrimental effects on the newborn cannot be excluded, women should not breast-feed whilst receiving Prograf.

4.7 Effects on ability to drive and use machines

Tacrolimus may cause visual and neurological disturbances. This effect may be enhanced if Prograf is administered in association with alcohol.

4.8 Undesirable effects

The adverse drug reaction profile associated with immunosuppressive agents is often difficult to establish owing to the underlying disease and the concurrent use of multiple medications.

Many of the adverse drug reactions stated below are reversible and/or respond to dose reduction. Oral administration appears to be associated with a lower incidence of adverse drug reactions compared with intravenous use. Adverse drug reactions are listed below in descending order by frequency of occurrence: very common (≥1/10); common (≥1/100, <1/10); uncommon (≥1/1,000, <1/100); rare (≥1/10,000, <1/1,000); very rare (<1/10,000); not known (cannot be estimated from the available data).

Cardiac disorders

common: ischaemic coronary artery disorders, tachycardia

uncommon: ventricular arrhythmias and cardiac arrest, heart failures, cardiomyopathies, ventricular hypertrophy, supraventricular arrhythmias, palpitations, ECG investigations abnormal, heart rate and pulse investigations abnormal

rare: pericardial effusion

very rare: echocardiogram abnormal

Blood and lymphatic system disorders

common: anaemia, leukopenia, thrombocytopenia, leukocytosis, red blood cell analyses abnormal

uncommon: coagulopathies, coagulation and bleeding analyses abnormal, pancytopenia, neutropenia

rare: thrombotic thrombocytopenic purpura, hypoprothrombinaemia

Nervous system disorders

very common: tremor, headache

common: seizures, disturbances in consciousness, paraesthesias and dysaesthesias, peripheral neuropathies, dizziness, writing impaired, nervous system disorders

uncommon: coma, central nervous system haemorrhages and cerebrovascular accidents, paralysis and paresis, encephalopathy, speech and language abnormalities, amnesia

rare: hypertonia

very rare: myasthenia

Eye disorders

common: vision blurred, photophobia, eye disorders

uncommon: cataract

rare: blindness

Ear and labyrinth disorders

common: tinnitus

uncommon: hypoacusis

rare: deafness neurosensory

very rare: hearing impaired

Respiratory, thoracic and mediastinal disorders

common: dyspnoea, parenchymal lung disorders, pleural effusion, pharyngitis, cough, nasal congestion and inflammations

uncommon: respiratory failures, respiratory tract disorders, asthma

rare: acute respiratory distress syndrome

Gastrointestinal disorders

very common: diarrhoea, nausea

common: gastrointestinal inflammatory conditions, gastrointestinal ulceration and perforation, gastrointestinal haemorrhages, stomatitis and ulceration, ascites, vomiting, gastrointestinal and abdominal pains, dyspeptic signs and symptoms, constipation, flatulence, bloating and distension, loose stools, gastrointestinal signs and symptoms

uncommon: ileus paralytic, peritonitis, acute and chronic pancreatitis, blood amylase increased, gastrooesophageal reflux disease, impaired gastric emptying

rare: subileus, pancreatic pseudocyst

Renal and urinary disorders

very common: renal impairment

common: renal failure, renal failure acute, oliguria, renal tubular necrosis, nephropathy toxic, urinary abnormalities, bladder and urethral symptoms

uncommon: anuria, haemolytic uraemic syndrome

very rare: nephropathy, cystitis haemorrhagic

Skin and subcutaneous tissue disorders

common: pruritus, rash, alopecias, acne, sweating increased

uncommon: dermatitis, photosensitivity

rare: toxic epidermal necrolysis (Lyell's syndrome)

very rare: Stevens Johnson syndrome

Musculoskeletal and connective tissue disorders

common: arthralgia, muscle cramps, pain in limb, back pain

uncommon: joint disorders

Endocrine disorders

rare: hirsutism

Metabolism and nutrition disorders

very common: hyperglycaemic conditions, diabetes mellitus, hyperkalaemia

common: hypomagnesaemia, hypophosphataemia, hypokalaemia, hypocalcaemia, hyponatraemia, fluid overload, hyperuricaemia, appetite decreased, anorexia, metabolic acidoses, hyperlipidaemia, hypercholesterolaemia, hypertriglyceridaemia, other electrolyte abnormalities

uncommon: dehydration, hypoproteinaemia, hyperphosphataemia, hypoglycaemia

Infections and infestations

As is well known for other potent immunosuppressive agents, patients receiving tacrolimus are frequently at increased risk for infections (viral, bacterial, fungal, protozoal). The course of pre-existing infections may be aggravated. Both generalised and localised infections can occur.

Cases of BK virus associated nephropathy, as well as cases of JC virus associated progressive multifocal leukoencephalopathy (PML), have been reported in patients treated with immunosuppressants, including Prograf.

Injury, poisoning and procedural complications

common: primary graft dysfunction

Medication errors, including inadvertent, unintentional or unsupervised substitution of immediate- or prolonged-release tacrolimus formulations, have been observed. A number of associated cases of transplant rejection have been reported (frequency cannot be estimated from available data).

Neoplasms benign, malignant and unspecified (incl. cysts and polyps)

Patients receiving immunosuppressive therapy are at increased risk of developing malignancies. Benign as well as malignant neoplasms including EBV-associated lymphoproliferative disorders and skin malignancies have been reported in association with tacrolimus treatment.

Vascular disorders

very common: hypertension

common: haemorrhage, thrombembolic and ischaemic events, peripheral vascular disorders, vascular hypotensive disorders

uncommon: infarction, venous thrombosis deep limb, shock

General disorders and administration site conditions

common: asthenic conditions, febrile disorders, oedema, pain and discomfort, blood alkaline phosphatase increased, weight increased, body temperature perception disturbed

uncommon: multi-organ failure, influenza like illness, temperature intolerance, chest pressure sensation, feeling jittery, feeling abnormal, blood lactate dehydrogenase increased, weight decreased

rare: thirst, fall, chest tightness, mobility decreased, ulcer

very rare: fat tissue increased

Immune system disorders

Allergic and anaphylactoid reactions have been observed in patients receiving tacrolimus (see section 4.4).

Hepatobiliary disorders

common: hepatic enzymes and function abnormalities, cholestasis and jaundice, hepatocellular damage and hepatitis, cholangitis

rare: hepatic artery thrombosis, venoocclusive liver disease

very rare: hepatic failure, bile duct stenosis

Reproductive system and breast disorders

uncommon: dysmenorrhoea and uterine bleeding

Psychiatric disorders

very common: insomnia

common: anxiety symptoms, confusion and disorientation, depression, depressed mood, mood disorders and disturbances, nightmare, hallucination, mental disorders

uncommon: psychotic disorder

4.9 Overdose

Experience with overdosage is limited. Several cases of accidental overdosage have been reported; symptoms have included tremor, headache, nausea and vomiting, infections, urticaria, lethargy, increased blood urea nitrogen and elevated serum creatinine concentrations, and increase in alanine aminotransferase levels.

No specific antidote to Prograf therapy is available. If overdosage occurs, general supportive measures and symptomatic treatment should be conducted.

Based on its high molecular weight, poor aqueous solubility, and extensive erythrocyte and plasma protein binding, it is anticipated that tacrolimus will not be dialysable. In isolated patients with very high plasma levels, haemofiltration or -diafiltration have been effective in reducing toxic concentrations. In cases of oral intoxication, gastric lavage and/or the use of adsorbents (such as activated charcoal) may be helpful, if used shortly after intake.

5. PHARMACOLOGICAL PROPERTIES

5.1 Pharmacodynamic properties

Pharmacotherapeutic group: Calcineurin inhibitors, ATC code: L04AD02

Mechanism of action and pharmacodynamic effects

At the molecular level, the effects of tacrolimus appear to be mediated by binding to a cytosolic protein (FKBP12) which is responsible for the intracellular accumulation of the compound. The FKBP12-tacrolimus complex specifically and competitively binds to and inhibits calcineurin, leading to a calcium-dependent inhibition of T-cell signal transduction pathways, thereby preventing transcription of a discrete set of lymphokine genes.

Tacrolimus is a highly potent immunosuppressive agent and has proven activity in both *in vitro* and *in vivo* experiments.

In particular, tacrolimus inhibits the formation of cytotoxic lymphocytes, which are mainly responsible for graft rejection. Tacrolimus suppresses T-cell activation and T-helper-cell dependent B-cell proliferation, as well as the formation of lymphokines (such as interleukins-2, -3, and γ-interferon) and the expression of the interleukin-2 receptor.

Results from published data in other primary organ transplantation

Prograf has evolved into an accepted treatment as primary immunosuppressive medicinal product following pancreas, lung and intestinal transplantation. In prospective published studies tacrolimus was investigated as primary immunosuppressant in approximately 175 patients following lung, 475 patients following pancreas and 630 patients following intestinal transplantation. Overall, the safety profile of tacrolimus in these published studies appeared to be similar to what was reported in the large studies, where tacrolimus was used as primary treatment in liver, kidney and heart transplantation. Efficacy results of the largest studies in each indication are summarised below.

Lung transplantation

The interim analysis of a recent multicentre study discussed 110 patients who underwent 1:1 randomisation to either tacrolimus or ciclosporin. Tacrolimus was started as continuous intravenous infusion at a dose of 0.01 to 0.03 mg/kg/day and oral tacrolimus was administered at a dose of 0.05 to 0.3 mg/kg/day. A lower incidence of acute rejection episodes for tacrolimus- versus ciclosporin-treated patients (11.5% versus 22.6%) and a lower incidence of chronic rejection, the bronchiolitis obliterans syndrome (2.86% versus 8.57%), was reported within the first year after transplantation. The 1-year patient survival rate was 80.8% in the tacrolimus and 83% in the ciclosporin group (Treede et al., 3rd ICI San Diego, US, 2004;Abstract 22).

Another randomised study included 66 patients on tacrolimus versus 67 patients on ciclosporin. Tacrolimus was started as continuous intravenous infusion at a dose of 0.025 mg/kg/day and oral tacrolimus was administered at a dose of 0.15 mg/kg/day with subsequent dose adjustments to target trough levels of 10 to 20 ng/ml. The 1-year patient survival was 83% in the tacrolimus and 71% in the ciclosporin group, the 2-year survival rates were 76% and 66%, respectively. Acute rejection episodes per 100 patient-days were numerically fewer in the tacrolimus (0.85 episodes) than in the ciclosporin group (1.09 episodes). Obliterative bronchiolitis developed in 21.7% of patients in the tacrolimus group compared with 38.0% of patients in the ciclosporin group ($p = 0.025$). Significantly more ciclosporin-treated patients ($n = 13$) required a switch to tacrolimus than tacrolimus-treated patients to ciclosporin ($n = 2$) ($p = 0.02$) (Keenan et al., Ann Thoracic Surg 1995;60:580).

In an additional two-centre study, 26 patients were randomised to the tacrolimus versus 24 patients to the ciclosporin group. Tacrolimus was started as continuous intravenous infusion at a dose of 0.05 mg/kg/day and oral tacrolimus was administered at a dose of 0.1 to 0.3 mg/kg/day with subsequent dose adjustments to target trough levels of 12 to 15 ng/ml. The 1-year survival rates were 73.1% in the tacrolimus versus 79.2% in the ciclosporin group. Freedom from acute rejection was higher in the tacrolimus group at 6 months (57.7% versus 45.8%) and at 1 year after lung transplantation (50% versus 33.3%) (Treede et al., J Heart Lung Transplant 2001;20:511).

The three studies demonstrated similar survival rates. The incidences of acute rejection were numerically lower with tacrolimus in all three studies and one of the studies reported a significantly lower incidence of bronchiolitis obliterans syndrome with tacrolimus.

Pancreas transplantation

A multicentre study included 205 patients undergoing simultaneous pancreas-kidney transplantation who were randomised to tacrolimus (n=103) or to ciclosporin (n=102). The initial oral per protocol dose of tacrolimus was 0.2 mg/kg/day with subsequent dose adjustments to target trough levels of 8 to 15 ng/ml by Day 5 and 5 to 10 ng/mL after Month 6. Pancreas survival at 1 year was significantly superior with tacrolimus: 91.3% versus 74.5% with ciclosporin ($p < 0.0005$), whereas renal graft survival was similar in both groups. In total 34 patients switched treatment from ciclosporin to tacrolimus, whereas only 6 tacrolimus patients required alternative therapy (Bechstein et al., Transplantation 2004;77:1221).

Intestinal transplantation

Published clinical experience from a single centre on the use of tacrolimus for primary treatment following intestinal transplantation showed that the actuarial survival rate of 155 patients (65 intestine alone, 75 liver and intestine, and 25 multivisceral) receiving tacrolimus and prednisone was 75% at 1 year, 54% at 5 years, and 42% at 10 years. In the early years the initial oral dose of tacrolimus was 0.3 mg/kg/day. Results continuously improved with increasing experience over the course of 11 years. A variety of innovations, such as techniques for early detection of Epstein-Barr (EBV) and CMV infections, bone marrow augmentation, the adjunct use of the interleukin-2 antagonist daclizumab, lower initial tacrolimus doses with target trough levels of 10 to 15 ng/ml, and most recently allograft irradiation were considered to have contributed to improved results in this indication over time (Abu-Elmagd et al., Ann Surg 2001;234:404).

5.2 Pharmacokinetic properties

Absorption

In man tacrolimus has been shown to be able to be absorbed throughout the gastrointestinal tract. Following oral administration of Prograf capsules peak concentrations (C_{max}) of tacrolimus in blood are achieved in approximately 1 - 3 hours. In some patients, tacrolimus appears to be continuously absorbed over a prolonged period yielding a relatively flat absorption profile. The mean oral bioavailability of tacrolimus is in the range of 20% - 25%.

After oral administration (0.30 mg/kg/day) to liver transplant patients, steady-state concentrations of Prograf were achieved within 3 days in the majority of patients.

In healthy subjects, Prograf 0.5 mg, Prograf 1 mg and Prograf 5 mg Capsules, hard have been shown to be bioequivalent, when administered as equivalent dose.

The rate and extent of absorption of tacrolimus is greatest under fasted conditions. The presence of food decreases both the rate and extent of absorption of tacrolimus, the effect being most pronounced after a high-fat meal. The effect of a high-carbohydrate meal is less pronounced.

In stable liver transplant patients, the oral bioavailability of Prograf was reduced when it was administered after a meal of moderate fat (34% of calories) content. Decreases in AUC (27%) and C_{max} (50%), and an increase in t_{max} (173%) in whole blood were evident.

In a study of stable renal transplant patients who were administered Prograf immediately after a standard continental breakfast the effect on oral bioavailability was less pronounced. Decreases in AUC (2 to 12%) and C_{max} (15 to 38%), and an increase in t_{max} (38 to 80%) in whole blood were evident.

Bile flow does not influence the absorption of Prograf.

A strong correlation exists between AUC and whole blood trough levels at steady-state. Monitoring of whole blood trough levels therefore provides a good estimate of systemic exposure.

Distribution and elimination

In man, the disposition of tacrolimus after intravenous infusion may be described as biphasic.

In the systemic circulation, tacrolimus binds strongly to erythrocytes resulting in an approximate 20:1 distribution ratio of whole blood/plasma concentrations. In plasma, tacrolimus is highly bound (> 98.8%) to plasma proteins, mainly to serum albumin and α-1-acid glycoprotein.

Tacrolimus is extensively distributed in the body. The steady-state volume of distribution based on plasma concentrations is approximately 1300 l (healthy subjects). Corresponding data based on whole blood averaged 47.6 l.

Tacrolimus is a low-clearance substance. In healthy subjects, the average total body clearance (TBC) estimated from whole blood concentrations was 2.25 l/h. In adult liver, kidney and heart transplant patients, values of 4.1 l/h, 6.7 l/h and 3.9 l/h, respectively, have been observed. Paediatric liver transplant recipients have a TBC approximately twice that of adult liver transplant patients. Factors such as low haematocrit and protein levels, which result in an increase in the unbound fraction of tacrolimus, or corticosteroid-induced increased metabolism are considered to be responsible for the higher clearance rates observed following transplantation.

The half-life of tacrolimus is long and variable. In healthy subjects, the mean half-life in whole blood is approximately 43 hours. In adult and paediatric liver transplant patients, it averaged 11.7 hours and 12.4 hours, respectively, compared with 15.6 hours in adult kidney transplant recipients. Increased clearance rates contribute to the shorter half-life observed in transplant recipients.

Metabolism and biotransformation

Tacrolimus is widely metabolised in the liver, primarily by the cytochrome P450-3A4. Tacrolimus is also considerably metabolised in the intestinal wall. There are several metabolites identified. Only one of these has been shown *in vitro* to have immunosuppressive activity similar to that of tacrolimus. The other metabolites have only weak or no immunosuppressive activity. In systemic circulation only one of the inactive metabolites is present at low concentrations. Therefore, metabolites do not contribute to pharmacological activity of tacrolimus.

Excretion

Following intravenous and oral administration of ^{14}C-labelled tacrolimus, most of the radioactivity was eliminated in the faeces. Approximately 2% of the radioactivity was eliminated in the urine. Less than 1% of unchanged tacrolimus was detected in the urine and faeces, indicating that tacrolimus is almost completely metabolised prior to elimination: bile being the principal route of elimination.

5.3 Preclinical safety data

The kidneys and the pancreas were the primary organs affected in toxicity studies performed in rats and baboons. In rats, tacrolimus caused toxic effects to the nervous system and the eyes. Reversible cardiotoxic effects were observed in rabbits following intravenous administration of tacrolimus.

Embryofoetal toxicity was observed in rats and rabbits and was limited to doses that caused significant toxicity in maternal animals. In rats, female reproductive function including birth was impaired at toxic dosages and the offspring showed reduced birth weights, viability and growth.

A negative effect of tacrolimus on male fertility in the form of reduced sperm counts and motility was observed in rats.

6. PHARMACEUTICAL PARTICULARS

6.1 List of excipients

Prograf 0.5 mg hard capsules

Capsule content:

Hypromellose

Croscarmellose sodium

Lactose monohydrate

Magnesium stearate

Capsule shell:

Titanium dioxide (E 171)

Yellow iron oxide (E 172)

Gelatine

Printing ink of capsule shell: Shellac, lecithin (soya), hydroxypropyl cellulose, simeticone, red iron oxide (E 172).

Prograf 1 mg hard capsules

Capsule content:

Hypromellose

Croscarmellose sodium

Lactose monohydrate

Magnesium stearate

Capsule shell:

Titanium dioxide (E 171)

Gelatine

Printing ink of capsule shell: Shellac, lecithin (soya), hydroxypropyl cellulose, simeticone, red iron oxide (E 172).

Prograf 5 mg hard capsules

Capsule content:

Hypromellose

Croscarmellose sodium

Lactose monohydrate

Magnesium stearate

Capsule shell:

Titanium dioxide (E 171)

Red iron oxide (E 172)

Gelatine

Printing ink of capsule shell: Shellac, lecithin (soya), simeticone, titanium dioxide (E 171).

6.2 Incompatibilities

Tacrolimus is not compatible with PVC. Tubing, syringes and other equipment used to prepare or administer a suspension of Prograf capsule contents should not contain PVC.

6.3 Shelf life

3 years

After opening the aluminium wrapper: 1 year

6.4 Special precautions for storage

This medicinal product does not require any special temperature storage conditions.

Store in the original package in order to protect from moisture.

Hard capsules should be taken immediately following removal from the blister.

6.5 Nature and contents of container

PVC/PVDC/Aluminium blisters. Ten capsules per blister. Two, three, five, six, nine or ten blisters with a desiccant in an aluminium wrapper.

Prograf 0.5 mg hard capsules
Packs of 20, 30, 50, 60 and 100 hard capsules.
Prograf 1 mg hard capsules
Packs of 20, 30, 50, 60, 90 and 100 hard capsules.
Prograf 5 mg hard capsules
Packs of 30, 50, 60 and 100 hard capsules.
Not all pack sizes may be marketed.

6.6 Special precautions for disposal and other handling
No special requirements.

7. MARKETING AUTHORISATION HOLDER
Astellas Pharma Ltd.
Lovett House,
Lovett Road,
Staines
TW18 3AZ
United Kingdom

8. MARKETING AUTHORISATION NUMBER(S)
Prograf 0.5 mg hard capsules
PL 00166/0206
Prograf 1 mg hard capsules
PL 00166/0203
Prograf 5 mg hard capsules
PL 00166/0204

9. DATE OF FIRST AUTHORISATION/RENEWAL OF THE AUTHORISATION
Prograf 0.5 mg hard capsules
Date of first authorisation: 15th September 1999
Date of last renewal: 27th November 2007
Prograf 1 mg hard capsules
Date of first authorisation: 7th June 1994
Date of last renewal: 27th November 2007
Prograf 5 mg hard capsules
Date of first authorisation: 7th June 1994
Date of last renewal: 27th November 2007

10. DATE OF REVISION OF THE TEXT
15th May 2009

11. LEGAL CATEGORY
POM

Prograf 5mg/ml Concentrate for Solution for Infusion

(Astellas Pharma Ltd)

1. NAME OF THE MEDICINAL PRODUCT
Prograf 5 mg/ml concentrate for solution for infusion

2. QUALITATIVE AND QUANTITATIVE COMPOSITION
1 ml concentrate for solution for infusion contains 5 mg of tacrolimus.

Excipients: 200 mg of polyoxyethylene hydrogenated castor oil and 638 mg of dehydrated alcohol.

For a full list of excipients, see section 6.1.

3. PHARMACEUTICAL FORM
Concentrate for solution for infusion

The concentrate is a clear colourless solution.

4. CLINICAL PARTICULARS
4.1 Therapeutic indications
Prophylaxis of transplant rejection in liver, kidney or heart allograft recipients.

Treatment of allograft rejection resistant to treatment with other immunosuppressive medicinal products.

4.2 Posology and method of administration
Prograf therapy requires careful monitoring by adequately qualified and equipped personnel. The medicinal product should only be prescribed, and changes in immunosuppressive therapy initiated, by physicians experienced in immunosuppressive therapy and the management of transplant patients.

General considerations

The recommended initial dosages presented below are intended to act solely as a guideline. Prograf dosing should primarily be based on clinical assessments of rejection and tolerability in each patient individually aided by blood level monitoring (see below for recommended target whole blood trough concentrations). If clinical signs of rejection are apparent, alteration of the immunosuppressive regimen should be considered.

Prograf can be administered intravenously or orally. In general, dosing may commence orally; if necessary, by administering the capsule contents suspended in water, via nasogastric tubing.

Prograf is routinely administered in conjunction with other immunosuppressive agents in the initial post-operative period. The Prograf dose may vary depending upon the immunosuppressive regimen chosen.

Method of administration

The concentrate should be used for intravenous infusion only after it is diluted with suitable carrier media.

The concentration of a solution for infusion should be within the range 0.004 - 0.100 mg/ml. The total volume of infusion during a 24-hour period should be in the range 20 – 500 ml.

The diluted solution should not be given as a bolus (see section 6.6).

Duration of dosing

Patients should be converted from intravenous to oral medication as soon as individual circumstances permit. Intravenous therapy should not be continued for more than 7 days.

Dosage recommendations – Liver transplantation

Prophylaxis of transplant rejection - adults

Oral Prograf therapy should commence at 0.10 - 0.20 mg/kg/day administered as two divided doses (e.g. morning and evening). Administration should commence approximately 12 hours after the completion of surgery.

If the dose cannot be administered orally as a result of the clinical condition of the patient, intravenous therapy of 0.01 - 0.05 mg/kg/day should be initiated as a continuous 24-hour infusion.

Prophylaxis of transplant rejection - children

An initial oral dose of 0.30 mg/kg/day should be administered in two divided doses (e.g. morning and evening). If the clinical condition of the patient prevents oral dosing, an initial intravenous dose of 0.05 mg/kg/day should be administered as a continuous 24-hour infusion.

Dose adjustment during post-transplant period in adults and children

Prograf doses are usually reduced in the post-transplant period. It is possible in some cases to withdraw concomitant immunosuppressive therapy, leading to Prograf monotherapy. Post-transplant improvement in the condition of the patient may alter the pharmacokinetics of tacrolimus and may necessitate further dose adjustments.

Rejection therapy – adults and children

Increased Prograf doses, supplemental corticosteroid therapy, and introduction of short courses of mono-/polyclonal antibodies have all been used to manage rejection episodes. If signs of toxicity are noted (e.g. pronounced adverse reactions - see section 4.8) the dose of Prograf may need to be reduced.

For conversion to Prograf, treatment should begin with the initial oral dose recommended for primary immunosuppression.

For information on conversion from ciclosporin to Prograf, see below under "Dose adjustments in specific patient populations".

Dosage recommendations - Kidney transplantation

Prophylaxis of transplant rejection – adults

Oral Prograf therapy should commence at 0.20 - 0.30 mg/kg/day administered as two divided doses (e.g. morning and evening). Administration should commence within 24 hours after the completion of surgery.

If the dose cannot be administered orally as a result of the clinical condition of the patient, intravenous therapy of 0.05 - 0.10 mg/kg/day should be initiated as a continuous 24-hour infusion.

Prophylaxis of transplant rejection – children

An initial oral dose of 0.30mg/kg/day should be administered in two divided doses (e.g. morning and evening). If the clinical condition of the patient prevents oral dosing, an initial intravenous dose of 0.075–0.100 mg/kg/day should be administered as a continuous 24-hour infusion.

Dose adjustment during post-transplant period in adults and children

Prograf doses are usually reduced in the post-transplant period. It is possible in some cases to withdraw concomitant immunosuppressive therapy, leading to Prograf-based dual-therapy. Post-transplant improvement in the condition of the patient may alter the pharmacokinetics of tacrolimus and may necessitate further dose adjustments.

Rejection therapy – adults and children

Increased Prograf doses, supplemental corticosteroid therapy, and introduction of short courses of mono-/polyclonal antibodies have all been used to manage rejection episodes. If signs of toxicity are noted (e.g. pronounced adverse reactions - see section 4.8) the dose of Prograf may need to be reduced.

For conversion to Prograf, treatment should begin with the initial oral dose recommended for primary immunosuppression.

For information on conversion from ciclosporin to Prograf, see below under "Dose adjustments in specific patient populations".

Dosage recommendations - Heart transplantation

Prophylaxis of transplant rejection – adults

Prograf can be used with antibody induction (allowing for delayed start of Prograf therapy) or alternatively in clinically stable patients without antibody induction.

Following antibody induction, oral Prograf therapy should commence at a dose of 0.075 mg/kg/day administered as two divided doses (e.g. morning and evening). Administration should commence within 5 days after the completion of surgery as soon as the patient's clinical condition is stabilised. If the dose cannot be administered orally as a result of the clinical condition of the patient, intravenous therapy of 0.01 to 0.02 mg/kg/day should be initiated as a continuous 24-hour infusion.

An alternative strategy was published where oral tacrolimus was administered within 12 hours post transplantation. This approach was reserved for patients without organ dysfunction (e.g. renal dysfunction). In that case, an initial oral tacrolimus dose of 2 to 4 mg per day was used in combination with mycophenolate mofetil and corticosteroids or in combination with sirolimus and corticosteroids.

Prophylaxis of transplant rejection – children

Prograf has been used with or without antibody induction in paediatric heart transplantation.

In patients without antibody induction, if Prograf therapy is initiated intravenously, the recommended starting dose is 0.03 - 0.05 mg/kg/day as a continuous 24-hour infusion targeted to achieve tacrolimus whole blood concentrations of 15 - 25 ng/ml. Patients should be converted to oral therapy as soon as clinically practicable. The first dose of oral therapy should be 0.30 mg/kg/day starting 8 to 12 hours after discontinuing intravenous therapy.

Following antibody induction, if Prograf therapy is initiated orally, the recommended starting dose is 0.10 - 0.30 mg/kg/day administered as two divided doses (e.g. morning and evening).

Dose adjustment during post-transplant period in adults and children

Prograf doses are usually reduced in the post-transplant period. Post-transplant improvement in the condition of the patient may alter the pharmacokinetics of tacrolimus and may necessitate further dose adjustments.

Rejection therapy – adults and children

Increased Prograf doses, supplemental corticosteroid therapy, and introduction of short courses of mono-/polyclonal antibodies have all been used to manage rejection episodes.

In adult patients converted to Prograf, an initial oral dose of 0.15 mg/kg/day should be administered in two divided doses (e.g. morning and evening).

In paediatric patients converted to Prograf, an initial oral dose of 0.20 - 0.30 mg/kg/day should be administered in two divided doses (e.g. morning and evening).

For information on conversion from ciclosporin to Prograf, see below under "Dose adjustments in specific patient populations".

Dosage recommendations - Rejection therapy, other allografts

The dose recommendations for lung, pancreas and intestinal transplantation are based on limited prospective clinical trial data. In lung-transplanted patients Prograf has been used at an initial oral dose of 0.10 - 0.15 mg/kg/day, in pancreas-transplanted patients at an initial oral dose of 0.2 mg/kg/day and in intestinal transplantation at an initial oral dose of 0.3 mg/kg/day.

Dosage adjustments in specific patient populations

Patients with liver impairment

Dose reduction may be necessary in patients with severe liver impairment in order to maintain the blood trough levels within the recommended target range.

Patients with kidney impairment

As the pharmacokinetics of tacrolimus are unaffected by renal function, no dose adjustment should be required. However, owing to the nephrotoxic potential of tacrolimus careful monitoring of renal function is recommended (including serial serum creatinine concentrations, calculation of creatinine clearance and monitoring of urine output).

Paediatric patients

In general, paediatric patients require doses 1 ½ - 2 times higher than the adult doses to achieve similar blood levels.

Elderly patients

There is no evidence currently available to indicate that dosing should be adjusted in elderly patients.

Conversion from ciclosporin

Care should be taken when converting patients from ciclosporin-based to Prograf-based therapy (see sections 4.4 and 4.5). Prograf therapy should be initiated after considering ciclosporin blood concentrations and the clinical condition of the patient. Dosing should be delayed in the presence of elevated ciclosporin blood levels. In practice, Prograf therapy has been initiated 12 - 24 hours after discontinuation of ciclosporin. Monitoring of ciclosporin blood levels should be continued following conversion as the clearance of ciclosporin might be affected.

Target whole blood trough concentration recommendations

Dosing should primarily be based on clinical assessments of rejection and tolerability in each individual patient.

As an aid to optimise dosing, several immunoassays are available for determining tacrolimus concentrations in whole blood including a semi-automated microparticle enzyme immunoassay (MEIA). Comparisons of concentrations from the published literature to individual values in clinical practice should be assessed with care and knowledge of the assay methods employed. In current clinical practice, whole blood levels are monitored using immunoassay methods.

Blood trough levels of tacrolimus should be monitored during the post-transplantation period. When dosed orally, blood trough levels should be drawn approximately 12 hours post-dosing, just prior to the next dose. The frequency of blood level monitoring should be based on clinical needs. As Prograf is a medicinal product with low clearance, adjustments to the dosage regimen may take several days before changes in blood levels are apparent. Blood trough levels should be monitored approximately twice weekly during the early post-transplant period and then periodically during maintenance therapy. Blood trough levels of tacrolimus should also be monitored following dose adjustment, changes in the immunosuppressive regimen, or following co-administration of substances which may alter tacrolimus whole blood concentrations (see section 4.5).

Clinical study analysis suggests that the majority of patients can be successfully managed if tacrolimus blood trough levels are maintained below 20 ng/ml. It is necessary to consider the clinical condition of the patient when interpreting whole blood levels.

In clinical practice, whole blood trough levels have generally been in the range 5 - 20 ng/ml in liver transplant recipients and 10 - 20 ng/ml in kidney and heart transplant patients in the early post-transplant period. Subsequently, during maintenance therapy, blood concentrations have generally been in the range of 5 - 15 ng/ml in liver, kidney and heart transplant recipients.

4.3 Contraindications

Hypersensitivity to tacrolimus or other macrolides.

Hypersensitivity to any of the excipients - in particular polyoxyethylene hydrogenated castor oil or structurally related compounds.

4.4 Special warnings and precautions for use

During the initial post-transplant period, monitoring of the following parameters should be undertaken on a routine basis: blood pressure, ECG, neurological and visual status, fasting blood glucose levels, electrolytes (particularly potassium), liver and renal function tests, haematology parameters, coagulation values, and plasma protein determinations. If clinically relevant changes are seen, adjustments of the immunosuppressive regimen should be considered.

Herbal preparations containing St. John's wort (Hypericum perforatum) or other herbal preparations should be avoided when taking Prograf due to the risk of interactions that lead to decrease in blood concentrations of tacrolimus and reduced clinical effect of tacrolimus (see section 4.5 Interactions with other medicinal products and other forms of interactions).

Since levels of tacrolimus in blood may significantly change during diarrhoea episodes, extra monitoring of tacrolimus concentrations is recommended during episodes of diarrhoea.

The combined administration of ciclosporin and tacrolimus should be avoided and care should be taken when administering tacrolimus to patients who have previously received ciclosporin (see sections 4.2 and 4.5).

Ventricular hypertrophy or hypertrophy of the septum, reported as cardiomyopathies, have been observed on rare occasions. Most cases have been reversible, occurring primarily in children with tacrolimus blood trough concentrations much higher than the recommended maximum levels. Other factors observed to increase the risk of these clinical conditions included pre-existing heart disease, corticosteroid usage, hypertension, renal or hepatic dysfunction, infections, fluid overload, and oedema. Accordingly, high-risk patients, particularly young children and those receiving substantial immunosuppression should be monitored, using such procedures as echocardiography or ECG pre- and post-transplant (e.g. initially at three months and then at 9-12 months). If abnormalities develop, dose reduction of Prograf therapy, or change of treatment to another immunosuppressive agent should be considered. Tacrolimus may prolong the QT interval but at this time lacks substantial evidence for causing Torsades de Pointes. Caution should be exercised in patients with diagnosed or suspected Congenital Long QT Syndrome.

Patients treated with Prograf have been reported to develop EBV-associated lymphoproliferative disorders. Patients switched to Prograf therapy should not receive anti-lymphocyte treatment concomitantly. Very young (< 2 years), EBV-VCA-negative children have been reported to have an increased risk of developing lymphoproliferative disorders. Therefore, in this patient group, EBV-VCA serology should be ascertained before starting treatment with Prograf. During treatment, careful monitoring with EBV-PCR is recommended. Positive EBV-PCR may persist for months and is per se not indicative of lymphoproliferative disease or lymphoma.

Patients treated with tacrolimus have been reported to develop posterior reversible encephalopathy syndrome (PRES). If patients taking tacrolimus present with symptoms indicating PRES such as headache, altered mental status, seizures, and visual disturbances, a radiological procedure (e.g. MRI) should be performed. If PRES is diagnosed, adequate blood pressure control and immediate discontinuation of systemic tacrolimus is advised. Most patients completely recover after appropriate measures are taken.

Patients treated with immunosuppressants, including Prograf are at increased risk of opportunistic infections (bacterial, fungal, viral and protozoal). Among these conditions are BK virus associated nephropathy and JC virus associated progressive multifocal leukoencephalopathy (PML). These infections are often related to a high total immunosuppressive burden and may lead to serious or fatal conditions that physicians should consider in patients with deteriorating renal function or neurological symptoms.

As with other immunosuppressive agents, owing to the potential risk of malignant skin changes, exposure to sunlight and UV light should be limited by wearing protective clothing and using a sunscreen with a high protection factor.

As with other potent immunosuppressive compounds, the risk of secondary cancer is unknown (see section 4.8).

If administered accidentally either arterially or perivasally, the reconstituted Prograf 5 mg/ml concentrate for solution for infusion may cause irritation at the injection site.

Prograf 5 mg/ml concentrate for solution for infusion contains polyoxyethylene hydrogenated castor oil, which has been reported to cause anaphylactoid reactions. Caution is therefore necessary in patients who have previously received preparations containing polyoxyethylene castor oil derivatives either by intravenous injection or infusion, and in patients with an allergenic predisposition. The risk of anaphylaxis may be reduced by slow infusion of reconstituted Prograf 5 mg/ml concentrate for solution for infusion or by the prior administration of an antihistamine.

The ethanol content (638 mg per ml) of Prograf 5 mg/ml concentrate for solution for infusion should be taken into account.

4.5 Interaction with other medicinal products and other forms of interaction

Metabolic interactions

Systemically available tacrolimus is metabolised by hepatic CYP3A4. There is also evidence of gastrointestinal metabolism by CYP3A4 in the intestinal wall. Concomitant use of medicinal products or herbal remedies known to inhibit or induce CYP3A4 may affect the metabolism of tacrolimus and thereby increase or decrease tacrolimus blood levels. It is therefore recommended to monitor tacrolimus blood levels whenever substances which have the potential to alter CYP3A metabolism are used concomitantly and to adjust the tacrolimus dose as appropriate in order to maintain similar tacrolimus exposure (see sections 4.2 and 4.4).

Inhibitors of metabolism

Clinically the following substances have been shown to increase tacrolimus blood levels:

Strong interactions have been observed with antifungal agents such as ketoconazole, fluconazole, itraconazole and voriconazole, the macrolide antibiotic erythromycin or HIV protease inhibitors (e.g. ritonavir). Concomitant use of these substances may require decreased tacrolimus doses in nearly all patients.

Weaker interactions have been observed with clotrimazole, clarithromycin, josamycin, nifedipine, nicardipine, diltiazem, verapamil, danazol, ethinylestradiol, omeprazole and nefazodone.

In vitro the following substances have been shown to be potential inhibitors of tacrolimus metabolism: bromocriptine, cortisone, dapsone, ergotamine, gestodene, lidocaine, mephenytoin, miconazole, midazolam, nilvadipine, norethisterone, quinidine, tamoxifen, troleandomycin.

Grapefruit juice has been reported to increase the blood level of tacrolimus and should therefore be avoided.

Inducers of metabolism

Clinically the following substances have been shown to decrease tacrolimus blood levels:

Strong interactions have been observed with rifampicin, phenytoin or St. John's Wort (Hypericum perforatum) which may require increased tacrolimus doses in almost all patients. Clinically significant interactions have also been observed with phenobarbital. Maintenance doses of corticosteroids have been shown to reduce tacrolimus blood levels.

High dose prednisolone or methylprednisolone administered for the treatment of acute rejection have the potential to increase or decrease tacrolimus blood levels.

Carbamazepine, metamizole and isoniazid have the potential to decrease tacrolimus concentrations.

Effect of tacrolimus on the metabolism of other medicinal products

Tacrolimus is a known CYP3A4 inhibitor; thus concomitant use of tacrolimus with medicinal products known to be metabolised by CYP3A4 may affect the metabolism of such medicinal products.

The half-life of ciclosporin is prolonged when tacrolimus is given concomitantly. In addition, synergistic/additive nephrotoxic effects can occur. For these reasons, the combined administration of ciclosporin and tacrolimus is not recommended and care should be taken when administering tacrolimus to patients who have previously received ciclosporin (see sections 4.2 and 4.4).

Tacrolimus has been shown to increase the blood level of phenytoin.

As tacrolimus may reduce the clearance of steroid-based contraceptives leading to increased hormone exposure, particular care should be exercised when deciding upon contraceptive measures.

Limited knowledge of interactions between tacrolimus and statins is available. Available data suggests that the pharmacokinetics of statins are largely unaltered by the co-administration of tacrolimus.

Animal data have shown that tacrolimus could potentially decrease the clearance and increase the half-life of pentobarbital and phenazone.

Other interactions which have led to clinically detrimental effects

Concurrent use of tacrolimus with medicinal products known to have nephrotoxic or neurotoxic effects may increase these effects (e.g., aminoglycosides, gyrase inhibitors, vancomycin, sulfamethoxazole+trimethoprim, NSAIDs, ganciclovir or aciclovir).

Enhanced nephrotoxicity has been observed following the administration of amphotericin B and ibuprofen in conjunction with tacrolimus.

As tacrolimus treatment may be associated with hyperkalaemia, or may increase pre-existing hyperkalaemia, high potassium intake, or potassium-sparing diuretics (e.g., amiloride, triamterene, or spironolactone) should be avoided.

Immunosuppressants may affect the response to vaccination and vaccination during treatment with tacrolimus may be less effective. The use of live attenuated vaccines should be avoided.

Protein binding considerations

Tacrolimus is extensively bound to plasma proteins. Possible interactions with other medicinal products known to have high affinity for plasma proteins should be considered (e.g., NSAIDs, oral anticoagulants, or oral antidiabetics).

4.6 Pregnancy and lactation

Human data show that tacrolimus is able to cross the placenta. Limited data from organ transplant recipients show no evidence of an increased risk of adverse effects on the course and outcome of pregnancy under tacrolimus treatment compared with other immunosuppressive medicinal products. To date, no other relevant epidemiological data are available. Due to the need of treatment, tacrolimus can be considered in pregnant women when there is no safer alternative and when the perceived benefit justifies the potential risk to the foetus. In case of *in utero* exposure, monitoring of the newborn for the potential adverse effects of tacrolimus is recommended (in particular the effects on the kidneys). There is a risk for premature delivery (<37 week) as well as for hyperkalaemia in the newborn, which, however, normalizes spontaneously.

In rats and rabbits, tacrolimus caused embryofoetal toxicity at doses which demonstrated maternal toxicity (see section 5.3). Tacrolimus affected male fertility in rats (see section 5.3).

Lactation

Human data demonstrate that tacrolimus is excreted into breast milk. As detrimental effects on the newborn cannot be excluded, women should not breast-feed whilst receiving Prograf.

4.7 Effects on ability to drive and use machines

Not relevant.

4.8 Undesirable effects

The adverse drug reaction profile associated with immunosuppressive agents is often difficult to establish owing to the underlying disease and the concurrent use of multiple medications.

Many of the adverse drug reactions stated below are reversible and/or respond to dose reduction. Oral administration appears to be associated with a lower incidence of adverse drug reactions compared with intravenous use. Adverse drug reactions are listed below in descending order by frequency of occurrence: very common (≥1/10); common (≥1/100, <1/10); uncommon (≥1/1,000, <1/100); rare (≥1/10,000, <1/1,000); very rare (<1/10,000); not known (cannot be estimated from the available data).

Cardiac disorders

common: ischaemic coronary artery disorders, tachycardia

uncommon: ventricular arrhythmias and cardiac arrest, heart failures, cardiomyopathies, ventricular hypertrophy, supraventricular arrhythmias, palpitations, ECG investigations abnormal, heart rate and pulse investigations abnormal

rare: pericardial effusion

very rare: echocardiogram abnormal

Blood and lymphatic system disorders

common: anaemia, leukopenia, thrombocytopenia, leukocytosis, red blood cell analyses abnormal

uncommon: coagulopathies, coagulation and bleeding analyses abnormal, pancytopenia, neutropenia rare: thrombotic thrombocytopenic purpura, hypoprothrombinaemia

Nervous system disorders

very common: tremor, headache

common: seizures, disturbances in consciousness, paraesthesias and dysaesthesias, peripheral neuropathies, dizziness, writing impaired, nervous system disorders

uncommon: coma, central nervous system haemorrhages and cerebrovascular accidents, paralysis and paresis, encephalopathy, speech and language abnormalities, amnesia

rare: hypertonia

very rare: myasthenia

Eye disorders

common: vision blurred, photophobia, eye disorders

uncommon: cataract

rare: blindness

Ear and labyrinth disorders

common: tinnitus

uncommon: hypoacusis

rare: deafness neurosensory

very rare: hearing impaired

Respiratory, thoracic and mediastinal disorders

common: dyspnoea, parenchymal lung disorders, pleural effusion, pharyngitis, cough, nasal congestion and inflammations

uncommon: respiratory failures, respiratory tract disorders, asthma

rare: acute respiratory distress syndrome

Gastrointestinal disorders

very common: diarrhoea, nausea

common: gastrointestinal inflammatory conditions, gastrointestinal ulceration and perforation, gastrointestinal haemorrhages, stomatitis and ulceration, ascites, vomiting, gastrointestinal and abdominal pains, dyspeptic signs and symptoms, constipation, flatulence, bloating and distension, loose stools, gastrointestinal signs and symptoms

uncommon: ileus paralytic, peritonitis, acute and chronic pancreatitis, blood amylase increased, gastrooesophageal reflux disease, impaired gastric emptying

rare: subileus, pancreatic pseudocyst

Renal and urinary disorders

very common: renal impairment

common: renal failure, renal failure acute, oliguria, renal tubular necrosis, nephropathy toxic, urinary abnormalities, bladder and urethral symptoms

uncommon: anuria, haemolytic uraemic syndrome

very rare: nephropathy, cystitis haemorrhagic

Skin and subcutaneous tissue disorders

common: pruritus, rash, alopecias, acne, sweating increased

uncommon: dermatitis, photosensitivity

rare: toxic epidermal necrolysis (Lyell's syndrome)

very rare: Stevens Johnson syndrome

Musculoskeletal and connective tissue disorders

common: arthralgia, muscle cramps, pain in limb, back pain

uncommon: joint disorders

Endocrine disorders

rare: hirsutism

Metabolism and nutrition disorders

very common: hyperglycaemic conditions, diabetes mellitus, hyperkalaemia

common: hypomagnesaemia, hypophosphataemia, hypokalaemia, hypocalcaemia, hyponatraemia, fluid overload, hyperuricaemia, appetite decreased, anorexia, metabolic acidoses, hyperlipidaemia, hypercholesterolaemia, hypertriglyceridaemia, other electrolyte abnormalities

uncommon: dehydration, hypoproteinaemia, hyperphosphataemia, hypoglycaemia

Infections and infestations

As is well known for other potent immunosuppressive agents, patients receiving tacrolimus are frequently at increased risk for infections (viral, bacterial, fungal, protozoal). The course of pre-existing infections may be aggravated. Both generalised and localised infections can occur.

Cases of BK virus associated nephropathy, as well as cases of JC virus associated progressive multifocal leukoencephalopathy (PML), have been reported in patients treated with immunosuppressants, including Prograf.

Injury, poisoning and procedural complications

common: primary graft dysfunction

Neoplasms benign, malignant and unspecified (incl. cysts and polyps)

Patients receiving immunosuppressive therapy are at increased risk of developing malignancies. Benign as well as malignant neoplasms including EBV-associated lymphoproliferative disorders and skin malignancies have been reported in association with tacrolimus treatment.

Vascular disorders

very common: hypertension

common: haemorrhage, thrombembolic and ischaemic events, peripheral vascular disorders, vascular hypotensive disorders

uncommon: infarction, venous thrombosis deep limb, shock

General disorders and administration site conditions

common: asthenic conditions, febrile disorders, oedema, pain and discomfort, blood alkaline phosphatase increased, weight increased, body temperature perception disturbed

uncommon: multi-organ failure, influenza like illness, temperature intolerance, chest pressure sensation, feeling jittery, feeling abnormal, blood lactate dehydrogenase increased, weight decreased

rare: thirst, fall, chest tightness, mobility decreased, ulcer

very rare: fat tissue increased

Immune system disorders

Allergic and anaphylactoid reactions have been observed in patients receiving tacrolimus (see section 4.4).

Hepatobiliary disorders

common: hepatic enzymes and function abnormalities, cholestasis and jaundice, hepatocellular damage and hepatitis, cholangitis

rare: hepatic artery thrombosis, venoocclusive liver disease

very rare: hepatic failure, bile duct stenosis

Reproductive system and breast disorders

uncommon: dysmenorrhoea and uterine bleeding

Psychiatric disorders

very common: insomnia

common: anxiety symptoms, confusion and disorientation, depression, depressed mood, mood disorders and disturbances, nightmare, hallucination, mental disorders

uncommon: psychotic disorder

4.9 Overdose

Experience with overdosage is limited. Several cases of accidental overdosage have been reported; symptoms have included tremor, headache, nausea and vomiting, infections, urticaria, lethargy, increased blood urea nitrogen and elevated serum creatinine concentrations, and increase in alanine aminotransferase levels.

No specific antidote to Prograf therapy is available. If overdosage occurs, general supportive measures and symptomatic treatment should be conducted.

Based on its high molecular weight, poor aqueous solubility, and extensive erythrocyte and plasma protein binding, it is anticipated that tacrolimus will not be dialysable. In isolated patients with very high plasma levels, haemofiltration or -diafiltration have been effective in reducing toxic concentrations. In cases of oral intoxication, gastric lavage and/or the use of adsorbents (such as activated charcoal) may be helpful, if used shortly after intake.

5. PHARMACOLOGICAL PROPERTIES

5.1 Pharmacodynamic properties

Pharmacotherapeutic group: Calcineurin inhibitors, ATC code: L04AD02

Mechanism of action and pharmacodynamic effects

At the molecular level, the effects of tacrolimus appear to be mediated by binding to a cytosolic protein (FKBP12) which is responsible for the intracellular accumulation of the compound. The FKBP12-tacrolimus complex specifically and competitively binds to and inhibits calcineurin, leading to a calcium-dependent inhibition of T-cell signal transduction pathways, thereby preventing transcription of a discrete set of lymphokine genes.

Tacrolimus is a highly potent immunosuppressive agent and has proven activity in both *in vitro* and *in vivo* experiments.

In particular, tacrolimus inhibits the formation of cytotoxic lymphocytes, which are mainly responsible for graft rejection. Tacrolimus suppresses T-cell activation and T-helper-cell dependent B-cell proliferation, as well as the formation of lymphokines (such as interleukins-2, -3, and γ-interferon) and the expression of the interleukin-2 receptor.

Results from published data in other primary organ transplantation

Prograf has evolved into an accepted treatment as primary immunosuppressive medicinal product following pancreas, lung and intestinal transplantation. In prospective published studies tacrolimus was investigated as primary immunosuppressant in approximately 175 patients following lung, 475 patients following pancreas and 630 patients following intestinal transplantation. Overall, the safety profile of tacrolimus in these published studies appeared to be similar to what was reported in the large studies, where tacrolimus was used as primary treatment in liver, kidney and heart transplantation. Efficacy results of the largest studies in each indication are summarised below.

Lung transplantation

The interim analysis of a recent multicentre study discussed 110 patients who underwent 1:1 randomisation to either tacrolimus or ciclosporin. Tacrolimus was started as continuous intravenous infusion at a dose of 0.01 to 0.03 mg/kg/day and oral tacrolimus was administered at a dose of 0.05 to 0.3 mg/kg/day. A lower incidence of acute rejection episodes for tacrolimus- versus ciclosporin-treated patients (11.5% versus 22.6%) and a lower incidence of chronic rejection, the bronchiolitis obliterans syndrome (2.86% versus 8.57%), was reported within the first year after transplantation. The 1-year patient survival rate was 80.8% in the tacrolimus and 83% in the ciclosporin group (Treede et al., 3rd ICI San Diego, US, 2004;Abstract 22).

Another randomised study included 66 patients on tacrolimus versus 67 patients on ciclosporin. Tacrolimus was started as continuous intravenous infusion at a dose of 0.025 mg/kg/day and oral tacrolimus was administered at a dose of 0.15 mg/kg/day with subsequent dose adjustments to target trough levels of 10 to 20 ng/ml. The 1-year patient survival was 83% in the tacrolimus and 71% in the ciclosporin group, the 2-year survival rates were 76% and 66%, respectively. Acute rejection episodes per 100 patient-days were numerically fewer in the tacrolimus (0.85 episodes) than in the ciclosporin group (1.09 episodes). Obliterative bronchiolitis developed in 21.7% of patients in the tacrolimus group compared with 38.0% of patients in the ciclosporin group (p = 0.025). Significantly more ciclosporin-treated patients (n = 13) required a switch to tacrolimus than tacrolimus-treated patients to ciclosporin (n = 2) (p = 0.02) (Keenan et al., Ann Thoracic Surg 1995;60:580).

In an additional two-centre study, 26 patients were randomised to the tacrolimus versus 24 patients to the ciclosporin group. Tacrolimus was started as continuous intravenous infusion at a dose of 0.05 mg/kg/day and oral tacrolimus was administered at a dose of 0.1 to 0.3 mg/kg/day with subsequent dose adjustments to target trough levels of 12 to 15 ng/ml. The 1-year survival rates were 73.1% in the tacrolimus versus 79.2% in the ciclosporin group. Freedom from acute rejection was higher in the tacrolimus group at 6 months (57.7% versus 45.8%) and at 1 year after lung transplantation (50% versus 33.3%) (Treede et al., J Heart Lung Transplant 2001;20:511).

The three studies demonstrated similar survival rates. The incidences of acute rejection were numerically lower with tacrolimus in all three studies and one of the studies reported a significantly lower incidence of bronchiolitis obliterans syndrome with tacrolimus.

Pancreas transplantation

A multicentre study included 205 patients undergoing simultaneous pancreas-kidney transplantation who were randomised to tacrolimus (n=103) or to ciclosporin (n=102). The initial oral per protocol dose of tacrolimus was 0.2 mg/kg/day with subsequent dose adjustments to target trough levels of 8 to 15 ng/ml by Day 5 and 5 to 10 ng/mL after Month 6. Pancreas survival at 1 year was significantly superior with tacrolimus: 91.3% versus 74.5% with ciclosporin ($p < 0.0005$), whereas renal graft survival was similar in both groups. In total 34 patients switched treatment from ciclosporin to tacrolimus, whereas only 6 tacrolimus patients required alternative therapy (Bechstein et al., Transplantation 2004;77:1221).

Intestinal transplantation

Published clinical experience from a single centre on the use of tacrolimus for primary treatment following intestinal transplantation showed that the actuarial survival rate of 155 patients (65 intestine alone, 75 liver and intestine, and 25 multivisceral) receiving tacrolimus and prednisone was 75% at 1 year, 54% at 5 years, and 42% at 10 years. In the early years the initial oral dose of tacrolimus was 0.3 mg/kg/day. Results continuously improved with increasing experience over the course of 11 years. A variety of innovations, such as techniques for early detection of Epstein-Barr (EBV) and CMV infections, bone marrow augmentation, the adjunct use of the interleukin-2 antagonist daclizumab, lower initial tacrolimus doses with target trough levels of 10 to 15 ng/ml, and most recently allograft irradiation were considered to have contributed to improved results in this indication over time (Abu-Elmagd et al., Ann Surg 2001;234:404).

5.2 Pharmacokinetic properties

Absorption

In man tacrolimus has been shown to be able to be absorbed throughout the gastrointestinal tract. Following oral administration of Prograf capsules peak concentrations (C_{max}) of tacrolimus in blood are achieved in approximately 1 - 3 hours. In some patients, tacrolimus appears to be continuously absorbed over a prolonged period yielding a relatively flat absorption profile. The mean oral bioavailability of tacrolimus is in the range of 20% - 25%.

After oral administration (0.30 mg/kg/day) to liver transplant patients, steady-state concentrations of Prograf were achieved within 3 days in the majority of patients.

In healthy subjects, Prograf 0.5 mg, Prograf 1 mg and Prograf 5 mg Capsules, hard have been shown to be bioequivalent, when administered as equivalent dose.

The rate and extent of absorption of tacrolimus is greatest under fasted conditions. The presence of food decreases both the rate and extent of absorption of tacrolimus, the effect being most pronounced after a high-fat meal. The effect of a high-carbohydrate meal is less pronounced.

In stable liver transplant patients, the oral bioavailability of Prograf was reduced when it was administered after a meal of moderate fat (34% of calories) content. Decreases in AUC (27%) and C_{max} (50%), and an increase in t_{max} (173%) in whole blood were evident.

In a study of stable renal transplant patients who were administered Prograf immediately after a standard continental breakfast the effect on oral bioavailability was less pronounced. Decreases in AUC (2 to 12%) and C_{max} (15 to 38%), and an increase in t_{max} (38 to 80%) in whole blood were evident.

Bile flow does not influence the absorption of Prograf.

A strong correlation exists between AUC and whole blood trough levels at steady-state. Monitoring of whole blood trough levels therefore provides a good estimate of systemic exposure.

Distribution and elimination

In man, the disposition of tacrolimus after intravenous infusion may be described as biphasic.

In the systemic circulation, tacrolimus binds strongly to erythrocytes resulting in an approximate 20:1 distribution ratio of whole blood/plasma concentrations. In plasma, tacrolimus is highly bound (> 98.8%) to plasma proteins, mainly to serum albumin and α-1-acid glycoprotein.

Tacrolimus is extensively distributed in the body. The steady-state volume of distribution based on plasma concentrations is approximately 1300 l (healthy subjects). Corresponding data based on whole blood averaged 47.6 l.

Tacrolimus is a low-clearance substance. In healthy subjects, the average total body clearance (TBC) estimated from whole blood concentrations was 2.25 l/h. In adult liver, kidney and heart transplant patients, values of 4.1 l/h, 6.7 l/h and 3.9 l/h, respectively, have been observed. Paediatric liver transplant recipients have a TBC approximately twice that of adult liver transplant patients. Factors such as low haematocrit and protein levels, which result in an increase in the unbound fraction of tacrolimus, or corticosteroid-induced increased metabolism are considered to be responsible for the higher clearance rates observed following transplantation.

The half-life of tacrolimus is long and variable. In healthy subjects, the mean half-life in whole blood is approximately 43 hours. In adult and paediatric liver transplant patients, it averaged 11.7 hours and 12.4 hours, respectively, compared with 15.6 hours in adult kidney transplant recipients. Increased clearance rates contribute to the shorter half-life observed in transplant recipients.

Metabolism and biotransformation

Tacrolimus is widely metabolised in the liver, primarily by the cytochrome P450-3A4. Tacrolimus is also considerably metabolised in the intestinal wall. There are several metabolites identified. Only one of these has been shown *in vitro* to have immunosuppressive activity similar to that of tacrolimus. The other metabolites have only weak or no immunosuppressive activity. In systemic circulation only one of the inactive metabolites is present at low concentrations. Therefore, metabolites do not contribute to pharmacological activity of tacrolimus.

Excretion

Following intravenous and oral administration of ^{14}C-labelled tacrolimus, most of the radioactivity was eliminated in the faeces. Approximately 2% of the radioactivity was eliminated in the urine. Less than 1% of unchanged tacrolimus was detected in the urine and faeces, indicating that tacrolimus is almost completely metabolised prior to elimination: bile being the principal route of elimination.

5.3 Preclinical safety data

The kidneys and the pancreas were the primary organs affected in toxicity studies performed in rats and baboons. In rats, tacrolimus caused toxic effects to the nervous system and the eyes. Reversible cardiotoxic effects were observed in rabbits following intravenous administration of tacrolimus.

Embryofoetal toxicity was observed in rats and rabbits and was limited to doses that caused significant toxicity in maternal animals. In rats, female reproductive function including birth was impaired at toxic dosages and the offspring showed reduced birth weights, viability and growth.

A negative effect of tacrolimus on male fertility in the form of reduced sperm counts and motility was observed in rats.

6. PHARMACEUTICAL PARTICULARS

6.1 List of excipients

Polyoxyethylene hydrogenated castor oil

Dehydrated alcohol

6.2 Incompatibilities

When diluting, this medicinal product must not be mixed with other medicinal products except those mentioned in section 6.6.

Tacrolimus is absorbed by PVC plastics. Tubing, syringes and any other equipment used to prepare and administer Prograf 5 mg/ml concentrate for solution for infusion should not contain PVC.

Tacrolimus is unstable under alkaline conditions. Combination of the reconstituted Prograf 5 mg/ml concentrate for solution for infusion with other pharmaceutical products that produce a marked alkaline solution (e.g. aciclovir and ganciclovir) should be avoided.

6.3 Shelf life

2 years

Chemical and physical in-use stability has been demonstrated for 24 hours at 25°C.

From a microbiological point of view, the product should be used immediately. If not used immediately, in-use storage times and conditions prior to use are the responsibility of the user and would normally not be longer than 24 hours at 2 to 8°C, unless the dilution has taken place in controlled and validated aseptic conditions.

6.4 Special precautions for storage

Store ampoule in the original package in order to protect from light.

Do not store above 25°C.

For storage conditions of the diluted medicinal product, see section 6.3.

6.5 Nature and contents of container

1 ml concentrate for solution for infusion in 2 ml, type I Ph. Eur. clear colourless glass ampoules.

Each carton contains 10 ampoules.

6.6 Special precautions for disposal and other handling

Prograf 5 mg/ml concentrate for solution for infusion must not be injected undiluted.

Prograf 5 mg/ml concentrate for solution for infusion should be diluted in 5 % w/v glucose solution or physiological saline solution in polyethylene, polypropylene or glass bottles, but not in PVC containers (see section 6.2). Only transparent and colourless solutions should be used.

The concentration of a solution for infusion should be within the range 0.004 - 0.100 mg/ml. The total volume of infusion during a 24-hour period should be in the range 20 – 500 ml.

The diluted solution should not be given as a bolus.

Unused concentrate in an opened ampoule or unused reconstituted solution should be disposed of immediately to avoid contamination.

7. MARKETING AUTHORISATION HOLDER

Astellas Pharma Ltd.

Lovett House,

Lovett Road,

Staines

TW18 3AZ

United Kingdom

8. MARKETING AUTHORISATION NUMBER(S)

PL: 00166/0205

9. DATE OF FIRST AUTHORISATION/RENEWAL OF THE AUTHORISATION

Date of first authorisation: 7 June 1994

Date of last renewal: 27th November 2007

10. DATE OF REVISION OF THE TEXT

15th May 2009

ProHance Syringes

(Bracco UK Limited)

1. NAME OF THE MEDICINAL PRODUCT

ProHance®

2. QUALITATIVE AND QUANTITATIVE COMPOSITION

Gadoteridol 279.3mg per ml (0.5M)

3. PHARMACEUTICAL FORM

Sterile solution for intravenous injection

4. CLINICAL PARTICULARS

4.1 Therapeutic indications

Using Magnetic Resonance Imaging (MRI), ProHance provides contrast enhancement of the brain, spine and surrounding tissues resulting in improved visualization (compared with unenhanced MRI) of lesions with abnormal vascularity or those thought to cause a disruption of the normal blood-brain barrier.

ProHance can also be used for whole body MRI including the head, neck, liver, breast, muscoloskeletal system and soft tissue pathologies.

4.2 Posology and method of administration

Adults

The recommended dose of ProHance® for imaging most brain and spinal pathologies is 0.1 mmol/kg. However, doses of 0.3 mmol/kg have been shown to be useful in patients suspected of having cerebral metastases or other poorly enhancing lesions.

The recommended dose for whole body MRI is 0.1 mmol/kg.

Children (2 years and above)

The recommended dose of ProHance® for brain imaging and spine pathologies is 0.1 mmol/kg (0.2 ml/kg).

ProHance®has been used in only a limited number of children aged between 6 months and 2 years. If an MRI procedure must be performed in this group, particular caution should be exercised.

The safety and efficacy of doses higher than 0.1 mmol/kg and sequential or repeat procedures have not been established.

Elderly

Caution should be exercised in elderly patients.

To ensure complete injection of the contrast medium, the injection should be followed by a 5 ml normal saline flush. The imaging procedure should be completed within 1 hour after injecting ProHance®.

4.3 Contraindications

A history of previous hypersensitivity to ProHance®, its constituents or other gadolinium-based contrast media.

ProHance®is contraindicated in children under 6 months of age.

4.4 Special warnings and precautions for use

Since Gadoteridol is renally cleared from the body, caution should be exercised in patients with severely impaired renal function.

There have been reports of nephrogenic systemic fibrosis (NSF) associated with use of some gadolinium-containing contrast agents in patients with severe renal impairment (GFR <30ml/min/1.73m^2). As there is a possibility that NSF may occur with ProHance®, it should only be used in these patients after careful consideration. Haemodialysis shortly after ProHance administration in patients currently receiving haemodialysis may be useful at removing Prohance from the body. There is no evidence to support the initiation of haemodialysis for prevention or treatment of NSFin patients not already undergoing haemodialysis.

Transitory changes in serum iron (within normal range in the majority of cases) have been observed in some patients after administration of ProHance® and these changes were shown not to be clinically significant.

Anaphylactic reactions have been observed following the use of gadoteridol. Appropriate drugs and instruments for emergency measures must be readily available.

4.5 Interaction with other medicinal products and other forms of interaction

There are no known drug interactions with Gadoteridol. No clinically significant changes or trends in laboratory tests were seen in clinical trials with ProHance®.

4.6 Pregnancy and lactation

There are no adequate and well controlled studies in pregnant women. ProHance should be used during pregnancy only if the potential benefit justifies the potential risk to the foetus.

It is not known to what extent ProHance is excreted in human milk. Because many drugs are excreted in human milk, breast feeding should be discontinued prior to administration and should not be recommenced until at least 24 hours after the administration of ProHance.

4.7 Effects on ability to drive and use machines

There are no known effects of ProHance® on the ability to drive or operate machinery.

4.8 Undesirable effects

The accepted safety considerations and procedures that are required for Magnetic Resonance Imaging are applicable when ProHance® is used for contrast enhancement.

Side effects: Taste disturbance (primarily metallic taste) nausea, urticaria, pain at injection site, *convulsions* and hypotension have been reported. Headache and chest pain have been rarely reported. These occurrences were transient and resolved without residual effect. The occurrences were not related to age, gender, rate of injection or dose administered.

4.9 Overdose

There have been no cases of overdose reported to date, consequently, neither signs nor symptoms of overdosage have been identified. In the event of overdosage occurring, the patient should be observed and treated symptomatically.

5. PHARMACOLOGICAL PROPERTIES

5.1 Pharmacodynamic properties

Gadoteridol is a non-ionic paramagnetic contrast medium for magnetic resonance imaging.

When placed in a magnetic field, gadoteridol decreases T1 relaxation times in targeted areas. At recommended doses, the effect is observed with greatest sensitivity in the T1-weighted sequences.

Gadoteridol does not cross the intact blood-brain barrier and, therefore, does not accumulate in normal brain or in lesions that have a normal blood-brain barrier, e.g. cysts, mature post-operative scars, etc. However, disruption of the blood-brain barrier or normal vascularity allows penetration of gadoteridol into lesions such as neoplasms, abscesses, and subacute infarcts.

5.2 Pharmacokinetic properties

The pharmacokinetics of intravenously administered gadoteridol in normal subjects conforms to a two- compartment open model with mean distribution and elimination half-lives (reported as mean ± SD) of about 0.20 ± 10.04 hours and 1.57 ± 10.08 hours, respectively.

Gadoteridol is exclusively eliminated in the urine with 94.4 ± 4.8% (mean ± SD) of the dose excreted within 24 hours post injection. There is no detectable biotransformation or decomposition of gadoteridol.

The renal and plasma clearance rates (1.41 ± 0.33 ml/min/kg and 1.50 ± 0.35 ml/min/kg, respectively) of gadoteridol are essentially identical, indicating no alteration in elimination kinetics on passage through the kidneys and that the drug is essentially cleared through the kidney. The volume of distribution (204 ± 58 ml 1 kg) is equal to that of extra cellular water, and clearance is similar to that of substances which are subject to glomerular filtration.

No serum protein binding was detected in rats.

5.3 Preclinical safety data

Toxicity

Single-dose studies in mice and rats showed that the maximum non-lethal dose were 7 mmol/kg and 10 mmol/kg respectively (more than 20 and 30 times the maximum clinical dose, respectively).

Some vacuolative changes in the renal cortical epithelium, reversible upon cessation of treatment, were noted both in rats and dogs in the 28 day studies in doses greater than 0.3 mmol/kg and 1 mmol/kg respectively.

Mutagenesis

ProHance did not show any mutagenic effects in a series of in vitro and in vivo tests. No genetic, chromosomal, nor DNA damage was shown even in presence of metabolic activation.

Carcinogenesis

Since ProHance is for single dose administration and is devoid of any mutagenic potential, no carcinogenicity studies have been conducted.

Reproduction

No effect on reproductive function was demonstrated after ProHance administration.

Teratogenicity

ProHance exerted no untoward effects on embryonic or foetal development, at daily doses in rabbits at least 60 times and in rats at least 100 times the recommended human dose of 0.1 mmol/kg.

No potential to cause irritation after intraarterial administration has been demonstrated.

6. PHARMACEUTICAL PARTICULARS

6.1 List of excipients

Calteridol Calcium

Tromethamine USP

Hydrochloric Acid Ph Eur

Sodium Hydroxide Ph Eur

Water for Injections Ph Eur

6.2 Incompatibilities

ProHance® should not be **admixed** with any other drug.

6.3 Shelf life

36 months

6.4 Special precautions for storage

Store at room temperature (15-30°C.), protect from light. Frozen syringes should be discarded.

6.5 Nature and contents of container

Syringes: Type I glass syringes with rubber stoppers and polypropylene plunger rods containing

5, 10, 15 or 17 ml.

6.6 Special precautions for disposal and other handling

a. Screw the threaded tip of the plunger rod clockwise into the cartridge plunger and push forward a few millimeters to break any friction between the cartridge plunger and syringe barrel.

b. Holding syringe erect, aseptically remove the rubber cap from the tip of the syringe and attach either a sterile, disposable needle or tubing with a compatible luer lock using a push-twist action.

c. Hold the syringe erect and push plunger forward until all the air is evacuated and fluid either appears at the tip of the needle or the tubing is filled. Following the usual aspiration procedure, complete the injection. To ensure complete delivery of the contrast medium, the injection should be followed by a normal saline flush.

d. Properly dispose of the syringe and any other material used.

7. MARKETING AUTHORISATION HOLDER

Bracco International B.V.

Strawinskylaan 3051

1077 ZX Amsterdam

The Netherlands

8. MARKETING AUTHORISATION NUMBER(S)

14447/0002

9. DATE OF FIRST AUTHORISATION/RENEWAL OF THE AUTHORISATION

28 February 1997

10. DATE OF REVISION OF THE TEXT

11/12/2007

ProHance Vials

(Bracco UK Limited)

1. NAME OF THE MEDICINAL PRODUCT

ProHance®

2. QUALITATIVE AND QUANTITATIVE COMPOSITION

Gadoteridol 279.3mg/ml (0.5M)

3. PHARMACEUTICAL FORM

Sterile solution for intravenous injection

4. CLINICAL PARTICULARS

4.1 Therapeutic indications

Using Magnetic Resonance Imaging (MRI), ProHance provides contrast enhancement of the brain, spine and surrounding tissues resulting in improved visualization (compared with unenhanced MRI) of lesions with abnormal vascularity or those thought to cause a disruption of the normal blood-brain barrier.

ProHance can also be used for whole body MRI including the head, neck, liver, breast, muscoloskeletal system and soft tissue pathologies.

4.2 Posology and method of administration

Adults

The recommended dose of ProHance® for imaging most brain and spinal pathologies is 0.1 mmol/kg. However, doses of 0.3 mmol/kg have been shown to be useful in patients suspected of having cerebral metastases or other poorly enhancing lesions.

The recommended dose for whole body MRI is 0.1 mmol/kg.

Children (2 years and above)

The recommended dose of ProHance® for brain imaging and spine pathologies is 0.1 mmol/kg (0.2 ml/kg).

ProHance® has been used in only a limited number of children aged between 6 months and 2 years. If an MRI procedure must be performed in this group, particular caution should be exercised.

The safety and efficacy of doses higher than 0.1 mmol/kg and sequential or repeat procedures have not been established.

Elderly

Caution should be exercised in elderly patients.

To ensure complete injection of the contrast medium, the injection should be followed by a 5 ml normal saline flush. The imaging procedure should be completed within 1 hour after injecting ProHance®.

4.3 Contraindications

A history of previous hypersensitivity to ProHance®, its constituents or other gadolinium-based contrast.

ProHance® is contraindicated in children under 6 months of age.

4.4 Special warnings and precautions for use

Since Gadoteridol is renally cleared from the body, caution should be exercised in patients with severely impaired renal function.

There have been reports of nephrogenic systemic fibrosis (NSF) associated with use of some gadolinium-containing contrast agents in patients with severe renal impairment (GFR <30ml/min/1.73m^2). As there is a possibility that NSF may occur with ProHance®, it should only be used in these patients after careful consideration. Haemodialysis shortly after ProHance administration in patients currently receiving haemodialysis may be useful at removing Prohance from the body. There is no evidence to support the initiation of haemodialysis for prevention or treatment of NSFin patients not already undergoing haemodialysis.

Transitory changes in serum iron (within normal range in the majority of cases) have been observed in some patients after administration of ProHance® and these changes were shown not to be clinically significant.

Anaphylactic reactions have been observed following the use of gadoteridol. Appropriate drugs and instruments for emergency measures must be readily available.

4.5 Interaction with other medicinal products and other forms of interaction

There are no known drug interactions with Gadoteridol. No clinically significant changes or trends in laboratory tests were seen in clinical trials with ProHance®.

4.6 Pregnancy and lactation

ProHance exerted no untoward effects on embryonic or foetal development, at daily doses in rabbits at least 60 times and in rats at least 100 times the usual human dose of 0.1 mmol/kg. There are no adequate and well controlled studies in pregnant women. ProHance should be used during pregnancy only if the potential benefit justifies the potential risk to the foetus.

It is not known to what extent ProHance is excreted in human milk. Because many drugs are excreted in human milk, breast feeding should be discontinued prior to administration and should not be recommended until at least 24 hours after the administration of ProHance.

4.7 Effects on ability to drive and use machines

There are no known effects of ProHance® on the ability to drive or operate machinery.

4.8 Undesirable effects

The accepted safety considerations and procedures that are required for Magnetic Resonance Imaging are applicable when ProHance® is used for contrast enhancement.

Side effects: Taste disturbance (primarily metallic taste) nausea, urticaria, pain at injection site, *convulsions* and hypotension have been reported. Headache and chest pain have been rarely reported. These occurrences were transient and resolved without residual effect. The occurrences were not related to age, gender, rate of injection or dose administered.

4.9 Overdose

There have been no cases of overdose reported to date, consequently, neither signs nor symptoms of overdosage have been identified. In the event of overdosage occurring, the patient should be observed and treated symptomatically.

5. PHARMACOLOGICAL PROPERTIES

5.1 Pharmacodynamic properties

Gadoteridol is a non-ionic paramagnetic contrast medium for Magnetic Resonance Imaging.

When placed in a magnetic field, gadoteridol decreases T1 relaxation times in targeted areas. At recommended doses, the effect is observed with greatest sensitivity in the T1-weighted sequences.

Gadoteridol does not cross the intact blood-brain barrier and, therefore, does not accumulate in normal brain or in lesions that have a normal blood-brain barrier, e.g. cysts, mature post-operative scars, etc. However, disruption of the blood-brain barrier or normal vascularity allows penetration of gadoteridol into lesions such as neoplasms, abscesses, and subacute infarcts.

5.2 Pharmacokinetic properties

The pharmacokinetics of intravenously administered gadoteridol in normal subjects conforms to a two- compartment open model with mean distribution and elimination half-lives (reported as mean ± SD) of about 0.20 ± 10.04 hours and 1.57 ± 10.08 hours, respectively.

Gadoteridol is exclusively eliminated in the urine with 94.4 ± 4.8% (mean ± SD) of the dose excreted within 24 hours post injection. There is no detectable biotransformation or decomposition of gadoteridol.

The renal and plasma clearance rates (1.41 ± 0.33 ml/min/kg and 1.50 ± 0.35 ml/min/kg, respectively) of gadoteridol are essentially identical, indicating no alteration in elimination kinetics on passage through the kidneys and that the drug is essentially cleared through the kidney. The volume of distribution (204 ± 58 ml 1 kg) is equal to that of extra cellular water, and clearance is similar to that of substances which are subject to glomerular filtration.

No serum protein binding was detected in rats.

6. PHARMACEUTICAL PARTICULARS

6.1 List of excipients

Calteridol Calcium

Tromethamine USP

Hydrochloric Acid Ph Eur

Sodium Hydroxide Ph Eur

Water for Injections Ph Eur

6.2 Incompatibilities

ProHance® should not be **admixed** with any other drug.

6.3 Shelf life

36 months

6.4 Special precautions for storage

Store at room temperature (15-30°C.), protect from light. ProHance should not be frozen.

6.5 Nature and contents of container

Vials: Type 1 glass vials with grey butyl stoppers and aluminium seals containing 5,10, 15 or 20ml.

6.6 Special precautions for disposal and other handling

None.

7. MARKETING AUTHORISATION HOLDER

Bracco International B.V.

Strawinskylaan 3051

1077 ZX Amsterdam

The Netherlands

8. MARKETING AUTHORISATION NUMBER(S)

14447/0001

9. DATE OF FIRST AUTHORISATION/RENEWAL OF THE AUTHORISATION

29/10/1992

10. DATE OF REVISION OF THE TEXT

11/12/2007

Promixin 1 million International Units (IU) Powder for Nebuliser Solution

(Profile Pharma Limited)

1. NAME OF THE MEDICINAL PRODUCT

Promixin, 1 million International Units (IU) Powder for Nebuliser Solution

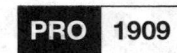

2. QUALITATIVE AND QUANTITATIVE COMPOSITION
Each vial contains 1 million International Units (IU) which is approximately equivalent to 80 mg of colistimethate sodium.

3. PHARMACEUTICAL FORM
Powder for nebuliser solution. The powder is white to off-white

4. CLINICAL PARTICULARS
4.1 Therapeutic indications
Promixin is indicated for the treatment by nebulisation of colonisation and infections of the lung due to susceptible *Pseudomonas aeruginosa* in patients with cystic fibrosis.

Consideration should be given to official guidance on the appropriate use of antibacterial agents.

4.2 Posology and method of administration
Sputum cultures should be obtained to confirm colonisation with *Pseudomonas aeruginosa* sensitive to colistimethate sodium prior to initiating treatment with Promixin.

The following information provides guidance on recommended doses and the dose should be adjusted according to clinical response.

Recommended doses are:

Children >2 years and adults: 1-2 million IU two or three times daily

The dosage is determined by the severity and type of infection, and renal function of the patient.

The dose may be varied across this range depending on the condition being treated.

Initial colonisation with *Pseudomonas aeruginosa* sensitive to colistimethate sodium may be treated with a 3-week course of 2 million IU twice daily in conjunction with other parenteral or oral antibiotics.

For frequent, recurrent infections (Less than three positive cultures of *Pseudomonas aeruginosa* sensitive to colistimethate sodium in a six month period) the dose may be increased up to a maximum of 2 million IU three times daily for up to 3 months, in conjunction with other parenteral or oral antibiotics.

Chronic colonisation (Three or more positive cultures of *Pseudomonas aeruginosa* sensitive to colistimethate sodium in a six month period) may require long-term therapy with 1 to 2 million IU twice daily. Additional parenteral or oral antibiotics may need to be administered to treat acute exacerbations of pulmonary infection.

Nebulised Promixin should be administered after physiotherapy and other inhaled treatments, where used. Other inhaled therapies may include agents to reduce the viscoelasticity of sputum and bronchodilators (see Section 4.4).

Colistimethate sodium is renally excreted and is nephrotoxic if high serum concentrations are achieved. Whilst this is unlikely during inhalation therapy, serum concentration estimations are recommended especially in patients with renal impairment.

Where there is renal impairment, excretion may be delayed and the daily dosage (magnitude of dose and dose interval) must be adjusted in relation to renal function to prevent accumulation of colistimethate sodium as indicated in the table.

Suggested modification of dosage of Promixin for patients with impaired renal function
(see Table 1 below)

Promixin is administered by nebulisation using a suitable nebuliser. For instructions on reconstitution of the product before administration see section 6.6. Once reconstituted use immediately.

4.3 Contraindications
Promixin is contraindicated in patients with known hypersensitivity to colistimethate sodium.

Colistimethate sodium is known to reduce the amount of acetylcholine released from the pre-synaptic neuromuscular junction and therefore should not be used in patients with myasthenia gravis.

4.4 Special warnings and precautions for use
Nebulisation of colistimethate sodium may induce coughing or bronchospasm. It is advisable to administer the first dose under medical supervision. Pre-dosing with a bronchodilator is recommended and should be routine, especially if this is part of the patient's current therapeutic regimen. FEV_1 should be evaluated pre and post dosing. If there is evidence of colistimethate sodium induced bronchial hyperreactivity in a patient not receiving pre-treatment bronchodilators the test should be repeated on a separate occasion using a bronchodilator. Evidence of bronchial hyperreactivity in the presence of a bronchodilator may indicate an allergic response and Promixin should be discontinued. Bronchospasm that occurs should be treated as medically indicated.

Bronchial hyperreactivity in response to colistimethate sodium may develop with continued use over time and it is recommended that pre and post treatment FEV_1s are evaluated at regular clinic visits.

Use with caution in renal impairment as colistimethate sodium is renally excreted.

Impairment of renal function has been reported, usually following use of higher than recommended intravenous or intramuscular doses in patients with normal renal function, or failure to reduce the intravenous or intramuscular dosage in patients with renal impairment or when used concomitantly with other nephrotoxic antibiotics. The effect is usually reversible on discontinuation of therapy.

High serum concentrations of colistimethate sodium after intravenous or intramuscular administration, may be associated with overdosage or failure to reduce the dosage in patients with renal impairment, and this may lead to neurotoxicity. Concomitant use with either non-depolarising muscle relaxants or antibiotics with similar neurotoxic effects can also lead to neurotoxicity. Dose reduction of colistimethate sodium may relieve symptoms. Neurotoxic effects that have been reported include: vertigo, transient facial paraesthesia, slurred speech, vasomotor instability, visual disturbances, confusion, psychosis and apnoea. (see also section 4.5)

Use with extreme caution in patients with porphyria.

4.5 Interaction with other medicinal products and other forms of interaction
Due to the effects of colistimethate sodium on the release of acetylcholine, non-depolarising muscle relaxants should be used with extreme caution in patients receiving Promixin as their effects could be prolonged.

Concomitant use of inhaled colistimethate sodium with other medications that are nephrotoxic or neurotoxic (e.g. cephalothin sodium, aminoglycosides, non-depolarising muscle relaxants) including those which are administered by the i.v. or i.m. routes should only be undertaken with the greatest caution.

4.6 Pregnancy and lactation
Safety in human pregnancy has not been established. There is evidence that colistimethate sodium crosses the placenta and consequently there is potential for foetal toxicity if administered during pregnancy. Animal studies are insufficient with respect to effects on reproduction. Promixin should only be given during pregnancy if the benefits outweigh any potential risk.

Colistimethate sodium is excreted in breast milk; breast feeding is not recommended during therapy.

4.7 Effects on ability to drive and use machines
Neurotoxicity, characterised by dizziness, confusion or visual disturbances have been reported following parenteral administration of colistimethate sodium. If these effects occur patients should be warned against driving or operating machinery.

4.8 Undesirable effects
The commonest undesirable effects following nebulisation of colistimethate sodium are coughing and bronchospasm (indicated by chest tightness which may be detected by a decrease in FEV_1) in approximately 10% of patients. (See also Section 4.4)

Adverse reactions are tabulated below by system organ class and frequency. Frequencies are defined as Very common (≥1/10): common (≥1/100 to <1/10): uncommon (≥1/1,000 to <1/100): rare (≥1/10,000 to <1/1,000) and very rare (<1/10,000), not known (cannot be estimated from the available data)

Body System	Frequency	Reported adverse reaction
Immune system disorders	Not known	Hypersensitivity reactions such as skin rash
Respiratory, thoracic and mediastinal disorders	Very common	Cough, chest tightness, bronchoconstriction or bronchospasm
General disorders and administration site conditions	Not known	Sore throat and sore mouth.

Should hypersensitivity reactions such as skin rash occur treatment with colistimethate sodium should be withdrawn.

Cases of sore throat or sore mouth may be due to hypersensitivity or superinfection with *Candida* species.

4.9 Overdose
Overdosage may cause apnoea, muscle weakness, vertigo, transient facial paraesthesia, slurred speech, vasomotor instability, visual disturbances, confusion, psychosis and renal insufficiency.

No antidote is available. Management of overdose is by means of supportive treatment and measures designed to increase clearance of colistimethate sodium such as inducing an osmotic diuresis with mannitol, peritoneal dialysis or prolonged haemodialysis.

5. PHARMACOLOGICAL PROPERTIES
5.1 Pharmacodynamic properties
Pharmacotherapeutic group: other antibacterials, Polymyxins.

ATC code: J01XB01

General properties
Colistimethate sodium is a polymyxin antibiotic and is derived from *Bacillus polymyxa var. colistinus*. It is a polypeptide and is active against a number of aerobic, Gram-negative bacteria.

The polymyxin antibiotics are surface active agents and act by binding to and changing the permeability of the bacterial cell membrane causing bacterial cell death. Polymyxins are bactericidal against Gram-negative bacteria with a hydrophobic outer membrane.

Breakpoints
Susceptible (S) ≤ 4 mg/L Resistant (R) ≥ 8 mg/L

Susceptibility
The table below lists bacterial species which are regarded as susceptible to colistimethate sodium. Bacterial resistance may vary according to region and information on resistant species in a specific area is desirable, particularly when treating severe infections. Only bacteria likely to be relevant to the clinical indication are listed.

SUSCEPTIBLE BACTERIA	RESISTANT BACTERIA
Acinetobacter species *Haemophilus influenzae* *Klebsiella* species *Pseudomonas aeruginosa*	*Brucella* species *Burkholderia cepacia* and related species *Serratia* species *Proteus mirabilis*

Resistance
Colistimethate sodium acquired resistance in mucoid *Pseudomonas aeruginosa* has been reported to be approximately 3%. Susceptibility testing should be performed on patients who are treated on a long term basis.

Cross resistance
Polymyxins including colistimethate sodium differ in their mechanism of action compared with other antibiotics and there is evidence to show that Gram-negative bacteria resistant to other antibiotics may be susceptible to colistimethate sodium. The resistance to polymyxins is not crossed with other antibiotic families.

5.2 Pharmacokinetic properties
Absorption
Gastrointestinal absorption is negligible hence the swallowing of colistimethate sodium deposited in the nasopharynx is unlikely to add to the systemic exposure. Absorption following lung administration appears to be variable and clinical work has shown that resultant serum concentrations may range from undetectable to rarely exceeding 4 mg/L (50,000 IU/L) compared to serum concentrations of 10–20 mg/L (approx. 125,000-250,000 IU/L) following intravenous use. Absorption following lung administration is influenced by the nebuliser system, aerosol droplet size and disease state of the lungs. A study in cystic fibrosis patients showed that colistimethate sodium was undetectable in the urine after 1 million IU were inhaled twice daily for 3 months. This is despite the fact that excretion is known to be primarily via the urine.

Distribution
Colistimethate sodium shows a low level of protein binding. Polymyxin antibiotics are known to persist in muscle tissue, liver, kidney, heart and brain.

Table 1

	Degree of Renal Impairment			
	Normal	Mild	Moderate	Severe
Creatinine (μmol/L)	60 – 105	106 - 129	130 - 214	215 – 340
Creatinine Clearance (% of normal)	76 to 100	40 to 75	25 to 40	Less than 25
Dose				
Unit dose (Million IU)	1.3 to 2	1 to 1.5	1	1 to 1.5
Frequency (Times per day)	3	2	1 or 2	Every 36 hours
Total Daily Dose (Million IU)	4 to 6	2 to 3	1 to 2	0.6 to 1

Pharmacokinetics

Serum concentrations and pharmacokinetics in 5 patients receiving inhaled colistimethate sodium

Parameter	160 mg (Approximately 2 million IU) Nebulised Colistimethate Sodium
AUC_{0-4} (h/mg/L)	165.9 ± 76.5
C_{max} (mg/L)	0.051 ± 0.0244
T_{max} (h)	1.9 ± 1.2
Ka (h^{-1})	3.0 ± 1.8
$t_{½}$ (h)	10.4 ± 3.6
Cl/F	0.27 ± 0.15

Volume of distribution has been calculated to be 0.09 L/Kg in a single study in patients with cystic fibrosis (CF).

Biotransformation

Colistimethate sodium undergoes conversion to its base *in vivo*. Approximately 80% of the parenteral dose is recoverable unchanged in the urine. There is no biliary excretion.

Elimination

There is no information on the elimination of colistimethate sodium following nebulisation.

Following i.v. administration excretion is primarily renal with 40% of a parenteral dose recovered in the urine within 8 hours and around 80% in 24 hours. It follows that dose should be reduced in the renally impaired in order to prevent accumulation. Refer to Section 4.2.

The elimination half-life is approximately 1.5 hours following i.v. administration to healthy adults. This compares with an elimination half-life of 3.4 ± 1.4 hours when CF patients were given a single 30 minute i.v. infusion.

Colistimethate sodium kinetics appear to be similar in all patient groups provided renal function is normal.

5.3 Preclinical safety data

Animal studies are insufficient with respect to effects on reproduction.

Data on potential genotoxicity are limited and carcinogenicity data for colistimethate sodium are lacking. Colistimethate sodium has been shown to induce chromosomal aberrations in human lymphocytes, *in vitro*. This effect may be related to a reduction in mitotic index, which was also observed.

6. PHARMACEUTICAL PARTICULARS

6.1 List of excipients

None

6.2 Incompatibilities

The addition of other antibiotics to solutions of Promixin may lead to precipitation.

6.3 Shelf life

Unopened: 2 years.

Once reconstituted: Use immediately.

6.4 Special precautions for storage

No special precautions for storage

6.5 Nature and contents of container

The product is supplied in clear type I glass vials sealed with a siliconised chlorobutyl type I rubber stopper and protected by a 20 mm aluminium tear-off cap incorporating a red flip-up central plastic top. The product is supplied in packs of 30 vials. Each pack contains a Promixin Disc to enable use with the I-neb AAD System.

6.6 Special precautions for disposal and other handling

Promixin may be reconstituted with Water for Injections (WFI) to produce a clear colourless to pale yellow hypotonic solution or a 50:50 mixture of WFI and 0.9% saline to produce a clear colourless to pale yellow isotonic solution. When reconstituted, Promixin may be used with any conventional nebuliser suitable for delivery of antibiotic solutions.

Solutions should be used immediately after reconstitution (see section 4.2). Any unused solution remaining in the nebuliser must be discarded following treatment. Promixin is supplied with a Promixin Disc, for use with the I-neb AAD System. For instructions on the use of Promixin with the I-neb AAD System, please refer to detailed instructions provided with the device.

Conventional nebulisers operate on a continuous flow basis and it is likely that some nebulised drug will be released into the local environment. When used with a conventional nebuliser, Promixin should be administered in a well-ventilated room, particularly in hospitals where several patients may be using nebulisers at the same time. Tubing or filters may be used to prevent waste aerosol from entering the environment.

7. MARKETING AUTHORISATION HOLDER

Profile Pharma Limited
Chichester Business Park
City Fields Way
Tangmere
Chichester
West Sussex
PO20 2FT
United Kingdom

8. MARKETING AUTHORISATION NUMBER(S)

PL 19419/0001

9. DATE OF FIRST AUTHORISATION/RENEWAL OF THE AUTHORISATION

20th February 2003 / 13th August 2008

10. DATE OF REVISION OF THE TEXT

09/01/2009

11. Legal category

POM

Promixin 1 MIU Powder for Solution for Injection

(Profile Pharma Limited)

1. NAME OF THE MEDICINAL PRODUCT

Promixin, 1 MIU (1 million International Units), Powder for Solution for Injection

2. QUALITATIVE AND QUANTITATIVE COMPOSITION

Each vial contains 1 million International Units (1 MIU) which is approximately equivalent to 80 mg of colistimethate sodium.

For excipients, see section 6.1

3. PHARMACEUTICAL FORM

Sterile powder for solution for injection

The powder is white to off white

4. CLINICAL PARTICULARS

4.1 Therapeutic indications

Promixin is indicated for intravenous use in the treatment of serious infections where sensitivity testing indicates that they are caused by susceptible Gram-negative bacteria. These include infections of the lower respiratory tract and urinary tract, where routine antibiotics may be contraindicated or ineffective because of resistance.

Consideration should be given to official guidance on the appropriate use of antibacterial agents.

4.2 Posology and method of administration

Administration is by intravenous infusion. Each dose of Promixin can be diluted in 50 mL and administered by intravenous infusion over 30 minutes. Patients fitted with a totally implantable venous access device (TIVAD) may tolerate an injection of up to 2 MIU in 10 mL given over a minimum of 5 minutes.

Solutions should be used immediately after reconstitution. For instructions on dilution of the product before administration see section 6.6.

The dose of Promixin is dependent upon the sensitivity of the causative bacteria, the severity and type of infection, the weight and renal function of the patient.

Up to 60 Kg: 50,000 IU/Kg (4 mg/Kg) bodyweight, to a maximum of 75,000 IU/Kg (6 mg/Kg), in 24 hours. The total daily dose should be administered as three equal doses at 8 hourly intervals.

Over 60 Kg: 1-2 MIU every 8 hours. The maximum dose is 6 MIU (480 mg) in 24 hours.

A minimum of 5 days treatment is recommended.

Serum concentration estimations are recommended, especially in patients with renal impairment or cystic fibrosis and in neonates. Peak serum concentrations of 10–15 mg/L (approximately 0.125-0.2 MIU/L) should be adequate, for the treatment of most infections.

Dosage may be increased up to a maximum of 6 MIU per 24 hours according to the patient's condition, if clinical or bacteriological response is slow.

Where there is renal impairment, excretion is delayed and the daily dosage (magnitude of dose and dose interval) must be adjusted in relation to renal function as indicated in the table, to prevent accumulation of colistimethate sodium. Further dose adjustment may be required according to the needs of an individual patient.

Suggested modification of dosage of Promixin for adults with impaired renal function

(see Table 1 below)

4.3 Contraindications

Promixin is contraindicated in patients with known hypersensitivity to colistimethate sodium.

Colistimethate sodium is known to reduce the amount of acetylcholine released from the pre-synaptic neuromuscular junction and therefore should not be used in patients with myasthenia gravis.

4.4 Special warnings and precautions for use

Use with caution in patients with renal impairment as colistimethate sodium is renally excreted.

Nephrotoxicity or neurotoxicity may rarely occur especially if the recommended dose is exceeded (see also section 4.5).

Do not use concomitantly with other medications with nephrotoxic or neurotoxic effects except with the greatest caution.

Use with extreme caution in patients with porphyria.

4.5 Interaction with other medicinal products and other forms of interaction

Due to the effects of colistimethate sodium on the release of acetylcholine, non-depolarising muscle relaxants should be used with extreme caution in patients receiving Promixin as their effects could be prolonged.

Concomitant use of colistimethate sodium with other medications that are nephrotoxic or neurotoxic (eg. cephalothin sodium, aminoglycosides, non-depolarising muscle relaxants) should only be undertaken with the greatest caution.

4.6 Pregnancy and lactation

Safety in human pregnancy has not been established. There is evidence that colistimethate sodium crosses the placenta and consequently there is potential for foetal toxicity if administered during pregnancy. Animal studies are insufficient with respect to effects on reproduction. Promixin should only be given during pregnancy if the benefits outweigh any potential risk.

Colistimethate sodium is excreted in breast milk; breast feeding is not recommended during therapy.

4.7 Effects on ability to drive and use machines

Neurotoxicity, characterised by dizziness, confusion or visual disturbances have been reported following parenteral administration of colistimethate sodium. If these effects occur patients should be warned against driving or operating machinery.

4.8 Undesirable effects

Hypersensitivity reactions such as skin rash have been known to occur. In the event such reactions occur, treatment with colistimethate sodium should be withdrawn.

Impairment of renal function has been reported, usually following use of higher than recommended doses in patients with normal renal function, or failure to reduce the dosage in patients with renal impairment or when used concomitantly with other nephrotoxic antibiotics. The effect is usually reversible on discontinuation of therapy.

High serum concentrations of colistimethate sodium, which may be associated with overdosage or failure to reduce the dosage in patients with renal impairment, have been known to lead to neurotoxicity. Concomitant use with either non-depolarising muscle relaxants or antibiotics with similar neurotoxic effects can also lead to neurotoxicity. Dose reduction of colistimethate sodium may relieve symptoms. Neurotoxic effects that have been reported include: vertigo, transient facial paraesthesia, slurred speech, vasomotor instability, visual disturbances, confusion, psychosis and apnoea.

Local irritation at the site of injection may occur.

4.9 Overdose

Overdosage may cause apnoea, muscle weakness and renal insufficiency. No antidote is available.

Management of overdose is by means of supportive treatment and measures designed to increase clearance of colistimethate sodium such as inducing an osmotic diuresis with mannitol, peritoneal dialysis or prolonged haemodialysis.

Table 1

	Degree of Renal Impairment			
	Normal	Mild	Moderate	Severe
Creatinine (μmol/L)	60 - 105	106 - 129	130 - 214	215 - 340
Creatinine Clearance (% of normal)	76 to 100	40 to 75	25 to 40	Less than 25
Dose				
Unit dose (MIU)	1.3 to 2	1 to 1.5	1	1 to 1.5
Frequency (Times per day)	3	2	1 or 2	Every 36 hours
Total Daily Dose (MIU)	4 to 6	2 to 3	1 to 2	0.6 to 1

5. PHARMACOLOGICAL PROPERTIES

5.1 Pharmacodynamic properties

Pharmacotherapeutic group: other antibacterials, Polymyxins

ATC code: J01XB01

General properties

Colistimethate sodium is a polymyxin antibiotic and is derived from Bacillus polymyxa var. colistinus. It is a polypeptide and is active against a number of aerobic, Gram-negative bacteria.

The polymyxin antibiotics are surface active agents and act by binding to and changing the permeability of bacterial cell membrane causing bacterial cell death. Polymyxins are bactericidal against Gram-negative bacteria with a hydrophobic outer membrane.

Breakpoints

Susceptible (S) $\leq$ 4 mg/L Resistant (R) $\geq$ 8 mg/L

Susceptibility

The table below lists bacterial species which are regarded as susceptible to colistimethate sodium. Bacterial resistance may vary according to region and information on resistant species in a specific area is desirable, particularly when treating severe infections.

SUSCEPTIBLE BACTERIA	RESISTANT BACTERIA
Gram-negative aerobes:	Gram-negative aerobes:
Acinetobacter species	*Brucella* species
Citrobacter species	*Burkholderia cepacia* and related species
Escherichia coli	*Neisseria* species
Enterobacter species	*Providencia* species
Haemophilus influenzae	*Serratia* species
Klebsiella species	*Proteus mirabilis*
Pseudomonas aeruginosa	Gram-negative anaerobes:
Salmonella species	*Bacteroides* fragilis
Shigella species	

Resistance

Colistimethate sodium acquired resistance in *Pseudomonas aeruginosa* appears to be rare. However, *in vitro* studies with *Salmonella* and *E. coli* have shown that resistance may occur with modification of the cell wall lipopolysaccharide phosphate groups. Modification is achieved by substitution of the phosphate groups with ethanolamine or aminoarabinose. *Proteus mirabilis*, *Burkholderia cepacia* and other naturally resistant Gram-negative bacteria, show complete substitution of their lipopolysaccharide groups.

Cross resistance

Polymyxins including colistimethate sodium differ in their mechanism of action compared with other antibiotics and there is evidence to show that Gram-negative bacteria resistant to other antibiotics may be susceptible to colistimethate sodium. The resistance to polymyxins is not crossed with other antibiotic families.

5.2 Pharmacokinetic properties

Distribution

Colistimethate sodium shows a low level of protein binding. Polymyxin antibiotics are known to persist in muscle tissue, liver, kidney, heart and brain.

In a study where cystic fibrosis patients received 5 to 7 mg/Kg/day in divided doses given as a 30 minute intravenous infusion, Cmax was 21.4 ± 5 mg/L and the Cmin at 8 hours was 2.8 ± 1.8 mg/L. Steady state Cmax was 23 ± 6 mg/L and Cmin at 8 hours was 4.5 ± 4 mg/L.

In another study where cystic fibrosis patients received 2 MIU every 8 hours for 12 days, Cmax was 12.9 mg/L (5.7 – 29.6 mg/L) and Cmin was 2.76 mg/L (1.0 – 6.2 mg/L).

In healthy volunteers given 150 mg (2 MIU approximately) intravenously, peak serum levels of 18 mg/L were observed after 10 minutes.

Volume of distribution has been calculated to be 0.09 L/Kg in a single study in patients with cystic fibrosis.

Biotransformation

Colistimethate sodium undergoes conversion to its base *in vivo*. Approximately 80% of the dose is recoverable unchanged in the urine. There is no biliary excretion and any remaining drug is believed to be inactivated in the tissues.

Elimination

Following intravenous administration excretion is primarily renal with 40% of a dose recovered in the urine within 8 hours and around 80% in 24 hours. It follows that doses should be reduced in the renally impaired in order to prevent accumulation (see section 4.2).

The elimination half-life is approximately 1.5 hours following intravenous administration to healthy adults. This compares with an elimination half-life of 3.4 ± 1.4 hours when cystic fibrosis patients were given a single 30 minute intravenous infusion.

Colistimethate sodium kinetics appears to be similar in all patient age groups provided renal function is normal.

5.3 Preclinical safety data

Animal studies are insufficient with respect to effects on reproduction.

Data on potential genotoxicity are limited and carcinogenicity data for colistimethate sodium are lacking. Colistimethate sodium has been shown to induce chromosomal aberrations in human lymphocytes, *in vitro*. This effect may be related to a reduction in mitotic index, which was also observed.

6. PHARMACEUTICAL PARTICULARS

6.1 List of excipients

None

6.2 Incompatibilities

Mixing drugs in solutions of Promixin should be avoided. The addition of other antibiotics such as erythromycin, tetracycline or cephalothin sodium to solutions of Promixin may lead to precipitation

6.3 Shelf life

Unopened: Two years

Once reconstituted: Use immediately.

6.4 Special precautions for storage

No special precautions for storage.

6.5 Nature and contents of container

The product is supplied in clear type I glass vials sealed with a siliconised chlorobutyl type I rubber stopper and protected by a 20 mm aluminium tear-off cap incorporating a red flip-up central plastic top. The product is supplied in packs of 10 vials.

6.6 Special precautions for disposal and other handling

Promixin may be reconstituted with 0.9% saline or Water for Injections (WFI) to produce a clear solution. Following reconstitution, the solution should be diluted to a suitable volume for infusion over 30 minutes. Suitable diluents are 0.9% saline, 5% dextrose, 5% fructose and Ringer's Solution. Solutions should be used immediately after reconstitution (see section 4.2)

Any unused medicinal product or waste material should be disposed of in accordance with local requirements.

7. MARKETING AUTHORISATION HOLDER

Profile Pharma Limited

Chichester Business Park

City Fields Way

Tangmere

Chichester

West Sussex

PO20 2FT

United Kingdom

8. MARKETING AUTHORISATION NUMBER(S)

PL 19419/0002

9. DATE OF FIRST AUTHORISATION/RENEWAL OF THE AUTHORISATION

Date of first authorisation: 24th June 2003

Date of latest renewal: 13th March 2009

10. DATE OF REVISION OF THE TEXT

13/03/2009

11. Legal category

POM

Propecia 1mg tablets

(Merck Sharp & Dohme Limited)

1. NAME OF THE MEDICINAL PRODUCT

PROPECIA® 1 mg Film-Coated Tablets

2. QUALITATIVE AND QUANTITATIVE COMPOSITION

Each tablet of 'Propecia' contains 1 mg of finasteride as the active ingredient.

3. PHARMACEUTICAL FORM

Film-coated tablet. Tan octagonal, film-coated, convex tablets, marked with a 'P' logo on one side and 'PROPECIA' on the other.

4. CLINICAL PARTICULARS

4.1 Therapeutic indications

'Propecia' is indicated for the treatment of men with male pattern hair loss (androgenetic alopecia) to increase hair growth and prevent further hair loss.

'Propecia' is **not** indicated for use in women or children and adolescents.

4.2 Posology and method of administration

The recommended dosage is one 1 mg tablet daily. 'Propecia' may be taken with or without food.

There is no evidence that an increase in dosage will result in increased efficacy.

Efficacy and duration of treatment should continuously be assessed by the treating physician. Generally, three to six months of once daily treatment are required before evidence of stabilisation of hair loss can be expected. Continuous use is recommended to sustain benefit. If treatment is stopped, the beneficial effects begin to reverse by six months and return to baseline by 9 to 12 months.

No dosage adjustment is required in patients with renal insufficiency.

No data are available on the concomitant use of 'Propecia' and topical minoxidil in male pattern hair loss.

4.3 Contraindications

'Propecia' is contraindicated for use in women due to the risk in pregnancy (see 4.6 'Pregnancy and lactation') and in patients with hypersensitivity to any component of this product.

'Propecia' is not indicated for use in women or children and adolescents.

'Propecia' should not be taken by men who are taking 'Proscar' (finasteride 5 mg) or any other 5α-reductase inhibitor for benign prostatic hyperplasia or any other condition.

4.4 Special warnings and precautions for use

In clinical studies with 'Propecia' in men 18-41 years of age, the mean value of serum prostate-specific antigen (PSA) decreased from 0.7 ng/ml at baseline to 0.5 ng/ml at month 12. This decrease in serum PSA concentrations needs to be considered, if during treatment with 'Propecia', a patient requires a PSA assay. In this case the PSA value should be doubled before making a comparison with the results from untreated men.

Excipients

Patients with rare hereditary problems of galactose intolerance, the Lapp lactase deficiency or glucose-galactose malabsorption should not take this medicine.

4.5 Interaction with other medicinal products and other forms of interaction

No drug interactions of clinical importance have been identified. Finasteride does not appear to affect the cytochrome P450-linked drug metabolising enzyme system. Compounds which have been tested in man have included antipyrine, digoxin, glibenclamide, propranolol, theophylline and warfarin and no interactions were found.

Although specific interaction studies were not performed, in clinical studies finasteride doses of 1 mg or more were used concomitantly with ACE inhibitors, paracetamol, alpha blockers, benzodiazepines, beta blockers, calcium-channel blockers, cardiac nitrates, diuretics, H_2 antagonists, HMG-CoA reductase inhibitors, prostaglandin synthetase inhibitors (NSAIDs), and quinolones, without evidence of clinically significant adverse interactions.

4.6 Pregnancy and lactation

Use during pregnancy

'Propecia' is contra-indicated for use in women due to the risk in pregnancy.

Because of the ability of type II 5α-reductase inhibitors to inhibit conversion of testosterone to dihydrotestosterone (DHT) in some tissues, these drugs, including finasteride, may cause abnormalities of the external genitalia of a male foetus when administered to a pregnant woman.

Exposure to finasteride: risk to male foetus

A small amount of finasteride, less than 0.001% of the 1 mg dose per ejaculation, has been detected in the seminal fluid of men taking 'Propecia'. Studies in Rhesus monkeys have indicated that this amount is unlikely to constitute a risk to the developing male foetus (see Section 5.3).

During continual collection of adverse experiences, post-marketing reports of exposure to finasteride during pregnancy via semen of men taking 1 mg or higher doses have been received for eight live male births, and one retrospectively-reported case concerned an infant with simple hypospadias. Causality cannot be assessed on the basis of this single retrospective report and hypospadias is a relatively common congenital anomaly with an incidence ranging from 0.8 to 8 per 1000 live male births. In addition, a further nine live male births occurred during clinical trials following exposure to finasteride via semen, during pregnancy, and no congenital anomalies have been reported.

Crushed or broken tablets of 'Propecia' should not be handled by women when they are or may potentially be pregnant because of the possibility of absorption of finasteride and the subsequent potential risk to a male foetus. 'Propecia' tablets are coated to prevent contact with the active ingredient during normal handling, provided that the tablets are not broken or crushed.

Use during lactation

'Propecia' is contraindicated for use in lactation.

4.7 Effects on ability to drive and use machines

There are no data to suggest that 'Propecia' affects the ability to drive or use machines.

4.8 Undesirable effects

Side effects, which usually have been mild, generally have not required discontinuation of therapy.

Finasteride for male pattern hair loss has been evaluated for safety in clinical studies involving more than 3,200 men. In three 12-month, placebo-controlled, double-blind, multicentre studies of comparable design, the overall safety profiles of 'Propecia' and placebo were similar. Discontinuation of therapy due to any clinical adverse experience occurred in 1.7% of 945 men treated with 'Propecia' and 2.1% of 934 men treated with placebo.

In these studies, the following drug-related adverse experiences were reported in $\geqslant$1% of men treated with 'Propecia': decreased libido ('Propecia', 1.8% vs. placebo, 1.3%) and erectile dysfunction (1.3%, 0.7%). In addition, decreased volume of ejaculate was reported in 0.8% of men treated with 'Propecia' and 0.4% of men treated with placebo. Resolution of these side effects occurred in men who discontinued therapy with 'Propecia' and in many who continued therapy. The effect of 'Propecia' on ejaculate volume was measured in a separate study and was not different from that seen with placebo.

By the fifth year of treatment with 'Propecia', the proportion of patients reporting each of the above side effects decreased to $\leq$0.3%.

Finasteride has also been studied for prostate cancer risk reduction at 5 times the dosage recommended for male pattern hair loss. In a 7-year placebo-controlled trial that enrolled 18,882 healthy men, of whom 9060 had prostate needle biopsy data available for analysis, prostate cancer was detected in 803 (18.4%) men receiving finasteride 5 mg and 1147 (24.4%) men receiving placebo. In the finasteride 5 mg group, 280 (6.4%) men had prostate cancer with Gleason scores of 7-10 detected on needle biopsy vs. 237 (5.1%) men in placebo group. Of the total cases of prostate cancer diagnosed in this study, approximately 98% were classified as intracapsular (stage T1 or T2). The relationship between long-term use of finasteride 5 mg and tumours with Gleason scores of 7-10 is unknown.

The following undesirable effects have been reported in post-marketing use: ejaculation disorder; breast tenderness and enlargement; hypersensitivity reactions including rash, pruritus, urticaria and swelling of the lips and face; and testicular pain.

4.9 Overdose

In clinical studies, single doses of finasteride up to 400 mg and multiple doses of finasteride up to 80 mg/day for three months did not result in side effects.

No specific treatment of overdosage with 'Propecia' is recommended.

5. PHARMACOLOGICAL PROPERTIES

5.1 Pharmacodynamic properties

Finasteride is a competitive and specific inhibitor of type II 5α-reductase. Finasteride has no affinity for the androgen receptor and has no androgenic, anti-androgenic, oestrogenic, anti-oestrogenic, or progestational effects. Inhibition of this enzyme blocks the peripheral conversion of testosterone to the androgen DHT, resulting in significant decreases in serum and tissue DHT concentrations. Finasteride produces a rapid reduction in serum DHT concentration, reaching significant suppression within 24 hours of dosing.

Hair follicles contain type II 5α-reductase. In men with male pattern hair loss, the balding scalp contains miniaturised hair follicles and increased amounts of DHT. Administration of finasteride decreases scalp and serum DHT concentrations in these men. Men with a genetic deficiency of type II 5α-reductase do not suffer from male pattern hair loss. Finasteride inhibits a process responsible for miniaturisation of the scalp hair follicles, which can lead to reversal of the balding process.

Studies in men

Clinical studies were conducted in 1879 men aged 18 to 41 with mild to moderate, but not complete, vertex hair loss and/or frontal/mid-area hair loss. In the two studies in men with vertex hair loss (n=1553), 290 men completed 5 years of treatment with Propecia vs. 16 patients on placebo. In these two studies, efficacy was assessed by the following methods: (i) hair count in a representative 5.1cm^2 area of scalp, (ii) patient self assessment questionnaire, (iii) investigator assessment using a seven point scale, and (iv) photographic assessment of standardised paired photographs by a blinded expert panel of dermatologists using a seven point scale.

In these 5- year studies men treated with 'Propecia' improved compared to both baseline and placebo beginning as early as 3 months, as determined by both the patient and investigator assessments of efficacy. With regard to hair count, the primary endpoint in these studies, increases compared to baseline were demonstrated starting at 6 months (the earliest time point assessed) through to the end of the study. In men treated with 'Propecia' these increases were greatest at 2 years and gradually declined thereafter to the end of 5 years; whereas hair loss in the placebo group progressively worsened compared to baseline over the entire 5 year period. In 'Propecia' treated patients, a mean increase from baseline of 88 hairs *[$p<0.01$; 95% CI (77.9, 97.80; n=433]* in the representative 5.1 cm^2 area was observed at 2 years and an increase from baseline of 38 hairs *[$p<0.01$; 95% CI (20.8, 55.6); n=219]* was observed at 5 years, compared with a decrease from baseline of 50 hairs *[$p<0.01$; 95% CI (-80.5, -20.6);n=47]* at 2 years and a decrease from baseline of 239 hairs *[$p<0.01$; 95% CI (-304.4, -173.4); n=15]* at 5 years in patients who received placebo. Standardised photographic assessment of efficacy demonstrated that 48% of men treated with finasteride for 5 years were rated as improved, and an additional 42% were rated as unchanged. This is in comparison to 25% of men treated with placebo for 5 years who were rated as improved or unchanged. These data demonstrate that treatment with 'Propecia' for 5 years resulted in a stabilisation of the hair loss that occurred in men treated with placebo.

An additional 48-week, placebo-controlled study designed to assess the effect of 'Propecia' on the phases of the hair-growth cycle (growing phase [anagen] and resting phase [telogen]) in vertex baldness enrolled 212 men with androgenetic alopecia. At baseline and 48 weeks, total, anagen and telogen hair counts were obtained in a 1-cm^2 target area of the scalp. Treatment with 'Propecia' led to improvements in anagen hair counts, while men in the placebo group lost anagen hair. At 48 weeks, men treated with 'Propecia' showed net increases in total and anagen hair counts of 17 hairs and 27 hairs, respectively, compared to placebo. This increase in anagen hair count, compared to total hair count, led to a net improvement in the anagen-to-telogen ratio of 47% at 48 weeks for men treated with 'Propecia', compared to placebo. These data provide direct evidence that treatment with 'Propecia' promotes the conversion of hair follicles into the actively growing phase.

Studies in women

Lack of efficacy was demonstrated in post-menopausal women with androgenetic alopecia who were treated with 'Propecia' in a 12 month, placebo-controlled study (n=137). These women did not show any improvement in hair count, patient self-assessment, investigator assessment, or ratings based on standardised photographs, compared with the placebo group.

5.2 Pharmacokinetic properties

Absorption

Relative to an intravenous reference dose, the oral bioavailability of finasteride is approximately 80%. The bioavailability is not affected by food. Maximum finasteride plasma concentrations are reached approximately two hours after dosing and the absorption is complete after six to eight hours.

Distribution

Protein binding is approximately 93%. The volume of distribution of finasteride is approximately 76 litres.

At steady state following dosing with 1 mg/day, maximum finasteride plasma concentration averaged 9.2 ng/ml and was reached 1 to 2 hours postdose; AUC $_{(0\text{-}24\ hr)}$ was 53 ng•hr/ml.

Finasteride has been recovered in the cerebrospinal fluid (CSF), but the drug does not appear to concentrate preferentially to the CSF. A small amount of finasteride has also been detected in the seminal fluid of subjects receiving the drug.

Biotransformation

Finasteride is metabolised primarily via the cytochrome P450 3A4 enzyme subfamily. Following an oral dose of ^{14}C-finasteride in man, two metabolites of the drug were identified that possess only a small fraction of the 5α-reductase inhibitory activity of finasteride.

Elimination

Following an oral dose of ^{14}C-finasteride in man, 39% of the dose was excreted in the urine in the form of metabolites (virtually no unchanged drug was excreted in the urine) and 57% of total dose was excreted in the faeces.

Plasma clearance is approximately 165 ml/min.

The elimination rate of finasteride decreases somewhat with age. Mean terminal half-life is approximately 5-6 hours in men 18-60 years of age and 8 hours in men more than 70 years of age. These findings are of no clinical significance and hence, a reduction in dosage in the elderly is not warranted.

Characteristics in patients

No adjustment in dosage is necessary in non-dialysed patients with renal impairment.

5.3 Preclinical safety data

In general, the findings in laboratory animal studies with oral finasteride were related to the pharmacological effects of 5α-reductase inhibition.

Intravenous administration of finasteride to pregnant rhesus monkeys at doses as high as 800 ng/day during the entire period of embryonic and foetal development resulted in no abnormalities in male foetuses. This represents at least 750 times the highest estimated exposure of pregnant women to finasteride from semen. In confirmation of the relevance of the Rhesus model for human foetal development, oral administration of finasteride 2 mg/kg/day (100 times the recommended human dose or approximately 12 million times the highest estimated exposure to finasteride from semen) to pregnant monkeys resulted in external genital abnormalities in male foetuses. No other abnormalities were observed in male foetuses and no finasteride-related abnormalities were observed in female foetuses at any dose.

6. PHARMACEUTICAL PARTICULARS

6.1 List of excipients

Lactose, microcrystalline cellulose E460, pregelatinised maize starch, sodium starch glycollate, docusate sodium, magnesium stearate E572, hypromellose E464, hydroxypropyl cellulose E463, titanium dioxide, talc, yellow iron oxide E172, red iron oxide E172.

6.2 Incompatibilities

Not applicable.

6.3 Shelf life

36 months.

6.4 Special precautions for storage

Do not store above 30°C. Store in original package.

6.5 Nature and contents of container

Aluminium blisters lidded with aluminium foil, containing 28 tablets or 84 tablets.

6.6 Special precautions for disposal and other handling

Crushed or broken tablets of 'Propecia' should not be handled by women when they are or may potentially be pregnant (see 4.6 'Pregnancy and lactation').

7. MARKETING AUTHORISATION HOLDER

Merck Sharp & Dohme Limited

Hertford Road, Hoddesdon, Hertfordshire EN11 9BU, UK.

8. MARKETING AUTHORISATION NUMBER(S)

PL 0025/0351

9. DATE OF FIRST AUTHORISATION/RENEWAL OF THE AUTHORISATION

20 September 1999/ 21 July 2005

10. DATE OF REVISION OF THE TEXT

September 2008

LEGAL CATEGORY

POM

® denotes registered trademark of Merck & Co., Inc., Whitehouse Station, NJ, USA.

SPC.PPC.07.UK.2802 F.T.031008

Propess 10mg vaginal delivery system

(Ferring Pharmaceuticals Ltd)

1. NAME OF THE MEDICINAL PRODUCT

PROPESS 10mg vaginal delivery system

2. QUALITATIVE AND QUANTITATIVE COMPOSITION

Each vaginal delivery system consists of a non-biodegradable polymeric drug delivery device containing 10mg dinoprostone (Prostaglandin E_2) dispersed throughout its matrix.

For a full list of excipients, see 6.1

3. PHARMACEUTICAL FORM

Vaginal delivery system

PROPESS is presented as a thin, flat semi-opaque polymeric vaginal delivery system which is rectangular in shape with radiused corners contained within a knitted polyester retrieval system.

4. CLINICAL PARTICULARS

4.1 Therapeutic indications

Initiation of cervical ripening in patients, at term (from 38th week of gestation).

4.2 Posology and method of administration

One vaginal delivery system is administered high into the posterior vaginal fornix.

If there has been insufficient cervical ripening in 24 hours, the vaginal delivery system should be removed.

A dosing interval of at least 30 minutes is recommended for the sequential use of oxytocin following the removal of the vaginal delivery system.

Administration

PROPESS should be removed from the freezer in direct connection with the insertion.

The vaginal delivery system should be inserted high into the posterior vaginal fornix using only small amounts of water soluble lubricants to aid insertion. After the vaginal delivery system has been inserted, the withdrawal tape may be cut with scissors always ensuring there is sufficient tape outside the vagina to allow removal. No attempt should be made to tuck the end of the tape into the vagina as this may make retrieval more difficult.

The patient should be recumbent for 20 minutes to 30 minutes after insertion. As dinoprostone will be released continuously over a period of 24 hours, it is important to monitor uterine contractions and fetal condition at frequent regular intervals.

Removal

The vaginal delivery system can be removed quickly and easily by gentle traction on the retrieval tape.

It is necessary to remove the vaginal delivery system to terminate drug administration when cervical ripening is judged to be complete or for any of the reasons listed below.

1. Onset of labour. For the purposes of induction of labour with PROPESS, the onset of labour is defined as the presence of regular painful uterine contractions occurring every 3 minutes irrespective of any cervical change. There are two important points to note:

(i) Once regular, painful contractions have been established with PROPESS they will not reduce in frequency or intensity as long as PROPESS remains *in situ* because dinoprostone is still being administered.

(ii) Patients, particularly multigravidae, may develop regular painful contractions without any apparent cervical change.

Effacement and dilatation of the cervix may not occur until uterine activity is established. Because of this, once regular painful uterine activity is established with PROPESS *in situ*, the vaginal delivery system should be removed irrespective of cervical state to avoid the risk of uterine hyperstimulation.

2. Spontaneous rupture of the membranes or amniotomy.
3. Any suggestion of uterine hyperstimulation or hypertonic uterine contractions.
4. Evidence of fetal distress.
5. Evidence of maternal systemic adverse dinoprostone effects such as nausea, vomiting, hypotension or tachycardia.
6. At least 30 minutes prior to starting an intravenous infusion of oxytocin.

The opening on one side of the retrieval device is present only to allow the manufacturer to enclose the vaginal delivery system into the retrieval device during manufacture. The vaginal delivery system should NEVER be removed from the retrieval device.

On removal of the product from the vagina, the vaginal delivery system will have swollen to 2-3 times its original size and be pliable.

4.3 Contraindications

PROPESS should not be used or left in place:

1. When labour has started.
2. When oxytocic drugs are being given.
3. When strong prolonged uterine contractions would be inappropriate such as in patients:

a. who have had previous major uterine surgery, e.g. caesarean section, myomectomy etc (see sections 4.4 and 4.8)

b. with cephalopelvic disproportion

c. with fetal malpresentation

d. with suspicion or evidence of fetal distress

e. who have had more than three full term deliveries

f. previous surgery or rupture of the cervix

4. When there is current pelvic inflammatory disease, unless adequate prior treatment has been instituted.
5. When there is hypersensitivity to dinoprostone or to any of the excipients.
6. When there is placenta previa or unexplained vaginal bleeding during the current pregnancy.

4.4 Special warnings and precautions for use

The condition of the cervix should be assessed carefully before PROPESS is used. After insertion, uterine activity and fetal condition must be monitored regularly. PROPESS must only be used if facilities for continuous fetal and uterine monitoring are available. If there is any suggestion of maternal or fetal complications or if adverse effects occur, the vaginal delivery system should be removed from the vagina.

The experience of PROPESS in patients with ruptured membranes is limited. Therefore, PROPESS should be used with caution in those patients. Since the release of dinoprostone from the insert can be affected in the presence of amniotic fluid, special attention should be given to uterine activity and fetal condition.

PROPESS should be used with caution in patients with a previous history of uterine hypertony, glaucoma or asthma.

Medication with non-steroidal anti-inflammatory drugs, including acetylsalicylic acid, should be stopped before administration of dinoprostone.

If uterine contractions are prolonged or excessive, there is possibility of uterine hypertonus or rupture and the vaginal delivery system should be removed immediately.

Uterine rupture has been reported in association with the use of PROPESS, mainly in patients with contra-indicated conditions (see section 4.3). Therefore, PROPESS should not be administered to patients with a history of previous caesarean section or uterine surgery given the potential risk for uterine rupture and associated obstetrical complications.

PROPESS should be used with caution when there is a multiple pregnancy. No studies in multiple pregnancy have been performed.

A second dose of PROPESS is not recommended, as the effects of a second dose have not been studied.

The use of the product in patients with diseases which could affect the metabolism or excretion of dinoprostone, e.g. lung, liver or renal disease, has not been specifically studied. The use of the product in such patients is not recommended.

Women aged 35 and over, women with complications during pregnancy, such as gestational diabetes, arterial hypertension and hypothyroidism, and women at gestational age above 40 weeks have a higher post-partum risk for developing disseminated intravascular coagulation (DIC). These factors may additionally enhance the risk of disseminated intravascular coagulation in women with pharmacologically induced labour (see section 4.8). Therefore, dinoprostone and oxytocin should be used with caution in these women. In the immediate post-partum phase the physician should look out carefully for early signs of a developing DIC (e.g fibrinolysis).

4.5 Interaction with other medicinal products and other forms of interaction

Prostaglandins potentiate the uterotonic effect of oxytocic drugs. Therefore, PROPESS should not be used concurrently with the use of oxytocic drugs.

4.6 Pregnancy and lactation

The product is for the initiation of cervical ripening in pregnant patients at term only where labour induction is indicated.

PROPESS is not indicated for use during early or other phases of pregnancy or during lactation.

4.7 Effects on ability to drive and use machines

Not relevant.

4.8 Undesirable effects

The occasional effects seen have been those normally associated with intravaginal dinoprostone administration.

CTG changes and unspecified fetal distress have been reported during and after administration of intravaginal dinoprostone. Increased uterine activity with hypertonic contractions with or without fetal distress has been reported. There is a much greater risk of hyperstimulation if the dinoprostone source is not removed before administration of oxytocin because prostaglandins are known to potentiate the uterotonic effects of oxytocic drugs.

Frequency	MedDRA System Organ Class	Adverse Events (MedDRA Preferred Term)
Common (>1/100, <1/10)	Pregnancy, puerperium and perinatal conditions	Abnormal labour affecting fetus Fetal heart rate disorder Fetal distress syndrome Uterine hypertonus
Uncommon (>1/1,000, <1/100)	Gastro-intestinal disorders	Nausea, vomiting, diarrhoea
Rare (>1/10,000, <1/1,000)	Blood and lymphatic system disorders Pregnancy, puerperium and perinatal conditions	Disseminated intravascular coagulation Uterine rupture
Very rare (<1/10,000) including isolated reports	Immune system disorders Reproductive system and breast disorders	Anaphylactic reaction Genital oedema

In the pivotal efficacy study, five (4.9%) of 102 patients had hyperstimulation. Of these, three cases were associated with fetal distress. Of the five cases, uterine hypertonus was resolved in four after removal of the insert.

In post-marketing experience reports, uterine rupture has been reported rarely in association with the use of PROPESS (see sections 4.3 and 4.4).

An increased risk of post-partum disseminated intravascular coagulation has been reported in patients whose labour was induced by pharmacological means, either with dinoprostone or oxytocin (see section 4.4).

PGE_2 is known to be responsible for the patency of the ductus arteriosus in pregnancy but there have been no reports of "blue babies" in the neonatal period after the use of PROPESS.

4.9 Overdose

Overdosage or hypersensitivity may lead to hyperstimulation of the uterine muscle or fetal distress. The PROPESS vaginal delivery system should be removed immediately and the patient should be managed in accordance with local protocol.

5. PHARMACOLOGICAL PROPERTIES

5.1 Pharmacodynamic properties

Pharmacotherapeutic group: oxytocics, ATC-code: G02AD02

Prostaglandin E_2 (PGE_2) is a naturally occurring compound found in low concentrations in most tissues of the body. It functions as a local hormone.

Prostaglandin E_2 plays an important role in the complex set of biochemical and structural alterations involved in cervical ripening. Cervical ripening involves a marked relaxation of the cervical smooth muscle fibres of the uterine cervix which must be transformed from a rigid structure to a soft, dilated configuration to allow passage of the fetus through the birth canal. This process involves activation of the enzyme collagenase which is responsible for the breakdown of the collagen.

Local administration of dinoprostone to the cervix results in cervical ripening which then induces the subsequent events which complete labour.

5.2 Pharmacokinetic properties

PGE_2 is rapidly metabolised primarily in the tissue of synthesis. Any which escapes local inactivation is rapidly cleared from the circulation with a half-life generally estimated as 1-3 minutes.

No correlation could be established between PGE_2 release and plasma concentrations of its metabolite, PGE_m. The relative contributions of endogenously and exogenously released PGE_2 to the plasma levels of the metabolite PGE_m could not be determined.

The reservoir of 10mg dinoprostone serves to maintain a controlled and constant release. The release rate is approximately 0.3mg per hour over 24 hours in women with intact membranes whereas release is higher and more variable in women with premature rupture of membranes. PROPESS releases dinoprostone to the cervical tissue continuously at a rate which allows cervical ripening to progress until complete, and with the facility to remove the dinoprostone source when the clinician decides that cervical ripening is complete or labour has started, at which point no further dinoprostone is required.

5.3 Preclinical safety data

Preclinical studies have demonstrated that dinoprostone is a locally acting substance which is rapidly inactivated and thus it has no significant systemic toxicity.

The hydrogel and polyester polymers are inert compounds with good local tolerability.

Reproduction toxicity, genotoxic or carcinogenic effects of the polymers have not been investigated but systemic exposure is negligible.

6. PHARMACEUTICAL PARTICULARS

6.1 List of excipients

Crosslinked polyethylene glycol (hydrogel)

Polyester yarn.

6.2 Incompatibilities

Not applicable

6.3 Shelf life

3 Years

6.4 Special precautions for storage

Store in a freezer. Store in the original container in order to protect from moisture.

6.5 Nature and contents of container

PROPESS vaginal delivery systems are presented in individual, sealed aluminium/polyethylene laminate sachets in packs of 5 vaginal delivery systems.

6.6 Special precautions for disposal and other handling

PROPESS should be removed from the freezer in direct connection with the insertion.

After usage, the whole product should be disposed of as clinical waste.

7. MARKETING AUTHORISATION HOLDER

Ferring Pharmaceuticals Ltd.

The Courtyard

Waterside Drive

Langley

Berkshire SL3 6EZ

United Kingdom

8. MARKETING AUTHORISATION NUMBER(S)

PL 03194/0084

9. DATE OF FIRST AUTHORISATION/RENEWAL OF THE AUTHORISATION

15th February 2001

10. DATE OF REVISION OF THE TEXT

16th February 2007

Propine

(Allergan Ltd)

1. NAME OF THE MEDICINAL PRODUCT

PROPINE®

2. QUALITATIVE AND QUANTITATIVE COMPOSITION

Dipivefrin hydrochloride 0.1% w/v.

3. PHARMACEUTICAL FORM

Eye drops.

4. CLINICAL PARTICULARS

4.1 Therapeutic indications

To control intraocular pressure in patients with chronic open angle glaucoma or ocular hypertensive patients with anterior chamber open angles.

4.2 Posology and method of administration

The usual dosage is one drop in the affected eye(s) every 12 hours.

4.3 Contraindications

a) Patients suffering from closed angle glaucoma

b) Hypersensitivity to any component of the formulation

4.4 Special warnings and precautions for use

Dipivefrin should be used with caution in patients with narrow angles since dilation of the pupil may trigger an attack of angle closure glaucoma.

Macular oedema is a rare occurrence with adrenaline use in aphakic patients. Prompt reversal generally follows discontinuance of the drug. Macular oedema with dipivefrin does present as a possibility in the aphakic patient.

PROPINE® should be used in caution with patients who have hypertension, heart disease or hyperthyroidism.

This product contains benzalkonium chloride and should not be used by patients continuing to wear soft (hydrophilic) contact lenses.

4.5 Interaction with other medicinal products and other forms of interaction

Systemic absorption is a possibility for PROPINE® and consequently there is potential for the following interactions to occur:

Mono-amine oxidase inhibitors: There is an elevated risk of adrenergic reactions with concomitant use of MAOIs. These interactions may occur up to 14 days after ceasing the concomitant MAOI therapy.

Tricyclic antidepressants: The pressor response to adrenergic agents and the risk of cardiac arrhythmia may be exacerbated in those patients receiving concomitant tricyclic antidepressants. Upon their cessation the pressor response may persist for up to several days.

Halogenated anaesthetics: PROPINE® should not be administered during general anaesthesia with those anaesthetic agents which sensitise the myocardium to sympathomimetics since under these circumstances there is an elevated risk of ventricular fibrillation.

4.6 Pregnancy and lactation

The safety of intensive or protracted use of dipivefrin during pregnancy has not been substantiated. Caution should be exercised when PROPINE® is administered to a nursing mother.

4.7 Effects on ability to drive and use machines

Mydriasis may occur in some patients. Do not drive or operate machinery if affected.

4.8 Undesirable effects

a) Cardiovascular: tachycardia, arrhythmias and hypertension have been reported with ocular administration of adrenaline, and may occur rarely with dipivefrin therapy.

b) Ocular: the most frequently reported side effects are conjunctival hyperaemia, and burning and stinging on instillation.

Rebound vasodilation, mydriasis and allergic reactions, including blepharoconjunctivitis have been reported occasionally.

Adrenochrome deposits in the conjunctiva and cornea have been associated rarely with the use of dipivefrin.

Follicular conjunctivitis has been reported during long term therapy with dipivefrin. The condition is reversible upon discontinuance of the drug.

c) Body as a Whole: headache may occur rarely with dipivefrin (and is occasionally associated with hypertension and tachycardia).

4.9 Overdose

There are no data available on overdosage with PROPINE®, which is unlikely to occur via the ocular route.

5. PHARMACOLOGICAL PROPERTIES

5.1 Pharmacodynamic properties

Dipivefrin is a prodrug that is converted inside the eye to adrenaline. Conversion takes place by enzyme hydrolysis.

Adrenaline, an adrenergic agonist, appears to exert its action by decreasing aqueous production and enhancing aqueous outflow facility.

5.2 Pharmacokinetic properties

Onset of action after instillation is about 30 minutes. Time to peak effect is about 1 hour.

5.3 Preclinical safety data

-

6. PHARMACEUTICAL PARTICULARS

6.1 List of excipients

Benzalkonium chloride

Disodium edetate

Sodium chloride

Hydrochloric acid (to adjust pH)

Purified water

6.2 Incompatibilities

None known

6.3 Shelf life

The shelf life of the unopened bottle is 18 months. Once opened, the shelf life is 28 days.

6.4 Special precautions for storage

Store at 25°C or less.

6.5 Nature and contents of container

White, low density polyethylene 5 ml and 10 ml fill dropper bottle and tip in single or triple packs; white, medium impact polystyrene (MIPS) screw cap or compliance screw cap (C-cap®).

6.6 Special precautions for disposal and other handling

No special instructions required.

7. MARKETING AUTHORISATION HOLDER

Allergan Ltd

Marlow International

The Parkway

Marlow

Bucks

SL7 1YL

UK

8. MARKETING AUTHORISATION NUMBER(S)

PL 00426/0040

9. DATE OF FIRST AUTHORISATION/RENEWAL OF THE AUTHORISATION

27th May 2002

10. DATE OF REVISION OF THE TEXT

20th December 2007

Proscar 5mg film-coated Tablets

(Merck Sharp & Dohme Limited)

1. NAME OF THE MEDICINAL PRODUCT

PROSCAR® 5mg film-coated Tablets

(finasteride)

2. QUALITATIVE AND QUANTITATIVE COMPOSITION

Each tablet contains 5 mg of finasteride.

3. PHARMACEUTICAL FORM

Blue-coloured, apple-shaped, film-coated tablets marked 'Proscar' on one side and 'MSD 72' on the other.

4. CLINICAL PARTICULARS

4.1 Therapeutic indications

'Proscar' is indicated for the treatment and control of benign prostatic hyperplasia (BPH) in patients with an enlarged prostate to:

– cause regression of the enlarged prostate, improve urinary flow and improve the symptoms associated with BPH

– reduce the incidence of acute urinary retention and the need for surgery including transurethral resection of the prostate (TURP) and prostatectomy.

4.2 Posology and method of administration

The recommended adult dose is one 5 mg tablet daily, with or without food.

'Proscar' can be administered alone or in combination with the alpha-blocker doxazosin (see section 5.1 'Pharmacodynamic properties').

Although early improvement in symptoms may be seen, treatment for at least six months may be necessary to assess whether a beneficial response has been achieved. Thereafter, treatment should be continued long term.

No dosage adjustment is required in the elderly or in patients with varying degrees of renal insufficiency (creatinine clearances as low as 9 ml/min).

There are no data available in patients with hepatic insufficiency.

'Proscar' is contra-indicated in children.

4.3 Contraindications

Hypersensitivity to any component of this product; women who are or may potentially be pregnant; children.

4.4 Special warnings and precautions for use

General

Patients with large residual urine volume and/or severely diminished urinary flow should be carefully monitored for obstructive uropathy.

Effects on prostate-specific antigen (PSA) and prostate cancer detection

No clinical benefit has yet been demonstrated in patients with prostate cancer treated with 'Proscar'.

Digital rectal examination, as well as other evaluations for prostate cancer, should be carried out on patients with BPH prior to initiating therapy with 'Proscar' and periodically thereafter. Generally, when PSA assays are performed a baseline PSA >10 ng/ml (Hybritech) prompts further evaluation and consideration of biopsy; for PSA levels between 4 and 10 ng/ml, further evaluation is advisable. There is considerable overlap in PSA levels among men with and without prostate cancer. Therefore, in men with BPH, PSA values within the normal reference range do not rule out prostate cancer regardless of treatment with 'Proscar'. A baseline PSA <4 ng/ml does not exclude prostate cancer.

'Proscar' causes a decrease in serum PSA concentrations by approximately 50% in patients with BPH even in the presence of prostate cancer. This decrease in serum PSA levels in patients with BPH treated with 'Proscar' should be considered when evaluating PSA data and does not rule out concomitant prostate cancer. This decrease is predictive over the entire range of PSA values, although it may vary in individual patients. In patients treated with 'Proscar' for six months or more, PSA values should be doubled for comparison with normal ranges in untreated men. This adjustment preserves the sensitivity and specificity of the PSA assay and maintains its ability to detect prostate cancer.

Any sustained increase in PSA levels of patients treated with finasteride should be carefully evaluated, including consideration of non-compliance to therapy with 'Proscar'.

Percent free PSA (free to total PSA ratio) is not significantly decreased by 'Proscar' and remains constant even under the influence of 'Proscar'. When percent free PSA is used as an aid in the detection of prostate cancer, no adjustment is necessary.

Excipients

Patients with rare hereditary problems of galactose intolerance, the Lapp lactase deficiency or glucose-galactose malabsorption should not take this medicine.

4.5 Interaction with other medicinal products and other forms of interaction

No clinically important drug interactions have been identified. 'Proscar' does not appear to significantly affect the cytochrome P450-linked drug metabolising enzyme system. Compounds which have been tested in man include propranolol, digoxin, glibenclamide, warfarin, theophylline, and antipyrine and no clinically meaningful interactions were found.

Other concomitant therapy: Although specific interaction studies were not performed in clinical studies, 'Proscar' was used concomitantly with ACE inhibitors, alpha-blockers, beta-blockers, calcium channel blockers, cardiac nitrates, diuretics, H_2 antagonists, HMG-CoA reductase inhibitors, non-steroidal anti-inflammatory drugs (NSAIDs) including aspirin and paracetamol, quinolones and benzodiazepines without evidence of clinically significant adverse interactions.

4.6 Pregnancy and lactation

Pregnancy: 'Proscar' is contra-indicated in women who are or may potentially be pregnant.

Because of the ability of Type II 5 α-reductase inhibitors to inhibit conversion of testosterone to dihydrotestosterone, these drugs, including finasteride, may cause abnormalities of the external genitalia of a male foetus when administered to a pregnant woman.

In animal developmental studies, dose-dependent development of hypospadias were observed in the male offspring of pregnant rats given finasteride at doses ranging from 100 μg/kg/day to 100 mg/kg/day, at an incidence of 3.6% to 100%. Additionally, pregnant rats produced male offspring with decreased prostatic and seminal vesicular weights, delayed preputial separation, transient nipple development and decreased anogenital distance, when given finasteride at doses below the recommended human dose. The critical period during which these effects can be induced has been defined in rats as days 16-17 of gestation.

The changes described above are expected pharmacological effects of Type II 5 α-reductase inhibitors. Many of the changes, such as hypospadias, observed in male rats exposed *in utero* to finasteride are similar to those reported in male infants with a genetic deficiency of Type II 5 α-reductase. It is for these reasons that 'Proscar' is contra-indicated in women who are or may potentially be pregnant.

No effects were seen in female offspring exposed *in utero* to any dose of finasteride.

Exposure to finasteride - risk to male foetus

Women should not handle crushed or broken tablets of 'Proscar' when they are or may potentially be pregnant because of the possibility of absorption of finasteride and the subsequent potential risk to a male foetus (see 'Pregnancy'). 'Proscar' tablets are coated and will prevent contact with the active ingredient during normal handling, provided that the tablets have not been broken or crushed.

Small amounts of finasteride have been recovered from the semen in subjects receiving finasteride 5 mg/day. It is not known whether a male foetus may be adversely affected if his mother is exposed to the semen of a patient being treated with finasteride. When the patient's sexual partner is or may potentially be pregnant, the patient is recommended to minimise exposure of his partner to semen.

Lactation: 'Proscar' is not indicated for use in women. It is not known whether finasteride is excreted in human milk.

4.7 Effects on ability to drive and use machines

None reported.

4.8 Undesirable effects

'Proscar' is well tolerated. In controlled clinical studies where patients received 5 mg of finasteride over periods of up to four years, the following adverse reactions were considered possibly, probably or definitely drug-related and occurred with a frequency greater than placebo and greater than or equal to 1%: impotence, decreased libido, ejaculation disorder, decreased volume of ejaculate; breast enlargement, breast tenderness and rash. There was no evidence of increased adverse experiences with increased duration of treatment with 'Proscar' and the incidence of new drug-related sexual adverse experiences decreased with duration of treatment.

Medical therapy of prostatic symptoms (MTOPS)

The MTOPS study compared finasteride 5 mg/day (n=768), doxazosin 4 or 8 mg/day (n=756), combination therapy of finasteride 5 mg/day and doxazosin 4 or 8 mg/day (n=786), and placebo (n=737). In this study, the safety and tolerability profile of the combination therapy was generally consistent with the profiles of the individual components. The incidence of ejaculation disorder events without regard to drug relationship were: finasteride 8.3%, doxazosin 5.3%, combination 15.0%, placebo 3.9%.

Other long-term data

In a 7 year placebo-controlled trial that enrolled 18,882 healthy men, of 9060 had prostate needle biopsy data available for analysis, prostate cancer was detected in 803 (18.4%) men receiving 'Proscar' and 1147 (24.4%) men receiving placebo. In the 'Proscar' group, 280 (6.4%) of men had prostate cancer with Gleason scores of 7-10 detected on needle biopsy vs 237 (5.1%). Of the total cases of prostate cancer diagnosed in this study, approximately 98% were classified as intracapsular (stage T1 or T2). The relationship between long-term use of 'Proscar' and tumours with Gleason scores of 7-10 is unknown.

Post Marketing Experience

The following additional adverse experiences have been reported in post-marketing experience:

– hypersensitivity reactions, including pruritus, urticaria and swelling of the lips and face

– testicular pain.

Laboratory test findings

Serum PSA concentration is correlated with patient age and prostatic volume, and prostatic volume is correlated with patient age. When PSA laboratory determinations are evaluated, consideration should be given to the fact that PSA levels generally decrease in patients treated with 'Proscar'. In most patients, a rapid decrease in PSA is seen within the first months of therapy, after which time PSA levels stabilise to a new baseline. The post-treatment baseline approximates half of the pre-treatment value. Therefore, in typical patients treated with 'Proscar' for six months or more, PSA values should be doubled for comparison to normal ranges in untreated men.

For clinical interpretation see 'Special warnings and precautions for use', *Effects on prostate-specific antigen (PSA) and prostate cancer detection.*

No other difference was observed in patients treated with placebo or 'Proscar' in standard laboratory tests.

4.9 Overdose

No specific treatment of overdosage with 'Proscar' is recommended. Patients have received single doses of 'Proscar' up to 400 mg and multiple doses of 'Proscar' up to 80 mg/day for up to three months without any adverse effects.

5. PHARMACOLOGICAL PROPERTIES

5.1 Pharmacodynamic properties

Finasteride is a competitive inhibitor of human 5 α-reductase, an intracellular enzyme which metabolises testosterone into the more potent androgen, dihydrotestosterone (DHT). In benign prostatic hyperplasia (BPH), enlargement of the prostate gland is dependent upon the conversion of testosterone to DHT within the prostate. 'Proscar' is highly effective in reducing circulating and intraprostatic DHT. Finasteride has no affinity for the androgen receptor.

In clinical studies of patients with moderate to severe symptoms of BPH, an enlarged prostate on digital rectal examination and low residual urinary volumes, 'Proscar' reduced the incidence of acute retention of urine from 7/100 to 3/100 over four years and the need for surgery (TURP or prostatectomy) from 10/100 to 5/100. These reductions were associated with a 2-point improvement in QUASI-AUA symptom score (range 0-34), a sustained regression in prostate volume of approximately 20% and a sustained increase in urinary flow rate.

Medical therapy of prostatic symptoms

The Medical Therapy of Prostatic Symptoms (MTOPS) Trial was a 4- to 6-year study in 3047 men with symptomatic BPH who were randomised to receive finasteride 5 mg/day, doxazosin 4 or 8 mg/day*, the combination of finasteride 5 mg/day and doxazosin 4 or 8 mg/day*, or placebo. The primary endpoint was time to clinical progression of BPH, defined as a ≥4 point confirmed increase from baseline in symptom score, acute urinary retention, BPH-related renal insufficiency, recurrent urinary tract infections or urosepsis, or incontinence. Compared to placebo, treatment with finasteride, doxazosin, or combination therapy resulted in a significant reduction in the risk of clinical progression of BPH by 34(p=0.002), 39 (p<0.001), and 67% (p<0.001), respectively. The majority of the events (274 out of 351) that constituted BPH progression were confirmed ≥4 point increases in symptom score; the risk of symptom score progression was reduced by 30 (95% CI 6 to 48%), 46 (95% CI 25 to 60%), and 64% (95% CI 48 to 75%) in the finasteride, doxazosin, and combination groups, respectively, compared to placebo. Acute urinary retention accounted for 41 of the 351 events of BPH progression; the risk of developing acute urinary retention was reduced by 67(p=0.011), 31 (p=0.296), and 79% (p=0.001) in the finasteride, doxazosin, and combination groups, respectively, compared to placebo. Only the finasteride and combination therapy groups were significantly different from placebo.

* Titrated from 1 mg to 4 or 8 mg as tolerated over a 3-week period

5.2 Pharmacokinetic properties

After an oral dose of ^{14}C-finasteride in man, 39% of the dose was excreted in the urine in the form of metabolites (virtually no unchanged drug was excreted in the urine), and 57% of total dose was excreted in the faeces. Two metabolites have been identified which possess only a small fraction of the Type II 5 α-reductase activity of finasteride.

The oral bioavailability of finasteride is approximately 80%, relative to an intravenous reference dose, and is unaffected by food. Maximum plasma concentrations are reached approximately two hours after dosing and the absorption is complete within 6-8 hours. Protein binding is approximately 93%. Plasma clearance and the volume of distribution are approximately 165 ml/min and 76 l, respectively.

In the elderly, the elimination rate of finasteride is somewhat decreased. Half-life is prolonged from a mean half-life of approximately six hours in men aged 18-60 years to eight hours in men aged more than 70 years. This is of no clinical significance and does not warrant a reduction in dosage.

In patients with chronic renal impairment, whose creatinine clearance ranged from 9-55 ml/min, the disposition of a single dose of ^{14}C-finasteride was not different from that in healthy volunteers. Protein binding also did not differ in patients with renal impairment. A portion of the metabolites which normally is excreted renally was excreted in the faeces. It therefore appears that faecal excretion increases commensurate to the decrease in urinary excretion of metabolites. Dosage adjustment in non-dialysed patients with renal impairment is not necessary.

There are no data available in patients with hepatic insufficiency.

Finasteride has been found to cross the blood-brain barrier. Small amounts of finasteride have been recovered in the seminal fluid of treated patients.

5.3 Preclinical safety data

Non-clinical data reveal no special hazard for humans based on conventional studies of repeated dose toxicity, genotoxicity, and carcinogenic potential. Reproduction toxicology studies in male rats have demonstrated reduced prostate and seminal vesicular weights, reduced secretion from accessory genital glands and reduced fertility index (caused by the primary pharmacological effect of finasteride). The clinical relevance of these findings is unclear.

As with other 5-alpha-reductase inhibitors, femininisation of male rat foetuses has been seen with administration of finasteride in the gestation period. Intravenous administration of finasteride to pregnant rhesus monkeys at doses up to 800 ng/day during the entire period of embryonic and foetal development resulted in no abnormalities in male foetuses. This dose is about 60-120 times higher than the estimated amount in semen of a man who have taken 5 mg finasteride, and to which a woman could be exposed via semen. In confirmation of the relevance of the Rhesus model for human foetal development, oral administration of finasteride 2 mg/kg/day (the systemic exposure (AUC) of monkeys was slightly higher (3x) than that of men who have taken 5 mg finasteride, or approximately 1-2 million times the estimated amount of finasteride in semen) to pregnant monkeys resulted in external genital abnormalities in male foetuses. No other abnormalities were observed in male foetuses and no finasteride-related abnormalities were observed in female foetuses at any dose."

6. PHARMACEUTICAL PARTICULARS

6.1 List of excipients

Cellulose, Microcrystalline (E460)

Docusate sodium

Lactose monohydrate

Magnesium stearate (E572)

Pregelatinised maize starch

Sodium starch glycollate Type A

Yellow iron oxide (E172)

Hydroxypropylcellulose (E463)

Indigo carmine aluminium lake (E132)

Hypromellose (E464)

Talc

Titanium dioxide (E171)

6.2 Incompatibilities

None reported.

6.3 Shelf life

Three years.

6.4 Special precautions for storage

Do not store above 30°C. Store in the original package.

6.5 Nature and contents of container

Opaque PVC/PE/PVDC blisters lidded with aluminium foil; packs of 28 tablets.

6.6 Special precautions for disposal and other handling

Women should not handle crushed or broken 'Proscar' Tablets when they are or may potentially be pregnant (see 'Contra-indications, 'Pregnancy and lactation', *Exposure to finasteride - risk to male foetus).*

7. MARKETING AUTHORISATION HOLDER

Merck Sharp & Dohme Limited

Hertford Road, Hoddesdon, Hertfordshire EN11 9BU, UK.

8. MARKETING AUTHORISATION NUMBER(S)

PL 0025/0279.

9. DATE OF FIRST AUTHORISATION/RENEWAL OF THE AUTHORISATION

July 1997.

10. DATE OF REVISION OF THE TEXT

March 2008.

LEGAL CATEGORY

POM

® denotes registered trademark of Merck & Co., Inc., Whitehouse Station, NJ, USA.

SPC.PSC.07.UK.2810 F.T. 240608

Prostin E2 Sterile Solution 10 mg/ml Intravenous

(Pharmacia Limited)

1. NAME OF THE MEDICINAL PRODUCT

Prostin E2 Sterile Solution 10 mg/ml

2. QUALITATIVE AND QUANTITATIVE COMPOSITION

Each ml contains 10 mg dinoprostone.

3. PHARMACEUTICAL FORM

Colourless, sterile solution, which after appropriate dilution is intended for intravenous administration to human beings

4. CLINICAL PARTICULARS

4.1 Therapeutic indications

Oxytocic agent. Therapeutic termination of pregnancy, missed abortion and hydatidiform mole by the intravenous route.

4.2 Posology and method of administration

Adults: Ampoule contents must be diluted before use and full instructions on method of dilution and dosage are given on the package insert which should be consulted prior to initiation of therapy. The following is a guide to dosage:

Dilute with normal saline or 5% dextrose according to the package insert to produce a 5 micrograms/ml solution. The 5 micrograms/ml solution is infused at 2.5 micrograms/minute for 30 minutes and then maintained or increased to 5 micrograms/minute. The rate should be maintained for at least 4 hours before increasing further.

Elderly: Not applicable

Children: Not applicable

4.3 Contraindications

Prostin E2 Sterile Solution should not be used where the patient is sensitive to prostaglandins.

Prostin E2 Sterile Solution 10 mg/ml is not recommended in the following circumstances:

1. For patients in whom oxytocic drugs are generally contra-indicated or where prolonged contractions of the uterus are considered inappropriate such as:

Cases with a history of Caesarean section or major uterine surgery;

Cases where there is evidence of a potential for obstructed labour;

2. In patients with a past history of, or existing, pelvic inflammatory disease, unless adequate prior treatment has been instituted.

3. Patients with active cardiac, pulmonary, renal or hepatic disease.

4.4 Special warnings and precautions for use

This product is only available to hospitals and clinics with specialised obstetric units and should only be used where 24-hour resident medical cover is provided

Use caution in handling this product to prevent contact with skin. Wash hands thoroughly with soap and water after administration.

It is advised that Prostin E2 Sterile Solution should not be administered by the intramyometrial route since there have been reports of a possible association between this route of administration and cardiac arrest in severely ill patients.

Caution should be exercised in the administration of Prostin E2 Sterile Solution in patients with:

(i) asthma or a history of asthma;

(ii) epilepsy or a history of epilepsy;

(iii) glaucoma or raised intra-ocular pressure;

(iv) compromised cardiovascular, hepatic, or renal function;

(v) hypertension.

As with any oxytocic agent, Prostin E2 Sterile Solution should be used with caution in patients with compromised (scarred) uteri.

Animal studies lasting several weeks at high doses have shown that prostaglandins of the E and F series can induce proliferation of bone. Such effects have also been noted in newborn infants who received prostaglandin E_1 during prolonged treatment. There is no evidence that short-term administration of prostaglandin E_2 can cause similar bone effects.

4.5 Interaction with other medicinal products and other forms of interaction

Since it has been found that prostaglandins potentiate the effect of oxytocin, it is not recommended that these drugs are used together. If used in sequence, the patient's uterine activity should be carefully monitored.

4.6 Pregnancy and lactation

Prostin E2 Sterile Solution 10 mg/ml is only used during pregnancy for therapeutic termination of pregnancy, missed abortion and hydatidiform mole. There has been some evidence in animals of a low order of teratogenic activity, therefore, if abortion does not occur or is suspected to be incomplete as a result of prostaglandin therapy, (as in spontaneous abortion, where the process is sometimes incomplete), the appropriate treatment for complete evacuation of the pregnant uterus should be instituted in all instances.

Prostaglandins are excreted in breast milk. This is not expected to be a hazard given the circumstances in which the product is used.

4.7 Effects on ability to drive and use machines

Not applicable

4.8 Undesirable effects

The most commonly reported events are vomiting, nausea and diarrhoea. Certain rare events that should be especially noted are: hypersensitivity to the drug; uterine rupture; and cardiac arrest. Other adverse events, in decreasing order of severity, reported with use of dinoprostone are:

Pulmonary/amniotic fluid embolism; Uterine hypercontractility or hypertonus; Hypertension - systemic (maternal); Bronchospasm/asthma; Rapid cervical dilation; Fever; Back ache; Rash.

In addition, with intravenous use, transient vasovagal symptoms, including flushing, shivering, headache and dizziness, have been recorded. Local tissue irritation and erythema have occurred. No evidence of thrombophlebitis has been recorded and local tissue erythema at the infusion site has disappeared within two to five hours after infusion. A temporary pyrexia and elevated WBC are not unusual, but both have reverted after termination of infusion.

4.9 Overdose

Uterine hypertonus or unduly severe uterine contractions have rarely been encountered, but might be anticipated to result from overdosage. Treatment of overdosage must be, at this time, symptomatic, as clinical studies with prostaglandin antagonists have not progressed to the point where recommendations may be made. If evidence of excessive uterine activity or side-effects appears, the rate of infusion should be decreased or discontinued. In cases of massive overdosage resulting in extreme uterine hypertonus, appropriate obstetric procedures are indicated.

5. PHARMACOLOGICAL PROPERTIES

5.1 Pharmacodynamic properties

Dinoprostone is a prostaglandin of the E series with actions on smooth muscle. It induces contraction of uterine muscle at any stage of pregnancy.

5.2 Pharmacokinetic properties

5.2a General characteristics of active substance

Dinoprostone is rapidly metabolised in the body. Intravenous administration results in very rapid distribution and metabolism, with only 3% of unchanged drug remaining in the blood after 15 minutes. At least nine prostaglandin E_2 metabolites have been identified in human blood and urine.

5.2b Characteristics in patients

No special characteristics. See "Special warnings and special precautions for use" for further information.

5.3 Preclinical safety data

There are no pre-clinical data of relevance to the prescriber which are additional to that already included in other sections of the SPC.

6. PHARMACEUTICAL PARTICULARS

6.1 List of excipients

Dehydrated alcohol.

6.2 Incompatibilities

None known

6.3 Shelf life

24 months.

6.4 Special precautions for storage

Store in a refrigerator at 4°C. Once diluted, the diluted solution should be stored in a refrigerator at 4°C and used within 24 hours.

6.5 Nature and contents of container

Ph. Eur. Type I glass ampoule, containing 0.5 ml sterile solution, packed in a carton.

6.6 Special precautions for disposal and other handling

Use caution in handling this product to prevent contact with skin. Wash hands thoroughly with soap and water after administration.

7. MARKETING AUTHORISATION HOLDER

Pharmacia Limited
Ramsgate Road
Sandwich
Kent
CT13 9NJ
UK

8. MARKETING AUTHORISATION NUMBER(S)

PL 0032/0021R

9. DATE OF FIRST AUTHORISATION/RENEWAL OF THE AUTHORISATION

27 June 1986/17 November 1998

10. DATE OF REVISION OF THE TEXT

January 2008

Legal Category:

POM

Prostin E2 Sterile Solution 10mg/ml Extra-Amniotic

(Pharmacia Limited)

1. NAME OF THE MEDICINAL PRODUCT

Prostin E2 Sterile Solution 10 mg/ml.

2. QUALITATIVE AND QUANTITATIVE COMPOSITION

Each ml contains 10 mg dinoprostone.

3. PHARMACEUTICAL FORM

Colourless, sterile solution, which after appropriate dilution is intended for extra-amniotic administration to human beings.

4. CLINICAL PARTICULARS

4.1 Therapeutic indications

Oxytocic agent. The therapeutic termination of pregnancy, by the extra-amniotic route.

4.2 Posology and method of administration

Adults: Ampoule contents must be diluted before use and full instructions on method of dilution and dosage are given on the package insert which should be consulted prior to initiation of therapy. The following is a guide to dosage:

Dilute with the 50ml of diluent provided according to the package insert to produce a 100 micrograms/ml solution. The 100 micrograms/ml solution is instilled via a 12-14 French gauge Foley catheter. Initial instillation is 1ml, then dependent on uterine response, 1 or 2 ml usually at two hour intervals.

Elderly: Not applicable

Children: Not applicable

4.3 Contraindications

Prostin E2 Sterile Solution should not be used where the patient is sensitive to prostaglandins.

Prostin E2 Sterile Solution 10 mg/ml is not recommended in the following circumstances:

1. For patients in whom oxytocic drugs are generally contra-indicated or where prolonged contractions of the uterus are considered inappropriate such as: Cases with a history of Caesarean section or major uterine surgery; Cases where there is evidence of a potential for obstructed labour;
2. In patients with a past history of; or existing, pelvic inflammatory disease, unless adequate prior treatment has been instituted.
3. In patients with cervicitis or vaginal infections.
4. Patients with active cardiac, pulmonary, renal or hepatic disease.

4.4 Special warnings and precautions for use

This product is only available to hospitals and clinics with specialised obstetric units and should only be used where 24-hour resident medical cover is provided

Use caution in handling this product to prevent contact with skin. Wash hands thoroughly with soap and water after administration.

It is advised that Prostin E2 Sterile Solution should not be administered by the intramyometrial route since there have been reports of a possible association between this route of administration and cardiac arrest in severely ill patients.

Caution should be exercised in the administration of Prostin E2 Sterile Solution to patients with:

(i) asthma or a history of asthma;
(ii) epilepsy or a history of epilepsy;
(iii) glaucoma or raised intra-ocular pressure;
(iv) compromised cardiovascular, hepatic, or renal function.
(v) hypertension

As with any oxytocic agent, Prostin E2 Sterile Solution should be used with caution in patients with compromised (scarred) uteri.

Animal studies lasting several weeks at high doses have shown that prostaglandins of the E and F series can induce proliferation of bone. Such effects have also been noted in newborn infants who received prostaglandin E1 during prolonged treatment. There is no evidence that short-term administration of prostaglandin E2 can cause similar bone effects.

4.5 Interaction with other medicinal products and other forms of interaction

Since it has been found that prostaglandins potentiate the effect of oxytocin, it is not recommended that these drugs are used together. If used in sequence, the patient's uterine activity should be carefully monitored.

4.6 Pregnancy and lactation

Pregnancy Code D

Prostin E2 Sterile Solution 10 mg/ml is only used during pregnancy for therapeutic termination of pregnancy. There has been some evidence in animals of a low order of teratogenic activity, therefore, if abortion does not occur or is suspected to be incomplete as a result of prostaglandin therapy, (as in spontaneous abortion, where the process is sometimes incomplete), the appropriate treatment for complete evacuation of the pregnant uterus should be instituted in all instances.

Prostaglandins are excreted in breast milk. This is not expected to be a hazard given the circumstances in which the product is used.

4.7 Effects on ability to drive and use machines

Not applicable

4.8 Undesirable effects

The most commonly reported events are vomiting, nausea and diarrhoea. Certain rare events that should be especially noted are: hypersensitivity to the drug; uterine rupture; and cardiac arrest. Other adverse effects, in decreasing order of severity reported with use of dinoprostone are:

Pulmonary/amniotic fluid embolism;

Uterine hypercontractility or hypertonus;

Hypertension - systemic (maternal);

Bronchospasm/asthma;

Rapid cervical dilation;

Fever;

Back ache;

Rash.

A temporary pyrexia and elevated WBC are not unusual, but both have reverted after termination of therapy. In extra-amniotic therapy, the possibility of local infection must be considered and appropriate therapy initiated if necessary.

4.9 Overdose

Uterine hypertonus or unduly severe uterine contractions have rarely been encountered, but might be anticipated to result from overdosage. Treatment of overdosage must be, at this time, symptomatic, as clinical studies with prostaglandin antagonists have not progressed to the point where recommendations may be made. If evidence of excessive uterine activity or side-effects appears, the rate of infusion should be decreased or discontinued. In cases of massive overdosage resulting in extreme uterine hypertonus, appropriate obstetric procedures are indicated.

5. PHARMACOLOGICAL PROPERTIES

5.1 Pharmacodynamic properties

Dinoprostone is a prostaglandin of the E series with actions on smooth muscle. It induces contraction of uterine muscle at any stage of pregnancy.

5.2 Pharmacokinetic properties

General characteristics of active substance

Dinoprostone is rapidly metabolised in the body. Intravenous administration results in very rapid distribution and metabolism, with only 3% of unchanged drug remaining in the blood after 15 minutes. At least nine prostaglandin E2 metabolites have been identified in human blood and urine.

Characteristics in Patients

No special characteristics. See "Special Warnings and Precautions for use" for further information.

5.3 Preclinical safety data

In mice and rats, the oral LD50 values were >500mg/kg and 141-513 mg/kg respectively.

Three month oral administration to rats resulted in significantly heavier stomach weights for treated compared with untreated rats, which effect was reversible on treatment cessation. Treated rats had a dose related acanthotic squamous glandular junction and thickened glandular gastric mucosal epithelium. No significant alterations were recognized in routine evaluation of the stemebrae and the femur.

A fourteen day oral toxicity study in dogs showed a maximum tolerated dose of 6-20 mg/kg/day. All treated dogs had microscopic evidence of increased fundic and pyloric mucus. The fundic and pyloric mucosa were thickened, having a cobblestone appearance and had an increased gastric mucus in both 20 mg/kg/day treated dogs and the

60 mg/kg/day male dog. These were the only gross and microscopic drug related changes observed.

Satisfactory results were obtained in intravenous and intramuscular tolerability tests performed in dog and monkey.

Teratogenic effects were observed in rats injected subcutaneously with 0.5 mg/animal. No teratogenic effects were seen in the rabbit at dosage levels of up to 1.5 mg/kg day.

No evidence of mutagenicity was obtained using the Ames Assay, the DNA Damage/Alkaline Elution Assay and the micronucleus test.

6. PHARMACEUTICAL PARTICULARS

6.1 List of excipients

Dehydrated alcohol - BP

6.2 Incompatibilities

None known

6.3 Shelf life

24 months.

6.4 Special precautions for storage

Store in a refrigerator at 4°C. The product after dilution should be stored in a refrigerator at 4°C and should not be kept for more than 48 hours.

6.5 Nature and contents of container

Ph. Eur. Type I glass ampoule, containing 0.5 ml sterile solution, packed in a carton, together with a vial containing diluent.

6.6 Special precautions for disposal and other handling

Use caution in handling this product to prevent contact with skin. Wash hands thoroughly with soap and water after administration.

7. MARKETING AUTHORISATION HOLDER

Pharmacia Limited

Ramsgate Road

Sandwich

Kent

CT13 9NJ

UK

8. MARKETING AUTHORISATION NUMBER(S)

PL 0032/0026R

9. DATE OF FIRST AUTHORISATION/RENEWAL OF THE AUTHORISATION

1 July 1991 / 18 March 1997

10. DATE OF REVISION OF THE TEXT

January 2008

Prostin E2 Sterile Solution 1mg/ml Intravenous

(Pharmacia Limited)

1. NAME OF THE MEDICINAL PRODUCT

Prostin E2 Sterile Solution 1 mg/ml.

2. QUALITATIVE AND QUANTITATIVE COMPOSITION

Each ml contains 1 mg dinoprostone.

3. PHARMACEUTICAL FORM

Colourless, sterile solution, which after appropriate dilution is intended for intravenous administration to human beings.

4. CLINICAL PARTICULARS

4.1 Therapeutic indications

The induction of labour by the intravenous route.

4.2 Posology and method of administration

Adults: Ampoule contents must be diluted before use and full instructions on method of dilution and dosage are given on the package insert which should be consulted prior to initiation of therapy. The following is a guide to dosage:

Dilute with normal saline or 5% dextrose according to the package insert to produce a 1.5 micrograms/ml solution. The 1.5 micrograms/ml solution is infused at 0.25 micrograms/minute for 30 minutes and then maintained or increased. Cases of fetal death *in utero* may require higher doses. An initial rate of 0.5 micrograms/minute may be used with stepwise increases, at intervals of not less than one hour.

Elderly: Not applicable

Children: Not applicable

4.3 Contraindications

Prostin E2 Sterile Solution should not be used where the patient is sensitive to prostaglandins.

Prostin E2 Sterile Solution 1 mg/ml is not recommended in the following circumstances:

1. For patients in whom oxytocic drugs are generally contra-indicated or where prolonged contractions of the uterus are considered inappropriate such as:

Cases with a history of Caesarean section or major uterine surgery;

Cases where there is cephalopelvic disproportion;

Cases in which fetal malpresentation is present;

Cases where there is clinical suspicion or definite evidence of pre-existing fetal distress;

Cases in which there is a history of difficult labour and/or traumatic delivery;

Grand multiparae with over five previous term pregnancies.

2. In patients with a past history of, or existing, pelvic inflammatory disease, unless adequate prior treatment has been instituted.

3. In patients where there is clinical suspicion or definite evidence of placenta praevia or unexplained vaginal bleeding during this pregnancy.

4. Patients with active cardiac, pulmonary, renal or hepatic disease.

4.4 Special warnings and precautions for use

This product is only available to hospitals and clinics with specialised obstetric units and should only be used where 24-hour resident medical cover is provided

Use caution in handling this product to prevent contact with skin. Wash hands thoroughly with soap and water after administration.

It is advised that Prostin E2 Sterile Solution should not be administered by the intramyometrial route since there have been reports of a possible association between this route of administration and cardiac arrest in severely ill patients.

Caution should be exercised in the administration of Prostin E2 Sterile Solution 1 mg/ml for the induction of labour in patients with:

(i) asthma or a history of asthma;

(ii) epilepsy or a history of epilepsy;

(iii) glaucoma or raised intra-ocular pressure;

(iv) compromised cardiovascular, hepatic, or renal function;

(v) hypertension

As with any oxytocic agent, Prostin E2 Sterile Solution should be used with caution in patients with compromised (scarred) uteri.

In labour induction, cephalopelvic relationships should be carefully evaluated before use of Prostin E2 Sterile Solution. During use, uterine activity, fetal status and the progression of cervical dilation should be carefully monitored to detect possible evidence of undesired responses, e.g. hypertonus, sustained uterine contractions, or fetal distress. In cases where there is a known history of hypertonic uterine contractility or tetanic uterine contractions, it is recommended that uterine activity and the state of the fetus (where applicable) should be continuously monitored throughout labour. The possibility of uterine rupture should be borne in mind where high-tone uterine contractions are sustained.

Animal studies lasting several weeks at high doses have shown that prostaglandins of the E and F series can induce proliferation of bone. Such effects have also been noted in newborn infants who received prostaglandin E_1 during prolonged treatment. There is no evidence that short-term administration of prostaglandin E_2 can cause similar bone effects.

4.5 Interaction with other medicinal products and other forms of interaction

Since it has been found that prostaglandins potentiate the effect of oxytocin, it is not recommended that these drugs are used together. If used in sequence, the patient's uterine activity should be carefully monitored.

4.6 Pregnancy and lactation

Prostin E2 Sterile Solution 1 mg/ml is only used during pregnancy, to induce labour.

Prostaglandins are excreted in breast milk. This is not expected to be a hazard given the circumstances in which the product is used.

4.7 Effects on ability to drive and use machines

Not applicable

4.8 Undesirable effects

The most commonly reported events are vomiting, nausea and diarrhoea. Certain rare events that should be especially noted are: hypersensitivity to the drug; uterine rupture; and cardiac arrest. Other adverse effects, reported in decreasing order of severity are:

Pulmonary/amniotic fluid embolism;

Abruptio placenta;

Stillbirth, neonatal death;

Uterine hypercontractility or hypertonus;

Fetal distress;

Hypertension - systemic (maternal);

Bronchospasm/asthma;

Rapid cervical dilation;

Fever;

Back ache;

Rash.

Transient vasovagal symptoms, including flushing, shivering, headache and dizziness, have been recorded with intravenous use of prostaglandin E_2. Local tissue irritation and erythema have occurred. No evidence of thrombophlebitis has been recorded and local tissue erythema at the infusion site has disappeared within two to five hours after infusion. A temporary pyrexia and elevated WBC are not unusual, but both have reverted after termination of infusion.

In addition, other adverse reactions that have been seen with the use of Prostin E2 for term labour induction have included: uterine hypercontractility with fetal bradycardia; uterine hypercontractility without fetal bradycardia; and low Apgar scores in the newborn.

4.9 Overdose

Uterine hypertonus or unduly severe uterine contractions have rarely been encountered, but might be anticipated to result from overdosage. In the rare instance where temporary discontinuation of therapy is not effective in reversing fetal distress or uterine hypertonus, then prompt delivery is indicated. Treatment of overdosage must be, at this time, symptomatic, since clinical studies with prostaglandin antagonists have not progressed to the point where recommendations may be made.

5. PHARMACOLOGICAL PROPERTIES

5.1 Pharmacodynamic properties

Dinoprostone is a prostaglandin of the E series with actions on smooth muscle. It induces contraction of uterine muscle at any stage of pregnancy.

5.2 Pharmacokinetic properties

5.2a General characteristics of active substance

Dinoprostone is rapidly metabolised in the body. Intravenous administration results in very rapid distribution and metabolism, with only 3% of unchanged drug remaining in the blood after 15 minutes. At least nine prostaglandin E_2 metabolites have been identified in human blood and urine.

5.2b Characteristics in patients

No special characteristics. See "Special warnings and special precautions for use" for further information.

5.3 Preclinical safety data

There are no pre-clinical data of relevance which are additional to that already included in other sections of the SPC.

6. PHARMACEUTICAL PARTICULARS

6.1 List of excipients

Dehydrated alcohol

6.2 Incompatibilities

None known

6.3 Shelf life

24 months.

6.4 Special precautions for storage

Store in a refrigerator at 4°C. The product after dilution should be stored in a refrigerator at 4°C and should not be kept for more than 24 hours.

6.5 Nature and contents of container

Ph. Eur. Type I glass ampoule, containing 0.75 ml sterile solution, packed in a carton.

6.6 Special precautions for disposal and other handling

Use caution in handling this product to prevent contact with skin. Wash hands thoroughly with soap and water after administration.

7. MARKETING AUTHORISATION HOLDER

Pharmacia Limited

Ramsgate Road

Sandwich

Kent

CT13 9NJ

UK

8. MARKETING AUTHORISATION NUMBER(S)

PL 0032/0020R

9. DATE OF FIRST AUTHORISATION/RENEWAL OF THE AUTHORISATION

27 June 1986/17 November 1998

10. DATE OF REVISION OF THE TEXT

January 2008

Prostin E2 Vaginal Gel 1mg, 2mg

(Pharmacia Limited)

1. NAME OF THE MEDICINAL PRODUCT

Prostin E2 Vaginal Gel 1 mg or 2 mg.

2. QUALITATIVE AND QUANTITATIVE COMPOSITION

Each 3 g gel (2.5 ml) contains 1 mg or 2mg dinoprostone.

3. PHARMACEUTICAL FORM

Translucent, thixotropic gel.

4. CLINICAL PARTICULARS

4.1 Therapeutic indications

Oxytocic. Prostin E2 Vaginal Gel is indicated for the induction of labour, when there are no fetal or maternal contra-indications.

4.2 Posology and method of administration

Adults: In primigravida patients with unfavourable induction features (Bishop score of 4 or less), an initial dose of 2 mg should be administered vaginally. In other patients an initial dose of 1 mg should be administered vaginally.

In both groups of patients, a second dose of 1 mg or 2 mg may be administered after 6 hours as follows:

1 mg should be used where uterine activity is insufficient for satisfactory progress of labour.

2 mg may be used where response to the initial dose has been minimal.

Maximum dose 4 mg in unfavourable primigravida patients or 3 mg in other patients (see "Precautions").

The gel should be inserted high into the posterior fornix avoiding administration into the cervical canal. The patient should be instructed to remain recumbent for at least 30 minutes.

Elderly: Not applicable

Children: Not applicable

4.3 Contraindications

Prostin E2 Vaginal Gel should not be used where the patient is sensitive to prostaglandins or other constituents of the gel.

Prostin E2 Vaginal Gel is not recommended in the following circumstances:

1. For patients in whom oxytocic drugs are generally contra-indicated or where prolonged contractions of the uterus are considered inappropriate such as:

Cases with a history of Caesarean section or major uterine surgery;

Cases where there is cephalopelvic disproportion;

Cases in which fetal malpresentation is present;

Cases where there is clinical suspicion or definite evidence of pre-existing fetal distress;

Cases in which there is a history of difficult labour and/or traumatic delivery;

Grand multiparae with over five previous term pregnancies.

2. Patients with ruptured membranes.

3. In patients with a past history of, or existing, pelvic inflammatory disease, unless adequate prior treatment has been instituted.

4. In patients where there is clinical suspicion or definite evidence of placenta praevia or unexplained vaginal bleeding during this pregnancy.

5. Patients with active cardiac, pulmonary, renal or hepatic disease.

This product is only available to hospitals and clinics with specialised obstetric units and should only be used where 24-hour resident medical cover is provided.

4.4 Special warnings and precautions for use

Use the total contents of the syringe for one patient only. Discard after use. Use caution in handling the product to prevent contact with skin. Wash hands thoroughly with soap and water after administration.

Prostin E2 Vaginal Gel and Prostin E2 Vaginal Tablets are not bioequivalent.

Caution should be exercised in the administration of Prostin E2 Vaginal Gel for the induction of labour in patients with:

(i) asthma or a history of asthma;

(ii) epilepsy or a history of epilepsy;

(iii) glaucoma or raised intra-ocular pressure;

(iv) compromised cardiovascular, hepatic, or renal function;

(v) hypertension

As with any oxytocic agent, Prostin E2 Vaginal Gel should be used with caution in patients with compromised (scarred) uteri.

In labour induction, cephalopelvic relationships should be carefully evaluated before use of Prostin E2 Vaginal Gel. During use, uterine activity, fetal status and the progression of cervical dilation should be carefully monitored to detect possible evidence of undesired responses, e.g. hypertonus, sustained uterine contractions, or fetal distress.

In cases where there is a known history of hypertonic uterine contractility or tetanic uterine contractions, it is recommended that uterine activity and the state of the fetus (where applicable) should be continuously monitored throughout labour. The possibility of uterine rupture should be borne in mind where high-tone uterine contractions are sustained.

Animal studies lasting several weeks at high doses have shown that prostaglandins of the E and F series can induce proliferation of bone. Such effects have also been noted in newborn infants who received prostaglandin E_1 during prolonged treatment. There is no evidence that short-term administration of prostaglandin E_2 can cause similar bone effects.

4.5 Interaction with other medicinal products and other forms of interaction

Since it has been found that prostaglandins potentiate the effect of oxytocin, it is not recommended that these drugs are used together. If used in sequence, the patient's uterine activity should be carefully monitored.

4.6 Pregnancy and lactation

Pregnancy Code A

Prostin E2 Vaginal Gel is only used during pregnancy, to induce labour.

Prostaglandins are excreted in breast milk. This is not expected to be a hazard given the circumstances in which the product is used.

4.7 Effects on ability to drive and use machines

Not applicable

4.8 Undesirable effects

The most commonly reported events are vomiting, nausea and diarrhoea. Certain rare events that should be especially noted are: hypersensitivity to the drug; uterine rupture; and cardiac arrest. Other adverse events, in decreasing order of severity, reported with use of dinoprostone are:

Pulmonary/amniotic fluid embolism;

Abruptio placenta;

Stillbirth, neonatal death;

Uterine hypercontractility or hypertonus;

Fetal distress;

Hypertension - systemic (maternal);

Bronchospasm/asthma;

Rapid cervical dilation;

Fever;

Backache;

Rash;

Vaginal symptoms - warmth, irritation, pain.

In addition, other adverse reactions that have been seen with the use of prostaglandin E_2 for term labour induction have included: uterine hypercontractility with fetal bradycardia; uterine hypercontractility without fetal bradycardia; and low Apgar scores in the newborn.

4.9 Overdose

Uterine hypertonus or unduly severe uterine contractions have rarely been encountered, but might be anticipated to result from overdosage. Where there is evidence of fetal distress or uterine hypertonus, then prompt delivery is indicated. Treatment of overdosage must be, at this time, symptomatic, since clinical studies with prostaglandin antagonists have not progressed to the point where recommendations may be made.

5. PHARMACOLOGICAL PROPERTIES

5.1 Pharmacodynamic properties

Dinoprostone is a prostaglandin of the E series which induces myometrial contractions and promotes cervical ripening.

5.2 Pharmacokinetic properties

General characteristics of active substance

When given vaginally, PGE_2 is rapidly absorbed. Plasma levels of 15-keto PGE_2 equivalents peak at 1.5 hours after administration of a 5 mg dose. *In vitro* work indicates that PGE_2 is 73% bound to human plasma albumin. It is rapidly metabolised in the lungs, kidneys, spleen and liver, with a single pass of the circulatory system converting 90% of an injected PGE_2 dose to metabolites.

Characteristics in patients

No special characteristics. See "Special warnings and special precautions for use" for further information.

5.3 Preclinical safety data

There are no pre-clinical data of relevance which are additional to those already included in other sections of the SPC.

6. PHARMACEUTICAL PARTICULARS

6.1 List of excipients

Triacetin and colloidal silicon dioxide

6.2 Incompatibilities

None known

6.3 Shelf life

Prostin E2 Vaginal Gel has a shelf-life of 24 months when stored in a refrigerator at 2-8°C.

6.4 Special precautions for storage

Store in a refrigerator at 2-8°C.

6.5 Nature and contents of container

Polyethylene syringe containing 3 g or 2.5 ml of gel.

6.6 Special precautions for disposal and other handling

Use the total contents of the syringe for one patient only. Discard after use. Use caution in handling this product to prevent contact with skin. Wash hands thoroughly with soap and water after administration.

7. MARKETING AUTHORISATION HOLDER

Pharmacia Limited

Ramsgate Road

Sandwich

Kent

CT13 9NJ

UK

8. MARKETING AUTHORISATION NUMBER(S)

1mg - PL 0032/0123

2mg - PL 0032/0124

9. DATE OF FIRST AUTHORISATION/RENEWAL OF THE AUTHORISATION

30 April 1986/17 November 1998

10. DATE OF REVISION OF THE TEXT

January 2008

Prostin E2 Vaginal Tablets

(Pharmacia Limited)

1. NAME OF THE MEDICINAL PRODUCT

Prostin E2 Vaginal Tablets 3mg

2. QUALITATIVE AND QUANTITATIVE COMPOSITION

Dinoprostone HSE 3 mg

3. PHARMACEUTICAL FORM

Tablet for vaginal administration

4. CLINICAL PARTICULARS

4.1 Therapeutic indications

Oxytocic. Prostin E2 Vaginal Tablets 3mg are indicated for the induction of labour, especially in patients with favourable induction features, when there are no fetal or maternal contra-indications.

4.2 Posology and method of administration

Method of administration: Vaginal tablets are administered by insertion high into the posterior fornix.

One tablet to be inserted high into the posterior fornix. A second tablet may be inserted after six to eight hours if labour is not established. Maximum dose 6 mg.

Children: Not applicable

Elderly: Not applicable

4.3 Contraindications

Prostin E2 Vaginal Tablets should not be used where the patient is sensitive to prostaglandins or other constituents of the tablet.

Prostin E2 Vaginal Tablets are not recommended in the following circumstances:

1. For patients in whom oxytocic drugs are generally contra-indicated or where prolonged contractions of the uterus are considered inappropriate such as:

- Cases with a history of Caesarean section or major uterine surgery;
- Cases where there is cephalopelvic disproportion;
- Cases in which fetal malpresentation is present;
- Cases where there is clinical suspicion or definite evidence of pre-existing fetal distress;
- Cases in which there is a history of difficult labour and/or traumatic delivery;
- Grand multiparae with over five previous term pregnancies.

2. Patients with ruptured membranes.

3. In patients with a past history of, or existing, pelvic inflammatory disease, unless adequate prior treatment has been instituted.

4. In patients where there is clinical suspicion or definite evidence of placenta praevia or unexplained vaginal bleeding during this pregnancy.

5. Patients with active cardiac, pulmonary, renal or hepatic disease.

4.4 Special warnings and precautions for use

This product is only available to hospitals and clinics with specialised obstetric units and should only be used where 24-hour resident medical cover is provided

Use caution in handling this product to prevent contact with skin. Wash hands thoroughly with soap and water after administration.

Caution should be exercised in the administration of Prostin E2 Vaginal Tablets for the induction of labour in patients with:

(i) asthma or a history of asthma;

(ii) epilepsy or a history of epilepsy;

(iii) glaucoma or raised intra-ocular pressure;

(iv) compromised cardiovascular, hepatic, or renal function;

(v) hypertension

As with any oxytocic agent, Prostin E2 Vaginal Tablets should be used with caution in patients with compromised (scarred) uteri.

In labour induction, cephalopelvic relationships should be carefully evaluated before use of Prostin E2 Vaginal Tablets. During use, uterine activity, fetal status and the progression of cervical dilation should be carefully monitored to detect possible evidence of undesired responses, e.g. hypertonus, sustained uterine contractions, or fetal distress.

In cases where there is a known history of hypertonic uterine contractility or tetanic uterine contractions, it is recommended that uterine activity and the state of the fetus (where applicable) should be continuously monitored throughout labour. The possibility of uterine rupture should be borne in mind where high-tone uterine contractions are sustained.

4.5 Interaction with other medicinal products and other forms of interaction
Since it has been found that prostaglandins potentiate the effect of oxytocin, it is not recommended that these drugs are used together. If used in sequence, the patient's uterine activity should be carefully monitored.

4.6 Pregnancy and lactation
Prostin E2 Vaginal Tablets are only used during pregnancy, to induce labour.

Prostaglandins are excreted in breast milk. This is not expected to be a hazard given the circumstances in which the product is used.

4.7 Effects on ability to drive and use machines
Not applicable

4.8 Undesirable effects
The most commonly reported events are vomiting, nausea and diarrhoea. Certain rare events that should be especially noted are: hypersensitivity to the drug; uterine rupture; and cardiac arrest. Other adverse events, in decreasing order of severity, reported with use of dinoprostone are:

Pulmonary/amniotic fluid embolism;

Abruptio placenta;

Stillbirth, neonatal death;

Uterine hypercontractility or hypertonus;

Fetal distress;

Hypertension - systemic (maternal);

Bronchospasm/asthma;

Rapid cervical dilation;

Fever;

Backache;

Rash;

Vaginal symptoms - warmth, irritation, pain.

In addition, other adverse reactions that have been seen with the use of prostaglandin E_2 for term labour induction have included: altered fetal heart rate patterns; uterine hypercontractility with fetal bradycardia; uterine hypercontractility without fetal bradycardia; and low Apgar scores in the newborn.

4.9 Overdose
Uterine hypertonus or unduly severe uterine contractions have rarely been encountered, but might be anticipated to result from overdosage. Where there is evidence of fetal distress or uterine hypertonus, then prompt delivery is indicated. Treatment of overdosage must be, at this time, symptomatic, since clinical studies with prostaglandin antagonists have not progressed to the point where recommendations may be made. It is currently believed that vomiting produced by overdosage may act as a self-limiting factor in protecting the patient.

5. PHARMACOLOGICAL PROPERTIES

5.1 Pharmacodynamic properties
Dinoprostone is a prostaglandin of the E series with actions on smooth muscle; the endogenous substance is termed prostaglandin E2 (PGE_2). It induces contraction of uterine muscle at any stage of pregnancy and is reported to act predominantly as a vasodilator on blood vessels and as a bronchodilator on bronchial muscle. It is postulated that vaginal absorption of PGE_2 stimulates endogenous PGE_2 and $PGF_{2\alpha}$ production, similar to that which is seen in spontaneous labour.

5.2 Pharmacokinetic properties
Following insertion of the tablet, PGE_2 absorption (as measured by the presence of PGE_2 metabolites) increases to reach a peak at about 40 minutes. PGE_2 is rapidly metabolised to 13, 14-dihydro, 15-keto PGE_2 which is converted to 13, 14-dihydro, 15-keto PGA_2 which binds covalently to albumen.

There has been found to be inter-patient variability regarding systemic absorption of PGE_2. This can be attributed to different conditions of the vaginal mucosa between patients.

5.3 Preclinical safety data
Animal studies lasting several weeks at high doses have shown that prostaglandins of the E and F series can induce proliferation of bone. Such effects have also been noted in newborn infants who received prostaglandin E_1 during prolonged treatment. There is no evidence that short-term administration of prostaglandin E_2 can cause similar bone effects.

6. PHARMACEUTICAL PARTICULARS

6.1 List of excipients
Lactose

Microcrystalline Cellulose

Colloidal Silicon Dioxide

Maize Starch

Magnesium Stearate

6.2 Incompatibilities
None known

6.3 Shelf life
24 months.

6.4 Special precautions for storage
Store in a refrigerator.

Where the tablets are pack in a bottle, the tablets should be used within one month of opening the bottle.

6.5 Nature and contents of container
Amber glass bottle with screw cap and tac seal. Each bottle contains a desiccant capsule and 4 tablets.

Aluminium foil strip of 4 tablets, each box containing 4 or 8 tablets.

6.6 Special precautions for disposal and other handling
Wash hands thoroughly with soap and water after administration.

7. MARKETING AUTHORISATION HOLDER
Pharmacia Limited

Ramsgate Road

Sandwich

Kent

CT13 9NJ

UK

8. MARKETING AUTHORISATION NUMBER(S)
PL 0032/0074

9. DATE OF FIRST AUTHORISATION/RENEWAL OF THE AUTHORISATION
15 March 1982/15 March 1998

10. DATE OF REVISION OF THE TEXT
January 2008

Prostin VR Sterile Solution

(Pharmacia Limited)

1. NAME OF THE MEDICINAL PRODUCT
Prostin VR Sterile Solution.

2. QUALITATIVE AND QUANTITATIVE COMPOSITION
Each 1 ml contains 500 micrograms (0.5 mg) alprostadil.

3. PHARMACEUTICAL FORM
Sterile solution for injection.

4. CLINICAL PARTICULARS

4.1 Therapeutic indications
Prostin VR is indicated to temporarily maintain the patency of the ductus arteriosus until corrective or palliative surgery can be performed in infants who have congenital defects and who depend upon the patent ductus for survival. Such congenital heart defects include pulmonary atresia, pulmonary stenosis, tricuspid atresia, tetralogy of Fallot, interruption of the aortic arch, co-arctation of the aorta, aortic stenosis, aortic atresia, mitral atresia, or transposition of the great vessels with or without other defects.

4.2 Posology and method of administration
For administration by intravenous drip or constant rate infusion pump.

In infants with lesions restricting pulmonary blood flow (blood is flowing through the ductus arteriosus from the aorta to the pulmonary artery), Prostin VR may be administered by continuous infusion through an umbilical artery catheter placed at or just above the junction of the descending aorta and the ductus arteriosus, or intravenously. Adverse effects have occurred with both routes of administration, but the types of reactions are different. A higher incidence of flushing has been associated with intra-arterial than with intravenous administration.

The infusion is generally initiated at a rate of 0.05 to 0.1 micrograms alprostadil per kilogram of body weight per minute. The most experience has been with 0.1 micrograms/kg/min. After a therapeutic response (an increase in pO_2 in neonates with restricted pulmonary blood flow or an increase in systemic blood pressure and blood pH in neonates with restricted systemic blood flow) has been obtained, the infusion rate should be reduced to the lowest possible dosage that will maintain the desired response.

Dilution Instructions: To prepare infusion solutions, dilute 1 ml of Prostin VR Sterile Solution with sterile 0.9% Sodium Chloride Intravenous Infusion or sterile 5% Dextrose Intravenous Infusion. If undiluted Prostin VR Sterile Solution comes in direct contact with a plastic container, plasticisers are leached from the sidewalls. The solution may turn hazy and the appearance of the container may change. Should this occur, the solution should be discarded and the plastic container should be replaced. This appears to be a concentration-dependent phenomenon. To minimise the possibility of haze formation, Prostin VR Sterile Solution should be added directly to the intravenous infusion solution, avoiding contact with the walls of plastic containers. Dilute to volumes appropriate for the delivery system available. Prepare fresh infusion solutions every 24 hours. Discard any solution more than 24 hours old.

PARTICULAR CARE SHOULD BE TAKEN IN CALCULATING AND PREPARING DILUTIONS OF PROSTIN VR

4.3 Contraindications
None

4.4 Special warnings and precautions for use
Warnings: Only the recommended Prostin VR dosages should be administered and only by medically trained personnel in hospitals or other facilities with immediately available intensive care.

Apnoea has been reported in neonates with congenital heart defects treated with Prostin VR Sterile Solution. In clinical studies the rate of apnoea reported has generally been between 8 and 38%. One study reported the rate as high as 52%. There is some evidence that apnoea is dose related. Apnoea is most often seen in neonates weighing less than 2kg at birth and usually appears during the first hour of drug infusion. Therefore Prostin VR Sterile Solution should be used where ventilatory assistance is immediately available.

Precautions: Prostin VR Sterile Solution (alprostadil) should be infused for the shortest time and at the lowest dose which will produce the desired effects. The risk of long-term infusion of Prostin VR should be weighed against the possible benefits that critically ill infants may derive from its administration.

Cortical proliferation of the long bones has followed long-term infusions of alprostadil in infants and dogs. The proliferation in infants regressed after withdrawal of the drug.

Use Prostin VR Sterile Solution cautiously in neonates with histories of bleeding tendencies.

Care should be taken to avoid the use of Prostin VR Sterile Solution in neonates with respiratory distress syndrome (hyaline membrane disease), which sometimes can be confused with cyanotic heart disease. If full diagnostic facilities are not immediately available, cyanosis (pO_2 less than 40 mm Hg) and restricted pulmonary blood flow apparent on an X-ray are good indicators of congenital heart defects.

In all infants, commencing when infusion starts, intermittently monitor arterial pressure by umbilical artery catheter, auscultation, or with a Doppler transducer. Should arterial pressure fall significantly, decrease the rate of infusion immediately.

A weakening of the wall of the ductus arteriosus and pulmonary artery has been reported, particularly during prolonged administration.

The administration of alprostadil to neonates may result in gastric outlet obstruction secondary to antral hyperplasia. This effect appears to be related to duration of therapy and cumulative dose of the drug. Neonates receiving alprostadil at recommended doses for more than 120 hours should be closely monitored for evidence of antral hyperplasia and gastric outlet obstruction.

Long-term carcinogenicity and fertility studies have not been done. The Ames and Alkaline Elution assays reveal no potential for mutagenesis.

4.5 Interaction with other medicinal products and other forms of interaction
No drug interactions have been reported to occur between Prostin VR and the standard therapy employed in neonates with congenital heart defects. Standard therapy includes antibiotics, such as penicillin or gentamicin; vasopressors, such as dopamine or isoproterenol; cardiac glycosides; and diuretics, such as furosemide.

4.6 Pregnancy and lactation
This product is for use in children only.

4.7 Effects on ability to drive and use machines
Not applicable

4.8 Undesirable effects
The most frequent adverse reactions observed with Prostin VR infusion in neonates with ductal-dependent congenital heart defects are related to the drug's known pharmacological effects. These include, in decreasing frequency, transient pyrexia, apnoea, bradycardia, seizures, hypotension, tachycardia, and diarrhoea. The relationship of the following adverse events, in decreasing frequency, to the drug is unknown: sepsis, cardiac arrest, disseminated intravascular coagulation, hypokalaemia, and oedema. Cutaneous vasodilation (flushing) is the only event related to the route of administration, occurring more frequently during intra-arterial administration.

4.9 Overdose
Apnoea, bradycardia, pyrexia, hypotension and flushing may be signs of drug overdose. If apnoea or bradycardia occur, the infusion should be discontinued and the appropriate medical treatment initiated. Caution should be used if the infusion is restarted. If pyrexia or hypotension occur, the infusion rate should be reduced until these symptoms subside. Flushing is usually attributed to incorrect intra-arterial catheter placement and is usually alleviated by repositioning the tip of the catheter.

5. PHARMACOLOGICAL PROPERTIES

5.1 Pharmacodynamic properties
Prostaglandins are potent vasoactive derivatives of arachadonic acid that exert vasomotor, metabolic and cellular effects on the pulmonary and coronary circulation. The E series of prostaglandins produces vasodilation of the systemic and coronary circulation in most species: these prostaglandins have been used for maintaining the patency of the ductus arteriosus in children.

Doses lower than 0.05microgram/kg/min (as low as 0.005 microgram/kg/min) alprostadil have been used

successfully in neonates, specifically when transport of the infant is necessary. No comparative trials exist and the efficacy and safety of this approach when compared to initiating dosing according to section 4.2 is currently unclear.

5.2 Pharmacokinetic properties

Based on studies in several animal species, intravenous or arterially administered prostaglandin E_1 is very rapidly metabolised and distributed throughout the entire body, with the exception of the CNS, where distribution, though detectable, is markedly reduced. The primary organisms for metabolism and inactivation of prostaglandin E_1 are probably the lung, liver and kidney which remove and metabolise 40-95% of the prostaglandin E_1 in a single pass through the organ. A number of other tissues possess lesser, but significant, capacity to metabolise prostaglandin E_1. The predominant metabolites found in plasma, 15-oxo-prostaglandin E_1 and 13,14-dihydro-15 oxo-prostaglandin E_1 are extensively metabolised by β and ω-oxidation prior to excretion, primarily by the kidney. Few urinary metabolites of prostaglandin E_1 have been characterised, but are widely believed to be analogous to those reported in detail for prostaglandin E_2 and prostaglandin $F_{2\alpha}$. Excretion is essentially complete within 24 hours after dosing, with no intact prostaglandin E_1 being found in urine and no evidence of tissue retention of prostaglandin E_1 or metabolites. In three species, rat, rabbit and lamb, the prostaglandin metabolising activity of lung from near-term fetal animals has been shown to be at least as effective as that of adults.

5.3 Preclinical safety data

See section 4.8 "Undesirable effects".

6. PHARMACEUTICAL PARTICULARS

6.1 List of excipients

Dehydrated ethanol

6.2 Incompatibilities

Diluted solutions of Prostin VR should be infused from glass or hard plastic containers, or PVC infusion bags. If undiluted Prostin VR Sterile Solution comes in direct contact with a plastic container, plasticisers are leached from the sidewalls. This appears to be a concentration-dependent phenomenon.

6.3 Shelf life

Three years.

6.4 Special precautions for storage

Store in a refrigerator.

6.5 Nature and contents of container

Glass ampoule, containing 1 ml solution.

6.6 Special precautions for disposal and other handling

Diluted solutions should be used within 24 hours.

7. MARKETING AUTHORISATION HOLDER

Pharmacia Limited

Ramsgate Road

Sandwich

Kent

CT13 9NJ

UK

8. MARKETING AUTHORISATION NUMBER(S)

PL 0032/0083

9. DATE OF FIRST AUTHORISATION/RENEWAL OF THE AUTHORISATION

Date of Grant: 23 July 1981

Date of Renewal: 17 April 1997

10. DATE OF REVISION OF THE TEXT

January 2008

Protamine Sulphate Injection BP

(UCB Pharma Limited)

1. NAME OF THE MEDICINAL PRODUCT

Protamine Sulphate Injection BP

2. QUALITATIVE AND QUANTITATIVE COMPOSITION

Protamine Sulphate Salmine 10mg/ml

3. PHARMACEUTICAL FORM

Sterile Solution

4. CLINICAL PARTICULARS

4.1 Therapeutic indications

Neutralisation of the anticoagulant effect of heparin therapy and the treatment of heparin overdose.

4.2 Posology and method of administration

Adults: Protamine Sulphate Injection should be administered by slow intravenous injection (max rate 5 mg/min) over a period of 10 minutes. The dose is dependent on the amount of heparin to be neutralised. One mg of Protamine Sulphate will usually neutralise at least 100 IU of mucous heparin or 80 IU of lung heparin if given within 15 minutes of heparin administration. If more than 15 minutes has elapsed since heparin administration then less Protamine is required due to the rapid excretion of heparin.

Not more than 50 milligrams of Protamine Sulphate should be administered in a ten minute period.

The requirement for protamine may be monitored by APTT (Activated Partial Thromboplastin Time) or other appropriate test of clotting ability.

To antagonise heparin bolus:

Time Elapsed	Protamine dose needed/100 IU Heparin
30 min	1.00 -1.5 mg
30-60 min	0.50- 0.7 mg
2 hours	0.25- 0.375 mg

To antagonise heparin infusion:

25-50mg after stopping infusion

To antagonise heparin subcutaneous injection:

1-1.5 mg/ 100 IU heparin. 25-50 mg can be given by slow IV injection and the remainder by slow IV infusion over 8-16 hours (or the expected duration of absorption of heparin), or 2 hourly divided doses.

To antagonise heparin during extracorporeal circulation:

1.5 mg per 100 IU heparin. Sequential APTTs may be needed to calculate correct dosage.

Children and Elderly: There are no reports to suggest that the recommended adult dose should not also be used in children and the elderly.

4.3 Contraindications

Previous life threatening reaction to protamine.

4.4 Special warnings and precautions for use

Not more than 50 milligrams of Protamine Sulphate (5 ml Protamine Sulphate Injection BP) should be administered in a 10 minute period.

Protamine Sulphate only partially reverses the effects of low molecular weight heparins. Consult the relevant manufacturer's product information for anti-Xa neutralisation, as the extent and time of neutralisation are dependent on the individual low molecular weight heparin.

Hypersensitivity reactions can occur: patients at risk include those who have received protamine-insulin preparations (Isophane insulin) and those with allergy to residual fish antigens that remain after purification and those who have had protamine before. There are reports of vasectomised or infertile men who have anti-protamine antibodies making them potential reactors to protamine.

When insufficient protamine is administered a heparin rebound occurs within 5 hours of neutralisation, which may be associated with clinical bleeding. This phenomenon has been described mainly in patients undergoing extra-corporeal circulation in arterial and cardiac surgery or in dialysis procedures.

It responds to further doses of protamine

Protamine sulphate is not suitable for reversing the effect of oral anti-coagulants.

4.5 Interaction with other medicinal products and other forms of interaction

Protamine interferes with fluorescence methods of estimating plasma catecholamines.

4.6 Pregnancy and lactation

There is insufficient information as to whether this drug may affect fertility in humans or have a teratogenic potential or other adverse affects on the foetus. Reproduction studies have not been performed in animals. It is not known whether protamine sulphate is distributed into breast milk.

4.7 Effects on ability to drive and use machines

Not applicable.

4.8 Undesirable effects

Intravenous injections of Protamine Sulphate, particularly if administered rapidly, may cause a sensation of warmth, flushing of the skin, hypotension, bradycardia and dyspnoea. Nausea, vomiting and lassitude may also occur.

Urticaria and other hypersensitivity reactions including severe cardiovascular collapse, bronchospasm and death may occur rarely. Therefore this drug should only be given when resuscitation techniques and measures for the treatment of anaphylactic shock are readily available. Catastrophic pulmonary vasoconstriction and oedema may be associated with protamine use following cardiac surgery. Cases of acute thrombosis have been reported with Protamine Sulphate during cardiac interventions (cardiac surgery or stent implantation).

4.9 Overdose

Overdose of protamine sulphate may cause bleeding. Protamine has a weak anticoagulant effect due to an interaction with platelets and with many proteins including fibrinogen.

5. PHARMACOLOGICAL PROPERTIES

5.1 Pharmacodynamic properties

When administered alone, protamine sulphate has a weak anticoagulant effect. However, when given in the presence of heparin (which is strongly acidic), a stable salt is formed which results in the loss of anticoagulant activity of both drugs.

5.2 Pharmacokinetic properties

When used with heparin, protamine sulphate's effects are almost immediate and persist for approximately 2 hours.

5.3 Preclinical safety data

None available

6. PHARMACEUTICAL PARTICULARS

6.1 List of excipients

Water for Injections BP, Sulphuric Acid BP and Sodium Hydroxide BP

6.2 Incompatibilities

Protamine Sulphate is incompatible with certain antibiotics, including several of the cephalosporins and penicillins.

6.3 Shelf life

36 months

6.4 Special precautions for storage

Store below 25°C

6.5 Nature and contents of container

5 ml neutral glass ampoules

6.6 Special precautions for disposal and other handling

No special requirements

7. MARKETING AUTHORISATION HOLDER

UCB Pharma Limited

208 Bath Road

Slough

Berkshire

SL1 3WE

UK

8. MARKETING AUTHORISATION NUMBER(S)

PL 00039/5697R

9. DATE OF FIRST AUTHORISATION/RENEWAL OF THE AUTHORISATION

24 January 1991

10. DATE OF REVISION OF THE TEXT

Drafted: August 2009

Protelos

(Servier Laboratories Limited)

1. NAME OF THE MEDICINAL PRODUCT

▼ PROTELOS 2 g granules for oral suspension

2. QUALITATIVE AND QUANTITATIVE COMPOSITION

Each sachet contains 2 g of strontium ranelate.

Excipient: also contains 20 mg of aspartame (E951).

For a full list of excipients, see section 6.1.

3. PHARMACEUTICAL FORM

Granules for oral suspension

Yellow granules

4. CLINICAL PARTICULARS

4.1 Therapeutic indications

Treatment of postmenopausal osteoporosis to reduce the risk of vertebral and hip fractures (see section 5.1).

4.2 Posology and method of administration

The recommended daily dose is one 2 g sachet once daily by oral administration.

Due to the nature of the treated disease, strontium ranelate is intended for long-term use.

The absorption of strontium ranelate is reduced by food, milk and derivative products and therefore, PROTELOS should be administered in-between meals. Given the slow absorption, PROTELOS should be taken at bedtime, preferably at least two hours after eating (see sections 4.5 and 5.2).

The granules in the sachets must be taken as a suspension in a glass of water. Although in-use studies have demonstrated that strontium ranelate is stable in suspension for 24 hours after preparation, the suspension should be drunk immediately after being prepared.

Patients treated with strontium ranelate should receive vitamin D and calcium supplements if dietary intake is inadequate.

Use in the elderly

The efficacy and safety of strontium ranelate have been established in a broad age range (up to 100 years at inclusion) of postmenopausal women with osteoporosis. No dosage adjustment is required in relation to age.

Use in renal impairment

No dosage adjustment is required in patients with mild-to-moderate renal impairment (30-70 ml/min creatinine clearance) (see section 5.2). Strontium ranelate is not recommended for patients with severe renal impairment (creatinine clearance below 30 ml/min) (see sections 4.4 and 5.2).

Use in hepatic impairment

As strontium ranelate is not metabolised, no dosage adjustment is required in patients with hepatic impairment.

Use in children and adolescents

PROTELOS is not recommended for use in children and adolescents due to a lack of data on safety and efficacy.

4.3 Contraindications

Hypersensitivity to the active substance or to any of the excipients.

4.4 Special warnings and precautions for use

In the absence of bone safety data in patients with severe renal impairment treated with strontium ranelate, PROTELOS is not recommended in patients with a creatinine clearance below 30 ml/min (see section 5.2). In accordance with good medical practice, periodic assessment of renal function is recommended in patients with chronic renal impairment. Continuation of treatment with PROTELOS in patients developing severe renal impairment should be considered on an individual basis.

In phase III placebo-controlled studies, strontium ranelate treatment was associated with an increase in the annual incidence of venous thromboembolism (VTE), including pulmonary embolism (see section 4.8). The cause of this finding is unknown. PROTELOS should be used with caution in patients at increased risk of VTE, including patients with a past history of VTE. When treating patients at risk, or developing risk of VTE, particular attention should be given to possible signs and symptoms of VTE and adequate preventive measures taken.

Strontium interferes with colorimetric methods for the determination of blood and urinary calcium concentrations. Therefore, in medical practice, inductively coupled plasma atomic emission spectrometry or atomic absorption spectrometry methods should be used to ensure an accurate assessment of blood and urinary calcium concentrations.

PROTELOS contains a source of phenylalanine, which may be harmful for people with phenylketonuria.

Treatment with PROTELOS should be discontinued in case of serious allergic reaction.

Cases of severe hypersensitivity syndromes, including, in particular, drug rash with eosinophilia and systemic symptoms (DRESS), sometimes fatal, have been reported with the use of PROTELOS (see section 4.8). The DRESS syndrome is characterised by rash, fever, eosinophilia and systemic involvement (e.g. adenopathy, hepatitis, interstitial nephropathy, interstitial lung disease). Time to onset was usually around 3-6 weeks and the outcome in most cases favourable upon discontinuation of PROTELOS and after initiation of corticosteroid therapy. Recovery could be slow and recurrences of the syndrome have been reported in some cases after discontinuation of corticosteroid therapy.

Patients should be informed to stop PROTELOS immediately and permanently when a rash occurs and to seek medical advice. Patients who have stopped treatment due to hypersensitivity reactions should not re-start therapy with PROTELOS.

4.5 Interaction with other medicinal products and other forms of interaction

Food, milk and derivative products, and medicinal products containing calcium may reduce the bioavailability of strontium ranelate by approximately 60-70%. Therefore, administration of PROTELOS and such products should be separated by at least two hours (see section 5.2).

An *in vivo* clinical interaction study showed that the administration of aluminium and magnesium hydroxides either two hours before or together with strontium ranelate caused a slight decrease in the absorption of strontium ranelate (20-25% AUC decrease), while absorption was almost unaffected when the antacid was given two hours after strontium ranelate. It is therefore preferable to take antacids at least two hours after PROTELOS. However, when this dosing regimen is impractical due to the recommended administration of PROTELOS at bedtime, concomitant intake remains acceptable.

As divalent cations can form complexes with oral tetracycline and quinolone antibiotics at the gastro-intestinal level and thereby reduce their absorption, simultaneous administration of strontium ranelate with these medicinal products is not recommended. As a precautionary measure, PROTELOS treatment should be suspended during treatment with oral tetracycline or quinolone antibiotics.

No interaction was observed with oral supplementation of vitamin D.

No evidence of clinical interactions or relevant increase of blood strontium levels with medicinal products expected to be commonly prescribed concomitantly with PROTELOS in the target population were found during clinical trials. These included: nonsteroidal anti-inflammatory agents (including acetylsalicylic acid), anilides (such as paracetamol), H_2 blockers and proton pump inhibitors, diuretics, digoxin and cardiac glycosides, organic nitrates and other vasodilators for cardiac diseases, calcium channel blockers, beta blockers, ACE inhibitors, angiotensin II antagonists, selective beta-2 adrenoceptor agonists, oral anticoagulants, platelet aggregation inhibitors, statins, fibrates and benzodiazepine derivatives.

4.6 Pregnancy and lactation

PROTELOS is only intended for use in postmenopausal women.

No clinical data on exposed pregnancies are available for strontium ranelate. At high doses, animal studies have shown reversible bone effects in the offspring of rats and rabbits treated during pregnancy (see section 5.3). If PROTELOS is used inadvertently during pregnancy, treatment must be stopped.

Strontium is excreted in milk. Strontium ranelate should not be given to nursing women.

4.7 Effects on ability to drive and use machines

Strontium ranelate has no or negligible influence on the ability to drive and use machines.

4.8 Undesirable effects

PROTELOS has been studied in clinical trials involving nearly 8,000 participants. Long-term safety has been evaluated in postmenopausal women with osteoporosis treated for up to 60 months with strontium ranelate 2 g/day (n=3,352) or placebo (n=3,317) in phase III studies. Mean age was 75 years at inclusion and 23% of the patients enrolled were 80 to 100 years of age.

Overall incidence rates for adverse events with strontium ranelate did not differ from placebo and adverse events were usually mild and transient. The most common adverse events consisted of nausea and diarrhoea, which were generally reported at the beginning of treatment with no noticeable difference between groups afterwards. Discontinuation of therapy was mainly due to nausea (1.3% and 2.2% in the placebo and strontium ranelate groups respectively).

Adverse reactions, defined as adverse events considered at least possibly attributable to strontium ranelate treatment in phase III studies are listed below using the following convention (frequencies *versus* placebo): very common (>1/10); common (>1/100, <1/10); uncommon (>1/1,000, <1/100); rare (>1/10,000, <1/1,000); very rare (<1/10,000).

Nervous system disorders

Common: headache (3.3% vs. 2.7%)

Gastrointestinal disorders

Common: nausea (7.1% vs. 4.6%), diarrhoea (7.0% vs. 5.0%), loose stools (1.0% vs. 0.2%)

Skin and subcutaneous tissue disorders

Common: dermatitis (2.3% vs. 2.0%), eczema (1.8% vs. 1.4%)

There were no differences in the nature of adverse events between treatment groups regardless of whether patients were aged below or above 80 at inclusion.

In phase III studies, the annual incidence of venous thromboembolism (VTE) observed over 5 years was approximately 0.7%, with a relative risk of 1.4 (95% CI = [1.0; 2.0]) in strontium ranelate treated patients as compared to placebo (see section 4.4).

In phase III studies, over 5 years, nervous system disorders were reported with higher frequency in patients treated with strontium ranelate, compared with placebo: disturbances in consciousness (2.6% vs. 2.1%), memory loss (2.5% vs. 2.0%) and seizures (0.4% vs. 0.1%).

Laboratory test findings

Transient emergent increases (> 3 times the upper limit of the normal range) in creatine kinase (CK) activity (musculo-skeletal fraction) were reported in 1.4% and 0.6% of the strontium ranelate and placebo groups respectively. In most cases, these values spontaneously reverted to normal without change in treatment.

The following events have been reported in post-marketing experience:

Gastrointestinal disorders

Frequency unknown: vomiting, abdominal pain, oral mucosal irritation including stomatitis and/or mouth ulceration

Skin and subcutaneous tissue disorders

Frequency unknown: hypersensitivity skin reactions including rash, pruritus, urticaria, angioedema, Stevens-Johnson syndrome. Cases of severe hypersensitivity syndromes including drug rash with eosinophilia and systemic symptoms (DRESS) (see section 4.4).

Musculoskeletal and connective tissue disorders

Frequency unknown: musculoskeletal pain including muscle spasm, myalgia, bone pain, arthralgia and pain in extremity.

General disorders and administration site conditions

Frequency unknown: peripheral oedema

Psychiatric disorders

Frequency unknown: confusional state

4.9 Overdose

Good tolerance was shown in a clinical study investigating the repeated administration of 4 g strontium ranelate per day over 25 days in healthy postmenopausal women. Single administration of doses up to 11 g in healthy young male volunteers did not cause any particular symptoms.

Following episodes of overdoses during clinical trials (up to 4 g/day for a maximal duration of 147 days), no clinically relevant events were observed.

Administration of milk or antacids may be helpful to reduce the absorption of the active substance. In the event of substantial overdose, vomiting may be considered to remove unabsorbed active substance.

5. PHARMACOLOGICAL PROPERTIES

5.1 Pharmacodynamic properties

Pharmacotherapeutic group: Drugs for the treatment of bone diseases - Other drugs affecting bone structure and mineralisation

ATC code: M05BX03

In vitro, strontium ranelate:

- increases bone formation in bone tissue culture as well as osteoblast precursor replication and collagen synthesis in bone cell culture;

- reduces bone resorption by decreasing osteoclast differentiation and resorbing activity.

This results in a rebalance of bone turnover in favour of bone formation.

The activity of strontium ranelate was studied in various non-clinical models. In particular, in intact rats, strontium ranelate increases trabecular bone mass, trabeculae number and thickness; this results in an improvement of bone strength.

In bone tissue of treated animals and humans, strontium is mainly adsorbed onto the crystal surface and only slightly substitutes for calcium in the apatite crystal of newly formed bone. Strontium ranelate does not modify the bone crystal characteristics. In iliac crest bone biopsies obtained after up to 60 months of treatment with strontium ranelate 2 g/day in phase III trials, no deleterious effects on bone quality or mineralisation were observed.

The combined effects of strontium distribution in bone (see section 5.2) and increased X-ray absorption of strontium as compared to calcium, leads to an amplification of bone mineral density (BMD) measurement by dual-photon X-ray absorptiometry (DXA). Available data indicate that these factors account for approximately 50% of the measured change in BMD over 3 years of treatment with PROTELOS 2 g/day. This should be taken into account when interpreting BMD changes during treatment with PROTELOS. In phase III studies, which demonstrated the anti-fracture efficacy of PROTELOS treatment, measured mean BMD increased from baseline with PROTELOS by approximately 4% per year at the lumbar spine and 2% per year at the femoral neck, reaching 13% to 15% and 5% to 6% respectively after 3 years, depending on the study.

In phase III studies, as compared to placebo, biochemical markers of bone formation (bone-specific alkaline phosphatase and C-terminal propeptide of type I procollagen) increased and those of bone resorption (serum C-telopeptide and urinary N-telopeptide cross links) decreased from the third month of treatment up to 3 years.

Secondary to the pharmacological effects of strontium ranelate, slight decreases in calcium and parathyroid hormone (PTH) serum concentrations, increases in blood phosphorus concentrations and in total alkaline phosphatase activity were observed, with no observed clinical consequences.

Clinical efficacy

Osteoporosis is defined as BMD of the spine or hip 2.5 SD or more below the mean value of a normal young population. A number of risk factors are associated with postmenopausal osteoporosis including low bone mass, low bone mineral density, early menopause, a history of smoking and a family history of osteoporosis. The clinical consequence of osteoporosis is fractures. The risk of fractures is increased with the number of risk factors.

Treatment of postmenopausal osteoporosis:

The anti-fracture studies program of PROTELOS was made up of two placebo-controlled phase III studies: SOTI study and TROPOS study. SOTI involved 1,649 postmenopausal women with established osteoporosis (low lumbar BMD and prevalent vertebral fracture) and a mean age of 70 years. TROPOS involved 5,091 postmenopausal women with osteoporosis (low femoral neck BMD and prevalent fracture in more than half of them) and a mean age of 77 years. Together, SOTI and TROPOS enrolled 1,556 patients over 80 years at inclusion (23.1% of the study population). In addition to their treatment (2 g/day strontium ranelate or placebo), the patients received adapted calcium and vitamin D supplements throughout both studies.

PROTELOS reduced the relative risk of new vertebral fracture by 41% over 3 years in the SOTI study (table 1). The effect was significant from the first year. Similar benefits were demonstrated in women with multiple fractures at baseline. With respect to clinical vertebral fractures (defined as fractures associated with back pain and/or a body height loss of at least 1 cm), the relative risk was reduced by 38%. PROTELOS also decreased the number of patients with a body height loss of at least 1 cm as compared to placebo. Quality of life assessment on the QUALIOST specific scale as well as the General Health perception score of the SF-36 general scale indicated benefit of PROTELOS, compared with placebo.

Efficacy of PROTELOS to reduce the risk of new vertebral fracture was confirmed in the TROPOS study, including for osteoporotic patients without fragility fracture at baseline.

Table 1 Incidence of patients with vertebral fracture and relative risk reduction

	Placebo	PROTELOS	Relative Risk Reduction vs. placebo (95%CI), p value
SOTI	N=723	N=719	
New vertebral fracture over 3 years	32.8%	20.9%	41% (27-52), p<0.001
New vertebral fracture over the 1st year	11.8%	6.1%	49% (26-64), p<0.001
New clinical vertebral fracture over 3 years	17.4%	11.3%	38% (17-53), p<0.001
TROPOS	N=1823	N=1817	
New vertebral fracture over 3 years	20.0%	12.5%	39% (27-49), p<0.001

Table 2 Incidence of patients with hip fracture and relative risk reduction in patients with BMD ⩽ -2.4 SD (NHANES III) and age ⩾ 74 years

	Placebo	PROTELOS	Relative Risk Reduction vs. placebo (95%CI), p value
TROPOS	N=995	N=982	
Hip fracture over 3 years	6.4%	4.3%	36% (0-59), p=0.046

(see Table 1 above)

In patients over 80 years of age at inclusion, a pooled analysis of SOTI and TROPOS studies showed that PROTELOS reduced the relative risk of experiencing new vertebral fractures by 32% over 3 years (incidence of 19.1% with strontium ranelate vs. 26.5% with placebo).

In an *a-posteriori* analysis of patients from the pooled SOTI and TROPOS studies with baseline lumbar spine and / or femoral neck BMD in the osteopenic range and without prevalent fracture but with at least one additional risk factor for fracture (N=176), PROTELOS reduced the risk of a first vertebral fracture by 72% over 3 years (incidence of vertebral fracture 3.6% with strontium ranelate vs. 12.0% with placebo).

An *a-posteriori* analysis was performed on a subgroup of patients from the TROPOS study of particular medical interest and at high-risk of fracture [defined by a femoral neck BMD T-score ⩽ -3 SD (manufacturer's range corresponding to -2.4 SD using NHANES III) and an age ⩾ 74 years (n=1,977, i.e. 40% of the TROPOS study population)]. In this group, over 3 years of treatment, PROTELOS reduced the risk of hip fracture by 36% relative to the placebo group (table 2).

(see Table 2 above)

5.2 Pharmacokinetic properties

Strontium ranelate is made up of 2 atoms of stable strontium and 1 molecule of ranelic acid, the organic part permitting the best compromise in terms of molecular weight, pharmacokinetics and acceptability of the medicinal product. The pharmacokinetics of strontium and ranelic acid have been assessed in healthy young men and healthy postmenopausal women, as well as during long-term exposure in postmenopausal osteoporotic women including elderly women.

Due to its high polarity, the absorption, distribution and binding to plasma proteins of ranelic acid are low. There is no accumulation of ranelic acid and no evidence of metabolism in animals and humans. Absorbed ranelic acid is rapidly eliminated unchanged via the kidneys.

Absorption

The absolute bioavailability of strontium is about 25% (range 19-27%) after an oral dose of 2 g strontium ranelate. Maximum plasma concentrations are reached 3-5 hours after a single dose of 2 g. Steady state is reached after 2 weeks of treatment. Intake of strontium ranelate with calcium or food reduces the bioavailability of strontium by approximately 60-70%, compared with administration 3 hours after a meal. Due to the relatively slow absorption of strontium, food and calcium intake should be avoided both before and after administration of PROTELOS. Oral supplementation with vitamin D has no effect on strontium exposure.

Distribution

Strontium has a volume of distribution of about 1 l/kg. The binding of strontium to human plasma proteins is low (25%) and strontium has a high affinity for bone tissue. Measurement of strontium concentration in iliac crest bone biopsies from patients treated for up to 60 months with strontium ranelate 2 g/day indicate that bone strontium concentrations may reach a plateau after about 3 years of treatment. There are no data in patients to demonstrate elimination kinetics of strontium from bone off-therapy.

Biotransformation

As a divalent cation, strontium is not metabolised. Strontium ranelate does not inhibit cytochrome P450 enzymes.

Elimination

The elimination of strontium is time and dose independent. The effective half-life of strontium is about 60 hours. Strontium excretion occurs via the kidneys and the gastrointestinal tract. Its plasma clearance is about 12 ml/min (CV 22%) and its renal clearance about 7 ml/min (CV 28%).

Pharmacokinetics in special clinical situations

Elderly

Population pharmacokinetic data showed no relationship between age and apparent clearance of strontium in the target population.

Patients with renal impairment

In patients with mild-to-moderate renal impairment (30-70 ml/min creatinine clearance), strontium clearance decreases as creatinine clearance decreases (approximately 30% decrease over the creatinine clearance range 30 to 70 ml/min) and thereby induces an increase in strontium plasma levels. In phase III studies, 85% of the patients had a creatinine clearance between 30 and 70 ml/min and 6% below 30 ml/min at inclusion, and the mean creatinine clearance was about 50 ml/min. No dosage adjustment is therefore required in patients with mild-to-moderate renal impairment.

There is no pharmacokinetic data in patients with severe renal impairment (creatinine clearance below 30 ml/min).

Patients with hepatic impairment

There is no pharmacokinetic data in patients with hepatic impairment. Due to the pharmacokinetic properties of strontium, no effect is expected.

5.3 Preclinical safety data

Non-clinical data revealed no special hazard for humans based on conventional studies of safety pharmacology, genotoxicity and carcinogenic potential.

Chronic oral administration of strontium ranelate at high doses in rodents induced bone and tooth abnormalities, mainly consisting of spontaneous fractures and delayed mineralisation. These effects were reported at bone strontium levels 2-3 times higher than long-term clinical bone strontium levels and were reversible after cessation of treatment.

Developmental toxicity studies in rats and rabbits resulted in bone and tooth abnormalities (e.g. bent long bones and wavy ribs) in the offspring. In rats, these effects were reversible 8 weeks after cessation of treatment.

6. PHARMACEUTICAL PARTICULARS

6.1 List of excipients

Aspartame (E951)

Maltodextrin

Mannitol (E421)

6.2 Incompatibilities

Not applicable.

6.3 Shelf life

3 years.

6.4 Special precautions for storage

This medicinal product does not require any special storage conditions.

6.5 Nature and contents of container

Paper/polyethylene/aluminium/polyethylene sachets.

Pack sizes

Boxes containing 7, 14, 28, 56, 84 or 100 sachets.

Not all pack sizes may be marketed.

6.6 Special precautions for disposal and other handling

No special requirements.

7. MARKETING AUTHORISATION HOLDER

LES LABORATOIRES SERVIER

22, rue Garnier

92200 Neuilly-sur-Seine

France

8. MARKETING AUTHORISATION NUMBER(S)

EU/1/04/288/001

EU/1/04/288/002

EU/1/04/288/003

EU/1/04/288/004

EU/1/04/288/005

EU/1/04/288/006

9. DATE OF FIRST AUTHORISATION/RENEWAL OF THE AUTHORISATION

21/09/2004

10. DATE OF REVISION OF THE TEXT

6 March 2009

Detailed information on this medicinal product is available on the website of the European Medicines Agency (EMEA) http://www.emea.europa.eu

Protirelin Ampoules

(Cambridge Laboratories)

1. NAME OF THE MEDICINAL PRODUCT

Protirelin Ampoules

2. QUALITATIVE AND QUANTITATIVE COMPOSITION

Each ampoule contains 200micrograms of Protirelin (Thyrotrophin-releasing hormone, TRH) in 2ml of solution.

3. PHARMACEUTICAL FORM

Solution for Injection

4. CLINICAL PARTICULARS

4.1 Therapeutic indications

The administration of Protirelin provides a means of assessing thyroid function and the reserve of TSH in the pituitary gland and is recommended as a test procedure where such assessment is indicated.

It is particularly useful as a diagnostic test for:

1. Mild hyperthyroidism
2. Ophthalmic Graves' disease
3. Mild or preclinical hypothyroidism
4. Hypopituitarism
5. Hypothalamic disease

It may also be used in place of the T_3 suppression test.

4.2 Posology and method of administration

Protirelin ampoules are for intravenous injection.

Intravenous injection

Tests employing intravenous Protirelin are based on the serum TSH response to a standard dose. They provide a means of both quantitative and qualitative assessment of thyroid function. It is essential for each laboratory to establish its own normal range of values for serum TSH before attempting quantitative assessment of Protirelin responses by this means.

Intravenous Protirelin test

a) Blood sample taken for control TSH assay.

b) Protirelin 200μg given as a single bolus injection.

c) Blood sample taken 20 minutes after injection for peak TSH assay.

d) If necessary, a further blood sample may be taken 60 minutes after injection to detect a delayed TSH response.

The ampoule solution should not be diluted.

The elderly

The use of Protirelin in the elderly has been well documented. Dosage requirements and the side-effects are similar to those of younger adults. The response may be decreased in elderly subjects, but this does not interfere with the interpretation of the test results.

Children up to the age of 12

The procedures for administering Protirelin to children are identical to those outlined above. An intravenous dose of 1μg/kg bodyweight may be used.

Interpretation of results

Interpretation of the responses to Protirelin is based on the increase in TSH and/or PBI, T_3 or T_4 levels from the basal values. In normal subjects, there is a prompt rise in serum levels of TSH. The changes observed in various conditions are briefly outlined below:

1. Hyperthyroidism - no rise in serum TSH or thyroid hormone levels.

2. Ophthalmic Graves' disease - often no rise in serum TSH or thyroid hormone levels.

3. Primary hypothyroidism - exaggerated and prolonged rise in serum TSH but no change in thyroid hormone levels.

4. Hypopituitarism - absent or impaired TSH or thyroid hormone response implies diminished TSH reserve.

5. Hypothalamic disease - a rise in serum TSH or thyroid hormone levels can occur in the presence of hypothyroidism; delayed responses are common.

The Protirelin test provides, in most instances, information similar to that obtained from a T_3 suppression test in that an absent or impaired response usually correlates with an absent or impaired response to T_3 suppression.

4.3 Contraindications
There are no absolute contra-indications to Protirelin.

4.4 Special warnings and precautions for use
In view of the postulated effect of bolus injections of Protirelin on smooth muscle, patients with bronchial asthma or other types of obstructive airways disease should be closely monitored. Caution should always be observed in patients with myocardial ischaemia and severe hypopituitarism.

4.5 Interaction with other medicinal products and other forms of interaction
The secretion of thyrotrophin appears to be modulated by dopaminergic and noradrenergic pathways. The TSH response to Protirelin may be reduced by thyroid hormones, levodopa, phenothiazines, salicylates, bromocriptine, carbamazepine, lithium and by pharmacological doses of corticosteroids.

An increased response may be seen in subjects taking metoclopramide, amiodarone or theophyllines and in men taking oestrogens. Over-treatment with antithyroid drugs may also cause an enhanced response.

4.6 Pregnancy and lactation
Animal studies and clinical experience have shown no evidence of hazard in human pregnancy at the recommended dosage. Nevertheless, the established medical principle of not administering drugs during early pregnancy should be observed.

Breast enlargement and leaking of milk have been reported following the administration of protirelin to lactating women.

4.7 Effects on ability to drive and use machines
None known.

4.8 Undesirable effects
Protirelin is well tolerated. Following rapid intravenous injection, side-effects of a mild and transient nature may be experienced. These comprise nausea, a desire to micturate, a feeling of flushing, slight dizziness and a peculiar taste, and have been attributed to a local action of the bolus of Protirelin on the muscle of the gastro-intestinal and genito-urinary tracts. A transient increase in pulse rate and blood pressure may also be noted.

4.9 Overdose
No symptoms of overdosage have been noted in patients receiving up to 1mg i.v.

5. PHARMACOLOGICAL PROPERTIES

5.1 Pharmacodynamic properties
Pharmacotherapeutic group: V04CJ.

Protirelin stimulates the secretion of thyroid stimulating hormone (TSH). Intravenous injection results in a prompt rise in serum TSH levels in normal subjects, peak levels being observed about twenty minutes after administration. There is a concomitant rise in serum levels of prolactin.

5.2 Pharmacokinetic properties
TSH rapidly disappears from the plasma after intravenous injection. Over 90% is removed within 20 minutes with a half life of about 5.3 minutes. About 5.5% of the dose is excreted in the urine, mostly within 30 minutes.

5.3 Preclinical safety data
There are no pre-clinical data of relevance to the prescriber which are additional to that already included in other sections of the SPC.

6. PHARMACEUTICAL PARTICULARS

6.1 List of excipients
Mannitol Ph.Eur

Glacial acetic acid Ph.Eur

Water for Injections Ph.Eur

6.2 Incompatibilities
None known.

6.3 Shelf life
Three years.

6.4 Special precautions for storage
The recommended maximum storage temperature is 30°C.

6.5 Nature and contents of container
Clear glass ampoules coded with orange and black colour rings each containing 2ml of solution, in packs of 10 ampoules.

6.6 Special precautions for disposal and other handling
None.

Administrative Data

7. MARKETING AUTHORISATION HOLDER
Cambridge Laboratories Limited

Deltic House

Kingfisher Way

Silverlink Business Park

Wallsend

Tyne & Wear

NE28 9NX

8. MARKETING AUTHORISATION NUMBER(S)
PL 12070/0009

9. DATE OF FIRST AUTHORISATION/RENEWAL OF THE AUTHORISATION
October 2002

10. DATE OF REVISION OF THE TEXT
July 2003

Protium 20 mg gastro-resistant tablet

(Nycomed UK Ltd)

1. NAME OF THE MEDICINAL PRODUCT
Protium® 20 mg gastro-resistant tablets.

2. QUALITATIVE AND QUANTITATIVE COMPOSITION
One gastro-resistant tablet contains

20 mg Pantoprazole (as pantoprazole sodium sesquihydrate 22.6 mg).

For excipients see 6.1.

3. PHARMACEUTICAL FORM
Gastro-resistant tablet.

A yellow, oral biconvex film coated tablet imprinted with "P20" in brown ink on one side.

4. CLINICAL PARTICULARS

4.1 Therapeutic indications
For the treatment of mild reflux disease and associated symptoms (e.g. heartburn, acid regurgitation, pain on swallowing).

For long-term management and prevention of relapse in reflux oesophagitis.

Prevention of gastroduodenal ulcers induced by non-selective non-steroidal anti-inflammatory drugs (NSAIDs) in patients at risk with a need for continuous NSAID treatment (see section 4.4).

4.2 Posology and method of administration
Recommended dosage:

Adults and adolescents 12 years of age and above:

Mild reflux disease and associated symptoms (e.g. heartburn, acid regurgitation, pain on swallowing)

The recommended oral dosage is one gastro-resistant tablet Protium® 20 mg per day. Symptom relief is generally accomplished within 2-4 weeks, and a 4-week treatment period is usually required for healing of associated oesophagitis. If this is not sufficient, healing will normally be achieved within a further 4 weeks. When symptom relief has been achieved, reoccurring symptoms can be controlled using an on-demand regimen of 20 mg once daily, when required. A switch to continuous therapy may be considered in case satisfactory symptom control cannot be maintained with on-demand treatment.

Long-term management and prevention of relapse in reflux oesophagitis

For long-term management, a maintenance dose of one gastro-resistant tablet Protium® 20 mg per day is recommended, increasing to 40 mg pantoprazole per day if a relapse occurs. Protium® 40 mg is available for this case. After healing of the relapse the dosage can be reduced again to 20 mg pantoprazole.

Adults:

Prevention of gastroduodenal ulcers induced by non-selective non-steroidal anti-inflammatory drugs (NSAIDs) in patients at risk with a need for continuous NSAID treatment

The recommended oral dosage is one gastro-resistant tablet Protium® 20 mg per day.

Children below 12 years of age:

Protium® is not recommended for use in children below 12 years of age due to limited data in this age group.

Note:

A daily dose of 20 mg pantoprazole should not be exceeded in patients with severe liver impairment.

No dose adjustment is necessary in elderly patients or in those with impaired renal function.

General instructions:

Protium® 20 mg gastro-resistant tablets should not be chewed or crushed, and should be swallowed whole with liquid before a meal.

4.3 Contraindications
Protium® 20 mg should not be used in cases of known hypersensitivity to the active ingredient or/and any of the other constituents of Protium® 20 mg.

Pantoprazole, like other PPIs, should not be co-administered with atazanavir (see Section 4.5).

4.4 Special warnings and precautions for use
Special warnings

None.

Special precautions for use

In patients with severe liver impairment the liver enzymes should be monitored regularly during treatment with pantoprazole, particularly on long-term use. In the case of a rise of the liver enzymes Protium® 20 mg should be discontinued.

The use of Protium® 20 mg as a preventive of gastroduodenal ulcers induced by non-selective non-steroidal anti-inflammatory drugs (NSAIDs) should be restricted to patients who require continued NSAID treatment and have an increased risk to develop gastrointestinal complications.

The increased risk should be assessed according to individual risk factors, e.g. high age (>65 years), history of gastric or duodenal ulcer or upper gastrointestinal bleeding.

Pantoprazole, as all acid-blocking medicines, may reduce the absorption of vitamin B12 (cyanocobalamin) due to hypo- or achlorhydria. This should be considered in patients with reduced body stores or risk factors for reduced vitamin B12 absorption on long-term therapy.

In long term treatment, especially when exceeding a treatment period of 1 year, patients should be kept under regular surveillance.

Note:

Prior to treatment a malignant disease of the oesophagus or stomach should be excluded as the treatment with pantoprazole may alleviate the symptoms of malignant diseases and can thus delay diagnosis.

Patients who do not respond after 4 weeks should be investigated.

4.5 Interaction with other medicinal products and other forms of interaction
Protium® 20 mg may reduce or increase the absorption of drugs whose bioavailability is pH-dependent (e.g. ketoconazole).

It has been shown that co-administration of atazanavir 300 mg/ritonavir 100 mg with omeprazole (40 mg once daily) or atazanavir 400 mg with lansoprazole (60 mg single dose) to healthy volunteers resulted in a substantial reduction in the bioavailability of atazanavir. The absorption of atazanavir is pH dependent. Therefore PPIs, including pantoprazole, should not be co-administered with atazanavir (see Section 4.3).

Pantoprazole is metabolized in the liver via the cytochrome P450 enzyme system. An interaction of pantoprazole with other drugs or compounds which are metabolized using the same enzyme system cannot be excluded. However, no clinically significant interactions were observed in specific tests with a number of such drugs or compounds, namely carbamazepine, caffeine, diazepam, diclofenac, digoxin, ethanol, glibenclamide, metoprolol, naproxen, nifedipine, phenytoin, piroxicam, theophylline and an oral contraceptive.

Although no interaction during concomitant administration of phenprocoumon or warfarin has been observed in clinical pharmacokinetic studies, a few isolated cases of changes in INR have been reported during concomitant treatment in the post-marketing period. Therefore, in patients treated with coumarin anticoagulants, monitoring of prothrombin time/INR is recommended after initiation, termination or during irregular use of pantoprazole.

There were also no interactions with concomitantly administered antacids.

4.6 Pregnancy and lactation
Clinical experience in pregnant women is limited. In animal reproduction studies, signs of slight foetotoxicity were observed at doses above 5 mg/kg. There is no information on the excretion of pantoprazole into human breast milk. Pantoprazole tablets should only be used when the benefit to the mother is considered greater than the potential risk to the foetus/baby.

4.7 Effects on ability to drive and use machines
There are no known effects on the ability to drive and use machines.

4.8 Undesirable effects
(see Table 1 on next page)

4.9 Overdose
There are no known symptoms of over-dosage in man. Doses up to 240 mg i.v. were administered over 2 minutes and were well tolerated.

In the case of over-dosage with clinical signs of intoxication, the usual rules of intoxication therapy apply.

5. PHARMACOLOGICAL PROPERTIES

5.1 Pharmacodynamic properties
Proton pump inhibitors

ATC Code: AO2BC02

Pantoprazole is a substituted benzimidazole which inhibits the secretion of hydrochloric acid in the stomach by specific action on the proton pumps of the parietal cells.

Pantoprazole is converted to its active form in the acidic canaliculi of the parietal cells where it inhibits the H^+, K^+-ATPase enzyme, i. e. the final stage in the production of hydrochloric acid in the stomach. The inhibition is dose-dependent and affects both basal and stimulated acid secretion. In most patients, freedom from symptoms is achieved in 2 weeks. As with other proton pump inhibitors and H_2 receptor inhibitors, treatment with pantoprazole causes a reduced acidity in the stomach and thereby an increase in gastrin in proportion to the reduction in acidity. The increase in gastrin is reversible. Since pantoprazole binds to the enzyme distal to the cell receptor level, the

Table 1 Undesirable effects

Frequency / Organ system	Common (>1/100, <1/10)	Uncommon (>1/1000, <1/100)	Rare (>1/1000, <1/10,000)	Very rare (<1/10,000, incl. isolated reports)
Blood and lymphatic system				Leukopenia; Thrombocytopenia
Gastrointestinal Disorders	Upper abdominal pain; Diarrhoea; Constipation; Flatulence	Nausea/Vomiting	Dry mouth	
General disorders and administration site conditions				Peripheral edema
Hepatobiliary disorders				Severe hepatocellular damage leading to jaundice with or without hepatic failure
Immune system disorders				Anaphylactic reactions including anaphylactic shock
Investigations				Increased liver enzymes (transaminases, γ-GT); Elevated triglycerides; Increased body temperature
Musculoskeletal, connective tissue disorders			Athralgia	Myalgia
Nervous system disorders	Headache	Dizziness; Disturbances in vision (blurred vision)		
Psychiatric disorders			Depression, Hallucination, Disorientation and Confusion, especially in pre-disposed patients, as well as the aggravation of these symptoms in case of pre-existence	
Renal and urinary disorders				Interstitial nephritis
Skin and subcutaneous tissue disorders		Allergic reactions such as pruritus and skin rash		Urticaria; Angioedema; Severe skin reactions such as Stevens Johnson Syndrome, Erythema Multiforme, Lyell-Syndrome; Photosensitivity

substance can affect hydrochloric acid secretion independently of stimulation by other substances (acetylcholine, histamine, gastrin). The effect is the same whether the product is given orally or intravenously.

The fasting gastrin values increase under pantoprazole. On short-term use, in most cases they do not exceed the normal upper limit. During long-term treatment, gastrin levels double in most cases. An excessive increase, however, occurs only in isolated cases. As a result, a mild to moderate increase in the number of specific endocrine (ECL) cells in the stomach is observed in a minority of cases during long-term treatment (simple to adenomatoid hyperplasia). However, according to the studies conducted so far, the formation of carcinoid precursors (atypical hyperplasia) or gastric carcinoids as were found in animal experiments (see Section 5.3) can be ruled out for humans for a 1-year treatment period.

An influence of a long term treatment with pantoprazole exceeding one year cannot be completely ruled out on endocrine parameters of the thyroid and liver enzymes according to results in animal studies.

5.2 Pharmacokinetic properties

General pharmacokinetics

Pantoprazole is rapidly absorbed and the maximal plasma concentration is achieved even after one single 20 mg oral dose. On average at about 2.0 h - 2.5 h p.a. the maximum serum concentrations of about 1-1.5 µg/ml are achieved, and these values remain constant after multiple administration. Volume of distribution is about 0.15 l/kg and clearance is about 0.1 l/h/kg.

Terminal half-life is about 1 h. There were a few cases of subjects with delayed elimination. Because of the specific binding of pantoprazole to the proton pumps of the parietal cell the elimination half-life does not correlate with the much longer duration of action (inhibition of acid secretion).

Pharmacokinetics do not vary after single or repeated administration. In the dose range of 10 to 80 mg, the plasma kinetics of pantoprazole are linear after both oral and intravenous administration.

Pantoprazole's serum protein binding is about 98%. The substance is almost exclusively metabolized in the liver. Renal elimination represents the major route of excretion (about 80%) for the metabolites of pantoprazole, the rest is excreted with the faeces. The main metabolite in both the serum and urine is desmethylpantoprazole which is conjugated with sulphate. The half-life of the main metabolite (about 1.5 h) is not much longer than that of pantoprazole.

Bioavailability

Pantoprazole is completely absorbed after oral administration. The absolute bioavailability from the tablet was found to be about 77%. Concomitant intake of food had no influence on AUC, maximum serum concentration and thus bioavailability. Only the variability of the lag-time will be increased by concomitant food intake.

Characteristics in patients/special groups of subjects

No dose reduction is requested when pantoprazole is administered to patients with restricted kidney function (incl. dialysis patients). As with healthy subjects, pantoprazole's half-life is short. Only very small amounts of pantoprazole can be dialyzed. Although the main metabolite has a moderately delayed half-life (2 - 3h), excretion is still rapid and thus accumulation does not occur.

Although for patients with liver cirrhosis (classes A and B according to Child) the half-life values increased to between 3 and 6 h and the AUC values increased by a factor of 3 - 5, the maximum serum concentration only increased slightly by a factor of 1.3 compared with healthy subjects.

A slight increase in AUC and Cmax in elderly volunteers compared with younger counterparts is also not clinically relevant.

Children

Following administration of single oral doses of 20 or 40 mg pantoprazole to children aged 5 – 16 years AUC and Cmax were in the range of corresponding values in adults. Following administration of single i.v. doses of 0.8 or 1.6 mg/kg pantoprazole to children aged 2 – 16 years there was no significant association between pantoprazole clearance and age or weight. AUC and volume of distribution were in accordance with data from adults.

5.3 Preclinical safety data

Preclinical data reveal no special hazard to humans based on conventional studies of safety pharmacology, repeated dose toxicity and genotoxicity.

In the 2-year carcinogenicity studies (corresponding to lifetime treatment) in rats, neuroendocrine neoplasms were found. In addition, squamous cell papillomas were found in the forestomach of rats in one study. The mechanism leading to the formation of gastric carcinoids by substituted benzimidazoles has been carefully investigated and allows the conclusion that it is a secondary reaction to the massively elevated serum gastrin levels occurring in the rat during chronic high-dose treatment.

In the two-year rodent studies an increased number of liver tumors was observed in rats (in one rat study only) and in female mice and was interpreted as being due to pantoprazole's high metabolic rate in the liver.

A slight increase of neoplastic changes of the thyroid was observed in the group of rats receiving the highest dose (200 mg/kg) in one 2 year study. The occurrence of these neoplasms is associated with the pantoprazole-induced changes in the breakdown of thyroxine in the rat liver. As the therapeutic dose in man is low, no side effects on the thyroid glands are expected.

From mutagenicity studies, cell transformation tests and a DNA binding study it is concluded that pantoprazole has no genotoxic potential.

Investigations revealed no evidence of impaired fertility or teratogenic effects.

Penetration of the placenta was investigated in the rat and was found to increase with advanced gestation. As a result, concentration of pantoprazole in the foetus is increased shortly before birth.

6. PHARMACEUTICAL PARTICULARS

6.1 List of excipients

sodium carbonate
mannitol
crospovidone
povidone K90
calcium stearate
hypromellose
povidone K25
propylene glycol
methacrylic acid-ethylacrylate-copolymer (1:1)
polysorbate 80
sodium laurilsulfate
triethyl citrate
titanium dioxide E 171
yellow ferric oxide E 172
printing ink (shellac, red, black and yellow ferric oxide E172, soya lecithin, titanium dioxide E171, antifoam DC 1510)

6.2 Incompatibilities

Not applicable

6.3 Shelf life

3 years

6.4 Special precautions for storage

No special precautions for storage.

6.5 Nature and contents of container

Packs: bottles (HDPE container with LDPE closure) and blisters (ALU/ALU blisters without cardboard reinforcement, ALU/ALU blisters with cardboard reinforcement (blister wallet)) with:

7 - gastro-resistant tablets
14 and 15* - gastro-resistant tablets
28 and 30* - gastro-resistant tablets
56 and 60* - gastro-resistant tablets
84 - gastro-resistant tablets
100* - gastro-resistant tablets
112 - gastro-resistant tablets

Hospital packs: bottles (HDPE container with LDPE closure) and blisters (ALU/ALU blisters without cardboard reinforcement, ALU/ALU blisters with cardboard reinforcement (blister wallet)) with:

50 - gastro-resistant tablets
84 - gastro-resistant tablets
90 - gastro-resistant tablets
112 - gastro-resistant tablets
140* - gastro-resistant tablets
140 (10x14*) (5x28*) - gastro-resistant tablets
700 (5x140*) - gastro-resistant tablets
280 (20x14*), (10x28*) - gastro-resistant tablets
500 - gastro-resistant tablets

*authorised in the Reference Member State

Note: Not all pack sizes may be marketed.

6.6 Special precautions for disposal and other handling

No special requirements.

7. MARKETING AUTHORISATION HOLDER

Nycomed GmbH
Byk-Gulden-Str. 2
D-78467 Konstanz
Germany

8. MARKETING AUTHORISATION NUMBER(S)
PL 31752/0001

9. DATE OF FIRST AUTHORISATION/RENEWAL OF THE AUTHORISATION
7 January 1999/CRD 27 July 2003

10. DATE OF REVISION OF THE TEXT
February 2008

Protium 40 mg i.v. Powder for Solution for Injection

(Nycomed UK Ltd)

1. NAME OF THE MEDICINAL PRODUCT
Protium® i.v. Powder for Solution for Injection.

2. QUALITATIVE AND QUANTITATIVE COMPOSITION
One vial contains:

40mg pantoprazole (as pantoprazole sodium).

For excipients see 6.1.

3. PHARMACEUTICAL FORM
Powder for Solution for Injection. A white to almost white dry substance.

4. CLINICAL PARTICULARS

4.1 Therapeutic indications
For symptomatic improvement and healing of gastrointestinal diseases which require a reduction in acid secretion:

Duodenal ulcer

Gastric ulcer

Moderate and severe reflux oesophagitis

Zollinger-Ellison Syndrome and other pathological hypersecretory conditions

Note: Prior to treatment of gastric ulcer, the possibility of malignancy should be excluded as treatment with Protium® i.v. may alleviate the symptoms of malignant ulcers and can thus delay diagnosis.

4.2 Posology and method of administration
Protium® i.v. is for intravenous administration ONLY and must NOT be given by any other route. Protium® i.v. is recommended only if oral application is not appropriate.

Duodenal ulcer, gastric ulcer, moderate and severe reflux oesophagitis

The recommended intravenous dosage is one vial (40 mg pantoprazole) of Protium® i.v. per day.

Long-term management of Zollinger-Ellison Syndrome and other pathological hypersecretory conditions

Patients should start their treatment with a daily dose of 80 mg Protium® i.v. Thereafter, the dosage can be titrated up or down as needed using measurements of gastric acid secretion to guide. With doses above 80 mg daily, the dose should be divided and given twice daily. A temporary increase of the dosage above 160 mg pantoprazole is possible but should not be applied longer than required for adequate acid control.

In case a rapid acid control is required, a starting dose of 2 × 80 mg Protium® i.v. is sufficient to manage a decrease of acid output into the target range (<10 mEq/h) within one hour in the majority of patients. Transition from Protium® i.v. to the oral formulation of Protium® should be performed as soon as it is clinically justified.

A ready-to-use intravenous solution is prepared by injecting 10 ml of 0.9% sodium chloride injection into the vial containing the lyophilised powder.

This freshly prepared solution should be administered intravenously over 2 to 15 minutes, either as a slow injection or it may be further diluted with 100 ml of 0.9% sodium chloride injection, or 5% glucose injection, and administered as a short-term infusion.

Protium® i.v. should not be reconstituted with diluents other than those stated.

After preparation, the solution must be used within 12 hours and the unused portion discarded.

In most patients, freedom from symptoms is achieved rapidly.

As soon as oral therapy is possible, treatment with Protium® i.v. should be discontinued.

Data are available on i.v. use for up to 7 days. Thereafter, oral Protium® treatment should be administered in compliance with the approved dosage regimen.

Duodenal ulcer:

Duodenal ulcers generally heal within 2 weeks. If a 2-week period of treatment is not sufficient, healing will be achieved in almost all cases within a further 2 weeks.

Gastric ulcer:

A 4-week period is usually required for the treatment of gastric ulcers. If this is not sufficient, healing will usually be achieved within a further 4 weeks.

Gastro-Oesophageal Reflux:

A 4-week period is usually required for the treatment of gastro-oesophageal reflux. If this is not sufficient, healing will usually be achieved within a further 4 weeks.

Elderly:

No dose adjustment is necessary in the elderly.

Patients with impaired renal function:

No dose adjustment is necessary in patients with renal impairment.

Patients with severe liver impairment:

In patients with severe liver impairment, the daily dose should be reduced to 20 mg pantoprazole. Furthermore, in these patients the liver enzymes should be monitored during Protium® i.v. therapy. In case of a rise in the liver enzymes, Protium® i.v. should be discontinued.

Children:

The experience in children is limited. Therefore, Protium® i.v. Powder for Solution for Injection is not recommended for use in patients below 18 years of age until further data become available.

4.3 Contraindications
Protium® i.v. should not be used in cases of known hypersensitivity to pantoprazole.

Pantoprazole like other PPIs, should not be co-administered with atazanavir (see Section 4.5).

4.4 Special warnings and precautions for use
Protium® i.v. is for intravenous administration ONLY and must NOT be given by any other route. Protium® i.v. is recommended only if oral application is not appropriate.

4.5 Interaction with other medicinal products and other forms of interaction
As with other acid secretion inhibitors, changes in absorption may be observed when drugs whose absorption is pH-dependent, e.g. ketoconazole, are taken concomitantly.

It has been shown that co-administration of atazanavir 300 mg/ritonavir 100 mg with omeprazole (40 mg once daily) or atazanavir 400 mg with lansoprazole (60 mg single dose) to healthy volunteers resulted in a substantial reduction in the bioavailability of atazanavir. The absorption of atazanavir is pH dependent. Therefore, PPIs, including pantoprazole, should not be co-administered with atazanavir (see Section 4.3).

Pantoprazole is metabolised in the liver via the cytochrome P450 enzyme system. Although studies have shown that pantoprazole has no significant effect on cytochrome P450, an interaction of pantoprazole with other drugs or compounds which are metabolised using the same enzyme system cannot be excluded.

However, no clinically significant interactions were observed in specific tests with a number of such drugs/compounds, namely antipyrine, caffeine, carbamazepine, diazepam, diclofenac, digoxin, ethanol, glibenclamide, metoprolol, naproxen, nifedipine, phenytoin, piroxicam, theophylline and an oral contraceptive. There were also no interactions with concomitantly administered antacids.

Although no interaction during concomitant administration of phenprocoumon or warfarin has been observed in clinical pharmacokinetic studies, a few isolated cases of changes in INR have been reported during concomitant treatment in the post-marketing period. Therefore, in patients treated with coumarin anticoagulants, monitoring of prothrombin time/INR is recommended after initiation, termination or during irregular use of pantoprazole.

4.6 Pregnancy and lactation
Use during pregnancy:

There is no information about the safety of pantoprazole during pregnancy in humans. Animal experiments have revealed no signs of foetal damage, but reproduction studies have revealed reduced litter weight and delayed development of the skeleton at doses above 15 mg/kg.

During pregnancy, Protium® i.v. should not be used unless the benefit exceeds the potential risk.

Use during lactation:

There is no information about the safety of pantoprazole during breast-feeding in humans. In the rat, not more than 0.02% of the administered dose is excreted via the breast milk.

During breast-feeding, Protium® i.v. should not be used unless the benefit exceeds the potential risk.

4.7 Effects on ability to drive and use machines
Pantoprazole does not affect the ability to drive and use machines.

4.8 Undesirable effects
(see Table 1 below)

4.9 Overdose
There are no known symptoms of overdosage in man. However, pantoprazole is very specific in action and no

Table 1 Undesirable effects

Frequency Organ System	Common (>1/100, <1/10)	Uncommon (>1/1000, <1/100)	Rare (<1/1000, >1/10,000)	Very rare (<1/10,000, incl. Isolated reports)
Blood and lymphatic system				Leukopenia; Thrombocytopenia
Gastrointestinal disorders	Upper abdominal pain; Diarrhoea; Constipation; Flatulence	Nausea/Vomiting	Dry mouth	
General disorders and administration site conditions				Injection site thrombophlebitis; Peripheral edema
Hepatobiliary disorders				Severe hepatocellular damage leading to jaundice with or without hepatic failure
Immune system disorders				Anaphylactic reactions including anaphylactic shock
Investigations				Increased liver enzymes (transaminases, γ-GT); Elevated triglycerides; Increased body temperature
Musculoskeletal, connective tissue disorders			Athralgia	Myalgia
Nervous system disorders	Headache	Dizziness; Disturbances in vision (blurred vision)		
Psychiatric disorders			Depression, Hallucination, Disorientation and confusion, especially in predisposed patients, as well as the aggravation of these symptoms in case of pre-existence	
Renal and urinary disorders				Interstitial nephritis
Skin and sub-cutaneous tissue disorders		Allergic reactions such as pruritus and skin rash		Urticaria; Angioedema; Severe skin reactions such as Stevens Johnson Syndrome; Erythema Multi-forme; Lyell-Syndrome; Photosensitivity

particular problems are anticipated. Doses up to 240 mg i.v. were administered without obvious adverse effects.

As pantoprazole is extensively protein bound, it is not readily dialysable. Apart from symptomatic and supportive treatment, no specific therapeutic recommendations can be made.

5. PHARMACOLOGICAL PROPERTIES

5.1 Pharmacodynamic properties

Proton pump inhibitors

ATC code: A02BC02

Pantoprazole is a proton pump inhibitor, i.e. it inhibits specifically and dose-proportionally the gastric H^+/K^+-ATPase enzyme which is responsible for acid secretion in the parietal cells of the stomach.

The substance is a substituted benzimidazole which accumulates in the acidic environment of the parietal cells after absorption. There it is converted into the active form, a cyclic sulphenamide, which binds to the H^+/K^+-ATPase, thus inhibiting the proton pump and causing potent and long-lasting suppression of basal and stimulated gastric acid secretion. As pantoprazole acts distally to the receptor level, it can inhibit gastric acid secretion irrespective of the nature of the stimulus (acetylcholine, histamine, gastrin).

Pantoprazole's selectivity is due to the fact that it can only exert its full effect in a strongly acidic environment (pH$<$3), remaining mostly inactive at higher pH values. As a result, its complete pharmacological and thus therapeutic effect can only be achieved in the acid-secretory parietal cells. By means of a feedback mechanism, this effect is diminished at the same rate as acid secretion is inhibited.

Pantoprazole has the same effect whether administered orally or intravenously.

Following intravenous or oral administration, pantoprazole inhibits the pentagastrin-stimulated gastric acid secretion. In volunteers, acid secretion was inhibited by 56% following the first i.v. administration of 30 mg and by 99% after 5 days. With an oral dose of 40 mg, inhibition was 51% on day 1 and 85% on day 7. Basal 24 hour acidity was reduced by 37% and 98%, respectively.

The fasting gastrin values increased under pantoprazole but in most cases they did not exceed the normal upper limit. Following completion of a course of oral treatment, the median gastrin levels clearly declined again.

5.2 Pharmacokinetic properties

General Pharmacokinetics

Terminal half-life is about 1 hour. Volume of distribution is about 0.15 L/kg, clearance is about 0.1 L/h/kg and Cmax is approximately 5.53 mg/l.

Pharmacokinetics do not vary after single or repeated administration. The plasma kinetics of pantoprazole are linear after both oral and intravenous administration.

Studies with pantoprazole in humans reveal no interaction with the cytochrome P450-system of the liver. There was no induction of the P450-system seen as tested after chronic administration with antipyrine as a marker. Also, no inhibition of metabolism was observed after concomitant administration of pantoprazole with either antipyrine, caffeine, carbamazepine, diazepam, diclofenac, digoxin, ethanol, glibenclamide, metropolol, naproxen, nifedipine, phenprocoumon, phenytoin, piroxicam, theophylline, or oral contraceptives. Concomitant administration of pantoprazole with warfarin has no influence on warfarin's effect on the coagulation factors.

Pantoprazole's plasma protein binding is about 98%. The substance is almost exclusively metabolised in the liver. Renal elimination represents the major route of excretion (about 80%) for the metabolites of pantoprazole; the rest are excreted in the faeces. The main metabolite in both the plasma and urine is desmethylpantoprazole which is conjugated with sulphate. The half-life of the main metabolites (about 1.5 hours) is not much longer than that of pantoprazole.

Characteristics in patients/special groups of subjects:

Although for patients with hepatic cirrhosis (classes A and B according to Child) the half-time values increased to between 7 and 9 hours and the AUC values increased by a factor of 5 to 7, the maximum plasma concentration only increased slightly by a factor of 1.5 compared with healthy subjects. As pantoprazole has a good safety profile and is well tolerated it can be given to patients with mild to moderate liver impairment.

No dose reduction is required when pantoprazole is administered to patients with impaired kidney function (including dialysis patients). As with healthy subjects, pantoprazole's half-life is short. Only very small amounts of pantoprazole are dialysed. Although the main metabolite has a moderately delayed half-life (2-3 hours), excretion is still rapid and thus accumulation does not occur.

A slight increase in AUC and Cmax in elderly volunteers compared with younger counterparts is also not clinically relevant.

Children

Following administration of single i.v. doses of 0.8 or 1.6 mg/kg pantoprazole to children aged 2 – 16 years there was no significant association between pantoprazole clearance and age and weight. AUC and volume of distribution were in accordance with data from adults.

5.3 Preclinical safety data

Acute toxicity

In acute toxicity studies in mice, the LD_{50} values were found to be 370 mg/kg bodyweight for i.v. administration and around 700 mg/kg bodyweight for oral administration.

In the rat, the corresponding values were around 240 mg/kg for i.v. administration and 900 mg/kg for oral administration.

Chronic toxicity

Hypergastrinaemia and morphologic changes of the mucosa were observed in studies investigating repeated administration for up to 12 months in the rat and dog. Most of the effects were reversible and attributable solely to the drug action, i.e. suppression of acid secretion.

In long-term studies in the rat and dog, there was an increase in stomach and liver weights, the increase being reversible after the substance was discontinued. The increase in liver weight following highly toxic doses was seen as a result of the induction of drug-metabolising enzymes.

Thyroid activation in two rat experiments is due to the rapid metabolism of thyroid hormones in the liver and has also been described in a similar form for other drugs. Changes in the thyroid and associated reduced degradation of cholesterol have been observed in one-year studies in the rat and dog. Hypertrophy of the thyroid and increases in cholesterol levels are reversible.

In studies in the dog, a species-species specific pulmonary oedema was observed. The animal-specific metabolite which was responsible for the oedema could not be identified in man.

Carcinogenicity

In a 2-year carcinogenicity study in rats - which corresponds to lifetime treatment for rats - ECL cell carcinoids were found. The mechanism leading to the formation of gastric carcinoids by substituted benzimidazoles has been carefully investigated and allows the conclusion that it is a secondary reaction to the massively elevated serum gastrin levels occurring in the rat during treatment. In addition, rats have more ECL cells in the mucosa of the glandular stomach than man, so that a larger number of responder cells for the increased gastrin values can become active.

ECL cell neoplasms were not observed in either the study in mice (24 months) or in long-term studies in the dog. In clinical studies (40 - 80 mg for 1 year), ECL cell density slightly increased.

In the two-year studies, an increased number of neoplastic changes of the liver was observed in rats and female mice and was interpreted as being due to pantoprazole's high rate of metabolism in the liver.

A slight increase of neoplastic changes of the thyroid was observed in the group of rats receiving the highest dose. The occurrence of these neoplasms is associated with the pantoprazole-induced changes in the breakdown of thyroxine in the rat liver. In man, no changes in the thyroid hormones T3, T4 and TSH were observed. This high dose phenomenon in the rat is therefore not relevant for man.

Mutagenicity

In mutagenicity studies, there were no indications of a mutagenic action in vivo or in vitro.

Reproduction toxicology

Investigations revealed no evidence of impaired fertility or teratogenic effects. Penetration of the placenta was investigated in the rat and was found to increase with advanced gestation. As a result, the concentration of pantoprazole in the foetus is increased shortly before birth, regardless of the route of administration.

In humans, there is no experience of the use of the drug during pregnancy.

6. PHARMACEUTICAL PARTICULARS

6.1 List of excipients

Edetate disodium dihydrate, sodium hydroxide.

6.2 Incompatibilities

Protium® i.v. is not compatible with acidic solutions.

6.3 Shelf life

2 years.

The reconstituted solution must be used within 12 hours after preparation.

Any unused portion should be discarded.

6.4 Special precautions for storage

Do not store above 25°C. Keep container in outer carton.

6.5 Nature and contents of container

10 ml glass vial (type 1 acc. to Ph.Eur.), with an aluminium cap and rubber stopper.

Dose units: 1, 5 and 20 vials.

6.6 Special precautions for disposal and other handling

A ready-to-use intravenous solution is prepared by injecting 10 ml of physiological sodium chloride solution into the vial containing the lyophilised powder. The reconstituted solution has a pH of 9 - 10.

This freshly prepared solution should be administered intravenously over 2 to 15 minutes, either as a slow injection or it may be further diluted with 100 ml of 0.9% sodium chloride injection, or 5% glucose injection, and administered as a short-term infusion.

Protium® i.v. should not be reconstituted with diluents other than those stated.

Once reconstituted, from a microbiological point of view, the product should be used immediately. If not used immediately, in-use storage times and conditions prior to use are the responsibility of the user and would normally not be longer than 12 hours at not more than 25°C.

Any product that has remained in the container or the visual appearance of which has changed (e.g. if cloudiness or precipitation is observed) has to be discarded. The content of the vial is for single use only.

7. MARKETING AUTHORISATION HOLDER

Nycomed GmbH

Byk-Gulden Straβe 2

D-78467 Konstanz, Germany

8. MARKETING AUTHORISATION NUMBER(S)

PL 31752/0003

9. DATE OF FIRST AUTHORISATION/RENEWAL OF THE AUTHORISATION

1 April 2003.

10. DATE OF REVISION OF THE TEXT

January 2008

Protium 40 mg tablet

(Nycomed UK Ltd)

1. NAME OF THE MEDICINAL PRODUCT

Protium® (or Panselect) 40 mg gastroresistant tablets.

2. QUALITATIVE AND QUANTITATIVE COMPOSITION

One gastro-resistant tablet contains:

40mg Pantoprazole (as pantoprazole sodium sesquihydrate).

For excipients see 6.1.

3. PHARMACEUTICAL FORM

Gastro-resistant coated tablet for oral use.

A yellow, oval, biconvex, film-coated tablet imprinted with "P 40" in brown ink on one side.

4. CLINICAL PARTICULARS

4.1 Therapeutic indications

For symptomatic improvement and healing of gastrointestinal diseases which require a reduction in acid secretion:

Moderate and severe reflux oesophagitis

Duodenal ulcer

Gastric ulcer

Zollinger-Ellison-Syndrome and other pathological hypersecretory conditions

Eradication of *Helicobacter pylori*, in combination with two antibiotics in patients with duodenal ulcer or gastritis.

In the case of combination therapy for the eradication of *Helicobacter pylori*, the Summaries of Product Characteristics of the respective drugs should be observed.

4.2 Posology and method of administration

Recommended dosage:

Adults and adolescents 12 years of age and above:

Treatment of moderate and severe reflux oesophagitis

One tablet of Protium 40 mg per day. Protium® should not be chewed or crushed, and should be swallowed whole with water either before or during breakfast.

Adults:

Treatment of duodenal ulcer and gastric ulcer

One tablet of Protium 40 mg per day. Protium® should not be chewed or crushed, and should be swallowed whole with water either before or during breakfast.

In combination therapy for the eradication of *Helicobacter pylori*, the recommended dose is one tablet taken twice daily. The second Protium® tablet should be taken before the evening meal. Combination therapy should be implemented for 7 days. At the end of the 7 days' combination period, pantoprazole may be continued to ensure the healing of the ulcer. For duodenal ulcers, this may require an additional 1 to 3 weeks.

The safety of longer-term use is generally well established. Long-term administration of pantoprazole has a safety profile similar to that observed with short-term treatment, and is well tolerated.

In most patients, freedom from symptoms is achieved rapidly. In a few instances, there may be benefit in extending treatment beyond 8 weeks to ensure healing.

Duodenal ulcer:

Duodenal ulcers generally heal within 2 weeks. If a 2-week period of treatment is not sufficient, healing will be achieved in almost all cases within a further 2 weeks.

Gastric ulcer:

A 4-week period is usually required for the treatment of gastric ulcers. If this is not sufficient, healing will usually be achieved within a further 4 weeks.

Gastro-Oesophageal Reflux:

A 4-week period is usually required for the treatment of gastro-oesophageal reflux. If this is not sufficient, healing will usually be achieved within a further 4 weeks.

Long-term management of Zollinger-Ellison-Syndrome and other pathological hypersecretory conditions:

For the long-term management of Zollinger-Ellison-Syndrome and other pathological hypersecretory conditions patients should start their treatment with a daily dose of 80 mg (2 tablets of Protium® 40 mg). Thereafter, the dosage can be titrated up or down as needed using measurements of gastric acid secretion to guide. With doses above 80 mg daily, the dose should be divided and given twice daily. A temporary increase of the dosage above 160 mg pantoprazole is possible but should not be applied longer than required for adequate acid control.

Treatment duration in Zollinger-Ellison-Syndrome and other pathological hypersecretory conditions is not limited and should be adapted according to clinical needs.

Eradication of *Helicobacter pylori* (*H. pylori*):

The use of Protium® in combination with two antibiotics (triple therapy) is recommended. The following combinations have been shown to be effective:

(a) Protium® 40 mg twice daily,
plus 1000 mg amoxycillin twice daily
and 500 mg clarithromycin twice daily

(b) Protium® 40 mg twice daily,
plus 400 mg metronidazole twice daily
and 250 mg clarithromycin twice daily

The second Protium® tablet should be taken before the evening meal. Combination therapy should be implemented for 7 days.

Elderly:

No dose adjustment is necessary in the elderly. However, the daily dose of 40 mg pantoprazole should not be exceeded. An exception is combination therapy for eradication of *H. pylori*, where elderly patients should receive the usual pantoprazole dose (2 × 40 mg/day) during 1 week treatment.

Children below 12 years of age:

Protium® 40 mg is not recommended for use in children below 12 years of age due to limited data in this age group.

Patients with impaired renal function:

No dose adjustment is necessary in patients with impaired renal function. However, the daily dose of 40mg pantoprazole should not be exceeded. For this reason, H. pylori triple therapy is not appropriate in these patients.

Patients with hepatic cirrhosis:

Due to an increased AUC and a modified metabolism of pantoprazole in patients with hepatic cirrhosis, the dose regimen should be reduced to one tablet every other day. For this reason, H. pylori triple therapy is not appropriate in these patients.

4.3 Contraindications

Protium® may not be used in cases of known hypersensitivity to any of its constituents.

Pantoprazole like other PPIs, should not be co-administered with atazanavir (see Section 4.5).

4.4 Special warnings and precautions for use

In patients with severe liver impairment, particularly those on long-term use, liver enzymes should be monitored regularly during treatment with pantoprazole. In the case of a rise in liver enzymes, Protium® should be discontinued.

Note:

Prior to treatment of gastric ulcer, the possibility of malignancy should be excluded as treatment with Protium® may alleviate the symptoms of malignant ulcers and can thus delay diagnosis.

Decreased gastric acidity due to any means – including proton pump inhibitors – increases gastric counts of bacteria normally present in the gastrointestinal tract. Treatment with acid-reducing drugs may lead to a slightly increased risk of gastrointestinal infections, such as *Salmonella* and *Campylobacter*.

In patients with Zollinger-Ellison-Syndrome and other pathological hypersecretory conditions requiring long-term treatment, pantoprazole, as all acid-blocking medicines, may reduce the absorption of vitamin B12 (cyanocobalamin) due to hypo- or achlorhydria. This should be considered if respective clinical symptoms are observed.

4.5 Interaction with other medicinal products and other forms of interaction

As with other acid secretion inhibitors, changes in absorption may be observed when drugs whose absorption is pH-dependent, e.g. ketoconazole, are taken concomitantly.

It has been shown that co-administration of atazanavir 300 mg/ritonavir 100 mg with omeprazole (40 mg once daily) or atazanavir 400 mg with lansoprazole (60 mg single dose) to healthy volunteers resulted in a substantial reduction in the bioavailability of atazanavir. The absorption of atazanavir is pH dependent. Therefore, PPIs, including pantoprazole, should not be co-administered with atazanavir (see Section 4.3).

Pantoprazole is metabolised in the liver via the cytochrome P450 enzyme system. Although studies have shown that pantoprazole has no significant effect on cytochrome P450, an interaction of pantoprazole with other drugs or compounds, which are metabolised using the same enzyme system, cannot be excluded.

However, no clinically significant interactions were observed in specific tests with a number of such drugs/compounds, namely antipyrine, carbamazepine, caffeine, diazepam, diclofenac, digoxin, ethanol, glibenclamide, metoprolol, naproxen, nifedipine, phenytoin, piroxicam, theophyllineand an oral contraceptive. There were also no interactions with concomitantly administered antacids.

Although no interaction during concomitant administration of phenprocoumon or warfarin has been observed in clinical pharmacokinetic studies, a few isolated cases of changes in INR have been reported during concomitant treatment in the post-marketing period. Therefore, in patients treated with coumarin anticoagulants, monitoring of prothrombin time/INR is recommended after initiation, termination or during irregular use of pantoprazole.

4.6 Pregnancy and lactation

Clinical experience in pregnant women is limited. In animal reproduction studies, signs of slight foetotoxicity were observed at doses above 5 mg/kg. There is no information on the excretion of pantoprazole into human breast milk.

During pregnancy and breast feeding, Protium® should only be used when the benefit exceeds the potential risk.

4.7 Effects on ability to drive and use machines

Pantoprazole does not affect the ability to drive and use machines.

4.8 Undesirable effects

(see Table 1 below)

4.9 Overdose

There are no known symptoms of over dosage in man. However, pantoprazole is very specific in action and no particular problems are anticipated. Doses up to 240 mg i.v. were administered without obvious adverse effects. As pantoprazole is extensively protein bound, it is not readily dialysable.

Apart from symptomatic and supportive treatment, no specific therapeutic recommendations can be made.

5. PHARMACOLOGICAL PROPERTIES

5.1 Pharmacodynamic properties

Proton Pump Inhibitors.

ATC code: A02BC02.

Pantoprazole is a proton pump inhibitor, i.e. it inhibits specifically and dose-proportionally the gastric H^+/K^+-ATPase enzyme, which is responsible for acid secretion in the parietal cells of the stomach.

The substance is a substituted benzimidazole, which accumulates, in the acidic environment of the parietal cells after absorption. There it is converted into the active form, a cyclic sulphenamide, which binds to the H^+/K^+-ATPase, thus inhibiting the proton pump and causing potent and long-lasting suppression of basal and stimulated gastric acid secretion. As pantoprazole acts distally to the receptor level, it can inhibit gastric acid secretion irrespective of the nature of the stimulus (acetylcholine, histamine, gastrin).

Pantoprazole's selectivity is due to the fact that it can only exert its full effect in a strongly acidic environment (pH < 3), remaining mostly inactive at higher pH values. As a result, its complete pharmacological and thus therapeutic effect can only be achieved in the acid-secretory parietal cells. By means of a feedback mechanism, this effect is diminished at the same rate as acid secretion is inhibited.

Pantoprazole has the same effect whether administered orally or intravenously.

Following intravenous or oral administration, pantoprazole inhibits the pentagastrin-stimulated gastric acid secretion. In volunteers, acid secretion was inhibited by 56% following the first i.v. administration of 30 mg and by 99% after 5 days. With an oral dose of 40 mg, inhibition was 51% on day 1 and 85% on day 7. Basal 24-hour acidity was reduced by 37% and 98%, respectively.

Table 1 Undesirable effects

Frequency Organ system	Common (>1/100, <1/10)	Uncommon (>1/1000, <1/100)	Rare (<1/1000 >1/10,000)	Very rare (<1/10,000, incl. isolated reports)
Blood and lymphatic system				Leukopenia; Thrombocytopenia
Gastrointestinal Disorders	Upper abdominal pain; Diarrhoea; Constipation; Flatulence	Nausea/Vomiting	Dry mouth	
General disorders and administration site conditions				Peripheral oedema
Hepatobiliary disorders				Severe hepatocellular damage leading to jaundice with or without hepatic failure
Immune system disorders				Anaphylactic reactions including anaphylactic shock
Investigations				Increased liver enzymes (transaminases, γ-GT); Elevated triglycerides; Increased body temperature
Musculoskeletal, connective tissue disorders			Arthralgia	Myalgia
Nervous system disorders	Headache	Dizziness; Disturbances in vision (blurred vision)		
Psychiatric disorders			Depression. Hallucination, Disorientation and Confusion, especially in pre-disposed patients, as well as the aggravation of these symptoms in case of pre-existence	
Renal and urinary disorders				Interstitial nephritis
Skin and sub-cutaneous tissue disorders		Allergic reactions such as pruritus and skin rash		Urticaria; Angioedema; Severe skin reactions such as Stevens Johnson Syndrome, Erythema Multi-forme, Lyell-Syndrome; Photosensitivity

The fasting gastrin values increased under pantoprazole but in most cases they did not exceed the normal upper limit. Following completion of a course of oral treatment, the median gastrin levels clearly declined again.

5.2 Pharmacokinetic properties

General Pharmacokinetics

Pantoprazole is rapidly absorbed and the maximal plasma concentration is achieved even after one single 40 mg oral dose. On average, the maximum serum concentrations are approximately 2-3 μg/ml about 2.5 hours post-administration and these values remain constant after multiple administration. Terminal half-life is about 1 hour. Volume of distribution is about 0.15 l/kg and clearance is about 0.1 l/h/kg. There were a few cases of subjects with delayed elimination. Because of the specific activation within the parietal cell, the elimination half-life does not correlate with the much longer duration of action (inhibition of acid secretion).

Pharmacokinetics does not vary after single or repeated administration. The plasma kinetics of pantoprazole are linear after both oral and intravenous administration.

Studies with pantoprazole in humans reveal no interaction with the cytochrome P450-system of the liver. There was no induction of the P450-system seen as tested after chronic administration with antipyrine as a marker. Also, no inhibition of metabolism was observed after concomitant administration of pantoprazole with either antipyrine, caffeine, carbamazepine, diazepam, diclofenac, digoxin, ethanol, glibenclamide, metoprolol, naproxen, nifedipine, phenprocoumon, phenytoin, piroxicam, theophylline and oral contraceptives. Concomitant administration of pantoprazole with warfarin has no influence on warfarin's effect on the coagulation factors.

The absolute bioavailability of the tablet is about 77%. Concomitant intake of food or antacids had no influence on AUC, maximum serum concentrations and thus bioavailability.

Pantoprazole's plasma protein binding is about 98%. The substance is almost exclusively metabolised in the liver. Renal elimination represents the major route of excretion (about 80%) for the metabolites of pantoprazole; the rest are excreted in the faeces. The main metabolite in both the plasma and urine is desmethylpantoprazole, which is conjugated with sulphate. The half-life of the main metabolites (about 1.5 hours) is not much longer than that of pantoprazole.

Characteristics in patients/special groups of subjects

Although for patients with hepatic cirrhosis (classes A and B according to *Child*) the half-time values increased to between 7 and 9 hours and the AUC values increased by a factor of 5 to 7, the maximum plasma concentration only increased slightly by a factor of 1.5 compared with healthy subjects. Therefore the dose regimen in patients with hepatic cirrhosis should be reduced to one tablet every other day.

No dose reduction is required when pantoprazole is administered to patients with impaired kidney function (including dialysis patients). As with healthy subjects, pantoprazole's half-life is short. Only very small amounts of pantoprazole are dialysed. Although the main metabolite has a moderately delayed half-life (2-3 hours), excretion is still rapid and thus accumulation does not occur.

A slight increase in AUC and Cmax in elderly volunteers compared with younger counterparts is also not clinically relevant.

Children

Following administration of single oral doses of 20 or 40 mg pantoprazole to children aged 5-16 years AUC and Cmax were in the range of corresponding values in adults. Following administration of single i.v. doses of 0.8 or 1.6 mg/kg pantoprazole to children aged 2 - 16 years there was no significant association between pantoprazole clearance and age or weight. AUC and volume of distribution were in accordance with data from adults.

5.3 Preclinical safety data

Acute toxicity

In acute toxicity studies in mice, the LD_{50} values were found to be 370 mg/kg bodyweight for i.v. administration and around 700 mg/kg bodyweight for oral administration.

In the rat, the corresponding values were around 240 mg/kg for i.v. administration and 900 mg/kg for oral administration.

Chronic toxicity

Hypergastrinaemia and morphologic changes of the mucosa were observed in studies investigating repeated administration for up to 12 months in the rat and dog. Most of the effects were reversible and attributable solely to the drug action, i.e. suppression of acid secretion.

In long-term studies in the rat and dog, there was an increase in stomach and liver weights; the increase being reversible after the substance was discontinued. The increase in liver weight following highly toxic doses was seen as a result of the induction of drug-metabolising enzymes.

Thyroid activation in two rat experiments is due to the rapid metabolism of thyroid hormones in the liver and has also been described in a similar form for other drugs. Changes in the thyroid and associated reduced degradation of cholesterol have been observed in one-year studies in the rat and dog. Hypertrophy of the thyroid and increases in cholesterol levels are reversible.

In studies in the dog, a species-species specific pulmonary oedema was observed. The animal-specific metabolite, which was responsible for the oedema, could not be identified in man.

Carcinogenicity

In a 2-year carcinogenicity study in rats - which corresponds to lifetime treatment for rats - ECL cell carcinoids were found. The mechanism leading to the formation of gastric carcinoids by substituted benzimidazoles has been carefully investigated and allows the conclusion that it is a secondary reaction to the massively elevated serum gastrin levels occurring in the rat during treatment. In addition, rats have more ECL cells in the mucosa of the glandular stomach than man, so that a larger number of responder cells for the increased gastrin values can become active.

ECL cell neoplasms were not observed in either the study in mice (24 months) or in long-term studies in the dog. In clinical studies (40 - 80 mg for 1 year), ECL cell density slightly increased.

In the two-year studies, an increased number of neoplastic changes of the liver was observed in rats and female mice and was interpreted as being due to pantoprazole's high rate of metabolism in the liver.

A slight increase of neoplastic changes of the thyroid was observed in the group of rats receiving the highest dose. The occurrence of these neoplasms is associated with the pantoprazole-induced changes in the breakdown of thyroxine in the rat liver. In man, no changes in the thyroid hormones T3, T4 and TSH were observed. This high dose phenomenon in the rat is therefore not relevant for man.

Mutagenicity

In mutagenicity studies, there were no indications of a mutagenic action *in vivo* or *in vitro*.

Reproduction toxicology

Investigations revealed no evidence of impaired fertility or teratogenic effects. Penetration of the placenta was investigated in the rat and was found to increase with advanced gestation. As a result, the concentration of pantoprazole in the foetus is increased shortly before birth, regardless of the route of administration.

In humans, there is no experience of the use of the drug during pregnancy.

6. PHARMACEUTICAL PARTICULARS

6.1 List of excipients

Crospovidone

Mannitol (=0.0036 BU)

Hypromellose

Methylacrylic acid-ethyl acrylate copolymer (1:1)

Sodium carbonate

Propylene glycol

Povidone K90

Calcium stearate

Triethyl citrate

Povidone K25

Titanium dioxide (E 171)

Polysorbate 80

Sodium lauril sulfate

Yellow iron oxide (E 172)

Printing ink

6.2 Incompatibilities

Not applicable.

6.3 Shelf life

Pantoprazole tablets are stable over a period of 3 years.

6.4 Special precautions for storage

Blister packaging: Do not store above 25°C

PE-bottle: Do not store above 30°C

6.5 Nature and contents of container

Protium® is distributed in PE-bottles or ALU/ALU blisters without cardboard reinforcement or ALU/ALU blisters with cardboard reinforcement (blister wallet), packed in carton boxes.

Dose units: 7, 14, 28 gastro-resistant coated tablets

2 tablet starter pack

6.6 Special precautions for disposal and other handling

No special requirements.

7. MARKETING AUTHORISATION HOLDER

Nycomed GmbH

Byk Gulden Straβe 2

D-78467 Konstanz

Germany

8. MARKETING AUTHORISATION NUMBER(S)

PL 31752/0002

9. DATE OF FIRST AUTHORISATION/RENEWAL OF THE AUTHORISATION

13 August 2003

10. DATE OF REVISION OF THE TEXT

January 2008

Protopic 0.03% ointment

(Astellas Pharma Ltd)

1. NAME OF THE MEDICINAL PRODUCT

Protopic 0.03% ointment

2. QUALITATIVE AND QUANTITATIVE COMPOSITION

1 g of Protopic 0.03% ointment contains 0.3 mg of tacrolimus as tacrolimus monohydrate (0.03%).

For a full list of excipients, see section 6.1.

3. PHARMACEUTICAL FORM

Ointment

A white to slightly yellowish ointment.

4. CLINICAL PARTICULARS

4.1 Therapeutic indications

Treatment of moderate to severe atopic dermatitis in adults who are not adequately responsive to or are intolerant of conventional therapies such as topical corticosteroids. Treatment of moderate to severe atopic dermatitis in children (2 years of age and above) who failed to respond adequately to conventional therapies such as topical corticosteroids.

Maintenance treatment of moderate to severe atopic dermatitis for the prevention of flares and the prolongation of flare-free intervals in patients experiencing a high frequency of disease exacerbations (i.e. occurring 4 or more times per year) who have had an initial response to a maximum of 6 weeks treatment of twice daily tacrolimus ointment (lesions cleared, almost cleared or mildly affected).

4.2 Posology and method of administration

Protopic should be initiated by physicians with experience in the diagnosis and treatment of atopic dermatitis.

Protopic can be used for short-term and intermittent long-term treatment. Treatment should not be continuous.

Protopic ointment should be applied as a thin layer to affected or commonly affected areas of the skin. Protopic ointment may be used on any part of the body, including face, neck and flexure areas, except on mucous membranes. Protopic ointment should not be applied under occlusion (see section 4.4).

Protopic is not recommended for use in children below the age of 2 years until further data are available.

Specific studies have not been conducted in elderly patients. However, the clinical experience available in this patient population has not shown the necessity for any dosage adjustment.

Treatment

Protopic treatment should begin at the first appearance of signs and symptoms. Each affected region of the skin should be treated with Protopic until lesions are cleared, almost cleared or mildly affected. Thereafter, patients are considered suitable for maintenance treatment (see below). At the first signs of recurrence (flares) of the disease symptoms, treatment should be re-initiated.

Use in children (2 years of age and above)

Treatment should be started twice a day for up to three weeks. Afterwards the frequency of application should be reduced to once a day until clearance of the lesion (see section 4.4).

Use in adults (16 years of age and above)

Protopic is available in two strengths, Protopic 0.03% and Protopic 0.1% ointment. Treatment should be started with Protopic 0.1% twice a day and treatment should be continued until clearance of the lesion. If symptoms recur, twice daily treatment with Protopic 0.1% should be restarted. An attempt should be made to reduce the frequency of application or to use the lower strength Protopic 0.03% ointment if the clinical condition allows.

Generally, improvement is seen within one week of starting treatment. If no signs of improvement are seen after two weeks of treatment, further treatment options should be considered.

Maintenance

Patients who are responding to up to 6 weeks treatment using tacrolimus ointment twice daily (lesions cleared, almost cleared or mildly affected) are suitable for maintenance treatment.

Protopic ointment should be applied once a day twice weekly (e.g. Monday and Thursday) to areas commonly affected by atopic dermatitis to prevent progression to flares. Between applications there should be 2–3 days without Protopic treatment.

Adult patients (16 years of age and above) should use Protopic 0.1% ointment, children (2 years of age and above) should use the lower strength Protopic 0.03% ointment.

If signs of a flare reoccur, twice daily treatment should be re-initiated (see treatment section above).

After 12 months, a review of the patient's condition should be conducted by the physician and a decision taken whether to continue maintenance treatment in the absence of safety data for maintenance treatment beyond 12 months. In children, this review should include suspension of treatment to assess the need to continue this regimen and to evaluate the course of the disease.

4.3 Contraindications
Hypersensitivity to macrolides in general, to tacrolimus or to any of the excipients.

4.4 Special warnings and precautions for use
Protopic should not be used in patients with congenital or acquired immunodeficiencies or in patients on therapy that cause immunosuppression.

The effect of treatment with Protopic ointment on the developing immune system of children, especially the young, has not yet been established and this should be taken into account when prescribing to this age group (see section 4.1).

Exposure of the skin to sunlight should be minimised and the use of ultraviolet (UV) light from a solarium, therapy with UVB or UVA in combination with psoralens (PUVA) should be avoided during use of Protopic ointment (see section 5.3). Physicians should advise patients on appropriate sun protection methods, such as minimisation of the time in the sun, use of a sunscreen product and covering of the skin with appropriate clothing. Protopic ointment should not be applied to lesions that are considered to be potentially malignant or pre-malignant.

Emollients should not be applied to the same area within 2 hours of applying Protopic ointment. Concomitant use of other topical preparations has not been assessed. There is no experience with concomitant use of systemic steroids or immunosuppressive agents.

Protopic ointment has not been evaluated for its efficacy and safety in the treatment of clinically infected atopic dermatitis. Before commencing treatment with Protopic ointment, clinical infections at treatment sites should be cleared. Patients with atopic dermatitis are predisposed to superficial skin infections. Treatment with Protopic may be associated with an increased risk of herpes viral infections (herpes simplex dermatitis [eczema herpeticum], herpes simplex [cold sores], Kaposi's varicelliform eruption). In the presence of these infections, the balance of risks and benefits associated with Protopic use should be evaluated.

The potential for local immunosuppression (possibly resulting in infections or cutaneous malignancies) in the long term (i.e. over a period of years) is unknown (see section 5.1).

Protopic contains the active substance tacrolimus, a calcineurin inhibitor. In transplant patients, prolonged systemic exposure to intense immunosuppression following systemic administration of calcineurin inhibitors has been associated with an increased risk of developing lymphomas and skin malignancies. In patients using tacrolimus ointment, cases of malignancies, including cutaneous and other types of lymphoma, and skin cancers have been reported (see section 4.8). Patients with atopic dermatitis treated with Protopic have not been found to have significant systemic tacrolimus levels.

Lymphadenopathy was uncommonly (0.8%) reported in clinical trials. The majority of these cases related to infections (skin, respiratory tract, tooth) and resolved with appropriate antibiotic therapy. Transplant patients receiving immunosuppressive regimens (e.g. systemic tacrolimus) are at increased risk for developing lymphoma; therefore patients who receive Protopic and who develop lymphadenopathy should be monitored to ensure that the lymphadenopathy resolves. Lymphadenopathy present at initiation of therapy should be investigated and kept under review. In case of persistent lymphadenopathy, the aetiology of the lymphadenopathy should be investigated. In the absence of a clear aetiology for the lymphadenopathy or in the presence of acute infectious mononucleosis, discontinuation of Protopic should be considered.

Care should be taken to avoid contact with eyes and mucous membranes. If accidentally applied to these areas, the ointment should be thoroughly wiped off and/or rinsed off with water.

The use of Protopic ointment under occlusion has not been studied in patients. Occlusive dressings are not recommended.

As with any topical medicinal product, patients should wash their hands after application if the hands are not intended for treatment.

Tacrolimus is extensively metabolised in the liver and although blood concentrations are low following topical therapy, the ointment should be used with caution in patients with hepatic failure (see section 5.2).

The use of Protopic ointment in patients with genetic epidermal barrier defects such as Netherton's syndrome is not recommended due to the potential for permanently increased systemic absorption of tacrolimus. The safety of Protopic ointment has not been established in patients with generalised erythroderma.

Care should be exercised if applying Protopic to patients with extensive skin involvement over an extended period of time, especially in children (see section 4.2).

The development of any new change different from previous eczema within a treated area should be reviewed by the physician.

4.5 Interaction with other medicinal products and other forms of interaction
Formal topical drug interaction studies with tacrolimus ointment have not been conducted.

Tacrolimus is not metabolised in human skin, indicating that there is no potential for percutaneous interactions that could affect the metabolism of tacrolimus.

Systemically available tacrolimus is metabolised via the hepatic Cytochrome P450 3A4 (CYP3A4). Systemic exposure from topical application of tacrolimus ointment is low (< 1.0 ng/ml) and is unlikely to be affected by concomitant use of substances known to be inhibitors of CYP3A4. However, the possibility of interactions cannot be ruled out and the concomitant systemic administration of known CYP3A4 inhibitors (e.g. erythromycin, itraconazole, ketoconazole and diltiazem) in patients with widespread and/or erythrodermic disease should be done with caution.

A potential interaction between vaccination and application of Protopic ointment has not been investigated. Because of the potential risk of vaccination failure, vaccination should be administered prior to commencement of treatment, or during a treatment-free interval with a period of 14 days between the last application of Protopic and the vaccination. In case of live attenuated vaccination, this period should be extended to 28 days or the use of alternative vaccines should be considered.

4.6 Pregnancy and lactation
There are no adequate data from the use of tacrolimus ointment in pregnant women. Studies in animals have shown reproductive toxicity following systemic administration (see section 5.3). The potential risk for humans is unknown.

Protopic ointment should not be used during pregnancy unless clearly necessary.

Human data demonstrate that, after systemic administration, tacrolimus is excreted into breast milk. Although clinical data have shown that systemic exposure from application of tacrolimus ointment is low, breast-feeding during treatment with Protopic ointment is not recommended.

4.7 Effects on ability to drive and use machines
No studies on the effects on the ability to drive and use machines have been performed. Protopic ointment is administered topically and is unlikely to have an effect on the ability to drive or use machines.

4.8 Undesirable effects
In clinical studies approximately 50% of patients experienced some type of skin irritation adverse reaction at the site of application. Burning sensation and pruritus were very common, usually mild to moderate in severity and tended to resolve within one week of starting treatment. Erythema was a common skin irritation adverse reaction. Sensation of warmth, pain, paraesthesia and rash at the site of application were also commonly observed. Alcohol intolerance (facial flushing or skin irritation after consumption of an alcoholic beverage) was common.

Patients may be at an increased risk of folliculitis, acne and herpes viral infections.

Adverse reactions with suspected relationship to treatment are listed below by system organ class. Frequencies are defined as very common (⩾ 1/10), common (⩾ 1/100 to < 1/10) and uncommon (⩾ 1/1,000 to < 1/100). Within each frequency grouping, undesirable effects are presented in order of decreasing seriousness.

<u>General disorders and administration site conditions</u>

Very common: Application site burning, application site pruritus
Common: Application site warmth, application site erythema, application site pain, application site irritation, application site paraesthesia, application site rash

<u>Infections and infestations</u>

Common: Herpes viral infections (herpes simplex dermatitis [eczema herpeticum], herpes simplex [cold sores], Kaposi's varicelliform eruption)

<u>Skin and subcutaneous tissue disorders</u>

Common: Folliculitis, pruritus

Uncommon: Acne

<u>Nervous system disorders</u>

Common: Paraesthesias and dysaesthesias (hyperaesthesia, burning sensation)

<u>Metabolism and nutrition disorders</u>

Common: Alcohol intolerance (facial flushing or skin irritation after consumption of an alcoholic beverage)

The following adverse reactions have been reported during post-marketing experience:

Skin and subcutaneous tissue disorders: Rosacea

In a study of maintenance treatment (twice weekly treatment) in adults and children with moderate and severe atopic dermatitis the following adverse events were noted to occur more frequently than in the control group: application site impetigo (7.7% in children) and application site infections (6.4% in children and 6.3% in adults).

Post-marketing: cases of malignancies, including cutaneous and other types of lymphoma, and skin cancers, have been reported in patients using tacrolimus ointment (see section 4.4).

4.9 Overdose
Overdosage following topical administration is unlikely.

If ingested, general supportive measures may be appropriate. These may include monitoring of vital signs and observation of clinical status. Due to the nature of the ointment vehicle, induction of vomiting or gastric lavage is not recommended.

5. PHARMACOLOGICAL PROPERTIES

5.1 Pharmacodynamic properties
Pharmacotherapeutic group: Other dermatologicals, ATC code: D11AX14

<u>Mechanism of action and pharmacodynamic effects</u>

The mechanism of action of tacrolimus in atopic dermatitis is not fully understood. While the following have been observed, the clinical significance of these observations in atopic dermatitis is not known.

Via its binding to a specific cytoplasmic immunophilin (FKBP12), tacrolimus inhibits calcium-dependent signal transduction pathways in T cells, thereby preventing the transcription and synthesis of IL-2, IL-3, IL-4, IL-5 and other cytokines such as GM-CSF, TNF-α and IFN-γ.

In vitro, in Langerhans cells isolated from normal human skin, tacrolimus reduced the stimulatory activity towards T cells. Tacrolimus has also been shown to inhibit the release of inflammatory mediators from skin mast cells, basophils and eosinophils.

In animals, tacrolimus ointment suppressed inflammatory reactions in experimental and spontaneous dermatitis models that resemble human atopic dermatitis. Tacrolimus ointment did not reduce skin thickness and did not cause skin atrophy in animals.

In patients with atopic dermatitis, improvement of skin lesions during treatment with tacrolimus ointment was associated with reduced Fc receptor expression on Langerhans cells and a reduction of their hyperstimulatory activity towards T cells. Tacrolimus ointment does not affect collagen synthesis in humans.

<u>Results from clinical studies in patients</u>

The efficacy and safety of Protopic was assessed in more than 18,500 patients treated with tacrolimus ointment in Phase I to Phase III clinical trials. Data from six major trials are presented here.

In a six-month multicentre double-blind randomised trial, 0.1% tacrolimus ointment was administered twice-a-day to adults with moderate to severe atopic dermatitis and compared to a topical corticosteroid based regimen (0.1% hydrocortisone butyrate on trunk and extremities, 1% hydrocortisone acetate on face and neck). The primary endpoint was the response rate at month 3 defined as the proportion of patients with at least 60% improvement in the mEASI (modified Eczema Area and Severity Index) between baseline and month 3. The response rate in the 0.1% tacrolimus group (71.6%) was significantly higher than that in the topical corticosteroid based treatment group (50.8%; p < 0.001; Table 1). The response rates at month 6 were comparable to the 3-month results.

Table 1 Efficacy at month 3

	Topical corticosteroid regimen§ (N=485)	Tacrolimus 0.1% (N=487)
Response rate of ⩾ 60% improvement in mEASI (Primary Endpoint)§§	50.8%	71.6%
Improvement ⩾ 90% in Physician's Global Evaluation	28.5%	47.7%

§ Topical corticosteroid regimen = 0.1% hydrocortisone butyrate on trunk and extremities, 1% hydrocortisone acetate on face and neck

§§ higher values = greater improvement

The incidence and nature of most adverse events were similar in the two treatment groups. Skin burning, herpes simplex, alcohol intolerance (facial flushing or skin sensitivity after alcohol intake), skin tingling, hyperaesthesia, acne and fungal dermatitis occurred more often in the tacrolimus treatment group. There were no clinically relevant changes in the laboratory values or vital signs in either treatment group throughout the study.

In the second trial, children aged from 2 to 15 years with moderate to severe atopic dermatitis received twice daily treatment for three weeks of 0.03% tacrolimus ointment, 0.1% tacrolimus ointment or 1% hydrocortisone acetate ointment. The primary endpoint was the area-under-the-curve (AUC) of the mEASI as a percentage of baseline averaged over the treatment period. The results of this multicentre, double-blind, randomised trial showed that tacrolimus ointment, 0.03% and 0.1%, is significantly more effective (p < 0.001 for both) than 1% hydrocortisone acetate ointment (Table 2).

Table 2 Efficacy at week 3

(see Table 2 on next page)

The incidence of local skin burning was higher in the tacrolimus treatment groups than in the hydrocortisone group. Pruritus decreased over time in the tacrolimus groups but not in the hydrocortisone group. There were no clinically relevant changes in the laboratory values or vital signs in either treatment group throughout the clinical trial.

Table 2 Efficacy at week 3

	Hydrocortisone acetate 1% (N=185)	Tacrolimus 0.03% (N=189)	Tacrolimus 0.1% (N=186)
Median mEASI as Percentage of Baseline mean AUC (Primary Endpoint)§	64.0%	44.8%	39.8%
Improvement ⩾ 90% in Physician's Global Evaluation	15.7%	38.5%	48.4%

§ lower values = greater improvement

The purpose of the third multicentre, double-blind, randomised study was the assessment of efficacy and safety of 0.03% tacrolimus ointment applied once or twice a day relative to twice daily administration of 1% hydrocortisone acetate ointment in children with moderate to severe atopic dermatitis. Treatment duration was for up to three weeks.

Table 3 Efficacy at week 3

(see Table 3 below)

The primary endpoint was defined as the percentage decrease in mEASI from the baseline to end of treatment. A statistically significant better improvement was shown for once daily and twice daily 0.03% tacrolimus ointment compared to twice daily hydrocortisone acetate ointment ($p<0.001$ for both). Twice daily treatment with 0.03% tacrolimus ointment was more effective than once daily administration (Table 3). The incidence of local skin burning was higher in the tacrolimus treatment groups than in the hydrocortisone group. There were no clinically relevant changes in the laboratory values or vital signs in either treatment group throughout the study.

In the fourth trial, approximately 800 patients (aged ⩾ 2 years) received 0.1% tacrolimus ointment intermittently or continuously in an open-label, long-term safety study for up to four years, with 300 patients receiving treatment for at least three years and 79 patients receiving treatment for a minimum of 42 months. Based on changes from baseline in EASI score and body surface area affected, patients regardless of age had improvement in their atopic dermatitis at all subsequent time points. In addition, there was no evidence of loss of efficacy throughout the duration of the clinical trial. The overall incidence of adverse events tended to decrease as the study progressed for all patients independent of age. The three most common adverse events reported were flu-like symptoms (cold, common cold, influenza, upper respiratory infection, etc.), pruritus and skin burning. No adverse events previously unreported in shorter duration and/or previous studies were observed in this long-term study.

The efficacy and safety of tacrolimus ointment in maintenance treatment of mild to severe atopic dermatitis was assessed in 524 patients in two Phase III multicentre clinical trials of similar design, one in adult patients (⩾ 16 years) and one in paediatric patients (2-15 years). In both studies, patients with active disease entered an open-label period (OLP) during which they treated affected lesions with tacrolimus ointment twice daily until improvement had reached a predefined score (Investigator's Global Assessment [IGA] ⩽ 2, i.e. clear, almost clear or mild disease) for a maximum of 6 weeks. Thereafter, patients entered a double-blind disease control period (DCP) for up to 12 months. Patients were randomised to receive either tacrolimus ointment (0.1% adults; 0.03% children) or vehicle, once a day twice weekly on Mondays and Thursdays. If a disease exacerbation occurred, patients were treated with open-label tacrolimus ointment twice daily for a maximum of 6 weeks until the IGA score returned to ⩽ 2.

The primary endpoint in both studies was the number of disease exacerbations requiring a "substantial therapeutic intervention" during the DCP, defined as an exacerbation with an IGA of 3-5 (i.e. moderate, severe and very severe disease) on the first day of the flare, and requiring more than 7 days treatment. Both studies showed significant benefit with twice weekly treatment with tacrolimus ointment with regard to the primary and key secondary endpoints over a period of 12 months in a pooled population of patients with mild to severe atopic dermatitis. In a subanalysis of a pooled population of patients with moderate to severe atopic dermatitis these differences remained statistically significant (Table 4). No adverse events not reported previously were observed in these studies.

Table 4 Efficacy (moderate to severe subpopulation)

(see Table 4 below)

5.2 Pharmacokinetic properties

Clinical data have shown that tacrolimus concentrations in systemic circulation after topical administration are low and, when measurable, transient.

Absorption

Data from healthy human subjects indicate that there is little or no systemic exposure to tacrolimus following single or repeated topical application of tacrolimus ointment.

Most atopic dermatitis patients (adults and children) treated with single or repeated application of tacrolimus ointment (0.03-0.1%), and infants from age of 5 months treated with tacrolimus ointment (0.03%) had blood concentrations < 1.0 ng/ml. When observed, blood concentrations exceeding 1.0 ng/ml were transient. Systemic exposure increases with increasing treatment areas. However, both the extent and the rate of topical absorption of tacrolimus decrease as the skin heals. In both adults and children with an average of 50% body surface area treated, systemic exposure (i.e. AUC) of tacrolimus from Protopic is approximately 30-fold less than that seen with oral immunosuppressive doses in kidney and liver transplant patients. The lowest tacrolimus blood concentration at which systemic effects can be observed is not known.

There was no evidence of systemic accumulation of tacrolimus in patients (adults and children) treated for prolonged periods (up to one year) with tacrolimus ointment.

Distribution

As systemic exposure is low with tacrolimus ointment, the high binding of tacrolimus (> 98.8%) to plasma proteins is considered not to be clinically relevant.

Following topical application of tacrolimus ointment, tacrolimus is selectively delivered to the skin with minimal diffusion into the systemic circulation.

Metabolism

Metabolism of tacrolimus by human skin was not detectable. Systemically available tacrolimus is extensively metabolised in the liver via CYP3A4.

Elimination

When administered intravenously, tacrolimus has been shown to have a low clearance rate. The average total body clearance is approximately 2.25 l/h. The hepatic clearance of systemically available tacrolimus could be reduced in subjects with severe hepatic impairment, or in subjects who are co-treated with drugs that are potent inhibitors of CYP3A4.

Following repeated topical application of the ointment the average half-life of tacrolimus was estimated to be 75 hours for adults and 65 hours for children.

5.3 Preclinical safety data

Repeated dose toxicity and local tolerance

Repeated topical administration of tacrolimus ointment or the ointment vehicle to rats, rabbits and micropigs was associated with slight dermal changes such as erythema, oedema and papules.

Long-term topical treatment of rats with tacrolimus led to systemic toxicity including alterations of kidneys, pancreas, eyes and nervous system. The changes were caused by high systemic exposure of rodents resulting from high transdermal absorption of tacrolimus. Slightly lower body weight gain in females was the only systemic change observed in micropigs at high ointment concentrations (3%).

Rabbits were shown to be especially sensitive to intravenous administration of tacrolimus, reversible cardiotoxic effects being observed.

Mutagenicity

In vitro and *in vivo* tests did not indicate a genotoxic potential of tacrolimus.

Carcinogenicity

Systemic carcinogenicity studies in mice (18 months) and rats (24 months) revealed no carcinogenic potential of tacrolimus.

In a 24-month dermal carcinogenicity study performed in mice with 0.1% ointment, no skin tumours were observed. In the same study an increased incidence of lymphoma was detected in association with high systemic exposure.

In a photocarcinogenicity study, albino hairless mice were chronically treated with tacrolimus ointment and UV radiation. Animals treated with tacrolimus ointment showed a statistically significant reduction in time to skin tumour (squamous cell carcinoma) development and an increase in the number of tumours. It is unclear whether the effect of tacrolimus is due to systemic immunosuppression or a local effect. The risk for humans cannot be completely ruled out as the potential for local immunosuppression with the long-term use of tacrolimus ointment is unknown.

Reproduction toxicity

Embryo/foetal toxicity was observed in rats and rabbits, but only at doses that caused significant toxicity in maternal animals. Reduced sperm function was noted in male rats at high subcutaneous doses of tacrolimus.

6. PHARMACEUTICAL PARTICULARS

6.1 List of excipients

White soft paraffin

Liquid paraffin

Propylene carbonate

White beeswax

Hard paraffin

6.2 Incompatibilities

Not applicable.

6.3 Shelf life

3 years

6.4 Special precautions for storage

Do not store above 25°C.

6.5 Nature and contents of container

Laminate tube with an inner lining of low-density-polyethylene fitted with a white polypropylene screw cap.

Package sizes: 10 g, 30 g and 60 g. Not all pack sizes may be marketed.

Table 3 Efficacy at week 3

	Hydrocortisone acetate 1% Twice daily (N=207)	Tacrolimus 0.03% Once daily (N=207)	Tacrolimus 0.03% Twice daily (N=210)
Median mEASI Percentage Decrease (Primary Endpoint)§	47.2%	70.0%	78.7%
Improvement ⩾ 90% in Physician's Global Evaluation	13.6%	27.8%	36.7%

§ higher values = greater improvement

Table 4 Efficacy (moderate to severe subpopulation)

	Adults, ⩾ 16 years		Children, 2-15 years	
	Tacrolimus 0.1% Twice weekly (N=80)	Vehicle Twice weekly (N=73)	Tacrolimus 0.03% Twice weekly (N=78)	Vehicle Twice weekly (N=75)
Median number of DEs requiring substantial intervention adjusted for time at risk (% of patients without DE requiring substantial intervention)	1.0 (48.8%)	5.3 (17.8%)	1.0 (46.2%)	2.9 (21.3%)
Median time to first DE requiring substantial intervention	142 days	15 days	217 days	36 days
Median number of DEs adjusted for time at risk (% of patients without any DE periods)	1.0 (42.5%)	6.8 (12.3%)	1.5 (41.0%)	3.5 (14.7%)
Median time to first DE	123 days	14 days	146 days	17 days
Mean (SD) percentage of days of DE exacerbation treatment	16.1 (23.6)	39.0 (27.8)	16.9 (22.1)	29.9 (26.8)

DE: disease exacerbation

$P<0.001$ in favour of tacrolimus ointment 0.1% (adults) and 0.03% (children) for the primary and key secondary endpoints

6.6 Special precautions for disposal and other handling
No special requirements.

Any unused product or waste material should be disposed of in accordance with local requirements.

7. MARKETING AUTHORISATION HOLDER
Astellas Pharma Europe B.V.

Elisabethhof 19

2353 EW Leiderdorp

Netherlands

8. MARKETING AUTHORISATION NUMBER(S)
EU/1/02/201/001

EU/1/02/201/002

EU/1/02/201/005

9. DATE OF FIRST AUTHORISATION/RENEWAL OF THE AUTHORISATION
Date of first authorisation: 28/02/2002

Date of renewal: 20/11/2006

10. DATE OF REVISION OF THE TEXT
07/04/09

Detailed information on this medicinal product is available on the website of the European Medicines Agency (EMEA) http://www.emea.europa.eu/.

Protopic 0.1% ointment

(Astellas Pharma Ltd)

1. NAME OF THE MEDICINAL PRODUCT
Protopic 0.1% ointment

2. QUALITATIVE AND QUANTITATIVE COMPOSITION
1 g of Protopic 0.1% ointment contains 1.0 mg of tacrolimus as tacrolimus monohydrate (0.1%).

For a full list of excipients, see section 6.1.

3. PHARMACEUTICAL FORM
Ointment

A white to slightly yellowish ointment.

4. CLINICAL PARTICULARS

4.1 Therapeutic indications
Treatment of moderate to severe atopic dermatitis in adults who are not adequately responsive to or are intolerant of conventional therapies such as topical corticosteroids.

Maintenance treatment of moderate to severe atopic dermatitis for the prevention of flares and the prolongation of flare-free intervals in patients experiencing a high frequency of disease exacerbations (i.e. occurring 4 or more times per year) who have had an initial response to a maximum of 6 weeks treatment of twice daily tacrolimus ointment (lesions cleared, almost cleared or mildly affected).

4.2 Posology and method of administration
Protopic should be initiated by physicians with experience in the diagnosis and treatment of atopic dermatitis.

Protopic can be used for short-term and intermittent long-term treatment. Treatment should not be continuous.

Protopic ointment should be applied as a thin layer to affected or commonly affected areas of the skin. Protopic ointment may be used on any part of the body, including face, neck and flexure areas, except on mucous membranes. Protopic ointment should not be applied under occlusion (see section 4.4).

Protopic is not recommended for use in children below the age of 2 years until further data are available.

Specific studies have not been conducted in elderly patients. However, the clinical experience available in this patient population has not shown the necessity for any dosage adjustment.

Treatment

Protopic treatment should begin at the first appearance of signs and symptoms. Each affected region of the skin should be treated with Protopic until lesions are cleared, almost cleared or mildly affected. Thereafter, patients are considered suitable for maintenance treatment (see below). At the first signs of recurrence (flares) of the disease symptoms, treatment should be re-initiated.

Use in adults (16 years of age and above)

Protopic is available in two strengths, Protopic 0.03% and Protopic 0.1% ointment. Treatment should be started with Protopic 0.1% twice a day and treatment should be continued until clearance of the lesion. If symptoms recur, twice daily treatment with Protopic 0.1% should be restarted. An attempt should be made to reduce the frequency of application or to use the lower strength Protopic 0.03% ointment if the clinical condition allows.

Generally, improvement is seen within one week of starting treatment. If no signs of improvement are seen after two weeks of treatment, further treatment options should be considered.

Maintenance

Patients who are responding to up to 6 weeks treatment using tacrolimus ointment twice daily (lesions cleared, almost cleared or mildly affected) are suitable for maintenance treatment.

Protopic ointment should be applied once a day twice weekly (e.g. Monday and Thursday) to areas commonly affected by atopic dermatitis to prevent progression to flares. Between applications there should be 2–3 days without Protopic treatment.

Adult patients (16 years of age and above) should use Protopic 0.1% ointment.

If signs of a flare reoccur, twice daily treatment should be re-initiated (see treatment section above).

After 12 months, a review of the patient's condition should be conducted by the physician and a decision taken whether to continue maintenance treatment in the absence of safety data for maintenance treatment beyond 12 months. In children, this review should include suspension of treatment to assess the need to continue this regimen and to evaluate the course of the disease.

4.3 Contraindications
Hypersensitivity to macrolides in general, to tacrolimus or to any of the excipients.

4.4 Special warnings and precautions for use
Protopic should not be used in patients with congenital or acquired immunodeficiencies or in patients on therapy that cause immunosuppression.

Exposure of the skin to sunlight should be minimised and the use of ultraviolet (UV) light from a solarium, therapy with UVB or UVA in combination with psoralens (PUVA) should be avoided during use of Protopic ointment (see section 5.3). Physicians should advise patients on appropriate sun protection methods, such as minimisation of the time in the sun, use of a sunscreen product and covering of the skin with appropriate clothing. Protopic ointment should not be applied to lesions that are considered to be potentially malignant or pre-malignant.

Emollients should not be applied to the same area within 2 hours of applying Protopic ointment. Concomitant use of other topical preparations has not been assessed. There is no experience with concomitant use of systemic steroids or immunosuppressive agents.

Protopic ointment has not been evaluated for its efficacy and safety in the treatment of clinically infected atopic dermatitis. Before commencing treatment with Protopic ointment, clinical infections at treatment sites should be cleared. Patients with atopic dermatitis are predisposed to superficial skin infections. Treatment with Protopic may be associated with an increased risk of herpes viral infections (herpes simplex dermatitis [eczema herpeticum], herpes simplex [cold sores], Kaposi's varicelliform eruption). In the presence of these infections, the balance of risks and benefits associated with Protopic use should be evaluated.

The potential for local immunosuppression (possibly resulting in infections or cutaneous malignancies) in the long term (i.e. over a period of years) is unknown (see section 5.1).

Protopic contains the active substance tacrolimus, a calcineurin inhibitor. In transplant patients, prolonged systemic exposure to intense immunosuppression following systemic administration of calcineurin inhibitors has been associated with an increased risk of developing lymphomas and skin malignancies. In patients using tacrolimus ointment, cases of malignancies, including cutaneous and other types of lymphoma, and skin cancers have been reported (see section 4.8). Patients with atopic dermatitis treated with Protopic have not been found to have significant systemic tacrolimus levels.

Lymphadenopathy was uncommonly (0.8%) reported in clinical trials. The majority of these cases related to infections (skin, respiratory tract, tooth) and resolved with appropriate antibiotic therapy. Transplant patients receiving immunosuppressive regimens (e.g. systemic tacrolimus) are at increased risk for developing lymphoma; therefore patients who receive Protopic and who develop lymphadenopathy should be monitored to ensure that the lymphadenopathy resolves. Lymphadenopathy present at initiation of therapy should be investigated and kept under review. In case of persistent lymphadenopathy, the aetiology of the lymphadenopathy should be investigated. In the absence of a clear aetiology for the lymphadenopathy or in the presence of acute infectious mononucleosis, discontinuation of Protopic should be considered.

Care should be taken to avoid contact with eyes and mucous membranes. If accidentally applied to these areas, the ointment should be thoroughly wiped off and/or rinsed off with water.

The use of Protopic ointment under occlusion has not been studied in patients. Occlusive dressings are not recommended.

As with any topical medicinal product, patients should wash their hands after application if the hands are not intended for treatment.

Tacrolimus is extensively metabolised in the liver and although blood concentrations are low following topical therapy, the ointment should be used with caution in patients with hepatic failure (see section 5.2).

The use of Protopic ointment in patients with genetic epidermal barrier defects such as Netherton's syndrome is not recommended due to the potential for permanently increased systemic absorption of tacrolimus. The safety of Protopic ointment has not been established in patients with generalised erythroderma.

Care should be exercised if applying Protopic to patients with extensive skin involvement over an extended period of time, especially in children (see section 4.2).

The development of any new change different from previous eczema within a treated area should be reviewed by the physician.

4.5 Interaction with other medicinal products and other forms of interaction
Formal topical drug interaction studies with tacrolimus ointment have not been conducted.

Tacrolimus is not metabolised in human skin, indicating that there is no potential for percutaneous interactions that could affect the metabolism of tacrolimus.

Systemically available tacrolimus is metabolised via the hepatic Cytochrome P450 3A4 (CYP3A4). Systemic exposure from topical application of tacrolimus ointment is low ($<$ 1.0 ng/ml) and is unlikely to be affected by concomitant use of substances known to be inhibitors of CYP3A4. However, the possibility of interactions cannot be ruled out and the concomitant systemic administration of known CYP3A4 inhibitors (e.g. erythromycin, itraconazole, ketoconazole and diltiazem) in patients with widespread and/or erythrodermic disease should be done with caution.

A potential interaction between vaccination and application of Protopic ointment has not been investigated. Because of the potential risk of vaccination failure, vaccination should be administered prior to commencement of treatment, or during a treatment-free interval with a period of 14 days between the last application of Protopic and the vaccination. In case of live attenuated vaccination, this period should be extended to 28 days or the use of alternative vaccines should be considered.

4.6 Pregnancy and lactation
There are no adequate data from the use of tacrolimus ointment in pregnant women. Studies in animals have shown reproductive toxicity following systemic administration (see section 5.3). The potential risk for humans is unknown.

Protopic ointment should not be used during pregnancy unless clearly necessary.

Human data demonstrate that, after systemic administration, tacrolimus is excreted into breast milk. Although clinical data have shown that systemic exposure from application of tacrolimus ointment is low, breast-feeding during treatment with Protopic ointment is not recommended.

4.7 Effects on ability to drive and use machines
No studies on the effects on the ability to drive and use machines have been performed. Protopic ointment is administered topically and is unlikely to have an effect on the ability to drive or use machines.

4.8 Undesirable effects
In clinical studies approximately 50% of patients experienced some type of skin irritation adverse reaction at the site of application. Burning sensation and pruritus were very common, usually mild to moderate in severity and tended to resolve within one week of starting treatment. Erythema was a common skin irritation adverse reaction. Sensation of warmth, pain, paraesthesia and rash at the site of application were also commonly observed. Alcohol intolerance (facial flushing or skin irritation after consumption of an alcoholic beverage) was common.

Patients may be at an increased risk of folliculitis, acne and herpes viral infections.

Adverse reactions with suspected relationship to treatment are listed below by system organ class. Frequencies are defined as very common ($\geqslant$ 1/10), common ($\geqslant$ 1/100 to $<$ 1/10) and uncommon ($\geqslant$1/1,000 to $<$ 1/100). Within each frequency grouping, undesirable effects are presented in order of decreasing seriousness.

General disorders and administration site conditions

Very common: Application site burning, application site pruritus

Common: Application site warmth, application site erythema, application site pain, application site irritation, application site paraesthesia, application site rash

Infections and infestations

Common: Herpes viral infections (herpes simplex dermatitis [eczema herpeticum], herpes simplex [cold sores], Kaposi's varicelliform eruption)

Skin and subcutaneous tissue disorders

Common: Folliculitis, pruritus

Uncommon: Acne

Nervous system disorders

Common: Paraesthesias and dysaesthesias (hyperaesthesia, burning sensation)

Metabolism and nutrition disorders

Common: Alcohol intolerance (facial flushing or skin irritation after consumption of an alcoholic beverage)

The following adverse reactions have been reported during post-marketing experience:

Skin and subcutaneous tissue disorders: Rosacea

In a study of maintenance treatment (twice weekly treatment) in adults and children with moderate and severe atopic dermatitis the following adverse events were noted to occur more frequently than in the control group: application site impetigo (7.7% in children) and application site infections (6.4% in children and 6.3% in adults).

Post-marketing: cases of malignancies, including cutaneous and other types of lymphoma, and skin cancers, have been reported in patients using tacrolimus ointment (see section 4.4).

4.9 Overdose

Overdosage following topical administration is unlikely.

If ingested, general supportive measures may be appropriate. These may include monitoring of vital signs and observation of clinical status. Due to the nature of the ointment vehicle, induction of vomiting or gastric lavage is not recommended.

5. PHARMACOLOGICAL PROPERTIES

5.1 Pharmacodynamic properties

Pharmacotherapeutic group: Other dermatologicals, ATC code: D11AX14

Mechanism of action and pharmacodynamic effects

The mechanism of action of tacrolimus in atopic dermatitis is not fully understood. While the following have been observed, the clinical significance of these observations in atopic dermatitis is not known.

Via its binding to a specific cytoplasmic immunophilin (FKBP12), tacrolimus inhibits calcium-dependent signal transduction pathways in T cells, thereby preventing the transcription and synthesis of IL-2, IL-3, IL-4, IL-5 and other cytokines such as GM-CSF, TNF-α and IFN-γ.

In vitro, in Langerhans cells isolated from normal human skin, tacrolimus reduced the stimulatory activity towards T cells. Tacrolimus has also been shown to inhibit the release of inflammatory mediators from skin mast cells, basophils and eosinophils.

In animals, tacrolimus ointment suppressed inflammatory reactions in experimental and spontaneous dermatitis models that resemble human atopic dermatitis. Tacrolimus ointment did not reduce skin thickness and did not cause skin atrophy in animals.

In patients with atopic dermatitis, improvement of skin lesions during treatment with tacrolimus ointment was associated with reduced Fc receptor expression on Langerhans cells and a reduction of their hyperstimulatory activity towards T cells. Tacrolimus ointment does not affect collagen synthesis in humans.

Results from clinical studies in patients

The efficacy and safety of Protopic was assessed in more than 18,500 patients treated with tacrolimus ointment in Phase I to Phase III clinical trials. Data from six major trials are presented here.

In a six-month multicentre double-blind randomised trial, 0.1% tacrolimus ointment was administered twice-a-day to adults with moderate to severe atopic dermatitis and compared to a topical corticosteroid based regimen (0.1% hydrocortisone butyrate on trunk and extremities, 1% hydrocortisone acetate on face and neck). The primary endpoint was the response rate at month 3 defined as the proportion of patients with at least 60% improvement in the mEASI (modified Eczema Area and Severity Index) between baseline and month 3. The response rate in the 0.1% tacrolimus group (71.6%) was significantly higher than that in the topical corticosteroid based treatment group (50.8%; p<0.001; Table 1). The response rates at month 6 were comparable to the 3-month results.

Table 1 Efficacy at month 3

	Topical corticosteroid regimen§ (N=485)	Tacrolimus 0.1% (N=487)
Response rate of ⩾ 60% improvement in mEASI (Primary Endpoint)§§	50.8%	71.6%
Improvement ⩾ 90% in Physician's Global Evaluation	28.5%	47.7%

§ Topical corticosteroid regimen = 0.1% hydrocortisone butyrate on trunk and extremities, 1% hydrocortisone acetate on face and neck

§§ higher values = greater improvement

The incidence and nature of most adverse events were similar in the two treatment groups. Skin burning, herpes simplex, alcohol intolerance (facial flushing or skin sensitivity after alcohol intake), skin tingling, hyperaesthesia, acne and fungal dermatitis occurred more often in the tacrolimus treatment group. There were no clinically relevant changes in the laboratory values or vital signs in either treatment group throughout the study.

In the second trial, children aged from 2 to 15 years with moderate to severe atopic dermatitis received twice daily treatment for three weeks of 0.03% tacrolimus ointment, 0.1% tacrolimus ointment or 1% hydrocortisone acetate ointment. The primary endpoint was the area-under-the-curve (AUC) of the mEASI as a percentage of baseline averaged over the treatment period. The results of this multicentre, double-blind, randomised trial showed that tacrolimus ointment, 0.03% and 0.1%, is significantly more effective (p < 0.001 for both) than 1% hydrocortisone acetate ointment (Table 2).

Table 2 Efficacy at week 3

(see Table 2 below)

The incidence of local skin burning was higher in the tacrolimus treatment groups than in the hydrocortisone group. Pruritus decreased over time in the tacrolimus groups but not in the hydrocortisone group. There were no clinically relevant changes in the laboratory values or vital signs in either treatment group throughout the clinical trial.

The purpose of the third multicentre, double-blind, randomised study was the assessment of efficacy and safety of 0.03% tacrolimus ointment applied once or twice a day relative to twice daily administration of 1% hydrocortisone acetate ointment in children with moderate to severe atopic dermatitis. Treatment duration was for up to three weeks.

Table 3 Efficacy at week 3

(see Table 3 below)

The primary endpoint was defined as the percentage decrease in mEASI from the baseline to end of treatment. A statistically significant better improvement was shown for once daily and twice daily 0.03% tacrolimus ointment compared to twice daily hydrocortisone acetate ointment (p<0.001 for both). Twice daily treatment with 0.03% tacrolimus ointment was more effective than once daily administration (Table 3). The incidence of local skin burning was higher in the tacrolimus treatment groups than in the hydrocortisone group. There were no clinically relevant changes in the laboratory values or vital signs in either treatment group throughout the study.

In the fourth trial, approximately 800 patients (aged ⩾ 2 years) received 0.1% tacrolimus ointment intermittently or continuously in an open-label, long-term safety study for up to four years, with 300 patients receiving treatment for at least three years and 79 patients receiving treatment for a minimum of 42 months. Based on changes from baseline in EASI score and body surface area affected, patients regardless of age had improvement in their atopic dermatitis at all subsequent time points. In addition, there was no evidence of loss of efficacy throughout the duration of the clinical trial. The overall incidence of adverse events tended to decrease as the study progressed for all patients independent of age. The three most common adverse events reported were flu-like symptoms (cold, common cold, influenza, upper respiratory infection, etc.), pruritus and skin burning. No adverse events previously unreported in shorter duration and/or previous studies were observed in this long-term study.

The efficacy and safety of tacrolimus ointment in maintenance treatment of mild to severe atopic dermatitis was assessed in 524 patients in two Phase III multicentre clinical trials of similar design, one in adult patients (⩾ 16 years) and one in paediatric patients (2-15 years). In both studies, patients with active disease entered an open-label period (OLP) during which they treated affected lesions with tacrolimus ointment twice daily until improvement had reached a predefined score (Investigator's Global Assessment [IGA] ⩽ 2, i.e. clear, almost clear or mild disease) for a maximum of 6 weeks. Thereafter, patients entered a double-blind disease control period (DCP) for up to 12 months. Patients were randomised to receive either tacrolimus ointment (0.1% adults; 0.03% children) or vehicle, once a day twice weekly on Mondays and Thursdays. If a disease exacerbation occurred, patients were treated with open-label tacrolimus ointment twice daily for a maximum of 6 weeks until the IGA score returned to ⩽ 2.

The primary endpoint in both studies was the number of disease exacerbations requiring a "substantial therapeutic intervention" during the DCP, defined as an exacerbation with an IGA of 3-5 (i.e. moderate, severe and very severe disease) on the first day of the flare, and requiring more than 7 days treatment. Both studies showed significant benefit with twice weekly treatment with tacrolimus ointment with regard to the primary and key secondary endpoints over a period of 12 months in a pooled population of patients with mild to severe atopic dermatitis. In a subanalysis of a pooled population of patients with moderate to severe atopic dermatitis these differences remained statistically significant (Table 4). No adverse events not reported previously were observed in these studies.

Table 4 Efficacy (moderate to severe subpopulation)

(see Table 4 below)

5.2 Pharmacokinetic properties

Clinical data have shown that tacrolimus concentrations in systemic circulation after topical administration are low and, when measurable, transient.

Table 2 Efficacy at week 3

	Hydrocortisone acetate 1% (N=185)	Tacrolimus 0.03% (N=189)	Tacrolimus 0.1% (N=186)
Median mEASI as Percentage of Baseline mean AUC (Primary Endpoint)§	64.0%	44.8%	39.8%
Improvement ⩾ 90% in Physician's Global Evaluation	15.7%	38.5%	48.4%

§ lower values = greater improvement

Table 3 Efficacy at week 3

	Hydrocortisone acetate 1% Twice daily (N=207)	Tacrolimus 0.03% Once daily (N=207)	Tacrolimus 0.03% Twice daily (N=210)
Median mEASI Percentage Decrease (Primary Endpoint)§	47.2%	70.0%	78.7%
Improvement ⩾ 90% in Physician's Global Evaluation	13.6%	27.8%	36.7%

§ higher values = greater improvement

Table 4 Efficacy (moderate to severe subpopulation)

	Adults, ⩾ 16 years		Children, 2-15 years	
	Tacrolimus 0.1% Twice weekly (N=80)	Vehicle Twice weekly (N=73)	Tacrolimus 0.03% Twice weekly (N=78)	Vehicle Twice weekly (N=75)
Median number of DEs requiring substantial intervention adjusted for time at risk (% of patients without DE requiring substantial intervention)	1.0 (48.8%)	5.3 (17.8%)	1.0 (46.2%)	2.9 (21.3%)
Median time to first DE requiring substantial intervention	142 days	15 days	217 days	36 days
Median number of DEs adjusted for time at risk (% of patients without any DE periods)	1.0 (42.5%)	6.8 (12.3%)	1.5 (41.0%)	3.5 (14.7%)
Median time to first DE	123 days	14 days	146 days	17 days
Mean (SD) percentage of days of DE exacerbation treatment	16.1 (23.6)	39.0 (27.8)	16.9 (22.1)	29.9 (26.8)

DE: disease exacerbation

P<0.001 in favour of tacrolimus ointment 0.1% (adults) and 0.03% (children) for the primary and key secondary endpoints

Absorption

Data from healthy human subjects indicate that there is little or no systemic exposure to tacrolimus following single or repeated topical application of tacrolimus ointment.

Most atopic dermatitis patients (adults and children) treated with single or repeated application of tacrolimus ointment (0.03-0.1%), and infants from age of 5 months treated with tacrolimus ointment (0.03%) had blood concentrations < 1.0 ng/ml. When observed, blood concentrations exceeding 1.0 ng/ml were transient. Systemic exposure increases with increasing treatment areas. However, both the extent and the rate of topical absorption of tacrolimus decrease as the skin heals. In both adults and children with an average of 50% body surface area treated, systemic exposure (i.e. AUC) of tacrolimus from Protopic is approximately 30-fold less than that seen with oral immunosuppressive doses in kidney and liver transplant patients. The lowest tacrolimus blood concentration at which systemic effects can be observed is not known.

There was no evidence of systemic accumulation of tacrolimus in patients (adults and children) treated for prolonged periods (up to one year) with tacrolimus ointment.

Distribution

As systemic exposure is low with tacrolimus ointment, the high binding of tacrolimus (> 98.8%) to plasma proteins is considered not to be clinically relevant.

Following topical application of tacrolimus ointment, tacrolimus is selectively delivered to the skin with minimal diffusion into the systemic circulation.

Metabolism

Metabolism of tacrolimus by human skin was not detectable. Systemically available tacrolimus is extensively metabolised in the liver via CYP3A4.

Elimination

When administered intravenously, tacrolimus has been shown to have a low clearance rate. The average total body clearance is approximately 2.25 l/h. The hepatic clearance of systemically available tacrolimus could be reduced in subjects with severe hepatic impairment, or in subjects who are co-treated with drugs that are potent inhibitors of CYP3A4.

Following repeated topical application of the ointment the average half-life of tacrolimus was estimated to be 75 hours for adults and 65 hours for children.

5.3 Preclinical safety data

Repeated dose toxicity and local tolerance

Repeated topical administration of tacrolimus ointment or the ointment vehicle to rats, rabbits and micropigs was associated with slight dermal changes such as erythema, oedema and papules.

Long-term topical treatment of rats with tacrolimus led to systemic toxicity including alterations of kidneys, pancreas, eyes and nervous system. The changes were caused by high systemic exposure of rodents resulting from high transdermal absorption of tacrolimus. Slightly lower body weight gain in females was the only systemic change observed in micropigs at high ointment concentrations (3%).

Rabbits were shown to be especially sensitive to intravenous administration of tacrolimus, reversible cardiotoxic effects being observed.

Mutagenicity

In vitro and *in vivo* tests did not indicate a genotoxic potential of tacrolimus.

Carcinogenicity

Systemic carcinogenicity studies in mice (18 months) and rats (24 months) revealed no carcinogenic potential of tacrolimus.

In a 24-month dermal carcinogenicity study performed in mice with 0.1% ointment, no skin tumours were observed. In the same study an increased incidence of lymphoma was detected in association with high systemic exposure.

In a photocarcinogenicity study, albino hairless mice were chronically treated with tacrolimus ointment and UV radiation. Animals treated with tacrolimus ointment showed a statistically significant reduction in time to skin tumour (squamous cell carcinoma) development and an increase in the number of tumours. It is unclear whether the effect of tacrolimus is due to systemic immunosuppression or a local effect. The risk for humans cannot be completely ruled out as the potential for local immunosuppression with the long-term use of tacrolimus ointment is unknown.

Reproduction toxicity

Embryo/foetal toxicity was observed in rats and rabbits, but only at doses that caused significant toxicity in maternal animals. Reduced sperm function was noted in male rats at high subcutaneous doses of tacrolimus.

6. PHARMACEUTICAL PARTICULARS

6.1 List of excipients

White soft paraffin

Liquid paraffin

Propylene carbonate

White beeswax

Hard paraffin

6.2 Incompatibilities

Not applicable.

6.3 Shelf life

3 years

6.4 Special precautions for storage

Do not store above 25°C.

6.5 Nature and contents of container

Laminate tube with an inner lining of low-density-polyethylene fitted with a white polypropylene screw cap.

Package sizes: 10 g, 30 g and 60 g. Not all pack sizes may be marketed.

6.6 Special precautions for disposal and other handling

No special requirements.

Any unused product or waste material should be disposed of in accordance with local requirements.

7. MARKETING AUTHORISATION HOLDER

Astellas Pharma Europe B.V.

Elisabethhof 19

2353 EW Leiderdorp

Netherlands

8. MARKETING AUTHORISATION NUMBER(S)

EU/1/02/201/003

EU/1/02/201/004

EU/1/02/201/006

9. DATE OF FIRST AUTHORISATION/RENEWAL OF THE AUTHORISATION

Date of first authorisation: 28/02/2002

Date of renewal: 20/11/2006

10. DATE OF REVISION OF THE TEXT

07/04/09

Detailed information on this medicinal product is available on the website of the European Medicines Agency (EMEA) http://www.emea.europa.eu/.

Provera Tablets 100 mg, Provera Tablets 200 mg & Provera Tablets 400 mg

(Pharmacia Limited)

1. NAME OF THE MEDICINAL PRODUCT

Provera Tablets 100 mg or Medroxyprogesterone Acetate Tablets 100 mg.

Provera Tablets 200 mg or Medroxyprogesterone Acetate Tablets 200 mg.

Provera® Tablets 400 mg

2. QUALITATIVE AND QUANTITATIVE COMPOSITION

1 tablet contains 100mg medroxyprogesterone acetate.

1 tablet contains 200 mg medroxyprogesterone acetate.

1 tablet contains 400 mg medroxyprogesterone acetate.

For excipients, see 6.1.

3. PHARMACEUTICAL FORM

Tablet.

4. CLINICAL PARTICULARS

4.1 Therapeutic indications

Progestogen indicated for the treatment of certain hormone dependant neoplasms, such as:

1. Endometrial carcinoma.
2. Renal cell carcinoma.
3. Carcinoma of breast in post menopausal women.

4.2 Posology and method of administration

Route of administration: Oral.

Adults

Endometrial and renal cell carcinoma	200 - 600 mg daily
Breast carcinoma	400 - 1500 mg daily

The incidence of minor side-effects, such as indigestion and weight gain, increase with the increase in dose.

Response to hormonal therapy may not be evident until after at least 8-10 weeks of therapy.

Elderly patients: This product has been used primarily in the older age group for the treatment of malignancies. There is no evidence to suggest that the older age group is any less prepared to handle the drug metabolically than is the younger patient. Therefore the same dosage, contraindications, and precautions would apply to either age group.

Children: The product is not anticipated for paediatric use in the indications recommended.

4.3 Contraindications

Medroxyprogesterone acetate is contraindicated in the following conditions:

- thrombophlebitis, thrombo-embolic disorders, and where there is a high risk of developing such manifestations [presence or history of atrial fibrillation, valvular disorders, endocarditis, heart failure, pulmonary embolism; thrombo-embolic ischaemic attack (TIA), cerebral infarction; atherosclerosis; immediate post surgery period]
- hypercalcaemia in patients with osseous metastases
- known sensitivity to medroxyprogesterone acetate or any component of the drug.
- impaired liver function or active liver disease.
- missed abortion, metrorrhagia, known or suspected pregnancy.
- undiagnosed vaginal bleeding.
- previous idiopathic or current venous thromboembolism (deep vein thrombosis, pulmonary embolism).
- active or recent arterial thromboembolic disease (e.g., angina, myocardial infarction).
- suspected or early breast carcinoma

Progestogens are known to be porphyrogenic. Patients with a history of attacks or aged under 30 are at greatest risk of an acute attack while on progesterone treatment. A careful assessment of potential benefit should be made where this risk is present.

4.4 Special warnings and precautions for use

Warnings:

In the treatment of carcinoma of breast occasional cases of hypercalcaemia have been reported.

Unexpected vaginal bleeding during therapy with medroxyprogesterone acetate should be investigated.

Medication should not be readministered pending examination if there is sudden partial or complete loss of vision or if there is a sudden onset of proptosis, diplopia or migraine. If examination reveals papilloedema or retinal vascular lesions, medication should not be readministered.

Medroxyprogesterone acetate may produce Cushingoid symptoms.

Some patients receiving medroxyprogesterone acetate may exhibit suppressed adrenal function. Medroxyprogesterone acetate may decrease ACTH and hydrocortisone blood levels.

Treatment with medroxyprogesterone acetate should be discontinued in the event of:

- jaundice or deterioration in liver function
- significant increase in blood pressure
- new onset of migraine-type headache

Precautions:

Animal studies show that Provera possesses adrenocorticoid activity. This has also been reported in man, therefore patients receiving large doses continuously and for long periods should be observed closely for signs normally associated with adrenocorticoid therapy, such as hypertension, sodium retention, oedema, etc. Care is needed in treating patients with diabetes and/or arterial hypertension.

Before using Provera the general medical condition of the patient should be carefully evaluated.

This product should be used under the supervision of a specialist and the patient kept under regular surveillance.

Patients with the following conditions should be carefully monitored while taking progestogens:

- Conditions which may be influenced by potential fluid retention
- o Epilepsy
- o Migraine
- o Asthma
- o Cardiac dysfunction
- o Renal dysfunction
- History of mental depression
- Diabetes (a decrease in glucose tolerance has been observed in some patients).
- Hyperlipidaemia

The pathologist (laboratory) should be informed of the patient's use of medroxyprogesterone acetate if endometrial or endocervical tissue is submitted for examination.

The physician/laboratory should be informed that medroxyprogesterone acetate may decrease the levels of the following endocrine biomarkers:

- Plasma/urinary steroids (e.g., cortisol, oestrogen, pregnanediol, progesterone, testosterone)
- Plasma/urinary gonadotrophins (e.g., LH and FSH)
- Sex-hormone-binding-globulin

The use of medroxyprogesterone acetate in oncology indications may also cause partial adrenal insufficiency (decrease in pituitary-adrenal axis response) during Metyrapone testing. Thus the ability of adrenal cortex to respond to ACTH should be demonstrated before metyrapone is administered.

Although medroxyprogesterone acetate has not been causally associated with the induction of thromboembolic disorders, any patient with a history or who develops this kind of event while undergoing therapy with medroxyprogesterone acetate should have her status and need for treatment carefully assessed before continuing therapy.

Risk of venous thromboembolism (VTE)

The risk of VTE has not been assessed for progesterone alone. However, VTE is a known risk factor of oestrogen-only and combined hormone replacement therapy. When prescribing medroxyprogesterone acetate for oncology indications the following precautions and risk factors should be considered in the light of the patient's condition, the dose of medroxyprogesterone acetate and the duration of therapy:

- Generally recognised risk factors for VTE include a personal or family history of VTE or known thromboembolic states, severe obesity (BMI > 30 kg/m^2) and systemic lupus erythematosus

- The risk of VTE may be temporarily increased with prolonged immobilisation, major trauma or major surgery.
- If VTE develops after initiating therapy, medroxyprogesterone acetate should be discontinued. Patients should be told to contact their doctor immediately if they become aware of a symptom suggestive of potential thromboembolism (e.g. painful swelling of a leg, sudden pain in the chest, dyspnoea).

4.5 Interaction with other medicinal products and other forms of interaction

Interaction with other medicaments

The metabolism of progestogens may be increased by concomitant administration of compounds known to induce drug-metabolising enzymes, specifically cytochrome P450 enzymes. These compounds include anticonvulsants (e.g., phenobarbital, phenytoin, carbamazepine) and anti-infectives (e.g., rifampicin, rifabutin, nevirapine, efavirenz,).

Ritonavir and nelfinavir, although known as strong inhibitors, by contrast exhibit inducing properties when used concomitantly with steroid hormones. Herbal preparations containing St John's Wort (Hypericum Perforatum) may induce the metabolism of progestogens. Progestogen levels may therefore be reduced.

Aminoglutethimide has been reported to decrease plasma levels of some progestogens.

Concurrent administration of ciclosporin and MPA has been reported to lead to increased plasma ciclosporin levels and/or decreased plasma MPA levels.

Interactions with oral anti-coagulants have been reported rarely, but causality has not been established.

When used in combination with cytotoxic drugs, it is possible that progestogens may reduce the haematological toxicity of chemotherapy.

Special care should be taken when progestogens are administered with other drugs which also cause fluid retention, such as NSAIDs and vasodilators.

Other forms of interaction

Progestogens can influence certain laboratory tests (e.g., tests for hepatic function, thyroid function and coagulation).

4.6 Pregnancy and lactation

Pregnancy

Medroxyprogesterone acetate is contraindicated in women who are pregnant. If medroxyprogesterone acetate is used during pregnancy, or if the patient becomes pregnant while using this drug, the patient should be apprised of the potential hazard to the foetus.

Some reports suggest an association between intrauterine exposure to progestational drugs in the first trimester of pregnancy and genital abnormalities in male and female foetuses.

Infants from unintentional pregnancies that occur 1 to 2 months after injection of medroxyprogesterone acetate injectable suspension may be at an increased risk of low birth weight, which, in turn, is associated with an increased risk of neonatal death. The attributable risk is low because pregnancies while on medroxyprogesterone acetate are uncommon.

Lactation

Medroxyprogesterone acetate and/or its metabolites are secreted in breast milk. Therefore, the use of Provera whilst breast-feeding is not recommended.

4.7 Effects on ability to drive and use machines

No adverse effect has been reported.

4.8 Undesirable effects

Reactions occasionally associated with the use of progestogens, particularly in high doses, are:

Breast: Tenderness, mastodynia or galactorrhoea.

Genitourinary: Abnormal uterine bleeding (irregular, increase, decrease), amenorrhoea, alterations of cervical secretions, cervical erosions, prolonged anovulation.

Central nervous system: Confusion, euphoria, loss of concentration, nervousness, insomnia, somnolence, fatigue, dizziness, depression, vision disorders and headache.

Skin and mucous membranes: Sensitivity reactions ranging from pruritus, urticaria, angioneurotic oedema, to generalised rash and anaphylaxis have occasionally been reported. Acne, alopecia or hirsutism have been reported in a few cases.

Allergy: Hypersensitivity reactions (e.g., anaphylaxis or anaphylactoid reactions, angioedema).

Gastro-intestinal/hepatobiliary: Constipation, diarrhoea, dry mouth, disturbed liver function, jaundice, vomiting, nausea and indigestion.

Metabolic and nutritional: Adrenergic-like effects (e.g., fine hand tremors, sweating, tremors, cramps in calves at night), corticoid-like effects (e.g., Cushingoid Syndrome), decreased glucose tolerance, diabetic cataract, exacerbation of diabetes mellitus, glycosuria.

Cardiovascular: Cerebral and myocardial infarction, congestive heart failure, increased blood pressure, palpitations, pulmonary embolism, retinal thrombosis, tachycardia, thromboembolic disorders, thrombophlebitis.

Haematological: Elevation of white blood cells and platelet count.

Miscellaneous: Change in appetite, change in libido, oedema/fluid retention, hypercalcaemia, malaise, hyperpyrexia, weight gain, moon facies.

4.9 Overdose

No action required other than cessation of therapy.

5. PHARMACOLOGICAL PROPERTIES

5.1 Pharmacodynamic properties

Pharmacotherapeutic group: Progestogens. ATC Code: L02A B

Medroxyprogesterone acetate has the pharmacological action of a progestogen.

5.2 Pharmacokinetic properties

Medroxyprogesterone acetate is absorbed from the gastro intestinal tract with a single oral dose of 10-250 mg. The time taken to reach the peak serum concentration (T_{max}) was 2-6 hours and the average peak serum concentration (C_{max}) was 13-46.89 mg/ml.

Unmetabolised medroxyprogesterone acetate is highly plasma protein bound. Medroxyprogesterone acetate is metabolised in the liver.

Medroxyprogesterone acetate is primarily metabolised by faecal excretion as glucuronide conjugated metabolite.

Metabolised medroxyprogesterone acetate is excreted more rapidly and in a greater percentage following oral doses than after aqueous intramuscular injection

400 mg only:

The comparative bioavailability of medroxyprogesterone acetate (MPA) in sixteen healthy male volunteers was determined following the oral ingestion of 400 mg MPA as two Provera 200 mg tablets or as one Provera 400mg tablet. It is concluded that the bioavailability appeared to be equivalent in this group of volunteers.

5.3 Preclinical safety data

No further preclinical safety data available.

6. PHARMACEUTICAL PARTICULARS

6.1 List of excipients

Microcrystalline cellulose

Maize Starch

Byco C

Macrogol 400

Sodium starch glycollate

Docusate sodium

Sodium benzoate

Magnesium stearate

Isopropyl alcohol

Purified water

6.2 Incompatibilities

Not applicable.

6.3 Shelf life

Provera 100mg: 36 months if stored in glass/HDPE bottles, or 24 month in blister packs.

Provera 200mg: 36 months if stored in glass/HDPE bottles, or 24 month in blister packs.

Provera 400mg: The shelf-life for Provera Tablets 400 mg is 36 months

6.4 Special precautions for storage

Provera 100mg: Store below 25°C. Bottle packs only: keep in a well closed container.

Provera 200mg: Store below 25°C. Bottle packs only: keep in a well closed container.

Provera 400mg: Store at controlled room temperature (15 - 30°C). Bottle packs only: keep in a well closed container.

6.5 Nature and contents of container

Provera 100mg: Amber glass bottle with screw cap containing 100 tablets. HDPE bottle with tamper evident cap containing 100 tablets. PVC/aluminium strip containing 30, 60 or 100 tablets.

Provera 200mg: Amber glass bottle with screw cap containing 100 tablets. HDPE bottle with tamper evident cap containing 100 tablets. PVC/aluminium strip containing 30, 60 or 100 tablets.

Provera 400mg: Glass/HDPE bottles of 60 tablets. PVC aluminium blisters of 30 tablets

6.6 Special precautions for disposal and other handling

None stated.

7. MARKETING AUTHORISATION HOLDER

Pharmacia Limited

Ramsgate Road

Sandwich

Kent

CT13 9NJ

UK

8. MARKETING AUTHORISATION NUMBER(S)

Provera 100mg: PL 0032/0111

Provera 200mg: PL 0032/0112

Provera 400mg: PL 0032/0131

9. DATE OF FIRST AUTHORISATION/RENEWAL OF THE AUTHORISATION

Provera 100mg: 7 November 1983/30 January 1996

Provera 200mg: 7 November 1983/30 January 1996

Provera 400mg: Date of first authorisation: 29 April 1986. Date of renewal of authorisation: 21 May 1998

10. DATE OF REVISION OF THE TEXT

August 2007

LEGAL CATEGORY

POM

Company Reference: PVB1_0

Provera Tablets 2.5 mg, Provera Tablets 5 mg & Provera Tablets 10 mg

(Pharmacia Limited)

1. NAME OF THE MEDICINAL PRODUCT

Provera Tablets 2.5 mg

Provera Tablets 5 mg

Provera Tablets 10 mg

2. QUALITATIVE AND QUANTITATIVE COMPOSITION

Each tablet contains 2.5 mg medroxyprogesterone acetate Ph. Eur.

Each tablet contains 5 mg medroxyprogesterone acetate Ph. Eur.

Each tablet contains 10 mg medroxyprogesterone acetate Ph. Eur.

3. PHARMACEUTICAL FORM

Tablets for oral use

4. CLINICAL PARTICULARS

4.1 Therapeutic indications

Progestogen. Indicated for dysfunctional (anovulatory) uterine bleeding, secondary amenorrhoea and for mild to moderate endometriosis.

4.2 Posology and method of administration

Oral.

Adults:

Dysfunctional (anovulatory) uterine bleeding: 2.5 - 10 mg daily for 5 - 10 days commencing on the assumed or calculated 16th - 21st day of the cycle. Treatment should be given for two consecutive cycles. When bleeding occurs from a poorly developed proliferative endometrium, conventional oestrogen therapy may be employed in conjunction with medroxyprogesterone acetate in doses of 5 - 10 mg for 10 days.

Secondary amenorrhoea: 2.5 - 10 mg daily for 5 - 10 days beginning on the assumed or calculated 16th to 21st day of the cycle. Repeat the treatment for three consecutive cycles. In amenorrhoea associated with a poorly developed proliferative endometrium, conventional oestrogen therapy may be employed in conjunction with medroxyprogesterone acetate in doses of 5 - 10 mg for 10 days.

Mild to moderate endometriosis: Beginning on the first day of the menstrual cycle, 10 mg three times a day for 90 consecutive days.

5 mg & 10 mg only

Breakthrough bleeding, which is self-limiting, may occur. No additional hormonal therapy is recommended for the management of this bleeding.

All strengths

Elderly: Not applicable

Children: Not applicable

4.3 Contraindications

Use in patients with a known sensitivity to medroxyprogesterone acetate.

Use in patients with impaired liver function or with active liver disease.

Before using Provera, the general medical condition of the patient should be carefully evaluated. This evaluation should exclude the presence of genital or breast neoplasia before considering the use of Provera.

4.4 Special warnings and precautions for use

Whether administered alone or in conjunction with oestrogens, Provera should not be employed in patients with abnormal uterine bleeding until a definite diagnosis has been established and the possibility of genital malignancy eliminated.

Rare cases of thrombo-embolism have been reported with use of Provera, especially at higher doses. Causality has not been established.

Doses of up to 30 mg a day may not suppress ovulation and patients should be advised to take adequate contraceptive measures, where appropriate.

Provera, especially in high doses, may cause weight gain and fluid retention. With this in mind, caution should be exercised in treating any patient with a pre-existing medical condition, such as epilepsy, migraine, asthma, cardiac or renal dysfunction, that might be adversely affected by weight gain or fluid retention.

Some patients receiving Provera may exhibit a decreased glucose tolerance. The mechanism for this is not known. This fact should be borne in mind when treating all patients and especially known diabetics.

Patients with a history of treatment for mental depression should be carefully monitored while receiving Provera therapy. Some patients may complain of premenstrual like depression while on Provera therapy.

4.5 Interaction with other medicinal products and other forms of interaction

Aminoglutethimide administered concurrently with Provera may significantly depress the bioavailability of Provera.

Interactions with other medicinal treatments (including oral anti-coagulants) have rarely been reported, but causality has not been determined. The possibility of interaction should be borne in mind in patients receiving concurrent treatment with other drugs.

4.6 Pregnancy and lactation

A negative pregnancy test should be demonstrated before starting therapy.

Medroxyprogesterone acetate and its metabolites are secreted in breast milk, but there is no evidence to suggest that this presents any hazard to the child.

4.7 Effects on ability to drive and use machines

No adverse effect has been reported.

4.8 Undesirable effects

The following medical events, listed in order of seriousness rather than frequency of occurrence, have been occasionally to rarely associated with the use of progestogens:

Rare anaphylactoid-like reactions.

Psychic: nervousness, insomnia, somnolence, fatigue, depression, dizziness and headache.

Skin and mucous membranes: urticaria, pruritus, rash, acne, hirsutism and alopecia.

Gastro-intestinal: nausea.

Breast: tenderness and galactorrhoea.

Miscellaneous: change in weight.

4.9 Overdose

In animals Provera has been shown to be capable of exerting an adreno-corticoid effect, but this has not been reported in the human, following usual dosages. The oral administration of Provera at a rate of 100 mg per day has been shown to have no effect on adrenal function.

5. PHARMACOLOGICAL PROPERTIES

5.1 Pharmacodynamic properties

Medroxyprogesterone acetate has actions and uses similar to those of progesterone.

MPA has minimal androgenic activity compared to progesterone and virtually no oestrogenic activity.

Progestogens are used in the treatment of dysfunctional uterine bleeding, secondary amenorrhoea and endometriosis.

5.2 Pharmacokinetic properties

MPA is rapidly absorbed from the G-I tract with a single oral dose of 10-250 mg. The time taken to reach the peak serum concentration (Tmax) was 2-6 hours and the average peak serum concentration (Cmax) was 13-46.89 mg/ml.

Unmetabolised MPA is highly plasma protein bound. MPA is metabolised in the liver.

MPA is primarily metabolised by faecal excretion as glucuronide conjugated metabolite.

Metabolised MPA is excreted more rapidly and in a greater percentage following oral doses than after aqueous intramuscular injection.

5.3 Preclinical safety data

None stated

6. PHARMACEUTICAL PARTICULARS

6.1 List of excipients

2.5 mg: Lactose Ph.Eur., Sucrose Ph.Eur., Maize starch Ph.Eur., Liquid Paraffin

Ph.Eur., Talc Ph.Eur., Calcium Stearate NF, E110,

Purified Water Ph.Eur.

5 mg: Lactose Ph.Eur., Starch Ph.Eur., Sucrose Ph.Eur., Liquid Paraffin

Ph.Eur., Calcium Stearate NF, Talc, FD & C Blue No. 2 Aluminium Lake,

Purified Water Ph.Eur.

10 mg: Lactose Ph.Eur., Sucrose Ph.Eur., Maize starch Ph.Eur., Liquid Paraffin

Ph.Eur., Talc Ph.Eur., Calcium Stearate NF, Purified Water Ph.Eur.

6.2 Incompatibilities

None known.

6.3 Shelf life

2.5 mg: 36 months

5 mg: 24 months if stored in blister strips

60 months if stored in either amber glass bottles with screw caps of

HDPE bottles with tamper evident caps.

10 mg: 5 years

6.4 Special precautions for storage

2.5mg & 5mg: Store bottle pack at controlled room temperature (15-30°C)

Store blister pack below 25°C

10mg: Glass bottles: None

Blister packs: Store below 25°C

6.5 Nature and contents of container

2.5 mg: HDPE tamper-evident bottles with LDPE push-fit tamper evident caps, containing 100 tablets.

Aluminium foil/PVC blisters, containing 10, 30, 50 or 100 tablets.

5 mg: Blister strips of 250 micron opaque PVC/20 micron aluminium foil containing 10, 20 or 100 tablets or amber glass bottles with screw caps or HDPE bottles with tamper evident caps containing

100 tablets.

10 mg: HDPE tamper-evident bottles with LDPE push-fit tamper evident caps, containing 50 tablets.

Aluminium foil/PVC blisters, containing 10, 20, 30, 50, 90 or 100 tablets.

6.6 Special precautions for disposal and other handling

None.

Administrative Data

7. MARKETING AUTHORISATION HOLDER

Pharmacia Limited

Ramsgate road

Sandwich

CT13 9NJ

UK

8. MARKETING AUTHORISATION NUMBER(S)

2.5 mg: PL 0032/0168

5 mg: PL 0032/5035R

10 mg: PL 0032/0151

9. DATE OF FIRST AUTHORISATION/RENEWAL OF THE AUTHORISATION

2.5 mg: Date of first authorisation: 28 May 1992

Renewal of authorisation: 06 January 2009

5 mg: Date of first authorisation: 8 January 1988

Renewal of authorisation: 01 December 2008

10 mg: Date of first authorisation: 8 January 1991

Renewal of authorisation: 11 March 2009

10. DATE OF REVISION OF THE TEXT

March 2009

Company Reference: PVA2_0

Provigil 100 mg Tablets, Provigil 200 mg Tablets

(Cephalon (UK) Limited)

1. NAME OF THE MEDICINAL PRODUCT

PROVIGIL®▼ 100 mg tablets

PROVIGIL®▼200 mg tablets

2. QUALITATIVE AND QUANTITATIVE COMPOSITION

Modafinil 100 mg per tablet.

Modafinil 200 mg per tablet.

For excipients, see 6.1.

3. PHARMACEUTICAL FORM

Tablet

White to off-white, capsule-shaped tablets, debossed with "PROVIGIL" on one side and "100 MG" on the other.

White to off-white, scored, capsule-shaped tablets, debossed with "PROVIGIL" on one side and "200 MG" on the other.

4. CLINICAL PARTICULARS

4.1 Therapeutic indications

PROVIGIL is indicated for the symptomatic relief of excessive sleepiness associated with:

- Narcolepsy
- Obstructive sleep apnoea/hypopnoea syndrome (OSAHS)
- Moderate to severe chronic shift work sleep disorder (SWSD).

Excessive sleepiness is defined as difficulty maintaining wakefulness and an increased likelihood of falling asleep in inappropriate situations.

Diagnosis of SWSD should be made according to the International Classification of Sleep Disorders (ICSD) guideline. The moderate to severe subgroup of patients with SWSD for whom Provigil is indicated is defined by the inclusion criteria in the pivotal clinical trials. See section 5.1 (Pharmacodynamic properties) for further details on these criteria.

4.2 Posology and method of administration

For oral use. Tablets should be swallowed whole.

Adults

Narcolepsy and Obstructive Sleep Apnoea / Hypopnoea Syndrome

The recommended daily dose is 200-400 mg, commencing at 200 mg and titrated according to clinical response. PROVIGIL may be taken as two divided doses in the morning and at noon, or as a single dose in the morning, according to physician assessment of the patient and the patient's response.

For patients with OSAHS, PROVIGIL treats the symptom of excessive daytime sleepiness associated with the condition. In addition to this symptomatic treatment, disease-modifying interventions (e.g., Continuous Positive Airway Pressure) should be commenced or continued.

Moderate to Severe Chronic Shift Work Sleep Disorder

The recommended daily dose is 200 mg. PROVIGIL should be taken as a single dose approximately 1 hour prior to the start of the work shift. PROVIGIL should be taken intermittently (i.e. only on the shifts worked).

Elderly

There are limited data available on the use of PROVIGIL in elderly patients. In view of the generally lower hepatic and renal clearance expected in an elderly population, it is recommended that patients over 65 years of age should commence therapy at 100 mg daily. The maximum dose of 400 mg per day should only be used in the absence of renal or hepatic impairment.

Hepatic and renal failure

The dose in patients with severe hepatic or renal failure should be reduced by half (100-200 mg per day).

Children

Because safety and effectiveness in controlled studies in children have not been established the use of PROVIGIL is not recommended in children (see section 4.4).

Additional information for the safe use of this product

Treatment should be initiated by or under the supervision of a physician with appropriate knowledge of relevant sleep disorders.

PROVIGIL treats the symptom of excessive sleepiness associated with the above conditions. Where appropriate, every effort should be made to treat the underlying condition prior to initiating treatment with PROVIGIL.

In patients with excessive sleepiness due to moderate to severe chronic SWSD, appropriate steps to ensure adequate sleep should be taken prior to determining the requirement for PROVIGIL.

4.3 Contraindications

PROVIGIL is contraindicated for use during pregnancy and lactation, or in patients with uncontrolled moderate to severe hypertension, or arrhythmia. PROVIGIL is also contraindicated in patients with known hypersensitivity to PROVIGIL or any component of the preparation.

4.4 Special warnings and precautions for use

Serious rash requiring hospitalisation and discontinuation of treatment has been reported with the use of modafinil, occurring within 1 to 5 weeks after treatment initiation (isolated cases have been reported after prolonged treatment (e.g., 3 months). In clinical trials of modafinil, the incidence of rash resulting in discontinuation was approximately 0.8% (13 per 1,585) in paediatric patients (age <17 years)); this includes serious rash. No serious skin rashes have been reported in adult clinical trials (0 per 4,264) of modafinil. Modafinil should be discontinued at the first sign of rash and not re-started (see section 4.8).

Patients with major anxiety should only receive treatment with PROVIGIL in a specialist unit.

Psychiatric adverse experiences, including suicidal ideation, have been reported in patients treated with modafinil. In such circumstances, Modafinil should be discontinued and not re-started. Caution should be exercised in administering modafinil to patients with a history of psychosis, depression or mania, given the possible emergence or exacerbation of psychiatric symptoms (see section 4.8).

Caution should also be exercised in administering modafinil to patients with history of alcohol, drug or illicit substance abuse.

Sexually active women of child-bearing potential should be established on a contraceptive programme before taking PROVIGIL. Since the effectiveness of steroidal contraceptives may be reduced when used with PROVIGIL, alternative or concomitant methods of contraception are recommended, and for two months after discontinuation of PROVIGIL (also see 4.5 with respect to potential interaction with steroidal contraceptives).

Blood pressure and heart rate should be monitored in hypertensive patients.

It is recommended that PROVIGIL tablets not be used in patients with a history of left ventricular hypertrophy or cor pulmonale. PROVIGIL should not be used in patients with mitral valve prolapse who have experienced the mitral valve prolapse syndrome when previously receiving CNS stimulants. This syndrome may present with ischaemic ECG changes, chest pain or arrhythmia.

In patients with obstructive sleep apnoea / hypopnoea syndrome, the underlying condition and any associated cardiovascular pathology should be monitored.

Patients should be advised that PROVIGIL is not a replacement for sleep and good sleep hygiene should be maintained. Steps to ensure good sleep hygiene may include a review of caffeine intake.

Whilst studies with modafinil have demonstrated a low potential for dependence, the possibility of dependence with long-term use cannot be entirely excluded.

PROVIGIL tablets contain lactose and therefore should not be used in patients with rare hereditary problems of galactose intolerance, the Lapp lactase deficiency, or glucose-galactose malabsorption.

4.5 Interaction with other medicinal products and other forms of interaction

Modafinil may increase its own metabolism via induction of CYP3A4/5 activity but the effect is modest and unlikely to have significant clinical consequences.

Anticonvulsants: Co-administration of potent inducers of CYP activity, such as carbamazepine and phenobarbital, could reduce the plasma levels of modafinil. Due to a possible inhibition of CYP2C19 by modafinil and suppression of CYP2C9 the clearance of phenytoin may be decreased when PROVIGIL is administered concomitantly. Patients should be monitored for signs of phenytoin toxicity, and repeated measurements of phenytoin plasma levels may be appropriate upon initiation or discontinuation of treatment with PROVIGIL.

Steroidal contraceptives: The effectiveness of steroidal contraceptives may be impaired due to induction of CYP3A4/5 by modafinil. Alternative or concomitant methods of contraception are recommended for patients treated with PROVIGIL. Adequate contraception will require continuation of these methods for two months after stopping PROVIGIL.

Antidepressants: A number of tricyclic antidepressants and selective serotonin reuptake inhibitors are largely metabolised by CYP2D6. In patients deficient in CYP2D6 (approximately 10% of a Caucasian population) a normally ancillary metabolic pathway involving CYP2C19 becomes more important. As modafinil may inhibit CYP2C19, lower doses of antidepressants may be required in such patients.

Anticoagulants: Due to possible suppression of CYP2C9 by modafinil the clearance of warfarin may be decreased when PROVIGIL is administered concomitantly. Prothrombin times should be monitored regularly during the first 2 months of PROVIGIL use and after changes in PROVIGIL dosage.

Other drugs: Drugs that are largely eliminated via CYP2C19 metabolism, such as diazepam, propranolol and omeprazole may have reduced clearance upon co-administration of PROVIGIL and may thus require dosage reduction. In addition, *in vitro* induction of CYP1A2, CYP2B6 and CYP3A4/5 activities has been observed in human hepatocytes, which were it to occur *in vivo*, could decrease the blood levels of drugs metabolised by these enzymes, thereby possibly decreasing their therapeutic effectiveness. Results from clinical interaction studies suggest that the largest effects may be on substrates of CYP3A4/5 that undergo significant presystemic elimination, particularly via CYP3A enzymes in the gastrointestinal tract. Examples include ciclosporin, HIV-protease inhibitors, buspirone, triazolam, midazolam and most of the calcium channel blockers and statins. In a case report, a 50% reduction in ciclosporin concentration was observed in a patient receiving ciclosporin in whom concurrent treatment with modafinil was initiated.

4.6 Pregnancy and lactation

There are no adequate data from the use of modafinil in pregnant women.

Modafinil was non-teratogenic in rats and rabbits at doses greater than the maximum clinical dose. However, plasma levels in preclinical studies, due to metabolic auto-induction, were less than or similar to that expected in patients.

Modafinil and its acid and sulphone metabolites pass into milk of lactating rats (see 5.3). It is not known whether modafinil passes into human milk.

Modafinil use during pregnancy and lactation is contra-indicated.

4.7 Effects on ability to drive and use machines

There is no information available concerning the effects of PROVIGIL on vehicle driving and/or the ability to use machinery. Undesirable effects such as blurred vision or dizziness might affect ability to drive (see 4.8 Undesirable Effects).

4.8 Undesirable effects

The following undesirable effects have been reported in clinical trials and/or post-marketing experience. The frequency of undesirable effects considered at least possibly related to treatment, in clinical trials involving 1561 patients taking PROVIGIL were as follows: very common $\geqslant$ 1/10, common $\geqslant$ 1/100 to $\leqslant$ 1/10, uncommon $\geqslant$ 1/1000 to $\leqslant$ 1/100, unknown (cannot be estimated from available data).

The most commonly reported adverse drug reaction is headache, affecting approximately 21% of patients. This is usually mild or moderate, dose-dependent and disappears within a few days.

Investigations

Common: abnormal liver function tests, dose related increases in alkaline phosphatase and gamma glutamyl transferase have been observed.

Uncommon: abnormal ECG, weight increase, weight decrease

Cardiac disorders

Common: tachycardia, palpitation

Uncommon: extrasystoles, arrhythmia, bradycardia

Blood and lymphatic system disorders

Uncommon: eosinophilia, leucopenia

Nervous system disorders

Very common: headache

Common: dizziness, somnolence, paraesthesia

Uncommon: dyskinesia, hypertonia, hyperkinesia, amnesia, migraine, tremor, vertigo, CNS stimulation, hypoaesthesia, incoordination, movement disorder, speech disorder, taste perversion

Eye disorders

Common: blurred vision

Uncommon: abnormal vision, dry eye

Respiratory, thoracic and mediastinal disorders

Uncommon: dyspnoea, increased cough, asthma, epistaxis, rhinitis

Gastrointestinal disorders

Common: abdominal pain, nausea, dry mouth, diarrhoea, dyspepsia, constipation

Uncommon: flatulence, reflux, vomiting, dysphagia, glossitis, mouth ulcers

Renal and urinary disorders

Uncommon: abnormal urine, urinary frequency

Skin and subcutaneous tissue disorders

Uncommon: sweating, rash, acne, pruritis

Unknown: serious skin reactions, including erythema multiforme, Stevens-Johnson Syndrome, Toxic Epidermal Necrolysis, and Drug Rash with Eosinophilia and Systemic Symptoms (DRESS).

Musculoskeletal and connective tissue disorders

Uncommon: back pain, neck pain, myalgia, myasthenia, leg cramps, arthralgia, twitch

Metabolism and nutrition disorders

Common: decreased appetite

Uncommon: hypercholesterolaemia, hyperglycaemia, diabetes mellitus, increased appetite,

Infections and infestations

Uncommon: pharyngitis, sinusitis

Vascular disorders:

Common: vasodilatation

Uncommon: hypertension, hypotension

General disorders and administration site conditions

Common: asthenia, chest pain

Uncommon: peripheral oedema, thirst

Immune system disorders

Uncommon: minor allergic reaction (e.g., hayfever symptoms)

Unknown: Angioedema, urticaria (hives). Hypersensitivity reactions (characterised by features such as fever, rash, lymphadenopathy and evidence of other concurrent organ involvement).

Reproductive system and breast disorders

Uncommon: menstrual disorder

Psychiatric disorders

Common: nervousness, insomnia, anxiety, depression, abnormal thinking, confusion

Uncommon: sleep disorder, emotional lability, decreased libido, hostility, depersonalisation, personality disorder, agitation, abnormal dreams, aggression.

Unknown: psychosis, mania, delusions, hallucinations and suicidal ideation.

4.9 Overdose

Symptoms most often accompanying modafinil overdose, alone or in combination with other drugs have included: insomnia; central nervous system symptoms such as restlessness, disorientation, confusion, excitation and hallucination; digestive changes such as nausea and diarrhoea; and cardiovascular changes such as tachycardia, bradycardia, hypertension and chest pain.

Management:

Induced emesis or gastric lavage should be considered. Hospitalisation and surveillance of psychomotor status; cardiovascular monitoring or surveillance until the patient's symptoms have resolved are recommended.

5. PHARMACOLOGICAL PROPERTIES

5.1 Pharmacodynamic properties

Therapeutic class: centrally acting sympathomimetic (ATC Code: N06BA07).

Modafinil promotes wakefulness in a variety of species, including man. The precise mechanism(s) through which modafinil promotes wakefulness is unknown.

In pre-clinical models, modafinil does not appear to be a direct or indirect acting alpha$_1$-adrenoceptor or dopamine receptor agonist. The wakefulness induced by amfetamine, but not by modafinil, is antagonised by the dopamine receptor antagonist haloperidol. Equal wakefulness-promoting doses of methylphenidate and amfetamine increase neuronal activation throughout the brain, but modafinil selectively and prominently increases neuronal activation in more discrete regions of the brain, especially in the hypothalamus.

In man, modafinil restores and/or improves the level and duration of wakefulness and daytime alertness in a dose-related manner. Administration of modafinil results in electrophysiological changes indicative of increased alertness and improvements in objective measures of ability to sustain wakefulness. Modafinil opposes the impairment of cognitive, psychomotor and neurosensorial performance induced by sleep deprivation. These changes are produced without any adverse changes in behaviour and appetite.

In patients with narcolepsy, morning administration of 400 mg modafinil or administration of 200 mg modafinil in the morning and at noon does not adversely affect nocturnal sleep.

Excessive sleepiness (ES) is defined as difficulty maintaining wakefulness and an increased likelihood of falling asleep in inappropriate situations. ES can be demonstrated by an Epworth Sleepiness Scale score of 11 or more.

Moderate sleepiness describes sleep episodes that are present daily and occur during very mild physical activity requiring, at most, a moderate degree of attention. Onset of sleep may occur for example during concerts, films at the cinema, theatre performances, group meetings and driving. This degree of sleepiness is usually associated with a Multiple Sleep Latency Test (MSLT) mean sleep latency of 5 to 10 minutes. Severe sleepiness describes sleep episodes that are present daily and occur during very mild physical activity requiring mild to moderate attention. Onset of sleep may occur for example during eating, direct personal conversation, driving, walking and physical activities. This degree of sleepiness is usually associated with an MSLT mean sleep latency of less than 5 minutes.

Shift Work Sleep Disorder (SWSD) is recognised as a clinical situation where persistent inability to adjust to changes in work schedules produces transient symptoms of insomnia or excessive sleepiness. All subjects in the pivotal clinical trials for SWSD had a clinical diagnosis made according to ICSD criteria (first edition). Essential criteria include a primary complaint of excessive sleepiness or insomnia which is temporally associated with a work period (usually night work) that occurs during the habitual sleep phase. The symptoms are not accounted for by any other medical or mental disorder and do not meet criteria for any other sleep disorder producing insomnia or excessive sleepiness. Polysomnography and the MSLT demonstrate loss of a normal sleep-wake pattern (i.e., disturbed chronobiological rhythmicity).

In the pivotal clinical trials subjects worked at least 5 night shifts per month of which at least 3 were consecutive and complained of excessive sleepiness in relation to these shifts over a period of at least 3 months. The moderate to severe subgroup of patients with SWSD for whom Provigil is indicated is defined by the inclusion criteria in the pivotal clinical trials. These criteria included a CGI-S (Clinical Global Impression of Severity) rating of at least "moderately ill" (relating to ES on shift nights) at baseline, a mean sleep latency of no more than 6 minutes on the Multiple Sleep Latency Test (MSLT) and no more than 87.5% sleep efficiency (time sleeping/time in bed).

5.2 Pharmacokinetic properties

Modafinil is a racemic compound, whose enantiomers have different pharmacokinetics. The half-life of *l*-modafinil is approximately three times that of the *d* enantiomer, as is the total systemic exposure (AUC) to *l*-modafinil. Apparent steady state is reached after 2-4 days of dosing.

Absorption

Modafinil is readily absorbed, with peak plasma concentrations occurring at 2-4 hours. Food has no effect on overall modafinil bioavailability but t_{max} may be delayed by approximately one hour if PROVIGIL is taken with food.

Distribution

Modafinil is well distributed in body tissue with an apparent volume of distribution larger than the volume of total body water. In human plasma, *in vitro*, modafinil is moderately bound to plasma protein (approximately 60%, mainly to albumin). This degree of protein binding is such that the risk of interaction with strongly bound drugs is unlikely.

Biotransformation

Modafinil is metabolised in the liver to two major metabolites, modafinil acid and modafinil sulphone, by esterase enzymes and CYP3A4/5, respectively. In preclinical models, the metabolites did not appear to contribute to the arousal effects of modafinil. *In vitro* studies using human hepatocytes have demonstrated that modafinil slightly induces the following in a concentration-dependent manner: CYP1A2, CYP2B6 and CYP3A4. In addition, the activity of CYP2C9 was suppressed in the hepatocytes. In human liver microsomes, modafinil and modafinil sulphone produced partial competitive, reversible inhibition of CYP2C19 at concentrations expected during clinical use (see 4.5).

Elimination

The excretion of modafinil and its metabolites is chiefly renal, with a small proportion being eliminated unchanged (< 10%). The elimination half-life of modafinil after multiple doses is 15 hours and enables a treatment regimen based upon 1 or 2 doses per day.

Linearity/non-linearity

The pharmacokinetics of modafinil are linear and independent of the dose administered in the dose range of 200 to 600 mg once daily. Systemic exposure increases in proportion to doses administered.

Renal failure/hepatic impairment

In severe chronic renal failure the pharmacokinetics of modafinil were unaltered but exposure to modafinil acid was increased 9 fold (see 4.2). There is minimal information available regarding the safety of such levels of this metabolite. In patients with severe hepatic impairment, oral clearance of modafinil was decreased by about 60% and the steady state concentration of modafinil was doubled. The dose of PROVIGIL should be reduced by half in patients with severe hepatic or renal impairment (see 4.2).

Elderly

Elderly patients may have diminished renal and/or hepatic function and dosage reductions should be considered (see 4.2).

5.3 Preclinical safety data

Toxicology studies by single and repeated dosing have revealed no particular toxic action in animals.

Reproduction function studies have revealed no effect on fertility, nor any teratogenic effect, nor any effect on viability, growth or development of the offspring.

Modafinil is not considered to be mutagenic or carcinogenic.

Animal exposure to modafinil, based on actual plasma levels in the general toxicology, reproductive and carcinogenicity studies, was less than or similar to that expected in humans. This circumstance is the result of metabolic autoinduction noted in the pre-clinical studies. However, animal exposure on a mg/kg dose basis to modafinil in the general toxicology, reproductive and carcinogenicity studies was greater than the expected exposure, calculated on a similar basis, in humans.

In the rat peri-post-natal study, modafinil concentration in milk was about 11.5 times higher than in plasma.

6. PHARMACEUTICAL PARTICULARS

6.1 List of excipients

Lactose monohydrate

Pregelatinised starch

Microcrystalline cellulose

Croscarmellose sodium

Povidone K29/32

Magnesium stearate

6.2 Incompatibilities

Not applicable

6.3 Shelf life

Three years.

6.4 Special precautions for storage

No special precautions for storage.

6.5 Nature and contents of container

Opaque PVC/PVDC/Aluminium blisters containing 10 tablets

Packs containing 30, 60 or 90 tablets.

Not all pack sizes may be marketed.

6.6 Special precautions for disposal and other handling

Not applicable

7. MARKETING AUTHORISATION HOLDER

Cephalon UK Limited

1 Albany Place

Hyde Way

Welwyn Garden City

Hertfordshire

AL7 3BT

United Kingdom

8. MARKETING AUTHORISATION NUMBER(S)

Provigil 100 mg tablets - PL 16260/0001

Provigil 200 mg tablets - PL 16260/0002

9. DATE OF FIRST AUTHORISATION/RENEWAL OF THE AUTHORISATION

PL 16260/0001 - 14 October 1997 / 14 October 2002

PL 16260/0002 – 2 December 2002 / 23 January 2009

10. DATE OF REVISION OF THE TEXT

PL 16260/0001 - February 2008

PL 16260/0002 – 23 January 2009

Provigil and Cephalon are registered trademarks.

Prozac 20mg hard capsules, and 20mg per 5ml oral liquid

(Eli Lilly and Company Limited)

1. NAME OF THE MEDICINAL PRODUCT

PROZAC* 20mg hard capsules.

PROZAC 20mg per 5ml oral liquid.

2. QUALITATIVE AND QUANTITATIVE COMPOSITION

Each capsule contains fluoxetine hydrochloride equivalent to 20mg of fluoxetine.

Each 5ml of oral liquid contains fluoxetine hydrochloride equivalent to 20mg of fluoxetine.

Oral liquid excipients: contains 3g of sucrose per 5ml dose. This should be taken into account in patients with diabetes mellitus.

For a full list of excipients, see section 6.1.

3. PHARMACEUTICAL FORM

Hard capsules.

The capsules are green and yellow, printed 'Lilly 3105'.

Oral liquid (clear, colourless, mint odoured).

4. CLINICAL PARTICULARS

4.1 Therapeutic indications

Adults:

Major depressive episodes.

Obsessive-compulsive disorder.

Bulimia nervosa: PROZAC is indicated as a complement of psychotherapy for the reduction of binge-eating and purging activity.

Children and Adolescents Aged 8 Years and Above:

Moderate to severe major depressive episode, if depression is unresponsive to psychological therapy after 4-6 sessions. Antidepressant medication should be offered to a child or young person with moderate to severe depression only in combination with a concurrent psychological therapy.

4.2 Posology and method of administration

For oral administration.

Major depressive episodes

Adults and the elderly: The recommended dose is 20mg daily. Dosage should be reviewed and adjusted if necessary, within 3 to 4 weeks of initiation of therapy and thereafter as judged clinically appropriate. Although there may be an increased potential for undesirable effects at higher doses, in some patients, with insufficient response to 20mg, the dose may be increased gradually up to a maximum of 60mg (see section 5.1). Dosage adjustments should be made carefully on an individual patient basis, to maintain the patients at the lowest effective dose.

Patients with depression should be treated for a sufficient period of at least 6 months to ensure that they are free from symptoms.

Obsessive-compulsive disorder

Adults and the elderly: The recommended dose is 20mg daily. Although there may be an increased potential for undesirable effects at higher doses, in some patients, if after two weeks there is insufficient response to 20mg, the dose may be increased gradually up to a maximum of 60mg.

If no improvement is observed within 10 weeks, treatment with fluoxetine should be reconsidered. If a good therapeutic response has been obtained, treatment can be continued at a dosage adjusted on an individual basis. While there are no systematic studies to answer the question of how long to continue fluoxetine treatment, OCD is a chronic condition and it is reasonable to consider continuation beyond 10 weeks in responding patients. Dosage adjustments should be made carefully on an individual patient basis, to maintain the patient at the lowest effective dose. The need for treatment should be reassessed periodically. Some clinicians advocate concomitant behavioural psychotherapy for patients who have done well on pharmacotherapy.

Long-term efficacy (more than 24 weeks) has not been demonstrated in OCD.

Bulimia nervosa: Adults and the elderly: A dose of 60mg/day is recommended. Long-term efficacy (more than 3 months) has not been demonstrated in bulimia nervosa.

All indications: Adults: The recommended dose may be increased or decreased. Doses above 80mg/day have not been systematically evaluated.

Fluoxetine may be administered as a single or divided dose, during or between meals.

When dosing is stopped, active drug substances will persist in the body for weeks. This should be borne in mind when starting or stopping treatment.

The capsule and liquid dosage forms are bioequivalent.

Children and adolescents aged 8 years and above (moderate to severe major depressive episode):

Treatment should be initiated and monitored under specialist supervision. The starting dose is 10mg/day given as 2.5ml of the PROZAC liquid formulation. Dose adjustments should be made carefully, on an individual basis, to maintain the patient at the lowest effective dose.

After one to two weeks, the dose may be increased to 20mg/day. Clinical trial experience with daily doses greater than 20mg is minimal. There is only limited data on treatment beyond 9 weeks.

Lower-weight children: Due to higher plasma levels in lower-weight children, the therapeutic effect may be achieved with lower doses (see section 5.2).

For paediatric patients who respond to treatment, the need for continued treatment after 6 months should be reviewed.

If no clinical benefit is achieved within 9 weeks, treatment should be reconsidered.

Elderly: Caution is recommended when increasing the dose, and the daily dose should generally not exceed 40mg. Maximum recommended dose is 60mg/day.

A lower or less frequent dose (eg, 20mg every second day) should be considered in patients with hepatic impairment (see section 5.2), or in patients where concomitant medication has the potential for interaction with PROZAC (see section 4.5).

Withdrawal symptoms seen on discontinuation of PROZAC: Abrupt discontinuation should be avoided. When stopping treatment with PROZAC the dose should be gradually reduced over a period of at least one to two weeks in order to reduce the risk of withdrawal reactions (see section 4.4 and section 4.8). If intolerable symptoms occur following a decrease in the dose or upon discontinuation of treatment, then resuming the previously prescribed dose may be considered. Subsequently, the physician may continue decreasing the dose, but at a more gradual rate.

4.3 Contraindications

Hypersensitivity to fluoxetine or to any of its excipients.

Monoamine oxidase inhibitors: Cases of serious and sometimes fatal reactions have been reported in patients receiving an SSRI in combination with a monoamine oxidase inhibitor (MAOI), and in patients who have recently discontinued an SSRI and have been started on a MAOI. Treatment of fluoxetine should only be started 2 weeks after discontinuation of an irreversible MAOI and the following day after discontinuation of a reversible MAOI-A.

Some cases presented with features resembling serotonin syndrome (which may resemble and be diagnosed as neuroleptic malignant syndrome). Cyproheptadine or dantrolene may benefit patients experiencing such reactions. Symptoms of a drug interaction with a MAOI include: hyperthermia, rigidity, myoclonus, autonomic instability with possible rapid fluctuations of vital signs, mental status changes that include confusion, irritability and extreme agitation, progressing to delirium and coma.

Therefore, fluoxetine is contra-indicated in combination with a non-selective MAOI. Similarly, at least 5 weeks should elapse after discontinuing fluoxetine treatment before starting a MAOI. If fluoxetine has been prescribed chronically and/or at a high dose, a longer interval should be considered.

The combination of fluoxetine with a reversible MAOI (eg, moclobemide) is not recommended. Treatment with fluoxetine can be initiated the following day after discontinuation of a reversible MAOI.

4.4 Special warnings and precautions for use

Use in children and adolescents under 18 years of age: Suicide-related behaviours (suicide attempt and suicidal thoughts) and hostility (predominantly aggression, oppositional behaviour and anger) were more frequently observed in clinical trials among children and adolescents treated with antidepressants compared to those treated with placebo. PROZAC should only be used in children and adolescents aged 8 to 18 years for the treatment of moderate to severe major depressive episodes and it should not be used in other indications. If, based on clinical need, a decision to treat is nevertheless taken, the patient should be carefully monitored for the appearance of suicidal symptoms. In addition, only limited evidence is available concerning long-term effect on safety in children and adolescents, including effects on growth, sexual maturation and cognitive, emotional and behavioural developments (see section 5.3).

In a 19-week clinical trial, decreased height and weight gain was observed in children and adolescents treated with fluoxetine (see section 4.8). It has not been established whether there is an effect on achieving normal adult height. The possibility of a delay in puberty cannot be ruled out (see sections 5.3 and 4.8). Growth and pubertal development (height, weight, and TANNER staging) should therefore be monitored during and after treatment with fluoxetine. If either is slowed, referral to a paediatrician should be considered.

In paediatric trials, mania and hypomania were commonly reported (see section 4.8). Therefore, regular monitoring for the occurrence of mania/hypomania is recommended. Fluoxetine should be discontinued in any patient entering a manic phase.

It is important that the prescriber discusses carefully the risks and benefits of treatment with the child/young person and/or their parents.

Rash and allergic reactions: Rash, anaphylactoid events and progressive systemic events, sometimes serious (involving skin, kidney, liver or lung), have been reported. Upon the appearance of rash or of other allergic phenomena for which an alternative aetiology cannot be identified, fluoxetine should be discontinued.

Seizures: Seizures are a potential risk with antidepressant drugs. Therefore, as with other antidepressants, fluoxetine should be introduced cautiously in patients who have a history of seizures. Treatment should be discontinued in any patient who develops seizures or where there is an increase in seizure frequency. Fluoxetine should be avoided in patients with unstable seizure disorders/

epilepsy and patients with controlled epilepsy should be carefully monitored.

Mania: Antidepressants should be used with caution in patients with a history of mania/hypomania. As with all antidepressants, fluoxetine should be discontinued in any patient entering a manic phase.

Hepatic/Renal function: Fluoxetine is extensively metabolised by the liver and excreted by the kidneys. A lower dose, eg, alternate day dosing, is recommended in patients with significant hepatic dysfunction. When given fluoxetine 20mg/day for 2 months, patients with severe renal failure (GFR <10ml/min) requiring dialysis showed no difference in plasma levels of fluoxetine or norfluoxetine compared to controls with normal renal function.

Cardiac disease: No conduction abnormalities that resulted in heart block were observed in the ECG of 312 patients who received fluoxetine in double-blind clinical trials. However, clinical experience in acute cardiac disease is limited; therefore, caution is advisable.

Weight loss: Weight loss may occur in patients taking fluoxetine but it is usually proportional to baseline body weight.

Diabetes: In patients with diabetes, treatment with an SSRI may alter glycaemic control. Hypoglycaemia has occurred during therapy with fluoxetine and hyperglycaemia has developed following discontinuation. Insulin and/or oral hypoglycaemic dosage may need to be adjusted.

Suicide/suicidal thoughts or clinical worsening: Depression is associated with an increased risk of suicidal thoughts, self-harm and suicide (suicide-related events). This risk persists until significant remission occurs. As improvement may not occur during the first few weeks or more of treatment, patients should be closely monitored until such improvement occurs. It is general clinical experience that the risk of suicide may increase in the early stages of recovery.

Other psychiatric conditions for which PROZAC is prescribed can also be associated with an increased risk of suicide-related events. In addition, these conditions may be co-morbid with major depressive disorder. The same precautions observed when treating patients with major depressive disorder should therefore be observed when treating patients with other psychiatric disorders.

Patients with a history of suicide-related events, those exhibiting a significant degree of suicidal ideation prior to commencement of treatment are known to be at greater risk of suicidal thoughts or suicide attempts, and should receive careful monitoring during treatment. A meta-analysis of placebo-controlled clinical trials of antidepressants drugs in adult patients with psychiatric disorders showed an increased risk of suicidal behaviour with antidepressants compared to placebo in patients less than 25 years old.

Close supervision of patients and in particular those at high risk should accompany drug therapy especially in early treatment and following dose changes.

Patients (and caregivers of patients) should be alerted about the need to monitor for any clinical worsening, suicidal behaviour or thoughts and unusual changes in behaviour and to seek medical advice immediately if these symptoms present.

Akathisia/psychomotor restlessness: The use of fluoxetine has been associated with the development of akathisia, characterised by a subjectively unpleasant or distressing restlessness and need to move, often accompanied by an inability to sit or stand still. This is most likely to occur within the first few weeks of treatment. In patients who develop these symptoms, increasing the dose may be detrimental.

Withdrawal symptoms seen on discontinuation of SSRI treatment: Withdrawal symptoms when treatment is discontinued are common, particularly if discontinuation is abrupt (see section 4.8). In clinical trials, adverse events seen on treatment discontinuation occurred in approximately 60% of patients in both the fluoxetine and placebo groups. Of these adverse events, 17% in the fluoxetine group and 12% in the placebo group were severe in nature.

The risk of withdrawal symptoms may be dependent on several factors, including the duration and dose of therapy and the rate of dose reduction. Dizziness, sensory disturbances (including paraesthesia), sleep disturbances (including insomnia and intense dreams), asthenia, agitation or anxiety, nausea and/or vomiting, tremor, and headache are the most commonly reported reactions. Generally, these symptoms are mild to moderate; however, in some patients they may be severe in intensity. They usually occur within the first few days of discontinuing treatment. Generally, these symptoms are self-limiting and usually resolve within 2 weeks, though in some individuals they may be prolonged (2-3 months or more). It is therefore advised that PROZAC should be gradually tapered when discontinuing treatment over a period of at least one to two weeks, according to the patient's needs (see '*Withdrawal symptoms seen on discontinuation of PROZAC*', section 4.2).

Haemorrhage: There have been reports of cutaneous bleeding abnormalities, such as ecchymosis and purpura with SSRIs. Ecchymosis has been reported as an infrequent event during treatment with fluoxetine. Other haemorrhagic manifestations (eg, gynaecological haemorrhages, gastro-intestinal bleedings and other cutaneous or mucous bleedings) have been reported rarely. Caution is advised in patients taking SSRIs, particularly in concomitant use with oral anticoagulants, drugs known to affect platelet function (eg, atypical antipsychotics, such as clozapine, phenothiazines, most TCAs, aspirin, NSAIDs), or other drugs that may increase risk of bleeding, as well as in patients with a history of bleeding disorders.

Electroconvulsive therapy (ECT): There have been rare reports of prolonged seizures in patients on fluoxetine receiving ECT treatment; therefore, caution is advisable.

St John's Wort: An increase in serotonergic effects, such as serotonin syndrome, may occur when selective serotonin reuptake inhibitors and herbal preparations containing St John's Wort (*Hypericum perforatum*) are used together.

On rare occasions, development of a serotonin syndrome or neuroleptic malignant syndrome-like events have been reported in association with treatment of fluoxetine, particularly when given in combination with other serotonergic (among others, L-tryptophan) and/or neuroleptic drugs. As these syndromes may result in potentially life-threatening conditions, treatment with fluoxetine should be discontinued if such events (characterised by clusters of symptoms, such as hyperthermia, rigidity, myoclonus, autonomic instability with possible rapid fluctuations of vital signs, mental status changes, including confusion, irritability, extreme agitation, progressing to delirium and coma) occur and supportive symptomatic treatment should be initiated.

PROZAC oral liquid contains sucrose: Patients with rare hereditary problems of fructose intolerance, glucose-galactose malabsorption or sucrase-isomaltase insufficiency should not take this medicine.

4.5 Interaction with other medicinal products and other forms of interaction

Interaction studies have only been performed in adults.

Half-life: The long elimination half-lives of both fluoxetine and norfluoxetine should be borne in mind (see section 5.2) when considering pharmacodynamic or pharmacokinetic drug interactions (eg, when switching from fluoxetine to other antidepressants).

Monoamine oxidase inhibitors: See section 4.3.

Not recommended combinations: MAOI-A (see section 4.3).

Combinations requiring precautions for use: MAOI-B (selegeline): Risk of serotonin syndrome. Clinical monitoring is recommended.

Phenytoin: Changes in blood levels have been observed when combined with fluoxetine. In some cases manifestations of toxicity have occurred. Consideration should be given to using conservative titration schedules of the concomitant drug and to monitoring clinical status.

Serotonergic drugs: Co-administration with serotonergic drugs (eg, tramadol, triptans) may increase the risk of serotonin syndrome. Use with triptans carries the additional risk of coronary vasoconstriction and hypertension.

Lithium and tryptophan: There have been reports of serotonin syndrome when SSRIs have been given with lithium or tryptophan and, therefore, the concomitant use of fluoxetine with these drugs should be undertaken with caution. When fluoxetine is used in combination with lithium, closer and more frequent clinical monitoring is required.

CYP2D6 isoenzyme: Because fluoxetine's metabolism (like tricyclic antidepressants and other selective serotonin antidepressants) involves the hepatic cytochrome CYP2D6 isoenzyme system, concomitant therapy with drugs also metabolised by this enzyme system may lead to drug interactions. Concomitant therapy with drugs predominantly metabolised by this isoenzyme, and which have a narrow therapeutic index (such as flecainide, encainide, carbamazepine and tricyclic antidepressants), should be initiated at or adjusted to the low end of their dose range. This will also apply if fluoxetine has been taken in the previous 5 weeks.

Oral anticoagulants: Altered anticoagulant effects (laboratory values and/or clinical signs and symptoms), with no consistent pattern, but including increased bleeding, have been reported uncommonly when fluoxetine is co-administered with oral anticoagulants. Patients receiving warfarin therapy should receive careful coagulation monitoring when fluoxetine is initiated or stopped (see section 4.4, '*Haemorrhage*').

Electroconvulsive therapy (ECT): There have been rare reports of prolonged seizures in patients on fluoxetine receiving ECT treatment; therefore, caution is advisable.

Alcohol: In formal testing, fluoxetine did not raise blood alcohol levels or enhance the effects of alcohol. However, the combination of SSRI treatment and alcohol is not advisable.

St John's Wort: In common with other SSRIs, pharmacodynamic interactions between fluoxetine and the herbal remedy St John's Wort (*Hypericum perforatum*) may occur, which may result in an increase of undesirable effects.

4.6 Pregnancy and lactation

Pregnancy: Data on a large number of exposed pregnancies do not indicate a teratogenic effect of fluoxetine. Fluoxetine can be used during pregnancy, but caution should be exercised, especially during late pregnancy or just prior to the onset of labour, since the following effects have been reported in neonates: irritability, tremor, hypotonia, persistent crying, difficulty in sucking or in sleeping. These symptoms may indicate either serotonergic effects or a withdrawal syndrome. The time to occur and the duration of these symptoms may be related to the long half-life of fluoxetine (4-6 days) and its active metabolite, norfluoxetine (4-16 days).

Lactation: Fluoxetine and its metabolite, norfluoxetine, are known to be excreted in human breast milk. Adverse events have been reported in breast-feeding infants. If treatment with fluoxetine is considered necessary, discontinuation of breast-feeding should be considered; however, if breast-feeding is continued, the lowest effective dose of fluoxetine should be prescribed.

4.7 Effects on ability to drive and use machines

Although fluoxetine has been shown not to affect psychomotor performance in healthy volunteers, any psychoactive drug may impair judgement or skills. Patients should be advised to avoid driving a car or operating hazardous machinery until they are reasonably certain that their performance is not affected.

4.8 Undesirable effects

Undesirable effects may decrease in intensity and frequency with continued treatment and do not generally lead to cessation of therapy.

In common with other SSRIs, the following undesirable effects have been seen:

Body as a whole: Hypersensitivity (eg, pruritus, rash, urticaria, anaphylactoid reaction, vasculitis, serum sickness-like reaction, angioedema) (see sections 4.3 and 4.4), chills, serotonin syndrome, photosensitivity and very rarely Erythema Multiforme that could progress to Stevens-Johnson syndrome or Toxic Epidermal Necrolysis (Lyell syndrome).

Digestive system: Gastro-intestinal disorders (eg, diarrhoea, nausea, vomiting, dyspepsia, dysphagia, taste perversion), dry mouth. Abnormal liver function tests have been reported rarely. Very rare cases of idiosyncratic hepatitis.

Nervous system: Headache, sleep abnormalities (eg, abnormal dreams, insomnia), dizziness, anorexia, fatigue (eg, somnolence, drowsiness), euphoria, transient abnormal movement (eg, twitching, ataxia, tremor, myoclonus), seizures and rarely, psychomotor restlessness/akathisia (see section 4.4). Hallucinations, manic reaction, confusion, agitation, anxiety and associated symptoms (eg, nervousness), impaired concentration and thought process (eg, depersonalisation), panic attacks, very rarely serotonin syndrome, suicidal thoughts and behaviour (these symptoms may be due to the underlying disease). Cases of suicidal ideation and suicidal behaviour have been reported during fluoxetine therapy or early after treatment discontinuation (see section 4.4).

Urogenital system: Urinary retention, urinary frequency.

Reproductive disorders: Sexual dysfunction (delayed or absent ejaculation, anorgasmia), priapism, galactorrhoea.

Miscellaneous: Alopecia, yawn, abnormal vision (eg, blurred vision, mydriasis), sweating, vasodilatation, arthralgia, myalgia, postural hypotension, ecchymosis. Other haemorrhagic manifestations (eg, gynaecological haemorrhages, gastro-intestinal bleedings and other cutaneous or mucous bleedings) have been reported rarely (see section 4.4, '*Haemorrhage*').

Hyponatraemia: Hyponatraemia (including serum sodium below 110mmol/l) has been rarely reported and appeared to be reversible when fluoxetine was discontinued. Some cases were possibly due to the syndrome of inappropriate antidiuretic hormone secretion. The majority of reports were associated with older patients, and patients taking diuretics or otherwise volume depleted.

Respiratory system: Pharyngitis, dyspnoea. Pulmonary events (including inflammatory processes of varying histopathology and/or fibrosis) have been reported rarely. Dyspnoea may be the only preceding symptom.

Withdrawal symptoms seen on discontinuation of fluoxetine treatments: Discontinuation of fluoxetine commonly leads to withdrawal symptoms. Dizziness, sensory disturbances (including paraesthesia), sleep disturbances (including insomnia and intense dreams), asthenia, agitation or anxiety, nausea and/or vomiting, tremor and headache are the most commonly reported reactions. Generally, these events are mild to moderate and are self-limiting; however, in some patients they may be severe and/or prolonged (see section 4.4). It is therefore advised that when PROZAC treatment is no longer required, gradual discontinuation by dose tapering should be carried out (see section 4.2 and section 4.4).

Children and adolescents (see section 4.4): In paediatric clinical trials, suicide-related behaviours (suicide attempt and suicidal thoughts) and hostility were more frequently observed among children and adolescents treated with antidepressants compared to those treated with placebo.

The safety of fluoxetine has not been systematically assessed for chronic treatment longer than 19 weeks.

In paediatric clinical trials, manic reactions, including mania and hypomania, were reported (2.6% of fluoxetine-treated patients versus 0% in placebo-controls), leading to discontinuation in the majority of cases. These patients had no prior episodes of hypomania/mania.

After 19 weeks of treatment, paediatric subjects treated with fluoxetine in a clinical trial gained an average of 1.1 cm less in height ($P = 0.004$) and 1.1 kg less in weight ($P = 0.008$) than subjects treated with placebo. Isolated cases of growth retardation have also been reported from clinical use.

Isolated cases of adverse events potentially indicating delayed sexual maturation or sexual dysfunction have been reported from paediatric clinical use (see also section 5.3).

In paediatric clinical trials, fluoxetine treatment was associated with a decrease in alkaline phosphatase levels.

4.9 Overdose

Cases of overdose of fluoxetine alone usually have a mild course. Symptoms of overdose have included nausea, vomiting, seizures, cardiovascular dysfunction ranging from asymptomatic arrhythmias to cardiac arrest, pulmonary dysfunction, and signs of altered CNS status ranging from excitation to coma. Fatality attributed to overdose of fluoxetine alone has been extremely rare. Cardiac and vital signs monitoring are recommended, along with general symptomatic and supportive measures. No specific antidote is known.

Forced diuresis, dialysis, haemoperfusion, and exchange transfusion are unlikely to be of benefit. Activated charcoal, which may be used with sorbitol, may be as or more effective than emesis or lavage. In managing overdosage, consider the possibility of multiple drug involvement. An extended time for close medical observation may be needed in patients who have taken excessive quantities of a tricyclic antidepressant if they are also taking, or have recently taken, fluoxetine.

5. PHARMACOLOGICAL PROPERTIES

5.1 Pharmacodynamic properties

Pharmacotherapeutic group: Selective serotonin reuptake inhibitors. *ATC code:* N06A B03.

Fluoxetine is a selective inhibitor of serotonin reuptake, and this probably accounts for the mechanism of action. Fluoxetine has practically no affinity to other receptors such as α_1-, α_2-, and β-adrenergic; serotonergic; dopaminergic; histaminergic$_1$; muscarinic; and GABA receptors.

Major depressive episodes: Clinical trials in patients with major depressive episodes have been conducted versus placebo and active controls. PROZAC has been shown to be significantly more effective than placebo, as measured by the Hamilton Depression Rating Scale (HAM-D). In these studies, PROZAC produced a significantly higher rate of response (defined by a 50% decrease in the HAM-D score) and remission compared to placebo.

Dose response: In the fixed dose studies of patients with major depression there is a flat dose response curve, providing no suggestion of advantage in terms of efficacy for using higher than the recommended doses. However, it is clinical experience that uptitrating might be beneficial for some patients.

Obsessive-compulsive disorder: In short-term trials (under 24 weeks), fluoxetine was shown to be significantly more effective than placebo. There was a therapeutic effect at 20mg/day, but higher doses (40 or 60mg/day) showed a higher response rate. In long-term studies (three short-term studies extension phase and a relapse prevention study), efficacy has not been shown.

Bulimia nervosa: In short-term trials (under 16 weeks), in out-patients fulfilling DSM-III-R-criteria for bulimia nervosa, fluoxetine 60mg/day was shown to be significantly more effective than placebo for the reduction of bingeing and purging activities. However, for long-term efficacy no conclusion can be drawn.

Two placebo-controlled studies were conducted in patients meeting pre-menstrual dysphoric disorder (PMDD) diagnostic criteria according to DSM-IV. Patients were included if they had symptoms of sufficient severity to impair social and occupational function and relationships with others. Patients using oral contraceptives were excluded. In the first study of continuous 20mg daily dosing for 6 cycles, improvement was observed in the primary efficacy parameter (irritability, anxiety and dysphoria). In the second study, with intermittent luteal phase dosing (20mg daily for 14 days) for 3 cycles, improvement was observed in the primary efficacy parameter (Daily Record of Severity of Problems score). However, definitive conclusions on efficacy and duration of treatment cannot be drawn from these studies.

Major depressive episodes (children and adolescents): Clinical trials in children and adolescents aged 8 years and above have been conducted versus placebo. PROZAC, at a dose of 20mg, has been shown to be significantly more effective than placebo in two short-term pivotal studies, as measured by the reduction of Childhood Depression Rating Scale-Revised (CDRS-R) total scores and Clinical Global Impression of Improvement (CGI-I) scores. In both studies, patients met criteria for moderate to severe MDD (DSM-III or DSM-IV) at three different evaluations by practising child psychiatrists. Efficacy in the fluoxetine trials may depend on the inclusion of a selective patient population (one that has not spontaneously recovered within a period of 3-5 weeks and whose depression persisted in the face of considerable attention). There is only limited data on safety and efficacy beyond 9 weeks. In general, efficacy of fluoxetine was modest. Response rates (the primary endpoint, defined as a 30% decrease in the CDRS-R score) demonstrated a statistically significant difference in one of the two pivotal studies (58% for fluoxetine versus 32% for placebo, $P = 0.013$; and 65% for fluoxetine versus 54% for placebo, $P = 0.093$). In these two studies, the mean absolute changes in CDRS-R from baseline to endpoint were 20 for fluoxetine versus 11 for placebo, $P = 0.002$; and 22 for fluoxetine versus 15 for placebo, $P < 0.001$.

5.2 Pharmacokinetic properties

Absorption: Fluoxetine is well absorbed from the gastro-intestinal tract after oral administration. The bioavailability is not affected by food intake.

Distribution: Fluoxetine is extensively bound to plasma proteins (about 95%) and it is widely distributed (volume of distribution: 20-40 l/kg). Steady-state plasma concentrations are achieved after dosing for several weeks. Steady-state concentrations after prolonged dosing are similar to concentrations seen at 4 to 5 weeks.

Metabolism: Fluoxetine has a non-linear pharmacokinetic profile with first pass liver effect. Maximum plasma concentration is generally achieved 6 to 8 hours after administration. Fluoxetine is extensively metabolised by the polymorphic enzyme CYP2D6. Fluoxetine is primarily metabolised by the liver to the active metabolite norfluoxetine (desmethylfluoxetine), by desmethylation.

Elimination: The elimination half-life of fluoxetine is 4 to 6 days and for norfluoxetine 4 to 16 days. These long half-lives are responsible for persistence of the drug for 5-6 weeks after discontinuation. Excretion is mainly (about 60%) via the kidney. Fluoxetine is secreted into breast milk.

At-Risk Populations

Elderly: Kinetic parameters are not altered in healthy elderly when compared to younger subjects.

Children and adolescents: The mean fluoxetine concentration in children is approximately 2-fold higher than that observed in adolescents and the mean norfluoxetine concentration 1.5-fold higher. Steady-state plasma concentrations are dependent on body weight and are higher in lower weight children (see section 4.2). As in adults, fluoxetine and norfluoxetine accumulated extensively following multiple oral dosing; steady-state concentrations were achieved within 3 to 4 weeks of daily dosing.

Hepatic insufficiency: In case of hepatic insufficiency (alcoholic cirrhosis), fluoxetine and norfluoxetine half-lives are increased to 7 and 12 days, respectively. A lower or less frequent dose should be considered.

Renal insufficiency: After single-dose administration of fluoxetine in patients with mild, moderate, or complete (anuria) renal insufficiency, kinetic parameters have not been altered when compared to healthy volunteers. However, after repeated administration, an increase in steady-state plateau of plasma concentrations may be observed.

5.3 Preclinical safety data

There is no evidence of carcinogenicity or mutagenicity from *in vitro* or animal studies.

In a juvenile toxicology study in CD rats, administration of 30mg/kg/day of fluoxetine hydrochloride on postnatal days 21 to 90 resulted in irreversible testicular degeneration and necrosis, epididymal epithelial vacuolation, immaturity and inactivity of the female reproductive tract and decreased fertility. Delays in sexual maturation occurred in males (10 and 30mg/kg/day) and females (30mg/kg/day). The significance of these findings in humans is unknown. Rats administered 30mg/kg also had decreased femur lengths compared with controls and skeletal muscle degeneration, necrosis and regeneration. At 10mg/kg/day, plasma levels achieved in animals were approximately 0.8 to 8.8-fold (fluoxetine) and 3.6 to 23.2-fold (norfluoxetine) those usually observed in paediatric patients. At 3mg/kg/day, plasma levels achieved in animals were approximately 0.04 to 0.5-fold (fluoxetine) and 0.3 to 2.1-fold (norfluoxetine) those usually achieved in paediatric patients.

A study in juvenile mice has indicated that inhibition of the serotonin transporter prevents the accrual of bone formation. This finding would appear to be supported by clinical findings. The reversibility of this effect has not been established.

Another study in juvenile mice (treated on postnatal days 4 to 21) has demonstrated that inhibition of the serotonin transporter had long-lasting effects on the behaviour of the mice. There is no information on whether the effect was reversible. The clinical relevance of this finding has not been established.

6. PHARMACEUTICAL PARTICULARS

6.1 List of excipients

The liquid contains:

Benzoic acid

Sucrose

Glycerin

Mint flavour (containing 0.23% alcohol)

Purified water

The capsules contain:

Starch flowable

Dimeticone

Capsule components:

Patent blue V (E131)

Yellow iron oxide (E172)

Titanium dioxide (E171)

Gelatin

Pharmaceutical grade edible printing ink: containing shellac and hydrated ferric oxide (black) E172

6.2 Incompatibilities

Not applicable.

6.3 Shelf life

20 mg capsules: 3 years.

Liquid: 2 years.

6.4 Special precautions for storage

Do not store above 30°C.

Liquid: Store in the original bottle to protect from light.

6.5 Nature and contents of container

20 mg capsules: PVC/aluminium blister packs of 2, 7, 12, 14, 20, 28, 30, 50, 56, 70, 98, 100 and 500 capsules.

Liquid: Brown glass bottles containing 60ml or 70ml with dosing syringe or 140ml oral liquid. The pack may include a measuring cup or syringe.

Not all pack/bottle sizes may be marketed.

6.6 Special precautions for disposal and other handling

No special requirements.

7. MARKETING AUTHORISATION HOLDER

Eli Lilly and Company Limited

Lilly House

Priestley Road

Basingstoke

Hampshire

RG24 9NL

England

8. MARKETING AUTHORISATION NUMBER(S)

20mg capsules: PL 0006/0195

Liquid: PL 0006/0272

9. DATE OF FIRST AUTHORISATION/RENEWAL OF THE AUTHORISATION

Capsules:

Date of first authorisation: 25 November 1988

Date of latest renewal: 02 April 2008

Liquid:

Date of first authorisation: 25 November 1988

Date of latest renewal: 02 April 2008

10. DATE OF REVISION OF THE TEXT

18 February 2009

LEGAL CATEGORY

POM

*PROZAC (fluoxetine hydrochloride) is a trademark of Eli Lilly and Company.

PZ53M

Psoriderm Cream

(Dermal Laboratories Limited)

1. NAME OF THE MEDICINAL PRODUCT

PSORIDERM™ CREAM

2. QUALITATIVE AND QUANTITATIVE COMPOSITION

Distilled Coal Tar 6.0% w/w; Lecithin 0.4% w/w.

3. PHARMACEUTICAL FORM

Buff coloured cream.

4. CLINICAL PARTICULARS

4.1 Therapeutic indications

For the topical treatment of sub-acute and chronic psoriasis, including psoriasis of the scalp and flexures.

4.2 Posology and method of administration

For adults, children and the elderly. Apply to the affected area once or twice daily, or as recommended by the physician. Wash hands after use.

4.3 Contraindications

Not to be used for acute, sore or pustular psoriasis or in the presence of infection. Not to be used in cases of sensitivity to any of the ingredients.

4.4 Special warnings and precautions for use

Keep away from the eyes and mucous membranes, genital or rectal areas. Avoid cuts and grazes or infected skin. The excipient propylene glycol may on rare occasions cause skin irritation in sensitive people. Replace cap after use. Avoid spillage.

4.5 Interaction with other medicinal products and other forms of interaction

None known.

4.6 Pregnancy and lactation

No special precautions.

4.7 Effects on ability to drive and use machines
None known.

4.8 Undesirable effects
Local side-effects do not normally occur. In rare cases of skin irritation, acne-like eruptions or photosensitivity, discontinue treatment. Rarely, Psoriderm Cream may stain skin, hair or fabric.

4.9 Overdose
There are no known toxic effects resulting from excessive use of Psoriderm Cream.

5. PHARMACOLOGICAL PROPERTIES
5.1 Pharmacodynamic properties
Coal tar has been used dermatologically for hundreds of years and has been shown to be safe and effective in the treatment of scaly skin conditions such as psoriasis. The British Pharmacopoeia contains monographs on coal tar and coal tar solution, and many formulations of coal tar are used in hospitals throughout the country. The coal tar used in Psoriderm Cream has been specially distilled and is based on a neutral fraction which has been shown to be effective in the treatment of psoriasis.

The precise mechanism of action of coal tar is not understood, largely as a result of it comprising up to 10,000 components. There is evidence that topical application of coal tar improves psoriasis by reducing the excessive rate of mitotic epidermal cell division.

Lecithin is a well known phospholipid which is present in foodstuffs. It is added to Psoriderm Cream to soften psoriasis scales and thereby enhance the absorption of the coal tar.

5.2 Pharmacokinetic properties
Not applicable.

5.3 Preclinical safety data
No relevant information additional to that contained elsewhere in the SPC.

6. PHARMACEUTICAL PARTICULARS
6.1 List of excipients
Stearic Acid; Isopropyl Palmitate; Propylene Glycol; Triethanolamine; Phenoxyethanol; Purified Water.

6.2 Incompatibilities
None known.

6.3 Shelf life
36 months.

6.4 Special precautions for storage
Do not store above 25°C.

6.5 Nature and contents of container
Amber glass jar containing 225 ml. This is supplied as an original pack (OP).

6.6 Special precautions for disposal and other handling
Not applicable.

7. MARKETING AUTHORISATION HOLDER
Dermal Laboratories

Tatmore Place, Gosmore

Hitchin, Herts SG4 7QR, UK.

8. MARKETING AUTHORISATION NUMBER(S)
00173/5000R.

9. DATE OF FIRST AUTHORISATION/RENEWAL OF THE AUTHORISATION
16 February 2006.

10. DATE OF REVISION OF THE TEXT
February 2006.

Psoriderm Emulsion 40% w/v Bath Additive

(Dermal Laboratories Limited)

1. NAME OF THE MEDICINAL PRODUCT
PSORIDERM^{TM} EMULSION 40% w/v BATH ADDITIVE

2. QUALITATIVE AND QUANTITATIVE COMPOSITION
Distilled Coal Tar 40.0% w/v.

3. PHARMACEUTICAL FORM
Bath additive. Buff coloured liquid emulsion.

4. CLINICAL PARTICULARS
4.1 Therapeutic indications
For use topically as an aid in the treatment of sub-acute and chronic psoriasis.

4.2 Posology and method of administration
For adults, children and the elderly. Add 30 ml of the emulsion to a standard bath of warm water. Soak for 5 minutes, pat dry.

4.3 Contraindications
Not to be used for acute, sore or pustular psoriasis or in the presence of infection.

Not to be used in cases of sensitivity to any of the ingredients.

4.4 Special warnings and precautions for use
Do not use product undiluted. Keep away from the eyes and broken or inflamed skin. Replace cap after use. Avoid spillage.

4.5 Interaction with other medicinal products and other forms of interaction
None known.

4.6 Pregnancy and lactation
No special precautions.

4.7 Effects on ability to drive and use machines
None known.

4.8 Undesirable effects
Local side-effects do not normally occur. In rare cases of skin irritation, acne-like eruptions or photosensitivity, discontinue treatment. Rarely, Psoriderm Bath Additive may stain skin, hair or fabric.

4.9 Overdose
There are no known toxic effects resulting from excessive use of Psoriderm Bath Additive. If accidentally swallowed, patients should contact a doctor or hospital immediately.

5. PHARMACOLOGICAL PROPERTIES
5.1 Pharmacodynamic properties
Coal tar has been used dermatologically for hundreds of years and has been shown to be safe and effective in the treatment of scaly skin conditions such as psoriasis. The British Pharmacopoeia contains monographs on coal tar and coal tar solution, and many formulations of coal tar are used in hospitals throughout the country. The coal tar used in Psoriderm Bath Additive has been specially distilled and is based on a neutral fraction which has been shown to be effective in the treatment of psoriasis.

The precise mechanism of action of coal tar is not understood, largely as a result of it comprising up to 10,000 components. There is evidence that topical application of coal tar improves psoriasis by reducing the excessive rate of mitotic epidermal cell division.

5.2 Pharmacokinetic properties
Dry scales, which are a common feature of psoriasis, generally reduce the effectiveness of topically applied treatments by reducing absorption of the active ingredient. An established means of overcoming this problem is to add a mild softening agent such as lecithin. In the case of Psoriderm Bath Additive, however, no such softening agent is included because the dosage and administration regime involves prolonged soaking (5 minutes) in a warm water emulsion which achieves a similar effect.

5.3 Preclinical safety data
None.

6. PHARMACEUTICAL PARTICULARS
6.1 List of excipients
Polysorbate 20; Triethanolamine; Phenoxyethanol; Water.

6.2 Incompatibilities
None known.

6.3 Shelf life
36 months.

6.4 Special precautions for storage
Do not store above 25°C.

6.5 Nature and contents of container
Amber glass bottle containing 200 ml. This is supplied as an original pack (OP).

6.6 Special precautions for disposal and other handling
Not applicable.

7. MARKETING AUTHORISATION HOLDER
Dermal Laboratories

Tatmore Place, Gosmore

Hitchin, Herts SG4 7QR, UK.

8. MARKETING AUTHORISATION NUMBER(S)
00173/5003R.

9. DATE OF FIRST AUTHORISATION/RENEWAL OF THE AUTHORISATION
4 January 2007.

10. DATE OF REVISION OF THE TEXT
August 2007.

Psoriderm Scalp Lotion Shampoo

(Dermal Laboratories Limited)

1. NAME OF THE MEDICINAL PRODUCT
PSORIDERM^{TM} SCALP LOTION SHAMPOO

2. QUALITATIVE AND QUANTITATIVE COMPOSITION
Distilled Coal Tar 2.5% w/v; Lecithin 0.3% w/v.

3. PHARMACEUTICAL FORM
Golden brown coloured foaming therapeutic shampoo.

4. CLINICAL PARTICULARS
4.1 Therapeutic indications
For the topical treatment of psoriasis of the scalp.

4.2 Posology and method of administration
For adults, children and the elderly. Wet the hair thoroughly. Apply a small amount of the shampoo to the scalp, and massage gently until a rich lather has been generated. Retain on the scalp for a few minutes. Remove excess lather with the hands before rinsing with warm water. Repeat the above procedure.

4.3 Contraindications
Not to be used for acute, sore or pustular psoriasis or in the presence of infection. Not to be used in cases of sensitivity to any of the ingredients.

4.4 Special warnings and precautions for use
Keep away from the eyes and mucous membranes. Replace cap after use. Avoid spillage.

4.5 Interaction with other medicinal products and other forms of interaction
None known.

4.6 Pregnancy and lactation
No special precautions.

4.7 Effects on ability to drive and use machines
None known.

4.8 Undesirable effects
Local side-effects do not normally occur. In rare cases of skin irritation, acne-like eruptions or photosensitivity, discontinue treatment. Rarely, Psoriderm Scalp Lotion may stain skin, hair or fabric.

4.9 Overdose
There are no known toxic effects resulting from excessive use of Psoriderm Scalp Lotion.

5. PHARMACOLOGICAL PROPERTIES
5.1 Pharmacodynamic properties
Coal tar has been used dermatologically for hundreds of years and has been shown to be safe and effective in the treatment of scaly scalp conditions such as psoriasis. The British Pharmacopoeia contains monographs on coal tar and coal tar solution, and many formulations of coal tar are used in hospitals throughout the country. The coal tar used in Psoriderm Scalp Lotion has been specially distilled and is based on a neutral fraction which has been shown to be effective in the treatment of psoriasis.

The precise mechanism of action of coal tar is not understood, largely as a result of it comprising up to 10,000 components. There is evidence that topical application of coal tar improves psoriasis by reducing the excessive rate of mitotic epidermal cell division.

Lecithin is a well known phospholipid which is present in foodstuffs. It is added to Psoriderm Scalp Lotion to soften psoriasis scales and thereby enhance the absorption of the coal tar.

5.2 Pharmacokinetic properties
Not applicable.

5.3 Preclinical safety data
Not applicable.

6. PHARMACEUTICAL PARTICULARS
6.1 List of excipients
Triethanolamine Lauryl Sulphate; Lauric Acid Diethanolamide; Disodium Edetate; Sodium Chloride; Phenoxyethanol; Purified Water.

6.2 Incompatibilities
None known.

6.3 Shelf life
36 months.

6.4 Special precautions for storage
Do not store above 25°C.

6.5 Nature and contents of container
White plastic bottle containing 250 ml. This is supplied as an original pack (OP).

6.6 Special precautions for disposal and other handling
Not applicable.

7. MARKETING AUTHORISATION HOLDER
Dermal Laboratories

Tatmore Place, Gosmore

Hitchin, Herts SG4 7QR, UK.

8. MARKETING AUTHORISATION NUMBER(S)
00173/5001R.

9. DATE OF FIRST AUTHORISATION/RENEWAL OF THE AUTHORISATION
4 January 2007.

10. DATE OF REVISION OF THE TEXT
July 2007.

Pulmicort CFC-free Inhaler 100 micrograms

(AstraZeneca UK Limited)

1. NAME OF THE MEDICINAL PRODUCT
Pulmicort CFC-free Inhaler 100 micrograms. ▼

2. QUALITATIVE AND QUANTITATIVE COMPOSITION

Each metered dose (ex-valve)/actuation contains budesonide 100 micrograms.

For full list of excipients, see Section 6.1.

3. PHARMACEUTICAL FORM

Pressurised inhalation, suspension.

The NebuChamber™ spacer device is the **only** spacer device to be used with Pulmicort CFC-free Inhaler.

4. CLINICAL PARTICULARS

4.1 Therapeutic indications

Asthma.

4.2 Posology and method of administration

For inhalation use.

Adults, including the elderly: 200 micrograms twice daily, in the morning and in the evening. During periods of severe asthma the daily dosage can be increased up to 1600 micrograms.

In patients whose asthma is well controlled, the daily dose may be reduced below 400 micrograms but should not go below 200 micrograms.

The dose should be reduced to the minimum needed to maintain good asthma control.

Children 2-12 years: 200 to 800 micrograms daily in divided doses.

A higher strength inhaler (200 microgram) is available for use in children with moderately severe/severe asthma and requiring a dose regimen of Pulmicort CFC-free Inhaler of 800 micrograms as a total daily dose.

The dose should be reduced to the minimum needed to maintain good asthma control.

Pulmicort CFC-free Inhaler is not recommended for use in children less than 2 years of age.

Patients maintained on oral glucocorticosteroids

Pulmicort CFC-free Inhaler may permit replacement or significant reduction in the dosage of oral glucocorticosteroids while maintaining asthma control. For further information on the withdrawal of oral corticosteroids see Section 4.4 (*Special warnings and precautions for use*).

Method of Administration

Instructions for the correct use of Pulmicort CFC-free Inhaler

Note: It is important to instruct the patient to:

- Carefully read the detailed instructions for use and refer to the accompanying pictograms in the Patient Information Leaflet which is packed with each inhaler.
- Take his/her time when using the inhaler and not to rush through the individual steps.
- To practise using the inhaler in front of the mirror. Advise the patient that if any mist is seen coming from the top of the inhaler or from the mouthpiece it may mean that he/she has not inhaled the medicine properly.
- Shake the inhaler thoroughly for a few seconds to mix the contents of the inhaler properly.
- Prime the inhaler by actuating it twice into the air when the inhaler is new, if it has been dropped, or when it has not been used for more than 7 days.
- Place the mouthpiece in the mouth. While breathing in slowly and deeply, press the canister firmly to release the medication. Advise the patient that he/she may need to use both hands to operate the inhaler. Continue to breathe in and hold the breath for as long as is comfortable.
- Remove the inhaler from the mouth before breathing out; the patient must be advised that he/she must not breathe out through the inhaler.
- If a second or subsequent actuation is required the patient should be advised to wait for about half a minute and then replace the mouthpiece in the mouth and repeat the instructions at the preceding two bullet points, the sixth and seventh bullet points as listed.
- Rinse the mouth out with water after inhaling the prescribed dose to minimise the risk of oropharyngeal thrush.
- Clean the mouthpiece of the inhaler regularly, at least once a week. Remove the dust cap and the aerosol canister. Clean the plastic actuator and dust cap with a dry cloth or tissue. Refer to the detailed instructions for cleaning in the Patient Information Leaflet, which is packed with each inhaler. Advise the patient that the metal aerosol canister should **not** be put into water or be cleaned with water.
- Always store Pulmicort CFC-free Inhaler so that it stands upright on its brown plastic base (with the valve downwards).

The use of Pulmicort CFC-free Inhaler with the NebuChamber™ spacer device is recommended to enable patients with difficulty in co-ordinating inhalation with actuation, such as infants, young children, the poorly co-operative or the elderly, to derive greater therapeutic benefit. The mouthpiece of Pulmicort CFC-free Inhaler fits directly into the NebuChamber spacer device. Pulmicort CFC-free Inhaler should only be used with the NebuChamber spacer device, it should NOT be used with any other spacer device as an alternative device may alter the pulmonary deposition of budesonide.

A spacer device should always be available together with a pressurised metered dose inhaler when a pressurised metered dose inhaler is prescribed for use by a child.

Instructions for the correct use of Pulmicort CFC-free Inhaler with the NebuChamber™ spacer device.

Note: It is important to instruct the patient to:

- Carefully read the instructions for use in the Patient Information Leaflet, which is packed with each inhaler.
- Carefully read the instructions for use in the instruction leaflet, which is packed with each spacer device.

On actuation of the aerosol the dose is released into the inhalation chamber. The inhalation chamber is then emptied by two slow deep breaths. Young children may need to breathe 5–10 times through the mouthpiece. For further doses the procedure is repeated. It is important to explain that when a small child is using the NebuChamber spacer device a parent or carer should hold and support the spacer device in the child's mouth to ensure that the child breathes through the spacer device properly. For young children who are unable to breathe through the mouthpiece, a face mask can be used. Compatible face masks are available separately and care should be taken to ensure a good fit is achieved.

4.3 Contraindications

History of hypersensitivity to budesonide or any of the excipients.

4.4 Special warnings and precautions for use

Special caution is necessary in patients with active or quiescent pulmonary tuberculosis, and in patients with fungal or viral infections in the airways.

Patients not dependent on steroids: Treatment with the recommended doses of budesonide usually gives a therapeutic benefit within 7 days. However, certain patients may have an excessive collection of mucus secretion in the bronchi. In these cases, a short course of oral corticosteroids (usually 1 to 2 weeks) should be given in addition to the aerosol. After the course of the oral drug, the inhaler alone should be sufficient therapy.

Steroid-dependent patients: Transfer of patients on oral steroids to treatment with Pulmicort CFC-free Inhaler demands special care, mainly due to the slow restitution of the disturbed hypothalamic-pituitary adrenocortical axis function, caused by extended treatment with oral corticosteroids. When the Pulmicort CFC-free Inhaler treatment is initiated the patient should be in a relatively stable phase. A high dose of budesonide, in combination with the previously used oral steroid dose, should be given for about 10 days.

The down titration dose should be selected at the discretion of the physician, based on the patient's disease and former steroid intake. For example, a down titration with 5 mg prednisolone per day, on a weekly basis; this reduction will mean that a daily dose of 20 mg per day would be reduced to 15 mg per day in the first week, 10 mg per day in the second week etc. The oral dose is thus reduced to the lowest level that, in combination with budesonide, provides maintained or improved asthma control.

In many cases it may be possible to completely substitute the oral steroid with inhaled budesonide; however some patients may have to be maintained on a low dose of oral steroid together with inhaled budesonide.

During the withdrawal of oral steroids some patients may experience uneasiness and may feel generally unwell in a non-specific way even though respiratory function is maintained or improved. Patients should be encouraged to continue with inhaled budesonide whilst withdrawing the oral steroid unless there are clinical signs to indicate the contrary.

Patients who have previously been dependent on oral steroids may, as a result of prolonged systemic steroid therapy, experience the effects of impaired adrenal function. Recovery may take a considerable amount of time after cessation of oral steroid therapy and hence oral steroid-dependent patients transferred to inhaled budesonide may remain at risk from impaired adrenal function for some considerable time. In such circumstances HPA axis function should be monitored regularly. These patients should be instructed to carry a steroid warning card indicating their needs.

Prolonged treatment with high doses of inhaled corticosteroids, particularly higher than recommended doses, may also result in clinically significant adrenal suppression. Therefore additional systemic corticosteroid cover should be considered during periods of stress such as severe infections or elective surgery. Such patients should be instructed to carry a steroid warning card indicating their needs (See also Section 4.8.*Undesirable effects*). Rapid reduction in the dose of steroids can induce acute adrenal crisis. Symptoms and signs which might be seen in acute adrenal crisis may be somewhat vague but may include anorexia, abdominal pain, weight loss, tiredness, headache, nausea, vomiting, decreased level of consciousness, seizures, hypotension and hypoglycaemia.

Treatment with supplementary systemic steroids or inhaled budesonide should not be stopped abruptly.

During transfer from oral therapy to Pulmicort CFC-free Inhaler, a generally lower systemic steroid action will be experienced which may result in the appearance of allergic or arthritic symptoms such as rhinitis, eczema and muscle and joint pain. Specific treatment should be initiated for these conditions. A general insufficient glucocorticosteroid effect should be suspected if, in rare cases, symptoms such as tiredness, headache, nausea and vomiting should occur. In these cases a temporary increase in the dose of oral glucocorticosteroids is sometimes necessary.

Exacerbations of asthma caused by bacterial infections are usually controlled by appropriate antibiotic treatment and possibly increasing the budesonide dosage or, if necessary, by giving systemic steroids.

As with other inhalation therapy paradoxical bronchospasm may occur with an immediate increase in wheezing and shortness of breath after dosing. Paradoxical bronchospasm responds to a rapid-acting inhaled bronchodilator and should be treated straightaway. Pulmicort CFC-free Inhaler should be discontinued immediately, the patient should be assessed and an alternative therapy instituted if necessary.

Systemic effects of inhaled corticosteroids may occur, particularly at high doses prescribed for prolonged periods. These effects are much less likely to occur than with oral corticosteroids. Possible systemic effects include Cushing's Syndrome, Cushingoid features, adrenal suppression, growth retardation in children and adolescents, decrease in bone mineral density, cataract and glaucoma.

It is important, therefore, that the patient is reviewed regularly and the dose of inhaled corticosteroid is titrated to the lowest dose at which effective control of asthma is maintained.

It is recommended that the height of children receiving prolonged treatment with inhaled corticosteroids be regularly monitored. If growth is slowed therapy should be reviewed with the aim of reducing the dose of inhaled corticosteroid, if possible, to the lowest dose at which effective control of asthma is maintained. In addition, consideration should be given to referring the patient to a paediatric respiratory specialist.

Pulmicort CFC-free Inhaler is not intended for rapid relief of acute episodes of asthma or symptoms of asthma. In these situations an inhaled short-acting bronchodilator is required. Patients should be advised to have such 'rescue' medication with them at all times.

If patients find short-acting bronchodilator treatment ineffective, or they need more inhalations than usual and respiratory symptoms persist, medical attention must be sought. In this situation consideration should be given to the need for or an increase in their regular therapy e.g. higher doses of inhaled budesonide, the addition of a long-acting beta agonist or a course of oral glucocorticosteroids.

Patients should be reminded of the importance of taking prophylactic therapy regularly, even when they are asymptomatic. Patients should also be reminded of the risk of oropharyngeal Candida infection, due to drug deposition in the oropharynx. Advising the patient to rinse the mouth out with water after each dose will minimise the risk. Oropharyngeal Candida infection usually responds to topical anti-fungal treatment without the need to discontinue the inhaled corticosteroid.

Patients should be instructed in the proper use of their inhaler and their technique should be checked to ensure that the patient can synchronise aerosol actuation with inspiration of breath to obtain optimum delivery of the inhaled drug to the lungs.

Reduced liver function may affect the elimination of glucocorticosteroids. The plasma clearance following an intravenous dose of budesonide however was similar in cirrhotic patients and in healthy subjects. After oral ingestion systemic availability of budesonide was increased by compromised liver function due to decreased first pass metabolism. The clinical relevance of this to treatment with Pulmicort CFC-free Inhaler is unknown as no data exist for inhaled budesonide, but increases in plasma levels and hence an increased risk of systemic adverse effects could be expected.

In vivo studies have shown that oral administration of ketoconazole and itraconazole (known inhibitors of CYP3A4 activity in the liver and in the intestinal mucosa) causes an increase in the systemic exposure to budesonide. Concomitant treatment with ketoconazole and itraconazole or other potent CYP3A4 inhibitors should be avoided (see Section 4.5 *Interactions with other medicinal products and other forms of interaction*). If this is not possible the time interval between administration of the interacting drugs should be as long as possible. A reduction in the dose of budesonide should also be considered.

4.5 Interaction with other medicinal products and other forms of interaction

The metabolism of budesonide is primarily mediated by CYP3A4, one of the cytochrome p450 enzymes. Inhibitors of this enzyme, e.g. ketoconazole and itraconazole, can therefore increase systemic exposure to budesonide, (see Section 4.4 *Special warnings and precautions for use* and Section 5.2 *Pharmacokinetic properties*). Other potent inhibitors of CYP3A4 are also likely to markedly increase plasma levels of budesonide.

4.6 Pregnancy and lactation

There is no experience with or evidence of safety of propellant HFA 134a in human pregnancy or lactation. However studies of the effect of HFA 134a on reproductive function and embryofetal development in animals have revealed no clinically relevant adverse effects.

Pregnancy

Results from a large prospective epidemiological study and from worldwide post marketing experience indicate no adverse effects of inhaled budesonide during pregnancy on the health of the fetus / newborn child. Animal studies have shown reproductive toxicity (see Section 5.3 *Preclinical safety data*). The potential risk for humans is unknown.

There are no relevant clinical data on the use of Pulmicort CFC-free Inhaler in human pregnancy.

Administration of Pulmicort CFC-free Inhaler during pregnancy requires that the benefits for the mother be weighed against the risks for the fetus. Pulmicort CFC-free Inhaler should only be used during pregnancy if the expected benefits outweigh the potential risks.

Lactation

Budesonide is excreted in breast milk. However, at therapeutic doses of Pulmicort CFC-free Inhaler, no budesonide related effects on the suckling child are anticipated.

There is no experience with or evidence of safety of propellant HFA 134a in human lactation. The use of budesonide formulated with propellant HFA 134a (as Pulmicort CFC-free Inhaler) should only be considered in situations where it is felt that the expected benefits to the mother will outweigh any potential risks to the neonate.

4.7 Effects on ability to drive and use machines

Pulmicort CFC-free Inhaler has no or negligible influence on the ability to drive and use machines.

4.8 Undesirable effects

Clinical trials, literature reports and post-marketing experience of orally inhaled budesonide suggest that the following adverse drug reactions may occur:

Common (>1/100, <1/10)	• Mild irritation in the throat • Candida infection in the oropharynx • Hoarseness • Coughing
Rare (>1/10 000, <1/1 000)	• Nervousness, restlessness, depression, behavioural disturbances • Immediate and delayed hypersensitivity reactions including rash, contact dermatitis, urticaria, angioedema, bronchospasm and anaphylactic reaction • Skin bruising

Candida infection in the oropharynx is due to drug deposition. Advising the patient to rinse the mouth out with water after each dose will minimise the risk. The incidence should be less with the use of the NebuChamber™ spacer device since this reduces oral deposition.

As with other inhalation therapy, paradoxical bronchospasm may occur, with an immediate increase in wheezing and shortness of breath after dosing. Paradoxical bronchospasm responds to a rapid-acting inhaled bronchodilator and should be treated straightaway. Pulmicort CFC-free Inhaler should be discontinued immediately, the patient should be assessed and an alternative therapy instituted if necessary.

Systemic effects of inhaled corticosteroids may occur, particularly at high doses prescribed for prolonged periods. These effects are much less likely to occur than with oral corticosteroids. Possible systemic effects include Cushing's Syndrome, Cushingoid features, adrenal suppression, growth retardation in children and adolescents, decrease in bone mineral density, cataract and glaucoma. Increased susceptibility to infections and impairment of the ability to adapt to stress may also occur. Effects are probably dependent on dose, exposure time, concomitant and previous steroid exposure and individual sensitivity.

Prolonged treatment with high doses of inhaled corticosteroids, particularly higher than recommended doses, may also result in clinically significant adrenal suppression. Therefore additional systemic corticosteroid cover should be considered during periods of stress, such as severe infections or elective surgery. Such patients should be instructed to carry a steroid warning card indicating their needs. (See also Section 4.4 *Special warnings and precautions for use*)

4.9 Overdose

The only harmful effect that follows inhalation of large amounts of the drug over a short period is suppression of HPA axis function. No special emergency action needs to be taken. Treatment with Pulmicort CFC-free Inhaler should be continued at the recommended dose to control the asthma.

5. PHARMACOLOGICAL PROPERTIES

5.1 Pharmacodynamic properties

Budesonide is a glucocorticosteroid that possesses a high local anti-inflammatory action, with a lower incidence and severity of adverse effects than those seen with oral corticosteroids.

Pharmacotherapeutic group: Other drugs for obstructive airway diseases, inhalants, glucocorticoids. ATC Code: RO3B A02.

Topical anti-inflammatory effect

The exact mechanism of action of glucocorticosteroids in the treatment of asthma is not fully understood. Anti-inflammatory actions such as inhibition of inflammatory mediator release and inhibition of cytokine-mediated immune response are probably important.

A clinical study in asthmatics comparing inhaled and oral budesonide at doses calculated to achieve similar systemic bioavailability demonstrated statistically significant evidence of efficacy with inhaled but not oral budesonide, compared with placebo. Thus, the therapeutic effect of conventional doses of inhaled budesonide may be largely explained by its direct action on the respiratory tract.

In a provocation study, pre-treatment with budesonide for four weeks has shown decreased bronchial constriction in immediate as well as late asthmatic reactions.

Onset of effect

After a single dose of orally inhaled budesonide delivered via dry powder inhaler, improvement of lung function is achieved within a few hours. After therapeutic use of orally inhaled budesonide delivered via dry powder inhaler, improvement in lung function has been shown to occur within 2 days of initiation of treatment although maximum benefit may not be achieved for up to 4 weeks.

Airway reactivity

Budesonide has also been shown to decrease airway reactivity to histamine and methacholine in hyperreactive patients.

Exercise-induced asthma

Therapy with inhaled budesonide has effectively been used for prevention of exercise-induced asthma.

Growth

Limited data from long-term studies suggest that most children and adolescents treated with inhaled budesonide ultimately achieve their adult target height. However, an initial small but transient reduction in growth (approximately 1 cm) has been observed. This generally occurs within the first year of treatment (see Section 4.4 *Special warnings and precautions for use*).

HPA axis function

Studies in healthy volunteers with inhaled budesonide (administered as a dry powder via Turbohaler) have shown dose-related effects on plasma and urinary cortisol. At recommended doses Pulmicort Turbohaler causes less effect on adrenal function than prednisolone 10 mg, as shown by ACTH tests.

5.2 Pharmacokinetic properties

After inhalation of budesonide via pressurised metered dose inhaler, approximately 10% to 15% of the metered dose is deposited in the lungs.

The maximal plasma concentration after oral inhalation of a single dose of 400 or 800 micrograms budesonide was 0.84 and 1.53 nmol/L respectively, and was reached after about 35 minutes.

Budesonide undergoes an extensive degree (approximately 90%) of biotransformation in the liver, to metabolites of low glucocorticosteroid activity.

The glucocorticosteroid activity of the major metabolites, 6β-hydroxybudesonide and 16α-hydroxyprednisolone, is less than 1% of that of budesonide. The metabolism of budesonide is primarily mediated by CYP3A4, one of the cytochrome p450 enzymes.

In a study, 100 mg ketoconazole taken twice daily increased plasma levels of concomitantly administered oral budesonide (single dose of 10 mg) on average by 7.8-fold. Information about this interaction is lacking for inhaled budesonide, but marked increases in plasma levels could be expected.

5.3 Preclinical safety data

The acute toxicity of budesonide is low and of the same order of magnitude and type as that of the reference glucocorticoids studied (beclometasone dipropionate, fluocinolone acetonide).

Results from subacute and chronic toxicity studies show that the systemic effects of budesonide are less severe than, or similar to, those observed after administration of the other glucocorticosteroids e.g. decreased body-weight gain and atrophy of lymphoid tissues and adrenal cortex.

An increased incidence of brain gliomas in male rats, in a carcinogenicity study, could not be verified in a repeat study in which the incidence of gliomas did not differ between any of the groups on active treatment (budesonide, prednisolone, triamcinolone acetonide) and the control groups.

Liver changes (primary hepatocellular neoplasms) found in male rats in the original carcinogenicity study were noted again in the repeat study with budesonide, as well as with the reference glucocorticosteroids. These effects are most probably related to a receptor effect and thus represent a class effect.

Available clinical experience shows no indication that budesonide or other glucocorticosteroids induce brain gliomas or primary hepatocellular neoplasms in man.

In animal reproduction studies, corticosteroids such as budesonide have been shown to induce malformations (cleft palate, skeletal malformations). However, these animal experimental results do not appear to be relevant in humans at the recommended doses.

Animal studies have also identified an involvement of excess prenatal glucocorticosteroids in increased risk for intrauterine growth retardation, adult cardiovascular disease and permanent changes in glucocorticoid receptor density, neurotransmitter turnover and behaviour at exposures below the teratogenic dose range.

The safe use of norflurane has been fully evaluated in preclinical studies. It is well accepted and used in several pressurised metered dose inhalers, and is essentially non-toxic. Magnesium stearate has a history of safe use in man for many years, which supports the view that magnesium stearate is essentially biologically inert. The safe use of magnesium stearate for inhalation has been fully evaluated in preclinical studies. Inhalation toxicity studies conducted with magnesium stearate in rats (26 weeks) and dogs (4 weeks) did not show signs of toxicity up to doses about 490 and 11000 times higher, respectively, than the maximum exposure achievable during the daily treatment with the new formulation. Furthermore, toxicity studies carried out using Pulmicort pressurised metered dose inhaler have shown no evidence of any local or systemic toxicity or irritation attributable to the excipients.

6. PHARMACEUTICAL PARTICULARS

6.1 List of excipients

Norflurane (HFA 134a) - a CFC-free propellant

Magnesium stearate.

6.2 Incompatibilities

Not applicable.

6.3 Shelf life

2 years.

6.4 Special precautions for storage

Do not store above 30°C.

Always store Pulmicort CFC-free Inhaler so that it stands upright on its brown plastic base (with the valve downwards).

The canister contains a pressurised liquid. Do not expose to temperatures higher than 50°C. Do not pierce the canister.

6.5 Nature and contents of container

The immediate container is an aluminium can which is sealed with a metering valve.

The container is assembled with an actuator containing a mouthpiece. The actuator and the mouthpiece are made of polypropylene.

Each inhaler delivers 120 metered doses/actuations after initial priming.

6.6 Special precautions for disposal and other handling

The canister should not be broken, punctured or burnt, even when apparently empty.

7. MARKETING AUTHORISATION HOLDER

AstraZeneca UK Ltd.,

600 Capability Green

Luton

LU1 3LU, UK.

8. MARKETING AUTHORISATION NUMBER(S)

PL 17901/0247

9. DATE OF FIRST AUTHORISATION/RENEWAL OF THE AUTHORISATION

24th September 2008

10. DATE OF REVISION OF THE TEXT

13th August 2009

Pulmicort CFC-free Inhaler 200 micrograms

(AstraZeneca UK Limited)

1. NAME OF THE MEDICINAL PRODUCT

Pulmicort CFC-free Inhaler 200 micrograms. ▼

2. QUALITATIVE AND QUANTITATIVE COMPOSITION

Each metered dose (ex-valve)/actuation contains budesonide 200 micrograms.

For full list of excipients, see Section 6.1.

3. PHARMACEUTICAL FORM

Pressurised inhalation, suspension.

The NebuChamber™ spacer device is the **only** spacer device to be used with Pulmicort CFC-free Inhaler.

4. CLINICAL PARTICULARS

4.1 Therapeutic indications

Asthma.

4.2 Posology and method of administration

For inhalation use.

Adults, including the elderly: 200 micrograms twice daily, in the morning and in the evening. During periods of severe asthma the daily dosage can be increased up to 1600 micrograms.

A lower strength inhaler (Pulmicort CFC-free Inhaler 100 micrograms) is available and should be used in patients whose asthma is deemed to be well-controlled and in whom the total daily dose may be reduced to less than 400 micrograms. The daily dose should not go below 200 micrograms. The dose should be reduced to the minimum needed to maintain good asthma control.

Children 2-12 years: 200 to 800 micrograms daily in divided doses.

A lower strength inhaler (100 microgram) is available for use in children with mild/moderately severe asthma.

Pulmicort CFC-free Inhaler is not recommended for use in children less than 2 years of age.

The dose should be reduced to the minimum needed to maintain good asthma control.

Patients maintained on oral glucocorticosteroids

Pulmicort CFC-free Inhaler may permit replacement or significant reduction in the dosage of oral glucocorticosteroids while maintaining asthma control. For further information on the withdrawal of oral corticosteroids see Section 4.4 (*Special warnings and precautions for use*).

Method of Administration

Instructions for the correct use of Pulmicort CFC-free Inhaler

Note: It is important to instruct the patient to:

- Carefully read the detailed instructions for use and refer to the accompanying pictograms in the Patient Information Leaflet that is packed with each inhaler.
- Take his/her time when using the inhaler and not to rush through the individual steps.
- To practise using the inhaler in front of the mirror. Advise the patient that if any mist is seen coming from the top of the inhaler or from the mouthpiece it may mean that he/she has not inhaled the medicine properly.
- Shake the inhaler thoroughly for a few seconds to mix the contents of the inhaler properly.
- Prime the inhaler by actuating it twice into the air when the inhaler is new, if it has been dropped, or when it has not been used for more than 7 days.
- Place the mouthpiece in the mouth. While breathing in slowly and deeply, press the canister firmly to release the medication. Advise the patient that he/she may need to use both hands to operate the inhaler. Continue to breathe in and hold the breath for as long as is comfortable.
- Remove the inhaler from the mouth before breathing out; the patient must be advised that he/she must not breathe out through the inhaler.
- If a second or subsequent actuation is required the patient should be advised to wait for about half a minute and then replace the mouthpiece in the mouth and repeat the instructions at the preceding two bullet points, the sixth and seventh bullet points as listed.
- Rinse the mouth out with water after inhaling the prescribed dose to minimise the risk of oropharygeal thrush.
- Clean the mouthpiece of the inhaler regularly, at least once a week. Remove the dust cap and the aerosol canister. Clean the plastic actuator and dust cap with a dry cloth or tissue. Refer to the detailed instructions for cleaning in the Patient Information Leaflet, which is packed with each inhaler. Advise the patient that the metal aerosol canister should **not** be put into water or be cleaned with water.
- Always store Pulmicort CFC-free Inhaler so that it stands upright on its brown plastic base (with the valve downwards).

The use of Pulmicort CFC-free Inhaler with the NebuChamber[TM] spacer device is recommended to enable patients with difficulty in co-ordinating inhalation with actuation, such as infants, young children, the poorly co-operative or the elderly, to derive greater therapeutic benefit. The mouthpiece of Pulmicort CFC-Free Inhaler fits directly into the NebuChamber spacer device. Pulmicort CFC-free Inhaler should only be used with the NebuChamber spacer device, it should NOT be used with any other spacer device as an alternative device may alter the pulmonary deposition of budesonide.

A spacer device should always be available together with a pressurised metered dose inhaler when a pressurised metered dose inhaler is prescribed for use by a child.

Instructions for the correct use of Pulmicort CFC-free Inhaler with the NebuChamber[TM] spacer device.

Note: It is important to instruct the patient to:

- Carefully read the instructions for use in the Patient Information Leaflet, which is packed with each inhaler.
- Carefully read the instructions for use in the instruction leaflet, which is packed with each spacer device.

On actuation of the aerosol the dose is released into the inhalation chamber. The inhalation chamber is then emptied by two slow deep breaths. Young children may need to breathe 5–10 times through the mouthpiece. For further doses the procedure is repeated. It is important to explain that when a small child is using the NebuChamber spacer device a parent or carer should hold and support the spacer device in the child's mouth to ensure that the child breathes through the spacer device properly. For young children who are unable to breathe through the mouthpiece, a face mask can be used. Compatible face masks are available separately and care should be taken to ensure a good fit is achieved.

4.3 Contraindications

History of hypersensitivity to budesonide or any of the excipients.

4.4 Special warnings and precautions for use

Special caution is necessary in patients with active or quiescent pulmonary tuberculosis, and in patients with fungal or viral infections in the airways.

Patients not dependent on steroids: Treatment with the recommended doses of budesonide usually gives a therapeutic benefit within 7 days. However, certain patients may have an excessive collection of mucus secretion in the bronchi. In these cases, a short course of oral corticosteroids (usually 1 to 2 weeks) should be given in addition to the aerosol. After the course of the oral drug, the inhaler alone should be sufficient therapy.

Steroid-dependent patients: Transfer of patients on oral steroids to treatment with Pulmicort CFC-free Inhaler demands special care, mainly due to the slow restitution of the disturbed hypothalamic-pituitary adrenocortical axis function, caused by extended treatment with oral corticosteroids. When the Pulmicort CFC-free Inhaler treatment is initiated the patient should be in a relatively stable phase. A high dose of budesonide, in combination with the previously used oral steroid dose, should be given for about 10 days.

The down titration dose should be selected at the discretion of the physician, based on the patient's disease and former steroid intake. For example, a down titration with 5 mg prednisolone per day, on a weekly basis; this reduction will mean that a daily dose of 20 mg per day would be reduced to 15 mg per day in the first week, 10 mg per day in the second week etc. The oral dose is thus reduced to the lowest level that, in combination with budesonide, provides maintained or improved asthma control.

In many cases it may be possible to completely substitute the oral steroid with inhaled budesonide; however some patients may have to be maintained on a low dose of oral steroid together with inhaled budesonide.

During the withdrawal of oral steroids some patients may experience uneasiness and may feel generally unwell in a non-specific way even though respiratory function is maintained or improved. Patients should be encouraged to continue with inhaled budesonide whilst withdrawing the oral steroid unless there are clinical signs to indicate the contrary.

Patients who have previously been dependent on oral steroids may, as a result of prolonged systemic steroid therapy, experience the effects of impaired adrenal function. Recovery may take a considerable amount of time after cessation of oral steroid therapy and hence oral steroid-dependent patients transferred to inhaled budesonide may remain at risk from impaired adrenal function for some considerable time. In such circumstances HPA axis function should be monitored regularly. These patients should be instructed to carry a steroid warning card indicating their needs.

Prolonged treatment with high doses of inhaled corticosteroids, particularly higher than recommended doses, may also result in clinically significant adrenal suppression. Therefore additional systemic corticosteroid cover should be considered during periods of stress such as severe infections or elective surgery. Such patients should be instructed to carry a steroid warning card indicating their needs (See also Section 4.8.*Undesirable effects*). Rapid reduction in the dose of steroids can induce acute adrenal crisis. Symptoms and signs which might be seen in acute adrenal crisis may be somewhat vague but may include anorexia, abdominal pain, weight loss, tiredness, headache, nausea, vomiting, decreased level of consciousness, seizures, hypotension and hypoglycaemia.

Treatment with supplementary systemic steroids or inhaled budesonide should not be stopped abruptly.

During transfer from oral therapy to Pulmicort CFC-free Inhaler, a generally lower systemic steroid action will be experienced which may result in the appearance of allergic or arthritic symptoms such as rhinitis, eczema and muscle and joint pain. Specific treatment should be initiated for these conditions. A general insufficient glucocorticosteroid effect should be suspected if, in rare cases, symptoms such as tiredness, headache, nausea and vomiting should occur. In these cases a temporary increase in the dose of oral glucocorticosteroids is sometimes necessary.

Exacerbations of asthma caused by bacterial infections are usually controlled by appropriate antibiotic treatment and possibly increasing the budesonide dosage or, if necessary, by giving systemic steroids.

As with other inhalation therapy paradoxical bronchospasm may occur with an immediate increase in wheezing and shortness of breath after dosing. Paradoxical bronchospasm responds to a rapid-acting inhaled bronchodilator and should be treated straightaway. Pulmicort CFC-free Inhaler should be discontinued immediately, the patient should be assessed and an alternative therapy instituted if necessary.

Systemic effects of inhaled corticosteroids may occur, particularly at high doses prescribed for prolonged periods. These effects are much less likely to occur than with oral corticosteroids. Possible systemic effects include Cushing's Syndrome, Cushingoid features, adrenal suppression, growth retardation in children and adolescents, decrease in bone mineral density, cataract and glaucoma.

It is important, therefore, that the patient is reviewed regularly and the dose of inhaled corticosteroid is titrated to the lowest dose at which effective control of asthma is maintained.

It is recommended that the height of children receiving prolonged treatment with inhaled corticosteroids be regularly monitored. If growth is slowed therapy should be reviewed with the aim of reducing the dose of inhaled corticosteroid, if possible, to the lowest dose at which effective control of asthma is maintained. In addition, consideration should be given to referring the patient to a paediatric respiratory specialist.

Pulmicort CFC-free Inhaler is not intended for rapid relief of acute episodes of asthma or symptoms of asthma. In these situations an inhaled short-acting bronchodilator is required. Patients should be advised to have such 'rescue' medication with them at all times.

If patients find short-acting bronchodilator treatment ineffective, or they need more inhalations than usual and respiratory symptoms persist, medical attention must be sought. In this situation consideration should be given to the need for or an increase in their regular therapy e.g. higher doses of inhaled budesonide, the addition of a long-acting beta agonist or a course of oral glucocorticosteroids.

Patients should be reminded of the importance of taking prophylactic therapy regularly, even when they are asymptomatic. Patients should also be reminded of the risk of oropharyngeal Candida infection, due to drug deposition in the oropharynx. Advising the patient to rinse the mouth out with water after each dose will minimise the risk. Oropharyngeal Candida infection usually responds to topical anti-fungal treatment without the need to discontinue the inhaled corticosteroid.

Patients should be instructed in the proper use of their inhaler and their technique should be checked to ensure that the patient can synchronise aerosol actuation with inspiration of breath to obtain optimum delivery of the inhaled drug to the lungs.

Reduced liver function may affect the elimination of glucocorticosteroids. The plasma clearance following an intravenous dose of budesonide however was similar in cirrhotic patients and in healthy subjects. After oral ingestion systemic availability of budesonide was increased by compromised liver function due to decreased first pass metabolism. The clinical relevance of this to treatment with Pulmicort CFC-free Inhaler is unknown as no data exist for inhaled budesonide, but increases in plasma levels and hence an increased risk of systemic adverse effects could be expected.

In vivo studies have shown that oral administration of ketoconazole and itraconazole (known inhibitors of CYP3A4 activity in the liver and in the intestinal mucosa) causes an increase in the systemic exposure to budesonide. Concomitant treatment with ketoconazole and itraconazole or other potent CYP3A4 inhibitors should be avoided (see Section 4.5 *Interactions with other medicinal products and other forms of interaction*). If this is not possible the time interval between administration of the interacting drugs should be as long as possible. A reduction in the dose of budesonide should also be considered.

4.5 Interaction with other medicinal products and other forms of interaction

The metabolism of budesonide is primarily mediated by CYP3A4, one of the cytochrome p450 enzymes. Inhibitors of this enzyme, e.g. ketoconazole and itraconazole, can therefore increase systemic exposure to budesonide, (see Section 4.4 *Special warnings and precautions for use* and Section 5.2 *Pharmacokinetic properties*). Other potent inhibitors of CYP3A4 are also likely to markedly increase plasma levels of budesonide.

4.6 Pregnancy and lactation

There is no experience with or evidence of safety of propellant HFA 134a in human pregnancy or lactation. However studies of the effect of HFA 134a on reproductive function and embryofetal development in animals have revealed no clinically relevant adverse effects.

Pregnancy

Results from a large prospective epidemiological study and from worldwide post marketing experience indicate no adverse effects of inhaled budesonide during pregnancy on the health of the fetus / newborn child. Animal studies have shown reproductive toxicity (see Section 5.3 *Preclinical safety data*). The potential risk for humans is unknown.

There are no relevant clinical data on the use of Pulmicort CFC-free Inhaler in human pregnancy.

Administration of Pulmicort CFC-free Inhaler during pregnancy requires that the benefits for the mother be weighed against the risks for the fetus. Pulmicort CFC-free Inhaler should only be used during pregnancy if the expected benefits outweigh the potential risks.

Lactation

Budesonide is excreted in breast milk. However, at therapeutic doses of Pulmicort CFC-free Inhaler, no budesonide related effects on the suckling child are anticipated.

There is no experience with or evidence of safety of propellant HFA 134a in human lactation. The use of budesonide formulated with propellant HFA 134a (as Pulmicort CFC-free Inhaler) should only be considered in situations where it is felt that the expected benefits to the mother will outweigh any potential risks to the neonate.

4.7 Effects on ability to drive and use machines
Pulmicort CFC-free Inhaler has no or negligible influence on the ability to drive and use machines.

4.8 Undesirable effects
Clinical trials, literature reports and post-marketing experience of orally inhaled budesonide suggest that the following adverse drug reactions may occur:

Common (>1/100, <1/10)	• Mild irritation in the throat • Candida infection in the oropharynx • Hoarseness • Coughing
Rare (>1/10 000, <1/1 000)	• Nervousness, restlessness, depression, behavioural disturbances • Immediate and delayed hypersensitivity reactions including rash, contact dermatitis, urticaria, angioedema, bronchospasm and anaphylactic reaction • Skin bruising

Candida infection in the oropharynx is due to drug deposition. Advising the patient to rinse the mouth out with water after each dose will minimise the risk. The incidence should be less with the use of the NebuChamber™ spacer device since this reduces oral deposition.

As with other inhalation therapy, paradoxical bronchospasm may occur, with an immediate increase in wheezing and shortness of breath after dosing. Paradoxical bronchospasm responds to a rapid-acting inhaled bronchodilator and should be treated straightaway. Pulmicort CFC-free Inhaler should be discontinued immediately, the patient should be assessed and an alternative therapy instituted if necessary.

Systemic effects of inhaled corticosteroids may occur, particularly at high doses prescribed for prolonged periods. These effects are much less likely to occur than with oral corticosteroids. Possible systemic effects include Cushing's Syndrome, Cushingoid features, adrenal suppression, growth retardation in children and adolescents, decrease in bone mineral density, cataract and glaucoma. Increased susceptibility to infections and impairment of the ability to adapt to stress may also occur. Effects are probably dependent on dose, exposure time, concomitant and previous steroid exposure and individual sensitivity.

Prolonged treatment with high doses of inhaled corticosteroids, particularly higher than recommended doses, may also result in clinically significant adrenal suppression. Therefore additional systemic corticosteroid cover should be considered during periods of stress, such as severe infections or elective surgery. Such patients should be instructed to carry a steroid warning card indicating their needs. (See also Section 4.4 *Special warnings and precautions for use*)

4.9 Overdose
The only harmful effect that follows inhalation of large amounts of the drug over a short period is suppression of HPA axis function. No special emergency action needs to be taken. Treatment with Pulmicort CFC-free Inhaler should be continued at the recommended dose to control the asthma.

5. PHARMACOLOGICAL PROPERTIES

5.1 Pharmacodynamic properties
Budesonide is a glucocorticosteroid that possesses a high local anti-inflammatory action, with a lower incidence and severity of adverse effects than those seen with oral corticosteroids.

Pharmacotherapeutic group: Other drugs for obstructive airway diseases, inhalants, glucocorticoids. ATC Code: RO3B A02.

Topical anti-inflammatory effect
The exact mechanism of action of glucocorticosteroids in the treatment of asthma is not fully understood. Anti-inflammatory actions such as inhibition of inflammatory mediator release and inhibition of cytokine-mediated immune response are probably important.

A clinical study in asthmatics comparing inhaled and oral budesonide at doses calculated to achieve similar systemic bioavailability demonstrated statistically significant evidence of efficacy with inhaled but not oral budesonide, compared with placebo. Thus, the therapeutic effect of conventional doses of inhaled budesonide may be largely explained by its direct action on the respiratory tract.

In a provocation study, pre-treatment with budesonide for four weeks has shown decreased bronchial constriction in immediate as well as late asthmatic reactions.

Onset of effect
After a single dose of orally inhaled budesonide delivered via dry powder inhaler, improvement of lung function is achieved within a few hours. After therapeutic use of orally inhaled budesonide delivered via dry powder inhaler, improvement in lung function has been shown to occur within 2 days of initiation of treatment although maximum benefit may not be achieved for up to 4 weeks.

Airway reactivity
Budesonide has also been shown to decrease airway reactivity to histamine and methacholine in hyperreactive patients.

Exercise-induced asthma
Therapy with inhaled budesonide has effectively been used for prevention of exercise-induced asthma.

Growth
Limited data from long-term studies suggest that most children and adolescents treated with inhaled budesonide ultimately achieve their adult target height. However, an initial small but transient reduction in growth (approximately 1 cm) has been observed. This generally occurs within the first year of treatment (see Section 4.4 *Special warnings and precautions for use*).

HPA axis function
Studies in healthy volunteers with inhaled budesonide (administered as a dry powder via Turbohaler) have shown dose-related effects on plasma and urinary cortisol. At recommended doses Pulmicort Turbohaler causes less effect on adrenal function than prednisolone 10 mg, as shown by ACTH tests.

5.2 Pharmacokinetic properties
After inhalation of budesonide via pressurised metered dose inhaler, approximately 10% to 15% of the metered dose is deposited in the lungs.

The maximal plasma concentration after oral inhalation of a single dose of 800 or 1600 micrograms budesonide was 1.32 and 2.41 nmol/L respectively, and was reached after about 40 minutes.

Budesonide undergoes an extensive degree (approximately 90%) of biotransformation in the liver, to metabolites of low glucocorticosteroid activity.

The glucocorticosteroid activity of the major metabolites, 6β-hydroxybudesonide and 16α-hydroxyprednisolone, is less than 1% of that of budesonide. The metabolism of budesonide is primarily mediated by CYP3A4, of the cytochrome p450 enzymes.

In a study, 100 mg ketoconazole taken twice daily increased plasma levels of concomitantly administered oral budesonide (single dose of 10 mg) on average by 7.8-fold. Information about this interaction is lacking for inhaled budesonide, but marked increases in plasma levels could be expected.

5.3 Preclinical safety data
The acute toxicity of budesonide is low and of the same order of magnitude and type as that of the reference glucocorticoids studied (beclometasone dipropionate, fluocinolone acetonide).

Results from subacute and chronic toxicity studies show that the systemic effects of budesonide are less severe than, or similar to, those observed after administration of the other glucocorticosteroids e.g. decreased body-weight gain and atrophy of lymphoid tissues and adrenal cortex.

An increased incidence of brain gliomas in male rats, in a carcinogenicity study, could not be verified in a repeat study in which the incidence of gliomas did not differ between any of the groups on active treatment (budesonide, prednisolone, triamcinolone acetonide) and the control groups.

Liver changes (primary hepatocellular neoplasms) found in male rats in the original carcinogenicity study were noted again in the repeat study with budesonide, as well as with the reference glucocorticosteroids. These effects are most probably related to a receptor effect and thus represent a class effect.

Available clinical experience shows no indication that budesonide or other glucocorticosteroids induce brain gliomas or primary hepatocellular neoplasms in man.

In animal reproduction studies, corticosteroids such as budesonide have been shown to induce malformations (cleft palate, skeletal malformations). However, these animal experimental results do not appear to be relevant in humans at the recommended doses.

Animal studies have also identified an involvement of excess prenatal glucocorticosteroids in increased risk for intrauterine growth retardation, adult cardiovascular disease and permanent changes in glucocorticoid receptor density, neurotransmitter turnover and behaviour at exposures below the teratogenic dose range.

The safe use of norflurane has been fully evaluated in preclinical studies. It is well accepted and used in several pressurised metered dose inhalers, and is essentially non-toxic. Magnesium stearate has a history of safe use in man for many years, which supports the view that magnesium stearate is essentially biologically inert. The safe use of magnesium stearate for inhalation has been fully evaluated in preclinical studies. Inhalation toxicity studies conducted with magnesium stearate in rats (26 weeks) and dogs (4 weeks) did not show signs of toxicity up to doses about 490 and 11000 times higher, respectively, than the maximum exposure achievable during the daily treatment with the new formulation. Furthermore, toxicity studies carried out using Pulmicort pressurised metered dose inhaler have shown no evidence of any local or systemic toxicity or irritation attributable to the excipients.

6. PHARMACEUTICAL PARTICULARS

6.1 List of excipients
Norflurane (HFA 134a) - a CFC-free propellant
Magnesium stearate.

6.2 Incompatibilities
Not applicable.

6.3 Shelf life
2 years.

6.4 Special precautions for storage
Do not store above 30°C.

Always store Pulmicort CFC-free Inhaler so that it stands upright on its brown plastic base (with the valve downwards).

The canister contains a pressurised liquid. Do not expose to temperatures higher than 50°C. Do not pierce the canister.

6.5 Nature and contents of container
The immediate container is an aluminium can which is sealed with a metering valve.

The container is assembled with an actuator containing a mouthpiece. The actuator and the mouthpiece are made of polypropylene.

Each inhaler delivers 120 metered doses/actuations after initial priming.

6.6 Special precautions for disposal and other handling
The canister should not be broken, punctured or burnt, even when apparently empty.

7. MARKETING AUTHORISATION HOLDER
AstraZeneca UK Ltd.,
600 Capability Green
Luton
LU1 3LU, UK.

8. MARKETING AUTHORISATION NUMBER(S)
PL 17901/0246

9. DATE OF FIRST AUTHORISATION/RENEWAL OF THE AUTHORISATION
24th September 2008

10. DATE OF REVISION OF THE TEXT
13th August 2009

Pulmicort Inhaler
(AstraZeneca UK Limited)

1. NAME OF THE MEDICINAL PRODUCT
Pulmicort® Inhaler

200 micrograms per actuation, pressurised inhalation suspension

2. QUALITATIVE AND QUANTITATIVE COMPOSITION
Pulmicort Inhaler contains budesonide 200 micrograms per actuation (puff).

For excipients, see 6.1.

3. PHARMACEUTICAL FORM
Pulmicort Inhaler is a pressurised inhalation suspension. The suspension is delivered via a pressurised metered dose inhaler (pMDI).

Pulmicort Inhaler may also be administered via Nebuhaler® and Nebuchamber®.

4. CLINICAL PARTICULARS

4.1 Therapeutic indications
Bronchial asthma.

4.2 Posology and method of administration
For oral inhalation.

Adults, including the elderly: 200 micrograms twice daily, in the morning and in the evening. During periods of severe asthma, the daily dosage can be increased up to 1600 micrograms.

In patients whose asthma is well controlled, the daily dose may be reduced below 400 micrograms, but should not go below 200 micrograms.

The dose should be reduced to the minimum needed to maintain good asthma control.

Children: 50 to 400 micrograms, to be given twice daily. During periods of severe asthma, the daily dose can be increased up to 800 micrograms.

The dose should be reduced to the minimum needed to maintain good asthma control.

Patients maintained on oral glucocorticosteroids
Pulmicort Inhaler may permit replacement or significant reduction in the dosage of oral glucocorticosteroids while maintaining asthma control. For further information on the withdrawal of oral corticosteroids, see section 4.4.

Pulmicort Inhaler with NebuChamber®.
Pulmicort Inhaler with NebuChamber consists of a Pulmicort Inhaler attached to a 250ml, non-electrostatic metal

spacer, with uni-directional inspiratory and expiratory valves.

The use of Pulmicort Inhaler with NebuChamber {*CE mark*} is recommended to enable patients with difficulty in co-ordinating inhalation with actuation, such as infants, young children, the poorly co-operative or the elderly, to derive greater therapeutic benefit. The use of the NebuChamber spacer device obviates the need to co-ordinate breathing and actuation, whilst also reducing oropharyngeal absorption of budesonide. NebuChamber has been designed to maximise the deposition from a pressurised metered dose inhaler in these patient groups.

Use of Pulmicort Inhaler with Nebuhaler ®:

Nebuhaler is a spacer device available separately that is compatible for use with Pulmicort. Nebuhaler is a Medical Device. Nebuhaler is a 750ml plastic cone with a one-way valve. The use of the Nebuhaler spacer device is recommended to enable patients with difficulty co-ordinating conventional aerosols to derive greater delivery and subsequent therapeutic benefits.

Method of Administration

Instructions for the correct use of Pulmicort Inhaler:

Note: It is important to instruct the patient

• To carefully read the instructions for use in the patient information leaflet, which is packed with each inhaler.

• To shake the inhaler thoroughly before each actuation, in order to mix the contents of the inhaler properly.

• To breathe in slowly and deeply through the mouthpiece and to release the dose whilst continuing to breathe in.

On actuation of Pulmicort Inhaler, a suspension of the substance is pumped out of the canister at a high velocity. When the patient inhales through the mouthpiece at the same time as releasing a dose, the substance will follow the inspired air into the airways.

Instructions for the correct use of Pulmicort Inhaler with NebuChamber:

Note: It is important to instruct the patient:

• To carefully read the instructions for use in the patient information leaflet, which is packed with each inhaler.

• To shake the inhaler thoroughly, in order to mix the contents of the inhaler properly.

On actuation of the aerosol, the dose is released into the inhalation chamber. The inhalation chamber is then emptied by two slow deep breaths. Young children may need to breathe 5 - 10 times through the mouthpiece. For further doses, the procedure is repeated. For young children who are unable to breathe through the mouthpiece, a face mask can be used. Compatible face masks are available separately and care should be taken to ensure a good fit is achieved.

4.3 Contraindications

History of hypersensitivity to budesonide or any of the excipients. No other specific contraindications are known, but special care is needed in patients with lung tuberculosis, fungal and viral infections in the airways.

4.4 Special warnings and precautions for use

Patients not dependent on steroids: Treatment with the recommended doses of Pulmicort usually gives a therapeutic benefit within 7 days. However, certain patients may have an excessive collection of mucus secretion in the bronchi. In these cases, a short course of oral corticosteroids (usually 1 to 2 weeks) should be given in addition to the aerosol. After the course of the oral drug, the inhaler alone should be sufficient therapy. Exacerbations of asthma caused by bacterial infections are usually controlled by appropriate antibiotic treatment and possibly increasing the Pulmicort dosage or, if necessary, by giving systemic steroids.

Steroid-dependent patients: Transfer of patients on oral steroids to treatment with Pulmicort demands special care, mainly due to the slow restitution of the disturbed hypothalamic-pituitary function, caused by extended treatment with oral corticosteroids. When the Pulmicort treatment is initiated, the patient should be in a relatively stable phase. Pulmicort is then given, in combination with the previously used oral steroid dose, for about 10 days.

After this period of time, the reduction of oral steroid dose can be started, with a dose reduction corresponding to about 1 mg prednisolone per day, every week. The oral dose is thus reduced to the lowest level which, in combination with Pulmicort, gives a stable respiratory capacity.

In many cases, it may eventually be possible to completely substitute the oral steroid with Pulmicort treatment, but other cases may have to be maintained on a low oral steroid dosage.

Some patients may experience uneasiness during the withdrawal period due to a decreased steroid effect. The physician may have to explain the reason for the Pulmicort treatment in order to encourage the patient to continue. The length of time needed for the body to regain its natural production of corticosteroid in sufficient amounts is often extensive. Prolonged treatment with high doses of inhaled corticosteroids, particularly higher than the recommended doses, may result in clinically significant adrenal suppression. Additional systemic corticosteroid cover should be considered during periods of stress or elective surgery.

During transfer from oral therapy to Pulmicort, a generally lower systemic steroid action will be experienced which may result in the appearance of allergic or arthritic symptoms such as rhinitis, eczema and muscle and joint pain. Specific treatment should be initiated for these conditions. A general insufficient glucocorticosteroid effect should be suspected if, in rare cases, symptoms such as tiredness, headache, nausea and vomiting should occur. In these cases a temporary increase in the dose of oral glucocorticosteroids is sometimes necessary.

As with other inhalation therapy, paradoxical bronchospasm may occur, with an immediate increase in wheezing after dosing. If a severe reaction occurs, treatment should be reassessed and an alternative therapy instituted if necessary.

Systemic effects of inhaled corticosteroids may occur, particularly at high doses prescribed for prolonged periods. These effects are much less likely to occur than with oral corticosteroids. Possible systemic effects include adrenal suppression, growth retardation in children and adolescents, decrease in bone mineral density, cataract and glaucoma.

It is important, therefore, that the dose of inhaled corticosteroid is titrated to the lowest dose at which effective control of asthma is maintained.

It is recommended that the height of children receiving prolonged treatment with inhaled corticosteroids is regularly monitored. If growth is slowed, therapy should be reviewed with the aim of reducing the dose of inhaled corticosteroid, if possible, to the lowest dose at which effective control of asthma is maintained. In addition, consideration should be given to referring the patient to a paediatric respiratory specialist.

If patients find short-acting bronchodilator treatment ineffective, or they need more inhalations than usual, medical attention must be sought. In this situation consideration should be given to the need for or an increase in their regular therapy, e.g., higher doses of inhaled budesonide, the addition of a long-acting beta agonist or a course of oral glucocorticosteroid.

Reduced liver function may affect the elimination of glucocorticosteroids. The plasma clearance following an intravenous dose of budesonide however was similar in cirrhotic patients and in healthy subjects. After oral ingestion systemic availability of budesonide was increased by compromised liver function due to decreased first pass metabolism. The clinical relevance of this to treatment with Pulmicort is unknown as no data exist for inhaled budesonide, but increases in plasma levels and hence an increased risk of systemic adverse effects could be expected.

In vivo studies have shown that oral administration of ketoconazole and itraconazole (known inhibitors of CYP3A4 activity in the liver and in the intestinal mucosa) causes an increase in the systemic exposure to budesonide. Concomitant treatment with ketoconazole and itraconazole or other potent CYP3A4 inhibitors should be avoided (see section 4.5 Interactions). If this is not possible, the time interval between administration of the interacting drugs should be as long as possible. A reduction in the dose of budesonide should also be considered.

4.5 Interaction with other medicinal products and other forms of interaction

The metabolism of budesonide is primarily mediated by CYP3A4, one of the cytochrome p450 enzymes. Inhibitors of this enzyme, e.g. ketoconazole and itraconazole, can therefore increase systemic exposure to budesonide, (see Section 4.4 Special Warnings and Special Precautions for Use and Section 5.2 Pharmacokinetic Properties). Other potent inhibitors of CYP3A4 are also likely to markedly increase plasma levels of budesonide.

4.6 Pregnancy and lactation

Data on approximately 2000 exposed pregnancies indicate no increased teratogenic risk associated with the use of inhaled budesonide. In animal studies, glucocorticosteroids have been shown to induce malformations (see Section 5.3). This is not likely to be relevant for humans given recommended doses, but therapy with inhaled budesonide should be regularly reviewed and maintained at the lowest effective dose.

The administration of budesonide during pregnancy requires that the benefits for the mother be weighed against the risk for the foetus. Inhaled glucocorticosteroids should be considered in preference to oral glucocorticosteroids because of the lower systemic effects at the doses required to achieve similar pulmonary responses. There is no information regarding the passage of budesonide into breast milk.

4.7 Effects on ability to drive and use machines

Pulmicort Inhaler does not affect the ability to drive or operate machinery.

4.8 Undesirable effects

Clinical trials, literature reports and post-marketing experience suggest that the following adverse drug reactions may occur:

Common (>1/100, <1/10)	• Mild irritation in the throat • Candida infection in the oropharynx • Hoarseness • Coughing
Rare (>1/10 000, <1/1 000)	• Nervousness, restlessness, depression, behavioural disturbances • Immediate and delayed hypersensitivity reactions including rash, contact dermatitis, urticaria, angioedema and bronchospasm • Skin bruising

The candida infection in the oropharynx is due to drug deposition. Advising the patient to rinse the mouth out with water after each dosing will minimise the risk. The incidence should be less with the NebuChamber® and Nebuhaler®, as these reduce oral deposition.

As with other inhalation therapy, paradoxical bronchospasm may occur in very rare cases (see Section 4.4).

Systemic effects of inhaled corticosteroids may occur, particularly at high doses prescribed for prolonged periods. These effects are much less likely to occur than with oral corticosteroids. Possible systemic effects include adrenal suppression, growth retardation in children and adolescents, decrease in bone mineral density, cataract and glaucoma. The effect is probably dependent on dose, exposure time, concomitant and previous steroid exposure, and individual sensitivity.

4.9 Overdose

The only harmful effect that follows inhalation of large amounts of the drug over a short period is suppression of hypothalamic-pituitary-adrenal (HPA) axis function. No special emergency action needs to be taken. Treatment with Pulmicort Inhaler should be continued at the recommended dose to control the asthma.

5. PHARMACOLOGICAL PROPERTIES

5.1 Pharmacodynamic properties

Budesonide is a glucocorticosteroid which possesses a high local anti-inflammatory action, with a lower incidence and severity of adverse effects than those seen with oral corticosteroids.

Pharmacotherapeutic group: Other drugs for obstructive airway diseases, inhalants, glucocorticoids. ATC Code: RO3B A02.

Topical anti-inflammatory effect

The exact mechanism of action of glucocorticosteroids in the treatment of asthma is not fully understood. Anti-inflammatory actions, such as inhibition of inflammatory mediator release and inhibition of cytokine-mediated immune response are probably important.

A clinical study in asthmatics comparing inhaled and oral budesonide at doses calculated to achieve similar systemic bioavailability demonstrated statistically significant evidence of efficacy with inhaled but not oral budesonide compared with placebo. Thus, the therapeutic effect of conventional doses of inhaled budesonide may be largely explained by its direct action on the respiratory tract.

In a provocation study pre-treatment with budesonide for four weeks has shown decreased bronchial constriction in immediate as well as late asthmatic reactions.

Onset of effect

After a single dose of orally inhaled budesonide, delivered via dry powder inhaler, improvement of the lung function is achieved within a few hours. After therapeutic use of orally inhaled budesonide delivered via dry powder inhaler, improvement in lung function has been shown to occur within 2 days of initiation of treatment, although maximum benefit may not be achieved for up to 4 weeks.

Airway reactivity

Budesonide has also been shown to decrease airway reactivity to histamine and methacholine in hyper-reactive patients.

Exercise-induced asthma

Therapy with inhaled budesonide has effectively been used for prevention of exercise-induced asthma.

Growth

Limited data from long term studies suggest that most children and adolescents treated with inhaled budesonide ultimately achieve their adult target height. However, an initial small but transient reduction in growth (approximately 1 cm) has been observed. This generally occurs within the first year of treatment (see section 4.4).

HPA axis function

Studies in healthy volunteers with inhaled budesonide (administered as a dry powder via Turbohaler) have shown dose-related effects on plasma and urinary cortisol. At recommended doses, Pulmicort Turbohaler, causes less effect on the adrenal function than prednisolone 10mg, as shown by ACTH tests.

5.2 Pharmacokinetic properties

In healthy volunteers, inhalation of tritium radiolabelled budesonide quickly gives a high plasma concentration and shows good lung deposition and minimal lung biotransformation, thus prolonging duration of action. Systemic availability after inhalation is approximately 70%.

Plasma concentration decreases exponentially with a plasma half-life of 2±0.2 hours.

The metabolism of budesonide is primarily mediated by CYP3A4, one of the cytochrome p450 enzymes. Rapid systemic biotransformation, with relatively inactive metabolites, thereby minimises the risk of systemic effects.

In a study, 100 mg ketoconazole taken twice daily, increased plasma levels of concomitantly administered oral budesonide (single dose of 10 mg) on average, by 7.8-fold. Information about this interaction is lacking for inhaled budesonide, but marked increases in plasma levels could be expected.

5.3 Preclinical safety data

The acute toxicity of budesonide is low and of the same order of magnitude and type as that of the reference glucocorticoids studied (beclomethasone dipropionate, fluocinolone acetonide).

Results from subacute and chronic toxicity studies show that the systemic effects of budesonide are less severe than, or similar to, those observed after administration of the other glucocorticosteroids, e.g. decreased body weight gain and atrophy of lymphoid tissues and adrenal cortex.

An increased incidence of brain gliomas in male rats, in a carcinogenicity study, could not be verified in a repeat study in which the incidence of gliomas did not differ between any of the groups on active treatment (budesonide, prednisolone, triamcinolone acetonide) and the control groups.

Liver changes (primary hepatocellular neoplasms) found in male rats in the original carcinogenicity study were noted again in the repeat study with budesonide, as well as with the reference glucocorticosteroids. These effects are most probably related to a receptor effect and thus represent a class effect.

Available clinical experience shows no indication that budesonide, or other glucocorticosteroids, induce brain gliomas or primary heptocellular neoplasms in man.

In animal reproduction studies, corticosteroids such as budesonide have been shown to induce malformations (cleft palate, skeletal malformations). However, these animal experimental results do not appear to be relevant in humans at the recommended doses.

Animal studies have also identified an involvement of excess prenatal glucocorticosteroids, in increased risk for intrauterine growth retardation, adult cardiovascular disease and permanent changes in glucocorticoid receptor density, neurotransmitter turnover and behaviour at exposures below the teratogenic dose range.

6. PHARMACEUTICAL PARTICULARS

6.1 List of excipients

Sorbitan trioleate, trichlorodifluoromethane (CFC 12), dichlorotetrafluoroethane (CFC 114) and trichlorofluoromethane (CFC 11).

6.2 Incompatibilities

None known.

6.3 Shelf life

2 years.

6.4 Special precautions for storage

Do not store above 30°C.

Do not puncture or expose the canister to high temperatures (40°C) or direct sunlight, even when empty.

6.5 Nature and contents of container

Pulmicort Inhaler is a pressurised metered dose inhaler delivering 200 micrograms budesonide in each actuation.

Pulmicort Inhaler consists of an aluminium vial with a metering valve which is fitted into a plastic device through which the dose is released.

100 and 200 actuation packs are available.

Pulmicort Inhaler is also available with NebuChamber. NebuChamber is a medical device. NebuChamber is a non-electrostatic metal spacer consisting of a 250ml inhalation chamber with unidirectional inspiratory and expiratory valves.

NebuChamber is constructed of stainless steel, it is entirely free of electrostatic forces. Drug delivery will not be affected by any electrostatic forces in the NebuChamber.

6.6 Special precautions for disposal and other handling

See *Section 4.2 Posology and Method of Administration*.

Pulmicort Inhaler may also be used in conjunction with a Nebuhaler spacer device. Nebuhaler is a Medical Device supplied separately with full instructions for use.

7. MARKETING AUTHORISATION HOLDER

AstraZeneca UK Ltd.,

600 Capability Green

Luton

LU1 3LU, UK.

8. MARKETING AUTHORISATION NUMBER(S)

PL 17901/0158

9. DATE OF FIRST AUTHORISATION/RENEWAL OF THE AUTHORISATION

12th August 2002

10. DATE OF REVISION OF THE TEXT

4th April 2005

Pulmicort LS Inhaler

(AstraZeneca UK Limited)

1. NAME OF THE MEDICINAL PRODUCT

Pulmicort® LS Inhaler, 50 micrograms per actuation, pressurised inhalation suspension.

2. QUALITATIVE AND QUANTITATIVE COMPOSITION

Pulmicort LS Inhaler contains budesonide, 50 micrograms per actuation (puff).

For excipients see 6.1.

3. PHARMACEUTICAL FORM

Pulmicort LS Inhaler is a pressurised inhalation suspension. The suspension is delivered via a pressurised metered dose inhaler (pMDI).

Pulmicort LS inhaler may also be administered via the Nebuhaler®.

4. CLINICAL PARTICULARS

4.1 Therapeutic indications

Pulmicort LS Inhaler is recommended in patients with bronchial asthma.

4.2 Posology and method of administration

Adults: 200 micrograms twice daily, in the morning and in the evening. During periods of severe asthma, the daily dosage can be increased up to 1600 micrograms.

In patients whose asthma is well controlled, the daily dose may be reduced below 400 micrograms, but should not go below 200 micrograms.

The dose should be reduced to the minimum needed to maintain good asthma control.

Children: 50 to 400 micrograms to be given twice daily. During periods of severe asthma, the daily dose can be increased up to 800 micrograms.

The dose should be reduced to the minimum needed to maintain good asthma control.

Elderly: Dosage as for adults.

Patients maintained on oral glucocorticosteroids

Pulmicort Inhaler may permit replacement or significant reduction in the dosage of oral glucocorticosteroids while maintaining asthma control. For further information on the withdrawal of oral corticosteroids, see section 4.4

Instructions for the correct use of Pulmicort LS Inhaler:

Note: It is important to instruct the patient

- To carefully read the instructions for use in the patient information leaflet, which is packed with each inhaler.
- To shake the inhaler thoroughly before each actuation, in order to mix the contents of the inhaler properly.
- To breathe in slowly and deeply through the mouthpiece and to release the dose whilst continuing to breathe in.

On actuation of Pulmicort LS Inhaler, a suspension of the substance is pumped out of the canister at a high velocity. When the patient inhales through the mouthpiece at the same time as releasing a dose, the substance will follow the inspired air into the airways.

4.3 Contraindications

History of hypersensitivity to budesonide or any of the excipients. No other specific contraindications are known, but special care is needed in patients with lung tuberculosis, fungal and viral infections in the airways.

4.4 Special warnings and precautions for use

Patients not dependent on steroids: Treatment with the recommended doses of Pulmicort LS Inhaler usually gives a therapeutic benefit within 7 days. However, certain patients may have an excessive collection of mucous secretion in the bronchi, which reduces penetration of the active substance into the airways. In these cases, a short course of oral corticosteroids (usually 1 to 2 weeks) should be given in addition to the aerosol. After the course of the oral drug, the inhaler alone should be sufficient therapy. Exacerbations of asthma caused by bacterial infections are usually controlled by appropriate antibiotic treatment and possibly increasing the Pulmicort LS Inhaler dosage or, if necessary, by giving systemic steroids.

Steroid-dependent patients: Transfer of patients dependent upon oral steroids to treatment with Pulmicort LS Inhaler demands special care, mainly due to the slow restitution of the disturbed hypothalamic-pituitary function, caused by extended treatment with oral corticosteroids. When the Pulmicort LS Inhaler treatment is initiated, the patient should be in a relatively stable phase. Pulmicort LS Inhaler is then given in combination with the previously used oral steroid dose, for about 10 days.

After this period of time, the reduction of the oral corticosteroid dose can be started, with a dose reduction corresponding to about 1 mg prednisolone per day, every week. The oral dose is thus reduced to the lowest level which, in combination with Pulmicort LS Inhaler, gives a stable respiratory capacity.

In many cases, it may eventually be possible to completely substitute the oral steroid with Pulmicort LS Inhaler, but other cases may have to be maintained on a low steroid dosage.

Some patients may experience unease during the withdrawal period due to a decreased steroid effect. The physician may have to explain the reason for the Pulmicort LS Inhaler treatment in order to encourage the patient to continue. The length of time needed for the body to regain its natural production of corticosteroid in sufficient amounts is often extensive. Prolonged treatment with high doses of inhaled corticosteroids, particularly higher than the recommended doses, may result in clinically significant adrenal suppression. Additional systemic corticosteroid cover should be considered during periods of stress or elective surgery.

During transfer from oral therapy to Pulmicort LS Inhaler, a generally lower systemic steroid action will be experienced which may result in the appearance of allergic or arthritic symptoms such as rhinitis, eczema, and muscle and joint pain. Specific treatment should be initiated for these conditions. A general insufficient glucocorticosteroid effect should be suspected if, in rare cases, symptoms such as tiredness, headache, nausea and vomiting should occur. In these cases a temporary increase in the dose of oral glucocorticosteroids is sometimes necessary.

As with other inhalation therapy, paradoxical bronchospasm may occur, with an immediate increase in wheezing after dosing. If a severe reaction occurs, treatment should be reassessed and an alternative therapy instituted if necessary.

Systemic effects of inhaled corticosteroids may occur, particularly at high doses prescribed for prolonged periods. These effects are much less likely to occur than with oral corticosteroids. Possible systemic effects include adrenal suppression, growth retardation in children and adolescents, decrease in bone mineral density, cataract and glaucoma.

It is important, therefore, that the dose of inhaled corticosteroid is titrated to the lowest dose at which effective control of asthma is maintained.

It is recommended that the height of children receiving prolonged treatment with inhaled corticosteroids is regularly monitored. If growth is slowed, therapy should be reviewed with the aim of reducing the dose of inhaled corticosteroid, if possible, to the lowest dose at which effective control of asthma is maintained. In addition, consideration should be given to referring the patient to a paediatric respiratory specialist.

If patients find short-acting bronchodilator treatment ineffective, or they need more inhalations than usual, medical attention must be sought. In this situation consideration should be given to the need for or an increase in their regulartherapy, e.g., higher doses of inhaled budesonide, the addition of a long-acting beta agonist or a course of oral glucocorticosteroid.

Reduced liver function may affect the elimination of glucocorticosteroids. The plasma clearance following an intravenous dose of budesonide however was similar in cirrhotic patients and in healthy subjects. After oral ingestion systemic availability of budesonide was increased by compromised liver function due to decreased first pass metabolism. The clinical relevance of this to treatment with Pulmicort is unknown as no data exist for inhaled budesonide, but increases in plasma levels and hence an increased risk of systemic adverse effects could be expected.

In vivo studies have shown that oral administration of ketoconazole and itraconazole (known inhibitors of CYP3A4 activity in the liver and in the intestinal mucosa) causes an increase in the systemic exposure to budesonide. Concomitant treatment with ketoconazole and itraconazole or other potent CYP3A4 inhibitors should be avoided (see section 4.5 Interactions). If this is not possible, the time interval between administration of the interacting drugs should be as long as possible. A reduction in the dose of budesonide should also be considered.

4.5 Interaction with other medicinal products and other forms of interaction

The metabolism of budesonide is primarily mediated by CYP3A4, one of the cytochrome p450 enzymes. Inhibitors of this enzyme, e.g. ketoconazole and itraconazole, can therefore increase systemic exposure to budesonide, (see Section 4.4 Special Warnings and Special Precautions for Use and Section 5.2 Pharmacokinetic Properties). Other potent inhibitors of CYP3A4 are also likely to markedly increase plasma levels of budesonide.

4.6 Pregnancy and lactation

Data on approximately 2000 exposed pregnancies indicate no increased teratogenic risk associated with the use of inhaled budesonide. In animal studies, glucocorticosteroids have been shown to induce malformations (see Section 5.3). This is not likely to be relevant for humans given recommended doses, but therapy with inhaled budesonide should be regularly reviewed and maintained at the lowest effective dose.

The administration of budesonide during pregnancy requires that the benefits for the mother be weighed against the risk for the foetus. Inhaled glucocorticosteroids should be considered in preference to oral glucocorticosteroids because of the lower systemic effects at the doses required to achieve similar pulmonary responses. There is no information regarding the passage of budesonide into breast milk.

4.7 Effects on ability to drive and use machines

Pulmicort LS Inhaler does not affect ability to drive or use machines.

4.8 Undesirable effects

Clinical trials, literature reports and post-marketing experience suggest that the following adverse drug reactions may occur:

Common (>1/100, <1/10)	• Mild irritation in the throat • Candida infection in the oropharynx • Hoarseness • Coughing
Rare (>1/10 000, <1/1 000)	• Nervousness, restlessness, depression, behavioural disturbances • Immediate and delayed hypersensitivity reactions including rash, contact dermatitis, urticaria, angioedema and bronchospasm • Skin bruising

The candida infection in the oropharynx is due to drug deposition. Advising the patient to rinse the mouth out with water after each dosing will minimise the risk. The incidence should be less with the Nebuhaler®, as this reduces oral deposition.

As with other inhalation therapy, paradoxical bronchospasm may occur in very rare cases (see Section 4.4).

Systemic effects of inhaled corticosteroids may occur, particularly at high doses prescribed for prolonged periods. These effects are much less likely to occur than with oral corticosteroids. Possible systemic effects include adrenal suppression, growth retardation in children and adolescents, decrease in bone mineral density, cataract and glaucoma. The effect is probably dependent on dose, exposure time, concomitant and previous steroid exposure, and individual sensitivity.

4.9 Overdose

The only harmful effect that follows inhalation of large amounts of the drug over a short period is suppression of hypothalamic-pituitary-adrenal (HPA) function. No special emergency action needs to be taken. Treatment with Pulmicort LS Inhaler should be continued at the recommended dose to control the asthma.

5. PHARMACOLOGICAL PROPERTIES

5.1 Pharmacodynamic properties

Budesonide is a glucocorticosteroid which possesses a high local anti-inflammatory action, with a lower incidence and severity of adverse effects than those seen with oral corticosteroids

Pharmacotherapeutic group: Other drugs for obstructive airway diseases, inhalants, glucocorticoids. ATC Code: RO3B A02.

Topical anti-inflammatory effect

The exact mechanism of action of glucocorticosteroids in the treatment of asthma is not fully understood. Anti-inflammatory actions, such as inhibition of inflammatory mediator release and inhibition of cytokine-mediated immune response are probably important.

A clinical study in asthmatics comparing inhaled and oral budesonide at doses calculated to achieve similar systemic bioavailability demonstrated statistically significant evidence of efficacy with inhaled but not oral budesonide compared with placebo. Thus, the therapeutic effect of conventional doses of inhaled budesonide may be largely explained by its direct action on the respiratory tract.

In a provocation study pre-treatment with budesonide for four weeks has shown decreased bronchial constriction in immediate as well as late asthmatic reactions.

Onset of effect

After a single dose of orally inhaled budesonide, delivered via dry powder inhaler, improvement of the lung function is achieved within a few hours. After therapeutic use of orally inhaled budesonide delivered via dry powder inhaler, improvement in lung function has been shown to occur within 2 days of initiation of treatment, although maximum benefit may not be achieved for up to 4 weeks.

Airway reactivity

Budesonide has also been shown to decrease airway reactivity to histamine and methacholine in hyper-reactive patients.

Exercise-induced asthma

Therapy with inhaled budesonide has effectively been used for prevention of exercise-induced asthma.

Growth

Limited data from long term studies suggest that most children and adolescents treated with inhaled budesonide ultimately achieve their adult target height. However, an initial small but transient reduction in growth (approximately 1 cm) has been observed. This generally occurs within the first year of treatment (see section 4.4).

HPA axis function

Studies in healthy volunteers with inhaled budesonide (administered as a dry powder via Turbohaler) have shown dose-related effects on plasma and urinary cortisol. At recommended doses, Pulmicort Turbohaler, causes less effect on the adrenal function than prednisolone 10mg, as shown by ACTH tests.

5.2 Pharmacokinetic properties

Budesonide is a glucocorticosteroid with high local anti-inflammatory effect.

Budesonide undergoes extensive biotransformation in the liver, to metabolites of low glucocorticosteroid activity. The glucocorticosteroid activity of the major metabolites 6β-hydroxybudesonide and 16α-hydroxyprednisolone, is less than 1% of that of budesonide. The metabolism of budesonide is primarily mediated by CYP3A4, one of the cytochrome p450 enzymes.

In a study, 100 mg ketoconazole taken twice daily, increased plasma levels of concomitantly administered oral budesonide (single dose of 10 mg) on average, by 7.8-fold. Information about this interaction is lacking for inhaled budesonide, but marked increases in plasma levels could be expected.

About 10% of the dose is deposited in the lungs. Of the fraction of budesonide which is swallowed, approximately 90% is inactivated at first passage through the liver. The maximal plasma concentration after inhalation of 1 mg budesonide is about 2.1 nmol/L and is reached after about 10 minutes.

5.3 Preclinical safety data

The acute toxicity of budesonide is low and of the same order of magnitude and type as that of the reference glucocorticosteroids studied (beclomethasone dipropionate, fluocinolone acetonide).

Results from subacute and chronic toxicity studies show that the systemic effects of budesonide are less severe than, or similar to, those observed after administration of the other glucocorticosteroids, e.g. decreased body-weight gain and atrophy of lymphoid tissues and adrenal cortex.

An increased incidence of brain gliomas in male rats, in a carcinogenicity study, could not be verified in a repeat study in which the incidence of gliomas did not differ between any of the groups on active treatment (budesonide, prednisolone, triamcinolone acetonide) and the control groups.

Liver changes (primary hepatocellular neoplasms) found in male rats in the original carcinogenicity study were noted again in the repeat study with budesonide, as well as with the reference glucocorticosteroids. These effects are most probably related to a receptor effect and thus represent a class effect.

Available clinical experience shows no indication that budesonide, or other glucocorticosteroids, induce brain gliomas or primary hepatocellular neoplasms in man.

In animal reproduction studies, corticosteroids such as budesonide have been shown to induce malformations (cleft palate, skeletal malformations). However, these animal experimental results do not appear to be relevant in humans at the recommended doses.

Animal studies have also identified an involvement of excess prenatal glucocorticosteroids, in increased risk for intrauterine growth retardation, adult cardiovascular disease and permanent changes in glucocorticoid receptor density, neurotransmitter turnover and behaviour at exposures below the teratogenic dose range.

6. PHARMACEUTICAL PARTICULARS

6.1 List of excipients

Sorbitan trioleate, trichlorofluoromethane, dichlorotetrafluoroethane, dichlorodifluoromethane.

6.2 Incompatibilities

None known.

6.3 Shelf life

24 months

6.4 Special precautions for storage

Do not store above 30°C.

Do not puncture or expose the canister to high temperatures (40°C) or direct sunlight, even when empty.

6.5 Nature and contents of container

Aluminium canister containing 200 metered doses of budesonide, fitted with a valve to deliver 50 micrograms budesonide per actuation. The canister fits into a plastic adaptor made of polypropylene, with a removable cover made of polypropylene or polyethylene.

6.6 Special precautions for disposal and other handling

See Section 4.2 Posology and Method of Administration.

7. MARKETING AUTHORISATION HOLDER

AstraZeneca UK Ltd.,

600 Capability Green,

Luton, LU1 3LU, UK.

8. MARKETING AUTHORISATION NUMBER(S)

PL 17901/0159

9. DATE OF FIRST AUTHORISATION/RENEWAL OF THE AUTHORISATION

28th June 2002

10. DATE OF REVISION OF THE TEXT

4th April 2004

Pulmicort Respules 0.5mg & 1mg Nebuliser Suspension

(AstraZeneca UK Limited)

1. NAME OF THE MEDICINAL PRODUCT

Pulmicort® Respules® 0.5 mg, nebuliser suspension

Pulmicort®Respules®1 mg, nebuliser suspension

2. QUALITATIVE AND QUANTITATIVE COMPOSITION

Pulmicort®Respules®0.5 mg, nebuliser suspension:

Budesonide, 0.25 mg/ml. Each 2 ml Respule contains 0.5 mg of budesonide.

Pulmicort®Respules®1 mg, nebuliser suspension:

Budesonide 0.5 mg/ml. Each 2 ml Respule contains 1 mg budesonide.

For excipients, see 6.1.

3. PHARMACEUTICAL FORM

Sterile nebuliser suspension. White to off-white suspension in plastic single dose units.

4. CLINICAL PARTICULARS

4.1 Therapeutic indications

Pulmicort Respules contain the potent, non-halogenated, corticosteroid, budesonide, for use in bronchial asthma, in patients where use of a pressurised inhaler or dry powder formulation is unsatisfactory or inappropriate.

Pulmicort Respules are also recommended for use in infants and children with acute laryngotracheobronchitis - croup.

4.2 Posology and method of administration

Dosage schedules: Pulmicort Respules should be administered from suitable nebulisers. The dose delivered to the patient varies depending on the nebulising equipment used. The nebulisation time and the dose delivered is dependent on flow rate, volume of nebuliser chamber and fill volume. An air-flow rate of 6 - 8 litres per minute through the device should be employed. A suitable fill volume for most nebulisers is 2 - 4 ml. The dosage of Pulmicort Respules should be adjusted to the need of the individual. The dose should be reduced to the minimum needed to maintain good asthma control. The highest dose (2 mg per day) for children under 12 years should only be considered in children with severe asthma and during limited periods.

Bronchial asthma

Initiation of therapy

When treatment is started, during periods of severe asthma and while reducing or discontinuing oral glucocorticosteroids, the recommended dose of Pulmicort Respules is:

Adults (including elderly): Usually 1 - 2 mg twice daily. In very severe cases the dosage may be further increased.

Children 12 years and older: Dosage as for adults.

Children 3 months to 12 years: 0.5 – 1 mg twice daily.

Maintenance

The maintenance dose should be individualised and be the lowest dose which keeps the patient symptom-free.

Adults (including elderly and children 12 years and older): 0.5 - 1 mg twice daily.

Children 3 months to 12 years: 0.25 - 0.5 mg twice daily.

Patients maintained on oral glucocorticosteroids

Pulmicort Respules may permit replacement or significant reduction in dosage of oral glucocorticosteroids while maintaining asthma control. For further information on the withdrawal of oral corticosteroids, see section 4.4.

Dose division and miscibility

Pulmicort Respules can be mixed with 0.9% saline and with solutions for nebulisation of terbutaline, salbutamol, fenoterol, acetylcysteine, sodium cromoglycate or ipratropium bromide. The admixture should be used within 30 minutes.

Recommended Dosage Table

Dose (mg)	Pulmicort Respules 0.5 mg nebuliser solution (0.25 mg/ml) Volume (ml)	Pulmicort Respules 1 mg nebuliser solution (0.5 mg/ml) Volume (ml)
0.25	1	-
0.5	2	1
0.75	3	-
1.0	4	2
1.5	6	3
2.0	8	4

Where an increased therapeutic effect is desired, especially in those patients without major mucus secretion in the airways, an increased dose of Pulmicort is recommended, rather than combined treatment with oral corticosteroids, because of the lower risk of systemic effects.

Acute laryngotracheobronchitis – croup

In infants and children with croup, the usual dose is 2 mg of nebulised budesonide. This dose is given as a single administration, or as two 1 mg doses separated by 30 minutes.

Instruction for correct use of Pulmicort Respules

The Respule should be detached from the strip, shaken gently and opened by twisting off the wing tab. The contents of the Respule should be gently squeezed into the nebuliser cup. The empty Respule should be thrown away and the top of the nebuliser cup replaced.

Pulmicort Respules should be administered via a jet nebuliser equipped with a mouthpiece or suitable face mask. The nebuliser should be connected to an air compressor with an adequate air flow (6-8 L/min), and the fill volume should be 2-4ml.

Note: It is important to instruct the patient

• to carefully read the instructions for use in the patient information leaflet which are packed together with each nebuliser

• that Ultrasonic nebulisers are not suitable for the administration of Pulmicort Respules and therefore are not recommended

• Pulmicort Respules can be mixed with 0.9% saline and with solutions for nebulisation of terbutaline, salbutamol, fenoterol, acetylcysteine, sodium cromoglycate and ipratropium bromide. The admixture should be used within 30 minutes.

• to rinse the mouth out with water after inhaling the prescribed dose to minimise the risk of oropharyngeal thrush

• to wash the facial skin with water after using the face mask to prevent irritation

• to adequately clean and maintain the nebuliser according to the manufacturer's instructions

The dosage of Pulmicort Respules should be adjusted to the need of the individual.

4.3 Contraindications

History of hypersensitivity to budesonide or any of the excipients.

4.4 Special warnings and precautions for use

Special care is needed in patients with pulmonary tuberculosis and viral infections of the airways.

Non steroid-dependent patients: A therapeutic effect is usually reached within 10 days. In patients with excessive mucus secretion in the bronchi, a short (about 2 weeks) additional oral corticosteroid regimen can be given initially. After the course of the oral drug, Pulmicort Respules alone should be sufficient therapy.

Steroid-dependent patients: When transfer from oral corticosteroid to treatment with Pulmicort is initiated, the patient should be in a relatively stable phase. Pulmicort is then given, in combination with the previously used oral steroid dose, for about 10 days.

After that, the oral steroid dose should be gradually reduced (by, for example, 2.5 mg prednisolone or the equivalent each month), to the lowest possible level. In many cases, it is possible to completely substitute Pulmicort for the oral corticosteroid.

During transfer from oral therapy to Pulmicort, a generally lower systemic corticosteroid action will be experienced, which may result in the appearance of allergic or arthritic symptoms such as rhinitis, eczema and muscle and joint pain. Specific treatment should be initiated for these conditions. A general insufficient glucocorticosteroid effect should be suspected if, in rare cases, symptoms such as tiredness, headache, nausea and vomiting should occur. In these cases a temporary increase in the dose of oral glucocorticosteroids is sometimes necessary.

As with other inhalation therapy, paradoxical bronchospasm may occur, with an immediate increase in wheezing after dosing. If a severe reaction occurs, treatment should be reassessed and an alternative therapy instituted if necessary.

Prolonged treatment with high doses of inhaled corticosteroids, particularly higher than the recommended doses, may result in clinically significant adrenal suppression. Additional systemic corticosteroid cover should be considered during periods of stress or elective surgery.

Systemic effects of inhaled corticosteroids may occur, particularly at high doses prescribed for prolonged periods. These effects are much less likely to occur than with oral corticosteroids. Possible systemic effects include adrenal suppression, growth retardation in children and adolescents, decrease in bone mineral density, cataract and glaucoma.

It is important, therefore, that the dose of inhaled corticosteroid is titrated to the lowest dose at which effective control of asthma is maintained.

It is recommended that the height of children receiving prolonged treatment with inhaled corticosteroids is regularly monitored. If growth is slowed, therapy should be reviewed, with the aim of reducing the dose of inhaled corticosteroid, if possible, to the lowest dose at which effective control of asthma is maintained. In addition, consideration should be given to referring the patient to a paediatric respiratory specialist.

Pulmicort Respules is not intended for rapid relief of acute episodes of asthma where an inhaled short-acting bronchodilator is required. If patients find short-acting bronchodilator treatment ineffective, or they need more inhalations than usual, medical attention must be sought. In this situation consideration should be given to the need for or an increase in their regular therapy, e.g., higher doses of inhaled budesonide or the addition of a long-acting beta agonist, or for a course of oral glucocorticosteroid.

Reduced liver function may affect the elimination of glucocorticosteroids. The plasma clearance following an intravenous dose of budesonide however was similar in cirrhotic patients and in healthy subjects. After oral ingestion systemic availability of budesonide was increased by compromised liver function due to decreased first pass metabolism. The clinical relevance of this to treatment with Pulmicort is unknown as no data exist for inhaled budesonide, but increases in plasma levels and hence an increased risk of systemic adverse effects could be expected.

In vivo studies have shown that oral administration of ketoconazole and itraconazole (known inhibitors of CYP3A4 activity in the liver and in the intestinal mucosa causes an increase in the systemic exposure to budesonide. Concomitant treatment with ketoconazole and itraconazole or other potent CYP3A4 inhibitors should be avoided (see section 4.5 Interactions). If this is not possible, the time interval between administration of the interacting drugs should be as long as possible. A reduction in the dose of budesonide should also be considered.

The nebuliser chamber should be cleaned after every administration. Wash the nebuliser chamber and mouthpiece or face-mask in hot water using a mild detergent. Rinse well and dry, by connecting the nebuliser chamber to the compressor or air inlet.

4.5 Interaction with other medicinal products and other forms of interaction

The metabolism of budesonide is primarily mediated by CYP3A4, one of the cytochrome p450 enzymes. Inhibitors of this enzyme, e.g. ketoconazole and itraconazole, can therefore increase systemic exposure to budesonide, (see Section 4.4 Special Warnings and Special Precautions for Use and Section 5.2 Pharmacokinetic Properties). Other potent inhibitors of CYP3A4 are also likely to markedly increase plasma levels of budesonide.

4.6 Pregnancy and lactation

Data on approximately 2000 exposed pregnancies indicate no increased teratogenic risk associated with the use of inhaled budesonide. In animal studies, glucocorticosteroids have been shown to induce malformations (see Section 5.3). This is not likely to be relevant for humans given recommended doses, but therapy with inhaled budesonide should be regularly reviewed and maintained at the lowest effective dose.

The administration of budesonide during pregnancy requires that the benefits for the mother be weighed against the risk for the foetus. Inhaled glucocorticosteroids should be considered in preference to oral glucocorticosteroids because of the lower systemic effects at the doses required to achieve similar pulmonary responses.

Budesonide is excreted in breast milk. However, at therapeutic doses of Pulmicort Respules no effects on the suckling child are anticipated. Pulmicort Respules can be used during breast feeding.

4.7 Effects on ability to drive and use machines

Pulmicort does not affect the ability to drive or use machinery.

4.8 Undesirable effects

Clinical trials, literature reports and post-marketing experience suggest that the following adverse drug reactions may occur:

Common (>1/100, <1/10)	• Mild irritation in the throat • Candida infection in the oropharynx • Hoarseness • Coughing
Rare (>1/10 000, <1/1 000)	• Nervousness, restlessness, depression, behavioural disturbances • Immediate and delayed hypersensitivity reactions including rash, contact dermatitis, urticaria, angioedema, bronchospasm and anaphylactic reaction. • Skin bruising

The candida infection in the oropharynx is due to drug deposition. Advising the patient to rinse the mouth out with water after each dosing will minimise the risk.

As with other inhalation therapy, paradoxical bronchospasm may occur in very rare cases (see Section 4.4).

Systemic effects of inhaled corticosteroids may occur, particularly at high doses prescribed for prolonged periods. These effects are much less likely to occur than with oral corticosteroids. Possible systemic effects include adrenal suppression, growth retardation in children and adolescents, decrease in bone mineral density, cataract and glaucoma. The effect is probably dependent on dose, exposure time, concomitant and previous steroid exposure, and individual sensitivity.

Facial skin irritation has occurred in some cases when a nebuliser with a face mask has been used. To prevent irritation, the facial skin should be washed with water after use of the face mask.

4.9 Overdose

Pulmicort Respules contains 0.1 mg/ml disodium edetate which has been shown to cause bronchoconstriction at levels above 1.2 mg/ml. Acute overdose with Pulmicort should not present a clinical problem.

5. PHARMACOLOGICAL PROPERTIES

5.1 Pharmacodynamic properties

Budesonide is a glucocorticosteroid which possesses a high local anti-inflammatory action, with a lower incidence and severity of adverse effects than those seen with oral corticosteroids.

Pharmacotherapeutic group: Other drugs for obstructive airway diseases, inhalants, glucocorticoids. ATC Code: RO3B A02.

Topical anti-inflammatory effect

The exact mechanism of action of glucocorticosteroids in the treatment of asthma is not fully understood. Anti-inflammatory actions, such as inhibition of inflammatory mediator release and inhibition of cytokine-mediated immune response are probably important.

A clinical study in asthmatics comparing inhaled and oral budesonide at doses calculated to achieve similar systemic bioavailability demonstrated statistically significant evidence of efficacy with inhaled but not oral budesonide compared with placebo. Thus, the therapeutic effect of conventional doses of inhaled budesonide may be largely explained by its direct action on the respiratory tract.

In a provocation study pre-treatment with budesonide for four weeks has shown decreased bronchial constriction in immediate as well as late asthmatic reactions.

Onset of effect

After a single dose of orally inhaled budesonide, delivered via dry powder inhaler, improvement of the lung function is achieved within a few hours. After therapeutic use of orally inhaled budesonide delivered via dry powder inhaler, improvement in lung function has been shown to occur within 2 days of initiation of treatment although maximum benefit may not be achieved for up to 4 weeks.

Airway reactivity

Budesonide has also been shown to decrease airway reactivity to histamine and methacholine in hyperreactive patients.

Exercise-induced asthma

Therapy with inhaled budesonide has effectively been used for prevention of exercise-induced asthma.

Growth

Limited data from long-term studies suggest that most children and adolescents treated with inhaled budesonide ultimately achieve their adult target height. However, an initial small but transient reduction in growth (approximately 1 cm) has been observed. This generally occurs within the first year of treatment (see section 4.4).

5.2 Pharmacokinetic properties

Budesonide undergoes an extensive biotransformation in the liver, to metabolites of low glucocorticosteroid activity. The glucocorticosteroid activity of the major metabolites, 6β-hydroxybudesonide and 16α-hydroxyprednisolone, is less than 1% of that of budesonide. The metabolism of budesonide is primarily mediated by CYP3A4, one of the cytochrome p450 enzymes.

In a study, 100 mg ketoconazole taken twice daily, increased plasma levels of concomitantly administered oral budesonide (single dose of 10 mg) on average, by 7.8-fold. Information about this interaction is lacking for inhaled budesonide, but marked increases in plasma levels could be expected.

Of the fraction of budesonide which is swallowed, approximately 90% is inactivated at first passage through the liver. The maximal plasma concentration after inhalation of 1 mg budesonide, delivered via dry powder inhaler, is about 3.5 nmol/L and is reached after about 20 minutes.

5.3 Preclinical safety data

The acute toxicity of budesonide is low and of the same order of magnitude and type as that of the reference glucocorticosteroids studied (beclomethasone dipropionate, fluocinolone acetonide).

Results from subacute and chronic toxicity studies show that the systemic effects of budesonide are less severe than, or similar to, those observed after administration of other glucocorticosteroids, e.g. decreased body-weight gain and atrophy of lymphoid tissues and adrenal cortex.

An increased incidence of brain gliomas in male rats, in a carcinogenicity study, could not be verified in a repeat study in which the incidence of gliomas did not differ between any of the groups on active treatment (budesonide, prednisolone, triamcinolone acetonide) and the control groups.

Liver changes (primary hepatocellular neoplasms) found in male rats in the original carcinogenicity study were noted again in the repeat study with budesonide, as well as with the reference glucocorticosteroids. These effects are most probably related to a receptor effect and thus represent a class effect.

Available clinical experience shows that there are no indications that budesonide, or other glucocorticosteroids, induce brain gliomas or primary hepatocellular neoplasms in man.

In animal reproduction studies, corticosteroids such as budesonide have been shown to induce malformations (cleft palate, skeletal malformations). However, these animal experimental results do not appear to be relevant in humans at the recommended doses.

Animal studies have also identified an involvement of excess prenatal glucocorticosteroids, in increased risk for intrauterine growth retardation, adult cardiovascular disease and permanent changes in glucocorticoid receptor density, neurotransmitter turnover and behaviour at exposures below the teratogenic dose range.

6. PHARMACEUTICAL PARTICULARS

6.1 List of excipients

Disodium edetate, sodium chloride, polysorbate 80, citric acid anhydrous, sodium citrate, water for injections.

6.2 Incompatibilities

None known.

6.3 Shelf life

24 months

Use within 3 months of opening the foil envelope.

If only 1ml of suspension is used, the remaining suspension is not sterile and should be discarded immediately.

See section 6.4

6.4 Special precautions for storage

Do not store above 30°C. Store the Respules in the foil envelope to protect them from light.

6.5 Nature and contents of container

Single dose unit made of LD-polyethylene. Each single dose unit contains 2 ml of suspension. Sheets of 5 units are packed in a heat sealed envelope of foil laminate. 4 heat sealed envelopes are packed into a carton.

6.6 Special precautions for disposal and other handling

See section 4.2

7. MARKETING AUTHORISATION HOLDER

AstraZeneca UK Ltd,

600 Capability Green,

Luton, LU1 3LU, UK.

8. MARKETING AUTHORISATION NUMBER(S)

Pulmicort®Respules®0.5 mg, nebuliser suspension: PL 17901/0160

Pulmicort®Respules®1 mg, nebuliser suspension: PL 17901/0161

9. DATE OF FIRST AUTHORISATION/RENEWAL OF THE AUTHORISATION

11th June 2002/ 15th Oct 2003

10. DATE OF REVISION OF THE TEXT

21st July 2009

Pulmicort Turbohaler 100

(AstraZeneca UK Limited)

1. NAME OF THE MEDICINAL PRODUCT

Pulmicort® Turbohaler® 100.

2. QUALITATIVE AND QUANTITATIVE COMPOSITION

Budesonide 100 micrograms/actuation.

There are no inactive ingredients.

3. PHARMACEUTICAL FORM

Breath-actuated metered dose powder inhaler.

4. CLINICAL PARTICULARS

4.1 Therapeutic indications

Pulmicort is recommended in patients with bronchial asthma.

4.2 Posology and method of administration

Pulmicort Turbohaler is for oral inhalation

When transferring patients to Turbohaler from other devices, treatment should be individualised, whether once or twice daily dosing is being used. The drug and method of delivery should be considered.

Divided doses (twice daily):

The dosage should be individualised.

The dose should always be reduced to the minimum needed to maintain good asthma control.

Adults (including elderly) and children over 12 years of age: When starting treatment, during periods of severe asthma and while reducing or discontinuing oral glucocorticosteroids, the dosage in adults should be 200 - 1600 micrograms daily, in divided doses.

In less severe cases and children over 12 years of age, 200 - 800 micrograms daily, in divided doses, may be used. During periods of severe asthma, the daily dosage can be increased to up to 1600 micrograms, in divided doses.

Children 5 - 12 years of age: 200 - 800 micrograms daily, in divided doses. During periods of severe asthma, the daily dose can be increased up to 800 micrograms.

Once daily dosage:

The dosage should be individualised.

The dose should always be reduced to the minimum needed to maintain good asthma control.

Adults (including elderly) and children over 12 years of age: 200 micrograms to 400 micrograms may be used in patients with mild to moderate asthma who have not previously received inhaled glucocorticosteroids.

Up to 800 micrograms may be used by patients with mild to moderate asthma already controlled on inhaled steroids (e.g. budesonide or beclomethasone dipropionate), administered twice daily.

Children 5 - 12 years of age: 200 micrograms to 400 micrograms may be used in children with mild to moderate asthma who have not previously received inhaled glucocorticosteroids, or who are already controlled on inhaled steroids (e.g. budesonide or beclomethasone dipropionate), administered twice daily.

The patient should be transferred to once daily dosing at the same equivalent total daily dose; the drug and method of delivery should be considered. The dose should subsequently be reduced to the minimum needed to maintain good asthma control.

Patients should be instructed to take the once daily dose in the evening. It is important that the dose is taken consistently and at a similar time each evening.

There are insufficient data to make recommendations for the transfer of patients from newer inhaled steroids to once daily Pulmicort Turbohaler.

Patients, in particular those receiving once daily treatment, should be advised that if their asthma deteriorates (e.g. increased frequency of bronchodilator use or persistent respiratory symptoms) they should double their steroid dose, by administering it twice daily, and should contact their doctor as soon as possible.

In patients where an increased therapeutic effect is desired, an increased dose of Pulmicort is recommended because of the lower risk of systemic effects as compared with a combined treatment with oral glucocorticosteroids.

Patients maintained on oral glucocorticosteroids

Pulmicort Turbohaler may permit replacement or significant reduction in dosage of oral glucocorticosteroids while maintaining asthma control. For further information on the withdrawal of oral corticosteroids, see section 4.4.

Patients should be reminded of the importance of taking prophylactic therapy regularly, even when they are asymptomatic. A short-acting inhaled bronchodilator should be made available for the relief of acute asthma symptoms.

Instructions for the correct use of Pulmicort Turbohaler

Turbohaler is inspiratory flow-driven which means that, when the patient inhales through the mouthpiece, the substance will follow the inspired air into the airways.

Note: It is important to instruct the patient:

- To carefully read the instructions for use in the patient information leaflet, which is packed with each Turbohaler
- To breathe in forcefully and deeply through the mouthpiece to ensure that an optimal dose is delivered to the lungs
- Never to breathe out through the mouthpiece
- To rinse the mouth out with water and spit it out, or to brush the teeth after inhaling the prescribed dose, to minimise the risk of oropharyngeal thrush

The patient may not taste or feel any medication when using Turbohaler due to the small amount of drug dispensed.

4.3 Contraindications

Hypersensitivity to budesonide.

4.4 Special warnings and precautions for use

Special caution is necessary in patients with active or quiescent pulmonary tuberculosis, and in patients with fungal or viral infections in the airways.

Non steroid-dependent patients: A therapeutic effect is usually reached within 10 days. In patients with excessive mucus secretion in the bronchi, a short (about 2 weeks) additional oral corticosteroid regimen can be given initially.

Steroid-dependent patients: When transferral from oral steroids to Pulmicort Turbohaler is started, the patient should be in a relatively stable phase. A high dose of Pulmicort Turbohaler is then given in combination with the previously used oral steroid dose for about 10 days.

After that, the oral steroid dose should be gradually reduced (by for example 2.5 milligrams prednisolone or the equivalent each month) to the lowest possible level. In many cases, it is possible to completely substitute Pulmicort for the oral steroid.

During transfer from oral therapy to Pulmicort, a generally lower systemic steroid action will be experienced which may result in the appearance of allergic or arthritic symptoms such as rhinitis, eczema and muscle and joint pain. Specific treatment should be initiated for these conditions. During the withdrawal of oral steroids, patients may feel unwell in a non-specific way, even though respiratory function is maintained or improved. Patients should be encouraged to continue with Pulmicort therapy whilst withdrawing the oral steroid, unless there are clinical signs to indicate the contrary. A general insufficient glucocorticosteroid effect should be suspected if, in rare cases, symptoms such as tiredness, headache, nausea and vomiting should occur. In these cases a temporary increase in the dose of oral glucocorticosteroids is sometimes necessary.

As with other inhalation therapy, paradoxical bronchospasm may occur, with an immediate increase in wheezing after dosing. If a severe reaction occurs, treatment should be reassessed and an alternative therapy instituted if necessary.

Patients who have previously been dependent on oral steroids may, as a result of prolonged systemic steroid therapy, experience the effects of impaired adrenal function. Recovery may take a considerable amount of time after cessation of oral steroid therapy, hence oral steroid-dependent patients transferred to budesonide may remain at risk from impaired adrenal function for some considerable time. In such circumstances, HPA axis functions should be monitored regularly.

Acute exacerbations of asthma may need an increase in the dose of Pulmicort or additional treatment with a short course of oral corticosteroid and/or an antibiotic, if there is an infection. The patient should be advised to use a short-acting inhaled bronchodilator as rescue medication to relieve acute asthma symptoms.

If patients find short-acting bronchodilator treatment ineffective or they need more inhalations than usual, medical attention must be sought. In this situation consideration should be given to the need for or an increase in their regular therapy, e.g., higher doses of inhaled budesonide or the addition of a long-acting beta agonist, or for a course of oral glucocorticosteroid.

Prolonged treatment with high doses of inhaled corticosteroids, particularly higher than the recommended doses, may result in clinically significant adrenal suppression. Additional systemic corticosteroid cover should be considered during periods of stress or elective surgery. These patients should be instructed to carry a steroid warning card indicating their needs. Treatment with supplementary systemic steroids or Pulmicort should not be stopped abruptly.

Systemic effects of inhaled corticosteroids may occur, particularly at high doses prescribed for prolonged periods. These effects are much less likely to occur than with oral corticosteroids. Possible systemic effects include adrenal suppression, growth retardation in children and adolescents, decrease in bone mineral density, cataract and glaucoma.

It is important, therefore, that the dose of inhaled corticosteroid is titrated to the lowest dose at which effective control of asthma is maintained.

It is recommended that the height of children receiving prolonged treatment with inhaled corticosteroids is regularly monitored. If growth is slowed, therapy should be reviewed with the aim of reducing the dose of inhaled corticosteroid, if possible, to the lowest dose at which effective control of asthma is maintained. In addition, consideration should be given to referring the patient to a paediatric respiratory specialist.

Reduced liver function may affect the elimination of glucocorticosteroids. The plasma clearance following an intravenous dose of budesonide however was similar in cirrhotic patients and in healthy subjects. After oral ingestion systemic availability of budesonide was increased by compromised liver function due to decreased first pass metabolism. The clinical relevance of this to treatment with Pulmicort is unknown as no data exist for inhaled budesonide, but increases in plasma levels and hence an increased risk of systemic adverse effects could be expected.

In vivo studies have shown that oral administration of ketoconazole and itraconazole (known inhibitors of CYP3A4 activity in the liver and in the intestinal mucosa causes an increase in the systemic exposure to budesonide. Concomitant treatment with ketoconazole and itraconazole or other potent CYP3A4 inhibitors should be avoided (see section 4.5 Interactions). If this is not possible, the time interval between administration of the interacting drugs should be as long as possible. A reduction in the dose of budesonide should also be considered.

4.5 Interaction with other medicinal products and other forms of interaction

The metabolism of budesonide is primarily mediated by CYP3A4, one of the cytochrome p450 enzymes. Inhibitors of this enzyme, e.g. ketoconazole and itraconazole, can therefore increase systemic exposure to budesonide, (see Section 4.4 Special Warnings and Special Precautions for Use and Section 5.2 Pharmacokinetic Properties). Other potent inhibitors of CYP3A4 are also likely to markedly increase plasma levels of budesonide.

4.6 Pregnancy and lactation

Data on approximately 2000 exposed pregnancies indicate no increased teratogenic risk associated with the use of inhaled budesonide. In animal studies, glucocorticosteroids have been shown to induce malformations (see Section 5.3). This is not likely to be relevant for humans given recommended doses, but therapy with inhaled budesonide should be regularly reviewed and maintained at the lowest effective dose.

The administration of budesonide during pregnancy requires that the benefits for the mother be weighed against the risk for the foetus. Inhaled glucocorticosteroids should be considered in preference to oral glucocorticosteroids because of the lower systemic effects at the doses required to achieve similar pulmonary responses.

Budesonide is excreted in breast milk. However, at therapeutic doses of Pulmicort Turbohaler no effects on the suckling child are anticipated. Pulmicort Turbohaler can be used during breast feeding.

4.7 Effects on ability to drive and use machines

Pulmicort Turbohaler does not affect the ability to drive or to use machines.

4.8 Undesirable effects

Clinical trials, literature reports and post-marketing experience suggest that the following adverse drug reactions may occur:

Common (>1/100, <1/10)	• Mild irritation in the throat • Candida infection in the oropharynx • Hoarseness • Coughing
Rare (>1/10 000, <1/1 000)	• Nervousness, restlessness, depression, behavioural disturbances • Immediate and delayed hypersensitivity reactions including rash, contact dermatitis, urticaria, angioedema, bronchospasm and anaphylactic reaction. • Skin bruising

The candida infection in the oropharynx is due to drug deposition. Advising the patient to rinse the mouth out with water after each dosing will minimise the risk.

As with other inhalation therapy, paradoxical bronchospasm may occur in very rare cases (see Section 4.4).

Systemic effects of inhaled corticosteroids may occur, particularly at high doses prescribed for prolonged periods. These effects are much less likely to occur than with oral corticosteroids. Possible systemic effects include adrenal suppression, growth retardation in children and adolescents, decrease in bone mineral density, cataract and glaucoma. The effect is probably dependent on dose, exposure time, concomitant and previous steroid exposure, and individual sensitivity.

4.9 Overdose

The only harmful effect that follows inhalation of large amounts of the drug over a short period is suppression of hypothalamic-pituitary-adrenal (HPA) function. No special emergency action needs to be taken. Treatment with Pulmicort Turbohaler should be continued at the recommended dose to control the asthma.

5. PHARMACOLOGICAL PROPERTIES

5.1 Pharmacodynamic properties

Budesonide is a glucocorticosteroid which possesses a high local anti-inflammatory action, with a lower incidence and severity of adverse effects than those seen with oral corticosteroids.

Pharmacotherapeutic group: Other drugs for obstructive airway diseases, inhalants, glucocorticoids. ATC Code: RO3B A02.

Topical anti-inflammatory effect

The exact mechanism of action of glucocorticosteroids in the treatment of asthma is not fully understood. Anti-inflammatory actions, such as inhibition of inflammatory mediator release and inhibition of cytokine-mediated immune response are probably important.

A clinical study in asthmatics comparing inhaled and oral budesonide at doses calculated to achieve similar systemic bioavailability demonstrated statistically significant evidence of efficacy with inhaled but not oral budesonide compared with placebo. Thus, the therapeutic effect of conventional doses of inhaled budesonide may be largely explained by its direct action on the respiratory tract.

In a provocation study pre-treatment with budesonide for four weeks has shown decreased bronchial constriction in immediate as well as late asthmatic reactions.

Onset of effect

After a single dose of orally inhaled budesonide, delivered via dry powder inhaler, improvement of the lung function is achieved within a few hours. After therapeutic use of orally inhaled budesonide delivered via dry powder inhaler, improvement in lung function has been shown to occur within 2 days of initiation of treatment, although maximum benefit may not be achieved for up to 4 weeks.

Airway reactivity

Budesonide has also been shown to decrease airway reactivity to histamine and methacholine in hyper-reactive patients.

Exercise-induced asthma

Therapy with inhaled budesonide has effectively been used for prevention of exercise-induced asthma.

Growth

Limited data from long term studies suggest that most children and adolescents treated with inhaled budesonide ultimately achieve their adult target height. However, an initial small but transient reduction in growth (approximately 1 cm) has been observed. This generally occurs within the first year of treatment (see section 4.4).

HPA axis function

Studies in healthy volunteers with Pulmicort Turbohaler have shown dose-related effects on plasma and urinary cortisol. At recommended doses, Pulmicort Turbohaler, causes less effect on the adrenal function than prednisolone 10mg, as shown by ACTH tests.

5.2 Pharmacokinetic properties

After inhalation via Turbohaler, about 25 - 30% of the metered dose is deposited in the lungs.

Of the fraction which is swallowed, approximately 90% is inactivated by first pass metabolism in the liver.

The maximal plasma concentration after inhalation of 1 milligram budesonide is about 3.5 nmol/L and is reached after about 20 minutes.

Budesonide undergoes an extensive degree (approximately 90%) of biotransformation in the liver, to metabolites of low glucocorticosteroid activity. The glucocorticosteroid activity of the major metabolites, 6β-hydroxybudesonide and 16α-hydroxyprednisolone, is less than 1% of that of budesonide. The metabolism of budesonide is primarily mediated by CYP3A4, one of the cytochrome p450 enzymes.

In a study, 100 mg ketoconazole taken twice daily, increased plasma levels of concomitantly administered oral budesonide (single dose of 10 mg) on average, by 7.8-fold. Information about this interaction is lacking for inhaled budesonide, but marked increases in plasma levels could be expected.

5.3 Preclinical safety data

The acute toxicity of budesonide is low and of the same order of magnitude and type as that of the reference glucocorticosteroids studied (beclomethasone dipropionate, fluocinolone acetonide).

Results from subacute and chronic toxicity studies show that the systemic effects of budesonide are less severe than, or similar to, those observed after administration of the other glucocorticosteroids, e.g. decreased body-weight gain and atrophy of lymphoid tissues and adrenal cortex.

An increased incidence of brain gliomas in male rats, in a carcinogenicity study, could not be verified in a repeat study in which the incidence of gliomas did not differ between any of the groups on active treatment (budesonide, prednisolone, triamcinolone acetonide) and the control groups.

Liver changes (primary hepatocellular neoplasms) found in male rats in the original carcinogenicity study were noted again in the repeat study with budesonide, as well as with the reference glucocorticosteroids. These effects are most probably related to a receptor effect and thus represent a class effect.

Available clinical experience shows no indication that budesonide, or other glucocorticosteroids, induce brain gliomas or primary hepatocellular neoplasms in man.

In animal reproduction studies, corticosteroids such as budesonide have been shown to induce malformations (cleft palate, skeletal malformations). However, these animal experimental results do not appear to be relevant in humans at the recommended doses.

Animal studies have also identified an involvement of excess prenatal glucocorticosteroids, in increased risk for intrauterine growth retardation, adult cardiovascular disease and permanent changes in glucocorticoid receptor density, neurotransmitter turnover and behaviour at exposures below the teratogenic dose range.

6. PHARMACEUTICAL PARTICULARS

6.1 List of excipients

Pulmicort Turbohaler contains only active drug, budesonide. There are no propellants, lubricants, preservatives, carrier substances or other additives.

6.2 Incompatibilities

None known.

6.3 Shelf life

24 months.

6.4 Special precautions for storage

Do not store above 30°C.

6.5 Nature and contents of container

Polyethylene container consisting of a cover screwed onto a bottom plate. Inside this is the inhaler with its main parts: a mouthpiece, a dosing mechanism and a substance store.

The device also contains a desiccant.

100 micrograms/actuation. 200 actuations.

6.6 Special precautions for disposal and other handling

See section 4.2

7. MARKETING AUTHORISATION HOLDER

AstraZeneca UK Ltd
600 Capability Green,
Luton, LU1 3LU, UK.

8. MARKETING AUTHORISATION NUMBER(S)

PL 17901/0162

9. DATE OF FIRST AUTHORISATION/RENEWAL OF THE AUTHORISATION

18th June 2002

10. DATE OF REVISION OF THE TEXT

13th August 2009

Pulmicort Turbohaler 200

(AstraZeneca UK Limited)

1. NAME OF THE MEDICINAL PRODUCT

Pulmicort® Turbohaler® 200.

2. QUALITATIVE AND QUANTITATIVE COMPOSITION

Budesonide 200 micrograms/actuation.

There are no inactive ingredients.

3. PHARMACEUTICAL FORM

Breath-actuated metered dose powder inhaler.

4. CLINICAL PARTICULARS

4.1 Therapeutic indications

Pulmicort is recommended in patients with bronchial asthma.

4.2 Posology and method of administration

Pulmicort Turbohaler is for oral inhalation.

When transferring patients to Turbohaler from other devices, treatment should be individualised, whether once or twice daily dosing is being used. The drug and method of delivery should be considered.

Divided doses (twice daily):

The dosage should be individualised.

The dose should always be reduced to the minimum needed to maintain good asthma control.

Adults (including elderly) and children over 12 years of age: When starting treatment, during periods of severe asthma and while reducing or discontinuing oral glucocorticosteroids, the dosage in adults should be 200 - 1600 micrograms daily, in divided doses.

In less severe cases and children over 12 years of age, 200 - 800 micrograms daily, in divided doses, may be used. During periods of severe asthma, the daily dosage can be increased to up to 1600 micrograms, in divided doses.

Children 5 - 12 years of age: 200 - 800 micrograms daily, in divided doses. During periods of severe asthma, the daily dose can be increased up to 800 micrograms.

Once daily dosage:

The dosage should be individualised.

The dose should always be reduced to the minimum needed to maintain good asthma control.

Adults (including elderly) and children over 12 years of age: 200 micrograms to 400 micrograms may be used in patients with mild to moderate asthma who have not previously received inhaled glucocorticosteroids.

Up to 800 micrograms may be used by patients with mild to moderate asthma already controlled on inhaled steroids (e.g. budesonide or beclomethasone dipropionate), administered twice daily.

Children 5 - 12 years of age: 200 micrograms to 400 micrograms may be used in children with mild to moderate asthma who have not previously received inhaled glucocorticosteroids, or who are already controlled on inhaled steroids (e.g. budesonide or beclomethasone dipropionate), administered twice daily.

The patient should be transferred to once daily dosing at the same equivalent total daily dose; the drug and method of delivery should be considered. The dose should subsequently be reduced to the minimum needed to maintain good asthma control.

Patients should be instructed to take the once daily dose in the evening. It is important that the dose is taken consistently and at a similar time each evening.

There are insufficient data to make recommendations for the transfer of patients from newer inhaled steroids to once daily Pulmicort Turbohaler.

Patients, in particular those receiving once daily treatment, should be advised that if their asthma deteriorates (e.g. increased frequency of bronchodilator use or persistent respiratory symptoms) they should double their steroid dose, by administering it twice daily, and should contact their doctor as soon as possible.

In patients where an increased therapeutic effect is desired, an increased dose of Pulmicort is recommended because of the lower risk of systemic effects as compared with a combined treatment with oral glucocorticosteroids.

Patients maintained on oral glucocorticosteroids

Pulmicort Turbohaler may permit replacement or significant reduction in dosage of oral glucocorticosteroids while maintaining asthma control. For further information on the withdrawal of oral corticosteroids, see section 4.4.

Patients should be reminded of the importance of taking prophylactic therapy regularly, even when they are asymptomatic. A short-acting inhaled bronchodilator should be made available for the relief of acute asthma symptoms.

Instructions for the correct use of Pulmicort Turbohaler

Turbohaler is inspiratory flow-driven which means that, when the patient inhales through the mouthpiece, the substance will follow the inspired air into the airways.

Note: It is important to instruct the patient:

- To carefully read the instructions for use in the patient information leaflet, which is packed with each Turbohaler
- To breathe in forcefully and deeply through the mouthpiece to ensure that an optimal dose is delivered to the lungs
- Never to breathe out through the mouthpiece
- To rinse the mouth out with water and spit it out, or to brush the teeth after inhaling the prescribed dose, to minimise the risk of oropharyngeal thrush

The patient may not taste or feel any medication when using Turbohaler due to the small amount of drug dispensed.

4.3 Contraindications

Hypersensitivity to budesonide.

4.4 Special warnings and precautions for use

Special caution is necessary in patients with active or quiescent pulmonary tuberculosis, and in patients with fungal or viral infections in the airways.

Non steroid-dependent patients: A therapeutic effect is usually reached within 10 days. In patients with excessive mucus secretion in the bronchi, a short (about 2 weeks) additional oral corticosteroid regimen can be given initially.

Steroid-dependent patients: When transferral from oral steroids to Pulmicort Turbohaler is started, the patient should be in a relatively stable phase. A high dose of Pulmicort Turbohaler is then given in combination with the previously used oral steroid dose for about 10 days.

After that, the oral steroid dose should be gradually reduced (by for example 2.5 milligrams prednisolone or the equivalent each month) to the lowest possible level. In many cases, it is possible to completely substitute Pulmicort for the oral steroid.

During transfer from oral therapy to Pulmicort, a generally lower systemic steroid action will be experienced which may result in the appearance of allergic or arthritic symptoms such as rhinitis, eczema and muscle and joint pain. Specific treatment should be initiated for these conditions. During the withdrawal of oral steroids, patients may feel unwell in a non-specific way, even though respiratory function is maintained or improved. Patients should be encouraged to continue with Pulmicort therapy whilst withdrawing the oral steroid, unless there are clinical signs to indicate the contrary. A general insufficient glucocorticosteroid effect should be suspected if, in rare cases, symptoms such as tiredness, headache, nausea and vomiting should occur. In these cases a temporary increase in the dose of oral glucocorticosteroids is sometimes necessary.

As with other inhalation therapy, paradoxical bronchospasm may occur, with an immediate increase in wheezing after dosing. If a severe reaction occurs, treatment should be reassessed and an alternative therapy instituted if necessary.

Patients who have previously been dependent on oral steroids may, as a result of prolonged systemic steroid therapy, experience the effects of impaired adrenal function. Recovery may take a considerable amount of time after cessation of oral steroid therapy, hence oral steroid-dependent patients transferred to budesonide may remain at risk from impaired adrenal function for some considerable time. In such circumstances, HPA axis functions should be monitored regularly.

Acute exacerbations of asthma may need an increase in the dose of Pulmicort or additional treatment with a short course of oral corticosteroid and/or an antibiotic, if there is an infection. The patient should be advised to use a short-acting inhaled bronchodilator as rescue medication to relieve acute asthma symptoms.

If patients find short-acting bronchodilator treatment ineffective or they need more inhalations than usual, medical attention must be sought. In this situation consideration should be given to the need for or an increase in their regular therapy, e.g., higher doses of inhaled budesonide or the addition of a long-acting beta agonist, or for a course of oral glucocorticosteroid.

Prolonged treatment with high doses of inhaled corticosteroids, particularly higher than the recommended doses, may result in clinically significant adrenal suppression. Additional systemic corticosteroid cover should be considered during periods of stress or elective surgery. These patients should be instructed to carry a steroid warning card indicating their needs. Treatment with supplementary systemic steroids or Pulmicort should not be stopped abruptly.

Systemic effects of inhaled corticosteroids may occur, particularly at high doses prescribed for prolonged periods. These effects are much less likely to occur than with oral corticosteroids. Possible systemic effects include adrenal suppression, growth retardation in children and adolescents, decrease in bone mineral density, cataract and glaucoma.

It is important, therefore, that the dose of inhaled corticosteroid is titrated to the lowest dose at which effective control of asthma is maintained.

It is recommended that the height of children receiving prolonged treatment with inhaled corticosteroids is regularly monitored. If growth is slowed, therapy should be reviewed with the aim of reducing the dose of inhaled corticosteroid, if possible, to the lowest dose at which effective control of asthma is maintained. In addition, consideration should be given to referring the patient to a paediatric respiratory specialist.

Reduced liver function may affect the elimination of glucocorticosteroids. The plasma clearance following an intravenous dose of budesonide however was similar in cirrhotic patients and in healthy subjects. After oral ingestion systemic availability of budesonide was increased by compromised liver function due to decreased first pass metabolism. The clinical relevance of this to treatment with Pulmicort is unknown as no data exist for inhaled budesonide, but increases in plasma levels and hence an increased risk of systemic adverse effects could be expected.

In vivo studies have shown that oral administration of ketoconazole and itraconazole (known inhibitors of CYP3A4 activity in the liver and in the intestinal mucosa causes an increase in the systemic exposure to budesonide. Concomitant treatment with ketoconazole and itraconazole or other potent CYP3A4 inhibitors should be avoided (see section 4.5 Interactions). If this is not possible, the time interval between administration of the interacting drugs should be as long as possible. A reduction in the dose of budesonide should also be considered.

4.5 Interaction with other medicinal products and other forms of interaction

The metabolism of budesonide is primarily mediated by CYP3A4, one of the cytochrome p450 enzymes. Inhibitors of this enzyme, e.g. ketoconazole and itraconazole, can therefore increase systemic exposure to budesonide, (see Section 4.4 Special Warnings and Special Precautions for Use and Section 5.2 Pharmacokinetic Properties). Other potent inhibitors of CYP3A4 are also likely to markedly increase plasma levels of budesonide.

4.6 Pregnancy and lactation

Data on approximately 2000 exposed pregnancies indicate no increased teratogenic risk associated with the use of inhaled budesonide. In animal studies, glucocorticosteroids have been shown to induce malformations (see Section 5.3). This is not likely to be relevant for humans given recommended doses, but therapy with inhaled budesonide should be regularly reviewed and maintained at the lowest effective dose.

The administration of budesonide during pregnancy requires that the benefits for the mother be weighed against the risk for the foetus. Inhaled glucocorticosteroids should be considered in preference to oral glucocorticosteroids because of the lower systemic effects at the doses required to achieve similar pulmonary responses.

Budesonide is excreted in breast milk. However, at therapeutic doses of Pulmicort Turbohaler no effects on the suckling child are anticipated. Pulmicort Turbohaler can be used during breast feeding.

4.7 Effects on ability to drive and use machines

Pulmicort Turbohaler does not affect the ability to drive or to use machines.

4.8 Undesirable effects

Clinical trials, literature reports and post-marketing experience suggest that the following adverse drug reactions may occur:

Common ($>$1/100, $<$1/10)	• Mild irritation in the throat • Candida infection in the oropharynx • Hoarseness • Coughing
Rare ($>$1/10 000, $<$1/1 000)	• Nervousness, restlessness, depression, behavioural disturbances • Immediate and delayed hypersensitivity reactions including rash, contact dermatitis, urticaria, angioedema, bronchospasm and anaphylactic reaction. • Skin bruising

The candida infection in the oropharynx is due to drug deposition. Advising the patient to rinse the mouth out with water after each dosing will minimise the risk.

As with other inhalation therapy, paradoxical bronchospasm may occur in very rare cases (see Section 4.4).

Systemic effects of inhaled corticosteroids may occur, particularly at high doses prescribed for prolonged periods. These effects are much less likely to occur than with oral corticosteroids. Possible systemic effects include adrenal suppression, growth retardation in children and adolescents, decrease in bone mineral density, cataract and glaucoma. The effect is probably dependent on dose, exposure time, concomitant and previous steroid exposure, and individual sensitivity.

4.9 Overdose

The only harmful effect that follows inhalation of large amounts of the drug over a short period is suppression of hypothalamic-pituitary-adrenal (HPA) function. No special emergency action needs to be taken. Treatment with Pulmicort Turbohaler should be continued at the recommended dose to control the asthma.

5. PHARMACOLOGICAL PROPERTIES

5.1 Pharmacodynamic properties

Budesonide is a glucocorticosteroid which possesses a high local anti-inflammatory action, with a lower incidence and severity of adverse effects than those seen with oral corticosteroids.

Pharmacotherapeutic group: Other drugs for obstructive airway diseases, inhalants, glucocorticoids. ATC Code: RO3B A02.

Topical anti-inflammatory effect

The exact mechanism of action of glucocorticosteroids in the treatment of asthma is not fully understood. Anti-inflammatory actions, such as inhibition of inflammatory mediator release and inhibition of cytokine-mediated immune response are probably important.

A clinical study in asthmatics comparing inhaled and oral budesonide at doses calculated to achieve similar systemic bioavailability demonstrated statistically significant evidence of efficacy with inhaled but not oral budesonide compared with placebo. Thus, the therapeutic effect of conventional doses of inhaled budesonide may be largely explained by its direct action on the respiratory tract.

In a provocation study pre-treatment with budesonide for four weeks has shown decreased bronchial constriction in immediate as well as late asthmatic reactions.

Onset of effect

After a single dose of orally inhaled budesonide, delivered via dry powder inhaler, improvement of the lung function is achieved within a few hours. After therapeutic use of orally inhaled budesonide delivered via dry powder inhaler, improvement in lung function has been shown to occur within 2 days of initiation of treatment, although maximum benefit may not be achieved for up to 4 weeks.

Airway reactivity

Budesonide has also been shown to decrease airway reactivity to histamine and methacholine in hyper-reactive patients.

Exercise-induced asthma

Therapy with inhaled budesonide has effectively been used for prevention of exercise-induced asthma.

Growth

Limited data from long term studies suggest that most children and adolescents treated with inhaled budesonide ultimately achieve their adult target height. However, an initial small but transient reduction in growth (approximately 1 cm) has been observed. This generally occurs within the first year of treatment (see section 4.4).

HPA axis function

Studies in healthy volunteers with Pulmicort Turbohaler have shown dose-related effects on plasma and urinary cortisol. At recommended doses, Pulmicort Turbohaler, causes less effect on the adrenal function than prednisolone 10mg, as shown by ACTH tests.

5.2 Pharmacokinetic properties

After inhalation via Turbohaler, about 25 - 30% of the metered dose is deposited in the lungs.

Of the fraction which is swallowed, approximately 90% is inactivated by first pass metabolism in the liver.

The maximal plasma concentration after inhalation of 1 milligram budesonide is about 3.5 nmol/L and is reached after about 20 minutes.

Budesonide undergoes an extensive degree (approximately 90%) of biotransformation in the liver, to metabolites of low glucocorticosteroid activity. The glucocorticosteroid activity of the major metabolites, 6β-hydroxybudesonide and 16α-hydroxyprednisolone, is less than 1% of that of budesonide. The metabolism of budesonide is primarily mediated by CYP3A4, one of the cytochrome p450 enzymes.

In a study, 100 mg ketoconazole taken twice daily, increased plasma levels of concomitantly administered oral budesonide (single dose of 10 mg) on average, by 7.8-fold. Information about this interaction is lacking for inhaled budesonide, but marked increases in plasma levels could be expected.

5.3 Preclinical safety data

The acute toxicity of budesonide is low and of the same order of magnitude and type as that of the reference glucocorticosteroids studied (beclomethasone dipropionate, fluocinolone acetonide).

Results from subacute and chronic toxicity studies show that the systemic effects of budesonide are less severe than, or similar to, those observed after administration of the other glucocorticosteroids, e.g. decreased body-weight gain and atrophy of lymphoid tissues and adrenal cortex.

An increased incidence of brain gliomas in male rats, in a carcinogenicity study, could not be verified in a repeat study in which the incidence of gliomas did not differ between any of the groups on active treatment (budesonide, prednisolone, triamcinolone acetonide) and the control groups.

Liver changes (primary hepatocellular neoplasms) found in male rats in the original carcinogenicity study were noted again in the repeat study with budesonide, as well as with the reference glucocorticosteroids. These effects are most probably related to a receptor effect and thus represent a class effect.

Available clinical experience shows no indication that budesonide, or other glucocorticosteroids, induce brain gliomas or primary hepatocellular neoplasms in man.

In animal reproduction studies, corticosteroids such as budesonide have been shown to induce malformations (cleft palate, skeletal malformations). However, these animal experimental results do not appear to be relevant in humans at the recommended doses.

Animal studies have also identified an involvement of excess prenatal glucocorticosteroids, in increased risk for intrauterine growth retardation, adult cardiovascular disease and permanent changes in glucocorticoid receptor density, neurotransmitter turnover and behaviour at exposures below the teratogenic dose range.

6. PHARMACEUTICAL PARTICULARS

6.1 List of excipients

Pulmicort Turbohaler contains only active drug, budesonide. There are no propellants, lubricants, preservatives, carrier substances or other additives.

6.2 Incompatibilities

None known.

6.3 Shelf life

24 months.

6.4 Special precautions for storage

Do not store above 30°C.

6.5 Nature and contents of container

Polyethylene container consisting of a cover screwed onto a bottom plate. Inside this is the inhaler with its main parts: a mouthpiece, a dosing mechanism and a substance store.

The device also contains a desiccant.

200 micrograms/actuation, 100 actuations.

6.6 Special precautions for disposal and other handling

See section 4.2

7. MARKETING AUTHORISATION HOLDER

AstraZeneca UK Ltd.

600 Capability Green,

Luton, LU1 3LU, UK.

8. MARKETING AUTHORISATION NUMBER(S)

PL 17901/0163

9. DATE OF FIRST AUTHORISATION/RENEWAL OF THE AUTHORISATION

18th June 2002

10. DATE OF REVISION OF THE TEXT

13th August 2009

Pulmicort Turbohaler 400

(AstraZeneca UK Limited)

1. NAME OF THE MEDICINAL PRODUCT

Pulmicort® Turbohaler® 400.

2. QUALITATIVE AND QUANTITATIVE COMPOSITION

Budesonide 400 micrograms/actuation.

There are no inactive ingredients.

3. PHARMACEUTICAL FORM

Breath-actuated metered dose powder inhaler.

4. CLINICAL PARTICULARS

4.1 Therapeutic indications

Pulmicort is recommended in patients with bronchial asthma.

4.2 Posology and method of administration

Pulmicort Turbohaler is for oral inhalation.

When transferring patients to Turbohaler from other devices, treatment should be individualised, whether once or twice daily dosing is being used. The drug and method of delivery should be considered.

Divided doses (twice daily):

The dosage should be individualised.

The dose should always be reduced to the minimum needed to maintain good asthma control.

Adults (including elderly) and children over 12 years of age: When starting treatment, during periods of severe asthma and while reducing or discontinuing oral glucocorticosteroids, the dosage in adults should be 200 - 1600 micrograms daily, in divided doses.

In less severe cases and children over 12 years of age, 200 - 800 micrograms daily, in divided doses, may be used. During periods of severe asthma, the daily dosage can be increased to up to 1600 micrograms, in divided doses.

Children 5 - 12 years of age: 200 - 800 micrograms daily, in divided doses. During periods of severe asthma, the daily dose can be increased up to 800 micrograms.

Once daily dosage:

The dosage should be individualised.

The dose should always be reduced to the minimum needed to maintain good asthma control.

Adults (including elderly) and children over 12 years of age: 200 micrograms to 400 micrograms may be used in patients with mild to moderate asthma who have not previously received inhaled glucocorticosteroids.

Up to 800 micrograms may be used by patients with mild to moderate asthma already controlled on inhaled steroids (e.g. budesonide or beclomethasone dipropionate), administered twice daily.

Children 5 - 12 years of age: 200 micrograms to 400 micrograms may be used in children with mild to moderate asthma who have not previously received inhaled glucocorticosteroids, or who are already controlled on inhaled steroids (e.g. budesonide or beclomethasone dipropionate), administered twice daily.

The patient should be transferred to once daily dosing at the same equivalent total daily dose; the drug and method of delivery should be considered. The dose should subsequently be reduced to the minimum needed to maintain good asthma control.

Patients should be instructed to take the once daily dose in the evening. It is important that the dose is taken consistently and at a similar time each evening.

There are insufficient data to make recommendations for the transfer of patients from newer inhaled steroids to once daily Pulmicort Turbohaler.

Patients, in particular those receiving once daily treatment, should be advised that if their asthma deteriorates (e.g. increased frequency of bronchodilator use or persistent respiratory symptoms) they should double their steroid dose, by administering it twice daily, and should contact their doctor as soon as possible.

In patients where an increased therapeutic effect is desired, an increased dose of Pulmicort is recommended because of the lower risk of systemic effects as compared with a combined treatment with oral glucocorticosteroids.

Patients maintained on oral glucocorticosteroids

Pulmicort Turbohaler may permit replacement or significant reduction in dosage of oral glucocorticosteroids while maintaining asthma control. For further information on the withdrawal of oral corticosteroids, see section 4.4.

Patients should be reminded of the importance of taking prophylactic therapy regularly, even when they are asymptomatic. A short-acting inhaled bronchodilator should be made available for the relief of acute asthma symptoms.

Instructions for the correct use of Pulmicort Turbohaler

Turbohaler is inspiratory flow-driven which means that, when the patient inhales through the mouthpiece, the substance will follow the inspired air into the airways.

Note: It is important to instruct the patient:

- To carefully read the instructions for use in the patient information leaflet, which is packed with each Turbohaler
- To breathe in forcefully and deeply through the mouthpiece to ensure that an optimal dose is delivered to the lungs
- Never to breathe out through the mouthpiece
- To rinse the mouth out with water and spit it out, or to brush the teeth after inhaling the prescribed dose, to minimise the risk of oropharyngeal thrush

The patient may not taste or feel any medication when using Turbohaler due to the small amount of drug dispensed.

4.3 Contraindications

Hypersensitivity to budesonide.

4.4 Special warnings and precautions for use

Special caution is necessary in patients with active or quiescent pulmonary tuberculosis, and in patients with fungal or viral infections in the airways.

Non steroid-dependent patients: A therapeutic effect is usually reached within 10 days. In patients with excessive mucus secretion in the bronchi, a short (about 2 weeks) additional oral corticosteroid regimen can be given initially.

Steroid-dependent patients: When transferral from oral steroids to Pulmicort Turbohaler is started, the patient should be in a relatively stable phase. A high dose of Pulmicort Turbohaler is then given in combination with the previously used oral steroid dose for about 10 days.

After that, the oral steroid dose should be gradually reduced (by for example 2.5 milligrams prednisolone or the equivalent each month) to the lowest possible level. In many cases, it is possible to completely substitute Pulmicort for the oral steroid.

During transfer from oral therapy to Pulmicort, a generally lower systemic steroid action will be experienced which may result in the appearance of allergic or arthritic symptoms such as rhinitis, eczema and muscle and joint pain. Specific treatment should be initiated for these conditions. During the withdrawal of oral steroids, patients may feel unwell in a non-specific way, even though respiratory function is maintained or improved. Patients should be encouraged to continue with Pulmicort therapy whilst withdrawing the oral steroid, unless there are clinical signs to indicate the contrary. A general insufficient glucocorticosteroid effect should be suspected if, in rare cases, symptoms such as tiredness, headache, nausea and vomiting should occur. In these cases a temporary increase in the dose of oral glucocorticosteroids is sometimes necessary.

As with other inhalation therapy, paradoxical bronchospasm may occur, with an immediate increase in wheezing after dosing. If a severe reaction occurs, treatment should be reassessed and an alternative therapy instituted if necessary.

Patients who have previously been dependent on oral steroids may, as a result of prolonged systemic steroid therapy, experience the effects of impaired adrenal function. Recovery may take a considerable amount of time after cessation of oral steroid therapy, hence oral steroid-dependent patients transferred to budesonide may remain at risk from impaired adrenal function for some considerable time. In such circumstances, HPA axis functions should be monitored regularly.

Acute exacerbations of asthma may need an increase in the dose of Pulmicort or additional treatment with a short course of oral corticosteroid and/or an antibiotic, if there is an infection. The patient should be advised to use a short-acting inhaled bronchodilator as rescue medication to relieve acute asthma symptoms.

If patients find short-acting bronchodilator treatment ineffective or they need more inhalations than usual, medical attention must be sought. In this situation consideration should be given to the need for or an increase in their regular therapy, e.g., higher doses of inhaled budesonide or the addition of a long-acting beta agonist, or for a course of oral glucocorticosteroid.

Prolonged treatment with high doses of inhaled corticosteroids, particularly higher than the recommended doses, may result in clinically significant adrenal suppression. Additional systemic corticosteroid cover should be considered during periods of stress or elective surgery. These patients should be instructed to carry a steroid warning card indicating their needs. Treatment with supplementary systemic steroids or Pulmicort should not be stopped abruptly.

Systemic effects of inhaled corticosteroids may occur, particularly at high doses prescribed for prolonged periods. These effects are much less likely to occur than with oral corticosteroids. Possible systemic effects include adrenal suppression, growth retardation in children and adolescents, decrease in bone mineral density, cataract and glaucoma.

It is important, therefore, that the dose of inhaled corticosteroid is titrated to the lowest dose at which effective control of asthma is maintained.

It is recommended that the height of children receiving prolonged treatment with inhaled corticosteroids is regularly monitored. If growth is slowed, therapy should be reviewed with the aim of reducing the dose of inhaled corticosteroid, if possible, to the lowest dose at which effective control of asthma is maintained. In addition, consideration should be given to referring the patient to a paediatric respiratory specialist.

Reduced liver function may affect the elimination of glucocorticosteroids. The plasma clearance following an intravenous dose of budesonide however was similar in cirrhotic patients and in healthy subjects. After oral ingestion systemic availability of budesonide was increased by compromised liver function due to decreased first pass metabolism. The clinical relevance of this to treatment with Pulmicort is unknown as no data exist for inhaled budesonide, but increases in plasma levels and hence an increased risk of systemic adverse effects could be expected.

In vivo studies have shown that oral administration of ketoconazole and itraconazole (known inhibitors of CYP3A4 activity in the liver and in the intestinal mucosa causes an increase in the systemic exposure to budesonide. Concomitant treatment with ketoconazole and itraconazole or other potent CYP3A4 inhibitors should be avoided (see section 4.5 Interactions). If this is not possible, the time interval between administration of the interacting drugs should be as long as possible. A reduction in the dose of budesonide should also be considered.

4.5 Interaction with other medicinal products and other forms of interaction

The metabolism of budesonide is primarily mediated by CYP3A4, one of the cytochrome p450 enzymes. Inhibitors of this enzyme, e.g. ketoconazole and itraconazole, can therefore increase systemic exposure to budesonide, (see Section 4.4 Special Warnings and Special Precautions for Use and Section 5.2 Pharmacokinetic Properties). Other potent inhibitors of CYP3A4 are also likely to markedly increase plasma levels of budesonide.

4.6 Pregnancy and lactation

Data on approximately 2000 exposed pregnancies indicate no increased teratogenic risk associated with the use of inhaled budesonide. In animal studies, glucocorticosteroids have been shown to induce malformations (see Section 5.3). This is not likely to be relevant for humans given recommended doses, but therapy with inhaled budesonide should be regularly reviewed and maintained at the lowest effective dose.

The administration of budesonide during pregnancy requires that the benefits for the mother be weighed against the risk for the foetus. Inhaled glucocorticosteroids should be considered in preference to oral glucocorticosteroids because of the lower systemic effects at the doses required to achieve similar pulmonary responses.

Budesonide is excreted in breast milk. However, at therapeutic doses of Pulmicort Turbohaler no effects on the suckling child are anticipated. Pulmicort Turbohaler can be used during breast feeding.

4.7 Effects on ability to drive and use machines

Pulmicort Turbohaler does not affect the ability to drive or to use machines.

4.8 Undesirable effects

Clinical trials, literature reports and post-marketing experience suggest that the following adverse drug reactions may occur:

Common (>1/100, <1/10)	• Mild irritation in the throat • Candida infection in the oropharynx • Hoarseness • Coughing
Rare (>1/10 000, <1/1 000)	• Nervousness, restlessness, depression, behavioural disturbances • Immediate and delayed hypersensitivity reactions including rash, contact dermatitis, urticaria, angioedema, bronchospasm and anaphylactic reaction. • Skin bruising

The candida infection in the oropharynx is due to drug deposition. Advising the patient to rinse the mouth out with water after each dosing will minimise the risk.

As with other inhalation therapy, paradoxical bronchospasm may occur in very rare cases (see Section 4.4).

Systemic effects of inhaled corticosteroids may occur, particularly at high doses prescribed for prolonged periods. These effects are much less likely to occur than with oral corticosteroids. Possible systemic effects include adrenal suppression, growth retardation in children and adolescents, decrease in bone mineral density, cataract and glaucoma. The effect is probably dependent on dose, exposure time, concomitant and previous steroid exposure, and individual sensitivity.

4.9 Overdose

The only harmful effect that follows inhalation of large amounts of the drug over a short period is suppression of hypothalamic-pituitary-adrenal (HPA) function. No special emergency action needs to be taken. Treatment with Pulmicort Turbohaler should be continued at the recommended dose to control the asthma.

5. PHARMACOLOGICAL PROPERTIES

5.1 Pharmacodynamic properties

Budesonide is a glucocorticosteroid which possesses a high local anti-inflammatory action, with a lower incidence and severity of adverse effects than those seen with oral corticosteroids.

Pharmacotherapeutic group: Other drugs for obstructive airway diseases, inhalants, glucocorticoids. ATC Code: RO3B A02.

Topical anti-inflammatory effect

The exact mechanism of action of glucocorticosteroids in the treatment of asthma is not fully understood. Anti-inflammatory actions, such as inhibition of inflammatory mediator release and inhibition of cytokine-mediated immune response are probably important.

A clinical study in asthmatics comparing inhaled and oral budesonide at doses calculated to achieve similar systemic bioavailability demonstrated statistically significant evidence of efficacy with inhaled but not oral budesonide compared with placebo. Thus, the therapeutic effect of conventional doses of inhaled budesonide may be largely explained by its direct action on the respiratory tract.

In a provocation study pre-treatment with budesonide for four weeks has shown decreased bronchial constriction in immediate as well as late asthmatic reactions.

Onset of effect

After a single dose of orally inhaled budesonide, delivered via dry powder inhaler, improvement of the lung function is achieved within a few hours. After therapeutic use of orally inhaled budesonide delivered via dry powder inhaler, improvement in lung function has been shown to occur within 2 days of initiation of treatment, although maximum benefit may not be achieved for up to 4 weeks.

Airway reactivity

Budesonide has also been shown to decrease airway reactivity to histamine and methacholine in hyper-reactive patients.

Exercise-induced asthma

Therapy with inhaled budesonide has effectively been used for prevention of exercise-induced asthma.

Growth

Limited data from long term studies suggest that most children and adolescents treated with inhaled budesonide ultimately achieve their adult target height. However, an initial small but transient reduction in growth (approximately 1 cm) has been observed. This generally occurs within the first year of treatment (see section 4.4).

HPA axis function

Studies in healthy volunteers with Pulmicort Turbohaler have shown dose-related effects on plasma and urinary cortisol. At recommended doses, Pulmicort Turbohaler, causes less effect on the adrenal function than prednisolone 10mg, as shown by ACTH tests.

5.2 Pharmacokinetic properties

After inhalation via Turbohaler, about 25 - 30% of the metered dose is deposited in the lungs.

Of the fraction which is swallowed, approximately 90% is inactivated by first pass metabolism in the liver.

The maximal plasma concentration after inhalation of 1 milligram budesonide is about 3.5 nmol/L and is reached after about 20 minutes.

Budesonide undergoes an extensive degree (approximately 90%) of biotransformation in the liver, to metabolites of low glucocorticosteroid activity. The glucocorticosteroid activity of the major metabolites, 6β-hydroxybudesonide and 16α-hydroxyprednisolone, is less than 1% of that of budesonide. The metabolism of budesonide is primarily mediated by CYP3A4, one of the cytochrome p450 enzymes.

In a study, 100 mg ketoconazole taken twice daily, increased plasma levels of concomitantly administered oral budesonide (single dose of 10 mg) on average, by 7.8-fold. Information about this interaction is lacking for inhaled budesonide, but marked increases in plasma levels could be expected.

5.3 Preclinical safety data

The acute toxicity of budesonide is low and of the same order of magnitude and type as that of the reference glucocorticosteroids studied (beclomethasone dipropionate, fluocinolone acetonide).

Results from subacute and chronic toxicity studies show that the systemic effects of budesonide are less severe than, or similar to, those observed after administration of the other glucocorticosteroids, e.g. decreased body-weight gain and atrophy of lymphoid tissues and adrenal cortex.

An increased incidence of brain gliomas in male rats, in a carcinogenicity study, could not be verified in a repeat study in which the incidence of gliomas did not differ between any of the groups on active treatment (budesonide, prednisolone, triamcinolone acetonide) and the control groups.

Liver changes (primary hepatocellular neoplasms) found in male rats in the original carcinogenicity study were noted again in the repeat study with budesonide, as well as with the reference glucocorticosteroids. These effects are most probably related to a receptor effect and thus represent a class effect.

Available clinical experience shows no indication that budesonide, or other glucocorticosteroids, induce brain gliomas or primary hepatocellular neoplasms in man.

In animal reproduction studies, corticosteroids such as budesonide have been shown to induce malformations (cleft palate, skeletal malformations). However, these animal experimental results do not appear to be relevant in humans at the recommended doses.

Animal studies have also identified an involvement of excess prenatal glucocorticosteroids, in increased risk for intrauterine growth retardation, adult cardiovascular disease and permanent changes in glucocorticoid receptor density, neurotransmitter turnover and behaviour at exposures below the teratogenic dose range.

6. PHARMACEUTICAL PARTICULARS

6.1 List of excipients

Pulmicort Turbohaler contains only active drug, budesonide. There are no propellants, lubricants, preservatives, carrier substances or other additives.

6.2 Incompatibilities

None known.

6.3 Shelf life

24 months.

6.4 Special precautions for storage

Do not store above 30°C.

6.5 Nature and contents of container

Polyethylene container consisting of a cover screwed onto a bottom plate. Inside this is the inhaler with its main parts: a mouthpiece, a dosing mechanism and a substance store.

The device also contains a desiccant.

400 micrograms/actuation, 50 actuations.

6.6 Special precautions for disposal and other handling

See section 4.2

7. MARKETING AUTHORISATION HOLDER

AstraZeneca UK Ltd

600 Capability Green,

Luton, LU1 3LU, UK.

8. MARKETING AUTHORISATION NUMBER(S)

PL 17901/0164

9. DATE OF FIRST AUTHORISATION/RENEWAL OF THE AUTHORISATION

18th June 2002

10. DATE OF REVISION OF THE TEXT

13th August 2009

Pulmo Bailly

(DDD Limited)

1. NAME OF THE MEDICINAL PRODUCT

Pulmo Bailly

2. QUALITATIVE AND QUANTITATIVE COMPOSITION

Codeine BP	7.0 mg/5 ml
Guaiacol (1949) BPC	75.0 mg/5 ml

For excipients, see 6.1

3. PHARMACEUTICAL FORM

Oral solution.

Pale amber solution.

4. CLINICAL PARTICULARS

4.1 Therapeutic indications

For the symptomatic relief of coughs associated with colds, bronchial catarrh, influenza and upper respiratory tract infections such as laryngitis and pharyngitis.

4.2 Posology and method of administration

Adults: Up to two 5 ml teaspoonfuls should be taken in half a small glass of water three times daily before meals. A further two teaspoonfuls should be taken at bedtime to encourage undisturbed sleep. Sugar or fruit squash may be added if desired.

Elderly: As adult dosage unless hepatic or renal dysfunction is present when a reduction in dosage is appropriate.

Children: One 5 ml teaspoonful to be taken as above. Not recommended to children under 5 years old.

4.3 Contraindications

Hypersensitivity to the ingredients. Severe respiratory dysfunction or bronchial asthma, severe hepatic dysfunction, head injuries or raised intracranial pressure. Toxic megacolon, paralytic ileus or obstructive bowel disease.

4.4 Special warnings and precautions for use

Prolonged use of codeine-containing products can lead to a morphine-type of dependance. Pulmo Bailly should be used with caution in patients with a history of alcoholism, hepatic, renal or respiratory dysfunction, ulcerative colitis or prostatic hypertrophy.

Prolonged use of codeine in the elderly carries the risk of faecal impaction. Codeine suppresses cough and therefore the use of Pulmo Bailly in patients with chronic bronchitis or bronchietasis may result in retention of bronchial secretions.

1. Do not exceed the stated dose
2. Pulmo Bailly may cause drowsiness or constipation
3. Consult your doctor if symptoms persist for 5 days or longer
4. Before using Pulmo Bailly consult your doctor if you are receiving other medicine
5. Not recommended for pregnant or nursing women

4.5 Interaction with other medicinal products and other forms of interaction

Codeine may delay the absorption of a number of drugs. The effect of other CNS depressants, e.g. hypnotics, sedatives or alcohol may be potentiated by codeine. Codeine may antagonise the effects of metoclopramide on gastro-intestinal motility.

4.6 Pregnancy and lactation

Pulmo Bailly is not recommended for use in pregnancy because a possible association between the use of codeine in early pregnancy and respiratory malformation has been suggested. In late pregnancy there is a risk that the use of codeine may cause neonatal withdrawal symptoms or respiratory depression. Since codeine has been detected in human milk, nursing mothers should not use Pulmo Bailly unless the benefits strongly outweigh the risks.

4.7 Effects on ability to drive and use machines

Pulmo Bailly may produce drowsiness. Patients, if so affected, should not drive or operate machinery.

4.8 Undesirable effects

Pulmo Bailly may cause constipation or drowsiness. The following side effects have also been seen with codeine: nausea, vomiting, biliary spasm, euphoria, hallucinations, orthostatic hypotension, oliguria, allergic reactions (pruritis, skin rash, facial oedema), syncope, dizziness, sedation, visual disturbances, tachycardia, bradycardia and palpitations.

4.9 Overdose

The effects in overdosage will be potentiated by simultaneous ingestion of alcohol and psychotropic drugs.

Symptoms

Central nervous system depression, including respiratory depression, may develop but is unlikely to be severe unless other sedative agents have been co-ingested, including alcohol, or the overdose is very large. The pupils may be pin-point in size; nausea and vomiting are common. Hypotension and tachycardia are possible but unlikely.

Management

This should include general symptomatic and supportive measures including a clear airway and monitoring of vital signs until stable. Consider activated charcoal if an adult presents within one hour of ingestion of more than 350 mg or a child more than 5 mg/kg.

Give naloxone if coma or respiratory depression is present. Naloxone is a competitive antagonist and has a short half-life so large and repeated doses may be required in a seriously poisoned patient. Observe for at least four hours after ingestion.

5. PHARMACOLOGICAL PROPERTIES

5.1 Pharmacodynamic properties

ATC code: Cough Suppressants and Expectorants, Combinations: Opium derivatives and Expectorants (RO5F A).

Codeine is a well-known centrally acting cough suppressant. Guaiacol acts as an expectorant, loosening bronchial secretions in the respiratory tract.

5.2 Pharmacokinetic properties

The pharmacokinetics of codeine are well known and have been documented in Martindale's The Extra Pharmacopoeia 28th Edition, 1982

Codeine and its salts are absorbed from the gastrointestinal tract. Ingestion of codeine phosphate produced peak plasma-codeine concentrations in about one hour. Codeine is metabolised by O- and N- dimethylation in the liver to morphine and norcodeine. Codeine and its metabolites are excreted almost entirely by the kidney, mainly as conjugates with glucuronic acid. The plasma half-life has been reported to be between 3 and 4 hours after administration by mouth or intramuscular injection.

The pharmacokinetics of guaiacol are less well documented. In rats, guaiacol is rapidly absorbed, being present in the blood 5 minutes after oral administration, and reaching its peak plasma concentration in about 10 minutes. Its elimination from the blood is usually as rapid.

5.3 Preclinical safety data

Not applicable.

6. PHARMACEUTICAL PARTICULARS

6.1 List of excipients

Phosphoric acid

Sucrose

Chloroform

Glycerol

Burnt sugar solution (1959)

Purified water

6.2 Incompatibilities

None known.

6.3 Shelf life

2 years.

6.4 Special precautions for storage

Do not store above 25°C and protect from light.

6.5 Nature and contents of container

Amber type III soda glass bottle with aluminium wadded cap or wadded polypropylene cap.

Round amber glass bottle with HDPE/PP child resistant closure and paper/PVDC liner.

Pack size: 90 ml.

6.6 Special precautions for disposal and other handling

No special requirements.

7. MARKETING AUTHORISATION HOLDER

DDD Limited

94 Rickmansworth Road

Watford

Hertfordshire WD18 7JJ

United Kingdom.

8. MARKETING AUTHORISATION NUMBER(S)

PL 00133/0033

9. DATE OF FIRST AUTHORISATION/RENEWAL OF THE AUTHORISATION

Date of last renewal: 27/10/2006

10. DATE OF REVISION OF THE TEXT

July 2009

Pulmozyme

(Roche Products Limited)

1. NAME OF THE MEDICINAL PRODUCT

Pulmozyme 2500 U/ 2.5ml, nebuliser solution

2. QUALITATIVE AND QUANTITATIVE COMPOSITION

Each ampoule contains 2500 U (corresponding to 2.5mg) of dornase alfa* per 2.5ml corresponding to 1000 U/ml or 1mg/ml**.

*phosphorylated glycosylated protein human deoxyribonuclease 1 produced in Chinese Hamster Ovary Cell Line CHO A14.16-1 MSB #757 by recombinant DNA technology

**1 Genentech unit/ml = 1µg/ml

For a full list of excipients, see section 6.1.

3. PHARMACEUTICAL FORM

Nebuliser solution

Clear, colourless to slightly yellowish solution

4. CLINICAL PARTICULARS

4.1 Therapeutic indications

Management of cystic fibrosis patients with a forced vital capacity (FVC) of greater than 40% of predicted and over 5 years of age to improve pulmonary function.

4.2 Posology and method of administration

2.5mg (corresponding to 2500 U) deoxyribonuclease I by inhalation once daily. Inhale the contents of one ampoule (2.5ml of solution) undiluted using a recommended jet nebuliser/compressor system (see section 6.6).

Some patients over the age of 21 years may benefit from twice daily dosage.

Most patients gain optimal benefit from regular daily use of Pulmozyme. In studies in which Pulmozyme was given in an intermittent regimen, improvement in pulmonary function was lost on cessation of therapy. Patients should therefore be advised to take their medication every day without a break.

Patients should continue their regular medical care, including their standard regimen of chest physiotherapy.

Administration can be safely continued in patients who experience exacerbation of respiratory tract infection.

Safety and efficacy have not yet been demonstrated in patients under the age of 5 years, or in patients with forced vital capacity less than 40% of predicted.

4.3 Contraindications

Hypersensitivity to the active substance or to any of the excipients.

4.4 Special warnings and precautions for use

None.

4.5 Interaction with other medicinal products and other forms of interaction

Pulmozyme can be effectively and safely used in conjunction with standard cystic fibrosis therapies such as antibiotics, bronchodilators, pancreatic enzymes, vitamins, inhaled and systemic corticosteroids, and analgesics.

4.6 Pregnancy and lactation

Pregnancy

The safety of dornase alfa has not been established in pregnant women. Animal studies do not indicate direct or indirect harmful effects with respect to pregnancy, or embryofoetal development (see section 5.3). Caution should be exercised when prescribing dornase alfa to pregnant women.

Lactation

As it is not known whether dornase alfa is excreted in human milk, caution should be exercised when dornase alfa is administered to a breast-feeding woman (see section 5.3).

4.7 Effects on ability to drive and use machines

Pulmozyme has no or negligible influence on the ability to drive and use machines.

4.8 Undesirable effects

The adverse event data reflect the clinical trial and post-marketing experience of using Pulmozyme at the recommended dose regimen.

Adverse reactions attributed to Pulmozyme are rare (< 1/1000). In most cases, the adverse reactions are mild and transient in nature and do not require alterations in Pulmozyme dosing.

Eye disorders:

Conjunctivitis

Respiratory, thoracic and mediastinal disorders:

Dysphonia, dyspnoea, pharyngitis, laryngitis, rhinitis (all non-infectious).

Gastrointestinal disorders:

Dyspepsia.

Skin and subcutaneous tissue disorders:

Rash, urticaria.

General disorders:

Chest pain (pleuritic/non-cardiac), pyrexia.

Investigations:

Pulmonary function tests decreased.

Patients who experience adverse events common to cystic fibrosis can, in general, safely continue administration of Pulmozyme as evidenced by the high percentage of patients completing clinical trials with Pulmozyme.

In clinical trials, few patients experienced adverse events resulting in permanent discontinuation from dornase alfa, and the discontinuation rate was observed to be similar between placebo (2%) and dornase alfa (3%).

Upon initiation of dornase alfa therapy, as with any aerosol, pulmonary function may decline and expectoration of sputum may increase.

Less than 5% of patients treated with dornase alfa have developed antibodies to dornase alpha and none of these patients have developed IgE antibodies to dornase alfa. Improvement in pulmonary function tests has still occurred even after the development of antibodies to dornase alfa.

4.9 Overdose

Pulmozyme overdosage has not been established. Single-dose inhalation studies in rats and monkeys at doses up to 180-fold higher than doses routinely used in clinical studies are well tolerated. Oral administration of dornase alfa in doses up to 200mg/kg are also well tolerated by rats.

In clinical studies, CF patients have received up to 20mg dornase alfa BID for up to six days and 10mg BID intermittently (2 weeks on/2 weeks off drug) for 168 days. Both dose regimens were shown to be well tolerated.

5. PHARMACOLOGICAL PROPERTIES

5.1 Pharmacodynamic properties

Pharmacotherapeutic group: respiratory system, ATC code: R 05 C B13.

Recombinant human DNase is a genetically engineered version of a naturally occurring human enzyme which cleaves extracellular DNA.

Retention of viscous purulent secretions in the airways contributes both to reduced pulmonary function and to exacerbations of infection. Purulent secretions contain very high concentrations of extracellular DNA, a viscous polyanion released by degenerating leukocytes, which accumulate in response to infection. *In vitro*, dornase alfa hydrolyses DNA in sputum and greatly reduces the viscoelasticity of cystic fibrosis sputum.

5.2 Pharmacokinetic properties

Absorption

Inhalation studies conducted in rats and non-human primates show a low percentage of dornase alfa systemic absorption, < 15% for rats and < 2% for monkeys. Consistent with the results of these animal studies, dornase alfa administered to patients as an inhaled aerosol shows low systemic exposure.

Absorption of dornase alfa from the gastrointestinal tract following oral administration to rats is negligible.

DNase is normally present in human serum. Inhalation of up to 40mg of dornase alfa for up to 6 days did not result in a significant elevation of serum DNase concentration above normal endogenous levels. No increase in serum DNase concentration greater than 10ng/ml was observed. Following administration of 2500 U (2.5mg) of dornase alfa twice daily for 24 weeks, mean serum DNase concentrations were no different from the mean pre-treatment baseline value of 3.5 ± 0.1ng/ml; suggesting low systemic absorption or accumulation.

Distribution

Studies in rats and monkeys have shown that, following intravenous administration, dornase alfa was cleared rapidly from the serum. The initial volume of distribution was similar to serum volume in these studies.

Inhalation of 2500 U (2.5mg) dornase alfa results in a mean sputum concentration of dornase alfa of approximately 3µg/ml within 15 minutes in CF patients. Concentrations of dornase alfa in sputum rapidly decline following inhalation.

Elimination

Studies in rats indicate that, following aerosol administration the disappearance half-life of dornase alfa from the lungs is 11 hours.

No pharmacokinetic data are available in very young or geriatric animals.

5.3 Preclinical safety data

Studies of dornase alfa in rabbits and rodents show no evidence of impaired fertility, teratogenicity, or effects on development.

In a study performed in lactating cynomolgus monkeys, receiving high doses of dornase alfa by the intravenous route, low concentrations (< 0.1% of the concentrations seen in the serum of pregnant cynomolgus monkeys), were detectable in the maternal milk. When administered to humans according to the dosage recommendation, there is minimal systemic absorption of dornase alfa; therefore no measurable concentrations of dornase alfa would be expected in human milk.

6. PHARMACEUTICAL PARTICULARS

6.1 List of excipients

Sodium Chloride

Calcium Chloride Dihydrate

Water for Injections

6.2 Incompatibilities

Pulmozyme is an unbuffered aqueous solution and should not be diluted or mixed with other drugs or solutions in the nebuliser bowl. Mixing of this solution could lead to adverse structural and/or functional changes in Pulmozyme or the admixed compound.

6.3 Shelf life
2 years.

6.4 Special precautions for storage
Store in a refrigerator (2°C - 8°C).

Keep the ampoule in the outer carton in order to protect from light.

A single brief exposure to elevated temperatures (less than or equal to 24 hours at up to 30°C) does not affect product stability.

6.5 Nature and contents of container
2.5 ml of nebuliser solution in an ampoule (low density polyethylene plastic).

Pack sizes of 6 and 30.

Not all pack sizes may be marketed.

6.6 Special precautions for disposal and other handling
The contents of one 2.5mg (2500 U) single-use ampoule of Pulmozyme sterile solution for inhalation should be inhaled once a day using a recommended jet nebuliser.

- Pulmozyme should not be mixed with other drugs or solutions in the nebuliser (see section 6.2).
- The complete contents of a single ampoule should be placed in the bowl of a jet nebuliser/compressor system, such as the Hudson T Up-draft II/Pulmo-Aide, Airlife Misty/Pulmo-Aide, customised Respirgard/Pulmo-Aide, or Acorn II/Pulmo-Aide.
- Pulmozyme may also be used in conjunction with a reusable jet nebuliser/compressor system, such as the Pari LL/Inhalierboy, Pari LC/Inhalierboy or Master, Aiolos/2 Aiolos, Side Stream/CR50 or MobilAire or Porta-Neb.
- Ultrasonic nebulisers may be unsuitable for delivery of Pulmozyme because they may inactivate Pulmozyme or have unacceptable aerosol delivery characteristics.
- The manufacturers' instructions on the use and maintenance of the nebuliser and compressor should be followed.
- Containment of the aerosol is not necessary.
- Pulmozyme ampoules are for single administration only. Any unused product or waste material should be disposed of in accordance with local requirements.

7. MARKETING AUTHORISATION HOLDER
Roche Products Limited
6 Falcon Way
Shire Park
Welwyn Garden City
AL7 1TW
United Kingdom

8. MARKETING AUTHORISATION NUMBER(S)
PL 00031/0335

9. DATE OF FIRST AUTHORISATION/RENEWAL OF THE AUTHORISATION
Date of first authorisation: 12 January 1994

Date of last renewal: 11 March 2009

10. DATE OF REVISION OF THE TEXT
11 March 2009

LEGAL STATUS
POM

Puri-Nethol Tablets
(GlaxoSmithKline UK)

1. NAME OF THE MEDICINAL PRODUCT
Puri-Nethol 50 mg tablets

2. QUALITATIVE AND QUANTITATIVE COMPOSITION
Mercaptopurine 50.0 mg/tab

3. PHARMACEUTICAL FORM
Tablets

4. CLINICAL PARTICULARS

4.1 Therapeutic indications
Cytotoxic agent.

Puri-Nethol is indicated for the treatment of acute leukaemia. It may be utilised in remission induction and it is particularly indicated for maintenance therapy in: acute lymphoblastic leukaemia; acute myelogenous leukaemia. Puri-Nethol may be used in the treatment of chronic granulocytic leukaemia.

4.2 Posology and method of administration
For oral administration

Dosage in adults and children:

For adults and children the usual starting dose is 2.5 mg/kg bodyweight per day, or 50-75 mg/m^2 body surface area per day, but the dose and duration of administration depend on the nature and dosage of other cytotoxic agents given in conjunction with Puri-Nethol.

The dosage should be carefully adjusted to suit the individual patient.

Puri-Nethol has been used in various combination therapy schedules for acute leukaemia and the literature should be consulted for details.

Dosage in the elderly:

No specific studies have been carried out in the elderly. However, it is advisable to monitor renal and hepatic function in these patients, and if there is any impairment, consideration should be given to reducing the Puri-Nethol dosage.

Dosage in renal impairment:

Consideration should be given to reducing the dosage in patients with impaired renal function.

Dosage in hepatic function:

Consideration should be given to reducing the dosage in patients with impaired hepatic function.

In general:

When Zyloric (allopurinol) and 6-mercaptopurine are administered concomitantly it is essential that only a quarter of the usual dose of 6-mercaptopurine is given since Zyloric (allopurinol) decreases the rate of catabolism of 6-mercaptopurine.

4.3 Contraindications
Hypersensitivity to any component of the preparation.

In view of the seriousness of the indications there are no other absolute contra-indications.

4.4 Special warnings and precautions for use
Puri-Nethol is an active cytotoxic agent for use only under the direction of physicians experienced in the administration of such agents.

Immunisation using a live organism vaccine has the potential to cause infection in immunocompromised hosts. Therefore, immunisations with live organism vaccines are not recommended.

Safe handling of Puri-Nethol Tablets:

See section 6.6 Instructions for Use/Handling

Monitoring:

Treatment with Puri-Nethol causes bone marrow suppression leading to leucopenia and thrombocytopenia and, less frequently, to anaemia. Full blood counts must be taken daily during remission induction and careful monitoring of haematological parameters should be conducted during maintenance therapy.

The leucocyte and platelet counts continue to fall after treatment is stopped, so at the first sign of an abnormally large fall in the counts, treatment should be interrupted immediately.

Bone marrow suppression is reversible if Puri-Nethol is withdrawn early enough.

During remission induction in acute myelogenous leukaemia the patient may frequently have to survive a period of relative bone marrow aplasia and it is important that adequate supportive facilities are available.

There are individuals with an inherited deficiency of the enzyme thiopurine methyltransferase (TPMT) who may be unusually sensitive to the myelosuppresive effect of 6-mercaptopurine and prone to developing rapid bone marrow depression following the initiation of treatment with Puri-Nethol. This problem could be exacerbated by coadministration with drugs that inhibit TPMT, such as olsalazine, mesalazine or sulfazalazine. Also a possible association between decreased TPMT activity and secondary leukaemias and myelodysplasia has been reported in individuals receiving 6–mercaptopurine in combination with other cytotoxics (see Section 4.8 Undesirable Effects). Some laboratories offer testing for TPMT deficiency, although these tests have not been shown to identify all patients at risk of severe toxicity. Therefore close monitoring of blood counts is still necessary.

Puri-Nethol is hepatotoxic and liver function tests should be monitored weekly during treatment. More frequent monitoring may be advisable in those with pre-existing liver disease or receiving other potentially hepatotoxic therapy. The patient should be instructed to discontinue Puri-Nethol immediately if jaundice becomes apparent.

During remission induction when rapid cell lysis is occurring, uric acid levels in blood and urine should be monitored as hyperuricaemia and/or hyperuricosuria may develop, with the risk of uric acid nephropathy.

Cross resistance usually exists between 6-mercaptopurine and 6-tioguanine.

The dosage of 6-mercaptopurine may need to be reduced when this agent is combined with other drugs whose primary or secondary toxicity is myelosuppression.

Mutagenicity and carcinogenicity:

Increases in chromosomal aberrations were observed in the peripheral lymphocytes of leukaemic patients, in a hypernephroma patient who received an unstated dose of 6-mercaptopurine and in patients with chronic renal disease treated at doses of 0.4 – 1.0 mg/kg/day.

In view of its action on cellular deoxyribonucleic acid (DNA) 6-mercaptopurine is potentially carcinogenic and consideration should be given to the theoretical risk of carcinogenisis with this treatment.

Two cases have been documented of the occurrence of acute nonlymphatic leukaemia in patients who received 6-mercaptopurine, in combination with other drugs, for non-neoplastic disorders. A single case has been reported where a patient was treated for pyoderma gangrenosum with 6-mercaptopurine and later developed acute nonlymphatic leukaemia, but it is not clear whether this was part of the natural history of the disease or if the 6-mercaptopurine played a causative role.

A patient with Hodgkins Disease treated with 6-mercaptopurine and multiple additional cytotoxic agents developed acute myelogenous leukaemia.

Twelve and a half years after 6-mercaptopurine treatment for myasthenia gravis a female patient developed chronic myeloid leukaemia.

4.5 Interaction with other medicinal products and other forms of interaction
Vaccinations with live organism vaccines are not recommended in immunocompromised individuals (see Section 4.4 Special Warnings and Precautions for Use).

When Zyloric (allopurinol) and Puri-Nethol are administered concomitantly it is essential that only a quarter of the usual dose of Puri-Nethol is given since Zyloric decreases the rate of catabolism of Puri-Nethol.

Inhibition of the anticoagulant effect of warfarin, when given with Puri-Nethol, has been reported.

As there is *in vitro* evidence that aminosalicylate derivatives (eg. olsalazine, mesalazine or sulfazalazine) inhibit the TPMT enzyme, they should be administered with caution to patients receiving concurrent Puri-Nethol therapy (see Section 4.4 Special Warnings and Precautions for Use).

4.6 Pregnancy and lactation
Pregnancy:

6-mercaptopurine is potentially teratogenic. The use of Puri-Nethol should be avoided whenever possible during pregnancy. In any individual case the potential hazard to the foetus must be balanced against the expected benefit to the mother.

As with all cytotoxic chemotherapy, adequate contraceptive precautions should be advised if either partner is receiving Puri-Nethol tablets.

Maternal Exposure:

Studies of 6-mercaptopurine in animals have shown reproductive toxicity (see Section 5.3 Preclinical Safety Data). The potential risk for humans is unclear.

Normal offspring have been born after mercaptopurine therapy administered as a single chemotherapy agent during human pregnancy. Abortions and prematurity have been reported after maternal exposure. Multiple congenital abnormalities have been reported following maternal 6-mercatopurine treatment in combination with other chemotherapy agents.

Paternal Exposure:

Congenital abnormalities and spontaneous abortion have been reported after paternal exposure to 6-mercaptopurine.

Effects on fertility:

The effect of Puri-Nethol therapy on human fertility is largely unknown but there are reports of successful fatherhood/motherhood after receiving treatment during childhood or adolescence. Transient profound oligospermia was observed in a young man who received 6-mercaptopurine 150 mg/day plus prednisone 80 mg/day for acute leukaemia. Two years after cessation of the chemotherapy, he had a normal sperm count and he fathered a normal child.

Lactation:

6-Mercaptopurine has been detected in the breast milk of renal transplant patients receiving immunosuppressive therapy with azathioprine, a pro-drug of 6-mercaptopurine and thus mothers receiving Puri-Nethol should not breast-feed.

4.7 Effects on ability to drive and use machines
There are no data on the effect of 6-mercaptopurine on driving performance or the ability to operate machinery. A detrimental effect on these activities cannot be predicted from the pharmacology of the drug.

4.8 Undesirable effects
For mercaptopurine there is a lack of modern clinical documentation which can serve as support for accurately determining the frequency of undesirable effects.

The following convention has been utilised for the classification of undesirable effects:- Very common $\geqslant 1/10$, common $\geqslant 1/100$, $< 1/10$, uncommon $\geqslant 1/1000$ and $< 1/100$, rare $\geqslant 1/10{,}000$ and $< 1/1000$, very rare $< 1/10{,}000$.

Neoplasms benign, malignant and unspecified (including cysts and polyps)

Very Rare: secondary leukaemia and myelodysplasia (see Section 4.4 Special Warnings and Precautions for Use)

Blood and lymphatic system disorders

Very common Bone marrow suppression; leucopenia and thrombocytopenia.

The main side effect of treatment with 6-mercaptopurine is bone marrow suppression leading to leucopenia and thrombocytopenia.

Uncommon anaemia

Immune system disorders

Hypersensitivity reactions with the following manifestations have been reported:

Rare: Arthralgia; skin rash; drug fever

Very Rare: Facial oedema

Metabolism and nutrition disorders

Uncommon Anorexia

Gastrointestinal disorders

Common Nausea; vomiting; pancreatitis in the IBD population* (an unlicensed indication)

Rare Oral ulceration; pancreatitis (in the licensed indications)

Very rare Intestinal ulceration

Hepato-biliary disorders

Common Biliary stasis; hepatotoxicity

Rare Hepatic necrosis

6-mercaptopurine is hepatotoxic in animals and man. The histological findings in man have shown hepatic necrosis and biliary stasis

The incidence of hepatotoxicity varies considerably and can occur with any dose but more frequently when the recommended dose of 2.5 mg/kg bodyweight daily or 75 mg/m^2 body surface area per day is exceeded.

Monitoring of liver function tests may allow early detection of hepatotoxicity. This is usually reversible if 6-mercaptopurine therapy is stopped soon enough but fatal liver damage has occurred.

Skin and subcutaneous tissue disorders

Rare alopecia

Reproductive system and breast disorders

Very Rare Transient oligospermia

4.9 Overdose

Symptoms and signs:

Gastrointestinal effects, including nausea, vomiting and diarrhoea and anorexia may be early symptoms of overdosage having occurred. The principal toxic effect is on the bone marrow, resulting in myelosuppression. Haematological toxicity is likely to be more profound with chronic overdosage than with a single ingestion of Puri-Nethol. Liver dysfunction and gastroenteritis may also occur.

The risk of overdosage is also increased when Zyloric is being given concomitantly with Puri-Nethol (see Section 4.5 Interactions with other Medicaments and other forms of Interaction).

Management:

As there is no known antidote the blood picture should be closely monitored and general supportive measures, together with appropriate blood transfusion, instituted if necessary. Active measures (such as the use of activated charcoal or gastric lavage) may not be effective in the event of 6-mercaptopurine overdose unless the procedure can be undertaken within 60 minutes of ingestion.

5. PHARMACOLOGICAL PROPERTIES

5.1 Pharmacodynamic properties

Pharmacotherapeutic group:

6-Mercaptopurine is sulphydryl analogue of the purine base hypoxanthine and acts as a cytotoxic antimetabolite.

Mode of Action:

6-Mercaptopurine is an inactive pro-drug which acts as a purine antagonist but requires cellular uptake and intracellular anabolism to tioguanine nucleotides for cytotoxicity. The 6-mercaptopurine metabolites inhibit *de novo* purine synthesis and purine nucleotide interconversions. The tioguanine nucleotides are also incorporated into nucleic acids and this contributes to the cytotoxic effects of the drug.

5.2 Pharmacokinetic properties

The bioavailability of oral 6-mercaptopurine shows considerable inter-individual variability, which probably results from its first-pass metabolism (when administered orally at a dosage of 75 mg/m^2 to 7 paediatric patients, the bioavailability averaged 16% of the administered dose, with a range of 5 to 37%).

The elimination half-life of 6-mercaptopurine is 90 ± 30 minutes, but the active metabolites have a longer half-life (approximately 5 hours) than the parent drug. The apparent body clearance is 4832 ± 2562 ml/min/m^2. There is low entry of 6-mercaptopurine into the cerebrospinal fluid.

The main method of elimination for 6-mercaptopurine is by metabolic alteration. The kidneys eliminate approximately 7% of 6-mercaptopurine unaltered within 12 hours of the drug being administered. Xanthine oxidase is the main catabolic enzyme of 6-mercaptopurine and it converts the drug into the inactive metabolite, 6-thiouric acid. This is excreted in the urine.

5.3 Preclinical safety data

6-Mercaptopurine, in common with other antimetabolites, is potentially mutagenic in man and chromosome damage has been reported in mice, rats and man.

Teratogenicity

6-Mercaptopurine causes embryolethality and severe teratogenic effects in the mouse, rat, hamster and rabbit at doses that are non-toxic to the mother. In all species, the degree of embryotoxicity and the type of malformations are dependent on the dose and stage of the gestation at the time of administration.

6. PHARMACEUTICAL PARTICULARS

6.1 List of excipients

Lactose

Maize Starch

Hydrolysed Starch

Stearic Acid

Magnesium Stearate

Purified Water

6.2 Incompatibilities

None known

6.3 Shelf life

60 months

6.4 Special precautions for storage

Store below 25°C. Keep the bottle tightly closed.

6.5 Nature and contents of container

Amber glass bottles with child resistant high density polyethylene closures with induction heat seal liners.

Pack size: 25 tablets

6.6 Special precautions for disposal and other handling

Safe handling:

It is recommended that the handling of Puri-Nethol tablets follows the "Guidelines for the Handling of Cytotoxic Drugs", according to prevailing local recommendations and/or regulations.

It is advisable that care be taken when handling or halving these tablets not to contaminate hands or inspire drug.

Disposal:

Puri-Nethol tablets surplus to requirements should be destroyed in a manner appropriate to the prevailing local regulations for the destruction of dangerous substances.

Administrative Data

7. MARKETING AUTHORISATION HOLDER

The Wellcome Foundation Ltd

Glaxo Wellcome House Berkeley Avenue

Greenford

Middlesex UB6 0NN

trading as

GlaxoSmithKline UK

Stockley Park West

Uxbridge

Middlesex UB11 1BT

8. MARKETING AUTHORISATION NUMBER(S)

PL 00003/5227R

9. DATE OF FIRST AUTHORISATION/RENEWAL OF THE AUTHORISATION

27 April 1998

10. DATE OF REVISION OF THE TEXT

12 July 2007

11. Legal Status

POM

Pyralvex

(Norgine Limited)

1. NAME OF THE MEDICINAL PRODUCT

PYRALVEX

2. QUALITATIVE AND QUANTITATIVE COMPOSITION

PYRALVEX contains the following active ingredients in each 1ml of solution.

Rhubarb extract	50 mg (equivalent to 5 mg anthraquinone glycosides)
Salicylic Acid	10mg

3. PHARMACEUTICAL FORM

Oromucosal solution.

4. CLINICAL PARTICULARS

4.1 Therapeutic indications

For the symptomatic relief of pain associated with recurrent mouth ulcers and denture irritation.

4.2 Posology and method of administration

Adults (including the elderly): To be applied to the inflamed oral mucosa (after removing any dentures) three or four times daily using the brush provided.

Children: Not recommended below the age of 12 years.

4.3 Contraindications

Hypersensitivity to any of the constituents.

4.4 Special warnings and precautions for use

Each bottle of PYRALVEX should be used by only one person.

4.5 Interaction with other medicinal products and other forms of interaction

None known.

4.6 Pregnancy and lactation

Animal studies are insufficient with respect to effects on pregnancy and-or embryonal/foetal development. The potential risk for humans is unknown. Caution should be exercised when prescribing to pregnant women.

Anthranoid glycosides derived from rhubarb may be excreted in breast milk. However, at therapeutic doses of Pyralvex, it is not known whether these, or salicylic acid are excreted in breast milk. A decision on whether to continue breast-feeding or to continue therapy with Pyralvex should be made taking into account the benefit of breast-feeding to the child and benefit of Pyralvex therapy to the woman.

4.7 Effects on ability to drive and use machines

None.

4.8 Undesirable effects

Gastrointestinal Disorders

A transient local burning sensation at the site of application occurs very commonly (>1/10).

Temporary discolouration of teeth or oral mucosa have been described commonly (>1/100, <1/10) following administration of PYRALVEX.

4.9 Overdose

Overdose associated with local application is unlikely, although the extent of systemic absorption of salicylic acid and anthranoid derivatives is not known. Systemic overdose following ingestion might lead to abdominal cramping, diarrhoea and possibly salicylism (presenting as hyperventilation, tinnitus, deafness, vasodilation, sweating).

5. PHARMACOLOGICAL PROPERTIES

5.1 Pharmacodynamic properties

Pharmacological studies have shown that the active ingredients of PYRALVEX display anti-inflammatory, analgesic and anti-microbial properties, which are the basis of its clinical efficacy.

5.2 Pharmacokinetic properties

Systemic availability of PYRALVEX is unlikely to be significant, owing to the low levels of ingredients administered.

5.3 Preclinical safety data

Preclinical studies indicate that at clinically effective doses, the ingredients in PYRALVEX are unlikely to have any potential for toxic effects.

6. PHARMACEUTICAL PARTICULARS

6.1 List of excipients

Ethanol

Water

6.2 Incompatibilities

None known.

6.3 Shelf life

The shelf life is 3 years.

6.4 Special precautions for storage

Store below 25°C.

6.5 Nature and contents of container

An amber glass bottle with brush applicator containing 10ml of solution.

6.6 Special precautions for disposal and other handling

No special requirements.

7. MARKETING AUTHORISATION HOLDER

Norgine Limited,

Chaplin House,

Widewater Place,

Moorhall Road,

Harefield,

UXBRIDGE,

Middlesex, UB9 6NS

United Kingdom

8. MARKETING AUTHORISATION NUMBER(S)

PL 00322/5013R

9. DATE OF FIRST AUTHORISATION/RENEWAL OF THE AUTHORISATION

May 1972

10. DATE OF REVISION OF THE TEXT

04 January 2008.

Rabipur

(Novartis Vaccines)

1. NAME OF THE MEDICINAL PRODUCT

Rabipur ⩾ 2.5 IU/ml, powder and solvent for solution for injection

Rabies vaccine for human use prepared in cell cultures

2. QUALITATIVE AND QUANTITATIVE COMPOSITION

After reconstitution, 1 dose (1 ml) contains:

Rabies virus* (Inactivated, strain Flury LEP) .... ⩾ 2.5 IU

* produced on purified chick embryo cells

For excipients, see Section 6.1.

3. PHARMACEUTICAL FORM

Powder and solvent for solution for injection.

A clear colourless solution results after reconstitution of the white freeze-dried powder with the clear and colourless solvent.

4. CLINICAL PARTICULARS

4.1 Therapeutic indications

a) Pre-exposure prophylaxis (before possible risk of exposure to rabies)

b) Post-exposure treatment (after known or possible exposure to rabies)

Consideration should be given to national and/or WHO guidance regarding the prevention of rabies.

4.2 Posology and method of administration

Posology

The recommended single intramuscular dose is 1 ml in all age groups.

Whenever possible according to vaccine availablility, it is recommended that one type of cell culture vaccine should be used throughout the course of pre- or post-exposure immunisation. However, adherence to the recommended schedules is of critical importance for post-exposure treatment, even if another type of cell culture vaccine has to be used.

PRE-EXPOSURE PROPHYLAXIS

Primary immunisation

In previously unvaccinated persons, an initial course of pre-exposure prophylaxis consists of three doses (each of 1 ml) administered on days 0, 7 and 21 or 28.

Booster doses

The need of intermittent serological testing for the presence of antibody ⩾ 0.5 IU/ml (as assessed by the Rapid Focus-Fluorescent inhibition Test) and the administration of booster doses should be assessed in accordance with official recommendations.

The following provides general guidance:

• Testing for neutralising antibodies at 6-month intervals is usually recommended if the risk of exposure is high (e. g. Laboratory staff working with rabies virus).

• In persons who are considered to be at continuing risk of exposure to rabies (e. g. veterinarians and their assistants, wildlife workers, hunters), a serological test should usually be performed at least every 2 years, with shorter intervals if appropriate to the perceived degree of risk.

• In above mentioned cases, a booster dose should be given should the antibody titre fall below 0.5 IU/ml.

• Alternatively, booster doses may be given at official recommended intervals without prior serological testing, according to the perceived risk. Experience shows that reinforcing doses are generally required every 2-5 years.

Rabipur may be used for booster vaccination after prior immunisation with human diploid cell rabies vaccine.

POST-EXPOSURE TREATMENT

Post-exposure immunisation should begin as soon as possible after exposure and should be accompanied by local measures to the site of inoculation so as to reduce the risk of infection. Official guidance should be sought regarding the appropriate concomitant measures that should be taken to prevent establishment of infection (see also section 4.4).

Previously fully immunised individuals:

For WHO exposure categories II and III, and in category I cases where there is uncertainty regarding the correct classification of exposure (see Table 1 below), two doses (each of 1 ml) should be administered, one each on days 0 and 3. On a case by case basis, schedule A (see Table 2 below) may be applied if the last dose of vaccine was given more than two years previously.

Table 1: Immunisation schedules appropriate to different types of exposure (WHO 2002)

(see Table 1 below)

Individuals unimmunised or with uncertain immune status

Depending on the WHO category as in Table 1, treatment according to schedules A or B (see Table 2 below) may be required for previously unimmunised persons and for those who have received fewer than 3 doses of vaccine or who have received a vaccine of doubtful potency.

Table 2: Post-exposure treatment of subjects with no or uncertain immune status

Schedule A Active immunisation after exposure is required	Schedule B Active and passive immunisation after exposure are required
One injection of Rabipur i.m. on days: 0, 3, 7, 14, 28 (5-doses schedule) Or One dose of Rabipur is given into the right deltoid muscle and one dose into the left deltoid muscle on day 0, and one dose is applied into the deltoid muscle on days 7 and 21 (2-1-1 regimen). In small children the vaccine is to be given into the thighs.	Give Rabipur as in schedule A + 1 × 20 IU/kg body weight human rabies immunoglobulin* concomitantly with the first dose of Rabipur. If HRIG is not available at the time of the first vaccination it must be administered not later than 7 days after the first vaccination.

* Observe manufacturer's instructions regarding administration

Table 1: Immunisation schedules appropriate to different types of exposure (WHO 2002)

Exposure Category	Type of contact with suspect or confirmed rabid domestic or wild animal, or animal unavailable for observation[(a)]	Recommended treatment
I	Touching or feeding of animals Licks on intact skin Touching of inoculated animal lure with intact skin	None, if reliable case history is available. In case of unreliable case history, treat according to schedule A (see Table 2).
II	Nibbling of uncovered skin Minor scratches or abrasions without bleeding Licks on broken skin Touching of inoculated animal lure with skin damaged	Administer vaccine immediately [(b)] as in schedule A (see Table 2). In case of uncertainty and/or exposure in a high-risk area, administer active and passive treatment as in schedule B (see Table 2). (See also footnote [c])
III	Single or multiple transdermal bites or scratches Contamination of mucous membrane with saliva (i. e. licks) Touching of inoculated animal lure with mucous membrane or fresh skin wound	Administer rabies immunoglobulin and vaccine immediately [(b)] as in schedule B (see Table 2). (See also footnote [c])

[a)] Exposure to rodents, rabbits and hares seldom, if ever, requires specific anti-rabies treatment.

[b)] If an apparently healthy dog or cat in or from a low-risk area is placed under observation, it may be justified to delay specific treatment.

[c)] Stop treatment if animal is a cat or dog and remains healthy throughout an observation period of 10 days or if animal is euthanised and found to be negative for rabies by appropriate laboratory techniques. Except in the case of threatened or endangered species, other domestic and wild animals suspected as rabid should be euthanised and their tissues examined using appropriate laboratory techniques.

Immunocompromised patients and patients with a particularly high risk of contracting rabies

For immunocompromised patients, those with multiple wounds and/or wounds on the head or other highly innervated areas, and those for whom there is a delay before initiation of treatment, it is recommended that:

- The days 0, 3, 7, 14 and 28 immunisation regimen should be used for these cases

- Two doses of vaccine may be given on day 0. That is, a single dose of 1 ml vaccine should be injected into the right deltoid and another single dose into the left deltoid muscle. In small children, one dose should be given into the anterolateral region of each thigh.

Severely immunosuppressed patients may not develop an immunologic response after rabies vaccination. Therefore, prompt and appropriate wound care after an exposure is an essential step in preventing death. In addition, rabies immune globulin should be administered in all immunosuppressed patients experiencing Category II and Category III wounds.

In immunocompromised patients, the neutralising antibody titre should be measured 14 days after the first injection. Patients with a titre that is less than 0.5 IU/ml should be given another two doses of vaccine simultaneously and as soon as possible. Further checks on the antibody titre should be made and further doses of vaccine should be administered as necessary.

In all cases, the immunisation schedule must be followed exactly as recommended, even if the patient does not present for treatment until a considerable time has elapsed since exposure.

Method of Administration

The vaccine should be given by intramuscular injection into the deltoid muscle, or into the anterolateral region of the thigh in small children.

It must not be given by intra-gluteal injection.

Do not administer by intravascular injection (see Section 4.4).

4.3 Contraindications

Post-exposure treatment

There are no contraindications to vaccination when post-exposure treatment is indicated. However, subjects considered to be at risk of a severe hypersensitivity reaction should receive an alternative rabies vaccine if a suitable product is available (see also section 4.4 regarding previous hypersensitivity reactions).

Pre-exposure prophylaxis

Rabipur should not be administered to subjects with a history of a severe hypersensitivity reaction to any of the ingredients in the vaccine. Note that the vaccine may contain polygeline, traces of neomycin, chlortetracycline, amphotericin B and chick proteins (see also section 4.4).

Vaccination should be delayed in subjects suffering from an acute febrile illness. Minor infections are not a contraindication to vaccination.

4.4 Special warnings and precautions for use

As with all vaccines, appropriate medical treatment should be immediately available for use in the rare event of an anaphylactic reaction to the vaccine.

A history of allergy to eggs or a positive skin test to ovalbumin does not necessarily indicate that a subject will be allergic to Rabipur. However, subjects who have a history of a severe hypersensitivity reaction to eggs or egg products should not receive the vaccine for pre-exposure prophylaxis. Such subjects should not receive the vaccine for post-exposure treatment unless a suitable alternative vaccine is not available, in which case all injections should be administered with close monitoring and with facilities for emergency treatment.

Similarly, subjects with a history of a severe hypersensitivity reaction to any of the other ingredients in Rabipur such as polygeline (stabilizer), or to amphotericin B, chlortetracycline or neomycin (which may be present as trace residues) should not receive the vaccine for pre-exposure prophylaxis. The vaccine should not be given to such persons for post-exposure treatment unless a suitable alternative vaccine is not available, in which case precautions should be taken as above.

Do not administer by intravascular injection.

If the vaccine is inadvertently administered into a blood vessel there is a risk of severe adverse reactions, including shock

After contact with animals which are suspected carriers of rabies, it is essential to observe the following procedures (according to WHO 1997):

Immediate wound treatment

In order to remove rabies virus, immediately cleanse wound with soap and flush thoroughly with water. Then treat with alcohol (70%) or iodine solution. Where possible, bite injuries should not be closed with a suture, or only sutured to secure apposition.

Tetanus vaccination and rabies immunoglobulin administration

Prophylaxis against tetanus should be implemented when necessary.

In cases of indicated passive immunisation, as much of the recommended dose of human rabies immunoglobulin (HRIG) as anatomically feasible should be applied as deeply as possible in and around the wound. Any remaining HRIG should be injected intramuscularly at a site distant from the vaccination site, preferably intragluteally. For detailed information plesase refer to the SmPC and/or package insert of HRIG.

4.5 Interaction with other medicinal products and other forms of interaction

Patients who are immunocompromised, including those receiving immunosuppressive therapy, may not mount an adequate response to rabies vaccine. Therefore, it is recommended that serological responses should be monitored in such patients and additional doses given as necessary (see section 4.2 for details).

Administration of rabies immunoglobulin may be necessary for management but may attenuate the effects of concomitantly administered rabies vaccine. Therefore, it is important that rabies immunoglobulin should be administered once only for treating each at-risk exposure and with adherence to the recommended dose.

Other essential inactivated vaccines may be given at the same time as Rabipur. Different injectable inactivated vaccines should be administered into separate injection sites.

4.6 Pregnancy and lactation

No cases of harm attributable to use of Rabipur during pregnancy have been observed. While it is not known whether Rabipur enters breast milk, no risk to the breastfeeding infant has been identified. Rabipur may be administered to pregnant and breastfeeding women when post-exposure treatment is required.

The vaccine may also be used for pre-exposure prophylaxis during pregnancy and in breastfeeding women if it is considered that the potential benefit outweighs any possible risk to the fetus/infant.

4.7 Effects on ability to drive and use machines

The vaccine is unlikely to produce an effect on ability to drive and use machines.

4.8 Undesirable effects

In clinical studies the most commonly reported solicited adverse reactions were injection site pain (30 –85 %, mainly pain due to injection) or injection site induration (15 - 35 %). Most injection site reactions were not severe and resolved within 24 to 48 hours after injection. Furthermore, the following undesirable effects were observed in clinical trials and/or during the post-marketing period:

Standard system organ class	Frequency	Adverse reactions
General disorders and administration site condition	Very common > 1/10	Injection site pain, injection site reaction, injection site induration
	Common > 1/100, < 1/10	Asthenia, malaise, fever, fatigue, influenza like illness, injection site erythema
Cardiac disorders	Rare > 1/10.000, < 1/1.000	Circulatory reactions (such as palpitations or hot flush)
Blood and lymphatic system disorders	Common > 1/100, < 1/10	Lymphadenopathy
Ear and labyrinth disorders	Very rare < 1/10.000	Vertigo
Eye disorders	Rare > 1/10.000, < 1/1.000	Visual disturbance
Nervous system disorders*	Common > 1/100, < 1/10	Headache
	Rare > 1/10.000, < 1/1.000	Paraesthesia
	Very rare < 1/10.000	Nervous system disorders (such as paresis or Guillain-Barré-Syndrome)
Skin disorders	Common > 1/100, < 1/10	Rash
Immune system disorders	Rare > 1/10.000, < 1/1.000	Allergic reactions (such as anaphylaxis, bronchospasm, oedema, urticaria or pruritus)
Musculosceletal and connective tissue disorders	Common > 1/100, < 1/10	Myalgia, arthralgia
Gastrointestinal disorders	Common > 1/100, < 1/10	Gastrointestinal disorder (such as nausea or abdominal pain)

* Statistically there is no indication of increasing frequencies of primary manifestations or triggered attacks of autoimmune diseases (e.g. multiple sclerosis) after vaccination. However, in individual cases it cannot be absolutely excluded that a vaccination may trigger an episode in patients with corresponding genetic disposition. According to the current state of scientific knowledge vaccinations are not the cause of autoimmune diseases.

4.9 Overdose

No symptoms of overdose are known.

5. PHARMACOLOGICAL PROPERTIES

5.1 Pharmacodynamic properties

ATC-Code: J07B G01

Pre-exposure Prophylaxis

In clinical trials with previously unimmunised subjects, almost all subjects achieve a protective antibody titre (⩾ 0.5 IU/ml) by day 28 of a primary series of three injections of Rabipur when given according to the recommended schedule by the intramuscular route.

As antibody titres slowly decrease, booster doses are required to maintain antibody levels above 0.5 IU/ml. However, persistence of protective antibody titres for 2 years after immunisation with Rabipur without additional booster has been found to be 100 % in clinical trials.

In clinical trials, a booster dose of Rabipur elicited a 10-fold or higher increase in Geometric Mean Titres (GMTs) by day 30. It has also been demonstrated that individuals who had previously been immunised with Human Diploid Cell Vaccine (HDCV) developed a rapid anamnestic response when boosted with Rabipur.

Persistence of antibody titres has been shown for 14 years in a limited number (n = 28) of subjects tested.

Nevertheless, the need for and timing of boosting should be assessed on a case by case basis, taking into account official guidance (see also section 4.2).

Post-exposure Treatment

In clinical studies, Rabipur elicited neutralising antibodies (⩾ 0.5 IU/ml) in 98% of patients within 14 days and in 99-100% of patients by day 28 – 38, when administered according to the WHO-recommended schedule of five intramuscular injections of 1 ml, one each on days 0, 3, 7, 14 and 28.

Concomitant administration of either Human Rabies Immunoglobulin (HRIG) or Equine Rabies Immunoglobulin (ERIG) with the first dose of rabies vaccine caused a slight decrease in GMTs. However, this was not considered to be clinically relevant.

5.2 Pharmacokinetic properties

Not applicable.

5.3 Preclinical safety data

Preclinical data including single-dose, repeated dose and local tolerance studies revealed no unexpected findings and no target organ toxicity. No genotoxicity and reproductive toxicity studies have been performed.

6. PHARMACEUTICAL PARTICULARS

6.1 List of excipients

Powder:

TRIS-(hydroxymethyl)-aminomethane

Sodium chloride

Disodium edetate (Titriplex III)

Potassium-L-glutamate

Polygeline

Sucrose

Solvent:

Water for injections

6.2 Incompatibilities

This vaccine should not be mixed with other medicinal products.

6.3 Shelf life

4 years

6.4 Special precautions for storage

Store at +2 to +8° C (in a refrigerator).

6.5 Nature and contents of container

Pack containing

Powder in a vial (type I glass) with stopper (chlorobutyl)

1 ml solvent for solution in an ampoule (type I glass)

with or without disposable syringe (polypropylene with polyethylene plunger)

Not all pack sizes may be marketed.

6.6 Special precautions for disposal and other handling

The vaccine should be visually inspected both before and after reconstitution for any foreign particulate matter and or change in physical appearance. The vaccine must not be used if any change in the appearance of the vaccine has taken place. For appearance see Section 3.

The powder for solution should be reconstituted using the solvent for solution supplied and carefully agitated prior to injection. The reconstituted vaccine should be used immediately.

Any unused vaccine or waste material should be disposed of in accordance with local requirements.

Administrative Data

7. MARKETING AUTHORISATION HOLDER

Novartis Vaccines and Diagnostics GmbH & Co. KG

P.O. Box 16 30

D-35006 Marburg

Germany

8. MARKETING AUTHORISATION NUMBER(S)

PL 16033/0008

9. DATE OF FIRST AUTHORISATION/RENEWAL OF THE AUTHORISATION

24 September 2003

10. DATE OF REVISION OF THE TEXT

January 2007

Ranexa prolonged-release tablets

(A. Menarini Pharma U.K. S.R.L.)

1. NAME OF THE MEDICINAL PRODUCT

Ranexa 375 mg ▼ prolonged-release tablets

Ranexa 500 mg ▼ prolonged-release tablets

Ranexa 750 mg ▼ prolonged-release tablets

2. QUALITATIVE AND QUANTITATIVE COMPOSITION

Each tablet contains 375 mg of ranolazine.

Each tablet contains 500 mg of ranolazine.

Each tablet contains 750 mg of ranolazine.

< 500 mg tablet >

Excipient: Each tablet contains 0.12 mg azo colouring agent E110.

< 750 mg tablet >

Excipients: Each tablet contains 0.04 mg azo colouring agent E102 and 12.0 mg lactose monohydrate.

For a full list of excipients see section 6.1.

3. PHARMACEUTICAL FORM

Prolonged-release tablet

Pale blue oval-shaped tablet engraved with CVT375 on one side.

Light orange oval-shaped tablet engraved with CVT500 on one side.

Pale green oval-shaped tablet engraved with CVT750 on one side.

4. CLINICAL PARTICULARS

4.1 Therapeutic indications

Ranexa is indicated as add-on therapy for the symptomatic treatment of patients with stable angina pectoris who are inadequately controlled or intolerant to first-line antianginal therapies (such as beta-blockers and/or calcium antagonists).

4.2 Posology and method of administration

Patients should be given the Ranexa package leaflet and the Patient Alert Card and instructed to present their Patient Alert Card and medication list to their health care professional at each visit.

Ranexa is available as 375 mg, 500 mg, and 750 mg prolonged-release tablets.

Adults: The recommended initial dose of Ranexa is 375 mg twice daily. After 2–4 weeks, the dose should be titrated to 500 mg twice daily and, according to the patient's response, further titrated to a recommended maximum dose of 750 mg twice daily (see section 5.1).

If a patient experiences treatment-related adverse events (e.g. dizziness, nausea, or vomiting), down-titration of Ranexa to 500 mg or 375 mg twice daily may be required. If symptoms do not resolve after dose reduction, treatment should be discontinued.

Concomitant treatment with CYP3A4 and P-glycoprotein (P-gp) inhibitors: Careful dose titration is recommended in patients treated with moderate CYP3A4 inhibitors (e.g. diltiazem, fluconazole, erythromycin) or P-gp inhibitors (e.g. verapamil, ciclosporin) (see sections 4.4 and 4.5).

Concomitant administration of potent CYP3A4 inhibitors is contraindicated (see sections 4.3 and 4.5).

Renal impairment: Careful dose titration is recommended in patients with mild to moderate renal impairment (creatinine clearance 30–80 ml/min) (see sections 4.4, 4.8, and 5.2). Ranexa is contraindicated in patients with severe renal impairment (creatinine clearance < 30 ml/min) (see sections 4.3 and 5.2).

Hepatic impairment: Careful dose titration is recommended in patients with mild hepatic impairment (see sections 4.4 and 5.2). Ranexa is contraindicated in patients with moderate or severe hepatic impairment (see sections 4.3 and 5.2).

Elderly: Dose titration in elderly patients should be exercised with caution (see section 4.4). Elderly may have increased ranolazine exposure due to age-related decrease in renal function (see section 5.2). The incidence of adverse events was higher in the elderly (see section 4.8).

Low weight: The incidence of adverse events was higher in patients with low weight (⩽ 60 kg). Dose titration in patients with low weight should be exercised with caution (see sections 4.4, 4.8, and 5.2).

Congestive heart failure (CHF): Dose titration in patients with moderate to severe CHF (NYHA Class III–IV) should be exercised with caution (see sections 4.4 and 5.2).

Paediatric patients: Ranexa is not recommended for use in children below the age of 18 years due to a lack of data on safety and efficacy.

Ranexa tablets should be swallowed whole and not crushed, broken, or chewed. They may be taken with or without food.

4.3 Contraindications

Hypersensitivity to the active substance or to any of the excipients (see section 6.1).

Severe renal impairment (creatinine clearance < 30 ml/min) (see sections 4.2 and 5.2).

Moderate or severe hepatic impairment (see sections 4.2 and 5.2).

Concomitant administration of potent CYP3A4 inhibitors (e.g. itraconazole, ketoconazole, voriconazol, posaconazol, HIV protease inhibitors, clarithromycin, telithromycin, nefazodone) (see sections 4.2 and 4.5).

Concomitant administration of Class Ia (e.g. quinidine) or Class III (e.g. dofetilide, sotalol) antiarrhythmics other than amiodarone.

4.4 Special warnings and precautions for use

Caution should be exercised when prescribing or uptitrating ranolazine to patients in whom an increased exposure is expected:

- Concomitant administration of moderate CYP3A4 inhibitors (see sections 4.2 and 4.5).
- Concomitant administration of P-gp inhibitors (see sections 4.2 and 4.5).
- Mild hepatic impairment (see sections 4.2 and 5.2).
- Mild to moderate renal impairment (creatinine clearance 30–80 ml/min) (see sections 4.2, 4.8, and 5.2).
- Elderly (see sections 4.2, 4.8, and 5.2).
- Patients with low weight (⩽ 60 kg) (see sections 4.2, 4.8, and 5.2).
- Patients with moderate to severe CHF (NYHA Class III–IV) (see sections 4.2 and 5.2).

In patients with a combination of these factors, additional exposure increases are expected. Dose- dependent side effects are likely to occur. If Ranexa is used in patients with a combination of several of these factors, monitoring of adverse events should be frequent, the dose reduced, and treatment discontinued, if needed.

The risk for increased exposure leading to adverse events in these different subgroups is higher in patients lacking CYP2D6 activity (poor metabolisers, PM) than subjects with CYP2D6 metabolising capacity (extensive metabolisers, EM) (see section 5.2). The above precautions are based on the risk in a CYP2D6 PM patient, and are needed when the CYP2D6 status is unknown. There is a lower need for precautions in patients with CYP2D6 EM status. If the CYP2D6 status of the patient has been determined (e.g. by genotyping) or is previously known to be EM, Ranexa can be used with caution in these patients when they have a combination of several of the above risk factors.

QT prolongation: A population-based analysis of combined data from patients and healthy volunteers demonstrated that the slope of the plasma concentration-QTc relationship was estimated to be 2.4 msec per 1000 ng/ml, which is approximately equal to a 2- to 7-msec increase over the plasma concentration range for ranolazine 500 to 1000 mg twice daily. Therefore, caution should be observed when treating patients with a history of congenital or a family history of long QT syndrome, in patients with known acquired QT interval prolongation, and in patients treated with drugs affecting the QTc interval (see section 4.5 also).

Drug-drug interactions: Co-administration with CYP3A4 inducers is expected to lead to lack of efficacy. Ranexa should not be used in patients treated with CYP3A4 inducers (e.g. rifampicin, phenytoin, phenobarbital, carbamazepine, St. John's Wort) (see section 4.5).

Renal impairment: Renal function decreases with age and it is therefore important to check renal function at regular intervals during treatment with ranolazine (see sections 4.2, 4.3, 4.8, and 5.2).

< 500 mg tablet >

Azo colouring agent E110: This medicinal product contains the azo colouring agent E110 which may cause allergic reactions.

< 750 mg tablet >

Lactose: This medicinal product contains lactose. Patients with rare hereditary problems of galactose intolerance, the Lapp lactase deficiency, or glucose-galactose malabsorption should not take this medicinal product.

Azo colouring agent E102: This medicinal product contains the azo colouring agent E102 which may cause allergic reactions.

4.5 Interaction with other medicinal products and other forms of interaction

Effects of other medicinal products on ranolazine

CYP3A4 or P-gp inhibitors: Ranolazine is a substrate of cytochrome CYP3A4. Inhibitors of CYP3A4 increase plasma concentrations of ranolazine. The potential for dose-related adverse events (e.g. nausea, dizziness) may also increase with increased plasma concentrations. Concomitant treatment with ketoconazole 200 mg twice daily increased the AUC of ranolazine by 3.0- to 3.9-fold during ranolazine treatment. Combining ranolazine with potent CYP3A4 inhibitors (e.g. itraconazole, ketoconazole, voriconazole, posaconazole, HIV protease inhibitors, clarithromycin, telithromycin, nefazodone) is contraindicated (see section 4.3). Grapefruit juice is also a potent CYP3A4 inhibitor.

Diltiazem (180 to 360 mg once daily), a moderately potent CYP3A4 inhibitor, causes dose-dependent increases in average ranolazine steady-state concentrations of 1.5- to 2.4-fold. Careful dose titration of Ranexa is recommended in patients treated with diltiazem and other moderately potent CYP3A4 inhibitors (e.g. erythromycin, fluconazole). Down-titration of Ranexa may be required (see sections 4.2 and 4.4).

Ranolazine is a substrate for P-gp. Inhibitors of P-gp (e.g. ciclosporin, quinidine, verapamil) increase plasma levels of ranolazine. Verapamil (120 mg three times daily) increases ranolazine steady-state concentrations 2.2-fold. Careful dose titration of Ranexa is recommended in patients treated with P-gp inhibitors. Down-titration of Ranexa may be required (see sections 4.2 and 4.4).

CYP3A4 inducers: Rifampicin (600 mg once daily) decreases ranolazine steady-state concentrations by approximately 95%. Initiation of treatment with Ranexa should be avoided during administration of inducers of CYP3A4 (e.g. rifampicin, phenytoin, phenobarbital, carbamazepine, St. John's Wort) (see section 4.4).

CYP2D6 inhibitors: Ranolazine is partially metabolised by CYP2D6; therefore, inhibitors of this enzyme may increase plasma concentrations of ranolazine. The potent CYP2D6 inhibitor paroxetine, at a dose of 20 mg once daily, increased steady-state plasma concentrations of ranolazine 1000 mg twice daily by an average of 1.2-fold. No dose adjustment is required. At the dose level 500 mg twice daily, co-administration of a potent inhibitor of CYP2D6 could result in an increase in ranolazine AUC of about 62%.

Effects of ranolazine on other medicinal products

Ranolazine is a moderate to potent inhibitor of P-gp and a mild inhibitor of CYP3A4, and may increase plasma concentrations of P-gp or CYP3A4 substrates. Tissue distribution of drugs which are transported by P-gp may be increased.

Available data suggest that ranolazine is a mild inhibitor of CYP2D6. The exposure of CYP2D6 substrates (e.g. tricyclic antidepressants and antipsychotics) may be increased during co-administration of Ranexa, and lower doses of these medicinal products may be required.

The potential for inhibition of CYP2B6 has not been evaluated. Caution is advised during co-administration with CYP2B6 substrates (e.g. bupropion, efavirenz, cyclophosphamide).

Digoxin: An increase in plasma digoxin concentrations by an average of 1.5-fold has been reported when Ranexa and digoxin are co-administered. Therefore, digoxin levels should be monitored following initiation and termination of Ranexa therapy.

Simvastatin: Simvastatin metabolism and clearance are highly dependent on CYP3A4. Ranexa 1000 mg twice daily increased plasma concentrations of simvastatin lactone, simvastatin acid, and the HMG-CoA reductase inhibitor activity by 1.4- to 1.6-fold.

There is a theoretical risk that concomitant treatment of ranolazine with other drugs known to prolong the QTc interval may give rise to a pharmacodynamic interaction and increase the possible risk of ventricular arrhythmias. Examples of such drugs include certain antihistamines (e.g. terfenadine, astemizole, mizolastine), certain antiarrhythmics (e.g. quinidine, disopyramide, procainamide), erythromycin, and tricyclic antidepressants (e.g. imipramine, doxepin, amitriptyline).

4.6 Pregnancy and lactation

Pregnancy: There are no adequate data from the use of ranolazine in pregnant women. Animal studies are insufficient with respect to effects on pregnancy and embryo-foetal development (see section 5.3). The potential risk for humans is unknown. Ranexa should not be used during pregnancy unless clearly necessary.

Lactation: It is unknown whether ranolazine is excreted in human breast milk. The excretion of ranolazine in milk has not been studied in animals. Ranexa should not be used during breast-feeding.

4.7 Effects on ability to drive and use machines

No studies on the effects of Ranexa on the ability to drive and use machines have been performed. Ranexa may cause dizziness and blurred vision (see section 4.8), which may affect the ability to drive and use machines.

4.8 Undesirable effects

Undesirable effects in patients receiving Ranexa are generally mild to moderate in severity and often develop within the first 2 weeks of treatment. These were reported during the Phase 3 clinical development programme, which included a total of 1,030 chronic angina patients treated with Ranexa.

The adverse events, considered to be at least possibly related to treatment, are listed below by body system, organ class, and absolute frequency. Frequencies are defined as very common (⩾ 1/10), common (⩾ 1/100 to < 1/10), uncommon (⩾ 1/1,000 to < 1/100), rare (⩾ 1/10,000 to < 1/1,000), and very rare (< 1/10,000).

Metabolism and nutrition disorders

Uncommon: anorexia, decreased appetite, dehydration.

Psychiatric disorders

Uncommon: anxiety, insomnia.

Rare: disorientation.

Nervous system disorders

Common: dizziness, headache.

Uncommon: lethargy, syncope, hypoaesthesia, somnolence, tremor, postural dizziness.

Rare: amnesia, depressed level of consciousness, loss of consciousness, parosmia.

Eye disorders

Uncommon: blurred vision, visual disturbance.

Ear and labyrinth disorders

Uncommon: vertigo, tinnitus.

Rare: impaired hearing.

Vascular disorders

Uncommon: hot flush, hypotension.

Rare: peripheral coldness, orthostatic hypotension.

Respiratory, thoracic, and mediastinal disorders

Uncommon: dyspnoea, cough, epistaxis.

Rare: throat tightness.

Gastrointestinal disorders

Common: constipation, vomiting, nausea.

Uncommon: abdominal pain, dry mouth, dyspepsia, flatulence, stomach discomfort.

Rare: pancreatitis, erosive duodenitis, oral hypoaesthesia.

Skin and subcutaneous tissue disorders

Uncommon: pruritus, hyperhydrosis.

Rare: allergic dermatitis, urticaria, cold sweat, rash.

Musculoskeletal and connective tissue disorders

Uncommon: pain in extremity, muscle cramp, joint swelling.

Renal and urinary disorders

Uncommon: dysuria, haematuria, chromaturia.

Reproductive system and breast disorders

Rare: erectile dysfunction.

General disorders and administration site conditions

Common: asthenia.

Uncommon: fatigue, peripheral oedema.

Investigations

Uncommon: increased blood creatinine, increased blood urea, prolonged QT corrected interval, increased platelet or white blood cell count, decreased weight.

Rare: elevated levels of hepatic enzyme.

The adverse event profile was generally similar in the MERLIN-TIMI 36 study. In this long term study, acute renal failure was also reported with an incidence less than 1% in placebo and ranolazine patients. Evaluations in patients who may be considered at higher risk of adverse events when treated with other antianginal medicinal products, e.g. patients with diabetes, Class I and II heart failure, or obstructive airway disease, confirmed that these conditions were not associated with clinically meaningful increases in the incidence of adverse events.

Elderly, renal impairment, and low weight: In general, adverse events occurred more frequently among elderly patients and patients with renal impairment; however, the types of events in these subgroups were similar to those observed in the general population. Of the most commonly reported, the following events occurred more often with Ranexa (placebo-corrected frequencies) in elderly (⩾ 75 years of age) than younger patients (< 75 years of age): constipation (8% versus 5%), nausea (6% versus 3%), hypotension (5% versus 1%), and vomiting (4% versus 1%).

In patients with mild or moderate renal impairment (creatinine clearance ⩾ 30–80 ml/min) compared to those with normal renal function (creatinine clearance > 80 ml/min), the most commonly reported events and their placebo-corrected frequencies included: constipation (8% versus 4%), dizziness (7% versus 5%), and nausea (4% versus 2%).

In general, the type and frequency of adverse events reported in patients with low body weight (⩽ 60 kg) were similar to those of patients with higher weight (> 60 kg); however, the placebo-corrected frequencies of the following common adverse events were higher in low body weight than heavier patients: nausea (14% versus 2%), vomiting (6% versus 1%), and hypotension (4% versus 2%).

Laboratory findings: Small, clinically insignificant, reversible elevations in serum creatinine levels have been observed in healthy subjects and patients treated with Ranexa. There was no renal toxicity related to these findings. A renal function study in healthy volunteers demonstrated a reduction in creatinine clearance with no change in glomerular filtration rate consistent with inhibition of renal tubular secretion of creatinine.

Post-marketing experience: In post-marketing experience, there have been reports of acute renal failure, including in patients with pre-existing mild to moderate renal impairment and/or taking concomitant medications that are known to interact with ranolazine (see section 4.4 and 4.5).

4.9 Overdose

In an oral high-dose tolerability study in angina patients, the incidence of dizziness, nausea, and vomiting increased in a dose-dependent manner. In addition to these adverse events, diplopia, lethargy, and syncope were observed in an intravenous overdose study in healthy volunteers. In the event of overdose, the patient should be closely monitored and the treatment should be symptomatic and supportive.

Approximately 62% of ranolazine is bound to plasma proteins, and therefore, complete clearance by haemodialysis is unlikely.

5. PHARMACOLOGICAL PROPERTIES

5.1 Pharmacodynamic properties

Pharmacotherapeutic group: Other cardiac preparations, ATC code: C01EB18

Mechanism of action: The mechanism of action of ranolazine is largely unknown. Ranolazine may have some anti-anginal effects by inhibition of the late sodium current in cardiac cells. This reduces intracellular sodium accumulation and consequently decreases intracellular calcium overload. Ranolazine, via its action to decrease the late sodium current, is considered to reduce these intracellular ionic imbalances during ischaemia. This reduction in cellular calcium overload is expected to improve myocardial relaxation and thereby decrease left ventricular diastolic stiffness. Clinical evidence of inhibition of the late sodium current by ranolazine is provided by a significant shortening of the QTc interval and an improvement in diastolic relaxation in an open-label study of 5 patients with a long QT syndrome (LQT3 having the SCN5A ΔKPQ gene mutation).

These effects do not depend upon changes in heart rate, blood pressure, or vasodilation.

Pharmacodynamic effects

Haemodynamic effects: Minimal decreases in mean heart rate (< 2 beats per minute) and mean systolic blood pressure (< 3 mm Hg) were observed in patients treated with ranolazine either alone or in combination with other antianginal medicinal products in controlled studies.

Electrocardiographic effects: Dose and plasma concentration-related increases in the QTc interval (about 6 msec at 1000 mg twice daily), reductions in T wave amplitude, and in some cases notched T waves, have been observed in patients treated with Ranexa. These effects of ranolazine on the surface electrocardiogram are believed to result from inhibition of the fast-rectifying potassium current, which prolongs the ventricular action potential, and from inhibition of the late sodium current, which shortens the ventricular action potential. A population analysis of combined data from 1,308 patients and healthy volunteers demonstrated a mean increase in QTc from baseline of 2.4 msec per 1000 ng/ml ranolazine plasma concentration. This value is consistent with data from pivotal clinical studies, where mean changes from baseline in QTcF (Fridericia's correction) after doses of 500 and 750 mg twice daily were 1.9 and 4.9 msec, respectively. The slope is higher in patients with clinically significant hepatic impairment.

In a large outcome study (MERLIN-TIMI 36) in 6,560 patients with UA/NSTEMI ACS, there was no difference between Ranexa and placebo in the risk of all-cause mortality (relative risk ranolazine:placebo 0.99), sudden cardiac death (relative risk ranolazine:placebo 0.87), or the frequency of symptomatic documented arrhythmias (3.0% versus 3.1%).

No proarrhythmic effects were observed in 3,162 patients treated with Ranexa based on 7-day Holter monitoring in the MERLIN-TIMI 36 study. There was a significantly lower incidence of arrhythmias in patients treated with Ranexa (74%) versus placebo (83%), including ventricular tachycardia ⩾ 8 beats (5% versus 8%).

Clinical efficacy: Clinical studies have demonstrated the efficacy and safety of Ranexa in the treatment of patients with chronic angina, either alone or when the benefit from other antianginal medicinal products was sub-optimal.

In the pivotal study, CARISA, Ranexa was added to treatment with atenolol 50 mg once daily, amlodipine 5 mg once daily, or diltiazem 180 mg once daily. Eight-hundred and twenty-three patients (23% women) were randomised to receive 12 weeks of treatment with Ranexa 750 mg twice daily, 1000 mg twice daily, or placebo. Ranexa demonstrated greater efficacy than placebo in prolonging exercise time at trough at 12 weeks for both doses studied when used as an add-on therapy. However, there was no difference in exercise duration between the two doses (24 seconds compared to placebo; p ⩽ 0.03).

Ranexa resulted in significant decreases in the number of angina attacks per week and consumption of short-acting nitroglycerin compared to placebo. Tolerance to ranolazine did not develop during treatment and a rebound increase in angina attacks was not observed following abrupt discontinuation.

The improvement in exercise duration in women was about 33% of the improvement in men at the 1000 mg twice-daily dose level. However, men and women had similar reductions in frequency of angina attacks and nitroglycerin consumption. Given the dose-dependent side effects and similar efficacy at 750 and 1000 mg twice daily, a maximum dose of 750 mg twice daily is recommended.

In a second study, ERICA, Ranexa was added to treatment with amlodipine 10 mg once daily (the maximum labelled dose). Five-hundred and sixty-five patients were randomised to receive an initial dose of Ranexa 500 mg twice daily or placebo for 1 week, followed by 6 weeks of treatment with Ranexa 1000 mg twice daily or placebo, in addition to concomitant treatment with amlodipine 10 mg once daily. Additionally, 45% of the study population also received long-acting nitrates. Ranexa resulted in significant decreases in the number of angina attacks per week (p = 0.028) and consumption of short-acting nitroglycerin (p = 0.014) compared to placebo. Both the average number of angina attacks and nitroglycerin tablets consumed decreased by approximately one per week.

In the main dose-finding study, MARISA, ranolazine was used as monotherapy. One-hundred and ninety-one patients were randomised to treatment with Ranexa 500 mg twice daily, 1000 mg twice daily, 1500 mg twice daily, and matching placebo, each for 1 week in a cross-over design. Ranexa was significantly superior to placebo in prolonging exercise time, time to angina, and time to 1 mm ST segment depression at all doses studied with an observed dose-response relationship. Improvement of exercise duration was statistically significant compared to placebo for all three doses of ranolazine from 24 seconds at 500 mg twice daily to 46 seconds at 1500 mg twice daily, showing a dose-related response. In this study, exercise duration was longest in the 1500 mg group; however, there was a disproportional increase in side effects, and the 1500 mg dose was not studied further.

In a large outcome study (MERLIN-TIMI 36) in 6,560 patients with UA/NSTEMI ACS, there was no difference in the risk of all-cause mortality (relative risk ranolazine:-placebo 0.99), sudden cardiac death (relative risk ranolazine:placebo 0.87), or the frequency of symptomatic documented arrhythmias (3.0% versus 3.1%) between Ranexa and placebo when added to standard medical therapy (including beta-blockers, calcium channel blockers, nitrates, anti-platelet agents, lipid-lowering medicinal products, and ACE inhibitors). Approximately one-half of the patients in MERLIN-TIMI 36 had a history of angina. The results showed that exercise duration was 31 seconds longer in ranolazine patients versus placebo patients (p = 0.002). The Seattle Angina Questionnaire showed significant effects on several dimensions, including angina frequency (p < 0.001), compared to placebo-treated patients.

A small proportion of non-Caucasians was included in the controlled clinical studies; therefore, no conclusions can be drawn regarding the effect and safety in non-Caucasians.

5.2 Pharmacokinetic properties

After oral administration of Ranexa, peak plasma concentrations (C_{max}) are typically observed between 2 and 6 hours. Steady state is generally achieved within 3 days of twice-daily dosing.

Absorption: The mean absolute bioavailability of ranolazine after oral administration of immediate-release ranolazine tablets ranged from 35–50%, with large inter-individual variability. Ranexa exposure increases more than in proportion to dose. There was a 2.5- to 3-fold increase in steady-state AUC as the dose was increased from 500 mg to 1000 mg twice daily. In a pharmacokinetic study in healthy volunteers, steady-state C_{max} was, on average, approximately 1770 (SD 1040) ng/ml, and steady-state AUC_{0-12} was, on average, 13,700 (SD 8290) ng × h/ml following a dose of 500 mg twice daily. Food does not affect the rate and extent of absorption of ranolazine.

Distribution: Approximately 62% of ranolazine is bound to plasma proteins, mainly alpha-1 acid glycoprotein and weakly to albumin. The mean steady-state volume of distribution (V_{ss}) is about 180 l.

Elimination: Ranolazine is eliminated primarily by metabolism. Less than 5% of the dose is excreted unchanged in the urine and faeces. Following oral administration of a single 500 mg dose of [^{14}C]-ranolazine to healthy subjects, 73% of the radioactivity was recovered in urine and 25% in faeces.

Clearance of ranolazine is dose-dependent, decreasing with increased dose. The elimination half-life is about 2–3 hours after intravenous administration. The terminal half-life at steady state after oral administration of ranolazine is about 7 hours, due to the absorption rate-limited elimination.

Biotransformation: Ranolazine undergoes rapid and extensive metabolism. In healthy young adults, ranolazine accounts for approximately 13% of the radioactivity in plasma following a single oral 500 mg dose of [^{14}C]-ranolazine. A large number of metabolites has been identified in human plasma (47 metabolites), urine (> 100 metabolites), and faeces (25 metabolites). Fourteen primary pathways have been identified of which O-demethylation and N-dealkylation are the most important. *In vitro* studies using human liver microsomes indicate that ranolazine is metabolised primarily by CYP3A4, but also by CYP2D6. At 500 mg twice daily, subjects lacking CYP2D6 activity (poor metabolisers, PM) had 62% higher AUC than subjects with CYP2D6 metabolising capacity (extensive metabolisers, EM). The corresponding difference at the 1000 mg twice-daily dose was 25%.

Special populations

The influence of various factors on the pharmacokinetics of ranolazine was assessed in a population pharmacokinetic evaluation in 928 angina patients and healthy subjects.

Gender effects: Gender had no clinically relevant effect on pharmacokinetic parameters.

Elderly patients: Age alone had no clinically relevant effect on pharmacokinetic parameters. However, the elderly may have increased ranolazine exposure due to age-related decrease in renal function.

Body weight: Compared to subjects weighing 70 kg, exposure was estimated to be about 1.4-fold higher in subjects weighing 40 kg.

CHF: CHF NYHA Class III and IV were estimated to have about 1.3-fold higher plasma concentrations.

Renal impairment: In a study evaluating the influence of renal function on ranolazine pharmacokinetics, ranolazine AUC was on average 1.7- to 2-fold higher in subjects with mild, moderate, and severe renal impairment compared with subjects with normal renal function. There was a large inter-individual variability in AUC in subjects with renal impairment. The AUC of metabolites increased with decreased renal function. The AUC of one pharmacologically active ranolazine metabolite was 5-fold increased in patients with severe renal impairment.

In the population pharmacokinetic analysis, a 1.2-fold increase in ranolazine exposure was estimated in subjects with moderate impairment (creatinine clearance 40 ml/min). In subjects with severe renal impairment (creatinine clearance 10–30 ml/min), a 1.3- to 1.8-fold increase in ranolazine exposure was estimated.

The influence of dialysis on the pharmacokinetics of ranolazine has not been evaluated.

Hepatic impairment: The pharmacokinetics of ranolazine have been evaluated in patients with mild or moderate hepatic impairment. There are no data in patients with severe hepatic impairment. Ranolazine AUC was unaffected in patients with mild hepatic impairment but increased 1.8-fold in patients with moderate impairment. QT prolongation was more pronounced in these patients.

Paediatrics: The pharmacokinetic parameters of ranolazine have not been studied in the paediatric population (< 18 years).

5.3 Preclinical safety data

Adverse reactions not observed in clinical studies, but seen in animals at levels similar to clinical exposure, were as follows: Ranolazine was associated with convulsions and increased mortality in rats and dogs at plasma concentrations approximately 3-fold higher than at the proposed maximum clinical dose.

Chronic toxicity studies in rats indicated that treatment was associated with adrenal changes at exposures slightly greater than those seen in clinical patients. This effect is associated with increased plasma cholesterol concentrations. No similar changes have been identified in humans. No effect on the adreno-cortical axis was noted in humans.

In long-term carcinogenicity studies at doses of ranolazine up to 50 mg/kg/day (150 mg/m^2/day) in mice and 150 mg/kg/day (900 mg/m^2/day) in rats, no relevant increases in the incidence of any tumour types were seen. These doses are equivalent to 0.1 and 0.8 times, respectively, the maximum recommended human dose of 2 grams on a mg/m^2 basis, and represent the maximum tolerated doses in these species.

Signs of embryonal and maternal toxicity, but not teratogenicity, were seen at doses of ranolazine up to 400 mg/kg/day (2400 mg/m^2/day) in rats and 150 mg/kg/day (1275 mg/m^2/day) in rabbits. These doses represent 2 and 1 times, respectively, the maximum recommended human dose.

6. PHARMACEUTICAL PARTICULARS

6.1 List of excipients

Excipients for all ranolazine prolonged-release tablets:

Carnauba wax
Hypromellose
Magnesium stearate
Methacrylic acid-ethyl acrylate copolymer (1:1)
Microcrystalline cellulose
Sodium hydroxide
Titanium dioxide

Additional excipients for 375 mg tablet:

Polyethylene glycol

Polysorbate 80

Blue #2/Indigo Carmine Aluminium Lake (E132)

Additional excipients for 500 mg tablet:

Polyethylene glycol

Polysorbate 80

Yellow #6/Sunset Yellow FCF Aluminium Lake (E110)

Additional excipients for 750 mg tablet:

Glycerol triacetate

Lactose monohydrate

Blue #1/Brilliant Blue FCF Aluminium Lake (E133) and Yellow #5/Tartrazine Aluminium Lake (E102)

6.2 Incompatibilities

Not applicable

6.3 Shelf life

4 years

6.4 Special precautions for storage

This medicinal product does not require any special storage conditions.

6.5 Nature and contents of container

PVC/PVDC/Aluminium blisters of 10 tablets per blister card. Each carton contains 3, 6 or 10 blister cards (30, 60 or 100 tablets) or one HDPE bottle containing 60 tablets.

Not all pack-sizes may be marketed.

6.6 Special precautions for disposal and other handling

No special requirements

7. MARKETING AUTHORISATION HOLDER

Menarini International Operations Luxembourg S.A.

1, Avenue de la Gare, L-1611 Luxembourg

Luxembourg

8. MARKETING AUTHORISATION NUMBER(S)

Ranexa 375 mg prolonged-release tablets:

EU/1/08/462/001 60 tablets in blister pack

EU/1/08/462/002 60 tablets in bottle

EU/1/08/462/007 30 tablets in blister pack

EU/1/08/462/008 100 tablets in blister pack

Ranexa 500 mg prolonged-release tablets:

EU/1/08/462/003 60 tablets in blister pack

EU/1/08/462/004 60 tablets in bottle

EU/1/08/462/009 30 tablets in blister pack

EU/1/08/462/010 100 tablets in blister pack

Ranexa 750 mg prolonged-release tablets:

EU/1/08/462/005 60 tablets in blister pack

EU/1/08/462/006 60 tablets in bottle

EU/1/08/462/011 30 tablets in blister pack

EU/1/08/462/012 100 tablets in blister pack

9. DATE OF FIRST AUTHORISATION/RENEWAL OF THE AUTHORISATION

Date of first authorisation: 09 July 2008

10. DATE OF REVISION OF THE TEXT

25 August 2009

Detailed information on this medicinal product is available on the website of the European Medicines Agency (EMEA) http://www.emea.europa.eu/.

Rapamune

(Wyeth Pharmaceuticals)

1. NAME OF THE MEDICINAL PRODUCT

Rapamune®▼ 1 mg coated tablets

Rapamune®▼ 2 mg coated tablets

Rapamune®▼ 1 mg/ml oral solution

2. QUALITATIVE AND QUANTITATIVE COMPOSITION

Each 1mg tablet contains 1 mg sirolimus.

Each 2mg tablet contains 2 mg sirolimus.

Each ml contains 1 mg sirolimus.

Excipients:

For a full list of excipients, see section 6.1

3. PHARMACEUTICAL FORM

1mg: White coloured, triangular-shaped coated tablet marked "RAPAMUNE 1 mg" on one side.

2mg: Yellow to beige coloured, triangular-shaped coated tablet marked "RAPAMUNE 2 mg" on one side.

or

Oral solution.

4. CLINICAL PARTICULARS

4.1 Therapeutic indications

Rapamune is indicated for the prophylaxis of organ rejection in adult patients at low to moderate immunological risk receiving a renal transplant. It is recommended that Rapamune be used initially in combination with ciclosporin microemulsion and corticosteroids for 2 to 3 months. Rapamune may be continued as maintenance therapy with corticosteroids only if ciclosporin microemulsion can be progressively discontinued (see sections 4.2 and 5.1).

4.2 Posology and method of administration

Rapamune is for oral use only.

Bioavailability has not been determined for tablets after they have been crushed, chewed or split and therefore this cannot be recommended.

Treatment should be initiated by and remain under the guidance of an appropriately qualified specialist in transplantation.

Use in adults

Initial therapy (2 to 3 months post-transplantation): The usual dosage regimen for Rapamune is a 6 mg oral loading dose, administered as soon as possible after transplantation, followed by 2 mg once daily. The Rapamune dose should then be individualised, to obtain whole blood trough levels of 4 to 12 ng/ml (chromatographic assay; see *Therapeutic drug monitoring*). Rapamune therapy should be optimised with a tapering regimen of steroids and ciclosporin microemulsion. Suggested ciclosporin trough concentration ranges for the first 2-3 months after transplantation are 150-400 ng/ml (monoclonal assay or equivalent technique).

Maintenance Therapy: Ciclosporin should be progressively discontinued over 4 to 8 weeks and the Rapamune dose should be adjusted to obtain whole blood trough levels of 12 to 20 ng/ml (chromatographic assay; see *Therapeutic drug monitoring*). Rapamune should be given with corticosteroids. In patients for whom ciclosporin withdrawal is either unsuccessful or cannot be attempted, the combination of ciclosporin and Rapamune should not be maintained for more than 3 months post-transplantation. In such patients, when clinically appropriate, Rapamune should be discontinued and an alternative immunosuppressive regimen instituted.

Use in black recipients: There is limited information indicating that black renal transplant recipients (predominantly African-American) require higher doses and trough levels of sirolimus to achieve the same efficacy as observed in non-black patients. Currently, the efficacy and safety data are too limited to allow specific recommendations for use of sirolimus in black recipients.

Use in children and adolescents($<$18 years): The available data on safety and efficacy are not sufficient to recommend the use of Rapamune in children and adolescents less than 18 years of age (see sections 4.8 and 5.1). Limited pharmacokinetic information is available in children and adolescents (see section 5.2).

Use in elderly patients ($>$ 65 years): Clinical studies of Rapamune did not include a sufficient number of patients $>$65 years of age to determine whether they will respond differently than younger patients. Sirolimus trough concentration data in 35 renal transplant patients $>$65 years of age were similar to those in the adult population (n=822) from 18 to 65 years of age.

Use in patients with renal impairment: No dosage adjustment is required (see section 5.2).

Use in patients with hepatic impairment: The clearance of sirolimus may be reduced in patients with impaired hepatic function (see section 5.2). In patients with severe hepatic impairment, it is recommended that the maintenance dose of Rapamune be reduced by approximately one half.

It is recommended that sirolimus whole blood trough levels be closely monitored in patients with impaired hepatic function (see *Therapeutic drug monitoring*). It is not necessary to modify the Rapamune loading dose.

Therapeutic drug monitoring: Most patients who received 2 mg of Rapamune 4 hours after ciclosporin had whole blood trough concentrations of sirolimus within the 4 to 12 ng/ml target range (expressed as chromatographic assay values). Optimal therapy requires therapeutic drug concentration monitoring in all patients. Whole blood sirolimus levels should be closely monitored in the following populations: (1) in patients with hepatic impairment; (2) when inducers or inhibitors of CYP3A4 are concurrently administered and after their discontinuation (see section 4.5); and/or (3) if ciclosporin dosing is markedly reduced or discontinued, as these populations are most likely to have special dosing requirements.

Therapeutic drug monitoring should not be the sole basis for adjusting sirolimus therapy. Careful attention should be made to clinical signs/symptoms, tissue biopsies, and laboratory parameters.

To minimise variability, Rapamune should be taken at the same time in relation to ciclosporin, 4 hours after the ciclosporin dose, and consistently either with or without food (see section 5.2). Optimally, adjustments in Rapamune dosage should be based on more than a single trough level obtained $>$5 days after a previous dosing change.

Following the discontinuation of ciclosporin therapy, a target trough range of 12 to 20 ng/ml (chromatographic assay) is recommended. Ciclosporin inhibits the metabolism of sirolimus, and consequently, sirolimus levels will decrease when ciclosporin is discontinued unless the sirolimus dose is increased. On average, the sirolimus dose will need to be 4-fold higher to account for both the absence of the pharmacokinetic interaction (2-fold increase) and the augmented immunosuppressive requirement in the absence of ciclosporin (2-fold increase). The rate at which the dose of sirolimus is increased should correspond to the rate of ciclosporin elimination.

If further dose adjustment(s) are required during maintenance therapy (after discontinuation of ciclosporin), in most patients these adjustments can be based on simple proportion: new Rapamune dose = current dose × (target concentration/current concentration). A loading dose should be considered in addition to a new maintenance dose when it is necessary to considerably increase sirolimus trough concentrations: Rapamune loading dose = 3 × (new maintenance dose − current maintenance dose). The maximum Rapamune dose administered on any day should not exceed 40 mg. If an estimated daily dose exceeds 40 mg due to the addition of a loading dose, the loading dose should be administered over 2 days. Sirolimus trough concentrations should be monitored at least 3 to 4 days after a loading dose(s).

In patients with severe hepatic impairment, monitoring should be performed every 5 to 7 days until 3 consecutive trough levels have shown stable concentrations of sirolimus after dose adjustment or after loading dose due to the delay in reaching steady state because of the prolonged half-life.

The recommended 24-hour trough concentration ranges for sirolimus are based on chromatographic methods. Several assay methodologies have been used to measure the whole blood concentrations of sirolimus. Currently in clinical practice, sirolimus whole blood concentration are being measured by both chromatographic and immunoassay methodologies. The concentration values obtained by these different methodologies are not interchangeable. When using a proprietary immunoassay system, always refer to the manufacturer's information to correlate values to a reference chromatographic assay. All sirolimus concentrations reported in this Summary of Product Characteristics were either measured using chromatographic methods or have been converted to chromatographic method equivalents. Adjustments to the targeted range should be made according to the assay being utilised to determine the sirolimus trough concentrations.

Other considerations for use: Ciclosporin (microemulsion) and other medicinal or non-medicinal products may interact with sirolimus (see section 4.5).

4.3 Contraindications

Hypersensitivity to the active substance or to any of the excipients.

4.4 Special warnings and precautions for use

Rapamune has not been adequately studied in patients at high immunological risk (see section 5.1).

Concomitant use with other immunosuppressive agents

Sirolimus has been administered concurrently with the following agents in clinical studies: ciclosporin, azathioprine, mycophenolate mofetil, corticosteroids and cytotoxic antibodies. Sirolimus in combination with other immunosuppressive agents has not been extensively investigated.

Based on information from subsequent clinical trials, the use of Rapamune, mycophenolate mofetil, and corticosteroids, in combination with IL-2 receptor antibody (IL2R Ab) induction, is not recommended in the *de novo* renal transplant setting (see section 5.1).

Immunosuppressants may affect response to vaccination. During treatment with immunosuppressants, including Rapamune, vaccination may be less effective. The use of live vaccines should be avoided during treatment with Rapamune.

In hepatically impaired patients, it is recommended that sirolimus whole blood trough levels be closely monitored. In patients with severe hepatic impairment, reduction in maintenance dose by one half is recommended based on decreased clearance (see sections 4.2 and 5.2). Since half-life is prolonged in these patients, therapeutic drug monitoring after a loading dose or a change of dose should be performed for a prolonged period of time until stable concentrations are reached (see sections 4.2 and 5.2).

Co-administration of sirolimus with strong inhibitors of CYP3A4 (such as ketoconazole, voriconazole, itraconazole, telithromycin or clarithromycin) or inducers of CYP3A4 (such as rifampin, rifabutin) is not recommended (see section 4.5).

Increased susceptibility to infection and the possible development of lymphoma and other malignancies, particularly of the skin, may result from immunosuppression (see section 4.8). Oversuppression of the immune system can also increase susceptibility to infection including opportunistic infections, fatal infections, and sepsis.

Patients treated with immunosuppressants, including Rapamune, are at increased risk for opportunistic infections (bacterial, fungal, viral and protozoal). Among these conditions are BK virus associated nephropathy and JC virus associated progressive multifocal leukoencephalopathy (PML). These infections are often related to a high total immunosuppressive burden and may lead to serious or fatal conditions that physicians should consider in the differential diagnosis in immunosuppressed patients with deteriorating renal function or neurological symptoms.

The safety and efficacy of Rapamune as immunosuppressive therapy have not been established in liver or lung transplant patients, and therefore, such use is not recommended.

In two clinical studies in de novo liver transplant patients the use of sirolimus plus ciclosporin or tacrolimus was associated with an increase in hepatic artery thrombosis, mostly leading to graft loss or death.

A clinical study in liver transplant patients randomised to conversion from a CNI-based regimen to a sirolimus-based regimen versus continuation of a CNI-based regimen 6-144 months post-liver transplantation failed to demonstrate superiority in baseline-adjusted GFR at 12 months (-4.45 mL/min and -3.07 mL/min, respectively). The study also failed to demonstrate non-inferiority of the rate of combined graft loss, missing survival data, or death for the sirolimus conversion group compared to the CNI continuation group. The rate of death in the sirolimus conversion group was higher than the CNI continuation group, although the rates were not significantly different. The rates of premature study discontinuation, adverse events overall (and infections, specifically), and biopsy-proven acute liver graft rejection at 12 months were all significantly greater in the sirolimus conversion group compared to the CNI continuation group.

There have been reports of impaired or delayed wound healing in patients receiving Rapamune, including lymphocele and wound dehiscence. Patients with a BMI greater than 30 kg/m^2 may be at increased risk of abnormal wound healing based on data from the medical literature.

There have also been reports of fluid accumulation, including peripheral oedema, lymphoedema, pleural effusion, and pericardial effusions (including haemodynamically significant effusions in children and adults), in patients receiving Rapamune.

Cases of bronchial anastomotic dehiscence, most fatal, have been reported in de novo lung transplant patients when sirolimus has been used as part of an immunosuppressive regimen.

Hypersensitivity reactions, including anaphylactic/anaphylactoid reactions, angioedema, exfoliative dermatitis, and hypersensitivity vasculitis, have been associated with the administration of sirolimus (see section 4.8).

In rare cases, the concomitant administration of sirolimus and ACE inhibitors has resulted in angioneurotic oedema-type reactions.

As usual for patients with increased risk for skin cancer, exposure to sunlight and UV light should be limited by wearing protective clothing and using a sunscreen with a high protection factor.

Cases of *Pneumocystis carinii* pneumonia have been reported in patients not receiving antimicrobial prophylaxis. Therefore, antimicrobial prophylaxis for *Pneumocystis carinii* pneumonia should be administered for the first 12 months following transplantation.

Cytomegalovirus (CMV) prophylaxis is recommended for 3 months after transplantation, particularly for patients at increased risk for CMV disease.

The use of Rapamune in renal transplant patients was associated with increased serum cholesterol and triglycerides that may require treatment. Patients administered Rapamune should be monitored for hyperlipidemia using laboratory tests and if hyperlipidemia is detected, subsequent interventions such as diet, exercise, and lipid-lowering agents should be initiated. The risk/benefit should be considered in patients with established hyperlipidemia before initiating an immunosuppressive regimen including Rapamune. Similarly the risk/benefit of continued Rapamune therapy should be re-evaluated in patients with severe refractory hyperlipidemia.

In clinical trials, the concomitant administration of Rapamune and HMG-CoA reductase inhibitors and/or fibrates was well tolerated. During Rapamune therapy, patients administered an HMG-CoA reductase inhibitor and/or fibrate, should be monitored for the possible development of rhabdomyolysis and other adverse effects as described in the respective Summary of Product Characteristics of these agents.

Renal function should be monitored during concomitant administration of Rapamune and ciclosporin. Appropriate adjustment of the immunosuppression regimen should be considered in patients with elevated serum creatinine levels. Caution should be exercised when co-administering other agents that are known to have a deleterious effect on renal function.

Patients treated with ciclosporin and Rapamune beyond 3 months had higher serum creatinine levels and lower calculated glomerular filtration rates compared to patients treated with ciclosporin and placebo or azathioprine controls. Patients who were successfully withdrawn from ciclosporin had lower serum creatinine levels and higher calculated glomerular filtration rates, as well as lower incidence of malignancy, compared to patients remaining on ciclosporin. The continued co-administration of ciclosporin and Rapamune as maintenance therapy cannot be recommended.

In patients with delayed graft function, sirolimus may delay recovery of renal function.

Periodic quantitative monitoring of urinary protein excretion is recommended. In a study evaluating conversion from calcineurin inhibitors to Rapamune in maintenance renal transplant patients, increased urinary protein excretion was commonly observed at 6 to 24 months after conversion to Rapamune (see section 5.1). New onset nephrosis (nephrotic syndrome) was also reported in 2% of the patients in the study (see section 4.8). The safety and efficacy of conversion from calcineurin inhibitors to Rapamune in maintenance renal transplant patients have not been established.

The concomitant use of Rapamune with a calcineurin inhibitor may increase the risk of calcineurin inhibitor-induced haemolytic uraemic syndrome/thrombotic thrombocytopenic purpura/thrombotic microangiopathy (HUS/TTP/TMA).

Sirolimus tablets contain sucrose and lactose. In those patients with a history of sucrase insufficiency, isomaltase insufficiency, fructose intolerance, glucose malabsorption, galactose intolerance (e.g. galactosemia), or Lapp lactase deficiency, a careful risk/benefit assessment should be performed prior to prescribing sirolimus tablets.

4.5 Interaction with other medicinal products and other forms of interaction

Sirolimus is extensively metabolised by the CYP3A4 isozyme in the intestinal wall and liver. Sirolimus is also a substrate for the multidrug efflux pump, P-glycoprotein (P-gp) located in the small intestine. Therefore, absorption and the subsequent elimination of sirolimus may be influenced by substances that affect these proteins. Inhibitors of CYP3A4 (such as ketoconazole, voriconazole, itraconazole, telithromycin, or clarithromycin) decrease the metabolism of sirolimus and increase sirolimus levels. Inducers of CYP3A4 (such as rifampin or rifabutin) increase the metabolism of sirolimus and decrease sirolimus levels. Co-administration of sirolimus with strong inhibitors of CYP3A4 or inducers of CYP3A4 is not recommended (see section 4.4).

Ciclosporin (CYP3A4 substrate): The rate and extent of sirolimus absorption was significantly increased by ciclosporin A (CsA). Sirolimus administered concomitantly (5 mg), and at 2h (5 mg) and 4h (10 mg) after CsA (300 mg) resulted in increased sirolimus AUC by approximately 183%, 141% and 80% respectively. The effect of CsA was also reflected by increases in sirolimus C_{max} and t_{max}. When given 2 hours before CsA administration, sirolimus C_{max} and AUC were not affected. Single-dose sirolimus did not affect the pharmacokinetics of ciclosporin (microemulsion) in healthy volunteers when administered simultaneously or 4 hours apart. It is recommended that Rapamune be administered 4 hours after ciclosporin (microemulsion).

Rifampicin (CYP3A4 inducer): Administration of multiple doses of rifampicin decreased sirolimus whole blood concentrations following a single 10 mg dose of Rapamune oral solution. Rifampicin increased the clearance of sirolimus by approximately 5.5-fold and decreased AUC and C_{max} by approximately 82% and 71%, respectively. Co-administration of sirolimus and rifampicin is not recommended (see section 4.4).

Ketoconazole (CYP3A4 inhibitor): Multiple-dose ketoconazole administration significantly affected the rate and extent of absorption and sirolimus exposure as reflected by increases in sirolimus C_{max}, t_{max}, and AUC of 4.4-fold, 1.4-fold, and 10.9-fold, respectively. Co-administration of sirolimus and ketoconazole is not recommended (see section 4.4).

Voriconazole (CYP3A4 inhibitor): Co-administration of sirolimus (2 mg single dose) with multiple-dose administration of oral voriconazole (400 mg every 12 hours for 1 day, then 100 mg every 12 hours for 8 days) in healthy subjects has been reported to increase sirolimus C_{max} and AUC by an average of 7-fold and 11-fold respectively. Co-administration of sirolimus and voriconazole is not recommended (see section 4.4).

Diltiazem (CYP3A4 inhibitor): The simultaneous oral administration of 10 mg of Rapamune oral solution and 120 mg of diltiazem significantly affected the bioavailability of sirolimus. Sirolimus C_{max}, t_{max}, and AUC were increased 1.4-fold, 1.3-fold, and 1.6-fold, respectively. Sirolimus did not affect the pharmacokinetics of either diltiazem or its metabolites desacetyldiltiazem and desmethyldiltiazem. If diltiazem is administered, sirolimus blood levels should be monitored and a dose adjustment may be necessary.

Verapamil (CYP3A4 inhibitor): Multiple-dose administration of verapamil and sirolimus oral solution significantly affected the rate and extent of absorption of both drugs. Whole blood sirolimus C_{max}, t_{max}, and AUC were increased 2.3-fold, 1.1-fold, and 2.2-fold, respectively. Plasma S-(-) verapamil C_{max} and AUC were both increased 1.5-fold, and t_{max} was decreased 24%. Sirolimus levels should be monitored and appropriate dose reductions of both medications should be considered.

Erythromycin (CYP3A4 inhibitor): Multiple-dose administration of erythromycin and sirolimus oral solution significantly increased the rate and extent of absorption of both drugs. Whole blood sirolimus C_{max}, t_{max}, and AUC were increased 4.4-fold, 1.4-fold, and 4.2-fold, respectively. The C_{max}, t_{max}, and AUC of plasma erythromycin base were increased 1.6-fold, 1.3-fold, and 1.7-fold, respectively. Sirolimus levels should be monitored and appropriate dose reductions of both medications should be considered.

Oral contraceptives: No clinically significant pharmacokinetic interaction was observed between sirolimus and 0.3 mg norgestrel/ 0.03 mg ethinyl estradiol. Although the results of a single dose drug interaction study with an oral contraceptive suggest the lack of a pharmacokinetic interaction, the results cannot exclude the possibility of changes in the pharmacokinetics that might affect the efficacy of the oral contraceptive during long term treatment with Rapamune.

Other possible interactions

Moderate and weak inhibitors of CYP3A4 may decrease the metabolism of sirolimus and increase sirolimus blood levels (e.g. **calcium channel blockers:** nicardipine; **antifungal agents**: clotrimazole, fluconazole; **antibiotics:** troleandomycin; **other substances:** bromocriptine, cimetidine, danazol, **protease inhibitors**).

Inducers of CYP3A4 may increase the metabolism of sirolimus and decrease sirolimus blood levels (e.g. St. John's wort (*Hypericum perforatum*), **anticonvulsants:** carbamazepine, phenobarbital, phenytoin).

Although sirolimus inhibits human liver microsomal cytochrome P_{450} CYP2C9, CYP2C19, CYP2D6, and CYP3A4/5 *in vitro*, the active substance is not expected to inhibit the activity of these isozymes *in vivo* since the sirolimus concentrations necessary to produce inhibition are much higher than those observed in patients receiving therapeutic doses of Rapamune. Inhibitors of P-gp may decrease the efflux of sirolimus from intestinal cells and increase sirolimus levels.

Grapefruit juice affects CYP3A4 mediated metabolism and should therefore be avoided.

Pharmacokinetic interactions may be observed with gastrointestinal prokinetic agents such as cisapride and metoclopramide.

No clinically significant pharmacokinetic interaction was observed between sirolimus and any of the following substances: acyclovir, atorvastatin, digoxin, glibenclamide, methylprednisolone, nifedipine, prednisolone, and trimethoprim/sulphamethoxazole.

4.6 Pregnancy and lactation

There are no adequate data from the use of sirolimus in pregnant women. Studies in animals have shown reproductive toxicity (see section 5.3). The potential risk for humans is unknown. Rapamune should not be used during pregnancy unless clearly necessary. Effective contraception must be used during Rapamune therapy and for 12 weeks after Rapamune has been stopped.

Following administration of radiolabelled sirolimus, radioactivity is excreted in the milk of lactating rats. It is not known whether sirolimus is excreted in human milk. Because of the potential for adverse reactions in nursing infants from sirolimus, nursing should be discontinued during therapy.

Impairments of sperm parameters have been observed among some patients treated with Rapamune. These effects have been reversible upon discontinuation of Rapamune in most cases (see section 5.3).

4.7 Effects on ability to drive and use machines

No studies on the effects on the ability to drive and use machines have been performed.

4.8 Undesirable effects

The most commonly reported adverse drug reactions (occurring in >10% of patients) are thrombocytopenia, anaemia, pyrexia, hypertension, hypokalaemia, hypophosphataemia, urinary tract infection, hypercholesterolaemia, hyperglycaemia, hypertriglyceridaemia, abdominal pain, lymphocoele, peripheral oedema, arthralgia, acne, diarrhoea, pain, constipation, nausea, headache, increased blood creatinine, and increased blood lactate dehydrogenase (LDH).

The incidence of any adverse event(s) may increase as the trough sirolimus level increases.

Adverse reactions based on experience from clinical trials and postmarketing experience are presented in the following table by system organ class and frequency of occurrence. Within each frequency grouping, undesirable effects are presented in order of decreasing seriousness. Only events for which there is at least reasonable suspicion of a causal relationship to Rapamune treatment are listed.

Most patients were on immunosuppressive regimens which included Rapamune in combination with other immunosuppressive agents.

(see Table 1 on next page)

Immunosuppression increases the susceptibility to the development of lymphoma and other malignancies, particularly of the skin (see section 4.4).

Cases of BK virus associated nephropathy, as well as cases of JC virus associated progressive multifocal leukoencephalopathy (PML), have been reported in patients treated with immunosuppressants, including Rapamune.

Hepatotoxicity has been reported, the risk may increase as the trough sirolimus level increases. There have been rare reports of fatal hepatic necrosis with elevated trough sirolimus levels.

Cases of interstitial lung disease (including pneumonitis and infrequently bronchiolitis obliterans organising pneumonia (BOOP) and pulmonary fibrosis), some fatal, with no identified infectious etiology have occurred in patients receiving immunosuppressive regimens including

Table 1

System Organ Class	Very common (≥ 1/10)	Common (≥ 1/100 to < 1/10)	Uncommon (≥ 1/1000 to < 1/100)	Rare (≥ 1/10000 to < 1/1000)
Infections and infestations	Urinary tract infection	Sepsis Pneumonia Pyelonephritis Herpes simplex Fungal, viral, and bacterial infections (such as mycobacterial infections, including tuberculosis, Epstein-Barr virus, CMV, and Herpes zoster)		
Neoplasms benign, malignant and unspecified (including cysts and polyps)		Skin Cancer	Lymphoma / post transplant lymphoproliferative disorder	
Blood and lymphatic system disorders	Thrombocytopenia Anaemia	Thrombotic thrombocytopenic purpura/haemolytic uraemic syndrome Leukopenia Neutropenia	Pancytopenia	
Immune system disorders				Hypersensitivity reactions, including anaphylactic/ anaphylactoid reactions, angioedema, exfoliative dermatitis, and hypersensitivity vasculitis (see section 4.4)
Metabolism and nutrition disorders	Hypokalaemia Hypophosphataemia Hypercholesterolaemia Hyperglycaemia Hypertriglyceridaemia			
Nervous system disorders	Headache			
Cardiac disorders		Tachycardia	Pericardial effusion (including haemodynamically significant effusions in children and adults)	
Vascular disorders	Lymphocele Hypertension	Deep vein thrombosis	Pulmonary embolism	Lymphoedema
Respiratory, thoracic, and mediastinal disorders		Pneumonitis Pleural effusion Epistaxis	Pulmonary haemorrhage	Alveolar proteinosis
Gastrointestinal disorders	Abdominal pain Diarrhoea Constipation Nausea	Stomatitis	Pancreatitis	
Hepatobiliary disorders		Liver function tests abnormal		
Skin and subcutaneous tissue disorders	Acne	Rash		
Musculoskeletal and connective tissue disorders	Arthralgia	Osteonecrosis		
Renal and urinary disorders		Proteinuria	Nephrotic syndrome (see section 4.4)	
General disorders and administration site conditions	Oedema peripheral Pyrexia Pain	Impaired healing Oedema		
Investigations	Blood lactate dehydrogenase increased Blood creatinine increased	Aspartate aminotransferase increased Alanine aminotransferase increased		

Rapamune. In some cases, the interstitial lung disease has resolved upon discontinuation or dose reduction of Rapamune. The risk may be increased as the trough sirolimus level increases.

Impaired healing following transplant surgery has been reported, including fascial dehiscence, incisional hernia, and anastomotic disruption (e.g. wound, vascular, airway, ureteral, biliary).

Impairments of sperm parameters have been observed among some patients treated with Rapamune. These effects have been reversible upon discontinuation of Rapamune in most cases (see section 5.3).

In patients with delayed graft function, sirolimus may delay recovery of renal function.

The concomitant use of sirolimus with a calcineurin inhibitor may increase the risk of calcineurin inhibitor-induced HUS/TTP/TMA.

Focal segmental glomerulosclerosis has been reported.

In an ongoing study evaluating the safety and efficacy of conversion from calcineurin inhibitors to sirolimus (target levels of 12 - 20 ng/mL) in maintenance renal transplant patients, enrollment was stopped in the subset of patients (n=90) with a baseline glomerular filtration rate of less than 40 mL/min. There was a higher rate of serious adverse events including pneumonia, acute rejection, graft loss and death in this sirolimus treatment arm (n=60, median time post-transplant 36 months).

Paediatric population

Controlled clinical trials with posology comparable to that currently indicated for the use of Rapamune in adults—that is, use in combination with ciclosporin and corticosteroids for 2 to 3 months post-transplantation followed by withdrawal of ciclosporin thereafter—have not been conducted in children or adolescents (< 18 years of age).

Safety was assessed in a controlled clinical trial enrolling renal transplant patients < 18 years of age considered of high-immunologic risk, defined as a history of one or more acute allograft rejection episodes and/or the presence of chronic allograft nephropathy on a renal biopsy (see section 5.1). The use of Rapamune in combination with calcineurin inhibitors and corticosteroids was associated with an increased risk of deterioration of renal function, serum lipid abnormalities (including but not limited to increased serum triglycerides and cholesterol), and urinary tract infections. The treatment regimen studied (continuous use of Rapamune in combination with calcineurin inhibitor) is not indicated for adult or paediatric patients (see section 4.1).

In another study enrolling renal transplant patients ≤20 years of age that was intended to assess the safety of progressive corticosteroid withdrawal (beginning at six months post-transplantation) from an immunosuppressive regimen initiated at transplantation that included full-dose immunosuppression with both Rapamune and a calcineurin inhibitor in combination with basiliximab induction, of the 274 patients enrolled, 19 (6.9%) were reported to have developed post-transplant lymphoproliferative disorder (PTLD). Among 89 patients known to be EBV seronegative prior to transplantation, 13 (15.6%) were reported to have developed PTLD. All patients who developed PTLD were aged < 18 years.

There is insufficient experience to recommend the use of Rapamune in children and adolescents (see section 4.2).

4.9 Overdose

At present, there is minimal experience with overdose. One patient experienced an episode of atrial fibrillation after ingestion of 150 mg of Rapamune. In general, the adverse effects of overdose are consistent with those listed in Section 4.8. General supportive measures should be initiated in all cases of overdose. Based on the poor aqueous solubility and high erythrocyte and plasma protein binding of Rapamune, it is anticipated that Rapamune will not be dialysable to any significant extent.

5. PHARMACOLOGICAL PROPERTIES

5.1 Pharmacodynamic properties

Pharmacotherapeutic group: selective immunosuppressant agents. ATC code: L04A A10.

Sirolimus inhibits T cell activation induced by most stimuli, by blocking calcium dependent and calcium independent intracellular signal transduction. Studies demonstrated that its effects are mediated by a mechanism that is different from that of ciclosporin, tacrolimus, and other immunosuppressive agents. Experimental evidence suggests that sirolimus binds to the specific cytosolic protein FKPB-12 and that the FKPB 12-sirolimus complex inhibits the activation of the mammalian Target Of Rapamycin (mTOR), a critical kinase for cell cycle progression. The inhibition of mTOR results in blockage of several specific signal transduction pathways. The net result is the inhibition of lymphocyte activation, which results in immunosuppression.

In animals, sirolimus has a direct effect on T and B cell activation suppressing immune mediated reactions such as allograft rejection.

<u>*Clinical Trials*</u>

Patients at low to moderate immunological risk were studied in the phase 3 ciclosporin elimination Rapamune maintenance trials which included patients receiving a renal allograft from a cadaveric or living donor. In addition, re-transplant recipients whose previous grafts survived for at least 6 months after transplantation were included. Ciclosporin was not withdrawn in patients experiencing Banff Grade 3 acute rejection episodes, who were dialysis-dependent, who had a serum creatinine > 400 µmol/l, or who had inadequate renal function to support ciclosporin withdrawal. Patients at high immunological risk of graft loss were not studied in sufficient number in the ciclosporin elimination Rapamune maintenance trials and are not recommended for this treatment regimen.

At 12, 24 and 36 months, graft and patient survival were similar for both groups. At 48 months, there was a statistically significant difference in graft survival in favour of the Rapamune following ciclosporin elimination group compared to the Rapamune with ciclosporin therapy group (including and excluding loss to follow-up). There was a significantly higher rate of first biopsy-proven rejection in the ciclosporin elimination group compared to the ciclosporin maintenance group during the period post-randomisation to 12 months (9.8% vs. 4.2%, respectively). Thereafter, the difference between the two groups was not significant.

The mean calculated glomerular filtration rate (GFR) at 12, 24, 36, 48 and 60 months was significantly higher for patients receiving Rapamune following ciclosporin elimination than for those in the Rapamune with ciclosporin therapy group. Based upon the analysis of data from 36 months and beyond, which showed a growing difference in graft survival and renal function, as well as significantly lower blood pressure in the ciclosporin elimination group, it was decided to discontinue subjects from the Rapamune with ciclosporin group. By 60 months, the incidence of non-skin malignancies was significantly higher in the cohort who continued ciclosporin as compared with the cohort who had ciclosporin withdrawn (8.4% vs. 3.8%, respectively). For skin carcinoma, the median time to first occurrence was significantly delayed.

The safety and efficacy of conversion from calcineurin inhibitors to Rapamune in maintenance renal transplant patients (6-120 months after transplantation) was assessed in a randomised, multicentre, controlled trial, stratified by calculated GFR at baseline (20-40 mL/min vs >40 mL/min). Concomitant immunosuppressive agents included mycophenolate mofetil, azathioprine, and corticosteroids. Enrollment in the patient stratum with baseline calculated GFR <40 mL/min was discontinued due to an imbalance in safety events (see section 4.8).

In the patient stratum with baseline calculated GFR>40 mL/min, renal function was not improved overall. The rates of acute rejection, graft loss, and death were similar at 1 and 2 years. Treatment emergent adverse events occurred more frequently during the first 6 months after Rapamune conversion. In the stratum with baseline calculated GFR>40 mL/min, the mean and median urinary protein to creatinine ratios were significantly higher in the Rapamune conversion group as compared to those of the calcineurin inhibitors continuation group at 24 months (see section 4.4). New onset nephrosis (nephrotic syndrome) was also reported (see section 4.8).

At 2 years, the rate of non-melanoma skin malignancies was significantly lower in the Rapamune conversion group as compared to the calcineurin inhibitors continuation group (1.8% and 6.9%). In a subset of the study patients with a baseline GFR>40 mL/min and normal urinary protein excretion, calculated GFR was higher at 1 and 2 years in patients converted to Rapamune than for the corresponding subset of calcineurin inhibitor continuation patients. The rates of acute rejection, graft loss, and death were similar, but urinary protein excretion was increased in the Rapamune treatment arm of this subset.

In two multi-centre clinical studies, de novo renal transplant patients treated with Rapamune, mycophenolate mofetil (MMF), corticosteroids, and an IL-2 receptor antagonist had significantly higher acute rejection rates and numerically higher death rates compared to patients treated with a calcineurin inhibitor, MMF, corticosteroids, and an IL-2 receptor antagonist (see section 4.4). Renal function was not better in the treatment arms with de novo Rapamune without a calcineurin inhibitor. An abbreviated dosing schedule of daclizumab was used in one of the studies.

Rapamune was assessed in a 36-month controlled clinical trial enrolling renal transplant patients <18 years of age considered at high-immunologic risk, defined as having a history of one or more acute allograft rejection episodes and/or the presence of chronic allograft nephropathy on a renal biopsy. Subjects were to receive Rapamune (sirolimus target concentrations of 5 to 15 ng/mL) in combination with a calcineurin inhibitor and corticosteroids or to receive calcineurin-inhibitor-based immunosuppression without Rapamune. The Rapamune group failed to demonstrate superiority to the control group in terms of the first occurrence of biopsy confirmed acute rejection, graft loss, or death. One death occurred in each group. The use of Rapamune in combination with calcineurin inhibitors and corticosteroids was associated with an increased risk of deterioration of renal function, serum lipid abnormalities (including but not limited to increased serum triglycerides and total cholesterol), and urinary tract infections (see section 4.8).

An unacceptably high frequency of PTLD was seen in a paediatric clinical transplant study when full dose Rapamune was administered to children and adolescents in addition to full dose calcineurin inhibitors with basiliximab and corticosteroids (see section 4.8).

5.2 Pharmacokinetic properties

Much of the general pharmacokinetic information was obtained using the oral solution, which is summarised first. Information directly related to the tablet formulation is summarised specifically in the *Oral Tablet* section.

Oral solution

Following administration of the oral solution, sirolimus is rapidly absorbed, with a time to peak concentration of 1 hour in healthy subjects receiving single doses and 2 hours in patients with stable renal allografts receiving multiple doses. The systemic availability of sirolimus in combination with simultaneously administered ciclosporin (Sandimune) is approximately 14%. Upon repeated administration, the average blood concentration of sirolimus is increased approximately 3-fold. The terminal half-life in stable renal transplant patients after multiple oral doses was 62±16h. The effective half-life, however, is shorter and mean steady-state concentrations were achieved after 5 to 7 days. The blood to plasma ratio (B/P) of 36 indicates that sirolimus is extensively partitioned into formed blood elements.

Pharmacokinetic parameters for sirolimus obtained from 19 renal transplant patients receiving microemulsion ciclosporin (4 hours prior to Rapamune) and corticosteroids, following daily doses of 2 mg Rapamune solution in a phase III clinical trial, were; $C_{max,ss}$ 12.2±6.2 ng/ml, $t_{max,ss}$ 3.01±2.40h, $AUC_{\tau,ss}$ 158±70 ng·h/ml, CL/F/W 182±72 ml/h/kg (parameters calculated from LC-MS/MS assay results). There was no significant difference in any of these parameters over time up to 6 months after transplantation. Mean sirolimus whole blood trough levels from the same phase III trial were 7.2 ng/ml (4.0 to 11 ng/ml, expressed as chromatographic assay values; n=226) for the 2 mg per day dose and 14 ng/ml (8.0 to 22 ng/ml, expressed as chromatographic assay values; n=219) for the 5 mg per day dose (see section 4.2).

Sirolimus is a substrate for both cytochrome P450 IIIA4 (CYP3A4) and P-glycoprotein. Sirolimus is extensively metabolised by O-demethylation and/or hydroxylation. Seven major metabolites, including hydroxyl, demethyl, and hydroxydemethyl, are identifiable in whole blood. Sirolimus is the major component in human whole blood and contributes to greater than 90% of the immunosuppressive activity. After a single dose of [^{14}C] sirolimus in healthy volunteers, the majority (91.1%) of radioactivity was recovered from the faeces, and only a minor amount (2.2%) was excreted in urine.

Clinical studies of Rapamune did not include a sufficient number of patients >65 years of age to determine whether they will respond differently than younger patients. Sirolimus trough concentration data in 35 renal transplant patients >65 years of age were similar to those in the adult population (n=822) from 18 to 65 years of age.

In healthy volunteers, a high fat meal altered the bioavailability characteristics of oral liquid sirolimus. There was a 34% decrease in the peak blood sirolimus concentration (C_{max}), a 3.5-fold increase in the time to peak concentration (t_{max}), and a 35% increase in total exposure (AUC). It is recommended that Rapamune be taken consistently either with or without food. The use of orange juice and water to dilute Rapamune were equivalent with respect to C_{max}, and AUC. Grapefruit juice affects CYP3A4 mediated metabolism and must therefore be avoided.

In paediatric patients on dialysis (30% to 50% reduction in glomerular filtration rate) within age ranges of 5 to 11 years and 12 to 18 years, the mean weight-normalised CL/F was larger for younger paediatric patients (580 ml/h/kg) than for older paediatric patients (450 ml/h/kg) as compared with adults (287 ml/h/kg). There was a large variability for individuals within the age groups.

Sirolimus concentrations were measured in concentration-controlled trials of paediatric renal-transplant patients who were also receiving ciclosporin and corticosteroids. The target for trough concentrations was 10-20 ng/mL. At steady state, 8 children aged 6-11 years received mean ± SD doses of 1.75 ± 0.71 mg/day (0.064 ± 0.018 mg/kg, 1.65 ± 0.43 mg/m^2) while 14 adolescents aged 12-18 years received mean ± SD doses of 2.79 ± 1.25 mg/day (0.053 ± 0.0150 mg/kg, 1.86 ± 0.61 mg/m^2). The younger children had a higher weight-normalized Cl/F (214 mL/h/kg) compared with the adolescents (136 mL/h/kg). These data indicate that younger children might require higher body-weight-adjusted doses than adolescents and adults to achieve similar target concentrations. However, the development of such special dosing recommendations for children requires more data to be definitely confirmed.

In mild and moderate hepatically impaired patients (Child-Pugh classification A or B), mean values for sirolimus AUC and $t_{1/2}$ were increased 61% and 43%, respectively, and CL/F was decreased 33% compared to normal healthy subjects. In severe hepatically impaired patients (Child-Pugh classification C), mean values for sirolimus AUC and $t_{1/2}$ were increased 210% and 170% respectively, and CL/F was decreased by 67% compared to normal healthy subjects. The longer half-lives observed in hepatically impaired patients delay reaching steady state.

The pharmacokinetics of sirolimus were similar in various populations with renal function ranging from normal to absent (dialysis patients).

Oral Tablet

In healthy subjects, the mean extent of bioavailability of sirolimus after single-dose administration of the tablet formulation is about 27% higher relative to the oral solution. The mean C_{max} was decreased by 35% and mean t_{max} increased by 82%. The difference in bioavailability was less marked upon steady-state administration to renal transplant recipients, and therapeutic equivalence has been demonstrated in randomised study of 477 patients. When switching patients between oral solution and tablet formulations, it is recommended to give the same dose and to verify the sirolimus trough concentration 1 to 2 weeks later to assure that it remains within recommended target ranges. Also when switching between different tablet strengths, verification of trough concentrations is recommended.

In 24 healthy volunteers receiving Rapamune tablets with a high-fat meal, C_{max}, t_{max} and AUC showed increases of 65%, 32%, and 23%, respectively. To minimise variability, Rapamune tablets should be taken consistently with or without food. Grapefruit juice affects CYP3A4-mediated metabolism and must, therefore, be avoided.

Sirolimus concentrations, following the administration of Rapamune tablets (5 mg) to healthy subjects as single doses are dose proportional between 5 and 40 mg.

Initial Therapy (2 to 3 months post-transplant): In most patients receiving Rapamune tablets with a loading dose of 6 mg followed by an initial maintenance dose of 2 mg, whole blood sirolimus trough concentrations rapidly achieved steady-state concentrations within the recommended target range (4 to 12 ng/ml, chromatographic assay). Sirolimus pharmacokinetic parameters following daily doses of 2 mg Rapamune tablets administered in combination with ciclosporin microemulsion (4 hours prior to Rapamune tablets) and corticosteroids in 13 renal transplant patients, based on data collected at months 1 and 3 after transplantation, were: $C_{min,ss}$, 7.39 ± 2.18 ng/ml; $C_{max,ss}$, 15.0 ± 4.9 ng/ml; $t_{max,ss}$, 3.46 ± 2.40 h; $AUC_{\tau,ss}$, 230 ± 67 ng·h/ml; CL/F/WT, 139 ± 63 ml/h/kg (parameters calculated from LC-MS/MS assay results). The corresponding results for the oral solution in the same clinical trial were $C_{min,ss}$ 5.40 ± 2.50 ng/ml, $C_{max,ss}$ 14.4 ± 5.3 ng/ml, $t_{max,ss}$ 2.12 ± 0.84 h, $AUC_{\tau,ss}$ 194 ± 78 ng·h/ml, CL/F/W 173 ± 50 ml/h/kg. Whole blood trough sirolimus concentrations, as measured by LC/MS/MS, were significantly correlated (r^2 = 0.85) with $AUC_{\tau,ss}$.

Based on monitoring in all patients during the period of concomitant therapy with ciclosporin, mean (10th, 90th percentiles) troughs (expressed as chromatographic assay values) and daily doses were 8.6 ± 3.0 ng/ml (5.0 to 13 ng/ml) and 2.1 ± 0.70 mg (1.5 to 2.7 mg), respectively (see section 4.2).

Maintenance therapy: From month 3 to month 12, following discontinuation of ciclosporin, mean (10th, 90th percentiles) troughs (expressed as chromatographic assay values) and daily doses were 19 ± 4.1 ng/ml (14 to 24 ng/mL) and 8.2 ± 4.2 mg (3.6 to 13.6 mg), respectively (see section 4.2). Therefore, the sirolimus dose was approximately 4-fold higher to account for both the absence of the pharmacokinetic interaction with ciclosporin (2-fold increase) and the augmented immunosuppressive requirement in the absence of ciclosporin (2-fold increase).

5.3 Preclinical safety data

Adverse reactions not observed in clinical studies, but seen in animals at exposure levels similar to clinical exposure levels and with possible relevance to clinical use were as follows: pancreatic islet cell vacuolation, testicular tubular degeneration, gastrointestinal ulceration, bone fractures and calluses, hepatic haematopoiesis, and pulmonary phospholipidosis.

Sirolimus was not mutagenic in the *in vitro* bacterial reverse mutation assays, the Chinese Hamster Ovary cell chromosomal aberration assay, the mouse lymphoma cell forward mutation assay, or the *in vivo* mouse micronucleus assay.

Carcinogenicity studies conducted in mouse and rat showed increased incidences of lymphomas (male and female mouse), hepatocellular adenoma and carcinoma (male mouse) and granulocytic leukaemia (female mouse). It is known that malignancies (lymphoma) secondary to the chronic use of immunosuppressive agents can occur and have been reported in patients in rare instances. In mouse, chronic ulcerative skin lesions were increased. The changes may be related to chronic immunosuppression. In rat, testicular interstitial cell adenomas were likely indicative of a species dependent response to lutenising hormone levels and are usually considered of limited clinical relevance.

In reproduction toxicity studies decreased fertility in male rats was observed. Partly reversible reductions in sperm counts were reported in a 13-week rat study. Reductions in testicular weights and/or histological lesions (e.g. tubular atrophy and tubular giant cells) were observed in rats and in a monkey study. In rats, sirolimus caused embryo/foetotoxicity that was manifested as mortality and reduced foetal weights (with associated delays in skeletal ossification). (see section 4.6).

6. PHARMACEUTICAL PARTICULARS

6.1 List of excipients

Tablet core:

Lactose monohydrate

Macrogol

Magnesium stearate

Talc

1 mg Tablet coating:

Macrogol

Glyceryl monooleate

Pharmaceutical glaze

Anhydrous calcium sulphate

Microcrystalline cellulose

Sucrose

Titanium dioxide

Poloxamer 188

α-tocopherol

Povidone

Carnauba wax:

Red opacode S-1-15095 (shellac glaze ~45% in ethanol, red iron oxide (E172), isopropyl alcohol, n-butyl alcohol, propylene glycol, ammonium hydroxide, simethicone).

2 mg Tablet coating:
Macrogol
Glyceryl monooleate
Pharmaceutical glaze
Anhydrous calcium sulphate
Microcrystalline cellulose
Sucrose
Titanium dioxide
Brown iron oxide (E172)
Yellow iron oxide (E172)
Poloxamer 188
α-tocopherol
Povidone
Carnauba wax
Red opacode S-1-15095 (shellac glaze ~45% in ethanol, red iron oxide (E172), isopropyl alcohol, n-butyl alcohol, propylene glycol, ammonium hydroxide, simethicone).

Solution: Polysorbate 80

Phosal 50 PG (phosphatidylcholine, propylene glycol, mono-, di-glycerides, ethanol (1.5% to 2.5%), soya fatty acids and ascorbyl palmitate).

6.2 Incompatibilities

Rapamune must not be diluted in grapefruit juice or any other liquid other than water or orange juice (see section 6.6).

Rapamune oral solution contains polysorbate-80, which is known to increase the rate of di-(2-ethylhexyl)phthalate (DEHP) extraction from polyvinyl chloride (PVC). It is important to follow the instructions to administer Rapamune oral solution at once when a plastic container is used for the dilution and/or administration (see section 6.6).

6.3 Shelf life

1mg/ml oral solution

2 years.

30 days for opened bottle.

24 hours in the dosing syringe (at room temperature, but not to exceed 25°C).

After dilution, (see section 6.6) the preparation should be used immediately.

1mg tablet

2 years

2mg tablet

23 months

6.4 Special precautions for storage

1mg tablet

Keep the blister in the outer carton in order to protect from light.

2mg tablet

Keep the blister in the outer carton in order to protect from light. Do not store above 25°C.

Bottle

Store in a refrigerator at 2°C to 8°C. Store in the original bottle in order to protect from light.

If necessary, the patient may store the bottles at room temperatures up to 25°C for a short period of time (24 hours).

6.5 Nature and contents of container

Tablet

Clear polyvinyl chloride (PVC)/polyethylene (PE)/polychlorotrifluoroethylene (Aclar) aluminium blister packages of 30 and 100 tablets. Not all pack sizes may be marketed.

Bottles

60 ml type III amber glass bottles with syringe adapter and 30 amber, plastic dosing syringes.

6.6 Special precautions for disposal and other handling

Any unused product or waste material should be disposed of in accordance with local requirements.

Tablets

No special requirements

Bottles

Instructions for use and handling:

The dosing syringe should be used to withdraw the prescribed amount of Rapamune from the bottle. Empty the correct amount of Rapamune from the syringe into only a glass or plastic container with at least 60 ml of water or orange juice. No other liquids, including grapefruit juice, should be used for dilution. Stir vigorously and drink at once. Refill the container with an additional volume (minimum of 120 ml) of water or orange juice, stir vigorously, and drink at once.

7. MARKETING AUTHORISATION HOLDER

Wyeth Europa Ltd.
Huntercombe Lane South
Taplow, Maidenhead
Berkshire, SL6 0PH
United Kingdom

8. MARKETING AUTHORISATION NUMBER(S)

EU/1/01/171/007-8 – 1mg Tablet (pack of 30)
EU/1/01/171/009-10 – 2mg Tablet (pack of 30)
EU/1/01/171/001 – 60ml bottle

9. DATE OF FIRST AUTHORISATION/RENEWAL OF THE AUTHORISATION

Date of first authorisation: 14 March 2001

Date of latest renewal: 15 March 2006

10. DATE OF REVISION OF THE TEXT

29 April 2009

Detailed information on this product is available on the website of the European Medicines Agency (EMEA) http://www.emea.europa.eu

Rapifen

(Janssen-Cilag Ltd)

1. NAME OF THE MEDICINAL PRODUCT

Rapifen®

2. QUALITATIVE AND QUANTITATIVE COMPOSITION

Each ml of Rapifen contains alfentanil hydrochloride 544 micrograms, equivalent to 500 micrograms alfentanil base.

3. PHARMACEUTICAL FORM

Aqueous injection.

4. CLINICAL PARTICULARS

4.1 Therapeutic indications

As an analgesic supplement for use before and during anaesthesia.

It is indicated for:

1. Short procedures and outpatient surgery.

2. Procedures of medium and long duration when given as a bolus followed by supplemental doses or by continuous infusion.

At very high doses, Rapifen may be used as an anaesthetic induction agent in ventilated patients.

4.2 Posology and method of administration

For intravenous administration.

Rapifen by the intravenous route can be administered to both adults and children. The dosage of Rapifen should be individualised according to age, bodyweight, physical status, underlying pathological condition, use of other drugs and type of surgery and anaesthesia. The usual recommended dosage regimen is as follows:

Adults	*Initial*	*Supplemental*
Spontaneous respiration	500 µg (1 ml)	250 µg (0.5 ml)
Assisted ventilation	30-50 µg/kg	15 µg/kg
Children	*Initial*	*Supplemental*
Assisted ventilation	*30-50 µg/kg*	15 µg/kg

If desired, Rapifen can be mixed with sodium chloride injection BP, dextrose injection BP or compound sodium lactate injection BP (Hartmann's solution). Such dilutions are compatible with plastic bags and giving sets. These dilutions should be used within 24 hours of preparation.

Children may require higher or more frequent dosing owing to a shorter half-life of Rapifen in this age group. The elderly and debilitated may require lower or less frequent dosing owing to a longer half-life of Rapifen in this age group (dilution may be helpful).

In spontaneously breathing patients, the initial bolus dose should be given slowly over about 30 seconds (dilution may be helpful).

After intravenous administration in unpremedicated adult patients, 1 ml Rapifen may be expected to have a peak effect in 90 seconds and to provide analgesia for 5-10 minutes. Periods of more painful stimuli may be overcome by the use of small increments of Rapifen. For procedures of longer duration, additional increments will be required.

In ventilated patients, the last dose of alfentanil should not be given later than about 10 minutes before the end of surgery to avoid the continuation of respiratory depression after surgery is complete.

In ventilated patients undergoing longer procedures, Rapifen may be infused at a rate of 0.5-1 microgram/kg/minute. Adequate plasma concentrations of alfentanil will only be achieved rapidly if this infusion is preceded by a loading dose of 50-100 microgram/kg given as a bolus or fast infusion over 10 minutes.

Lower doses may be adequate, for example, in geriatric patients or where anaesthesia is being supplemented by other agents.

The infusion should be discontinued up to 30 minutes before the anticipated end of surgery.

Increasing the infusion rate may prolong recovery. Supplementation of the anaesthetic, if required, for periods of painful stimuli, is best managed by extra bolus doses of Rapifen (1-2 ml) or low concentrations of a volatile agent for brief periods.

Patients with severe burns presenting for dressing, etc, have received a loading dose of 18-28 µg/kg/min for up to 30 minutes without requiring mechanical ventilation. In heart surgery, when used as a sole anaesthetic, doses in the range of 12-50 mg/hour have been used.

4.3 Contraindications

Obstructive airways disease or respiratory depression if not ventilating.

Concurrent administration with monoamine oxidase inhibitors or within 2 weeks of their discontinuation.

Administration in labour or before clamping of the cord during caesarean section due to the possibility of respiratory depression in the newborn infant.

Patients with a known intolerance to alfentanil and other morphinomimetics.

4.4 Special warnings and precautions for use

Warnings:

Following administration of Rapifen, a fall in blood pressure may occur. The magnitude of this effect may be exaggerated in the hypovolaemic patient or in the presence of concomitant sedative medication. Appropriate measures to maintain a stable arterial pressure should be taken.

Significant respiratory depression and loss of consciousness will occur following administration of Rapifen in doses in excess of 1 mg and is dose-related. This and the other pharmacological effects of Rapifen are usually of short duration and can be reversed by the specific opioid antagonists (e.g. naloxone). Additional doses of the antagonists may be necessary because the respiratory depression may last longer than the duration of action of the opioid antagonist.

Like other opioids, alfentanil may cause bradycardia, an effect that may be marked and rapid in onset but which can be antagonised by atropine. Particular care must be taken following treatment with drugs which may depress the heart or increase vagal tone, such as anaesthetic agents or beta-blockers, since they may predispose to bradycardia or hypotension. Heart rate and blood pressure should therefore be monitored carefully. If hypotension or bradycardia occur, appropriate measures should be instituted.

Cardiac arrest following bradycardia has been reported on very rare occasions in non-atropinised patients. Therefore it is advisable to be prepared to administer an anticholinergic drug.

Precautions:

It is wise to reduce the dosage in the elderly and debilitated patients. In hypothyroidism, pulmonary disease, decreased respiratory reserve, alcoholism and liver or renal impairment the dosage should be titrated with care and prolonged monitoring may be required.

Patients on chronic opioid therapy or with a history of opioid abuse may require higher doses.

Rapifen may induce muscle rigidity during induction. Rigidity, which may also involve the thoracic muscles, can be avoided by the following measures:

- Slow IV injection (usually sufficient for lower doses);
- Premedication with a benzodiazepine;
- Administration of a muscle relaxant just prior to administration of Rapifen.
- Non-epileptic (myo)clonic movements can occur.

As with all potent opioids, profound analgesia is accompanied by marked respiratory depression, which may persist into or recur in the early postoperative period. Care should be taken after infusions or large doses of alfentanil to ensure that adequate spontaneous breathing has been established and maintained in the absence of stimulation before discharging the patient from the recovery area. Resuscitation equipment and narcotic antagonists should be readily available. Hyperventilation during anaesthesia may alter the patient's response to CO_2, thus affecting respiration postoperatively.

The use of rapid bolus injections of opioids should be avoided in patients with compromised intracerebral compliance; in such patients a transient decrease in the mean arterial pressure has occasionally been accompanied by a transient reduction of the cerebral perfusion pressure.

This medicinal product contains less than 1 mmol sodium (23 mg) per 5 mg dose, i.e. essentially 'sodium-free'.

4.5 Interaction with other medicinal products and other forms of interaction

Alfentanil is metabolised mainly via the human cytochrome P450 3A4 enzyme. Available human pharmacokinetic data indicate that the metabolism of alfentanil may be inhibited by fluconazole, erythromycin, diltiazem and cimetidine (known cytochrome P450 3A4 enzyme inhibitors). *In vitro* data suggest that other potent cytochrome P450 3A4 enzyme inhibitors (e.g. ketoconazole, itraconazole, ritonavir) may also inhibit the metabolism of alfentanil. This could increase the risk of prolonged or delayed respiratory depression. The concomitant use of such drugs requires special patient care and observation; in particular, it may be necessary to lower the dose of Rapifen.

Treatment with drugs which may depress the heart or increase vagal tone, such as beta-blockers and anaesthetic agents, may predispose to bradycardia or hypotension. Bradycardia and possibly asystole can occur when Rapifen is combined with non-vagolytic muscle relaxants.

The use of opioid premedication, barbiturates, benzodiazepines, neuroleptics, halogenic gases and other non-selective CNS depressants may enhance or prolong the respiratory depressant effects of alfentanil.

If other narcotic or CNS depressant drugs are used concurrently with alfentanil, the effects of the drugs can be expected to be additive. When patients have received such drugs the dose of alfentanil required will be less than usual. Likewise, following the administration of alfentanil, the dose of other CNS depressant drugs should be reduced.

4.6 Pregnancy and lactation

Although no teratogenic or acute embryotoxic effects have been observed in animal experiments, insufficient data are available to evaluate any harmful effects in man.

Consequently, it is necessary to consider possible risks and potential advantages before administering this drug to pregnant patients.

IV administration during childbirth (including Caesarian section) is not recommended, because alfentanil crosses the placenta and because the foetal respiratory centre is particularly sensitive to opiates. If, however, Rapifen is administered, an antidote should always be at hand for the child.

Alfentanil may appear in breast milk. It is therefore recommended that breast feeding is not initiated within 24 hours of treatment.

4.7 Effects on ability to drive and use machines

Where early discharge is envisaged, patients should be advised not to drive or operate machinery for the 24 hours following administration.

4.8 Undesirable effects

Adverse Drug Reactions

The most frequently reported ADRs (incidence ⩾10%) are: nausea and vomiting. Undesirable effects listed below in Table 1 have been reported in a clinical trial and/or from spontaneous reports from post-marketing experience. The following terms and frequencies are applied: very common (⩾ 1/10), common (⩾ 1/100 to < 1/10), uncommon (⩾ 1/1000 to < 1/100), rare (⩾ 1/10,000 to < 1/1000), very rare (< 1/10,000), and not known (frequency cannot be estimated from the available data). Adverse drug reactions from spontaneous reports during worldwide postmarketing experience with Alfentanil that met threshold criteria are included. Unlike for clinical trials, precise frequencies cannot be provided for spontaneous reports. The frequency for these reports is therefore classified as 'not known'.

Table 1
Adverse drug reactions reported in clinical trials and/or postmarketing

Body System/ Organ Class *Frequency Category*	Clinical trials	Spontaneous Reports[a]
Immune system disorders		
Uncommon	Allergic reactions (such as anaphylaxis, bronchospasm, urticaria)	
Psychiatric Disorders		
Common	Somnolence	
Uncommon	Disorientation, Agitation, Euphoria	
Nervous system disorders		
Common	Muscle rigidity (may also involve thoracic muscles), Myoclonic movements, Dizziness	
Uncommon	Headache	
Not known		Loss of consciousness (Postoperative period), Convulsion
Eye disorders		
Uncommon	Blurred/double vision	
Not known		Miosis
Cardiac disorders		
Common	Bradycardia, Tachycardia	
Uncommon	Arrhythmia	
Not known		Cardiac arrest
Vascular Disorders		
Common	Hypotension, Hypertension	
Respiratory, thoracic, and mediastinal disorders		
Common	Apnoea, Respiratory depression	
Uncommon	Cough, Recurrence of respiratory depression, Laryngospasm, Hiccup	
Not known		Respiratory arrest (including fatal outcome)
Gastrointestinal disorders		
Very common	Nausea, Vomiting	
Skin and subcutaneous tissue disorders		
Uncommon	Pruritis, Sweating	
General disorders and administration site conditions		
Uncommon	Injection site pain, Shivering	
Not known		Pyrexia

a: Listed are only those adverse drug reactions that were not identified in clinical trials

4.9 Overdose

The manifestations of alfentanil overdose are generally an extension of its pharmacological action, which include the following:

	Action
Bradycardia	Anticholinergics such as atropine or glycopyrrolate.
Hypoventilation or apnoea	O_2 administration, assisted or controlled respiration and an opioid antagonist may be required.
Muscle rigidity	Intravenous neuromuscular blocking agent may be given.

If hypotension is severe or persists, the possibility of hypovolaemia should be considered and controlled with appropriate parenteral fluid administration.

The suggested treatments given above do not preclude the use of other clinically indicated counter measures.

Body temperature and adequate fluid intake should be maintained and the patient observed for 24 hours. A specific opioid antagonist (e.g. naloxone) should be available to treat respiratory depression.

5. PHARMACOLOGICAL PROPERTIES

5.1 Pharmacodynamic properties

The analgesic potency of Rapifen is one quarter that of fentanyl. The duration of action of Rapifen is one third that on an equianalgesic dose of fentanyl and is clearly dose-related. Its depressant effects on respiratory rate and alveolar ventilation are also of shorter duration than those of fentanyl.

The onset of action of Rapifen is four times more rapid than that of an equianalgesic dose of fentanyl. The peak analgesic and respiratory depressant effects occur within 90 seconds.

In man, alfentanil at therapeutic doses had no detrimental effects of myocardial performance. The cardiovascular stability is remarkable both in healthy and poor-risk patients. The only changes seen in blood pressure and heart rate are transient, slight decreases occurring immediately after induction. The incidence and degree of respiratory depression is less and of shorter duration after alfentanil than with fentanyl. Like other narcotic analgesics, alfentanil increases the amplitude of the EEG and reduces its frequency. Alfentanil reduces intraocular pressure by about 45%. It blocks increases in plasma cortisol and in plasma antidiuretic and growth hormones throughout surgery and prevents increases in plasma catecholamines up to but not during or after cardiopulmonary bypass in patients undergoing open heart surgery.

5.2 Pharmacokinetic properties

Alfentanil is a synthetic opioid with μ-agonist pharmacological effects.

After bolus injections ranging from 2.4 to 125 μg/kg, plasma levels in man decay triexponentially with a terminal half life of approximately 90 minutes. Total distribution volume varies from 0.4 to 1.0 L/kg, indicating a limited distribution of alfentanil to the tissues. Plasma clearance, varying from 3.3 to 8.3 ml/kg/min represents approximately one third of liver plasma flow indicating that elimination of alfentanil is not flow dependent. Since only 0.4% of the dose is excreted with the urine as unchanged drug, elimination of alfentanil occurs mainly by metabolism.

These main parameters in patients undergoing surgery are similar to those in healthy volunteers. Only when the drug was given as the sole anaesthetic in a continuous high infusion over about 5 hours was the clearance of alfentanil reduced resulting in a plasma half-life of about 200 minutes, the distribution volume not being markedly changed.

Plasma protein binding of alfentanil is 92%, mainly due to a strong binding to the 'acute phase' α_1 acid-glycoprotein. It is not bound to the blood cells. Pharmacokinetics were comparable in rats, dogs and man. The elderly show a longer half-life for Rapifen after IV bolus doses.

Special Populations

Paediatric patients

Protein binding in newborns is 75% and increases in children to 85%. The plasma clearance in newborns is approximately 7.2 ± 3.2mL/kg/min and 4.7 ± 1.7 mL/kg/min in children between 4.5 to 7.75 years. The volume of distribution at steady state was 1230 ± 520 mL/kg in newborns and 163.5 ± 110 mL/kg in children. The half-life is 146 ± 57 minutes in newborns and 40.2 ± 8.9 minutes in children.

Hepatic Impairment

After administration of a single intravenous dose of 50 μg/kg, the terminal half-life in cirrhotic patients is significantly longer than in controls. The volume of distribution remains unchanged. The free fraction of alfentanil increases in cirrhotic patients to 18.5% compared with 11.5% in controls. This increase in free fraction together with a reduction in clearance from 3.06 mL/min/kg in controls to 1.60 mL/min/kg in cirrhotic patients will result in a more prolonged and pronounced effect (see Section 4.4.).

Renal Impairment

The volume of distribution and clearance of the free fraction is similar in renal failure patients and healthy controls. The free fraction of alfentanil in patients with renal failure is increased to 12.4 to 19 % compared with 10.3 to 11% in controls. This may result in an increase in clinical effects of alfentanil (see Section 4.4.).

5.3 Preclinical safety data

Preclinical effects observed were only at exposures considered sufficiently in excess of the maximum human exposure indicating little relevance to clinical use.

6. PHARMACEUTICAL PARTICULARS

6.1 List of excipients

Sodium chloride

Water for injection

6.2 Incompatibilities

See 'Dosage and dosage schedules'.

6.3 Shelf life

5 years.

6.4 Special precautions for storage

Store in a controlled drug store, at or below 25°C.

6.5 Nature and contents of container

Colourless glass one-point-cut ampoules (PhEur, Type I).

Pack size: packs of 10 × 2 ml ampoules; packs of 5 and 10 × 10 ml ampoules.

6.6 Special precautions for disposal and other handling

For single use only. Discard any unused contents.

7. MARKETING AUTHORISATION HOLDER

Janssen-Cilag Limited

50-100 Holmers Farm Way

High Wycombe

Buckinghamshire

HP12 4EG

UK

8. MARKETING AUTHORISATION NUMBER(S)

PL 0242/0091

9. DATE OF FIRST AUTHORISATION/RENEWAL OF THE AUTHORISATION

27 July 1983/30 March 2004

10. DATE OF REVISION OF THE TEXT

10th July 2009

Legal category POM

Rapifen Intensive Care

(Janssen-Cilag Ltd)

1. NAME OF THE MEDICINAL PRODUCT

Rapifen® Intensive Care

2. QUALITATIVE AND QUANTITATIVE COMPOSITION

Alfentanil hydrochloride 5.44 mg equivalent to 5 mg alfentanil base per ml.

3. PHARMACEUTICAL FORM

Solution for injection.

4. CLINICAL PARTICULARS

4.1 Therapeutic indications

Rapifen Intensive Care is a potent opioid analgesic with a very rapid onset of action. It is indicated for analgesia and suppression of respiratory activity in mechanically ventilated patients on intensive care and to provide analgesic cover for painful manoeuvres. It will aid compliance with mechanical ventilation, and tolerance of the endotracheal tube. Intravenous bolus doses of Rapifen (0.5 mg/ml) may be used to provide additional pain relief during brief painful procedures such as physiotherapy, endotracheal suction, etc. Despite being mechanically ventilated, patients may be awake in the presence of adequate analgesia.

At the proposed doses, Rapifen Intensive Care has no sedative activity. Therefore supplementation with an appropriate hypnotic or sedative agent is recommended. Admixture is not advisable due to the need to individually titrate both agents.

Alfentanil given by infusion should only be given in areas where facilities are available to deal with respiratory depression and where continuous monitoring is performed. Alfentanil should only be prescribed by physicians familiar with the use of potent opioids when given by continuous IV infusion.

4.2 Posology and method of administration

Method of Administration

For intravenous infusions.

Dosage

Rapifen Intensive Care should be diluted with sodium chloride intravenous infusion BP, glucose intravenous infusion BP, or compound sodium lactate intravenous infusion BP (Hartmann's solution). Such dilutions are compatible with plastic bags and giving sets. These dilutions should be used within 24 hours of preparation.

Once the patient has been intubated, mechanical ventilation can be initiated using the following dosage regimen:

The recommended initial infusion rate for mechanically ventilated adult patients is 2 mg per hour (equivalent to 0.4 ml per hour of undiluted Rapifen Intensive Care). For a 70 kg patient, this corresponds to approximately 30 micrograms per kilogram per hour.

More rapid control may initially be gained by using a loading dose. For example, a dose of 5 mg may be given in divided doses over a period of 10 minutes, during which time careful monitoring of blood pressure and heart rate should be performed. If hypotension or bradycardia occurs, the rate of administration should be reduced accordingly and other appropriate measures instituted.

The dose to produce the desired effects should then be individually determined and reassessed regularly to ensure that the optimum dose is being used.

In clinical trials, patient requirements have generally been met with doses of 0.5 to 10 mg alfentanil per hour.

Additional bolus doses of 0.5-1.0 mg alfentanil may be given to provide analgesia during short painful procedures.

The elderly and those patients with liver impairment and hypothyroidism will require lower doses. Obese patients may require a dose based on their lean body mass.

Adolescents and young adults will require higher than average doses. There is little experience of use of alfentanil to treat children in intensive care.

The maximum recommended duration of treatment with alfentanil infusions is 4 days.

Present data suggest that clearance of alfentanil is unaltered in renal failure. However there is an increased free fraction and hence dosage requirements may be less than in the patient with normal renal function.

4.3 Contraindications

Known intolerance of alfentanil or other morphinomimetics. Pregnancy, and concurrent administration with monoamine oxidase inhibitors.

4.4 Special warnings and precautions for use

Warnings:

Following administration of Rapifen Intensive Care, a fall in blood pressure may occur. The magnitude of this effect may be exaggerated in the hypovolaemic patient or in the presence of concomitant sedative medication. Appropriate measures to maintain a stable arterial pressure should be taken.

Like other opioids, alfentanil may cause bradycardia, an effect which may be marked and rapid in onset but which can be antagonised by atropine.

Particular care must be taken following treatment with drugs which may depress the heart or increase vagal tone, such as anaesthetic agents or beta-blockers since they may predispose to bradycardia or hypotension. Heart rate and blood pressure should therefore be monitored carefully. If hypotension or bradycardia occurs, the rate of administration of alfentanil should be reduced and other appropriate measures instituted.

Cardiac arrest following bradycardia has been reported on very rare occasions in non-atropinised patients. Therefore it is advisable to be prepared to administer an anticholinergic drug.

Care must be taken if the patient has received monoamine oxidase inhibitors within the previous 2 weeks.

Significant respiratory depression and loss of consciousness will occur following administration of alfentanil in doses in excess of 1 mg and is dose-related. If necessary for assessment purposes, naloxone or other specific antagonists may be administered to reverse the opioid respiratory depression and other pharmacological effects of alfentanil. More than one dose of naloxone may be required in view of its short half life.

Muscle rigidity (morphine-like effect) may occur, in which case neuromuscular blocking drugs may be helpful.

Precautions:

It is wise to reduce the dosage in the elderly and debilitated patient. In hypothyroidism, pulmonary disease, decreased respiratory reserve, alcoholism and liver or renal impairment the dosage should be titrated with care and prolonged monitoring may be required.

Patients on chronic opioid therapy or with a history of opioid abuse may require higher doses.

Non-epileptic (myo)clonic movements can occur.

As with all potent opioids, profound analgesia is accompanied by marked respiratory depression, which may persist into or recur in the early post infusion period. Care should therefore be taken throughout the weaning period and adequate spontaneous respiration should be established and maintained in the absence of stimulation or ventilatory support. Following cessation of the infusion, the patient should be closely observed for at least 6 hours. Prior use of opioid medication may enhance or prolong the respiratory depressant effects of alfentanil.

The use of rapid bolus injections of opioids should be avoided in patients with compromised intracerebral compliance; in such patients a transient decrease in the mean arterial pressure has occasionally been accompanied by a transient reduction of the cerebral perfusion pressure.

This medicinal product contains less than 1 mmol sodium (23 mg) per 5 mg dose, i.e. essentially 'sodium-free'.

4.5 Interaction with other medicinal products and other forms of interaction

Alfentanil is metabolised mainly via the human cytochrome P450 3A4 enzyme. Available human pharmacokinetic data indicate that the metabolism of alfentanil may be inhibited by fluconazole, erythromycin, diltiazem and cimetidine (known cytochrome P450 3A4 enzyme inhibitors). *In vitro* data suggest that other potent cytochrome P450 3A4 enzyme inhibitors (e.g. ketoconazole, itraconazole, ritonavir) may also inhibit the metabolism of alfentanil. This could increase the risk of prolonged or delayed respiratory depression. The concomitant use of such drugs requires special patient care and observation; in particular, it may be necessary to lower the dose of Rapifen.

Treatment with drugs which may depress the heart or increase vagal tone, such as beta-blockers and anaesthetic agents, may predispose to bradycardia or hypotension. Bradycardia and possibly asystole can occur when Rapifen Intensive Care is combined with non-vagolytic muscle relaxants.

Prior use of opioid premedication, barbiturates, benzodiazepines, neuroleptics, halogenic gases and other non-selective CNS depressants may enhance or prolong the respiratory depressant effects of alfentanil.

If other narcotic or CNS depressant drugs are used concurrently with alfentanil, the effects of the drugs can be expected to be additive. When patients have received such drugs, the dose of alfentanil required will be less than usual. Likewise, following the administration of alfentanil, the dose of other CNS depressant drugs should be reduced.

4.6 Pregnancy and lactation

Although no teratogenic or acute embryotoxic effects have been observed in animal experiments, insufficient data are available to evaluate any harmful effects in man.

Consequently, it is necessary to consider possible risks and potential advantages before administering this drug to pregnant patients.

IV administration during childbirth (including Caesarian section) is not recommended, because alfentanil crosses the placenta and because the foetal respiratory centre is particularly sensitive to opiates. If, however, Rapifen is administered, an antidote should always be at hand for the child.

Alfentanil may appear in breast milk. It is therefore recommended that breast feeding is not initiated within 24 hours of treatment.

4.7 Effects on ability to drive and use machines

Where early discharge is envisaged, patients should be advised not to drive or operate machinery for the 24 hours following administration.

4.8 Undesirable effects

Adverse Drug Reactions

The most frequently reported ADRs (incidence ⩾10%) are: nausea and vomiting. Undesirable effects listed below in Table 1 have been reported in a clinical trial and/or from spontaneous reports from post-marketing experience. The following terms and frequencies are applied: very common (⩾ 1/10), common (⩾ 1/100 to < 1/10), uncommon (⩾ 1/1000 to < 1/100), rare (⩾ 1/10,000 to < 1/1000), very rare (< 1/10,000), and not known (frequency cannot be estimated from the available data). Adverse drug reactions from spontaneous reports during worldwide postmarketing experience with Alfentanil that met threshold criteria are included. Unlike for clinical trials, precise frequencies cannot be provided for spontaneous reports. The frequency for these reports is therefore classified as 'not known'.

Table 1
Adverse drug reactions reported in clinical trials and/or postmarketing

Body System/ Organ Class *Frequency Category*	Clinical trials	Spontaneous Reports[a]
Immune system disorders		
Uncommon	Allergic reactions (such as anaphylaxis, bronchospasm, urticaria)	
Psychiatric Disorders		
Common	Somnolence	
Uncommon	Disorientation, Agitation, Euphoria	
Nervous system disorders		
Common	Muscle rigidity (may also involve thoracic muscles), Myoclonic movements, Dizziness	
Uncommon	Headache	
Not known		Loss of consciousness (Postoperative period), Convulsion
Eye disorders		
Uncommon	Blurred/double vision	
Not known		Miosis
Cardiac disorders		
Common	Bradycardia, Tachycardia	
Uncommon	Arrhythmia	
Not known		Cardiac arrest
Vascular Disorders		
Common	Hypotension, Hypertension	
Respiratory, thoracic, and mediastinal disorders		
Common	Apnoea, Respiratory depression	
Uncommon	Cough, Recurrence of respiratory depression, Laryngospasm, Hiccup	
Not known		Respiratory arrest (including fatal outcome)
Gastrointestinal disorders		
Very common	Nausea, Vomiting	

Skin and subcutaneous tissue disorders		
Uncommon	Pruritis, Sweating	
General disorders and administration site conditions		
Uncommon	Injection site Pain, Shivering	
Not known		Pyrexia

a: Listed are only those adverse drug reactions that were not identified in clinical trials

4.9 Overdose
The manifestations of alfentanil overdose are generally an extension of its pharmacological action, which include the following:-

	Action:
Bradycardia:	Anticholinergics such as atropine or glycopyrrolate;
Hypoventilation or apnoea:	O_2 administration, assisted or controlled respiration and an opioid antagonist may be required;
Muscle rigidity:	Intravenous neuromuscular blocking agent may be given.

The suggested treatments given above do not preclude the use of other clinically indicated counter measures.

Body temperature and adequate fluid intake should be maintained and the patient observed for 24 hours.

A specific narcotic antagonist (e.g. naloxone) should be available to treat respiratory depression.

5. PHARMACOLOGICAL PROPERTIES
5.1 Pharmacodynamic properties
In man, alfentanil at therapeutic doses has no detrimental effects on myocardial performance. The cardiovascular stability is remarkable both in healthy and poor-risk patients. The only changes seen in blood pressure and heart rate were transient, slight decreases occurring immediately after induction. The incidence and degree of respiratory depression is less and of shorter duration after alfentanil than with fentanyl. Like other narcotic analgesics, alfentanil increases the amplitude of the EEG and reduces its frequency. Alfentanil reduces intraocular pressure by about 45%. It blocks increases in plasma cortisol and in plasma antidiuretic and growth hormones throughout surgery, and prevents increases in plasma catecholamines up to, but not during or after, cardiopulmonary bypass in patients undergoing open heart surgery.

5.2 Pharmacokinetic properties
Alfentanil is a synthetic opioid with μ-agonist pharmacological effects.

After bolus injections ranging from 2.4 to 125 μg/kg, plasma levels in man decay triexponentially with a terminal half life of approx. 90 minutes. Total distribution volume varies from 0.4 to 1.0 l/kg, indicating a limited distribution of alfentanil to the tissues. Plasma clearance, varying from 3.3 to 8.3 ml/kg/min represents approximately one third of liver plasma flow indicating that elimination of alfentanil is not flow dependent. Since only 0.4% of the dose is excreted with the urine as unchanged drug, elimination of alfentanil occurs mainly by metabolism.

These main parameters in patients undergoing surgery are similar to those in healthy volunteers. Only when the drug was given as the sole anaesthetic in a continuous high infusion over about 5 hours was the clearance of alfentanil reduced resulting in a plasma half-life of about 200 minutes, the distribution volume not being markedly changed.

Plasma protein binding of alfentanil is 92%, mainly due to a strong binding to the 'acute phase' α_1-acid-glycoprotein. It is not bound to the blood cells. Pharmacokinetics were comparable in rats, dogs and man. The elderly show a longer half-life for alfentanil, after IV bolus doses.

Special Populations
Paediatric patients
Protein binding in newborns is 75% and increases in children to 85%. The plasma clearance in newborns is approximately 7.2 ± 3.2mL/kg/min and 4.7 ± 1.7 mL/kg/min in children between 4.5 to 7.75 years. The volume of distribution at steady state was 1230 ± 520 mL/kg in newborns and 163.5 ± 110 mL/kg in children. The half-life is 146 ± 57 minutes in newborns and 40.2 ± 8.9 minutes in children.
Hepatic Impairment
After administration of a single intravenous dose of 50 μg/kg, the terminal half-life in cirrhotic patients is significantly longer than in controls. The volume of distribution remains unchanged. The free fraction of alfentanil increases in cirrhotic patients to 18.5% compared with 11.5% in controls. This increase in free fraction together with a reduction in clearance from 3.06 mL/min/kg in controls to 1.60 mL/min/kg in cirrhotic patients will result in a more prolonged and pronounced effect (see Section 4.4.).
Renal Impairment
The volume of distribution and clearance of the free fraction is similar in renal failure patients and healthy controls. The free fraction of alfentanil in patients with renal failure is increased to 12.4 to 19 % compared with 10.3 to 11% in controls. This may result in an increase in clinical effects of alfentanil (see Section 4.4.).

5.3 Preclinical safety data
Preclinical effects observed were only at exposures considered sufficiently in excess of the maximum human exposure indicating little relevance to clinical use.

6. PHARMACEUTICAL PARTICULARS
6.1 List of excipients
Sodium chloride
Water for injections
Sodium hydroxide 0.1 N
Hydrochloric acid 0.1 N

6.2 Incompatibilities
See Section 4.2 Posology and Method of administration.

6.3 Shelf life
60 months.

6.4 Special precautions for storage
Store in the controlled drug store, at or below 25°C.

6.5 Nature and contents of container
Type I USP clear glass ampoules containing 1 ml, packed in 5s or 10s.

6.6 Special precautions for disposal and other handling
For single use only. Discard any unused contents.

7. MARKETING AUTHORISATION HOLDER
Janssen-Cilag Limited
50-100 Holmers Farm Way
High Wycombe
Buckinghamshire
HP12 4EG
UK

8. MARKETING AUTHORISATION NUMBER(S)
PL 0242/0137

9. DATE OF FIRST AUTHORISATION/RENEWAL OF THE AUTHORISATION
Date of first Authorisation: 31/07/89
Date of Renewal: 23/06/05

10. DATE OF REVISION OF THE TEXT
10th July 2009

Rapilysin 10 U
(Actavis UK Ltd)

1. NAME OF THE MEDICINAL PRODUCT
Rapilysin 10 U powder and solvent for solution for injection.

2. QUALITATIVE AND QUANTITATIVE COMPOSITION
1 vial contains 10 U* reteplase ** in 0.56 g powder
1 prefilled syringe contains 10 ml water for injections.
The reconstituted solution contains 1 U reteplase per ml.
For a full list of excipients see section 6.1.
* Potency of reteplase is expressed in units (U) by using a reference standard which is specific for reteplase and is not comparable with units used for other thrombolytic agents.
** Recombinant plasminogen activator produced in Escherichia coli by recombinant DNA technology.

3. PHARMACEUTICAL FORM
Powder and solvent for solution for injection.
White powder and clear colourless liquid (water for injections).

4. CLINICAL PARTICULARS
4.1 Therapeutic indications
Rapilysin is indicated for the thrombolytic treatment of suspected myocardial infarction with persistent ST elevation or recent left Bundle Branch Block within 12 hours after the onset of acute myocardial infarction AMI symptoms.

4.2 Posology and method of administration
Treatment with reteplase should be initiated as soon as possible after the onset of AMI symptoms.

Rapilysin should be prescribed by physicians experienced in the use of thrombolytic treatment and with the facilities to monitor its use.

Reteplase is supplied as a freeze-dried substance in vials. The lyophilisate is reconstituted with the contents of the accompanying syringe (see section 6.6).

Rapilysin should be injected preferably through an intravenous line whose sole purpose is the injection of Rapilysin. No other medicines should be injected through the line reserved for Rapilysin, neither at the same time, nor prior to, nor following Rapilysin injection. This applies to all products including heparin, and acetylsalicylic acid, which should be administered before and following the administration of reteplase to reduce the risk of re-thrombosis.

In those patients where the same line has to be used, this line (including Y-line) must be flushed thoroughly with 0.9 % sodium chloride or 5 % dextrose solution prior to and following the Rapilysin injection.

Dosage of Rapilysin
Rapilysin is administered as a 10 U bolus dose followed by a second 10 U bolus dose 30 minutes later (double bolus).

Each bolus is administered as a slow intravenous injection within 2 minutes. Ensure that the injection is not mistakenly given paravenously.

Heparin and acetylsalicylic acid should be administered before and following the administration of Rapilysin to reduce the risk of rethrombosis.

Dosage of Heparin
The recommended dose of heparin is 5000 I.U. given as a bolus injection prior to reteplase therapy followed by an infusion of 1000 I.U. per hour starting after the second reteplase bolus. Heparin should be administered for at least 24 hours, preferably for 48 – 72 hours, aiming to keep aPTT values 1.5 to 2 times normal.

Dosage of Acetylsalicylic Acid
The initial dose of acetylsalicylic acid prior to thrombolysis should be at least 250 mg (250 – 350 mg) followed by 75 – 150 mg/day at least until discharge.

Use in children
There is no experience in children

4.3 Contraindications
Hypersensitivity to reteplase, polysorbate 80 or any of the other ingredients.

Because thrombolytic therapy increases the risk of bleeding, reteplase is contra-indicated in the following situations:

- known haemorrhagic diathesis
- patients with current concomitant therapy with oral anticoagulants (e.g. warfarin sodium)
- intracranial neoplasm, arteriovenous malformation or aneurysm
- neoplasm with increased bleeding risk
- history of cerebrovascular accident
- recent (< 10 days) prolonged and vigorous external heart massage
- severe uncontrolled hypertension
- active peptic ulceration
- portal hypertension (oesophageal varices)
- severe liver or renal dysfunction
- acute pancreatitis, pericarditis, bacterial endocarditis
- within 3 months of severe bleeding, major trauma or major surgery (e.g. coronary artery bypass graft, intracranial or intraspinal surgery or trauma), obstetrical delivery, organ biopsy, previous puncture of non-compressible vessels.

4.4 Special warnings and precautions for use
Each patient being considered for therapy with reteplase should be carefully evaluated.

For information on product incompatibilities see section 6.2

Bleeding
The most common complication encountered during reteplase therapy is bleeding. In the following conditions the risks of reteplase therapy may be increased and should be weighed against the anticipated benefits:

- cerebrovascular disease
- systolic blood pressure at entry > 160 mmHg
- recent gastrointestinal or genitourinary bleeding (within 10 days)
- high likelihood of left heart thrombus, e.g. mitral stenosis with atrial fibrillation
- septic thrombophlebitis or occluded arteriovenous cannula at seriously infected site
- age over 75 years
- any other condition in which bleeding constitutes a significant hazard or would be particularly difficult because of its location

The concomitant use of heparin anticoagulation may contribute to bleeding. As fibrin is lysed during reteplase therapy, bleeding from recent puncture sites may occur. Therefore, thrombolytic therapy requires careful attention to all possible bleeding sites (including catheter insertion sites, arterial and venous puncture sites, cut down sites and needle puncture sites). The use of rigid catheter as well as intramuscular injections and nonessential handling of the patient should be avoided during treatment with reteplase.

Caution should be employed when used with other medicinal products affecting haemostasis such as heparin, low-molecular-weight heparins, heparinoids, oral anticoagulants and antiplatelet agents other than acetylsalicylic acid, such as dipyridamole, ticlopidine, clopidogrel or glycoprotein IIb/IIIa receptor antagonists.

Should serious bleeding, in particular cerebral haemorrhage, occur any concomitant heparin should be terminated immediately. In addition, the second bolus of reteplase should not be given if the serious bleeding occurs before it is administered. In general, however, it is not necessary to replace the coagulation factors because of the relatively short half-life of reteplase. Most patients who have bleeding can be managed by interruption of thrombolytic and anticoagulant therapy, volume replacement and manual pressure applied to an incompetent vessel. Protamine should be considered if heparin has been administered within 4 hours of the onset of bleeding. In the patients who fail to respond to these conservative measures, judicious use of transfusion products may be indicated. Transfusions of cryoprecipitate, fibrinogen, fresh frozen plasma and platelets should be considered with clinical and laboratory reassessment after each administration. A target fibrinogen level of 1 g/l is desirable with cryoprecipitate or fibrinogen infusion.

At present, insufficient data in patients with a diastolic blood pressure > 100 mmHg prior to thrombolytic therapy are available for reteplase.

Arrhythmias

Coronary thrombolysis may result in arrhythmias associated with reperfusion. It is strongly recommended that antiarrhythmic therapy for bradycardia and/or ventricular tachyarrhythmias (e.g. ventricular tachycardia or fibrillation) be available when reteplase is administered.

Readministration

Since at present there is no experience with readministration of reteplase, the readministration is not recommended. However, no antibody formation to the reteplase molecule has been observed.

If an anaphylactoid reaction occurs, the injection should be discontinued immediately and appropriate therapy should be initiated.

4.5 Interaction with other medicinal products and other forms of interaction

No interaction studies with reteplase and medicinal product commonly administered in patients with AMI have been performed. Retrospective analyses of clinical studies did not reveal any clinically relevant interactions with medicinal product used concomitantly with reteplase in patients with acute myocardial infarction. Heparin, vitamin K antagonists and medicinal product that alter platelet function (such as acetylsalicylic acid, dipyridamole and abciximab) may increase the risk of bleeding if administered prior to, during or after reteplase therapy.

Attention should be paid to this effect especially during periods of low plasma fibrinogen (up to about 2 days after fibrinolytic therapy of AMI).

For information on product incompatibilities see section 4.2.

4.6 Pregnancy and lactation

There are no adequate data on the use of reteplase in pregnant women. The only relevant available animal data refer to studies performed in rabbits, which showed vaginal bleedings associated with abortions (see section 5.3) The potential risk for humans is unknown.

Except in life-threatening situations, Rapilysin should not be used in pregnant women.

It is not known whether reteplase is excreted into breast milk. Breast milk should be discarded within the first 24 hours after thrombolytic therapy.

4.7 Effects on ability to drive and use machines

Not relevant

4.8 Undesirable effects

The most commonly reported adverse drug reaction associated with reteplase treatment is haemorrhage, predominantly at the injection site. Local reactions at injection site can also occur.

As with other thrombolytic agents, recurrent ischaemia / angina, hypotension and heart failure / pulmonary oedema have been reported frequently as sequelae of myocardial infarction and / or thrombolytic administration.

The frequency of the adverse drug reactions is described using the following convention:

Very common $\geqslant$ 1/10

Common $\geqslant$ 1/100, < 1/10

Uncommon $\geqslant$ 1/1,000, < 1/100

Rare $\geqslant$ 1/10,000, < 1/1,000

Very rare < 1/10,000, (including isolated reports)

Haemorrhage

The most frequent adverse drug reaction associated with reteplase treatment is haemorrhage.

- very common: bleeding at the injection site (e.g. haematoma)
- common: as gastrointestinal (haematemesis, melena), gingival or genitourinary bleeding
- uncommon: haemopericardium, retroperitoneal bleeding, cerebral haemorrhage, epistaxis, haemoptysis, eye haemorrhage and ecchymosis were observed.

Reports of intracranial bleeding, many of which are fatal, are of particular concern.

Systolic blood pressure over 160 mmHg before thrombolysis with reteplase was associated with greater risk for cerebral bleeding. The risk of intracranial bleeding and fatal intracranial bleeding increases with increasing age. Blood transfusions were rarely required. Death and permanent disability are not uncommonly reported in patients who have experienced stroke (including intracranial bleeding) and other serious bleeding episodes.

Cardiovascular disorders

As with other thrombolytic agents, the following events have been reported as sequelae of myocardial infarction and / or thrombolytic administration.

- *very common*: recurrent ischaemia / angina, hypotension and heart failure / pulmonary oedema
- *common*: arrhythmias (e.g. AV block, atrial fibrillation / flutter, ventricular tachycardia / fibrillation, electromechanical dissociation (EMD)), cardiac arrest, cardiogenic shock and reinfarction
- *uncommon*: mitral regurgitation, pulmonary embolism, other systemic embolism / cerebral embolism and ventricular septal defect

These cardiovascular events can be life-threatening and may lead to death.

Nervous system disorders

- *uncommon:* cerebral haemorrhage was observed.
- very rare *:* events related to the nervous system (e.g. epileptic seizure, convulsion, aphasia, speech disorder, delirium, acute brain syndrome, agitation, confusion, depression, psychosis)

Ischaemic or haemorrhagic cerebrovascular events may be contributing or underlying conditions.

General disorders and administration site conditions

- *very common*: haemorrhage at the injection site (e.g. haematoma); a local reaction at injection site for example a burning sensation can occur.

Immune system disorders

- *uncommon*: hypersensitivity reactions (e.g. allergic reactions)
- *very rare*: serious anaphylaxis/ anaphylactoid reactions

Available evidence on reteplase does not indicate an antibody-mediated origin of these hypersensitivity reactions.

4.9 Overdose

In the event of overdosage one might expect depletion of fibrinogen and other blood coagulation components (e.g. coagulation factor V) with a consequent risk of bleeding.

For further information see section 4.4, section bleeding.

5. PHARMACOLOGICAL PROPERTIES

5.1 Pharmacodynamic properties

Pharmaco-therapeutic group: antithrombotic agent, ATC Code: **B01AD**

Reteplase is a recombinant plasminogen activator that catalyzes the cleavage of endogenous plasminogen to generate plasmin. This plasminogenolysis occurs preferentially in the presence of fibrin. Plasmin in turn degrades fibrin, which is the main component of the matrix of thrombi, thereby exerting its thrombolytic action.

Reteplase (10+10 U) dose-dependently reduces plasma fibrinogen levels by about 60 to 80 %. The fibrinogen level normalises within 2 days. As with other plasminogen activators a rebound phenomenon then occurs during which fibrinogen levels reach a maximum within 9 days and remain elevated for up to 18 days.

Reductions of plasma levels of plasminogen and α2-antiplasmin normalise within 1 to 3 days. Coagulation factor V, clotting factor VIII, α2-macroglobulin, and C1-esterase inhibitor are only slightly reduced and normalise within 1 to 2 days. Plasminogen activator inhibitor 1 (PAI-1) activity can be reduced to around zero, but rapidly normalises within two hours showing a rebound phenomenon. Prothrombin activation fragment 1 levels and thrombin-antithrombin III-complexes increase during thrombolysis indicating thrombin production of which the clinical relevance is unknown.

A large comparative mortality trial (INJECT) in approx. 6000 patients showed that reteplase reduced the incidence of heart failure (secondary efficacy criterion) in a significant manner and was at least equally effective in terms of reducing mortality (primary efficacy criterion) when compared to streptokinase. In two clinical trials aiming primarily at coronary artery patency (RAPID I and II) reteplase was associated with higher early patency rates (primary efficacy criterion), as well as with a lower incidence of heart failure (secondary efficacy criterion) than alteplase (3 hour and "accelerated" dosage regimens). A clinical trial in approximately 15 000 patients comparing reteplase with the accelerated dose regimen of alteplase (GUSTO III) (2:1 randomisation reteplase: alteplase) did not show statistically different results for the primary endpoint of 30-day mortality (reteplase: 7.47 %, alteplase 7.23 %, p = 0.61) or for the combined endpoint of 30-day mortality and non-fatal disabling stroke (reteplase: 7.89 %, alteplase 7.88 %, p = 0.99). Overall stroke rates were 1.64 % in the reteplase and 1.79 % in the alteplase group. In the reteplase group, 49.4 % of these strokes were fatal and 27.1 % were disabling. In the alteplase group 33.0 % were fatal and 39.8 % were disabling.

5.2 Pharmacokinetic properties

Following intravenous bolus injection of 10 + 10 U in patients with acute myocardial infarction reteplase antigen is distributed in plasma with a dominant half-life ($t1/2\alpha$) of 18±5 min and eliminated with a terminal half-life ($t1/2\beta$) of 5.5 hours±12.5 min at a clearance rate of 121±25 ml/min. Reteplase activity is cleared from the plasma at a rate of 283±101 ml/min, resulting in a dominant half-life ($t1/2\alpha$) of 14.6±6.7 min and a terminal half-life ($t1/2\beta$) of 1.6 hours±39 min. Only minor amounts of reteplase were immunologically detected in the urine. Exact data on the main elimination routes for reteplase in humans are not available and the consequences of hepatic or renal insufficiency are not known. Experiments in rats indicate that the liver and the kidneys are the main organs of active uptake and lysosomal degradation.

Additional studies in human plasma samples *in vitro* suggest that complexation with C1-inactivator, α2-antiplasmin and α2-antitrypsin contributes to the inactivation of reteplase in plasma. The relative contribution of the inhibitors to inactivation of reteplase decreases as follows: C1-inactivator > α2-antiplasmin > α2-antitrypsin.

The half-life of reteplase was increased in patients with AMI as compared to healthy volunteers. An additional increase of half-life of activity in patients with myocardial infarction and severely impaired liver and renal function cannot be excluded, but no clinical data of pharmacokinetics of reteplase in these patients are available. Animal data show that in case of severely impaired renal function with a pronounced increase in serum creatinine and serum urea an increase in half-life of reteplase has to be expected. Mild impairment of renal function did not significantly affect the pharmacokinetic properties of reteplase.

5.3 Preclinical safety data

Acute toxicity studies were performed in rats, rabbits and monkeys Subacute toxicity studies were performed in rats, dogs and monkeys. The predominant acute symptom after single high doses of reteplase in rats and rabbits was transient apathy shortly after injection. In cynomolgus monkeys, the sedative effect ranged from slight apathy to unconsciousness, caused by a reversible dose-related drop in blood pressure. There was increased local haemorrhage at the injection site.

Subacute toxicity studies did not reveal any unexpected adverse events. In dogs repeated dosing of the human peptide reteplase led to immunologic-allergic reactions. Genotoxicity of reteplase was excluded by a complete battery of tests at different genetic end points in vitro and in vivo.

Reproductive toxicity studies were performed in rats (fertility and embryo-foetotoxicity study including a littering phase) and in rabbits (embryo-foetotoxicity study, dose-range finding only). In rats, a species insensitive to the pharmacological effects of reteplase, there were no adverse effects on fertility, embryo-foetal development and offspring. In rabbits, vaginal bleedings and abortions possibly associated to prolonged haemostasis, but no foetal abnormalities were noted. A pre- and postnatal toxicity study was not performed with reteplase.

6. PHARMACEUTICAL PARTICULARS

6.1 List of excipients

Powder:

Tranexamic acid

di potassium-hydrogen phosphate

phosphoric acid

sucrose

Polysorbate 80

Solvent:

Water for injections

6.2 Incompatibilities

This medicinal product should not be mixed with Heparin and/or acetylsalicylic acid.

In the absence of compatibility studies with other medicinal products, this medicinal product must not be mixed with other medicinal products.

Heparin and Rapilysin are incompatible when combined in solution. Other incompatibilities may also exist. No other medicines should be added to the injection solution.

6.3 Shelf life

Shelf-life as package for sale:
3 years.

Reconstituted product:

Chemical and physical in-use stability has been demonstrated for 8 hours between 2° and 30 °C after dissolving with water for injection.

From a microbiological point of view, the product should be used immediately. If not used immediately, in-use storage times and conditions prior to use are the responsibility of the user.

6.4 Special precautions for storage

Do not store above 25 °C.

Keep the vial in the outer carton in order to protect from light.

For storage conditions of the reconstituted medicinal product, see section 6.3.

6.5 Nature and contents of container
Each pack contains:

2 colorless vials of 10 U of powder with a rubber closure

2 prefilled syringes with 10 ml solvent for single use 2 reconstitution **Spikes**

2 needles 19 G1

6.6 Special precautions for disposal and other handling
Incompatibility of some prefilled glass syringes (including Rapilysin) with certain needle free connectors has been reported. Therefore, the compatibility of the glass syringe and intravenous access should be ensured before use. In case of incompatibility an adaptor can be used and removed together with the glass syringe immediately after administration

Use aseptic technique throughout.

1. Remove the protective flip-cap from the vial of Rapilysin 10 U and clean the rubber closure with an alcohol wipe.

2. Open the package containing the reconstitution spike, remove both protective caps from the reconstitution spike.

3. Insert the spike through the rubber closure into the vial of Rapilysin 10 U.

4. Take the 10 ml syringe out of the package. Remove the tip cap from the syringe. Connect the syringe to the reconstitution spike and transfer the 10 ml of solvent into the vial of Rapilysin 10 U.

5. With the reconstitution spike and syringe still attached to the vial, swirl the vial gently to dissolve the Rapilysin 10 U powder. DO NOT SHAKE.

6. The reconstituted preparation results in a clear, colourless solution. If the solution is not clear and colourless it should be discarded.

7. Withdraw 10 ml of Rapilysin 10 U solution back into the syringe. A small amount of solution may remain in the vial due to overfill.

8. Disconnect the syringe from the reconstitution spike. The dose is now ready for intravenous administration

9. The reconstituted solution must be used immediately. Visual inspection of the solution is necessary after reconstitution. Only clear, colourless solutions should be injected. If the solution is not clear and colourless it should be discarded.

10. No other medicines should be injected through the line reserved for Rapilysin either at the same time, or prior to, or following Rapilysin injection. This applies to all products including heparin and acetylsalicylic acid, which should be administered before and following the administration of reteplase to reduce the risk of re-thrombosis

11. In those patients where the same line has to be used, this line (including Y-line) must be flushed thoroughly with a 0.9 % sodium chloride or 5 % dextrose solution prior to and following the Rapilysin injection (see section 4.2 Posology and method of administration).

Precaution for disposal:

Any unused product or waste material should be disposed of in accordance with local requirements.

7. MARKETING AUTHORISATION HOLDER
Actavis Group PTC ehf

Reykjavíkurvegi 76-78

220 Hafnarfjordur

Iceland.

8. MARKETING AUTHORISATION NUMBER(S)
EU/1/96/018/001

9. DATE OF FIRST AUTHORISATION/RENEWAL OF THE AUTHORISATION
Date of first authorisation: 29 August 1996

Date of last renewal: 29 August 2006

10. DATE OF REVISION OF THE TEXT

Rapitil Eye Drops

(sanofi-aventis)

1. NAME OF THE MEDICINAL PRODUCT
Rapitil™ Eye Drops

2. QUALITATIVE AND QUANTITATIVE COMPOSITION
Nedocromil sodium 2.0% w/v.

3. PHARMACEUTICAL FORM
Presented as a 5 ml sterile, preserved, aqueous solution containing 2% nedocromil sodium in a dropper bottle for administration to the eye.

4. CLINICAL PARTICULARS
4.1 Therapeutic indications
For the prevention, relief and treatment of allergic conjunctivitis, including seasonal allergic conjunctivitis, allergic conjunctivitis and vernal-kerato conjunctivitis.

4.2 Posology and method of administration
Adults (including the elderly) and children aged 6 years and over:

In seasonal allergic conjunctivitis: one drop into each eye twice daily, increasing when necessary to four times daily.

In seasonal allergic conjunctivitis therapy should be restricted to 12 weeks.

In vernal kerato-conjunctivitis: one drop into each eye four times daily.

Adults (including the elderly):

In perennial allergic conjunctivitis: one drop into each eye twice daily, increasing when necessary to four times daily.

Rapitil should be used regularly to ensure optimum control of symptoms.

There is only limited clinical trial evidence with Rapitil in children aged below 6 years, therefore use in this age range cannot be recommended.

4.3 Contraindications
Contraindicated in patients with known hypersensitivity to any constituent of the formulation.

4.4 Special warnings and precautions for use
Patients who use soft contact lenses should be advised not to wear them during the treatment period. In patients who continue to use hard or gas-permeable contact lenses during treatment with the eye drops, the lenses should be taken out of the eye prior to instillation and not inserted again for at least 10 minutes.

4.5 Interaction with other medicinal products and other forms of interaction
None has been reported.

4.6 Pregnancy and lactation
Studies in pregnant and lactating animals have failed to reveal a hazard with nedocromil sodium. However, as with all medications caution should be exercised during pregnancy (especially during the first trimester) and whilst breast feeding.

On the basis of animal studies and its physicochemical properties it is considered that only negligible amounts of nedocromil sodium may pass into human breast milk. There is no information to suggest that the use of nedocromil sodium by nursing mothers has any undesirable effects upon the baby.

4.7 Effects on ability to drive and use machines
No sedative effects have been reported.

4.8 Undesirable effects
Transient stinging and burning may occur after instillation. Other symptoms of local irritation have been reported rarely. Some patients have reported a distinctive taste.

4.9 Overdose
Animal studies have not shown evidence of toxic effects of nedocromil sodium even at high dosage, nor have extended human studies revealed any safety hazard with the drug. Overdosage is unlikely, therefore, to cause problems. However, if suspected, treatment should be supportive and directed to the control of the relevant symptoms.

5. PHARMACOLOGICAL PROPERTIES
5.1 Pharmacodynamic properties
Rapitil, the ophthalmic preparation of nedocromil sodium, displays specific anti-allergic and anti-inflammatory properties. Nedocromil sodium has been shown to prevent the release of inflammatory mediators from a range of inflammatory cell types.

5.2 Pharmacokinetic properties
Following topical ophthalmic administration, less than 4% of the dose is absorbed following multiple dosing. Absorption occurs primarily through the nasal mucosa as approximately 80% of the ophthalmic dose drains into the nose via the naso-lachrymal duct, although 1-2% of the dose may be absorbed orally.

Nedocromil sodium is reversibly bound to plasma proteins and is not metabolised, but is excreted unchanged in bile and urine. The drug is rapidly cleared from the plasma (plasma clearance 10.2 $\pm$ 1.3 ml/min/kg - elimination half-life 5.3 $\pm$ 0.9 min) and accumulation does not occur.

5.3 Preclinical safety data
Animal studies have failed to reveal toxic effects with nedocromil sodium even at high doses.

6. PHARMACEUTICAL PARTICULARS
6.1 List of excipients
benzalkonium chloride,

sodium chloride,

disodium edetate.

6.2 Incompatibilities
None known.

6.3 Shelf life
36 months.

6.4 Special precautions for storage
Store below 25°C, away from direct sunlight. Discard any remaining contents four weeks after opening the bottle.

6.5 Nature and contents of container
A plastic dropper bottle containing 5ml of sterile, aqueous solution for administration to the eye.

6.6 Special precautions for disposal and other handling
Please refer to enclosed package insert.

7. MARKETING AUTHORISATION HOLDER
Sanofi-aventis

One Onslow Street

Guildford

Surrey

GU1 4YS

UK

8. MARKETING AUTHORISATION NUMBER(S)
PL 04425/0285

9. DATE OF FIRST AUTHORISATION/RENEWAL OF THE AUTHORISATION
26 February 2004

10. DATE OF REVISION OF THE TEXT
December 2006

Legal category
POM

Rebif 22 micrograms solution for injection in pre-filled syringe

(Merck Serono)

1. NAME OF THE MEDICINAL PRODUCT
Rebif 22 micrograms solution for injection in pre-filled syringe

2. QUALITATIVE AND QUANTITATIVE COMPOSITION
Each pre-filled syringe (0.5 ml) contains 22 micrograms (6 MIU*) of interferon beta-1a**.

* Million International Units, measured by cytopathic effect (CPE) bioassay against the in-house IFN beta-1a standard which is calibrated against the current international NIH standard (GB-23-902-531).

** produced in Chinese hamster ovary Cells (CHO-K1) by recombinant DNA technology.

Excipient: 2.5 mg benzyl alcohol

For a full list of excipients, see section 6.1.

3. PHARMACEUTICAL FORM
Solution for injection in pre-filled syringe.

Clear to opalescent solution, with pH 3.5 to 4.5 and osmolarity 250 to 450 mOsm/l.

4. CLINICAL PARTICULARS
4.1 Therapeutic indications
Rebif is indicated for the treatment of relapsing multiple sclerosis.

In clinical trials, this was characterised by two or more acute exacerbations in the previous two years (see section 5.1).

Efficacy has not been demonstrated in patients with secondary progressive multiple sclerosis without ongoing relapse activity (see section 5.1).

4.2 Posology and method of administration
Treatment should be initiated under supervision of a physician experienced in the treatment of the disease.

Rebif is available in three strengths: 8.8 micrograms, 22 micrograms and 44 micrograms. For patients initiating treatment with Rebif, Rebif 8.8 micrograms and Rebif 22 micrograms are available in a package that corresponds to the patient needs for the first month of therapy.

The recommended posology of Rebif is 44 micrograms given three times per week by subcutaneous injection. A lower dose of 22 micrograms, also given three times per week by subcutaneous injection, is recommended for patients who cannot tolerate the higher dose in view of the treating specialist.

When first starting treatment with Rebif, the dose should be gradually escalated in order to allow tachyphylaxis to develop thus reducing adverse reactions. The Rebif initiation package corresponds to the patient needs for the first month of treatment.

Method of administration

Prior to injection and for an additional 24 hours after each injection, an antipyretic analgesic is advised to decrease flu-like symptoms associated with Rebif administration.

At the present time, it is not known for how long patients should be treated. Safety and efficacy with Rebif have not been demonstrated beyond 4 years of treatment. It is recommended that patients should be evaluated at least every second year in the 4-year period after initiation of treatment with Rebif and a decision for longer term treatment should then be made on an individual basis by the treating physician.

Paediatric use

No formal clinical trials or pharmacokinetic studies have been conducted in children or adolescents. However, limited published data suggest that the safety profile in adolescents from 12 to 16 years of age receiving Rebif 22 micrograms subcutaneously three times per week is similar to that seen in adults. There is very limited information on the use of Rebif in children under 12 years of age and therefore Rebif should not be used in this population.

4.3 Contraindications

• Initiation of treatment in pregnancy (see section 4.6).

• Hypersensitivity to natural or recombinant interferon-β, or to any excipients.

• Current severe depression and/or suicidal ideation (see sections 4.4 and 4.8).

4.4 Special warnings and precautions for use

Patients should be informed of the most frequent adverse reactions associated with interferon beta administration, including symptoms of the flu-like syndrome (see section 4.8). These symptoms tend to be most prominent at the initiation of therapy and decrease in frequency and severity with continued treatment.

Rebif should be administered with caution to patients with previous or current depressive disorders in particular to those with antecedents of suicidal ideation (see section 4.3). Depression and suicidal ideation are known to occur in increased frequency in the multiple sclerosis population and in association with interferon use. Patients treated with Rebif should be advised to immediately report any symptoms of depression and/or suicidal ideation to their prescribing physician. Patients exhibiting depression should be monitored closely during therapy with Rebif and treated appropriately. Cessation of therapy with Rebif should be considered (see sections 4.3 and 4.8).

Rebif should be administered with caution to patients with a history of seizures, to those receiving treatment with anti-epileptics, particularly if their epilepsy is not adequately controlled with anti-epileptics (see sections 4.5 and 4.8).

Patients with cardiac disease, such as angina, congestive heart failure or arrhythmia, should be closely monitored for worsening of their clinical condition during initiation of therapy with interferon beta-1a. Symptoms of the flu-like syndrome associated with interferon beta-1a therapy may prove stressful to patients with cardiac conditions.

Injection site necrosis (ISN) has been reported in patients using Rebif (see section 4.8). To minimise the risk of injection site necrosis patients should be advised to:

• use an aseptic injection technique,

• rotate the injection sites with each dose.

The procedure for the self-administration by the patient should be reviewed periodically especially if injection site reactions have occurred.

If the patient experiences any break in the skin, which may be associated with swelling or drainage of fluid from the injection site, the patient should be advised to consult with their physician before continuing injections with Rebif. If the patient has multiple lesions, Rebif should be discontinued until healing has occurred. Patients with single lesions may continue provided that the necrosis is not too extensive.

In clinical trials with Rebif, asymptomatic elevations of hepatic transaminases (particularly alanine aminotransferase (ALT)) were common and 1-3% of patients developed elevations of hepatic transaminases above 5 times the upper limit of normal (ULN). In the absence of clinical symptoms, serum ALT levels should be monitored prior to the start of therapy, at months 1, 3 and 6 on therapy and periodically thereafter. Dose reduction of Rebif should be considered if ALT rises above 5 times the ULN, and gradually re-escalated when enzyme levels have normalized. Rebif should be initiated with caution in patients with a history of significant liver disease, clinical evidence of active liver disease, alcohol abuse or increased serum ALT (>2.5 times ULN). Treatment with Rebif should be stopped if icterus or other clinical symptoms of liver dysfunction appear (see section 4.8).

Rebif, like other interferons beta, has a potential for causing severe liver injury (see section 4.8) including acute hepatic failure. The mechanism for the rare symptomatic hepatic dysfunction is not known. No specific risk factors have been identified.

Laboratory abnormalities are associated with the use of interferons. Therefore, in addition to those laboratory tests normally required for monitoring patients with multiple sclerosis, liver enzyme monitoring and complete and differential blood cell counts and platelet counts are recommended at regular intervals (1, 3 and 6 months) following introduction of Rebif therapy and then periodically thereafter in the absence of clinical symptoms.

Patients being treated with Rebif may occasionally develop new or worsening thyroid abnormalities. Thyroid function testing is recommended at baseline and if abnormal, every 6-12 months following initiation of therapy. If tests are normal at baseline, routine testing is not needed but should be performed if clinical findings of thyroid dysfunction appear (see section 4.8).

Caution should be used, and close monitoring considered when administering interferon beta-1a to patients with severe renal and hepatic failure and to patients with severe myelosuppression.

Serum neutralising antibodies against interferon beta-1a may develop. The precise incidence of antibodies is as yet uncertain. Clinical data suggest that after 24 to 48 months of treatment with Rebif 22 micrograms, approximately 24% of patients develop persistent serum antibodies to interferon beta-1a. The presence of antibodies has been shown to attenuate the pharmacodynamic response to interferon beta-1a (Beta-2 microglobulin and neopterin). Although the clinical significance of the induction of antibodies has not been fully elucidated, the development of neutralising antibodies is associated with reduced efficacy on clinical and MRI variables. If a patient responds poorly to therapy with Rebif, and has neutralising antibodies, the treating physician should reassess the benefit/risk ratio of continued Rebif therapy.

The use of various assays to detect serum antibodies and differing definitions of antibody positivity limits the ability to compare antigenicity among different products.

Only sparse safety and efficacy data are available from non-ambulatory patients with multiple sclerosis. Rebif has not yet been investigated in patients with primary progressive multiple sclerosis and should not be used in such patients.

This medicinal product contains 2.5 mg benzyl alcohol per dose. Must not be given to premature babies or neonates. May cause toxic reactions and anaphylactoid reactions in infants and children up to 3 years old.

4.5 Interaction with other medicinal products and other forms of interaction

No interaction studies have been performed with interferon beta-1a in humans.

Interferons have been reported to reduce the activity of hepatic cytochrome P450-dependent enzymes in humans and animals. Caution should be exercised when administering Rebif in combination with medicinal products that have a narrow therapeutic index and are largely dependent on the hepatic cytochrome P450 system for clearance, e.g. antiepileptics and some classes of antidepressants.

The interaction of Rebif with corticosteroids or adrenocorticotropic hormone (ACTH) has not been studied systematically. Clinical studies indicate that multiple sclerosis patients can receive Rebif and corticosteroids or ACTH during relapses.

4.6 Pregnancy and lactation

There is limited information on the use of Rebif in pregnancy. Available data indicates that there may be an increased risk of spontaneous abortion. Therefore initiation of treatment is contraindicated during pregnancy (see section 4.3).

Women of child-bearing potential should take appropriate contraceptive measures. If the patient becomes pregnant or plans to become pregnant while taking Rebif she should be informed of the potential hazards and discontinuation of therapy should be considered (see section 5.3). In patients with a high relapse rate before treatment has started, the risk of a severe relapse following discontinuation of Rebif in the event of pregnancy should be weighed against a possible increased risk of spontaneous abortion.

It is not known whether Rebif is excreted in human milk. Because of the potential for serious adverse reactions in breast-fed infants, a decision should be made whether to discontinue breast-feeding or Rebif therapy.

4.7 Effects on ability to drive and use machines

Central nervous system-related adverse events associated with the use of interferon beta (e.g. dizziness) might influence the patient's ability to drive or use machines (see section 4.8).

4.8 Undesirable effects

The highest incidence of adverse reactions associated with Rebif therapy is related to flu-like syndrome. Flu-like symptoms tend to be most prominent at the initiation of therapy and decrease in frequency with continued treatment. Approximately 70% of patients treated with Rebif can expect to experience the typical interferon flu-like syndrome within the first six months after starting treatment. Approximately 30% of patients will also experience reactions at the injection site, predominantly mild inflammation or erythema. Asymptomatic increases in laboratory parameters of hepatic function and decreases in white blood cells (WBC) are also common.

The majority of adverse reactions observed with IFN beta-1a are usually mild and reversible, and respond well to dose reductions. In case of severe or persistent undesirable effects, the dose of Rebif may be temporarily lowered or interrupted, at the discretion of the physician.

The adverse reactions reported below are classified according to frequency of occurrence as follows:

Very Common	≥ 1/10
Common	≥1/100 to <1/10
Uncommon	≥1/1,000 to <1/100
Rare	≥1/10,000 to <1/1,000
Very rare	<1/10,000
Not known	Cannot be estimated from the available data

Within each frequency grouping, undesirable effects are presented in order of decreasing seriousness.

The data presented is obtained from pooled clinical studies in multiple sclerosis (placebo=824 patients; Rebif 22 micrograms three times per week (TIW)=398 patients; Rebif 44 micrograms TIW=727 patients) and shows the frequency of adverse reactions observed at six months (excess over placebo). Adverse reactions are listed below by frequency of occurrence and by MedDRA System Organ Class.

(see Table 1 on next page)

Interferon beta has a potential for causing severe liver injury. The mechanism for the rare symptomatic hepatic dysfunction is not known. The majority of the cases of severe liver injury occurred within the first six months of treatment. No specific risk factors have been identified. Treatment with Rebif should be stopped if icterus or other clinical symptoms of liver dysfunction appear (see section 4.4).

The administration of interferons has been associated with anorexia, dizziness, anxiety, arrhythmias, vasodilation and palpitation, menorrhagia and metrorrhagia.

An increased formation of auto-antibodies may occur during treatment with interferon beta.

4.9 Overdose

In case of overdose, patients should be hospitalised for observation and appropriate supportive treatment should be given.

5. PHARMACOLOGICAL PROPERTIES

5.1 Pharmacodynamic properties

Pharmacotherapeutic group: Immunostimulants, Interferons, ATC code: L03AB07.

Interferons (IFNs) are a group of endogenous glycoproteins endowed with immunomodulatory, antiviral and antiproliferative properties.

Rebif (interferon beta-1a) shares the same amino acid sequence with endogenous human interferon beta. It is produced in mammalian cells (Chinese hamster ovary) and is therefore glycosylated like the natural protein.

The precise mechanism of action of Rebif in multiple sclerosis is still under investigation.

The safety and efficacy of Rebif has been evaluated in patients with relapsing-remitting multiple sclerosis at doses ranging from 11 to 44 micrograms (3-12 million IU), administered subcutaneously three times per week. At licensed posology, Rebif 22 micrograms has been demonstrated to decrease the incidence (approximately 30% over 2 years) and severity of clinical relapses in patients with at least 2 exacerbations in the previous 2 years and with an EDSS of 0-5.0 at entry. The proportion of patients with disability progression, as defined by at least one point increase in EDSS confirmed three months later, was reduced from 39% (placebo) to 30% (Rebif 22 micrograms). Over 4 years, the reduction in the mean exacerbation rate was 22% in patients treated with Rebif 22 micrograms, and 29% in patients treated with Rebif 44 micrograms group compared with a group of patients treated with placebo for 2 years and then either Rebif 22 or Rebif 44 micrograms for 2 years.

In a 3-year study in patients with secondary progressive multiple sclerosis (EDSS 3-6.5) with evidence of clinical progression in the preceding two years and who had not experienced relapses in the preceding 8 weeks, Rebif had no significant effect on progression of disability, but relapse rate was reduced by approximately 30%. If the patient population was divided into 2 subgroups (those with and those without relapses in the 2-year period prior to study entry), there was no effect on disability in patients without relapses, but in patients with relapses, the proportion with progression in disability at the end of the study was reduced from 70% (placebo) to 57% (Rebif 22 micrograms and 44 micrograms combined). These results obtained in a subgroup of patients a posteriori should be interpreted cautiously.

Rebif has not yet been investigated in patients with primary progressive multiple sclerosis, and should not be used in such patients.

5.2 Pharmacokinetic properties

In healthy volunteers after intravenous administration, interferon beta-1a exhibits a sharp multi-exponential decline, with serum levels proportional to the dose. The initial half-life is in the order of minutes and the terminal half-life is several hours, with the possible presence of a deep compartment. When administered by the subcutaneous or intramuscular routes, serum levels of interferon beta remain low, but are still measurable up to 12 to 24 hours post-dose. Subcutaneous and intramuscular administrations of Rebif produce equivalent exposure to interferon beta. Following a single 60 microgram dose, the maximum peak concentration, as measured by immunoassay, is around 6 to 10 IU/ml, occurring on average around 3 hours after the dose. After subcutaneous administration at the same dose repeated every 48 hours for 4 doses, a moderate accumulation occurs (about 2.5 × for AUC).

Regardless of the route of dosing, pronounced pharmacodynamic changes are associated with the administration of Rebif. After a single dose, intracellular and serum activity of 2-5A synthetase and serum concentrations of beta-2 microglobulin and neopterin increase within 24 hours, and start to decline within 2 days. Intramuscular and subcutaneous administrations produce fully superimposable responses. After repeated subcutaneous administration every 48 hours for 4 doses, these biological responses remain elevated, with no signs of tolerance development.

Table 1

System Organ Class	Very common	Common	Uncommon	Not known*
Infections and infestations			Injection site abscess	Injection site infections, including cellulitis
Blood and lymphatic system disorders	Neutropenia, lymphopenia, leucopenia, thrombocytopenia, anaemia			Thrombotic thrombocytopenic purpura/Haemolytic uremic syndrome
Endocrine Disorders			Thyroid dysfunction most often presenting as hypothyroidism or hyperthyroidism	
Psychiatric disorders		Depression, insomnia		Suicide attempt
Nervous system disorders	Headache			Seizures, transient neurological symptoms (i.e. hypoesthesia, muscle spasm, paraesthesia, difficulty in walking, musculoskeletal stiffness) that may mimic multiple sclerosis exacerbations
Eye disorders				Retinal vascular disorders (e.g. retinopathy, cotton wool spots and obstruction of retinal artery or vein)
Gastrointestinal disorders		Diarrhoea, vomiting, nausea		
Skin and subcutaneous tissue disorders		Pruritus, rash, erythematous rash, maculo-papular rash		Angioedema, urticaria, erythema multiforme, erythema multiforme-like skin reactions, Stevens-Johnson syndrome, hair loss
Musculoskeletal and connective tissue disorders		Myalgia, arthralgia		
General disorders and administration site conditions	Injection site inflammation, injection site reaction, influenza-like symptoms	Injection site pain, fatigue, rigors, fever	Injection site necrosis, injection site mass	
Investigations	Asymptomatic transaminase increase	Severe elevations of transaminase		
Respiratory, thoracic and mediastinal disorders				Dyspnoea
Immune system disorders				Anaphylactic reactions
Vascular disorders				Thromboembolic events
Hepatobiliary disorders				Hepatitis with or without icterus

*Adverse reactions identified during post marketing surveillance (frequency not known)

Interferon beta-1a is mainly metabolised and excreted by the liver and the kidneys.

5.3 Preclinical safety data

Non-clinical data reveal no special hazard for humans based on conventional studies of safety pharmacology, repeated-dose toxicity, and genotoxicity.

Rebif has not been investigated for carcinogenicity.

A study on embryo/foetal toxicity in monkeys showed no evidence of reproductive disturbances. Based on observations with other alpha and beta interferons, an increased risk of abortions cannot be excluded. No information is available on the effects of the interferon beta-1a on male fertility.

6. PHARMACEUTICAL PARTICULARS

6.1 List of excipients

Mannitol

Poloxamer 188

L-methionine

Benzyl alcohol

Sodium acetate

Acetic acid for pH adjustment

Sodium hydroxide for pH adjustment

Water for injections

6.2 Incompatibilities

Not applicable.

6.3 Shelf life

18 months.

6.4 Special precautions for storage

Store in a refrigerator (2°C – 8°C) away from the cooling element. Do not freeze. Store in the original package in order to protect from light.

6.5 Nature and contents of container

One ml type 1glass syringe, with a stainless steel needle, containing 0.5 ml solution.

Rebif 22 micrograms is available as a package of 1, 3 or 12 syringes.

Not all pack sizes may be marketed.

6.6 Special precautions for disposal and other handling

The solution for injection in a pre-filled syringe is ready for use. It may also be administered with a suitable auto-injector.

For single use only. Only clear to opalescent solution without particles should be used and without visible signs of deterioration.

Any unused product or waste material should be disposed of in accordance with local requirements.

7. MARKETING AUTHORISATION HOLDER

Merck Serono Europe Limited

56, Marsh Wall

London E14 9TP

United Kingdom

8. MARKETING AUTHORISATION NUMBER(S)

EU/1/98/063/001

EU/1/98/063/002

EU/1/98/063/003

9. DATE OF FIRST AUTHORISATION/RENEWAL OF THE AUTHORISATION

Date of first authorisation: 4th May 1998

Date of first renewal: 4th May 2003

Date of latest renewal: 4th May 2008

10. DATE OF REVISION OF THE TEXT

24th July 2009

Rebif 22 micrograms/0.5 ml solution for injection in cartridge

(Merck Serono)

1. NAME OF THE MEDICINAL PRODUCT

Rebif 22 micrograms/0.5 ml solution for injection in cartridge

2. QUALITATIVE AND QUANTITATIVE COMPOSITION

Each pre-filled cartridge contains 66 micrograms (18 MIU*) of interferon beta-1a** in 1.5 ml solution, corresponding to 44 micrograms/ml.

* Million International Units, measured by cytopathic effect (CPE) bioassay against the in-house IFN beta-1a standard which is calibrated against the current international NIH standard (GB-23-902-531).

** produced in Chinese hamster ovary Cells (CHO-K1) by recombinant DNA technology.

Excipient: 7.5 mg benzyl alcohol

For a full list of excipients, see section 6.1.

3. PHARMACEUTICAL FORM

Solution for injection in cartridge.

Clear to opalescent solution, with pH 3.7 to 4.1 and osmolarity 250 to 450 mOsm/l.

4. CLINICAL PARTICULARS

4.1 Therapeutic indications

Rebif is indicated for the treatment of relapsing multiple sclerosis.

In clinical trials, this was characterised by two or more acute exacerbations in the previous two years (see section 5.1).

Efficacy has not been demonstrated in patients with secondary progressive multiple sclerosis without ongoing relapse activity (see section 5.1).

4.2 Posology and method of administration

Treatment should be initiated under supervision of a physician experienced in the treatment of the disease.

The recommended posology of Rebif is 44 micrograms given three times per week by subcutaneous injection. A lower dose of 22 micrograms, also given three times per week by subcutaneous injection, is recommended for patients who cannot tolerate the higher dose in view of the treating specialist.

When first starting treatment with Rebif, the dose should be gradually escalated in order to allow tachyphylaxis to develop thus reducing adverse reactions. The Rebif initiation package corresponds to the patient needs for the first month of treatment.

Method of administration

Rebif solution for injection in cartridge is intended for multidose use and should only be used with the RebiSmart autoinjector device following adequate training of the patient and/or carer.

For administration, the instructions provided in the package leaflet and in the instruction manual provided with the RebiSmart autoinjector device should be followed.

Prior to injection and for an additional 24 hours after each injection, an antipyretic analgesic is advised to decrease flu-like symptoms associated with Rebif administration.

At the present time, it is not known for how long patients should be treated. Safety and efficacy with Rebif have not been demonstrated beyond 4 years of treatment. It is recommended that patients should be evaluated at least every second year in the 4-year period after initiation of treatment with Rebif and a decision for longer term treatment should then be made on an individual basis by the treating physician.

Paediatric use

No formal clinical trials or pharmacokinetic studies have been conducted in children or adolescents. However, limited published data suggest that the safety profile in adolescents from 12 to 16 years of age receiving Rebif 22 micrograms subcutaneously three times per week is similar to that seen in adults. There is very limited information on the use of Rebif in children under 12 years of age and therefore Rebif should not be used in this population.

4.3 Contraindications

- Initiation of treatment in pregnancy (see section 4.6).
- Hypersensitivity to natural or recombinant interferon-β, or to any excipients.
- Current severe depression and/or suicidal ideation (see sections 4.4 and 4.8).

4.4 Special warnings and precautions for use

Patients should be informed of the most frequent adverse reactions associated with interferon beta administration, including symptoms of the flu-like syndrome (see section 4.8). These symptoms tend to be most prominent at the initiation of therapy and decrease in frequency and severity with continued treatment.

Rebif should be administered with caution to patients with previous or current depressive disorders in particular to those with antecedents of suicidal ideation (see section 4.3). Depression and suicidal ideation are known to occur in increased frequency in the multiple sclerosis population and in association with interferon use. Patients treated with Rebif should be advised to immediately report any symptoms of depression and/or suicidal ideation to their prescribing physician. Patients exhibiting depression should be monitored closely during therapy with Rebif and treated appropriately. Cessation of therapy with Rebif should be considered (see sections 4.3 and 4.8).

Rebif should be administered with caution to patients with a history of seizures, to those receiving treatment with anti-epileptics, particularly if their epilepsy is not adequately controlled with anti-epileptics (see sections 4.5 and 4.8).

Patients with cardiac disease, such as angina, congestive heart failure or arrhythmia, should be closely monitored for worsening of their clinical condition during initiation of therapy with interferon beta-1a. Symptoms of the flu-like syndrome associated with interferon beta-1a therapy may prove stressful to patients with cardiac conditions.

Injection site necrosis (ISN) has been reported in patients using Rebif (see section 4.8). To minimise the risk of injection site necrosis patients should be advised to:

- use an aseptic injection technique,
- rotate the injection sites with each dose.

The procedure for the self-administration by the patient should be reviewed periodically especially if injection site reactions have occurred.

If the patient experiences any break in the skin, which may be associated with swelling or drainage of fluid from the injection site, the patient should be advised to consult with their physician before continuing injections with Rebif. If the patient has multiple lesions, Rebif should be discontinued until healing has occurred. Patients with single lesions may continue provided that the necrosis is not too extensive.

In clinical trials with Rebif, asymptomatic elevations of hepatic transaminases (particularly alanine aminotransferase (ALT)) were common and 1-3% of patients developed elevations of hepatic transaminases above 5 times the upper limit of normal (ULN). In the absence of clinical symptoms, serum ALT levels should be monitored prior to the start of therapy, at months 1, 3 and 6 on therapy and periodically thereafter. Dose reduction of Rebif should be considered if ALT rises above 5 times the ULN, and gradually re-escalated when enzyme levels have normalized. Rebif should be initiated with caution in patients with a history of significant liver disease, clinical evidence of active liver disease, alcohol abuse or increased serum ALT (>2.5 times ULN). Treatment with Rebif should be stopped if icterus or other clinical symptoms of liver dysfunction appear (see section 4.8).

Rebif, like other interferons beta, has a potential for causing severe liver injury (see section 4.8) including acute hepatic failure. The mechanism for the rare symptomatic hepatic dysfunction is not known. No specific risk factors have been identified.

Laboratory abnormalities are associated with the use of interferons. Therefore, in addition to those laboratory tests normally required for monitoring patients with multiple sclerosis, liver enzyme monitoring and complete and differential blood cell counts and platelet counts are recommended at regular intervals (1, 3 and 6 months) following introduction of Rebif therapy and then periodically thereafter in the absence of clinical symptoms.

Patients being treated with Rebif may occasionally develop new or worsening thyroid abnormalities. Thyroid function testing is recommended at baseline and if abnormal, every 6-12 months following initiation of therapy. If tests are normal at baseline, routine testing is not needed but should be performed if clinical findings of thyroid dysfunction appear (see section 4.8).

Caution should be used, and close monitoring considered when administering interferon beta-1a to patients with severe renal and hepatic failure and to patients with severe myelosuppression.

Serum neutralising antibodies against interferon beta-1a may develop. The precise incidence of antibodies is as yet uncertain. Clinical data suggest that after 24 to 48 months of treatment with Rebif 22 micrograms, approximately 24% of patients develop persistent serum antibodies to interferon beta-1a. The presence of antibodies has been shown to attenuate the pharmacodynamic response to interferon beta-1a (Beta-2 microglobulin and neopterin). Although the clinical significance of the induction of antibodies has not been fully elucidated, the development of neutralising antibodies is associated with reduced efficacy on clinical and MRI variables. If a patient responds poorly to therapy with Rebif, and has neutralising antibodies, the treating physician should reassess the benefit/risk ratio of continued Rebif therapy.

The use of various assays to detect serum antibodies and differing definitions of antibody positivity limits the ability to compare antigenicity among different products.

Only sparse safety and efficacy data are available from non-ambulatory patients with multiple sclerosis. Rebif has not yet been investigated in patients with primary progressive multiple sclerosis and should not be used in such patients.

This medicinal product contains 2.5 mg benzyl alcohol per dose of 0.5 ml. Must not be given to premature babies or neonates. May cause toxic reactions and anaphylactoid reactions in infants and children up to 3 years old.

4.5 Interaction with other medicinal products and other forms of interaction

No interaction studies have been performed with interferon beta-1a in humans.

Interferons have been reported to reduce the activity of hepatic cytochrome P450-dependent enzymes in humans and animals. Caution should be exercised when administering Rebif in combination with medicinal products that have a narrow therapeutic index and are largely dependent on the hepatic cytochrome P450 system for clearance, e.g. antiepileptics and some classes of antidepressants.

The interaction of Rebif with corticosteroids or adrenocorticotropic hormone (ACTH) has not been studied systematically. Clinical studies indicate that multiple sclerosis patients can receive Rebif and corticosteroids or ACTH during relapses.

4.6 Pregnancy and lactation

There is limited information on the use of Rebif in pregnancy. Available data indicates that there may be an increased risk of spontaneous abortion. Therefore initiation of treatment is contraindicated during pregnancy (see section 4.3).

Women of child-bearing potential should take appropriate contraceptive measures. If the patient becomes pregnant or plans to become pregnant while taking Rebif she should be informed of the potential hazards and discontinuation of therapy should be considered (see section 5.3). In patients with a high relapse rate before treatment has started, the risk of a severe relapse following discontinuation of Rebif in the event of pregnancy should be weighed against a possible increased risk of spontaneous abortion.

It is not known whether Rebif is excreted in human milk. Because of the potential for serious adverse reactions in breast-fed infants, a decision should be made whether to discontinue breast-feeding or Rebif therapy.

4.7 Effects on ability to drive and use machines

Central nervous system-related adverse events associated with the use of interferon beta (e.g. dizziness) might influence the patient's ability to drive or use machines (see section 4.8).

4.8 Undesirable effects

The highest incidence of adverse reactions associated with Rebif therapy is related to flu-like syndrome. Flu-like symptoms tend to be most prominent at the initiation of therapy and decrease in frequency with continued treatment. Approximately 70% of patients treated with Rebif can expect to experience the typical interferon flu-like syndrome within the first six months after starting treatment. Approximately 30% of patients will also experience reactions at the injection site, predominantly mild inflammation or erythema. Asymptomatic increases in laboratory parameters of hepatic function and decreases in white blood cells (WBC) are also common.

The majority of adverse reactions observed with IFN beta-1a are usually mild and reversible, and respond well to dose reductions. In case of severe or persistent undesirable effects, the dose of Rebif may be temporarily lowered or interrupted, at the discretion of the physician.

The adverse reactions reported below are classified according to frequency of occurrence as follows:

Very Common	⩾1/10
Common	⩾1/100 to <1/10
Uncommon	⩾1/1,000 to <1/100
Rare	⩾1/10,000 to <1/1,000
Very rare	<1/10,000
Not known	Cannot be estimated from the available data

Within each frequency grouping, undesirable effects are presented in order of decreasing seriousness.

The data presented is obtained from pooled clinical studies in multiple sclerosis (placebo=824 patients; Rebif 22 micrograms three times per week (TIW)=398 patients; Rebif 44 micrograms TIW=727 patients) and shows the frequency of adverse reactions observed at six months (excess over placebo). Adverse reactions are listed below by frequency of occurrence and by MedDRA System Organ Class.

(see Table 1 on next page)

Interferon beta has a potential for causing severe liver injury. The mechanism for the rare symptomatic hepatic dysfunction is not known. The majority of the cases of severe liver injury occurred within the first six months of treatment. No specific risk factors have been identified. Treatment with Rebif should be stopped if icterus or other clinical symptoms of liver dysfunction appear (see section 4.4).

The administration of interferons has been associated with anorexia, dizziness, anxiety, arrhythmias, vasodilation and palpitation, menorrhagia and metrorrhagia.

An increased formation of auto-antibodies may occur during treatment with interferon beta.

4.9 Overdose

In case of overdose, patients should be hospitalised for observation and appropriate supportive treatment should be given.

5. PHARMACOLOGICAL PROPERTIES

5.1 Pharmacodynamic properties

Pharmacotherapeutic group: Immunostimulants, Interferon, ATC code: L03AB07.

Interferons (IFNs) are a group of endogenous glycoproteins endowed with immunomodulatory, antiviral and antiproliferative properties.

Rebif (interferon beta-1a) shares the same amino acid sequence with endogenous human interferon beta. It is produced in mammalian cells (Chinese hamster ovary) and is therefore glycosylated like the natural protein.

The precise mechanism of action of Rebif in multiple sclerosis is still under investigation.

The safety and efficacy of Rebif has been evaluated in patients with relapsing-remitting multiple sclerosis at doses ranging from 11 to 44 micrograms (3-12 million IU), administered subcutaneously three times per week. At licensed posology, Rebif 22 micrograms has been demonstrated to decrease the incidence (approximately 30% over 2 years) and severity of clinical relapses in patients with at least 2 exacerbations in the previous 2 years and with an EDSS of 0-5.0 at entry. The proportion of patients with disability progression, as defined by at least one point increase in EDSS confirmed three months later, was reduced from 39% (placebo) to 30% (Rebif 22 micrograms). Over 4 years, the reduction in the mean exacerbation rate was 22% in patients treated with Rebif 22 micrograms, and 29% in patients treated with Rebif 44 micrograms group compared with a group of patients treated with placebo for 2 years and then either Rebif 22 or Rebif 44 micrograms for 2 years.

In a 3-year study in patients with secondary progressive multiple sclerosis (EDSS 3-6.5) with evidence of clinical progression in the preceding two years and who had not experienced relapses in the preceding 8 weeks, Rebif had no significant effect on progression of disability, but relapse rate was reduced by approximately 30%. If the patient population was divided into 2 subgroups (those with and those without relapses in the 2-year period prior to study entry), there was no effect on disability in patients without relapses, but in patients with relapses, the proportion with progression in disability at the end of the study was reduced from 70% (placebo) to 57% (Rebif 22 micrograms and 44 micrograms combined). These results obtained in a subgroup of patients a posteriori should be interpreted cautiously.

Rebif has not yet been investigated in patients with primary progressive multiple sclerosis, and should not be used in such patients.

5.2 Pharmacokinetic properties

In healthy volunteers after intravenous administration, interferon beta-1a exhibits a sharp multi-exponential decline, with serum levels proportional to the dose. The initial half-life is in the order of minutes and the terminal half-life is several hours, with the possible presence of a deep compartment. When administered by the subcutaneous or intramuscular routes, serum levels of interferon beta remain low, but are still measurable up to 12 to 24 hours post-dose. Subcutaneous and intramuscular administrations of Rebif produce equivalent exposure to interferon beta. Following a single 60 microgram dose, the maximum peak concentration, as measured by immunoassay, is around 6 to 10 IU/ml, occurring on average around 3 hours after the dose. After subcutaneous administration at the same dose repeated every 48 hours for 4 doses, a moderate accumulation occurs (about 2.5 × for AUC).

Regardless of the route of dosing, pronounced pharmacodynamic changes are associated with the administration of Rebif. After a single dose, intracellular and serum activity of 2-5A synthetase and serum concentrations of beta-2 microglobulin and neopterin increase within 24 hours, and start to decline within 2 days. Intramuscular and subcutaneous administrations produce fully superimposable responses. After repeated subcutaneous administration every 48 hours for 4 doses, these biological responses remain elevated, with no signs of tolerance development.

Interferon beta-1a is mainly metabolised and excreted by the liver and the kidneys.

5.3 Preclinical safety data

Non-clinical data reveal no special hazard for humans based on conventional studies of safety pharmacology, repeated-dose toxicity, and genotoxicity.

Rebif has not been investigated for carcinogenicity.

Table 1

System Organ Class	Very common	Common	Uncommon	*Not known
Infections and infestations			Injection site abscess	Injection site infections, including cellulitis
Blood and lymphatic system disorders	Neutropenia, lymphopenia, leucopenia, thrombocytopenia, anaemia			Thrombotic thrombocytopenic purpura/Haemolytic uremic syndrome
Endocrine Disorders			Thyroid dysfunction most often presenting as hypothyroidism or hyperthyroidism	
Psychiatric disorders		Depression, insomnia		Suicide attempt
Nervous system disorders	Headache			Seizures, transient neurological symptoms (i.e. hypoesthesia, muscle spasm, paraesthesia, difficulty in walking, musculoskeletal stiffness) that may mimic multiple sclerosis exacerbations
Eye disorders				Retinal vascular disorders (e.g. retinopathy, cotton wool spots and obstruction of retinal artery or vein)
Gastrointestinal disorders		Diarrhoea, vomiting, nausea		
Skin and subcutaneous tissue disorders		Pruritus, rash, erythematous rash, maculo-papular rash		Angioedema, urticaria, erythema multiforme, erythema multiforme-like skin reactions, Stevens-Johnson syndrome, hair loss
Musculoskeletal and connective tissue disorders		Myalgia, arthralgia		
General disorders and administration site conditions	Injection site inflammation, injection site reaction, influenza-like symptoms	Injection site pain, fatigue, rigors, fever	Injection site necrosis, injection site mass	
Investigations	Asymptomatic transaminase increase	Severe elevations of transaminase		
Respiratory, thoracic and mediastinal disorders				Dyspnoea
Immune system disorders				Anaphylactic reactions
Vascular disorders				Thromboembolic events
Hepatobiliary disorders				Hepatitis with or without icterus

*Adverse reactions identified during post marketing surveillance (frequency not known)

A study on embryo/foetal toxicity in monkeys showed no evidence of reproductive disturbances. Based on observations with other alpha and beta interferons, an increased risk of abortions cannot be excluded. No information is available on the effects of the interferon beta-1a on male fertility.

6. PHARMACEUTICAL PARTICULARS

6.1 List of excipients

Mannitol

Poloxamer 188

L-methionine

Benzyl alcohol

Sodium acetate

Acetic acid for pH adjustment

Sodium hydroxide for pH adjustment

Water for injections

6.2 Incompatibilities

Not applicable.

6.3 Shelf life

18 months.

After first injection use within 28 days.

6.4 Special precautions for storage

Store in a refrigerator (2°C – 8°C) away from the cooling element. Do not freeze. Store the cartridge in the original package in order to protect from light.

The RebiSmart autoinjector device containing a pre-filled cartridge of Rebif must be stored in the device storage box in a refrigerator (2°C – 8°C).

Should refrigeration be temporarily unavailable, Rebif can be stored by the patient at or below 25°C for up to 14 days then put back in the refrigerator and used before the expiry date.

6.5 Nature and contents of container

Cartridges (type 1 glass) with a plunger stopper (rubber) and crimp cap (aluminium and halobutyl rubber) containing 1.5 ml solution for injection.

Pack size of 4 cartridges.

6.6 Special precautions for disposal and other handling

The solution for injection in a pre-filled cartridge is ready for use with the RebiSmart autoinjector device. For storage of the autoinjector device with the cartridge, see section 6.4.

For multidose use. Only clear to opalescent solution without particles should be used and without visible signs of deterioration.

Any unused product or waste material should be disposed of in accordance with local requirements.

7. MARKETING AUTHORISATION HOLDER

Merck Serono Europe Limited

56, Marsh Wall

London E14 9TP

United Kingdom

8. MARKETING AUTHORISATION NUMBER(S)

EU/1/98/063/008

9. DATE OF FIRST AUTHORISATION/RENEWAL OF THE AUTHORISATION

Date of first authorisation: 4th May 1998

Date of first renewal: 4th May 2003

Date of latest renewal: 4th May 2008

10. DATE OF REVISION OF THE TEXT

24th July 2009

Rebif 44 micrograms solution for injection in pre-filled syringe

(Merck Serono)

1. NAME OF THE MEDICINAL PRODUCT

Rebif 44 micrograms solution for injection in pre-filled syringe

2. QUALITATIVE AND QUANTITATIVE COMPOSITION

Each pre-filled syringe (0.5 ml) contains 44 micrograms (12 MIU*) of interferon beta-1a**.

* Million International Units, measured by cytopathic effect (CPE) bioassay against the in house IFN beta-1a standard which is calibrated against the current international NIH standard (GB-23-902-531).

** produced in Chinese hamster ovary Cells (CHO-K1) by recombinant DNA technology.

Excipient: 2.5 mg benzyl alcohol

For a full list of excipients, see section 6.1.

3. PHARMACEUTICAL FORM

Solution for injection in pre-filled syringe.

Clear to opalescent solution, with pH 3.5 to 4.5 and osmolarity 250 to 450 mOsm/l.

4. CLINICAL PARTICULARS

4.1 Therapeutic indications

Rebif is indicated for the treatment of relapsing multiple sclerosis.

In clinical trials, this was characterised by two or more acute exacerbations in the previous two years (see section 5.1).

Efficacy has not been demonstrated in patients with secondary progressive multiple sclerosis without ongoing relapsing activity (see section 5.1).

4.2 Posology and method of administration

Treatment should be initiated under supervision of a physician experienced in the treatment of the disease.

Rebif is available in three strengths: 8.8 micrograms, 22 micrograms and 44 micrograms. For patients initiating treatment with Rebif, Rebif 8.8 micrograms and Rebif 22 micrograms are available in a package that corresponds to the patient needs for the first month of therapy.

The recommended posology of Rebif is 44 micrograms given three times per week by subcutaneous injection. A lower dose of 22 micrograms, also given three times per week by subcutaneous injection, is recommended for patients who cannot tolerate the higher dose in view of the treating specialist.

When first starting treatment with Rebif, the dose should be gradually escalated in order to allow tachyphylaxis to develop thus reducing adverse reactions. The Rebif initiation package corresponds to the patient needs for the first month of treatment.

Method of administration

Prior to injection and for an additional 24 hours after each injection, an antipyretic analgesic is advised to decrease flu-like symptoms associated with Rebif administration.

At the present time, it is not known for how long patients should be treated. Safety and efficacy with Rebif have not been demonstrated beyond 4 years of treatment. It is recommended that patients should be evaluated at least every second year in the 4-year period after initiation of treatment with Rebif and a decision for longer term treatment should then be made on an individual basis by the treating physician.

Paediatric use

No formal clinical trials or pharmacokinetic studies have been conducted in children or adolescents. However, limited published data suggest that the safety profile in adolescents from 12 to 16 years of age receiving Rebif 22 micrograms subcutaneous three times per week is similar to that seen in adults. There is very limited information on the use of Rebif in children under 12 years of age and therefore Rebif should not be used in this population.

4.3 Contraindications

- Initiation of treatment in pregnancy (see section 4.6).
- Hypersensitivity to natural or recombinant interferon-β, or to any excipients.
- Current severe depression and/or suicidal ideation (see sections 4.4 and 4.8).

4.4 Special warnings and precautions for use

Patients should be informed of the most frequent adverse reactions associated with interferon beta administration, including symptoms of the flu-like syndrome (see section 4.8). These symptoms tend to be most prominent at the initiation of therapy and decrease in frequency and severity with continued treatment.

Rebif should be administered with caution to patients with previous or current depressive disorders in particular to those with antecedents of suicidal ideation (see section 4.3). Depression and suicidal ideation are known to occur in increased frequency in the multiple sclerosis population and in association with interferon use. Patients treated with Rebif should be advised to immediately report any symptoms of depression and/or suicidal ideation to their prescribing physician. Patients exhibiting depression should be monitored closely during therapy with Rebif and treated appropriately. Cessation of therapy with Rebif should be considered (see sections 4.3 and 4.8).

Rebif should be administered with caution to patients with a history of seizures, to those receiving treatment with anti-epileptics, particularly if their epilepsy is not adequately controlled with anti-epileptics (see sections 4.5 and 4.8).

Patients with cardiac disease, such as angina, congestive heart failure or arrhythmia, should be closely monitored for worsening of their clinical condition during initiation of therapy with interferon beta-1a. Symptoms of the flu-like syndrome associated with interferon beta-1a therapy may prove stressful to patients with cardiac conditions.

Injection site necrosis (ISN) has been reported in patients using Rebif (see section 4.8). To minimise the risk of injection site necrosis patients should be advised to:

- use an aseptic injection technique,
- rotate the injection sites with each dose.

The procedure for the self-administration by the patient should be reviewed periodically especially if injection site reactions have occurred.

If the patient experiences any break in the skin, which may be associated with swelling or drainage of fluid from the injection site, the patient should be advised to consult with their physician before continuing injections with Rebif. If the patient has multiple lesions, Rebif should be discontinued until healing has occurred. Patients with single lesions may continue provided that the necrosis is not too extensive.

In clinical trials with Rebif, asymptomatic elevations of hepatic transaminases (particularly alanine aminotransferase (ALT)) were common and 1-3% of patients developed elevations of hepatic transaminases above 5 times the upper limit of normal (ULN). In the absence of clinical symptoms, serum ALT levels should be monitored prior to the start of therapy, at months 1, 3 and 6 on therapy and periodically thereafter. Dose reduction of Rebif should be considered if ALT rises above 5 times the ULN, and gradually re-escalated when enzyme levels have normalized. Rebif should be initiated with caution in patients with a history of significant liver disease, clinical evidence of active liver disease, alcohol abuse or increased serum ALT (>2.5 times ULN). Treatment with Rebif should be stopped if icterus or other clinical symptoms of liver dysfunction appear (see section 4.8).

Rebif, like other interferons beta, has a potential for causing severe liver injury (see section 4.8) including acute hepatic failure. The mechanism for the rare symptomatic hepatic dysfunction is not known. No specific risk factors have been identified.

Laboratory abnormalities are associated with the use of interferons. The overall incidence of these is slightly higher with Rebif 44 than Rebif 22 micrograms. Therefore, in addition to those laboratory tests normally required for monitoring patients with multiple sclerosis, liver enzyme monitoring and complete and differential blood cell counts and platelet counts are recommended at regular intervals (1, 3 and 6 months) following introduction of Rebif therapy and then periodically thereafter in the absence of clinical symptoms. These should be more frequent when initiating Rebif 44 micrograms.

Patients being treated with Rebif may occasionally develop new or worsening thyroid abnormalities. Thyroid function testing is recommended at baseline and if abnormal, every 6-12 months following initiation of therapy. If tests are normal at baseline, routine testing is not needed but should be performed if clinical findings of thyroid dysfunction appear (see section 4.8).

Caution should be used, and close monitoring considered when administering interferon beta-1a to patients with severe renal and hepatic failure and to patients with severe myelosuppression.

Serum neutralising antibodies against interferon beta-1a may develop. The precise incidence of antibodies is as yet uncertain. Clinical data suggest that after 24 to 48 months of treatment with Rebif 44 micrograms, approximately 13 to 14% of patients develop persistent serum antibodies to interferon beta-1a. The presence of antibodies has been shown to attenuate the pharmacodynamic response to interferon beta-1a (Beta-2 microglobulin and neopterin). Although the clinical significance of the induction of antibodies has not been fully elucidated, the development of neutralising antibodies is associated with reduced efficacy on clinical and MRI variables. If a patient responds poorly to therapy with Rebif, and has neutralising antibodies, the treating physician should reassess the benefit/risk ratio of continued Rebif therapy.

The use of various assays to detect serum antibodies and differing definitions of antibody positivity limits the ability to compare antigenicity among different products.

Only sparse safety and efficacy data are available from non-ambulatory patients with multiple sclerosis. Rebif has not yet been investigated in patients with primary progressive multiple sclerosis and should not be used in such patients.

This medicinal product contains 2.5 mg benzyl alcohol per dose. Must not be given to premature babies or neonates. May cause toxic reactions and anaphylactoid reactions in infants and children up to 3 years old.

4.5 Interaction with other medicinal products and other forms of interaction

No interaction studies have been performed with interferon beta-1a in humans.

Interferons have been reported to reduce the activity of hepatic cytochrome P450-dependent enzymes in humans and animals. Caution should be exercised when administering Rebif in combination with medicinal products that have a narrow therapeutic index and are largely dependent on the hepatic cytochrome P450 system for clearance, e.g. antiepileptics and some classes of antidepressants.

The interaction of Rebif with corticosteroids or adrenocorticotropic hormone (ACTH) has not been studied systematically. Clinical studies indicate that multiple sclerosis patients can receive Rebif and corticosteroids or ACTH during relapses.

4.6 Pregnancy and lactation

There is limited information on the use of Rebif in pregnancy. Available data indicates that there may be an increased risk of spontaneous abortion. Therefore initiation of treatment is contraindicated during pregnancy (see section 4.3).

Women of child-bearing potential should take appropriate contraceptive measures. If the patient becomes pregnant or plans to become pregnant while taking Rebif she should be informed of the potential hazards and discontinuation of therapy should be considered (see section 5.3). In patients with a high relapse rate before treatment has started, the risk of a severe relapse following discontinuation of Rebif in the event of pregnancy should be weighed against a possible increased risk of spontaneous abortion.

It is not known whether Rebif is excreted in human milk. Because of the potential for serious adverse reactions in breast-fed infants, a decision should be made whether to discontinue breast-feeding or Rebif therapy.

4.7 Effects on ability to drive and use machines

Central nervous system-related adverse events associated with the use of interferon beta (e.g. dizziness) might influence the patient's ability to drive or use machines (see section 4.8).

4.8 Undesirable effects

The highest incidence of adverse reactions associated with Rebif therapy is related to flu-like syndrome. Flu-like symptoms tend to be most prominent at the initiation of therapy and decrease in frequency with continued treatment. Approximately 70% of patients treated with Rebif can expect to experience the typical interferon flu-like syndrome within the first six months after starting treatment. Approximately 30% of patients will also experience reactions at the injection site, predominantly mild inflammation or erythema. Asymptomatic increases in laboratory parameters of hepatic function and decreases in white blood cells (WBC) are also common.

The majority of adverse reactions observed with IFN beta-1a are usually mild and reversible, and respond well to dose reductions. In case of severe or persistent undesirable effects, the dose of Rebif may be temporarily lowered or interrupted, at the discretion of the physician.

The adverse reactions reported below are classified according to frequency of occurrence as follows:

Very Common	⩾ 1/10
Common	⩾1/100 to <1/10
Uncommon	⩾1/1,000 to <1/100
Rare	⩾1/10,000 to <1/1,000
Very rare	<1/10,000
Not known	Cannot be estimated from the available data

Within each frequency grouping, undesirable effects are presented in order of decreasing seriousness.

The data presented is obtained from pooled clinical studies in multiple sclerosis (placebo=824 patients; Rebif 22 micrograms three times per week (TIW)=398 patients; Rebif 44 micrograms TIW=727 patients) and shows the frequency of adverse reactions observed at six months (excess over placebo). Adverse reactions are listed below by frequency of occurrence and by MedDRA System Organ Class.

(see Table 1 on next page)

Interferon beta has a potential for causing severe liver injury. The mechanism for the rare symptomatic hepatic dysfunction is not known. The majority of the cases of severe liver injury occurred within the first six months of treatment. No specific risk factors have been identified. Treatment with Rebif should be stopped if icterus or other clinical symptoms of liver dysfunction appear (see section 4.4).

The administration of interferons has been associated with anorexia, dizziness, anxiety, arrhythmias, vasodilation and palpitation, menorrhagia and metrorrhagia.

An increased formation of auto-antibodies may occur during treatment with interferon beta.

4.9 Overdose

In case of overdose, patients should be hospitalised for observation and appropriate supportive treatment should be given.

5. PHARMACOLOGICAL PROPERTIES

5.1 Pharmacodynamic properties

Pharmacotherapeutic group: Immunostimulants, Interferons, ATC code: L03AB07.

Interferons (IFNs) are a group of endogenous glycoproteins endowed with immunomodulatory, antiviral and antiproliferative properties.

Rebif (interferon beta-1a) shares the same amino acid sequence with endogenous human interferon beta. It is produced in mammalian cells (Chinese hamster ovary) and is therefore glycosylated like the natural protein.

The precise mechanism of action of Rebif in multiple sclerosis is still under investigation.

The safety and efficacy of Rebif has been evaluated in patients with relapsing-remitting multiple sclerosis at doses ranging from 11 to 44 micrograms (3-12 million IU), administered subcutaneously three times per week. At licensed posology, Rebif 44 micrograms has been demonstrated to decrease the incidence (approximately 30% over 2 years) and severity of clinical relapses in patients with at least 2 exacerbations in the previous 2 years and with an EDSS of 0-5.0 at entry. The proportion of patients with disability progression, as defined by at least one point increase in EDSS confirmed three months later, was reduced from 39% (placebo) to 27% (Rebif 44 micrograms). Over 4 years, the reduction in the mean exacerbation rate was 22% in patients treated with Rebif 22 micrograms, and 29% in patients treated with Rebif 44 micrograms group compared with a group of patients treated with placebo for 2 years and then either Rebif 22 or Rebif 44 micrograms for 2 years.

In a 3-year study in patients with secondary progressive multiple sclerosis (EDSS 3-6.5) with evidence of clinical progression in the preceding two years and who had not experienced relapses in the preceding 8 weeks, Rebif had no significant effect on progression of disability, but relapse rate was reduced by approximately 30%. If the patient population was divided into 2 subgroups (those with and those without relapses in the 2-year period prior to study entry), there was no effect on disability in patients without relapses, but in patients with relapses, the proportion with progression in disability at the end of the study was reduced from 70% (placebo) to 57% (Rebif 22 micrograms and 44 micrograms combined). These results obtained in a subgroup of patients a posteriori should be interpreted cautiously.

Rebif has not yet been investigated in patients with primary progressive multiple sclerosis, and should not be used in such patients.

5.2 Pharmacokinetic properties

In healthy volunteers after intravenous administration, interferon beta-1a exhibits a sharp multi-exponential decline, with serum levels proportional to the dose. The initial half-life is in the order of minutes and the terminal half-life is several hours, with the possible presence of a deep compartment. When administered by the subcutaneous or intramuscular routes, serum levels of interferon beta remain low, but are still measurable up to 12 to 24 hours post-dose. Subcutaneous and intramuscular administrations of Rebif produce equivalent exposure to interferon beta. Following a single 60 microgram dose, the maximum peak concentration, as measured by immunoassay, is around 6 to 10 IU/ml, occurring on average around 3 hours after the dose. After subcutaneous administration at the same dose repeated every 48 hours for 4 doses, a moderate accumulation occurs (about 2.5 × for AUC).

Regardless of the route of dosing, pronounced pharmacodynamic changes are associated with the administration of Rebif. After a single dose, intracellular and serum activity of 2-5A synthetase and serum concentrations of beta-2 microglobulin and neopterin increase within 24 hours, and start to decline within 2 days. Intramuscular and subcutaneous administrations produce fully superimposable responses. After repeated subcutaneous administration every 48 hours for 4 doses, these biological responses remain elevated, with no signs of tolerance development.

Interferon beta-1a is mainly metabolised and excreted by the liver and the kidneys.

5.3 Preclinical safety data

Non-clinical data reveal no special hazard for humans based on conventional studies of safety pharmacology, repeated-dose toxicity, and genotoxicity.

Table 1

System Organ Class	Very common	Common	Uncommon	Not known*
Infections and infestations			Injection site abscess	Injection site infections, including cellulitis
Blood and lymphatic system disorders	Neutropenia, lymphopenia, leucopenia, thrombocytopenia, anaemia			Thrombotic thrombocytopenic purpura/Haemolytic uremic syndrome
Endocrine Disorders			Thyroid dysfunction most often presenting as hypothyroidism or hyperthyroidism	
Psychiatric disorders		Depression, insomnia		Suicide attempt
Nervous system disorders	Headache			Seizures, transient neurological symptoms (i.e. hypoesthesia, muscle spasm, paraesthesia, difficulty in walking, musculoskeletal stiffness) that may mimic multiple sclerosis exacerbations
Eye disorders				Retinal vascular disorders (e.g. retinopathy, cotton wool spots and obstruction of retinal artery or vein)
Gastrointestinal disorders		Diarrhoea, vomiting, nausea		
Skin and subcutaneous tissue disorders		Pruritus, rash, erythematous rash, maculo-papular rash		Angioedema, urticaria, erythema multiforme, erythema multiforme-like skin reactions, Stevens-Johnson syndrome, hair loss
Musculoskeletal and connective tissue disorders		Myalgia, arthralgia		
General disorders and administration site conditions	Injection site inflammation, injection site reaction, influenza-like symptoms	Injection site pain, fatigue, rigors, fever	Injection site necrosis, injection site mass	
Investigations	Asymptomatic transaminase increase	Severe elevations of transaminase		
Respiratory, thoracic and mediastinal disorders				Dyspnoea
Immune system disorders				Anaphylactic reactions
Vascular disorders				Thromboembolic events
Hepatobiliary disorders				Hepatitis with or without icterus

*Adverse reactions identified during post marketing surveillance (frequency not known)

Rebif has not been investigated for carcinogenicity.

A study on embryo/foetal toxicity in monkeys showed no evidence of reproductive disturbances. Based on observations with other alpha and beta interferons, an increased risk of abortions cannot be excluded. No information is available on the effects of the interferon beta-1a on male fertility.

6. PHARMACEUTICAL PARTICULARS

6.1 List of excipients

Mannitol

Poloxamer 188

L-methionine

Benzyl alcohol

Sodium acetate

Acetic acid for pH adjustment

Sodium hydroxide for pH adjustment

Water for injections

6.2 Incompatibilities

Not applicable.

6.3 Shelf life

18 months.

6.4 Special precautions for storage

Store in a refrigerator (2°C – 8°C) away from the cooling element. Do not freeze. Store in the original package in order to protect from light.

6.5 Nature and contents of container

One ml type 1 glass syringe, with a stainless steel needle, containing 0.5 ml solution.

Rebif 44 micrograms is available as a package of 1, 3 or 12 syringes.

Not all pack sizes may be marketed.

6.6 Special precautions for disposal and other handling

The solution for injection in a pre-filled syringe is ready for use. It may also be administered with a suitable auto-injector.

For single use only. Only clear to opalescent solution without particles should be used and without visible signs of deterioration.

Any unused product or waste material should be disposed of in accordance with local requirements.

7. MARKETING AUTHORISATION HOLDER

Merck Serono Europe Limited

56, Marsh Wall

London E14 9TP

United Kingdom

8. MARKETING AUTHORISATION NUMBER(S)

EU/1/98/063/004

EU/1/98/063/005

EU/1/98/063/006

9. DATE OF FIRST AUTHORISATION/RENEWAL OF THE AUTHORISATION

Date of first authorisation: 4th May 1998

Date of first renewal: 4th May 2003

Date of latest renewal: 4th May 2008

10. DATE OF REVISION OF THE TEXT

24th July 2009

Rebif 44 micrograms/0.5ml solution for injection in cartridge

(Merck Serono)

1. NAME OF THE MEDICINAL PRODUCT

Rebif 44 micrograms/0.5ml solution for injection in cartridge

2. QUALITATIVE AND QUANTITATIVE COMPOSITION

Each pre-filled cartridge contains 132 micrograms (36 MIU*) of interferon beta-1a** in 1.5 ml solution, corresponding to 88 micrograms/ml.

* Million International Units, measured by cytopathic effect (CPE) bioassay against the in house IFN beta-1a standard which is calibrated against the current international NIH standard (GB-23-902-531).

** produced in Chinese hamster ovary Cells (CHO-K1) by recombinant DNA technology.

Excipient: 7.5 mg benzyl alcohol

For a full list of excipients, see section 6.1.

3. PHARMACEUTICAL FORM

Solution for injection in cartridge.

Clear to opalescent solution, with pH 3.7 to 4.1 and osmolarity 250 to 450 mOsm/l.

4. CLINICAL PARTICULARS

4.1 Therapeutic indications

Rebif is indicated for the treatment of relapsing multiple sclerosis.

In clinical trials, this was characterised by two or more acute exacerbations in the previous two years (see section 5.1).

Efficacy has not been demonstrated in patients with secondary progressive multiple sclerosis without ongoing relapsing activity (see section 5.1).

4.2 Posology and method of administration

Treatment should be initiated under supervision of a physician experienced in the treatment of the disease.

The recommended posology of Rebif is 44 micrograms given three times per week by subcutaneous injection. A lower dose of 22 micrograms, also given three times per week by subcutaneous injection, is recommended for patients who cannot tolerate the higher dose in view of the treating specialist.

When first starting treatment with Rebif, the dose should be gradually escalated in order to allow tachyphylaxis to develop thus reducing adverse reactions. The Rebif initiation package corresponds to the patient needs for the first month of treatment.

Method of administration

Rebif solution for injection in cartridge is intended for multi-dose use and should only be used with the RebiSmart autoinjector device following adequate training of the patient and/or carer.

For administration, the instructions provided in the package leaflet and in the instruction manual provided with the RebiSmart autoinjector device should be followed.

Prior to injection and for an additional 24 hours after each injection, an antipyretic analgesic is advised to decrease flu-like symptoms associated with Rebif administration.

At the present time, it is not known for how long patients should be treated. Safety and efficacy with Rebif have not been demonstrated beyond 4 years of treatment. It is recommended that patients should be evaluated at least every second year in the 4-year period after initiation of treatment with Rebif and a decision for longer term treatment should then be made on an individual basis by the treating physician.

Paediatric use

No formal clinical trials or pharmacokinetic studies have been conducted in children or adolescents. However, limited published data suggest that the safety profile in adolescents from 12 to 16 years of age receiving Rebif 22 micrograms subcutaneous three times per week is similar to that seen in adults. There is very limited information on the use of Rebif in children under 12 years of age and therefore Rebif should not be used in this population.

4.3 Contraindications

• Initiation of treatment in pregnancy (see section 4.6).

• Hypersensitivity to natural or recombinant interferon-β, or to any excipients.

• Current severe depression and/or suicidal ideation (see sections 4.4 and 4.8).

4.4 Special warnings and precautions for use

Patients should be informed of the most frequent adverse reactions associated with interferon beta administration, including symptoms of the flu-like syndrome (see section 4.8). These symptoms tend to be most prominent at the initiation of therapy and decrease in frequency and severity with continued treatment.

Rebif should be administered with caution to patients with previous or current depressive disorders in particular to those with antecedents of suicidal ideation (see section 4.3). Depression and suicidal ideation are known to occur in increased frequency in the multiple sclerosis population and in association with interferon use. Patients treated with Rebif should be advised to immediately report any symptoms of depression and/or suicidal ideation to their prescribing physician. Patients exhibiting depression should be monitored closely during therapy with Rebif and treated appropriately. Cessation of therapy with Rebif should be considered (see sections 4.3 and 4.8).

Rebif should be administered with caution to patients with a history of seizures, to those receiving treatment with anti-epileptics, particularly if their epilepsy is not adequately controlled with anti-epileptics (see sections 4.5 and 4.8).

Patients with cardiac disease, such as angina, congestive heart failure or arrhythmia, should be closely monitored for worsening of their clinical condition during initiation of therapy with interferon beta-1a. Symptoms of the flu-like syndrome associated with interferon beta-1a therapy may prove stressful to patients with cardiac conditions.

Injection site necrosis (ISN) has been reported in patients using Rebif (see section 4.8). To minimise the risk of injection site necrosis patients should be advised to:

- use an aseptic injection technique,
- rotate the injection sites with each dose.

The procedure for the self-administration by the patient should be reviewed periodically especially if injection site reactions have occurred.

If the patient experiences any break in the skin, which may be associated with swelling or drainage of fluid from the injection site, the patient should be advised to consult with their physician before continuing injections with Rebif. If the patient has multiple lesions, Rebif should be discontinued until healing has occurred. Patients with single lesions may continue provided that the necrosis is not too extensive.

In clinical trials with Rebif, asymptomatic elevations of hepatic transaminases (particularly alanine aminotransferase (ALT)) were common and 1-3% of patients developed elevations of hepatic transaminases above 5 times the upper limit of normal (ULN). In the absence of clinical symptoms, serum ALT levels should be monitored prior to the start of therapy, at months 1, 3 and 6 on therapy and periodically thereafter. Dose reduction of Rebif should be considered if ALT rises above 5 times the ULN, and gradually re-escalated when enzyme levels have normalized. Rebif should be initiated with caution in patients with a history of significant liver disease, clinical evidence of active liver disease, alcohol abuse or increased serum ALT (>2.5 times ULN). Treatment with Rebif should be stopped if icterus or other clinical symptoms of liver dysfunction appear (see section 4.8).

Rebif, like other interferons beta, has a potential for causing severe liver injury (see section 4.8) including acute hepatic failure. The mechanism for the rare symptomatic hepatic dysfunction is not known. No specific risk factors have been identified.

Laboratory abnormalities are associated with the use of interferons. The overall incidence of these is slightly higher with Rebif 44 than Rebif 22 micrograms. Therefore, in addition to those laboratory tests normally required for monitoring patients with multiple sclerosis, liver enzyme monitoring and complete and differential blood cell counts and platelet counts are recommended at regular intervals (1, 3 and 6 months) following introduction of Rebif therapy and then periodically thereafter in the absence of clinical symptoms. These should be more frequent when initiating Rebif 44 micrograms.

Patients being treated with Rebif may occasionally develop new or worsening thyroid abnormalities. Thyroid function testing is recommended at baseline and if abnormal, every 6-12 months following initiation of therapy. If tests are normal at baseline, routine testing is not needed but should be performed if clinical findings of thyroid dysfunction appear (see section 4.8).

Caution should be used, and close monitoring considered when administering interferon beta-1a to patients with severe renal and hepatic failure and to patients with severe myelosuppression.

Serum neutralising antibodies against interferon beta-1a may develop. The precise incidence of antibodies is as yet uncertain. Clinical data suggest that after 24 to 48 months of treatment with Rebif 44 micrograms, approximately 13 to 14% of patients develop persistent serum antibodies to interferon beta-1a. The presence of antibodies has been shown to attenuate the pharmacodynamic response to interferon beta-1a (Beta-2 microglobulin and neopterin). Although the clinical significance of the induction of antibodies has not been fully elucidated, the development of neutralising antibodies is associated with reduced efficacy on clinical and MRI variables. If a patient responds poorly to therapy with Rebif, and has neutralising antibodies, the treating physician should reassess the benefit/risk ratio of continued Rebif therapy.

The use of various assays to detect serum antibodies and differing definitions of antibody positivity limits the ability to compare antigenicity among different products.

Only sparse safety and efficacy data are available from non-ambulatory patients with multiple sclerosis. Rebif has not yet been investigated in patients with primary progressive multiple sclerosis and should not be used in such patients

This medicinal product contains 2.5 mg benzyl alcohol per dose of 0.5 ml. Must not be given to premature babies or neonates. May cause toxic reactions and anaphylactoid reactions in infants and children up to 3 years old.

4.5 Interaction with other medicinal products and other forms of interaction

No interaction studies have been performed with interferon beta-1a in humans.

Interferons have been reported to reduce the activity of hepatic cytochrome P450-dependent enzymes in humans and animals. Caution should be exercised when administering Rebif in combination with medicinal products that have a narrow therapeutic index and are largely dependent on the hepatic cytochrome P450 system for clearance, e.g. antiepileptics and some classes of antidepressants.

The interaction of Rebif with corticosteroids or adrenocorticotropic hormone (ACTH) has not been studied systematically. Clinical studies indicate that multiple sclerosis patients can receive Rebif and corticosteroids or ACTH during relapses.

4.6 Pregnancy and lactation

There is limited information on the use of Rebif in pregnancy. Available data indicates that there may be an increased risk of spontaneous abortion. Therefore initiation of treatment is contraindicated during pregnancy (see section 4.3).

Women of child-bearing potential should take appropriate contraceptive measures. If the patient becomes pregnant or plans to become pregnant while taking Rebif she should be informed of the potential hazards and discontinuation of therapy should be considered (see section 5.3). In patients with a high relapse rate before treatment has started, the risk of a severe relapse following discontinuation of Rebif in the event of pregnancy should be weighed against a possible increased risk of spontaneous abortion.

It is not known whether Rebif is excreted in human milk. Because of the potential for serious adverse reactions in breast-fed infants, a decision should be made whether to discontinue breast-feeding or Rebif therapy.

4.7 Effects on ability to drive and use machines

Central nervous system-related adverse events associated with the use of interferon beta (e.g. dizziness) might influence the patient's ability to drive or use machines (see section 4.8).

4.8 Undesirable effects

The highest incidence of adverse reactions associated with Rebif therapy is related to flu-like syndrome. Flu-like symptoms tend to be most prominent at the initiation of therapy and decrease in frequency with continued treatment. Approximately 70% of patients treated with Rebif can expect to experience the typical interferon flu-like syndrome within the first six months after starting treatment. Approximately 30% of patients will also experience reactions at the injection site, predominantly mild inflammation or erythema. Asymptomatic increases in laboratory parameters of hepatic function and decreases in white blood cells (WBC) are also common.

The majority of adverse reactions observed with IFN beta-1a are usually mild and reversible, and respond well to dose reductions. In case of severe or persistent undesirable effects, the dose of Rebif may be temporarily lowered or interrupted, at the discretion of the physician.

The adverse reactions reported below are classified according to frequency of occurrence as follows:

Very Common	≥ 1/10
Common	≥1/100 to <1/10
Uncommon	≥1/1,000 to <1/100
Rare	≥1/10,000 to <1/1,000
Very rare	<1/10,000
Not known	Cannot be estimated from the available data

Within each frequency grouping, undesirable effects are presented in order of decreasing seriousness.

The data presented is obtained from pooled clinical studies in multiple sclerosis (placebo=824 patients; Rebif 22 micrograms three times per week (TIW)=398 patients; Rebif 44 micrograms TIW=727 patients) and shows the frequency of adverse reactions observed at six months (excess over placebo). Adverse reactions are listed below by frequency of occurrence and by MedDRA System Organ Class.

(see Table 1 on next page)

Interferon beta has a potential for causing severe liver injury. The mechanism for the rare symptomatic hepatic dysfunction is not known. The majority of the cases of severe liver injury occurred within the first six months of treatment. No specific risk factors have been identified. Treatment with Rebif should be stopped if icterus or other clinical symptoms of liver dysfunction appear (see section 4.4).

The administration of interferons has been associated with anorexia, dizziness, anxiety, arrhythmias, vasodilation and palpitation, menorrhagia and metrorrhagia.

An increased formation of auto-antibodies may occur during treatment with interferon beta.

4.9 Overdose

In case of overdose, patients should be hospitalised for observation and appropriate supportive treatment should be given.

5. PHARMACOLOGICAL PROPERTIES

5.1 Pharmacodynamic properties

Pharmacotherapeutic group: Immunostimulants, Interferons, ATC code: L03AB07.

Interferons (IFNs) are a group of endogenous glycoproteins endowed with immunomodulatory, antiviral and antiproliferative properties.

Rebif (interferon beta-1a) shares the same amino acid sequence with endogenous human interferon beta. It is produced in mammalian cells (Chinese hamster ovary) and is therefore glycosylated like the natural protein.

The precise mechanism of action of Rebif in multiple sclerosis is still under investigation.

The safety and efficacy of Rebif has been evaluated in patients with relapsing-remitting multiple sclerosis at doses ranging from 11 to 44 micrograms (3-12 million IU), administered subcutaneously three times per week. At licensed posology, Rebif 44 micrograms has been demonstrated to decrease the incidence (approximately 30% over 2 years) and severity of clinical relapses in patients with at least 2 exacerbations in the previous 2 years and with an EDSS of 0-5.0 at entry. The proportion of patients with disability progression, as defined by at least one point increase in EDSS confirmed three months later, was reduced from 39% (placebo) to 27% (Rebif 44 micrograms). Over 4 years, the reduction in the mean exacerbation rate was 22% in patients treated with Rebif 22 micrograms, and 29% in patients treated with Rebif 44 micrograms group compared with a group of patients treated with placebo for 2 years and then either Rebif 22 or Rebif 44 micrograms for 2 years.

In a 3-year study in patients with secondary progressive multiple sclerosis (EDSS 3-6.5) with evidence of clinical progression in the preceding two years and who had not experienced relapses in the preceding 8 weeks, Rebif had no significant effect on progression of disability, but relapse rate was reduced by approximately 30%. If the patient population was divided into 2 subgroups (those with and those without relapses in the 2-year period prior to study entry), there was no effect on disability in patients without relapses, but in patients with relapses, the proportion with progression in disability at the end of the study was reduced from 70% (placebo) to 57% (Rebif 22 micrograms and 44 micrograms combined). These results obtained in a subgroup of patients a posteriori should be interpreted cautiously.

Rebif has not yet been investigated in patients with primary progressive multiple sclerosis, and should not be used in such patients.

5.2 Pharmacokinetic properties

In healthy volunteers after intravenous administration, interferon beta-1a exhibits a sharp multi-exponential decline, with serum levels proportional to the dose. The initial half-life is in the order of minutes and the terminal half-life is several hours, with the possible presence of a deep compartment. When administered by the subcutaneous or intramuscular routes, serum levels of interferon beta remain low, but are still measurable up to 12 to 24 hours post-dose. Subcutaneous and intramuscular administrations of Rebif produce equivalent exposure to interferon beta. Following a single 60 microgram dose, the maximum peak concentration, as measured by immunoassay, is around 6 to 10 IU/ml, occurring on average around 3 hours after the dose. After subcutaneous administration at the same dose repeated every 48 hours for 4 doses, a moderate accumulation occurs (about 2.5 × for AUC).

Regardless of the route of dosing, pronounced pharmacodynamic changes are associated with the administration of Rebif. After a single dose, intracellular and serum activity of 2-5A synthetase and serum concentrations of beta-2 microglobulin and neopterin increase within 24 hours, and start to decline within 2 days. Intramuscular and subcutaneous administrations produce fully superimposable responses. After repeated subcutaneous administration every 48 hours for 4 doses, these biological responses remain elevated, with no signs of tolerance development.

Interferon beta-1a is mainly metabolised and excreted by the liver and the kidneys.

5.3 Preclinical safety data

Non-clinical data reveal no special hazard for humans based on conventional studies of safety pharmacology, repeated-dose toxicity, and genotoxicity.

Table 1

System Organ Class	Very common	Common	Uncommon	Not known*
Infections and infestations			Injection site abscess	Injection site infections, including cellulitis
Blood and lymphatic system disorders	Neutropenia, lymphopenia, leucopenia, thrombocytopenia, anaemia			Thrombotic thrombocytopenic purpura/Haemolytic uremic syndrome
Endocrine Disorders			Thyroid dysfunction most often presenting as hypothyroidism or hyperthyroidism	
Psychiatric disorders		Depression, insomnia		Suicide attempt
Nervous system disorders	Headache			Seizures, transient neurological symptoms (i.e. hypoesthesia, muscle spasm, paraesthesia, difficulty in walking, musculoskeletal stiffness) that may mimic multiple sclerosis exacerbations
Eye disorders				Retinal vascular disorders (e.g. retinopathy, cotton wool spots and obstruction of retinal artery or vein)
Gastrointestinal disorders		Diarrhoea, vomiting, nausea		
Skin and subcutaneous tissue disorders		Pruritus, rash, erythematous rash, maculo-papular rash		Angioedema, urticaria, erythema multiforme, erythema multiforme-like skin reactions, Stevens-Johnson syndrome, hair loss
Musculoskeletal and connective tissue disorders		Myalgia, arthralgia		
General disorders and administration site conditions	Injection site inflammation, injection site reaction, influenza-like symptoms	Injection site pain, fatigue, rigors, fever	Injection site necrosis, injection site mass	
Investigations	Asymptomatic transaminase increase	Severe elevations of transaminase		
Respiratory, thoracic and mediastinal disorders				Dyspnoea
Immune system disorders				Anaphylactic reactions
Vascular disorders				Thromboembolic events
Hepatobiliary disorders				Hepatitis with or without icterus

*Adverse reactions identified during post marketing surveillance (frequency not known)

Rebif has not been investigated for carcinogenicity.

A study on embryo/foetal toxicity in monkeys showed no evidence of reproductive disturbances. Based on observations with other alpha and beta interferons, an increased risk of abortions cannot be excluded. No information is available on the effects of the interferon beta-1a on male fertility.

6. PHARMACEUTICAL PARTICULARS

6.1 List of excipients

Mannitol

Poloxamer 188

L-methionine

Benzyl alcohol

Sodium acetate

Acetic acid for pH adjustment

Sodium hydroxide for pH adjustment

Water for injections

6.2 Incompatibilities

Not applicable.

6.3 Shelf life

18 months.

After first injection use within 28 days.

6.4 Special precautions for storage

Store in a refrigerator (2°C – 8°C) away from the cooling element. Do not freeze. Store the cartridge in the original package in order to protect from light.

The RebiSmart autoinjector device containing a pre-filled cartridge of Rebif must be stored in the device storage box in a refrigerator (2°C – 8°C).

Should refrigeration be temporarily unavailable, Rebif can be stored by the patient at or below 25°C for up to 14 days then put back in the refrigerator and used before the expiry date.

6.5 Nature and contents of container

Cartridges (type 1 glass) with a plunger stopper (rubber) and crimp cap (aluminium and halobutyl rubber) containing 1.5 ml solution for injection.

Pack size of 4 cartridges.

6.6 Special precautions for disposal and other handling

The solution for injection in a pre-filled cartridge is ready for use with the RebiSmart autoinjector device. For storage of the RebiSmart autoinjector device with the cartridge, see section 6.4.

For multidose use. Only clear to opalescent solution without particles should be used and without visible signs of deterioration.

Any unused product or waste material should be disposed of in accordance with local requirements.

7. MARKETING AUTHORISATION HOLDER

Merck Serono Europe Limited

56, Marsh Wall

London E14 9TP

United Kingdom

8. MARKETING AUTHORISATION NUMBER(S)

EU/1/98/063/009

9. DATE OF FIRST AUTHORISATION/RENEWAL OF THE AUTHORISATION

Date of first authorisation: 4th May 1998

Date of first renewal: 4th May 2003

Date of latest renewal: 4th May 2008

10. DATE OF REVISION OF THE TEXT

24th July 2009

Rebif 8.8 micrograms and 22 micrograms solution for injection in pre-filled syringe initiation pack

(Merck Serono)

1. NAME OF THE MEDICINAL PRODUCT

Rebif 8.8 micrograms solution for injection in pre-filled syringe

Rebif 22 micrograms solution for injection in pre-filled syringe

2. QUALITATIVE AND QUANTITATIVE COMPOSITION

Each pre-filled syringe (0.2 ml) contains 8.8 micrograms (2.4 MIU*) of interferon beta-1a**.

* Million International Units, measured by cytopathic effect (CPE) bioassay against the in-house IFN beta-1a standard which is calibrated against the current international NIH standard (GB-23-902-531).

** produced in Chinese hamster ovary Cells (CHO-K1) by recombinant DNA technology.

Excipient: 1.0 mg benzyl alcohol

For a full list of excipients, see section 6.1.

Each pre-filled syringe (0.5 ml) contains 22 micrograms (6 MIU*) of interferon beta-1a**.

* Million International Units, measured by cytopathic effect (CPE) bioassay against the in-house IFN beta-1a standard which is calibrated against the current international NIH standard (GB-23-902-531).

** produced in Chinese hamster ovary Cells (CHO-K1) by recombinant DNA technology.

Excipient: 2.5 mg benzyl alcohol

For a full list of excipients, see section 6.1.

3. PHARMACEUTICAL FORM

Solution for injection in pre-filled syringe.

Clear to opalescent solution, with pH 3.5 to 4.5 and osmolarity 250 to 450 mOsm/l.

4. CLINICAL PARTICULARS

4.1 Therapeutic indications

Rebif is indicated for the treatment of relapsing multiple sclerosis.

In clinical trials, this was characterised by two or more acute exacerbations in the previous two years (see section 5.1).

Efficacy has not been demonstrated in patients with secondary progressive multiple sclerosis without ongoing relapse activity (see section 5.1).

4.2 Posology and method of administration

Treatment should be initiated under supervision of a physician experienced in the treatment of the disease.

The Rebif initiation package corresponds to the patient needs for the first month of treatment. When first starting treatment with Rebif, in order to allow tachyphylaxis to develop thus reducing adverse reactions, it is recommended that 8.8 micrograms be administered by subcutaneous injection three times per week during the initial 2 weeks of therapy. Thereafter, 22 micrograms be administered by subcutaneous injection three times per week in weeks 3 and 4, and the total of the 44 micrograms strength be administered from the fifth week onwards.

Method of administration

Prior to injection and for an additional 24 hours after each injection, an antipyretic analgesic is advised to decrease flu-like symptoms associated with Rebif administration.

At the present time, it is not known for how long patients should be treated. Safety and efficacy with Rebif have not been demonstrated beyond 4 years of treatment. It is recommended that patients should be evaluated at least every second year in the 4-year period after initiation of treatment with Rebif and a decision for longer term treatment should then be made on an individual basis by the treating physician.

Paediatric use

No formal clinical trials or pharmacokinetic studies have been conducted in children or adolescents. However, limited published data suggest that the safety profile in adolescents from 12 to 16 years of age receiving Rebif 22 micrograms subcutaneous three times per week is similar to that seen in adults. There is very limited information on the use of Rebif in children under 12 years of age and therefore Rebif should not be used in this population.

4.3 Contraindications

• Initiation of treatment in pregnancy (see section 4.6).

• Hypersensitivity to natural or recombinant interferon-β, or to any excipients.

• Current severe depression and/or suicidal ideation (see sections 4.4 and 4.8).

4.4 Special warnings and precautions for use

Patients should be informed of the most frequent adverse reactions associated with interferon beta administration, including symptoms of the flu-like syndrome (see section 4.8). These symptoms tend to be most prominent at the initiation of therapy and decrease in frequency and severity with continued treatment.

Rebif should be administered with caution to patients with previous or current depressive disorders in particular to those with antecedents of suicidal ideation (see section 4.3). Depression and suicidal ideation are known to occur in increased frequency in the multiple sclerosis population and in association with interferon use. Patients treated with Rebif should be advised to immediately report any symptoms of depression and/or suicidal ideation to their prescribing physician. Patients exhibiting depression should be monitored closely during therapy with Rebif and treated appropriately. Cessation of therapy with Rebif should be considered (see sections 4.3 and 4.8).

Rebif should be administered with caution to patients with a history of seizures, to those receiving treatment with anti-epileptics, particularly if their epilepsy is not adequately controlled with anti-epileptics (see sections 4.5 and 4.8).

Patients with cardiac disease, such as angina, congestive heart failure or arrhythmia, should be closely monitored for worsening of their clinical condition during initiation of therapy with interferon beta-1a. Symptoms of the flu-like syndrome associated with interferon beta-1a therapy may prove stressful to patients with cardiac conditions.

Injection site necrosis (ISN) has been reported in patients using Rebif (see section 4.8). To minimise the risk of injection site necrosis patients should be advised to:

• use an aseptic injection technique,

• rotate the injection sites with each dose.

The procedure for the self-administration by the patient should be reviewed periodically especially if injection site reactions have occurred.

If the patient experiences any break in the skin, which may be associated with swelling or drainage of fluid from the injection site, the patient should be advised to consult with their physician before continuing injections with Rebif. If the patient has multiple lesions, Rebif should be discontinued until healing has occurred. Patients with single lesions may continue provided that the necrosis is not too extensive.

In clinical trials with Rebif, asymptomatic elevations of hepatic transaminases (particularly alanine aminotransferase (ALT)) were common and 1-3% of patients developed elevations of hepatic transaminases above 5 times the upper limit of normal (ULN). In the absence of clinical symptoms, serum ALT levels should be monitored prior to the start of therapy, at months 1, 3 and 6 on therapy and periodically thereafter. Dose reduction of Rebif should be considered if ALT rises above 5 times the ULN, and gradually re-escalated when enzyme levels have normalized. Rebif should be initiated with caution in patients with a history of significant liver disease, clinical evidence of active liver disease, alcohol abuse or increased serum ALT (>2.5 times ULN). Treatment with Rebif should be stopped if icterus or other clinical symptoms of liver dysfunction appear (see section 4.8).

Rebif, like other interferons beta, has a potential for causing severe liver injury (see section 4.8) including acute hepatic failure. The mechanism for the rare symptomatic hepatic dysfunction is not known. No specific risk factors have been identified.

Laboratory abnormalities are associated with the use of interferons. Therefore, in addition to those laboratory tests normally required for monitoring patients with multiple sclerosis, liver enzyme monitoring and complete and differential blood cell counts and platelet counts are recommended at regular intervals (1, 3 and 6 months) following introduction of Rebif therapy and then periodically thereafter in the absence of clinical symptoms.

Patients being treated with Rebif may occasionally develop new or worsening thyroid abnormalities. Thyroid function testing is recommended at baseline and if abnormal, every 6-12 months following initiation of therapy. If tests are normal at baseline, routine testing is not needed but should be performed if clinical findings of thyroid dysfunction appear (see section 4.8).

Caution should be used, and close monitoring considered when administering interferon beta-1a to patients with severe renal and hepatic failure and to patients with severe myelosuppression.

Serum neutralising antibodies against interferon beta-1a may develop. The precise incidence of antibodies is as yet uncertain. Clinical data suggest that after 24 to 48 months of treatment with Rebif 22 micrograms, approximately 24% of patients develop persistent serum antibodies to interferon beta-1a. The presence of antibodies has been shown to attenuate the pharmacodynamic response to interferon beta-1a (Beta-2 microglobulin and neopterin). Although the clinical significance of the induction of antibodies has not been fully elucidated, the development of neutralising antibodies is associated with reduced efficacy on clinical and MRI variables. If a patient responds poorly to therapy with Rebif, and has neutralising antibodies, the treating physician should reassess the benefit/risk ratio of continued Rebif therapy.

The use of various assays to detect serum antibodies and differing definitions of antibody positivity limits the ability to compare antigenicity among different products.

Only sparse safety and efficacy data are available from non-ambulatory patients with multiple sclerosis. Rebif has not yet been investigated in patients with primary progressive multiple sclerosis and should not be used in such patients.

This medicinal product contains 1.0 mg benzyl alcohol per dose of 0.2 ml and 2.5 mg benzyl alcohol per dose of 0.5 ml. Must not be given to premature babies or neonates. May cause toxic reactions and anaphylactoid reactions in infants and children up to 3 years old.

4.5 Interaction with other medicinal products and other forms of interaction

No interaction studies have been performed with interferon beta-1a in humans.

Interferons have been reported to reduce the activity of hepatic cytochrome P450-dependent enzymes in humans and animals. Caution should be exercised when administering Rebif in combination with medicinal products that have a narrow therapeutic index and are largely dependent on the hepatic cytochrome P450 system for clearance, e.g. antiepileptics and some classes of antidepressants.

The interaction of Rebif with corticosteroids or adrenocorticotropic hormone (ACTH) has not been studied systematically. Clinical studies indicate that multiple sclerosis patients can receive Rebif and corticosteroids or ACTH during relapses.

4.6 Pregnancy and lactation

There is limited information on the use of Rebif in pregnancy. Available data indicates that there may be an increased risk of spontaneous abortion. Therefore initiation of treatment is contraindicated during pregnancy (see section 4.3).

Women of child-bearing potential should take appropriate contraceptive measures. If the patient becomes pregnant or plans to become pregnant while taking Rebif she should be informed of the potential hazards and discontinuation of therapy should be considered (see section 5.3). In patients with a high relapse rate before treatment has started, the risk of a severe relapse following discontinuation of Rebif in the event of pregnancy should be weighed against a possible increased risk of spontaneous abortion.

It is not known whether Rebif is excreted in human milk. Because of the potential for serious adverse reactions in breast-fed infants, a decision should be made either to discontinue nursing or to discontinue Rebif therapy.

4.7 Effects on ability to drive and use machines

Central nervous system-related adverse events associated with the use of interferon beta (e.g. dizziness) might influence the patient's ability to drive or use machines (see section 4.8).

4.8 Undesirable effects

The highest incidence of adverse reactions associated with Rebif therapy is related to flu-like syndrome. Flu-like symptoms tend to be most prominent at the initiation of therapy and decrease in frequency with continued treatment. Approximately 70% of patients treated with Rebif can expect to experience the typical interferon flu-like syndrome within the first six months after starting treatment. Approximately 30% of patients will also experience reactions at the injection site, predominantly mild inflammation or erythema. Asymptomatic increases in laboratory parameters of hepatic function and decreases in white blood cells (WBC) are also common.

The majority of adverse reactions observed with IFN beta-1a are usually mild and reversible, and respond well to dose reductions. In case of severe or persistent undesirable effects, the dose of Rebif may be temporarily lowered or interrupted, at the discretion of the physician.

The adverse reactions reported below are classified according to frequency of occurrence as follows:

Very Common	⩾1/10
Common	⩾1/100 to <1/10
Uncommon	⩾1/1,000 to <1/100
Rare	⩾1/10,000 to <1/1,000
Very rare	<1/10,000
Not known	Cannot be estimated from the available data

Within each frequency grouping, undesirable effects are presented in order of decreasing seriousness.

The data presented is obtained from pooled clinical studies in multiple sclerosis (placebo=824 patients; Rebif 22 micrograms three times per week (TIW)=398 patients; Rebif 44 micrograms TIW=727 patients) and shows the frequency of adverse reactions observed at six months (excess over placebo). Adverse reactions are listed below by frequency of occurrence and by MedDRA System Organ Class.

(see Table 1 on next page)

Interferon beta has a potential for causing severe liver injury. The mechanism for the rare symptomatic hepatic dysfunction is not known. The majority of the cases of severe liver injury occurred within the first six months of treatment. No specific risk factors have been identified. Treatment with Rebif should be stopped if icterus or other clinical symptoms of liver dysfunction appear (see section 4.4).

The administration of interferons has been associated with anorexia, dizziness, anxiety, arrhythmias, vasodilation and palpitation, menorrhagia and metrorrhagia.

An increased formation of auto-antibodies may occur during treatment with interferon beta.

4.9 Overdose

In case of overdose, patients should be hospitalised for observation and appropriate supportive treatment should be given.

5. PHARMACOLOGICAL PROPERTIES

5.1 Pharmacodynamic properties

Pharmacotherapeutic group: Immunostimulants, Interferons, ATC code: L03AB07.

Interferons (IFNs) are a group of endogenous glycoproteins endowed with immunomodulatory, antiviral and antiproliferative properties.

Rebif (interferon beta-1a) shares the same amino acid sequence with endogenous human interferon beta. It is produced in mammalian cells (Chinese hamster ovary) and is therefore glycosylated like the natural protein.

The precise mechanism of action of Rebif in multiple sclerosis is still under investigation.

The safety and efficacy of Rebif has been evaluated in patients with relapsing-remitting multiple sclerosis at doses ranging from 11 to 44 micrograms (3-12 million IU), administered subcutaneously three times per week. At licensed posology, Rebif 22 micrograms has been demonstrated to decrease the incidence (approximately 30% over 2 years) and severity of clinical relapses in patients with at least 2 exacerbations in the previous 2 years and with an EDSS of 0-5.0 at entry. The proportion of patients with disability progression, as defined by at least one point increase in EDSS confirmed three months later, was reduced from 39% (placebo) to 30% (Rebif 22 micrograms). Over 4 years, the reduction in the mean exacerbation rate was 22% in patients treated with Rebif 22 micrograms, and 29% in patients treated with Rebif 44 micrograms group compared with a group of patients treated with placebo for 2 years and then either Rebif 22 or Rebif 44 micrograms for 2 years.

In a 3-year study in patients with secondary progressive multiple sclerosis (EDSS 3-6.5) with evidence of clinical progression in the preceding two years and who had not experienced relapses in the preceding 8 weeks, Rebif had no significant effect on progression of disability, but relapse rate was reduced by approximately 30%. If the patient population was divided into 2 subgroups (those with and those without relapses in the 2-year period prior to study entry), there was no effect on disability in patients without relapses, but in patients with relapses, the proportion with progression in disability at the end of the study was reduced from 70% (placebo) to 57% (Rebif 22 micrograms and 44 micrograms combined). These results obtained in a subgroup of patients a posteriori should be interpreted cautiously.

Rebif has not yet been investigated in patients with primary progressive multiple sclerosis, and should not be used in such patients.

5.2 Pharmacokinetic properties

In healthy volunteers after intravenous administration, interferon beta-1a exhibits a sharp multi-exponential decline, with serum levels proportional to the dose. The initial half-life is in the order of minutes and the terminal half-life is several hours, with the possible presence of a deep compartment. When administered by the subcutaneous or intramuscular routes, serum levels of interferon beta remain low, but are still measurable up to 12 to 24 hours post-dose. Subcutaneous and intramuscular administrations of Rebif produce equivalent exposure to interferon beta. Following a single 60 microgram dose, the maximum peak concentration, as measured by immunoassay, is around 6 to 10 IU/ml, occurring on average around 3 hours after the dose. After subcutaneous administration at the same dose repeated every 48 hours for 4 doses, a moderate accumulation occurs (about 2.5 × for AUC).

Regardless of the route of dosing, pronounced pharmacodynamic changes are associated with the administration of Rebif. After a single dose, intracellular and serum activity of 2-5A synthetase and serum concentrations of beta-2 microglobulin and neopterin increase within 24 hours, and start to decline within 2 days. Intramuscular and subcutaneous administrations produce fully superimposable responses. After repeated subcutaneous administration every 48 hours for 4 doses, these biological responses remain elevated, with no signs of tolerance development.

Table 1

System Organ Class	Very common	Common	Uncommon	Not known*
Infections and infestations			Injection site abscess	Injection site infections, including cellulitis
Blood and lymphatic system disorders	Neutropenia, lymphopenia, leucopenia, thrombocytopenia, anaemia			Thrombotic thrombocytopenic purpura/Haemolytic uremic syndrome
Endocrine Disorders			Thyroid dysfunction most often presenting as hypothyroidism or hyperthyroidism	
Psychiatric disorders		Depression, insomnia		Suicide attempt
Nervous system disorders	Headache			Seizures, transient neurological symptoms (i.e. hypoesthesia, muscle spasm, paraesthesia, difficulty in walking, musculoskeletal stiffness) that may mimic multiple sclerosis exacerbations
Eye disorders				Retinal vascular disorders (e.g. retinopathy, cotton wool spots and obstruction of retinal artery or vein)
Gastrointestinal disorders		Diarrhoea, vomiting, nausea		
Skin and subcutaneous tissue disorders		Pruritus, rash, erythematous rash, maculo-papular rash		Angioedema, urticaria, erythema multiforme, erythema multiforme-like skin reactions, Stevens-Johnson syndrome, hair loss
Musculoskeletal and connective tissue disorders		Myalgia, arthralgia		
General disorders and administration site conditions	Injection site inflammation, injection site reaction, influenza-like symptoms	Injection site pain, fatigue, rigors, fever	Injection site necrosis, injection site mass	
Investigations	Asymptomatic transaminase increase	Severe elevations of transaminase		
Respiratory, thoracic and mediastinal disorders				Dyspnoea
Immune system disorders				Anaphylactic reactions
Vascular disorders				Thromboembolic events
Hepatobiliary disorders				Hepatitis with or without icterus

*Adverse reactions identified during post marketing surveillance (frequency not known)

Interferon beta-1a is mainly metabolised and excreted by the liver and the kidneys.

5.3 Preclinical safety data

Non-clinical data reveal no special hazard for humans based on conventional studies of safety pharmacology, repeated-dose toxicity, and genotoxicity.

Rebif has not been investigated for carcinogenicity.

A study on embryo/foetal toxicity in monkeys showed no evidence of reproductive disturbances. Based on observations with other alpha and beta interferons, an increased risk of abortions cannot be excluded. No information is available on the effects of the interferon beta-1a on male fertility.

6. PHARMACEUTICAL PARTICULARS

6.1 List of excipients

Mannitol

Poloxamer 188

L-methionine

Benzyl alcohol

Sodium acetate

Acetic acid for pH adjustment

Sodium hydroxide for pH adjustment

Water for injections

6.2 Incompatibilities

Not applicable.

6.3 Shelf life

18 months.

6.4 Special precautions for storage

Store in a refrigerator (2°C – 8°C) away from the cooling element. Do not freeze. Store in the original package in order to protect from light.

6.5 Nature and contents of container

For patients initiating treatment with Rebif, Rebif 8.8 micrograms and Rebif 22 micrograms are available in an initiation pack composed of 6 individual doses of a 1 ml type 1 glass syringe with a stainless steel needle containing 0.2 ml of Rebif 8.8 micrograms solution for injection and 6 individual doses of a 1 ml type 1 glass syringe with a stainless steel needle containing 0.5 ml of Rebif 22 micrograms solution for injection.

This package corresponds to the patient needs for the first month of therapy.

6.6 Special precautions for disposal and other handling

The solution for injection in a pre-filled syringe is ready for use. It may also be administered with a suitable auto-injector.

For single use only. Only clear to opalescent solution without particles should be used and without visible signs of deterioration.

Any unused product or waste material should be disposed of in accordance with local requirements.

7. MARKETING AUTHORISATION HOLDER

Merck Serono Europe Limited

56, Marsh Wall

London E14 9TP

United Kingdom

8. MARKETING AUTHORISATION NUMBER(S)

EU/1/98/063/007

9. DATE OF FIRST AUTHORISATION/RENEWAL OF THE AUTHORISATION

Date of first authorisation: 4th May 1998

Date of first renewal: 4th May 2003

Date of latest renewal: 4th May 2008

10. DATE OF REVISION OF THE TEXT

24th July 2009

Rebif 8.8 micrograms/0.1 ml solution for injection in cartridge and Rebif 22 micrograms/0.25 ml solution for injection in cartridge

(Merck Serono)

1. NAME OF THE MEDICINAL PRODUCT

Rebif 8.8 micrograms/0.1 ml solution for injection in cartridge

Rebif 22 micrograms/0.25 ml solution for injection in cartridge

2. QUALITATIVE AND QUANTITATIVE COMPOSITION

Each pre-filled cartridge contains 132 micrograms (36 MIU*) of interferon beta-1a** in 1.5 ml solution, corresponding to 88 micrograms/ml.

* Million International Units measured by cytopathic effect (CPE) bioassay against the in-house IFN beta-1a standard which is calibrated against the current international NIH standard (GB-23-902-531).

** produced in Chinese hamster ovary Cells (CHO-K1) by recombinant DNA technology.

Excipient: 7.5 mg benzyl alcohol

For a full list of excipients, see section 6.1.

3. PHARMACEUTICAL FORM

Solution for injection in cartridge.

Clear to opalescent solution, with pH 3.7 to 4.1 and osmolarity 250 to 450 mOsm/l.

4. CLINICAL PARTICULARS

4.1 Therapeutic indications

Rebif is indicated for the treatment of relapsing multiple sclerosis.

In clinical trials, this was characterised by two or more acute exacerbations in the previous two years (see section 5.1).

Efficacy has not been demonstrated in patients with secondary progressive multiple sclerosis without ongoing relapse activity (see section 5.1).

4.2 Posology and method of administration

Treatment should be initiated under supervision of a physician experienced in the treatment of the disease.

The Rebif initiation package corresponds to the patient needs for the first month of treatment. When first starting treatment with Rebif, in order to allow tachyphylaxis to develop thus reducing adverse reactions, it is recommended that 8.8 micrograms be administered by subcutaneous injection three times per week during the initial 2 weeks of therapy. Thereafter, 22 micrograms be administered by subcutaneous injection three times per week in weeks 3 and 4, and the total of the 44 micrograms strength be administered from the fifth week onwards.

Method of administration

Rebif solution for injection in cartridge is intended for multidose use and should only be used with the RebiSmart autoinjector device following adequate training of the patient and/or carer.

For administration, the instructions provided in the package leaflet and in the instruction manual provided with the RebiSmart autoinjector device should be followed.

Prior to injection and for an additional 24 hours after each injection, an antipyretic analgesic is advised to decrease flu-like symptoms associated with Rebif administration.

At the present time, it is not known for how long patients should be treated. Safety and efficacy with Rebif have not been demonstrated beyond 4 years of treatment. It is recommended that patients should be evaluated at least every second year in the 4-year period after initiation of treatment with Rebif and a decision for longer term treatment should then be made on an individual basis by the treating physician.

Paediatric use

No formal clinical trials or pharmacokinetic studies have been conducted in children or adolescents. However, limited published data suggest that the safety profile in adolescents from 12 to 16 years of age receiving Rebif 22 micrograms subcutaneous three times per week is similar to that seen in adults. There is very limited information on the use of Rebif in children under 12 years of age and therefore Rebif should not be used in this population.

4.3 Contraindications

- Initiation of treatment in pregnancy (see section 4.6).

• Hypersensitivity to natural or recombinant interferon-β, or to any excipients.

• Current severe depression and/or suicidal ideation (see sections 4.4 and 4.8).

4.4 Special warnings and precautions for use

Patients should be informed of the most frequent adverse reactions associated with interferon beta administration, including symptoms of the flu-like syndrome (see section 4.8). These symptoms tend to be most prominent at the initiation of therapy and decrease in frequency and severity with continued treatment.

Rebif should be administered with caution to patients with previous or current depressive disorders in particular to those with antecedents of suicidal ideation (see section 4.3). Depression and suicidal ideation are known to occur in increased frequency in the multiple sclerosis population and in association with interferon use. Patients treated with Rebif should be advised to immediately report any symptoms of depression and/or suicidal ideation to their prescribing physician. Patients exhibiting depression should be monitored closely during therapy with Rebif and treated appropriately. Cessation of therapy with Rebif should be considered (see sections 4.3 and 4.8).

Rebif should be administered with caution to patients with a history of seizures, to those receiving treatment with anti-epileptics, particularly if their epilepsy is not adequately controlled with anti-epileptics (see sections 4.5 and 4.8).

Patients with cardiac disease, such as angina, congestive heart failure or arrhythmia, should be closely monitored for worsening of their clinical condition during initiation of therapy with interferon beta-1a. Symptoms of the flu-like syndrome associated with interferon beta-1a therapy may prove stressful to patients with cardiac conditions.

Injection site necrosis (ISN) has been reported in patients using Rebif (see section 4.8). To minimise the risk of injection site necrosis patients should be advised to:

• use an aseptic injection technique,

• rotate the injection sites with each dose.

The procedure for the self-administration by the patient should be reviewed periodically especially if injection site reactions have occurred.

If the patient experiences any break in the skin, which may be associated with swelling or drainage of fluid from the injection site, the patient should be advised to consult with their physician before continuing injections with Rebif. If the patient has multiple lesions, Rebif should be discontinued until healing has occurred. Patients with single lesions may continue provided that the necrosis is not too extensive.

In clinical trials with Rebif, asymptomatic elevations of hepatic transaminases (particularly alanine aminotransferase (ALT)) were common and 1-3% of patients developed elevations of hepatic transaminases above 5 times the upper limit of normal (ULN). In the absence of clinical symptoms, serum ALT levels should be monitored prior to the start of therapy, at months 1, 3 and 6 on therapy and periodically thereafter. Dose reduction of Rebif should be considered if ALT rises above 5 times the ULN, and gradually re-escalated when enzyme levels have normalized. Rebif should be initiated with caution in patients with a history of significant liver disease, clinical evidence of active liver disease, alcohol abuse or increased serum ALT (>2.5 times ULN). Treatment with Rebif should be stopped if icterus or other clinical symptoms of liver dysfunction appear (see section 4.8).

Rebif, like other interferons beta, has a potential for causing severe liver injury (see section 4.8) including acute hepatic failure. The mechanism for the rare symptomatic hepatic dysfunction is not known. No specific risk factors have been identified.

Laboratory abnormalities are associated with the use of interferons. Therefore, in addition to those laboratory tests normally required for monitoring patients with multiple sclerosis, liver enzyme monitoring and complete and differential blood cell counts and platelet counts are recommended at regular intervals (1, 3 and 6 months) following introduction of Rebif therapy and then periodically thereafter in the absence of clinical symptoms.

Patients being treated with Rebif may occasionally develop new or worsening thyroid abnormalities. Thyroid function testing is recommended at baseline and if abnormal, every 6-12 months following initiation of therapy. If tests are normal at baseline, routine testing is not needed but should be performed if clinical findings of thyroid dysfunction appear (see section 4.8).

Caution should be used, and close monitoring considered when administering interferon beta-1a to patients with severe renal and hepatic failure and to patients with severe myelosuppression.

Serum neutralising antibodies against interferon beta-1a may develop. The precise incidence of antibodies is as yet uncertain. Clinical data suggest that after 24 to 48 months of treatment with Rebif 22 micrograms, approximately 24% of patients develop persistent serum antibodies to interferon beta-1a. The presence of antibodies has been shown to attenuate the pharmacodynamic response to interferon beta-1a (Beta-2 microglobulin and neopterin). Although the clinical significance of the induction of antibodies has not been fully elucidated, the development of neutralising antibodies is associated with reduced efficacy on clinical and MRI variables. If a patient responds poorly to therapy with Rebif, and has neutralising antibodies, the treating physician should reassess the benefit/risk ratio of continued Rebif therapy.

The use of various assays to detect serum antibodies and differing definitions of antibody positivity limits the ability to compare antigenicity among different products.

Only sparse safety and efficacy data are available from non-ambulatory patients with multiple sclerosis. Rebif has not yet been investigated in patients with primary progressive multiple sclerosis and should not be used in such patients.

This medicinal product contains 0.5 mg benzyl alcohol per dose of 0.1 ml and 1.25 mg benzyl alcohol per dose of 0.25 ml. Must not be given to premature babies or neonates. May cause toxic reactions and anaphylactoid reactions in infants and children up to 3 years old.

4.5 Interaction with other medicinal products and other forms of interaction

No interaction studies have been performed with interferon beta-1a in humans.

Interferons have been reported to reduce the activity of hepatic cytochrome P450-dependent enzymes in humans and animals. Caution should be exercised when administering Rebif in combination with medicinal products that have a narrow therapeutic index and are largely dependent on the hepatic cytochrome P450 system for clearance, e.g. antiepileptics and some classes of antidepressants.

The interaction of Rebif with corticosteroids or adrenocorticotropic hormone (ACTH) has not been studied systematically. Clinical studies indicate that multiple sclerosis patients can receive Rebif and corticosteroids or ACTH during relapses.

4.6 Pregnancy and lactation

There is limited information on the use of Rebif in pregnancy. Available data indicates that there may be an increased risk of spontaneous abortion. Therefore initiation of treatment is contraindicated during pregnancy (see section 4.3).

Women of child-bearing potential should take appropriate contraceptive measures. If the patient becomes pregnant or plans to become pregnant while taking Rebif she should be informed of the potential hazards and discontinuation of therapy should be considered (see section 5.3). In patients with a high relapse rate before treatment has started, the risk of a severe relapse following discontinuation of Rebif in the event of pregnancy should be weighed against a possible increased risk of spontaneous abortion.

It is not known whether Rebif is excreted in human milk. Because of the potential for serious adverse reactions in breast-fed infants, a decision should be made either to discontinue nursing or to discontinue Rebif therapy.

4.7 Effects on ability to drive and use machines

Central nervous system-related adverse events associated with the use of interferon beta (e.g. dizziness) might influence the patient's ability to drive or use machines (see section 4.8).

4.8 Undesirable effects

The highest incidence of adverse reactions associated with Rebif therapy is related to flu-like syndrome. Flu-like symptoms tend to be most prominent at the initiation of therapy and decrease in frequency with continued treatment. Approximately 70% of patients treated with Rebif can expect to experience the typical interferon flu-like syndrome within the first six months after starting treatment. Approximately 30% of patients will also experience reactions at the injection site, predominantly mild inflammation or erythema. Asymptomatic increases in laboratory parameters of hepatic function and decreases in white blood cells (WBC) are also common.

The majority of adverse reactions observed with IFN beta-1a are usually mild and reversible, and respond well to dose reductions. In case of severe or persistent undesirable effects, the dose of Rebif may be temporarily lowered or interrupted, at the discretion of the physician.

The adverse reactions reported below are classified according to frequency of occurrence as follows:

Very Common	⩾1/10
Common	⩾1/100 to <1/10
Uncommon	⩾1/1,000 to <1/100
Rare	⩾1/10,000 to <1/ 1,000
Very rare	<1/10,000
Not known	Cannot be estimated from the available data

Within each frequency grouping, undesirable effects are presented in order of decreasing seriousness.

The data presented is obtained from pooled clinical studies in multiple sclerosis (placebo=824 patients; Rebif 22 micrograms three times per week (TIW)=398 patients; Rebif 44 micrograms TIW=727 patients) and shows the frequency of adverse reactions observed at six months (excess over placebo). Adverse reactions are listed below by frequency of occurrence and by MedDRA System Organ Class.

(see Table 1 on next page)

Interferon beta has a potential for causing severe liver injury. The mechanism for the rare symptomatic hepatic dysfunction is not known. The majority of the cases of severe liver injury occurred within the first six months of treatment. No specific risk factors have been identified. Treatment with Rebif should be stopped if icterus or other clinical symptoms of liver dysfunction appear (see section 4.4).

The administration of interferons has been associated with anorexia, dizziness, anxiety, arrhythmias, vasodilation and palpitation, menorrhagia and metrorrhagia.

An increased formation of auto-antibodies may occur during treatment with interferon beta.

4.9 Overdose

In case of overdose, patients should be hospitalised for observation and appropriate supportive treatment should be given.

5. PHARMACOLOGICAL PROPERTIES

5.1 Pharmacodynamic properties

Pharmacotherapeutic group: Immunostimulants, Interferons, ATC code: L03AB07.

Interferons (IFNs) are a group of endogenous glycoproteins endowed with immunomodulatory, antiviral and antiproliferative properties.

Rebif (interferon beta-1a) shares the same amino acid sequence with endogenous human interferon beta. It is produced in mammalian cells (Chinese hamster ovary) and is therefore glycosylated like the natural protein.

The precise mechanism of action of Rebif in multiple sclerosis is still under investigation.

The safety and efficacy of Rebif has been evaluated in patients with relapsing-remitting multiple sclerosis at doses ranging from 11 to 44 micrograms (3-12 million IU), administered subcutaneously three times per week. At licensed posology, Rebif 22 micrograms has been demonstrated to decrease the incidence (approximately 30% over 2 years) and severity of clinical relapses in patients with at least 2 exacerbations in the previous 2 years and with an EDSS of 0-5.0 at entry. The proportion of patients with disability progression, as defined by at least one point increase in EDSS confirmed three months later, was reduced from 39% (placebo) to 30% (Rebif 22 micrograms). Over 4 years, the reduction in the mean exacerbation rate was 22% in patients treated with Rebif 22 micrograms, and 29% in patients treated with Rebif 44 micrograms group compared with a group of patients treated with placebo for 2 years and then either Rebif 22 or Rebif 44 micrograms for 2 years.

In a 3-year study in patients with secondary progressive multiple sclerosis (EDSS 3-6.5) with evidence of clinical progression in the preceding two years and who had not experienced relapses in the preceding 8 weeks, Rebif had no significant effect on progression of disability, but relapse rate was reduced by approximately 30%. If the patient population was divided into 2 subgroups (those with and those without relapses in the 2-year period prior to study entry), there was no effect on disability in patients without relapses, but in patients with relapses, the proportion with progression in disability at the end of the study was reduced from 70% (placebo) to 57% (Rebif 22 micrograms and 44 micrograms combined). These results obtained in a subgroup of patients a posteriori should be interpreted cautiously.

Rebif has not yet been investigated in patients with primary progressive multiple sclerosis, and should not be used in such patients.

5.2 Pharmacokinetic properties

In healthy volunteers after intravenous administration, interferon beta-1a exhibits a sharp multi-exponential decline, with serum levels proportional to the dose. The initial half-life is in the order of minutes and the terminal half-life is several hours, with the possible presence of a deep compartment. When administered by the subcutaneous or intramuscular routes, serum levels of interferon beta remain low, but are still measurable up to 12 to 24 hours post-dose. Subcutaneous and intramuscular administrations of Rebif produce equivalent exposure to interferon beta. Following a single 60 microgram dose, the maximum peak concentration, as measured by immunoassay, is around 6 to 10 IU/ml, occurring on average around 3 hours after the dose. After subcutaneous administration at the same dose repeated every 48 hours for 4 doses, a moderate accumulation occurs (about 2.5 × for AUC).

Regardless of the route of dosing, pronounced pharmacodynamic changes are associated with the administration of Rebif. After a single dose, intracellular and serum activity of 2-5A synthetase and serum concentrations of beta-2 microglobulin and neopterin increase within 24 hours, and start to decline within 2 days. Intramuscular and subcutaneous administrations produce fully superimposable responses. After repeated subcutaneous administration every 48 hours for 4 doses, these biological responses remain elevated, with no signs of tolerance development.

Interferon beta-1a is mainly metabolised and excreted by the liver and the kidneys.

Table 1

System Organ Class	Very common	Common	Uncommon	Not known*
Infections and infestations			Injection site abscess	Injection site infections, including cellulitis
Blood and lymphatic system disorders	Neutropenia, lymphopenia, leucopenia, thrombocytopenia, anaemia			Thrombotic thrombocytopenic purpura/Haemolytic uremic syndrome
Endocrine Disorders			Thyroid dysfunction most often presenting as hypothyroidism or hyperthyroidism	
Psychiatric disorders		Depression, insomnia		Suicide attempt
Nervous system disorders	Headache			Seizures, transient neurological symptoms (i.e. hypoesthesia, muscle spasm, paraesthesia, difficulty in walking, musculoskeletal stiffness) that may mimic multiple sclerosis exacerbations
Eye disorders				Retinal vascular disorders (e.g. retinopathy, cotton wool spots and obstruction of retinal artery or vein)
Gastrointestinal disorders		Diarrhoea, vomiting, nausea		
Skin and subcutaneous tissue disorders		Pruritus, rash, erythematous rash, maculo-papular rash		Angioedema, urticaria, erythema multiforme, erythema multiforme-like skin reactions, Stevens-Johnson syndrome, hair loss
Musculoskeletal and connective tissue disorders		Myalgia, arthralgia		
General disorders and administration site conditions	Injection site inflammation, injection site reaction, influenza-like symptoms	Injection site pain, fatigue, rigors, fever	Injection site necrosis, injection site mass	
Investigations	Asymptomatic transaminase increase	Severe elevations of transaminase		
Respiratory, thoracic and mediastinal disorders				Dyspnoea
Immune system disorders				Anaphylactic reactions
Vascular disorders				Thromboembolic events
Hepatobiliary disorders				Hepatitis with or without icterus

*Adverse reactions identified during post marketing surveillance (frequency not known)

5.3 Preclinical safety data

Non-clinical data reveal no special hazard for humans based on conventional studies of safety pharmacology, repeated-dose toxicity, and genotoxicity.

Rebif has not been investigated for carcinogenicity.

A study on embryo/foetal toxicity in monkeys showed no evidence of reproductive disturbances. Based on observations with other alpha and beta interferons, an increased risk of abortions cannot be excluded. No information is available on the effects of the interferon beta-1a on male fertility.

6. PHARMACEUTICAL PARTICULARS

6.1 List of excipients

Mannitol

Poloxamer 188

L-methionine

Benzyl alcohol

Sodium acetate

Acetic acid for pH adjustment

Sodium hydroxide for pH adjustment

Water for injections

6.2 Incompatibilities

Not applicable.

6.3 Shelf life

18 months.

After first injection use within 28 days.

6.4 Special precautions for storage

Store in a refrigerator (2°C – 8°C) away from the cooling element. Do not freeze. Store the cartridge in the original package in order to protect from light.

The RebiSmart autoinjector device containing a pre-filled cartridge of Rebif must be stored in the device storage box in a refrigerator (2°C – 8°C).

Should refrigeration be temporarily unavailable, Rebif can be stored by the patient at or below 25°C for up to 14 days then put back in the refrigerator and used before the expiry date.

6.5 Nature and contents of container

Cartridges (type 1 glass) with a plunger stopper (rubber) and crimp cap (aluminium and halobutyl rubber) containing 1.5 ml solution for injection.

Pack size of 2 cartridges.

This package corresponds to the patient needs for the first month of therapy.

6.6 Special precautions for disposal and other handling

The solution for injection in a pre-filled cartridge is ready for use with the RebiSmart autoinjector device. For storage of the RebiSmart autoinjector device with the cartridge, see section 6.4.

For multidose use. Only clear to opalescent solution without particles should be used and without visible signs of deterioration.

Any unused product or waste material should be disposed of in accordance with local requirements.

7. MARKETING AUTHORISATION HOLDER

Merck Serono Europe Limited

56, Marsh Wall

London E14 9TP

United Kingdom

8. MARKETING AUTHORISATION NUMBER(S)

EU/1/98/063/010

9. DATE OF FIRST AUTHORISATION/RENEWAL OF THE AUTHORISATION

Date of first authorisation: 4th May 1998

Date of first renewal: 4th May 2003

Date of latest renewal: 4th May 2008

10. DATE OF REVISION OF THE TEXT

24th July 2009

Rectogesic 4 mg/g Rectal Ointment

(ProStrakan)

1. NAME OF THE MEDICINAL PRODUCT

Rectogesic 4 mg/g Rectal Ointment.

2. QUALITATIVE AND QUANTITATIVE COMPOSITION

Glyceryl trinitrate: 4 mg/g.

One gram of rectal ointment contains 40 mg Glyceryl trinitrate in propylene glycol corresponding to 4 mg Glyceryl trinitrate (GTN). The delivered dose from 375 mg of this formulation is approximately 1.5 mg GTN.

The ointment also contains 36 mg Propylene Glycol, and 140 mg Lanolin, per gram rectal ointment.

For a full list of excipients, see section 6.1.

3. PHARMACEUTICAL FORM

Rectal ointment.

Off-white smooth opaque ointment formulation.

4. CLINICAL PARTICULARS

4.1 Therapeutic indications

Rectogesic 4 mg/g Rectal Ointment is indicated for relief of pain associated with chronic anal fissure.

In the clinical development of the drug, a modest effect has been shown on improvements in average daily pain intensity (see Section 5.1).

4.2 Posology and method of administration

Route of administration: rectal use

Adults:

A finger covering, such as cling film or a finger cot, may be placed on the finger to be used to apply the ointment. (Finger cots to be obtained separately from local pharmacy or surgical supplies retailer or cling film from local store.) The finger is placed along side a 2.5cm dosing line which is provided on the outside carton in which Rectogesic is supplied, and a strip of ointment the length of the line is expressed onto the end of the finger by gently squeezing the tube. The amount of ointment expressed is approximately 375 mg (1.5 mg GTN). The covered finger is then gently inserted into the anal canal to the distal interphalangeal joint of the finger and applied circumferentially to the anal canal.

The dose delivered from the 4 mg/g ointment is 1.5 mg glyceryl trinitrate. The dose is to be applied intra-anally every twelve hours. Treatment may be continued until the pain abates, up to a maximum of 8 weeks.

Rectogesic should be used following conservative treatment failure for acute symptoms of anal fissure.

Elderly:

No specific information concerning the usage of Rectogesic in the elderly is available

Patients with Hepatic or Renal Impairment

No specific information concerning the usage of Rectogesic in patients with hepatic or renal impairment is available

Children and Adolescents:

Rectogesic is not recommended for use in children and adolescents below 18 years of age due to a lack of data on safety and efficacy.

4.3 Contraindications

Hypersensitivity to the active substance "glyceryl trinitrate" or to any of the excipients or idiosyncratic reactions to other organic nitrates.

Concomitant treatment with sildenafil citrate, tadalafil, vardenafil and with nitric oxide (NO) donors, such as other long-acting GTN products, isosorbide dinitrate and amyl or butyl-nitrite.

Postural hypotension, hypotension or uncorrected hypovolaemia as the use of glyceryl trinitrate in such states could produce severe hypotension or shock.

Increased intracranial pressure (e.g. head trauma or cerebral haemorrhage) or inadequate cerebral circulation.

Migraine or recurrent headache.

Aortic or mitral stenosis.

Hypertrophic obstructive cardiomyopathy.

Constrictive pericarditis or pericardial tamponade.

Marked anaemia.

Closed-angle glaucoma.

4.4 Special warnings and precautions for use

The risk/benefit ratio of Rectogesic has to be established on an individual basis. In some patients, following treatment with Rectogesic, severe headache can occur. In some cases re-evaluation of the correct dosing is suggested. In patients where the risk benefit ratio is deemed to be negative, treatment with Rectogesic should be withdrawn under the guidance of a physician and other therapeutic or surgical interventions should be initiated.

Rectogesic should be used with caution in patients who have severe hepatic or renal disease.

Excessive hypotension, especially for prolonged periods of time, must be avoided because of possible deleterious effects on the brain, heart, liver and kidney from poor perfusion and the attendant risk of ischaemia, thrombosis and altered function of these organs. Patients should be advised to change position slowly when changing from lying or sitting to upright to minimize postural hypotension. This advice is particularly important for those patients with low blood volume and under diuretic treatment. Paradoxical bradycardia and increased angina pectoris may accompany glyceryl trinitrate-induced hypotension. The elderly may be more susceptible to the development of postural hypotension, particularly on sudden rising. No specific information concerning the usage of Rectogesic in the elderly is available.

Alcohol may enhance the hypotensive effects of glyceryl trinitrate.

If the physician elects to use glyceryl trinitrate ointment for patients with acute myocardial infarction or congestive heart failure, careful clinical and haemodynamic monitoring must be used to avoid the potential hazards of hypotension and tachycardia.

If bleeding associated with haemorrhoids increases, treatment should be stopped.

This formulation contains propylene glycol and lanolin which may cause skin irritations and skin reactions (e.g. contact dermatitis).

If anal pain persists, differential diagnosis may be required to exclude other causes of the pain.

Glyceryl trinitrate can interfere with the measurement of catecholamines and vanilmandelic acid in urine as it increases the excretion of these substances.

Concomitant treatment with a number of other medicinal products should be handled with caution. Please refer to section 4.5 for specific information.

4.5 Interaction with other medicinal products and other forms of interaction

Concomitant treatment with other vasodilators, calcium channel blockers, ACE inhibitors, beta blockers, diuretics, anti-hypertensives, tricyclic anti-depressants and major tranquillisers, as well as the consumption of alcohol, may potentiate the blood pressure lowering effects of Rectogesic. Therefore, concomitant treatment with these medications should be carefully considered before treatment with Rectogesic is initiated.

The hypotensive effect of nitrates are potentiated by concurrent administration of phosphodiesterase inhibitors, e.g. sildenafil, tadalafil and vardenafil (see Section 4.3).

Rectogesic is contraindicated for concomitant treatment with, nitric oxide (NO) donors such as isosorbide dinitrate and amyl or butyl-nitrite (see Section 4.3).

Acetyl cysteine may potentiate the vasodilatory effects of glyceryl trinitrate.

Concomitant treatment with heparin leads to a decrease in heparin efficacy. Close monitoring of blood coagulation parameters is necessary and the dose of heparin has to be adapted accordingly. After withdrawal of Rectogesic there may be an abrupt increase in PTT. In this case reduction of heparin dosage may be necessary.

Concurrent administration of glyceryl trinitrate may cause a reduction of the thrombolytic activity of alteplase.

Co-administration of Rectogesic with dihydroergotamine may increase the bioavailability of dihydroergotamine and lead to coronary vasoconstriction. The possibility that the ingestion of acetylsalicylic acid and non-steroidal anti-inflammatory drugs might diminish the therapeutic response to Rectogesic cannot be excluded.

4.6 Pregnancy and lactation

Pregnancy: There are no adequate data from the use of glyceryl trinitrate in pregnant women. Animal studies are inconclusive with respect to effects on pregnancy embryonal/foetal parturition and postnatal development (see Section 5.3). Rectogesic should not be used during pregnancy.

Lactation: It is not known whether glyceryl trinitrate is excreted in human milk. Due to the potential harmful effects on the breast fed child (see Section 5.3), the use of Rectogesic is not recommended during breast feeding.

4.7 Effects on ability to drive and use machines

No studies on the effect on the ability to drive and use machines have been performed with Rectogesic. Rectogesic may cause dizziness, light-headedness, blurred vision, headache or tiredness in some patients, especially on first use. Patients should be cautioned about driving or operating machinery while using Rectogesic.

4.8 Undesirable effects

In patients treated with Rectogesic 4 mg/g Rectal Ointment, the most common treatment related adverse reaction was dose-related headache which occurred with an incidence of 57%.

Adverse reactions from clinical studies are displayed by system organ class in the table below. Within the system organ class, the adverse reactions are listed by frequency using the following groupings: very common (> 1/10), common (>1/100 <1/10), uncommon (>1/1000 <1/100).

System Organ Class	Frequency	Adverse Reaction
Nervous system disorder	Very common	Headache
	Common	Dizziness
Gastrointestinal disorders	Common	Nausea
	Uncommon	Diarrhoea, anal discomfort, vomiting, rectal bleeding, rectal disorder
Skin and subcutaneous tissue disorders	Uncommon	Pruritus, anal burning and itching
Cardiovascular system disorders	Uncommon	Tachycardia

Adverse reactions to glyceryl trinitrate 2% ointment (used in the prophylaxis of angina pectoris) are generally dose-related and almost all of these reactions are the result of vasodilator activity. Headache, which may be severe, is the most commonly reported side effect. In the Phase III clinical trials with Rectogesic 4 mg/g Rectal Ointment the incidence of mild, moderate and severe headache was 18%, 25% and 20%. Patients with a previous history of migraine or recurrent headache were at a higher risk of developing headache during treatment (see Section 4.3). Headache may be recurrent with each daily dose, especially at higher doses. Headache can be treated with mild analgesics e.g. paracetamol and in general is reversible on discontinuation of treatment.

Transient episodes of light-headedness, occasionally related to blood pressure changes, also may occur. Hypotension (including orthostatic hypotension) occurs infrequently, but in some patients may be severe enough to warrant discontinuation of therapy. Syncope, crescendo angina and rebound hypertension have been reported but are uncommon. Allergic reactions to glyceryl trinitrate are uncommon, and the great majority of those reported have been cases of contact dermatitis or fixed drug eruptions occurring in patients receiving glyceryl trinitrate in ointments or patches. There have been a few reports of genuine anaphylactoid reactions and these reactions can probably occur in patients receiving glyceryl trinitrate by any route. Extremely rarely, ordinary doses of organic nitrates have caused methaemoglobinaemia in normal-seeming patients. Flush has been observed as a rare adverse reaction for other products containing glyceryl trinitrate.

4.9 Overdose

Accidental overdose of Rectogesic may result in hypotension and reflex tachycardia. No specific antagonist of the vasodilator effects of nitroglycerin is known, and no intervention has been subjected to controlled study as a therapy for nitroglycerin overdose. Because the hypotension associated with nitroglycerin overdose is the result of venodilation and arterial hypovolaemia, prudent therapy in this situation should be directed toward increasing central fluid volume. Passive elevation of the patient's legs may be sufficient, but intravenous infusion of normal saline or similar fluid may also be necessary. In exceptional cases of severe hypotension or shock, resuscitation measures may be needed.

Excessive dosage may also give rise to methaemoglobinaemia. This should be treated with methylene blue infusion.

5. PHARMACOLOGICAL PROPERTIES

5.1 Pharmacodynamic properties

Pharmacotherapeutic group: Muscle relaxants

ATC Code: C05AE01

The principal pharmacologic action of glyceryl trinitrate is mediated via the release of nitric oxide. When glyceryl trinitrate ointment is applied by the intra-anal route, the internal anal sphincter becomes relaxed.

Hypertonicity of the internal but not the external anal sphincter is a predisposing factor in the formation of anal fissures. The blood vessels to the anoderm course through the internal anal sphincter (IAS). Therefore hypertonicity of the IAS may thereby decrease blood flow and cause ischaemia to this region.

Distension of the rectum results in the anorector inhibitory reflex and relaxation of the internal anal sphincter. The nerves mediating this reflex lie in the wall of the gut. Release of the neurotransmitter NO from nerves of this type play a significant role in the physiology of the internal anal sphincter. Specifically, NO mediates the anorector inhibitory reflex in man, relaxing the IAS.

The link between IAS hypertonicity and spasm and the presence of an anal fissure has been established. Patients with chronic anal fissure have a significantly higher mean maximum resting anal pressure than controls and anodermal blood flow in chronic anal fissure patients was significantly lower than in controls. In patients whose fissures healed following a sphincterotomy, a reduction in anal pressure and improvement in anodermal blood flow was demonstrated, providing further evidence for the ischaemic nature of anal fissure. Topical application of a NO donor (glyceryl trinitrate) relaxes the anal sphincter, resulting in a reduction of anal pressure and an improvement in anoderm blood flow.

Effect on pain

In three Phase III clinical trials Rectogesic 4 mg/g Rectal Ointment has been shown to improve the average daily pain intensity associated with chronic anal fissure compared with placebo, measured using a 100mm visual analogue scale. In the first study, Rectogesic 4 mg/g Rectal Ointment decreased average daily pain intensity over 21 days by 13.3mm (baseline 39.2mm) compared to 4.3mm (baseline 25.7mm) for placebo ($p<0.0063$) and over 56 days by 18.8mm compared to 6.9mm ($p<0.0001$), respectively. This corresponds to a treatment effect (difference between the percentage change for Rectogesic and placebo) of 17.2% over 21 days and 21.1% over 56 days. In the second study, Rectogesic 4 mg/g Rectal Ointment decreased average daily pain intensity over 21 days by 11.1mm (baseline 33.4mm) compared to 7.7mm (baseline 34.0mm) for placebo ($p<0.0388$) and over 56 days by 17.2mm compared to 13.8mm ($p<0.0039$), respectively. This corresponds to a treatment effect of 10.6% over 21 days and 10.9% over 56 days. In the third study, Rectogesic 4 mg/g Rectal Ointment decreased average daily pain intensity over 21 days by 28.1mm (baseline 55.0mm) compared to 24.9mm (baseline 54.1mm) for placebo ($p<0.0489$) and over 56 days by 35.2mm compared to 33.8mm ($p<0.0447$), respectively. This corresponds to a treatment effect of 5.1% over 21 days and 1.5% over 56 days.

Effect on healing

In all three studies, healing of anal fissures in patients treated with Rectogesic 4 mg/g Rectal Ointment was not statistically different from placebo. Rectogesic is not indicated for healing of chronic anal fissure.

5.2 Pharmacokinetic properties

The volume of distribution of glyceryl trinitrate is about 3 L/kg and is cleared from this volume at extremely rapid rates, with a resulting serum half-life of about 3 minutes. The observed clearance rates (close to 1 L/kg/min) greatly exceed hepatic blood flow. The known sites of extrahepatic metabolism include red blood cells and vascular walls. The initial products in the metabolism of glyceryl trinitrate are inorganic nitrate and the 1,2 and 1,3-dinitroglycerols. The dinitrates are less effective vasodilators than glyceryl trinitrate, but they are longer lived in the serum. Their contribution to the relaxation of the internal anal sphincter is unknown. The dinitrates are further metabolised to non-vasoactive mononitrates and ultimately to glycerol and carbon dioxide. In six healthy subjects, the average bioavailability of glyceryl trinitrate applied to the anal canal as a 0.2% ointment was approximately 50% of the 0.75 mg dose.

5.3 Preclinical safety data

Repeat Dose Toxicity

No systemic toxicity studies have been conducted with Rectogesic. Published data suggest that high oral doses of glyceryl trinitrate may have toxic effects (methaemoglobinaemia, testicular atrophy and aspermatogenesis) in long term treatment. However, these findings represent no special hazards for humans under the conditions of therapeutic use.

Mutagenicity and carcinogenicity

Data from preclinical studies with GTN indicate genotoxic effects in the repair deficient S. typhimurium strain TA1535 only and carcinogenic effects. However, an increased carcinogenic risk under the conditions of therapeutic use is considered very unlikely.

Reproductive Toxicity

Reproductive toxicity studies, in rats and rabbits with intravenous, intraperitoneal, and dermal administration of glyceryl trinitrate did not show any adverse effects on fertility or embryonic development at dosages which did not induce parental toxicity. No teratogenicity had been observed. In rats foetotoxic effects (decreased birth weights) were seen at dosages above 1 mg/kg/d (i.p.) and 28 mg/kg/d (dermal) after in utero exposure during foetal development.

6. PHARMACEUTICAL PARTICULARS

6.1 List of excipients

Propylene glycol

Lanolin

Sorbitan sesquioleate

Hard paraffin

White soft paraffin

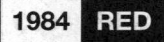

6.2 Incompatibilities
Not applicable.

6.3 Shelf life
15 months

After first opening: 8 weeks

6.4 Special precautions for storage
Do not store above 25°C.

Do not freeze.

Keep the tube tightly closed.

6.5 Nature and contents of container
30 g

Aluminium tubes with white polyethylene non-piercing screw caps

6.6 Special precautions for disposal and other handling
No special requirements.

7. MARKETING AUTHORISATION HOLDER
ProStrakan Limited

Galabank Business Park

Galashiels

TD1 1QH

UK

8. MARKETING AUTHORISATION NUMBER(S)
PL 16508/0037

9. DATE OF FIRST AUTHORISATION/RENEWAL OF THE AUTHORISATION
28/08/2009

10. DATE OF REVISION OF THE TEXT
28/08/2009

Reductil 10mg & 15mg

(Abbott Laboratories Limited)

1. NAME OF THE MEDICINAL PRODUCT
Reductil 10 mg capsules, hard

Reductil 15 mg capsules, hard

2. QUALITATIVE AND QUANTITATIVE COMPOSITION
One capsule of Reductil 10 mg contains 10 mg of sibutramine hydrochloride monohydrate (equivalent to 8.37 mg of sibutramine).

One capsule of Reductil 15 mg contains 15 mg of sibutramine hydrochloride monohydrate (equivalent to 12.55 mg of sibutramine).

For excipients, see 6.1

3. PHARMACEUTICAL FORM
10 mg Hard capsule with a blue cap and yellow body

15 mg Hard capsule with a blue cap and white body

4. CLINICAL PARTICULARS

4.1 Therapeutic indications
Reductil 10 mg / 15 mg is indicated as adjunctive therapy within a weight management programme for:

- Patients with nutritional obesity and a body mass index (BMI) of 30 kg/m^2 or higher

- Patients with nutritional excess weight and a BMI of 27 kg/m^2 or higher, if other obesity-related risk factors such as type 2 diabetes or dyslipidaemia are present.

Note:

Reductil may only be prescribed to patients who have not adequately responded to an appropriate weight-reducing regimen alone, ie patients who have difficulty achieving or maintaining >5% weight loss within 3 months.

Treatment with Reductil 10 mg / 15 mg should only be given as part of a long-term integrated therapeutic approach for weight reduction under the care of a physician experienced in the treatment of obesity. An appropriate approach to obesity management should include dietary and behavioural modification as well as increased physical activity. This integrated approach is essential for a lasting change in eating habits and behaviour which is fundamental to the long-term maintenance of the reduced weight level once Reductil is stopped. Patients should change their lifestyle while on Reductil so that they are able to maintain their weight once drug treatment has ceased. They should be informed that, if they fail to do so, they may regain weight. Even after cessation of Reductil continued monitoring of the patient by the physician should be encouraged.

4.2 Posology and method of administration
Adults: The initial dose is one (1) capsule of Reductil 10 mg swallowed whole, once daily, in the morning, with liquid (eg a glass of water). The capsule can be taken with or without food.

In those patients with an inadequate response to Reductil 10 mg (defined as less than 2 kg weight loss after four (4) weeks treatment), the dose may be increased to one (1) capsule of Reductil 15 mg once daily, provided that Reductil 10 mg was well tolerated.

Treatment must be discontinued in patients who have responded inadequately to Reductil 15 mg (defined as less than 2 kg weight loss after four (4) weeks treatment). Non-responders are at a higher risk of undesirable effects (see section 4.8 "Undesirable Effects").

Duration of treatment:

Treatment must be discontinued in patients who have not responded adequately, ie whose weight loss stabilises at less than 5% of their initial bodyweight or whose weight loss within three (3) months after starting therapy has been less than 5% of their initial bodyweight. Treatment should not be continued in patients who regain 3 kg or more after previously achieved weight loss.

In patients with associated co-morbid conditions, it is recommended that treatment with Reductil 10 mg / 15 mg should only be continued if it can be shown that the weight loss induced is associated with other clinical benefits, such as improvements in lipid profile in patients with dyslipidaemia or glycaemic control of type 2 diabetes.

Reductil 10 mg / 15 mg should only be given for periods up to one year. Data on use over one year is limited.

4.3 Contraindications
- Known hypersensitivity to sibutramine hydrochloride monohydrate or to any of the excipients

- Organic causes of obesity

- History of major eating disorders

- Psychiatric illness. Sibutramine has shown potential antidepressant activity in animal studies and, therefore it cannot be excluded that sibutramine could induce a manic episode in bipolar patients.

- Gilles de la Tourette's syndrome

- Concomitant use, or use during the past two weeks, of monoamine oxidase inhibitors or of other centrally-acting drugs for the treatment of psychiatric disorders (such as antidepressants, antipsychotics) or for weight reduction, or tryptophan for sleep disturbances.

- History of coronary artery disease, congestive heart failure, tachycardia, peripheral arterial occlusive disease, arrhythmia or cerebrovascular disease (stroke or TIA)

- Inadequately controlled hypertension (>145/90 mmHg; see section 4.4 "Special warnings and special precautions")

- Hyperthyroidism

- Severe hepatic impairment

- Severe renal impairment and in patients with end stage renal disease on dialysis

- Benign prostatic hyperplasia with urinary retention

- Phaeochromocytoma

- Narrow angle glaucoma

- History of drug, medication or alcohol abuse

- Pregnancy and lactation (see section 4.6 "Pregnancy and lactation")

- Children and young adults up to the age of 18 years, owing to insufficient data

- Patients above 65 years of age, owing to insufficient data.

4.4 Special warnings and precautions for use
Warnings:

Blood pressure and pulse rate should be monitored in all patients on Reductil 10 mg / 15mg, as sibutramine has caused clinically relevant increases in blood pressure in some patients. In the first three months of treatment, these parameters should be checked every 2 weeks; between month 4 and 6 these parameters should be checked once monthly and regularly thereafter, at maximum intervals of three months. Treatment should be discontinued in patients who have an increase, at two consecutive visits, in resting heart rate of ≥10 bpm or systolic/diastolic blood pressure of ≥ 10 mmHg. In previously well-controlled hypertensive patients, if blood pressure exceeds 145/90 mmHg at two consecutive readings, treatment should be discontinued (see section 4.8 "Undesirable effects, cardiovascular system"). In patients with sleep apnoea syndrome particular care should be taken in monitoring blood pressure.

- For use of sibutramine concomitantly with sympathomimetics, please refer to section 4.5.

- Although sibutramine has not been associated with primary pulmonary hypertension, it is important, in view of general concerns with anti-obesity drugs, to be on the look out for symptoms such as progressive dyspnoea, chest pain and ankle oedema in the course of routine check-ups. The patient should be advised to consult a doctor immediately if these symptoms occur.

- Reductil 10 mg / 15 mg should be given with caution to patients with epilepsy.

- Increased plasma levels have been observed in the assessment of sibutramine in patients with mild to moderate hepatic impairment. Although no adverse effects have been reported, Reductil 10 mg / 15 mg should be used with caution in these patients.

- Although only inactive metabolites are excreted by the renal route, Reductil 10 mg / 15 mg should be used with caution in patients with mild to moderate renal impairment.

- Reductil 10 mg / 15 mg should be given with caution to patients who have a family history of motor or verbal tics.

- Women of child-bearing potential should employ adequate contraception whilst taking Reductil 10 mg / 15 mg.

- There is the possibility of drug abuse with CNS-active drugs. However, available clinical data have shown no evidence of drug abuse with sibutramine.

- There are general concerns that certain anti-obesity drugs are associated with an increased risk of cardiac valvulopathy. However, clinical data show no evidence of an increased incidence with sibutramine.

- Patients with a history of major eating disorders, such as anorexia nervosa and bulimia nervosa, are contraindicated. No data are available for sibutramine in the treatment of patients with binge (compulsive) eating disorder.

- Sibutramine should be given with caution to patients with open angle glaucoma and those who are at risk of raised intraocular pressure, e.g. family history.

- In common with other agents that inhibit serotonin reuptake, there is a potential for an increased risk of bleeding (including gynaecological, gastrointestinal and other cutaneous or mucous bleeding) in patients taking sibutramine. Sibutramine should, therefore, be used with caution in patients predisposed to bleeding events and those taking concomitant medications known to affect haemostasis or platelet function.

- Cases of depression, suicidal ideation and suicide have been reported rarely in patients on sibutramine treatment. Special attention is therefore required in patients with a history of depression. If signs or symptoms of depression occur during the treatment with sibutramine, the discontinuation of sibutramine and commencement of an appropriate treatment should be considered.

- Reductil 10 mg / 15 mg contains lactose and therefore should not be used in patients with rare hereditary problems of galactose intolerance, Lapp lactase deficiency or glucose-galactose malabsorption.

4.5 Interaction with other medicinal products and other forms of interaction
Sibutramine and its active metabolites are eliminated by hepatic metabolism; the main enzyme involved is CYP3A4, and CYP2C9 and CYP1A2 can also contribute. Caution should be exercised on concomitant administration of Reductil 10 mg / 15 mg with drugs which affect CYP3A4 enzyme activity (see section 5.2 "Pharmacokinetic properties"). CYP3A4 inhibitors include ketoconazole, itraconazole, erythromycin, clarithromycin, troleandomycin and cyclosporin. Co-administration of ketoconazole or erythromycin with sibutramine increased plasma concentrations (AUC) of sibutramine active metabolites (23% or 10% respectively) in an interaction study. Mean heart rate increased by up to 2.5 beats per minute more than on sibutramine alone.

Rifampicin, phenytoin, carbamazepine, phenobarbital and dexamethasone are CYP3A4 enzyme inducers and may accelerate sibutramine metabolism, although this has not been studied experimentally.

The simultaneous use of several drugs, each of which increases levels of serotonin in the brain, may give rise to serious interactions. This phenomenon is called serotonin syndrome and may occur in rare cases in connection with the simultaneous use of a selective serotonin reuptake inhibitor [SSRI] together with certain antimigraine drugs (such as sumatriptan, dihydroergotamine), or along with certain opioids (such as pentazocine, pethidine, fentanyl, dextromethorphan), or in the case of simultaneous use of two SSRIs.

As sibutramine inhibits serotonin reuptake (among other effects), Reductil 10 mg / 15mg should not be used concomitantly with other drugs which also raise serotonin levels in the brain.

Concomitant use of Reductil 10 mg / 15 mg with other drugs which may raise the blood pressure or heart rate (e.g. sympathomimetics) has not been systematically evaluated. Drugs of this type include certain cough, cold and allergy medications (eg ephedrine, pseudoephedrine), and certain decongestants (eg xylometazoline). Caution should be used when prescribing Reductil 10 mg / 15 mg to patients who use these medicines.

Reductil 10 mg / 15 mg does not impair the efficacy of oral contraceptives.

At single doses, there was no additional impairment of cognitive or psychomotor performance when sibutramine was administered concomitantly with alcohol. However, the consumption of alcohol is not compatible with the recommended dietary measures as a general rule.

No data on the concomitant use of Reductil 10 mg / 15 mg with orlistat are available.

Two weeks should elapse between stopping sibutramine and starting monoamine oxidase inhibitors.

4.6 Pregnancy and lactation
Use in pregnancy: Sibutramine should not be used during pregnancy. It is generally considered inappropriate for weight-reducing drugs to be used during pregnancy, so women of childbearing potential should employ an adequate method of contraception while taking sibutramine and notify their physician if they become pregnant or intend to become pregnant during therapy. No controlled studies with Reductil have been conducted in pregnant women. Studies in pregnant rabbits have shown effects on reproduction at maternally toxic doses (see section 5.3 "Preclinical safety data"). The relevance of these findings to humans is unknown.

Use in lactation: It is not known whether sibutramine is excreted in human breast milk and therefore administration of Reductil 10 mg / 15 mg is contraindicated during lactation.

4.7 Effects on ability to drive and use machines

Although sibutramine did not affect psychomotor or cognitive performance in healthy volunteers, any centrally-acting drug may impair judgement, thinking or motor skills. Therefore, patients should be cautioned that their ability to drive a vehicle, operate machinery or work in a hazardous environment may be impaired when taking Reductil 10 mg / 15 mg.

4.8 Undesirable effects

Most side effects reported with sibutramine occurred at the start of treatment (during the first 4 weeks). Their severity and frequency diminished over time. They were generally not serious, did not entail discontinuation of treatment, and were reversible.

The side effects observed in phase II/III clinical trials are listed below by body system (very common > 1/10, common ≤1/10 and > 1/100):

Body system	Frequency	Undesirable effects
Cardiovascular system (see detailed information below)	Common	Tachycardia Palpitations Raised blood pressure/ hypertension Vasodilation (hot flush)
Gastrointestinal system	Very common	Constipation
	Common	Nausea Haemorrhoid aggravation
Central nervous system	Very common	Dry mouth Insomnia
	Common	Light-headedness Paraesthesia Headache Anxiety
Skin	Common	Sweating
Sensory functions	Common	Taste perversion

Cardiovascular system

A mean increase in resting systolic and diastolic blood pressure of 2-3 mmHg, and a mean increase in heart rate of 3-7 beats per minute have been observed. Higher increases in blood pressure and heart rate cannot be excluded in isolated cases.

Any clinically significant increase in blood pressure and pulse rate tends to occur early on in treatment (first 4-12 weeks). Therapy should be discontinued in such cases (see Section 4.4 "Special warnings and special precautions.").

For use of Reductil 10 mg / 15 mg in patients with hypertension, see section 4.3 "Contraindications" and 4.4 "Special warnings and special precautions".

Clinically significant adverse events seen in clinical studies and during postmarketing surveillance are listed below by body system:

Blood and lymphatic system disorders:

Thrombocytopenia, Henoch-Schonlein purpura

Cardiovascular disorders:

Atrial fibrillation, paroxysmal supraventricular tachycardia

Immune system disorders:

Allergic hypersensitivity reactions ranging from mild skin eruptions and urticaria to angioedema and anaphylaxis have been reported

Psychiatric disorders:

Agitation

Depression in patients both with and without a prior history of depression (see section 4.4).

Nervous system disorders:

Seizures

Serotonin syndrome in combination with other agents affecting serotonin release (section 4.5).

Transient short-term memory disturbance

Eye disorders:

Blurred vision

Gastrointestinal disorders:

Diarrhoea, vomiting, gastrointestinal haemorrhage

Skin and subcutaneous tissue disorders:

Alopecia, rash, urticaria, cutaneous bleeding reactions (ecchmosis, petechiae)

Renal and urinary disorders:

Acute interstitial nephritis, mesangiocapillary glomerulonephritis, urinary retention

Reproductive system and breast disorders:

Abnormal ejaculation/orgasm, impotence, menstrual cycle disorders, metrorrhagia

Investigations:

Reversible increases in liver enzymes

Other:

Withdrawal symptoms such as headache and increased appetite have rarely been observed.

4.9 Overdose

There is limited experience of overdosing with sibutramine. The most frequently noted adverse events associated with overdose are tachycardia, hypertension, headache and dizziness. Treatment should consist of the general measures employed in the management of overdosing, such as keeping airways unobstructed as needed, monitoring of cardiovascular functions and general symptomatic and supportive measures. Early administration of activated charcoal may delay the absorption of sibutramine. Gastric lavage may also be of benefit. Cautious use of beta-blockers may be indicated in patients with elevated blood pressure or tachycardia. The results from a study in patients with end-stage renal disease on dialysis showed that sibutramine metabolites were not eliminated to a significant degree with hemodialysis.

5. PHARMACOLOGICAL PROPERTIES

5.1 Pharmacodynamic properties

Pharmacotherapeutic group: anti-obesity drug, ATC code A08A A10.

Sibutramine produces its therapeutic effects predominantly via its active secondary and primary amine metabolites (metabolite 1 and metabolite 2) which are inhibitors of noradrenaline, serotonin (5-hydroxytryptamine; 5-HT) and dopamine reuptake. In human brain tissue, metabolite 1 and metabolite 2 are ~3-fold more potent as in vitro inhibitors of noradrenaline and serotonin reuptake than of dopamine reuptake. Plasma samples taken from sibutramine-treated volunteers caused significant inhibition of both noradrenaline reuptake (73%) and serotonin reuptake (54%) with no significant inhibition of dopamine reuptake (16%). Sibutramine and its metabolites are neither monoamine-releasing agents nor are they monoamine oxidase inhibitors. They have no affinity with a large number of neurotransmitter receptors, including serotonergic (5-HT_1, 5-HT_{1A}, 5-HT_{1B}, 5-HT_{2A}, 5-HT_{2C}), adrenergic (β_1, β_2, β_3, α_1, α_2), dopaminergic (D_1-like, D_2-like), muscarinic, histaminergic (H_1), benzodiazepine and NMDA receptors.

In animal models using lean growing and obese rats, sibutramine produces a reduction in bodyweight gain. This is believed to result from its impact on food intake, ie by enhancing satiety, but enhanced thermogenesis also contributes to weight loss. These effects have been shown to be mediated by the inhibition of serotonin and noradrenaline re-uptake.

In clinical trials in man, Reductil was shown to effect weight loss by enhancing satiety. Data are also available which demonstrate a thermogenic effect of Reductil by attenuating the adaptive decline in resting metabolic rate during weight loss. Weight loss induced by Reductil is accompanied by beneficial changes in serum lipids and glycaemic control in patients with dyslipidaemia and type 2 diabetes, respectively.

In obese patients with type 2 diabetes mellitus weight loss with sibutramine was associated with mean reductions of 0.6% (unit) in HbA_{1c}. Similarly, in obese patients with dyslipidaemia, weight loss was associated with increases in HDL cholesterol of 12-22% and reductions in triglycerides of 9-21%.

5.2 Pharmacokinetic properties

Sibutramine is well absorbed and undergoes extensive first-pass metabolism. Peak plasma levels (C_{max}) were achieved 1.2 hours after a single oral dose of 20 mg of sibutramine hydrochloride monohydrate. The half-life of the parent compound is 1.1 hours. The pharmacologically active metabolites 1 and 2 reach C_{max} in three hours with elimination half-lives of 14 and 16 hours, respectively. Linear kinetics have been demonstrated over the dose range of 10 to 30 mg, with no dose-related change in the elimination half-lives but a dose-proportionate increase in plasma concentrations. On repeated dosing, steady-state concentrations of metabolites 1 and 2 are achieved within 4 days, with an approximately 2-fold accumulation. The pharmacokinetics of sibutramine and its metabolites in obese subjects are similar to those in normal weight subjects. The relatively limited data available so far provide no evidence of a clinically relevant difference in the pharmacokinetics of males and females. The pharmacokinetic profile observed in elderly healthy subjects (mean age 70 years) was similar to that seen in young healthy subjects.

<u>Renal Impairment</u>

The disposition of sibutramine metabolites 1, 2, 5 and 6 was studied in patients with varying degrees of renal function. Sibutramine itself was not measurable.

The AUCs of active metabolites 1 and 2 were generally not affected by renal impairment, except that the AUC of metabolite 2 in end-stage renal disease patients on dialysis was approximately half of that measured in normal subjects (CLcr ⩾ 80 mL/min). The AUCs of inactive metabolites 5 and 6 increased 2-3 fold in patients with moderate impairment (30 mL/min < CLcr ⩽ 60 mL/min), 8-11 fold in patients with severe impairment (CLcr ⩽ 30 mL/min), and 22-33 fold in patients with end-stage renal disease on dialysis as compared to normal subjects. Approximately 1% of the oral dose was recovered in the dialysate as a combination of metabolites 5 and 6 during hemodialysis process, while metabolites 1 and 2 were not measurable in the dialysate.

Sibutramine should not be used in patients with severe renal impairment, including end-stage renal disease patients on dialysis.

Hepatic impairment

In subjects with moderate hepatic impairment, bioavailability of the active metabolites was 24% higher after a single dose of sibutramine. Plasma protein binding of sibutramine and its metabolites 1 and 2 amounts to approximately 97%, 94% and 94%, respectively. Hepatic metabolism is the major route of elimination of sibutramine and its active metabolites 1 and 2. Other (inactive) metabolites are excreted primarily via the urine, at a urine: faeces ratio of 10: 1.

In vitro hepatic microsome studies indicated that CYP3A4 is the major cytochrome P450 isoenzyme responsible for sibutramine metabolism. In vitro, there was no indication of an affinity with CYP2D6, a low capacity enzyme involved in pharmacokinetic interactions with various drugs. Further in vitro studies have revealed that sibutramine has no significant effect on the activity of the major P450 isoenzymes, including CYP3A4. The CYP450s involved in the further metabolism of metabolite 2 were shown (in vitro) to be CYP3A4 and CYP2C9. Although there are no data at present, it is likely that CYP3A4 is also involved in further metabolism of metabolite 1.

5.3 Preclinical safety data

The toxicity of sibutramine seen after single doses in experimental animals has generally been a result of exaggerated pharmacodynamic effects. Longer-term treatment was associated with only mild pathological changes and secondary or species-related findings. It follows that they are unlikely to present concerns during the proper clinical use of sibutramine. Reproduction studies were conducted in rats and rabbits. In rabbits, one study showed a slightly higher incidence of fetal cardiovascular anomalies in the treatment groups than in the control group, while another study showed a lower incidence than in controls. In addition, in the latter study but not in the former, the treatment group had slightly more fetuses with two minor anomalies (a tiny thread-like ossified connection between the maxilla and jugal bones, and very slight differences in the spacing of the roots of some small arteries from the aortic arch). The relevance of these findings to humans is unknown. Sibutramine's use in human pregnancy has not been investigated. Extensive genetic toxicity tests disclosed no evidence of sibutramine-induced mutagenicity. Studies in rodents have shown that sibutramine has no carcinogenic potential relevant to man.

6. PHARMACEUTICAL PARTICULARS

6.1 List of excipients

Capsule content: lactose monohydrate, magnesium stearate, microcrystalline cellulose, colloidal anhydrous silica.

Capsule shell (10 mg): indigo carmine (E 132), titanium dioxide (E 171), gelatin, sodium lauryl sulphate, quinoline yellow (E 104).

Capsule shell (15 mg): indigo carmine (E 132), titanium dioxide (E 171), gelatin, sodium lauryl sulphate.

Printing ink: dimethicone, propylene glycol, iron oxides and hydroxides (E 172), shellac glaze, lecithin (E 322), titanium dioxide (E 171).

6.2 Incompatibilities

Not applicable

6.3 Shelf life

3 years

6.4 Special precautions for storage

Do not store above 25°C. Store in the original package.

6.5 Nature and contents of container

Reductil 10 mg / 15 mg, capsules in a PVC/PVDC blister strip pack.

Calendar pack containing 28 capsules (4 weeks)

6.6 Special precautions for disposal and other handling

No special requirements

7. MARKETING AUTHORISATION HOLDER

Abbott Laboratories Limited

Queenborough

Kent ME11 5EL

United Kingdom

8. MARKETING AUTHORISATION NUMBER(S)

Reductil 10 mg: PL 0037/0326

Reductil 15 mg: PL 0037/0327

9. DATE OF FIRST AUTHORISATION/RENEWAL OF THE AUTHORISATION

14 January 2004

10. DATE OF REVISION OF THE TEXT

9 October 2007

ReFacto AF

(Wyeth Pharmaceuticals)

1. NAME OF THE MEDICINAL PRODUCT

ReFacto AF®▼250 IU powder and solvent for solution for injection.

ReFacto AF®▼500 IU powder and solvent for solution for injection.

ReFacto AF®▼1000 IU powder and solvent for solution for injection.

ReFacto AF®▼2000 IU powder and solvent for solution for injection.

2. QUALITATIVE AND QUANTITATIVE COMPOSITION

Each vial contains nominally 250 IU*, 500 IU*, 1000 IU* or 2000 IU* moroctocog alfa**

ReFacto AF 250 IU: After reconstitution, each ml of solution contains approximately 62.5 IU/ml moroctocog alfa.

ReFacto AF 500 IU: After reconstitution, each ml of the solution contains approximately 125 IU/ml moroctocog alfa.

ReFacto AF 1000 IU: After reconstitution, each ml of the solution contains approximately 250 IU/ml moroctocog alfa.

ReFacto AF 2000 IU: After reconstitution, each ml of the solution contains approximately 500 IU/ml moroctocog alfa.

* The potency (International Units) is determined using the European Pharmacopoeia chromogenic assay. The specific activity of ReFacto AF is 7,600-13,800 IU/mg protein.

** Human coagulation factor VIII produced by recombinant DNA technology in Chinese hamster ovary (CHO) cells. Moroctocog alfa is a glycoprotein with 1438 amino acids with a sequence that is comparable to the 90 + 80 kDa form of factor VIII (i.e. B-domain deleted) and similar post-translational modifications to those of the plasma-derived molecule.

The manufacturing process for ReFacto has been modified to eliminate any exogenous human- or animal-derived protein in the cell culture process, purification, or final formulation; and at the same time the invented name has been changed to ReFacto AF.

Excipients:

After reconstitution, 1.23 mmol (29 mg) sodium per vial.

For a full list of excipients, see section 6.1.

3. PHARMACEUTICAL FORM

Powder and solvent for solution for injection.

White to off-white cake/powder.

Clear, colourless solvent.

4. CLINICAL PARTICULARS

4.1 Therapeutic indications

Treatment and prophylaxis of bleeding in patients with haemophilia A (congenital factor VIII deficiency).

ReFacto AF is appropriate for use in adults and children of all ages, including newborns.

ReFacto AF does not contain von Willebrand factor, and hence is not indicated in von Willebrand's disease.

4.2 Posology and method of administration

Treatment should be initiated under the supervision of a physician experienced in the treatment of haemophilia A.

Posology

The labelled potency of ReFacto AF is based on the European Pharmacopoeial chromogenic substrate assay, in which the manufacturing potency standard has been calibrated to the WHO International Standard using the chromogenic substrate assay. When monitoring patients' factor VIII activity levels during treatment with ReFacto AF, use of the European Pharmacopoeial chromogenic substrate assay is strongly recommended. The chromogenic assay yields results which are higher than those observed with use of the one-stage clotting assay. Typically, one-stage clotting assay results are 20-50% lower than the chromogenic substrate assay results. The ReFacto AF laboratory standard can be used to correct for this discrepancy (see section 5.2).

Another moroctocog alfa product approved for use outside Europe has a different potency assigned using a manufacturing potency standard that has been calibrated to the WHO International Standard using a one-stage clotting assay; this product is identified by the tradename XYNTHA. Due to the difference in methods used to assign product potency of XYNTHA and ReFacto AF, 1 IU of the XYNTHA product (one-stage assay calibrated) is approximately equivalent to 1.38 IU of the ReFacto AF product (chromogenic assay calibrated). If a patient normally treated with XYNTHA is prescribed ReFacto AF, the treating physician may consider adjustment of dosing recommendations based on factor VIII recovery values.

Based on their current regimen, individuals with haemophilia A should be advised to bring an adequate supply of factor VIII product for anticipated treatment when travelling. Patients should be advised to consult with their healthcare provider prior to travel.

The dosage and duration of the substitution therapy depend on the severity of the factor VIII deficiency, on the location and extent of bleeding, and on the patient's clinical condition. Doses administered should be titrated to the patient's clinical response. In the presence of an inhibitor, higher doses or appropriate specific treatment may be required.

The number of units of factor VIII administered is expressed in International Units (IUs), which are related to the current WHO standard for factor VIII products. Factor VIII activity in plasma is expressed either as a percentage (relative to normal human plasma) or in International Units (relative to an International Standard for factor VIII in plasma). One International Unit (IU) of factor VIII activity is equivalent to the quantity of factor VIII in one ml of normal human plasma. The calculation of the required dosage of factor VIII is based upon the empirical finding that 1 International Unit (IU) of factor VIII per kg body weight raises the plasma factor VIII activity by 2 IU/dl. The required dosage is determined using the following formula:

Required units (IU) = body weight (kg) × desired factor VIII rise (% or IU/dl) × 0.5 (IU/kg per IU/dl), where 0.5 IU/kg per IU/dl represents the reciprocal of the incremental recovery generally observed following infusions of factor VIII.

The amount to be administered and the frequency of administration should always be oriented to the clinical effectiveness in the individual case.

In the case of the following haemorrhagic events, the factor VIII activity should not fall below the given plasma levels (in % of normal or in IU/dl) in the corresponding period. The following table can be used to guide dosing in bleeding episodes and surgery:

Degree of haemorrhage/ Type of surgical procedure	Factor VIII level required (% or IU/dl)	Frequency of doses (hours)/ Duration of therapy (days)
Haemorrhage		
Early haemarthrosis, muscle bleeding or oral bleeding	20-40	Repeat every 12-24 hours. At least 1 day until the bleeding episode as indicated by pain is resolved or healing is achieved.
More extensive haemarthrosis, muscle bleeding or haematoma	30-60	Repeat infusion every 12-24 hours for 3-4 days or more until pain and acute disability are resolved.
Life-threatening haemorrhages	60-100	Repeat infusion every 8-24 hours until threat is resolved.
Surgery		
Minor, including tooth extraction	30-60	Every 24 hours, at least 1 day, until healing is achieved.
Major	80-100 (pre- and post-operative)	Repeat infusion every 8-24 hours until adequate wound healing, then therapy for at least another 7 days to maintain a factor VIII activity of 30% to 60% (IU/dl).

During the course of treatment, appropriate determination of factor VIII levels is advised to guide the dose to be administered and the frequency of repeated infusions. In the case of major surgical interventions in particular, precise monitoring of the substitution therapy by means of coagulation analysis (plasma factor VIII activity) is indispensable. Individual patients may vary in their response to factor VIII, achieving different levels of *in vivo* recovery and demonstrating different half-lives.

For long-term prophylaxis against bleeding in patients with severe haemophilia A, the usual doses are 20 to 40 IU of factor VIII per kg body weight at intervals of 2 to 3 days. In some cases, especially in younger patients, shorter dosage intervals or higher doses may be necessary.

Patients using factor-VIII replacement therapy are to be monitored for the development of factor VIII inhibitors. If expected factor VIII activity plasma levels are not attained, or if bleeding is not controlled with an appropriate dose, an assay should be performed to determine if factor VIII inhibitors are present. Data from clinical trials indicated that if inhibitors are present at levels less than 10 Bethesda Units (BUs), administration of additional antihaemophilic factor may neutralise the inhibitors. In patients with levels of inhibitor above 10 BU, factor VIII therapy may not be effective and other therapeutic options should be considered. Management of such patients should be directed by physicians with experience in the care of patients with haemophilia (see section 4.4).

Special populations

Renal or hepatic impairment

Dosage adjustment for patients with renal or hepatic impairment has not been studied in clinical trials.

Paediatric patients

Safety and efficacy studies with ReFacto have been performed both in previously treated children and adolescents (n=31, ages 8-18 years) and in previously untreated neonates, infants and children (n=101, ages < 1-52 months).

The need for an increased dose relative to that used for adults and older children should be anticipated when treating younger children with ReFacto AF. In a study of ReFacto in children less than 6 years of age, pharmacokinetic analysis revealed half-life and recovery less than that observed in older children and adults (see section 5.2). During the clinical trials, children less than 6 years of age on a prophylaxis regimen used an average dose of 50 IU/kg of ReFacto and experienced an average of 6.1 bleeding episodes per year. Older children and adults on a prophylaxis regimen used an average dose of 27 IU/kg and experienced an average of 10 bleeding episodes per year. In a clinical trial setting the mean dose per infusion of ReFacto for bleeding episodes in children less than 6 years of age was higher than the mean dose administered to older children and adults (51.3 IU/kg and 29.3 IU/kg, respectively).

Method of administration

ReFacto AF is administered by intravenous injection over several minutes after reconstitution of the lyophilised powder for injection with sodium chloride 9 mg/ml (0.9%) solution for injection (provided). The rate of administration should be determined by the patient's comfort level.

Appropriate training is recommended for non-healthcare professionals administering the product.

In the interest of patients, it is recommended that every time ReFacto AF is administered, the name and batch number of the product should be recorded.

For reconstitution instructions prior to administration, see section 6.6.

4.3 Contraindications

Hypersensitivity to the active substance or to any of the excipients.

Hypersensitivity to hamster proteins.

4.4 Special warnings and precautions for use

As with any intravenous protein product, allergic-type hypersensitivity reactions are possible. The product contains traces of hamster proteins. Patients should be informed of the early signs of hypersensitivity reactions (including hives, generalised urticaria, tightness of the chest, wheezing, hypotension) and anaphylaxis. If allergic or anaphylactic reactions occur, administration of ReFacto AF is to be discontinued immediately, and an appropriate treatment must be initiated. In case of shock, the current medical standards for treatment of shock are to be observed. Patients are to be advised to discontinue use of the product and contact their physician or seek immediate emergency care, depending on the type and severity of the reaction, if any of these symptoms occur.

The formation of neutralising antibodies (inhibitors) to factor VIII is a known complication in the management of individuals with haemophilia A. These inhibitors are usually IgG immunoglobulins directed against the factor VIII procoagulant activity, which are quantified in Bethesda Units (BUs) per ml of plasma using the Nijmegen modification of the Bethesda assay. The risk of developing inhibitors is correlated to the exposure to factor VIII, this risk being highest within the first 20 exposure days. Inhibitors have been observed in previously treated patients receiving factor VIII products, including ReFacto AF. Cases of recurrence of inhibitors (low titre) have been observed after switching from one recombinant factor VIII product to another in previously treated patients with more than 100 exposure days who have a history of inhibitor development. Patients treated with recombinant coagulation factor VIII should be carefully monitored for the development of inhibitors by appropriate clinical observations and laboratory tests (see also section 4.8).

Reports of lack of effect, mainly in prophylaxis patients, have been received in the clinical trials and in the post-marketing setting for ReFacto. The reported lack of effect with ReFacto has been described as bleeding into target joints, bleeding into new joints or a subjective feeling by the patient of new onset bleeding. When prescribing ReFacto AF it is important to individually titrate and monitor each patient's factor level in order to ensure an adequate therapeutic response.

In the interest of patient safety, it is recommended that every time ReFacto AF is administered, the name on the carton and batch number of the product are recorded. Patients can affix one of the peel-off labels found on the vial to document the batch number in their diary or for reporting any side effects.

After reconstitution this medicinal product contains 1.23 mmol (29 mg) sodium per vial, to be taken into consideration by patients on a controlled sodium diet.

4.5 Interaction with other medicinal products and other forms of interaction

No interaction studies have been performed.

4.6 Pregnancy and lactation

Animal reproduction studies have not been conducted with factor VIII. Because of the rare occurrence of haemophilia A in women, experience regarding the use of factor VIII during pregnancy and breast-feeding is not available. Therefore, factor VIII should be used during pregnancy and lactation only if clearly indicated.

4.7 Effects on ability to drive and use machines
No studies on the effects on the ability to drive and use machines have been performed.

4.8 Undesirable effects
Factor VIII inhibition
The occurrence of neutralising antibodies (inhibitors) to factor VIII is well known in the treatment of patients with haemophilia A. As with all coagulation factor VIII products, patients are to be monitored for the development of inhibitors that are to be titrated in Bethesda Units (BUs) using the Nijmegen modification of the Bethesda assay. If such inhibitors occur, the condition may manifest itself as an insufficient clinical response. In such cases, it is recommended that a specialised haemophilia centre be contacted.

In a clinical study with ReFacto AF in previously treated patients (PTPs), the incidence of factor VIII inhibitors was the primary safety endpoint. Two clinically silent, low-titre, transient inhibitors were observed in 94 patients with a median exposure of 76 exposure days (ED, range 1-92), corresponding to 2.2% of the 89 patients with at least 50 ED. In a supporting study of ReFacto AF, 1 *de novo* and 2 recurrent inhibitors (all low-titre, central laboratory determination) were observed in 110 patients; median exposure of 58 ED (range 5-140) and 98 patients had at least 50 ED to ReFacto AF. Ninety-eight (98) of the original 110 patients continued treatment in a second supportive study and had subsequent extended exposure to ReFacto AF with a median of 169 additional ED (range 9-425). One (1) additional low-titre *de novo* inhibitor was observed. The frequency of inhibitors observed in these studies is within the expected range.

In a clinical study with ReFacto in PTPs, 1 inhibitor was observed in 113 patients. Also, there have been spontaneous post-marketing reports of high-titre inhibitors involving previously treated patients.

There are no clinical data on previously untreated patients (PUPs) with ReFacto AF. However, clinical trials are planned in previously untreated patients (PUPs) with ReFacto AF. In a clinical trial, 32 out of 101 (32%) previously untreated patients (PUPs) treated with ReFacto developed inhibitors: 16 out of 101 (16%) with a titre > 5 BU and 16 out of 101 (16%) with a titre ≤ 5 BU. The median number of exposure days up to inhibitor development in these patients was 12 (range 3-49). Of the 16 patients with high titres, 15 received immune tolerance (IT) treatment. Of the 16 patients with low titres, IT treatment was started in 10. IT had an efficacy of 73% for patients with high titres and 90% for those with low titres. For all 101 treated PUPs, regardless of inhibitor development, the median number of exposure days is 197 (range 1-1299).

Table 1

System Organ Class	Frequency of Occurrence per Patient with ReFacto or ReFacto AF		
	Very common (≥1/10)	Common (≥1/100 to <1/10)	Uncommon (≥1/1,000 to <1/100)
Blood and lymphatic disorders	Factor VIII inhibitors - PUPs	Factor VIII inhibitors - PTPs	
Metabolism and nutrition disorders			Anorexia
Nervous system disorders		Headache	Neuropathy, dizziness, somnolence, dysgeusia
Cardiac disorders			Angina pectoris, tachycardia, palpitations
Vascular disorders		Haemorrhage/ Haematoma	Hypotension, thrombophlebitis, vasodilatation, flushing
Respiratory, thoracic and mediastinal disorders			Dyspnoea, cough
Gastrointestinal disorders	Vomiting	Nausea	Abdominal pain, diarrhoea
Skin and subcutaneous tissue disorders			Urticaria, pruritis, rash, hyperhidrosis
Musculoskeletal, connective tissue and bone disorders		Arthralgia	Myalgia
General disorders and administration site conditions		Asthenia, pyrexia	Chills/feeling cold, injection site inflammation, injection site reaction, injection site pain
Investigations			Aspartate aminotransferase increased, alanine aminotransferase increased, blood bilirubin increased, blood creatine phosphokinase increased
Surgical and medical procedures		Vascular access complication	

Table 2

Pharmacokinetic parameter estimates for ReFacto in previously treated patients with haemophilia A

PK parameter	Mean	SD	Median
AUC_t (IU·h/ml)	19.9	4.9	19.9
$t_{1/2}$ (h)	14.8	5.6	12.7
CL (ml/h·kg)	2.4	0.75	2.3
MRT (h)	20.2	7.4	18.0
K-value (IU/dl increase in FVIII:C per IU/kg FVIII given)	2.4	0.38	2.5

Abbreviations: AUC_t = area under the plasma concentration-time curve from zero to the last measurable concentration; $t_{½}$ = half-life; CL = clearance; MRT = mean residence time; K-value = incremental recovery; SD = standard deviation

Adverse reactions based on experience from clinical trials with ReFacto or ReFacto AF are presented in the table below by system organ class. These frequencies have been estimated on a per-patient basis and are described using the following categories: very common (≥1/10); common (≥1/100 to <1/10); and uncommon (≥1/1,000 to <1/100).

Within each frequency grouping, undesirable effects are presented in order of decreasing seriousness.

(see Table 1 below)

One event of cyst in an 11-year old patient and one event described as confusion in a 13-year old patient have been reported as possibly related to ReFacto AF treatment.

Safety of ReFacto AF was evaluated in previously treated children and adolescents (n=18, age 12-16 in a study and n=49, age 7-16 in a supporting study). Although a limited number of children have been studied, there is a tendency for higher frequencies of adverse events in children aged 7-16 as compared to adults. A clinical trial evaluating use of moroctocog alfa (AF-CC) in children less than 6 years of age is on going.

The following adverse events have also been reported for ReFacto: paraesthesia, fatigue, blurred vision, acne, gastritis, gastroenteritis, and pain.

Hypersensitivity or allergic reactions (which may include angioedema, burning and stinging at the infusion site, chills, flushing, generalised urticaria, headache, hives, hypotension, lethargy, nausea, restlessness, tachycardia, tightness of the chest, tingling, vomiting, wheezing) have been observed infrequently for ReFacto, and may in some cases progress to severe anaphylaxis including shock (see section 4.4).

Trace amounts of hamster protein may be present in ReFacto AF. Very rarely, development of antibodies to hamster protein has been observed, but there were no clinical sequelae. In a study of ReFacto, twenty of 113 (18%) PTPs had an increase in anti-CHO antibody titre, without any apparent clinical effect.

If any reaction takes place that is thought to be related to the administration of ReFacto AF, the rate of infusion is to be decreased or the infusion stopped, as dictated by the response of the patient (see section 4.4).

4.9 Overdose
No case of overdose has been reported.

5. PHARMACOLOGICAL PROPERTIES

5.1 Pharmacodynamic properties
Pharmacotherapeutic group: antihaemorrhagics, blood coagulation factor VIII; ATC code: B02BD02.

ReFacto AF contains B-domain deleted recombinant coagulation factor VIII (moroctocog alfa). It is a glycoprotein with an approximate molecular mass of 170,000 Da consisting of 1438 amino acids. ReFacto AF has functional characteristics comparable to those of endogenous factor VIII. Factor VIII activity is greatly reduced in patients with haemophilia A, and, therefore, replacement therapy is necessary.

When infused into a haemophiliac patient, factor VIII binds to the von Willebrand factor present in the patient's circulation.

Activated factor VIII acts as a cofactor for activated factor IX, accelerating the conversion of factor X to activated factor X. Activated factor X converts prothrombin into thrombin. Thrombin then converts fibrinogen into fibrin, and a clot is formed. Haemophilia A is a sex-linked hereditary disorder of blood coagulation due to decreased levels of factor VIII:C and results in profuse bleeding into joints, muscles or internal organs, either spontaneously or as a result of accidental or surgical trauma. By replacement therapy, the plasma levels of factor VIII are increased, thereby enabling a temporary correction of the factor deficiency and correction of the bleeding tendencies.

5.2 Pharmacokinetic properties
Pharmacokinetic properties of ReFacto, derived from a cross-over study of ReFacto and a plasma-derived FVIII concentrate, using the chromogenic substrate assay (see section 4.2), in 18 previously treated patients are listed in the table above.

(see Table 2 above)

In a study in which the potency of ReFacto AF, ReFacto and FVIII activity in patient plasma were measured using the chromogenic substrate assay, ReFacto AF was shown to be bioequivalent to ReFacto. The ratios of geometric least-square means of ReFacto AF-to-ReFacto were 100.6%, 99.5% and 98.1% for K-value, AUC_t and AUC_∞ (area under the plasma concentration curve from time zero to infinity), respectively. The corresponding 90% confidence intervals about the ratios of ReFacto AF to ReFacto geometric means were within the bioequivalence window of 80% to 125%, demonstrating bioequivalence of ReFacto AF to ReFacto.

In a cross-over pharmacokinetic study, the pharmacokinetic parameters for ReFacto AF were determined at baseline and followed-up in 25 previously treated patients (≥ 12 years) after repeated administration of ReFacto AF for six months. The ratios of geometric least-square means of month 6-to-baseline pharmacokinetic were 107%, 100% and 104% for K-value, AUC_t and AUC_∞, respectively. The corresponding 90% confidence intervals about the ratios of month 6-to-baseline for the above pharmacokinetic parameters were within the equivalence window of 80% to 125%. This indicates no time-dependent changes in the pharmacokinetic properties of ReFacto AF.

In the same study, in which the drug potency of ReFacto AF and a full-length recombinant factor VIII (FLrFVIII) comparator, and the FVIII activity measured in patient plasma samples were all determined using the same one-stage clotting assay at a central laboratory, ReFacto AF was shown to be pharmacokinetically equivalent to FLrFVIII in 30 previously treated patients (≥ 12 years) using the standard bioequivalence approach.

In PUPs, pharmacokinetic parameters of ReFacto were evaluated using the chromogenic assay. These patients (n=59; median age 10 ± 8.3 months) had a mean incremental recovery at Week 0 of 1.5 ± 0.6 IU/dl per IU/kg (range 0.2 to 2.8 IU/dl per IU/kg) which was lower than that obtained in PTPs treated with ReFacto at Week 0 with a mean K-value of 2.4 ± 0.4 IU/dl per IU/kg (range 1.1 to 3.8 IU/dl per IU/kg). In the PUPs, the mean incremental recovery was stable over time (5 visits during a 2-year period) and ranged from 1.5 to 1.8 IU/dl per IU/kg. Population pharmacokinetic modeling using data from 44 PUPs led to a mean estimated half-life of 8.0 ± 2.2 hours.

5.3 Preclinical safety data

Non-clinical data reveal no special hazard for humans based on conventional studies of safety pharmacology, repeated dose toxicity, and genotoxicity.

No investigations on carcinogenic potential or toxicity to reproduction have been conducted.

6. PHARMACEUTICAL PARTICULARS

6.1 List of excipients

Powder

Sucrose

Calcium chloride dihydrate

L-Histidine

Polysorbate 80

Sodium chloride

Solvent

Sodium chloride

Water for injections

6.2 Incompatibilities

In the absence of compatibility studies, this medicinal product must not be mixed with other medicinal products, including other infusion solutions.

Only the provided infusion set is to be used, because treatment failure can occur as a consequence of human-coagulation factor VIII adsorption to the internal surfaces of some infusion equipment.

6.3 Shelf life

Unopened powder vial

2 years.

After reconstitution

Chemical and physical in-use stability has been demonstrated for 3 hours at temperatures up to 25°C.

The product does not contain a preservative, and the reconstituted product should be used immediately, or within 3 hours after reconstitution. Other in-use storage times and conditions are the responsibility of the user.

6.4 Special precautions for storage

Store and transport refrigerated (2°C - 8°C). Do not freeze, in order to prevent damage to the pre-filled syringe.

The product may be removed from refrigerated storage for one single period of maximum 3 months at room temperature (up to 25°C). At the end of this period of room temperature storage, the product must not be returned to refrigerated storage, but is to be used or discarded.

Keep the vial in the outer carton in order to protect from light.

For storage conditions of the reconstituted medicinal product, see section 6.3.

6.5 Nature and contents of container

250 IU, 500 IU, 1000 IU or 2000 IU powder in a 10 ml vial (type 1 glass) with a stopper (butyl) and a flip-off seal (aluminum) and 4 ml of solvent in a pre-filled syringe (type 1 glass) with a plunger stopper (butyl), a tip-cap (butyl) and a sterile vial adapter reconstitution device, a sterile infusion set, alcohol swabs, a plaster and a gauze pad.

6.6 Special precautions for disposal and other handling

The vial of lyophilised product powder for injection must be reconstituted with the supplied solvent [sodium chloride 9 mg/ml (0.9%) solution] from the pre-filled syringe using the sterile vial adapter reconstitution device. The vial should be gently rotated until all of the powder is dissolved.

The product, when reconstituted, contains polysorbate-80, which is known to increase the rate of di-(2-ethylhexyl)phthalate (DEHP) extraction from polyvinyl chloride (PVC). This is to be considered during the preparation and administration of the product, including storage time elapsed in a PVC container following reconstitution. It is important that the recommendations in section 6.3 be followed closely.

After reconstitution, the solution is drawn back into the syringe. The solution will be clear or slightly opalescent and colourless. The solution is to be discarded if visible particulate matter or discolouration is observed.

Any unused product or waste material is to be disposed of in accordance with local requirements.

7. MARKETING AUTHORISATION HOLDER

Wyeth Europa Ltd.

Huntercombe Lane South

Taplow, Maidenhead

Berkshire, SL6 0PH

United Kingdom

8. MARKETING AUTHORISATION NUMBER(S)

ReFacto AF 250 IU powder and solvent for solution for injection: EU/1/99/103/001

ReFacto AF 500 IU powder and solvent for solution for injection: EU/1/99/103/002

ReFacto AF 1000 IU powder and solvent for solution for injection: EU/1/99/103/003

ReFacto AF 2000 IU powder and solvent for solution for injection: EU/1/99/103/004

9. DATE OF FIRST AUTHORISATION/RENEWAL OF THE AUTHORISATION

Date of first authorisation: 13 Apr 1999

Date of last renewal: 15 Apr 2009

10. DATE OF REVISION OF THE TEXT

15 April 2009

Detailed information on this medicinal product is available on the website of the European Medicines Agency (EMEA) http://www.emea.europa.eu/.

Refolinon Injection 2 ml / 10 ml

(Pharmacia Limited)

1. NAME OF THE MEDICINAL PRODUCT

Refolinon Injection

2. QUALITATIVE AND QUANTITATIVE COMPOSITION

Clear pale yellow liquid for injection containing leucovorin 3 mg/ml in ampoules of 2 ml and 10 ml, as the calcium salt

3. PHARMACEUTICAL FORM

Solution for injection

4. CLINICAL PARTICULARS

4.1 Therapeutic indications

Leucovorin (folinic acid) is the formyl derivative of tetrahydrofolic acid and is an intermediate product of the metabolism of folic acid. Leucovorin is used in cytotoxic therapy as an antidote to folic acid antagonists such as methotrexate. Leucovorin is effective in the treatment of megaloblastic anaemia due to folate deficiency.

Warning: Leucovorin should not be given simultaneously with a folic acid antagonist, for the purpose of reducing or preventing clinical toxicity, as the therapeutic effect of the antagonist may be nullified.

4.2 Posology and method of administration

Leucovorin calcium should not be administered intrathecally.

Adults and Children:

Leucovorin rescue: Depending upon the dose of methotrexate administered, dosage regimens of leucovorin calcium vary. Up to 120 mg leucovorin calcium are generally given, usually in divided doses over 12-24 hours by intramuscular injection, bolus intravenous injection or intravenous infusion in normal saline. This is followed by 12-15 mg intramuscularly or 15 mg orally every 6 hours for 48 hours. Rescue therapy is usually started 24 hours after the commencement of methotrexate administration.

If overdosage of methotrexate is suspected, the dose of leucovorin calcium should be equal to or greater than the dose of methotrexate and should be administered within one hour of the methotrexate administration.

4.3 Contraindications

Leucovorin calcium should not be used in patients who have a known hypersensitivity to any of the constituents of the product.

Calcium folinate should not be used for the treatment of pernicious anaemia or other megaloblastic anaemia where vitamin B_{12} is deficient.

Calcium folinate should only be given by intramuscular or intravenous injection and must not be administered intrathecally. When folinic acid has been administered intrathecally following intrathecal overdose of methotrexate, death has been reported.

4.4 Special warnings and precautions for use

Calcium folinate should only be used with methotrexate and 5-fluorouracil by clinicians experienced in the use of cancer chemotherapeutic agents.

4.5 Interaction with other medicinal products and other forms of interaction

Leucovorin should not be given simultaneously with a folic acid antagonist, for the purpose of reducing or preventing clinical toxicity, as the therapeutic effect of the antagonist may be nullified.

Folic acid in large amounts may counteract the antiepileptic effect of phenobarbital, phenytoin, as well as primidone and increase the frequency of seizures.

Concurrent administration of chloramphenicol and folic acid in folate-deficient patients may result in antagonism of the haematopoietic response to folic acid.

Calcium folinate may enhance the toxicity of fluorouracil.

4.6 Pregnancy and lactation

Pregnancy:

There are no adequate and well-controlled clinical studies conducted in pregnant or breast feeding women. No formal animal reproductive toxicity studies with calcium folinate have been conducted. There are no indications that folic acid induces harmful effects if administered during pregnancy. During pregnancy, methotrexate should only be administered on strict indications, where the benefits of the drug to the mother should be weighed against possible hazards to the foetus. Should treatment with methotrexate or other folate antagonists take place despite pregnancy or lactation, there are no limitations as to the use of calcium folinate to diminish toxicity or counteract the effects.

5-fluorouracil use is generally contraindicated during pregnancy and contraindicated during breastfeeding; this applies also to the combined use of calcium folinate with 5-fluorouracil.

Please refer to the SPC for methotrexate, other folate antagonists (and 5-fluorouracil) containing medicinal products.

Lactation:

It is not known whether calcium folinate is excreted into human breast milk. Calcium folinate can be used during breast feeding when considered necessary according to the therapeutic indications.

4.7 Effects on ability to drive and use machines

None stated.

4.8 Undesirable effects

Adverse reactions to leucovorin calcium are rare, but following intravenous and intramuscular administration occasional pyrexial reactions have been reported.

The most common dose-limiting adverse reaction occurring in patients receiving combination of calcium folinate and 5-fluorouracil are stomatitis and diarrhoea. In addition, haematological adverse reactions, such as leucocytopenia and thrombocytopenia, may occur. These adverse reactions are dose-dependent and their occurrence can usually be decreased by reducing the dosage of cytotoxic drugs. These adverse reactions can be controlled by close monitoring of haematological values, e.g. blood leucocyte and thrombocyte levels, and serum electrolyte (e.g. Na, K, Ca) and creatinine levels.

Anaphylactoid and urticaria allergic reactions have also been reported with the use of leucovorin.

4.9 Overdose

There have been no reported sequelae in patients who have received significantly more calcium folinate then the recommended dosage. However, excessive amounts of calcium folinate may nullify the chemotherapeutic effect of folic acid antagonists.

Should overdosage of the combination of 5-fluorouracil and calcium folinate occur, the overdosage instructions for 5-FU should be followed.

5. PHARMACOLOGICAL PROPERTIES

5.1 Pharmacodynamic properties

Methotrexate rescue: Leucovorin (5-formyltetrahydrofolate) acts partly by providing a fresh supply of tetrahydrofolate and also by competitively displacing methotrexate from dihydrofolate reductase so that its excretion is accelerated (methotrexate binds to the enzyme dihydrofolate reductase which is responsible for reducing dietary folic acid to dihydrofolate and tetrahydrofolate thus inhibiting its action).

Megaloblastic anaemia: Leucovorin is an active folic acid derivative and it can therefore relieve pathological conditions associated with folic acid deficiency, e.g. megaloblastic anaemia.

5.2 Pharmacokinetic properties

The bioavailability of leucovorin following administration of both tablet and parenteral formulations is comparable. After 30 minutes approximately 90% of the total reduced folates were assayed as 5-methyltetrahydrofolate following oral administration compared with only 72% following i.m. administration. The half-life of leucovorin after reaching peak plasma levels was 35-45 minutes by both routes. Peak serum tetrahydrofolate levels were reached 2 hours after oral administration and approximately 40 minutes after i.m. administration.

5.3 Preclinical safety data

None stated.

6. PHARMACEUTICAL PARTICULARS

6.1 List of excipients

Sodium Chloride

Sodium Hydroxide

Hydrochloric Acid

Water for injections

6.2 Incompatibilities

None stated.

6.3 Shelf life

24 Months

6.4 Special precautions for storage

Store at 2°C – 8°C and protect from light.

6.5 Nature and contents of container

Type 1 colourless glass ampoules containing 2 or 10 ml. Packs of 5 or 10 ampoules.

6.6 Special precautions for disposal and other handling

Protect from light.

7. MARKETING AUTHORISATION HOLDER
Pharmacia Limited
Ramsgate Road
Sandwich
Kent
CT13 9NJ
United Kingdom

8. MARKETING AUTHORISATION NUMBER(S)
PL 00032/0346

9. DATE OF FIRST AUTHORISATION/RENEWAL OF THE AUTHORISATION
17th July 2002

10. DATE OF REVISION OF THE TEXT
August 2009
Ref: REA 4.0

Refolinon Tablets

(Pharmacia Limited)

1. NAME OF THE MEDICINAL PRODUCT
Refolinon Tablets

2. QUALITATIVE AND QUANTITATIVE COMPOSITION
Leucovorin calcium equivalent to
leucovorin (folinic acid) 15.0 mg

3. PHARMACEUTICAL FORM
Uncoated tablet for oral use

4. CLINICAL PARTICULARS

4.1 Therapeutic indications
Leucovorin (folinic acid) is the formyl derivative of tetrahydrofolic acid and is an intermediate product of the metabolism of folic acid. Leucovorin is used in cytotoxic therapy as an antidote to folic acid antagonists such as methotrexate. Leucovorin is effective in the treatment of megaloblastic anaemia.

4.2 Posology and method of administration
To be given orally.

Although leucovorin calcium may also be available as a solution for injection, leucovorin calcium should not be administered intrathecally.

Adults and children:

Leucovorin rescue: Depending upon the dose of methotrexate administered, dosage regimens of leucovorin calcium vary. Up to 120 mg leucovorin calcium are generally given, usually in divided doses over 12-24 hours by intramuscular injection, bolus intravenous injection or intravenous infusion in normal saline. This is followed by 12-15 mg intramuscularly or 15 mg orally every 6 hours for 48 hours. Rescue therapy is usually started 24 hours after the commencement of methotrexate administration.

If overdosage of methotrexate is suspected, the dose of leucovorin calcium should be equal to or greater than the dose of methotrexate and should be administered within one hour of the methotrexate administration.

Megaloblastic anaemia (folate deficiency): 15 mg (one tablet) leucovorin per day.

4.3 Contraindications
Leucovorin calcium should not be used in patients who have a known hypersensitivity to any of the constituents of the product.

Calcium folinate should not be used for the treatment of pernicious anaemia or other megaloblastic anaemia where vitamin B_{12} is deficient.

4.4 Special warnings and precautions for use
Calcium folinate should only be used with methotrexate and 5-fluorouracil by clinicians experienced in the use of cancer chemotherapeutic agents.

Patients with rare hereditary problems of galacatose intolerance, the Lapp lactose deficiency or glucose-galactose malabsorption should not take this medicine.

4.5 Interaction with other medicinal products and other forms of interaction
Leucovorin should not be given simultaneously with a folic acid antagonist, for the purpose of reducing or preventing clinical toxicity, as the therapeutic effect of the antagonist may be nullified.

Folic acid in large amounts may counteract the antiepileptic effect of phenobarbital, phenytoin, as well as primidone and increase the frequency of seizures.

Concurrent administration of chloramphenicol and folic acid in folate-deficient patients may result in antagonism of the haematopoietic response to folic acid.

Calcium folinate may enhance the toxicity of fluorouracil.

4.6 Pregnancy and lactation
Pregnancy

There are no adequate and well-controlled clinical studies conducted in pregnant or breast feeding women. No formal animal reproductive toxicity studies with calcium folinate have been conducted. There are no indications that folic acid induces harmful effects if administered during pregnancy. During pregnancy, methotrexate should only be administered on strict indications, where the benefits of the drug to the mother should be weighed against possible hazards to the foetus. Should treatment with methotrexate or other folate antagonists take place despite pregnancy or lactation, there are no limitations as to the use of calcium folinate to diminish toxicity or counteract the effects.

5-fluorouracil use is generally contraindicated during pregnancy and contraindicated during breastfeeding; this applies also to the combined use of calcium folinate with 5-fluorouracil.

Please refer to the SPC for methotrexate, other folate antagonists (and 5-fluorouracil) containing medicinal products.

Lactation

It is not known whether calcium folinate is excreted into human breast milk. Calcium folinate can be used during breast feeding when considered necessary according to the therapeutic indications.

4.7 Effects on ability to drive and use machines
None known.

4.8 Undesirable effects
Adverse reactions to leucovorin calcium are rare, but following intravenous and intramuscular administration occasional pyrexial reactions have been reported.

The most common dose-limiting adverse reaction occurring in patients receiving combination of calcium folinate and 5-fluorouracil are stomatitis and diarrhoea. In addition, haematological adverse reactions, such as leucocytopenia and thrombocytopenia, may occur. These adverse reactions are dose-dependent and their occurrence can usually be decreased by reducing the dosage of cytotoxic drugs. These adverse reactions can be controlled by close monitoring of haematological values, e.g. blood leucocyte and thrombocyte levels, and serum electrolyte (e.g. Na, K, Ca) and creatinine levels.

Anaphylactoid and urticaria allergic reactions have also been reported with the use of leucovorin.

4.9 Overdose
There have been no reported sequelae in patients who have received significantly more calcium folinate then the recommended dosage. However, excessive amounts of calcium folinate may nullify the chemotherapeutic effect of folic acid antagonists.

Should overdosage of the combination of 5-fluorouracil and calcium folinate occur, the overdosage instructions for 5-FU should be followed.

5. PHARMACOLOGICAL PROPERTIES

5.1 Pharmacodynamic properties
Methotrexate rescue: Leucovorin (5-formyltetrahydrofolinate) acts partly by providing a fresh supply of tetrahydrofolate and also by competitively displacing methotrexate from dihydrofolate reductase so that its excretion is accelerated (methotrexate binds to the enzyme dihydrofolate reductase which is responsible for reducing dietary folic acid to dihydrofolate and tetrahydrofolate thus inhibiting its action.

Megaloblastic anaemia: Leucovorin is an active folic acid derivative and it can therefore relieve pathological conditions associated with folic acid deficiency e.g. megaloblastic anaemia.

5.2 Pharmacokinetic properties
The bioavailability of leucovorin following administration of both tablet and parenteral formulations is comparable. After 30 minutes approximately 90% of the total reduced folates were assayed as 5-methyltetrahydrofolate following oral administration compared with only 72% following i.m. administration. The half-life of leucovorin after reaching peak plasma levels was 35-45 minutes by both routes. Peak serum tetrahydrofolate levels were reached 2 hours after oral administration and approximately 40 minutes after i.m administration.

5.3 Preclinical safety data
None stated.

6. PHARMACEUTICAL PARTICULARS

6.1 List of excipients
Avicel PH101 NF
Magnesium stearate Ph. Eur
Lactose Ph. Eur

6.2 Incompatibilities
None known.

6.3 Shelf life
60 months.

6.4 Special precautions for storage
Store below 25 °C. Do not refrigerate or freeze. Keep out of the reach and sight of children.

6.5 Nature and contents of container
The tablets are contained in white high density polyethylene containers with polyethylene screw closures. The bottles contain 30 or 100 tablets.

6.6 Special precautions for disposal and other handling
The tablets are contained in white high density polyethylene containers with polyethylene screw closures. The bottles contain 30 or 100 tablets.

7. MARKETING AUTHORISATION HOLDER
Pharmacia Ltd
Ramsgate Road
Sandwich
Kent
CT13 9NJ

8. MARKETING AUTHORISATION NUMBER(S)
PL 00032/0347

9. DATE OF FIRST AUTHORISATION/RENEWAL OF THE AUTHORISATION
02/12/2005

10. DATE OF REVISION OF THE TEXT
August 2009
V6.0

Regranex 0.01% gel

(Janssen-Cilag Ltd)

1. NAME OF THE MEDICINAL PRODUCT
REGRANEX 0.01% gel

2. QUALITATIVE AND QUANTITATIVE COMPOSITION
Each gram of gel contains100 µg of becaplermin*.

*Recombinant human Platelet Derived Growth Factor-BB (rhPDGF-BB) produced in *Saccharomyces cerevisiae* by recombinant DNA technology.

Excipients:

Each gram contains E218 (methyl parahydroxybenzoate) 1.56mg and E216 (propyl parahydroxybenzoate) 0.17mg, see section 4.4

For a full list of excipients, see section see 6.1.

3. PHARMACEUTICAL FORM
Gel

REGRANEX is a clear colourless to straw-coloured preserved gel.

4. CLINICAL PARTICULARS

4.1 Therapeutic indications
REGRANEX is indicated, in association with other good wound care measures, to promote granulation and thereby the healing of full-thickness, neuropathic, chronic, diabetic ulcers less than or equal to 5 cm^2.

4.2 Posology and method of administration
Treatment with REGRANEX should be initiated and monitored by physicians (specialists or non-specialists) who are experienced in the management of diabetic wounds.

REGRANEX should always be used in conjunction with good wound care consisting of initial debridement (to remove all the necrotic and/or infected tissue), additional debridement as necessary and a non-weight-bearing regimen to alleviate pressure on the ulcer. REGRANEX should be applied as a continuous thin layer to the entire ulcerated area(s) once daily using a clean application aid. The site(s) of application should then be covered by a moist saline gauze dressing that maintains a moist wound-healing environment. REGRANEX should not be used in conjunction with occlusive dressings.

- A tube of REGRANEX should be used on a single patient only
- Care should be taken during use to avoid microbial contamination and spoilage
- Hands should be washed thoroughly before applying REGRANEX
- The tip of the tube should not come into contact with the wound or any other surface
- The use of a clean application aid is recommended and contact with other parts of the body should be avoided
- Before application, the ulcer should be gently rinsed with saline or water to remove residual gel.
- The tube should be closed tightly after each use.

REGRANEX should not be used for more than 20 weeks in any individual patient.

If during treatment with REGRANEX no meaningful healing progress is evident after the first ten weeks of continuous therapy, treatment should be re- evaluated, and factors known to compromise healing (such as osteomyelitis, ischaemia, infection) should be re- assessed. Therapy should be continued to the maximum of 20 weeks as long as healing progress is seen on periodic evaluations.

Special population

Paediatric population

Safety and effectiveness in children and adolescents below the age of 18years have not been established.

REGRANEX has not been studied in children.

4.3 Contraindications
- Known hypersensitivity to the active substance or to any of the excipients.
- Known neoplasm(s) at or near the site(s) of application.
- In patients with clinically infected ulcers. (See section 4.4).

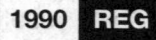

Table 1 Serious adverse reactions reported in clinical trials

System organ class	Very Common	Common	Rare
Infections and infestations	Infections Cellulitis	Osteomyelitis	
Skin and subcutaneous tissue disorders	Skin ulceration	Skin disorder (including erythema)	Dermatitis bullous Excessive granulation tissue*
General disorders and administration sites conditions		Pain	Oedema

*Based on post marketing experience

4.4 Special warnings and precautions for use

In view of the lack of data, and since becaplermin is a growth factor, it should be used with caution in patients with known malignancies.

Prior to the use of REGRANEX, related underlying conditions such as osteomyelitis and peripheral arteriopathy should be excluded or treated if present. Osteomyelitis should be assessed by X-ray examination. Peripheral arteriopathy should be excluded by the assessment of the pedal pulses or other techniques. Ulcers with a suspicious appearance should be biopsied to exclude malignancy.

Infection should be treated prior to the use of REGRANEX. If a wound becomes infected during REGRANEX therapy, the product should be discontinued until the infection has cleared.

REGRANEX should not be used in patients with ulcers that are not of primarily neuropathic origin, such as those due to arteriopathy or other factors.

REGRANEX should not be used in ulcers of baseline surface area > 5 cm^2, or for more than 20 weeks in any individual. There are insufficient data to support safe use of the product for more than 20 weeks (see 5.1 Pharmacodynamic properties). Efficacy has not been demonstrated for ulcers of baseline surface area > 5 cm^2.

REGRANEX contains E218 (methyl parahydroxybenzoate) and E216 (propyl parahydroxybenzoate). These may cause allergic reactions (possibly delayed).

4.5 Interaction with other medicinal products and other forms of interaction

No interaction studies have been performed. Consequently, it is recommended that REGRANEX should not be applied to the ulcer site in conjunction with other topical medications.

4.6 Pregnancy and lactation

Pregnancy

There are no adequate data from the use of becaplermin in pregnant women. Consequently, REGRANEX should not be used in pregnant women.

Breast Feeding

It is not known whether becaplermin is excreted in human milk. Therefore, REGRANEX should not be used in nursing mothers.

4.7 Effects on ability to drive and use machines

No studies on the effects on the ability to drive and use machines have been performed.

4.8 Undesirable effects

The following list of adverse reactions is based on experience from clinical trials and on postmarketing experience.

Adverse reactions are listed under headings of frequency (number of patients expected to experience the reaction), using the following categories: very common (>1/10); common (>1/100, <1/10); uncommon (>1/1000, <1/100); rare (>1/10,000, <1/1000); very rare (<1/10,000); not known.

Serious adverse reactions reported in clinical trials.

(see Table 1 above)

4.9 Overdose

Since absorption is insignificant from the site of topical application, no untoward systemic events are expected.

5. PHARMACOLOGICAL PROPERTIES

5.1 Pharmacodynamic properties

Pharmacotherapeutic group: Preparation for treatment of wounds and ulcers, ATC code: D 03 AX06

REGRANEX contains becaplermin, a recombinant human Platelet Derived Growth Factor-BB (rhPDGF-BB). Becaplermin is produced by insertion of the gene for the B chain of human platelet derived growth factor into the yeast, *Saccharomyces cerevisiae*. The biological activity of becaplermin includes promoting the chemotactic recruitment and proliferation of cells involved in wound repair. Thus it helps the growth of normal tissue for healing. In animal wound models, the predominant effect of becaplermin is to enhance the formation of granulation tissue. From data combined from 4 clinical trials conducted over a 20 week treatment phase for ulcers of baseline surface area less than or equal to 5 cm^2, 47% of ulcers treated with becaplermin 100 µg/g gel completely healed, compared to 35% which were treated with placebo gel alone. Subjects recruited into these studies were diabetic adults aged 19 years or over who were suffering from at least one stage III or IV diabetic ulcer of at least 8 weeks duration.

5.2 Pharmacokinetic properties

Absorption

Clinical absorption studies were conducted in patients with a mean diabetic ulcer area of 10.5 cm^2 (range 2.3 - 43.5 cm^2). Following 14 consecutive daily topical applications of REGRANEX, only insignificant systemic absorption of becaplermin occurred.

5.3 Preclinical safety data

Becaplermin was not mutagenic in a battery of *in vitro* and *in vivo* tests. Since absorption is insignificant from the site of topical application in man, carcinogenesis and reproductive toxicity studies have not been conducted with REGRANEX. In the process of healing the wound, becaplermin induces cell proliferation. However, skin tumours have not been reported in the clinical trials at the site of application or in close proximity.

In a preclinical study designed to determine the effects of PDGF on exposed bone, rats injected at the metatarsals with 3 or 10 µg/site (concentration of 30 or 100 µg/ml/site) of becaplermin every other day for 13 days displayed histological changes indicative of accelerated bone remodelling consisting of periosteal hyperplasia and subperiosteal bone resorption and exostosis. The soft tissue adjacent to the injection site had fibroplasia with accompanying mononuclear cell infiltration reflective of the ability of PDGF to stimulate connective tissue growth.

Preclinical absorption studies through full-thickness wounds were conducted in rats with a wound area of 1.4 - 1.6 cm^2. Systemic absorption of a single dose and multiple applications for 5 consecutive days of becaplermin to those wounds was insignificant.

6. PHARMACEUTICAL PARTICULARS

6.1 List of excipients

carmellose sodium (E466)

sodium chloride

sodium acetate

glacial acetic acid (E260)

methyl parahydroxybenzoate (methylparaben) (E218)

propyl parahydroxybenzoate (propylparaben) (E216)

metacresol

lysine hydrochloride

water for injections

6.2 Incompatibilities

There are no known incompatibilities.

6.3 Shelf life

1 year.

Use within 6 weeks after first opening.

6.4 Special precautions for storage

Store in a refrigerator (2°C - 8°C).

Do not freeze.

Close tightly after each use

6.5 Nature and contents of container

15 g of gel in a multidose tube (laminated polyethylene-lined). Pack size of 1.

6.6 Special precautions for disposal and other handling

After treatment is completed, any unused gel should be discarded in accordance with local requirements.

7. MARKETING AUTHORISATION HOLDER

JANSSEN-CILAG INTERNATIONAL NV

Turnhoutseweg, 30

B-2340 Beerse

Belgium

8. MARKETING AUTHORISATION NUMBER(S)

EU/1/99/101/001

9. DATE OF FIRST AUTHORISATION/RENEWAL OF THE AUTHORISATION

March 29, 1999/ March 19,2009

10. DATE OF REVISION OF THE TEXT

March 19, 2009

Regurin 20mg tablets

(Speciality European Pharma)

1. NAME OF THE MEDICINAL PRODUCT

Regurin 20mg tablets

2. QUALITATIVE AND QUANTITATIVE COMPOSITION

The active ingredient is trospium chloride. Each coated tablet contains 20 mg trospium chloride.

Excipients:

For excipients, see 6.1.

3. PHARMACEUTICAL FORM

Coated tablet

Brownish-yellow, glossy coated, biconvex tablets

4. CLINICAL PARTICULARS

4.1 Therapeutic indications

Symptomatic treatment of urge incontinence and/or increased urinary frequency and urgency as may occur in patients with overactive bladder (e.g. idiopathic or neurologic detrusor overactivity).

4.2 Posology and method of administration

One coated tablet twice daily (equivalent to 40 mg of trospium chloride per day).

In patients with severe renal impairment (creatinine clearance between 10 and 30 ml/min.1.73 m^2) the recommended dosage is one coated tablet per day or every second day (equivalent to 20mg of trospium chloride per day or every second day).

The coated table should be swallowe whole with a glass of water before meals on an empty stomach.

The need for continued treatment should be reassessed at regular intervals of 3-6 months.

Since no data are available, use in children under 12 years of age is contra-indicated.

4.3 Contraindications

Trospium chloride is contraindicated in patients with urinary retention, severe gastro-intestinal condition (including toxic megacolon), myasthenia gravis, narrow-angle glaucoma, and tachyarrhythmia.

Trospium chloride is also contraindicated in patients who have demonstrated hypersensitivity to the active substance or to any of the excipients.

4.4 Special warnings and precautions for use

Trospium chloride should be used with caution by patients:

- with obstructive conditions of the gastrointestinal tract such as pyloric stenosis
- with obstruction of the urinary flow with the risk of formation of urinary retention
- with autonomic neuropathy
- with hiatus hernia associated with reflux oesophagitis
- in whom fast heart rates are undesirable e.g. those with hyperthyroidism, coronary artery disease and congestive heart failure.

As there are no data in patients with severe hepatic impairment, treatment of these patients with trospium chloride is not recommended. In patients with mild to moderate liver impairment caution should be exercised.

Trospium chloride is mainly eliminated by renal excretion. Marked elevations in the plasma levels have been observed in patients with severe renal impairment.

Therefore, in this population but also in patients with mild to moderate renal impairment caution should be exercised (see 4.2).

Before commencing therapy organic causes of urinary frequency, urgency, and urge incontinence, such as heart diseases, diseases of the kidneys, polydipsia, or infections, or tumours of urinary organs should be excluded.

Regurin contains lactose monohydrate, sucrose and wheat starch. Patients with rare hereditary problems of galactose intolerance, the Lapp lactase deficiency or glucose-galactose malabsorption should not take this medicine.

Patients with rare hereditary problems of fructose intolerance or sucrose-isomaltase insufficiency should not take this medicine.

Patients with wheat allergy (different from coeliac disease) should not take this medicine. Apart from that, trospium chloride is suitable for people with coeliac disease.

4.5 Interaction with other medicinal products and other forms of interaction

Pharmacodynamic interactions:

The following potential pharmacodynamic interactions may occur: Potentiation of the effect of drugs with anticholinergic action (such as amantadine, tricyclic antidepressants), enhancement of the tachycardic action of β-sympathomimetics; decrease in efficacy of pro-kinetic agents (e.g. metoclopramide).

Since trospium chloride may influence gastro-intestinal motility and secretion, the possibility cannot be excluded that the absorption of other concurrently administered medicinal products may be altered.

Pharmacokinetic interactions:

An inhibition of the absorption of trospium chloride with drugs like guar, cholestyramine and colestipol cannot be excluded. Therefore the simultaneous administration of these drugs with trospium chloride is not recommended.

Metabolic interactions of trospium chloride have been investigated in vitro on cytochrome P450 enzymes involved in active substance metabolism (P450 1A2, 2A6, 2C9, 2C19, 2D6, 2E1, 3A4). No influence on their metabolic activities were observed. Since trospium chloride is metabolised only to a low extent and since ester hydrolysis is the only relevant metabolic pathway, no metabolic interactions are expected.

4.6 Pregnancy and lactation
Animal studies do not indicate direct or indirect harmful effects with respect to pregnancy, embryonal/foetal development, parturition or postnatal development (see section 5.3). In rats, placental transfer and passage into the maternal milk of trospium chloride occurs.

For Regurin 20mg no clinical data on exposed pregnancies are available.

Caution should be exercised when prescribing to pregnant or breastfeeding women.

4.7 Effects on ability to drive and use machines
Principally, disorders of accommodation can lower the ability to actively participate in road traffic and to use machines.

However, examinations of parameters characterising the ability to participate in road traffic (visual orientation, general ability to react, reaction under stress, concentration and motor coordination) have not revealed any effects of trospium chloride.

4.8 Undesirable effects
Anticholinergic effects such as dry mouth, dyspepsia and constipation may occur during treatment with trospium chloride.

Very common (>10%)

gastrointestinal system: dry mouth

Common (>1%)

gastrointestinal system: dyspepsia, constipation, abdominal pain, nausea

Uncommon (<1%)

gastrointestinal system: flatulence

Rare (<0.1%)

urinary system: micturition disorders (e.g. formation of residual urine)

cardiovascular system: tachycardia

vision disorders: disorders of accommodation (this applies in particular to patients who are hypometropic and whose vision has not been adequately corrected)

gastro-intestinal system: diarrhoea

respiratory system: dyspnoea

skin: rash

body as a whole: asthenia, chest pain

Very Rare (<0.01%)

urinary system: urinary retention

cardiovascular system: tachyarrhythmia

musculoskeletal system: myalgia, arthralgia

skin: angio-oedema

liver and biliary system: mild to moderate increase in serum transaminase levels

body as a whole: anaphylaxis

central nervous system: headache, dizziness

4.9 Overdose
After administration of a maximum single dose of 360 mg trospium chloride to healthy volunteers, dryness of the mouth, tachycardia and disorders of micturition were observed to an increased extent. No manifestations of severe overdose or intoxication in humans have been reported to date. Increased anticholinergic symptoms are to be expected as signs of intoxication.

In the case of intoxication the following measures should be taken:

- gastric lavage and reduction of absorption (e.g. activated charcoal)
- local administration of pilocarpine to glaucoma patients
- catheterisation in patients with urinary retention
- treatment with a parasympathomimetic agent (e.g. neostigmine) in the case of severe symptoms
- administration of beta blockers in the case of insufficient response, pronounced tachycardia and/or circulatory instability (e.g. initially 1 mg propranolol intravenously along with monitoring of ECG and blood pressure).

5. PHARMACOLOGICAL PROPERTIES

5.1 Pharmacodynamic properties
Pharmacotherapeutic group: Urinary Antispasmodic, ATC code: G04BD15

Trospium chloride is a quaternary derivative of nortropane and therefore belongs to the class of parasympatholytic or anticholinergic active drugs, as it competes concentration-dependently with acetylcholine, the body's endogenous transmitter at postsynaptic, parasympathic binding sites.

Trospium chloride binds with high affinity to muscarinic receptors of the so called M_1-, M_2- and M_3- subtypes and demonstrates negligible affinity to nicotinic receptors.

Consequently, the anticholinercic effect of trospium chloride exerts a relaxing action on smooth muscle tissue and organ functions mediated by muscarinic receptors. Both in preclinical as well as in clinical experiments, trospium chloride diminishes the contractile tone of smooth muscle in the gastrointestinal and genito-urinary tract.

Furthermore, it can inhibit the secretion of bronchial mucus, saliva, sweat and the occular accommodation. No effects on the central nervous system have so far been observed.

In two specific safety studies in healthy volunteers trospium chloride has been proven not to affect cardiac repolarisation, but has been shown to have consistent and dose dependent heart rate accelerating effect.

A long term clinical trial with trospium chloride 20mg bid found an increase of QT> 60 ms in 1.5% (3/197) of included patients. The clinical relevance of these findings has not been established. Routine safety monitoring in two other placebo-controlled clinical trials of three months duration do not support such an influence of trospium chloride: In the first study an increase of QTcF >= 60 msec was seen in 4/258 (1.6%) in trospium-treated patients vs. 9/256 (3.5%)in placebo-treated patients. Corresponding figures in the second trial were 8/325 (2.5%) in trospium-treated patients vs. 8/325 (2.5%) in placebo-treated patients.

An increase in ECG heart rate of about 6 bpm was observed during two pivotal phase-III studies (IP631-018, IP631-022) in patients given the prolonged release formulation of trospium chloride (total number of patients exposed to drug substance N= 948, duration of trials = 9 months). No other significant ECG abnormality was found.

5.2 Pharmacokinetic properties
After oral administration of trospium chloride maximum plasma levels are reached at 4-6 hours. Following a single dose of 20mg the maximum plasma level is about 4ng/ml. Within the tested interval, 20 to 60mg as a single dose, the plasma levels are proportional to the administered dose. The absolute bioavailability of a single oral dose of 20 mg of trospium chloride (1 coated tablet Regurin 20mg) is 9.6 ± 4.5% (mean value ± standard deviation). At steady state the intraindividual variability is 16%, the interindividual variability is 36%.

Simultaneous intake of food, especially high fat diets, reduces the bioavailability of trospium chloride. After a high fat meal mean C_{max} and AUC are reduced to 15-20% of the values in the fasted state.

Trospium chloride exhibits diurnal variability in exposure with a decrease of both C_{max} and AUC for evening relative to morning doses.

Most of the systemically available trospium chloride is excreted unchanged by the kidneys, though a small portion (10% of the renal excretion) appears in the urine as the spiroalcohol, a metabolite formed by ester hydrolysis. The terminal elimination half life is in the range of 10-20 hours. No accumulation occurs. The plasma protein binding is 50-80%.

Pharmacokinetic data in elderly patients suggests no major differences. There are also no gender differences.

In a study in patients with severe renal impairment (creatinine clearance 8-32 ml/min) mean AUC was 4-fold higher, C_{max} was 2-fold higher and the mean half-life was prolonged 2-fold compared with healthy subjects.

Pharmacokinetic results of a study with mildly and moderately hepatically impaired patients do not suggest a need for dose adjustment in patients with hepatic impairment, and are consistent with the limited role of hepatic metabolism in the elimination of trospium chloride.

5.3 Preclinical safety data
Preclinical data reveal no special hazard to humans based on conventional studies of safety pharmacology, repeated dose toxicity, genotoxicity, carcinogenicity, and toxicity to reproduction.

Placental transfer and passage of trospium chloride into the maternal milk occurs in rats.

6. PHARMACEUTICAL PARTICULARS

6.1 List of excipients
Tablet core: Wheat starch

Microcrystalline cellulose

Lactose monohydrate

Povidone

Croscarmellose sodium

Stearic acid

Silica colloidal anhydrous

Talc

Tablet Coat: Sucrose

Carmellose sodium

Talc

Silica colloidal anhydrous

Calcium carbonate E170

Macrogol 8000

Titanium dioxide (E171)

Iron oxide hydrate yellow (E172)

Beeswax white

Carnauba wax

Note for diabetics: 1 coated tablet corresponds to 0.06g of carbohydrate (equivalent to 0.005 bread units).

6.2 Incompatibilities
Not applicable.

6.3 Shelf life
5 years

6.4 Special precautions for storage
This medicinal product does not require any special storage conditions.

6.5 Nature and contents of container
PVC foiled aluminium blister.

Pack sizes approved: 2, 20, 28, 30, 40, 50, 56, 60, 90, 100, 120, 150, 200, 500, 600, 1000, 1200, 2000.

Not all pack sizes may be marketed.

6.6 Special precautions for disposal and other handling
No special requirements.

7. MARKETING AUTHORISATION HOLDER
MADAUS GmbH

51101 Cologne

Germany

Tel.: 0221/8998-0

Fax: 0221 / 8998-711

e-mail: info@madaus.de

8. MARKETING AUTHORISATION NUMBER(S)
PL 25843/0002

9. DATE OF FIRST AUTHORISATION/RENEWAL OF THE AUTHORISATION
24 July 2007

10. DATE OF REVISION OF THE TEXT
10 June 2009

Regurin XL 60mg

(Speciality European Pharma)

1. NAME OF THE MEDICINAL PRODUCT
Regurin XL 60 mg prolonged-release capsule, hard

2. QUALITATIVE AND QUANTITATIVE COMPOSITION
Each prolonged-release capsule, hard contains 60 mg trospium chloride.

Excipients:

Each prolonged-release capsule, hard contains 154.5 mg sucrose.

For a full list of excipients, see section 6.1.

3. PHARMACEUTICAL FORM
Prolonged-release capsule, hard

The Regurin XL 60 mg prolonged-release capsule, hard has an opaque orange cap and an opaque white body imprinted with SAN 60 and contains white to off-white pellets.

4. CLINICAL PARTICULARS

4.1 Therapeutic indications
Symptomatic treatment of urge incontinence and/or increased urinary frequency and urgency as may occur in patients with overactive bladder.

4.2 Posology and method of administration
One capsule once daily (equivalent to 60 mg of trospium chloride per day).

Regurin XL 60 mg should be taken with water on an empty stomach one hour before a meal.

Renal impairment:

Data on the use of Regurin XL 60 mg are not available for patients with renal impairment. Trospium chloride is mainly excreted unchanged by the kidneys. An increase in plasma levels is documented for the immediate release formulation. For the prolonged release formulation an appropriate level of dose adjustment is not known for renally impaired patients and the product is therefore not recommended for use in renally impaired patients (see section 4.4 and 5.2).

Hepatic impairment:

Data on patients with mild and moderate impairment of liver function are only available for the immediate release formulation of trospium chloride, but not for the prolonged release formulation. These patients should be treated with caution. Regurin XR 60 mg should not be given to patients with severe hepatic impairment (see section 4.4 and 5.2).

The need for continued treatment should be reassessed at regular intervals of 3-6 months.

Regurin XL 60 mg is not recommended for use in children and adolescents below 18 years due to lack of data on safety and efficacy.

4.3 Contraindications
Trospium chloride is contraindicated in patients with urinary retention, severe gastro-intestinal condition (including toxic megacolon), myasthenia gravis, narrow-angle glaucoma, and tachyarrhythmia.

Trospium chloride is also contraindicated in patients who have demonstrated hypersensitivity to the active substance or to any of the excipients.

4.4 Special warnings and precautions for use
Trospium chloride should be used with caution by patients:

- with obstructive conditions of the gastrointestinal tract such as pyloric stenosis

- with obstruction of the urinary flow with the risk of formation of urinary retention

- with autonomic neuropathy

- with hiatus hernia associated with reflux oesophagitis

- in whom fast heart rates are undesirable e.g. those with hyperthyroidism, coronary artery disease and congestive heart failure.

Data on the use of the prolonged-release formulation of trospium chloride are not available for patients with hepatic impairment. Based on data available for the immediate release formulation of trospium chloride, Regurin XL 60 mg is not recommended for patients with severe hepatic impairment and caution should be exercised in patients with mild to moderate liver impairment (see section 4.2 and 5.2).

Trospium chloride is mainly eliminated by renal excretion. For the immediate release formulation marked elevations in plasma levels have been observed in patients with severe renal impairment and lead to dose adjustment.

For the prolonged release formulation an appropriate level of dose adjustment is not known. Therefore, it is recommended not to treat renally impaired patients with Regurin XL 60 mg (see section 4.2 and 5.2).

Before commencing therapy organic causes of urinary frequency, urgency, and urge incontinence, such as heart diseases, diseases of the kidneys, polydipsia, or infections, or tumours of urinary organs should be excluded.

Regurin XL 60 mg contains sucrose.

Patients with rare hereditary problems of fructose intolerance, glucose-galactose malabsorption or sucrase-isomaltase insufficiency should not take this medicine.

4.5 Interaction with other medicinal products and other forms of interaction
Pharmacodynamic interactions:

The following potential pharmacodynamic interactions may occur: Potentiation of the effect of medicinal products with anticholinergic action (such as amantadine, tricyclic antidepressants), enhancement of the tachycardic action of β-sympathomimetics; decrease in efficacy of pro-kinetic agents (e.g. metoclopramide).

Since trospium chloride may influence gastro-intestinal motility and secretion, the possibility cannot be excluded that the absorption of other concurrently administered medicinal products may be altered.

Pharmacokinetic interactions:

An inhibition of the absorption of trospium chloride with active substances like guar, cholestyramine and colestipol cannot be excluded. Therefore the simultaneous administration of medicinal products containing these active substances with trospium chloride is not recommended.

Though trospium chloride was shown not to affect pharmacokinetics of digoxin, an interaction with other active substances eliminated by active tubular secretion cannot be excluded.

Metabolic interactions of trospium chloride have been investigated in vitro on cytochrome P450 enzymes involved in active substance metabolism (P450 1A2, 2A6, 2C9, 2C19, 2D6, 2E1, 3A4). No influence on their metabolic activities were observed. Since trospium chloride is metabolised only to a low extent and since ester hydrolysis is the only relevant metabolic pathway, no metabolic interactions are expected.

4.6 Pregnancy and lactation
Animal studies do not indicate direct or indirect harmful effects with respect to pregnancy, embryonal/foetal development, parturition or postnatal development (see section 5.3). In rats, placental transfer and passage into the maternal milk of trospium chloride occurs.

Clinical data on exposure during pregnancy or lactation are not available for Regurin XL 60 mg.

Caution should be exercised when prescribing to pregnant or breastfeeding women.

4.7 Effects on ability to drive and use machines
Principally, disorders of accommodation can lower the ability to actively participate in road traffic and to use machines.

However, examinations of parameters characterising the ability to participate in road traffic (visual orientation, general ability to react, reaction under stress, concentration and motor coordination) have not revealed any effects of trospium chloride.

4.8 Undesirable effects
Undesirable effects observed with trospium chloride are caused mainly by typical anticholinergic effects such as dry mouth, dyspepsia and constipation.

In two Phase 3, placebo-controlled, double-blind clinical studies 1165 patients were treated for 12 weeks with either Regurin XL 60 mg or placebo. The following table lists possibly related adverse events reported for patients treated with Regurin XL 60 mg:

(see Table 1 below)

In ensuing open-label phases of the two Phase 3 clinical studies the most common adverse events constipation (6.8%) and dry mouth (6.5%) were reported less frequently.

For immediate-release formulations of trospium chloride the following undesirable effects have been observed in post-marketing surveillance:

Cardiac disorders: tachyarrhythmia; Gastrointestinal disorders: diarrhoea; General disorders and administration site conditions: chest pain; Immune system disorders: anaphylaxis; Investigations: mild to moderate increase in serum transaminase levels; Muscoloskeletal and connective tissue disorders: myalgia, arthralgia; Nervous system disorders: dizziness; Respiratory, thoracic and mediastinal disorders: dyspnoea; Skin and subcutaneous tissue disorders: angio-oedema, Stevens-Johnson Syndrom (SJS) / Toxic Epidermal Necrolysis (TEN).

The frequencies for the prolonged-release capsule Regurin XL 60 mg are not known.

4.9 Overdose
After administration of a maximum single dose of 360 mg trospium chloride as immediate release preparation to healthy volunteers, dryness of the mouth, tachycardia and disorders of micturition were observed to an increased extent. No manifestations of severe overdose or intoxication in humans have been reported to date. Exaggerated anticholinergic symptoms are to be expected as signs of intoxication following administration of trospium chloride as an extended release preparation as well.

In the case of intoxication the following measures should be taken:

- gastric lavage and reduction of absorption (e.g. activated charcoal)

- local administration of pilocarpine to glaucoma patients

- catheterisation in patients with urinary retention

- treatment with a parasympathomimetic agent (e.g. neostigmine) in the case of severe symptoms

- administration of beta blockers in the case of insufficient response, pronounced tachycardia and/or circulatory instability (e.g. initially 1 mg propranolol intravenously along with monitoring of ECG and blood pressure).

5. PHARMACOLOGICAL PROPERTIES

5.1 Pharmacodynamic properties
Pharmacotherapeutic group: Urinary Antispasmodic, ATC code: G04BD09

Trospium chloride is a quaternary derivative of nortropane and therefore belongs to the class of parasympatholytic or anticholinergic active substances, as it competes concentration-dependently with acetylcholine, the body's endogenous transmitter at postsynaptic, parasympathic binding sites.

Trospium chloride binds with high affinity to muscarinic receptors of the so called M_1-, M_2- and M_3- subtypes and demonstrates negligible affinity to nicotinic receptors.

Consequently, the anticholinercic effect of trospium chloride exerts a relaxing action on smooth muscle tissue and organ functions mediated by muscarinic receptors. Both in preclinical as well as in clinical experiments, trospium chloride diminishes the contractile tone of smooth muscle in the gastrointestinal and genito-urinary tract.

Furthermore, it can inhibit the secretion of bronchial mucus, saliva, sweat and the occular accommodation. No effects on the central nervous system have so far been observed.

In two specific safety studies in healthy volunteers trospium chloride has been proven not to affect cardiac repolarisation, but has been shown to have consistent and dose dependent heart rate accelerating effect.

A long term clinical trial with the immediate release formulation of trospium chloride 20mg bid found an increase of QT> 60 ms in 1.5% (3/197) of included patients. The clinical relevance of these findings has not been established. Routine safety monitoring in two other placebo-controlled clinical trials of three months duration do not support such an influence of the immediate release formulation of trospium chloride: In the first study an increase of QTcF >= 60 msec was seen in 4/258 (1.6%)in trospium-treated patients vs. 9/256 (3.5%)in placebo-treated patients. Corresponding figures in the second trial were 8/326 (2.5%) in trospium-treated patients vs. 8/325 (2.5%)in placebo-treated patients.

An increase in ECG heart rate of about 6 bpm was observed during two pivotal phase-III studies (IP631-018, IP631-022) in patients given the prolonged release formulation of trospium chloride (total number of patients exposed to drug substance N= 948, duration of trials = 9 months). No other significant ECG abnormality was found.

5.2 Pharmacokinetic properties
Absorption

The absolute bioavailability of a single oral dose of 20 mg of trospium chloride as immediate release formulation is 9.6 ± 4.5% (mean value ± standard deviation).

Compared to an immediate release formulation, Regurin XL 60 mg following multiple oral dosing resulted in a further reduction of peak exposure (Cmax) and relative overall systemic exposure (AUC) by approximately 28% and 33% respectively.

Oral administration (single and multiple dosing) of trospium chloride 60 mg prolonged release formulation as once daily dosing achieved maximum plasma levels of approximately 2 ng/ml and 1.9 ng/ml (C_{max}) respectively. Following single and multiple dosing of 20 mg of trospium chloride as immediate release formulation corresponding values revealed to be higher indicating plasma levels of 2 -4 ng/mL (C_{max}). Time to maximum concentration (T_{max}) was

Table 1

	Very common (>1/10)	Common (≥1/100, <1/10)	Uncommon (≥1/1000, <1/100)	Rare (≥1/10.000, <1/1000)	Very Rare (<1/10.000)
Cardiac disorders				Tachycardia	
Eye disorders		Dry eye		Vision disorders	
Gastrointestinal disorders	Dry mouth	Dyspepsia Constipation Constipation aggravated Abdominal pain Abdominal distension Nausea	Flatulence		
General disorders and administration site conditions				Asthenia	
Infections and infestations					Urinary tract infection
Nervous system disorders					Headache
Renal and urinary disorders				Micturition disorders Urinary retention	
Respiratory, thoracic and mediastinal disorders		Nasal dryness			
Skin and subcutaneous disorders				Rash	

around 5 hrs with both preparations, whereas steady state concentration differed slightly resulting at day 8 by multiple dosing of the 60 mg prolonged release formulation.

Administration of Regurin XL 60 mg immediately after a high (50%) fat-content meal reduced the oral bioavailability of trospium chloride by 35% for $AUC_{(0-Tlast)}$ and by 60% for C_{max}. Other pharmacokinetic parameters such as T_{max} and $t_{½}$ were unchanged in the presence of food. Coadministration with antacid, however, had no effect on the oral bioavailability of Regurin XL 60 mg.

Distribution

Protein binding ranged from 48 to 78%, depending upon the assessment method used, when a range of concentration levels of trospium chloride (0.5-100 μg/L) were incubated *in vitro* with human serum.

The ratio of ^3H-trospium chloride in plasma to whole blood was 1.6:1. This ratio indicates that the majority of ^3H- trospium chloride is distributed in plasma.

Trospium chloride is highly distributed to non-CNS tissues, with an apparent volume of distribution > 600 L.

Biotransformation

Of a trospium chloride dose absorbed following oral administration, metabolites account for approximately 40% of the excreted dose. The major metabolic pathway of trospium is hypothesized as ester hydrolysis with subsequent conjugation of benzylic acid to form azoniaspironortropanol with glucuronic acid. Cytochrome P450 does not contribute significantly to the elimination of trospium. Data taken from in vitro studies of human liver microsomes, investigating the inhibitory effect of trospium on seven cytochrome P450 isoenzyme substrates (CYP1A2, 2A6, 2C9, 2C19, 2D6, 2E1, and 3A4), suggest a lack of inhibition at clinically relevant concentrations.

Elimination

The terminal elimination half-life was extended after multiple dosing of trospium chloride 60 mg prolonged release formulation to approximately 38,5 hours in comparison to about 20hrs after immediate release formulations. Most of the systemically available trospium chloride is excreted unchanged mainly by glomerular filtration and tubular secretion. A small portion (10 % of the renal excretion) appears in the urine as spiroalcohol, a metabolite formed by ester hydrolysis.

Special patient groups

Pharmacokinetic data of trospium chloride in elderly patients suggest no major differences. There are also no gender differences.

Severe renal impairment may significantly alter the disposition of Regurin XL 60 mg. In a study in patients with severe renal impairment (creatinine clearance 8-32 ml/min) after administration of trospium chloride as 20 mg immediate release formulation, mean AUC was 4-fold higher, C_{max} was 2-fold higher and the mean half-life was prolonged 2-fold compared with healthy subjects.

Pharmacokinetic studies have not been done on patients with renal impairment using the prolonged-release formulation of trospium chloride.

Therefore, Regurin XL 60 mg is not recommended for patients with renal impairment (see sections 4.2 and 4.4).

After a single dose of 40mg of the immediate-release formulation of trospium chloride given to patients with mild (Child-Pugh 5-6) and moderate to severe (Child-Pugh 7-12) hepatic impairment, Cmax was increased 12% and 63%, respectively, in comparison to healthy controls. The AUC was, however, decreased by 5% and 15%, respectively. Mean oral and mean renal clearance were 5% and 7% higher in subjects with mild and 17% and 51% higher in patients with moderate/severe hepatic impairment. Pharmacokinetic studies have not been done on patients with hepatic impairment using the prolonged-release formulation of trospium chloride.

5.3 Preclinical safety data

Preclinical data on trospium chloride reveal no special hazard to humans based on conventional studies of safety pharmacology, repeated dose toxicity, genotoxicity, carcinogenicity, and toxicity to reproduction.

Placental transfer and passage of trospium chloride into the maternal milk occurs in rats.

6. PHARMACEUTICAL PARTICULARS

6.1 List of excipients

Capsule content: Sucrose

Maize starch

Methyl acrylate-methyl methacrylate-methacrylic acid-copolymer

Ammonium hydroxide

Triglycerides, medium chain

Oleic acid

Ethylcellulose

Titanium dioxide (E 171),

Hypromellose

Macrogol 400

Polysorbate 80

Triethyl citrate

Talc

Capsule Shell: Gelatin

Titanium dioxide (E 171),

Iron oxide yellow (E 172)

Iron oxide red (E 172)

Printing ink:

Shellac (20% esterified),

Iron oxide black (E 172),

Propylene glycol

6.2 Incompatibilities

Not applicable.

6.3 Shelf life

3 years packaged in PVC/Aclar/aluminium blister or PVC/aluminium blister

18 months packaged in PVC/PVDC/aluminium blister

6.4 Special precautions for storage

This medicinal product does not require any special storage conditions.

6.5 Nature and contents of container

Polyvinylchloride (PVC)/aluminium blister, Polyvinylchloride/Polyvinylidenchloride (PVC/PVDC)/aluminium blister or PVC/Aclar®/aluminium blister.

Packs of 4, 7, 10, 14, 28, 30, 56, 60, 84, 90 and 10x28 capsules.

Sample packs of 4.

Not all pack sizes may be marketed.

6.6 Special precautions for disposal and other handling

No special requirements.

Any unused product or waste material should be disposed of in accordance with local requirements.

7. MARKETING AUTHORISATION HOLDER

MADAUS GmbH

51101 Cologne

Germany

Tel.: 0221/8998-0

Fax: 0221 / 8998-711

e-mail: info@madaus.de

8. MARKETING AUTHORISATION NUMBER(S)

PL25843/0003

9. DATE OF FIRST AUTHORISATION/RENEWAL OF THE AUTHORISATION

06/11/2008

10. DATE OF REVISION OF THE TEXT

11/2008

Relenza 5mg/dose inhalation powder.

(GlaxoSmithKline UK)

1. NAME OF THE MEDICINAL PRODUCT

Relenza ▼ 5mg/dose, inhalation powder, pre-dispensed.

2. QUALITATIVE AND QUANTITATIVE COMPOSITION

Each pre-dispensed quantity of inhalation powder (one blister) contains 5 mg zanamivir. Each delivered inhalation (the amount that leaves the mouthpiece of the Diskhaler) contains 4.0 mg zanamivir.

Excipients: Lactose monohydrate (approximately 20 mg which contains milk protein).

For a full list of excipients, see section 6.1.

3. PHARMACEUTICAL FORM

Inhalation powder, pre-dispensed. White to off-white powder.

4. CLINICAL PARTICULARS

4.1 Therapeutic indications

Treatment of influenza

Relenza is indicated for treatment of both influenza A and B in adults and children (≥ 5 years) who present with symptoms typical of influenza when influenza is circulating in the community.

Prevention of influenza

Relenza is indicated for post-exposure prophylaxis of influenza A and B in adults and children (≥ 5 years) following contact with a clinically diagnosed case in a household (see section 5.1 for children aged 5-11 years). In exceptional circumstances, Relenza may be considered for seasonal prophylaxis of influenza A and B during a community outbreak (e.g. in case of a mismatch between circulating and vaccine strains and a pandemic situation).

Relenza is not a substitute for influenza vaccination. The appropriate use of Relenza for prevention of influenza should be determined on a case-by-case basis depending on the circumstances and the population requiring protection.

The use of antivirals for the treatment and prevention of influenza should take into consideration official recommendations, the variability of epidemiology, and the impact of the disease in different geographical areas and patient populations.

4.2 Posology and method of administration

Inhaled drugs, e.g. asthma medication, should be administered prior to administration of Relenza (see section 4.4).

Treatment of influenza

Treatment should begin as soon as possible, within 48 hours after onset of symptoms for adults, and within 36 hours after onset of symptoms for children.

Relenza is for administration to the respiratory tract by oral inhalation only, using the Diskhaler device provided. One blister should be utilised for each inhalation.

The recommended dose of Relenza for treatment of influenza in adults and children from the age of 5 years is two inhalations (2 × 5 mg) twice daily for five days, providing a total daily inhaled dose of 20 mg.

Prevention of influenza

Post-exposure prophylaxis

The recommended dose of Relenza for prevention of influenza, following close contact with an individual, is two inhalations (2 × 5 mg) once daily for 10 days. Therapy should begin as soon as possible and within 36 hours of exposure to an infected person.

Seasonal prophylaxis

The recommended dose of Relenza for prevention of influenza during a community outbreak is 2 inhalations (2 × 5 mg) once daily for up to 28 days.

Impaired Renal or Hepatic Function: No dose modification is required. (See section 5.2).

Elderly patients: No dose modification is required. (See section 5.2).

4.3 Contraindications

Hypersensitivity to the active substance or to any of the excipients.

4.4 Special warnings and precautions for use

Due to the limited number of patients with severe asthma or with other chronic respiratory disease, patients with unstable chronic illnesses or immunocompromised patients (see Section 5.1) who have been treated, it has not been possible to demonstrate the efficacy and safety of Relenza in these groups. Due to limited and inconclusive data, the efficacy of Relenza in the prevention of influenza in the nursing home setting has not been demonstrated. The efficacy of zanamivir for the treatment of elderly patients ≥ 65 years has also not been established (see section 5.1).

There have been very rare reports of patients being treated with Relenza who have experienced bronchospasm and/or decline in respiratory function which may be acute and/or serious. Some of these patients did not have any previous history of respiratory disease. Any patients experiencing such reactions should discontinue Relenza and seek medical evaluation immediately.

Due to the limited experience, patients with severe asthma require a careful consideration of the risk in relation to the expected benefit, and Relenza should not be administered unless close medical monitoring and appropriate clinical facilities are available in case of bronchoconstriction. In patients with persistent asthma or severe COPD, management of the underlying disease should be optimised during therapy with Relenza.

Should zanamivir be considered appropriate for patients with asthma or chronic obstructive pulmonary disease, the patient should be informed of the potential risk of bronchospasm with Relenza and should have a fast acting bronchodilator available. Patients on maintenance inhaled bronchodilating therapy should be advised to use their bronchodilators before taking Relenza (see section 4.2).

This medicinal product contains lactose. Patients with rare hereditary problems of galactose intolerance, the Lapp lactase deficiency or glucose-galactose malabsorption should not take this medicine.

Relenza is not a substitute for influenza vaccination and the use of Relenza must not affect the evaluation of individuals for annual vaccination. The protection against influenza only lasts as long as Relenza is administered. Relenza should be used for the treatment and prevention of influenza only when reliable epidemiological data indicate that influenza is circulating in the community.

Relenza is effective only against illness caused by influenza viruses. There is no evidence for the efficacy of Relenza in any illness caused by agents other than influenza viruses.

Neuropsychiatric events have been reported during administration of Relenza in patients with influenza, especially in children and adolescents. Therefore, patients should be closely monitored for behavioural changes and the benefits and risks of continuing treatment should be carefully evaluated for each patient (see section 4.8).

4.5 Interaction with other medicinal products and other forms of interaction

Zanamivir is not protein bound and not hepatically metabolised or modified. Clinically significant drug interactions are unlikely. Zanamivir, when given for 28 days, did not impair the immune response to influenza vaccine.

4.6 Pregnancy and lactation

Pregnancy: The safe use of Relenza during pregnancy has not been established.

In rats and rabbits zanamivir has been shown to cross the placenta. High doses of zanamivir were not associated with malformations in rats or rabbits and only minor alterations were reported. The potential risk for humans is unknown. Relenza should not be used in pregnancy unless the expected benefit to the mother is thought to outweigh any possible risk to the foetus.

Lactation: In rats zanamivir has been shown to be secreted into milk. There is no information on secretion into breast milk in humans.

The use of zanamivir is not recommended in mothers who are breast feeding.

4.7 Effects on ability to drive and use machines

Zanamivir has no or negligible effect on ability to drive and use machines.

4.8 Undesirable effects

There have been rare reports of patients with previous history of respiratory disease (asthma, COPD) and very rare reports of patients without previous history of respiratory disease, who have experienced acute bronchospasm and/or serious decline in respiratory function after use of Relenza (see section 4.4).

The adverse events considered at least possibly related to the treatment are listed below by body system, organ class and absolute frequency. Frequencies are defined as very common (>1/10), common (>1/100, <1/10), uncommon (>1/1000, <1/100), rare (>1/10,000, <1/1000), very rare (<1/10,000).

Within each frequency grouping, undesirable effects are presented in order of decreasing seriousness.

Immune system disorders

Very rare: allergic-type reaction including facial and oropharyngeal oedema

Respiratory, thoracic and mediastinal disorders:

Very rare: bronchospasm, dyspnea, throat tightness or constriction

Skin and subcutaneous tissue disorders:

Very rare: rash, urticaria

Psychiatric and nervous system disorders:

Convulsions and psychiatric events such as depressed level of consciousness, abnormal behaviour, hallucinations and delirium have been reported during Relenza administration in patients with influenza. The symptoms were mainly reported in children and adolescents. Convulsions and psychiatric symptoms have also been reported in patients with influenza not taking Relenza.

4.9 Overdose

Accidental overdose is unlikely due to the physical limitations of the presentation, the route of administration and the poor oral bioavailability (2 to 3%) of zanamivir. Doses of zanamivir up to 64 mg/day (approximately 3 times the maximum daily recommended dose) have been administered by oral inhalation (by nebuliser) without adverse effects. Additionally, systemic exposure by intravenous administration of up to 1200 mg/day for five days showed no adverse effect.

5. PHARMACOLOGICAL PROPERTIES

5.1 Pharmacodynamic properties

Pharmacotherapeutic group: Antiviral, neuraminidase inhibitor

ATC code J05AH01

Mechanism of action

Zanamivir is a selective inhibitor of neuraminidase, the influenza virus surface enzyme. Neuraminidase inhibition occurred in vitro at very low zanamivir concentrations (50% inhibition at 0.64nM – 7.9nM against influenza A and B strains). Viral neuraminidase aids the release of newly formed virus particles from infected cells, and may facilitate access of virus through mucus to epithelial cell surfaces, to allow viral infection of other cells. The inhibition of this enzyme is reflected in both *in vitro* and *in vivo* activity against influenza A and B virus replication, and encompasses all of the known neuraminidase subtypes of influenza A viruses.

The activity of zanamivir is extracellular. It reduces the propagation of both influenza A and B viruses by inhibiting the release of infectious influenza virions from the epithelial cells of the respiratory tract. Influenza viral replication occurs in the superficial epithelium of the respiratory tract. The efficacy of topical administration of zanamivir to this site has been confirmed in clinical studies. To date, virus with reduced susceptibility to zanamivir has not been detected in samples obtained pre and post treatment from patients in clinical studies.

Cross-resistance has been observed between some zanamivir-resistant and some oseltamivir-resistant influenza virus mutants generated in vitro. No studies have been performed to assess risk of emergence of cross-resistance during clinical use.

Clinical experience

Treatment of influenza

Relenza alleviates the symptoms of influenza and reduces their median duration by 1.5 days (range 1.0 – 2.5 days) in adults as detailed in the table below. The median time to alleviation of influenza symptoms in elderly subjects (≥65 years) and in children aged 5-6 years, was not significantly reduced. The efficacy of Relenza has been demonstrated in otherwise healthy adults when treatment is initiated within 48 hours, and in otherwise healthy children when treatment is initiated within 36 hours, after the onset of symptoms. No treatment benefit has been documented for patients with afebrile disease (< 37.8°C).

1. Six key Phase III randomised, placebo-controlled, parallel-group, multicentre treatment studies (NAIB3001, NAIA3002, NAIB3002, NAI30008, NAI30012 and NAI30009) have been conducted with zanamivir for the treatment of naturally acquired influenza A and B. Study NAI30008 recruited only patients with asthma (n=399), COPD (n=87), or asthma and COPD (n=32), study NAI30012 recruited only elderly (≥65 years) patients (n=358) and study NAI30009 (n=471) recruited paediatric patients, 5-12 years. The Intent to Treat population of these six studies comprised 2942 patients of which 1490 received 10 mg zanamivir b.i.d by oral inhalation. The primary endpoint was identical for all six Phase III studies, i.e. time to alleviation of clinically significant signs and symptoms of influenza. For all six phase III studies, alleviation was defined as no fever, i.e. temperature <37.8°C and feverishness score of 'none'('same as normal/none' in NAI30012), and headache, myalgia, cough and sore throat recorded as 'none' ('same as normal/none' in NAI30012) or 'mild' and maintained for 24 hours.

Comparison of Median Time (Days) to Alleviation of Influenza Symptoms:

Influenza Positive Population

(see Table 1 below)

In the Intent to Treat (ITT) population the difference in time to alleviation of symptoms was 1.0 day (95% CI: 0.5 to 1.5) in the combined analysis of NAIB3001, NAIA3002 and NAIB3002, 1.0 day (95% CI: 0 to 2) in study NAI30008, 1.0 day (95% CI –1.0 to 3.0) in study NAI30012 and 0.5 days (95% CI: 0 to 1.5) in study NAI30009. There are limited data in high risk children.

In a combined analysis of patients with influenza B (n=163), including 79 treated with zanamivir, a 2.0 day treatment benefit was observed (95%CI: 0.50 to 3.50).

In the pooled analysis of 3 phase III studies in influenza positive, predominantly healthy adults, the incidence of complications was 152/558 (27%) in placebo recipients and 119/609 (20%) in zanamivir recipients (relative risk zanamivir:placebo 0.73; 95% CI 0.59 to 0.90, p=0.004). In study NAI30008 enrolling patients with asthma and COPD the incidence of complications was 56/153 (37%) in influenza-positive placebo recipients and 52/160 (33%) in influenza positive zanamivir recipients (relative risk zanamivir:placebo 0.89; 95% CI: 0.65 to 1.21, p=0.520). In study NAI30012 enrolling elderly patients the incidence of complications was 46/114 (40%) in influenza positive placebo recipients and 39/120 (33%) in influenza positive zanamivir recipients (relative risk zanamivir:placebo 0.80, 95% CI: 0.57 to 1.13, p=0.256). In the paediatric study NAI30009, the incidence of complications was 41/182 (23%) in influenza-positive placebo recipients and 26/164 (16%) in influenza-positive zanamivir recipients (relative risk zanamivir:placebo 0.70; 95% CI: 0.45 to 1.10, p=0.151).

In a placebo controlled study in patients with predominantly mild/moderate asthma and/or Chronic Obstructive Pulmonary Disease (COPD) there was no clinically significant difference between zanamivir and placebo in forced expiratory volume in one second (FEV_1) or peak expiratory flow rate (PEFR) measured during treatment or after the end of treatment.

Prevention of influenza

The efficacy of Relenza in preventing naturally occurring influenza illness has been demonstrated in two post-exposure prophylaxis studies in households and two seasonal prophylaxis studies during community outbreaks of influenza. The primary efficacy endpoint in these studies was the incidence of symptomatic, laboratory-confirmed influenza, defined as the presence of two or more of the following symptoms: oral temperature 37.8C or feverishness, cough, headache, sore throat, and myalgia; and laboratory confirmation of influenza by culture, PCR, or seroconversion (defined as a 4-fold increase in convalescent antibody titer from baseline).

Post exposure prophylaxis

Two studies assessed post-exposure prophylaxis in household contacts of an index case. Within 1.5 days of onset of symptoms in an index case, each household (including all family members ≥ 5 years of age) was randomized to Relenza 10 mg or placebo inhaled once daily for 10 days. In the first study only, each index case was randomized to the same treatment (Relenza or placebo) as the other household members. In this study, the proportion of households with at least one new case of symptomatic influenza was reduced from 19% (32 of 168 households) with placebo to 4% (7 of 169 households) with Relenza (79% protective efficacy; 95% CI: 57% to 89%, p<0.001). In the second study, index cases were not treated and the incidence of symptomatic influenza was reduced from 19% (46 of 242 households) with placebo to 4% (10 of 245 households) with Relenza (81% protective efficacy; 95% CI: 64% to 90%, p<0.001). Results were similar in the subgroups with influenza A or B. In these studies, which included a total of 2128 contact cases, 553 children were aged 5-11 years, of which 123 children were 5-6 years. The incidence of symptomatic laboratory confirmed influenza in the 5- to 6-year-old group (placebo vs. zanamivir) was 4/33 (12%) vs. 1/28 (4%) in the first study and 4/26 (15%) vs. 1/36 (3%) in the second study, which seems to be consistent with older age categories. However, as the studies were not powered to establish protective efficacy in individual age categories, a formal subgroup analysis has not been performed.

Seasonal Prophylaxis

Two seasonal prophylaxis studies assessed Relenza 10 mg versus placebo inhaled once daily for 28 days during community outbreaks. In the first study, which involved unvaccinated, otherwise healthy adults aged ≥ 18 years, the incidence of symptomatic influenza was reduced from 6.1% (34 of 554) with placebo to 2.0% (11 of 553) with Relenza (67% protective efficacy; 95% CI: 39% to 83%, p<0.001). The second study involved community-dwelling subjects aged ≥ 12 years at high risk of complications from influenza, where 67% of participants had received vaccine in the season of the study. High risk was defined as subjects ≥ 65 years of age and subjects with chronic disorders of the pulmonary or cardiovascular systems or with diabetes mellitus. In this study, the incidence of

Table 1 Influenza Positive Population

Study	Placebo	Zanamivir 10mg inhaled twice daily	Difference in Days	(95% CI) p-value
NAIB3001	n=160 6.0	n=161 4.5	1.5	(0.5, 2.5) 0.004
NAIA3002	n=257 6.0	n=312 5.0	1.0	(0.0, 1.5) 0.078
NAIB3002	n=141 7.5	n=136 5.0	2.5	(1.0, 4.0) <0.001
Combined analysis of NAIB3001, NAIA3002, and NAIB3002	n=558 6.5	n=609 5.0	1.5	(1.0, 2.0) <0.001
Asthma/COPD study				
NAI30008	n=153 7.0	n=160 5.5	1.5	(0.5, 3.25) 0.009
Elderly study				
NAI30012	n=114 7.5	n=120 7.25	0.25	(-2.0 to 3.25) 0.609
Paediatric study				
NAI30009	n=182 5.0	n=164 4.0	1.0	(0.5, 2.0) <0.001

symptomatic influenza was reduced from 1.4% (23 of 1,685) with placebo to 0.2% (4 of 1,678) with Relenza (83% protective efficacy; 95% CI: 56% to 93%, $p<0.001$).

Due to limited and inconclusive data, the efficacy of Relenza in the prevention of influenza in the nursing home setting has not been established.

5.2 Pharmacokinetic properties

Absorption: Pharmacokinetic studies in humans have shown that the absolute oral bioavailability of the drug is low (mean (min, max) is 2%(1%, 5%)). Similar studies of orally inhaled zanamivir indicate that approximately 10-20% of the dose is systemically absorbed, with serum concentrations generally peaking within 1-2 hours. The poor absorption of the drug results in low systemic concentrations and therefore there is no significant systemic exposure to zanamivir after oral inhalation. There is no evidence of modification in the kinetics after repeated dosing with oral inhaled administration.

Distribution: After oral inhalation, zanamivir is widely deposited at high concentrations throughout the respiratory tract, thus delivering the drug to the site of influenza infection. Following a single 10mg dose the concentrations of zanamivir were measured in induced sputum. Zanamivir concentrations of 337 (range 58-1593) and 52 (range 17-286) fold above the median viral neuraminidase IC_{50} were measured at 12h and 24h respectively. The high concentrations of zanamivir in the respiratory tract will result in the rapid onset of inhibition of the viral neuraminidase. The major immediate site of deposition is the oropharynx (mean 78%) from where zanamivir was rapidly eliminated to the GI-tract. The early deposition in total lungs ranged between 8 and 21%.

Metabolism: Zanamivir has been shown to be renally excreted as unchanged drug, and does not undergo metabolism. *In vitro* studies demonstrated that zanamivir did not affect the activity of a range of probe substrates for cytochrome P450 isoenzymes (CYP1A/2, A6, 2C9, 2C18, 2D6, 2E1, 3A4) in human hepatic microsomes, nor did it induce cytochrome P450 expression in rats, suggesting that metabolic interactions between zanamivir and other drugs are unlikely *in vivo*.

Elimination: The serum half-life of zanamivir following administration by oral inhalation ranges from 2.6 to 5.05 hours. It is entirely excreted unchanged in the urine. Total clearance ranges from 2.5 to 10.9 L/h as approximated by urinary clearance. Renal elimination is completed within 24 hours.

Patients with renal impairment: Inhaled zanamivir results in approximately 10%-20% of the inhaled dose being absorbed. In the severe renal impairment group from the single IV zanamivir dose trial subjects were sampled after a dose of 2 mg or twice to four times the expected exposure from inhalation. Using the normal dosing regimen (10mg bid), the predicted exposure at Day 5 is 40 fold lower than what was tolerated in healthy subjects after repeated iv administration. Given the importance of local concentrations, the low systemic exposure, and the previous tolerance of much higher exposures no dose adjustment is advised.

Patients with hepatic impairment: Zanamivir is not metabolised, therefore dose adjustment in patients with hepatic impairment is not required.

Elderly patients: At the therapeutic daily dose of 20mg, bioavailabilty is low (10-20%), and as a result there is no significant systemic exposure of patients to zanamivir. Any alteration of pharmacokinetics that may occur with age is unlikely to be of clinical consequence and no dose modification is recommended.

Paediatric patients: In an open-label single-dose study the pharmacokinetics of zanamivir was evaluated in 16 paediatric subjects, aged 6 to12 years, using dry powder (10 mg) inhalation formulation (Diskhaler device). The systemic exposure was similar to 10 mg of inhaled powder in adults, but the variability was large in all age groups and more pronounced in the youngest children. Five patients were excluded due to undetectable serum concentrations at all time points or 1.5 hours post-dose, suggesting inadequate drug delivery.

5.3 Preclinical safety data

General toxicity studies did not indicate any significant toxicity of zanamivir. Zanamivir was not genotoxic and no clinically relevant findings were observed in long term carcinogenicity studies in rats and mice.

6. PHARMACEUTICAL PARTICULARS

6.1 List of excipients

Lactose monohydrate (which contains milk protein).

6.2 Incompatibilities

Not applicable

6.3 Shelf life-LIFE

7 years

6.4 Special precautions for storage

Do not store above 30°C.

6.5 Nature and contents of container

Relenza inhalation powder is packed in a circular aluminium foil disk (a Rotadisk) with four regularly distributed blisters. An inspiration driven inhaler made of plastic (a Diskhaler) is used for administration of doses (the contents of 2 blisters constitute a dose) from these foil disks, and is provided in the pack.

The pack contains 1 or 5 foil disks and a Diskhaler.

6.6 Special precautions for disposal and other handling

The inhaler (Diskhaler) is loaded with a disk containing inhalation powder packed in individual blisters. These blisters are pierced when the inhaler is used, and with a deep inhalation the powder can then be inhaled through the mouthpiece down into the respiratory tract. Detailed instructions for use are enclosed in the pack.

7. MARKETING AUTHORISATION HOLDER

Glaxo Wellcome UK Ltd trading as GlaxoSmithKline UK

Stockley Park West

Uxbridge

Middlesex

UB11 1BT

8. MARKETING AUTHORISATION NUMBER(S)

PL 10949/0327

9. DATE OF FIRST AUTHORISATION/RENEWAL OF THE AUTHORISATION

24th June 1999

10. DATE OF REVISION OF THE TEXT

20th May 2009

POM

Relestat 0.5 mg/ml, eye drops, solution

(Allergan Ltd)

1. NAME OF THE MEDICINAL PRODUCT

Relestat, 0.5 mg/ml, eye drops, solution.

2. QUALITATIVE AND QUANTITATIVE COMPOSITION

One ml of eye drops, solution, contains 0.5 mg of epinastine hydrochloride.

(equivalent to 0.436 mg epinastine)

Excipient: benzalkonium chloride 0.1 mg/ml

For a full list of excipients, see section 6.1.

3. PHARMACEUTICAL FORM

Eye drops, solution.

A clear colourless solution.

4. CLINICAL PARTICULARS

4.1 Therapeutic indications

Treatment of the symptoms of seasonal allergic conjunctivitis.

4.2 Posology and method of administration

The recommended dose for adults is one drop instilled in each affected eye twice daily, during the symptomatic period.

There is no experience with the use of Relestat for more than 8 weeks.

The contents of the bottle remain sterile until the original closure is broken by twisting the cap to pierce the dropper tip. To avoid contamination do not touch any surface with the dropper tip.

If more than one topical ophthalmic medicinal product is being used, the medicinal products should be administered at least 10 minutes apart.

Elderly patients

Relestat has not been studied in elderly patients. Post-marketing safety data from the tablet formulation of epinastine hydrochloride (up to 20 mg once daily) indicates that there are no particular safety issues for elderly patients compared with adult patients. As such, no dosage adjustment is considered to be necessary.

Children and Adolescents

Relestat may be used in adolescents (12 years of age and older) at the same dosage as in adults.

Hepatic impairment

Relestat has not been studied in patients with hepatic impairment. Post-marketing safety data from the tablet formulation of epinastine hydrochloride (up to 20 mg once daily) indicates that the incidence of adverse reactions was higher in this group compared with adult patients without hepatic impairment. The daily dose of a 10 mg epinastine hydrochloride tablet is more than 100-fold higher than the daily dose following Relestat. In addition, the metabolism of epinastine in humans is minimal (<10%). Therefore, no dosage adjustment is considered to be necessary.

Renal impairment

Relestat has not been studied in patients with renal impairment. Post-marketing safety data from the tablet formulation of epinastine hydrochloride (up to 20 mg once daily) indicate that there are no particular safety issues for patients with renal impairment. As such, no dosage adjustment is considered to be necessary.

4.3 Contraindications

Hypersensitivity to epinastine or to any of the excipients.

4.4 Special warnings and precautions for use

Benzalkonium chloride is commonly used as a preservative in ophthalmic products and has been reported rarely to cause punctate keratopathy and/or toxic ulcerative keratopathy.

Benzalkonium chloride may be absorbed by and discolour soft contact lenses and therefore patients should be instructed to wait until 10-15 minutes after instillation of Relestat before inserting contact lenses. Relestat should not be administered while wearing contact lenses.

4.5 Interaction with other medicinal products and other forms of interaction

No interaction studies have been performed.

No drug-drug interactions are anticipated in humans since systemic concentrations of epinastine are extremely low following ocular dosing. In addition, epinastine is mainly excreted unchanged in humans indicating a low level of metabolism.

4.6 Pregnancy and lactation

Pregnancy

Data on a limited number (11) of exposed pregnancies indicate no adverse effects of epinastine on pregnancy or on the health of the foetus/newborn child. To date, no other relevant epidemiological data are available. Animal studies do not indicate direct or indirect harmful effects with respect to pregnancy, embryonic/foetal development, parturition or postnatal development (see section 5.3).

Caution should be exercised when prescribing to pregnant women.

Lactation

Epinastine is excreted in the breast milk of rats, but it is not known if epinastine is excreted in human milk. Due to the lack of experience, caution should be exercised when prescribing to breast-feeding women.

4.7 Effects on ability to drive and use machines

Based on the pharmacodynamic profile, reported adverse reactions and specific psychometric studies, epinastine has no or negligible influence on the ability to drive and use machines.

If transient blurred vision occurs at instillation, the patient should wait until the vision clears before driving or using machinery.

4.8 Undesirable effects

In clinical studies, the overall incidence of adverse drug reactions following Relestat was less than 10%. No serious adverse reactions occurred. Most were ocular and mild. The most common adverse reaction was burning sensation in eye (mostly mild); all other adverse reactions were uncommon.

The following adverse drug reactions were reported during clinical trials with Relestat:

Eye disorders

Common (≥1/100 to <1/10): burning sensation

Uncommon (≥1/1000 to <1/100): allergic conjunctivitis, blepharoptosis, conjunctival oedema, conjunctival hyperaemia, eye discharge, eye dryness, irritation, itching, increased sensitivity, photophobia, visual disturbance

Nervous system disorders

Uncommon (≥1/1000 to <1/100): headache

Respiratory, thoracic and mediastinal disorders

Uncommon (≥1/1000 to <1/100): asthma, nasal irritation, rhinitis

Gastrointestinal disorders

Uncommon (≥1/1000 to <1/100): oral dryness, taste alteration

Skin and subcutaneous tissue disorders

Uncommon (≥1/1000 to <1/100): pruritus

4.9 Overdose

After instillation of 0.3% epinastine hydrochloride eye drops 3 times daily (corresponds to 9 times the recommended daily dose) reversible miosis, without influence on visual acuity or other ocular parameters, was observed.

The 5 ml bottle of Relestat contains 2.5 mg of epinastine hydrochloride. A tablet formulation is marketed at a once daily dose of up to 20 mg epinastine hydrochloride, as such, intoxication after oral ingestion of the ophthalmic formulation is not expected even if the whole content of the bottle is swallowed.

No case of overdose has been reported.

5. PHARMACOLOGICAL PROPERTIES

5.1 Pharmacodynamic properties

Pharmacotherapeutic group: Ophthalmologicals; Decongestants and Antiallergics; Other antiallergics

ATC code: S01G X10

Epinastine is a topically active, direct H_1-receptor antagonist. Epinastine has a high binding affinity for the histamine H_1-receptor and a 400 times lower affinity for the histamine H_2-receptor. Epinastine also possesses affinity for the α_1-, α_2-, and the 5-HT_2-receptor. It has low affinity for cholinergic, dopaminergic and a variety of other receptor sites. Epinastine does not penetrate the blood/brain barrier and, therefore, does not induce side effects of the central nervous system, i.e., it is non-sedative.

Following topical eye application in animals, epinastine showed evidence for antihistaminic activity, a modulating effect on the accumulation of inflammatory cells, and mast cell stabilising activity.

In provocation studies with allergens in humans, epinastine was able to ameliorate ocular symptoms following ocular antigen challenge. The duration of the effect was at least 8 hours.

5.2 Pharmacokinetic properties
Following administration of one drop of Relestat in each eye twice daily, an average maximum plasma concentration of 0.042 ng/ml is reached after about two hours. Epinastine has a volume of distribution of 417 litres and is 64% bound to plasma proteins. The clearance is 928 ml/min and the terminal plasma elimination half-life is about 8 hours. Less than 10% is metabolised. Epinastine is mainly excreted renally unchanged. The renal elimination is mainly via active tubular secretion.

Preclinical studies *in vitro* and *in vivo* show that epinastine binds to melanin and accumulates in the pigmented ocular tissues of rabbits and monkeys. *In vitro* data indicate that the binding to melanin is moderate and reversible.

5.3 Preclinical safety data
Non clinical data revealed no special hazard for humans based on conventional studies of safety pharmacology, repeated dose toxicity, genotoxicity, carcinogenic potential and toxicity to reproduction.

6. PHARMACEUTICAL PARTICULARS
6.1 List of excipients
Benzalkonium chloride,

Disodium edetate,

Sodium chloride,

Sodium dihydrogen phosphate dihydrate,

Sodium hydroxide/hydrochloric acid,

Purified water.

6.2 Incompatibilities
Not applicable.

6.3 Shelf life
2 years.

After first opening: 4 weeks.

6.4 Special precautions for storage
Keep the bottle in the outer carton in order to protect from light.

Do not store above 25°C.

6.5 Nature and contents of container
5 ml polyethylene bottle with a white polystyrene screw cap with spike device for opening the bottle.

6.6 Special precautions for disposal and other handling
No special requirements

Any unused product or waste material should be disposed of in accordance with local requirements.

7. MARKETING AUTHORISATION HOLDER
Allergan Pharmaceuticals Ireland

Castlebar Road

Westport

Co. Mayo

Ireland

8. MARKETING AUTHORISATION NUMBER(S)
PL 05179/0004

9. DATE OF FIRST AUTHORISATION/RENEWAL OF THE AUTHORISATION
18/10/2007

10. DATE OF REVISION OF THE TEXT
18/10/2007

Relistor
(Wyeth Pharmaceuticals)

1. NAME OF THE MEDICINAL PRODUCT
RELISTOR▼ 12 mg /0.6 ml solution for injection.

2. QUALITATIVE AND QUANTITATIVE COMPOSITION
Each vial of 0.6 ml contains 12 mg methylnaltrexone bromide.

One ml of solution contains 20 mg methylnaltrexone bromide.

For a full list of excipients, see section 6.1.

3. PHARMACEUTICAL FORM
Solution for injection.

Sterile, clear solution, colourless to pale-yellow, essentially free from visible particulates.

4. CLINICAL PARTICULARS
4.1 Therapeutic indications
Treatment of opioid-induced constipation in advanced illness patients who are receiving palliative care when response to usual laxative therapy has not been sufficient.

4.2 Posology and method of administration
For adults only.

RELISTOR should be added to induce prompt bowel movements when response to usual laxative therapy has been insufficient.

The recommended dose of methylnaltrexone bromide is 8 mg (0.4 ml RELISTOR) (for patients weighing 38-61 kg) or 12 mg (0.6 ml RELISTOR) (for patients weighing 62-114 kg).

The usual administration schedule is one single dose every other day. Doses may also be given with longer intervals, as per clinical need.

Patients may receive two consecutive doses 24 hours apart, only when there has been no response (bowel movement) to the dose on the preceding day.

Patients whose weight falls outside of the ranges should be dosed at 0.15 mg/kg. The injection volume for these patients should be calculated:

Dose (ml) = patient weight (kg) × 0.0075

Renal patients

In patients with severe renal impairment (creatinine clearance less than 30 ml/min), the dose of methylnaltrexone bromide should be reduced from 12 mg to 8 mg (0.4 ml RELISTOR) for those weighing 62 to 114 kg, or from 0.15 mg/kg to 0.075 mg/kg for those whose weight falls outside the 62 to 114 kg range (see section 5.2). There are no data available from patients with end-stage renal impairment on dialysis, and RELISTOR is not recommended in these patients (see section 4.4).

Hepatic impairment

No dose adjustment is necessary in patients with mild to moderate hepatic impairment (see section 5.2).

There are no data available from patients with severe hepatic impairment (Child-Pugh Class C), and RELISTOR is not recommended in these patients (see section 4.4).

Paediatric patients

There is no experience in children under the age of 18 (see section 5.2). Therefore, methylnaltrexone should not be used in the paediatric age group until further data become available.

Elderly patients

No dose adjustment is recommended based on age (see section 5.2).

Administration

RELISTOR is given as a subcutaneous injection.

It is recommended to rotate injection sites. It is not recommended to inject into areas where the skin is tender, bruised, red, or hard. Areas with scars or stretch marks should be avoided.

The three areas of the body recommended for injection of RELISTOR are upper legs, abdomen, and upper arms.

RELISTOR can be injected without regard to food.

4.3 Contraindications
Hypersensitivity to the active substance or to any of the excipients.

Use of methylnaltrexone bromide in patients with known or suspected mechanical gastrointestinal obstruction or acute surgical abdomen is contraindicated.

4.4 Special warnings and precautions for use
The activity of methylnaltrexone bromide has been studied in patients with constipation induced by opioids. Therefore, RELISTOR should not be used for treatment of patients with constipation not related to opioid use. If severe or persistent diarrhoea occurs during treatment, patients should be advised not to continue therapy with RELISTOR and consult their physician.

Data from clinical trials suggest treatment with methylnaltrexone bromide can result in the rapid onset (within 30 to 60 minutes on average) of a bowel movement.

Methylnaltrexone bromide treatment has not been studied in clinical trials for longer than 4 months, and should therefore only be used for a limited period (see section 5.2).

RELISTOR should only be used in patients who are receiving palliative care. It is added to usual laxative treatment.

RELISTOR is not recommended in patients with severe hepatic impairment or with end-stage renal impairment requiring dialysis (see section 4.2).

Use of methylnaltrexone bromide in patients with colostomy, peritoneal catheter, active diverticular disease or fecal impaction has not been studied. Therefore, RELISTOR should only be administered with caution in these patients.

This medicinal product contains less than 1 mmol sodium (23 mg) per dose, i.e., essentially sodium-free).

4.5 Interaction with other medicinal products and other forms of interaction
Methylnaltrexone does not affect the pharmacokinetics of medicinal products metabolised by cytochrome P450 (CYP) isozymes. Methylnaltrexone is minimally metabolised by CYP isozymes. *In vitro* metabolism studies suggest that methylnaltrexone does not inhibit the activity of CYP1A2, CYP2E1, CYP2B6, CYP2A6, CYP2C9, CYP2C19 or CYP3A4, while it is a weak inhibitor of the metabolism of a model CYP2D6 substrate. In a clinical drug interaction study in healthy adult male subjects, a subcutaneous dose of 0.3 mg/kg of methylnaltrexone did not significantly affect the metabolism of dextromethorphan, a CYP2D6 substrate.

The organic cation transporter (OCT)-related drug-drug interaction potential between methylnaltrexone and an OCT inhibitor was studied in 18 healthy subjects by comparing the single-dose pharmacokinetic profiles of methylnaltrexone before and after multiple 400 mg doses of cimetidine. The renal clearance of methylnaltrexone was reduced following multiple-dose administration of cimetidine (from 31 l/h to 18 L/h). However, this resulted in a small reduction in total clearance (from 107 L/h to 95 l/h). Consequently, no meaningful change in AUC of methylnaltrexone, in addition to C_{max}, was observed before and after multiple-dose administration of cimetidine.

4.6 Pregnancy and lactation
Pregnancy

There are no adequate data with the use of methylnaltrexone bromide in pregnant women. Studies in animals have shown reproductive toxicity at high doses (see section 5.3). The potential risk for humans is unknown. RELISTOR should not be used during pregnancy unless clearly necessary.

Lactation

It is unknown whether methylnaltrexone bromide is excreted in human breast milk. Animal studies have shown excretion of methylnaltrexone bromide in breast milk. A decision on whether to continue/discontinue breast-feeding or to continue/discontinue therapy with RELISTOR should be made, taking into account the benefit of breast-feeding to the child and the benefit of RELISTOR therapy to the woman.

4.7 Effects on ability to drive and use machines
No studies on the effects on the ability to drive and use machines have been performed. However, as a pure peripherally restricted opioid antagonist, the likelihood that methylnaltrexone will affect such activities is low.

Dizziness may occur, and this may have an effect on driving and use of machines (see section 4.8).

4.8 Undesirable effects
The most common drug-related adverse reactions in all patients exposed to methylnaltrexone bromide during all phases of placebo-controlled studies were abdominal pain, nausea, diarrhoea and flatulence. Generally, these reactions were mild or moderate.

The adverse reactions are classified as: Very common (≥1/10); Common (≥1/100 to <1/10); Uncommon (≥1/1,000 to <1/100); Rare (≥1/10,000 to <1/1,000); Very rare (<1/10,000), unknown (cannot be estimated from the available data). Within each frequency grouping, undesirable effects are presented in order of decreasing seriousness:

Nervous system disorders

Common: Dizziness

Gastrointestinal disorders

Very common: Abdominal pain, nausea, flatulence, diarrhoea

Skin and subcutaneous tissue disorders

Common: Injection site reactions (e.g. stinging, burning, pain, redness, oedema)

4.9 Overdose
No case of overdose has been reported during clinical trials.

A study of healthy volunteers noted orthostatic hypotension associated with a dose of 0.64 mg/kg administered as an intravenous bolus.

In the event of an overdose, signs and symptoms of orthostatic hypotension should be monitored and reported to a physician. Treatment should be initiated as appropriate.

5. PHARMACOLOGICAL PROPERTIES
5.1 Pharmacodynamic properties
Pharmacotherapeutic group: Peripheral opioid receptor antagonists, ATC code: A06AH01.

Mode of action

Methylnaltrexone bromide is a selective antagonist of opioid binding at the mu-receptor. *In vitro* studies have shown methylnaltrexone to be a mu-opioid receptor antagonist (inhibition constant [K_i] = 28 nM), with 8-fold less potency for kappa opioid receptors (K_i = 230 nM) and much reduced affinity for delta opioid receptors.

As a quaternary amine, the ability of methylnaltrexone to cross the blood-brain barrier is restricted. This allows methylnaltrexone to function as a peripherally acting mu-opioid antagonist in tissues such as the gastrointestinal tract, without impacting opioid-mediated analgesic effects on the central nervous system.

Clinical efficacy and safety

The efficacy and safety of methylnaltrexone bromide in the treatment of opioid-induced constipation in patients receiving palliative care was demonstrated in two randomised, double-blind, placebo-controlled studies. In these studies, the median age was 68 years (range 21-100); 51 % were females. In both studies, patients had advanced terminal illness and limited life expectancy, with the majority having a primary diagnosis of incurable cancer; other primary diagnoses included end-stage COPD/emphysema, cardiovascular disease/heart failure, Alzheimer's disease/dementia, HIV/AIDS, or other advanced illnesses. Prior to screening, patients had opioid-induced constipation defined as either <3 bowel movements in the preceding week or no bowel movement for >2 days.

Study 301 compared methylnaltrexone bromide given as a single, double-blind, subcutaneous dose of 0.15 mg/kg or 0.3 mg/kg versus placebo. The double-blind dose was followed by an open-label, 4-week dosing period, where methylnaltrexone bromide could be used as needed, no more frequently than 1 dose in a 24-hour period. Throughout both study periods, patients maintained their usual laxative regimen. A total of 154 patients (methylnaltrexone bromide 0.15 mg/kg, n=47, methylnaltrexone bromide 0.3 mg/kg, n=55, placebo, n=52) were treated in the double-blind period. The primary endpoint was the proportion of patients with a rescue-free laxation within 4 hours of the double-blind dose of study medicinal product. Methylnaltrexone bromide-treated patients had a significantly higher rate of laxation within 4 hours of the double-blind dose (62 % for 0.15 mg/kg and 58 % for 0.3 mg/kg) than placebo-treated patients (14 %); $p<0.0001$ for each dose versus placebo.

Study 302 compared double-blind, subcutaneous doses of methylnaltrexone bromide given every other day for 2 weeks versus placebo. During the first week (days 1, 3, 5, 7), patients received either methylnaltrexone bromide 0.15 mg/kg or placebo. In the second week, a patient's assigned dose could be increased to 0.30 mg/kg if the patient had 2 or fewer rescue-free laxations up to day 8. At any time, the patient's assigned dose could be reduced based on tolerability. Data from 133 (62 methylnaltrexone bromide, 71 placebo) patients were analysed. There were 2 primary endpoints: proportion of patients with a rescue-free laxation within 4 hours of the first dose of study medicinal product and proportion of patients with a rescue-free laxation within 4 hours after at least 2 of the first 4 doses of medicinal product. Methylnaltrexone bromide-treated patients had a higher rate of laxation within 4 hours of the first dose (48 %) than placebo-treated patients (16 %); $p<0.0001$. Methylnaltrexone bromide-treated patients also had significantly higher rates of laxation within 4 hours after at least 2 of the first 4 doses (52 %) than did placebo-treated patients (9 %); $p<0.0001$. Stool consistency was not meaningfully improved in patients who had soft stool at baseline.

In both studies, there was no evidence to suggest differential effects of age or gender on safety or efficacy.

The effect on race could not be analysed because the study population was predominantly Caucasian (88%).

Durability of response was demonstrated in Study 302, in which the laxation response rate was consistent from dose 1 through dose 7 over the course of the 2-week, double-blind period.

The efficacy and safety of methylnaltrexone bromide were also demonstrated in open-label treatment administered from Day 2 through Week 4 in Study 301, and in two open-label extension studies (301EXT and 302EXT) in which methylnaltrexone bromide was given as needed for up to 4 months (only 8 patients up to this point). A total of 136, 21, and 82 patients received at least one open-label dose in studies 301, 301EXT, and 302EXT, respectively. RELISTOR was administered every 3.2 days (median dosing interval, with a range of 1-39 days).

The rate of laxation response was maintained throughout the extension studies for those patients who continued treatment.

There was no significant relationship between baseline opioid dose and laxation response in methylnaltrexone bromide-treated patients in these studies. In addition, median daily opioid dose did not vary meaningfully from baseline in either methylnaltrexone bromide-treated patients or in placebo-treated patients. There were no clinically relevant changes in pain scores from baseline in either the methylnaltrexone bromide or placebo-treated patients.

Effect on cardiac repolarisation

In a double-blind, randomised, parallel-group ECG study of single, subcutaneous doses of methylnaltrexone bromide (0.15, 0.30 and 0.50 mg/kg), in 207 healthy volunteers, no signal of QT/QTc prolongation or any evidence of an effect on secondary ECG parameters or waveform morphology was detected as compared to placebo and a positive control (orally administered 400 mg moxifloxacin).

5.2 Pharmacokinetic properties

Absorption

Methylnaltrexone bromide is absorbed rapidly, with peak concentrations (C_{max}) achieved at approximately 0.5 hours following subcutaneous administration. The C_{max} and area under the plasma concentration-time curve (AUC) increase with dose increase from 0.15 mg/kg to 0.5 mg/kg in a dose-proportional manner. Absolute bioavailability of a 0.30 mg/kg subcutaneous dose versus a 0.30 mg/kg intravenous dose is 82 %.

Distribution

Methylnaltrexone undergoes moderate tissue distribution. The steady-state volume of distribution (Vss) is approximately 1.1 l/kg. Methylnaltrexone is minimally bound to human plasma proteins (11.0 % to 15.3 %) as determined by equilibrium dialysis.

Metabolism

Methylnaltrexone is metabolised to a modest extent in humans based on the amount of methylnaltrexone metabolites recovered from excreta. Conversion to methyl-6-naltrexol isomers and methylnaltrexone sulphate appears to be the primary pathway to metabolism. Each of the methyl-6-naltrexol isomers has somewhat less antagonist activity than parent compound, and a low exposure in plasma of approximately 8% of the drug-related materials. Methylnaltrexone sulphate is an inactive metabolite and present in plasma at a level of approximately 25 % of drug related materials. N-demethylation of methylnaltrexone to produce naltrexone is not significant, accounting for 0.06 % of the administered dose.

Excretion

Methylnaltrexone is eliminated primarily as the unchanged active substance. Approximately half of the dose is excreted in the urine and somewhat less in faeces. The terminal disposition half-life ($t_{1/2}$) is approximately 8 hours.

Special populations

Hepatic insufficiency

The effect of mild and moderate hepatic impairment on the systemic exposure to methylnaltrexone has been studied in 8 subjects each, with Child-Pugh Class A and B, compared to healthy subjects. Results showed no meaningful effect of hepatic impairment on the AUC or C_{max} of methylnaltrexone. The effect of severe hepatic impairment on the pharmacokinetics of methylnaltrexone has not been studied.

Renal insufficiency

In a study of volunteers with varying degrees of renal impairment receiving a single dose of 0.30 mg/kg methylnaltrexone bromide, renal impairment had a marked effect on the renal excretion of methylnaltrexone. The renal clearance of methylnaltrexone decreased with increasing severity of renal impairment. Severe renal impairment decreased the renal clearance of methylnaltrexone by 8- to 9-fold; however, this resulted in only a 2-fold increase in total methylnaltrexone exposure (AUC). C_{max} was not significantly changed. No studies were performed in patients with end-stage renal impairment requiring dialysis.

Paediatric patients

No studies have been performed in the paediatric population (see section 4.2).

Elderly patients

In a study comparing single and multiple-dose pharmacokinetic profiles of intravenous methylnaltrexone at a dose of 24 mg between healthy, young (18 to 45 years of age n=10) and elderly (65 years of age and over n=10) subjects, the effect of age on exposure to methylnaltrexone was found to be minor. The mean steady-state C_{max} and AUC for the elderly were 545 ng/ml and 412 ng·h/ml, approximately 8.1 % and 20 %, respectively, greater than those for young subjects. Therefore, no dose adjustment is recommended based on age.

Gender

No meaningful gender differences have been observed.

Weight

An integrated analysis of pharmacokinetic data from healthy subjects indicated that methylnaltrexone mg/kg dose-adjusted exposure increased as body weight increased. The mean methylnaltrexone exposure at 0.15 mg/kg over a weight range of 38 to 114 kg was 179 (range=139-240) ng·h/ml. This exposure for the 0.15 mg/kg dose can be achieved with a weight-band-based dose adjustment using an 8 mg dose for body weight 38 to less than 62 kg and a 12 mg dose for body weight 62 to 114 kg, yielding a mean exposure of 187 (range =148-220) ng·h/ml. In addition, the analysis showed that 8 mg dose for body weight 38 to less than 62 kg and a 12 mg dose for body weight 62 to 114 kg correspond to mean doses of 0.16 (range=0.21-0.13) mg/kg and 0.16 (range=0.19-0.11) mg/kg, respectively, based on the body weight distribution of patients participating in studies 301 and 302.

5.3 Preclinical safety data

Non-clinical data reveal no special hazard for humans based on conventional studies of safety pharmacology, repeated dose toxicity, and genotoxicity. Cardiac effects were observed in some non-clinical studies in canines (prolongation of action potentials in Purkinje fibers or prolongation of the QTc interval). The mechanism of this effect is unknown; however, the human cardiac potassium ion channel (hERG) appears not to be involved.

Subcutaneous injections of RELISTOR at 150 mg/kg/day decreased fertility in rats. Doses up to 25 mg/kg/day (18 times the exposure [AUC] in humans at a subcutaneous dose of 0.3 mg/kg) did not affect fertility or general reproductive performance.

There was no evidence of teratogenicity in rats or rabbits. Subcutaneous injections of RELISTOR at 150/100 mg/kg/day to rats resulted in decreased offspring weights; doses up to 25 mg/kg/day (18 times the exposure [AUC] in humans at a subcutaneous dose of 0.3 mg/kg) had no effect on labour, delivery, or offspring survival and growth.

Methylnaltrexone bromide is excreted via the milk of lactating rats.

Carcinogenicity studies have not been conducted with RELISTOR.

6. PHARMACEUTICAL PARTICULARS

6.1 List of excipients

Sodium chloride

Sodium calcium edetate

Glycine hydrochloride

Water for injections

Hydrochloric acid (to adjust pH)

Sodium hydroxide (to adjust pH)

6.2 Incompatibilities

In the absence of compatibility studies, this medicinal product must not be mixed with other medicinal products.

6.3 Shelf life

2 years.

After withdrawl in the injection syringe:

Due to light sensitivity, the solution for injection should be used within 24 hours.

6.4 Special precautions for storage

Store below 30°C.

Keep the vial in the outer carton in order to protect from light.

For storage of the medicinal product in the syringe, see section 6.3.

6.5 Nature and contents of container

Clear, Type I, flint glass, single-use vial, grey butyl rubber stopper, and aluminium overseal with flip-off-cap.

Each vial contains 0.6 ml of solution for injection.

The presentations of RELISTOR are:

1 vial of solution for injection

2 vials of solution for injection

2 sterile 1 ml injection syringes with retractable injection needle

4 alcohol swabs

7 vials of solution for injection

7 sterile 1 ml injection syringes with retractable injection needle

14 alcohol swabs

Not all pack sizes may be marketed.

6.6 Special precautions for disposal and other handling

Any unused product or waste material should be disposed of in accordance with local requirements.

7. MARKETING AUTHORISATION HOLDER

Wyeth Europa Limited

Huntercombe Lane South

Taplow, Maidenhead

Berkshire SL6 0PH

United Kingdom

Tel: 44-1628 604 377

Fax 44-1628 666 368

8. MARKETING AUTHORISATION NUMBER(S)

EU/1/08/463/001 - 1 vial of solution for injection

EU/1/08/463/002 - 2 vials of solution for injection, with syringes with retractable needles and swabs

EU/1/08/463/003 - 7 vials of solution for injection, with syringes with retractable needles and swabs

9. DATE OF FIRST AUTHORISATION/RENEWAL OF THE AUTHORISATION

Date of first authorisation: 02 July 2008

10. DATE OF REVISION OF THE TEXT

03 July 2009

Detailed information on this medicinal product is available on the website of the European Medicines Agency (EMEA) http://www.emea.europa.eu/.

Relpax - 20 mg and 40 mg

(Pfizer Limited)

1. NAME OF THE MEDICINAL PRODUCT

RELPAX 20mg and 40mg Film-Coated Tablets.

2. QUALITATIVE AND QUANTITATIVE COMPOSITION

Each film-coated tablet contains 20mg, and 40mg eletriptan (as hydrobromide).

Excipients: 23.000 mg Lactose
0.036 mg Sunset yellow

Excipients: 46.000 mg Lactose
0.072 mg Sunset yellow

For full list of excipients, see section 6.1.

3. PHARMACEUTICAL FORM

Film-coated tablet.

Round, convex orange tablets debossed with 'REP 20' and 'REP 40' on one side and 'Pfizer' on the other.

4. CLINICAL PARTICULARS

4.1 Therapeutic indications

Acute treatment of the headache phase of migraine attacks, with or without aura.

4.2 Posology and method of administration

RELPAX tablets should be taken as early as possible after the onset of migraine headache but they are also effective if taken at a later stage during a migraine attack.

RELPAX, if taken during the aura phase, has not been demonstrated to prevent migraine headache and therefore RELPAX should only be taken during the headache phase of migraine.

RELPAX tablets should not be used prophylactically.

The tablets should be swallowed whole with water.

Adults (18-65 years of age):

The recommended initial dose is 40mg.

If headache returns within 24 hours: If the migraine headache recurs within 24 hours of an initial response, a second dose of the same strength of RELPAX has been shown to be effective in treating the recurrence. If a second dose is required, it should not be taken within 2 hours of the initial dose.

If no response is obtained: If a patient does not achieve a headache response to the first dose of RELPAX within 2 hours, a second dose should not be taken for the same attack as clinical trials have not adequately established efficacy with the second dose. Clinical trials show that patients who do not respond to the treatment of an attack are still likely to respond to the treatment of a subsequent attack.

Patients who do not obtain satisfactory efficacy after an appropriate trial of 40mg, (e.g. good tolerability and failure to respond in 2 out of 3 attacks), may be effectively treated with 80mg (2 × 40mg) in subsequent migraine attacks (see section 5.1 Pharmacodynamic Properties – Further information on Clinical Trials). A second dose of 80mg should not be taken within 24 hours.

The maximum daily dose should not exceed 80mg (see section 4.8 Undesirable effects).

Elderly (over 65 years of age)

The safety and effectiveness of eletriptan in patients over 65 years of age have not been systematically evaluated due to the small number of such patients in clinical trials. Use of RELPAX in the elderly is therefore not recommended.

Adolescents (12-17 years of age)

The efficacy of RELPAX has not been established in this population and its use is therefore not recommended in this age group.

Children (6-11 years of age)

The safety and efficacy of RELPAX in children have not been evaluated. Therefore the use of RELPAX is not recommended in this age group (see 5.2 Pharmacokinetic Properties).

Hepatic Impairment

No dose adjustment is required in patients with mild or moderate hepatic impairment. As RELPAX has not been studied in patients with severe hepatic impairment, it is contra-indicated in these patients.

Renal Impairment

As the blood pressure effects of RELPAX are amplified in renal impairment (see 4.4 Special Warnings and Precautions for Use), a 20mg initial dose, is recommended in patients with mild or moderate renal impairment. The maximum daily dose should not exceed 40mg. RELPAX is contra-indicated, in patients with severe renal impairment.

4.3 Contraindications

Hypersensitivity to eletriptan hydrobromide or to any of the excipients.

Patients with severe hepatic or severe renal impairment.

Moderately severe or severe hypertension, or untreated mild hypertension.

Patients with confirmed coronary heart disease, including ischaemic heart disease (angina pectoris, previous myocardial infarction or confirmed silent ischaemia), objective or subjective symptoms of ischaemic heart disease or Prinzmetal's angina.

Patients with significant arrhythmias or heart failure.

Patients with peripheral vascular disease.

Patients with a history of cerebrovascular accident (CVA) or transient ischaemic attack (TIA).

Administration of ergotamine, or derivatives of ergotamine (including methysergide), within 24hr before or after treatment with eletriptan (see 4.5 Interactions with other medicinal products and other forms of interaction). Concomitant administration of other 5-HT_1 receptor agonists with eletriptan.

4.4 Special warnings and precautions for use

This medicinal product contains lactose. Patients with rare hereditary problems of galactose intolerance, the Lapp lactase deficiency or glucose-galactose malabsorption should not take this medicine.

This medicinal product also contains sunset yellow which may cause allergic reactions.

RELPAX should not be used together with potent CYP3A4 inhibitors eg. ketoconazole, itraconazole, erythromycin, clarithromycin, josamycin and protease inhibitors (ritonavir, indinavir and nelfinavir).

RELPAX should only be used where a clear diagnosis of migraine has been established. RELPAX is not indicated for the management of hemiplegic, ophthalmoplegic, or basilar migraine.

RELPAX should not be given for the treatment of 'atypical' headaches, i.e. headaches, which may be related to a possibly serious condition (stroke, aneurysm rupture) where cerebrovascular vasoconstriction may be harmful.

Eletriptan can be associated with transient symptoms including chest pain and tightness, which may be intense and involve the throat (see 4.8 Undesirable effects). Where such symptoms are thought to indicate ischaemic heart disease, no further dose should be taken and appropriate evaluation should be carried out.

RELPAX should not be given without prior evaluation, to patients in whom unrecognised cardiac disease is likely, or to patients at risk of coronary artery disease (CAD) [e.g. patients with hypertension, diabetes, smokers or users of nicotine substitution therapy, men over 40 years of age, post-menopausal women and those with a strong family history of CAD]. Cardiac evaluations may not identify every patient who has cardiac disease and, in very rare cases, serious cardiac events have occurred, in patients without underlying cardiovascular disease when 5-HT_1 agonists have been administered. Patients in whom CAD is established, should not be given RELPAX (see 4.3 Contra-indications).

5-HT_1 receptor agonists have been associated with coronary vasospasm. In rare cases, myocardial ischaemia or infarction, have been reported with 5-HT_1 receptor agonists.

Undesirable effects may be more common during concomitant use of triptans and herbal preparations containing St. John's wort (Hypericum perforatum)

Within the clinical dose range, slight and transient increases in blood pressure have been seen with eletriptan doses of 60mg or greater. However, these increases have not been associated with clinical sequelae in the clinical trial programme. The effect was much more pronounced in renally impaired and elderly subjects. In renally impaired subjects, the range of mean maximum increases in systolic blood pressure was 14 -17mmHg (normal 3mmHg) and for diastolic blood pressure was 14 -21mmHg (normal 4mmHg). In elderly subjects, the mean maximum increase in systolic blood pressure was 23mmHg compared with 13mmHg in young adults (placebo 8mmHg). Post-marketing reports of increases in blood pressure have also been received for patients taking 20 and 40 mg doses of eletriptan, and in non-renally impaired and non-elderly patients.

Excessive use of any anti-migraine medicinal product can lead to daily chronic headaches requiring a therapeutic window.

Serotonin syndrome (including altered mental status, autonomic instability and neuromuscular abnormalities) has been reported following concomitant treatment with triptans and selective serotonin reuptake inhibitors (SSRIs) or serotonin noradrenaline reuptake inhibitors (SNRIs). These reactions can be severe. If concomitant treatment with eletriptan and an SSRI or SNRI is clinically warranted, appropriate observation of the patient is advised, particularly during treatment initiation, with dose increases, or with addition of another serotonergic medication (see section 4.5).

4.5 Interaction with other medicinal products and other forms of interaction

Effect of other medicinal products on eletriptan

In the pivotal clinical trials of eletriptan no evidence of interaction with beta-blockers, tricyclic antidepressants, selective serotonin re-uptake inhibitors and flunarizine was reported but data from formal clinical interaction studies with these medicinal products are not available (other than propranolol, see below).

Population pharmacokinetic analysis of clinical studies has suggested that the following medicinal products (beta-blockers, tricyclic antidepressants, selective serotonin re-uptake inhibitors, oestrogen based hormone replacement therapy, oestrogen containing oral contraceptives and calcium channel blockers) are unlikely to have an effect on the pharmacokinetic properties of eletriptan.

Eletriptan is not a substrate for MAO. Therefore there is no expectation of an interaction between eletriptan and MAO inhibitors. Therefore no formal interaction study has been undertaken.

In clinical studies with propranolol (160mg), verapamil (480mg) and fluconazole (100mg) the C_{max} of eletriptan was increased 1.1 fold, 2.2 fold and 1.4 fold respectively. The increase in eletriptan's AUC being 1.3 fold, 2.7 fold and 2.0 fold respectively. These effects are not considered clinically significant as there were no associated increases in blood pressure or adverse events compared to administering eletriptan alone.

In clinical studies with erythromycin (1000mg) and ketoconazole (400mg), specific and potent inhibitors of CYP3A4, significant increases in eletriptan C_{max} (2 and 2.7- fold) and AUC (3.6 and 5.9- fold) respectively, were observed. This increased exposure was associated with an increase in eletriptan $t_{1/2}$ from 4.6 to 7.1 hours for erythromycin and from 4.8 to 8.3 hours for ketoconazole (see 5.2 Pharmacokinetic Properties). Therefore, RELPAX should not be used together with potent CYP3A4 inhibitors eg. ketoconazole, itraconazole, erythromycin, clarithromycin, josamycin and protease inhibitors (ritonavir, indinavir and nelfinavir).

In clinical studies with oral (caffeine/ergotamine) administered 1 and 2 hours after eletriptan, minor though additive increases in blood pressure were observed which are predictable based on the pharmacology of the two drugs. Therefore it is recommended that either ergotamine-containing or ergot-type medications (e.g. dihydroergotamine) should not be taken within 24 hours of eletriptan dosing. Conversely, at least 24 hours should elapse after the administration of an ergotamine-containing preparation before eletriptan is given.

Effect of eletriptan on other medicinal products

There is no *in vitro* or *in vivo* evidence that clinical doses (and associated concentrations) of eletriptan will inhibit or induce cytochrome P450 enzymes including CYP3A4 drug metabolising enzymes and therefore it is considered that eletriptan is unlikely to cause clinically important drug interactions mediated by these enzymes.

Selective Serotonin Reuptake Inhibitors (SSRIs) /Serotonin Norepinephrine Reuptake Inhibitors (SNRIs) and Serotonin Syndrome:

There have been reports describing patients with symptoms compatible with serotonin syndrome (including altered mental status, autonomic instability and neuromuscular abnormalities) following the use of selective serotonin reuptake inhibitors (SSRIs) or serotonin noradrenaline reuptake inhibitors (SNRIs) and triptans (see section 4.4).

4.6 Pregnancy and lactation

Pregnancy: For RELPAX no clinical data on exposed pregnancies are available. Animal studies do not indicate direct or indirect harmful effects with respect to pregnancy, embryonal/fetal development, parturition or postnatal development. RELPAX should be used during pregnancy only if clearly needed.

Lactation: Eletriptan is excreted in human breast milk. In one study of 8 women given a single dose of 80mg, the mean total amount of eletriptan in breast milk over 24 hours in this group was 0.02% of the dose. Nevertheless, caution should be exercised when considering the administration of RELPAX to women who are breast-feeding. Infant exposure can be minimised by avoiding breast-feeding for 24 hours after treatment.

4.7 Effects on ability to drive and use machines

Migraine or treatment with RELPAX may cause drowsiness or dizziness in some patients. Patients should be advised to evaluate their ability to perform complex tasks such as driving during migraine attacks and following administration of RELPAX.

4.8 Undesirable effects

RELPAX has been administered in clinical trials to over 5000 subjects, taking one or two doses of RELPAX 20 or 40 or 80mg. The most common adverse reactions noted were asthenia, somnolence, nausea and dizziness. In randomised clinical studies using doses of 20, 40 and 80mg, a trend for a dose-dependency of the incidence of adverse events has been shown. The following adverse reactions (with an incidence $\geqslant$1% and higher than placebo) were reported in patients treated with therapeutic doses in clinical trials. Events are categorized by frequency as common ($\geqslant$1/100 to $<$1/10), uncommon ($\geqslant$1/1,000 to $<$1/100), or rare ($\geqslant$1/10,000 to $<$1/1,000).

Infections and infestations:

Common: pharyngitis, and rhinitis

Rare: respiratory tract infection

Blood and the lymphatic system disorders:

Rare: lymphadenopathy

Metabolism and nutrition disorders:

Uncommon: anorexia

Psychiatric disorders:

Uncommon: thinking abnormal, agitation, confusion, depersonalisation, euphoria, depression, and insomnia

Rare: emotional lability

Nervous system disorders:

Common: somnolence, headache, dizziness, tingling or abnormal sensation, hypertonia, hypoaesthesia, and myasthenia

Uncommon: tremor, hyperaesthesia, ataxia, hypokinesia, speech disorder, stupor, and taste perversion

Eye disorders:

Uncommon: abnormal vision, eye pain, photophobia, and lacrimation disorder

Rare: conjuntivitis

Ear and labyrinth disorders:

Common: vertigo

Uncommon: ear pain, tinnitus

Cardiac disorders:

Common: palpitation, and tachycardia

Rare: bradycardia

Vascular disorders:

Common: flushing

Uncommon: peripheral vascular disorder

Rare: shock

Respiratory, thoracic and mediastinal disorders:

Common: throat tightness

Uncommon: dyspnea, respiratory disorder and yawning

Rare: asthma and voice alteration

Gastrointestinal disorders:

Common: abdominal pain, nausea, dry mouth, and dyspepsia

Uncommon: diarrhoea, and glossitis

Rare: constipation, oesophagitis, tongue oedema and eructation

Hepato-biliary disorders:

Rare: bilirubinaemia, and increased AST

Skin and subcutaneous tissue disorders:

Common: sweating

Uncommon: rash and pruritis

Rare: skin disorder and urticaria

Musculoskeletal, connective tissue and bone disorders:

Common: back pain, myalgia

Uncommon: arthralgia, arthrosis and bone pain

Rare: arthritis, myopathy and twitching

Renal and urinary disorders:

Uncommon: urinary frequency, urinary tract disorder and polyuria

Reproductive system and breast disorders:

Rare: breast pain and menorrhagia

General disorders and administration site conditions:

Common: sensation of warmth, asthenia, chest symptoms (pain, tightness, pressure), and chills

Uncommon: malaise, face oedema, thirst, oedema and peripheral oedema

The common adverse events seen with eletriptan are typical of adverse events reported with 5-HT1 agonists as a class.

In post-marketing experience, the following undesirable effects have been reported:

- Immune System Disorders: Allergic reactions, some of which may be serious
- Nervous system disorders: Serotonin syndrome, Rare cases of syncope
- Vascular Disorders: hypertension
- Gastrointestinal disorders: As with some other 5HT 1B/1D agonists, rare reports of ischaemic colitis have been received., vomiting

4.9 Overdose

Subjects have received single doses of 120mg without significant adverse effects. However, based on the pharmacology of this class, hypertension or other more serious cardiovascular symptoms could occur on overdose.

In cases of overdose, standard supportive measures should be adopted as required. The elimination half-life of eletriptan is about 4 hours, and therefore monitoring of patients and provision of general supportive therapy after overdose with eletriptan should continue for at least 20 hours or while signs and symptoms persist.

It is unknown what effect haemodialysis or peritoneal dialysis has on the serum concentrations of eletriptan.

5. PHARMACOLOGICAL PROPERTIES

5.1 Pharmacodynamic properties

Pharmacotherapeutic group: Selective Serotonin ($5HT_1$) receptor agonists ATC code: NO2CC06

Mode of action/pharmacology: Eletriptan is a selective agonist at the vascular $5\text{-}HT_{1B}$ and neuronal $5\text{-}HT_{1D}$ receptors. Eletriptan also exhibits high affinity for the $5\text{-}HT_{1F}$ receptor which may contribute to its anti-migraine mechanism of action. Eletriptan has modest affinity for the human recombinant $5\text{-}HT_{1A}$, $5\text{-}HT_{2B}$, $5\text{-}HT_{1E}$ and $5\text{-}HT_7$ receptors.

Further Information on Clinical Trials

The efficacy of RELPAX in the acute treatment of migraine has been evaluated in 10 placebo-controlled trials that included about 4000 patients who received RELPAX at doses of 20 to 80mg. Headache relief occurred as early as 30 minutes following oral dosing. Response rates (i.e. reduction of moderate or severe headache pain to no or mild pain) 2 hours after dosing were 59-77% for the 80mg dose, 54-65% for the 40mg dose, 47-54% for the 20mg dose, and 19-40% following placebo. RELPAX was also effective in the treatment of associated symptoms of migraine such as vomiting, nausea, photophobia and phonophobia.

The recommendation for dose titration to 80mg, is derived from open label long term studies and from a short term double blind study, where only a trend towards statistical significance was observed.

RELPAX remains effective in menstrually associated migraine. RELPAX, if taken during the aura phase, has not been demonstrated to prevent migraine headache and therefore RELPAX should only be taken during the headache phase of migraine.

In a non placebo controlled pharmacokinetic study of patients with renal impairment, larger elevations in blood pressure were recorded after an 80mg dose of RELPAX than with normal volunteers (see Section 4.4). This cannot be explained by any pharmacokinetic changes and so may represent a specific pharmacodynamic response to eletriptan in patients with renal impairment.

5.2 Pharmacokinetic properties

Absorption:

Eletriptan is rapidly and well absorbed across the gastrointestinal tract (at least 81%) after oral administration. Absolute oral bioavailability across males and females is approximately 50%. The median T_{max} is 1.5 hours after oral dosing. Linear pharmacokinetics were demonstrated over the clinical dose range (20-80mg).

The AUC and C_{max} of eletriptan were increased by approximately 20-30% following oral administration with a high fat meal. Following oral administration during a migraine attack, there was a reduction of approximately 30% in AUC and T_{max} was increased to 2.8 hours.

Following repeated doses (20mg tid) for 5-7 days, the pharmacokinetics of eletriptan remained linear and accumulation was predictable. On multiple dosing of larger doses (40mg tid and 80mg bid), the accumulation of eletriptan over 7 days was greater than predicted (approximately 40%).

Distribution:

The volume of distribution of eletriptan following IV administration is 138L indicating distribution into the tissues. Eletriptan is only moderately protein bound (approximately 85%).

Metabolism:

In vitro studies indicate that eletriptan is primarily metabolised by hepatic cytochrome P-450 enzyme CYP3A4. This finding is substantiated by increased plasma concentrations of eletriptan following co-administration with erythromycin and ketoconazole, known selective and potent CYP3A4 inhibitors. *In vitro* studies also indicate a small involvement of CYP2D6 although clinical studies do not indicate any evidence of polymorphism with this enzyme.

There are two major circulating metabolites identified that significantly contribute to plasma radioactivity following administration of C^{14}-labelled eletriptan. The metabolite formed by N-oxidation, has demonstrated no activity in animal *in vitro* models. The metabolite formed by N-demethylation, has been demonstrated to have similar activity to eletriptan in animal *in vitro* models. A third area of radioactivity in plasma has not been formally identified, but is most likely to be a mixture of hydroxylated metabolites which have also been observed excreted in urine and faeces.

The plasma concentrations of the N-demethylated active metabolite are only 10-20% of those of parent and so would not be expected to significantly contribute to the therapeutic action of eletriptan.

Elimination:

Mean total plasma clearance of eletriptan following IV administration is 36 L/h with a resultant plasma half-life of approximately 4 hours. The mean renal clearance following oral administration is approximately 3.9 L/h. Non-renal clearance accounts for approximately 90% of the total clearance indicating that eletriptan is eliminated primarily by metabolism.

Pharmacokinetics in Special Patient Groups

Gender

A meta analysis across clinical pharmacology studies and a population pharmacokinetic analysis of clinical trial data indicate that gender does not have any clinically significant influence on plasma concentrations of eletriptan.

Elderly (over 65 years of age)

Though not statistically significant, there is a small reduction (16%) in clearance associated with a statistically significant increased half-life (from approximately 4.4 hours to 5.7 hours) between elderly (65-93 years) and younger adult subjects.

Adolescents (12-17 years of age)

The pharmacokinetics of eletriptan (40mg and 80mg) in adolescent migraine patients dosed between attacks, were similar to those seen in healthy adults.

Children (6-11 years of age)

The clearance of eletriptan is unchanged in children relative to adolescents. However the volume of distribution is lower in children resulting in higher plasma levels than would be predicted following the same dose in adults.

Hepatic Impairment

Subjects with hepatic impairment (Child-Pugh A and B) demonstrated a statistically significant increase in both AUC (34%) and half-life. There was a small increase in C_{max} (18%). This small change in exposure is not considered clinically relevant.

Renal Impairment

Subjects with mild (creatinine clearance 61-89ml/min), moderate (creatinine clearance 31-60ml/min) or severe (creatinine clearance <30ml/min) renal impairment did not have any statistically significant alterations in their eletriptan pharmacokinetics or plasma protein binding. Blood pressure elevations were observed in this group.

5.3 Preclinical safety data

Preclinical data, revealed no special hazard for humans based on conventional studies of safety pharmacology, repeated dose toxicity, genotoxicity, carcinogenicity and toxicity to reproduction.

6. PHARMACEUTICAL PARTICULARS

6.1 List of excipients

Core Tablet: Microcrystalline cellulose, lactose monohydrate, croscarmellose sodium and magnesium stearate.

Film Coat: titanium dioxide (E171), hypromellose, lactose monohydrate, triacetin and Sunset Yellow Aluminium Lake (E110).

6.2 Incompatibilities

Not Applicable.

6.3 Shelf life

3 years

6.4 Special precautions for storage

Opaque PVC/Aclar/Aluminium blister: this medicinal product does not require any special storage conditions

HDPE bottles: keep the container tightly closed, in order to protect from moisture

6.5 Nature and contents of container

Opaque PVC/Aclar/Aluminium blister packs containing 2, 3, 4, 6, 10, 18, 30 and 100 tablets (20, 40mg).

HDPE bottles with child-resistant HDPE/PP closures containing 30 and 100 tablets (20, 40mg).

Not all pack sizes may be marketed.

6.6 Special precautions for disposal and other handling

No special requirements.

7. MARKETING AUTHORISATION HOLDER

Pfizer Limited

Sandwich

Kent, CT13 9NJ

United Kingdom

8. MARKETING AUTHORISATION NUMBER(S)

PL 00057/0452

PL 00057/0453

9. DATE OF FIRST AUTHORISATION/RENEWAL OF THE AUTHORISATION

Date of First Authorisation: 12 February 2001

Date of Last Renewal: First Renewal

10. DATE OF REVISION OF THE TEXT

2nd February 2008

LEGAL CATEGORY

POM

Company reference: RP5_1

Remedeine and Remedeine forte tablets

(Napp Pharmaceuticals Limited)

1. NAME OF THE MEDICINAL PRODUCT

REMEDEINE® and REMEDEINE FORTE® tablets

2. QUALITATIVE AND QUANTITATIVE COMPOSITION

REMEDEINE tablets contain Paracetamol 500 mg and Dihydrocodeine Tartrate BP 20 mg.

REMEDEINE FORTE tablets contain Paracetamol 500 mg and Dihydrocodeine Tartrate BP 30 mg.

3. PHARMACEUTICAL FORM

White to off-white, circular, flat faced tablets with a bevelled edge.

REMEDEINE tablets are engraved PD/20 on one side.

REMEDEINE FORTE tablets are engraved PD/30 on one side.

4. CLINICAL PARTICULARS

4.1 Therapeutic indications

REMEDEINE tablets

For the treatments of severe pain.

REMEDEINE FORTE tablets

For the treatment of severe pain where there is a higher analgesic

4.2 Posology and method of administration

Route of Administration

Oral.

REMEDEINE\REMEDEINE FORTE tablets should, if possible, be taken during or after meals.

Adults and children over 12 years

1 or 2 tablets every four to six hours.

Do not exceed eight tablets in any 24-hour period.

Children under 12 years

Not recommended.

Elderly

One tablet every 4 - 6 hours increasing to two tablets every 4 - 6 hours if required and tolerated. Caution should be exercised when increasing the dose in the elderly.

4.3 Contraindications

Respiratory depression, obstructive airways disease, hypersensitivity to paracetamol, dihydrocodeine or other tablet constituents.

4.4 Special warnings and precautions for use

REMEDEINE\REMEDEINE FORTE tablets should be given with caution in patients with allergic disorders and should not be given during an attack of asthma. Caution should also be observed if there is marked impairment of liver function, advanced kidney disease and in chronic alcoholics.

Do not exceed the recommended dose.

Patients should be advised not to take other paracetamol-containing products concurrently.

Dosage should be reduced in the elderly, in hypothyroidism and in chronic hepatic disease. An overdose can cause hepatic necrosis.

Dihydrocodeine should be used with caution in patients taking monoamine oxidase inhibitors and should be avoided in those patients with raised intracranial pressure or head injury.

Use with caution in patients with prostatic hypertrophy since dihydrocodeine may cause urinary retention.

The risk-benefit of continued use should be assessed regularly by the prescriber, and in particular the prescriber should take care to avoid any unnecessary increase in dosage especially where there is evidence of a previous history of drug dependence or abuse.

4.5 Interaction with other medicinal products and other forms of interaction

Additive CNS depression may occur with alcohol, and other CNS depressants such as anxiolytics, anti-depressants, hypnotics and anti-psychotics. The rate of absorption of paracetamol may be increased by metoclopramide or domperidone and absorption of paracetamol may be reduced by cholestyramine.

The anti-coagulant effect of warfarin and other coumarins may be enhanced by prolonged regular use of paracetamol with increased risk of bleeding.

4.6 Pregnancy and lactation

Epidemiological studies in human pregnancy have shown no effects due to paracetamol or dihydrocodeine. However, both drugs should be avoided during pregnancy unless considered essential by the physician.

Paracetamol is excreted in breast milk but not in a clinically significant amount. Available published data do not contra-indicate breast feeding.

4.7 Effects on ability to drive and use machines

Dihydrocodeine may cause drowsiness and, if affected, patients should not drive or operate machinery.

4.8 Undesirable effects

Constipation, if it occurs, is readily treated with a mild laxative.

Other side-effects of dihydrocodeine, which may occur in a few patients, are nausea, vomiting, headache, vertigo, giddiness, urinary retention, pruritus, sedation, dysphoria, hallucinations and allergic reactions including skin rashes.

Adverse effects of paracetamol are rare but hypersensitivity reactions including skin rash, blood dyscrasias, acute pancreatitis have been reported.

Dependence may occur. Regular prolonged use of dihydrocodeine is known to lead to addiction and tolerance. Symptoms of restlessness and irritability may result when treatment is then stopped.

Prolonged use of a painkiller can make conditions such as headache worse.

4.9 Overdose

Paracetamol

Liver damage is possible in adults who have taken 10g or more of paracetamol. Ingestion of 5g or more of paracetamol may lead to liver damage if the patient has risk factors (see below).

Risk factors

If the patient

a) Is on long term treatment with carbamazepine, phenobarbitone, phenytoin, primidone, rifampicin, St John's Wort or other drugs that induce liver enzymes.

Or

b) Regularly consumes ethanol in excess of recommended amounts.

Or

c) Is likely to be glutathione depleted e.g. eating disorders, cystic fibrosis, HIV infection, starvation, cachexia.

Symptoms

Symptoms of paracetamol overdosage in the first 24 hours are pallor, nausea, vomiting, anorexia and abdominal pain. Liver damage may become apparent 12 to 48 hours after ingestion. Abnormalities of glucose metabolism and metabolic acidosis may occur. In severe poisoning, hepatic failure may progress to encephalopathy, haemorrhage, hypoglycaemia, cerebral oedema, and death. Acute renal failure with acute tubular necrosis, strongly suggested by loin pain, haematuria and proteinuria, may develop even in the absence of severe liver damage. Cardiac arrhythmias and pancreatitis have been reported.

Management

Immediate treatment is essential in the management of paracetamol overdose. Despite a lack of significant early symptoms, patients should be referred to hospital urgently for immediate medical attention. Symptoms may be limited to nausea or vomiting and may not reflect the severity of overdose or the risk of organ damage. Management should be in accordance with established treatment guidelines, see BNF overdose section.

Treatment with activated charcoal should be considered if the overdose has been taken within 1 hour. Plasma paracetamol concentration should be measured at 4 hours or later after ingestion (earlier concentrations are unreliable). Treatment with N-acetylcysteine may be used up to 24 hours after ingestion of paracetamol, however, the maximum protective effect is obtained up to 8 hours post-ingestion. The effectiveness of the antidote declines sharply after this time. If required the patient should be given intravenous N-acetylcysteine, in line with the established dosage schedule. If vomiting is not a problem, oral methionine may be a suitable alternative for remote areas, outside hospital. Management of patients who present with serious hepatic dysfunction beyond 24 hours from ingestion should be discussed with the NPIS or a liver unit.

Dihydrocodeine

Symptoms

Acute overdosage with dihydrocodeine can be manifested by somnolence progressing to stupor or coma, miotic pupils, rhabdomyolysis, non-cardiac pulmonary oedema, bradycardia, hypotension and respiratory depression or apnoea.

Management

Primary attention should be given to the establishment of a patent airway and institution of assisted or controlled ventilation.

In the case of massive overdosage, administer naloxone intravenously (0.4 to 2 mg for an adult and 0.01 mg/kg body weight for children) if the patient is in a coma or respiratory depression is present. Repeat the dose at 2 minute intervals if there is no response, or by an infusion. An infusion of 60% of the initial dose per hour is a useful starting point. A solution of 10 mg made up in 50 ml dextrose will produce 200 micrograms/ml for infusion using an IV pump (dose adjusted to the clinical response). Infusions are not a substitute for frequent review of the patient's clinical state. Intramuscular naloxone is an alternative in the event that IV access is not possible.

As the duration of action of naloxone is relatively short, the patient must be carefully monitored until spontaneous respiration is reliably re-established. Naloxone is a competitive antagonist and large doses (4 mg) may be required in seriously poisoned patients. For less severe overdosage, administer naloxone 0.2 mg intravenously followed by increments of 0.1 mg every 2 minutes if required.

Naloxone should not be administered in the absence of clinically significant respiratory or circulatory depression secondary to dihydrocodeine overdosage. Naloxone should be administered cautiously to persons who are known, or suspected, to be physically dependent on dihydrocodeine. In such cases, an abrupt or complete reversal of opioid effects may precipitate pain and an acute withdrawal syndrome.

Consider activated charcoal (50 g for adults, 10-15 g for children), if a substantial amount has been ingested within 1 hour, provided the airway can be protected.

5. PHARMACOLOGICAL PROPERTIES

5.1 Pharmacodynamic properties

Paracetamol is an effective analgesic possessing a remarkably low level of side effects. Its broad clinical utility has been extensively reported, and it now largely replaces aspirin for routine use. Paracetamol is well tolerated; having a bland effect on gastric mucosa, unlike aspirin, it neither exacerbates symptoms of peptic ulcer nor precipitates bleeding. Dihydrocodeine tartrate has been widely used for a number of years as a powerful analgesic.

In addition the compound exhibits well-defined anti-tussive activity.

Fortifying paracetamol with dihydrocodeine tartrate provides an effective combination of drugs for the treatment of severe pain.

5.2 Pharmacokinetic properties

Dihydrocodeine is well absorbed from the gastrointestinal tract. Like other phenanthrene derivatives, dihydrocodeine is mainly metabolised in the liver with the resultant metabolites being excreted mainly in the urine.

Metabolism of dihydrocodeine includes 0-demethylation, N-demethylation and 6-keto reduction.

Paracetamol is readily absorbed from the gastrointestinal tract with peak plasma concentrations occurring 30 minutes to 2 hours after ingestion. It is metabolised in the liver and excreted in the urine as the glucuronide and sulphate conjugates.

5.3 Preclinical safety data

There are no pre-clinical data of relevance to the prescriber which are additional to that already included in other sections of the SPC.

6. PHARMACEUTICAL PARTICULARS

6.1 List of excipients

Magnesium Stearate Ph Eur

Starch Maize Special Ph Eur

6.2 Incompatibilities

None known.

6.3 Shelf life

Three years.

6.4 Special precautions for storage

Store at or below 30°C protected from moisture.

6.5 Nature and contents of container

REMEDEINE tablets are available in polyethylene containers with polypropylene lids containing 56 or 112 tablets.

REMEDEINE FORTE tablets are available in polyethylene containers with polypropylene lids containing 56 tablets.

6.6 Special precautions for disposal and other handling

None

7. MARKETING AUTHORISATION HOLDER

Napp Pharmaceuticals Ltd

Cambridge Science Park

Milton Road

Cambridge CB4 0GW

Tel: 01223 424444

8. MARKETING AUTHORISATION NUMBER(S)

PL 16950/0059, 0060

9. DATE OF FIRST AUTHORISATION/RENEWAL OF THE AUTHORISATION

20 November 1991/14 January 1998

10. DATE OF REVISION OF THE TEXT

28th January 2009

11. DOSIMETRY

POM

® The Napp device, REMEDEINE and REMEDEINE FORTE are Registered Trade Marks.

Reminyl Oral Solution

(Shire Pharmaceuticals Limited)

1. NAME OF THE MEDICINAL PRODUCT

Reminyl® 4 mg/ml oral solution

2. QUALITATIVE AND QUANTITATIVE COMPOSITION

1 ml oral solution contains 4 mg galantamine (as hydrobromide).

Excipients: methyl parahydroxybenzoate and propyl parahydroxybenzoate.

For a full list of excipients, see section 6.1.

3. PHARMACEUTICAL FORM

Oral solution.

Clear and colourless oral solution.

4. CLINICAL PARTICULARS

4.1 Therapeutic indications

Reminyl is indicated for the symptomatic treatment of mild to moderately severe dementia of the Alzheimer type.

4.2 Posology and method of administration

Adults/Elderly

Administration

Reminyl oral solution should be administered twice a day, preferably with morning and evening meals. Ensure adequate fluid intake during treatment (See section 4.8).

Before start of treatment

The diagnosis of probable Alzheimer type of dementia should be adequately confirmed according to current clinical guidelines (see section 4.4).

Starting dose

The recommended starting dose is 8 mg/day (4 mg twice a day) for four weeks.

Maintenance dose

- The tolerance and dosing of galantamine should be reassessed on a regular basis, preferably within three months after start of treatment. Thereafter, the clinical benefit of galantamine and the patient's tolerance of treatment should be reassessed on a regular basis according to current clinical guidelines. Maintenance treatment can be continued for as long as therapeutic benefit is favourable and the patient tolerates treatment with galantamine. Discontinuation of galantamine should be considered when evidence of a therapeutic effect is no longer present or if the patient does not tolerate treatment.
- The initial maintenance dose is 16 mg/day (8 mg twice a day) and patients should be maintained on 16 mg/day for at least 4 weeks.
- An increase to the maintenance dose of 24 mg/day (12 mg twice a day) should be considered on an individual basis after appropriate assessment including evaluation of clinical benefit and tolerability.

• In individual patients not showing an increased response or not tolerating 24 mg/day, a dose reduction to 16 mg/day should be considered.

• There is no rebound effect after abrupt discontinuation of treatment (e.g. in preparation for surgery).

Children

Galantamine is not recommended for use in children due to a lack of data on safety and efficacy.

Hepatic and renal impairment

Galantamine plasma levels may be increased in patients with moderate to severe hepatic or renal impairment. In patients with moderately impaired hepatic function, based on pharmacokinetic modelling, it is recommended that dosing should begin with 4 mg once daily, preferably taken in the morning, for at least one week. Thereafter, patients should proceed with 4 mg twice-daily for at least 4 weeks. In these patients, daily doses should not exceed 8 mg twice-daily. In patients with severe hepatic impairment (Child-Pugh score greater than 9), the use of galantamine is contraindicated (see section 4.3). No dosage adjustment is required for patients with mild hepatic impairment.

For patients with a creatinine clearance greater than 9 ml/min no dosage adjustment is required. In patients with severe renal impairment (creatinine clearance less than 9 ml/min), the use of galantamine is contraindicated (see section 4.3).

Concomitant treatment

In patients treated with potent CYP2D6 or CYP3A4 inhibitors dose reductions can be considered (see section 4.5).

4.3 Contraindications

Hypersensitivity to the active substance or to any of the excipients.

Since no data are available on the use of galantamine in patients with severe hepatic (Child-Pugh score greater than 9) and severe renal (creatinine clearance less than 9 ml/min) impairment, galantamine is contraindicated in these populations. Galantamine is contra-indicated in patients who have both significant renal and hepatic dysfunction.

4.4 Special warnings and precautions for use

Reminyl is indicated for a patient with mild to moderately severe dementia of the Alzheimer type. The benefit of galantamine in patients with other types of dementia or other types of memory impairment has not been demonstrated. In 2 clinical trials of two years duration in individuals with so called mild cognitive impairment (milder types of memory impairment not fulfilling the criteria of Alzheimer dementia), galantamine therapy failed to demonstrate any benefit either in slowing cognitive decline or reducing the clinical conversion to dementia. The mortality rate in the galantamine group was significantly higher than in the placebo group, 14/1026 (1.4%) patients on galantamine and 3 /1022 (0.3%) patients on placebo. The deaths were due to various causes. About half of the galantamine deaths appeared to result from various vascular causes (myocardial infarction, stroke, and sudden death). The relevance of this finding for the treatment of patients with Alzheimer dementia is unknown. In Alzheimer dementia, placebo-controlled studies of only 6 months duration have been conducted. In these studies no increased mortality in the galantamine groups appeared.

A diagnosis of Alzheimer's dementia should be made according to current guidelines by an experienced physician. Therapy with galantamine should occur under the supervision of a physician and should only be initiated if a caregiver is available who will regularly monitor medicinal product intake by the patient.

Patients with Alzheimer's disease lose weight. Treatment with cholinesterase inhibitors, including galantamine, has been associated with weight loss in these patients. During therapy, patient's weight should be monitored.

As with other cholinomimetics, galantamine should be given with caution in the following conditions:

Cardiac disorders

Because of their pharmacological action, cholinomimetics may have vagotonic effects on heart rate (e.g. bradycardia). The potential for this action may be particularly important to patients with 'sick sinus syndrome' or other supraventricular cardiac conduction disturbances or in those who use medicinal products that significantly reduce heart rate concomitantly, such as digoxin and beta blockers or for patients with an uncorrected electrolyte disturbance (e.g. hyperkalaemia, hypokalaemia). Caution should therefore be exercised when administering galantamine to patients with cardiovascular diseases, e.g. immediate post-myocardial infarction period, new-onset atrial fibrillation, second degree heart block or greater, unstable angina pectoris, or congestive heart failure, especially NYHA group III – IV.

In a pooled analysis of placebo-controlled studies in patients with Alzheimer dementia treated with galantamine an increased incidence of certain cardiovascular adverse events were observed (see section 4.8).

Gastrointestinal disorders

Patients at increased risk of developing peptic ulcers, e.g. those with a history of ulcer disease or those predisposed to these conditions, including those receiving concurrent non-steroidal anti-inflammatory drugs (NSAIDs), should be monitored for symptoms. The use of galantamine is not recommended in patients with gastro-intestinal obstruction or recovering from gastro-intestinal surgery.

Nervous system disorders

Although cholinomimetics are believed to have some potential to cause seizures, seizure activity may also be a manifestation of Alzheimer's disease. In rare cases an increase in cholinergic tone may worsen Parkinsonian symptoms.

In a pooled analysis of placebo-controlled studies in patients with Alzheimer's dementia treated with galantamine cerebrovascular events were uncommonly observed (see section 4.8 Undesirable effects). This should be considered when administering galantamine to patients with cerebrovascular disease.

Respiratory, thoracic and mediastinal disorders

Cholinomimetics should be prescribed with care for patients with a history of severe asthma or obstructive pulmonary disease or active pulmonary infections (e.g. pneumonia).

Renal and urinary disorders

The use of galantamine is not recommended in patients with urinary outflow obstruction or recovering from bladder surgery.

Surgical and medical procedures

Galantamine, as a cholinomimetic is likely to exaggerate succinylcholinetype muscle relaxation during anaesthesia, especially in cases of pseudocholinesterase deficiency.

Other

Reminyl oral solution contains methyl parahydroxybenzoate and propyl parahydroxybenzoate which may cause allergic reactions (possibly delayed).

4.5 Interaction with other medicinal products and other forms of interaction

Pharmacodynamic interactions

Because of its mechanism of action, galantamine should not be given concomitantly with other cholinomimetics, (such as ambenonium, donepezil, neostigmine, pyridostigmine, rivastigmine or systemically administered pilocarpine). Galantamine has the potential to antagonise the effect of anticholinergic medication. Should anticholinergic medication such as atropine be abruptly stopped there is a potential risk that galantamine's effects could be exacerbated. As expected with cholinomimetics, a pharmacodynamic interaction is possible with medicinal products that significantly reduce the heart rate such as digoxin, beta blockers, certain calcium-channel blocking agents and amiodarone. Caution should be taken with medicinal products that have potential to cause torsades de pointes. In such cases an ECG should be considered.

Galantamine, as a cholinomimetic, is likely to exaggerate succinylcholine-type muscle relaxation during anaesthesia, especially in cases of pseudocholinesterase deficiency.

Pharmacokinetic interactions

Multiple metabolic pathways and renal excretion are involved in the elimination of galantamine. The possibility of clinically relevant interactions is low. However, the occurrence of significant interactions may be clinically relevant in individual cases.

Concomitant administration with food slows the absorption rate of galantamine but does not affect the extent of absorption. It is recommended that Reminyl be taken with food in order to minimise cholinergic side effects.

Other medicinal products affecting the metabolism of galantamine

Formal drug interaction studies showed an increase in galantamine bioavailability of about 40% during co-administration of paroxetine (a potent CYP2D6 inhibitor) and of 30% and 12% during co-treatment with ketoconazole and erythromycin (both CYP3A4 inhibitors). Therefore, during initiation of treatment with potent inhibitors of CYP2D6 (e.g. quinidine, paroxetine, or fluoxetine) or CYP3A4 (e.g. ketoconazole or ritonavir) patients may experience an increased incidence of cholinergic adverse reactions, predominantly nausea and vomiting. Under these circumstances, based on tolerability, a reduction of the galantamine maintenance dose can be considered (see section 4.2).

Memantine, an N-methyl-D-aspartate (NMDA) receptor antagonist, at a dose of 10 mg once a day for 2 days followed by 10 mg twice a day for 12 days, had no effect on the pharmacokinetics of galantamine (as Reminyl XL prolonged-release capsules 16 mg once a day) at steady state.

Effect of galantamine on the metabolism of other medicinal products

Therapeutic doses of galantamine 24mg/day had no effect on the kinetics of digoxin although pharmacodynamic interactions may occur (see also pharmacodynamic interactions).

Therapeutic doses of galantamine 24 mg/day had no effect on the kinetics and prothrombin time of warfarin.

4.6 Pregnancy and lactation

Pregnancy

For galantamine no clinical data on exposed pregnancies are available. Studies in animals have shown reproductive toxicity (see section 5.3). Caution should be exercised when prescribing to pregnant women.

Lactation

It is not known whether galantamine is excreted in human breast milk and there are no studies in lactating women. Therefore, women on galantamine should not breast-feed.

4.7 Effects on ability to drive and use machines

Galantamine has minor or moderate influence on the ability to drive and use machines. Symptoms include dizziness and somnolence, especially during the first weeks after initiation of treatment.

4.8 Undesirable effects

The most common adverse events observed in clinical trials (incidence ⩾ 5% and twice the frequency of placebo) were nausea, vomiting, diarrhoea, abdominal pain, dyspepsia, anorexia, fatigue, dizziness, headache, somnolence and weight decrease. Nausea, vomiting and anorexia were more commonly observed in women.

Other common adverse events observed in clinical trials (incidence ⩾ 5% and ⩾ placebo) were confusion, depression, fall, injury, insomnia, rhinitis and urinary tract infection.

The majority of these adverse events occurred during the titration period. Nausea and vomiting, the most frequent adverse events, lasted less than a week in most cases and the majority of patients had only one episode. Prescription of anti-emetics and ensuring adequate fluid intake may be useful in these instances.

Adverse events observed during clinical trials and post marketing experience.

(see Table 1 on next page)

Some of these adverse events may be attributable to cholinomimetic properties of galantamine or in some cases may represent manifestations or exacerbations of the underlying disease processes common in the elderly population.

4.9 Overdose

Symptoms

Signs and symptoms of significant overdosing of galantamine are predicted to be similar to those of overdosing of other cholinomimetics. These effects generally involve the central nervous system, the parasympathetic nervous system, and the neuromuscular junction. In addition to muscle weakness or fasciculations, some or all of the signs of a cholinergic crisis may develop: severe nausea, vomiting, gastro-intestinal cramping, salivation, lacrimation, urination, defecation, sweating, bradycardia, hypotension, collapse and convulsions. Increasing muscle weakness together with tracheal hypersecretions and bronchospasm, may lead to vital airway compromise.

There have been post-marketing reports of torsade de pointes, QT prolongation, bradycardia, ventricular tachycardia and brief loss of consciousness in association with inadvertent overdoses of galantamine. In one case where the dose was known, eight 4 mg tablets (32 mg total) were ingested on a single day.

Two additional cases of accidental ingestion of 32 mg (nausea, vomiting, and dry mouth; nausea, vomiting, and substernal chest pain) and one of 40 mg (vomiting) resulted in brief hospitalisations for observation with full recovery. One patient, who was prescribed 24 mg/day and had a history of hallucinations over the previous two years, mistakenly received 24 mg twice- daily for 34 days and developed hallucinations requiring hospitalisation. Another patient, who was prescribed 16 mg/day of oral solution, inadvertently ingested 160 mg (40 ml) and experienced sweating, vomiting, bradycardia, and near-syncope one hour later, which necessitated hospital treatment. His symptoms resolved within 24 hours.

Treatment

As in any case of overdose, general supportive measures should be used. In severe cases, anticholinergics such as atropine can be used as a general antidote for cholinomimetics. An initial dose of 0.5 to 1.0 mg i.v. is recommended, with subsequent doses based on the clinical response.

Because strategies for the management of overdose are continually evolving, it is advisable to contact a poison control centre to determine the latest recommendations for the management of an overdose.

5. PHARMACOLOGICAL PROPERTIES

5.1 Pharmacodynamic properties

Pharmacotherapeutic group: Antidementia drugs

ATC-code: N06DA04

Galantamine, a tertiary alkaloid is a selective, competitive and reversible inhibitor of acetylcholinesterase. In addition, galantamine enhances the intrinsic action of acetylcholine on nicotinic receptors, probably through binding to an allosteric site of the receptor. As a consequence, an increased activity in the cholinergic system associated with improved cognitive function can be achieved in patients with dementia of the Alzheimer type.

Clinical studies

The dosages of galantamine effective in placebo-controlled clinical trials with a duration of 5 to 6 months were 16, 24 and 32 mg/day. Of these doses 16 and 24 mg/day were determined to have the best benefit/risk relationship and are the recommended maintenance doses. The

Table 1 Adverse events observed during clinical trials and post marketing experience

System Organ Class	Very Common	Common	Uncommon	Rare	Very Rare
Infections and infestations		Rhinitis Urinary tract infections			
Metabolism and nutrition disorders		Anorexia Weight decrease		Dehydration (leading to renal insufficiency and renal failure) Hypokalaemia	
Psychiatric disorders		Confusion Depression (very rarely with suicidality) Insomnia		Aggression Agitation Hallucinations	
Nervous system disorders		Dizziness Somnolence Syncope Tremor	Paraesthesia	Seizures	Worsening of Parkinsonism
Ear and labyrinth disorders			Tinnitus		
Cardiac disorders			Atrial arrhythmia Myocardial infarction Myocardial ischaemia Palpitation	Bradycardia (severe)	AV block
Vascular disorders		Hypertension	Cerebrovascular disease Transient ischaemic attack		Hypotension
Gastrointestinal disorders	Vomiting Nausea	Abdominal pain Diarrhoea Dyspepsia			Dysphagia Gastrointestinal bleeding
Hepatobiliary disorders					Elevated liver enzymes Hepatitis
Skin and subcutaneous tissue disorders				Rash	Increased sweating
Musculoskeletal and connective tissue disorders			Leg Cramps		
General disorders and administration site conditions		Asthenia Fatigue Fever Headache Malaise			
Injury, poisoning and procedural complications		Fall Injury			

Frequencies are defined as: very common (≥ 1/10), common (≥ 1/100, to < 1/10), uncommon (≥ 1/1,000 to, < 1/100), rare (≥ 1/10,000, to < 1/1,000) and very rare (< 1/10,000).

efficacy of galantamine has been shown using outcome measures which evaluate the three major symptom complexes of the disease and a global scale: the ADAS-Cog (a performance based measure of cognition), DAD and ADCS-ADL-Inventory (measurements of basic and instrumental Activities of Daily Living), the Neuropsychiatric Inventory (a scale that measures behavioural disturbances) and the CIBIC-plus (a global assessment by an independent physician based on a clinical interview with the patient and caregiver).

Composite responder analysis based on at least 4 points improvement in ADAS-Cog/11 compared to baseline and CIBIC-plus unchanged + improved (1-4), and DAD/ADL score unchanged + improved. See table below.

(see Table 2 below)

The results of a 26-week double-blind placebo-controlled trial, in which patients with vascular dementia and patients with Alzheimer's disease and concomitant cerebrovascular disease ("mixed dementia") were included, indicate that the symptomatic effect of galantamine is maintained in patients with Alzheimer's disease and concomitant cerebrovascular disease (see section 4.4, Nervous system disorders). In a post-hoc subgroup analysis, no statistically significant effect was observed in the subgroup of patients with vascular dementia alone.

In a second 26-week placebo-controlled trial in patients with probable vascular dementia, no clinical benefit of galantamine treatment was demonstrated.

5.2 Pharmacokinetic properties

Galantamine is an alkalinic compound with one ionisation constant (pKa 8.2). It is slightly lipophilic and has a partition coefficient (Log P) between n-octanol/buffer solution (pH 12) of 1.09. The solubility in water (pH 6) is 31 mg/ml. Galantamine has three chiral centres, the S, R, S-form is the naturally occurring form. Galantamine is partially metabolised by various cytochromes, mainly CYP2D6 and CYP3A4. Some of the metabolites formed during the degradation of galantamine have been shown to be active *in vitro* but are of no importance *in vivo*.

GENERAL CHARACTERISTICS OF GALANTAMINE

Absorption

The absorption is rapid, with a t_{max} of about 1 hour after both tablets and oral solution. The absolute bioavailability of galantamine is high, 88.5 ± 5.4%. The presence of food delays the rate of absorption and reduces Cmax by about 25%, without affecting the extent of absorption (AUC).

Distribution

The mean volume of distribution is 175 L. Plasma protein binding is low, 18%.

Metabolism

Up to 75% of galantamine dosed is eliminated via metabolism. *In vitro* studies indicate that CYP2D6 is involved in the formation of O-desmethylgalantamine and CYP3A4 is involved in the formation of N-oxide-galantamine. The levels of excretion of total radioactivity in urine and faeces were not different between poor and extensive CYP2D6 metabolisers. In plasma from poor and extensive metabolisers, unchanged galantamine and its glucuronide accounted for most of the sample radioactivity. None of the active metabolites of galantamine (norgalantamine, O-desmethylgalantamine and O-desmethyl-norgalantamine) could be detected in their unconjugated form in plasma from poor and extensive metabolisers after single dosing.

Table 2 Composite responder analysis based on at least 4 points improvement in ADAS-Cog/11 compared to baseline and CIBIC-plus unchanged + improved (1-4), and DAD/ADL score unchanged + improved

Treatment	At least 4 points improvement from baseline in ADAS-Cog/11 and CIBIC-plus Unchanged+Improved							
	Change in DAD≥0 GAL-USA-1 and GAL-INT-1(Month 6)				Change in ADCS/ADLInventory≥0 GAL-USA-10(Month 5)			
	N	n (%) of responder	Comparison with placebo		N	n (%) of responder	Comparison with placebo	
			Diff (95%CI)	p-value†			Diff (95%CI)	p-value†
Classical ITT#								
Placebo	422	21 (5.0)	–	–	273	18 (6.6)	–	–
Gal 16 mg/day	–	–	–	–	266	39 (14.7)	8.1 (3, 13)	0.003
Gal 24 mg/day	424	60 (14.2)	9.2 (5, 13)	<0.001	262	40 (15.3)	8.7 (3, 14)	0.002
Traditional LOCF*								
Placebo	412	23 (5.6)	–	–	261	17 (6.5)	–	–
Gal 16 mg/day	–	–	–	–	253	36 (14.2)	7.7 (2, 13)	0.005
Gal 24 mg/day	399	58 (14.5)	8.9 (5, 13)	<0.001	253	40 (15.8)	9.3 (4, 15)	0.001

ITT Intent To Treat

†CMH test of difference from placebo.

* LOCF: Last Observation Carried Forward.

Norgalantamine was detectable in plasma from patients after multiple dosing, but did not represent more than 10% of the galantamine levels. *In vitro* studies indicated that the inhibition potential of galantamine with respect to the major forms of human cytochrome P450 is very low.

Elimination

Galantamine plasma concentration declines bi-exponentially, with a terminal half-life in the order of 7-8 h in healthy subjects. Typical oral clearance in the target population is about 200 ml/min with intersubject variability of 30% as derived from the population analysis. Seven days after a single oral dose of 4 mg ^{3}H-galantamine, 90-97% of the radioactivity is recovered in urine and 2.2 – 6.3% in faeces. After i.v. infusion and oral administration, 18-22% of the dose was excreted as unchanged galantamine in the urine in 24 hours, with a renal clearance of 68.4 ± 22.0 ml/min, which represents 20-25% of the total plasma clearance.

Dose-linearity

After repeated oral dosing of 12 and 16 mg galantamine twice-daily as tablets, mean trough and peak plasma concentrations fluctuated between 29 – 97 ng/ml and 42 – 137 ng/ml. The pharmacokinetics of galantamine are linear in the dose range of 4 - 16 mg twice-daily. In patients taking 12 or 16 mg twice-daily, no accumulation of galantamine was observed between months 2 and 6.

Characteristics in patients

Data from clinical trials in patients indicate that the plasma concentrations of galantamine in patients with Alzheimer's disease are 30-40% higher than in healthy young subjects. Based upon the population pharmacokinetic analysis, clearance in female subjects is 20% lower as compared to males. No major effects of age per se or race are found on the galantamine clearance. The galantamine clearance in poor metabolisers of CYP2D6 is about 25% lower than in extensive metabolisers, but no bimodality in the population is observed. Therefore, the metabolic status of the patient is not considered to be of clinical relevance in the overall population.

The pharmacokinetics of galantamine in subjects with mild hepatic impairment (Child-Pugh score of 5-6) were comparable to those in healthy subjects. In patients with moderate hepatic impairment (Child-Pugh score of 7-9), AUC and half-life of galantamine were increased by about 30% (see section 4.2).

Elimination of galantamine decreases with decreasing creatinine clearance as observed in a study with renally impaired subjects. Compared to Alzheimer patients, peak and trough plasma concentrations are not increased in patients with a creatinine clearance of ≥9 ml/min. Therefore, no increase in adverse events is expected and no dosage adjustments are needed (see section 4.2).

Pharmacokinetic/pharmacodynamic relationship

No apparent correlation between average plasma concentrations and efficacy parameters (i.e. Change in ADAS-Cog11 and CIBIC-plus at Month 6) were observed in the large Phase III trials with a dose-regimen of 12 and 16 mg twice-daily. Plasma concentrations in patients experiencing syncope were within the same range as in the other patients at the same dose.

The occurrence of nausea is shown to correlate with higher peak plasma concentrations (see section 4.5).

5.3 Preclinical safety data

Non-clinical data suggest no special hazard for humans based on conventional studies of safety pharmacology, repeated dose toxicity, genotoxicity and carcinogenic potential.

Reproduction toxicity studies showed a slight delay in development in rats and rabbits, at doses which are below the threshold of toxicity in the pregnant females.

6. PHARMACEUTICAL PARTICULARS

6.1 List of excipients

Methyl parahydroxybenzoate

Propyl parahydroxybenzoate

Sodium saccharin

Sodium hydroxide

Purified water

6.2 Incompatibilities

Not applicable.

6.3 Shelf life

2 years.

After first opening: 3 months.

6.4 Special precautions for storage

Do not freeze

6.5 Nature and contents of container

The oral solution is packaged in a 100 ml amber glass bottle with a LDPE insert, a PP/LDPE child resistant closure and a HDPE/LDPE/PS pipette of 6 ml, calibrated in millilitres. The pipette has a minimum volume of 0.5 ml and a maximum volume of 4 ml.

6.6 Special precautions for disposal and other handling

To open the bottle and use the pipette:

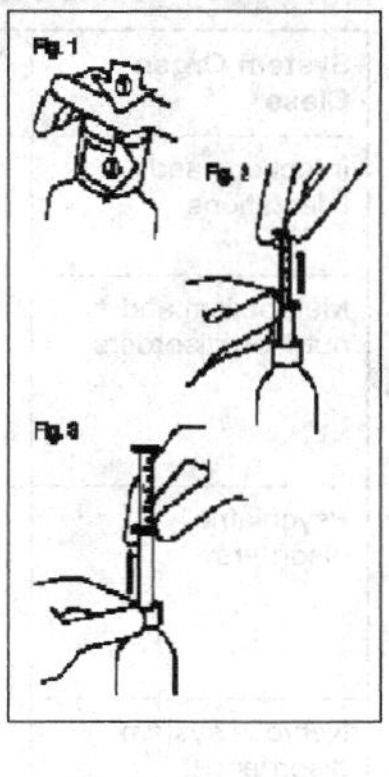

Fig. 1: The bottle comes with a child-resistant cap, and should be opened as follows:

- Push the plastic screw cap down while turning it counter clockwise.
- Remove the unscrewed cap.

Fig. 2: Insert the pipette into the bottle.

While holding the bottom ring, pull the top ring up to the mark corresponding to the number of millilitres you need to give.

Fig. 3: Holding the bottom ring, remove the entire pipette from the bottle.

Empty the pipette into any non-alcoholic drink by sliding the upper ring down and drink it immediately.

Close the bottle.

Rinse the pipette with some water.

7. MARKETING AUTHORISATION HOLDER

Shire Pharmaceuticals Limited, Hampshire International Business Park, Chineham, Basingstoke, Hampshire RG24 8EP, UK.

8. MARKETING AUTHORISATION NUMBER(S)

PL 08557/0042

9. DATE OF FIRST AUTHORISATION/RENEWAL OF THE AUTHORISATION

Date of first authorisation: 14 September 2000

Date of last renewal: 01 March 2005

10. DATE OF REVISION OF THE TEXT

September 2007

Reminyl Tablets

(Shire Pharmaceuticals Limited)

1. NAME OF THE MEDICINAL PRODUCT

Reminyl 4 mg Tablets

Reminyl 8 mg Tablets

Reminyl 12 mg Tablets

2. QUALITATIVE AND QUANTITATIVE COMPOSITION

Each 4 mg tablet contains 4 mg galantamine (as hydrobromide).

Excipients: Lactose monohydrate 38.59 mg

Each 8 mg tablet contains 8 mg galantamine (as hydrobromide).

Excipients: Lactose monohydrate 77.18 mg

Each 12 mg tablet contains 12 mg galantamine (as hydrobromide).

Excipients: Lactose monohydrate 115.77 mg and orange yellow S aluminium lake (E110) 0.45mg.

For a full list of excipients, see section 6.1.

3. PHARMACEUTICAL FORM

Film-coated tablet.

Reminyl 4 mg tablet: Off-white, circular, biconvex tablets with the inscription "JANSSEN" on one side and "G4" on the other side

Reminyl 8 mg tablet: Pink, circular, biconvex tablets with the inscription "JANSSEN" on one side and "G8" on the other side

Reminyl 12 mg tablet: Orange-brown, circular, biconvex tablets with the inscription "JANSSEN" on one side and "G12" on the other side

4. CLINICAL PARTICULARS

4.1 Therapeutic indications

Reminyl is indicated for the symptomatic treatment of mild to moderately severe dementia of the Alzheimer type.

4.2 Posology and method of administration

Adults/Elderly

Administration

Reminyl tablets should be administered twice a day, preferably with morning and evening meals. Ensure adequate fluid intake during treatment (See section 4.8).

Before start of treatment

The diagnosis of probable Alzheimer type of dementia should be adequately confirmed according to current clinical guidelines (see section 4.4).

Starting dose

The recommended starting dose is 8 mg/day (4 mg twice a day) for four weeks.

Maintenance dose

- The tolerance and dosing of galantamine should be reassessed on a regular basis, preferably within three months after start of treatment. Thereafter, the clinical benefit of galantamine and the patient's tolerance of treatment should be reassessed on a regular basis according to current clinical guidelines. Maintenance treatment can be continued for as long as therapeutic benefit is favourable and the patient tolerates treatment with galantamine. Discontinuation of galantamine should be considered when evidence of a therapeutic effect is no longer present or if the patient does not tolerate treatment.
- The initial maintenance dose is 16 mg/day (8 mg twice a day) and patients should be maintained on 16 mg/day for at least 4 weeks.
- An increase to the maintenance dose of 24 mg/day (12 mg twice a day) should be considered on an individual basis after appropriate assessment including evaluation of clinical benefit and tolerability.
- In individual patients not showing an increased response or not tolerating 24 mg/day, a dose reduction to 16 mg/day should be considered.
- There is no rebound effect after abrupt discontinuation of treatment (e.g. in preparation for surgery).

Children

Galantamine is not recommended for use in children due to a lack of data on safety and efficacy.

Hepatic and renal impairment

Galantamine plasma levels may be increased in patients with moderate to severe hepatic or renal impairment. In patients with moderately impaired hepatic function, based on pharmacokinetic modelling, it is recommended that dosing should begin with 4 mg once daily, preferably taken in the morning, for at least one week. Thereafter, patients should proceed with 4 mg twice-daily for at least 4 weeks. In these patients, daily doses should not exceed 8 mg twice-daily. In patients with severe hepatic impairment (Child-Pugh score greater than 9), the use of galantamine is contraindicated (see section 4.3). No dosage adjustment is required for patients with mild hepatic impairment.

For patients with a creatinine clearance greater than 9 ml/min no dosage adjustment is required. In patients with severe renal impairment (creatinine clearance less than 9 ml/min), the use of galantamine is contraindicated (see section 4.3).

Concomitant treatment

In patients treated with potent CYP2D6 or CYP3A4 inhibitors dose reductions can be considered (see section 4.5).

4.3 Contraindications

Hypersensitivity to the active substance or to any of the excipients.

Since no data are available on the use of galantamine in patients with severe hepatic (Child-Pugh score greater than 9) and severe renal (creatinine clearance less than 9 ml/min) impairment, galantamine is contraindicated in these populations. Galantamine is contra-indicated in patients who have both significant renal and hepatic dysfunction.

4.4 Special warnings and precautions for use

Reminyl is indicated for a patient with mild to moderately severe dementia of the Alzheimer type. The benefit of galantamine in patients with other types of dementia or other types of memory impairment has not been demonstrated. In 2 clinical trials of two years duration in individuals with so called mild cognitive impairment (milder types of memory impairment not fulfilling the criteria of Alzheimer dementia), galantamine therapy failed to demonstrate any benefit either in slowing cognitive decline or reducing the clinical conversion to dementia. The mortality rate in the galantamine group was significantly higher than in the placebo group, 14/1026 (1.4%) patients on galantamine and 3 /1022 (0.3%) patients on placebo. The deaths were due to various causes. About half of the galantamine deaths appeared to result from various vascular causes (myocardial infarction, stroke, and sudden death). The relevance of this finding for the treatment of patients with Alzheimer dementia is unknown. In Alzheimer dementia, placebo-controlled studies of only 6 months duration have been conducted. In these studies no increased mortality in the galantamine groups appeared.

A diagnosis of Alzheimer's dementia should be made according to current guidelines by an experienced physician. Therapy with galantamine should occur under the supervision of a physician and should only be initiated if a caregiver is available who will regularly monitor medicinal product intake by the patient.

Patients with Alzheimer's disease lose weight. Treatment with cholinesterase inhibitors, including galantamine, has been associated with weight loss in these patients. During therapy, patient's weight should be monitored.

As with other cholinomimetics, galantamine should be given with caution in the following conditions:

Cardiac disorders

Because of their pharmacological action, cholinomimetics may have vagotonic effects on heart rate (e.g. bradycardia). The potential for this action may be particularly important to patients with 'sick sinus syndrome' or other supraventricular cardiac conduction disturbances or in those who use medicinal products that significantly reduce heart rate concomitantly, such as digoxin and beta blockers or for patients with an uncorrected electrolyte disturbance (e.g. hyperkalaemia, hypokalaemia). Caution should therefore be exercised when administering galantamine to patients with cardiovascular diseases, e.g. immediate post-myocardial infarction period, new-onset atrial fibrillation, second degree heart block or greater, unstable angina pectoris, or congestive heart failure, especially NYHA group III – IV.

In a pooled analysis of placebo-controlled studies in patients with Alzheimer dementia treated with galantamine an increased incidence of certain cardiovascular adverse events were observed (see section 4.8).

Gastrointestinal disorders

Patients at increased risk of developing peptic ulcers, e.g. those with a history of ulcer disease or those predisposed to these conditions, including those receiving concurrent non-steroidal anti-inflammatory drugs (NSAIDs), should be monitored for symptoms. The use of galantamine is not recommended in patients with gastro-intestinal obstruction or recovering from gastro-intestinal surgery.

Nervous system disorders

Although cholinomimetics are believed to have some potential to cause seizures, seizure activity may also be a manifestation of Alzheimer's disease. In rare cases an increase in cholinergic tone may worsen Parkinsonian symptoms.

In a pooled analysis of placebo-controlled studies in patients with Alzheimer's dementia treated with galantamine cerebrovascular events were uncommonly observed (see section 4.8 Undesirable effects). This should be considered when administering galantamine to patients with cerebrovascular disease.

Respiratory, thoracic and mediastinal disorders

Cholinomimetics should be prescribed with care for patients with a history of severe asthma or obstructive pulmonary disease or active pulmonary infections (e.g. pneumonia).

Renal and urinary disorders

The use of galantamine is not recommended in patients with urinary outflow obstruction or recovering from bladder surgery.

Surgical and medical procedures

Galantamine, as a cholinomimetic is likely to exaggerate succinylcholinetype muscle relaxation during anaesthesia, especially in cases of pseudocholinesterase deficiency.

Other

Orange yellow S aluminium lake (E110), present in the 12 mg tablet, may cause allergic reactions.

Reminyl tablets contain lactose monohydrate. Patients with rare hereditary problems of galactose intolerance, the Lapp lactase deficiency or glucose-galactose malabsorption should not take this medicine.

4.5 Interaction with other medicinal products and other forms of interaction

Pharmacodynamic interactions

Because of its mechanism of action, galantamine should not be given concomitantly with other cholinomimetics (such as ambenonium, donepezil, neostigmine, pyridostigmine, rivastigmine or systemically administered pilocarpine). Galantamine has the potential to antagonise the effect of anticholinergic medication. Should anticholinergic medication such as atropine be abruptly stopped there is a potential risk that galantamine's effects could be exacerbated. As expected with cholinomimetics, a pharmacodynamic interaction is possible with medicinal products that significantly reduce the heart rate such as digoxin, beta blockers, certain calcium-channel blocking agents and amiodarone. Caution should be taken with medicinal products that have potential to cause torsades de pointes. In such cases an ECG should be considered. Galantamine, as a cholinomimetic, is likely to exaggerate succinylcholine-type muscle relaxation during anaesthesia, especially in cases of pseudocholinesterase deficiency.

Pharmacokinetic interactions

Multiple metabolic pathways and renal excretion are involved in the elimination of galantamine. The possibility of clinically relevant interactions is low. However, the occurrence of significant interactions may be clinically relevant in individual cases.

Concomitant administration with food slows the absorption rate of galantamine but does not affect the extent of absorption. It is recommended that Reminyl be taken with food in order to minimise cholinergic side effects.

Other medicinal products affecting the metabolism of galantamine

Formal drug interaction studies showed an increase in galantamine bioavailability of about 40% during co-administration of paroxetine (a potent CYP2D6 inhibitor) and of 30% and 12% during co-treatment with ketoconazole and erythromycin (both CYP3A4 inhibitors). Therefore, during initiation of treatment with potent inhibitors of CYP2D6 (e.g. quinidine, paroxetine, or fluoxetine) or CYP3A4 (e.g. ketoconazole or ritonavir) patients may experience an increased incidence of cholinergic adverse reactions, predominantly nausea and vomiting. Under these circumstances, based on tolerability, a reduction of the galantamine maintenance dose can be considered (see section 4.2).

Table 1 Adverse events observed during clinical trials and post marketing experience

System Organ Class	Very Common	Common	Uncommon	Rare	Very Rare
Infections and infestations		Rhinitis Urinary tract infections			
Metabolism and nutrition disorders		Anorexia Weight decrease		Dehydration (leading to renal insufficiency and renal failure) Hypokalaemia	
Psychiatric disorders		Confusion Depression(very rarely with suicidality) Insomnia		Aggression Agitation Hallucinations	
Nervous system disorders		Dizziness Somnolence Syncope Tremor	Paraesthesia	Seizures	Worsening of Parkinsonism
Ear and labyrinth disorders			Tinnitus		
Cardiac disorders			Atrial arrhythmia Myocardial infarction Myocardial ischaemia Palpitation	Bradycardia (severe)	AV block
Vascular disorders		Hypertension	Cerebrovascular disease Transient ischaemic attack		Hypotension
Gastrointestinal disorders	Vomiting Nausea	Abdominal pain Diarrhoea Dyspepsia			Dysphagia Gastrointestinal bleeding
Hepatobiliary disorders					Elevated liver enzymes Hepatitis
Skin and subcutaneous tissue disorders				Rash	Increased sweating
Musculoskeletal and connective tissue disorders			Leg Cramps		
General disorders and administration site conditions		Asthenia Fatigue Fever Headache Malaise			
Injury, poisoning and procedural complications		Fall Injury			

Frequencies are defined as: very common (⩾ 1/10), common (⩾ 1/100, to < 1/10), uncommon (⩾ 1/1,000, to < 1/100), rare (⩾ 1/10,000, to <1/1,000) and very rare (<1/10,000).

Memantine, an N-methyl-D-aspartate (NMDA) receptor antagonist, at a dose of 10 mg once a day for 2 days followed by 10 mg twice a day for 12 days, had no effect on the pharmacokinetics of galantamine (as Reminyl XL prolonged-release capsules 16 mg once a day) at steady state.

Effect of galantamine on the metabolism of other medicinal products

Therapeutic doses of galantamine 24mg/day had no effect on the kinetics of digoxin although pharmacodynamic interactions may occur (see also pharmacodynamic interactions).

Therapeutic doses of galantamine 24 mg/day had no effect on the kinetics and prothrombin time of warfarin.

4.6 Pregnancy and lactation

Pregnancy

For galantamine no clinical data on exposed pregnancies are available. Studies in animals have shown reproductive toxicity (see section 5.3). Caution should be exercised when prescribing to pregnant women.

Lactation

It is not known whether galantamine is excreted in human breast milk and there are no studies in lactating women. Therefore, women on galantamine should not breast-feed.

4.7 Effects on ability to drive and use machines

Galantamine has minor or moderate influence on the ability to drive and use machines. Symptoms include dizziness and somnolence, especially during the first weeks after initiation of treatment.

4.8 Undesirable effects

The most common adverse events observed in clinical trials (incidence ⩾ 5% and twice the frequency of placebo) were nausea, vomiting, diarrhoea, abdominal pain, dyspepsia, anorexia, fatigue, dizziness, headache, somnolence and weight decrease. Nausea, vomiting and anorexia were more commonly observed in women.

Other common adverse events observed in clinical trials (incidence ⩾ 5% and ⩾ placebo) were confusion, depression, fall, injury, insomnia, rhinitis and urinary tract infection.

The majority of these adverse events occurred during the titration period. Nausea and vomiting, the most frequent adverse events, lasted less than a week in most cases and the majority of patients had only one episode. Prescription of anti-emetics and ensuring adequate fluid intake may be useful in these instances.

Adverse events observed during clinical trials and post marketing experience.

(see Table 1 above)

Some of these adverse events may be attributable to cholinomimetic properties of galantamine or in some cases may represent manifestations or exacerbations of the underlying disease processes common in the elderly population.

4.9 Overdose

Symptoms

Signs and symptoms of significant overdosing of galantamine are predicted to be similar to those of overdosing of other cholinomimetics. These effects generally involve the central nervous system, the parasympathetic nervous system, and the neuromuscular junction. In addition to muscle weakness or fasciculations, some or all of the signs of a cholinergic crisis may develop: severe nausea, vomiting, gastro-intestinal cramping, salivation, lacrimation, urination, defecation, sweating, bradycardia, hypotension, collapse and convulsions. Increasing muscle weakness together with tracheal hypersecretions and bronchospasm, may lead to vital airway compromise.

There have been post-marketing reports of torsade de pointes, QT prolongation, bradycardia, ventricular tachycardia and brief loss of consciousness in association with inadvertent overdoses of galantamine. In one case where the dose was known, eight 4 mg tablets (32 mg total) were ingested on a single day.

Table 2 Composite responder analysis based on at least 4 points improvement in ADAS-Cog/11 compared to baseline and CIBIC-plus unchanged + improved (1-4), and DAD/ADL score unchanged + improved

Treatment	At least 4 points improvement from baseline in ADAS-Cog/11 and CIBIC-plus Unchanged+Improved							
	Change in DAD ≥ 0 GAL-USA-1 and GAL-INT-1 (Month 6)				Change in ADCS/ADLInventory ≥ 0 GAL-USA-10 (Month 5)			
	N	n (%) of responder	Comparison with placebo		N	n (%) of responder	Comparison with placebo	
			Diff (95%CI)	p-value†			Diff (95%CI)	p-value†
Classical ITT #								
Placebo	422	21 (5.0)	–	–	273	18 (6.6)	–	–
Gal 16 mg/day	–	–	–	–	266	39 (14.7)	8.1 (3, 13)	0.003
Gal 24 mg/day	424	60 (14.2)	9.2 (5, 13)	<0.001	262	40 (15.3)	8.7 (3, 14)	0.002
Traditional. LOCF*								
Placebo	412	23 (5.6)	–	–	261	17 (6.5)		
Gal 16 mg/day	–	–	–	–	253	36 (14.2)	7.7 (2, 13)	0.005
Gal 24 mg/day	399	58 (14.5)	8.9 (5, 13)	<0.001	253	40 (15.8)	9.3 (4, 15)	0.001

ITT: Intent To Treat

†CMH test of difference from placebo.

* LOCF: Last Observation Carried Forward.

Two additional cases of accidental ingestion of 32 mg (nausea, vomiting, and dry mouth; nausea, vomiting, and substernal chest pain) and one of 40 mg (vomiting) resulted in brief hospitalisations for observation with full recovery. One patient, who was prescribed 24 mg/day and had a history of hallucinations over the previous two years, mistakenly received 24 mg twice daily for 34 days and developed hallucinations requiring hospitalisation. Another patient, who was prescribed 16 mg/day of oral solution, inadvertently ingested 160 mg (40 ml) and experienced sweating, vomiting, bradycardia, and near-syncope one hour later, which necessitated hospital treatment. His symptoms resolved within 24 hours.

Treatment

As in any case of overdose, general supportive measures should be used. In severe cases, anticholinergics such as atropine can be used as a general antidote for cholinomimetics. An initial dose of 0.5 to 1.0 mg i.v. is recommended, with subsequent doses based on the clinical response.

Because strategies for the management of overdose are continually evolving, it is advisable to contact a poison control centre to determine the latest recommendations for the management of an overdose.

5. PHARMACOLOGICAL PROPERTIES

5.1 Pharmacodynamic properties

Pharmacotherapeutic group: Antidementia drugs

ATC-code: N06DA04

Galantamine, a tertiary alkaloid is a selective, competitive and reversible inhibitor of acetylcholinesterase. In addition, galantamine enhances the intrinsic action of acetylcholine on nicotinic receptors, probably through binding to an allosteric site of the receptor. As a consequence, an increased activity in the cholinergic system associated with improved cognitive function can be achieved in patients with dementia of the Alzheimer type.

Clinical studies

The dosages of galantamine effective in placebo-controlled clinical trials with a duration of 5 to 6 months were 16, 24 and 32 mg/day. Of these doses 16 and 24 mg/day were determined to have the best benefit/risk relationship and are the recommended maintenance doses. The efficacy of galantamine has been shown using outcome measures which evaluate the three major symptom complexes of the disease and a global scale: the ADAS-Cog (a performance based measure of cognition), DAD and ADCS-ADL-Inventory (measurements of basic and instrumental Activities of Daily Living), the Neuropsychiatric Inventory (a scale that measures behavioural disturbances) and the CIBIC-plus (a global assessment by an independent physician based on a clinical interview with the patient and caregiver).

Composite responder analysis based on at least 4 points improvement in ADAS-Cog/11 compared to baseline and CIBIC-plus unchanged + improved (1-4), and DAD/ADL score unchanged + improved. See table above.

(see Table 2 above)

The results of a 26-week double-blind placebo-controlled trial, in which patients with vascular dementia and patients with Alzheimer's disease and concomitant cerebrovascular disease ("mixed dementia") were included, indicate that the symptomatic effect of galantamine is maintained in patients with Alzheimer's disease and concomitant cerebrovascular disease (see section 4.4, Nervous system disorders). In a post-hoc subgroup analysis, no statistically significant effect was observed in the subgroup of patients with vascular dementia alone.

In a second 26-week placebo-controlled trial in patients with probable vascular dementia, no clinical benefit of galantamine treatment was demonstrated.

5.2 Pharmacokinetic properties

Galantamine is an alkalinic compound with one ionisation constant (pKa 8.2). It is slightly lipophilic and has a partition coefficient (Log P) between n-octanol/buffer solution (pH 12) of 1.09. The solubility in water (pH 6) is 31 mg/ml. Galantamine has three chiral centres, the S, R, S-form is the naturally occurring form. Galantamine is partially metabolised by various cytochromes, mainly CYP2D6 and CYP3A4. Some of the metabolites formed during the degradation of galantamine have been shown to be active *in vitro* but are of no importance *in vivo*.

GENERAL CHARACTERISTICS OF GALANTAMINE

Absorption

The absorption is rapid, with a t_{max} of about 1 hour after both tablets and oral solution. The absolute bioavailability of galantamine is high, 88.5 ± 5.4%. The presence of food delays the rate of absorption and reduces Cmax by about 25%, without affecting the extent of absorption (AUC).

Distribution

The mean volume of distribution is 175 L. Plasma protein binding is low, 18%.

Metabolism

Up to 75% of galantamine dosed is eliminated via metabolism. *In vitro* studies indicate that CYP2D6 is involved in the formation of O-desmethylgalantamine and CYP3A4 is involved in the formation of N-oxide-galantamine. The levels of excretion of total radioactivity in urine and faeces were not different between poor and extensive CYP2D6 metabolisers. In plasma from poor and extensive metabolisers, unchanged galantamine and its glucuronide accounted for most of the sample radioactivity. None of the active metabolites of galantamine (norgalantamine, O-desmethylgalantamine and O-desmethyl-norgalantamine) could be detected in their unconjugated form in plasma from poor and extensive metabolisers after single dosing. Norgalantamine was detectable in plasma from patients after multiple dosing, but did not represent more than 10% of the galantamine levels. *In vitro* studies indicated that the inhibition potential of galantamine with respect to the major forms of human cytochrome P450 is very low.

Elimination

Galantamine plasma concentration declines bi-exponentially, with a terminal half-life in the order of 7-8 h in healthy subjects. Typical oral clearance in the target population is about 200 mL/min with intersubject variability of 30% as derived from the population analysis. Seven days after a single oral dose of 4 mg ^{3}H-galantamine, 90-97% of the radioactivity is recovered in urine and 2.2 – 6.3% in faeces. After i.v. infusion and oral administration, 18-22% of the dose was excreted as unchanged galantamine in the urine in 24 hours, with a renal clearance of 68.4 ± 22.0 ml/min, which represents 20-25% of the total plasma clearance.

Dose-linearity

After repeated oral dosing of 12 and 16 mg galantamine twice-daily as tablets, mean trough and peak plasma concentrations fluctuated between 29 – 97 ng/ml and 42 – 137 ng/ml. The pharmacokinetics of galantamine are linear in the dose range of 4 - 16 mg twice-daily. In patients taking 12 or 16 mg twice-daily, no accumulation of galantamine was observed between months 2 and 6.

CHARACTERISTICS IN PATIENTS

Data from clinical trials in patients indicate that the plasma concentrations of galantamine in patients with Alzheimer's disease are 30-40% higher than in healthy young subjects. Based upon the population pharmacokinetic analysis, clearance in female subjects is 20% lower as compared to males. No major effects of age per se or race are found on the galantamine clearance. The galantamine clearance in poor metabolisers of CYP2D6 is about 25% lower than in extensive metabolisers, but no bimodality in the population is observed. Therefore, the metabolic status of the patient is not considered to be of clinical relevance in the overall population.

The pharmacokinetics of galantamine in subjects with mild hepatic impairment (Child-Pugh score of 5-6) were comparable to those in healthy subjects. In patients with moderate hepatic impairment (Child-Pugh score of 7-9), AUC and half-life of galantamine were increased by about 30% (see section 4.2).

Elimination of galantamine decreases with decreasing creatinine clearance as observed in a study with renally impaired subjects. Compared to Alzheimer patients, peak and trough plasma concentrations are not increased in patients with a creatinine clearance of ≥9 ml/min. Therefore, no increase in adverse events is expected and no dosage adjustments are needed (see section 4.2).

PHARMACOKINETIC/PHARMACODYNAMIC RELATIONSHIP

No apparent correlation between average plasma concentrations and efficacy parameters (i.e. Change in ADAS-Cog11 and CIBIC-plus at Month 6) were observed in the large Phase III trials with a dose-regimen of 12 and 16 mg twice-daily.

Plasma concentrations in patients experiencing syncope were within the same range as in the other patients at the same dose.

The occurrence of nausea is shown to correlate with higher peak plasma concentrations (see section 4.5).

5.3 Preclinical safety data

Non-clinical data suggest no special hazard for humans based on conventional studies of safety pharmacology, repeated dose toxicity, genotoxicity and carcinogenic potential.

Reproduction toxicity studies showed a slight delay in development in rats and rabbits, at doses, which are below the threshold of toxicity in the pregnant females.

6. PHARMACEUTICAL PARTICULARS

6.1 List of excipients

Tablet core:

Colloidal anhydrous silica

Crospovidone

Lactose monohydrate

Magnesium stearate

Microcrystalline cellulose

Film-coating:

Hypromellose

Propylene glycol

Talc

Titanium dioxide (E171)

The 4 mg tablet also contains yellow ferric oxide (E172).

The 8 mg tablet also contains red ferric oxide (E172).

The 12 mg tablet also contains red ferric oxide (E172) and orange yellow S aluminium lake (E110).

6.2 Incompatibilities

Not applicable.

6.3 Shelf life

2 years.

6.4 Special precautions for storage

This medicinal product does not require any special storage conditions.

6.5 Nature and contents of container

Available pack sizes:

4 mg

56 film-coated tablets (PVC-PE-PVDC/Aluminium blister)

8 mg

56 film-coated tablets (PVC-PE-PVDC/Aluminium blister)

12 mg

56 film-coated tablets (PVC-PE-PVDC/Aluminium blister)

6.6 Special precautions for disposal and other handling

No special requirements.

7. MARKETING AUTHORISATION HOLDER

Shire Pharmaceuticals Limited, Hampshire International Business Park, Chineham, Basingstoke, Hampshire RG24 8EP, UK.

8. MARKETING AUTHORISATION NUMBER(S)

4mg tablets: PL 08557/0039

8mg tablets: PL 08557/0040

12mg tablets: PL 08557/0041

9. DATE OF FIRST AUTHORISATION/RENEWAL OF THE AUTHORISATION

Date of first authorisation: 14 September 2000

Date of last renewal: 01 March 2005

10. DATE OF REVISION OF THE TEXT

September 2007

Reminyl XL 8mg, 16mg and 24mg prolonged release capsules

(Shire Pharmaceuticals Limited)

1. NAME OF THE MEDICINAL PRODUCT

Reminyl XL 8 mg prolonged release capsules

Reminyl XL 16 mg prolonged release capsules

Reminyl XL 24 mg prolonged release capsules

2. QUALITATIVE AND QUANTITATIVE COMPOSITION

Each 8 mg capsule contains 8 mg galantamine (as hydrobromide).

Each 16 mg capsule contains 16 mg galantamine (as hydrobromide).

Each 24 mg capsule contains 24 mg galantamine (as hydrobromide).

Excipients:

8mg: sucrose 59 mg

16mg: sucrose 117 mg

24mg: sucrose 176 mg

For a full list of excipients, see section 6.1.

3. PHARMACEUTICAL FORM

Prolonged release capsule, hard

8mg: White opaque, size 4 hard capsules with the inscription "G8", containing white to off-white pellets.

16mg: Pink opaque, size 2 hard capsules with the inscription "G16", containing white to off-white pellets.

24mg: Caramel opaque, size 1 hard capsules with the inscription "G24", containing white to off-white pellets.

4. CLINICAL PARTICULARS

4.1 Therapeutic indications

Reminyl XL is indicated for the symptomatic treatment of mild to moderately severe dementia of the Alzheimer type.

4.2 Posology and method of administration

Adults/Elderly

Administration

Reminyl XL prolonged release capsules should be administered once daily in the morning, preferably with food. The capsules should be swallowed whole together with some liquid. The capsules must not be chewed or crushed.

Ensure adequate fluid intake during treatment (see section 4.8).

Before start of treatment

The diagnosis of probable Alzheimer type of dementia should be adequately confirmed according to current clinical guidelines (see section 4.4).

Starting dose

The recommended starting dose is 8 mg/day for 4 weeks.

Maintenance dose

• The tolerance and dosing of galantamine should be reassessed on a regular basis, preferably within three months after start of treatment. Thereafter, the clinical benefit of galantamine and the patient's tolerance of treatment should be reassessed on a regular basis according to current clinical guidelines. Maintenance treatment can be continued for as long as therapeutic benefit is favourable and the patient tolerates treatment with galantamine. Discontinuation of galantamine should be considered when evidence of a therapeutic effect is no longer present or if the patient does not tolerate treatment.

• The initial maintenance dose is 16 mg/day and patients should be maintained on 16 mg/day for at least 4 weeks.

• An increase to the maintenance dose of 24 mg/day should be considered on an individual basis after appropriate assessment including evaluation of clinical benefit and tolerability.

• In individual patients not showing an increased response or not tolerating 24 mg/day, a dose reduction to 16 mg/day should be considered.

• There is no rebound effect after abrupt discontinuation of treatment (e.g. in preparation for surgery).

Switching to Reminyl XL prolonged release capsules from Reminyl tablets or Reminyl oral solution

It is recommended that the same total daily dose of galantamine is administered to patients. Patients switching to the once-daily regimen should take their last dose of Reminyl tablets or oral solution in the evening and start Reminyl XL prolonged release capsules once daily the following morning.

Children

Galantamine is not recommended for use in children due to a lack of data on safety and efficacy.

Hepatic and renal impairment

Galantamine plasma levels may be increased in patients with moderate to severe hepatic or renal impairment. In patients with moderately impaired hepatic function, based on pharmacokinetic modelling, it is recommended that dosing should begin with 8 mg prolonged release capsule once every other day, preferably taken in the morning, for one week. Thereafter, patients should proceed with 8 mg once daily for four weeks. In these patients, daily doses should not exceed 16 mg. In patients with severe hepatic impairment (Child-Pugh score greater than 9), the use of galantamine is contraindicated (see section 4.3). No dosage adjustment is required for patients with mild hepatic impairment.

For patients with a creatinine clearance greater than 9 ml/min no dosage adjustment is required. In patients with severe renal impairment (creatinine clearance less than 9 ml/min), the use of galantamine is contraindicated (see section 4.3).

Concomitant treatment

In patients treated with potent CYP2D6 or CYP3A4 inhibitors, dose reductions can be considered (see section 4.5).

4.3 Contraindications

Hypersensitivity to the active substance or to any of the excipients.

Since no data are available on the use of galantamine in patients with severe hepatic (Child-Pugh score greater than 9) and severe renal (creatinine clearance less than 9 ml/min) impairment, galantamine is contraindicated in these populations. Galantamine is contraindicated in patients who have both significant renal and hepatic dysfunction.

4.4 Special warnings and precautions for use

Reminyl XL is indicated for a patient with mild to moderately severe dementia of the Alzheimer type. The benefit of galantamine in patients with other types of dementia or other types of memory impairment has not been demonstrated. In 2 clinical trials of two years duration in individuals with so called mild cognitive impairment (milder types of memory impairment not fulfilling the criteria of Alzheimer dementia), galantamine therapy failed to demonstrate any benefit either in slowing cognitive decline or reducing the clinical conversion to dementia. The mortality rate in the galantamine group was significantly higher than in the placebo group, 14/1026 (1.4%) patients on galantamine and 3 /1022 (0.3%) patients on placebo. The deaths were due to various causes. About half of the galantamine deaths appeared to result from various vascular causes (myocardial infarction, stroke, and sudden death). The relevance of this finding for the treatment of patients with Alzheimer dementia is unknown. In Alzheimer dementia, placebo-controlled studies of only 6 months duration have been conducted. In these studies no increased mortality in the galantamine groups appeared.

A diagnosis of Alzheimer's dementia should be made according to current guidelines by an experienced physician. Therapy with galantamine should occur under the supervision of a physician and should only be initiated if a caregiver is available who will regularly monitor medicinal product intake by the patient.

Patients with Alzheimer's disease lose weight. Treatment with cholinesterase inhibitors, including galantamine, has been associated with weight loss in these patients. During therapy, patient's weight should be monitored.

As with other cholinomimetics, galantamine should be given with caution in the following conditions:

Cardiac disorders

Because of their pharmacological action, cholinomimetics may have vagotonic effects on heart rate (e.g. bradycardia). The potential for this action may be particularly important to patients with 'sick sinus syndrome' or other supraventricular cardiac conduction disturbances or in those who use medicinal products that significantly reduce heart rate concomitantly, such as digoxin and beta blockers or for patients with an uncorrected electrolyte disturbance (e.g. hyperkalaemia, hypokalaemia).

Caution should therefore be exercised when administering galantamine to patients with cardiovascular diseases, e.g. immediate post-myocardial infarction period, new-onset atrial fibrillation, second degree heart block or greater, unstable angina pectoris, or congestive heart failure, especially NYHA group III – IV.

In a pooled analysis of placebo-controlled studies in patients with Alzheimer dementia treated with galantamine an increased incidence of certain cardiovascular adverse events were observed (see section 4.8).

Gastrointestinal disorders

Patients at increased risk of developing peptic ulcers, e.g. those with a history of ulcer disease or those predisposed to these conditions, including those receiving concurrent non-steroidal anti-inflammatory drugs (NSAIDs), should be monitored for symptoms. The use of galantamine is not recommended in patients with gastrointestinal obstruction or recovering from gastrointestinal surgery.

Nervous system disorders

Although cholinomimetics are believed to have some potential to cause seizures, seizure activity may also be a manifestation of Alzheimer's disease. In rare cases an increase in cholinergic tone may worsen Parkinsonian symptoms.

In a pooled analysis of placebo-controlled studies in patients with Alzheimer's dementia treated with galantamine cerebrovascular events were uncommonly observed (see section 4.8 Undesirable effects). This should be considered when administering galantamine to patients with cerebrovascular disease.

Respiratory, thoracic and mediastinal disorders

Cholinomimetics should be prescribed with care for patients with a history of severe asthma or obstructive pulmonary disease or active pulmonary infections (e.g. pneumonia).

Renal and urinary disorders

The use of galantamine is not recommended in patients with urinary outflow obstruction or recovering from bladder surgery.

Surgical and medical procedures

Galantamine, as a cholinomimetic is likely to exaggerate succinylcholine-type muscle relaxation during anaesthesia, especially in cases of pseudocholinesterase deficiency.

Other

Reminyl XL prolonged release capsules contain sucrose. Patients with rare hereditary problems of fructose intolerance, glucose-galactose malabsorption or sucrase-isomaltase insufficiency should not take this medicine.

4.5 Interaction with other medicinal products and other forms of interaction

Pharmacodynamic interactions

Because of its mechanism of action, galantamine should not be given concomitantly with other cholinomimetics (such as ambenonium, donepezil, neostigmine, pyridostigmine, rivastigmine or systemically administered pilocarpine). Galantamine has the potential to antagonise the effect of anticholinergic medication. Should anticholinergic medication such as atropine be abruptly stopped there is a potential risk that galantamine's effect could be exacerbated. As expected with cholinomimetics, a pharmacodynamic interaction is possible with medicinal products that significantly reduce the heart rate such as digoxin, beta-blockers, certain calcium-channel blocking agents and amiodarone. Caution should be taken with medicinal products that have potential to cause torsades de pointes. In such cases an ECG should be considered.

Galantamine, as a cholinomimetic, is likely to exaggerate succinylcholine-type muscle relaxation during anaesthesia, especially in cases of pseudocholinesterase deficiency.

Pharmacokinetic interactions

Multiple metabolic pathways and renal excretion are involved in the elimination of galantamine. The possibility of clinically relevant interactions is low. However, the occurrence of significant interactions may be clinically relevant in individual cases.

Concomitant administration with food slows the absorption rate of galantamine but does not affect the extent of absorption. It is recommended that Reminyl XL be taken with food in order to minimise cholinergic side effects.

Other medicinal products affecting the metabolism of galantamine

Formal drug interaction studies showed an increase in galantamine bioavailability of about 40% during co-administration of paroxetine (a potent CYP2D6 inhibitor) and of 30% and 12% during co-treatment with ketoconazole and erythromycin (both CYP3A4 inhibitors). Therefore, during initiation of treatment with potent inhibitors of CYP2D6 (e.g. quinidine, paroxetine or fluoxetine) or CYP3A4 (e.g. ketoconazole or ritonavir) patients may experience an increased incidence of cholinergic adverse reactions, predominantly nausea and vomiting. Under these circumstances, based on tolerability, a reduction of the galantamine maintenance dose can be considered (see section 4.2).

Memantine, an N-methyl-D-aspartate (NMDA) receptor antagonist, at a dose of 10 mg once a day for 2 days followed by 10 mg twice a day for 12 days, had no effect on the pharmacokinetics of galantamine (as Reminyl XL prolonged-release capsules 16 mg once a day) at steady state.

Effect of galantamine on the metabolism of other medicinal products

Therapeutic doses of galantamine 24 mg/day had no effect on the kinetics of digoxin, although pharmacodynamic interactions may occur (see also pharmacodynamic interactions).

Therapeutic doses of galantamine 24 mg/day had no effect on the kinetics and prothrombin time of warfarin.

4.6 Pregnancy and lactation

Pregnancy

For galantamine no clinical data on exposed pregnancies are available. Studies in animals have shown reproductive toxicity (see section 5.3). Caution should be exercised when prescribing to pregnant women.

Lactation

It is not known whether galantamine is excreted in human breast milk and there are no studies in lactating women. Therefore, women on galantamine should not breast-feed.

4.7 Effects on ability to drive and use machines

Galantamine has minor or moderate influence on the ability to drive and use machines. Symptoms include dizziness and somnolence, especially during the first weeks after initiation of treatment.

4.8 Undesirable effects

The most common adverse events observed in clinical trials (incidence ⩾ 5% and twice the frequency of placebo) were nausea, vomiting, diarrhoea, abdominal pain, dyspepsia, anorexia, fatigue, dizziness, headache, somnolence and weight decrease. Nausea, vomiting and anorexia were more commonly observed in women.

Other common adverse events observed in clinical trials (incidence ⩾ 5% and ⩾ placebo) were confusion, depression, fall, injury, insomnia, rhinitis and urinary tract infection.

In a randomised, double-blind, placebo controlled, clinical trial, adverse events that occurred with once-daily treatment with Reminyl XL prolonged release capsules were similar in frequency and nature to those seen with Reminyl tablets.

The majority of these adverse events occurred during the titration period. Nausea and vomiting, the most frequent adverse events, lasted less than a week in most cases and the majority of patients had only one episode. Prescription of anti-emetics and ensuring adequate fluid intake may be useful in these instances.

Adverse events observed during clinical trials and post marketing experience.

(see Table 1 opposite)

Some of these adverse events may be attributable to cholinomimetic properties of galantamine or in some cases may represent manifestations or exacerbations of the underlying disease processes common in the elderly population.

Table 1 Adverse events observed during clinical trials and post marketing experience

System Organ Class	Very Common	Common	Uncommon	Rare	Very Rare
Infections and infestations		Rhinitis Urinary tract infections			
Metabolism and nutrition disorders		Anorexia Weight decrease		Dehydration (leading to renal insufficiency and renal failure) Hypokalaemia	
Psychiatric disorders		Confusion Depression (very rarely with suicidality) Insomnia		Aggression Agitation Hallucinations	
Nervous system disorders		Dizziness Somnolence Syncope Tremor	Paraesthesia	Seizures	Worsening of Parkinsonism
Ear and labyrinth disorders			Tinnitus		
Cardiac disorders			Atrial arrhythmia Myocardial infarction Myocardial ischaemia Palpitation	Bradycardia (severe)	AV block
Vascular disorders		Hypertension	Cerebrovascular disease Transient ischaemic attack		Hypotension
Gastrointestinal disorders	Vomiting Nausea	Abdominal pain Diarrhoea Dyspepsia			Dysphagia Gastrointestinal bleeding
Hepatobiliary disorders					Elevated liver enzymes Hepatitis
Skin and subcutaneous tissue disorders				Rash	Increased sweating
Musculoskeletal and connective tissue disorders			Leg Cramps		
General disorders and administration site conditions		Asthenia Fatigue Fever Headache Malaise			
Injury, poisoning and procedural complications		Fall Injury			

Frequencies are defined as: very common (⩾ 1/10), common (⩾ 1/100 to < 1/10), uncommon (⩾ 1/1,000 to < 1/100), rare (⩾ 1/10,000 to < 1/1,000) and very rare (< 1/10,000).

4.9 Overdose

Symptoms

Signs and symptoms of significant overdosing of galantamine are predicted to be similar to those of overdosing of other cholinomimetics. These effects generally involve the central nervous system, the parasympathetic nervous system, and the neuromuscular junction. In addition to muscle weakness or fasciculations, some or all of the signs of a cholinergic crisis may develop: severe nausea, vomiting, gastrointestinal cramping, salivation, lacrimation, urination, defecation, sweating, bradycardia, hypotension, collapse and convulsions. Increasing muscle weakness together with tracheal hypersecretions and bronchospasm, may lead to vital airway compromise.

There have been post-marketing reports of torsade de pointes, QT prolongation, bradycardia, ventricular tachycardia and brief loss of consciousness in association with inadvertent overdoses of galantamine. In one case where the dose was known, eight Reminyl 4 mg tablets (32 mg total) were ingested on a single day.

Two additional cases of accidental ingestion of 32 mg (nausea, vomiting, and dry mouth; nausea, vomiting, and

Table 2 Composite Responder Analysis Based on at Least 4 Points Improvement in ADAS-cog/11 Compared to Baseline and CIBIC-plus Unchanged + Improved (1-4), and DAD/ADL Score Unchanged + Improved

At least 4 points improvement from baseline in ADAS-cog/11 and CIBIC-plus Unchanged + Improved								
Treatment	Change in DAD ⩾ 0 GAL-USA-1 and GAL-INT-1 (Month 6)				Change in ADCS/ADL-Inventory ⩾ 0 GAL-USA-10 (Month 5)			
	n	n (%) of responder	Comparison with placebo		n	n (%) of responder	Comparison with placebo	
			Diff (95%CI)	p-value†			Diff (95%CI)	p-value†
Classical ITT#								
Placebo	422	21 (5.0)	–	–	273	18 (6.6)	–	–
Gal 16 mg/day	–	–	–	–	266	39 (14.7)	8.1 (3, 13)	0.003
Gal 24 mg/day	424	60 (14.2)	9.2 (5, 13)	<0.001	262	40 (15.3)	8.7 (3, 14)	0.002
*Traditional LOCF**								
Placebo	412	23 (5.6)	–	–	261	17 (6.5)	–	–
Gal 16 mg/day	–	–	–	–	253	36 (14.2)	7.7 (2, 13)	0.005
Gal 24 mg/day	399	58 (14.5)	8.9 (5, 13)	<0.001	253	40 (15.8)	9.3 (4, 15)	0.001

ITT: Intent To Treat

†CMH test of difference from placebo.

* LOCF: Last Observation Carried Forward.

substernal chest pain) and one of 40 mg (vomiting) resulted in brief hospitalisations for observation with full recovery. One patient, who was prescribed 24 mg/day and had a history of hallucinations over the previous two years, mistakenly received 24 mg twice daily for 34 days and developed hallucinations requiring hospitalisation. Another patient, who was prescribed 16 mg/day of oral solution, inadvertently ingested 160 mg (40 ml) and experienced sweating, vomiting, bradycardia, and near-syncope one hour later, which necessitated hospital treatment. His symptoms resolved within 24 hours.

Treatment

As in any case of overdose, general supportive measures should be used. In severe cases, anticholinergics such as atropine can be used as a general antidote for cholinomimetics. An initial dose of 0.5 to 1.0 mg i.v. is recommended, with subsequent doses based on the clinical response.

Because strategies for the management of overdose are continually evolving, it is advisable to contact a poison control centre to determine the latest recommendations for the management of an overdose.

5. PHARMACOLOGICAL PROPERTIES

5.1 Pharmacodynamic properties

Pharmacotherapeutic group: Antidementia drugs

ATC-code: N06DA04

Galantamine, a tertiary alkaloid is a selective, competitive and reversible inhibitor of acetylcholinesterase. In addition, galantamine enhances the intrinsic action of acetylcholine on nicotinic receptors, probably through binding to an allosteric site of the receptor. As a consequence, an increased activity in the cholinergic system associated with improved cognitive function can be achieved in patients with dementia of the Alzheimer type.

Clinical studies

Reminyl XL was originally developed in the form of immediate-release tablets (Reminyl) for twice-daily administration. The dosages of galantamine effective in these placebo-controlled clinical trials with a duration of 5 to 6 months were 16, 24 and 32 mg/day. Of these doses 16 and 24 mg/day were determined to have the best benefit/risk relationship and are the recommended maintenance doses. The efficacy of galantamine has been shown using outcome measures which evaluate the three major symptom complexes of the disease and a global scale: the ADAS-cog/11 (a performance based measure of cognition), DAD and ADCS-ADL-Inventory (measurements of basic and instrumental Activities of Daily Living), the Neuropsychiatric Inventory (a scale that measures behavioural disturbances) and the CIBIC-plus (a global assessment by an independent physician based on a clinical interview with the patient and caregiver).

Composite Responder Analysis Based on at Least 4 Points Improvement in ADAS-cog/11 Compared to Baseline and CIBIC-plus Unchanged + Improved (1-4), and DAD/ADL Score Unchanged + Improved. See Table below.

(see Table 2 on previous page)

The efficacy of Reminyl XL prolonged release capsules was studied in a randomised, double-blind, placebo-controlled trial, GAL-INT-10, using a 4-week dose escalation, flexible dosing regimen of 16 or 24 mg/day for a treatment duration of 6 months. Reminyl immediate-release tablets (Gal-IR) were added as a positive control arm. Efficacy was evaluated using the ADAS-cog/11 and the CIBIC-plus scores as co-primary efficacy criteria, and ADCS-ADL and NPI scores as secondary end-points. Reminyl XL prolonged release capsules (Gal-PR) demonstrated statistically significant improvements in the ADAS-cog/11 score compared to placebo, but were not statistically different in the CIBIC-plus score compared to placebo. The results of the ADCS-ADL score were statistically significantly better compared to placebo at week 26.

Composite Responder Analysis at Week 26 Based on at Least 4 Points Improvement from Baseline in ADAS-cog/11, Total ADL Score Unchanged + Improved (⩾0) and No Worsening in CIBIC-plus Score (1-4). See Table below.

(see Table 3 below)

The results of a 26-week double-blind placebo-controlled trial, in which patients with vascular dementia and patients with Alzheimer's disease and concomitant cerebrovascular disease ("mixed dementia") were included, indicate that the symptomatic effect of galantamine is maintained in patients with Alzheimer's disease and concomitant cerebrovascular disease (see section 4.4, Nervous system disorders). In a post-hoc subgroup analysis, no statistically significant effect was observed in the subgroup of patients with vascular dementia alone.

In a second 26-week placebo-controlled trial in patients with probable vascular dementia, no clinical benefit of galantamine treatment was demonstrated.

5.2 Pharmacokinetic properties

Galantamine is an alkalinic compound with one ionisation constant (pKa 8.2). It is slightly lipophilic and has a partition coefficient (Log P) between n-octanol/buffer solution (pH 12) of 1.09. The solubility in water (pH 6) is 31 mg/ml. Galantamine has three chiral centres. The S, R, S-form is the naturally occurring form. Galantamine is partially metabolised by various cytochromes, mainly CYP2D6 and CYP3A4. Some of the metabolites formed during the degradation of galantamine have been shown to be active *in vitro* but are of no importance *in vivo*.

General characteristics of galantamine

Absorption

The absolute bioavailability of galantamine is high, 88.5 ± 5.4%. Reminyl XL prolonged release capsules are bioequivalent to the twice-daily immediate-release tablets with respect to AUC_{24h} and C_{min}. The C_{max} value is reached after 4.4 hours and is about 24% lower than that of the tablet. Food has no significant effect on AUC of the prolonged release capsules. C_{max} was increased by about 12% and T_{max} increased by about 30 minutes when the capsule was given after food. However, these changes are unlikely to be clinically significant.

Distribution

The mean volume of distribution is 175 l. Plasma protein binding is low, 18%.

Metabolism

Up to 75% of galantamine dosed is eliminated via metabolism. *In vitro* studies indicate that CYP2D6 is involved in the formation of O-desmethylgalantamine and CYP3A4 is involved in the formation of N-oxide-galantamine. The levels of excretion of total radioactivity in urine and faeces were not different between poor and extensive CYP2D6 metabolisers. In plasma from poor and extensive metabolisers, unchanged galantamine and its glucuronide accounted for most of the sample radioactivity. None of the active metabolites of galantamine (norgalantamine, O-desmethylgalantamine and O-desmethyl-norgalantamine) could be detected in their unconjugated form in plasma from poor and extensive metabolisers after single dosing. Norgalantamine was detectable in plasma from patients after multiple dosing, but did not represent more than 10% of the galantamine levels. *In vitro* studies indicated that the inhibition potential of galantamine with respect to the major forms of human cytochrome P450 is very low.

Elimination

Galantamine plasma concentration declines bi-exponentially, with a terminal half-life around 8-10 hours in healthy subjects. Typical oral clearance in the target population is about 200 ml/min with intersubject variability of 30% as derived from the population analysis of immediate-release tablets. Seven days after a single oral dose of 4 mg ^{3}H-galantamine, 90-97% of the radioactivity is recovered in urine and 2.2-6.3% in faeces. After i.v. infusion and oral administration, 18-22% of the dose was excreted as unchanged galantamine in the urine in 24 hours, with a renal clearance of 68.4 ±22.0 ml/min, which represents 20-25% of the total plasma clearance.

Dose-linearity

Galantamine pharmacokinetics of Reminyl XL prolonged release capsules are dose proportional within the studied dose range of 8 mg to 24 mg once-daily in elderly and young age groups.

Characteristics in patients

Data from clinical trials in patients indicate that the plasma concentrations of galantamine in patients with Alzheimer's disease are 30% to 40% higher than in healthy young subjects primarily due to the advanced age and reduced kidney function. Based upon the population pharmacokinetic analysis, clearance in female subjects is 20% lower as compared to males. The galantamine clearance in poor metabolisers of CYP2D6 is about 25% lower than in extensive metabolisers, but no bimodality in the population is observed. Therefore, the metabolic status of the patient is not considered to be of clinical relevance in the overall population.

The pharmacokinetics of galantamine in subjects with mild hepatic impairment (Child-Pugh score of 5 to 6) were comparable to those in healthy subjects. In patients with moderate hepatic impairment (Child-Pugh score of 7 to 9), AUC and half-life of galantamine were increased by about 30% (see section 4.2).

Elimination of galantamine decreases with decreasing creatinine clearance as observed in a study with renally impaired subjects. Compared to Alzheimer patients, peak and trough plasma concentrations are not increased in patients with a creatinine clearance of ⩾ 9 ml/min. Therefore, no increase in adverse events is expected and no dosage adjustments are needed (see section 4.2).

Pharmacokinetic/pharmacodynamic relationship

No apparent correlation between average plasma concentrations and efficacy parameters (i.e. change in ADAS-cog/11 and CIBIC-plus at month 6) were observed in the large Phase III trials with a dose-regimen of 12 and 16 mg twice-daily.

Plasma concentrations in patients experiencing syncope were within the same range as in the other patients at the same dose.

The occurrence of nausea is shown to correlate with higher peak plasma concentrations (see section 4.5).

5.3 Preclinical safety data

Non-clinical data suggest no special hazard for humans based on conventional studies of safety pharmacology, repeated dose toxicity, genotoxicity and carcinogenic potential.

Reproduction toxicity studies showed a slight delay in development in rats and rabbits, at doses that are below the threshold of toxicity in the pregnant females.

6. PHARMACEUTICAL PARTICULARS

6.1 List of excipients

Prolonged release pellets

Diethyl phthalate

Ethylcellulose

Hypromellose

Macrogol 400

Maize starch

Sucrose

Capsules

Gelatin

Titanium dioxide (E171)

The 16 mg capsule also contains red ferric oxide (E172).

The 24 mg capsule also contains red ferric oxide (E172) and yellow ferric oxide (E172).

Imprinting ink

Benzoic acid (E210)

Black ferric oxide (E172)

Dimethyl siloxanes

Glycerides

Lecithin (soya) (E322)

Methylcellulose

Macrogol

Macrogol stearate

Shellac

Sorbic acid

Xanthan gum

6.2 Incompatibilities

Not applicable.

6.3 Shelf life

2 years.

6.4 Special precautions for storage

Do not store above 30°C.

6.5 Nature and contents of container

Available pack sizes:

8 mg

28 prolonged release capsules, hard (PVC-PE-PVDC/Aluminium blister)

16 mg

28 prolonged release capsules, hard (PVC-PE-PVDC/Aluminium blister)

24 mg

28 prolonged release capsules, hard (PVC-PE-PVDC/Aluminium blister)

6.6 Special precautions for disposal and other handling

No special requirements.

7. MARKETING AUTHORISATION HOLDER

Shire Pharmaceuticals Limited

Hampshire International Business Park

Chineham

Basingstoke

Hampshire RG24 8EP

United Kingdom

8. MARKETING AUTHORISATION NUMBER(S)

8mg : PL 08557/0052

16mg : PL 08557/0053

24mg : PL 08557/0054

Table 3 Composite Responder Analysis at Week 26 Based on at Least 4 Points Improvement from Baseline in ADAS-cog/11, Total ADL Score Unchanged + Improved (⩾0) and No Worsening in CIBIC-plus Score (1-4)

GAL-INT-10	Placebo	Gal-IR†	Gal-PR*	p-value (Gal-PR* vs. Placebo)
	(n = 245)	(n = 225)	(n = 238)	
Composite Response: n (%)	20 (8.2)	43 (19.1)	38 (16.0)	0.008

†Immediate release tablets

* Prolonged release capsules

9. DATE OF FIRST AUTHORISATION/RENEWAL OF THE AUTHORISATION

Date of first authorisation: 06 January 2005

Date of last renewal: 01 March 2005

10. DATE OF REVISION OF THE TEXT

January 2008

Replagal 1mg/ml concentrate for solution for infusion

(Shire Human Genetic Therapies)

1. NAME OF THE MEDICINAL PRODUCT

Replagal 1 mg/ml concentrate for solution for infusion.

2. QUALITATIVE AND QUANTITATIVE COMPOSITION

1 ml of concentrate for solution for infusion contains 1 mg of agalsidase alfa.

Each vial of 1 ml of concentrate contains 1 mg of agalsidase alfa.

Each vial of 3.5 ml of concentrate contains 3.5 mg of agalsidase alfa.

Agalsidase alfa is the human protein α-galactosidase A produced in a human cell line by genetic engineering technology.

For a full list of excipients, see section 6.1.

3. PHARMACEUTICAL FORM

Concentrate for solution for infusion.

A clear and colourless solution.

4. CLINICAL PARTICULARS

4.1 Therapeutic indications

Replagal is indicated for long-term enzyme replacement therapy in patients with a confirmed diagnosis of Fabry Disease (α-galactosidase A deficiency).

4.2 Posology and method of administration

Replagal treatment should be supervised by a physician experienced in the management of patients with Fabry Disease or other inherited metabolic diseases.

Replagal is administered at a dose of 0.2 mg/kg body weight every other week by intravenous infusion over 40 minutes. For preparation and administration instructions, see section 6.6.

Patients aged over 65 years

Studies in patients over the age of 65 have not been performed and no dosage regimen can presently be recommended in these patients as safety and efficacy have not yet been established.

Patients with hepatic impairment

No studies have been performed in patients with hepatic impairment.

Patients with renal impairment

No dose adjustment is necessary in patients with renal impairment.

The presence of extensive renal damage (eGFR <60mL/min) may limit the renal response to enzyme replacement therapy. Limited data are available in patients on dialysis or post-kidney transplantation, no dose adjustment is recommended.

Paediatric Patients

The experience in children is limited. Studies in children (0-6 years) have not been performed and no dosage regimen can presently be recommended in the patients as safety and efficacy have not yet been established. Limited clinical data in children (7-18 years) do not permit to recommend an optimal dosage regimen presently (see section 5.2). Because no unexpected safety issues were encountered in the 6 month study with Replagal administered at 0.2 mg/kg in this population, this dose regimen is suggested for children between 7– 18 years of age.

4.3 Contraindications

Hypersensitivity to the active substance or any of the excipients.

4.4 Special warnings and precautions for use

Idiosyncratic infusion related reactions

13.7% of patients treated with Replagal in clinical trials have experienced idiosyncratic infusion related reactions. Overall, the percentage of infusion related reactions was significantly lower in females than males. The most common symptoms have been rigors, headache, nausea, pyrexia, flushing and fatigue. Serious infusion reactions have been reported uncommonly; symptoms reported include pyrexia, rigors, tachycardia, urticaria, nausea/vomiting, angioneurotic oedema with throat tightness, stridor and swollen tongue. Other infusion-related symptoms may include dizziness and hyperhidrosis. The onset of infusion related reactions has generally occurred within the first 2-4 months after initiation of treatment with Replagal although later onset (after 1 year) has been reported as well. These effects have decreased with time. If mild or moderate acute infusion reactions occur, medical attention must be sought immediately and appropriate actions instituted. The infusion can be temporarily interrupted (5 to 10 minutes) until symptoms subside and the infusion may then be restarted. Mild and transient effects may not require medical treatment or discontinuation of the infusion. In addition, oral or intravenous pre-treatment with antihistamines and/or corticosteroids, from 1 to 24 hours prior to infusion may prevent subsequent reactions in those cases where symptomatic treatment was required.

Allergic-type hypersensitivity reactions

As with any intravenous protein product, allergic-type hypersensitivity reactions are possible. If severe allergic or anaphylactic-type reactions occur, the administration of Replagal should be discontinued immediately and appropriate treatment initiated. The current medical standards for emergency treatment are to be observed.

IgG antibodies to the protein

As with all protein pharmaceutical products, patients may develop IgG antibodies to the protein. A low titre IgG antibody response has been observed in approximately 24% of the male patients treated with Replagal. Based on limited data this percentage has been found to be lower (7%) in the male paediatric population. These IgG antibodies appeared to develop following approximately 3-12 months of treatment. After 12 to 54 months of therapy, 17% of Replagal treated patients were still antibody positive whereas 7% showed evidence for the development of immunologic tolerance, based on the disappearance of IgG antibodies over time. The remaining 76% remained antibody negative throughout. No IgE antibodies have been detected in any patient receiving Replagal.

Patients with renal impairment

The presence of extensive renal damage may limit the renal response to enzyme replacement therapy, possibly due to underlying irreversible pathological changes. In such cases, the loss of renal function remains within the expected range of the natural progression of disease.

4.5 Interaction with other medicinal products and other forms of interaction

Replagal should not be co-administered with chloroquine, amiodarone, benoquin or gentamicin since these substances have the potential to inhibit intra-cellular α-galactosidase activity.

As α-galactosidase A is itself an enzyme, it would be an unlikely candidate for cytochrome P450 mediated drug-drug interactions. In clinical studies, neuropathic pain medicinal products (such as carbamazepine, phenytoin and gabapentin) were administered concurrently to most patients without any evidence of interaction.

4.6 Pregnancy and lactation

Very limited clinical data on pregnancies exposed to Replagal (n=4) have shown no adverse effects on the mother and newborn child. Animal studies do not indicate direct or indirect harmful effects with respect to pregnancy or embryonal/foetal development when exposed during organogenesis (see Section 5.3).

It is not known whether Replagal is excreted in human milk. Caution should be exercised when prescribing to pregnant or breast-feeding women.

4.7 Effects on ability to drive and use machines

Replagal has no or negligible influence on the ability to drive and use machines.

4.8 Undesirable effects

The most commonly reported undesirable effects were infusion associated reactions, which occurred in 13.7% of patients treated with Replagal in clinical trials. Most undesirable effects were mild to moderate in severity. Table 1 lists adverse drug reactions (ADRs) reported for the 153 patients treated with Replagal in clinical trials, including 21 patients with history of endstage renal disease and 17 female patients. Information is presented by system organ class and frequency (very common >1/10; common >1/100, <1/10; uncommon >1/1000, <1/100). Within each frequency grouping, undesirable effects are presented in order of decreasing seriousness. The occurrence of an event in a single patient is defined as uncommon in view of the number of patients treated. A single patient could be affected by several ADRs.

Table 1	
Metabolism and nutrition disorders	
Common:	peripheral oedema
Nervous system disorders	
Very common:	headache
Common:	dizziness, dysgeusia, neuropathic pain, tremor, hypersomnia, hypoesthesia, paraesthesia
Uncommon:	parosmia
Eye disorders	
Common:	lacrimation increased
Ear and labyrinth disorders	
Common:	tinnitus, tinnitus aggravated
Cardiac disorders	
Common:	tachycardia, palpitations
Vascular disorders	
Very Common:	flushing
Common:	hypertension
Respiratory, thoracic and mediastinal disorders	
Common:	cough, hoarseness, throat tightness, dyspnoea, nasopharyngitis, pharyngitis, throat secretion increased, rhinorrhoea
Gastrointestinal disorders	
Very common:	nausea
Common:	diarrhoea, vomiting, abdominal pain/discomfort
Skin and subcutaneous tissue disorders	
Common:	acne, erythema, pruritus, rash, livedo reticularis
Uncommon:	angioneurotic oedema, urticaria
Musculoskeletal, connective tissue and bone disorders	
Common:	musculoskeletal discomfort, myalgia, back pain, limb pain, peripheral swelling, arthralgia, joint swelling
Uncommon:	sensation of heaviness
General disorders and administration site conditions	
Very common:	rigors pyrexia, pain and discomfort, fatigue
Common:	fatigue aggravated, feeling hot, feeling cold, asthenia, chest pain, chest tightness, influenza like illness, injection site rash, malaise
Investigations	
Common:	corneal reflex decreased
Uncommon:	oxygen saturation decreased

See also section 4.4.

Adverse drug reactions reported in patients with history of end stage renal disease were similar to those reported in the general patient population.

Adverse drug reactions reported in the paediatric population (children and adolescents) were, in general, similar to those reported in adults. However, infusion related reactions and pain exacerbation occurred more frequently. The most frequent were mild infusion-related reactions that mainly included rigors, pyrexia, flushing, headache, nausea, and dyspnoea.

4.9 Overdose

No case of overdose has been reported.

5. PHARMACOLOGICAL PROPERTIES

5.1 Pharmacodynamic properties

Pharmacotherapeutic group: Other alimentary tract and metabolism products - Enzymes.

ATC code: A16AB03 agalsidase alfa.

Fabry Disease is a glycosphingolipid storage disorder that is caused by deficient activity of the lysosomal enzyme α-galactosidase A, resulting in accumulation of globotriaosylceramide (also referred to as Gb3 or CTH), the glycosphingolipid substrate for this enzyme. Agalsidase alfa catalyses the hydrolysis of Gb3, cleaving a terminal galactose residue from the molecule. Treatment with the enzyme has been shown to reduce accumulation of Gb3 in many cell types including endothelial and parenchymal cells. Agalsidase alfa has been produced in a human cell line to provide for a human glycosylation profile that can influence uptake by mannose-6-phosphate receptors on the surface of target cells.

The safety and efficacy of Replagal was assessed in two randomised, double blind, placebo controlled studies and open label extension studies, in a total of forty patients with a diagnosis of Fabry Disease based on clinical and biochemical evidence. Patients received the recommended dosage of 0.2 mg/kg of Replagal. Twenty-five patients completed the first study and entered an extension study. After 6 months of therapy there was a significant reduction in pain in the Replagal treated patients compared with placebo (p=0.021), as measured by the Brief Pain Inventory (a validated pain measurement scale). This was associated with a significant reduction in chronic neuropathic pain medication use and number of days on pain medication. In subsequent studies, in male paediatric patients, a reduction in pain was observed after 9 and 12 months of Replagal therapy compared to pre-treatment baseline.

Twelve to 18 months of treatment with Replagal resulted in improvement in quality of life (QoL), as measured by validated instruments.

After 6 months of therapy Replagal stabilised renal function compared with a decline in placebo treated patients. Kidney biopsy specimens revealed a significant increase in the fraction of normal glomeruli and a significant decrease in the fraction of glomeruli with mesangial widening in patients treated with Replagal in contrast to the patients treated with placebo. After 12 to 18 months of maintenance therapy, Replagal improved renal function as measured by inulin based glomerular filtration rate by 8.7 ± 3.7 ml/min. (p=0.030). Longer term therapy (48-54 months) resulted in stabilisation of GFR in male patients with normal baseline GFR (≥ 90 mL/min/1.73 m^2) and with mild to moderate renal dysfunction (GFR 60 to < 90 mL/min/1.73 m^2), and in slowing of the rate of decline in renal function and progression to end-stage renal disease in male Fabry patients with more severe renal dysfunction (GFR 30 to < 60 mL/min/1.73 m^2).

In male paediatric Fabry patients, hyperfiltration can be the earliest manifestation of renal involvement in the disease. Reduction in their hypernormal eGFRs was observed within 6 months of initiating Replagal therapy.

In a second study, fifteen patients with left ventricular hypertrophy completed a 6 month placebo-controlled study and entered an extension study. Treatment with Replagal resulted in an 11.5 g decrease in left ventricular mass as measured by magnetic resonance imaging (MRI) in the controlled study, while patients receiving placebo exhibited an increase in left ventricular mass of 21.8 g. In addition, in the first study involving 25 patients, Replagal effected a significant reduction in cardiac mass after 12 to 18 months of maintenance therapy ($p<0.001$). Replagal was also associated with improved myocardial contractility, a decrease in mean QRS duration and a concomitant decrease in septal thickness on echocardiography. Two patients with right bundle branch block in the studies conducted reverted to normal following therapy with Replagal. Subsequent open label studies demonstrated significant reduction from baseline in left ventricular mass by echocardiography in both male and female Fabry patients over 24 to 36 months of Replagal treatment. The reductions in LV mass observed by echocardiography in both male and female Fabry patients over 24 to 36 months of Replagal treatment were associated with meaningful symptom improvement as measured using the NYHA and CCS in Fabry patients with severe heart failure or anginal symptoms at baseline.

Compared with placebo, treatment with Replagal also reduced accumulation of Gb3. After the first 6 months of therapy mean decreases of approximately 20 - 50 % were observed in plasma, urine sediment and liver, kidney and heart biopsy samples. After 12 to 18 months treatment a reduction of 50 – 80% was observed in plasma and urine sediment. The metabolic effects were also associated with clinically significant weight gain, increased sweating and increased energy. Consistent with the clinical effects of Replagal, treatment with the enzyme reduced accumulation of Gb3 in many cell types, including renal glomerular and tubular epithelial cells, renal capillary endothelial cells (cardiac and dermal capillary endothelial cells were not examined) and cardiac myocytes. In male paediatric Fabry patients plasma Gb3 decreased 40-50% after 6 months of Replagal therapy and this reduction persisted after a total of 12 months of treatment.

Antibodies to agalsidase alfa have not been shown to be associated with any clinically significant effects on safety (e.g. infusion reactions) or efficacy.

Infusion of Replagal at home may be considered for patients who are tolerating their infusions well.

This medicinal product has been authorised under "Exceptional Circumstances". This means that due to the rarity of the disease it has not been possible to obtain complete information on this medicinal product.

The European Medicines Agency (EMEA) will review any new information which may become available every year and this SPC will be updated as necessary.

5.2 Pharmacokinetic properties

Single doses ranging from 0.007 - 0.2 mg enzyme per kg body weight were administered to adult male patients as 20 - 40 minute intravenous infusions while female patients received 0.2 mg enzyme per kg body weight as 40 minute infusions. The pharmacokinetic properties were essentially unaffected by the dose of the enzyme. Following a single intravenous dose of 0.2 mg/kg, agalsidase alfa had a biphasic distribution and elimination profile from the circulation. Pharmacokinetic parameters were not significantly different between male and female patients. Elimination half-lives were 108 ± 17 minutes in males compared to 89 ± 28 minutes in females and volume of distribution was approximately 17% body weight in both sexes. Clearance normalised for body weight was 2.66 and 2.10 ml/min/kg for males and females, respectively. Based on the similarity of pharmacokinetic properties of agalsidase alfa in both males and females, tissue distribution in major tissues and organs is also expected to be comparable in male and female patients.

In children (aged 7-18 years), Replagal administered at 0.2 mg/kg was cleared faster from the circulation than in adults. Mean clearance of Replagal in children aged (7-11 years), in adolescents (aged 12-18 years), and adults was 4.2 ml/min/kg, 3.1 ml/min/kg, and 2.3 ml/min/kg, respectively. Pharmacodynamic data suggest that at a dose of 0.2 mg/kg Replagal, the reductions in plasma Gb3 are more or less comparable between adolescents and young children (see section 5.1).

Following six months of Replagal treatment 12 of 28 male patients showed altered pharmacokinetics including an apparent increase in clearance. These changes were associated with the development of low titre antibodies to agalsidase alfa but no clinically significant effects on safety or efficacy were observed in the patients studied.

Based on the analysis of pre- and post-dose liver biopsies in males with Fabry Disease, the tissue half-life has been estimated to be in excess of 24 hours and hepatic uptake of the enzyme estimated to be 10% of administered dose.

Agalsidase alfa is a protein and is therefore: 1) not expected to bind to proteins, 2) expected that metabolic degradation will follow the pathways of other proteins, i.e. peptide hydrolysis, 3) unlikely to be a candidate for drug-drug interactions.

Renal elimination of agalsidase alfa is considered to be a minor clearance pathway since pharmacokinetic parameters are not altered by impaired renal function. As metabolism is expected to occur by peptide hydrolysis, impaired liver function is not expected to affect the pharmacokinetics of agalsidase alfa in a clinically significant manner.

5.3 Preclinical safety data

Non-clinical data reveal no special hazard for humans based on studies of repeated dose toxicity. Genotoxic and carcinogenic potential are not expected. Reproduction toxicity studies in female rats and rabbits have shown no effect on pregnancy or the developing foetus. No studies have been conducted with respect to parturition or peri/post-natal development. It is not known whether Replagal crosses the placenta.

6. PHARMACEUTICAL PARTICULARS

6.1 List of excipients

Sodium phosphate monobasic, monohydrate

Polysorbate 20

Sodium chloride

Sodium hydroxide

Water for injections

6.2 Incompatibilities

In the absence of compatibility studies this medicinal product must not be mixed with other medicinal products.

6.3 Shelf life

2 years

Chemical and physical in use stability has been demonstrated for 24 hours at 25°C.

From a microbiological point of view, the product should be used immediately. If not used immediately, in-use storage times and conditions prior to use are the responsibility of the user and would normally not be longer than 24 hours at 2 to 8°C, unless dilution has taken place in controlled and validated aseptic conditions.

6.4 Special precautions for storage

Store in a refrigerator (2°C – 8°C).

6.5 Nature and contents of container

1 ml of concentrate for solution for infusion in a 3 ml vial (Type I glass) with a stopper (fluoro-resin coated butyl rubber), a one piece seal (aluminium) and flip-off cap. Pack sizes of 1, 4 or 10 vials.

3.5 ml of concentrate for solution for infusion in a 5 ml vial (Type I glass) with a stopper (fluoro-resin coated butyl rubber), a one piece seal (aluminium) and flip-off cap. Pack sizes of 1, 4 or 10 vials.

Not all pack sizes may be marketed.

6.6 Special precautions for disposal and other handling

• Calculate the dose and number of Replagal vials needed.

• Dilute the total volume of Replagal concentrate required in 100 ml of 9 mg/ml (0.9%) sodium chloride solution for infusion. Care must be taken to ensure the sterility of the prepared solutions since Replagal does not contain any preservative or bacteriostatic agent; aseptic technique must be observed. Once diluted, the solution should be mixed gently but not shaken.

• The solution should be inspected visually for particulate matter and discolouration prior to administration.

• Administer the infusion solution over a period of 40 minutes using an intravenous line with an integral filter. Since no preservative is present, it is recommended that administration is started as soon as possible and within 3 hours of dilution.

• Do not infuse Replagal concomitantly in the same intravenous line with other agents.

• For single use only. Any unused product or waste material should be disposed of in accordance with local requirements.

7. MARKETING AUTHORISATION HOLDER

Shire Human Genetic Therapies AB, Svärdvägen 11D, 182 33 Danderyd, Sweden

Tel: +46 8 5449 6400

Fax: +46 8 5449 6429

8. MARKETING AUTHORISATION NUMBER(S)

EU/1/01/189/001-006

9. DATE OF FIRST AUTHORISATION/RENEWAL OF THE AUTHORISATION

Date of first authorisation: 03/08/2001

Date of last renewal: 03/08/2006

10. DATE OF REVISION OF THE TEXT

30/10/2008

Detailed information on this medicinal product is available on the website of the European Medicines Agency (EMEA) http://www.emea.europa.eu/.

Requip Tablets

(GlaxoSmithKline UK)

1. NAME OF THE MEDICINAL PRODUCT

Requip®

2. QUALITATIVE AND QUANTITATIVE COMPOSITION

Ropinirole hydrochloride equivalent to 0.25, 0.5, 1.0, 2.0 or 5.0 mg ropinirole free base.

For a full list of excipients, see section 6.1.

3. PHARMACEUTICAL FORM

Film-coated, pentagonal-shaped tablets for oral administration. The tablet strengths are distinguished by colour; 0.25 mg (white), 0.5mg (yellow), 1.0 mg (green), 2.0 mg (pink) and 5.0 mg (blue).

4. CLINICAL PARTICULARS

4.1 Therapeutic indications

Treatment of idiopathic Parkinson's Disease:

Ropinirole may be used alone (without levodopa) in the treatment of idiopathic Parkinson's disease.

Addition of ropinirole to levodopa may be used to control "on-off" fluctuations and permit a reduction in the total daily dose of levodopa.

4.2 Posology and method of administration

Individual dose titration against efficacy and tolerability is recommended.

Ropinirole should be taken three times a day, preferably with meals to improve gastrointestinal tolerance.

Treatment initiation: The initial dose should be 0.25 mg t.i.d. A guide for the titration regimen for the first four weeks of treatment is given in the table below:

	Week			
	1	2	3	4
Unit dose (mg)	0.25	0.5	0.75	1.0
Unit dose presentation (mg)	0.25	0.5	0.25, 0.5	1.0
Total daily dose (mg)	0.75	1.5	2.25	3.0

Therapeutic regimen: After the initial titration, weekly increments of up to 3 mg/day may be given. Ropinirole is usually given in divided doses three times per day.

If using the "Follow on Titration" pack, follow the proposed titration regime:

	Week			
	5	6	7	8
Unit dose (mg)	1.5	2.0	2.5	3.0
Unit dose presentation (mg)	0.5, 1.0	2.0	0.5, 2.0	1.0, 2.0
Total daily dose (mg)	4.5	6.0	7.5	9.0

A therapeutic response may be seen between 3 and 9 mg/day, although adjunct therapy patients may require higher doses. If sufficient symptomatic control is not achieved, or maintained, the dose of ropinirole may be increased until an acceptable therapeutic response is established. Doses above 24 mg/day have not been investigated in clinical trials and this dose should not be exceeded.

When ropinirole is administered as adjunct therapy to L-dopa, the concurrent dose of L-dopa may be reduced gradually by around 20% in total. In patients with advanced Parkinson's disease receiving ropinirole in combination with L-dopa, dyskinesias can occur during the initial titration of ropinirole. In clinical trials it was shown that a reduction of the L-dopa dose may ameliorate dyskinesia (see also section 4.8).

When switching treatment from another dopamine agonist to ropinirole, the manufacturer's guidance on discontinuation should be followed before initiating ropinirole.

Ropinirole should be discontinued gradually by reducing the number of daily doses over the period of one week.

In parkinsonian patients with mild to moderate renal impairment (creatinine clearance 30-50 ml/min) no change in the clearance of ropinirole was observed, indicating that no dosage adjustment is necessary in this population

The use of ropinirole in patients with severe renal (creatinine clearance <30 ml/min) or hepatic impairment has not been studied. Administration of ropinirole to such patients is not recommended.

Elderly: The clearance of ropinirole is decreased in patients over 65 years of age, but the dose of ropinirole for elderly patients can be titrated in the normal manner.

Children: Parkinson's disease does not occur in children. The use of ropinirole in this population has therefore not been studied and it should not be given to children.

4.3 Contraindications

Hypersensitivity to ropinirole or to any of the excipients.

In light of the results of animal studies and the lack of studies in human pregnancy, ropinirole is contra-indicated in pregnancy, lactation and in women of child-bearing potential unless adequate contraception is used.

4.4 Special warnings and precautions for use

Due to the pharmacological action of ropinirole, patients with severe cardiovascular disease should be treated with caution.

Co-administration of ropinirole with anti-hypertensive and anti-arrhythmic agents has not been studied. Caution should be exercised when these compounds are given concomitantly with ropinirole because of the unknown potential for the occurrence of hypotension, bradycardias or other arrhythmias.

Patients with a history or presence of major psychotic disorders should only be treated with dopamine agonists if the potential benefits outweigh the risks (see also Section 4.5).

Pathological gambling, increased libido and hypersexuality have been reported in patients treated with dopamine agonists for Parkinson's disease, including ropinirole.

Ropinirole has been associated with somnolence and episodes of sudden sleep onset, particularly in patients with Parkinson's Disease. Sudden onset of sleep during daily activities, in some cases without awareness or warning signs, has been reported uncommonly. Patients must be informed of this and advised to exercise caution while driving or operating machines during treatment with ropinirole. Patients who have experienced somnolence and/or an episode of sudden sleep onset must refrain from driving or operating machines. Furthermore, a reduction of dosage or termination of therapy may be considered.

Patients with rare hereditary problems of galactose intolerance, the Lapp lactase deficiency or glucose-galactose malabsorption should not take this medicine.

4.5 Interaction with other medicinal products and other forms of interaction

Neuroleptics and other centrally active dopamine antagonists, such as sulpiride or metoclopramide, may diminish the effectiveness of ropinirole and, therefore, concomitant use of these drugs with ropinirole should be avoided.

No pharmacokinetic interaction has been seen between ropinirole and L-dopa or domperidone which would necessitate dosage adjustment of either drug. No interaction has been seen between ropinirole and other drugs commonly used to treat Parkinson's disease but, as is common practice, care should be taken when adding a new drug to a treatment regimen. Other dopamine agonists may be used with caution.

In a study in parkinsonian patients receiving concurrent digoxin, no interaction was seen which would require dosage adjustment.

It has been established from in vitro experiments that ropinirole is metabolised by the cytochrome P450 enzyme CYP1A2. There is, therefore, the potential for an interaction between ropinirole and substrates (such as theophylline) or inhibitors (such as ciprofloxacin, fluvoxamine and cimetidine) of this enzyme. In patients already receiving ropinirole, the dose of ropinirole may need to be adjusted when these drugs are introduced or withdrawn.

Increased plasma concentrations of ropinirole have been observed in patients treated with high doses of oestrogens. In patients already receiving hormone replacement therapy (HRT), ropinirole treatment may be initiated in the normal manner. However, if HRT is stopped or introduced during treatment with ropinirole, dosage adjustment may be required.

No information is available on the potential for interaction between ropinirole and alcohol. As with other centrally active medications, patients should be cautioned against taking ropinirole with alcohol.

Smoking is known to induce CYP1A2 metabolism, therefore if patients stop or start smoking during treatment with ropinirole, adjustment of dose may be required.

4.6 Pregnancy and lactation

Ropinirole should not be used during pregnancy. In animal studies, administration of ropinirole to pregnant rats at maternally toxic doses resulted in decreased foetal body weight at 60 mg/kg (approximately three times the AUC of the maximum dose in man), increased foetal death at 90 mg/kg (~x5) and digit malformations at 150 mg/kg (~x9).

There was no teratogenic effect in the rat at 120 mg/kg (~x7) and no indication of an effect on development in the rabbit. There have been no studies of ropinirole in human pregnancy.

Ropinirole should not be used in nursing mothers as it may inhibit lactation.

4.7 Effects on ability to drive and use machines

Patients should be warned about the possibility of dizziness (including vertigo). Patients being treated with ropinirole and presenting with somnolence and/or sudden sleep episodes must be informed to refrain from driving or engaging in activities where impaired alertness may put themselves or others at risk of serious injury or death (e.g. operating machines) until such recurrent episodes and somnolence have resolved (see also Section 4.4).

4.8 Undesirable effects

Adverse events are listed below by system organ class and frequency. Frequencies are defined as: very common (>1/10), common (>1/100, <1/10), uncommon (>1/1,000, <1/100), rare (>1/10,000, <1/1,000) very rare (<1/10,000), including isolated reports. Common and uncommon events were generally determined from pooled safety data from clinical trial populations of ropinirole and are quoted as excess incidence over placebo. Rare and very rare events were generally determined from post-marketing data and refer to reporting rate rather than true frequency.

The most commonly reported undesirable effects are nausea, somnolence, dyskinesia and syncope.

Adverse Drug Reactions Reported from Patients taking ropinirole

Immune system disorders	
very rare	Hypersensitivity reactions (including urticaria, angioedema, rash, pruritus)[3]
Psychiatric disorders	
common	confusion[1], hallucinations
uncommon	Psychotic reactions (other than hallucinations), including delusion, paranoia, delirium. Patients treated with dopamine agonists for treatment of Parkinson's disease, including ropinirole, especially at high doses, have been reported as exhibiting signs of pathological gambling, increased libido and hypersexuality, generally reversible upon reduction of the dose or treatment discontinuation[3].
Nervous system disorders	
very common	somnolence[2], dyskinesia[1*]
common	dizziness (including vertigo)[1,2], syncope[2]
uncommon	extreme somnolence[3], sudden onset of sleep[3]
Vascular disorders	
common	hypotension, postural hypotension
Gastrointestinal disorders	
very common	nausea
common	abdominal pain[2], vomiting[2], dyspepsia[2]
General disorders and administrative site conditions	
common	leg oedema[2]
Hepatobiliary disorders	
very rare	hepatic enzymes increased[3]

1 Adjunct therapy studies

2 Monotherapy studies

3 Post-marketing data (see Section 4.4)

* In patients with advanced Parkinson's disease, dyskinesias can occur during the initial titration of ropinirole. In clinical trials it was shown that a reduction of the L-dopa dose may ameliorate dyskinesia (see also section 4.2)

4.9 Overdose

The symptoms of ropinirole overdose are generally related to its dopaminergic activity. These symptoms may be alleviated by appropriate treatment with dopamine antagonists such as neuroleptics or metoclopramide.

5. PHARMACOLOGICAL PROPERTIES

5.1 Pharmacodynamic properties

Ropinirole is a non-ergoline dopamine agonist.

Parkinson's disease is characterised by a marked dopamine deficiency in the nigral striatal system. Ropinirole alleviates this deficiency by stimulating striatal dopamine receptors.

Ropinirole acts in the hypothalamus and pituitary to inhibit the secretion of prolactin.

5.2 Pharmacokinetic properties

Oral absorption of ropinirole is rapid and essentially complete. Bioavailability of ropinirole is approximately 50% and average peak concentrations of the drug are achieved at a median time of 1.5 hours post-dose. Wide inter-individual variability in the pharmacokinetic parameters has been seen but, overall, there is a proportional increase in the systemic exposure (Cmax and AUC) to the drug with an increase in dose, over the therapeutic dose range. Consistent with its high lipophilicity, ropinirole exhibits a large volume of distribution (approx. 8 l/kg) and is cleared from the systemic circulation with an average elimination half-life of about six hours. Plasma protein binding of the drug is low (10-40%). Ropinirole is metabolised primarily by oxidative metabolism and ropinirole and its metabolites are mainly excreted in the urine. The major metabolite is at least 100 times less potent than ropinirole in animal models of dopaminergic function.

No change in the oral clearance of ropinirole is observed following single and repeated oral administration. As expected for a drug being administered approximately every half life, there is, on average, two-fold higher steady-state plasma concentrations of ropinirole following the recommended t.i.d. regimen compared to those observed following a single oral dose.

5.3 Preclinical safety data

General toxicology: Ropinirole caused no serious or irreversible toxicity in laboratory animals at 15mg/kg (monkey), 20mg/kg (mouse) or 50mg/kg (rat). The toxicology profile is principally determined by the pharmacological activity of the drug (behavioural changes, hypoprolactinaemia, decrease in blood pressure and heart rate, ptosis and salivation).

Genotoxicity: Genotoxicity was not observed in a battery of in vitro and in vivo tests.

Carcinogenicity: Two-year studies have been conducted in the mouse and rat at dosages up to 50 mg/kg. The mouse study did not reveal any carcinogenic effect. In the rat, the only drug-related lesions were Leydig cell hyperplasia/adenoma in the testis resulting from the hypoprolactinaemic effect of ropinirole. These lesions are considered to be a species specific phenomenon and do not constitute a hazard with regard to the clinical use of ropinirole.

6. PHARMACEUTICAL PARTICULARS

6.1 List of excipients

Tablet cores: hydrous lactose, microcrystalline cellulose, croscarmellose sodium, magnesium stearate.

The five tablet strengths of ropinirole are distinguished by colour. The composition of the film coat therefore varies. All film coats contain hydroxypropyl methylcellulose and polyethylene glycol. The variations are shown in the table below:

(see Table 1 below)

6.2 Incompatibilities

None known

6.3 Shelf life

Two years

6.4 Special precautions for storage

This product should be stored in a dry place at or below 25°C and protected from light.

Table 1

	Tablet strength (mg) and colour				
	0.25	0.5	1.0	2.0	5.0
Tablet Colour	White	Yellow	Green	Pink	Blue
Titanium Dioxide	√	√	√	√	√
Iron Oxide Yellow		√	√	√	
Iron Oxide Red		√		√	
Indigo Carmine Aluminium		√	√		√
Polysorbate 80	√				√

6.5 Nature and contents of container

Opaque PVC/PVdC or PVC/Aclar or PVC/Aclar/PVC blister starter pack of 105. (Each pack contains 42 ReQuip 0.25mg tablets, 42 ReQuip 0.5mg tablets and 21 ReQuip 1mg tablets.)

Opaque PVC/PVdC or PVC/Aclar or PVC/Aclar/PVC blister follow on pack of 147. (Each pack contains 42 ReQuip 0.5mg tablets, 42 Requip 1mg tablets, 63 Requip 2mg tablets.)

Tablets 1 mg, in 60 ml HPDE bottle of 84.

Tablets 2 mg, in 60 ml HPDE bottle of 84.

Tablets 5 mg, in 60 ml HPDE bottle of 84.

NOT ALL PACK SIZES MAY BE MARKETED

6.6 Special precautions for disposal and other handling

None

Administrative Data

7. MARKETING AUTHORISATION HOLDER

SmithKline Beecham plc

Trading as:

GlaxoSmithKline UK,

Stockley Park West,

Uxbridge,

Middlesex UB11 1BT

8. MARKETING AUTHORISATION NUMBER(S)

Requip Tablets 0.25 mg 10592/0085

Requip Tablets 0.5 mg 10592/0086

Requip Tablets 1 mg 10592/0087

Requip Tablets 2 mg 10592/0088

Requip Tablets 5 mg 10592/0089

9. DATE OF FIRST AUTHORISATION/RENEWAL OF THE AUTHORISATION

24th January 2002

10. DATE OF REVISION OF THE TEXT

17 September 2009

11. Legal Status

POM

Requip XL prolonged-release tablets

(GlaxoSmithKline UK)

1. NAME OF THE MEDICINAL PRODUCT

Requip® XL▼ 2, 4 or 8 mg prolonged-release tablets.

2. QUALITATIVE AND QUANTITATIVE COMPOSITION

2 / 4 / 8 mg ropinirole (as hydrochloride).

Excipient(s):

Lactose

Sunset yellow (E110) - 4 mg only

For a full list of excipients, see section 6.1.

3. PHARMACEUTICAL FORM

Prolonged-release tablet.

2 mg: Pink capsule-shaped, film-coated tablets marked "GS" on one side and "3V2" on the other.

4 mg: Light brown capsule-shaped, film-coated tablets marked "GS" on one side and "WXG" on the other.

8 mg: Red capsule-shaped, film-coated tablets marked "GS" on one side and "5CC" on the other.

4. CLINICAL PARTICULARS

4.1 Therapeutic indications

Treatment of idiopathic Parkinson's disease in patients already taking ropinirole immediate release tablets and in whom adequate symptomatic control has been established.

Substitution of ropinirole prolonged-release tablets (Requip XL) for ropinirole immediate release tablets may be used as:

(i) Monotherapy, alone (without levodopa) in idiopathic Parkinson's disease or as

(ii) Adjunctive therapy in addition to levodopa to control "on-off" fluctuations which might permit a reduction in the total daily dose of levodopa.

Substitution of Requip XL for ropinirole immediate release tablets should be supervised by appropriate specialists in Parkinson's disease.

4.2 Posology and method of administration

Oral use.

Ropinirole prolonged-release tablets should be taken once a day and at a similar time each day. The tablets must be swallowed whole and must not be chewed, crushed or divided. The tablets may be taken with or without food.

Adults

Switching from ropinirole immediate release tablets to ropinirole prolonged-release tablets

Patients should be considered for switching to ropinirole prolonged-release tablets only after they have achieved sufficient symptomatic control on ropinirole immediate release tablets.

Patients may be switched overnight from ropinirole immediate release tablets to ropinirole prolonged-release tablets.

The dose of ropinirole prolonged-release tablets should be based on the total daily dose of immediate release formulation that the patient was receiving. The recommended dose for switching from ropinirole immediate release tablets to ropinirole prolonged-release tablets are provided in the following table. If patients are taking a different total daily dose of ropinirole immediate release tablets to those typically prescribed doses as shown in the table, they should be switched to the nearest available dose of ropinirole prolonged-release tablets as stated in the table:

Ropinirole immediate release tablets (Requip) Total daily dose (mg)	Ropinirole prolonged-release tablets (Requip XL) Total daily dose (mg)
3 - 4.5	4
6	6
7.5 - 9	8
12	12
15 - 18	16
21	20
24	24

After switching to Requip XL prolonged-release tablets, patients will initially require more frequent and careful monitoring in order to adjust the dose if necessary.

If sufficient symptomatic control is not maintained after switching to a dose of less than 8 mg once daily of ropinirole prolonged-release tablets, the daily dose may be increased by 2 mg at weekly or longer intervals up to a dose of 8 mg once daily of ropinirole prolonged-release tablets.

If sufficient symptomatic control is not achieved or maintained at a dose of 8 mg or greater once daily of ropinirole prolonged-release tablets, the daily dose may be increased by 2 mg at two weekly or longer intervals.

Individual dose titration against efficacy and tolerability is recommended.

Patients should be maintained on the lowest dose of ropinirole prolonged-release tablets that achieves symptomatic control.

The maximum daily dose of Requip XL is 24 mg. Doses above 24 mg/day have not been studied in clinical trials.

When ropinirole prolonged-release tablets are administered as adjunct therapy to levodopa, it may be possible to gradually reduce the levodopa dose, depending on the clinical response. In patients with advanced Parkinson's disease receiving ropinirole in combination with L-dopa, dyskinesias can occur during the initial titration of ropinirole. In clinical trials it was shown that a reduction of the L-dopa dose may ameliorate dyskinesia (see also 4.8 Undesirable effects).

The dose in patients experiencing disabling somnolence should be down titrated; for some other adverse events, down-titration followed by more gradual up-titration has been shown to be beneficial.

Dose interruption or discontinuation

If treatment is interrupted for one day or more, re-initiation by dose titration on ropinirole immediate release tablets should be considered.

If it is necessary to discontinue ropinirole treatment, this should be done gradually by reducing the daily dose over the period of one week.

When switching treatment from another dopamine agonist to ropinirole, the manufacturer's guidance on discontinuation should be followed before initiating ropinirole immediate release tablets according to the recommended titration regimen. Patients can be switched to ropinirole prolonged-release tablets once sufficient symptomatic control is achieved (see 'Starting dose').

Renal and hepatic impairment

In parkinsonian patients with mild to moderate renal impairment (creatinine clearance between 30 and 50 ml/min) no change in the clearance of ropinirole was observed, indicating that no dosage adjustment is necessary in this population.

The use of ropinirole in patients with severe renal (creatinine clearance less than 30 ml/min) impairment or hepatic impairment has not been studied. Administration of ropinirole to such patients is not recommended.

Elderly

The clearance of ropinirole is decreased in patients over 65 years of age. The increase in dosage should be gradual and titrated against the symptomatic response.

Children and adolescents

Ropinirole has not been studied in patients under 18 years of age therefore, ropinirole is not recommended for use in patients within this age group.

4.3 Contraindications

Hypersensitivity to ropinirole or to any of the excipients.

In light of the results of animal studies and the lack of studies in human pregnancy, ropinirole is contraindicated in pregnancy, lactation and in women of child-bearing potential unless adequate contraception is used (see Section 4.6).

4.4 Special warnings and precautions for use

Due to the pharmacological action of ropinirole, patients with severe cardiovascular disease should be treated with caution.

Co-administration of ropinirole with anti-hypertensive and anti-arrhythmic agents has not been studied. Caution should be exercised when these compounds are given concomitantly with ropinirole because of the unknown potential for the occurrence of hypotension, bradycardias or other arrhythmias.

Patients with a history or presence of major psychotic disorders should only be treated with dopamine agonists if the potential benefits outweigh the risks (see also section 4.5).

Pathological gambling, increased libido and hypersexuality have been reported in patients treated with dopamine agonists for Parkinson's disease, including ropinirole.

Ropinirole has been associated with somnolence and episodes of sudden sleep onset, particularly in patients with Parkinson's disease. Sudden onset of sleep during daily activities, in some cases without awareness or warning signs, has been reported uncommonly. Patients must be informed of this and advised to exercise caution while driving or operating machines during treatment with ropinirole. Patients who have experienced somnolence and/or an episode of sudden sleep onset must refrain from driving or operating machines. Furthermore, a reduction of dosage or termination of therapy may be considered.

Patients with rare hereditary problems of galactose intolerance, the Lapp lactase deficiency or glucose-galactose malabsorption should not take this medicine.

The 4 mg tablets contain the azo colouring agent sunset yellow (E110), which may cause allergic reactions.

4.5 Interaction with other medicinal products and other forms of interaction

Neuroleptics and other centrally active dopamine antagonists, such as sulpiride or metoclopramide, may diminish the effectiveness of ropinirole and, therefore, concomitant use of these drugs with ropinirole should be avoided.

There is no pharmacokinetic interaction between ropinirole and L-dopa or domperidone which would necessitate dosage adjustment of these drugs. No interaction has been seen between ropinirole and other drugs commonly used to treat Parkinson's disease but, as is common practice, care should be taken when adding a new drug to a treatment regimen. Other dopamine agonists may be used with caution.

In a study in parkinsonian patients receiving concurrent digoxin, no interaction was seen which would require dosage adjustment.

It has been established from *in vitro* experiments that ropinirole is metabolised by the cytochrome P450 enzyme CYP1A2. There is, therefore, the potential for an interaction between ropinirole and substrates (such as theophylline) or inhibitors (such as ciprofloxacin, fluvoxamine and cimetidine) of this enzyme. In patients already receiving ropinirole, the dose of ropinirole may need to be adjusted when these drugs are introduced or withdrawn.

Increased plasma concentrations of ropinirole have been observed in patients treated with high doses of oestrogens. In patients already receiving hormone replacement therapy (HRT), ropinirole treatment may be initiated in the normal manner. However, if HRT is stopped or introduced during treatment with ropinirole, dosage adjustment may be required.

No information is available on the potential for interaction between ropinirole and alcohol. As with other centrally active medications, patients should be made aware of the effects of taking ropinirole with alcohol.

Smoking is known to induce CYP1A2 metabolism, therefore if patients stop or start smoking during treatment with ropinirole, adjustment of dose may be required.

4.6 Pregnancy and lactation

Ropinirole should not be used during pregnancy. In animal studies, administration of ropinirole to pregnant rats at maternally toxic doses resulted in decreased foetal body weight at 60 mg/kg (approximately three times the AUC of the maximum dose in man), increased foetal death at 90 mg/kg (~x5) and digit malformations at 150 mg/kg (~x9). There was no teratogenic effect in the rat at 120 mg/kg (~x7) and no indication of an effect on development in the rabbit. There have been no studies of ropinirole in human pregnancy.

Ropinirole should not be used in nursing mothers as it may inhibit lactation.

4.7 Effects on ability to drive and use machines

Patients should be warned about the possibility of dizziness (including vertigo). Patients being treated with ropinirole and presenting with somnolence and/or sudden sleep episodes must be informed to refrain from driving or engaging in activities where impaired alertness may put themselves or others at risk of serious injury or death (e.g. operating machines) until such recurrent episodes and somnolence have resolved (see also section 4.4).

4.8 Undesirable effects

Adverse events are listed below by system organ class and frequency. Frequencies are defined as: very common (>1/10), common (>1/100, <1/10), uncommon (>1/1,000, <1/100), rare (>1/10,000, <1/1,000) very rare (<1/10,000), including isolated reports.

Data are presented for adverse drug reactions reported at a higher rate with ropinirole than placebo or a higher or comparable rate to comparator in clinical trials.

During clinical trials, the most commonly reported undesirable effects for ropinirole prolonged-release tablets were nausea and somnolence during monotherapy and dyskinesia during adjunctive therapy with levodopa.

The following adverse events were reported during clinical trials up to 24 mg/day and other post-marketing experience with ropinirole tablets in the treatment of Parkinson's disease.

Immune system disorders	
Very rare	Hypersensitivity reactions (including urticaria, angioedema, rash, pruritus)[5].
Psychiatric disorders	
Common	Hallucinations, confusion[1]
Uncommon	Psychotic reactions (other than hallucinations), including delusion, paranoia, delirium. Patients treated with dopamine agonists for treatment of Parkinson's disease, including ropinirole, especially at high doses, have been reported as exhibiting signs of pathological gambling, increased libido and hypersexuality, generally reversible upon reduction of the dose or treatment discontinuation[5]
Nervous system disorders	
Very common	Dyskinesia[1,3,6], somnolence[2,4], syncope[2]
Common	Dizziness (including vertigo)[3,4], somnolence[3]
Uncommon	Extreme somnolence[5], sudden onset of sleep[5]
Vascular disorders	
Common	Postural hypotension[3,5], hypotension[3,5]
Uncommon	Postural hypotension[4], hypotension[4]
Gastrointestinal disorders	
Very common	Nausea[2,4]
Common	Nausea[1,3], constipation[3,4], abdominal pain[2], vomiting[2], dyspepsia[2]
General disorders and administrative site conditions	
Common	Peripheral oedema[2,3,4]
Hepatobiliary disorders	
Very rare	Hepatic enzymes increased[5]

1. Ropinirole immediate release tablets adjunct therapy clinical trial data only
2. Ropinirole immediate release tablets monotherapy clinical trial data only
3. Ropinirole prolonged-release tablets adjunct therapy clinical trial data only
4. Ropinirole prolonged-release tablets monotherapy clinical trial data only
5. Post-marketing data
6. In patients with advanced Parkinson's disease, dyskinesias can occur during the initial titration of ropinirole. In clinical trials it was shown that a reduction of the L-dopa dose may ameliorate dyskinesia (see 4.2 Posology and method of administration).

4.9 Overdose

The symptoms of ropinirole overdose are generally related to its dopaminergic activity. These symptoms may be alleviated by appropriate treatment with dopamine antagonists such as neuroleptics or metoclopramide.

5. PHARMACOLOGICAL PROPERTIES

5.1 Pharmacodynamic properties

Pharmacotherapeutic group

Non-ergoline dopamine agonist.

ATC code: N04BC04

Mechanism of action

Parkinson's disease is characterised by a marked dopamine deficiency in the nigral striatal system. Ropinirole is a non-ergoline D2/D3 dopamine agonist that alleviates this deficiency by stimulating striatal dopamine receptors.

Ropinirole acts in the hypothalamus and pituitary to inhibit the secretion of prolactin.

Clinical efficacy

A 36-week, double-blind, three-period crossover study, in monotherapy with a primary end point of change from period baseline in Unified Parkinson's Disease Rating Scale (UPDRS) total motor score was conducted in 161 patients with early phase Parkinson's disease. A subgroup analysis of patients initiated on monotherapy treatment with ropinirole immediate release tablets and switched overnight to the nearest equivalent dose of ropinirole prolonged-release tablets was consistent with similar efficacy from equivalent mg for mg doses. In separate pharmacokinetic studies the AUCs for these two formulations were found to be similar.

A 24-week, double-blind, placebo-controlled, parallel group study in patients with Parkinson's disease who were not optimally controlled on levodopa demonstrated that adjunctive therapy of ropinirole prolonged-release tablets results in clinically relevant and statistically significant superiority over placebo in a change from baseline in awake time "off" (adjusted mean treatment difference -1.7 hours, $p<0.0001$).

5.2 Pharmacokinetic properties

Wide inter-individual variability in the pharmacokinetic parameters has been seen. Bioavailability of ropinirole is approximately 50% (36–57%).

Absorption

Following oral administration of ropinirole prolonged-release tablets, plasma concentrations of ropinirole increase slowly, with a median time to Cmax of six hours. The bioavailability of ropinirole following administration of ropinirole prolonged-release tablets was similar in both the fed and fasted state.

Distribution

Plasma protein binding of the drug is low (10–40%). Consistent with its high lipophilicity, ropinirole exhibits a large volume of distribution (approximately 8 l/kg).

Metabolism

Ropinirole is primarily cleared by CYP1A2 metabolism and its metabolites are mostly excreted in the urine. The major metabolite is at least 100-times less potent than ropinirole in animal models of dopaminergic function.

Elimination

Ropinirole is cleared from the systemic circulation with an average elimination half-life of about six hours. The increase in systemic exposure (Cmax and AUC) to ropinirole is approximately proportional over the therapeutic dose range. No change in the oral clearance of ropinirole is observed following single and repeated oral administration.

5.3 Preclinical safety data

General toxicology

Ropinirole is well tolerated in laboratory animals in the dose range of 15-50 mg/kg. The toxicology profile is principally determined by the pharmacological activity of the drug (behavioural changes, hypoprolactinaemia, decrease in blood pressure and heart rate, ptosis and salivation).

Genotoxicity

Genotoxicity was not observed in a battery of *in vitro* and *in vivo* tests.

Carcinogenicity

Two-year studies have been conducted in the mouse and rat at dosages up to 50 mg/kg. The mouse study did not reveal any carcinogenic effect. In the rat, the only drug-related lesions were Leydig cell hyperplasia/adenoma in the testis resulting from the hypoprolactinaemic effect of ropinirole. These lesions are considered to be a species specific phenomenon and do not constitute a hazard with regard to the clinical use of ropinirole.

6. PHARMACEUTICAL PARTICULARS

6.1 List of excipients

Tablet core

Hypromellose 2208, hydrogenated castor oil, carmellose sodium, povidone K29-32, maltodextrin, magnesium stearate, lactose monohydrate, anhydrous colloidal silica, mannitol (E421), ferric oxide yellow (E172) and glycerol dibehenate.

Film coat

2 mg: Hypromellose 2910, ferric oxide yellow (E172), titanium dioxide (E171), macrogol 400 and ferric oxide red (E172).

4 mg: Hypromellose 2910, titanium dioxide (E171), macrogol 400, sunset yellow (E110) and indigo carmine (E132).

8 mg: Hypromellose 2910, ferric oxide yellow (E172), titanium dioxide (E171), ferric oxide black (E172), macrogol 400 and ferric oxide red (E172).

6.2 Incompatibilities

Not applicable.

6.3 Shelf life

ReQuip XL 2mg prolonged-release tablets 2 years.

ReQuip XL 4mg prolonged-release tablets 3 years.

ReQuip XL 8mg prolonged-release tablets 3 years.

6.4 Special precautions for storage

Do not store above 25°C. Store in the original package.

6.5 Nature and contents of container

PVC/PCTFE/Aluminium blister packs.

Packs of 28 prolonged-release tablets.

6.6 Special precautions for disposal and other handling

No special requirements.

7. MARKETING AUTHORISATION HOLDER

SmithKline Beecham plc
Great West Road,
Brentford,
Middlesex TW8 9GS
Trading as:
GlaxoSmithKline UK
Stockley Park West,
Uxbridge,
Middlesex UB11 1BT

8. MARKETING AUTHORISATION NUMBER(S)

Requip XL 2 mg prolonged-release tablets PL 10592/0293

Requip XL 4 mg prolonged-release tablets PL 10592/0295

Requip XL 8 mg prolonged-release tablets PL 10592/0296

9. DATE OF FIRST AUTHORISATION/RENEWAL OF THE AUTHORISATION

07/05/2008

10. DATE OF REVISION OF THE TEXT

05/06/2009

Resonium A

(sanofi-aventis)

1. NAME OF THE MEDICINAL PRODUCT

Resonium A.

2. QUALITATIVE AND QUANTITATIVE COMPOSITION

Contains Sodium Polystyrene Sulphonate 99.934% w/w.

3. PHARMACEUTICAL FORM

Buff coloured powder.

4. CLINICAL PARTICULARS

4.1 Therapeutic indications

Resonium A is an ion-exchange resin that is recommended for the treatment of hyperkalaemia associated with anuria or severe oliguria. It is also used to treat hyperkalaemia in patients requiring dialysis and in patients on regular haemodialysis or on prolonged peritoneal dialysis.

4.2 Posology and method of administration

Resonium A is for oral or rectal administration only.

The dosage recommendations detailed in this section are a guide only; the precise requirements should be decided on the basis of regular serum electrolyte determinations.

Adults, including the elderly:

Oral

The usual dose is 15g, three or four times a day. The resin is given by mouth in a little water, or it may be made into a paste with some sweetened vehicle.

Rectal

In cases where vomiting may make oral administration difficult, the resin may be given rectally as a suspension of 30g resin in 100ml 2% methylcellulose (medium viscosity) and 100ml water, as a daily retention enema. In the initial stages administration by this route as well as orally may help to achieve a more rapid lowering of the serum potassium level.

The enema should if possible be retained for at least nine hours following which the colon should be irrigated to remove the resin. If both routes are used initially it is probably unnecessary to continue rectal administration once the oral resin has reached the rectum.

Children:

Oral

1g/kg body weight daily in divided doses for acute hyperkalaemia. Dosage may be reduced to 0.5g/kg of body weight daily in divided doses for maintenance therapy.

The resin is given orally, preferably with a drink (not a fruit squash because of the high potassium content) or a little jam or honey.

Rectal

When refused by mouth it should be given rectally, using a dose at least as great as that which would have been given orally, diluted in the same ratio as described for adults.

Following retention of the enema, the colon should be irrigated to ensure adequate removal of the resin.

Neonates:

Resonium A should not be given by the oral route. With rectal administration, the minimum effective dosage within the range 0.5g/kg to 1g/kg should be employed diluted as for adults and with adequate irrigation to ensure recovery of the resin.

4.3 Contraindications

• In patients with plasma potassium levels below 5mmol/litre.

- History of hypersensitivity to polystyrene sulphonate resins.
- Obstructive bowel disease.
- Resonium A should not be administered ***orally*** to neonates and is contraindicated in neonates with reduced gut motility (post-operatively or drug-induced).

4.4 Special warnings and precautions for use

Hypokalaemia: The possibility of severe potassium depletion should be considered, and adequate clinical and biochemical control is essential during treatment, especially in patients on digitalis. Administration of the resin should be stopped when the serum potassium falls to 5mmol/litre.

Other electrolyte disturbances: Because the resin may bind calcium and magnesium ions, deficiencies of these electrolytes may occur. Accordingly, patients should be monitored for all applicable electrolyte disturbances.

Other risks: In the event of clinically significant constipation, treatment should be discontinued until normal bowel movement has resumed. Magnesium-containing laxatives should not be used (see section 4.5 Interactions).

The patient should be positioned carefully when ingesting the resin, in order to avoid aspiration, which may lead to bronchopulmonary complications.

Children and neonates: In neonates, sodium polystyrene sulphonate should not be given by the oral route. In children and neonates particular care is needed with rectal administration as excessive dosage or inadequate dilution could result in impaction of the resin. Due to the risk of digestive haemorrhage or colonic necrosis, particular care should be observed in premature infants or low birth weight infants.

Patients at risk from an increase in sodium load: Care should be taken when administering to patients in whom an increase in sodium load may be detrimental (i.e. congestive heart failure, hypertension, renal damage or oedema). In such cases, Calcium Resonium (calcium polystyrene sulphonate) may be used in place of Resonium A.

4.5 Interaction with other medicinal products and other forms of interaction

Concomitant use not recommended

Sorbitol (oral or rectal): Concomitant use of sorbitol with sodium polystyrene sulphonate may cause colonic necrosis. Therefore concomitant administration is not recommended.

To be used with caution

- Cation-donating agents: may reduce the potassium binding effectiveness of Resonium A.
- Non-absorbable cation-donating antacids and laxatives: There have been reports of systemic alkalosis following concurrent administration of cation-exchange resins and non-absorbable cation-donating antacids and laxatives such as magnesium hydroxide and aluminium carbonate.
- Aluminium hydroxide: Intestinal obstruction due to concretions of aluminium hydroxide has been reported when aluminium hydroxide has been combined with the resin.
- Digitalis-like drugs: The toxic effects of digitalis on the heart, especially various ventricular arrhythmias and A-V nodal dissociation, are likely to be exaggerated if hypokalaemia is allowed to develop. (see 4.4 Special warnings and special precautions for use).
- Lithium: Possible decrease of lithium absorption.
- Levothyroxine: Possible decrease of levothyroxine absorption.

4.6 Pregnancy and lactation

No data are available regarding the use of polystyrene sulphonate resins in pregnancy and lactation. The administration of Resonium A in pregnancy and during breast feeding therefore, is not advised unless, in the opinion of the physician, the potential benefits outweigh any potential risks.

4.7 Effects on ability to drive and use machines

There are no specific warnings.

4.8 Undesirable effects

In accordance with its pharmacological actions, the resin may give rise to sodium retention, hypokalaemia and hypocalcaemia and their related clinical manifestations (see Warnings and Precautions and Overdosage).

•Gastrointestinal disorders

Gastric irritation, anorexia, nausea, vomiting, constipation and occasionally diarrhoea may occur. Faecal impaction following rectal administration particularly in children, and gastrointestinal concretions (bezoars) following oral administration have been reported. Intestinal obstruction has also been reported although this has been extremely rare and, possibly, a reflection of co-existing pathology or inadequate dilution of resin.

Gastro-intestinal tract ulceration or necrosis which could lead to intestinal perforation have been reported following administration of sodium polystyrene sulphonate.

•Respiratory disorders

Some cases of acute bronchitis and/or bronco-pneumonia associated with inhalation of particles of sodium polystyrene sulphonate have been described.

4.9 Overdose

Biochemical disturbances from overdosage may give rise to clinical signs of symptoms of hypokalaemia, including irritability, confusion, delayed thought processes, muscle weakness, hyporeflexia and eventual paralysis. Apnoea may be a serious consequence of this progression. Electrocardiographic changes may be consistent with hypokalaemia; cardiac arrhythmia may occur. Hypocalcaemic tetany may occur. Appropriate measures should be taken to correct serum electrolytes and the resin should be removed from the alimentary tract by appropriate use of laxatives or enemas.

5. PHARMACOLOGICAL PROPERTIES

5.1 Pharmacodynamic properties

Resonium A is a cation exchange resin for the treatment of hyperkalaemia.

5.2 Pharmacokinetic properties

Ion exchange resins with a particle size ranging from 5 - 10 micrometres (as in Resonium A) are not absorbed from the gastro-intestinal tract and are wholly excreted in the faeces.

5.3 Preclinical safety data

There are no pre-clinical data of relevance to the prescriber which are additional to that already included in other sections of the SPC.

6. PHARMACEUTICAL PARTICULARS

6.1 List of excipients

Resonium A also contains: saccharin and vanillin.

6.2 Incompatibilities

There are no specific incompatibilities.

6.3 Shelf life

60 months.

6.4 Special precautions for storage

None stated.

6.5 Nature and contents of container

Supplied in HDPE containers with LDPE tamper evident closures containing 454g Resonium A together with a plastic scoop, which, when filled level, contains approximately 15g.

6.6 Special precautions for disposal and other handling

Refer to 4.2. Posology and method of administration.

7. MARKETING AUTHORISATION HOLDER

Sanofi-aventis

One Onslow Street

Guildford

Surrey

GU1 4YS

UK

8. MARKETING AUTHORISATION NUMBER(S)

11723/0070

9. DATE OF FIRST AUTHORISATION/RENEWAL OF THE AUTHORISATION

2 April 2003

10. DATE OF REVISION OF THE TEXT

27 April 2009

Legal category: P

Respontin Nebules

(Allen & Hanburys)

1. NAME OF THE MEDICINAL PRODUCT

Respontin$_{TM}$ Nebules$_{TM}$

2. QUALITATIVE AND QUANTITATIVE COMPOSITION

1ml or 2ml plastic ampoules containing 0.25mg/ml of Ipratropium Bromide Ph.Eur.

3. PHARMACEUTICAL FORM

Oral inhalation solution via a nebuliser.

4. CLINICAL PARTICULARS

4.1 Therapeutic indications

Respontin Nebules are indicated for the treatment of reversible airways obstruction.

4.2 Posology and method of administration

The recommended dose is:

Adults: 0.4 to 2ml solution (100-500 micrograms) up to four times daily.

Children (3 to 14 years): 0.4 to 2ml solution (100-500 micrograms) up to three times daily.

The volume of ipratropium bromide solution may need to be diluted in order to obtain a final volume suitable for the particular nebuliser used. If dilution is necessary use only sterile sodium chloride 0.9% solution.

There is no specific information on the use of the isotonic nebuliser solution in the elderly. Clinical trials with the previously available hypotonic formulation included patients over 65 years and no adverse reactions specific to this age group were reported.

4.3 Contraindications

Known hypersensitivity to any components of the formulation or to atropine.

4.4 Special warnings and precautions for use

Use of the nebuliser solution should be subject to close medical supervision during initial dosing. There have been rare reports of paradoxical bronchospasm associated with the administration of ipratropium bromide nebuliser solution. The patient should be advised to seek medical advice should a reduced response become apparent.

Patients must be instructed in the correct administration of Respontin Nebules and warned not to allow the solution or mist to enter the eyes. Acute angle-closure glaucoma has been reported rarely when ipratropium bromide has been used in conjunction with nebulised β_2-agonist bronchodilators. Protection of the eyes appears to prevent any increase in intra-ocular pressure and patients who may be susceptible to glaucoma should be warned specifically of the need for ocular protection. Inhaled doses of ipratropium bromide up to 1mg have not been associated with elevation of intra-ocular pressure.

Use anticholinergic agents with caution in patients with prostatic hypertrophy.

4.5 Interaction with other medicinal products and other forms of interaction

There is evidence that the concurrent administration of ipratropium bromide and sympathomimetic drugs produces a greater relief of bronchospasm than either drug given alone. Ipratropium bromide has been shown to produce effective bronchodilatation in patients receiving β-adrenergic blocking agents.

4.6 Pregnancy and lactation

Ipratropium bromide has been in general use for several years and there is no definite evidence of ill-consequence during pregnancy. Animal studies have shown no hazard. Nevertheless, medicines should not be used in pregnancy, especially during the first trimester, unless the expected benefit is thought to outweigh any possible risk to the fetus.

4.7 Effects on ability to drive and use machines

None stated.

4.8 Undesirable effects

Anticholinergic side-effects are unlikely at therapeutic doses, but some patients may experience a dry mouth. Urinary retention and constipation have only rarely been reported with ipratropium bromide. There is no evidence that in the therapeutic dose range, ipratropium bromide has any adverse effect on bronchial secretion.

4.9 Overdose

Inhaled doses of 5mg produce an increase in heart rate and palpitation but single doses at 2mg have been given to adults and 1mg to children without causing side-effects. Single doses of ipratropium bromide 30mg by mouth cause anticholinergic side effects but these are not severe and do not require specific reversal.

5. PHARMACOLOGICAL PROPERTIES

5.1 Pharmacodynamic properties

Ipratropium bromide is an anticholinergic bronchodilater which affects airways function primarily through its neural effects on the parasympathetic nervous system. Ipratropium bromide blocks the acetylcholine receptors on smooth muscle in the lung. Stimulation of these receptors normally produces contraction and depending on the degree of activation, bronchoconstriction. Thus ipratropium bromide will cause bronchodilatation.

5.2 Pharmacokinetic properties

Ipratoprium bromide is a quaternary ammonium compound which is poorly absorbed from the gastro-intestinal tract, and is slow to cross mucous membranes and the blood/brain barrier. Following, inhalation, uptake into the plasma is minimal, a peak blood concentration is obtained 1½ to 3 hours after inhalation. Excretion is chiefly via the kidneys.

5.3 Preclinical safety data

There are no pre-clinical data of relevance to the prescriber which are additional to that already included in other sections of the SmPC.

6. PHARMACEUTICAL PARTICULARS

6.1 List of excipients

Sodium Chloride	Ph.Eur
Diluted Phosphoric Acid	Ph.Eur
Purified Water	Ph.Eur

6.2 Incompatibilities

None stated.

6.3 Shelf life

24 months.

6.4 Special precautions for storage

Store below 25°C. Protect from light.

This product contains no preservative. A new Nebule should be used for each dose. A Nebule should be opened immediately before administration and any remaining solution should be discarded. Any unused Nebules should be discarded four weeks after opening the foil pack.

6.5 Nature and contents of container

1 or 2 ml low density polyethylene ampoules in boxes of 20 in strips of 5 or 10.

6.6 Special precautions for disposal and other handling

The nebulised solution may be inhaled through a face mask, T-piece or via an endotracheal tube. Intermittent positive pressure ventilation (IPPV) may be used but is rarely necessary. When there is a risk of anoxia through hypoventilation, oxygen should be added to the inspired air.

As many nebulisers operate on a continuous flow basis, it is likely that some nebulised drug will be released into the local environment. Ipratropium bromide should therefore be administered in a well-ventilated room, particularly in hospitals where several patients may be using nebulisers at the same time. Do not allow the solution or mist to enter the eyes.

Administrative Data

7. MARKETING AUTHORISATION HOLDER

Glaxo Wellcome UK Limited, trading as Allen & Hanburys,

Stockley Park West,

Uxbridge,

Middlesex,

UB11 1BT.

8. MARKETING AUTHORISATION NUMBER(S)

PL10949/0275

9. DATE OF FIRST AUTHORISATION/RENEWAL OF THE AUTHORISATION

15th April 2003

10. DATE OF REVISION OF THE TEXT

September 1997

11. Legal Status

POM.

Retin-A Gel 0.01%

(Janssen-Cilag Ltd)

1. NAME OF THE MEDICINAL PRODUCT

RETIN-A® Gel 0.01%.

2. QUALITATIVE AND QUANTITATIVE COMPOSITION

Tretinoin 0.01% w/w.

3. PHARMACEUTICAL FORM

Gel.

4. CLINICAL PARTICULARS

4.1 Therapeutic indications

Treatment of acne vulgaris. Suitable for use on oily skin.

4.2 Posology and method of administration

Retin-A should be applied once or twice daily to the area of skin where acne lesions occur.

Only apply sufficient to cover the affected areas lightly, using a gauze swab, cotton wool or the tips of clean fingers. Avoid over-saturation to the extent that excess medication could run into the eyes, angles of the nose or other areas where treatment is not intended.

Initial application may cause transitory stinging and a feeling of warmth. The correct frequency of administration should produce a slight erythema similar to that of mild sunburn.

If Retin-A is applied excessively, no more rapid or better results will be obtained and marked redness, peeling or discomfort may occur. Should this occur accidentally or through over enthusiastic use, application should be discontinued for a few days.

Patience is needed in this treatment, since the therapeutic effects will not usually be observed until after 6-8 weeks of treatment. During the early weeks of treatment, an apparent exacerbation of inflammatory lesions may occur. This is due to the action of the medication on deep, previously unseen comedones and papules.

Once the acne lesions have responded satisfactorily, it should be possible to maintain the improvement with less frequent applications.

Moisturisers and cosmetics may be used during treatment with Retin-A but should not be applied to the skin at the same time. The skin should be thoroughly washed before application of Retin-A. Astringent toiletries should be avoided.

Method of administration

For cutaneous administration.

4.3 Contraindications

Retin-A Gel is contraindicated in patients with:

- A history of sensitivity/hypersensitivity reactions to any of the components

- Pregnancy

- Personal or familial history of cutaneous epithelioma

- Acute eczemas (as tretinoin has been reported to cause severe irritation on eczematous skin)

- Rosacea and perioral dermatitis.

4.4 Special warnings and precautions for use

Local irritation

The presence of cutaneous irritative signs (eg erythema, peeling, pruritus, sunburn, etc) should prohibit initiation or recommencement of treatment with Retin-A until the symptoms resolve.

In certain sensitive individuals, topical use may induce severe local erythema, swelling, pruritus, warmth, burning or stinging, blistering, crusting and/or peeling at the site of application. If the degree of local irritation warrants, the patient should be directed to apply the medication less frequently or discontinue its use temporarily. If a patient experiences severe or persistent irritation, the patient should be advised to discontinue application of Retin-A completely and, if necessary, consult a physician.

Weather extremes, such as wind or cold, also may be irritating to patients being treated with Retin-A.

Exposure to sunlight

Exposure to sunlight, including ultraviolet sunlamps, should be avoided or minimised during the use of tretinoin. Patients with sunburn should be advised not to use the product until fully recovered because of potential severe irritation to skin. A patient who experiences considerable sun exposure due to occupational duties and/or anyone inherently sensitive to the sun should exercise particular caution. When exposure to sunlight cannot be avoided, use of sunscreen products and protective clothing over treated areas is recommended.

General precautions for use

Before application of Retin-A, areas to be treated should be cleansed thoroughly.

Abstain from washing the treated area frequently: twice daily is sufficient. Use of mild soap is recommended. Dry skin without rubbing.

Avoid contact with eyes, eyelids, nostrils, mouth and mucous membranes. If contact in these areas occurs, careful washing with water is recommended.

Warning

The weight of evidence indicates that topical tretinoin is not carcinogenic. In a lifetime study of CD-1 mice, a low incidence of skin tumours was seen at 100 and 200 times the estimated clinical dose but, although no such tumours were seen in the study controls, the incidence in these treated animals was within the historic control range for CD-1 mice.

Studies in hairless albino mice suggest that tretinoin may accelerate the tumorigenic potential of UVB light from a solar simulator. In other studies, when lightly pigmented hairless mice treated with tretinoin were exposed to carcinogenic doses of UVB light, the photocarcinogenic effects of tretinoin were not observed. Due to significantly different experimental conditions, no strict comparison of this disparate data is possible. Although the significance of these studies in man is not clear, patients should avoid or minimise exposure to sunlight.

The weight of evidence indicates that topical tretinoin is not mutagenic. The mutagenic potential of tretinoin was evaluated in the Ames assay and the *in vivo* mouse micronucleus assay, both of which showed negative findings.

4.5 Interaction with other medicinal products and other forms of interaction

Retin-A should be used with caution in the presence of:

– concomitant topical medications

– toiletry preparations having a strong drying, abrasive or desquamative effect.

Following prolonged use of a peeling agent it is advisable to 'rest' a patient's skin until the effects of the peeling agent subside before the use of Retin-A is begun. When Retin-A and peeling agents are alternated contact dermatitis may result and the frequency of application may have to be reduced.

4.6 Pregnancy and lactation

The topical human dose used in a 50 kg adult applying a maximum volume of 500 mg of 0.05% Retin-A cream is 0.005 mg/kg. In animal reproductive studies, oral tretinoin is known to be teratogenic and has been shown to be foetotoxic in rats when given in doses 500 times the topical human dose. In reproduction studies in rats and rabbits, topical tretinoin, when used at doses 500 and 320 times the topical human dose, respectively, induced minor skeletal abnormalities, eg irregularly contoured or partially ossified skull bones. These changes may be considered variants of normal development and are usually corrected after weaning. Retin-A should not be used during pregnancy.

It is not known whether tretinoin is excreted in human milk, therefore caution should be exercised when Retin-A is administered to a nursing mother.

4.7 Effects on ability to drive and use machines

Retin-A is administered topically and is unlikely to have an effect on one's ability to drive or operate machinery.

4.8 Undesirable effects

Local reactions frequently reported during therapy included: dry or peeling skin, burning, stinging, warmth, erythema, pruritus, rash and temporary hypo- and hyperpigmentation. These skin reactions were usually mild to moderate and were generally well-tolerated. They usually occurred early in therapy and, except for dry or peeling skin which persisted during therapy, generally decreased over the course of therapy.

Rarely reported undesirable effects are blistering and crusting of the skin, eye irritation and oedema.

True contact allergy to topical tretinoin is rarely encountered. Heightened susceptibility to either sunlight or other sources of UVB light has been reported.

4.9 Overdose

Excessive application of Retin-A does not improve the results of treatment and may induce marked irritation, eg erythema, peeling, pruritus, etc. Oral ingestion of Retin-A may lead to the same effects associated with excessive oral intake of vitamin A (eg pruritus, dry skin, arthralgias, anorexia, vomiting). In the event of accidental ingestion, if the ingestion is recent an appropriate method of gastric emptying should be used as soon as possible.

5. PHARMACOLOGICAL PROPERTIES

5.1 Pharmacodynamic properties

Tretinoin (β-all *trans* retinoic acid, vitamin A acid) produces profound metabolic changes in keratinizing epithelia. Tretinoin increases the proliferative activity of epidermal cells in *in vivo* and *in vitro* studies, and cellular differentiation (keratinization and cornification) is also altered.

5.2 Pharmacokinetic properties

Topical administration of Retin-A products produces dose-dependent erythema, peeling and irritation and excessive use of the products should be avoided. Retin-A 0.1% w/w did not produce an allergic response when tested in 160 subjects by the Draize test. The percutaneous absorption of 0.1% w/w C^{14} labelled retinoic acid was studied in 6 adult male volunteers; between 0.3% and 2.18% of the retinoic acid was absorbed through the skin following a single topical application of the ^{14}C retinoic acid formulation. No systemic toxic effects have been reported following topical application of Retin-A formulations.

5.3 Preclinical safety data

See Sections 4.4 (Special warnings and precautions) and 4.6 (Pregnancy and lactation).

6. PHARMACEUTICAL PARTICULARS

6.1 List of excipients

Butylated hydroxytoluene

Hydroxypropyl cellulose

Undenatured ethanol

6.2 Incompatibilities

Avoid or minimise exposure of Retin-A areas to sunlight or sunlamps during the course of treatment.

6.3 Shelf life

36 months.

6.4 Special precautions for storage

Do not store above 25°C.

6.5 Nature and contents of container

Aluminium tube lined with epoxy resin or epoxy resin with wax. Tube cap of polyethylene or urea resin.

Aluminium tube may contain 20 or 60 g of gel per pack.

(Not all pack sizes are marketed.)

6.6 Special precautions for disposal and other handling

Not applicable.

7. MARKETING AUTHORISATION HOLDER

Janssen-Cilag Ltd

50-100 Holmers Farm Way

High Wycombe

Buckinghamshire

HP12 4EG

UK

8. MARKETING AUTHORISATION NUMBER(S)

PL 00242/0265

9. DATE OF FIRST AUTHORISATION/RENEWAL OF THE AUTHORISATION

1 September 1995/November 2004

10. DATE OF REVISION OF THE TEXT

29 June 2009

Legal category POM.

Retin-A Gel 0.025%

(Janssen-Cilag Ltd)

1. NAME OF THE MEDICINAL PRODUCT

RETIN-A® Gel 0.025% w/w

2. QUALITATIVE AND QUANTITATIVE COMPOSITION

Tretinoin BP 0.025% w/w.

3. PHARMACEUTICAL FORM

Gel.

4. CLINICAL PARTICULARS

4.1 Therapeutic indications

Treatment of acne vulgaris.

Retin-A Gel is suitable for use on oily skin.

4.2 Posology and method of administration

Retin-A should be applied once or twice daily to the area of skin where acne lesions occur.

Only apply sufficient to cover the affected areas lightly, using a gauze swab, cotton wool or the tips of clean fingers. Avoid over-saturation to the extent that excess medication could run into the eyes, angles of the nose or other areas where treatment is not intended.

Initial application may cause transitory stinging and a feeling of warmth. The correct frequency of administration should produce a slight erythema similar to that of mild sunburn.

If Retin-A is applied excessively, no more rapid or better results will be obtained and marked redness, peeling or discomfort may occur. Should this occur accidentally or through over enthusiastic use, application should be discontinued for a few days.

Patience is needed in this treatment, since the therapeutic effects will not usually be observed until after 6-8 weeks of treatment. During the early weeks of treatment, an apparent exacerbation of inflammatory lesions may occur. This is due to the action of the medication on deep, previously unseen comedones and papules.

Once the acne lesions have responded satisfactorily, it should be possible to maintain the improvement with less frequent applications.

Moisturisers and cosmetics may be used during treatment with Retin-A but should not be applied to the skin at the same time. The skin should be thoroughly washed before application of Retin-A. Astringent toiletries should be avoided.

Method of Administration

Cutaneous use.

4.3 Contraindications

Retin-A is contraindicated in patients with:

- A history of sensitivity/hypersensitivity reactions to any of the components
- Pregnancy
- Personal or familial history of cutaneous epithelioma
- Acute eczemas (as tretinoin has been reported to cause severe irritation on eczematous skin)
- Rosacea and perioral dermatitis.

4.4 Special warnings and precautions for use

Local irritation

The presence of cutaneous irritative signs (eg erythema, peeling, pruritus, sunburn etc) should prohibit initiation or recommencement of treatment with Retin-A until the symptoms resolve.

In certain sensitive individuals, topical use may induce severe local erythema, swelling, pruritus, warmth, burning or stinging, blistering, crusting and/or peeling at the site of application. If the degree of local irritation warrants, the patient should be directed to apply the medication less frequently or discontinue its use temporarily. If a patient experiences severe or persistent irritation, the patient should be advised to discontinue application of Retin-A completely and, if necessary, consult a physician.

Weather extremes, such as wind or cold, also may be irritating to patients being treated with Retin-A.

Exposure to sunlight, including ultraviolet sunlamps, should be avoided or minimised during the use of tretinoin. Patients with sunburn should be advised not to use the product until fully recovered because of potential severe irritation to skin. A patient who experiences considerable sun exposure due to occupational duties and/or anyone inherently sensitive to the sun should exercise particular caution. When exposure to sunlight cannot be avoided, use of sunscreen products and protective clothing over treated areas is recommended.

General precautions for use:

Before application of Retin-A, areas to be treated should be cleansed thoroughly.

Abstain from washing the treated area frequently: twice daily is sufficient. Use of mild soap is recommended. Dry skin without rubbing.

Avoid contact with eyes, eyelids, nostrils, mouth and mucous membranes. If contact in these areas occurs, careful washing with water is recommended.

Warning:

The weight of evidence indicates that topical tretinoin is not carcinogenic. In a lifetime study of CD-1 mice, a low incidence of skin tumours was seen at 100 and 200 times the estimated clinical dose but, although no such tumours were seen in the study controls, the incidence in these treated animals was within the historic control range for CD-1 mice.

Studies in hairless albino mice suggest that tretinoin may accelerate the tumorigenic potential of UVB light from a solar simulator. In other studies, when lightly pigmented hairless mice treated with tretinoin were exposed to carcinogenic doses of UVB light, the photocarcinogenic effects of tretinoin were not observed. Due to significantly different experimental conditions, no strict comparison of this disparate data is possible. Although the significance of these studies in man is not clear, patients should avoid or minimise exposure to sunlight.

The weight of evidence indicates that topical tretinoin is not mutagenic. The mutagenic potential of tretinoin was evaluated in the Ames assay and the *in-vivo* mouse micronucleus assay, both of which showed negative findings.

4.5 Interaction with other medicinal products and other forms of interaction

Retin-A should be used with caution in the presence of:

– concomitant topical medications

– toiletry preparations having a strong drying, abrasive or desquamative effect.

Following prolonged use of a peeling agent it is advisable to 'rest' a patients skin until the effects of the peeling agent subside before the use of Retin-A is begun. When Retin-A and peeling agents are alternated contact dermatitis may result and the frequency of application may have to be reduced.

4.6 Pregnancy and lactation

The topical human dose used in a 50 kg adult applying a maximum volume of 500 mg of 0.05% Retin-A cream is 0.005 mg/kg. In animal reproductive studies, oral tretinoin is known to be teratogenic and has been shown to be foetotoxic in rats when given in doses 500 times the topical human dose. In reproduction studies in rats and rabbits, topical tretinoin, when used at doses 500 and 320 times the topical human dose, respectively, induced minor skeletal abnormalities, eg irregularly contoured or partially ossified skull bones. These changes may be considered variants of normal development and are usually corrected after weaning. Retin-A should not be used during pregnancy.

It is not known whether tretinoin is excreted in human milk, therefore caution should be exercised when Retin-A is administered to a nursing mother.

4.7 Effects on ability to drive and use machines

Retin-A is administered topically and is unlikely to have an effect on one's ability to drive or operate machinery.

4.8 Undesirable effects

Local reactions frequently reported during therapy included: dry or peeling skin, burning, stinging, warmth, erythema, pruritus, rash and temporary hypo- and hyperpigmentation. These skin reactions were usually mild to moderate and were generally well-tolerated. They usually occurred early in therapy and, except for dry or peeling skin which persisted during therapy, generally decreased over the course of therapy.

Rarely reported undesirable effects are blistering and crusting of the skin, eye irritation and oedema.

True contact allergy to topical tretinoin is rarely encountered. Heightened susceptibility to either sunlight or other sources of UVB light has been reported.

4.9 Overdose

Excessive application of Retin-A does not improve the results of treatment and may induce marked irritation, e.g. erythema, peeling, pruritus etc. Oral ingestion of Retin-A may lead to the same effects associated with excessive oral intake of vitamin A (e.g. pruritus, dry skin, arthralgias, anorexia, vomiting). In the event of accidental ingestion, if the ingestion is recent an appropriate method of gastric emptying should be used as soon as possible.

5. PHARMACOLOGICAL PROPERTIES

5.1 Pharmacodynamic properties

Tretinoin (β-all *trans* retinoic acid, vitamin A acid) produces profound metabolic changes in keratinizing epithelia. Tretinoin increases the proliferative activity of epidermal cells in *in vivo* and *in vitro* studies, and cellular differentiation (keratinization and cornification) is also altered.

5.2 Pharmacokinetic properties

Topical administration of Retin-A products produces dose-dependent erythema, peeling and irritation and excessive use of the products should be avoided. Retin-A 0.025% w/w did not produce an allergic response when tested in 160 subjects by the Draize test. The percutaneous absorption of 0.1% w/w C^{14} labelled Retinoic Acid was studied in 6 adult male volunteers; between 0.3% and 2.18% of the retinoic acid was absorbed through the skin following a single topical application of the ^{14}C retinoic acid formulation. No systemic toxic effects have been reported following topical application of Retin-A formulations.

5.3 Preclinical safety data

See Sections 4.4 (Special warnings and precautions) and 4.6 (Pregnancy and lactation).

6. PHARMACEUTICAL PARTICULARS

6.1 List of excipients

Butylated hydroxytoluene

Hydroxypropyl cellulose

Undenatured ethanol

6.2 Incompatibilities

None known.

6.3 Shelf life

24 months.

6.4 Special precautions for storage

Do not store above 25°C.

6.5 Nature and contents of container

Aluminium tube lined with epoxy resin or epoxy resin with wax. Tube cap of polyethylene or urea resin.

Aluminium tube may contain 10, 15, 20 or 60 g of gel per pack.

6.6 Special precautions for disposal and other handling

Not applicable.

7. MARKETING AUTHORISATION HOLDER

Janssen-Cilag Limited

50-100 Holmers Farm Way

High Wycombe

Buckinghamshire

HP12 4EG

UK

8. MARKETING AUTHORISATION NUMBER(S)

PL 0242/0268

9. DATE OF FIRST AUTHORISATION/RENEWAL OF THE AUTHORISATION

1 September 1995/21 May 2003

10. DATE OF REVISION OF THE TEXT

29 June 2009

Legal category POM.

Retrovir 10 mg/ml IV for Infusion

(GlaxoSmithKline UK)

1. NAME OF THE MEDICINAL PRODUCT

Retrovir 10 mg/ml IV Concentrate for Solution for Infusion

2. QUALITATIVE AND QUANTITATIVE COMPOSITION

Vials containing zidovudine 200 mg in 20ml solution (10 mg zidovudine/ml)

For a full list of excipients, see section 6.1.

3. PHARMACEUTICAL FORM

Concentrate for solution for infusion (Sterile concentrate)

Retrovir IV for Infusion is a clear, nearly colourless, sterile aqueous solution with a pH of approximately 5.5.

4. CLINICAL PARTICULARS

4.1 Therapeutic indications

Retrovir IV for Infusion is indicated for the short-term management of serious manifestations of Human Immunodeficiency Virus (HIV) infection in patients with Acquired Immune Deficiency Syndrome (AIDS) who are unable to take Retrovir oral formulations. If at all possible Retrovir IV should not be used as monotherapy for this indication (see section 5.1).

Retrovir chemoprophylaxis, is indicated for use in HIV-positive pregnant women (over 14 weeks of gestation) for prevention of maternal-foetal HIV transmission and for primary prophylaxis of HIV infection in newborn infants. Retrovir IV should only be used when oral treatment is not possible (except during labour and delivery – see section 4.2).

4.2 Posology and method of administration

Retrovir should be prescribed by physicians who are experienced in the treatment of HIV infection.

The required dose of Retrovir IV for Infusion must be administered by slow intravenous infusion of the diluted product over a one-hour period.

Retrovir IV for Infusion must **NOT** be given intramuscularly.

Dilution: Retrovir IV for Infusion **must** be diluted prior to administration (see section 6.6).

Dosage in adults: A dose for Retrovir IV for Infusion of 1 or 2 mg zidovudine/kg bodyweight every 4 hours provides similar exposure (AUC) to an oral dose of 1.5 or 3.0 mg zidovudine/kg every 4 hours (600 or 1200 mg/day for a 70 kg patient). The current recommended oral dose of Retrovir is 250 or 300 mg twice daily. This current dose is used as part of a multi-drug treatment regimen.

Patients should receive Retrovir IV for Infusion only until oral therapy can be administered.

Dosage in children: Limited data are available on the use of Retrovir IV for Infusion in children. A range of intravenous dosages between 80-160 mg/m^2 every 6 hours (320-640 mg/ m^2/day) have been used. Exposure following the 120 mg/ m^2 dose every 6 hours approximately corresponds to an oral dose of 180 mg/m^2 every 6 hours. An oral dose of Retrovir of 360 to 480 mg/m^2 per day approximately corresponds to an intravenous dose of 240-320 mg/m^2/day.

Dosage in the prevention of maternal-foetal transmission: Pregnant women (over 14 weeks of gestation) should be given 500 mg/day orally (100 mg five times per day) until the beginning of labour. During labour and delivery Retrovir should be administered intravenously at 2 mg/kg bodyweight given over one hour followed by a continuous intravenous infusion at 1 mg/kg/h until the umbilical cord is clamped.

The newborn infants should be given 2 mg/kg bodyweight orally every 6 hours starting within 12 hours after birth and continuing until 6 weeks-old (e.g. a 3 kg neonate would require a 0.6 ml dose of oral solution every 6 hours). Infants unable to receive oral dosing should be given Retrovir intravenously at 1.5 mg/kg bodyweight infused over 30 minutes every 6 hours.

In case of planned caesarean, the infusion should be started 4 hours before the operation. In the event of a false labour, the Retrovir infusion should be stopped and oral dosing restarted.

Dosage adjustments in patients with haematological adverse reactions: Substitution of zidovudine should be considered in patients whose haemoglobin level or neutrophil count fall to clinically significant levels. Other potential causes of anaemia or neutropenia should be excluded. Retrovir dose reduction or interruption should be considered in the absence of alternative treatments (see sections 4.3 and 4.4).

Dosage in the elderly: Zidovudine pharmacokinetics have not been studied in patients over 65 years of age and no specific data are available. However, since special care is advised in this age group due to age-associated changes such as the decrease in renal function and alterations in haematological parameters, appropriate monitoring of patients before and during use of Retrovir is advised.

Dosage in renal impairment: In patients with severe renal impairment, the recommended IV dosage is 1 mg/kg 3-4 times daily. This is equivalent to the current recommended oral daily dosage for this patient group of 300 – 400 mg allowing for oral bioavailability of 60-70%. Haematological parameters and clinical response may influence the need for subsequent dosage adjustment. For patients with end-stage renal disease maintained on haemodialysis or peritoneal dialysis, the recommended dose is 100 mg every 6-8 hrs (300 mg – 400 mg daily) (see section 5.2).

Dosage in hepatic impairment: Data in patients with cirrhosis suggest that accumulation of zidovudine may occur in patients with hepatic impairment because of decreased glucuronidation. Dosage reductions may be necessary but, due to the large variability in zidovudine exposures in patients with moderate to severe liver disease, precise recommendations cannot be made. If monitoring of plasma zidovudine levels is not feasible, physicians will need to monitor for signs of intolerance, such as the development of haematological adverse reactions (anaemia, leucopenia, neutropenia) and reduce the dose and/or increase the interval between doses as appropriate (see section 4.4).

4.3 Contraindications

Retrovir IV for Infusion is contra-indicated in patients known to be hypersensitive to zidovudine, or to any of the excipients.

Retrovir IV for infusion should not be given to patients with abnormally low neutrophil counts (less than 0.75×10^9/litre) or abnormally low haemoglobin levels (less than 7.5 g/decilitre or 4.65 mmol/litre).

Retrovir is contra-indicated in newborn infants with hyperbilirubinaemia requiring treatment other than phototherapy, or with increased transaminase levels of over five times the upper limit of normal.

4.4 Special warnings and precautions for use

Retrovir is not a cure for HIV infection or AIDS. Patients receiving Retrovir or any other antiretroviral therapy may continue to develop opportunistic infections and other complications of HIV infection.

The concomitant use of rifampicin stavudine with zidovudine should be avoided (see section 4.5).

Haematological Adverse Reactions: Anaemia (usually not observed before six weeks of Retrovir therapy but occasionally occurring earlier), neutropenia (usually not observed before four weeks' therapy but sometimes occurring earlier) and leucopenia (usually secondary to neutropenia) can be expected to occur in patients receiving Retrovir IV for Infusion; These occurred more frequently at high dosages (1200-1500 mg/day orally) and in patients with poor bone marrow reserve prior to treatment, particularly with advanced HIV disease (see section 4.8).

Haematological parameters should be carefully monitored. It is recommended that blood tests are performed at least weekly in patients receiving Retrovir IV for Infusion.

If the haemoglobin level falls to between 7.5 g/dl (4.65 mmol/l) and 9 g/dl (5.59 mmol/l) or the neutrophil count falls to between 0.75×10^9/l and 1.0×10^9/l, the daily dosage may be reduced until there is evidence of marrow recovery; alternatively, recovery may be enhanced by brief (2-4 weeks) interruption of Retrovir therapy. Marrow recovery is usually observed within 2 weeks after which time Retrovir therapy at a reduced dosage may be reinstituted. Data on the use of Retrovir for periods in excess of 2 weeks are limited. In patients with significant anaemia, dosage adjustments do not necessarily eliminate the need for transfusions (see section 4.3).

> *Lactic acidosis*: lactic acidosis usually associated with hepatomegaly and hepatic steatosis has been reported with the use of nucleoside analogues. Early symptoms (symptomatic hyperlactatemia) include benign digestive symptoms (nausea, vomiting and abdominal pain), non-specific malaise, loss of appetite, weight loss, respiratory symptoms (rapid and/or deep breathing) or neurological symptoms (including motor weakness).
>
> Lactic acidosis has a high mortality and may be associated with pancreatitis, liver failure, or renal failure.
>
> Lactic acidosis generally occurred after a few or several months of treatment.
>
> Treatment with nucleoside analogues should be discontinued in the setting of symptomatic hyperlactatemia and metabolic/lactic acidosis, progressive hepatomegaly, or rapidly elevating aminotransferase levels.
>
> Caution should be exercised when administering nucleoside analogues to any patient (particularly obese women) with hepatomegaly, hepatitis or other known risk factors for liver disease and hepatic steatosis (including certain medicinal products and alcohol). Patients co-infected with hepatitis C and treated with alpha interferon and ribavirin may constitute a special risk.
>
> Patients at increased risk should be followed closely.

Mitochondrial toxicity: Nucleoside and nucleotide analogues have been demonstrated in vitro and in vivo to cause a variable degree of mitochondrial damage. There have been reports of mitochondrial dysfunction in HIV-negative infants exposed in utero and/or post-natally to nucleoside analogues. The main adverse events reported are haematological disorders (anaemia, neutropenia), metabolic disorders (hyperlactataemia, hyperlipasaemia). These events are often transitory. Some late-onset neurological disorders have been reported (hypertonia, convulsion, abnormal behaviour). Whether the neurological disorders are transient or permanent is currently unknown. Any child exposed in utero to nucleoside and nucleotide analogues, even HIV-negative children, should have clinical and laboratory follow-up and should be fully investigated for possible mitochondrial dysfunction in case of relevant signs or symptoms. These findings do not affect current recommendations to use antiretroviral therapy in pregnant women to prevent vertical transmission of HIV.

Lipodystrophy: Combination antiretroviral therapy has been associated with the redistribution of body fat (lipodystrophy) in HIV patients. The long-term consequences of these events are currently unknown. Knowledge about the mechanism is incomplete. A connection between visceral lipomatosis and PIs and lipoatrophy and NRTIs has been hypothesised. A higher risk of lipodystrophy has been associated with individual factors such as older age, and with drug related factors such as longer duration of antiretroviral treatment and associated metabolic disturbances. Clinical examination should include evaluation for physical signs of fat redistribution. Consideration should be given to the measurement of fasting serum lipids and blood glucose. Lipid disorders should be managed as clinically appropriate (see section 4.8).

Liver disease: Zidovudine clearance in patients with mild hepatic impairment without cirrhosis [Child-Pugh scores of 5-6] is similar to that seen in healthy subjects, therefore no zidovudine dose adjustment is required. In patients with moderate to severe liver disease [Child-Pugh scores of 7-15], specific dosage recommendations cannot be made due to the large variability in zidovudine exposure observed, therefore zidovudine use in this group of patients is not recommended.

Patients with chronic hepatitis B or C and treated with combination antiretroviral therapy are at an increased risk of severe and potentially fatal hepatic adverse events. In case of concomitant antiviral therapy for hepatitis B or C, please also refer to the relevant product information for these medicinal products.

Patients with pre-existing liver dysfunction, including chronic active hepatitis, have an increased frequency of liver function abnormalities during combination antiretroviral therapy and should be monitored according to standard practice. If there is evidence of worsening liver disease in such patients, interruption or discontinuation of treatment must be considered (see section 4.2).

Immune Reactivation Syndrome: In HIV-infected patients with severe immune deficiency at the time of institution of combination antiretroviral therapy (CART), an inflammatory reaction to asymptomatic or residual opportunistic pathogens may arise and cause serious clinical conditions, or aggravation of symptoms. Typically, such reactions have been observed within the first few weeks or months of initiation of CART. Relevant examples are cytomegalovirus retinitis, generalized and/or focal mycobacterial infections and Pneumocystis carinii pneumonia. Any inflammatory symptoms should be evaluated and treatment instituted when necessary.

Patients should be cautioned about the concomitant use of self-administered medications (see section 4.5).

Patients should be advised that Retrovir therapy has not been proven to prevent the transmission of HIV to others through sexual contact or contamination with blood.

Osteonecrosis: Although the etiology is considered to be multifactorial (including corticosteroid use, alcohol consumption, severe immunosuppression, higher body mass index), cases of osteonecrosis have been reported particularly in patients with advanced HIV-disease and/or long-term exposure to combination antiretroviral therapy (CART). Patients should be advised to seek medical advice if they experience joint aches and pain, joint stiffness or difficulty in movement.

4.5 Interaction with other medicinal products and other forms of interaction

Limited data suggests that co-administration of zidovudine with rifampicin decreases the AUC (area under the plasma concentration curve) of zidovudine by 48% ± 34%. This may result in a partial loss or total loss of efficacy of zidovudine. The concomitant use of rifampicin with zidovudine should be avoided (see section 4.4).

Zidovudine in combination with stavudine is antagonistic in vitro. The concomitant use of stavudine with zidovudine should be avoided (see section 4.4).

Probenecid increases the AUC of zidovudine by 106% (range 100 to 170%). Patients receiving both drugs should be closely monitored for haematological toxicity.

A modest increase in Cmax (28%) was observed for zidovudine when administered with lamivudine, however overall exposure (AUC) was not significantly altered. Zidovudine has no effect on the pharmacokinetics of lamivudine.

Phenytoin blood levels have been reported to be low in some patients receiving Retrovir, while in one patient a high level was noted. These observations suggest that phenytoin levels should be carefully monitored in patients receiving both drugs.

In a pharmacokinetic study co-administration of zidovudine and atovaquone showed a decrease in zidovudine clearance after oral dosing leading to a 35%±23% increase in plasma zidovudine AUC. The mode of interaction is unknown and as higher concentrations of atovaquone can be achieved with atovaquone suspension it is possible that greater changes in the AUC values for zidovudine might be induced when atovaquone is administered as a suspension. Given the limited data available the clinical significance of this is unknown.

Valproic acid, fluconazole or methadone when co-administered with zidovudine have been shown to increase the AUC with a corresponding decrease in its clearance. As only limited data are available the clinical significance of these findings is unclear but if zidovudine is used concurrently with either valproic acid, fluconazole or methadone, patients should be monitored closely for potential toxicity of zidovudine.

Concomitant treatment, especially acute therapy, with potentially nephrotoxic or myelosuppressive drugs (e.g. systemic pentamidine, dapsone, pyrimethamine, co-trimoxazole, amphotericin, flucytosine, ganciclovir, interferon, vincristine, vinblastine and doxorubicin) may also increase the risk of adverse reactions to zidovudine. If concomitant therapy with any of these drugs is necessary then extra care should be taken in monitoring renal function and haematological parameters and, if required, the dosage of one or more agents should be reduced.

Limited data from clinical trials do not indicate a significantly increased risk of adverse reactions to zidovudine with cotrimoxazole, aerosolised pentamidine, pyrimethamine and aciclovir at doses used in prophylaxis.

4.6 Pregnancy and lactation

Pregnancy:

The use of Retrovir in pregnant women over 14 weeks of gestation, with subsequent treatment of their newborn infants, has been shown to significantly reduce the rate of maternal-foetal transmission of HIV based on viral cultures in infants.

The results from the pivotal U.S. placebo-controlled study indicated that Retrovir reduced maternal-foetal transmission by approximately 70%. In this study, pregnant women had CD4 cell counts of 200 to 1818/mm^3 (median in treated group 560/mm^3) and began treatment therapy between weeks 14 and 34 of gestation and had no clinical indications for Retrovir therapy; their newborn infants received Retrovir until 6-weeks old.

A decision to reduce the risk of maternal transmission of HIV should be based on the balance of potential benefits and potential risk. Pregnant women considering the use of Retrovir during pregnancy for prevention of HIV transmission to their infants should be advised that transmission may still occur in some cases despite therapy.

The efficacy of zidovudine to reduce the maternal-foetal transmission in women with previously prolonged treatment with zidovudine or other antiretroviral agents or women infected with HIV strains with reduced sensitivity to zidovudine is unknown.

It is unknown whether there are any long-term consequences of in utero and infant exposure to Retrovir.

Based on the animal carcinogenicity/mutagenicity findings a carcinogenic risk to humans cannot be excluded (see section 5.3). The relevance of these findings to both infected and uninfected infants exposed to Retrovir is unknown. However, pregnant women considering using Retrovir during pregnancy should be made aware of these findings.

Given the limited data on the general use of Retrovir in pregnancy, Retrovir should only be used prior to the 14th week of gestation when the potential benefit to the mother and foetus outweigh the risks. Studies in pregnant rats and rabbits given zidovudine orally at dosage levels up to 450 and 500 mg/kg/day respectively during the major period of organogenesis have revealed no evidence of teratogenicity. There was, however, a statistically significant increase in foetal resorptions in rats given 150 to 450 mg/kg/day and in rabbits given 500 mg/kg/day.

A separate study, reported subsequently, found that rats given a dosage of 3000 mg/kg/day, which is very near the oral median lethal dose (3683 mg/kg), caused marked maternal toxicity and an increase in the incidence of foetal malformations. No evidence of teratogenicity was observed in this study at the lower dosages tested (600 mg/kg/day or less).

Fertility:

Zidovudine did not impair male or female fertility in rats given oral doses of up to 450 mg/kg/day. There are no data on the effect of Retrovir on human female fertility. In men, Retrovir has not been shown to affect sperm count, morphology or motility.

Lactation:

Health experts recommend that women infected with HIV do not breast feed their infants in order to avoid the transmission of HIV. After administration of a single dose of 200 mg zidovudine to HIV-infected women, the mean concentration of zidovudine was similar in human milk and serum. Therefore, since the drug and the virus pass into breast milk it is recommended that mothers taking Retrovir do not breast feed their infants.

4.7 Effects on ability to drive and use machines

Retrovir IV for Infusion is generally used in an in-patient hospital population and information on ability to drive and use machinery is not usually relevant. There have been no studies to investigate the effect of Retrovir on driving performance or the ability to operate machinery. Furthermore, a detrimental effect on such activities cannot be predicted from the pharmacology of the drug. Nevertheless, the clinical status of the patient and the adverse reaction profile of Retrovir should be borne in mind when considering the patient's ability to drive or operate machinery.

4.8 Undesirable effects

The adverse reaction profile appears similar for adults and children. The most serious adverse reactions include anaemia (which may require transfusions), neutropenia and leucopenia. These occurred more frequently at higher dosages (1200-1500 mg/day) and in patients with advanced HIV disease (especially when there is poor bone marrow reserve prior to treatment), and particularly in patients with CD4 cell counts less than 100/mm^3. Dosage reduction or cessation of therapy may become necessary (see section 4.4).

The incidence of neutropenia was also increased in those patients whose neutrophil counts, haemoglobin levels and serum vitamin B_{12} levels were low at the start of Retrovir therapy.

The following events have been reported in patients treated with Retrovir.

The adverse events considered at least possibly related to the treatment (adverse drug reactions, ADR) are listed below by body system, organ class and absolute frequency. Frequencies are defined as Very common (greater than 10%), Common (1 - 10%), Uncommon (0.1-1%), Rare (0.01-0.1%) and Very rare (less than 0.01%).

Blood and lymphatic system disorders

Common: Anaemia, neutropenia and leucopenia

Uncommon: Pancytopenia with bone marrow hypoplasia, thrombocytopenia

Rare: Pure red cell aplasia

Very rare: Aplastic anaemia

Metabolism and nutrition disorders

Rare: Lactic acidosis in the absence of hypoxaemia, anorexia

Psychiatric disorders

Rare: Anxiety and depression

Nervous system disorders

Very common: Headache

Common: Dizziness

Rare: Convulsions, loss of mental acuity, insomnia, paraesthesia, somnolence

Cardiac disorders

Rare: Cardiomyopathy

Respiratory, thoracic and mediastinal disorders

Uncommon: Dyspnoea

Rare: Cough

Gastrointestinal disorders

Very common: Nausea

Common: Vomiting, diarrhoea and abdominal pain

Uncommon: Flatulence

Rare: Oral mucosa pigmentation, taste disturbance and dyspepsia. Pancreatitis.

Hepatobiliary disorders

Common: Raised blood levels of liver enzymes and bilirubin

Rare: Liver disorders such as severe hepatomegaly with steatosis

Skin and subcutaneous tissue disorders

Uncommon: Rash and pruritis

Rare: Urticaria, nail and skin pigmentation, and sweating

Musculoskeletal and connective tissue disorders

Common: Myalgia

Uncommon: Myopathy

Renal and urinary disorders

Rare: Urinary frequency

Reproductive system and breast disorders

Rare: Gynaecomastia

General disorders and administration site disorders

Common: Malaise

Uncommon: Asthenia, fever, and generalised pain

Rare: Chest pain and influenza-like syndrome, chills

Experience with Retrovir IV for Infusion treatment for periods in excess of two weeks is limited, although some patients have received treatment for up to 12 weeks. The most frequent adverse reactions were anaemia, neutropenia and leucopenia. Local reactions were infrequent.

The available data from studies of Retrovir Oral Formulations indicate that the incidence of nausea and other frequently reported clinical adverse reactions consistently decreased over time during the first few weeks of therapy with Retrovir.

Adverse reactions with Retrovir for the prevention of maternal-foetal transmission:

In a placebo-controlled trial, overall clinical adverse reactions and laboratory test abnormalities were similar for women in the Retrovir and placebo groups. However, there was a trend for mild and moderate anaemia to be seen more commonly prior to delivery in the zidovudine treated women.

In the same trial, haemoglobin concentrations in infants exposed to Retrovir for this indication were marginally lower than in infants in the placebo group, but transfusion was not required. Anaemia resolved within 6 weeks after completion of Retrovir therapy. Other clinical adverse reactions and laboratory test abnormalities were similar in the Retrovir and placebo groups. It is unknown whether there are any long-term consequences of in utero and infant exposure to Retrovir.

Within each frequency grouping, undesirable effects are presented in order of decreasing seriousness.

Cases of lactic acidosis, sometimes fatal, usually associated with severe hepatomegaly and hepatic steatosis, have been reported with the use of nucleoside analogues (see section 4.4).

Combination antiretroviral therapy has been associated with redistribution of body fat (lipodystrophy) in HIV patients including the loss of peripheral and facial subcutaneous fat, increased intra-abdominal and visceral fat, breast hypertrophy and dorsocervical fat accumulation (buffalo hump).

Combination antiretroviral therapy has been associated with metabolic abnormalities such as hypertriglyceridaemia, hypercholesterolaemia, insulin resistance, hyperglycaemia and hyperlactataemia (see section 4.4).

In HIV-infected patients with severe immune deficiency at the time of initiation of combination antiretroviral therapy (CART), an inflammatory reaction to asymptomatic or residual opportunistic infections may arise (see section 4.4).

Cases of osteonecrosis have been reported, particularly in patients with generally acknowledged risk factors, advanced HIV disease or long-term exposure to combination antiretroviral therapy (CART). The frequency of this is unknown (see section 4.4).

4.9 Overdose

Symptoms and signs:

Dosages as high as 7.5 mg/kg by infusion every four hours for two weeks have been administered to five patients. One patient experienced an anxiety reaction while the other four had no untoward effects.

No specific symptoms or signs have been identified following acute oral overdose with zidovudine apart from those listed as undesirable effects such as fatigue, headache, vomiting, and occasional reports of haematological disturbances. Following a report where a patient took an unspecified quantity of zidovudine with serum levels consistent with an overdose of greater than 17 g there were no short term clinical, biochemical or haematological sequelae identified.

Treatment:

Patients should be observed closely for evidence of toxicity (see section 4.8) and given the necessary supportive therapy.

Haemodialysis and peritoneal dialysis appear to have a limited effect on elimination of zidovudine but enhance the elimination of the glucuronide metabolite.

5. PHARMACOLOGICAL PROPERTIES

5.1 Pharmacodynamic properties

Pharmacotherapeutic group: nucleoside analogue, ATC code: J05A F01

Mode of action:

Zidovudine is an antiviral agent which is highly active in vitro against retroviruses including the Human Immunodeficiency Virus (HIV).

Zidovudine is phosphorylated in both infected and uninfected cells to the monophosphate (MP) derivative by cellular thymidine kinase. Subsequent phosphorylation of zidovudine-MP to the diphosphate (DP), and then the triphosphate (TP) derivative is catalysed by cellular thymidylate kinase and non-specific kinases respectively. Zidovudine-TP acts as an inhibitor of and substrate for the viral reverse transcriptase. The formation of further proviral DNA is blocked by incorporation of zidovudine-MP into the chain and subsequent chain termination. Competition by zidovudine-TP for HIV reverse transcriptase is approximately 100-fold greater than for cellular DNA polymerase alpha.

Clinical virology:

The relationships between in vitro susceptibility of HIV to zidovudine and clinical response to therapy remain under investigation. In vitro sensitivity testing has not been standardised and results may therefore vary according to methodological factors. Reduced in vitro sensitivity to zidovudine has been reported for HIV isolates from patients who have received prolonged courses of Retrovir therapy. The available information indicates that for early HIV disease, the frequency and degree of reduction of in vitro sensitivity is notably less than for advanced disease.

The reduction of sensitivity with the emergence of zidovudine resistant strains limits the usefulness of zidovudine monotherapy clinically. In clinical studies, clinical endpoint data indicate that zidovudine, particularly in combination with lamivudine, and also with didanosine or zalcitabine results in a significant reduction in the risk of disease progression and mortality. The use of a protease inhibitor in a combination of zidovudine and lamivudine, has been shown to confer additional benefit in delaying disease progression, and improving survival compared to the double combination on its own.

The anti-viral effectiveness in vitro of combinations of antiretroviral agents are being investigated. Clinical and in vitro studies of zidovudine in combination with lamivudine indicate that zidovudine-resistant virus isolates can become zidovudine sensitive when they simultaneously acquire resistance to lamivudine. Furthermore there is clinical evidence that zidovudine plus lamivudine delays the emergence of zidovudine resistance in anti-retroviral naive patients.

In some in vitro studies zidovudine has been shown to act additively or synergistically with a number of anti-HIV agents, such as lamivudine, didanosine, and interferon-alpha, inhibiting the replication of HIV in cell culture. However, in vitro studieswith triple combinations of nucleoside analogues or two nucleoside analogues and a protease inhibitor have been shown to bemore effective in inhibiting HIV-1 induced cytopathic effects than one or two drug combinations.

Resistance to thymidine analogues (of which zidovudine is one) is well characterised and is conferred by the stepwise accumulation of up to six specific mutations in the HIV reverse transcriptase at codons 41, 67, 70, 210, 215 and 219. Viruses acquire phenotypic resistance to thymidine analogues through the combination of mutations at codons 41 and 215 or by the accumulation of at least four of the six mutations. These thymidine analogue mutations alone do not cause high-level cross-resistance to any of the other nucleosides, allowing for the subsequent use of any of the other approved reverse transcriptase inhibitors.

Two patterns of multi-drug resistance mutations, the first characterised by mutations in the HIV reverse transcriptase at codons 62, 75, 77, 116 and 151 and the second involving a T69S mutation plus a 6-base pair insert at the same position, result in phenotypic resistance to AZT as well as to the other approved nucleoside reverse transcriptase inhibitors. Either of these two patterns of multinucleoside resistance mutations severely limits future therapeutic options.

In the US ACTGO76 trial, Retrovir was shown to be effective in reducing the rate of maternal-foetal transmission of HIV-1 (23% infection rate for placebo versus 8% for zidovudine) when administered (100 mg five times a day) to HIV-positive pregnant women (from week 14-34 of pregnancy) and their newborn infants (2 mg/kg every 6 hours) until 6 weeks of age. In the shorter duration 1998 Thailand CDC study, use of oral Retrovir therapy only (300 mg twice daily), from week 36 of pregnancy until delivery, also reduced the rate of maternal-foetal transmission of HIV (19% infection rate for placebo versus 9% for zidovudine). These data, and data from a published study comparing zidovudine regimens to prevent maternal-foetal HIV transmission have shown that short maternal treatments (from week 36 of pregnancy) are less efficacious than longer maternal treatments (from week 14-34 of pregnancy) in the reduction of perinatal HIV transmission.

5.2 Pharmacokinetic properties

Adults:

Absorption:

Dose-independent kinetics were observed in patients receiving one-hour infusions of 1 to 5 mg/kg 3 to 6 times daily. Mean steady state peak (C^{ss}max) and trough (C^{ss}min) plasma concentrations in adults following a one-hour infusion of 2.5 mg/kg every 4 hours were 4.0 and 0.4 μM, respectively (or 1.1 and 0.1 μg/ml).

Distribution:

The mean terminal plasma half-life was 1.1 hours, the mean total body clearance was 27.1 ml/min/kg and the apparent volume of distribution was 1.6 litres/kg.

In adults, the average cerebrospinal fluid/plasma zidovudine concentration ratio 2 to 4 hours after chronic intermittent oral dosing was found to be approximately 0.5. Data indicate that zidovudine crosses the placenta and is found in amniotic fluid and foetal blood. Zidovudine has also been detected in semen and milk.

Plasma protein binding is relatively low (34 to 38%) and drug interactions involving binding site displacement are not anticipated.

Metabolism:

Zidovudine is primarily eliminated by hepatic conjugation to an inactive glucoronidated metabolite. The 5'-glucuronide of zidovudine is the major metabolite in both plasma and urine, accounting for approximately 50-80% of the administered dose eliminated by renal excretion. 3'-amino-3'-deoxythymidine (AMT) has been identified as a metabolite of zidovudine following intravenous dosing.

Excretion:

Renal clearance of zidovudine greatly exceeds creatinine clearance, indicating that significant tubular secretion takes place.

Paediatrics:

Absorption:

In children over the age of 5-6 months, the pharmacokinetic profile of zidovudine is similar to that in adults. C^{ss}max levels were 1.46 μg/ml following an intravenous dose of 80 mg zidovudine/m^2 body surface area, 2.26 μg/ml following 120 mg/m^2 and 2.96 μg/ml following 160 mg/m^2.

Distribution:

With intravenous dosing, the mean terminal plasma half-life and total body clearance were 1.5 hours and 30.9 ml/min/kg respectively.

In children the mean cerebrospinal fluid/plasma zidovudine concentration ratio ranged from 0.52-0.85, as determined during oral therapy 0.5 to 4 hours after dosing and was 0.87 as determined during intravenous therapy 1-5 hours after a 1 hour infusion. During continuous intravenous infusion, the mean steady-state cerebrospinal fluid/plasma concentration ratio was 0.24.

Metabolism:

The major metabolite is 5'-glucuronide. After intravenous dosing, 29% of the dose was recovered unchanged in the urine and 45% excreted as the glucuronide.

Excretion:

Renal clearance of zidovudine greatly exceeds creatinine clearance indicating that significant tubular secretion takes place.

The data available on the pharmacokinetics in neonates and young infants indicate that glucuronidation of zidovudine is reduced with a consequent increase in bioavailability, reduction in clearance and longer half-life in infants less than 14 days old but thereafter the pharmacokinetics appear similar to those reported in adults.

Pregnancy:

The pharmacokinetics of zidovudine has been investigated in a study of eight women during the third trimester of pregnancy. As pregnancy progressed, there was no evidence of drug accumulation. The pharmacokinetics of zidovudine was similar to that of non-pregnant adults. Consistent with passive transmission of the drug across the placenta, zidovudine concentrations in infant plasma at birth were essentially equal to those in maternal plasma at delivery.

Elderly:

No specific data are available on the pharmacokinetics of zidovudine in the elderly.

Renal impairment:

Compared to healthy subjects, patients with advanced renal failure have a 50% higher peak plasma concentration after oral administration. Systemic exposure (measured as area under the zidovudine concentration time curve) is increased 100%; the half-life is not significantly altered. In renal failure there is substantial accumulation of the major glucuronide metabolite but this does not appear to cause toxicity. Haemodialysis and peritoneal dialysis have no significant effect on zidovudine elimination whereas elimination of the inactive glucuronide metabolite is increased. (see section 4.2).

Hepatic impairment:

There are limited data concerning the pharmacokinetics of zidovudine in patients with hepatic impairment (see section 4.2). No specific data are available on the pharmacokinetics of zidovudine in the elderly.

5.3 Preclinical safety data

Mutagenicity:

No evidence of mutagenicity was observed in the Ames test. However, zidovudine was weakly mutagenic in a mouse lymphoma cell assay and was positive in an in vitro cell transformation assay. Clastogenic effects (chromosome damage) were observed in an in vitro study in human lymphocytes and in in vivo oral repeat dose micronucleus studies in rats and mice. An in vivo cytogenetic study in rats did not show chromosomal damage. A study of the peripheral blood lymphocytes of eleven AIDS patients showed a higher chromosome breakage frequency in those who had received Retrovir than in those who had not. A pilot study has demonstrated that zidovudine is incorporated into leukocyte nuclear DNA of adults, including pregnant women, taking zidovudine as treatment for HIV-1 infection, or for the prevention of mother to child viral transmission. Zidovudine was also incorporated into DNA from cord blood leukocytes of infants from zidovudine-treated mothers. A transplacental genotoxicity study conducted in monkeys compared zidovudine alone with the combination of zidovudine and lamivudine at human-equivalent exposures. The study demonstrated that foetuses exposed in utero to the combination sustained a higher level of nucleoside analogue-DNA incorporation into multiple foetal organs, and showed evidence of more telomere shortening than in those exposed to zidovudine alone. The clinical significance of these findings is unknown.

Carcinogenicity:

In oral carcinogenicity studies with zidovudine in mice and rats, late appearing vaginal epithelial tumours were observed. A subsequent intravaginal carcinogenicity study confirmed the hypothesis that the vaginal tumours were the result of long term local exposure of the rodent vaginal epithelium to high concentrations of unmetabolised zidovudine in urine. There were no other drug-related tumours observed in either sex of either species.

In addition, two transplacental carcinogenicity studies have been conducted in mice. One study, by the US National Cancer Institute, administered zidovudine at maximum tolerated doses to pregnant mice from day 12 to 18 of gestation. One year post-natally, there was an increase in the incidence of tumours in the lung, liver and female reproductive tract of offspring exposed to the highest dose level (420 mg/kg term body weight).

In a second study, mice were administered zidovudine at doses up to 40 mg/kg for 24 months, with exposure beginning prenatally on gestation day 10. Treatment related findings were limited to late-occurring vaginal epithelial tumours, which were seen with a similar incidence and time of onset as in the standard oral carcinogenicity study. The second study thus provided no evidence that zidovudine acts as a transplacental carcinogen.

It is concluded that the transplacental carcinogenicity data from the first study represents a hypothetical risk, whereas the reduction in risk of maternal transfection of HIV to the uninfected child by the use of zidovudine in pregnancy has been well proven.

6. PHARMACEUTICAL PARTICULARS

6.1 List of excipients

Hydrochloric acid (pH for adjustment)

Sodium hydroxide (pH for adjustment)

Water for injection

6.2 Incompatibilities

In the absence of compatibility studies, this medicinal product must not be mixed with other medicinal products

6.3 Shelf life

3 years. (Refer to Section 6.6 for shelf life after opening)

6.4 Special precautions for storage

Do not store above 30°C.

Keep the vial in the outer carton.

6.5 Nature and contents of container

Type I glass vial (amber, neutral glass) with rubber stopper containing 20ml sterile concentrate, available in pack sizes of 5.

6.6 Special precautions for disposal and other handling

Retrovir I.V. for Infusion must be diluted prior to administration. Since no antimicrobial preservative is included, dilution must be carried out under full aseptic conditions, preferably immediately prior to administration, and any unused portion of the vial should be discarded.

The required dose should be added to and mixed with Glucose Intravenous Infusion 5% w/v to give a final zidovudine concentration of either 2 mg/ml or 4 mg/ml. These dilutions are chemically and physically stable for up to 48 hours at both 5°C and 25°C. Should any visible turbidity appear in the product either before or after dilution or during infusion, the preparation should be discarded.

Any unused product or waste material should be disposed of in accordance with local requirements.

7. MARKETING AUTHORISATION HOLDER

The Wellcome Foundation Limited

trading as:

Glaxo Wellcome and/or GlaxoSmithKline UK

Stockley Park West

Uxbridge

Middlesex

UB11 1BT

8. MARKETING AUTHORISATION NUMBER(S)

PL 00003/0332

9. DATE OF FIRST AUTHORISATION/RENEWAL OF THE AUTHORISATION

Date of first authorisation: 20 April 1993

Date of last renewal: 08 December 2006

10. DATE OF REVISION OF THE TEXT

01 December 2008

Retrovir 100 mg/10 ml, oral solution

(GlaxoSmithKline UK)

1. NAME OF THE MEDICINAL PRODUCT

Retrovir 100 mg/10 ml oral solution

2. QUALITATIVE AND QUANTITATIVE COMPOSITION

10 ml of solution contains 100 mg zidovudine.

10 ml of solution contains 6.4 g of maltitol

For a full list of excipients, see section 6.1.

3. PHARMACEUTICAL FORM

Retrovir 100 mg/10ml oral solution/syrup

A clear, pale yellow, strawberry-flavoured, sugar-free oral solution.

The pack contains an oral-dosing syringe which should be fitted to the bottle before use.

4. CLINICAL PARTICULARS

4.1 Therapeutic indications

Retrovir oral formulations are indicated in anti-retroviral combination therapy for Human Immunodeficiency Virus (HIV) infected adults and children.

Retrovir chemoprophylaxis is indicated for use in HIV-positive pregnant women (over 14 weeks of gestation) for prevention of maternal-foetal HIV transmission and for primary prophylaxis of HIV infection in newborn infants.

4.2 Posology and method of administration

Retrovir should be prescribed by physicians who are experienced in the treatment of HIV infection.

Dosage in adults and adolecents weighing at least 30 kg: The usual recommended dose of Retrovir in combination with other anti-retroviral agents is 250 or 300 mg twice daily.

Dosage in children: Retrovir 100 mg capsules are also available for use in children.

Children weighing at least 9 kg and less than 30 kg: The recommended dose of Retrovir is 9 mg/kg twice daily in combination with other antiretroviral agents. The maximum dosage should not exceed 300 mg twice daily.

Children weighing at least 4 kg and less than 9 kg: The recommended dose of Retrovir is 12 mg/kg twice daily in combination with other antiretroviral agents.

Available data are insufficient to propose specific dosage recommendations for children weighing less than 4 kg (See below -maternal foetal transmission and section 5.2).

Dosage in the prevention of maternal-foetal transmission: Pregnant women (over 14 weeks of gestation) should be given 500 mg/day orally (100 mg five times per day) until the beginning of labour. During labour and delivery Retrovir should be administered intravenously at 2 mg/kg bodyweight given over one hour followed by a continuous intravenous infusion at 1 mg/kg/h until the umbilical cord is clamped.

The newborn infants should be given 2 mg/kg bodyweight orally every 6 hours starting within 12 hours after birth and continuing until 6 weeks old (e.g. a 3 kg neonate would require a 0.6 ml dose of oral solution every 6 hours). Infants unable to receive oral dosing should be given Retrovir intravenously at 1.5 mg/kg bodyweight infused over 30 minutes every 6 hours.

Due to the small volumes of oral solution required, care should be taken when calculating neonate doses. To facilitate dosing precision a 1 ml syringe is included in the neonate pack.

In case of planned caesarean, the infusion should be started 4 hours before the operation. In the event of a false labour, the Retrovir infusion should be stopped and oral dosing restarted.

Dosage adjustments in patients with haematological adverse reactions: Substitution of zidovudine should be considered in patients whose haemoglobin level or neutrophil count fall to clinically significant levels. Other potential causes of anaemia or neutropenia should be excluded. Retrovir dose reduction or interruption should be considered in the absence of alternative treatments (see sections 4.3 and 4.4).

Dosage in the elderly: Zidovudine pharmacokinetics have not been studied in patients over 65 years of age and no specific data are available. However, since special care is advised in this age group due to age-associated changes such as the decrease in renal function and alterations in haematological parameters, appropriate monitoring of patients before and during use of Retrovir is advised.

Dosage in renal impairment: The recommended dose for patients with severe renal impairment (creatinine clearance < 10 ml/min) and patients with end-stage renal disease maintained on haemodialysis or peritoneal dialysis is 100 mg every 6 to 8 hrs (300-400 mg daily). Haematological parameters and clinical response may influence the need for subsequent dosage adjustment (see section 5.2).

Dosage in hepatic impairment: Data in patients with cirrhosis suggest that accumulation of zidovudine may occur in patients with hepatic impairment because of decreased glucuronidation. Dosage reductions may be necessary but, due to the large variability in zidovudine exposures in patients with moderate to severe liver disease, precise recommendations cannot be made. If monitoring of plasma zidovudine levels is not feasible, physicians will need to monitor for signs of intolerance, such as the development of haematological adverse reactions (anaemia, leucopenia, neutropenia) and reduce the dose and/or increase the interval between doses as appropriate (see section 4.4).

4.3 Contraindications

Retrovir Oral Formulations are contra-indicated in patients known to be hypersensitive to zidovudine, or to any of the excipients.

Retrovir Oral Formulations should not be given to patients with abnormally low neutrophil counts (less than 0.75×10^9/litre) or abnormally low haemoglobin levels (less than 7.5 g/decilitre or 4.65 mmol/litre).

Retrovir is contra-indicated in new born infants with hyperbilirubinaemia requiring treatment other than phototherapy, or with increased transaminase levels of over five times the upper limit of normal.

4.4 Special warnings and precautions for use

Retrovir is not a cure for HIV infection or AIDS. Patients receiving Retrovir or any other antiretroviral therapy may continue to develop opportunistic infections and other complications of HIV infection.

The concomitant use of rifampicin or stavudine with zidovudine should be avoided (see section 4.5).

Haematological Adverse Reactions: Anaemia (usually not observed before six weeks of Retrovir therapy but occasionally occurring earlier), neutropenia (usually not observed before four weeks' therapy but sometimes occurring earlier) and leucopenia (usually secondary to neutropenia) can be expected to occur in patients receiving Retrovir; These occurred more frequently at higher dosages (1200-1500 mg/day) and in patients with poor bone marrow reserve prior to treatment, particularly with advanced HIV disease (see section 4.8).

Haematological parameters should be carefully monitored. For patients with advanced symptomatic HIV disease it is generally recommended that blood tests are performed at least every two weeks for the first three months of therapy and at least monthly thereafter. Depending on the overall condition of the patient, blood tests may be performed less often, for example every 1 to 3 months.

If the haemoglobin level falls to between 7.5 g/dl (4.65 mmol/l) and 9 g/dl (5.59 mmol/l) or the neutrophil count falls to between 0.75×10^9/l and 1.0×10^9/l, the daily dosage may be reduced until there is evidence of marrow recovery; alternatively, recovery may be enhanced by brief (2-4 weeks) interruption of Retrovir therapy. Marrow recovery is usually observed within 2 weeks after which time Retrovir therapy at a reduced dosage may be reinstituted. In patients with significant anaemia, dosage adjustments do not necessarily eliminate the need for transfusions (see section 4.3).

Lactic acidosis: lactic acidosis usually associated with hepatomegaly and hepatic steatosis has been reported with the use of nucleoside analogues. Early symptoms (symptomatic hyperlactatemia) include benign digestive symptoms (nausea, vomiting and abdominal pain), non-specific malaise, loss of appetite, weight loss, respiratory symptoms (rapid and/or deep breathing) or neurological symptoms (including motor weakness).

Lactic acidosis has a high mortality and may be associated with pancreatitis, liver failure, or renal failure.

Lactic acidosis generally occurred after a few or several months of treatment.

Treatment with nucleoside analogues should be discontinued in the setting of symptomatic hyperlactatemia and metabolic/lactic acidosis, progressive hepatomegaly, or rapidly elevating aminotransferase levels.

Caution should be exercised when administering nucleoside analogues to any patient (particularly obese women) with hepatomegaly, hepatitis or other known risk factors for liver disease and hepatic steatosis (including certain medicinal products and alcohol). Patients co-infected with hepatitis C and treated with alpha interferon and ribavirin may constitute a special risk.

Patients at increased risk should be followed closely.

Mitochondrial toxicity: Nucleoside and nucleotide analogues have been demonstrated in vitro and in vivo to cause a variable degree of mitochondrial damage. There have been reports of mitochondrial dysfunction in HIV-negative infants exposed in utero and/or post-natally to nucleoside analogues. The main adverse events reported are haematological disorders (anaemia, neutropenia), metabolic disorders (hyperlactataemia, hyperlipasaemia). These events are often transitory. Some late-onset neurological disorders have been reported (hypertonia, convulsion, abnormal behaviour). Whether the neurological disorders are transient or permanent is currently unknown. Any child exposed in utero to nucleoside and nucleotide analogues, even HIV-negative children, should have clinical and laboratory follow-up and should be fully investigated for possible mitochondrial dysfunction in case of relevant signs or symptoms. These findings do not affect current recommendations to use antiretroviral therapy in pregnant women to prevent vertical transmission of HIV.

Lipodystrophy: Combination antiretroviral therapy has been associated with the redistribution of body fat (lipodystrophy) in HIV patients. The long-term consequences of these events are currently unknown. Knowledge about the mechanism is incomplete. A connection between visceral lipomatosis and PIs and lipoatrophy and NRTIs has been hypothesised. A higher risk of lipodystrophy has been associated with individual factors such as older age, and with drug related factors such as longer duration of antiretroviral treatment and associated metabolic disturbances. Clinical examination should include evaluation for physical signs of fat redistribution. Consideration should be given to the measurement of fasting serum lipids and blood glucose. Lipid disorders should be managed as clinically appropriate (see section 4.8).

Liver disease: Zidovudine clearance in patients with mild hepatic impairment without cirrhosis [Child-Pugh scores of 5-6] is similar to that seen in healthy subjects, therefore no zidovudine dose adjustment is required. In patients with moderate to severe liver disease [Child-Pugh scores of 7-15], specific dosage recommendations cannot be made due to the large variability in zidovudine exposure observed, therefore zidovudine use in this group of patients is not recommended.

Patients with chronic hepatitis B or C and treated with combination antiretroviral therapy are at an increased risk of severe and potentially fatal hepatic adverse events. In case of concomitant antiviral therapy for hepatitis B or C, please also refer to the relevant product information for these medicinal products.

Patients with pre-existing liver dysfunction, including chronic active hepatitis, have an increased frequency of liver function abnormalities during combination antiretroviral therapy and should be monitored according to standard practice. If there is evidence of worsening liver disease in such patients, interruption or discontinuation of treatment must be considered (see section 4.2).

Immune Reactivation Syndrome: In HIV-infected patients with severe immune deficiency at the time of institution of combination antiretroviral therapy (CART), an inflammatory reaction to asymptomatic or residual opportunistic pathogens may arise and cause serious clinical conditions, or aggravation of symptoms. Typically, such reactions have been observed within the first few weeks or months of initiation of CART. Relevant examples are cytomegalovirus retinitis, generalized and/or focal mycobacterial infections and Pneumocystis carinii pneumonia. Any inflammatory symptoms should be evaluated and treatment instituted when necessary.

Patients should be cautioned about the concomitant use of self-administered medications (see section 4.5).

Patients with rare hereditary problems of fructose intolerance should not take this medicine.

Patients should be advised that Retrovir therapy has not been proven to prevent the transmission of HIV to others through sexual contact or contamination with blood.

Use in Elderly and in Patients with Renal or Hepatic Impairment: see section 4.2.

Osteonecrosis: Although the etiology is considered to be multifactorial (including corticosteroid use, alcohol consumption, severe immunosuppression, higher body mass index), cases of osteonecrosis have been reported particularly in patients with advanced HIV-disease and/or long-term exposure to combination antiretroviral therapy (CART). Patients should be advised to seek medical advice if they experience joint aches and pain, joint stiffness or difficulty in movement.

4.5 Interaction with other medicinal products and other forms of interaction

Limited data suggests that co-administration of zidovudine with rifampicin decreases the AUC (area under the plasma concentration curve) of zidovudine by 48% ± 34%. This may result in a partial loss or total loss of efficacy of zidovudine. The concomitant use of rifampicin with zidovudine should be avoided (see section 4.4).

Zidovudine in combination with stavudine is antagonistic in vitro. The concomitant use of stavudine with zidovudine should be avoided (see section 4.4).

Probenecid increases the AUC of zidovudine by 106% (range 100 to 170%). Patients receiving both drugs should be closely monitored for haematological toxicity.

A modest increase in Cmax (28%) was observed for zidovudine when administered with lamivudine, however overall exposure (AUC) was not significantly altered. Zidovudine has no effect on the pharmacokinetics of lamivudine.

Phenytoin blood levels have been reported to be low in some patients receiving Retrovir, while in one patient a high level was noted. These observations suggest that phenytoin levels should be carefully monitored in patients receiving both drugs.

In a pharmacokinetic study co-administration of zidovudine and atovaquone showed a decrease in zidovudine clearance after oral dosing leading to a 35%±23% increase in plasma zidovudine AUC. The mode of interaction is unknown and as higher concentrations of atovaquone can be achieved with atovaquone suspension it is possible that greater changes in the AUC values for zidovudine might be induced when atovaquone is administered as a suspension. Given the limited data available the clinical significance of this is unknown.

Valproic acid, fluconazole or methadone when co-administered with zidovudine have been shown to increase the AUC with a corresponding decrease in its clearance. As only limited data are available the clinical significance of these findings is unclear but if zidovudine is used concurrently with either valproic acid, fluconazole or methadone, patients should be monitored closely for potential toxicity of zidovudine.

Concomitant treatment, especially acute therapy, with potentially nephrotoxic or myelosuppressive drugs (eg. systemic pentamidine, dapsone, pyrimethamine, co-trimoxazole, amphotericin, flucytosine, ganciclovir, interferon, vincristine, vinblastine and doxorubicin) may also increase the risk of adverse reactions to zidovudine. If concomitant therapy with any of these drugs is necessary then extra care should be taken in monitoring renal function and haematological parameters and, if required, the dosage of one or more agents should be reduced.

Limited data from clinical trials do not indicate a significantly increased risk of adverse reactions to zidovudine with cotrimoxazole, aerosolised pentamidine, pyrimethamine and aciclovir at doses used in prophylaxis.

Clarithromycin tablets reduce the absorption of zidovudine. This can be avoided by separating the administration of zidovudine and clarithromycin by at least two hours.

4.6 Pregnancy and lactation

Pregnancy:

The use of Retrovir in pregnant women over 14 weeks of gestation, with subsequent treatment of their newborn infants, has been shown to significantly reduce the rate of maternal-foetal transmission of HIV based on viral cultures in infants.

The results from the pivotal U.S. placebo-controlled study indicated that Retrovir reduced maternal-foetal transmission by approximately 70%. In this study, pregnant women had CD4 cell counts of 200 to 1818/mm^3 (median in treated group 560/mm^3) and began treatment therapy between weeks 14 and 34 of gestation and had no clinical indications for Retrovir therapy; their newborn infants received Retrovir until 6-weeks old.

A decision to reduce the risk of maternal transmission of HIV should be based on the balance of potential benefits and potential risk. Pregnant women considering the use of Retrovir during pregnancy for prevention of HIV transmission to their infants should be advised that transmission may still occur in some cases despite therapy.

The efficacy of zidovudine to reduce the maternal-foetal transmission in women with previously prolonged treatment with zidovudine or other antiretroviral agents or women infected with HIV strains with reduced sensitivity to zidovudine is unknown.

It is unknown whether there are any long-term consequences of in utero and infant exposure to Retrovir.

Based on the animal carcinogenicity/mutagenicity findings a carcinogenic risk to humans cannot be excluded (see section 5.3). The relevance of these findings to both infected and uninfected infants exposed to Retrovir is unknown. However, pregnant women considering using Retrovir during pregnancy should be made aware of these findings.

Given the limited data on the general use of Retrovir in pregnancy, Retrovir should only be used prior to the 14th week of gestation when the potential benefit to the mother and foetus outweigh the risks. Studies in pregnant rats and rabbits given zidovudine orally at dosage levels up to 450 and 500 mg/kg/day respectively during the major period of organogenesis have revealed no evidence of teratogenicity. There was, however, a statistically significant increase in foetal resorptions in rats given 150 to 450 mg/kg/day and in rabbits given 500 mg/kg/day.

A separate study, reported subsequently, found that rats given a dosage of 3000 mg/kg/day, which is very near the oral median lethal dose (3683 mg/kg), caused marked maternal toxicity and an increase in the incidence of foetal malformations. No evidence of teratogenicity was observed in this study at the lower dosages tested (600 mg/kg/day or less).

Fertility:

Zidovudine did not impair male or female fertility in rats given oral doses of up to 450 mg/kg/day. There are no data on the effect of Retrovir on human female fertility. In men, Retrovir has not been shown to affect sperm count, morphology or motility.

Lactation:

Health experts recommend that women infected with HIV do not breast feed their infants in order to avoid the transmission of HIV. After administration of a single dose of 200 mg zidovudine to HIV-infected women, the mean concentration of zidovudine was similar in human milk and serum. Therefore, since the drug and the virus pass into breast milk it is recommended that mothers taking Retrovir do not breast feed their infants.

4.7 Effects on ability to drive and use machines

There have been no studies to investigate the effect of Retrovir on driving performance or the ability to operate machinery. Furthermore, a detrimental effect on such activities cannot be predicted from the pharmacology of the drug. Nevertheless, the clinical status of the patient and the adverse reaction profile of Retrovir should be borne in mind when considering the patient's ability to drive or operate machinery.

4.8 Undesirable effects

The adverse reaction profile appears similar for adults and children. The most serious adverse reactions include anaemia (which may require transfusions), neutropenia and leucopenia. These occurred more frequently at higher dosages (1200-1500 mg/day) and in patients with advanced HIV disease (especially when there is poor bone marrow reserve prior to treatment), and particularly in patients with CD4 cell counts less than 100/mm^3. Dosage reduction or cessation of therapy may become necessary (see section 4.4).

The incidence of neutropenia was also increased in those patients whose neutrophil counts, haemoglobin levels and serum vitamin B_{12} levels were low at the start of Retrovir therapy.

The following events have been reported in patients treated with Retrovir.

The adverse events considered at least possibly related to the treatment (adverse drug reactions, ADR) are listed below by body system, organ class and absolute frequency. Frequencies are defined as Very common (greater than 10%), Common (1 - 10%), Uncommon (0.1-1%), Rare (0.01-0.1%) and Very rare (less than 0.01%).

Blood and lymphatic system disorders

Common: Anaemia, neutropenia and leucopenia

Uncommon: Pancytopenia with bone marrow hypoplasia, thrombocytopenia

Rare: Pure red cell aplasia

Very rare: Aplastic anaemia

Metabolism and nutrition disorders

Rare: Lactic acidosis in the absence of hypoxaemia, anorexia

Psychiatric disorders

Rare: Anxiety and depression

Nervous system disorders

Very common: Headache

Common: Dizziness

Rare: Convulsions, loss of mental acuity, insomnia, paraesthesia, somnolence

Cardiac disorders

Rare: Cardiomyopathy

Respiratory, thoracic and mediastinal disorders

Uncommon: Dyspnoea

Rare: Cough

Gastrointestinal disorders

Very common: Nausea

Common: Vomiting, diarrhoea and abdominal pain

Uncommon: Flatulence

Rare: Pancreatitis. Oral mucosa pigmentation, taste disturbance and dyspepsia.

Hepatobiliary disorders

Common: Raised blood levels of liver enzymes and bilirubin

Rare: Liver disorders such as severe hepatomegaly with steatosis

Skin and subcutaneous tissue disorders

Uncommon: Rash and pruritis

Rare: Urticaria, nail and skin pigmentation, and sweating

Musculoskeletal and connective tissue disorders

Common: Myalgia

Uncommon: Myopathy

Renal and urinary disorders

Rare: Urinary frequency

Reproductive system and breast disorders

Rare: Gynaecomastia

General disorders and administration site disorders

Common: Malaise

Uncommon: Asthenia, fever, and generalised pain

Rare: Chest pain and influenza-like syndrome, chills

The available data from both placebo-controlled and open-label studies indicate that the incidence of nausea and other frequently reported clinical adverse reactions consistently decreases over time during the first few weeks of therapy with Retrovir.

Adverse reactions with Retrovir for the prevention of maternal-foetal transmission:

In a placebo-controlled trial, overall clinical adverse reactions and laboratory test abnormalities were similar for women in the Retrovir and placebo groups. However, there was a trend for mild and moderate anaemia to be seen more commonly prior to delivery in the zidovudine treated women.

In the same trial, haemoglobin concentrations in infants exposed to Retrovir for this indication were marginally lower than in infants in the placebo group, but transfusion was not required. Anaemia resolved within 6 weeks after completion of Retrovir therapy. Other clinical adverse reactions and laboratory test abnormalities were similar in the Retrovir and placebo groups. It is unknown whether there are any long-term consequences of in utero and infant exposure to Retrovir.

Cases of lactic acidosis, sometimes fatal, usually associated with severe hepatomegaly and hepatic steatosis, have been reported with the use of nucleoside analogues (see section 4.4).

Combination antiretroviral therapy has been associated with redistribution of body fat (lipodystrophy) in HIV patients including the loss of peripheral and facial subcutaneous fat, increased intra-abdominal and visceral fat, breast hypertrophy and dorsocervical fat accumulation (buffalo hump).

Combination antiretroviral therapy has been associated with metabolic abnormalities such as hypertriglyceridaemia, hypercholesterolaemia, insulin resistance, hyperglycaemia and hyperlactataemia (see section 4.4).

In HIV-infected patients with severe immune deficiency at the time of initiation of combination antiretroviral therapy (CART), an inflammatory reaction to asymptomatic or residual opportunistic infections may arise (see section 4.4).

Cases of osteonecrosis have been reported, particularly in patients with generally acknowledged risk factors, advanced HIV disease or long-term exposure to combination antiretroviral therapy (CART). The frequency of this is unknown (see section 4.4).

4.9 Overdose

Symptoms and signs:

No specific symptoms or signs have been identified following acute overdose with zidovudine apart from those listed as undesirable effects such as fatigue, headache, vomiting, and occasional reports of haematological disturbances. Following a report where a patient took an unspecified quantity of zidovudine with serum levels consistent with an overdose of greater than 17 g there were no short term clinical, biochemical or haematological sequelae identified.

Treatment:

Patients should be observed closely for evidence of toxicity (see section 4.8) and given the necessary supportive therapy.

Haemodialysis and peritoneal dialysis appear to have a limited effect on elimination of zidovudine but enhance the elimination of the glucuronide metabolite.

5. PHARMACOLOGICAL PROPERTIES

5.1 Pharmacodynamic properties

Pharmacotherapeutic group: nucleoside analogue, ATC code: J05A F01

Mode of action:

Zidovudine is an antiviral agent which is highly active in vitro against retroviruses including the Human Immunodeficiency Virus (HIV).

Zidovudine is phosphorylated in both infected and uninfected cells to the monophosphate (MP) derivative by cellular thymidine kinase. Subsequent phosphorylation of zidovudine-MP to the diphosphate (DP), and then the triphosphate (TP) derivative is catalysed by cellular thymidylate kinase and non-specific kinases respectively. Zidovudine-TP acts as an inhibitor of and substrate for the viral reverse transcriptase. The formation of further proviral DNA is blocked by incorporation of zidovudine-MP into the chain and subsequent chain termination. Competition by zidovudine-TP for HIV reverse transcriptase is approximately 100-fold greater than for cellular DNA polymerase alpha.

Clinical virology:

The relationships between in vitro susceptibility of HIV to zidovudine and clinical response to therapy remain under investigation. In vitro sensitivity testing has not been standardised and results may therefore vary according to methodological factors. Reduced in vitro sensitivity to zidovudine has been reported for HIV isolates from patients who have received prolonged courses of Retrovir therapy. The available information indicates that for early HIV disease, the frequency and degree of reduction of in vitro sensitivity is notably less than for advanced disease.

The reduction of sensitivity with the emergence of zidovudine resistant strains limits the usefulness of zidovudine monotherapy clinically. In clinical studies, clinical endpoint data indicate that zidovudine, particularly in combination with lamivudine, and also with didanosine or zalcitabine results in a significant reduction in the risk of disease progression and mortality. The use of a protease inhibitor in a combination of zidovudine and lamivudine, has been shown to confer additional benefit in delaying disease progression, and improving survival compared to the double combination on its own.

The anti-viral effectiveness in vitro of combinations of antiretroviral agents are being investigated. Clinical and in vitro studies of zidovudine in combination with lamivudine indicate that zidovudine-resistant virus isolates can become zidovudine sensitive when they simultaneously acquire resistance to lamivudine. Furthermore there is clinical evidence that zidovudine plus lamivudine delays the emergence of zidovudine resistance in anti-retroviral naive patients.

In some in vitro studies zidovudine has been shown to act additively or synergistically with a number of anti-HIV agents, such as lamivudine, didanosine, and interferon-alpha, inhibiting the replication of HIV in cell culture. However, in vitro studies with triple combinations of nucleoside analogues or two nucleoside analogues and a protease inhibitor have been shown to be more effective in inhibiting HIV-1 induced cytopathic effects than one or two drug combinations.

Resistance to thymidine analogues (of which zidovudine is one) is well characterised and is conferred by the stepwise accumulation of up to six specific mutations in the HIV reverse transcriptase at codons 41, 67, 70, 210, 215 and 219. Viruses acquire phenotypic resistance to thymidine analogues through the combination of mutations at codons 41 and 215 or by the accumulation of at least four of the six mutations. These thymidine analogue mutations alone do not cause high-level cross-resistance to any of the other nucleosides, allowing for the subsequent use of any of the other approved reverse transcriptase inhibitors.

Two patterns of multi-drug resistance mutations, the first characterised by mutations in the HIV reverse transcriptase at codons 62, 75, 77, 116 and 151 and the second involving a T69S mutation plus a 6-base pair insert at the same position, result in phenotypic resistance to AZT as well as to the other approved nucleoside reverse transcriptase inhibitors. Either of these two patterns of multinucleoside resistance mutations severely limits future therapeutic options.

In the US ACTGO76 trial, Retrovir was shown to be effective in reducing the rate of maternal-foetal transmission of HIV-1 (23% infection rate for placebo versus 8% for zidovudine) when administered (100 mg five times a day) to HIV-positive pregnant women (from week 14-34 of pregnancy) and their newborn infants (2 mg/kg every 6 hours) until 6 weeks of age. In the shorter duration 1998 Thailand CDC study, use of oral Retrovir therapy only (300 mg twice daily), from week 36 of pregnancy until delivery, also reduced the rate of maternal-foetal transmission of HIV (19% infection rate for placebo versus 9% for zidovudine). These data, and data from a published study comparing zidovudine regimens to prevent maternal-foetal HIV transmission have shown that short maternal treatments (from week 36 of pregnancy) are less efficacious than longer maternal treatments (from week 14-34 of pregnancy) in the reduction of perinatal HIV transmission.

5.2 Pharmacokinetic properties

Adults:

Absorption:

Zidovudine is well absorbed from the gut and, at all dose levels studied, the bioavailability was 60-70%. From a bioequivalence study, steady-state mean (CV%) C[ss]max, C[ss]min, and AUC[ss] values in 16 patients receiving zidovudine 300 mg tablets twice daily were 8.57 (54%) microM (2.29 μg/ml), 0.08 (96%) microM (0.02 μg/ml), and 8.39 (40%) h*microM (2.24 h*μg/ml), respectively.

Distribution:

From studies with intravenous Retrovir, the mean terminal plasma half-life was 1.1 hours, the mean total body clearance was 27.1 ml/min/kg and the apparent volume of distribution was 1.6 Litres/kg.

In adults, the average cerebrospinal fluid/plasma zidovudine concentration ratio 2 to 4 hours after dosing was found to be approximately 0.5. Data indicate that zidovudine crosses the placenta and is found in amniotic fluid and foetal blood. Zidovudine has also been detected in semen and milk.

Plasma protein binding is relatively low (34 to 38%) and drug interactions involving binding site displacement are not anticipated.

Metabolism:

Zidovudine is primarily eliminated by hepatic conjugation to an inactive glucoronidated metabolite. The 5'-glucuronide of zidovudine is the major metabolite in both plasma and urine, accounting for approximately 50-80% of the administered dose eliminated by renal excretion. 3'-amino-3'-deoxythymidine (AMT) has been identified as a metabolite of zidovudine following intravenous dosing.

Excretion:

Renal clearance of zidovudine greatly exceeds creatinine clearance, indicating that significant tubular secretion takes place.

Paediatrics:

Absorption:

In children over the age of 5-6 months, the pharmacokinetic profile of zidovudine is similar to that in adults. Zidovudine is well absorbed from the gut and, at all dose levels studied, its bioavailability was 60-74% with a mean of 65%. $C^{ss}max$ levels were 4.45μM (1.19 μg/ml) following a dose of 120 mg Retrovir (in solution)/m^2 body surface area and 7.7 μM (2.06 μg/ml) at 180 mg/m^2 body surface area. Dosages of 180 mg/m^2 four times daily in children produced similar systemic exposure (24 hour AUC 40.0 hr μM or 10.7 hr μg/ml) as doses of 200 mg six times daily in adults (40.7 hr μM or 10.9 hr μg/ml).

Distribution:

With intravenous dosing, the mean terminal plasma half-life and total body clearance were 1.5 hours and 30.9 ml/min/kg respectively.

In children the mean cerebrospinal fluid/plasma zidovudine concentration ratio ranged from 0.52-0.85, as determined during oral therapy 0.5 to 4 hours after dosing and was 0.87 as determined during intravenous therapy 1-5 hours after a 1 hour infusion. During continuous intravenous infusion, the mean steady-state cerebrospinal fluid/plasma concentration ratio was 0.24.

Metabolism:

The major metabolite is 5'-glucuronide. After intravenous dosing, 29% of the dose was recovered unchanged in the urine and 45% excreted as the glucuronide.

Excretion:

Renal clearance of zidovudine greatly exceeds creatinine clearance indicating that significant tubular secretion takes place.

The data available on the pharmacokinetics in neonates and young infants indicate that glucuronidation of zidovudine is reduced with a consequent increase in bioavailability, reduction in clearance and longer half-life in infants less than 14 days old but thereafter the pharmacokinetics appear similar to those reported in adults.

Pregnancy:

The pharmacokinetics of zidovudine has been investigated in a study of eight women during the third trimester of pregnancy. As pregnancy progressed, there was no evidence of drug accumulation. The pharmacokinetics of zidovudine was similar to that of non-pregnant adults. Consistent with passive transmission of the drug across the placenta, zidovudine concentrations in infant plasma at birth were essentially equal to those in maternal plasma at delivery.

Elderly:

No specific data are available on the pharmacokinetics of zidovudine in the elderly.

Renal impairment:

In patients with severe renal impairment, apparent zidovudine clearance after oral zidovudine administration was approximately 50% of that reported in healthy subjects with normal renal function. Haemodialysis and peritoneal dialysis have no significant effect on zidovudine elimination whereas elimination of the inactive glucuronide metabolite is increased (see section 4.2).

Hepatic impairment:

There are limited data on the pharmacokinetics of zidovudine in patients with hepatic impairment (see section 4.2).

5.3 Preclinical safety data

Mutagenicity:

No evidence of mutagenicity was observed in the Ames test. However, zidovudine was weakly mutagenic in a mouse lymphoma cell assay and was positive in an in vitro cell transformation assay. Clastogenic effects were observed in an in vitro study in human lymphocytes and in in vivo oral repeat dose micronucleus studies in rats and mice. An in vivo cytogenetic study in rats did not show chromosomal damage. A study of the peripheral blood lymphocytes of eleven AIDS patients showed a higher chromosome breakage frequency in those who had received Retrovir than in those who had not. A pilot study has demonstrated that zidovudine is incorporated into leukocyte nuclear DNA of adults, including pregnant women, taking zidovudine as treatment for HIV-1 infection, or for the prevention of mother to child viral transmission. Zidovudine was also incorporated into DNA from cord blood leukocytes of infants from zidovudine-treated mothers. A transplacental genotoxicity study conducted in monkeys compared zidovudine alone with the combination of zidovudine and lamivudine at human-equivalent exposures. The study demonstrated that foetuses exposed in utero to the combination sustained a higher level of nucleoside analogue-DNA incorporation into multiple foetal organs, and showed evidence of more telomere shortening than in those exposed to zidovudine alone. The clinical significance of these findings is unknown.

Carcinogenicity:

In oral carcinogenicity studies with zidovudine in mice and rats, late appearing vaginal epithelial tumours were observed. A subsequent intravaginal carcinogenicity study confirmed the hypothesis that the vaginal tumours were the result of long term local exposure of the rodent vaginal epithelium to high concentrations of unmetabolised zidovudine in urine. There were no other drug-related tumours observed in either sex of either species.

In addition, two transplacental carcinogenicity studies have been conducted in mice. One study, by the US National Cancer Institute, administered zidovudine at maximum tolerated doses to pregnant mice from day 12 to 18 of gestation. One year post-natally, there was an increase in the incidence of tumours in the lung, liver and female reproductive tract of offspring exposed to the highest dose level (420 mg/kg term body weight).

In a second study, mice were administered zidovudine at doses up to 40 mg/kg for 24 months, with exposure beginning prenatally on gestation day 10. Treatment related findings were limited to late-occurring vaginal epithelial tumours, which were seen with a similar incidence and time of onset as in the standard oral carcinogenicity study. The second study thus provided no evidence that zidovudine acts as a transplacental carcinogen.

It is concluded that the transplacental carcinogenicity data from the first study represents a hypothetical risk, whereas the reduction in risk of maternal transfection of HIV to the uninfected child by the use of zidovudine in pregnancy has been well proven.

6. PHARMACEUTICAL PARTICULARS

6.1 List of excipients

Maltitol solution

Glycerol

Citric Acid

E211 Sodium Benzoate

Saccharin Sodium

Flavour Strawberry

Flavour White Sugar

Purified Water.

6.2 Incompatibilities

In the absence of compatibility studies, this medicinal product must not be mixed with other medicinal products.

6.3 Shelf life

2 years.

Discard oral solution 1 month after first opening bottle.

6.4 Special precautions for storage

Do not store above 30°C.

Keep the bottle in the outer carton.

6.5 Nature and contents of container

Retrovir Oral Solution/Syrup:

200 ml amber glass bottle with a plastic or metal cap and polyethylene wad. A 10 ml oral-dosing syringe is included in the pack, with an adaptor, which should be fitted to the bottle before use.

Retrovir Oral Solution/Syrup (Neonate Pack):

200 ml amber glass bottle with a plastic or metal cap and polyethylene wad. A 1 ml oral-dosing syringe is included in the pack, with an adaptor, which should be fitted to the bottle before use.

Not all pack sizes may be marketed.

6.6 Special precautions for disposal and other handling

No special requirements.

7. MARKETING AUTHORISATION HOLDER

The Wellcome Foundation Limited

trading as:

Glaxo Wellcome and/or GlaxoSmithKline UK

Stockley Park West

Uxbridge

Middlesex

UB11 1BT

8. MARKETING AUTHORISATION NUMBER(S)

PL 00003/0288

9. DATE OF FIRST AUTHORISATION/RENEWAL OF THE AUTHORISATION

Date of first authorisation: 16 August 1991

Date of last renewal: 08 December 2006

10. DATE OF REVISION OF THE TEXT

01 December 2008

Retrovir 100mg Capsules

(GlaxoSmithKline UK)

1. NAME OF THE MEDICINAL PRODUCT

Retrovir 100 mg capsules, hard

2. QUALITATIVE AND QUANTITATIVE COMPOSITION

Each capsule contains 100 mg zidovudine

For a full list of excipients, see section 6.1.

3. PHARMACEUTICAL FORM

Capsules, hard

Hard gelatin capsules with opaque white cap and body and a central blue band, printed "Wellcome", "100" and coded Y9C.

4. CLINICAL PARTICULARS

4.1 Therapeutic indications

Retrovir oral formulations are indicated in anti-retroviral combination therapy for Human Immunodeficiency Virus (HIV) infected adults and children.

Retrovir chemoprophylaxis is indicated for use in HIV-positive pregnant women (over 14 weeks of gestation) for prevention of maternal-foetal HIV transmission and for primary prophylaxis of HIV infection in newborn infants.

4.2 Posology and method of administration

Retrovir should be prescribed by physicians who are experienced in the treatment of HIV infection.

An oral solution of Retrovir is also available.

Dosage in adults and adolecents weighing at least 30 kg: The usual recommended dose of Retrovir in combination with other anti-retroviral agents is 250 or 300 mg twice daily.

Dosage in children:

Children weighing more than 21 kg and less than 30 kg: The recommended dose of Retrovir is two 100 mg capsules twice daily in combination with other antiretroviral agents.

Children weighing at least 14 kg and less than or equal to 21 kg: The recommended dose of Retrovir is one 100 mg capsule taken in the morning and two 100 mg capsules taken in the evening.

Children weighing at least 8 kg and less than 14 kg: The recommended dose of zidovudone is one 100 mg capsule twice daily.

Available data are insufficient to propose specific dosage recommendations for children weighing less than 4 kg (See below -maternal foetal transmission and section 5.2).

(see Table 1 below)

Oral solution is available for dosing children less than 8kg and for those children above 8kg unable to swallow capsules (see Oral Solution SPC)

Dosage in the prevention of maternal-foetal transmission: Pregnant women (over 14 weeks of gestation) should be given 500 mg/day orally (100 mg five times per day) until the beginning of labour. During labour and delivery Retrovir should be administered intravenously at 2 mg/kg bodyweight given over one hour followed by a continuous intravenous infusion at 1 mg/kg/h until the umbilical cord is clamped.

The newborn infants should be given 2 mg/kg bodyweight orally every 6 hours starting within 12 hours after birth and continuing until 6 weeks old (e.g. a 3 kg neonate would require a 0.6 ml dose of oral solution every 6 hours). Infants unable to receive oral dosing should be given Retrovir intravenously at 1.5 mg/kg bodyweight infused over 30 minutes every 6 hours.

In case of planned caesarean, the infusion should be started 4 hours before the operation. In the event of a false labour, the Retrovir infusion should be stopped and oral dosing restarted.

Dosage adjustments in patients with haematological adverse reactions: Substitution of zidovudine should be considered in patients whose haemoglobin level or neutrophil count fall to clinically significant levels. Other potential causes of anaemia or neutropenia should be excluded. Retrovir dose reduction or interruption should be considered in the absence of alternative treatments (see sections 4.3 and 4.4).

Dosage in the elderly: Zidovudine pharmacokinetics have not been studied in patients over 65 years of age and no specific data are available. However, since special care is advised in this age group due to age-associated changes such as the decrease in renal function and alterations in haematological parameters, appropriate monitoring of patients before and during use of Retrovir is advised.

Dosage in renal impairment: The recommended dose for patients with severe renal impairment (creatinine clearance < 10 ml/min) and patients with end-stage renal disease maintained on haemodialysis or peritoneal dialysis is 100 mg every 6 to 8 hrs (300-400 mg daily). Haematological parameters and clinical response may influence the need for subsequent dosage adjustment (see section 5.2).

Dosage in hepatic impairment: Data in patients with cirrhosis suggest that accumulation of zidovudine may occur in patients with hepatic impairment because of decreased glucuronidation. Dosage reductions may be necessary but, due to the large variability in zidovudine exposures

Table 1

Weight (kg)	In the morning	In the evening	Daily dose (mg)
8-13	one 100 mg capsule	one 100 mg capsule	200
14-21	one 100 mg capsule	two 100 mg capsules	300
22-30	two 100 mg capsules	two 100 mg capsules	400
Alternatively children weighing at least 28 kg to 30 kg (included) could take:			
28-30	one 250 mg capsule	one 250 mg capsule	500

in patients with moderate to severe liver disease, precise recommendations cannot be made. If monitoring of plasma zidovudine levels is not feasible, physicians will need to monitor for signs of intolerance, such as the development of haematological adverse reactions (anaemia, leucopenia, neutropenia) and reduce the dose and/or increase the interval between doses as appropriate (see section 4.4).

4.3 Contraindications

Retrovir Oral Formulations are contra-indicated in patients known to be hypersensitive to zidovudine, or to any of the excipients.

Retrovir Oral Formulations should not be given to patients with abnormally low neutrophil counts (less than 0.75×10^9/litre) or abnormally low haemoglobin levels (less than 7.5 g/decilitre or 4.65 mmol/litre).

Retrovir is contra-indicated in new born infants with hyperbilirubinaemia requiring treatment other than phototherapy, or with increased transaminase levels of over five times the upper limit of normal.

4.4 Special warnings and precautions for use

Retrovir is not a cure for HIV infection or AIDS. Patients receiving Retrovir or any other antiretroviral therapy may continue to develop opportunistic infections and other complications of HIV infection.

The concomitant use of rifampicin or stavudine with zidovudine should be avoided (see section 4.5).

Haematological Adverse Reactions: Anaemia (usually not observed before six weeks of Retrovir therapy but occasionally occurring earlier), neutropenia (usually not observed before four weeks' therapy but sometimes occurring earlier) and leucopenia (usually secondary to neutropenia) can be expected to occur in patients receiving Retrovir; These occurred more frequently at higher dosages (1200-1500 mg/day) and in patients with poor bone marrow reserve prior to treatment, particularly with advanced HIV disease (see section 4.8).

Haematological parameters should be carefully monitored. For patients with advanced symptomatic HIV disease it is generally recommended that blood tests are performed at least every two weeks for the first three months of therapy and at least monthly thereafter. Depending on the overall condition of the patient, blood tests may be performed less often, for example every 1 to 3 months.

If the haemoglobin level falls to between 7.5 g/dl (4.65 mmol/l) and 9 g/dl (5.59 mmol/l) or the neutrophil count falls to between 0.75×10^9/l and 1.0×10^9/l, the daily dosage may be reduced until there is evidence of marrow recovery; alternatively, recovery may be enhanced by brief (2-4 weeks) interruption of Retrovir therapy. Marrow recovery is usually observed within 2 weeks after which time Retrovir therapy at a reduced dosage may be reinstituted. In patients with significant anaemia, dosage adjustments do not necessarily eliminate the need for transfusions (see section 4.3).

Lactic acidosis: lactic acidosis usually associated with hepatomegaly and hepatic steatosis has been reported with the use of nucleoside analogues. Early symptoms (symptomatic hyperlactatemia) include benign digestive symptoms (nausea, vomiting and abdominal pain), non-specific malaise, loss of appetite, weight loss, respiratory symptoms (rapid and/or deep breathing) or neurological symptoms (including motor weakness).

Lactic acidosis has a high mortality and may be associated with pancreatitis, liver failure, or renal failure.

Lactic acidosis generally occurred after a few or several months of treatment.

Treatment with nucleoside analogues should be discontinued in the setting of symptomatic hyperlactatemia and metabolic/lactic acidosis, progressive hepatomegaly, or rapidly elevating aminotransferase levels.

Caution should be exercised when administering nucleoside analogues to any patient (particularly obese women) with hepatomegaly, hepatitis or other known risk factors for liver disease and hepatic steatosis (including certain medicinal products and alcohol). Patients co-infected with hepatitis C and treated with alpha interferon and ribavirin may constitute a special risk.

Patients at increased risk should be followed closely.

Mitochondrial toxicity: Nucleoside and nucleotide analogues have been demonstrated in vitro and in vivo to cause a variable degree of mitochondrial damage. There have been reports of mitochondrial dysfunction in HIV-negative infants exposed in utero and/or post-natally to nucleoside analogues. The main adverse events reported are haematological disorders (anaemia, neutropenia), metabolic disorders (hyperlactataemia, hyperlipasaemia). These events are often transitory. Some late-onset neurological disorders have been reported (hypertonia, convulsion, abnormal behaviour). Whether the neurological disorders are transient or permanent is currently unknown. Any child exposed in utero to nucleoside and nucleotide analogues, even HIV-negative children, should have clinical and laboratory follow-up and should be fully investigated for possible mitochondrial dysfunction in case of relevant signs or symptoms. These findings do not affect current recommendations to use antiretroviral therapy in pregnant women to prevent vertical transmission of HIV.

Lipodystrophy: Combination antiretroviral therapy has been associated with the redistribution of body fat (lipodystrophy) in HIV patients. The long-term consequences of these events are currently unknown. Knowledge about the mechanism is incomplete. A connection between visceral lipomatosis and PIs and lipoatrophy and NRTIs has been hypothesised. A higher risk of lipodystrophy has been associated with individual factors such as older age, and with drug related factors such as longer duration of antiretroviral treatment and associated metabolic disturbances. Clinical examination should include evaluation for physical signs of fat redistribution. Consideration should be given to the measurement of fasting serum lipids and blood glucose. Lipid disorders should be managed as clinically appropriate (see section 4.8).

Liver disease: Zidovudine clearance in patients with mild hepatic impairment without cirrhosis [Child-Pugh scores of 5-6] is similar to that seen in healthy subjects, therefore no zidovudine dose adjustment is required. In patients with moderate to severe liver disease [Child-Pugh scores of 7-15], specific dosage recommendations cannot be made due to the large variability in zidovudine exposure observed, therefore zidovudine use in this group of patients is not recommended.

Patients with chronic hepatitis B or C and treated with combination antiretroviral therapy are at an increased risk of severe and potentially fatal hepatic adverse events. In case of concomitant antiviral therapy for hepatitis B or C, please also refer to the relevant product information for these medicinal products.

Patients with pre-existing liver dysfunction, including chronic active hepatitis, have an increased frequency of liver function abnormalities during combination antiretroviral therapy and should be monitored according to standard practice. If there is evidence of worsening liver disease in such patients, interruption or discontinuation of treatment must be considered (see section 4.2).

Immune Reactivation Syndrome: In HIV-infected patients with severe immune deficiency at the time of institution of combination antiretroviral therapy (CART), an inflammatory reaction to asymptomatic or residual opportunistic pathogens may arise and cause serious clinical conditions, or aggravation of symptoms. Typically, such reactions have been observed within the first few weeks or months of initiation of CART. Relevant examples are cytomegalovirus retinitis, generalized and/or focal mycobacterial infections and Pneumocystis carinii pneumonia. Any inflammatory symptoms should be evaluated and treatment instituted when necessary.

Patients should be cautioned about the concomitant use of self-administered medications (see section 4.5).

Patients should be advised that Retrovir therapy has not been proven to prevent the transmission of HIV to others through sexual contact or contamination with blood.

Use in Elderly and in Patients with Renal or Hepatic Impairment: see section 4.2.

Osteonecrosis: Although the etiology is considered to be multifactorial (including corticosteroid use, alcohol consumption, severe immunosuppression, higher body mass index), cases of osteonecrosis have been reported particularly in patients with advanced HIV-disease and/or long-term exposure to combination antiretroviral therapy (CART). Patients should be advised to seek medical advice if they experience joint aches and pain, joint stiffness or difficulty in movement.

4.5 Interaction with other medicinal products and other forms of interaction

Limited data suggests that co-administration of zidovudine with rifampicin decreases the AUC (area under the plasma concentration curve) of zidovudine by 48% ± 34%. This may result in a partial loss or total loss of efficacy of zidovudine. The concomitant use of rifampicin with zidovudine should be avoided (see section 4.4).

Zidovudine in combination with stavudine is antagonistic in vitro. The concomitant use of stavudine with zidovudine should be avoided (see section 4.4).

Probenecid increases the AUC of zidovudine by 106% (range 100 to 170%). Patients receiving both drugs should be closely monitored for haematological toxicity.

A modest increase in Cmax (28%) was observed for zidovudine when administered with lamivudine, however overall exposure (AUC) was not significantly altered. Zidovudine has no effect on the pharmacokinetics of lamivudine.

Phenytoin blood levels have been reported to be low in some patients receiving Retrovir, while in one patient a high level was noted. These observations suggest that phenytoin levels should be carefully monitored in patients receiving both drugs.

In a pharmacokinetic study co-administration of zidovudine and atovaquone showed a decrease in zidovudine clearance after oral dosing leading to a 35%±23% increase in plasma zidovudine AUC. The mode of interaction is unknown and as higher concentrations of atovaquone can be achieved with atovaquone suspension it is possible that greater changes in the AUC values for zidovudine might be induced when atovaquone is administered as a suspension. Given the limited data available the clinical significance of this is unknown.

Valproic acid, fluconazole or methadone when co-administered with zidovudine have been shown to increase the AUC with a corresponding decrease in its clearance. As only limited data are available the clinical significance of these findings is unclear but if zidovudine is used concurrently with either valproic acid, fluconazole or methadone, patients should be monitored closely for potential toxicity of zidovudine.

Concomitant treatment, especially acute therapy, with potentially nephrotoxic or myelosuppressive drugs (eg. systemic pentamidine, dapsone, pyrimethamine, co-trimoxazole, amphotericin, flucytosine, ganciclovir, interferon, vincristine, vinblastine and doxorubicin) may also increase the risk of adverse reactions to zidovudine. If concomitant therapy with any of these drugs is necessary then extra care should be taken in monitoring renal function and haematological parameters and, if required, the dosage of one or more agents should be reduced.

Limited data from clinical trials do not indicate a significantly increased risk of adverse reactions to zidovudine with cotrimoxazole, aerosolised pentamidine, pyrimethamine and aciclovir at doses used in prophylaxis.

Clarithromycin tablets reduce the absorption of zidovudine. This can be avoided by separating the administration of zidovudine and clarithromycin by at least two hours.

4.6 Pregnancy and lactation

Pregnancy:

The use of Retrovir in pregnant women over 14 weeks of gestation, with subsequent treatment of their newborn infants, has been shown to significantly reduce the rate of maternal-foetal transmission of HIV based on viral cultures in infants.

The results from the pivotal U.S. placebo-controlled study indicated that Retrovir reduced maternal-foetal transmission by approximately 70%. In this study, pregnant women had CD4 cell counts of 200 to 1818/mm^3 (median in treated group 560/mm^3) and began treatment therapy between weeks 14 and 34 of gestation and had no clinical indications for Retrovir therapy; their newborn infants received Retrovir until 6-weeks old.

A decision to reduce the risk of maternal transmission of HIV should be based on the balance of potential benefits and potential risk. Pregnant women considering the use of Retrovir during pregnancy for prevention of HIV transmission to their infants should be advised that transmission may still occur in some cases despite therapy.

The efficacy of zidovudine to reduce the maternal-foetal transmission in women with previously prolonged treatment with zidovudine or other antiretroviral agents or women infected with HIV strains with reduced sensitivity to zidovudine is unknown.

It is unknown whether there are any long-term consequences of in utero and infant exposure to Retrovir.

Based on the animal carcinogenicity/mutagenicity findings a carcinogenic risk to humans cannot be excluded (see section 5.3). The relevance of these findings to both infected and uninfected infants exposed to Retrovir is unknown. However, pregnant women considering using Retrovir during pregnancy should be made aware of these findings.

Given the limited data on the general use of Retrovir in pregnancy, Retrovir should only be used prior to the 14th week of gestation when the potential benefit to the mother and foetus outweigh the risks. Studies in pregnant rats and rabbits given zidovudine orally at dosage levels up to 450 and 500 mg/kg/day respectively during the major period of organogenesis have revealed no evidence of teratogenicity. There was, however, a statistically significant increase in foetal resorptions in rats given 150 to 450 mg/kg/day and in rabbits given 500 mg/kg/day.

A separate study, reported subsequently, found that rats given a dosage of 3000 mg/kg/day, which is very near the oral median lethal dose (3683 mg/kg), caused marked maternal toxicity and an increase in the incidence of foetal malformations. No evidence of teratogenicity was observed in this study at the lower dosages tested (600 mg/kg/day or less).

Fertility:

Zidovudine did not impair male or female fertility in rats given oral doses of up to 450 mg/kg/day. There are no data on the effect of Retrovir on human female fertility. In men, Retrovir has not been shown to affect sperm count, morphology or motility.

Lactation:

Health experts recommend that women infected with HIV do not breast feed their infants in order to avoid the transmission of HIV. After administration of a single dose of 200 mg zidovudine to HIV-infected women, the mean concentration of zidovudine was similar in human milk and serum. Therefore, since the drug and the virus pass into breast milk it is recommended that mothers taking Retrovir do not breast feed their infants.

4.7 Effects on ability to drive and use machines

There have been no studies to investigate the effect of Retrovir on driving performance or the ability to operate machinery. Furthermore, a detrimental effect on such activities cannot be predicted from the pharmacology of the drug. Nevertheless, the clinical status of the patient and the adverse reaction profile of Retrovir should be borne in mind when considering the patient's ability to drive or operate machinery.

4.8 Undesirable effects

The adverse reaction profile appears similar for adults and children. The most serious adverse reactions include anaemia (which may require transfusions), neutropenia and leucopenia. These occurred more frequently at higher dosages (1200-1500 mg/day) and in patients with advanced HIV disease (especially when there is poor bone marrow reserve prior to treatment), and particularly in patients with CD4 cell counts less than 100/mm^3. Dosage reduction or cessation of therapy may become necessary (see section 4.4).

The incidence of neutropenia was also increased in those patients whose neutrophil counts, haemoglobin levels and serum vitamin B_{12} levels were low at the start of Retrovir therapy.

The following events have been reported in patients treated with Retrovir.

The adverse events considered at least possibly related to the treatment (adverse drug reactions, ADR) are listed below by body system, organ class and absolute frequency. Frequencies are defined as Very common (greater than 10%), Common (1 - 10%), Uncommon (0.1-1%), Rare (0.01-0.1%) and Very rare (less than 0.01%).

Blood and lymphatic system disorders

Common: Anaemia, neutropenia and leucopenia

Uncommon: Pancytopenia with bone marrow hypoplasia, thrombocytopenia

Rare: Pure red cell aplasia

Very rare: Aplastic anaemia

Metabolism and nutrition disorders

Rare: Lactic acidosis in the absence of hypoxaemia, anorexia

Psychiatric disorders

Rare: Anxiety and depression

Nervous system disorders

Very common: Headache

Common: Dizziness

Rare: Convulsions, loss of mental acuity, insomnia, paraesthesia, somnolence

Cardiac disorders

Rare: Cardiomyopathy

Respiratory, thoracic and mediastinal disorders

Uncommon: Dyspnoea

Rare: Cough

Gastrointestinal disorders

Very common: Nausea

Common: Vomiting, diarrhoea and abdominal pain

Uncommon: Flatulence

Rare: Pancreatitis. Oral mucosa pigmentation, taste disturbance and dyspepsia.

Hepatobiliary disorders

Common: Raised blood levels of liver enzymes and bilirubin

Rare: Liver disorders such as severe hepatomegaly with steatosis

Skin and subcutaneous tissue disorders

Uncommon: Rash and pruritis

Rare: Urticaria, nail and skin pigmentation, and sweating

Musculoskeletal and connective tissue disorders

Common: Myalgia

Uncommon: Myopathy

Renal and urinary disorders

Rare: Urinary frequency

Reproductive system and breast disorders

Rare: Gynaecomastia

General disorders and administration site disorders

Common: Malaise

Uncommon: Asthenia, fever, and generalised pain

Rare: Chest pain and influenza-like syndrome, chills

The available data from both placebo-controlled and open-label studies indicate that the incidence of nausea and other frequently reported clinical adverse reactions consistently decreases over time during the first few weeks of therapy with Retrovir.

Adverse reactions with Retrovir for the prevention of maternal-foetal transmission:

In a placebo-controlled trial, overall clinical adverse reactions and laboratory test abnormalities were similar for women in the Retrovir and placebo groups. However, there was a trend for mild and moderate anaemia to be seen more commonly prior to delivery in the zidovudine treated women.

In the same trial, haemoglobin concentrations in infants exposed to Retrovir for this indication were marginally lower than in infants in the placebo group, but transfusion was not required. Anaemia resolved within 6 weeks after completion of Retrovir therapy. Other clinical adverse reactions and laboratory test abnormalities were similar in the Retrovir and placebo groups. It is unknown whether there are any long-term consequences of in utero and infant exposure to Retrovir.

Cases of lactic acidosis, sometimes fatal, usually associated with severe hepatomegaly and hepatic steatosis, have been reported with the use of nucleoside analogues (see section 4.4).

Combination antiretroviral therapy has been associated with redistribution of body fat (lipodystrophy) in HIV patients including the loss of peripheral and facial subcutaneous fat, increased intra-abdominal and visceral fat, breast hypertrophy and dorsocervical fat accumulation (buffalo hump).

Combination antiretroviral therapy has been associated with metabolic abnormalities such as hypertriglyceridaemia, hypercholesterolaemia, insulin resistance, hyperglycaemia and hyperlactataemia (see section 4.4).

In HIV-infected patients with severe immune deficiency at the time of initiation of combination antiretroviral therapy (CART), an inflammatory reaction to asymptomatic or residual opportunistic infections may arise (see section 4.4).

Cases of osteonecrosis have been reported, particularly in patients with generally acknowledged risk factors, advanced HIV disease or long-term exposure to combination antiretroviral therapy (CART). The frequency of this is unknown (see section 4.4).

4.9 Overdose

Symptoms and signs:

No specific symptoms or signs have been identified following acute overdose with zidovudine apart from those listed as undesirable effects such as fatigue, headache, vomiting, and occasional reports of haematological disturbances. Following a report where a patient took an unspecified quantity of zidovudine with serum levels consistent with an overdose of greater than 17 g there were no short term clinical, biochemical or haematological sequelae identified.

Treatment:

Patients should be observed closely for evidence of toxicity (see section 4.8) and given the necessary supportive therapy.

Haemodialysis and peritoneal dialysis appear to have a limited effect on elimination of zidovudine but enhance the elimination of the glucuronide metabolite.

5. PHARMACOLOGICAL PROPERTIES

5.1 Pharmacodynamic properties

Pharmacotherapeutic group: nucleoside analogue, ATC code: J05A F01

Mode of action:

Zidovudine is an antiviral agent which is highly active in vitro against retroviruses including the Human Immunodeficiency Virus (HIV).

Zidovudine is phosphorylated in both infected and uninfected cells to the monophosphate (MP) derivative by cellular thymidine kinase. Subsequent phosphorylation of zidovudine-MP to the diphosphate (DP), and then the triphosphate (TP) derivative is catalysed by cellular thymidylate kinase and non-specific kinases respectively. Zidovudine-TP acts as an inhibitor of and substrate for the viral reverse transcriptase. The formation of further proviral DNA is blocked by incorporation of zidovudine-MP into the chain and subsequent chain termination. Competition by zidovudine-TP for HIV reverse transcriptase is approximately 100-fold greater than for cellular DNA polymerase alpha.

Clinical virology:

The relationships between in vitro susceptibility of HIV to zidovudine and clinical response to therapy remain under investigation. In vitro sensitivity testing has not been standardised and results may therefore vary according to methodological factors. Reduced in vitro sensitivity to zidovudine has been reported for HIV isolates from patients who have received prolonged courses of Retrovir therapy. The available information indicates that for early HIV disease, the frequency and degree of reduction of in vitro sensitivity is notably less than for advanced disease.

The reduction of sensitivity with the emergence of zidovudine resistant strains limits the usefulness of zidovudine monotherapy clinically. In clinical studies, clinical endpoint data indicate that zidovudine, particularly in combination with lamivudine, and also with didanosine or zalcitabine results in a significant reduction in the risk of disease progression and mortality. The use of a protease inhibitor in a combination of zidovudine and lamivudine, has been shown to confer additional benefit in delaying disease progression, and improving survival compared to the double combination on its own.

The anti-viral effectiveness in vitro of combinations of antiretroviral agents are being investigated. Clinical and in vitro studies of zidovudine in combination with lamivudine indicate that zidovudine-resistant virus isolates can become zidovudine sensitive when they simultaneously acquire resistance to lamivudine. Furthermore there is clinical evidence that zidovudine plus lamivudine delays the emergence of zidovudine resistance in anti-retroviral naive patients.

In some in vitro studies zidovudine has been shown to act additively or synergistically with a number of anti-HIV agents, such as lamivudine, didanosine, and interferon-alpha, inhibiting the replication of HIV in cell culture. However, in vitro studies with triple combinations of nucleoside analogues or two nucleoside analogues and a protease inhibitor have been shown to be more effective in inhibiting HIV-1 induced cytopathic effects than one or two drug combinations.

Resistance to thymidine analogues (of which zidovudine is one) is well characterised and is conferred by the stepwise accumulation of up to six specific mutations in the HIV reverse transcriptase at codons 41, 67, 70, 210, 215 and 219. Viruses acquire phenotypic resistance to thymidine analogues through the combination of mutations at codons 41 and 215 or by the accumulation of at least four of the six mutations. These thymidine analogue mutations alone do not cause high-level cross-resistance to any of the other nucleosides, allowing for the subsequent use of any of the other approved reverse transcriptase inhibitors.

Two patterns of multi-drug resistance mutations, the first characterised by mutations in the HIV reverse transcriptase at codons 62, 75, 77, 116 and 151 and the second involving a T69S mutation plus a 6-base pair insert at the same position, result in phenotypic resistance to AZT as well as to the other approved nucleoside reverse transcriptase inhibitors. Either of these two patterns of multinucleoside resistance mutations severely limits future therapeutic options.

In the US ACTGO76 trial, Retrovir was shown to be effective in reducing the rate of maternal-foetal transmission of HIV-1 (23% infection rate for placebo versus 8% for zidovudine) when administered (100 mg five times a day) to HIV-positive pregnant women (from week 14-34 of pregnancy) and their newborn infants (2 mg/kg every 6 hours) until 6 weeks of age. In the shorter duration 1998 Thailand CDC study, use of oral Retrovir therapy only (300 mg twice daily), from week 36 of pregnancy until delivery, also reduced the rate of maternal-foetal transmission of HIV (19% infection rate for placebo versus 9% for zidovudine). These data, and data from a published study comparing zidovudine regimens to prevent maternal-foetal HIV transmission have shown that short maternal treatments (from week 36 of pregnancy) are less efficacious than longer maternal treatments (from week 14-34 of pregnancy) in the reduction of perinatal HIV transmission.

5.2 Pharmacokinetic properties

Adults:

Absorption:

Zidovudine is well absorbed from the gut and, at all dose levels studied, the bioavailability was 60-70%. From a bioequivalence study, steady-state mean (CV%) C[ss]max, C[ss]min, and AUC[ss] values in 16 patients receiving zidovudine 300 mg tablets twice daily were 8.57 (54%) microM (2.29 μg/ml), 0.08 (96%) microM (0.02 μg/ml), and 8.39 (40%) h*microM (2.24 h*μg/ml), respectively.

Distribution:

From studies with intravenous Retrovir, the mean terminal plasma half-life was 1.1 hours, the mean total body clearance was 27.1 ml/min/kg and the apparent volume of distribution was 1.6 Litres/kg.

In adults, the average cerebrospinal fluid/plasma zidovudine concentration ratio 2 to 4 hours after dosing was found to be approximately 0.5. Data indicate that zidovudine crosses the placenta and is found in amniotic fluid and foetal blood. Zidovudine has also been detected in semen and milk.

Plasma protein binding is relatively low (34 to 38%) and drug interactions involving binding site displacement are not anticipated.

Metabolism:

Zidovudine is primarily eliminated by hepatic conjugation to an inactive glucoronidated metabolite. The 5'-glucuronide of zidovudine is the major metabolite in both plasma and urine, accounting for approximately 50-80% of the administered dose eliminated by renal excretion. 3'-amino-3'-deoxythymidine (AMT) has been identified as a metabolite of zidovudine following intravenous dosing.

Excretion:

Renal clearance of zidovudine greatly exceeds creatinine clearance, indicating that significant tubular secretion takes place.

Paediatrics:

Absorption:

In children over the age of 5-6 months, the pharmacokinetic profile of zidovudine is similar to that in adults. Zidovudine is well absorbed from the gut and, at all dose levels studied, its bioavailability was 60-74% with a mean of 65%. $C^{ss}max$ levels were 4.45μM (1.19 μg/ml) following a dose of 120 mg Retrovir (in solution)/m^2 body surface area and 7.7 μM (2.06 μg/ml) at 180 mg/m^2 body surface area. Dosages of 180 mg/m^2 four times daily in children produced similar systemic exposure (24 hour AUC 40.0 hr μM or 10.7 hr μg/ml) as doses of 200 mg six times daily in adults (40.7 hr μM or 10.9 hr μg/ml).

Distribution:

With intravenous dosing, the mean terminal plasma half-life and total body clearance were 1.5 hours and 30.9 ml/min/kg respectively.

In children the mean cerebrospinal fluid/plasma zidovudine concentration ratio ranged from 0.52-0.85, as determined during oral therapy 0.5 to 4 hours after dosing and was 0.87 as determined during intravenous therapy 1-5 hours after a 1 hour infusion. During continuous intravenous infusion, the mean steady-state cerebrospinal fluid/plasma concentration ratio was 0.24.

Metabolism:

The major metabolite is 5'-glucuronide. After intravenous dosing, 29% of the dose was recovered unchanged in the urine and 45% excreted as the glucuronide.

Excretion:

Renal clearance of zidovudine greatly exceeds creatinine clearance indicating that significant tubular secretion takes place.

The data available on the pharmacokinetics in neonates and young infants indicate that glucuronidation of zidovudine is reduced with a consequent increase in bioavailability, reduction in clearance and longer half-life in infants less than 14 days old but thereafter the pharmacokinetics appear similar to those reported in adults.

Pregnancy:

The pharmacokinetics of zidovudine has been investigated in a study of eight women during the third trimester of pregnancy. As pregnancy progressed, there was no evidence of drug accumulation. The pharmacokinetics of zidovudine was similar to that of non-pregnant adults. Consistent with passive transmission of the drug across the placenta, zidovudine concentrations in infant plasma at birth were essentially equal to those in maternal plasma at delivery.

Elderly:

No specific data are available on the pharmacokinetics of zidovudine in the elderly.

Renal impairment:

In patients with severe renal impairment, apparent zidovudine clearance after oral zidovudine administration was approximately 50% of that reported in healthy subjects with normal renal function. Haemodialysis and peritoneal dialysis have no significant effect on zidovudine elimination whereas elimination of the inactive glucuronide metabolite is increased (see section 4.2).

Hepatic impairment:

There are limited data on the pharmacokinetics of zidovudine in patients with hepatic impairment (see section 4.2).

5.3 Preclinical safety data

Mutagenicity:

No evidence of mutagenicity was observed in the Ames test. However, zidovudine was weakly mutagenic in a mouse lymphoma cell assay and was positive in an in vitro cell transformation assay. Clastogenic effects were observed in an in vitro study in human lymphocytes and in in vivo oral repeat dose micronucleus studies in rats and mice. An in vivo cytogenetic study in rats did not show chromosomal damage. A study of the peripheral blood lymphocytes of eleven AIDS patients showed a higher chromosome breakage frequency in those who had received Retrovir than in those who had not. A pilot study has demonstrated that zidovudine is incorporated into leukocyte nuclear DNA of adults, including pregnant women, taking zidovudine as treatment for HIV-1 infection, or for the prevention of mother to child viral transmission. Zidovudine was also incorporated into DNA from cord blood leukocytes of infants from zidovudine-treated mothers. A transplacental genotoxicity study conducted in monkeys compared zidovudine alone with the combination of zidovudine and lamivudine at human-equivalent exposures. The study demonstrated that foetuses exposed in utero to the combination sustained a higher level of nucleoside analogue-DNA incorporation into multiple foetal organs, and showed evidence of more telomere shortening than in those exposed to zidovudine alone. The clinical significance of these findings is unknown.

Carcinogenicity:

In oral carcinogenicity studies with zidovudine in mice and rats, late appearing vaginal epithelial tumours were observed. A subsequent intravaginal carcinogenicity study confirmed the hypothesis that the vaginal tumours were the result of long term local exposure of the rodent vaginal epithelium to high concentrations of unmetabolised zidovudine in urine. There were no other drug-related tumours observed in either sex of either species.

In addition, two transplacental carcinogenicity studies have been conducted in mice. One study, by the US National Cancer Institute, administered zidovudine at maximum tolerated doses to pregnant mice from day 12 to 18 of gestation. One year post-natally, there was an increase in the incidence of tumours in the lung, liver and female reproductive tract of offspring exposed to the highest dose level (420 mg/kg term body weight).

In a second study, mice were administered zidovudine at doses up to 40 mg/kg for 24 months, with exposure beginning prenatally on gestation day 10. Treatment related findings were limited to late-occurring vaginal epithelial tumours, which were seen with a similar incidence and time of onset as in the standard oral carcinogenicity study. The second study thus provided no evidence that zidovudine acts as a transplacental carcinogen.

It is concluded that the transplacental carcinogenicity data from the first study represents a hypothetical risk, whereas the reduction in risk of maternal transfection of HIV to the uninfected child by the use of zidovudine in pregnancy has been well proven.

6. PHARMACEUTICAL PARTICULARS

6.1 List of excipients

Capsule core:

Maize starch

Microcrystalline Cellulose

Sodium Starch Glycollate

Magnesium Stearate.

Capsule coating:

E171 Titanium dioxide

Gelatin

Indigo carmine E132

Polysorbate 80

Printing ink:

Opacode S-IR-8100 HV Black (contains Black Iron Oxide E172)

6.2 Incompatibilities

Not applicable.

6.3 Shelf life

5 years

6.4 Special precautions for storage

Do not store above 30°C.

Store in the original package.

6.5 Nature and contents of container

HDPE or glass bottle containing 100 capsules.

PVC/aluminium foil blister pack containing 100 capsules.

Not all pack sizes may be marketed.

6.6 Special precautions for disposal and other handling

No special requirements.

7. MARKETING AUTHORISATION HOLDER

The Wellcome Foundation Limited

trading as:

Glaxo Wellcome and/or GlaxoSmithKline UK

Stockley Park West

Uxbridge

Middlesex

UB11 1BT

8. MARKETING AUTHORISATION NUMBER(S)

PL 00003/0239

9. DATE OF FIRST AUTHORISATION/RENEWAL OF THE AUTHORISATION

Date of first authorisation: 03 March 1987

Date of last renewal: 08 December 2006

10. DATE OF REVISION OF THE TEXT

01 December 2008

Retrovir 250mg Capsules

(GlaxoSmithKline UK)

1. NAME OF THE MEDICINAL PRODUCT

Retrovir 250 mg capsules, hard

2. QUALITATIVE AND QUANTITATIVE COMPOSITION

Each capsule contains 250 mg zidovudine.

For a full list of excipients, see section 6.1.

3. PHARMACEUTICAL FORM

Capsules, hard

Hard gelatin capsules with opaque blue cap, opaque white body and a central blue band, printed "Wellcome", "250" and coded H2F.

4. CLINICAL PARTICULARS

4.1 Therapeutic indications

Retrovir oral formulations are indicated in anti-retroviral combination therapy for Human Immunodeficiency Virus (HIV) infected adults and children.

Retrovir chemoprophylaxis is indicated for use in HIV-positive pregnant women (over 14 weeks of gestation) for prevention of maternal-foetal HIV transmission and for primary prophylaxis of HIV infection in newborn infants.

4.2 Posology and method of administration

Retrovir should be prescribed by physicians who are experienced in the treatment of HIV infection.

Dosage in adults and adolecents weighing at least 30 kg: The usual recommended dose of Retrovir in combination with other anti-retroviral agents is 250 or 300 mg twice daily.

Dosage in children: Retrovir 100 mg capsules and Retrovir 100 mg/10 ml oral solution are available for use in children.

(see Table 1 below)

Oral solution is available for dosing children less than 8kg and for those children above 8kg unable to swallow capsules (see Oral Solution SPC)

Dosage in the prevention of maternal-foetal transmission: Pregnant women (over 14 weeks of gestation) should be given 500 mg/day orally (100 mg five times per day) until the beginning of labour. During labour and delivery Retrovir should be administered intravenously at 2 mg/kg bodyweight given over one hour followed by a continuous intravenous infusion at 1 mg/kg/h until the umbilical cord is clamped.

The newborn infants should be given 2 mg/kg bodyweight orally every 6 hours starting within 12 hours after birth and continuing until 6 weeks old (e.g. a 3 kg neonate would require a 0.6 ml dose of oral solution every 6 hours). Infants unable to receive oral dosing should be given Retrovir intravenously at 1.5 mg/kg bodyweight infused over 30 minutes every 6 hours.

In case of planned caesarean, the infusion should be started 4 hours before the operation. In the event of a false labour, the Retrovir infusion should be stopped and oral dosing restarted.

Dosage adjustments in patients with haematological adverse reactions: Substitution of zidovudine should be considered in patients whose haemoglobin level or neutrophil count fall to clinically significant levels. Other potential causes of anaemia or neutropenia should be excluded. Retrovir dose reduction or interruption should be considered in the absence of alternative treatments (see sections 4.3 and 4.4).

Dosage in the elderly: Zidovudine pharmacokinetics have not been studied in patients over 65 years of age and no specific data are available. However, since special care is advised in this age group due to age-associated changes such as the decrease in renal function and alterations in haematological parameters, appropriate monitoring of patients before and during use of Retrovir is advised.

Dosage in renal impairment: The recommended dose for patients with severe renal impairment (creatinine clearance < 10 ml/min) and patients with end-stage renal disease maintained on haemodialysis or peritoneal dialysis is 100 mg every 6 to 8 hrs (300-400 mg daily). Haematological parameters and clinical response may influence the need for subsequent dosage adjustment (see section 5.2).

Dosage in hepatic impairment: Data in patients with cirrhosis suggest that accumulation of zidovudine may occur in patients with hepatic impairment because of decreased glucuronidation. Dosage reductions may be necessary but, due to the large variability in zidovudine exposures in patients with moderate to severe liver disease, precise recommendations cannot be made. If monitoring of plasma zidovudine levels is not feasible, physicians will need to monitor for signs of intolerance, such as the development of haematological adverse reactions (anaemia, leucopenia, neutropenia) and reduce the dose and/or increase the interval between doses as appropriate (see section 4.4).

4.3 Contraindications

Retrovir Oral Formulations are contra-indicated in patients known to be hypersensitive to zidovudine, or to any of the excipients.

Retrovir Oral Formulations should not be given to patients with abnormally low neutrophil counts (less than

Table 1

Weight (kg)	In the morning	In the evening	Daily dose (mg)
8-13	one 100 mg capsule	one 100 mg capsule	200
14-21	one 100 mg capsule	two 100 mg capsules	300
22-30	two 100 mg capsules	two 100 mg capsules	400
Alternatively children weighing at least 28 kg to 30 kg (included) could take:			
28-30	one 250 mg capsule	one 250 mg capsule	500

0.75×10^9/litre) or abnormally low haemoglobin levels (less than 7.5 g/decilitre or 4.65 mmol/litre).

Retrovir is contra-indicated in new born infants with hyperbilirubinaemia requiring treatment other than phototherapy, or with increased transaminase levels of over five times the upper limit of normal.

4.4 Special warnings and precautions for use

Retrovir is not a cure for HIV infection or AIDS. Patients receiving Retrovir or any other antiretroviral therapy may continue to develop opportunistic infections and other complications of HIV infection.

The concomitant use of rifampicin or stavudine with zidovudine should be avoided (see section 4.5).

Haematological Adverse Reactions: Anaemia (usually not observed before six weeks of Retrovir therapy but occasionally occurring earlier), neutropenia (usually not observed before four weeks' therapy but sometimes occurring earlier) and leucopenia (usually secondary to neutropenia) can be expected to occur in patients receiving Retrovir; These occurred more frequently at higher dosages (1200-1500 mg/day) and in patients with poor bone marrow reserve prior to treatment, particularly with advanced HIV disease (see section 4.8).

Haematological parameters should be carefully monitored. For patients with advanced symptomatic HIV disease it is generally recommended that blood tests are performed at least every two weeks for the first three months of therapy and at least monthly thereafter. Depending on the overall condition of the patient, blood tests may be performed less often, for example every 1 to 3 months.

If the haemoglobin level falls to between 7.5 g/dl (4.65 mmol/l) and 9 g/dl (5.59 mmol/l) or the neutrophil count falls to between 0.75×10^9/l and 1.0×10^9/l, the daily dosage may be reduced until there is evidence of marrow recovery; alternatively, recovery may be enhanced by brief (2-4 weeks) interruption of Retrovir therapy. Marrow recovery is usually observed within 2 weeks after which time Retrovir therapy at a reduced dosage may be reinstituted. In patients with significant anaemia, dosage adjustments do not necessarily eliminate the need for transfusions (see section 4.3).

Lactic acidosis: lactic acidosis usually associated with hepatomegaly and hepatic steatosis has been reported with the use of nucleoside analogues. Early symptoms (symptomatic hyperlactatemia) include benign digestive symptoms (nausea, vomiting and abdominal pain), non-specific malaise, loss of appetite, weight loss, respiratory symptoms (rapid and/or deep breathing) or neurological symptoms (including motor weakness).

Lactic acidosis has a high mortality and may be associated with pancreatitis, liver failure, or renal failure.

Lactic acidosis generally occurred after a few or several months of treatment.

Treatment with nucleoside analogues should be discontinued in the setting of symptomatic hyperlactatemia and metabolic/lactic acidosis, progressive hepatomegaly, or rapidly elevating aminotransferase levels.

Caution should be exercised when administering nucleoside analogues to any patient (particularly obese women) with hepatomegaly, hepatitis or other known risk factors for liver disease and hepatic steatosis (including certain medicinal products and alcohol). Patients co-infected with hepatitis C and treated with alpha interferon and ribavirin may constitute a special risk.

Patients at increased risk should be followed closely.

Mitochondrial toxicity: Nucleoside and nucleotide analogues have been demonstrated in vitro and in vivo to cause a variable degree of mitochondrial damage. There have been reports of mitochondrial dysfunction in HIV-negative infants exposed in utero and/or post-natally to nucleoside analogues. The main adverse events reported are haematological disorders (anaemia, neutropenia), metabolic disorders (hyperlactataemia, hyperlipasaemia). These events are often transitory. Some late-onset neurological disorders have been reported (hypertonia, convulsion, abnormal behaviour). Whether the neurological disorders are transient or permanent is currently unknown. Any child exposed in utero to nucleoside and nucleotide analogues, even HIV-negative children, should have clinical and laboratory follow-up and should be fully investigated for possible mitochondrial dysfunction in case of relevant signs or symptoms. These findings do not affect current recommendations to use antiretroviral therapy in pregnant women to prevent vertical transmission of HIV.

Lipodystrophy: Combination antiretroviral therapy has been associated with the redistribution of body fat (lipodystrophy) in HIV patients. The long-term consequences of these events are currently unknown. Knowledge about the mechanism is incomplete. A connection between visceral lipomatosis and PIs and lipoatrophy and NRTIs has been hypothesised. A higher risk of lipodystrophy has been associated with individual factors such as older age, and with drug related factors such as longer duration of antiretroviral treatment and associated metabolic disturbances. Clinical examination should include evaluation for physical signs of fat redistribution. Consideration should be given to the measurement of fasting serum lipids and blood glucose. Lipid disorders should be managed as clinically appropriate (see section 4.8).

Liver disease: Zidovudine clearance in patients with mild hepatic impairment without cirrhosis [Child-Pugh scores of 5-6] is similar to that seen in healthy subjects, therefore no zidovudine dose adjustment is required. In patients with moderate to severe liver disease [Child-Pugh scores of 7-15], specific dosage recommendations cannot be made due to the large variability in zidovudine exposure observed, therefore zidovudine use in this group of patients is not recommended.

Patients with chronic hepatitis B or C and treated with combination antiretroviral therapy are at an increased risk of severe and potentially fatal hepatic adverse events. In case of concomitant antiviral therapy for hepatitis B or C, please also refer to the relevant product information for these medicinal products.

Patients with pre-existing liver dysfunction, including chronic active hepatitis, have an increased frequency of liver function abnormalities during combination antiretroviral therapy and should be monitored according to standard practice. If there is evidence of worsening liver disease in such patients, interruption or discontinuation of treatment must be considered (see section 4.2).

Immune Reactivation Syndrome: In HIV-infected patients with severe immune deficiency at the time of institution of combination antiretroviral therapy (CART), an inflammatory reaction to asymptomatic or residual opportunistic pathogens may arise and cause serious clinical conditions, or aggravation of symptoms. Typically, such reactions have been observed within the first few weeks or months of initiation of CART. Relevant examples are cytomegalovirus retinitis, generalized and/or focal mycobacterial infections and Pneumocystis carinii pneumonia. Any inflammatory symptoms should be evaluated and treatment instituted when necessary.

Patients should be cautioned about the concomitant use of self-administered medications (see section 4.5).

Patients should be advised that Retrovir therapy has not been proven to prevent the transmission of HIV to others through sexual contact or contamination with blood.

Use in Elderly and in Patients with Renal or Hepatic Impairment: see section 4.2.

Osteonecrosis: Although the etiology is considered to be multifactorial (including corticosteroid use, alcohol consumption, severe immunosuppression, higher body mass index), cases of osteonecrosis have been reported particularly in patients with advanced HIV-disease and/or long-term exposure to combination antiretroviral therapy (CART). Patients should be advised to seek medical advice if they experience joint aches and pain, joint stiffness or difficulty in movement.

4.5 Interaction with other medicinal products and other forms of interaction

Limited data suggests that co-administration of zidovudine with rifampicin decreases the AUC (area under the plasma concentration curve) of zidovudine by 48% ± 34%. This may result in a partial loss or total loss of efficacy of zidovudine. The concomitant use of rifampicin with zidovudine should be avoided (see section 4.4).

Zidovudine in combination with stavudine is antagonistic in vitro. The concomitant use of stavudine with zidovudine should be avoided (see section 4.4).

Probenecid increases the AUC of zidovudine by 106% (range 100 to 170%). Patients receiving both drugs should be closely monitored for haematological toxicity.

A modest increase in Cmax (28%) was observed for zidovudine when administered with lamivudine, however overall exposure (AUC) was not significantly altered. Zidovudine has no effect on the pharmacokinetics of lamivudine.

Phenytoin blood levels have been reported to be low in some patients receiving Retrovir, while in one patient a high level was noted. These observations suggest that phenytoin levels should be carefully monitored in patients receiving both drugs.

In a pharmacokinetic study co-administration of zidovudine and atovaquone showed a decrease in zidovudine clearance after oral dosing leading to a 35%±23% increase in plasma zidovudine AUC. The mode of interaction is unknown and as higher concentrations of atovaquone can be achieved with atovaquone suspension it is possible that greater changes in the AUC values for zidovudine might be induced when atovaquone is administered as a suspension. Given the limited data available the clinical significance of this is unknown.

Valproic acid, fluconazole or methadone when co-administered with zidovudine have been shown to increase the AUC with a corresponding decrease in its clearance. As only limited data are available the clinical significance of these findings is unclear but if zidovudine is used concurrently with either valproic acid, fluconazole or methadone, patients should be monitored closely for potential toxicity of zidovudine.

Concomitant treatment, especially acute therapy, with potentially nephrotoxic or myelosuppressive drugs (eg. systemic pentamidine, dapsone, pyrimethamine, co-trimoxazole, amphotericin, flucytosine, ganciclovir, interferon, vincristine, vinblastine and doxorubicin) may also increase the risk of adverse reactions to zidovudine. If concomitant therapy with any of these drugs is necessary then extra care should be taken in monitoring renal function and haematological parameters and, if required, the dosage of one or more agents should be reduced.

Limited data from clinical trials do not indicate a significantly increased risk of adverse reactions to zidovudine with cotrimoxazole, aerosolised pentamidine, pyrimethamine and aciclovir at doses used in prophylaxis.

Clarithromycin tablets reduce the absorption of zidovudine. This can be avoided by separating the administration of zidovudine and clarithromycin by at least two hours.

4.6 Pregnancy and lactation

Pregnancy:

The use of Retrovir in pregnant women over 14 weeks of gestation, with subsequent treatment of their newborn infants, has been shown to significantly reduce the rate of maternal-foetal transmission of HIV based on viral cultures in infants.

The results from the pivotal U.S. placebo-controlled study indicated that Retrovir reduced maternal-foetal transmission by approximately 70%. In this study, pregnant women had CD4 cell counts of 200 to 1818/mm^3 (median in treated group 560/mm^3) and began treatment therapy between weeks 14 and 34 of gestation and had no clinical indications for Retrovir therapy; their newborn infants received Retrovir until 6-weeks old.

A decision to reduce the risk of maternal transmission of HIV should be based on the balance of potential benefits and potential risk. Pregnant women considering the use of Retrovir during pregnancy for prevention of HIV transmission to their infants should be advised that transmission may still occur in some cases despite therapy.

The efficacy of zidovudine to reduce the maternal-foetal transmission in women with previously prolonged treatment with zidovudine or other antiretroviral agents or women infected with HIV strains with reduced sensitivity to zidovudine is unknown.

It is unknown whether there are any long-term consequences of in utero and infant exposure to Retrovir.

Based on the animal carcinogenicity/mutagenicity findings a carcinogenic risk to humans cannot be excluded (see section 5.3). The relevance of these findings to both infected and uninfected infants exposed to Retrovir is unknown. However, pregnant women considering using Retrovir during pregnancy should be made aware of these findings.

Given the limited data on the general use of Retrovir in pregnancy, Retrovir should only be used prior to the 14th week of gestation when the potential benefit to the mother and foetus outweigh the risks. Studies in pregnant rats and rabbits given zidovudine orally at dosage levels up to 450 and 500 mg/kg/day respectively during the major period of organogenesis have revealed no evidence of teratogenicity. There was, however, a statistically significant increase in foetal resorptions in rats given 150 to 450 mg/kg/day and in rabbits given 500 mg/kg/day.

A separate study, reported subsequently, found that rats given a dosage of 3000 mg/kg/day, which is very near the oral median lethal dose (3683 mg/kg), caused marked maternal toxicity and an increase in the incidence of foetal malformations. No evidence of teratogenicity was observed in this study at the lower dosages tested (600 mg/kg/day or less).

Fertility:

Zidovudine did not impair male or female fertility in rats given oral doses of up to 450 mg/kg/day. There are no data on the effect of Retrovir on human female fertility. In men, Retrovir has not been shown to affect sperm count, morphology or motility.

Lactation:

Health experts recommend that women infected with HIV do not breast feed their infants in order to avoid the transmission of HIV. After administration of a single dose of 200 mg zidovudine to HIV-infected women, the mean concentration of zidovudine was similar in human milk and serum. Therefore, since the drug and the virus pass into breast milk it is recommended that mothers taking Retrovir do not breast feed their infants.

4.7 Effects on ability to drive and use machines

There have been no studies to investigate the effect of Retrovir on driving performance or the ability to operate machinery. Furthermore, a detrimental effect on such activities cannot be predicted from the pharmacology of the drug. Nevertheless, the clinical status of the patient and the adverse reaction profile of Retrovir should be borne in mind when considering the patient's ability to drive or operate machinery.

4.8 Undesirable effects

The adverse reaction profile appears similar for adults and children. The most serious adverse reactions include anaemia (which may require transfusions), neutropenia and leucopenia. These occurred more frequently at higher dosages (1200-1500 mg/day) and in patients with advanced HIV disease (especially when there is poor bone marrow reserve prior to treatment), and particularly in patients with CD4 cell counts less than 100/mm^3. Dosage reduction or cessation of therapy may become necessary (see section 4.4).

The incidence of neutropenia was also increased in those patients whose neutrophil counts, haemoglobin levels and serum vitamin B_{12} levels were low at the start of Retrovir therapy.

The following events have been reported in patients treated with Retrovir.

The adverse events considered at least possibly related to the treatment (adverse drug reactions, ADR) are listed below by body system, organ class and absolute frequency. Frequencies are defined as Very common (greater than 10%), Common (1 - 10%), Uncommon (0.1-1%), Rare (0.01-0.1%) and Very rare (less than 0.01%).

Blood and lymphatic system disorders

Common: Anaemia, neutropenia and leucopenia

Uncommon: Pancytopenia with bone marrow hypoplasia, thrombocytopenia

Rare: Pure red cell aplasia

Very rare: Aplastic anaemia

Metabolism and nutrition disorders

Rare: Lactic acidosis in the absence of hypoxaemia, anorexia

Psychiatric disorders

Rare: Anxiety and depression

Nervous system disorders

Very common: Headache

Common: Dizziness

Rare: Convulsions, loss of mental acuity, insomnia, paraesthesia, somnolence

Cardiac disorders

Rare: Cardiomyopathy

Respiratory, thoracic and mediastinal disorders

Uncommon: Dyspnoea

Rare: Cough

Gastrointestinal disorders

Very common: Nausea

Common: Vomiting, diarrhoea and abdominal pain

Uncommon: Flatulence

Rare: Pancreatitis. Oral mucosa pigmentation, taste disturbance and dyspepsia.

Hepatobiliary disorders

Common: Raised blood levels of liver enzymes and bilirubin

Rare: Liver disorders such as severe hepatomegaly with steatosis

Skin and subcutaneous tissue disorders

Uncommon: Rash and pruritis

Rare: Urticaria, nail and skin pigmentation, and sweating

Musculoskeletal and connective tissue disorders

Common: Myalgia

Uncommon: Myopathy

Renal and urinary disorders

Rare: Urinary frequency

Reproductive system and breast disorders

Rare: Gynaecomastia

General disorders and administration site disorders

Common: Malaise

Uncommon: Asthenia, fever, and generalised pain

Rare: Chest pain and influenza-like syndrome, chills

The available data from both placebo-controlled and open-label studies indicate that the incidence of nausea and other frequently reported clinical adverse reactions consistently decreases over time during the first few weeks of therapy with Retrovir.

Adverse reactions with Retrovir for the prevention of maternal-foetal transmission:

In a placebo-controlled trial, overall clinical adverse reactions and laboratory test abnormalities were similar for women in the Retrovir and placebo groups. However, there was a trend for mild and moderate anaemia to be seen more commonly prior to delivery in the zidovudine treated women.

In the same trial, haemoglobin concentrations in infants exposed to Retrovir for this indication were marginally lower than in infants in the placebo group, but transfusion was not required. Anaemia resolved within 6 weeks after completion of Retrovir therapy. Other clinical adverse reactions and laboratory test abnormalities were similar in the Retrovir and placebo groups. It is unknown whether there are any long-term consequences of in utero and infant exposure to Retrovir.

Cases of lactic acidosis, sometimes fatal, usually associated with severe hepatomegaly and hepatic steatosis, have been reported with the use of nucleoside analogues (see section 4.4).

Combination antiretroviral therapy has been associated with redistribution of body fat (lipodystrophy) in HIV patients including the loss of peripheral and facial subcutaneous fat, increased intra-abdominal and visceral fat, breast hypertrophy and dorsocervical fat accumulation (buffalo hump).

Combination antiretroviral therapy has been associated with metabolic abnormalities such as hypertriglyceridaemia, hypercholesterolaemia, insulin resistance, hyperglycaemia and hyperlactataemia (see section 4.4).

In HIV-infected patients with severe immune deficiency at the time of initiation of combination antiretroviral therapy (CART), an inflammatory reaction to asymptomatic or residual opportunistic infections may arise (see section 4.4).

Cases of osteonecrosis have been reported, particularly in patients with generally acknowledged risk factors, advanced HIV disease or long-term exposure to combination antiretroviral therapy (CART). The frequency of this is unknown (see section 4.4).

4.9 Overdose

Symptoms and signs:

No specific symptoms or signs have been identified following acute overdose with zidovudine apart from those listed as undesirable effects such as fatigue, headache, vomiting, and occasional reports of haematological disturbances. Following a report where a patient took an unspecified quantity of zidovudine with serum levels consistent with an overdose of greater than 17 g there were no short term clinical, biochemical or haematological sequelae identified.

Treatment:

Patients should be observed closely for evidence of toxicity (see section 4.8) and given the necessary supportive therapy.

Haemodialysis and peritoneal dialysis appear to have a limited effect on elimination of zidovudine but enhance the elimination of the glucuronide metabolite.

5. PHARMACOLOGICAL PROPERTIES

5.1 Pharmacodynamic properties

Pharmacotherapeutic group: nucleoside analogue, ATC code: J05A F01

Mode of action:

Zidovudine is an antiviral agent which is highly active in vitro against retroviruses including the Human Immunodeficiency Virus (HIV).

Zidovudine is phosphorylated in both infected and uninfected cells to the monophosphate (MP) derivative by cellular thymidine kinase. Subsequent phosphorylation of zidovudine-MP to the diphosphate (DP), and then the triphosphate (TP) derivative is catalysed by cellular thymidylate kinase and non-specific kinases respectively. Zidovudine-TP acts as an inhibitor of and substrate for the viral reverse transcriptase. The formation of further proviral DNA is blocked by incorporation of zidovudine-MP into the chain and subsequent chain termination. Competition by zidovudine-TP for HIV reverse transcriptase is approximately 100-fold greater than for cellular DNA polymerase alpha.

Clinical virology:

The relationships between in vitro susceptibility of HIV to zidovudine and clinical response to therapy remain under investigation. In vitro sensitivity testing has not been standardised and results may therefore vary according to methodological factors. Reduced in vitro sensitivity to zidovudine has been reported for HIV isolates from patients who have received prolonged courses of Retrovir therapy. The available information indicates that for early HIV disease, the frequency and degree of reduction of in vitro sensitivity is notably less than for advanced disease.

The reduction of sensitivity with the emergence of zidovudine resistant strains limits the usefulness of zidovudine monotherapy clinically. In clinical studies, clinical endpoint data indicate that zidovudine, particularly in combination with lamivudine, and also with didanosine or zalcitabine results in a significant reduction in the risk of disease progression and mortality. The use of a protease inhibitor in a combination of zidovudine and lamivudine, has been shown to confer additional benefit in delaying disease progression, and improving survival compared to the double combination on its own.

The anti-viral effectiveness in vitro of combinations of antiretroviral agents are being investigated. Clinical and in vitro studies of zidovudine in combination with lamivudine indicate that zidovudine-resistant virus isolates can become zidovudine sensitive when they simultaneously acquire resistance to lamivudine. Furthermore there is clinical evidence that zidovudine plus lamivudine delays the emergence of zidovudine resistance in anti-retroviral naive patients.

In some in vitro studies zidovudine has been shown to act additively or synergistically with a number of anti-HIV agents, such as lamivudine, didanosine, and interferon-alpha, inhibiting the replication of HIV in cell culture. However, in vitro studies with triple combinations of nucleoside analogues or two nucleoside analogues and a protease inhibitor have been shown to be more effective in inhibiting HIV-1 induced cytopathic effects than one or two drug combinations.

Resistance to thymidine analogues (of which zidovudine is one) is well characterised and is conferred by the stepwise accumulation of up to six specific mutations in the HIV reverse transcriptase at codons 41, 67, 70, 210, 215 and 219. Viruses acquire phenotypic resistance to thymidine analogues through the combination of mutations at codons 41 and 215 or by the accumulation of at least four of the six mutations. These thymidine analogue mutations alone do not cause high-level cross-resistance to any of the other nucleosides, allowing for the subsequent use of any of the other approved reverse transcriptase inhibitors.

Two patterns of multi-drug resistance mutations, the first characterised by mutations in the HIV reverse transcriptase at codons 62, 75, 77, 116 and 151 and the second involving a T69S mutation plus a 6-base pair insert at the same position, result in phenotypic resistance to AZT as well as to the other approved nucleoside reverse transcriptase inhibitors. Either of these two patterns of multinucleoside resistance mutations severely limits future therapeutic options.

In the US ACTGO76 trial, Retrovir was shown to be effective in reducing the rate of maternal-foetal transmission of HIV-1 (23% infection rate for placebo versus 8% for zidovudine) when administered (100 mg five times a day) to HIV-positive pregnant women (from week 14-34 of pregnancy) and their newborn infants (2 mg/kg every 6 hours) until 6 weeks of age. In the shorter duration 1998 Thailand CDC study, use of oral Retrovir therapy only (300 mg twice daily), from week 36 of pregnancy until delivery, also reduced the rate of maternal-foetal transmission of HIV (19% infection rate for placebo versus 9% for zidovudine). These data, and data from a published study comparing zidovudine regimens to prevent maternal-foetal HIV transmission have shown that short maternal treatments (from week 36 of pregnancy) are less efficacious than longer maternal treatments (from week 14-34 of pregnancy) in the reduction of perinatal HIV transmission.

5.2 Pharmacokinetic properties

Adults:

Absorption:

Zidovudine is well absorbed from the gut and, at all dose levels studied, the bioavailability was 60-70%. From a bioequivalence study, steady-state mean (CV%) C[ss]max, C[ss]min, and AUC[ss] values in 16 patients receiving zidovudine 300 mg tablets twice daily were 8.57 (54%) microM (2.29 µg/ml), 0.08 (96%) microM (0.02 µg/ml), and 8.39 (40%) h*microM (2.24 h*µg/ml), respectively.

Distribution:

From studies with intravenous Retrovir, the mean terminal plasma half-life was 1.1 hours, the mean total body clearance was 27.1 ml/min/kg and the apparent volume of distribution was 1.6 Litres/kg.

In adults, the average cerebrospinal fluid/plasma zidovudine concentration ratio 2 to 4 hours after dosing was found to be approximately 0.5. Data indicate that zidovudine crosses the placenta and is found in amniotic fluid and foetal blood. Zidovudine has also been detected in semen and milk.

Plasma protein binding is relatively low (34 to 38%) and drug interactions involving binding site displacement are not anticipated.

Metabolism:

Zidovudine is primarily eliminated by hepatic conjugation to an inactive glucoronidated metabolite. The 5'-glucuronide of zidovudine is the major metabolite in both plasma and urine, accounting for approximately 50-80% of the administered dose eliminated by renal excretion. 3'-amino-3'-deoxythymidine (AMT) has been identified as a metabolite of zidovudine following intravenous dosing.

Excretion:

Renal clearance of zidovudine greatly exceeds creatinine clearance, indicating that significant tubular secretion takes place.

Paediatrics:

Absorption:

In children over the age of 5-6 months, the pharmacokinetic profile of zidovudine is similar to that in adults. Zidovudine is well absorbed from the gut and, at all dose levels studied, its bioavailability was 60-74% with a mean of 65%. C^{ss}max levels were 4.45µM (1.19 µg/ml) following a dose of 120 mg Retrovir (in solution)/m^2 body surface area and 7.7 µM (2.06 µg/ml) at 180 mg/m^2 body surface area. Dosages of 180 mg/m^2 four times daily in children produced similar systemic exposure (24 hour AUC 40.0 hr µM or 10.7 hr µg/ml) as doses of 200 mg six times daily in adults (40.7 hr µM or 10.9 hr µg/ml).

Distribution:

With intravenous dosing, the mean terminal plasma half-life and total body clearance were 1.5 hours and 30.9 ml/min/kg respectively.

In children the mean cerebrospinal fluid/plasma zidovudine concentration ratio ranged from 0.52-0.85, as determined during oral therapy 0.5 to 4 hours after dosing and was 0.87 as determined during intravenous therapy 1-5 hours after a 1 hour infusion. During continuous intravenous infusion, the mean steady-state cerebrospinal fluid/plasma concentration ratio was 0.24.

Metabolism:

The major metabolite is 5'-glucuronide. After intravenous dosing, 29% of the dose was recovered unchanged in the urine and 45% excreted as the glucuronide.

Excretion:

Renal clearance of zidovudine greatly exceeds creatinine clearance indicating that significant tubular secretion takes place.

The data available on the pharmacokinetics in neonates and young infants indicate that glucuronidation of zidovudine is reduced with a consequent increase in bioavailability, reduction in clearance and longer half-life in infants less than 14 days old but thereafter the pharmacokinetics appear similar to those reported in adults.

Pregnancy:

The pharmacokinetics of zidovudine has been investigated in a study of eight women during the third trimester of pregnancy. As pregnancy progressed, there was no evidence of drug accumulation. The pharmacokinetics of zidovudine was similar to that of non-pregnant adults. Consistent with passive transmission of the drug across the placenta, zidovudine concentrations in infant plasma at birth were essentially equal to those in maternal plasma at delivery.

Elderly:

No specific data are available on the pharmacokinetics of zidovudine in the elderly.

Renal impairment:

In patients with severe renal impairment, apparent zidovudine clearance after oral zidovudine administration was approximately 50% of that reported in healthy subjects with normal renal function. Haemodialysis and peritoneal dialysis have no significant effect on zidovudine elimination whereas elimination of the inactive glucuronide metabolite is increased (see section 4.2).

Hepatic impairment:

There are limited data on the pharmacokinetics of zidovudine in patients with hepatic impairment (see section 4.2).

5.3 Preclinical safety data

Mutagenicity:

No evidence of mutagenicity was observed in the Ames test. However, zidovudine was weakly mutagenic in a mouse lymphoma cell assay and was positive in an in vitro cell transformation assay. Clastogenic effects were observed in an in vitro study in human lymphocytes and in in vivo oral repeat dose micronucleus studies in rats and mice. An in vivo cytogenetic study in rats did not show chromosomal damage. A study of the peripheral blood lymphocytes of eleven AIDS patients showed a higher chromosome breakage frequency in those who had received Retrovir than in those who had not. A pilot study has demonstrated that zidovudine is incorporated into leukocyte nuclear DNA of adults, including pregnant women, taking zidovudine as treatment for HIV-1 infection, or for the prevention of mother to child viral transmission. Zidovudine was also incorporated into DNA from cord blood leukocytes of infants from zidovudine-treated mothers. A transplacental genotoxicity study conducted in monkeys compared zidovudine alone with the combination of zidovudine and lamivudine at human-equivalent exposures. The study demonstrated that foetuses exposed in utero to the combination sustained a higher level of nucleoside analogue-DNA incorporation into multiple foetal organs, and showed evidence of more telomere shortening than in those exposed to zidovudine alone. The clinical significance of these findings is unknown.

Carcinogenicity:

In oral carcinogenicity studies with zidovudine in mice and rats, late appearing vaginal epithelial tumours were observed. A subsequent intravaginal carcinogenicity study confirmed the hypothesis that the vaginal tumours were the result of long term local exposure of the rodent vaginal epithelium to high concentrations of unmetabolised zidovudine in urine. There were no other drug-related tumours observed in either sex of either species.

In addition, two transplacental carcinogenicity studies have been conducted in mice. One study, by the US National Cancer Institute, administered zidovudine at maximum tolerated doses to pregnant mice from day 12 to 18 of gestation. One year post-natally, there was an increase in the incidence of tumours in the lung, liver and female reproductive tract of offspring exposed to the highest dose level (420 mg/kg term body weight).

In a second study, mice were administered zidovudine at doses up to 40 mg/kg for 24 months, with exposure beginning prenatally on gestation day 10. Treatment related findings were limited to late-occurring vaginal epithelial tumours, which were seen with a similar incidence and time of onset as in the standard oral carcinogenicity study. The second study thus provided no evidence that zidovudine acts as a transplacental carcinogen.

It is concluded that the transplacental carcinogenicity data from the first study represents a hypothetical risk, whereas the reduction in risk of maternal transfection of HIV to the uninfected child by the use of zidovudine in pregnancy has been well proven.

6. PHARMACEUTICAL PARTICULARS

6.1 List of excipients

Capsule core:

Maize starch

Microcrystalline Cellulose

Sodium Starch Glycollate

Magnesium Stearate.

Capsule coating:

E171 Titanium dioxide

Gelatin

Indigo carmine E132

Polysorbate 80

Printing ink:

Opacode S-IR-8100 HV Black (contains Black Iron Oxide E172)

6.2 Incompatibilities

Not applicable.

6.3 Shelf life

5 years

6.4 Special precautions for storage

Do not store above 30°C.

Store in the original package.

6.5 Nature and contents of container

PVC/aluminium foil blister pack containing 40 capsules.

6.6 Special precautions for disposal and other handling

No special requirements.

7. MARKETING AUTHORISATION HOLDER

The Wellcome Foundation Limited

trading as:

Glaxo Wellcome and/or GlaxoSmithKline UK

Stockley Park West

Uxbridge

Middlesex

UB11 1BT

8. MARKETING AUTHORISATION NUMBER(S)

PL 00003/0240

9. DATE OF FIRST AUTHORISATION/RENEWAL OF THE AUTHORISATION

Date of first authorisation: 03 March 1987

Date of last renewal: 08 December 2006

10. DATE OF REVISION OF THE TEXT

01 December 2008

Revatio 20 mg film-coated tablets

(Pfizer Limited)

1. NAME OF THE MEDICINAL PRODUCT

Revatio ®▼20 mg film-coated tablets

2. QUALITATIVE AND QUANTITATIVE COMPOSITION

Each film-coated tablet contains 20 mg of sildenafil (as citrate). Revatio tablets also contain lactose.

For a full list of excipients, see section 6.1.

3. PHARMACEUTICAL FORM

Film-coated tablet.

White, round, biconvex film-coated tablets marked "PFIZER" on one side and "RVT 20" on the other.

4. CLINICAL PARTICULARS

4.1 Therapeutic indications

Treatment of patients with pulmonary arterial hypertension classified as WHO functional class II and III, to improve exercise capacity. Efficacy has been shown in primary pulmonary hypertension and pulmonary hypertension associated with connective tissue disease.

4.2 Posology and method of administration

Revatio is intended for oral use.

Treatment should only be initiated and monitored by a physician experienced in the treatment of pulmonary arterial hypertension. In case of clinical deterioration in spite of Revatio treatment, alternative therapies should be considered.

Use in adults (⩾ 18 years):

The recommended dose is 20 mg three times a day. Tablets should be taken approximately 6 to 8 hours apart with or without food.

Use in the elderly (⩾ 65 years):

Dosage adjustments are not required in elderly patients. Clinical efficacy as measured by 6-minute walk distance could be less in elderly patients.

Use in patients with impaired renal function:

Initial dose adjustments are not required in patients with renal impairment, including severe renal impairment (creatinine clearance < 30 ml/min). A downward dose adjustment to 20 mg twice daily should be considered after a careful benefit-risk assessment only if therapy is not well-tolerated.

Use in patients with impaired hepatic function:

Initial dose adjustments are not required in patients with hepatic impairment (Child-Pugh class A and B). A downward dose adjustment to 20 mg twice daily should be considered after a careful benefit-risk assessment only if therapy is not well-tolerated.

Revatio is contraindicated in patients with severe hepatic impairment (Child-Pugh class C), (see section 4.3).

Use in children and adolescents (< 18 years):

The safety and efficacy in children and adolescents have not been studied in large controlled clinical trials. Therefore, the use of sildenafil is not recommended in these patients.

Discontinuation of treatment:

Limited data suggests that the abrupt discontinuation of Revatio is not associated with rebound worsening of pulmonary arterial hypertension. However to avoid the possible occurrence of sudden clinical deterioration during withdrawal, a gradual dose reduction should be considered. Intensified monitoring is recommended during the discontinuation period.

Use in patients using other medicines:

Co-administration of sildenafil and intravenous epoprostenol has been evaluated (see section 4.8 and 5.1).

The efficacy and safety of sildenafil co-administered with other treatments for pulmonary arterial hypertension (eg. bosentan, iloprost) has not been studied in controlled clinical trials. Therefore caution is recommended in case of co-administration.

The safety and efficacy of Revatio when co-administered with other PDE5 inhibitors has not been studied in pulmonary arterial hypertension patients.

4.3 Contraindications

Hypersensitivity to the active substance or to any of the excipients.

Consistent with its known effects on the nitric oxide/cyclic guanosine monophosphate (cGMP) pathway (see section 5.1), sildenafil was shown to potentiate the hypotensive effects of nitrates, and its co-administration with nitric oxide donors (such as amyl nitrite) or nitrates in any form is therefore contraindicated.

Combination with potent CYP3A4 inhibitors (eg. ketoconazole, itraconazole, ritonavir) (see section 4.5).

Revatio is contraindicated in patients who have loss of vision in one eye because of non-arteritic anterior ischaemic optic neuropathy (NAION), regardless of whether this episode was in connection or not with previous PDE5 inhibitor exposure (see section 4.4).

The safety of sildenafil has not been studied in the following sub-groups of patients and its use is therefore contraindicated: severe hepatic impairment, recent history of stroke or myocardial infarction, severe hypotension (blood pressure < 90/50 mmHg) at initiation.

4.4 Special warnings and precautions for use

The efficacy of Revatio has not been established in patients with severe pulmonary arterial hypertension (functional class IV). If the clinical situation deteriorates, therapies that are recommended at the severe stage of the disease (e.g. epoprostenol) should be considered (see section 4.2).

The benefit-risk balance of sildenafil has not been established in patients with class I functional classification of pulmonary arterial hypertension. No studies have been performed in related forms of pulmonary arterial hypertension other than related to connective tissue disease and surgical repair.

The safety of sildenafil has not been studied in patients with known hereditary degenerative retinal disorders such as *Retinitis pigmentosa* (a minority of these patients have genetic disorders of retinal phosphodiesterases) and therefore its use is not recommended.

In general, any dose adjustment should be administered only after a careful benefit-risk assessment.

A downward dose adjustment to 20 mg twice daily should be considered when sildenafil is co-administered to patients already receiving medium potency CYP3A4 inhibitors like erythromycin or saquinavir. A downward dose adjustment to 20 mg once daily is recommended in case of co-administration with CYP3A4 inhibitors of intermediate potency like clarithromycin, telithromycin and nefazodone. Co-administration of potent CYP3A4 inhibitors (e.g. ketoconazole, itraconazole, ritonavir) with sildenafil for pulmonary arterial hypertension is contraindicated (see section 4.3). Dose adjustments of sildenafil may be required when co-administered with CYP3A4 inducers (see section 4.5).

When prescribing sildenafil, physicians should carefully consider whether patients with certain underlying conditions could be adversely affected by sildenafil's mild to moderate vasodilatory effects, for example patients with hypotension, patients with fluid depletion, severe left ventricular outflow obstruction or autonomic dysfunction (see section 4.4).

Sildenafil potentiates the hypotensive effect of nitrates therefore concomitant use of Revatio with nitrates is contraindicated (see section 4.3).

In post-marketing experience with sildenafil for male erectile dysfunction, serious cardiovascular events, including myocardial infarction, unstable angina, sudden cardiac death, ventricular arrhythmia, cerebrovascular haemorrhage, transient ischaemic attack, hypertension and hypotension have been reported in temporal association with the use of sildenafil. Most, but not all, of these patients had pre-existing cardiovascular risk factors. Many events were reported to occur during or shortly after sexual intercourse and a few were reported to occur shortly after the use of sildenafil without sexual activity. It is not possible to determine whether these events are related directly to these factors or to other factors.

Sildenafil should be used with caution in patients with anatomical deformation of the penis (such as angulation, cavernosal fibrosis or Peyronie's disease), or in patients who have conditions which may predispose them to priapism (such as sickle cell anaemia, multiple myeloma or leukaemia).

Visual defects and cases of non-arteritic anterior ischaemic optic neuropathy have been reported in connection with the intake of sildenafil and other PDE5 inhibitors. The patient should be advised that in case of sudden visual defect, he should stop taking Revatio and consult a physician immediately (see section 4.3).

Caution is advised when sildenafil is administered to patients taking an alpha-blocker as the co-administration may lead to symptomatic hypotension in susceptible individuals (see section 4.5). In order to minimize the potential for developing postural hypotension, patients should be haemodynamically stable on alpha-blocker therapy prior to initiating sildenafil treatment. Physicians should advise patients what to do in the event of postural hypotensive symptoms.

Studies with human platelets indicate that sildenafil potentiates the antiaggregatory effect of sodium nitroprusside *in vitro*. There is no safety information on the administration of sildenafil to patients with bleeding disorders or active peptic ulceration. Therefore sildenafil should be administered to these patients only after careful benefit-risk assessment.

In pulmonary arterial hypertension patients, there may be a potential for increased risk of bleeding when sildenafil is initiated in patients already using a Vitamin K antagonist, particularly in patients with pulmonary arterial hypertension secondary to connective tissue disease.

No data are available with sildenafil in patients with pulmonary hypertension associated with pulmonary veno-occlusive disease. However, cases of life threatening pulmonary oedema have been reported with vasodilators (mainly prostacyclin) when used in those patients. Consequently, should signs of pulmonary oedema occur when sildenafil is administered in patients with pulmonary hypertension, the possibility of associated veno-occlusive disease should be considered.

Lactose monohydrate is present in the tablet film coat. Patients with rare hereditary problems of galactose intolerance, the Lapp lactase deficiency or glucose-galactose malabsorption should not take this medicine.

4.5 Interaction with other medicinal products and other forms of interaction

<u>Effects of other medicinal products on sildenafil</u>

In vitro studies:

Sildenafil metabolism is principally mediated by the cytochrome P450 (CYP) isoforms 3A4 (major route) and 2C9 (minor route). Therefore, inhibitors of these isoenzymes may reduce sildenafil clearance and inducers of these isoenzymes may increase sildenafil clearance.

In vivo studies:

Population pharmacokinetic analysis of pulmonary arterial hypertension clinical trial data indicated a reduction in sildenafil clearance and/or an increase of oral bioavailability when co-administered with CYP3A4 substrates and the combination of CYP3A4 substrates and beta-blockers. These were the only factors with a statistically significant impact on sildenafil pharmacokinetics in patients with pulmonary arterial hypertension. The exposure to sildenafil in patients on CYP3A4 substrates and CYP3A4 substrates plus beta-blockers was 43 % and 66 % higher, respectively, compared to patients not receiving these classes of medicines. Sildenafil exposure was 5-fold higher at a dose of 80 mg three times a day compared to the exposure at a dose of 20 mg three times a day. This concentration range covers the increase in sildenafil exposure observed in specifically designed drug interaction studies with CYP3A4 inhibitors (except more potent CYP3A4 inhibitors e.g. ketoconazole, itraconazole, ritonavir).

CYP3A4 inducers seemed to have a substantial impact on the pharmacokinetics of sildenafil in pulmonary arterial hypertension patients, which was confirmed in the in-vivo interaction study with CYP3A4 inducer bosentan.

Co-administration of bosentan (a moderate inducer of CYP3A4, CYP2C9 and possibly of CYP2C19) 125mg twice daily with sildenafil 80 mg three times a day (at steady state) concomitantly administered during 6 days in healthy volunteers resulted in a 63% decrease of sildenafil AUC. Caution is recommended in case of co-administration.

Efficacy of sildenafil should be closely monitored in patients using concomitant potent CYP3A4 inducers, such as carbamazepine, phenytoin, phenobarbital, St John's Wort and rifampicine.

Co-administration of the HIV protease inhibitor ritonavir, which is a highly potent P450 inhibitor, at steady state (500 mg twice daily) with sildenafil (100 mg single dose) resulted in a 300 % (4-fold) increase in sildenafil C_{max} and a 1,000 % (11-fold) increase in sildenafil plasma AUC. At 24 hours, the plasma levels of sildenafil were still approximately 200 ng/ml, compared to approximately 5 ng/ml when sildenafil was administered alone. This is consistent with ritonavir's marked effects on a broad range of P450 substrates. Based on these pharmacokinetic results co-administration of sildenafil with ritonavir is contraindicated in pulmonary arterial hypertension patients (see section 4.3).

Co-administration of the HIV protease inhibitor saquinavir, a CYP3A4 inhibitor, at steady state (1200 mg three times a day) with sildenafil (100 mg single dose) resulted in a 140 % increase in sildenafil C_{max} and a 210 % increase in sildenafil AUC. Sildenafil had no effect on saquinavir pharmacokinetics.

When a single 100 mg dose of sildenafil was administered with erythromycin, a specific CYP3A4 inhibitor, at steady state (500 mg twice daily for 5 days), there was a 182 % increase in sildenafil systemic exposure (AUC). In normal healthy male volunteers, there was no evidence of an effect of azithromycin (500 mg daily for 3 days) on the AUC, C_{max}, T_{max}, elimination rate constant, or subsequent half-life of sildenafil or its principal circulating metabolite. Cimetidine (800 mg), a cytochrome P450 inhibitor and non-specific CYP3A4 inhibitor, caused a 56 % increase in plasma sildenafil concentrations when co-administered with sildenafil (50 mg) to healthy volunteers.

Potent CYP3A4 inhibitors such as ketoconazole and itraconazole would be expected to have effects similar to ritonavir (see section 4.3). CYP3A4 inhibitors of intermediate potency (e.g. clarithromycin, telithromycin and nefazodone) are expected to have an effect in between that of ritonavir and CYP3A4 inhibitors of medium potency (e.g. saquinavir/erythromycin), a seven-fold increase in exposure is assumed. Therefore dose adjustments are recommended when using CYP3A4 inhibitors of intermediate potency (see section 4.4).

The population pharmacokinetic analysis in pulmonary arterial hypertension patients suggested that co-administration of beta-blockers in combination with CYP3A4 substrates might result in an additional increase in sildenafil exposure compared with administration of CYP3A4 substrates alone.

Grapefruit juice is a weak inhibitor of CYP3A4 gut wall metabolism and may give rise to modest increases in plasma levels of sildenafil.

Single doses of antacid (magnesium hydroxide/aluminium hydroxide) did not affect the bioavailability of sildenafil.

Co-administration of oral contraceptives (ethinyloestradiol 30 μg and levonorgestrel 150 μg) did not affect the pharmacokinetics of sildenafil.

Nicorandil is a hybrid of potassium channel activator and nitrate. Due to the nitrate component it has the potential to have serious interaction with sildenafil.

<u>Effects of sildenafil on other medicinal products</u>

In vitro studies:

Sildenafil is a weak inhibitor of the cytochrome P450 isoforms 1A2, 2C9, 2C19, 2D6, 2E1 and 3A4 ($IC_{50} > 150$ μM). There are no data on the interaction of sildenafil and non-specific phosphodiesterase inhibitors such as theophylline or dipyridamole.

In vivo studies:

No significant interactions were shown when sildenafil (50 mg) was co-administered with tolbutamide (250 mg) or warfarin (40 mg), both of which are metabolised by CYP2C9.

Sildenafil had no significant effect on atorvastatin exposure (AUC increased 11%), suggesting that sildenafil does not have a clinically relevant effect on CYP3A4.

No interactions were observed between sildenafil (100 mg single dose) and acenocoumarol.

Sildenafil (50 mg) did not potentiate the increase in bleeding time caused by acetyl salicylic acid (150 mg).

Sildenafil (50 mg) did not potentiate the hypotensive effects of alcohol in healthy volunteers with mean maximum blood alcohol levels of 80 mg/dl.

In a study of healthy volunteers sildenafil at steady state (80 mg three times a day) resulted in a 50% increase in bosentan AUC (125 mg twice daily). Caution is recommended in case of co-administration.

In a specific interaction study, where sildenafil (100 mg) was co-administered with amlodipine in hypertensive patients, there was an additional reduction on supine systolic blood pressure of 8 mmHg. The corresponding additional reduction in supine diastolic blood pressure was 7 mmHg. These additional blood pressure reductions were of a similar magnitude to those seen when sildenafil was administered alone to healthy volunteers.

In three specific drug-drug interaction studies, the alpha-blocker doxazosin (4 mg and 8 mg) and sildenafil (25 mg, 50 mg, or 100 mg) were administered simultaneously to patients with benign prostatic hyperplasia (BPH) stabilized on doxazosin therapy. In these study populations, mean additional reductions of supine systolic and diastolic blood pressure of 7/7 mmHg, 9/5 mmHg, and 8/4 mmHg, respectively, and mean additional reductions of standing blood pressure of 6/6 mmHg, 11/4 mmHg, and 4/5 mmHg, respectively were observed. When sildenafil and doxazosin were administered simultaneously to patients stabilized on doxazosin therapy, there were infrequent reports of patients who experienced symptomatic postural hypotension. These reports included dizziness and light-headedness, but not syncope. Concomitant administration of sildenafil to patients taking alpha-blocker therapy may lead to symptomatic hypotension in susceptible individuals (see section 4.4).

Sildenafil (100 mg single dose) did not affect the steady state pharmacokinetics of the HIV protease inhibitor saquinavir, which is a CYP3A4 substrate/inhibitor.

Consistent with its known effects on the nitric oxide/cGMP pathway (see section 5.1), sildenafil was shown to potentiate the hypotensive effects of nitrates, and its co-administration with nitric oxide donors or nitrates in any form is therefore contraindicated (see section 4.3).

Sildenafil had no clinically significant impact on the plasma levels of oral contraceptives (ethinyloestradiol 30 μg and levonorgestrel 150 μg).

4.6 Pregnancy and lactation

There are no data from the use of sildenafil in pregnant women. Animal studies do not indicate direct or indirect harmful effects with respect to pregnancy and embryonal/foetal development. Studies in animals have shown toxicity with respect to postnatal development (see section 5.3).

Due to lack of data, Revatio should not be used in pregnant women unless strictly necessary.

It is not known whether sildenafil enters the breast milk. Revatio should not be administered to breast-feeding mothers.

4.7 Effects on ability to drive and use machines

As dizziness and altered vision were reported in clinical trials with sildenafil, patients should be aware of how they might be affected by Revatio, before driving or operating machinery. No studies on the effects on the ability to drive and use machines have been performed.

4.8 Undesirable effects

In the pivotal placebo-controlled study of Revatio in pulmonary arterial hypertension, a total of 207 patients were treated with Revatio at daily doses ranging from 20 mg to 80 mg three times a day and 70 patients were treated with placebo. The duration of treatment was 12 weeks. 259 subjects who completed the pivotal study entered a long-term extension study. Doses up to 80 mg three times a day (4 times the recommended dose of 20 mg three times a day) were studied (N=149 patients treated for at least 1 year, 101 on 80 mg three times a day). The overall frequency of discontinuation in sildenafil treated patients at the recommended daily dose of 20 mg three times a day (2.9 %) was low and the same as placebo (2.9 %).

In a placebo-controlled study of Revatio as an adjunct to intravenous epoprostenol in pulmonary arterial hypertension, a total of 134 patients were treated with Revatio (in a fixed titration starting from 20 mg, to 40 mg and then 80 mg, three times a day) and epoprostenol, and 131 patients were treated with placebo and epoprostenol. The duration of treatment was 16 weeks. The overall frequency of discontinuations in sildenafil/epoprostenol treated patients due to adverse events was 5.2 % compared to 10.7 % in the placebo/epoprostenol treated patients. Newly reported adverse drug reactions, which occurred more frequently in the sildenafil/ epoprostenol group, were bloodshot eyes/red eyes, blurred vision, nasal congestion, night sweats, back pain and dry mouth. The known adverse events headache, flushing, pain in extremity and oedema were noted in a higher frequency in sildenafil/epoprostenol treated patients compared to placebo/epoprostenol treated patients.

In the two placebo controlled studies adverse events were generally mild to moderate in severity. The most commonly reported adverse reactions that occurred (greater or equal to 10 %) on Revatio compared to placebo were headache, flushing, dyspepsia, diarrhoea and limb pain.

Adverse reactions which occurred in ≥1 % of Revatio-treated patients and were more frequent (≥1 % difference) on Revatio in the study or in the Revatio combined data set of both placebo-controlled studies in pulmonary arterial hypertension at doses of 20, 40 or 80 mg three times a day, listed in the table below by class and frequency grouping (very common (≥1/10), common (≥1/100, <1/10), uncommon (≥1/1000, <1/100) and not known (cannot be estimated from the available data). Within each frequency grouping, undesirable effects are presented in order of decreasing seriousness.

Reports from post-marketing experience are in italics.

MedDRA System Organ Class	Adverse Drug Reaction
Infections and infestations	
Common	Cellulitis, influenza, sinusitis not otherwise specified (NOS)
Blood and the lymphatic system disorders	
Common	Anaemia NOS
Metabolism and nutrition disorders	
Common	Fluid retention
Psychiatric disorders	
Common	Insomnia, anxiety

Nervous system disorders	
Very Common	Headache
Common	Migraine NOS, tremor, paraesthesia, burning sensation NOS, hypoaesthesia
Eye disorders	
Common	Retinal haemorrhage, visual disturbance NOS, blurred vision, photophobia, chromatopsia, cyanopsia, eye irritation, blood shot eyes/red eyes
Uncommon	Visual acuity reduced, diplopia, abnormal sensation in eye
Ear and labyrinth disorders	
Common	Vertigo
Not known	*Sudden deafness**
Vascular disorders	
Very Common	Flushing
Respiratory, thoracic and mediastinal disorders	
Common	Bronchitis NOS, epistaxis, rhinitis NOS, cough, nasal congestion
Gastrointestinal disorders	
Very Common	Diarrhoea, dyspepsia
Common	Gastritis NOS, gastroenteritis NOS, gastrooesophageal reflux disease, haemorrhoids, abdominal distension, dry mouth
Skin and subcutaneous tissue disorders	
Common	Alopecia, erythema, night sweats
Not known	*Skin rash*
Musculoskeletal, connective tissue and bone disorders	
Very Common	Limb pain
Common	Myalgia, back pain
Reproductive system and breast disorders	
Uncommon	Gynaecomastia
Not known	*Priapism, prolonged erection*
General disorders and administration site conditions	
Common	Pyrexia

• Sudden decrease or loss of hearing has been reported in a small number of post-marketing and clinical trial cases with the use of all PDE5 inhibitors, including sildenafil.

In post marketing surveillance, adverse events/reactions that have been reported with an unknown frequency in the treatment of male erectile dysfunction (MED) include: Eye disorders: Non-arteritic anterior ischaemic optic neuropathy (NAION), retinal vascular occlusion and visual field defect.

4.9 Overdose

In single dose volunteer studies of doses up to 800 mg, adverse reactions were similar to those seen at lower doses, but the incidence rates and severities were increased. At single doses of 200 mg the incidence of adverse reactions (headache, flushing, dizziness, dyspepsia, nasal congestion, altered vision) was increased.

In cases of overdose, standard supportive measures should be adopted as required. Renal dialysis is not expected to accelerate clearance as sildenafil is highly bound to plasma proteins and not eliminated in the urine.

5. PHARMACOLOGICAL PROPERTIES

5.1 Pharmacodynamic properties

Pharmacotherapeutic group: Drugs used in erectile dysfunction, ATC code: G04B E03

Sildenafil is a potent and selective inhibitor of cyclic guanosine monophosphate (cGMP) specific phosphodiesterase type 5 (PDE5), the enzyme that is responsible for degradation of cGMP. Apart from the presence of this enzyme in the corpus cavernosum of the penis, PDE5 is also present in the pulmonary vasculature. Sildenafil, therefore, increases cGMP within pulmonary vascular smooth muscle cells resulting in relaxation. In patients with pulmonary arterial hypertension this can lead to vasodilation of the pulmonary vascular bed and, to a lesser degree, vasodilatation in the systemic circulation.

Studies *in vitro* have shown that sildenafil is selective for PDE5. Its effect is more potent on PDE5 than on other known phosphodiesterases. There is a 10-fold selectivity over PDE6 which is involved in the phototransduction pathway in the retina. There is an 80-fold selectivity over PDE1, and over 700-fold over PDE 2, 3, 4, 7, 8, 9, 10 and 11. In particular, sildenafil has greater than 4,000-fold selectivity for PDE5 over PDE3, the cAMP-specific phosphodiesterase isoform involved in the control of cardiac contractility.

Sildenafil causes mild and transient decreases in systemic blood pressure which, in the majority of cases, do not translate into clinical effects. After chronic dosing of 80 mg three times a day to patients with systemic hypertension the mean change from baseline in systolic and diastolic blood pressure was a decrease of 9.4 mmHg and 9.1 mm Hg respectively. After chronic dosing of 80 mg three times a day to patients with pulmonary arterial hypertension lesser effects in blood pressure reduction were observed (a reduction in both systolic and diastolic pressure of 2 mmHg). At the recommended dose of 20 mg three times a day no reductions in systolic or diastolic pressure were seen.

Single oral doses of sildenafil up to 100 mg in healthy volunteers produced no clinically relevant effects on ECG. After chronic dosing of 80 mg three times a day to patients with pulmonary arterial hypertension no clinically relevant effects on the ECG were reported.

In a study of the hemodynamic effects of a single oral 100 mg dose of sildenafil in 14 patients with severe coronary artery disease (CAD) (> 70 % stenosis of at least one coronary artery), the mean resting systolic and diastolic blood pressures decreased by 7 % and 6 % respectively compared to baseline. Mean pulmonary systolic blood pressure decreased by 9 %. Sildenafil showed no effect on cardiac output, and did not impair blood flow through the stenosed coronary arteries.

Mild and transient differences in colour discrimination (blue/green) were detected in some subjects using the Farnsworth-Munsell 100 hue test at 1 hour following a 100 mg dose, with no effects evident after 2 hours post-dose. The postulated mechanism for this change in colour discrimination is related to inhibition of PDE6, which is involved in the phototransduction cascade of the retina. Sildenafil has no effect on visual acuity or contrast sensitivity. In a small size placebo-controlled study of patients with documented early age-related macular degeneration (n=9), sildenafil (single dose, 100 mg) demonstrated no significant changes in visual tests conducted (visual acuity, Amsler grid, colour discrimination simulated traffic light, Humphrey perimeter and photostress).

Efficacy in adult patients with pulmonary arterial hypertension (PAH)

A randomised, double-blind, placebo-controlled study was conducted in 278 patients with primary pulmonary hypertension, PAH associated with connective tissue disease (CTD), and PAH following surgical repair of congenital heart lesions. Patients were randomised to one of four treatment groups: placebo, sildenafil 20 mg, sildenafil 40 mg or sildenafil 80 mg, three times a day. Of the 278 patients randomised, 277 patients received at least 1 dose of study drug. The study population consisted of 68 (25 %) men and 209 (75 %) women with a mean age of 49 years (range: 18-81 years) and baseline 6-minute walk test distance between 100 and 450 metres inclusive (mean: 344 metres). 175 patients (63%) included were diagnosed with primary pulmonary hypertension, 84 (30%) were diagnosed with PAH associated with connective tissue disease (CTD) and 18 (7%) of the patients were diagnosed with PAH following surgical repair of congenital heart lesions. Most patients were WHO Functional Class II (107/277, 39%) or III (160/277, 58%) with a mean baseline 6 minute walking distance of 378 meters and 326 meters respectively; fewer patients were Class I (1/277, 0.4%) or IV (9/277, 3%) at baseline. Patients with left ventricular ejection fraction < 45 % or left ventricular shortening fraction < 0.2 were not studied.

Sildenafil (or placebo) was added to patients' background therapy which could have included a combination of anticoagulation, digoxin, calcium channel blockers, diuretics or oxygen. The use of prostacyclin, prostacyclin analogues and endothelin receptor antagonists was not permitted as add-on therapy, and neither was arginine supplementation. Patients who previously failed bosentan therapy were excluded from the study.

The primary efficacy endpoint was the change from baseline at week 12 in 6-minute walk distance. A statistically significant increase in 6-minute walk distance was observed in all 3 sildenafil dose groups compared to those on placebo. Placebo corrected increases in walk distance were 45 metres ($p < 0.0001$), 46 metres ($p < 0.0001$) and 50 metres ($p < 0.0001$) for sildenafil 20 mg, 40 mg and 80 mg respectively. There was no significant difference in effect between sildenafil doses.

When analysed by WHO functional class, a statistically significant increase in 6-minute walk distance was observed in the 20 mg dose group. For class II and class III, placebo corrected increases of 49 metres (p = 0.0007) and 45 metres (p = 0.0031) were observed respectively.

The improvement in walk distance was apparent after 4 weeks of treatment and this effect was maintained at weeks 8 and 12. Results were generally consistent in subgroups according to baseline walking distance, aetiology (primary and CTD-associated PAH), WHO functional class, gender, race, location, mean PAP and PVRI.

Patients on all sildenafil doses achieved a statistically significant reduction in mean pulmonary arterial pressure (mPAP) compared to those on placebo. The placebo-corrected treatment was –2.7 mmHg (p=0.04) for sildenafil 20 mg three times a day. There was no evidence of a difference in effect between sildenafil 20 mg and the higher doses tested. The mean change from baseline in pulmonary vascular resistance (PVR) was –122 dyne.sec/cm^5 for sildenafil 20 mg three times a day. The percent reduction at 12 weeks for sildenafil 20 mg in PVR (11.2%) was proportionally greater than the reduction in systemic vascular resistance (SVR) (7.2%). The effect of sildenafil on mortality is unknown.

Long-term Survival Data

Patient enrolled into the pivotal study were eligible to enter a long term open label extension study. A study of 207 patients were treated with Revatio in the pivotal study, and their long term survival status was assessed for a minimum of 3 years. In this population, Kaplan-Meier estimates of 1, 2 and 3 year survival were 96%, 91% and 82%, respectively. Survival in patients of WHO functional class II at baseline at 1, 2 and 3 years was 99%, 91% and 84% respectively, and for patients of WHO functional class III at baseline was 94%, 90% and 81% respectively.

Efficacy in adult patients with PAH (when used in combination with epoprostenol)

A randomised, double-blind, placebo controlled study was conducted in 267 patients with PAH who were stabilised on intravenous epoprostenol. The PAH patients included those with Primary Pulmonary Arterial Hypertension (212/267, 79%) and PAH associated with CTD (55/267, 21%). Most patients were WHO Functional Class II (68/267, 26%) or III (175/267, 66%); fewer patients were Class I (3/267, 1%) or IV (16/267, 6%) at baseline; for a few patients (5/267, 2%), the WHO Functional Class was unknown. Patients were randomised to placebo or sildenafil (in a fixed titration starting from 20 mg, to 40 mg and then 80 mg, three times a day) when used in combination with intravenous epoprostenol.

The primary efficacy endpoint was the change from baseline at week 16 in 6-minute walk distance. There was a statistically significant benefit of sildenafil compared to placebo in 6-minute walk distance. A mean placebo corrected increase in walk distance of 26 metres was observed in favour of sildenafil (95% CI: 10.8, 41.2) (p=0.0009). For patients with a baseline walking distance ⩾325 metres, the treatment effect was 38.4 metres in favour of sildenafil; for patients with a baseline walking distance <325 metres, the treatment effect was 2.3 metres in favour of placebo. For patients with primary PAH, the treatment effect was 31.1 metres compared to 7.7 metres for patients with PAH associated with CTD. The difference in results between these randomisation subgroups may have arisen by chance in view of their limited sample size.

Patients on sildenafil achieved a statistically significant reduction in mean Pulmonary Arterial Pressure (mPAP) compared to those on placebo. A mean placebo-corrected treatment effect of -3.9 mmHg was observed in favour of sildenafil (95% CI: -5.7, -2.1) (p=0.00003).

5.2 Pharmacokinetic properties

Absorption:

Sildenafil is rapidly absorbed. Maximum observed plasma concentrations are reached within 30 to 120 minutes (median 60 minutes) of oral dosing in the fasted state. The mean absolute oral bioavailability is 41 % (range 25-63 %). After oral three times a day dosing of sildenafil, AUC and C_{max} increase in proportion with dose over the dose range of 20-40 mg. After oral doses of 80 mg three times a day a more than dose proportional increase in sildenafil plasma levels has been observed. In pulmonary arterial hypertension patients, the oral bioavailability of sildenafil after 80 mg three times a day was on average 43 % (90 % CI: 27% - 60%) higher compared to the lower doses.

When sildenafil is taken with food, the rate of absorption is reduced with a mean delay in T_{max} of 60 minutes and a mean reduction in C_{max} of 29 % however, the extent of absorption was not significantly affected (AUC decreased by 11%).

Distribution:

The mean steady state volume of distribution (V_d) for sildenafil is 105 l, indicating distribution into the tissues. After oral doses of 20 mg three times a day, the mean maximum total plasma concentration of sildenafil at steady state is approximately 113 ng/ml. Sildenafil and its major circulating N-desmethyl metabolite are approximately 96 % bound to plasma proteins. Protein binding is independent of total drug concentrations.

Metabolism:

Sildenafil is cleared predominantly by the CYP3A4 (major route) and CYP2C9 (minor route) hepatic microsomal isoenzymes. The major circulating metabolite results from N-demethylation of sildenafil. This metabolite has a phosphodiesterase selectivity profile similar to sildenafil and an *in vitro* potency for PDE5 approximately 50 % that of the parent drug. The N-desmethyl metabolite is further metabolised, with a terminal half-life of approximately 4 h. In patients with pulmonary arterial hypertension, plasma concentrations of N-desmethyl metabolite are approximately 72 % those of sildenafil after 20 mg three times a day dosing (translating into a 36 % contribution to sildenafil's pharmacological effects). The subsequent effect on efficacy is unknown.

Elimination:

The total body clearance of sildenafil is 41 l/h with a resultant terminal phase half-life of 3-5 h. After either oral or intravenous administration, sildenafil is excreted as metabolites predominantly in the faeces (approximately 80 % of administered oral dose) and to a lesser extent in the urine (approximately 13 % of administered oral dose).

Pharmacokinetics in special patient groups

Elderly:

Healthy elderly volunteers (65 years or over) had a reduced clearance of sildenafil, resulting in approximately 90 % higher plasma concentrations of sildenafil and the active N-desmethyl metabolite compared to those seen in healthy younger volunteers (18-45 years). Due to age-differences in plasma protein binding, the corresponding increase in free sildenafil plasma concentration was approximately 40 %.

Renal insufficiency:

In volunteers with mild to moderate renal impairment (creatinine clearance = 30-80 ml/min), the pharmacokinetics of sildenafil were not altered after receiving a 50 mg single oral dose. In volunteers with severe renal impairment (creatinine clearance <30 ml/min), sildenafil clearance was reduced, resulting in mean increases in AUC and C_{max} of 100 % and 88 % respectively compared to age-matched volunteers with no renal impairment. In addition, N-desmethyl metabolite AUC and C_{max} values were significantly increased 200 % and 79 % respectively in subjects with severe renal impairment compared to subjects with normal renal function.

Hepatic insufficiency:

In volunteers with mild to moderate hepatic cirrhosis (Child-Pugh class A and B) sildenafil clearance was reduced, resulting in increases in AUC (85 %) and C_{max} (47 %) compared to age-matched volunteers with no hepatic impairment. In addition, N-desmethyl metabolite AUC and C_{max} values were significantly increased by 154 % and 87 %, respectively in cirrhotic subjects compared to subjects with normal hepatic function. The pharmacokinetics of sildenafil in patients with severely impaired hepatic function have not been studied.

Population pharmacokinetics:

In patients with pulmonary arterial hypertension, the average steady state concentrations were 20 – 50 % higher over the investigated dose range of 20–80 mg three times a day compared to healthy volunteers. There was a doubling of the C_{min} compared to healthy volunteers. Both findings suggest a lower clearance and/or a higher oral bioavailability of sildenafil in patients with pulmonary arterial hypertension compared to healthy volunteers.

5.3 Preclinical safety data

Non clinical data revealed no special hazard for humans based on conventional studies of safety pharmacology, repeated dose toxicity, genotoxicity and carcinogenic potential, fertility and embryonal/foetal development.

In pups of rats which were pre- and postnatally treated with 60 mg/kg sildenafil, a decreased litter size, a lower pup weight on day 1 and a decreased 4-day survival were seen at exposures which were approximately fifty times the expected human exposure at 20 mg three times a day. These effects were observed at exposures considered sufficiently in excess of the maximum human exposure indicating little relevance to clinical use.

6. PHARMACEUTICAL PARTICULARS

6.1 List of excipients

Tablet core:

microcrystalline cellulose

calcium hydrogen phosphate (anhydrous)

croscarmellose sodium

magnesium stearate

Film coat:

hypromellose

titanium dioxide (E171)

lactose monohydrate

glycerol triacetate

6.2 Incompatibilities

Not applicable.

6.3 Shelf life

5 years.

6.4 Special precautions for storage

Do not store above 30 °C. Store in the original package in order to protect from moisture.

6.5 Nature and contents of container

PVC/Aluminium blisters of 90 tablets (15 tablets per blister strip) in a carton.

6.6 Special precautions for disposal and other handling

No special requirements.

7. MARKETING AUTHORISATION HOLDER

Pfizer Limited, Sandwich, Kent CT13 9NJ, United Kingdom.

8. MARKETING AUTHORISATION NUMBER(S)

EU/1/05/318/001

9. DATE OF FIRST AUTHORISATION/RENEWAL OF THE AUTHORISATION

Date of first authorisation: 28 October 2005

10. DATE OF REVISION OF THE TEXT

07/2009

11. LEGAL CATEGORY

POM

Ref: RV8_0

Detailed information on this product is available on the website of the European Medicines Agency (EMEA) http://www.emea.europa.eu

Rhinocort Aqua 64 micrograms, nasal spray

(AstraZeneca UK Limited)

1. NAME OF THE MEDICINAL PRODUCT

Rhinocort® Aqua, 64 micrograms, nasal spray

2. QUALITATIVE AND QUANTITATIVE COMPOSITION

Each actuation contains: Budesonide 64 micrograms (1.28 mg/ml).

For excipients, see 6.1.

3. PHARMACEUTICAL FORM

Nasal spray, suspension.

4. CLINICAL PARTICULARS

4.1 Therapeutic indications

Seasonal and perennial allergic rhinitis and vasomotor rhinitis. Treatment of nasal polyps.

4.2 Posology and method of administration

For nasal inhalation. Dosage should be individualised.

Rhinitis (Adults including elderly)

Recommended start dose	Once daily dosing	Twice daily dosing
256 micrograms per day	Two applications of 64 micrograms into each nostril each morning **or** If good effect is achieved, one application of 64 micrograms	One application of 64 micrograms into each nostril morning and evening

Nasal Polyps (Adults including elderly)

Recommended start dose	Once daily dosing	Twice daily dosing
256 micrograms per day	Not applicable	One application of 64 micrograms into each nostril morning and evening.

Treatment can be continued for up to 3 months.

Patients should be reminded of the importance of taking this medicine regularly.

The dose should be titrated to the lowest dose at which effective control of symptoms is achieved.

Children: There are insufficient data to recommend the use of Rhinocort Aqua in children. However, it is unlikely that the risk/benefit ratio in children is different from that in adults.

4.3 Contraindications

Hypersensitivity to any of the ingredients.

4.4 Special warnings and precautions for use

Special care is demanded in treatment of patients transferred from oral steroids to Rhinocort where disturbances of the hypothalamic-pituitary-adrenal (HPA) axis could be expected.

Special care is needed in patients with fungal and viral infections of the airways and in patients with lung tuberculosis.

The patient should be informed that the full effect of Rhinocort is not achieved until after a few days treatment. Treatment of seasonal rhinitis should, if possible, start before exposure to the allergens. Concomitant treatment may sometimes be necessary to counteract eye symptoms caused by the allergy. In continuous long-term treatment, the nasal mucosa should be inspected regularly e.g. every 6 months.

Systemic effects of nasal corticosteroids may occur, particularly at high doses prescribed for prolonged periods. Growth retardation has been reported in children receiving nasal corticosteroids at licensed doses.

It is recommended that the height of children receiving prolonged treatment with nasal corticosteroids is regularly monitored. If growth is slowed, therapy should be reviewed with the aim of reducing the dose of nasal corticosteroid, if possible, to the lowest dose at which effective control of symptoms is maintained. In addition, consideration should also be given to referring the patient to a paediatric specialist.

Treatment with higher than recommended doses may result in clinically significant adrenal suppression. If there is evidence for higher than recommended doses being used, additional systemic corticosteroid cover should be considered during periods of stress or elective surgery.

In vivo studies have shown that oral administration of itraconazole and ketoconazole (known inhibitors of CYP3A4 activity in the liver and in the intestinal mucosa, see also section 4.5 Interactions) may cause an increase in the systemic exposure to budesonide. This is of limited clinical importance for short-term (1-2 weeks) treatment with itraconazole or ketoconazole, but should be taken into consideration during long-term treatment.

4.5 Interaction with other medicinal products and other forms of interaction

The metabolism of budesonide is primarily mediated by CYP3A4, a subfamily of cytochrome P450. Inhibitors of this enzyme, e.g. itraconazole and ketoconazole, can therefore increase systemic exposure to budesonide. However, the use of itraconazole or ketoconazole concomitant with Rhinocort Aqua for shorter periods is of limited importance, see section 4.4 Special warnings and precautions for use.

4.6 Pregnancy and lactation

Administration during pregnancy should be avoided unless there are compelling reasons. Results from prospective epidemiological studies and from worldwide post marketing experience indicate no increased risk for overall congenital malformations from the use of inhaled or intranasal budesonide during early pregnancy. Budesonide is excreted in breast milk. However, at therapeutic doses of Rhinocort no effects on the breast fed child are anticipated. Rhinocort can be used during breastfeeding.

4.7 Effects on ability to drive and use machines

Rhinocort Aqua does not affect the ability to drive or operate machinery.

4.8 Undesirable effects

Adverse reactions, which have been associated with budesonide, are given below, listed by system organ class and frequency. Frequency is defined as: very common (⩾1/10), common (⩾1/100 and <1/10), uncommon (⩾1/1000 and <1/100), rare (⩾1/10 000 and <1/1000), very rare (<1/10 000) and not known (reported spontaneously and cannot be estimated from available post marketing data).

Immune system disorders	Uncommon	Immediate and delayed hypersensitivity reactions including urticaria, rash, dermatitis angioedema and pruritus
	Not Known	Anaphylactic reaction
Eye disorders	Rare	Raised intraocular pressure or glaucoma
Respiratory, thoracic and mediastinal disorders	Common	Haemorrhagic secretion and epistaxis Nasal Irritation (sneezing, stinging and dryness)
	Very rare	Nasal septum perforation Ulceration of mucus membrane

Systemic effects of nasal corticosteroids may occur, particularly when prescribed at high doses for prolonged periods (see section 4.4).

4.9 Overdose

Acute overdose with Rhinocort should not present clinical problems.

Inhalation of high doses of corticosteroids may lead to suppression of the hypothalamic-pituitary-adrenal (HPA) axis function.

5. PHARMACOLOGICAL PROPERTIES

5.1 Pharmacodynamic properties

Budesonide is a non-halogenated glucocorticosteroid with a high local anti-inflammatory action within the respiratory tract.

ATC code: R01A D05

5.2 Pharmacokinetic properties

Bioavailablity of oral budesonide in man is low (11-13%) due to an extensive first-pass metabolism in the liver.

The systemic availability of budesonide from Rhinocort Aqua, with reference to the metered dose is 33%. In adults, the maximal plasma concentration after administration of 256 micrograms budesonide from Rhinocort Aqua is 0.64 nM and is reached within 0.7 hours. The AUC after administration of 256 micrograms budesonide from Rhinocort Aqua is 2.7 nmolxh/L in adults.

5.3 Preclinical safety data

The acute toxicity of budesonide is low and of the same order of magnitude and type as that of the reference glucocorticoids studied (beclomethasone dipropionate, flucinolone acetonide). Results from subacute and chronic toxicity studies show that the systemic effects of budesonide are less severe than or similar to those observed after administration of the other glucocorticosteroids e.g. decreased body weight gain and atrophy of lymphoid tissues and adrenal cortex. An increased incidence of brain gliomas in male rats in a carcinogenicity study could not be verified in a repeat study, in which the incidence of gliomas did not differ between any of the groups on active treatment (budesonide, prednisolone, triamcinolone acetonide) and the control groups. Liver changes (primary hepatocellular neoplasms) found in male rats in the original carcinogenicity study were noted again in the repeat study with budesonide, as well as with the reference glucocorticosteroids. These effects are most probably related to a receptor effect and thus represent a class effect.

Available clinical experience shows no indication that budesonide or other glucocorticosteroids induce brain gliomas or primary heptocellular neoplasms in man. Budesonide has been used successfully in the treatment of seasonal allergic rhinitis for several years.

In animal reproduction studies, corticosteroids such as budesonide have been shown to induce malformations (cleft plate, skeletal malformations). However these animal experimental results do not appear to be relevant in humans at the recommended doses.

Animal studies have also identified an involvement of excess prenatal glucocorticosteroids in increased risk for intrauterine growth retardation, adult cardiovascular disease and permanent changes in glucocorticoid receptor density, neurotransmitter turnover and behaviour at exposures below the teratogenic dose range.

6. PHARMACEUTICAL PARTICULARS

6.1 List of excipients

Disodium edetate

Potassium sorbate (E202)

Glucose anhydrous

Microcrystalline cellulose (E460)

Carboxymethylcellulose sodium (E466)

Polysorbate 80 (E433)

Hydrochloric acid

Purified water

6.2 Incompatibilities

None known.

6.3 Shelf life

2 years.

6.4 Special precautions for storage

Use within 2 months of starting treatment.

Do not store above 30°C. Do not refrigerate or freeze.

6.5 Nature and contents of container

Rhinocort Aqua is an aqueous solution of budesonide in either a 10 ml or 20 ml amber/brown glass (type II) bottle. Each bottle is fitted with a spray pump and contains either 120 or 240 actuations. Not all pack sizes may be available in the UK.

6.6 Special precautions for disposal and other handling

Before using Rhinocort Aqua for the first time the nozzle must be primed (filled with the medicine). To do this the bottle is shaken and the protective cap removed. The bottle is then held upright and the nozzle pumped up and down several times (5-10 times) spraying into the air, until an even mist is seen. The priming effect remains for approximately 24 hours. If a longer period of time passes before the next dose is taken, the nozzle must be loaded with medicine again. This time it is sufficient to spray just once into the air.

a. The patient is then instructed to blow their nose. Next, the bottle needs to be shaken and the protective cap removed.

b. The bottle is then held upright, with one finger held on either side of the nozzle.

c. The tip of the nozzle is inserted into the nostril and the nozzle pressed down once (or more as instructed by the doctor). The spray is then administered into the other nostril in the same way. Note: it is not necessary to inhale at the same time as spraying.

d. The nozzle needs to be wiped with a clean tissue after use and the protective cap replaced. The bottle should be stored in an upright position.

e. **Keeping the Rhinocort Aqua nozzle clean**

The plastic nozzle of Rhinocort Aqua should be cleaned regularly and at any time the spray of medicine is not coming out as it should. If this happens, first the nozzle should be checked to ensure that it is primed with medicine (see earlier). If, after the nozzle is primed again, the pump is still not working, the nozzle should be cleaned by using the following instructions:

The plastic nozzle is removed with a clean tissue and washed in warm, not hot, water. The nozzle is then rinsed thoroughly, dried and then replaced onto the top of the bottle. The nozzle should not be unblocked with a pin or other sharp object. After cleaning, the nozzle must be primed (filled with medicine) again before use.

7. MARKETING AUTHORISATION HOLDER

AstraZeneca UK Ltd.,

600 Capability Green,

Luton, LU1 3LU, UK.

8. MARKETING AUTHORISATION NUMBER(S)

PL 17901/0074

9. DATE OF FIRST AUTHORISATION/RENEWAL OF THE AUTHORISATION

12 December 2003

10. DATE OF REVISION OF THE TEXT

8th April 2009

Rhophylac 300 (1500 IU)

(CSL Behring UK Limited)

1. NAME OF THE MEDICINAL PRODUCT

Rhophylac 300 micrograms / 2 ml, solution for injection in pre-filled syringe

2. QUALITATIVE AND QUANTITATIVE COMPOSITION

Human Anti-D immunoglobulin

Each 2 ml solution in pre-filled syringe contains:

Human anti-D immunoglobulin 1500 IU (300 micrograms)

Corresponding to a concentration of 750 IU (150 micrograms) per ml

The product contains a maximum of 30 mg/ml of human plasma proteins of which 10 mg/ml is human albumin as stabiliser. At least 95 % of the other plasma proteins are IgG.

Rhophylac contains not more than 5 micrograms/ml IgA.

For a full list of excipients, see section 6.1

3. PHARMACEUTICAL FORM

Solution for injection in pre-filled syringe

4. CLINICAL PARTICULARS

4.1 Therapeutic indications

Prevention of Rh(D) immunisation in Rh(D)-negative women

- Pregnancy/delivery of a Rh(D)-positive baby

- Abortion/threatened abortion, ectopic pregnancy or hydatidiform mole

- Transplacental haemorrhage (TPH) resulting from antepartum haemorrhage (AMH), amniocentesis, chorionic biopsy or obstetric manipulative procedures e.g. external version, or abdominal trauma.

Treatment of Rh(D)-negative persons after incompatible transfusions of Rh(D)-positive blood or other products containing red blood cells

4.2 Posology and method of administration

Posology

The following dose schedules are recommended based on the clinical studies performed with Rhophylac, however consideration must be given to professional guidelines for the use of anti-D IgG in the individual EU member states.

Prevention of Rh(D) immunisation in Rh(D)-negative women:

• Antepartum prophylaxis: The recommended dose is a single dose of 300 micrograms (1500 IU) administered by intravenous or intramuscular injection at 28 - 30 weeks of gestation.

• Postpartum prophylaxis: For intravenous administration, 200 micrograms (1000 IU) is a sufficient dose. If administered intramuscularly, 200 micrograms (1000 IU) to 300 micrograms (1500 IU) is recommended. Rhophylac should be administered as soon as possible within 72 hours of delivery. The post partum dose must be given even when antepartum prophylaxis has been administered. If a large foeto-maternal haemorrhage (greater than 4 ml (0.7% - 0.8% of women)) is suspected, e.g., in the event of foetal anaemia or intrauterine foetal death, its extent should be determined by a suitable method, e.g., Kleihauer-Betke test, and additional doses of anti-D should be administered as indicated (20 micrograms/100IU for each 1 ml of foetal red blood cells).

• Prophylaxis following complications of pregnancy:

- Interventions and incidents occurring up to 12 weeks gestation: 200 micrograms (1000 IU) should be administered by intravenous or intramuscular injection as soon as possible and not later than 72 hours after the at-risk event.

- Interventions and incidents occurring after 12 weeks of gestation: at least 200 micrograms (1000 IU) should be administered by intravenous or intramuscular injection as soon as possible and not later than 72 hours after the at-risk event.

- Chorionic villus sampling: 200 micrograms (1000 IU) should be administered by intravenous or intramuscular injection as soon as possible and not later than 72 hours after the at-risk event.

Incompatible transfusions:

The recommended dose is 20 micrograms (100 IU) anti-D immunoglobulin per 2 ml of transfused Rh(D)-positive blood or per 1 ml of erythrocyte concentrate. The intravenous administration is recommended. If given by intramuscular administration the large doses should be applied over a period of several days. A maximum dose of 3000 micrograms is sufficient in the case of larger incompatible transfusions independent of whether the transfusion volume is greater than 300 ml of Rh(D)-positive blood.

Method of administration

Rhophylac can be administered by intravenous or intramuscular injection. In case of haemorrhagic disorders where intramuscular injections are contraindicated, Rhophylac should be administered intravenously. If large doses (>5 ml) are required and intramuscular injection is chosen, it is advisable to administer them in divided doses at different sites.

4.3 Contraindications

Hypersensitivity to any of the components.

The intramuscular injection is contraindicated in persons with severe thrombocytopenia or other disorders of haemostasis.

4.4 Special warnings and precautions for use

In the case of postpartum use, anti-D immunoglobulin is intended for maternal administration. It should not be given to the newborn infant.

The product is not intended for use in Rh(D)-positive individuals.

Patients should be observed for at least 20 minutes after administration. If symptoms of allergic or anaphylactic type reactions occur, immediate discontinuation of the administration is required.

Allergic responses to anti-D immunoglobulin may occur. Patients should be informed of the early signs of hypersensitivity reactions including hives, generalised urticaria, tightness of the chest, wheezing, hypotension and anaphylaxis. The treatment required depends on the nature and severity of the side effect. If necessary, the current medical standards for shock treatment should be observed.

The concentration of IgA in Rhophylac was found to be below the detection limit of 5 micrograms/ml. Nevertheless, the product may contain trace amounts of IgA. Although anti-D immunoglobulin has been used successfully to treat selected IgA deficient patients, individuals who are deficient in IgA have the potential for developing IgA antibodies and may have anaphylactic reactions after administration of blood components containing IgA. The physician must therefore weigh the benefit of treatment with Rhophylac against the potential risks of hypersensitivity reactions.

Information on safety with respect to transmissible agents

Standard measures to prevent infections resulting from the use of medicinal products prepared from human blood or plasma include selection of donors, screening of individual donations and plasma pools for specific markers of infection and the inclusion of effective manufacturing steps for the inactivation/removal of viruses. Despite this, when medicinal products prepared from human blood or plasma are administered, the possibility of transmitting infective agents cannot be totally excluded. This also applies to unknown or emerging viruses and other pathogens.

The measures taken are considered effective for HIV, HBV and HCV.

They may be of limited value against non-enveloped viruses such as HAV or parvovirus B19.

There is reassuring clinical experience regarding the lack of hepatits A or parvovirus B19 transmission with immunoglobulins and it is also assumed that the antibody content makes an important contribution to the viral safety.

It is strongly recommended that every time that Rhophylac is administered to a patient, the name and batch number of the product are recorded in order to maintain a link between the patient and the batch of the product.

4.5 Interaction with other medicinal products and other forms of interaction

Interactions of Rhophylac with other treatments have not been investigated. The information given in this section is derived from the literature and current guidelines.

Active immunisation with live virus vaccines (e.g. measles, mumps, rubella or varicella) should be postponed until 3 months after the last administration of anti-D immunoglobulin, as the efficacy of the live virus vaccine may be impaired. If anti-D immunoglobulin needs to be administered within 2- 4 weeks of a live virus vaccination, then the efficacy of such a vaccination may be impaired.

After injection of immunoglobulin the transitory rise of the various passively transferred antibodies in the patients blood may result in misleading positive results in serological testing for red blood cell antibodies e.g. Coomb's test in the neonate.

Rhophylac can contain antibodies to other Rh antigens, e.g. anti-Rh(C) antibodies, which might be detected by sensitive serological test methods following administration of the product.

4.6 Pregnancy and lactation

This medicinal product is used in pregnancy.

No study drug-related adverse events were reported for the children delivered of 432 patients who received antepartum administration of Rhophylac.

4.7 Effects on ability to drive and use machines
No effects on ability to drive and use machines have been observed.

4.8 Undesirable effects
When anti-D immunoglobulins are administered by the intramuscular route, local pain and tenderness can be observed at the injection site.

Occasionally fever, malaise, headache, cutaneous reactions and chills occur. In rare cases, nausea, vomiting, hypotension, tachycardia, and allergic or anaphylactic type reactions, including dyspnoea and shock, are reported, even when the patient has shown no hypersensitivity to previous administration.

For viral safety with respect to transmissible agents, see section 4.4.

4.9 Overdose
No data are available on overdosage. Patients in receipt of an incompatible transfusion who receive very large doses of anti-D immunoglobulin should be monitored clinically and by biological parameters because of the risk of haemolytic reaction. In other Rh(D)-negative individuals overdosage should not lead to more frequent or more severe undesirable effects than the normal dose.

5. PHARMACOLOGICAL PROPERTIES
5.1 Pharmacodynamic properties
Pharmacotherapeutic group: immune sera and immunoglobulins: Anti-D (Rh) immunoglobulin. ATC Code: J06BB01.

Rhophylac contains specific IgG antibodies against the Rh(D) antigen of human erythrocytes.

During pregnancy, and especially at the time of childbirth, foetal red blood cells may enter the maternal circulation. When the woman is Rh(D)-negative and the foetus Rh(D)-positive, the women might become immunised to the Rh(D) antigen and may produce anti-Rh(D) antibodies which cross the placenta and may cause haemolytic disease of the newborn. Passive immunisation with anti-D immunoglobulin prevents Rh(D) immunisation in more than 99% of cases provided that a sufficient dose of anti-D immunoglobulin is administered early enough after exposure to Rh(D)-positive foetal red blood cells.

The mechanism by which anti-D immunoglobulin suppresses immunisation to Rh(D)-positive red cells is not known. Suppression may be related to the clearance of the red cells from the circulation before they reach immunocompetent sites or, it may be due to more complex mechanisms involving recognition of foreign antigen and antigen presentation by the appropriate cells at the appropriate sites in the presence or absence of antibody.

In Rh(D)-negative healthy male volunteers, both the intravenous and intramuscular administration of 200 micrograms (1000 IU) of Rhophylac at 48 hours after injection of 5 ml of Rh(D)-positive red blood cells resulted in an almost complete clearance of Rh(D)-positive red blood cells within 24 hours. While the intravenous administration of Rhophylac caused an instant onset of red blood cell disappearance, the onset of elimination of red blood cells following intramuscular administration was delayed as anti-D IgG had to be first absorbed from the injection site. On an average, 70% of injected red cells were cleared 2 hours after intravenous administration of Rhophylac. After intramuscular administration, a similar degree of red cell clearance was measured after 12 hours.

Furthermore, the efficacy, safety and pharmacokinetics of Rhophylac are supported by the results of three clinical studies in patients. Rhophylac 200 micrograms (1000 IU) was administered postpartum in 139 per protocol patients. Rhophylac 300 micrograms (1500 IU) was administered antepartum as well as postpartum in 446 and 256 per protocol patients, respectively. None of the patients included in these studies developed antibodies against the Rh(D) antigen.

Clinical studies with Rhophylac at doses below 200 micrograms (1000 IU) have not been performed.

5.2 Pharmacokinetic properties
Measurable levels of antibodies are obtained approximately 4 hours after intramuscular injection. Peak serum levels are usually achieved 5 days later.

Measurable levels of antibodies are obtained immediately after intravenous injection. The mean half-life in the circulation of pregnant women with normal IgG levels was 17 days. IgG and IgG-complexes are broken down in cells of the reticuloendothelial system.

5.3 Preclinical safety data
There are no preclinical data of relevance for anti-D immunoglobulin. Repeated dose testing and embryo-foetal toxicity studies have not been conducted and are impracticable due to induction of, and interference with antibodies. The potential for mutagenic effects of immunoglobulins have not been studied.

6. PHARMACEUTICAL PARTICULARS
6.1 List of excipients
Human albumin
Glycine
Sodium chloride

6.2 Incompatibilities
In the absence of compatibility studies, this medicinal product must not be mixed with other medicinal products.

6.3 Shelf life
3 years

6.4 Special precautions for storage
Store in a refrigerator(+2°C to +8°C). Do not freeze.

Keep the syringe (originally blistered) in the outer carton in order to protect from light.

Store out of the reach and sight of children.

6.5 Nature and contents of container
Glass syringe (type I glass) pre-filled with 2 ml solution for injection (1500 IU anti-D IgG).

Pack size: 1 blister pack contains 1 pre-filled syringe and 1 injection needle.

6.6 Special precautions for disposal and other handling
Rhophylac should be brought to room or body temperature before use.

The solution should be clear or slightly opalescent. Do not use solutions which are cloudy or have deposits.

Use only once (one syringe – one patient).

Any unused product or waste material should be disposed of in accordance with local requirements.

7. MARKETING AUTHORISATION HOLDER
CSL Behring GmbH

Emil-von-Behring-Strasse 76

35041 Marburg

Germany

8. MARKETING AUTHORISATION NUMBER(S)
PL 15036/0019

9. DATE OF FIRST AUTHORISATION/RENEWAL OF THE AUTHORISATION
01 June 2006

10. DATE OF REVISION OF THE TEXT
21 September 2007

Ridaura Tiltab Tablets 3mg

(Astellas Pharma Ltd)

1. NAME OF THE MEDICINAL PRODUCT
RIDAURA TILTAB TABLETS 3 MG

2. QUALITATIVE AND QUANTITATIVE COMPOSITION
Auranofin HSE 3mg

3. PHARMACEUTICAL FORM
Tablet

4. CLINICAL PARTICULARS
4.1 Therapeutic indications
Ridaura is an orally active gold preparation. It is indicated in the management of adults with active progressive rheumatoid arthritis only when non-steroidal anti-inflammatory drugs have been found to be inadequate alone to control the disease, i.e. when second-line therapy is required. In patients with adult rheumatoid arthritis Ridaura has been shown to reduce disease activity reflected by synovitis, associated symptoms, and appropriate laboratory parameters. Gold cannot reverse structural damage to joints caused by previous disease. Ridaura does not produce an immediate response and therapeutic effects may be seen after three to six months of treatment.

4.2 Posology and method of administration
For Adults and the Elderly only:

For Adults:

The usual starting dose is 6 mg daily as one 3 mg tablet twice a day, in the morning and the evening with meals. If this is well tolerated a single daily dose may be given as two 3 mg tablets with breakfast or with the evening meal.

Treatment should be continued for a minimum of three to six months to assess response, as Ridaura is a slow-acting drug. If the response is inadequate after six months an increase to 9 mg (one tablet three times a day) may be tolerated. If response remains inadequate after a three month trial of 9 mg daily, Ridaura therapy should be discontinued. Safety at dosages exceeding 9 mg daily has not been studied.

Absorption of gold from Ridaura tablets is rapid but incomplete. Although mean blood gold levels are proportional to dose, no correlation between blood gold levels and safety or efficacy has been established. Dosage adjustments should therefore depend on monitoring clinical response and adverse events rather than on monitoring blood gold concentrations.

Anti-inflammatory drugs and analgesics may be prescribed as necessary with Ridaura.

The Elderly:

Dosage as for adults. As with all drugs extra caution should be exercised in administration to the elderly.

4.3 Contraindications
Contraindicated in pregnancy.

Contraindicated where hypersensitivity to gold compounds or other heavy metals exists.

Although not necessarily reported in association with Ridaura, do not use in patients with a history of any of the following gold-induced disorders: enterocolitis, pulmonary fibrosis, exfoliate dermatitis, bone marrow aplasia, or other severe blood dyscrasias or toxicity to other heavy metals. Use should also be avoided in progressive renal disease or severe active hepatic disease and in systemic lupus erythromatosus.

4.4 Special warnings and precautions for use
Use with caution in patients with any degree of renal impairment or hepatic dysfunction, inflammatory bowel disease, rash, or history of bone marrow depression.

Close monitoring is essential. Full blood count with differential and platelet counts (which should be plotted) and tests for urinary protein must be performed prior to Ridaura therapy and at least monthly thereafter, see also section 4.8. Ridaura should be withdrawn if the platelet count falls below 100,000 per ml or if signs and symptoms suggestive of thrombocytopenia, leucopenia and aplastic anaemia occur. The occurrence of purpura, ecchymoses or petechia would suggest the presence of thrombocytopenia and may indicate a need for additional platelet count determinations. Patients with gastrointestinal symptoms, with rash, with pruritus (which may precede rash), with stomatitis, or a metallic taste in the mouth (which might precede stomatitis), should also be closely monitored as such symptoms may indicate a need for modification of dosage or withdrawal, see also section 4.8. Pulmonary fibrosis may rarely occur and chest X-ray is recommended at least annually.

Prior to initiating treatment patients must be advised of the potential side effects associated with Ridaura. They should be warned to report promptly any unusual signs or symptoms during treatment such as pruritus, rash, metallic taste, sore throat or tongue, mouth ulceration, easy bruising, purpura, epistaxis, bleeding gums, menorrhagia, or diarrhoea.

Gold has been shown to be carcinogenic in rodents although there was no evidence of carcinogenicity in a 7-year dog study.

Patients should be cautioned to minimise exposure to ultraviolet light.

Auranofin has not been co-administered with other disease modifying agents such as penicillamine, levamisole and chloroquine/hydrochloroquine and, therefore, concomitant use cannot be recommended.

Patients with rare hereditary problems of galactose intolerance, the Lapp lactase deficiency or glucose-galactose malabsorption should not take this medicine.

Enterocolitis is a rare but potentially serious side effect, the development of diarrhoea with rectal bleeding or rectal bleeding alone unless rapidly explained otherwise mandates the immediate cessation of therapy. Patients should be warned to seek medical advice as soon as possible if they develop these symptoms.

4.5 Interaction with other medicinal products and other forms of interaction
Specific experience of interactions with auranofin is lacking. However, the theoretical potential for interaction with gold therapy, both oral and parenteral, should be considered.

Concomitant therapy with metal antagonists and potentially nephrotoxic or haemotoxic drugs should be administered with caution. Such drugs include penicillamine, aminoglycosides, amphotericin B, penicillins, phenylbutazone, phenytoin, sulfonamides, NSAIDs, acyclovir and alcohol.

Drugs affecting GI motility and those which are highly protein-bound may alter the absorption and binding, respectively, of auranofin.

4.6 Pregnancy and lactation
Gold is teratogenic in some animal species. Ridaura should not be used in pregnancy. Women of child-bearing potential should not be treated with Ridaura without full consideration of the benefits of treatment against the potential risk of teratogenicity; they should practise effective contraception during treatment and for at least six months after. Patients should be fully informed of the teratogenic risk, and termination of any pregnancy occurring during treatment should be considered in view of the possibility of foetal malformation. If women are to be treated post-partum with Ridaura, breast-feeding should be avoided.

4.7 Effects on ability to drive and use machines
None stated.

4.8 Undesirable effects
Adverse reactions can occur throughout treatment with Ridaura, although the highest incidence can be expected during the first six months of treatment. The most common reaction to Ridaura is diarrhoea or loose stools, occurring in about 30% of patients according to the literature. Up to about one patient in twenty will be unable to tolerate Ridaura because of diarrhoea.

Blood and lymphatic system	
Blood dyscrasias including leucopenia*, granulocytopenia and thrombocytopenia*, anaemia, eosinophilia	**Common** (>1/100, <1/10)
Agranulocytosis, aplastic anaemia*, red cell aplasia	**Very rare** (<1/10,000)
Nervous system disorders	
Headache	**Uncommon** (>1/1000, <1/100)
Dizziness	**Very rare** (<1/10,000)/not known cannot be estimated from the available data)
Peripheral neuropathy	**Very rare** (<1/10,000)
Eye disorders	
Conjunctivitis	**Common** (>1/100, <1/10)
Gold deposits in the lens/ corneas	**Very rare** (<1/10,000)
Respiratory, thoracic and Mediastinal disorders	
Interstitial pneumonitis	**Rare** (>1/10,000, <1/1,000)
Pulmonary fibrosis	**Very rare** (<1/10,000)
Gastrointestinal disorders	
Diarrhoea or loose stools	**Very Common** (>1/10)
Oral mucous membrane disorder and stomatitis, disturbed taste	**Uncommon** (>1/1000, <1/100)
Nausea and vomiting, abdominal pain	**Uncommon** (>1/1000, <1/100)
Enterocolitis	**Very rare** (<1/10,000)
Colitis	**Very rare (<1/10,000)**
Skin and subcutaneous tissue disorders	
Rashes and pruritis	**Very Common** (>1/10)
Exfoliative dermatitis and alopecia	**Very rare** (<1/10,000)
Renal and urinary disorders	
Proteinuria	**Common** (>1/100, <1/10)
Glomerular disease/nephrotic syndrome/membranous glomerulonephritis	**Very rare** (<1/10,000)
Investigations	
Decrease in haemoglobin Decrease in haematocrit Changes in liver function Changes in renal function	**Common** (>1/100, <1/10)

* Please see section 4.4 for monitoring requirements and cessation of therapy

The frequencies are taken from adverse events reported in controlled studies and post-marketing experience.

Treatment with Ridaura should be stopped in cases of persistent rash, especially if accompanied by pruritus. In cases of clinically significant proteinuria treatment with Ridaura should be stopped promptly. Treatment may be restarted after the proteinuria has cleared, however, under close supervision in patients who have experienced only minimal proteinuria.

Transient decreases in haemoglobin or haematocrit early in treatment have been reported. Occasional decreases in white blood counts have been reported during auranofin treatment.

There have been some reports of gold deposits in the lens or corneas of patients treated with auranofin. These deposits have not led to any eye disorders or any degree of visual impairment.

4.9 Overdose

Ridaura overdosage experience is limited. One patient who took 27 mg daily for 10 days developed an encephalopathy and peripheral neuropathy. Ridaura was discontinued and the patient eventually recovered.

In case of acute overdosage, immediate induction of vomiting or gastric lavage and appropriate supportive therapy are recommended. Chelating agents such as BAL have been used in injectable gold overdosage, and may be considered, although there has been no specific experience with Ridaura.

5. PHARMACOLOGICAL PROPERTIES

5.1 Pharmacodynamic properties

Auranofin is a disease-modifying slow-acting immunomodulating agent.

5.2 Pharmacokinetic properties

About 20% to 30% of the gold in a dose of Ridaura is absorbed and, although there is considerable variation in absorption, this is less than that seen with parenteral gold. Steady state blood concentrations are achieved 8 to 12 weeks after starting and are on average 5 to 10 times less than those following parenteral gold, with no correlation with clinical response or adverse events. About 70% of the gold administered in Ridaura appears in the faeces during the first week following a single dose, and at six months after dosing, less than 1% of the gold administered remains in the body, in contrast to around 30% of gold given parenterally. In contrast to parenteral gold, which does not become cell-associated, 40% of the gold in the blood of Ridaura-treated patients is associated with blood cells.

The metabolism of Ridaura is not fully understood, although it is clear from both animal and in-vitro studies with human blood that both the sulphur and the phosphorus ligands of Ridaura are rapidly dissociated from the gold.

5.3 Preclinical safety data

No relevant pre-clinical safety data has been generated.

6. PHARMACEUTICAL PARTICULARS

6.1 List of excipients

Lactose

Microcrystalline cellulose

Maize starch

Sodium starch glycollate

Magnesium stearate

Hydroxypropylmethylcellulose

Propylene glycol

Opaspray M-1-6054

6.2 Incompatibilities

None

6.3 Shelf life

Five years

6.4 Special precautions for storage

None

6.5 Nature and contents of container

Standard SKand F polypropylene securitainers or HDPE containers with wadless polypropylene screw caps containing 60 tablets.

6.6 Special precautions for disposal and other handling

None

Administrative Data

7. MARKETING AUTHORISATION HOLDER

Astellas Pharma Ltd

Lovett House

Lovett Road

Staines

TW18 3AZ

United Kingdom

8. MARKETING AUTHORISATION NUMBER(S)

PL0166/0176

9. DATE OF FIRST AUTHORISATION/RENEWAL OF THE AUTHORISATION

31/10/97

10. DATE OF REVISION OF THE TEXT

28 January 2008

11. Legal category

POM

Rifadin 150mg Capsules

(sanofi-aventis)

1. NAME OF THE MEDICINAL PRODUCT

Rifadin Capsules 150mg

2. QUALITATIVE AND QUANTITATIVE COMPOSITION

Rifampicin Ph Eur 150 mg

3. PHARMACEUTICAL FORM

Blue and red hard gelatin capsules.

4. CLINICAL PARTICULARS

4.1 Therapeutic indications

Indications for use

Tuberculosis: In combination with other active anti-tuberculosis drugs in the treatment of all forms of tuberculosis, including fresh, advanced, chronic and drug-resistant cases. Rifadin is also effective against most atypical strains of Mycobacteria.

Leprosy: In combination with at least one other active anti-leprosy drug in the management of multibacillary and paucibacillary leprosy to effect conversion of the infectious state to a non-infectious state.

Other Infections: In the treatment of Brucellosis, Legionnaires Disease, and serious staphylococcal infections. To prevent emergence of resistant strains of the infecting organisms, Rifadin should be used in combination with another antibiotic appropriate for the infection.

Prophylaxis of meningococcal meningitis: For the treatment of asymptomatic carriers of *N. meningitidis* to eliminate meningococci from the nasopharynx.

Haemophilus influenzae: For the treatment of asymptomatic carriers of *H.influenzae* and as chemoprophylaxis of exposed children, 4 years of age or younger.

4.2 Posology and method of administration

Recommended Dosage

For oral administration

The daily dose of Rifadin, calculated from the patient's body weight, should preferably be taken at least 30 minutes before a meal or 2 hours after a meal to ensure rapid and complete absorption.

Tuberculosis:

Rifadin should be given with other effective anti-tuberculosis drugs to prevent the possible emergence of rifampicin-resistant strains of Mycobacteria.

Adults: The recommended single daily dose in tuberculosis is 8-12 mg/kg.

Usual Daily dose: Patients weighing less than 50 kg - 450 mg. Patients weighing 50 kg or more - 600 mg.

Children: In children, oral doses of 10-20 mg/kg body weight daily are recommended, although a total daily dose should not usually exceed 600 mg.

Leprosy:

600 mg doses of rifampicin should be given once per month. Alternatively, a daily regimen may be used. The recommended single daily dose is 10 mg/kg.

Usual daily dose: Patients weighing less than 50 kg - 450 mg. Patients weighing

50 kg or more - 600 mg.

In the treatment of leprosy, rifampicin should always be used in conjunction with at least one other antileprosy drug,

Brucellosis, Legionnaires Disease or serious staphylococcal infections

Adults: The recommended daily dose is 600-1200 mg given in 2 to 4 divided doses, together with another appropriate antibiotic to prevent the emergence of resistant strains of the infecting organisms.

Prophylaxis of meningococcal meningitis

Adults: 600 mg twice daily for 2 days.

Children (1 - 12 years): 10 mg/kg twice daily for 2 days.

Children (3 months - 1 year): 5 mg/kg twice daily for 2 days.

Prophylaxis of Haemophilus influenzae

Adults and children: For members of households exposed to H. influenzae B disease when the household contains a child 4 years of age or younger, it is recommended that all members (including the child) receive rifampicin 20 mg/kg once daily (maximum daily dose 600 mg) for 4 days.

Index cases should be treated prior to discharge from hospital.

Neonates (1 month): 10 mg/kg daily for 4 days.

Impaired liver function:

A daily dose of 8 mg/kg should not be exceeded in patients with impaired liver function.

Use in the elderly:

In elderly patients, the renal excretion of rifampicin is decreased proportionally with physiological decrease of renal function; due to compensatory increase of liver excretion, the terminal half-life in serum is similar to that of younger patients. However, as increased blood levels have been noted in one study of rifampicin in elderly patients, caution should be exercised in using rifampicin in such patients, especially if there is evidence of impaired liver function.

4.3 Contraindications

Rifadin is contra-indicated in the presence of jaundice, and in patients who are hypersensitive to the rifamycins or any of the excipients.

Rifadin use is contraindicated when given concurrently with the combination of saquinavir/ritonavir (see section 4.5 Interactions).

4.4 Special warnings and precautions for use

Rifampicin should be given under the supervision of a respiratory or other suitably qualified physician.

Cautions should be taken in case of renal impairment if dose > 600 mg/day.

All tuberculosis patients should have pre-treatment measurements of liver function.

Adults treated for tuberculosis with rifampicin should have baseline measurements of hepatic enzymes, bilirubin, serum creatinine, a complete blood count, and a platelet count (or estimate).

Patients with impaired liver function should only be given rifampicin in cases of necessity, and then with caution and under close medical supervision. In these patients, lower doses of rifampicin are recommended and careful monitoring of liver function, especially serum glutamic pyruvic transaminase (SGPT) and serum glutamic oxaloacetic transaminase (SGOT) should initially be carried out prior to therapy, weekly for two weeks, then every two weeks for the next six weeks. If signs of hepatocellular damage occur, rifampicin should be withdrawn.

Rifampicin should also be withdrawn if clinically significant changes in hepatic function occur. The need for other forms of antituberculosis therapy and a different regimen should be considered. Urgent advice should be obtained from a specialist in the management of tuberculosis. If rifampicin is re-introduced after liver function has returned to normal, liver function should be monitored daily.

In patients with impaired liver function, elderly patients, malnourished patients, and possibly, children under two years of age, caution is particularly recommended when instituting therapeutic regimens in which isoniazid is to be used concurrently with Rifadin. If the patient has no evidence of pre-existing liver disease and normal pre-treatment liver function, liver function tests need only be repeated if fever, vomiting, jaundice or other deterioration in the patient's condition occur.

Patients should be seen at least monthly during therapy and should be specifically questioned concerning symptoms associated with adverse reactions.

In some patients hyperbilirubinaemia can occur in the early days of treatment. This results from competition between rifampicin and bilirubin for hepatic excretion.

An isolated report showing a moderate rise in bilirubin and/or transaminase level is not in itself an indication for interrupting treatment; rather the decision should be made after repeating the tests, noting trends in the levels and considering them in conjunction with the patient's clinical condition.

Because of the possibility of immunological reaction including anaphylaxis (see section 4.8 Undesirable effects) occurring with intermittent therapy (less than 2 to 3 times per week) patients should be closely monitored. Patients should be cautioned against interrupting treatment.

Rifampicin has enzyme induction properties that can enhance the metabolism of endogenous substrates including adrenal hormones, thyroid hormones and vitamin D. Isolated reports have associated porphyria exacerbation with rifampicin administration.

4.5 Interaction with other medicinal products and other forms of interaction

Cytochrome P-450 enzyme interaction

Rifampicin is a potent inducer of certain cytochrome P-450 enzymes. Coadministration of rifampicin with other drugs that are also metabolised through these cytochrome P-450 enzymes may accelerate the metabolism and reduce the activity of these other drugs. Therefore, caution should be used when prescribing rifampicin with drugs metabolised by cytochrome P-450. To maintain optimum therapeutic blood levels, dosages of drugs metabolised by these enzymes may require adjustment when starting or stopping concomitantly administered rifampicin.

Examples of drugs metabolised by cytochrome P-450 enzymes are:

- Antiarrhythmics (e.g. disopyramide, mexiletine, quinidine, propafenone, tocainide),
- Antiepileptics (e.g. phenytoin),
- Hormone antagonist (antiestrogens e.g. tamoxifen, toremifene, gestinone),
- Antipsychotics (e.g. haloperidol, aripiprazole),
- Anticoagulants (e.g. coumarins),
- Antifungals (e.g. fluconazole, itraconazole, ketoconazole, voriconazole),
- Antivirals (e.g. saquinavir, indinavir, efavirenz, amprenavir, nelfinavir, atazanavir, lopinavir, nevirapine),
- Barbiturates
- Beta-blockers (e.g. bisoprolol, propanolol),
- Anxiolytics and hypnotics (e.g. diazepam, benzodiazepines, zolpicolone, zolpidem),
- Calcium channel blockers (e.g. diltiazem, nifedipine, verapamil, nimodipine, isradipine, nicardipine, nisoldipine),
- Antibacterials (e.g. chloramphenicol, clarithromycin, dapsone, doxycycline, fluoroquinolones, telithromycin),
- Corticosteroids
- Cardiac glycosides (digitoxin, digoxin),
- Clofibrate,
- Systemic hormonal contraceptives
- Oestrogen,
- Antidiabetic (e.g. chlorpropamide, tolbutamide, sulfonylureas, rosiglitazone),
- Immunosuppressive agents (e.g. ciclosporin, sirolimus, tacrolimus)
- Irinotecan,
- Thyroid hormone (e.g. levothyroxine),
- Losartan,
- Analgestics (e.g. methadone, narcotic analgesics),
- Praziquantel,
- Progestogens,
- Quinine,
- Riluzole,
- Selective 5-HT3 receptor antagonists (e.g. ondansetron)
- Statins metabolised by CYP 3A4 (e.g. simvastatin),
- Theophylline,
- Tricyclic antidepressants (e.g. amitriptyline, nortriptyline),
- Cytotoxics (e.g. imatinib),
- Diuretics (e.g. eplerenone)

Patients on oral contraceptives should be advised to use alternative, non-hormonal methods of birth control during Rifadin therapy. Also diabetes may become more difficult to control.

Other Interactions

When rifampicin is given concomitantly with the combination saquinavir/ritonavir, the potential for hepatotoxicity is increased. Therefore, concomitant use of Rifadin with saquinvir/ritonavir is contraindicated (see section 4.3 Contraindications).

When the two drugs were taken concomitantly, decreased concentrations of atovaquone and increased concentrations of rifampicin were observed.

Concurrent use of ketoconazole and rifampicin has resulted in decreased serum concentrations of both drugs.

Concurrent use of rifampicin and enalapril has resulted in decreased concentrations of enalaprilat, the active metabolite of enalapril. Dosage adjustments should be made if indicated by the patient's clinical condition.

Concomitant antacid administration may reduce the absorption of rifampicin. Daily doses of rifampicin should be given at least 1 hour before the ingestion of antacids.

When rifampicin is given concomitantly with either halothane or isoniazid, the potential for hepatotoxicity is increased. The concomitant use of rifampicin and halothane should be avoided. Patients receiving both rifampicin and isoniazid should be monitored closely for hepatotoxicity.

If *p*-aminosalicylic acid and rifampicin are both included in the treatment regimen, they should be given not less than eight hours apart to ensure satisfactory blood levels.

Interference with laboratory and diagnostic tests

Therapeutic levels of rifampicin have been shown to inhibit standard microbiological assays for serum folate and Vitamin B12. Thus alternative assay methods should be considered. Transient elevation of BSP and serum bilirubin has been reported. Rifampicin may impair biliary excretion of contrast media used for visualization of the gallbladder, due to competition for biliary excretion. Therefore, these tests should be performed before the morning dose of rifampicin.

4.6 Pregnancy and lactation

Pregnancy

At very high doses in animals rifampicin has been shown to have teratogenic effects. There are no well controlled studies with rifampicin in pregnant women. Although rifampicin has been reported to cross the placental barrier and appear in cord blood, the effect of rifampicin, alone or in combination with other antituberculosis drugs, on the human foetus is not known. Therefore, Rifadin should be used in pregnant women or in women of child bearing potential only if the potential benefit justifies the potential risk to the foetus. When Rifadin is administered during the last few weeks of pregnancy it may cause post-natal haemorrhages in the mother and infant for which treatment with Vitamin K1 may be indicated.

Lactation

Rifampicin is excreted in breast milk, patients receiving rifampicin should not breast feed unless in the physician's judgement the potential benefit to the patient outweighs the potential risk to the infant.

4.7 Effects on ability to drive and use machines

None stated

4.8 Undesirable effects

Reactions occurring with either daily or intermittent dosage regimens include:

Cutaneous reactions which are mild and self-limiting and do not appear to be hypersensitivity reactions. Typically they consist of flushing and itching with or without a rash. Urticaria and more serious hypersensitivity cutaneous reactions have occurred but are uncommon. Exfoliate dermatitis, pemphigoid reaction, erythema multiforme including Stevens-Johnson syndrome, Lyells syndrome and vasculitis have been reported rarely.

Gastrointestinal reactions consist of anorexia, nausea, vomiting, abdominal discomfort and diarrhoea. Pseudomembranous colitis has been reported with rifampicin therapy.

Hepatitis can be caused by rifampicin and liver function tests should be monitored (see section 4.4. Special warnings and precautions for use).

Central Nervous System: Psychoses have been rarely reported.

Thrombocytopenia with or without purpura may occur, usually associated with intermittent therapy, but is reversible if drug is discontinued as soon as purpura occurs. Cerebral haemorrhage and fatalities have been reported when rifampicin administration has been continued or resumed after the appearance of purpura.

Disseminated intravascular coagulation has also been rarely reported.

Eosinophilia, leucopenia, oedema, muscle weakness and myopathy have been reported to occur in a small percentage of patients treated with rifampicin.

Agranulocytosis has been reported very rarely reported.

Rare reports of adrenal insufficiency in patients with compromised adrenal function have been observed.

Reactions usually occurring with intermittent dosage regimens and probably of immunological origin include:

- 'Flu Syndrome' consisting of episodes of fever, chills, headache, dizziness, and bone pain appearing most commonly during the 3rd to the 6th monthly of therapy. The frequency of the syndrome varies but may occur in up to 50 % of patients given once-weekly regimens with a dose of rifampicin of 25 mg/kg or more.
- Shortness of breath and wheezing.
- Decrease in blood pressure and shock.
- Anaphylaxis.
- Acute haemolytic anaemia.
- Acute renal failure usually due to acute tubular necrosis or acute interstitial nephritis.

If serious complications arise, e.g. renal failure, thrombocytopenia or haemolytic anaemia, rifampicin should be stopped and never restarted.

Occasional disturbances of the menstrual cycle have been reported in women receiving long-term anti-tuberculosis therapy with regimens containing rifampicin.

Rifampicin may produce a reddish colouration of the urine, sweat, sputum and tears. The patient should be forewarned of this. Soft contact lenses may be permanently stained.

4.9 Overdose

In cases of overdose with Rifadin, gastric lavage should be performed as soon as possible. Intensive supportive measures should be instituted and individual symptoms treated as they arise.

5. PHARMACOLOGICAL PROPERTIES

5.1 Pharmacodynamic properties

Rifampicin is an active bactericidial antituberculosis drug which is particularly active against the rapidly growing extracellular organisms and also has bactericidial activity intracellularly. Rifampicin has activity against slow and intermittently-growing *M. Tuberculosis*.

Rifampicin inhibits DNA-dependent RNA polymerase activity in susceptible cells. Specifically, it interacts with bacterial RNA polymerase but does not inhibit the mammalian enzyme. Cross-resistance to rifampicin has only been shown with other rifamycins.

5.2 Pharmacokinetic properties

Rifampicin is readily absorbed from the gastrointestinal tract. Peak serum concentrations of the order of 10 µg/ml occur about 2 to 4 hours after a dose of 10 mg/kg body weight on an empty stomach.

Absorption of rifampicin is reduced when the drug is ingested with food.

The pharmacokinetics (oral and intravenous) in children are similar to adults.

In normal subjects the biological half-life of rifampicin in serum averages about 3 hours after a 600 mg dose and increases to 5.1 hours after a 900 mg dose. With repeated administration, the half-life decreases and reaches average values of approximately 2-3 hours. At a dose of up to 600 mg/day, it does not differ in patients with renal failure and consequently, no dosage adjustment is required.

Rifampicin is rapidly eliminated in the bile and an enterophepatic circulation ensues. During this process, rifampicin undergoes progressive deacetylation, so that nearly all the drug in the bile is in this form in about 6 hours. This metabolite retains essentially complete antibacterial activity. Intestinal reabsorption is reduced by deacetylation and elimination is facilitated. Up to 30 % of a dose is excreted in the urine, with about half of this being unchanged drug.

Rifampicin is widely distributed throughout the body. It is present in effective concentrations in many organs and body fluids, including cerebrospinal fluid. Rifampicin is about 80 % protein bound. Most of the unbound fraction is not ionized and therefore is diffused freely in tissues.

5.3 Preclinical safety data

Not applicable

6. PHARMACEUTICAL PARTICULARS

6.1 List of excipients

Corn starch Ph Eur

Magnesium stearate Ph Eur

6.2 Incompatibilities

None stated

6.3 Shelf life

4 years from date of manufacture

6.4 Special precautions for storage

Store below 25°C.

Protect from light and moisture.

6.5 Nature and contents of container

Blister packs of 100 capsules in cardboard cartons. Blister material is aluminium foil / PVDC (Aluminium 0.025 mm; PVDC 20 gsm) and transparent PVC / PVDC foil (PVC 0.25 mm; PVDC 60 gsm).

6.6 Special precautions for disposal and other handling

Not applicable

7. MARKETING AUTHORISATION HOLDER

Sanofi-aventis

One Onslow Street

Guildford

Surrey

GU1 4YS

UK

8. MARKETING AUTHORISATION NUMBER(S)

PL 04425/5915R

9. DATE OF FIRST AUTHORISATION/RENEWAL OF THE AUTHORISATION

9th April 2005

10. DATE OF REVISION OF THE TEXT

13 March 2009

Legal category

POM

Rifadin 300mg Capsules

(sanofi-aventis)

1. NAME OF THE MEDICINAL PRODUCT

Rifadin Capsules 300mg

2. QUALITATIVE AND QUANTITATIVE COMPOSITION

Rifampicin Ph Eur 300 mg

3. PHARMACEUTICAL FORM

Red hard gelatin capsules.

4. CLINICAL PARTICULARS

4.1 Therapeutic indications

Indications for use

Tuberculosis: In combination with other active anti-tuberculosis drugs in the treatment of all forms of tuberculosis, including fresh, advanced, chronic and drug-resistant cases. Rifadin is also effective against most atypical strains of Mycobacteria.

Leprosy: In combination with at least one other active anti-leprosy drug in the management of multibacillary and paucibacillary leprosy to effect conversion of the infectious state to a non-infectious state.

Other Infections: In the treatment of Brucellosis, Legionnaires Disease, and serious staphylococcal infections. To prevent emergence of resistant strains of the infecting organisms, Rifadin should be used in combination with another antibiotic appropriate for the infection.

Prophylaxis of meningococcal meningitis: For the treatment of asymptomatic carriers of *N. meningitidis* to eliminate meningococci from the nasopharynx.

Haemophilus influenzae: For the treatment of asymptomatic carriers of *H.influenzae* and as chemoprophylaxis of exposed children, 4 years of age or younger.

4.2 Posology and method of administration

Recommended Dosage

For oral administration

The daily dose of Rifadin, calculated from the patient's body weight, should preferably be taken at least 30 minutes before a meal or 2 hours after a meal to ensure rapid and complete absorption.

Tuberculosis:

Rifadin should be given with other effective anti-tuberculosis drugs to prevent the possible emergence of rifampicin-resistant strains of Mycobacteria.

Adults: The recommended single daily dose in tuberculosis is 8-12 mg/kg.

Usual Daily dose: Patients weighing less than 50 kg - 450 mg. Patients weighing 50 kg or more – 600 mg.

Children: In children, oral doses of 10-20 mg/kg body weight daily are recommended, although a total daily dose should not usually exceed 600 mg.

Leprosy:

600 mg doses of rifampicin should be given once per month. Alternatively, a daily regimen may be used. The recommended single daily dose is 10 mg/kg.

Usual daily dose: Patients weighing less than 50 kg - 450 mg. Patients weighing 50 kg or more – 600 mg.

In the treatment of leprosy, rifampicin should always be used in conjunction with at least one other antileprosy drug,

Brucellosis, Legionnaires Disease or serious staphylococcal infections

Adults: The recommended daily dose is 600-1200 mg given in 2 to 4 divided doses, together with another appropriate antibiotic to prevent the emergence of resistant strains of the infecting organisms.

Prophylaxis of meningococcal meningitis

Adults: 600 mg twice daily for 2 days.

Children (1 - 12 years): 10 mg/kg twice daily for 2 days.

Children (3 months - 1 year): 5 mg/kg twice daily for 2 days.

Prophylaxis of Haemophilus influenzae

Adults and children: For members of households exposed to H. influenzae B disease when the household contains a child 4 years of age or younger, it is recommended that all members (including the child) receive rifampicin 20 mg/kg once daily (maximum daily dose 600 mg) for 4 days.

Index cases should be treated prior to discharge from hospital.

Neonates (1 month): 10 mg/kg daily for 4 days.

Impaired liver function:

A daily dose of 8 mg/kg should not be exceeded in patients with impaired liver function.

Use in the elderly:

In elderly patients, the renal excretion of rifampicin is decreased proportionally with physiological decrease of renal function; due to compensatory increase of liver excretion, the terminal half-life in serum is similar to that of younger patients. However, as increased blood levels have been noted in one study of rifampicin in elderly patients, caution should be exercised in using rifampicin in such patients, especially if there is evidence of impaired liver function.

4.3 Contraindications

Rifadin is contra-indicated in the presence of jaundice, and in patients who are hypersensitive to the rifamycins or any of the excipients.

Rifadin use is contraindicated when given concurrently with the combination of saquinavir/ritonavir (see section 4.5 Interactions).

4.4 Special warnings and precautions for use

Rifampicin should be given under the supervision of a respiratory or other suitably qualified physician.

Cautions should be taken in case of renal impairment if dose > 600 mg/day.

All tuberculosis patients should have pre-treatment measurements of liver function.

Patients with impaired liver function should only be given rifampicin in cases of necessity, and then with caution and under close medical supervision. In these patients, lower doses of rifampicin are recommended and careful monitoring of liver function, especially serum glutamic pyruvic transaminase (SGPT) and serum glutamic oxaloacetic transaminase (SGOT) should initially be carried out prior to therapy, weekly for two weeks, then every two weeks for the next six weeks. If signs of hepatocellular damage occur, rifampicin should be withdrawn.

Rifampicin should also be withdrawn if clinically significant changes in hepatic function occur. The need for other forms of antituberculosis therapy and a different regimen should be considered. Urgent advice should be obtained from a specialist in the management of tuberculosis. If rifampicin is re-introduced after liver function has returned to normal, liver function should be monitored daily.

In patients with impaired liver function, elderly patients, malnourished patients, and possibly, children under two years of age, caution is particularly recommended when instituting therapeutic regimens in which isoniazid is to be used concurrently with Rifadin. If the patient has no evidence of pre-existing liver disease and normal pre-treatment liver function, liver function tests need only be repeated if fever, vomiting, jaundice or other deterioration in the patient's condition occur.

Patients should be seen at least monthly during therapy and should be specifically questioned concerning symptoms associated with adverse reactions.

In some patients hyperbilirubinaemia can occur in the early days of treatment. This results from competition between rifampicin and bilirubin for hepatic excretion.

An isolated report showing a moderate rise in bilirubin and/or transaminase level is not in itself an indication for interrupting treatment; rather the decision should be made after repeating the tests, noting trends in the levels and considering them in conjunction with the patient's clinical condition.

Adults treated for tuberculosis with rifampicin should have baseline measurements of hepatic enzymes, bilirubin, serum creatinine, a complete blood count, and a platelet count (or estimate).

Because of the possibility of immunological reaction including anaphylaxis (see section 4.8 Undesirable effects) occurring with intermittent therapy (less than 2 to 3 times per week) patients should be closely monitored. Patients should be cautioned against interrupting treatment.

Rifampicin has enzyme induction properties that can enhance the metabolism of endogenous substrates including adrenal hormones, thyroid hormones and vitamin D. Isolated reports have associated porphyria exacerbation with rifampicin administration.

4.5 Interaction with other medicinal products and other forms of interaction

Cytochrome P-450 enzyme interaction

Rifampicin is a potent inducer of certain cytochrome P-450 enzymes. Coadministration of rifampicin with other drugs that are also metabolised through these cytochrome P-450 enzymes may accelerate the metabolism and reduce the activity of these other drugs. Therefore, caution should be used when prescribing rifampicin with drugs metabolised by cytochrome P-450. To maintain optimum therapeutic blood levels, dosages of drugs metabolised by these enzymes may require adjustment when starting or stopping concomitantly administered rifampicin.

Examples of drugs metabolised by cytochrome P-450 enzymes are:

- Antiarrhythmics (e.g. disopyramide, mexiletine, quinidine, propafenone, tocainide),
- Antiepileptics (e.g. phenytoin),
- Hormone antagonist (antiestrogens e.g. tamoxifen, toremifene, gestinone),
- Antipsychotics (e.g. haloperidol, aripiprazole),
- Anticoagulants (e.g. coumarins),
- Antifungals (e.g. fluconazole, itraconazole, ketoconazole, voriconazole),
- Antivirals (e.g. saquinavir, indinavir, efavirenz, amprenavir, nelfinavir, atazanavir, lopinavir, nevirapine),
- Barbiturates
- Beta-blockers (e.g. bisoprolol, propanolol),
- Anxiolytics and hypnotics (e.g. diazepam, benzodiazepines, zolpicolone, zolpidem),
- Calcium channel blockers (e.g. diltiazem, nifedipine, verapamil, nimodipine, isradipine, nicardipine, nisoldipine),
- Antibacterials (e.g. chloramphenicol, clarithromycin, dapsone, doxycycline, fluoroquinolones, telithromycin),
- Corticosteroids
- Cardiac glycosides (digitoxin, digoxin),
- Clofibrate,
- Systemic hormonal contraceptives
- Oestrogen,
- Antidiabetic (e.g. chlorpropamide, tolbutamide, sulfonylureas, rosiglitazone),
- Immunosuppressive agents (e.g. ciclosporin, sirolimus, tacrolimus)
- Irinotecan,
- Thyroid hormone (e.g. levothyroxine),
- Losartan,
- Analgestics (e.g. methadone, narcotic analgesics),
- Praziquantel,
- Progestogens,
- Quinine,
- Riluzole,
- Selective 5-HT3 receptor antagonists (e.g. ondansetron)
- Statins metabolised by CYP 3A4 (e.g. simvastatin),
- Theophylline,
- Tricyclic antidepressants (e.g. amitriptyline, nortriptyline),
- Cytotoxics (e.g. imatinib),
- Diuretics (e.g. eplerenone)

Patients on oral contraceptives should be advised to use alternative, non-hormonal methods of birth control during Rifadin therapy. Also diabetes may become more difficult to control.

Other Interactions

When rifampicin is given concomitantly with the combination saquinavir/ritonavir, the potential for hepatotoxicity is increased. Therefore, concomitant use of Rifadin with saquinvir/ritonavir is contraindicated (see section 4.3 Contraindications).

When the two drugs were taken concomitantly, decreased concentrations of atovaquone and increased concentrations of rifampicin were observed.

Concurrent use of ketoconazole and rifampicin has resulted in decreased serum concentrations of both drugs.

Concurrent use of rifampicin and enalapril has resulted in decreased concentrations of enalaprilat, the active metabolite of enalapril. Dosage adjustments should be made if indicated by the patient's clinical condition.

Concomitant antacid administration may reduce the absorption of rifampicin. Daily doses of rifampicin should be given at least 1 hour before the ingestion of antacids.

When rifampicin is given concomitantly with either halothane or isoniazid, the potential for hepatotoxicity is increased. The concomitant use of rifampicin andhalothane should be avoided. Patients receiving both rifampicin and isoniazid should be monitored closely for hepatotoxicity.

If *p*-aminosalicylic acid and rifampicin are both included in the treatment regimen, they should be given not less than eight hours apart to ensure satisfactory blood levels.

Interference with laboratory and diagnostic tests

Therapeutic levels of rifampicin have been shown to inhibit standard microbiological assays for serum folate and

Vitamin B12. Thus alternative assay methods should be considered. Transient elevation of BSP and serum bilirubin has been reported. Rifampicin may impair biliary excretion of contrast media used for visualization of the gallbladder, due to competition for biliary excretion. Therefore, these tests should be performed before the morning dose of rifampicin.

4.6 Pregnancy and lactation

Pregnancy

At very high doses in animals rifampicin has been shown to have teratogenic effects. There are no well controlled studies with rifampicin in pregnant women. Although rifampicin has been reported to cross the placental barrier and appear in cord blood, the effect of rifampicin, alone or in combination with other antituberculosis drugs, on the human foetus is not known. Therefore, Rifadin should be used in pregnant women or in women of child bearing potential only if the potential benefit justifies the potential risk to the foetus. When Rifadin is administered during the last few weeks of pregnancy it may cause post-natal haemorrhages in the mother and infant for which treatment with Vitamin K1 may be indicated.

Lactation

Rifampicin is excreted in breast milk, patients receiving rifampicin should not breast feed unless in the physician's judgement the potential benefit to the patient outweighs the potential risk to the infant.

4.7 Effects on ability to drive and use machines

None stated

4.8 Undesirable effects

Reactions occurring with either daily or intermittent dosage regimens include:

Cutaneous reactions which are mild and self-limiting and do not appear to be hypersensitivity reactions. Typically they consist of flushing and itching with or without a rash. Urticaria and more serious hypersensitivity cutaneous reactions have occurred but are uncommon. Exfoliate dermatitis, pemphigoid reaction, erythema multiforme including Stevens-Johnson syndrome, Lyells syndrome and vasculitis have been reported rarely.

Gastrointestinal reactions consist of anorexia, nausea, vomiting, abdominal discomfort, and diarrhoea. Pseudomembranous colitis has been reported with rifampicin therapy.

Hepatitis can be caused by rifampicin and liver function tests should be monitored (see section 4.4. Special warnings and precautions for use).

Central Nervous System: Psychoses have been rarely reported.

Thrombocytopenia with or without purpura may occur, usually associated with intermittent therapy, but is reversible if drug is discontinued as soon as purpura occurs. Cerebral haemorrhage and fatalities have been reported when rifampicin administration has been continued or resumed after the appearance of purpura.

Disseminated intravascular coagulation has also been rarely reported.

Eosinophilia, leucopenia, oedema, muscle weakness and myopathy have been reported to occur in a small percentage of patients treated with rifampicin.

Agranulocytosis has been reported very rarely reported.

Rare reports of adrenal insufficiency in patients with compromised adrenal function have been observed.

Reactions usually occurring with intermittent dosage regimens and probably of immunological origin include:

- 'Flu Syndrome' consisting of episodes of fever, chills, headache, dizziness, and bone pain appearing most commonly during the 3rd to the 6th monthly of therapy. The frequency of the syndrome varies but may occur in up to 50 % of patients given once-weekly regimens with a dose of rifampicin of 25 mg/kg or more.
- Shortness of breath and wheezing.
- Decrease in blood pressure and shock.
- Anaphylaxis.
- Acute haemolytic anaemia.
- Acute renal failure usually due to acute tubular necrosis or acute interstitial nephritis.

If serious complications arise, e.g. renal failure, thrombocytopenia or haemolytic anaemia, rifampicin should be stopped and never restarted.

Occasional disturbances of the menstrual cycle have been reported in women receiving long-term anti-tuberculosis therapy with regimens containing rifampicin.

Rifampicin may produce a reddish colouration of the urine, sweat, sputum and tears. The patient should be forewarned of this. Soft contact lenses may be permanently stained.

4.9 Overdose

Human Experience

• Signs and Symptoms:

Nausea, vomiting, abdominal pain, pruritus, headache and increasing lethargy will probably occur within a short time after acute ingestion; unconsciousness may occur when there is severe hepatic disease. Transient increases in liver enzymes and/or bilirubin may occur. Brownish-red or orange colouration of the skin, urine, sweat, saliva, tears and faeces will occur, and its intensity is proportional to the amount ingested. Facial or periorbital oedema has also been reported in paediatric patients. Hypotension, sinus tachycardia, ventricular arrhythmias, seizures and cardiac arrest were reported in some fatal cases.

The minimum acute lethal or toxic dose is not well established. However, nonfatal acute overdoses in adults have been reported with doses ranging from 9 to 12 g rifampicin. Fatal acute overdoses in adults have been reported with doses ranging from 14-60 g. Alcohol or a history of alcohol abuse was involved in some of the fatal and nonfatal reports.

Nonfatal overdoses in paediatric patients ages 1 to 4 years old of 100 mg/kg for one to two doses have been reported.

• Management:

Intensive supportive measures should be instituted and individual symptoms treated as they arise. Since nausea and vomiting are likely to be present, gastric lavage is probably preferable to induction of emesis. Following evacuation of the gastric contents, the instillation of activated charcoal slurry into the stomach may help absorb any remaining drug from the gastrointestinal tract. Antiemetic medication may be required to control severe nausea and vomiting. Active diuresis (with measured intake and output) will help promote excretion of the drug. Haemodialysis may be of value in some patients.

5. PHARMACOLOGICAL PROPERTIES

5.1 Pharmacodynamic properties

Rifampicin is an active bactericidial antituberculosis drug which is particularly active against the rapidly growing extracellular organisms and also has bactericidial activity intracellularly. Rifampicin has activity against slow and intermittently-growing *M. Tuberculosis*.

Rifampicin inhibits DNA-dependent RNA polymerase activity in susceptible cells. Specifically, it interacts with bacterial RNA polymerase but does not inhibit the mammalian enzyme. Cross-resistance to rifampicin has only been shown with other rifamycins.

5.2 Pharmacokinetic properties

Rifampicin is readily absorbed from the gastrointestinal tract. Peak serum concentrations of the order of 10 μg/ml occur about 2 to 4 hours after a dose of 10 mg/kg body weight on an empty stomach.

Absorption of rifampicin is reduced when the drug is ingested with food.

The pharmacokinetics (oral and intravenous) in children are similar to adults.

In normal subjects the biological half-life of rifampicin in serum averages about 3 hours after a 600 mg dose and increases to 5.1 hours after a 900 mg dose. With repeated administration, the half-life decreases and reaches average values of approximately 2-3 hours. At a dose of up to 600 mg/day, it does not differ in patients with renal failure and consequently, no dosage adjustment is required.

Rifampicin is rapidly eliminated in the bile and an enterophepatic circulation ensues. During this process, rifampicin undergoes progressive deacetylation, so that nearly all the drug in the bile is in this form in about 6 hours. This metabolite retains essentially complete antibacterial activity. Intestinal reabsorption is reduced by deacetylation and elimination is facilitated. Up to 30 % of a dose is excreted in the urine, with about half of this being unchanged drug.

Rifampicin is widely distributed throughout the body. It is present in effective concentrations in many organs and body fluids, including cerebrospinal fluid. Rifampicin is about 80 % protein bound. Most of the unbound fraction is not ionized and therefore is diffused freely in tissues.

5.3 Preclinical safety data

Not applicable

6. PHARMACEUTICAL PARTICULARS

6.1 List of excipients

Corn starch Ph Eur

Magnesium stearate Ph Eur

6.2 Incompatibilities

None stated

6.3 Shelf life

4 years from date of manufacture

6.4 Special precautions for storage

Store below 25°C.

Protect from light and moisture.

6.5 Nature and contents of container

Blister packs of 100 capsules in cardboard cartons. Blister material is aluminium foil / PVDC (Aluminium 0.025 mm; PVDC 20 gsm) and transparent PVC / PVDC foil (PVC 0.25 mm; PVDC 60 gsm).

6.6 Special precautions for disposal and other handling

Not applicable

7. MARKETING AUTHORISATION HOLDER

Sanofi-aventis

One Onslow Street

Guildford

Surrey

GU1 4YS

UK

8. MARKETING AUTHORISATION NUMBER(S)

PL 04425/5916R

9. DATE OF FIRST AUTHORISATION/RENEWAL OF THE AUTHORISATION

09/04/2005

10. DATE OF REVISION OF THE TEXT

13 March 2009

Legal category

POM

Rifadin For Infusion 600mg

(sanofi-aventis)

1. NAME OF THE MEDICINAL PRODUCT

Rifadin for Infusion 600mg

2. QUALITATIVE AND QUANTITATIVE COMPOSITION

Rifampicin BP 600mg

3. PHARMACEUTICAL FORM

Lyophilisate (for reconstitution prior to use) and accompanying ampoule of solvent.

4. CLINICAL PARTICULARS

4.1 Therapeutic indications

Rifadin for Infusion is indicated for acutely ill patients who are unable to tolerate oral therapy e.g. post operative or comatose patients or patients in whom gastrointestinal absorption is impaired.

Tuberculosis: Rifadin, used in combination with other active anti-tuberculosis drugs, is indicated in the treatment of all forms of tuberculosis, including fresh, advanced, chronic and drug-resistant cases. Rifadin is also effective against most atypical strains of Mycobacteria.

Leprosy: Rifadin, used in combination with at least one other active anti-leprosy drug, is indicated in the management of multibacillary and paucibacillary leprosy to effect conversion of the infectious state to a non-infectious state.

Other infections: Rifadin is indicated in the treatment of Brucellosis, Legionnaires Disease, and serious staphylococcal infections. To prevent emergence of resistant strains of the infecting organisms, Rifadin should be used in combination with another antibiotic appropriate for the infection.

4.2 Posology and method of administration

Treatment with Rifadin for Infusion should include concomitant use of other appropriate antibacterials to prevent the emergence of resistant strains of the causative organism.

<u>Tuberculosis</u>:

Adults: A single daily administration of 600mg given by intravenous infusion over 2 to 3 hours has been found to be effective and well tolerated for adult patients. Serum concentrations following this dosage regimen are similar to those obtained after 600mg by mouth.

Children: The usual paediatric regimen is a single daily dose of up to 20mg/kg bodyweight; the total daily dose should not normally exceed 600mg.

<u>Leprosy</u>:

The recommended daily dose is 10 mg/kg.

Usual daily dose:	Patients weighing less than 50 kg - 450 mg
	Patients weighing 50 kg or more - 600 mg.

Alternatively, 600 mg doses of rifampicin may be given once per month.

In the treatment of leprosy, rifampicin should always be used in conjunction with at least one other antileprosy drug.

<u>Brucellosis, Legionnaires Disease or serious staphylococcal infections</u>:

Adults: The recommended daily dose is 600 - 1200mg given in 2 to 4 divided doses, together with another antibacterial agent with similar properties to prevent the emergence of resistant strains.

<u>Impaired liver function</u>:

A daily dose of 8mg/kg should not be exceeded in patients with impaired liver function.

<u>Use in the elderly</u>:

In elderly patients, the renal excretion of rifampicin is decreased proportionally with physiological decrease of renal function; due to compensatory increase of liver excretion, the serum terminal half-life is similar to that of younger patients. However, as increased blood levels have been noted in one study of rifampicin in elderly patients, caution should be exercised in using rifampicin in such patients, especially if there is evidence of liver function impairment.

When patients are able to accept oral medication, they should be transferred to Rifadin Capsules or Syrup (for further information on these products see their separate data sheets).

4.3 Contraindications

Rifadin for Infusion is contraindicated in patients who are hypersensitive to rifamycins or any of the excipients.

Although not recommended for use in patients with jaundice, the therapeutic benefit of Rifadin for Infusion should be weighed against the possible risks.

Rifadin for Infusion use is contraindicated when given concurrently with the combination of saquinavir/ritonavir (see section 4.5 Interactions).

4.4 Special warnings and precautions for use

Rifampicin should be given under the supervision of a respiratory or other suitably qualified physician.

Cautions should be taken in case of renal impairment if dose $>$ 600 mg/day.

All tuberculosis patients should have pre-treatment measurements of liver function.

Adults treated for tuberculosis with rifampicin should have baseline measurements of hepatic enzymes, bilirubin, serum creatinine, a complete blood count, and a platelet count (or estimate).

Patients with impaired liver function should only be given rifampicin in cases of necessity, and then with caution and under close medical supervision. In these patients, lower doses of rifampicin are recommended and careful monitoring of liver function, especially serum glutamic pyruvic transaminase (SGPT) and serum glutamic oxaloacetic transaminase (SGOT) should initially be carried out prior to therapy, weekly for two weeks, then every two weeks for the next six weeks. If signs of hepatocellular damage occur, rifampicin should be withdrawn.

Rifampicin should also be withdrawn if clinically significant changes in hepatic function occur. The need for other forms of antituberculosis therapy and a different regimen should be considered. Urgent advice should be obtained from a specialist in the management of tuberculosis. If rifampicin is re-introduced after liver function has returned to normal, liver function should be monitored daily.

In patients with impaired liver function, elderly patients, malnourished patients, and possibly, children under two years of age, caution is particularly recommended when instituting therapeutic regimens in which isoniazid is to be used concurrently with rifampicin. If the patient has no evidence of pre-existing liver disease and normal pre-treatment liver function, liver function tests need only be repeated if fever, vomiting, jaundice or other deterioration in the patient's condition occur.

Patients should be seen at least monthly during therapy and should be specifically questioned concerning symptoms associated with adverse reactions.

In some patients hyperbilirubinaemia can occur in the early days of treatment. This results from competition between rifampicin and bilirubin for hepatic excretion. An isolated report showing a moderate rise in bilirubin and/or transaminase level is not in itself an indication for interrupting treatment; rather the decision should be made after repeating the tests, noting trends in the levels and considering them in conjunction with the patient's clinical condition.

Because of the possibility of immunological reaction including anaphylaxis (see section 4.8 Undesirable effects) occurring with intermittent therapy (less than 2 to 3 times per week) patients should be closely monitored. Patients should be cautioned against interrupting treatment since these reactions may occur.

Rifampicin has enzyme induction properties that can enhance the metabolism of endogenous substrates including adrenal hormones, thyroid hormones and vitamin D. Isolated reports have associated porphyria exacerbation with rifampicin administration.

Rifadin infusion is for intravenous infusion only and must not be administered by intramuscular or subcutaneous route. Avoid extravasation during injection; local irritation and inflammation due to extravascular infiltration of the infusion have been observed. If these occur, the infusion should be discontinued and restarted at another site.

4.5 Interaction with other medicinal products and other forms of interaction

Cytochrome P-450 enzyme interaction

Rifampicin is a potent inducer of certain cytochrome P-450 enzymes. Coadministration of rifampicin with other drugs that are also metabolised through these cytochrome P-450 enzymes may accelerate the metabolism and reduce the activity of these other drugs. Therefore, caution should be used when prescribing rifampicin with drugs metabolised by cytochrome P-450. To maintain optimum therapeutic blood levels, dosages of drugs metabolised by these enzymes may require adjustment when starting or stopping concomitantly administered rifampicin.

Examples of drugs metabolised by cytochrome P-450 enzymes are:

- Antiarrhythmics (e.g. disopyramide, mexiletine, quinidine, propafenone, tocainide),
- Antiepileptics (e.g. phenytoin),
- Hormone antagonist (antiestrogens e.g. tamoxifen, toremifene, gestinone),
- Antipsychotics (e.g. haloperidol, aripiprazole),
- Anticoagulants (e.g. coumarins),
- Antifungals (e.g. fluconazole, itraconazole, ketoconazole, voriconazole),
- Antivirals (e.g. saquinavir, indinavir, efavirenz, amprenavir, nelfinavir, atazanavir, lopinavir, nevirapine),
- Barbiturates
- Beta-blockers (e.g. bisoprolol, propanolol),
- Anxiolytics and hypnotics (e.g. diazepam, benzodiazepines, zolpicolone, zolpidem),
- Calcium channel blockers (e.g. diltiazem, nifedipine, verapamil, nimodipine, isradipine, nicardipine, nisoldipine),
- Antibacterials (e.g. chloramphenicol, clarithromycin, dapsone, doxycycline, fluoroquinolones, telithromycin),
- Corticosteroids
- Cardiac glycosides (digitoxin, digoxin),
- Clofibrate,
- Systemic hormonal contraceptives
- Oestrogen,
- Antidiabetic (e.g. chlorpropamide, tolbutamide, sulfonylureas, rosiglitazone),
- Immunosuppressive agents (e.g. ciclosporin, sirolimus, tacrolimus)
- Irinotecan,
- Thyroid hormone (e.g. levothyroxine),
- Losartan,
- Analgestics (e.g. methadone, narcotic analgesics),
- Praziquantel,
- Progestogens,
- Quinine,
- Riluzole,
- Selective 5-HT3 receptor antagonists (e.g. ondansetron)
- Statins metabolised by CYP 3A4 (e.g. simvastatin),
- Theophylline,
- Tricyclic antidepressants (e.g. amitriptyline, nortriptyline),
- Cytotoxics (e.g. imatinib),
- Diuretics (e.g. eplerenone)

Patients on oral contraceptives should be advised to use alternative, non-hormonal methods of birth control during Rifadin therapy. Also diabetes may become more difficult to control.

Other Interactions

When rifampicin is given concomitantly with the combination saquinavir/ritonavir, the potential for hepatotoxicity is increased. Therefore, concomitant use of Rifadin with saquinavir/ritonavir is contraindicated (see section 4.3 Contraindications).

When the two drugs were taken concomitantly, decreased concentrations of atovaquone and increased concentrations of rifampicin were observed.

Concurrent use of ketoconazole and rifampicin has resulted in decreased serum concentrations of both drugs.

Concurrent use of rifampicin and enalapril has resulted in decreased concentrations of enalaprilat, the active metabolite of enalapril. Dosage adjustments should be made if indicated by the patient's clinical condition.

Concomitant antacid administration may reduce the absorption of rifampicin. Daily doses of rifampicin should be given at least 1 hour before the ingestion of antacids.

When rifampicin is given concomitantly with either halothane or isoniazid, the potential for hepatotoxicity is increased. The concomitant use of rifampicin and halothane should be avoided. Patients receiving both rifampicin and isoniazid should be monitored closely for hepatotoxicity.

If *p*-aminosalicylic acid and rifampicin are both included in the treatment regimen, they should be given not less than eight hours apart to ensure satisfactory blood levels.

Interference with laboratory and diagnostic tests

Therapeutic levels of rifampicin have been shown to inhibit standard microbiological assays for serum folate and Vitamin B12. Thus alternative assay methods should be considered. Transient elevation of BSP and serum bilirubin has been reported. Rifampicin may impair biliary excretion of contrast media used for visualization of the gallbladder, due to competition for biliary excretion. Therefore, these tests should be performed before the daily administration of Rifadin for Infusion.

4.6 Pregnancy and lactation

Pregnancy

At very high doses in animals rifampicin has been shown to have teratogenic effects. There are no well controlled studies with rifampicin in pregnant women. Although rifampicin has been reported to cross the placental barrier and appear in cord blood, the effect of rifampicin, alone or in combination with other antituberculosis drugs, on the human foetus is not known. Therefore, Rifadin for Infusion should be used in pregnant women or in women of child bearing potential only if the potential benefit justifies the potential risk to the foetus. When Rifadin is administered during the last few weeks of pregnancy it may cause post-natal haemorrhages in the mother and infant for which treatment with Vitamin K1 may be indicated.

Lactation

Rifampicin is excreted in breast milk and infants should not be breast fed by a patient receiving rifampicin unless in the physician's judgement the potential benefit to the patient outweighs the potential risk to the infant.

4.7 Effects on ability to drive and use machines

None known.

4.8 Undesirable effects

Rifadin for Infusion is generally well tolerated and accepted by patients, although hypersensitivity reactions have been described and occasionally patients have experienced fever, skin rashes and nausea/vomiting.

Occasional instances of phlebitis and pain at the infusion site have been reported.

Reactions occurring with either daily or intermittent dosage regimens include:

Cutaneous reactions which are mild and self-limiting may occur and do not appear to be hypersensitivity reactions. Typically they consist of flushing and itching with or without a rash. Urticaria and more serious hypersensitivity cutaneous reactions have occurred but are uncommon. Exfoliate dermatitis, pemphigoid reaction, erythema multiforme including Stevens-Johnson syndrome, Lyells syndrome and vasculitis have been reported rarely.

Gastrointestinal reactions consist of anorexia, nausea, vomiting, abdominal discomfort, and diarrhoea. Pseudomembranous colitis has been reported with rifampicin therapy.

Hepatitis can be caused by rifampicin and liver function tests should be monitored (see section 4.4. Special warnings and precautions for use).

Central Nervous System: Psychoses have been rarely reported.

Thrombocytopenia with or without purpura may occur, usually associated with intermittent therapy, but is reversible if drug is discontinued as soon as purpura occurs. Cerebral haemorrhage and fatalities have been reported when rifampicin administration has been continued or resumed after the appearance of purpura.

Disseminated intravascular coagulation has also been rarely reported.

Eosinophilia, leucopenia, oedema, muscle weakness and myopathy have been reported to occur in a small percentage of patients treated with rifampicin.

Agranulocytosis has been reported very rarely reported.

Rare reports of adrenal insufficiency in patients with compromised adrenal function have been observed.

Reactions usually occurring with intermittent dosage regimens and probably of immunological origin include:

- 'Flu Syndrome' consisting of episodes of fever, chills, headache, dizziness, and bone pain appearing most commonly during the 3rd to the 6th month of therapy. The frequency of the syndrome varies but may occur in up to 50 % of patients given once-weekly regimens with a dose of rifampicin of 25 mg/kg or more.
- Shortness of breath and wheezing.
- Decrease in blood pressure and shock.
- Anaphylaxis.
- Acute haemolytic anaemia.
- Acute renal failure usually due to acute tubular necrosis or acute interstitial nephritis.

If serious complications arise, e.g. renal failure, thrombocytopenia or haemolytic anaemia, rifampicin should be stopped and never restarted.

Occasional disturbances of the menstrual cycle have been reported in women receiving long-term anti-tuberculosis therapy with regimens containing rifampicin.

Rifampicin may produce a reddish colouration of the urine, sweat, sputum and tears. The patient should be forewarned of this. Soft contact lenses may be permanently stained.

4.9 Overdose

Human Experience

- Signs and Symptoms:

Nausea, vomiting, abdominal pain, pruritus, headache and increasing lethargy will probably occur within a short time after acute ingestion; unconsciousness may occur when there is severe hepatic disease. Transient increases in liver enzymes and/or bilirubin may occur. Brownish-red or orange colouration of the skin, urine, sweat, saliva, tears and faeces will occur, and its intensity is proportional to the amount ingested. Facial or periorbital oedema has also been reported in paediatric patients. Hypotension, sinus tachycardia, ventricular arrhythmias, seizures and cardiac arrest were reported in some fatal cases.

The minimum acute lethal or toxic dose is not well established. However, nonfatal acute overdoses in adults have been reported with doses ranging from 9 to 12 g rifampicin. Fatal acute overdoses in adults have been reported with doses ranging from 14-60 g. Alcohol or a history of alcohol abuse was involved in some of the fatal and nonfatal reports.

Nonfatal overdoses in paediatric patients ages 1 to 4 years old of 100 mg/kg for one to two doses have been reported.

• Management:

Intensive supportive measures should be instituted and individual symptoms treated as they arise. Since nausea and vomiting are likely to be present, gastric lavage is probably preferable to induction of emesis. Following evacuation of the gastric contents, the instillation of activated charcoal slurry into the stomach may help absorb any remaining drug from the gastrointestinal tract. Antiemetic medication may be required to control severe nausea and vomiting. Active diuresis (with measured intake and output) will help promote excretion of the drug. Haemodialysis may be of value in some patients.

5. PHARMACOLOGICAL PROPERTIES

5.1 Pharmacodynamic properties

Rifampicin is an active bactericidial antituberculosis drug which is particularly active against the rapidly growing extracellular organisms and also has bactericidial activity intracellularly. Rifampicin has activity against slow and intermittently-growing *M. Tuberculosis*.

Rifampicin inhibits DNA-dependent RNA polymerase activity in susceptible cells. Specifically, it interacts with bacterial RNA polymerase but does not inhibit the mammalian enzyme. Cross-resistance to rifampicin has only been shown with other rifamycins.

5.2 Pharmacokinetic properties

After intravenous administration of a 300 or 600 mg dose of Rifadin infusion infused over 30 minutes to healthy male volunteers (n = 12), mean peak plasma concentrations were 9.0 and 17.5 μg/ml, respectively. The average plasma concentrations in these volunteers remained detectable for 8 and 12 hours, respectively.

The pharmacokinetics (oral and intravenous) in children are similar to adults.

In normal subjects the biological half-life of rifampicin in serum averages about 3 hours after a 600 mg dose and increases to 5.1 hours after a 900 mg dose. With repeated administration, the half-life decreases and reaches average values of approximately 2-3 hours. At a dose of up to 600 mg/day, it does not differ in patients with renal failure and consequently, no dosage adjustment is required.

Rifampicin is rapidly eliminated in the bile and an enterohepatic circulation ensues. During this process, rifampicin undergoes progressive deacetylation, so that nearly all the drug in the bile is in this form in about 6 hours. This metabolite retains essentially complete antibacterial activity. Intestinal reabsorption is reduced by deacetylation and elimination is facilitated. Up to 30 % of a dose is excreted in the urine, with about half of this being unchanged drug.

Rifampicin is widely distributed throughout the body. It is present in effective concentrations in many organs and body fluids, including cerebrospinal fluid. Rifampicin is about 80 % protein bound. Most of the unbound fraction is not ionized and therefore is diffused freely in tissues.

5.3 Preclinical safety data

Not applicable

6. PHARMACEUTICAL PARTICULARS

6.1 List of excipients

Sodium sulfoxylate formaldehyde

Sodium hydroxide

Solvent

Polysorbate 81 (Tween 81)

Water for Injections.

6.2 Incompatibilities

Compatibilities: Rifadin for Infusion is compatible with the following infusion solutions for up to 6 hours: Mannitol 10% and 20%, Macrodex with Saline Solution, Macrodex with Glucose Solution, Rheomacrodex, Sodium Bicarbonate 1.4%, Laevulose 5% and 10%, Ringer Lactate, Ringer Acetate, Dextrose 5% and 10%, Saline Solution.

Incompatibilities: Rifadin for Infusion is incompatible with the following: Perfudex, Sodium Bicarbonate 5%, Sodium Lactate 0.167M, Ringer Acetate with Dextrose.

6.3 Shelf life

Unopened vial of lyophilisate: 48 months

Unopened ampoule of solvent: 60 months

Reconstituted Solution: 6 hours

6.4 Special precautions for storage

Store below 25°C.

6.5 Nature and contents of container

20ml clear neutral glass vial sealed with butyl rubber stopper and aluminium/plastic "flip-off" cap (colour coded blue) containing 600mg Rifampicin and 10ml clear glass ampoule containing solvent.

Pack size: combination of 1 vial of lyophilisate and 1 ampoule of solvent.

6.6 Special precautions for disposal and other handling

Not applicable.

7. MARKETING AUTHORISATION HOLDER

Sanofi-aventis

One Onslow Street

Guildford

Surrey

GU1 4YS

UK

8. MARKETING AUTHORISATION NUMBER(S)

PL 04425/0051

9. DATE OF FIRST AUTHORISATION/RENEWAL OF THE AUTHORISATION

7th December 1982 / 9th April 2005

10. DATE OF REVISION OF THE TEXT

13 March 2009

LEGAL STATUS

POM

Rifadin syrup 100mg/5ml

(sanofi-aventis)

1. NAME OF THE MEDICINAL PRODUCT

Rifadin Syrup 100mg/5ml

2. QUALITATIVE AND QUANTITATIVE COMPOSITION

Rifampicin Ph Eur 100 mg

3. PHARMACEUTICAL FORM

Raspberry coloured and flavoured suspension.

4. CLINICAL PARTICULARS

4.1 Therapeutic indications

Indications for use

Tuberculosis: In combination with other active anti-tuberculosis drugs in the treatment of all forms of tuberculosis, including fresh, advanced, chronic and drug-resistant cases. Rifadin is also effective against most atypical strains of Mycobacteria.

Leprosy: In combination with at least one other active anti-leprosy drug in the management of multibacillary and paucibacillary leprosy to effect conversion of the infectious state to a non-infectious state.

Other Infections: In the treatment of Brucellosis, Legionnaires Disease, and serious staphylococcal infections. To prevent emergence of resistant strains of the infecting organisms, Rifadin should be used in combination with another antibiotic appropriate for the infection.

Prophylaxis of meningococcal meningitis: For the treatment of asymptomatic carriers of *N. meningitidis* to eliminate meningococci from the nasopharynx.

Haemophilus influenzae: For the treatment of asymptomatic carriers of *H.influenzae* and as chemoprophylaxis of exposed children, 4 years of age or younger.

4.2 Posology and method of administration

Recommended Dosage

For oral administration

The daily dose of Rifadin, calculated from the patient's body weight, should preferably be taken at least 30 minutes before a meal or 2 hours after a meal to ensure rapid and complete absorption.

Tuberculosis:

Rifadin should be given with other effective anti-tuberculosis drugs to prevent the possible emergence of rifampicin-resistant strains of Mycobacteria.

Adults: The recommended single daily dose in tuberculosis is 8-12 mg/kg.

Usual Daily dose: Patients weighing less than 50 kg - 450 mg. Patients weighing 50 kg or more - 600 mg.

Children: In children, oral doses of 10-20 mg/kg body weight daily are recommended, although a total daily dose should not usually exceed 600 mg.

Leprosy:

600 mg doses of rifampicin should be given once per month. Alternatively, a daily regimen may be used. The recommended single daily dose is 10 mg/kg.

Usual daily dose: Patients weighing less than 50 kg - 450 mg. Patients weighing 50 kg or more - 600 mg.

In the treatment of leprosy, rifampicin should always be used in conjunction with at least one other antileprosy drug,

Brucellosis, Legionnaires Disease or serious staphylococcal infections

Adults: The recommended daily dose is 600-1200 mg given in 2 to 4 divided doses, together with another appropriate antibiotic to prevent the emergence of resistant strains of the infecting organisms.

Prophylaxis of meningococcal meningitis

Adults: 600 mg twice daily for 2 days.

Children (1 - 12 years): 10 mg/kg twice daily for 2 days.

Children (3 months - 1 year): 5 mg/kg twice daily for 2 days.

Prophylaxis of Haemophilus influenzae

Adults and children: For members of households exposed to H. influenzae B disease when the household contains a child 4 years of age or younger, it is recommended that all members (including the child) receive rifampicin 20 mg/kg once daily (maximum daily dose 600 mg) for 4 days.

Index cases should be treated prior to discharge from hospital.

Neonates (1 month): 10 mg/kg daily for 4 days.

Impaired liver function:

A daily dose of 8 mg/kg should not be exceeded in patients with impaired liver function.

Use in the elderly:

In elderly patients, the renal excretion of rifampicin is decreased proportionally with physiological decrease of renal function; due to compensatory increase of liver excretion, the terminal half-life in serum is similar to that of younger patients. However, as increased blood levels have been noted in one study of rifampicin in elderly patients, caution should be exercised in using rifampicin in such patients, especially if there is evidence of impaired liver function.

4.3 Contraindications

Rifadin is contra-indicated in the presence of jaundice, and in patients who are hypersensitive to the rifamycins or any of the excipients.

Rifadin use is contraindicated when given concurrently with the combination of saquinavir/ritonavir (see section 4.5 Interactions).

4.4 Special warnings and precautions for use

Rifampicin should be given under the supervision of a respiratory or other suitably qualified physician.

Cautions should be taken in case of renal impairment if dose > 600 mg/day.

All tuberculosis patients should have pre-treatment measurements of liver function.

Adults treated for tuberculosis with rifampicin should have baseline measurements of hepatic enzymes, bilirubin, serum creatinine, a complete blood count, and a platelet count (or estimate).

Patients with impaired liver function should only be given rifampicin in cases of necessity, and then with caution and under close medical supervision. In these patients, lower doses of rifampicin are recommended and careful monitoring of liver function, especially serum glutamic pyruvic transaminase (SGPT) and serum glutamic oxaloacetic transaminase (SGOT) should initially be carried out prior to therapy, weekly for two weeks, then every two weeks for the next six weeks. If signs of hepatocellular damage occur, rifampicin should be withdrawn.

Rifampicin should also be withdrawn if clinically significant changes in hepatic function occur. The need for other forms of antituberculosis therapy and a different regimen should be considered. Urgent advice should be obtained from a specialist in the management of tuberculosis. If rifampicin is re-introduced after liver function has returned to normal, liver function should be monitored daily.

In patients with impaired liver function, elderly patients, malnourished patients, and possibly, children under two years of age, caution is particularly recommended when instituting therapeutic regimens in which isoniazid is to be used concurrently with Rifadin. If the patient has no evidence of pre-existing liver disease and normal pre-treatment liver function, liver function tests need only be repeated if fever, vomiting, jaundice or other deterioration in the patient's condition occur.

Patients should be seen at least monthly during therapy and should be specifically questioned concerning symptoms associated with adverse reactions.

In some patients hyperbilirubinaemia can occur in the early days of treatment. This results from competition between rifampicin and bilirubin for hepatic excretion.

An isolated report showing a moderate rise in bilirubin and/or transaminase level is not in itself an indication for interrupting treatment; rather the decision should be made after repeating the tests, noting trends in the levels and considering them in conjunction with the patient's clinical condition.

Because of the possibility of immunological reaction including anaphylaxis (see section 4.8 Undesirable effects) occurring with intermittent therapy (less than 2 to 3 times per week) patients should be closely monitored. Patients should be cautioned against interrupting treatment.

Rifampicin has enzyme induction properties that can enhance the metabolism of endogenous substrates including adrenal hormones, thyroid hormones and vitamin D. Isolated reports have associated porphyria exacerbation with rifampicin administration.

Rifadin syrup contains sodium metabisulfite which may cause allergic type reactions including anaphylactic symptoms and life threatening or less severe asthmatic episodes in certain susceptible people.

4.5 Interaction with other medicinal products and other forms of interaction

Cytochrome P-450 enzyme interaction

Rifampicin is a potent inducer of certain cytochrome P-450 enzymes. Coadministration of rifampicin with other drugs that are also metabolised through these cytochrome P-450 enzymes may accelerate the metabolism and reduce the activity of these other drugs. Therefore, caution should be used when prescribing rifampicin with drugs metabolised by cytochrome P-450. To maintain optimum therapeutic blood levels, dosages of drugs metabolised by these enzymes may require adjustment when starting or stopping concomitantly administered rifampicin.

Examples of drugs metabolised by cytochrome P-450 enzymes are:

- Antiarrhythmics (e.g. disopyramide, mexiletine, quinidine, propafenone, tocainide),
- Antiepileptics (e.g. phenytoin),
- Hormone antagonist (antiestrogens e.g. tamoxifen, toremifene, gestinone),
- Antipsychotics (e.g. haloperidol, aripiprazole),
- Anticoagulants (e.g. coumarins),
- Antifungals (e.g. fluconazole, itraconazole, ketoconazole, voriconazole),
- Antivirals (e.g. saquinavir, indinavir, efavirenz, amprenavir, nelfinavir, atazanavir, lopinavir, nevirapine),
- Barbiturates
- Beta-blockers (e.g. bisoprolol, propanolol),
- Anxiolytics and hypnotics (e.g. diazepam, benzodiazepines, zolpicolone, zolpidem),
- Calcium channel blockers (e.g. diltiazem, nifedipine, verapamil, nimodipine, isradipine, nicardipine, nisoldipine),
- Antibacterials (e.g. chloramphenicol, clarithromycin, dapsone, doxycycline, fluoroquinolones, telithromycin),
- Corticosteroids
- Cardiac glycosides (digitoxin, digoxin),
- Clofibrate,
- Systemic hormonal contraceptives
- Oestrogen,
- Antidiabetic (e.g. chlorpropamide, tolbutamide, sulfonylureas, rosiglitazone),
- Immunosuppressive agents (e.g. ciclosporin, sirolimus, tacrolimus)
- Irinotecan,
- Thyroid hormone (e.g. levothyroxine),
- Losartan,
- Analgestics (e.g. methadone, narcotic analgesics),
- Praziquantel,
- Progestogens,
- Quinine,
- Riluzole,
- Selective 5-HT3 receptor antagonists (e.g. ondansetron)
- Statins metabolised by CYP 3A4 (e.g. simvastatin),
- Theophylline,
- Tricyclic antidepressants (e.g. amitriptyline, nortriptyline),
- Cytotoxics (e.g. imatinib),
- Diuretics (e.g. eplerenone)

Patients on oral contraceptives should be advised to use alternative, non-hormonal methods of birth control during Rifadin therapy. Also diabetes may become more difficult to control.

Other Interactions

When rifampicin is given concomitantly with the combination saquinavir/ritonavir, the potential for hepatotoxicity is increased. Therefore, concomitant use of Rifadin with saquinvir/ritonavir is contraindicated (see section 4.3 Contraindications).

When the two drugs were taken concomitantly, decreased concentrations of atovaquone and increased concentrations of rifampicin were observed.

Concurrent use of ketoconazole and rifampicin has resulted in decreased serum concentrations of both drugs.

Concurrent use of rifampicin and enalapril has resulted in decreased concentrations of enalaprilat, the active metabolite of enalapril. Dosage adjustments should be made if indicated by the patient's clinical condition.

Concomitant antacid administration may reduce the absorption of rifampicin. Daily doses of rifampicin should be given at least 1 hour before the ingestion of antacids.

When rifampicin is given concomitantly with either halothane or isoniazid, the potential for hepatotoxicity is increased. The concomitant use of rifampicin and halothane should be avoided. Patients receiving both rifampicin and isoniazid should be monitored closely for hepatotoxicity.

If *p*-aminosalicylic acid and rifampicin are both included in the treatment regimen, they should be given not less than eight hours apart to ensure satisfactory blood levels.

Interference with laboratory and diagnostic tests

Therapeutic levels of rifampicin have been shown to inhibit standard microbiological assays for serum folate and Vitamin B12. Thus alternative assay methods should be considered. Transient elevation of BSP and serum bilirubin has been reported. Rifampicin may impair biliary excretion of contrast media used for visualization of the gallbladder, due to competition for biliary excretion. Therefore, these tests should be performed before the morning dose of rifampicin.

4.6 Pregnancy and lactation

Pregnancy

At very high doses in animals rifampicin has been shown to have teratogenic effects. There are no well controlled studies with rifampicin in pregnant women. Although rifampicin has been reported to cross the placental barrier and appear in cord blood, the effect of rifampicin, alone or in combination with other antituberculosis drugs, on the human foetus is not known. Therefore, Rifadin should be used in pregnant women or in women of child bearing potential only if the potential benefit justifies the potential risk to the foetus. When Rifadin is administered during the last few weeks of pregnancy it may cause post-natal haemorrhages in the mother and infant for which treatment with Vitamin K1 may be indicated.

Lactation

Rifampicin is excreted in breast milk, patients receiving rifampicin should not breast feed unless in the physician's judgement the potential benefit to the patient outweighs the potential risk to the infant.

4.7 Effects on ability to drive and use machines

None stated

4.8 Undesirable effects

Reactions occurring with either daily or intermittent dosage regimens include:

Cutaneous reactions which are mild and self-limiting and do not appear to be hypersensitivity reactions. Typically they consist of flushing and itching with or without a rash. Urticaria and more serious hypersensitivity cutaneous reactions have occurred but are uncommon. Exfoliate dermatitis, pemphigoid reaction, erythema multiforme including Stevens-Johnson syndrome, Lyells syndrome and vasculitis have been reported rarely.

Gastrointestinal reactions consist of anorexia, nausea, vomiting, abdominal discomfort, and diarrhoea. Pseudomembranous colitis has been reported with rifampicin therapy.

Hepatitis can be caused by rifampicin and liver function tests should be monitored (see section 4.4. Special warnings and precautions for use).

Central Nervous System: Psychoses have been rarely reported.

Thrombocytopenia with or without purpura may occur, usually associated with intermittent therapy, but is reversible if drug is discontinued as soon as purpura occurs. Cerebral haemorrhage and fatalities have been reported when rifampicin administration has been continued or resumed after the appearance of purpura.

Disseminated intravascular coagulation has also been rarely reported.

Eosinophilia, leucopenia, oedema, muscle weakness and myopathy have been reported to occur in a small percentage of patients treated with rifampicin.

Agranulocytosis has been reported very rarely reported.

Rare reports of adrenal insufficiency in patients with compromised adrenal function have been observed.

Reactions usually occurring with intermittent dosage regimens and probably of immunological origin include:

- 'Flu Syndrome' consisting of episodes of fever, chills, headache, dizziness, and bone pain appearing most commonly during the 3rd to the 6th monthly of therapy. The frequency of the syndrome varies but may occur in up to 50 % of patients given once-weekly regimens with a dose of rifampicin of 25 mg/kg or more.
- Shortness of breath and wheezing.
- Decrease in blood pressure and shock.
- Anaphylaxis.
- Acute haemolytic anaemia.
- Acute renal failure usually due to acute tubular necrosis or acute interstitial nephritis.

If serious complications arise, e.g. renal failure, thrombocytopenia or haemolytic anaemia, rifampicin should be stopped and never restarted.

Occasional disturbances of the menstrual cycle have been reported in women receiving long-term anti-tuberculosis therapy with regimens containing rifampicin.

Rifampicin may produce a reddish colouration of the urine, sweat, sputum and tears. The patient should be forewarned of this. Soft contact lenses may be permanently stained.

4.9 Overdose

Human Experience

- Signs and Symptoms:

Nausea, vomiting, abdominal pain, pruritus, headache and increasing lethargy will probably occur within a short time after acute ingestion; unconsciousness may occur when there is severe hepatic disease. Transient increases in liver enzymes and/or bilirubin may occur. Brownish-red or orange colouration of the skin, urine, sweat, saliva, tears and faeces will occur, and its intensity is proportional to the amount ingested. Facial or periorbital oedema has also been reported in paediatric patients. Hypotension, sinus tachycardia, ventricular arrhythmias, seizures and cardiac arrest were reported in some fatal cases.

The minimum acute lethal or toxic dose is not well established. However, nonfatal acute overdoses in adults have been reported with doses ranging from 9 to 12 g rifampicin. Fatal acute overdoses in adults have been reported with doses ranging from 14-60 g. Alcohol or a history of alcohol abuse was involved in some of the fatal and nonfatal reports.

Nonfatal overdoses in paediatric patients ages 1 to 4 years old of 100 mg/kg for one to two doses have been reported.

- Management:

Intensive supportive measures should be instituted and individual symptoms treated as they arise. Since nausea and vomiting are likely to be present, gastric lavage is probably preferable to induction of emesis. Following evacuation of the gastric contents, the instillation of activated charcoal slurry into the stomach may help absorb any remaining drug from the gastrointestinal tract. Antiemetic medication may be required to control severe nausea and vomiting. Active diuresis (with measured intake and output) will help promote excretion of the drug. Haemodialysis may be of value in some patients.

5. PHARMACOLOGICAL PROPERTIES

5.1 Pharmacodynamic properties

Rifampicin is an active bactericidial antituberculosis drug which is particularly active against the rapidly growing extracellular organisms and also has bactericidial activity intracellularly. Rifampicin has activity against slow and intermittently-growing *M. Tuberculosis*.

Rifampicin inhibits DNA-dependent RNA polymerase activity in susceptible cells. Specifically, it interacts with bacterial RNA polymerase but does not inhibit the mammalian enzyme. Cross-resistance to rifampicin has only been shown with other rifamycins.

5.2 Pharmacokinetic properties

Rifampicin is readily absorbed from the gastrointestinal tract. Peak serum concentrations of the order of 10 µg/ml occur about 2 to 4 hours after a dose of 10 mg/kg body weight on an empty stomach.

Absorption of rifampicin is reduced when the drug is ingested with food.

The pharmacokinetics (oral and intravenous) in children are similar to adults.

In normal subjects the biological half-life of rifampicin in serum averages about 3 hours after a 600 mg dose and increases to 5.1 hours after a 900 mg dose. With repeated administration, the half-life decreases and reaches average values of approximately 2-3 hours. At a dose of up to 600 mg/day, it does not differ in patients with renal failure and consequently, no dosage adjustment is required.

Rifampicin is rapidly eliminated in the bile and an enterophepatic circulation ensues. During this process, rifampicin undergoes progressive deacetylation, so that nearly all the drug in the bile is in this form in about 6 hours. This metabolite retains essentially complete antibacterial activity. Intestinal reabsorption is reduced by deacetylation and elimination is facilitated. Up to 30 % of a dose is excreted in the urine, with about half of this being unchanged drug.

Rifampicin is widely distributed throughout the body. It is present in effective concentrations in many organs and body fluids, including cerebrospinal fluid. Rifampicin is about 80 % protein bound. Most of the unbound fraction is not ionized and therefore is diffused freely in tissues.

5.3 Preclinical safety data

Not applicable

6. PHARMACEUTICAL PARTICULARS

6.1 List of excipients

Agar Ph Eur

Sucrose Ph Eur

Methyl-p-hydroxybenzoate Ph Eur

Propyl-p-hydroxybenzoate Ph Eur

Potassium sorbate Ph Eur

Sodium metabisulphite Ph Eur

Tween 80 Ph Eur

Raspberry essence HSE

Saccharin USNF

Diethanolamine USNF

Purified water Ph Eur

6.2 Incompatibilities

None stated

6.3 Shelf life

3 years from date of manufacture

6.4 Special precautions for storage

Store below 30°C.

Do not dilute.

Dispense in clear or amber glass bottles.

6.5 Nature and contents of container

120ml in amber glass bottles

6.6 Special precautions for disposal and other handling

Not applicable

7. MARKETING AUTHORISATION HOLDER
Sanofi-aventis
One Onslow Street
Guildford
Surrey
GU1 4YS
UK

8. MARKETING AUTHORISATION NUMBER(S)
PL 04425/5917R

9. DATE OF FIRST AUTHORISATION/RENEWAL OF THE AUTHORISATION
23/03/05

10. DATE OF REVISION OF THE TEXT
13 March 2009

LEGAL CLASSIFICATION
POM

Rifater Tablets

(sanofi-aventis)

1. NAME OF THE MEDICINAL PRODUCT
Rifater Tablets

2. QUALITATIVE AND QUANTITATIVE COMPOSITION
Rifampicin Ph Eur 120 mg
Isoniazid Ph Eur 50 mg
Pyrazinamide Ph Eur 300 mg

3. PHARMACEUTICAL FORM
Tablets

4. CLINICAL PARTICULARS

4.1 Therapeutic indications
Rifater is indicated in the treatment of pulmonary tuberculosis.

4.2 Posology and method of administration
Rifater is recommended in the initial intensive phase of the short-course treatment of pulmonary tuberculosis. During this phase, which lasts for 2 months, Rifater should be administered on a daily continuous basis. The concomitant administration of ethambutol or intramuscular streptomycin over the same period of time is advised.

Each Rifater tablet contains isoniazid (INH), pyrazinamide (Z) and rifampicin (RAMP) in such a ratio that the administration of 9-12mg/kg RAMP, 4-5mg/kg INH and 23-30mg/kg Z can be achieved by giving 3 tablets daily to patients weighing less than 40kg, 4 tablets to patients weighing 40-49kg, 5 tablets to patients weighing 50-64kg and 6 tablets to patients weighing 65kg or more.

Rifater should be given as a single dose and preferably on an empty stomach at least 30 minutes before a meal, or 2 hours after a meal to ensure rapid and complete absorption.

Once the initial intensive phase of treatment has been completed treatment can be continued with the combination rifampicin-isoniazid (Rifinah) always on a daily basis.

This regimen, if correctly applied, is 100% effective with very few, if any, relapses. The clinical evidence indicates that these occur generally in the first 6 months after stopping treatment with bacilli fully sensitive to the drugs employed, so that changes in the drugs to be utilised for further treatment are not required. The regimen has been found to be fully effective also in the presence of a bacillary population resistant to isoniazid, to streptomycin or to both drugs.

Children: The ratio of the three drugs in Rifater may not be appropriate in children (eg higher mg/kg doses of INH are usually given in children than in adults). Rifater can be used only in special cases, after careful consideration of the mg/kg dose of each component.

Use in the Elderly: Caution should be exercised in such patients, in view of the possible decrease of the excretory function of the kidney and of the liver.

4.3 Contraindications
Rifater is contra-indicated in patients who are hypersensitive to any one of the components of the combination or any of the excipients. Rifater is contra-indicated in the presence of jaundice.

Rifater use is contraindicated when given concurrently with the combination of saquinavir/ritonavir (see section 4.5 Interactions).

4.4 Special warnings and precautions for use
The precautions for the use of Rifater are the same as those considered when a triple individual administration of rifampicin, isoniazid and pyrazinamide is required. Rifater should only be given under supervision. Each of these drugs has been associated with liver dysfunction.

Rifater should be given under the supervision of a respiratory or other suitably qualified physician.

All tuberculosis patients should have pre-treatment measurements of liver function.

Adults treated for tuberculosis with Rifater should have baseline measurements of hepatic enzymes, bilirubin, serum creatinine, a complete blood count and a platelet count (or estimate).

Patients should be seen at least monthly during therapy and should be questioned specifically about symptoms associated with adverse reactions. All patients with abnormalities should have follow-up, including laboratory testing, if necessary.

However, because there is a higher frequency of isoniazid-associated hepatitis among persons older than 35 years of age, a transaminase measurement should be obtained at baseline and at least monthly during therapy in this age group. Other factors associated with an increased risk of hepatitis include daily use of alcohol, chronic liver disease, intravenous drug use and being a black or Hispanic woman.

If the patient has no evidence of pre-existing liver disease and normal pre-treatment liver function, liver function tests need only be repeated if fever, vomiting, jaundice or other deterioration in the patient's condition occur.

Patients with impaired liver function should only be given Rifater in cases of necessity and then with caution and under strict medical supervision. In these patients, careful monitoring of liver function, especially serum glutamic pyruvic transaminase (SGPT) and serum glutamic oxaloacetic transaminase (SGOT) should be carried out prior to therapy and then every two to four weeks during therapy.

If signs of hepatocellular damage or clinically significant changes in hepatic function occur, Rifater should be withdrawn. The need for other forms of antituberculosis therapy and a different regimen should be considered. Urgent advice should be obtained from a specialist in the management of tuberculosis. If Rifater is reintroduced after liver function has returned to normal, liver function should be monitored daily.

<u>Rifampicin</u>

Cautions should be taken in cases of renal impairment if dose > 600 mg/day.

In patients with impaired liver function, elderly patients, malnourished patients and possibly children under two years of age, caution is particularly recommended when instituting therapeutic regimens in which isoniazid is to be used concurrently with rifampicin.

In some cases, hyperbilirubinaemia resulting from competition between rifampicin and bilirubin for excretory pathways of the liver at the cell level can occur in the early days of treatment. An isolated report showing a moderate rise in bilirubin and/or transaminase level is not in itself an indication for interrupting treatment; rather, the decision should be made after repeating the tests, noting trends in the levels and considering them in conjunction with the patient's clinical condition.

Because of the possibility of immunological reaction including anaphylaxis (see section 4.8 Undesirable effects) occurring with intermittent rifampicin therapy (less than 2 or 3 per week) patients should be closely monitored. Patients should be cautioned against interruption of dosage regimens since these reactions may occur.

Rifampicin has enzyme induction properties that can enhance the metabolism of endogenous substrates including adrenal hormones, thyroid hormones and vitamin D. Isolated reports have associated porphyria exacerbation with rifampicin administration.

<u>Isoniazid</u>

Use of isoniazid should be carefully monitored in patients with current chronic liver disease or severe renal dysfunction.

Severe and sometimes fatal hepatitis associated with isoniazid therapy may occur and may develop even after many months of treatment. The risk of developing hepatitis is age related. Therefore, patients should be monitored for the prodromal symptoms of hepatitis; such as fatigue, weakness, malaise, anorexia, nausea or vomiting. If these symptoms appear or if signs suggestive of hepatic damage are detected, isoniazid should be discontinued promptly, since continued use of the drug in these cases has been reported to cause a more severe form of liver damage.

Care should be exercised in the treatment of elderly or malnourished patients who may also require Vitamin B6 supplementation with the isoniazid therapy.

Use of isoniazid should be carefully monitored in patients with slow acetylator status, epilepsy, history of psychosis, history of peripheral neuropathy, diabetes, alcohol dependence, HIV infection or porphyria.

<u>Pyrazinamide</u>

Rifater should be used with caution in patients with a history of gout. If hyperuricaemia accompanied by an acute gouty arthritis occurs, the patient should be transferred to a regimen not containing pyrazinamide (e.g. Rifinah 150 or 300).

The possibility of pyrazinamide having an adverse effect on blood clotting time or vascular integrity should be borne in mind in patients with haemoptysis.

4.5 Interaction with other medicinal products and other forms of interaction

Food Interaction

Because isoniazid has some monoamine oxidase inhibiting activity, an interaction with tyramine-containing foods (cheese, red wine) may occur. Diamine oxidase may also be inhibited, causing exaggerated response (e.g. headache, sweating, palpitations, flushing, hypotension) to foods containing histamine (e.g. skipjack, tuna, other tropical fish). Tyramine- and histamine-containing foods should be avoided by patients receiving Rifater.

Interactions with other medicinal products

Cytochrome P-450 enzyme interaction

Rifampicin is known to induce and isoniazid is known to inhibit certain cytochrome P-450 enzymes. In general, the impact of the competing effects of rifampicin and isoniazid on the metabolism of drugs that undergo biotransformation through the affected pathways is unknown. Therefore, caution should be used when prescribing Rifater with drugs metabolised by cytochrome P-450. To maintain optimum therapeutic blood levels, dosages of drugs metabolised by these enzymes may require adjustment when starting or stopping Rifater.

Interactions with Rifampicin

Examples of drugs metabolised by cytochrome P-450 enzymes are:

- Antiarrhythmics (e.g. disopyramide, mexiletine, quinidine, propafenone, tocainide),
- Antiepileptics (e.g. phenytoin),
- Hormone antagonist (antiestrogens e.g. tamoxifen, toremifene, gestinone),
- Antipsychotics (e.g. haloperidol, aripiprazole),
- Anticoagulants (e.g. coumarins),
- Antifungals (e.g. fluconazole, itraconazole, ketoconazole, voriconazole),
- Antivirals (e.g. saquinavir, indinavir, efavirenz, amprenavir, nelfinavir, atazanavir, lopinavir, nevirapine),
- Barbiturates
- Beta-blockers (e.g. bisoprolol, propanolol),
- Anxiolytics and hypnotics (e.g. diazepam, benzodiazepines, zopiclone, zolpidem),
- Calcium channel blockers (e.g. diltiazem, nifedipine, verapamil, nimodipine, isradipine, nicardipine, nisoldipine),
- Antibacterials (e.g. chloramphenicol, clarithromycin, dapsone, doxycycline, fluoroquinolones, telithromycin),
- Corticosteroids
- Cardiac glycosides (digitoxin, digoxin),
- Clofibrate,
- Systemic hormonal contraceptives
- Oestrogen,
- Antidiabetic (e.g. chlorpropamide, tolbutamide, sulfonylureas, rosiglitazone),
- Immunosuppressive agents (e.g. ciclosporin, sirolimus, tacrolimus)
- Irinotecan,
- Thyroid hormone (e.g. levothyroxine),
- Losartan,
- Analgesics (e.g. methadone, narcotic analgesics),
- Praziquantel,
- Progestogens,
- Quinine,
- Riluzole,
- Selective 5-HT3 receptor antagonists (e.g. ondansetron)
- Statins metabolised by CYP 3A4 (e.g. simvastatin),
- Theophylline,
- Tricyclic antidepressants (e.g. amitriptyline, nortriptyline),
- Cytotoxics (e.g. imatinib),
- Diuretics (e.g. eplerenone)

Patients using oral contraceptives should be advised to change to non-hormonal methods of birth control during Rifater therapy. Also diabetes may become more difficult to control.

When rifampicin is given concomitantly with the combination saquinavir/ritonavir, the potential for hepatotoxicity is increased. Therefore, concomitant use of Rifater with saquinavir/ritonavir is contraindicated (see section 4.3 Contraindications).

Other Interactions

Rifampicin may reduce the effect of ACE inhibitors (e.g. enalapril, imidapril), antiemetics (e.g. aprepitant), antineoplastic agents (e.g. imatinib), diuretics (e.g. eplerenone), drugs used in erectile dysfunction (e.g. tadalafil), oral hypoglycemic agents (e.g. nateglinide, repaglinide) and NSAIDS (e.g. etoricoxib).

When the two drugs were taken concomitantly, decreased concentrations of atovaquone and increased concentrations of rifampicin were observed.

Concurrent use of ketoconazole and rifampicin has resulted in decreased serum concentrations of both drugs.

Concomitant antacid administration may reduce the absorption of rifampicin. Daily doses of rifampicin should be given at least 1 hour before the ingestion of antacids.

The potential for hepatotoxicity is increased with an anaesthetic.

When rifampicin is given concomitantly with either halothane or isoniazid, the potential for hepatotoxicity is increased. The concomitant use of rifampicin and halothane should be avoided. Patients receiving both rifampicin and isoniazid should be monitored closely for hepatotoxicity.

If p-aminosalicylic acid and rifampicin are both included in the treatment regimen, they should be given not less than eight hours apart to ensure satisfactory blood levels.

Interactions with Isoniazid

The following drugs may interact with isoniazid:

- Antiepileptics (e.g. carbamazepine and phenytoin)

There may be an increased risk of distal sensory neuropathy when isoniazid is used in patients taking stavudine.

Concomitant use of zalcitabine with isoniazid has been shown to approximately double the renal clearance if isoniazid in HIV infected patients.

Administration of prednisolone 20mg to 13 slow acetylators and 13 fast acetylators for receiving isoniazid 10mg/kg reduced plasma concentrations of isoniazid by 25% and 40%, respectively. The clinical significance of this effect has not been established.

The effect of acute alcohol intake (serum levels 1g/L maintained for 12 hours) on the metabolism of isoniazid (300mg/d for 2 days) was studies in 10 healthy volunteers in a controlled cross over design. The metabolism of isoniazid and its metabolite, acetyl isoniazid, was not modified by this acute alcohol intake. The metabolism of isoniazid may be increased in chronic alcoholics; however this effect has not been quantified.

Other Interactions

Para-aminosalicylic acid may increase the plasma concentration and elimination half-life of isoniazid by competing for acetylating enzymes.

General anaesthetics may increase the hepatotoxicity of isoniazid.

The absorption of isoniazid is reduced by antacids.

The risk of CNS toxicity is increased when isoniazid is given with cycloserine.

Isoniazid may reduce plasma concentration of ketoconazole and increase plasma concentration of theophylline.

Pyrazinamide

Pyrazinamide antagonizes the effects of probenecid and sulfinpyrazone.

Interference with laboratory and diagnostic tests

Therapeutic levels of rifampicin have been shown to inhibit standard microbiological assays for serum folate and Vitamin B12. Thus alternative assay methods should be considered. Transient elevation of BSP and serum bilirubin has been reported. Rifampicin may impair biliary excretion of contrast media used for visualization of the gallbladder, due to competition for biliary excretion. Therefore, these tests should be performed before the morning dose of rifampicin.

4.6 Pregnancy and lactation

Pregnancy

Rifampicin

At very high doses in animals rifampicin has been shown to have teratogenic effects. There are no well controlled studies with Rifater in pregnant women. Although rifampicin has been reported to cross the placental barrier and appear in cord blood, the effect of rifampicin, alone or in combination with other antituberculosis drugs, on the human foetus is not known. When administered during the last few weeks of pregnancy, rifampicin may cause post-natal haemorrhages in the mother and infant, for which treatment with Vitamin K1 may be indicated.

Isoniazid

It has been reported that in both rats and rabbits, isoniazid may exert an embryocardial effect when administered orally during pregnancy, although no isoniazid-related congenital anomalies have been found in reproduction studies in mammalian species (mice, rats, rabbits).

Therefore, Rifater should be used in pregnant women or in women of child-bearing potential only if the potential benefit justifies the potential risk to the foetus.

Lactation

Rifampicin, isoniazid and pyrazinamide are excreted in breast milk and infants should not be breast fed by a patient receiving Rifater unless in the physician's judgement the potential benefit to the patient outweighs the potential risk to the infant.

In breast-fed infants whose mothers are taking isoniazid, there is a theoretical risk of convulsions and neuropathy (associated with vitamin B6 deficiency), therefore they should be monitored for early signs of these effects and consideration should be given to treating both mother and infant prophylactically with pyridoxine.

4.7 Effects on ability to drive and use machines

Isoniazid has been associated with vertigo, visual disorders and psychotic reactions (see section 4.8). Patients should be informed of these, and advised that if affected, they should not drive, operate machinery or take part in any activities where these symptoms may put either themselves or others at risk.

4.8 Undesirable effects

Rifampicin

Reactions occurring with either daily or intermittent dosage regimens include:

Cutaneous reactions which are mild and self-limiting may appear and do not appear to be hypersensitivity reactions. Typically they consist of flushing and itching with or without a rash. Urticaria and more serious hypersensitivity cutaneous reactions have occurred but are uncommon. Exfoliate dermatitis, pemphigoid reaction, erythema multiforme including Stevens-Johnson syndrome, Lyells syndrome and vasculitis have been reported rarely.

Gastro-intestinal reactions consist of anorexia, nausea, vomiting, abdominal discomfort, and diarrhoea. Pseudomembranous colitis has been reported with rifampicin therapy.

Hepatitis can be caused by rifampicin and liver function tests should be monitored. (See section 4.4. Special warnings and precautions for use).

Central Nervous System: Psychoses have been rarely reported.

Thrombocytopenia with or without purpura may occur, usually associated with intermittent therapy, but is reversible if drug is discontinued as soon as purpura occurs. Cerebral haemorrhage and fatalities have been reported when rifampicin administration has been continued or resumed after the appearance of purpura.

Disseminated intravascular coagulation has also been rarely reported.

Eosinophilia, leucopenia, oedema, muscle weakness and myopathy have been reported to occur in a small percentage of patients treated with rifampicin.

Agranulocytosis has been reported very rarely.

Rare reports of adrenal insufficiency in patients with compromised adrenal function have been observed.

Reactions usually occurring with intermittent dosage regimens and probably of immunological origin include:

- 'Flu Syndrome' consisting of episodes of fever, chills, headache, dizziness, and bone pain appearing most commonly during the 3rd to 6th month of therapy. The frequency of the syndrome varies but may occur in up to 50% of patients given once-weekly regimens with a dose of rifampicin of 25mg/kg or more.
- Shortness of breath and wheezing.
- Decrease in blood pressure and shock.
- Anaphylaxis.
- Acute haemolytic anaemia.
- Acute renal failure usually due to acute tubular necrosis or to acute interstitial nephritis.

If serious complications arise, (renal failure, thrombocytopenia or haemolytic anaemia), Rifater should be stopped and never restarted.

Occasional disturbances of the menstrual cycle have been reported in women receiving long term anti-tuberculosis therapy with regimens containing rifampicin.

Rifampicin may produce a reddish colouration of the urine, sputum, sweat and tears. The patient should be forewarned of this. Soft contact lenses may be permanently stained.

Isoniazid

Severe and sometimes fatal hepatitis may occur with isoniazid therapy. Hypersensitivity reactions including fever and anaphylactic reactions have been reported with isoniazid treatment. Nervous system disorders include vertigo; polyneuritis associated with isoniazid, presenting as paraesthesia, muscle weakness, loss of tendon reflexes etc, is unlikely to occur with the recommended daily dose of Rifater. Various haematological disturbances have been identified during treatment with isoniazid, including eosinophilia, agranulocytosis, thrombocytopenia and anaemia, aplastic anaemia, haemolytic anaemia. High doses of isoniazid can cause convulsions, toxic encephalopathy, optic neuritis and atrophy, memory impairment and toxic psychosis. The possibility that the frequency of seizures may be increased in patients with epilepsy should be borne in mind. Systemic lupus erythromatosus-like syndrome and pellagra have also been reported with isoniazid therapy. Cutaneous reactions (rash, acne, Stevens-Johnson syndrome, exfoliative dermatitis, pemphigus) and gastrointestinal reactions (pancreatitis, constipation, dry mouth, nausea, vomiting, epigastric distress) have been reported.

Other adverse reactions associated with isoniazid therapy are; hyperglycaemia, gynaecomastia and anti-nuclear antibodies

Pyrazinamide

Adverse reactions, other than hepatic reactions, which have been attributed to pyrazinamide are active gout (pyrazinamide has been reported to reduce urate excretion), sideroblastic anaemia, thrombocytopenia with or without purpura, arthralgia, anorexia, nausea and vomiting, dysuria, malaise, fever and aggravation of peptic ulcer. The hepatic reaction is the most common adverse reaction and varies from a symptomless abnormality of hepatic cell function detected only through laboratory liver function tests, through a mild syndrome of fever, malaise and liver tenderness, to more serious reactions such as clinical jaundice and rare cases of acute yellow atrophy and death.

Skin and subcutaneous tissue disorders: Urticaria, pruritus, erythema, rash.

Very rarely, angioedema has been reported.

4.9 Overdose

There is limited overdose information involving rifampicin, isoniazid and pyrazinamide in combination.

Signs and Symptoms

Rifampicin

Nausea, vomiting, abdominal pain, pruritus, headache and increasing lethargy will probably occur within a short time after acute ingestion; unconsciousness may occur when there is severe hepatic disease. Transient increases in liver enzymes and/or bilirubin may occur. Brownish-red or orange colouration of the skin, urine, sweat, saliva, tears and faeces will occur, and its intensity is proportional to the amount ingested. Facial or periorbital oedema has also been reported in paediatric patients. Hypotension, sinus tachycardia, ventricular arrhythmias, seizures and cardiac arrest were reported in some fatal cases.

The minimum acute lethal or toxic dose is not well established. However, nonfatal acute overdoses in adults have been reported with doses ranging from 9 to 12 g rifampicin. Fatal acute overdoses in adults have been reported with doses ranging from 14 to 60 g. Alcohol or a history of alcohol abuse was involved in some of the fatal and nonfatal reports. Nonfatal overdoses in paediatrics patients ages 1 to 4 years old of 100 mg/kg for one to two doses have been reported.

Isoniazid

Isoniazid overdosage produces signs and symptoms within 30 minutes to 3 hours after ingestion. Nausea, vomiting, dizziness, slurring of speech, blurring of vision and visual hallucinations (including bright colours and strange designs), are among the early manifestations. With marked overdosage, respiratory distress and CNS depression, progressing rapidly from stupor to profound coma are to be expected, along with severe, intractable seizures. Severe metabolic acidosis, acetonuria and hyperglycaemia are typical laboratory findings.

Pyrazinamide

There is limited information related to pyrazinamide overdose. Liver toxicity and hyperuricemia may occur with overdosage.

Management

In cases of overdosage with Rifater, gastric lavage should be performed as soon as possible. Following evacuation of the gastric contents, the instillation of activated charcoal slurry into the stomach may help absorb any remaining drug from the gastrointestinal tract. Antiemetic medication may be required to control severe nausea and vomiting.

Intensive supportive measures should be instituted, including airway patency and individual symptoms treated as they arise.

Isoniazid

If acute isoniazid overdose is suspected, even in asymptomatic patients, the administration of intravenous pyridoxine (vitamin B6) should be considered. In patients with seizures not controlled with pyridoxine (vitamin B6), anticonvulsant therapy should be administered. Sodium bicarbonate should be given to control metabolic acidosis. Haemodialysis is advised for refractory cases; if this is not available, peritoneal dialysis can be used along with forced diuresis.

5. PHARMACOLOGICAL PROPERTIES

5.1 Pharmacodynamic properties

Rifampicin, isoniazid and pyrazinamide are all active bactericidal antituberculosis drugs. Rifampicin and isoniazid are particularly active against the rapidly growing extracellular organisms. Pyrazinamide is active against intracellular organisms, particularly in the acid pH environment of macrophages. Rifampicin and isoniazid also have bactericidal activity intracellularly. Rifampicin has activity against slow and intermittently-growing M tuberculosis. Thus, the three agents, rifampicin, isoniazid and pyrazinamide have activity against the three different bacterial populations.

Rifampicin inhibits DNA-dependent RNA polymerase activity in susceptible cells. Specifically, it interacts with bacterial RNA polymerase but does not inhibit the mammalian enzyme. Cross-resistance to rifampicin has only been shown after the development of resistance to other rifamycins.

5.2 Pharmacokinetic properties

Rifampicin

Rifampicin is readily absorbed from the stomach and the duodenum. Peak serum concentrations of the order of 10 µg/ml occur about 2-4 hours after a dose of 10mg/kg body weight on an empty stomach.

In normal subjects the biological half-life of rifampicin in serum averages about 3 hours after a 600mg dose and increases to 5.1 hours after 900mg dose. With repeated administration, the half-life decreases and reaches average values of approximately 2-3 hours. At a dose of up to 600 mg/day the half-life does not differ in patients with renal failure and, consequently, no dosage adjustment is required. The half-life of rifampicin may be decreased when isoniazid is administered concurrently.

After absorption, rifampicin is rapidly eliminated in the bile and an enterohepatic circulation ensues. During this process, rifampicin undergoes progressive deacetylation, so that nearly all the drug in the bile is in this form in about 6 hours. This metabolite retains essentially complete antibacterial activity. Intestinal reabsorption is reduced by deacetylation and elimination is facilitated. Up to 30% of a dose is excreted in the urine with about half of this being unchanged drug. Absorption of rifampicin is reduced when the drug is ingested with food.

Rifampicin is widely distributed throughout the body. It is present in effective concentrations in many organs and body fluids, including cerebrospinal fluid. Rifampicin is about 80% protein bound. Most of the unbound fraction is not ionized and therefore is diffused freely in tissues.

Isoniazid

After oral administration, isoniazid produces peak blood levels within 1 to 2 hours, which decline to 50% or less within 6 hours. Ingestion of isoniazid with food may reduce its absorption. It diffuses readily into all body fluids (cerebrospinal, pleural, and ascitic fluids), tissues, organs and excreta (saliva, sputum and faeces). The drug also passes through the placental barrier and into the milk in concentrations comparable to those in the plasma. From 50 to 70% of a dose of isoniazid is excreted in the urine in 24 hours.

Isoniazid is metabolised primarily by acetylation and dehydrazination. The rate of acetylation is genetically determined. Approximately 50% of Black and Europeans are 'Slow inactivators', the majority of Asians are 'rapid inactivators'.

Pyridoxine deficiency (B_6) is sometimes observed in adults with high doses of isoniazid, probably due to its competition with pyridoxal phosphate of the enzyme apotryptophanase.

Pyrazinamide

Pyrazinamide is well absorbed from the gastrointestinal tract and rapidly distributed throughout the body, with peak plasma levels in 2 hours. It is hydrolysed to pyrazinoic acid and then metabolised to 5-hydroxypyrazinoic acid. Glomerular filtration is the primary route of excretion. It is bactericidal in acid pH, and has intracellular antibacterial activity against *M. tuberculosis*.

Pharmacokinetic studies in normal volunteers have shown that the three ingredients in Rifater have comparable bioavailability whether they are given together as individual dose forms or as Rifater.

5.3 Preclinical safety data

Not applicable

6. PHARMACEUTICAL PARTICULARS

6.1 List of excipients

Polyvinylpyrrolidone

Sodium Carboxymethylcellulose

Sodium Lauryl Sulphate

Calcium Stearate

Sucrose

Acacia Gum

Talc

Light Magnesium Carbonate

Kaolin

Titanum Dioxide

Colloidal Silicon Dioxide

Aluminium Hydroxide Gel

Iron Oxide

6.2 Incompatibilities

None stated

6.3 Shelf life

4 years from date of manufacture

6.4 Special precautions for storage

Do not store above 25°C. Store in the original container.

6.5 Nature and contents of container

PDVC and PVC/PVDC aluminium foil blisters packed in cardboard cartons.

Pack size: 100 tablets

6.6 Special precautions for disposal and other handling

Not applicable

7. MARKETING AUTHORISATION HOLDER

Sanofi-aventis

One Onslow Street

Guildford

Surrey

GU1 4YS

UK

8. MARKETING AUTHORISATION NUMBER(S)

PL 04425/0060

9. DATE OF FIRST AUTHORISATION/RENEWAL OF THE AUTHORISATION

27 April 1984/10 May 1995

10. DATE OF REVISION OF THE TEXT

13 March 2009

LEGAL STATUS

POM

Rifinah 150 and 300

(sanofi-aventis)

1. NAME OF THE MEDICINAL PRODUCT

Rifinah™ 150

Rifinah™ 300

2. QUALITATIVE AND QUANTITATIVE COMPOSITION

Rifinah 150: Rifampicin PhEur 150mg, Isoniazid PhEur 100mg

Rifinah 300: Rifampicin PhEur 300mg, Isoniazid PhEur 150mg

3. PHARMACEUTICAL FORM

Rifinah 150: Cyclamen, smooth, shiny, round, curved sugar coated tablet.

Rifinah 300: Orange, smooth, shiny capsule shaped sugar coated tablet.

4. CLINICAL PARTICULARS

4.1 Therapeutic indications

Rifinah is indicated in the treatment of all forms of tuberculosis, including fresh, advanced and chronic cases.

4.2 Posology and method of administration

For oral administration.

Another antituberculosis drug may be given concurrently with Rifinah until the susceptibility of the infecting organism to rifampicin and isoniazid has been confirmed.

Adults: Patients should be given the following single daily dose preferably on an empty stomach at least 30 minutes before a meal or 2 hours after a meal:

Rifinah 150: Patients weighing less than 50kg - 3 tablets.

Rifinah 300: Patients weighing 50kg or more - 2 tablets.

Use in the elderly: Caution should be exercised in such patients especially if there is evidence of liver impairment.

4.3 Contraindications

Rifinah is contraindicated in the presence of jaundice. Rifinah is contraindicated in patients who are hypersensitive to rifamycins or isoniazid or any of the excipients.

Rifinah use is contraindicated when given concurrently with the combination of saquinavirr/ritonavir (see section 4.5 Interactions).

4.4 Special warnings and precautions for use

Rifinah is a combination of 2 drugs, each of which has been associated with liver dysfunction.

All tuberculosis patients should have pre-treatment measurements of liver function.

Adults treated for tuberculosis with Rifinah should have baseline measurements of hepatic enzymes, bilirubin, serum creatinine, a complete blood count and a platelet count (or estimate).

Patients should be seen at least monthly during therapy and should be questioned specifically about symptoms associated with adverse reactions.

All patients with abnormalities should have follow-up, including laboratory testing, if necessary. However, because there is a higher frequency of isoniazid-associated hepatitis among persons older than 35 years of age, a transaminase measurement should be obtained at baseline and at least monthly during therapy in this age group. Other factors associated with an increased risk of hepatitis include daily use of alcohol, chronic liver disease, intravenous drug use and being a black or Hispanic woman.

If the patient has no evidence of pre-existing liver disease and normal pre-treatment liver function, liver function tests need only be repeated if fever, vomiting, jaundice or other deterioration in the patient's condition occurs.

Rifampicin

Rifampicin should be given under the supervision of a respiratory or other suitably qualified physician.

Patients with impaired liver function should only be given rifampicin in cases of necessity, and then with caution and under close medical supervision. In these patients, lower doses of rifampicin are recommended and careful monitoring of liver function, especially serum glutamic pyruvic transaminase (SGPT) and serum glutamic oxaloacetic transaminase (SGOT) should initially be carried out prior to therapy, weekly for two weeks, then every two weeks for the next six weeks. If signs of hepatocellular damage occur, rifampicin should be withdrawn.

Rifampicin should also be withdrawn if clinically significant changes in hepatic function occur. The need for other forms of antituberculosis therapy and a different regimen should be considered. Urgent advice should be obtained from a specialist in the management of tuberculosis. If rifampicin is re-introduced after liver function has returned to normal, liver function should be monitored daily.

In patients with impaired liver function, elderly patients, malnourished patients and possibly children under two years of age, caution is particularly recommended when instituting therapeutic regimens in which isoniazid is to be used concurrently with rifampicin.

In some patients, hyperbilirubinaemia can occur in the early days of treatment. This results from competition between rifampicin and bilirubin for hepatic excretion. An isolated report showing a moderate rise in bilirubin and/or transaminase level is not in itself an indication for interrupting treatment; rather the decision should be made after repeating the tests, noting trends in the levels and considering them in conjunction with the patient's clinical condition.

Because of the possibility of immunological reaction including anaphylaxis (see section 4.8 Undesirable effects) occurring with intermittent therapy (less than 2 to 3 times per week) patients should be closely monitored. Patients should be cautioned against interruption of dosage regimens since these reactions may occur.

Rifampicin has enzyme induction properties that can enhance the metabolism of endogenous substrates including adrenal hormones, thyroid hormones and vitamin D. Isolated reports have associated porphyria exacerbation with rifampicin administration.

Isoniazid

Use of isoniazid should be carefully monitored in patients with current chronic liver disease or severe renal dysfunction.

Severe and sometimes fatal hepatitis associated with isoniazid therapy may occur and may develop even after many months of treatment. The risk of developing hepatitis is age related. Therefore, patients should be monitored for the prodromal symptoms of hepatitis, such as fatigue, weakness, malaise, anorexia, nausea or vomiting. If these symptoms appear or if signs suggestive of hepatic damage are detected, isoniazid should be discontinued promptly, since continued use of the drug in these cases has been reported to cause a more severe form of liver damage.

Care should be exercised in the treatment of elderly or malnourished patients who may also require vitamin B6 supplementation with the isoniazid therapy.

Use of isoniazid should be carefully monitored in patients with slow acetylator status, epilepsy, history of psychosis, history of peripheral neuropathy, diabetes, alcohol dependence, HIV infection or porphyria.

4.5 Interaction with other medicinal products and other forms of interaction

Food Interaction

Because isoniazid has some monoamine oxidase inhibiting activity, an interaction with tyramine-containing foods (cheese, red wine) may occur. Diamine oxidase may also be inhibited, causing exaggerated response (e.g. headache, sweating, palpitations, flushing, hypotension) to foods containing histamine (e.g. skipjack, tuna, other tropical fish). Tyramine- and histamine-containing foods should be avoided by patients receiving Rifinah.

Interactions with Other Medicinal Products

Cytochrome P-450 enzyme interaction

Rifampicin is known to induce and isoniazid is known to inhibit certain cytochrome P-450 enzymes. In general, the impact of the competing effects of rifampicin and isoniazid on the metabolism of drugs that undergo biotransformation through the affected pathways is unknown. Therefore, caution should be used when prescribing Rifinah with drugs metabolised by cytochrome P-450. To maintain optimum therapeutic blood levels, dosages of drugs metabolised by these enzymes may require adjustment when starting or stopping Rifinah.

Rifampicin

Examples of drugs metabolised by cytochrome P-450 enzymes are:

- Antiarrhythmics (e.g. disopyramide, mexiletine, quinidine, propafenone, tocainide),
- Antiepileptics (e.g. phenytoin),
- Hormone antagonist (antiestrogens e.g. tamoxifen, toremifene, gestinone),
- Antipsychotics (e.g. haloperidol, aripiprazole),
- Anticoagulants (e.g. coumarins),
- Antifungals (e.g. fluconazole, itraconazole, ketoconazole, voriconazole),
- Antivirals (e.g. saquinavir, indinavir, efavirenz, amprenavir, nelfinavir, atazanavir, lopinavir, nevirapine),
- Barbiturates
- Beta-blockers (e.g. bisoprolol, propanolol),
- Anxiolytics and hypnotics (e.g. diazepam, benzodiazepines, zopiclone, zolpidem),
- Calcium channel blockers (e.g. diltiazem, nifedipine, verapamil, nimodipine, isradipine, nicardipine, nisoldipine),
- Antibacterials (e.g. chloramphenicol, clarithromycin, dapsone, doxycycline, fluoroquinolones, telithromycin),
- Corticosteroids
- Cardiac glycosides (digitoxin, digoxin),
- Clofibrate,
- Systemic hormonal contraceptives
- Oestrogen,
- Antidiabetic (e.g. chlorpropamide, tolbutamide, sulfonylureas, rosiglitazone),

- Immunosuppressive agents (e.g. ciclosporin, sirolimus, tacrolimus)
- Irinotecan,
- Thyroid hormone (e.g. levothyroxine),
- Losartan,
- Analgesics (e.g. methadone, narcotic analgesics),
- Praziquantel,
- Progestogens,
- Quinine,
- Riluzole,
- Selective 5-HT3 receptor antagonists (e.g. ondansetron)
- Statins metabolised by CYP 3A4 (e.g. simvastatin),
- Theophylline,
- Tricyclic antidepressants (e.g. amitriptyline, nortriptyline),
- Cytotoxics (e.g. imatinib),
- Diuretics (e.g. eplerenone)

Patients using oral contraceptives should be advised to change to non-hormonal methods of birth control during Rifinah therapy. Also, diabetes may become more difficult to control.

When rifampicin is given concomitantly with the combination saquinavir/ritonavir, the potential for hepatotoxicity is increased. Therefore, concomitant use of Rifinah with saquinavir/ritonavir is contraindicated (see section 4.3 Contraindications).

Other Interactions

When the two drugs were taken concomitantly, decreased concentrations of atovaquone and increased concentrations of rifampicin were observed.

Concurrent use of ketoconazole and rifampicin has resulted in decreased serum concentrations of both drugs.

Concurrent use of rifampicin and enalapril has resulted in decreased concentrations of enalaprilat, the active metabolite of enalapril. Dosage adjustments should be made if indicated by the patient's clinical condition.

Concomitant antacid administration may reduce the absorption of rifampicin.

Daily doses of rifampicin should be given at least 1 hour before the ingestion of antacids.

When rifampicin is given concomitantly with either halothane or isoniazid, the potential for hepatotoxicity is increased. The concomitant use of rifampicin and halothane should be avoided. Patients receiving both rifampicin and isoniazid should be monitored closely for hepatotoxicity.

When rifampicin is taken with para-aminosalicylic acid (PAS), rifampicin levels in the serum may decrease. Therefore, the drugs should be taken at least eight hours apart.

Interactions with Isoniazid

The following drugs may interact with isoniazid:

- Antiepileptics (e.g. carbamazepine and phenytoin

There may be an increased risk of distal sensory neuropathy when isoniazid is used in patients taking stavudine.

Concomitant use of zalcitabine with isoniazid has been shown to approximately double the renal clearance if isoniazid in HIV infected patients.

Administration of prednisolone 20mg to 13 slow acetylators and 13 fast acetylators for receiving isoniazid 10mg/kg reduced plasma concentrations of isoniazid by 25% and 40%, respectively. The clinical significance of this effect has not been established.

The effect of acute alcohol intake (serum levels 1g/L maintained for 12 hours) on the metabolism of isoniazid (300mg/d for 2 days) was studies in 10 healthy volunteers in a controlled cross over design. The metabolism of isoniazid and its metabolite, acetyl isoniazid, was not modified by this acute alcohol intake. The metabolism of isoniazid may be increased in chronic alcoholics; however this effect has not been quantified.

Appropriate adjustments of these drugs should be made.

Other Interactions

Para-aminosalicylic acid may increase the plasma concentration and elimination half-life of isoniazid by competing for acetylating enzymes.

General anaesthetics may increase the hepatotoxicity of isoniazid.

The absorption of isoniazid is reduced by antacids.

The risk of CNS toxicity is increased when isoniazid is given with cycloserine.

Isoniazid may reduce plasma concentration of ketoconazole and increase plasma concentration of theophylline.

Interference with laboratory and diagnostic tests

Therapeutic levels of rifampicin have been shown to inhibit standard microbiological assays for serum folate and Vitamin B12. Thus, alternative assay methods should be considered. Transient elevation of BSP and serum bilirubin has been reported. Rifampicin may impair biliary excretion of contrast media used for visualization of the gallbladder, due to competition for biliary excretion. Therefore, these tests should be performed before the morning dose of rifampicin.

4.6 Pregnancy and lactation

Pregnancy

Rifampicin

Rifampicin has been shown to be teratogenic in rodents when given in large doses. There are no well controlled studies with Rifinah in pregnant women. Although rifampicin has been reported to cross the placental barrier and appear in cord blood, the effect of rifampicin, alone or in combination with other antituberculosis drugs, on the human foetus is not known.

When administered during the last few weeks of pregnancy, rifampicin can cause post-natal haemorrhages in the mother and infant, for which treatment with Vitamin K1 may be indicated.

Isoniazid

It has been reported that in both rats and rabbits, isoniazid may exert an embryocardial effect when administered orally during pregnancy, although no isoniazid-related congenital anomalies have been found in reproduction studies in mammalian species (mice, rats, rabbits).

Therefore, Rifinah should be used in pregnant women or in women of child bearing potential only if the potential benefit justifies the potential risk to the foetus.

Lactation

Rifampicin and isoniazid are excreted in breast milk and infants should not be breast fed by a patient receiving Rifinah unless in the physician's judgement the potential benefit to the patient outweighs the potential risk to the infant.

In breast-fed infants whose mothers are taking isoniazid, there is a theoretical risk of convulsions and neuropathy (associated with vitamin B6 deficiency), therefore they should be monitored for early signs of these effects and consideration should be given to treating both mother and infant prophylactically with pyridoxine.

4.7 Effects on ability to drive and use machines

Isoniazid has been associated with vertigo, visual disorders and psychotic reactions (see section 4.8). Patients should be informed of these, and advised that if affected, they should not drive, operate machinery or take part in any activities where these symptoms may put either themselves or others at risk

4.8 Undesirable effects

Rifampicin

Reactions to rifampicin occurring with either daily or intermittent dosage regimens include:

Cutaneous reactions which are mild and self-limiting may occur and do not appear to be hypersensitivity reactions. Typically they consist of flushing and itching with or without a rash. Urticaria and more serious hypersensitivity reactions occur but are uncommon. Exfoliative dermatitis, pemphigoid reaction, erythema multiforme including Stevens-Johnson syndrome, Lyells syndrome and vasculitis have been reported rarely.

Gastrointestinal reactions consist of anorexia, nausea, vomiting, abdominal discomfort, and diarrhoea. Pseudomembranous colitis has been reported with rifampicin therapy.

Hepatitis can be caused by rifampicin and liver function tests should be monitored (see section 4.4. Special warnings and precautions for use).

Central Nervous System: Psychoses have been rarely reported.

Thrombocytopenia with or without purpura may occur, usually associated with intermittent therapy, but is reversible if drug is discontinued as soon as purpura occurs. Cerebral haemorrhage and fatalities have been reported when rifampicin administration has been continued or resumed after the appearance of purpura.

Disseminated intravascular coagulation has also been rarely reported.

Eosinophilia, leucopenia, oedema, muscle weakness and myopathy have been reported to occur in a small percentage of patients treated with rifampicin.

Agranulocytosis has been reported very rarely reported.

Rare reports of adrenal insufficiency in patients with compromised adrenal function have been observed.

Reactions usually occurring with intermittent dosage regimens and probably of immunological origin include:

- 'Flu Syndrome' consisting of episodes of fever, chills, headache, dizziness, and bone pain appearing most commonly during the 3rd to the 6th month of therapy. The frequency of the syndrome varies but may occur in up to 50 % of patients given once-weekly regimens with a dose of rifampicin of 25 mg/kg or more.
- Shortness of breath and wheezing.
- Decrease in blood pressure and shock.
- Anaphylaxis.
- Acute haemolytic anaemia.
- Acute renal failure usually due to acute tubular necrosis or acute interstitial nephritis.

If serious complications arise, e.g. renal failure, thrombocytopenia or haemolytic anaemia, rifampicin should be stopped and never restarted.

Occasional disturbances of the menstrual cycle have been reported in women receiving long-term antituberculosis therapy with regimens containing rifampicin.

Rifampicin may produce a reddish colouration of the urine, sweat, sputum and tears. The patient should be forewarned of this. Soft contact lenses may be permanently stained.

Isoniazid

Hypersensitivity reactions: Fever, anaphylactic reactions.

Nervous system: Vertigo; polyneuritis, presenting as paresthesia, muscle weakness, loss of tendon reflexes, etc, is unlikely to occur with the recommended daily dose of Rifinah. The incidence is higher in "slow acetylators". Other neurotoxic effects, which are uncommon with conventional doses, are convulsions, toxic encephalopathy, optic neuritis and atrophy, memory impairment and toxic psychosis. The possibility that the frequency of seizures may be increased in patients with epilepsy should be borne in mind.

Cutaneous: Rash, acne, Stevens-Johnson syndrome, exfoliative dermatitis and pemphigus.

Hematologic: Eosinophilia, agranulocytosis, thrombocytopenia, anemia, aplastic anaemia and haemolytic anaemia

Gastrointestinal: Pancreatitis, constipation, dry mouth, nausea, vomiting and epigastric distress.

Hepatic: Severe and sometimes fatal hepatitis may occur with isoniazid therapy.

Reproductive system and breast disorders: gynaecomastia

Investigations: anti-nuclear antibodies

Metabolism and Nutrition Disorders: hyperglycaemia

Miscellaneous: Pellagra, systemic lupus erythematosus-like syndrome.

4.9 Overdose

- Signs and Symptoms

Rifampicin

Nausea, vomiting, abdominal pain, pruritus, headache and increasing lethargy will probably occur within a short time after acute ingestion; unconsciousness may occur when there is severe hepatic disease. Transient increases in liver enzymes and/or bilirubin may occur. Brownish-red or orange colouration of the skin, urine, sweat, saliva, tears and faeces will occur, and its intensity is proportional to the amount ingested. Facial or periorbital oedema has also been reported in paediatric patients. Hypotension; sinus tachycardia, ventricular arrhythmias, seizures and cardiac arrest were reported in some fatal cases.

The minimum acute lethal or toxic dose is not well established. However, nonfatal acute overdoses in adults have been reported with doses ranging from 9 to 12 g rifampicin. Fatal acute overdoses in adults have been reported with doses ranging from 14 to 60 g. Alcohol or a history of alcohol abuse was involved in some of the fatal and nonfatal reports. Nonfatal overdoses in paediatric patients ages 1 to 4 years old of 100 mg/kg for one to two doses have been reported.

Isoniazid

Isoniazid overdosage produces signs and symptoms within 30 minutes to 3 hours after ingestion. Nausea, vomiting, dizziness, slurring of speech, blurring of vision, and visual hallucinations (including bright colours and strange designs) are among the early manifestations. With marked overdosage, respiratory distress and CNS depression, progressing rapidly from stupor to profound coma are to be expected, along with severe, intractable seizures. Severe metabolic acidosis, acetonuria and hyperglycaemia are typical laboratory findings.

- Management:

In cases of overdosage with Rifinah, gastric lavage should be performed as soon as possible. Following evacuation of the gastric contents, the instillation of activated charcoal slurry into the stomach may help absorb any remaining drug from the gastrointestinal tract. Antiemetic medication may be required to control severe nausea and vomiting.

Intensive supportive measures should be instituted, including airway patency, and individual symptoms treated as they arise.

If acute isoniazide overdose is suspected, even in asymptomatic patients, the administration of intravenous pyridoxine (vitamin B6) should be considered. In patients with seizures not controlled with pyridoxine, anticonvulsant therapy should be administered. Sodium bicarbonate should be given to control metabolic acidosis. Haemodialysis is advised for refractory cases; if this is not available, peritoneal dialysis can be used along with forced diuresis.

5. PHARMACOLOGICAL PROPERTIES

5.1 Pharmacodynamic properties

Rifampicin and isoniazid are active bactericidial antituberculosis drugs which are particularly active against the rapidly growing extracellular organisms and also have bactericidal activity intracellularly. Rifampicin has activity against slow- and intermittently-growing *M. Tuberculosis*.

Rifampicin inhibits DNA-dependent RNA polymerase activity in susceptible cells. Specifically, it interacts with bacterial RNA polymerase but does not inhibit the mammalian enzyme. Cross-resistance to rifampicin has only been shown with other rifamycins.

Isoniazid acts against actively growing tubercle bacilli.

5.2 Pharmacokinetic properties

Rifampicin

Rifampicin is readily absorbed from the stomach and the duodenum. Peak serum concentrations of the order of 10 μg/ml occur about 2-4 hours after a dose of 10mg/kg body weight on an empty stomach.

In normal subjects the biological half-life of rifampicin in serum averages about 3 hours after a 600mg dose and increases to 5.1 hours after a 900mg dose. With repeated administration, the half-life decreases and reaches average values of approximately 2-3 hours. At a dose of up to 600 mg/day, the half-life does not differ in patients with renal failure and consequently, no dosage adjustment is required.

After absorption, rifampicin is rapidly eliminated in the bile and an enterohepatic circulation ensues. During this process, rifampicin undergoes progressive deacetylation, so that nearly all the drug in the bile is in this form in about 6 hours. This metabolite retains essentially complete antibacterial activity. Intestinal reabsorption is reduced by deacetylation and elimination is facilitated. Up to 30 % of a dose is excreted in the urine, with about half of this being unchanged drug. Absorption of rifampicin is reduced when the drug is ingested with food.

Rifampicin is widely distributed throughout the body. It is present in effective concentrations in many organs and body fluids, including cerebrospinal fluid. Rifampicin is about 80 % protein bound. Most of the unbound fraction is not ionized and therefore is diffused freely in tissues.

Isoniazid

After oral administration isoniazid produces peak blood levels within 1 to 2 hours which decline to 50% or less within 6 hours. Ingestion of isoniazid with food may reduce its absorption. It diffuses readily into all body fluids (cerebrospinal, pleural and ascitic fluids), tissues, organs and excreta (saliva, sputum and faeces). From 50 to 70% of a dose of isoniazid is excreted in the urine in 24 hours.

Isoniazid is metabolised primarily by acetylation and dehydrazination. The rate of acetylation is genetically determined.

Pharmacokinetic studies in normal volunteers have been shown that the two ingredients in Rifinah have comparable bioavailability whether they are given together as individual dose forms or as Rifinah.

5.3 Preclinical safety data

None stated.

6. PHARMACEUTICAL PARTICULARS

6.1 List of excipients

Sodium lauryl sulphate, calcium stearate, sodium carboxymethylcellulose, magnesium stearate, microcrystalline cellulose, acacia, gelatin, kaolin, magnesium carbonate - light, talc, titanium dioxide (E171), colloidal silicon dioxide, polyvinylpyrollidone K30, sucrose, carnauba wax, colophony, white beeswax, hard paraffin and erythrosine (E127) (Rifinah 150) or sunset yellow (E110) (Rifinah 300).

6.2 Incompatibilities

None stated.

6.3 Shelf life

48 months.

6.4 Special precautions for storage

Store below 25°C. If it proves necessary to open a blister pack, Rifinah should be dispensed in amber glass or plastic containers. Protect from moisture.

6.5 Nature and contents of container

Rifinah 150: Original packs of 84 tablets (4 weeks calendar packs).

Rifinah 300: Original packs of 56 tablets (4 weeks calendar packs).

6.6 Special precautions for disposal and other handling

None stated.

7. MARKETING AUTHORISATION HOLDER

Sanofi-aventis

One Onslow Street

Guildford

Surrey

GU1 4YS

UK

8. MARKETING AUTHORISATION NUMBER(S)

Rifinah 150: PL 04425/0041

Rifinah 300: PL 04425/0042

9. DATE OF FIRST AUTHORISATION/RENEWAL OF THE AUTHORISATION

19 April 1999

10. DATE OF REVISION OF THE TEXT

13 March 2009

LEGAL CLASSIFICATION

POM

Rilutek 50 mg film-coated tablets

(sanofi-aventis)

1. NAME OF THE MEDICINAL PRODUCT

RILUTEK 50 mg film-coated tablets

2. QUALITATIVE AND QUANTITATIVE COMPOSITION

Each film-coated tablet contains 50 mg of riluzole

For a full list of excipients, see section 6.1.

3. PHARMACEUTICAL FORM

Film-coated tablet

The tablets are capsule-shaped, white and engraved with "RPR 202" on one side.

4. CLINICAL PARTICULARS

4.1 Therapeutic indications

RILUTEK is indicated to extend life or the time to mechanical ventilation for patients with amyotrophic lateral sclerosis (ALS).

Clinical trials have demonstrated that RILUTEK extends survival for patients with ALS (see section 5.1). Survival was defined as patients who were alive, not intubated for mechanical ventilation and tracheotomy-free.

There is no evidence that RILUTEK exerts a therapeutic effect on motor function, lung function, fasciculations, muscle strength and motor symptoms. RILUTEK has not been shown to be effective in the late stages of ALS.

Safety and efficacy of RILUTEK has only been studied in ALS. Therefore, RILUTEK should not be used in patients with any other form of motor neurone disease.

4.2 Posology and method of administration

Treatment with RILUTEK should only be initiated by specialist physicians with experience in the management of motor neurone diseases.

The recommended daily dose in adults or elderly is 100 mg (50 mg every 12 hours).

No significant increased benefit can be expected from higher daily doses.

Special populations

Children: RILUTEK is not recommended for use in children, due to a lack of data on the safety and efficacy of riluzole in any neurodegenerative diseases occurring in children or adolescents.

Patients with impaired renal function: RILUTEK is not recommended for use in patients with impaired renal function, as studies at repeated doses have not been conducted in this population (see section 4.4).

Elderly: based on pharmacokinetic data, there are no special instructions for the use of RILUTEK in this population.

Patients with impaired hepatic function: (see section 4.3, section 4.4, and section 5.2).

4.3 Contraindications

Hypersensitivity to the active substance or to any of the excipients.

Hepatic disease or baseline transaminases greater than 3 times the upper limit of normal.

Patients who are pregnant or breast-feeding.

4.4 Special warnings and precautions for use

Liver impairment:

Riluzole should be prescribed with care in patients with a history of abnormal liver function, or in patients with slightly elevated serum transaminases (ALT/SGPT; AST/SGOT up to 3 times the upper limit of the normal range (ULN)), bilirubin and/or gamma-glutamyl transferase (GGT) levels. Baseline elevations of several liver function tests (especially elevated bilirubin) should preclude the use of riluzole (see section 4.8).

Because of the risk of hepatitis, serum transaminases, including ALT, should be measured before and during therapy with riluzole. ALT should be measured every month during the first 3 months of treatment, every 3 months during the remainder of the first year, and periodically thereafter. ALT levels should be measured more frequently in patients who develop elevated ALT levels.

Riluzole should be discontinued if the ALT levels increase to 5 times the ULN. There is no experience with dose reduction or rechallenge in patients who have developed an increase of ALT to 5 times ULN. Readministration of riluzole to patients in this situation cannot be recommended.

Neutropenia:

Patients should be warned to report any febrile illness to their physicians. The report of a febrile illness should prompt physicians to check white blood cell counts and to discontinue riluzole in case of neutropenia (see section 4.8).

Interstitial lung disease

Cases of interstitial lung disease have been reported in patients treated with riluzole, some of them were severe (see section 4.8). If respiratory symptoms develop such as dry cough and/or dyspnea, chest radiography should be performed, and in case of findings suggestive of interstitial lung disease (e.g. bilateral diffuse lung opacities), riluzole should be discontinued immediately. In the majority of the reported cases, symptoms resolved after drug discontinuation and symptomatic treatment.

Renal impairment:

Studies at repeated doses have not been conducted in patients with impaired renal function (see section 4.2).

4.5 Interaction with other medicinal products and other forms of interaction

There have been no clinical studies to evaluate the interactions of riluzole with other medicinal products.

In vitro studies using human liver microsomal preparations suggest that CYP 1A2 is the principal isozyme involved in the initial oxidative metabolism of riluzole. Inhibitors of CYP 1A2 (e.g. caffeine, diclofenac, diazepam, nicergoline, clomipramine, imipramine, fluvoxamine, phenacetin, theophylline, amitriptyline and quinolones) could potentially decrease the rate of riluzole elimination, while inducers of CYP 1A2 (e.g. cigarette smoke, charcoal-broiled food, rifampicin and omeprazole) could increase the rate of riluzole elimination.

4.6 Pregnancy and lactation

RILUTEK is contraindicated (see section 4.3) in pregnancy (see section 5.3).

Clinical experience with riluzole in pregnant women is lacking.

RILUTEK is contraindicated (see section 4.3) in breast-feeding women (see section 5.3).

It is not known whether riluzole is excreted in human milk.

4.7 Effects on ability to drive and use machines

Patients should be warned about the potential for dizziness or vertigo, and advised not to drive or operate machinery if these symptoms occur.

No studies on the effects on the ability to drive and use machines have been performed.

4.8 Undesirable effects

In phase III clinical studies conducted in ALS patients treated with riluzole, the most commonly reported adverse reactions were asthenia, nausea and abnormal liver function tests.

Undesirable effects ranked under headings of frequency are listed below, using the following convention: very common (⩾1/10), common (⩾1/100 to <1/10), uncommon (⩾1/1,000 to <1/100), rare (⩾1/10,000 to <1/1,000), very rare (<1/10,000), not known (cannot be estimated from the available data).

Blood and the lymphatic system disorders

Uncommon: anaemia

Not known: severe neutropenia (see section 4.4)

Immune system disorders

Uncommon: anaphylactoid reaction, angioedema

Nervous system disorder

Common: headache, dizziness, oral paraesthesia and somnolence

Cardiac disorders

Common: tachycardia

Respiratory, thoracic and mediastinal disorders

Uncommon: interstitial lung disease (see section 4.4)

Gastrointestinal disorders

Very common: nausea

Common: diarrhoea, abdominal pain, vomiting

Uncommon: pancreatitis

Hepato-biliary disorders

Very common: abnormal liver function tests*. Increased alanine aminotransferase usually appeared within 3 months after the start of therapy with riluzole; they were usually transient and levels returned to below twice the ULN after 2 to 6 months while treatment was continued. These increases could be associated with jaundice. In patients (n=20) from clinical studies with increases in ALT to more than 5 times the ULN, treatment was discontinued and the levels returned to less than 2 times the ULN within 2 to 4 months in most cases (see section 4.4)

Not known: hepatitis

General disorders and administration site conditions

Very common: asthenia

Common: pain

* study data indicate that Asian patients may be more susceptible to liver function test abnormalities - 3.2% (194/5995) of Asian patients and 1.8% (100/5641) of Caucasian patients.

4.9 Overdose

Neurological and psychiatric symptoms, acute toxic encephalopathy with stupor, coma, and methemoglobinemia have been observed in isolated cases.

In case of overdose, treatment is symptomatic and supportive.

5. PHARMACOLOGICAL PROPERTIES

5.1 Pharmacodynamic properties

Pharmacotherapeutic group: other nervous system drugs, ATC code: N07XX02.

Although the pathogenesis of ALS is not completely elucidated, it is suggested that glutamate (the primary excitatory neurotransmitter in the central nervous system) plays a role for cell death in the disease.

Riluzole is proposed to act by inhibiting glutamate processes. The mode of action is unclear.

Clinical trials

In a trial, 155 patients were randomised to riluzole 100 mg/day (50 mg twice daily) or placebo and were followed-up for 12 to 21 months. Survival, as defined in the second paragraph of section 4.1, was significantly extended for patients who received riluzole as compared to patients who received placebo. The median survival time was 17.7 months versus 14.9 months for riluzole and placebo, respectively.

In a dose-ranging trial, 959 patients with ALS were randomised to one of four treatment groups: riluzole 50, 100, 200 mg/day, or placebo and were followed-up for 18 months. In patients treated with riluzole 100 mg/day, survival was significantly higher compared to patients who received placebo. The effect of riluzole 50 mg/day was not statistically significant compared to placebo and the effect of 200 mg/day was essentially comparable to that of 100 mg/day. The median survival time approached 16.5 months versus 13.5 months for riluzole 100 mg/day and placebo, respectively.

In a parallel group study designed to assess the efficacy and safety of riluzole in patients at a late stage of the disease, survival time and motor function under riluzole did not differ significantly from that of placebo. In this study the majority of patients had a vital capacity less than 60%.

In a double-blind placebo-controlled trial designed to assess the efficacy and safety of riluzole in Japanese patients, 204 patients were randomised to riluzole 100 mg/day (50 mg twice daily) or placebo and were followed-up for 18 months. In this study, the efficacy was assessed on inability to walk alone, loss of upper limb function, tracheostomy, need for artificial ventilation, gastric tube feeding or death. Tracheostomy-free survival in patients treated with riluzole did not differ significantly from placebo. However, the power of this study to detect differences between treatment groups was low. Meta-analysis including this study and those described above showed a less striking effect on survival for riluzole as compared to placebo although the differences remained statistically significant.

5.2 Pharmacokinetic properties

The pharmacokinetics of riluzole have been evaluated in healthy male volunteers after single oral administration of 25 to 300 mg and after multiple-dose oral administration of 25 to 100 mg bid. Plasma levels increase linearly with the dose and the pharmacokinetic profile is dose-independent.

With multiple dose administration (10 day-treatment at 50 mg riluzole bid), unchanged riluzole accumulates in plasma by about 2 fold and steady-state is reached in less than 5 days.

Absorption

Riluzole is rapidly absorbed after oral administration with maximal plasma concentrations occurring within 60 to 90 minutes (C_{max} = 173 ± 72 (sd) ng/ml). About 90% of the dose is absorbed and the absolute bioavailability is 60 ± 18%.

The rate and extent of absorption is reduced when riluzole is administered with high-fat meals (decrease in C_{max} of 44%, decrease in AUC of 17%).

Distribution

Riluzole is extensively distributed throughout the body and has been shown to cross the blood brain barrier. The volume of distribution of riluzole is about 245 ± 69 l (3.4 l/kg). Riluzole is about 97% protein bound and it binds mainly to serum albumin and to lipoproteins.

Metabolism

Unchanged riluzole is the main component in plasma and is extensively metabolised by cytochrome P450 and subsequent glucuronidation. In vitro studies using human liver preparations demonstrated that cytochrome P450 1A2 is the principal isoenzyme involved in the metabolism of riluzole. The metabolites identified in urine are three phenolic derivatives, one ureido-derivative and unchanged riluzole.

The primary metabolic pathway for riluzole is initial oxidation by cytochrome P450 1A2 producing N-hydroxy-riluzole (RPR112512), the major active metabolite of riluzole. This metabolite is rapidly glucuronoconjugated to O- and N-glucuronides.

Elimination

The elimination half-life ranges from 9 to 15 hours. Riluzole is eliminated mainly in the urine.

The overall urinary excretion accounts for about 90% of the dose. Glucuronides accounted for more than 85% of the metabolites in the urine. Only 2% of a riluzole dose was recovered unchanged in the urine.

Special populations

Patients with impaired renal function: there is no significant difference in pharmacokinetic parameters between patients with moderate or severe chronic renal insufficiency (creatinine clearance between 10 and 50 ml.min^{-1}) and healthy volunteers after a single oral dose of 50 mg riluzole.

Elderly: the pharmacokinetic parameters of riluzole after multiple dose administration (4.5 days of treatment at 50 mg riluzole bid) are not affected in the elderly (> 70 years).

Patients with impaired hepatic function: the AUC of riluzole after a single oral dose of 50 mg increases by about 1.7 fold in patients with mild chronic liver insufficiency and by about 3 fold in patients with moderate chronic liver insufficiency.

Race: a clinical study conducted to evaluate the pharmacokinetics of riluzole and its metabolite N-hydroxyriluzole following repeated oral administration twice daily for 8 days in 16 healthy Japanese and 16 Caucasian adult males showed in the Japanese group a lower exposure of riluzole (Cmax 0.85 [90% CI 0.68-1.08] and AUC inf. 0.88 [90% CI 0.69-1.13]) and similar exposure to the metabolite. The clinical significance of these results is not known.

5.3 Preclinical safety data

Riluzole did not show any carcinogenicity potential in either rats or mice.

Standard tests for genotoxicity performed with riluzole were negative. Tests on the major active metabolite of riluzole gave positive results in two in vitro tests. Intensive testing in seven other standard *in vitro* or *in vivo* assays did not show any genotoxic potential of the metabolite. On the basis of these data, and taking into consideration the negative studies on the carcinogenesis of riluzole in the mouse and rat, the genotoxic effect of this metabolite is not considered to be of relevance in humans.

Reductions in red blood cell parameters and/or alterations in liver parameters were noted inconsistently in subacute and chronic toxicity studies in rats and monkeys. In dogs, haemolytic anaemia was observed.

In a single toxicity study, the absence of corpora lutea was noted at a higher incidence in the ovary of treated compared to control female rats. This isolated finding was not noted in any other study or species.

All these findings were noted at doses which were 2-10 times higher than the human dose of 100 mg/day.

Fertility studies in rats revealed slight impairment of reproductive performance and fertility at doses of 15 mg/kg/day (which is higher than the therapeutic dose), probably due to sedation and lethargy.

In the pregnant rat, the transfer of ^{14}C- riluzole across the placenta to the foetus has been detected. In rats, riluzole decreased the pregnancy rate and the number of implantations at exposure levels at least twice the systemic exposure of humans given clinical therapy. No malformations were seen in animal reproductive studies.

In lactating rats, ^{14}C-riluzole was detected in milk.

6. PHARMACEUTICAL PARTICULARS

6.1 List of excipients

Core:

Dibasic calcium phosphate, anhydrous

Micro crystalline cellulose

Colloidal silica, anhydrous

Magnesium stearate

Croscarmellose sodium

Coating:

Hypromellose

Macrogol 6000

Titanium dioxide (E171)

6.2 Incompatibilities

Not applicable.

6.3 Shelf life

3 years

6.4 Special precautions for storage

This medicinal product does not require any special storage conditions.

6.5 Nature and contents of container

Tablets are packaged in opaque pvc/aluminium blister cards.

Each package contains 56 tablets (4 blister cards of 14 tablets each).

6.6 Special precautions for disposal and other handling

No special requirements.

7. MARKETING AUTHORISATION HOLDER

Aventis Pharma S.A.

20 avenue Raymond Aron

F-92165 Antony Cedex

France

8. MARKETING AUTHORISATION NUMBER(S)

EU/1/96/010/001

9. DATE OF FIRST AUTHORISATION/RENEWAL OF THE AUTHORISATION

Date of first authorisation: 10 June 1996

Date of last renewal: 10 June 2006

10. DATE OF REVISION OF THE TEXT

May 2009

Legal category: POM

Risperdal Consta 25 mg, 37.5 mg, 50 mg.

(Janssen-Cilag Ltd)

1. NAME OF THE MEDICINAL PRODUCT

RISPERDAL CONSTA ▼ 25 mg powder and solvent for prolonged-release suspension for intramuscular injection

RISPERDAL CONSTA ▼ 37.5 mg powder and solvent for prolonged-release suspension for intramuscular injection

RISPERDAL CONSTA ▼ 50 mg powder and solvent for prolonged-release suspension for intramuscular injection

2. QUALITATIVE AND QUANTITATIVE COMPOSITION

1 vial contains 25 mg, 37.5 mg or 50 mg risperidone.

1 ml reconstituted suspension contains 12.5 mg, 18.75 mg or 25 mg of risperidone.

For a full list of excipients, see section 6.1.

3. PHARMACEUTICAL FORM

Powder and solvent for prolonged-release suspension for injection.

Vial with powder.

White to off-white free flowing powder.

Pre-filled syringe of solvent for reconstitution.

Clear, colourless aqueous solution.

4. CLINICAL PARTICULARS

4.1 Therapeutic indications

RISPERDAL CONSTA is indicated for the maintenance treatment of schizophrenia in patients currently stabilised with oral antipsychotics.

4.2 Posology and method of administration

Adults

Starting dose:

For most patients the recommended dose is 25 mg intramuscular every two weeks. For those patients on a fixed dose of oral risperidone for two weeks or more, the following conversion scheme should be considered. Patients treated with a dosage of 4 mg or less oral risperidone should receive 25 mg RISPERDAL CONSTA, while patients treated with higher oral doses should be considered for the higher RISPERDAL CONSTA dose of 37.5 mg.

Where patients are not currently taking oral risperidone, the oral pre-treatment dosage should be considered when choosing the i.m. starting dose. The recommended starting dose is 25 mg RISPERDAL CONSTA every two weeks. Patients on higher dosages of the used oral antipsychotic should be considered for the higher RISPERDAL CONSTA dose of 37.5 mg.

Sufficient antipsychotic coverage with oral risperidone or the previous antipsychotic should be ensured during the three-week lag period following the first RISPERDAL CONSTA injection (see section 5.2).

RISPERDAL CONSTA should not be used in acute exacerbations of schizophrenia without ensuring sufficient antipsychotic coverage with oral risperidone or the previous antipsychotic during the three-week lag period following the first RISPERDAL CONSTA injection.

Maintenance dose:

For most patients the recommended dose is 25 mg intramuscular every two weeks. Some patients may benefit from the higher doses of 37.5 mg or 50 mg. Upward dosage adjustment should not be made more frequently than every 4 weeks. The effect of this dose adjustment should not be anticipated earlier than 3 weeks after the first injection with the higher dose. No additional benefit was observed with 75 mg in clinical trials. Doses higher than 50 mg every 2 weeks are not recommended.

Elderly

No dose adjustment is required. The recommended dose is 25 mg intramuscularly every two weeks. Where patients are not currently taking oral risperidone, the recommended dose is 25 mg RISPERDAL CONSTA every two weeks. For those patients on a fixed dose of oral risperidone for two weeks or more, the following conversion scheme should be considered. Patients treated with a dosage of 4 mg or less oral risperidone should receive 25 mg RISPERDAL CONSTA, while patients treated with higher oral doses should be considered for the higher RISPERDAL CONSTA dose of 37.5 mg.

Sufficient antipsychotic coverage should be ensured during the three-week lag period following the first RISPERDAL CONSTA injection (see section 5.2). RISPERDAL CONSTA clinical data in elderly are limited. RISPERDAL CONSTA should be used with caution in elderly.

Hepatic and renal impairment

RISPERDAL CONSTA has not been studied in hepatically and renally impaired patients. If hepatically or renally impaired patients require treatment with RISPERDAL CONSTA, a starting dose of 0.5 mg twice daily oral risperidone is recommended during the first week. The second week 1 mg twice daily or 2 mg once daily can be given. If an oral total daily dose of at least 2 mg is well tolerated, an injection of 25 mg RISPERDAL CONSTA can be administered every 2 weeks.

Sufficient antipsychotic coverage should be ensured during the three-week lag period following the first RISPERDAL CONSTA injection (see section 5.2).

Paediatric population

RISPERDAL CONSTA is not recommended for use in children below 18 years of age due to a lack of data on safety and efficacy.

Method of administration

RISPERDAL CONSTA should be administered every two weeks by deep intramuscular gluteal injection using the enclosed safety needle. Injections should alternate between the buttocks. Do not administer intravenously (see section 4.4 and section 6.6).

For instructions on preparation and handling RISPERDAL CONSTA, see section 6.6.

4.3 Contraindications

Hypersensitivity to the active substance or to any of the excipients.

4.4 Special warnings and precautions for use

For risperidone-naive patients, it is recommended to establish tolerability with oral risperidone prior to initiating treatment with RISPERDAL CONSTA (see section 4.2).

Elderly patients with dementia

RISPERDAL CONSTA has not been studied in elderly patients with dementia, hence it is not indicated for use in this group of patients.

Overall mortality

Elderly patients with dementia treated with atypical antipsychotics have an increased mortality compared to placebo in a meta-analysis of 17 controlled trials of atypical antipsychotics, including oral RISPERDAL. In placebo-controlled trials with oral RISPERDAL in this population, the incidence of mortality was 4.0% for RISPERDAL-treated patients compared to 3.1% for placebo-treated patients. The odds ratio (95% exact confidence interval) was 1.21 (0.7, 2.1). The mean age (range) of patients who died was 86 years (range 67-100).

Concomitant use with furosemide

In the oral RISPERDAL placebo-controlled trials in elderly patients with dementia, a higher incidence of mortality was observed in patients treated with furosemide plus risperidone (7.3%; mean age 89 years, range 75-97) when compared to patients treated with risperidone alone (3.1%; mean age 84 years, range 70-96) or furosemide alone (4.1%; mean age 80 years, range 67-90). The increase in mortality in patients treated with furosemide plus risperidone was observed in two of the four clinical trials. Concomitant use of risperidone with other diuretics (mainly thiazide diuretics used in low dose) was not associated with similar findings.

No pathophysiological mechanism has been identified to explain this finding, and no consistent pattern for cause of death observed. Nevertheless, caution should be exercised and the risks and benefits of this combination or co-treatment with other potent diuretics should be considered prior to the decision to use. There was no increased incidence of mortality among patients taking other diuretics as concomitant treatment with risperidone. Irrespective of treatment, dehydration was an overall risk factor for mortality and should therefore be carefully avoided in elderly patients with dementia.

Cerebrovascular adverse events (CVAE)

In placebo-controlled trials in elderly patients with dementia there was a significantly higher incidence (approximately 3-fold increased) of CVAEs, such as stroke (including fatalities) and transient ischaemic attack in patients treated with RISPERDAL compared with patients treated with placebo (mean age 85 years; range 73 to 97). The pooled data from six placebo-controlled studies in mainly elderly patients (>65 years of age) with dementia showed that CVAEs (serious and non-serious, combined) occurred in 3.3% (33/1009) of patients treated with risperidone and 1.2% (8/712) of patients treated with placebo. The odds ratio (95% exact confidence interval) was 2.96 (1.34, 7.50). The mechanism for this increased risk is not known. An increased risk cannot be excluded for other antipsychotics or other patient populations. RISPERDAL CONSTA should be used with caution in patients with risk factors for stroke.

Orthostatic hypotension

Due to the alpha-blocking activity of risperidone, (orthostatic) hypotension can occur, especially during initiation of treatment. Clinically significant hypotension has been observed postmarketing with concomitant use of risperidone and antihypertensive treatment. Risperidone should be used with caution in patients with known cardiovascular disease (e.g. heart failure, myocardial infarction, conduction abnormalities, dehydration, hypovolemia, or cerebrovascular disease). The risk/benefit of further treatment with RISPERDAL CONSTA should be assessed if clinically relevant orthostatic hypotension persists.

Tardive dyskinesia/extrapyramidal symptoms (TD/EPS)

Medicines with dopamine receptor antagonistic properties have been associated with the induction of tardive dyskinesia characterised by rhythmical involuntary movements, predominantly of the tongue and/or face. The onset of extrapyramidal symptoms is a risk factor for tardive dyskinesia. If signs and symptoms of tardive dyskinesia appear, the discontinuation of all antipsychotics should be considered.

Neuroleptic malignant syndrome (NMS)

Neuroleptic Malignant Syndrome, characterised by hyperthermia, muscle rigidity, autonomic instability, altered consciousness and elevated serum creatine phosphokinase levels has been reported to occur with antipsychotics. Additional signs may include myoglobinuria (rhabdomyolysis) and acute renal failure. In this event, all antipsychotics, including RISPERDAL CONSTA, should be discontinued.

Parkinson's disease and dementia with Lewy bodies

Physicians should weigh the risks versus the benefits when prescribing antipsychotics, including RISPERDAL CONSTA, to patients with Parkinson's Disease or Dementia with Lewy Bodies (DLB). Parkinson's Disease may worsen with risperidone. Both groups may be at increased risk of Neuroleptic Malignant Syndrome as well as having an increased sensitivity to antipsychotic medicinal products; these patients were excluded from clinical trials. Manifestation of this increased sensitivity can include confusion, obtundation, postural instability with frequent falls, in addition to extrapyramidal symptoms.

Hyperglycemia

Hyperglycemia or exacerbation of pre-existing diabetes has been reported in very rare cases during treatment with RISPERDAL CONSTA. Appropriate clinical monitoring is advisable in diabetic patients and in patients with risk factors for the development of diabetes mellitus.

Hyperprolactinaemia

Tissue culture studies suggest that cell growth in human breast tumours may be stimulated by prolactin. Although no clear association with the administration of antipsychotics has so far been demonstrated in clinical and epidemiological studies, caution is recommended in patients with relevant medical history. RISPERDAL CONSTA should be used with caution in patients with pre-existing hyperprolactinaemia and in patients with possible prolactin-dependent tumours.

QT prolongation

QT prolongation has very rarely been reported postmarketing. As with other antipsychotics, caution should be exercised when risperidone is prescribed in patients with known cardiovascular disease, family history of QT prolongation, bradycardia, or electrolyte disturbances (hypokalaemia, hypomagnesaemia), as it may increase the risk of arrhythmogenic effects, and in concomitant use with medicines known to prolong the QT interval.

Seizures

RISPERDAL CONSTA should be used cautiously in patients with a history of seizures or other conditions that potentially lower the seizure threshold.

Priapism

Priapism may occur with RISPERDAL CONSTA treatment due to its alpha-adrenergic blocking effects.

Body temperature regulation

Disruption of the body's ability to reduce core body temperature has been attributed to antipsychotic medicines. Appropriate care is advised when prescribing RISPERDAL CONSTA to patients who will be experiencing conditions which may contribute to an elevation in core body temperature, e.g., exercising strenuously, exposure to extreme heat, receiving concomitant treatment with anticholinergic activity, or being subject to dehydration.

Weight gain

As with other antipsychotics, patients should be advised of the potential for weight gain. Weight should be measured regularly.

Renal or hepatic impairment

Although oral risperidone has been studied, RISPERDAL CONSTA has not been studied in patients with renal or liver insufficiency. RISPERDAL CONSTA should be administered with caution in this group of patients (see section 4.2).

Administration

Care must be taken to avoid inadvertent injection of RISPERDAL CONSTA into a blood vessel.

Excipients

This medicinal product contains less than 1 mmol sodium (23 mg) per dose, i.e., essentially 'sodium-free'.

4.5 Interaction with other medicinal products and other forms of interaction

Interaction studies were performed with oral RISPERDAL.

As with other antipsychotics, caution is advised when prescribing risperidone with medicinal products known to prolong the QT interval, e.g., class Ia antiarrhythmics (e.g., quinidine, dysopiramide, procainamide), class III antiarrhythmics (e.g., amiodarone, sotalol), tricyclic antidepressants (i.e., amitriptyline), tetracyclic antidepressant (i.e., maprotiline), some antihistaminics, other antipsychotics, some antimalarials (i.e., chinice and mefloquine), and with medicines causing electrolyte imbalance (hypokalaemia, hypomagnesiaemia), bradycardia, or those which inhibit the hepatic metabolism of risperidone. This list is indicative and not exhaustive.

Potential for RISPERDAL CONSTA to affect other medicinal products

Risperidone should be used with caution in combination with other centrally-acting substances notably including alcohol, opiates, antihistamines and benzodiazepines due to the increased risk of sedation.

RISPERDAL CONSTA may antagonise the effect of levodopa and other dopamine agonists. If this combination is deemed necessary, particularly in end-stage Parkinson's disease, the lowest effective dose of each treatment should be prescribed.

Clinically significant hypotension has been observed postmarketing with concomitant use of risperidone and antihypertensive treatment.

RISPERDAL does not show a clinically relevant effect on the pharmacokinetics of lithium, valproate, digoxin or topiramate.

Potential for other medicinal products to affect RISPERDAL CONSTA

Carbamazepine has been shown to decrease the plasma concentrations of the active antipsychotic fraction of risperidone. Similar effects may be observed with e.g. rifampicin, phenytoin and phenobarbital which also induce CYP 3A4 hepatic enzyme as well as P-glycoprotein. When carbamazepine or other CYP 3A4 hepatic enzyme/P-glycoprotein (P-gp) inducers are initiated or discontinued, the physician should re-evaluate the dosing of RISPERDAL CONSTA.

Fluoxetine and paroxetine, CYP 2D6 inhibitors, increase the plasma concentration of risperidone, but less so of the active antipsychotic fraction. It is expected that other CYP 2D6 inhibitors, such as quinidine, may affect the plasma concentrations of risperidone in a similar way. When concomitant fluoxetine or paroxetine is initiated or discontinued, the physician should re-evaluate the dosing of RISPERDAL CONSTA.

Verapamil, an inhibitor of CYP 3A4 and P-gp, increases the plasma concentration of risperidone.

Galantamine and donepezil do not show a clinically relevant effect on the pharmacokinetics of risperidone and on the active antipsychotic fraction.

Phenothiazines, tricyclic antidepressants, and some beta-blockers may increase the plasma concentrations of risperidone but not those of the active antipsychotic fraction. Amitriptyline does not affect the pharmacokinetics of risperidone or the active antipsychotic fraction. Cimetidine and ranitidine increase the bioavailability of risperidone, but only marginally that of the active antipsychotic fraction. Erythromycin, a CYP 3A4 inhibitor, does not change the pharmacokinetics of risperidone and the active antipsychotic fraction.

See section 4.4 regarding increased mortality in elderly patients with dementia concomitantly receiving furosemide.

4.6 Pregnancy and lactation

Pregnancy

There are no adequate data from the use of risperidone in pregnant women. According to postmarketing data reversible extrapyramidal symptoms in the neonate were observed following the use of risperidone during the last trimester of pregnancy. Consequently, newborns should be monitored carefully. Risperidone was not teratogenic in animal studies but other types of reproductive toxicity were seen (see section 5.3). The potential risk for humans is unknown. Therefore, RISPERDAL CONSTA should not be used during pregnancy unless clearly necessary.

Lactation

In animal studies, risperidone and 9-hydroxy-risperidone are excreted in the milk. It has been demonstrated that risperidone and 9-hydroxy-risperidone are also excreted in human breast milk in small quantities. There are no data available on adverse effects in breast-feeding infants. Therefore, the advantage of breast-feeding should be weighed against the potential risks for the child.

4.7 Effects on ability to drive and use machines

RISPERDAL CONSTA has minor or moderate influence on the ability to drive and use machines due to potential nervous system and visual effects (see section 4.8). Therefore, patients should be advised not to drive or operate machinery until their individual susceptibility is known.

4.8 Undesirable effects

The most frequently reported adverse drug reactions (ADRs) (incidence $\geqslant$ 1/10) are: Insomnia, anxiety, headache, upper respiratory tract infection, parkinsonism, depression, and akathisia.

Serious injections site reactions including injection site necrosis, abscess, cellulitis, ulcer, haematoma, cyst, and nodule were reported postmarketing. The frequency is considered not known (cannot be estimated from the available data). Isolated cases required surgical intervention.

The following are all the ADRs that were reported in clinical trials and postmarketing. The following terms and frequencies are applied: very common ($\geqslant$1/10), common ($\geqslant$1/100 to <1/10), uncommon ($\geqslant$1/1000 to <1/100), rare ($\geqslant$1/10,000 to <1/1,000), very rare (<1/10,000), and not known (cannot be estimated from the available clinical trial data).

Within each frequency grouping, undesirable effects are presented in order of decreasing seriousness.

Adverse Drug Reactions by System Organ Class and Frequency Category	
Investigations	
Common	Electrocardiogram abnormal, Blood prolactin increased[a], Blood glucose increased, Hepatic enzyme increased, Transaminases increased, Gamma-glutamyltransferase increased, Weight increased, Weight decreased
Uncommon	Electrocardiogram QT prolonged
Cardiac disorders	
Common	Atrioventricular block, Tachycardia
Uncommon	Bundle branch block, Atrial fibrillation, Bradycardia, Sinus bradycardia, Palpitations
Blood and lymphatic system disorders	
Common	Anaemia
Uncommon	Thrombocytopenia, Neutropenia
Not known	Agranulocytosis
Nervous system disorders	
Very common	Parkinsonism[b], Akathisia[b], Headache
Common	Tardive dyskinesia, Dystonia[b], Dyskinesia[b], Tremor, Somnolence, Sedation, Dizziness
Uncommon	Convulsion, Syncope, Dizziness postural, Hypoaesthesia, Paraesthesia, Lethargy, Hypersomnia
Eye disorders	
Common	Vision blurred, Conjunctivitis
Not known	Retinal artery occlusion
Ear and labyrinth disorders	
Common	Vertigo
Uncommon	Ear pain
Respiratory, thoracic and mediastinal disorders	
Common	Dyspnoea, Cough, Nasal congestion, Pharyngolaryngeal pain
Rare	Sleep apnea syndrome
Gastrointestinal disorders	
Common	Vomiting, Diarrhoea, Constipation, Nausea, Abdominal pain, Dyspepsia, Toothache, Dry mouth, Stomach discomfort, Gastritis
Rare	Intestinal obstruction, Pancreatitis
Renal and urinary disorders	
Common	Urinary incontinence
Skin and subcutaneous tissue disorders	
Common	Rash, Eczema
Uncommon	Angioedema, Pruritus, Acne, Alopecia, Dry skin
Musculoskeletal and connective tissue disorders	
Common	Arthralgia, Back pain, Pain in extremity, Myalgia
Uncommon	Muscular weakness, Neck pain, Buttock pain, Musculoskeletal chest pain
Endocrine disorders	
Rare	Inappropriate antidiuretic hormone secretion
Metabolism and nutrition disorders	
Uncommon	Increased appetite, Decreased appetite
Very rare	Diabetic ketoacidosis
Not known	Water intoxication
Infections and infestations	
Very common	Upper respiratory tract infection
Common	Pneumonia, Influenza, Lower respiratory tract infection, Bronchitis, Urinary tract infection, Ear infection, Sinusitis, Viral infection
Uncommon	Cystitis, Gastroenteritis, Infection, Localised infection, Subcutaneous abscess
Injury, poisoning and procedural complications	
Common	Fall
Uncommon	Procedural pain
Vascular disorders	
Common	Hypertension, Hypotension
Uncommon	Orthostatic hypotension
General disorders and administration site conditions	
Common	Pyrexia, Peripheral oedema, Chest pain, Fatigue, Pain, Injection site pain, Asthenia, Influenza like illness
Uncommon	Injection site induration, induration, injection site reaction, chest discomfort, sluggishness, feeling abnormal
Rare	Hypothermia
Immune system disorders	
Uncommon	Hypersensitivity
Not known	Anaphylactic reaction
Hepatobiliary disorders	
Rare	Jaundice
Reproductive system and breast disorders	
Common	Amenorrhoea, Erectile dysfunction, Galactorrhoea
Uncommon	Sexual dysfunction, Gynaecomastia
Not known	Priapism
Psychiatric disorders	
Very common	Depression, Insomnia, Anxiety
Common	Agitation, Sleep disorder
Uncommon	Mania, Libido decreased, Nervousness

[a] Hyperprolactinemia can in some cases lead to gynaecomastia, menstrual disturbances, amenorrhoea, galactorrhea.

[b] Extrapyramidal disorder may occur: Parkinsonism (salivary hypersecretion, musculoskeletal stiffness, parkinsonism, drooling, cogwheel rigidity, bradykinesia, hypokinesia, masked facies, muscle tightness, akinesia, nuchal rigidity, muscle rigidity, parkinsonian gait, and glabellar reflex abnormal), akathisia (akathisia, restlessness, hyperkinesia, and restless leg syndrome), tremor, dyskinesia (dyskinesia, muscle twitching, choreoathetosis, athetosis, and myoclonus), dystonia.

Dystonia includes dystonia, muscle spasms, hypertonia, torticollis, muscle contractions involuntary, muscle contracture, blepharospasm, oculogyration, tongue paralysis, facial spasm, laryngospasm, myotonia, opisthotonus, oropharyngeal spasm, pleurothotonus, tongue spasm, and trismus. Tremor includes tremor and parkinsonian rest tremor. It should be noted that a broader spectrum of symptoms are included, that do not necessarily have an extrapyramidal origin.

The following is a list of additional ADRs associated with risperidone that have been identified as ADRs during clinical trials investigating the oral risperidone formulation (RISPERDAL) but were not determined to be ADRs in the clinical trials investigating RISPERDAL CONSTA.

Additional Adverse Drug Reactions Reported With Oral RISPERDAL but not With RISPERDAL CONSTA by System Organ Class
Investigations
Body temperature increased, Eosinophil count increased, White blood cell count decreased, Haemoglobin decreased, Blood creatine phosphokinase increased, Body temperature decreased
Infections and Infestations
Tonsillitis, Cellulitis, Otitis media, Eye infection, Acarodermatitis, Respiratory tract infection, Onychomycosis, Otitis media chronic
Blood and Lymphatic Disorders
Granulocytopenia
Immune System Disorders
Drug hypersensitivity
Metabolism and Nutrition Disorders
Anorexia, Polydipsia
Psychiatric Disorders
Confusional state, Listless, Anorgasmia, Blunted affect
Nervous System Disorders
Unresponsive to stimuli, Loss of consciousness, Neuroleptic malignant syndrome, Diabetic coma, Cerebrovascular accident, Depressed level of consciousness, Cerebral ischemia, Cerebrovascular disorder, Transient ischemic attack, Dysarthria, Disturbance in attention, Balance disorder, Speech disorder, Coordination abnormal, Movement disorder
Eye Disorders
Ocular hyperemia, Eye discharge, Eye swelling, Dry eye, Lacrimation increased, Photophobia, Visual acuity reduced, Eye rolling, Glaucoma
Ear and Labyrinth Disorders
Tinnitus
Vascular Disorders
Flushing
Respiratory, Thoracic, and Mediastinal Disorders
Wheezing, Pneumonia aspiration, Pulmonary congestion, Respiratory disorder, Rales, Epistaxis, Respiratory tract congestion, Hyperventilation, Dysphonia
Gastrointestinal Disorders
Dysphagia, Faecal incontinence, Faecaloma, Lip swelling, Cheilitis
Skin and Subcutaneous Tissue Disorders
Skin lesion, Skin disorder, Skin discoloration, Seborrheic dermatitis, Hyperkeratosis, Dandruff, Erythema
Musculoskeletal, Connective Tissue, and Bone Disorders
Rhabdomyolysis, Joint swelling, Posture abnormal, Joint stiffness
Renal and Urinary Disorders
Enuresis, Dysuria, Pollakiuria
Reproductive System and Breast Disorders
Ejaculation disorder, Vaginal discharge, Menstrual disorder
General Disorders and Administration Site Conditions
Generalised oedema, Face oedema, Gait disturbance, Thirst, Chills, Peripheral coldness, Drug withdrawal syndrome

Class effects

As with other antipsychotics, very rare cases of QT prolongation have been reported postmarketing with risperidone. Other class-related cardiac effects reported with antipsychotics which prolong QT interval include ventricular arrhythmia, ventricular fibrillation, ventricular tachycardia, sudden death, cardiac arrest and Torsades de Pointes.

Weight gain

In the 12-week double-blind, placebo-controlled trial, 9% of patients treated with RISPERDAL CONSTA, compared with 6% of patients treated with placebo, experienced a weight gain of ⩾ 7% of body weight at endpoint. In the 1-year, open-label study of RISPERDAL CONSTA, changes in body weight in individual patients were generally within ±7% from baseline; 25% of patients had an increase in body weight of ⩾ 7%.

4.9 Overdose

While overdose is less likely to occur with parenteral than with oral medicinal products, information pertaining to oral is presented.

Symptoms

In general, reported signs and symptoms have been those resulting from an exaggeration of the known pharmacological effects of risperidone. These include drowsiness and sedation, tachycardia and hypotension, and extrapyramidal symptoms. In overdose, QT-prolongation and convulsions have been reported. Torsade de Pointes has been reported in association with combined overdose of oral RISPERDAL and paroxetine.

In case of acute overdose, the possibility of multiple drug involvement should be considered.

Treatment

Establish and maintain a clear airway and ensure adequate oxygenation and ventilation. Cardiovascular monitoring should commence immediately and should include continuous electrocardiographic monitoring to detect possible arrhythmias.

There is no specific antidote to RISPERDAL. Therefore appropriate supportive measures should be instituted. Hypotension and circulatory collapse should be treated with appropriate measures such as intravenous fluids and/or sympathomimetic agents. In case of severe extrapyramidal symptoms, anticholinergic medicinal product should be administered. Close medical supervision and monitoring should continue until the patient recovers.

5. PHARMACOLOGICAL PROPERTIES

5.1 Pharmacodynamic properties

Pharmacotherapeutic group: Other antipsychotics, ATC code: N05AX08

Figure 1 Mean in total PANSS score over time (LOCF) in patients with schizophrenia

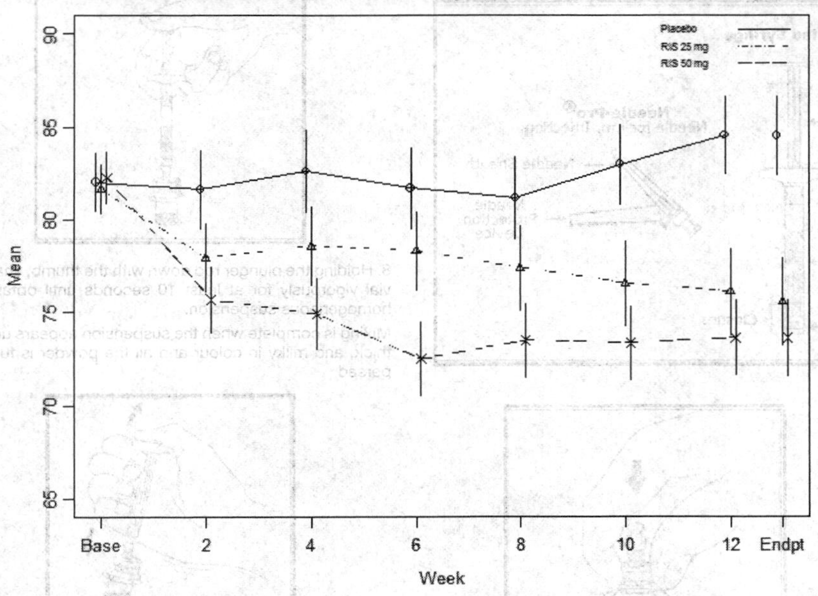

Mechanism of action

Risperidone is a selective monoaminergic antagonist with unique properties. It has a high affinity for serotoninergic 5-HT2 and dopaminergic D2 receptors. Risperidone binds also to alpha1-adrenergic receptors, and, with lower affinity, to H1-histaminergic and alpha2-adrenergic receptors. Risperidone has no affinity for cholinergic receptors. Although risperidone is a potent D2 antagonist, that is considered to improve the positive symptoms of schizophrenia, it causes less depression of motor activity and induction of catalepsy than classical antipsychotics. Balanced central serotonin and dopamine antagonism may reduce extrapyramidal side effect liability and extend the therapeutic activity to the negative and affective symptoms of schizophrenia.

Clinical efficacy

The effectiveness of RISPERDAL CONSTA (25 mg and 50 mg) in the management of the manifestations of psychotic disorders (schizophrenia/schizoaffective disorder) was established in one 12-week, placebo-controlled trial in adult psychotic inpatients and outpatients who met the DSM-IV criteria for schizophrenia.

In a 12-week comparative trial in stable patients with schizophrenia, RISPERDAL CONSTA was shown to be as effective as the oral tablet formulation. The long-term (50 weeks) safety and efficacy of RISPERDAL CONSTA was also evaluated in an open-label trial of stable psychotic inpatients and outpatients who met the DSM-IV criteria for schizophrenia or schizoaffective disorder. Over time efficacy was maintained with RISPERDAL CONSTA (Figure 1).

Figure 1. Mean in total PANSS score over time (LOCF) in patients with schizophrenia.

(see Figure 1 above)

5.2 Pharmacokinetic properties

Absorption

The absorption of risperidone from RISPERDAL CONSTA is complete.

After a single intramuscular injection with RISPERDAL CONSTA, the release profile consists of a small initial release of risperidone (<1% of the dose), followed by a lag time of 3 weeks. The main release of risperidone starts from Week 3 onwards, is maintained from 4 to 6 weeks, and subsides by Week 7. Oral antipsychotic supplementation should therefore be given during the first 3 weeks of RISPERDAL CONSTA treatment (see section 4.2).

The combination of the release profile and the dosage regimen (intramuscular injection every two weeks) results in sustained therapeutic plasma concentrations. Therapeutic plasma concentrations remain until 4 to 6 weeks after the last RISPERDAL CONSTA injection.

After repeated intramuscular injections with 25 or 50 mg RISPERDAL CONSTA every two weeks, median trough and peak plasma concentrations of the active antipsychotic fraction fluctuated between 9.9-19.2 ng/ml and 17.9-45.5 ng/ml respectively. No accumulation of risperidone was observed during long term use (12 months) in patients who were injected with 25–50 mg every two weeks.

Distribution

Risperidone is rapidly distributed. The volume of distribution is 1-2 l/kg. In plasma, risperidone is bound to albumin and alpha-1-acid glycoprotein. The plasma protein binding of risperidone is 90%; that of the active metabolite 9-hydroxy-risperidone is 77%.

Biotransformation and elimination

Risperidone is metabolised by CYP 2D6 to 9-hydroxy-risperidone, which has a similar pharmacological activity as risperidone. Risperidone plus 9-hydroxy-risperidone form the active antipsychotic fraction. CYP 2D6 is subject to genetic polymorphism. Extensive CYP 2D6 metabolisers convert risperidone rapidly into 9-hydroxy-risperidone, whereas poor CYP 2D6 metabolisers convert it much more slowly. Although extensive metabolisers have lower risperidone and higher 9-hydroxy-risperidone concentrations than poor metabolisers, the pharmacokinetics of risperidone and 9-hydroxy-risperidone combined (i.e., the active antipsychotic fraction), after single and multiple doses, are similar in extensive and poor metabolisers of CYP 2D6.

Another metabolic pathway of risperidone is N-dealkylation. *In vitro* studies in human liver microsomes showed that risperidone at clinically relevant concentration does not substantially inhibit the metabolism of medicines metabolised by cytochrome P450 isozymes, including CYP 1A2, CYP 2A6, CYP 2C8/9/10, CYP 2D6, CYP 2E1, CYP 3A4, and CYP 3A5. One week after oral risperidone administration, 70% of the dose is excreted in the urine and 14% in the faeces. In urine, risperidone plus 9-hydroxy-risperidone represent 35-45% of the orally administered dose. The remainder is inactive metabolites. The elimination phase is complete approximately 7 to 8 weeks after the last RISPERDAL CONSTA injection.

Linearity

The pharmacokinetics of risperidone are linear in the dose range of 25-50 mg injected every 2 weeks.

Elderly, hepatic and renal impairment

A single-dose pharmacokinetic study with oral risperidone showed on average a 43% higher active antipsychotic fraction plasma concentrations, a 38% longer half-life and a reduced clearance of the active antipsychotic fraction by 30% in the elderly. Higher active antipsychotic fraction plasma concentrations and a reduced clearance of the active antipsychotic fraction by on average 60% were observed in patients with renal insufficiency. Risperidone plasma concentrations were normal in patients with liver insufficiency, but the mean free fraction of risperidone in plasma was increased by about 35%.

Pharmacokinetic/pharmacodynamic relationship

There was no relationship between the plasma concentrations of the active antipsychotic fraction and the change in total PANSS (Positive And Negative Syndrome Scale) and total ESRS (Extrapyramidal Symptom Rating Scale) scores across the assessment visits in any of the phase-III trials where efficacy and safety was examined.

Gender, race and smoking habits

A population pharmacokinetic analysis revealed no apparent effect of gender, race or smoking habits on the pharmacokinetics of risperidone or the active antipsychotic fraction.

5.3 Preclinical safety data

Similar to the (sub)chronic toxicity studies with oral risperidone in rats and dogs, the major effects of treatment with RISPERDAL CONSTA (up to 12 months of intramuscular administration) were prolactin-mediated mammary gland stimulation, male and female genital tract changes, and central nervous system (CNS) effects, related to the pharmacodynamic activity of risperidone.

Risperidone was not teratogenic in rat and rabbit. In rat reproduction studies with risperidone, adverse effects were seen on mating behaviour of the parents, and on birth weight and survival of the offspring. In rats, intrauterine exposure to risperidone was associated with cognitive deficits in adulthood. Other dopamine antagonists, when administered to pregnant animals, have caused negative effects on learning and motor development in the offspring.

RISPERDAL CONSTA administration to male and female rats for 12 and 24 months produced osteodystrophy at a dose of 40 mg/kg/2 weeks. The effect dose for osteodystrophy in rats was on a mg/m^2 basis 8 times the maximum recommended human dose and is associated with a plasma exposure 2 times the maximum anticipated exposure in humans at the maximum recommended dose. No osteodystrophy was observed in dogs treated for 12 months with RISPERDAL CONSTA up to 20 mg/kg/2 weeks. This dose yielded plasma exposures up to 14 times the maximum recommended human dose.

There was no evidence of genotoxic potential.

As expected for a potent dopamine D2-antagonist, in oral carcinogenicity studies of risperidone in rats and mice, increases in pituitary gland adenomas (mouse), endocrine pancreas adenomas (rat), and mammary gland adenomas (both species) were seen.

In an intramuscular carcinogenicity study with RISPERDAL CONSTA in Wistar (Hannover) rats (doses of 5 and 40 mg/kg/2 weeks), increased incidences of endocrine pancreas, pituitary gland, and adrenal medullary tumours were observed at 40 mg/kg, while mammary gland tumours were present at 5 and 40 mg/kg. These tumours observed upon oral and intramuscular dosing can be related to prolonged dopamine D_2 antagonism and hyperprolactinaemia. Tissue culture studies suggest that cell growth in human breast tumours may be stimulated by prolactin. Hypercalcemia, postulated to contribute to an increased incidence of adrenal medullary tumours in RISPERDAL CONSTA-treated rats, was observed in both dose groups. There is no evidence to suggest that hypercalcemia might cause phaeochromocytomas in humans.

Renal tubular adenomas occurred in male rats treated with RISPERDAL CONSTA at 40 mg/kg/2 weeks. No renal tumours occurred in the low dose, the NaCl 0.9%, or the microspheres vehicle control group. The mechanism underlying the renal tumours in RISPERDAL CONSTA-treated male Wistar (Hannover) rats is unknown. A treatment-related increase in renal tumour incidence did not occur in the oral carcinogenicity studies with Wistar (Wiga) rats or in Swiss mice administered oral risperidone. Studies conducted to explore the substrain differences in the tumour organ profile suggest that the Wistar (Hannover) substrain employed in the carcinogenicity study differs substantially from the Wistar (Wiga) substrain employed in the oral carcinogenicity study with respect to spontaneous age-related non-neoplastic renal changes, serum prolactin increases, and renal changes in response to risperidone. There are no data suggesting kidney-related changes in dogs treated chronically with RISPERDAL CONSTA.

The relevance of the osteodystrophy, the prolactin-mediated tumours and of the presumed rat substrain-specific renal tumours in terms of human risk is unknown.

Local irritation at the injection site in dogs and rats was observed after administration of high doses of RISPERDAL CONSTA. In a 24-month intramuscular carcinogenicity study in rats, no increased incidence of injection site tumours was seen in either the vehicle or active groups.

In vitro and in vivo, animal models show that at high doses risperidone may cause QT interval prolongation, which has been associated with a theoretically increased risk of torsade de pointes in patients.

6. PHARMACEUTICAL PARTICULARS

6.1 List of excipients

Microspheres

[poly-(d,l-lactide-co-glycolide)]

Solvent

Polysorbate 20

Carmellose sodium

Disodium hydrogen phosphate dihydrate

Citric acid anhydrous

Sodium chloride

Sodium hydroxide

Water for injection.

6.2 Incompatibilities

This medicinal product must not be mixed with other medicinal products except those mentioned in section 6.6.

6.3 Shelf life

3 years at 2-8°C.

After reconstitution: Chemical and physical in-use stability has been demonstrated for 24 hours at 25°C.

From a microbiological point of view, the product should be used immediately. If not used immediately, in-use storage times and conditions prior to use are the responsibility of the user and would normally not be longer than 6 hours at 25°C, unless reconstitution has taken place in controlled and validated aseptic conditions.

6.4 Special precautions for storage

The entire dose pack should be stored in the refrigerator.
Do not store above 25°C.

If refrigeration is unavailable, RISPERDAL CONSTA can be stored at temperatures not exceeding 25°C for no more than 7 days prior to administration. Do not expose unrefrigerated product to temperatures above 25°C.

Figure 2

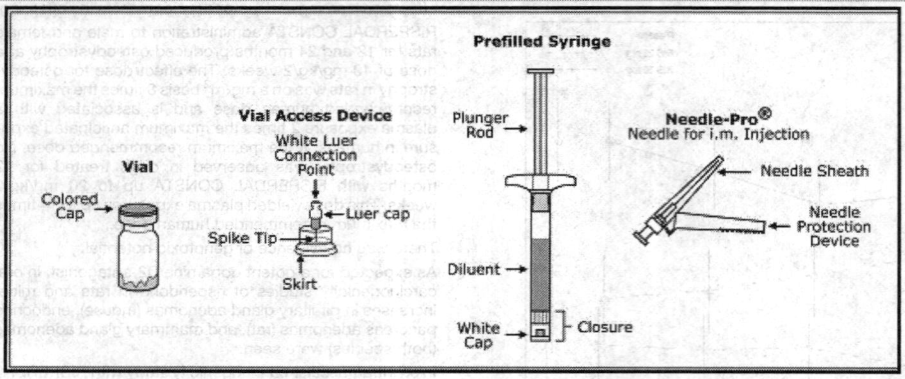

Store in the original package.

For storage conditions of the reconstituted medicinal product, see section 6.3.

Not all packs may be marketed.

6.5 Nature and contents of container

Not all packs may be marketed.

Needle-Free Vial Access Device

One vial containing RISPERDAL CONSTA extended release microspheres

One prefilled syringe containing 2 ml solvent for RISPERDAL CONSTA

One Alaris SmartSite Needle-Free Vial Access Device for reconstitution

One Needle-Pro needle for intramuscular injection (safety 20G 2'' TW needle with needle protection device)

6.6 Special precautions for disposal and other handling Instructions for Needle-Free Vial Access Device

RISPERDAL CONSTA extended release microspheres in the vial must be reconstituted **only** in the solvent in the syringe supplied in the dose pack, and must be administered **only** with the Needle-Pro safety needle supplied in the dose pack. Do not substitute any components in the dose pack. To assure that the intended dose of risperidone is delivered, the full contents from the vial must be administered. Administration of partial contents may not deliver the intended dose of risperidone.

(see Figure 2 above)

Remove the dose pack of RISPERDAL CONSTA from the refrigerator and allow it to come to room temperature prior to reconstitution.

Contents of the dose pack:

One vial containing RISPERDAL CONSTA extended release microspheres

One Alaris SmartSite needle-free vial access device for reconstitution

One prefilled syringe containing the solvent for RISPERDAL CONSTA

One Needle-Pro needle for intramuscular injection (safety 20G 2'' TW needle-with needle protection device)

1. Flip off the plastic coloured cap from the vial.

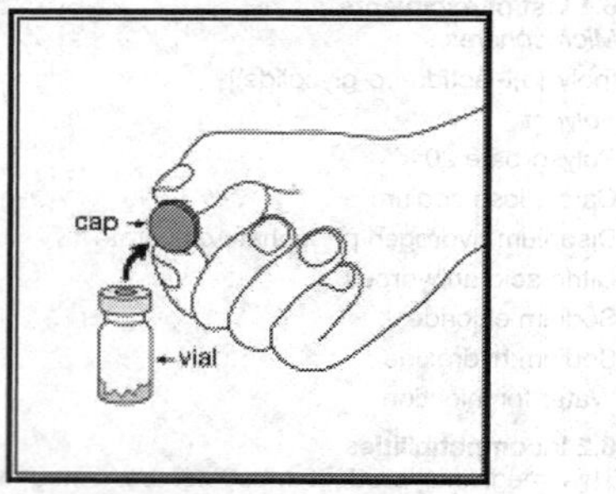

2. Peel back the blister pouch and remove the vial access device by holding the white luer cap.

Do not touch the spike tip of the access device at any time.

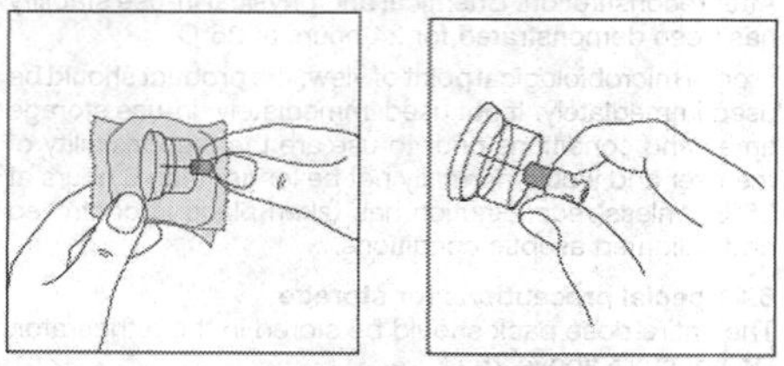

3. Place vial on a hard surface. With a straight push down movement press the spike tip of the vial access device through the centre of the vial's rubber stopper until the device securely snaps onto the vial top.

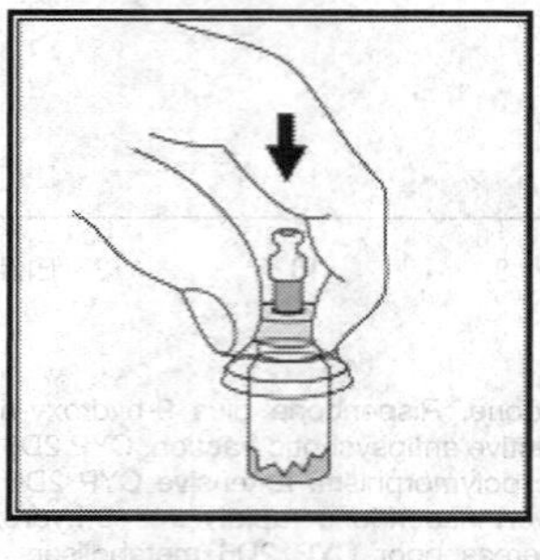

4. Swab the connection point of the vial access device with preferred antiseptic prior to attaching the syringe to the vial access device.

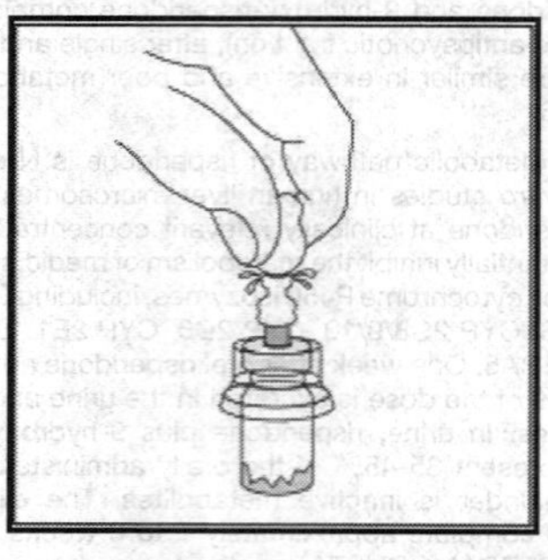

5. Open the prefilled syringe by breaking the seal of the closure and remove the white cap together with the rubber tip cap inside.

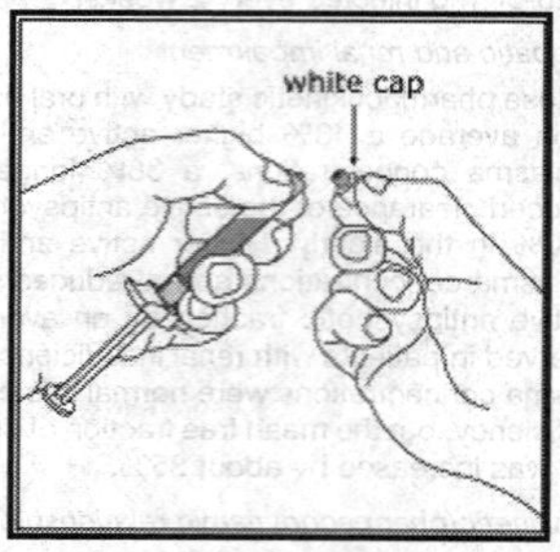

6. Press the syringe tip into the vial access device and twist in a clockwise motion to ensure that the syringe is securely attached to the white luer cap of the vial access device.

Hold the skirt of the vial access device during attachment to prevent spinning.

Keep the syringe and the vial access device aligned.

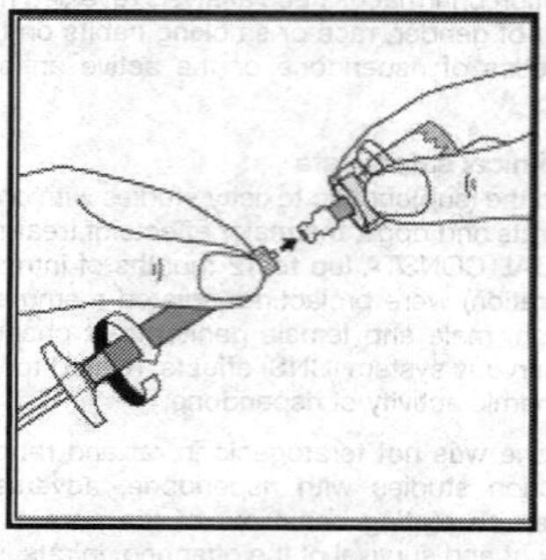

7. Inject the entire contents (solvent) of the syringe into the vial.

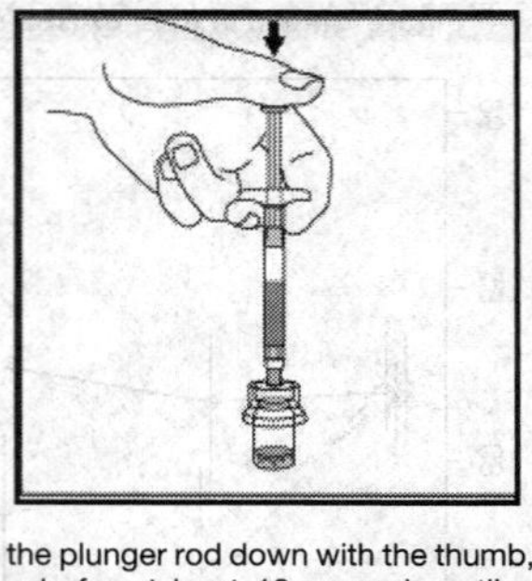

8. Holding the plunger rod down with the thumb, shake the vial vigorously for at least 10 seconds until obtaining a homogeneous suspension.

Mixing is complete when the suspension appears uniform, thick, and milky in colour and all the powder is fully dispersed.

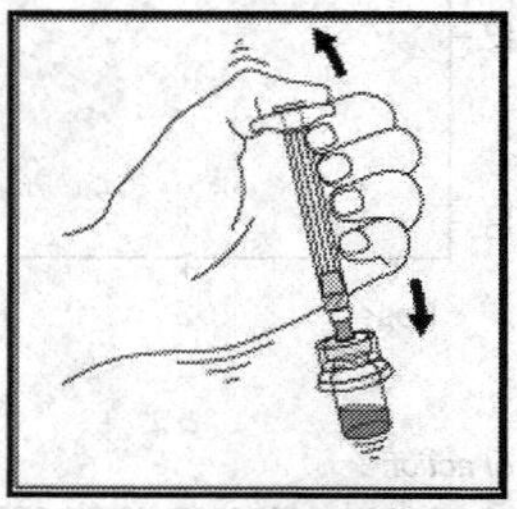

DO NOT STORE THE VIAL AFTER RECONSTITUTION OR THE SUSPENSION MAY SETTLE.

9. Invert the vial completely and slowly withdraw the entire contents of the suspension from the vial.

For identification purposes, tear section of the vial label at the perforation and apply detached section to the syringe.

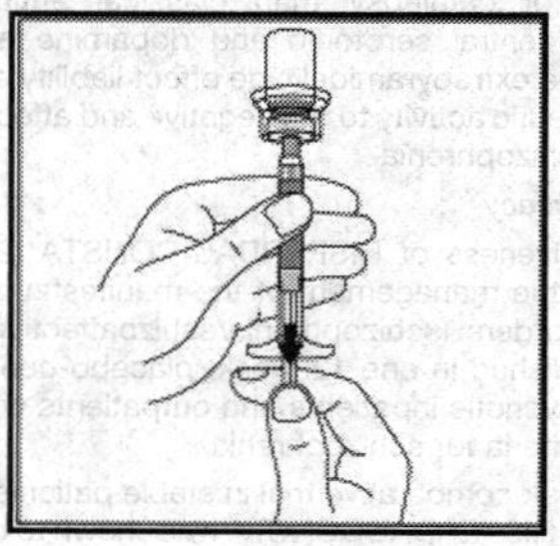

10. Unscrew the syringe from the vial access device. Discard the vial and the vial access device appropriately.

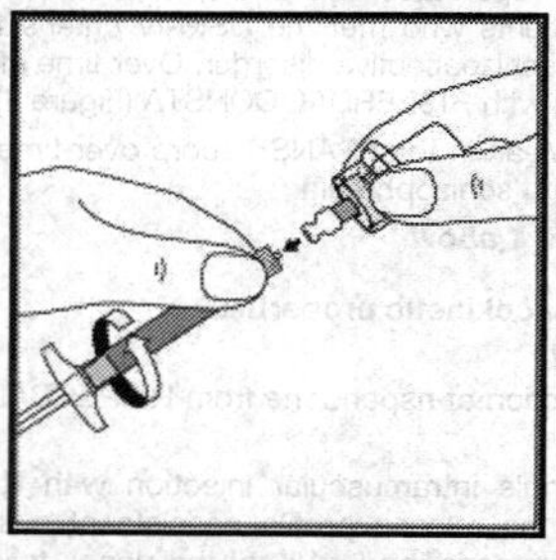

11. Peel the blister pouch of the Needle-Pro device open half way. Grasp sheath using the plastic peel pouch.

Attach the luer connection of the Needle-Pro device with an easy clockwise twisting motion to the syringe. Seat the needle firmly on the Needle-Pro device with a push and clockwise twist.

Prepare the patient for injection.

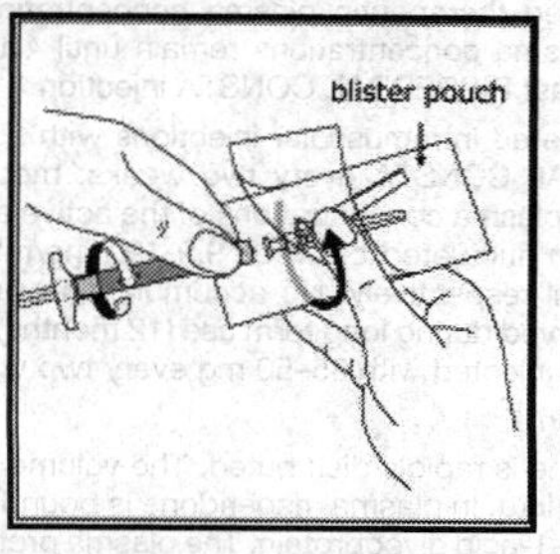

RESUSPENSION OF RISPERDAL CONSTA WILL BE NECESSARY PRIOR TO ADMINISTRATION AS SETTLING WILL OCCUR OVER TIME ONCE PRODUCT IS RECONSTITUTED. RESUSPEND THE MICROSPHERES IN THE SYRINGE BY SHAKING VIGOROUSLY.

12. Pull sheath away from the needle – do not twist sheath as needle may be loosened from Needle-Pro device.

Tap the syringe gently to make any air bubbles rise to the top.

Remove air bubbles from the syringe barrel by moving the plunger rod forward with the needle in an upright position. Inject the entire contents of the syringe intramuscularly into the buttock of the patient.

DO NOT ADMINISTER INTRAVENOUSLY.

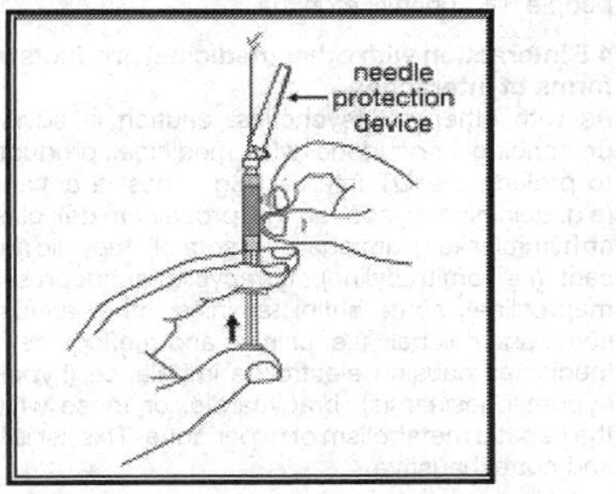

WARNING:
To avoid a needle stick injury with a contaminated needle, do not:
- Intentionally disengage the Needle-Pro device
- Attempt to straighten the needle or engage the Needle-Pro device if the needle is bent or damaged
- Mishandle the needle protection device that could lead to protrusion of the needle from it

After procedure is completed, press the needle into the needle protection device. Perform a one-handed technique by GENTLY pressing the needle protection device against a flat surface. As the needle protection device is pressed, the needle is firmly engaged into it. Visually confirm that the needle is fully engaged into the needle protection device. Immediately discard appropriately.

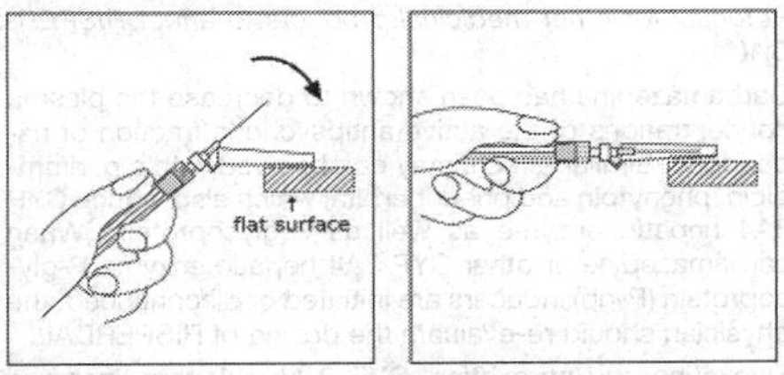

Any unused product or waste material should be disposed of in accordance with local requirements.

7. MARKETING AUTHORISATION HOLDER

Janssen-Cilag Ltd
50-100 Holmers Farm Way
High Wycombe
Bucks
HP12 4EG
UK

8. MARKETING AUTHORISATION NUMBER(S)

PL 00242/0375
PL 00242/0376
PL 00242/0377

9. DATE OF FIRST AUTHORISATION/RENEWAL OF THE AUTHORISATION

8 August 2002/28 February 2004

10. DATE OF REVISION OF THE TEXT

01 April 2009

Risperdal Tablets, Liquid & Quicklet

(Janssen-Cilag Ltd)

1. NAME OF THE MEDICINAL PRODUCT

RISPERDAL▼* 0.5,1, 2, 3, 4 and 6 mg film-coated tablets
RISPERDAL▼* 1mg/ml oral solution
RISPERDAL Quicklet▼* 0.5,1, 2, 3 & 4 mg orodispersible tablets

**Intensive monitoring is requested only when used for the recently licensed indications of short-term treatment of persistent aggression in Alzheimer's dementia and conduct disorder in children*

2. QUALITATIVE AND QUANTITATIVE COMPOSITION

Film-coated Tablets:

Each film-coated tablet contains 0.5,1, 2, 3, 4 or 6 mg of risperidone

Excipients:

Each 0.5 mg film-coated tablet contains 91 mg lactose

Each 1 mg film-coated tablet contains 131 mg lactose

Each 2 mg film-coated tablet contains 130 mg lactose and 0.05 mg orange yellow S aluminium lake (E110)

Each 3 mg film-coated tablet contains 195 mg lactose

Each 4 mg film-coated tablet contains 260 mg lactose

Each 6 mg film-coated tablet contains 115 mg lactose and 0.01 mg orange yellow S aluminium lake (E110)

Oral Solution:

1 ml oral solution contains 1 mg of risperidone

Orodispersible Tablets:

Each orodispersible tablet contains 0.5,1,2,3 or 4 mg of risperidone

Excipients:

Each 0.5 mg orodispersible tablet contains 0.25 mg aspartame (E951)

Each 1 mg orodispersible tablet contains 0.5 mg aspartame (E951)

Each 2 mg orodispersible tablet contains 0.75 mg aspartame (E951)

Each 3 mg orodispersible tablet contains 1.125 mg aspartame (E951)

Each 4 mg orodispersible tablet contains 1.5 mg aspartame (E951)

For a full list of excipients, see section 6.1.

3. PHARMACEUTICAL FORM

Film-coated Tablets:

Film-coated tablet

0.5 mg risperidone as brownish-red half-scored oblong biconvex tablets.

1 mg risperidone as white half-scored oblong tablets.

2 mg risperidone as orange half-scored oblong tablets.

3 mg risperidone as yellow half-scored oblong tablets.

4 mg risperidone as green half-scored oblong tablets.

6 mg risperidone as yellow circular biconvex tablets.

The score line is only to facilitate breaking for ease of swallowing and not to divide into equal doses.

Oral Solution:

Oral solution.

The solution is clear and colourless

Orodispersible Tablets:

Orodispersible tablet

0.5 mg risperidone as light coral, round, biconvex tablets

1 mg risperidone as light coral, square, biconvex tablets

2 mg risperidone as coral, square, biconvex tablets

3 mg risperidone as coral, round, biconvex tablets

4 mg risperidone as coral, round, biconvex tablets

Oro-dispersible tablets are etched on one side with R 0.5, R1, R2, R3, and R4 respectively.

4. CLINICAL PARTICULARS

4.1 Therapeutic indications

RISPERDAL is indicated for the treatment of schizophrenia.

RISPERDAL is indicated for the treatment of moderate to severe manic episodes associated with bipolar disorders.

RISPERDAL is indicated for the short-term treatment (up to 6 weeks) of persistent aggression in patients with moderate to severe Alzheimer's dementia unresponsive to non-pharmacological approaches and when there is a risk of harm to self or others.

RISPERDAL is indicated for the short-term symptomatic treatment (up to 6 weeks) of persistent aggression in conduct disorder in children from the age of 5 years and adolescents with subaverage intellectual functioning or mental retardation diagnosed according to DSM-IV criteria, in whom the severity of aggressive or other disruptive behaviours require pharmacologic treatment. Pharmacological treatment should be an integral part of a more comprehensive treatment programme, including psychosocial and educational intervention. It is recommended that risperidone be prescribed by a specialist in child neurology and child and adolescent psychiatry or physicians well familiar with the treatment of conduct disorder of children and adolescents.

4.2 Posology and method of administration

Schizophrenia

Adults

RISPERDAL may be given once daily or twice daily.

Patients should start with 2 mg/day risperidone. The dosage may be increased on the second day to 4 mg. Subsequently, the dosage can be maintained unchanged, or further individualised, if needed. Most patients will benefit from daily doses between 4 and 6 mg. In some patients, a slower titration phase and a lower starting and maintenance dose may be appropriate.

Doses above 10 mg/day have not demonstrated superior efficacy to lower doses and may cause increased incidence of extrapyramidal symptoms. Safety of doses above 16 mg/day has not been evaluated, and are therefore not recommended.

Elderly

A starting dose of 0.5 mg twice daily is recommended. This dosage can be individually adjusted with 0.5 mg twice daily increments to 1 to 2 mg twice daily.

Paediatric population

Risperidone is not recommended for use in children below age 18 with schizophrenia due to a lack of data on efficacy.

Manic episodes in bipolar disorder

Adults

RISPERDAL should be administered on a once daily schedule, starting with 2 mg risperidone. Dosage adjustments, if indicated, should occur at intervals of not less than 24 hours and in dosage increments of 1 mg per day. Risperidone can be administered in flexible doses over a range of 1 to 6 mg per day to optimize each patient's level of efficacy and tolerability. Daily doses over 6 mg risperidone have not been investigated in patients with manic episodes.

As with all symptomatic treatments, the continued use of RISPERDAL must be evaluated and justified on an ongoing basis.

Elderly

A starting dose of 0.5 mg twice daily is recommended. This dosage can be individually adjusted with 0.5 mg twice daily increments to 1 to 2 mg twice daily. Since clinical experience in elderly is limited, caution should be exercised.

Paediatric population

Risperidone is not recommended for use in children below age 18 with bipolar mania due to a lack of data on efficacy.

Persistent aggression in patients with moderate to severe Alzheimer's dementia

A starting dose of 0.25 mg twice daily is recommended. This dosage can be individually adjusted by increments of 0.25 mg twice daily, not more frequently than every other day, if needed. The optimum dose is 0.5 mg twice daily for most patients. Some patients, however, may benefit from doses up to 1 mg twice daily.

RISPERDAL should not be used more than 6 weeks in patients with persistent aggression in Alzheimer's dementia. During treatment, patients must be evaluated frequently and regularly, and the need for continuing treatment reassessed.

Conduct disorder

Children and adolescents from 5 to 18 years of age

For subjects $\geqslant$50 kg, a starting dose of 0.5 mg once daily is recommended. This dosage can be individually adjusted by increments of 0.5 mg once daily not more frequently than every other day, if needed. The optimum dose is 1 mg once daily for most patients. Some patients, however, may benefit from 0.5 mg once daily while others may require 1.5 mg once daily. For subjects $<$50 kg, a starting dose of 0.25 mg once daily is recommended. This dosage can be individually adjusted by increments of 0.25 mg once daily not more frequently than every other day, if needed. The optimum dose is 0.5 mg once daily for most patients. Some patients, however, may benefit from 0.25 mg once daily while others may require 0.75 mg once daily.

As with all symptomatic treatments, the continued use of RISPERDAL must be evaluated and justified on an ongoing basis.

RISPERDAL is not recommended in children less than 5 years of age, as there is no experience in children less than 5 years of age with this disorder.

Renal and hepatic impairment

Patients with renal impairment have less ability to eliminate the active antipsychotic fraction than in adults with normal renal function. Patients with impaired hepatic function have increases in plasma concentration of the free fraction of risperidone.

Irrespective of the indication, starting and consecutive dosing should be halved, and dose titration should be slower for patients with renal or hepatic impairment.

RISPERDAL should be used with caution in these groups of patients.

Method of administration

RISPERDAL is for oral use. Food does not affect the absorption of RISPERDAL.

Upon discontinuation, gradual withdrawal is advised. Acute withdrawal symptoms, including nausea, vomiting, sweating, and insomnia have very rarely been described after abrupt cessation of high doses of antipsychotic medicines (see section 4.8). Recurrence of psychotic symptoms may also occur, and the emergence of involuntary movement disorders (such as akathisia, dystonia and dyskinesia) has been reported.

Switching from other antipsychotics.

When medically appropriate, gradual discontinuation of the previous treatment while RISPERDAL therapy is initiated is recommended. Also, if medically appropriate, when switching patients from depot antipsychotics, initiate RISPERDAL therapy in place of the next scheduled injection. The need for continuing existing anti-Parkinson medicines should be re-evaluated periodically.

RISPERDAL oral solution:

For instructions on handling RISPERDAL oral solution see section 6.6.

RISPERDAL orodispersible tablets:

Do not open the blister until ready to administer. Peel open the blister to expose the tablet. Do not push the tablet through the foil because it may break. Remove the tablet from the blister with dry hands.

Immediately place the tablet on the tongue. The tablet will begin disintegrating within seconds. Water may be used if desired.

4.3 Contraindications

Hypersensitivity to the active substance or to any of the excipients.

4.4 Special warnings and precautions for use

Elderly patients with dementia

Overall mortality

Elderly patients with dementia treated with atypical antipsychotics have an increased mortality compared to placebo in a meta-analysis of 17 controlled trials of atypical antipsychotics, including RISPERDAL. In placebo-controlled trials with RISPERDAL in this population, the incidence of mortality was 4.0% for RISPERDAL-treated patients compared to 3.1% for placebo-treated patients. The odds ratio (95% exact confidence interval) was 1.21 (0.7, 2.1). The mean age (range) of patients who died was 86 years (range 67-100).

Concomitant use with furosemide

In the RISPERDAL placebo-controlled trials in elderly patients with dementia, a higher incidence of mortality was observed in patients treated with furosemide plus risperidone (7.3%; mean age 89 years, range 75-97) when compared to patients treated with risperidone alone (3.1%; mean age 84 years, range 70-96) or furosemide alone (4.1%; mean age 80 years, range 67-90). The increase in mortality in patients treated with furosemide plus risperidone was observed in two of the four clinical trials. Concomitant use of risperidone with other diuretics (mainly thiazide diuretics used in low dose) was not associated with similar findings.

No pathophysiological mechanism has been identified to explain this finding, and no consistent pattern for cause of death observed. Nevertheless, caution should be exercised and the risks and benefits of this combination or co-treatment with other potent diuretics should be considered prior to the decision to use. There was no increased incidence of mortality among patients taking other diuretics as concomitant treatment with risperidone. Irrespective of treatment, dehydration was an overall risk factor for mortality and should therefore be carefully avoided in elderly patients with dementia.

Cerebrovascular Adverse Events (CVAE)

In placebo-controlled trials in elderly patients with dementia there was a significantly higher incidence (approximately 3-fold increased) of CVAEs, such as stroke (including fatalities) and transient ischaemic attack in patients treated with RISPERDAL compared with patients treated with placebo (mean age 85 years; range 73 to 97). The pooled data from six placebo-controlled studies in mainly elderly patients (>65 years of age) with dementia showed that CVAEs (serious and non-serious, combined) occurred in 3.3% (33/1009) of patients treated with risperidone and 1.2% (8/712) of patients treated with placebo. The odds ratio (95% exact confidence interval) was 2.96 (1.34, 7.50). The mechanism for this increased risk is not known. An increased risk cannot be excluded for other antipsychotics or other patient populations. RISPERDAL should be used with caution in patients with risk factors for stroke.

The risk of CVAEs was significantly higher in patients with mixed or vascular type of dementia when compared to Alzheimer's dementia. Therefore, patients with other types of dementias than Alzheimer's should not be treated with risperidone.

Physicians are advised to assess the risks and benefits of the use of RISPERDAL in elderly patients with dementia, taking into account risk predictors for stroke in the individual patient. Patients/caregivers should be cautioned to immediately report signs and symptoms of potential CVAEs such as sudden weakness or numbness in the face, arms or legs, and speech or vision problems. All treatment options should be considered without delay, including discontinuation of risperidone.

RISPERDAL should only be used short term for persistent aggression in patients with moderate to severe Alzheimer's dementia to supplement non-pharmacological approaches which have had limited or no efficacy and when there is potential risk of harm to self or others.

Patients should be reassessed regularly, and the need for continuing treatment reassessed.

Orthostatic hypotension

Due to the alpha-blocking activity of risperidone, (orthostatic) hypotension can occur, especially during the initial dose-titration period. Clinically significant hypotension has been observed postmarketing with concomitant use of risperidone and antihypertensive treatment. RISPERDAL should be used with caution in patients with known cardiovascular disease (e.g. heart failure, myocardial infarction, conduction abnormalities, dehydration, hypovolemia, or cerebrovascular disease), and the dosage should be gradually titrated as recommended (see section 4.2). A dose reduction should be considered if hypotension occurs.

Tardive dyskinesia/extrapyramidal symptoms (TD/EPS)

Medicines with dopamine receptor antagonistic properties have been associated with the induction of tardive dyskinesia characterised by rhythmical involuntary movements, predominantly of the tongue and/or face. The onset of extrapyramidal symptoms is a risk factor for tardive dyskinesia. If signs and symptoms of tardive dyskinesia appear, the discontinuation of all antipsychotics should be considered.

Neuroleptic malignant syndrome (NMS)

Neuroleptic Malignant Syndrome, characterised by hyperthermia, muscle rigidity, autonomic instability, altered consciousness and elevated serum creatine phosphokinase levels has been reported to occur with antipsychotics. Additional signs may include myoglobinuria (rhabdomyolysis) and acute renal failure. In this event, all antipsychotics, including RISPERDAL, should be discontinued.

Parkinson's disease and dementia with Lewy bodies

Physicians should weigh the risks versus the benefits when prescribing antipsychotics, including RISPERDAL, to patients with Parkinson's Disease or Dementia with Lewy Bodies (DLB). Parkinson's Disease may worsen with risperidone. Both groups may be at increased risk of Neuroleptic Malignant Syndrome as well as having an increased sensitivity to antipsychotic medicinal products; these patients were excluded from clinical trials. Manifestation of this increased sensitivity can include confusion, obtundation, postural instability with frequent falls, in addition to extrapyramidal symptoms.

Hyperglycemia

Hyperglycemia or exacerbation of pre-existing diabetes has been reported in very rare cases during treatment with RISPERDAL. Appropriate clinical monitoring is advisable in diabetic patients and in patients with risk factors for the development of diabetes mellitus.

Hyperprolactinaemia

Tissue culture studies suggest that cell growth in human breast tumours may be stimulated by prolactin. Although no clear association with the administration of antipsychotics has so far been demonstrated in clinical and epidemiological studies, caution is recommended in patients with relevant medical history. RISPERDAL should be used with caution in patients with pre-existing hyperprolactinaemia and in patients with possible prolactin-dependent tumours.

QT prolongation

QT prolongation has very rarely been reported postmarketing. As with other antipsychotics, caution should be exercised when risperidone is prescribed in patients with known cardiovascular disease, family history of QT prolongation, bradycardia, or electrolyte disturbances (hypokalaemia, hypomagnesaemia), as it may increase the risk of arrhythmogenic effects, and in concomitant use with medicines known to prolong the QT interval.

Seizures

RISPERDAL should be used cautiously in patients with a history of seizures or other conditions that potentially lower the seizure threshold.

Priapism

Priapism may occur with RISPERDAL treatment due to its alpha-adrenergic blocking effects.

Body temperature regulation

Disruption of the body's ability to reduce core body temperature has been attributed to antipsychotic medicines. Appropriate care is advised when prescribing RISPERDAL to patients who will be experiencing conditions which may contribute to an elevation in core body temperature, e.g. exercising strenuously, exposure to extreme heat, receiving concomitant treatment with anticholinergic activity, or being subject to dehydration.

Children and adolescents

Before risperidone is prescribed to a child or adolescent with conduct disorder they should be fully assessed for physical and social causes of the aggressive behaviour such as pain or inappropriate environmental demands.

The sedative effect of risperidone should be closely monitored in this population because of possible consequences on learning ability. A change in the time of administration of risperidone could improve the impact of the sedation on attention faculties of children and adolescents.

Risperidone was associated with mean increases in body weight and body mass index (BMI). Changes in height in the long-term open-label extension studies were within expected age-appropriate norms. The effect of long-term risperidone treatment on sexual maturation and height have not been adequately studied.

Because of the potential effects of prolonged hyperprolactinemia on growth and sexual maturation in children and adolescents, regular clinical evaluation of endocrinological status should be considered, including measurements of height, weight, sexual maturation, monitoring of menstrual functioning, and other potential prolactin-related effects.

During treatment with risperidone regular examination for extrapyramidal symptoms and other movement disorders should also be conducted.

For specific posology recommendations in children and adolescents see Section 4.2.

Excipients

The film-coated tablets contain lactose. Patients with rare hereditary problems of galactose intolerance, the Lapp lactase deficiency or glucose-galactose malabsorption should not take this medicine.

The 2 mg and 6 mg film-coated tablets contain sunset yellow (E110). May cause allergic reactions.

The orodispersible tablets contain aspartame. Aspartame is a source of phenylalanine which may be harmful for people with phenylketonuria.

4.5 Interaction with other medicinal products and other forms of interaction

As with other antipsychotics, caution is advised when prescribing risperidone with medicinal products known to prolong the QT interval, e.g. class Ia antiarrhythmics (e.g. quinidine, dysopiramide, procainamide), class III antiarrhythmics (e.g. amiodarone, sotalol), tricyclic antidepressant (i.e. amitriptyline), tetracyclic antidepressants (i.e. maprotiline), some antihistaminics, other antipsychotics, some antimalarials (i.e. chinice and mefloquine), and with medicines causing electrolyte imbalance (hypokalaemia, hypomagnesiaemia), bradycardia, or those which inhibit the hepatic metabolism of risperidone. This list is indicative and not exhaustive.

Potential for RISPERDAL to affect other medicinal products

Risperidone should be used with caution in combination with other centrally-acting substances notably including alcohol, opiates, antihistamines and benzodiazepines due to the increased risk of sedation.

RISPERDAL may antagonise the effect of levodopa and other dopamine agonists. If this combination is deemed necessary, particularly in end-stage Parkinson's disease, the lowest effective dose of each treatment should be prescribed.

Clinically significant hypotension has been observed postmarketing with concomitant use of risperidone and antihypertensive treatment.

RISPERDAL does not show a clinically relevant effect on the pharmacokinetics of lithium, valproate, digoxin or topiramate.

Potential for other medicinal products to affect RISPERDAL

Carbamazepine has been shown to decrease the plasma concentrations of the active antipsychotic fraction of risperidone. Similar effects may be observed with e.g. rifampicin, phenytoin and phenobarbital which also induce CYP 3A4 hepatic enzyme as well as P-glycoprotein. When carbamazepine or other CYP 3A4 hepatic enzyme/P-glycoprotein (P-gp) inducers are initiated or discontinued, the physician should re-evaluate the dosing of RISPERDAL.

Fluoxetine and paroxetine, CYP 2D6 inhibitors, increase the plasma concentration of risperidone, but less so of the active antipsychotic fraction. It is expected that other CYP 2D6 inhibitors, such as quinidine, may affect the plasma concentrations of risperidone in a similar way. When concomitant fluoxetine or paroxetine is initiated or discontinued, the physician should re-evaluate the dosing of RISPERDAL.

Verapamil, an inhibitor of CYP 3A4 and P-gp, increases the plasma concentration of risperidone.

Galantamine and donepezil do not show a clinically relevant effect on the pharmacokinetics of risperidone and on the active antipsychotic fraction.

Phenothiazines, tricyclic antidepressants, and some betablockers may increase the plasma concentrations of risperidone but not those of the active antipsychotic fraction. Amitriptyline does not affect the pharmacokinetics of risperidone or the active antipsychotic fraction. Cimetidine and ranitidine increase the bioavailability of risperidone, but only marginally that of the active antipsychotic fraction. Erythromycin, a CYP 3A4 inhibitor, does not change the pharmacokinetics of risperidone and the active antipsychotic fraction.

The combined use of psychostimulants (e.g. methylphenidate) with RISPERDAL in children and adolescents did not alter the pharmacokinetics and efficacy of RISPERDAL.

See section 4.4 regarding increased mortality in elderly patients with dementia concomitantly receiving furosemide.

Concomitant use of oral RISPERDAL with paliperidone is not recommended as paliperidone is the active metabolite of risperidone and the combination of the two may lead to additive active antipsychotic fraction exposure.

4.6 Pregnancy and lactation

Pregnancy

There are no adequate data from the use of risperidone in pregnant women. According to postmarketing data reversible extrapyramidal symptoms in the neonate were observed following the use of risperidone during the last trimester of pregnancy. Consequently newborns should be monitored carefully. Risperidone was not teratogenic in animal studies but other types of reproductive toxicity were seen (see section 5.3). The potential risk for humans is unknown. Therefore, RISPERDAL should not be used during pregnancy unless clearly necessary. If discontinuation during pregnancy is necessary, it should not be done abruptly.

Lactation

In animal studies, risperidone and 9-hydroxy-risperidone are excreted in the milk. It has been demonstrated that risperidone and 9-hydroxy-risperidone are also excreted in human breast milk in small quantities. There are no data available on adverse reactions in breast-feeding infants. Therefore, the advantage of breast-feeding should be weighed against the potential risks for the child.

4.7 Effects on ability to drive and use machines

RISPERDAL can have minor or moderate influence on the ability to drive and use machines due to potential nervous system and visual effects (see section 4.8). Therefore, patients should be advised not to drive or operate machinery until their individual susceptibility is known.

4.8 Undesirable effects

The most frequently reported adverse drug reactions (ADRs) (incidence ⩾10%) are: Parkinsonism, headache, and insomnia.

The following are all the ADRs that were reported in clinical trials and postmarketing. The following terms and frequencies are applied:

very common (⩾1/10), common (⩾1/100 to <1/10), uncommon (⩾1/1000 to <1/100), rare (⩾1/10,000 to <1/1000),

very rare (<1/10,000), and not known (cannot be estimated from the available clinical trial data).

Within each frequency grouping, undesirable effects are presented in order of decreasing seriousness.

Adverse Drug Reactions by System Organ Class and Frequency

Investigations	
Common	Blood prolactin increased[a], Weight increased
Uncommon	Electrocardiogram QT prolonged, Electrocardiogram abnormal, Blood glucose increased, Transaminases increased, White blood cell count decreased Body temperature increased, Eosinophil count increased, Haemoglobin decreased, Blood creatine phosphokinase increased
Rare	Body temperature decreased
Cardiac disorders	
Common	Tachycardia
Uncommon	Atrioventricular block, Bundle branch block, Atrial fibrillation, Sinus bradycardia, Palpitations
Blood and lymphatic system disorders	
Uncommon	Anaemia, Thrombocytopenia
Rare	Granulocytopenia
Not known	Agranulocytosis
Nervous system disorders	
Very common	Parkinsonism[b], Headache
Common	Akathisia[b], Dizziness, Tremor[b], Dystonia[b], Somnolence, Sedation, Lethargy, Dyskinesia[b]
Uncommon	Unresponsive to stimuli, Loss of consciousness, Syncope, Depressed level of consciousness, Cerebrovascular accident, Transient ischaemic attack, Dysarthria, Disturbance in attention, Hypersomnia, Dizziness postural, Balance disorder, Tardive dyskinesia, Speech disorder, Coordination abnormal, Hypoaesthesia
Rare	Neuroleptic malignant syndrome, Diabetic coma, Cerebrovascular disorder, Cerebral ischaemia, Movement disorder
Eye disorders	
Common	Vision blurred
Uncommon	Conjunctivitis, Ocular hyperaemia, Eye discharge, Eye swelling, Dry eye, Lacrimation increased, Photophobia
Rare	Visual acuity reduced, Eye rolling, Glaucoma
Ear and labyrinth disorders	
Uncommon	Ear pain, Tinnitus
Respiratory, thoracic and mediastinal disorders	
Common	Dyspnoea, Epistaxis, Cough, Nasal congestion, Pharyngolaryngeal pain
Uncommon	Wheezing, Pneumonia aspiration, Pulmonary congestion, Respiratory disorder, Rales, Respiratory tract congestion, Dysphonia
Rare	Sleep apnea syndrome, Hyperventilation
Gastrointestinal disorders	
Common	Vomiting, Diarrhoea, Constipation, Nausea, Abdominal pain, Dyspepsia, Dry mouth, Stomach discomfort
Uncommon	Dysphagia, Gastritis, Faecal incontinence, Faecaloma
Rare	Intestinal obstruction, Pancreatitis, Lip swelling, Cheilitis
Renal and urinary disorders	
Common	Enuresis
Uncommon	Dysuria, Urinary incontinence, Pollakiuria
Skin and subcutaneous tissue disorders	
Common	Rash, Erythema
Uncommon	Angioedema, Skin lesion, Skin disorder, Pruritus, Acne, Skin discolouration, Alopecia, Seborrhoeic dermatitis, Dry skin, Hyperkeratosis
Rare	Dandruff
Musculoskeletal and connective tissue disorders	
Common	Arthralgia, Back pain, Pain in extremity
Uncommon	Muscular weakness, Myalgia, Neck pain, Joint swelling, Posture abnormal, Joint stiffness, Musculoskeletal chest pain
Rare	Rhabdomyolysis
Endocrine disorders	
Rare	Inappropriate antidiuretic hormone secretion
Metabolism and nutrition disorders	
Common	Increased appetite, Decreased appetite
Uncommon	Anorexia, Polydipsia
Very rare	Diabetic ketoacidosis
Not known	Water intoxication
Infections and infestations	
Common	Pneumonia, Influenza, Bronchitis, Upper respiratory tract infection, Urinary tract infection
Uncommon	Sinusitis, Viral infection, Ear infection, Tonsillitis, Cellulitis, Otitis media, Eye infection, Localised infection, Acarodermatitis, Respiratory tract infection, Cystitis, Onychomycosis
Rare	Otitis media chronic
Vascular disorders	
Uncommon	Hypotension, Orthostatic hypotension, Flushing
General disorders and administration site conditions	
Common	Pyrexia, Fatigue, Peripheral oedema, Asthenia, Chest pain
Uncommon	Face oedema, Gait disturbance, Feeling abnormal, Sluggishness, Influenza like illness, Thirst, Chest discomfort, Chills
Rare	Generalised oedema, Hypothermia, Drug withdrawal syndrome, Peripheral coldness
Immune system disorders	
Uncommon	Hypersensitivity
Rare	Drug hypersensitivity
Not known	Anaphylactic reaction
Hepatobiliary disorders	
Rare	Jaundice
Reproductive system and breast disorders	
Uncommon	Amenorrhoea, Sexual dysfunction, Erectile dysfunction, Ejaculation disorder, Galactorrhoea, Gynaecomastia, Menstrual disorder, Vaginal discharge,
Not known	Priapism
Psychiatric disorders	
Very common	Insomnia
Common	Anxiety, Agitation, Sleep disorder
Uncommon	Confusional state, Mania, Libido decreased, Listless, Nervousness
Rare	Anorgasmia, Blunted affect

[a] Hyperprolactinemia can in some cases lead to gynaecomastia, menstrual disturbances, amenorrhoea, galactorrhea.

[b] Extrapyramidal disorder may occur: Parkinsonism (salivary hypersecretion, musculoskeletal stiffness, parkinsonism, drooling, cogwheel rigidity, bradykinesia, hypokinesia, masked facies, muscle tightness, akinesia, nuchal rigidity, muscle rigidity, parkinsonian gait, and glabellar reflex abnormal), akathisia (akathisia, restlessness, hyperkinesia, and restless leg syndrome), tremor, dyskinesia (dyskinesia, muscle twitching, choreoathetosis, athetosis, and myoclonus), dystonia.

Dystonia includes dystonia, muscle spasms, hypertonia, torticollis, muscle contractions involuntary, muscle contracture, blepharospasm, oculogyration, tongue paralysis, facial spasm, laryngospasm, myotonia, opisthotonus, oropharyngeal spasm, pleurothotonus, tongue spasm, and trismus. Tremor includes tremor and parkinsonian rest tremor. It should be noted that a broader spectrum of symptoms are included, that do not necessarily have an extrapyramidal origin.

The following is a list of additional ADRs associated with risperidone that have been identified as ADRs during clinical trials investigating the long-acting injectable risperidone formulation (RISPERDAL CONSTA) but were not determined to be ADRs in the clinical trials investigating oral RISPERDAL. This table excludes those ADRs specifically associated with the formulation or injection route of administration of RISPERDAL CONSTA.

Additional Adverse Drug Reactions Reported With RISPERDAL CONSTA but Not With Oral RISPERDAL by System Organ Class
Investigations
Weight decreased, Gamma-glutamyltransferase increased, Hepatic enzyme increased
Cardiac Disorders
Bradycardia
Blood and Lymphatic Disorders
Neutropenia
Nervous System Disorders
Paresthesia, Convulsion
Eye Disorders
Blepharospasm
Ear and Labyrinth Disorders
Vertigo
Gastrointestinal Disorders
Toothache, Tongue spasm
Skin and Subcutaneous Tissue Disorders
Eczema
Musculoskeletal, Connective Tissue, and Bone Disorders
Buttock pain
Infections and Infestations
Lower respiratory tract infection, Infection, Gastroenteritis, Subcutaneous abscess
Injury and Poisoning
Fall
Vascular Disorders
Hypertension
General Disorders and Administration Site Conditions
Pain
Psychiatric Disorders
Depression

Class effects

As with other antipsychotics, very rare cases of QT prolongation have been reported postmarketing with risperidone. Other class-related cardiac effects reported with antipsychotics which prolong QT interval include ventricular arrhythmia, ventricular fibrillation, ventricular tachycardia, sudden death, cardiac arrest and Torsades de Pointes.

Weight gain

The proportions of RISPERDAL and placebo-treated adult patients with schizophrenia meeting a weight gain criterion of ⩾ 7% of body weight were compared in a pool of 6- to 8-week, placebo-controlled trials, revealing a statistically significantly greater incidence of weight gain for RISPERDAL (18%) compared to placebo (9%). In a pool of placebo-controlled 3-week studies in adult patients with acute mania, the incidence of weight increase of ⩾ 7% at endpoint was comparable in the RISPERDAL (2.5%) and placebo (2.4%) groups, and was slightly higher in the active-control group (3.5%).

In a population of children and adolescents with conduct and other disruptive behaviour disorders, in long-term studies, weight increased by a mean of 7.3 kg after 12 months of treatment. The expected weight gain for normal children between 5-12 years of age is 3 to 5 kg per year. From 12-16 years of age, this magnitude of gaining 3 to 5 kg per year is maintained for girls, while boys gain approximately 5 kg per year.

Additional information on special populations

Adverse drug reactions that were reported with higher incidence in elderly patients with dementia or paediatric patients than in adult populations are described below:

Elderly patients with dementia

Transient ischaemic attack and cerebrovascular accident were ADRs reported in clinical trials with a frequency of 1.4% and 1.5%, respectively, in elderly patients with dementia. In addition, the following ADRs were reported with a frequency ⩾5% in elderly patients with dementia and with at least twice the frequency seen in other adult populations: urinary tract infection, peripheral oedema, lethargy, and cough.

Paediatric patients

The following ADRs were reported with a frequency ⩾5% in paediatric patients (5 to 17 years) and with at least twice the frequency seen in clinical trials in adults: somnolence/sedation, fatigue, headache, increased appetite, vomiting, upper respiratory tract infection, nasal congestion, abdominal pain, dizziness, cough, pyrexia, tremor, diarrhoea, and enuresis.

4.9 Overdose

Symptoms

In general, reported signs and symptoms have been those resulting from an exaggeration of the known pharmacological effects of risperidone. These include drowsiness and sedation, tachycardia and hypotension, and extrapyramidal symptoms. In overdose, QT-prolongation and convulsions have been reported. Torsade de Pointes has been reported in association with combined overdose of RISPERDAL and paroxetine.

In case of acute overdose, the possibility of multiple drug involvement should be considered.

Treatment

Establish and maintain a clear airway and ensure adequate oxygenation and ventilation. Gastric lavage (after intubation, if the patient is unconscious) and administration of activated charcoal together with a laxative should be considered only when drug intake was less than one hour before. Cardiovascular monitoring should commence immediately and should include continuous electrocardiographic monitoring to detect possible arrhythmias.

There is no specific antidote to RISPERDAL. Therefore, appropriate supportive measures should be instituted. Hypotension and circulatory collapse should be treated with appropriate measures such as intravenous fluids and/or sympathomimetic agents. In case of severe extrapyramidal symptoms, an anticholinergic medicinal product should be administered. Close medical supervision and monitoring should continue until the patient recovers.

5. PHARMACOLOGICAL PROPERTIES

5.1 Pharmacodynamic properties

Pharmacotherapeutic group: Other antipsychotics, ATC code: N05AX08

Mechanism of action

Risperidone is a selective monoaminergic antagonist with unique properties. It has a high affinity for serotoninergic 5-HT_2 and dopaminergic D_2 receptors. Risperidone binds also to alpha$_1$-adrenergic receptors, and, with lower affinity, to H_1-histaminergic and alpha$_2$-adrenergic receptors. Risperidone has no affinity for cholinergic receptors. Although risperidone is a potent D_2 antagonist, which is considered to improve the positive symptoms of schizophrenia, it causes less depression of motor activity and induction of catalepsy than classical antipsychotics. Balanced central serotonin and dopamine antagonism may reduce extrapyramidal side effect liability and extend the therapeutic activity to the negative and affective symptoms of schizophrenia.

Pharmacodynamic effects

Schizophrenia

The efficacy of risperidone in the short-term treatment of schizophrenia was established in four studies, 4- to 8-weeks in duration, which enrolled over 2500 patients who met DSM-IV criteria for schizophrenia. In a 6-week, placebo-controlled trial involving titration of risperidone in doses up to 10 mg/day administered twice daily, risperidone was superior to placebo on the Brief Psychiatric Rating Scale (BPRS) total score. In an 8-week, placebo-controlled trial involving four fixed doses of risperidone (2, 6, 10, and 16 mg/day, administered twice daily), all four risperidone groups were superior to placebo on the Positive and Negative Syndrome Scale (PANSS) total score. In an 8-week, dose comparison trial involving five fixed doses of risperidone (1, 4, 8, 12, and 16 mg/day administered twice-daily), the 4, 8, and 16 mg/day risperidone dose groups were superior to the 1 mg risperidone dose group on PANSS total score. In a 4-week, placebo-controlled dose comparison trial involving two fixed doses of risperidone (4 and 8 mg/day administered once daily), both risperidone dose groups were superior to placebo on several PANSS measures, including total PANSS and a response measure (>20% reduction in PANSS total score). In a longer-term trial, adult outpatients predominantly meeting DSM-IV criteria for schizophrenia and who had been clinically stable for at least 4 weeks on an antipsychotic medicinal product were randomised to risperidone 2 to 8 mg/day or to haloperidol for 1 to 2 years of observation for relapse. Patients receiving risperidone experienced a significantly longer time to relapse over this time period compared to those receiving haloperidol.

Manic episodes in bipolar disorder

The efficacy of risperidone monotherapy in the acute treatment of manic episodes associated with bipolar I disorder was demonstrated in three double-blind, placebo-controlled monotherapy studies in approximately 820 patients who had bipolar I disorder, based on DSM-IV criteria. In the three studies, risperidone 1 to 6 mg/day (starting dose 3 mg in two studies and 2 mg in one study) was shown to be significantly superior to placebo on the pre-specified primary endpoint, i.e. the change from baseline in total Young Mania Rating Scale (YMRS) score at Week 3. Secondary efficacy outcomes were generally consistent with the primary outcome. The percentage of patients with a decrease of ⩾ 50% in total YMRS score from baseline to the 3-week endpoint was significantly higher for risperidone than for placebo. One of the three studies included a haloperidol arm and a 9-week double-blind maintenance phase. Efficacy was maintained throughout the 9-week maintenance treatment period. Change from baseline in total YMRS showed continued improvement and was comparable between risperidone and haloperidol at Week 12.

The efficacy of risperidone in addition to mood stabilisers in the treatment of acute mania was demonstrated in one of two 3-week double-blind studies in approximately 300 patients who met the DSM-IV criteria for bipolar I disorder. In one 3-week study, risperidone 1 to 6 mg/day starting at 2 mg/day in addition to lithium or valproate was superior to lithium or valproate alone on the pre-specified primary endpoint, i.e. the change from baseline in YMRS total score at Week 3. In a second 3-week study, risperidone 1 to 6 mg/day starting at 2 mg/day, combined with lithium, valproate, or carbamazepine was not superior to lithium, valproate, or carbamazepine alone in the reduction of YMRS total score. A possible explanation for the failure of this study was induction of risperidone and 9-hydroxy-risperidone clearance by carbamazepine, leading to subtherapeutic levels of risperidone and 9-hydroxy-risperidone. When the carbamazepine group was excluded in a post-hoc analysis, risperidone combined with lithium or valproate was superior to lithium or valproate alone in the reduction of YMRS total score.

Persistent aggression in dementia

The efficacy of risperidone in the treatment of Behavioural and Psychological Symptoms of Dementia (BPSD), which includes behavioural disturbances, such as aggressiveness, agitation, psychosis, activity, and affective disturbances was demonstrated in three double-blind, placebo-controlled studies in 1150 elderly patients with moderate to severe dementia. One study included fixed risperidone doses of 0.5, 1, and 2 mg/day. Two flexible-dose studies included risperidone dose groups in the range of 0.5 to 4 mg/day and 0.5 to 2 mg/day, respectively. Risperidone showed statistically significant and clinically important effectiveness in treating aggression and less consistently in treating agitation and psychosis in elderly dementia patients (as measured by the Behavioural Pathology in Alzheimer's Disease Rating Scale [BEHAVE-AD] and the Cohen-Mansfield Agitation Inventory [CMAI]). The treatment effect of risperidone was independent of Mini-Mental State Examination (MMSE) score (and consequently of the severity of dementia); of sedative properties of risperidone; of the presence or absence of psychosis; and of the type of dementia, Alzheimer's, vascular, or mixed. (See also section 4.4)

Conduct disorder

The efficacy of risperidone in the short-term treatment of disruptive behaviours was demonstrated in two double-blind placebo-controlled studies in approximately 240 patients 5 to 12 years of age with a DSM-IV diagnosis of disruptive behaviour disorders (DBD) and borderline intellectual functioning or mild or moderate mental retardation/learning disorder. In the two studies, risperidone 0.02 to 0.06 mg/kg/day was significantly superior to placebo on the pre-specified primary endpoint, i.e. the change from baseline in the Conduct Problem subscale of the Nisonger-Child Behaviour Rating Form (N-CBRF) at Week 6.

5.2 Pharmacokinetic properties

RISPERDAL orodispersible tablets and oral solutionare bio-equivalent to RISPERDAL film-coated tablets.

Risperidone is metabolised to 9-hydroxy-risperidone, which has a similar pharmacological activity to risperidone (see *Biotransformation and Elimination*).

Absorption

Risperidone is completely absorbed after oral administration, reaching peak plasma concentrations within 1 to 2 hours. The absolute oral bioavailability of risperidone is 70% (CV=25%). The relative oral bioavailability of risperidone from a tablet is 94% (CV=10%) compared with a solution. The absorption is not affected by food and thus risperidone can be given with or without meals. Steady-state of risperidone is reached within 1 day in most patients. Steady-state of 9-hydroxy-risperidone is reached within 4-5 days of dosing.

Distribution

Risperidone is rapidly distributed. The volume of distribution is 1-2 l/kg. In plasma, risperidone is bound to albumin and alpha$_1$-acid glycoprotein. The plasma protein binding of risperidone is 90%, that of 9-hydroxy-risperidone is 77%.

Biotransformation and elimination

Risperidone is metabolised by CYP 2D6 to 9-hydroxy-risperidone, which has a similar pharmacological activity as risperidone. Risperidone plus 9-hydroxy-risperidone form the active antipsychotic fraction. CYP 2D6 is subject to genetic polymorphism. Extensive CYP 2D6 metabolisers convert risperidone rapidly into 9-hydroxy-risperidone, whereas poor CYP 2D6 metabolisers convert it much more slowly. Although extensive metabolisers have lower risperidone and higher 9-hydroxy-risperidone concentrations than poor metabolisers, the pharmacokinetics of risperidone and 9-hydroxy-risperidone combined (i.e. the active antipsychotic fraction), after single and multiple doses, are similar in extensive and poor metabolisers of CYP 2D6.

Another metabolic pathway of risperidone is N-dealkylation. *In vitro* studies in human liver microsomes showed that risperidone at clinically relevant concentration does not substantially inhibit the metabolism of medicines metabolised by cytochrome P450 isozymes, including CYP 1A2, CYP 2A6, CYP 2C8/9/10, CYP 2D6, CYP 2E1, CYP 3A4, and CYP 3A5. One week after administration, 70% of the dose is excreted in the urine and 14% in the faeces. In urine, risperidone plus 9-hydroxy-risperidone represent 35-45% of the dose. The remainder is inactive metabolites. After oral administration to psychotic patients, risperidone is eliminated with a half-life of about 3 hours. The elimination half-life of 9-hydroxy-risperidone and of the active antipsychotic fraction is 24 hours.

Linearity

Risperidone plasma concentrations are dose-proportional within the therapeutic dose-range.

Elderly, hepatic and renal impairment

A single-dose study showed on average a 43% higher active antipsychotic fraction plasma concentrations, a 38% longer half-life and a reduced clearance of the active antipsychotic fraction by 30% in the elderly. Higher active antipsychotic fraction plasma concentrations and a reduced clearance of the active antipsychotic fraction by on average 60% were observed in patients with renal insufficiency. Risperidone plasma concentrations were normal in patients with liver insufficiency, but the mean free fraction of risperidone in plasma was increased by about 35%.

Paediatric patients

The pharmacokinetics of risperidone, 9-hydroxy-risperidone and the active antipsychotic fraction in children are similar to those in adults.

Gender, race and smoking habits

A population pharmacokinetic analysis revealed no apparent effect of gender, race or smoking habits on the pharmacokinetics of risperidone or the active antipsychotic fraction.

5.3 Preclinical safety data

In (sub)chronic toxicity studies, in which dosing was started in sexually immature rats and dogs, dose-dependant effects were present in male and female genital tract and mammary gland. These effects were related to the increased serum prolactin levels, resulting from the dopamine D_2-receptor blocking activity of risperidone. In addition, tissue culture studies suggest that cell growth in human breast tumours may be stimulated by prolactin. Risperidone was not teratogenic in rat and rabbit. In rat reproduction studies with risperidone, adverse effects were seen on mating behaviour of the parents, and on the birth weight and survival of the offspring. In rats, intrauterine exposure to risperidone was associated with cognitive deficits in adulthood. Other dopamine antagonists, when administered to pregnant animals, have caused negative effects on learning and motor development in the offspring. Risperidone was not genotoxic in a battery of tests. In oral carcinogenicity studies of risperidone in rats and mice, increases in pituitary gland adenomas (mouse), endocrine pancreas adenomas (rat), and mammary gland adenomas (both species) were seen. These tumours can be related to prolonged dopamine D_2 antagonism and hyperprolactinaemia. The relevance of these tumour findings in rodents in terms of human risk is unknown. In vitro and in vivo, animal models show that at high doses risperidone may cause QT interval prolongation, which has been associated with a theoretically increased risk of torsade de pointes in patients.

6. PHARMACEUTICAL PARTICULARS

6.1 List of excipients

RISPERDAL 0.5,1,2, 3, 4 & 6 mg film-coated tablets:

Tablet core

Lactose monohydrate

Maize starch

Cellulose microcrystalline (E460)

Hypromellose (E464)

Magnesium stearate

Silica colloidal anhydrous

Sodium laurilsulfate

Film-coating

Hypromellose (E464)

Propylene glycol (E490)

Titanium dioxide (E171): 0.5, 2, 3, 4 & 6 mg

Talc (E553B): 0.5, 2, 3, 4 & 6 mg

Red Ferric Oxide (E172): 0.5 mg

Orange yellow S aluminium lake (E110): 2 & 6 mg

Quinoline yellow (E104): 3, 4 & 6 mg

Indigotindisulfonate aluminium lake (E132): 4 mg

RISPERDAL oral solution:

Tartaric acid (E334)

Benzoic acid (E210)

Sodium hydroxide

Purified water

RISPERDAL 0.5,1, 2,3 & 4 mg orodispersible tablets:

Polacrilex resin

Gelatin (E485)

Mannitol (E421)

Glycine (E640)

Simeticone

Carbomer

Sodium hydroxide

Aspartame (E951)

Red Ferric Oxide (E172)

Peppermint oil

Xanthan Gum (2, 3 & 4 mg orodispersible tablets)

6.2 Incompatibilities

RISPERDAL oral solution: incompatible with tea.

6.3 Shelf life

2 years (0.5 & 6 mg film-coated tablet, 0.5,1, 2,3 & 4 mg orodispersible tablet)

3 years (1,2,3 &4 mg film-coated tablet).

RISPERDAL oral solution: 3 years. Chemical and physical in-use stability has been demonstrated for 3 months at 25°C.

6.4 Special precautions for storage

Do not store above 30°C.

RISPERDAL orodispersible tablets: Do not store above 30°C. Store in the original package.

RISPERDAL oral solution: Do not store above 30°C. Do not freeze. Store in the original package.

6.5 Nature and contents of container

Film-coated Tablets

Blister strips consisting of 200 μm polyvinylchloride (PVC)/ 25 μm low density polyethylene (LDPE)/90 g/m^2 polyvinylidene chloride (PVDC) and 20 μm aluminium foil. The strips are packed in cardboard cartons to contain either 6[a], 20, 28[b] or 60 tablets per pack.

[a]1mg film-coated tablet only

[b]6 mg film-coated tablet only

Oral Solution

Amber glass bottle with a plastic child-resistant and tamper-evident cap. Risperdal Liquid may be presented in bottle sizes of 30 and 100 ml.

The pipette supplied with the 30 ml bottle is calibrated in milligrams and milliliters with a minimum volume of 0.25 ml and a maximum volume of 3 ml. Calibration marks every 0.25 ml up to 3 ml are printed on this pipette.

The pipette supplied with the 100 ml bottle is calibrated in milligrams and milliliters with a minimum volume of 0.25 ml and a maximum volume of 3 ml. Calibration marks every 0.25 ml up to 3 ml are printed on this pipette.

Note: not all bottle sizes are marketed.

Orodispersible Tablets

Blister strips consisting of polychlorotrifluoroethylene/ polyvinylchloride/polyethylene film and aluminium foil (film/foil) or aluminium foil and aluminium foil (foil/foil). The strips are packed in cardboard cartons to contain 8, 28 or 56 tablets per pack.

6.6 Special precautions for disposal and other handling

Film-coated Tablets: No special requirement.

Oro-dispersible Tablets (see section 4.2)

Oral Solution

Fig. 1: The bottle comes with a child-resistant cap, and should be opened as follows:
- Push the plastic screw cap down while turning it counter clockwise.
- Remove the unscrewed cap.

Fig. 2: Insert the pipette into the bottle. While holding the bottom ring, pull the top ring up to the mark that corresponds to the number of millilitres or milligrams you need to give.

Fig.3: Holding the bottom ring, remove the entire pipette from the bottle. Empty the pipette into any non-alcoholic drink, except for tea, by sliding the upper ring down. Close the bottle. Rinse the pipette with some water.

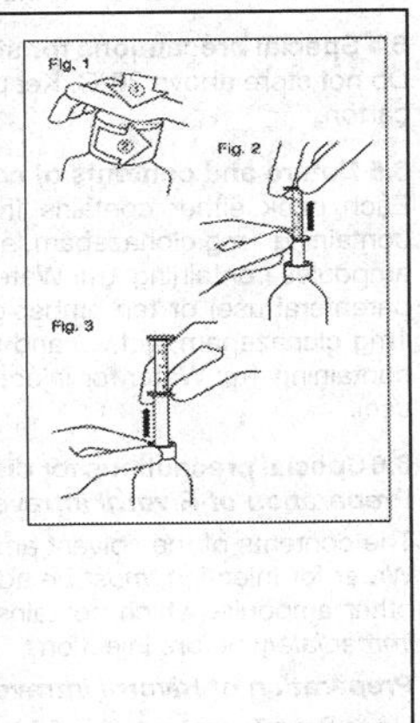

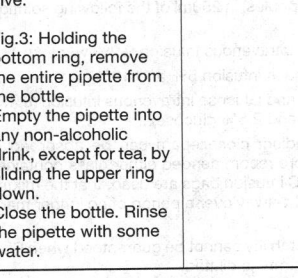

7. MARKETING AUTHORISATION HOLDER

Janssen-Cilag Ltd

50-100 Holmers Farm Way

High Wycombe

Buckinghamshire

HP12 4EG

UK

8. MARKETING AUTHORISATION NUMBER(S)

PL 00242/0347

PL 00242/0186

PL 00242/0187

PL 00242/0188

PL 00242/0189

PL 00242/0317

PL 00242/0199

PL 00242/0378

PL 00242/0379

PL 00242/0380

PL 00242/0407

PL 00242/0408

9. DATE OF FIRST AUTHORISATION/RENEWAL OF THE AUTHORISATION

30 June 2000/28 February 2004 (0.5 mg film-coated tablet)

8 December 1992/ 28 February 2004 (1,2,3 & 4 mg film-coated tablet)

15 July 1997/28 February 2004 (6 mg film-coated tablet)

7 January 2003/28 February 2004 (0.5 &1 mg orodispersible tablet)

7 December 2006 (3 & 4 mg orodispersible tablet)

21 November 1995/ 28 February 2004 (oral solution)

10. DATE OF REVISION OF THE TEXT

8 December 2008.

Rivotril Ampoules

(Roche Products Limited)

1. NAME OF THE MEDICINAL PRODUCT

Rivotril 1mg/ml Concentrate for Solution for Injection or Infusion

(Rivotril 1mg/ml Sterile Concentrate)

2. QUALITATIVE AND QUANTITATIVE COMPOSITION

Each ampoule contains 1mg of the active ingredient clonazepam.

For excipients, see 6.1.

3. PHARMACEUTICAL FORM

Concentrate for solution for injection or infusion.

Clear, colourless to slightly green-yellow solution.

4. CLINICAL PARTICULARS

4.1 Therapeutic indications

Administered intravenously, Rivotril quickly controls status epilepticus in all clinical forms.

4.2 Posology and method of administration

Rivotril sterile concentrate is for intravenous administration. For the treatment of status epilepticus, the dose and rate of administration are governed by the response of the patient.

Adults

1mg (one ampoule of active substance mixed with one ampoule of solvent for parenteral use) by slow intravenous injection.

Elderly

Care should be taken with the elderly.

Children

0.5mg (equivalent to half an ampoule of active substance mixed with half an ampoule of solvent for parenteral use) by slow intravenous injection.

Special dosage instructions

Rivotril can be administered with one or several other antiepileptic agents, in which case the dosage of each drug must be adjusted to achieve optimum effect.

As with all antiepileptic agents, treatment with Rivotril must not be stopped abruptly, but must be reduced in a stepwise fashion (see section *4.8 Undesirable effects*).

Mode of administration

Rivotril must be diluted prior to administration in order to avoid irritation of the veins, see section *6.6 Instructions for use/handling*.

Intravenous injection of Rivotril should be into a large vein of the antecubital fossa. The injection should be given slowly - in adults, the rate of injection must not exceed 0.25mg – 0.5mg (0.5 – 1.0ml of the prepared solution) per minute – and should be administered with continuous monitoring of EEG, respiration and blood pressure. This will greatly diminish the rare possibility of hypotension or apnoea occurring. Nevertheless, facilities for resuscitation should always be available. A total dose of 20mg should not be exceeded.

Rivotril sterile concentrate may be diluted when given in intravenous infusions of saline or glucose, such as are customary in the treatment of status epilepticus, see section *6.6 Instructions for use/handling*.

4.3 Contraindications

Patients with known sensitivity to benzodiazepines or any of the drugs excipients; acute pulmonary insufficiency, severe respiratory insufficiency, sleep apnoea syndrome, myasthenia gravis, severe hepatic insufficiency.

Rivotril sterile concentrate contains benzyl alcohol. Since there have been reports of permanent neuropsychiatric deficits and multiple system organ failure associated with benzyl alcohol, administration to neonates, and especially to premature infants, must be avoided.

4.4 Special warnings and precautions for use

Suicidal ideation and behaviour have been reported in patients treated with anti-epileptic agents in several indications. A meta-analysis of randomised placebo controlled trials of anti-epileptic drugs has also shown a small increased risk of suicidal ideation and behaviour. The mechanism of this risk is not known and the available data do not exclude the possibility of an increased risk for clonazepam.

Therefore patients should be monitored for signs of suicidal ideation and behaviours and appropriate treatment should be considered. Patients (and caregivers of patients) should be advised to seek medical advice should signs of suicidal ideation or behaviour emerge.

Patients with a history of depression and/or suicide attempts should be kept under close supervision.

Rivotril should be used with caution in patients with chronic pulmonary insufficiency, or with impairment of renal or hepatic function, and in the elderly or the debilitated. In these cases dosage should generally be reduced.

As with all other anti-epileptic drugs, treatment with Rivotril even if of short duration, must not be abruptly interrupted, but must be withdrawn by gradually reducing the dose in view of the risk of precipitating status epilepticus. This precaution must also be taken when withdrawing another drug while the patient is still receiving Rivotril therapy.

Rivotril may be used only with particular caution in patients with spinal or cerebellar ataxia, in the event of acute intoxication with alcohol or drugs and in patients with severe liver damage (e.g. cirrhosis of the liver).

Benzodiazepines should be used with extreme caution in patients with a history of alcohol or drug abuse.

In infants and small children Rivotril may cause increased production of saliva and bronchial secretion. Therefore special attention must be paid to maintaining patency of the airways.

The dosage of Rivotril must be carefully adjusted to individual requirements in patients with pre-existing disease of the respiratory system (e.g. chronic obstructive pulmonary disease) or liver and in patients undergoing treatment with other centrally acting medications or anticonvulsant (antiepileptic) agents (see section *4.5 Interaction with other medicaments and other forms of interaction*).

Like all drugs of this type, Rivotril may, depending on dosage, administration and individual susceptibility, modify the patient's reactions (e.g. driving ability, behaviour in traffic).

In cases of loss or bereavement, psychological adjustment may be inhibited by benzodiazepines.

During I.V. administration, a vein of sufficient calibre must be chosen and the injection administered very slowly, with continuous monitoring of respiration and blood pressure. If the injection is rapid or the calibre of the vein is insufficient, there is a risk of thrombophlebitis, which may in turn lead to thrombosis.

4.5 Interaction with other medicinal products and other forms of interaction

Since alcohol can provoke epileptic seizures, irrespective of therapy, patients must under no circumstances drink alcohol while under treatment. In combination with Rivotril, alcohol may modify the effects of the drug, compromise the success of therapy or give rise to unpredictable side-effects.

When Rivotril is used in conjunction with other anti-epileptic drugs, side-effects such as sedation and apathy, and toxicity may be more evident, particularly with hydantoins or phenobarbital and combinations including them. This requires extra care in adjusting dosage in the initial stages of treatment. The combination of Rivotril and sodium valproate has, rarely, been associated with the development of absence status epilepticus. Although some patients tolerate and benefit from this combination of drugs, this potential hazard should be borne in mind when its use is considered.

The antiepileptic drugs phenytoin, phenobarbital, carbamazepine and valproate may induce the metabolism of clonazepam causing higher clearance and lower plasma concentrations of the latter during combined treatment.

The selective serotonine reuptake inhibitors sertraline and fluoxetine do not affect the pharmacokinetics of clonazepam when administered concomitantly.

Known inhibitors of hepatic enzymes, e.g. cimetidine, have been shown to reduce the clearance of benzodiazepines and may potentiate their action and known inducers of hepatic enzymes, e.g. rifampicin, may increase the clearance of benzodiazepines.

In concurrent treatment with phenytoin or primidone, a change, usually a rise in the serum concentration of these two substances has occasionally been observed.

Concurrent use of Rivotril and other centrally acting medications, e.g. other anticonvulsant (antiepileptic) agents, anaesthetics, hypnotics, psychoactive drugs and some analgesics as well as muscle-relaxants may result in mutual potentiation of drug effects. This is especially true in the presence of alcohol. In combination therapy with centrally-acting medications, the dosage of each drug must be adjusted to achieve the optimum effect.

4.6 Pregnancy and lactation

Preclinical studies in animals have shown reproductive toxicity (see section *5.3 Preclinical safety data*). From epidemiological evaluations there is evidence that anticonvulsant drugs act as teratogens.

Rivotril has harmful pharmacological effects on pregnancy and the foetus/newborn child. Administration of high doses in the last trimester of pregnancy or during labour can cause irregularities in the heart beat of the unborn child and hypothermia, hypotonia, mild respiratory depression and poor sucking in the neonate. Infants born to mothers who took benzodiazepines chronically during the later stages of pregnancy may have developed physical dependence and may be at some risk for developing withdrawal symptoms in the post-natal period. Therefore Rivotril should not be used in pregnancy unless clearly necessary.

The active ingredient of Rivotril has been found to pass into the maternal milk in small amounts. Therefore Rivotril should not be used in mothers who breastfeed unless clearly necessary.

4.7 Effects on ability to drive and use machines

As a general rule, epileptic patients are not allowed to drive. Even when adequately controlled on Rivotril, it should be remembered that any increase in dosage or alteration in timings of dosage may modify patients' reactions, depending on individual susceptibility. Even if taken as directed, clonazepam can slow reactions to such an extent that the ability to drive a vehicle or operate machinery is impaired. This effect is aggravated by consumption of alcohol. Driving, operating machinery and other hazardous activities should therefore be avoided altogether or at least during the first few days of treatment. The decision on this question rests with the patient's physician and should be based on the patient's response to treatment and the dosage involved.

4.8 Undesirable effects

The side-effects observed consist of fatigue, muscle weakness, dizziness, ataxia, light-headedness, somnolence, occasional muscular hypotonia and co-ordination disturbances. Such effects are usually transitory and disappear spontaneously as treatment continues or with dosage reduction. They tend to occur early in treatment and can be greatly reduced, if not avoided, by commencing with low dosages followed by progressive increases.

Poor concentration, restlessness, confusion and disorientation have been observed. Anterograde amnesia may occur using benzodiazepines at therapeutic dosage, the risk increasing at higher dosages. Amnestic effects may be associated with inappropriate behaviour.

Depression may occur in patients treated with Rivotril, but it may be also associated with the underlying disease.

In rare cases, urticaria, pruritus, transient hair loss, pigmentation changes, nausea, gastrointestinal symptoms, headache, decrease in sexual drive (loss of libido), impotence and urinary incontinence may occur. Isolated cases of reversible development of premature secondary sex characteristics in children (incomplete precocious puberty) have been reported. Allergic reactions and a very few cases of anaphylaxis and angioedema have been reported to occur with benzodiazepines.

Particularly in long-term or high-dose treatment, reversible disorders such as a slowing or slurring of speech (dysarthria), reduced co-ordination of movements and gait (ataxia) and disorders of vision (double vision, nystagmus) may occur.

Rarely respiratory depression may occur with intravenous Rivotril, particularly if other depressant drugs have been administered. As a rule, this effect can be avoided by careful adjustment of the dose in individual requirements.

Use of benzodiazepines may lead to the development of physical and psychological dependence upon these products. The risk of dependence increases with dose and duration of treatment and is particularly pronounced in predisposed patients with a history of alcoholism or drug abuse.

Once physical dependence has developed, abrupt termination of treatment will be accompanied by withdrawal symptoms. During long-term treatment, withdrawal symptoms may develop, especially with high doses or if the daily dose is reduced rapidly or abruptly discontinued. The symptoms include tremor, sweating, agitation, sleep disturbances and anxiety, headaches, muscle pain, extreme anxiety, tension, restlessness, confusion, irritability and epileptic seizures which may be associated with the underlying disease. In severe cases the following symptoms may occur: derealisation, depersonalisation, hyperacusis, numbness and tingling of the extremities, hypersensitivity to light, noise and physical contact or hallucinations. Since the risk of withdrawal symptoms is greater after abrupt discontinuation of treatment, abrupt withdrawal of the drug should therefore be avoided and treatment - even if only of short duration - should be terminated by gradually reducing the daily dose.

In infants and small children, and particularly those with a degree of mental impairment, Rivotril may give rise to salivary or bronchial hypersecretion with drooling. Supervision of the airway may be required.

With certain forms of epilepsy, an increase in the frequency of seizures during long-term treatment is possible.

As with other benzodiazepines, isolated cases of blood dyscrasias and abnormal liver function tests have been reported.

Rivotril generally has a beneficial effect on behaviour disturbances in epileptic patients. In certain cases, paradoxical effects such as aggressiveness, excitability, nervousness, hostility, anxiety, sleep disturbances, nightmares, vivid dreams, irritability, agitation, psychotic disorders and activation of new types of seizures may be precipitated. If these occur, the benefit of continuing the drug should be weighed against the adverse effect. The addition to the regimen of another suitable drug may be necessary or, in some cases, it may be advisable to discontinue Rivotril therapy.

Although Rivotril has been given uneventfully to patients with porphyria, rarely it may induce convulsions in these patients.

During IV administration, a vein of sufficient calibre must be chosen and the injection administered very slowly, with continuous monitoring of respiration and blood pressure. In adults, the rate of injection must not exceed 0.25 – 0.5mg (0.5 – 1ml of the prepared solution) per minute (see section *4.2*). If the injection is rapid or the calibre of the vein is insufficient, there is a risk of thrombophlebitis, which may in turn lead to thrombosis.

An increased risk of falls and fractures has been recorded in elderly benzodiazepine users.

4.9 Overdose

As with other benzodiazepine drugs, overdosage should not present undue problems of management or threat to life. Patients have recovered from overdoses in excess of 60mg without special treatment. Severe somnolence with muscle hypotonia will be present.

Symptoms:

The symptoms of overdosage or intoxication vary greatly from person to person depending on age, bodyweight and individual response. Benzodiazepines commonly cause drowsiness, ataxia, dysarthria and nystagmus. Overdose of Rivotril is seldom life-threatening if the drug is taken alone, but may lead to coma, areflexia, apnoea, hypotension and cardiorespiratory depression. Coma usually lasts only a few hours but in elderly people it may be more protracted and cyclical. Benzodiazepine respiratory depressant effects are more serious in patients with severe chronic obstructive airways disease.

Benzodiazepines potentiate the effects of other central nervous system depressants, including alcohol.

Management:

1. Maintain a clear airway and adequate ventilation if indicated.

2. The benefit of gastric decontamination is uncertain. Consider activated charcoal (50g for an adult, 10-15g for a child) in adults or children who have taken more than 0.4mg/kg within 1 hour, provided they are not too drowsy.

3. Gastric lavage is unnecessary if these drugs have been taken alone.

4. Patients who are asymptomatic at 4 hours are unlikely to develop symptoms.

5. Supportive measures as indicated by the patient's clinical state. In particular, patients may require symptomatic treatment for cardiorespiratory effects or central nervous system effects.

6. Flumazenil (Anexate), a benzodiazepine antagonist is available but should rarely be required. It has a short half-life (about an hour) Flumazenil is **NOT TO BE USED IN MIXED OVERDOSE OR AS A "DIAGNOSTIC TEST"** (see separate prescribing information).

Warning

The use of flumazenil is not recommended in epileptic patients who have been receiving benzodiazepine treatment for a prolonged period. Although flumazenil exerts a slight intrinsic anticonvulsant effect, its abrupt suppression of the protective effect of a benzodiazepine agonist can give rise to convulsions in epileptic patients.

If excitation occurs, barbiturates should not be used.

5. PHARMACOLOGICAL PROPERTIES

5.1 Pharmacodynamic properties

Clonazepam exhibits pharmacological properties which are common to benzodiazepines and include anticonvulsive, sedative, muscle relaxing and anxiolytic effects. Animal data and electroencephalographic investigations in man have shown that clonazepam rapidly suppresses many types of paroxysmal activity including the spike and wave discharge in absences seizures (petit mal), slow spike wave, generalised spike wave, spikes with temporal or other locations as well as irregular spikes and waves.

Generalised EEG abnormalities are more readily suppressed by clonazepam than are focal EEG abnormalities such as focal spikes. Clonazepam has beneficial effects in generalised and focal epilepsies.

5.2 Pharmacokinetic properties

Absorption

Clonazepam is quickly and completely absorbed after oral administration of Rivotril. Peak plasma concentrations are reached in most cases within 1 - 4 hours after an oral dose. Bioavailability is 90% after oral administration.

Routine monitoring of plasma concentrations of Rivotril is of unproven value since this does not appear to correlate well with either therapeutic response or side-effects.

Distribution

The mean volume of distribution of clonazepam is estimated at about 3 l/kg. Clonazepam must be assumed to cross the placental barrier and has been detected in maternal milk.

Metabolism

The biotransformation of clonazepam involves oxidative hydroxylation and reduction of the 7-nitro group by the liver with formation of 7-amino or 7-acetylamino compounds, with trace amounts of 3-hydroxy derivatives of all three compounds, and their glucuronide and sulphate conjugates. The nitro compounds are pharmacologically active, whereas the amino compounds are not.

Within 4 - 10 days 50 - 70% of the total radioactivity of a radiolabeled oral dose of clonazepam is excreted in the urine and 10 - 30% in the faeces, almost exclusively in the form of free or conjugated metabolites. Less than 0.5% appears as unchanged clonazepam in the urine.

Elimination

The elimination half-life is between 20 and 60 hours (mean 30 hours).

Pharmacokinetics in special clinical situations

Based on kinetic criteria no dose adjustment is required in patients with renal failure.

5.3 Preclinical safety data

In pre-clinical murine studies there was at least a two fold increase in teratogenic birth defects at dose levels of 3, 9 and 18 times the human therapeutic dose compared to the controls.

6. PHARMACEUTICAL PARTICULARS

6.1 List of excipients

Active substance ampoule: Ethanol absolute, glacial acetic acid, benzyl alcohol, propylene glycol, nitrogen pure.

Solvent ampoule: Water for injections.

6.2 Incompatibilities

Do not prepare Rivotril infusions using sodium bicarbonate solution, as otherwise precipitation of the solution may occur.

6.3 Shelf life

Unopened ampoules: 60 months.

Shelf-life of diluted product: From a chemical and physical stability point of view the diluted product is stable for up to 12 hours. However, it should be used immediately after dilution in order to reduce the possibility of microbial contamination unless it is diluted under validated aseptic conditions. See section 6.6 for instructions for dilution.

6.4 Special precautions for storage

Do not store above 30°C. Keep the ampoules in the outer carton.

6.5 Nature and contents of container

Each pack either contains five amber glass ampoules containing 1mg clonazepam (active) and five amber glass ampoules containing 1ml Water for Injections (solvent for parenteral use) or ten amber glass ampoules containing 1mg clonazepam (active) and ten amber glass ampoules containing 1ml Water for Injections (solvent for parenteral use).

6.6 Special precautions for disposal and other handling

Preparation of Rivotril intravenous injection:

The contents of the solvent ampoule, which contains 1ml Water for Injection, *must* be added to the contents of the other ampoule, which contains 1mg clonazepam in 1ml, *immediately* before injection.

Preparation of Rivotril intravenous infusion:

Up to 3mg (3 ampoules) in 250ml of the following solutions is permissible:

Sodium chloride intravenous infusion 0.9% w/v

Glucose intravenous infusion 5% and 10%

Sodium chloride and Glucose intravenous infusion (0.45% sodium chloride and 2.5% glucose)

The active ingredient clonazepam can be absorbed on PVC. It is therefore recommended either glass containers be used or, if PVC infusion bags are used, that the mixture be infused straight-away over a period of no longer than 2 hours.

Maintenance of stability cannot be guaranteed when Rivotril sterile concentrate is diluted.

7. MARKETING AUTHORISATION HOLDER

Roche Products Limited
6 Falcon Way
Shire Park
Welwyn Garden City
AL7 1TW
United Kingdom

8. MARKETING AUTHORISATION NUMBER(S)

PL 0031/0078R

9. DATE OF FIRST AUTHORISATION/RENEWAL OF THE AUTHORISATION

20 February 1991/24 September 1996

10. DATE OF REVISION OF THE TEXT

October 2008

Rivotril is a registered trade mark

Item Code

Rivotril Tablets

(Roche Products Limited)

1. NAME OF THE MEDICINAL PRODUCT

Rivotril 0.5mg Tablets

Rivotril 2mg Tablets

2. QUALITATIVE AND QUANTITATIVE COMPOSITION

Rivotril 0.5mg Tablets:

Each tablet contains 0.5mg clonazepam.

Excipients: Also contains 40mg lactose monohydrate.

Rivotril 2mg Tablets:

Each tablet contains 2mg clonazepam.

Excipients: Also contains 121.5mg lactose anhydrous.

For excipients, see 6.1.

3. PHARMACEUTICAL FORM

Tablets.

Rivotril 0.5mg Tablets:

Round, dull pinkish-buff tablets with 'ROCHE 0,5' imprinted on one face and a single break mark on the other.

The Tablets can be broken into equal halves to facilitate dosing.

Rivotril 2mg Tablets:

Round, white tablets with 'ROCHE 2' imprinted on one face and cross break marks on the other.

The tablets can be broken into equal halves or quarters to facilitate dosing.

4. CLINICAL PARTICULARS

4.1 Therapeutic indications

Tablets: All clinical forms of epileptic disease and seizures in infants, children and adults, especially absence seizures (petit mal) including atypical absence; primary or secondarily generalised tonic-clonic (grand mal), tonic or clonic seizures; partial (focal) seizures with elementary or complex symptomatology; various forms of myoclonic seizures, myoclonus and associated abnormal movements.

4.2 Posology and method of administration

The scored 0.5mg tablets facilitate the administration of lower daily doses in the initial stages of treatment.

Adults

Initial dosage should not exceed 1mg/day. The maintenance dosage for adults normally falls within the range 4 to 8mg.

Elderly

The elderly are particularly sensitive to the effects of centrally depressant drugs and may experience confusion. It is recommended that the initial dosage of Rivotril should not exceed 0.5mg/day.

These are total daily dosages which should be divided into 3 or 4 doses taken at intervals throughout the day. If necessary, larger doses may be given at the discretion of the physician, up to a maximum of 20mg daily. The maintenance dose should be attained after 2 to 4 weeks of treatment.

Infants and children

To ensure optimum dosage adjustment, children should be given the 0.5mg tablets.

Initial dosage should not exceed 0.25mg/day for infants and small children (1 to 5 years) and 0.5mg/day for older children. The maintenance dosage normally falls within the ranges:

School children (5 to 12 years) 3 to 6mg

Small children (1 to 5 years) 1 to 3mg

Infants (0 to 1 year) 0.5 to 1mg

In some forms of childhood epilepsy, certain patients may cease to be adequately controlled by Rivotril. Control may be re-established by increasing the dose, or interrupting treatment with Rivotril for 2 or 3 weeks. During the interruption in therapy, careful observation and other drugs may be needed.

Mode of administration

Treatment should be started with low doses. The dose may be increased progressively until the maintenance dose suited to the individual patient has been found.

The dosage of Rivotril must be adjusted to the needs of each individual and depends on the individual response to therapy. The maintenance dosage must be determined according to clinical response and tolerance.

The daily dose should be divided into 3 equal doses. If doses are not equally divided, the largest dose should be given before retiring. Once the maintenance dose level has been reached, the daily amount may be given in a single dose in the evening.

Simultaneous administration of more than one antiepileptic drug is a common practice in the treatment of epilepsy and may be undertaken with Rivotril. The dosage of each drug may be required to be adjusted to obtain the optimum effect. If status epilepticus occurs in a patient receiving oral Rivotril, intravenous Rivotril may still control the status. Before adding Rivotril to an existing anticonvulsant regimen, it should be considered that the use of multiple anticonvulsants may result in an increase of undesired effects.

4.3 Contraindications

Patients with known sensitivity to benzodiazepines; or any of the drugs excipients; acute pulmonary insufficiency; severe respiratory insufficiency, sleep apnoea syndrome, myasthenia gravis, severe hepatic insufficiency.

4.4 Special warnings and precautions for use

Suicidal ideation and behaviour have been reported in patients treated with anti-epileptic agents in several indications. A meta-analysis of randomised placebo controlled trials of anti-epileptic drugs has also shown a small increased risk of suicidal ideation and behaviour. The mechanism of this risk is not known and the available data do not exclude the possibility of an increased risk for clonazepam.

Therefore patients should be monitored for signs of suicidal ideation and behaviours and appropriate treatment should be considered. Patients (and caregivers of patients) should be advised to seek medical advice should signs of suicidal ideation or behaviour emerge.

Patients with a history of depression and/or suicide attempts should be kept under close supervision.

Rivotril should be used with caution in patients with chronic pulmonary insufficiency, or with impairment of renal or hepatic function, and in the elderly or the debilitated. In these cases dosage should generally be reduced.

As with all other antiepileptic drugs, treatment with Rivotril even if of short duration, must not be abruptly interrupted, but must be withdrawn by gradually reducing the dose in view of the risk of precipitating status epilepticus. This precaution must also be taken when withdrawing another drug while the patient is still receiving Rivotril therapy.

Prolonged use of benzodiazepines may result in dependence development with withdrawal symptoms on cessation of use.

Rivotril may be used only with particular caution in patients with spinal or cerebellar ataxia, in the event of acute intoxication with alcohol or drugs and in patients with severe liver damage (e.g. cirrhosis of the liver).

Benzodiazepines should be used with extreme caution in patients with a history of alcohol or drug abuse.

In infants and small children Rivotril may cause increased production of saliva and bronchial secretion. Therefore special attention must be paid to maintaining patency of the airways.

The dosage of Rivotril must be carefully adjusted to individual requirements in patients with pre-existing disease of the respiratory system (e.g. chronic obstructive pulmonary disease) or liver and in patients undergoing treatment with other centrally acting medications or anticonvulsant (antiepileptic) agents (see *section 4.5*).

Like all drugs of this type, Rivotril may, depending on dosage, administration and individual susceptibility, modify the patient's reactions (e.g. driving ability, behaviour in traffic).

In cases of loss or bereavement, psychological adjustment may be inhibited by benzodiazepines.

Patients with rare hereditary problems of galactose intolerance, the Lapp lactase deficiency or glucose-galactose malabsorption, should not take this medicine.

4.5 Interaction with other medicinal products and other forms of interaction

Since alcohol can provoke epileptic seizures, irrespective of therapy, patients must under no circumstances drink alcohol while under treatment. In combination with Rivotril, alcohol may modify the effects of the drug, compromise the success of therapy or give rise to unpredictable side-effects.

When Rivotril is used in conjunction with other antiepileptic drugs, side-effects such as sedation and apathy, and toxicity may be more evident, particularly with hydantoins or phenobarbital and combinations including them. This requires extra care in adjusting dosage in the initial stages of treatment. The combination of Rivotril and sodium valproate has, rarely, been associated with the development of absence status epilepticus. Although some patients tolerate and benefit from this combination of drugs, this potential hazard should be borne in mind when its use is considered.

The antiepileptic drugs phenytoin, phenobarbital, carbamazepine and valproate may induce the metabolism of clonazepam causing higher clearance and lower plasma concentrations of the latter during combined treatment.

The selective serotonine reuptake inhibitors sertraline and fluoxetine do not affect the pharmacokinetics of clonazepam when administered concomitantly.

Known inhibitors of hepatic enzymes, e.g. cimetidine, have been shown to reduce the clearance of benzodiazepines and may potentiate their action and known inducers of hepatic enzymes, e.g. rifampicin, may increase the clearance of benzodiazepines.

In concurrent treatment with phenytoin or primidone, a change, usually a rise in the serum concentration of these two substances has occasionally been observed.

Concurrent use of Rivotril and other centrally acting medications, e.g. other anticonvulsant (antiepileptic) agents, anaesthetics, hypnotics, psychoactive drugs and some analgesics as well as muscle-relaxants may result in mutual potentiation of drug effects. This is especially true in the presence of alcohol. In combination therapy with centrally-acting medications, the dosage of each drug must be adjusted to achieve the optimum effect.

4.6 Pregnancy and lactation

Preclinical studies in animals have shown reproductive toxicity (see *section 5.3 Preclinical safety data*). From epidemiological evaluations there is evidence that anticonvulsant drugs act as teratogens.

Rivotril has harmful pharmacological effects on pregnancy and the foetus/newborn child. Administration of high doses in the last trimester of pregnancy or during labour can cause irregularities in the heart beat of the unborn child and hypothermia, hypotonia, mild respiratory depression and poor sucking in the neonate. Infants born to mothers who took benzodiazepines chronically during the later stages of pregnancy may have developed physical dependence and may be at some risk for developing withdrawal symptoms in the post-natal period. Therefore Rivotril should not be used in pregnancy unless clearly necessary.

The active ingredient of Rivotril has been found to pass into the maternal milk in small amounts. Therefore Rivotril should not be used in mothers who breastfeed unless clearly necessary.

4.7 Effects on ability to drive and use machines

As a general rule, epileptic patients are not allowed to drive. Even when adequately controlled on Rivotril, it should be remembered that any increase in dosage or alteration in timings of dosage may modify patients' reactions, depending on individual susceptibility. Even if taken as directed, clonazepam can slow reactions to such an extent that the ability to drive a vehicle or operate machinery is impaired. This effect is aggravated by consumption of alcohol. Driving, operating machinery and other hazardous activities should therefore be avoided altogether or at least during the first few days of treatment. The decision on this question rests with the patient's physician and should be based on the patient's response to treatment and the dosage involved.

4.8 Undesirable effects

The side-effects observed consist of fatigue, muscle weakness, dizziness, ataxia, light-headedness, somnolence, occasional muscular hypotonia and co-ordination disturbances. Such effects are usually transitory and disappear spontaneously as treatment continues or with dosage reduction. They tend to occur early in treatment and can be greatly reduced, if not avoided, by commencing with low dosages followed by progressive increases.

Poor concentration, restlessness, confusion and disorientation have been observed. Anterograde amnesia may occur using benzodiazepines at therapeutic dosage, the risk increasing at higher dosages. Amnestic effects may be associated with inappropriate behaviour.

Depression may occur in patients treated with Rivotril, but it may be also associated with the underlying disease.

In rare cases, urticaria, pruritus, transient hair loss, pigmentation changes, nausea, gastrointestinal symptoms, headache, decrease in sexual drive (loss of libido), impotence and urinary incontinence may occur. Isolated cases of reversible development of premature secondary sex characteristics in children (incomplete precocious puberty) have been reported. Allergic reactions and a very few cases of anaphylaxis and angioedema have been reported to occur with benzodiazepines.

Particularly in long-term or high-dose treatment, reversible disorders such as a slowing or slurring of speech (dysarthria), reduced co-ordination of movements and gait (ataxia) and disorders of vision (double vision, nystagmus) may occur.

Rarely respiratory depression may occur with intravenous Rivotril, particularly if other depressant drugs have been administered. As a rule, this effect can be avoided by careful adjustment of the dose in individual requirements.

Use of benzodiazepines may lead to the development of physical and psychological dependence upon these products. The risk of dependence increases with dose and duration of treatment and is particularly pronounced in predisposed patients with a history of alcoholism or drug abuse.

Once physical dependence has developed, abrupt termination of treatment will be accompanied by withdrawal symptoms. During long-term treatment, withdrawal symptoms may develop, especially with high doses or if the daily dose is reduced rapidly or abruptly discontinued. The symptoms include tremor, sweating, agitation, sleep disturbances and anxiety, headaches, muscle pain, extreme anxiety, tension, restlessness, confusion, irritability and epileptic seizures which may be associated with the underlying disease. In severe cases the following symptoms may occur: derealisation, depersonalisation, hyperacusis, numbness and tingling of the extremities, hypersensitivity to light, noise and physical contact or hallucinations. Since the risk of withdrawal symptoms is greater after abrupt discontinuation of treatment, abrupt withdrawal of the drug should therefore be avoided and treatment - even if only of short duration - should be terminated by gradually reducing the daily dose.

In infants and small children, and particularly those with a degree of mental impairment, Rivotril may give rise to salivary or bronchial hypersecretion with drooling. Supervision of the airway may be required.

With certain forms of epilepsy, an increase in the frequency of seizures during long-term treatment is possible.

As with other benzodiazepines, isolated cases of blood dyscrasias and abnormal liver function tests have been reported.

Rivotril generally has a beneficial effect on behaviour disturbances in epileptic patients. In certain cases, paradoxical effects such as aggressiveness, excitability, nervousness, hostility, anxiety, sleep disturbances, nightmares, vivid dreams, irritability, agitation, psychotic disorders and activation of new types of seizures may be precipitated. If these occur, the benefit of continuing the drug should be weighed against the adverse effect. The addition to the regimen of another suitable drug may be necessary or, in some cases, it may be advisable to discontinue Rivotril therapy.

Although Rivotril has been given uneventfully to patients with porphyria, rarely it may induce convulsions in these patients.

An increased risk of falls and fractures has been recorded in elderly benzodiazepine users.

4.9 Overdose

As with other benzodiazepine drugs, overdosage should not present undue problems of management or threat to life. Patients have recovered from overdoses in excess of 60mg without special treatment. Severe somnolence with muscle hypotonia will be present.

Symptoms:

The symptoms of overdosage or intoxication vary greatly from person to person depending on age, bodyweight and individual response. Benzodiazepines commonly cause drowsiness, ataxia, dysarthria and nystagmus. Overdose of Rivotril is seldom life-threatening if the drug is taken alone, but may lead to coma, areflexia, apnoea, hypotension and cardiorespiratory depression. Coma usually lasts only a few hours but in elderly people it may be more protracted and cyclical. Benzodiazepine respiratory depressant effects are more serious in patients with severe chronic obstructive airways disease.

Benzodiazepines potentiate the effects of other central nervous system depressants, including alcohol.

Management:

1. Maintain a clear airway and adequate ventilation if indicated.

2. The benefit of gastric decontamination is uncertain. Consider activated charcoal (50g for an adult, 10-15g for a child) in adults or children who have taken more than 0.4mg/kg within 1 hour, provided they are not too drowsy.

3. Gastric lavage is unnecessary if these drugs have been taken alone.

4. Patients who are asymptomatic at 4 hours are unlikely to develop symptoms.

5. Supportive measures as indicated by the patient's clinical state. In particular, patients may require symptomatic treatment for cardiorespiratory effects or central nervous system effects.

6. Flumazenil (Anexate), a benzodiazepine antagonist is available but should rarely be required. It has a short half-life (about an hour). Flumazenil is **NOT TO BE USED IN MIXED OVERDOSE OR AS A "DIAGNOSTIC TEST"** (see separate prescribing information).

Warning

The use of flumazenil is not recommended in epileptic patients who have been receiving benzodiazepine treatment for a prolonged period. Although flumazenil exerts a slight intrinsic anticonvulsant effect, its abrupt suppression of the protective effect of a benzodiazepine agonist can give rise to convulsions in epileptic patients.

If excitation occurs, barbiturates should not be used.

5. PHARMACOLOGICAL PROPERTIES

5.1 Pharmacodynamic properties

Clonazepam exhibits pharmacological properties which are common to benzodiazepines and include anticonvulsive, sedative, muscle relaxing and anxiolytic effects. Animal data and electroencephalographic investigations in man have shown that clonazepam rapidly suppresses many types of paroxysmal activity including the spike and wave discharge in absence seizures (petit mal), slow spike wave, generalised spike wave, spikes with temporal or other locations as well as irregular spikes and waves.

Generalised EEG abnormalities are more readily suppressed by clonazepam than are focal EEG abnormalities such as focal spikes. Clonazepam has beneficial effects in generalised and focal epilepsies.

5.2 Pharmacokinetic properties

Absorption

Clonazepam is quickly and completely absorbed after oral administration of Rivotril. Peak plasma concentrations are reached in most cases within 1 - 4 hours after an oral dose. Bioavailability is 90% after oral administration.

Routine monitoring of plasma concentrations of Rivotril is of unproven value since this does not appear to correlate well with either therapeutic response or side-effects.

Distribution

The mean volume of distribution of clonazepam is estimated at about 3 l/kg. Clonazepam must be assumed to cross the placental barrier and has been detected in maternal milk.

Metabolism

The biotransformation of clonazepam involves oxidative hydroxylation and reduction of the 7-nitro group by the liver with formation of 7-amino or 7-acetylamino compounds, with trace amounts of 3-hydroxy derivatives of all three compounds, and their glucuronide and sulphate conjugates. The nitro compounds are pharmacologically active, whereas the amino compounds are not.

Within 4 - 10 days 50 - 70% of the total radioactivity of a radiolabelled oral dose of clonazepam is excreted in the urine and 10 - 30% in the faeces, almost exclusively in the form of free or conjugated metabolites. Less than 0.5% appears as unchanged clonazepam in the urine.

Elimination

The elimination half-life is between 20 and 60 hours (mean 30 hours).

Pharmacokinetics in special clinical situations

Based on kinetic criteria no dose adjustment is required in patients with renal failure.

5.3 Preclinical safety data

In preclinical murine studies there was at least a two fold increase in teratogenic birth defects at dose levels of 3, 9 and 18 times the human therapeutic dose compared to the controls.

6. PHARMACEUTICAL PARTICULARS

6.1 List of excipients

Rivotril 0.5mg tablets:

Lactose (monohydrate)

Maize starch

Pregelatinised potato starch

Talc

Magnesium stearate

Deionised water

Dye iron oxide red E172

Dye iron oxide yellow E172.

Rivotril 2mg tablets:

Lactose (anhydrous)

Pregelatinised maize starch

Magnesium stearate

Microcrystalline cellulose.

6.2 Incompatibilities

Not applicable.

6.3 Shelf life

60 months

6.4 Special precautions for storage

Store in the original container and in the outer carton, in order to protect from light.

6.5 Nature and contents of container

Rivotril 0.5mg Tablets:

Amber glass bottles with polyethylene screw closures, containing 50, 100 or 150 tablets.

Rivotril 2mg Tablets:

Amber glass bottles with polyethylene screw closures, containing 30 or 100 tablets.

Not all pack sizes may be marketed.

6.6 Special precautions for disposal and other handling

There are no special instructions.

Administrative Data

7. MARKETING AUTHORISATION HOLDER

Roche Products Limited
6 Falcon Way
Shire Park
Welwyn Garden City
AL7 1TW
United Kingdom

8. MARKETING AUTHORISATION NUMBER(S)

Rivotril 0.5mg Tablets: PL 00031/0076R

Rivotril 2mg Tablets: PL 00031/0077R

9. DATE OF FIRST AUTHORISATION/RENEWAL OF THE AUTHORISATION

26 July 1983/27 May 2005

10. DATE OF REVISION OF THE TEXT

October 2008

legal status

POM

Rivotril is a registered trade mark

Roaccutane 10mg Soft Capsules

(Roche Products Limited)

1. NAME OF THE MEDICINAL PRODUCT

Roaccutane 10 mg soft capsules

2. QUALITATIVE AND QUANTITATIVE COMPOSITION

Each soft capsule contains 10 mg of isotretinoin.

Excipients: Contains soya bean oil (refined, hydrogenated and partially hydrogenated) and sorbitol (E420).

For a full list of excipients, see section 6.1.

3. PHARMACEUTICAL FORM

Capsules, soft

10 mg capsules: Oval, opaque, brown-red capsules imprinted with ROA 10 in black ink.

4. CLINICAL PARTICULARS

4.1 Therapeutic indications

Severe forms of acne (such as nodular or conglobate acne or acne at risk of permanent scarring) resistant to adequate courses of standard therapy with systemic anti-bacterials and topical therapy.

4.2 Posology and method of administration

Isotretinoin should only be prescribed by or under the supervision of physicians with expertise in the use of systemic retinoids for the treatment of severe acne and a full understanding of the risks of isotretinoin therapy and monitoring requirements.

The capsules should be taken with food once or twice daily.

Adults including adolescents and the elderly:

Isotretinoin therapy should be started at a dose of 0.5 mg/kg daily. The therapeutic response to isotretinoin and some of the adverse effects are dose-related and vary between patients. This necessitates individual dosage adjustment during therapy. For most patients, the dose ranges from 0.5-1.0 mg/kg per day.

Long-term remission and relapse rates are more closely related to the total dose administered than to either duration of treatment or daily dose. It has been shown that no substantial additional benefit is to be expected beyond a cumulative treatment dose of 120-150 mg/kg. The duration of treatment will depend on the individual daily dose. A treatment course of 16-24 weeks is normally sufficient to achieve remission.

In the majority of patients, complete clearing of the acne is obtained with a single treatment course. In the event of a definite relapse a further course of isotretinoin therapy may be considered using the same daily dose and cumulative treatment dose. As further improvement of the acne can be observed up to 8 weeks after discontinuation of treatment, a further course of treatment should not be considered until at least this period has elapsed.

Patients with severe renal insufficiency

In patients with severe renal insufficiency treatment should be started at a lower dose (e.g. 10 mg/day). The dose should then be increased up to 1 mg/kg/day or until the patient is receiving the maximum tolerated dose (see section 4.4).

Children

Roaccutane is not indicated for the treatment of prepubertal acne and is not recommended in patients less than 12 years of age due to a lack of data on efficacy and safety.

Patients with intolerance

In patients who show severe intolerance to the recommended dose, treatment may be continued at a lower dose with the consequences of a longer therapy duration and a higher risk of relapse. In order to achieve the maximum possible efficacy in these patients the dose should normally be continued at the highest tolerated dose.

4.3 Contraindications

Isotretinoin is contraindicated in women who are pregnant or breastfeeding (see section 4.6).

Isotretinoin is contraindicated in women of childbearing potential unless all of the conditions of the Pregnancy Prevention Programme are met (see section 4.4).

Isotretinoin is also contraindicated in patients with hypersensitivity to isotretinoin or to any of the excipients. Roaccutane 10 mg contains soya oil, partially hydrogenated soya oil, and hydrogenated soya oil. Therefore,

Roaccutane 10 mg is contraindicated in patients allergic to peanut or soya.

Isotretinoin is also contraindicated in patients

- With hepatic insufficiency
- With excessively elevated blood lipid values
- With hypervitaminosis A
- Receiving concomitant treatment with tetracyclines (see section 4.5).

4.4 Special warnings and precautions for use

Pregnancy Prevention Programme

This medicinal product is TERATOGENIC

Isotretinoin is contraindicated in women of childbearing potential unless all of the following conditions of the Pregnancy Prevention Programme are met:

- She has severe acne (such as nodular or conglobate acne or acne at risk of permanent scarring) resistant to adequate courses of standard therapy with systemic anti-bacterials and topical therapy (see section 4.1).
- She understands the teratogenic risk.
- She understands the need for rigorous follow-up, on a monthly basis.
- She understands and accepts the need for effective contraception, without interruption, 1 month before starting treatment, throughout the duration of treatment and 1 month after the end of treatment. At least one and preferably two complementary forms of contraception including a barrier method should be used.
- Even if she has amenorrhea she must follow all of the advice on effective contraception.
- She should be capable of complying with effective contraceptive measures.
- She is informed and understands the potential consequences of pregnancy and the need to rapidly consult if there is a risk of pregnancy.
- She understands the need and accepts to undergo pregnancy testing before, during and 5 weeks after the end of treatment.
- She has acknowledged that she has understood the hazards and necessary precautions associated with the use of isotretinoin.

These conditions also concern women who are not currently sexually active unless the prescriber considers that there are compelling reasons to indicate that there is no risk of pregnancy.

The prescriber must ensure that:

- The patient complies with the conditions for pregnancy prevention as listed above, including confirmation that she has an adequate level of understanding.
- The patient has acknowledged the aforementioned conditions.
- The patient has used at least one and preferably two methods of effective contraception including a barrier method for at least 1 month prior to starting treatment and is continuing to use effective contraception throughout the treatment period and for at least 1 month after cessation of treatment.
- Negative pregnancy test results have been obtained before, during and 5 weeks after the end of treatment. The dates and results of pregnancy tests should be documented.

Contraception

Female patients must be provided with comprehensive information on pregnancy prevention and should be referred for contraceptive advice if they are not using effective contraception.

As a minimum requirement, female patients at potential risk of pregnancy must use at least one effective method of contraception. Preferably the patient should use two complementary forms of contraception including a barrier method. Contraception should be continued for at least 1 month after stopping treatment with isotretinoin, even in patients with amenorrhea.

Pregnancy testing

According to local practice, medically supervised pregnancy tests with a minimum sensitivity of 25mIU/mL are recommended to be performed in the first 3 days of the menstrual cycle, as follows.

Prior to starting therapy:

In order to exclude the possibility of pregnancy prior to starting contraception, it is recommended that an initial medically supervised pregnancy test should be performed and its date and result recorded. In patients without regular menses, the timing of this pregnancy test should reflect the sexual activity of the patient and should be undertaken approximately 3 weeks after the patient last had unprotected sexual intercourse. The prescriber should educate the patient about contraception.

A medically supervised pregnancy test should also be performed during the consultation when isotretinoin is prescribed or in the 3 days prior to the visit to the prescriber, and should have been delayed until the patient had been using effective contraception for at least 1 month. This test should ensure the patient is not pregnant when she starts treatment with isotretinoin.

Follow-up visits

Follow-up visits should be arranged at 28 day intervals. The need for repeated medically supervised pregnancy tests every month should be determined according to local practice including consideration of the patient's sexual activity and recent menstrual history (abnormal menses, missed periods or amenorrhea). Where indicated, follow-up pregnancy tests should be performed on the day of the prescribing visit or in the 3 days prior to the visit to the prescriber.

End of treatment

Five weeks after stopping treatment, women should undergo a final pregnancy test to exclude pregnancy.

Prescribing and dispensing restrictions

Prescriptions of isotretinoin for women of childbearing potential should be limited to 30 days of treatment and continuation of treatment requires a new prescription. Ideally, pregnancy testing, issuing a prescription and dispensing of isotretinoin should occur on the same day. Dispensing of isotretinoin should occur within a maximum of 7 days of the prescription.

Male patients:

The available data suggest that the level of maternal exposure from the semen of the patients receiving isotretinoin, is not of a sufficient magnitude to be associated with the teratogenic effects of isotretinoin.

Male patients should be reminded that they must not share their medication with anyone, particularly not females.

Additional precautions

Patients should be instructed never to give this medicinal product to another person, and to return any unused capsules to their pharmacist at the end of treatment.

Patients should not donate blood during therapy and for 1 month following discontinuation of isotretinoin because of the potential risk to the foetus of a pregnant transfusion recipient.

Educational material

In order to assist prescribers, pharmacists and patients in avoiding foetal exposure to isotretinoin the Marketing Authorisation Holder will provide educational material to reinforce the warnings about the teratogenicity of isotretinoin, to provide advice on contraception before therapy is started and to provide guidance on the need for pregnancy testing.

Full patient information about the teratogenic risk and the strict pregnancy prevention measures as specified in the Pregnancy Prevention Programme should be given by the physician to all patients, both male and female.

Psychiatric disorders

Depression, depression aggravated, anxiety, aggressive tendencies, mood alterations, psychotic symptoms, and very rarely, suicidal ideation, suicide attempts and suicide have been reported in patients treated with isotretinoin (see section 4.8). Particular care needs to be taken in patients with a history of depression and all patients should be monitored for signs of depression and referred for appropriate treatment if necessary. However, discontinuation of isotretinoin may be insufficient to alleviate symptoms and therefore further psychiatric or psychological evaluation may be necessary.

Skin and subcutaneous tissues disorders

Acute exacerbation of acne is occasionally seen during the initial period but this subsides with continued treatment, usually within 7 - 10 days, and usually does not require dose adjustment.

Exposure to intense sunlight or to UV rays should be avoided. Where necessary a sun-protection product with a high protection factor of at least SPF 15 should be used.

Aggressive chemical dermabrasion and cutaneous laser treatment should be avoided in patients on isotretinoin for a period of 5-6 months after the end of the treatment because of the risk of hypertrophic scarring in atypical areas and more rarely post inflammatory hyper or hypopigmentation in treated areas. Wax depilation should be avoided in patients on isotretinoin for at least a period of 6 months after treatment because of the risk of epidermal stripping.

Concurrent administration of isotretinoin with topical keratolytic or exfoliative anti-acne agents should be avoided as local irritation may increase (see section 4.5).

Patients should be advised to use a skin moisturising ointment or cream and a lip balm from the start of treatment as isotretinoin is likely to cause dryness of the skin and lips.

Eye disorders

Dry eyes, corneal opacities, decreased night vision and keratitis usually resolve after discontinuation of therapy. Dry eyes can be helped by the application of a lubricating eye ointment or by the application of tear replacement therapy. Intolerance to contact lenses may occur which may necessitate the patient to wear glasses during treatment.

Decreased night vision has also been reported and the onset in some patients was sudden (see section 4.7). Patients experiencing visual difficulties should be referred for an expert ophthalmological opinion. Withdrawal of isotretinoin may be necessary.

Musculo-skeletal and connective tissue disorders

Myalgia, arthralgia and increased serum creatine phosphokinase values have been reported in patients receiving isotretinoin, particularly in those undertaking vigorous physical activity (see section 4.8).

Bone changes including premature epiphyseal closure, hyperostosis, and calcification of tendons and ligaments have occurred after several years of administration at very high doses for treating disorders of keratinisation. The dose levels, duration of treatment and total cumulative dose in these patients generally far exceeded those recommended for the treatment of acne.

Benign intracranial hypertension

Cases of benign intracranial hypertension have been reported, some of which involved concomitant use of tetracyclines (see section 4.3 and section 4.5). Signs and symptoms of benign intracranial hypertension include headache, nausea and vomiting, visual disturbances and papilloedema. Patients who develop benign intracranial hypertension should discontinue isotretinoin immediately.

Hepatobiliary disorders

Liver enzymes should be checked before treatment, 1 month after the start of treatment, and subsequently at 3 monthly intervals unless more frequent monitoring is clinically indicated. Transient and reversible increases in liver transaminases have been reported. In many cases these changes have been within the normal range and values have returned to baseline levels during treatment. However, in the event of persistent clinically relevant elevation of transaminase levels, reduction of the dose or discontinuation of treatment should be considered.

Renal insufficiency

Renal insufficiency and renal failure do not affect the pharmacokinetics of isotretinoin. Therefore, isotretinoin can be given to patients with renal insufficiency. However, it is recommended that patients are started on a low dose and titrated up to the maximum tolerated dose (see section 4.2).

Lipid Metabolism

Serum lipids (fasting values) should be checked before treatment, 1 month after the start of treatment, and subsequently at 3 monthly intervals unless more frequent monitoring is clinically indicated. Elevated serum lipid values usually return to normal on reduction of the dose or discontinuation of treatment and may also respond to dietary measures.

Isotretinoin has been associated with an increase in plasma triglyceride levels. Isotretinoin should be discontinued if hypertriglyceridaemia cannot be controlled at an acceptable level or if symptoms of pancreatitis occur (see section 4.8). Levels in excess of 800mg/dL or 9mmol/L are sometimes associated with acute pancreatitis, which may be fatal.

Gastrointestinal disorders

Isotretinoin has been associated with inflammatory bowel disease (including regional ileitis) in patients without a prior history of intestinal disorders. Patients experiencing severe (hemorrhagic) diarrhoea should discontinue isotretinoin immediately.

Allergic reactions

Anaphylactic reactions have been rarely reported, in some cases after previous topical exposure to retinoids. Allergic cutaneous reactions are reported infrequently. Serious cases of allergic vasculitis, often with purpura (bruises and red patches) of the extremities and extracutaneous involvement have been reported. Severe allergic reactions necessitate interruption of therapy and careful monitoring.

Fructose intolerance

Roaccutane contains sorbitol. Patients with rare hereditary problems of fructose intolerance should not take this medicine.

High Risk Patients

In patients with diabetes, obesity, alcoholism or a lipid metabolism disorder undergoing treatment with isotretinoin, more frequent checks of serum values for lipids and/or blood glucose may be necessary. Elevated fasting blood sugars have been reported, and new cases of diabetes have been diagnosed during isotretinoin therapy.

4.5 Interaction with other medicinal products and other forms of interaction

Patients should not take vitamin A as concurrent medication due to the risk of developing hypervitaminosis A.

Cases of benign intracranial hypertension (pseudotumor cerebri) have been reported with concomitant use of isotretinoin and tetracyclines. Therefore, concomitant treatment with tetracyclines must be avoided (see section 4.3 and section 4.4).

Concurrent administration of isotretinoin with topical keratolytic or exfoliative anti-acne agents should be avoided as local irritation may increase (see section 4.4).

4.6 Pregnancy and lactation

Pregnancy is an absolute contraindication to treatment with isotretinoin (see section 4.3). If pregnancy does occur in spite of these precautions during treatment with isotretinoin or in the month following there is a great risk of very severe and serious malformation of the foetus.

The foetal malformations associated with exposure to isotretinoin include central nervous system abnormalities (hydrocephalus, cerebellar malformation/abnormalities, microcephaly), facial dysmorphia, cleft palate, external ear abnormalities (absence of external ear, small or absent external auditory canals), eye abnormalities (microphthalmia), cardiovascular abnormalities (conotruncal malformations such as tetralogy of Fallot, transposition of great vessels, septal defects), thymus gland abnormality and parathyroid gland abnormalities. There is also an increased incidence of spontaneous abortion.

If pregnancy occurs in a woman treated with isotretinoin, treatment must be stopped and the patient should be referred to a physician specialised or experienced in teratology for evaluation and advice.

Lactation:

Isotretinoin is highly lipophilic, therefore the passage of isotretinoin into human milk is very likely. Due to the potential for adverse effects in the child exposed via mothers' milk, the use of isotretinoin is contraindicated in nursing mothers.

4.7 Effects on ability to drive and use machines

A number of cases of decreased night vision have occurred during isotretinoin therapy and in rare instances have persisted after therapy (see section 4.4 and section 4.8). Because the onset in some patients was sudden, patients should be advised of this potential problem and warned to be cautious when driving or operating machines.

Drowsiness, dizziness and visual disturbances have been reported very rarely. Patients should be warned that if they experience these effects, they should not drive, operate machinery or take part in any other activities where the symptoms could put either themselves or others at risk.

4.8 Undesirable effects

Some of the side effects associated with the use of isotretinoin are dose-related. The side effects are generally reversible after altering the dose or discontinuation of treatment, however some may persist after treatment has stopped. The following symptoms are the most commonly reported undesirable effects with isotretinoin: dryness of the skin, dryness of the mucosae e.g. of the lips (cheilitis), the nasal mucosa (epistaxis) and the eyes (conjunctivitis).

Infections:	
Very Rare (≤ 1/10 000)	Gram positive (mucocutaneous) bacterial infection
Blood and lymphatic system disorders:	
Very common (≥ 1/10)	Anaemia, red blood cell sedimentation rate increased, thrombocytopenia, thrombocytosis
Common (≥ 1/100, < 1/10)	Neutropenia
Very Rare (≤ 1/10 000)	Lymphadenopathy
Immune system disorders:	
Rare (≥ 1/10 000, < 1/1000)	Allergic skin reaction, anaphylactic reactions, hypersensitivity
Metabolism and nutrition disorders:	
Very Rare (≤ 1/10 000)	Diabetes mellitus, hyperuricaemia
Psychiatric disorders:	
Rare (≥ 1/10 000, < 1/1000)	Depression, depression aggravated, aggressive tendencies, anxiety, mood alterations.
Very Rare (≤ 1/10 000)	Abnormal behaviour, psychotic disorder, suicidal ideation suicide attempt, suicide
Nervous system disorders:	
Common (≥ 1/100, < 1/10)	Headache
Very Rare (≤ 1/10 000)	Benign intracranial hypertension, convulsions, drowsiness, dizziness
Eye disorders:	
Very common (≥ 1/10)	Blepharitis, conjunctivitis, dry eye, eye irritation
Very Rare (≤ 1/10 000)	Blurred vision, cataract, colour blindness (colour vision deficiencies), contact lens intolerance, corneal opacity, decreased night vision, keratitis, papilloedema (as sign of benign intracranial hypertension), photophobia, visual disturbances.
Ear and labyrinth disorders:	
Very Rare (≤ 1/10 000)	Hearing impaired
Vascular disorders:	
Very Rare (≤ 1/10 000)	Vasculitis (for example Wegener's granulomatosis, allergic vasculitis)
Respiratory, thoracic and mediastinal disorders:	
Common (≥ 1/100, < 1/10)	Epistaxis, nasal dryness, nasopharyngitis
Very Rare (≤ 1/10 000)	Bronchospasm (particularly in patients with asthma), hoarseness
Gastrointestinal disorders:	
Very Rare (≤ 1/10 000)	Colitis, ileitis, dry throat, gastrointestinal haemorrhage, haemorrhagic diarrhoea and inflammatory bowel disease, nausea, pancreatitis (see section 4.4)
Hepatobiliary disorders:	
Very common (≥ 1/10)	Transaminase increased (see section 4.4)
Very Rare (≤ 1/10 000)	Hepatitis
Skin and subcutaneous tissues disorders:	
Very common (≥ 1/10)	Cheilitis, dermatitis, dry skin, localised exfoliation, pruritus, rash erythematous, skin fragility (risk of frictional trauma)
Rare (≥ 1/10 000, < 1/1000)	Alopecia
Very Rare (≤ 1/10 000)	Acne fulminans, acne aggravated (acne flare), erythema (facial), exanthema, hair disorders, hirsutism, nail dystrophy, paronychia, photosensitivity reaction, pyogenic granuloma, skin hyperpigmentation, sweating increased
Musculo-skeletal and connective tissue disorders:	
Very common (≥ 1/10)	Arthralgia, myalgia, back pain (particularly in children and adolescent patients)
Very Rare (≤ 1/10 000)	Arthritis, calcinosis (calcification of ligaments and tendons), epiphyses premature fusion, exostosis, (hyperostosis), reduced bone density, tendonitis
Renal and urinary disorders:	
Very Rare (≤ 1/10 000)	Glomerulonephritis
General disorders and administration site conditions:	
Very Rare (≤ 1/10 000)	Granulation tissue (increased formation of), malaise
Investigations:	
Very common (≥ 1/10)	Blood triglycerides increased, high density lipoprotein decreased
Common (≥ 1/100, < 1/10)	Blood cholesterol increased, blood glucose increased, haematuria, proteinuria
Very Rare (≤ 1/10 000)	Blood creatine phosphokinase increased

The incidence of the adverse events was calculated from pooled clinical trial data involving 824 patients and from post-marketing data.

4.9 Overdose

Isotretinoin is a derivative of vitamin A. Although the acute toxicity of isotretinoin is low, signs of hypervitaminosis A could appear in cases of accidental overdose. Manifestations of acute vitamin A toxicity include severe headache, nausea or vomiting, drowsiness, irritability and pruritus. Signs and symptoms of accidental or deliberate overdosage with isotretinoin would probably be similar. These symptoms would be expected to be reversible and to subside without the need for treatment.

5. PHARMACOLOGICAL PROPERTIES

5.1 Pharmacodynamic properties

Pharmacotherapeutic group: Retinoid for treatment of acne.

ATC code: D10B A01

Mechanism of action

Isotretinoin is a stereoisomer of all-trans retinoic acid (tretinoin). The exact mechanism of action of isotretinoin has not yet been elucidated in detail, but it has been established that the improvement observed in the clinical picture of severe acne is associated with suppression of sebaceous gland activity and a histologically demonstrated reduction in the size of the sebaceous glands. Furthermore, a dermal anti-inflammatory effect of isotretinoin has been established.

Efficacy

Hypercornification of the epithelial lining of the pilosebaceous unit leads to shedding of corneocytes into the duct and blockage by keratin and excess sebum. This is followed by formation of a comedone and, eventually, inflammatory lesions. Isotretinoin inhibits proliferation of sebocytes and appears to act in acne by re-setting the orderly program of differentiation. Sebum is a major substrate for the growth of Propionibacterium acnes so that reduced sebum production inhibits bacterial colonisation of the duct.

5.2 Pharmacokinetic properties

Absorption

The absorption of isotretinoin from the gastro-intestinal tract is variable and dose-linear over the therapeutic range. The absolute bioavailability of isotretinoin has not been determined, since the compound is not available as an intravenous preparation for human use, but extrapolation from dog studies would suggest a fairly low and variable systemic bioavailability. When isotretinoin is taken with food, the bioavailability is doubled relative to fasting conditions.

Distribution

Isotretinoin is extensively bound to plasma proteins, mainly albumin (99.9 %). The volume of distribution of isotretinoin in man has not been determined since isotretinoin is not available as an intravenous preparation for human use. In humans little information is available on the distribution of isotretinoin into tissue. Concentrations of isotretinoin in the epidermis are only half of those in serum. Plasma concentrations of isotretinoin are about 1.7 times those of whole blood due to poor penetration of isotretinoin into red blood cells.

Metabolism

After oral administration of isotretinoin, three major metabolites have been identified in plasma: 4-oxo-isotretinoin, tretinoin, (all-trans retinoic acid), and 4-oxo-tretinoin. These metabolites have shown biological activity in several in vitro tests. 4-oxo-isotretinoin has been shown in a clinical study to be a significant contributor to the activity of isotretinoin (reduction in sebum excretion rate despite no effect on plasma levels of isotretinoin and tretinoin). Other minor metabolites includes glucuronide conjugates. The major metabolite is 4-oxo-isotretinoin with plasma concentrations at steady state, that are 2.5 times higher than those of the parent compound.

Isotretinoin and tretinoin (all-trans retinoic acid) are reversibly metabolised (interconverted), and the metabolism of tretinoin is therefore linked with that of isotretinoin. It has been estimated that 20-30 % of an isotretinoin dose is metabolised by isomerisation.

Enterohepatic circulation may play a significant role in the pharmacokinetics of isotretinoin in man. In vitro metabolism studies have demonstrated that several CYP enzymes are involved in the metabolism of isotretinoin to 4-oxo-isotretinoin and tretinoin. No single isoform appears to have a predominant role. Isotretinoin and its metabolites do not significantly affect CYP activity.

Elimination

After oral administration of radiolabelled isotretinoin approximately equal fractions of the dose were recovered in urine and faeces. Following oral administration of isotretinoin, the terminal elimination half-life of unchanged drug in patients with acne has a mean value of 19 hours. The terminal elimination half-life of 4-oxo-isotretinoin is longer, with a mean value of 29 hours.

Isotretinoin is a physiological retinoid and endogenous retinoid concentrations are reached within approximately two weeks following the end of isotretinoin therapy.

Pharmacokinetics in special populations

Since isotretinoin is contraindicated in patients with hepatic impairment, limited information on the kinetics of isotretinoin is available in this patient population. Renal failure does not significantly reduce the plasma clearance of isotretinoin or 4-oxo-isotretinoin.

5.3 Preclinical safety data

Acute toxicity

The acute oral toxicity of isotretinoin was determined in various animal species. LD50 is approximately 2000 mg/kg in rabbits, approximately 3000 mg/kg in mice, and over 4000 mg/kg in rats.

Chronic toxicity

A long-term study in rats over 2 years (isotretinoin dosage 2, 8 and 32 mg/kg/d) produced evidence of partial hair loss and elevated plasma triglycerides in the higher dose groups. The side effect spectrum of isotretinoin in the rodent thus closely resembles that of vitamin A, but does not include the massive tissue and organ calcifications observed with vitamin A in the rat. The liver cell changes observed with vitamin A did not occur with isotretinoin.

All observed side effects of hypervitaminosis A syndrome were spontaneously reversible after withdrawal of isotretinoin. Even experimental animals in a poor general state had largely recovered within 1–2 weeks.

Teratogenicity

Like other vitamin A derivatives, isotretinoin has been shown in animal experiments to be teratogenic and embryotoxic.

Due to the teratogenic potential of isotretinoin there are therapeutic consequences for the administration to women of a childbearing age (see section 4.3, section 4.4, and section 4.6).

Fertility

Isotretinoin, in therapeutic dosages, does not affect the number, motility and morphology of sperm and does not jeopardise the formation and development of the embryo on the part of the men taking isotretinoin.

Mutagenicity

Isotretinoin has not been shown to be mutagenic in *in vitro* or *in vivo* animal tests.

6. PHARMACEUTICAL PARTICULARS

6.1 List of excipients

Capsule filling:

Beeswax, yellow;

Soya-bean oil, refined;

Soya-bean oil, hydrogenated;

Soya-bean oil, partially hydrogenated.

Capsule shell:

Gelatin;

Glycerol 85%;

Karion 83 containing sorbitol, mannitol, hydrogenated hydrolysed starch;

Titanium dioxide (E171);

Red iron oxide (E172).

Dry printing ink:

Shellac, modified;

Black iron oxide (E172);

Propylene Glycol.

6.2 Incompatibilities

Not applicable.

6.3 Shelf life

3 years

6.4 Special precautions for storage

Triplex (PVC/PE/PVDC)-aluminium blisters:

Do not store above 25 °C.

Store in the original package and keep blister in the outer carton in order to protect from moisture and light.

Aluminium-aluminium blisters:

Do not store above 30 °C.

Store in the original package in order to protect from moisture and light.

6.5 Nature and contents of container

Triplex-aluminium blister packs containing 20, 30, 50 or 100 capsules

Aluminium-aluminium blister packs containing 20, 30, 50 or 100 capsules

Not all pack sizes or pack types may be marketed.

6.6 Special precautions for disposal and other handling

Return any unused Roaccutane capsules to the Pharmacist.

7. MARKETING AUTHORISATION HOLDER

Roche Products Limited,
6 Falcon Way, Shire Park
Welwyn Garden City,
AL7 1TW
United Kingdom

8. MARKETING AUTHORISATION NUMBER(S)

PL 00031/0617

9. DATE OF FIRST AUTHORISATION/RENEWAL OF THE AUTHORISATION

10 July 2009

10. DATE OF REVISION OF THE TEXT

October 2009

Roaccutane 20mg Soft Capsules

(Roche Products Limited)

1. NAME OF THE MEDICINAL PRODUCT

Roaccutane 20 mg soft capsules

2. QUALITATIVE AND QUANTITATIVE COMPOSITION

Each soft capsule contains 20 mg of isotretinoin.

Excipients: Contains soya bean oil (refined, hydrogenated and partially hydrogenated) and sorbitol (E420).

For a full list of excipients, see section 6.1.

3. PHARMACEUTICAL FORM

Capsules, soft

20 mg capsules: Oval, opaque, brown-red and white capsules imprinted with ROA 20 in black ink.

4. CLINICAL PARTICULARS

4.1 Therapeutic indications

Severe forms of acne (such as nodular or conglobate acne or acne at risk of permanent scarring) resistant to adequate courses of standard therapy with systemic anti-bacterials and topical therapy.

4.2 Posology and method of administration

Isotretinoin should only be prescribed by or under the supervision of physicians with expertise in the use of systemic retinoids for the treatment of severe acne and a full understanding of the risks of isotretinoin therapy and monitoring requirements.

The capsules should be taken with food once or twice daily.

Adults including adolescents and the elderly:

Isotretinoin therapy should be started at a dose of 0.5 mg/kg daily. The therapeutic response to isotretinoin and some of the adverse effects are dose-related and vary between patients. This necessitates individual dosage adjustment during therapy. For most patients, the dose ranges from 0.5-1.0 mg/kg per day.

Long-term remission and relapse rates are more closely related to the total dose administered than to either duration of treatment or daily dose. It has been shown that no substantial additional benefit is to be expected beyond a cumulative treatment dose of 120-150 mg/kg. The duration of treatment will depend on the individual daily dose. A treatment course of 16-24 weeks is normally sufficient to achieve remission.

In the majority of patients, complete clearing of the acne is obtained with a single treatment course. In the event of a definite relapse a further course of isotretinoin therapy may be considered using the same daily dose and cumulative treatment dose. As further improvement of the acne can be observed up to 8 weeks after discontinuation of treatment, a further course of treatment should not be considered until at least this period has elapsed.

Patients with severe renal insufficiency

In patients with severe renal insufficiency treatment should be started at a lower dose (e.g. 10 mg/day). The dose should then be increased up to 1 mg/kg/day or until the patient is receiving the maximum tolerated dose (see section 4.4).

Children

Roaccutane is not indicated for the treatment of prepubertal acne and is not recommended in patients less than 12 years of age due to a lack of data on efficacy and safety.

Patients with intolerance

In patients who show severe intolerance to the recommended dose, treatment may be continued at a lower dose with the consequences of a longer therapy duration and a higher risk of relapse. In order to achieve the maximum possible efficacy in these patients the dose should normally be continued at the highest tolerated dose.

4.3 Contraindications

Isotretinoin is contraindicated in women who are pregnant or breastfeeding (see section 4.6).

Isotretinoin is contraindicated in women of childbearing potential unless all of the conditions of the Pregnancy Prevention Programme are met (see section 4.4).

Isotretinoin is also contraindicated in patients with hypersensitivity to isotretinoin or to any of the excipients. Roaccutane 20 mg contains soya oil, partially hydrogenated soya oil, and hydrogenated soya oil. Therefore, Roaccutane 20 mg is contraindicated in patients allergic to peanut or soya.

Isotretinoin is also contraindicated in patients

- With hepatic insufficiency
- With excessively elevated blood lipid values
- With hypervitaminosis A
- Receiving concomitant treatment with tetracyclines (see section 4.5).

4.4 Special warnings and precautions for use

Pregnancy Prevention Programme

This medicinal product is TERATOGENIC

Isotretinoin is contraindicated in women of childbearing potential unless all of the following conditions of the Pregnancy Prevention Programme are met:

- She has severe acne (such as nodular or conglobate acne or acne at risk of permanent scarring) resistant to adequate courses of standard therapy with systemic anti-bacterials and topical therapy (see section 4.1).
- She understands the teratogenic risk.
- She understands the need for rigorous follow-up, on a monthly basis.
- She understands and accepts the need for effective contraception, without interruption, 1 month before starting treatment, throughout the duration of treatment and 1 month after the end of treatment. At least one and preferably two complementary forms of contraception including a barrier method should be used.
- Even if she has amenorrhea she must follow all of the advice on effective contraception.
- She should be capable of complying with effective contraceptive measures.
- She is informed and understands the potential consequences of pregnancy and the need to rapidly consult if there is a risk of pregnancy.
- She understands the need and accepts to undergo pregnancy testing before, during and 5 weeks after the end of treatment.
- She has acknowledged that she has understood the hazards and necessary precautions associated with the use of isotretinoin.

These conditions also concern women who are not currently sexually active unless the prescriber considers that there are compelling reasons to indicate that there is no risk of pregnancy.

The prescriber must ensure that:

- The patient complies with the conditions for pregnancy prevention as listed above, including confirmation that she has an adequate level of understanding.
- The patient has acknowledged the aforementioned conditions.
- The patient has used at least one and preferably two methods of effective contraception including a barrier method for at least 1 month prior to starting treatment and is continuing to use effective contraception throughout the treatment period and for at least 1 month after cessation of treatment.
- Negative pregnancy test results have been obtained before, during and 5 weeks after the end of treatment. The dates and results of pregnancy tests should be documented.

Contraception

Female patients must be provided with comprehensive information on pregnancy prevention and should be referred for contraceptive advice if they are not using effective contraception.

As a minimum requirement, female patients at potential risk of pregnancy must use at least one effective method of contraception. Preferably the patient should use two complementary forms of contraception including a barrier method. Contraception should be continued for at least 1 month after stopping treatment with isotretinoin, even in patients with amenorrhea.

Pregnancy testing

According to local practice, medically supervised pregnancy tests with a minimum sensitivity of 25mIU/mL are recommended to be performed in the first 3 days of the menstrual cycle, as follows.

Prior to starting therapy:

In order to exclude the possibility of pregnancy prior to starting contraception, it is recommended that an initial medically supervised pregnancy test should be performed and its date and result recorded. In patients without regular menses, the timing of this pregnancy test should reflect the sexual activity of the patient and should be undertaken approximately 3 weeks after the patient last had unprotected sexual intercourse. The prescriber should educate the patient about contraception.

A medically supervised pregnancy test should also be performed during the consultation when isotretinoin is prescribed or in the 3 days prior to the visit to the prescriber, and should have been delayed until the patient had been using effective contraception for at least 1 month. This test should ensure the patient is not pregnant when she starts treatment with isotretinoin.

Follow-up visits

Follow-up visits should be arranged at 28 day intervals. The need for repeated medically supervised pregnancy tests every month should be determined according to local practice including consideration of the patient's sexual activity and recent menstrual history (abnormal menses, missed periods or amenorrhea). Where indicated, follow-up pregnancy tests should be performed on the day of the prescribing visit or in the 3 days prior to the visit to the prescriber.

End of treatment

Five weeks after stopping treatment, women should undergo a final pregnancy test to exclude pregnancy.

Prescribing and dispensing restrictions

Prescriptions of isotretinoin for women of childbearing potential should be limited to 30 days of treatment and continuation of treatment requires a new prescription. Ideally, pregnancy testing, issuing a prescription and dispensing of isotretinoin should occur on the same day. Dispensing of isotretinoin should occur within a maximum of 7 days of the prescription.

Male patients:

The available data suggest that the level of maternal exposure from the semen of the patients receiving isotretinoin, is not of a sufficient magnitude to be associated with the teratogenic effects of isotretinoin.

Male patients should be reminded that they must not share their medication with anyone, particularly not females.

Additional precautions

Patients should be instructed never to give this medicinal product to another person, and to return any unused capsules to their pharmacist at the end of treatment.

Patients should not donate blood during therapy and for 1 month following discontinuation of isotretinoin because of the potential risk to the foetus of a pregnant transfusion recipient.

Educational material

In order to assist prescribers, pharmacists and patients in avoiding foetal exposure to isotretinoin the Marketing Authorisation Holder will provide educational material to reinforce the warnings about the teratogenicity of isotretinoin, to provide advice on contraception before therapy is started and to provide guidance on the need for pregnancy testing.

Full patient information about the teratogenic risk and the strict pregnancy prevention measures as specified in the Pregnancy Prevention Programme should be given by the physician to all patients, both male and female.

Psychiatric disorders

Depression, depression aggravated, anxiety, aggressive tendencies, mood alterations, psychotic symptoms, and very rarely, suicidal ideation, suicide attempts and suicide have been reported in patients treated with isotretinoin (see section 4.8). Particular care needs to be taken in patients with a history of depression and all patients should be monitored for signs of depression and referred for appropriate treatment if necessary. However, discontinuation of isotretinoin may be insufficient to alleviate symptoms and therefore further psychiatric or psychological evaluation may be necessary.

Skin and subcutaneous tissues disorders

Acute exacerbation of acne is occasionally seen during the initial period but this subsides with continued treatment, usually within 7 - 10 days, and usually does not require dose adjustment.

Exposure to intense sunlight or to UV rays should be avoided. Where necessary a sun-protection product with a high protection factor of at least SPF 15 should be used.

Aggressive chemical dermabrasion and cutaneous laser treatment should be avoided in patients on isotretinoin for a period of 5-6 months after the end of the treatment because of the risk of hypertrophic scarring in atypical areas and more rarely post inflammatory hyper or hypopigmentation in treated areas. Wax depilation should be avoided in patients on isotretinoin for at least a period of 6 months after treatment because of the risk of epidermal stripping.

Concurrent administration of isotretinoin with topical keratolytic or exfoliative anti-acne agents should be avoided as local irritation may increase (see section 4.5).

Patients should be advised to use a skin moisturising ointment or cream and a lip balm from the start of treatment as isotretinoin is likely to cause dryness of the skin and lips.

Eye disorders

Dry eyes, corneal opacities, decreased night vision and keratitis usually resolve after discontinuation of therapy. Dry eyes can be helped by the application of a lubricating eye ointment or by the application of tear replacement therapy. Intolerance to contact lenses may occur which may necessitate the patient to wear glasses during treatment.

Decreased night vision has also been reported and the onset in some patients was sudden (see section 4.7). Patients experiencing visual difficulties should be referred for an expert ophthalmological opinion. Withdrawal of isotretinoin may be necessary.

Musculo-skeletal and connective tissue disorders

Myalgia, arthralgia and increased serum creatine phosphokinase values have been reported in patients receiving isotretinoin, particularly in those undertaking vigorous physical activity (see section 4.8).

Bone changes including premature epiphyseal closure, hyperostosis, and calcification of tendons and ligaments have occurred after several years of administration at very high doses for treating disorders of keratinisation. The dose levels, duration of treatment and total cumulative dose in these patients generally far exceeded those recommended for the treatment of acne.

Benign intracranial hypertension

Cases of benign intracranial hypertension have been reported, some of which involved concomitant use of tetracyclines (see section 4.3 and section 4.5). Signs and symptoms of benign intracranial hypertension include headache, nausea and vomiting, visual disturbances and papilloedema. Patients who develop benign intracranial hypertension should discontinue isotretinoin immediately.

Hepatobiliary disorders

Liver enzymes should be checked before treatment, 1 month after the start of treatment, and subsequently at 3 monthly intervals unless more frequent monitoring is clinically indicated. Transient and reversible increases in liver transaminases have been reported. In many cases these changes have been within the normal range and values have returned to baseline levels during treatment. However, in the event of persistent clinically relevant elevation of transaminase levels, reduction of the dose or discontinuation of treatment should be considered.

Renal insufficiency

Renal insufficiency and renal failure do not affect the pharmacokinetics of isotretinoin. Therefore, isotretinoin can be given to patients with renal insufficiency. However, it is recommended that patients are started on a low dose and titrated up to the maximum tolerated dose (see section 4.2).

Lipid Metabolism

Serum lipids (fasting values) should be checked before treatment, 1 month after the start of treatment, and subsequently at 3 monthly intervals unless more frequent monitoring is clinically indicated. Elevated serum lipid values usually return to normal on reduction of the dose or discontinuation of treatment and may also respond to dietary measures.

Isotretinoin has been associated with an increase in plasma triglyceride levels. Isotretinoin should be discontinued if hypertriglyceridaemia cannot be controlled at an acceptable level or if symptoms of pancreatitis occur (see section 4.8). Levels in excess of 800mg/dL or 9mmol/L are sometimes associated with acute pancreatitis, which may be fatal.

Gastrointestinal disorders

Isotretinoin has been associated with inflammatory bowel disease (including regional ileitis) in patients without a prior history of intestinal disorders. Patients experiencing severe (hemorrhagic) diarrhoea should discontinue isotretinoin immediately.

Allergic reactions

Anaphylactic reactions have been rarely reported, in some cases after previous topical exposure to retinoids. Allergic cutaneous reactions are reported infrequently. Serious cases of allergic vasculitis, often with purpura (bruises and red patches) of the extremities and extracutaneous involvement have been reported. Severe allergic reactions necessitate interruption of therapy and careful monitoring.

Fructose intolerance

Roaccutane contains sorbitol. Patients with rare hereditary problems of fructose intolerance should not take this medicine.

High Risk Patients

In patients with diabetes, obesity, alcoholism or a lipid metabolism disorder undergoing treatment with isotretinoin, more frequent checks of serum values for lipids and/or blood glucose may be necessary. Elevated fasting blood sugars have been reported, and new cases of diabetes have been diagnosed during isotretinoin therapy.

4.5 Interaction with other medicinal products and other forms of interaction

Patients should not take vitamin A as concurrent medication due to the risk of developing hypervitaminosis A.

Cases of benign intracranial hypertension (pseudotumor cerebri) have been reported with concomitant use of isotretinoin and tetracyclines. Therefore, concomitant treatment with tetracyclines must be avoided (see section 4.3 and section 4.4).

Concurrent administration of isotretinoin with topical keratolytic or exfoliative anti-acne agents should be avoided as local irritation may increase (see section 4.4).

4.6 Pregnancy and lactation

Pregnancy is an <u>absolute</u> contraindication to treatment with isotretinoin (see section 4.3). If pregnancy does occur in spite of these precautions during treatment with isotretinoin or in the month following there is a great risk of very severe and serious malformation of the foetus.

The foetal malformations associated with exposure to isotretinoin include central nervous system abnormalities (hydrocephalus, cerebellar malformation/abnormalities, microcephaly), facial dysmorphia, cleft palate, external ear abnormalities (absence of external ear, small or absent external auditory canals), eye abnormalities (microphthalmia), cardiovascular abnormalities (conotruncal malformations such as tetralogy of Fallot, transposition of great vessels, septal defects), thymus gland abnormality and parathyroid gland abnormalities. There is also an increased incidence of spontaneous abortion.

If pregnancy occurs in a woman treated with isotretinoin, treatment must be stopped and the patient should be referred to a physician specialised or experienced in teratology for evaluation and advice.

<u>Lactation</u>:

Isotretinoin is highly lipophilic, therefore the passage of isotretinoin into human milk is very likely. Due to the potential for adverse effects in the child exposed via mothers' milk, the use of isotretinoin is contraindicated in nursing mothers.

4.7 Effects on ability to drive and use machines

A number of cases of decreased night vision have occurred during isotretinoin therapy and in rare instances have persisted after therapy (see section 4.4 and section 4.8). Because the onset in some patients was sudden, patients should be advised of this potential problem and warned to be cautious when driving or operating machines.

Drowsiness, dizziness and visual disturbances have been reported very rarely. Patients should be warned that if they experience these effects, they should not drive, operate machinery or take part in any other activities where the symptoms could put either themselves or others at risk.

4.8 Undesirable effects

Some of the side effects associated with the use of isotretinoin are dose-related. The side effects are generally reversible after altering the dose or discontinuation of treatment, however some may persist after treatment has stopped. The following symptoms are the most commonly reported undesirable effects with isotretinoin: dryness of the skin, dryness of the mucosae e.g. of the lips (cheilitis), the nasal mucosa (epistaxis) and the eyes (conjunctivitis).

Infections:	
Very Rare (≤ 1/10 000)	Gram positive (mucocutaneous) bacterial infection
Blood and lymphatic system disorders:	
Very common (≥ 1/10)	Anaemia, red blood cell sedimentation rate increased, thrombocytopenia, thrombocytosis
Common (≥ 1/100, < 1/10)	Neutropenia
Very Rare (≤ 1/10 000)	Lymphadenopathy
Immune system disorders:	
Rare (≥ 1/10 000, < 1/1000)	Allergic skin reaction, anaphylactic reactions, hypersensitivity
Metabolism and nutrition disorders:	
Very Rare (≤ 1/10 000)	Diabetes mellitus, hyperuricaemia
Psychiatric disorders:	
Rare (≥ 1/10 000, < 1/1000)	Depression, depression aggravated, aggressive tendencies, anxiety, mood alterations.
Very Rare (≤ 1/10 000)	Abnormal behaviour, psychotic disorder, suicidal ideation suicide attempt, suicide
Nervous system disorders:	
Common (≥ 1/100, < 1/10)	Headache
Very Rare (≤ 1/10 000)	Benign intracranial hypertension, convulsions, drowsiness, dizziness
Eye disorders:	
Very common (≥ 1/10)	Blepharitis, conjunctivitis, dry eye, eye irritation
Very Rare (≤ 1/10 000)	Blurred vision, cataract, colour blindness (colour vision deficiencies), contact lens intolerance, corneal opacity, decreased night vision, keratitis, papilloedema (as sign of benign intracranial hypertension), photophobia, visual disturbances.
Ear and labyrinth disorders:	
Very Rare (≤ 1/10 000)	Hearing impaired
Vascular disorders:	
Very Rare (≤ 1/10 000)	Vasculitis (for example Wegener's granulomatosis, allergic vasculitis)
Respiratory, thoracic and mediastinal disorders:	
Common (≥ 1/100, < 1/10)	Epistaxis, nasal dryness, nasopharyngitis
Very Rare (≤ 1/10 000)	Bronchospasm (particularly in patients with asthma), hoarseness

Gastrointestinal disorders:	
Very Rare (≤ 1/10 000)	Colitis, ileitis, dry throat, gastrointestinal haemorrhage, haemorrhagic diarrhoea and inflammatory bowel disease, nausea, pancreatitis (see section 4.4)
Hepatobiliary disorders:	
Very common (≥ 1/10)	Transaminase increased (see section 4.4)
Very Rare (≤ 1/10 000)	Hepatitis
Skin and subcutaneous tissues disorders:	
Very common (≥ 1/10)	Cheilitis, dermatitis, dry skin, localised exfoliation, pruritus, rash erythematous, skin fragility (risk of frictional trauma)
Rare (≥ 1/10 000, < 1/1000)	Alopecia
Very Rare (≤ 1/10 000)	Acne fulminans, acne aggravated (acne flare), erythema (facial), exanthema, hair disorders, hirsutism, nail dystrophy, paronychia, photosensitivity reaction, pyogenic granuloma, skin hyperpigmentation, sweating increased
Musculo-skeletal and connective tissue disorders:	
Very common (≥ 1/10)	Arthralgia, myalgia, back pain (particularly in children and adolescent patients)
Very Rare (≤ 1/10 000)	Arthritis, calcinosis (calcification of ligaments and tendons), epiphyses premature fusion, exostosis, (hyperostosis), reduced bone density, tendonitis
Renal and urinary disorders:	
Very Rare (≤ 1/10 000)	Glomerulonephritis
General disorders and administration site conditions:	
Very Rare (≤ 1/10 000)	Granulation tissue (increased formation of), malaise
Investigations:	
Very common (≥ 1/10)	Blood triglycerides increased, high density lipoprotein decreased.
Common (≥ 1/100, < 1/10)	Blood cholesterol increased, blood glucose increased, haematuria, proteinuria
Very Rare (≤ 1/10 000)	Blood creatine phosphokinase increased

The incidence of the adverse events was calculated from pooled clinical trial data involving 824 patients and from post-marketing data.

4.9 Overdose

Isotretinoin is a derivative of vitamin A. Although the acute toxicity of isotretinoin is low, signs of hypervitaminosis A could appear in cases of accidental overdose. Manifestations of acute vitamin A toxicity include severe headache, nausea or vomiting, drowsiness, irritability and pruritus. Signs and symptoms of accidental or deliberate overdosage with isotretinoin would probably be similar. These symptoms would be expected to be reversible and to subside without the need for treatment.

5. PHARMACOLOGICAL PROPERTIES

5.1 Pharmacodynamic properties

Pharmacotherapeutic group: Retinoid for treatment of acne.

ATC code: D10B A01

Mechanism of action

Isotretinoin is a stereoisomer of all-trans retinoic acid (tretinoin). The exact mechanism of action of isotretinoin has not yet been elucidated in detail, but it has been established that the improvement observed in the clinical picture of severe acne is associated with suppression of sebaceous gland activity and a histologically demonstrated reduction in the size of the sebaceous glands. Furthermore, a dermal anti-inflammatory effect of isotretinoin has been established.

Efficacy

Hypercornification of the epithelial lining of the pilosebaceous unit leads to shedding of corneocytes into the duct and blockage by keratin and excess sebum. This is followed by formation of a comedone and, eventually, inflammatory lesions. Isotretinoin inhibits proliferation of sebocytes and appears to act in acne by re-setting the orderly program of differentiation. Sebum is a major substrate for the growth of Propionibacterium acnes so that reduced sebum production inhibits bacterial colonisation of the duct.

5.2 Pharmacokinetic properties

Absorption

The absorption of isotretinoin from the gastro-intestinal tract is variable and dose-linear over the therapeutic range. The absolute bioavailability of isotretinoin has not been determined, since the compound is not available as an intravenous preparation for human use, but extrapolation from dog studies would suggest a fairly low and variable systemic bioavailability. When isotretinoin is taken with food, the bioavailability is doubled relative to fasting conditions.

Distribution

Isotretinoin is extensively bound to plasma proteins, mainly albumin (99.9 %). The volume of distribution of isotretinoin in man has not been determined since isotretinoin is not available as an intravenous preparation for human use. In humans little information is available on the distribution of isotretinoin into tissue. Concentrations of isotretinoin in the epidermis are only half of those in serum. Plasma concentrations of isotretinoin are about 1.7 times those of whole blood due to poor penetration of isotretinoin into red blood cells.

Metabolism

After oral administration of isotretinoin, three major metabolites have been identified in plasma: 4-oxo-isotretinoin, tretinoin, (all-trans retinoic acid), and 4-oxo-tretinoin. These metabolites have shown biological activity in several in vitro tests. 4-oxo-isotretinoin has been shown in a clinical study to be a significant contributor to the activity of isotretinoin (reduction in sebum excretion rate despite no effect on plasma levels of isotretinoin and tretinoin). Other minor metabolites includes glucuronide conjugates. The major metabolite is 4-oxo-isotretinoin with plasma concentrations at steady state, that are 2.5 times higher than those of the parent compound.

Isotretinoin and tretinoin (all-trans retinoic acid) are reversibly metabolised (interconverted), and the metabolism of tretinoin is therefore linked with that of isotretinoin. It has been estimated that 20-30 % of an isotretinoin dose is metabolised by isomerisation.

Enterohepatic circulation may play a significant role in the pharmacokinetics of isotretinoin in man. In vitro metabolism studies have demonstrated that several CYP enzymes are involved in the metabolism of isotretinoin to 4-oxo-isotretinoin and tretinoin. No single isoform appears to have a predominant role. Isotretinoin and its metabolites do not significantly affect CYP activity.

Elimination

After oral administration of radiolabelled isotretinoin approximately equal fractions of the dose were recovered in urine and faeces. Following oral administration of isotretinoin, the terminal elimination half-life of unchanged drug in patients with acne has a mean value of 19 hours. The terminal elimination half-life of 4-oxo-isotretinoin is longer, with a mean value of 29 hours.

Isotretinoin is a physiological retinoid and endogenous retinoid concentrations are reached within approximately two weeks following the end of isotretinoin therapy.

Pharmacokinetics in special populations

Since isotretinoin is contraindicated in patients with hepatic impairment, limited information on the kinetics of isotretinoin is available in this patient population. Renal failure does not significantly reduce the plasma clearance of isotretinoin or 4-oxo-isotretinoin.

5.3 Preclinical safety data

Acute toxicity

The acute oral toxicity of isotretinoin was determined in various animal species. LD50 is approximately 2000 mg/kg in rabbits, approximately 3000 mg/kg in mice, and over 4000 mg/kg in rats.

Chronic toxicity

A long-term study in rats over 2 years (isotretinoin dosage 2, 8 and 32 mg/kg/d) produced evidence of partial hair loss and elevated plasma triglycerides in the higher dose groups. The side effect spectrum of isotretinoin in the rodent thus closely resembles that of vitamin A, but does not include the massive tissue and organ calcifications observed with vitamin A in the rat. The liver cell changes observed with vitamin A did not occur with isotretinoin.

All observed side effects of hypervitaminosis A syndrome were spontaneously reversible after withdrawal of isotretinoin. Even experimental animals in a poor general state had largely recovered within 1–2 weeks.

Teratogenicity

Like other vitamin A derivatives, isotretinoin has been shown in animal experiments to be teratogenic and embryotoxic.

Due to the teratogenic potential of isotretinoin there are therapeutic consequences for the administration to women of a childbearing age (see section 4.3, section 4.4, and section 4.6).

Fertility

Isotretinoin, in therapeutic dosages, does not affect the number, motility and morphology of sperm and does not jeopardise the formation and development of the embryo on the part of the men taking isotretinoin.

Mutagenicity

Isotretinoin has not been shown to be mutagenic in *in vitro* or *in vivo* animal tests.

6. PHARMACEUTICAL PARTICULARS

6.1 List of excipients

Capsule filling:

Beeswax, yellow;

Soya-bean oil, refined;

Soya-bean oil, hydrogenated;

Soya-bean oil, partially hydrogenated.

Capsule shell:

Gelatin;

Glycerol 85%;

Karion 83 containing sorbitol, mannitol, hydrogenated hydrolysed starch;

Titanium dioxide (E171);

Red iron oxide (E172).

Dry printing ink:

Shellac, modified;

Black iron oxide (E172);

Propylene Glycol.

6.2 Incompatibilities

Not applicable.

6.3 Shelf life

3 years

6.4 Special precautions for storage

Triplex (PVC/PE/PVDC)-aluminium blisters:

Do not store above 25°C.

Store in the original package and keep blister in the outer carton in order to protect from moisture and light.

Aluminium-aluminium blisters:

Do not store above 30°C.

Store in the original package in order to protect from moisture and light.

6.5 Nature and contents of container

Triplex-aluminium blister packs containing 20, 30, 50 or 100 capsules

Aluminium-aluminium blister packs containing 20, 30, 50 or 100 capsules

Not all pack sizes or pack types may be marketed.

6.6 Special precautions for disposal and other handling

Return any unused Roaccutane capsules to the Pharmacist.

7. MARKETING AUTHORISATION HOLDER

Roche Products Limited,

6 Falcon Way, Shire Park

Welwyn Garden City,

AL7 1TW

United Kingdom

8. MARKETING AUTHORISATION NUMBER(S)

PL 00031/0160

9. DATE OF FIRST AUTHORISATION/RENEWAL OF THE AUTHORISATION

10 July 2009

10. DATE OF REVISION OF THE TEXT

October 2009

RoActemra 20mg/ml Concentrate for Solution for Infusion

(Roche Products Limited)

1. NAME OF THE MEDICINAL PRODUCT

RoActemra▼ 20 mg/ml concentrate for solution for infusion.

2. QUALITATIVE AND QUANTITATIVE COMPOSITION

Each ml concentrate contains 20 mg tocilizumab*.

Each vial contains 80 mg of tocilizumab* in 4 ml (20 mg/ml).

Each vial contains 200 mg of tocilizumab* in 10 ml (20 mg/ml).

Each vial contains 400 mg of tocilizumab* in 20 ml (20 mg/ml).

*humanised IgG1 monoclonal antibody against the human interleukin-6 (IL-6) receptor produced in Chinese hamster ovary (CHO) cells by recombinant DNA technology.

Excipients:

Each 80 mg vial contains 0.10 mmol (2.21 mg) sodium.

Each 200 mg vial contains 0.20 mmol (4.43 mg) sodium.

Each 400 mg vial contains 0.39 mmol (8.85 mg) sodium.

For a full list of excipients, see section 6.1.

3. PHARMACEUTICAL FORM

Concentrate for solution for infusion (sterile concentrate).

Clear to opalescent, colourless to pale yellow solution.

4. CLINICAL PARTICULARS

4.1 Therapeutic indications

RoActemra, in combination with methotrexate (MTX), is indicated for the treatment of moderate to severe active rheumatoid arthritis (RA) in adult patients who have either responded inadequately to, or who were intolerant to, previous therapy with one or more disease-modifying anti-rheumatic drugs (DMARDs) or tumour necrosis factor (TNF) antagonists. In these patients, RoActemra can be given as monotherapy in case of intolerance to MTX or where continued treatment with MTX is inappropriate.

4.2 Posology and method of administration

Treatment should be initiated by healthcare professionals experienced in the diagnosis and treatment of RA. Patients treated with RoActemra should be given the Patient Alert Card.

Posology

The recommended posology is 8 mg/kg body weight, but no lower than 480 mg, given once every four weeks.

Doses above 1.2 g have not been evaluated in clinical studies (see section 5.1).

Dose adjustments due to laboratory abnormalities (see section 4.4).

- Liver enzyme abnormalities

Laboratory Value	Action
> 1 to 3 × Upper Limit of Normal (ULN)	Dose modify concomitant MTX if appropriate For persistent increases in this range, reduce RoActemra dose to 4 mg/kg or interrupt RoActemra until alanine aminotransferase (ALT) or aspartate aminotransferase (AST) have normalised Restart with 4 mg/kg or 8 mg/kg, as clinically appropriate
> 3 to 5 × ULN (confirmed by repeat testing, see section 4.4).	Interrupt RoActemra dosing until < 3 × ULN and follow recommendations above for >1 to 3 × ULN For persistent increases >3 × ULN, discontinue RoActemra
> 5 × ULN	Discontinue RoActemra

- Low absolute neutrophil count (ANC)

Laboratory Value (cells × 10^9/l)	Action
ANC >1	Maintain dose
ANC 0.5 to 1	Interrupt RoActemra dosing When ANC increases >1 × 10^9/l resume RoActemra at 4 mg/kg and increase to 8 mg/kg as clinically appropriate
ANC <0.5	Discontinue RoActemra

- Low platelet count

Laboratory Value (cells × 10^3/µl)	Action
50 to 100	Interrupt RoActemra dosing When platelet count >100 × 10^3/µl resume RoActemra at 4 mg/kg and increase to 8 mg/kg as clinically appropriate
<50	Discontinue RoActemra

Special populations

Paediatric patients: RoActemra is not recommended for use in children below 18 years of age due to insufficient data on safety and efficacy.

Elderly patients: No dose adjustment is required in patients aged 65 years and older.

Renal impairment: No dose adjustment is required in patients with mild renal impairment. RoActemra has not been studied in patients with moderate to severe renal impairment (see section 5.2). Renal function should be monitored closely in these patients.

Hepatic impairment: RoActemra has not been studied in patients with hepatic impairment. Therefore, no dose recommendations can be made.

Method of administration

After dilution, RoActemra should be administered as an intravenous infusion over 1 hour.

RoActemra should be diluted to a final volume of 100 ml with sterile, non-pyrogenic sodium chloride 9 mg/ml (0.9%) solution for injection using aseptic technique.

For further information on dilution prior to administration, see section 6.6.

4.3 Contraindications

Hypersensitivity to the active substance or to any of the excipients.

Active, severe infections (see section 4.4).

4.4 Special warnings and precautions for use

Infections

RoActemra treatment should not be initiated in patients with active infections (see section 4.3). Administration of RoActemra should be interrupted if a patient develops a serious infection until the infection is controlled (see section 4.8). Healthcare professionals should exercise caution when considering the use of RoActemra in patients with a history of recurring or chronic infections or with underlying conditions (e.g. diverticulitis, diabetes) which may predispose patients to infections.

Vigilance for the timely detection of serious infection is recommended for patients receiving biological treatments for moderate to severe RA as signs and symptoms of acute inflammation may be lessened, associated with suppression of the acute phase reaction. The effects of tocilizumab on C-reactive protein (CRP), neutrophils and signs and symptoms of infection should be considered when evaluating a patient for a potential infection. Patients should be instructed to contact their healthcare professional immediately when any symptoms suggesting infection appear, in order to assure rapid evaluation and appropriate treatment.

Tuberculosis

As recommended for other biological treatments in RA, patients should be screened for latent tuberculosis (TB) infection prior to starting RoActemra therapy. Patients with latent TB should be treated with standard anti-mycobacterial therapy before initiating RoActemra.

Complications of diverticulitis

Events of diverticular perforations as complications of diverticulitis have been reported uncommonly with RoActemra (see section 4.8). RoActemra should be used with caution in patients with previous history of intestinal ulceration or diverticulitis. Patients presenting with symptoms potentially indicative of complicated diverticulitis, such as abdominal pain, haemorrhage and/or unexplained change in bowel habits with fever should be evaluated promptly for early identification of diverticulitis which can be associated with gastrointestinal perforation.

Hypersensitivity reactions

Serious hypersensitivity reactions have been reported in association with infusion of RoActemra in approximately 0.3% of patients (see section 4.8). Appropriate treatment should be available for immediate use in the event of an anaphylactic reaction during administration of RoActemra.

Active hepatic disease and hepatic impairment

Treatment with RoActemra, particularly when administered concomitantly with MTX, may be associated with elevations in hepatic transaminases (see section 4.8). Therefore, caution should be exercised when considering treatment of patients with active hepatic disease or hepatic impairment, as the safety of RoActemra in these patients has not been adequately studied (see section 4.2).

Hepatic transaminase elevations

In clinical trials, transient or intermittent mild and moderate elevations of hepatic transaminases have been reported commonly with RoActemra treatment, without progression to hepatic injury (see section 4.8). An increased frequency of these elevations was observed when potentially hepatotoxic drugs (e.g. MTX) were used in combination with RoActemra.

Caution should be exercised when considering initiation of RoActemra treatment in patients with elevated ALT or AST >1.5 × ULN. In patients with baseline ALT or AST >5 × ULN, treatment is not recommended.

ALT and AST levels should be monitored every 4 to 8 weeks for the first 6 months of treatment followed by every 12 weeks thereafter. For recommended modifications based on transaminases see section 4.2. For ALT or AST elevations >3–5 × ULN, confirmed by repeat testing, RoActemra treatment should be interrupted.

Haematological abnormalities

Decreases in neutrophil and platelet counts have occurred following treatment with tocilizumab 8 mg/kg in combination with MTX (see section 4.8). There may be an increased risk of neutropenia in patients who have previously been treated with a TNF antagonist.

Caution should be exercised when considering initiation of RoActemra treatment in patients with a low neutrophil or platelet count (i.e. ANC <2 × 10^9/ l or platelet count below 100 × 10^3/µl). In patients with an ANC <0.5 × 10^9/ l or a platelet count <50 × 10^3/µl treatment is not recommended.

Neutrophils and platelets should be monitored 4 to 8 weeks after start of therapy and thereafter according to standard clinical practice. For recommended dose modifications based on ANC and platelet counts, see section 4.2.

Lipid parameters

Elevations in lipid parameters including total cholesterol, low-density lipoprotein (LDL), high-density lipoprotein (HDL) and triglycerides were observed in patients treated with tocilizumab (see section 4.8). In the majority of patients, there was no increase in atherogenic indices, and elevations in total cholesterol responded to treatment with lipid lowering agents.

Assessment of lipid parameters should be performed 4 to 8 weeks following initiation of RoActemra therapy. Patients should be managed according to local clinical guidelines for management of hyperlipidaemia.

Neurological disorders

Physicians should be vigilant for symptoms potentially indicative of new-onset central demyelinating disorders. The potential for central demyelination with RoActemra is currently unknown.

Malignancy

The risk of malignancy is increased in patients with RA. Immunomodulatory medicinal products may increase the risk of malignancy.

Vaccinations

Live and live attenuated vaccines should not be given concurrently with RoActemra as clinical safety has not been established.

Cardiovascular risk

RA patients have an increased risk for cardiovascular disorders and should have risk factors (e.g. hypertension, hyperlipidaemia) managed as part of usual standard of care.

Combination with TNF antagonists

There is no experience with the use of RoActemra with TNF antagonists or other biological treatments for RA. RoActemra is not recommended for use with other biological agents.

Sodium

This medicinal product contains 1.17 mmol (or 26.55 mg) sodium per maximum dose of 1200 mg. To be taken into consideration by patients on a controlled sodium diet. Doses below 1025 mg of this medicinal product contain less than 1 mmol sodium (23 mg), i.e. essentially 'sodium free'.

4.5 Interaction with other medicinal products and other forms of interaction

Concomitant administration of a single dose of 10 mg/kg tocilizumab with 10-25 mg MTX once weekly had no clinically significant effect on MTX exposure.

Population pharmacokinetic analyses did not detect any effect of MTX, non-steroidal anti-inflammatory drugs (NSAIDs) or corticosteroids on tocilizumab clearance.

The expression of hepatic CYP450 enzymes is suppressed by cytokines, such as IL-6, that stimulate chronic inflammation. Thus, CYP450 expression may be reversed when potent cytokine inhibitory therapy, such as tocilizumab, is introduced.

In vitro studies with cultured human hepatocytes demonstrated that IL-6 caused a reduction in CYP1A2, CYP2C9, CYP2C19, and CYP3A4 enzyme expression. Tocilizumab normalises expression of these enzymes.

In a study in RA patients, levels of simvastatin (CYP3A4) were decreased by 57% one week following a single dose of tocilizumab, to the level similar to, or slightly higher than, those observed in healthy subjects.

When starting or stopping therapy with tocilizumab, patients taking medicinal products which are individually adjusted and are metabolised via CYP450 3A4, 1A2 or 2C9 (e.g. atorvastatin, calcium channel blockers, theophylline, warfarin, phenytoin, ciclosporin, or benzodiazepines) should be monitored as doses may need to be increased to maintain therapeutic effect. Given its long elimination half-life ($t_{1/2}$), the effect of tocilizumab on CYP450 enzyme activity may persist for several weeks after stopping therapy.

4.6 Pregnancy and lactation

Pregnancy

There are no adequate data from the use of tocilizumab in pregnant women. A study in animals has shown an increased risk of spontaneous abortion/embryo-foetal death at a high dose (see section 5.3). The potential risk for humans is unknown. Women of childbearing potential must use effective contraception during and up to 6 months after treatment.

RoActemra should not be used during pregnancy unless clearly necessary.

Lactation

It is unknown whether tocilizumab is excreted in human breast milk. The excretion of tocilizumab in milk has not been studied in animals. A decision on whether to continue/discontinue breast-feeding or to continue/discontinue therapy with RoActemra should be made taking into account the benefit of breast-feeding to the child and the benefit of RoActemra therapy to the woman.

4.7 Effects on ability to drive and use machines

No studies on the effects on the ability to drive and use machines have been performed. However, given that dizziness has been commonly reported, patients who

Table 1. Summary of ADRs occurring in patients with RA receiving tocilizumab as monotherapy or in combination with MTX or other DMARDs

System Organ Class	Very Common	Common	Uncommon
Infections and infestations	Upper respiratory tract infections	Cellulitis, Pneumonia, Oral herpes simplex, Herpes zoster	Diverticulitis
Gastrointestinal disorders		Mouth ulceration, Gastritis	Stomatitis
Skin and subcutaneous tissue disorders		Rash, Pruritus	Urticaria
Nervous system disorders		Headache, Dizziness	
Investigations		Hepatic transaminases increased	Total bilirubin increased
Vascular disorders		Hypertension	
Blood and lymphatic system disorders		Leucopoenia, Neutropenia	
Metabolism and nutrition disorders		Hypercholesterolaemia	Hypertriglyceridaemia
General disorders and administration site conditions			Hypersensitivity reactions
Eye disorders		Conjunctivitis	

experience this adverse reaction should be advised not to drive or use machines until it has resolved.

4.8 Undesirable effects

A total of 3,778 patients received at least one dose of RoActemra 4 mg/kg or 8 mg/kg.

The adverse drug reactions (ADRs) presented in Table 1 are based on the safety of tocilizumab studied in 4 placebo-controlled studies (studies II, III, IV and V) and 1 MTX-controlled study (study I) (see section 5.1). In these studies, 774 patients received tocilizumab 4 mg/kg in combination with MTX, 1,582 patients received tocilizumab 8 mg/kg in combination with MTX or other DMARDs and 288 patients received tocilizumab 8 mg/kg monotherapy.

The long-term open label extension studies included 2,562 patients who received tocilizumab 8 mg/kg with or without DMARDs. The total exposure in the long-term safety analysis was 3,685 patient years.

The most commonly reported ADRs (occurring in ≥5% of patients treated with tocilizumab monotherapy or in combination with DMARDs) were upper respiratory tract infections, nasopharyngitis, headache, hypertension and increased ALT.

The ADRs listed in Table 1 are presented by system organ class and frequency categories, defined using the following convention: very common (≥1/10); common (≥1/100 to <1/10) or uncommon (≥1/1,000 to <1/100). Within each frequency grouping, undesirable effects are presented in order of decreasing seriousness.

Table 1. Summary of ADRs occurring in patients with RA receiving tocilizumab as monotherapy or in combination with MTX or other DMARDs

(see Table 1 above)

Infections

In the controlled studies the rate of all infections reported with tocilizumab 8 mg/kg plus DMARD treatment was 127 events per 100 patient years compared to 112 events per 100 patient years in the placebo plus DMARD group. In the long-term open label extension studies, the rate of infections with RoActemra plus DMARDs was 116 events per 100 patient years exposure.

In controlled clinical studies, the rate of serious infections with tocilizumab 8 mg/kg plus DMARDs was 5.3 events per 100 patient years exposure compared to 3.9 events per 100 patient years exposure in the placebo plus DMARD group. In the monotherapy study the rate of serious infections was 3.6 events per 100 patient years of exposure in the tocilizumab group and 1.5 events per 100 patient years of exposure in the MTX group.

In the long-term safety population (core and extension studies), the rate of serious infections observed with tocilizumab plus DMARD treatment was 3.9 events per 100 patient years exposure. Reported serious infections included pneumonia, cellulitis, herpes zoster, gastroenteritis, diverticulitis, sepsis and bacterial arthritis. Serious infections were rarely fatal. Cases of opportunistic infections have been reported.

Complications of diverticulitis

During the six month controlled trials, complications of diverticulitis including generalised purulent peritonitis, lower gastrointestinal perforation, fistulae and abscess have been reported uncommonly with tocilizumab therapy.

Infusion reactions

Adverse events associated with infusion (selected events occurring during or within 24 hours of infusion) were reported by 6.9% of patients in the tocilizumab 8 mg/kg plus DMARD group and 5.1% of patients in the placebo plus DMARD group. Events reported during the infusion were primarily episodes of hypertension; events reported within 24 hours of finishing an infusion were headache and skin reactions (rash, urticaria). These events were not treatment limiting.

The rate of anaphylactic reactions (occurring in a total of 6/3,778 patients, 0.2%) was several fold higher with the 4 mg/kg dose, compared to the 8 mg/kg dose. Clinically significant hypersensitivity reactions associated with tocilizumab and requiring treatment discontinuation were reported in a total of 13 out of 3,778 patients (0.3%) treated with tocilizumab during the controlled and open label clinical studies. These reactions were generally observed during the second to fifth infusions of tocilizumab (see section 4.4).

Immunogenicity

A total of 2,876 patients have been tested for anti-tocilizumab antibodies in the controlled clinical trials. Of the 46 patients (1.6%) who developed anti-tocilizumab antibodies, 6 had an associated medically significant hypersensitivity reaction, of which 5 led to permanent discontinuation of treatment. In 30 patients (1.1%) who developed neutralising antibodies, no apparent correlation to clinical response was observed.

Haematological abnormalities

Decreases in neutrophil counts below 1×10^9/l occurred in 3.4% of patients on tocilizumab 8 mg/kg plus DMARDs compared to <0.1% of patients on placebo plus DMARDs. Approximately half of the patients who developed an ANC $<1 \times 10^9$/l did so within 8 weeks after starting therapy. Decreases below 0.5×10^9/l were reported in 0.3% patients receiving tocilizumab 8 mg/kg plus DMARDs. There was no clear association between decreases in neutrophils and the occurrence of serious infections.

Decreases in platelet counts below 100×10^3/μl occurred in 1.7% of patients on tocilizumab 8 mg/kg plus DMARDs compared to <1% on placebo plus DMARDs. These decreases occurred without associated bleeding events.

Hepatic transaminase elevations

Transient elevations in ALT/AST >3 × ULN were observed in 2.1% of patients on tocilizumab 8 mg/kg compared to 4.9% of patients on MTX and in 6.5% of patients who received 8 mg/kg tocilizumab plus DMARDs compared to 1.5% of patients on placebo plus DMARDs.

The addition of potentially hepatotoxic drugs (e.g. MTX) to tocilizumab monotherapy resulted in increased frequency of these elevations. Elevations of ALT/AST >5 × ULN were observed in 0.7% of tocilizumab monotherapy patients and 1.4% of tocilizumab plus DMARD patients, the majority of whom were discontinued permanently from tocilizumab treatment. These elevations were not associated with clinically relevant increase in direct bilirubin, nor were they associated with clinical evidence of hepatitis or hepatic impairment.

Lipid parameters

During the six month controlled trials, increases of lipid parameters such as total cholesterol, triglycerides, LDL cholesterol, and/or HDL cholesterol have been reported commonly. Approximately 24% of patients receiving RoActemra in clinical trials experienced sustained elevations in total cholesterol ≥6.2 mmol/l, with 15% experiencing a sustained increase in LDL to ≥4.1 mmol/l. Elevations in lipid parameters responded to treatment with lipid-lowering agents.

Malignancies

The clinical data are insufficient to assess the potential incidence of malignancy following exposure to tocilizumab. Long-term safety evaluations are ongoing.

4.9 Overdose

There are limited data available on overdose with RoActemra. One case of accidental overdose was reported in

Table 2. ACR responses in placebo-/MTX-/DMARDs-controlled studies (% patients)

	Study I AMBITION		Study II LITHE		Study III OPTION		Study IV TOWARD		Study V RADIATE	
Week	TCZ 8 mg/kg	MTX	TCZ 8 mg/kg + MTX	PBO + MTX	TCZ 8 mg/kg + MTX	PBO + MTX	TCZ 8 mg/kg + DMARD	PBO + DMARD	TCZ 8 mg/kg + MTX	PBO + MTX
	N = 286	N = 284	N = 398	N = 393	N = 205	N = 204	N = 803	N = 413	N = 170	N = 158
ACR 20										
24	70%***	53%	56%***	27%	59%***	27%	61%***	25%	50%***	10%
52			56%***	25%						
ACR 50										
24	44%**	34%	32%***	10%	44%***	11%	38%***	9%	29%***	4%
52			36%***	10%						
ACR 70										
24	28%**	15%	13%***	2%	22%***	2%	21%***	3%	12%**	1%
52			20%***	4%						

TCZ - Tocilizumab

MTX - Methotrexate

PBO - Placebo

DMARD - Disease modifying anti-rheumatic drug

** - p< 0.05 , TCZ vs. PBO + MTX/DMARD*

*** - p< 0.01, TCZ vs. PBO + MTX/DMARD*

**** - p< 0.0001, TCZ vs. PBO + MTX/DMARD*

which a patient with multiple myeloma received a single dose of 40 mg/kg. No adverse reactions were observed.

No serious adverse reactions were observed in healthy volunteers who received a single dose up to 28 mg/kg, although dose limiting neutropenia was observed.

5. PHARMACOLOGICAL PROPERTIES

5.1 Pharmacodynamic properties

Pharmacotherapeutic group: Immunosupressants, Interleukin inhibitors; ATC code: L04AC07.

Mechanism of action

Tocilizumab binds specifically to both soluble and membrane-bound IL-6 receptors (sIL-6R and mIL-6R). Tocilizumab has been shown to inhibit sIL-6R and mIL-6R-mediated signalling. IL-6 is a pleiotropic pro-inflammatory cytokine produced by a variety of cell types including T- and B-cells, monocytes and fibroblasts. IL-6 is involved in diverse physiological processes such as T-cell activation, induction of immunoglobulin secretion, induction of hepatic acute phase protein synthesis and stimulation of haemopoiesis. IL-6 has been implicated in the pathogenesis of diseases including inflammatory diseases, osteoporosis and neoplasia.

In clinical studies with tocilizumab, rapid decreases in CRP, erythrocyte sedimentation rate (ESR) and serum amyloid A (SAA) were observed. Consistent with the effect on acute phase reactants, treatment with tocilizumab was associated with reduction in platelet count within the normal range. Increases in haemoglobin levels were observed, through tocilizumab decreasing the IL-6 driven effects on hepcidin production to increase iron availability. In tocilizumab-treated patients, decreases in the levels of CRP to within normal ranges were seen as early as week 2, with decreases maintained while on treatment.

Clinical efficacy

The efficacy of tocilizumab in alleviating the signs and symptoms of RA was assessed in five randomised, double-blind, multi-centre studies. Studies I-V enrolled patients ≥18 years of age with active RA diagnosed according to the American College of Rheumatology (ACR) criteria and who had at least eight tender and six swollen joints at baseline.

In Study I, tocilizumab was administered intravenously every four weeks as monotherapy. In Studies II, III and V, tocilizumab was administered intravenously every four weeks in combination with MTX vs. placebo and MTX. In Study IV, tocilizumab was administered intravenously every 4 weeks in combination with other DMARDs vs. placebo and other DMARDs. The primary endpoint for each of the five studies was the proportion of patients who achieved an ACR 20 response at week 24.

Study I evaluated 673 patients who had not been treated with MTX within six months prior to randomisation and who had not discontinued previous MTX treatment as a result of clinically important toxic effects or lack of response. The majority (67%) of patients were MTX-naïve. Doses of 8 mg/kg of tocilizumab were given every four weeks as monotherapy. The comparator group was weekly MTX (dose titrated from 7.5 mg to a maximum of 20 mg weekly over an eight week period).

Study II, a two year study with planned analyses at week 24 and week 52, evaluated 1196 patients who had an inadequate clinical response to MTX. Doses of 4 or 8 mg/kg of tocilizumab or placebo were given every four weeks as blinded therapy for 52 weeks in combination with stable MTX (10 mg to 25 mg weekly). The primary endpoint at week 24 was the proportion of patients who achieved an ACR 20 response. At week 52 the co-primary endpoints were prevention of joint damage and improvement in physical function.

Study III evaluated 623 patients who had an inadequate clinical response to MTX. Doses of 4 or 8 mg/kg tocilizumab or placebo were given every four weeks, in combination with stable MTX (10 mg to 25 mg weekly).

Study IV evaluated 1,220 patients who had an inadequate response to their existing rheumatologic therapy, including one or more DMARDs. Doses of 8 mg/kg tocilizumab or placebo were given every four weeks in combination with stable DMARDs.

Study V evaluated 499 patients who had an inadequate clinical response or were intolerant to one or more TNF antagonist therapies. The TNF antagonist therapy was discontinued prior to randomisation. Doses of 4 or 8 mg/kg tocilizumab or placebo were given every four weeks in combination with stable MTX (10 mg to 25 mg weekly).

Clinical response

In all studies, patients treated with tocilizumab 8 mg/kg had statistically significant higher ACR 20, 50, 70 response rates at 6 months compared to control (Table 2). In study I, superiority of tocilizumab 8 mg/kg was demonstrated against the active comparator MTX.

The treatment effect was similar in patients independent of rheumatoid factor status, age, gender, race, number of prior treatments or disease status. Time to onset was rapid (as early as week 2) and the magnitude of response continued to improve with duration of treatment. Continued durable responses were seen for over 24 months in the ongoing open label extension studies I, III, IV and V.

In patients treated with tocilizumab 8 mg/kg, significant improvements were noted on all individual components of the ACR response including: tender and swollen joint counts; patients and physician global assessment; disability index scores; pain assessment and CRP compared to patients receiving placebo plus MTX or other DMARDs in all studies.

Patients in studies I – V had a mean Disease Activity Score (DAS28) of 6.5–6.8 at baseline. Significant reduction in DAS28 from baseline (mean improvement) of 3.1–3.4 were observed in tocilizumab-treated patients compared to control patients (1.3-2.1). The proportion of patients achieving a DAS28 clinical remission (DAS28 <2.6) was significantly higher in patients receiving tocilizumab (28–34%) compared to 1–12% of control patients at 24 weeks. In study II, 47% of patients achieved a DAS28 <2.6 at 52 weeks compared to 33% of patients at week 24.

In a pooled analysis of studies II, III and IV, the proportion of patients achieving an ACR 20, 50 and 70 response was significantly higher (59% vs. 50%, 37% vs. 27%, 18% vs. 11%, respectively) in the tocilizumab 8 mg/kg plus DMARD vs. the tocilizumab 4 mg/kg plus DMARD group ($p < 0.03$). Similarly the proportion of patients achieving a DAS 28 remission (DAS28 <2.6) was significantly higher (31% vs. 16% respectively) in patients receiving tocilizumab 8 mg/kg plus DMARD than in patients receiving tocilizumab 4 mg/kg plus DMARD ($p < 0.0001$).

Table 2. ACR responses in placebo-/MTX-/DMARDs-controlled studies (% patients)

(see Table 2 on previous page)

Radiographic response

In Study II, in patients with an inadequate response to MTX, inhibition of structural joint damage was assessed radiographically and expressed as change in modified Sharp score and its components, the erosion score and joint space narrowing score. Inhibition of joint structural damage was shown with significantly less radiographic progression in patients receiving tocilizumab compared to control (Table 3).

Table 3. Radiographic mean changes over 52 weeks in Study II

	PBO + MTX (+ TCZ from week 24) N = 393	TCZ 8 mg/kg + MTX N = 398
Total Sharp-Genant score	1.13	0.29*
Erosion score	0.71	0.17*
JSN score	0.42	0.12**

PBO - Placebo

MTX - Methotrexate

TCZ - Tocilizumab

JSN - Joint space narrowing

** - p≤ 0.0001, TCZ vs. PBO + MTX*

*** - p< 0.005, TCZ vs. PBO + MTX*

Health-related and quality of life outcomes

Tocilizumab-treated patients reported an improvement in all patient-reported outcomes (Health Assessment Questionnaire Disability Index - HAQ-DI), Short Form-36 and Functional Assessment of Chronic Illness Therapy questionnaires. Statistically significant improvements in HAQ-DI scores were observed in patients treated with RoActemra compared with patients treated with DMARDs.

Haemoglobin levels

Statistically significant improvements in haemoglobin levels were observed with tocilizumab compared with DMARDs ($p < 0.0001$) at week 24. Mean haemoglobin levels increased by week 2 and remained within normal range through to week 24.

5.2 Pharmacokinetic properties

The pharmacokinetics of tocilizumab were determined using a population pharmacokinetic analysis on a database composed of 1,793 RA patients treated with a one-hour infusion of 4 and 8 mg/kg tocilizumab every 4 weeks for 24 weeks.

The following parameters (predicted mean ± SD) were estimated for a dose of 8 mg/kg tocilizumab given every 4 weeks: steady-state area under curve (AUC) = 35000 ± 15500 h μg/ml, trough concentration (C_{min}) = 9.74 ± 10.5 μg/ml and maximum concentration (C_{max}) = 183 ± 85.6 μg/ml, and the accumulation ratios for AUC and C_{max} were small, 1.22 and 1.06, respectively. The accumulation ratio was higher for C_{min} (2.35), which was expected based on the non-linear clearance contribution at lower concentrations. Steady-state was reached following the first administration for C_{max} and after 8 and 20 weeks for AUC and C_{min}, respectively.

Distribution

In RA patients the central volume of distribution was 3.5 l, the peripheral volume of distribution was 2.9 l resulting in a volume of distribution at steady state of 6.4 l.

Elimination

Following intravenous administration, tocilizumab undergoes biphasic elimination from the circulation. The total clearance of tocilizumab was concentration-dependent and is the sum of the linear and non-linear clearance. The linear clearance was estimated as a parameter in the population pharmacokinetic analysis and was 12.5 ml/h. The concentration-dependent non-linear clearance plays a major role at low tocilizumab concentrations. Once the non-linear clearance pathway is saturated, at higher tocilizumab concentrations, clearance is mainly determined by the linear clearance.

The $t_{1/2}$ of tocilizumab was concentration-dependent. At steady-state following a dose of 8 mg/kg every 4 weeks, the effective $t_{1/2}$ decreased with decreasing concentrations within a dosing interval from 14 days to 8 days.

Linearity

Pharmacokinetic parameters of tocilizumab did not change with time. A more than dose-proportional increase in the AUC and C_{min} was observed for doses of 4 and 8 mg/kg every 4 weeks. C_{max} increased dose-proportionally. At steady-state, predicted AUC and C_{min} were 2.7 and 6.5 fold higher at 8 mg/kg as compared to 4 mg/kg, respectively.

Special populations

Renal impairment: No formal study of the effect of renal impairment on the pharmacokinetics of tocilizumab has been conducted. Most of the patients in the population pharmacokinetic analysis had normal renal function or mild renal impairment. Mild renal impairment (creatinine clearance based on Cockcroft-Gault <80 ml/min and ≥50 ml/min) did not impact the pharmacokinetics of tocilizumab.

Hepatic impairment: No formal study of the effect of hepatic impairment on the pharmacokinetics of tocilizumab has been conducted.

Age, gender and ethnicity: Population pharmacokinetic analyses in adult RA patients, showed that age, gender and ethnic origin did not affect the pharmacokinetics of tocilizumab.

5.3 Preclinical safety data

Non-clinical data reveal no special hazard for humans based on conventional studies of safety pharmacology, repeated dose toxicity and genotoxicity.

Carcinogenicity and fertility studies were not performed with tocilizumab due to the lack of appropriate models for an antibody with no reactivity to rodent IL-6 receptors.

Available non-clinical data demonstrated the effect of IL-6 on malignant progression and apoptosis resistance to various cancer types. This data does not suggest a relevant risk for cancer initiation and progression under tocilizumab treatment. Additionally, proliferative lesions were not observed in a 6-month chronic toxicity study in cynomolgus monkeys or in IL-6 deficient mice.

Available non-clinical data do not suggest an effect on fertility under tocilizumab treatment. Effects on endocrine active and reproductive system organs were not observed in a chronic cynomolgus monkey toxicity study and reproductive performance was not affected in IL-6 deficient mice. Tocilizumab administered to cynomolgus monkeys during early gestation, was observed to have no direct or indirect harmful effect on pregnancy or embryonal-foetal development. However, a slight increase in abortion/embryonal-foetal death was observed with high systemic exposure (>100 × human exposure) in the 50 mg/kg/day high-dose group compared to placebo and other low-dose groups. Although IL-6 does not seem to be a critical cytokine for foetal growth or the immunological control of the maternal/foetal interface, a relation of this finding to tocilizumab cannot be excluded.

6. PHARMACEUTICAL PARTICULARS

6.1 List of excipients

Sucrose

Polysorbate 80

Disodium phosphate dodecahydrate

Sodium dihydrogen phosphate dihydrate

Water for injections

6.2 Incompatibilities

This medicinal product must not be mixed with other medicinal products except those mentioned in section 6.6.

6.3 Shelf life

Unopened vial: 30 months

Diluted product: After dilution, the prepared solution for infusion is physically and chemically stable in sodium chloride 9 mg/ml (0.9%) solution for injection at 30°C for 24 hours.

From a microbiological point of view, the prepared solution for infusion should be used immediately. If not used immediately, in use storage times and conditions prior to use are the responsibility of the user and would normally not be longer than 24 hours at 2°C–8°C, unless dilution has taken place in controlled and validated aseptic conditions.

RoActemra is supplied as a sterile concentrate that does not contain preservatives.

6.4 Special precautions for storage

Store vials in a refrigerator (2°C–8°C). Do not freeze.

Keep the vial(s) in the outer carton in order to protect from light.

For storage conditions of the diluted medicinal product see section 6.3.

6.5 Nature and contents of container

RoActemra is supplied in a vial (type I glass) with a stopper (butyl rubber) containing 4 ml, 10 ml or 20 ml concentrate. Pack sizes of 1 and 4 vials.

Not all pack sizes may be marketed.

6.6 Special precautions for disposal and other handling

Instructions for dilution prior to administration

Parenteral medicinal products should be inspected visually for particulate matter or discoloration prior to administration. Only solutions which are clear to opalescent, colourless to pale yellow and free of visible particles should be diluted.

Withdraw a volume of sterile, non-pyrogenic sodium chloride 9 mg/ml (0.9%) solution for injection from a 100 ml infusion bag, equal to the volume of RoActemra concentrate required for the patients dose, under aseptic conditions. The required amount of RoActemra concentrate (0.4 ml/kg) should be withdrawn from the vial and placed in the 100 ml infusion bag. This should be a final volume of 100 ml. To mix the solution, gently invert the infusion bag to avoid foaming.

RoActemra is for single-use only.

Any unused product or waste material should be disposed of in accordance with local requirements.

7. MARKETING AUTHORISATION HOLDER

Roche Registration Limited
6 Falcon Way
Shire Park
Welwyn Garden City
AL7 1TW
United Kingdom

8. MARKETING AUTHORISATION NUMBER(S)

EU/1/08/492/001
EU/1/08/492/003
EU/1/08/492/005

9. DATE OF FIRST AUTHORISATION/RENEWAL OF THE AUTHORISATION

Date of first authorisation: 16th January 2009

10. DATE OF REVISION OF THE TEXT

28 October 2009

Detailed information on this medicinal product is available on the website of the European Medicines Agency (EMEA) http://www.emea.europa.eu/.

Rocaltrol

(Roche Products Limited)

1. NAME OF THE MEDICINAL PRODUCT

Rocaltrol 0.25 microgram Capsules.

Rocaltrol 0.5 microgram Capsules.

2. QUALITATIVE AND QUANTITATIVE COMPOSITION

Each capsule contains either 0.25 or 0.5 microgram of calcitriol.

For excipients, see 6.1.

3. PHARMACEUTICAL FORM

Soft capsules.

0.25 microgram: One length brown-orange to red-orange opaque and the other white to grey-yellow or grey-orange opaque.

0.5 microgram: Both lengths brown-orange to red-orange opaque.

4. CLINICAL PARTICULARS

4.1 Therapeutic indications

Rocaltrol is indicated for the correction of the abnormalities of calcium and phosphate metabolism in patients with renal osteodystrophy.

Rocaltrol is also indicated for the treatment of established post-menopausal osteoporosis.

4.2 Posology and method of administration

The dose of Rocaltrol should be carefully adjusted for each patient according to the biological response so as to avoid hypercalcaemia.

The effectiveness of treatment depends in part on an adequate daily intake of calcium, which should be augmented by dietary changes or supplements if necessary. The capsules should be swallowed with a little water.

Adults

Renal Osteodystrophy

The initial daily dose is 0.25 mcg of Rocaltrol. In patients with normal or only slightly reduced calcium levels, doses of 0.25 mcg every other day are sufficient. If no satisfactory response in the biochemical parameters and clinical manifestations of the disease is observed within 2 - 4 weeks, the daily dosage may be increased by 0.25 mcg at 2 - 4 week intervals. During this period, serum calcium levels should be determined at least twice weekly. Should the serum calcium levels rise to 1 mg/ 100ml (250 μmol/l) above normal (9 to 11 mg/100 ml or 2250 - 2750 μmol/l), or serum creatinine rises to > 120 μmol/l, treatment with Rocaltrol should be stopped immediately until normocalcaemia ensues. Most patients respond to between 0.5 mcg and 1.0 mcg daily. See section 4.5 for details of dose adjustments related to drug interactions.

An oral Rocaltrol pulse therapy with an initial dosage of 0.1 mcg/kg/week split into two or three equal doses given at the end of the dialysis has been shown to be effective in patients with osteodystrophy refractory to continuous therapy. A maximum total cumulative dosage of 12 mcg per week should not be exceeded.

Post-menopausal Osteoporosis

The recommended dose of Rocaltrol is 0.25 mcg twice daily.

Serum calcium and creatinine levels should be determined at 1, 3 and 6 months and at 6 monthly intervals thereafter.

Elderly

Clinical experience with Rocaltrol in elderly patients indicates that the dosage recommended for use in younger adults may be given without apparent ill-consequence.

Children

Dosage in children has not been established.

Rocaltrol capsules are for oral administration only.

4.3 Contraindications

Rocaltrol should not be given to patients with hypercalcaemia or evidence of metastatic calcification. The use of Rocaltrol in patients with known hypersensitivity to calcitriol (or drugs of the same class) and any of the constituent excipients is contraindicated.

Rocaltrol is contraindicated if there is evidence of vitamin D toxicity.

Owing to the presence of sorbitol, patients with rare hereditary problems of fructose intolerance should not take this medicine.

4.4 Special warnings and precautions for use

All other vitamin D compounds and their derivatives, including proprietary compounds or foodstuffs which may be "fortified" with vitamin D, should be withheld during treatment with Rocaltrol.

If the patient is switched from a long acting vitamin D preparation (e.g. ergocalciferol or colecalciferol) to calcitriol, it may take several months for the level in the blood to return to the baseline value, thereby increasing the risk of hypercalcaemia.

An abrupt increase in calcium intake as a result of changes in diet (e.g. increased consumption of dairy products) or uncontrolled intake of calcium preparations may trigger hypercalcaemia. Patients and families should be advised that strict adherence to prescribed diets is mandatory and they should be instructed on how to recognise the symptoms of hypercalcaemia.

In patients with end-stage renal failure, treatment does not obviate the need to control plasma phosphate with phosphate-binding agents. Since Rocaltrol affects phosphate transport in the gut and bone, the dose of phosphate-binding agent may need to be modified. The value for serum calcium multiplied by phosphorus (Ca × P) should not be allowed to exceed 70 mg^2/dl^2 or 5.6 $mmol^2/l^2$.

Immobilised patients, e.g. those who have undergone surgery, are particularly exposed to the risk of hypercalcaemia.

Patients with normal renal function who are taking Rocaltrol should avoid dehydration. Adequate fluid intake should be maintained.

4.5 Interaction with other medicinal products and other forms of interaction

Concomitant treatment with a thiazide diuretic increases the risk of hypercalcaemia. Calcitriol dosage must be determined with care in patients undergoing treatment with digitalis, as hypercalcaemia in such patients may precipitate cardiac arrhythmias.

Vitamin D derivatives can increase magnesium absorption, although magnesium balance is generally not affected, owing to a compensatory increase in urinary excretion. It is therefore recommended that magnesium-containing drugs (e.g. antacids) are not taken by patients with chronic renal failure on dialysis during therapy with Rocaltrol since, under these circumstances, hypermagnesaemia could occur.

Administration of enzyme inducers such as phenytoin or phenobarbital may lead to increased metabolism and hence reduced serum concentrations of calcitriol. Therefore higher doses of calcitriol may be necessary if these drugs are administered simultaneously.

A relationship of functional antagonism exists between vitamin D analogues, which promote calcium absorption, and corticosteroids, which inhibit it.

Colestyramine can reduce intestinal absorption of fat-soluble vitamins and therefore may impair intestinal absorption of calcitriol.

4.6 Pregnancy and lactation

The safety of Rocaltrol during pregnancy has not been established. Studies of reproductive toxicology in animals have not yielded unequivocal findings, and no controlled studies on the effect of exogenous calcitriol on pregnancy and foetal development have been performed in human subjects. Consequently Rocaltrol should be given only when the potential benefit has been weighed against the possible hazard to the foetus. The usual caution in prescribing any drug for women of childbearing age should be observed.

It should be assumed that exogenous calcitriol passes into breast milk. Mothers may breastfeed while taking Rocaltrol, provided that the serum calcium levels of the mother and infant are monitored.

4.7 Effects on ability to drive and use machines

Not relevant.

4.8 Undesirable effects

The number of adverse effects reported from clinical use of Rocaltrol over a period of 15 years in all indications is very low with each individual effect, including hypercalcaemia, occurring rarely (≤ 0.001%).

Hypercalcaemia and hypercalcuria are the major side effects of Rocaltrol and indicate excessive dosage. Patients with tertiary hyperparathyroidism, renal failure, or on regular haemodialysis are particularly prone to develop hypercalcaemia. The clinical features of hypercalcaemia include anorexia, constipation, nausea, vomiting, headache, weakness, apathy and somnolence. More severe manifestations may include fever, thirst/polydipsia, dehydration, polyuria, nocturia, abdominal pain, paralytic ileus, cardiac arrhythmias and psychiatric disturbances. Rarely, overt psychosis and metastatic calcification (particularly nephrocalcinosis and renal stones) may occur. The relatively short biological half-life of Rocaltrol permits rapid elimination of the compound when treatment is stopped and hypercalcaemia will recede within 2 - 7 days. This rate of reversal of biological effects is more rapid than when other vitamin D derivatives are used.

In patients with normal renal function, chronic hypercalcaemia may be associated with an increase in serum creatinine.

Mild, non-progressive and reversible elevations in levels of liver enzymes (SGOT, SGPT) have been noted in a few patients treated with Rocaltrol, but no pathological changes in the liver have been reported.

Hypersensitivity reactions (pruritus, rash, urticaria and, very rarely, severe erythematous skin disorders) may occur in susceptible individuals.

4.9 Overdose

In acute overdosage, toxic features are unlikely to arise, and the recommended treatment is liberal fluids only.

Should hypercalcaemia occur following prolonged treatment, Rocaltrol should be discontinued until plasma calcium levels have returned to normal. A low-calcium diet will speed this reversal. Rocaltrol can then be restarted at a lower dose or given in the same dose but at less frequent intervals than previously. Severe or persistent hypercalcaemia may be treated by administering corticosteroids, ensuring adequate hydration, inducing a diuresis where practicable and by general supportive measures. Calcitonin may increase the rate of fall of serum calcium when bone resorption is increased.

In patients treated by intermittent haemodialysis, a low concentration of calcium in the dialysate may also be used. However, a high concentration of calcium in the dialysate may contribute to the development of hypercalcaemia.

5. PHARMACOLOGICAL PROPERTIES

5.1 Pharmacodynamic properties

Calcitriol has the greatest biological activity of the known vitamin D metabolites and is normally formed in the kidneys from its immediate precursor, 25-hydroxycholecalciferol. In physiological amounts it augments the intestinal absorption of calcium and phosphate and plays a significant part in the regulation of bone mineralisation. The defective production of calcitriol in chronic renal failure contributes to the abnormalities of mineral metabolism found in that disorder.

Rocaltrol is a synthetic preparation of calcitriol. Oral administration of Rocaltrol to patients with chronic renal failure compensates for impaired endogenous production of calcitriol which is decreased when the glomerular filtration rate falls below 30 ml/min. Consequently, intestinal malabsorption of calcium and phosphate and the resulting hypocalcaemia are improved, thereby reversing the signs and symptoms of bone disease.

In patients with established post-menopausal osteoporosis, Rocaltrol increases calcium absorption, elevates circulating levels of calcitriol and reduces vertebral fracture frequency.

The onset and reversal of the effects of Rocaltrol are more rapid than those of other compounds with vitamin D activity and adjustment of the dose can be achieved sooner and more precisely. The effects of inadvertent overdosage can also be reversed more readily.

5.2 Pharmacokinetic properties

Absorption

Calcitriol is rapidly absorbed from the intestine. Peak serum concentrations following a single oral dose of 0.25-0.75 mcg Rocaltrol were found within 2-4 hours in healthy subjects.

After a single oral dose of 0.5 mcg Rocaltrol in healthy subjects, the average serum concentrations of calcitriol rose from a baseline value of 40.0 ± 4.4 pg/ml to 60.0 ± 4.4 pg/ml after two hours, and then fell to 53.0 ± 6.9 after four hours, to 50.0 ± 7.0 after eight hours, to 44 ± 4.6 after twelve hours and to 41.5 ± 5.1 pg/ml after 24 hours.

Distribution

During transport in the blood at physiological concentrations, calcitriol is mostly bound to a specific vitamin D binding protein (DBP), but also, to a lesser degree, to lipoproteins and albumin. At higher blood calcitriol concentrations, DBP appears to become saturated, and increased binding to lipoproteins and albumin occurs.

Metabolism

Calcitriol is inactivated in both the kidney and the intestine, through the formation of a number of intermediates.

Elimination

The reported elimination half-life of calcitriol in serum is between 5 and 17 hours in normal subjects, but may extend to between 18 and 44 hours in patients with severe chronic renal failure. However, the pharmacological effect of a single dose of calcitriol lasts at least 4 days. Calcitriol is excreted in the bile and is subject to enterohepatic circulation.

5.3 Preclinical safety data

Acute toxicity studies of calcitriol in mice and rats indicated oral approximate median lethal doses of 3.9 and 3.2 mg/kg, respectively. These values are several orders of magnitude higher than the proposed clinical dose of 0.25 mcg twice daily (approximately 8-10 ng/kg/day).

Subchronic toxicity studies in rats and dogs indicated that calcitriol at an oral dose of 20 ng/kg/day (twice the usual human dosage) for up to 6 months produced no or minimal adverse effects. A dose of 80 ng/kg/day (8 times the usual human dosage) for up to 6 months produced moderate adverse effects; changes seen appeared to be primarily the result of prolonged hypercalcaemia.

Reproductive toxicity studies in rats indicated that oral doses up to 300 ng/kg/day (30 times the usual human dose) did not adversely affect reproduction. In rabbits, multiple foetal abnormalities were observed in one litter from each group at oral doses of 300 ng/kg/day and 80 ng/kg/day, but not at 20 ng/kg/day (twice the usual human dose). Although there were no statistically significant differences between treated groups and controls in the numbers of litters or foetuses showing abnormalities, the possibility that these findings were due to calcitriol administration could not be discounted.

6. PHARMACEUTICAL PARTICULARS

6.1 List of excipients

Content

Butylhydroxyanisole

Butylhydroxytoluene

Medium-chain triglycerides

Shell

Gelatin

Glycerol

Karion 83 (Sorbitol, Mannitol, Hydrogenated hydrolysed starch)

Titanium dioxide E171

Iron oxide red E172

Iron oxide yellow E172

6.2 Incompatibilities

None.

6.3 Shelf life

3 years.

6.4 Special precautions for storage

Do not store above 25°C. Store in the original package and keep the blisters in the outer carton in order to protect from light and moisture.

6.5 Nature and contents of container

PVC opaque blisters containing 100 capsules (5 strips of 20 capsules).

6.6 Special precautions for disposal and other handling

Not applicable.

7. MARKETING AUTHORISATION HOLDER

Roche Products Limited, 6 Falcon Way, Shire Park, Welwyn Garden City, AL7 1TW, United Kingdom.

8. MARKETING AUTHORISATION NUMBER(S)

Rocaltrol 0.25 microgram Capsules: PL 00031/0122

Rocaltrol 0.5 microgram Capsules: PL 00031/0123

9. DATE OF FIRST AUTHORISATION/RENEWAL OF THE AUTHORISATION

13 January 2003

10. DATE OF REVISION OF THE TEXT

May 2008

Rocaltrol is a registered trade mark

Rocephin 250mg, 1g and 2g vials

(Roche Products Limited)

1. NAME OF THE MEDICINAL PRODUCT

Rocephin 250mg vials.

2. QUALITATIVE AND QUANTITATIVE COMPOSITION

Each 250mg vial contains 250mg ceftriaxone as 298.3mg hydrated disodium ceftriaxone.

Each 1g vial contains 1g ceftriaxone as 1.19g hydrated disodium ceftriaxone.

Each 2g vial contains 2g ceftriaxone as 2.39g hydrated disodium ceftriaxone.

3. PHARMACEUTICAL FORM

Powder for solution for injection.

4. CLINICAL PARTICULARS

4.1 Therapeutic indications

Ceftriaxone is indicated for the treatment of the following infections when known or likely to be due to one or more susceptible micro-organisms (see section *5.1*) and when parenteral therapy is required:

Pneumonia.

septicaemia.

Meningitis.

Bone, skin and soft tissue infections.

Infections in neutropenic patients.

Gonorrhoea.

Peri-operative prophylaxis of infections associated with surgery.

Treatment may be started before the results of susceptibility tests are known.

Consideration should be given to official guidance on the appropriate use of antibacterial agents.

4.2 Posology and method of administration

Rocephin may be administered by deep intramuscular injection, slow intravenous injection, or as a slow intravenous infusion, after reconstitution of the solution according to the directions given below. Dosage and mode of administration should be determined by the severity of the infection, susceptibility of the causative organism and the patient's condition. Under most circumstances a once-daily dose - or, in the specified indications, a single dose - will give satisfactory therapeutic results.

Adults and children 12 years and over

Standard therapeutic dosage: 1g once daily.

Severe infections: 2 - 4g daily, normally as a single dose every 24 hours.

The duration of therapy varies according to the course of the disease. As with antibiotic therapy in general, administration of Rocephin should be continued for a minimum of 48 to 72 hours after the patient has become afebrile or evidence of bacterial eradication has been obtained.

Acute, uncomplicated gonorrhoea: A single dose of 250mg intramuscularly should be administered. Simultaneous administration of probenecid is not indicated.

Peri-operative prophylaxis: Usually 1g as a single intramuscular or slow intravenous dose. In colorectal surgery, 2g should be given intramuscularly (dosages greater than 1g should be divided and injected at more than one site), or by slow intravenous infusion, in conjunction with a suitable agent against anaerobic bacteria.

Elderly

These dosages do not require modification in elderly patients provided that renal and hepatic function are satisfactory (see below).

Neonates, infants and children up to 12 years

The following dosage schedules are recommended for once daily administration:

Neonates

A daily dose of 20 - 50mg/kg body weight, not to exceed 50mg/kg. In the neonate, the intravenous dose should be given over 60 minutes to reduce the displacement of bilirubin from albumin, thereby reducing the potential risk of bilirubin encephalopathy (see section *4.4*).

Infants and children of up to 12 years

Standard therapeutic dosage: 20 - 50mg/kg body weight once daily.

In severe infections up to 80mg/kg body weight daily may be given. For children with body weights of 50kg or more, the usual adult dosage should be used. Doses of 50mg/kg or over should be given by slow intravenous infusion over at least 30 minutes. Doses greater than 80mg/kg body weight should be avoided because of the increased risk of biliary precipitates.

Renal and hepatic impairment

In patients with impaired renal function, there is no need to reduce the dosage of Rocephin provided liver function is intact. Only in cases of pre-terminal renal failure (creatinine clearance < 10ml per minute) should the daily dosage be limited to 2g or less.

In patients with liver damage there is no need for the dosage to be reduced provided renal function is intact.

In severe renal impairment accompanied by hepatic insufficiency, the plasma concentration of Rocephin should be determined at regular intervals and dosage adjusted.

In patients undergoing dialysis, no additional supplementary dosing is required following the dialysis. Serum concentrations should be monitored, however, to determine whether dosage adjustments are necessary, since the elimination rate in these patients may be reduced.

4.3 Contraindications

Hypersensitivity to ceftriaxone or to any of the cephalosporins.

Previous immediate and/or severe hypersensitivity reaction to a penicillin or to any other type of beta-lactam drug.

Rocephin should not be given to neonates with jaundice or to those who are hypoalbuminaemic or acidotic or have other conditions, such as prematurity, in which bilirubin binding is likely to be impaired.

4.4 Special warnings and precautions for use

Before therapy with ceftriaxone is instituted, careful inquiry should be made to determine whether the patient has had any previous hypersensitivity reactions to ceftriaxone, any other cephalosporin, or to any penicillin or other beta-lactam drug. Ceftriaxone is contraindicated in patients who have had a previous hypersensitivity reaction to any cephalosporin. It is also contraindicated in patients who have had a previous immediate and/or any severe hypersensitivity reaction to any penicillin or to any other beta-lactam drug. Ceftriaxone should be given with caution to patients who have had any other type of hypersensitivity reaction to a penicillin or any other beta-lactam drug.

Ceftriaxone should be given with caution to patients who have other allergic diatheses.

Antibiotic-associated diarrhoea, colitis and pseudomembranous colitis have all been reported with the use of ceftriaxone. These diagnoses should be considered in any patient who develops diarrhoea during or shortly after treatment. Ceftriaxone should be discontinued if severe and/or bloody diarrhoea occurs during treatment and appropriate therapy instituted.

Ceftriaxone should be used with caution in individuals with a previous history of gastro-intestinal disease, particularly colitis.

As with other cephalosporins, prolonged use of ceftriaxone may result in the overgrowth of non-susceptible organisms, such as *enterococci* and *Candida spp*.

In severe renal impairment accompanied by hepatic insufficiency, dosage reduction is required as outlined under section *4.2*.

In vivo and *in vitro* studies have shown that ceftriaxone, like some other cephalosporins, can displace bilirubin from serum albumin. Clinical data obtained in neonates have confirmed this finding. Rocephin should therefore not be used in jaundiced new-borns or in those who are hypoalbuminaemic or acidotic, in whom bilirubin binding is likely to be impaired. Particular caution should be exercised in babies born prematurely.

Rocephin may precipitate in the gallbladder and then be detectable as shadows on ultrasound (see section *4.8*). This can happen in patients of any age, but is more likely in infants and small children who are usually given a larger dose of Rocephin on a body weight basis. In children, doses greater than 80mg/kg body weight should be avoided because of the increased risk of biliary precipitates. There is no clear evidence of gallstones or of acute cholecystitis developing in children or infants treated with Rocephin. As the condition appears to be transient and reversible upon discontinuation, therapeutic procedures are not normally indicated.

Cephalosporins as a class tend to be absorbed onto the surface of the red cell membranes and react with antibodies directed against the drug to produce a positive Coombs' test and occasionally a rather mild haemolytic anaemia. In this respect, there may be some cross-reactivity with penicillins.

Cases of pancreatitis, possibly of biliary obstruction aetiology, have been rarely reported in patients treated with Rocephin. Most patients presented with risk factors for biliary stasis and biliary sludge, e.g. preceding major therapy, severe illness and total parenteral nutrition. A trigger or cofactor role of Rocephin-related biliary precipitation can not be ruled out.

The stated dosage should not be exceeded.

Each gram of Rocephin contains approximately 3.6mmol sodium. To be taken into consideration by patients on a controlled sodium diet.

4.5 Interaction with other medicinal products and other forms of interaction

No impairment of renal function has been observed in man after simultaneous administration of Rocephin with diuretics.

No interference with the action or increase in nephrotoxicity of aminoglycosides has been observed during simultaneous administration with Rocephin.

The ceftriaxone molecule does not contain the N-methylthio-tetrazole substituent which has been associated with a disulfiram-like effect when alcohol is taken during therapy with certain cephalosporins.

In vitro, chloramphenicol has been shown to be antagonistic with respect to ceftriaxone and other cephalosporins. The clinical relevance of this finding is unknown, but caution is advised if concurrent administration of ceftriaxone with chloramphenicol is proposed.

In patients treated with Rocephin, the Coombs' test may rarely become false-positive. Rocephin, like other antibiotics, may result in false-positive tests for galactosaemia. Likewise, non-enzymatic methods for glucose determination in urine may give false-positive results. For this reason, urine-glucose determination during therapy with Rocephin should be done enzymatically.

Ceftriaxone may adversely affect the efficacy of oral hormonal contraceptives. Consequently, it is advisable to use supplementary (non-hormonal) contraceptive measures during treatment and in the month following treatment.

4.6 Pregnancy and lactation

Pregnancy

For ceftriaxone, limited clinical data on exposed pregnancies are available. Ceftriaxone crosses the placental barrier. Reproductive studies in animals have shown no evidence of embryotoxicity, foetotoxicity, teratogenicity or adverse effects on male or female fertility, birth or perinatal and postnatal development. In primates, no embryotoxicity or teratogenicity has been observed. Since safety in human pregnancy is not established ceftriaxone should not be used unless absolutely indicated.

Lactation

Low concentrations of ceftriaxone are excreted in human milk. Caution should be exercised when ceftriaxone is administered to a nursing woman.

4.7 Effects on ability to drive and use machines

Not applicable

4.8 Undesirable effects

The most frequently reported adverse events for ceftriaxone are diarrhoea, nausea and vomiting. Other reported adverse events include hypersensitivity reactions such as allergic skin reactions and anaphylactic reactions, secondary infections with yeast, fungi or resistant organisms as well as changes in blood cell counts.

Infections and infestations

Rare (⩾ 0.01% - < 0.1%): Mycosis of the genital tract.

Superinfections of various sites with yeasts, fungi or other resistant organisms are possible.

Blood and lymphatic system disorders

Rare (⩾ 0.01% - < 0.1%): Neutropenia, leucopenia, eosinophilia, thrombocytopenia, anaemia (including haemolytic anaemia), slight prolongation of prothrombin time.

Very rare (< 0.01 %) including isolated reports: Positive Coombs' test, coagulation disorders, agranulocytosis (< 500/m^3), mostly after 10 days of treatment and following total doses of 20g ceftriaxone and more.

Immune system disorders

Rare (⩾ 0.01% - < 0.1%): Anaphylactic (e.g. bronchospasm) and anaphylactoid reactions (see section *4.4*)

Nervous system disorders

Rare (⩾ 0.01% - < 0.1%): Headache, dizziness.

Gastrointestinal disorders

Common (⩾ 1% - < 10%): Loose stools or diarrhoea, nausea, vomiting.

Rare (⩾ 0.01% - < 0.1%): Stomatitis, glossitis. These side effects are usually mild and commonly disappear during treatment or after discontinuation of treatment.

Very rare (< 0.01%) including isolated reports: Pseudomembranous colitis (mostly caused by *Clostridium difficile*), pancreatitis (possibly caused by obstruction of bile ducts).

Hepato-biliary disorders

Rare (⩾ 0.01% - < 0.1%): Increase in serum liver enzymes (AST, ALT, alkaline phosphatase).

Precipitation of ceftriaxone calcium salt in the gallbladder has been observed (see section *4.4*), mostly in patients treated with doses higher than the recommended standard dose. In children, prospective studies have shown a variable incidence of precipitation with intravenous application, in some studies to above 30 %. The incidence seems to be lower with slow infusion (20-30 minutes). This effect is usually asymptomatic, but in rare cases, the precipitations have been accompanied by clinical symptoms such as pain, nausea and vomiting. Symptomatic treatment is recommended in these cases. Precipitation is usually reversible upon discontinuation of ceftriaxone.

Skin and subcutaneous tissue disorders

Uncommon (⩾ 0.1% - < 1%): Allergic skin reactions such as maculopapular rash or exanthema, urticaria, dermatitis, pruritus, oedema.

Very rare (< 0.01%) including isolated reports: Erythema multiforme, Stevens Johnson Syndrome, Lyell's Syndrome/toxic epidermal necrolysis.

Renal and urinary disorders

Rare (⩾ 0.01% - < 0.1%): Increase in serum creatinine, oliguria, glycosuria, haematuria.

Very rare (< 0.01%) including isolated reports: Renal precipitation, mostly in children older than 3 years who have been treated with either high daily doses (80 mg/kg/day and more) or total doses exceeding 10g and with other risk factors such as dehydration or immobilisation. Renal precipitation is reversible upon discontinuation of ceftriaxone. Anuria and renal impairment have been reported in association.

General disorders and administration site conditions

Rare (⩾ 0.01% - < 0.1%): Phlebitis and injection site pain following intravenous administration. This can be minimised by slow injection over at least 2-4 minutes. Rigors, pyrexia.

An intramuscular injection without lidocaine is painful.

4.9 Overdose

In the case of overdosage, drug concentrations would not be reduced by haemodialysis or peritoneal dialysis. There is no specific antidote. Treatment should be symptomatic.

5. PHARMACOLOGICAL PROPERTIES

5.1 Pharmacodynamic properties

ATC classification

Pharmacotherapeutic group: cephalosporins and related substances, ATC code: J01DA13

Mode of action

Ceftriaxone has bactericidal activity resulting from the inhibition of bacterial cell wall synthesis ultimately leading to cell death. Ceftriaxone is stable to a broad range of bacterial β-lactamases and is active against a broad spectrum of bacterial pathogens including both Gram-positive and Gram-negative species.

Mechanism of resistance

Ceftriaxone is stable to a wide range of both Gram-positive and Gram-negative beta-lactamases, including those which are able to hydrolyse advanced generation penicillin derivatives and other cephalosporins. Resistance to ceftriaxone is encoded mainly by the production of some beta-lactam hydrolysing enzymes (including carbapenemases and some ESBLs) especially in Gram-negative organisms. For Gram-positive organisms such as *S. aureus* and *S. pneumoniae*, acquired resistance is mainly encoded by cell wall target site alterations. Outside of the advanced generation parenteral cephalosporins, cross-resistance to other drug classes is generally not encountered.

Breakpoints

Current MIC breakpoints used to interpret ceftriaxone susceptibility data are shown below. The use of NCCLS breakpoints predominate and are the breakpoints used in data presented in the Table. Values quoted comprise mg/L (MIC testing) or mm (disk diffusion testing) using a 30mg/L drug concentration.

National Committee for Clinical Laboratory Standards (NCCLS) (M100-S12) – 2002

(see Table 1 below)

Susceptibility

The prevalence of acquired resistance may vary geographically and with time for selected species and local information on resistance is desirable, particularly when treating severe infections. As necessary, expert advice should be sought when the local prevalence of resistance is such that the utility of the agent in at least some types of infections is questionable.

Ceftriaxone susceptibility among Gram-positive and Gram-negative bacterial species in Europe from January 1999-December 2001:

Commonly susceptible species (i.e. resistance < 10% in all EU Member States)

Gram-Positive aerobes:
MS[a] coagulase negative *Staphylococcus* spp. (including *S. epidermis*)*
MS[b] *Staphylococcus aureus**
Group B (*Streptococcus agalactiae*)
Streptococcus bovis
*Streptococcus pneumoniae**
Group A *Streptococcus (Streptococcus pyogenes)**
*Streptococcus viridans**

Gram-Negative aerobes:
Citrobacter spp. (including *C. freundii*)
*Escherichia coli**
Haemophilus influenzae (including beta-lactamase positive isolates)[c]*
*Haemophilus para-influenzae**
Klebsiella spp. (including *K. pneumoniae* and *K. oxytoca*)*
*Moraxella catarrhalis**
*Morganella morganii**
Neisseria gonorrhoea (including penicillin-resistant isolates)*
*Neisseria meningitidis**
Proteus spp. (including *P. mirabilis* and *P. vulgaris*)*
Salmonella spp. (including *S. typhimurium*)
Serratia spp. (including *Serratia marsescens*)*
Shigella spp.

Anaerobes:
Clostridium spp.*

Species for which acquired resistance may be a problem (i.e. resistance ⩾ 10% in at least one EU Member State)

Gram-Negative aerobes:
Pseudomonas aeruginosa +
Enterobacter spp. (including *E. aerogenes* and *E. cloacae*)*+
Acinetobacter spp. (including *A. baumanii* and *A. calcoaceticus*)*+

Anaerobes:
Bacteroides spp.*
Peptostreptococcus spp.*

Inherently resistant organisms

Gram-Positive aerobes:
MR[d] coagulase negative *Staphylococcus* spp. (including *S. epidermidis*)
MR[e] *Staphylococcus aureus*
Enterococcus spp.

Gram-Negative aerobes:
Listeria monocytogenes
Mycoplasma spp.
Stenotrophomonas maltophilia
Ureaplasma urealyticum

Others:
Chlamydia spp.

[a]Methicillin-susceptible Coagulase-Negative *Staphylococcus*

[b]Methicillin-susceptible *Staphylococcus aureus*

[c]Non-susceptible range (no resistant breakpoints defined)

[d]Methicillin-resistant Coagulase-Negative *Staphylococcus*

[e]Methicillin-resistant *Staphylococcus aureus*

* Species for which the efficacy of ceftriaxone has been demonstrated both *in vitro* and *in vivo*

+ Species for which high rates of resistance have been observed in one or more regions within the EU approximate guidance on probabilities whether micro-organisms will be susceptible The table above comprises current levels of susceptibility according to routinely produced susceptibility test results in France, Germany, Greece, Italy, the Netherlands, Spain, and the United Kingdom. All data is presented using contemporary NCCLS derived susceptibility breakpoints except France (CA-SFM). Data is derived from The Surveillance Network(TM) (TSN) Databases in each respective region. The prevalence of resistance may vary geographically and with time for selected species and local information on resistance is desirable, particularly when treating severe infections. This information gives only to ceftriaxone or not.

5.2 Pharmacokinetic properties

The pharmacokinetics of Rocephin are largely determined by its concentration-dependent binding to serum albumin. The plasma free (unbound) fraction of the drug in man is approximately 5% over most of the therapeutic concentration range, increasing to 15% at concentrations of 300mg/l. Owing to the lower albumin content, the proportion of free ceftriaxone in interstitial fluid is correspondingly higher than in plasma.

Table 1 National Committee for Clinical Laboratory Standards (NCCLS) (M100-S12) – 2002

	Susceptible	Intermediate	Resistant
Enterobacteriaceae, P. aeruginosa and other non-Enterobacteriaceae, Staphylococcus spp.	⩽ 8 Disk: ⩽ 13	16-32 Disk: 14 – 20	⩾ 64 Disk: ⩾ 21
Haemophilus spp.	⩽ 2 Disk: ⩾ 26	-	-
Neisseria spp.	⩽ 0.25 Disk: ⩾ 35	-	-
Streptococcus pneumoniae *	⩽ 0.5	1	⩾ 2
Other *Streptococcus* spp.**	Beta strep ⩽ 0.5 Disk: ⩾ 24 Viridans group: ⩽ 0.5 Disk: ⩾ 27	- Viridans group: 1 Disk: 25-26	- Viridans group: ⩾ 2 Disk: ⩽ 24

* Recent 2002 *S. pneumoniae* breakpoints (NCCLS M100-S12) defined as ⩽ 1 (Sensitive), 2 (Intermediate) and ⩾ 4 (Resistant) for non-meningitis specimens and ⩽ 0.5 (Sensitive), 1 (Intermediate), and ⩾ 2 (Resistant) for meningitis specimens.

** Recent 2002 *Streptococcus viridans* group breakpoints (NCCLS M100-S12) defined ⩽ 1 (Sensitive), 2 (Intermediate), and ⩾ 4 (Resistant)

Plasma concentrations: Mean peak concentrations after bolus intravenous injection are about 120mg/l following a 500mg dose and about 200mg/l following a 1g dose; mean levels of 250mg/l are achieved after infusion of 2g over 30 minutes. Intramuscular injection of 500mg Rocephin in 1.06% Lidocaine produces mean peak plasma concentrations of 40 - 70mg/l within 1 hour. Bioavailability after intramuscular injection is 100%.

Excretion: Rocephin is eliminated mainly as unchanged ceftriaxone, approximately 60% of the dose being excreted in the urine (almost exclusively by glomerular filtration) and the remainder via the biliary and intestinal tracts. The total plasma clearance is 10 - 22ml/min. The renal clearance is 5 - 12ml/min. The elimination half-life in adults is about 8 hours. The half-life is not significantly affected by the dose, the route of administration or by repeated administration.

Pharmacokinetics in special clinical situations

In the first week of life, 80% of the dose is excreted in the urine; over the first month, this falls to levels similar to those in the adult.

In elderly persons aged over 75 years, the average elimination half-life is usually 2 to 3 times longer than in the young adult group. As with all cephalosporins, a decrease in renal function in the elderly may lead to an increase in half-life. Evidence gathered to date with ceftriaxone however, suggests that no modification of the dosage regimen is needed.

In patients with *renal* or *hepatic dysfunction*, the pharmacokinetics of ceftriaxone are only minimally altered and the elimination half-life is only slightly increased. If kidney function alone is impaired, biliary elimination of ceftriaxone is increased; if liver function alone is impaired, renal elimination is increased.

Cerebrospinal fluid: Rocephin crosses non-inflamed and inflamed meninges, attaining concentrations 4 - 17% of the simultaneous plasma concentration.

5.3 Preclinical safety data

There are no preclinical data of relevance to the prescriber which are additional to that already included in other sections of the SPC.

6. PHARMACEUTICAL PARTICULARS

6.1 List of excipients

None

6.2 Incompatibilities

Solutions containing Rocephin should not be mixed with or added to solutions containing other agents. In particular, Rocephin is not compatible with calcium-containing solutions such as Hartmann's solution and Ringer's solution. Based on literature reports, ceftriaxone is not compatible with amsacrine, vancomycin, fluconazole, aminoglycosides and labetalol.

6.3 Shelf life

3 years.

For shelf life of diluted product see section *6.6*.

6.4 Special precautions for storage

Do not store above 25°C. Keep vial in the outer carton.

For shelf life of diluted product see section *6.6*.

6.5 Nature and contents of container

Type 1 Ph. Eur 15ml glass vial with teflonised rubber stopper and aluminium cap, containing a sterile, white to yellowish-orange crystalline powder.

Packs of 1 vial.

Each gram of Rocephin contains approximately 3.6mmol sodium.

6.6 Special precautions for disposal and other handling Instructions for use, handling and disposal

Preparation of solutions for injection and infusion

The use of freshly prepared solutions is recommended. These maintain potency for at least 6 hours at or below 25°C or 24 hours at 2-8°C. Protect from light.

Rocephin should not be mixed in the same syringe with any drug other than 1.06% Lidocaine Hydrochloride BP solution (for intramuscular injection only).

Intramuscular injection: 250mg Rocephin should be dissolved in 1ml of 1.06% Lidocaine Hydrochloride BP solution, or 1g in 3.5ml of 1.06% Lidocaine Hydrochloride BP solution. The solution should be administered by deep intramuscular injection. Dosages greater than 1g should be divided and injected at more than one site.

Solutions in Lidocaine should not be administered intravenously.

Intravenous injection: 250mg Rocephin should be dissolved in 5ml of Water for Injections BP or 1g in 10ml of Water for Injections BP. The injection should be administered over at least 2 - 4 minutes, directly into the vein or via the tubing of an intravenous infusion.

Intravenous infusion: 2g of Rocephin should be dissolved in 40ml of one of the following calcium-free solutions: Dextrose Injection BP 5% or 10%, Sodium Chloride Injection BP, Sodium Chloride and Dextrose Injection BP (0.45% Sodium Chloride and 2.5% Dextrose), Dextran 6% in Dextrose Injection BP 5%, Hydroxyethyl Starch 6 - 10% infusions. The infusion should be administered over at least 30 minutes.

The displacement value of 250mg of Rocephin is 0.194ml.

7. MARKETING AUTHORISATION HOLDER

Roche Products Limited, 6 Falcon Way, Shire Park, Welwyn Garden City, AL7 1TW, United Kingdom.

8. MARKETING AUTHORISATION NUMBER(S)

Vials 250mg PL 0031/0169

Vials 1g PL0031/0171

Vials 2g PL0031/0172

9. DATE OF FIRST AUTHORISATION/RENEWAL OF THE AUTHORISATION

23 October 2003

10. DATE OF REVISION OF THE TEXT

July 2007

Roferon-A 18MIU/0.6ml Cartridge

(Roche Products Limited)

1. NAME OF THE MEDICINAL PRODUCT

Roferon-A 18 million international units (MIU) solution for injection in cartridge

2. QUALITATIVE AND QUANTITATIVE COMPOSITION

Each cartridge contains 18 Million International Units interferon alfa-2a* per 0.6 millilitres** (18MIU/0.6ml).

* produced in Escherichia coli by recombinant DNA technology.

** Contains volume overages

For a full list of excipients, see section 6.1.

Excipients recognized to have a known effect:

Benzyl alcohol (10mg/1ml)

3. PHARMACEUTICAL FORM

Solution for injection in cartridge.

Solution is clear and colourless to light yellow.

4. CLINICAL PARTICULARS

4.1 Therapeutic indications

Roferon-A is indicated for the treatment of:

- Hairy cell leukaemia.

- AIDS patients with progressive, asymptomatic Kaposi's sarcoma who have a CD4 count > 250/mm^3.

- Chronic phase Philadelphia-chromosome positive chronic myelogenous leukaemia. Roferon-A is not an alternative treatment for CML patients who have an HLA-identical relative and for whom allogeneic bone marrow transplantation is planned or possible in the immediate future. It is still unknown whether Roferon-A can be considered as a treatment with a curative potential in this indication.

- Cutaneous T-cell lymphoma. Interferon alfa-2a (Roferon-A) may be active in patients who have progressive disease and who are refractory to, or unsuitable for, conventional therapy.

- Adult patients with histologically proven chronic hepatitis B who have markers for viral replication, i.e., those who are positive for HBV DNA or HBeAg.

- Adult patients with histologically proven chronic hepatitis C who are positive for HCV antibodies or HCV RNA and have elevated serum alanine aminotransferase (ALT) without liver decompensation.

The efficacy of interferon alfa-2a in the treatment of hepatitis C is enhanced when combined with ribavirin. Roferon-A should be given alone mainly in case of intolerance or contraindication to ribavirin.

- Follicular non-Hodgkin's lymphoma.

- Advanced renal cell carcinoma.

- Patients with AJCC stage II malignant melanoma (Breslow tumour thickness > 1.5 mm, no lymph node involvement or cutaneous spread) who are free of disease after surgery.

4.2 Posology and method of administration

Not all available Roferon-A strengths can be used for all indications mentioned in section 4.1 Therapeutic indications. The prescribed strength should correspond with the recommended dose for each individual indication.

- HAIRY CELL LEUKAEMIA

Initial dosage:

Three million IU daily, given by subcutaneous injection for 16 - 24 weeks. If intolerance develops, either the daily dose should be lowered to 1.5 million IU or the schedule changed to three times per week, or both.

Maintenance dosage:

Three million IU, given three times per week by subcutaneous injection. If intolerance develops, the dose should be lowered to 1.5 million IU three times per week.

Duration of treatment:

Patients should be treated for approximately six months before the physician decides whether to continue treatment in responding patients or to discontinue treatment in non-responding patients. Patients have been treated for up to 20 consecutive months. The optimal duration of Roferon-A treatment for hairy cell leukaemia has not been determined.

The minimum effective dose of Roferon-A in hairy cell leukaemia has not been established.

- AIDS-RELATED KAPOSI'S SARCOMA

Roferon-A is indicated for the treatment of AIDS patients with progressive, asymptomatic Kaposi's sarcoma who have a CD4 count > 250/mm^3. AIDS patients with CD4 counts < 250/mm^3, or those with a history of opportunistic infections or constitutional symptoms, are unlikely to respond to Roferon-A therapy and therefore should not be treated. The optimal posology has not yet been well established.

Roferon-A should not be used in conjunction with protease inhibitors. With the exception of zidovudine, there is a lack of safety data for the combination of Roferon-A with reverse transcriptase inhibitors.

Initial dosage:

Roferon-Ashould be given by subcutaneous injection, and escalated to at least 18 million IU daily and if possible to 36 million IU daily for a total of ten to twelve weeks in patients of 18 years or older. The recommended escalation schedule is as follows:

days 1-3	3 million IU daily
days 4-6	9 million IU daily
days 7-9	18 million IU daily - and, if tolerated, increase to:
days 10-84	36 million IU daily

Maintenance dosage:

Roferon-A should be given by subcutaneous injection three times per week at the maximum dose which is acceptable to the patient, but not exceeding 36 million IU.

Patients with AIDS-related Kaposi's sarcoma treated with 3 million IU of Roferon-A given daily showed a lower response rate than those treated with the recommended dosage.

Duration of treatment:

The evolution of lesions should be documented to determine response to therapy. Patients should be treated for a minimum of 10 weeks and preferably for at least twelve weeks before the physician decides whether to continue treatment in responding patients or to discontinue treatment in non-responding patients. Patients generally showed evidence of response after approximately three months of therapy. Patients have been treated for up to 20 consecutive months. If a response to treatment occurs, treatment should continue at least until there is no further evidence of tumour. The optimal duration of Roferon-A treatment for AIDS-related Kaposi's sarcoma has not been determined.

Note:

Lesions of Kaposi's sarcoma frequently reappear when Roferon-A treatment is discontinued.

- CHRONIC MYELOGENOUS LEUKAEMIA

Roferon-A is indicated for the treatment of patients with chronic phase Philadelphia-chromosome positive chronic myelogenous leukaemia. Roferon-A is not an alternative treatment for CML patients who have an HLA-identical relative and for whom allogeneic bone marrow transplantation is planned or possible in the immediate future.

Roferon-A produces haematological remissions in 60% of patients with chronic phase CML, independent of prior treatment. Two thirds of these patients have complete haematological responses which occur as late as 18 months after treatment start.

In contrast to cytotoxic chemotherapy, interferon alfa-2a is able to generate sustained, ongoing cytogenetic responses beyond 40 months. It is still unkown whether Roferon-A can be considered as a treatment with a curative potential in this indication.

Dosage:

It is recommended that Roferon-A should be given by subcutaneous injection for eight to 12 weeks to patients 18 years or more. The recommended schedule is:

Days 1-3	3 million IU daily
Days 4-6	6 million IU daily
Days 7-84	9 million IU daily

Duration of treatment:

Patients should be treated for a minimum of eight weeks, preferably for at least twelve weeks before the physician decides whether or not to continue treatment in responding patients or to discontinue treatment in patients not showing any changes in haematological parameters. Responding patients should be treated until complete haematological response is achieved or for a maximum of 18 months. All patients with complete haematologic responses should continue treatment with 9 million IU daily (optimum) or 9 million IU three times a week (minimum) in order to achieve a cytogenetic response in the shortest possible time. The optimal duration of Roferon-A treatment for chronic myelogenous leukaemia has not been determined, although cytogenetic responses have been observed two years after treatment start.

The safety, efficacy and optimal dosage of Roferon-A in children with CML has not yet been established.

- CUTANEOUS T-CELL LYMPHOMA (CTCL)

Interferon alfa-2a (Roferon-A) may be active in patients with progressive cutaneous T-cell lymphoma and who are refractory to, or unsuitable for conventional therapy.

The optimal dosage has not been established.

Initial dosage:

Roferon-A should be given by subcutaneous injection, and escalated to 18 million IU daily for a total of 12 weeks in patients of 18 years or older. The recommended escalation schedule is as follows:

Days 1 to 3; 3 million IU daily

Days 4 to 6; 9 million IU daily

Days 7 to 84; 18 million IU daily

Maintenance dosage:

Roferon-A should be given by subcutaneous injection three times per week at the maximum dose which is acceptable to the patient, but not exceeding 18 million IU.

Duration of treatment:

Patients should be treated for a minimum of eight weeks and preferably for at least twelve weeks before the physician decides whether to continue treatment in responding patients or to discontinue treatment in non-responding patients. Minimum treatment duration in responding patients should be 12 months in order to maximise the chance to achieve a complete response and improve the chance for a prolonged response. Patients have been treated for up to 40 consecutive months. The optimal duration of Roferon-A treatment for cutaneous T-cell lymphoma has not been determined.

Warning:

Objective tumor responses have not been observed in approximately 40% of patients with CTCL. Partial responses are usually seen within 3 months and complete responses within 6 months, although it may occasionally take more than one year to reach the best response.

- CHRONIC HEPATITIS B

Roferon-A is indicated for the treatment of adult patients with histologically proven chronic hepatitis B who have markers for viral replication, i.e., those who are positive for HBV DNA or HBeAg.

Dosage recommendation:

The optimal schedule of treatment has not been established yet. The dose is usually in the range of 2.5 million IU to 5.0 million IU/m^2 body surface administered subcutaneously three times per week for a period of 4 to 6 months.

The dosage may be adjusted accordingto the patient's tolerance to the medication. If no improvement has been observed after 3-4 months of treatment, discontinuation of therapy should be considered.

Children: up to 10 million IU/m^2 has been safely administered to children with chronic hepatitis B. However efficacy of therapy has not been demonstrated.

- CHRONIC HEPATITIS C

ROFERON-A IN COMBINATION WITH RIBAVIRIN

RELAPSED PATIENTS

Roferon-A is given in combination with ribavirin for adult patients with chronic hepatitis C who have previously responded to interferon alpha monotherapy, but who have relapsed after treatment was stopped.

Dosage:

Roferon-A: 4.5 MIU 3 times per week by subcutaneous injection for a period of 6 months.

Dosage of Ribavirin:

Ribavirin dose: 1000 mg to 1200 mg/day in two divided doses (once in the morning with breakfast and once with the evening meal). Please refer to the SmPC for ribavirin for further details on the posology and method of administration of ribavirin.

NAÏVE PATIENTS

The efficacy of interferon alfa-2a in the treatment of hepatitis C is enhanced when combined with ribavirin. Roferon-A should be given alone mainly in case of intolerance or contraindication to ribavirin.

Dosage:

Roferon-A: 3 to 4.5 MIU 3 times per week by subcutaneous injection for a period of at least 6 months. Treatment should be continued for an additional 6 months in patients who have negative HCV RNA at month 6, and are infected with genotype 1 and have high pretreatment viral load.

Dosage of Ribavirin: see above

Other negative prognostic factors (age > 40 years, male gender, bridging fibrosis) should be taken into account in order to extend therapy to 12 months.

Patients who failed to show a virologic response after 6 months of treatment (HCV-RNA below lower limit of detection) do generally not become sustained virologic responders (HCV-RNA below lower limit of detection six months after withdrawal of treatment).

Roferon-A monotherapy

Roferon-A monotherapy should be given mainly in case of intolerance or contraindication to ribavirin.

Initial dosage:

Roferon-Ashould be administered at a dose of 3 to 6 million IU by subcutaneous injection three times a week for six months as induction therapy, patient tolerance permitting. In patients who fail to respond after three to four months of treatment, discontinuation of Roferon-A should be considered.

Maintenance dosage:

Patients whose serum ALT has normalized and/or HCV RNA has become undetectable require maintenance therapy with 3 million IU Roferon-A three times a week for an additional six months or longer to consolidate the complete response. The optimal duration of treatment has not yet been determined but a therapy of at least 12 months is advised.

Note:

The majority of patients who relapse after adequate treatment with Roferon-A alone do so within four months of the end of treatment.

- FOLLICULAR NON-HODGKINS LYMPHOMA

Roferon-A prolongs disease-free and progression-free survival when used as adjunctive treatment to CHOP-like chemotherapy regimens in patients with advanced (high tumour burden) follicular non-Hodgkin's lymphoma. However, the efficacy of adjunctive interferon alfa-2a treatment on overall long-term survival of these patients has not yet been established.

Dosage Recommendation:

Roferon-Ashould be administered concomitantly to a conventional chemotherapy regimen (such as the combination of cyclophosphamide, prednisone, vincristine and doxorubicin) according to a schedule such as 6 million IU/m^2 given subcutaneously from day 22 to day 26 of each 28-day cycle.

- ADVANCED RENAL CELL CARCINOMA

Therapy with Roferon-A in combination with vinblastine induces overall response rates of approximately 17-26%, delays disease progression, and prolongs overall survival in patients with advanced renal cell carcinoma.

Dosage recommendation:

Roferon-A should be given by subcutaneous injection at a dose of 3 million IU three times weekly for one week, 9 million IU three times weekly for the following week and 18 million IU three times weekly thereafter. Concomitantly vinblastine should be given intravenously according to the manufacturer's instructions at a dose of 0.1 mg/kg once every 3 weeks.

If the Roferon-A dosage of 18 million IU three times per week is not tolerated the dose may be reduced to 9 million IU three times per week.

Treatment should be given for a minimum of three months, up to a maximum of 12 months or until the development of progressive disease. Patients who achieve a complete response may stop treatment three months after the response is established.

- SURGICALLY RESECTED MALIGNANT MELANOMA.

Adjuvant therapy with a low dose of Roferon-A prolongs disease-free interval in patients with no nodal or distant metastases following resection of a melanoma (tumour thickness > 1.5 mm).

Dosage recommendation:

Roferon-A should be administered subcutaneously at a dose of 3 million IU three times a week for 18 months, starting no later than six weeks post surgery. If intolerance develops, the dose should be lowered to 1.5 million IU three times a week.

4.3 Contraindications

Roferon-A is contraindicated in patients with:

1) A history of hypersensitivity to recombinant interferon alfa-2a or to any of the excipients,

2) Patients with severe pre-existing cardiac disease or with any history of cardiac illness. No direct cardiotoxic effect has been demonstrated, but it is likely that acute, self-limiting toxicities (i.e., fever, chills) frequently associated with administration of Roferon-A may exacerbate pre-existing cardiac conditions,

3) Severe renal, hepatic or myeloid dysfunction,

4) Uncontrolled seizure disorders and/or compromised central nervous system function (see section 4.4.),

5) Chronic hepatitis with advanced, decompensated hepatic disease or cirrhosis of the liver,

6) Chronic hepatitis patients who are being or have recently been treated with immunosuppressive agents,

7) Benzyl alcohol, which is an excipient in Roferon-A solution for injection has on rare occasions been associated with potentially fatal toxicities and anaphylactoid reactions in children up to 3 years old. Therefore, Roferon-A solution for injection should not be used in premature babies, neonates, infants or children up to 3 years old. Roferon-A solution contains 10 mg / ml Benzyl alcohol.

Combination therapy with ribavirin: Also see ribavirin labelling if interferon alfa-2a is to be administered in combination with ribavirin in patients with chronic hepatitis C.

4.4 Special warnings and precautions for use

Roferon-A should be administered under the supervision of a qualified physician experienced in the management of the respective indication. Appropriate management of the therapy and its complications is possible only when adequate diagnostic and treatment facilities are readily available.

Patients should be informed not only of the benefits of therapy but also that they will probably experience adverse reactions.

Hypersensitivity: If a hypersensitivity reaction occurs during treatment with Roferon-A or in the combination therapy with ribavirin, treatment has to be discontinued and appropriate medical therapy has to be instituted immediately. Transient rashes do not necessitate interruption of treatment.

In transplant patients (e.g., kidney or bone marrow transplant) therapeutic immunosuppression may be weakened because interferons also exert an immunostimulatory action.

Fever/Infections: While fever may be associated with the flu-like syndrome reported commonly during interferon therapy, other causes of persistent fever, particularly serious infections (bacterial, viral, fungal) must be ruled out, especially in patients with neutropenia. Serious infections (bacterial, viral, fungal) have been reported during treatment with alfa interferons including Roferon-A. Appropriate anti-infective therapy should be started immediately and discontinuation of therapy should be considered.

Psychiatric: Severe psychiatric adverse reactions may manifest in patients receiving therapy with interferons, including Roferon-A. Depression, suicidal ideation, suicidal attempt, and suicide may occur in patients with and without previous psychiatric illness. Physicians should monitor all patients treated with Roferon-A for evidence of depression. Physicians should inform patients of the possible development of depression prior to initiation of therapy, and patients should report any sign or symptom of depression immediately. Psychiatric intervention and/ or drug discontinuation should be considered in such cases.

Ophthalmologic: As with other interferons, retinopathy including retinal haemorrhages, cotton wool spots, papilloedema, retinal artery or vein thrombosis and optic neuropathy which may result in loss of vision, have been reported after treatment with Roferon-A. Any patient complaining of decrease or loss of vision must have an eye examination. Because these ocular events may occur in conjunction with other disease states, a visual examination prior to initiation of Roferon-A monotherapy or in the combination therapy with ribavirin is recommended in patients with diabetes mellitus or hypertension. Roferon-A monotherapy or the combination therapy with ribavirin should be discontinued in patients who develop new or worsening ophthalmologic disorders.

Endocrine: Hyperglycemia has been observed rarely in patients treated with Roferon-A. All patients who develop symptoms of hyperglycemia should have their blood glucose measured and followed-up accordingly. Patients with diabetes mellitus may require adjustment of their antidiabetic regimen.

When mild to moderate renal, hepatic or myeloid dysfunction is present, close monitoring of these functions is required.

Hepatic function: In rare cases interferon alpha has been suspected of causing an exacerbation of an underlying autoimmune disease in hepatitis patients. Therefore, when treating hepatitis patients with a history of autoimmune disease caution is recommended. If a deterioration in liver function in these patients develops a determination of autoimmune antibodies should be considered. If necessary treatment should be discontinued.

Bone marrow suppression: Extreme caution should be exercised when administering Roferon-A to patients with severe myelosuppression as it has a suppressive effect on the bone marrow, leading to a fall in the white blood count, particularly granulocytes, platelet count and, less commonly, hemoglobin concentration. This can lead to an increased risk of infection or of haemorrhage. It is important to monitor closely these events in patients and periodic complete blood counts should be performed during the course of Roferon-Atreatment, both prior to therapy and at appropriate periods during therapy.

Autoimmune: The development of different auto-antibodies has been reported during treatment with alpha interferons. Clinical manifestations of autoimmune disease during interferon therapy occur more frequently in subjects predisposed to the development of autoimmune disorders. In patients with an underlying or clinical history of autoimmune disorders, monitoring of symptoms suggestive of these disorders, as well as measurement of auto antibodies and TSH level, is recommended.

The use of Roferon-A in children is not recommended as the safety and effectiveness of Roferon-A in children have not been established.

Efficacy in patients with chronic hepatitis B or C who are on hemodialysis or have hemophilia or are coinfected with human immunodeficiency virus has not been demonstrated.

This product contains less than 1 mmol sodium (23 mg) per 0.6 ml, i.e. essentially 'sodium-free'.

Combination therapy with ribavirin: Also see ribavirin labelling if interferon alfa-2a is to be administered in combination with ribavirin in patients with chronic hepatitis C.

Patients co-infected with HIV and receiving Highly Active Anti-Retroviral Therapy (HAART) may be at increased risk of developing lactic acidosis. Caution should be used when adding Roferon-A and ribavirin to HAART therapy (see ribavirin SPC).

Co-infected patients with advanced cirrhosis receiving HAART may be at increased risk of hepatic decompensation and death. Adding treatment with alfa interferons alone or in combination with ribavirin may increase the risk in this patient subset.

4.5 Interaction with other medicinal products and other forms of interaction

Since alpha-interferons alter cellular metabolism, the potential to modify the activity of other drugs exists. In a small study, Roferon-A was shown to have an effect on specific microsomal enzyme systems. The clinical relevance of these findings is unknown.

Alpha-interferons may affect the oxidative metabolic process; this should be borne in mind when prescribing concomitant therapy with drugs metabolised by this route. However, as yet no specific information is available.

Roferon-A has been reported to reduce the clearance of theophylline.

As Roferon-A may affect central nervous system functions, interactions could occur following concurrent administration of centrally-acting drugs. The neurotoxic, haematotoxic or cardiotoxic effects of previously or concurrently administered drugs may be increased by interferons.

Combination therapy with ribavirin: Also see ribavirin labelling if interferon alfa-2a is to be administered in combination with ribavirin in patients with chronic hepatitis C.

4.6 Pregnancy and lactation

Men and women receiving Roferon-A should practise effective contraception. There are no adequate data on the use of Roferon-A in pregnant women. When doses greatly in excess of the recommended clinical dose were administered to pregnant rhesus monkeys in the early to mid-fetal period, an abortifacient effect was observed (see section 5.3). Although animal tests do not indicate that Roferon-A is a teratogen, harm to the fetus from use during pregnancy cannot be excluded. In pregnancy, Roferon-A should be administered only if the benefit to the woman justifies the potential risk to the fetus.

It is not known whether this drug is excreted in human milk. A decision must be taken whether to suspend breast feeding or to discontinue the drug, taking into account the importance of the drug to the mother.

Use with ribavirin in patients with chronic hepatitis C

Significant teratogenic and/or embryocidal effects have been demonstrated in all animal species exposed to ribavirin. Ribavirin therapy is contraindicated in women who are pregnant. Extreme care must be taken to avoid pregnancy in female patients or in partners of male patients taking Roferon-A in combination with ribavirin. Female patients of childbearing potential and their partners must each use an effective contraceptive during treatment and for 4 months after treatment has been concluded. Male patients and their female partners must each use an effective contraceptive during treatment and for 7 months after treatment has been concluded. Please refer to the ribavirin SPC.

4.7 Effects on ability to drive and use machines

No studies on the effects on the ability to drive and use machines have been performed. However depending on dose and schedule as well as the sensitivity of the individual patient, Roferon-A may have an effect on the speed of reaction which could impair certain operations, e.g., driving, operation of machinery etc.

4.8 Undesirable effects

Combination therapy with ribavirin: Also see ribavirin labeling if interferon alfa-2a is to be administered in combination with ribavirin in patients with chronic hepatitis C.

The following data on adverse reactions are based on information derived from the treatment of cancer patients with a wide variety of malignancies and often refractory to previous therapy and suffering from advanced disease, patients with chronic hepatitis B, and patients with chronic hepatitis C.

Approximately two thirds of cancer patients experienced anorexia and one half nausea. Cardiovascular and pulmonary disorders were seen in about one fifth of cancer patients and consisted of transient hypotension, hypertension, edema, cyanosis, arrhythmias, palpitations and chest pain. Most cancer patients received doses that were significantly higher than the dose now recommended and may explain the higher frequency and severity of adverse reactions in this patient group compared with patients with hepatitis B where adverse reactions are usually transient, and patients return to pre-treatment status within 1 to 2 weeks after the end of therapy. Cardiovascular disorders were very rarely seen in patients with hepatitis B. In hepatitis B patients, changes in transaminases usually signal an improvement in the clinical state of the patient.

The majority of the patients experienced flu-like symptoms such as fatigue, pyrexia, rigors, decreased appetite, myalgia, headache, arthralgia and diaphoresis. These acute side-effects can usually be reduced or eliminated by concurrent administration of paracetamol and tend to diminish with continued therapy or dose modification although continuing therapy can lead to lethargy, asthenia and fatigue.

Within each frequency grouping, undesirable effects are presented in order of decreasing seriousness:

(see Table 1 on next page)

Rarely, alpha interferons including Roferon-A used alone or in combination with ribavirin, may be associated with pancytopenia, and very rarely, aplastic anemia has been reported.

Neutralizing antibodies to interferons may form in some patients. In certain clinical conditions (cancer, systemic lupus erythematosus, herpes zoster) antibodies to human leukocyte interferon may also occur spontaneously in patients who have never received exogenous interferons. The clinical significance of the development of antibodies has not been fully clarified.

In clinical trials where lyophilised Roferon-A which had been stored at 25°C was used, neutralizing antibodies to Roferon-A have been detected in approximately one fifth of patients. In patients with hepatitis C, a trend for responding patients who develop neutralizing antibodies to lose response while still on treatment and to lose it earlier than patients who do not develop such antibodies, has been seen. No other clinical sequelae of the presence of antibodies to Roferon-A have been documented. The clinical significance of the development of antibodies has not been fully clarified.

No data on neutralizing antibodies yet exist from clinical trials in which lyophilized Roferon-A or Roferon-A solution for injection which is stored at 4°C has been used. In a mouse model, the relative immunogenicity of lyophilized Roferon-A increases with time when the material is stored at 25°C - no such increase in immunogenicity is observed when lyophilised Roferon-A is stored at 4°C, the recommended storage conditions.

4.9 Overdose

There are no reports of overdosage but repeated large doses of interferon can be associated with profound lethargy, fatigue, prostration and coma. Such patients should be hospitalised for observation and appropriate supportive treatment given.

Patients who experience severe reactions to Roferon-A will usually recover within days after discontinuation of therapy, given appropriate supportive care. Coma has been observed in 0.4% of cancer patients in clinical trials.

5. PHARMACOLOGICAL PROPERTIES

5.1 Pharmacodynamic properties

Pharmacotherapeutic group: Antineoplastic and immunomodulating agents, *Interferons*

ATC Code L03AB04

Roferon-A has been shown to possess many of the activities of the so-called natural human alpha-interferon preparations. Roferon-A exerts its antiviral effects by inducing a state of resistance to viral infections in cells and by modulating the effector arm of the immune system to neutralize viruses or eliminate virus infected cells. The essential mechanism for the antitumour action of Roferon-A is not yet known. However, several changes are described in human tumoural cells treated with Roferon-A: HT 29 cells show a significant reduction of DNA, RNA and protein synthesis. Roferon-A has been shown to exert antiproliferative activity against a variety of human tumours *in vitro* and to inhibit the growth of some human tumour xenografts in nude mice. A limited number of human tumour cell lines grown *in vivo* in immunocompromised nude mice has been tested for the susceptibility to Roferon-A. *In vivo* antiproliferative activity of Roferon-A has been studied on tumours including breast mucoid carcinoma, adenocarcinoma of the caecum, colon carcinoma and prostatic carcinoma. The degree of antiproliferative activity is variable.

Unlike other human proteins, many of the effects of interferon alfa-2a are partially or completely suppressed when it is tested in other animal species. However, significant antivaccinia virus activity was induced in rhesus monkeys pre-treated with interferon alfa-2a.

Clinical Trials

Hairy Cell Leukaemia

The therapeutic efficacy of Roferon-A in the treatment of hairy cell leukaemia has been demonstrated in a large trial of 218 patients, of whom 174 were evaluable for efficacy after 16-24 weeks of therapy. Response was observed in 88% of patients (complete response 33%, partial response 55%).

AIDS-related Kaposi's Sarcoma

The efficacy of Roferon-A in the treatment of Kaposi's sarcoma was assessed in 364 patients receiving of 3 to 54 MIU per day. Objective response rates were dose-related, ranging from 14% to 50%, with a daily dose of 36 MIU producing the best overall therapeutic benefit (13.3% complete response, 12.2% partial response). High baseline CD4 lymphocyte count was a favorable prognostic factor for response, with 46% of patients with a CD4 count $>400/mm^3$ responding to Roferon-A. Response to Roferon-A therapy was the strongest prognostic factor for survival.

Chronic Myelogenous Leukaemia (CML)

The efficacy of Roferon-A was assessed in 226 patients with chronic phase CML, and compared with 109 patients receiving chemotherapy (hydroxyurea or busulfan). Both groups had favourable features at diagnosis (less than 10% blasts in the blood) and treatment was initiated with interferon within 6 months of diagnosis. Treatment of patients with CML in the chronic phase leads to the same proportion of patients (85-90%) achieving a haematologic response as treatment with the standard chemotherapy regimens. In addition patients treated with Roferon-A resulted in 8% complete cytogenetic response and 38% partial cytogenetic response versus 9% partial cytogenetic response during chemotherapy. Time to progression from the chronic phase of leukaemia to an accelerated or a blastic phase was longer in the Roferon-A group (69 months) than in the conventional chemo-therapy group (46 months) ($p<0.001$) as was median overall survival (72.8 months versus 54.5 months, $p=0.002$).

Cutaneous T-cell Lymphoma (CTCL)

The efficacy of Roferon-A was assessed in 169 patients with CTCL, the majority of whom (78%) were resistant to, or had relapsed on, standard therapy. Among the 85 patients evaluable, overall response to treatment was 58% (20% complete response, 38% partial response). Patients with all stages of disease responded to therapy. Median duration of complete response from start of treatment was 22 months, with 94% of complete responders remaining in remission at 9 months.

Chronic Hepatitis B

The efficacy of Roferon-A in the treatment of chronic hepatitis B was assessed in trials involving over 900 patients. In the pivotal controlled study 238 patients were randomised into four groups: patients received either 2.5 MIU / m^2, 5.0 MIU / m^2, 10 MIU / m^2, tiw of Roferon-A or no treatment. Treatment duration was 12-24 weeks depending on response i. e. clearance of HBeAg and HBV DNA from serum. Patients were followed for up to 12 months after treatment was discontinued. There was a statistically significant difference in sustained response [clearance of hepatitis B e antigen (HBeAg) and hepatitis B viral DNA (HBV DNA)] between treated and untreated patients (37% versus 13%). Response differences between various dose groups did not reach statistical significance (33%, 34% and 43% for the 2.5, 5.0 and 10.0 MIU / m^2 groups). Serological and virological responses were associated with marked improvement in liver histology after 12 months of treatment free-follow up.

Chronic Hepatitis C

The efficacy of Roferon-A in the treatment of chronic hepatitis C has been assessed in 1701 patients, with 130 untreated or placebo treated controls. At recommended doses, Roferon-A induces complete biochemical response in up to 85% of patients, with response rates maintained for at least 6 months after treatment ranging from 11 to 44% depending on pre-treatment disease characteristics, IFN dose and treatment duration. Biochemical response to Roferon-A is associated with significant improvement of liver disease as shown by evaluation of pre-and post-liver biopsies. For those patients who have a sustained response 3-6 months after end of therapy, response has been reported to be maintained for up to 4 years.

The therapeutic efficacy of Interferon alfa-2a alone and in combination with ribavirin was compared in a double-blind randomised clinical trial in naive (previously untreated) and relapsed patients with virologically, biochemically and histologically documented chronic hepatitis C. Six months after end of treatment sustained biochemical and virological response as well as histological improvement were assessed.

A statistically significant 10-fold increase (from 4% to 43%; $p<0.01$) in sustained virological and biochemical response was observed in relapsed patients. The favourable profile of the combination therapy was also reflected in the response rates relative to HCV genotype or baseline viral load. Although the sustained response rates in patients with HCV genotype-1 were lower than in the overall population (approx. 30% versus 0% in the monotherapy arm) the relative benefit of ribavirin in combination with interferon alfa-2a is particularly significant in this group of patients. In addition the histological improvement favoured the combination therapy.

Supportive favourable results from a small study in naïve patients were reported using interferon alfa-2a (3 MIU 3 times per week) with ribavirin.

For other information on pharmacodynamic properties please refer to the SmPC for Ribavirin.

Follicular Non-Hodgkin's lymphoma

The efficacy of Roferon-A in addition to cytotoxic chemotherapy (CHOP-like regimen of cyclophosphamide, vincristine, prednisone and doxorubicin) was assessed in 122 patients with clinically aggressive low-grade or intermediate-grade non-Hodgkin's lymphoma and compared with 127 controls receiving the same chemotherapy regimen. The two regimens produced comparable objective responses, but the regimen including Roferon-A had a greater effect in prolonging the time to treatment failure ($p<0.001$), the duration of complete response ($p<0.003$).

Table 1

Body System	Very common (≥1/10)	Common (≥1/100 to <1/10)	Uncommon (≥1/1 000 to ≤1/100)	Rare (≥1/10 000 to ≤1/1 000)	Very rare (≤1/10 000)
Infections and infestations				Pneumonia Herpes simplex[1]	
Blood and lymphatic system disorders[2]	Leukopenia	Thrombocytopenia Anemia		Agranulocytosis Hemolytic anemia	Idiopathic thrombocytopenic purpura
Immune system disorders				Autoimmune disorder Acute hypersensivity reactions[3]	Sarcoidosis
Endocrine disorders				Hypothyroidism Hyperthyroidism Thyroid dysfunction	
Metabolism and nutrition disorders	Anorexia Nausea Inconsequential hypocalcemia		Dehydration Electrolyte imbalance	Diabete mellitus Hyperglycemia	Hyper-triglyceridemia Hyperlipidemia
Psychiatric disorders			Depression Anxiety Mental status changes Confusional state Abnormal behavior Nervousness Memory impairment Sleep disorder	Suicide Suicide attempt Suicidal ideation	
Nervous system disorders	Headache	Dysgeusia	Neuropathy Dizziness Hypoasthesia Parasthesia Tremor Somnolence	Coma Cerebrovascular accident Convulsions Transient erectile dysfunction	Encephalopathy
Eye disorders			Visual disturbance Conjunctivitis	Ischemic retinopathy	Retinal artery thrombosis Optic neuropathy Retinal hemorrhage Retinal vein thrombosis Retinal exudates Retinopathy Papilledema
Ear and labyrinth disorders			Vertigo		
Cardiac disorders		Arrhythmias[4] Palpitations Cyanosis		Cardiorespiratory arrest Myocardial infarction Congestive heart failure Pulmonary edema	
Vascular disorders			Hypertension Hypotension	Vasculitis	
Respiratory, thoracic and mediastinal disorders				Dyspnea Cough	
Gastrointestinal disorders	Diarrhea	Vomiting Abdominal pain Nausea Dry mouth		Pancreatitis Intestinal hypermotility Constipation Dyspepsia Flatulence	Reactivation of peptic ulcer gastrointestinal bleeding (non life threatening)
Hepato-biliary disorders				Hepatic failure Hepatitis Hepatic dysfunction	
Skin and subcutaneous tissue disorders	Alopecia[5] Sweating increased		Psoriasis[6] Pruritus	Rash Dry skin Epistaxis Mucosal dryness Rhinorrhea	
Musculoskeletal, connective tissue and bone disorders	Myalgia Arthralgia			Systemic lupus erythematosus Arthritis	
Renal and urinary disorders			Proteinuria Increased cell count in urine	Acute renal failure[7] Renal impairment	
General disorders and administration site conditions	Flu like illness Appetite decreased Pyrexia Rigors Fatigue	Chest pain Edema			Injection site necrosis Injection site reaction
Investigations		Weight loss	Increased ALT Increased transaminase Increased blood alkaline phosphatase	Increased blood creatinine Increased blood urea Increased blood bilirubin Increased blood uric acid Increased blood LDH	

[1] (including exacerbations of herpes labialis)

[2] In myelosuppressed patients, thrombocytopenia and decreased haemoglobin occurred more frequently. Recovery of severe haematological deviations to pre-treatment levels usually occurred within seven to ten days after discontinuing Roferon-A treatment.

[3] (e.g. urticaria, angioedema, bronchospasm and anaphylaxis)

[4] including atrioventricular block

[5] (reversible upon discontinuation; increased hair loss may continue for several weeks after end of treatment)

[6] exacerbation of, or provocation of psoriasis

[7] (mainly in cancer patients with renal disease)

Renal Cell Carcinoma

The efficacy of Roferon-A, given in combination with vinblastine, was compared with vinblastine alone. The combination of Roferon-A plus vinblastine is superior to vinblastine alone in the treatment of patients with locally advanced or metastatic renal cell carcinoma. Median survival was 67.8 weeks for the 79 patients receiving Roferon-A plus vinblastine and 37.8 weeks for the 81 patients treated with vinblastine (p=.0049). Overall response rates were 16.5% for patients treated Roferon-A plus vinblastine and 2.5% for patients treated with vinblastine alone (p=.0025).

Surgically Resected Malignant Melanoma

The efficacy of Roferon-A in patients with primary cutaneous melanoma thicker than 1.5 mm and without clinically detectable node metastasis was assessed in a large randomised study involving 253 patients receiving Roferon-A at a dose of 3 MIU three times a week for 18 months, compared with 246 untreated controls. After a median follow-up of 4.4 years a significant extension of relapse-free interval (p=0.035) but no statistically significant difference in overall survival (p=0.059) in Roferon-A treated patients compared with controls have been shown. The overall treatment effect was a 25% reduction in the risk of relapse.

5.2 Pharmacokinetic properties

The serum concentrations of interferon alfa-2a reflected a large intersubject variation in both healthy volunteers and patients with disseminated cancer. The pharmacokinetics of Roferon-A in animals (monkey, dog and mouse) were similar to those seen in man. The pharmacokinetics of Roferon-A in man were linear over a 3 million to 198 million IU dose range. In healthy man, interferon alfa-2a exhibited an elimination half-life of 3.7 - 8.5 hours (mean: 5.1 hours), a volume of distribution at steady state of 0.223 - 0.748 l/kg (mean: 0.4 l/kg) and a total body clearance of 2.14 - 3.62 ml/min/kg (mean: 2.79 ml/min/kg) after a 36 million IU intravenous infusion. After intramuscular administration of 36 million IU, peak serum concentrations ranged from 1500 to 2580 pg/ml (mean: 2020 pg/ml) at a mean time to peak of 3.8 hours, and after subcutaneous administration of 36 million IU from 1250 to 2320 pg/ml (mean: 1730 pg/ml) at a mean time to peak of 7.3 hours.

The apparent fraction of the dose absorbed after intramuscular or subcutaneous injection is greater than 80%.

The pharmacokinetics of interferon alfa-2a after single intramuscular doses to patients with disseminated cancer and chronic hepatitis B were similar to those found in healthy volunteers. Dose-proportional increases in serum concentrations were observed after single doses up to 198 million IU. There were no changes in the distribution or elimination of interferon alfa-2a during twice daily (0.5 - 36 million IU), once daily (1 - 54 million IU), or three times weekly (1 - 136 million IU) dosing regimens up to 28 days of dosing. Renal catabolism is the major pathway for Roferon-A elimination. Biliary excretion and liver metabolism are considered to be minor pathways of elimination of Roferon-A.

Intramuscular administration of Roferon-A one or more times daily for up to 28 days to some patients with disseminated cancer resulted in peak plasma concentrations of two to four times greater than those seen after single doses. However, multiple dosing caused no changes in its distribution or elimination parameters during several dosage regimens studied.

For other information on pharmacokinetic properties please refer to the SmPC for Ribavirin.

5.3 Preclinical safety data

Because of species specificity of human interferon, only limited toxicological studies have been carried out with Roferon-A. The acute parenteral toxicity of Roferon-A has been studied in mice rats, rabbits and ferrets at doses up to 30 million IU/kg intravenously, and 500 million IU/kg intramuscularly. No treatment-related mortality was noted in any species studied given Roferon-A by any of the routes of administration. With doses greatly exceeding the recommended clinical dose no significant adverse effects were observed except for an abortifacient effect when administered to pregnant rhesus monkeys in the early to mid-foetal period and transient menstrual cycle irregularities including prolonged menstrual periods in non-pregnant monkeys. The relevance of these findings in man has not been established.

Mutagenic effects of Roferon-A have not been observed experimentally.

For other information on preclinical safety data please refer to the SmPC for Ribavirin.

6. PHARMACEUTICAL PARTICULARS

6.1 List of excipients

Ammonium acetate

Sodium Chloride

Benzyl alcohol (10mg/1ml)

Polysorbate 80

Glacial Acetic acid

Sodium Hydroxide

Water for Injections

6.2 Incompatibilities

In the absence of compatibility studies, this medicinal product must not be mixed with other medicinal products.

6.3 Shelf life

2 years

Chemical and physical in use stability has been demonstrated for 28 days at 25°C.

From a microbiological point of view, once opened, the product may be stored for a maximum of 28 days at 25°C. Other in-use storage times and conditions are the responsibility of the user.

However, it is recommended that the Roferon-Pen/cartridge combination be returned to the fridge after each injection.

6.4 Special precautions for storage

Store in a refrigerator (2°C - 8°C). Do not freeze. Keep cartridge in the outer carton.

The 18 MIU/0.6 ml solution for injection is suitable for multiple-dose use.

For storage conditions of the reconstituted medicinal product, see section 6.3.

6.5 Nature and contents of container

0.6 ml of solution in cartridge (type I glass), with a plunger stopper (PTFE laminated), aluminium crimp cap with PTFE laminated butyl rubber stopper inner seal. Pack sizes of 1, 3 and 6. Not all pack sizes may be marketed.

6.6 Special precautions for disposal and other handling

Roferon®-A cartridges are for multi-dose and single patient use only and should be used exclusively with the Roferon®-Pen. A new, sterile needle must be used for every injection.

Each Roferon®Pen is provided with a user manual which fully describes the use of the pen/cartridge combination. Penfine® needles are recommended for use with Roferon®-Pen. However, a limited range of other needle types can also be used.

Always discard cartridges containing residual drug after expiry of the in-use shelf life. Needles should be discarded safely after use.

Any unused product or waste material should be disposed of in accordance with local requirements.

7. MARKETING AUTHORISATION HOLDER

Roche Products Limited

6 Falcon Way, Shire Park

Welwyn Garden City

AL7 1TW, United Kingdom

8. MARKETING AUTHORISATION NUMBER(S)

PL 00031/0510

9. DATE OF FIRST AUTHORISATION/RENEWAL OF THE AUTHORISATION

Date of first authorisation: 25 July 1996

Date of last renewal: 22 July 2009

10. DATE OF REVISION OF THE TEXT

19 December 2008

Roferon-A Pre-Filled Syringe

(Roche Products Limited)

1. NAME OF THE MEDICINAL PRODUCT

Roferon-A 3 million international units (MIU) solution for injection in pre-filled syringe

Roferon-A 4.5 million international units (MIU) solution for injection in pre-filled syringe

Roferon-A 6 million international units (MIU) solution for injection in pre-filled syringe

Roferon-A 9 million international units (MIU) solution for injection in pre-filled syringe

Roferon-A 18 million international units (MIU) solution for injection in pre-filled syringe

2. QUALITATIVE AND QUANTITATIVE COMPOSITION

Each pre-filled syringe contains 3 Million International Units interferon alfa-2a* per 0.5 millilitres** (3MIU/0.5ml).

4.5 Million International Units interferon alfa-2a* per 0.5 millilitres** (4.5MIU/0.5ml).

6 Million International Units interferon alfa-2a* per 0.5 millilitres** (6MIU/0.5ml).

9 Million International Units interferon alfa-2a* per 0.5 millilitres** (9MIU/0.5ml).

18 Million International Units interferon alfa-2a* per 0.5 millilitres** (18MIU/0.5ml).

* produced in Escherichia coli by recombinant DNA technology

** Contains volume overages

For a full list of excipients, see section 6.1.

Excipients recognized to have a known effect:

Benzyl alcohol (10mg/1ml)

3. PHARMACEUTICAL FORM

Solution for injection in pre-filled syringe.

Solution is clear and colourless to light yellow.

4. CLINICAL PARTICULARS

4.1 Therapeutic indications

Roferon-A is indicated for the treatment of:

- Hairy cell leukaemia.

- AIDS patients with progressive, asymptomatic Kaposi's sarcoma who have a CD4 count > 250/mm^3.

- Chronic phase Philadelphia-chromosome positive chronic myelogenous leukaemia. Roferon-A is not an alternative treatment for CML patients who have an HLA-identical relative and for whom allogeneic bone marrow transplantation is planned or possible in the immediate future. It is still unknown whether Roferon-A can be considered as a treatment with a curative potential in this indication.

- Cutaneous T-cell lymphoma. Interferon alfa-2a (Roferon-A) may be active in patients who have progressive disease and who are refractory to, or unsuitable for, conventional therapy.

- Adult patients with histologically proven chronic hepatitis B who have markers for viral replication, i.e., those who are positive for HBV DNA or HBeAg.

- Adult patients with histologically proven chronic hepatitis C who are positive for HCV antibodies or HCV RNA and have elevated serum alanine aminotransferase (ALT) without liver decompensation.

The efficacy of interferon alfa-2a in the treatment of hepatitis C is enhanced when combined with ribavirin. Roferon-A should be given alone mainly in case of intolerance or contraindication to ribavirin.

- Follicular non-Hodgkin's lymphoma.

- Advanced renal cell carcinoma.

- Patients with AJCC stage II malignant melanoma (Breslow tumour thickness > 1.5 mm, no lymph node involvement or cutaneous spread) who are free of disease after surgery.

4.2 Posology and method of administration

Not all available Roferon-A strengths can be used for all indications mentioned in section *4.1 Therapeutic indications*. The prescribed strength should correspond with the recommended dose for each individual indication.

- HAIRY CELL LEUKAEMIA

Initial dosage:

Three million IU daily, given by subcutaneous injection for 16 - 24 weeks. If intolerance develops, either the daily dose should be lowered to 1.5 million IU or the schedule changed to three times per week, or both.

Maintenance dosage:

Three million IU, given three times per week by subcutaneous injection. If intolerance develops, the dose should be lowered to 1.5 million IU three times per week.

Duration of treatment:

Patients should be treated for approximately six months before the physician decides whether to continue treatment in responding patients or to discontinue treatment in non-responding patients. Patients have been treated for up to 20 consecutive months. The optimal duration of Roferon-A treatment for hairy cell leukaemia has not been determined.

The minimum effective dose of Roferon-A in hairy cell leukaemia has not been established.

- AIDS-RELATED KAPOSI'S SARCOMA

Roferon-A is indicated for the treatment of AIDS patients with progressive, asymptomatic Kaposi's sarcoma who have a CD4 count > 250/mm^3. AIDS patients with CD4 counts < 250/mm^3, or those with a history of opportunistic infections or constitutional symptoms, are unlikely to respond to Roferon-A therapy and therefore should not be treated. The optimal posology has not yet been well established.

Roferon-A should not be used in conjunction with protease inhibitors. With the exception of zidovudine, there is a lack of safety data for the combination of Roferon-A with reverse transcriptase inhibitors.

Initial dosage:

Roferon-A should be given by subcutaneous injection, and escalated to at least 18 million IU daily and if possible to 36 million IU daily for a total of ten to twelve weeks in patients of 18 years or older. The recommended escalation schedule is as follows:

days 1-3	3 million IU daily
days 4-6	9 million IU daily
days 7-9	18 million IU daily - and, if tolerated, increase to:
days 10-84	36 million IU daily

Maintenance dosage:

Roferon-A should be given by subcutaneous injection three times per week at the maximum dose which is acceptable to the patient, but not exceeding 36 million IU.

Patients with AIDS-related Kaposi's sarcoma treated with 3 million IU of Roferon-A given daily showed a lower response rate than those treated with the recommended dosage.

Duration of treatment:

The evolution of lesions should be documented to determine response to therapy. Patients should be treated for a minimum of 10 weeks and preferably for at least twelve weeks before the physician decides whether to continue treatment in responding patients or to discontinue treatment in non-responding patients. Patients generally showed evidence of response after approximately three months of therapy. Patients have been treated for up to 20 consecutive months. If a response to treatment occurs, treatment should continue at least until there is no further evidence of tumour. The optimal duration of Roferon-A treatment for AIDS-related Kaposi's sarcoma has not been determined.

Note:

Lesions of Kaposi's sarcoma frequently reappear when Roferon-A treatment is discontinued.

- CHRONIC MYELOGENOUS LEUKAEMIA

Roferon-A is indicated for the treatment of patients with chronic phase Philadelphia-chromosome positive chronic myelogenous leukaemia. Roferon-A is not an alternative treatment for CML patients who have an HLA-identical relative and for whom allogeneic bone marrow transplantation is planned or possible in the immediate future.

Roferon-A produces haematological remissions in 60% of patients with chronic phase CML, independent of prior treatment. Two thirds of these patients have complete haematological responses which occur as late as 18 months after treatment start.

In contrast to cytotoxic chemotherapy, interferon alfa-2a is able to generate sustained, ongoing cytogenetic responses beyond 40 months. It is still unknown whether Roferon-A can be considered as a treatment with a curative potential in this indication.

Dosage:

It is recommended that Roferon-A should be given by subcutaneous injection for eight to 12 weeks to patients 18 years or more. The recommended schedule is:

Days 1-3	3 million IU daily
Days 4-6	6 million IU daily
Days 7-84	9 million IU daily

Duration of treatment:

Patients should be treated for a minimum of eight weeks, preferably for at least twelve weeks before the physician decides whether or not to continue treatment in responding patients or to discontinue treatment in patients not showing any changes in haematological parameters. Responding patients should be treated until complete haematological response is achieved or for a maximum of 18 months. All patients with complete haematologic responses should continue treatment with 9 million IU daily (optimum) or 9 million IU three times a week (minimum) in order to achieve a cytogenetic response in the shortest possible time. The optimal duration of Roferon-A treatment for chronic myelogenous leukaemia has not been determined, although cytogenetic responses have been observed two years after treatment start.

The safety, efficacy and optimal dosage of Roferon-A in children with CML has not yet been established.

- CUTANEOUS T-CELL LYMPHOMA (CTCL)

Interferon alfa-2a (Roferon-A) may be active in patients with progressive cutaneous T-cell lymphoma and who are refractory to, or unsuitable for conventional therapy.

The optimal dosage has not been established.

Initial dosage:

Roferon-A should be given by subcutaneous injection, and escalated to 18 million IU daily for a total of 12 weeks in patients of 18 years or older. The recommended escalation schedule is as follows:

Days 1 to 3;	3 million IU daily
Days 4 to 6;	9 million IU daily
Days 7 to 84;	18 million IU daily

Maintenance dosage:

Roferon-A should be given by subcutaneous injection three times per week at the maximum dose which is acceptable to the patient, but not exceeding 18 million IU.

Duration of treatment:

Patients should be treated for a minimum of eight weeks and preferably for at least twelve weeks before the physician decides whether to continue treatment in responding patients or to discontinue treatment in non-responding patients. Minimum treatment duration in responding patients should be 12 months in order to maximise the chance to achieve a complete response and improve the chance for a prolonged response. Patients have been treated for up to 40 consecutive months. The optimal duration of Roferon-A treatment for cutaneous T-cell lymphoma has not been determined.

Warning:

Objective tumor responses have not been observed in approximately 40% of patients with CTCL. Partial responses are usually seen within 3 months and complete responses within 6 months, although it may occasionally take more than one year to reach the best response.

- CHRONIC HEPATITIS B

Roferon-A is indicated for the treatment of adult patients with histologically proven chronic hepatitis B who have markers for viral replication, i.e., those who are positive for HBV DNA or HBeAg.

Dosage recommendation:

The optimal schedule of treatment has not been established yet. The dose is usually in the range of 2.5 million IU to 5.0 million IU/m^2 body surface administered subcutaneously three times per week for a period of 4 to 6 months. The dosage may be adjusted according to the patient's tolerance to the medication. If no improvement has been observed after 3-4 months of treatment, discontinuation of therapy should be considered.

Children: up to 10 million IU/m^2 has been safely administered to children with chronic hepatitis B. However efficacy of therapy has not been demonstrated.

- CHRONIC HEPATITIS C

ROFERON-A IN COMBINATION WITH RIBAVIRIN

RELAPSED PATIENTS

Roferon-A is given in combination with ribavirin for adult patients with chronic hepatitis C who have previously responded to interferon alpha monotherapy, but who have relapsed after treatment was stopped.

Dosage:

Roferon-A: 4.5 MIU 3 times per week by subcutaneous injection for a period of 6 months.

Dosage of Ribavirin:

Ribavirin dose: 1000 mg to 1200 mg/day in two divided doses (once in the morning with breakfast and once with the evening meal). Please refer to the SmPC for ribavirin for further details on the posology and method of administration of ribavirin.

NAÏVE PATIENTS

The efficacy of interferon alfa-2a in the treatment of hepatitis C is enhanced when combined with ribavirin. Roferon-A should be given alone mainly in case of intolerance or contraindication to ribavirin.

Dosage:

Roferon-A: 3 to 4.5 MIU 3 times per week by subcutaneous injection for a period of at least 6 months. Treatment should be continued for an additional 6 months in patients who have negative HCV RNA at month 6, and are infected with genotype 1 and have high pretreatment viral load.

Dosage of Ribavirin: see above

Other negative prognostic factors (age > 40 years, male gender, bridging fibrosis) should be taken into account in order to extend therapy to 12 months.

Patients who failed to show a virologic response after 6 months of treatment (HCV-RNA below lower limit of detection) do generally not become sustained virologic responders (HCV-RNA below lower limit of detection six months after withdrawal of treatment).

Roferon-A monotherapy

Roferon-A monotherapy should be given mainly in case of intolerance or contraindication to ribavirin.

Initial dosage:

Roferon-A should be administered at a dose of 3 to6 million IU by subcutaneous injection three times a week for six months as induction therapy, patient tolerance permitting. In patients who fail to respond after three to four months of treatment, discontinuation of Roferon-A should be considered.

Maintenance dosage:

Patients whose serum ALT has normalized and/or HCV RNA has become undetectable require maintenance therapy with 3 million IU Roferon-A three times a week for an additional six months or longer to consolidate the complete response. The optimal duration of treatment has not yet been determined but a therapy of at least 12 months is advised.

Note:

The majority of patients who relapse after adequate treatment with Roferon-A alone do so within four months of the end of treatment.

- FOLLICULAR NON-HODGKINS LYMPHOMA

Roferon-A prolongs disease-free and progression-free survival when used as adjunctive treatment to CHOP-like chemotherapy regimens in patients with advanced (high tumour burden) follicular non-Hodgkin's lymphoma. However, the efficacy of adjunctive interferon alfa-2a treatment on overall long-term survival of these patients has not yet been established.

Dosage Recommendation:

Roferon-A should be administered concomitantly to a conventional chemotherapy regimen (such as the combination of cyclophosphamide, prednisone, vincristine and doxorubicin) according to a schedule such as 6 million IU/m^2 given subcutaneously from day 22 to day 26 of each 28-day cycle.

- ADVANCED RENAL CELL CARCINOMA

Therapy with Roferon-A in combination with vinblastine induces overall response rates of approximately 17-26%, delays disease progression, and prolongs overall survival in patients with advanced renal cell carcinoma.

Dosage recommendation:

Roferon-A should be given by subcutaneous injection at a dose of 3 million IU three times weekly for one week, 9 million IU three times weekly for the following week and 18 million IU three times weekly thereafter. Concomitantly vinblastine should be given intravenously according to the manufacturer's instructions at a dose of 0.1 mg/kg once every 3 weeks.

If the Roferon-A dosage of 18 million IU three times per week is not tolerated the dose may be reduced to 9 million IU three times per week.

Treatment should be given for a minimum of three months, up to a maximum of 12 months or until the development of progressive disease. Patients who achieve a complete response may stop treatment three months after the response is established.

- SURGICALLY RESECTED MALIGNANT MELANOMA.

Adjuvant therapy with a low dose of Roferon-A prolongs disease-free interval in patients with no nodal or distant metastases following resection of a melanoma (tumour thickness > 1.5 mm).

Dosage recommendation:

Roferon-A should be administered subcutaneously at a dose of 3 million IU three times a week for 18 months, starting no later than six weeks post surgery. If intolerance develops, the dose should be lowered to 1.5 million IU three times a week.

4.3 Contraindications

Roferon-A is contraindicated in patients with:

1) A history of hypersensitivity to recombinant interferon alfa-2a or to any of the excipients,

2) Patients with severe pre-existing cardiac disease or with any history of cardiac illness. No direct cardiotoxic effect has been demonstrated, but it is likely that acute, self-limiting toxicities (i.e., fever, chills) frequently associated with administration of Roferon-A may exacerbate pre-existing cardiac conditions,

3) Severe renal, hepatic or myeloid dysfunction,

4) Uncontrolled seizure disorders and/or compromised central nervous system function (see section 4.4.),

5) Chronic hepatitis with advanced, decompensated hepatic disease or cirrhosis of the liver,

6) Chronic hepatitis who are being or have recently been treated with immunosuppressive agents,

7) Benzyl alcohol, which is an excipient in Roferon-A solution for injectionhas on rare occasions been associated with potentially fatal toxicities and anaphylactoid reactions in children up to 3 years old. Therefore, Roferon-A solution for injection should not be used in premature babies, neonates, infants or children up to 3 years old Roferon-A solution contains 10 mg / ml Benzyl alcohol.

Combination therapy with ribavirin: Also see ribavirin labelling if interferon alfa-2a is to be administered in combination with ribavirin in patients with chronic hepatitis C.

4.4 Special warnings and precautions for use

Roferon-A should be administered under the supervision of a qualified physician experienced in the management of the respective indication. Appropriate management of the therapy and its complications is possible only when adequate diagnostic and treatment facilities are readily available.

Patients should be informed not only of the benefits of therapy but also that they will probably experience adverse reactions.

Hypersensitivity: If a hypersensitivity reaction occurs during treatment with Roferon-A or in the combination therapy with ribavirin, treatment has to be discontinued and appropriate medical therapy has to be instituted immediately. Transient rashes do not necessitate interruption of treatment.

In transplant patients (e.g., kidney or bone marrow transplant) therapeutic immunosuppression may be weakened because interferons also exert an immunostimulatory action.

Fever/Infections: While fever may be associated with the flu-like syndrome reported commonly during interferon therapy, other causes of persistent fever, particularly serious infections (bacterial, viral, fungal) must be ruled out, especially in patients with neutropenia. Serious infections (bacterial, viral, fungal) have been reported during treatment with alfa interferons including Roferon-A. Appropriate anti-infective therapy should be started immediately and discontinuation of therapy should be considered.

Psychiatric: Severe psychiatric adverse reactions may manifest in patients receiving therapy with interferons, including Roferon-A. Depression, suicidal ideation, suicidal attempt, and suicide may occur in patients with and without previous psychiatric illness. Physicians should monitor all patients treated with Roferon-A for evidence of depression. Physicians should inform patients of the possible development of depression prior to initiation of therapy, and patients should report any sign or symptom of depression immediately. Psychiatric intervention and/or drug discontinuation should be considered in such cases.

Ophthalmologic: As with other interferons, retinopathy including retinal haemorrhages, cotton wool spots, papilloedema, retinal artery or vein thrombosis and optic neuropathy which may result in loss of vision, have been reported after treatment with Roferon-A. Any patient complaining of decrease or loss of vision must have an eye examination. Because these ocular events may occur in conjunction with other disease states, a visual examination prior to initiation of Roferon-A monotherapy or in the combination therapy with ribavirin is recommended in patients with diabetes mellitus or hypertension. Roferon-A monotherapy or the combination therapy with ribavirin should be discontinued in patients who develop new or worsening ophthalmologic disorders.

Endocrine: Hyperglycaemia has been observed rarely in patients treated with Roferon-A. All patients who develop symptoms of hyperglycaemia should have their blood glucose measured and followed-up accordingly. Patients with diabetes mellitus may require adjustment of their antidiabetic regimen.

When mild to moderate renal, hepatic or myeloid dysfunction is present, close monitoring of these functions is required.

Hepatic function: In rare cases interferon alpha has been suspected of causing an exacerbation of an underlying autoimmune disease in hepatitis patients. Therefore, when treating hepatitis patients with a history of autoimmune disease caution is recommended. If a deterioration in liver function in these patients develops a determination of autoimmune antibodies should be considered. If necessary treatment should be discontinued.

Bone marrow suppression: Extreme caution should be exercised when administering Roferon-A to patients with severe myelosuppression as it has a suppressive effect on the bone marrow, leading to a fall in the white blood count, particularly granulocytes, platelet count and, less commonly, haemoglobin concentration. This can lead to an increased risk of infection or of haemorrhage. It is important to monitor closely these events in patients and periodic complete blood counts should be performed during the course of Roferon-A treatment, both prior to therapy and at appropriate periods during therapy.

Autoimmune: The development of different auto-antibodies has been reported during treatment with alpha interferons. Clinical manifestations of autoimmune disease during interferon therapy occur more frequently in subjects predisposed to the development of autoimmune disorders. In patients with an underlying or clinical history of autoimmune disorders, monitoring of symptoms suggestive of these disorders, as well as measurement of auto antibodies and TSH level, is recommended.

The use of Roferon-A in children is not recommended as the safety and effectiveness of Roferon-Ain children have not been established.

Efficacy in patients with chronic hepatitis B or C who are on haemodialysis or have haemophilia or are coinfected with human immunodeficiency virus has not been demonstrated.

This product contains less than 1 mmol sodium (23 mg) per 0.5 ml, i.e. essentially 'sodium-free'.

Combination therapy with ribavirin: Also see ribavirin labelling if interferon alfa-2a is to be administered in combination with ribavirin in patients with chronic hepatitis C.

Patients co-infected with HIV and receiving Highly Active Anti-Retroviral Therapy (HAART) may be at increased risk of developing lactic acidosis. Caution should be used when adding Roferon-A and ribavirin to HAART therapy (see ribavirin SPC).

Co-infected patients with advanced cirrhosis receiving HAART may be at increased risk of hepatic decompensation and death. Adding treatment with alfa interferons alone or in combination with ribavirin may increase the risk in this patient subset.

4.5 Interaction with other medicinal products and other forms of interaction

Since alpha-interferons alter cellular metabolism, the potential to modify the activity of other drugs exists. In a small study, Roferon-A was shown to have an effect on specific microsomal enzyme systems. The clinical relevance of these findings is unknown.

Alpha-interferons may affect the oxidative metabolic process; this should be borne in mind when prescribing concomitant therapy with drugs metabolised by this route. However, as yet no specific information is available.

Roferon-A has been reported to reduce the clearance of theophylline.

As Roferon-A may affect central nervous system functions, interactions could occur following concurrent administration of centrally-acting drugs. The neurotoxic, haematotoxic or cardiotoxic effects of previously or concurrently administered drugs may be increased by interferons.

Combination therapy with ribavirin: Also see ribavirin labelling if interferon alfa-2a is to be administered in combination with ribavirin in patients with chronic hepatitis C.

4.6 Pregnancy and lactation

Men and women receiving Roferon-A should practise effective contraception. There are no adequate data on the use of Roferon-A in pregnant women. When doses greatly in excess of the recommended clinical dose were administered to pregnant rhesus monkeys in the early to mid-fetal period, an abortifacient effect was observed (see section 5.3). Although animal tests do not indicate that Roferon-A is a teratogen, harm to the fetus from use during pregnancy cannot be excluded. In pregnancy, Roferon-A should be administered only if the benefit to the woman justifies the potential risk to the fetus.

It is not known whether this drug is excreted in human milk. A decision must be taken whether to suspend breast feeding or to discontinue the drug, taking into account the importance of the drug to the mother.

Use with ribavirin in patients with chronic hepatitis C

Significant teratogenic and/or embryocidal effects have been demonstrated in all animal species exposed to ribavirin. Ribavirin therapy is contraindicated in women who are pregnant. Extreme care must be taken to avoid pregnancy in female patients or in partners of male patients taking Roferon-A in combination with ribavirin. Female patients of childbearing potential and their partners must each use an effective contraceptive during treatment and for 4 months after treatment has been concluded. Male patients and their female partners must each use an effective contraception during treatment and for 7 months after treatment has been concluded. Please refer to the ribavirin SPC.

4.7 Effects on ability to drive and use machines

No studies on the effects on the ability to drive and use machines have been performed. However depending on dose and schedule as well as the sensitivity of the individual patient, Roferon-A may have an effect on the speed of reaction which could impair certain operations, e.g., driving, operation of machinery etc.

4.8 Undesirable effects

Combination therapy with ribavirin: Also see ribavirin labeling if interferon alfa-2a is to be administered in combination with ribavirin in patients with chronic hepatitis C.

The following data on adverse reactions are based on information derived from the treatment of cancer patients with a wide variety of malignancies and often refractory to previous therapy and suffering from advanced disease, patients with chronic hepatitis B, and patients with chronic hepatitis C.

Approximately two thirds of cancer patients experienced anorexia and one half nausea. Cardiovascular and pulmonary disorders were seen in about one fifth of cancer patients and consisted of transient hypotension, hypertension, edema, cyanosis, arrhythmias, palpitations and chest pain. Most cancer patients received doses that were significantly higher than the dose now recommended and may explain the higher frequency and severity of adverse reactions in this patient group compared with patients with hepatitis B where adverse reactions are usually transient, and patients return to pre-treatment status within 1 to 2 weeks after the end of therapy. Cardiovascular disorders were very rarely seen in patients with hepatitis B. In hepatitis B patients, changes in transaminases usually signal an improvement in the clinical state of the patient.

The majority of the patients experienced flu-like symptoms such as fatigue, pyrexia, rigors, decreased appetite, myalgia, headache, arthralgia and diaphoresis. These acute side-effects can usually be reduced or eliminated by concurrent administration of paracetamol and tend to diminish with continued therapy or dose modification although continuing therapy can lead to lethargy, asthenia and fatigue.

Within each frequency grouping, undesirable effects are presented in order of decreasing seriousness:

(see Table 1 on next page)

Rarely, alpha interferons including Roferon-A used alone or in combination with ribavirin, may be associated with pancytopenia, and very rarely, aplastic anemia has been reported.

Neutralizing antibodies to interferons may form in some patients. In certain clinical conditions (cancer, systemic lupus erythematosus, herpes zoster) antibodies to human leukocyte interferon may also occur spontaneously in patients who have never received exogenous interferons. The clinical significance of the development of antibodies has not been fully clarified.

In clinical trials where lyophilised Roferon-A which had been stored at 25°C was used, neutralizing antibodies to Roferon-A have been detected in approximately one fifth of patients. In patients with hepatitis C, a trend for responding patients who develop neutralizing antibodies to lose response while still on treatment and to lose it earlier than patients who do not develop such antibodies, has been seen. No other clinical sequelae of the presence of antibodies to Roferon-A have been documented. The clinical significance of the development of antibodies has not been fully clarified.

No data on neutralizing antibodies yet exist from clinical trials in which lyophilized Roferon-A or Roferon-A solution for injection which is stored at 4°C has been used. In a mouse model, the relative immunogenicity of lyophilized Roferon-A increases with time when the material is stored at 25°C - no such increase in immunogenicity is observed when lyophilised Roferon-A is stored at 4°C, the recommended storage conditions.

4.9 Overdose

There are no reports of overdosage but repeated large doses of interferon can be associated with profound lethargy, fatigue, prostration and coma. Such patients should be hospitalised for observation and appropriate supportive treatment given.

Patients who experience severe reactions to Roferon-A will usually recover within days after discontinuation of therapy, given appropriate supportive care. Coma has been observed in 0.4% of cancer patients in clinical trials.

5. PHARMACOLOGICAL PROPERTIES

5.1 Pharmacodynamic properties

Pharmacotherapeutic group: Antineoplastic and immunomodulating agents, *Interferons*

ATC Code L03AB04

Roferon-A has been shown to possess many of the activities of the so-called natural human alpha-interferon preparations. Roferon-A exerts its antiviral effects by inducing a state of resistance to viral infections in cells and by modulating the effector arm of the immune system to neutralize viruses or eliminate virus infected cells. The essential mechanism for the antitumour action of Roferon-A is not yet known. However, several changes are described in human tumoural cells treated with Roferon-A: HT 29 cells show a significant reduction of DNA, RNA and protein synthesis. Roferon-A has been shown to exert antiproliferative activity against a variety of human tumours *in vitro* and to inhibit the growth of some human tumour xenografts in nude mice. A limited number of human tumour cell lines grown *in vivo* in immunocompromised nude mice has been tested for the susceptibility to Roferon-A. *In vivo* antiproliferative activity of Roferon-A has been studied on tumours including breast mucoid carcinoma, adenocarcinoma of the caecum, colon carcinoma and prostatic carcinoma. The degree of antiproliferative activity is variable.

Unlike other human proteins, many of the effects of interferon alfa-2a are partially or completely suppressed when it is tested in other animal species. However, significant antivaccinia virus activity was induced in rhesus monkeys pre-treated with interferon alfa-2a.

Clinical Trials

Hairy Cell Leukemia

The therapeutic efficacy of Roferon-A in the treatment of hairy cell leukemia has been demonstrated in a large trial of 218 patients, of whom 174 were evaluable for efficacy after 16-24 weeks of therapy. Response was observed in 88% of patients (complete response 33%, partial response 55%).

AIDS-related Kaposi's Sarcoma

The efficacy of Roferon-A in the treatment of Kaposi's sarcoma was assessed in 364 patients receiving of 3 to 54 MIU per day. Objective response rates were dose-related, ranging from 14% to 50%, with a daily dose of 36 MIU producing the best overall therapeutic benefit (13.3% complete response, 12.2% partial response). High baseline CD4 lymphocyte count was a favorable prognostic factor for response, with 46% of patients with a CD4 count $>400/mm^3$ responding to Roferon-A. Response to Roferon-A therapy was the strongest prognostic factor for survival.

Chronic Myelogenous Leukemia (CML)

The efficacy of Roferon-A was assessed in 226 patients with chronic phase CML, and compared with 109 patients receiving chemotherapy (hydroxyurea or busulfan). Both groups had favorable features at diagnosis (less than 10% blasts in the blood) and treatment was initiated with interferon within 6 months of diagnosis. Treatment of patients with CML in the chronic phase leads to the same proportion of patients (85-90%) achieving a haematologic response as treatment with the standard chemotherapy regimens. In addition patients treated with Roferon-A resulted in 8% complete cytogenetic response and 38% partial cytogenetic response versus 9% partial cytogenetic response during chemotherapy. Time to progression from the chronic phase of leukemia to an accelerated or a blastic phase was longer in the Roferon-A group (69 months) than in the conventional chemo-therapy group (46 months) ($p<0.001$) as was median overall survival (72.8 months versus 54.5 months, $p=0.002$).

Cutaneous T-cell Lymphoma (CTCL)

The efficacy of Roferon-A was assessed in 169 patients with CTCL, the majority of whom (78%) were resistant to, or had relapsed on, standard therapy. Among the 85 patients evaluable, overall response to treatment was 58% (20% complete response, 38% partial response). Patients with all stages of disease responded to therapy. Median duration of complete response from start of treatment was 22 months, with 94% of complete responders remaining in remission at 9 months.

Chronic Hepatitis B

The efficacy of Roferon-A in the treatment of chronic hepatitis B was assessed in trials involving over 900 patients. In the pivotal controlled study 238 patients were randomised into four groups: patients received either 2.5 MIU / m^2, 5.0 MIU / m^2, 10 MIU / m^2, tiw of Roferon-A or no treatment. Treatment duration was 12-24 weeks depending on response i. e. clearance of HBeAg and HBV DNA from serum. Patients were followed for up to 12 months after treatment was discontinued. There was a statistically significant difference in sustained response [clearance of hepatitis B e antigen (HBeAg) and hepatitis B viral DNA (HBV DNA)] between treated and untreated patients (37%

Table 1

Body System	Very common (≥1/10)	Common (≥1/100 to <1/10)	Uncommon (≥1/1 000 to ≤1/100)	Rare (≥1/10 000 to ≤1/1 000)	Very rare (≤1/10 000)
Infections and infestations				Pneumonia Herpes simplex[1]	
Blood and lymphatic system disorders[2]	Leukopenia	Thrombocytopenia Anemia		Agranulocytosis Hemolytic anemia	Idiopathic thrombocytopenic purpura
Immune system disorders				Autoimmune disorder Acute hypersensivity reactions[3]	Sarcoidosis
Endocrine disorders				Hypothyroidism Hyperthyroidism Thyroid dysfunction	
Metabolism and nutrition disorders	Anorexia Nausea Inconsequential hypocalcemia		Dehydration Electrolyte imbalance	Diabete mellitus Hyperglycemia	Hyper-triglyceridemia Hyperlipidemia
Psychiatric disorders			Depression Anxiety Mental status changes Confusional state Abnormal behavior Nervousness Memory impairment Sleep disorder	Suicide Suicide attempt Suicidal ideation	
Nervous system disorders	Headache	Dysgeusia	Neuropathy Dizziness Hypoasthesia Parasthesia Tremor Somnolence	Coma Cerebrovascular accident Convulsions Transient erectile dysfunction	Encephalopathy
Eye disorders			Visual disturbance Conjunctivitis	Ischemic retinopathy	Retinal artery thrombosis Optic neuropathy Retinal hemorrhage Retinal vein thrombosis Retinal exudates Retinopathy Papilledema
Ear and labyrinth disorders			Vertigo		
Cardiac disorders		Arrhythmias[4] Palpitations Cyanosis		Cardiorespiratory arrest Myocardial infarction Congestive heart failure Pulmonary edema	
Vascular disorders			Hypertension Hypotension	Vasculitis	
Respiratory, thoracic and mediastinal disorders				Dyspnea Cough	
Gastrointestinal disorders	Diarrhea	Vomiting Abdominal pain Nausea Dry mouth		Pancreatitis Intestinal hypermotility Constipation Dyspepsia Flatulence	Reactivation of peptic ulcer gastrointestinal bleeding (non life threatening)
Hepato-biliary disorders				Hepatic failure Hepatitis Hepatic dysfunction	
Skin and subcutaneous tissue disorders	Alopecia[5] Sweating increased		Psoriasis[6] Pruritus	Rash Dry skin Epistaxis Mucosal dryness Rhinorrhea	
Musculoskeletal, connective tissue and bone disorders	Myalgia Arthralgia			Systemic lupus erythematosus Arthritis	
Renal and urinary disorders			Proteinuria Increased cell count in urine	Acute renal failure[7] Renal impairment	
General disorders and administration site conditions	Flu like illness Appetite decreased Pyrexia Rigors Fatigue	Chest pain Edema			Injection site necrosis Injection site reaction
Investigations		weight loss	Increased ALT Increased transaminase Increased blood alkaline phosphatase	Increased blood creatinine Increased blood urea Increased blood bilirubin Increased blood uric acid Increased blood LDH	

1 (including exacerbations of herpes labialis)

[2] In myelosuppressed patients, thrombocytopenia and decreased haemoglobin occurred more frequently. Recovery of severe haematological deviations to pre-treatment levels usually occurred within seven to ten days after discontinuing Roferon-A treatment.

[3] (e.g. urticaria, angioedema, bronchospasm and anaphylaxis)

[4] including atrioventricular block

[5] (reversible upon discontinuation; increased hair loss may continue for several weeks after end of treatment)

[6] exacerbation of, or provocation of psoriasis

[7] (mainly in cancer patients with renal disease)

versus 13%). Response differences between various dose groups did not reach statistical significance (33%, 34% and 43% for the 2.5, 5.0 and 10.0 MIU / m^2 groups). Serological and virological responses were associated with marked improvement in liver histology after 12 months of treatment free-follow up.

Chronic Hepatitis C

The efficacy of Roferon-A in the treatment of chronic hepatitis C has been assessed in 1701 patients, with 130 untreated or placebo treated controls. At recommended doses, Roferon-A induces complete biochemical response in up to 85% of patients, with response rates maintained for at least 6 months after treatment ranging from 11 to 44% depending on pre-treatment disease characteristics, IFN dose and treatment duration. Biochemical response to Roferon-A is associated with significant improvement of liver disease as shown by evaluation of pre-and post-liver biopsies. For those patients who have a sustained response 3-6 months after end of therapy, response has been reported to be maintained for up to 4 years.

The therapeutic efficacy of Interferon alfa-2a alone and in combination with ribavirin was compared in a double-blind randomised clinical trial in naive (previously untreated) and relapsed patients with virologically, biochemically and histologically documented chronic hepatitis C. Six months after end of treatment sustained biochemical and virological response as well as histological improvement were assessed.

A statistically significant 10-fold increase (from 4% to 43%; $p<0.01$) in sustained virological and biochemical response was observed in relapsed patients. The favourable profile of the combination therapy was also reflected in the response rates relative to HCV genotype or baseline viral load. Although the sustained response rates in patients with HCV genotype-1 were lower than in the overall population (approx. 30% versus 0% in the monotherapy arm) the relative benefit of ribavirin in combination with interferon alfa-2a is particularly significant in this group of patients. In addition the histological improvement favoured the combination therapy.

Supportive favourable results from a small study in naïve patients were reported using interferon alfa-2a (3 MIU 3 times per week) with ribavirin.

For other information on pharmacodynamic properties please refer to the SmPC for Ribavirin.

Follicular Non-Hodgkin's lymphoma

The efficacy of Roferon-A in addition to cytotoxic chemotherapy (CHOP-like regimen of cyclophosphamide, vincristine, prednisone and doxorubicin) was assessed in 122 patients with clinically aggressive low-grade or intermediate-grade non-Hodgkin's lymphoma and compared with 127 controls receiving the same chemotherapy regimen. The two regimens produced comparable objective responses, but the regimen including Roferon-A had a greater effect in prolonging the time to treatment failure ($p<0.001$), the duration of complete response ($p<0.003$).

Renal Cell Carcinoma

The efficacy of Roferon-A, given in combination with vinblastine, was compared with vinblastine alone. The combination of Roferon-A plus vinblastine is superior to vinblastine alone in the treatment of patients with locally advanced or metastatic renal cell carcinoma. Median survival was 67.8 weeks for the 79 patients receiving Roferon-A plus vinblastine and 37.8 weeks for the 81 patients treated with vinblastine (p=.0049). Overall response rates were 16.5% for patients treated Roferon-A plus vinblastine and 2.5% for patients treated with vinblastine alone (p=.0025).

Surgically Resected Malignant Melanoma

The efficacy of Roferon-A in patients with primary cutaneous melanoma thicker than 1.5 mm and without clinically detectable node metastasis was assessed in a large randomised study involving 253 patients receiving Roferon-A at a dose of 3 MIU three times a week for 18 months, compared with 246 untreated controls. After a median follow-up of 4.4 years a significant extension of relapse-free interval (p=0.035) but no statistically significant difference in overall survival (p=0.059) in Roferon-A treated patients compared with controls have been shown. The overall treatment effect was a 25% reduction in the risk of relapse.

5.2 Pharmacokinetic properties

The serum concentrations of interferon alfa-2a reflected a large intersubject variation in both healthy volunteers and patients with disseminated cancer. The pharmacokinetics of Roferon-A in animals (monkey, dog and mouse) were similar to those seen in man. The pharmacokinetics of Roferon-A in man were linear over a 3 million to 198 million IU dose range. In healthy man, interferon alfa-2a exhibited an elimination half-life of 3.7 - 8.5 hours (mean: 5.1 hours), a volume of distribution at steady state of 0.223 - 0.748 l/kg (mean: 0.4 l/kg) and a total body clearance of 2.14 - 3.62 ml/min/kg (mean: 2.79 ml/min/kg) after a 36 million IU intravenous infusion. After intramuscular administration of 36 million IU, peak serum concentrations ranged from 1500 to 2580 pg/ml (mean: 2020 pg/ml) at a mean time to peak of 3.8 hours, and after subcutaneous administration of 36 million IU from 1250 to 2320 pg/ml (mean: 1730 pg/ml) at a mean time to peak of 7.3 hours.

The apparent fraction of the dose absorbed after intramuscular or subcutaneous injection is greater than 80%.

The pharmacokinetics of interferon alfa-2a after single intramuscular doses to patients with disseminated cancer and chronic hepatitis B were similar to those found in healthy volunteers. Dose-proportional increases in serum concentrations were observed after single doses up to 198 million IU. There were no changes in the distribution or elimination of interferon alfa-2a during twice daily (0.5 - 36 million IU), once daily (1 - 54 million IU), or three times weekly (1 - 136 million IU) dosing regimens up to 28 days of dosing. Renal catabolism is the major pathway for Roferon-A elimination. Biliary excretion and liver metabolism are considered to be minor pathways of elimination of Roferon-A.

Intramuscular administration of Roferon-A one or more times daily for up to 28 days to some patients with disseminated cancer resulted in peak plasma concentrations of two to four times greater than those seen after single doses. However, multiple dosing caused no changes in its distribution or elimination parameters during several dosage regimens studied.

For other information on pharmacokinetic properties please refer to the SmPC for Ribavirin.

5.3 Preclinical safety data

Because of species specificity of human interferon, only limited toxicological studies have been carried out with Roferon-A. The acute parenteral toxicity of Roferon-A has been studied in mice rats, rabbits and ferrets at doses up to 30 million IU/kg intravenously, and 500 million IU/kg intramuscularly. No treatment-related mortality was noted in any species studied given Roferon-A by any of the routes of administration. With doses greatly exceeding the recommended clinical dose no significant adverse effects were observed except for an abortifacient effect when administered to pregnant rhesus monkeys in the early to mid-foetal period and transient menstrual cycle irregularities including prolonged menstrual periods in non-pregnant monkeys. The relevance of these findings in man has not been established.

Mutagenic effects of Roferon-A have not been observed experimentally.

For other information on preclinical safety data please refer to the SmPC for Ribavirin.

6. PHARMACEUTICAL PARTICULARS

6.1 List of excipients

Ammonium acetate

Sodium Chloride

Benzyl alcohol (10mg/1ml)

Polysorbate 80

Glacial Acetic acid

Sodium Hydroxide

Water for Injections

6.2 Incompatibilities

In the absence of compatibility studies, this medicinal product must not be mixed with other medicinal products.

6.3 Shelf life

2 years

6.4 Special precautions for storage

Store in a refrigerator (2°C - 8°C). Do not freeze. Keep the pre-filled syringe in the outer carton.

6.5 Nature and contents of container

0.5 ml of solution in pre-filled syringe (type I glass) with a plunger stopper (butyl rubber), a tip cap (butyl rubber), plunger rod (plastic), needle (stainless steel); pack sizes of 1, 5, 6, 12 and 30.

Not all pack sizes may be marketed.

6.6 Special precautions for disposal and other handling

For single use only.

Any unused product or waste material should be disposed of in accordance with local requirements.

7. MARKETING AUTHORISATION HOLDER

Roche Products Limited

6 Falcon Way, Shire Park

Welwyn Garden City

AL7 1TW, United Kingdom

8. MARKETING AUTHORISATION NUMBER(S)

PL 00031/0485

PL 00031/0486

PL 00031/0487

PL 00031/0488

PL 00031/0602

9. DATE OF FIRST AUTHORISATION/RENEWAL OF THE AUTHORISATION

Date of first authorisation: 25 July 1996

Date of last renewal: 22 July 2009

10. DATE OF REVISION OF THE TEXT

19 December 2008

Rogitine Ampoules 10mg

(Alliance Pharmaceuticals)

1. NAME OF THE MEDICINAL PRODUCT

Rogitine® ampoules 10mg

2. QUALITATIVE AND QUANTITATIVE COMPOSITION

Phentolamine mesilate PhEur 10mg.

3. PHARMACEUTICAL FORM

Colourless to pale yellow solution in 1ml Water for Injections PhEur

4. CLINICAL PARTICULARS

4.1 Therapeutic indications

Management of hypertensive episodes that may occur in patients with phaeochromocytoma, for example during pre-operative preparation and surgical manipulation.

Diagnosis of phaeochromocytoma by Rogitine blocking test if other more specific tests are not available.

4.2 Posology and method of administration

Adults

Management of hypertensive episodes in patients with phaeochromocytoma

For the management of hypertensive crises that arise during the pre-operative phase or during induction of anaesthesia, intubation, or surgical removal of the tumour, 2 to 5mg of Rogitine is injected intravenously and repeated if necessary. The blood pressure response should be monitored.

Diagnosis of phaeochromocytoma - Rogitine blocking test

The test is most reliable in detecting phaeochromocytoma in patients with sustained hypertension and least reliable in those with paroxysmal hypertension. False-positive tests may occur in patients with hypertension without phaeochromocytoma.

Preparation for the test:

Sedatives, analgesics and all other medications except those that might be deemed essential (such as digitalis and insulin) are withheld for at least 24 hours, and preferably 48 to 72 hours, prior to the test. Antihypertensive drugs are withheld until blood pressure returns to the untreated, hypertensive level. This test is not performed on a patient who is normotensive.

Procedure: (intravenous) The patient is kept at rest in the supine position throughout the test, preferably in a quiet, darkened room. Injection of Rogitine is delayed until blood pressure is stabilised, as evidenced by blood pressure readings taken every 10 minutes for at least 30 minutes.

The dose for adults is 5mg. The syringe needle is inserted into the vein and injection delayed until the pressor response to venepuncture has subsided.

Rogitine is injected rapidly. Blood pressure is recorded immediately after injection, at 30-second intervals for the first 3 minutes, and at 60-second intervals for the next 7 minutes.

Interpretation: A positive response, suggestive of phaeochromocytoma, is indicated when the blood pressure is reduced by more than 35mmHg systolic and by 25mmHg diastolic. A typical positive response is a reduction in pressure of 60mmHg systolic and 25mmHg diastolic. Usually, the maximal effect is evident within 2 minutes after injection. A return to preinjection pressure commonly occurs within 15 to 20 minutes but may occur more rapidly.

If blood pressure decreases to a dangerous level, the patient should be treated as outlined under Section 4.9 "Overdose".

A negative response is indicated when the blood pressure is elevated, unchanged, or reduced by less than 35mmHg systolic and 25mmHg diastolic after injection of Rogitine. A negative response to this test does not exclude the diagnosis of phaeochromocytoma, especially in patients with paroxysmal hypertension, in whom the incidence of false-negative responses is high.

Procedure: (intramuscular) A dose of 5mg is administered intramuscularly.

Interpretation: Blood pressure is recorded every 5 minutes for 30 to 45 minutes following injection. A positive response is indicated when the blood pressure is reduced by 35mmHg systolic and by 25mmHg diastolic, or more, within 20 minutes following injection.

Children:

Management of hypertensive episodes in patients with phaeochromocytoma: The dosage is 1mg given intravenously.

Diagnosis of phaeochromocytoma - Rogitine blocking test: The dosage is 1mg given intravenously or 3mg given intramuscularly.

Elderly: In elderly patients, it is advisable to use the lowest dose or a low infusion rate in case of undiagnosed coronary insufficiency, (see Section 4.3 "Contra-indications").

Patients with renal impairment: Since no pharmacokinetic studies with Rogitine have been performed in patients with renal impairment, use caution in administering Rogitine to these patients.

4.3 Contraindications

Known hypersensitivity to phentolamine and related compounds. Known hypersensitivity to sulphites. Hypotension. Myocardial infarction, history of myocardial infarction, coronary insufficiency, angina, or other evidence of coronary artery disease.

4.4 Special warnings and precautions for use

Monitoring of the blood pressure is necessary for appropriate selection of patient, dosage, and duration of therapy. Myocardial infarction, cerebrovascular spasm, and cerebrovascular occlusion have been reported following the administration of Rogitine, usually in association with marked hypotensive episodes.

The presence of sulphites in Rogitine ampoules can lead to isolated hypersensitivity reactions especially in patients with bronchial asthma, which may become manifest as an acute asthma attack, shock, or clouding of consciousness.

For screening tests in patients with hypertension, the generally available urinary assay of catecholamines or other biochemical assays have largely replaced the Rogitine blocking test and other pharmacological tests for reasons of accuracy and safety. Therefore the Rogitine blocking test is not the procedure of choice and should be used only when these other specific tests are not available.

Tachycardia and cardiac arrhythmias may occur with the use of Rogitine.

Due to its stimulatory effect on the gastro-intestinal tract, including gastric secretion, Rogitine should be used with caution in patients with gastritis and peptic ulcer. Excessive cardiac stimulation and hypertensive crisis may occur during surgical removal of a tumour due to manipulation of the phaeochromocytoma, despite the fact that phentolamine had been given as pre-medication to prevent such an occurrence. In the event of this complication, use a $_1$-selective, -adrenergic blocking agent in slow i.v. injection.

4.5 Interaction with other medicinal products and other forms of interaction

Rogitine may augment the hypotensive effect of other antihypertensive agents. Antipsychotics may enhance the hypotensive effect of -adrenergic blocking agents.

4.6 Pregnancy and lactation

Experience with Rogitine in pregnant women is not available. Do not use in pregnancy unless treatment is considered essential.

No information is available as to whether phentolamine passes into breast milk. For safety reasons, it is not recommended to use Rogitine during lactation.

4.7 Effects on ability to drive and use machines

Patients should be warned of the potential hazards of driving or operating machinery if they experience side effects such as dizziness and sedation.

4.8 Undesirable effects

Cardiovascular system: Frequent: Orthostatic hypotension and tachycardia. Occasional: Acute or prolonged hypotensive episodes (flushing, sweating and feelings of apprehension). Myocardial infarction, cerebrospasm, and cerebrovascular occlusion may occur under these circumstances. Rare: Anginal pain and cardiac arrhythmias.

Central nervous system: Occasional: Dizziness and weakness.

Gastro-intestinal tract: Occasional: Nausea, vomiting and diarrhoea.

Other organ systems: Occasional: Nasal stuffiness and flushing. Rare: Chest pain.

4.9 Overdose

Symptoms: Arterial hypotension, reflex tachycardia, cardiac stimulation, arrhythmia, increase of systemic venous capacity, and possibly shock. These effects may be accompanied by headache, hyperexcitability and disturbances of vision, sweating, increased gastric motility, vomiting and diarrhoea, hypoglycaemia.

Treatment: *Hypotension, excessive peripheral vasodilation*: noradrenaline, in cautiously titrated continuous i.v. infusion, can be considered the physiological antagonist; the effect of Rogitine may wear off in a short time, and administration of noradrenaline may have to be adjusted accordingly. When a pressor agent is used, ECG should be monitored, as major arrhythmias may occur. Alternative measures such as keeping the patient's legs raised and administering a plasma expander should be implemented concomitantly. Do not use adrenaline since this may cause a further fall of blood pressure under the given conditions.

Disturbances of cardiac rhythm: adjust treatment to the nature of the arrhythmia.

Hypoglycaemia: Provide glucose iv until reaction is compensated.

5. PHARMACOLOGICAL PROPERTIES

5.1 Pharmacodynamic properties

Phentolamine is a competitive non-selective $_1$ and $_2$-adrenergic receptor blocker of relatively short duration. It causes vasodilation and a fall in blood pressure which is based upon the blockade of both postjunctional vascular $_1$ and $_2$-adrenoceptors. It also antagonises the vasoconstrictor response to noradrenaline and adrenaline infusions. Enhanced neural release of noradrenaline due to presynaptic $_2$-blockade may contribute to the positive inotropic and chronotropic effects of Rogitine on cardiac muscle.

The administration of Rogitine intravenously to man produces transient declines in mean systemic vascular resistance and mean systemic arterial pressure as a result of dilatation in the arterial as well as in the venous vascular bed. These effects of Rogitine are accompanied by tachycardia, triggered by the baroreceptor reflex system and the autonomic nervous system.

5.2 Pharmacokinetic properties

The elimination of phentolamine from blood is rapid and does not follow first order kinetics. After two to four hours the concentration has fallen to about 15% of the peak value. At concentrations of 0.02 to 109μg/ml, 54% of phentolamine is bound to human serum proteins. Phentolamine is extensively metabolised, on average about 13% of a dose given by intravenous infusion is excreted unchanged in the urine. Phentolamine metabolism is more pronounced following oral administration than after intravenous administration.

5.3 Preclinical safety data

According to the experimental data available, phentolamine did not reveal either a mutagenic or a teratogenic potential. Long-term carcinogenicity studies have not been conducted with phentolamine.

6. PHARMACEUTICAL PARTICULARS

6.1 List of excipients

Water, sodium metabisulphite and glucose.

6.2 Incompatibilities

Rogitine should not be mixed with alkaline solutions.

6.3 Shelf life

5 Years

6.4 Special precautions for storage

Store ampoules in the outer carton at 2 to 8°C. Do not freeze.

6.5 Nature and contents of container

Glass ampoules in boxes of 5.

6.6 Special precautions for disposal and other handling

None

Administrative Data

7. MARKETING AUTHORISATION HOLDER

Alliance Pharmaceuticals Ltd

Avonbridge House

Bath Road

Chippenham

Wiltshire

SN15 2BB

8. MARKETING AUTHORISATION NUMBER(S)

PL16853/0012

9. DATE OF FIRST AUTHORISATION/RENEWAL OF THE AUTHORISATION

25 June 1998

10. DATE OF REVISION OF THE TEXT

17/02/2006

Alliance, Alliance Pharmaceuticals and associated devices are registered Trademarks of Alliance Pharmaceuticals Ltd.

Rotarix

(GlaxoSmithKline UK)

1. NAME OF THE MEDICINAL PRODUCT

Rotarix ▼ powder and solvent for **oral** suspension

Rotavirus vaccine, live

2. QUALITATIVE AND QUANTITATIVE COMPOSITION

After reconstitution, 1 dose (1ml) contains:

Human rotavirus RIX4414 strain (live, attenuated)* not less than $10^{6.0}$ $CCID_{50}$

*Produced on Vero cells

Excipients:

This product contains sucrose 9 mg and sorbitol 13.5 mg (see section 4.4)

For a full list of excipients, see section 6.1.

3. PHARMACEUTICAL FORM

Powder and solvent for **oral** suspension.

The powder is white.

The solvent is a turbid liquid with a slow settling white deposit and a colourless supernatant.

4. CLINICAL PARTICULARS

4.1 Therapeutic indications

Rotarix is indicated for the active immunisation of infants from the age of 6 weeks for prevention of gastro-enteritis due to rotavirus infection (see section 4.2).

In clinical trials, efficacy was demonstrated against gastro-enteritis due to rotavirus of types G1P[8], G2P[4], G3P[8], G4P[8] and G9P[8] (see sections 4.4 and 5.1).

The use of Rotarix should be based on official recommendations.

4.2 Posology and method of administration

<u>*Posology*</u>

The vaccination course consists of two doses. The first dose may be administered from the age of 6 weeks. There should be an interval of at least 4 weeks between doses. The vaccination course should preferably be given before 16 weeks of age, but must be completed by the age of 24 weeks.

Rotarix may be given with the same posology to preterm infants born after at least 27 weeks of gestational age (see sections 4.8 and 5.1).

In clinical trials, spitting or regurgitation of the vaccine has rarely been observed and, under such circumstances, a replacement dose was not given. However, in the unlikely event that an infant spits out or regurgitates most of the vaccine dose, a single replacement dose may be given at the same vaccination visit.

It is recommended that infants who receive a first dose of Rotarix complete the 2-dose regimen with Rotarix. There are no data on safety, immunogenicity or efficacy when Rotarix is administered for the first dose and another rotavirus vaccine is administered for the second dose or vice versa.

<u>*Method of administration*</u>

Rotarix is for **oral** use only.

Rotarix should under no circumstances be injected.

4.3 Contraindications

Hypersensitivity to the active substance or to any of the excipients.

Hypersensitivity after previous administration of rotavirus vaccines.

Previous history of intussusception.

Subjects with uncorrected congenital malformation of the gastrointestinal tract that would predispose for intussusception.

Administration of Rotarix should be postponed in subjects suffering from acute severe febrile illness. The presence of a minor infection is not a contra-indication for immunisation.

The administration of Rotarix should be postponed in subjects suffering from diarrhoea or vomiting.

4.4 Special warnings and precautions for use

It is good clinical practice that vaccination should be preceded by a review of the medical history especially with regard to the contraindications and by a clinical examination.

There are no data on the safety and efficacy of Rotarix in infants with gastrointestinal illnesses or growth retardation. Administration of Rotarix may be considered with caution in such infants when, in the opinion of the physician, withholding the vaccine entails a greater risk.

Asymptomatic and mildly symptomatic HIV infections are not expected to affect the safety or efficacy of Rotarix. A clinical study in a limited number of asymptomatic or mildly symptomatic HIV positive infants showed no apparent safety problems (see section 4.8).

Administration of Rotarix to infants who have known or suspected immunodeficiency should be based on careful consideration of potential benefits and risks.

Excretion of the vaccine virus in the stools is known to occur after vaccination with peak excretion around the 7th day. Viral antigen particles detected by ELISA were found in 50% of stools after the first dose and 4% of stools after the second dose. When these stools were tested for the presence of live vaccine strain, only 17% were positive.

Cases of transmission of this excreted vaccine virus to seronegative contacts of vaccinees have been observed without causing any clinical symptom.

Rotarix should be administered with caution to individuals with immunodeficient close contacts, such as individuals with malignancies, or who are otherwise immunocompromised or individuals receiving immunosuppressive therapy.

Contacts of recent vaccinees should observe personal hygiene (e.g. wash their hands after changing child's nappies).

The potential risk of apnoea and the need for respiratory monitoring for 48-72h should be considered when administering the primary immunisation series to very premature infants (born ⩽ 28 weeks of gestation) and particularly for those with a previous history of respiratory immaturity.

As the benefit of the vaccination is high in this group of infants, vaccination should not be withheld or delayed.

A protective immune response may not be elicited in all vaccinees (see section 5.1).

In clinical trials, efficacy was demonstrated against gastro-enteritis due to rotavirus of types G1P[8], G2P[4], G3P[8], G4P[8] and G9P[8]. The extent of protection that Rotarix might provide against other serotypes is unknown. Clinical studies from which efficacy data were derived were conducted in Europe and Central and South America (see section 5.1).

Rotarix does not protect against gastro-enteritis due to other pathogens than rotavirus.

No data are available on the use of Rotarix for post-exposure prophylaxis.

Rotarix should under no circumstances be injected.

The vaccine contains sucrose and sorbitol as excipients. Patients with rare hereditary problems of fructose intolerance, glucose-galactose malabsorption or sucrase-isomaltase insufficiency should not take this vaccine.

4.5 Interaction with other medicinal products and other forms of interaction

Rotarix can be given concomitantly with any of the following monovalent or combination vaccines [including hexavalent vaccines (DTPa-HBV-IPV/Hib)]: diphtheria-tetanus-whole cell pertussis vaccine (DTPw), diphtheria-tetanus-acellular pertussis vaccine (DTPa), *Haemophilus influenzae* type b vaccine (Hib), inactivated polio vaccine (IPV), hepatitis B vaccine (HBV), pneumococcal conjugate vaccine and meningococcal serogroup C conjugate vaccine. Clinical studies demonstrated that the immune responses and the safety profiles of the administered vaccines were unaffected.

Concominant administration of Rotarix and oral polio vaccine (OPV) does not affect the immune response to the polio antigens. Although concomitant administration of OPV may slightly reduce the immune response to rotavirus vaccine, clinical protection against severe rotavirus gastro-enteritis was shown to be maintained in a clinical trial involving more than 4200 subjects who received Rotarix concomitantly with OPV.

There are no restrictions on the infant's consumption of food or liquid, either before or after vaccination.

4.6 Pregnancy and lactation

Rotarix is not intended for use in adults. Thus human data on use during pregnancy or lactation are not available and animal reproduction studies have not been performed.

Based on evidence generated in clinical trials, breast-feeding does not reduce the protection against rotavirus gastro-enteritis afforded by Rotarix. Therefore, breast-feeding may be continued during the vaccination schedule.

4.7 Effects on ability to drive and use machines

Not relevant.

4.8 Undesirable effects

• *Clinical trials*

In a total of eleven placebo-controlled clinical trials, approximately 77800 doses of Rotarix were administered to approximately 40200 infants.

In two clinical trials (Finland), Rotarix was administered alone (administration of routine paediatric vaccines was staggered). The incidence of diarrhoea, vomiting, loss of appetite, fever and irritability was not different in the group receiving Rotarix when compared to the group receiving placebo. No increase in the incidence or severity of these reactions was seen with the second dose.

In the remaining nine trials (Europe, Canada, USA, Latin America, Singapore, South-Africa), Rotarix was co-administered with routine paediatric vaccines (see section 4.5). The adverse reaction profile observed in these subjects was similar to the adverse reaction profile observed in subjects receiving the same paediatric vaccines and placebo.

Adverse reactions are listed below per system organ class and frequency.

Within each frequency grouping, undesirable effects are presented in order of decreasing seriousness.

Frequencies are reported as:

Very common (≥1/10)

Common (≥1/100, <1/10)

Uncommon (≥1/1,000, <1/100)

Rare (≥1/10,000, <1/1,000)

Nervous system disorders

Uncommon: somnolence

Respiratory, thoracic and mediastinal disorders

Rare: hoarseness, rhinorrhoea

Gastrointestinal disorders

Very common: loss of appetite

Common: diarrhoea, vomiting, abdominal pain, flatulence, regurgitation of food

Uncommon: constipation

Skin and subcutaneous tissue disorders

Rare: dermatitis, rash

Musculoskeletal and connective tissue disorders

Rare: muscle cramp

Infections and infestations

Rare: upper respiratory tract infection

General disorders and administration site conditions

Common: fever, fatigue

Psychiatric disorders

Very common: irritability

Uncommon: sleep disorder, crying

The risk of intussusception has been evaluated in a large safety trial conducted in Latin America and Finland where 63225 subjects were enrolled. This trial gave evidence of no increased risk of intussusception in the Rotarix group when compared with the placebo group as shown in the table below.

(see Table 1 below)

Safety in preterm infants

In a clinical study, 670 pre-term infants from 27 to 36 weeks of gestational age were administered Rotarix and 339 received placebo. The first dose was administered from 6 weeks after birth. Serious adverse events were observed in 5.1% of recipients of Rotarix as compared with 6.8% of placebo recipients. Similar rates of other adverse events were observed in Rotarix and placebo recipients. No cases of intussusception were reported.

Safety in infants with human immunodeficiency (HIV) infection

In a clinical study, 100 infants with HIV infection were administered Rotarix or placebo. The safety profile was similar between Rotarix and placebo recipients.

• *Post marketing surveillance:*

Respiratory, thoracic and mediastinal disorders:

Apnoea in very premature infants (≤ 28 weeks of gestation) (see section 4.4)

4.9 Overdose

No case of overdose has been reported.

5. PHARMACOLOGICAL PROPERTIES

5.1 Pharmacodynamic properties

Pharmaco-therapeutic group: rotavirus diarrhoea vaccines, ATC code: J07BH01

Protective efficacy

Clinical studies have been conducted in Europe and Latin America to evaluate the protective efficacy of Rotarix against any and severe rotavirus gastro-enteritis.

A clinical study performed in Europe evaluated Rotarix given according to different European schedules (2, 3 months; 2, 4 months; 3, 4 months; 3, 5 months) in 4000 subjects. Severity of gastro-enteritis was defined according to the Vesikari 20-point scale which evaluates the full clinical picture of rotavirus gastro-enteritis by taking into account the severity and duration of diarrhoea and vomiting, the severity of fever and dehydration as well as the need for treatment.

After two doses of Rotarix, the protective vaccine efficacy observed during the first and second year of life is presented in the following table:

(see Table 2 opposite)

Vaccine efficacy during the first year of life progressively increased with increasing disease severity, reaching 100% (95% CI: 84.7;100) for Vesikari scores ≥17.

A clinical study performed in Latin America evaluated Rotarix in more than 20000 subjects. Severity of gastro-enteritis was defined according to WHO criteria. The protective vaccine efficacy against severe rotavirus gastro-enteritis requiring hospitalisation and/or rehydration therapy in a medical facility and the type specific vaccine efficacy after two doses of Rotarix are presented in the table below:

Type	Severe rotavirus gastro-enteritis (1st year of life) Rotarix N=9009; Placebo N=8858 (§)	Severe rotavirus gastro-enteritis (2nd year of life) Rotarix N=7175; Placebo N=7062 (§)
	Efficacy (%) [95% CI]	Efficacy (%) [95% CI]
All RVGE	84.7* [71.7;92.4]	79.0* [66.4;87.4]
G1P[8]	91.8* [74.1;98.4]	72.4* [34.5;89.9]
G3P[8]	87.7* [8.3;99.7]	71.9 [<0.0;97.1]
G4P[8]	50.8# [<0.0;99.2]	63.1* [0.7;88.2]
G9P[8]	90.6* [61.7;98.9]	87.7* [72.9;95.3]
Strains with P[8] genotype	90.9* [79.2;96.8]	79.5* [67.0;87.9]

(§) ATP cohort for efficacy

* Statistically significant ($p < 0.05$)

The numbers of cases, on which the estimates of efficacy against G4P[8] were based, were very small (1 case in the Rotarix group and 2 cases in the placebo group).

Table 1

Intussusception within 31 days after administration of:	Rotarix N=31673	Placebo N=31552	Relative risk (95% CI*)
First dose	1	2	0.50 (0.07;3.80)
Second dose	5	5	0.99 (0.31;3.21)

*CI: confidence interval

Table 2

	1st year of life Rotarix N=2572; Placebo N=1302 (§)		2nd year of life Rotarix N=2554; Placebo N=1294 (§)	
Vaccine efficacy (%) against any and severe rotavirus gastro-enteritis [95% CI]				
Type	**Any severity**	**Severe†**	**Any severity**	**Severe†**
G1P[8]	95.6* [87.9;98.8]	96.4* [85.7;99.6]	82.7* [67.8;91.3]	96.5* [86.2;99.6]
G2P[4]	62.0 [<0.0;94.4]	74.7 [<0.0;99.6]	57.1* [<0.0;82.6]	89.9* [9.4;99.8]
G3P[8]	89.9* [9.5;99.8]	100* [44.8;100]	79.7* [<0.0;98.1]	83.1 [<0.0;99.7]
G4P[8]	88.3* [57.5;97.9]	100* [64.9;100]	69.6 [<0.0;95.3]	87.3* [<0.0;99.7]
G9P[8]	75.6* [51.1;88.5]	94.7* [77.9;99.4]	70.5* [50.7;82.8]	76.8* [50.8;89.7]
Strains with P[8] genotype	88.2* [80.8;93.0]	96.5* [90.6;99.1]	75.7* [65.0;83.4]	87.5* [77.8;93.4]
Circulating rotavirus strains	87.1* [79.6;92.1]	95.8* [89.6;98.7]	71.9* [61.2;79.8]	85.6* [75.8;91.9]
Vaccine efficacy (%) against rotavirus gastro-enteritis requiring medical attention [95% CI]				
Circulating rotavirus strains	91.8* [84;96.3]		76.2* [63.0;85.0]	
Vaccine efficacy (%) against hospitalisation due to rotavirus gastro-enteritis [95% CI]				
Circulating rotavirus strains	100* [81.8;100]		92.2* [65.6;99.1]	

† Severe gastro-enteritis defined as a score ≥11 on the Vesikari scale

(§) ATP cohort for efficacy

* Statistically significant ($p < 0.05$)

A pooled analysis of five efficacy studies*, showed a 71.4% (95% CI:20.1;91.1) efficacy against severe rotavirus gastro-enteritis (Vesikari score ⩾11) caused by rotavirus G2P[4] type during the first year of life.

* In these studies, the point estimates and confidence intervals were respectively: 100% (95% CI: -1858.0;100), 100% (95% CI: 21.1;100), 45.4% (95% CI: -81.5;86.6), 74.7 (95% CI:-386.2;99.6). No point estimate was available for the remaining study.

Immune response

The immunologic mechanism by which Rotarix protects against rotavirus gastro-enteritis is not completely understood. A relationship between antibody responses to rotavirus vaccination and protection against rotavirus gastro-enteritis has not been established.

The following table shows the percentage of subjects with serum anti-rotavirus IgA antibody titers ⩾ 20U/ml (by ELISA) one to two months after the second dose of vaccine or placebo as observed in different studies.

(see Table 3 below)

Immune response in preterm infants

In a clinical study conducted in preterm infants, born after at least 27 weeks of gestational age, the immunogenicity of Rotarix was assessed in a subset of 147 subjects and showed that Rotarix is immunogenic in this population; 85.7% (95% CI: 79.0;90.9) of subjects achieved serum anti-rotavirus IgA antibody titers ⩾ 20U/ml (by ELISA) one month after the second dose of vaccine.

5.2 Pharmacokinetic properties

Evaluation of pharmacokinetic properties is not required for vaccines.

5.3 Preclinical safety data

Non-clinical data reveal no special hazard for humans based on conventional studies of repeated dose toxicity.

6. PHARMACEUTICAL PARTICULARS

6.1 List of excipients

Powder

Sucrose

Dextran

Sorbitol

Amino acids

Dulbecco's Modified Eagle Medium (DMEM)

Solvent

Calcium carbonate

Xanthan gum

Sterile water

6.2 Incompatibilities

In the absence of compatibility studies, this medicinal product must not be mixed with other medicinal products.

6.3 Shelf life

3 years.

After reconstitution:

After the reconstitution, the vaccine should be administered immediately. If not used immediately, in-use storage should not be longer than 24 hours and at a temperature between 2-25°C.

6.4 Special precautions for storage

Store in a refrigerator (2°C – 8°C).

Do not freeze.

Store in the original package, in order to protect from light.

For storage conditions of the reconstituted product, see section 6.3.

6.5 Nature and contents of container

1 dose of powder in a glass container (type I glass) with a stopper (rubber butyl)

1ml of solvent in an **oral** applicator (type I glass) with a plunger stopper and a protective tip cap (rubber butyl).

Transfer adapter for reconstitution (1/dose)

in the following pack sizes:

- pack size of 1 glass container of powder plus 1 **oral** applicator of solvent

Figure 1

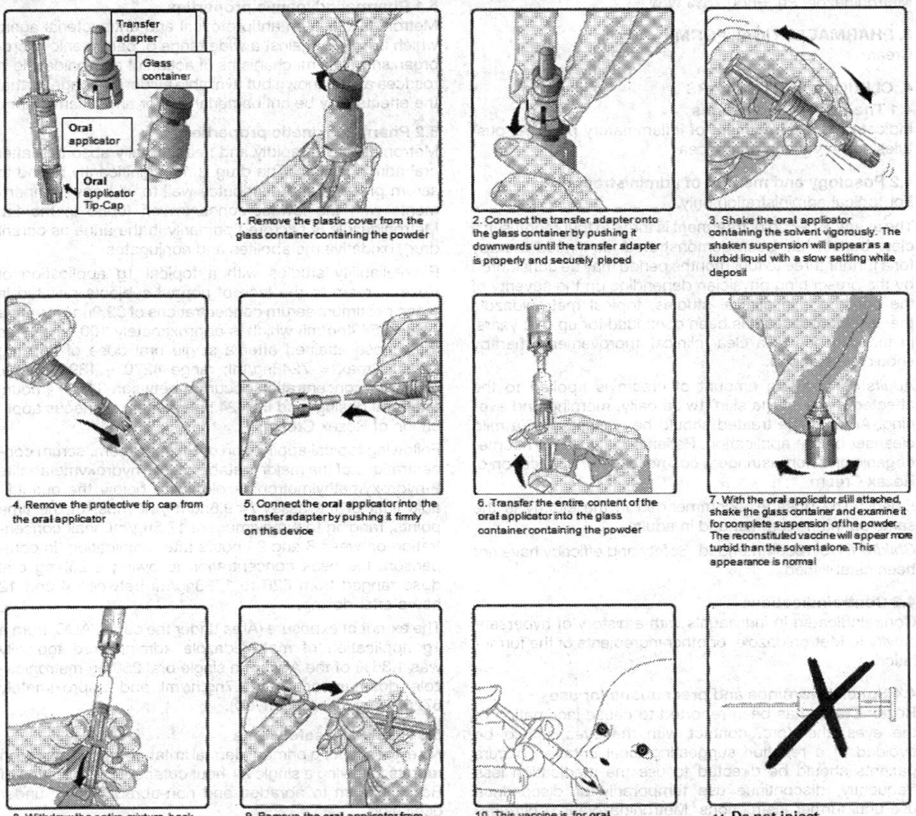

1. Remove the plastic cover from the glass container containing the powder

2. Connect the transfer adapter onto the glass container by pushing it downwards until the transfer adapter is properly and securely placed

3. Shake the oral applicator containing the solvent vigorously. The shaken suspension will appear as a turbid liquid with a slow settling white deposit

4. Remove the protective tip cap from the oral applicator

5. Connect the oral applicator into the transfer adapter by pushing it firmly on this device

6. Transfer the entire content of the oral applicator into the glass container containing the powder

7. With the oral applicator still attached, shake the glass container and examine it for complete suspension of the powder. The reconstituted vaccine will appear more turbid than the solvent alone. This appearance is normal

8. Withdraw the entire mixture back into the oral applicator

9. Remove the oral applicator from the transfer adapter

10. This vaccine is for oral administration only. The child should be seated in a reclining position. Administer the entire content of the oral applicator orally (by administering the entire content of the oral applicator on the inside of the cheek)

11. Do not inject.

- pack size of 5 glass containers of powder plus 5 **oral** applicators of solvent

- pack size of 10 glass containers of powder plus 10 **oral** applicators of solvent

- pack size of 25 glass containers of powder plus 25 **oral** applicators of solvent

Not all pack sizes may be marketed.

6.6 Special precautions for disposal and other handling

A white deposit and clear supernatant is observed upon storage of the **oral** applicator containing the solvent. The solvent should be inspected visually both before and after shaking for any foreign particulate matter and/or abnormal physical appearance prior to reconstitution.

The reconstituted vaccine is slightly more turbid than the solvent and is milky white in appearance.

The reconstituted vaccine should also be inspected visually for any foreign particulate matter and/or abnormal physical appearance prior to administration. In the event of either being observed, discard the vaccine. Any unused vaccine or waste material should be disposed of in accordance with local requirements.

Instructions for reconstitution and administration of the vaccine:

1. Remove the plastic cover from the glass container containing the powder.

2. Connect the transfer adapter onto the glass container by pushing it downwards until the transfer adapter is properly and securely placed.

3. Shake the **oral** applicator containing the solvent vigorously. The shaken suspension will appear as a turbid liquid with a slow settling white deposit.

4. Remove the protective tip cap from the **oral** applicator.

5. Connect the **oral** applicator into the transfer adapter by pushing it firmly on this device.

6. Transfer the entire content of the **oral** applicator into the glass container containing the powder.

7. With the **oral** applicator still attached, shake the glass container and examine it for complete suspension of the powder. The reconstituted vaccine will appear more turbid than the solvent alone. This appearance is normal.

8. Withdraw the entire mixture back into the **oral** applicator.

9. Remove the **oral** applicator from the transfer adapter.

10. This vaccine is for **oral administration only**. The child should be seated in a reclining position. Administer the entire content of the **oral** applicator **orally** (by administering the entire content of the **oral** applicator on the inside of the cheek).

11. **Do not inject.**

If the reconstituted vaccine is to be stored temporarily before administration, replace the protective tip cap on the **oral** applicator. The **oral** applicator containing the reconstituted vaccine should be shaken gently again before **oral** administration. **Do not inject.**

(see Figure 1 above)

Table 3

Schedule	Studies conducted in	Vaccine		Placebo	
		N	% ⩾ 20U/ml [95% CI]	N	% ⩾ 20U/ml [95% CI]
2, 3 months	France, Germany	239	82.8 [77.5;87.4]	127	8.7 [4.4;15.0]
2, 4 months	Spain	186	85.5 [79.6;90.2]	89	12.4 [6.3;21.0]
3, 5 months	Finland, Italy	180	94.4 [90.0;97.3]	114	3.5 [1.0;8.7]
3, 4 months	Czech Republic	182	84.6 [78.5;89.5]	90	2.2 [0.3;7.8]
2, 3 to 4 months	Latin America; 11 countries	393	77.9% [73.8;81.6]	341	15.1% [11.7;19.0]

7. MARKETING AUTHORISATION HOLDER

GlaxoSmithKline Biologicals s.a.

Rue de l'Institut 89

B-1330 Rixensart, Belgium

8. MARKETING AUTHORISATION NUMBER(S)

EU/1/05/330/001

9. DATE OF FIRST AUTHORISATION/RENEWAL OF THE AUTHORISATION

Date of first authorisation: 21 February 2006

10. DATE OF REVISION OF THE TEXT

21/08/2009

Rozex Cream

(Galderma (U.K) Ltd)

1. NAME OF THE MEDICINAL PRODUCT

Rozex Cream

2. QUALITATIVE AND QUANTITATIVE COMPOSITION
Metronidazole Ph. Eur 0.75% w/w

3. PHARMACEUTICAL FORM
Cream

4. CLINICAL PARTICULARS

4.1 Therapeutic indications
Indicated in the treatment of inflammatory papules, pustules and erythema of rosacea

4.2 Posology and method of administration
For topical administration only.

The average period of treatment is three to four months. If a clear benefit has been demonstrated, continued therapy for a further three to four months period may be considered by the prescribing physician depending on the severity of the condition. In clinical studies, topical metronidazole therapy for rosacea has been continued for up to 2 years. In the absence of a clear clinical improvement, therapy should be stopped.

Adults: A pea-size amount of cream is applied to the affected areas of the skin, twice daily, morning and evening. Areas to be treated should be washed with a mild cleanser before application. Patients may use non-comedogenic and non-astringent cosmetics after application of Rozex Cream.

Elderly: The dosage recommended in the elderly is the same as that recommended in adults.

Children: Not recommended. Safety and efficacy have not been established.

4.3 Contraindications
Contraindicated in individuals with a history of hypersensitivity to Metronidazole, or other ingredients of the formulation.

4.4 Special warnings and precautions for use
Rozex Cream has been reported to cause lacrimation of the eyes, therefore, contact with the eyes should be avoided. If a reaction suggesting local irritation occurs patients should be directed to use the medication less frequently, discontinue use temporarily or discontinue use until further instructions. Metronidazole is a nitroimidazole and should be used with care in patients with evidence of, or history of, blood dyscrasia. Exposure of treated sites to ultraviolet or strong sunlight should be avoided during use of metronidazole. Unnecessary and prolonged use of this medication should be avoided.

4.5 Interaction with other medicinal products and other forms of interaction
Interaction with systemic medication is unlikely because absorption of metronidazole following cutaneous application of Rozex Cream is low. Oral metronidazole has been reported to potentiate the effect of warfarinand other coumarin anticoagulants, resulting in a prolongation of prothrombin time. The effect of topical metronidazole on prothrombin is not known. However, very rare cases of modification of the INR values have been reported with concomitant use of Rozex and coumarin anticoagulants.

4.6 Pregnancy and lactation
There is no experience to date with the use of Rozex Cream in pregnancy. Metronidazole crosses the placental barrier and rapidly enters the foetal circulation. There is inadequate evidence of the safety of Metronidazole in human pregnancy. In animals, Metronidazole was not teratogenic or embryotoxic unless administered at extremely high doses. Rozex Cream should only be used in pregnancy when there is no safer alternative.

After oral administration, Metronidazole is excreted in breast milk in concentrations similar to those found in the plasma. Even though Metronidazole blood levels from topical administration are significantly lower than those achieved after oral administration, in nursing mothers a decision should be made to discontinue nursing or to discontinue the drug, taking into account the importance of the drug to the mother.

4.7 Effects on ability to drive and use machines
Not applicable

4.8 Undesirable effects
Because of the minimal absorption of metronidazole and consequently its insignificant plasma concentration after topical administration, the adverse experiences reported with the oral form of the drug have not been reported with Rozex Cream. Adverse reactions reported with Rozex Cream have been only local and mild, and include skin discomfort (burning and stinging), erythema, pruritis, skin irritation, worsening of rosacea, nausea, metallic taste and tingling or numbness of the extremities, and watery eyes if applied too closely to this area.

4.9 Overdose
No data exists about overdosage in humans. Acute oral toxicity studies with a topical gel formulation containing 0.75% w/w metronidazole in rats have shown no toxic action with doses of up to 5 g of finished product per kilogram body weight, the highest dose used. This dose is equivalent to the oral intake of 12 tubes of 30g packaging Rozex Cream for an adult weighing 72 kg, and 2 tubes of Cream for a child weighing 12 kg.

5. PHARMACOLOGICAL PROPERTIES

5.1 Pharmacodynamic properties
Metronidazole is an antiprotozoal and antibacterial agent which is active against a wide range of pathogenic microorganisms. The mechanisms of action of metronidazole in rosacea are unknown but available evidence suggests that the effects may be antibacterial and/or anti-inflammatory.

5.2 Pharmacokinetic properties
Metronidazole is rapidly and nearly totally absorbed after oral administration. The drug is not significantly bound to serum proteins and distributes well to all body compartments with the lowest concentration found in the fat. Metronidazole is excreted primarily in the urine as parent drug, oxidative metabolites and conjugates.

Bioavailability studies with a topical 1g application of Rozex Cream to the face of normal subjects resulted in mean maximum serum concentrations of 32.9ng/ml (range 14.8 to 54.4ng/ml) which is approximately 100 times less than those attained after a single oral dose of 250 mg (mean Cmax = 7248ng/ml; range 4270 – 13970ng/ml). The peak concentration occurred between 0.25 – 4 hours after oral dosing, and 6 to 24 hours after cutaneous application of Rozex Cream.

Following topical application of Rozex Cream, serum concentrations of the major metabolite (the hydroxymetabolite 2-hydroxymethylmetronidazole) were below the quantifiable limit of the assay (<9.6ng/ml) at most of the time points, ranging to a maximum of 17.5ng/ml peak concentration between 8 and 24 hours after application. In comparison, the peak concentration following a 250mg oral dose ranged from 626 to 1788ng/ml between 4 and 12 hours after dosing.

The extent of exposure (Area under the curve, AUC) from a 1g application of metronidazole administered topically was 1.36% of the AUC of a single oral 250mg metronidazole dose (mean + 912.7ng.hr/ml and approximately 67207ng.ml/hr respectively).

5.3 Preclinical safety data
No evidence for a primary dermal irritation was observed in rabbits following a single 24-hour cutaneous application of Rozex Cream to abraded and non-abraded skin, under occlusion.

Metronidazole has shown mutagenic activity in several in vitro bacterial assay systems. In addition, a dose-response increase in the frequency of micronuclei was observed in mice after intraperitoneal injection and an increase in chromosome aberrations have been reported in patients with Crohn's disease who were treated with 200 to 1200mg/day of oral metronidazole for 1 to 24 months. However, the preponderance of evidence from these studies suggests that although metronidazole has a potential for producing mutations, this should not occur in well oxygenated mammalian cells, i.e., under normal aerobic conditions.

The carcinogenicity of metronidazole by the oral route of administration has been evaluated in rats, mice and hamsters. These studies showed that oral metronidazole caused an increased incidence of pulmonary tumours in mice and possibly other tumours, including liver tumours, in the rat. Conversely, two lifetime studies in hamsters produced negative results. Moreover, one study showed a significant enhancement of UV-induced skin tumours in hairless mice treated with metronidazole intraperitoneally (15µg per g body weight and per day for 28 weeks).

Although the significance of these results to the cutaneous use of metronidazole for the treatment of rosacea is unclear, patients should be advised to avoid or minimise exposure of metronidazole cream-treated sites to sun. After several decades of systemic use, no evidence has been published to suggest that metronidazole is associated with carcinogenic potential in humans.

6. PHARMACEUTICAL PARTICULARS

6.1 List of excipients
Emulsifying Wax, Benzyl alcohol, Isopropyl palmitate, Glycerol, Sorbitol 70% (non-crystallising), lactic acid and/or Sodium Hydroxide, Purified Water.

6.2 Incompatibilities
None known

6.3 Shelf life
Rozex Cream has a shelf life when unopened of 36 months

6.4 Special precautions for storage
Store at a temperature not exceeding 25°C. Do not refrigerate.

6.5 Nature and contents of container
Aluminium tubes with epoxy phenolic lining, fitted with white polypropylene screw caps; pack sizes: 30g, 40g & 50g

6.6 Special precautions for disposal and other handling
Replace cap tightly after use.

7. MARKETING AUTHORISATION HOLDER
Galderma (UK.) Limited
Meridien House
69-71 Clarendon Road
Watford
Herts.
WD17 1DS
UK

8. MARKETING AUTHORISATION NUMBER(S)
PL 10590/0028

9. DATE OF FIRST AUTHORISATION/RENEWAL OF THE AUTHORISATION
18th June 1997

10. DATE OF REVISION OF THE TEXT
February 2006

Rozex Gel

(Galderma (U.K) Ltd)

1. NAME OF THE MEDICINAL PRODUCT
Rozex Gel

2. QUALITATIVE AND QUANTITATIVE COMPOSITION
Metronidazole Ph. Eur 0.75% w/w

3. PHARMACEUTICAL FORM
Gel

4. CLINICAL PARTICULARS

4.1 Therapeutic indications
Indicated in the treatment of inflammatory papules, pustules and erythema of rosacea

4.2 Posology and method of administration
For topical administration only.

Adults: Apply and rub in a film of Gel twice daily, morning and evening, to entire affected area after washing.

Elderly: The dosage recommended in the elderly is the same as that recommended in adults.

Children: Not recommended

4.3 Contraindications
Contraindicated in individuals with a history of hypersensitivity to Metronidazole, or other ingredients of the formulation.

4.4 Special warnings and precautions for use
Rozex Gel has been reported to cause lacrimation of the eyes, therefore, contact with the eyes should be avoided. If a reaction suggesting local irritation occurs patients should be directed to use the medication less frequently, discontinue use temporarily or discontinue use until further instructions. Metronidazole is a nitroimidazole and should be used with care in patients with evidence of, or history of, blood dyscrasia. Exposure of treated sites to ultraviolet or strong sunlight should be avoided during use of metronidazole. Unnecessary and prolonged use of this medication should be avoided.

4.5 Interaction with other medicinal products and other forms of interaction
Interaction with systemic medication is unlikely because absorption of metronidazole following cutaneous application of Rozex Gel is low. Oral metronidazole has been reported to potentiate the effect of warfarin and other coumarin anticoagulants, resulting in a prolongation of prothrombin time. The effect of topical metronidazole on prothrombin is not known. However, very rare cases of modification of the INR values have been reported with concomitant use of Rozex and coumarin anticoagulants.

4.6 Pregnancy and lactation
There is no experience to date with the use of Rozex Gel in pregnancy. Metronidazole crosses the placental barrier and rapidly enters the foetal circulation. There is inadequate evidence of the safety of Metronidazole in human pregnancy. In animals, Metronidazole was not teratogenic or embryotoxic unless administered at extremely high doses. Rozex Gel should only be used in pregnancy where there is no safer alternative.

After oral administration, Metronidazole is excreted in breast milk in concentrations similar to those found in the plasma, Metronidazole blood levels from topical administration are significantly lower than those achieved after oral administration. A decision should be made to discontinue nursing or to discontinue the drug, taking into account the importance of the drug to the mother.

4.7 Effects on ability to drive and use machines
Not applicable

4.8 Undesirable effects
Because of the minimal absorption of metronidazole and consequently its insignificant plasma concentration after topical administration, the adverse experiences reported with the oral form of the drug have not been reported with Rozex Gel. Adverse reactions reported with Rozex Gel have been only local and mild, and include skin discomfort (burning and stinging), erythema, pruritis, skin irritation, worsening of rosacea, nausea, metallic taste and tingling or numbness of the extremities, and watery eyes if applied too closely to this area.

4.9 Overdose
No data exists about overdosage in humans. Acute oral toxicity studies with a topical gel formulation containing 0.75% w/w metronidazole in rats have shown no toxic action with doses of up to 5 g of finished product per kilogram body weight, the highest dose used. This dose is equivalent to the oral intake of 12 tubes of 30g packaging

Rozex Gel for an adult weighing 72 kg, and 2 tubes of Gel for a child weighing 12 kg.

5. PHARMACOLOGICAL PROPERTIES

5.1 Pharmacodynamic properties

Metronidazole is an antiprotozoal and antibacterial agent which is active against a wide range of pathogenic micro-organisms. The mechanisms of action of metronidazole in rosacea are unknown but available evidence suggests that the effects may be antibacterial and/or anti-inflammatory.

5.2 Pharmacokinetic properties

Metronidazole is rapidly and nearly totally absorbed after oral administration. The drug is not significantly bound to serum proteins and distributes well to all body compartments with the lowest concentration found in the fat. Metronidazole is excreted primarily in the urine as parent drug, oxidative metabolites and conjugates.

Bioavailability studies with Rozex Gel in rosacea patients treated with 7.5 mg metronidazole applied topically to the face resulted in maximum serum concentrations of 66 ng/ml which is approximately 100 times less than those attained after a single oral dose of 250 mg. In most patients at most time points after Rozex Gel application, serum concentrations of metronidazole were below the detectable limits of the assay (25 ng/ml).

5.3 Preclinical safety data

The toxicity studies conducted with the Metronidazole 0.75% Topical Gel formulation demonstrate that the product is non-toxic in rats after acute oral administration 5g/kg and produced no ocular irritation in rabbit eyes. The formulation produced no observable effects in rabbits after dermal application of 13 mg /kg for 90 days.

No compound-related dermal or systemic effects were observed in a 13-week cutaneous route toxicity study, in which Rozex gel containing Metronidazole 0.75% w/w was applied daily to rabbits at doses ranging between 0.13 and 13 mg/kg.

Metronidazole has shown evidence of carcinogenic activity in a number of studies involving chronic, oral administration in mice and rats but not in studies involving hamsters.

One study showed a significant enhancement of UV induced skin tumours in hairless mice treated with Metronidazole intraperitoneally (15µg per g body weight and per day for 28 weeks). Although the significance of these studies to man is not clear, patients should be advised to avoid or minimise exposure of metronidazole treated sites to sun.

Metronidazole has shown mutagenic activity in several in vitro bacterial assay systems. In addition, a dose-response increase in the frequency of micronuclei was observed in mice after intraperitoneal injection and an increase in chromosome aberrations have been reported in patients with Crohn's disease who were treated with 200 to 1200mg/day of metronidazole for 1 to 24 months. However, no excess chromosomal aberrations in circulating human lymphocytes have been observed in patients treated for 8 months.

6. PHARMACEUTICAL PARTICULARS

6.1 List of excipients

Carbomer 940 (Carbopol 980) Ph. Eur

Disodium Edetate Ph. Eur.

Methyl Hydroxybenzoate Ph. Eur.

Propyl Hydroxybenzoate Ph. Eur.

Propylene Glycol Ph. Eur.

Sodium Hydroxide Ph. Eur.

Purified Water Ph. Eur.

6.2 Incompatibilities

None known

6.3 Shelf life

Rozex Gel has a shelf life when unopened of 36 months

6.4 Special precautions for storage

Store at a temperature not exceeding 25°C, away from direct heat. Do not freeze.

6.5 Nature and contents of container

Aluminium tubes with epoxy phenolic lining, and white polypropylene or polyethylene screw caps; pack sizes: 5, 30g, 40g & 50.

6.6 Special precautions for disposal and other handling

Not applicable

7. MARKETING AUTHORISATION HOLDER

Galderma (UK.) Limited

Meridien House

69-71 Clarendon Road

Watford

Herts.

WD17 1DS

UK

8. MARKETING AUTHORISATION NUMBER(S)

PL 10590/0016

9. DATE OF FIRST AUTHORISATION/RENEWAL OF THE AUTHORISATION

16/03/2006

10. DATE OF REVISION OF THE TEXT

February 2006

Rupafin 10mg Tablets

(GlaxoSmithKline UK)

1. NAME OF THE MEDICINAL PRODUCT

Rupafin▼ 10 mg Tablets

2. QUALITATIVE AND QUANTITATIVE COMPOSITION

Each tablet contains:

10 mg of rupatadine (as fumarate)

Excipients: lactose

For a full list of excipients, see section 6.1.

3. PHARMACEUTICAL FORM

Tablet.

Round, light salmon coloured tablets.

4. CLINICAL PARTICULARS

4.1 Therapeutic indications

Symptomatic treatment of allergic rhinitis and chronic idiopathic urticaria in adults and adolescents (over 12 years of age).

4.2 Posology and method of administration

Adults and adolescents (over 12 years of age)

The recommended dose is 10 mg (one tablet) once a day, with or without food.

Elderly

Rupafin should be used with caution in elderly people (see section 4.4).

Paediatric patients

Rupafin 10 mg Tablets is not recommended for use in children below age 12 due to a lack of data on safety and efficacy.

Patients with renal or hepatic insufficiency

As there is no clinical experience in patients with impaired kidney or liver functions, the use of Rupafin 10 mg Tablets is at present not recommended in these patients.

4.3 Contraindications

Hypersensitivity to rupatadine or to any of the excipients.

4.4 Special warnings and precautions for use

The administration of Rupafin with grapefruit juice is not recommended (see section 4.5).

Cardiac safety of rupatadine was assessed in a thorough QT/QTc study. Rupatadine up to 10 times therapeutic dose did not produce any effect on the ECG and hence raises no cardiac safety concerns. However rupatadine should be used with caution in patients with known prolongation of the QT interval, patients with uncorrected hypokalemia, patients with ongoing pro-arrhythmic conditions, such as clinically significant bradycardia, acute myocardial ischemia.

Rupafin 10 mg Tablets should be used with caution in elderly patients (65 years and older). Although no overall differences in effectiveness or safety were observed in clinical trials, higher sensitivity of some older individuals cannot be excluded due to the low number of elderly patients enrolled (see section 5.2).

Regarding use in children less than 12 years old and in patients with renal or hepatic impairment, see section 4.2.

Due to the presence of lactose monohydrate in Rupafin 10 mg tablets, patients with rare hereditary problems of galactose intolerance, the Lapp lactase deficiency or glucose-galactose malabsorption should not take this medicine.

4.5 Interaction with other medicinal products and other forms of interaction

Interaction with ketoconazole or erythromycin: The concomitant administration of rupatadine 20 mg and ketoconazole or erythromycin increases the systemic exposure to rupatadine 10 times and 2-3 times respectively. These modifications were not associated with an effect on the QT interval or with an increase of the adverse reactions in comparison with the drugs when administered separately. However, rupatadine should be used with caution when it is administered concomitantly with these drug substances and other inhibitors of the isozyme CYP3A4.

Interaction with grapefruit: The concomitant administration of grapefruit juice increased 3.5 times the systemic exposure of rupatadine. Grapefruit juice should not be taken simultaneously.

Interaction with alcohol: After administration of alcohol, a dose of 10 mg of rupatadine produced marginal effects in some psychomotor performance tests although they were not significantly different from those induced by intake of alcohol only. A dose of 20 mg increased the impairment caused by the intake of alcohol.

Interaction with CNS depressants: As with other antihistamines, interactions with CNS depressants cannot be excluded.

Interaction with statins: Asymptomatic CPK increases have been uncommonly reported in rupatadine clinical trials. The risk of interactions with statins, some of which are also metabolised by the cytochrome P450 CYP3A4 isoenzyme, is unknown. For these reasons, rupatadine should be used with caution when it is coadministered with statins.

4.6 Pregnancy and lactation

Data on a limited number (2) exposed pregnancies indicate no adverse effects of rupatadine on pregnancy or on the health of the foetus/newborn child. To date, no other relevant epidemiological data are available. Animal studies do not indicate direct or indirect harmful effects with respect to pregnancy, embryonal/foetal development, parturition or postnatal development (see section 5.3). Caution should be exercised when prescribing rupatadine to pregnant women.

Rupatadine is excreted in animal milk. It is unknown whether rupatadine is excreted into breast milk. Due to the lack of human data, caution should be exercised when prescribing rupatadine to lactating milk.

4.7 Effects on ability to drive and use machines

Rupatadine 10 mg had no influence on the ability to drive and use machines. Nevertheless, care should be taken before driving or using machinery until the patient's individual reaction on rupatadine has been established.

4.8 Undesirable effects

Rupatadine 10 mg has been administered to over 2025 patients in clinical studies, 120 of whom received rupatadine for at least 1 year.

The most common adverse reactions in controlled clinical studies were somnolence (9.5%), headache (6.9%) and fatigue (3.2%).

The majority of adverse reactions observed in clinical trials were mild to moderate in severity and usually did not require cessation of therapy. The frequencies are summarised according to the following scheme:

System Organ Class	Common (⩾ 1/100 to < 1/10)	Uncommon (⩾ 1/1000 to < 1/100)
Investigations		Blood creatine phosphokinase increased, Alanine aminotransferase increased, Aspartate aminotransferase increased, Liver function test abnormal, Weight increased
Nervous system disorders	Somnolence, Headache, Dizziness	Disturbance in attention
Respiratory, thoracic and mediastinal disorders		Epistaxis, Nasal dryness, Pharyngitis, Cough, Dry throat, Pharyngolaryngeal pain, Rhinitis
Gastrointestinal disorders	Dry mouth	Nausea, Abdominal pain upper, Diarrhoea, Dyspepsia, Vomiting, Abdominal pain, Constipation
Skin and subcutaneous tissue disorders		Rash
Musculoskeletal and connective tissue disorders		Back pain, Arthralgia, Myalgia
Metabolism and nutrition disorders		Increased appetite
General disorders and administration site conditions	Fatigue, Asthenia	Thirst, Malaise, Pyrexia
Psychiatric disorders		Irritability

4.9 Overdose

No case of overdose has been reported. In a clinical safety study rupatadine at daily dose of 100 mg during 6 days was well tolerated. The most common adverse reaction was somnolence. If accidental ingestion of very high doses occurs symptomatic treatment together with the required supportive measures should be given.

5. PHARMACOLOGICAL PROPERTIES

5.1 Pharmacodynamic properties

Pharmacotherapeutic group: other antihistamines for systemic use, ATC code: R06A X28.

Rupatadine is a second generation antihistamine, long-acting histamine antagonist, with selective peripheral H_1-receptor antagonist activity. Some of the metabolites (desloratadine and its hydroxylated metabolites) retain an antihistaminic activity and may partially contribute to the overall efficacy of the drug.

In vitro studies with rupatadine at high concentration have shown an inhibition of the degranulation of mast cells induced by immunological and non-immunological stimuli as well as the release of cytokines, particularly of the TNF_{α} in human mast cells and monocytes. The clinical relevance of the observed experimental data remains to be confirmed.

Clinical trials in volunteers (n= 375) and patients (n=2650) with allergic rhinitis and chronic idiopathic urticaria did not show significant effect on the electrocardiogram when rupatadine was administered at doses ranging from 2 mg to 100 mg.

In a placebo-controlled trials in patients with Chronic Idiopathic Urticaria, rupatadine was effective reducing the mean pruritus score from baseline over the 4 week treatment period (change vs baseline: rupatadine 57.5%, placebo 44.9%) and decreasing the mean number of wheals (54.3% vs 39.7%).

5.2 Pharmacokinetic properties

Absorption and bioavailability

Rupatadine is rapidly absorbed after oral administration, with a t_{max} of approximately 0.75 hours after intake. The mean C_{max} was 2.6 ng/ml after a single oral dose of 10 mg and 4.6 ng/ml after a single oral dose of 20 mg. Pharmacokinetics of rupatadine was linear for a dose between 10 and 40 mg. After a dose of 10 mg once a day for 7 days, the mean C_{max} was 3.8 ng/ml. The plasma concentration followed a bi-exponential drop-off with a mean elimination half-life of 5.9 hours. The binding-rate of rupatadine to plasma proteins was 98.5-99%.

As rupatadine has never been administered to humans by intravenous route, no data is available on its absolute bioavailability.

Effect of the intake of food

Intake of food increased the systemic exposure (AUC) to rupatadine by about 23%. The exposure to one of its active metabolites and to the main inactive metabolite was practically the same (reduction of about 5% and 3% respectively). The time taken to reach the maximum plasma concentration (t_{max}) of rupatadine was delayed by 1 hour. The maximum plasma concentration (C_{max}) was not affected by food intake. These differences had no clinical significance.

Metabolism and elimination

In a study of excretion in humans (40 mg of ^{14}C-rupatadine), 34.6% of the radioactivity administered was recovered in urine and 60.9% in faeces collected over 7 days. Rupatadine undergoes considerable pre-systemic metabolism when administered by oral route. The amounts of unaltered active substance found in urine and faeces were insignificant. This means that rupatadine is almost completely metabolised. *In vitro* metabolism studies in human liver microsomes indicate that rupatadine is mainly metabolised by the cytochrome P450 (CYP 3A4).

Specific patient groups

In a study on healthy volunteers to compare the results in young adults and elderly patients, the values for AUC and C_{max} for rupatadine were higher in the elderly than in young adults. This is probably due to a decrease of the first-pass hepatic metabolism in the elderly. These differences were not observed in the metabolites analysed. The mean elimination half-life of rupatadine in elderly and young volunteers was 8.7 hours and 5.9 hours respectively. As these results for rupatadine and for its metabolites were not clinically significant, it was concluded that it is not necessary to make any adjustment when using a dose of 10 mg in the elderly.

5.3 Preclinical safety data

Preclinical data reveal no special hazard for humans based on conventional studies of pharmacology, repeated dose toxicity, genotoxicity, and carcinogenic potential.

More than 100 times the clinically recommended dose (10 mg) of rupatadine did neither extend the QTc or QRS interval nor produce arrhythmia in various species of animals such as rats, guinea pigs and dogs. Rupatadine and one of its main active metabolites in humans, 3-hydroxydesloratadine, did not affect the cardiac action potential in isolated dog Purkinje fibres at concentrations at least 2000 times greater than the C_{max} reached after the administration of a dose of 10 mg in humans. In a study that evaluated the effect on cloned human HERG channel, rupatadine inhibited that channel at a concentration 1685 times greater than the C_{max} obtained after the administration of 10 mg of rupatadine. Desloratadine, the metabolite with the greatest activity, had no effect at a 10 micromolar concentration. Studies of tissue distribution in rats with radiolabelled rupatadine showed that rupatadine does not accumulate in heart tissue.

In the rat, a significant reduction of male and female fertility occurred at the high dose of 120 mg/kg/day, providing C_{max} 268 times those measured in humans at the therapeutic dose (10 mg/day). Foetal toxicity (growth delay, incomplete ossification, minor skeletal findings) was reported in rats at maternotoxic dose-levels only (25 and 120 mg/kg/day). In rabbits, no evidence of developmental toxicity was noted at doses up to 100 mg/kg. The developmental No Adverse Effect Levels were determined at 5 mg/kg/day in rats and 100 mg/kg/day in rabbits, yielding C_{max} 45 and 116 times higher, respectively, than those measured in humans at the therapeutic dose (10 mg/day).

6. PHARMACEUTICAL PARTICULARS

6.1 List of excipients

Pregelatinised maize starch

Microcrystalline cellulose

Red iron oxide (E-172)

Yellow iron oxide (E-172)

Lactose monohydrate

Magnesium stearate

6.2 Incompatibilities

Not applicable

6.3 Shelf life

3 years

6.4 Special precautions for storage

Keep the blister in the outer carton in order to protect from light.

6.5 Nature and contents of container

PVC/PVDC/aluminium blister.

Packs of 3, 7, 10, 15, 20, 30, 50 and 100 tablets. Not all pack sizes may be marketed.

6.6 Special precautions for disposal and other handling

No special requirements.

Any unused product or waste material should be disposed of in accordance with local requirements.

7. MARKETING AUTHORISATION HOLDER

J. Uriach & Cía., S.A.

Av. Camí Reial, 51-57

08184 Palau-solità i Plegamans (Spain)

8. MARKETING AUTHORISATION NUMBER(S)

PL 11906/0007

9. DATE OF FIRST AUTHORISATION/RENEWAL OF THE AUTHORISATION

24/10/2007

10. DATE OF REVISION OF THE TEXT

11/12/2007

Rynacrom 4% Nasal Spray

(sanofi-aventis)

1. NAME OF THE MEDICINAL PRODUCT

Rynacrom 4% Nasal Spray

2. QUALITATIVE AND QUANTITATIVE COMPOSITION

Sodium Cromoglicate BP 4% w/v

3. PHARMACEUTICAL FORM

Rynacrom 4% Nasal Spray is presented as an aqueous solution, containing 4% w/v sodium cromoglicate in a metered dose spray pack, for nasal administration.

4. CLINICAL PARTICULARS

4.1 Therapeutic indications

Rynacrom 4% Nasal Spray is indicated for the preventative treatment of allergic rhinitis (seasonal and perennial).

4.2 Posology and method of administration

For nasal administration

Adults (including the Elderly) and Children:

One spray into each nostril two to four times daily.

Each actuation of the pump unit delivers approximately 5.2mg of sodium cromoglicate.

Since therapy is essentially preventative, regular doses, distinct from using the drug intermittently to relieve symptoms, should be observed.

4.3 Contraindications

Rynacrom 4% Nasal Spray is contraindicated in patients with known sensitivity to sodium cromoglicate, or any of the ingredients.

4.4 Special warnings and precautions for use

None known.

4.5 Interaction with other medicinal products and other forms of interaction

There are no known interactions between sodium cromoglicate and other drugs. A reduction in concomitant antihistamine therapy will often be possible during treatment with Rynacrom 4% Nasal Spray.

4.6 Pregnancy and lactation

Cumulative experience with sodium cromoglicate suggests that it has no effect on foetal development. It should only be used in pregnancy if there is a clear need.

On the basis of animal studies and its physico-chemical properties, sodium cromoglicate is unlikely to pass into human breast milk. There is no evidence to suggest that the use of sodium cromoglicate by nursing mothers has any undesirable effects on the baby.

4.7 Effects on ability to drive and use machines

None known.

4.8 Undesirable effects

Occasional irritation of the nasal mucosa may occur during the first days of use. In rare cases wheezing or tightness of the chest have been reported by patients.

4.9 Overdose

No action other than medical supervision should be necessary.

5. PHARMACOLOGICAL PROPERTIES

5.1 Pharmacodynamic properties

Sodium cromoglicate inhibits the release of mediators of the allergic reaction from sensitised mast cells. In the nose, the inhibition of mediator release prevents the symptoms of rhinitis.

5.2 Pharmacokinetic properties

After instillation of Rynacrom 4% Nasal Spray into the nose, less than 7% of the total dose administered is absorbed via the nasal mucosa. This fraction is excreted unchanged in the bile and urine. The remainder of the dose is expelled from the nose, or swallowed and excreted via the alimentary tract.

5.3 Preclinical safety data

There are no pre-clinical safety data of relevance to the prescriber which are additional to those already included in other sections of the Summary of Product Characteristics.

6. PHARMACEUTICAL PARTICULARS

6.1 List of excipients

Disodium edetate

Benzalkonium chloride

Purified water

6.2 Incompatibilities

None known.

6.3 Shelf life

36 months.

6.4 Special precautions for storage

Store below 25°C. Protect from direct sunlight.

6.5 Nature and contents of container

Rynacrom 4% Nasal Spray is presented as a transparent, colourless to pale yellow liquid in a 22ml high density polyethylene bottle, fitted with a metered dose pump unit, protected by a polypropylene cover.

6.6 Special precautions for disposal and other handling

A patient information leaflet is included in each pack.

7. MARKETING AUTHORISATION HOLDER

Sanofi-aventis

One Onslow Street

Guildford

Surrey

GU1 4YS

UK

8. MARKETING AUTHORISATION NUMBER(S)

PL 04425/0371

9. DATE OF FIRST AUTHORISATION/RENEWAL OF THE AUTHORISATION

1st May 2005

10. DATE OF REVISION OF THE TEXT

December 2006

11. LEGAL CATEGORY

P

Rythmodan Capsules

(sanofi-aventis)

1. NAME OF THE MEDICINAL PRODUCT

Rythmodan 100mg Capsules.

Rythmodan 150mg Capsules.

2. QUALITATIVE AND QUANTITATIVE COMPOSITION

Capsule containing Disopyramide 100mg.

Capsule containing Disopyramide 150mg.

For excipients, see section 6.1.

3. PHARMACEUTICAL FORM

Capsule.

4. CLINICAL PARTICULARS

4.1 Therapeutic indications

Rythmodan is used in the treatment of cardiac arrhythmias as follows:-

1. The prevention and treatment of arrhythmias occurring after myocardial infarction.

2. Maintenance of normal rhythm following electroconversion eg atrial fibrillation, atrial flutter.

3. Persistent ventricular extrasystoles.

4. Control of arrhythmias following the use of digitalis or similar glycosides.

5. Suppression of arrhythmias during surgical procedures eg cardiac catheterisation.

6. The prevention of paraxysmal supraventricular tachycardia.

7. Other types of arrhythmias e.g. atrial extrasystoles, Wolff-Parkinson-White Syndrome.

4.2 Posology and method of administration

Route of administration

Oral

300 mg to 800mg daily in divided doses.

Children:

Not recommended as insufficient data available.

Elderly

A dose reduction due to reduced renal and hepatic function in the elderly (especially elderly non-smokers) should be considered (see section 4.4)

4.3 Contraindications

Disopyramide is contra–indicated in un–paced second or third degree atrioventricular block; bundle–branch block associated with first–degree atrioventricular block; unpaced bifascicular block; pre-existing long QT syndromes; severe sinus node dysfunction; severe heart failure, unless of secondary to cardiac arrhythmia; hypersensitivity to disopyramide. It is also contra–indicated in concomitant administration with other anti–arrhythmics or other drugs liable to provoke ventricular arrhythmias, especially Torsade de Pointes (see section 4.5). The sustained release formulation is contra–indicated in patients with renal or hepatic impairment.

4.4 Special warnings and precautions for use

In view of the serious nature of many of the conditions being treated it is suggested that Rythmodan Injection should only be used when facilities exist for cardiac monitoring or defibrillation, should the need arise.

Antiarrhythmic drugs belonging to the class 1c (Vaughan Williams Classification) were included in the Cardiac Arrhythmia Suppression Trial (CAST), a long term multicentre randomised, double blind study in patients with asymptomatic non life–threatening ventricular arrhythmia who have had a myocardial infarction more than six days but less than two years previously. A significant increase in mortality and non–fatal cardiac arrest rate was seen in patients treated with class 1c antiarrhythmic drugs when compared with a matched placebo group. The applicability of the CAST results to other antiarrhythmic and other populations (eg. those without recent infarction) is uncertain. At present, it is best to assume that the risk extends to other antiarrhythmic agents for patients with structural heart disease.

There is no evidence that prolonged suppression of ventricular premature contractions with antiarrhythmic drugs prevents sudden death.

All antiarrhythmic drugs can produce unwanted effects when they are used to treat symptomatic but not life threatening arrhythmia; the expected benefits should be balanced against their risks.

In patients with structural heart disease, proarrhythmia and cardiac decompensation are special risks associated with antiarrhythmic drugs. Special caution should be exercised when prescribing in this context.

Disopyramide should not be used in patients with uncompensated congestive heart failure, unless this heart failure is secondary to cardiac arrhythmia. If disopyramide is to be given under these circumstances, special care and monitoring are essential.

Haemodynamically significant arrhythmias are difficult to treat and affected patients have a high mortality risk. Treatment of these arrhythmias, by whatever modality, must be initiated in hospital.

Owing to its negative inotropic effect, disopyramide should be used with caution in patients suffering from significant cardiac failure. This group may be specially sensitive to the negative inotropic properties of disopyramide. Such patients should be fully digitalised or controlled with other therapy before treatment with disopyramide is commenced.

Aggravation of existing arrhythmia, or emergence of a new type of arrhythmia, demands urgent review of disopyramide treatment.

Similarly, if an atrioventricular block or a bifascicular block occurs during treatment, the use of disopyramide should be reviewed.

There have been reports of ventricular tachycardia, ventricular fibrillation and Torsade de Pointes in patients receiving disopyramide. These have usually, but not always, been associated with significant widening of the QRS complex or prolonged QT interval. The QT interval and QRS duration must be monitored and disopyramide should be stopped if these are increased by more than 25%. If these changes or arrhythmias develop the drug should be discontinued. Disopyramide should be used only with caution in patients with atrial flutter or atrial tachycardia with block as conversion of a partial AV block to a 1:1 response may occur, leading to a potentially more serious tachyarrhythmia.

The occurrence of hypotension following disopyramide administration requires prompt discontinuation of the drug. This has been observed especially in patients with cardiomyopathy or uncompensated congestive heart failure. Any resumption of therapy should be at a lower dose with close patient monitoring. Disopyramide should be used with caution in the treatment of digitalis intoxication.

Potassium imbalance: Antiarrhythmic drugs may be hazardous in patients with potassium imbalance, as potassium abnormalities can induce arrhythmias.

During treatment with disopyramide, potassium levels should be checked regularly. Patients treated with diuretics or stimulant laxatives are at particular risk of hypokalaemia.

Renal insufficiency: In renal insufficiency, the dosage of disopyramide should be reduced by adjusting the interval between administrations.

Hepatic insufficiency: Hepatic impairment causes an increase in the plasma half–life of Rythmodan and a reduced dosage may be required.

Hypoglycaemia: Hypoglycaemia has been reported in association with disopyramide administration. The risk of hypoglycaemia, sometimes severe, occurs particularly in elderly or malnourished subjects, treated diabetics and patients with renal insufficiency or cardiac failure. Blood sugar levels should be monitored in all patients. Strict adherence to the dosing recommendations is advised. If hypoglycaemia occurs then treatment with disopyramide should be stopped.

Hypoglycaemia may be associated with interactions wit drugs metabolised by hepatic CYP3A (see Section 4.5 Interactions with other medicines).

Atropine–like effects: There is a risk of:

– ocular hypertension in patients with narrow–angle glaucoma,

– acute urinary retention in patients with prostatic enlargement,

– aggravation of myasthenia gravis.

4.5 Interaction with other medicinal products and other forms of interaction

Combination with other antiarrhythmic drugs: Combinations of antiarrhythmic drugs are not well researched and their effect may be unpredictable. Thus, antiarrhythmic combination should be avoided except under certain circumstances, eg. beta–blockers for angina pectoris; digoxin with beta–blocker and verapamil for the control of atrial fibrillation, when defined as effective for an individual.

Interaction with drugs associated with risk of Torsade de Pointes, such as

– tricyclic and tetracyclic antidepressants

– All macrolide antibiotics (e.g. erythromycin, clarithromycin, azithromycin etc)

– astemizole; cisapride; pentamidine; pimozide; sparfloxacin; terfenadine and thioridazone.

Phosphodiesterase Type 5 Inhibitors:

There is evidence that phosphodiesterase Type 5 inhibitors may be potentially associated with a risk of QT prolongation. Concomitant administration of disopyramide with such drugs may potentially enhance this QT prolongation effect and is not recommended.

The concomitant use of these medications whilst undergoing treatment with disopyramide increases the chance of cardiac arrhythmia.

There is some evidence that disopyramide is metabolised by hepatic CYP3A. Concomitant administration of significant inhibitors of this isozyme (e.g. certain macrolide or azole antifungal antibiotics) may therefore increase the serum levels of disopyramide. On the other hand, inducers of CYP3A (e.g. rifampicin and certain anticonvulsants such as phenytoin, primidone and phenobarbital) may reduce disopyramide and increase MN–disopyramide serum levels. Since the magnitude of such potential effects is not foreseeable, such drug combinations are not recommended.

When prescribing a drug metabolised by CYP3A [such as theophylline, HIV protease inhibitors (e.g. ritonavir, indinavir, saquinavir), ciclosporin A, warfarin] it should be kept in mind that disopyramide is probably also a substrate of this isozyme and thus competitive inhibition of metabolism might occur, possibly increasing serum levels of these drugs.

Interactions with hypokalaemia inducing drugs: Concomitant use with drugs can induce hypokalaemia such as: diuretics, amphotericin B, tetracosactide (corticotropin analogue), gluco and mineralo–corticoids may reduce the action of the drug, or potentiate proarrhythmic effects. Stimulant laxatives are not recommended to be given concomitantly, due to their potassium lowering potential.

Other drug interactions:

Atropine and other anticholinergic drugs, including phenothiazines, may potentiate the atropine–like effects of disopyramide.

4.6 Pregnancy and lactation

Pregnancy: Although Rythmodan has undergone animal tests for teratogenicity without evidence of any effect on the developing foetus, its safety in human pregnancy has not been established. Rythmodan has been reported to stimulate contractions of the pregnant uterus. The drug should only be used during pregnancy if benefits clearly outweigh the possible risks to the mother and foetus.

Lactation: Studies have shown that oral Rythmodan is secreted in breast milk, although no adverse effects to the infant have been noted. However, clinical experience is limited and Rythmodan should only be used in lactation if, in the clinician's judgement, it is essential for the welfare of the patient. The infant should be closely supervised, particularly for anticholinergic effects and drug levels determined if necessary. Ideally, if the drug is considered essential, an alternative method of feeding should be used.

4.7 Effects on ability to drive and use machines

Some adverse reactions may impair the patients ability to concentrate and react, and hence the ability to drive or operate machinery. (See section 4.8).

4.8 Undesirable effects

Cardiac: It is accepted that the arrhythmogenic potential of disopyramide is weak. However, as with all antiarrhythmic drugs, disopyramide may worsen or provoke arrhythmias. This proarrhythmic effect is more likely to occur in the presence of hypokalemia with the associated use of antiarrhythmic drugs, in patients with severe structural heart disease with prolongation of the QT interval.

Intra–cardiac conduction abnormalities may occur: QT interval prolongation, widening of the QRS complex, atrioventricular block and bundle–branch block.

Other types of arrhythmia have been reported: Bradycardia, sinus block, ventricular fibrillation, ventricular tachycardia and torsades de pointes.

Episodes of severe heart failure or even cardiogenic shock have also been described particularly in patients with severe structural heart disease. The resulting low cardiac output can cause hypotension, renal insufficiency and/or acute hepatic ischemia.

Other adverse reactions include:

Atropine like: Urinary (dysuria; acute urinary retention); ocular (disorders of accommodation; diplopia); gastrointestinal - (dry mouth; abdominal pain; nausea, vomiting, anorexia, diarrhoea; constipation); impotence; psychiatric disorders.

Skin reactions: very rarely, rashes; isolated reports of anaphylactic–type reactions possibly culminating in shock (only reported in association with the injectable formulation).

Rarely: Hypoglycaemia, sometimes severe (see Section 4.4 Special Warnings and Precautions for Use). In some cases, severe hypoglycaemia resulted in coma.

Very rarely: cholestatic jaundice, headache, dizzy sensation, neutropenia.

Rapid infusion may cause profuse sweating.

4.9 Overdose

There is no specific antidote for disopyramide. Prostigmine derivatives can be used to treat anticholinergic effects. Symptomatic supportive measures may include: early gastric lavage; administration of a cathartic followed by activated charcoal by mouth or stomach tube; IV administration of isoprenaline, other vasopressors and/or positive inotropic agents; if needed - infusion of lactate and/or magnesium, electro–systolic assistance, cardioversion, insertion of an intra–aortic balloon for counterpulsion and mechanically assisted ventilation. Haemodialysis, haemofiltration or haemoperfusion with activated charcoal has been employed to lower the serum concentrations of the drug.

5. PHARMACOLOGICAL PROPERTIES

5.1 Pharmacodynamic properties

Class 1 anti-arrhythmic agent.

It decreases membrane responsiveness, prolongs the effective refractory period (ERP) and slows automaticity in cells with augmented automaticity. Effective refractory period of the atrium is lengthened, ERP of the A-V node is shortened and conduction in accessory pathways is prolonged.

Disopyramide is a myocardial depressant and has anticholinergic effects.

5.2 Pharmacokinetic properties

Elimination phase of plasma t1/2: 5-8 hours. Increased in hepatic impairment, cardiac and hepatic disease.

Protein binding: 50 - 60%. Saturable and concentration dependent.

Volume of distribution: Variable according to method of determination.

Metabolism: Approximately 25% of a dose metabolised to a mono-N-dealkylated derivative. Additional 10% as other metabolites.

Excretion: 75% unchanged drug via urine, remainder in faeces mono-N-dealkylated metabolite 25% in urine, 64% via faeces.

5.3 Preclinical safety data

Not applicable.

6. PHARMACEUTICAL PARTICULARS

6.1 List of excipients

Maize starch

Magnesium stearate

STA-RX 1500 (pregelatinised starch)

Talc.

Capsule shell:

Gelatin

Indigo carmine,

Iron oxide and

Titanium dioxide (E171)

6.2 Incompatibilities
Not known.

6.3 Shelf life
PVC Blister: 36 months

6.4 Special precautions for storage
Do not store above 25°C

6.5 Nature and contents of container
PVC/PVdC blister strips in cardboard cartons containing 84 capsules.

6.6 Special precautions for disposal and other handling
None.

7. MARKETING AUTHORISATION HOLDER
Sanofi-aventis

One Onslow Street

Guildford

Surrey

GU1 4YS

8. MARKETING AUTHORISATION NUMBER(S)
Rythmodan 100mg capsules: PL 04425/0607

Rythmodan 150mg capsules: PL 04425/0608

9. DATE OF FIRST AUTHORISATION/RENEWAL OF THE AUTHORISATION
12 February 2009

10. DATE OF REVISION OF THE TEXT
February 2009

Legal Category: POM

Rythmodan Injection

(sanofi-aventis)

1. NAME OF THE MEDICINAL PRODUCT
Rythmodan Injection.

2. QUALITATIVE AND QUANTITATIVE COMPOSITION
Each glass ampoule contains 12.88mg disopyramide phosphate (equivalent to 10mg of disopyramide) per 1ml of solution.

For excipients, see section 6.1.

3. PHARMACEUTICAL FORM
Intravenous.

4. CLINICAL PARTICULARS

4.1 Therapeutic indications
Conversion of ventricular and supraventricular arrhythmias after myocardial infarction, including patients not responding to lignocaine or other intravenous treatment.

Control of ventricular and atrial extrasystoles, supraventricular tachycardia, and Wolff–Parkinson–White syndrome.

Control of arrhythmias following digitalis or similar glycosides when Rythmodan cannot be given orally.

4.2 Posology and method of administration
Route of Administration: Rythmodan Injection is intended for intravenous use only.

__Adults__

The recommended dosage can be given by two different regimes:

1. An initial direct intravenous injection of 2mg/kg (but not exceeding 150mg (15ml) irrespective of body weight) should be given slowly over not less than five minutes, ie, the rate of injection must not exceed 30mg (3ml) per minute in order to reduce or avoid unwanted haemodynamic effects. If conversion occurs during this time the injection should be stopped. If the arrhythmia is to respond to Rythmodan it will usually do so within 10–15 minutes after completion of the injection.

If conversion is achieved by intravenous Rythmodan but the arrhythmia subsequently recurs, a further slow direct intravenous injection over not less than five minutes may be administered cautiously and preferably under ECG control. The total administration by the intravenous route should not exceed 4mg/kg (maximum 300mg) in the first hour, nor should the combined administration by the intravenous and oral routes exceed 800mg in 24 hours.

2. An initial direct intravenous injection as above, ie over not less than five minutes, maintained by intravenous infusion by drip of 20–30mg/hour (or 0.4mg/kg/hour) up to a maximum of 800mg daily. This regime should be employed if the patient is unable to take oral medication or in particularly serious arrhythmias being treated in coronary care units.

__Children__

Not applicable.

Rythmodan Injection is not intended for use in children.

__Elderly__

A dose reduction due to reduced renal and hepatic function in the elderly (especially elderly non-smokers) should be considered (see section 4.4).

4.3 Contraindications
Disopyramide is contra–indicated in un–paced second or third degree atrioventricular block; bundle–branch block associated with first degree atrioventricular block; un-paced bifascicular block; pre-existing long QT syndromes; severe sinus node dysfunction; severe heart failure, unless secondary to cardiac arrhythmia; and hypersensitivity to disopyramide. It is also contra–indicated in concomitant administration with other anti–arrhythmics or other drugs liable to provoke ventricular arrhythmias, especially Torsade de Pointes (see section 4.5). The sustained release formulation is contra–indicated in patients with renal or hepatic impairment.

4.4 Special warnings and precautions for use
In view of the serious nature of many of the conditions being treated it is suggested that Rythmodan Injection should only be used when facilities exist for cardiac monitoring or defibrillation, should the need arise.

Antiarrhythmic drugs belonging to the class 1c (Vaughan Williams Classification) were included in the Cardiac Arrhythmia Suppression Trial (CAST), a long term multi-centre randomised, double blind study in patients with asymptomatic non life–threatening ventricular arrhythmia who had a myocardial infarction more than six days but less than two years previously. A significant increase in mortality and non–fatal cardiac arrest rate was seen in patients treated with class 1c antiarrhythmic drugs when compared with a matched placebo group. The applicability of the CAST results to other antiarrhythmics and other populations (eg. those without recent infarction) is uncertain. At present, it is best to assume that the risk extends to other antiarrhythmic agents for patients with structural heart disease.

There is no evidence that prolonged suppression of ventricular premature contractions with antiarrhythmic drugs prevents sudden death.

All antiarrhythmic drugs can produce unwanted effects when they are used to treat symptomatic but not life threatening arrhythmia; the expected benefits should be balanced against their risks.

In patients with structural heart disease, proarrhythmia and cardiac decompensation are special risks associated with antiarrhythmic drugs. Special caution should be exercised when prescribing in this taken context.

Disopyramide should not be used in patients with uncompensated congestive heart failure, unless this heart failure is secondary to cardiac arrhythmia. If disopyramide is to be given under these circumstances, special care and monitoring are essential.

Haemodynamically significant arrhythmias are difficult to treat and affected patients have a high mortality risk. Treatment of these arrhythmias, by whatever modality, must be initiated in hospital.

Owing to its negative inotropic effect, disopyramide should be used with caution in patients suffering from significant cardiac failure. This group may be specially sensitive to the negative inotropic properties of disopyramide. Such patients should be fully digitalised or controlled with other therapy before treatment with disopyramide is commenced.

Aggravation of existing arrhythmia, or emergence of a new type of arrhythmia, demands urgent review of disopyramide treatment.

Similarly, if an atrioventricular block or a bifascicular block occurs during treatment, the use of disopyramide should be reviewed.

There have been reports of ventricular tachycardia, ventricular fibrillation and Torsade de Pointes in patients receiving disopyramide. These have usually, but not always, been associated with significant widening of the QRS complex or prolonged QT interval. The QT interval and QRS duration must be monitored and disopyramide should be stopped if these are increased by more than 25%. If these changes or arrhythmias develop the drug should be discontinued. Disopyramide should be used with caution in patients with atrial flutter or atrial tachycardia with block as conversion of a partial AV block to a 1:1 response may occur, leading to a potentially more serious tachyarrhythmia.

The occurrence of hypotension following disopyramide administration, requires prompt discontinuation of the drug. This has been observed especially in patients with cardiomyopathy or uncompensated congestive heart failure. Any resumption of therapy should be at a lower dose with close patient monitoring. Disopyramide should be used with caution in the treatment of digitalis intoxication.

__Potassium imbalance:__ Antiarrhythmic drugs may be hazardous in patients with potassium imbalance, as potassium abnormalities can induce arrhythmias.

During treatment with disopyramide, potassium levels should be checked regularly. Patients treated with diuretics or stimulant laxatives are at particular risk of hypokalaemia.

__Renal insufficiency:__ In renal insufficiency, the dosage of disopyramide should be reduced by adjusting the interval between administrations.

__Hepatic insufficiency:__ Hepatic impairment causes an increase in the plasma half–life of Rythmodan and a reduced dosage may be required.

__Hypoglycaemia:__Hypoglycaemia has been reported in association with disopyramide administration. The risk of hypoglycaemia, sometimes severe, occurs particularly in elderly or malnourished subjects, treated diabetics and patients with renal insufficiency or cardiac failure. Blood sugar levels should be monitored in all patients. Strict adherence to the dosing recommendations is advised. If hypoglycaemia occurs, then treatment with disopyramide should be stopped.

Hypoglycaemia may be associated with interactions with drugs metabolised by hepatic CYP3A (see Section 4.5 Interactions with other medicines).

__Atropine–like effect:__ There is a risk of:

- ocular hypertension in patients with narrow–angle glaucoma,

- acute urinary retention in patients with prostatic enlargement,

- aggravation of myasthenia gravis.

4.5 Interaction with other medicinal products and other forms of interaction

__Combination with other antiarrhythmic drugs:__ Combinations of antiarrhythmic drugs are not well researched and their effect may be unpredictable. Thus, antiarrhythmic combination should be avoided except under certain circumstances, eg. beta–blockers for angina pectoris; digoxin with beta–blocker and/or verapamil for the control of atrial fibrillation, when defined as effective for an individual.

__Interaction with drugs associated with risk of Torsade de Pointes, such as:__

– tricyclic and tetracyclic antidepressants

– All macrolide antibiotics (e.g. erythromycin, clarithromycin, azithromycin etc)

– astemizole; cisapride; pentamidine; pimozide; sparfloxacin; terfenadine and thioridazone.

Phosphodiesterase Type 5 Inhibitors:

There is evidence that phosphodiesterase Type 5 inhibitors may be potentially associated with a risk of QT prolongation. Concomitant administration of disopyramide with such drugs may potentially enhance this QT prolongation effect and is not recommended.

The concomitant use of these medications whilst undergoing treatment with disopyramide increases the chance of cardiac arrhythmia.

There is some evidence that disopyramide is metabolised by hepatic CYP3A. Concomitant administration of significant inhibitors of this isozyme (e.g. certain macrolide or azole antifungal antibiotics) may therefore increase the serum levels of disopyramide. On the other hand, inducers of CYP3A (e.g. rifampicin and certain anticonvulsants such as phenytoin, primidone and phenobarbital) may reduce disopyramide and increase MN–disopyramide serum levels. Since the magnitude of such potential effects is not foreseeable, such drug combinations are not recommended.

When prescribing a drug metabolised by CYP3A [such as theophylline, HIV protease inhibitors (e.g. ritonavir, indinavir, saquinavir), ciclosporin A, warfarin] it should be kept in mind that disopyramide is probably also a substrate of this isozyme and thus competitive inhibition of metabolism might occur, possibly increasing serum levels of these drugs.

__Interactions with hypokalaemia inducing drugs:__ Concomitant use with drugs that can induce hypokalaemia such as: diuretics, amphotericin B, tetracosactide (corticotropin analogue), gluco and mineralo–corticoids may reduce the action of the drug, or potentiate proarrhythmic effects. Stimulant laxatives are not recommended to be given concomitantly, due to their potassium lowering potential.

__Other drug interactions:__

Atropine and other anticholinergic drugs, including phenothiazines, may potentiate the atropine–like effects of disopyramide.

4.6 Pregnancy and lactation
Pregnancy: Although Rythmodan has undergone animal tests for teratogenicity without evidence of any effect on the developing foetus, its safety in human pregnancy has not been established. Rythmodan has been reported to stimulate contractions of the pregnant uterus. The drug should only be used during pregnancy if benefits clearly outweigh the possible risks to the mother and foetus.

Lactation: No data for Rythmodan Injection, but studies have shown that oral disopyramide is secreted in breast milk, although no adverse effects to the infant have been noted. However, clinical experience is limited and disopyramide should only be used in lactation if, in the clinician's judgement, it is essential for the welfare of the patient. The infant should be closely supervised, particularly for anticholinergic effects and drug levels determined if necessary. Ideally, if the drug is considered essential, an alternative method of feeding should be used.

4.7 Effects on ability to drive and use machines
Some adverse reactions may impair the patients' ability to concentrate and react, and hence the ability to drive or operate machinery. (See section 4.8).

4.8 Undesirable effects

Cardiac: It is accepted that the arrhythmogenic potential of disopyramide is weak. However, as with all antiarrhythmic drugs, disopyramide may worsen or provoke arrhythmias. This proarrhythmic effect is more likely to occur in the presence of hypokalaemia with the associated use of antiarrhythmic drugs, in patients with severe structural heart disease or prolongation of the QT interval.

Intra–cardiac conduction abnormalities may occur: QT interval prolongation, widening of the QRS complex, atrioventricular block and bundle–branch block.

Other types of arrhythmia have been reported: Bradycardia, sinus block, ventricular fibrillation, ventricular tachycardia and torsades de pointes.

Episodes of severe heart failure or even cardiogenic shock have also been described particularly in patients with severe structural heart disease. The resulting low cardiac output can cause hypotension, renal insufficiency and/or acute hepatic ischemia.

Other adverse reactions include:

Atropine like: Urinary (dysuria; acute urinary retention); ocular (disorders of accommodation; diplopia); gastrointestinal - (dry mouth; abdominal pain; nausea, vomiting, anorexia, diarrhoea; constipation); impotence; psychiatric disorders.

Skin reactions: very rarely, rashes; isolated reports of anaphylactic–type reactions possibly culminating in shock (only reported in association with the injectable formulation).

Rarely: Hypoglycaemia, sometimes severe (see Section 4.4 Special Warnings and Precautions for Use). In some cases, severe hypoglycaemia resulted in coma.

Very rarely: cholestatic jaundice, headache, dizzy sensation, neutropenia.

Rapid infusion may cause profuse sweating.

4.9 Overdose

There is no specific antidote for disopyramide. Prostigmine derivatives can be used to treat anticholinergic effects. Symptomatic supportive measures may include: early gastric lavage; administration of a cathartic followed by activated charcoal by mouth or stomach tube; IV administration of isoprenaline, other vasopressors and/or positive inotropic agents; if needed - infusion of lactate and/or magnesium, electro–systolic assistance, cardioversion, insertion of an intra–aortic balloon for counterpulsion and mechanically assisted ventilation. Haemodialysis, haemofiltration or haemoperfusion with activated charcoal has been employed to lower the serum concentration of the drug.

5. PHARMACOLOGICAL PROPERTIES

5.1 Pharmacodynamic properties

Class 1 antiarrhythmic agent.

5.2 Pharmacokinetic properties

Following intravenous administration, disopyramide is rapidly distributed. Doses of 1.5–2mg/kg produce plasma levels of about 10microg/ml, declining rapidly to 3.8–4.2microg/ml at 5 minutes and to less than 3microg/ml at 15 minutes.

In multidose studies, direct slow intravenous injection of 2mg/kg followed by an infusion of 20mg/hr, maintained plasma levels of disopyramide between 2.5 and 2.8microg/ml from the first hour onwards.

Distribution T1/2: 2–4 minutes in healthy volunteers. Longer (15 minutes) in patients with acute myocardial infarct.

Elimination Phase Of Plasma T1/2: 5–8 hours. Increased in renal impairment, cardiac and hepatic disease.

Protein Binding: 50–60%. Saturable and concentration dependent.

Volume Of Distribution: Variable according to method of determination

Metabolism: Approximately 25% of a dose metabolised to a mono–n–dealkylated derivative. Additional 10% as other metabolites.

Excretion: 75% unchanged drug via urine, remainder in faeces. Mono–n–dealkylated metabolite 25% in urine, 64% via faeces.

5.3 Preclinical safety data

Not applicable.

6. PHARMACEUTICAL PARTICULARS

6.1 List of excipients

Benzyl Alcohol

Sorbitol

Water for Injection.

6.2 Incompatibilities

Not applicable.

6.3 Shelf life

60 months.

6.4 Special precautions for storage

Store below 25°C

6.5 Nature and contents of container

Colourless neutral glass ampoules are available as 5ml.

6.6 Special precautions for disposal and other handling

Not Applicable.

7. MARKETING AUTHORISATION HOLDER

Hoechst Marion Roussel Ltd

Broadwater Park

Denham

Uxbridge

Middlesex UB9 5HP

UK

8. MARKETING AUTHORISATION NUMBER(S)

PL 13402/0112

9. DATE OF FIRST AUTHORISATION/RENEWAL OF THE AUTHORISATION

15th June 1998

10. DATE OF REVISION OF THE TEXT

17 June 2008

Legal category: POM

Sabril Sachets 0.5g and Tablets 500mg

(sanofi-aventis)

1. NAME OF THE MEDICINAL PRODUCT

Sabril 500 mg granules for oral solution

Sabril 500 mg film-coated tablets.

2. QUALITATIVE AND QUANTITATIVE COMPOSITION

Each sachet or tablet contains 500mg vigabatrin

For a full list of excipients, see section 6.1.

3. PHARMACEUTICAL FORM

Film-coated tablet:

White to off-white, oval, biconvex, tablets with a break-line on one side and "Sabril" engraved on the other side. The scoreline is only to facilitate breaking for ease of swallowing and not to divide into equal doses.

Granules for oral solution:

White to off-white granular powder.

4. CLINICAL PARTICULARS

4.1 Therapeutic indications

Treatment in combination with other anti-epileptic drugs for patients with resistant partial epilepsy with or without secondary generalisation, that is where all other appropriate drug combinations have proved inadequate or have not been tolerated.

Monotherapy in the treatment of infantile spasms (West's syndrome).

4.2 Posology and method of administration

Sabril treatment may only be initiated by a specialist in epileptology, neurology or paediatric neurology. Follow-up should be arranged under supervision of a specialist in epileptology, neurology or paediatric neurology.

Sabril is for oral administration once or twice daily and may be taken before or after meals. Sachet contents may be placed in beverage (e.g. water, fruit juice or milk) immediately before oral administration.

If the control of epilepsy is not clinically significantly improved after an adequate trial, vigabatrin treatment should not be continued. Vigabatrin should be gradually withdrawn under close medical supervision.

Adults

Maximal efficacy is usually seen in the 2-3g/day range. A starting dose of 1g daily should be added to the patient's current anti-epileptic drug regimen. The daily dose should then be titrated in 0.5g increments at weekly intervals depending on clinical response and tolerability. The highest recommended dose is 3g/day.

No direct correlation exists between the plasma concentration and the efficacy. The duration of the effect of the drug is dependent on the rate of GABA transaminase resynthesis rather than the concentration of the drug in the plasma (see also Sections 5.1 Pharmacodynamic properties and 5.2 Pharmacokinetic properties).

Children

The recommended starting dose in children is 40mg/kg/day. Maintenance recommendations in relation to bodyweight are:

Bodyweight:	10 to 15kg:	0.5-1g/day
	15 to 30kg:	1-1.5g/day
	30 to 50kg:	1.5-3g/day
	>50kg:	2-3g/day

The maximum recommended dose in each of these categories should not be exceeded.

Infants - Monotherapy for infantile spasms (West's Syndrome). The recommended starting dose is 50mg/kg/day. This may be titrated over a period of one week if necessary. Doses of up to 150mg/kg/day have been used with good tolerability.

Elderly and Patients with Renal Impairment

Since vigabatrin is eliminated via the kidney, caution should be exercised when administering the drug to the elderly and more particularly in patients with creatinine clearance less than 60ml/min. Adjustment of dose or frequency of administration should be considered. Such patients may respond to a lower maintenance dose. Patients should be monitored for undesirable effects such as sedation or confusion (see Sections 4.4 Special warnings and special precautions for use, and 4.8 Undesirable effects).

4.3 Contraindications

Hypersensitivity to vigabatrin or to any excipient in the medicinal product.

4.4 Special warnings and precautions for use

Except for the treatment of infantile spasms, Sabril should not be initiated as monotherapy.

Visual field defects have been reported in patients receiving vigabatrin with a high prevalence (about 1/3 of patients). Frequencies found in an open clinical study are present in section 5.1. The onset is usually after months to years of vigabatrin therapy. The degree of visual field restriction may be severe and this may have practical consequences for the patient. Most of the patients with perimetry-confirmed defects have been asymptomatic. Hence, this undesirable effect can only be reliably detected by systematic perimetry which is usually possible only in patients with a developmental age of more than 9 years. A specifically developed method based on field specific Visual Evoked Potentials (VEP) is available from the company on request to test the presence of peripheral vision in children aged 3 years and above. At present this method has not been validated in the detection of vigabatrin attributed visual field defects. Electroretinography may be useful but should be used only in adults who are unable to cooperate with perimetry or in the very young (see Visual Field Defects).

Available data suggests that visual field defects are irreversible even after discontinuation of vigabatrin. A deterioration of VFD after the treatment is discontinued cannot be excluded.

Therefore, vigabatrin should only be used after a careful assessment of the balance of benefits and risk compared with alternatives.

Vigabatrin is not recommended for use in patients with any pre-existing clinically significant visual field defect.

Patients should undergo systematic screening examination when starting vigabatrin and at regular intervals for detection of visual field defects. Visual field testing should continue at 6 month intervals for the whole duration of treatment (see Visual Field Defects).

Visual Field Defects (VFD)

Based on available data, the usual pattern is a concentric constriction of the visual field of both eyes, which is generally more marked nasally than temporally. In the central visual field (within 30 degree of eccentricity), frequently an annular nasal defect is seen. Central visual acuity is not impaired. However, the VFDs reported in patients receiving vigabatrin have ranged from mild to severe. Severe cases are potentially disabling.

Most patients with perimetry-confirmed defects had not previously spontaneously noticed any symptoms, even in cases where a severe defect was observed in perimetry. Available evidence suggests that the VFD is irreversible even after discontinuation of vigabatrin. A deterioration of VFD after the treatment is discontinued cannot be excluded.

Pooled data from prevalence surveys suggest that as many as 1/3 of patients receiving vigabatrin therapy have VFDs. Males may be at greater risk than females. Frequencies found in an open clinical study are presented in section 5.1. A possible association between the risk of visual field defects and the extent of vigabatrin exposure, both in terms of daily dose (from 1 gram to more than 3 grams) and in terms of duration of treatment (maximum during the first three years) has been shown in this study.

All patients should have ophthalmological consultation with visual field examination before the initiation of vigabatrin treatment.

Appropriate visual field testing (perimetry) by using a standardised static perimetry (Humphrey or Octopus) or kinetic perimetry (Goldmann) must be performed before treatment initiation and at six-month intervals for the whole duration of treatment. Static perimetry is the preferred method for detecting vigabatrin associated visual field defect.

Electroretinography may be useful but should only be used in adults who are unable to cooperate with perimetry. Based on the available data the first oscillatory potential and 30 Hz flicker responses of the electroretinogram appear to be correlated with a vigabatrin associated VFD. These responses are delayed and reduced beyond the normal limits. Such changes have not been seen in vigabatrin treated patients without a VFD.

The patient and/or caregiver must be given a thorough description of the frequency and implications of the development of VFD during vigabatrin treatment. Patients should be instructed to report any new visual problems and symptoms which may be associated with visual field constriction. If visual symptoms develop, the patient should be referred to an ophthalmologist.

If a visual field constriction is observed during follow-up, consideration should be given to gradual discontinuation of vigabatrin. If the decision to continue treatment is made, consideration should be given to more frequent follow-up (perimetry) in order to detect progression or sight threatening defects.

Vigabatrin should not be used concomitantly with other retinotoxic drugs.

Children

Perimetry is seldom possible in children less than 9 years of developmental age. The risks of treatment must be very carefully weighed against possible benefit in children. Currently, there is no established method to diagnose or exclude visual field defects in children in whom a standardised perimetry cannot be performed. A specifically developed method based on field specific Visual Evoked Potentials (VEP) is available from the company on request to test the presence of peripheral vision in children aged 3 years and above. At present this method has not been validated in the detection of vigabatrin attributed visual field defects. If the method reveals normal central visual field response but an absent peripheral response, benefit-risk of vigabatrin must be reviewed and consideration given to gradual discontinuation. The presence of peripheral vision does not exclude the possibility of developing VFD. Electroretinography may be useful but should be used only in children less than 3 years of age.

Neurological and psychiatric conditions

In view of the results of the animal safety studies (see Section 5.3 Preclinical safety data), it is recommended that patients treated with vigabatrin are closely observed for adverse effects on neurological function.

Rare reports of encephalopathic symptoms such as marked sedation, stupor and confusion in association with non-specific slow wave activity on electroencephalogram have been described soon after the initiation of vigabatrin treatment. Risk factors for the development of these reactions include higher than recommended starting dose, faster dose escalation at higher steps than recommended, and renal failure. These events have been reversible following dose reduction or discontinuation of vigabatrin. (See Section 4.8 Undesirable effects).

As with other antiepileptic drugs some patients may experience an increase in seizure frequency or the onset of new types of seizures with vigabatrin (see Section 4.8 Undesirable effects). These phenomena may also be the consequence of an overdosage, a decrease in plasma concentrations of concomitant antiepileptic treatment, or a paradoxical effect.

As with other antiepileptic drugs, abrupt withdrawal may lead to rebound seizures. If a patient is to be withdrawn from vigabatrin treatment, it is recommended that this is done by gradual dose reduction over a 2- to 4-week period.

Vigabatrin should be used with caution in patients with a history of psychosis, depression or behavioural problems. Psychiatric events (e.g., agitation, depression, abnormal thinking, paranoid reactions) have been reported during vigabatrin treatment. These events occurred in patients with and without a psychiatric history, and were usually reversible when vigabatrin doses were reduced or gradually discontinued.

Suicidal ideation and behaviour

Suicidal ideation and behaviour have been reported in patients treated with anti-epileptic agents in several indications. A meta-analysis of randomised placebo-controlled trials of anti-epileptic drugs has also shown a small increased risk of suicidal ideation and behaviour. The mechanism of this risk is not known and the available data do not exclude the possibility of an increased risk for vigabatrin.

Therefore, patients should be monitored for signs of suicidal ideation and behaviour, and appropriate treatment should be considered. Patients (and caregivers of patients) should be advised to seek medical advice immediately should signs of suicidal ideation or behaviour emerge.

Elderly and patients with renal impairment

Since vigabatrin is eliminated via the kidney, caution should be exercised in patients with a creatinine clearance of less than 60ml/min and in elderly patients. These patients should be monitored closely for undesirable effects such as sedation and confusion. (See Section 4.2 Posology and method of administration).

4.5 Interaction with other medicinal products and other forms of interaction

As vigabatrin is neither metabolised, nor protein bound and is not an inducer of hepatic cytochrome P450 drug metabolising-enzymes, interactions with other drugs are unlikely. However, during controlled clinical studies, a gradual reduction of 16-33% in the plasma concentration of phenytoin has been observed. The exact nature of this interaction is presently not understood, however, in the majority of cases it is unlikely to be of therapeutic significance.

The plasma concentrations of carbamazepine, phenobarbitone, and sodium valproate have also been monitored during controlled clinical trials and no clinically significant interactions have been detected.

Vigabatrin may lead to a decrease in measured plasma activity of alanine aminotransferase (ALT) and to a lesser extent, aspartate aminotransferase (AST). The magnitude of suppression for ALT has been reported to vary between

30% and 100%. Therefore, these liver tests may be quantitatively unreliable in patients taking vigabatrin. (See Section 4.8 Undesirable effects)

Vigabatrin may increase the amount of amino acids in the urine possibly leading to a false positive test for certain rare genetic metabolic disorders (eg, alpha aminoadipic aciduria).

4.6 Pregnancy and lactation

Vigabatrin should only be used during pregnancy if clearly necessary.

Based on data on a limited number of exposed pregnancies with vigabatrin, available from spontaneous reports, abnormal outcomes (congenital anomalies or spontaneous abortion) were reported in the offspring of mothers taking vigabatrin. No definite conclusion can be drawn as to whether vigabatrin produces an increased risk of malformation when taken during pregnancy because of limited data, and the presence of concomitant antiepilepsy medicinal products during each reported pregnancy.

Women of child bearing potential/ contraception

Specialized advice should be provided to all patients who could begin a pregnancy or who are in the fertile age. The need of antiepileptic treatment must be re-evaluated when a patient plans a pregnancy.

Pregnancy

The risk of congenital defects is increased from 2 to 3 fold in children born from mothers treated with an antiepileptic; those more frequently reported are cleft lip, cardiovascular defects and neural tube defects.

Polytherapy with antiepileptic drugs may be associated with a higher risk of congenital malformation than monotherapy.

If a patient becomes pregnant, treatment should be reviewed. Sudden interruption of effective antiepileptic treatment may lead to aggravation of the condition in the mother that is detrimental to the foetus.

There is no information on the possible occurrence of visual field defect in children who have been exposed to vigabatrin in utero.

Fertility

Studies in animals have shown reproductive toxicity (see Section 5.3 Preclinical safety data).

Lactation

Vigabatrin is excreted into breast milk. Breast feeding is not recommended during vigabatrin treatment.

4.7 Effects on ability to drive and use machines

As a general rule, patients with uncontrolled epilepsy are not allowed to drive or handle potentially dangerous machinery. In view of the fact that drowsiness has been observed in clinical trials with Sabril, patients should be warned of this possibility at the start of treatment.

Visual field defects which can significantly affect the ability to drive and use machines have been frequently reported in association with Sabril. Patients should be evaluated for the presence of visual field defect (see also Section 4.4 Special Warnings and special precautions for use). Special care should be taken by patients driving, operating machinery or performing any hazardous task.

4.8 Undesirable effects

Visual field defects ranging from mild to severe have been reported frequently in patients receiving vigabatrin. Severe cases are potentially disabling. The onset is usually after months to years of vigabatrin therapy. Pooled data from prevalence surveys suggest that as many as 1/3 of patients receiving vigabatrin therapy develop visual field defects (see also Section 4.4 Special warnings and special precautions for use).

Approximately 50% of patients in controlled clinical studies have experienced undesirable effects during vigabatrin treatment. In adults, these were mostly central nervous system related such as sedation, drowsiness, fatigue and impaired concentration. However, in children excitation or agitation is frequent. The incidence of these undesirable effects is generally higher at the beginning of treatment and decreases with time.

As with other antiepileptic drugs, some patients may experience an increase in seizure frequency, including status epilepticus with vigabatrin. Patients with myoclonic seizures may be particularly liable to this effect. New onset myoclonus and exacerbation of existing myoclonus may occur in rare cases.

Undesirable effects ranked under headings of frequency are listed below, using the following convention:

Very common (>=1/10); common (>=1/100 to <1/10); uncommon (>=1/1,000 to <1/100); rare (>=1/10,000 to <1/1,000); very rare (<1/10,000); Not known (cannot be estimated from the available data).

*Investigations**

Common: weight increased

Nervous system disorders

Very common: somnolence

Common: speech disorder, headache, dizziness, paraesthesia, disturbance in attention and memory impairment, mental impairment (thought disturbance), tremor

Uncommon: coordination abnormal (ataxia)

Rare: encephalopathy**

Very rare: optic neuritis

Eye disorders

Very common: visual field defect

Common: vision blurred, diplopia, nystagmus,

Rare: retinal disorder (such as peripheral retinal atrophy)

Very rare: optic atrophy

Gastrointestinal disorders

Common: nausea, abdominal pain

Skin and subcutaneous tissue disorders

Uncommon: rash

Rare: angioedema, urticaria

General disorders and administration site conditions

Very common: fatigue

Common: oedema, irritability

Hepato-biliary disorders

Very rare: hepatitis

*Psychiatric disorders****

Very common: excitation (children), agitation (children)

Common: agitation, aggression, nervousness, depression, paranoid reaction

Uncommon: hypomania, mania, psychotic disorder

Rare: suicide attempt

Very rare: hallucination

*Laboratory data indicate that vigabatrin treatment does not lead to renal toxicity. Decreases in ALT and AST, which are considered to be a result of inhibition of these aminotransferases by vigabatrin, have been observed. Chronic treatment with vigabatrin may be associated with a slight decrease in haemoglobin which rarely attains clinical significance.

**Rare reports of encephalopathic symptoms such as marked sedation, stupor and confusion in association with non-specific slow wave activity on electroencephalogram have been described soon after the initiation of vigabatrin treatment. Such reactions have been fully reversible following dose reduction or discontinuation of vigabatrin (see Section 4.4 Special warnings and special precautions for use).

***Psychiatric reactions have been reported during vigabatrin therapy. These reactions occurred in patients with and without a psychiatric history and were usually reversible when vigabatrin doses were reduced or gradually discontinued (see Section 4.4 Special warnings and special precautions for use). Depression was a common psychiatric reaction in clinical trials but seldom required discontinuation of vigabatrin.

4.9 Overdose

Symptoms

Vigabatrin overdose has been reported. When provided, doses most commonly were between 7.5 to 30g; however, ingestions up to 90g have been reported. Nearly half of the cases involved multiple drug ingestions. When reported, the most common symptoms included drowsiness or coma. Other less frequently reported symptoms included vertigo, headache, psychosis, respiratory depression or apnea, bradycardia, hypotension, agitation, irritability, confusion, abnormal behaviour, and speech disorder. None of the overdoses resulted in death.

Management

There is no specific antidote. The usual supportive measures should be employed. Measures to remove unabsorbed drug should be considered. Activated charcoal has been shown to not significantly adsorb vigabatrin in an in vitro study. The effectiveness of hemodialysis in the treatment of vigabatrin overdose is unknown. In isolated case reports in renal failure patients receiving therapeutic doses of vigabatrin, hemodialysis reduced vigabatrin plasma concentrations by 40% to 60%.

5. PHARMACOLOGICAL PROPERTIES

5.1 Pharmacodynamic properties

Pharmaco-therapeutic group: Antiepileptics, ATC code: N03AG04

Vigabatrin is an antiepileptic drug with a clearly defined mechanism of action. Treatment with vigabatrin leads to an increase in the concentration of GABA (gamma aminobutyric acid), the major inhibitory neurotransmitter in the brain. This is because vigabatrin was designed rationally as a selective irreversible inhibitor of GABA-transaminase, the enzyme responsible for the breakdown of GABA.

Controlled and long-term clinical trials have shown that vigabatrin is an effective anticonvulsant agent when given as add-on therapy in patients with epilepsy not controlled satisfactorily by conventional therapy. This efficacy is particularly marked in patients with seizures of partial origin.

Epidemiology of VFD in patients with refractory partial epilepsy was examined in an observational, open-label, multicentre, comparative, parallel group, Phase IV study, including 734 patients, at least 8 years old, with refractory partial epilepsy for at least one year.

Patients were split in three treatment groups: patients currently treated with vigabatrin (group I), patients previously exposed to vigabatrin (group II) and patients never exposed to vigabatrin (group III). The following table presents the main findings at inclusion and at the first and last conclusive evaluations in the evaluable population (n=524):

(see Table 1 below)

5.2 Pharmacokinetic properties

Vigabatrin is a water soluble compound and it is rapidly and completely absorbed from the gastrointestinal tract. Food administration does not alter the extent of vigabatrin absorption. The drug is widely distributed with an apparent volume of distribution slightly greater than total body water. Plasma and cerebrospinal fluid concentrations are linearly related to dose over the recommended dose range.

There is no direct correlation between plasma concentration and efficacy. The duration of the effect of the drug is dependent on the GABA transaminase re-synthesis rate.

Vigabatrin is eliminated from the plasma with a terminal half-life of 5-8 hours with approximately 70% of a single oral dose being recovered as unchanged drug in the urine in the first 24 hours post-dose. No metabolites have been identified.

Vigabatrin does not induce the hepatic cytochrome P450 enzymes nor is it metabolised or protein bound. Therefore drug interactions are unlikely.

5.3 Preclinical safety data

Animal safety studies carried out in the rat, mouse, dog and monkey have indicated that vigabatrin has no significant adverse effects on the liver, kidney, lung, heart or gastrointestinal tract.

In the brain, microvacuolation has been observed in white matter tracts of rat, mouse and dog at doses of 30-50mg/kg/day. In the monkey these lesions are minimal or equivocal. This effect is caused by a separation of the outer lamellar sheath of myelinated fibres, a change characteristic of intramyelinic oedema. In both rat and dog the intramyelinic oedema was reversible on stopping vigabatrin treatment and even with continued treatment histologic regression was observed. However, in rodents, minor residual changes consisting of swollen axons (eosinophilic spheroids) and mineralised microbodies have been observed. In the dog, the results of an electrophysiological study indicate that intramyelinic oedema is associated with an increase in the latency of the somatosensory evoked potential which is reversible when the drug is withdrawn.

In humans, there is no evidence of intramyelinic oedema. Tests done to confirm lack of significant adverse effect on neurological function include evoked potentials, CAT scans, magnetic resonance imaging, CSF analyses and in a small number of cases, neuropathological examinations of brain specimens.

Vigabatrin-associated retinotoxicity has only been observed in albino rats, but not in pigmented rats, dogs or monkeys. The retinal changes in albino rats were characterised as focal or multifocal disorganisation of the outer nuclear layer with displacement of nuclei into the rod and cone area. The other layers of retina were not affected. These lesions were observed in 80-100% of animals at the dose of 300mg/kg/day orally. The histologic appearance of these lesions was similar to that found in albino rats following excessive exposure to light. However, the retinal changes may also represent a direct drug-induced effect.

Animal experiments have shown that vigabatrin has no negative influence on fertility or pup development. No teratogenicity was seen in rats in doses up to 150mg/kg (3 times the human dose) or in rabbits in doses up to 100mg/kg. However, in rabbits, a slight increase in the incidence of cleft palate at doses of 150-200mg/kg was seen.

Studies with vigabatrin revealed no evidence of mutagenic or carcinogenic effects.

Table 1

	Children (from 8 to 12 years old)			Adults (> 12 years old)		
	Group I[1]	Group II[2]	Group III	Group I[3]	Group II[4]	Group III
	N=38	N=47	N=41	N=150	N=151	N=97
Visual field defect with non-identified aetiology						
Observed at inclusion	1 (4.4%)	3 (8.8%)	2 (7.1%)	31 (34.1%)	20 (19.2%)	1 (1.4%)
Observed at first conclusive evaluation	4 (10.5%)	6 (12.8%)	2 (4.9%)	59 (39.3%)	39 (25.8%)	4 (4.1%)
Observed at last conclusive evaluation	10 (26.3%)	7 (14.9%)	3 (7.3%)	70 (46.7%)	47 (31.1%)	5 (5.2%)

[1] Median treatment duration: 44.4 months, mean daily dose 1.48 g
[2] Median treatment duration: 20.6 months, mean daily dose 1.39 g
[3] Median treatment duration: 48.8 months, mean daily dose 2.10 g
[4] Median treatment duration: 23.0 months, mean daily dose 2.18 g

6. PHARMACEUTICAL PARTICULARS

6.1 List of excipients

Sachets: Povidone K30 (E1201)

Tablet core:

Povidone K30 (E1201)

Microcrystalline cellulose (E460)

Magnesium stearate

Sodium starch glycollate (Type A)

Tablet coating:

Hypromellose 15 mPa.s (E464)

Titanium dioxide (E171)

Macrogol 8000

6.2 Incompatibilities

Not applicable

6.3 Shelf life

Sachets: 3 years

Use immediately following reconstitution

Tablets: 5 years

6.4 Special precautions for storage

The tablets and sachets do not require any special storage conditions.

6.5 Nature and contents of container

Sachets: Laminated (polyethylene/aluminium foil/polyethylene/paper) heat-sealed sachet packs containing 50 sachets.

Tablets: Clear colourless PVC-aluminium blisters of 10 film-coated tablets.

Each blister pack contains 100 tablets.

6.6 Special precautions for disposal and other handling

Sachets: No special requirements. The content of the recommended number of sachets is dissolved in at least 100 ml of water, fruit juice or milk just before administration. Upon reconstitution with water, the solution has a clear and yellow appearance.

Tablets: No special requirements

7. MARKETING AUTHORISATION HOLDER

Sanofi-aventis

One Onslow Street

Guildford

Surrey

GU1 4Y

8. MARKETING AUTHORISATION NUMBER(S)

Sachets: PL 04425/0170

Tablets: PL 04425/0171

9. DATE OF FIRST AUTHORISATION/RENEWAL OF THE AUTHORISATION

Sachets: 26th January, 2001/19th June 2006

Tablets: 26th January 2001/19th June 2006

10. DATE OF REVISION OF THE TEXT

21 February 2009

LEGAL STATUS

POM

SAFLUTAN 15 micrograms/ml eye drops, solution, single-dose container

(Merck Sharp & Dohme Limited)

1. NAME OF THE MEDICINAL PRODUCT

SAFLUTAN™▼ 15 micrograms/ml eye drops, solution, single-dose container

2. QUALITATIVE AND QUANTITATIVE COMPOSITION

One ml of eye drops, solution, contains 15 micrograms of tafluprost.

One single-dose container (0.3 ml) of eye drops, solution, contains 4.5 micrograms of tafluprost.

For a full list of excipients, see section 6.1.

3. PHARMACEUTICAL FORM

Eye drops, solution, single-dose container (eye drops).

A clear, colourless solution.

4. CLINICAL PARTICULARS

4.1 Therapeutic indications

Reduction of elevated intraocular pressure in open angle glaucoma and ocular hypertension.

As monotherapy in patients:

o who would benefit from preservative free eye drops

o insufficiently responsive to first line therapy

o intolerant or contra-indicated to first line therapy.

As adjunctive therapy to beta-blockers.

4.2 Posology and method of administration

Posology

The recommended dose is one drop of SAFLUTAN in the conjunctival sac of the affected eye(s) once daily in the evening.

The dose should not exceed once daily as more frequent administration may lessen the intraocular pressure lowering effect.

For single use only, one container is sufficient to treat both eyes. Any unused solution should be discarded immediately after use.

Use in elderly:

No dosage alteration in elderly patients is necessary.

Use in children and adolescents:

Tafluprost is not recommended for use in children or adolescents below age 18 due to a lack of data on safety and efficacy.

Use in renal/hepatic impairment

Tafluprost has not been studied in patients with renal/hepatic impairment and should therefore be used with caution in such patients.

Method of administration

To reduce the risk of darkening of the eyelid skin the patients should wipe off any excess solution from the skin. As with any other eye drops, nasolacrimal occlusion or gently closing the eyelid after administration is recommended. This may reduce the systemic absorption of medicinal products administered via the ocular route.

If more than one topical ophthalmic medicinal product is being used, each one should be administered at least 5 minutes apart.

4.3 Contraindications

Hypersensitivity to tafluprost or to any of the excipients.

4.4 Special warnings and precautions for use

Before treatment is initiated, patients should be informed of the possibility of eyelash growth, darkening of the eyelid skin and increased iris pigmentation. Some of these changes may be permanent, and may lead to differences in appearance between the eyes when only one eye is treated.

The change in iris pigmentation occurs slowly and may not be noticeable for several months. The change in eye colour has predominantly been seen in patients with mixed coloured irises, e.g. blue-brown, grey-brown, yellow-brown and green-brown. The risk of lifelong heterochromia between the eyes in unilateral cases is obvious.

There is no experience with tafluprost in neovascular, angle-closure, narrow-angle or congenital glaucoma. There is only limited experience with tafluprost in aphakic patients and in pigmentary or pseudoexfoliative glaucoma.

Caution is recommended when using tafluprost in aphakic patients, pseudophakic patients with torn posterior lens capsule or anterior chamber lenses, or in patients with known risk factors for cystoid macular oedema or iritis/uveitis.

There is no experience in patients with severe asthma. Such patients should therefore be treated with caution.

4.5 Interaction with other medicinal products and other forms of interaction

No interactions are anticipated in humans, since systemic concentrations of tafluprost are extremely low following ocular dosing. Therefore, specific interaction studies with other medicinal products have not been performed with tafluprost.

In clinical studies tafluprost was used concomitantly with timolol without evidence of interaction.

4.6 Pregnancy and lactation

Women of childbearing potential/contraception

SAFLUTAN must not be used in women of childbearing age/potential unless adequate contraceptive measures are in place (see section 5.3).

Pregnancy

There are no adequate data from the use of tafluprost in pregnant women. Tafluprost can have harmful pharmacologic effects on pregnancy and/or the fetus/newborn child. Studies in animals have shown reproductive toxicity (see section 5.3). Therefore, SAFLUTAN should not be used during pregnancy unless clearly necessary (in case no other treatment options are available).

Lactation

It is unknown whether tafluprost is excreted in human milk. A study in rats has shown excretion of tafluprost in breast milk after topical administration (see section 5.3). Therefore, tafluprost should not be used during breast-feeding.

4.7 Effects on ability to drive and use machines

Tafluprost has no influence on the ability to drive and use machines. As with any ocular treatment, if transient blurred vision occurs at instillation, the patient should wait until the vision clears before driving or using machinery.

4.8 Undesirable effects

In clinical studies, over 1200 patients have been treated with tafluprost either as monotherapy or as adjunctive therapy to timolol 0.5%. The most frequently reported treatment-related adverse event was ocular hyperaemia. It occurred in approximately 13% of the patients participating in the clinical studies with tafluprost in Europe and the US. It was mild in most cases and led to discontinuation on an average in 0.4% of patients participating in the pivotal studies.

The following undesirable effects related to treatment were reported during clinical trials with tafluprost in Europe and the US after a maximum follow-up of 12 months:

Within each frequency grouping, adverse reactions are presented in order of decreasing frequency.

Eye disorders

Very common ($\geqslant$1/10): conjunctival/ocular hyperaemia

Common ($\geqslant$1/100 to $<$1/10): eye pruritus, eye irritation, eye pain, changes in eyelashes (increased length, thickness and number of lashes), dry eye, eyelash discolouration, foreign body sensation in eyes, erythema of eye lid, blurred vision, increased lacrimation, blepharal pigmentation, eye discharge, reduced visual acuity, photophobia, eyelid oedema and increased iris pigmentation.

Uncommon ($\geqslant$1/1000 to $<$1/100): superficial punctate keratitis (SPK), asthenopia, conjunctival oedema, blepharitis, ocular discomfort, anterior chamber flare, conjunctival follicles, allergic conjunctivitis, anterior chamber cell, conjunctival pigmentation and abnormal sensation in eye.

Nervous system disorders

Common ($\geqslant$1/100 to $<$1/10): headache

Skin and subcutaneous tissue disorders

Uncommon ($\geqslant$1/1000 to $<$1/100): hypertrichosis of eyelid

4.9 Overdose

No case of overdose has been reported. Overdose is unlikely to occur after ocular administration.

If overdose occurs, treatment should be symptomatic.

5. PHARMACOLOGICAL PROPERTIES

5.1 Pharmacodynamic properties

Pharmacotherapeutic group: Antiglaucoma preparations and miotics, prostaglandin analogues

ATC code: S01EE05

Mechanism of action

Tafluprost is a fluorinated analogue of prostaglandin $F_{2\alpha}$. Tafluprost acid, the biologically active metabolite of tafluprost, is a highly potent and selective agonist of the human prostanoid FP receptor. Tafluprost acid has a 12-fold higher affinity for the FP receptor than latanoprost. Pharmacodynamic studies in monkeys indicate that tafluprost reduces intraocular pressure by increasing the uveoscleral outflow of aqueous humour.

Clinical effects on intraocular pressure

Reduction of intraocular pressure starts between 2 and 4 hours after the first administration and maximum effect is reached at around 12 hours after instillation. The duration of effect is maintained for at least 24 hours. Pivotal studies with a tafluprost formulation containing the preservative benzalkonium chloride have demonstrated that tafluprost is effective as monotherapy and has an additive effect when administered as adjunctive therapy to timolol: In a 6-month study, tafluprost showed a significant IOP lowering effect of 6 to 8 mmHg at different time points of the day as compared to 7 to 9 mmHg with latanoprost. In a second 6-month clinical study, tafluprost reduced IOP by 5 to 7 mmHg as compared to 4 to 6 mmHg with timolol. The IOP lowering effect of tafluprost was maintained in the extension of these studies up to 12 months. In a 6-week study, the IOP-lowering effect of tafluprost was compared with its vehicle when used adjunctively with timolol. Compared to baseline values (measured after a 4-week run in on timolol), the additional IOP-lowering effects were 5 to 6 mmHg in the timolol-tafluprost group and 3 to 4 mmHg in the timolol-vehicle group. The preserved and the non-preserved formulations of tafluprost showed a similar IOP-lowering effect of over 5 mmHg in a small cross-over study with a 4-week treatment period.

Secondary pharmacodynamics

When rabbits were treated for 4 weeks with a tafluprost 0.0015% ophthalmic solution once daily, the optic nerve head blood flow was significantly increased compared to baseline when measured by the laser speckle flowgraphy on Days 14 and 28.

5.2 Pharmacokinetic properties

After once daily ocular administration of one drop of unpreserved tafluprost 0.0015% eye drops in single-dose container to both eyes for 8 days, plasma concentrations were low and had similar profiles on days 1 and 8. The plasma concentrations peaked at 10 minutes after dosing and declined to below the lower limit of detection (10 pg/mL) before one hour after dosing. Mean C_{max} (26.2 and 26.6 pg/mL) and $AUC_{0\text{-}last}$ (394.3 and 431.9 pg*min/mL) values were similar on days 1 and 8, indicating that a steady drug concentration was reached during the first week of ocular dosing. No statistically significant differences in the systemic bioavailability between the preserved and unpreserved formulation were detected.

In a rabbit study, the absorption of tafluprost into the aqueous humour was comparable after a single ocular instillation of unpreserved or preserved tafluprost 0.0015% ophthalmic solution.

In monkeys, there was no specific distribution of radiolabelled tafluprost in the iris-ciliary body or choroid including retinal pigment epithelium, which suggested low affinity for melanin pigment.

The principle metabolic pathway of tafluprost in humans is the hydrolysis to tafluprost acid and further beta-oxidation to the pharmacologically inactive 1,2-dinor and 1,2,3,4-tetranor tafluprost acids, which may be glucuronated or hydroxylated. Cytochrome P450 (CYP) enzyme system is not involved in the metabolism of tafluprost acid.

5.3 Preclinical safety data

Non-clinical data reveal no special hazard for humans based on conventional studies of safety pharmacology, systemic repeated dose toxicity, genotoxicity and carcinogenic potential. As with other PGF2 agonists, repeated dose topical ocular administration of tafluprost to monkeys produced irreversible effects on iris pigmentation and reversible enlargement of the palpebral fissure.

Increased contraction of rat and rabbit uteri *in vitro* was observed at tafluprost acid concentrations that exceeded 4 to 40 times, respectively, the maximum plasma concentrations of tafluprost acid in humans. Uterotonic activity of tafluprost has not been tested in human uterus preparations.

Reproduction toxicity studies were performed in the rat and rabbit with intravenous administration. In rats, no adverse effects on fertility or early embryonic development were observed at systemic exposure over 12 000 times the maximum clinical exposure based on C_{max} or greater than 75 times based on AUC.

In conventional embryo-foetal development studies, tafluprost caused reductions in foetal body weights and increases in post-implantation losses. Tafluprost increased the incidence of skeletal abnormalities in rats as well as the incidence of skull, brain and spine malformations in rabbits. In the rabbit study, plasma levels of tafluprost and its metabolites were below the level of quantification.

In a pre- and postnatal development study in rats, increased mortality of newborns, decreased body weights and delayed pinna unfolding were observed in offspring at tafluprost doses greater than 20 times the clinical dose.

The experiments in rats with radiolabelled tafluprost showed that around 0.1% of the topically applied dose on eyes was transferred into milk. As the half-life of active metabolite (tafluprost acid) in plasma is very short (not detectable after 30 minutes in humans), most of the radioactivity probably represented metabolites with little, or no pharmacologic activity. Based on metabolism of the drug and natural prostaglandins, the oral bioavailability is expected to be very low.

6. PHARMACEUTICAL PARTICULARS

6.1 List of excipients

Glycerol

Sodium dihydrogen phosphate dihydrate

Disodium edetate

Polysorbate 80

Hydrochloric acid and/or sodium hydroxide for pH adjustment

Water for injections.

6.2 Incompatibilities

Not applicable

6.3 Shelf life

2 years.

After first opening a foil pouch: 28 days.

6.4 Special precautions for storage

Store in a refrigerator (2°C - 8°C).

After opening the foil pouch:

- Keep the single-dose containers in the original foil pouch
- Do not store above 25°C
- Discard an opened single-dose container with any remaining solution immediately after use.

6.5 Nature and contents of container

Low-density polyethylene (LDPE) single-dose containers packed in foil pouch. Each single-dose container has a fill volume of 0.3 ml and there are 10 containers in each foil pouch.

The following pack sizes are available: 30 × 0.3 ml single-dose containers and 90 × 0.3 ml single-dose containers.

Not all pack sizes may be marketed.

6.6 Special precautions for disposal and other handling

No special requirements.

7. MARKETING AUTHORISATION HOLDER

Merck Sharp & Dohme Limited

Hertford Road

Hoddesdon

Hertfordshire

EN11 9BU, UK

8. MARKETING AUTHORISATION NUMBER(S)

PL 00025/0529

9. DATE OF FIRST AUTHORISATION/RENEWAL OF THE AUTHORISATION

17 October 2008

10. DATE OF REVISION OF THE TEXT

06/2009

LEGAL CATEGORY

POM

Ⓜ denotes trademark of Merck & Co., Inc., Whitehouse Station, NJ, USA.

SPC.SAF.09.UK.3038

Saizen 1.33mg

(Merck Serono)

1. NAME OF THE MEDICINAL PRODUCT

SAIZEN® 1.33mg, powder and solvent for solution for injection

2. QUALITATIVE AND QUANTITATIVE COMPOSITION

Each vial of Saizen 1.33 mg contains Somatropin* (recombinant human growth hormone).

*produced by recombinant DNA technology in mammalian cells

For excipients, see section 6.1.

3. PHARMACEUTICAL FORM

Powder and solvent for solution for injection

White lyophilised powder and clear, colourless solvent.

4. CLINICAL PARTICULARS

4.1 Therapeutic indications

Saizen is indicated in the treatment of:

- growth failure in children caused by decreased or absent secretion of endogenous growth hormone.
- growth failure in girls with gonadal dysgenesis (Turner Syndrome), confirmed by chromosomal analysis.
- growth failure in prepubertal children due to chronic renal failure (CRF).
- growth disturbance (current height SDS < -2.5 and parental adjusted height SDS < -1) in short children born small for gestational age (SGA) with a birth weight and/or length below – 2 SD, who failed to show catch-up growth (HV SDS < 0 during the last year) by 4 years of age or later.
- replacement therapy in adults with pronounced growth hormone deficiency as diagnosed by a single dynamic test for growth hormone deficiency. Patients must also fulfil the following criteria:

Childhood Onset:

Patients who were diagnosed as growth hormone deficient during childhood, must be retested and their growth hormone deficiency confirmed before replacement therapy with Saizen is started.

Adult Onset:

Patients must have growth hormone deficiency as a result of hypothalamic or pituitary disease and at least one other hormone deficiency diagnosed (except for prolactin) and adequate replacement therapy instituted, before replacement therapy using growth hormone may begin.

4.2 Posology and method of administration

Saizen 1.33 mg is intended for single dose use.

Saizen dosage should be individualised for each patient based on body surface area (BSA) or on body weight (BW).

It is recommended that Saizen be administered at bedtime according to the following dosage:

Growth failure due to inadequate endogenous growth hormone secretion:

0.7-1.0 mg/m^2 body surface area (BSA) per day or 0.025-0.035 mg/kg body weight (BW) per day by subcutaneous or intramuscular administration.

Growth failure in girls due to gonadal dysgenesis (Turner Syndrome)

1.4 mg/m^2 body surface area (BSA) per day or 0.045-0.050 mg/kg body weight (BW) per day by subcutaneous administration.

Concomitant therapy with non-androgenic anabolic steroids in patients with Turner Syndrome can enhance the growth response.

Growth failure in prepubertal children due to chronic renal failure (CRF):

1.4 mg/m^2 body surface area (BSA), approximately equal to 0.045-0.050 mg/kg body weight (BW), per day by subcutaneous administration.

Growth failure in short children born small for gestational age (SGA):

The recommended daily dose is 0.035 mg/kg body weight (or 1 mg/m^2/day, equal to 0.1 IU/kg/day or 3 IU/m^2/day) per day, by subcutaneous administration.

Duration of treatment

Treatment should be discontinued when the patient has reached a satisfactory adult height, or the epiphyses are fused.

For growth disturbance in short children born SGA, treatment is usually recommended until final height is reached. Treatment should be discontinued after the first year if height velocity SDS is below +1. Treatment should be discontinued when final height is reached (defined as height velocity < 2 cm/year), and if confirmation is required if bone age is > 14 years (girls) or > 16 years (boys), corresponding to closure of the epiphyseal growth plates.

Growth Hormone Deficiency in adults

At the start of somatropin therapy, low doses of 0.15-0.3mg are recommended, given as a daily subcutaneous injection. The dose should be adjusted stepwise, controlled by Insulin-like Growth Factor 1 (IGF-1) values. The recommended final GH dose seldom exceeds 1.0mg/day. In general the lowest efficacious dose should be administered. In older or overweight patients, lower doses may be necessary.

4.3 Contraindications

Saizen should not be used in children in whom epiphyseal fusion occurred.

Saizen is contraindicated in patients known to be hypersensitive to Somatropin and any of the excipients in the powder for solution for injection or the solvent.

Saizen is contraindicated in patients with active neoplasia. Any anti-tumor therapy must be completed prior to starting treatment with Somatropin.

Saizen should not be used in cases with evidence of any progression or recurrence of an underlying intra-cranial lesion.

Patients with acute critical illness suffering complications following open heart surgery, abdominal surgery, multiple accidental trauma, acute respiratory failure or similar conditions should not be treated with Somatropin. (Regarding patients undergoing Somatropin therapy and becoming critically ill, see 4.4 "Special warnings and special precautions for use".)

4.4 Special warnings and precautions for use

Treatment should be carried out under the regular guidance of a physician who is experienced in the diagnosis and management of patients with growth hormone deficiency.

Patients with an intra or extracranial neoplasia in remission who are receiving treatment with growth hormone should be examined carefully and at regular intervals by the physician.

Patients with growth hormone deficiency secondary to an intracranial tumour should be examined frequently for progression or recurrence of the underlying disease process.

Some cases of leukaemia have been reported in growth hormone deficient children, untreated as well as treated with growth hormone, and might possibly represent a slightly increased incidence compared with non-growth hormone deficient children. A causal relationship to growth hormone therapy has not been established.

Growth Hormone administration is followed by a transient phase of hypoglycemia of approximately 2 hours, then from 2-4 hours onward by an increase in blood glucose levels despite high insulin concentrations. Somatropin may induce a state of insulin resistance, which can result in hyperinsulinism and in some patients hyperglycemia. To detect insulin resistance, patients should be monitored for evidence of glucose intolerance.

Saizen should be used with caution in patients with diabetes mellitus or with a family history of diabetes mellitus. Patients with diabetes mellitus may require adjustment of their antidiabetic therapy.

Stable background retinopathy should not lead to discontinuation of Somatropin replacement therapy. In case of development of preproliferative changes and the presence of proliferative retinopathy Somatropin replacement therapy should be discontinued.

During treatment with Somatropin an enhanced T4 to T3 conversion has been found which may result in a reduction in serum T4 and an increase in serum T3 concentrations. In general, the peripheral thyroid hormone levels have remained within the reference ranges for healthy subjects. The effects of Somatropin on thyroid hormone levels may be of clinical relevance in patients with central subclinical hypothyroidism in whom overt hypothyroidism theoretically may develop. Conversely, in patients receiving replacement therapy with thyroxine mild hyperthyroidism may occur. It is therefore particularly advisable to test thyroid function after starting treatment with Somatropin and after dose adjustments.

Fluid retention is expected during growth hormone replacement therapy in adults.

In case of persistent oedema or severe paraesthesia the dosage should be decreased in order to avoid the development of carpal tunnel syndrome.

In case of severe or recurrent headache, visual problems, nausea and/or vomiting, funduscopy for papilloedema is recommended. If papilloedema is confirmed a diagnosis of benign intracranial hypertension (or pseudotumor cerebri) should be considered and Saizen treatment should be discontinued. At present there is insufficient evidence to guide clinical decision-making in patients with resolved intracranial hypertension. If growth hormone treatment is restarted, careful monitoring for symptoms of intracranial hypertension is necessary and treatment should be discontinued if intracranial hypertension recurs.

Slipped capital femoral epiphysis is often associated with endocrine disorders such as GHD and hypothyroidism, and with growth spurts. In children treated with growth hormone, slipped capital femoral epiphysis may either be due to underlying endocrine disorders or to the increased growth velocity caused by the treatment. Growth spurts may increase the risk of joint-related problems, the hip joint being under particular strain during the prepubertal growth spurt. Physicians and parents should be alert to the development of a limp or complaints of hip or knee pain in children treated with Saizen.

Patients with growth failure due to chronic renal failure should be examined periodically for evidence of progression of renal osteodystrophy. Slipped capitalfemoral epiphysis or avascular necrosis of the femoral head may be seen in children with advanced renal osteodystrophy and it is uncertain whether these problems are affected by growth hormone therapy. X-rays of the hip should be obtained prior to initiating therapy.

In children with chronic renal failure, renal function should have decreased to below 50% of normal before therapy is instituted. To verify the growth disturbance, growth should have been followed for a year before institution of therapy. Conservative treatment for renal insufficiency (which includes control of acidosis, hyperparathyroidism and nutritional status for one year prior to the treatment) should have been established and should be maintained during treatment. Treatment should be discontinued at the time of renal transplantation.

In short children born SGA other medical reasons or treatments that could explain growth disturbance should be ruled out before starting treatment.

For SGA patients it is recommended to measure fasting insulin and blood glucose before start of treatment and annually thereafter. In patients with increased risk for diabetes mellitus (e.g. familial history of diabetes, obesity, increased body mass index, severe insulin resistance, acanthosis nigricans) oral glucose tolerance testing (OGTT) should be performed. If overt diabetes occurs, growth hormone should not be administered.

For SGA patients it is recommended to measure IGF-I level before start of treatment and twice a year thereafter. If on repeated measurements IGF-I levels exceed +2 SD compared to references for age and pubertal status, the IGF-I/IGFBP-3 ratio could be taken into account to consider dose adjustment.

Experience in initiating treatment in SGA patients near onset of puberty is limited. It is therefore not recommended to initiate treatment near onset of puberty. Experience with SGA patients with Silver-Russel syndrome is limited.

Some of the height gain obtained with treating short children born SGA with Somatropin may be lost if treatment is stopped before final height is reached.

The injection site should be varied to prevent lipoatrophy.

Growth Hormone Deficiency in the Adult is a lifelong condition and should be treated accordingly, however experience with patients over sixty years and experience with prolonged treatment is limited.

In all patients developing acute critical illness, the possible benefit of treatment with somatropin must be weighed against the potential risk involved.

Cases of sleep apnoea and sudden death in patients with Prader-Willi-Syndrome under treatment with Somatropin have been reported. Saizen is not indicated for the treatment of patients with Prader-Willi-Syndrome.

4.5 Interaction with other medicinal products and other forms of interaction

Concomitant corticosteroid therapy may inhibit the response to Saizen.

Somatropin has been reported to induce a modest reduction of serum cortisol levels in GH deficient patients receiving adrenal substitution treatment. Therefore, it is recommended to monitor serum cortisol levels in patients on corticosteroid replacement therapy in whom Somatropin therapy is started and adjust the dose of corticosteroids if necessary.

Published in vitro data indicate that growth hormone may be an inducer of cytochrome P450 3A4. The clinical significance of this observation is unknown. However, when Somatropin is administered in combination with drugs known to be metabolised by CYP P450 3A4 hepatic enzymes, it is advisable to monitor the clinical effectiveness of such drugs.

4.6 Pregnancy and lactation

Pregnancy: For Saizen no clinical data on exposed pregnancies are available. Thus, the risk for humans is unknown. Although animal studies do not point to a potential risk during pregnancy, Saizen should be discontinued if pregnancy occurs.

Lactation: It is not known if exogenous peptide hormones are excreted into breast milk but absorption of intact protein from the gastrointestinal tract of the infant is unlikely.

4.7 Effects on ability to drive and use machines

Saizen does not interfere with the patient's ability to drive or use machinery.

4.8 Undesirable effects

Up to 10 % of patients may experience redness and itching at the site of injection, particularly when the subcutaneous route is used.

Fluid retention is expected during growth hormone replacement therapy in adults. Oedema, joint swelling, arthralgias, myalgias and paresthesias may be clinical manifestations of fluid retention. However, these symptoms / signs are usually transient and dose dependent.

Adult patients with growth hormone deficiency, following diagnosis of growth hormone deficiency in childhood, reported side-effects less frequently than those with adult onset growth hormone deficiency.

Antibodies to Somatropin can form in some patients; the clinical significance of these antibodies is unknown, though to date the antibodies have been of low binding capacity and have not been associated with growth attenuation except in patients with gene deletions. In very rare instances, where short stature is due to deletion of the growth hormone gene complex, treatment with growth hormone may induce growth attenuating antibodies.

The adverse reactions reported below are classified according to frequency of occurrence as follows:

Very Common	⩾ 1/10
Common	> 1/100 - < 1/10
Uncommon	> 1/1000 - < 1/100
Rare	> 1/10000 - < 1/1000
Very rare	⩽ 1/10000

Application site disorders

Common

Injection site reactions

Localized lipoatrophy, which can be avoided by varying the site of injection

Body as a whole – General disorders

Common (in adults) ***Uncommon*** (in children)

Fluid retention: peripheral oedema, stiffness, arthralgia, myalgia, paresthesia.

Uncommon

Carpal tunnel syndrome

CNS

Uncommon

Idiopathic intracranial hypertension (benign intracranial hypertension)

Endocrine Disorders

Very rare

Hypothyroidism

Musculo-skeletal disorders

Very rare

Slipped capital femoral epiphysis (Epiphysiolysis capitis femoris), or avascular necrosis of the femoral head

Metabolism disorders

Insulin resistance can result in hyperinsulinism and in rare cases in hyperglycemia.

4.9 Overdose

No cases of acute overdosage have been reported. However, exceeding the recommended doses can cause side effects. Overdosage can lead to hypoglycaemia and subsequently to hyperglycaemia. Moreover, Somatropin overdose is likely to cause manifestations of fluid retention.

5. PHARMACOLOGICAL PROPERTIES

5.1 Pharmacodynamic properties

Pharmaco-therapeutic group: Anterior pituitary lobe hormones and analogues, ATC code: HO1A.

Saizen contains recombinant human growth hormone produced by genetically engineered mammalian cells.

It is a peptide of 191 amino acids identical to human pituitary growth hormone with respect to aminoacid sequence and composition as well as peptide map, isoelectric point, molecular weight, isomeric structure and bioactivity.

Growth hormone is synthesised in a transformed murine cell line that has been modified by the addition of the gene for pituitary growth hormone.

Saizen is an anabolic and anticatabolic agent which exerts effects not only on growth but also on body composition and metabolism. It interacts with specific receptors on a variety of cell types including myocytes, hepatocytes, adipocytes, lymphocytes and hematopoietic cells. Some, but not all of its effects are mediated through another class of hormones known as somatomedins (IGF-1 and IGF-2).

Depending on the dose, the administration of Saizen elicits a rise in IGF-1, IGFBP-3, non-esterified fatty acids and glycerol, a decrease in blood urea, and decreases in urinary nitrogen, sodium and potassium excretion. The duration of the increase in GH levels may play a role in determining the magnitude of the effects. A relative saturation of the effects of Saizen at high doses is probable. This is not the case for glycemia and urinary C-peptide excretion, which are significantly elevated only after high doses (20 mg).

In a randomised clinical trial, three years treatment of prepubertal short children born SGA with a dose of 0.067 mg/kg/day resulted in a mean gain of +1.8 height-SDS. In those children who did not receive treatment beyond 3 years, part of the treatment benefit was lost, but the patients retained a significant gain of +0.7 height-SDS at final height ($p<0.01$ compared to baseline). Patients who received a second treatment course after a variable period of observation experienced a total gain of +1.3 height-SDS (p=0.001 compared to baseline) at final height. (The mean cumulative treatment duration in the latter group was 6.1 years). The gain in height-SDS (+1.3 ± 1.1) at final height in this group was significantly ($p<0.05$) different from the gain in height-SDS obtained in the first group (+0.7±0.8) that received only 3.0 years of treatment on average.

A second clinical trial investigated two different dose regimens over four years. One group was treated with 0.067 mg/kg/day for 2 years and then observed without treatment for 2 years. The second group received 0.067mg/kg/day in the first and third year and no treatment in the second and fourth year. Either treatment regimen resulted in a cumulative administered dose of 0.033/mg/kg/day over the four-year study period. Both groups showed a comparable acceleration of growth and a significant improvement of +1.55 ($p<0.0001$) and + 1.43 ($p<0.0001$) height-SDS respectively at the end of the four year study period. Long-term safety data are still limited.

5.2 Pharmacokinetic properties

The pharmacokinetics of Saizen are linear at least up to doses of 8 IU (2.67 mg). At higher doses (60 IU/20 mg) some degree of non-linearity cannot be ruled out, however with no clinical relevance.

Following IV administration in healthy volunteers the volume of distribution at steady-state is around 7 L, total metabolic clearance is around 15 L/h while the renal clearance is negligible, and the drug exhibits an elimination half-life of 20 to 35 min.

Following single-dose SC and IM administration of Saizen, the apparent terminal half-life is much longer, around 2 to 4 hours. This is due to a rate limiting absorption process.

Maximum serum growth hormone (GH) concentrations are reached after approximately 4 hours and serum GH levels return to baseline within 24 hours, indicating that no accumulation of GH will occur during repeated administrations.

The absolute bioavailability of both routes is 70-90 %.

5.3 Preclinical safety data

Preclinical data reveal no special hazard for humans based on conventional studies of safety pharmacology, repeated dose toxicity and genotoxicity. Reproductive toxicology studies do not indicate any adverse effect on fertility and reproduction, despite administration of doses sufficiently high to produce some pharmacological effects on growth.

6. PHARMACEUTICAL PARTICULARS

6.1 List of excipients

Powder for solution for injection

Mannitol, Disodium phosphate dihydrate, Sodium dihydrogen phosphate monohydrate, Sodium Chloride

Solvent for parenteral use

0.9 % w/v sodium chloride in water for injections

6.2 Incompatibilities

No incompatibilities of Saizen with other pharmaceutical preparations are known at present.

6.3 Shelf life

2 years.

After reconstitution: Immediate use is recommended. However, in use stability has been demonstrated up to 24 hours in a refrigerator (2°C to 8°C).

6.4 Special precautions for storage

Store in a refrigerator (2°C to 8°C) in the original package.

Store the reconstituted product in a refrigerator (2°C to 8°C) in the original package.

Do not freeze.

6.5 Nature and contents of container

The 5 ml vials of SAIZEN® 1.33 mg and the 2 ml ampoules containing 1 ml of the solvent are of neutral glass (Type I). The vials are closed by rubber stoppers.

SAIZEN® 1.33 mg is available in the following pack sizes:

1 vial of SAIZEN® 1.33 mg product and 1 ampoule of solvent

5 vials of SAIZEN® 1.33 mg product and 5 ampoules of solvent.

10 vials of SAIZEN® 1.33 mg product and 10 ampoules of solvent.

Not all pack sizes may be marketed.

6.6 Special precautions for disposal and other handling

Reconstitution:

The powder for solution for injection should be used with the enclosed solvent for parenteral use. The reconstituted solution for injection should be clear with no particles. If the solution contains particles, it must not be injected.

Use with a syringe:

To reconstitute SAIZEN®, inject 0.5 – 1 ml of the solvent into the vial of SAIZEN® 1.33 mg aiming the liquid against the glass wall. Swirl the vial with a GENTLE rotary motion until the content is dissolved completely. Avoid vigorous shaking.

Discard any unused solvent.

7. MARKETING AUTHORISATION HOLDER
Serono Ltd.

Bedfont Cross, Stanwell Road

Feltham, Middlesex.

TW14 8NX

Telephone: +44(0)20 8818 7200

8. MARKETING AUTHORISATION NUMBER(S)
Product Licence Numbers

Saizen 1.33 mg PL 03400/0023

Sodium chloride injection PL 03400/0024

9. DATE OF FIRST AUTHORISATION/RENEWAL OF THE AUTHORISATION
First Authorised in UK: 10 November 1989

Renewed:19 April 2005

10. DATE OF REVISION OF THE TEXT
April 2005

LEGAL STATUS
POM

Saizen 3.33mg

(Merck Serono)

1. NAME OF THE MEDICINAL PRODUCT
Saizen® 3.33 mg powder and solvent for solution for injection

2. QUALITATIVE AND QUANTITATIVE COMPOSITION
Each vial of Saizen 3.33 mg contains Somatropin* (recombinant human growth hormone).

*produced by recombinant DNA technology in mammalian cells

For excipients, see section 6.1.

3. PHARMACEUTICAL FORM
Powder and solvent for solution for injection.

White lyophilised powder and clear, colourless solvent.

4. CLINICAL PARTICULARS

4.1 Therapeutic indications
Saizen is indicated in the treatment of:

• growth failure in children caused by decreased or absent secretion of endogenous growth hormone.

• growth failure in girls with gonadal dysgenesis (Turner Syndrome), confirmed by chromosomal analysis.

• growth failure in prepubertal children due to chronic renal failure (CRF).

• growth disturbance (current height SDS $<$ -2.5 and parental adjusted height SDS $<$ -1) in short children born small for gestational age (SGA) with a birth weight and/or length below – 2 SD, who failed to show catch-up growth (HV SDS $<$ 0 during the last year) by 4 years of age or later.

• replacement therapy in adults with pronounced growth hormone deficiency as diagnosed by a single dynamic test for growth hormone deficiency. Patients must also fulfil the following criteria:

Childhood Onset:

Patients who were diagnosed as growth hormone deficient during childhood, must be retested and their growth hormone deficiency confirmed before replacement therapy with Saizen is started.

Adult Onset:

Patients must have growth hormone deficiency as a result of hypothalamic or pituitary disease and at least one other hormone deficiency diagnosed (except for prolactin) and adequate replacement therapy instituted, before replacement therapy using growth hormone may begin.

4.2 Posology and method of administration
Saizen 3.33 mg is intended for multiple dose use.

Saizen dosage should be individualised for each patient based on body surface area (BSA) or on body weight (BW).

It is recommended that Saizen be administered at bedtime according to the following dosage:

Growth failure due to inadequate endogenous growth hormone secretion:

0.7-1.0 mg/m^2 body surface area (BSA) per day or 0.025-0.035 mg/kg body weight (BW) per day by subcutaneous or intramuscular administration.

Growth failure in girls due to gonadal dysgenesis (Turner Syndrome)

1.4 mg/m^2 body surface area (BSA) per day or 0.045-0.050 mg/kg body weight (BW) per day by subcutaneous administration.

Concomitant therapy with non-androgenic anabolic steroids in patients with Turner Syndrome can enhance the growth response.

Growth failure in prepubertal children due to chronic renal failure (CRF):

1.4 mg/m^2 body surface area (BSA), approximately equal to 0.045-0.050 mg/kg body weight (BW), per day by subcutaneous administration.

Growth failure in short children born small for gestational age (SGA):

The recommended daily dose is 0.035 mg/kg body weight (or 1 mg/m^2/day, equal to 0.1 IU/kg/day or 3 IU/m^2/day) per day, by subcutaneous administration.

Duration of treatment

Treatment should be discontinued when the patient has reached a satisfactory adult height, or the epiphyses are fused.

For growth disturbance in short children born SGA, treatment is usually recommended until final height is reached. Treatment should be discontinued after the first year if height velocity SDS is below +1. Treatment should be discontinued when final height is reached (defined as height velocity $<$ 2 cm/year), and if confirmation is required if bone age is $>$ 14 years (girls) or $>$ 16 years (boys), corresponding to closure of the epiphyseal growth plates.

Growth Hormone Deficiency in adults:

At the start of somatropin therapy, low doses of 0.15-0.3mg are recommended, given as a daily subcutaneous injection. The dose should be adjusted stepwise, controlled by Insulin-like Growth Factor 1 (IGF-1) values. The recommended final GH dose seldom exceeds 1.0mg/day. In general the lowest efficacious dose should be administered. In older or overweight patients, lower doses may be necessary.

4.3 Contraindications
Saizen should not be used in children in whom epiphyseal fusion occurred.

Saizen is contraindicated in patients known to be hypersensitive to Somatropin and any of the excipients in the powder for solution for injection or the solvent.

Saizen is contraindicated in patients with active neoplasia. Any anti-tumor therapy must be completed prior to starting treatment with Somatropin.

Saizen should not be used in cases with evidence of any progression or recurrence of an underlying intra-cranial lesion.

Patients with acute critical illness suffering complications following open heart surgery, abdominal surgery, multiple accidental trauma, acute respiratory failure or similar conditions should not be treated with Somatropin. (Regarding patients undergoing Somatropin therapy and becoming critically ill, see 4.4 "Special warnings and special precautions for use".)

4.4 Special warnings and precautions for use
Treatment should be carried out under the regular guidance of a physician who is experienced in the diagnosis and management of patients with growth hormone deficiency.

Patients with an intra or extracranial neoplasia in remission who are receiving treatment with growth hormone should be examined carefully and at regular intervals by the physician.

Patients with growth hormone deficiency secondary to an intracranial tumour should be examined frequently for progression or recurrence of the underlying disease process.

Some cases of leukaemia have been reported in growth hormone deficient children, untreated as well as treated with growth hormone, and might possibly represent a slightly increased incidence compared with non-growth hormone deficient children. A causal relationship to growth hormone therapy has not been established.

Growth Hormone administration is followed by a transient phase of hypoglycemia of approximately 2 hours, then from 2-4 hours onward by an increase in blood glucose levels despite high insulin concentrations. Somatropin may induce a state of insulin resistance which can result in hyperinsulinism and in some patients hyperglycemia. To detect insulin resistance, patients should be monitored for evidence of glucose intolerance.

Saizen should be used with caution in patients with diabetes mellitus or with a family history of diabetes mellitus. Patients with diabetes mellitus may require adjustment of their antidiabetic therapy.

Stable background retinopathy should not lead to discontinuation of Somatropin replacement therapy. In case of development of preproliferative changes and the presence of proliferative retinopathy Somatropin replacement therapy should be discontinued.

During treatment with Somatropin an enhanced T4 to T3 conversion has been found which may result in a reduction in serum T4 and an increase in serum T3 concentrations. In general, the peripheral thyroid hormone levels have remained within the reference ranges for healthy subjects. The effects of Somatropin on thyroid hormone levels may be of clinical relevance in patients with central subclinical hypothyroidism in whom overt hypothyroidism theoretically may develop. Conversely, in patients receiving replacement therapy with thyroxine mild hyperthyroidism may occur. It is therefore particularly advisable to test thyroid function after starting treatment with Somatropin and after dose adjustments.

Fluid retention is expected during growth hormone replacement therapy in adults.

In case of persistent oedema or severe paraesthesia the dosage should be decreased in order to avoid the development of carpal tunnel syndrome.

In case of severe or recurrent headache, visual problems, nausea and/or vomiting, funduscopy for papilloedema is recommended. If papilloedema is confirmed a diagnosis of benign intracranial hypertension (or pseudotumor cerebri) should be considered and Saizen treatment should be discontinued. At present there is insufficient evidence to guide clinical decision-making in patients with resolved intracranial hypertension. If growth hormone treatment is restarted, careful monitoring for symptoms of intracranial hypertension is necessary and treatment should be discontinued if intracranial hypertension recurs.

Slipped capital femoral epiphysis is often associated with endocrine disorders such as GHD and hypothyroidism, and with growth spurts. In children treated with growth hormone, slipped capital femoral epiphysis may either be due to underlying endocrine disorders or to the increased growth velocity caused by the treatment. Growth spurts may increase the risk of joint-related problems, the hip joint being under particular strain during the prepubertal growth spurt. Physicians and parents should be alert to the development of a limp or complaints of hip or knee pain in children treated with Saizen.

Patients with growth failure due to chronic renal failure should be examined periodically for evidence of progression of renal osteodystrophy. Slipped capitalfemoral epiphysis or avascular necrosis of the femoral head may be seen in children with advanced renal osteodystrophy and it is uncertain whether these problems are affected by growth hormone therapy. X-rays of the hip should be obtained prior to initiating therapy.

In children with chronic renal failure, renal function should have decreased to below 50% of normal before therapy is instituted. To verify the growth disturbance, growth should have been followed for a year before institution of therapy. Conservative treatment for renal insufficiency (which includes control of acidosis, hyperparathyroidism and nutritional status for one year prior to the treatment) should have been established and should be maintained during treatment. Treatment should be discontinued at the time of renal transplantation.

In short children born SGA other medical reasons or treatments that could explain growth disturbance should be ruled out before starting treatment.

For SGA patients it is recommended to measure fasting insulin and blood glucose before start of treatment and annually thereafter. In patients with increased risk for diabetes mellitus (e.g. familial history of diabetes, obesity, increased body mass index, severe insulin resistance, acanthosis nigricans) oral glucose tolerance testing (OGTT) should be performed. If overt diabetes occurs, growth hormone should not be administered.

For SGA patients it is recommended to measure IGF-I level before start of treatment and twice a year thereafter. If on repeated measurements IGF-I levels exceed +2 SD compared to references for age and pubertal status, the IGF-I/IGFBP-3 ratio could be taken into account to consider dose adjustment.

Experience in initiating treatment in SGA patients near onset of puberty is limited. It is therefore not recommended to initiate treatment near onset of puberty. Experience with SGA patients with Silver-Russel syndrome is limited.

Some of the height gain obtained with treating short children born SGA with Somatropin may be lost if treatment is stopped before final height is reached.

The injection site should be varied to prevent lipoatrophy.

Benzyl alcohol as a preservative in bacteriostatic sodium chloride solution may cause toxic reactions and anaphylactoid reactions in infants and children up to 3 years old and must not be given to premature babies or neonates. Saizen may be reconstituted with Sodium Chloride Injection BP or Sterile Water for Injections for immediate use when administering to children under 3 years of age.

Growth Hormone Deficiency in the Adult is a lifelong condition and should be treated accordingly, however experience with patients over sixty years and experience with prolonged treatment is limited

In all patients developing acute critical illness, the possible benefit of treatment with somatropin must be weighed against the potential risk involved.

Cases of sleep apnoea and sudden death in patients with Prader-Willi-Syndrome under treatment with Somatropin have been reported. Saizen is not indicated for the treatment of patients with Prader-Willi-Syndrome.

4.5 Interaction with other medicinal products and other forms of interaction
Concomitant corticosteroid therapy may inhibit the response to Saizen.

Somatropin has been reported to induce a modest reduction of serum cortisol levels in GH deficient patients receiving adrenal substitution treatment. Therefore, it is recommended to monitor serum cortisol levels in patients on corticosteroid replacement therapy in whom Somatropin therapy is started and adjust the dose of corticosteroids if necessary.

Published in vitro data indicate that growth hormone may be an inducer of cytochrome P450 3A4. The clinical significance of this observation is unknown. However, when Somatropin is administered in combination with drugs known to be metabolised by CYP P450 3A4 hepatic enzymes, it is advisable to monitor the clinical effectiveness of such drugs.

4.6 Pregnancy and lactation

Pregnancy: For Saizen no clinical data on exposed pregnancies are available. Thus, the risk for humans is unknown. Although animal studies do not point to a potential risk during pregnancy, Saizen should be discontinued if pregnancy occurs.

Lactation: It is not known if exogenous peptide hormones are excreted into breast milk but absorption of intact protein from the gastrointestinal tract of the infant is unlikely.

4.7 Effects on ability to drive and use machines

Saizen does not interfere with the patient's ability to drive or use machinery.

4.8 Undesirable effects

Up to 10 % of patients may experience redness and itching at the site of injection, particularly when the subcutaneous route is used.

Fluid retention is expected during growth hormone replacement therapy in adults. Oedema, joint swelling, arthralgias, myalgias and paresthesias may be clinical manifestations of fluid retention. However, these symptoms / signs are usually transient and dose dependent.

Adult patients with growth hormone deficiency, following diagnosis of growth hormone deficiency in childhood, reported side-effects less frequently than those with adult onset growth hormone deficiency.

Antibodies to Somatropin can form in some patients; the clinical significance of these antibodies is unknown, though to date the antibodies have been of low binding capacity and have not been associated with growth attenuation except in patients with gene deletions. In very rare instances, where short stature is due to deletion of the growth hormone gene complex, treatment with growth hormone may induce growth attenuating antibodies.

The adverse reactions reported below are classified according to frequency of occurrence as follows:

Very Common	⩾ 1/10
Common	> 1/100 - < 1/10
Uncommon	> 1/1000 - < 1/100
Rare	> 1/10000 - < 1/1000
Very rare	⩽ 1/10000

Application site disorders

Common

Injection site reactions

Localized lipoatrophy, which can be avoided by varying the site of injection

Body as a whole – General disorders

Common (in adults) ***Uncommon*** (in children)

Fluid retention: peripheral oedema, stiffness, arthralgia, myalgia, paresthesia.

Uncommon

Carpal tunnel syndrome

CNS

Uncommon

Idiopathic intracranial hypertension (benign intracranial hypertension)

Endocrine Disorders

Very rare

Hypothyroidism

Musculo-skeletal disorders

Very rare

Slipped capital femoral epiphysis (Epiphysiolysis capitis femoris), or avascular necrosis of the femoral head

Metabolism disorders

Insulin resistance can result in hyperinsulinism and in rare cases in hyperglycemia.

4.9 Overdose

No cases of acute overdosage have been reported. However, exceeding the recommended doses can cause side effects. Overdosage can lead to hypoglycaemia and subsequently to hyperglycaemia. Moreover, Somatropin overdose is likely to cause manifestations of fluid retention.

5. PHARMACOLOGICAL PROPERTIES

5.1 Pharmacodynamic properties

Pharmaco-therapeutic group: Anterior pituitary lobe hormones and analogues, ATC code: HO1A.

Saizen contains recombinant human growth hormone produced by genetically engineered mammalian cells.

It is a peptide of 191 amino acids identical to human pituitary growth hormone with respect to aminoacid sequence and composition as well as peptide map, isoelectric point, molecular weight, isomeric structure and bioactivity.

Growth hormone is synthesised in a transformed murine cell line that has been modified by the addition of the gene for pituitary growth hormone.

Saizen is an anabolic and anticatabolic agent, which exerts effects not only on growth but also on body composition and metabolism. It interacts with specific receptors on a variety of cell types including myocytes, hepatocytes, adipocytes, lymphocytes and hematopoietic cells. Some, but not all of its effects are mediated through another class of hormones known as somatomedins (IGF-1 and IGF-2).

Depending on the dose, the administration of Saizen elicits a rise in IGF-1, IGFBP-3, non-esterified fatty acids and glycerol, a decrease in blood urea, and decreases in urinary nitrogen, sodium and potassium excretion. The duration of the increase in GH levels may play a role in determining the magnitude of the effects. A relative saturation of the effects of Saizen at high doses is probable. This is not the case for glycemia and urinary C-peptide excretion, which are significantly elevated only after high doses (20 mg).

In a randomised clinical trial, three years treatment of prepubertal short children born SGA with a dose of 0.067 mg/kg/day resulted in a mean gain of +1.8 height-SDS. In those children who did not receive treatment beyond 3 years, part of the treatment benefit was lost, but the patients retained a significant gain of +0.7 height-SDS at final height ($p < 0.01$ compared to baseline). Patients who received a second treatment course after a variable period of observation experienced a total gain of +1.3 height-SDS (p=0.001 compared to baseline) at final height. (The mean cumulative treatment duration in the latter group was 6.1 years). The gain in height-SDS (+1.3 ± 1.1) at final height in this group was significantly ($p < 0.05$) different from the gain in height-SDS obtained in the first group (+0.7±0.8) that received only 3.0 years of treatment on average.

A second clinical trial investigated two different dose regimens over four years. One group was treated with 0.067 mg/kg/day for 2 years and then observed without treatment for 2 years. The second group received 0.067mg/kg/day in the first and third year and no treatment in the second and fourth year. Either treatment regimen resulted in a cumulative administered dose of 0.033/mg/kg/day over the four-year study period. Both groups showed a comparable acceleration of growth and a significant improvement of +1.55 ($p < 0.0001$) and + 1.43 ($p < 0.0001$) height-SDS respectively at the end of the four year study period. Long-term safety data are still limited.

5.2 Pharmacokinetic properties

The pharmacokinetics of Saizen are linear at least up to doses of 8 IU (2.67 mg). At higher doses (60 IU/20 mg) some degree of non-linearity cannot be ruled out, however with no clinical relevance.

Following IV administration in healthy volunteers the volume of distribution at steady-state is around 7 L, total metabolic clearance is around 15 L/h while the renal clearance is negligible, and the drug exhibits an elimination half-life of 20 to 35 min.

Following single-dose SC and IM administration of Saizen, the apparent terminal half-life is much longer, around 2 to 4 hours. This is due to a rate limiting absorption process.

Maximum serum growth hormone (GH) concentrations are reached after approximately 4 hours and serum GH levels return to baseline within 24 hours, indicating that no accumulation of GH will occur during repeated administrations.

The absolute bioavailability of both routes is 70-90 %.

5.3 Preclinical safety data

Preclinical data reveal no special hazard for humans based on conventional studies of safety pharmacology, repeated dose toxicity and genotoxicity. Reproductive toxicology studies do not indicate any adverse effect on fertility and reproduction, despite administration of doses sufficiently high to produce some pharmacological effects on growth.

6. PHARMACEUTICAL PARTICULARS

6.1 List of excipients

Powder for solution for injection

Mannitol, Disodium phosphate dihydrate, Sodium dihydrogen phosphate monohydrate

Solvent for parenteral use

0.9 % w/v sodium chloride in water for injections and 0.9 % w/v benzyl alcohol

6.2 Incompatibilities

No incompatibilities of Saizen with other pharmaceutical preparations are known at present.

6.3 Shelf life

2 years.

After reconstitution, the product may be stored for a maximum of 7 days in a refrigerator (2°C to 8°C).

6.4 Special precautions for storage

Store in a refrigerator (2°C to 8°C) in the original package.

Store the reconstituted product in a refrigerator (2°C to 8°C) in the original package.

Do not freeze.

6.5 Nature and contents of container

The 10 ml vials containing 3.33 mg of powder and the 5 ml vials containing 5 ml of solvent are of neutral glass (Type I). The vials are closed by rubber stoppers.

Saizen 3.33 mg is available in the following pack sizes:

1 vial of Saizen 3.33 mg product and 1 vial of bacteriostatic solvent.

5 vials of Saizen 3.33 mg product and 5 vials of bacteriostatic solvent.

Not all pack sizes may be marketed.

6.6 Special precautions for disposal and other handling

Reconstitution:

The powder for solution for injection should be used with the enclosed solvent for parenteral use. The reconstituted solution for injection should be clear with no particles. If the solution contains particles, it must not be injected.

Use with a syringe:

To reconstitute Saizen, inject 1 ml of the bacteriostatic solvent into the vial of Saizen 3.33 mg aiming the liquid against the glass wall. Swirl the vial with a GENTLE rotary motion until the content is dissolved completely. Avoid vigorous shaking.

Discard any unused solvent.

7. MARKETING AUTHORISATION HOLDER

Serono Ltd.

Bedfont Cross, Stanwell Road

Feltham, Middlesex.

TW14 8NX

Telephone: +44(0)20 8818 7200

8. MARKETING AUTHORISATION NUMBER(S)

Product Licence Numbers

Saizen 3.33 mg PL 03400/0034

Bacteriostatic solvent PL 03400/0035

9. DATE OF FIRST AUTHORISATION/RENEWAL OF THE AUTHORISATION

First authorisation in UK: 27th August 1991

Renewed: 19 April 2005

10. DATE OF REVISION OF THE TEXT

April 2005

LEGAL STATUS

POM

Saizen 8mg click.easy

(Merck Serono)

1. NAME OF THE MEDICINAL PRODUCT

Saizen® 8 mg click.easy® powder and solvent for solution for injection

2. QUALITATIVE AND QUANTITATIVE COMPOSITION

Each vial of Saizen 8 mg click.easy contains Somatropin* (recombinant human growth hormone).

*produced by recombinant DNA technology in mammalian cells

Reconstitution with the contents of the bacteriostatic solvent cartridge gives a concentration of 5.83 mg per ml.

For excipients, see section 6.1.

3. PHARMACEUTICAL FORM

Powder and solvent for solution for injection.

White lyophilised powder and clear, colourless solvent

4. CLINICAL PARTICULARS

4.1 Therapeutic indications

Saizen is indicated in the treatment of:

- growth failure in children caused by decreased or absent secretion of endogenous growth hormone.
- growth failure in girls with gonadal dysgenesis (Turner Syndrome), confirmed by chromosomal analysis.
- growth failure in prepubertal children due to chronic renal failure (CRF).
- growth disturbance (current height SDS < -2.5 and parental adjusted height SDS < -1) in short children born small for gestational age (SGA) with a birth weight and/or length below – 2 SD, who failed to show catch-up growth (HV SDS < 0 during the last year) by 4 years of age or later.
- replacement therapy in adults with pronounced growth hormone deficiency as diagnosed by a single dynamic test for growth hormone deficiency. Patients must also fulfil the following criteria:

Childhood Onset:

Patients who were diagnosed as growth hormone deficient during childhood, must be retested and their growth hormone deficiency confirmed before replacement therapy with Saizen is started.

Adult Onset:

Patients must have growth hormone deficiency as a result of hypothalamic or pituitary disease and at least one other hormone deficiency diagnosed (except for prolactin) and adequate replacement therapy instituted, before replacement therapy using growth hormone may begin.

4.2 Posology and method of administration

Saizen 8 mg click.easy is intended for multiple dose use.

Saizen dosage should be individualised for each patient based on body surface area (BSA) or on body weight (BW).

It is recommended that Saizen be administered at bedtime according to the following dosage:

Growth failure due to inadequate endogenous growth hormone secretion:

0.7-1.0 mg/m2 body surface area (BSA) per day or 0.025-0.035 mg/kg body weight (BW) per day by subcutaneous administration.

Growth failure in girls due to gonadal dysgenesis (Turner Syndrome):

1.4 mg/m2 body surface area (BSA) per day or 0.045-0.050 mg/kg body weight (BW) per day by subcutaneous administration.

Concomitant therapy with non-androgenic anabolic steroids in patients with Turner Syndrome can enhance the growth response.

Growth failure in prepubertal children due to chronic renal failure (CRF):

1.4 mg/m2 body surface area (BSA), approximately equal to 0.045-0.050 mg/kg body weight (BW), per day by subcutaneous administration.

Growth failure in short children born small for gestational age (SGA):

The recommended daily dose is 0.035 mg/kg body weight (or 1 mg/m2/day, equal to 0.1 IU/kg/day or 3 IU/m2/day) per day, by subcutaneous administration.

Duration of treatment

Treatment should be discontinued when the patient has reached a satisfactory adult height, or the epiphyses are fused.

For growth disturbance in short children born SGA, treatment is usually recommended until final height is reached. Treatment should be discontinued after the first year if height velocity SDS is below +1. Treatment should be discontinued when final height is reached (defined as height velocity < 2 cm/year), and if confirmation is required if bone age is > 14 years (girls) or > 16 years (boys), corresponding to closure of the epiphyseal growth plates.

Growth Hormone Deficiency in adults

At the start of somatropin therapy, low doses of 0.15-0.3mg are recommended, given as a daily subcutaneous injection. The dose should be adjusted stepwise, controlled by Insulin-like Growth Factor 1 (IGF-1) values. The recommended final GH dose seldom exceeds 1.0mg/day. In general the lowest efficacious dose should be administered. In older or overweight patients, lower doses may be necessary.

Method of administration

For administration of the reconstituted solution for injection of Saizen 8 mg click.easy, follow the instructions given in the package leaflet and in the instruction manual provided with the selected auto-injector: one.click auto-injector, cool.click needle-free auto-injector or easypod auto-injector. See also section 6.6 for instructions for use/handling.

4.3 Contraindications

Saizen should not be used in children in whom epiphyseal fusion occurred.

Saizen is contraindicated in patients known to be hypersensitive to Somatropin and any of the excipients in the powder for solution for injection or the solvent.

Saizen is contraindicated in patients with active neoplasia. Any anti-tumor therapy must be completed prior to starting treatment with Somatropin.

Saizen should not be used in cases with evidence of any progression or recurrence of an underlying intra-cranial lesion.

Patients with acute critical illness suffering complications following open heart surgery, abdominal surgery, multiple accidental trauma, acute respiratory failure or similar conditions should not be treated with Somatropin. (Regarding patients undergoing Somatropin therapy and becoming critically ill, see 4.4 "Special warnings and special precautions for use".)

4.4 Special warnings and precautions for use

Treatment should be carried out under the regular guidance of a physician who is experienced in the diagnosis and management of patients with growth hormone deficiency.

Patients with an intra or extracranial neoplasia in remission who are receiving treatment with growth hormone should be examined carefully and at regular intervals by the physician.

Patients with growth hormone deficiency secondary to an intracranial tumour should be examined frequently for progression or recurrence of the underlying disease process.

Some cases of leukaemia have been reported in growth hormone deficient children, untreated as well as treated with growth hormone, and might possibly represent a slightly increased incidence compared with non-growth hormone deficient children. A causal relationship to growth hormone therapy has not been established.

Growth Hormone administration is followed by a transient phase of hypoglycemia of approximately 2 hours, then from 2-4 hours onward by an increase in blood glucose levels despite high insulin concentrations. Somatropin may induce a state of insulin resistance which can result in hyperinsulinism and in some patients in hyperglycemia. To detect insulin resistance, patients should be monitored for evidence of glucose intolerance.

Saizen should be used with caution in patients with diabetes mellitus or with a family history of diabetes mellitus. Patients with diabetes mellitus may require adjustment of their antidiabetic therapy.

Stable background retinopathy should not lead to discontinuation of Somatropin replacement therapy. In case of development of preproliferative changes and the presence of proliferative retinopathy Somatropin replacement therapy should be discontinued.

During treatment with Somatropin an enhanced T4 to T3 conversion has been found which may result in a reduction in serum T4 and an increase in serum T3 concentrations. In general, the peripheral thyroid hormone levels have remained within the reference ranges for healthy subjects. The effects of Somatropin on thyroid hormone levels may be of clinical relevance in patients with central subclinical hypothyroidism in whom overt hypothyroidism theoretically may develop. Conversely, in patients receiving replacement therapy with thyroxine mild hyperthyroidism may occur. It is therefore particularly advisable to test thyroid function after starting treatment with Somatropin and after dose adjustments.

Fluid retention is expected during growth hormone replacement therapy in adults.

In case of persistent oedema or severe paraesthesia the dosage should be decreased in order to avoid the development of carpal tunnel syndrome.

In case of severe or recurrent headache, visual problems, nausea and/or vomiting, funduscopy for papilloedema is recommended. If papilloedema is confirmed a diagnosis of benign intracranial hypertension (or pseudotumor cerebri) should be considered and Saizen treatment should be discontinued. At present there is insufficient evidence to guide clinical decision-making in patients with resolved intracranial hypertension. If growth hormone treatment is restarted, careful monitoring for symptoms of intracranial hypertension is necessary and treatment should be discontinued if intracranial hypertension recurs.

Slipped capital femoral epiphysis is often associated with endocrine disorders such as GHD and hypothyroidism, and with growth spurts. In children treated with growth hormone, slipped capital femoral epiphysis may either be due to underlying endocrine disorders or to the increased growth velocity caused by the treatment. Growth spurts may increase the risk of joint-related problems, the hip joint being under particular strain during the prepubertal growth spurt. Physicians and parents should be alert to the development of a limp or complaints of hip or knee pain in children treated with Saizen.

Patients with growth failure due to chronic renal failure should be examined periodically for evidence of progression of renal osteodystrophy. Slipped capital femoral epiphysis or avascular necrosis of the femoral head may be seen in children with advanced renal osteodystrophy and it is uncertain whether these problems are affected by growth hormone therapy. X-rays of the hip should be obtained prior to initiating therapy.

In children with chronic renal failure, renal function should have decreased to below 50% of normal before therapy is instituted. To verify the growth disturbance, growth should have been followed for a year before institution of therapy. Conservative treatment for renal insufficiency (which includes control of acidosis, hyperparathyroidism and nutritional status for one year prior to the treatment) should have been established and should be maintained during treatment. Treatment should be discontinued at the time of renal transplantation.

In short children born SGA other medical reasons or treatments that could explain growth disturbance should be ruled out before starting treatment.

For SGA patients it is recommended to measure fasting insulin and blood glucose before start of treatment and annually thereafter. In patients with increased risk for diabetes mellitus (e.g. familial history of diabetes, obesity, increased body mass index, severe insulin resistance, acanthosis nigricans) oral glucose tolerance testing (OGTT) should be performed. If overt diabetes occurs, growth hormone should not be administered.

For SGA patients it is recommended to measure IGF-I level before start of treatment and twice a year thereafter. If on repeated measurements IGF-I levels exceed +2 SD compared to references for age and pubertal status, the IGF-I/IGFBP-3 ratio could be taken into account to consider dose adjustment.

Experience in initiating treatment in SGA patients near onset of puberty is limited. It is therefore not recommended to initiate treatment near onset of puberty. Experience with SGA patients with Silver-Russel syndrome is limited.

Some of the height gain obtained with treating short children born SGA with Somatropin may be lost if treatment is stopped before final height is reached.

The injection site should be varied to prevent lipoatrophy.

Growth Hormone Deficiency in the Adult is a lifelong condition and should be treated accordingly, however experience with patients over sixty years and experience with prolonged treatment is limited.

In all patients developing acute critical illness, the possible benefit of treatment with somatropin must be weighed against the potential risk involved.

Cases of sleep apnoea and sudden death in patients with Prader-Willi-Syndrome under treatment with Somatropin have been reported. Saizen is not indicated for the treatment of patients with Prader-Willi-Syndrome.

4.5 Interaction with other medicinal products and other forms of interaction

Concomitant corticosteroid therapy may inhibit the response to Saizen.

Somatropin has been reported to induce a modest reduction of serum cortisol levels in GH deficient patients receiving adrenal substitution treatment. Therefore, it is recommended to monitor serum cortisol levels in patients on corticosteroid replacement therapy in whom Somatropin therapy is started and adjust the dose of corticosteroids if necessary.

Published in vitro data indicate that growth hormone may be an inducer of cytochrome P450 3A4. The clinical significance of this observation is unknown. However, when Somatropin is administered in combination with drugs known to be metabolised by CYP P450 3A4 hepatic enzymes, it is advisable to monitor the clinical effectiveness of such drugs.

4.6 Pregnancy and lactation

Pregnancy: For Saizen no clinical data on exposed pregnancies are available. Thus, the risk for humans is unknown. Although animal studies do not point to a potential risk during pregnancy, Saizen should be discontinued if pregnancy occurs.

Lactation: It is not known if exogenous peptide hormones are excreted into breast milk but absorption of intact protein from the gastrointestinal tract of the infant is unlikely.

4.7 Effects on ability to drive and use machines

Saizen does not interfere with the patient's ability to drive or use machinery.

4.8 Undesirable effects

Up to 10% of patients may experience redness and itching at the site of injection, particularly when the subcutaneous route is used.

Fluid retention is expected during growth hormone replacement therapy in adults. Oedema, joint swelling, arthralgias, myalgias and paresthesias may be clinical manifestations of fluid retention. However, these symptoms / signs are usually transient and dose dependent.

Adult patients with growth hormone deficiency, following diagnosis of growth hormone deficiency in childhood, reported side-effects less frequently than those with adult onset growth hormone deficiency.

Antibodies to Somatropin can form in some patients; the clinical significance of these antibodies is unknown, though to date the antibodies have been of low binding capacity and have not been associated with growth attenuation except in patients with gene deletions. In very rare instances, where short stature is due to deletion of the growth hormone gene complex, treatment with growth hormone may induce growth attenuating antibodies.

The adverse reactions reported below are classified according to frequency of occurrence as follows:

Very Common	≥ 1/10
Common	> 1/100 - < 1/10
Uncommon	> 1/1000 - < 1/100
Rare	> 1/10000 - < 1/1000
Very rare	≤ 1/10000

Application site disorders

Common

Injection site reactions

Localized lipoatrophy, which can be avoided by varying the site of injection

Body as a whole – General disorders

Common (in adults) ***Uncommon*** (in children)

Fluid retention: peripheral oedema, stiffness, arthralgia, myalgia, paresthesia.

Uncommon

Carpal tunnel syndrome

CNS

Uncommon

Idiopathic intracranial hypertension (benign intracranial hypertension)

Endocrine Disorders

Very rare

Hypothyroidism

Musculo-skeletal disorders

Very rare

Slipped capital femoral epiphysis (Epiphysiolysis capitis femoris)), or avascular necrosis of the femoral head

Metabolism disorders

Insulin resistance can result in hyperinsulinism and in rare cases in hyperglycemia.

4.9 Overdose

No cases of acute overdosage have been reported. However, exceeding the recommended doses can cause side effects. Overdosage can lead to hypoglycaemia and subsequently to hyperglycaemia. Moreover, Somatropin overdose is likely to cause manifestations of fluid retention.

5. PHARMACOLOGICAL PROPERTIES

5.1 Pharmacodynamic properties

Pharmaco-therapeutic group: Anterior pituitary lobe hormones and analogues, ATC code: HO1A.

Saizen contains recombinant human growth hormone produced by genetically engineered mammalian cells.

It is a peptide of 191 amino acids identical to human pituitary growth hormone with respect to aminoacid sequence and composition as well as peptide map, isoelectric point, molecular weight, isomeric structure and bioactivity.

Growth hormone is synthesised in a transformed murine cell line that has been modified by the addition of the gene for pituitary growth hormone.

Saizen is an anabolic and anticatabolic agent which exerts effects not only on growth but also on body composition and metabolism. It interacts with specific receptors on a variety of cell types including myocytes, hepatocytes, adipocytes, lymphocytes and hematopoietic cells. Some, but not all of its effects are mediated through another class of hormones known as somatomedins (IGF-1 and IGF-2).

Depending on the dose, the administration of Saizen elicits a rise in IGF-1, IGFBP-3, non-esterified fatty acids and glycerol, a decrease in blood urea, and decreases in urinary nitrogen, sodium and potassium excretion. The duration of the increase in GH levels may play a role in determining the magnitude of the effects. A relative saturation of the effects of Saizen at high doses is probable. This is not the case for glycemia and urinary C-peptide excretion, which are significantly elevated only after high doses (20 mg).

In a randomised clinical trial, three years treatment of prepubertal short children born SGA with a dose of 0.067 mg/kg/day resulted in a mean gain of +1.8 height-SDS. In those children who did not receive treatment beyond 3 years, part of the treatment benefit was lost, but the patients retained a significant gain of +0.7 height-SDS at final height ($p<0.01$ compared to baseline). Patients who received a second treatment course after a variable period of observation experienced a total gain of +1.3 height-SDS ($p=0.001$ compared to baseline) at final height. (The mean cumulative treatment duration in the latter group was 6.1 years). The gain in height-SDS ($+1.3 \pm 1.1$) at final height in this group was significantly ($p<0.05$) different from the gain in height-SDS obtained in the first group ($+0.7\pm0.8$) that received only 3.0 years of treatment on average.

A second clinical trial investigated two different dose regimens over four years. One group was treated with 0.067 mg/kg/day for 2 years and then observed without treatment for 2 years. The second group received 0.067mg/kg/day in the first and third year and no treatment in the second and fourth year. Either treatment regimen resulted in a cumulative administered dose of 0.033/mg/kg/day over the four-year study period. Both groups showed a comparable acceleration of growth and a significant improvement of +1.55 ($p<0.0001$) and + 1.43 ($p<0.0001$) height-SDS respectively at the end of the four year study period. Long-term safety data are still limited.

5.2 Pharmacokinetic properties

The pharmacokinetics of Saizen are linear at least up to doses of 8 IU (2.67 mg). At higher doses (60 IU/20 mg) some degree of non-linearity cannot be ruled out, however with no clinical relevance.

Following IV administration in healthy volunteers the volume of distribution at steady-state is around 7 L, total metabolic clearance is around 15 L/h while the renal clearance is negligible, and the drug exhibits an elimination half-life of 20 to 35 min.

Following single-dose SC and IM administration of Saizen, the apparent terminal half-life is much longer, around 2 to 4 hours. This is due to a rate limiting absorption process.

Maximum serum growth hormone (GH) concentrations are reached after approximately 4 hours and serum GH levels return to baseline within 24 hours, indicating that no accumulation of GH will occur during repeated administrations.

The absolute bioavailability of both routes is 70-90 %.

5.3 Preclinical safety data

The local tolerability of Saizen solutions containing 0.3% metacresol when injected in animals was considered good and found suitable for SC or IM administration.

Preclinical data reveal no special hazard for humans based on conventional studies of safety pharmacology, repeated dose toxicity and genotoxicity. Reproductive toxicology studies do not indicate any adverse effect on fertility and reproduction, despite administration of doses sufficiently high to produce some pharmacological effects on growth.

6. PHARMACEUTICAL PARTICULARS

6.1 List of excipients

Powder for solution for injection

Sucrose

Phosphoric acid

Sodium Hydroxide

Solvent for parenteral use

Metacresol 0.3% (w/v) in water for injections

6.2 Incompatibilities

No incompatibilities of Saizen with other pharmaceutical preparations are known at present.

6.3 Shelf life

3 years.

After reconstitution, the product may be stored for a maximum of 28 days in a refrigerator (2°C to 8°C).

When containing a cartridge of reconstituted Saizen, the easypod and one.click auto-injectors have to be stored in a refrigerator (2°C-8°C). When using the cool.click needle-free auto-injector, only the cartridge of reconstituted Saizen should be stored in a refrigerator (2°C-8°C).

6.4 Special precautions for storage

Do not store above 25°C. Do not freeze. Store in the original package.

For storage of the reconstituted product, see section 6.3.

6.5 Nature and contents of container

The DIN 2R 3 ml vials containing 8 mg of powder and the 3 ml cartridges containing 1.37 ml of solvent are of neutral glass (Type I). The vials and cartridges are closed by rubber stoppers.

Saizen 8 mg click.easy is available in the following pack sizes:

1 vial of Saizen 8 mg product and 1 cartridge of bacteriostatic solvent pre-assembled in 1 reconstitution device (click.easy) comprising of 1 device housing and 1 sterile transfer cannula.

5 vials of Saizen 8 mg product and 5 cartridges of bacteriostatic solvent pre-assembled in 5 reconstitution devices (click.easy) comprising each of 1 device housing and 1 sterile transfer cannula.

Not all pack sizes may be marketed.

6.6 Special precautions for disposal and other handling

The cartridge containing the reconstituted solution of Saizen 8 mg click.easy is for use only with the one.click auto-injector, the cool.click needle-free auto-injector, or the easypod auto-injector.

For storage of the auto-injectors containing the cartridge, see section 6.3.

For administration of Saizen 8 mg click.easy, follow the instructions given in the package leaflet and in the instruction manual provided with each appropriate auto-injector. Intended users of easypod are primarily children starting from the age of 7 up to adults. Use of the devices by children should always be made under adult's supervision.

The powder for solution for injection must be reconstituted with the enclosed bacteriostatic solvent (0.3% (w/v) metacresol in water for injections) for parenteral use, using the click.easy reconstitution device. The reconstituted solution for injection should be clear with no particles. If the solution contains particles, it must not be injected.

Any unused product or waste material should be disposed of in accordance with local requirements.

7. MARKETING AUTHORISATION HOLDER

Serono Ltd

Bedfont Cross, Stanwell Road

Feltham, Middlesex

TW14 8NX

Telephone: +44 (0)20 8818 7200

8. MARKETING AUTHORISATION NUMBER(S)

Product Licence Numbers

SAIZEN® 8 mg click.easy® PL 03400/0079

Bacteriostatic Solvent cartridge PL 03400/0076

9. DATE OF FIRST AUTHORISATION/RENEWAL OF THE AUTHORISATION

First authorisation in UK: 30th July 1998

Renewed: 19th April 2005

10. DATE OF REVISION OF THE TEXT

17th October 2006

LEGAL STATUS

POM

Salactol Collodion

(Dermal Laboratories Limited)

1. NAME OF THE MEDICINAL PRODUCT

SALACTOL™ COLLODION

2. QUALITATIVE AND QUANTITATIVE COMPOSITION

Salicylic Acid 16.7% w/w; Lactic Acid 16.7% w/w.

3. PHARMACEUTICAL FORM

Colourless or pale yellow/brown evaporative collodion paint.

4. CLINICAL PARTICULARS

4.1 Therapeutic indications

For the topical treatment of warts, verrucas, corns and calluses.

4.2 Posology and method of administration

For adults, children and the elderly. Salactol should be applied once daily usually at night. It can take up to twelve (12) weeks for resistant lesions to disappear, and it is necessary to persevere with the treatment. Soak the affected site in warm water and pat dry. Gently rub the surface of the wart, verruca, corn or callus with a pumice stone or manicure emery board to remove any hard skin. Using the applicator provided, carefully apply a few drops of Salactol to the lesion, allowing each drop to dry before applying the next one. Take care to localise the application to the affected area. Plantar warts should be covered with an adhesive plaster. Leave for 24 hours. Repeat the procedure daily, after first removing any plaster.

4.3 Contraindications

Not to be used on or near the face, intertriginous or anogenital regions or by diabetics or individuals with impaired peripheral blood circulation. Not to be used on moles, birthmarks, hairy warts or on any other skin lesions for which Salactol is not indicated. Not to be used in cases of sensitivity to any of the ingredients.

4.4 Special warnings and precautions for use

Keep away from the eyes and mucous membranes. The gel should be applied carefully to the wart, verruca, corn or callus only, to avoid possible irritation of surrounding normal skin. Some mild, transient irritation may be expected, but in cases of more severe or persistent pain/irritation, the treatment should be suspended and/or discontinued. See also Section 4.8. Extremely flammable. Avoid spillage. Avoid inhaling vapour. Replace cap tightly after use.

4.5 Interaction with other medicinal products and other forms of interaction

None known.

4.6 Pregnancy and lactation

No special precautions.

4.7 Effects on ability to drive and use machines

None known.

4.8 Undesirable effects

Salactol may be irritant in certain patients, which in rare instances may appear as a temporary blemish on the skin. See also Section 4.4.

4.9 Overdose

Any excessive use of Salactol could cause irritation of the skin. If this occurs, Salactol should be used more sparingly or applied less frequently. Accidental oral ingestion should be treated immediately by gastric lavage with a 2 to 5% aqueous sodium bicarbonate solution. Fluid and electrolyte balance should be monitored and appropriate supportive measures should be provided. Symptoms include headache, nausea, vomiting, diarrhoea and respiratory depression.

5. PHARMACOLOGICAL PROPERTIES

5.1 Pharmacodynamic properties

The combination of salicylic acid and lactic acid in flexible collodion has been shown to be particularly efficacious in treating warts, verrucas, corns and calluses.

Salicylic acid has bacteriostatic and fungicidal actions as well as keratolytic properties. Its effectiveness for topical treatment of hyperkeratotic skin lesions is based on mild keratolytic action which produces slow and painless destruction of the epithelium. In the treatment of warts, a mild irritant reaction, which may render the virus more prone to immunologic stimulation or response, may add to the mechanical removal of infected cells. Apart from its antiseptic and caustic properties, lactic acid enhances the availability of salicylic acid from the dried collodion.

5.2 Pharmacokinetic properties

Salactol contains 16.7% salicylic acid and 16.7% lactic acid in flexible collodion. The bioavailability of salicylic acid is reduced as the collodion film dries on the skin due to entrapment of the drug which inhibits release. The addition of lactic acid to salicylic acid collodion provides more efficient release of the salicylic acid, since the non-volatile lactic acid remains in the film, thus permitting continued release of the keratolytic which may otherwise be entrapped within the dried collodion film. Systemic absorption of salicylic acid or lactic acid after application to small circumscribed areas is exceedingly unlikely.

5.3 Preclinical safety data

No special information.

6. PHARMACEUTICAL PARTICULARS

6.1 List of excipients

Pyroxylin; Colophony; Castor Oil; IMS; Ether.

6.2 Incompatibilities

None known.

6.3 Shelf life
36 months.

6.4 Special precautions for storage
Do not store above 25°C.

6.5 Nature and contents of container
Amber glass bottle containing 10 ml, incorporating a specially designed spatula for ease of application. This is supplied as an original pack (OP).

6.6 Special precautions for disposal and other handling
Not applicable.

7. MARKETING AUTHORISATION HOLDER
Dermal Laboratories

Tatmore Place, Gosmore

Hitchin, Herts SG4 7QR, UK.

8. MARKETING AUTHORISATION NUMBER(S)
00173/5006R.

9. DATE OF FIRST AUTHORISATION/RENEWAL OF THE AUTHORISATION
2 May 2006.

10. DATE OF REVISION OF THE TEXT
April 2007.

Salatac Gel

(Dermal Laboratories Limited)

1. NAME OF THE MEDICINAL PRODUCT
SALATAC™ GEL

2. QUALITATIVE AND QUANTITATIVE COMPOSITION
Salicylic Acid 12.0% w/w; Lactic Acid 4.0% w/w.

3. PHARMACEUTICAL FORM
Clear, colourless, collodion-like wart gel.

4. CLINICAL PARTICULARS

4.1 Therapeutic indications
For the topical treatment of warts, verrucas, corns and calluses.

4.2 Posology and method of administration
For adults, children and the elderly. Salatac Gel should be applied once daily. The gel should be applied once every night. Treatment can take up to twelve (12) weeks for resistant lesions to disappear, and it is necessary to persevere with treatment.

1. Every night, soak the affected site in warm water for 2 to 3 minutes.

2. Dry thoroughly with the patient's own towel.

3. Carefully apply one or two drops of the gel to the lesion and allow to dry over its surface. Take care to avoid spreading on to surrounding normal skin. No adhesive plaster is necessary.

4. The following evening, carefully remove and discard the elastic film formed from the previous application, and reapply the gel. Occasionally, if removal of the elastic film proves difficult, carefully reapply the gel over it and allow to dry. This should help thicken the film to assist removal. If necessary, such re-application may be made on two or three successive days.

5. Once a week, gently rub away the treated surface using an emery board, as provided, or pumice stone used only for this purpose, before re-applying the gel.

6. The wart, verruca, corn or callus may take up to twelve (12) weeks to disappear and it is important to persevere with the treatment.

7. At the end of treatment, if the elastic film is difficult to remove, it may be allowed to remain on the skin until it sheds.

4.3 Contraindications
Not to be used on or near the face, intertriginous or anogenital regions, or by diabetics or individuals with impaired peripheral blood circulation. Not to be used on moles or on any other skin lesions for which the gel is not indicated. Not to be used in cases of sensitivity to any of the ingredients.

4.4 Special warnings and precautions for use
Keep away from the eyes, mucous membranes and from cuts and grazes. The gel should be applied carefully to the wart, verruca, corn or callus only, to avoid possible irritation of surrounding normal skin. Do not use excessively. Some mild, transient irritation may be expected, but in cases of more severe or persistent pain/irritation, treatment should be suspended and/or discontinued. See also Section 4.8. Avoid inhaling vapour, and keep cap firmly closed when not in use. Contact with clothing, fabrics, plastics and other materials may cause damage, and should be avoided. For external use only. Keep all medicines out of the reach of children.

4.5 Interaction with other medicinal products and other forms of interaction
None known.

4.6 Pregnancy and lactation
No special precautions.

4.7 Effects on ability to drive and use machines
None known.

4.8 Undesirable effects
Salatac Gel may be irritant in certain patients, which in rare instances may appear as a temporary blemish on the skin. See also Section 4.4.

4.9 Overdose
Any excessive use of Salatac Gel could cause irritation of the skin. If this occurs, Salatac Gel should be used more sparingly or applied less frequently.

5. PHARMACOLOGICAL PROPERTIES

5.1 Pharmacodynamic properties
The active ingredients, salicylic acid and lactic acid, are well-established pharmacopoeial substances. In combination, they are routinely used in the treatment of verrucas, warts, corns and calluses for their keratolytic properties.

When applied topically, and in high enough concentrations, salicylic acid acts by achieving a slow, painless destruction of the thickened stratum corneum. It softens and destroys the stratum corneum of the affected tissue by reducing the adhesiveness of the corneocytes while causing the cornified epithelium to swell, soften, macerate and finally desquamate. In the treatment of warts, a mild irritant reaction, which may render the virus more prone to immunologic stimulation or response, may add to the mechanical removal of infected cells. The other active ingredient, lactic acid, enhances the availability of the salicylic acid from the dried collodion, in addition to having antiseptic and caustic properties.

5.2 Pharmacokinetic properties
Salatac Gel contains 12% salicylic acid and 4% lactic acid in an evaporative collodion-like gel which forms a cohesive and adhesive film on the skin.

The formulation is presented in a collapsible aluminium tube fitted with a special applicator nozzle allowing the formulation to be dispensed precisely to the affected areas only. This minimises the spread of the preparation onto the surrounding healthy skin which could otherwise lead to inflammation, irritation and poor patient compliance. The film-forming characteristics of the collodion-like gel vehicle also offer distinct advantages in clinical usage.

The gel quickly forms a surface film, well before it dries completely, thereby prolonging the period during which the keratolytic solution can properly infiltrate and achieve intimate contact with the surface layers of the thickened stratum corneum.

Furthermore, even when the film appears to have dried completely, the inclusion of the non-evaporative lactic acid ensures that a proportion of the salicylic acid remains in solution within the vehicle, thus permitting continued release of the keratolytic, which may otherwise be entrapped within the collodion-like film.

Systemic absorption of salicylic acid or lactic acid after application of the recommended daily dose of one or two drops of the preparation to small, circumscribed areas is exceedingly unlikely.

5.3 Preclinical safety data
No special information.

6. PHARMACEUTICAL PARTICULARS

6.1 List of excipients
Camphor; Pyroxylin; Ethanol (96%); Ethyl Acetate.

6.2 Incompatibilities
None known.

6.3 Shelf life
36 months.

6.4 Special precautions for storage
Highly flammable - keep away from flames. Do not store above 25°C.

6.5 Nature and contents of container
Collapsible tube containing 8 g, complete with special applicator, emery board and instructions. This is supplied as an original pack (OP).

6.6 Special precautions for disposal and other handling
Not applicable.

7. MARKETING AUTHORISATION HOLDER
Dermal Laboratories

Tatmore Place, Gosmore

Hitchin, Herts SG4 7QR, UK.

8. MARKETING AUTHORISATION NUMBER(S)
00173/0046.

9. DATE OF FIRST AUTHORISATION/RENEWAL OF THE AUTHORISATION
29 July 2008.

10. DATE OF REVISION OF THE TEXT
July 2008.

Salazopyrin En-Tabs

(Pharmacia Limited)

1. NAME OF THE MEDICINAL PRODUCT
Salazopyrin En-Tabs

2. QUALITATIVE AND QUANTITATIVE COMPOSITION
Sulfasalazine EP 500mg

3. PHARMACEUTICAL FORM
Yellow film-coated, ovoid gastro-resistant tablets embossed "Kph" on one side and "102" on the other.

4. CLINICAL PARTICULARS

4.1 Therapeutic indications
a) Induction and maintenance of remission of ulcerative colitis; treatment of active Crohn's Disease.

b) Treatment of rheumatoid arthritis which has failed to respond to non-steroidal anti-inflammatory drugs (NSAIDs).

4.2 Posology and method of administration
EN-Tablets should be used where there is gastro-intestinal intolerance of plain tablets. They should not be crushed or broken.

The dose is adjusted according to the severity of the disease and the patient's tolerance to the drug, as detailed below.

Elderly Patients: No special precautions are necessary.

a) Ulcerative colitis

Adults

Severe Attack: Salazopyrin 2-4 tablets four times a day may be given in conjunction with steroids as part of an intensive management regime. Rapid passage of the tablets may reduce effect of the drug.

Night-time interval between doses should not exceed 8 hours.

Moderate Attack: 2-4 tablets four times a day may be given in conjunction with steroids.

Mild Attack: 2 tablets four times a day with or without steroids.

Maintenance Therapy: With induction of remission reduce the dose gradually to 4 tablets per day. This dosage should be continued indefinitely, since discontinuance even several years after an acute attack is associated with a four fold increase in risk of relapse.

Children

The dose is reduced in proportion to body weight.

Acute Attack or relapse: 40 - 60mg/kg per day

Maintenance Dosage: 20 - 30mg/kg per day

Salazopyrin Suspension may provide a more flexible dosage form.

b) Crohn's Disease

In active Crohn's Disease, Salazopyrin should be administered as in attacks of ulcerative colitis (see above).

c) Rheumatoid Arthritis

Patients with rheumatoid arthritis, and those treated over a long period with NSAIDs, may have sensitive stomachs and for this reason enteric-coated Salazopyrin (EN-Tabs) are recommended for this disease, as follows:

The patient should start with one tablet daily, increasing his dosage by a tablet a day each week until one tablet four times a day, or two three times a day are reached, according to tolerance and response. Onset of effect is slow and a marked effect may not be seen for six weeks. A reduction in ESR and C-reactive protein should accompany an improvement in joint mobility. $NSAID_s$ may be taken concurrently with Salazopyrin.

4.3 Contraindications
Sulfasalazine is contraindicated in:

Infants under the age of 2 years.

Patients with a known hypersensitivity to sulfasalazine, its metabolites or any of the excipients as well as sulfonamides or salicylates.

Patients with porphyria.

4.4 Special warnings and precautions for use
Complete blood counts (including differential white cell count), liver function tests and assessment of renal function (including urinalysis) should be performed in all patients before starting therapy with sulfasalazine, and frequently during the first 3 months of therapy. Thereafter, monitoring should be performed as clinically indicated. The patient should also be counselled to report immediately with any sore throat, fever, malaise malaise, pallor, purpura, jaundice or unexpected non-specific illness during sulfasalazine treatment, this may indicate myelosuppression, haemolysis or hepatoxicity. Treatment should be stopped immediately while awaiting the results of blood tests.

Sulfasalazine should not be given to patients with impaired hepatic or renal function or with blood dyscrasias, unless the potential benefit outweighs the risk.

Sulfasalazine should be given with caution to patients with severe allergy or bronchial asthma.

Use in children with the concomitant condition systemic onset juvenile rheumatoid arthritis may result in a serum sickness like reaction; therefore sulfasalazine is not recommended in these patients.

Since sulfasalazine may cause haemolytic anaemia, it should be used with caution in patients with G-6-PD deficiency.

Oral sulfasalazine inhibits the absorption and metabolism of folic acid and may cause folic acid deficiency potentially resulting in serious blood disorders (e.g., macrocytosis and pancytopenia), this can be normalised by administration of folic acid or folinic acid (leucovorin).

Because sulfasalazine causes crystalluria and kidney stone formation, adequate fluid intake should be ensured during treatment.

Oligospermia and infertility may occur in men treated with sulfasalazine. Discontinuation of the drug appears to reverse these effects within 2 to 3 months.

4.5 Interaction with other medicinal products and other forms of interaction

Reduced absorption of digoxin, resulting in non-therapeutic serum levels, has been reported when used concomitantly with oral sulfasalazine.

Sulfonamides bear certain chemical similarities to some oral hypoglycemic agents. Hypoglycemia has occurred in patients receiving sulfonamides. Patients receiving sulfasalazine and hypoglycemic agents should be closely monitored.

Due to inhibition of thiopurine methyltransferase by salazopyrin, bone marrow suppression and leucopenia have been reported when the thiopurine 6-mercaptopurine or it's prodrug, azathioprine, and oral salazopyrin were used concomitantly.

Due to inhibition of thiopurine methyltransferase by salazopyrin, bone marrow suppression and leucopenia have been reported when the thiopurine 6-mercaptopurine or it's prodrug, azathioprine, and oral salazopyrin were used concomitantly.

Coadministration of oral sulfasalazine and methotrexate to rheumatoid arthritis patients did not alter the pharmacokinetic disposition of the drugs. However, an increased incidence of gastrointestinal adverse events, especially nausea, was reported.

4.6 Pregnancy and lactation

Pregnancy

Reproduction studies in rats and rabbits have revealed no evidence of harm to the fetus. Published data regarding use of sulfasalazine in pregnant women have revealed no evidence of teratogenic hazards. If sulfasalazine is used during pregnancy, the possibility of fetal harm appears remote. Oral sulfasalazine inhibits the absorption and metabolism of folic acid and may cause folic acid deficiency. Because the possibility of harm cannot be completely ruled out, sulfasalazine should be used during pregnancy only if clearly needed.

Lactation

Sulfasalazine and sulfapyridine are found in low levels in breast milk. Caution should be used, particularly if breastfeeding premature infants or those deficient in G-6-PD.

4.7 Effects on ability to drive and use machines

No specific effects.

4.8 Undesirable effects

Overall, about 75% of ADRs occur within 3 months of starting therapy, and over 90% by 6 months. Some undesirable effects are dose-dependent and symptoms can often be alleviated by reduction of the dose.

General

Sulfasalazine is split by intestinal bacteria to sulfapyridine and 5-amino salicylate so ADRs to either sulfonamide or salicylate are possible. Patients with slow acetylator status are more likely to experience ADRs related to sulfapyridine. The most commonly encountered ADRs are nausea, headache, rash, loss of appetite and raised temperature.

Specific

The following reactions have been recorded in patients taking sulfasalazine:

Haematological. Potentially fatal leucopenia, neutropenia, agranulocytosis, aplastic anaemia and thrombocytopenia. Leucopenia, which is normally mild and transient, may occur in up to 1.5% of patients and agranulocytosis in up to one in 700 patients during the second month of therapy.

The risk of sulfasalazine associated blood disorders is substantially higher in patients treated for rheumatoid arthritis than it is for patients treated for inflammatory bowel disease.

Heinz body anaemia, methaemoglobinaemia, hypoprothrombinaemia, haemolytic anaemia, megaloblastic anaemia.

Hypersensitivity reactions

Generalised skin eruptions, Stevens-Johnson Syndrome, exfoliative dermatitis, epidermal necrolysis, pruritis, urticaria, photosensitisation, anaphylaxis, serum sickness, drug fever, lymphadenopathy, periorbital oedema, conjuctivial and scleral polyarteritis nodosa, LE-phenomenon and lung complications with dyspnoea, fever, cough, eosinophilia, fibrosing alveolitis, pericarditis, vasculitis, nephritis, alopecia.

Gastro-intestinal reactions

Stomatitis, parotitis, pancreatitis, hepatitis.

CNS Reactions

Vertigo, tinnitus, peripheral neuropathy, aseptic meningitis, ataxia, convulsions, insomnia, mental depression and hallucinations.

Fertility

Oligospermia, reversible on discontinuance of drug.

Renal Reactions

Crystalluria, haematuria, proteinuria and nephrotic syndrome.

4.9 Overdose

The drug has low acute per oral toxicity in the absence of hyper-sensitivity. There is no specific antidote and treatment should be supportive.

5. PHARMACOLOGICAL PROPERTIES

5.1 Pharmacodynamic properties

Pharmacological particulars: around 90% of a dose reaches the colon where bacteria split the drug into sulfapyridine (SP) and mesalazine (ME). These are also active, and the unsplit sulfasalazine (SASP) is also active on a variety of symptoms. Most SP is absorbed, hydroxylated or glucuronidated and a mix of unchanged and metabolised SP appears in the urine. Some ME is taken up and acetylated in the colon wall, such that renal excretion is mainly AC-ME. SASP is excreted unchanged in the bile and urine.

Overall the drug and its metablites exert immunimodulatory effects, antibacterial effects, effects on the arachidonic acid cascade and alteration of activity of certain enzymes. The net result clinically is a reduction in activity of the inflammatory bowel disease. In rheumatoid arthritis a disease modifying effect is evident in 1-3 months, with characteristics falls in CRP and other indicators of inflammation. ME is not believed to be responsible for this effect.

Radiographic studies show marked reduction in progression (larsen or sharp index) compared with placebo or hydroxychloroquine over two years in early patients. If drug is stopped the benefit appears to be maintained.

5.2 Pharmacokinetic properties

Pharmacokinetic particulars: studies with en-tabs show no statistically significant differences in main parameters compared with an equivalent dose of SASP powder, and the figures produced below relate to ordinary tablets. With regard to the use of Salazopyrin in bowel disease there is no evidence that systemic levels are of any relevance other than with regard to ADR incidence. Here levels of SP over about 50μg/ml are associated with a substantial risk of ADRS, especially in slow acetylators.

For SASP given as a single 3g oral dose, peak serum levels of SASP occured in 3-5 hours, elimination half life was 5.7±0.7 hours, lag time 1.5 hours. During maintenance therapy renal clearance of SASP was 7.3±1.7ml/min, for SP 9.9±1.9 and AC-ME 100±20. Free SP first appears in plasma in 4.3 hours after a single dose with an absorption half life of 2.7 hours. The elimination half life was calculated as 18 hours.

Turning to mesalazine, in urine only AC-ME (not free ME) was demonstrable, the acetylation probably largely achieved in the colon mucosa. After a 3g SASP dose lag time was 6.1±2.3 hours and plasma levels kept below 2μg/ml total ME. Urinary excretion half life was 6.0±3.1 hours and absorption half life based on these figures 3.0±1.5 hours. Renal clearance constant was 125ml/min corresponding to the GFR.

With regard to rheumatoid arthritis there is no data which suggests any differences from those above.

5.3 Preclinical safety data

In two-year carcinogenicity studies in rats and mice, sulfasalazine showed some evidence of carcinogenicity. In rats, there was a small increase in the incidence of transitional cell papillomas in the urinary bladder and kidney. The tumours were judged to be induced mechanically by calculi formed in the urine rather than through a direct genotoxic mechanism. In the mouse study, there was a significant increase in the incidence of hepatocellular adenoma or carcinoma. The mechanism of induction of hepatocellular neoplasia has been investigated and attributed to species-specific effects of sulfasalazine that are not relevant to humans.

Sulfasalazine did not show mutagenicity in the bacterial reverse mutation assay (Ames test) or in the L51784 mouse lymphoma cell assay at the HGPRT gene. It did not induce sister chromatid exchanges or chromosomal aberrations in cultured Chinese hamster ovary cells, and in vivo mouse bone marrow chromosomal aberration tests were negative. However, sulfasalazine showed positive or equivocal mutagenic responses in rat and mouse micronucleus assays, and in human lymphocyte sister chromatid exchange, chromosomal aberration and micronucleus assays. The ability of sulfasalazine to induce chromosome damage has been attributed to perturbation of folic acid levels rather than to a direct genotoxic mechanism.

Based on information from non-clinical studies, sulfasalazine is judged to pose no carcinogenic risk to humans. Sulfasalazine use has not been associated with the development of neoplasia in human epidemiology studies.

6. PHARMACEUTICAL PARTICULARS

6.1 List of excipients

Povidone; maize starch; magnesium stearate; colloidal silicon dioxide; cellulose acetate phthalate; propylene glycol; traces of beeswax, carnauba wax, glyceryl monostearate, talc.

6.2 Incompatibilities

Certain types of extended wear soft contact lenses may be permanently stained during therapy.

6.3 Shelf life

The tablets are stable for five years.

6.4 Special precautions for storage

Store in a dry place

6.5 Nature and contents of container

Polyolefin Square pot with screw cap. To contain 112 tablets

6.6 Special precautions for disposal and other handling

Take the tablets whole: Do not break

7. MARKETING AUTHORISATION HOLDER

Pharmacia Ltd

Ramsgate Road

Sandwich

Kent CT13 9NJ

United Kingdom

8. MARKETING AUTHORISATION NUMBER(S)

PL 00032/0387

9. DATE OF FIRST AUTHORISATION/RENEWAL OF THE AUTHORISATION

16 September 2002

10. DATE OF REVISION OF THE TEXT

28 July 2009

11. LEGAL CATEGORY

POM.

SZ 4_0 En-Tabs UK

Salazopyrin Suppositories

(Pharmacia Limited)

1. NAME OF THE MEDICINAL PRODUCT

Salazopyrin Suppositories

2. QUALITATIVE AND QUANTITATIVE COMPOSITION

Sulfasalazine EP 0.5 g

3. PHARMACEUTICAL FORM

Suppository

4. CLINICAL PARTICULARS

4.1 Therapeutic indications

Ulcerative colitis or Crohn's Disease affecting the rectum.

4.2 Posology and method of administration

The dose is adjusted according to the severity of the disease and the patient's tolerance of the drug.

Acute attack or relapse - Adults and the Elderly

Two suppositories are to be inserted in the morning and two at bedtime after defecation. After three weeks the dosage is gradually reduced as improvement occurs.

Adjustment to oral therapy - Adults and the Elderly

In severe generalised ulcerative colitis of the rectum or recto sigmoid, or in cases who are responding slowly to oral therapy, one or two suppositories may be given in the morning and at bedtime additional to oral therapy.

Children

The adult dose is reduced on the basis of body weight.

4.3 Contraindications

General

Because of lower absorption levels and shorter retention time in the body, Salazopyrin Suppositories give rise to fewer adverse events than equivalent treatment by mouth. However, because of the theoretical possibility that serious adverse events can arise from treatment from either route, the details below are based on adverse event reports to both oral and rectal treatment.

i) A known hypersensitivity to sulfasalazine, its metabolites or any of the excipients as well as sulfonamides or salicylates.

ii) Use in infants under two years old.

iii) Porphyria.

4.4 Special warnings and precautions for use

Complete blood counts (including differential white cell count), liver function tests and assessment of renal function (including urinalysis) should be performed in all patients before starting therapy with sulfasalazine, and frequently during the first 3 months of therapy. Thereafter, monitoring should be performed as clinically indicated. The patient should also be counselled to report immediately with any sore throat, fever, malaise, pallor, purpura, jaundice or unexpected non-specific illness during sulfasalazine treatment, this may indicate myelosuppression, haemolysis or hepatoxicity. Treatment should be stopped immediately while awaiting the results of blood tests.

Sulfasalazine should not be given to patients with impaired hepatic or renal function or with blood dyscrasias, unless the potential benefit outweighs the risk.

Sulfasalazine should be given with caution to patients with severe allergy or bronchial asthma.

Use in children with the concomitant condition systemic onset juvenile rheumatoid arthritis may result in a serum sickness like reaction; therefore sulfasalazine is not recommended in these patients.

Since sulfasalazine may cause haemolytic anaemia, it should be used with caution in patients with G-6-PD deficiency.

Oral sulfasalazine inhibits the absorption and metabolism of folic acid and may cause folic acid deficiency potentially resulting in serious blood disorders (e.g., macrocytosis and pancytopenia), this can be normalised by administration of folic acid or folinic acid (leucovorin).

Because sulfasalazine causes crystalluria and kidney stone formation, adequate fluid intake should be ensured during treatment.

Oligospermia and infertility may occur in men treated with sulfasalazine. Discontinuation of the drug appears to reverse these effects within 2 to 3 months. As far as is know oligospermia has not occurred during therapy per rectum.

4.5 Interaction with other medicinal products and other forms of interaction

There have been no adverse interactions reported, due to the drug largely remaining confined to the rectum. However, there is a potential for interaction as follows:

Reduced absorption of digoxin, resulting in non-therapeutic serum levels, has been reported when used concomitantly with oral sulfasalazine.

Sulfonamides bear certain chemical similarities to some oral hypoglycemic agents. Hypoglycemia has occurred in patients receiving sulfonamides. Patients receiving sulfasalazine and hypoglycemic agents should be closely monitored.

Due to inhibition of thiopurine methyltransferase by salazopyrin, bone marrow suppression and leucopenia have been reported when the thiopurine 6-mercaptopurine or it's prodrug, azathioprine, and oral salazopyrin were used concomitantly.

Coadministration of oral sulfasalazine and methotrexate to rheumatoid arthritis patients did not alter the pharmacokinetic disposition of the drugs. However, an increased incidence of gastrointestinal adverse events, especially nausea, was reported.

4.6 Pregnancy and lactation

Pregnancy

Reproduction studies in rats and rabbits have revealed no evidence of harm to the fetus. Published data regarding use of sulfasalazine in pregnant women have revealed no evidence of teratogenic hazards. If sulfasalazine is used during pregnancy, the possibility of fetal harm appears remote. Oral sulfasalazine inhibits the absorption and metabolism of folic acid and may cause folic acid deficiency. Because the possibility of harm cannot be completely ruled out, sulfasalazine should be used during pregnancy only if clearly needed.

Lactation

Sulfasalazine and sulfapyridine are found in low levels in breast milk. Caution should be used, particularly if breast-feeding premature infants or those deficient in G-6-PD.

4.7 Effects on ability to drive and use machines

No specific effects.

4.8 Undesirable effects

The following have been reported to sulfasalazine given orally or rectally. The drug rectally is well tolerated. Overall, about 75% of adverse drug reactions occur within three months of starting therapy and over 90% by six months. Some undesirable effects are dose-dependent and symptoms can often be alleviated by reduction of the dose.

General

Sulfasalazine is split by intestinal bacteria to sulfapyridine and 5-amino salicylate so adverse drugs reactions to either sulfonamide or salicylate are possible. Patients with slow acetylator status are more likely to experience adverse drug reactions related to sulfapyridine. The most commonly encountered adverse drugs reactions are nausea, headache, rash, loss of appetite and raised temperature.

Specific

The following reactions have been recorded in patients taking sulfasalazine:

Haematological

Potentially fatal leucopenia, neutropenia, agranulocytosis, aplastic anaemia and thrombocytopenia. Leucopenia which is normally mild and transient, may occur in up to 1.5% of patients and agranulocytosis in up to one in 700 patients during the second month of therapy.

Heinz body anaemia, methaemoglobinaemia, hypoprothrombinaemia, haemolytic anaemia, megaloblastic anaemia.

Hypersensitivity Reactions

Generalised skin eruptions, Stevens-Johnson syndrome, exfoliative dermatitis, epidermal necrolysis, pruritus, urticaria, photosensitisation, anaphylaxis, serum sickness, drug fever, lymphadenopathy, periorbital oedema, conjunctival and scleral injection, arthralgia, allergic myocarditis, polyarteritis nodosa, LE-phenomenon and lung complications with dyspnoea, fever, cough, eosinophilia, fibrosing alveolitis, pericarditis, vasculitis, nephritis, alopecia.

Gastro-intestinal Reactions

Stomatitis, parotitis, pancreatitis, hepatitis.

CNS Reactions

Vertigo, tinnitus, peripheral neuropathy, aseptic meningitis, ataxia, convulsions, insomnia, mental depression and hallucinations.

Fertility

Oligospermia, reversible on discontinuance of drug.

Renal Reactions

Crystalluria, haematuria, proteinuria and nephrotic syndrome.

4.9 Overdose

Overdose with suppositories is unlikely. In the event, evacuate the bowel and treat supportively. The toxicity of sulphasalazine is low in acute dosage. There is no specific antidote.

5. PHARMACOLOGICAL PROPERTIES

5.1 Pharmacodynamic properties

Therapeutic benefit of sulfasalazine in ulcerative colitis and Crohn's Disease appears to be due to a local action of the sulfasalazine and its split product 5-aminosalicylic acid on the mucous membrane and deeper colonic structures. Pharmacological actions noted for these compounds include inhibition of neutrophil activation, free radical scavenging, inhibition of superoxide production, inhibition of bacterial growth. Sulfasalazine inhibits 15-Prostaglandin dehydrogenase and slows prostaglandin metabolism. Lipoxygenase release in inflammatory cells is also depressed. NK cells and T cell proliferation are inhibited.

5.2 Pharmacokinetic properties

There are considerable individual differences in the retention time of suppositories in volunteer studies. Consequently uptake values vary widely also. Given that the effect of the drug is almost certainly due to a local effect pharmacokinetics becomes less relevant to therapeutic action than to possible adverse effects related to systemic levels.

A study of five volunteers over three days following insertion of 2 × 0.5 g suppositories gave the following results: Retention time: mean 8.9 hours (s.d. 5.2), serum concentration at 10 hours: sulfasalazine 1.7 mcg/ml (s.d. 0.46), sulfapyridine less than 1 mcg/ml. Percentage renal excretion: 10.2 (s.d. 4.3). Uptake as reflected by excretion is much below that of the oral rate and may explain the good tolerance of the dose form.

5.3 Preclinical safety data

In two-year carcinogenicity studies in rats and mice, sulfasalazine showed some evidence of carcinogenicity. In rats, there was a small increase in the incidence of transitional cell papillomas in the urinary bladder and kidney. The tumours were judged to be induced mechanically by calculi formed in the urine rather than through a direct genotoxic mechanism. In the mouse study, there was a significant increase in the incidence of hepatocellular adenoma or carcinoma. The mechanism of induction of hepatocellular neoplasia has been investigated and attributed to species-specific effects of sulfasalazine that are not relevant to humans.

Sulfasalazine did not show mutagenicity in the bacterial reverse mutation assay (Ames test) or in the L51784 mouse lymphoma cell assay at the HGPRT gene. It did not induce sister chromatid exchanges or chromosomal aberrations in cultured Chinese hamster ovary cells, and in vivo mouse bone marrow chromosomal aberration tests were negative. However, sulfasalazine showed positive or equivocal mutagenic responses in rat and mouse micronucleus assays, and in human lymphocyte sister chromatid exchange, chromosomal aberration and micronucleus assays. The ability of sulfasalazine to induce chromosome damage has been attributed to perturbation of folic acid levels rather than to a direct genotoxic mechanism.

Based on information from non-clinical studies, sulfasalazine is judged to pose no carcinogenic risk to humans. Sulfasalazine use has not been associated with the development of neoplasia in human epidemiology studies.

6. PHARMACEUTICAL PARTICULARS

6.1 List of excipients

Povidone

Adepa Solidus

6.2 Incompatibilities

Certain types of extended wear soft contact lenses may be permanently stained during therapy.

6.3 Shelf life

Five years

6.4 Special precautions for storage

Do not store above 25°C.

6.5 Nature and contents of container

PVC/Polyethylene laminate moulds

6.6 Special precautions for disposal and other handling

As the suppositories melt at body temperature they should be kept below 25°C and handled as little as possible before insertion so that they are firm.

Sulfasalazine is an orange dye, and care should thus be taken with clothing, bedding etc with regard to seepage or spillage.

Insertion

Empty the bowel if possible. Push the suppository through the anus with a finger, as far as possible. The urge to expel them will pass in a few minutes, once they have melted.

7. MARKETING AUTHORISATION HOLDER

Pharmacia Limited

Ramsgate Road

Sandwich

Kent, CT13 9NJ

United Kingdom

8. MARKETING AUTHORISATION NUMBER(S)

PL 00022/0156

9. DATE OF FIRST AUTHORISATION/RENEWAL OF THE AUTHORISATION

17 January 1994 /16th September 2002

10. DATE OF REVISION OF THE TEXT

28th July 2009

11. LEGAL CATEGORY

POM.

Ref: SZ 4_0 Supp UK

Salazopyrin Suspension

(Pharmacia Limited)

1. NAME OF THE MEDICINAL PRODUCT

Salazopyrin Suspension.

2. QUALITATIVE AND QUANTITATIVE COMPOSITION

Sulfasalazine Ph.Eur., 250 mg in 5 mL.

3. PHARMACEUTICAL FORM

Oral suspension.

4. CLINICAL PARTICULARS

4.1 Therapeutic indications

Induction and maintenance of remission of ulcerative colitis and treatment of active Crohn's disease.

4.2 Posology and method of administration

The dose is adjusted according to the severity of the disease and the patient's tolerance of the drug, as detailed below.

Adults and the Elderly

Severe attacks: 20 to 40 ml four times a day may be given in conjunction with steroids as part of an intensive management regime. Rapid passage of the suspension may reduce the effect of the drug.

The night time interval between doses should not exceed 8 hours.

Moderate attacks: 20 ml four times a day may be taken with or without steroids.

Maintenance therapy: With induction of remission, reduce the dose gradually to 40 ml per day. This dosage should be continued indefinitely, since discontinuance even several years after an acute attack is associated with a four-fold increase in relapse.

Children

The dose is reduced in proportion to body weight.

Acute attack or relapse: 0.8 - 1.2 ml/kg/day.

Maintenance dosage: 0.4 - 0.6 ml/kg/day.

4.3 Contraindications

- Use in infants under the age of two years.
- Use in patients where there is a significant hypersensitivity to sulfasalazine, sulfonamides, salicylates or the sodium benzoate preservative.
- Acute intermittent porphyria.

4.4 Special warnings and precautions for use

Haematological and hepatic side effects may occur. Differential white cell, red cell and platelet cells should be performed initially and at least monthly for a minimum of the first three months of treatment. The patient should also be counselled to report immediately with any sore throat, fever, malaise or unexpected non-specific illness. Treatment should be stopped immediately if there is a suspicion or laboratory evidence of a potentially serious blood dyscrasia.

Liver function tests should be carried out at monthly intervals for the first three months of treatment. Patients with liver disease should be treated with caution.

Kidney function should be checked initially and at regular intervals during the treatment. Since sulfasalazine may cause haemolytic anaemia, it should be used with caution in patients with glucose-6-phosphate dehydrogenase deficiency.

Changes in blood picture (e.g. macrocytosis and pancytopenia) can be normalised by the administration of folic acid or folinic acid (leucovorin).

Sulfasalazine may colour the urine orange-yellow.

4.5 Interaction with other medicinal products and other forms of interaction
Certain types of extended wear soft contact lenses may be permanently stained during therapy.

Uptake of digoxin and folate may be reduced.

Adequate fluid intake and avoidance of acidification of the urine (such as with concomitant use of methenamine) may minimise crystalluria and stone formation.

Sulfonamides bear certain chemical similarities to some oral hypoglycemic agents. Hypoglycemia has occurred in patients receiving sulfonamides. Patients receiving sulfasalazine and hypoglycemic agents should be closely monitored.

Due to inhibition of thiopurine methyltransferase by salazopyrin, bone marrow suppression and leucopenia have been reported when the thiopurine 6-mercaptopurine or it's prodrug, azathioprine, and oral salazopyrin were used concomitantly.

4.6 Pregnancy and lactation
Long-term clinical usage and experimental studies have failed to reveal any teratogenic or icteric hazards. The amounts of drug circulating in breast milk should not present a risk to a healthy infant.

4.7 Effects on ability to drive and use machines
No specific effects.

4.8 Undesirable effects
Overall, about 75% of ADRs occur within three months of treatment and over 90% by six months. Some unwanted effects are dose-dependent and symptoms can often be alleviated by reduction of the dose.

General

Sulfasalazine is split by intestinal bacteria to sulfapyridine and 5-amino salicylate so ADRs to either sulfonamide or salicylate are possible. Patients with slow acetylator status are more likely to experience ADRs related to sulfapyridine. The most commonly encountered ADRs are nausea, headache, rash loss of appetite and raised temperature.

Specific

The following reactions have been recorded in patients taking sulfasalazine:

Haematological

Potentially fatal leucopenia, neutropenia, agranulocytosis, aplastic anaemia and thrombocytopenia. Leucopenia, which is normally mild and transient, may occur in up to 1.5% of patients and agranulocytosis in up to one in 700 patients during the second month of therapy.

The risk of sulfasalazine-associated blood disorders is substantially higher in patients treated for rheumatoid arthritis than it is in patients treated for inflammatory bowel disease.

Heinz body anaemia, methaemoglobinaemia, hypoprothrombinaemia, haemolytic anaemia, megaloblastic anaemia.

Hypersensitivity reactions

Generalised skin eruptions, Stevens-Johnson Syndrome, exfoliative dermatitis, epidermal necrolysis, pruritis, urticaria, photosensitisation, anaphylaxis, serum sickness, drug fever, lymphadenopathy, periorbital oedema, conjunctival and scleral injection, arthralgia, allergic myocarditis, polyarteritis nodosa, LE-phenomenon and lung complications with dyspnoea, fever, cough, eosinophilia, fibrosing alveolitis, pericarditis, vasculitis, nephritis, alopecia.

Gastro-intestinal reactions

Stomatitis, parotitis, pancreatitis, hepatitis.

CNS reactions

Vertigo, tinnitus, peripheral neuropathy, aseptic meningitis, ataxia, convulsions, insomnia, mental depression and hallucinations.

Fertility

Oligospermia, reversible on discontinuance of drug.

Renal Reactions

Crystalluria, haematuria, proteinurea and nephrotic syndrome.

4.9 Overdose
The drug has low acute per oral toxicity in the absence of hypersensitivity. There is no specific antidote and treatment should be supportive.

5. PHARMACOLOGICAL PROPERTIES

5.1 Pharmacodynamic properties
Sulfasalazine has beneficial effects in the treatment of ulcerative colitis and maintenance of remission, and in the treatment of acute Crohn's disease. Around 90% of a dose reaches the colon where bacteria split the drug into sulpyapyridine and mesalazine. These are active, and the unsplit sulfasalazine is also active on a variety of systems. Most Sulfapyridine is absorbed, hydroxylated or glucuronidated and a mix of unchanged and metabolised sulfapyridine appears in the urine.

Some mesalazine is taken up and acetylated in the colon wall, such that renal excretion is mainly acetyl-mesalazine. Sulfasalazine is excreted unchanged in the bile and urine. Overall the drug and its metabolites exert immunomodulatory effects, antibacterial effects, effects on the arachidonic acid cascade and alteration of activity of certain enzymes. The net result clinically is a reduction in activity of the inflammatory bowel disease.

The enteric coated sulfasalazine is registered for the treatment of rheumatoid arthritis, where the effect resembles penicillamine or gold.

5.2 Pharmacokinetic properties
With regard to the use of Salazopyrin in bowel disease there is no evidence that systemic levels are of any relevance other than with regard to ADR incidence. Here levels of sulfapyridine over about 50μg/ml are associated with a substantial risk of ADRs, especially in slow acetylators.

For sulfasalazine given as a single 3g oral dose, peak serum levels of sulfasalazine occurred in 3-5 hours, elimination half life was 5.7 ±0.7 hours, lag time 1.5 hours. During maintenance therapy renal clearance of sulfasalazine was 7.3 ±1.7ml/min, for sulfapyridine 9.9 ±1.9 and acetyl-mesalazine 100 ±20. Free sulfasalazine first appears in plasma in 4.3 hours after a single dose with an absorption half life of 2.7 hours. The elimination half life was calculated as 18 hours. For mesalazine, only acetyl-mesalazine (not free mesalazine) was demonstrable, the acetylation probably largely achieved in the colon mucosa. After 3g sulfasalazine dose lag time was 6.1 ±2.3 hours and plasma levels kept below 2μg/ml. total mesalazine. Urinary excretion half life was 6.0 ±3.1 hours and absorption half life based on these figures 3.0 ±1.5 hours. Renal clearance constant was 125 ml/min corresponding to the GFR. Studies in volunteers suggest that sulfasalazine is handled in a similar manner whether given as suspension or tablets.

5.3 Preclinical safety data
In two-year carcinogenicity studies in rats and mice, sulfasalazine showed some evidence of carcinogenicity. In rats, there was a small increase in the incidence of transitional cell papillomas in the urinary bladder and kidney. The tumours were judged to be induced mechanically by calculi formed in the urine rather than through a direct genotoxic mechanism. In the mouse study, there was a significant increase in the incidence of hepatocellular adenoma or carcinoma. The mechanism of induction of hepatocellular neoplasia has been investigated and attributed to species-specific effects of sulfasalazine that are not relevant to humans.

Sulfasalazine did not show mutagenicity in the bacterial reverse mutation assay (Ames test) or in the L51784 mouse lymphoma cell assay at the HGPRT gene. It did not induce sister chromatid exchanges or chromosomal aberrations in cultured Chinese hamster ovary cells, and in vivo mouse bone marrow chromosomal aberration tests were negative. However, sulfasalazine showed positive or equivocal mutagenic responses in rat and mouse micronucleus assays, and in human lymphocyte sister chromatid exchange, chromosomal aberration and micronucleus assays. The ability of sulfasalazine to induce chromosome damage has been attributed to perturbation of folic acid levels rather than to a direct genotoxic mechanism.

Based on information from non-clinical studies, sulfasalazine is judged to pose no carcinogenic risk to humans. Sulfasalazine use has not been associated with the development of neoplasia in human epidemiology studies.

6. PHARMACEUTICAL PARTICULARS

6.1 List of excipients
Xanthan gum, sodium benzoate, polysorbate 80, orange/lemon flavour, microcrystalline cellulose, sucrose, purified water.

6.2 Incompatibilities
None relevant.

6.3 Shelf life
30 months

6.4 Special precautions for storage
Do not store at above 25°C.

6.5 Nature and contents of container
Natural HDPE bottle with a tamper evident cap or child resistant cap and containing 500 ml of suspension.

6.6 Special precautions for disposal and other handling
Take the suspension with food.

7. MARKETING AUTHORISATION HOLDER
Pharmacia Limited

Ramsgate Road

Sandwich

Kent CT13 9NJ

8. MARKETING AUTHORISATION NUMBER(S)
PL 00032/0389

9. DATE OF FIRST AUTHORISATION/RENEWAL OF THE AUTHORISATION
15 January 1994 / 25th March 2002

10. DATE OF REVISION OF THE TEXT
19th October 2005

11. LEGAL CATEGORY
POM.

Ref: SZD 2_0 UK

Salazopyrin Tablets

(Pharmacia Limited)

1. NAME OF THE MEDICINAL PRODUCT
Salazopyrin Tablets

2. QUALITATIVE AND QUANTITATIVE COMPOSITION
Sulfasalazine EP 500 mg

3. PHARMACEUTICAL FORM
Yellow round tablets embossed "KPh" on one side and "101" and a score line on the other.

4. CLINICAL PARTICULARS

4.1 Therapeutic indications
Induction and maintenance of remission of ulcerative colitis; treatment of active Crohn's Disease.

4.2 Posology and method of administration
The dose is adjusted according to the severity of the disease and the patient's tolerance to the drug, as detailed below.

Elderly Patients

No special precautions are necessary.

A) Ulcerative colitis

Adults

Severe Attacks

Salazopyrin 2-4 tablets four times a day may be given in conjunction with steroids as part of an intensive management regime. Rapid passage of the tablets may reduce effect of the drug.

Night-time interval between doses should not exceed 8 hours.

Moderate Attack

2-4 tablets four times a day may be given in conjunction with steroids.

Maintenance Therapy

With induction of remission reduce the dose gradually to 4 tablets per day. This dosage should be continued indefinitely since discontinuance even several years after an acute attack is associated with a four fold increase in risk of relapse.

Children

The dose is reduced in proportion to body weight.

Acute Attack or Relapse

40-60mg/kg per day

Maintenance Dosage

20-30mg/kg per day

Salazopyrin Suspension may provide a more flexible dosage form.

B) Crohn's Disease

In active Crohn's Disease, Salazopyrin should be administered as in attacks of ulcerative colitis (see above).

4.3 Contraindications
Sulfasalazine is contraindicated in:

Infants under the age of 2 years.

Patients with a known hypersensitivity to sulfasalazine, its metabolites or any of the excipients as well as sufonamides or salicylates.

Patients with porphyria.

4.4 Special warnings and precautions for use
Complete blood counts (including differential white cell count), liver function tests and assessment of renal function (including urinalysis) should be performed in all patients before starting therapy with sulfasalazine, and frequently during the first 3 months of therapy. Thereafter, monitoring should be performed as clinically indicated. The patient should also be counselled to report immediately with any sore throat, fever, malaise, pallor, purpura, jaundice or unexpected non-specific illness during sulfasalazine treatment, this may indicate myelosuppression, haemolysis or hepatoxicity. Treatment should be stopped immediately while awaiting the results of blood tests.

Sulfasalazine should not be given to patients with impaired hepatic or renal function or with blood dyscrasias, unless the potential benefit outweighs the risk.

Sulfasalazine should be given with caution to patients with severe allergy or bronchial asthma.

Use in children with the concomitant condition sysemic onset juvenile rheumatoid arthritis may result in a serum sickness like reaction; therefore sulfasalazine is not recommended in these patients.

Since sulfasalazine may cause haemolytic anaemia, it should be used with caution in patients with G-6-PD deficiency.

Oral sulfasalazine inhibits the absorption and metabolism of folic acid and may cause folic acid deficiency potentially resulting in serious blood disorders (e.g., macrocytosis and pancytopenia), this can be normalised by administration of folic acid or folinic acid (leucovorin).

Because sulfasalazine causes crystalluria and kidney stone formation, adequate fluid intake should be ensured during treatment.

Oligospermia and infertility may occur in men treated with sulfasalazine. Discontinuation of the drug appears to reverse these effects within 2 to 3 months.

4.5 Interaction with other medicinal products and other forms of interaction

Reduced absorption of digoxin, resulting in non-therapeutic serum levels, has been reported when used concomitantly with oral sulfasalazine.

Sulfonamides bear certain chemical similarities to some oral hypoglycemic agents. Hypoglycemia has occurred in patients receiving sulfonamides. Patients receiving sulfasalazine and hypoglycemic agents should be closely monitored.

Due to inhibition of thiopurine methyltransferase by salazopyrin, bone marrow suppression and leucopenia have been reported when the thiopurine 6-mercaptopurine or it's prodrug, azathioprine, and oral salazopyrin were used concomitantly.

Coadministration of oral sulfasalazine and methotrexate to rheumatoid arthritis patients did not alter the pharmacokinetic disposition of the drugs. However, an increased incidence of gastrointestinal adverse events, especially nausea, was reported.

4.6 Pregnancy and lactation

Pregnancy

Reproduction studies in rats and rabbits have revealed no evidence of harm to the fetus. Published data regarding use of sulfasalazine in pregnant women have revealed no evidence of teratogenic hazards. If sulfasalazine is used during pregnancy, the possibility of fetal harm appears remote. Oral sulfasalazine inhibits the absorption and metabolism of folic acid and may cause folic acid deficiency. Because the possibility of harm cannot be completely ruled out, sulfasalazine should be used during pregnancy only if clearly needed.

Lactation

Sulfasalazine and sulfapyridine are found in low levels in breast milk. Caution should be used, particularly if breast-feeding premature infants or those deficient in G-6-PD.

4.7 Effects on ability to drive and use machines

No specific effects.

4.8 Undesirable effects

Overall, about 75% of ADRs occur within 3 months of starting therapy, and over 90% by 6 months. Some undesirable effects are dose-dependent and symptoms can often be alleviated by reduction of the dose.

General

Sulfasalazine is split by intestinal bacteria to sulfapyridine and 5-amino salicylate so ADRs to either sulfonamide or salicylate are possible. Patients with slow acetylator status are more likely to experience ADRs related to sulfapyridine. The most commonly encountered ADRs are nausea, headache, rash, loss of appetite and raised temperature.

Specific

The following reactions have been recorded in patients taking sulfasalazine:

Haematological

Potentially fatal leucopenia, neutropenia, agranulocytosis, aplastic anaemia and thrombocytopenia Leucopenia, which is normally mild and transient, may occur in up to 1.5% of patients and agranulocytosis in up to one in 700 patients during the second month of therapy.

Heinz body anaemia, methaemoglobinaemia, hypoprothrombinaemia, haemolytic anaemia, megaloblastic anaemia.

Hypersensitivity Reactions

Generalised skin eruptions, Stevens-Johnson Syndrome, exfoliative dermatitis, epidermal necrolysis, pruritis, urticaria, photosensitisation, anaphylaxis, serum sickness, drug fever, lymphadenopathy, periorbital oedema, conjuctivial and scleral infection, arthralgia, allergic myocarditis, polyarteritis nodosa, LE-phenomenon and lung complications with dyspnoea, fever, cough, eosinophilia, fibrosing alveolitis, pericarditis, vasculitis, nephritis, alopecia.

Gastro-Intestinal Reactions

Stomatitis, parotitis, pancreatitis, hepatitis.

CNS Reactions

Vertigo, tinnitus, peripheral neuropathy, aseptic meningitis, ataxia, convulsions, insomnia, mental depression and hallucinations.

Fertility

Oligospermia, reversible on discontinuance of drug.

Renal Reactions

Crystalluria, haematuria, proteinuria and nephrotic syndrome.

4.9 Overdose

The drug has low acute per oral toxicity in the absence of hypersensitivity. There is no specific antidote and treatment should be supportive.

5. PHARMACOLOGICAL PROPERTIES

5.1 Pharmacodynamic properties

Around 90% of a dose reaches the colon where bacteria split the drug into sulfapyridine (SP) and mesalazine (ME). These are active, and the unsplit sulfasalazine (SASP) is also active on a variety of symptoms. Most SP is absorbed, hydroxylated or glucuronidated and a mix of unchanged and metabolised SP appears in the urine. Some ME is taken up and acetylated in the colon wall, such that renal excretion is mainly ac-me. SASP is excreted unchanged in the bile and urine. Overall the drug and its metabolites exert immunomodulatory effects, antibacterial effects, effects on the arachidonic acid cascade and alteration of activity of certain enzymes. The net result clinically is a reduction in activity of the inflammatory bowel disease. The enteric coated SASP is registered for the treatment of rheumatoid arthritis, where the effect resembles penicillamine or gold.

5.2 Pharmacokinetic properties

With regard to the use of salazopyrin in bowel disease there is no evidence that systemic levels are of any relevance other than with regard to ADR incidence. Here levels of SP over about 50μg/ml are associated with a substantial risk of ADRs, especially in slow acetylators. For SASP given as a single 3g oral dose, peak serum levels of SASP occurred in 3-5 hours, elimination half life was 5.7 ±0.7 hours, lag time 1.5 hours. During maintenance therapy renal clearance of SASP was 7.3 ±1.7ml/min, for SP 9.9 ±1.9 and AC-ME 100 ±20. Free SP first appears in plasma in 4.3 hours after a single dose with an absorption half life of 2.7 hours. The elimination half life was calculated as 18 hours. Turning to mesalazine, in urine only AC-ME (not free ME) was demonstrable, the acetylation probably largely achieved in the colon mucosa. After a 3g SASP dose lag time was 6.1 ±2.3 hours and plasma levels kept below 2μg/ml total ME. Urinary excretion half-life was 6.0 ±3.1 hours and absorption half life based on these figures 3.0 ±1.5 hours. Renal clearance constant was 125 ml/min corresponding to the GFR.

5.3 Preclinical safety data

In two-year carcinogenicity studies in rats and mice, sulfasalazine showed some evidence of carcinogenicity. In rats, there was a small increase in the incidence of transitional cell papillomas in the urinary bladder and kidney. The tumours were judged to be induced mechanically by calculi formed in the urine rather than through a direct genotoxic mechanism. In the mouse study, there was a significant increase in the incidence of hepatocellular adenoma or carcinoma. The mechanism of induction of hepatocellular neoplasia has been investigated and attributed to species-specific effects of sulfasalazine that are not relevant to humans.

Sulfasalazine did not show mutagenicity in the bacterial reverse mutation assay (Ames test) or in the L51784 mouse lymphoma cell assay at the HGPRT gene. It did not induce sister chromatid exchanges or chromosomal aberrations in cultured Chinese hamster ovary cells, and in vivo mouse bone marrow chromosomal aberration tests were negative. However, sulfasalazine showed positive or equivocal mutagenic responses in rat and mouse micronucleus assays, and in human lymphocyte sister chromatid exchange, chromosomal aberration and micronucleus assays. The ability of sulfasalazine to induce chromosome damage has been attributed to perturbation of folic acid levels rather than to a direct genotoxic mechanism.

Based on information from non-clinical studies, sulfasalazine is judged to pose no carcinogenic risk to humans. Sulfasalazine use has not been associated with the development of neoplasia in human epidemiology studies.

6. PHARMACEUTICAL PARTICULARS

6.1 List of excipients

Povidone; maize starch; magnesium stearate; colloidal silicon dioxide.

6.2 Incompatibilities

Certain types of extended wear soft contact lenses may be permanently stained during therapy.

6.3 Shelf life

The tablets are stable for 5 years.

6.4 Special precautions for storage

None

6.5 Nature and contents of container

Square or rectangular HDPE jar with easy to open tamper-evisent polypropylene screw-cap. To contain 112 tablets.

6.6 Special precautions for disposal and other handling

Take with water

7. MARKETING AUTHORISATION HOLDER

Pharmacia Limited

Ramsgate Road

Sandwich

Kent, CT13 9NJ

United Kingdom

8. MARKETING AUTHORISATION NUMBER(S)

PL 00032/0390

9. DATE OF FIRST AUTHORISATION/RENEWAL OF THE AUTHORISATION

02/04/2002

10. DATE OF REVISION OF THE TEXT

14th July 2009

11. LEGAL CATEGORY

POM.

SZ 4_0 Tabs UK

Salofalk 1.5g granules

(Dr. Falk Pharma UK Ltd)

1. NAME OF THE MEDICINAL PRODUCT

Salofalk 1.5 g gastro-resistant prolonged release granules

2. QUALITATIVE AND QUANTITATIVE COMPOSITION

Each sachet of Salofalk 1.5g granules contains 1.5g mesalazine.

Excipient:

Each sachet of Salofalk 1.5g granules contains 3.0mg aspartame.

For a full list of excipients, see section 6.1.

3. PHARMACEUTICAL FORM

Gastro-resistant prolonged release granules.

Description: Stick-formed or round, greyish white granules.

4. CLINICAL PARTICULARS

4.1 Therapeutic indications

For the treatment of acute episodes and the maintenance of remission of ulcerative colitis.

4.2 Posology and method of administration

Adults and elderly:

For the treatment of acute episodes of ulcerative colitis:

Once daily 1 or 2 sachets of Salofalk 1.5g granules or 3 sachets of Salofalk 1000mg granules or 3 sachets of Salofalk 500mg granules (equivalent to 1.5 – 3.0g mesalazine daily) preferably to be taken in the morning according to the individual clinical requirement.

It is also possible to take the prescribed daily dose in three divided doses (1 sachet of Salofalk 500mg granules three times daily, or 1 sachet of Salofalk 1000mg granules three times daily), if this is more convenient to the patient.

For the maintenance of remission of ulcerative colitis:

1 sachet of Salofalk 500mg granules three times daily (equivalent to 1.5g mesalazine daily).

Children below 6 years of age:

Salofalk granules should not be used in children under 6 years of age because there is very limited experience with this age group.

Children older than 6 years of age and adolescents:

In acute attacks, depending on disease severity, 30-50 mg mesalazine/kg/day should be given once daily preferably in the morning or in 3 divided doses. For **maintenance of remission**, 15-30 mg mesalazine/kg/day may be given in 2 divided doses. It is generally recommended that half the adult dose may be given to children up to a body weight of 40 kg; and the normal adult dose to those above 40 kg.

All patients:

The contents of the sachets of Salofalk granules should not be chewed. The granules should be taken on the tongue and swallowed, without chewing, with plenty of liquid.

Both in the treatment of acute inflammatory episodes and during long term treatment, Salofalk granules should be used on a regular basis and consistently in order to achieve the desired therapeutic effects.

In general, an acute episode of ulcerative colitis subsides after 8-12 weeks; the dosage can then, in most patients, be reduced to the maintenance dose.

4.3 Contraindications

Salofalk granules are contra-indicated in cases of:

- Pre-existing hypersensitivity to salicylic acid and its derivatives or to any of the other constituents.
- Severe impairment of hepatic and renal function.
- Pre-existing gastric or duodenal ulcer.
- Haemorrhagic diathesis.

4.4 Special warnings and precautions for use

Blood tests (differential blood count; liver function parameters like ALT or AST; serum creatinine) and urinary status (dip sticks) should be determined prior to and during treatment, at the discretion of the treating physician. As a guideline, controls are recommended 14 days after commencement of treatment, then a further two to three times at intervals of 4 weeks.

If the findings are normal, control examinations should be carried out every 3 months. If additional symptoms occur, control examinations should be performed immediately.

Caution is recommended in patients with impaired hepatic function.

Salofalk granules are not recommended in patients with impaired renal function.

Mesalazine-induced renal toxicity should be considered if renal function deteriorates during treatment.

Patients with pulmonary disease, in particular asthma, should be very carefully monitored during a course of treatment with Salofalk granules.

Patients with a history of adverse drug reactions to preparations containing sulfasalazine should be kept under close medical surveillance on commencement of a course of treatment with Salofalk granules. Should Salofalk granules cause acute intolerability reactions such as cramps, acute abdominal pain, fever, severe headache and rash, therapy should be discontinued immediately.

In patients with phenylketonuria it should be kept in mind that Salofalk 1.5g granules contain aspartame as a sweetening agent, equivalent to 1.68 mg phenylalanine.

Salofalk granules should not be used for the treatment of children below the age of 6 years.

4.5 Interaction with other medicinal products and other forms of interaction

Specific interaction studies have not been performed.

Interactions may occur during treatment with Salofalk granules and concomitant administration of the following medicinal products. Most of these possible interactions are based on theoretical reasons:

- Coumarin-type anticoagulants:

possible potentiation of the anticoagulant effects (increasing the risk of gastrointestinal haemorrhage)

- Glucocorticoids:

possible increase in undesirable gastric effects

- Sulphonylureas:

possible increase in the blood glucose-lowering effects

- Methotrexate:

possible increase in the toxic potential of methotrexate

- Probenecid/sulphinpyrazone:

possible attenuation of the uricosuric effects

- Spironolactone/frusemide:

possible attenuation of the diuretic effects

- Rifampicin:

possible attenuation of the tuberculostatic effects

- Lactulose or similar preparations, which lower stool pH:

possible reduction of mesalazine release from granules due to decreased pH caused by bacterial metabolism

In patients who are concomitantly treated with azathioprine or 6-mercaptopurine, possible enhanced myelosuppressive effects of azathioprine or 6-mercaptopurine should be taken into account.

4.6 Pregnancy and lactation

There are no adequate data from the use of Salofalk granules in pregnant woman. However, data on a limited number of exposed pregnancies indicate no adverse effect of mesalazine on pregnancy or on the health of the foetus/newborn child. To date no other relevant epidmiologic data are available. In one single case after long-term use of a high dose mesalazine (2-4 g, orally) during pregnancy, renal failure in a neonate was reported.

Animal studies on oral mesalazine do not indicate direct or indirect harmful effects with respect to pregnancy, embryonal / foetal development, parturition or postnatal development.

Salofalk granules should only be used during pregnancy if the potential benefit outweighs the possible risk.

N-acetyl-5-aminosalicylic acid and to a lesser degree mesalazine are excreted in breast milk. Only limited experience during lactation in woman is available to date. Hypersensitivity reactions like diarrhoea can not be excluded. Therefore, Salofalk granules should only be used during breast-feeding if the potential benefit outweighs the possible risk. If the suckling neonate develops diarrhoea, the breast-feeding should be discontinued.

4.7 Effects on ability to drive and use machines

No effects on ability to drive and use machines have been observed

4.8 Undesirable effects

system organ class	*frequency due to MedDRA convention*	
	rare (≥ 1/10,000; < 1/1,000)	*very rare* (< 1/ 10,000)
Blood and lymphatic system disorders		Altered blood counts (aplastic anaemia, agranulocytosis, pancytopenia, neutropenia, leukopenia, thrombocytopenia)
Nervous system disorders	Headache, dizziness	peripheral neuropathy
Gastrointestinal disorders	Abdominal pain, diarrhoea, flatulence, nausea, vomiting	
Renal and urinary disorders		Impairment of renal function including acute and chronic interstitial nephritis and renal insufficiency
Skin and subcutaneous tissue disorders		Alopecia
Musculoskeletal and connective tissue disorders		Myalgia, arthralgia
Immune system disorders		Hypersensitivity reactions such as allergic exanthema, drug fever, bronchospasm, peri- and myocarditis, acute pancreatitis, allergic alveolitis, lupus erythematosus syndrome, pancolitis
Hepatobiliary disorders		Changes in hepatic function parameters (increase in transaminases and parameters of cholestasis), hepatitis, cholestatic hepatitis
Reproductive system disorders		Oligospermia (reversible)

4.9 Overdose

No cases of intoxication have been reported to date and no specific antidotes are known.

If necessary, intravenous infusion of electrolytes (forced diuresis) should be considered in cases of overdose.

5. PHARMACOLOGICAL PROPERTIES

5.1 Pharmacodynamic properties

Pharmacotherapeutic group: Intestinal ant-inflammatory agent

ATC code: A07EC02

The mechanism of the anti-inflammatory action is unknown. The results of *in vitro* studies indicate that inhibition of lipoxygenase may play a role.

Effects on prostaglandin concentrations in the intestinal mucosa have also been demonstrated. Mesalazine (5-aminosalicylic acid / 5-ASA) may also function as a radical scavenger of reactive oxygen compounds.

Mesalazine, orally administered, acts predominantly locally at the gut mucosa and in the submucous tissue from the luminal side of the intestine. It is important, therefore, that mesalazine is available at the regions of inflammation. Systemic bioavailability / plasma concentrations of mesalazine therefore are of no relevance for therapeutic efficacy, but rather a factor for safety. In order to realise this, Salofalk granules are gastric juice resistant and release mesalazine in a pH dependent manner due to an Eudragit L coating, and prolonged manner due to the matrix granule structure.

5.2 Pharmacokinetic properties

General considerations of mesalazine:

Absorption:

Mesalazine absorption is highest in proximal gut regions and lowest in distal gut areas.

Biotransformation:

Mesalazine is metabolised both pre-systemically by the intestinal mucosa and the liver to the pharmacologically inactive N-acetyl-5-aminosalicylic acid (N-Ac-5-ASA). The acetylation seems to be independent of the acetylator phenotype of the patient. Some acetylation also occurs through the action of colonic bacteria. Protein binding of mesalazine and N-Ac-5-ASA is 43 % and 78 %, respectively.

Elimination:

Mesalazine and its metabolite N-Ac-5-ASA are eliminated via the faeces (major part), renally (varies between 20 and 50 %, dependent on kind of application, pharmaceutical preparation and route of mesalazine release, respectively), and biliary (minor part). Renal excretion predominantly occurs as N-Ac-5-ASA. About 1 % of total orally administered mesalazine dose is excreted into the breast milk mainly as N-Ac-5-ASA.

Salofalk Granules specific:

Distribution:

Owing to the granule size of about 1 mm, transit from the stomach to the small intestine is fast.

A combined pharmacoscintigraphic/pharmacokinetic study showed that the compound reaches the ileocaecal region within approx. 3 hours and the ascending colon within approx. 4 hours. The total transit time in the colon amounts to about 20 hours. Approximately 80 % of an administered oral dose is estimated to be available in the colon, sigmoid and rectum.

Absorption:

Mesalazine release from Salofalk granules starts after a lag phase of about 2-3 hours, peak plasma concentrations are reached at about 4-5 hours. The systemic bioavailability of mesalazine after oral administration is estimated to be approximately 15-25 %.

Food intake delays absorption for 1 to 2 hours but does not change the rate and extent of absorption.

Elimination:

From a 3 × 500 mg daily mesalazine dose, a total renal elimination of mesalazine and N-Ac-5-ASA under steady state condition was calculated to be about 25 %. The unmetabolised excreted mesalazine part was less than 1 % of the oral dose. The elimination half-life in this study was 4.4 hours.

5.3 Preclinical safety data

Preclinical data reveal no special hazard for humans based on conventional studies of safety pharmacology, genotoxicity, carcinogenicity (rat) or toxicity to reproduction.

Kidney toxicity (renal papillary necrosis and epithelial damage in the proximal convoluted tubule or the whole nephron) has been seen in repeat-dose toxicity studies with high oral doses of mesalazine. The clinical relevance of this finding is unknown.

6. PHARMACEUTICAL PARTICULARS

6.1 List of excipients

Aspartame (E951)

Carmellose sodium

Cellulose, microcrystalline

Citric acid, anhydrous

Silica, colloidal anhydrous

Hypromellose

Magnesium stearate

Methacrylic acid-methyl methacrylate copolymer (1:1) (Eudragit L 100)

Methylcellulose

Polyacrylate dispersion 40 % (Eudragit NE 40 D containing 2 % Nonoxynol 100)

Povidone K 25

Simeticone

Sorbic acid

Talc

Titanium dioxide (E 171)

Triethyl citrate

Vanilla custard flavouring (containing propylene glycol)

6.2 Incompatibilities

Not applicable.

6.3 Shelf life

4 years.

6.4 Special precautions for storage

No special precautions for storage.

6.5 Nature and contents of container

Container: Polyester/ Aluminium/ Polyethylene-Foil

Package sizes: 20, 30, 35, 45, 50, 60, 70, 90, 100 and 150 sachets Salofalk 1.5 g granules.

Not all package sizes will be marketed.

6.6 Special precautions for disposal and other handling

No special requirements.

7. MARKETING AUTHORISATION HOLDER

Dr. Falk Pharma GmbH

Leinenweberstr. 5

79108 Freiburg

Germany

Tel: +49 (0)761 1514-0

8. MARKETING AUTHORISATION NUMBER(S)

PL 08637/0016

9. DATE OF FIRST AUTHORISATION/RENEWAL OF THE AUTHORISATION

Date of first authorisation: May 2008

Renewal of the authorisations:

10. DATE OF REVISION OF THE TEXT

11 DOSIMETRY (IF APPLICABLE)

Not applicable.

12 INSTRUCTIONS FOR PREPARATION OF RADIOPHARMACEUTICALS (IF APPLICABLE)

Not applicable.

Salofalk 1000mg Granules

(Dr. Falk Pharma UK Ltd)

1. NAME OF THE MEDICINAL PRODUCT

Salofalk 1000mg gastro-resistant prolonged release granules

2. QUALITATIVE AND QUANTITATIVE COMPOSITION

Each sachet of Salofalk 1000mg granules contains 1000 mg mesalazine.

Excipient:

Each sachet of Salofalk 1000mg granules contains 2.0 mg aspartame.

For a full list of excipients, see section 6.1.

3. PHARMACEUTICAL FORM

Gastro-resistant prolonged release granules.

Description: Stick-formed or round, greyish white granules.

4. CLINICAL PARTICULARS

4.1 Therapeutic indications

For the treatment of acute episodes and the maintenance of remission of ulcerative colitis.

4.2 Posology and method of administration

Adults and elderly:

For the treatment of acute episodes of ulcerative colitis:

Once daily 3 sachets of Salofalk 500mg granules or 3 sachets of Salofalk 1000mg granules (equivalent to 1.5 – 3.0 g mesalazine daily) preferably to be taken in the morning according to the individual clinical necessities.

It is also possible to take the prescribed daily dose in three divided doses (1 sachet of Salofalk 500mg granules three times daily, or 1 sachet of Salofalk 1000mg granules three times daily), if this is more convenient to the patient.

For the maintenance of remission of ulcerative colitis:

1 sachet of Salofalk 500mg granules three times daily (equivalent to 1.5 g mesalazine daily).

Children below 6 years of age:

Salofalk granules should not be used in children under 6 years of age because there is very limited experience with this age group.

Children older than 6 years of age and adolescents:

In acute attacks, depending on disease severity, 30-50 mg mesalazine/kg/day should be given once daily preferably in the morning or in 3 divided doses. For **maintenance of remission**, 15-30 mg mesalazine/kg/day may be given in 2 divided doses. It is generally recommended that half the adult dose may be given to children up to a body weight of 40 kg; and the normal adult dose to those above 40 kg.

All patients:

The contents of the sachets of Salofalk granules should not be chewed. The granules should be taken on the tongue and swallowed, without chewing, with plenty of liquid.

Both in the treatment of acute inflammatory episodes and during long term treatment, Salofalk granules should be used on a regular basis and consistently in order to achieve the desired therapeutic effects.

In general, an acute episode of ulcerative colitis subsides after 8-12 weeks; the dosage can then, in most patients, be reduced to the maintenance dose.

4.3 Contraindications

Salofalk granules are contra-indicated in cases of:

- Pre-existing hypersensitivity to salicylic acid and its derivatives or to any of the other constituents.
- Severe impairment of hepatic and renal function.
- Pre-existing gastric or duodenal ulcer.
- Haemorrhagic diathesis.

4.4 Special warnings and precautions for use

Blood tests (differential blood count; liver function parameters like ALT or AST; serum creatinine) and urinary status (dip sticks) should be determined prior to and during treatment, at the discretion of the treating physician. As a guideline, controls are recommended 14 days after commencement of treatment, then a further two to three times at intervals of 4 weeks.

If the findings are normal, control examinations should be carried out every 3 months. If additional symptoms occur, control examinations should be performed immediately.

Caution is recommended in patients with impaired hepatic function.

Salofalk granules are not recommended in patients with impaired renal function.

Mesalazine-induced renal toxicity should be considered if renal function deteriorates during treatment.

Patients with pulmonary disease, in particular asthma, should be very carefully monitored during a course of treatment with Salofalk granules.

Patients with a history of adverse drug reactions to preparations containing sulfasalazine should be kept under close medical surveillance on commencement of a course of treatment with Salofalk granules. Should Salofalk granules cause acute intolerability reactions such as cramps, acute abdominal pain, fever, severe headache and rash, therapy should be discontinued immediately.

In patients with phenylketonuria it should be kept in mind that Salofalk 1000mg granules contain aspartame as a sweetening agent, equivalent to 1.12 mg phenylalanine.

Salofalk granules should not be used for the treatment of children below the age of 6 years.

4.5 Interaction with other medicinal products and other forms of interaction

Specific interaction studies have not been performed.

Interactions may occur during treatment with Salofalk granules and concomitant administration of the following medicinal products. Most of these possible interactions are based on theoretical reasons:

- Coumarin-type anticoagulants:

possible potentiation of the anticoagulant effects (increasing the risk of gastrointestinal haemorrhage)

- Glucocorticoids:

possible increase in undesirable gastric effects

- Sulphonylureas:

possible increase in the blood glucose-lowering effects

- Methotrexate:

possible increase in the toxic potential of methotrexate

- Probenecid/sulphinpyrazone:

possible attenuation of the uricosuric effects

- Spironolactone/frusemide:

possible attenuation of the diuretic effects

- Rifampicin:

possible attenuation of the tuberculostatic effects

- Lactulose or similar preparations, which lower stool pH:

possible reduction of mesalazine release from granules due to decreased pH caused by bacterial metabolism

In patients who are concomitantly treated with azathioprine or 6-mercaptopurine, possible enhanced myelosuppressive effects of azathioprine or 6-mercaptopurine should be taken into account.

4.6 Pregnancy and lactation

There are no adequate data from the use of Salofalk granules in pregnant woman. However, data on a limited number of exposed pregnancies indicate no adverse effect of mesalazine on pregnancy or on the health of the foetus/newborn child. To date no other relevant epidemiologic data are available. In one single case after long-term use of a high dose mesalazine (2-4 g, orally) during pregnancy, renal failure in a neonate was reported.

Animal studies on oral mesalazine do not indicate direct or indirect harmful effects with respect to pregnancy, embryonal / foetal development, parturition or postnatal development.

Salofalk granules should only be used during pregnancy if the potential benefit outweighs the possible risk.

N-acetyl-5-aminosalicylic acid and to a lesser degree mesalazine are excreted in breast milk. Only limited experience during lactation in woman is available to date. Hypersensitivity reactions like diarrhoea can not be excluded. Therefore, Salofalk granules should only be used during breast-feeding if the potential benefit outweighs the possible risk. If the suckling neonate develops diarrhoea, the breast-feeding should be discontinued.

4.7 Effects on ability to drive and use machines

No effects on ability to drive and use machines have been observed.

4.8 Undesirable effects

Gastrointestinal undesirable effects (rare, ⩾ 0.01 % - < 0.1 %):

Abdominal pain, diarrhoea, flatulence, nausea, vomiting

Nervous system disorders:

Headache, dizziness (rare, ⩾ 0.01 % - < 0.1 %)

peripheral neuropathy (very rare, < 0.01 %)

Renal undesirable effects (very rare, < 0.01 %):

Impairment of renal function including acute and chronic interstitial nephritis and renal insufficiency

Hypersensitivity reactions (very rare, < 0.01 %):

Allergic exanthema, drug fever, bronchospasm, peri- and myocarditis, acute pancreatitis, allergic alveolitis, lupus erythematosus syndrome, pancolitis

Musculoskeletal disorders (very rare, < 0.01 %):

Myalgia, arthralgia

Blood and the lymphatic system disorders (very rare, < 0.01 %):

Altered blood counts (aplastic anaemia, agranulocytosis, pancytopenia, neutropenia, leukopenia, thrombocytopenia)

Hepato-biliary disorders (very rare, < 0.01 %):

Changes in hepatic function parameters (increase in transaminases and parameters of cholestasis), hepatitis, cholestatic hepatitis

Skin and appendages disorders (very rare, < 0.01 %):

Alopecia

Reproductive system disorders (very rare, < 0.01 %):

Oligospermia (reversible)

4.9 Overdose

No cases of intoxication have been reported to date and no specific antidotes are known.

If necessary, intravenous infusion of electrolytes (forced diuresis) should be considered in cases of overdose.

5. PHARMACOLOGICAL PROPERTIES

5.1 Pharmacodynamic properties

Pharmacotherapeutic group: Intestinal anti-inflammatory agent

ATC code: A07EC02

The mechanism of the anti-inflammatory action is unknown. The results of *in vitro* studies indicate that inhibition of lipoxygenase may play a role.

Effects on prostaglandin concentrations in the intestinal mucosa have also been demonstrated. Mesalazine (5-aminosalicylic acid / 5-ASA) may also function as a radical scavenger of reactive oxygen compounds.

Mesalazine, orally administered, acts predominantly locally at the gut mucosa and in the submucous tissue from the luminal side of the intestine. It is important, therefore, that mesalazine is available at the regions of inflammation. Systemic bioavailability / plasma concentrations of mesalazine therefore are of no relevance for therapeutic efficacy, but rather a factor for safety. In order to realise this, Salofalk granules are gastric juice resistant and release mesalazine in a pH dependent manner due to an Eudragit L coating, and prolonged manner due to the matrix granule structure.

5.2 Pharmacokinetic properties

General considerations of mesalazine:

Absorption:

Mesalazine absorption is highest in proximal gut regions and lowest in distal gut areas.

Biotransformation:

Mesalazine is metabolised both pre-systemically by the intestinal mucosa and the liver to the pharmacologically inactive N-acetyl-5-aminosalicylic acid (N-Ac-5-ASA). The acetylation seems to be independent of the acetylator phenotype of the patient. Some acetylation also occurs through the action of colonic bacteria. Protein binding of mesalazine and N-Ac-5-ASA is 43 % and 78 %, respectively.

Elimination:

Mesalazine and its metabolite N-Ac-5-ASA are eliminated via the faeces (major part), renally (varies between 20 and 50 %, dependent on kind of application, pharmaceutical preparation and route of mesalazine release, respectively), and biliary (minor part). Renal excretion predominantly occurs as N-Ac-5-ASA. About 1 % of total orally administered mesalazine dose is excreted into the breast milk mainly as N-Ac-5-ASA.

Salofalk Granules specific:

Distribution:

Owing to the granule size of about 1 mm, transit from the stomach to the small intestine is fast.

A combined pharmacoscintigraphic/pharmacokinetic study showed that the compound reaches the ileocaecal region within approx. 3 hours and the ascending colon within approx. 4 hours. The total transit time in the colon amounts to about 20 hours. Approximately 80 % of an administered oral dose is estimated to be available in the colon, sigmoid and rectum.

Absorption:

Mesalazine release from Salofalk granules starts after a lag phase of about 2-3 hours, peak plasma concentrations are reached at about 4-5 hours. The systemic bioavailability of mesalazine after oral administration is estimated to be approximately 15-25 %.

Food intake delays absorption for 1 to 2 hours but does not change the rate and extent of absorption.

Elimination:

From a 3 × 500 mg daily mesalazine dose, a total renal elimination of mesalazine and N-Ac-5-ASA under steady state condition was calculated to be about 25 %. The unmetabolised excreted mesalazine part was less than 1 % of the oral dose. The elimination half-life in this study was 4.4 hours.

5.3 Preclinical safety data

Preclinical data reveal no special hazard for humans based on conventional studies of safety pharmacology, genotoxicity, carcinogenicity (rat) or toxicity to reproduction.

Kidney toxicity (renal papillary necrosis and epithelial damage in the proximal convoluted tubule or the whole nephron) has been seen in repeat-dose toxicity studies with high oral doses of mesalazine. The clinical relevance of this finding is unknown.

6. PHARMACEUTICAL PARTICULARS

6.1 List of excipients

Aspartame (E 951)

Carmellose sodium

Cellulose, microcrystalline

Citric acid, anhydrous

Silica, colloidal anhydrous

Hypromellose

Magnesium stearate

Methacrylic acid-methyl methacrylate copolymer (1:1) (Eudragit L 100)

Methylcellulose

Polyacrylate dispersion 40 per cent (Eudragit NE 40 D containing 2 per cent Nonoxynol 100)

Povidone K 25

Simeticone

Sorbic acid

Talc

Titanium dioxide (E 171)

Triethyl citrate

Vanilla custard flavouring (containing propylene glycol)

6.2 Incompatibilities

Not applicable.

6.3 Shelf life

4 years.

6.4 Special precautions for storage

No special precautions for storage.

6.5 Nature and contents of container
Container: Polyester/ Aluminium/ Polyethylene-Foil

Package sizes: 20 sachets, 50 sachets, 60 sachets, 100 sachets or 150 sachets Salofalk 1000mg granules

Not all package sizes may be marketed.

6.6 Special precautions for disposal and other handling
No special requirements.

7. MARKETING AUTHORISATION HOLDER
Dr. Falk Pharma GmbH

Leinenweberstr. 5

P. O. Box 6529

79041 Freiburg

Germany

Tel: +49 (0)761 1514-0

8. MARKETING AUTHORISATION NUMBER(S)
PL 08637/0008

9. DATE OF FIRST AUTHORISATION/RENEWAL OF THE AUTHORISATION
Date of first authorisation: 15 October 2001

Date of renewal: 01 March 2007

10. DATE OF REVISION OF THE TEXT
February 2008

Salofalk 250mg Tablets

(Dr. Falk Pharma UK Ltd)

1. NAME OF THE MEDICINAL PRODUCT
Salofalk® 250mg Tablets

2. QUALITATIVE AND QUANTITATIVE COMPOSITION
Mesalazine 250mg.

For excipients, see 6.1

3. PHARMACEUTICAL FORM
Enteric coated tablet

4. CLINICAL PARTICULARS

4.1 Therapeutic indications
Treatment of mild to moderate acute exacerbations of ulcerative colitis and for the maintenance of remission of ulcerative colitis

4.2 Posology and method of administration
Method of Administration: Oral

Adults: Acute treatment: six tablets daily in three divided doses.

Maintenance Treatment: three to six tablets daily in divided doses.

Elderly: As for adults

4.3 Contraindications
Patients with an active peptic ulcer, blood clotting abnormalities, severe hepatic or severe renal impairment or where there is a pathological propensity to bleeding. Salofalk® should not be used in babies and young children

4.4 Special warnings and precautions for use
Serious blood dyscrasias have been reported very rarely with mesalazine. Haematological investigations should be performed if the patient develops unexplained bleeding, bruising, purpura, anaemia, fever or sore throat.

Reports of interstitial nephritis occurring with mesalazine treatment are uncommon, however it is advisable that renal function be monitored, with serum creatinine levels measured prior to treatment start, every 3 months for the first year, 6 monthly for the next 4 years, and then annually thereafter. Use with extreme caution in patients with mild to moderate renal impairment (see section 4.3). If dehydration develops, normal electrolyte levels and fluid balance should be restored as soon as possible.

Treatment should be stopped if there is suspicion or evidence of blood dyscrasia, or if renal function deteriorates

4.5 Interaction with other medicinal products and other forms of interaction
The hypoglycaemic action of sulphonylureas can be intensified, as can gastrointestinal haemorrhage caused by coumarins. The toxicity of methotrexate can be increased. The uricosuric action of probenecid and sulfinpyrazone can be decreased, as can the diuretic action of furosemide and the action of spironolactone. The antituberculosis action of rifampicin can also be diminished.

Concomitant use with other known nephrotoxic agents, such as NSAIDs and azathioprine, may increase the risk of renal reactions (see section 4.4)

4.6 Pregnancy and lactation
Animal experiments with mesalazine have produced no evidence of embryonic effects. All competent authors recommend to continue treatment with sulfasalazine, the parent drug of mesalazine, during pregnancy. Up to now, they didn't see any untoward effect on its course or on the foetus. Therefore there is no reason to prohibit Salofalk® treatment during pregnancy. No untoward effects were seen in a reproductive and fertility study with mesalazine in breast-fed rat pups. But up to now there is a limited experience in using mesalazine/ sulfasalazine during the lactation period in man. Therefore, it should be stated that the experience with Salofalk® 250 during lactation up to now is not sufficient. The acetylated form of mesalazine is found in the breast milk in slight amounts

4.7 Effects on ability to drive and use machines
Salofalk® is not expected to affect ability to drive and use machines

4.8 Undesirable effects
Salofalk® may cause hypersensitivity reactions. These are unrelated to dose. Mesalazine may be associated with an exacerbation of the symptoms of colitis in those patients who have previously had such problems with sulfasalazine. There have been rare reports of leucopenia, neutropenia, agranulocytosis, aplastic anaemia and thrombocytopenia, pancreatitis, abnormalities of hepatic function, hepatitis and cholestatic hepatitis, myocarditis and pericarditis, allergic lung reactions, lupus erythematosus-like reactions, bullous skin reactions including erythema multiforme, Stevens Johnson Syndrome and rash (including urticaria), interstitial nephritis, peripheral neuropathy and nephrotic syndrome with oral mesalazine treatment, usually reversible on withdrawal. Renal failure has been reported. Mesalazine-induced nephrotoxicity should be suspected in patients developing renal dysfunction during treatment. Increased methaemoglobin levels may occur

4.9 Overdose
Due to the enteric nature of the formulation of Salofalk® 250mg tablets and the particular pharmacokinetic properties of mesalazine, only small amounts of the drug are available for systemic action. Consequently signs of intoxication are unlikely even after large doses. However, in principle, symptoms consistent with salicylate intoxication may occur (management of which is shown in brackets).

– Mixed Acidosis-Alkalosis (reinstatement of the acid-base balance to match the situation and electrolyte substitutions).

– Hyperventilation

– Pulmonary Oedema

– Dehydration from perspiration and vomiting (fluid intake)

– Hypoglycaemia (glucose intake)

There is no specific antidote to mesalazine but in many cases of overdose, gastric lavage and intravenous transfusion of electrolytes to promote diuresis should be implemented

5. PHARMACOLOGICAL PROPERTIES

5.1 Pharmacodynamic properties
The main site of action of mesalazine is the inflamed musosa in the terminal ileum and colon. The pH dependent enteric coating applied to Salofalk® tablets (Eudragit L) disintegrates above pH 6.0 ensuring that the drug is released at the site of action, where it is absorbed to a certain degree. The absorbed portion is acetylated and excreted predominantly in the acetylated form via the kidneys. A small portion (about 5% of the absorbed quantity) is excreted in the bile. In faeces, mesalazine is found particularly in unchanged form and partially in acetylated form

5.2 Pharmacokinetic properties
The elimination half-lives are 0.7-2.4 hours (mean 1.4 ± 0.6 hours). The plasma protein binding of mesalazine is 43% and of acetylated mesalazine 78%. The rapid acetylation is not reversible and, in contrast to sulfapyridine, there is no difference between slow and rapid acetylation

5.3 Preclinical safety data
None Stated

6. PHARMACEUTICAL PARTICULARS

6.1 List of excipients
Sodium carbonate, glycine, povidone, microcrystalline cellulose (E460), colloidal anhydrous silica, calcium stearate, hydroxypropylmethylcellulose (E464), methacrylic acid copolymer (Eudragit L), talc, titanium dioxide (E171), iron oxide (E172), polyethylene glycol, polymethacrylate (Eudragit E).

6.2 Incompatibilities
None stated

6.3 Shelf life
Three years

6.4 Special precautions for storage
None.

6.5 Nature and contents of container
Orange PVC/PVDC/ Al blister strips packed in cartons containing 10†, 100 or 300† tablets.

† Not currently marketed

6.6 Special precautions for disposal and other handling
None stated

7. MARKETING AUTHORISATION HOLDER
Dr Falk Pharma UK Ltd

Bourne End Business Park

Cores End Road

Bourne End

Buckinghamshire

SL8 5AS

8. MARKETING AUTHORISATION NUMBER(S)
PL 10341/0004.

9. DATE OF FIRST AUTHORISATION/RENEWAL OF THE AUTHORISATION
13 September 1991.

10. DATE OF REVISION OF THE TEXT
August 2008

11. DOSIMETRY
Not applicable

12 INSTRUCTIONS FOR PREPARATION OF RADIOPHARMACEUTICALS (IF APPLICABLE)
Not applicable

Salofalk 500mg Granules

(Dr. Falk Pharma UK Ltd)

1. NAME OF THE MEDICINAL PRODUCT
Salofalk 500mg gastro-resistant prolonged release granules

2. QUALITATIVE AND QUANTITATIVE COMPOSITION
Each sachet of Salofalk 500mg granules contains 500 mg mesalazine.

Excipient:

Each sachet of Salofalk 500mg granules contains 1.0mg aspartame.

For a full list of excipients, see section 6.1.

3. PHARMACEUTICAL FORM
Gastro-resistant prolonged release granules.

Description: Stick-formed or round, greyish white granules.

4. CLINICAL PARTICULARS

4.1 Therapeutic indications
For the treatment of acute episodes and the maintenance of remission of ulcerative colitis.

4.2 Posology and method of administration
Adults and elderly:

For the treatment of acute episodes of ulcerative colitis:

Once daily 3 sachets of Salofalk 500mg granules or 3 sachets of Salofalk 1000mg granules (equivalent to 1.5 – 3.0 g mesalazine daily) preferably to be taken in the morning according to the individual clinical necessities.

It is also possible to take the prescribed daily dose in three divided doses (1 sachet of Salofalk 500mg granules three times daily, or 1 sachet of Salofalk 1000mg granules three times daily), if this is more convenient to the patient.

For the maintenance of remission of ulcerative colitis:

1 sachets of Salofalk 500mg granules three times daily (equivalent to 1.5 g mesalazine daily).

Children below 6 years of age:

Salofalk granules should not be used in children under 6 years of age because there is very limited experience with this age group.

Children older than 6 years of age and adolescents:

In acute attacks, depending on disease severity, 30-50 mg mesalazine/kg/day should be given once daily preferably in the morning or in 3 divided doses. For **maintenance of remission**, 15-30 mg mesalazine/kg/day may be given in 2 divided doses. It is generally recommended that half the adult dose may be given to children up to a body weight of 40 kg; and the normal adult dose to those above 40 kg.

All patients:

The contents of the sachets of Salofalk granules should not be chewed. The granules should be taken on the tongue and swallowed, without chewing, with plenty of liquid.

Both in the treatment of acute inflammatory episodes and during long term treatment, Salofalk granules should be used on a regular basis and consistently in order to achieve the desired therapeutic effects.

In general, an acute episode of ulcerative colitis subsides after 8-12 weeks; the dosage can then, in most patients, be reduced to the maintenance dose.

4.3 Contraindications
Salofalk granules are contra-indicated in cases of:

- Pre-existing hypersensitivity to salicylic acid and its derivatives or to any of the other constituents.
- Severe impairment of hepatic and renal function.
- Pre-existing gastric or duodenal ulcer.
- Haemorrhagic diathesis.

4.4 Special warnings and precautions for use
Blood tests (differential blood count; liver function parameters like ALT or AST; serum creatinine) and urinary status (dip sticks) should be determined prior to and during treatment, at the discretion of the treating physician. As a guideline, controls are recommended 14 days after commencement of treatment, then a further two to three times at intervals of 4 weeks.

If the findings are normal, control examinations should be carried out every 3 months. If additional symptoms occur, control examinations should be performed immediately.

Caution is recommended in patients with impaired hepatic function.

Salofalk granules are not recommended in patients with impaired renal function.

Mesalazine-induced renal toxicity should be considered if renal function deteriorates during treatment.

Patients with pulmonary disease, in particular asthma, should be very carefully monitored during a course of treatment with Salofalk granules.

Patients with a history of adverse drug reactions to preparations containing sulfasalazine should be kept under close medical surveillance on commencement of a course of treatment with Salofalk granules. Should Salofalk granules cause acute intolerability reactions such as cramps, acute abdominal pain, fever, severe headache and rash, therapy should be discontinued immediately.

In patients with phenylketonuria it should be kept in mind that Salofalk 500mg granules contain aspartame as a sweetening agent, equivalent to 0.56 mg phenylalanine.

Salofalk granules should not be used for the treatment of children below the age of 6 years.

4.5 Interaction with other medicinal products and other forms of interaction

Specific interaction studies have not been performed.

Interactions may occur during treatment with Salofalk granules and concomitant administration of the following medicinal products. Most of these possible interactions are based on theoretical reasons:

- Coumarin-type anticoagulants:

possible potentiation of the anticoagulant effects (increasing the risk of gastrointestinal haemorrhage)

- Glucocorticoids:

possible increase in undesirable gastric effects

- Sulphonylureas:

possible increase in the blood glucose-lowering effects

- Methotrexate:

possible increase in the toxic potential of methotrexate

- Probenecid/sulphinpyrazone:

possible attenuation of the uricosuric effects

- Spironolactone/frusemide:

possible attenuation of the diuretic effects

- Rifampicin:

possible attenuation of the tuberculostatic effects

- Lactulose or similar preparations, which lower stool pH:

possible reduction of mesalazine release from granules due to decreased pH caused by bacterial metabolism

In patients who are concomitantly treated with azathioprine or 6-mercaptopurine, possible enhanced myelosuppressive effects of azathioprine or 6-mercaptopurine should be taken into account.

4.6 Pregnancy and lactation

There are no adequate data from the use of Salofalk granules in pregnant woman. However, data on a limited number of exposed pregnancies indicate no adverse effect of mesalazine on pregnancy or on the health of the foetus/newborn child. To date no other relevant epidmiologic data are available. In one single case after long-term use of a high dose mesalazine (2-4 g, orally) during pregnancy, renal failure in a neonate was reported.

Animal studies on oral mesalazine do not indicate direct or indirect harmful effects with respect to pregnancy, embryonal / foetal development, parturition or postnatal development.

Salofalk granules should only be used during pregnancy if the potential benefit outweighs the possible risk.

N-acetyl-5-aminosalicylic acid and to a lesser degree mesalazine are excreted in breast milk. Only limited experience during lactation in woman is available to date. Hypersensitivity reactions like diarrhoea can not be excluded. Therefore, Salofalk granules should only be used during breast-feeding if the potential benefit outweighs the possible risk. If the suckling neonate develops diarrhoea, the breast-feeding should be discontinued.

4.7 Effects on ability to drive and use machines

No effects on ability to drive and use machines have been observed

4.8 Undesirable effects

Gastrointestinal undesirable effects (rare, $\geqslant$ 0.01 % - < 0.1 %):

Abdominal pain, diarrhoea, flatulence, nausea, vomiting

Nervous system disorders:

Headache, dizziness (rare, $\geqslant$0.01 % - < 0.1 %)

peripheral neuropathy (very rare, <0.01 %)

Renal undesirable effects (very rare, < 0.01 %):

Impairment of renal function including acute and chronic interstitial nephritis and renal insufficiency

Hypersensitivity reactions (very rare, < 0.01 %):

Allergic exanthema, drug fever, bronchospasm, peri- and myocarditis, acute pancreatitis, allergic alveolitis, lupus erythematosus syndrome, pancolitis

Musculoskeletal disorders (very rare, < 0.01 %):

Myalgia, arthralgia

Blood and the lymphatic system disorders (very rare, < 0.01 %):

Altered blood counts (aplastic anaemia, agranulocytosis, pancytopenia, neutropenia, leukopenia, thrombocytopenia)

Hepato-biliary disorders (very rare, <0.01 %):

Changes in hepatic function parameters (increase in transaminases and parameters of cholestasis), hepatitis, cholestatic hepatitis

Skin and appendages disorders (very rare, <0.01 %):

Alopecia

Reproductive system disorders (very rare, <0.01 %):

Oligospermia (reversible)

4.9 Overdose

No cases of intoxication have been reported to date and no specific antidotes are known.

If necessary, intravenous infusion of electrolytes (forced diuresis) should be considered in cases of overdose.

5. PHARMACOLOGICAL PROPERTIES

5.1 Pharmacodynamic properties

Pharmacotherapeutic group: Intestinal anti-inflammatory agent

ATC code: A07EC02

The mechanism of the anti-inflammatory action is unknown. The results of *in vitro* studies indicate that inhibition of lipoxygenase may play a role.

Effects on prostaglandin concentrations in the intestinal mucosa have also been demonstrated. Mesalazine (5-aminosalicylic acid / 5-ASA) may also function as a radical scavenger of reactive oxygen compounds.

Mesalazine, orally administered, acts predominantly locally at the gut mucosa and in the submucous tissue from the luminal side of the intestine. It is important, therefore, that mesalazine is available at the regions of inflammation. Systemic bioavailability / plasma concentrations of mesalazine therefore are of no relevance for therapeutic efficacy, but rather a factor for safety. In order to realise this, Salofalk granules are gastric juice resistant and release mesalazine in a pH dependent manner due to an Eudragit L coating, and prolonged manner due to the matrix granule structure.

5.2 Pharmacokinetic properties

General considerations of mesalazine:

Absorption:

Mesalazine absorption is highest in proximal gut regions and lowest in distal gut areas.

Biotransformation:

Mesalazine is metabolised both pre-systemically by the intestinal mucosa and the liver to the pharmacologically inactive N-acetyl-5-aminosalicylic acid (N-Ac-5-ASA). The acetylation seems to be independent of the acetylator phenotype of the patient. Some acetylation also occurs through the action of colonic bacteria. Protein binding of mesalazine and N-Ac-5-ASA is 43 % and 78 %, respectively.

Elimination:

Mesalazine and its metabolite N-Ac-5-ASA are eliminated via the faeces (major part), renally (varies between 20 and 50 %, dependent on kind of application, pharmaceutical preparation and route of mesalazine release, respectively), and biliary (minor part). Renal excretion predominantly occurs as N-Ac-5-ASA. About 1 % of total orally administered mesalazine dose is excreted into the breast milk mainly as N-Ac-5-ASA.

Salofalk Granules specific:

Distribution:

Owing to the granule size of about 1 mm, transit from the stomach to the small intestine is fast.

A combined pharmacoscintigraphic/pharmacokinetic study showed that the compound reaches the ileocaecal region within approx. 3 hours and the ascending colon within approx. 4 hours. The total transit time in the colon amounts to about 20 hours. Approximately 80 % of an administered oral dose is estimated to be available in the colon, sigmoid and rectum.

Absorption:

Mesalazine release from Salofalk granules starts after a lag phase of about 2-3 hours, peak plasma concentrations are reached at about 4-5 hours. The systemic bioavailability of mesalazine after oral administration is estimated to be approximately 15-25 %.

Food intake delays absorption for 1 to 2 hours but does not change the rate and extent of absorption.

Elimination:

From a 3 × 500 mg daily mesalazine dose, a total renal elimination of mesalazine and N-Ac-5-ASA under steady state condition was calculated to be about 25 %. The unmetabolised excreted mesalazine part was less than 1 % of the oral dose. The elimination half-life in this study was 4.4 hours.

5.3 Preclinical safety data

Preclinical data reveal no special hazard for humans based on conventional studies of safety pharmacology, genotoxicity, carcinogenicity (rat) or toxicity to reproduction.

Kidney toxicity (renal papillary necrosis and epithelial damage in the proximal convoluted tubule or the whole nephron) has been seen in repeat-dose toxicity studies with high oral doses of mesalazine. The clinical relevance of this finding is unknown.

6. PHARMACEUTICAL PARTICULARS

6.1 List of excipients

Aspartame (E951)

Carmellose sodium

Cellulose, microcrystalline

Citric acid, anhydrous

Silica, colloidal anhydrous

Hypromellose

Magnesium stearate

Methacrylic acid-methyl methacrylate copolymer (1:1) (Eudragit L 100)

Methylcellulose

Polyacrylate dispersion 40 per cent (Eudragit NE 40 D containing 2 per cent Nonoxynol 100)

Povidone K 25

Simeticone

Sorbic acid

Talc

Titanium dioxide (E 171)

Triethyl citrate

Vanilla custard flavouring (containing propylene glycol)

6.2 Incompatibilities

Not applicable.

6.3 Shelf life

4 years.

6.4 Special precautions for storage

No special precautions for storage.

6.5 Nature and contents of container

Container: Polyester/ Aluminium/ Polyethylene-Foil

Package sizes: 50 sachets, 100 sachets or 300 sachets Salofalk 500mg granules

Not all package sizes may be marketed.

6.6 Special precautions for disposal and other handling

No special requirements.

7. MARKETING AUTHORISATION HOLDER

Dr. Falk Pharma GmbH

Leinenweberstr. 5

P. O. Box 6529

79041 Freiburg

Germany

Tel: +49 (0)761 1514-0

8. MARKETING AUTHORISATION NUMBER(S)

PL 08637 / 0007

9. DATE OF FIRST AUTHORISATION/RENEWAL OF THE AUTHORISATION

Date of first authorisation: 15 October 2001

Date of renewal: 01 March 2007

10. DATE OF REVISION OF THE TEXT

12/2007

Salofalk Enema 2g

(Dr. Falk Pharma UK Ltd)

1. NAME OF THE MEDICINAL PRODUCT

Salofalk Enema 2g.

2. QUALITATIVE AND QUANTITATIVE COMPOSITION

Each enema contains the following active ingredient:

Mesalazine 2g in 59 ml of suspension.

3. PHARMACEUTICAL FORM

Enema.

4. CLINICAL PARTICULARS

4.1 Therapeutic indications

Therapy and prophylaxis of acute attacks of mild ulcerative colitis, especially in the rectum and sigmoid colon and also in the descending colon.

4.2 Posology and method of administration

Method of administration: Rectal

Adults and the Elderly: 1 enema once a day at bedtime. The action of Salofalk is enhanced if the patient lies on the left side when introducing the enema. The dosage should be adjusted to suit the progress of the condition. Do not discontinue treatment suddenly.

Children: There is no recommended dose for children. Mesalazine should not be used in babies and infants.

4.3 Contraindications

Severe renal and hepatic function disturbances. Active gastrointestinal ulcers. Hypersensitivity to salicylates.

4.4 Special warnings and precautions for use

The drug should not be prescribed for infants.

Serious blood dyscrasias have been reported rarely with mesalazine. Haematological investigations including methaemoglobin values should be performed regularly during the course of therapy and if the patient develops unexplained bleeding, bruising, purpura, anaemia, fever or sore throat. Treatment should be stopped if there is suspicion or evidence of blood dyscrasia, or if renal function deteriorates. Sulphite component as excipient in enema preparation may cause hypersensitivity reactions in patients suffering from bronchial asthma.

Reports of interstitial nephritis occurring with mesalazine treatment are uncommon; however, patients on oral forms may require renal monitoring. Use with extreme caution in patients with mild to moderate renal impairment (see section 4.3) and if dehydration develops, normal electrolyte levels and fluid balance should be restored as soon as possible.

4.5 Interaction with other medicinal products and other forms of interaction

Although the following interactions are theoretically possible, owing to the low degree of absorption of the rectally administered mesalazine, the risk of their onset is extremely low: mesalazine may potentiate the actions of sulphonylureas. Interactions with coumarin, methotrexate, probenecid, sulfinpyrazone, spironolactone, furosemide and rifampicin cannot be excluded. Mesalazine can theoretically potentiate the side effects of glucocorticoids on the stomach. Concurrent use with other known nephrotoxic agents such as NSAID's and azathioprine may increase the risk of renal reactions (see section 4.4).

4.6 Pregnancy and lactation

Animal experiments on mesalazine have produced no evidence of embryonic effects. No untoward effects were seen in a reproductive and fertility study with mesalazine in breast-fed rat pups. Mesalazine is acetylated in the body and passes in this form into breast milk. Limited use of mesalazine in pregnancy has shown no untoward effect on the foetus. However, it should not be used during the first trimester. It can be used with caution during pregnancy and only if the potential benefits outweigh the potential risks.

4.7 Effects on ability to drive and use machines

Salofalk Enema is not expected to affect ability to drive and use machines. If dizziness develops, the patient should not drive or operate machinery.

4.8 Undesirable effects

Rectal Salofalk may cause acute intolerance (sensitivity reactions). This is characterised by abdominal pain, bloody diarrhoea, fever, pruritus and rash. These are unrelated to dose.

The most common adverse effects following treatment with rectal mesalazine are:

- General symptoms such as dizziness, malaise, paraesthesia, arthralgia and pyrexia may develop following rectal administration of sulphasalazine.

- GI effects: abdominal pain, flatulence, nausea, worsening or development of diarrhoea.

- CNS effects: Headache, malaise, dizziness and peripheral neuropathy.

- Sensitivity reactions: Mesalazine may be associated with an exacerbation of the symptoms of colitis in those patients who have previously had such problems with sulfasalazine. Allergic skin reactions such as rash, bullous skin reactions including erythema multiforme and Stevens-Johnson syndrome.

- Other adverse effects: Fever, arthralgia, pericarditis, myocarditis, pancreatitis

Other adverse effects were reported following oral administration of mesalazine.

There have been rare reports of leucopenia, neutropenia, agranulocytosis, aplastic anaemia and thrombocytopenia, abnormalities of hepatic function, hepatitis, cholestatic hepatitis, allergic lung reactions, interstitial nephritis and nephrotic syndrome with oral mesalazine treatment, usually reversible on withdrawal. Renal failure has been reported. Mesalazine-induced nephrotoxicity should be suspected in patients developing renal dysfunction during treatment. Increased methaemoglobin levels may occur. Headache and digestive disturbances such as nausea and diarrhoea may occur. Isolated cases of hair loss have been reported.

4.9 Overdose

There have been no reported cases of overdosage.

5. PHARMACOLOGICAL PROPERTIES

5.1 Pharmacodynamic properties

Mesalazine is the biologically active metabolite of salicylazosulfapyridine that is used in the treatment of certain chronic inflammatory conditions of the intestine.

5.2 Pharmacokinetic properties

Following rectal administration the major fraction is recovered from the faeces, a small percentage (approximately 15%) is absorbed; the absorbed mesalazine is excreted mainly in the urine; biliary excretion is secondary. The acetylated and the non-acetylated forms of mesalazine bind slightly to plasma proteins.

5.3 Preclinical safety data

None stated.

6. PHARMACEUTICAL PARTICULARS

6.1 List of excipients

Salofalk Enema 2g contain the following excipients:

Carbomer

Disodium edetate

Potassium acetate

Potassium metabisulphite

Purified water

Sodium benzoate

Xanthan gum

6.2 Incompatibilities

None known.

6.3 Shelf life

24 months.

6.4 Special precautions for storage

Store at room temperature (15-25°C) and protect from light.

6.5 Nature and contents of container

Low density concertina shaped polythene bottle with a low density polythene application nozzle packed in cartons containing seven individually blister packed bottles.

6.6 Special precautions for disposal and other handling

None

Administrative Data

7. MARKETING AUTHORISATION HOLDER

Dr Falk Pharma UK Ltd

Unit k

Bourne End Business Park

Cores End Road

Bourne End

Bucks

SL8 5AS

United Kingdom

8. MARKETING AUTHORISATION NUMBER(S)

PL 10341/0008

9. DATE OF FIRST AUTHORISATION/RENEWAL OF THE AUTHORISATION

31st December 2004

10. DATE OF REVISION OF THE TEXT

August 2006

Salofalk Rectal Foam 1g

(Dr. Falk Pharma UK Ltd)

1. NAME OF THE MEDICINAL PRODUCT

Salofalk 1g/actuation Rectal Foam.

2. QUALITATIVE AND QUANTITATIVE COMPOSITION

1 actuation contains:

Mesalazine 1.0g

Excipients: cetostearyl alcohol, propylene glycol and meta bisulphite

For a full list of excipients, see section 6.1.

3. PHARMACEUTICAL FORM

Rectal foam.

White-greyish to slightly reddish-violet, creamy firm foam.

4. CLINICAL PARTICULARS

4.1 Therapeutic indications

Treatment of active, mild ulcerative colitis of the sigmoid colon and rectum.

4.2 Posology and method of administration

Method of Administration: rectal.

Adults and adolescents above 12 years of age:

Two administrations once a day at bedtime. The canister is first fitted with an applicator and then shaken for about 20 seconds before the applicator is inserted into the rectum as far as comfortable. To administer a dose of Salofalk®, the pump dome is fully pushed down and released. Note that the spray will only work properly when held with the pump dome pointing down. Following the first or second activation depending upon need (see below) the applicator should be held in position for 10-15 seconds before being withdrawn from the rectum. If the patient has difficulty in holding this amount of foam, the foam can also be administered in divided doses: one at bedtime and the other during the night (after evacuation of the first single dose) or in the early morning. The best results are obtained when the intestine is evacuated prior to administration of Salofalk®.

In general, an acute episode of a mild ulcerative colitis subsides after 4-6 weeks. It is recommended to continue the maintenance therapy with an oral mesalazine preparation e.g. Salofalk gastro-resistant prolonged release granules at a dosage recommended for this preparation.

Children below 12 years of age:

Salofalk rectal foam should not be used in children below 12 years of age because of insufficient experience with the rectal foam in this age group.

4.3 Contraindications

Salofalk® is contraindicated in cases of:

- pre-existing hypersensitivity to salicylic acid and its derivatives or to any of the other constituents.
- severe impairment of hepatic and renal function
- pre-existing gastric or duodenal ulcers
- haemorrhagic diathesis

Salofalk should not be used for the treatment of children below the age of 12 years.

Caution:

Asthmatics should be treated with care with Salofalk® since sulphite contained in the foam may cause hypersensitivity reactions.

4.4 Special warnings and precautions for use

Blood tests (differential blood counts; liver function parameters like ALT or AST; serum creatinine) and urinary status (dip sticks) should be determined prior to and during treatment, at the discretion of the treating physician. As a guideline, controls are recommended 14 days after commencement of treatment, then a further two to three times at intervals of 4 weeks.

If the findings are normal, control examinations should be carried out every 3 months. If additional symptoms occur, control examinations should be performed immediately. Caution is recommended in patients with impaired hepatic function. Salofalk is not recommended in patients with impaired renal function. Mesalazine-induced renal toxicity should be considered if renal function deteriorates during treatment.

Patients with pulmonary disease, in particular asthma, should be very carefully monitored during a course of treatment with Salofalk.

Patients with a history of adverse drug reactions to preparations containing sulphasalazine should be kept under close medical surveillance on commencement of a course of treatment with Salofalk. Should Salofalk cause acute intolerability reactions such as cramps, acute abdominal pain, fever, severe headache and rash, therapy should be discontinued immediately.

Special notes:

In isolated cases hypersensitivity reactions principally in the form of respiratory problems may be experienced also by non-asthmatics due to the content of sulphite. This medicine contains propylene glycol that may cause lactic acidosis, hyperosmolality, haemolysis and CNS depression. Slight to mild skin irritation due to propylene glycol may occur. This medicine contains cetostearyl alcohol that may cause local skin reactions (e.g contact dermatitis).

4.5 Interaction with other medicinal products and other forms of interaction

Specific interaction studies have not been performed.

Interactions may occur during treatment with Salofalk and concomitant administration of the following medicinal products. Most of these possible interactions are based on theoretical reasons:

- *Coumarin-type Anticoagulants:* possible potentiation of the anticoagulant effects (increasing the risk of gastro-intestinal haemorrhage)

- *Glucocorticoids:* possible increase in undesirable gastric effects

- *Sulphonylureas:* possible increase in the blood glucose-lowering effects.

- *Methotrexate:* possible increase in the toxic potential of methotrexate.

- *Probenecid/Sulphinpyrazone:* possible attenuation of the uricosuric effects.

- *Spironolactone/frusemide:* possible attenuation of the diuretic effects.

- *Rifampicin:* possible attenuation of the tuberculostatic effects.

In patients who are concomitantly treated with azathioprine or 6-mercaptopurine, possible enhanced myelosuppresive effects of azathioprine or 6-mercaptopurine should be taken into account.

4.6 Pregnancy and lactation

There are no adequate data from the use of Salofalk rectal foam in pregnant women.

However, data on a limited number of exposed pregnancies after oral application of mesalazine indicate no adverse effect on pregnancy or on the health of the fetus/newborn child. To date no other relevant epidemiological data are available. No animal reproductive studies with Salofalk rectal foam have been performed.

Previous animal studies on oral mesalazine do not indicate direct or indirect harmful effects with respect to pregnancy, embryonal/fetal development, parturition or postnatal development.

Salofalk rectal foam should not be used during pregnancy unless the potential benefit outweighs the possible risk.

N-acetyl-mesalazine (N-Ac-5-ASA) and to a lesser degree mesalazine are excreted in breast milk. Only limited experience during lactation in women after oral application is available to date. Hypersensitivity reactions like diarrhoea can not be excluded.

Therefore, Salofalk rectal foam is not recommended in breast-feeding women. If treatment is necessary, breast-feeding should be discontinued.

4.7 Effects on ability to drive and use machines

No effects on ability to drive and use machines have been observed.

4.8 Undesirable effects

(see Table 1 below)

Special note:

Care should be taken when administering Salofalk to patients with diminished renal function.

4.9 Overdose

No cases of intoxication have been reported to date and no specific antidotes are known. If necessary, intravenous infusion of electrolytes (forced diuresis) should be considered in cases of overdose.

5. PHARMACOLOGICAL PROPERTIES

5.1 Pharmacodynamic properties

Pharmacotherapeutic group:

Aminosalicylic acid and similar agents mesalazine ATC Code: A07EC02.

The mechanism of the anti-inflammatory action is unknown. The results of *in vitro* studies indicate that inhibition of lipoxygenase may play a role. Effects on prostaglandin concentrations in the intestinal mucosa have also been demonstrated. Mesalazine may also function as a radical scavenger of reactive oxygen compounds. Mesalazine acts predominantly locally at the gut mucosa and in the submucus tissue from the luminal side of the intestine. It is important therefore that mesalazine is available at the regions of inflammation. Systemic bioavailability / plasma concentrations of mesalazine therefore are of no relevance for therapeutic efficacy, but rather a factor for safety.

5.2 Pharmacokinetic properties

General considerations of mesalazine:

Absorption:

Mesalazine absorption is highest in the proximal gut regions and lowest in distal gut areas.

Biotransformation:

Mesalazine is metabolised both pre-systemically by the intestinal mucosa and the liver to the pharmacologically inactive N-acetyl-5-aminosalicylic acid (N-Ac-5-ASA). The acetylation seems to be independent of the acetylator phenotype of the patient. Some acetylation also occurs through the action of colonic bacteria. Protein binding of mesalazine and N-Ac-5-ASA is 43% and 78% respectively.

Elimination:

Mesalazine and its metabolite N-Ac-5-ASA are eliminated via the faeces (major part), renally (varies between 20 and 50%, dependant on kind of application, pharmaceutical preparation and route of mesalazine release, respectively), and biliary (minor part). Renal excretion predominantly occurs as N-Ac-5-ASA. About 1% of total orally administered mesalazine dose is excreted into the breast milk mainly as N-Ac-5-ASA.

Salofalk Foam Specific:

Distribution:

A combined pharmacoscintigraphic / pharmacokinetic study showed that spreading of Salofalk Foam is homogeneous and fast, and is almost complete within 1 hour. It reaches the gut regions rectum, sigmoid colon, and left-sided colon in dependence of extension of inflammation.

Absorption:

Absorption of mesalazine is fast, and peak plasma concentrations for mesalazine and its metabolite N-Ac-5-ASA are reached at about 4 hours. However, plasma concentrations of a 2g mesalazine rectal dose of foam are about comparable with an 250mg oral dose mesalazine, reaching maximum concentrations of about 0.4 µg/ml. Pre-systemic metabolisation is fast, and N-Ac-5-ASA reaches its maximum plasma concentrations also at about 4 hours, like mesalazine, but plasma concentrations are about 4-5 times higher, about 2µg/ml.

5.3 Preclinical safety data

With the exception of a local tolerance study in dogs, which showed good rectal tolerance, no preclinical studies have been performed with Salofalk Foam.

Preclinical data reveal no special hazard for humans based on conventional studies of safety pharmacology, genotoxicity, carcinogenicity (rat) or toxicity to reproduction. Kidney toxicity (renal papillary necrosis and epithelial damage in the proximal convoluted tubule or the whole nephron) has been seen in repeat-dose toxicity studies with high oral doses of mesalazine. The clinical relevance of this finding is unknown.

Table 1

system organ class	*frequency due to MedDRA convention*			
	Common (≥ 1/100 to < 1/10)	*Uncommon (≥ 1/1,000 to <1/100)*	*rare (≥ 1/10,000 to <1/1,000)*	*very rare (< 1/ 10,000)*
General disorders and administra-tion site conditions	Abdominal distension	Anal discomfort; application site irritation, rectal tenesmus		
Blood and lymphatic system disorders				Altered blood counts (aplastic anaemia, agranulocytosis, pancytopenia, neutropenia, leukopenia, thrombocytopenia)
Nervous system disorders			Headache, dizziness	peripheral neuropathy
Gastrointes-tinal disorders			Abdominal pain, diarrhoea, flatulence, nausea, vomiting	
Renal and urinary disorders				Impairment of renal function including acute and chronic interstitial nephritis and renal insufficiency
Skin and subcutaneous tissue disorders				Alopecia
Musculo-skeletal and connective tissue disorders				Myalgia, arthralgia
Immune system disorders				Hypersensitivity reactions such as allergic exanthema, drug fever, bronchospasm, peri- and myocarditis, acute pancreatitis, allergic alveolitis, lupus erythematosus syndrome, pancolitis
Hepatobiliary disorders				Changes in hepatic function parameters (increase in transaminases and parameters of cholestasis), hepatitis, cholestatic hepatitis
Reproductive system disorders				Oligospermia (reversible)

6. PHARMACEUTICAL PARTICULARS

6.1 List of excipients

Sodium metabisulphite (E223),

cetostearyl alcohol,

polysorbate 60,

disodium edetate,

propylene glycol,

Propellants:

propane,

n-butane,

isobutane.

6.2 Incompatibilities

Not applicable

6.3 Shelf life

3 years.

After first actuation: 12 weeks.

6.4 Special precautions for storage

Do not store above 25°C. Do not refrigerate or freeze. This is a pressurised container, containing 3.75% by mass of inflammable propellant. It should be kept away from any flames, sparks or incandescent material including cigarettes. It should be protected from direct sunlight and temperatures over 50°C and must not be pierced or burned even when empty.

6.5 Nature and contents of container

Aluminium pressurised container with metering valve containing 80g (14 actuations) of suspension together with 14 PVC applicators coated with white soft paraffin and liquid paraffin for administration of the foam.

6.6 Special precautions for disposal and other handling

Any unused product waste material should be disposed of in accordance with local requirements.

7. MARKETING AUTHORISATION HOLDER

Dr. Falk Pharma GmbH

Leinenweberstr. 5

P.O. Box 6529

D-79108 Freiburg

Germany

Phone: +49 (0) 761 1514-0

8. MARKETING AUTHORISATION NUMBER(S)

PL 08637/0003

9. DATE OF FIRST AUTHORISATION/RENEWAL OF THE AUTHORISATION

October 2006

10. DATE OF REVISION OF THE TEXT

July 2009

Salofalk Suppositories 500mg

(Dr. Falk Pharma UK Ltd)

1. NAME OF THE MEDICINAL PRODUCT

Salofalk Suppositories 500mg.

2. QUALITATIVE AND QUANTITATIVE COMPOSITION

Each suppository contains the following active ingredient: Mesalazine 500mg.

3. PHARMACEUTICAL FORM

Suppository.

4. CLINICAL PARTICULARS

4.1 Therapeutic indications

Management of mild and moderate attacks of ulcerative colitis, especially in the rectum and sigmoid colon and also in the descending colon.

4.2 Posology and method of administration

Method of administration: Rectal

Adults and the Elderly: 1 to 2 suppositories, 2 to 3 times daily. The action of Salofalk is enhanced if the patient lies on the left side when introducing the suppository. The dosage should be adjusted to suit the progress of the condition. Do not discontinue treatment suddenly.

Children: There is no recommended dose for children. Mesalazine should not be used in babies and infants.

4.3 Contraindications

Severe renal and hepatic function disturbances. Active gastrointestinal ulcers. Hypersensitivity to salicylates.

4.4 Special warnings and precautions for use

The drug should not be prescribed for infants.

Serious blood dyscrasias have been reported very rarely with mesalazine. Haematological investigations including methaemoglobin values should be performed regularly during the course of therapy and if the patient develops unexplained bleeding, bruising, purpura, anaemia, fever or sore throat. Treatment should be stopped if there is suspicion or evidence of blood dyscrasia or if renal function deteriorates.

Reports of interstitial nephritis occurring with mesalazine treatment are uncommon; However patients on oral formulations may require renal monitoring.

Use with extreme caution in patients with mild to moderate renal impairment (see section 4.4) and if dehydration develops, normal electrolyte levels and fluid balance should be restored as soon as possible.

4.5 Interaction with other medicinal products and other forms of interaction

Although the following interactions are theoretically possible, owing to the low degree of absorption of the rectally administered mesalazine, the risk of their onset is extremely low: mesalazine may potentiate the actions of sulfonylureas. Interactions with coumarin, methotrexate, probenecid, sulfinpyrazone, spironolactone, furosemide and rifampicin cannot be excluded. Mesalazine can theoretically potentiate the side effects of glucocorticoids on the stomach.

Concurrent use with other known nephrotoxic agents such as NSAID's and azathioprine may increase the risk of renal reactions (see section 4.4).

4.6 Pregnancy and lactation

Animal experiments on mesalazine have produced no evidence of embryonic effects. No untoward effects were seen in a reproductive and fertility study with mesalazine in breast-fed rat pups. Mesalazine is acetylated in the body and passes in this form into breast milk. Limited use of mesalazine in pregnancy has shown no untoward effect on the foetus. However, it should not be used in the first trimester. It can be used with caution during pregnancy and only if the potential benefits outweigh the potential risks.

4.7 Effects on ability to drive and use machines

Salofalk Suppositories are not expected to affect ability to drive and use machines. If dizziness develops, the patient should not drive or operate machinery.

4.8 Undesirable effects

Rectal Salofalk may cause acute intolerance (sensitivity reactions). This is characterised by abdominal pain, bloody diarrhoea, fever, pruritus and rash. These are unrelated to dose.

The most common adverse effects following treatment with rectal mesalazine are:

General symptoms such as dizziness, malaise, paraesthesia, arthralgia and pyrexia may develop following rectal administration of sulphasalazine.

GI effects: abdominal pain, flatulence, nausea, worsening or development of diarrhoea.

CNS effects: Headache, malaise, dizziness and peripheral neuropathy.

Sensitivity reactions: Mesalazine may be associated with an exacerbation of the symptoms of colitis in those patients who have previously had such problems with sulfasalazine. Allergic skin reactions such as rash, bullous skin reactions including erythema multiforme and Stevens-Johnson syndrome.

Other adverse effects: Fever, arthralgia, pericarditis, myocarditis, pancreatitis

Other adverse effects were reported following oral administration of mesalazine. There have been rare reports of leucopenia, neutropenia, agranulocytosis, aplastic anaemia and thrombocytopenia, abnormalities of hepatic function, hepatitis, cholestatic hepatitis, allergic lung reactions, interstitial nephritis and nephrotic syndrome with oral mesalazine treatment, usually reversible on withdrawal. Renal failure has been reported. Mesalazine-induced nephrotoxicity should be suspected in patients developing renal dysfunction during treatment. Increased methaemaglobin levels may occur. Headache and digestive disturbances such as nausea and diarrhoea may occur. Isolated cases of hair loss have been reported.

4.9 Overdose

There have been no reported cases of overdosage.

5. PHARMACOLOGICAL PROPERTIES

5.1 Pharmacodynamic properties

Mesalazine is the biologically active metabolite of salicylazosulfapyridine that is used in the treatment of certain chronic inflammatory conditions of the intestine.

5.2 Pharmacokinetic properties

Following rectal administration the major fraction is recovered from the faeces, a small percentage (approximately 15%) is absorbed; the absorbed mesalazine is excreted mainly in the urine; biliary excretion is secondary. The acetylated and the non-acetylated forms of mesalazine bind slightly to plasma proteins.

5.3 Preclinical safety data

None stated.

6. PHARMACEUTICAL PARTICULARS

6.1 List of excipients

Salofalk Suppositories 500mg contain the following excipients:

Hard Fat, Docusate sodium, Cetyl alcohol,

6.2 Incompatibilities

None known.

6.3 Shelf life

36 months.

6.4 Special precautions for storage

Store at room temperature (15-25° C) and protect from light.

6.5 Nature and contents of container

Cartons of ten or thirty suppositories in white, opaque PVC/PE moulded strips.

Each strip contains five suppositories

6.6 Special precautions for disposal and other handling

None

Administrative Data

7. MARKETING AUTHORISATION HOLDER

Dr Falk Pharma UK Ltd
Unit k
Bourne End Business Park
Cores End Road
Bourne End
Bucks
SL8 5AS
United Kingdom

8. MARKETING AUTHORISATION NUMBER(S)

PL 10341/0009

9. DATE OF FIRST AUTHORISATION/RENEWAL OF THE AUTHORISATION

31st December 2004

10. DATE OF REVISION OF THE TEXT

August 2006

Samsca 15 mg tablet

(Otsuka Pharmaceuticals (UK) Ltd)

1. NAME OF THE MEDICINAL PRODUCT

Samsca▼ 15 mg tablets

2. QUALITATIVE AND QUANTITATIVE COMPOSITION

Each tablet contains 15 mg tolvaptan.

Excipients:

Each tablet contains approximately 37 mg lactose monohydrate.

For a full list of excipients, see section 6.1.

3. PHARMACEUTICAL FORM

Tablet

Blue, triangular, shallow-convex, debossed with "OTSUKA" and "15" on one side.

4. CLINICAL PARTICULARS

4.1 Therapeutic indications

Treatment of adult patients with hyponatraemia secondary to syndrome of inappropriate antidiuretic hormone secretion (SIADH).

4.2 Posology and method of administration

Due to the need for a dose titration phase with close monitoring of serum sodium and volume status, treatment with Samsca should be initiated in hospital.

Posology

Treatment with tolvaptan should be initiated at a dose of 15 mg once daily. The dose may be increased to a maximum of 60 mg once daily as tolerated to achieve the desired level of serum sodium. During titration, patients should be monitored for serum sodium and volume status (see section 4.4). In case of inadequate improvement in serum sodium levels, other treatment options should be considered, either in place of or in addition to tolvaptan. For patients with an appropriate increase in serum sodium, the underlying disease and serum sodium levels should be monitored at regular intervals to evaluate further need of tolvaptan treatment. In the setting of hyponatraemia, the treatment duration is determined by the underlying disease and its treatment. Tolvaptan treatment is expected to last until the underlying disease is adequately treated or until such time that hyponatraemia is no longer a clinical issue.

Patients with renal impairment

Tolvaptan is contraindicated in anuric patients (see section 4.3).

Tolvaptan has not been studied in patients with severe renal failure. The efficacy and safety in this population is not well established.

Based on the data available, no dose adjustment is required in those with mild to moderate renal impairment.

Patients with hepatic impairment

No dose adjustment is needed in patients with mild or moderate hepatic impairment (Child-Pugh classes A and B). No information is available in patients with severe hepatic impairment (Child-Pugh class C). In these patients dosing should be managed cautiously and electrolytes and volume status should be monitored (see section 4.4).

Elderly population

No dose adjustment is needed in elderly patients.

Paediatric population

There is no experience in children and adolescents under the age of 18 years. Samsca is not recommended in the paediatric age group.

Method of administration

For oral use.

Administration preferably in the morning, without regard to meals. Tablets should be swallowed without chewing with a glass of water. Samsca should not be taken with grapefruit juice (see section 4.5).

4.3 Contraindications

- Hypersensitivity to the active substance or to any of the excipients
- Anuria
- Volume depletion
- Hypovolaemic hyponatraemia
- Hypernatraemia
- Patients who cannot perceive thirst
- Pregnancy (see section 4.6)
- Breastfeeding (see section 4.6)

4.4 Special warnings and precautions for use

Urgent need to raise serum sodium acutely

Tolvaptan has not been studied in a setting of urgent need to raise serum sodium acutely. For such patients, alternative treatment should be considered.

Access to water

Tolvaptan may cause undesirable effects related to water loss such as thirst, dry mouth and dehydration (see section 4.8). Therefore, patients should have access to water and be able to drink sufficient amounts of water. If fluid restricted patients are treated with tolvaptan, extra caution should be exercised to ensure that patients do not become overly dehydrated.

Urinary outflow obstruction

Urinary output must be secured. Patients with partial obstruction of urinary outflow, for example patients with prostatic hypertrophy or impairment of micturition, have an increased risk of developing acute retention.

Fluid and electrolyte balance

Tolvaptan may cause rapid increases in serum sodium. Therefore after initiation of treatment, patients should be closely monitored for serum sodium and volume status. The rate of sodium correction should be managed carefully in patients at risk for demyelinisation syndromes (e.g. hypoxia, alcoholism, malnutrition). Fluid and electrolyte status should be monitored in all patients and particularly in those with renal and hepatic impairment. In patients receiving tolvaptan who develop too rapid a rise in serum sodium (>12 mmol/l per 24 hours), treatment with tolvaptan should be discontinued and administration of hypotonic fluid should be considered.

Diabetes mellitus

Diabetic patients with an elevated glucose concentration (e.g. in excess of 300 mg/dl) may present with pseudohyponatraemia. This condition should be excluded prior and during treatment with tolvaptan.

Tolvaptan may cause hyperglycaemia (see section 4.8). Therefore, diabetic patients treated with tolvaptan should be managed cautiously. In particular this applies to patients with inadequately controlled type II diabetes.

Lactose and galactose intolerance

Samsca contains lactose as an excipient. Patients with rare hereditary problems of galactose intolerance, the Lapp lactase deficiency or glucose-galactose malabsorption should not take this medicine.

4.5 Interaction with other medicinal products and other forms of interaction

CYP3A4 inhibitors

Tolvaptan plasma concentrations have been increased by up to 5.4-fold area under time-concentration curve (AUC) after the administration of strong CYP3A4 inhibitors. Caution should be exercised in co-administering CYP3A4 inhibitors (e.g. ketoconazole, macrolide antibiotics, diltiazem) with tolvaptan (see section 4.4).

Co-administration of grapefruit juice and tolvaptan resulted in a 1.8-fold increase in exposure to tolvaptan. Patients taking tolvaptan should avoid ingesting grapefruit juice.

CYP3A4 inducers

Tolvaptan plasma concentrations have been decreased by up to 87% (AUC) after the administration of CYP3A4 inducers. Caution should be exercised in co-administering CYP3A4 inducers (e.g. rifampicin, barbiturates) with tolvaptan.

CYP3A4 substrates

In healthy subjects, tolvaptan, a CYP3A4 substrate, had no effect on the plasma concentrations of some other CYP3A4 substrates (e.g. warfarin or amiodarone). Tolvaptan increased plasma levels of lovastatin by 1.3 to 1.5-fold. Even though this increase has no clinical relevance, it indicates tolvaptan can potentially increase exposure to CYP3A4 substrates.

Diuretics

There is no evidence of clinically significant interactions with loop and thiazide diuretics.

Digoxin

Steady state digoxin concentrations have been increased (1.3-fold increase in maximum observed plasma concentration [C_{max}] and 1.2-fold increase in area under the plasma concentration-time curve over the dosing interval

[AUC_τ]) when co administered with multiple once daily 60 mg doses of tolvaptan. Patients receiving digoxin should therefore be evaluated for excessive digoxin effects when treated with tolvaptan.

Warfarin

There is no evidence of clinically significant interactions with warfarin.

Co-administration with hypertonic saline

There is no experience with concomitant use of Samsca and hypertonic saline. Concomitant use with hypertonic saline is not recommended.

4.6 Pregnancy and lactation

Pregnancy

There are no adequate data from the use of tolvaptan in pregnant women. Studies in animals have shown reproductive toxicity (see section 5.3). The potential risk for humans is unknown.

Women of childbearing potential should use adequate contraceptive measures during tolvaptan use. Samsca must not be used during pregnancy (see section 4.3).

Breastfeeding

It is unknown whether tolvaptan is excreted in human breast milk. Studies in rats have shown excretion of tolvaptan in breast milk.

The potential risk for humans is unknown. Samsca is contraindicated during breastfeeding (see section 4.3).

4.7 Effects on ability to drive and use machines

When driving vehicles or using machines it should be taken into account that occasionally dizziness, asthenia or syncope may occur.

4.8 Undesirable effects

The adverse reaction profile of tolvaptan is based on a clinical trials database of 3294 tolvaptan-treated patients and is consistent with the pharmacology of the active substance. The frequencies correspond with very common (≥1/10), common (≥1/100 to <1/10) and uncommon (≥1/1000 to <1/100). Within each frequency grouping, adverse reactions are presented in order of decreasing seriousness.

Adverse reactions reported in clinical trials in patients with hyponatraemia

The pharmacodynamically predictable and most commonly reported adverse reactions are thirst, dry mouth and pollakiuria occurring in approximately 18%, 9% and 6% of patients.

System Organ Class	Frequency
Metabolism and nutrition disorders	Common: polydipsia, dehydration, hyperkalaemia, hyperglycaemia, decreased appetite
Nervous system disorders	Uncommon: dysgeusia
Vascular disorders	Common: orthostatic hypotension
Gastrointestinal disorders	Very common: nausea Common: constipation, dry mouth
Skin and subcutaneous tissue disorders	Common: ecchymosis, pruritus
Renal and urinary disorders	Common: pollakiuria, polyuria
General disorders and administration site conditions	Very common: thirst Common: asthenia, pyrexia
Investigations	Common: increased blood creatinine

In clinical trials investigating other indications the following undesirable effects have been observed: Common: hypernatraemia, hypoglycaemia, hyperuricaemia, syncope, dizziness.

Uncommon: pruritic rash.

4.9 Overdose

No case of overdose has been reported. Single doses up to 480 mg and multiple doses up to 300 mg per day for 5 days have been well tolerated in clinical trials in healthy volunteers.

The oral median lethal dose (LD_{50}) of tolvaptan in rats and dogs is >2000 mg/kg. No mortality was observed in rats or dogs following single oral doses of 2000 mg/kg (maximum feasible dose). A single oral dose of 2000 mg/kg was lethal in mice and symptoms of toxicity in affected mice included decreased locomotor activity, staggering gait, tremor and hypothermia.

A profuse and prolonged aquaresis (free water clearance) is anticipated. Adequate fluid intake must be maintained.

5. PHARMACOLOGICAL PROPERTIES

5.1 Pharmacodynamic properties

Pharmacotherapeutic group: Vasopressin antagonists, ATC code C03XA01

Tolvaptan is a selective vasopressin V_2-receptor antagonist with an affinity for the V_2-receptor greater than that of native arginine vasopressin. When taken orally, 15 to 60 mg doses of tolvaptan cause an increase in urine excretion resulting in increased aquaresis, decreased urine osmolality and increased serum sodium concentrations. Urine excretion of sodium and potassium are not significantly affected. Tolvaptan metabolites do not appear to have relevant pharmacological activity at clinical concentrations in humans.

Oral administration of 15 to 120 mg doses of tolvaptan produced a significant increase in urine excretion rate within 2 hours of dosing. The increase in 24-hour urine volume was dose dependent. Following single oral doses of 15 to 60 mg, urine excretion rates returned to baseline levels after 24 hours. A mean of about 7 litres was excreted during 0 to 12 hours, independent of dose. Markedly higher doses of tolvaptan produce more sustained responses without affecting the magnitude of excretion, as active concentrations of tolvaptan are present for longer periods of time.

Hyponatraemia

In 2 pivotal, double-blind, placebo-controlled, clinical trials, a total of 424 patients with euvolaemic or hypervolaemic hyponatraemia (serum sodium <135 mEq/l) due to a variety of underlying causes (heart failure [HF], liver cirrhosis, SIADH and others) were treated for 30 days with tolvaptan (n=216) or placebo (n=208) at an initial dose of 15 mg/day. The dose could be increased to 30 and 60 mg/day depending on response using a 3 day titration scheme. The mean serum sodium concentration at trial entry was 129 mEq/l (range 114 - 136).

The primary endpoint for these trials was the average daily AUC for change in serum sodium from baseline to Day 4 and baseline to Day 30. Tolvaptan was superior to placebo ($p<0.0001$) for both periods in both studies. This effect was seen in all patients, the severe (serum sodium: <130 mEq/l) and mild (serum sodium: 130 - <135 mEq/l) subsets and for all disease aetiology subsets (e.g. HF, cirrhosis, SIADH/other). At 7 days after discontinuing treatment, sodium values decreased to levels of placebo treated patients.

Following 3 days of treatment, the pooled analysis of the two trials revealed five-fold more tolvaptan than placebo patients achieved normalisation of serum sodium concentrations (49% vs. 11%). This effect continued as on Day 30, when more tolvaptan than placebo patients still had normal concentrations (60% vs. 27%). These responses were seen in patients independent of the underlying disease. The results of self-assessed health status using the SF-12 Health Survey for the mental scores showed statistically significant and clinically relevant improvements for tolvaptan treatment compared to placebo.

Data on the long-term safety and efficacy of tolvaptan were assessed for up to 106 weeks in a clinical trial in patients (any aetiology) who had previously completed one of the pivotal hyponatraemia trials. A total of 111 patients started tolvaptan treatment in an open-label, extension trial, regardless of their previous randomisation. Improvements in serum sodium levels were observed as early as the first day after dosing and continued for on-treatment assessments up to Week 106. When treatment was discontinued, serum sodium concentrations decreased to approximately baseline values, despite the reinstatement of standard care therapy.

Clinical data from trials in other patient populations

EVEREST (Efficacy of Vasopressin Antagonism in Heart Failure Outcome Study with Tolvaptan) was a long-term outcome, double-blind, controlled clinical trial in patients hospitalised with worsening HF and signs and symptoms of volume overload. In the long-term outcome trial, a total of 2072 patients received 30 mg tolvaptan with standard of care (SC) and 2061 received placebo with SC. The primary objective of the study was to compare the effects of tolvaptan + SC with placebo + SC on the time to all-cause mortality and on the time to first occurrence of cardiovascular (CV) mortality or hospitalisation for HF. Tolvaptan treatment had no statistically significant favourable or unfavourable effects on overall survival or the combined endpoint of CV mortality or HF hospitalisation, and did not provide convincing evidence for clinically relevant benefit.

5.2 Pharmacokinetic properties

Absorption and distribution

After oral administration, tolvaptan is rapidly absorbed with peak plasma concentrations occurring about 2 hours after dosing. The absolute bioavailability of tolvaptan is about 56%. Co-administration with food has no effect on plasma concentrations. Following single oral doses of ≥300 mg, peak plasma concentrations appear to plateau, possibly due to saturation of absorption. The terminal elimination half-life is about 8 hours and steady-state concentrations of tolvaptan are obtained after the first dose. Tolvaptan binds reversibly (98%) to plasma proteins.

Biotransformation and elimination

Tolvaptan is extensively metabolised by the liver. Less than 1% of intact active substance is excreted unchanged in the urine. Radio labelled tolvaptan experiments showed that 40% of the radioactivity was recovered in the urine and 59% was recovered in the faeces where unchanged tolvaptan accounted for 32% of radioactivity. Tolvaptan is only a minor component in plasma (3%).

Linearity

Tolvaptan has linear pharmacokinetics for doses of 15 to 60 mg.

Pharmacokinetics in special populations

Clearance of tolvaptan is not significantly affected by age.

The effect of mildly or moderately impaired hepatic function (Child-Pugh classes A and B) on the pharmacokinetics of tolvaptan was investigated in 87 patients with liver disease of various origins. No clinically significant changes have been seen in clearance for doses ranging from 5 to 60 mg. Very limited information is available in patients with severe hepatic impairment (Child-Pugh class C).

In an analysis on population pharmacokinetics for patients with heart failure, tolvaptan concentrations of patients with mildly (creatinine clearance [C_{cr}] 50 to 80 ml/min) or moderately (C_{cr} 20 to 50 ml/min) impaired renal function were not significantly different to tolvaptan concentrations in patients with normal renal function (C_{cr} 80 to 150 ml/min). The efficacy and safety of tolvaptan in those with a creatinine clearance <10 ml/min has not been evaluated and is therefore unknown.

5.3 Preclinical safety data

Non-clinical data revealed no special hazard for humans based on conventional studies of safety pharmacology, repeated dose toxicity, genotoxicity or carcinogenic potential.

Teratogenicity was noted in rabbits given 1000 mg/kg/day (15 times the exposure from the recommended human dose on an AUC basis). No teratogenic effects were seen in rabbits at 300 mg/kg/day (about 2.5 to 5.3 times the exposure in humans at the recommended dose, based on AUC).

In a peri- and post-natal study in rats, delayed ossification and reduced pup bodyweight were seen at the high dose of 1000 mg/kg/day.

6. PHARMACEUTICAL PARTICULARS

6.1 List of excipients

Maize starch

Hydroxypropylcellulose

Lactose monohydrate

Magnesium stearate

Microcrystalline cellulose

Indigo carmine (E 132) aluminium lake

6.2 Incompatibilities

Not applicable.

6.3 Shelf life

4 years

6.4 Special precautions for storage

Store in the original package in order to protect from light and moisture.

6.5 Nature and contents of container

10 × 1 tablets in PVC/aluminium perforated unit dose blister.

30 × 1 tablets in PVC/aluminium perforated unit dose blister.

Not all pack sizes may be marketed.

6.6 Special precautions for disposal and other handling

No special requirements.

7. MARKETING AUTHORISATION HOLDER

Otsuka Pharmaceutical Europe Ltd

Hunton House

Highbridge Business Park

Oxford Road

Uxbridge

Middlesex, UB8 1HU

United Kingdom

8. MARKETING AUTHORISATION NUMBER(S)

EU/1/09/539/001-002

9. DATE OF FIRST AUTHORISATION/RENEWAL OF THE AUTHORISATION

Date of first authorisation: 03/08/2009

10. DATE OF REVISION OF THE TEXT

{MM/YYYY}

Detailed information on this product is available on the website of the European Medicines Agency (EMEA) http://www.emea.europa.eu

Samsca 30 mg tablet

(Otsuka Pharmaceuticals (UK) Ltd)

1. NAME OF THE MEDICINAL PRODUCT

Samsca▼ 30 mg tablets

2. QUALITATIVE AND QUANTITATIVE COMPOSITION

Each tablet contains 30 mg tolvaptan.

Excipients:

Each tablet contains approximately 74 mg lactose monohydrate.

For a full list of excipients, see section 6.1.

3. PHARMACEUTICAL FORM

Tablet

Blue, round, shallow-convex, debossed with "OTSUKA" and "30" on one side.

4. CLINICAL PARTICULARS

4.1 Therapeutic indications

Treatment of adult patients with hyponatraemia secondary to syndrome of inappropriate antidiuretic hormone secretion (SIADH).

4.2 Posology and method of administration

Due to the need for a dose titration phase with close monitoring of serum sodium and volume status, treatment with Samsca should be initiated in hospital.

Posology

Treatment with tolvaptan should be initiated at a dose of 15 mg once daily. The dose may be increased to a maximum of 60 mg once daily as tolerated to achieve the desired level of serum sodium. During titration, patients should be monitored for serum sodium and volume status (see section 4.4). In case of inadequate improvement in serum sodium levels, other treatment options should be considered, either in place of or in addition to tolvaptan. For patients with an appropriate increase in serum sodium, the underlying disease and serum sodium levels should be monitored at regular intervals to evaluate further need of tolvaptan treatment. In the setting of hyponatraemia, the treatment duration is determined by the underlying disease and its treatment. Tolvaptan treatment is expected to last until the underlying disease is adequately treated or until such time that hyponatraemia is no longer a clinical issue.

Patients with renal impairment

Tolvaptan is contraindicated in anuric patients (see section 4.3).

Tolvaptan has not been studied in patients with severe renal failure. The efficacy and safety in this population is not well established.

Based on the data available, no dose adjustment is required in those with mild to moderate renal impairment.

Patients with hepatic impairment

No dose adjustment is needed in patients with mild or moderate hepatic impairment (Child-Pugh classes A and B). No information is available in patients with severe hepatic impairment (Child-Pugh class C). In these patients dosing should be managed cautiously and electrolytes and volume status should be monitored (see section 4.4).

Elderly population

No dose adjustment is needed in elderly patients.

Paediatric population

There is no experience in children and adolescents under the age of 18 years. Samsca is not recommended in the paediatric age group.

Method of administration

For oral use.

Administration preferably in the morning, without regard to meals. Tablets should be swallowed without chewing with a glass of water. Samsca should not be taken with grapefruit juice (see section 4.5).

4.3 Contraindications

- Hypersensitivity to the active substance or to any of the excipients
- Anuria
- Volume depletion
- Hypovolaemic hyponatraemia
- Hypernatraemia
- Patients who cannot perceive thirst
- Pregnancy (see section 4.6)
- Breastfeeding (see section 4.6)

4.4 Special warnings and precautions for use

Urgent need to raise serum sodium acutely

Tolvaptan has not been studied in a setting of urgent need to raise serum sodium acutely. For such patients, alternative treatment should be considered.

Access to water

Tolvaptan may cause undesirable effects related to water loss such as thirst, dry mouth and dehydration (see section 4.8). Therefore, patients should have access to water and be able to drink sufficient amounts of water. If fluid restricted patients are treated with tolvaptan, extra caution should be exercised to ensure that patients do not become overly dehydrated.

Urinary outflow obstruction

Urinary output must be secured. Patients with partial obstruction of urinary outflow, for example patients with prostatic hypertrophy or impairment of micturition, have an increased risk of developing acute retention.

Fluid and electrolyte balance

Tolvaptan may cause rapid increases in serum sodium. Therefore after initiation of treatment, patients should be closely monitored for serum sodium and volume status. The rate of sodium correction should be managed carefully in patients at risk for demyelinisation syndromes (e.g. hypoxia, alcoholism, malnutrition). Fluid and electrolyte status should be monitored in all patients and particularly in those with renal and hepatic impairment. In patients receiving tolvaptan who develop too rapid a rise in serum sodium (>12 mmol/l per 24 hours), treatment with tolvaptan should be discontinued and administration of hypotonic fluid should be considered.

Diabetes mellitus

Diabetic patients with an elevated glucose concentration (e.g. in excess of 300 mg/dl) may present with pseudohyponatraemia. This condition should be excluded prior and during treatment with tolvaptan.

Tolvaptan may cause hyperglycaemia (see section 4.8). Therefore, diabetic patients treated with tolvaptan should be managed cautiously. In particular this applies to patients with inadequately controlled type II diabetes.

Lactose and galactose intolerance

Samsca contains lactose as an excipient. Patients with rare hereditary problems of galactose intolerance, the Lapp lactase deficiency or glucose-galactose malabsorption should not take this medicine.

4.5 Interaction with other medicinal products and other forms of interaction

CYP3A4 inhibitors

Tolvaptan plasma concentrations have been increased by up to 5.4-fold area under time-concentration curve (AUC) after the administration of strong CYP3A4 inhibitors. Caution should be exercised in co-administering CYP3A4 inhibitors (e.g. ketoconazole, macrolide antibiotics, diltiazem) with tolvaptan (see section 4.4).

Co-administration of grapefruit juice and tolvaptan resulted in a 1.8-fold increase in exposure to tolvaptan. Patients taking tolvaptan should avoid ingesting grapefruit juice.

CYP3A4 inducers

Tolvaptan plasma concentrations have been decreased by up to 87% (AUC) after the administration of CYP3A4 inducers. Caution should be exercised in co-administering CYP3A4 inducers (e.g. rifampicin, barbiturates) with tolvaptan.

CYP3A4 substrates

In healthy subjects, tolvaptan, a CYP3A4 substrate, had no effect on the plasma concentrations of some other CYP3A4 substrates (e.g. warfarin or amiodarone). Tolvaptan increased plasma levels of lovastatin by 1.3 to 1.5-fold. Even though this increase has no clinical relevance, it indicates tolvaptan can potentially increase exposure to CYP3A4 substrates.

Diuretics

There is no evidence of clinically significant interactions with loop and thiazide diuretics.

Digoxin

Steady state digoxin concentrations have been increased (1.3-fold increase in maximum observed plasma concentration [C_{max}] and 1.2-fold increase in area under the plasma concentration-time curve over the dosing interval [AUC_{τ}]) when co administered with multiple once daily 60 mg doses of tolvaptan. Patients receiving digoxin should therefore be evaluated for excessive digoxin effects when treated with tolvaptan.

Warfarin

There is no evidence of clinically significant interactions with warfarin.

Co-administration with hypertonic saline

There is no experience with concomitant use of Samsca and hypertonic saline. Concomitant use with hypertonic saline is not recommended.

4.6 Pregnancy and lactation

Pregnancy

There are no adequate data from the use of tolvaptan in pregnant women. Studies in animals have shown reproductive toxicity (see section 5.3). The potential risk for humans is unknown.

Women of childbearing potential should use adequate contraceptive measures during tolvaptan use. Samsca must not be used during pregnancy (see section 4.3).

Breastfeeding

It is unknown whether tolvaptan is excreted in human breast milk. Studies in rats have shown excretion of tolvaptan in breast milk.

The potential risk for humans is unknown. Samsca is contraindicated during breastfeeding (see section 4.3).

4.7 Effects on ability to drive and use machines

When driving vehicles or using machines it should be taken into account that occasionally dizziness, asthenia or syncope may occur.

4.8 Undesirable effects

The adverse reaction profile of tolvaptan is based on a clinical trials database of 3294 tolvaptan-treated patients and is consistent with the pharmacology of the active substance. The frequencies correspond with very common (≥1/10), common (≥1/100 to <1/10) and uncommon (≥1/1000 to <1/100). Within each frequency grouping, adverse reactions are presented in order of decreasing seriousness.

Adverse reactions reported in clinical trials in patients with hyponatraemia

The pharmacodynamically predictable and most commonly reported adverse reactions are thirst, dry mouth and pollakiuria occurring in approximately 18%, 9% and 6% of patients.

System Organ Class	Frequency
Metabolism and nutrition disorders	Common: polydipsia, dehydration, hyperkalaemia, hyperglycaemia, decreased appetite
Nervous system disorders	Uncommon: dysgeusia
Vascular disorders	Common: orthostatic hypotension
Gastrointestinal disorders	Very common: nausea Common: constipation, dry mouth
Skin and subcutaneous tissue disorders	Common: ecchymosis, pruritus
Renal and urinary disorders	Common: pollakiuria, polyuria
General disorders and administration site conditions	Very common: thirst Common: asthenia, pyrexia
Investigations	Common: increased blood creatinine

In clinical trials investigating other indications the following undesirable effects have been observed: Common: hypernatraemia, hypoglycaemia, hyperuricaemia, syncope, dizziness.

Uncommon: pruritic rash.

4.9 Overdose

No case of overdose has been reported. Single doses up to 480 mg and multiple doses up to 300 mg per day for 5 days have been well tolerated in clinical trials in healthy volunteers.

The oral median lethal dose (LD_{50}) of tolvaptan in rats and dogs is >2000 mg/kg. No mortality was observed in rats or dogs following single oral doses of 2000 mg/kg (maximum feasible dose). A single oral dose of 2000 mg/kg was lethal in mice and symptoms of toxicity in affected mice included decreased locomotor activity, staggering gait, tremor and hypothermia.

A profuse and prolonged aquaresis (free water clearance) is anticipated. Adequate fluid intake must be maintained.

5. PHARMACOLOGICAL PROPERTIES

5.1 Pharmacodynamic properties

Pharmacotherapeutic group: Vasopressin antagonists, ATC code C03XA01

Tolvaptan is a selective vasopressin V_2-receptor antagonist with an affinity for the V_2-receptor greater than that of native arginine vasopressin. When taken orally, 15 to 60 mg doses of tolvaptan cause an increase in urine excretion resulting in increased aquaresis, decreased urine osmolality and increased serum sodium concentrations. Urine excretion of sodium and potassium are not significantly affected. Tolvaptan metabolites do not appear to have relevant pharmacological activity at clinical concentrations in humans.

Oral administration of 15 to 120 mg doses of tolvaptan produced a significant increase in urine excretion rate within 2 hours of dosing. The increase in 24-hour urine volume was dose dependent. Following single oral doses of 15 to 60 mg, urine excretion rates returned to baseline levels after 24 hours. A mean of about 7 litres was excreted during 0 to 12 hours, independent of dose. Markedly higher doses of tolvaptan produce more sustained responses without affecting the magnitude of excretion, as active concentrations of tolvaptan are present for longer periods of time.

Hyponatraemia

In 2 pivotal, double-blind, placebo-controlled, clinical trials, a total of 424 patients with euvolaemic or hypervolaemic hyponatraemia (serum sodium <135 mEq/l) due to a variety of underlying causes (heart failure [HF], liver cirrhosis, SIADH and others) were treated for 30 days with tolvaptan (n=216) or placebo (n=208) at an initial dose of 15 mg/day. The dose could be increased to 30 and 60 mg/day depending on response using a 3 day titration scheme. The mean serum sodium concentration at trial entry was 129 mEq/l (range 114 - 136).

The primary endpoint for these trials was the average daily AUC for change in serum sodium from baseline to Day 4 and baseline to Day 30. Tolvaptan was superior to placebo (p<0.0001) for both periods in both studies. This effect was seen in all patients, the severe (serum sodium: <130 mEq/l) and mild (serum sodium: 130 - <135 mEq/l) subsets and for all disease aetiology subsets (e.g. HF, cirrhosis, SIADH/other). At 7 days after discontinuing treatment, sodium values decreased to levels of placebo treated patients.

Following 3 days of treatment, the pooled analysis of the two trials revealed five-fold more tolvaptan than placebo patients achieved normalisation of serum sodium concentrations (49% vs. 11%). This effect continued as on Day 30, when more tolvaptan than placebo patients still had normal concentrations (60% vs. 27%). These responses were seen in patients independent of the underlying disease. The results of self-assessed health status using the SF-12 Health Survey for the mental scores showed statistically significant and clinically relevant improvements for tolvaptan treatment compared to placebo.

Data on the long-term safety and efficacy of tolvaptan were assessed for up to 106 weeks in a clinical trial in patients (any aetiology) who had previously completed one of the pivotal hyponatraemia trials. A total of 111 patients started tolvaptan treatment in an open-label, extension trial, regardless of their previous randomisation. Improvements in serum sodium levels were observed as early as the first day after dosing and continued for on-treatment assessments up to Week 106. When treatment was discontinued, serum sodium concentrations decreased to approximately baseline values, despite the reinstatement of standard care therapy.

Clinical data from trials in other patient populations

EVEREST (Efficacy of Vasopressin Antagonism in Heart Failure Outcome Study with Tolvaptan) was a long-term outcome, double-blind, controlled clinical trial in patients hospitalised with worsening HF and signs and symptoms of volume overload. In the long-term outcome trial, a total of 2072 patients received 30 mg tolvaptan with standard of care (SC) and 2061 received placebo with SC. The primary objective of the study was to compare the effects of tolvaptan + SC with placebo + SC on the time to all-cause mortality and on the time to first occurrence of cardiovascular (CV) mortality or hospitalisation for HF. Tolvaptan treatment had no statistically significant favourable or unfavourable effects on overall survival or the combined endpoint of CV mortality or HF hospitalisation, and did not provide convincing evidence for clinically relevant benefit.

5.2 Pharmacokinetic properties

Absorption and distribution

After oral administration, tolvaptan is rapidly absorbed with peak plasma concentrations occurring about 2 hours after dosing. The absolute bioavailability of tolvaptan is about 56%. Co-administration with food has no effect on plasma concentrations. Following single oral doses of ⩾300 mg, peak plasma concentrations appear to plateau, possibly due to saturation of absorption. The terminal elimination half-life is about 8 hours and steady-state concentrations of tolvaptan are obtained after the first dose. Tolvaptan binds reversibly (98%) to plasma proteins.

Biotransformation and elimination

Tolvaptan is extensively metabolised by the liver. Less than 1% of intact active substance is excreted unchanged in the urine. Radio labelled tolvaptan experiments showed that 40% of the radioactivity was recovered in the urine and 59% was recovered in the faeces where unchanged tolvaptan accounted for 32% of radioactivity. Tolvaptan is only a minor component in plasma (3%).

Linearity

Tolvaptan has linear pharmacokinetics for doses of 15 to 60 mg.

Pharmacokinetics in special populations

Clearance of tolvaptan is not significantly affected by age.

The effect of mildly or moderately impaired hepatic function (Child-Pugh classes A and B) on the pharmacokinetics of tolvaptan was investigated in 87 patients with liver disease of various origins. No clinically significant changes have been seen in clearance for doses ranging from 5 to 60 mg. Very limited information is available in patients with severe hepatic impairment (Child-Pugh class C).

In an analysis on population pharmacokinetics for patients with heart failure, tolvaptan concentrations of patients with mildly (creatinine clearance [C_{cr}] 50 to 80 ml/min) or moderately (C_{cr} 20 to 50 ml/min) impaired renal function were not significantly different to tolvaptan concentrations in patients with normal renal function (C_{cr} 80 to 150 ml/min). The efficacy and safety of tolvaptan in those with a creatinine clearance <10 ml/min has not been evaluated and is therefore unknown.

5.3 Preclinical safety data

Non-clinical data revealed no special hazard for humans based on conventional studies of safety pharmacology, repeated dose toxicity, genotoxicity or carcinogenic potential.

Teratogenicity was noted in rabbits given 1000 mg/kg/day (15 times the exposure from the recommended human dose on an AUC basis). No teratogenic effects were seen in rabbits at 300 mg/kg/day (about 2.5 to 5.3 times the exposure in humans at the recommended dose, based on AUC).

In a peri- and post-natal study in rats, delayed ossification and reduced pup bodyweight were seen at the high dose of 1000 mg/kg/day.

6. PHARMACEUTICAL PARTICULARS

6.1 List of excipients

Maize starch

Hydroxypropylcellulose

Lactose monohydrate

Magnesium stearate

Microcrystalline cellulose

Indigo carmine (E 132) aluminium lake

6.2 Incompatibilities

Not applicable.

6.3 Shelf life

4 years

6.4 Special precautions for storage

Store in the original package in order to protect from light and moisture.

6.5 Nature and contents of container

10 × 1 tablets in PVC/aluminium perforated unit dose blister.

30 × 1 tablets in PVC/aluminium perforated unit dose blister.

Not all pack sizes may be marketed.

6.6 Special precautions for disposal and other handling

No special requirements.

7. MARKETING AUTHORISATION HOLDER

Otsuka Pharmaceutical Europe Ltd

Hunton House

Highbridge Business Park

Oxford Road

Uxbridge

Middlesex, UB8 1HU

United Kingdom

8. MARKETING AUTHORISATION NUMBER(S)

EU/1/09/539/003-004

9. DATE OF FIRST AUTHORISATION/RENEWAL OF THE AUTHORISATION

Date of first authorisation: 03/08/2009

10. DATE OF REVISION OF THE TEXT

{MM/YYYY}

Detailed information on this product is available on the website of the European Medicines Agency (EMEA) http://www.emea.europa.eu

Sandocal + D 1200 Effervescent Tablets

(Novartis Consumer Health)

1. NAME OF THE MEDICINAL PRODUCT

Sandocal®+D 1200 Effervescent tablets

2. QUALITATIVE AND QUANTITATIVE COMPOSITION

Each effervescent tablet contains:

2716 mg of calcium lactate gluconate and 2100 mg of calcium carbonate (equivalent to 1200 mg or 30 mmol of calcium).

8 mg of colecalciferol concentrate "powder form" equivalent to 800 I.U. or 20 µg colecalciferol (vitamin D3).

Also contains: Sucrose, sorbitol, aspartame (E951), 7.14 mmol (corresponding to 164.28 mg) of sodium per tablet.

For full list of excipients, see section 6.1.

3. PHARMACEUTICAL FORM

Effervescent tablets

White circular, flat faced, bevelled edge tablets with an orange odour.

4. CLINICAL PARTICULARS

4.1 Therapeutic indications

- Prevention and treatment of calcium and vitamin D deficiency.

- Calcium and vitamin D supplement as an adjunct to specific therapy in the prevention and treatment of osteoporosis for patients who are at risk of calcium and vitamin D deficiency.

4.2 Posology and method of administration

Adults and adolescents: take 1 effervescent tablet daily.

The effervescent tablets should be dissolved in a glass of water (approx. 200 ml) and drunk immediately. Sandocal+D 1200 effervescent tablets may be taken at anytime with or without food.

Oral use.

4.3 Contraindications

• Hypersensitivity to the active substances or to any of the excipients of the effervescent tablet

• Diseases and/or conditions resulting in hypercalcaemia and/or hypercalciuria

• Nephrocalcinosis, nephrolithiasis

• Hypervitaminosis D

4.4 Special warnings and precautions for use

During long-term treatment, serum calcium levels should be followed and renal function should be monitored through measurements of serum creatinine. Monitoring is especially important in patients on concomitant treatment with cardiac glycosides or thiazide diuretics (see section 4.5) and in patients with a high tendency to calculus formation. In case of hypercalcaemia or signs of impaired renal function, the dose should be reduced or the treatment discontinued.

In patients with impaired renal function, vitamin D should be used with caution. Serum and urinary calcium together with phosphate levels should be monitored during treatment. The risk of soft tissue calcification should also be taken into account.

In patients with severe renal insufficiency, vitamin D in the form of colecalciferol is not metabolised normally and other forms of vitamin D might be suitable as thought appropriate by the health professionals.

In patients suffering from sarcoidosis, Sandocal+D 1200 effervescent tablets should be prescribed with caution due to the risk of increased metabolism of vitamin D into its active form. Sarcoidosis patients should be monitored with regard to the calcium content in serum and urine if Sandocal+D 1200 effervescent tablets are prescribed.

In immobilized patients with osteoporosis, Sandocal+D 1200 effervescent tablets should be used cautiously due to increased risk of hypercalcaemia.

The content of vitamin D (800 IU) in Sandocal+D 1200 effervescent tablets should be considered when prescribing other medicinal products containing vitamin D. Additional doses of calcium or vitamin D should be taken under close medical supervision.

There have been literature reports alluding to possible increased absorption of aluminium with citrate salts. Sandocal+D 1200 effervescent tablet (which contains citric acid) should be used with caution in patients with severely impaired renal function, especially those also receiving aluminium-containing preparations.

Patients with rare hereditary problems of fructose intolerance, glucose-galactose malabsorption or sucrase-isomaltase insufficiency should not take this medicine.

Each Sandocal+D 1200 effervescent tablet contains aspartame, a source of phenylalanine equivalent to 15 mg/dose, and may be harmful for people with phenylketonuria.

Sandocal+D 1200 effervescent tablets contain 7.14 mmol (corresponding to 164.28 mg) of sodium per tablet.

Information for diabetics:

Sandocal+D 1200 effervescent tablets contain 0.003 Carbohydrate Units per tablet and are therefore suitable for diabetics.

4.5 Interaction with other medicinal products and other forms of interaction

Thiazide diuretics reduce the urinary excretion of calcium. Due to increased risk of hypercalcaemia, serum calcium should be regularly monitored during concomitant use of thiazide diuretics.

Systemic corticosteroids reduce calcium absorption. During concomitant use, it may be necessary to increase the dose of Sandocal+D 1200 effervescent tablets.

Ion exchange resins such as cholestyramine or laxatives such as paraffin oil may reduce the gastrointestinal absorption of vitamin D. Therefore Sandocal+D 1200 effervescent tablets are recommended to be taken at least one hour before or four to six hours after intake of these preparations.

Tetracycline preparations administered concomitantly with calcium preparations may not be well-absorbed. For this reason, tetracycline preparations should be administered at least two hours before or four to six hours after oral intake of calcium.

Cardiac glycoside toxicity may increase with hypercalcaemia resulting from treatment with calcium and vitamin D. Patients should be monitored with regard to electrocardiogram (ECG) and serum calcium levels.

If an oral bisphosphonate or sodium fluoride is used concomitantly, this preparation should be administered at least three hours before the intake of Sandocal+D 1200 effervescent tablets since gastrointestinal absorption of either oral bisphosphonate or sodium fluoride may be reduced.

Oxalic acid (found in spinach and rhubarb) and phytic acid (found in whole cereals) may inhibit calcium absorption through formation of insoluble compounds with calcium ions. The patient should not take calcium products within two hours of eating foods high in oxalic acid and phytic acid.

4.6 Pregnancy and lactation

Pregnancy:

Sandocal+D 1200 effervescent tablets can be used during pregnancy, in case of a calcium and vitamin D deficiency. However, for supplementation starting during the third trimester of pregnancy, the daily intake should not exceed 1500 mg calcium and 1000 IU vitamin D.

Studies in animals have shown reproductive toxicity of high doses of vitamin D.

In pregnant women, overdoses of calcium and vitamin D should be avoided as permanent hypercalcaemia has been related to adverse effects on the developing foetus. There are no indications that vitamin D at therapeutic doses is teratogenic in humans.

Breast-feeding:

Sandocal+D 1200 effervescent tablets can be used during breast-feeding. Calcium and vitamin D_3 pass into breast milk. This should be considered when giving additional vitamin D to the child.

4.7 Effects on ability to drive and use machines
Sandocal+D 1200 effervescent tablets has no influence on the ability to drive and use machines.

4.8 Undesirable effects
Adverse reactions are listed below, by system organ class and frequency. Frequencies are defined as: uncommon (>1/1000, <1/100), rare (>1/10 000, <1/1000), or very rare (1<10 000), including isolated reports.

Immune system disorders
Very Rare (<1/10,000): Hypersensitivity reactions such as angioedema or laryngeal oedema.

Metabolism and nutrition disorders
Rare (>1/10,000, <1/1,000): hypercalcaemia, hypercalciuria.

Gastrointestinal disorders
Uncommon (>1/1,000, <1/100): nausea, diarrhoea, abdominal pain, constipation, flatulence, abdominal distension.

Skin and subcutaneous tissue disorders
Uncommon (>1/1,000, <1/100): rash, pruritus, urticaria.

4.9 Overdose
Overdose leads to hypervitaminosis, hypercalciuria and hypercalcaemia. Symptoms of hypercalcaemia may include: nausea, vomiting, thirst, polydipsia, polyuria, dehydration and constipation. Chronic overdose with resulting hypercalcaemia can cause vascular and organ calcification.

The threshold for vitamin D intoxication is between 40,000 and 100,000 I.U per day and for calcium intoxication is from supplementation in excess of 2000 mg per day, taken for several months, in persons with normal parathyroid function.

Treatment of overdose:
In the case of an intoxication, treatment should be stopped immediately and the fluid deficiency should be corrected.

Where overdosage requires treatment it should be via hydration, including i.v. saline solution when needed. A loop diuretic (e.g., furosemide) may then be used to further increase calcium excretion and to prevent volume overload, but thiazide diuretics should be avoided. In patients with renal failure, hydration is ineffective and they should undergo dialysis. In the case of persistent hypercalcaemia, contributing factors should be excluded, e.g., vitamin A or D hypervitaminosis, primary hyperparathyroidism, malignancies, renal failure, or immobilisation.

5. PHARMACOLOGICAL PROPERTIES

5.1 Pharmacodynamic properties
Pharmacotherapeutic group:
- Minerals supplements
- Vitamins

ATC codes: Calcium carbonate (A 12 AA 04), Calcium lactate gluconate (A 12 AA 06) and Colecalciferol (A 11 CC 05)

Sandocal+D 1200 effervescent tablets are a fixed combination of calcium and vitamin D_3. Vitamin D_3 increases the intestinal absorption of calcium. Administration of calcium and vitamin D_3 counteracts the increase of parathyroid hormone (PTH) which causes increased bone resorption and results from calcium deficiency.

Human vitamin-D status depends on the latitude, the time spent outdoors and diet (vitamin-D containing food, food supplements, fish, cod liver oil). Vitamin-D hypovitaminosis - especially at winter and early spring - is common in many countries, including those in Europe, and affects all segments of the population, including children, adolescents and elderly people, due to less effective UV-radiation. People living indoors and not spending enough time in sunlight are prone to vitamin-D hypovitaminosis.

In a double-blind placebo controlled study of 18 months, 3270 women aged 84 ± 6 living in nursing homes were supplemented with colecalciferol (800 IU/day) + calcium (1.2 g/day), resulting in a significant decrease in PTH secretion. After 18 months, the results of the intent to treat analysis showed 80 hip fractures in the calcium vitamin D group as compared to 110 hip fractures in the placebo-group (p=0.004). In the conditions of this study, calcium and vitamin D treatment of 1387 women thus prevented 30 hip fractures. After 36 months of follow-up, 137 women presented with at least one hip fracture in the calcium-vitamin D group (n=1176) as compared to 178 in the placebo group (n=1127) (p≤0.02).

5.2 Pharmacokinetic properties
Calcium:
Sandocal+D 1200 effervescent tablets contains two calcium salts, calcium lactate gluconate and calcium carbonate, which readily dissolve in water to make the active ionised form of calcium freely usable.

Absorption:
Some 25-50% of the ingested dose of calcium is absorbed, predominantly in the proximal part of the small intestine and delivered to the exchangeable calcium pool. Vitamin D is required for calcium absorption and increases the capability of the absorptive mechanisms.

Distribution and metabolism:
99% of the calcium in the body is concentrated in the mineral component of bones and teeth. The remaining 1% is present in the intra- and extracellular fluids. About 50% of the total blood-calcium content is in the physiologically active ionised form with approximately 5% being complexed to citrate, phosphate or other anions. The remaining 45% being bound to proteins, principally albumin.

Elimination:
Calcium is excreted in the urine, faeces and sweat. Urinary excretion depends on glomerular filtration and tubular reabsorption.

Vitamin D_3:
Absorption:
Colecalciferol is absorbed in the intestine.

Distribution and metabolism:
Colecalciferol is transported by protein binding in the blood to the liver where it undergoes the first hydroxylation to 25-hydroxycolecalciferol. It is then further hydroxylated in the kidneys into 1,25-dihydroxycolecalciferol which is the actual active metabolite of vitamin D_3 responsible for increasing calcium absorption.

Non-hydroxylated vitamin D_3 is stored in muscle and adipose tissues.

Elimination:
The plasma half-life of vitamin D_3 is in the order of several days; elimination is through the faeces and urine.

5.3 Preclinical safety data
At doses far higher than the human therapeutic range teratogenicity has been observed in animal studies.

There is further no information of relevance to the safety assessment in addition to what is stated in other parts of the SPC.

6. PHARMACEUTICAL PARTICULARS

6.1 List of excipients
Citric acid
Sodium hydrogen carbonate
Macrogol 6000
Aspartame (E951)
Orange flavour (contains: orange essential oils, maltodextrin, arabic gum, sorbitol (E 420), dextrose)
Sucrose
Bovine gelatin
Maize starch
Partially hydrogenated soya oil
Alpha-tocopherol

6.2 Incompatibilities
Not applicable.

6.3 Shelf life
18 months.

6.4 Special precautions for storage
Do not store above 30°C.

Keep the tube tightly closed. Store in the original package.

6.5 Nature and contents of container
The effervescent tablets are packed in polypropylene tubes and tamperproof polyethylene stoppers with desiccant, each containing 10 tablets.

The tubes are packed in boxes containing 10, 20 (2 tubes of 10), 30 (3 tubes of 10), 40 (2 packs of 20), 60 (3 packs of 20), 80 (4 packs of 20) and 100 (5 packs of 20) tablets.

Not all pack sizes may be marketed.

6.6 Special precautions for disposal and other handling
No special requirements.

7. MARKETING AUTHORISATION HOLDER
Novartis Consumer Health UK Limited
Wimblehurst Road
Horsham
West Sussex
RH12 5AB
Trading as Novartis Consumer Health

8. MARKETING AUTHORISATION NUMBER(S)
PL 00030/217

9. DATE OF FIRST AUTHORISATION/RENEWAL OF THE AUTHORISATION
05/06/2008

10. DATE OF REVISION OF THE TEXT
06/02/2009

Legal category: P

Sandocal 1000
(Novartis Consumer Health)

1. NAME OF THE MEDICINAL PRODUCT
Sandocal® 1000 Effervescent Tablets

2. QUALITATIVE AND QUANTITATIVE COMPOSITION
Each effervescent tablet of 1000 mg contains:
2263 mg of calcium lactate gluconate and 1750 mg of calcium carbonate (equivalent to 1000 mg or 25 mmol of calcium).

For excipients, see section 6.1.

3. PHARMACEUTICAL FORM
Effervescent tablet

White, circular, flat faced, bevelled edge effervescent tablets with an orange odour

4. CLINICAL PARTICULARS

4.1 Therapeutic indications
- Prevention and treatment of calcium deficiency
- Calcium supplement as an adjunct to specific therapy in the prevention and treatment of osteoporosis
- Rickets and osteomalacia, in addition to vitamin D_3 therapy

4.2 Posology and method of administration
Adults and children: 1000mg per day.

The effervescent tablets should be dissolved in a glass of water (approx. 200 ml) and drunk immediately. Sandocal 1000 effervescent tablet may be taken with or without food.

4.3 Contraindications
- Hypersensitivity to the active substances or to any of the excipients of the effervescent tablet
- Diseases and/or conditions resulting in hypercalcaemia and/or hypercalciuria
- Nephrocalcinosis, nephrolithiasis

4.4 Special warnings and precautions for use
For patients with mild hypercalciuria (exceeding 300 mg/24 hours or 7.5 mmol/24 hours), or with a history of urinary calculi, monitoring of calcium excretion in the urine is required. If necessary, the calcium dose should be reduced or therapy should be discontinued. An increased fluid intake is recommended for patients prone to formation of calculi in the urinary tract.

In patients with impaired renal function, calcium salts should be taken under medical supervision with monitoring of calcium and phosphate serum levels.

During high dose therapy and especially during concomitant treatment with vitamin D, there is a risk of hypercalcaemia with subsequent kidney function impairment. In these patients serum calcium levels should be followed and renal function should be monitored.

There have been literature reports alluding to possible increased absorption of aluminium with citrate salts. Sandocal 1000 effervescent tablet (which contains citric acid) should be used with caution in patients with severely impaired renal function, especially those also receiving aluminium-containing preparations.

Each Sandocal 1000 effervescent tablet contains aspartame, a source of phenylalanine equivalent to 15 mg/dose, and may be harmful for people with phenylketonuria.

Patients with rare hereditary problems of fructose intolerance or glucose-galactose malabsorption should not take this medicine.

Sandocal 1000 contains 5.95 mmol (corresponding to 136.90 mg) of sodium per tablet.

Sandocal 1000 effervescent tablets should be kept out of the reach of children.

Information for diabetics:
One effervescent tablet contains 0.002 Carbohydrate Units and is therefore suitable for diabetics.

4.5 Interaction with other medicinal products and other forms of interaction
Thiazide diuretics reduce the urinary excretion of calcium. Due to increased risk of hypercalcaemia, serum calcium should be regularly monitored during concomitant use of thiazide diuretics.

Systemic corticosteroids reduce calcium absorption. During concomitant use, it may be necessary to increase the dose of Sandocal 1000.

Tetracycline preparations administered concomitantly with calcium preparations may not be well-absorbed. For this reason, tetracycline preparations should be administered at least two hours before or four to six hours after oral intake of calcium.

Cardiac glycoside toxicity may increase with hypercalcaemia resulting from treatment with calcium. Patients should be monitored with regard to electrocardiogram (ECG) and serum calcium levels.

If an oral bisphosphonate or sodium fluoride is used concomitantly, this preparation should be administered at least three hours before the intake of Sandocal 1000 since gastrointestinal absorption of either oral bisphosphonate or sodium fluoride may be reduced.

Oxalic acid (found in spinach and rhubarb) and phytic acid (found in whole cereals) may inhibit calcium absorption through formation of insoluble compounds with calcium ions. The patient should not take calcium products within two hours of eating foods high in oxalic acid and phytic acid.

4.6 Pregnancy and lactation

The adequate daily intake (including food and supplementation) for normal pregnant and lactating women is 1000-1300 mg calcium.

During pregnancy, the daily intake of calcium should not exceed 1500 mg. Significant amounts of calcium are secreted in milk during lactation but do not cause any adverse effects to the neonate.

Sandocal 1000 effervescent tablets can be used during pregnancy and lactation in case of a calcium deficiency

4.7 Effects on ability to drive and use machines

Sandocal 1000 has no influence on the ability to drive and use machines.

4.8 Undesirable effects

Adverse reactions are listed below, by system organ class and frequency. Frequencies are defined as: *uncommon* (>1/1,000, <1/100), *rare* (>1/10,000, <1/1,000) or *very rare* (<1/10,000), including isolated reports.

Immune system disorders:

Rare: Hypersensitivity, such as rash, pruritus, urticaria.

Very rare: Isolated cases of systemic allergic reactions (anaphylactic reaction, face oedema, angioneurotic oedema) have been reported

Metabolism and nutrition disorders:

Uncommon: Hypercalcaemia, hypercalciuria

Gastrointestinal disorders:

Rare: flatulence, constipation, diarrhoea, nausea, vomiting, abdominal pain

4.9 Overdose

Overdose leads to hypercalciuria and hypercalcaemia. Symptoms of hypercalcaemia may include: nausea, vomiting, thirst, polydipsia, polyuria, dehydration and constipation. Chronic overdose with resulting hypercalcaemia can cause vascular and organ calcification.

The threshold for calcium intoxication is from supplementation in excess of 2000 mg per day, taken for several months.

Treatment of overdose:

In the case of an intoxication, treatment should be stopped immediately and the fluid deficiency should be corrected.

In case of chronic overdose where hypercalcaemia is present, the initial therapeutic step is hydration with saline solution. A loop diuretic (e.g., furosemide) may then be used to further increase calcium excretion and to prevent volume overload, but thiazide diuretics should be avoided. In patients with renal failure, hydration is ineffective and they should undergo dialysis. In the case of persistent hypercalcaemia, contributing factors should be excluded, e.g., vitamin A or D hypervitaminosis, primary hyperparathyroidism, malignancies, renal failure, or immobilisation.

5. PHARMACOLOGICAL PROPERTIES

5.1 Pharmacodynamic properties

Pharmacotherapeutic group: Mineral supplements

ATC codes: Calcium carbonate (A 12 AA 04), Calcium lactate gluconate (A 12 AA 06)

Calcium is an essential mineral, necessary for bone formation and maintenance, for electrolyte equilibrium in the body and for the proper functioning of numerous regulatory mechanisms.

5.2 Pharmacokinetic properties

Sandocal 1000 contains two calcium salts, calcium lactate gluconate and calcium carbonate, which readily dissolve in water to make the active ionised form of calcium freely usable.

Absorption:

Some 25-50% of the ingested dose of calcium is absorbed, predominantly in the proximal part of the small intestine, and delivered to the exchangeable calcium pool.

Distribution and metabolism:

The mineral component of bones and teeth contains 99% of the body's calcium. The remaining 1% is present in the intra- and extracellular fluids. About 50% of the total blood-calcium content is in the physiologically active ionised form, with approximately 5% being complexed to citrate, phosphate or other anions. The remaining 45% of serum calcium is bound to proteins, principally albumin.

Elimination:

Calcium is excreted in the urine, faeces and sweat. Urinary excretion depends on glomerular filtration and tubular reabsorption.

5.3 Preclinical safety data

There is no information of relevance to the safety assessment in addition to what is stated in other parts of the SmPC.

6. PHARMACEUTICAL PARTICULARS

6.1 List of excipients

Citric acid anhydrous (fine granulate)

Orange flavour powder (contains: orange essential oils, maltodextrin, arabic gum, sorbitol (E 420), dextrose)

Aspartame (E951)

Macrogol 6000

Sodium hydrogen carbonate

6.2 Incompatibilities

Not applicable.

6.3 Shelf life

3 years.

6.4 Special precautions for storage

Keep the tube tightly closed. Store in the original package.

6.5 Nature and contents of container

The effervescent tablets are packed in polypropylene tubes and tamperproof polyethylene stoppers with desiccant, each containing 10 or 20 tablets. The tubes are packed in boxes containing 10, 20, 30, 40, 60, 80, 100 and 600 (for 500 mg only) tablets.

Not all pack sizes may be marketed.

6.6 Special precautions for disposal and other handling

No special requirements.

7. MARKETING AUTHORISATION HOLDER

Novartis Consumer Health (UK) Ltd

Wimblehurst Road

Horsham

West Sussex

RH12 5AB

UK

Trading as Novartis Consumer Health

8. MARKETING AUTHORISATION NUMBER(S)

PL 00030/0179

9. DATE OF FIRST AUTHORISATION/RENEWAL OF THE AUTHORISATION

4 September 2000

10. DATE OF REVISION OF THE TEXT

20 October 2006

Legal category

P

Sando-K

(HK Pharma Limited)

1. NAME OF THE MEDICINAL PRODUCT

SANDO-K®

2. QUALITATIVE AND QUANTITATIVE COMPOSITION

Effervescent Tablets containing 0.6g potassium chloride Ph.Eur., 0.4g potassium bicarbonate USP

3. PHARMACEUTICAL FORM

Flat, round, white effervescent tablet with a slightly rough surface, weighing 2.4g and of 22mm diameter and 4.25mm thick

4. CLINICAL PARTICULARS

4.1 Therapeutic indications

Prevention and treatment of hypokalaemic states such as those associated with:

i) Use of drugs which can induce potassium depletion eg. frusemide, thiazide diuretics, corticosteroids, carbenoxolone and cardiac glycosides, especially in combination with diuretics;

ii) Potassium loss resulting from severe diarrhoea, vomiting or fistulas;

iii) Acid-base disturbances e.g. alkalosis, renal tubular acidosis, states in which there is aldosterone excess, Cushing syndrome;

iv) Decreased intake of potassium e.g. malnutrition, alcoholism, some elderly patients with deficient diets;

v) Since SANDO-K Effervescent Tablets contain Cl^- they may be used in the treatment of hypokalaemia associated with hypochloraemic alkalosis.

4.2 Posology and method of administration

Oral administration, after dissolution of the tablet in water. May be taken with food if preferred.

Adults and children: Dosage is dependent upon the clinical conditions and diet of the patient, however the administration of 2 to 4 tablets daily (24 to 48 mmol K^+) is likely to provide an adequate prophylactic or therapeutic dose in most patients. Large doses may be indicated in more severe hypokalaemic conditions when the dose should be regulated by the patient's response as determined by serum electrolyte levels and acid-base studies.

Dosage guidelines: A drop in serum potassium level of 1 mmol/l represents a loss of about 100-200 mmol of potassium from body stores. While serum potassium levels below 2 mmol/l may warrant intravenous replacement therapy, following are approximate guidelines in less severe potassium depletion:

For serum levels between 2-3 mmol/l, a maximum daily dose of 100-200 mmol K^+ (8-16 tablets) and for serum levels between 3-4 mmol/l, a maximum daily dose of 50-100 mmol K^+ (4-8 tablets) should be considered.

Elderly: No evidence exists that elderly patients require different dosages or show different side-effects than younger patients. However, such patients should be carefully supervised as factors sometimes associated with ageing, such as poor diet or impaired renal function, may indirectly affect the dosage or tolerability.

4.3 Contraindications

Severe renal impairment with oliguria, inadequately treated Addison's disease, hyperkalaemia from any cause, crush injuries and acute dehydration.

4.4 Special warnings and precautions for use

Periodic evaluation of the patient's clinical status, serum electrolytes and the ECG should be carried out when replacement therapy is undertaken. This is particularly important in patients with cardiac disease and in those receiving digitalis. Care should be taken to avoid dosage in excess of requirements for patients with impaired renal function. Caution is also necessary in patients receiving potassium-sparing diuretics and ACE-inhibitors, and in patients with myotonia congenita or severe haemolysis. In patients with acidosis, the acid-base balance should be monitored. In patients with hypertension, it should be remembered that correction of hypokalaemia may lower blood pressure.

4.5 Interaction with other medicinal products and other forms of interaction

If co-administered with potassium-sparing diuretics and ACE-inhibitors, the risk of hyperkalaemia must be considered.

4.6 Pregnancy and lactation

No clinical problems have been encountered during pregnancy and lactation. Nevertheless, the benefit of treatment should be considered in relation to the risks before SANDO-K is given to pregnant or nursing women.

4.7 Effects on ability to drive and use machines

No effects known

4.8 Undesirable effects

Abdominal discomfort, diarrhoea, nausea and vomiting may occur. If there are any signs of gastric irritancy, SANDO-K, in common with all other potassium salts, should be given with or after food. Gastric irritancy has occurred but this is rare since the tablets dissolve in water and are taken in solution, thus preventing high local concentrations. A moderate hyperkalaemia may be asymptomatic; if suspected reference to the section on overdosage is recommended.

4.9 Overdose

Hyperkalaemia. Poisoning is usually minimal below 6.5 mmol per litre but may be severe above 8 mmol per litre. However, comparatively low doses may cause adverse effects when excretion is delayed as in renal insufficiency. The absolute toxicity is dependent on other electrolytes and acid-base levels.

Hyperkalaemic symptoms include paraesthesia of the extremities, listlessness, mental confusion, weakness, paralysis, hypotension, cardiac arrhythmias, heart block and cardiac arrest.

Hyperkalaemia is often asymptomatic. However, increasing serum potassium levels can be detected by changes in the ECG; initially the appearance of tall, peaked T waves, followed by a widening of the QRS complex bending into the abnormal T waves. P-wave voltage decreases and the PR interval is prolonged.

Severe cardiac toxicity may be treated with calcium gluconate (10-20ml of a 10% injection given over 1-5 minutes with ECG monitoring). The effect may be transient and the injection may need to be repeated.

Raised serum potassium levels respond to administration of dextrose (300-500ml/hr of 10 or 25% solution), dextrose and insulin (as for dextrose with 10 units of insulin per 20g dextrose), or sodium bicarbonate solution.

Cation exchange resins may be used, or in severe cases peritoneal dialysis or haemodialysis may be necessary.

Caution should be exercised in patients who are digitalised and who may experience acute digitalis intoxication in the course of potassium removal.

5. PHARMACOLOGICAL PROPERTIES

5.1 Pharmacodynamic properties

The potassium ion is essential to the maintenance of body function, being involved in the synthesis of protein, metabolism of carbohydrate and storage of energy reserves. It interacts with sodium in the operation of the trans- membrane pump and at the site of exchange in the kidney, exchanges with sodium ion to maintain body homeostasis. A close relationship between potassium ion and magnesium ion has also been noted; a deficit in one ion has been associated with low levels of the other.

The diet of a healthy adult will provide an adequate intake of potassium (considered to be 20.5 to 33.3 mmol potassium daily) from a total intake of 60-100 mmol potassium. Total body potassium in an adult is about 3,500 mmol depending on the non-fat body tissues. A deficient intake or failure to conserve potassium leads to symptoms of hypokalaemia.

5.2 Pharmacokinetic properties

Unless a deficiency is present, requiring a supplement, sufficient potassium is taken into the body through the daily diet. The chloride salt of potassium is readily absorbed from the gastro-intestinal tract. Potassium enters the intracellular fluid to maintain a concentration of about 150 mEq/l and the normal range of concentration of potassium in the plasma is considered to be 3.5 - 5 mEq/l. Excretion of potassium is mainly by the distal tubules of the kidney, by the faeces (5 to 10 mmol/day) and a smaller amount in perspiration.

Metabolic, drug induced, or dietary deficiencies in potassium intake may require administration of a supplement.

5.3 Preclinical safety data

SANDO-K Effervescent Tablets contain potassium chloride and postassium bicarbonate (both of which are the subject of pharmacopoeial monographs). The physiological, pharmacological and clinical toxicity of potassium salts are well documented and limited animal data are therefore available

6. PHARMACEUTICAL PARTICULARS

6.1 List of excipients

Dioctyle sodium sulphosuccinate BPC, Colloidal anhydrous silica EP, Talc (acid washed) EP, Sodium saccharin BP, Icing sugar, CP HSE, Pulverised sugar, EP, Citric acid anhydrous 30/60 EP, Polyethylene glycol 4000 EP, Purified water EP

6.2 Incompatibilities

Not applicable

6.3 Shelf life

36 months

6.4 Special precautions for storage

Do not store above 25°C. Store in the original container. Keep the container tightly closed.

6.5 Nature and contents of container

High density polypropylene tube with polyethylene bellowed stopper containing integral silica gel dessicant capsule. Pack size 20.

6.6 Special precautions for disposal and other handling

Not applicable

7. MARKETING AUTHORISATION HOLDER

HK Pharma

PO Box 105

Hitchin

Herts SG5 2DE

8. MARKETING AUTHORISATION NUMBER(S)

PL 16784/0002

9. DATE OF FIRST AUTHORISATION/RENEWAL OF THE AUTHORISATION

28 April 1998

10. DATE OF REVISION OF THE TEXT

November 2002

Scopoderm TTS

(Novartis Consumer Health)

1. NAME OF THE MEDICINAL PRODUCT

SCOPODERM® TTS®

2. QUALITATIVE AND QUANTITATIVE COMPOSITION

Each patch contains 1.5mg hyoscine U.S.P.

3. PHARMACEUTICAL FORM

Scopoderm TTS is a transdermal therapeutic system. Each patch is a flat system of laminates, sealed around the edge, containing a clear oily filling. The system is a thin circular disc, tan coloured and fitted with a transparent, hexagonal protective liner which projects over the edge of the disc. Viewed through the liner, the system appears silver in colour. Each system has a contact surface area measuring 2.5cm^2 and hyoscine content of 1.5mg. The average amount of hyoscine absorbed from each system in 72 hours is 1mg.

4. CLINICAL PARTICULARS

4.1 Therapeutic indications

For the prevention of symptoms of motion sickness such as nausea, vomiting and vertigo.

4.2 Posology and method of administration

Route of Administration

Transdermal

Dosage and Administration

Adults

To achieve the optimum protective effect, one system should be applied about 5-6 hours before embarking on a journey (or on the evening before). The system should be placed onto a clean, dry, hairless area of skin behind the ear, taking care to avoid any cuts or irritation. One system can provide protection for up to 72 hours. Should protection be required for longer periods of time, a fresh system should be placed behind the other ear after 72 hours. (No more than one system should be used at a time). Conversely, if protection is only required for shorter periods of time, the system should be removed at the end of the journey.

Patients should wash their hands thoroughly after handling the system. In addition, after removal of the system, the site of application should also be washed. These precautions are necessary to minimise any chance of hyoscine accidentally being transferred to the eyes (see side-effects).

Limited contact with water (i.e. during bathing or swimming), should not affect the system, although it should be kept as dry as possible.

If the Scopoderm TTS becomes accidentally detached, it should be replaced by a fresh system.

Use in Elderly

Scopoderm TTS may be used in the elderly (see dosage recommendations for adults) although the elderly may be more prone to suffer from the side-effects of hyoscine (see precautions).

Use in Children

Scopoderm TTS can be used in children age 10 years or over (see dosage recommendations for adults). Insufficient data are available to recommend the use of Scopoderm TTS for younger children.

4.3 Contraindications

Scopoderm TTS is contra-indicated in patients with glaucoma or with a history of the condition, and in patients with known hypersensitivity to hyoscine.

4.4 Special warnings and precautions for use

Scopoderm TTS should be used with caution in patients with pyloric stenosis, those who have bladder outflow obstruction, or in patients with intestinal obstruction.

Patients should not consume alcohol whilst using Scopoderm TTS.

Scopoderm TTS should also be used with caution in elderly patients, and in patients with impaired hepatic or renal function.

In rare cases, confusional states and visual hallucinations may occur. In such cases, Scopoderm TTS should be removed immediately. If severe symptoms persist, appropriate therapeutic measures should be taken (see overdosage section).

Idiosyncratic reactions may occur with ordinary therapeutic doses of hyoscine.

In isolated cases an increase in seizure frequency in epileptic patients has been reported.

Care should be taken after removal of the system as side-effects may persist for up to 24 hours or longer.

4.5 Interaction with other medicinal products and other forms of interaction

Scopoderm TTS should be used with caution in patients being treated with drugs that act on the central nervous system (including alcohol) or drugs with anticholinergic properties.

4.6 Pregnancy and lactation

Teratogenic studies have been performed in pregnant rats and rabbits with hyoscine administered by daily intravenous injection. No adverse effects were noted in rats. In rabbits, the drug had a marginal embryotoxic effect at a high dose (at drug plasma levels approximately 100 times those observed in humans using Scopoderm TTS).

Scopoderm TTS should only be used during pregnancy if the expected benefits to the mother outweigh the potential risks to the foetus.

It is not known if hyoscine passes into the breast milk. Therefore nursing mothers should refrain from breast feeding their infants whilst using Scopoderm TTS.

4.7 Effects on ability to drive and use machines

Scopoderm TTS may cause drowsiness, dizziness, confusion or visual disturbance in certain individuals. Patients using the system must not drive, operate machinery, pilot an aircraft, dive or engage in any other activities in which such symptoms could be dangerous (see side-effects).

4.8 Undesirable effects

The following side-effects may occur:

Eyes

In isolated cases pupillary dilatation may precipitate acute glaucoma, particularly narrow angle glaucoma

(see Contra-Indications).

Occasional: Irritation of the eyelids

If traces of hyoscine on the hands enter the eyes, transient cycloplegia and pupillary dilatation (occasionally unilateral) frequently occur.

Mouth

Frequent: Transient dryness of the mouth.

Central Nervous System

Occasional: Drowsiness.

Rare: Impairment of memory and concentration, restlessness, dizziness, disorientation, confusion and visual hallucinations. (see precautions).

Skin

Occasional: Local irritation

In isolated cases: A generalised skin rash

Urogenital system

Rare: Disturbances of micturition (i.e. urine retention)

Side-effects after removal of Scopoderm TTS

Rare: Unwanted effects, including headache, nausea, vomiting and disturbance of balance, occurring after removal of the system. These symptoms have occurred most often in patients who have used the system for several days. In such cases, patients should not drive or engage in other activities requiring concentration

(see warnings).

4.9 Overdose

Symptoms

Initially, restlessness, excitation and confusion may be observed. In response to higher doses, delirium, hallucinations and convulsions set in. At very high doses, coma and respiratory paralysis may occur.

Treatment

If symptoms of overdosage occur, the system(s) should be removed immediately. Physostigmine is the most effective antidote. Depending on the severity of poisoning, physostigmine should be given by slow intravenous injection in doses of 1-4mg (0.5mg in children). Repeated injections may be necessary since physostigmine is rapidly metabolised. Diazepam may be used to counter excitation and convulsions although at higher doses it may cause respiratory depression. In severe cases, artificial respiration may be necessary. If hyperthermia occurs, immediate action should be taken to dissipate heat.

5. PHARMACOLOGICAL PROPERTIES

5.1 Pharmacodynamic properties

The transdermal therapeutic system (TTS) is a novel form of drug delivery designed to achieve a continuous release of hyoscine through the intact skin to the systemic circulation for up to 72 hours.

Hyoscine has anticholinergic properties. It acts as a competitive antagonist to acetylchloline and other parasympathomimetic agents. Its mechanism of action in the central nervous system in preventing motion sickness has yet to be elucidated. Hyoscine produces classical symptoms of parasympathetic blockade.

5.2 Pharmacokinetic properties

Following Scopoderm TTS administration, measurement of the urinary excretion has shown the equilibrium between absorption and elimination to be reached within about 6 hours. Steady plasma concentrations of hyoscine in the range of 0.17-0.33nmol/litre are produced. Provided the system is not removed, this equilibrium is maintained and plasma hyoscine levels are within this therapeutic range for up to 72 hours.

After removal of Scopoderm TTS, the plasma concentration diminishes slowly to approximately one third over the following 24 hours because hyoscine in the skin continues to enter the blood stream.

5.3 Preclinical safety data

None stated

6. PHARMACEUTICAL PARTICULARS

6.1 List of excipients

Drug Reservoir

Light mineral oil

Polyisobutylene (1.200.000)

Polyisobutylene (35.000)

Backing Film

Pigmented MDPE/AL/PET/HS Film (vapour coated aluminised polyester with outer coating of pigmented medium density polyethylene (MDPE) and a heat sealable inner coating. Thickness 0.0686mm.

Release Controlling Membrane

Polypropylene Film. Thickness 0.0254mm.

Adhesive (to skin)

Light mineral oil

Polyisobutylene (1.200.000)

Polyisobutylene (35.000)

Release Liner (discarded before use)

Silicone/Polyester Film

Thickness 0.0762mm

6.2 Incompatibilities

None stated

6.3 Shelf life

36 months

6.4 Special precautions for storage

Store below 25°C. Do not freeze.

6.5 Nature and contents of container

Scopoderm TTS - Individually packed into sealed paper laminated aluminium foil pouches. Outer cardboard carton containing two patches.

6.6 Special precautions for disposal and other handling

Patients should wash their hands thoroughly after handling the system. In addition, after removal of the system, the site of application should also be washed. These precautions are necessary to minimise any chance of hyoscine accidentally being transferred to the eyes (see side-effects).

7. MARKETING AUTHORISATION HOLDER

Novartis Consumer Health UK Limited

Trading as: Novartis Consumer Health

Wimblehurst Road

Horsham

West Sussex

RH12 5AB

UK

8. MARKETING AUTHORISATION NUMBER(S)

00030/0180

9. DATE OF FIRST AUTHORISATION/RENEWAL OF THE AUTHORISATION

Date of first authorisation: 30 March 2001

Date of last renewal: 5 December 2008

10. DATE OF REVISION OF THE TEXT

5 December 2008.

Legal category: POM

Sebomin MR

(Actavis UK Ltd)

1. NAME OF THE MEDICINAL PRODUCT

Sebomin 100mg MR Capsules.

2. QUALITATIVE AND QUANTITATIVE COMPOSITION

Each capsule contains 100mg anhydrous minocycline (as the hydrochloride).

For excipients, see 6.1

3. PHARMACEUTICAL FORM

Prolonged-release capsule, hard.

Orange, opaque, hard gelatin capsules (size 2) printed "C" and "MR" in white.

4. CLINICAL PARTICULARS

4.1 Therapeutic indications

The treatment of acne.

4.2 Posology and method of administration

Dosage:

Adults: One 100mg capsule every 24 hours.

Children over 12 years: One 100mg capsule every 24 hours.

Children under 12 years: Sebomin MR is not recommended.

Elderly: No special dosing requirements.

Treatment of acne should be continued for a minimum of 6 weeks. If there is no satisfactory response to Sebomin MR after six months, the treatment should be discontinued and other therapies considered. If Sebomin MR is to be continued for longer than six months, patients should be monitored at least three monthly thereafter for signs and symptoms of hepatitis or SLE (see Special warnings and precautions for use).

Administration:

The capsules should be swallowed whole with plenty of fluid, while sitting or standing in order to reduce the risk of oesophageal irritation and ulceration. They should not be taken with food as this affects the absorption of minocycline.

4.3 Contraindications

- Known hypersensitivity to tetracyclines
- Pregnancy
- Lactation
- Children under the age of 12 years
- Complete renal failure.

4.4 Special warnings and precautions for use

Minocycline should be used with caution in patients with hepatic dysfunction and in conjunction with alcohol and other hepatotoxic drugs. It is recommended that alcohol consumption should remain within the Government's recommended limits.

Rare cases of auto-immune hepatotoxicity and isolated cases of systemic lupus erythematosus (SLE) and also exacerbation of pre-existing SLE have been reported. If patients develop signs or symptoms of SLE or hepatotoxicity, or suffer exacerbation of pre-existing SLE, minocycline should be discontinued.

Clinical studies have shown that in patients with renal impairment there is no significant drug accumulation when they are treated with minocycline in the recommended doses. However, reduction of dosage and monitoring of renal function may be required in cases of severe renal insufficiency.

Cross-resistance between tetracyclines may develop in micro-organisms and cross-sensitisation in patients. Minocycline should be discontinued if there are signs/symptoms of overgrowth of resistant organisms, e.g. enteritis, glossitis, stomatitis, vaginitis, pruritus ani or staphylococcal enteritis.

Patients taking oral contraceptives should be warned that there is a possibility of contraceptive failure if diarrhoea or breakthrough bleeding occurs.

Minocycline may cause hyperpigmentation at various body sites. Hyperpigmentation may be present regardless of dose or duration of treatment but develops more commonly during long term treatment. Patients should be advised to report any unusual pigmentation without delay and minocycline should be discontinued.

If a photosensitivity reaction occurs, patients should be warned to avoid direct exposure to natural or artificial light and to discontinue therapy at the first sign of skin discomfort.

The capsule shell contains sunset yellow (E110), which can cause allergic - type reactions including asthma. Allergy is more common in those people who are allergic to aspirin.

Use in children:

The use of tetracyclines during tooth development in children under the age of 12 years may cause permanent discolouration. Enamel hypoplasia has also been reported.

4.5 Interaction with other medicinal products and other forms of interaction

Minocycline should not be used with penicillins. Tetracyclines depress plasma prothrombin activity and reduced doses of concomitant anticoagulants may be necessary.

Absorption of minocycline is impaired by the concomitant administration of antacids, iron, calcium, magnesium, aluminium and zinc salts. It is recommended that any indigestion remedies, vitamins, or other supplements containing these salts are taken at least 3 hours before or after a dose of minocycline. The capsules should not be taken with food as this affects the absorption of minocycline.

4.6 Pregnancy and lactation

Pregnancy:

Results of animal studies indicate that tetracyclines cross the placenta, are found in foetal tissues and can have toxic effects on the developing foetus (often related to retardation of skeletal development). Evidence of embryotoxicity has also been noted in animals treated early in pregnancy.

Minocycline therefore, should not be used in pregnancy unless considered essential.

The use of drugs of the tetracycline class during tooth development (last half of pregnancy) may cause permanent discolouration of the teeth (yellow-grey-brown). This adverse reaction has been observed following repeated short term courses however it is more common during long term use of the drug. Enamel hypoplasia has also been reported.

Lactation:

Tetracyclines have been found in the milk of lactating women who are taking a drug in this class. Permanent tooth discolouration may occur in the developing infant and enamel hypoplasia has been reported.

4.7 Effects on ability to drive and use machines

Minocycline has been associated with headache, lightheadedness, dizziness and vertigo and rarely impaired hearing. Patients should be warned about the possible hazards of driving or operating machinery during treatment.

4.8 Undesirable effects

Common

As with other tetracyclines, gastrointestinal disturbances including nausea, anorexia, vomiting and diarrhoea may occur. Dermatological reactions such as erythema multiforme, erythema nodosum, Stevens Johnson syndrome, exfoliative dermatitis, hair loss and photosensitivity have been reported, as well as maculopapular and erythematous rashes. Hypersensitivity reactions can include urticaria, fever, arthralgia, myalgia, arthritis, pulmonary infiltration, wheezing, angioneurotic oedema, anaphylaxis and anaphylactoid purpura.

Cases of systemic lupus erythematosus (SLE) and also exacerbation of pre-existing SLE have been reported (see also Special warnings and precautions for use).

In common with other tetracyclines, bulging fontanelles in infants and benign intracranial hypertension in juveniles and adults have been reported. If evidence of raised intracranial pressure develops, treatment should cease.

Blood haemolytic anaemia, thrombocytopenia, neutropenia and eosinophilia have been reported with tetracyclines.

As with other tetracyclines, transient increases in liver function test values have been reported. Some hepatic reactions have an auto-immune basis, and may occur after several months of minocycline treatment (see Posology and method of administration). When given over prolonged periods, tetracyclines have been reported to produce brown-black microscopic discolouration of thyroid tissue.

Uncommon

There have been isolated incidences of pancreatitis.

Hyperpigmentation of skin, nails or discolouration of teeth and buccal mucosa have been reported occasionally. These are generally reversible on cessation of therapy.

There are isolated cases of discolouration of conjunctiva, lacrimal secretions, breast secretions and perspiration.

Rare

Hepatitis and acute liver failure have been reported.

Fixed drug eruptions have been observed.

Pericarditis, myocarditis, vasculitis and renal failure including interstitial nephritis have been reported.

Bone discolouration has been observed.

(See also Pregnancy and Lactation).

4.9 Overdose

No specific antidote. Gastric lavage plus appropriate supportive treatment.

5. PHARMACOLOGICAL PROPERTIES

5.1 Pharmacodynamic properties

Pharmacotheraputic group: Tetracycline, ATC code: J01A A08

Sebomin MR contain the active ingredient minocycline as minocycline hydrochloride, a semi-synthetic derivative of tetracycline.

Minocycline has a long serum half-life and can be administered at 12 hour intervals, the modified release form can be given once daily.

Minocycline interferes with the third stage of bacterial protein synthesis. After amino acids are activated and attached to t-RNA (transfer RNA), the resulting amino acyl-t-RNA migrates to the bacterial ribosome for synthesis of proteins. Minocycline binds to the 30s subunit on the ribosome and inhibits binding of the aminoacyl-t-RNA molecules.

There is also evidence that minocycline may cause alterations in the cytoplasmic membrane, thereby allowing leakage of nucleotides and other compounds from the cell. This would explain the rapid inhibition of DNA replication that ensues when cells are exposed to concentrations of minocycline greater than that needed to inhibit protein synthesis.

In higher concentration, minocycline inhibits mammalian protein synthesis and may aggravate pre-existing renal functional impairment. The drug may interfere with parenteral nutrition in post operative patients by inhibiting utilization of amino acids for protein synthesis.

Minocycline is reported to be active against both Gram negative and Gram positive organisms.

5.2 Pharmacokinetic properties

Absorption

Oral bioavailability for minocycline has been reported to be 90%.

One report has demonstrated that food did not significantly affect the absorption of minocycline following 50 mg oral doses. However, another study reported that minocycline absorption was decreased by 77%, 27% and 13% when given with iron, milk and food.

Distribution

Total protein binding of minocycline has been reported to be in the order of 76%.

Other sites of distribution of minocycline include the following:

AQUEOUS HUMOR

Minocycline administered orally with a loading dose of 200 mg followed by 2 doses of 100 mg 12 hours apart produce adequate drug concentration in the aqueous humor of noninflamed eyes. The plasma to aqueous humor ratio was approximately 2:1.

CEREBROSPINAL FLUID

Minocycline has been reported to cross the blood/brain barrier to a higher degree than doxycycline. However, passage of either drug has been shown to be significantly decreased in patients with uninflamed meninges.

GINGIVAL FLUID

The mean gingival crevicular fluid drug concentration of 8.03 +/- 1.64 mcg/ml was reported after 7 days of oral minocycline 200 mg in patients with moderate to severe periodontal disease. Mean serum concentration was 2.58 +/- 0.32 mcg/ml.

JOINT FLUID CONCENTRATIONS

Following 200 mg oral doses of minocycline, joint fluid levels 3 to 12 hours following the dose were 0.43 to 0.88 mcg/ml.

SALIVA/TEARS

Minocycline achieved significant levels in saliva and tears sufficient to inhibit most strains of meningococci. Following oral doses of 100 mg every 12 hours for 5 days, the concentration of drug in saliva and tear equalled or was greater than the average MIC for meningococci for up to 12 hours after the dose. Two hours following an oral dose, concentrations of minocycline in saliva and tears were at 0.3 mcg/mL and 0.4 mcg/mL, respectively.

SINUS SECRETIONS

Following a dose of 100 mg twice daily for 4 days in patients with sinusitis a sinus level of 1.06 mcg/5 mL was found. The mean minocycline serum level was 3.16 mcg/ml, giving a sinus secretion to serum level ratio of 0.34:1.

Metabolism

An inactive metabolite, 9-hydroxyminocycline has been isolated.

Elimination

Minocycline has a very low renal clearance as compared to other tetracyclines. However, urinary concentrations approximating 10 times that of serum are attained for the first 4 to 6 hours following an oral dose.

Minocycline is excreted 19% in the faeces, this level is much lower than most other tetracyclines.

5.3 Preclinical safety data

There are no preclinical data of relevance to the prescriber which are additional to that already included in other sections of the SPC.

6. PHARMACEUTICAL PARTICULARS

6.1 List of excipients

glycerol monostearate 40-55,

microcrystalline cellulose 101 (E460(i)),

povidone K-30 (E1201),

purified talc (E553b).

Capsule shell

gelatin,

purified water,

titanium dioxide (E171),

sunset yellow (E110),

quinoline yellow (E104).

Printing ink

shellac (E904),

ethyl alcohol,

isopropyl alcohol,

propylene glycol,

butyl alcohol,

povidone (E1201),

sodium hydroxide,

titanium dioxide (E171).

6.2 Incompatibilities

Not applicable.

6.3 Shelf life

24 months.

6.4 Special precautions for storage

Do not store above 30°C.

Polypropylene container - store in the original container,

PVC/aluminium blister pack - keep container in the outer carton.

6.5 Nature and contents of container

PVC/aluminium blister pack in outer cardboard container

28, 30, 56, 60, 84, 90

Polypropylene container with polyethylene cap

100, 112, 120, 200, 250, 500

Not all pack sizes may be marketed.

6.6 Special precautions for disposal and other handling

No special requirements.

7. MARKETING AUTHORISATION HOLDER

Actavis UK Limited

(Trading style: Actavis)

Whiddon Valley

Barnstaple

North Devon

EX32 8NS

United Kingdom

8. MARKETING AUTHORISATION NUMBER(S)

PL 00142/0526

9. DATE OF FIRST AUTHORISATION/RENEWAL OF THE AUTHORISATION

20 June 2003

Renewed – 19.03.09

10. DATE OF REVISION OF THE TEXT

19.03.09

Sectral 100mg and 200mg capsules

(sanofi-aventis)

1. NAME OF THE MEDICINAL PRODUCT

Sectral capsules 100mg

Sectral capsules 200mg

2. QUALITATIVE AND QUANTITATIVE COMPOSITION

The active component of SECTRAL Capsules 100mg is: Acebutolol hydrochloride 111.0mg (equivalent to 100mg of base).

The active component of SECTRAL Capsules 200mg is: Acebutolol hydrochloride 222.0mg (equivalent to 200mg of base).

For a full list of excipients, see section 6.1

3. PHARMACEUTICAL FORM

Sectral Capsules 100: Hard gelatin capsules, the bodies being opaque yellowish-buff and the caps opaque white in colour. Length approximately 17mm, diameter of body approximately 6mm. Both body and cap are printed in black: Sectral 100.

Sectral Capsules 200: Hard gelatin capsules, the bodies being opaque yellowish-buff and the caps opaque pink in colour. Length approximately 17mm, diameter of body approximately 6mm. Both body and cap are printed in black: Sectral 200

The capsules contain a white or almost white powder.

4. CLINICAL PARTICULARS

4.1 Therapeutic indications

The management of all grades of hypertension, angina pectoris and the control of tachyarrhythmias.

4.2 Posology and method of administration

Hypertension: Initial dosage of 400mg orally once daily at breakfast or 200mg orally twice daily. If response is not adequate within two weeks, dosage may be increased up to 400mg orally twice daily; if the hypertension is still not adequately controlled consideration should be given to adding a second antihypertensive agent such as the calcium antagonist nifedipine or small doses of a thiazide diuretic.

Angina pectoris: Initial dosage of 400mg orally once daily at breakfast or 200mg twice daily. In severe forms up to 300mg three times daily may be required. Up to 1200mg daily has been used.

Cardiac Arrhythmias: When given orally, an initial dose of 200mg is recommended. The daily dose requirement for long term anti arrhythmic activity should lie between 400 and 1200mg daily. The dose can be gauged by response, and better control may be achieved by divided doses rather than single doses. It may take up to three hours for maximal anti-arrhythmic effect to become apparent.

Elderly: There are no specific dosage recommendations for the elderly with normal glomerular filtration rate. Dose reduction is necessary if moderate to severe renal impairment is present (see Section 4.4)

Children: Paediatric dose has not been established.

For all indications, it is advised that the lowest recommended dosage be used initially.

4.3 Contraindications

Cardiogenic shock is an absolute contraindication. Extreme caution is required in patients with blood pressures of the order of 100/60 mmHg or below. SECTRAL is also contraindicated in patients with second and third degree heart block, sick sinus syndrome, marked bradycardia (< 45-50 bpm), uncontrolled heart failure, metabolic acidosis, severe.peripheral circulatory disorders, hypersensitivity to acebutolol, any of the excipients or to beta blockers, and untreated phaeochromocytoma.

4.4 Special warnings and precautions for use

Renal impairment is not a contraindication to the use of SECTRAL which has both renal and non-renal excretory pathways. Some caution should be exercised when administering high doses to patients with severe renal failure as accumulation could possibly occur in these circumstances.

The dosage frequency should not exceed once daily in patients with renal impairment. As a guide, the dosage should be reduced by 50% when glomerular filtration rates are between 25-50ml/min and by 75% when they are below 25ml/min (see Section 4.2).

Drug-induced bronchospasm is usually at least partially reversible by the use of a suitable agonist.

Although cardio-selective beta blockers may have less effect on lung function than non-selective beta blockers as with all beta blockers they should be avoided in patients with obstructive airways disease unless there are compelling clinical reasons for their use. Where such reasons exist, cardio-selective β-blockers should be used with the utmost care (from Section 4.3).

Beta-blockers may induce bradycardia. In such cases, the dosage should be reduced.

They may be used with care in patients with controlled heart failure (see Section 4.3).

Use with caution in patients with Prinzmetal's angina.

Beta blockers may aggravate peripheral circulatory disorders. They may mask signs of thyrotoxicosis and hypoglycaemia. They should only be used in patients with phaeochromocytoma with comcomitant alpha-adrenoceptor therapy

Patients with known psoriasis should take beta-blockers only after careful consideration.

Beta-blockers may increase both the sensitivity towards allergens and the seriousness of anaphylactic reactions.

Withdrawal of treatment by beta blockers should be achieved by gradual dosage reduction; this is especially important in patients with ischaemic heart disease

When it has been decided to interrupt beta-blockade prior to surgery, therapy should be discontinued for at least 24 hours. Continuation of therapy reduces the risk of arrhythmias but the risk of hypotension may be increased. If treatment is continued, caution should be observed with the use of certain anaesthetic drugs. The patient may be protected against vagal reactions by intravenous administration of atropine.

4.5 Interaction with other medicinal products and other forms of interaction

Sectral should not be used with Verapamil or within several days of Verapamil therapy (and vice versa). Use with great care with any other calcium antagonists, particularly Diltiazem.

Class I anti-arrhythmic drugs (such as disopyramide) and amiodarone may increase atrial conduction time and induce negative inotropic effects when used concomitantly with beta-blockers.

In patients with labile and insulin-dependent diabetes, the dosage of the hypoglycaemic agent (ie insulin or oral diabetic drugs) may need to be reduced. However beta-blockers have also been known to blunt the effect of glibenclamide. Beta-adrenergic blockade may also prevent the appearance of signs of hypoglycaemia (tachycardia, see Section 4.4).

Cross reactions due to displacement of other drugs from plasma protein binding sites are unlikely due to the low degree of plasma protein binding exhibited by acebutolol and diacetolol.

If a beta-blocker is used concurrently with clonidine the latter should not be withdrawn until several days after the former is discontinued.

Acebutolol may antagonize the effect of sympathomimetic and xanthine bronchodilators.

Concurrent use of digoxin and beta blockers may occasionally induce serious bradycardia. The anti-hypertensive effects of beta blockers may be attenuated by non-steroidal anti-inflammatory agents.

Concomitant administration of tricyclic antidepressants, barbiturates and phenothiazines as well as other anti-hypertensive agent- may increase the blood pressure lowering effect of beta-blockers.

There is a theoretical risk that concurrent administration of monoamine oxidase inhibitors and high doses of beta-blockers, even if they are cardio-selective can produce hypertension.

SECTRAL therapy should be brought to the attention of the anaesthetist prior to general anaesthesia (see Section 4.4). If treatment is continued, special care should be taken when using anaesthetic agents causing myocardial depression such as ether, cyclopropane and trichlorethylene.

4.6 Pregnancy and lactation

Pregnancy: SECTRAL should not be administered to female patients during the first trimester of pregnancy unless the physician considers it essential. In such cases the lowest possible dose should be used.

Beta blockers administered in late pregnancy may give rise to bradycardia, hypoglycaemia and cardiac or pulmonary complications in the foetus/neonate.

Beta-blockers can reduce placental perfusion, which may result in intrauterine foetal death, immature and premature deliveries

Animal studies have shown no teratogenic hazard.

Lactation: Acebutolol and its active metabolite are excreted in breast milk and the half life of acebutolol in the neonate is double that in adults. The risks of hypoglycaemia and bradycardia occurring in the nursing infant have not been evaluated. Therefore, breast-feeding is not recommended during treatment.

4.7 Effects on ability to drive and use machines

As with all beta-blockers, dizziness or fatigue may occur occasionally. This should be taken into account when driving or operating machinery.

4.8 Undesirable effects

SECTRAL possesses antihypertensive effects but these are unlikely to be noted in normotensive subjects. The side-effects common to beta-blockade include: bradycardia, heart failure, a slowing of AV conduction or increase of an existing AV block, hypotension, gastrointestinal effects (such as nausea, vomiting and diarrhoea), cold and cyanotic extremities, paraesthesia, Raynaud's syndrome, intermittent claudication, confusion, dizziness, impaired vision, headaches, shortness of breath, nightmares, hallucinations, psychoses and depression, loss of libido and lethargy. The low lipid solubility and lack of accumulation in CNS tissues of acebutolol and its active metabolite reduce the likelihood of sleep disturbances, depression or other central effects and such occurrences are rare.

Pulmonary infiltration and pneumonitis appear to be rare but potentially serious complications of beta-blockade therapy. Cases of pneumonitis have been reported with acebutolol.

There have been reports of skin rashes and/or dry eyes associated with the use of beta-adrenoceptor blocking drugs. The reported incidence is small and in most cases the symptoms have cleared when treatment was withdrawn. Discontinuation of the drug should be considered in such cases.

Cessation of therapy with a beta-blocker should be gradual. (see Section 4.4)

Although some patients have developed anti-nuclear factor titres, the incidence of associated clinical symptoms is rare and when present, these clear promptly on discontinuation of treatment. Rare cases of a Lupus-like syndrome have been reported.

Bronchospasm has occurred rarely during treatment with acebutolol.

4.9 Overdose

In the event of excessive bradycardia or hypotension, 1mg atropine sulphate administered intravenously should be given without delay. If this is insufficient it should be followed by a slow intravenous injection of isoprenaline (5mcg per minute) with constant monitoring until a response occurs. In severe cases of self-poisoning with circulatory collapse unresponsive to atropine and catecholamines the intravenous injection of glucagon 10-20mg may produce a dramatic improvement. Cardiac pacing may be employed if bradycardia becomes severe.

Judicious use of vasopressors, diazepam, phenytoin, lidocaine, digoxin and bronchodilators should be considered depending on the presentation of the patient. Acebutolol can be removed from blood by haemodialysis. Other symptoms and signs of overdosage include cardiogenic shock, AV block, conduction defects, pulmonary oedema, depressed level of consciousness, bronchospasm, hypoglycaemia and rarely hyperkalaemia.

5. PHARMACOLOGICAL PROPERTIES

5.1 Pharmacodynamic properties

Mode of action: SECTRAL is a beta adrenoceptor antagonist which is cardioselective, i.e. acts preferentially on beta-1 adrenergic receptors in the heart. Its principal effects are to reduce heart rate especially on exercise and to lower blood pressure in hypertensive subjects. SECTRAL and its equally active metabolite, diacetolol have anti-arrhythmic activity, the combined plasma half-life of the active drug and metabolite being 7-10 hours. Both have partial agonist activity (PAA) also known as intrinsic sympathomimetic activity (ISA). This property ensures that some degree of stimulation of beta receptors is maintained. Under conditions of rest, this tends to balance the negative chronotropic and negative inotropic effects. SECTRAL blocks the effects of excessive catecholamine stimulation resulting from stress.

5.2 Pharmacokinetic properties

After oral administration, acebutolol is rapidly and almost completely absorbed. Absorption appears to be unaffected by the presence of food in the gut. There is rapid formation of a major equiactive metabolite, diacetolol, which possesses a similar pharmacological profile to acebutolol. Peak plasma concentrations of active material (i.e. acebutolol plus diacetolol) are achieved within 2-4 hours and the terminal plasma elimination half-life is around 8-10 hours. Because of biliary excretion and direct transfer across the gut wall from the systemic circulation to the gut lumen, more than 50% of an oral dose of SECTRAL is recovered in the faeces with acebutolol and diacetolol in equal proportions; the rest of the dose is recovered in the urine, mainly as diacetolol. Both acebutolol and diacetolol are hydrophilic and exhibit poor penetration of the CNS.

5.3 Preclinical safety data

No particulars.

6. PHARMACEUTICAL PARTICULARS

6.1 List of excipients

Sectral capsules: Starch Potato, Silica colloidal anhydrous (E551), Magnesium Stearate (E572).

Sectral 100mg Capsule Shell:

Body: Yellow iron oxide (E172), Titanium dioxide (E171), Gelatin

Cap: Titanium dioxide (E171), Gelatin, Ink: Opacode S-1-8100 Black containing

Shellac, Iron oxide (E172), Lecithin, Antifoam DC 1501

Sectral 200mg Capsule Shell:

Body: Yellow iron oxide (E172), Titanium dioxide (E171), Gelatin

Cap: Titanium dioxide (E171), Gelatin, Red iron oxide (E172), Ink: Opacode S-1-8100 Black containing Shellac, Iron oxide (E172), Lecithin, Antifoam DC 1501.

6.2 Incompatibilities

Not applicable

6.3 Shelf life

The shelf-life of Sectral 100mg and 200mg capsules is 60 months.

6.4 Special precautions for storage

Store in a dry place below 25°C. Protect from light

6.5 Nature and contents of container

Sectral Capsules 100mg: Aluminium foil/UPVC blister strip packs of 84 tablets.

Sectral Capsules 200mg: Aluminium foil/UPVC blister strip packs of 56 tablets.

6.6 Special precautions for disposal and other handling

None

7. MARKETING AUTHORISATION HOLDER

Sanofi-aventis

One Onslow Street

Guildford

Surrey, GU1 4YS, UK

8. MARKETING AUTHORISATION NUMBER(S)

Sectral Capsules 100mg: PL 4425/0262

Sectral Capsules 200mg: PL 4425/0263

9. DATE OF FIRST AUTHORISATION/RENEWAL OF THE AUTHORISATION

13th July 2001

10. DATE OF REVISION OF THE TEXT

November 2006

LEGAL CLASSIFICATION

POM

Sectral 400mg tablets

(sanofi-aventis)

1. NAME OF THE MEDICINAL PRODUCT

SECTRAL TABLETS 400mg

2. QUALITATIVE AND QUANTITATIVE COMPOSITION

Acebutolol hydrochloride 443.40mg (equivalent to 400mg of base).

For a full list of excipients, see section 6.1.

3. PHARMACEUTICAL FORM

White to off-white, circular, biconvex, film-coated tablets with bevel edges, one face impressed SECTRAL 400 or ACB 400. Plain reverse.

4. CLINICAL PARTICULARS

4.1 Therapeutic indications

SECTRAL Tablets 400 mg Tablets are indicated for the following:

The management of hypertension, angina pectoris and the control of tachyarrhythmias.

4.2 Posology and method of administration

Hypertension: Initial dosage of 400mg orally once daily at breakfast or 200mg orally twice daily. If response is not adequate within two weeks, dosage may be increased up to 400mg orally twice daily; in some patients 1200mg orally daily, given as 800mg at breakfast and 400mg in the evening may be required. A further reduction in blood pressure may be obtained by the concurrent administration of a thiazide diuretic or other anti-hypertensive agent (except Rauwolfia and its alkaloids).

Angina pectoris: Initial dosage of 400mg orally once daily at breakfast or 200mg twice daily. In severe forms up to 300mg three times daily may be required. Up to 1200mg daily has been used.

Cardiac Arrhythmias: When given orally, an initial dose of 200mg is recommended. The daily dose requirement for long term anti arrhythmic activity should lie between 400 and 1200mg daily. The dose can be gauged by response, and better control may be achieved by divided doses rather than single doses. It may take up to three hours for maximal anti-arrhythmic effect to become apparent.

Elderly: There are no specific dosage recommendations for the elderly with normal glomerular filtration rate. Dose reduction is necessary if moderate to severe renal impairment is present (see Section 4.4)

Children: Paediatric dose has not been established.

For all indications, it is advised that the lowest recommended dosage be used initially.

4.3 Contraindications

Cardiogenic shock is an absolute contraindication. Extreme caution is required in patients with blood pressures of the order of 100/60 mmHg or below.

SECTRAL is also contraindicated in patients with second and third degree heart block, sick sinus syndrome, marked bradycardia (< 45 – 50 bpm) and uncontrolled heart failure, metabolic acidosis, severe peripheral circulatory disorders, hypersensitivity to Acebutolol, any of the excipients or to beta blockers, and untreated phaeochromocytoma.

4.4 Special warnings and precautions for use

Renal impairment is not contraindicated to the use of SECTRAL which has both renal and non-renal excretory pathways. Some caution should be exercised when administering high doses to patients with severe renal failure as accumulation could possibly occur in these circumstances.

The dosage frequency should not exceed once daily in patients with renal impairment. As a guide, the dosage should be reduced by 50% when glomerular filtration rates are between 25-50ml/min and by 75% when they are below 25ml/min (see section 4.2).

Drug-induced bronchospasm is usually at least partially reversible by the use of a suitable agonist.

Although cardio-selective beta blockers may have less effect on lung function than non-selective beta blockers as with all beta blockers these should be avoided in patients with obstructive airways disease unless there are compelling clinical reasons for their use. Where such reasons exist, cardio-selective β-blockers should be used with the utmost care. (from section 4.3)

Beta-blockers may induce bradycardia. In such cases, the dosage should be reduced. They may be used with patients with controlled heart failure. (see Section 4.3)

Use with caution in patients with Prinzmetal's angina.

Beta-blockers may aggravate peripheral circulatory disorders. They may mask signs of thyrotoxicosis and hypoglycaemia. They should only be used in patients with phaeochromocytoma with concomitant alpha-adrenoreceptor therapy.

Patients with known psoriasis should take beta-blockers only after careful consideration.

Beta-blockers may increase both the sensitivity towards allergens and the seriousness of anaphylactic reactions.

Withdrawal of treatment by beta-blockers should be achieved by gradual dosage reduction: this is especially important in patients with ischaemic heart disease.

When it has been decided to interrupt beta-blockade prior to surgery, therapy should be discontinued for at least 24 hours. Continuation of the therapy reduces the risk of arrhythmias but the risk of hypotension may be increased. If treatment is continued, caution should be observed with certain anaesthetic drugs. The patient may be protected against vagal reactions by intravenous administration of atropine

4.5 Interaction with other medicinal products and other forms of interaction

SECTRAL should not be used with Verapamil or within several days of Verapamil therapy (and vice versa). Use with great care with any other calcium antagonists, particularly Diltiazem

Class 1 anti-arrthythmic drugs (such as disopyramide) and amiodarone may increase atrial conduction time and induce negative inotropic effects when used concomitantly with beta-blockers.

In patients with labile and insulin-dependent diabetes, the dosage of the hypoglycaemic agent may need to be reduced. However beta-blockers have also been known to blunt the effect of glibenclamide. Beta-andrenergic blockade may also prevent the appearance of signs of hypoglycaemia (tachycardia, see section 4.4)

Cross reactions due to displacement of other drugs from plasma protein binding sites are unlikely due to the low degree of plasma protein binding exhibited by Acebutolol and Diacetolol.

If a beta-blocker is used concurrently with clonidine the latter should not be withdrawn until several days after the former is discontinued.

Acebutolol may antagonize the effect of sympathomimetic and xanthine bronchodilators.

Concurrent use of digoxin and beta-blockers may occasionally induce serious bradycardia. The anti-hypertensive effects of beta-blockers may be attenuated by non-steroidal anti-inflammatory agents.

Concomitant administration of tricyclic antidepressants, barbiturates and phenothiazines as well as other anti-hypertensive agents may increase the blood pressure lowering effects of beta-blockers.

There is a theoretical risk that concurrent administration of monoamine oxidase inhibitors and high doses of beta-blockers, even if they are cardio-selective can produce hypertension. SECTRAL therapy should be brought to the attention of the anaesthetist prior to general anaesthesia. (see Section 4.4). If treatment is continued, special care should be taken when using anaesthetic agents such as ether, cyclopropane and trichlorethylene.

4.6 Pregnancy and lactation

Pregnancy: As with all medicines, SECTRAL should not be given to female patients during the first trimester of pregnancy unless the physician considers it essential. In such cases the lowest possible dose should be used.

Beta-blockers administered in late pregnancy may give rise to bradycardia, hypoglycaemia and cardiac or pulmonary complications of the foetus/neonate.

Beta-blockers can reduce placental perfusion, which may result in intrauterine foetal death, immature and premature deliveries.

Animal studies have shown no teratogenic hazard.

Lactation: Acebutolol and its active metabolite are excreted in breast milk and the half-life of Acebutolol in the neonate is double that in adults. The risks of hypoglycaemia and bradycardia occurring in the nursing infant have not been evaluated. Therefore, breast-feeding is not recommended during treatment.

4.7 Effects on ability to drive and use machines

As with all beta-blockers, dizziness of fatigue may accur occasionally. This should be taken into account when driving or operating machinery.

4.8 Undesirable effects

SECTRAL possesses antihypertensive effects but these are unlikely to be noted in normotensive subjects. The side effects common to beta-blockade include bradycardia, heart failure, a slowing of AV conduction or increase of an existing AV block, hypotension, gastrointestinal effects (such as nausea, vomiting and diarrhoea), cold and cyanotic extremities, paraesthesia, Raynaud's syndrome, intermittent claudication, confusion dizziness, impaired vision, headaches, shortness of breath, nightmares, hallucinations, psychoses and depression, loss of libido and lethargy. The low lipid solubility and lack of cumulation in CNS tissues of Acebutolol and its active metabolite reduce the likelihood of sleep disturbances, depression or other central effects and such occurrences are rare.

Pulmonary infiltration and pneumonitis appear to be rare but potentially serious complications of beta-blockade therapy.

Cases of pneumonia have been reported with Acebutolol.

There have been reports of skin rashes and/or dry eyes associated with the use of beta-adrenoceptor blocking drugs. The reported incidence is small and in most cases the symptoms have cleared when treatment is withdrawn. Discontinuation of the drug should be considered in such cases. Cessation of therapy with beta-blocker should be gradual (see Section 4.4).

The exacerbation of psoriasis and psoriasiform skin reactions have been reported with beta-adrenoreceptor antagonists including acebutolol.

Although some patients have developed anti-nuclear factor titres, the incidence of associated clinical symptoms is rare and when present, these clear promptly on discontinuation of treatment. In rare cases, lupus-like syndrome have been reported.

Bronchospasm has occurred rarely during treatment with Acebutolol.

4.9 Overdose

In the event of excessive bradycardia or hypotension, 1mg atropine sulphate administered intravenously should be given without delay. If this is insufficient it should be followed by a slow intravenous injection of isoprenaline (5mcg per minute) with constant monitoring until a response occurs. In severe cases of self-poisoning with circulatory collapse unresponsive to atropine and catecholamines the intravenous injection of glucagon 10-20mg may produce a dramatic improvement. Cardiac pacing may be employed if bradycardia becomes severe.

Judicious use of vasopressors, diazepam, phenytoin, lidocaine, digoxin and bronchodilators should be considered depending on the presentation of the patient. Acebutolol can be removed from blood by haemodialysis. Other symptoms and signs of over dosage include cardiogenic shock, AV block, conduction defects, pulmonary oedema, depressed level of consciousness, bronchospasm, hypoglycaemia and rarely hyperkalaemia.

5. PHARMACOLOGICAL PROPERTIES

5.1 Pharmacodynamic properties

Mode of action: SECTRAL is a beta adrenoceptor antagonist which is cardio selective, i.e. acts preferentially on beta-1 adrenergic receptors in the heart. Its principal effects are to reduce heart rate especially on exercise and to lower blood pressure in hypertensive subjects. SECTRAL and its active metabolite, diacetolol have antiarrhythmic activity, the combined plasma half-life of the active drug and metabolite being 7-10 hours. Both have partial agonist activity (PAA) also known as intrinsic sympathomimetic activity (ISA). This property ensures that some degree of stimulation of beta-receptors is maintained. Under conditions of rest, this tends to balance the negative chronotropic and negative inotropic effects. SECTRAL blocks the effects of excessive catecholamine stimulation resulting from stress.

5.2 Pharmacokinetic properties

After oral administration, Acebutolol is rapidly and almost completely absorbed. Absorption appears to be unaffected by the presence of food in the gut. There is rapid formation of a major equiactive metabolite, diacetolol, which possesses a similar pharmacological profile to Acebutolol. Peak plasma concentrations of active material (i.e. Acebutolol plus diacetolol) are achieved within 2-4 hours and the terminal plasma elimination half-life is around 8-10 hours. Because of biliary excretion and direct transfer across the gut wall from the systemic circulation to the gut lumen, more than 50% of an oral dose of SECTRAL is recovered in the faeces with Acebutolol and diacetolol in equal proportions; the rest of the dose is recovered in the urine, mainly as diacetolol. Both Acebutolol and diacetolol are hydrophilic and exhibit poor penetration of the CNS.

5.3 Preclinical safety data

No particulars.

6. PHARMACEUTICAL PARTICULARS

6.1 List of excipients

Lactose monohydrate

Starch Maize

Talc (E553b)

Silica colloidal anhydrous (E551)

Povidone K30

Magnesium Stearate (E572)

Tablet coat:

Opadry OY-L-28900 containing

Titanium dioxide (E171)

Lactose monohydrate

Hypromellose (E464)

Macrogol

6.2 Incompatibilities

Not applicable

6.3 Shelf life

The shelf-life of SECTRAL Tablets 400mg is 36 months

6.4 Special precautions for storage

None

6.5 Nature and contents of container

SECTRAL is packed in aluminium foil/PVC blister strip packs of 28 tablets

6.6 Special precautions for disposal and other handling

None

7. MARKETING AUTHORISATION HOLDER

Sanofi-aventis

One Onslow Street

Guildford

Surrey, GU1 4YS, UK

8. MARKETING AUTHORISATION NUMBER(S)

PL 4425/0264

9. DATE OF FIRST AUTHORISATION/RENEWAL OF THE AUTHORISATION

13th July 2001

10. DATE OF REVISION OF THE TEXT

16 February 2007

LEGAL CLASSIFICATION

POM

Securon I.V.

(Abbott Laboratories Limited)

1. NAME OF THE MEDICINAL PRODUCT

Securon IV

2. QUALITATIVE AND QUANTITATIVE COMPOSITION

Verapamil Hydrochloride BP 2.5 mg/ml

3. PHARMACEUTICAL FORM

Aqueous solution for intravenous injection.

4. CLINICAL PARTICULARS

4.1 Therapeutic indications

Securon IV is indicated for the treatment of paroxysmal supraventricular tachycardia and the reduction of ventricular rate in atrial flutter/fibrillation.

4.2 Posology and method of administration

For slow intravenous injection.

Adults: 5-10 mg by slow intravenous injection over a period of 2 minutes. The patient should be observed continuously, preferably under ECG and blood pressure control. If necessary, *e.g.* in paroxysmal tachycardia, a further 5 mg may be given after 5 to 10 minutes.

Children: Securon IV must always be administered under ECG monitoring in young patients.

0-1 year: 0.1-0.2 mg/kg bodyweight (usual single dose range: 0.75-2 mg).

1-15 years: 0.1-0.3 mg/kg bodyweight (usual single dose range: 2-5 mg).

The dose may be repeated after 30 minutes if necessary. Many cases are controlled by doses at the lower end of the range. The injection should be stopped at the onset of the desired effect.

Elderly: The dosage should be administered over 3 minutes to minimise the risk of adverse effects.

Dosage in impaired liver and renal function: Significant hepatic and renal impairment should not increase the effects of a single intravenous dose but may prolong its duration of action.

For use with beta-blocker therapy, see 'Contra-indications' and 'Special Warnings and Precautions for Use'.

4.3 Contraindications

Hypersensitivity to the active substance or to any of the excipients.

Cardiogenic shock; acute myocardial infarction complicated by bradycardia, marked hypotension or left ventricular failure; second or third degree AV block (except in patients with a functioning artificial ventricular pacemaker); sino-atrial block; sick sinus syndrome (except in patients with a functioning artificial ventricular pacemaker); uncompensated heart failure; bradycardia of less than 50 beats/minute; hypotension of less than 90 mmHg systolic; simultaneous administration of intravenous beta-blockers.

Patients with atrial flutter/fibrillation in the presence of an accessory pathway (*e.g.* WPW syndrome) may develop increased conduction across the anomalous pathway and ventricular tachycardia may be precipitated.

4.4 Special warnings and precautions for use

Verapamil may affect impulse conduction. For this reason, Securon IV should be used with caution in patients with bradycardia or first degree AV block. Verapamil may affect left ventricular contractility; this effect is small and normally not important but cardiac failure may be precipitated or aggravated. In patients with poor ventricular function, therefore, Securon IV should only be given after cardiac failure has been controlled with appropriate therapy, *e.g.* digitalis.

Caution should be exercised in treatment with HMG CoA reductase inhibitors (e.g., simvastatin, atorvastatin or lovastatin) for patients taking verapamil. These patients should be started at the lowest possible dose of verapamil and titrated upwards. If verapamil treatment is to be added to patients already taking an HMG CoA reductase inhibitor (e.g., simvastatin, atorvastatin or lovastatin), refer to advice in the respective statin product information.

4.5 Interaction with other medicinal products and other forms of interaction

In rare instances, including when patients with severe cardiomyopathy, congestive heart failure or recent myocardial infarction were given intravenous beta-adrenergic blocking agents or disopyramide concomitantly with intravenous verapamil hydrochloride, serious adverse effects have occurred. Concomitant use of verapamil hydrochloride with agents that decrease adrenergic function may result in an exaggerated hypotensive response.

In vitro metabolic studies indicate that verapamil hydrochloride is metabolized by cytochrome P450 CYP3A4, CYP1A2, CYP2C8, CYP2C9 and CYP2C18. Verapamil has been shown to be an inhibitor of CYP3A4 enzymes and P-glycoprotein (P-gp). Clinically significant interactions have been reported with inhibitors of CYP3A4 causing elevation of plasma levels of verapamil hydrochloride while inducers of CYP3A4 have caused a lowering of plasma levels of verapamil hydrochloride, therefore, patients should be monitored for drug interactions.

The following are potential drug interactions associated with verapamil:

Acetylsalicylic acid

Concomitant use of verapamil with aspirin may increase the risk of bleeding

Alpha blockers

Verapamil may increase the plasma concentrations of *prazosin* and *terazosin* which may have an additive hypotensive effect.

Antiarrhythmics

Verapamil may slightly decrease the plasma clearance of *flecainide* whereas *flecainide* has no effect on the verapamil plasma clearance.

Verapamil may increase the plasma concentrations of *quinidine*.

The combination of verapamil and *antiarrhythmic agents* may lead to additive cardiovascular effects (e.g. AV block, bradycardia, hypotension, heart failure). Care must be exercised if Securon IV is combined with anti-arrhythmic agents by any route.

Anticonvulsants

Verapamil may increase the plasma concentrations of *carbamazepine*. This may produce side effects such as diplopia, headache, ataxia or dizziness. Verapamil may also increase the plasma concentrations of *phenytoin*.

Antidepressants

Verapamil may increase the plasma concentrations of *imipramine*.

Antidiabetics

Verapamil may increase the plasma concentrations of *glibenclamide (glyburide)*.

Anti-infectives

Rifampicin may reduce the plasma concentrations of verapamil which may produce a redcued blood pressure lowering effect. *Erythromycin* and *telithromycin* may increase the plasma concentrations of verapamil.

Antineoplastics

There is no significant difference between the pharmacokinetic parameters of *doxorubicin* with intravenous verapamil administration.

Barbiturates

Phenobarbital may reduce the plasma concentrations of verapamil.

Benzodiazepines and other anxiolytics

Verapamil may increase the plasma concentrations of *buspirone* and *midazolam*.

Beta blockers

Verapamil may increase the plasma concentrations of *metoprolol* and *propranolol* which may lead to additive cardiovascular effects (e.g. AV block, bradycardia, hypotension, heart failure).

Securon IV should not be given in combination with intravenous *beta-blocker* therapy and care must be exercised if Securon IV is combined with oral *beta-blocker* therapy.

Cardiac glycosides

Verapamil may increase the plasma concentrations of *digitoxin* and *digoxin*. Verapamil has been shown to increase the serum concentration of *digoxin* and caution should be exercised with regard to digitalis toxicity. The digitalis level should be determined and the glycoside dose reduced, if required.

Colchicine

Colchicine is a substrate for both CYP3A and the efflux transporter, P-glycoprotein (P-gp). Verapamil is known to inhibit CYP3A and P-gp. When verapamil and *colchicine* are administered together, inhibition of P-gp and/or CYP3A by verapamil may lead to increased exposure to *colchicine*. Combined use is not recommended.

H_2 Receptor antagonists

Cimetidine may increase the plasma concentrations of verapamil following intravenous verapamil administration.

HIV antiviral agents

Due to the metabolic inhibitory potential of some of the *HIV antiviral agents*, such as *ritonavir*, plasma concentrations of verapamil may increase. Caution should be used or dose of verapamil may be decreased.

Immunosuppressants

Verapamil may increase the plasma concentrations of *ciclosporin, everolimus, sirolimus* and *tacrolimus*.

Inhaled anaesthetics

When used concomitantly, *inhalation anaesthetics* and calcium antagonists, such as verapamil hydrochloride, should each be titrated carefully to avoid additive cardiovascular effects (e.g. AV block, bradycardia, hypotension, heart failure).

Lipid lowering agents

Verapamil may increase the plasma concentrations *atorvastatin, lovastatin* and *simvastatin*.

Treatment with *HMG CoA reductase inhibitors* (e.g., *simvastatin, atorvastatin* or *lovastatin*) in a patient taking verapamil should be started at the lowest possible dose and titrated upwards. If verapamil treatment is to be added to patients already taking an *HMG CoA reductase inhibitor* (e.g., *simvastatin, atorvastatin* or *lovastatin*), consider a reduction in the statin dose and retitrate against serum cholesterol concentrations.

Atorvastatin may increase verapamil levels. Although there is no direct in vivo clinical evidence, there is strong potential for verapamil to significantly affect *atorvastatin* pharmacokinetics in a similar manner to *simvastatin* or *lovastatin*. Consider using caution when *atorvastatin* and verapamil are concomitantly administered.

Fluvastatin, pravastatin and *rosuvastatin* are not metabolized by CYP3A4 and are less likely to interact with verapamil.

Lithium

Serum levels of *lithium* may be reduced. However there may be increased sensitivity to *lithium* causing enhanced neurotoxicity.

Neuromuscular blocking agents employed in anaesthesia

The effects may be potentiated.

Protein-bound drugs

As verapamil hydrochloride is highly bound to plasma proteins, it should be administered with caution to patients receiving other highly *protein-bound drugs*.

Serotonin receptor agonists

Verapamil may increase the plasma concentrations of *almotriptan*.

Theophylline

Verapamil may increase the plasma concentrations of *theophylline*.

Uricosurics

Sulfinpyrazone may reduce the plasma concentrations of verapamil which may produce a reduced blood pressure lowering effect.

Other

St. John's Wort may reduce the plasma concentrations of verapamil, whereas *grapefruit juice* may increase the plasma concentrations of verapamil.

4.6 Pregnancy and lactation

Although animal studies have not shown any teratogenic effects, verapamil should not be given during the first trimester of pregnancy unless, in the clinician's judgement, it is essential for the welfare of the patient.

Verapamil is excreted into the breast milk in small amounts and is unlikely to be harmful. However, rare hypersensitivity reactions have been reported with verapamil. For this reason, it should only be used during lactation if, in the clinician's judgement, it is essential for the welfare of the patient.

4.7 Effects on ability to drive and use machines

None stated.

4.8 Undesirable effects

Adverse events observed in clinical trials are depicted in the following table. Within each system organ class, the adverse drug reactions are ranked under headings of frequency, using the following convention: common (>1/100, <1/10), uncommon (>1/1,000, <1/100), rare (>1/10,000, <1/1,000), very rare (<1/10,000), including isolated reports.

System Organ Class	Frequency	Undesirable Effects
Nervous system disorders	common	- dizziness - headache
Cardiac disorders/ vascular disorders	common	- bradycardia - hypotension
	uncommon	- tachycardia
Gastrointestinal disorders	uncommon	- nausea - abdominal pain

Cases of seizures during verapamil hydrochloride injection have been reported.

In rare cases of hypersensitivity, bronchospasm accompanied by pruritis and urticaria has been reported.

Other Reactions from Postmarketing Surveillance or Phase IV Clinical Trials

Other adverse events reported with verapamil are listed below by system organ class:

Psychiatric disorders: on rare occasions, nervousness has been reported.

Nervous system disorders: somnolence and extrapyramidal syndrome.

Ear and labyrinth disorders: vertigo.

Cardiac disorders/vascular disorders: decreased myocardial contractility has been reported. On rare occasions, 2nd and 3rd block may occur and in extreme cases, this may lead to asystole. The asystole is usually of short duration and cardiac action returns spontaneously after a few seconds, usually in the form of sinus rhythm. If necessary, the procedures for the treatment of overdosage should be followed as described below. On rare occasions, flushing has been reported.

Gastrointestinal disorders: gingival hyperplasia may occur very rarely when the drug is administered over prolonged periods, and is fully reversible when the drug is discontinued. On rare occasions, vomiting has also been reported.

Skin and subcutaneous tissue disorders: Steven-Johnson syndrome, erythema and hyperhidrosis.

Reproductive system and breast disorders: On very rare occasions, gynaecomastia has been observed in elderly male patients under long-term verapamil treatment; this was fully reversible in all cases when the drug was discontinued.

Investigations: A reversible impairment of liver function characterized by an increase of transaminase and/or alkaline phosphatase may occur on very rare occasions during verapamil treatment and is most probably a hypersensitivity reaction.

4.9 Overdose

The symptoms of overdosage include hypotension, shock, loss of consciousness, first and second degree AV block (frequently as Wenckebach's phenomenon with or without escape rhythms), total AV block with total AV dissociation, escape rhythm, asystole, bradycardia up to high degree AV block and, sinus arrest, hyperglycaemia, stupor and metabolic acidosis. Fatalities have occurred as a result of overdose.

Treatment of overdosage depends on the type and severity of symptoms. The specific antidote is calcium, *e.g.* 10-20 ml of 10% calcium gluconate solution i.v. (2.25-4.5 mmol) if necessary by repeated injection or continuous infusion (*e.g.* 5 mmol/hour). The usual emergency measures for acute cardiovascular collapse should be applied and followed by intensive care. Verapamil hydrochloride cannot be removed by haemodialysis. Similarly, in the case of second or third degree AV block, atropine, orciprenaline, isoprenaline and if required, pacemaker therapy should be considered. If there are signs of myocardial insufficiency, dopamine, dobutamine, cardiac glycosides or calcium gluconate (10-20 ml of a 10% solution) can be administered.

In the case of hypotension, after appropriately positioning the patient, dopamine, dobutamine or noradrenaline may be given.

5. PHARMACOLOGICAL PROPERTIES

5.1 Pharmacodynamic properties

Verapamil is a calcium antagonist which blocks the inward movement of calcium ions in cardiac muscle cells, in smooth muscle cells of the coronary and systemic arteries and in cells of the intracardiac conduction system. Because of its effect on the movement of calcium in the intracardiac conduction system, verapamil reduces automaticity, decreases conduction velocity and increases the refractory period.

5.2 Pharmacokinetic properties

Following intravenous infusion in man, verapamil is eliminated bi-exponentially with a rapid distribution phase (half-life about 4 minutes) and a slower terminal elimination phase (half-life 2-5 hours). Plasma protein binding of verapamil is about 90%. Renal insufficiency does not affect the kinetics of verapamil. In patients with liver cirrhosis, elimination half-life is prolonged.

5.3 Preclinical safety data

Not applicable.

6. PHARMACEUTICAL PARTICULARS

6.1 List of excipients

Water for injections, sodium chloride (8.5 mg/ml), hydrochloric acid as pH adjuster.

6.2 Incompatibilities

Securon IV is incompatible with alkaline solutions.

6.3 Shelf life

Ampoule: 60 months.

Syringe: 36 months.

6.4 Special precautions for storage

Store at room temperature. Protect from light.

6.5 Nature and contents of container

2 ml glass ampoule (hydrolytic type 1) containing 5 mg verapamil. Pack size:

5 × 2 ml ampoules.

2 ml pre-filled glass syringe (borosilicate type 1) with tip cap and butyl rubber stopper and polystyrene plunger. Pack size: 5 × 2 ml syringes.

6.6 Special precautions for disposal and other handling

None.

7. MARKETING AUTHORISATION HOLDER

Abbott Laboratories Ltd

Queenborough

Kent

ME11 5EL

United Kingdom

8. MARKETING AUTHORISATION NUMBER(S)

PL 00037/0367

9. DATE OF FIRST AUTHORISATION/RENEWAL OF THE AUTHORISATION

17 June 2003

10. DATE OF REVISION OF THE TEXT

02nd April 2009

Securon SR

(Abbott Laboratories Limited)

1. NAME OF THE MEDICINAL PRODUCT

Securon SR

2. QUALITATIVE AND QUANTITATIVE COMPOSITION

Verapamil Hydrochloride Ph Eur – 240 mg

3. PHARMACEUTICAL FORM

Modified-release tablets.

The tablets are oblong, pale green, scored and embossed with two Knoll logos (triangles) on one side.

4. CLINICAL PARTICULARS

4.1 Therapeutic indications

Securon SR is indicated for:

The treatment of mild to moderate hypertension.

The treatment and prophylaxis of angina pectoris.

Secondary prevention of reinfarction after an acute myocardial infarction in patients without heart failure, and not receiving diuretics (apart from low-dose diuretics when used for indications other than heart failure), and where beta-blockers are not appropriate. Treatment is to be started at least one week after an acute myocardial infarction.

4.2 Posology and method of administration

Securon SR tablets should not be chewed. Securon SR tablets are scored and may be halved without damaging the modified-release formulation.

Adults

Hypertension: One tablet of Securon SR daily. For patients new to verapamil therapy, the physician should consider halving the initial dose to 120 mg (one tablet Half Securon SR). Most patients respond to 240 mg daily (one tablet Securon SR) given as a single dose. If control is not achieved after a period of at least one week, the dosage may be increased to a maximum of two Securon SR tablets daily (one in the morning and one in the evening at an interval of about twelve hours). A further reduction in blood pressure may be achieved by combining Securon SR with other antihypertensive agents, in particular diuretics. Half Securon SR may be used for dose titration purposes.

Angina pectoris: One tablet of Securon SR twice daily. A small number of patients respond to a lower dose and where indicated, adjustment down to one tablet of Securon SR daily could be made. Half Securon SR may be used for dose titration purposes.

Secondary prevention of reinfarction after an acute myocardial infarction in patients without heart failure, and not receiving diuretics (apart from low-dose diuretics when used for indications other than heart failure), and where beta-blockers are not appropriate: Treatment is to be started at least one week after an acute myocardial infarction. 360 mg/day in divided doses, to be taken either as one Half Securon SR (120 mg) tablet three times daily, or as one Securon SR (240 mg) tablet in the morning and one Half Securon SR (120 mg) tablet in the evening, on a daily basis.

Elderly patients

The adult dose is recommended unless renal or hepatic function is impaired (see Section 4.4, 'Special Warnings and Precautions for Use').

Children

Securon SR and Half Securon SR are not recommended for children.

4.3 Contraindications

Hypersensitivity to the active substance or to any of the excipients.

Cardiogenic shock; acute myocardial infarction complicated by bradycardia, marked hypotension or left ventricular failure; second or third degree atrioventricular (AV) block (except in patients with a functioning artificial pacemaker); sino-atrial block; sick sinus syndrome (except in patients with a functioning artificial pacemaker); uncompensated heart failure; bradycardia of less than 50 beats/minute; hypotension of less than 90 mmHg systolic.

Patients with atrial flutter/fibrillation in the presence of an accessory pathway (*e.g.* WPW syndrome) may develop increased conduction across the anomalous pathway and ventricular tachycardia may be precipitated.

4.4 Special warnings and precautions for use

Since verapamil is extensively metabolised in the liver, careful dose titration is required in patients with liver disease. The disposition of verapamil in patients with renal impairment has not been fully established and therefore careful patient monitoring is recommended. Verapamil is not removed during dialysis.

Verapamil may affect impulse conduction and should therefore be used with caution in patients with bradycardia or first degree AV block. Verapamil may affect left ventricular contractility; this effect is small and normally not important but cardiac failure may be precipitated or aggravated. In patients with incipient cardiac failure, therefore, verapamil should be given only after such cardiac failure has been controlled with appropriate therapy, e.g. digitalis.

When treating hypertension with verapamil, monitoring of the patient's blood pressure at regular intervals is required.

Caution should be exercised in treatment with HMG CoA reductase inhibitors (e.g., simvastatin, atorvastatin or lovastatin) for patients taking verapamil. These patients should be started at the lowest possible dose of verapamil and titrated upwards. If verapamil treatment is to be added to patients already taking an HMG CoA reductase inhibitor (e.g., simvastatin, atorvastatin or lovastatin), refer to advice in the respective statin product information.

4.5 Interaction with other medicinal products and other forms of interaction

In vitro metabolic studies indicate that verapamil hydrochloride is metabolized by cytochrome P450 CYP3A4, CYP1A2, CYP2C8, CYP2C9 and CYP2C18. Verapamil has been shown to be an inhibitor of CYP3A4 enzymes and P-glycoprotein (P-gp). Clinically significant interactions have been reported with inhibitors of CYP3A4 causing elevation of plasma levels of verapamil hydrochloride while inducers of CYP3A4 have caused a lowering of plasma levels of verapamil hydrochloride, therefore, patients should be monitored for drug interactions.

The following are potential drug interactions associated with verapamil:

Acetylsalicylic acid

Concomitant use of verapamil with aspirin may increase the risk of bleeding

Alcohol

Increase in blood *alcohol* has been reported.

Alpha blockers

Verapamil may increase the plasma concentrations of *prazosin* and *terazosin* which may have an additive hypotensive effect.

Antiarrhythmics

Verapamil may slightly decrease the plasma clearance of *flecainide* whereas *flecainide* has no effect on the verapamil plasma clearance.

Verapamil may increase the plasma concentrations of *quinidine*. Pulmonary oedema may occur in patients with hypertrophic cardiomyopathy

The combination of verapamil and *antiarrhythmic agents* may lead to additive cardiovascular effects (e.g. AV block, bradycardia, hypotension, heart failure).

Anticonvulsants

Verapamil may increase the plasma concentrations of *carbamazepine*. This may produce side effects such as diplopia, headache, ataxia or dizziness. Verapamil may also increase the plasma concentrations of *phenytoin*.

Antidepressants

Verapamil may increase the plasma concentrations of *imipramine*.

Antidiabetics

Verapamil may increase the plasma concentrations of *glibenclamide (glyburide)*.

Antihypertensives, diuretics, vasodilators

Potentiation of the hypotensive effect.

Anti-infectives

Rifampicin may reduce the plasma concentrations of verapamil which may produce a reduced blood pressure lowering effect. *Erythromycin* and *telithromycin* may increase the plasma concentrations of verapamil.

Antineoplastics

Verapamil may increase the plasma concentrations of *doxorubicin*.

Barbiturates

Phenobarbital may reduce the plasma concentrations of verapamil.

Benzodiazepines and other anxiolytics

Verapamil may increase the plasma concentrations of *buspirone* and *midazolam*.

Beta blockers

Verapamil may increase the plasma concentrations of *metoprolol* and *propranolol* which may lead to additive cardiovascular effects (e.g. AV block, bradycardia, hypotension, heart failure).

Intravenous *beta-blockers* should not be given to patients under treatment with verapamil.

Cardiac glycosides

Verapamil may increase the plasma concentrations of *digitoxin* and *digoxin*. Verapamil has been shown to increase the serum concentration of *digoxin* and caution should be exercised with regard to digitalis toxicity. The digitalis level should be determined and the glycoside dose reduced, if required.

Colchicine

Colchicine is a substrate for both CYP3A and the efflux transporter, P-glycoprotein (P-gp). Verapamil is known to inhibit CYP3A and P-gp. When verapamil and *colchicine* are administered together, inhibition of P-gp and/or CYP3A by verapamil may lead to increased exposure to *colchicine*. Combined use is not recommended.

H_2 Receptor antagonists

Cimetidine may increase the plasma concentrations of verapamil.

HIV antiviral agents

Due to the metabolic inhibitory potential of some of the *HIV antiviral agents*, such as *ritonavir*, plasma concentrations of verapamil may increase. Caution should be used or dose of verapamil may be decreased.

Immunosuppressants

Verapamil may increase the plasma concentrations of *ciclosporin, everolimus, sirolimus* and *tacrolimus*.

Inhaled anaesthetics

When used concomitantly, *inhalation anaesthetics* and calcium antagonists, such as verapamil hydrochloride, should each be titrated carefully to avoid additive cardiovascular effects (e.g. AV block, bradycardia, hypotension, heart failure).

Lipid lowering agents

Verapamil may increase the plasma concentrations *atorvastatin, lovastatin* and *simvastatin.*

Treatment with HMG *CoA reductase inhibitors* (e.g., *simvastatin, atorvastatin* or *lovastatin*) in a patient taking verapamil should be started at the lowest possible dose and titrated upwards. If verapamil treatment is to be added to patients already taking an *HMG CoA reductase inhibitor* (e.g., *simvastatin, atorvastatin* or *lovastatin*), consider a reduction in the statin dose and retitrate against serum cholesterol concentrations.

Atorvastatin may increase verapamil levels. Although there is no direct in vivo clinical evidence, there is strong potential for verapamil to significantly affect *atorvastatin* pharmacokinetics in a similar manner to *simvastatin* or *lovastatin.* Consider using caution when *atorvastatin* and verapamil are concomitantly administered.

Fluvastatin, pravastatin and *rosuvastatin* are not metabolized by CYP3A4 and are less likely to interact with verapamil.

Lithium

Serum levels of *lithium* may be reduced. However, there may be increased sensitivity to *lithium* causing enhanced neurotoxicity.

Neuromuscular blocking agents employed in anaesthesia

The effects may be potentiated.

Serotonin receptor agonists

Verapamil may increase the plasma concentrations of *almotriptan*.

Theophylline

Verapamil may increase the plasma concentrations of *theophylline*.

Uricosurics

Sulfinpyrazone may reduce the plasma concentrations of verapamil which may produce a reduced blood pressure lowering effect.

Other

St. John's Wort may reduce the plasma concentrations of verapamil, whereas *grapefruit juice* may increase the plasma concentrations of verapamil.

4.6 Pregnancy and lactation

Although animal studies have not shown any teratogenic effects, verapamil should not be given during the first trimester of pregnancy unless, in the clinician's judgement, it is essential for the welfare of the patient.

Verapamil is excreted into the breast milk in small amounts and is unlikely to be harmful. However, rare hypersensitivity reactions have been reported with verapamil and therefore it should only be used during lactation if, in the clinician's judgement, it is essential for the welfare of the patient.

4.7 Effects on ability to drive and use machines

Depending on individual susceptibility, the patient's ability to drive a vehicle, operate machinery or work under hazardous conditions may be impaired. This is particularly true in the initial stages of treatment, when changing over from another drug or when the dose is raised. Like many other common medicines, verapamil has been shown to increase the blood levels of alcohol and slow its elimination. Therefore, the effects of alcohol may be exaggerated.

4.8 Undesirable effects

Reactions from Postmarketing Surveillance or Phase IV Clinical Trials

The following adverse events reported with verapamil are listed below by system organ class:

Immune system disorders: allergic reactions (e.g. erythema, pruritus, urticaria) are very rarely seen.

Nervous system disorders: headache, dizziness, paresthesia, tremor and extrapyramidal syndrome.

Ear and labyrinth disorders: vertigo and tinnitus.

Cardiac disorders/vascular disorders: bradycardic arrhythmias such as sinus bradycardia, sinus arrest with asystole, 2nd and 3rd degree AV block, bradyarrhythmia in atrial fibrillation, peripheral oedema, palpitations, tachycardia, development or aggravation of heart failure and hypotension. There have been rare reports of flushing.

Gastrointestinal disorders: nausea, vomiting, constipation, ileus and abdominal pain/discomfort. Gingival hyperplasia may occur very rarely when the drug is administered over prolonged periods, and is fully reversible when the drug is discontinued.

Skin and subcutaneous tissue disorders: ankle oedema, Quincke's oedema, Steven-Johnson syndrome, erythema multiforme, erythromelalgia, alopecia and purpura.

Musculoskeletal and connective tissue disorders: muscular weakness, myalgia and arthralgia.

Reproductive system and breast disorders: impotence (erectile dysfunction) has been rarely reported and isolated cases of galactorrhoea. On very rare occasions, gynaecomastia has been observed in elderly male patients under long-term verapamil treatment, and is fully reversible in all cases when the drug was discontinued.

General disorders and administration site conditions: fatigue.

Investigations: A reversible impairment of liver function characterized by an increase of transaminase and/or alkaline phosphatase may occur on very rare occasions during verapamil treatment and is most probably a hypersensitivity reaction. Rises in blood prolactin levels have been reported.

4.9 Overdose

The course of symptoms in verapamil intoxication depends on the amount taken, the point in time at which detoxification measures are taken and myocardial contractility (age-related). The main symptoms are as follows: blood pressure fall (at times to values not detectable), shock symptoms, loss of consciousness, 1st and 2nd degree AV block (frequently as Wenckebach's phenomenon with or without escape rhythms), total AV block with total AV dissociation, escape rhythm, asystole, bradycardia up to high degree AV block and, sinus arrest, hyperglycaemia, stupor and metabolic acidosis. Fatalities have occurred as a result of overdose.

The therapeutic measures to be taken depend on the point in time at which verapamil was taken and the type and severity of intoxication symptoms. In intoxications with large amounts of slow-release preparations (Securon SR and Half Securon SR), it should be noted that the release of the active drug and the absorption in the intestine may take more than 48 hours. Verapamil hydrochloride cannot be removed by haemodialysis. Depending on the time of ingestion, it should be taken into account that there may be some lumps of incompletely dissolved tablets along the entire length of the gastrointestinal tract, which function as active drug depots.

General measures to be taken: Gastric lavage with the usual precautions, even later than 12 hours after ingestion, if no gastrointestinal motility (peristaltic sounds) is detectable. Where intoxication by Securon SR or Half Securon SR is suspected, extensive elimination measures are indicated, such as induced vomiting, removal of the contents of the stomach and the small intestine under endoscopy, intestinal lavage, laxative, high enemas. The usual intensive resuscitation measures apply, such as extrathoracic heart massage, respiration, defibrillation and/or pacemaker therapy.

Specific measures to be taken: Elimination of cardiodepressive effects, hypotension or bradycardia. The specific antidote is calcium, e.g. 10 -20 ml of a 10% calcium gluconate solution administered intravenously (2.25 - 4.5 mmol), repeated if necessary or given as a continuous drip infusion (e.g. 5 mmol/hour).

The following measures may also be necessary: In case of 2nd or 3rd degree AV block, sinus bradycardia, asystole - atropine, isoprenaline, orciprenaline or pacemaker therapy. In case of hypotension - dopamine, dobutamine, noradrenaline. If there are signs of continuing myocardial failure - dopamine, dobutamine, if necessary repeated calcium injections.

5. PHARMACOLOGICAL PROPERTIES

5.1 Pharmacodynamic properties

Verapamil, a phenylalkylamine calcium antagonist, has a balanced profile of cardiac and peripheral effects. It lowers heart rate, increases myocardial perfusion and reduces coronary spasm. In a clinical study in patients after myocardial infarction, verapamil reduced total mortality, sudden cardiac death and reinfarction rate.

Verapamil reduces total peripheral resistance and lowers high blood pressure by vasodilation, without reflex tachycardia. Because of its use-dependent action on the voltage-operated calcium channel, the effects of verapamil are more pronounced on high than on normal blood pressure.

As early as day one of treatment, blood pressure falls; the effect is found to persist also in long-term therapy. Verapamil is suitable for the treatment of all types of hypertension: for monotherapy in mild to moderate hypertension; combined with other antihypertensives (in particular with diuretics and, according to more recent findings, with ACE inhibitors) in more severe types of hypertension. In hypertensive diabetic patients with nephropathy, verapamil in combination with ACE inhibitors led to a marked reduction of albuminuria and to an improvement of creatinine clearance.

5.2 Pharmacokinetic properties

Absorption: More than 90% of an orally-administered dose of verapamil is absorbed. Due to an intensive hepatic first-pass metabolism, the absolute bioavailability is about 22% with a variability of about 10 - 35%. Under multiple dosing, bioavailability increases by about 30%. Bioavailability is not affected by food consumption.

Distribution, biotransformation and elimination: Plasma concentrations reach their peak 4 - 8 hours after drug intake. Plasma protein binding of verapamil is about 90%. The elimination half-life is about 5 - 8 hours. The mean residence time of modified-release verapamil is 13 hours. After repeated single daily doses, steady-state conditions are reached between 3 - 4 days.

Within 5 days, approximately 70% of an orally-administered dose is excreted in the urine and about 16% with the faeces. Only 3 - 4 % is eliminated renally as unchanged drug. The drug is extensively metabolized. A number of metabolites are generated in humans (twelve have been identified). Of these metabolites only norverapamil has any appreciable pharmacological effect (approximately 20% that of the parent compound, which was observed in a study with dogs). Norverapamil represents about 6% of the dose eliminated in urine. Norverapamil can reach steady-state plasma concentrations approximately equal to those of verapamil itself. Renal insufficiency does not affect the kinetics of verapamil.

At-risk patients: In patients with liver cirrhosis, bioavailability is increased and elimination half-life is prolonged. In patients with compensated hepatic insufficiency, no influence on the kinetics of verapamil was observed.

5.3 Preclinical safety data

None stated.

6. PHARMACEUTICAL PARTICULARS

6.1 List of excipients

Microcrystalline cellulose, sodium alginate, povidone, magnesium stearate, purified water, hydroxypropyl methylcellulose, polyethylene glycol 400, polyethylene glycol 6000, talc, titanium dioxide (E171), l-green lake [quinoline yellow (E104) and indigo carmine (E132)], montan glycol wax.

6.2 Incompatibilities

None stated.

6.3 Shelf life

5 years.

6.4 Special precautions for storage

Do not store above 25°C and store in the original package – blister pack.

Do not store above 25°C and keep the container tightly closed – bottle pack.

6.5 Nature and contents of container

Calendar pack consisting of a PVC/PVDC blister in a cardboard outer container. Pack size: 28 tablets.

Polypropylene bottle with polyethylene stopper. Pack size: 100 tablets.

6.6 Special precautions for disposal and other handling

There are no specific instructions for use/handling. The tablets should not be chewed, but may be halved without affecting the modified-release form.

7. MARKETING AUTHORISATION HOLDER

Abbott Laboratories Limited

Queenborough

Kent

ME11 5EL

United Kingdom

8. MARKETING AUTHORISATION NUMBER(S)

PL 00037/0369

9. DATE OF FIRST AUTHORISATION/RENEWAL OF THE AUTHORISATION

14 March 2002

10. DATE OF REVISION OF THE TEXT

02nd April 2009

Selexid Tablets

(Leo Laboratories Limited)

1. NAME OF THE MEDICINAL PRODUCT

Selexid® Tablets.

2. QUALITATIVE AND QUANTITATIVE COMPOSITION

Pivmecillinam hydrochloride 200mg

3. PHARMACEUTICAL FORM

Tablets.

4. CLINICAL PARTICULARS

4.1 Therapeutic indications

Treatment of infections due to mecillinam sensitive organisms, including:

- urinary tract infections
- salmonellosis

Preliminary experience in a small number of patients suggests that Selexid® Tablets may be a useful alternative antibiotic in the treatment of acute typhoid fever and in some carriers of salmonellae when antibiotic treatment is considered essential.

4.2 Posology and method of administration

Route of administration is oral. The tablets must be taken with at least half a glass of water and preferably taken with or immediately after a meal.

Adults and children weighing more than 40 kg:

Urinary tract infections:

- acute uncomplicated cystitis: 72 hour course of 2 tablets immediately followed by 1 tablet 3 times daily to a total of 10 tablets.
- Chronic or recurrent bacteriuria: 2 tablets 3 to 4 times daily.

Salmonellosis:

- Enteric fever: 1.2 - 2.4g daily for 14 days.
- Salmonella carriers: 1.2 - 2.4 g daily for 2-4 weeks.

Children weighing less than 40 kg:

- Urinary tract infections: 20-40 mg/kg body weight, daily, in 3 to 4 divided doses.
- Salmonellosis: 30-60 mg/kg body weight, daily, in 3 to 4 divided doses.

Dosage in the elderly:

Renal excretion of mecillinam is delayed in the elderly, but significant accumulation of the drug is not likely at the recommended adult dosage of Selexid® Tablets.

4.3 Contraindications

Selexid® Tablets are contra-indicated in patients with:

- Hypersensitivity to the drug substance or any of the other ingredients.
- Hypersensitivity to penicillins and/or cephalosporins
- Oesophageal strictures and/or obstructive changes in the gastrointestinal tract.
- A predisposition to carnitine deficiency.

Selexid® Tablets are contra-indicated in infants under 3 months.

4.4 Special warnings and precautions for use

During long term use, it is advisable to carry out routine liver and kidney function tests.

Selexid® Tablets should be used with caution in patients with porphyria since pivmecillinam has been associated with acute attacks of porphyria.

As with other antibiotics which are excreted mainly by the kidneys, raised blood levels of mecillinam may occur if repeated doses are given to patients with impaired renal function.

Selexid® Tablets should be used with caution for long-term or frequently-repeated treatment, due to the possibility of carnitine depletion.

Concurrent treatment with valproic acid, valproate or other medication liberating pivalic acid should be avoided.

4.5 Interaction with other medicinal products and other forms of interaction

Clearance of methotrexate from the body can be reduced by concurrent use of penicillins. The methotrexate dose may need to be adjusted.

Simultaneous administration of probenecid reduces the excretion of penicillins, and hence increases blood levels of the antibiotic.

Simultaneous administration of other beta-lactam antibiotics with Selexid® Tablets may produce a synergistic effect.

4.6 Pregnancy and lactation

The drug, as mecillinam, crosses the placenta. Although tests in two animal species have shown no teratogenic effects, in keeping with current practice, use during pregnancy should be avoided.

4.7 Effects on ability to drive and use machines

No effects on the ability to drive or use machines have been observed.

4.8 Undesirable effects

The most frequently reported undesirable effects are gastrointestinal disorders and various skin reactions. Oesophageal and mouth ulceration can occur if Selexid® Tablets are taken with insufficient amount of fluid. Allergic reactions, changes in blood counts and hepatic function disorders have been reported in isolated cases.

Based on a review of clinical studies in urinary tract infections, undesirable effects have been identified in $<10\%$ of patients. Therapy was rarely discontinued due to adverse events.

Blood and lymphatic system disorders

Thrombocytopenia

Granulocytopenia

Leucopenia

Eosinophilia

Immune system disorders

Anaphylactic reaction

Gastrointestinal disorders

Oesophageal ulcer

Oesophagitis

Antibiotic associated colitis

Diarrhoea

Vomiting

Mouth ulceration

Dysphagia

Nausea

Abdominal pain

Hepato-biliary disorders

Hepatic function abnormal

Reversible increase in ASAT, ALAT, alkaline phosphatase and bilirubin

Skin and subcutaneous tissue disorder

Rash (including erythematous or maculo-papular)

Urticaria

Pruritus

Angioneurotic oedema

Investigations

Carnitine decreased

4.9 Overdose

There has been no experience of overdosage with Selexid® Tablets. However, excessive doses are likely to induce nausea, vomiting and gastritis. Treatment should be restricted to symptomatic and supportive measures.

5. PHARMACOLOGICAL PROPERTIES

5.1 Pharmacodynamic properties

Selexid® is an orally active antibiotic. Chemically it is the pivaloyloxymethylester of the amidinopenicillanic acid, mecillinam. On oral administration it is well absorbed and subsequently hydrolysed in the body to mecillinam, the active antibacterial agent, by non-specific esterases present in blood, gastro-intestinal mucosa and other tissues.

Selexid® is highly active against most enterobacteriaceae, including *E. coli*, Klebsiella, Proteus, Enterobacter, Serratia, Salmonella, Shigella and Yersina.

Selexid® is less active against gram positive bacteria and organisms such as *Pseudomonas aeruginosa* and *Streptococcus faecalis* are practically resistant to mecillinam.

Whilst Selexid®, like the penicillins and cephalosporins, interferes with the biosynthesis of the bacterial cell wall, the target of the inhibition is different. This different mode of action is probably responsible for the synergistic action which has been found, both *in vitro* and *in vivo*, between Selexid® and various penicillins and cephalosporins.

5.2 Pharmacokinetic properties

Peak serum levels of mecillinam averaging 5 microgram/ml are reached after 1 hour following a dose of 10 mg/kg body weight in children and 400 mg in adults.

The serum half-life is 1.2 hours. The protein binding amounts to 5-10%. Approximately 50% of the administered dose is excreted as mecillinam in the urine within the first six hours. Mecillinam is partly excreted with bile, giving rise to biliary concentrations about 3 times the serum levels. Concurrent administration of probenecid delays the renal excretion of mecillinam, producing more sustained serum levels. The absorption of Selexid® is practically unaffected by taking the tablets with food.

5.3 Preclinical safety data

There are no pre-clinical data of relevance to the prescriber which are additional to that already included in other sections of the SPC.

6. PHARMACEUTICAL PARTICULARS

6.1 List of excipients

Cellulose microcrystalline

Hydroxypropyl cellulose

Magnesium stearate

Hypromellose

Simethicone

Paraffin, synthetic

6.2 Incompatibilities

Not applicable.

6.3 Shelf life

3 years.

6.4 Special precautions for storage

Store below 25°C in a dry place.

6.5 Nature and contents of container

Aluminium/Aluminium blister packs containing 10 tablets.

6.6 Special precautions for disposal and other handling

None.

Administrative Data

7. MARKETING AUTHORISATION HOLDER

LEO Laboratories Limited,

Longwick Road

Princes Risborough

Bucks. HP27 9RR, UK.

8. MARKETING AUTHORISATION NUMBER(S)

PL 0043/0048

9. DATE OF FIRST AUTHORISATION/RENEWAL OF THE AUTHORISATION

20 May 1977 / 29 October 2004

10. DATE OF REVISION OF THE TEXT

January 2008

LEGAL CATEGORY

POM

Septrin Adult Suspension

(GlaxoSmithKline UK)

1. NAME OF THE MEDICINAL PRODUCT

Septrin 80 mg/400 mg per 5 ml Adult Suspension

2. QUALITATIVE AND QUANTITATIVE COMPOSITION

Each 5 ml contains 400 mg Sulfamethoxazole and 80 mg Trimethoprim.

Excipients:

This product contains less than 1 mmol of sodium (23 mg) per dose, and therefore is essentially sodium free.

Also contains 2.5 g sucrose per 5 ml and less than 100 mg of ethanol per 5 ml.

For a full list of excipients, see Section 6.1.

3. PHARMACEUTICAL FORM

Suspension. Off-white in colour.

4. CLINICAL PARTICULARS

4.1 Therapeutic indications

Septrin Adult Suspension is indicated for the treatment of the following infections when owing to sensitive organisms (see section 5.1):

Treatment and prevention of *Pneumocystis jiroveci.(P. carinii)* pneumonitis

Treatment and prophylaxis of toxoplasmosis

Treatment of nocardiosis

The following infections may be treated with Septrin where there is bacterial evidence of sensitivity to Septrin and good reason to prefer the combination of antibiotics in Septrin to a single antibiotic:

Acute uncomplicated urinary tract infections

Acute otitis media

Acute exacerbation of chronic bronchitis

Consideration should be given to official guidance on the appropriate use of antibacterial agents.

4.2 Posology and method of administration

Method of administration: oral

It may be preferable to take Septrin with some food or drink to minimise the possibility of gastrointestinal disturbances.

Standard dosage recommendations for acute infections

Adults and children over 12 years:

Adult Suspension: 10ml every 12 hours

This dosage approximates to 6mg trimethoprim and 30mg sulfamethoxazole per kilogram body weight per 24 hours.

Treatment should be continued until the patient has been symptom free for two days; the majority will require treatment for at least 5 days. If clinical improvement is not evident after 7 days' therapy, the patient should be reassessed.

As an alternative to Standard Dosage for acute uncomplicated lower urinary tract infections, short-term therapy of 1 to 3 days' duration has been shown to be effective.

Where dosage is expressed as "tablets" this refers to the adult tablet, i.e. 80mg Trimethoprim BP and 400 mg Sulfamethoxazole BP. If other formulations are to be used appropriate adjustment should be made.

Special Dosage Recommendations

(Standard dosage applies unless otherwise specified)

Impaired renal function: Adults and children over 12 years: (no information is available for children under 12 years of age).

Creatinine Clearance (ml/min)	Recommended Dosage
>30	STANDARD DOSAGE
15 to 30	Half the STANDARD DOSAGE
<15	Not recommended

Measurements of plasma concentration of sulfamethoxazole at intervals of 2 to 3 days are recommended in samples obtained 12 hours after administration of Septrin. If the concentration of total sulfamethoxazole exceeds 150 microgram/ml then treatment should be interrupted until the value falls below 120 microgram/ml.

The elderly:

See Special Warnings and Precautions for Use. Unless otherwise specified standard dosage applies.

Impaired hepatic function:

No data are available relating to dosage in patients with impaired hepatic function.

Pneumocystis jiroveci (P. carinii) pneumonitis:

Treatment: A higher dosage is recommended using 20 mg trimethoprim and 100 mg sulfamethoxazole per kg of body weight per day in two or more divided doses for two weeks. The aim is to obtain peak plasma or serum levels of trimethoprim of greater than or equal to 5 microgram/ml (verified in patients receiving 1-hour infusions of intravenous Septrin). (See 4.8 Undesirable Effects).

Prevention:

Adults: The following dose schedules may be used:

- 160 mg trimethoprim/800mg sulfamethoxazole daily 7 days per week.
- 160 mg trimethoprim/800mg sulfamethoxazole three days per week on alternate days.
- 320 mg trimethoprim/1600mg sulfamethoxazole per day in two divided doses three days per week on alternate days

Children: The following dose schedules may be used for the duration of the period at risk (see Acute Infections subsection of 4.2):

– Standard dosage taken in two divided doses, seven days per week

– Standard dosage taken in two divided doses, three times per week on alternate days

– Standard dosage taken in two divided doses, three times per week on consecutive days

– Standard dosage taken as a single dose, three times per week on consecutive days

The daily dose given on a treatment day approximates to 150mg trimethoprim/m^2/day and 750mg sulfamethoxazole /m^2/day. The total daily dose should not exceed 320 trimethoprim and 1600 mg sulfamethoxazole.

Nocardiosis: This is no consensus on the most appropriate dosage. Adult doses of 6 to 8 tablets daily for up to 3 months have been used (one tablet contains 400 mg sulfamethoxazole and 80 mg trimethoprim).

Toxoplasmosis: There is no consensus on the most appropriate dosage for the treatment or prophylaxis of this condition. The decision should be based on clinical experience. For prophylaxis, however, the dosages suggested for prevention of *Pneumocystis jiroveci* pneumonitis may be appropriate.

4.3 Contraindications

Septrin should not be given to patients with a history of hypersensitivity to sulphonamides, trimethoprim, co-trimoxazole or any excipients of Septrin.

Contra-indicated in patients showing marked liver parenchymal damage.

Contra-indicated in severe renal insufficiency where repeated measurements of the plasma concentration cannot be performed.

Septrin should not be given to premature babies nor to full-term infants during the first 6 weeks of life except for the treatment/prophylaxis of PCP in infants 4 weeks of age or greater.

4.4 Special warnings and precautions for use

Fatalities, although very rare, have occurred due to severe reactions including Stevens-Johnson syndrome, Lyell's syndrome (toxic epidermal necrolysis), fulminant hepatic necrosis, agranulocytosis, aplastic anaemia, other blood dyscrasias and hypersensitivity of the respiratory tract.

Septrin should be discontinued at the first appearance of skin rash. (See 4.8 Undesirable Effects).

Particular care is *always* advisable when treating elderly patients because, as a group, they are more susceptible to adverse reactions and more likely to suffer serious effects as a result particularly when complicating conditions exist, e.g. impaired kidney and/or liver function and/or concomitant use of other drugs.

An adequate urinary output should be maintained at all times. Evidence of crystalluria *in vivo* is rare, although sulphonamide crystals have been noted in cooled urine from treated patients. In patients suffering from malnutrition the risk may be increased.

Regular monthly blood counts are advisable when Septrin is given for long periods, or to folate deficient patients or to the elderly; since there exists a possibility of asymptomatic changes in haematological laboratory indices due to lack of available folate. These changes may be reversed by administration of folinic acid (5 to 10 mg/day) without interfering with the antibacterial activity.

In glucose-6-phosphate dehydrogenase (G-6-PD) deficient patients haemolysis may occur.

Septrin should be given with caution to patients with severe allergy or bronchial asthma.

Septrin should not be used in the treatment of streptococcal pharayngitis due to Group A Beta-haemolytic streptococci; eradication of these organisms from the oropharynx is less effective than with penicillin.

Trimethoprim has been noted to impair phenylalanine metabolism but this is of no significance in phenylketonuric patients on appropriate dietary restriction.

The administration of Septrin to patients known or suspected to be at risk of acute porphyria should be avoided. Both trimethoprim and sulphonamides (although not specifically sulfamethoxazole) have been associated with clinical exacerbation of porphyria.

Close monitoring of serum potassium and sodium is warranted in patients at risk of hyperkalaemia and hyponatraemia.

Except under careful supervision Septrin should not be given to patients with serious haematological disorders (see 4.8 Undesirable Effects). Septrin has been given to patients receiving cytotoxic therapy with little or no additional effect on the bone marrow or peripheral blood.

The combination of antibiotics in Septrin should only be used where, in the judgement of the physician, the benefits of treatment outweigh any possible risks; consideration should be given to the use of a single effective antibacterial agent.

Patients with rare hereditary problems of fructose intolerance, glucose-galactose malabsorption or sucrase-isomaltase insufficiency should not take this medicine. See Section 2 Quantitative and Qualitative Composition.

This medicinal product contains methyl hydroxybenzoate, which may cause allergic reactions (possibly delayed).

This medicinal product contains small amounts of ethanol (alcohol), less than 100 mg per 5 ml.

This medicinal product contains less than 1 mmol of sodium (23 mg) per dose, and therefore is essentially sodium free.

4.5 Interaction with other medicinal products and other forms of interaction

Trimethoprim may interfere with the estimation of serum/plasma creatinine when the alkaline picrate reaction is used. This may result in overestimation of serum/plasma creatinine of the order of 10%. The creatinine clearance is reduced: the renal tubular secretion of creatinine is decreased from 23% to 9% whilst the glomerular filtration remains unchanged.

In some situations, concomitant treatment with zidovudine may increase the risk of haematological adverse reactions to co-trimoxazole. If concomitant treatment is necessary, consideration should be given to monitoring of haematological parameters.

Reversible deterioration in renal function has been observed in patients treated with co-trimoxazole and cyclosporin following renal transplantation.

Concurrent use of rifampicin and Septrin results in a shortening of the plasma half-life of trimethoprim after a period of about one week. This is not thought to be of clinical significance.

When trimethoprim is administered simultaneously with drugs that form cations at physiological pH, and are also partly excreted by active renal secretion (e.g. procainamide, amantadine), there is the possibility of competitive inhibition of this process which may lead to an increase in plasma concentration of one or both of the drugs.

In elderly patients concurrently receiving diuretics, mainly thiazides, there appears to be an increased risk of thrombocytopenia with or without purpura.

Occasional reports suggest that patients receiving pyrimethamine at doses in excess of 25 mg weekly may develop megaloblastic anaemia should co-trimoxazole be prescribed concurrently.

Co-trimoxazole has been shown to potentiate the anticoagulant activity of warfarin via stereo-selective inhibition of its metabolism. Sulfamethoxazole may displace warfarin from plasma-albumin protein-binding sites *in vitro*. Careful control of the anticoagulant therapy during treatment with Septrin is advisable.

Co-trimoxazole prolongs the half-life of phenytoin and if co-administered could result in excessive phenytoin effect.

Close monitoring of the patient's condition and serum phenytoin levels are advisable.

Concomitant use of trimethoprim with digoxin has been shown to increase plasma digoxin levels in a proportion of elderly patients.

Co-trimoxazole may increase the free plasma levels of methotrexate.

Trimethoprim interferes with assays for serum methotrexate when dihydrofolate reductase from *Lactobacillus casei* is used in the assay. No interference occurs if methotrexate is measured by radioimmuno assay.

Administration of trimethoprim/sulfamethoxazole 160mg/800mg (co-trimoxazole) causes a 40% increase in lamivudine exposure because of the trimethoprim component. Lamivudine has no effect on the pharmacokinetics of trimethoprim or sulfamethoxazole.

Interaction with sulphonylurea hypoglycaemic agents is uncommon but potentiation has been reported.

Caution should be exercised in patients taking any other drugs that can cause hyperkalaemia.

If Septrin is considered appropriate therapy in patients receiving other anti-folate drugs such as methotrexate, a folate supplement should be considered.

4.6 Pregnancy and lactation

Pregnancy

There are not any adequate data from the use of Septrin in pregnant women. Case-control studies have shown that there may be an association between exposure to folate antagonists and birth defects in humans.

Trimethoprim is a folate antagonist and, in animal studies, both agents have been shown to cause foetal abnormalities (see 5.3 Preclinical Safety Data).

Septrin should not be used in pregnancy, particularly in the first trimester, unless clearly necessary. Folate supplementation should be considered if Septrin is used in pregnancy.

Sulfamethoxazole competes with bilirubin for binding to plasma albumin. As significantly maternally derived drug levels persist for several days in the newborn, there may be a risk of precipitating or exacerbating neonatal hyperbilirubinaemia, with an associated theoretical risk of kernicterus, when Septrin is administered to the mother near the time of delivery. This theoretical risk is particularly relevant in infants at increased risk of hyperbilirubinaemia, such as those who are preterm and those with glucose-6-phosphate dehydrogenase deficiency.

Lactation

The components of Septrin (trimethoprim and sulphamethoxazole) are excreted in breast milk. Administration of Septrin should be avoided in late pregnancy and in lactating mothers where the mother or infant has, or is at particular risk of developing, hyperbilirubinaemia. Additionally, administration of Septrin should be avoided in infants younger than eight weeks in view of the predisposition of young infants to hyperbilirubinaemia.

4.7 Effects on ability to drive and use machines

There have been no studies to investigate the effect of Septrin on driving performance or the ability to operate machinery. Further a detrimental effect on such activities cannot be predicted from the pharmacology of the drug. Nevertheless the clinical status of the patient and the adverse events profile of Septrin should be borne in mind when considering the patients ability to operate machinery.

4.8 Undesirable effects

As co-trimoxazole contains trimethoprim and a sulphonamide the type and frequency of adverse reactions associated with such compounds are expected to be consistent with extensive historical experience.

Data from large published clinical trials were used to determine the frequency of very common to rare adverse events. Very rare adverse events were primarily determined from post-marketing experience data and therefore refer to reporting rate rather than a "true" frequency. In addition, adverse events may vary in their incidence depending on the indication.

The following convention has been used for the classification of adverse events in terms of frequency:- Very common ≥1/10, common ≥1/100 and <1/10, uncommon ≥1/1000 and <1/100, rare ≥1/10,000 and <1/1000, very rare <1/10,000.

Infections and Infestations

Common: Monilial overgrowth

Blood and lymphatic system disorders

Very rare: Leucopenia, neutropenia, thrombocytopenia, agranulocytosis, megaloblastic anaemia, aplastic anaemia, haemolytic anaemia, methaemoglobinaemia, eosinophilia, purpura, haemolysis in certain susceptible G-6-PD deficient patients

Immune system disorders

Very rare: Serum sickness, anaphylaxis, allergic myocarditis, angioedema, drug fever, allergic vasculitis resembling Henoch-Schoenlein purpura, periarteritis nodosa, systemic lupus erythematosus

Metabolism and nutrition disorders

Very common: Hyperkalaemia

Very rare: Hypoglycaemia, hyponatraemia, anorexia

Psychiatric disorders

Very rare: Depression, hallucinations

Nervous system disorders

Common: Headache

Very rare: Aseptic meningitis, convulsions, peripheral neuritis, ataxia, vertigo, tinnitus, dizziness

Aseptic meningitis was rapidly reversible on withdrawal of the drug, but recurred in a number of cases on re-exposure to either co-trimoxazole or to trimethoprim alone.

Respiratory, thoracic and mediastinal disorders

Very rare: Cough, shortness of breath, pulmonary infiltrates

Cough, shortness of breath and pulmonary infiltrates may be early indicators of respiratory hypersensitivity which, while very rare, has been fatal.

Gastrointestinal disorders

Common: Nausea, diarrhoea

Uncommon: Vomiting

Very rare: Glossitis, stomatitis, pseudomembranous colitis, pancreatitis

Eye Disorders

Very rare: Uveitis

Hepatobiliary disorders

Very rare: Elevation of serum transaminases, elevation of bilirubin levels, cholestatic jaundice, hepatic necrosis

Cholestatic jaundice and hepatic necrosis may be fatal.

Skin and subcutaneous tissue disorders

Common: Skin rashes

Very rare: Photosensitivity, exfoliative dermatitis, fixed drug eruption, erythema multiforme, Stevens-Johnson syndrome, Lyell's syndrome (toxic epidermal necrolysis)

Lyell's syndrome carries a high mortality.

Musculoskeletal and connective tissue disorders

Very rare: Arthralgia, myalgia

Renal and urinary disorders

Very rare: Impaired renal function (sometimes reported as renal failure), interstitial nephritis

Effects associated with *Pneumocystis jiroveci (P. carinii)* *Pneumonitis* (PCP) management

Very rare: Severe hypersensitivity reactions, rash, fever, neutropenia, thrombocytopenia, raised liver enzymes, hyperkalaemia, hyponatraemia, rhabdomyolysis.

At the high dosages used for PCP management severe hypersensitivity reactions have been reported, necessitating cessation of therapy. If signs of bone marrow depression occur, the patient should be given calcium folinate supplementation (5-10 mg/day). Severe hypersensitivity reactions have been reported in PCP patients on re-exposure to co-trimoxazole, sometimes after a dosage interval of a few days. Rhabdomyolysis has been reported in HIV positive patients receiving co-trimoxazole for prophylaxis or treatment of PCP.

4.9 Overdose

Nausea, vomiting, dizziness and confusion are likely signs/symptoms of overdosage. Bone marrow depression has been reported in acute trimethoprim overdosage.

If vomiting has not occurred, induction of vomiting may be desirable. Gastric lavage may be useful, though absorption from the gastrointestinal tract is normally very rapid and complete within approximately two hours. This may not be the case in gross overdosage. Dependant on the status of renal function administration of fluids is recommended if urine output is low.

Both trimethoprim and active sulfamethoxazole are moderately dialysable by haemodialysis. Peritoneal dialysis is not effective.

5. PHARMACOLOGICAL PROPERTIES

5.1 Pharmacodynamic properties

Pharmacotherapeutic group: Combinations of sulfonamides and trimethoprim, incl. derivatives; ATC code: J01EE01

Mode of Action

Septrin is an antibacterial drug composed of two active principles, sulfamethoxazole and trimethoprim. Sulfamethoxazole is a competitive inhibitor of dihydropteroate synthetase enzyme. Sulfamethoxazole competitively inhibits the utilisation of para-aminobenzoic acid (PABA) in the synthesis of dihydrofolate by the bacterial cell resulting in bacteriostasis. Trimethoprim binds to and reversibly inhibits bacterial dihydrofolate reductase (DHFR) and blocks the production of tetrahydrofolate. Depending on the conditions the effect may be bactericidal. Thus trimethoprim and sulfamethoxazole block two consecutive steps in the biosynthesis of purines and therefore nucleic acids essential to many bacteria. This action produces marked potentiation of activity *in vitro* between the two agents.

Mechanism of resistance

In vitro studies have shown that bacterial resistance can develop more slowly with both sulfamethoxazole and trimethoprim in combination that with either sulfamethoxazole or trimethoprim alone.

Resistance to sulfamethoxazole may occur by different mechanisms. Bacterial mutations cause an increase the concentration of PABA and thereby out-compete with sulfamethoxazole resulting in a reduction of the inhibitory effect on dihydropteroate synthetase enzyme. Another resistance mechanism is plasmid-mediated and results from production of an altered dihydropteroate synthetase enzyme, with reduced affinity for sulfamethoxazole compared to the wild-type enzyme.

Resistance to trimethoprim occurs through a plasmid-mediated mutation which results in production of an altered dihydrofolate reductase enzyme having a reduced affinity for trimethoprim compared to the wild-type enzyme.

Trimethoprim binds to plasmodial DHFR but less tightly than to bacterial enzyme. Its affinity for mammalian DHFR is some 50,000 times less than for the corresponding bacterial enzyme.

Many common pathogenic bacteria are susceptible *in vitro* to trimethoprim and sulfamethoxazole at concentrations well below those reached in blood, tissue fluids and urine after the administration of recommended doses. In common with other antibiotics, however, *in vitro* activity does not necessarily imply that clinical efficacy has been demonstrated and it must be noted that satisfactory susceptibility testing is achieved only with recommended media free from inhibitory substances, especially thymidine and thymine.

Breakpoints

EUCAST

Enterobacteriaceae: S≤ 2 R> 4

S. maltophilia: S≤ 4 R> 4

Acinetobacter: S≤ 2 R> 4

Staphylococcus: S≤ 2 R> 4

Enterococcus: S≤ 0.032 R> 1

Streptococcus ABCG: S≤ 1 R> 2

Streptococcus pneumoniae: S≤ 1 R> 2

Hemophilus influenza: S≤ 0.5 R> 1

Moraxella catarrhalis: S≤0.5 R>1

Psuedomonas aeruginosa and other non-enterobacteriaceae: S≤ 2* R> 4*

S = susceptible, R = resistant. *These are CLSI breakpoints since no EUCAST breakpoints are currently available for these organisms.

Trimethoprim: sulfamethoxazole in the ratio 1:19. Breakpoints are expressed as trimethoprim concentration.

Antibacterial Spectrum

The prevalence of resistance may vary geographically and with time for selected species and local information on resistance is desirable, particularly when treating severe infections. As necessary, expert advice should be sought when the local prevalence of resistance is such that the utility of the agent in at least some types of infections is questionable. This information gives only an approximate guidance on probabilities whether microorganisms will be susceptible to trimethoprim/sulfamethoxazole or not.

Trimethoprim/sulfamethoxazole susceptibility against a number of bacteria are shown in the table below:

Commonly susceptible species:
Gram-positive aerobes: *Staphylococcus aureus* *Staphylococcus saprophyticus* *Streptococcus pyogenes*
Gram-negative aerobes: *Enterobacter cloacae* *Haemophilus influenzae* *Klebsiella oxytoca* *Moraxella catarrhalis* *Salmonella* spp. *Stenotrophomonas maltophilia* *Yersinia* spp.
Species for which acquired resistance may be a problem:
Gram-positive aerobes: *Enterococcus faecalis* *Enterococcus faecium* *Nocardia* spp. *Staphylococcus epidermidis* *Streptococcus pneumoniae*

Gram-negative aerobes: *Citrobacter* spp. *Enterobacter aerogenes* *Escherichia coli* *Klebsiella pneumoniae* *Klebsiella pneumonia* *Proteus mirabilis* *Proteus vulgaris* *Providencia* spp. *Serratia marcesans*	
Inherently resistant organisms:	
Gram-negative aerobes: *Pseudomonas aeruginosa* *Shigella* spp. *Vibrio cholera*	

5.2 Pharmacokinetic properties

After oral administration trimethoprim and sulfamethoxazole are rapidly and nearly completely absorbed. The presence of food does not appear to delay absorption. Peak levels in the blood occur between one and four hours after ingestion and the level attained is dose related. Effective levels persist in the blood for up to 24 hours after a therapeutic dose. Steady state levels in adults are reached after dosing for 2-3 days. Neither component has an appreciable effect on the concentrations achieved in the blood by the other.

Trimethoprim is a weak base with a pKa of 7.4. It is lipophilic. Tissue levels of trimethoprim are generally higher than corresponding plasma levels, the lungs and kidneys showing especially high concentrations. Trimethoprim concentrations exceed those in plasma in the case of bile, prostatic fluid and tissue, saliva, sputum and vaginal secretions. Levels in the aqueous humor, breast milk, cerebrospinal fluid, middle ear fluid, synovial fluid and tissue (intestinal) fluid are adequate for antibacterial activity. Trimethoprim passes into amniotic fluid and foetal tissues reaching concentrations approximating those of maternal serum.

Approximately 50% of trimethoprim in the plasma is protein bound. The half-life in man is in the range 8.6 to 17 hours in the presence of normal renal function. It is increased by a factor of 1.5 to 3.0 when the creatinine clearance is less than 10 ml/minute. There appears to be no significant difference in the elderly compared with young patients.

The principal route of excretion of trimethoprim is renal and approximately 50% of the dose is excreted in the urine within 24 hours as unchanged drug. Several metabolites have been identified in the urine. Urinary concentrations of trimethoprim vary widely.

Sulfamethoxazole is a weak acid with a pKa of 6.0. The concentration of active sulphamethoxazole in a variety of body fluids is of the order of 20 to 50% of the plasma concentration.

Approximately 66% of sulfamethoxazole in the plasma is protein bound. The half-life in man is approximately 9 to 11 hours in the presence of normal renal function. There is no change in the half-life of active sulfamethoxazole with a reduction in renal function but there is prolongation of the half-life of the major, acetylated metabolite when the creatinine clearance is below 25 ml/minute.

The principal route of excretion of sulfamethoxazole is renal; between 15% and 30% of the dose recovered in the urine is in the active form. In elderly patients there is a reduced renal clearance of sulfamethoxazole.

5.3 Preclinical safety data

Reproductive toxicology:

At doses in excess of recommended human therapeutic dose, trimethoprim and sulfamethoxazole have been reported to cause cleft palate and other foetal abnormalities in rats, findings typical of a folate antagonist. Effects with trimethoprim were preventable by administration of dietary folate. In rabbits, foetal loss was seen at doses of trimethoprim in excess of human therapeutic doses.

6. PHARMACEUTICAL PARTICULARS

6.1 List of excipients

Syrup or sucrose

Glycerol (E422)

Dispersible Cellulose (E460)

Sodium carboxymethylcellulose (E467)

Methyl hydroxybenzoate (E218)

Saccharin sodium (E954)

Ammonium glycyrrhizinate

Anise Oil

Ethanol (96%)

Flavour, vanilla 407

Polysorbate 80 (E433)

Purified Water

6.2 Incompatibilities

See drug interactions.

6.3 Shelf life

4 years

6.4 Special precautions for storage

Store below 25°C

Protect from light

6.5 Nature and contents of container

Amber glass bottles with metal roll on pilfer proof caps or polypropylene child resistant caps.

Pack size: 100 ml

Septrin 80 mg/400 mg per 5 ml Adult Suspension comes with a double-ended polypropylene measuring spoon.

6.6 Special precautions for disposal and other handling

Trimethoprim interferes with assays for serum methotrexate when dihydrofolate reductase from *Lactobacillus casei* is used in the assay. No interference occurs if methotrexate is measured by radioimmunoassay.

Trimethoprim may interfere with the estimation of serum/plasma creatinine when the alkaline picrate reaction is used. This may result in overestimation of serum/plasma creatinine of the order of 10%. Functional inhibition of the renal tubular secretion of creatinine may produce a spurious fall in the estimated rate of creatinine clearance.

Septrin 80 mg/400 mg per 5 ml Adult Suspension may be diluted with Syrup BP. Although they may show some sedimentation such dilutions remain stable for at least a month. Shake thoroughly before use.

7. MARKETING AUTHORISATION HOLDER

The Wellcome Foundation Limited

Glaxo Wellcome House

Berkeley Avenue

Greenford

Middlesex

UB6 0NN

Trading as:

GlaxoSmithKline UK

Stockley Park West

Uxbridge

Middlesex UB11 1BT

8. MARKETING AUTHORISATION NUMBER(S)

PL 00003/5223R

9. DATE OF FIRST AUTHORISATION/RENEWAL OF THE AUTHORISATION

Date of first authorisation: 30 October 1986

Date of last renewal: 08 November 2006

10. DATE OF REVISION OF THE TEXT

21 July 2009

Septrin for Infusion

(GlaxoSmithKline UK)

1. NAME OF THE MEDICINAL PRODUCT

Septrin 16 mg/80 mg per ml for Infusion

2. QUALITATIVE AND QUANTITATIVE COMPOSITION

Each 5 ml of Septrin 16 mg/80 mg per ml for Infusion contains 80 mg Trimethoprim and 400 mg Sulfamethoxazole.

Excipients:

This product contains 1.7 mmoles of sodium and 13.2 vol % ethanol (alcohol) per 5 ml.

For a full list of excipients, see Section 6.1

3. PHARMACEUTICAL FORM

Solution for Infusion

A clear liquid.

4. CLINICAL PARTICULARS

4.1 Therapeutic indications

Septrin for Infusion is indicated for the treatment of the following infections when owing to sensitive organisms (see section 5.1):

Acute uncomplicated urinary tract infection.

It is recommended that initial episodes of uncomplicated urinary tract infections be treated with a single effective antibacterial agent rather than a combination such as Septrin for Infusion.

Treatment and prevention of *Pneumocystis jiroveci* pneumonitis (previously known as *Pneumocystis carinii* pneumonia or "PCP")

Treatment and prophylaxis of toxoplasmosis.

Treatment of nocardiosis.

In general, the indications for the use of Septrin for Infusion are the same as those for oral presentations.

Consideration should be given to official guidance on the appropriate use of antibacterial agents.

4.2 Posology and method of administration

Method of Administration: Septrin for Infusion is for administration only by the intravenous route and must be diluted before administration.

It is intended that Septrin for Infusion should be used only during such a period as the patient is unable to accept oral therapy, where initiation of treatment is particularly urgent or for convenience if the patient is already receiving intravenous fluids. Although Septrin for Infusion is useful in critically ill patients, there may be no therapeutic advantage over the oral preparation.

For instructions on dilution of the product before administration, see section 6.6.

Standard dosage recommendations for acute infections

Adults and children over 12 years:

2 ampoules (10 ml) every 12 hours.

Children aged 12 years and under:

The recommended dosage is approximately 6 mg trimethoprim and 30 mg sulfamethoxazole per kg bodyweight per 24 hours, given in two equally divided doses. As a guide the following schedules may be used diluted as described above.

6 weeks to 5 months:	1.25 ml every 12 hours
6 months to 5 years:	2.5 ml every 12 hours
6 to 12 years:	5.0 ml every 12 hours

For severe infections in all age groups, dosage may be increased by 50%.

Treatment should be continued until the patient has been symptom free for two days; the majority will require treatment for at least 5 days.

The elderly:

See Special Warnings and Precautions for Use.

Impaired hepatic function:

No data are available relating to dosage in patients with impaired hepatic function.

Special Dosage Recommendations

(Standard dosage applies unless otherwise specified)

Impaired renal function:

Adults and children over 12 years (no information is available for children under 12 years of age):

Creatinine Clearance (ml/min)	Recommended Dosage
More than 30	STANDARD DOSAGE
15-30	Half the STANDARD DOSAGE
Less than 15	Not recommended

Measurements of plasma concentrations of sulfamethoxazole at intervals of 2 to 3 days are recommended in samples obtained 12 hours after administration of Septrin 16 mg/80 mg per ml for Infusion. If the concentration of total sulfamethoxazole exceeds 150 micrograms/ml then treatment should be interrupted until the value falls below 120 micrograms/ml.

Pneumocystis jiroveci (P. carinii) pneumonitis:

Treatment

20 mg trimethoprim and 100 mg sulfamethoxazole per kg of bodyweight per day in two or more divided doses. Therapy should be changed to the oral route as soon as possible and continued for a total treatment period of two weeks. The aim is to obtain peak plasma or serum levels of trimethoprim of greater than or equal to 5 microgram/ml (verified in patients receiving 1-hour infusions of intravenous Septrin). (See 4.8 Undesirable Effects)

Prevention

Standard dosage for the duration of the period at risk.

Nocardiosis: There is no consensus on the most appropriate dosage. Adult doses of 6 to 8 tablets daily for up to 3 months have been used (one tablet contains 400 mg sulfamethoxazole and 80 mg trimethoprim).

Toxoplasmosis: There is no consensus on the most appropriate dosage for the treatment or prophylaxis of this condition. The decision should be based on clinical experience. For prophylaxis, however, the dosages suggested for prevention of *Pneumocystis jiroveci* pneumonitis may be appropriate.

4.3 Contraindications

Septrin 16 mg/80 mg per ml for Infusion should not be given to patients with a history of hypersensitivity to sulphonamides, trimethoprim, co-trimoxazole or any excipients of Septrin.

Septrin 16 mg/80 mg per ml for Infusion is contra-indicated in patients showing marked liver parenchymal damage.

Septrin 16 mg/80 mg per ml for Infusion is contra-indicated in severe renal insufficiency where repeated measurements of the plasma concentration cannot be performed.

Septrin 16 mg/80 mg per ml for Infusion should not be given to premature babies nor to full-term infants during the first six weeks of life except for the treatment/prophylaxis of PCP in infants 4 weeks of age or greater.

4.4 Special warnings and precautions for use

Fatalities, although very rare, have occurred due to severe reactions including Stevens-Johnson syndrome, Lyell's syndrome (toxic epidermal necrolysis), fulminant hepatic necrosis, agranulocytosis, aplastic anaemia, other blood dyscrasias and hypersensitivity of the respiratory tract.

Septrin 16 mg/80 mg per ml for Infusion should be discontinued at the first appearance of a skin rash (see 4.8 Undesirable Effects).

Fluid overload is possible, especially when very high doses are being administered to patients with underlying cardio-pulmonary disease.

An adequate urinary output should be maintained at all times. Evidence of crystalluria *in vivo* is rare, although sulphonamide crystals have been noted in cooled urine from treated patients. In patients suffering from malnutrition the risk may be increased.

For patients with known renal impairment special measures should be adopted (See 4.2 Posology and Method of Administration).

Regular monthly blood counts are advisable when Septrin is given for long periods, or to folate deficient patients or to the elderly since there exists a possibility of asymptomatic changes in haematological laboratory indices due to lack of available folate. These changes may be reversed by administration of folinic acid (5 to 10 mg/day) without interfering with the antibacterial activity.

Particular care is always advisable when treating elderly patients because, as a group, they are more susceptible to adverse reactions and more likely to suffer serious side effects as a result, particularly when complicating conditions exist, e.g. impaired kidney and/or liver function and/or concomitant drugs.

In glucose-6-phosphate dehydrogenase-deficient (G-6-PD) patients, haemolysis may occur.

Septrin should be given with caution to patients with severe allergy or bronchial asthma.

Septrin should not be used in the treatment of streptococcal pharyngitis due to Group A beta-haemolytic streptococci. Eradication of these organisms from the oropharynx is less effective than with penicillin.

Trimethoprim has been noted to impair phenylalanine metabolism but this is of no significance in phenylketonuric patients on appropriate dietary restriction.

The administration of Septrin to patients known or suspected to be at risk of acute porphyria should be avoided. Both trimethoprim and sulphonamides (although not specifically sulfamethoxazole) have been associated with clinical exacerbation of porphyria.

Close monitoring of serum potassium and sodium is warranted in patients at risk of hyperkalaemia and hyponatraemia.

This medicinal product contains 13.2 vol% ethanol (alcohol), i.e. up to 521 mg per dose. This is equivalent to 2.64 ml of beer, or 1.1 ml of wine. Harmful for those suffering from alcoholism. To be taken into account in pregnant or breast-feeding women, children and high-risk groups such as patients with liver disease, or epilepsy.

This medicinal product contains sodium metabisulphite, which may rarely cause severe hypersensitivity reaction and bronchospasm.

This medicinal product contains 1.7 mmoles (or 38.87 mg) of sodium. To be taken into consideration by patients on a sodium controlled diet.

Except under careful supervision Septrin for Infusion should not be given to patients with serious haematological disorders (see 4.8 Undesirable Effects). Septrin has been given to patients receiving cytotoxic therapy with little or no additional effect on the bone marrow or peripheral blood.

The combination of the antibiotics in Septrin for Infusion should only be used where, in the judgement of the physician, the benefits of treatment outweigh any possible risks; consideration should be given to the use of a single effective antibacterial agent.

4.5 Interaction with other medicinal products and other forms of interaction

Trimethoprim may interfere with the estimation of serum/plasma creatinine when the alkaline picrate reaction is used. This may result in overestimation of serum/plasma creatinine of the order of 10%. The creatinine clearance is reduced: the renal tubular secretion of creatinine is decreased from 23% to 9% whilst the glomerular filtration remains unchanged.

In some situations, concomitant treatment with zidovudine may increase the risk of haematological adverse reactions to co-trimoxazole. If concomitant treatment is necessary, consideration should be given to monitoring of haematological parameters.

Reversible deterioration in renal function has been observed in patients treated with co-trimoxazole and ciclosporin following renal transplantation.

Concurrent use of rifampicin and Septrin results in a shortening of the plasma half-life of trimethoprim after a period of about one week. This is not thought to be of clinical significance.

When trimethoprim is administered simultaneously with drugs that form cations at physiological pH, and are also partly excreted by active renal secretion (e.g. procainamide, amantadine), there is the possibility of competitive inhibition of this process which may lead to an increase in plasma concentration of one or both of the drugs.

In elderly patients concurrently receiving diuretics, mainly thiazides, there appears to be an increased risk of thrombocytopenia with or without purpura.

Occasional reports suggest that patients receiving pyrimethamine as malarial prophylaxis at doses in excess of 25 mg weekly may develop megaloblastic anaemia should co-trimoxazole be prescribed concurrently.

Co-trimoxazole has been shown to potentiate the anticoagulant activity of warfarin via stereo-selective inhibition of its metabolism. Sulfamethoxazole may displace warfarin from plasma-albumin protein-binding sites *in vitro*. Careful control of the anticoagulant therapy during treatment with Septrin is advisable.

Co-trimoxazole prolongs the half-life of phenytoin and if co-administered the prescriber should be alert for excessive phenytoin effect. Close monitoring of the patient's condition and serum phenytoin levels is advisable.

Concomitant use of trimethoprim with digoxin has been shown to increase plasma digoxin levels in a proportion of elderly patients.

Co-trimoxazole may increase the free plasma levels of methotrexate.

Trimethoprim interferes with assays for serum methotrexate when dihydrofolate reductase from *Lactobacillus casei* is used in the assay. No interference occurs if methotrexate is measured by radioimmuno assay.

Administration of trimethoprim/sulfamethoxazole 160mg/800mg (co-trimoxazole) causes a 40% increase in lamivudine exposure because of the trimethoprim component. Lamivudine has no effect on the pharmacokinetics of trimethoprim or sulfamethoxazole.

Interaction with sulphonylurea hypoglycaemic agents is uncommon but potentiation has been reported.

Caution should be exercised in patients taking any other drugs that can cause hyperkalaemia.

If Septrin is considered appropriate therapy in patients receiving other anti-folate drugs such as methotrexate, a folate supplement should be considered.

4.6 Pregnancy and lactation

Pregnancy

There are not any adequate data from the use of Septrin for Infusion in pregnant women. Case-control studies have shown that there may be an association between exposure to folate antagonists and birth defects in humans.

Trimethoprim is a folate antagonist and, in animal studies, both agents have been shown to cause foetal abnormalities (see 5.3 Preclinical Safety Data).

Septrin for Infusion should not be used in pregnancy, particularly in the first trimester, unless clearly necessary. Folate supplementation should be considered if Septrin for Infusion is used in pregnancy.

Sulfamethoxazole competes with bilirubin for binding to plasma albumin. As significantly maternally derived drug levels persist for several days in the newborn, there may be a risk of precipitating or exacerbating neonatal hyperbilirubinaemia, with an associated theoretical risk of kernicterus, when Septrin for Infusion is administered to the mother near the time of delivery. This theoretical risk is particularly relevant in infants at increased risk of hyperbilirubinaemia, such as those who are preterm and those with glucose-6-phosphate dehydrogenase deficiency.

Lactation

The components of Septrin for Infusion (trimethoprim and sulfamethoxazole) are excreted in breast milk. Administration of Septrin for Infusion should be avoided in late pregnancy and in lactating mothers where the mother or infant has, or is at particular risk of developing, hyperbilirubinaemia. Additionally, administration of Septrin for Infusion should be avoided in infants younger than eight weeks in view of the predisposition of young infants to hyperbilirubinaemia.

4.7 Effects on ability to drive and use machines

None known.

4.8 Undesirable effects

As co-trimoxazole contains trimethoprim and a sulphonamide the type and frequency of adverse reactions associated with such compounds are expected to be consistent with extensive historical experience.

Data from large published clinical trials were used to determine the frequency of very common to rare adverse events. Very rare adverse events were primarily determined from post-marketing experience data and therefore refer to reporting rate rather than a "true" frequency. In addition, adverse events may vary in their incidence depending on the indication.

The following convention has been used for the classification of adverse events in terms of frequency:- Very common $\geqslant 1/10$, common $\geqslant 1/100$ and $< 1/10$, uncommon $\geqslant 1/1000$ and $< 1/100$, rare $\geqslant 1/10{,}000$ and $< 1/1000$, very rare $< 1/10{,}000$.

Infections and Infestations

Common: Monilial overgrowth

Blood and lymphatic system disorders

Very rare: Leucopenia, neutropenia, thrombocytopenia, agranulocytosis, megaloblastic anaemia, aplastic anaemia, haemolytic anaemia, methaemoglobinaemia, eosinophilia, purpura, haemolysis in certain susceptible G-6-PD deficient patients

Immune system disorders

Very rare: Serum sickness, anaphylaxis, allergic myocarditis, angioedema, drug fever, allergic vasculitis resembling Henoch-Schoenlein purpura, periarteritis nodosa, systemic lupus erythematosus

Metabolism and nutrition disorders

Very common: Hyperkalaemia

Very rare: Hypoglycaemia, hyponatraemia, anorexia

Psychiatric disorders

Very rare: Depression, hallucinations

Nervous system disorders

Common: Headache

Very rare: Aseptic meningitis, convulsions, peripheral neuritis, ataxia, vertigo, tinnitus, dizziness

Aseptic meningitis was rapidly reversible on withdrawal of the drug, but recurred in a number of cases on re-exposure to either co-trimoxazole or to trimethoprim alone.

Respiratory, thoracic and mediastinal disorders

Very rare: Cough, shortness of breath, pulmonary infiltrates

Cough, shortness of breath and pulmonary infiltrates may be early indicators of respiratory hypersensitivity which, while very rare, has been fatal.

Gastrointestinal disorders

Common: Nausea, diarrhoea

Uncommon: Vomiting

Very rare: Glossitis, stomatitis, pseudomembranous colitis, pancreatitis

Eye Disorders

Very rare: Uveitis

Hepatobiliary disorders

Very rare: Elevation of serum transaminases, elevation of bilirubin levels, cholestatic jaundice, hepatic necrosis

Cholestatic jaundice and hepatic necrosis may be fatal.

Skin and subcutaneous tissue disorders

Common: Skin rashes

Very rare: Photosensitivity, exfoliative dermatitis, fixed drug eruption, erythema multiforme, Stevens-Johnson syndrome, Lyell's syndrome (toxic epidermal necrolysis)

Lyell's syndrome carries a high mortality.

Musculoskeletal and connective tissue disorders

Very rare: Arthralgia, myalgia

Renal and urinary disorders

Very rare: Impaired renal function (sometimes reported as renal failure),

interstitial nephritis

Effects associated with *Pneumocystis jiroveci (P.carinii)* Pneumonitis (PCP) management

Very rare: Severe hypersensitivity reactions, rash, fever, neutropenia, thrombocytopenia, raised liver enzymes, hyperkalaemia, hyponatraemia, rhabdomyolysis.

At the high dosages used for PCP management severe hypersensitivity reactions have been reported, necessitating cessation of therapy. If signs of bone marrow depression occur, the patient should be given calcium folinate supplementation (5-10 mg/day). Severe hypersensitivity reactions have been reported in PCP patients on re-exposure to co-trimoxazole, sometimes after a dosage interval of a few days. Rhabdomyolysis has been reported in HIV positive patients receiving co-trimoxazole for prophylaxis or treatment of PCP.

4.9 Overdose

The maximum tolerated dose in humans is unknown.

Nausea, vomiting, dizziness and confusion are likely symptoms of overdosage. Bone marrow depression has been reported in acute trimethoprim overdosage.

In cases of known, suspected or accidental overdosage, stop therapy.

Dependent on the status of renal function, administration of fluids is recommended if urine output is low.

Both trimethoprim and active sulfamethoxazole are dialysable by renal dialysis. Peritoneal dialysis is not effective.

5. PHARMACOLOGICAL PROPERTIES

5.1 Pharmacodynamic properties

Pharmacotherapeutic group: Combinations of sulfonamides and trimethoprim, incl. derivatives; ATC code: J01EE01

Mode of Action

Septrin is an antibacterial drug composed of two active principles, sulfamethoxazole and trimethoprim. Sulfamethoxazole is a competitive inhibitor of dihydropteroate synthetase enzyme. Sulfamethoxazole competitively inhibits the utilisation of para-aminobenzoic acid (PABA) in the synthesis of dihydrofolate by the bacterial cell resulting in bacteriostasis. Trimethoprim binds to and reversibly inhibits bacterial dihydrofolate reductase (DHFR) and blocks the production of tetrahydrofolate. Depending on the conditions the effect may be bactericidal. Thus trimethoprim and sulfamethoxazole block two consecutive steps in the biosynthesis of purines and therefore nucleic acids essential to many bacteria. This action produces marked potentiation of activity in vitro between the two agents.

Mechanism of resistance

In vitro studies have shown that bacterial resistance can develop more slowly with both sulfamethoxazole and trimethoprim in combination that with either sulfamethoxazole or trimethoprim alone.

Resistance to sulfamethoxazole may occur by different mechanisms. Bacterial mutations cause an increase the concentration of PABA and thereby out-compete with sulfamethoxazole resulting in a reduction of the inhibitory effect on dihydropteroate synthetase enzyme. Another resistance mechanism is plasmid-mediated and results from production of an altered dihydropteroate synthetase enzyme, with reduced affinity for sulfamethoxazole compared to the wild-type enzyme.

Resistance to trimethoprim occurs through a plasmid-mediated mutation which results in production of an altered dihydrofolate reductase enzyme having a reduced affinity for trimethoprim compared to the wild-type enzyme.

Trimethoprim binds to plasmodial DHFR but less tightly than to bacterial enzyme. Its affinity for mammalian DHFR is some 50,000 times less than for the corresponding bacterial enzyme.

Many common pathogenic bacteria are susceptible in vitro to trimethoprim and sulfamethoxazole at concentrations well below those reached in blood, tissue fluids and urine after the administration of recommended doses. In common with other antibiotics, however, in vitro activity does not necessarily imply that clinical efficacy has been demonstrated and it must be noted that satisfactory susceptibility testing is achieved only with recommended media free from inhibitory substances, especially thymidine and thymine.

Breakpoints

EUCAST

Enterobacteriaceae: S≤ 2 R> 4

S. maltophilia: S≤ 4 R> 4

Acinetobacter: S≤ 2 R> 4

Staphylococcus: S≤ 2 R> 4

Enterococcus: S≤ 0.032 R> 1

Streptococcus ABCG: S≤ 1 R> 2

Streptococcus pneumoniae: S≤ 1 R> 2

Hemophilus influenza: S≤ 0.5 R> 1

Moraxella catarrhalis: S≤0.5 R>1

Psuedomonas aeruginosa and other non-enterobacteriaceae: S≤ 2* R> 4*

S = susceptible, R = resistant. *These are CLSI breakpoints since no EUCAST breakpoints are currently available for these organisms.

Trimethoprim: sulfamethoxazole in the ratio 1:19. Breakpoints are expressed as trimethoprim concentration.

Antibacterial Spectrum

The prevalence of resistance may vary geographically and with time for selected species and local information on resistance is desirable, particularly when treating severe infections. As necessary, expert advice should be sought when the local prevalence of resistance is such that the utility of the agent in at least some types of infections is questionable. This information gives only an approximate guidance on probabilities whether microorganisms will be susceptible to trimethoprim/sulfamethoxazole or not.

Trimethoprim/sulfamethoxazole susceptibility against a number of bacteria are shown in the table below:

Commonly susceptible species:
Gram-positive aerobes: *Staphylococcus aureus* *Staphylococcus saprophyticus* *Streptococcus pyogenes*
Gram-negative aerobes: *Enterobacter cloacae* *Haemophilus influenzae* *Klebsiella oxytoca* *Moraxella catarrhalis* *Salmonella* spp. *Stenotrophomonas maltophilia* *Yersinia* spp.
Species for which acquired resistance may be a problem:
Gram-positive aerobes: *Enterococcus faecalis* *Enterococcus faecium* *Nocardia* spp. *Staphylococcus epidermidis* *Streptococcus pneumoniae*
Gram-negative aerobes: *Citrobacter* spp. *Enterobacter aerogenes* *Escherichia coli* *Klebsiella pneumoniae* *Klebsiella pneumonia* *Proteus mirabilis* *Proteus vulgaris* *Providencia* spp. *Serratia marcesans*
Inherently resistant organisms:
Gram-negative aerobes: *Pseudomonas aeruginosa* *Shigella* spp. *Vibrio cholera*

5.2 Pharmacokinetic properties

Peak plasma levels of trimethoprim and sulfamethoxazole are higher and achieved more rapidly after one hour of intravenous infusion of Septrin 16 mg/80 mg per ml for Infusion than after oral administration of an equivalent dose of a Septrin oral presentation. Plasma concentrations, elimination half-life and urinary excretion rates show no significant differences following either the oral or intravenous route of administration.

Trimethoprim is a weak base with a pKa of 7.3. It is lipophilic. Tissue levels of trimethoprim are generally higher than corresponding plasma levels, the lungs and kidneys showing especially high concentrations. Trimethoprim concentrations exceed those in plasma in the case of bile, prostatic fluid and tissue, sputum, and vaginal secretions. Levels in the aqueous humor, breast milk, cerebrospinal fluid, middle ear fluid, synovial fluid and tissue (interstitial) fluid are adequate for antibacterial activity. Trimethoprim passes into amniotic fluid and fetal tissues reaching concentrations approximating those of maternal serum.

Approximately 50% of trimethoprim in the plasma is protein bound. The half-life in man is in the range 8.6 to 17 hours in the presence of normal renal function. It is increased by a factor of 1.5 to 3.0 when the creatinine clearance is less than 10 ml/minute. There appears to be no significant difference in the elderly compared with young patients.

The principal route of excretion of trimethoprim is renal and approximately 50% of the dose is excreted in the urine within 24 hours as unchanged drug. Several metabolites have been identified in the urine. Urinary concentrations of trimethoprim vary widely.

Sulfamethoxazole is a weak acid with a pKa of 6.0. The concentration of active sulfamethoxazole in amniotic fluid, aqueous humor, bile, cerebrospinal fluid, middle ear fluid, sputum, synovial fluid and tissue (interstitial) fluid is of the order of 20 to 50% of the plasma concentration. Approximately 66% of sulfamethoxazole in the plasma is protein bound. The half-life in man is approximately 9 to 11 hours in the presence of normal renal function. There is no change in the half-life of active sulfamethoxazole with a reduction in renal function but there is prolongation of the half-life of the major, acetylated metabolite when the creatinine clearance is below 25 ml/minute.

The principal route of excretion of sulfamethoxazole is renal; between 15% and 30% of the dose recovered in the urine is in the active form. In elderly patients there is a reduced renal clearance of sulfamethoxazole.

5.3 Preclinical safety data

Reproductive toxicology: At doses in excess of recommended human therapeutic dose, trimethoprim and sulfamethoxazole have been reported to cause cleft palate and other foetal abnormalities in rats, findings typical of a folate antagonist. Effects with trimethoprim were preventable by administration of dietary folate. In rabbits, foetal loss was seen at doses of trimethoprim in excess of human therapeutic doses.

6. PHARMACEUTICAL PARTICULARS

6.1 List of excipients

Propylene Glycol (E1520)

Tromethamine

Sodium Hydroxide (E524)

Sodium Metabisulphite (E223)

Ethanol

Water for Injections

6.2 Incompatibilities

None known.

6.3 Shelf life

36 months

6.4 Special precautions for storage

Store below 30°C. Protect from light.

6.5 Nature and contents of container

Neutral glass ampoules (5ml nominal fill volume)

Pack size: 10 × 5ml ampoules

6.6 Special precautions for disposal and other handling

Septrin for Infusion must be diluted before administration.

Dilution should be carried out immediately before use. After adding Septrin 16 mg/80 mg per ml for Infusion to the infusion solution, shake thoroughly to ensure complete mixing. If visible turbidity or crystallisation appears at any time before or during an infusion, the mixture should be discarded.

It is recommended that Septrin16 mg/80 mg per ml for Infusion is diluted according to the following schedules:

One ampoule (5 ml) to 125 ml infusion solution.

Two ampoules (10 ml) to 250 ml infusion solution.

Three ampoules (15 ml) to 500 ml infusion solution.

Septrin 16 mg/80 mg per ml for Infusion is known to be compatible, when diluted as recommended above, with the following fluids:

Glucose Intravenous Infusion BP (5% w/v and 10% w/v).

Sodium Chloride Intravenous Infusion BP (0.9% w/v).

Sodium Chloride (0.18% w/v) and Glucose (4% w/v) Intravenous Infusion BP.

Dextran 70 Injection BP (6% w/v) in glucose (5% w/v) or normal saline.

Dextran 40 Injection BP (10% w/v) in glucose (5% w/v) or normal saline.

Ringer's Solution for Injection BPC 1959.

No other substance should be mixed with the infusion.

The duration of the infusion should be approximately one to one and a half hours, but this should be balanced against the fluid requirements of the patient.

When fluid restriction is necessary, Septrin 16 mg/80 mg per ml for Infusion may be administered at a higher concentration, 5 ml diluted with 75 ml of glucose 5% w/v in water. The resultant solution, whilst being clear to the naked eye, may on occasion exceed the BP limits set for particulate matter in large volume parenterals. The solution should be infused over a period not exceeding one hour. Discard any unused solution.

7. MARKETING AUTHORISATION HOLDER

The Wellcome Foundation Ltd.,

Glaxo Wellcome House,

Berkeley Avenue,

Greenford,

Middlesex

Trading as

GlaxoSmithKline UK

Stockley Park West

Uxbridge

Middlesex UB11 1BT

8. MARKETING AUTHORISATION NUMBER(S)

PL 00003/0095R

9. DATE OF FIRST AUTHORISATION/RENEWAL OF THE AUTHORISATION

Date of first authorisation: 18 March 1974

Date of last of renewal: 17 October 2006

10. DATE OF REVISION OF THE TEXT

21 July 2009

Septrin Forte Tablets

(GlaxoSmithKline UK)

1. NAME OF THE MEDICINAL PRODUCT

Septrin 160 mg/800 mg Forte Tablets

2. QUALITATIVE AND QUANTITATIVE COMPOSITION

Each tablet contains 800 mg Sulfamethoxazole and 160 mg of Trimethoprim.

Excipients:

For full list of excipients, see Section 6.1

3. PHARMACEUTICAL FORM

Tablet

White, elongated tablet marked "GX O2C" on one side and a scoreline on the other side.

4. CLINICAL PARTICULARS

4.1 Therapeutic indications

Septrin Forte tablets are indicated for the treatment of the following infections when owing to sensitive organisms (see section 5.1):

Treatment and prevention of *Pneumocystis jiroveci (P. carinii)* pneumonitis

Treatment and prophylaxis of toxoplasmosis

Treatment of nocardiosis

The following infections may be treated with Septrin where there is bacterial evidence of sensitivity to Septrin and good reason to prefer the combination of antibiotics in Septrin to a single antibiotic:

Acute uncomplicated urinary tract infection

Acute otitis media

Acute exacerbation of chronic bronchitis

Consideration should be given to official guidance on the appropriate use of antibacterial agents.

4.2 Posology and method of administration

Method of administration: oral.

It may be preferable to take Septrin with some food or drink to minimise the possibility of gastrointestinal disturbances.

Standard dosage recommendations for acute infections

Adults and children over 12 years:

Forte Tablets Standard Dose

1 every 12 hours

This dosage approximates to 6 mg trimethoprim and 30 mg sulfamethoxazole per kilogram body weight per 24 hours.

Treatment should be continued until the patient has been symptom free for two days; the majority will require treatment for at least 5 days. If clinical improvement is not evident after 7 days' therapy, the patient should be reassessed.

As an alternative to Standard Dosage for acute uncomplicated lower urinary tract infections, short-term therapy of 1 to 3 days' duration has been shown to be effective.

The elderly:

See Special Warnings and Precautions for Use. Unless otherwise specified standard dosage applies.

Impaired hepatic function:

No data are available relating to dosage in patients with impaired hepatic function.

Special Dosage Recommendations

(Standard dosage applies unless otherwise specified).

Where dosage is expressed as "tablets" this refers to the adult tablet, i.e 80 mg Trimethoprim BP and 400 mg Sulfamethoxazole BP. If other formulations are to be used appropriate adjustment should be made.

Impaired renal function:

Adults and children over 12 years: (no information is available for children under 12 years of age).

Creatinine Clearance (ml/min)	Recommended Dosage
>30	STANDARD DOSAGE
15 to 30	Half the STANDARD DOSAGE
<15	Not recommended

Measurements of plasma concentration of sulfamethoxazole at intervals of 2 to 3 days are recommended in samples obtained 12 hours after administration of Septrin. If the concentration of total sulfamethoxazole exceeds 150 microgram/ml then treatment should be interrupted until the value falls below 120 microgram/ml.

Pneumocystis jiroveci (P. carinii) pneumonitis: Treatment: A higher dosage is recommended using 20 mg trimethoprim and 100 mg sulfamethoxazole per kg of body weight per day in two or more divided doses for two weeks. The aim is to obtain peak plasma or serum levels of trimethoprim of greater than or equal to 5 microgram/ml (verified in patients receiving 1-hour infusions of intravenous Septrin). (See 4.8 Undesirable Effects).

Prevention: Adults: The following dose schedules may be used:

160 mg trimethoprim/800 mg sulfamethoxazole daily 7 days per week.

160 mg trimethoprim/800 mg sulfamethoxazole three times per week on alternative days.

320 mg trimethoprim/1600 mg sulfamethoxazole per day in two divided doses three times per week on alternative days.

Children:

The following dose schedules may be used for the duration of the period at risk (see Standard dosage recommendations for acute infections subsection of 4.2):

– Standard dosage taken in two divided doses, seven days per week

– Standard dosage taken in two divided doses, three times per week on alternate days

– Standard dosage taken in two divided doses, three times per week on consecutive days

– Standard dosage taken as a single dose, three times per week on consecutive days

The daily dose given on a treatment day approximates to 150 mg trimethoprim/m^2/day and 750 mg sulfamethoxazole/m^2/day. The total daily dose should not exceed 320 mg trimethoprim and 1600 mg sulfamethoxazole.

Nocardiosis: There is no consensus on the most appropriate dosage. Adult doses of 6 to 8 tablets daily for up to 3 months have been used (one tablet contains 400 mg sulfamethoxazole and 80 mg trimethoprim).

Toxoplasmosis: There is no consensus on the most appropriate dosage for the treatment or prophylaxis of this condition. The decision should be based on clinical experience. For prophylaxis, however, the dosages suggested for prevention of *Pneumocystis jiroveci* pneumonitis may be appropriate.

4.3 Contraindications

Septrin should not be given to patients with a history of hypersensitivity to sulphonamides, trimethoprim, co-trimoxazole or any excipients of Septrin.

Contra-indicated in patients showing marked liver parenchymal damage.

Contra-indicated in severe renal insufficiency where repeated measurements of the plasma concentration cannot be performed.

Septrin should not be given to premature babies nor to full-term infants during the first 6 weeks of life except for the treatment/prophylaxis of PCP in infants 4 weeks of age or greater.

4.4 Special warnings and precautions for use

Fatalities, although very rare, have occurred due to severe reactions including Stevens-Johnson syndrome, Lyell's syndrome (toxic epidermal necrolysis), fulminant hepatic necrosis, agranulocytosis, aplastic anaemia, other blood dyscrasias and hypersensitivity of the respiratory tract.

Septrin should be discontinued at the first appearance of skin rash. (See 4.8 Undesirable Effects).

Particular care is always advisable when treating elderly patients because, as a group, they are more susceptible to adverse reactions and more likely to suffer serious effects as a result particularly when complicating conditions exist, e.g. impaired kidney and/or liver function and/or concomitant use of other drugs.

An adequate urinary output should be maintained at all times. Evidence of crystalluria *in vivo* is rare, although sulphonamide crystals have been noted in cooled urine from treated patients. In patients suffering from malnutrition the risk may be increased.

Regular monthly blood counts are advisable when Septrin is given for long periods, or to folate deficient patients or to the elderly, since there exists a possibility of asymptomatic changes in haematological laboratory indices due to lack of available folate. These changes may be reversed by administration of folinic acid (5 to 10 mg/day) without interfering with the antibacterial activity.

In glucose-6-phosphate dehydrogenase (G-6-PD) deficient patients haemolysis may occur.

Septrin should be given with caution to patients with severe allergy or bronchial asthma.

Septrin should not be used in the treatment of streptococcal pharyngitis due to Group A beta-haemolytic streptococci; eradication of these organisms from the oropharynx is less effective than with penicillin.

Trimethoprim has been noted to impair phenylalanine metabolism but this is of no significance in phenylketonuric patients on appropriate dietary restriction.

The administration of Septrin to patients known or suspected to be at risk of acute porphyria should be avoided. Both trimethoprim and sulphonamides (although not specifically sulfamethoxazole) have been associated with clinical exacerbation of porphyria.

Close monitoring of serum potassium and sodium is warranted in patients at risk of hyperkalaemia and hyponatraemia.

Except under careful supervision Septrin should not be given to patients with serious haematological disorders (see 4.8 Undesirable Effects). Septrin has been given to patients receiving cytotoxic therapy with little or no additional effect on the bone marrow or peripheral blood.

The combination of antibiotics in Septrin should only be used where, in the judgement of the physician, the benefits of treatment outweigh any possible risks; consideration should be given to the use of a single effective antibacterial agent.

4.5 Interaction with other medicinal products and other forms of interaction

Trimethoprim may interfere with the estimation of serum/plasma creatinine when the alkaline picrate reaction is used. This may result in overestimation of serum/plasma creatinine of the order of 10%. The creatinine clearance is reduced: the renal tubular secretion of creatinine is decreased from 23% to 9% whilst the glomerular filtration remains unchanged.

In some situations, concomitant treatment with zidovudine may increase the risk of haematological adverse reactions to co-trimoxazole. If concomitant treatment is necessary, consideration should be given to monitoring of haematological parameters.

Reversible deterioration in renal function has been observed in patients treated with co-trimoxazole and cyclosporin following renal transplantation.

Concurrent use of rifampicin and Septrin results in a shortening of the plasma half-life of trimethoprim after a period of about one week. This is not thought to be of clinical significance.

When trimethoprim is administered simultaneously with drugs that form cations at physiological pH, and are also partly excreted by active renal secretion (e.g. procainamide, amantadine), there is the possibility of competitive inhibition of this process which may lead to an increase in plasma concentration of one or both of the drugs.

In elderly patients concurrently receiving diuretics, mainly thiazides, there appears to be an increased risk of thrombocytopenia with or without purpura.

Occasional reports suggest that patients receiving pyrimethamine at doses in excess of 25 mg weekly may develop megaloblastic anaemia should co-trimoxazole be prescribed concurrently.

Co-trimoxazole has been shown to potentiate the anticoagulant activity of warfarin via stereo-selective inhibition of its metabolism. Sulfamethoxazole may displace warfarin from plasma-albumin protein-binding sites *in vitro*. Careful control of the anticoagulant therapy during treatment with Septrin is advisable.

Co-trimoxazole prolongs the half-life of phenytoin and if co-administered could result in excessive phenytoin effect. Close monitoring of the patient's condition and serum phenytoin levels are advisable.

Concomitant use of trimethoprim with digoxin has been shown to increase plasma digoxin levels in a proportion of elderly patients.

Co-trimoxazole may increase the free plasma levels of methotrexate.

Trimethoprim interferes with assays for serum methotrexate when dihydrofolate reductase from *Lactobacillus casei* is used in the assay. No interference occurs if methotrexate is measured by radioimmuno assay.

Administration of trimethoprim/sulfamethoxazole 160mg/800mg (co-trimoxazole) causes a 40% increase in lamivudine exposure because of the trimethoprim component. Lamivudine has no effect on the pharmacokinetics of trimethoprim or sulfamethoxazole.

Interaction with sulphonylurea hypoglycaemic agents is uncommon but potentiation has been reported.

Caution should be exercised in patients taking any other drugs that can cause hyperkalaemia.

If Septrin is considered appropriate therapy in patients receiving other anti-folate drugs such as methotrexate, a folate supplement should be considered.

4.6 Pregnancy and lactation

Pregnancy

There are not any adequate data from the use of Septrin in pregnant women. Case-control studies have shown that there may be an association between exposure to folate antagonists and birth defects in humans.

Trimethoprim is a folate antagonist and, in animal studies, both agents have been shown to cause foetal abnormalities (see 5.3 Preclinical Safety Data). Septrin should not be used in pregnancy, particularly in the first trimester, unless clearly necessary. Folate supplementation should be considered if Septrin is used in pregnancy.

Sulfamethoxazole competes with bilirubin for binding to plasma albumin. As significantly maternally derived drug levels persist for several days in the newborn, there may be a risk of precipitating or exacerbating neonatal hyperbilirubinaemia, with an associated theoretical risk of kernicterus, when Septrin is administered to the mother near the time of delivery. This theoretical risk is particularly relevant in infants at increased risk of hyperbilirubinaemia, such as those who are preterm and those with glucose-6-phosphate dehydrogenase deficiency.

Lactation

The components of Septrin (trimethoprim and sulfamethoxazole) are excreted in breast milk. Administration of Septrin should be avoided in late pregnancy and in lactating mothers where the mother or infant has, or is at particular risk of developing, hyperbilirubinaemia. Additionally, administration of Septrin should be avoided in infants younger than eight weeks in view of the predisposition of young infants to hyperbilirubinaemia.

4.7 Effects on ability to drive and use machines

There have been no studies to investigate the effect of Septrin on driving performance or the ability to operate machinery. Further a detrimental effect on such activities cannot be predicted from the pharmacology of the drug. Nevertheless the clinical status of the patient and the adverse events profile of Septrin should be borne in mind when considering the patients ability to operate machinery.

4.8 Undesirable effects

As co-trimoxazole contains trimethoprim and a sulphonamide the type and frequency of adverse reactions associated with such compounds are expected to be consistent with extensive historical experience.

Data from large published clinical trials were used to determine the frequency of very common to rare adverse events. Very rare adverse events were primarily determined from post-marketing experience data and therefore refer to reporting rate rather than a "true" frequency. In addition, adverse events may vary in their incidence depending on the indication.

The following convention has been used for the classification of adverse events in terms of frequency:- Very common $\geqslant 1/10$, common $\geqslant 1/100$ and $< 1/10$, uncommon $\geqslant 1/1000$ and $< 1/100$, rare $\geqslant 1/10,000$ and $< 1/1000$, very rare $< 1/10,000$.

Infections and Infestations

Common: Monilial overgrowth

Blood and lymphatic system disorders

Very rare: Leucopenia, neutropenia, thrombocytopenia, agranulocytosis, megaloblastic anaemia, aplastic anaemia, haemolytic anaemia, methaemoglobinaemia, eosinophilia, purpura, haemolysis in certain susceptible G-6-PD deficient patients

Immune system disorders

Very rare: Serum sickness, anaphylaxis, allergic myocarditis, angioedema, drug fever, allergic vasculitis resembling Henoch-Schoenlein purpura, periarteritis nodosa, systemic lupus erythematosus

Metabolism and nutrition disorders

Very common: Hyperkalaemia

Very rare: Hypoglycaemia, hyponatraemia, anorexia

Psychiatric disorders

Very rare: Depression, hallucinations

Nervous system disorders

Common: Headache

Very rare: Aseptic meningitis, convulsions, peripheral neuritis, ataxia, vertigo, tinnitus, dizziness

Aseptic meningitis was rapidly reversible on withdrawal of the drug, but recurred in a number of cases on re-exposure to either co-trimoxazole or to trimethoprim alone.

Respiratory, thoracic and mediastinal disorders

Very rare: Cough, shortness of breath, pulmonary infiltrates

Cough, shortness of breath and pulmonary infiltrates may be early indicators of respiratory hypersensitivity which, while very rare, has been fatal.

Gastrointestinal disorders

Common: Nausea, diarrhoea

Uncommon: Vomiting

Very rare: Glossitis, stomatitis, pseudomembranous colitis, pancreatitis

Eye Disorders

Very rare: Uveitis

Hepatobiliary disorders

Very rare: Elevation of serum transaminases, elevation of bilirubin levels, cholestatic jaundice, hepatic necrosis

Cholestatic jaundice and hepatic necrosis may be fatal.

Skin and subcutaneous tissue disorders

Common: Skin rashes

Very rare: Photosensitivity, exfoliative dermatitis, fixed drug eruption, erythema multiforme, Stevens-Johnson syndrome, Lyell's syndrome (toxic epidermal necrolysis)

Lyell's syndrome carries a high mortality.

Musculoskeletal and connective tissue disorders

Very rare: Arthralgia, myalgia

Renal and urinary disorders

Very rare: Impaired renal function (sometimes reported as renal failure), interstitial nephritis

Effects associated with *Pneumocystis jiroveci (P.carinii)* Pneumonitis (PCP) management

Very rare: Severe hypersensitivity reactions, rash, fever, neutropenia, thrombocytopenia, raised liver enzymes, hyperkalaemia, hyponatraemia, rhabdomyolysis.

At the high dosages used for PCP management severe hypersensitivity reactions have been reported, necessitating cessation of therapy. If signs of bone marrow depression occur, the patient should be given calcium folinate supplementation (5-10 mg/day). Severe hypersensitivity reactions have been reported in PCP patients on re-exposure to co-trimoxazole, sometimes after a dosage interval of a few days. Rhabdomyolysis has been reported in HIV positive patients receiving co-tromixazole for prophylaxis or treatment of PCP.

4.9 Overdose

Nausea, vomiting, dizziness and confusion are likely signs/symptoms of overdosage. Bone marrow depression has been reported in acute trimethoprim overdosage.

If vomiting has not occurred, induction of vomiting may be desirable. Gastric lavage may be useful, though absorption from the gastrointestinal tract is normally very rapid and complete within approximately two hours. This may not be the case in gross overdosage. Dependant on the status of renal function administration of fluids is recommended if urine output is low.

Both trimethoprim and active sulphamethoxazole are moderately dialysable by haemodialysis. Peritoneal dialysis is not effective.

5. PHARMACOLOGICAL PROPERTIES

5.1 Pharmacodynamic properties

Pharmacotherapeutic group: Combinations of sulfonamides and trimethoprim, incl. derivatives; ATC code: J01EE01

Mode of Action

Septrin is an antibacterial drug composed of two active principles, sulfamethoxazole and trimethoprim. Sulfamethoxazole is a competitive inhibitor of dihydropteroate synthetase enzyme. Sulfamethoxazole competitively inhibits the utilisation of para-aminobenzoic acid (PABA) in the synthesis of dihydrofolate by the bacterial cell resulting in bacteriostasis. Trimethoprim binds to and reversibly inhibits bacterial dihydrofolate reductase (DHFR) and blocks the production of tetrahydrofolate. Depending on the conditions the effect may be bactericidal. Thus trimethoprim and sulfamethoxazole block two consecutive steps in the biosynthesis of purines and therefore nucleic acids essential to many bacteria. This action produces marked potentiation of activity *in vitro* between the two agents.

Mechanism of resistance

In vitro studies have shown that bacterial resistance can develop more slowly with both sulfamethoxazole and trimethoprim in combination that with either sulfamethoxazole or trimethoprim alone.

Resistance to sulfamethoxazole may occur by different mechanisms. Bacterial mutations cause an increase the concentration of PABA and thereby out-compete with sulfamethoxazole resulting in a reduction of the inhibitory effect on dihydropteroate synthetase enzyme. Another resistance mechanism is plasmid-mediated and results from production of an altered dihydropteroate synthetase enzyme, with reduced affinity for sulfamethoxazole compared to the wild-type enzyme.

Resistance to trimethoprim occurs through a plasmid-mediated mutation which results in production of an altered dihydrofolate reductase enzyme having a reduced affinity for trimethoprim compared to the wild-type enzyme.

Trimethoprim binds to plasmodial DHFR but less tightly than to bacterial enzyme. Its affinity for mammalian DHFR is some 50,000 times less than for the corresponding bacterial enzyme.

Many common pathogenic bacteria are susceptible *in vitro* to trimethoprim and sulfamethoxazole at concentrations well below those reached in blood, tissue fluids and urine after the administration of recommended doses. In common with other antibiotics, however, *in vitro* activity does not necessarily imply that clinical efficacy has been demonstrated and it must be noted that satisfactory susceptibility testing is achieved only with recommended media free from inhibitory substances, especially thymidine and thymine.

Breakpoints

EUCAST

Enterobacteriaceae: S≤ 2 R> 4

S. maltophilia: S≤ 4 R> 4

Acinetobacter: S≤ 2 R> 4

Staphylococcus: S≤ 2 R> 4

Enterococcus: S≤ 0.032 R> 1

Streptococcus ABCG: S≤ 1 R> 2

Streptococcus pneumoniae: S≤ 1 R> 2

Hemophilus influenza: S≤ 0.5 R> 1

Moraxella catarrhalis: S≤0.5 R>1

Psuedomonas aeruginosa and other non-enterobacteriaceae: S≤ 2* R> 4*

S = susceptible, R = resistant. *These are CLSI breakpoints since no EUCAST breakpoints are currently available for these organisms.

Trimethoprim: sulfamethoxazole in the ratio 1:19. Breakpoints are expressed as trimethoprim concentration.

Antibacterial Spectrum

The prevalence of resistance may vary geographically and with time for selected species and local information on resistance is desirable, particularly when treating severe infections. As necessary, expert advice should be sought when the local prevalence of resistance is such that the utility of the agent in at least some types of infections is questionable. This information gives only an approximate guidance on probabilities whether microorganisms will be susceptible to trimethoprim/sulfamethoxazole or not.

Trimethoprim/sulfamethoxazole susceptibility against a number of bacteria are shown in the table below:

Commonly susceptible species:
Gram-positive aerobes: *Staphylococcus aureus* *Staphylococcus saprophyticus* *Streptococcus pyogenes*
Gram-negative aerobes: *Enterobacter cloacae* *Haemophilus influenzae* *Klebsiella oxytoca* *Moraxella catarrhalis* *Salmonella* spp. *Stenotrophomonas maltophilia* *Yersinia* spp.
Species for which acquired resistance may be a problem:
Gram-positive aerobes: *Enterococcus faecalis* *Enterococcus faecium* *Nocardia* spp. *Staphylococcus epidermidis* *Streptococcus pneumoniae*
Gram-negative aerobes: *Citrobacter* spp. *Enterobacter aerogenes* *Escherichia coli* *Klebsiella pneumoniae* *Klebsiella pneumonia* *Proteus mirabilis* *Proteus vulgaris* *Providencia* spp. *Serratia marcesans*
Inherently resistant organisms:
Gram-negative aerobes: *Pseudomonas aeruginosa* *Shigella* spp. *Vibrio cholera*

5.2 Pharmacokinetic properties

After oral administration trimethoprim and sulfamethoxazole are rapidly and nearly completely absorbed. The presence of food does not appear to delay absorption. Peak levels in the blood occur between one and four hours after ingestion and the level attained is dose related. Effective levels persist in the blood for up to 24 hours after a therapeutic dose. Steady state levels in adults are reached after dosing for 2-3 days. Neither component has an appreciable effect on the concentrations achieved in the blood by the other.

Trimethoprim is a weak base with a pKa of 7.4. It is lipophilic. Tissue levels of trimethoprim are generally higher than corresponding plasma levels, the lungs and kidneys showing especially high concentrations. Trimethoprim concentrations exceed those in plasma in the case of bile, prostatic fluid and tissue, saliva, sputum and vaginal secretions. Levels in the aqueous humor, breast milk, cerebrospinal fluid, middle ear fluid, synovial fluid and tissue (intestinal) fluid are adequate for antibacterial activity. Trimethoprim passes into amniotic fluid and foetal tissues reaching concentrations approximating those of maternal serum.

Approximately 50% of trimethoprim in the plasma is protein bound. The halflife in man is in the range 8.6 to 17 hours in the presence of normal renal function. It is increased by a factor of 1.5 to 3.0 when the creatinine clearance is less than 10 ml/minute. There appears to be no significant difference in the elderly compared with young patients.

The principal route of excretion of trimethoprim is renal and approximately 50% of the dose is excreted in the urine within 24 hours as unchanged drug. Several metabolites have been identified in the urine. Urinary concentrations of trimethoprim vary widely.

Sulfamethoxazole is a weak acid with a pKa of 6.0. The concentration of active sulfamethoxazole in a variety of body fluids is of the order of 20 to 50% of the plasma concentration.

Approximately 66% of sulfamethoxazole in the plasma is protein bound. The half-life in man is approximately 9 to 11 hours in the presence of normal renal function. There is no change in the half-life of active sulfamethoxazole with a reduction in renal function but there is prolongation of the half-life of the major, acetylated metabolite when the creatinine clearance is below 25 ml/minute.

The principal route of excretion of sulfamethoxazole is renal; between 15% and 30% of the dose recovered in the urine is in the active form. In elderly patients there is a reduced renal clearance of sulphamethoxazole.

5.3 Preclinical safety data

Reproductive toxicology:

At doses in excess of recommended human therapeutic dose, trimethoprim and sulfamethoxazole have been reported to cause cleft palate and other foetal abnormalities in rats, findings typical of a folate antagonist. Effects with trimethoprim were preventable by administration of dietary folate. In rabbits, foetal loss was seen at doses of trimethoprim in excess of human therapeutic doses.

6. PHARMACEUTICAL PARTICULARS

6.1 List of excipients

Povidone

Sodium Starch Glycollate

Magnesium Stearate

Docusate Sodium

6.2 Incompatibilities

None Known

6.3 Shelf life

60 months

6.4 Special precautions for storage

Do not store above 25° C

Keep container in the outer carton.

6.5 Nature and contents of container

Polypropylene container with polyethylene snap-fit closure or PVC/Al Foil blister packs

Pack Size: 100

Round enamelled tin

Pack size: 2000

PVC/Aluminium foil blister pack (sample pack)

Pack size: 5

6.6 Special precautions for disposal and other handling

Trimethoprim interferes with assays for serum methotrexate when dihydrofolate reductase from *Lactobacillus casei* is used in the assay. No interference occurs if methotrexate is measured by radioimmuno assay.

Trimethoprim may interfere with the estimation of serum/plasma creatinine when the alkaline picrate reaction is used. This may result in overestimation of serum/plasma creatinine of the order of 10%. Functional inhibition of the renal tubular secretion of creatinine may produce a spurious fall in the estimated rate of creatinine clearance.

7. MARKETING AUTHORISATION HOLDER

The Wellcome Foundation Ltd

Glaxo Wellcome House

Berkeley Avenue

Greenford,

Middlesex, UB6 0NN

Trading as:
GlaxoSmithKline UK
Stockley Park West
Uxbridge
Middlesex UB11 1BT

8. MARKETING AUTHORISATION NUMBER(S)
PL 00003/0121

9. DATE OF FIRST AUTHORISATION/RENEWAL OF THE AUTHORISATION
Date of first authorisation: 14 April 1977
Date of last renewal: 15 July 2003

10. DATE OF REVISION OF THE TEXT
21 July 2009

Septrin Paediatric Suspension

(GlaxoSmithKline UK)

1. NAME OF THE MEDICINAL PRODUCT
Septrin 40 mg/200 mg per 5 ml Paediatric Suspension

2. QUALITATIVE AND QUANTITATIVE COMPOSITION
Each 5 ml contains 200 mg Sulfamethoxazole and 40 mg Trimethoprim

Excipients:

This product contains less than 1 mmol of sodium (23 mg) per dose, and therefore is essentially sodium free.

Also contains 3.25 g sorbitol per 5 ml and less than 100 mg of ethanol per 5 ml.

For a full list of excipients, see Section 6.1

3. PHARMACEUTICAL FORM
Suspension
Off white in colour.

4. CLINICAL PARTICULARS

4.1 Therapeutic indications
Septrin Paediatric Suspension is indicated for the treatment of the following infections when owing to sensitive organisms (see section 5.1):

Treatment and prevention of *Pneumocystis jiroveci (P. carinii)* pneumonitis

Treatment and prophylaxis of toxoplasmosis

Treatment of nocardiosis

The following infections may be treated with Septrin where there is bacterial evidence of sensitivity to Septrin and good reason to prefer the combination of antibiotics in Septrin to a single antibiotic:

Acute uncomplicated urinary tract infection

Acute otitis media

Acute exacerbation of chronic bronchitis

Consideration should be given to official guidance on the appropriate use of antibacterial agents.

4.2 Posology and method of administration
Method of administration: oral.

It may be preferable to take Septrin with some food or drink to minimise the possibility of gastrointestinal disturbances.

Standard dosage recommendations for acute infections

Children aged 12 years and under:

STANDARD DOSAGE	
Age	Paediatric Suspension
6 to 12 years	10 ml every 12 hours
6 months to 5 years	5 ml every 12 hours
6 weeks to 5 months	2.5 ml every 12 hours

This dosage approximates to 6 mg trimethoprim and 30 mg sulfamethoxazole per kilogram body weight per 24 hours.

Treatment should be continued until the patient has been symptom free for two days; the majority will require treatment for at least 5 days. If clinical improvement is not evident after 7 days' therapy, the patient should be reassessed.

As an alternative to Standard Dosage for acute uncomplicated lower urinary tract infections, short-term therapy of 1 to 3 days' duration has been shown to be effective.

Special dosage recommendations

(Standard dosage applies unless otherwise specified)

Pneumocystis jiroveci (P. carinii) pneumonitis:

Treatment: A higher dosage is recommended using 20 mg trimethoprim and 100 mg sulfamethoxazole per kg of body weight per day in two or more divided doses for two weeks. The aim is to obtain peak plasma or serum levels of trimethoprim of greater than or equal to 5 microgram/ml (verified in patients receiving 1-hour infusions of intravenous Septrin). (See 4.8 Undesirable Effects).

Prevention:

The following dose schedules may be used for the duration of the period at risk (see Standard dosage recommendations for acute infections subsection of 4.2):

– Standard dosage taken in two divided doses, seven days per week

– Standard dosage taken in two divided doses, three times per week on alternate days

– Standard dosage taken in two divided doses, three times per week on consecutive days

– Standard dosage taken as a single dose, three times per week on consecutive days

The daily dose given on a treatment day approximates to 150 mg trimethoprim/m^2/day and 750 mg sulfamethoxazole/m^2/day. The total daily dose should not exceed 320 mg trimethoprim and 1600 mg sulfamethoxazole.

Nocardiosis: There is no consensus on the most appropriate dosage. Adult doses of 6 to 8 tablets daily for up to 3 months have been used (one tablet contains 400 mg sulfamethoxazole and 80 mg trimethoprim).

Toxoplasmosis: There is no consensus on the most appropriate dosage for the treatment or prophylaxis of this condition. The decision should be based on clinical experience. For prophylaxis, however, the dosages suggested for prevention of *Pneumocystis jiroveci* pneumonitis may be appropriate.

Children aged 12 years and under with renal impairment:

No data are available relating to dosage in children aged 12 years and under with impaired renal function.

Children aged 12 years and under with hepatic impairment:

No data are available relating to dosage in children aged 12 years and under with impaired hepatic function.

4.3 Contraindications
Septrin should not be given to patients with a history of hypersensitivity to sulphonamides, trimethoprim, co-trimoxazole, or any excipients of Septrin.

Contra-indicated in patients showing marked liver parenchymal damage.

Contra-indicated in severe renal insufficiency where repeated measurements of the plasma concentration cannot be performed.

Septrin should not be given to premature babies nor to full-term infants during the first 6 weeks of life except for the treatment/prophylaxis of PCP in infants 4 weeks of age or greater.

4.4 Special warnings and precautions for use
Fatalities, although very rare, have occurred due to severe reactions including Stevens-Johnson syndrome, Lyell's syndrome (toxic epidermal necrolysis), fulminant hepatic necrosis, agranulocytosis, aplastic anaemia, other blood dyscrasias and hypersensitivity of the respiratory tract.

Septrin should be discontinued at the first appearance of skin rash. (See 4.8 Undesirable Effects).

Particular care is *always* advisable when treating elderly patients because, as a group, they are more susceptible to adverse reactions and more likely to suffer serious effects as a result particularly when complicating conditions exist, e.g. impaired kidney and/or liver function and/or concomitant use of other drugs.

An adequate urinary output should be maintained at all times. Evidence of crystalluria *in vivo* is rare, although sulphonamide crystals have been noted in cooled urine from treated patients. In patients suffering from malnutrition the risk may be increased.

Regular monthly blood counts are advisable when Septrin is given for long periods, or to folate deficient patients or to the elderly, since there exists a possibility of asymptomatic changes in haematological laboratory indices due to lack of available folate. These changes may be reversed by administration of folinic acid (5 to 10 mg/day) without interfering with the antibacterial activity.

In glucose-6-phosphate dehydrogenase (G-6-PD) deficient patients haemolysis may occur.

Septrin should be given with caution to patients with severe allergy or bronchial asthma.

Septrin should not be used in the treatment of streptococcal pharyngitis due to Group A beta-haemolytic streptococci; eradication of these organisms from the oropharynx is less effective than with penicillin.

Trimethoprim has been noted to impair phenylalanine metabolism but this is of no significance in phenylketonuric patients on appropriate dietary restriction.

The administration of Septrin to patients known or suspected to be at risk of acute porphyria should be avoided. Both trimethoprim and sulphonamides (although not specifically sulfamethoxazole) have been associated with clinical exacerbation of porphyria.

Close monitoring of serum potassium and sodium is warranted in patients at risk of hyperkalaemia and hyponatraemia.

Except under careful supervision Septrin should not be given to patients with serious haematological disorders (see 4.8 Undesirable Effects). Septrin has been given to patients receiving cytotoxic therapy with little or no additional effect on the bone marrow or peripheral blood.

The combination of antibiotics in Septrin should only be used where, in the judgement of the physician, the benefits of treatment outweigh any possible risks; consideration should be given to the use of a single effective antibacterial agent.

Patients with rare hereditary problems of fructose intolerance should not take this medicine. See Section 2 Quantitative and Qualitative Composition.

This medicinal product contains methyl hydroxybenzoate, which may cause allergic reactions (possibly delayed).

This medicinal product contains small amounts of ethanol (alcohol), less than 100 mg per 5 ml.

This medicinal product contains less than 1 mmol of sodium (23 mg) per dose, and therefore is essentially sodium free.

4.5 Interaction with other medicinal products and other forms of interaction
Trimethoprim may interfere with the estimation of serum/plasma creatinine when the alkaline picrate reaction is used. This may result in overestimation of serum/plasma creatinine of the order of 10%. The creatinine clearance is reduced: the renal tubular secretion of creatinine is decreased from 23% to 9% whilst the glomerular filtration remains unchanged.

In some situations, concomitant treatment with zidovudine may increase the risk of haematological adverse reactions to co-trimoxazole. If concomitant treatment is necessary, consideration should be given to monitoring of haematological parameters.

Reversible deterioration in renal function has been observed in patients treated with co-trimoxazole and cyclosporin following renal transplantation.

Concurrent use of rifampicin and Septrin results in a shortening of the plasma half-life of trimethoprim after a period of about one week. This is not thought to be of clinical significance.

When trimethoprim is administered simultaneously with drugs that form cations at physiological pH, and are also partly excreted by active renal secretion (e.g. procainamide, amantadine), there is the possibility of competitive inhibition of this process which may lead to an increase in plasma concentration of one or both of the drugs.

In elderly patients concurrently receiving diuretics, mainly thiazides, there appears to be an increased risk of thrombocytopenia with or without purpura.

Occasional reports suggest that patients receiving pyrimethamine at doses in excess of 25 mg weekly may develop megaloblastic anaemia should co-trimoxazole be prescribed concurrently.

Co-trimoxazole has been shown to potentiate the anticoagulant activity of warfarin via stereo-selective inhibition of its metabolism. Sulfamethoxazole may displace warfarin from plasma-albumin protein-binding sites *in vitro*. Careful control of the anticoagulant therapy during treatment with Septrin is advisable.

Co-trimoxazole prolongs the half-life of phenytoin and if co-administered could result in excessive phenytoin effect. Close monitoring of the patient's condition and serum phenytoin levels are advisable.

Concomitant use of trimethoprim with digoxin has been shown to increase plasma digoxin levels in a proportion of elderly patients.

Co-trimoxazole may increase the free plasma levels of methotrexate.

Trimethoprim interferes with assays for serum methotrexate when dihydrofolate reductase from *Lactobacillus casei* is used in the assay. No interference occurs if methotrexate is measured by radioimmuno assay.

Administration of trimethoprim/sulfamethoxazole 160mg/800mg (co-trimoxazole) causes a 40% increase in lamivudine exposure because of the trimethoprim component. Lamivudine has no effect on the pharmacokinetics of trimethoprim or sulfamethoxazole.

Interaction with sulphonylurea hypoglycaemic agents is uncommon but potentiation has been reported.

Caution should be exercised in patients taking any other drugs that can cause hyperkalaemia.

If Septrin is considered appropriate therapy in patients receiving other anti-folate drugs such as methotrexate, a folate supplement should be considered.

4.6 Pregnancy and lactation
Pregnancy

There are not any adequate data from the use of Septrin in pregnant women. Case-control studies have shown that there may be an association between exposure to folate antagonists and birth defects in humans.

Trimethoprim is a folate antagonist and, in animal studies, both agents have been shown to cause foetal abnormalities (see 5.3 Preclinical Safety Data).

Septrin should not be used in pregnancy, particularly in the first trimester, unless clearly necessary. Folate supplementation should be considered if Septrin is used in pregnancy.

Sulfamethoxazole competes with bilirubin for binding to plasma albumin. As significantly maternally derived drug levels persist for several days in the newborn, there may be a risk of precipitating or exacerbating neonatal hyperbilirubinaemia, with an associated theoretical risk of kernicterus, when Septrin is administered to the mother near the time of delivery. This theoretical risk is particularly relevant in infants at increased risk of hyperbilirubinaemia, such as those who are preterm and those with glucose-6-phosphate dehydrogenase deficiency.

Lactation

The components of Septrin (trimethoprim and sulfamethoxazole) are excreted in breast milk. Administration of Septrin should be avoided in late pregnancy and in lactating mothers where the mother or infant has, or is at particular risk of developing, hyperbilirubinaemia. Additionally, administration of Septrin should be avoided in infants younger than eight weeks in view of the predisposition of young infants to hyperbilirubinaemia.

4.7 Effects on ability to drive and use machines

There have been no studies to investigate the effect of Septrin on driving performance or the ability to operate machinery. Further a detrimental effect on such activities cannot be predicted from the pharmacology of the drug. Nevertheless the clinical status of the patient and the adverse events profile of Septrin should be borne in mind when considering the patients ability to operate machinery.

4.8 Undesirable effects

As co-trimoxazole contains trimethoprim and a sulphonamide the type and frequency of adverse reactions associated with such compounds are expected to be consistent with extensive historical experience.

Data from large published clinical trials were used to determine the frequency of very common to rare adverse events. Very rare adverse events were primarily determined from post-marketing experience data and therefore refer to reporting rate rather than a "true" frequency. In addition, adverse events may vary in their incidence depending on the indication.

The following convention has been used for the classification of adverse events in terms of frequency:- Very common $\geqslant 1/10$, common $\geqslant 1/100$ and $< 1/10$, uncommon $\geqslant 1/1000$ and $< 1/100$, rare $\geqslant 1/10{,}000$ and $< 1/1000$, very rare $< 1/10{,}000$.

Infections and Infestations

Common: Monilial overgrowth

Blood and lymphatic system disorders

Very rare: Leucopenia, neutropenia, thrombocytopenia, agranulocytosis, megaloblastic anaemia, aplastic anaemia, haemolytic anaemia, methaemoglobinaemia, eosinophilia, purpura, haemolysis in certain susceptible G-6-PD deficient patients

Immune system disorders

Very rare: Serum sickness, anaphylaxis, allergic myocarditis, angioedema, drug fever, allergic vasculitis resembling Henoch-Schoenlein purpura, periarteritis nodosa, systemic lupus erythematosus

Metabolism and nutrition disorders

Very common: Hyperkalaemia

Very rare: Hypoglycaemia, hyponatraemia, anorexia

Psychiatric disorders

Very rare: Depression, hallucinations

Nervous system disorders

Common: Headache

Very rare: Aseptic meningitis, convulsions, peripheral neuritis, ataxia, vertigo, tinnitus, dizziness

Aseptic meningitis was rapidly reversible on withdrawal of the drug, but recurred in a number of cases on re-exposure to either co-trimoxazole or to trimethoprim alone.

Respiratory, thoracic and mediastinal disorders

Very rare: Cough, shortness of breath, pulmonary infiltrates

Cough, shortness of breath and pulmonary infiltrates may be early indicators of respiratory hypersensitivity which, while very rare, has been fatal.

Gastrointestinal disorders

Common: Nausea, diarrhoea

Uncommon: Vomiting

Very rare: Glossitis, stomatitis, pseudomembranous colitis, pancreatitis

Eye Disorders

Very rare: Uveitis

Hepatobiliary disorders

Very rare: Elevation of serum transaminases, elevation of bilirubin levels, cholestatic jaundice, hepatic necrosis

Cholestatic jaundice and hepatic necrosis may be fatal.

Skin and subcutaneous tissue disorders

Common: Skin rashes

Very rare: Photosensitivity, exfoliative dermatitis, fixed drug eruption, erythema multiforme, Stevens-Johnson syndrome, Lyell's syndrome (toxic epidermal necrolysis)

Lyell's syndrome carries a high mortality.

Musculoskeletal and connective tissue disorders

Very rare: Arthralgia, myalgia

Renal and urinary disorders

Very rare: Impaired renal function (sometimes reported as renal failure), interstitial nephritis

Effects associated with *Pneumocystis jiroveci (P. carinii)* Pneumonitis (PCP) management

Very rare: Severe hypersensitivity reactions, rash, fever, neutropenia, thrombocytopenia, raised liver enzymes, hyperkalaemia, hyponatraemia, rhabdomyolysis.

At the high dosages used for PCP management severe hypersensitivity reactions have been reported, necessitating cessation of therapy. If signs of bone marrow depression occur, the patient should be given calcium folinate supplementation (5-10 mg/day). Severe hypersensitivity reactions have been reported in PCP patients on re-exposure to co-trimoxazole, sometimes after a dosage interval of a few days. Rhabdomyolysis has been reported in HIV positive patients receiving co-trimoxazole for prophylaxis or treatment of PCP.

4.9 Overdose

Nausea, vomiting, dizziness and confusion are likely signs/symptoms of overdosage. Bone marrow depression has been reported in acute trimethoprim overdosage.

If vomiting has not occurred, induction of vomiting may be desirable. Gastric lavage may be useful, though absorption from the gastrointestinal tract is normally very rapid and complete within approximately two hours. This may not be the case in gross overdosage. Dependant on the status of renal function administration of fluids is recommended if urine output is low.

Both trimethoprim and active sulfamethoxazole are moderately dialysable by haemodialysis. Peritoneal dialysis is not effective.

5. PHARMACOLOGICAL PROPERTIES

5.1 Pharmacodynamic properties

Pharmacotherapeutic group: Combinations of sulfonamides and trimethoprim, incl. derivatives; ATC code: J01EE01

Mode of Action

Septrin is an antibacterial drug composed of two active principles, sulfamethoxazole and trimethoprim. Sulfamethoxazole is a competitive inhibitor of dihydropteroate synthetase enzyme. Sulfamethoxazole competitively inhibits the utilisation of para-aminobenzoic acid (PABA) in the synthesis of dihydrofolate by the bacterial cell resulting in bacteriostasis. Trimethoprim binds to and reversibly inhibits bacterial dihydrofolate reductase (DHFR) and blocks the production of tetrahydrofolate. Depending on the conditions the effect may be bactericidal. Thus trimethoprim and sulfamethoxazole block two consecutive steps in the biosynthesis of purines and therefore nucleic acids essential to many bacteria. This action produces marked potentiation of activity *in vitro* between the two agents.

Mechanism of resistance

In vitro studies have shown that bacterial resistance can develop more slowly with both sulfamethoxazole and trimethoprim in combination that with either sulfamethoxazole or trimethoprim alone.

Resistance to sulfamethoxazole may occur by different mechanisms. Bacterial mutations cause an increase the concentration of PABA and thereby out-compete with sulfamethoxazole resulting in a reduction of the inhibitory effect on dihydropteroate synthetase enzyme. Another resistance mechanism is plasmid-mediated and results from production of an altered dihydropteroate synthetase enzyme, with reduced affinity for sulfamethoxazole compared to the wild-type enzyme.

Resistance to trimethoprim occurs through a plasmid-mediated mutation which results in production of an altered dihydrofolate reductase enzyme having a reduced affinity for trimethoprim compared to the wild-type enzyme.

Trimethoprim binds to plasmodial DHFR but less tightly than to bacterial enzyme. Its affinity for mammalian DHFR is some 50,000 times less than for the corresponding bacterial enzyme.

Many common pathogenic bacteria are susceptible *in vitro* to trimethoprim and sulfamethoxazole at concentrations well below those reached in blood, tissue fluids and urine after the administration of recommended doses. In common with other antibiotics, however, *in vitro* activity does not necessarily imply that clinical efficacy has been demonstrated and it must be noted that satisfactory susceptibility testing is achieved only with recommended media free from inhibitory substances, especially thymidine and thymine.

Breakpoints

EUCAST

Enterobacteriaceae: S$\leqslant$ 2 R> 4

S. maltophilia: S$\leqslant$ 4 R> 4

Acinetobacter: S$\leqslant$ 2 R> 4

Staphylococcus: S$\leqslant$ 2 R> 4

Enterococcus: S$\leqslant$ 0.032 R> 1

Streptococcus ABCG: S$\leqslant$ 1 R> 2

Streptococcus pneumoniae: S$\leqslant$ 1 R> 2

Hemophilus influenza: S$\leqslant$ 0.5 R> 1

Moraxella catarrhalis: S$\leqslant$0.5 R>1

Psuedomonas aeruginosa and other non-enterobacteriaceae: S$\leqslant$ 2* R> 4*

S = susceptible, R = resistant. *These are CLSI breakpoints since no EUCAST breakpoints are currently available for these organisms.

Trimethoprim: sulfamethoxazole in the ratio 1:19. Breakpoints are expressed as trimethoprim concentration.

Antibacterial Spectrum

The prevalence of resistance may vary geographically and with time for selected species and local information on resistance is desirable, particularly when treating severe infections. As necessary, expert advice should be sought when the local prevalence of resistance is such that the utility of the agent in at least some types of infections is questionable. This information gives only an approximate guidance on probabilities whether microorganisms will be susceptible to trimethoprim/sulfamethoxazole or not.

Trimethoprim/sulfamethoxazole susceptibility against a number of bacteria are shown in the table below:

Commonly susceptible species:
Gram-positive aerobes: *Staphylococcus aureus* *Staphylococcus saprophyticus* *Streptococcus pyogenes*
Gram-negative aerobes: *Enterobacter cloacae* *Haemophilus influenzae* *Klebsiella oxytoca* *Moraxella catarrhalis* *Salmonella* spp. *Stenotrophomonas maltophilia* *Yersinia* spp.
Species for which acquired resistance may be a problem:
Gram-positive aerobes: *Enterococcus faecalis* *Enterococcus faecium* *Nocardia* spp. *Staphylococcus epidermidis* *Streptococcus pneumoniae*
Gram-negative aerobes: *Citrobacter* spp. *Enterobacter aerogenes* *Escherichia coli* *Klebsiella pneumoniae* *Klebsiella pneumonia* *Proteus mirabilis* *Proteus vulgaris* *Providencia* spp. *Serratia marcesans*
Inherently resistant organisms:
Gram-negative aerobes: *Pseudomonas aeruginosa* *Shigella* spp. *Vibrio cholera*

5.2 Pharmacokinetic properties

After oral administration trimethoprim and sulfamethoxazole are rapidly and nearly completely absorbed. The presence of food does not appear to delay absorption. Peak levels in the blood occur between one and four hours after ingestion and the level attained is dose related. Effective levels persist in the blood for up to 24 hours after a therapeutic dose. Steady state levels in adults are reached after dosing for 2-3 days. Neither component has an appreciable effect on the concentrations achieved in the blood by the other.

Trimethoprim is a weak base with a pKa of 7.4. It is lipophilic. Tissue levels of trimethoprim are generally higher than corresponding plasma levels, the lungs and kidneys showing especially high concentrations. Trimethoprim concentrations exceed those in plasma in the case of bile, prostatic fluid and tissue, saliva, sputum and vaginal secretions. Levels in the aqueous humor, breast milk, cerebrospinal fluid, middle ear fluid, synovial fluid and tissue (intestinal) fluid are adequate for antibacterial activity. Trimethoprim passes into amniotic fluid and foetal tissues reaching concentrations approximating those of maternal serum.

Approximately 50% of trimethoprim in the plasma is protein bound. The half-life in man is in the range 8.6 to 17 hours in the presence of normal renal function. It is increased by a factor of 1.5 to 3.0 when the creatinine clearance is less than 10 ml/minute. There appears to be no significant difference in the elderly compared with young patients.

The principal route of excretion of trimethoprim is renal and approximately 50% of the dose is excreted in the urine within 24 hours as unchanged drug. Several metabolites have been identified in the urine. Urinary concentrations of trimethoprim vary widely.

Sulfamethoxazole is a weak acid with a pKa of 6.0. The concentration of active sulfamethoxazole in a variety of body fluids is of the order of 20 to 50% of the plasma concentration.

Approximately 66% of sulfamethoxazole in the plasma is protein bound and the principal route of excretion of sulfamethoxazole is renal. The half-life in man is approximately 9 to 11 hours in the presence of normal renal function. There is no change in the half-life of active sulfamethoxazole with a reduction in renal function but there is prolongation of the half-life of the major, acetylated metabolite when the creatinine clearance is below 25 ml/minute.

The principle route of excretion of sulphamethoxazole is renal; between 15% and 30% of the dose recovered in the urine is in the active form. In elderly patients there is a reduced renal clearance of sulfamethoxazole.

5.3 Preclinical safety data

Reproductive toxicology:

At doses in excess of recommended human therapeutic dose, trimethoprim and sulfamethoxazole have been reported to cause cleft palate and other foetal abnormalities in rats, findings typical of a folate antagonist. Effects with trimethoprim were preventable by administration of dietary folate. In rabbits, foetal loss was seen at doses of trimethoprim in excess of human therapeutic doses.

6. PHARMACEUTICAL PARTICULARS

6.1 List of excipients

Sorbitol solution 70% (non crystallising) (E420 ii)

Glycerol (E422)

Dispersible Cellulose (E460)

Sodium Carmellose

Polysorbate 80 (E433)

Methyl Hydroxybenzoate (E218)

Sodium Benzoate (E211)

Saccharin Sodium (E954)

Ethanol (96%)

Flavour, Banana 81.605P

Flavour, Vanilla 407

Purified Water to 5 ml

6.2 Incompatibilities

None Known

6.3 Shelf life

36 months

6.4 Special precautions for storage

Store below 25°C

Protect from light

6.5 Nature and contents of container

Amber glass bottles with metal roll-on closures.

Pack size: 100 and 30 ml

A double-ended 5mL/2.5mL measuring spoon is included.

Paper/Aluminium foil/ionomer resin sachet

Pack size: 5ml

6.6 Special precautions for disposal and other handling

Trimethoprim interferes with assays for serum methotrexate when dihydrofolate reductase from *Lactobacillus casei* is used in the assay. No interference occurs if methotrexate is measured by radioimmuno assay.

Trimethoprim may interfere with the estimation of serum/plasma creatinine when the alkaline picrate reaction is used. This may result in overestimation of serum/plasma creatinine of the order of 10%. Functional inhibition of the renal tubular secretion of creatinine may produce a spurious fall in the estimated rate of creatinine clearance.

7. MARKETING AUTHORISATION HOLDER

The Wellcome Foundation Ltd

Glaxo Wellcome House

Berkeley Avenue

Greenford,

Middlesex, UB6 0NN

Trading as:

GlaxoSmithKline UK

Stockley Park West

Uxbridge

Middlesex UB11 1BT

8. MARKETING AUTHORISATION NUMBER(S)

PL 00003/5222R

9. DATE OF FIRST AUTHORISATION/RENEWAL OF THE AUTHORISATION

Date of first authorisation: 09 January 1972

Date of last of renewal: 17 October 2006

10. DATE OF REVISION OF THE TEXT

21 July 2009

Septrin Tablets

(GlaxoSmithKline UK)

1. NAME OF THE MEDICINAL PRODUCT

Septrin 80 mg/400 mg Tablets

2. QUALITATIVE AND QUANTITATIVE COMPOSITION

Each tablet contains 400 mg Sulfamethoxazole and 80 mg Trimethoprim

Excipients,

For a full list of excipients, see Section 6.1

3. PHARMACEUTICAL FORM

Tablets.

White, biconvex tablets marked "GX Y2B" with scoreline on one side.

4. CLINICAL PARTICULARS

4.1 Therapeutic indications

Septrin tablets are indicated for the treatment of the following infections when owing to sensitive organisms (see section 5.1):

Treatment and prevention of *Pneumocystis jiroveci (P. carinii)* pneumonitis

Treatment and prophylaxis of toxoplasmosis

Treatment of nocardiosis

The following infections may be treated with Septrin where there is bacterial evidence of sensitivity to Septrin and good reason to prefer the combination of antibiotics in Septrin to a single antibiotic:

Acute uncomplicated urinary tract infection

Acute otitis media

Acute exacerbation of chronic bronchitis

Consideration should be given to official guidance on the appropriate use of antibacterial agents.

4.2 Posology and method of administration

Method of administration: oral

It may be preferable to take Septrin with some food or drink to minimise the possibility of gastrointestinal disturbances.

Standard dosage recommendations for acute infections

Adults and children over 12 years:

Tablets 2 every 12 hours

This dosage approximates to 6 mg trimethoprim and 30 mg sulfamethoxazole per kilogram body weight per 24 hours.

Treatment should be continued until the patient has been symptom free for two days; the majority will require treatment for at least 5 days. If clinical improvement is not evident after 7 days' therapy, the patient should be reassessed.

As an alternative to Standard Dosage for acute uncomplicated lower urinary tract infections, short-term therapy of 1 to 3 days' duration has been shown to be effective.

The elderly:

See Special Warnings and Precautions for Use. Unless otherwise specified standard dosage applies.

Impaired hepatic function:

No data are available relating to dosage in patients with impaired hepatic function.

Special Dosage Recommendations

(Standard dosage applies unless otherwise specified)

Where dosage is expressed as "tablets" this refers to the adult tablet, i.e. 80 mg Trimethoprim BP and 400 mg Sulfamethoxazole BP. If other formulations are to be used appropriate adjustment should be made.

Impaired renal function:

Adults and children over 12 years (no information is available for children under 12 years of age):

Creatinine Clearance (ml/min)	Recommended Dosage
>30	STANDARD DOSAGE
15 to 30	Half the STANDARD DOSAGE
<15	Not recommended

Measurements of plasma concentration of sulfamethoxazole at intervals of 2 to 3 days are recommended in samples obtained 12 hours after administration of Septrin. If the concentration of total sulfamethoxazole exceeds 150 microgram/ml then treatment should be interrupted until the value falls below 120 microgram/ml.

Pneumocystis jiroveci (P.carinii) pneumonitis:

Treatment: A higher dosage is recommended, using 20 mg trimethoprim and 100 mg sulfamethoxazole per kg of body weight per day in two or more divided doses for two weeks. The aim is to obtain peak plasma or serum levels of trimethoprim of greater than or equal to 5 microgram/ml (verified in patients receiving 1-hour infusions of intravenous Septrin). (See 4.8 Undesirable Effects).

Prevention:

Adults: The following dose schedules may be used:

160 mg trimethoprim/800 mg sulfamethoxazole daily 7 days per week.

160 mg trimethoprim/800 mg sulfamethoxazole three times per week on alternate days.

320 mg trimethoprim/1600 mg sulfamethoxazole per day in two divided doses three times per week on alternate days.

Children:

The following dose schedules may be used for the duration of the period at risk (see Standard dosage recommendations for acute infections subsection of 4.2):

– Standard dosage taken in two divided doses, seven days per week

– Standard dosage taken in two divided doses, three times per week on alternate days

– Standard dosage taken in two divided doses, three times per week on consecutive days

– Standard dosage taken as a single dose, three times per week on consecutive days

The daily dose given on a treatment day approximates to 150 mg trimethoprim/m^2/day and 750 mg sulfamethoxazole/m^2/day. The total daily dose should not exceed 320 mg trimethoprim and 1600 mg sulfamethoxazole.

Nocardiosis: There is no consensus on the most appropriate dosage. Adult doses of 6 to 8 tablets daily for up to 3 months have been used.

Toxoplasmosis: There is no consensus on the most appropriate dosage for the treatment or prophylaxis of this condition. The decision should be based on clinical experience. For prophylaxis, however, the dosages suggested for prevention of *Pneumocystis jiroveci* pneumonitis may be appropriate.

4.3 Contraindications

Septrin should not be given to patients with a history of hypersensitivity to sulphonamides, trimethoprim, co-trimoxazole or any excipients of Septrin.

Contra-indicated in patients showing marked liver parenchymal damage.

Contra-indicated in severe renal insufficiency where repeated measurements of the plasma concentration cannot be performed.

Septrin should not be given to premature babies nor to full-term infants during the first 6 weeks of life except for the treatment/prophylaxis of PCP in infants 4 weeks of age or greater.

4.4 Special warnings and precautions for use

Fatalities, although very rare, have occurred due to severe reactions including Stevens-Johnson syndrome, Lyell's syndrome (toxic epidermal necrolysis), fulminant hepatic necrosis, agranulocytosis, aplastic anaemia, other blood dyscrasias and hypersensitivity of the respiratory tract.

Septrin should be discontinued at the first appearance of skin rash.(see 4.8 Undesirable Effects).

Particular care is *always* advisable when treating elderly patients because, as a group, they are more susceptible to adverse reactions and more likely to suffer serious effects as a result particularly when complicating conditions exist, e.g. impaired kidney and/or liver function and/or concomitant use of other drugs.

An adequate urinary output should be maintained at all times. Evidence of crystalluria *in vivo* is rare, although sulphonamide crystals have been noted in cooled urine from treated patients. In patients suffering from malnutrition the risk may be increased.

Regular monthly blood counts are advisable when Septrin is given for long periods, or to folate deficient patients or to the elderly; since there exists a possibility of asymptomatic changes in haematological laboratory indices due to lack of available folate. These changes may be reversed by administration of folinic acid (5 to 10 mg/day) without interfering with the antibacterial activity.

In glucose-6-phosphate dehydrogenase (G-6-PD) deficient patients haemolysis may occur.

Septrin should be given with caution to patients with severe allergy or bronchial asthma.

Septrin should not be used in the treatment of streptococcal pharyngitis due to Group A beta-haemolytic streptococci; eradication of these organisms from the oropharynx is less effective than with penicillin.

Trimethoprim has been noted to impair phenylalanine metabolism but this is of no significance in phenylketonuric patients on appropriate dietary restriction.

The administration of Septrin to patients known or suspected to be at risk of acute porphyria should be avoided. Both trimethoprim and sulphonamides (although not specifically sulfamethoxazole) have been associated with clinical exacerbation of porphyria.

Close monitoring of serum potassium is warranted in patients at risk of hyperkalaemia.

Except under careful supervision Septrin should not be given to patients with serious haematological disorders (see 4.8 Undesirable Effects). Septrin has been given to patients receiving cytotoxic therapy with little or no additional effect on the bone marrow or peripheral blood.

The combination of antibiotics in Septrin should only be used where, in the judgement of the physician, the benefits of treatment outweigh any possible risks; consideration should be given to the use of a single effective antibacterial agent.

4.5 Interaction with other medicinal products and other forms of interaction

Trimethoprim may interfere with the estimation of serum/plasma creatinine when the alkaline picrate reaction is used. This may result in overestimation of serum/plasma creatinine of the order of 10%. The creatinine clearance is reduced: the renal tubular secretion of creatinine is decreased from 23% to 9% whilst the glomerular filtration remains unchanged.

In some situations, concomitant treatment with zidovudine may increase the risk of haematological adverse reactions to co-trimoxazole. If concomitant treatment is necessary, consideration should be given to monitoring of haematological parameters.

Reversible deterioration in renal function has been observed in patients treated with co-trimoxazole and cyclosporin following renal transplantation.

Concurrent use of rifampicin and Septrin results in a shortening of the plasma half-life of trimethoprim after a period of about one week. This is not thought to be of clinical significance.

When trimethoprim is administered simultaneously with drugs that form cations at physiological pH, and are also partly excreted by active renal secretion (e.g. procainamide, amantadine), there is the possibility of competitive inhibition of this process which may lead to an increase in plasma concentration of one or both of the drugs.

In elderly patients concurrently receiving diuretics, mainly thiazides, there appears to be an increased risk of thrombocytopenia with or without purpura.

Occasional reports suggest that patients receiving pyrimethamine at doses in excess of 25 mg weekly may develop megaloblastic anaemia should co-trimoxazole be prescribed concurrently.

Co-trimoxazole has been shown to potentiate the anticoagulant activity of warfarin via stereo-selective inhibition of its metabolism. Sulfamethoxazole may displace warfarin from plasma-albumin protein-binding sites *in vitro*. Careful control of the anticoagulant therapy during treatment with Septrin is advisable.

Co-trimoxazole prolongs the half-life of phenytoin and if co-administered could result in excessive phenytoin effect. Close monitoring of the patient's condition and serum phenytoin levels are advisable.

Concomitant use of trimethoprim with digoxin has been shown to increase plasma digoxin levels in a proportion of elderly patients.

Co-trimoxazole may increase the free plasma levels of methotrexate.

Trimethoprim interferes with assays for serum methotrexate when dihydrofolate reductase from *Lactobacillus casei* is used in the assay. No interference occurs if methotrexate is measured by radioimmuno assay.

Administration of trimethoprim/sulfamethoxazole 160mg/800mg (co-trimoxazole) causes a 40% increase in lamivudine exposure because of the trimethoprim component. Lamivudine has no effect on the pharmacokinetics of trimethoprim or sulfamethoxazole.

Interaction with sulphonylurea hypoglycaemic agents is uncommon but potentiation has been reported.

Caution should be exercised in patients taking any other drugs that can cause hyperkalaemia.

If Septrin is considered appropriate therapy in patients receiving other anti-folate drugs such as methotrexate, a folate supplement should be considered.

4.6 Pregnancy and lactation

Pregnancy

There are not any adequate data from the use of Septrin in pregnant women. Case-control studies have shown that there may be an association between exposure to folate antagonists and birth defects in humans.

Trimethoprim is a folate antagonist and, in animal studies, both agents have been shown to cause foetal abnormalities (see 5.3 Preclinical Safety Data).

Septrin should not be used in pregnancy, particularly in the first trimester, unless clearly necessary. Folate supplementation should be considered if Septrin is used in pregnancy.

Sulfamethoxazole competes with bilirubin for binding to plasma albumin. As significantly maternally derived drug levels persist for several days in the newborn, there may be a risk of precipitating or exacerbating neonatal hyperbilirubinaemia, with an associated theoretical risk of kernicterus, when Septrin is administered to the mother near the time of delivery. This theoretical risk is particularly relevant in infants at increased risk of hyperbilirubinaemia, such as those who are preterm and those with glucose-6-phosphate dehydrogenase deficiency.

Lactation

The components of Septrin (trimethoprim and sulfamethoxazole) are excreted in breast milk. Administration of Septrin should be avoided in late pregnancy and in lactating mothers where the mother or infant has, or is at particular risk of developing, hyperbilirubinaemia. Additionally, administration of Septrin should be avoided in infants younger than eight weeks in view of the predisposition of young infants to hyperbilirubinaemia.

4.7 Effects on ability to drive and use machines

There have been no studies to investigate the effect of Septrin on driving performance or the ability to operate machinery. Further a detrimental effect on such activities cannot be predicted from the pharmacology of the drug. Nevertheless the clinical status of the patient and the adverse events profile of Septrin should be borne in mind when considering the patients ability to operate machinery.

4.8 Undesirable effects

The frequency categories associated with the adverse events below are estimates. For most events, suitable data for estimating incidence were not available. In addition, adverse events may vary in their incidence depending on the indication.

Data from large published clinical trials were used to determine the frequency of very common to rare adverse events. Very rare adverse events were primarily determined from post-marketing experience data and therefore refer to reporting rate rather than a "true" frequency.

The following convention has been used for the classification of adverse events in terms of frequency:- Very common ⩾1/10, common ⩾1/100 and <1/10, uncommon ⩾1/1000 and <1/100, rare ⩾1/10,000 and <1/1000, very rare <1/10,000.

Infections and Infestations

Common:	Monilial overgrowth

Blood and lymphatic system disorders

Very rare:	Leucopenia, neutropenia, thrombocytopenia, agranulocytosis, megaloblastic anaemia, aplastic anaemia, haemolytic anaemia, methaemoglobinaemia, eosinophilia, purpura, haemolysis in certain susceptible G-6-PD deficient patients

The majority of haematological changes are mild and reversible when treatment is stopped. Most of the changes cause no clinical symptoms although they may become severe in isolated cases, especially in the elderly, in those with hepatic or renal dysfunction or in those with poor folate status. Fatalities have been recorded in at-risk patients and these patients should be observed carefully (see 4.3 Contra-indications).

Immune system disorders

Very rare:	Serum sickness, anaphylaxis, allergic myocarditis, angioedema, drug fever, allergic vasculitis resembling Henoch-Schoenlein purpura, periarteritis nodosa, systemic lupus erythematosus

Metabolism and nutrition disorders

Very common:	Hyperkalaemia
Very rare:	Hypoglycaemia, hyponatraemia, anorexia

Close supervision is recommended when co-trimoxazole is used in elderly patients or in patients taking high doses of co-trimoxazole as these patients may be more susceptible to hyperkalaemia and hyponatraemia.

Psychiatric disorders

Very rare:	Depression, hallucinations

Nervous system disorders

Common:	Headache
Very rare:	Aseptic meningitis, convulsions, peripheral neuritis, ataxia, vertigo, tinnitus, dizziness

Aseptic meningitis was rapidly reversible on withdrawal of the drug, but recurred in a number of cases on re-exposure to either co-trimoxazole or to trimethoprim alone.

Respiratory, thoracic and mediastinal disorders

Very rare:	Cough, shortness of breath, pulmonary infiltrates

Cough, shortness of breath and pulmonary infiltrates may be early indicators of respiratory hypersensitivity which, while very rare, has been fatal.

Gastrointestinal disorders

Common:	Nausea, diarrhoea
Uncommon:	Vomiting
Very rare:	Glossitis, stomatitis, pseudomembranous colitis, pancreatitis

Eye Disorders

Very rare:	Uveitis

Hepatobiliary disorders

Very rare:	Elevation of serum transaminases, elevation of bilirubin levels, cholestatic jaundice, hepatic necrosis

Cholestatic jaundice and hepatic necrosis may be fatal.

Skin and subcutaneous tissue disorders

Common:	Skin rashes
Very rare:	Photosensitivity, exfoliative dermatitis, fixed drug eruption, erythema multiforme, Stevens-Johnson syndrome, Lyell's syndrome (toxic epidermal necrolysis)

Lyell's syndrome carries a high mortality.

Musculoskeletal and connective tissue disorders

Very rare:	Arthralgia, myalgia

Renal and urinary disorders

Very rare:	Impaired renal function (sometimes reported as renal failure), interstitial nephritis

Effects associated with *Pneumocystis jiroveci (P.carinii)* Pneumonitis (PCP) management

Very rare:	Severe hypersensitivity reactions, rash, fever, neutropenia, thrombocytopenia, raised liver enzymes, hyperkalaemia, hyponatraemia

At the high dosages used for PCP management severe hypersensitivity reactions have been reported, necessitating cessation of therapy. If signs of bone marrow depression occur, the patient should be given calcium folinate supplementation (5-10 mg/day). Severe hypersensitivity reactions have been reported in PCP patients on re-exposure to co-trimoxazole, sometimes after a dosage interval of a few days.

4.9 Overdose

Nausea, vomiting, dizziness and confusion are likely signs/symptoms of overdosage. Bone marrow depression has been reported in acute trimethoprim overdosage.

If vomiting has not occurred, induction of vomiting may be desirable. Gastric lavage may be useful, though absorption from the gastrointestinal tract is normally very rapid and complete within approximately two hours. This may not be the case in gross overdosage. Dependant on the status of renal function administration of fluids is recommended if urine output is low.

Both trimethoprim and active sulfamethoxazole are moderately dialysable by haemodialysis. Peritoneal dialysis is not effective.

5. PHARMACOLOGICAL PROPERTIES

5.1 Pharmacodynamic properties

Pharmacotherapeutic group: Combinations of sulfonamides and trimethoprim, incl. derivatives; ATC code: J01EE01

Mode of Action

Septrin is an antibacterial drug composed of two active principles, sulfamethoxazole and trimethoprim. Sulfamethoxazole is a competitive inhibitor of dihydropteroate synthetase enzyme. Sulfamethoxazole competitively inhibits the utilisation of para-aminobenzoic acid (PABA) in the synthesis of dihydrofolate by the bacterial cell resulting in bacteriostasis. Trimethoprim binds to and reversibly inhibits bacterial dihydrofolate reductase (DHFR) and blocks the production of tetrahydrofolate. Depending on the conditions the effect may be bactericidal. Thus trimethoprim and sulfamethoxazole block two consecutive steps in the biosynthesis of purines and therefore nucleic acids essential to many bacteria. This action produces marked potentiation of activity *in vitro* between the two agents.

Mechanism of resistance

In vitro studies have shown that bacterial resistance can develop more slowly with both sulfamethoxazole and trimethoprim in combination that with either sulfamethoxazole or trimethoprim alone.

Resistance to sulfamethoxazole may occur by different mechanisms. Bacterial mutations cause an increase the concentration of PABA and thereby out-compete with sulfamethoxazole resulting in a reduction of the inhibitory effect on dihydropteroate synthetase enzyme. Another resistance mechanism is plasmid-mediated and results from production of an altered dihydropteroate synthetase enzyme, with reduced affinity for sulfamethoxazole compared to the wild-type enzyme.

Resistance to trimethoprim occurs through a plasmid-mediated mutation which results in production of an altered dihydrofolate reductase enzyme having a reduced affinity for trimethoprim compared to the wild-type enzyme.

Trimethoprim binds to plasmodial DHFR but less tightly than to bacterial enzyme. Its affinity for mammalian DHFR is some 50,000 times less than for the corresponding bacterial enzyme.

Many common pathogenic bacteria are susceptible *in vitro* to trimethoprim and sulfamethoxazole at concentrations well below those reached in blood, tissue fluids and urine after the administration of recommended doses. In common with other antibiotics, however, *in vitro* activity does not necessarily imply that clinical efficacy has been demonstrated and it must be noted that satisfactory susceptibility testing is achieved only with recommended media free from inhibitory substances, especially thymidine and thymine.

Breakpoints

EUCAST

Enterobacteriaceae: S⩽ 2 R> 4

S. maltophilia: S⩽ 4 R> 4

Acinetobacter: S⩽ 2 R> 4

Staphylococcus: S⩽ 2 R> 4

Enterococcus: S⩽ 0.032 R> 1

Streptococcus ABCG: S⩽ 1 R> 2

Streptococcus pneumoniae: S⩽ 1 R> 2

Hemophilus influenza: S⩽ 0.5 R> 1

Moraxella catarrhalis: S⩽0.5 R>1

Psuedomonas aeruginosa and other non-enterobacteriaceae: S⩽ 2* R> 4*

S = susceptible, R = resistant. *These are CLSI breakpoints since no EUCAST breakpoints are currently available for these organisms.

Trimethoprim: sulfamethoxazole in the ratio 1:19. Breakpoints are expressed as trimethoprim concentration.

Antibacterial Spectrum

The prevalence of resistance may vary geographically and with time for selected species and local information on resistance is desirable, particularly when treating severe infections. As necessary, expert advice should be sought when the local prevalence of resistance is such that the utility of the agent in at least some types of infections is questionable. This information gives only an approximate guidance on probabilities whether microorganisms will be susceptible to trimethoprim/sulfamethoxazole or not.

Trimethoprim/sulfamethoxazole susceptibility against a number of bacteria are shown in the table below:

Commonly susceptible species:
Gram-positive aerobes: *Staphylococcus aureus* *Staphylococcus saprophyticus* *Streptococcus pyogenes*
Gram-negative aerobes: *Enterobacter cloacae* *Haemophilus influenzae* *Klebsiella oxytoca* *Moraxella catarrhalis* *Salmonella* spp. *Stenotrophomonas maltophilia* *Yersinia* spp.
Species for which acquired resistance may be a problem:
Gram-positive aerobes: *Enterococcus faecalis* *Enterococcus faecium* *Nocardia* spp. *Staphylococcus epidermidis* *Streptococcus pneumoniae*
Gram-negative aerobes: *Citrobacter* spp. *Enterobacter aerogenes* *Escherichia coli* *Klebsiella pneumoniae* *Klebsiella pneumonia* *Proteus mirabilis* *Proteus vulgaris* *Providencia* spp. *Serratia marcesans*
Inherently resistant organisms:
Gram-negative aerobes: *Pseudomonas aeruginosa* *Shigella* spp. *Vibrio cholera*

5.2 Pharmacokinetic properties

After oral administration trimethoprim and sulfamethoxazole are rapidly and nearly completely absorbed. The presence of food does not appear to delay absorption. Peak levels in the blood occur between one and four hours after ingestion and the level attained is dose related. Effective levels persist in the blood for up to 24 hours after a therapeutic dose. Steady state levels in adults are reached after dosing for 2-3 days. Neither component has an appreciable effect on the concentrations achieved in the blood by the other.

Trimethoprim is a weak base with a pKa of 7.4. It is lipophilic. Tissue levels of trimethoprim are generally higher than corresponding plasma levels, the lungs and kidneys showing especially high concentrations. Trimethoprim concentrations exceed those in plasma in the case of bile, prostatic fluid and tissue, saliva, sputum and vaginal secretions. Levels in the aqueous humor, breast milk, cerebrospinal fluid, middle ear fluid, synovial fluid and tissue (intestinal) fluid are adequate for antibacterial activity. Trimethoprim passes into amniotic fluid and foetal tissues reaching concentrations approximating those of maternal serum.

Approximately 50% of trimethoprim in the plasma is protein bound. The half-life in man is in the range 8.6 to 17 hours in the presence of normal renal function. It is increased by a factor of 1.5 to 3.0 when the creatinine clearance is less than 10 ml/minute. There appears to be no significant difference in the elderly compared with young patients.

The principal route of excretion of trimethoprim is renal and approximately 50% of the dose is excreted in the urine within 24 hours as unchanged drug. Several metabolites have been identified in the urine. Urinary concentrations of trimethoprim vary widely.

Sulfamethoxazole is a weak acid with a pKa of 6.0. The concentration of active sulfamethoxazole in a variety of body fluids is of the order of 20 to 50% of the plasma concentration.

Approximately 66% of sulfamethoxazole in the plasma is protein bound. The half-life in man is approximately 9 to 11 hours in the presence of normal renal function. There is no change in the half-life of active sulfamethoxazole with a reduction in renal function but there is prolongation of the half-life of the major, acetylated metabolite when the creatinine clearance is below 25 ml/minute.

The principal route of excretion of sulfamethoxazole is renal; between 15% and 30% of the dose recovered in the urine is in the active form. In elderly patients there is a reduced renal clearance of sulphamethoxazole.

5.3 Preclinical safety data

Reproductive toxicology:

At doses in excess of recommended human therapeutic dose, trimethoprim and sulfamethoxazole have been reported to cause cleft palate and other foetal abnormalities in rats, findings typical of a folate antagonist. Effects with trimethoprim were preventable by administration of dietary folate. In rabbits, foetal loss was seen at doses of trimethoprim in excess of human therapeutic doses.

6. PHARMACEUTICAL PARTICULARS

6.1 List of excipients

Tablets

Sodium starch glycollate

Povidone

*Dioctyl sodium sulphosuccinate

*Docusate sodium

Magnesium stearate

*alternative ingredients

6.2 Incompatibilities

See drug interactions.

6.3 Shelf life

5 years.

6.4 Special precautions for storage

Do not store above 25°C. Keep container in the outer carton.

6.5 Nature and contents of container

Amber glass bottles with low density polyethylene snap-fit closures and PVC/Al foil blister pack.

Pack size: 50 and 100

Round enamelled tins with lever lids.

Pack size: 5000

6.6 Special precautions for disposal and other handling

Trimethoprim interferes with assays for serum methotrexate when dihydrofolate reductase from *Lactobacillus casei* is used in the assay. No interference occurs if methotrexate is measured by radioimmuno assay.

Trimethoprim may interfere with the estimation of serum/plasma creatinine when the alkaline picrate reaction is used. This may result in overestimation of serum/plasma creatinine of the order of 10%. Functional inhibition of the renal tubular secretion of creatinine may product a spurious fall in the estimated rate of creatinine clearance.

Administrative Data

7. MARKETING AUTHORISATION HOLDER

The Wellcome Foundation Ltd

Glaxo Wellcome House

Berkeley Avenue

Greenford

Middlesex UB6 ONN

Trading as:

GlaxoSmithKline UK

Stockley Park West

Uxbridge

Middlesex UB11 1BT

8. MARKETING AUTHORISATION NUMBER(S)

PL 00003/0109R

9. DATE OF FIRST AUTHORISATION/RENEWAL OF THE AUTHORISATION

Date of first authorisation: 30 October 1986

Date of last renewal: 8 July 2003

10. DATE OF REVISION OF THE TEXT

21 July 2009

Seractil 300mg Film-Coated Tablets

(Genus Pharmaceuticals)

1. NAME OF THE MEDICINAL PRODUCT

Seractil ▼ 300 mg film-coated tablets

2. QUALITATIVE AND QUANTITATIVE COMPOSITION

Each film-coated tablet contains 300 mg of dexibuprofen.

For excipients, see 6.1.

3. PHARMACEUTICAL FORM

Film-coated tablet

White, round, unscored film-coated tablet.

4. CLINICAL PARTICULARS

4.1 Therapeutic indications

Symptomatic treatment for the relief of pain and inflammation associated with osteoarthritis.

Acute symptomatic treatment of pain during menstrual bleeding (primary dysmenorrhoea).

Symptomatic treatment of other forms of mild to moderate pain, such as muscular-skeletal pain or dental pain.

4.2 Posology and method of administration

The dosage should be adjusted to the severity of the disorder and the complaints of the patient. During chronic administration, the dosage should be adjusted to the lowest maintenance dose that provides adequate control of symptoms.

For individual dosage film-coated tablets with 200, 300 and 400 mg dexibuprofen are available.

The recommended dosage is 600 to 900 mg dexibuprofen daily, divided in up to three single doses.

For the treatment of mild to moderate pain, initially single doses of 200 mg dexibuprofen and daily doses of 600 mg dexibuprofen are recommended.

The maximum single dose is 400 mg dexibuprofen.

The dose may be temporarily increased up to 1200 mg dexibuprofen per day in patients with acute conditions or exacerbations. The maximum daily dose is 1200 mg.

For dysmenorrhoea a daily dose of 600 to 900 mg dexibuprofen, divided in up to three single doses, is recommended. The maximum single dose is 300 mg, the maximum daily dose is 900 mg.

Dexibuprofen has not been studied in children and adolescents (< 18 years): Safety and efficacy have not been established and therefore it is not recommended in these age groups.

In elderly patients it is recommended to start the therapy at the lower end of the dosage range. The dosage may be increased to that recommended for general population only after good general tolerance has been ascertained.

Hepatic dysfunction: Patients with mild to moderate hepatic dysfunction should start therapy at reduced doses and be closely monitored. Dexibuprofen should not be used in patients with severe hepatic dysfunction (see 4.3. Contraindications).

Renal dysfunction: The initial dosage should be reduced in patients with mild to moderate impaired renal function. Dexibuprofen should not be used in patients with severe renal dysfunction (see 4.3. Contraindications).

The film coated tablets can be taken with or without a meal (see 5.2.). In general NSAIDs (non-steroidal anti-inflammatory drugs) are preferably taken with food to reduce gastrointestinal irritation, particularly during chronic use. However, a later onset of action in some patientsmay be anticipated when the tablets are taken with or directly after a meal.

The score in the 200 and 400 mg tablets makes it possible to divide the tablets before administration so as to assist with swallowing.

Dividing the tablets will not provide an exact "half" dose.

4.3 Contraindications

Dexibuprofen must not be administered in the following cases:

- Patients previously sensitive to dexibuprofen, to any other NSAID, or to any of the excipients of the product.
- Patients in whom substances with a similar action (e.g. aspirin or other NSAIDs)

precipitate attacks of asthma, bronchospasm, acute rhinitis, or cause nasal polyps, urticaria or angioneurotic oedema.

- Patients with active or suspected gastrointestinal ulcer or history of recurrent gastrointestinal ulcer.
- Patients who have gastrointestinal bleeding or other active bleedings or bleeding disorders.
- Patients with active Crohn's disease or active ulcerative colitis.
- Patients with severe heart failure.
- Patients with severe renal dysfunction (GFR < 30ml/min).
- Patients with severely impaired hepatic function.
- Patients with haemorrhagic diathesis and other coagulation disorders, or patients receiving anticoagulant therapy.
- From the beginning of 6th month of pregnancy (see 4.6).

4.4 Special warnings and precautions for use

Care is recommended in conditions that predispose patients to the gastrointestinal adverse effects of NSAIDs such as dexibuprofen, including existing gastrointestinal disorders, previous gastric or duodenal ulcer, ulcerative colitis, Crohn's disease and alcoholism.

These patients should be closely monitored for digestive disturbances, especially gastrointestinal bleeding, when taking dexibuprofen or any other NSAID.

Gastrointestinal bleeding or ulceration/perforation have in general more serious consequences in the elderly. They can occur at any time during treatment with or without warning symptoms or a previous history of serious gastrointestinal events.

In the rare instances where gastrointestinal bleeding or ulceration occurs in patients receiving dexibuprofen, treatment should be immediately discontinued (see 4.3. Contraindications).

As with other NSAIDs, allergic reactions, including anaphylactic/anaphylactoid reactions, can also occur without earlier exposure to the drug.

In the treatment of patients with heart failure, hypertension, renal or hepatic disease, especially during concomitant diuretic treatment, the risk of fluid retention and a deterioration in renal function must be taken into account. If used in these patients, the dose of dexibuprofen should be kept as low as possible and renal function should be regularly monitored.

Caution must be exercised in the treatment of elderly patients, who generally have a greater tendency to experience side effects to NSAIDs.

Dexibuprofen should only be given with care to patients with systemic lupus erythematosus and mixed connective tissue disease, because such patients may be predisposed to NSAID-induced CNS and renal side effects.

Caution is required in patients suffering from, or with a previous history of, bronchial asthma since NSAIDs can cause bronchospasm in such patients (see 4.3 Contraindications).

NSAIDs may mask the symptoms of infections.

As with all NSAIDs, dexibuprofen can increase plasma urea nitrogen and creatinine. As with other inhibitors of NSAIDs, dexibuprofen can be associated with adverse effects on the renal system, which can lead to glomerular nephritis, interstitial nephritis, renal papillary necrosis, nephrotic syndrome and acute renal failure (see 4.2. Posology, 4.3. Contraindications and 4.5 Interactions).

As with other NSAIDs, dexibuprofen can cause transient small increases in some liver parameters, and also significant increases in SGOT and SGPT. In case of a relevant increase in such parameters, therapy must be discontinued (see 4.2. Posology and 4.3. Contraindications).

In common with other NSAIDs dexibuprofen may reversibly inhibit platelet aggregation and function and prolong bleeding time. Caution should be exercised when dexibuprofen is given concurrently with oral anticoagulants (see section 4.5).

Patients receiving long-term treatment with dexibuprofen should be monitored as a precautionary measure (renal, hepatic functions and haematologic function/blood counts).

During long-term, high dose, off-label treatment with analgesic drugs, headaches can occur which must not be treated with higher doses of the medicinal product.

In general the habitual use of analgesics, especially the combination of different analgesic drug substances, can lead to lasting renal lesions with the risk of renal failure (analgesic nephropathy). Thus combinations with racemic ibuprofen or other NSAIDs (including OTC products) should be avoided.

The use of dexibuprofen, as with any other drug known to inhibit cyclooxygenase / prostaglandin synthesis, may impair fertility reversibly and is not recommended in women attempting to conceive. In women who have difficulty conceiving or who are undergoing investigation of infertility, withdrawal of Seractil should be considered.

Data of preclinical studies indicate that inhibition of platelet aggregation by low-dose acetylsalicylic acid may be impaired if ibuprofen is administrated concurrently;

this interaction could reduce the cardiovascular-protective effect. Therefore if concomitant administration of low-dose acetylsalicylic acid is indicated special precaution is required if duration of treatment exceeds short term use.

4.5 Interaction with other medicinal products and other forms of interaction

The information in this section is based upon previous experience with racemic ibuprofen and other NSAIDs.

In general, NSAIDs should be used with caution with other drugs that can increase the risk of gastrointestinal ulceration or gastrointestinal bleeding or renal impairment.

Concomitant use not recommended:

Anticoagulants: The effects of anticoagulants on bleeding time can be potentiated by NSAIDs. If concomitant treatment can not be avoidedblood coagulation tests (INR, bleeding time) should be performed during the initiation of dexibuprofen treatment and the dosage of the anticoagulant should be adjusted if necessary (see section 4.4).

Methotrexate used at doses of 15 mg/week or more: If NSAIDs and methotrexate are given within 24 hours of each other plasma levels of methotrexate may increase, via a reduction in its renal clearance thus increasing the potential for methotrexate toxicity. Therefore, in patients receiving high-dose treatment with methotrexate, the concomitant use of dexibuprofen is not recommended (see section 4.4).

Lithium: NSAIDs can increase the plasma levels of lithium, by reducing its renal clearance. The combination is not recommended (see section 4.4). Frequent lithium monitoring should be performed. The possibility of reducing the dose of lithium should be considered.

Other NSAIDs and salicylates (acetylsalicylic acid at doses above those used for anti-thrombotic treatment, approximately 100 mg/day): The concomitant use with other NSAIDs should be avoided, since simultanous administration of different NSAIDs can increase the risk of gastrointestinal ulceration and haemorrhage.

Precautions:

Acetylsalicylic acid: Concomitant administration of ibuprofen may impair inhibition of platelet aggregation by low-dose acetylsalicylic acid.

Antihypertensives: NSAIDs may reduce the efficacy of beta-blockers, possibly due to inhibition of the formation of vasodilatory prostaglandins.

The concomitant use of NSAIDs and ACE inhibitors or angiotensin-II receptor antagonists may be associated with an increased risk of acute renal failure, especially in patients with pre-existing impairment of renal function. When given to the elderly and/or dehydrated patients, such a combination can lead to acute renal failure by acting directly on glomerular filtration. At the beginning of the treatment, a careful monitoring of renal function is recommended.

Furthermore, chronic administration of NSAIDs can theoretically reduce the antihypertensive effect of angiotensin-II receptor antagonists, as reported with ACE inhibitors. Therefore, caution is required when using such a combination and at the start of treatment, renal function should be carefully monitored (and patients should be encouraged to maintain adequate fluid intake).

Ciclosporin, tacrolimus: Concomitant administration with NSAIDs may increase the risk of nephrotoxicity on account of reduced synthesis of prostaglandins in the kidney. During combination treatment renal function must be closely monitored, especially in the elderly.

Corticosteroids: The risk of gastrointestinal ulceration may be increased by the concomitant administration of NSAIDs and corticosteroids.

Digoxin: NSAIDs can increase the plasma levels of digoxin and increase the risk of digoxin toxicity.

Methotrexate used at doses lower than 15 mg/week: Ibuprofen has been reported to increase methotrexate levels. If dexibuprofen is used in combination with low doses of methotrexate, then the patient's blood count should be monitored carefully, particularly during the first weeks of coadministration. An increased surveillance is required in the presence of even mildly impaired renal function, notably in the elderly, and renal function should be monitored to anticipate any reductions in the clearance of methotrexate.

Phenytoin: Ibuprofen may displace phenytoin from protein-binding sites, possibly leading to increased phenytoin serum levels and toxicity. Although clinical evidence for this interaction is limited, phenytoin dosage adjustment, based on monitoring of plasma concentrations and/or observed signs of toxicity, is recommended.

Thiazides, thiazide-related substances, loop diuretics and potassium-sparing diuretics: Concurrent use of an NSAID and a diuretic may increase the risk of renal failure secondary to a reduction in renal blood flow.

Drugs increasing potassium plasma levels:

As with other NSAIDs, concomitant treatment with drugs increasing potassium plasma levels, like potassium-sparing diuretics, ACE inhibitors, angiotensin-II receptors antagonists, immunosuppressants like cyclosporin or tacrolimus, trimethoprime, heparins, etc... may be associated with increased serum potassium levels; hence serum potassium levels should be monitored.

Thrombolytics, ticlopidine and antiplatelet agents: Dexibuprofen inhibits platelet aggregation via inhibition of platelet cyclooxygenase. Therefore, caution is required when dexibuprofen is combined with thrombolytics, ticlopidine and other antiplatelet agents, because of the risk of increased antiplatelet effect.

4.6 Pregnancy and lactation

Pregnancy:

For dexibuprofen, no clinical data on exposed pregnancies are available. Animal studies with ibuprofen and other NSAIDs have shown reproductive toxicity (see 5.3 Preclinical Safety Data).

Inhibition of prostaglandin synthesis may adversely affect the pregnancy and/or the embryo/fetal development, and as the consequences of inhibiting the synthesis of prostaglandins are not fully known, dexibuprofen, like other drugs of this class, should only be administered in the first 5 months of pregnancy if clearly needed, in the lowest effective dose and as short as possible.

During the third trimester of pregnancy, all prostaglandin synthesis inhibitors may expose the fetus to:

- cardiopulmonary toxicity (with premature closure of the ductus arteriosus and pulmonary hypertension),
- renal dysfunction, which may progress to renal failure with oligo-hydroamniosis, the mother and the neonate, at the end of pregnancy, to:
- possible prolongation of bleeding time,
- inhibition of uterine contractions resulting in delayed or prolonged labour.

Therefore, from the beginning of the 6th month of pregnancy onward dexibuprofen is contraindicated.

The use of dexibuprofen, as with any drug substance known to inhibit cyclooxygenase / prostaglandin synthesis is not recommended in women attempting to conceive (see 4.4).

Lactation:

Ibuprofen is slightly excreted in human milk. Breast-feeding is possible with dexibuprofen if dosage is low and the treatment period is short.

4.7 Effects on ability to drive and use machines

During treatment with dexibuprofen the patient's reaction capacity may be reduced when dizziness or fatigue appear as side effects. This should be taken into consideration when increased alertness is required, e.g. when driving or operating machinery. For a single or short term use of Dexibuprofen no special precautions are necessary.

4.8 Undesirable effects

Clinical experience has shown that the risk of undesirable effects induced by dexibuprofen is comparable to that of racemic ibuprofen. The most common adverse events are gastrointestinal in nature.

It should be noted that the adverse events listed below include those reported predominantly for racemic ibuprofen, even though in some cases the adverse event has either not yet been observed with dexibuprofen or has not yet been reported in the frequency mentioned.

Gastrointestinal:

Very common (>1/10): Dyspepsia, diarrhoea.

Common (>1/100, <1/10): Nausea, vomiting, abdominal pain.

Uncommon (>1/1,000, <1/100): Gastrointestinal ulcers and bleeding, ulcerative stomatitis.

Rare (>1/10,000, <1/1,000): Gastrointestinal perforation, flatulence, constipation, esophagitis, esophageal strictures. Exacerbation of diverticular disease, unspecific haemorrhagic colitis, colitis ulcerosa or Crohn's disease.

If gastrointestinal blood loss occurs, this may cause anaemia and haematemesis.

Skin and hypersensitivity reaction:

Common: Rash.

Uncommon: Urticaria, pruritus, purpura (including allergic purpura), angiooedema, rhinitis, bronchospasm.

Rare: Anaphylactic reaction

Very rare (<1/10,000): Erythema multiforme, epidermal necrolysis, systemic lupus erythematosus, alopecia, photosensitivity reactions, severe skin reactions like Stevens-Johnson-Syndrome, acute toxic epidermal necrolysis (Lyell-Syndrome) and allergic vasculitis.

Generalized hypersensitivity reactions have not yet been reported with dexibuprofen but their occurrence cannot be excluded considering the clinical experience with racemic ibuprofen. The symptoms may include fever with rash, abdominal pain, headache, nausea and vomiting, signs of liver injury and even aseptic meningitis. In the majority of cases in which aseptic meningitis has been reported with ibuprofen, some form of underlying auto-immune disease (such as systemic lupus erythematosus or other collagen diseases) was present as a risk factor. In case of a severe generalized hypersensitivity reaction swelling of face, tongue and larynx, bronchospasm, asthma, tachycardia, hypotension and shock can occur.

Central nervous system:

Common: Fatigue or drowsiness, headache, dizziness, vertigo.

Uncommon: Insomnia, anxiety, restlessness, visual disturbances, tinnitus.

Rare: Psychotic reaction, agitation, irritability, depression, confusion or disorientation, reversible toxic amblyopia, impaired hearing.

Very rare: Aseptic meningitis (see hypersensitivity reactions).

Haematological:

Bleeding time may be prolonged. Rare cases of blood disorders include: Thrombocytopenia, leucopenia, granulocytopenia, pancytopenia, agranulocytosis, aplastic anemia or haemolytic anaemia.

Cardiovascular:

Peripheral oedema has been reported in association with dexibuprofen treatment.

Patients with hypertension or renal impairment seem to be predisposed to fluid retention.

Hypertension or cardiac failure (especially in the elderly) may occur.

Renal:

According to the experience with NSAIDs in general, interstitial nephritis, nephrotic syndrome or renal failure cannot be excluded.

Hepatic:

Rare cases of abnormal liver function, hepatitis and jaundice have been observed with racemic ibuprofen.

Others:

In very rare cases infection related inflammation may be aggravated.

4.9 Overdose

Dexibuprofen has a low acute toxicity and patients have survived after single doses as high as 54 g of racemic ibuprofen. Most overdoses have been asymptomatic.

There is a risk of symptoms at doses >80 - 100 mg/kg racemic ibuprofen.

The onset of symptoms usually occurs within 4 hours. Mild symptoms are most common, including abdominal pain, nausea, vomiting, lethargy, drowsiness, headache, nystagmus, tinnitus and ataxia. Rarely, moderate or severe symptoms include gastrointestinal bleeding, hypotension, hypothermia, metabolic acidosis, seizures, impaired kidney function, coma, adult respiratory distress syndrome and transient episodes of apnea (in very young children following large ingestions).

Treatment is symptomatic, and there is no specific antidote. Amounts not likely to produce symptoms (less than 50 mg/kg dexibuprofen) may be diluted with water to minimize gastrointestinal upset. In case of ingestion of a significant amount, activated charcoal should be administered.

Emptying of the stomach by emesis may only be considered if the procedure can be undertaken within 60 minutes of ingestion. Gastric lavage should not be considered unless a patient has ingested a potentially life-threatening amount of the drug and the procedure can be undertaken within 60 minutes of ingestion. Forced diuresis, hemodialysis or hemoperfusion are unlikely to be of assistance because dexibuprofen is strongly bound to plasma proteins.

5. PHARMACOLOGICAL PROPERTIES

Pharmacotherapeutic group: Antiinflammatory and antirheumatic products, non-steroids, propionic acid derivatives.

ATC code: M01AE14

5.1 Pharmacodynamic properties

Dexibuprofen (= S(+)-ibuprofen) is considered to be the pharmacologically active enantiomer of racemic ibuprofen. Racemic ibuprofen is a non-steroidal substance with antiinflammatory and analgesic effects. Its mechanism of action is thought to be due to inhibition of prostaglandin synthesis. Bridging studies in order to compare the efficacy of racemic ibuprofen and dexibuprofen in osteoarthritis over a treatment period of 15 days and in dysmenorrhea, including symptoms of pain, have demonstrated at least non-inferiority of dexibuprofen versus racemic ibuprofen at the recommended dosage.

5.2 Pharmacokinetic properties

Dexibuprofen is absorbed primarily from the small intestine. After metabolic transformation in the liver (hydroxylation, carboxylation), the pharmacologically inactive metabolites are completely excreted, mainly by the kidneys (90%), but also in the bile. The elimination half-life is 1.8 – 3.5 hours; the plasma protein binding is about 99 %. Maximum plasma levels are reached about 2 hours after oral administration.

The administration of dexibuprofen with a meal delays the time to reach maximum concentrations (from 2.1 hours after fasting conditions to 2.8 hours after non-fasting conditions) and decreases the maximum plasma concentrations (from 20.6 to 18.1 μg/ml, which is of no clinical relevance), but has no effect on the extent of absorption.

5.3 Preclinical safety data

Bridging studies on single and repeated dose toxicity, reproduction toxicity and mutagenicity have shown that the toxicological profile of dexibuprofen is comparable to that of racemic ibuprofen.

Racemic ibuprofen inhibited ovulation in the rabbit and impaired implantation in different animal species (rabbit, rat, mouse). Administration of prostaglandin synthesis inhibitors including ibuprofen (mostly in doses higher than used therapeutically) to pregnant animals has been shown to result in increased pre- and postimplantation loss, embryo-fetal lethality and increased incidences of malformations.

6. PHARMACEUTICAL PARTICULARS

6.1 List of excipients

Tablet core: Hypromellose, microcrystalline cellulose, carmellose calcium, colloidal anhydrous silica, talc.

Film-coating material: Hypromellose, titanium dioxide (E171), glycerol triacetate, talc, macrogol 6000.

6.2 Incompatibilities

Not applicable.

6.3 Shelf life

3 years (PVC/PVDC/aluminium blisters)

18 months (PE jars)

6.4 Special precautions for storage

Do not store above 25°C.

6.5 Nature and contents of container

10, 20, 30, 50, 60, 90, 100, 100x1 and 500x1 film-coated tablets in PVC/PVDC/aluminium blisters.

150 film-coated tablets in PE jars with dosing hole and hinged closure.

Not all pack sizes may be marketed.

6.6 Special precautions for disposal and other handling

No special requirements.

7. MARKETING AUTHORISATION HOLDER

Gebro Pharma GmbH, A-6391 Fieberbrunn

Austria

8. MARKETING AUTHORISATION NUMBER(S)

PL 04536/0006

9. DATE OF FIRST AUTHORISATION/RENEWAL OF THE AUTHORISATION

31 October 2000

10. DATE OF REVISION OF THE TEXT

April 2004

11. Legal Category

POM

Seractil 400mg Film-Coated Tablets

(Genus Pharmaceuticals)

1. NAME OF THE MEDICINAL PRODUCT

Seractil▼ 400 mg film-coated tablets

2. QUALITATIVE AND QUANTITATIVE COMPOSITION

Each film-coated tablet contains 400 mg of dexibuprofen. For excipients, see 6.1.

3. PHARMACEUTICAL FORM

Film-coated tablet

White, oblong, both-sided scored film-coated tablet.

4. CLINICAL PARTICULARS

4.1 Therapeutic indications

Symptomatic treatment for the relief of pain and inflammation associated with osteoarthritis.

Acute symptomatic treatment of pain during menstrual bleeding (primary dysmenorrhoea).

Symptomatic treatment of other forms of mild to moderate pain, such as muscular-skeletal pain or dental pain.

4.2 Posology and method of administration

The dosage should be adjusted to the severity of the disorder and the complaints of the patient. During chronic administration, the dosage should be adjusted to the lowest maintenance dose that provides adequate control of symptoms.

For individual dosage film-coated tablets with 200, 300 and 400 mg dexibuprofen are available.

The recommended dosage is 600 to 900 mg dexibuprofen daily, divided in up to three single doses.

For the treatment of mild to moderate pain, initially single doses of 200 mg dexibuprofen and daily doses of 600 mg dexibuprofen are recommended.

The maximum single dose is 400 mg dexibuprofen.

The dose may be temporarily increased up to 1200 mg dexibuprofen per day in patients with acute conditions or exacerbations. The maximum daily dose is 1200 mg.

For dysmenorrhoea a daily dose of 600 to 900 mg dexibuprofen, divided in up to three single doses, is recommended. The maximum single dose is 300 mg, the maximum daily dose is 900 mg.

Dexibuprofen has not been studied in children and adolescents (< 18 years): Safety and efficacy have not been established and therefore it is not recommended in these age groups.

In elderly patients it is recommended to start the therapy at the lower end of the dosage range. The dosage may be increased to that recommended for general population only after good general tolerance has been ascertained.

Hepatic dysfunction: Patients with mild to moderate hepatic dysfunction should start therapy at reduced doses and be closely monitored. Dexibuprofen should not be used in patients with severe hepatic dysfunction (see 4.3. Contraindications).

Renal dysfunction: The initial dosage should be reduced in patients with mild to moderate impaired renal function. Dexibuprofen should not be used in patients with severe renal dysfunction (see 4.3. Contraindications).

The film coated tablets can be taken with or without a meal (see 5.2.). In general NSAIDs (non-steroidal anti-inflammatory drugs) are preferably taken with food to reduce gastrointestinal irritation, particularly during chronic use. However, a later onset of action in some patients may be anticipated when the tablets are taken with or directly after a meal.

The score in the 200 and 400 mg tablets makes it possible to divide the tablets before administration so as to assist with swallowing.

Dividing the tablets will not provide an exact "half" dose.

4.3 Contraindications

Dexibuprofen must not be administered in the following cases:

- Patients previously sensitive to dexibuprofen, to any other NSAID, or to any of the excipients of the product.
- Patients in whom substances with a similar action (e.g. aspirin or other NSAIDs)

precipitate attacks of asthma, bronchospasm, acute rhinitis, or cause nasal polyps, urticaria or angioneurotic oedema.

- Patients with active or suspected gastrointestinal ulcer or history of recurrent gastrointestinal ulcer.
- Patients who have gastrointestinal bleeding or other active bleedings or bleeding disorders.
- Patients with active Crohn's disease or active ulcerative colitis.
- Patients with severe heart failure.
- Patients with severe renal dysfunction (GFR < 30ml/min).
- Patients with severely impaired hepatic function.
- Patients with haemorrhagic diathesis and other coagulation disorders, or patients receiving anticoagulant therapy.
- From the beginning of 6th month of pregnancy (see 4.6).

4.4 Special warnings and precautions for use

Care is recommended in conditions that predispose patients to the gastrointestinal adverse effects of NSAIDs such as dexibuprofen, including existing gastrointestinal disorders, previous gastric or duodenal ulcer, ulcerative colitis, Crohn's disease and alcoholism.

These patients should be closely monitored for digestive disturbances, especially gastrointestinal bleeding, when taking dexibuprofen or any other NSAID.

Gastrointestinal bleeding or ulceration/perforation have in general more serious consequences in the elderly. They can occur at any time during treatment with or without warning symptoms or a previous history of serious gastrointestinal events.

In the rare instances where gastrointestinal bleeding or ulceration occurs in patients receiving dexibuprofen, treatment should be immediately discontinued (see 4.3. Contraindications).

As with other NSAIDs, allergic reactions, including anaphylactic/anaphylactoid reactions, can also occur without earlier exposure to the drug.

In the treatment of patients with heart failure, hypertension, renal or hepatic disease, especially during concomitant diuretic treatment, the risk of fluid retention and a deterioration in renal function must be taken into account. If used in these patients, the dose of dexibuprofen should be kept as low as possible and renal function should be regularly monitored.

Caution must be exercised in the treatment of elderly patients, who generally have a greater tendency to experience side effects to NSAIDs.

Dexibuprofen should only be given with care to patients with systemic lupus erythematosus and mixed connective tissue disease, because such patients may be predisposed to NSAID-induced CNS and renal side effects.

Caution is required in patients suffering from, or with a previous history of, bronchial asthma since NSAIDs can cause bronchospasm in such patients (see 4.3 Contraindications).

NSAIDs may mask the symptoms of infections.

As with all NSAIDs, dexibuprofen can increase plasma urea nitrogen and creatinine. As with other NSAIDs, dexibuprofen can be associated with adverse effects on the renal system, which can lead to glomerular nephritis, interstitial nephritis, renal papillary necrosis, nephrotic syndrome and acute renal failure (see 4.2. Posology, 4.3. Contraindications and 4.5 Interactions).

As with other NSAIDs, dexibuprofen can cause transient small increases in some liver parameters, and also significant increases in SGOT and SGPT. In case of a relevant increase in such parameters, therapy must be discontinued (see 4.2. Posology and 4.3. Contraindications).

In common with other NSAIDs dexibuprofen may reversibly inhibit platelet aggregation and function and prolong bleeding time. Caution should be exercised when dexibuprofen is given concurrently with oral anticoagulants (see section 4.5).

Patients receiving long-term treatment with dexibuprofen should be monitored as a precautionary measure (renal, hepatic functions and haematologic function/blood counts).

During long-term, high dose, off-label treatment with analgesic drugs, headaches can occur which must not be treated with higher doses of the medicinal product.

In general the habitual use of analgesics, especially the combination of different analgesic drug substances, can lead to lasting renal lesions with the risk of renal failure (analgesic nephropathy). Thus combinations with racemic ibuprofen or other NSAIDs (including OTC products) should be avoided.

The use of dexibuprofen, as with any other drug known to inhibit cyclooxygenase / prostaglandin synthesis, may impair fertility reversibly and is not recommended in women attempting to conceive. In women who have difficulty conceiving or who are undergoing investigation of infertility, withdrawal of Seractil should be considered.

Data of preclinical studies indicate that inhibition of platelet aggregation by low-dose acetylsalicylic acid may be impaired if ibuprofen is administrated concurrently;

this interaction could reduce the cardiovascular-protective effect. Therefore if concomitant administration of low-dose acetylsalicylic acid is indicated special precaution is required if duration of treatment exceeds short term use.

4.5 Interaction with other medicinal products and other forms of interaction

The information in this section is based upon previous experience with racemic ibuprofen and other NSAIDs.

In general, NSAIDs should be used with caution with other drugs that can increase the risk of gastrointestinal ulceration or gastrointestinal bleeding or renal impairment.

Concomitant use not recommended:

Anticoagulants: The effects of anticoagulants on bleeding time can be potentiated by NSAIDs. If concomitant treatment can not be avoided blood coagulation tests (INR, bleeding time) should be performed during the initiation of dexibuprofen treatment and the dosage of the anticoagulant should be adjusted if necessary (see section 4.4).

Methotrexate used at doses of 15 mg/week or more: If NSAIDs and methotrexate are given within 24 hours of each other plasma levels of methotrexate may increase, via a reduction in its renal clearance thus increasing the potential for methotrexate toxicity. Therefore, in patients receiving high-dose treatment with methotrexate, the concomitant use of dexibuprofen is not recommended (see section 4.4).

Lithium: NSAIDs can increase the plasma levels of lithium, by reducing its renal clearance. The combination is not recommended (see section 4.4). Frequent lithium monitoring should be performed. The possibility of reducing the dose of lithium should be considered.

Other NSAIDs and salicylates (acetylsalicylic acid at doses above those used for anti-thrombotic treatment, approximately 100 mg/day): The concomitant use with other NSAIDs should be avoided, since simultanous administration of different NSAIDs can increase the risk of gastrointestinal ulceration and haemorrhage.

Precautions:

Acetylsalicylic acid: Concomitant administration of ibuprofen may impair inhibition of platelet aggregation by low-dose acetylsalicylic acid.

Antihypertensives: NSAIDs may reduce the efficacy of beta-blockers, possibly due to inhibition of the formation of vasodilatory prostaglandins.

The concomitant use of NSAIDs and ACE inhibitors or angiotensin-II receptor antagonists may be associated with an increased risk of acute renal failure, especially in patients with pre-existing impairment of renal function. When given to the elderly and/or dehydrated patients, such a combination can lead to acute renal failure by acting directly on glomerular filtration. At the beginning of the treatment, a careful monitoring of renal function is recommended.

Furthermore, chronic administration of NSAIDs can theoretically reduce the antihypertensive effect of angiotensin-II receptor antagonists, as reported with ACE inhibitors. Therefore, caution is required when using such a combination and at the start of treatment, renal function should be carefully monitored (and patients should be encouraged to maintain adequate fluid intake).

Ciclosporin, tacrolimus: Concomitant administration with NSAIDs may increase the risk of nephrotoxicity on account of reduced synthesis of prostaglandins in the kidney. During combination treatment renal function must be closely monitored, especially in the elderly.

Corticosteroids: The risk of gastrointestinal ulceration may be increased by the concomitant administration of NSAIDs and corticosteroids.

Digoxin: NSAIDs can increase the plasma levels of digoxin and increase the risk of digoxin toxicity.

Methotrexate used at doses lower than 15 mg/week: Ibuprofen has been reported to increase methotrexate levels. If dexibuprofen is used in combination with low doses of methotrexate, then the patient's blood count should be monitored carefully, particularly during the first weeks of coadministration. An increased surveillance is required in the presence of even mildly impaired renal function, notably in the elderly, and renal function should be monitored to anticipate any reductions in the clearance of methotrexate.

Phenytoin: Ibuprofen may displace phenytoin from protein-binding sites, possibly leading to increased phenytoin serum levels and toxicity. Although clinical evidence for this interaction is limited, phenytoin dosage adjustment, based on monitoring of plasma concentrations and/or observed signs of toxicity, is recommended.

Thiazides, thiazide-related substances, loop diuretics and potassium-sparing diuretics: Concurrent use of an NSAID and a diuretic may increase the risk of renal failure secondary to a reduction in renal blood flow.

Drugs increasing potassium plasma levels:

As with other NSAIDs, concomitant treatment with drugs increasing potassium plasma levels, like potassium-sparing diuretics, ACE inhibitors, angiotensin-II receptors antagonists, immunosuppressants like cyclosporin or tacrolimus, trimethoprime, heparins, etc... may be associated with increased serum potassium levels; hence serum potassium levels should be monitored.

Thrombolytics, ticlopidine and antiplatelet agents: Dexibuprofen inhibits platelet aggregation via inhibition of platelet cyclooxygenase. Therefore, caution is required when dexibuprofen is combined with thrombolytics, ticlopidine and other antiplatelet agents, because of the risk of increased antiplatelet effect.

4.6 Pregnancy and lactation

Pregnancy:

For dexibuprofen, no clinical data on exposed pregnancies are available. Animal studies with ibuprofen and other NSAIDs have shown reproductive toxicity (see 5.3 Preclinical Safety Data).

Inhibition of prostaglandin synthesis may adversely affect the pregnancy and/or the embryo/fetal development, and as the consequences of inhibiting the synthesis of prostaglandins are not fully known, dexibuprofen, like other drugs of this class, should only be administered in the first 5 months of pregnancy if clearly needed, in the lowest effective dose and as short as possible.

During the third trimester of pregnancy, all prostaglandin synthesis inhibitors may expose the fetus to:

- cardiopulmonary toxicity (with premature closure of the ductus arteriosus and pulmonary hypertension),
- renal dysfunction, which may progress to renal failure with oligo-hydroamniosis, the mother and the neonate, at the end of pregnancy, to:
- possible prolongation of bleeding time,
- inhibition of uterine contractions resulting in delayed or prolonged labour.

Therefore, from the beginning of the 6th month of pregnancy onward dexibuprofen is contraindicated.

The use of dexibuprofen, as with any drug substance known to inhibit cyclooxygenase / prostaglandin synthesis is not recommended in women attempting to conceive (see 4.4).

Lactation:

Ibuprofen is slightly excreted in human milk. Breast-feeding is possible with dexibuprofen if dosage is low and the treatment period is short.

4.7 Effects on ability to drive and use machines

During treatment with dexibuprofen the patient's reaction capacity may be reduced when dizziness or fatigue appear as side effects. This should be taken into consideration when increased alertness is required, e.g. when driving or operating machinery. For a single or short term use of Dexibuprofen no special precautions are necessary.

4.8 Undesirable effects

Clinical experience has shown that the risk of undesirable effects induced by dexibuprofen is comparable to that of racemic ibuprofen. The most common adverse events are gastrointestinal in nature.

It should be noted that the adverse events listed below include those reported predominantly for racemic ibuprofen, even though in some cases the adverse event has either not yet been observed with dexibuprofen or has not yet been reported in the frequency mentioned.

Gastrointestinal:

Very common (>1/10): Dyspepsia, diarrhoea.

Common (>1/100, <1/10): Nausea, vomiting, abdominal pain.

Uncommon (>1/1,000, <1/100): Gastrointestinal ulcers and bleeding, ulcerative stomatitis.

Rare (>1/10,000, <1/1,000): Gastrointestinal perforation, flatulence, constipation, esophagitis, esophageal strictures. Exacerbation of diverticular disease, unspecific haemorrhagic colitis, colitis ulcerosa or Crohn's disease.

If gastrointestinal blood loss occurs, this may cause anaemia and haematemesis.

Skin and hypersensitivity reaction:

Common: Rash.

Uncommon: Urticaria, pruritus, purpura (including allergic purpura), angioedema, rhinitis, bronchospasm.

Rare: Anaphylactic reaction

Very rare (<1/10,000): Erythema multiforme, epidermal necrolysis, systemic lupus erythematosus, alopecia, photosensitivity reactions, severe skin reactions like Stevens-Johnson-Syndrome, acute toxic epidermal necrolysis (Lyell-Syndrome) and allergic vasculitis.

Generalized hypersensitivity reactions have not yet been reported with dexibuprofen but their occurrence cannot be excluded considering the clinical experience with racemic ibuprofen. The symptoms may include fever with rash, abdominal pain, headache, nausea and vomiting, signs of liver injury and even aseptic meningitis. In the majority of cases in which aseptic meningitis has been reported with ibuprofen, some form of underlying auto-immune disease (such as systemic lupus erythematosus or other collagen diseases) was present as a risk factor. In case of a severe generalized hypersensitivity reaction swelling of face, tongue and larynx, bronchospasm, asthma, tachycardia, hypotension and shock can occur.

Central nervous system:

Common: Fatigue or drowsiness, headache, dizziness, vertigo.

Uncommon: Insomnia, anxiety, restlessness, visual disturbances, tinnitus.

Rare: Psychotic reaction, agitation, irritability, depression, confusion or disorientation, reversible toxic amblyopia, impaired hearing.

Very rare: Aseptic meningitis (see hypersensitivity reactions).

Haematological:

Bleeding time may be prolonged. Rare cases of blood disorders include: Thrombocytopenia, leucopenia, granulocytopenia, pancytopenia, agranulocytosis, aplastic anemia or haemolytic anaemia.

Cardiovascular:

Peripheral oedema has been reported in association with dexibuprofen treatment.

Patients with hypertension or renal impairment seem to be predisposed to fluid retention.

Hypertension or cardiac failure (especially in the elderly) may occur.

Renal:

According to the experience with NSAIDs in general, interstitial nephritis, nephrotic syndrome or renal failure cannot be excluded.

Hepatic:

Rare cases of abnormal liver function, hepatitis and jaundice have been observed with racemic ibuprofen.

Others:

In very rare cases infection related inflammation may be aggravated.

4.9 Overdose

Dexibuprofen has a low acute toxicity and patients have survived after single doses as high as 54 g of racemic ibuprofen. Most overdoses have been asymptomatic. There is a risk of symptoms at doses >80 - 100 mg/kg racemic ibuprofen.

The onset of symptoms usually occurs within 4 hours. Mild symptoms are most common, including abdominal pain, nausea, vomiting, lethargy, drowsiness, headache, nystagmus, tinnitus and ataxia. Rarely, moderate or severe symptoms include gastrointestinal bleeding, hypotension, hypothermia, metabolic acidosis, seizures, impaired kidney function, coma, adult respiratory distress syndrome and transient episodes of apnea (in very young children following large ingestions).

Treatment is symptomatic, and there is no specific antidote. Amounts not likely to produce symptoms (less than 50 mg/kg dexibuprofen) may be diluted with water to minimize gastrointestinal upset. In case of ingestion of a significant amount, activated charcoal should be administered.

Emptying of the stomach by emesis may only be considered if the procedure can be undertaken within 60 minutes of ingestion. Gastric lavage should not be considered unless a patient has ingested a potentially life-threatening amount of the drug and the procedure can be undertaken within 60 minutes of ingestion. Forced diuresis, hemodialysis or hemoperfusion are unlikely to be of assistance because dexibuprofen is strongly bound to plasma proteins.

5. PHARMACOLOGICAL PROPERTIES

Pharmacotherapeutic group: Antiinflammatory and antirheumatic products, non-steroids, propionic acid derivatives.

ATC code: M01AE14

5.1 Pharmacodynamic properties

Dexibuprofen (= S(+)-ibuprofen) is considered to be the pharmacologically active enantiomer of racemic ibuprofen. Racemic ibuprofen is a non-steroidal substance with anti-inflammatory and analgesic effects. Its mechanism of action is thought to be due to inhibition of prostaglandin synthesis. Bridging studies in order to compare the efficacy of racemic ibuprofen and dexibuprofen in osteoarthritis over a treatment period of 15 days and in dysmenorrhea, including symptoms of pain, have demonstrated at least non-inferiority of dexibuprofen versus racemic ibuprofen at the recommended dosage.

5.2 Pharmacokinetic properties

Dexibuprofen is absorbed primarily from the small intestine. After metabolic transformation in the liver (hydroxylation, carboxylation), the pharmacologically inactive metabolites are completely excreted, mainly by the kidneys (90%), but also in the bile. The elimination half-life is 1.8 – 3.5 hours; the plasma protein binding is about 99 %. Maximum plasma levels are reached about 2 hours after oral administration.

The administration of dexibuprofen with a meal delays the time to reach maximum concentrations (from 2.1 hours after fasting conditions to 2.8 hours after non-fasting conditions) and decreases the maximum plasma concentrations (from 20.6 to 18.1 μg/ml, which is of no clinical relevance), but has no effect on the extent of absorption.

5.3 Preclinical safety data

Bridging studies on single and repeated dose toxicity, reproduction toxicity and mutagenicity have shown that the toxicological profile of dexibuprofen is comparable to that of racemic ibuprofen.

Racemic ibuprofen inhibited ovulation in the rabbit and impaired implantation in different animal species (rabbit, rat, mouse). Administration of prostaglandin synthesis inhibitors including ibuprofen (mostly in doses higher than used therapeutically) to pregnant animals has been shown to result in increased pre- and postimplantation loss, embryo-fetal lethality and increased incidences of malformations.

6. PHARMACEUTICAL PARTICULARS

6.1 List of excipients

Tablet core: Hypromellose, microcrystalline cellulose, carmellose calcium, colloidal anhydrous silica, talc.

Film-coating material: Hypromellose, titanium dioxide (E171), glycerol triacetate, talc, macrogol 6000.

6.2 Incompatibilities

Not applicable.

6.3 Shelf life

3 years (PVC/PVDC/aluminium blisters)

18 months (PE jars)

6.4 Special precautions for storage

Do not store above 25°C.

6.5 Nature and contents of container

10, 20, 30, 50, 60, 90, 100, 100x1 and 500x1 film-coated tablets in PVC/PVDC/aluminium blisters.

150 film-coated tablets in PE jars with dosing hole and hinged closure.

Not all pack sizes may be marketed.

6.6 Special precautions for disposal and other handling

No special requirements.

7. MARKETING AUTHORISATION HOLDER

Gebro Pharma GmbH, A-6391 Fieberbrunn

Austria

8. MARKETING AUTHORISATION NUMBER(S)

PL 04536/0007

9. DATE OF FIRST AUTHORISATION/RENEWAL OF THE AUTHORISATION

31 October 2000

10. DATE OF REVISION OF THE TEXT

April 2004

11. Legal Category

POM

Serc-16mg

(Solvay Healthcare Limited)

1. NAME OF THE MEDICINAL PRODUCT

Serc®-16/Betahistine Tablets 16 mg

2. QUALITATIVE AND QUANTITATIVE COMPOSITION

Each tablet contains 16 mg betahistine dihydrochloride.

3. PHARMACEUTICAL FORM

Tablet:

Round, biconvex, scored, white to almost white tablets imprinted '267' on one face and 'S' on the reverse.

4. CLINICAL PARTICULARS

4.1 Therapeutic indications

Vertigo, tinnitus and hearing loss associated with Ménière's syndrome.

4.2 Posology and method of administration

Adults (including the elderly): initially 16 mg three times daily taken preferably with meals. Maintenance doses are generally in the range 24-48 mg daily.

Children: no dosage recommendations are made for children.

4.3 Contraindications

Phaeochromocytoma. Hypersensitivity to the active substance or to any of the excipients.

4.4 Special warnings and precautions for use

Caution is advised in the treatment of patients with a history of peptic ulcer. Clinical intolerance to Serc in bronchial asthma patients has been shown in a relatively few patients. These patients need to be carefully monitored during the therapy.

4.5 Interaction with other medicinal products and other forms of interaction

No *in-vivo* interaction studies have been performed. Based on *in-vitro* data no *in-vivo* inhibition on Cytochrome P450 enzymes is expected.

Although an antagonism between Serc and antihistamines could be expected on a theoretical basis, no such interactions have been reported.

4.6 Pregnancy and lactation

Pregnancy:

There are no adequate data from the use of betahistine in pregnant women.

Animal studies are insufficient with respect to effects on pregnancy, embryonal/foetal development, parturition and postnatal development. The potential risk for humans is unknown. Betahistine should not be used during pregnancy unless clearly necessary.

Lactation:

It is not known whether betahistine is excreted in human milk. There are no animal studies on the excretion of betahistine in milk. The importance of the drug to the mother should be weighed against the benefits of nursing and the potential risks for the child.

4.7 Effects on ability to drive and use machines

Betahistine is regarded to have no or negligible effects on the ability to drive and use machines as no effects potentially influencing this ability were found to be related to betahistine in clinical studies.

4.8 Undesirable effects

The following undesirable effects have been experienced with the below indicated frequencies in betahistine-treated patients in placebo-controlled clinical trials [very common ($\geq$1/10); common ($\geq$1/100 to <1/10); uncommon ($\geq$1/1,000 to <1/100); rare ($\geq$1/10,000 to <1/1,000); very rare (<1/10,000)].

Gastrointestinal disorders

Common: nausea and dyspepsia

In addition to those events reported during clinical trials, the following undesirable effects have been reported spontaneously during post-marketing use and in scientific literature. A frequency cannot be estimated from the available data and is therefore classified as "not known".

Immune System disorders

Hypersensitivity reactions, e.g. anaphylaxis have been reported.

Gastrointestinal disorders

Mild gastric complaints (e.g. vomiting, gastrointestinal pain, abdominal distension and bloating) have been observed. These can normally be dealt with by taking the dose during meals or by lowering the dose.

Nervous System disorders

Headache

Skin and subcutaneous tissue disorders

Cutaneous and subcutaneous hypersensitivity reactions have been reported, in particular angioneurotic oedema, urticaria, rash, and pruritus.

4.9 Overdose

A few overdose cases have been reported. Some patients experienced mild to moderate symptoms with doses up to 640 mg (e.g. nausea, somnolence, abdominal pain). More serious complications (e.g. convulsion, pulmonary or cardiac complications) were observed in cases of intentional overdose of betahistine especially in combination with other overdosed drugs. Treatment of overdose should include standard supportive measures.

5. PHARMACOLOGICAL PROPERTIES

5.1 Pharmacodynamic properties

The active ingredient is a specific histamine agonist with virtually no H_2-activity. It appears to act on the precapillary sphincter in the stria vascularis of the inner ear, thus reducing the pressure in the endolymphatic space.

5.2 Pharmacokinetic properties

Betahistine is rapidly and completely absorbed after oral administration of the drug in tablets. It is excreted almost quantitatively in urine as 2-pyridylacetic acid within 24 hours after administration. No unchanged betahistine has been detected.

5.3 Preclinical safety data

There are no pre-clinical data of relevance to the prescriber which are additional to that already included in other sections of the SPC.

6. PHARMACEUTICAL PARTICULARS

6.1 List of excipients

Microcrystalline cellulose, mannitol, citric acid monohydrate, colloidal anhydrous silica and talc.

6.2 Incompatibilities

Not applicable.

6.3 Shelf life

5 years.

6.4 Special precautions for storage

Do not store above 25°C. Store in the original package.

6.5 Nature and contents of container

PVC/PVdC blister packs containing 84 tablets.

HDPE tablet containers containing 500 or 1000 tablets.

6.6 Special precautions for disposal and other handling

None.

7. MARKETING AUTHORISATION HOLDER

Solvay Healthcare Limited/Solvay Healthcare Limited T/A Mansbridge Pharmaceuticals Ltd

Mansbridge Road

West End

Southampton

SO18 3JD

8. MARKETING AUTHORISATION NUMBER(S)

PL 00512/0088

9. DATE OF FIRST AUTHORISATION/RENEWAL OF THE AUTHORISATION

15 October 1997/ 14 October 2002

10. DATE OF REVISION OF THE TEXT

03/07/2009

Serc-8mg

(Solvay Healthcare Limited)

1. NAME OF THE MEDICINAL PRODUCT

Serc®-8 or Betahistine Tablets 8 mg.

2. QUALITATIVE AND QUANTITATIVE COMPOSITION

Each tablet contains 8 mg betahistine dihydrochloride.

3. PHARMACEUTICAL FORM

A round, flat, white to almost white tablet. Serc-8 is imprinted '256' on one face and 'S' on the reverse. Betahistine Tablets 8 mg are imprinted 'B HIST 8' on one face.

4. CLINICAL PARTICULARS

4.1 Therapeutic indications

Vertigo, tinnitus and hearing loss associated with Ménière's syndrome.

4.2 Posology and method of administration

Adults (including the elderly): initially two tablets three times daily taken preferably with meals. Maintenance doses are generally in the range 24-48 mg daily.

Children: No dosage recommendations.

4.3 Contraindications

Phaeochromocytoma. Hypersensitivity to the active substance or to any of the excipients.

4.4 Special warnings and precautions for use

Caution is advised in the treatment of patients with a history of peptic ulcer. Clinical intolerance to Serc in bronchial asthma patients has been shown in a relatively few patients. These patients need to be carefully monitored during the therapy.

4.5 Interaction with other medicinal products and other forms of interaction

No *in-vivo* interaction studies have been performed. Based on *in-vitro* data no *in-vivo* inhibition on Cytochrome P450 enzymes is expected.

Although an antagonism between Serc and antihistamines could be expected on a theoretical basis, no such interactions have been reported.

4.6 Pregnancy and lactation

Pregnancy:

There are no adequate data from the use of betahistine in pregnant women.

Animal studies are insufficient with respect to effects on pregnancy, embryonal/foetal development, parturition and postnatal development. The potential risk for humans is unknown. Betahistine should not be used during pregnancy unless clearly necessary.

Lactation:

It is not known whether betahistine is excreted in human milk. There are no animal studies on the excretion of betahistine in milk. The importance of the drug to the mother should be weighed against the benefits of nursing and the potential risks for the child.

4.7 Effects on ability to drive and use machines

Betahistine is regarded to have no or negligible effects on the ability to drive and use machines as no effects potentially influencing this ability were found to be related to betahistine in clinical studies.

4.8 Undesirable effects

The following undesirable effects have been experienced with the below indicated frequencies in betahistine-treated patients in placebo-controlled clinical trials [very common ($\geq$1/10); common ($\geq$1/100 to <1/10); uncommon ($\geq$1/1,000 to <1/100); rare ($\geq$1/10,000 to <1/1,000); very rare (<1/10,000)].

Gastrointestinal disorders

Common: nausea and dyspepsia

In addition to those events reported during clinical trials, the following undesirable effects have been reported spontaneously during post-marketing use and in scientific literature. A frequency cannot be estimated from the available data and is therefore classified as "not known".

Immune System disorders

Hypersensitivity reactions, e.g. anaphylaxis have been reported.

Gastrointestinal disorders

Mild gastric complaints (e.g. vomiting, gastrointestinal pain, abdominal distension and bloating) have been observed. These can normally be dealt with by taking the dose during meals or by lowering the dose.

Nervous System disorders

Headache

Skin and subcutaneous tissue disorders

Cutaneous and subcutaneous hypersensitivity reactions have been reported, in particular angioneurotic oedema, urticaria, rash, and pruritus.

4.9 Overdose

A few overdose cases have been reported. Some patients experienced mild to moderate symptoms with doses up to 640 mg (e.g. nausea, somnolence, abdominal pain). More serious complications (e.g. convulsion, pulmonary or cardiac complications) were observed in cases of intentional overdose of betahistine especially in combination with other overdosed drugs. Treatment of overdose should include standard supportive measures.

5. PHARMACOLOGICAL PROPERTIES

5.1 Pharmacodynamic properties

The active ingredient is a specific histamine agonist with virtually no H_2-activity. It appears to act on the precapillary sphincter in the stria vascularis of the inner ear, thus reducing the pressure in the endolymphatic space.

5.2 Pharmacokinetic properties

Betahistine is rapidly and completely absorbed after oral administration of the drug in tablets. It is excreted almost quantitatively in urine as 2-pyridylacetic acid within 24 hours after administration. No unchanged betahistine has been detected.

5.3 Preclinical safety data

There are no pre-clinical data of relevance to the prescriber which are additional to that already included in other sections of the SPC.

6. PHARMACEUTICAL PARTICULARS

6.1 List of excipients

Microcrystalline cellulose, mannitol, citric acid monohydrate, colloidal anhydrous silica and talc.

6.2 Incompatibilities

None.

6.3 Shelf life

5 years.

6.4 Special precautions for storage

Do not store above 25°C. Store in the original package.

6.5 Nature and contents of container

Blister strips of 15 tablets. The blister strips are made of PVC/PVdC film and aluminium foil. Each carton contains 120 tablets.

Grey polypropylene tablet container with white polypropylene tamper evident closure containing 500 or 1000 tablets.

6.6 Special precautions for disposal and other handling

None.

7. MARKETING AUTHORISATION HOLDER

Solvay Healthcare Limited

Mansbridge Road

West End

Southampton

SO18 3JD.

T/A Mansbridge Pharmaceuticals (Betahistine Tablets 8 mg ONLY)

8. MARKETING AUTHORISATION NUMBER(S)

PL 00512/0076

9. DATE OF FIRST AUTHORISATION/RENEWAL OF THE AUTHORISATION

7 October 98

10. DATE OF REVISION OF THE TEXT

03/07/2009

Seretide 100, 250, 500 Accuhaler

(Allen & Hanburys)

1. NAME OF THE MEDICINAL PRODUCT

Seretide Accuhaler 50 microgram /100 microgram /dose inhalation powder, pre-dispensed.

Seretide Accuhaler 50 microgram /250 microgram /dose inhalation powder, pre-dispensed.

Seretide Accuhaler 50 microgram /500 microgram /dose inhalation powder, pre-dispensed.

2. QUALITATIVE AND QUANTITATIVE COMPOSITION

Each single dose of Seretide provides:

50 micrograms of salmeterol (as salmeterol xinafoate) and 100, 250 or 500 micrograms of fluticasone propionate.

For a full list of excipients, see section 6.1.

3. PHARMACEUTICAL FORM

Inhalation powder, pre-dispensed.

4. CLINICAL PARTICULARS

4.1 Therapeutic indications

Asthma

Seretide is indicated in the regular treatment of asthma where use of a combination product (long-acting beta-2-agonist and inhaled corticosteroid) is appropriate:

- patients not adequately controlled with inhaled corticosteroids and 'as needed' inhaled short acting beta-2-agonist

or

- patients already adequately controlled on both inhaled corticosteroid and long-acting beta-2-agonist.

Note: Seretide 50 microgram /100 microgram strength is not appropriate in adults and children with severe asthma.

Chronic Obstructive Pulmonary Disease (COPD)

Seretide is indicated for the symptomatic treatment of patients with COPD, with a FEV_1 <60% predicted normal (pre-bronchodilator) and a history of repeated exacerbations, who have significant symptoms despite regular bronchodilator therapy.

4.2 Posology and method of administration

Seretide Accuhaler is for inhalation use only.

Patients should be made aware that Seretide Accuhaler must be used daily for optimum benefit, even when asymptomatic.

Patients should be regularly reassessed by a doctor, so that the strength of Seretide they are receiving remains optimal and is only changed on medical advice. **The dose should be titrated to the lowest dose at which effective control of symptoms is maintained. Where the control of symptoms is maintained with the lowest strength of the combination given twice daily then the next step could include a test of inhaled corticosteroid alone.** As an alternative, patients requiring a long acting beta-2-agonist could be titrated to Seretide given once daily if, in the opinion of the prescriber, it would be adequate to maintain disease control. In the event of once daily dosing when the patient has a history of nocturnal symptoms the dose should be given at night and when the patient has a history of mainly day-time symptoms the dose should be given in the morning.

Patients should be given the strength of Seretide containing the appropriate fluticasone propionate dosage for the severity of their disease. Prescribers should be aware that, in patients with asthma, fluticasone propionate is as effective as other inhaled steroids at approximately half the microgram daily dose. For example, 100mcg of fluticasone propionate is approximately equivalent to 200mcg of beclomethasone dipropionate (CFC containing) or budesonide. If an individual patient should require dosages outside the recommended regimen, appropriate doses of beta-agonist and/or corticosteroid should be prescribed.

Recommended Doses:

Asthma

Adults and adolescents 12 years and older:

One inhalation of 50 micrograms salmeterol and 100 micrograms fluticasone propionate twice daily.

or

One inhalation of 50 micrograms salmeterol and 250 micrograms fluticasone propionate twice daily.

or

One inhalation of 50 micrograms salmeterol and 500 micrograms fluticasone propionate twice daily.

A short term trial of Seretide may be considered as initial maintenance therapy in adults or adolescents with moderate persistent asthma (defined as patients with daily symptoms, daily rescue use and moderate to severe airflow limitation) for whom rapid control of asthma is essential. In these cases, the recommended initial dose is one inhalation of 50 micrograms salmeterol and 100 micrograms fluticasone propionate twice daily. Once control of asthma is attained treatment should be reviewed and consideration given as to whether patients should be stepped down to an inhaled corticosteroid alone. Regular review of patients as treatment is stepped down is important.

A clear benefit has not been shown as compared to inhaled fluticasone propionate alone used as initial maintenance therapy when one or two of the criteria of severity are missing. In general inhaled corticosteroids remain the first line treatment for most patients. Seretide is not intended for the initial management of mild asthma. Seretide 50 microgram/100 micrograms strength is not appropriate in adults and children with severe asthma; it is recommended to establish the appropriate dosage of inhaled corticosteroid before any fixed combination can be used in patients with severe asthma.

Children 4 years and older:

One inhalation of 50 micrograms salmeterol and 100 micrograms fluticasone propionate twice daily.

The maximum licensed dose of fluticasone propionate delivered by Seretide Accuhaler in children is 100 mcg twice daily.

There are no data available for use of Seretide in children aged under 4 years.

COPD

Adults:

One inhalation of 50 micrograms salmeterol and 500 micrograms fluticasone propionate twice daily.

Special patient groups:

There is no need to adjust the dose in elderly patients or in those with renal impairment. There are no data available for use of Seretide in patients with hepatic impairment.

Using the Accuhaler:

The device is opened and primed by sliding the lever. The mouthpiece is then placed in the mouth and the lips closed round it. The dose can then be inhaled and the device closed.

4.3 Contraindications

Seretide is contraindicated in patients with hypersensitivity (allergy) to any of the active substances or to the excipient (see section 6.1).

4.4 Special warnings and precautions for use

The management of asthma should normally follow a stepwise programme and patient response should be monitored clinically and by lung function tests.

Seretide Accuhaler should not be used to treat acute asthma symptoms for which a fast and short acting bronchodilator is required. Patients should be advised to have their medicinal product to be used for relief in an acute asthma attack available at all times.

Patients should not be initiated on Seretide during an exacerbation, or if they have significantly worsening or acutely deteriorating asthma.

Serious asthma-related adverse events and exacerbations may occur during treatment with Seretide. Patients should be asked to continue treatment but to seek medical advice if asthma symptoms remain uncontrolled or worsen after initiation on Seretide.

Increasing use of short-acting bronchodilators to relieve symptoms indicates deterioration of control and patients should be reviewed by a physician.

Sudden and progressive deterioration in control of asthma is potentially life threatening and the patient should undergo urgent medical assessment. Consideration should be given to increasing corticosteroid therapy. The patient should also be medically reviewed where the current dosage of Seretide has failed to give adequate control of asthma.

Once asthma symptoms are controlled, consideration may be given to gradually reducing the dose of Seretide. Regular review of patients as treatment is stepped down is important. The lowest effective dose of Seretide should be used (see section 4.2).

For patients with asthma or COPD, consideration should be given to additional corticosteroid therapies.

Treatment with Seretide should not be stopped abruptly in patients with asthma due to risk of exacerbation. Therapy should be down-titrated under physician supervision. For patients with COPD cessation of therapy may also be associated with symptomatic decompensation and should be supervised by a physician.

As with all inhaled medication containing corticosteroids, Seretide should be administered with caution in patients with pulmonary tuberculosis.

Rarely, Seretide may cause cardiac arrhythmias e.g. supraventricular tachycardia, extrasystoles and atrial fibrillation, and a mild transient reduction in serum potassium at high therapeutic doses. Therefore Seretide should be used with caution in patients with severe cardiovascular disorders, heart rhythm abnormalities, diabetes mellitus, thyrotoxicosis, uncorrected hypokalaemia or patients predisposed to low levels of serum potassium.

There have been very rare reports of increases in blood glucose levels (see section 4.8) and this should be considered when prescribing to patients with a history of diabetes mellitus.

As with other inhalation therapy paradoxical bronchospasm may occur with an immediate increase in wheezing after dosing. Seretide Accuhaler should be discontinued immediately, the patient assessed and alternative therapy instituted if necessary.

Seretide contains lactose up to 12.5 milligram/dose. This amount does not normally cause problems in lactose intolerant people.

Care should be taken when transferring patients to Seretide therapy, particularly if there is any reason to suppose that adrenal function is impaired from previous systemic steroid therapy.

Systemic effects may occur with any inhaled corticosteroid, particularly at high doses prescribed for long periods. These effects are much less likely to occur than with oral corticosteroids. Possible systemic effects include Cushing's syndrome, Cushingoid features, adrenal suppression, growth retardation in children and adolescents, decrease in bone mineral density, cataract and glaucoma. **It is important, therefore, that the patient is reviewed regularly and the dose of inhaled corticosteroid is reduced to the lowest dose at which effective control of asthma is maintained.**

It is recommended that the height of children receiving prolonged treatment with inhaled corticosteroid is regularly monitored.

Prolonged treatment of patients with high doses of inhaled corticosteroids may result in adrenal suppression and acute adrenal crisis. Children and adolescents <16years taking high doses of fluticasone propionate (typically ⩾ 1000mcg/day) may be at particular risk. Very rare cases of adrenal suppression and acute adrenal crisis have also been described with doses of fluticasone propionate between 500 and less than 1000mcg. Situations, which could potentially trigger acute adrenal crisis include trauma, surgery, infection or any rapid reduction in dosage. Presenting symptoms are typically vague and may include anorexia, abdominal pain, weight loss, tiredness, headache, nausea, vomiting, hypotension, decreased level of consciousness, hypoglycaemia, and seizures. Additional systemic corticosteroid cover should be considered during periods of stress or elective surgery.

The benefits of inhaled fluticasone propionate therapy should minimise the need for oral steroids, but patients transferring from oral steroids may remain at risk of impaired adrenal reserve for a considerable time. Patients who have required high dose emergency corticosteroid therapy in the past may also be at risk. This possibility of residual impairment should always be borne in mind in emergency and elective situations likely to produce stress, and appropriate corticosteroid treatment must be considered. The extent of the adrenal impairment may require specialist advice before elective procedures.

Ritonavir can greatly increase the concentration of fluticasone propionate in plasma. Therefore, concomitant use should be avoided, unless the potential benefit to the patient outweighs the risk of systemic corticosteroid side-effects. There is also an increased risk of systemic side effects when combining fluticasone propionate with other potent CYP3A inhibitors (see section 4.5).

There was an increased reporting of lower respiratory tract infections (particularly pneumonia and bronchitis) in the TORCH study in patients with COPD receiving Seretide compared with placebo (see section 4.8 and 5.1). In TORCH, older patients, patients with a lower body mass index ($<25kg/m^2$) and patients with very severe disease ($FEV_1 < 30\%$ predicted) were at greatest risk of developing pneumonia regardless of treatment. Physicians should remain vigilant for the possible development of pneumonia and other lower respiratory tract infections in patients with COPD as the clinical features of such infections and exacerbation frequently overlap. If a patient with severe COPD has experienced pneumonia the treatment with Seretide should be re-evaluated.

Data from a large clinical trial (the Salmeterol Multi-Center Asthma Research Trial, SMART) suggested African-American patients were at increased risk of serious respiratory-related events or deaths when using salmeterol compared with placebo (see section 5.1). It is not known if this was due to pharmacogenetic or other factors. Patients of black African or Afro-Caribbean ancestry should therefore be asked to continue treatment but to seek medical advice if asthma symptoms remained uncontrolled or worsen whilst using Seretide.

4.5 Interaction with other medicinal products and other forms of interaction

Both non-selective and selective beta-blockers should be avoided unless there are compelling reasons for their use.

Concomitant use of other beta-adrenergic containing drugs can have a potentially additive effect.

Under normal circumstances, low plasma concentrations of fluticasone propionate are achieved after inhaled dosing, due to extensive first pass metabolism and high systemic clearance mediated by cytochrome P450 3A4 in the gut and liver. Hence, clinically significant drug interactions mediated by fluticasone propionate are unlikely.

In an interaction study in healthy subjects with intranasal fluticasone propionate, ritonavir (a highly potent cytochrome P450 3A4 inhibitor) 100 mg b.i.d. increased the fluticasone propionate plasma concentrations several hundred fold, resulting in markedly reduced serum cortisol concentrations. Information about this interaction is lacking for inhaled fluticasone propionate, but a marked increase in fluticasone propionate plasma levels is expected. Cases of Cushing's syndrome and adrenal suppression have been reported. The combination should be avoided unless the benefit outweighs the increased risk of systemic glucocorticoid side-effects.

In a small study in healthy volunteers, the slightly less potent CYP3A inhibitor ketoconazole increased the exposure of fluticasone propionate after a single inhalation by 150%. This resulted in a greater reduction of plasma cortisol as compared with fluticasone propionate alone. Co-treatment with other potent CYP3A inhibitors, such as itraconazole, is also expected to increase the systemic fluticasone propionate exposure and the risk of systemic side-effects. Caution is recommended and long-term treatment with such drugs should if possible be avoided.

4.6 Pregnancy and lactation

There are insufficient data on the use of salmeterol and fluticasone propionate during pregnancy and lactation in man to assess the possible harmful effects. In animal studies foetal abnormalities occur after administration of beta-2-adrenoreceptor agonists and glucocorticosteroids (see section 5.3).

Administration of Seretide to pregnant women should only be considered if the expected benefit to the mother is greater than any possible risk to the foetus.

The lowest effective dose of fluticasone propionate needed to maintain adequate asthma control should be used in the treatment of pregnant women.

There are no data available for human breast milk. Both salmeterol and fluticasone propionate are excreted into breast milk in rats. Administration of Seretide to women who are breastfeeding should only be considered if the expected benefit to the mother is greater than any possible risk to the child.

4.7 Effects on ability to drive and use machines

No studies of the effect on the ability to drive and use machines have been performed.

4.8 Undesirable effects

As Seretide contains salmeterol and fluticasone propionate, the type and severity of adverse reactions associated with each of the compounds may be expected. There is no incidence of additional adverse events following concurrent administration of the two compounds.

Adverse events which have been associated with salmeterol/fluticasone propionate are given below, listed by system organ class and frequency. Frequencies are defined as: very common ($\geq 1/10$), common ($\geq 1/100$ and $< 1/10$), uncommon ($\geq 1/1000$ and $< 1/100$), rare ($\geq 1/10,000$ to $< 1/1000$), and very rare ($< 1/10,000$) including isolated reports. Very common, common and uncommon events were derived from clinical trial data. The incidence in placebo was not taken into account. Very rare events were derived from post-marketing spontaneous data.

System Organ Class	Adverse Event	Frequency
Cardiac Disorders	Palpitations	Common
	Tachycardia	Uncommon
	Cardiac arrhythmias (including atrial fibrillation, supraventricular tachycardia and extrasystoles).	Very Rare
Nervous System Disorders	Headache	*Very Common
	Tremor	Common
Eye Disorders	Cataract, Glaucoma	Very Rare
Respiratory, Thoracic & Mediastinal Disorders	Nasopharyngitis	**#Very Common
	Throat irritation	Common
	Hoarseness/dysphonia	Common
	Sinusitis	*#Common
	Paradoxical bronchospasm	Very Rare
Skin and subcutaneous tissue disorders	Contusions	*#Common
Musculoskeletal & Connective Tissue Disorders	Muscle cramps	Common
	Traumatic fractures	*#Common
	Arthralgia	Very Rare
	Myalgia	Very Rare
Endocrine Disorders	Cushing's syndrome, Cushingoid features, Adrenal suppression, Growth retardation in children and adolescents, Decreased bone mineral density	Very Rare
Metabolism & Nutrition Disorders	Hypokalaemia	#Common
	Hyperglycaemia	Very Rare
Infections & Infestations	Candidiasis of the mouth and throat	Common
	Pneumonia	*#Common
	Bronchitis	*#Common
Immune System Disorders	Hypersensitivity reactions with the following manifestations:	
	Cutaneous hypersensitivity reactions	Uncommon
	Angioedema (mainly facial and oropharyngeal oedema), Respiratory symptoms (dyspnoea and/or bronchospasm), Anaphylactic reactions including anaphylactic shock	Very Rare
Psychiatric Disorders	Anxiety, sleep disorders and behavioural changes, including hyperactivity and irritability (predominantly in children)	Very Rare

*Reported commonly in placebo

**Reported very commonly in placebo

#Reported over 3 years in a COPD study

The pharmacological side effects of beta-2-agonist treatment, such as tremor, palpitations and headache, have been reported, but tend to be transient and reduce with regular therapy.

Due to the fluticasone propionate component, hoarseness and candidiasis (thrush) of the mouth and throat can occur in some patients. Both hoarseness and incidence of candidiasis may be relieved by gargling with water after using the product. Symptomatic candidiasis can be treated with topical anti-fungal therapy whilst still continuing with the Seretide Accuhaler.

Pneumonia was reported in studies of patients with COPD (see section 5.1).

Possible systemic effects include Cushing's syndrome, Cushingoid features, adrenal suppression, growth retardation in children and adolescents, decrease in bone mineral density, cataract and glaucoma (see section 4.4).

There have been very rare reports of hyperglycaemia (see section 4.4).

As with other inhalation therapy, paradoxical bronchospasm may occur (see section 4.4).

4.9 Overdose

There are no data available from clinical trials on overdose with Seretide, however data on overdose with both drugs are given below:

The signs and symptoms of salmeterol overdose are tremor, headache and tachycardia. The preferred antidotes are cardioselective beta-blocking agents, which should be used with caution in patients with a history of bronchospasm. If Seretide therapy has to be withdrawn due to overdose of the beta agonist component of the drug, provision of appropriate replacement steroid therapy should be considered. Additionally, hypokalaemia can occur and potassium replacement should be considered.

Acute: Acute inhalation of fluticasone propionate doses in excess of those recommended may lead to temporary suppression of adrenal function. This does not need emergency action as adrenal function is recovered in a few days, as verified by plasma cortisol measurements.

Chronic overdose of inhaled fluticasone propionate: Refer to section 4.4: risk of adrenal suppression: Monitoring of adrenal reserve may be necessary. In cases of fluticasone propionate overdose Seretide therapy may still be continued at a suitable dosage for symptom control.

5. PHARMACOLOGICAL PROPERTIES

5.1 Pharmacodynamic properties

Pharmacotherapeutic Group: Adrenergics and other anti-asthmatics.

ATC Code: R03AK06

Seretide Asthma clinical trials

A twelve month study (Gaining Optimal Asthma ControL, GOAL), in 3416 adult and adolescent patients with persistent asthma, compared the safety and efficacy of Seretide versus inhaled corticosteroid (Fluticasone Propionate) alone to determine whether the goals of asthma management were achievable. Treatment was stepped up every 12 weeks until **Total control was achieved or the highest dose of study drug was reached. GOAL showed more patients treated with Seretide achieved asthma control than patients treated with ICS alone and this control was attained at a lower corticosteroid dose.

Well Controlled asthma was achieved more rapidly with Seretide than with ICS alone. The time on treatment for 50% of subjects to achieve a first individual Well Controlled week was 16 days for Seretide compared to 37 days for the ICS group. In the subset of steroid naive asthmatics the time to an individual Well Controlled week was 16 days in the Seretide treatment compared to 23 days following treatment with ICS.

The overall study results showed:

(see Table 1 on next page)

The results of this study suggest that Seretide 50/100mcg bd may be considered as initial maintenance therapy in patients with moderate persistent asthma for whom rapid control of asthma is deemed essential (see section 4.2).

A double-blind, randomised, parallel group study in 318 patients with persistent asthma aged ≥ 18 years evaluated the safety and tolerability of administering two inhalations twice daily (double dose) of Seretide for two weeks. The study showed that doubling the inhalations of each strength of Seretide for up to 14 days resulted in a small increase in beta-agonist-related adverse events (tremor; 1 patient [1%] vs 0, palpitations; 6 [3%] vs 1 [$<1\%$], muscle cramps; 6[3%] vs 1 [$<1\%$]) and a similar incidence of inhaled corticosteroid related adverse events (e.g. oral candidiasis; 6 [6%] vs 16 [8%], hoarseness; 2 [2%] vs 4 [2%]) compared to one inhalation twice daily. The small increase in beta-agonist-related adverse events should be taken into account if doubling the dose of Seretide is considered by the physician in adult patients requiring additional short-term (up to 14 days) inhaled corticosteroid therapy.

Seretide COPD clinical trials

TORCH was a 3-year study to assess the effect of treatment with Seretide Accuhaler 50/500mcg bd, salmeterol Accuhaler 50mcg bd, fluticasone propionate (FP) Accuhaler 500mcg bd or placebo on all-cause mortality in patients with COPD. COPD patients with a baseline (pre-bronchodilator) $FEV_1 < 60\%$ of predicted normal were randomised to double-blind medication. During the study, patients were permitted usual COPD therapy with the exception of other inhaled corticosteroids, long-acting bronchodilators and long-term systemic corticosteroids. Survival status at 3 years was determined for all patients regardless of withdrawal from study medication. The primary endpoint was reduction in all cause mortality at 3 years for Seretide vs Placebo.

(see Table 2 on next page)

There was a trend towards improved survival in subjects treated with Seretide compared with placebo over 3 years however this did not achieve the statistical significance level $p \leq 0.05$.

The percentage of patients who died within 3 years due to COPD-related causes was 6.0% for placebo, 6.1% for salmeterol, 6.9% for FP and 4.7% for Seretide.

Table 1 Percentage of Patients Attaining *Well Controlled (WC) and **Totally Controlled (TC) Asthma over 12 months

Pre-Study Treatment	Salmeterol/FP		FP	
	WC	TC	WC	TC
No ICS (SABA alone)	78%	50%	70%	40%
Low dose ICS (≤500mcg BDP or equivalent/day)	75%	44%	60%	28%
Medium dose ICS (>500-1000mcg BDP or equivalent/day)	62%	29%	47%	16%
Pooled results across the 3 treatment levels	71%	41%	59%	28%

*Well controlled asthma; occasional symptoms or SABA use or less than 80% predicted lung function plus no night-time awakenings, no exacerbations and no side effects enforcing a change in therapy

**Total control of asthma; no symptoms, no SABA use, greater than or equal to 80% predicted lung function, no night-time awakenings, no exacerbations and no side effects enforcing a change in therapy

Table 2

	Placebo N = 1524	Salmeterol 50 N = 1521	FP 500 N = 1534	Seretide 50/500 N = 1533
All cause mortality at 3 years				
Number of deaths (%)	231 (15.2%)	205 (13.5%)	246 (16.0%)	193 (12.6%)
Hazard Ratio vs Placebo (CIs) p value	N/A	0.879 (0.73, 1.06) 0.180	1.060 (0.89, 1.27) 0.525	0.825 (0.68, 1.00) 0.052[1]
Hazard Ratio Seretide 50/500 vs components (CIs) p value	N/A	0.932 (0.77, 1.13) 0.481	0.774 (0.64, 0.93) 0.007	N/A

1. Non significant P value after adjustment for 2 interim analyses on the primary efficacy comparison from a log-rank analysis stratified by smoking status

Table 3 Key findings from SMART: primary endpoint

Patient group	Number of primary endpoint events / number of patients		Relative Risk (95% confidence intervals)
	salmeterol	placebo	
All patients	50/13,176	36/13,179	1.40 (0.91, 2.14)
Patients using inhaled steroids	23/6,127	19/6,138	1.21 (0.66, 2.23)
Patients not using inhaled steroids	27/7,049	17/7,041	1.60 (0.87, 2.93)
African-American patients	**20/2,366**	**5/2,319**	**4.10 (1.54, 10.90)**

(Risk in bold is statistically significant at the 95% level.)

Table 4 Key findings from SMART by inhaled steroid use at baseline: secondary endpoints

	Number of secondary endpoint events / number of patients		Relative Risk (95% confidence intervals)
	salmeterol	placebo	
Respiratory -related death			
Patients using inhaled steroids	10/6127	5/6138	2.01 (0.69, 5.86)
Patients not using inhaled steroids	14/7049	6/7041	2.28 (0.88, 5.94)
Combined asthma-related death or life-threatening experience			
Patients using inhaled steroids	16/6127	13/6138	1.24 (0.60, 2.58)
Patients not using inhaled steroids	**21/7049**	**9/7041**	**2.39 (1.10, 5.22)**
Asthma-related death			
Patients using inhaled steroids	4/6127	3/6138	1.35 (0.30, 6.04)
Patients not using inhaled steroids	9/7049	0/7041	*

(*=could not be calculated because of no events in placebo group. Risk in bold figures is statistically significant at the 95% level. The secondary endpoints in the table above reached statistical significance in the whole population.) The secondary endpoints of combined all-cause death or life-threatening experience, all cause death, or all cause hospitalisation did not reach statistical significance in the whole population.

The mean number of moderate to severe exacerbations per year was significantly reduced with Seretide as compared with treatment with salmeterol, FP and placebo (mean rate in the Seretide group 0.85 compared with 0.97 in the salmeterol group, 0.93 in the FP group and 1.13 in the placebo). This translates to a reduction in the rate of moderate to severe exacerbations of 25% (95% CI: 19% to 31%; p<0.001) compared with placebo, 12% compared with salmeterol (95% CI: 5% to 19%, p=0.002) and 9% compared with FP (95% CI: 1% to 16%, p=0.024). Salmeterol and FP significantly reduced exacerbation rates compared with placebo by 15% (95% CI: 7% to 22%; p<0.001) and 18% (95% CI: 11% to 24%; p<0.001) respectively.

Health Related Quality of Life, as measured by the St George's Respiratory Questionnaire (SGRQ) was improved by all active treatments in comparison with placebo. The average improvement over three years for Seretide compared with placebo was -3.1 units (95% CI: -4.1 to -2.1; p<0.001), compared with salmeterol was -2.2 units (p<0.001) and compared with FP was -1.2 units (p=0.017). A 4-unit decrease is considered clinically relevant.

The estimated 3-year probability of having pneumonia reported as an adverse event was 12.3% for placebo, 13.3% for salmeterol, 18.3% for FP and 19.6% for Seretide (Hazard ratio for Seretide vs placebo: 1.64, 95% CI: 1.33 to 2.01, p<0.001). There was no increase in pneumonia related deaths; deaths while on treatment that were adjudicated as primarily due to pneumonia were 7 for placebo, 9 for salmeterol, 13 for FP and 8 for Seretide. There was no significant difference in probability of bone fracture (5.1% placebo, 5.1% salmeterol, 5.4% FP and 6.3% Seretide; Hazard ratio for Seretide vs placebo: 1.22, 95% CI: 0.87 to 1.72, p=0.248.

Placebo-controlled clinical trials, over 6 and 12 months, have shown that regular use of Seretide 50/500 micrograms improves lung function and reduces breathlessness and the use of relief medication.

<u>The Salmeterol Multi-center Asthma Research Trial (SMART)</u>

SMART was a multi-centre, randomised, double-blind, placebo-controlled, parallel group 28-week study in the US which randomised 13,176 patients to salmeterol (50μg twice daily) and 13,179 patients to placebo in addition to the patients' usual asthma therapy. Patients were enrolled if ≥12 years of age, with asthma and if currently using asthma medication (but not a LABA). Baseline ICS use at study entry was recorded, but not required in the study. The primary endpoint in SMART was the combined number of respiratory-related deaths and respiratory-related life-threatening experiences.

Key findings from SMART: primary endpoint

(see Table 3 below)

Key findings from SMART by inhaled steroid use at baseline: secondary endpoints

(see Table 4 below)

<u>Mechanism of action:</u>

Seretide contains salmeterol and fluticasone propionate which have differing modes of action. The respective mechanisms of action of both drugs are discussed below:

<u>Salmeterol:</u>

Salmeterol is a selective long-acting (12 hour) beta-2-adrenoceptor agonist with a long side chain which binds to the exo-site of the receptor.

Salmeterol produces a longer duration of bronchodilation, lasting for at least 12 hours, than recommended doses of conventional short-acting beta-2-agonists.

<u>Fluticasone propionate:</u>

Fluticasone propionate given by inhalation at recommended doses has a glucocorticoid anti-inflammatory action within the lungs, resulting in reduced symptoms and exacerbations of asthma, without the adverse effects observed when corticosteroids are administered systemically.

5.2 Pharmacokinetic properties

When salmeterol and fluticasone propionate were administered in combination by the inhaled route, the pharmacokinetics of each component were similar to those observed when the drugs were administered separately. For pharmacokinetic purposes therefore each component can be considered separately.

<u>Salmeterol:</u>

Salmeterol acts locally in the lung therefore plasma levels are not an indication of therapeutic effects. In addition there are only limited data available on the pharmacokinetics of salmeterol because of the technical difficulty of assaying the drug in plasma due to the low plasma concentrations at therapeutic doses (approximately 200 picogram/ml or less) achieved after inhaled dosing.

<u>Fluticasone propionate:</u>

The absolute bioavailability of a single dose of inhaled fluticasone propionate in healthy subjects varies between approximately 5-11% of the nominal dose depending on the inhalation device used. In patients with asthma or COPD a lesser degree of systemic exposure to inhaled fluticasone propionate has been observed.

Systemic absorption occurs mainly through the lungs and is initially rapid then prolonged. The remainder of the inhaled dose may be swallowed but contributes minimally to systemic exposure due to the low aqueous solubility and pre-systemic metabolism, resulting in oral availability of less than 1%. There is a linear increase in systemic exposure with increasing inhaled dose.

The disposition of fluticasone propionate is characterised by high plasma clearance (1150ml/min), a large volume of distribution at steady-state (approximately 300l) and a terminal half-life of approximately 8 hours.

Plasma protein binding is 91%.

Fluticasone propionate is cleared very rapidly from the systemic circulation. The main pathway is metabolism to an inactive carboxylic acid metabolite, by the cytochrome P450 enzyme CYP3A4. Other unidentified metabolites are also found in the faeces.

The renal clearance of fluticasone propionate is negligible. Less than 5% of the dose is excreted in urine, mainly as metabolites. The main part of the dose is excreted in faeces as metabolites and unchanged drug.

5.3 Preclinical safety data

The only safety concerns for human use derived from animal studies of salmeterol xinafoate and fluticasone propionate given separately were effects associated with exaggerated pharmacological actions.

In animal reproduction studies, glucocorticosteroids have been shown to induce malformations (cleft palate, skeletal malformations). However, these animal experimental results do not seem to be relevant for man given recommended doses. Animal studies with salmeterol xinafoate have shown embryofoetal toxicity only at high exposure levels. Following co-administration, increased incidences of transposed umbilical artery and incomplete ossification of occipital bone were found in rats at doses associated with known glucocorticoid-induced abnormalities.

6. PHARMACEUTICAL PARTICULARS

6.1 List of excipients

Lactose monohydrate (which contains milk proteins).

6.2 Incompatibilities

Not applicable.

6.3 Shelf life

18 months.

6.4 Special precautions for storage

Do not store above 30°C.

6.5 Nature and contents of container

The inhalation powder is contained in blisters held on a formed PVC coated base, with a peelable foil laminate lid. The strip is contained in a moulded plastic device.

The plastic devices are available in cardboard containers, which hold

1 × 28 dose Accuhaler

or 1 × 60 dose Accuhaler

or 2 × 60 dose Accuhaler

or 3 × 60 dose Accuhaler or 10 × 60 dose Accuhaler

Not all pack sizes may be marketed.

6.6 Special precautions for disposal and other handling

The Accuhaler releases a powder which is inhaled into the lungs. A dose indicator on the Accuhaler indicates the number of doses left. For detailed instructions for use see the Patient Information Leaflet.

7. MARKETING AUTHORISATION HOLDER

Glaxo Wellcome UK Ltd,

trading as Allen & Hanburys,

Stockley Park West,

Uxbridge,

Middlesex, UB11 1BT

8. MARKETING AUTHORISATION NUMBER(S)

Seretide 100 Accuhaler PL10949/0314

Seretide 250 Accuhaler PL10949/0315

Seretide 500 Accuhaler PL10949/0316

9. DATE OF FIRST AUTHORISATION/RENEWAL OF THE AUTHORISATION

Date of first authorisation:1 February 1999

Date of latest renewal:3 December 2008

10. DATE OF REVISION OF THE TEXT

11 December 2008

Seretide 50, 125, 250 Evohaler

(Allen & Hanburys)

1. NAME OF THE MEDICINAL PRODUCT

Seretide Evohaler 25 microgram /50 microgram/dose pressurised inhalation, suspension.

Seretide Evohaler 25 microgram /125 microgram/dose pressurised inhalation, suspension.

Seretide Evohaler 25 microgram /250 microgram/dose pressurised inhalation, suspension.

2. QUALITATIVE AND QUANTITATIVE COMPOSITION

25 micrograms of salmeterol (as salmeterol xinafoate) and 50, 125 or 250 micrograms of fluticasone propionate (delivered from the valve). This is equivalent to 21 micrograms of salmeterol and 44, 110 or 220 micrograms of fluticasone propionate delivered from the actuator (delivered dose).

For a full list of excipients, see section 6.1.

3. PHARMACEUTICAL FORM

Pressurised inhalation, suspension.

The canister contains a white to off white suspension.

4. CLINICAL PARTICULARS

4.1 Therapeutic indications

Seretide is indicated in the regular treatment of asthma where use of a combination product (long-acting beta-2-agonist and inhaled corticosteroid) is appropriate:

- patients not adequately controlled with inhaled corticosteroids and 'as needed' inhaled short acting beta-2-agonist

or

- patients already adequately controlled on both inhaled corticosteroid and long-acting beta-2-agonist.

4.2 Posology and method of administration

Seretide Evohaler is for inhalation use only.

Patients should be made aware that Seretide Evohaler must be used daily for optimum benefit, even when asymptomatic.

Patients should be regularly reassessed by a doctor, so that the strength of Seretide they are receiving remains optimal and is only changed on medical advice. **The dose should be titrated to the lowest dose at which effective control of symptoms is maintained. Where the control of symptoms is maintained with the lowest strength of the combination given twice daily then the next step could include a test of inhaled corticosteroid alone.** As an alternative, patients requiring a long acting beta-2-agonist could be titrated to Seretide given once daily if, in the opinion of the prescriber, it would be adequate to maintain disease control. In the event of once daily dosing when the patient has a history of nocturnal symptoms the dose should be given at night and when the patient has a history of mainly day-time symptoms the dose should be given in the morning.

Patients should be given the strength of Seretide containing the appropriate fluticasone propionate dosage for the severity of their disease. Note: Seretide 25 microgram /50 microgram strength is not appropriate in adults and children with severe asthma. Prescribers should be aware that, in patients with asthma, fluticasone propionate is as effective as other inhaled steroids at approximately half the microgram daily dose. For example, 100mcg of fluticasone propionate is approximately equivalent to 200mcg of beclomethasone dipropionate (CFC containing) or budesonide. If an individual patient should require dosages outside the recommended regimen, appropriate doses of beta-agonist and/or corticosteroid should be prescribed.

Recommended Doses:

Adults and adolescents 12 years and older:

Two inhalations of 25 micrograms salmeterol and 50 micrograms fluticasone propionate twice daily.

or

Two inhalations of 25 micrograms salmeterol and 125 micrograms fluticasone propionate twice daily.

or

Two inhalations of 25 micrograms salmeterol and 250 micrograms fluticasone propionate twice daily.

A short term trial of Seretide may be considered as initial maintenance therapy in adults or adolescents with moderate persistent asthma (defined as patients with daily symptoms, daily rescue use and moderate to severe airflow limitation) for whom rapid control of asthma is essential. In these cases, the recommended initial dose is two inhalations of 25 micrograms salmeterol and 50 micrograms fluticasone propionate twice daily. Once control of asthma is attained treatment should be reviewed and consideration given as to whether patients should be stepped down to an inhaled corticosteroid alone. Regular review of patients as treatment is stepped down is important.

A clear benefit has not been shown as compared to inhaled fluticasone propionate alone used as initial maintenance therapy when one or two of the criteria of severity are missing. In general inhaled corticosteroids remain the first line treatment for most patients. Seretide is not intended for the initial management of mild asthma. Seretide 25 microgram /50 micrograms strength is not appropriate in adults and children with severe asthma; it is recommended to establish the appropriate dosage of inhaled corticosteroid before any fixed combination can be used in patients with severe asthma.

Children 4 years and older:

Two inhalations of 25 micrograms salmeterol and 50 micrograms fluticasone propionate twice daily.

The maximum licensed dose of fluticasone propionate delivered by Seretide inhaler in children is 100mcg twice daily.

There are no data available for use of Seretide inhaler in children aged under 4 years.

Use of a spacer device with Seretide inhaler is recommended in patients who find it difficult to synchronise aerosol actuation with inspiration of breath. Either the Volumatic or AeroChamber Plus spacer device can be used (depending on National Guidance). Limited data are available that demonstrate an increase in systemic exposure when the AeroChamber Plus spacer device is used compared with the Volumatic spacer device (see section 4.4).

Patients should be instructed in the proper use and care of their inhaler and spacer and their technique checked to ensure optimum delivery of the inhaled drug to the lungs.

Patients should continue to use the same make of spacer device as switching between spacer devices can result in changes in the dose delivered to the lungs (see section 4.4).

Re-titration to the lowest effective dose should always follow the introduction or change of a spacer device.

Special patient groups:

There is no need to adjust the dose in elderly patients or in those with renal impairment. There are no data available for use of Seretide in patients with hepatic impairment.

Instructions for Use:

Patients should be instructed in the proper use of their inhaler (see patient information leaflet)

During inhalation, the patient should preferably sit or stand. The inhaler has been designed for use in a vertical position.

Testing the inhaler:

Before using for the first time patients should remove the mouthpiece cover by gently squeezing the sides of the cover, shake the inhaler well, hold the inhaler between the fingers and thumb with your thumb at the base, below the mouthpiece and release puffs into the air until the counter reads 120 to make sure that it works. The inhaler should be shaken immediately before releasing each puff. If the inhaler has not been used for a week or more remove the mouthpiece cover, the patients should shake the inhaler well and release two puffs into the air. Each time the inhaler is activated the number on the counter will count down by one.

Use of the inhaler:

1. Patients should remove the mouthpiece cover by gently squeezing the sides of the cover.

2. Patients should check inside and outside of the inhaler including the mouthpiece for the presence of loose objects.

3. Patients should shake the inhaler well to ensure that any lose objects are removed and that the contents of the inhaler are evenly mixed

4. Patients should hold the inhaler upright between fingers and thumb with their thumb on the base, below the mouthpiece.

5. Patients should breathe out as far as is comfortable and then place the mouthpiece in their mouth between their teeth and close their lips around it, Patients should be instructed not to bite the mouth piece.

6. Just after starting to breathe in through their mouth, patients should press firmly down on the top of the inhaler to release Seretide, while still breathing in steadily and deeply.

7. While holding their breath, patients should take the inhaler from their mouth and take their finger from the top of the inhaler. Patients should continue holding their breath for as long as is comfortable.

8. To take a second inhalation, patients should keep the inhaler upright and wait about half a minute before repeating steps 3 to 7.

9. Patients should immediately replace the mouthpiece cover in the correct orientation by firmly pushing and snapping the cap into position. The cover does not require excessive force and it will click into position

IMPORTANT

Patients should not rush stages 5, 6 and 7. It is important that patients start to breathe in as slowly as possible just before operating their inhaler. Patients should practise in front of a mirror for the first few times. If they see "mist" coming from the top of their inhaler or the sides of their mouth they should start again from stage 2.

Patients should consider getting a replacement when the counter shows the number 020. The counter will stop at 000 when all the recommended puffs have been used. Replace the inhaler when the counter reads 000.

Patients should never try to alter the numbers on the counter or detach the counter from the metal canister. The counter cannot be reset and is permanently attached to the canister.

Cleaning:

Your inhaler should be cleaned at least once a week.

1. Remove the mouth piece cover.

2. Do not remove the canister from the plastic casing.

3. Wipe the inside and outside of the mouthpiece and the plastic casing with a dry cloth or tissue.

4. Replace the mouthpiece cover in the correct orientation. The cover does not require excessive force and it will click into position.

DO NOT PUT THE METAL CONTAINER IN WATER

4.3 Contraindications

Seretide is contraindicated in patients with hypersensitivity to any of the active substances or to the excipient.

4.4 Special warnings and precautions for use

The management of asthma should normally follow a stepwise programme and patient response should be monitored clinically and by lung function tests.

Seretide Evohaler should not be used to treat acute asthma symptoms for which a fast and short acting bronchodilator is required. Patients should be advised to have their medicinal product to be used for relief in an acute asthma attack available at all times.

Patients should not be initiated on Seretide during an exacerbation, or if they have significantly worsening or acutely deteriorating asthma.

Serious asthma-related adverse events and exacerbations may occur during treatment with Seretide. Patients should be asked to continue treatment but to seek medical advice if asthma symptoms remain uncontrolled or worsen after initiation on Seretide.

Increasing use of short-acting bronchodilators to relieve asthma symptoms indicates deterioration of asthma control and patients should be reviewed by a physician.

Sudden and progressive deterioration in control of asthma is potentially life-threatening and the patient should undergo urgent medical assessment. Consideration should be given to increasing corticosteroid therapy. The patient should also be medically reviewed where the current dosage of Seretide has failed to give adequate control of asthma. Consideration should be given to additional corticosteroid therapies.

Once asthma symptoms are controlled, consideration may be given to gradually reducing the dose of Seretide. Regular review of patients as treatment is stepped down is important. The lowest effective dose of Seretide should be used (see section 4.2).

Treatment with Seretide should not be stopped abruptly.

As with all inhaled medication containing corticosteroids, Seretide should be administered with caution in patients with pulmonary tuberculosis.

Rarely, Seretide may cause cardiac arrhythmias e.g. supraventricular tachycardia, extrasystoles and atrial fibrillation, and a mild transient reduction in serum potassium at high therapeutic doses. Therefore Seretide should be used with caution in patients with severe cardiovascular disorders, heart rhythm abnormalities, diabetes mellitus, thyrotoxicosis, uncorrected hypokalaemia or patients predisposed to low levels of serum potassium.

There have been very rare reports of increases in blood glucose levels (See section 4.8) and this should be considered when prescribing to patients with a history of diabetes mellitus.

As with other inhalation therapy paradoxical bronchospasm may occur with an immediate increase in wheezing after dosing. Seretide Evohaler should be discontinued immediately, the patient assessed and alternative therapy instituted if necessary.

Care should be taken when transferring patients to Seretide therapy, particularly if there is any reason to suppose that adrenal function is impaired from previous systemic steroid therapy.

Systemic effects may occur with any inhaled corticosteroid, particularly at high doses prescribed for long periods. These effects are much less likely to occur than with oral corticosteroids. Possible systemic effects include Cushing's syndrome, Cushingoid features, adrenal suppression, growth retardation in children and adolescents, decrease in bone mineral density, cataract and glaucoma. **It is important, therefore, that the patient is reviewed regularly and the dose of inhaled corticosteroid is reduced to the lowest dose at which effective control of asthma is maintained.**

It is recommended that the height of children receiving prolonged treatment with inhaled corticosteroid is regularly monitored.

Prolonged treatment of patients with high doses of inhaled corticosteroids may result in adrenal suppression and acute adrenal crisis. Children and adolescents <16years taking high doses of fluticasone (typically ⩾ 1000mcg/day) may be at particular risk. Very rare cases of adrenal suppression and acute adrenal crisis have also been described with doses of fluticasone propionate between 500 and less than 1000mcg. Situations, which could potentially trigger acute adrenal crisis, include trauma, surgery, infection or any rapid reduction in dosage. Presenting symptoms are typically vague and may include anorexia, abdominal pain, weight loss, tiredness, headache, nausea, vomiting, hypotension, decreased level of consciousness, hypoglycaemia, and seizures. Additional systemic corticosteroid cover should be considered during periods of stress or elective surgery.

Systemic absorption of salmeterol and fluticasone propionate is largely through the lungs. As the use of a spacer device with a metered dose inhaler may increase drug delivery to the lungs it should be noted that this could potentially lead to an increase in the risk of systemic adverse effects. Single dose pharmacokinetic data have demonstrated that the systemic exposure to salmeterol and fluticasone propionate may be increased as much as two-fold when the AeroChamber Plus spacer device is used with Seretide inhaler as compared with the Volumatic spacer device.

The benefits of inhaled fluticasone propionate therapy should minimise the need for oral steroids, but patients transferring from oral steroids may remain at risk of impaired adrenal reserve for a considerable time. Patients who have required high dose emergency corticosteroid therapy in the past may also be at risk. This possibility of residual impairment should always be borne in mind in emergency and elective situations likely to produce stress, and appropriate corticosteroid treatment must be considered. The extent of the adrenal impairment may require specialist advice before elective procedures.

Ritonavir can greatly increase the concentration of fluticasone propionate in plasma. Therefore, concomitant use should be avoided, unless the potential benefit to the patient outweighs the risk of systemic corticosteroid side-effects. There is also an increased risk of systemic side effects when combining fluticasone propionate with other potent CYP3A inhibitors (see section 4.5).

There was an increased reporting of lower respiratory tract infections (particularly pneumonia and bronchitis) in a 3 year study in patients with Chronic Obstructive Pulmonary Disease (COPD) receiving Seretide compared with placebo (see section 4.8). In a 3 year COPD study, older patients, patients with a lower body mass index (<25kg/m^2) and patients with very severe disease (FEV_1 <30% predicted) were at greatest risk of developing pneumonia regardless of treatment. Physicians should remain vigilant for the possible development of pneumonia and other lower respiratory tract infections in patients with COPD as the clinical features of such infections and exacerbation frequently overlap. If a patient with severe COPD has experienced pneumonia the treatment with Seretide should be re-evaluated.

Data from a large clinical trial (the Salmeterol Multi-Center Asthma Research Trial, SMART) suggested African-American patients were at increased risk of serious respiratory-related events or deaths when using salmeterol compared with placebo (see section 5.1). It is not known if this was due to pharmacogenetic or other factors. Patients of black African or Afro-Caribbean ancestry should therefore be asked to continue treatment but to seek medical advice if asthma symptoms remained uncontrolled or worsen whilst using Seretide.

4.5 Interaction with other medicinal products and other forms of interaction

Both non-selective and selective beta-blockers should be avoided in patients with asthma, unless there are compelling reasons for their use.

Concomitant use of other beta-adrenergic containing drugs can have a potentially additive effect.

Under normal circumstances, low plasma concentrations of fluticasone propionate are achieved after inhaled dosing, due to extensive first pass metabolism and high systemic clearance mediated by cytochrome P450 3A4 in the gut and liver. Hence, clinically significant drug interactions mediated by fluticasone propionate are unlikely.

In an interaction study in healthy subjects with intranasal fluticasone propionate, ritonavir (a highly potent cytochrome P450 3A4 inhibitor) 100 mg b.i.d. increased the fluticasone propionate plasma concentrations several hundred fold, resulting in markedly reduced serum cortisol concentrations. Information about this interaction is lacking for inhaled fluticasone propionate, but a marked increase in fluticasone propionate plasma levels is expected. Cases of Cushing's syndrome and adrenal suppression have been reported. The combination should be avoided unless the benefit outweighs the increased risk of systemic glucocorticoid side-effects.

In a small study in healthy volunteers, the slightly less potent CYP3A inhibitor ketoconazole increased the exposure of fluticasone propionate after a single inhalation by 150%. This resulted in a greater reduction of plasma cortisol as compared with fluticasone propionate alone. Co-treatment with other potent CYP3A inhibitors, such as itraconazole, is also expected to increase the systemic fluticasone propionate exposure and the risk of systemic side-effects. Caution is recommended and long-term treatment with such drugs should if possible be avoided.

4.6 Pregnancy and lactation

There are insufficient data on the use of salmeterol and fluticasone propionate during pregnancy and lactation in man to assess the possible harmful effects. In animal studies foetal abnormalities occur after administration of beta-2-adrenoreceptor agonists and glucocorticosteroids (see section 5.3).

Administration of Seretide to pregnant women should only be considered if the expected benefit to the mother is greater than any possible risk to the foetus.

The lowest effective dose of fluticasone propionate needed to maintain adequate asthma control should be used in the treatment of pregnant women.

There are no data available for human breast milk. Both salmeterol and fluticasone propionate are excreted into breast milk in rats. Administration of Seretide to women who are breastfeeding should only be considered if the expected benefit to the mother is greater than any possible risk to the child.

4.7 Effects on ability to drive and use machines

No studies of the effect on the ability to drive and use machines have been performed.

4.8 Undesirable effects

As Seretide contains salmeterol and fluticasone propionate, the type and severity of adverse reactions associated with each of the compounds may be expected. There is no incidence of additional adverse events following concurrent administration of the two compounds.

Adverse events which have been associated with salmeterol/fluticasone propionate are given below, listed by system organ class and frequency. Frequencies are defined as: very common (⩾1/10), common (⩾1/100 and <1/10), uncommon (⩾1/1000 and <1/100), and very rare (<1/10,000) including isolated reports. Very common, common and uncommon events were derived from clinical trial data. The incidence in placebo was not taken into account. Very rare events were derived from post-marketing spontaneous data.

System Organ Class	Adverse Event	Frequency
Infections & Infestations	Candidiasis of the mouth and throat	Common
	Pneumonia	*#Common
	Bronchitis	*#Common
Immune System Disorders	Hypersensitivity reactions with the following manifestations:	
	Cutaneous hypersensitivity reactions	Uncommon
	Angioedema (mainly facial and oropharyngeal oedema), Respiratory symptoms (dyspnoea and/or bronchospasm), Anaphylactic reactions including anaphylactic shock	Very Rare
Endocrine Disorders	Cushing's syndrome, Cushingoid features, Adrenal suppression, Growth retardation in children and adolescents, Decreased bone mineral density, Cataract, Glaucoma	Very Rare
Metabolism & Nutrition Disorders	Hypokalaemia	#Common
	Hyperglycaemia	Very Rare
Psychiatric Disorders	Anxiety, sleep disorders and behavioural changes, including hyperactivity and irritability (predominantly in children)	Very Rare
Nervous System Disorders	Headache	*Very Common
	Tremor	Common
Cardiac Disorders	Palpitations	Common
	Tachycardia	Uncommon
	Cardiac arrhythmias (including atrial fibrillation, supraventricular tachycardia and extrasystoles).	Very Rare
Respiratory, Thoracic & Mediastinal Disorders	Nasopharyngitis	**#Very Common
	Throat irritation	Common
	Hoarseness/dysphonia	Common
	Sinusitis	*#Common
	Paradoxical bronchospasm	Very Rare
Skin and subcutaneous tissue disorders	Contusions	*#Common
Musculoskeletal & Connective Tissue Disorders	Muscle cramps	Common
	Traumatic fractures	*#Common
	Arthralgia	Very Rare
	Myalgia	Very Rare

*Reported commonly in placebo

** Reported very commonly in placebo

Reported over 3 years in a COPD study

The pharmacological side effects of beta-2-agonist treatment, such as tremor, palpitations and headache, have been reported, but tend to be transient and reduce with regular therapy.

Due to the fluticasone propionate component, hoarseness and candidiasis (thrush) of the mouth and throat can occur in some patients. Both hoarseness and incidence of candidiasis may be relieved by gargling with water after using the product. Symptomatic candidiasis can be treated with topical anti-fungal therapy whilst still continuing with the Seretide Evohaler.

Pneumonia was reported in studies of patients with Chronic Obstructive Pulmonary Disease (COPD).

Possible systemic effects include Cushing's syndrome, Cushingoid features, adrenal suppression, growth retardation in children and adolescents, decrease in bone mineral density, cataract and glaucoma (see section 4.4).

There have been very rare reports of hyperglycaemia (see section 4.4).

As with other inhalation therapy, paradoxical bronchospasm may occur (see section 4.4).

4.9 Overdose

There are no data available from clinical trials on overdose with Seretide, however data on overdose with both drugs are given below:

The signs and symptoms of salmeterol overdose are tremor, headache and tachycardia. The preferred antidotes are cardioselective beta-blocking agents, which should be used with caution in patients with a history of bronchospasm. If Seretide therapy has to be withdrawn due to overdose of the beta agonist component of the drug, provision of appropriate replacement steroid therapy should be considered. Additionally, hypokalaemia can occur and potassium replacement should be considered.

Acute: Acute inhalation of fluticasone propionate doses in excess of those recommended may lead to temporary suppression of adrenal function. This does not need emergency action as adrenal function is recovered in a few days, as verified by plasma cortisol measurements.

Chronic overdose of inhaled fluticasone propionate: Refer to section 4.4: risk of adrenal suppression.

Monitoring of adrenal reserve may be necessary. In cases of fluticasone propionate overdose Seretide therapy may still be continued at a suitable dosage for symptom control.

5. PHARMACOLOGICAL PROPERTIES

5.1 Pharmacodynamic properties

Pharmacotherapeutic Group: Adrenergics and other antiasthmatics.

ATC Code: R03AK06

Seretide Asthma clinical trials

A twelve month study (Gaining Optimal Asthma ControL, GOAL), in 3416 adult and adolescent patients with persistent asthma, compared the safety and efficacy of Seretide versus inhaled corticosteroid (Fluticasone Propionate) alone to determine whether the goals of asthma management were achievable. Treatment was stepped up every 12 weeks until **Total control was achieved or the highest dose of study drug was reached. GOAL showed more patients treated with Seretide achieved asthma control than patients treated with ICS alone and this control was attained at a lower corticosteroid dose

Well-Controlled asthma was achieved more rapidly with Seretide than with ICS alone. The time on treatment for 50% of subjects to achieve a first individual Well-Controlled week was 16 days for Seretide compared to 37 days for the ICS group. In the subset of steroid naive asthmatics the time to an individual Well Controlled week was 16 days in the Seretide treatment compared to 23 days following treatment with ICS.

The overall study results showed:

(see Table 1 below)

The results of this study suggest that Seretide 50/100mcg bd may be considered as initial maintenance therapy in patients with moderate persistent asthma for whom rapid control of asthma is deemed essential (see section 4.2).

A double-blind, randomised, parallel group study in 318 patients with persistent asthma aged ⩾18 years evaluated the safety and tolerability of administering two inhalations twice daily (double dose) of Seretide for two weeks. The study showed that doubling the inhalations of each strength of Seretide for up to 14 days resulted in a small increase in beta-agonist-related adverse events (tremor; 1 patient [1%] vs 0, palpitations; 6 [3%] vs 1 [<1%], muscle cramps; 6[3%] vs 1 [<1%]) and a similar incidence of inhaled corticosteroid related adverse events (e.g. oral candidiasis; 6 [6%] vs 16 [8%], hoarseness; 2 [2%] vs 4 [2%]) compared to one inhalation twice daily. The small increase in beta-agonist-related adverse events should be taken into account if doubling the dose of Seretide is considered by the physician in adult patients requiring additional short-term (up to 14 days) inhaled corticosteroid therapy.

The Salmeterol Multi-center Asthma Research Trial (SMART)

SMART was a multi-centre, randomised, double-blind, placebo-controlled, parallel group 28-week study in the US which randomised 13,176 patients to salmeterol (50μg twice daily) and 13,179 patients to placebo in addition to the patients' usual asthma therapy. Patients were enrolled if ⩾12 years of age, with asthma and if currently using asthma medication (but not a LABA). Baseline ICS use at study entry was recorded, but not required in the study. The primary endpoint in SMART was the combined number of respiratory-related deaths and respiratory-related life-threatening experiences.

Key findings from SMART: primary endpoint

(see Table 2 below)

Key findings from SMART by inhaled steroid use at baseline: secondary endpoints

(see Table 3 below)

Mechanism of action:

Seretide contains salmeterol and fluticasone propionate which have differing modes of action.

The respective mechanisms of action of both drugs are discussed below.

Salmeterol:

Salmeterol is a selective long-acting (12 hour) beta-2-adrenoceptor agonist with a long side chain which binds to the exo-site of the receptor.

Salmeterol produces a longer duration of bronchodilation, lasting for at least 12 hours, than recommended doses of conventional short-acting beta-2-agonists.

Fluticasone propionate:

Fluticasone propionate given by inhalation at recommended doses has a glucocorticoid anti-inflammatory action within the lungs, resulting in reduced symptoms and exacerbations of asthma, with less adverse effects than when corticosteroids are administered systemically.

5.2 Pharmacokinetic properties

When salmeterol and fluticasone propionate were administered in combination by the inhaled route, the pharmacokinetics of each component were similar to those observed when the drugs were administered separately. For pharmacokinetic purposes therefore each component can be considered separately.

Salmeterol:

Salmeterol acts locally in the lung therefore plasma levels are not an indication of therapeutic effects. In addition there are only limited data available on the pharmacokinetics of salmeterol because of the technical difficulty of assaying the drug in plasma due to the low plasma concentrations at therapeutic doses (approximately 200 picogram/ml or less) achieved after inhaled dosing.

Fluticasone propionate:

The absolute bioavailability of a single dose of inhaled fluticasone propionate in healthy subjects varies between approximately 5-11% of the nominal dose depending on the inhalation device used. In patients with asthma a lesser degree of systemic exposure to inhaled fluticasone propionate has been observed.

Systemic absorption occurs mainly through the lungs and is initially rapid then prolonged. The remainder of the inhaled dose may be swallowed but contributes minimally to systemic exposure due to the low aqueous solubility and pre-systemic metabolism, resulting in oral availability of less than 1%. There is a linear increase in systemic exposure with increasing inhaled dose.

The disposition of fluticasone propionate is characterised by high plasma clearance (1150ml/min), a large volume of

Table 1 Percentage of Patients Attaining *Well Controlled (WC) and **Totally Controlled (TC) Asthma over 12 months

Pre-Study Treatment	Salmeterol/FP		FP	
	WC	TC	WC	TC
No ICS (SABA alone)	78%	50%	70%	40%
Low dose ICS (⩽500mcg BDP or equivalent/day)	75%	44%	60%	28%
Medium dose ICS (>500-1000mcg BDP or equivalent/day)	62%	29%	47%	16%
Pooled results across the 3 treatment levels	71%	41%	59%	28%

*Well controlled asthma; occasional symptoms or SABA use or less than 80% predicted lung function plus no night-time awakenings, no exacerbations and no side effects enforcing a change in therapy

**Total control of asthma; no symptoms, no SABA use, greater than or equal to 80% predicted lung function, no night-time awakenings, no exacerbations and no side effects enforcing a change in therapy

Table 2 Key findings from SMART: primary endpoint

Patient group	Number of primary endpoint events / number of patients		Relative Risk (95% confidence intervals)
	salmeterol	placebo	
All patients	50/13,176	36/13,179	1.40 (0.91, 2.14)
Patients using inhaled steroids	23/6,127	19/6,138	1.21 (0.66, 2.23)
Patients not using inhaled steroids	27/7,049	17/7,041	1.60 (0.87, 2.93)
African-American patients	**20/2,366**	**5/2,319**	**4.10 (1.54, 10.90)**

(Risk in bold is statistically significant at the 95% level.)

Table 3 Key findings from SMART by inhaled steroid use at baseline: secondary endpoints

	Number of secondary endpoint events / number of patients		Relative Risk (95% confidence intervals)
	salmeterol	placebo	
Respiratory -related death			
Patients using inhaled steroids	10/6127	5/6138	2.01 (0.69, 5.86)
Patients not using inhaled steroids	14/7049	6/7041	2.28 (0.88, 5.94)
Combined asthma-related death or life-threatening experience			
Patients using inhaled steroids	16/6127	13/6138	1.24 (0.60, 2.58)
Patients not using inhaled steroids	**21/7049**	**9/7041**	**2.39 (1.10, 5.22)**
Asthma-related death			
Patients using inhaled steroids	4/6127	3/6138	1.35 (0.30, 6.04)
Patients not using inhaled steroids	9/7049	0/7041	*

(*=could not be calculated because of no events in placebo group. Risk in bold figures is statistically significant at the 95% level. The secondary endpoints in the table above reached statistical significance in the whole population.) The secondary endpoints of combined all-cause death or life-threatening experience, all cause death, or all cause hospitalisation did not reach statistical significance in the whole population.

distribution at steady-state (approximately 300l) and a terminal half-life of approximately 8 hours.

Plasma protein binding is 91%.

Fluticasone propionate is cleared very rapidly from the systemic circulation. The main pathway is metabolism to an inactive carboxylic acid metabolite, by the cytochrome P450 enzyme CYP3A4. Other unidentified metabolites are also found in the faeces.

The renal clearance of fluticasone propionate is negligible. Less than 5% of the dose is excreted in urine, mainly as metabolites. The main part of the dose is excreted as faeces as metabolites and unchanged drug.

5.3 Preclinical safety data

The only safety concerns for human use derived from animal studies of salmeterol xinafoate and fluticasone propionate given separately were effects associated with exaggerated pharmacological actions.

In animal reproduction studies, glucocorticosteroids have been shown to induce malformations (cleft palate, skeletal malformations). However, these animal experimental results do not seem to be relevant for man given recommended doses. Animal studies with salmeterol xinafoate have shown embryofoetal toxicity only at high exposure levels. Following co-administration, increased incidences of transposed umbilical artery and incomplete ossification of occipital bone were found in rats at doses associated with known glucocorticoid-induced abnormalities.

The non-CFC propellant, Norflurane, has been shown to have no toxic effect at very high vapour concentrations, far in excess of those likely to be experienced by patients, in a wide range of animal species exposed daily for periods of two years.

6. PHARMACEUTICAL PARTICULARS

6.1 List of excipients

Norflurane (HFA 134a).

6.2 Incompatibilities

Not applicable.

6.3 Shelf life

1 year

6.4 Special precautions for storage

Replace the mouthpiece cover firmly and snap it into position

The canister contains a pressurised liquid. Do not store above 25°C. The container should not be punctured, broken or burnt even when apparently empty.

As with most inhaled medicinal products in pressurised containers, the therapeutic effect of this medicinal product may decrease when the container is cold.

6.5 Nature and contents of container

The suspension is contained in an internally lacquered, 8ml aluminium alloy pressurised container sealed with a metering valve. The containers are fitted into plastic actuators incorporating an atomising mouthpiece and fitted with dustcaps. The canister has a counter attached to it, which shows how many actuations of medicine are left. The number will show through a window in the back of the plastic actuator. One pressurised container delivers 120 actuations.

The devices are available in cardboard containers, which hold

1 × 120 actuations Inhaler

or 3 × 120 actuations Inhaler

or 10 × 120 actuations Inhaler - hospital/pharmacy use only (for dispensing purposes)

Not all pack sizes may be marketed.

6.6 Special precautions for disposal and other handling

No special requirements.

7. MARKETING AUTHORISATION HOLDER

Glaxo Wellcome UK Limited

Trading as Allen & Hanburys

Stockley Park West

Uxbridge, Middlesex UB11 1BT.

8. MARKETING AUTHORISATION NUMBER(S)

PL 10949/0337 - Seretide Evohaler 25 microgram /50 microgram/dose pressurised inhalation, suspension.

PL 10949/0338 - Seretide Evohaler 25 microgram /125 microgram/dose pressurised inhalation, suspension.

PL 10949/ 0339 - Seretide Evohaler 25 microgram /250 microgram/dose pressurised inhalation, suspension

9. DATE OF FIRST AUTHORISATION/RENEWAL OF THE AUTHORISATION

16 June 2000 / 27 September 2005

10. DATE OF REVISION OF THE TEXT

January 2008

Serevent Accuhaler

(Allen & Hanburys)

1. NAME OF THE MEDICINAL PRODUCT

Serevent[TM] Accuhaler[TM]

2. QUALITATIVE AND QUANTITATIVE COMPOSITION

Serevent Accuhaler is a moulded plastic device containing a foil strip with regularly spaced blisters each containing 50 micrograms of salmeterol (as xinafoate).

For excipients, see 6.1

3. PHARMACEUTICAL FORM

Inhalation powder.

4. CLINICAL PARTICULARS

4.1 Therapeutic indications

Salmeterol is a selective β_2-agonist indicated for reversible airways obstruction in patients with asthma and chronic obstructive pulmonary disease (COPD).

In asthma (including nocturnal asthma and exercise induced symptoms) it is indicated for those treated with inhaled corticosteroids who require a long-acting beta agonist in accordance with current treatment guidelines.

Serevent Accuhaler is not a replacement for inhaled or oral corticosteroids which should be continued at the same dose, and not stopped or reduced, when treatment with Serevent Accuhaler is initiated.

4.2 Posology and method of administration

Serevent Accuhaler is for inhalation use only.

Serevent Accuhaler should be used regularly. The full benefits of treatment will be apparent after several doses of the drug.

In reversible airways obstruction such as asthma

Adults (including the elderly): One inhalation (50 micrograms) twice daily, increasing to two inhalations (2 × 50 micrograms) twice daily if required.

Children 4 years and over: One inhalation (50 micrograms) twice daily.

The dosage or frequency of administration should only be increased on medical advice.

There are insufficient clinical data to recommend the use of Serevent Accuhaler in children under the age of four.

In chronic obstructive pulmonary disease

Adults (including the elderly): One inhalation (50 micrograms) twice daily.

Children: Not appropriate.

Special patient groups: There is no need to adjust the dose in patients with impaired renal function.

Using the Accuhaler:

The Accuhaler should be used in a standing or sitting position. The device is opened and primed by sliding the lever. The mouthpiece is then placed in the mouth and the lips closed round it. The dose can then be inhaled and the device closed.

4.3 Contraindications

Hypersensitivity to any ingredient of the preparation (see section 6.1)

4.4 Special warnings and precautions for use

Salmeterol should not be used (and is not sufficient) as the first treatment for asthma

Serevent Accuhaler should not be initiated in patients with significantly worsening or acutely deteriorating asthma.

Sudden and progressive deterioration in asthma control is potentially life-threatening and consideration should be given to starting or increasing corticosteroid therapy. Under these circumstances, daily peak flow monitoring may be advisable. For maintenance treatment of asthma Serevent should be given in combination with inhaled or oral corticosteroids.

Although Serevent may be introduced as add-on therapy when inhaled corticosteroids do not provide adequate control of asthma symptoms, patients should not be initiated on Serevent during an acute severe asthma exacerbation, or if they have significantly worsening or acutely deteriorating asthma.

Serious asthma-related adverse events and exacerbations may occur during treatment with Serevent. Patients should be asked to continue treatment but to seek medical advice if asthma symptoms remain uncontrolled or worsen after initiation on Serevent.

Serevent Accuhaler is not a replacement for inhaled or oral corticosteroids (see section 4.1). Patients with asthma must be warned not to stop steroid therapy, and not to reduce it without medical advice, even if they feel better on Serevent Accuhaler.

With its relatively slow onset of action Serevent Accuhaler should not be used to relieve acute asthma symptoms, for which an inhaled short-acting bronchodilator is required. Patients should be advised to have such rescue medication available.

Long-acting bronchodilators should not be the only or the main treatment in maintenance asthma therapy (see section 4.1).

Increasing use of bronchodilators, in particular short-acting inhaled β_2-agonists to relieve symptoms, indicates deterioration of asthma control. The patient should be instructed to seek medical advice if short-acting relief bronchodilator treatment becomes less effective, or more inhalations than usual are required. In this situation the patient should be assessed and consideration given to the need for increased anti-inflammatory therapy (e.g. higher doses of inhaled corticosteroid or a course of oral corticosteroid). Severe exacerbations of asthma must be treated in the normal way.

Once asthma symptoms are controlled, consideration may be given to gradually reducing the dose of Serevent. Regular review of patients as treatment is stepped down is important. The lowest effective dose of Serevent should be used.

Salmeterol should be administered with caution in patients with thyrotoxicosis.

There have been very rare reports of increases in blood glucose levels (see section 4.8) and this should be considered when prescribing to patients with a history of diabetes mellitus.

Cardiovascular effects, such as increases in systolic blood pressure and heart rate, may occasionally be seen with all sympathomimetic drugs, especially at higher than therapeutic doses. For this reason, salmeterol should be used with caution in patients with pre-existing cardiovascular disease.

Potentially serious hypokalaemia may result from β_2-agonist therapy. Particular caution is advised in acute severe asthma as this effect may be potentiated by hypoxia and by concomitant treatment with xanthine derivatives, steroids and diuretics. Serum potassium levels should be monitored in such situations.

Data from a large clinical trial (the Salmeterol Multi-Center Asthma Research Trial, SMART) suggested African-American patients were at increased risk of serious respiratory-related events or deaths when using salmeterol compared with placebo (see section 5.1). It is not known if this was due to pharmacogenetic or other factors. Patients of black African or Afro-Caribbean ancestry should therefore be asked to continue treatment but to seek medical advice if asthma symptoms remained uncontrolled or worsen whilst using Serevent.

Concomitant use of systemic ketoconazole significantly increases systemic exposure to salmeterol. This may lead to an increase in the incidence of systemic effects (e.g. prolongation in the QTc interval and palpitations). Concomitant treatment with ketoconazole or other potent CYP3A4 inhibitors should therefore be avoided unless the benefits outweigh the potentially increased risk of systemic side effects of salmeterol treatment (see section 4.5).

Patients should be instructed in proper use and their technique checked to ensure that the drug is reaching the target areas within the lungs.

4.5 Interaction with other medicinal products and other forms of interaction

Both non-selective and selective β-blockers should be avoided in patients with reversible obstructive airways disease, unless there are compelling reasons for their use.

Potent CYP3A4 inhibitors

Co-administration of ketoconazole (400 mg orally once daily) and salmeterol (50 mcg inhaled twice daily) in 15 healthy subjects for 7 days resulted in a significant increase in plasma salmeterol exposure (1.4-fold Cmax and 15-fold AUC). This may lead to an increase in the incidence of other systemic effects of salmeterol treatment (e.g. prolongation of QTc interval and palpitations) compared with salmeterol or ketoconazole treatment alone (see Section 4.4).

Clinically significant effects were not seen on blood pressure, heart rate, blood glucose and blood potassium levels. Co-administration with ketoconazole did not increase the elimination half-life of salmeterol or increase salmeterol accumulation with repeat dosing.

The concomitant administration of ketoconazole should be avoided, unless the benefits outweigh the potentially increased risk of systemic side effects of salmeterol treatment. There is likely to be a similar risk of interaction with other potent CYP3A4 inhibitors (e.g. itraconazole, telithromycin, ritonavir).

Moderate CYP 3A4 inhibitors

Co-administration of erythromycin (500mg orally three times a day) and salmeterol (50μg inhaled twice daily) in 15 healthy subjects for 6 days resulted in a small but non-statistically significant increase in salmeterol exposure (1.4-fold Cmax and 1.2-fold AUC). Co-administration with erythromycin was not associated with any serious adverse effects.

4.6 Pregnancy and lactation

In animal studies, some effects on the fetus, typical for a β_2-agonist, occurred at exposure levels substantially higher than those that occur with therapeutic use. Extensive experience with other β_2-agonists has provided no evidence that such effects are relevant for women receiving clinical doses. As yet, experience of the use of salmeterol during pregnancy is limited. As with any medicine, use during pregnancy should be considered only if the expected benefit to the mother is greater than any possible risk to the fetus.

Plasma levels of salmeterol after inhaled therapeutic doses are negligible, and therefore levels in milk should be correspondingly low. Nevertheless, as there is limited experience of the use of salmeterol in nursing mothers, its use in such circumstances should only be considered if the expected benefit to the mother is greater than any possible risk to the infant.

Studies in lactating animals support the view that salmeterol is likely to be secreted in only very small amounts into breast milk.

4.7 Effects on ability to drive and use machines

None reported.

4.8 Undesirable effects

Adverse reactions are listed below by system organ class and frequency. Frequencies are defined as: very common ($\geq$ 1/10), common ($\geq$1/100 and <1/10), uncommon ($\geq$1/1000 and <1/100), rare ($\geq$1/10,000 and <1/1000), very rare (<1/10,000) and not known (cannot be estimated from the available data).

The following frequencies are estimated at the standard dose of 50mcg twice daily. Frequencies at the higher dose of 100mcg twice daily have also been taken to account where appropriate.

System Organ Class	Adverse Reaction	Frequency
Immune System Disorders	Hypersensitivity reactions with the following manifestations:	
	Rash (itching and redness)	Uncommon
	Bronchospasm and anaphylactic shock	Not known
	Oedema and angioedema,	Not known
Metabolism & Nutrition Disorders	Hypokalaemia	Rare
	Hyperglycaemia	Not known
Psychiatric Disorders	Nervousness	Uncommon
	Insomnia	Rare
Nervous System Disorders	Headache	Common
	Tremor	Common
	Dizziness	Rare
Cardiac Disorders	Palpitations	Common
	Tachycardia	Uncommon
	Cardiac arrhythmias (including atrial fibrillation, supraventricular tachycardia and extrasystoles).	Not known
Respiratory, Thoracic & Mediastinal Disorders	Oropharyngeal irritation	Not known
	Paradoxical bronchospasm	Not known
Gastro-Intestinal Disorders	Nausea	Not known
Musculoskeletal & Connective Tissue Disorders	Muscle cramps	Common
	Arthralgia	Not known
General Disorders and Administration Site Conditions	Non-specific chest pain	Not known

As with other inhalation therapy, paradoxical bronchospasm may occur with an immediate increase in wheezing and drop in peak expiratory flow rate (PEFR) after dosing. This responds to a fast-acting inhaled bronchodilator. Serevent Accuhaler should be discontinued immediately, the patient assessed, and if necessary an alternative presentation or therapy should be instituted (see section 4.4).

The pharmacological side effects of β_2-agonist treatment, such as tremor, subjective palpitations and headache, have been reported, but tend to be transient and to reduce with regular therapy. Tremor and tachycardia occur more commonly when administered at doses higher than 50mcg twice daily.

4.9 Overdose

The symptoms and signs of salmeterol overdosage are tremor, headache and tachycardia. Hypokalaemia may occur. Monitor serum potassium levels. The preferred antidote for overdosage with Serevent Accuhaler is a cardioselective β-blocking agent. Cardioselective β-blocking drugs should be used with caution in patients with a history of bronchospasm.

5. PHARMACOLOGICAL PROPERTIES

5.1 Pharmacodynamic properties

Salmeterol is a selective long-acting (usually 12 hours) β_2-adrenoceptor agonist with a long side-chain which binds to the exo-site of the receptor. These pharmacological properties of salmeterol offer more effective protection against histamine-induced bronchoconstriction and produce a longer duration of bronchodilatation, lasting for at least 12 hours, than recommended doses of conventional short-acting β_2-agonists. *In vitro* tests have shown that salmeterol is a potent and long-lasting inhibitor of the release from the human lung of mast cell mediators, such as histamine, leukotrienes and prostaglandin D2. In man, salmeterol inhibits the early and late phase response to inhaled allergen; the latter persisting for over 30 hours after a single dose when the bronchodilator effect is no longer evident. Single dosing with salmeterol attenuates bronchial hyper-responsiveness. These properties indicate that salmeterol has additional non-bronchodilator activity, but the full clinical significance is not yet clear. The mechanism is different from the anti-inflammatory effect of corticosteroids, which should not be stopped or reduced when Serevent Accuhaler is prescribed.

Salmeterol has been studied in the treatment of conditions associated with COPD, and has been shown to improve symptoms and pulmonary function, and quality of life. Salmeterol acts as a β_2-agonist on the reversible component of the disease. *In vitro* salmeterol has also been shown to increase cilial beat frequency of human bronchial epithelial cells, and also reduce a ciliotoxic effect of *Pseudomonas* toxin on the bronchial epithelium of patients with cystic fibrosis.

Asthma Clinical Trials

The Salmeterol Multi-centre Asthma Research Trial (SMART)

SMART was a multi-centre, randomised, double-blind, placebo-controlled, parallel group 28-week study in the US which randomised 13,176 patients to salmeterol (50μg twice daily) and 13,179 patients to placebo in addition to the patients' usual asthma therapy. Patients were enrolled if $\geq$12 years of age, with asthma and if currently using asthma medication (but not a LABA). Baseline ICS use at study entry was recorded, but not required in the study. The primary endpoint in SMART was the combined number of respiratory-related deaths and respiratory-related life-threatening experiences.

Key findings from SMART: primary endpoint

(see Table 1 below)

Key findings from SMART by inhaled steroid use at baseline: secondary endpoints

(see Table 2 below)

COPD clinical trials

TORCH study

TORCH was a 3-year study to assess the effect of treatment with Seretide Diskus 50/500mcg bd, salmeterol Diskus 50mcg bd, fluticasone propionate (FP) Diskus 500mcg bd or placebo on all-cause mortality in patients with COPD. COPD patients with a baseline (pre-bronchodilator) FEV1 <60% of predicted normal were randomised to double-blind medication. During the study, patients were permitted usual COPD therapy with the exception of other inhaled corticosteroids, long-acting bronchodilators and long-term systemic corticosteroids. Survival status at 3 years was determined for all patients regardless of withdrawal from study medication. The primary endpoint was reduction in all cause mortality at 3 years for Seretide vs Placebo.

(see Table 3 on next page)

There was a trend towards improved survival in subjects treated with Seretide compared with placebo over 3 years however this did not achieve the statistical significance level $p \leq 0.05$. The percentage of patients who died within 3 years due to COPD-related causes was 6.0% for placebo, 6.1% for salmeterol, 6.9% for FP and 4.7% for Seretide.

The mean number of moderate to severe exacerbations per year was significantly reduced with Seretide as compared with treatment with salmeterol, FP and placebo (mean rate in the Seretide group 0.85 compared with 0.97 in the salmeterol group, 0.93 in the FP group and 1.13 in the placebo). This translates to a reduction in the rate of moderate to severe exacerbations of 25% (95% CI: 19% to 31%; $p<0.001$) compared with placebo, 12% compared with salmeterol (95% CI: 5% to 19%, p=0.002) and 9% compared with FP (95% CI: 1% to 16%, p=0.024). Salmeterol and FP significantly reduced exacerbation rates compared with placebo by 15% (95% CI: 7% to 22%; $p<0.001$) and 18% (95% CI: 11% to 24%; $p<0.001$) respectively.

Health Related Quality of Life, as measured by the St George's Respiratory Questionnaire (SGRQ) was improved by all active treatments in comparison with placebo. The average improvement over three years for Seretide compared with placebo was -3.1 units (95% CI: -4.1 to -2.1; $p<0.001$), compared with salmeterol was -2.2 units ($p<0.001$) and compared with FP was -1.2 units (p=0.017). A 4-unit decrease is considered clinically relevant.

The estimated 3-year probability of having pneumonia reported as an adverse event was 12.3% for placebo, 13.3% for salmeterol, 18.3% for FP and 19.6% for Seretide (Hazard ratio for Seretide vs placebo: 1.64, 95% CI: 1.33 to 2.01, $p<0.001$). There was no increase in pneumonia related deaths; deaths while on treatment that were adjudicated as primarily due to pneumonia were 7 for placebo, 9 for salmeterol, 13 for FP and 8 for Seretide. There was no significant difference in probability of bone fracture (5.1% placebo, 5.1% salmeterol, 5.4% FP and 6.3% Seretide; Hazard ratio for Seretide vs placebo: 1.22, 95% CI: 0.87 to 1.72, p=0.248.

5.2 Pharmacokinetic properties

Salmeterol acts locally in the lung, therefore plasma levels are not predictive of therapeutic effects. In addition there are only limited data available on the pharmacokinetics of salmeterol because of the technical difficulty of assaying

Table 1 Key findings from SMART: primary endpoint

Patient group	Number of primary endpoint events / number of patients		Relative Risk (95% confidence intervals)
	salmeterol	placebo	
All patients	50/13,176	36/13,179	1.40 (0.91, 2.14)
Patients using inhaled steroids	23/6,127	19/6,138	1.21 (0.66, 2.23)
Patients not using inhaled steroids	27/7,049	17/7,041	1.60 (0.87, 2.93)
African-American patients	**20/2,366**	**5/2,319**	**4.10 (1.54, 10.90)**

(Risk in bold is statistically significant at the 95% level.)

Table 2 Key findings from SMART by inhaled steroid use at baseline: secondary endpoints

	Number of secondary endpoint events / number of patients		Relative Risk (95% confidence intervals)
	salmeterol	placebo	
Respiratory -related death			
Patients using inhaled steroids	10/6127	5/6138	2.01 (0.69, 5.86)
Patients not using inhaled steroids	14/7049	6/7041	2.28 (0.88, 5.94)
Combined asthma-related death or life-threatening experience			
Patients using inhaled steroids	16/6127	13/6138	1.24 (0.60, 2.58)
Patients not using inhaled steroids	**21/7049**	**9/7041**	**2.39 (1.10, 5.22)**
Asthma-related death			
Patients using inhaled steroids	4/6127	3/6138	1.35 (0.30, 6.04)
Patients not using inhaled steroids	9/7049	0/7041	*

(*=could not be calculated because of no events in placebo group. Risk in bold is statistically significant at the 95% level. The secondary endpoints in the table above reached statistical significance in the whole population.) The secondary endpoints of combined all-cause death or life-threatening experience, all cause death, or all cause hospitalisation did not reach statistical significance in the whole population.

Table 3

	Placebo N = 1524	Salmeterol 50 N = 1521	FP 500 N = 1534	Seretide 50/500 N = 1533
All cause mortality at 3 years				
Number of deaths (%)	231 (15.2%)	205 (13.5%)	246 (16.0%)	193 (12.6%)
Hazard Ratio vs Placebo (CIs)	N/A	0.879 (0.73, 1.06)	1.060 (0.89, 1.27)	0.825 (0.68, 1.00)
p value		0.180	0.525	0.052[1]
Hazard Ratio Seretide 50/500 vs components (CIs)	N/A	0.932 (0.77, 1.13)	0.774 (0.64, 0.93)	N/A
p value		0.481	0.007	

1. Non significant P value after adjustment for 2 interim analyses on the primary efficacy comparison from a log-rank analysis stratified by smoking status

the drug in plasma because of the very low plasma concentrations at therapeutic doses (approximately 200 pg/ml or less) achieved after inhaled dosing.

After regular dosing with salmeterol xinafoate, xinafoic acid can be detected in the systemic circulation, reaching steady state concentrations of approximately 100 ng/ml. These concentrations are up to 1000-fold lower than steady state levels observed in toxicity studies. These concentrations in long term regular dosing (more than 12 months) in patients with airways obstruction, have been shown to produce no ill effects.

5.3 Preclinical safety data
In reproduction studies in animals, some effects on the fetus, typical of a β_2-agonist, have been observed at very high doses.

Salmeterol xinafoate produced no genetic toxicity in a range of studies using either prokaryotic or eukaryotic cell systems *in vitro* or *in vivo* in the rat.

Long term studies with salmeterol xinafoate, induced class-related benign tumours of smooth muscle in the mesovarium of rats and the uterus of mice. The scientific literature and our own pharmacological studies provide good evidence that these effects are species-specific and have no relevance for clinical use.

6. PHARMACEUTICAL PARTICULARS

6.1 List of excipients
Lactose (which contains milk protein).

6.2 Incompatibilities
None reported.

6.3 Shelf life
24 months when not stored above 30°C for moderate climates.

18 months when not stored above 30°C for tropical climates.

6.4 Special precautions for storage
Do not store above 30°C.

Store in the original package.

6.5 Nature and contents of container
The powder mix of salmeterol xinafoate and lactose is filled into a blister strip consisting of a formed base foil with a peelable foil laminate lid. The foil strip is contained within the Accuhaler device. Pack sizes 28 or 60. Not all pack sizes may be marketed.

6.6 Special precautions for disposal and other handling
The powdered medicine is inhaled through the mouth into the lungs.

The Accuhaler device contains the medicine in individual blisters which are opened as the device is manipulated.

For detailed instructions for use refer to the Patient Information Leaflet in every pack.

Administrative Data

7. MARKETING AUTHORISATION HOLDER
Glaxo Wellcome UK Ltd
Trading as Allen & Hanburys
Stockley Park West
Uxbridge
Middlesex UB11 1BT.

8. MARKETING AUTHORISATION NUMBER(S)
10949/0214

9. DATE OF FIRST AUTHORISATION/RENEWAL OF THE AUTHORISATION
13 July 2000

10. DATE OF REVISION OF THE TEXT
14 August 2009

Serevent Diskhaler

(Allen & Hanburys)

1. NAME OF THE MEDICINAL PRODUCT
Serevent$_{TM}$ Diskhaler$_{TM}$

2. QUALITATIVE AND QUANTITATIVE COMPOSITION
Disks comprising four regularly spaced double-foil blisters each delivering a mixture of 50 micrograms salmeterol (as xinafoate) and lactose used in a Diskhaler device.

For excipients, see section 6.1

3. PHARMACEUTICAL FORM
Inhalation powder.

4. CLINICAL PARTICULARS

4.1 Therapeutic indications
Salmeterol is a selective β2-agonist indicated for reversible airways obstruction in patients with asthma and chronic obstructive pulmonary disease (COPD).

In asthma (including nocturnal asthma and exercise induced symptoms) it is indicated for those treated with inhaled corticosteroids who require a long-acting beta agonist in accordance with current treatment guidelines.

Serevent Diskhaler is not a replacement for inhaled or oral corticosteroids which should be continued at the same dose, and not stopped or reduced, when treatment with Serevent Diskhaler is initiated.

4.2 Posology and method of administration
Serevent Diskhaler is for inhalation use only.

Serevent Diskhaler should be used regularly. The full benefits of treatment will be apparent after several doses of the drug.

In reversible airways obstruction such as asthma

Adults (including the elderly): One blister (50 micrograms) twice daily, increasing to two blisters (2 × 50 micrograms) twice daily if required.

Children 4 years and over: One blister (50 micrograms) twice daily.

The dosage or frequency of administration should only be increased on medical advice.

There are insufficient clinical data to recommend the use of Serevent Diskhaler in children under the age of four.

In chronic obstructive pulmonary disease

Adults (including the elderly): One blister (50 micrograms) twice daily.

Children: Not appropriate.

Special patient groups: There is no need to adjust the dose in patients with impaired renal function.

4.3 Contraindications
Hypersensitivity to any ingredient of the preparation (see section 6.1)

4.4 Special warnings and precautions for use
Salmeterol should not be used (and is not sufficient) as the first treatment for asthma.

Serevent Diskhaler should not be initiated in patients with significantly worsening or acutely deteriorating asthma.

Sudden and progressive deterioration in asthma control is potentially life-threatening and consideration should be given to starting or increasing corticosteroid therapy. Under these circumstances, regular peak flow monitoring may be advisable. For maintenance treatment of asthma Serevent should be given in combination with inhaled or oral corticosteroids.

Serevent Diskhaler is not a replacement for inhaled or oral corticosteroids (see section 4.1). Patients with asthma must be warned not to stop steroid therapy, and not to reduce it without medical advice, even if they feel better on Serevent Diskhaler.

With its relatively slow onset of action Serevent Diskhaler should not be used to relieve acute asthma symptoms, for which an inhaled short-acting bronchodilator is required. Patients should be advised to have such rescue medication available.

Long-acting bronchodilators should not be the only or the main treatment in maintenance asthma therapy (see section 4.1.

Increasing use of bronchodilators, in particular short-acting inhaled β2-agonists to relieve symptoms, indicates deterioration of asthma control. The patient should be instructed to seek medical advice if short-acting relief bronchodilator treatment becomes less effective, or more inhalations than usual are required. In this situation the patient should be assessed and consideration given to the need for increased anti-inflammatory therapy (e.g. higher doses of inhaled corticosteroid or a course of oral corticosteroid). Severe exacerbations of asthma must be treated in the normal way.

Although Serevent may be introduced as add-on therapy when inhaled corticosteroids do not provide adequate control of asthma symptoms, patients should not be initiated on Serevent during an acute severe asthma exacerbation, or if they have significantly worsening or acutely deteriorating asthma.

Serious asthma-related adverse events and exacerbations may occur during treatment with Serevent. Patients should be asked to continue treatment but to seek medical advice if asthma symptoms remain uncontrolled or worsen after initiation on Serevent.

Once asthma symptoms are controlled, consideration may be given to gradually reducing the dose of Serevent. Regular review of patients as treatment is stepped down is important. The lowest effective dose of Serevent should be used.

Salmeterol should be administered with caution in patients with thyrotoxicosis.

There have been very rare reports of increases in blood glucose levels (see section 4.8) and this should be considered when prescribing to patients with a history of diabetes mellitus.

Cardiovascular effects, such as increases in systolic blood pressure and heart rate, may occasionally be seen with all sympathomimetic drugs, especially at higher than therapeutic doses. For this reason, salmeterol should be used with caution in patients with pre-existing cardiovascular disease.

Potentially serious hypokalaemia may result from β2-agonist therapy. Particular caution is advised in acute severe asthma as this effect may be potentiated by hypoxia and by concomitant treatment with xanthine derivatives, steroids and diuretics. Serum potassium levels should be monitored in such situations.

Data from a large clinical trial (the Salmeterol Multi-Center Asthma Research Trial, SMART) suggested African-American patients were at increased risk of serious respiratory-related events or deaths when using salmeterol compared with placebo (see section 5.1). It is not known if this was due to pharmacogenetic or other factors. Patients of black African or Afro-Caribbean ancestry should therefore be asked to continue treatment but to seek medical advice if asthma symptoms remained uncontrolled or worsen whilst using Serevent.

Concomitant use of systemic ketoconazole significantly increases systemic exposure to salmeterol. This may lead to an increase in the incidence of systemic effects (e.g. prolongation in the QTc interval and palpitations). Concomitant treatment with ketoconazole or other potent CYP3A4 inhibitors should therefore be avoided unless the benefits outweigh the potentially increased risk of systemic side effects of salmeterol treatment (see section 4.5).

4.5 Interaction with other medicinal products and other forms of interaction
Both non-selective and selective β-blockers should be avoided in patients with reversible obstructive airways disease, unless there are compelling reasons for their use.

Potent CYP3A4 inhibitors

Co-administration of ketoconazole (400 mg orally once daily) and salmeterol (50 mcg inhaled twice daily) in 15 healthy subjects for 7 days resulted in a significant increase in plasma salmeterol exposure (1.4-fold Cmax and 15-fold AUC). This may lead to an increase in the incidence of other systemic effects of salmeterol treatment (e.g. prolongation of QTc interval and palpitations) compared with salmeterol or ketoconazole treatment alone (see Section 4.4).

Clinically significant effects were not seen on blood pressure, heart rate, blood glucose and blood potassium levels. Co-administration with ketoconazole did not increase the elimination half-life of salmeterol or increase salmeterol accumulation with repeat dosing.

The concomitant administration of ketoconazole should be avoided, unless the benefits outweigh the potentially increased risk of systemic side effects of salmeterol treatment. There is likely to be a similar risk of interaction with other potent CYP3A4 inhibitors (e.g. itraconazole, telithromycin, ritonavir).

Moderate CYP 3A4 inhibitors

Co-administration of erythromycin (500mg orally three times a day) and salmeterol (50μg inhaled twice daily) in 15 healthy subjects for 6 days resulted in a small but non-statistically significant increase in salmeterol exposure (1.4-fold Cmax and 1.2-fold AUC). Co-administration with erythromycin was not associated with any serious adverse effects.

4.6 Pregnancy and lactation
In animal studies, some effects on the fetus, typical for a β2-agonist, occurred at exposure levels substantially higher than those that occur with therapeutic use. Extensive experience with other β2-agonists has provided no evidence that such effects are relevant for women receiving clinical doses. As yet, experience of the use of

salmeterol during pregnancy is limited. As with any medicine, use during pregnancy should be considered only if the expected benefit to the mother is greater than any possible risk to the fetus.

Plasma levels of salmeterol after inhaled therapeutic doses are negligible, and therefore levels in milk should be correspondingly low. Nevertheless, as there is limited experience of the use of salmeterol in nursing mothers, its use in such circumstances should only be considered if the expected benefit to the mother is greater than any possible risk to the infant.

Studies in lactating animals support the view that salmeterol is likely to be secreted in only very small amounts into breast milk.

4.7 Effects on ability to drive and use machines

None reported.

4.8 Undesirable effects

Adverse reactions are listed below by system organ class and frequency. Frequencies are defined as: very common (≥ 1/10), common (≥1/100 and <1/10), uncommon (≥1/1000 and <1/100), rare (≥1/10,000 and <1/1000), very rare (<1/10,000) and not known (cannot be estimated from the available data).

The following frequencies are estimated at the standard dose of 50mcg twice daily. Frequencies at the higher dose of 100mcg twice daily have also been taken to account where appropriate.

System Organ Class	Adverse Reaction	Frequency
Immune System Disorders	Hypersensitivity reactions with the following manifestations:	
	Rash (itching and redness)	Uncommon
	Bronchospasm and anaphylactic shock	Not known
	Oedema and angioedema,	Not known
Metabolism & Nutrition Disorders	Hypokalaemia	Rare
	Hyperglycaemia	Not known
Psychiatric Disorders	Nervousness	Uncommon
	Insomnia	Rare
Nervous System Disorders	Headache	Common
	Tremor	Common
	Dizziness	Rare
Cardiac Disorders	Palpitations	Common
	Tachycardia	Uncommon
	Cardiac arrhythmias (including atrial fibrillation, supraventricular tachycardia and extrasystoles).	Not known
Respiratory, Thoracic & Mediastinal Disorders	Oropharyngeal irritation	Not known
	Paradoxical bronchospasm	Not known
Gastro-Intestinal Disorders	Nausea	Not known
Musculoskeletal & Connective Tissue Disorders	Muscle cramps	Common
	Arthralgia	Not known
General Disorders and Administration Site Conditions	Non-specific chest pain	Not known

As with other inhalation therapy, paradoxical bronchospasm may occur with an immediate increase in wheezing and drop in peak expiratory flow rate (PEFR) after dosing. This responds to a fast-acting inhaled bronchodilator. Serevent Diskhaler should be discontinued immediately, the patient assessed, and if necessary an alternative presentation or therapy should be instituted (see section 4.4).

The pharmacological side-effects of β2-agonist treatment, such as tremor, palpitations and headache, have been reported, but tend to be transient and to reduce with regular therapy. Tremor and tachycardia occur more commonly when administered at doses higher than 50mcg twice daily.

4.9 Overdose

The symptoms and signs of salmeterol overdosage are tremor, headache and tachycardia. Hypokalaemia may occur. Monitor serum potassium levels. The preferred antidote for overdosage with Serevent Diskhaler is a cardioselective β-blocking agent. Cardioselective β-blocking drugs should be used with caution in patients with a history of bronchospasm.

5. PHARMACOLOGICAL PROPERTIES

5.1 Pharmacodynamic properties

Salmeterol is a selective long-acting (usually 12 hours) β2-adrenoceptor agonist with a long side-chain which binds to the exo-site of the receptor.

These pharmacological properties of salmeterol offer more effective protection against histamine-induced bronchoconstriction and produce a longer duration of bronchodilatation, lasting for at least 12 hours, than recommended doses of conventional short-acting β2-agonists. In vitro tests have shown that salmeterol is a potent and long-lasting inhibitor of the release from the human lung of mast cell mediators, such as histamine, leukotrienes and prostaglandin D2. In man, salmeterol inhibits the early and late phase response to inhaled allergen; the latter persisting for over 30 hours after a single dose when the bronchodilator effect is no longer evident. Single dosing with salmeterol attenuates bronchial hyper-responsiveness. These properties indicate that salmeterol has additional non-bronchodilator activity, but the full clinical significance is not yet clear. The mechanism is different from the anti-inflammatory effect of corticosteroids, which should not be stopped or reduced when Serevent Diskhaler is prescribed.

Salmeterol has been studied in the treatment of conditions associated with COPD, and has been shown to improve symptoms and pulmonary function, and quality of life. Salmeterol acts as a β2-agonist on the reversible component of the disease. In vitro salmeterol has also been shown to increase cilial beat frequency of human bronchial epithelial cells, and also reduce a ciliotoxic effect of Pseudomonas toxin on the bronchial epithelium of patients with cystic fibrosis.

Asthma clinical trials

The Salmeterol Multi- centre Asthma Research Trial (SMART)

SMART was a multi-centre, randomised, double-blind, placebo-controlled, parallel group 28-week study in the US which randomised 13,176 patients to salmeterol (50μg twice daily) and 13,179 patients to placebo in addition to the patients' usual asthma therapy. Patients were enrolled if ≥12 years of age, with asthma and if currently using asthma medication (but not a LABA). Baseline ICS use at study entry was recorded, but not required in the study. The primary endpoint in SMART was the combined number of respiratory-related deaths and respiratory-related life-threatening experiences.

Key findings from SMART: primary endpoint

(see Table 1 below)

Key findings from SMART by inhaled steroid use at baseline: secondary endpoints

(see Table 2 below)

COPD clinical trials

TORCH study

TORCH was a 3-year study to assess the effect of treatment with Seretide Diskus 50/500mcg bd, salmeterol Diskus 50mcg bd, fluticasone propionate (FP) Diskus 500mcg bd or placebo on all-cause mortality in patients with COPD. COPD patients with a baseline (pre-bronchodilator) FEV1 <60% of predicted normal were randomised to double-blind medication. During the study, patients were permitted usual COPD therapy with the exception of other inhaled corticosteroids, long-acting bronchodilators and long-term systemic corticosteroids. Survival status at 3 years was determined for all patients regardless of withdrawal from study medication. The primary endpoint was reduction in all cause mortality at 3 years for Seretide vs Placebo.

(see Table 3 on next page)

There was a trend towards improved survival in subjects treated with Seretide compared with placebo over 3 years however this did not achieve the statistical significance level $p \leq 0.05$. The percentage of patients who died within 3 years due to COPD-related causes was 6.0% for placebo, 6.1% for salmeterol, 6.9% for FP and 4.7% for Seretide.

The mean number of moderate to severe exacerbations per year was significantly reduced with Seretide as compared with treatment with salmeterol, FP and placebo (mean rate in the Seretide group 0.85 compared with 0.97 in the salmeterol group, 0.93 in the FP group and 1.13 in the placebo). This translates to a reduction in the rate of moderate to severe exacerbations of 25% (95% CI: 19% to 31%; $p<0.001$) compared with placebo, 12% compared with salmeterol (95% CI: 5% to 19%, $p=0.002$) and 9% compared with FP (95% CI: 1% to 16%, $p=0.024$). Salmeterol and FP significantly reduced exacerbation rates compared with placebo by 15% (95% CI: 7% to 22%; $p<0.001$) and 18% (95% CI: 11% to 24%; $p<0.001$) respectively.

Health Related Quality of Life, as measured by the St George's Respiratory Questionnaire (SGRQ) was improved by all active treatments in comparison with placebo. The average improvement over three years for Seretide compared with placebo was -3.1 units (95% CI: -4.1 to -2.1; $p<0.001$), compared with salmeterol was -2.2 units ($p<0.001$) and compared with FP was -1.2 units ($p=0.017$). A 4-unit decrease is considered clinically relevant.

The estimated 3-year probability of having pneumonia reported as an adverse event was 12.3% for placebo, 13.3% for salmeterol, 18.3% for FP and 19.6% for Seretide (Hazard ratio for Seretide vs placebo: 1.64, 95% CI: 1.33 to 2.01, $p<0.001$). There was no increase in pneumonia related deaths; deaths while on treatment that were

Table 1 Key findings from SMART: primary endpoint

Patient group	Number of primary endpoint events / number of patients		Relative Risk (95% confidence intervals)
	salmeterol	placebo	
All patients	50/13,176	36/13,179	1.40 (0.91, 2.14)
Patients using inhaled steroids	23/6,127	19/6,138	1.21 (0.66, 2.23)
Patients not using inhaled steroids	27/7,049	17/7,041	1.60 (0.87, 2.93)
African-American patients	**20/2,366**	**5/2,319**	**4.10 (1.54, 10.90)**

(Risk in bold is statistically significant at the 95% level.)

Table 2 Key findings from SMART by inhaled steroid use at baseline: secondary endpoints

	Number of secondary endpoint events / number of patients		Relative Risk (95% confidence intervals)
	salmeterol	placebo	
Respiratory -related death			
Patients using inhaled steroids	10/6127	5/6138	2.01 (0.69, 5.86)
Patients not using inhaled steroids	14/7049	6/7041	2.28 (0.88, 5.94)
Combined asthma-related death or life-threatening experience			
Patients using inhaled steroids	16/6127	13/6138	1.24 (0.60, 2.58)
Patients not using inhaled steroids	**21/7049**	**9/7041**	**2.39 (1.10, 5.22)**
Asthma-related death			
Patients using inhaled steroids	4/6127	3/6138	1.35 (0.30, 6.04)
Patients not using inhaled steroids	9/7049	0/7041	*

(*=could not be calculated because of no events in placebo group. Risk in bold is statistically significant at the 95% level. The secondary endpoints in the table above reached statistical significance in the whole population.) The secondary endpoints of combined all-cause death or life-threatening experience, all cause death, or all cause hospitalisation did not reach statistical significance in the whole population.

Table 3

	Placebo N = 1524	Salmeterol 50 N = 1521	FP 500 N = 1534	Seretide 50/500 N = 1533
All cause mortality at 3 years				
Number of deaths (%)	231 (15.2%)	205 (13.5%)	246 (16.0%)	193 (12.6%)
Hazard Ratio vs Placebo (CIs)	N/A	0.879 (0.73, 1.06)	1.060 (0.89, 1.27)	0.825 (0.68, 1.00)
p value		0.180	0.525	0.052[1]
Hazard Ratio Seretide 50/500 vs components (CIs)	N/A	0.932 (0.77, 1.13)	0.774 (0.64, 0.93)	N/A
p value		0.481	0.007	

1. Non significant P value after adjustment for 2 interim analyses on the primary efficacy comparison from a log-rank analysis stratified by smoking status

adjudicated as primarily due to pneumonia were 7 for placebo, 9 for salmeterol, 13 for FP and 8 for Seretide. There was no significant difference in probability of bone fracture (5.1% placebo, 5.1% salmeterol, 5.4% FP and 6.3% Seretide; Hazard ratio for Seretide vs placebo: 1.22, 95% CI: 0.87 to 1.72, p=0.248.

5.2 Pharmacokinetic properties

Salmeterol acts locally in the lung, therefore plasma levels are not predictive of therapeutic effect. In addition there are only limited data available on the pharmacokinetics of salmeterol because of the technical difficulty of assaying the drug in plasma because of the very low plasma concentrations (approximately 200 pg/ml or less) achieved after inhaled dosing.

After regular dosing with salmeterol xinafoate, xinafoic acid can be detected in the systemic circulation, reaching steady state concentrations of approximately 100 ng/ml. These concentrations are up to 1000-fold lower than steady state levels observed in toxicity studies. These concentrations in long term regular dosing (more than 12 months) in patients with airways obstruction, have been shown to produce no ill effects.

5.3 Preclinical safety data

In reproduction studies in animals, some effects on the fetus, typical of a β2-agonist, have been observed at very high doses.

Salmeterol xinafoate produced no genetic toxicity in a range of studies using either prokaryotic or eukaryotic cell systems in vitro or in vivo in the rat.

Long-term studies with salmeterol xinafoate, induced class-related benign tumours of smooth muscle in the mesovarium of rats and the uterus of mice. The scientific literature and our own pharmacological studies provide good evidence that these effects are species-specific and have no relevance for clinical use.

6. PHARMACEUTICAL PARTICULARS

6.1 List of excipients

Lactose (which contains milk protein).

6.2 Incompatibilities

None reported.

6.3 Shelf life

2 years when not stored above 25°C.

6.4 Special precautions for storage

Do not store above 25°C.

A disk may be kept in the Diskhaler device but the blisters must only be pierced immediately prior to use.

6.5 Nature and contents of container

A circular double-foil disk with four blisters containing the powder mix of salmeterol (as xinafoate) and lactose. The foil disk is inserted into the Diskhaler device.

The following packs are registered: 5, 7, 10, 14, 15 disks alone or with a Diskhaler. Starter pack consisting of a Diskhaler pre-loaded with one disk (with or without a spare disk, peak flow meter and diary card).

The following packs are available: 14 disks alone or with a Diskhaler. 5 disks with a Diskhaler (Hospital only).

6.6 Special precautions for disposal and other handling

The powdered medicine is inhaled through the mouth into the lungs. The Diskhaler device is loaded with a disk which contains the medicine in individual blisters which are opened as the device is manipulated.

For detailed instructions for use refer to the Patient Information Leaflet in every pack.

7. MARKETING AUTHORISATION HOLDER

Glaxo Wellcome UK Ltd, trading as Allen & Hanburys

Stockley Park West,

Uxbridge, Middlesex, UB11 1BT

8. MARKETING AUTHORISATION NUMBER(S)

PL 10949/0069

9. DATE OF FIRST AUTHORISATION/RENEWAL OF THE AUTHORISATION

14 October 1996

10. DATE OF REVISION OF THE TEXT

14 August 2009

Serevent Evohaler

(Allen & Hanburys)

1. NAME OF THE MEDICINAL PRODUCT

Serevent™ Evohaler™▼ 25 micrograms per actuation pressurised inhalation suspension.

2. QUALITATIVE AND QUANTITATIVE COMPOSITION

One metered dose (ex-valve) contains 25 micrograms salmeterol (as xinafoate). This is equivalent to a delivered dose (ex-actuator) of 21 micrograms salmeterol (as xinafoate).

For a full list of excipients, see section 6.1.

3. PHARMACEUTICAL FORM

Pressurised inhalation suspension.

White to off white suspension sealed in an aluminium canister in a green actuator.

4. CLINICAL PARTICULARS

4.1 Therapeutic indications

Regular symptomatic add-on treatment of reversible airways obstruction in patients with asthma, including those with nocturnal asthma, who are inadequately controlled on inhaled corticosteroids in accordance with current treatment guidelines. Treatment of chronic obstructive pulmonary disease (COPD). Prevention of exercise-induced asthma.

4.2 Posology and method of administration

Serevent Evohaler is for inhalation use only.

Serevent Evohaler should be used regularly. The full benefits of treatment will be apparent after several doses of the medicinal product. As there may be adverse reactions associated with excessive dosing with this class of medicinal product, the dosage or frequency of administration should only be increased on medical advice.

Recommended Doses:

Asthma

Adults and adolescents 12 years and older:

Two actuations of 25 micrograms salmeterol twice daily.

In asthma patients with more severe airways obstruction up to four inhalations of 25 micrograms of salmeterol twice daily may be of benefit.

Children aged 4 years and older:

Two actuations of 25 micrograms salmeterol twice daily.

Children below 4 years of age:

Serevent Evohaler is not recommended for use in children below four years of age due to insufficient data on safety and efficacy.

COPD

Adults: Two actuations of 25 micrograms salmeterol twice daily.

Children: There is no relevant indication for use of Serevent Evohaler in children.

Special patient groups:

There is no need to adjust the dose in elderly patients or in those with renal impairment. There are no data available on the use of Serevent Evohaler in patients with hepatic impairment.

INSTRUCTIONS FOR USE:

Patients should be carefully instructed in the proper use of their inhaler (see Patient Information Leaflet).

1. Patients should remove the mouthpiece cover by gently squeezing the sides of the cover.
2. Patients should check inside and outside of the inhaler including the mouthpiece for the presence of loose objects.
3. Patients should shake the inhaler well to ensure that any loose objects are removed and that the contents of the inhaler are evenly mixed. Before using for the first time or if the inhaler has not been used for a week patients should release one puff into the air to make sure that it works.
4. Patients should hold the inhaler upright between fingers and thumb with their thumb on the base, below the mouthpiece.
5. Patients should breathe out as far as is comfortable and then place the mouthpiece in their mouth between their teeth and close their lips around it. Patients should be instructed not to bite the mouthpiece.
6. Just after starting to breathe in through their mouth patients should press down on the top of the inhaler to release salmeterol while still breathing in steadily and deeply.
7. While holding their breath, patients should take the inhaler from their mouth and take their finger from the top of the inhaler. They should continue holding their breath for as long as is comfortable.
8. If patients are going to take a further puff, they should keep the inhaler upright and wait about half a minute before repeating steps 3 to7.
9. After use patients should always replace the mouthpiece cover to keep out dust and fluff.
10. Patients should replace the mouthpiece cover by firmly pushing and snapping the cap into position.

Important:

Patients should not rush stages5, 6 and 7. It is important that they start to breathe in as slowly as possible just before operating their inhaler.

Patients should practise in front of a mirror for the first few times. If they see "mist" coming from the top of their inhaler or the sides of their mouth they should start again from stage 2.

Serevent Evohaler should be used with a Volumatic spacer device by patients who find it difficult to synchronise aerosol actuation with inspiration of breath which is often the case for children and the elderly.

Cleaning:

The inhaler should be cleaned at least once a week by:

1. Removing the mouthpiece cover.
2. Wiping the inside and outside of the mouthpiece and the plastic casing with a dry cloth or tissue.
3. Replacing the mouthpiece cover.

The canister must not be removed from the plastic casing when cleaning the inhaler.

PATIENTS MUST NOT PUT THE METAL CANISTER INTO WATER.

4.3 Contraindications

Serevent Evohaler is contraindicated in patients with hypersensitivity to salmeterol xinafoate or to the excipient (see Section 6.1).

4.4 Special warnings and precautions for use

The management of asthma should normally follow a stepwise programme and patient response should be monitored clinically and by lung function tests.

Salmeterol should not be used (and is not sufficient) as the first treatment for asthma.

Salmeterol is not a replacement for oral or inhaled corticosteroids. Its use is complementary to them. Patients must be warned not to stop steroid therapy and not to reduce it without medical advice even if they feel better on salmeterol.

Salmeterol should not be used to treat acute asthma symptoms for which a fast and short-acting inhaled bronchodilator is required. Patients should be advised to have their medicinal product to be used for the relief of acute asthma symptoms available at all times.

Increasing use of short-acting bronchodilators to relieve asthma symptoms indicates deterioration of asthma control. The patient should be instructed to seek medical advice if short-acting relief bronchodilator treatment becomes less effective or more inhalations than usual are required. In this situation the patient should be assessed and consideration given to the need for increased anti-inflammatory therapy (e.g. higher doses of inhaled corticosteroid or a course of oral corticosteroid). Severe exacerbations of asthma must be treated in the normal way.

Although Serevent may be introduced as add-on therapy when inhaled corticosteroids do not provide adequate control of asthma symptoms, patients should not be initiated on Serevent during an acute severe asthma exacerbation, or if they have significantly worsening or acutely deteriorating asthma.

Serious asthma-related adverse events and exacerbations may occur during treatment with Serevent. Patients should be asked to continue treatment but to seek medical advice if asthma symptoms remain uncontrolled or worsen after initiation on Serevent.

Sudden and progressive deterioration in control of asthma is potentially life-threatening and the patient should undergo urgent medical assessment. Consideration should be given to increasing corticosteroid therapy. Under these circumstances daily peak flow monitoring may be advisable. For maintenance treatment of asthma salmeterol should be given in combination with inhaled or oral corticosteroids. Long-acting bronchodilators should not be the only or the main treatment in maintenance asthma therapy (see Section 4.1).

Once asthma symptoms are controlled, consideration may be given to gradually reducing the dose of Serevent. Regular review of patients as treatment is stepped down is important. The lowest effective dose of Serevent should be used.

Salmeterol should be administered with caution in patients with thyrotoxicosis.

There have been very rare reports of increases in blood glucose levels (see Section 4.8) and this should be considered when prescribing to patients with a history of diabetes mellitus.

Cardiovascular effects, such as increases in systolic blood pressure and heart rate, may occasionally be seen with all sympathomimetic drugs, especially at higher than therapeutic doses. For this reason, salmeterol should be used with caution in patients with pre-existing cardiovascular disease.

Potentially serious hypokalaemia may result from β_2 agonist therapy. Particular caution is advised in acute severe asthma as this effect may be potentiated by hypoxia and by concomitant treatment with xanthine derivatives, steroids and diuretics. Serum potassium levels should be monitored in such situations.

Data from a large clinical trial (the Salmeterol Multi-Center Asthma Research Trial, SMART) suggested African-American patients were at increased risk of serious respiratory-related events or deaths when using salmeterol compared with placebo (see section 5.1). It is not known if this was due to pharmacogenetic or other factors. Patients of black African or Afro-Caribbean ancestry should therefore be asked to continue treatment but to seek medical advice if asthma symptoms remained uncontrolled or worsen whilst using Serevent.

Concomitant use of systemic ketoconazole significantly increases systemic exposure to salmeterol. This may lead to an increase in the incidence of systemic effects (e.g. prolongation in the QTc interval and palpitations). Concomitant treatment with ketoconazole or other potent CYP3A4 inhibitors should therefore be avoided unless the benefits outweigh the potentially increased risk of systemic side effects of salmeterol treatment (see section 4.5).

Patients should be instructed in the proper use of their inhaler and their technique checked to ensure optimum delivery of the inhaled medicinal product to the lungs.

As systemic absorption is largely through the lungs, the use of a spacer plus metered dose inhaler may vary the delivery to the lungs. It should be noted that this could potentially lead to an increase in the risk of systemic adverse effects so that dose adjustment may be necessary.

4.5 Interaction with other medicinal products and other forms of interaction

Both non-selective and selective beta-blockers should be avoided in patients with asthma unless there are compelling reasons for their use.

Potentially serious hypokalaemia may result from β_2 agonist therapy. Particular caution is advised in acute severe asthma as this effect may be potentiated by concomitant treatment with xanthine derivatives, steroids and diuretics.

Potent CYP3A4 inhibitors

Co-administration of ketoconazole (400 mg orally once daily) and salmeterol (50 mcg inhaled twice daily) in 15 healthy subjects for 7 days resulted in a significant increase in plasma salmeterol exposure (1.4-fold Cmax and 15-fold AUC). This may lead to an increase in the incidence of other systemic effects of salmeterol treatment (e.g. prolongation of QTc interval and palpitations) compared with salmeterol or ketoconazole treatment alone (see Section 4.4).

Clinically significant effects were not seen on blood pressure, heart rate, blood glucose and blood potassium levels. Co-administration with ketoconazole did not increase the elimination half-life of salmeterol or increase salmeterol accumulation with repeat dosing.

The concomitant administration of ketoconazole should be avoided, unless the benefits outweigh the potentially increased risk of systemic side effects of salmeterol treatment. There is likely to be a similar risk of interaction with other potent CYP3A4 inhibitors (e.g. itraconazole, telithromycin, ritonavir).

Moderate CYP 3A4 inhibitors

Co-administration of erythromycin (500mg orally three times a day) and salmeterol (50µg inhaled twice daily) in 15 healthy subjects for 6 days resulted in a small but non-statistically significant increase in salmeterol exposure (Cmax mean ratio was 1.40). Co-administration with erythromycin was not associated with any serious adverse effects.

4.6 Pregnancy and lactation

There are insufficient data on the use of salmeterol or this medicinal product during pregnancy and lactation in women to assess the possible harmful effects. In animal studies fetal abnormalities occur after administration of beta-2-adrenoreceptor agonists (see Section 5.3).

Use of Serevent Evohaler during pregnancy should only be considered if the expected benefit to the mother is greater than any possible risk to the fetus.

It is unknown whether salmeterol is excreted in human breast milk. Animal studies in rats have shown excretion of salmeterol in breast milk. A decision on whether to continue/discontinue breast-feeding or to continue/discontinue therapy with Serevent Evohaler should be made taking into account the benefit of breast-feeding to the child and the benefit of Serevent Evohaler therapy to the woman.

Studies of HFA-134a revealed no effects on the reproductive performance and lactation of adult or two successive generations of rats or on the fetal development of rats or rabbits.

4.7 Effects on ability to drive and use machines

No studies on the effect on the ability to drive and use machines have been performed.

4.8 Undesirable effects

Adverse reactions are listed below by system organ class and frequency. Frequencies are defined as: very common ($\geq$ 1/10), common ($\geq$1/100 and $<$1/10), uncommon ($\geq$1/1000 and $<$1/100), rare ($\geq$1/10,000 and $<$1/1000) and very rare ($<$1/10,000) including isolated reports. Common and uncommon events were generally determined from clinical trial data. The incidence on placebo was not taken into account. Very rare events are generally determined from post-marketing spontaneous data.

The following frequencies are estimated at the standard dose of 50mcg twice daily. Frequencies at the higher dose of 100mcg twice daily have also been taken to account where appropriate.

System Organ Class	*Adverse Reaction*	*Frequency*
Immune System Disorders	*Hypersensitivity reactions with the following manifestations:*	
	Rash (itching and redness)	*Uncommon*
	Anaphylactic reactions including oedema and angioedema, bronchospasm and anaphylactic shock	*Very Rare*
Metabolism & Nutrition Disorders	*Hypokalaemia*	*Rare*
	Hyperglycaemia	*Very Rare*
Psychiatric Disorders	*Nervousness*	*Uncommon*
	Insomnia	*Rare*
Nervous System Disorders	*Headache*	*Common*
	Tremor	*Common*
	Dizziness	*Rare*
Cardiac Disorders	*Palpitations*	*Common*
	Tachycardia	*Uncommon*
	Cardiac arrhythmias (including atrial fibrillation, supraventricular tachycardia and extrasystoles)	*Very Rare*
Respiratory, Thoracic & Mediastinal Disorders	*Oropharyngeal irritation*	*Very Rare*
	Paradoxical bronchospasm	*Very Rare*
Gastro-Intestinal Disorders	*Nausea*	*Very Rare*
Musculoskeletal & Connective Tissue Disorders	*Muscle cramps*	*Common*
	Arthralgia	*Very Rare*
General Disorders and Administration Site Conditions	*Non-specific chest pain*	*Very Rare*

The pharmacological side effects of beta-2 agonist treatment, such as tremor, headache and palpitations have been reported, but tend to be transient and to reduce with regular therapy. Tremor and tachycardia occur more commonly when administered at doses higher than 50mcg twice daily.

As with other inhalational therapy paradoxical bronchospasm may occur with an immediate increase in wheezing and fall in peak expiratory flow rate (PEFR) after dosing. This should be treated immediately with a fast-acting inhaled bronchodilator. Serevent Evohaler should be discontinued immediately, the patient assessed, and if necessary alternative therapy instituted (see Section 4.4).

4.9 Overdose

The signs and symptoms of salmeterol overdose are tremor, headache and tachycardia. The preferred antidotes are cardioselective beta-blocking agents, which should be used with caution in patients with a history of bronchospasm.

Additionally hypokalaemia can occur and therefore serum potassium levels should be monitored. Potassium replacement should be considered.

5. PHARMACOLOGICAL PROPERTIES

5.1 Pharmacodynamic properties

Pharmacotherapeutic Group: Selective beta-2-adrenoreceptor agonists.

ATC Code: R03AC12

Salmeterol is a selective long-acting (12 hour) beta-2-adrenoceptor agonist with a long side chain which binds to the exo-site of the receptor.

These pharmacological properties of salmeterol offer more effective protection against histamine-induced bronchoconstriction and produce a longer duration of bronchodilation, lasting for at least 12 hours, than recommended doses of conventional short-acting β_2 agonists. In man salmeterol inhibits the early and late phase response to inhaled allergen; the latter persisting for over 30 hours after a single dose when the bronchodilator effect is no longer evident. Single dosing with salmeterol attenuates bronchial hyper-responsiveness. These properties indicate that salmeterol has additional non-bronchodilator activity, but the full clinical significance is not yet clear. The mechanism is different from the anti-inflammatory effect of corticosteroids which should not be stopped or reduced when salmeterol is prescribed.

Salmeterol has been studied in the treatment of conditions associated with COPD and has been shown to improve symptoms, pulmonary function and quality of life.

Asthma clinical trials

The Salmeterol Multi-center Asthma Research Trial (SMART)

SMART was a multi-centre, randomised, double-blind, placebo-controlled, parallel group 28-week study in the US which randomised 13,176 patients to salmeterol (50µg twice daily) and 13,179 patients to placebo in addition to the patients' usual asthma therapy. Patients were enrolled if $\geq$12 years of age, with asthma and if currently using asthma medication (but not a LABA). Baseline ICS use at study entry was recorded, but not required in the study. The primary endpoint in SMART was the combined number of respiratory-related deaths and respiratory-related life-threatening experiences.

Key findings from SMART: primary endpoint

(see Table 1 on next page)

Key findings from SMART by inhaled steroid use at baseline: secondary endpoints

(see Table 2 on next page)

COPD clinical trials

TORCH study

TORCH was a 3-year study to assess the effect of treatment with Seretide Diskus 50/500mcg bd, salmeterol Diskus 50mcg bd, fluticasone propionate (FP) Diskus 500mcg bd or placebo on all-cause mortality in patients with COPD. COPD patients with a baseline (pre-bronchodilator) FEV1 $<$60% of predicted normal were randomised to double-blind medication. During the study, patients were permitted usual COPD therapy with the exception of other inhaled corticosteroids, long-acting bronchodilators and long-term systemic corticosteroids. Survival status at 3 years was determined for all patients regardless of withdrawal from study medication. The primary endpoint was reduction in all cause mortality at 3 years for Seretide vs Placebo.

(see Table 3 on next page)

There was a trend towards improved survival in subjects treated with Seretide compared with placebo over 3 years however this did not achieve the statistical significance level $p \leq 0.05$.

The percentage of patients who died within 3 years due to COPD-related causes was 6.0% for placebo, 6.1% for salmeterol, 6.9% for FP and 4.7% for Seretide.

The mean number of moderate to severe exacerbations per year was significantly reduced with Seretide as compared with treatment with salmeterol, FP and placebo (mean rate in the Seretide group 0.85 compared with 0.97 in the salmeterol group, 0.93 in the FP group and 1.13 in the placebo). This translates to a reduction in the rate of moderate to severe exacerbations of 25% (95% CI: 19% to 31%; $p<0.001$) compared with placebo, 12% compared with salmeterol (95% CI: 5% to 19%, p=0.002) and 9% compared with FP (95% CI: 1% to 16%, p=0.024). Salmeterol and FP significantly reduced exacerbation rates compared with placebo by 15% (95% CI: 7% to 22%; $p<0.001$) and 18% (95% CI: 11% to 24%; $p<0.001$) respectively.

Table 1 Key findings from SMART: primary endpoint

Patient group	Number of primary endpoint events / number of patients		Relative Risk (95% confidence intervals)
	salmeterol	placebo	
All patients	50/13,176	36/13,179	1.40 (0.91, 2.14)
Patients using inhaled steroids	23/6,127	19/6,138	1.21 (0.66, 2.23)
Patients not using inhaled steroids	27/7,049	17/7,041	1.60 (0.87, 2.93)
African-American patients	***20/2,366***	***5/2,319***	***4.10 (1.54, 10.90)***

(Risk in bold is statistically significant at the 95% level.)

Table 2 Key findings from SMART by inhaled steroid use at baseline: secondary endpoints

	Number of secondary endpoint events / number of patients		Relative Risk (95% confidence intervals)
	salmeterol	placebo	
Respiratory -related death			
Patients using inhaled steroids	10/6127	5/6138	2.01 (0.69, 5.86)
Patients not using inhaled steroids	14/7049	6/7041	2.28 (0.88, 5.94)
Combined asthma-related death or life-threatening experience			
Patients using inhaled steroids	16/6127	13/6138	1.24 (0.60, 2.58)
Patients not using inhaled steroids	**21/7049**	**9/7041**	**2.39 (1.10, 5.22)**
Asthma-related death			
Patients using inhaled steroids	4/6127	3/6138	1.35 (0.30, 6.04)
Patients not using inhaled steroids	9/7049	0/7041	*

(*=could not be calculated because of no events in placebo group. Risk in bold is statistically significant at the 95% level. The secondary endpoints in the table above reached statistical significance in the whole population.) The secondary endpoints of combined all-cause death or life-threatening experience, all cause death, or all cause hospitalisation did not reach statistical significance in the whole population.

Table 3

	Placebo N = 1524	Salmeterol 50 N = 1521	FP 500 N = 1534	Seretide 50/500 N = 1533
All cause mortality at 3 years				
Number of deaths (%)	231 (15.2%)	205 (13.5%)	246 (16.0%)	193 (12.6%)
Hazard Ratio vs Placebo (CIs) p value	N/A	0.879 (0.73, 1.06) 0.180	1.060 (0.89, 1.27) 0.525	0.825 (0.68, 1.00) 0.052[1]
Hazard Ratio Seretide 50/500 vs components (CIs) p value	N/A	0.932 (0.77, 1.13) 0.481	0.774 (0.64, 0.93) 0.007	N/A

1. Non significant P value after adjustment for 2 interim analyses on the primary efficacy comparison from a log-rank analysis stratified by smoking status

Health Related Quality of Life, as measured by the St George's Respiratory Questionnaire (SGRQ) was improved by all active treatments in comparison with placebo. The average improvement over three years for Seretide compared with placebo was -3.1 units (95% CI: -4.1 to -2.1; $p<0.001$), compared with salmeterol was -2.2 units ($p<0.001$) and compared with FP was -1.2 units ($p=0.017$). A 4-unit decrease is considered clinically relevant.

The estimated 3-year probability of having pneumonia reported as an adverse event was 12.3% for placebo, 13.3% for salmeterol, 18.3% for FP and 19.6% for Seretide (Hazard ratio for Seretide vs placebo: 1.64, 95% CI: 1.33 to 2.01, $p<0.001$). There was no increase in pneumonia related deaths; deaths while on treatment that were adjudicated as primarily due to pneumonia were 7 for placebo, 9 for salmeterol, 13 for FP and 8 for Seretide. There was no significant difference in probability of bone fracture (5.1% placebo, 5.1% salmeterol, 5.4% FP and 6.3% Seretide; Hazard ratio for Seretide vs placebo: 1.22, 95% CI: 0.87 to 1.72, p=0.248.

5.2 Pharmacokinetic properties

Salmeterol acts locally in the lung therefore plasma levels are not an indication of therapeutic effects. In addition there are only limited data available on the pharmacokinetics of salmeterol because of the technical difficulty of assaying the active substance in plasma due to the low plasma concentrations at therapeutic doses (approximately 200 picogram/ml or less) achieved after inhaled dosing.

5.3 Preclinical safety data

The only findings in animal studies with relevance for clinical use were the effects associated with exaggerated pharmacological activity.

In reproduction and development toxicity studies with salmeterol xinafoate there were no effects in rats. In rabbits, typical beta-2 agonist embryo fetal toxicity (cleft palate, premature opening of the eye lids, sternebral fusion and reduced ossification rate of the frontal cranial bones) occurred at high exposure levels (approximately 20 times the maximum recommended human daily dose based on the comparison of AUCs).

Salmeterol xinafoate was negative in a range of standard genotoxicity studies.

The non-CFC propellant, norflurane, has been shown to have no toxic effect at very high vapour concentrations, far in excess of those likely to be experienced by patients, in a wide range of animal species exposed daily for periods of up to two years including no effects on the reproductive performance or embryofetal development.

6. PHARMACEUTICAL PARTICULARS

6.1 List of excipients

Norflurane (HFA 134a), a hydrofluoroalkane (non-chlorofluorocarbon) propellant

6.2 Incompatibilities

Not applicable.

6.3 Shelf life

2 years

6.4 Special precautions for storage

Replace the mouthpiece cover firmly and snap it into position.

Do not store above 30° C.

Pressurised container. Do not expose to temperatures higher than 50°C. Do not puncture, break or burn even when apparently empty.

6.5 Nature and contents of container

The suspension is contained in an internally lacquered, 8ml aluminium alloy pressurised container sealed with a metering valve. The containers are fitted into plastic actuators incorporating an atomising mouthpiece and fitted with dustcaps. One pressurised container delivers 120 actuations.

6.6 Special precautions for disposal and other handling

No special requirements.

7. MARKETING AUTHORISATION HOLDER

GlaxoWellcome UK Ltd
Trading as Allen & Hanburys
Stockley Park West
Uxbridge
Middlesex UB11 1BT

8. MARKETING AUTHORISATION NUMBER(S)

PL 10949/0369

9. DATE OF FIRST AUTHORISATION/RENEWAL OF THE AUTHORISATION

28 October 2005

10. DATE OF REVISION OF THE TEXT

15 January 2009

Seroquel

(AstraZeneca UK Limited)

1. NAME OF THE MEDICINAL PRODUCT

SEROQUEL™▼*

** Intensive monitoring is requested only when used for the recently licensed indication of bipolar depression.*

2. QUALITATIVE AND QUANTITATIVE COMPOSITION

25 mg tablet: Each tablet contains 25 mg (as 28.78 mg quetiapine fumarate).

Excipient: 18 mg lactose (anhydrous) per tablet.

100 mg tablet: Each tablet contains 100 mg (as 115.13 mg quetiapine fumarate).

Excipient: 20 mg lactose (anhydrous) per tablet.

150 mg tablet: Each tablet contains 150 mg (as 172.69 mg quetiapine fumarate).

Excipient: 29 mg lactose (anhydrous) per tablet.

200 mg tablet: Each tablet contains 200 mg (as 230.26 mg quetiapine fumarate).

Excipient: 39 mg lactose (anhydrous) per tablet.

300 mg tablet: Each tablet contains 300 mg (as quetiapine fumarate).

Excipient: 59 mg lactose (anhydrous) per tablet.

For a full list of excipients, see Section 6.1

3. PHARMACEUTICAL FORM

Film-coated tablet.

4. CLINICAL PARTICULARS

4.1 Therapeutic indications

Treatment of schizophrenia.

Treatment of manic episodes associated with bipolar disorder.

Treatment of major depressive episodes in bipolar disorder.

4.2 Posology and method of administration

SEROQUEL can be administered with or without food.

Adults

For the treatment of schizophrenia: Seroquel should be administered twice a day. The total daily dose for the first 4 days of therapy is 50 mg (Day 1), 100 mg (Day 2), 200 mg (Day 3) and 300 mg (Day 4).

From Day 4 onwards, the dose should be titrated to the usual effective dose range of 300 to 450 mg/day. Depending on the clinical response and tolerability of the individual patient, the dose may be adjusted within the range 150 to 750 mg/day.

For the treatment of manic episodes associated with bipolar disorder: Seroquel should be administered twice a day. As monotherapy or as adjunct therapy to mood stabilizers, the total daily dose for the first four days of therapy is 100 mg (Day 1), 200 mg (Day 2), 300 mg (Day 3) and 400 mg (Day 4). Further dosage adjustments up to 800 mg per day by Day 6 should be in increments of no greater than 200 mg per day.

The dose may be adjusted depending on clinical response and tolerability of the individual patient, within the range of 200 to 800 mg per day. The usual effective dose is in the range of 400 to 800 mg per day.

For the treatment of depressive episodes in bipolar disorder: Seroquel should be administered once daily at bedtime. The total daily dose for the first four days of therapy is 50 mg (Day 1), 100 mg (Day 2), 200 mg (Day 3) and 300 mg (Day 4). The recommended daily dose is 300 mg. In clinical trials, no additional benefit was seen in the 600 mg group compared to the 300 mg group. Individual patients may benefit from a 600 mg dose. In individual patients, in the event of tolerance concerns, clinical trials have indicated that dose reduction to a minimum of 200 mg could be considered. When treating depressive episodes in bipolar disorder, treatment should be initiated by physicians experienced in treating bipolar disorder.

Elderly

As with other antipsychotics, SEROQUEL should be used with caution in the elderly, especially during the initial dosing period. Elderly patients should be started on SEROQUEL 25 mg/day. The dose should be increased daily, in increments of 25 to 50 mg, to an effective dose, which is likely to be lower than that in younger patients.

Efficacy and safety have not been evaluated in patients over 65 years with depressive episodes in the framework of bipolar disorder.

Children and adolescents

The safety and efficacy of SEROQUEL have not been evaluated in children and adolescents.

Renal and hepatic impairment

The oral clearance of quetiapine is reduced by approximately 25% in patients with renal or hepatic impairment. Quetiapine is extensively metabolised by the liver, and therefore should be used with caution in patients with known hepatic impairment.

Patients with renal or hepatic impairment should be started on SEROQUEL 25 mg/day. The dose should be increased daily, in increments of 25 to 50 mg, to an effective dose.

4.3 Contraindications

SEROQUEL is contra-indicated in patients who are hypersensitive to any component of this product.

4.4 Special warnings and precautions for use

Suicide/suicidal thoughts or clinical worsening

Depression in bipolar disorder is associated with an increased risk of suicidal thoughts, self-harm and suicide (suicide-related events). This risk persists until significant remission occurs. As improvement may not occur during the first few weeks or more of treatment, patients should be closely monitored until such improvement occurs. It is general clinical experience that the risk of suicide may increase in the early stages of recovery.

In clinical studies of patients with major depressive episodes in bipolar disorder an increased risk of suicide-related events was observed in young adult patients less than 25 years of age who were treated with quetiapine as compared to those treated with placebo (3.0% vs. 0%, respectively).

Cardiovascular disease

SEROQUEL should be used with caution in patients with known cardiovascular disease, cerebrovascular disease, or other conditions predisposing to hypotension.

SEROQUEL may induce orthostatic hypotension, especially during the initial dose-titration period; this is more common in elderly patients than in younger patients.

QT Prolongation

In clinical trials and use in accordance with the SPC, quetiapine was not associated with a persistent increase in absolute QT intervals. However, with overdose (see Section 4.9) QT prolongation was observed. As with other antipsychotics, caution should be exercised when quetiapine is prescribed in patients with cardiovascular disease or family history of QT prolongation. Also, caution should be exercised when quetiapine is prescribed with medicines known to increase QTc interval, and concomitant neuroleptics, especially in the elderly, in patients with congenital long QT syndrome, congestive heart failure, heart hypertrophy, hypokalaemia or hypomagnesaemia (see Section 4.5 Interaction with other medicinal products and other forms of interaction).

Seizures

In controlled clinical trials there was no difference in the incidence of seizures in patients treated with SEROQUEL or placebo. As with other antipsychotics, caution is recommended when treating patients with a history of seizures.

Extrapyramidal symptoms

In placebo controlled clinical trials quetiapine was associated with an increased incidence of extrapyramidal symptoms (EPS) compared to placebo in patients treated for major depressive episodes in bipolar disorder (see Section 4.8 Undesirable effects).

Tardive dyskinesia

As with other antipsychotics, there is a potential for SEROQUEL to cause tardive dyskinesia after long-term treatment. If signs and symptoms of tardive dyskinesia appear, dose reduction or discontinuation of SEROQUEL should be considered.

Neuroleptic malignant syndrome

Neuroleptic malignant syndrome has been associated with antipsychotic treatment, including quetiapine (see Section 4.8 Undesirable effects). Clinical manifestations include hyperthermia, altered mental status, muscular rigidity, autonomic instability, and increased creatine phosphokinase. In such an event, SEROQUEL should be discontinued and appropriate medical treatment given.

Severe neutropenia

Severe neutropenia (neutrophil count $<0.5 \times 10^9$/L) has been uncommonly reported in quetiapine clinical trials. Most cases of severe neutropenia have occurred within a couple of months of starting therapy with quetiapine. There is no apparent dose relationship. Possible risk factors for neutropenia include pre-existing low white cell count (WBC) and history of drug induced neutropenia. Quetiapine should be discontinued in patients with a neutrophil count $<1.0 \times 10^9$/L. Patients should be observed for signs and symptoms of infection and neutrophil counts followed (until they exceed 1.5×10^9/L). (See Section 4.8 Undesirable effects).

Somnolence

Quetiapine treatment has been associated with somnolence and related symptoms, such as sedation (see Section 4.8 Undesirable effects). In clinical trials for treatment of patients with bipolar depression, onset was usually within the first 3 days of treatment and was predominantly of mild to moderate intensity. Bipolar depression patients experiencing somnolence of severe intensity may require more frequent contact for a minimum of 2 weeks from onset of somnolence, or until symptoms improve and treatment discontinuation may need to be considered.

Acute withdrawal reactions

Acute withdrawal symptoms such as insomnia, nausea, headache, diarrhoea, vomiting, dizziness and irritability have been described after abrupt cessation of Seroquel. Recurrence of psychotic symptoms may also occur, and the emergence of involuntary movement disorders (such as akathisia, dystonia and dyskinesia) has been reported. Gradual withdrawal over a period of at least one to two weeks is advisable (see Section 4.8 Undesirable effects).

Interactions

See also Section 4.5 Interactions with other medicinal products and other forms of interaction.

Concomitant use of quetiapine with hepatic enzyme inducers such as carbamazepine may substantially decrease systemic exposure to quetiapine. Depending on clinical response, higher doses of SEROQUEL may need to be considered if quetiapine is used concomitantly with a hepatic enzyme inducer.

During concomitant administration of drugs which are potent CYP3A4 inhibitors (such as azole antifungals, macrolide antibiotics and protease inhibitors), plasma concentrations of quetiapine can be significantly higher than observed in patients in clinical trials. (See also Section 5.2 Pharmacokinetics.) As a consequence of this, lower doses of SEROQUEL should be used. Special consideration should be given in elderly and debilitated patients. The risk-benefit ratio needs to be considered on an individual basis in all patients.

Hyperglycaemia

Hyperglycaemia or exacerbation of pre-existing diabetes has been reported during treatment with quetiapine. Appropriate clinical monitoring is advisable in diabetic patients and in patients with risk factors for the development of diabetes mellitus (see also Section 4.8 Undesirable effects).

Elderly patients with dementia-related psychosis

Seroquel is not approved for the treatment of patients with dementia-related psychosis.

An approximately 3-fold increased risk of cerebrovascular adverse events have been seen in randomised placebo controlled clinical trials in the dementia population with some atypical antipsychotics. The mechanism for this increased risk is not known. An increased risk cannot be excluded for other antipsychotics or other patient populations. Quetiapine should be used with caution in patients with risk factors for stroke.

Hepatic effects

If jaundice develops, Seroquel should be discontinued.

Lipids

Increases in triglycerides and cholesterol have been observed in clinical trials with quetiapine (see Section 4.8 Undesirable effects). Lipid increases should be managed as clinically appropriate.

Lactose

Seroquel tablets contain lactose. Patients with rare hereditary problems of galactose intolerance, the Lapp lactase deficiency, or glucose-galactose malabsorption should not take this medicine.

4.5 Interaction with other medicinal products and other forms of interaction

Given the primary central nervous system effects of quetiapine SEROQUEL should be used with caution in combination with other centrally acting drugs and alcohol.

The pharmacokinetics of lithium was not altered when co-administered with SEROQUEL

The pharmacokinetics of valproic acid and quetiapine were not altered to a clinically relevant extent when co-administered as valproate semisodium (also known as divalproex sodium (USAN)) and SEROQUEL (quetiapine fumarate). Valproate semisodium is a stable coordination compound comprised of sodium valproate and valproic acid in a 1:1 molar relationship.

The pharmacokinetics of quetiapine was not significantly altered following co-administration with the antipsychotics risperidone or haloperidol. However co-administration of SEROQUEL and thioridazine caused increases in the clearance of quetiapine.

Quetiapine did not induce the hepatic enzyme systems involved in the metabolism of antipyrine. However, in a multiple dose trial in patients to assess the pharmacokinetics of quetiapine given before and during treatment with carbamazepine (a known hepatic enzyme inducer), co-administration of carbamazepine significantly increased the clearance of quetiapine. This increase in clearance reduced systemic quetiapine exposure (as measured by AUC) to an average of 13% of the exposure during administration of quetiapine alone; although a greater effect was seen in some patients. As a consequence of this interaction, lower plasma concentrations can occur, and hence, in each patient, consideration for a higher dose of SEROQUEL, depending on clinical response, should be considered. It should be noted that the recommended maximum daily dose of SEROQUEL is 750mg/day for the treatment of schizophrenia and 800mg/day for the treatment of manic episodes associated with bipolar disorder. Continued treatment at higher doses should only be considered as a result of careful consideration of the benefit risk assessment for an individual patient. Co-administration of SEROQUEL with another microsomal enzyme inducer, phenytoin, also caused increases in the clearance of quetiapine. Increased doses of SEROQUEL may be required to maintain control of psychotic symptoms in patients co-administered SEROQUEL and phenytoin and other hepatic enzyme inducers (e.g. barbiturates, rifampicin etc.). The dose of SEROQUEL may need to be reduced if phenytoin or carbamazepine or other hepatic enzyme inducers are withdrawn and replaced with a non-inducer (e.g. sodium valproate).

CYP3A4 is the primary enzyme responsible for cytochrome P450 mediated metabolism of quetiapine. The pharmacokinetics of quetiapine was not altered following co-administration with cimetidine, a known P450 enzyme inhibitor. The pharmacokinetics of quetiapine were not significantly altered following co-administration with the antidepressants imipramine (a known CYP2D6 inhibitor) or fluoxetine (a known CYP3A4 and CYP2D6 inhibitor). However, caution is recommended when SEROQUEL is co-administered with potent CYP3A4 inhibitors (such as azole antifungals, macrolide antibiotics and protease inhibitors). (See also Section 4.4 Special Warnings & Special Precautions for Use and Section 5.2 Pharmacokinetics.)

Caution should be exercised when quetiapine is used concomitantly with drugs known to cause electrolyte imbalance or to increase QTc interval.

4.6 Pregnancy and lactation

The safety and efficacy of SEROQUEL during human pregnancy have not been established (see Section 5.3 Preclinical safety data, Reproduction studies, for animal reproductive toxicology data). Therefore, SEROQUEL should only be used during pregnancy if the benefits justify the potential risks.

The degree to which quetiapine is excreted into human milk is unknown. Women who are breast feeding should therefore be advised to avoid breast feeding while taking SEROQUEL.

4.7 Effects on ability to drive and use machines

Because SEROQUEL may cause somnolence, patients should be cautioned about operating hazardous machines, including motor vehicles.

4.8 Undesirable effects

The most commonly reported Adverse Drug Reactions (ADRs) with SEROQUEL are somnolence, dizziness, dry mouth, mild asthenia, constipation, tachycardia, orthostatic hypotension, and dyspepsia.

As with other antipsychotics, syncope, neuroleptic malignant syndrome, leucopenia, neutropenia and peripheral edema, have been associated with SEROQUEL.

The incidences of ADRs associated with SEROQUEL therapy, are tabulated below according to the format recommended by the Council for International Organizations of Medical Sciences (CIOMS III Working Group; 1995).

The frequencies of adverse events are ranked according to the following: Very common (>1/10), common (>1/100, <1/10), uncommon (>1/1000, <1/100), rare (>1/10,000, <1/1000) and very rare (<1/10,000).

Blood and lymphatic system disorders	
Common:	Leucopenia
Uncommon:	Eosinophilia
Immune system disorders	
Uncommon:	Hypersensitivity
Very rare:	Anaphylactic reaction

Endocrine disorders	
Common:	Hyperprolactinaemia[17]
Metabolism and nutritional disorders	
Common:	Increased appetite
Very rare:	Diabetes Mellitus[1, 6, 16]
Psychiatric disorders	
Common:	Abnormal dreams and nightmares
Nervous system disorders	
Very Common:	Dizziness[1, 5, 18], somnolence[2, 18]
Common:	Syncope[1, 5, 18], Extrapyramidal symptoms[1, 15]
Uncommon:	Seizure[1], Restless leg syndrome, Dysarthria
Cardiac disorders	
Common:	Tachycardia[1, 5]
Eye disorders	
Common:	Vision blurred
Vascular disorders	
Common:	Orthostatic hypotension[1, 5, 18]
Respiratory, thoracic and mediastinal disorders	
Common:	Rhinitis
Gastrointestinal disorders	
Very Common:	Dry mouth
Common:	Constipation, dyspepsia
Uncommon:	Dysphagia[12]
Reproductive system and breast disorders	
Rare:	Priapism, galactorrhoea
General disorders and administration site conditions	
Very Common:	Withdrawal (discontinuation) symptoms[1, 9]
Common:	Mild asthenia, peripheral oedema, irritability
Rare:	Neuroleptic malignant syndrome[1]
Investigations	
Very Common:	Elevations in serum triglyceride levels[10], elevations in total cholesterol (predominantly LDL cholesterol)[11], weight gain[3]
Common:	Elevations in serum transaminases (ALT, AST)[4], decreased neutrophil count[7], blood glucose increased to hyperglycaemic levels[8, 16]
Uncommon:	Elevations in gamma-GT levels[4], platelet count decreased[13]
Rare:	Elevations in blood creatine phosphokinase[14]

(1) See section 4.4 Special Warnings and Special Precautions for Use.

(2) Somnolence may occur, usually during the first two weeks of treatment and generally resolves with the continued administration of SEROQUEL.

(3) Based on >7% increase in body weight from baseline. Occurs predominantly during the early weeks of treatment.

(4) Asymptomatic elevations in serum transaminase (ALT, AST) or gamma-GT-levels have been observed in some patients administered SEROQUEL.

(5) As with other antipsychotics with alpha1 adrenergic blocking activity, SEROQUEL may induce orthostatic hypotension, associated with dizziness, tachycardia and, in some patients, syncope, especially during the initial dose-titration period.

(6) Exacerbation of pre-existing diabetes has been reported in very rare cases.

(7) In placebo-controlled monotherapy trials in patients with a baseline neutrophil count $\geqslant 1.5 \times 10^9$/L, the incidence of at least one occurrence of neutrophil count $<1.5 \times 10^9$/L was 1.72% in patients treated with SEROQUEL compared to 0.73% in placebo-treated patients. In all clinical trials (placebo-controlled, open-label, active comparator; patients with a baseline neutrophil count $\geqslant 1.5 \times 10^9$/L), the incidence of at least one occurrence of neutrophil count $<0.5 \times 10^9$/L was 0.21% in patients treated with SEROQUEL and 0% in placebo-treated patients and the incidence $\geqslant 0.5$ - $<1.0 \times 10^9$/L was 0.75% in patients treated with SEROQUEL and 0.11% in placebo-treated patients.

(8) Fasting blood glucose $\geqslant 7.0$ mmol/L or a non fasting blood glucose $\geqslant 11.1$.mmol/L on at least one occasion.

(9) The following withdrawal symptoms have been observed most frequently in acute placebo-controlled, monotherapy clinical trials, which evaluated discontinuation symptoms: insomnia, nausea, headache, diarrhoea, vomiting, dizziness, and irritability. The incidence of these reactions had decreased significantly after 1 week post-discontinuation.

(10) Triglycerides $\geqslant 200$ mg/dL ($\geqslant 2.258$ mmol/L) on at least one occasion.

(11) Cholesterol $\geqslant 240$ mg/dL ($\geqslant 6.2064$ mmol/L) on at least one occasion.

(12) An increase in the rate of dysphagia with SEROQUEL vs. placebo was only observed in the clinical trials in bipolar depression.

(13) Platelets $\leqslant 100 \times 10^9$/L on at least one occasion.

(14) Based on clinical trial adverse event reports of blood creatine phosphokinase increase not associated with neuroleptic malignant syndrome.

(15) See text below.

(16) Calculation of frequency for these ADRs have been taken from post-marketing data only.

(17) Prolactin levels (patients >18 years of age): >20 μg/L (>869.56 pmol/L) males; >30 μg/L (>1304.34 pmol/L) females at any time.

(18) May lead to falls.

In short-term, placebo-controlled clinical trials in bipolar depression the aggregated incidence of extrapyramidal symptoms was 8.9% for Seroquel compared to 3.8% for placebo, though the incidence of the individual adverse events were generally low and did not exceed 4% in any treatment group. In short-term, placebo-controlled clinical trials in schizophrenia and bipolar mania the aggregated incidence of extrapyramidal symptoms was similar to placebo (schizophrenia: 7.8% for Seroquel and 8.0% for placebo; bipolar mania: 11.2% for Seroquel and 11.4% for placebo).

Cases of QT prolongation, ventricular arrhythmia, sudden unexplained death, cardiac arrest and torsades de pointes have been reported very rarely with the use of neuroleptics and are considered class effects (see Section 4.4 Special warnings and special precautions for use).

Quetiapine treatment was associated with small dose-related decreases in thyroid hormone levels, particularly total T_4 and free T_4. The reduction in total and free T_4 was maximal within the first two to four weeks of quetiapine treatment, with no further reduction during long-term treatment. In nearly all cases, cessation of quetiapine treatment was associated with a reversal of the effects on total and free T_4, irrespective of the duration of treatment. Smaller decreases in total T_3 and reverse T_3 were seen only at higher doses. Levels of TBG were unchanged and in general, reciprocal increases in TSH were not observed, with no indication that SEROQUEL causes clinically relevant hypothyroidism.

Exacerbation of pre-existing diabetes has been reported in very rare cases during quetiapine treatment.

As with other antipsychotics, Seroquel may be associated with weight gain, predominantly during the early weeks of treatment.

Acute withdrawal reactions have been reported (see Section 4.4 Special warnings and special precautions for use).

Post-marketing

Reports of jaundice have been reported.

4.9 Overdose

Fatal outcome has been reported in clinical trials following an acute overdose at 13.6 grams, and in post-marketing on doses as low as 6 grams of Seroquel alone. However, survival has also been reported following acute overdoses of up to 30 grams.

In post-marketing experience, there have been very rare reports of overdose of quetiapine alone resulting in death or coma or QT-prolongation.

In general, reported signs and symptoms were those resulting from an exaggeration of the active substance's known pharmacological effects, i.e., drowsiness and sedation, tachycardia and hypotension.

Patients with pre-existing severe cardiovascular disease may be at an increased risk of the effects of overdose. (See Section 4.4 Special warnings and special precautions for use: Cardiovascular).

Management

There is no specific antidote to quetiapine. In cases of severe signs, the possibility of multiple drug involvement should be considered, and intensive care procedures are recommended, including establishing and maintaining a patent airway, ensuring adequate oxygenation and ventilation, and monitoring and support of the cardiovascular system. Whilst the prevention of absorption in overdose has not been investigated, gastric lavage can be indicated in severe poisonings and if possible to perform within one hour of ingestion. The administration of activated charcoal should be considered.

Close medical supervision and monitoring should be continued until the patient recovers.

5. PHARMACOLOGICAL PROPERTIES

5.1 Pharmacodynamic properties

Pharmacotherapeutic group: Antipsychotics

Therapeutic classification: N05A H04

Mechanism of action

Quetiapine is an atypical antipsychotic agent. Quetiapine and the active human plasma metabolite, N-desalkyl quetiapine interact with a broad range of neurotransmitter receptors. Quetiapine and N-desalkyl quetiapine exhibit affinity for brain serotonin ($5HT_2$) and dopamine D_1 and D_2 receptors. Quetiapine exhibits a higher affinity for serotonin ($5HT_2$) receptors in the brain than it does for dopamine D_1 and D_2 receptors in the brain. Additionally, N-desalkyl quetiapine has high affinity for the norepinephrine transporter (NET). Quetiapine and N-desalkyl quetiapine also have high affinity at histaminergic and adrenergic α_1 receptors, with a lower affinity at adrenergic α_2 and serotonin $5HT_1A$ receptors. Quetiapine has no appreciable affinity at cholinergic muscarinic or benzodiazepine receptors.

Pharmacodynamic effect

Quetiapine is active in tests for antipsychotic activity, such as conditioned avoidance. It also blocks the action of dopamine agonists, measured either behaviourally or electrophysiologically, and elevates dopamine metabolite concentrations, a neurochemical index of D_2-receptor blockade.

The results of animal studies predictive of EPS liability revealed that quetiapine causes only weak catalepsy at effective dopamine D_2 receptor blocking doses, that quetiapine causes selective reduction in the firing of mesolimbic A10 dopaminergic neurones versus the A9 nigrostriatal neurones involved in motor function, and that quetiapine exhibits minimal dystonic liability in neuroleptic-sensitised monkeys.

The extent to which the N-desalkyl quetiapine metabolite contributes to the pharmacological activity of Seroquel in humans is not known.

Clinical Efficacy

The results of three placebo-controlled clinical trials in patients with schizophrenia, including one that used a dose range of SEROQUEL of 75 to 750 mg/day, identified no difference between SEROQUEL and placebo in the incidence of EPS or use of concomitant anticholinergics.

In four controlled trials, evaluating doses of SEROQUEL up to 800 mg for the treatment of bipolar mania, two each in monotherapy and as adjunct therapy to lithium or valproate semisodium, there were no differences between the SEROQUEL and placebo treatment groups in the incidence of EPS or concomitant use of anticholinergics.

In clinical trials, SEROQUEL has been shown to be effective in the treatment of both positive and negative symptoms of schizophrenia. In one trial against chlorpromazine, and two against haloperidol, SEROQUEL showed similar short-term efficacy.

In clinical trials, SEROQUEL has been shown to be effective as monotherapy or as adjunct therapy in reducing manic symptoms in patients with bipolar mania. The mean last week median dose of SEROQUEL in responders, was approximately 600 mg and approximately 85% of the responders were in the dose range of 400 to 800 mg per day.

In a meta-analysis of atypical antipsychotic drugs, it has been reported that elderly patients with dementia-related psychosis are at an increased risk of death compared to placebo. However in two 10-week placebo-controlled Seroquel studies in the same patient population (n=710; mean age: 83 years; range: 56-99 years) the incidence of mortality in Seroquel-treated patients was 5.5% versus 3.2% in the placebo group. The patients in these trials died from a variety of causes that were consistent with expectations for this population. These data do not establish a causal relationship between Seroquel treatment and death in elderly patients with dementia.

In 4 clinical trials in patients with depressive episodes in bipolar I or bipolar II disorder, with and without rapid cycling courses, 51% of quetiapine treated patients had at least a 50% improvement in MADRS total score at week 8 compared to 37% of the placebo treated patients. The antidepressant effect was significant at Day 8 (week 1). There were fewer episodes of treatment-emergent mania with Seroquel than with placebo. In continuation treatment the anti-depressant effect was maintained for patients on Seroquel (mean duration of treatment 30 weeks). Seroquel reduced the risk of a recurrent mood (manic and depressed) event by 49 %. Seroquel was superior to placebo in treating the anxiety symptoms associated with bipolar depression as assessed by mean change from baseline to week 8 in HAM-A total score.

5.2 Pharmacokinetic properties

Quetiapine is well absorbed and extensively metabolised following oral administration. The bioavailability of quetiapine is not significantly affected by administration with food. Quetiapine is approximately 83% bound to plasma proteins. Steady-state peak molar concentrations of the active metabolite N-desalkyl quetiapine are 35% of that observed for quetiapine. The elimination half-lives of quetiapine and N-desalkyl quetiapine are approximately 7 and 12 hours, respectively.

Clinical trials have demonstrated that SEROQUEL is effective when given twice a day. This is further supported by data from a positron emission tomography (PET) study which identified that $5HT_2$ and D_2 receptor occupancy are maintained for up to 12 hours after dosing with quetiapine.

The pharmacokinetics of quetiapine and N-desalkyl quetiapine are linear across the approved dosing range. The kinetics of quetiapine do not differ between men and women.

The mean clearance of quetiapine in the elderly is approximately 30 to 50% lower than that seen in adults aged 18 to 65 years.

The mean plasma clearance of quetiapine was reduced by approximately 25% in subjects with severe renal impairment (creatinine clearance less than 30 ml/min/1.73m^2) and in subjects with hepatic impairment (stable alcoholic cirrhosis), but the individual clearance values are within the range for normal subjects. The average molar dose fraction of free quetiapine and the active human plasma metabolite N-desalkyl quetiapine is <5% excreted in the urine.

Quetiapine is extensively metabolised, with parent compound accounting for less than 5% of unchanged drug-related material in the urine or faeces, following the administration of radiolabelled quetiapine. Approximately 73% of the radioactivity is excreted in the urine and 21% in the faeces.

In vitro investigations established that CYP3A4 is the primary enzyme responsible for cytochrome P450 mediated metabolism of quetiapine. N-desalkyl quetiapine is primarily formed and eliminated via CYP3A4.

In a multiple-dose trial in healthy volunteers to assess the pharmacokinetics of quetiapine given before and during treatment with ketoconazole, co–administration of ketoconazole resulted in an increase in mean C_{max} and AUC of quetiapine of 235% and 522%, respectively, with a corresponding decrease in mean oral clearance of 84%. The mean half–life of quetiapine increased from 2.6 to 6.8 hours, but the mean t_{max} was unchanged.

Quetiapine and several of its metabolites (including N-desalkyl quetiapine) were found to be weak inhibitors of human cytochrome P450 1A2, 2C9, 2C19, 2D6 and 3A4 activities in vitro. In vitro CYP inhibition is observed only at concentrations approximately 5 to 50 fold higher than those observed at a dose range of 300 to 800 mg/day in humans. Based on these *in vitro* results, it is unlikely that co-administration of quetiapine with other drugs will result in clinically significant drug inhibition of cytochrome P450 mediated metabolism of the other drug.

5.3 Preclinical safety data

Acute toxicity studies

Quetiapine has low acute toxicity. Findings in mice and rats after oral (500 mg/kg) or intraperitoneal (100 mg/kg) dosing were typical of an effective neuroleptic agent and included decreased motor activity, ptosis, loss of righting reflex, fluid around the mouth and convulsions.

Repeat-dose toxicity studies

In multiple-dose studies in rats, dogs and monkeys, anticipated central nervous system effects of an antipsychotic drug were observed with quetiapine (eg, sedation at lower doses and tremor, convulsions or prostration at higher exposures).

Hyperprolactinaemia, induced through the dopamine D_2 receptor antagonist activity of quetiapine or its metabolites, varied between species but was most marked in the rat, and a range of effects consequent to this were seen in the 12-month study, including mammary hyperplasia, increased pituitary weight, decreased uterine weight and enhanced growth of females.

Reversible morphological and functional effects on the liver, consistent with hepatic enzyme induction, were seen in mouse, rat and monkey.

Thyroid follicular cell hypertrophy and concomitant changes in plasma thyroid hormone levels occurred in rat and monkey.

Pigmentation of a number of tissues, particularly the thyroid, was not associated with any morphological or functional effects.

Transient increases in heart rate, unaccompanied by an effect on blood pressure, occurred in dogs.

Posterior triangular cataracts seen after 6 months in dogs at 100 mg/kg/day were consistent with inhibition of cholesterol biosynthesis in the lens. No cataracts were observed in Cynomolgus monkeys dosed up to 225 mg/kg/day, nor in rodents. Monitoring in clinical studies did not reveal drug-related corneal opacities in man.

No evidence of neutrophil reduction or agranulocytosis was seen in any of the toxicity studies.

Carcinogenicity studies

In the rat study (doses 0, 20, 75 and 250 mg/kg/day) the incidence of mammary adenocarcinomas was increased at all doses in female rats, consequential to prolonged hyperprolactinaemia.

In male rat (250 mg/kg/day) and mouse (250 and 750 mg/kg/day), there was an increased incidence of thyroid follicular cell benign adenomas, consistent with known rodent-specific mechanisms resulting from enhanced hepatic thyroxine clearance.

Reproduction studies

Effects related to elevated prolactin levels (marginal reduction in male fertility and pseudopregnancy, protracted periods of diestrus, increased precoital interval and reduced pregnancy rate) were seen in rats, although these are not directly relevant to humans because of species differences in hormonal control of reproduction.

Quetiapine had no teratogenic effects.

Mutagenicity studies

Genetic toxicity studies with quetiapine show that it is not a mutagen or clastogen.

6. PHARMACEUTICAL PARTICULARS

6.1 List of excipients

Core	Coating
Povidone (Ph. Eur)	Hypromellose (Ph. Eur)
Calcium Hydrogen Phosphate dihydrate (Ph. Eur)	Macrogol 400 (Ph. Eur) Titanium Dioxide (Ph. Eur, E171)
Microcrystalline Cellulose (Ph. Eur)	Ferric Oxide, Yellow (Ph. Eur, E172) (25 mg, 100 mg & 150 mg tablets)
Sodium Starch Glycollate Type A (Ph. Eur)	Ferric Oxide, Red (Ph. Eur, E172) (25 mg tablets)
Lactose Monohydrate (Ph. Eur)	
Magnesium Stearate (Ph. Eur)	

6.2 Incompatibilities

None known

6.3 Shelf life

36 months.

6.4 Special precautions for storage

Do not store above 30°C. Store in the original package.

6.5 Nature and contents of container

25mg tablet: The tablets are round, 6mm, peach coloured, bi-convex and film-coated.

100mg tablet: The tablets are round, 8.5 mm, yellow coloured, bi-convex and film-coated.

150mg tablet: The tablets are round, 10mm, pale yellow coloured, biconvex and film-coated.

200mg tablets: The tablets are round, 11mm, white, bi-convex and film-coated.

300mg tablets: The tablets are capsule-shaped, white and film-coated.

The tablets are packed into PVC aluminium foil blister strips. The blister strips are themselves packed into cartons.

Tablet strength	Carton (pack) contents	Strips/blisters
25 mg tablets	6 tablets	1 strip of 6 blisters
	20 tablets	2 strips of 10 blisters
	30 tablets	3 strips of 10 blisters
	60 tablets	6 strips of 10 blisters
	50 tablets	10 strips of 5 blisters
	100 tablets	10 strips of 10 blisters
100 mg, 150mg, 200mg and 300mg tablets	20 tablets	2 strips of 10 blisters
	30 tablets	3 strips of 10 blisters
	60 tablets	6 strips of 10 blisters
	90 tablets	9 strips of 10 blisters
	50 tablets	10 strips of 5 blisters
	50 tablets	5 strips of 10 blisters
	100 tablets	10 strips of 10 blisters (100 mg, 150 mg and 200 mg tablets only)
Mixed pack	10 tablets	1 strip containing 6 × 25 mg, 2 × 100 mg and 2 × 150 mg tablets

Not all pack sizes may be marketed.

6.6 Special precautions for disposal and other handling

None stated.

7. MARKETING AUTHORISATION HOLDER

AstraZeneca UK Limited

600 Capability Green,

Luton, LU1 3LU, UK.

8. MARKETING AUTHORISATION NUMBER(S)

25 mg tablet PL 17901/0038

100 mg tablet PL 17901/0039

150 mg tablet PL 17901/0041

200 mg tablet PL 17901/0040

300 mg tablet PL 17901/0088

9. DATE OF FIRST AUTHORISATION/RENEWAL OF THE AUTHORISATION

25th June 2000 / 18th Sept 2003

10. DATE OF REVISION OF THE TEXT

9th September 2009

Seroquel XL 50 mg, 200 mg, 300 mg, 400 mg prolonged-release tablets

(AstraZeneca UK Limited)

1. NAME OF THE MEDICINAL PRODUCT

Seroquel XL 50 mg, 200 mg, 300 mg, 400 mg prolonged-release tablets ▼

2. QUALITATIVE AND QUANTITATIVE COMPOSITION

Each 50 mg tablet contains 50 mg quetiapine (as quetiapine fumarate)

Excipient: 119 mg lactose (anhydrous) per tablet.

Each 200 mg tablet contains 200 mg quetiapine (as quetiapine fumarate)

Excipient: 50 mg lactose (anhydrous) per tablet.

Each 300 mg tablet contains 300 mg quetiapine (as quetiapine fumarate)

Excipient: 47 mg lactose (anhydrous) per tablet.

Each 400 mg tablet contains 400 mg quetiapine (as quetiapine fumarate)

Excipient: 15 mg lactose (anhydrous) per tablet.

For a full list of excipients, see section 6.1.

3. PHARMACEUTICAL FORM

Prolonged-release tablet

50 mg: Peach, bi-convex, capsule shaped tablets, marked with XR50.

200 mg: Yellow, bi-convex, capsule shaped tablets, marked with XR200.

300 mg: Pale yellow, bi-convex, capsule shaped tablets, marked with XR300.

400 mg: White, bi-convex, capsule shaped tablets, marked with XR400.

4. CLINICAL PARTICULARS

4.1 Therapeutic indications

Seroquel XL is indicated for:

- the treatment of schizophrenia
- the treatment of manic episodes associated with bipolar disorder.
- the treatment of major depressive episodes in bipolar disorder

Seroquel XL is not indicated for the prevention of recurrence of manic or depressive episodes.

Seroquel XL is effective in preventing relapse in stable schizophrenic patients who have been maintained on Seroquel XL (see section 5.1 Pharmacodynamic properties).

4.2 Posology and method of administration

Seroquel XL should be administered once daily, without food (at least one hour before a meal). The tablets should be swallowed whole and not split, chewed or crushed.

Adults:

For the treatment of schizophrenia

The daily dose at the start of therapy is 300 mg on Day 1 and 600 mg on Day 2. The recommended daily dose is 600 mg. Enhanced efficacy at doses higher than 600 mg has not been demonstrated, although individual patients may benefit from a dose up to 800 mg daily. Doses greater than 600 mg should be initiated by a specialist. The dose should be adjusted within the effective dose range of 400 mg to 800 mg per day, depending on the clinical response and tolerability of the patient. For maintenance therapy in schizophrenia no dosage adjustment is necessary.

For the treatment of manic episodes associated with bipolar disorder

The daily dose at the start of therapy is 300 mg on Day 1, 600 mg on Day 2 and up to 800 mg after Day 2. The dose should be adjusted within the effective dose range of 400 mg to 800 mg per day, depending on the clinical response and tolerability of the patient.

For the treatment of depressive episodes associated with bipolar disorder

Seroquel XL should be administered once daily at bedtime. The total daily dose for the first four days of therapy is 50 mg (Day 1), 100 mg (Day 2), 200 mg (Day 3) and 300 mg (Day 4). The recommended daily dose is 300 mg. In clinical trials, no additional benefit was seen in the 600 mg group compared to the 300 mg group. Individual patients may benefit from a 600 mg dose. In individual patients, in the event of tolerance concerns, clinical trials have indicated that dose reduction to a minimum of 200 mg could be considered. When treating depressive episodes in bipolar disorder, treatment should be initiated by physicians experienced in treating bipolar disorder.

Switching from Seroquel immediate-release tablets:

For more convenient dosing, patients who are currently being treated with divided doses of immediate-release Seroquel tablets (Seroquel IR, tradename Seroquel®) may be switched to Seroquel XL at the equivalent total daily dose taken once daily. To ensure the maintenance of clinical response, a period of dose titration may be required.

Elderly:

As with other antipsychotics, Seroquel XL should be used with caution in the elderly, especially during the initial dosing period. The rate of dose titration of Seroquel XL may need to be slower, and the daily therapeutic dose lower, than that used in younger patients. The mean plasma clearance of quetiapine was reduced by 30% to 50% in elderly patients when compared to younger patients. Elderly patients should be started on 50 mg/day. The dose can be increased in increments of 50 mg/day to an effective dose, depending on the clinical response and tolerability of the individual patient.

Efficacy and safety have not been evaluated in patients over 65 years with depressive episodes in the framework of bipolar disorder.

Children and Adolescents:

The safety and efficacy of Seroquel XL have not been evaluated in children and adolescents.

Renal and hepatic impairment:

The oral clearance of quetiapine is reduced by approximately 25% in patients with renal or hepatic impairment. Quetiapine is extensively metabolized by the liver. Therefore, Seroquel XL should be used with caution in patients with known hepatic impairment.

Patients with hepatic or renal impairment should be started on 50 mg/day. The dose should be increased in increments of 50 mg/day to an effective dose, depending on the clinical response and tolerability of the individual patient.

4.3 Contraindications

Hypersensitivity to the active substance or to any of the excipients of this product.

4.4 Special warnings and precautions for use

Suicide/suicidal thoughts or clinical worsening:

Depression in bipolar disorder is associated with an increased risk of suicidal thoughts, self-harm and suicide (suicide-related events). This risk persists until significant remission occurs. As improvement may not occur during the first few weeks or more of treatment, patients should be closely monitored until such improvement occurs. It is general clinical experience that the risk of suicide may increase in the early stages of recovery.

In clinical studies of patients with major depressive episodes in bipolar disorder an increased risk of suicide-related events was observed in young adult patients less than 25 years of age who were treated with quetiapine as compared to those treated with placebo (3.0% vs. 0%, respectively).

Cardiovascular:

Seroquel XL should be used with caution in patients with known cardiovascular disease, cerebrovascular disease, or other conditions predisposing to hypotension. Quetiapine may induce orthostatic hypotension especially during the initial dose-titration period and therefore dose reduction or more gradual titration should be considered if this occurs.

Seizures:

In controlled clinical trials there was no difference in the incidence of seizures in patients treated with quetiapine or placebo. As with other antipsychotics, caution is recommended when treating patients with a history of seizures (see section 4.8 Undesirable effects).

Extrapyramidal symptoms:

In placebo controlled clinical trials quetiapine was associated with an increased incidence of extrapyramidal symptoms (EPS) compared to placebo in patients treated for major depressive episodes in bipolar disorder (see section 4.8 Undesirable effects).

Tardive Dyskinesia:

If signs and symptoms of tardive dyskinesia appear, dose reduction or discontinuation of Seroquel XL should be considered (see section 4.8 Undesirable effects).

Neuroleptic Malignant Syndrome:

Neuroleptic malignant syndrome has been associated with antipsychotic treatment, including quetiapine (see section 4.8 Undesirable effects). Clinical manifestations include hyperthermia, altered mental status, muscular rigidity, autonomic instability, and increased creatinine phosphokinase. In such an event, Seroquel XL should be discontinued and appropriate medical treatment given.

Severe neutropenia:

Severe neutropenia (neutrophil count $<0.5 \times 10^9$/L) has been uncommonly reported in quetiapine clinical trials. Most cases of severe neutropenia have occurred within a couple of months of starting therapy with quetiapine. There is no apparent dose relationship. Possible risk factors for neutropenia include pre-existing low white cell count (WBC) and history of drug induced neutropenia. Quetiapine should be discontinued in patients with a neutrophil count $<1.0 \times 10^9$/L. Patients should be observed for signs and symptoms of infection and neutrophil counts followed (until they exceed 1.5×10^9/L). (See section 4.8 Undesirable effects).

Somnolence:

Quetiapine treatment has been associated with somnolence and related symptoms, such as sedation (see section 4.8 Undesirable effects). In clinical trials for treatment of patients with bipolar depression, onset was usually within the first 3 days of treatment and was predominantly of mild to moderate intensity. Bipolar depression patients experiencing somnolence of severe intensity may require more frequent contact for a minimum of 2 weeks from onset of somnolence, or until symptoms improve and treatment discontinuation may need to be considered.

Interactions:

See also section 4.5 Interaction with other medicinal products and other forms of interaction.

Concomitant use of quetiapine with a strong hepatic enzyme inducer such as carbamazepine or phenytoin substantially decreases quetiapine plasma concentrations, which could affect the efficacy of quetiapine therapy. In patients receiving a hepatic enzyme inducer, initiation of Seroquel XL treatment should only occur if the physician considers that the benefits of Seroquel XL outweigh the risks of removing the hepatic enzyme inducer. It is important that any change in the inducer is gradual, and if required, replaced with a non-inducer (e.g. sodium valproate).

Hyperglycaemia:

Hyperglycaemia or exacerbation of pre-existing diabetes has been reported during treatment with quetiapine. Appropriate clinical monitoring is advisable in diabetic patients and in patients with risk factors for the development of diabetes mellitus (see section 4.8 Undesirable effects).

Lipids:

Increases in triglycerides and cholesterol have been observed in clinical trials with quetiapine (see section 4.8 Undesirable effects). Lipid increases should be managed as clinically appropriate.

QT Prolongation:

In clinical trials and use in accordance with the SPC, quetiapine was not associated with a persistent increase in absolute QT intervals. However, with overdose (see section 4.9 Overdose) QT prolongation was observed. As with other antipsychotics, caution should be exercised when quetiapine is prescribed in patients with cardiovascular disease or family history of QT prolongation. Also caution should be exercised when quetiapine is prescribed with medicines known to increase QTc interval, and concomitant neuroleptics, especially in the elderly, in patients with congenital long QT syndrome, congestive heart failure, heart hypertrophy, hypokalaemia or hypomagnesaemia (see section 4.5 Interaction with other medicinal products and other forms of interaction).

Withdrawal:

Acute withdrawal symptoms such as nausea, vomiting, insomnia, headache, diarrhoea, dizziness and irritability have been described after abrupt cessation of high doses of Seroquel. Gradual withdrawal over a period of at least one to two weeks is advisable (see section 4.8 Undesirable effects).

Elderly patients with dementia-related psychosis:

Seroquel XL is not approved for the treatment of dementia-related psychosis.

An approximately 3-fold increased risk of cerebrovascular adverse events has been seen in randomised placebo controlled trials in the dementia population with some atypical antipsychotics. The mechanism for this increased risk is not known. An increased risk cannot be excluded for other antipsychotics or other patient populations. Seroquel XL should be used with caution in patients with risk factors for stroke.

In a meta-analysis of atypical antipsychotic drugs, it has been reported that elderly patients with dementia-related psychosis are at an increased risk of death compared to placebo. However in two 10-week placebo controlled quetiapine studies in the same patient population (n=710; mean age: 83 years; range: 56-99 years) the incidence of mortality in quetiapine treated patients was 5.5% versus 3.2% in the placebo group. The patients in these trials died from a variety of causes that were consistent with expectations for this population. These data do not establish a causal relationship between quetiapine treatment and death in elderly patients with dementia.

Hepatic effects:

If jaundice develops, Seroquel XL should be discontinued.

Lactose:

Seroquel XL tablets contain lactose. Patients with rare hereditary problems of galactose intolerance, the Lapp lactase deficiency, or glucose-galactose malabsorption should not take this medicine.

Additional information:

Quetiapine data in combination with divalproex or lithium in moderate to severe manic episodes is limited; however, combination therapy was well tolerated (see section 4.8 Undesirable effects and 5.1 Pharmacodynamic properties). The data showed an additive effect at week 3. A second study did not demonstrate an additive effect at week 6. There are no combination data available beyond week 6.

4.5 Interaction with other medicinal products and other forms of interaction

Given the primary central nervous system effects of quetiapine, Seroquel XL should be used with caution in combination with other centrally acting drugs and alcohol.

Cytochrome P450 CYP3A4 is the enzyme that is primarily responsible for the cytochrome P450 mediated metabolism of quetiapine. In an interaction study in healthy volunteers, concomitant administration of quetiapine (dosage of 25 mg) with ketoconazole, a CYP3A4 inhibitor, caused a 5- to 8-fold increase in the AUC of quetiapine. On the basis of this, concomitant use of quetiapine with CYP3A4 inhibitors is contraindicated. It is also not recommended to take quetiapine together with grapefruit juice.

In a multiple dose trial in patients to assess the pharmacokinetics of quetiapine given before and during treatment with carbamazepine (a known hepatic enzyme inducer), co-administration of carbamazepine significantly increased the clearance of quetiapine. This increase in clearance reduced systemic quetiapine exposure (as measured by AUC) to an average of 13% of the exposure during administration of quetiapine alone; although a greater effect was seen in some patients. As a consequence of this interaction, lower plasma concentrations can occur, which could affect the efficacy of Seroquel XL therapy. Co-administration of quetiapine and phenytoin (another microsomal enzyme inducer) caused a greatly increased clearance of quetiapine by approx. 450%. In patients receiving a hepatic enzyme inducer, initiation of Seroquel XL treatment should only occur if the physician considers that the benefits of Seroquel XL outweigh the risks of removing the hepatic enzyme inducer. It is important that any change in the inducer is gradual, and if required, replaced with a non-inducer (e.g. sodium valproate) (see section 4.4 Special warnings and precautions for use).

The pharmacokinetics of quetiapine were not significantly altered by co-administration of the antidepressants imipramine (a known CYP2D6 inhibitor) or fluoxetine (a known CYP3A4 and CYP2D6 inhibitor).

The pharmacokinetics of quetiapine were not significantly altered by co-administration of the antipsychotics risperidone or haloperidol. Concomitant use of quetiapine and thioridazine caused an increased clearance of quetiapine of approx. 70%.

The pharmacokinetics of quetiapine were not altered following co-administration with cimetidine.

The pharmacokinetics of lithium were not altered when co-administered with quetiapine.

The pharmacokinetics of sodium valproate and quetiapine were not altered to a clinically relevant extent when co-administered.

Formal interaction studies with commonly used cardiovascular drugs have not been performed.

Caution should be exercised when quetiapine is used concomitantly with drugs known to cause electrolyte imbalance or to increase QTc interval.

4.6 Pregnancy and lactation

The safety and efficacy of quetiapine during human pregnancy have not yet been established. Up to now there are no indications for harmfulness in animal tests, possible effects on the foetal eye have not been examined, though. Therefore, Seroquel XL should only be used during pregnancy if the benefits justify the potential risks. Following pregnancies in which quetiapine was used, neonatal withdrawal symptoms were observed.

The degree to which quetiapine is excreted into human milk is unknown. Women who are breast-feeding should therefore be advised to avoid breast-feeding while taking Seroquel XL.

4.7 Effects on ability to drive and use machines

Given its primary central nervous system effects, quetiapine may interfere with activities requiring mental alertness. Therefore, patients should be advised not to drive or operate machinery, until individual susceptibility to this is known.

4.8 Undesirable effects

The most commonly reported Adverse Drug Reactions (ADRs) with quetiapine are somnolence, dizziness, dry mouth, mild asthenia, constipation, tachycardia, orthostatic hypotension and dyspepsia.

As with other antipsychotics, syncope, neuroleptic malignant syndrome, leucopenia, neutropenia and peripheral oedema, have been associated with quetiapine.

The incidences of ADRs associated with quetiapine therapy, are tabulated below according to the format recommended by the Council for International Organizations of Medical Sciences (CIOMS III Working Group 1995).

The frequencies of adverse events are ranked according to the following: Very common (>1/10), common (>1/100, <1/10), uncommon (>1/1000, <1/100), rare (>1/10,000, <1/1000) and very rare (<1/10,000).

Blood and lymphatic system disorders	
Common:	Leucopenia
Uncommon:	Eosinophilia
Immune system disorders	
Uncommon:	Hypersensitivity
Very rare:	Anaphylactic reaction [6]
Endocrine disorders	
Common:	Hyperprolactinaemia[16]
Metabolism and nutritional disorders	
Common:	Increased appetite
Very rare:	Diabetes Mellitus [1, 5, 6]
Psychiatric disorders	
Common:	Abnormal dreams and nightmares
Nervous system disorders	
Very Common:	Dizziness [4, 17], somnolence [2, 17], headache
Common:	Syncope [4, 17], Extrapyramidal symptoms [1,13]
Uncommon:	Seizure [1], restless leg syndrome, Dysarthria
Very rare	Tardive dyskinesia [6]
Cardiac disorders	
Common:	Tachycardia [4]
Eye disorders	
Common:	Vision blurred
Vascular disorders	
Common:	Orthostatic hypotension [4, 17]
Respiratory, thoracic and mediastinal disorder	
Common:	Rhinitis
Gastrointestinal disorders	
Very Common:	Dry mouth
Common:	Constipation, dyspepsia
Uncommon:	Dysphagia [7]
Hepato-biliary disorders	
Rare:	Jaundice [6]
Very rare:	Hepatitis [6]
Skin and subcutaneous tissue disorders	
Very rare:	Angioedema [6], Stevens-Johnson syndrome [6]
Reproductive system and breast disorders	
Rare:	Priapism, Galactorrhoea
General disorders and administration site conditions	
Very common	Withdrawal (discontinuation) symptoms [1, 10]
Common:	Mild asthenia, peripheral oedema, irritability
Rare:	Neuroleptic malignant syndrome [1]
Investigations	
Very common	Elevations in serum triglyceride levels [11] Elevations in total cholesterol (predominantly LDL cholesterol) [12], weight gain [8]
Common:	Elevations in serum transaminases (ALT, AST) [3], decreased neutrophil count, blood glucose increased to hyperglycaemic levels [9]
Uncommon:	Elevations in gamma-GT levels [3], Platelet count decreased [14]
Rare:	Elevations in blood creatine phosphokinase [15]

(1) See section 4.4 Special warnings and precautions for use.

(2) Somnolence may occur, usually during the first two weeks of treatment and generally resolves with the continued administration of quetiapine.

(3) Asymptomatic elevations in serum transaminase (ALT, AST) or gamma-GT-levels have been observed in some patients administered quetiapine.

(4) As with other antipsychotics with alpha1 adrenergic blocking activity, quetiapine may commonly induce orthostatic hypotension, associated with dizziness, tachycardia and, in some patients, syncope, especially during the initial dose-titration period. (See section 4.4 Special warnings and precautions for use).

(5) Exacerbation of pre-existing diabetes has been reported in very rare cases.

(6) Calculation of Frequency for these ADR's have only been taken from postmarketing data with the immediate-release formulation of Seroquel.

(7) An increase in the rate of dysphagia with quetiapine vs. placebo was only observed in the clinical trials in bipolar depression.

(8) Based on >7% increase in body weight from baseline. Occurs predominantly during the early weeks of treatment.

(9) Fasting blood glucose $\geqslant$ 7.0 mmol/L or a non fasting blood glucose $\geqslant$ 11.1 mmol/L on at least one occasion.

(10) The following withdrawal symptoms have been observed most frequently in acute placebo-controlled, monotherapy clinical trials, which evaluated discontinuation symptoms: insomnia, nausea, headache, diarrhoea, vomiting, dizziness, and irritability. The incidence of these reactions had decreased significantly after 1 week post-discontinuation.

(11) Triglycerides $\geqslant$200 mg/dL ($\geqslant$2.258 mmol/L) on at least one occasion.

(12) Cholesterol $\geqslant$240 mg/dL ($\geqslant$6.2064 mmol/L) on at least one occasion.

(13) See text below.

(14) Platelets $\leqslant 100 \times 10^9$/L on at least one occasion.

(15) Based on clinical trial adverse event reports of blood creatine phosphokinase increase not associated with neuroleptic malignant syndrome.

(16) Prolactin levels (patients >18 years of age): >20 μg/L (>869.56 pmol/L) males; >30 μg/L (>1304.34 pmol/L) females at any time.

(17) May lead to falls.

Cases of QT prolongation, ventricular arrhythmia, sudden unexplained death, cardiac arrest and torsades de pointes have been reported very rarely with the use of neuroleptics and are considered class effects.

In short-term, placebo-controlled clinical trials in bipolar depression the aggregated incidence of extrapyramidal symptoms was 8.9% for quetiapine compared to 3.8% for placebo, though the incidence of the individual adverse events were generally low and did not exceed 4% in any treatment group. In short-term, placebo-controlled clinical trials in schizophrenia and bipolar mania the aggregated incidence of extrapyramidal symptoms was similar to placebo (schizophrenia: 7.8% for quetiapine and 8.0% for placebo; bipolar mania: 11.2% for quetiapine and 11.4% for placebo).

Quetiapine treatment was associated with small dose-related decreases in thyroid hormone levels, particularly total T_4 and free T_4. The reduction in total and free T_4 was maximal within the first two to four weeks of quetiapine treatment, with no further reduction during long-term treatment. In nearly all cases, cessation of quetiapine treatment was associated with a reversal of the effects on total and free T_4, irrespective of the duration of treatment. Smaller decreases in total T_3 and reverse T_3 were seen only at higher doses. Levels of TBG were unchanged and in general, reciprocal increases in TSH were not observed, with no indication that quetiapine causes clinically relevant hypothyroidism.

4.9 Overdose

In clinical trials, survival has been reported in acute overdoses of up to 30 grams of quetiapine. Most patients who overdosed reported no adverse events or recovered fully from the reported events. Death has been reported in a clinical trial following an overdose of 13.6 grams of quetiapine alone. In post marketing experience, there have been very rare reports of overdose of quetiapine alone resulting in death or coma or QT-prolongation.

Patients with pre-existing severe cardiovascular disease may be at an increased risk of the effects of overdose. (See section 4.4 Special warnings and precautions for use: Cardiovascular).

In general, reported signs and symptoms were those resulting from an exaggeration of the drug's known pharmacological effects, i.e., drowsiness and sedation, tachycardia and hypotension.

There is no specific antidote to quetiapine. In cases of severe signs, the possibility of multiple drug involvement should be considered, and intensive care procedures are recommended, including establishing and maintaining a patent airway, ensuring adequate oxygenation and ventilation, and monitoring and support of the cardiovascular system. Whilst the prevention of absorption in overdose has not been investigated, gastric lavage (after intubation, if patient is unconscious) and administration of activated charcoal together with a laxative should be considered.

Close medical supervision and monitoring should be continued until the patient recovers.

5. PHARMACOLOGICAL PROPERTIES

5.1 Pharmacodynamic properties

Pharmacotherapeutic group: Antipsychotics

ATC code: N05A H04

Mechanism of action:

Quetiapine is an atypical antipsychotic agent. Quetiapine and the active human plasma metabolite, N-desalkyl quetiapine interact with a broad range of neurotransmitter receptors. Quetiapine and N-desalkyl quetiapine exhibit affinity for brain serotonin ($5HT_2$) and dopamine D_1- and D_2-receptors. It is this combination of receptor antagonism with a higher selectivity for $5HT_2$ relative to D_2-receptors, which is believed to contribute to the clinical antipsychotic properties and low extrapyramidal side effect (EPS) liability of Seroquel. Additionally, N-desalkyl quetiapine has high affinity at serotonin $5HT_1$ receptors. Quetiapine and N-desalkyl quetiapine also have high affinity at histaminergic and adrenergic α_1-receptors, with a lower affinity at adrenergic α_2-receptors. Quetiapine has no appreciable affinity at cholinergic muscarinic or benzodiazepine receptors.

Quetiapine is active in tests for antipsychotic activity, such as conditioned avoidance. It also blocks the action of dopamine agonists, measured either behaviourally or electrophysiologically, and elevates dopamine metabolite concentrations, a neurochemical index of D_2-receptor blockade. The extent to which the N-desalkyl quetiapine metabolite contributes to the pharmacological activity of Seroquel in humans is not known.

Pharmacodynamic effects:

In pre-clinical tests predictive of EPS, quetiapine is unlike standard antipsychotics and has an atypical profile. Quetiapine does not produce dopamine D_2-receptor supersensitivity after chronic administration. Quetiapine produces only weak catalepsy at effective dopamine D_2-receptor blocking doses. Quetiapine demonstrates selectivity for the limbic system by producing depolarisation blockade of the mesolimbic but not the nigrostriatal dopamine-containing neurones following chronic administration. Quetiapine exhibits minimal dystonic liability in haloperidol-sensitised or drug-naive Cebus monkeys after acute and chronic administration. The results of these tests predict that Seroquel XL should have minimal EPS liability, and it has been hypothesised that agents with a lower EPS liability may also have a lower liability to produce tardive dyskinesia (see section 4.8 Undesirable effects).

Clinical efficacy:

The efficacy of Seroquel XL in the treatment of schizophrenia was demonstrated in one 6-week placebo-controlled trial in patients who met DSM-IV criteria for schizophrenia, and one active-controlled Seroquel IR-to-Seroquel XL switching study in clinically stable outpatients with schizophrenia.

The primary outcome variable in the placebo-controlled trial was change from baseline to final assessment in the PANSS total score. Seroquel XL 400 mg/day, 600 mg/day and 800 mg/day were associated with statistically significant improvements in psychotic symptoms compared to placebo. The effect size of the 600 mg and 800 mg doses was greater than that of the 400 mg dose.

In the 6-week active-controlled switching study the primary outcome variable was the proportion of patients who showed lack of efficacy, i.e., who discontinued study treatment due to lack of efficacy or whose PANSS total score increased 20% or more from randomisation to any visit. In patients stabilised on Seroquel IR 400 mg to 800 mg, efficacy was maintained when patients were switched to an equivalent daily dose of Seroquel XL given once daily.

In a long-term study in stable schizophrenic patients who had been maintained on Seroquel XL for 16 weeks, Seroquel XL was more effective than placebo in preventing relapse. The estimated risks of relapse after 6 months treatments was 14.3% for the Seroquel XL treatment group compared to 68.2% for placebo. The average dose was 669 mg. There were no additional safety findings associated with treatment with Seroquel XL for up to 9 months (median 7 months). In particular, reports of adverse events related to EPS and weight gain did not increase with longer-term treatment with Seroquel XL.

In the treatment of moderate to severe manic episodes, quetiapine demonstrated superior efficacy to placebo in reduction of manic symptoms at 3 and 12 weeks, in two monotherapy trials. There are no data from long-term studies to demonstrate quetiapine's effectiveness in preventing subsequent manic or depressive episodes. Quetiapine data in combination with divalproex or lithium in moderate to severe manic episodes at 3 and 6 weeks is limited; however, combination therapy was well tolerated. The data showed an additive effect at week 3. A second study did not demonstrate an additive effect at week 6. There are no combination data available beyond week 6. The mean last week median dose of quetiapine in responders was approximately 600 mg/day and approximately 85% of the responders were in the dose range of 400 to 800 mg/day.

In a clinical trial, in patients with depressive episodes in bipolar I or bipolar II disorder, 300 mg/day Seroquel XL showed superior efficacy to placebo in reduction of MADRS total score. The antidepressant effect of Seroquel XL was significant at Day 8 (week 1) and was maintained through the end of the trial (week 8).

In 4 additional clinical trials in patients with depressive episodes in bipolar I or bipolar II disorder, with and without rapid cycling courses, 51% of quetiapine treated patients had at least a 50% improvement in MADRS total score at week 8 compared to 37% of the placebo treated patients. The antidepressant effect was significant at Day 8 (week 1). There were fewer episodes of treatment-emergent mania with Seroquel than with placebo. In continuation treatment the anti-depressant effect was maintained for patients on Seroquel (mean duration of treatment 30 weeks). Seroquel reduced the risk of a recurrent mood (manic and depressed) event by 49%. Seroquel was superior to placebo in treating the anxiety symptoms associated with bipolar depression as assessed by mean change from baseline to week 8 in HAM-A total score.

In placebo-controlled monotherapy trials in patients with a baseline neutrophil count $\geqslant 1.5 \times 10^9$/L, the incidence of at least one occurrence of neutrophil count $< 1.5 \times 10^9$/L, was 1.72% in patients treated with quetiapine compared to 0.73% in placebo-treated patients. In all clinical trials (placebo-controlled, open-label, active comparator; patients with a baseline neutrophil count $\geqslant 1.5 \times 10^9$/L), the incidence of at least one occurrence of neutrophil count $<0.5 \times 10^9$/L was 0.21% in patients treated with quetiapine and 0% in placebo treated patients and the incidence $\geqslant 0.5 - < 1.0 \times 10^9$/L was 0.75% in patients treated with quetiapine and 0.11% in placebo-treated patients.

In placebo-controlled studies in elderly patients with dementia-related psychosis, the incidence of cerebrovascular adverse events per 100 patient years was not higher in quetiapine-treated patients than in placebo-treated patients.

5.2 Pharmacokinetic properties

Quetiapine is well absorbed and extensively metabolised following oral administration. Quetiapine is approximately 83% bound to plasma proteins. Steady-state peak molar concentrations of the active metabolite N-desalkyl quetiapine are 35% of that observed for quetiapine.

The pharmacokinetics of quetiapine and N-desalkyl quetiapine are linear across the approved dosing range. The kinetics of quetiapine does not differ between men and women.

Seroquel XL achieves peak plasma concentrations at approximately 6 hours after administration (Tmax). Seroquel XL displays dose-proportional pharmacokinetics for doses of up to 800 mg administered once daily. The maximum plasma concentration (Cmax) and the area under the plasma concentration-time curve (AUC) for Seroquel XL administered once daily are comparable to those achieved for the same total daily dose of immediate-release quetiapine fumarate (Seroquel IR) administered twice daily. The elimination half lives of quetiapine and N-desalkyl quetiapine are approximately 7 and 12 hours, respectively.

The mean clearance of quetiapine in the elderly is approximately 30 to 50% lower than that seen in adults aged 18 to 65 years.

There are no clinically relevant differences in the observed apparent oral clearance (CL/F) and exposure of quetiapine between subjects with schizophrenia and bipolar disorder.

The mean plasma clearance of quetiapine was reduced by approximately 25% in subjects with severe renal impairment (creatinine clearance less than 30 ml/min/1.73m^2), but the individual clearance values are within the range for normal subjects. The average molar dose fraction of free quetiapine and the active human plasma metabolite N-desalkyl quetiapine is <5% excreted in the urine.

Quetiapine is extensively metabolised by the liver, with parent compound accounting for less than 5% of unchanged drug-related material in the urine or faeces, following the administration of radiolabelled quetiapine. Approximately 73% of the radioactivity is excreted in the urine and 21% in the faeces. The mean quetiapine plasma clearance decreases by approx. 25% in persons with known hepatic impairment (stable alcohol cirrhosis). As quetiapine is extensively metabolised by the liver, elevated plasma levels are expected in the population with hepatic impairment. Dose adjustments may be necessary in these patients (see section 4.2 Posology and method of administration).

In vitro investigations established that CYP3A4 is the primary enzyme responsible for cytochrome P450 mediated metabolism of quetiapine. N-desalkyl quetiapine is primarily formed and eliminated via CYP3A4.

Quetiapine and several of its metabolites (including N-desalkyl quetiapine) were found to be weak inhibitors of human cytochrome P450 1A2, 2C9, 2C19, 2D6 and 3A4 activities in vitro. In vitro CYP inhibition is observed only at concentrations approximately 5 to 50 fold higher than those observed at a dose range of 300 to 800 mg/day in humans. Based on these in vitro results, it is unlikely that co-administration of quetiapine with other drugs will result in clinically significant drug inhibition of cytochrome P450 mediated metabolism of the other drug. From animal studies it appears that quetiapine can induce cytochrome P450 enzymes. In a specific interaction study in psychotic patients, however, no increase in the cytochrome P450 activity was found after administration of quetiapine.

In a study examining the effects of food on the bioavailability of quetiapine, a high-fat meal was found to produce statistically significant increases in the Seroquel XL Cmax and AUC of 44% to 52% and 20% to 22%, respectively, for the 50 mg and 300 mg tablets. Seroquel XL should be taken at least one hour before a meal.

5.3 Preclinical safety data

There was no evidence of genotoxicity in a series of *in vitro* and *in vivo* genotoxicity studies. In laboratory animals at a clinically relevant exposure level the following deviations were seen, which as yet have not been confirmed in long-term clinical research:

In rats, pigment deposition in the thyroid gland has been observed; in cynomolgus monkeys thyroid follicular cell hypertrophy, a lowering in plasma T_3 levels, decreased haemoglobin concentration and a decrease of red and white blood cell count have been observed; and in dogs lens opacity and cataracts.

Taking these findings into consideration, the benefits of the treatment with quetiapine need to be balanced against the safety risks for the patient.

6. PHARMACEUTICAL PARTICULARS

6.1 List of excipients

Core

Microcrystalline cellulose

Sodium citrate

Lactose monohydrate

Magnesium stearate

Hypromellose

Coating

Hypromellose

Macrogol 400

Titanium dioxide (E171)

Ferric oxide, yellow (E172) (50mg, 200mg, 300mg only)

Ferric oxide, red (E172) (50 mg only)

6.2 Incompatibilities

Not applicable.

6.3 Shelf life

3 years

6.4 Special precautions for storage

Do not store above 30°C. Store in the original package.

6.5 Nature and contents of container

PVC+PCTFE/aluminium blisters

Carton (pack) contents	*Blisters*
10 tablets	*1 blister of 10 tablets*
30 tablets	*3 blisters of 10 tablets*
50 tablets	*10 blisters of 5 tablets*
60 tablets	*6 blisters of 10 tablets*
100 tablets	*10 blisters of 10 tablets*

Not all pack sizes may be marketed.

6.6 Special precautions for disposal and other handling

No special requirements.

7. MARKETING AUTHORISATION HOLDER

AstraZeneca UK Ltd

600 Capability Green

Luton

LU1 3LU

United Kingdom

8. MARKETING AUTHORISATION NUMBER(S)

50 mg: PL 17901/0249

200 mg: PL 17901/0250

300 mg: PL 17901/0251

400 mg: PL 17901/0252

9. DATE OF FIRST AUTHORISATION/RENEWAL OF THE AUTHORISATION

10th September 2008

10. DATE OF REVISION OF THE TEXT

9th September 2009

Seroxat 10mg, 20mg, 30mg tablets, 20mg/10ml oral suspension

(GlaxoSmithKline UK)

1. NAME OF THE MEDICINAL PRODUCT

Seroxat® 10 mg film-coated tablets.

Seroxat® 20 mg film-coated tablets.

Seroxat® 30 mg film-coated tablets.

Seroxat® 20 mg/10 ml oral suspension.

2. QUALITATIVE AND QUANTITATIVE COMPOSITION

Each film-coated tablet contains 10 mg/20 mg/30 mg paroxetine (as paroxetine hydrochloride hemihydrate).

Each 10 ml of oral suspension contains 20 mg paroxetine (as paroxetine hydrochloride hemihydrate).

For excipients, see section 6.1.

3. PHARMACEUTICAL FORM

Film-coated tablet.

Oral suspension.

10 mg tablet

White to pinkish-white, film-coated, oval tablets, debossed FC1 and break-line on one side and debossed GS and break-line on the other side.

The 10 mg film-coated tablet has a break-line, and can be divided into equal halves if required.

20 mg tablet

White, film-coated tablet, oval shaped biconvex tablets debossed with "Seroxat 20" / "20" on one side and a break bar on the other.

The 20 mg film-coated tablet has a break-line, and can be divided into equal halves if required.

30 mg tablet

Blue, oval shaped biconvex tablets debossed with "Seroxat 30" / "30" on one side and a break bar on the reverse.

Oral Suspension

A bright orange fairly viscous suspension having an odour of oranges, free from foreign matter.

4. CLINICAL PARTICULARS

4.1 Therapeutic indications

Treatment of

- Major Depressive Episode
- Obsessive Compulsive Disorder
- Panic Disorder with and without agoraphobia
- Social Anxiety Disorders/Social phobia
- Generalised Anxiety Disorder
- Post-traumatic Stress Disorder

4.2 Posology and method of administration

It is recommended that paroxetine is administered once daily in the morning with food.

The tablet should be swallowed rather than chewed.

Shake bottle before use.

MAJOR DEPRESSIVE EPISODE

The recommended dose is 20 mg daily. In general, improvement in patients starts after one week but may only become evident from the second week of therapy.

As with all antidepressant medicinal products, dosage should be reviewed and adjusted if necessary within 3 to 4 weeks of initiation of therapy and thereafter as judged clinically appropriate. In some patients, with insufficient response to 20 mg, the dose may be increased gradually up to a maximum of 50 mg a day in 10 mg steps according to the patient's response.

Patients with depression should be treated for a sufficient period of at least 6 months to ensure that they are free from symptoms.

OBSESSIVE COMPULSIVE DISORDER

The recommended dose is 40 mg daily. Patients should start on 20 mg/day and the dose may be increased gradually in 10 mg increments to the recommended dose. If after some weeks on the recommended dose insufficient response is seen some patients may benefit from having their dose increased gradually up to a maximum of 60 mg/day.

Patients with OCD should be treated for a sufficient period to ensure that they are free from symptoms. This period may be several months or even longer. (see section 5.1 Pharmacodynamic Properties)

PANIC DISORDER

The recommended dose is 40 mg daily. Patients should be started on 10 mg/day and the dose gradually increased in 10 mg steps according to the patient's response up to the recommended dose. A low initial starting dose is recommended to minimise the potential worsening of panic symptomatology, which is generally recognised to occur early in the treatment of this disorder. If after some weeks on the recommended dose insufficient response is seen some patients may benefit from having their dose increased gradually up to a maximum of 60 mg/day.

Patients with panic disorder should be treated for a sufficient period to ensure that they are free from symptoms. This period may be several months or even longer (see section 5.1 Pharmacodynamic Properties)

SOCIAL ANXIETY DISORDER/SOCIAL PHOBIA

The recommended dose is 20 mg daily. If after some weeks on the recommended dose insufficient response is seen some patients may benefit from having their dose increased gradually in 10 mg steps up to a maximum of 50 mg/day. Long-term use should be regularly evaluated (see section 5.1 Pharmacodynamic Properties).

GENERALISED ANXIETY DISORDER

The recommended dose is 20 mg daily. If after some weeks on the recommended dose insufficient response is seen some patients may benefit from having their dose increased gradually in 10 mg steps up to a maximum of 50 mg/day. Long-term use should be regularly evaluated (see section 5.1 Pharmacodynamic Properties).

POST-TRAUMATIC STRESS DISORDER

The recommended dose is 20 mg daily. If after some weeks on the recommended dose insufficient response is seen some patients may benefit from having their dose increased gradually in 10 mg steps up to a maximum of 50 mg/day. Long-term use should be regularly evaluated (see section 5.1 Pharmacodynamic Properties).

GENERAL INFORMATION

WITHDRAWAL SYMPTOMS SEEN ON DISCONTINUATION OF PAROXETINE

Abrupt discontinuation should be avoided (see section 4.4 Special Warnings and Special Precautions for Use and section 4.8 Undesirable Effects). The taper phase regimen used in clinical trials involved decreasing the daily dose by 10 mg at weekly intervals. If intolerable symptoms occur following a decrease in the dose or upon discontinuation of treatment, then resuming the previously prescribed dose may be considered. Subsequently, the physician may continue decreasing the dose, but at a more gradual rate.

Special Populations:

• **Elderly**

Increased plasma concentrations of paroxetine occur in elderly subjects, but the range of concentrations overlaps with that observed in younger subjects. Dosing should commence at the adult starting dose. Increasing the dose might be useful in some patients, but the maximum dose should not exceed 40 mg daily.

• **Children and adolescents (7-17 years)**

Paroxetine should not be used for the treatment of children and adolescents as controlled clinical trials have found paroxetine to be associated with increased risk for suicidal behaviour and hostility. In addition, in these trials efficacy has not been adequately demonstrated (see section 4.4 Special Warnings and Special Precautions for use and section 4.8 Undesirable Effects).

• **Children aged below 7 years**

The use of paroxetine has not been studied in children less than 7 years. Paroxetine should not be used, as long as safety and efficacy in this age group have not been established.

• **Renal/hepatic impairment**

Increased plasma concentrations of paroxetine occur in patients with severe renal impairment (creatinine clearance less than 30 ml/min) or in those with hepatic impairment. Therefore, dosage should be restricted to the lower end of the dosage range.

4.3 Contraindications

Known hypersensitivity to paroxetine or any of the excipients.

Paroxetine is contraindicated in combination with monoamine oxidase inhibitors (MAOIs). In exceptional circumstances, linezolid (an antibiotic which is a reversible non-selective MAOI) can be given in combination with paroxetine provided that there are facilities for close observation of symptoms of serotonin syndrome and monitoring of blood pressure (see section 4.5).

Treatment with paroxetine can be initiated:

- two weeks after discontinuation of an irreversible MAOI, or

- at least 24hrs after discontinuation of a reversible MAOI (e.g. moclobemide, linezolid).

At least one week should elapse between discontinuation of paroxetine and initiation of therapy with any MAOI.

Paroxetine should not be used in combination with thioridazine, because, as with other drugs which inhibit the hepatic enzyme CYP450 2D6, paroxetine can elevate plasma levels of thioridazine (see section 4.5 Interactions with other medicinal products and other forms of interaction). Administration of thioridazine alone can lead to QTc interval prolongation with associated serious ventricular arrhythmia such as torsades de pointes, and sudden death.

Paroxetine should not be used in combination with pimozide (see section 4.5 Interactions with other medicinal products and other forms of interaction).

4.4 Special warnings and precautions for use

Treatment with paroxetine should be initiated cautiously two weeks after terminating treatment with an irreversible MAOI or 24 hours after terminating treatment with a reversible MAO inhibitor. Dosage of paroxetine should be increased gradually until an optimal response is reached (see section 4.3 Contraindications and section 4.5 Interactions with other medicinal products and other forms of interaction).

Use in children and adolescents under 18 years of age

Paroxetine should not be used in the treatment of children and adolescents under the age of 18 years. Suicide-related behaviours (suicide attempt and suicidal thoughts), and hostility (predominantly aggression, oppositional behaviour and anger) were more frequently observed in clinical trials among children and adolescents treated with antidepressants compared to those treated with placebo. If, based on clinical need, a decision to treat is nevertheless taken, the patient should be carefully monitored for the appearance of suicidal symptoms. In addition, long-term safety data in children and adolescents concerning growth, maturation and cognitive and behavioural development are lacking.

Suicide/suicidal thoughts or clinical worsening

Depression is associated with an increased risk of suicidal thoughts, self harm and suicide (suicide-related events). This risk persists until significant remission occurs. As improvement may not occur during the first few weeks or more of treatment, patients should be closely monitored until such improvement occurs. It is general clinical experience that the risk of suicide may increase in the early stages of recovery.

Other psychiatric conditions for which paroxetine is prescribed can also be associated with an increased risk of suicide-related events. In addition, these conditions may be co-morbid with major depressive disorder. The same precautions observed when treating patients with major depressive disorder should therefore be observed when treating patients with other psychiatric disorders.

Patients with a history of suicide-related events, or those exhibiting a significant degree of suicidal ideation prior to commencement of treatment are known to be at greater risk of suicidal thoughts or suicide attempts, and should receive careful monitoring during treatment. A meta-analysis of placebo-controlled clinical trials of antidepressant drugs in adult patients with psychiatric disorders showed an increased risk of suicidal behaviour with antidepressants compared to placebo in patients less than 25 years old (see also section 5.1).

Close supervision of patients and in particular those at high risk should accompany drug therapy especially in early treatment and following dose changes. Patients (and caregivers of patients) should be alerted about the need to monitor for any clinical worsening, suicidal behaviour or thoughts and unusual changes in behaviour and to seek medical advice immediately if these symptoms present.

Akathisia/psychomotor restlessness

The use of paroxetine has been associated with the development of akathisia, which is characterized by an inner sense of restlessness and psychomotor agitation such as an inability to sit or stand still usually associated with subjective distress. This is most likely to occur within the first few weeks of treatment. In patients who develop these symptoms, increasing the dose may be detrimental.

Serotonin Syndrome/Neuroleptic Malignant Syndrome

On rare occasions development of a serotonin syndrome or neuroleptic malignant syndrome-like events may occur in association with treatment of paroxetine, particularly when given in combination with other serotonergic and/or neuroleptic drugs. As these syndromes may result in potentially life-threatening conditions, treatment with paroxetine should be discontinued if such events (characterised by clusters of symptoms such as hyperthermia, rigidity, myoclonus, autonomic instability with possible rapid fluctuations of vital signs, mental status changes including confusion, irritability, extreme agitation progressing to delirium and coma) occur and supportive symptomatic treatment should be initiated. Paroxetine should not be used in combination with serotonin-precursors (such as L-tryptophan, oxitriptan) due to the risk of serotonergic syndrome.

(See Sections 4.3 Contraindications and 4.5 Interactions with other medicinal products and other forms of interaction).

Mania

As with all antidepressants, paroxetine should be used with caution in patients with a history of mania. Paroxetine should be discontinued in any patient entering a manic phase.

Renal/hepatic impairment

Caution is recommended in patients with severe renal impairment or in those with hepatic impairment. (see section 4.2 Posology and Method of Administration)

Diabetes

In patients with diabetes, treatment with an SSRI may alter glycaemic control. Insulin and/or oral hypoglycaemic dosage may need to be adjusted.

Epilepsy

As with other antidepressants, paroxetine should be used with caution in patients with epilepsy.

Seizures

Overall the incidence of seizures is less than 0.1% in patients treated with paroxetine. The drug should be discontinued in any patient who develops seizures.

ECT

There is little clinical experience of the concurrent administration of paroxetine with ECT.

Glaucoma

As with other SSRIs, paroxetine can cause mydriasis and should be used with caution in patients with narrow angle glaucoma or history of glaucoma.

Cardiac Conditions

The usual precautions should be observed in patients with cardiac conditions.

Hyponatraemia

Hyponatraemia has been reported rarely, predominantly in the elderly. Caution should also be exercised in those patients at risk of hyponatraemia e.g. from concomitant medications and cirrhosis. The hyponatraemia generally reverses on discontinuation of paroxetine.

Haemorrhage

There have been reports of cutaneous bleeding abnormalities such as ecchymoses and purpura with SSRIs. Other haemorrhagic manifestations e.g. gastrointestinal haemorrhage have been reported. Elderly patients may be at an increased risk.

Caution is advised in patients taking SSRI's concomitantly with oral anticoagulants, drugs known to affect platelet function or other drugs that may increase risk of bleeding (e.g. atypical antipsychotics such as clozapine, phenothiazines, most TCA's, acetylsalicylic acid, NSAID's, COX-2 inhibitors) as well as in patients with a history of bleeding disorders or conditions which may predispose to bleeding.

Drugs affecting gastric pH

In patients receiving oral suspension, the paroxetine plasma concentration may be influenced by gastric pH. *In vitro* data have shown that an acidic environment is required for release of the active drug from the suspension, hence absorption may be reduced in patients with a high gastric pH or achlorhydria, such as after the use of certain drugs (antacid drugs, histamine H2-receptor antagonists, proton pump inhibitors), in certain disease states (e.g. atrophic gastritis, pernicious anemia, chronic Helicobacter pylori infection), and after surgery (vagotomy, gastrectomy). The pH dependency should be taken into account when changing paroxetine formulation (e.g. the plasma paroxetine concentration may decrease after changing from tablet to oral suspension in patients with a high gastric pH). Caution is therefore recommended in patients when initiating or ending treatment with drugs increasing gastric pH. Dose adjustments may be necessary in such situations.

Interaction with tamoxifen

Paroxetine may lead to reduced efficacy of tamoxifen (see section 4.5). It is recommended that prescribers consider using an alternative antidepressant with minimal CYP2D6 activity.

Withdrawal symptoms seen on discontinuation of paroxetine treatment

Withdrawal symptoms when treatment is discontinued are common, particularly if discontinuation is abrupt (see section 4.8 Undesirable effects). In clinical trials adverse events seen on treatment discontinuation occurred in 30% of patients treated with paroxetine compared to 20% of patients treated with placebo. The occurrence of withdrawal symptoms is not the same as the drug being addictive or dependence producing.

The risk of withdrawal symptoms may be dependent on several factors including the duration and dose of therapy and the rate of dose reduction.

Dizziness, sensory disturbances (including paraesthesia, electric shock sensations and tinnitus), sleep disturbances (including intense dreams), agitation or anxiety, nausea, tremor, confusion, sweating, headache, diarrhoea, palpitations, emotional instability, irritability, and visual disturbances have been reported. Generally these symptoms are mild to moderate, however, in some patients they may be severe in intensity. They usually occur within the first few days of discontinuing treatment, but there have been very rare reports of such symptoms in patients who have inadvertently missed a dose. Generally these symptoms are self-limiting and usually resolve within 2 weeks, though in some individuals they may be prolonged (2-3 months or more). It is therefore advised that paroxetine should be gradually tapered when discontinuing treatment over a period of several weeks or months, according to the patient's needs (see "Withdrawal Symptoms Seen on Discontinuation of Paroxetine", Section 4.2 Posology and Method of Administration).

Warnings for excipients

Parabens

Paroxetine oral suspension contains methyl and propyl parahydroxybenzoate (parabens), which are known to cause urticaria; generally delayed type reactions, such as contact dermatitis, but rarely immediate reaction with bronchospasm.

Sunset Yellow Colouring Agent

Paroxetine oral suspension contains the colouring agent FD&C Yellow No. 6 (sunset yellow, EEC No. 110), which may cause allergic reactions.

Sorbitol E420

Paroxetine oral suspension contains sorbitol (E420). Patients with rare hereditary problems of fructose intolerance should not take this medicine.

4.5 Interaction with other medicinal products and other forms of interaction

Serotonergic drugs

As with other SSRIs, co-administration with serotonergic drugs may lead to an incidence of 5-HT associated effects (serotonin syndrome: see Section 4.4 Special Warnings and Special Precautions for Use). Caution should be advised and a closer clinical monitoring is required when serotonergic drugs (such as L-tryptophan, triptans, tramadol, linezolid, SSRIs, lithium and St. John's Wort – Hypericum perforatum – preparations) are combined with paroxetine. Concomitant use of paroxetine and MAOIs is contraindicated because of the risk of serotonin syndrome (see Section 4.3 Contraindications).

Pimozide

Increased pimozide levels of on average 2.5 times have been demonstrated in a study of a single low dose pimozide (2 mg) when co-administered with 60 mg paroxetine. This may be explained by the known CYP2D6 inhibitory properties of paroxetine. Due to the narrow therapeutic index of pimozide and its known ability to prolong QT interval, concomitant use of pimozide and paroxetine is contraindicated (see Section 4.3 Contraindications).

Drug metabolising enzymes

The metabolism and pharmacokinetics of paroxetine may be affected by the induction or inhibition of drug metabolising enzymes.

When paroxetine is to be co-administered with a known drug metabolising enzyme inhibitor, consideration should be given to using paroxetine doses at the lower end of the range.

No initial dosage adjustment is considered necessary when the drug is to be co-administered with known drug metabolising enzyme inducers (e.g. carbamazepine, rifampicin, phenobarbital, phenytoin) or with fosamprenavir/ritonavir. Any paroxetine dosage adjustment (either after initiation or following discontinuation of an enzyme inducer) should be guided by clinical effect (tolerability and efficacy).

Fosamprenavir/ritonavir: Co-administration of fosamprenavir/ritonavir 700/100 mg twice daily with paroxetine 20 mg daily in healthy volunteers for 10 days significantly decreased plasma levels of paroxetine by approximately 55%. The plasma levels of fosamprenavir/ritonavir during co-administration of paroxetine were similar to reference values of other studies, indicating that paroxetine had no significant effect on metabolism of fosamprenavir/ritonavir. There are no data available about the effects of long-term co-administration of paroxetine and fosamprenavir/ritonavir exceeding 10 days.

Procyclidine: Daily administration of paroxetine increases significantly the plasma levels of procyclidine. If anti-cholinergic effects are seen, the dose of procyclidine should be reduced.

Anticonvulsants: carbamazepine, phenytoin, sodium valproate. Concomitant administration does not seem to show any effect on pharmacokinetic/dynamic profile in epileptic patients.

CYP2D6 inhibitory potency of paroxetine

As with other antidepressants, including other SSRIs, paroxetine inhibits the hepatic cytochrome P450 enzyme CYP2D6. Inhibition of CYP2D6 may lead to increased plasma concentrations of co-administered drugs metabolised by this enzyme. These include certain tricyclic antidepressants (e.g. clomipramine, nortriptyline, and desipramine), phenothiazine neuroleptics (e.g. perphenazine and thioridazine, see section 4.3 Contraindications), risperidone, atomoxetine, certain Type 1c antiarrhythmics (e.g. propafenone and flecainide) and metoprolol. It is not recommended to use paroxetine in combination with metoprolol when given in cardiac insufficiency, because of the narrow therapeutic index of metoprolol in this indication.

Tamoxifen is a pro-drug requiring metabolic activation by CYP2D6. Inhibition of CYP2D6 by paroxetine may lead to reduced plasma concentrations of an active metabolite and hence reduced efficacy of tamoxifen, especially in extensive metabolisers. It is recommended that prescribers consider using an alternative antidepressant with minimal CYP2D6 activity.

Alcohol

As with other psychotropic drugs patients should be advised to avoid alcohol use while taking paroxetine.

Oral anticoagulants

A pharmacodynamic interaction between paroxetine and oral anticoagulants may occur. Concomitant use of paroxetine and oral anticoagulants can lead to an increased anticoagulant activity and haemorrhagic risk. Therefore, paroxetine should be used with caution in patients who are treated with oral anticoagulants. (see section 4.4 Special Warnings and Special Precautions for use)

NSAIDs and acetylsalicylic acid, and other antiplatelet agents

A pharmacodynamic interaction between paroxetine and NSAIDs/acetylsalicylic acid may occur. Concomitant use of paroxetine and NSAIDs/acetylsalicylic acid can lead to an increased haemorrhagic risk. (see section 4.4 Special warnings and Special Precautions for use)

Caution is advised in patients taking SSRI's, concomitantly with oral anticoagulants, drugs known to affect platelet function or increase risk of bleeding (e.g. atypical antipsychotics such as clozapine, phenothiazines, most TCA's, acetylsalicylic acid, NSAID's, COX-2 inhibitors) as well as in patients with a history of bleeding disorders or conditions which may predispose to bleeding.

Drugs affecting gastric pH

In vitro data have shown that dissociation of paroxetine from the oral suspension is pH-dependant. Therefore, drugs that alter gastric pH (such as antacid drugs, proton pump inhibitors or histamine H2-receptor antagonists) may affect plasma paroxetine concentrations in patients taking the oral suspension (see section 4.4).

4.6 Pregnancy and lactation

Pregnancy

Some epidemiological studies suggest an increased risk of congenital malformations, particularly cardiovascular (e.g. ventricular and atrial septum defects) associated with the use of paroxetine during the first trimester. The mechanism is unknown. The data suggest that the risk of having an infant with a cardiovascular defect following maternal paroxetine exposure is less than 2/100 compared with an expected rate for such defects of approximately 1/100 in the general population.

Paroxetine should only be used during pregnancy when strictly indicated. The prescribing physician will need to weigh the option of alternative treatments in women who are pregnant or are planning to become pregnant. Abrupt discontinuation should be avoided during pregnancy (see "Withdrawal Symptoms Seen on Discontinuation of Paroxetine", section 4.2 Posology and Method of Administration).

Neonates should be observed if maternal use of paroxetine continues into the later stages of pregnancy, particularly the third trimester.

The following symptoms may occur in the neonate after maternal paroxetine use in later stages of pregnancy: respiratory distress, cyanosis, apnoea, seizures, temperature instability, feeding difficulty, vomiting, hypoglycaemia, hypertonia, hypotonia, hyperreflexia, tremor, jitteriness, irritability, lethargy, constant crying, somnolence and difficulty in sleeping. These symptoms could be due to either serotonergic effects or withdrawal symptoms. In a majority of instances the complications begin immediately or soon (<24 hours) after delivery.

Animal studies showed reproductive toxicity, but did not indicate direct harmful effects with respect to pregnancy, embryonal/foetal development, parturition or postnatal development (see Section 5.3 Preclinical Safety Data).

Lactation

Small amounts of paroxetine are excreted into breast milk. In published studies, serum concentrations in breast-fed infants were undetectable (<2 ng/ml) or very low (<4 ng/ml), and no signs of drug effects were observed in these infants. Since no effects are anticipated, breast-feeding can be considered.

4.7 Effects on ability to drive and use machines

Clinical experience has shown that therapy with paroxetine is not associated with impairment of cognitive or psychomotor function. However, as with all psychoactive drugs, patients should be cautioned about their ability to drive a car and operate machinery.

Although paroxetine does not increase the mental and motor skill impairments caused by alcohol, the concomitant use of paroxetine and alcohol is not advised.

4.8 Undesirable effects

Some of the adverse drug reactions listed below may decrease in intensity and frequency with continued treatment and do not generally lead to cessation of therapy. Adverse drug reactions are listed below by system organ class and frequency. Frequencies are defined as: very common ($\geqslant$ 1/10), common ($\geqslant$ 1/100, <1/10), uncommon ($\geqslant$ 1/1,000, <1/100), rare ($\geqslant$ 1/10,000, <1/1,000), very rare (<1/10,000), including isolated reports.

Blood and lymphatic system disorders

Uncommon: abnormal bleeding, predominantly of the skin and mucous membranes (mostly ecchymosis).

Very rare: thrombocytopenia.

Immune system disorders

Very rare: allergic reactions (including urticaria and angioedema).

Endocrine disorders

Very rare: syndrome of inappropriate anti-diuretic hormone secretion (SIADH).

Metabolism and nutrition disorders

Common: increases in cholesterol levels, decreased appetite.

Rare: hyponatraemia.

Hyponatraemia has been reported predominantly in elderly patients and is sometimes due to syndrome of inappropriate anti-diuretic hormone secretion (SIADH).

Psychiatric disorders

Common: somnolence, insomnia, agitation.

Uncommon: confusion, hallucinations.

Rare: manic reactions, anxiety, depersonalisation, panic attacks, akathisia (see section 4.4).

Frequency not known: suicidal ideation and suicidal behaviour.

Cases of suicidal ideation and suicidal behaviours have been reported during paroxetine therapy or early after treatment discontinuation (see section 4.4).

These symptoms may also be due to the underlying disease

Nervous system disorders

Common: dizziness, tremor, headache.

Uncommon: extrapyramidal disorders.

Rare: convulsions.

Very rare: serotonin syndrome (symptoms may include agitation, confusion, diaphoresis, hallucinations, hyperreflexia, myoclonus, shivering, tachycardia and tremor).

Reports of extrapyramidal disorder including oro-facial dystonia have been received in patients sometimes with underlying movement disorders or who were using neuroleptic medication.

Eye disorders

Common: blurred vision.

Uncommon: mydriasis (see section 4.4 Special Warnings and Special Precautions for Use).

Very rare: acute glaucoma.

Ear and labyrinth disorders

Frequency not known: tinnitus.

Cardiac disorders

Uncommon: sinus tachycardia.

Rare: bradycardia.

Vascular disorders

Uncommon: transient increases or decreases in blood pressure, postural hypotension. Transient increases or decreases of blood pressure have been reported following treatment with paroxetine, usually in patients with pre-existing hypertension or anxiety.

Respiratory, thoracic and mediastinal disorders

Common: yawning.

Gastrointestinal disorders

Very common: nausea.

Common: constipation, diarrhoea, dry mouth.

Very rare: gastrointestinal bleeding.

Hepato-biliary disorders

Rare: elevation of hepatic enzymes.

Very rare: hepatic events (such as hepatitis, sometimes associated with jaundice and/or liver failure). Elevation of hepatic enzymes have been reported. Post-marketing reports of hepatic events (such as hepatitis, sometimes associated with jaundice and/or liver failure) have also been received very rarely. Discontinuation of paroxetine should be considered if there is prolonged elevation of liver function test results.

Skin and subcutaneous tissue disorders

Common: sweating.

Uncommon: skin rashes, pruritus

Very rare: photosensitivity reactions.

Renal and urinary disorders

Uncommon: urinary retention, urinary incontinence.

Reproductive system and breast disorders

Very common: sexual dysfunction.

Rare: hyperprolactinaemia/galactorrhoea.

Very rare: priapism.

Musculoskeletal disorders

Rare: arthralgia, myalgia

General disorder and administration site conditions

Common: asthenia, body weight gain

Very rare: peripheral oedema.

WITHDRAWAL SYMPTOMS SEEN ON DISCONTINUATION OF PAROXETINE TREATMENT

Common: dizziness, sensory disturbances, sleep disturbances, anxiety, headache.

Uncommon: agitation, nausea, tremor, confusion, sweating, emotional instability, visual disturbances, palpitations, diarrhoea, irritability.

Discontinuation of paroxetine (particularly when abrupt) commonly leads to withdrawal symptoms. Dizziness, sensory disturbances (including paraesthesia, electric shock sensations and tinnitus), sleep disturbances (including intense dreams), agitation or anxiety, nausea, tremor, confusion, sweating, headache, diarrhoea, palpitations, emotional instability, irritability, and visual disturbances have been reported.

Generally these events are mild to moderate and are self-limiting, however, in some patients they may be severe and/or prolonged. It is therefore advised that when paroxetine treatment is no longer required, gradual discontinuation by dose tapering should be carried out (see section 4.2 Posology and Method of Administration and section 4.4 Special Warnings and Special Precautions for use).

ADVERSE EVENTS FROM PAEDIATRIC CLINICAL TRIALS

In short-term (up to 10-12 weeks) clinical trials in children and adolescents, the following adverse events were observed in paroxetine treated patients at a frequency of at least 2% of patients and occurred at a rate at least twice that of placebo were: increased suicidal related behaviours (including suicide attempts and suicidal thoughts), self-harm behaviours and increased hostility. Suicidal thoughts and suicide attempts were mainly observed in clinical trials of adolescents with Major Depressive Disorder. Increased hostility occurred particularly in children with obsessive compulsive disorder, and especially in younger children less than 12 years of age. Additional events that were more often seen in the paroxetine compared to placebo group were: decreased appetite, tremor, sweating, hyperkinesia, agitation, emotional lability (including crying and mood fluctuations).

In studies that used a tapering regimen, symptoms reported during the taper phase or upon discontinuation of paroxetine at a frequency of at least 2% of patients and occurred at a rate at least twice that of placebo were: emotional lability (including crying, mood fluctuations, self-harm, suicidal thoughts and attempted suicide), nervousness, dizziness, nausea and abdominal pain (see section 4.4 Special Warnings and Special Precautions for use).

4.9 Overdose

Symptoms and Signs

A wide margin of safety is evident from available overdose information on paroxetine.

Experience of paroxetine in overdose has indicated that, in addition to those symptoms mentioned under section 4.8 "Undesirable Effects", vomiting, fever and involuntary muscle contractions have been reported. Patients have generally recovered without serious sequelae even when doses of up to 2000 mg have been taken alone. Events such as coma or ECG changes have occasionally been reported and, very rarely with a fatal outcome, but generally when paroxetine was taken in conjunction with other psychotropic drugs, with or without alcohol.

Treatment

No specific antidote is known.

The treatment should consist of those general measures employed in the management of overdose with any antidepressant. Where appropriate, the stomach should be emptied either by the induction of emesis, lavage or both. Following evacuation, 20 to 30 g of activated charcoal may be administered every 4 to 6 h during the first 24 h after ingestion. Supportive care with frequent monitoring of vital signs and careful observation is indicated.

5. PHARMACOLOGICAL PROPERTIES

5.1 Pharmacodynamic properties

Pharmacotherapeutic group: Antidepressants – selective serotonin reuptake inhibitors, ATC code: N06A B05

Mechanism of Action

Paroxetine is a potent and selective inhibitor of 5-hydroxytryptamine (5-HT, serotonin) uptake and its antidepressant action and effectiveness in the treatment of OCD, Social Anxiety disorder/Social Phobia, General Anxiety Disorder, Post-traumatic Stress Disorder and Panic Disorder is thought to be related to its specific inhibition of 5-HT uptake in brain neurones.

Paroxetine is chemically unrelated to the tricyclic, tetracyclic and other available antidepressants. Paroxetine has low affinity for muscarinic cholinergic receptors and animal studies have indicated only weak anticholinergic properties.

In accordance with this selective action, *in vitro* studies have indicated that, in contrast to tricyclic antidepressants, paroxetine has little affinity for alpha1, alpha2 and beta-adrenoceptors, dopamine (D2), 5-HT1 like, 5-HT2 and histamine (H1) receptors. This lack of interaction with post-synaptic receptors *in vitro* is substantiated by *in vivo* studies which demonstrate lack of CNS depressant and hypotensive properties.

Pharmacodynamic Effects

Paroxetine does not impair psychomotor function and does not potentiate the depressant effects of ethanol.

As with other selective 5-HT uptake inhibitors, paroxetine causes symptoms of excessive 5-HT receptor stimulation when administered to animals previously given monoamine oxidase (MAO) inhibitors or tryptophan.

Behavioural and EEG studies indicate that paroxetine is weakly activating at doses generally above those required to inhibit 5-HT uptake. The activating properties are not "amphetamine-like" in nature.

Animal studies indicate that paroxetine is well tolerated by the cardiovascular system. Paroxetine produces no clinically significant changes in blood pressure, heart rate and ECG after administration to healthy subjects.

Studies indicate that, in contrast to antidepressants which inhibit the uptake of noradrenaline, paroxetine has a much reduced propensity to inhibit the antihypertensive effects of guanethidine.

In the treatment of depressive disorders, paroxetine exhibits comparable efficacy to standard antidepressants.

There is also some evidence that paroxetine may be of therapeutic value in patients who have failed to respond to standard therapy.

Morning dosing with paroxetine does not have any detrimental effect on either the quality or duration of sleep. Moreover, patients are likely to experience improved sleep as they respond to paroxetine therapy.

Adult suicidality analysis

A paroxetine-specific analysis of placebo controlled trials of adults with psychiatric disorders showed a higher frequency of suicidal behaviour in young adults (aged 18-24 years) treated with paroxetine compared with placebo (2.19% vs 0.92%). In the older age groups, no such increase was observed. In adults with major depressive disorder (all ages), there was an increase in the frequency of suicidal behaviour in patients treated with paroxetine compared with placebo (0.32% vs 0.05%); all of the events were suicide attempts. However, the majority of these attempts for paroxetine (8 of 11) were in younger adults (see also section 4.4).

Dose response

In the fixed dose studies there is a flat dose response curve, providing no suggestion of advantage in terms of efficacy for using higher than the recommended doses. However, there are some clinical data suggesting that up-titrating the dose might be beneficial for some patients.

Long-term efficacy

The long-term efficacy of paroxetine in depression has been demonstrated in a 52 week maintenance study with relapse prevention design: 12% of patients receiving paroxetine (20-40mg daily) relapsed, versus 28% of patients on placebo.

The long-term efficacy of paroxetine in treating obsessive compulsive disorder has been examined in three 24 week maintenance studies with relapse prevention design. One of the three studies achieved a significant difference in the proportion of relapsers between paroxetine (38%) compared to placebo (59%).

The long-term efficacy of paroxetine in treating panic disorder has been demonstrated in a 24 week maintenance study with relapse prevention design: 5% of patients receiving paroxetine (10-40mg daily) relapsed, versus 30% of patients on placebo. This was supported by a 36 week maintenance study.

The long-term efficacy of paroxetine in treating social anxiety disorder and generalised anxiety disorder and Post-traumatic Stress Disorderhas not been sufficiently demonstrated.

5.2 Pharmacokinetic properties

Absorption

Paroxetine is well absorbed after oral dosing and undergoes first-pass metabolism. Due to first-pass metabolism, the amount of paroxetine available to the systemic circulation is less than that absorbed from the gastrointestinal tract. Partial saturation of the first-pass effect and reduced plasma clearance occur as the body burden increases with higher single doses or on multiple dosing. This results in disproportionate increases in plasma concentrations of paroxetine and hence pharmacokinetic parameters are not constant, resulting in non-linear kinetics. However, the non-linearity is generally small and is confined to those subjects who achieve low plasma levels at low doses.

Steady state systemic levels are attained by 7 to 14 days after starting treatment with immediate or controlled release formulations and pharmacokinetics do not appear to change during long-term therapy.

Distribution

Paroxetine is extensively distributed into tissues and pharmacokinetic calculations indicate that only 1% of the paroxetine in the body resides in the plasma.

Approximately 95% of the paroxetine present is protein bound at therapeutic concentrations.

No correlation has been found between paroxetine plasma concentrations and clinical effect (adverse experiences and efficacy).

Transfer to human breast milk, and to the foetuses of laboratory animals, occurs in small amounts.

Metabolism

The principal metabolites of paroxetine are polar and conjugated products of oxidation and methylation which are readily cleared. In view of their relative lack of pharmacological activity, it is most unlikely that they contribute to paroxetine's therapeutic effects.

Metabolism does not compromise paroxetine's selective action on neuronal 5-HT uptake.

Elimination

Urinary excretion of unchanged paroxetine is generally less than 2% of dose whilst that of metabolites is about 64% of dose. About 36% of the dose is excreted in faeces, probably via the bile, of which unchanged paroxetine represents less than 1% of the dose. Thus paroxetine is eliminated almost entirely by metabolism.

Metabolite excretion is biphasic, being initially a result of first-pass metabolism and subsequently controlled by systemic elimination of paroxetine.

The elimination half-life is variable but is generally about 1 day.

Special Patient Populations

Elderly and Renal/Hepatic Impairment

Increased plasma concentrations of paroxetine occur in elderly subjects and in those subjects with severe renal impairment or in those with hepatic impairment, but the range of plasma concentrations overlaps that of healthy adult subjects.

5.3 Preclinical safety data

Toxicology studies have been conducted in rhesus monkeys and albino rats; in both, the metabolic pathway is similar to that described for humans. As expected with lipophilic amines, including tricyclic antidepressants, phospholipidosis was detected in rats. Phospholipidosis was not observed in primate studies of up to one-year duration at doses that were 6 times higher than the recommended range of clinical doses.

Carcinogenesis: In two-year studies conducted in mice and rats, paroxetine had no tumorigenic effect.

Genotoxicity: Genotoxicity was not observed in a battery of *in vitro* and *in vivo* tests.

Reproduction toxicity studies in rats have shown that paroxetine affects male and female fertility. In rats, increased pup mortality and delayed ossification were observed. The latter effects were likely related to maternal toxicity and are not considered a direct effect on the foetus/neonate.

6. PHARMACEUTICAL PARTICULARS

6.1 List of excipients

10 mg tablet

Tablet core:

Dibasic calcium phosphate dihydrate

Sodium starch glycolate (Type A)

Magnesium stearate.

Tablet coating:

Hypromellose

Macrogol 400

Polysorbate 80

Titanium dioxide (E171)

Iron oxide red (E172).

20 mg tablet

Tablet core:

Dibasic calcium phosphate dihydrate

Sodium starch glycolate (Type A)

Magnesium stearate.

Tablet coating:

Hypromellose

Macrogol 400

Polysorbate 80

Titanium dioxide (E171).

30 mg tablet

Tablet core:

Dibasic calcium phosphate dihydrate

Sodium starch glycolate (Type A)

Magnesium stearate.

Tablet coating:

Hypromellose

Macrogol 400

Polysorbate 80

Titanium dioxide (E171)

Indigo carmine (E132).

Oral suspension

Polacrilin potassium

Dispersible cellulose

Propylene glycol

Glycerol

Sorbitol (E420)

Methyl parahydroxybenzoate (E218)

Propyl parahydroxybenzoate (E216)

Sodium citrate dihydrate

Citric acid anhydrate

Sodium saccharin

Natural orange flavour

Natural lemon flavour

Yellow colouring (E110)

Simethicone emulsion

Purified water.

6.2 Incompatibilities

Not applicable.

6.3 Shelf life
10/20/30 mg tablet

3 years.

Oral suspension

2 years (1 month after opening).

6.4 Special precautions for storage
10/20/30 mg tablet

Do not store above 30°C.

Store in the original package (to protect from light).

Oral suspension

Do not store above 25°C.

6.5 Nature and contents of container
10 mg tablet

Blister packs comprising opaque polyvinyl (PVC) backed with aluminium foil.

Pack sizes: 14 and 28 tablets.

Not all pack sizes may be marketed.

20 mg tablet

Blister packs comprising opaque PVC/PVdC or opaque polyvinyl chloride (PVC) backed with aluminium foil. Plastic containers (bottles) made of polypropylene, with polyethylene closures, may also be used.

Pack sizes: 4, 10, 14, 20, 28, 30, 50, 56, 60, 98, 100, 250 and 500 tablets.

Not all pack sizes may be marketed.

30 mg tablet

Blister packs comprising opaque PVC/PVdC or opaque polyvinyl chloride (PVC) backed with aluminium foil. Plastic containers (bottles) made of polypropylene, with polyethylene closures, may also be used.

Pack sizes: 28, 30, 56 and 60 tablets.

Not all pack sizes may be marketed.

Oral suspension

Amber glass bottle sealed with polypropylene child-resistant cap lined with a polyethylene wad.

A polypropylene measuring cup is included.

Pack size: 150 ml.

6.6 Special precautions for disposal and other handling
No special requirements.

7. MARKETING AUTHORISATION HOLDER
SmithKline Beecham plc

Great West Road

Brentford

Middlesex TW8 9GS.

trading as:

SmithKline Beecham Pharmaceuticals

Welwyn Garden City

Hertfordshire AL7 1EY

And/or

GlaxoSmithKline UK,

StockleyPark West,

Uxbridge,

Middlesex UB11 1BT

8. MARKETING AUTHORISATION NUMBER(S)
Seroxat Tablets 10 mg: 10592/0218

Seroxat Tablets 20 mg: 10592/0001

Seroxat Tablets 30 mg: 10592/0002

Seroxat Oral suspension:10592/0092

9. DATE OF FIRST AUTHORISATION/RENEWAL OF THE AUTHORISATION
27/09/2005

10. DATE OF REVISION OF THE TEXT
22/5/2009

11. LEGAL STATUS
POM

Sevikar 20 mg/5 mg, 40 mg/5 mg, 40 mg/10 mg Film-Coated Tablets

(Daiichi Sankyo UK Limited)

1. NAME OF THE MEDICINAL PRODUCT
Sevikar 20 mg/5 mg film-coated tablets▼

Sevikar 40 mg/5 mg film-coated tablets▼

Sevikar 40 mg/10 mg film-coated tablets▼

2. QUALITATIVE AND QUANTITATIVE COMPOSITION
Sevikar 20 mg/5 mg film-coated tablets:

Each film-coated tablet of Sevikar contains 20 mg of olmesartan medoxomil and 5 mg of amlodipine (as amlodipine besilate).

Sevikar 40 mg/5 mg film-coated tablets:

Each film-coated tablet of Sevikar contains 40 mg of olmesartan medoxomil and 5 mg of amlodipine (as amlodipine besilate).

Sevikar 40 mg/10 mg film-coated tablets:

Each film-coated tablet of Sevikar contains 40 mg of olmesartan medoxomil and 10 mg of amlodipine (as amlodipine besilate).

For a full list of excipients, see section 6.1.

3. PHARMACEUTICAL FORM
Film-coated tablet.

Sevikar 20 mg/5 mg film-coated tablets:

White, round, film-coated tablet with C73 debossed on one side.

Sevikar 40 mg/5 mg film-coated tablets:

Cream, round, film-coated tablet with C75 debossed on one side.

Sevikar 40 mg/10 mg film-coated tablets:

Brownish-red, round, film-coated tablet with C77 debossed on one side.

4. CLINICAL PARTICULARS

4.1 Therapeutic indications
Treatment of essential hypertension.

Sevikar is indicated in patients whose blood pressure is not adequately controlled on olmesartan medoxomil or amlodipine monotherapy (see section 4.2 and section 5.1).

4.2 Posology and method of administration
Adults

The recommended dosage of Sevikar is 1 tablet per day.

Sevikar 20 mg/5 mg may be administered in patients whose blood pressure is not adequately controlled by 20 mg olmesartan medoxomil or 5 mg amlodipine alone.

Sevikar 40 mg/5 mg may be administered in patients whose blood pressure is not adequately controlled by Sevikar 20 mg/5 mg.

Sevikar 40 mg/10 mg may be administered in patients whose blood pressure is not adequately controlled by Sevikar 40 mg/5 mg.

A step-wise titration of the dosage of the individual components is recommended before changing to the fixed combination. When clinically appropriate, direct change from monotherapy to the fixed combination may be considered.

For convenience, patients receiving olmesartan medoxomil and amlodipine from separate tablets may be switched to Sevikar tablets containing the same component doses.

Method of administration:

The tablet should be swallowed with a sufficient amount of fluid (e.g. one glass of water). The tablet should not be chewed and should be taken at the same time each day.

Sevikar can be taken with or without food.

Elderly (age 65 years or over)

No adjustment of the recommended dose is generally required for elderly patients (see section 5.2).

If up-titration to the maximum dose of 40 mg olmesartan medoxomil daily is required, blood pressure should be closely monitored.

Renal impairment

The maximum dose of olmesartan medoxomil in patients with mild to moderate renal impairment (creatinine clearance of 20 – 60 mL/min) is 20 mg olmesartan medoxomil once daily, owing to limited experience of higher dosages in this patient group. The use of Sevikar in patients with severe renal impairment (creatinine clearance < 20 mL/min) is not recommended (see 4.4, 5.2).

Monitoring of potassium levels and creatinine is advised in patients with moderate renal impairment.

Hepatic impairment

Sevikar should be used with caution in patients with mild to moderate hepatic impairment (see sections 4.4, 5.2).

In patients with moderate hepatic impairment, an initial dose of 10 mg olmesartan medoxomil once daily is recommended and the maximum dose should not exceed 20 mg once daily. Close monitoring of blood pressure and renal function is advised in hepatically-impaired patients who are already receiving diuretics and/or other antihypertensive agents. There is no experience of olmesartan medoxomil in patients with severe hepatic impairment.

As with all calcium antagonists, amlodipine's half-life is prolonged in patients with impaired liver function and dosage recommendations have not been established. Sevikar should therefore be administered with caution in these patients.

Children and adolescents

Sevikar is not recommended for use in children and adolescents below 18 years of age due to a lack of data on safety and efficacy (see section 5.2).

4.3 Contraindications
Hypersensitivity to the active substances, to dihydropyridine derivatives or to any of the excipients (see section 6.1).

Second and third trimester of pregnancy (see section 4.4 and 4.6).

Lactation (see section 4.6).

Severe hepatic insufficiency and biliary obstruction (see section 5.2).

Due to the component amlodipine Sevikar is also contraindicated in patients with:

- Cardiogenic shock.
- Acute myocardial infarction (within the first 4 weeks).
- Unstable angina pectoris.

4.4 Special warnings and precautions for use
Patients with hypovolaemia or sodium depletion:

Symptomatic hypotension may occur in patients who are volume and/or sodium depleted by vigorous diuretic therapy, dietary salt restriction, diarrhoea or vomiting, especially after the first dose. Correction of this condition prior to administration of Sevikar or close medical supervision at the start of the treatment is recommended.

Other conditions with stimulation of the renin-angiotensin-aldosterone system:

In patients whose vascular tone and renal function depend predominantly on the activity of the renin-angiotensin-aldosterone system (e.g. patients with severe congestive heart failure or underlying renal disease, including renal artery stenosis), treatment with other medicinal products that affect this system, such as angiotensin II receptor antagonists, has been associated with acute hypotension, azotaemia, oliguria or, rarely, acute renal failure.

Renovascular hypertension:

There is an increased risk of severe hypotension and renal insufficiency when patients with bilateral renal artery stenosis or stenosis of the artery to a single functioning kidney are treated with medicinal products that affect the renin-angiotensin-aldosterone system.

Renal impairment and kidney transplantation:

When Sevikar is used in patients with impaired renal function, periodic monitoring of serum potassium and creatinine levels is recommended. Use of Sevikar is not recommended in patients with severe renal impairment (creatinine clearance < 20 mL/min) (see sections 4.2, 5.2). There is no experience of the administration of Sevikar in patients with a recent kidney transplant or in patients with end-stage renal impairment (i.e. creatinine clearance < 12 mL/min).

Hepatic impairment:

Exposure to amlodipine and olmesartan medoxomil is increased in patients with hepatic impairment (see section 5.2). Care should be taken when Sevikar is administered in patients with mild to moderate hepatic impairment. In moderately impaired patients, the dose of olmesartan medoxomil should not exceed 20 mg (see section 4.2). Use of Sevikar in patients with severe hepatic impairment is contraindicated (see section 4.3).

Hyperkalaemia:

As with other angiotensin II antagonists and ACE inhibitors, hyperkalaemia may occur during treatment, especially in the presence of renal impairment and/or heart failure (see section 4.5). Close monitoring of serum potassium levels in at-risk patients is recommended.

Concomitant use with potassium supplements, potassium-sparing diuretics, salt substitutes containing potassium, or other medicinal products that may increase potassium levels (heparin, etc.) should be undertaken with caution and with frequent monitoring of potassium levels.

Lithium:

As with other angiotensin II receptor antagonists, the concomitant use of Sevikar and lithium is not recommended (see section 4.5).

Aortic or mitral valve stenosis; obstructive hypertrophic cardiomyopathy:

Due to the amlodipine component of Sevikar, as with all other vasodilators, special caution is indicated in patients suffering from aortic or mitral valve stenosis, or obstructive hypertrophic cardiomyopathy.

Primary aldosteronism:

Patients with primary aldosteronism generally will not respond to antihypertensive medicinal products acting through inhibition of the renin-angiotensin system. Therefore, the use of Sevikar is not recommended in such patients.

Heart failure:

As a consequence of the inhibition of the renin-angiotensin-aldosterone system, changes in renal function may be anticipated in susceptible individuals. In patients with severe heart failure whose renal function may depend on the activity of the renin-angiotensin-aldosterone system, treatment with angiotensin-converting enzyme (ACE) inhibitors and angiotensin receptor antagonists has been associated with oliguria and/or progressive azotaemia and (rarely) with acute renal failure and/or death.

In a long-term, placebo controlled study (PRAISE-2) of amlodipine in patients with NYHA III and IV heart failure of nonischaemic aetiology, amlodipine was associated with increased reports of pulmonary oedema despite no significant difference in the incidence of worsening heart failure as compared to placebo (see section 5.1).

Ethnic differences:

As with all other angiotensin II antagonists, the blood pressure lowering effect of Sevikar can be somewhat less in black patients than in non-black patients, possibly because of a higher prevalence of low-renin status in the black hypertensive population.

Pregnancy:

Angiotensin II antagonists should not be initiated during pregnancy. Unless continued angiotensin II antagonist therapy is considered essential, patients planning pregnancy should be changed to alternative anti-hypertensive treatments which have an established safety profile for use in pregnancy. When pregnancy is diagnosed, treatment with angiotensin II antagonists should be stopped immediately, and, if appropriate, alternative therapy should be started (see section 4.3 and 4.6).

Other:

As with any antihypertensive agent, excessive blood pressure decrease in patients with ischaemic heart disease or ischaemic cerebrovascular disease could result in a myocardial infarction or stroke.

4.5 Interaction with other medicinal products and other forms of interaction

Potential interactions related to the Sevikar combination:

To be taken into account with concomitant use

Other antihypertensive agents:

The blood pressure lowering effect of Sevikar can be increased by concomitant use of other antihypertensive medicinal products (e.g. alpha blockers, diuretics).

Potential interactions related to the olmesartan medoxomil component of Sevikar:

Concomitant use not recommended

Medicinal products affecting potassium levels:

Concomitant use of potassium-sparing diuretics, potassium supplements, salt substitutes containing potassium or other medicinal products that may increase serum potassium levels (e.g. heparin, ACE inhibitors) may lead to increases in serum potassium (see section 4.4). If medicinal products which affect potassium levels are to be prescribed in combination with Sevikar, monitoring of serum potassium levels is recommended.

Lithium:

Reversible increases in serum lithium concentrations and toxicity have been reported during concomitant administration of lithium with angiotensin converting enzyme inhibitors and, rarely, with angiotensin II antagonists. Therefore concomitant use of Sevikar and lithium is not recommended (see section 4.4). If concomitant use of Sevikar and lithium proves necessary, careful monitoring of serum lithium levels is recommended.

Concomitant use requiring caution

Non-steroidal anti-inflammatory medicinal products (NSAIDs) including selective COX-2 inhibitors, acetylsalicylic acid (> 3 g/day) and non-selective NSAIDs:

When angiotensin II antagonists are administered simultaneously with NSAIDs, attenuation of the antihypertensive effect may occur. Furthermore, concomitant use of angiotensin II antagonists and NSAIDs may increase the risk of worsening of renal function and may lead to an increase in serum potassium. Therefore monitoring of renal function at the beginning of such concomitant therapy is recommended, as well as adequate hydration of the patient.

Additional information

After treatment with antacid (aluminium magnesium hydroxide), a modest reduction in bioavailability of olmesartan was observed.

Olmesartan medoxomil had no significant effect on the pharmacokinetics or pharmacodynamics of warfarin or the pharmacokinetics of digoxin. Coadministration of olmesartan medoxomil with pravastatin had no clinically relevant effects on the pharmacokinetics of either component in healthy subjects.

Olmesartan had no clinically relevant inhibitory effects on human cytochrome P450 enzymes 1A1/2, 2A6, 2C8/9, 2C19, 2D6, 2E1 and 3A4 *in vitro*, and had no or minimal inducing effects on rat cytochrome P450 activities. No clinically relevant interactions between olmesartan and medicinal products metabolised by the above cytochrome P450 enzymes are expected.

Potential interactions related to the amlodipine component of Sevikar:

Concomitant use requiring caution

CYP3A4 inhibitors:

A study in elderly patients showed that diltiazem inhibits the metabolism of amlodipine, probably via CYP3A4, since plasma concentrations of amlodipine increased by approximately 50% and its effect was increased. The possibility that more potent CYP3A4 inhibitors (e.g. ketoconazole, itraconazole, ritonavir) may increase the plasma concentration of amlodipine to a greater extent than diltiazem cannot be excluded.

CYP3A4 inducers (anticonvulsants [e.g. carbamazepine, phenobarbital, phenytoin, fosphenytoin, primidone], rifampicin, Hypericum perforatum):

Concomitant administration may decrease the plasma concentration of amlodipine. Clinical monitoring is indicated, with possible adjustment of amlodipine dosage during treatment with the CYP3A4 inducer and after its withdrawal.

Sildenafil: When amlodipine and sildenafil were used in combination, each agent independently exerted its own blood pressure lowering effect.

Additional information:

Concomitant administration of 240 ml of grapefruit juice with a single oral dose of 10 mg amlodipine in 20 healthy volunteers did not show a significant effect on the pharmacokinetic properties of amlodipine.

Co-administration of amlodipine with cimetidine had no significant effect on the pharmacokinetics of amlodipine.

Co-administration of amlodipine with atorvastatin, digoxin, warfarin or ciclosporin had no significant effect on the pharmacokinetics or pharmacodynamics of these agents.

4.6 Pregnancy and lactation

Pregnancy (see section 4.3)

There are no data about the use of Sevikar in pregnant patients. Animal reproductive toxicity studies with Sevikar have not been performed.

Olmesartan medoxomil (active ingredient of Sevikar)

The use of angiotensin II antagonists is not recommended during the first trimester of pregnancy (see section 4.4). The use of angiotensin II antagonists is contraindicated during the 2nd and 3rd trimester of pregnancy (see section 4.3. and 4.4).

Epidemiological evidence regarding the risk of teratogenicity following exposure to ACE inhibitors during the first trimester of pregnancy has not been conclusive; however a small increase in risk cannot be excluded. Whilst there is no controlled epidemiological data on the risk with angiotensin II antagonists, similar risks may exist for this class of drugs. Unless continued angiotensin receptor blocker therapy is considered essential, patients planning pregnancy should be changed to alternative anti-hypertensive treatments which have an established safety profile for use in pregnancy. When pregnancy is diagnosed, treatment with angiotensin II antagonists should be stopped immediately, and, if appropriate, alternative therapy should be started.

Angiotensin II antagonists therapy exposure during the second and third trimesters is known to induce human fetotoxicity (decreased renal function, oligohydramnios, skull ossification retardation) and neonatal toxicity (renal failure, hypotension, hyperkalaemia). (See also section 5.3.)

Should exposure to angiotensin II antagonists have occurred from the second trimester on, ultrasound examinations of the renal function and of the skull are recommended. Newborns exposed to angiotensin II antagonists *in utero* must be closely monitored for the occurrence of hypotension, oliguria and hyperkalaemia.

Amlodipine (active ingredient of Sevikar)

Data on a limited number of exposed pregnancies do not indicate that amlodipine or other calcium receptor antagonists have a harmful effect on the health of the fetus. However, there may be a risk of prolonged delivery.

As a consequence, Sevikar is not recommended during the first trimester of pregnancy and is contraindicated during the second and third trimesters of pregnancy (see section 4.3 and 4.4).

Lactation (see section 4.3)

Olmesartan is excreted into the milk of lactating rats. However, it is not known whether olmesartan passes into human milk. It is not known whether amlodipine is excreted in breast milk. Similar calcium channel blockers of the dihydropyridine type are excreted in breast milk. The risks to newborn infants of exposure to Sevikar in breast milk are unknown. Therefore, as a precaution, the use of Sevikar during lactation is contraindicated. A decision should be made whether to discontinue breast-feeding or discontinue Sevikar, taking into account the importance of Sevikar to the mother.

4.7 Effects on ability to drive and use machines

No studies on the effects on the ability to drive and use machines have been performed. However, it should be borne in mind that dizziness or fatigue may occasionally occur in patients taking antihypertensive therapy.

4.8 Undesirable effects

Sevikar:

The safety of Sevikar was investigated in controlled clinical trials in 2892 patients receiving olmesartan medoxomil in combination with amlodipine.

The following terminologies have been used in order to classify the occurrence of undesirable effects

Very common (⩾1/10)

Common (⩾1/100 to <1/10)

Uncommon (⩾1/1,000 to <1/100)

Rare (⩾1/10,000 to <1/1,000)

Very rare (<1/10,000), not known (cannot be estimated from the available data)

(see Table 1 below)

Additional information on the individual components

Adverse reactions previously reported with one of the individual components may be potential adverse reactions with Sevikar, even if not observed in clinical trials with this product.

Olmesartan medoxomil (active ingredient of Sevikar)

Further adverse events reported in clinical studies with olmesartan medoxomil monotherapy in hypertension were as follows: Angina pectoris, bronchitis, pharyngitis, rhinitis, abdominal pain, gastroenteritis, arthritis, skeletal pain, haematuria, urinary tract infection, chest pain, influenza-like symptoms, pain.

Table 1

System Organ Class	Common (⩾ 1/100 to < 1/10)	Uncommon (⩾ 1/1,000 to < 1/100)	Rare (⩾ 1/10,000 to < 1/1,000)
Immune system disorders			Drug hypersensitivity
Metabolism and nutrition disorders		Hyperkalaemia	
Psychiatric disorders		Libido decreased	
Nervous system disorders	Dizziness, headache	Postural dizziness, lethargy, paraesthesia, hypoaesthesia	Syncope
Ear and labyrinth disorders		Vertigo	
Cardiac disorders		Palpitations, Tachycardia	
Vascular disorders		Hypotension, orthostatic hypotension	
Respiratory, thoracic and mediastinal disorders		Dyspnoea, cough	
Gastro-intestinal disorders		Nausea, vomiting, dyspepsia, diarrhoea, constipation, dry mouth, upper abdominal pain	
Skin and subcutaneous tissue disorders		Rash	Urticaria
Musculoskeletal and connective tissue disorders		Muscle spasm, pain in extremity, back pain	
Renal and urinary disorders		Pollakiuria	
Reproductive system, and breast disorders		Erectile dysfunction	
General disorders and administration site conditions	Peripheral oedema, oedema, pitting oedema, fatigue	Asthenia	Face oedema
Investigations		Blood potassium decreased, blood creatinine increased, blood uric acid increased, gamma glutamyl transferase increased	

Further laboratory adverse events reported in clinical studies with olmesartan medoxomil monotherapy (irrespective of causality) were: Increased creatine phosphokinase, hypertriglyceridaemia, liver enzyme elevations.

In post-marketing experience with olmesartan medoxomil, additional adverse reactions reported, all at very rare frequency, were as follows: Thrombocytopenia, pruritus, exanthema, angioneurotic oedema, face oedema, allergic dermatitis, myalgia, acute renal failure, renal insufficiency, blood urea increased, malaise.

Single cases of rhabdomyolysis have been reported in temporal association with the intake of angiotensin II receptor blockers. A causal relationship, however, has not been established.

Additional information on special populations

In elderly patients the frequency of hypotension is slightly increased from rare to uncommon.

Amlodipine (active ingredient of Sevikar)

Further adverse reactions reported with amlodipine monotherapy were as follows:

Common additional adverse reactions are facial flushing and abdominal pain. Less common adverse reactions include: Leukocytopenia, thrombocytopenia, gynaecomastia, hyperglycaemia, sleep disorder, irritability, depression, confusion, mood changes including anxiety, malaise, tremor, increased sweating, taste changes, peripheral neuropathy, visual disturbances, tinnitus, chest pain, aggravation of angina pectoris, vasculitis, rhinitis, gingival hyperplasia, gastritis, elevated liver enzymes, jaundice, hepatitis, pancreatitis, increased micturition frequency, impotency, exanthema, pruritus, alopecia, skin discolouration, purpura, isolated cases of allergic reactions (pruritus, rash, angio-oedema, erythema exsudativum multiforme, exfoliative dermatitis, Stevens Johnson syndrome, Quincke oedema), myalgia, arthralgia, increase or decrease in weight. Isolated cases of myocardial infarction and arrhythmias (including extrasystole, ventricular tachycardia, bradycardia and atrial arrhythmias) and angina pectoris have been reported in patients with coronary artery disease, but a clear association with amlodipine has not been established.

4.9 Overdose

Symptoms:

There is no experience of overdose with Sevikar. The most likely effects of olmesartan medoxomil overdosage are hypotension and tachycardia; bradycardia could be encountered if parasympathetic (vagal) stimulation occurred. Amlodipine overdosage can be expected to lead to excessive peripheral vasodilatation with marked hypotension and possibly a reflex tachycardia. Marked and potentially prolonged systemic hypotension up to and including shock with fatal outcome has been reported.

Treatment:

If intake is recent, gastric lavage may be considered. In healthy subjects, the administration of activated charcoal immediately or up to 2 hours after ingestion of amlodipine has been shown to reduce substantially the absorption of amlodipine.

Clinically significant hypotension due to an overdose of Sevikar requires active support of the cardiovascular system, including close monitoring of heart and lung function, elevation of the extremities, and attention to circulating fluid volume and urine output. A vasoconstrictor may be helpful in restoring vascular tone and blood pressure, provided that there is no contraindication to its use. Intravenous calcium gluconate may be beneficial in reversing the effects of calcium channel blockade.

Since amlodipine is highly protein-bound, dialysis is not likely to be of benefit. The dialysability of olmesartan is unknown.

5. PHARMACOLOGICAL PROPERTIES

5.1 Pharmacodynamic properties

Pharmacotherapeutic group: Angiotensin II antagonists and calcium channel blockers, ATC code C09DB02.

Sevikar is a combination of an angiotensin II receptor antagonist, olmesartan medoxomil, and a calcium channel blocker, amlodipine besilate. The combination of these active ingredients has an additive antihypertensive effect, reducing blood pressure to a greater degree than either component alone.

Sevikar

In an 8-week, double-blind, randomised, placebo-controlled factorial design study in 1940 patients (71% Caucasian and 29% non-Caucasian patients), treatment with each combination dose of Sevikar resulted in significantly greater reductions in diastolic and systolic blood pressures than the respective monotherapy components. The mean change in systolic/diastolic blood pressure was dose-dependent: -24/-14 mmHg (20 mg/5 mg combination), -25/-16 mmHg (40 mg/5 mg combination) and -30/-19 mmHg (40 mg/10 mg combination).

Sevikar 40 mg/5 mg reduced seated systolic/diastolic blood pressure by an additional 2.5/1.7 mmHg over Sevikar 20 mg/5 mg. Similarly Sevikar 40 mg/10 mg reduced seated systolic/diastolic blood pressure by an additional 4.7/3.5 mmHg over Sevikar 40 mg/5 mg.

The proportions of patients reaching blood pressure goal (< 140/90 mmHg for non-diabetic patients and < 130/80 mmHg for diabetic patients) were 42.5%, 51.0% and 49.1% for Sevikar 20 mg/5 mg, 40 mg/5 mg and 40 mg/10 mg respectively.

The majority of the antihypertensive effect of Sevikar was generally achieved within the first 2 weeks of therapy.

A second double-blind, randomised, placebo-controlled study evaluated the effectiveness of adding amlodipine to the treatment in Caucasian patients whose blood pressure was inadequately controlled by 8 weeks of monotherapy with 20 mg olmesartan medoxomil.

In patients who continued to receive only 20 mg olmesartan medoxomil, systolic/diastolic blood pressure was reduced by -10.6/-7.8 mmHg after a further 8 weeks. The addition of 5 mg amlodipine for 8 weeks resulted in a reduction in systolic/diastolic blood pressure of -16.2/-10.6 mmHg ($p = 0.0006$).

The proportion of patients reaching blood pressure goal (< 140/90 mmHg for non-diabetic patients and < 130/80 mmHg for diabetic patients) was 44.5% for the 20 mg/5 mg combination compared to 28.5% for 20 mg olmesartan medoxomil.

A further study evaluated the addition of various doses of olmesartan medoxomil in Caucasian patients whose blood pressure was not adequately controlled by 8 weeks of monotherapy with 5 mg amlodipine.

In patients who continued to receive only 5 mg amlodipine, systolic/diastolic blood pressure was reduced by -9.9/-5.7 mmHg after a further 8 weeks. The addition of 20 mg olmesartan medoxomil resulted in a reduction in systolic/diastolic blood pressure of -15.3/-9.3 mmHg and the addition of 40 mg olmesartan medoxomil resulted in a reduction in systolic/diastolic blood pressure of -16.7/-9.5 mmHg ($p < 0.0001$).

The proportions of patients reaching blood pressure goal (< 140/90 mmHg for non-diabetic patients and < 130/80 mmHg for diabetic patients) was 29.9% for the group who continued to receive 5 mg amlodipine alone, 53.5% for Sevikar 20 mg/5 mg and 50.5% for Sevikar 40 mg/5 mg.

Randomised data in uncontrolled hypertensive patients, comparing the use of medium dose Sevikar combination therapy versus escalation to top dose monotherapy of amlodipine or olmesartan, are not available.

The three studies performed confirmed that the blood pressure lowering effect of Sevikar once daily was maintained throughout the 24-hour dose interval, with trough-to-peak ratios of 71% to 82% for systolic and diastolic response and with 24-hour effectiveness being confirmed by ambulatory blood pressure monitoring.

The antihypertensive effect of Sevikar was similar irrespective of age and gender, and was similar in patients with and without diabetes.

In two open-label, non-randomised extension studies, sustained efficacy using Sevikar 40 mg/5 mg was demonstrated at one year for 49 - 67% of patients.

Olmesartan medoxomil (active ingredient of Sevikar)

The olmesartan medoxomil component of Sevikar is a selective angiotensin II type 1 (AT_1) receptor antagonist. Olmesartan medoxomil is rapidly converted to the pharmacologically active metabolite, olmesartan. Angiotensin II is the primary vasoactive hormone of the renin-angiotensin-aldosterone system and plays a significant role in the pathophysiology of hypertension. The effects of angiotensin II include vasoconstriction, stimulation of the synthesis and release of aldosterone, cardiac stimulation and renal reabsorption of sodium. Olmesartan blocks the vasoconstrictor and aldosterone-secreting effects of angiotensin II by blocking its binding to the AT_1 receptor in tissues including vascular smooth muscle and the adrenal gland. The action of olmesartan is independent of the source or route of synthesis of angiotensin II. The selective antagonism of the angiotensin II (AT_1) receptors by olmesartan results in increases in plasma renin levels and angiotensin I and II concentrations, and some decrease in plasma aldosterone concentrations.

In hypertension, olmesartan medoxomil causes a dose-dependent, long-lasting reduction in arterial blood pressure. There has been no evidence of first-dose hypotension, of tachyphylaxis during long-term treatment, or of rebound hypertension after abrupt cessation of therapy.

Following once daily administration to patients with hypertension, olmesartan medoxomil produces an effective and smooth reduction in blood pressure over the 24 hour dose interval. Once daily dosing produced similar decreases in blood pressure as twice daily dosing at the same total daily dose.

With continuous treatment, maximum reductions in blood pressure are achieved by 8 weeks after the initiation of therapy, although a substantial proportion of the blood pressure lowering effect is already observed after 2 weeks of treatment.

The effect of olmesartan medoxomil on mortality and morbidity is not yet known.

Amlodipine (active ingredient of Sevikar)

The amlodipine component of Sevikar is a calcium channel blocker that inhibits the transmembrane influx of calcium ions through the potential-dependent L-type channels into the heart and smooth muscle. Experimental data indicate that amlodipine binds to both dihydropyridine and non-dihydropyridine binding sites. Amlodipine is relatively vessel-selective, with a greater effect on vascular smooth muscle cells than on cardiac muscle cells. The antihypertensive effect of amlodipine derives from a direct relaxant effect on arterial smooth muscle, which leads to a lowering of peripheral resistance and hence of blood pressure.

In hypertensive patients, amlodipine causes a dose-dependent, long-lasting reduction in arterial blood pressure. There has been no evidence of first-dose hypotension, of tachyphylaxis during long-term treatment, or of rebound hypertension after abrupt cessation of therapy.

Following administration of therapeutic doses to patients with hypertension, amlodipine produces an effective reduction in blood pressure in the supine, sitting and standing positions. Chronic use of amlodipine is not associated with significant changes in heart rate or plasma catecholamine levels. In hypertensive patients with normal renal function, therapeutic doses of amlodipine reduce renal vascular resistance and increase glomerular filtration rate and effective renal plasma flow, without changing filtration fraction or proteinuria.

In haemodynamic studies in patients with heart failure and in clinical studies based on exercise tests in patients with NYHA class II-IV heart failure, amlodipine was found not to cause any clinical deterioration, as measured by exercise tolerance, left ventricular ejection fraction and clinical signs and symptoms.

In a placebo-controlled study (PRAISE) designed to evaluate patients with NYHA class III-IV heart failure treated with digoxin, diuretics and ACE inhibitors, amlodipine was shown not to cause any increase in the risk of death or in the combined risk of mortality and morbidity in patients with heart failure.

A follow-up study (PRAISE 2) showed that amlodipine did not have an effect on the total or cardiovascular mortality of decompensatio cordis class III-IV patients without ischemic origin. In this study treatment with amlodipine was associated with an increase in pulmonary oedema, although this could not be related to an increase in symptoms.

5.2 Pharmacokinetic properties

Sevikar

Following oral intake of Sevikar, peak plasma concentrations of olmesartan and amlodipine are reached at 1.5 – 2 h and 6 – 8 hours, respectively. The rate and extent of absorption of the two active substances from Sevikar are equivalent to the rate and extent of absorption following intake of the two components as separate tablets. Food does not affect the bioavailability of olmesartan and amlodipine from Sevikar.

Olmesartan medoxomil (active ingredient of Sevikar)

Absorption and distribution:

Olmesartan medoxomil is a prodrug. It is rapidly converted to the pharmacologically active metabolite, olmesartan, by esterases in the gut mucosa and in portal blood during absorption from the gastrointestinal tract. No intact olmesartan medoxomil or intact side chain medoxomil moiety have been detected in plasma or excreta. The mean absolute bioavailability of olmesartan from a tablet formulation was 25.6%.

The mean peak plasma concentration (C_{max}) of olmesartan is reached within about 2 hours after oral dosing with olmesartan medoxomil, and olmesartan plasma concentrations increase approximately linearly with increasing single oral doses up to about 80 mg.

Food had minimal effect on the bioavailability of olmesartan and therefore olmesartan medoxomil may be administered with or without food.

No clinically relevant gender-related differences in the pharmacokinetics of olmesartan have been observed.

Olmesartan is highly bound to plasma protein (99.7%), but the potential for clinically significant protein binding displacement interactions between olmesartan and other highly bound coadministered active substances is low (as confirmed by the lack of a clinically significant interaction between olmesartan medoxomil and warfarin). The binding of olmesartan to blood cells is negligible. The mean volume of distribution after intravenous dosing is low (16 – 29 L).

Metabolism and elimination:

Total plasma clearance of olmesartan was typically 1.3 L/h (CV, 19%) and was relatively slow compared to hepatic blood flow (ca 90 L/h). Following a single oral dose of ^{14}C-labelled olmesartan medoxomil, 10% – 16% of the administered radioactivity was excreted in the urine (the vast majority within 24 hours of dose administration) and the remainder of the recovered radioactivity was excreted in the faeces. Based on the systemic availability of 25.6%, it can be calculated that absorbed olmesartan is cleared by both renal excretion (ca 40%) and hepato-biliary excretion (ca 60%). All recovered radioactivity was identified as olmesartan. No other significant metabolite was detected. Enterohepatic recycling of olmesartan is minimal. Since a large proportion of olmesartan is excreted via the biliary route, use in patients with biliary obstruction is contraindicated (see section 4.3).

The terminal elimination half life of olmesartan is between 10 and 15 hours after multiple oral dosing. Steady state is reached after the first few doses and no further accumulation is evident after 14 days of repeated dosing. Renal clearance is approximately 0.5 – 0.7 L/h and is independent of dose.

Amlodipine (active ingredient of Sevikar)

Absorption and distribution:

After oral administration of therapeutic doses, amlodipine is slowly absorbed from the gastrointestinal tract. The absorption of amlodipine is unaffected by the concomitant intake of food. The absolute bioavailability of the unchanged compound is estimated to be 64% – 80%. Peak plasma levels are reached 6 to 12 hours post-dose. The volume of distribution is about 20 L/kg. The pKa of amlodipine is 8.6. Plasma protein binding *in vitro* is approximately 98%.

Metabolism and elimination:

The plasma elimination half-life varies from 35 to 50 hours. Steady-state plasma levels are reached after 7 – 8 consecutive days. Amlodipine is extensively metabolised to inactive metabolites. About 60% of the administered dose is excreted in the urine, about 10% of which in the form of unchanged amlodipine.

Olmesartan medoxomil and amlodipine (active ingredients of Sevikar)

Special populations

Paediatric patients (age below 18 years):

No pharmacokinetic data in paediatric patients are available.

Elderly (age 65 years or over):

In hypertensive patients, the olmesartan AUC at steady state is increased by ca 35% in elderly patients (65 – 75 years old) and by ca 44% in very elderly patients (⩾ 75 years old) compared with the younger age group (see section 4.2). This may be at least in part related to a mean decrease in renal function in this group of patients. The recommended dosage regimen for elderly patients is, however, the same, although caution should be exercised when increasing the dosage.

Following oral intake of amlodipine, the time to peak plasma concentration is comparable in young and in elderly patients. In elderly patients, the clearance of amlodipine tends to decline, resulting in increases in AUC and in elimination half-life.

Renal impairment:

In renally impaired patients, the olmesartan AUC at steady state increased by 62%, 82% and 179% in patients with mild, moderate and severe renal impairment, respectively, compared to healthy controls (see sections 4.2, 4.4).

Amlodipine is extensively metabolised to inactive metabolites. Ten percent of the substance is excreted unchanged in the urine. Changes in amlodipine plasma concentration are not correlated with the degree of renal impairment. In these patients, amlodipine may be administered at the normal dosage. Amlodipine is not dialysable.

Hepatic impairment:

After single oral administration, olmesartan AUC values are 6% and 65% higher in mildly and moderately hepatically impaired patients, respectively, than in their corresponding matched healthy controls. The unbound fraction of olmesartan at 2 hours post-dose in healthy subjects, in patients with mild hepatic impairment and in patients with moderate hepatic impairment is 0.26%, 0.34% and 0.41%, respectively. Following repeated dosing in patients with moderate hepatic impairment, olmesartan mean AUC is again about 65% higher than in matched healthy controls. Olmesartan mean C_{max} values are similar in hepatically-impaired and healthy subjects. Olmesartan medoxomil has not been evaluated in patients with severe hepatic impairment (see sections 4.2, 4.4).

The clearance of amlodipine is decreased and the half-life is prolonged in patients with impaired hepatic function, resulting in an increase in AUC of about 40% – 60% (see sections 4.2, 4.4).

5.3 Preclinical safety data

Based on the non-clinical toxicity profile of each substance, no exacerbation of toxicities for the combination is expected, because each substance has different targets, i.e. the kidneys for olmesartan medoxomil and the heart for amlodipine.

In a 3-month, repeat-dose toxicity study of orally administered olmesartan medoxomil/amlodipine in combination in rats the following alterations were observed: decreases in red blood cell count-related parameters and kidney changes both of which might be induced by the olmesartan medoxomil component; alterations in the intestines (luminal dilatation and diffuse mucosal thickening of the ileum and colon), the adrenals (hypertrophy of the glomerular cortical cells and vacuolation of the fascicular cortical cells), and hypertrophy of the ducts in the mammary glands which might be induced by the amlodipine component. These alterations neither augmented any of the previously reported and existing toxicity of the individual agents nor induced any new toxicity, and no toxicologically synergistic effects were observed.

Olmesartan medoxomil (active ingredient of Sevikar)

In chronic toxicity studies in rats and dogs, olmesartan medoxomil showed similar effects to other AT_1 receptor antagonists and ACE inhibitors: raised blood urea (BUN) and creatinine; reduction in heart weight; reduction of red cell parameters (erythrocytes, haemoglobin, haematocrit); histological indications of renal damage (regenerative lesions of the renal epithelium, thickening of the basal membrane, dilatation of the tubules). These adverse effects caused by the pharmacological action of olmesartan medoxomil have also occurred in preclinical trials on other AT_1 receptor antagonists and ACE inhibitors and can be reduced by simultaneous oral administration of sodium chloride. In both species, increased plasma renin activity and hypertrophy/hyperplasia of the juxtaglomerular cells of the kidney were observed. These changes, which are a typical effect of the class of ACE inhibitors and other AT_1 receptor antagonists, would appear to have no clinical relevance.

Like other AT_1 receptor antagonists olmesartan medoxomil was found to increase the incidence of chromosome breaks in cell cultures *in vitro*. No relevant effects were observed in several *in vivo* studies using olmesartan medoxomil at very high oral doses of up to 2000 mg/kg. The overall data of a comprehensive genotoxicity testing programme suggest that olmesartan is very unlikely to exert genotoxic effects under conditions of clinical use.

Olmesartan medoxomil was not carcinogenic, in a 2-year study in rats nor in two 6-month carcinogenicity studies in transgenic mice.

In reproductive studies in rats, olmesartan medoxomil did not affect fertility and there was no evidence of a teratogenic effect. In common with other angiotensin II antagonists, survival of offspring was reduced following exposure to olmesartan medoxomil and pelvic dilatation of the kidney was seen after exposure of the dams in late pregnancy and lactation. In common with other antihypertensive agents, olmesartan medoxomil was shown to be more toxic to pregnant rabbits than to pregnant rats, however, there was no indication of a fetotoxic effect.

Amlodipine (active ingredient of Sevikar)

Preclinical data reveal no special hazard for humans based on conventional studies of safety pharmacology, repeated dose toxicity, genotoxicity and carcinogenic potential. In animal studies with respect to the reproduction in rats at high doses delayed parturition, difficult labour and impaired fetal and pup survival were seen.

6. PHARMACEUTICAL PARTICULARS

6.1 List of excipients

Tablet core:

Starch, pregelatinised maize

Silicified microcrystalline cellulose (microcrystalline cellulose with colloidal silicon dioxide)

Croscarmellose sodium

Magnesium stearate

Tablet coat:

Polyvinyl alcohol

Macrogol 3350

Talc

Titanium dioxide (E171)

Iron (III) oxide yellow (E172) (Sevikar 40 mg/5 mg and 40 mg/10 mg film-coated tablets only)

Iron (III) oxide red (E172) (Sevikar 40 mg/10 mg film-coated tablets only)

6.2 Incompatibilities

Not applicable.

6.3 Shelf life

3 years.

6.4 Special precautions for storage

This medicinal product does not require any special storage conditions.

6.5 Nature and contents of container

OPA / Aluminium / PVC / Aluminium blister.

Pack size: 28 film-coated tablets.

6.6 Special precautions for disposal and other handling

No special requirements.

7. MARKETING AUTHORISATION HOLDER

Daiichi Sankyo UK Ltd

Chiltern Place

Chalfont Park

Gerrards Cross

Buckinghamshire

SL9 0BG

UK

8. MARKETING AUTHORISATION NUMBER(S)

Sevikar 20 mg/5 mg film-coated tablet: PL 08265/0026

Sevikar 40 mg/5 mg film-coated tablet: PL 08265/0027

Sevikar 40 mg/10 mg film-coated tablet: PL 08265/0028

9. DATE OF FIRST AUTHORISATION/RENEWAL OF THE AUTHORISATION

29 October 2008

10. DATE OF REVISION OF THE TEXT

29 October 2008

Sevoflurane

(Abbott Laboratories Limited)

1. NAME OF THE MEDICINAL PRODUCT

Sevoflurane

2. QUALITATIVE AND QUANTITATIVE COMPOSITION

The finished product is comprised only of the active ingredient (Sevoflurane).

3. PHARMACEUTICAL FORM

Sevoflurane is a nonflammable volatile liquid. Sevoflurane is administered via inhalation of the vaporised liquid.

4. CLINICAL PARTICULARS

4.1 Therapeutic indications

Sevoflurane is indicated for induction and maintenance of general anaesthesia in adult and paediatric patients for inpatient and outpatient surgery.

4.2 Posology and method of administration

Sevoflurane should be delivered via a vaporiser specifically calibrated for use with Sevoflurane so that the concentration delivered can be accurately controlled. MAC (minimum alveolar concentration) values for Sevoflurane decrease with age and with the addition of nitrous oxide. The table below indicates average MAC values for different age groups.

MAC values for Adults and Paediatric patients according to age		
Age of Patient (years)	Sevoflurane in Oxygen	Sevoflurane in 65% N_2O/ 35% O_2 *
0 – 1 months	3.3%	2.0%**
1 - < 6 months	3.0%	
6 months - < 3 years	2.8%	
3 - 12	2.5%	
25	2.6%	1.4%
40	2.1%	1.1%
60	1.7%	0.9%
80	1.4%	0.7%

* Neonates are full term gestational age. MAC in premature infants has not been determined.

** In 1 – 3 year old paediatric patients, 60% N_2O/40% O_2 was used.

Induction:

Dosage should be individualised and titrated to the desired effect according to the patient's age and clinical status. A short acting barbiturate or other intravenous induction agent may be administered followed by inhalation of sevoflurane. Induction with sevoflurane may be achieved in oxygen or in combination with oxygen-nitrous oxide mixtures. In adults inspired concentrations of up to 5% Sevoflurane usually produce surgical anaesthesia in less than 2 minutes. In children, inspired concentrations of up to 7% Sevoflurane usually produce surgical anaesthesia in less than 2 minutes. Alternatively, for induction of anaesthesia in unpremedicated patients, inspired concentrations of up to 8% Sevoflurane may be used.

Maintenance:

Surgical levels of anaesthesia may be sustained with concentrations of 0.5 - 3% Sevoflurane with or without the concomitant use of nitrous oxide.

Elderly: As with other inhalation agents, lesser concentrations of Sevoflurane are normally required to maintain surgical anaesthesia.

Emergence:

Emergence times are generally short following Sevoflurane anaesthesia. Therefore, patients may require early post operative pain relief.

4.3 Contraindications

Sevoflurane should not be used in patients with known hypersensitivity to Sevoflurane or other halogenated anaesthetics. Sevoflurane is also contraindicated in patients with known or suspected genetic susceptibility to malignant hyperthermia.

Sevoflurane should not be used in patients with a history of unexplained moderate/severe hepatic dysfunction with jaundice, fever, and/or eosinophillia in association with halogenated anesthetics.

4.4 Special warnings and precautions for use

Sevoflurane should be administered only by persons trained in the administration of general anaesthesia. Facilities for maintenance of a patient airway, artificial ventilation, oxygen enrichment and circulatory resuscitation must be immediately available. Sevoflurane should be delivered via a vaporiser specifically calibrated for use with Sevoflurane so that the concentration delivered can be accurately controlled. Hypotension and respiratory depression increase as anaesthesia is deepened.

During the maintenance of anaesthesia, increasing the concentration of Sevoflurane produces dose-dependent decreases in blood pressure. Excessive decrease in blood pressure may be related to depth of anaesthesia and in such instances may be corrected by decreasing the inspired concentration of Sevoflurane.

As with all anaesthetics, particular care should be taken when selecting the dose for hypovolaemic, hypotensive or weakened patients.

As with all anaesthetics, maintenance of haemodynamic stability is important to avoid myocardial ischaemia in patients with coronary artery disease.

In patients at risk from elevation of intra-cranial pressure, Sevoflurane should be administered cautiously in conjunction with techniques to lower intra-cranial pressure (eg hyperventilation).

Caution should be observed when using Sevoflurane during obstetric anaesthesia because the relaxant effect on the uterus could increase the risk of uterine bleeding (see section 4.6).

Malignant Hyperthermia: In susceptible individuals, potent inhalation anaesthetic agents may trigger a skeletal muscle hypermetabolic state leading to high oxygen demand and the clinical syndrome known as malignant hyperthermia. Treatment includes discontinuation of triggering agents (e.g. Sevoflurane), administration of intravenous dantrolene sodium, and application of supportive therapy. Renal failure may appear later, and urine flow should be monitored and sustained if possible.

Use of inhaled anaesthetic agents has been associated with very rare increases in serum potassium levels that have resulted in cardiac arrhythmias and death in children during the postoperative period. The condition has been described in patients with latent as well as overt neuromuscular disease, particularly Duchenne muscular dystrophy. Use of suxamethonium has been associated with most, but not all of these cases. These patients showed evidence of muscle damage with increased serum creatine kinase concentration and myoglobinuria. These patients did NOT have classical signs of malignant hyperthermia such as muscle rigidity, rapid increase in body temperature, or increased oxygen uptake and carbon dioxide production. Prompt and vigorous treatment for hyperkalaemia and arrhythmias is recommended. Subsequent evaluation for latent neuromuscular disease is indicated.

Isolated cases of ventricular arrhythmia were reported in paediatric patients with Pompe's disease.

Observe caution in patients with underlying liver disease (see sections 4.3 and 4.8). Patients with repeated exposures to halogenated hydrocarbons, including Sevoflurane, within a relatively short interval may have an increased risk of hepatic injury.

Because of the small number of patients with renal insufficiency (baseline serum creatinine greater than 133μmol/litre) studied, the safety of Sevoflurane administration in this group has not been fully established. Therefore, Sevoflurane should be used with caution in patients with renal insufficiency. In some studies in rats, nephrotoxicity was seen in animals exposed to levels of Compound A (pentafluoroisopropenyl fluoromethyl ether (PIFE)) in excess of those usually seen in routine clinical practice. The mechanism of this renal toxicity in rats is unknown and its relevance to man has not been established. (See Section 5.3, Preclinical Safety Data for further details.)

Use of Sevoflurane has been an association with seizures occurring in children and young adults as well as older adults with and without predisposing risk factors. Clinical judgment is necessary before Sevoflurane is used in patients at risk of seizures. In children the depth of anaesthesia should be limited. EEG may permit the optimization of Sevoflurane dose and help avoid the development of seizure activity in patients with a predisposition for seizures (section 4.8).

Dystonic movements in children have been observed (see section 4.8).

The recovery from general anaesthesia should be assessed carefully before patients are discharged from the recovery room. Rapid emergence from anaesthesia is generally seen with Sevoflurane so early relief of post-operative pain may be required. Rapid emergence in children may be associated with agitation and lack of co-operation (in about 25% of cases).

Experience with repeat exposure to Sevoflurane is very limited. However, there were no obvious differences in adverse events between first and subsequent exposures.

Potential Interactions with CO_2 Absorbents

An exothermic reaction with degradation of volatile anaesthetics can occur when the carbon dioxide absorbent in the vaporizer becomes desiccated following an extended period of use as a result of dry gas flow through the circuit. Rare cases of extreme heat, smoke, and/or spontaneous fire in the anaesthesia machine have been reported during Sevoflurane use in conjunction with the use of desiccated CO_2 absorbent, specifically those containing potassium hydroxide (e.g Baralyme). An unusually delayed rise or unexpected decline of inspired Sevoflurane concentration compared to the vaporizer setting may be associated with excessive heating of the CO_2 absorbent canister.

Sevoflurane degradants were observed in the respiratory circuit of an experimental anaesthesia machine using desiccated CO_2 absorbents and maximum Sevoflurane concentrations (8%) for extended periods of time ($\geqslant$ 2 hours). Concentrations of formaldehyde observed at the anaesthesia respiratory circuit (using sodium hydroxide containing absorbents) were consistent with levels known to cause mild respiratory irritation. The clinical relevance of the degradants observed under this extreme experimental model is unknown.

It must be taken into account that the colour indicator does not always change after desiccation has taken place. If a health care professional suspects that the carbon dioxide absorbent has become desiccated, it must be replaced before subsequent use of volatile anesthetics (such as Sevoflurane).

4.5 Interaction with other medicinal products and other forms of interaction

The action of non-depolarising muscle relaxants is potentiated with Sevoflurane, therefore, when administered with Sevoflurane, dosage adjustments of these agents should be made.

Sevoflurane is similar to Isoflurane in the sensitisation of the myocardium to the arrhythmogenic effect of exogenously administered adrenaline.

MAC values for Sevoflurane decrease with the addition of nitrous oxide as indicated in the table on 'Effect of Age on MAC of Sevoflurane' (see Dosage and Method of Administration).

Benzodiazepines and opiates are expected to reduce Sevoflurane MAC. Opioids (e.g. alfentanil and sufentanil), used concomitantly with Sevoflurane, may lead to a synergistic fall in heart rate, blood pressure and respiratory rate.

As with other agents, lesser concentrations of Sevoflurane may be required following use of an intravenous anaesthetic e.g. propofol.

The metabolism of Sevoflurane may be increased by known inducers of CYP2E1 (e.g. isoniazid and alcohol), but it is not inducible by barbiturates.

Significant increases in plasma fluoride concentrations have been observed following the increased activity of CYP 2E1.

Sevoflurane may increase the negative inotropic, chronotropic and dromotropic effects of beta blockers (by blocking cardiovascular compensatory mechanisms).

4.6 Pregnancy and lactation

Pregnancy

Sevoflurane should only be used in pregnancy if clearly indicated.

It has a relaxant effect on the uterus, which can lead to increased uterine bleeding, as was reported in a study of its use during termination of pregnancy. Use during labour and delivery is limited to one small study in Caesarian section.

Animal studies indicate that Sevoflurane is not teratogenic.

Reproduction studies in rats and rabbits (doses up to 1 MAC) showed no effect on male and female reproductive capability. Reduced fetal body weight, with increased skeletal anomalies, were noted in rats at maternally toxic concentrations but no adverse fetal effects were noted in rabbit.

Lactation

Caution should be exercised when Sevoflurane is administered to nursing mothers as it is not known whether it is excreted in human milk.

4.7 Effects on ability to drive and use machines

As with other agents, patients should be advised that performance of activities requiring mental alertness, such as operating hazardous machinery, may be impaired for some time after general anaesthesia.

Patients should not be allowed to drive for a suitable period after Sevoflurane anaesthesia.

4.8 Undesirable effects

As with all potent inhaled anaesthetics, Sevoflurane may cause dose-dependent cardio-respiratory depression. Most adverse events are mild to moderate in severity and are transient in duration. Nausea and vomiting are commonly observed in the post-operative period, at a similar incidence to those found with other inhalation

Table 1

System Organ Class	Frequency	Adverse Reactions
Blood and lymphatic system disorders	Uncommon	Leukopenia Leukocytosis
Psychiatric disorders	Common*	Agitation
	Uncommon	Confusional state
Nervous system disorders	Common	Somnolence Dizziness Headache
Cardiac disorders	Very Common	Bradycardia
	Common	Tachycardia
	Uncommon	Atrioventricular block complete Atrial fibrillation Arrhythmia Ventricular extrasystoles Supraventricular extrasystoles Extrasystoles
Vascular disorders	Very Common	Hypotension
	Common	Hypertension
Respiratory, thoracic and mediastinal disorders	Very Common	Cough
	Common	Laryngospasm Respiratory disorder
	Uncommon	Apnoea Hypoxia Asthma
Gastrointestinal disorders	Very Common	Vomiting Nausea
	Common	Salivary hypersecretion
Renal and urinary disorders	Uncommon	Urinary retention Glycosuria
General disorders and administration site conditions	Common	Fever Hypothermia Chills
Investigations	Common	Aspartate aminotransferase increased Blood glucose abnormal Liver function test abnormal** White blood cell count abnormal Blood fluoride increased***
	Uncommon	Alanine aminotransferase increased Blood creatinine increased Blood lactate dehydrogenase increased

*Frequency is Very Common in paediatric population.

**Occasional cases of transient changes in hepatic function tests were reported with Sevoflurane and reference agents.

***Transient increases in serum inorganic fluoride levels may occur during and after Sevoflurane anaesthesia. Concentrations of inorganic fluoride generally peak within two hours of the end of Sevoflurane anaesthesia and return to normal within 48 hours to pre-operative levels. In clinical trials, elevated fluoride concentrations were not associated with impairment of renal function.

anaesthetics. These effects are common sequelae of surgery and general anaesthesia which may be due to the inhalational anaesthetic, other agents administered intra-operatively or post-operatively and to the patient's response to the surgical procedure.

Adverse event data are derived from controlled clinical trials conducted in the United States and Europe in over 3,200 patients. The type, severity and frequency of adverse events in Sevoflurane patients were comparable to adverse events in patients treated with other inhalation anaesthetics.

The most frequent adverse events associated with Sevoflurane overall were nausea (24%) and vomiting (17%). Agitation occurred frequently in children (23%).

All Adverse reactions at least possibly relating to Sevoflurane from clinical trials are presented in the following table by body system and frequency. The following frequency categories are used: Very common ($\geq$1/10); common ($\geq$1/100, <1/10); uncommon ($\geq$1/1,000, <1/100); rare ($\geq$1/10,000, <1/1,000); very rare (<1/10,000), including isolated reports. The type, severity and frequency of adverse reactions in Sevoflurane patients were comparable to adverse reactions in reference-drug patients.

(see Table 1 on previous page)

Post-marketing Experience

Adverse reactions have been spontaneously reported during post-approval use of Sevoflurane. These events are reported voluntarily from a population of an unknown rate of exposure. Therefore it is not possible to estimate the true incidence of adverse events.

Summary of Post-Marketing Adverse Drug Reactions

System Organ Class	Adverse Reactions
Immune system disorders	Anaphylactic reaction Anaphylactoid reaction Hypersensitivity
Nervous system disorders	Convulsion Dystonia
Respiratory, thoracic and mediastinal disorders	Pulmonary oedema Bronchospasm
Hepato-biliary disorders	Hepatitis Hepatic failure Hepatic necrosis
Skin and subcutaneous tissue disorders	Pruritus Rash Urticaria
Musculoskeletal and connective tissue disorders	Muscle twitching
Renal and Urinary disorders	Renal failure acute
General disorders and administration site conditions	Hyperthermia malignant

4.9 Overdose

In the event of overdosage, the following action should be taken: Stop drug administration, establish a clear airway and initiate assisted or controlled ventilation with pure oxygen and maintain adequate cardiovascular function.

5. PHARMACOLOGICAL PROPERTIES

5.1 Pharmacodynamic properties

Pharmaco-therapeutic group: Anaesthetics, general - ATC code: N01A

Changes in the clinical effects of Sevoflurane rapidly follow changes in the inspired concentration.

Cardiovascular Effects

As with all other inhalation agents Sevoflurane depresses cardiovascular function in a dose related fashion. In one volunteer study, increases in Sevoflurane concentration resulted in decrease in mean arterial pressure, but there was no change in heart rate. Sevoflurane did not alter plasma noradrenaline concentrations in this study.

Nervous System Effects

No evidence of seizure was observed during the clinical development programme.

In patients with normal intracranial pressure (ICP), Sevoflurane had minimal effect on ICP and preserved CO_2 responsiveness. The safety of Sevoflurane has not been investigated in patients with a raised ICP. In patients at risk for elevations of ICP, Sevoflurane should be administered cautiously in conjunction with ICP-reducing manoeuvres such as hyperventilation.

5.2 Pharmacokinetic properties

The low solubility of Sevoflurane in blood should result in alveolar concentrations which rapidly increase upon induction and rapidly decrease upon cessation of the inhaled agent.

In humans <5% of the absorbed Sevoflurane is metabolised. The rapid and extensive pulmonary elimination of Sevoflurane minimises the amount of anaesthetic available for metabolism. Sevoflurane is defluorinated via cytochrome p450(CYP)2E1 resulting in the production of hexafluoroisopropanol (HFIP) with release of inorganic fluoride and carbon dioxide (or a one carbon fragment). HFIP is then rapidly conjugated with glucuronic acid and excreted in the urine.

The metabolism of Sevoflurane may be increased by known inducers of CYP2E1 (e.g. isoniazid and alcohol), but it is not inducible by barbiturates.

Transient increases in serum inorganic fluoride levels may occur during and after Sevoflurane anaesthesia. Generally, concentrations of inorganic fluoride peak within 2 hours of the end of Sevoflurane anaesthesia and return within 48 hours to pre-operative levels.

5.3 Preclinical safety data

Animal studies have shown that hepatic and renal circulation are well maintained with Sevoflurane.

Sevoflurane decreases the cerebral metabolic rate for oxygen ($CMRO_2$) in a fashion analogous to that seen with isoflurane. An approximately 50% reduction of $CMRO_2$ is observed at concentrations approaching 2.0 MAC. Animal studies have demonstrated that Sevoflurane does not have a significant effect on cerebral blood flow.

In animals, Sevoflurane significantly suppresses electroencephalographic (EEG) activity comparable to equipotent doses of isoflurane. There is no evidence that Sevoflurane is associated with epileptiform activity during normocapnia or hypocapnia. In contrast to enflurane, attempts to elicit seizure-like EEG activity during hypocapnia with rhythmic auditory stimuli have been negative.

Compound A was minimally nephrotoxic at concentrations of 50-114 ppm for 3 hours in a range of studies in rats. The toxicity was characterised by sporadic single cell necrosis of the proximal tubule cells. The mechanism of this renal toxicity in rats is unknown and its relevance to man has not been established. Comparable human thresholds for Compound A-related nephrotoxicity would be predicted to be 150-200 ppm. The concentrations of Compound A found in routine clinical practice are on average 19 ppm in adults (maximum 32 ppm) with use of Soda lime as the CO_2 absorbent.

6. PHARMACEUTICAL PARTICULARS

6.1 List of excipients

Water (as a Lewis Acid Inhibitor).

6.2 Incompatibilities

Sevoflurane is stable when stored under normal room lighting conditions. No discernible degradation of Sevoflurane occurs in the presence of strong acids or heat. Sevoflurane is not corrosive to stainless steel, brass, aluminum, nickel-plated brass, chrome-plated brass or copper beryllium alloy.

Chemical degradation can occur upon exposure of inhaled anaesthetics to CO_2 absorbent within the anaesthesia machine. When used as directed with fresh absorbents, degradation of Sevoflurane is minimal and degradants are undetectable or non-toxic. Sevoflurane degradation and subsequent degradant formation are enhanced by increasing absorbent temperature, desiccated CO_2 absorbent (especially potassium hydroxide-containing, e.g. Baralyme®), increased Sevoflurane concentration and decreased fresh gas flow. Sevoflurane can undergo alkaline degradation by two pathways. The first results from the loss of hydrogen fluoride with the formation of pentafluoroisopropanyl fluoromethyl ether (PIFE or more commonly known as Compound A). The second pathway for degradation of Sevoflurane occurs only in the presence of desiccated CO_2 absorbents and leads to the dissociation of Sevoflurane into hexafluoroisopropanol (HFIP) and formaldehyde. HFIP is inactive, non-genotoxic, rapidly glucoronidated, cleared and has toxicity comparable to Sevoflurane. Formaldehyde is present during normal metabolic processes. Upon exposure to a highly desiccated absorbent, formaldehyde can further degrade into methanol and formate. Formate can contribute to the formation of carbon monoxide in the presence of high temperature. Methanol can react with compound A to form the methoxy addition product Compound B. Compound B can undergo further HF elimination to form Compounds C, D and E. With highly desiccated absorbents, especially those containing potassium hydroxide (e.g Baralyme®) the fomation of formaldehyde, methanol, carbon monoxide, Compound A and perhaps some of its degradants, Compounds B, C and D may occur.

6.3 Shelf life

The recommended shelf life is 36 months.

6.4 Special precautions for storage

Do not store above 25°C. Do not refrigerate. Keep cap tightly closed.

6.5 Nature and contents of container

100ml and 250ml amber polyethylene napthalate (PEN) bottles.

6.6 Special precautions for disposal and other handling

Sevoflurane should be administered via a vaporiser calibrated specifically for Sevoflurane using a key filling system designed for Sevoflurane specific vaporisers or other appropriate Sevoflurane specific vaporiser filling systems.

Carbon dioxide absorbents should not be allowed to dry out when inhalational anaesthetics are being administered. Some halogenated anaesthetics have been reported to interact with dry carbon dioxide absorbent to form carbon monoxide. However, in order to minimise the risk of formation of carbon monoxide in re-breathing circuits and the possibility of elevated carboxyhaemoglobin levels, CO_2 absorbents should not be allowed to dry out. There have been rare cases of excessive heat production, smoke and fire in the anaesthetic machine when Sevoflurane has been used in conjunction with a desiccated (dried out) CO_2 absorbent. If the CO_2 absorbent is suspected to be desiccated it should be replaced.

7. MARKETING AUTHORISATION HOLDER

Abbott Laboratories Ltd

Queenborough

Kent

ME11 5EL, UK.

8. MARKETING AUTHORISATION NUMBER(S)

PL 0037/0258

9. DATE OF FIRST AUTHORISATION/RENEWAL OF THE AUTHORISATION

1 September 1995

10. DATE OF REVISION OF THE TEXT

January 2009

Sevredol tablets 10mg, 20mg and 50mg

(Napp Pharmaceuticals Limited)

1. NAME OF THE MEDICINAL PRODUCT

Sevredol® tablets 10 mg, 20 mg, 50 mg.

2. QUALITATIVE AND QUANTITATIVE COMPOSITION

Morphine Sulphate 10 mg, 20 mg, 50 mg

For excipients see 6.1.

3. PHARMACEUTICAL FORM

Film-coated tablet.

10 mg

Blue, film-coated, capsule-shaped, biconvex tablet with a score line on one side. "IR" is marked on the left side and "10" on the right.

20 mg

Pink, film-coated, capsule-shaped, biconvex tablet with a score line on one side. "IR" is marked on the left side and "20" on the right.

50 mg

Pale, green film-coated, capsule-shaped, biconvex tablet with a score line on one side. "IR" is marked on the left side and "50" on the right.

4. CLINICAL PARTICULARS

4.1 Therapeutic indications

Sevredol tablets are indicated for the relief of severe pain.

4.2 Posology and method of administration

Route of administration

Oral.

Adults and children over 12 years.

The dosage of ***Sevredol*** tablets is dependent on the severity of pain and the patient's previous history of analgesic requirements. One tablet to be taken every four hours or as directed by a physician. Increasing severity of pain or tolerance to morphine will require increased dosage of ***Sevredol*** tablets using 10 mg, 20 mg or 50 mg alone or in combination to achieve the desired relief.

Patients receiving ***Sevredol*** tablets in place of parenteral morphine should be given a sufficiently increased dosage to compensate for any reduction in analgesic effects associated with oral administration. Usually such increased requirement is of the order of 100%. In such patients individual dose adjustments are required.

Elderly:

A reduction in adult dosage may be advisable.

Children 3 -12 years of age:

Only ***Sevredol*** 10 mg and 20 mg tablets are suitable for children:-

3 - 5 years	5 mg, 4-hourly
6 -12 years	5 -10 mg, 4-hourly

Sevredol tablets 50 mg are not recommended for children.

4.3 Contraindications

Hypersensitivity to any of the constituents, respiratory depression, head injury, obstructive airways disease, paralytic ileus, acute abdomen, delayed gastric emptying, known morphine sensitivity, acute hepatic disease, concurrent administration of mono-amine oxidase inhibitors or within two weeks of discontinuation of their use. Not recommended during pregnancy.

Not recommended for children below 3 years of age.

4.4 Special warnings and precautions for use

The major risk of opioid excess is respiratory depression.

As with all narcotics a reduction in dosage may be advisable in the elderly, in hypothyroidism, in renal and chronic hepatic disease. Use with caution in patients with impaired respiratory function, convulsive disorders, acute alcoholism, delirium tremens, raised intracranial pressure, hypotension with hypovolaemia, severe cor pulmonale, opioid dependent patients, patients with a history of substance abuse, diseases of the biliary tract, pancreatitis, inflammatory bowel disorders, prostatic hypertrophy, adrenocortical insufficiency, ***Sevredol*** tablets should not be used where there is a possibility of paralytic ileus occurring. Should paralytic ileus be suspected or occur during use, ***Sevredol*** tablets should be discontinued immediately.

Morphine may lower the seizure threshold in patients with a history of epilepsy.

Patients with rare hereditary problems of galactose intolerance, the Lapp lactase deficiency or glucose-galactose malabsorption should not take this medicine.

Patients about to undergo additional pain relieving procedures (e.g. surgery, plexus blockade) should not receive ***Sevredol*** tablets for 4 hours prior to the intervention. If further treatment with ***Sevredol*** tablets is indicated then the dosage should be adjusted to new post-operative requirements. ***Sevredol*** tablets should be used with caution pre-operatively and within the first 24 hours post-operatively. ***Sevredol*** tablets should also be used with caution following abdominal surgery as morphine impairs intestinal motility and should not be used until the physician is assured of normal bowel function.

The patient may develop tolerance to the drug with chronic use and require progressively higher doses to maintain pain control. Prolonged use of this product may lead to physical dependence and a withdrawal syndrome may occur upon abrupt cessation of therapy. When a patient no longer requires therapy with morphine, it may be advisable to taper the dose gradually to prevent symptoms of withdrawal

Morphine has an abuse profile similar to other strong agonist opioids. Morphine may be sought and abused by people with latent or manifest addiction disorders. The product should be used with particular care in patients with a history of alcohol and drug abuse.

Abuse of oral dosage forms by parenteral administration can be expected to result in serious adverse events, which may be fatal.

4.5 Interaction with other medicinal products and other forms of interaction

Morphine should be used with caution in patients who are concurrently receiving other central nervous system depressants including sedatives or hypnotics, general anaesthetics, phenothiazines, other tranquilisers, muscle relaxants, antihypertensives and alcohol. Interactive effects resulting in respiratory depression, hypotension, profound sedation, or coma may result if these drugs are taken in combination with the usual doses of morphine.

Mixed agonist/antagonist opioid analgesics (e.g. buprenorphine, nalbuphine, pentazocine) should not be administered to a patient who has received a course of therapy with a pure opioid agonist analgesic.

Cimetidine inhibits the metabolism of morphine.

Monoamine oxidase inhibitors are known to interact with narcotic analgesics producing CNS excitation or depression with hyper- or hypotensive crisis. Morphine should not be co-administered with monoamine oxidase inhibitors or within two weeks of such therapy.

Plasma concentrations of morphine may be reduced by rifampicin.

Although there are no pharmacokinetic data available for concomitant use of ritonavir with morphine, ritonavir induces the hepatic enzymes responsible for the glucuronidation of morphine, and may possibly decrease plasma concentrations of morphine.

4.6 Pregnancy and lactation

Sevredol tablets are not recommended during pregnancy and labour due to the risk of neonatal respiratory depression. Administration to nursing mothers is not recommended as morphine is excreted in breast milk. Withdrawal symptoms may be observed in the new born of mothers undergoing chronic treatment.

4.7 Effects on ability to drive and use machines

Treatment with ***Sevredol*** tablets may cause sedation and it is not recommended that patients drive or use machines if they experience drowsiness.

4.8 Undesirable effects

In normal doses, the commonest side effects of morphine are nausea, vomiting, constipation and drowsiness. With chronic therapy, nausea and vomiting are unusual with ***Sevredol*** tablets but should they occur the tablets can be readily combined with an anti-emetic if required. Constipation may be treated with appropriate laxatives.

Common (incidence of ⩾ 1%) and Uncommon (incidence of < 1%) adverse drug reactions are listed in the table below:

Body System	Common (⩾ 1%)	Uncommon (< 1%)
Immune system disorders		Allergic reaction Anaphylactic reaction Anaphylactoid reaction
Psychiatric disorders	Confusion Insomnia Thinking disturbances	Agitation Drug dependence Dysphoria Euphoria Hallucinations Mood altered
Nervous system disorders	Headache Involuntary muscle contractions Myoclonus Somnolence	Convulsions Hypertonia Paraesthesia Syncope Vertigo
Eye disorders		Miosis Visual disturbance
Cardiac disorders		Bradycardia Palpitations Tachycardia
Vascular disorders		Facial flushing Hypertension Hypotension
Respiratory, thoracic and mediastinal disorders	Bronchospasm Cough decreased	Pulmonary oedema Respiratory depression
Gastrointestinal disorders	Abdominal pain Anorexia Constipation Dry mouth Dyspepsia Nausea Vomiting	Gastrointestinal disorders Ileus Taste perversion
Hepatobiliary disorders	Exacerbation of pancreatitis	Biliary pain Increased hepatic enzymes
Skin and subcutaneous tissue disorders	Hyperhidrosis Rash	Urticaria
Renal and urinary disorders		Ureteric spasm Urinary retention
Reproductive system and breast disorders		Amenorrhoea Decreased libido Erectile dysfunction
General disorders and administration site conditions	Asthenia Pruritus	Drug tolerance Drug withdrawal syndrome Malaise Peripheral oedema

The effects of morphine have led to its abuse and dependence may develop with regular, inappropriate use. This is not a major concern in the treatment of patients with severe pain.

4.9 Overdose

Signs of morphine toxicity and overdosage are pin-point pupils, skeletal muscle flaccidity, bradycardia, respiratory depression and hypotension. Circulatory failure and deepening coma may occur in more severe cases. Rhabdomyolysis progressing to renal failure has been reported in opioid overdosage.

Treatment of morphine overdosage:

Primary attention should be given to the establishment of a patent airway and institution of assisted or controlled ventilation.

The pure opioid antagonists are specific antidotes against the effects of opioid overdose. Other supportive measures should be employed as needed.

In the case of massive overdosage, administer naloxone 0.8 mg intravenously. Repeat at 2-3 minute intervals as necessary, or by an infusion of 2 mg in 500 ml of normal saline or 5% dextrose (0.004 mg/ml).

The infusion should be run at a rate related to the previous bolus doses administered and should be in accordance with the patient's response. However, because the duration of action of naloxone is relatively short, the patient must be carefully monitored until spontaneous respiration is reliably re-established.

For less severe overdosage, administer naloxone 0.2 mg intravenously followed by increments of 0.1 mg every 2 minutes if required.

Naloxone should not be administered in the absence of clinically significant respiratory or circulatory depression secondary to morphine overdosage. Naloxone should be administered cautiously to persons who are known, or suspected, to be physically dependent on morphine. In such cases, an abrupt or complete reversal of opioid effects may precipitate an acute withdrawal syndrome.

Gastric contents may need to be emptied as this can be useful in removing unabsorbed drug.

5. PHARMACOLOGICAL PROPERTIES

5.1 Pharmacodynamic properties

Pharmacotherapeutic group: natural opium alkaloid

ATC code: N02A A01

Morphine acts as an agonist at opiate receptors in the CNS particularly mu and to a lesser extent kappa receptors. mu receptors are thought to mediate supraspinal analgesia, respiratory depression and euphoria and kappa receptors, spinal analgesia, miosis and sedation.

Central Nervous System

The principal actions of therapeutic value of morphine are analgesia and sedation (i.e., sleepiness and anxiolysis). Morphine produces respiratory depression by direct action on brain stem respiratory centers.

Morphine depresses the cough reflex by direct effect on the cough center in the medulla. Antitussive effects may occur with doses lower than those usually required for analgesia. Morphine causes miosis, even in total darkness. Pinpoint pupils are a sign of narcotic overdose but are not pathognomonic (e.g., pontine lesions of hemorrhagic or ischemic origin may produce similar findings). Marked mydriasis rather than miosis may be seen with hypoxia in the setting of morphine overdose.

Gastrointestinal Tract and Other Smooth Muscle

Morphine causes a reduction in motility associated with an increase in smooth muscle tone in the antrum of the stomach and duodenum. Digestion of food in the small intestine is delayed and propulsive contractions are decreased. Propulsive peristaltic waves in the colon are decreased, while tone is increased to the point of spasm resulting in constipation.

Morphine generally increases smooth muscle tone, especially the sphincters of the gastrointestinal and biliary tracts. Morphine may produce spasm of the sphincter of Oddi, thus raising intrabiliary pressure.

Cardiovascular System

Morphine may produce release of histamine with or without associated peripheral vasodilation. Manifestations of histamine release and/or peripheral vasodilation may include pruritus, flushing, red eyes, sweating, and/or orthostatic hypotension.

Endocrine System

Opioids may influence the hypothalamic-pituitary-adrenal or -gonadal axes. Some changes that can be seen include an increase in serum prolactin, and decreases in plasma cortisol, oestrogen and testosterone in association with inappropriately low or normal ACTH, LH or FSH levels. Clinical symptoms may be manifest from these hormonal changes.

Other Pharmacologic Effects

In vitro and animal studies indicate various effects of natural opioids, such as morphine, on components of the immune system; the clinical significance of these findings is unknown.

5.2 Pharmacokinetic properties

Morphine is well absorbed from ***Sevredol*** tablets, however first pass metabolism does occur. Apart from the liver, metabolism also occurs in the kidney and intestinal mucosa. The major urinary metabolite is morphine-3-glucuronide but morphine-6-glucuronide is also formed. The half life for morphine in the plasma is approximately 2.5 - 3.0 hours.

5.3 Preclinical safety data

There are no pre-clinical data of relevance to the prescriber which are additional to that already included in other sections of the SPC.

6. PHARMACEUTICAL PARTICULARS

6.1 List of excipients

<u>Tablet core</u>

Lactose (anhydrous)

Pregelatinised maize starch

Povidone

Purified water

Magnesium stearate

Talc

<u>Film coat</u>

10 mg tablet: Opadry (blue) 06B20843 containing Macrogol 400, E464, E133, E171
Purified water

20 mg tablet: Hypromellose (5 cps)
Hypromellose (15 cps)
Macrogol 400
Opaspray (pink) M-1-5503 containing E171, E127, E110
Purified water

50 mg tablet: Opadry OY-21037 Green (containing hypromellose E464, titanium dioxide E171, macrogol 400, quinoline yellow E104, indigo carmine E132, iron oxide yellow E172)

6.2 Incompatibilities

None known.

6.3 Shelf life

Three years.

6.4 Special precautions for storage

Do not store above 30°C.

6.5 Nature and contents of container

PVdC coated PVC blister packs and polypropylene containers with polyethylene lids containing 56 and 112 tablets.

Medical sample packs containing up to 24 tablets are also available.

6.6 Special precautions for disposal and other handling

None

7. MARKETING AUTHORISATION HOLDER

Napp Pharmaceuticals Ltd

Cambridge Science Park

Milton Road

Cambridge CB4 0GW

8. MARKETING AUTHORISATION NUMBER(S)

PL 16950/0063-0065

9. DATE OF FIRST AUTHORISATION/RENEWAL OF THE AUTHORISATION

1 May 1999/22 March 2003

10. DATE OF REVISION OF THE TEXT

November 2007

11 LEGAL CATEGORY

CD (Sch 2), POM

® The Napp device and ***Sevredol*** are Registered Trade Marks.

Silkis 3 micrograms per g ointment

(Galderma (U.K) Ltd)

1. NAME OF THE MEDICINAL PRODUCT

Silkis 3 micrograms per g ointment

2. QUALITATIVE AND QUANTITATIVE COMPOSITION

One gram of ointment contains 3 micrograms of calcitriol (INN).

For a full list of excipients, see section 6.1

3. PHARMACEUTICAL FORM

Ointment

White, translucent ointment

4. CLINICAL PARTICULARS

4.1 Therapeutic indications

Topical treatment of mild to moderately severe plaque psoriasis (psoriasis vulgaris) with up to 35% of body surface area involvement.

4.2 Posology and method of administration

Silkis Ointment should be applied to the psoriasis affected areas twice per day, once in the morning and once in the evening before retiring and after washing. It is recommended that not more than 35% of the body surface be exposed to daily treatment. Not more than 30 g of ointment should be used per day. There is limited clinical experience available for the use of this dosage regimen of more than 6 weeks.

There is no experience of the use of Silkis in children (see 4.4. Special Warnings and Precautions for Use). Patients with kidney or liver dysfunction should not use Silkis (see also 4.3. Contra-indications).

4.3 Contraindications

Patients on systemic treatment of calcium homeostasis.

Patients with kidney or liver dysfunction.

Patients with hypercalcaemia and patients known to suffer from abnormal calcium metabolism.

Silkis must not be used in patients known to be hypersensitive to the active substance or to any of the excipients.

4.4 Special warnings and precautions for use

The ointment can be applied to the face with caution, as there is an increased risk of irritation in this area. Contact with the eyes should be avoided. The hands should be washed after applying the ointment in order to avoid unintentional application to non lesional areas. Not more than 35% of the body surface should be exposed to daily treatment. Not more than 30g of ointment should be used per day.

Due to potential effects on calcium metabolism, substances which stimulate absorption must not be added to the ointment, and the ointment must not be covered with an occlusive dressing.

In case of severe irritation or contact allergy, the treatment with Silkis should be discontinued and the patient should obtain medical advice. If contact allergy is demonstrated this discontinuation is definitive.

In view of the particular sensitivity of neonatal versus adult rodents to the toxic effects of calcitriol, exposure of children to calcitriol ointment should be avoided (see also 4.2. Posology and Method of administration)

Although no clinically significant hypercalcaemia was observed in clinical studies with a dosage under 30 g/day of Silkis ointment, some absorption of calcitriol through the skin does occur and excessive use of the ointment can lead to systemic side-effects, such as an increase in urine and serum calcium levels.

There is no information about the use of Silkis in other clinical forms of psoriasis (other than plaque psoriasis) *i.e.* Psoriasis guttata acuta, pustular psoriasis, psoriasis erythrodermica and rapid progressive plaque psoriasis.

4.5 Interaction with other medicinal products and other forms of interaction

Silkis must be used with caution in patients receiving medications known to increase the serum calcium level, such as thiazide diuretics. Caution must also be exercised in patients receiving calcium supplements or high doses of vitamin D. There is no experience of the concurrent use of calcitriol and other medications for the treatment of psoriasis.

Information of interaction of systemic medications after the use of calcitriol ointment is limited. As no relevant elevation of plasma level is seen after the use of calcitriol on the skin, interaction with systemic medication is unlikely.

Silkis Ointment has a slight irritant potential, and therefore, it is possible that concomitant use of peeling agents, astringents or irritants products may produce additive irritant effects.

4.6 Pregnancy and lactation

Use during Pregnancy:

There are no adequate data from the use of Silkis in pregnant women. Studies in animals have shown developmental toxicity at doses which caused maternal toxicity (see section 5.3). The potential risk for humans is unknown.

Silkis should only be used during pregnancy in restricted amounts when clearly necessary. Calcium levels should be monitored.

Use during Lactation:

Calcitriol has been found in milk of lactating dams. Due to the lack of human data, it should not be used during breastfeeding.

4.7 Effects on ability to drive and use machines

No effects on ability to drive and use machines have been observed.

4.8 Undesirable effects

Between 10% and 20% of patients can be expected to experience adverse reactions. Adverse reactions are usually localised to the application site and mild to moderate in nature.

Very common adverse reactions: Adverse reactions occurring in ⩾1/10 of patients.
Common adverse reactions: Adverse reactions occurring in ⩾1/100, <1/10 of patients.
Uncommon adverse reactions: Adverse reactions occurring in ⩾1/1000, <1/100 of patients.
Rare adverse reactions: Adverse reactions occurring in ⩾1/10000; <1/1000 of patients.
Very rare adverse reactions: Adverse reactions occurring in <1/10000 of patients
Adverse reactions reported by more than two patients in the clinical studies are included.

System Organ Class	Frequency	Preferred term
Skin and Subcutaneous disorders	Common	Pruritus, Skin discomfort, Skin irritation, Erythema
	Uncommon	Dry skin, Psoriasis (aggravated)

In case of severe irritation or contact allergy, the treatment with Silkis should be discontinued and the patient should obtain medical advice. If contact allergy is demonstrated this discontinuation is definitive.

4.9 Overdose

The most common symptoms which may occur after accidental administration are anorexia, nausea, vomiting, constipation, hypotonia and depression. Lethargy and coma are occasionally observed. If hypercalcaemia or hypercalciuria occurs, the use of Silkis should be discontinued until the serum or urinary calcium levels have returned to normal.

If the medication is applied excessively no more rapid or better results will be obtained and marked redness, peeling or discomfort may occur.

5. PHARMACOLOGICAL PROPERTIES

5.1 Pharmacodynamic properties

ATC code: D 05AX03

Calcitriol inhibits the proliferation and stimulates differentiation of keratinocytes. Calcitriol inhibits proliferation of T-cells and normalises the production of various inflammation factors.

Topical administration of Silkis Ointment to patients with plaque psoriasis results in an improvement of the skin lesions. This effect is noted from 4 weeks after the start of treatment.

5.2 Pharmacokinetic properties

The mean absorption of calcitriol is estimated at around 10%. Following absorption, both unchanged calcitriol and metabolites have been demonstrated in plasma. The effect of the metabolites on calcium homeostasis is negligible. In most patients, circulating levels of exogenous calcitriol are below the level of detection (2pg/ml).

In clinical trials, no relevant increase in plasma calcitriol levels after treatment of large body surface areas of up to 6000 cm^2 (35% body surface area) was noted.

5.3 Preclinical safety data

Animal studies show that repeated excessive exposure to calcitriol leads to renal failure and tissue calcification due to hypervitaminosis D associated with hypercalciuria, hypercalcaemia, and hyperphosphataemia.

No indication of teratogenicity was observed in embryo-foetal toxicity studies designed to assess the teratogenic potential of calcitriol. Some evidence of developmental toxicity was obtained in a cutaneous rabbit study at doses which caused maternal toxicity. No such effect was found in rats.

Local toxicity studies in animals with Calcitriol showed slight skin and eye irritation.

6. PHARMACEUTICAL PARTICULARS

6.1 List of excipients

Liquid paraffin, white soft paraffin and alpha- tocopherol.

6.2 Incompatibilities

There are no relevant data on the compatibility of Silkis with other medicinal products. Therefore, Silkis should be used according to the posology and method of administration provided above (Section 4.2), and should not be mixed with other medicinal products.

6.3 Shelf life

3 years

Shelf life after first opening: 8 weeks.

6.4 Special precautions for storage

No special precautions for storage.

6.5 Nature and contents of container

The product is packaged in collapsible aluminium tubes coated internally with an epoxy - phenolic resin and fitted with a white high density polyethylene or polypropylene screw cap. Tubes contain either 15, 30 or 100g of ointment.

Not all pack sizes may be marketed.

6.6 Special precautions for disposal and other handling

None.

7. MARKETING AUTHORISATION HOLDER

Galderma (UK) Limited

Meridien House

69-71 Clarendon Road

Watford

Herts

WD17 1DS

UK

8. MARKETING AUTHORISATION NUMBER(S)

PL 10590/0047

9. DATE OF FIRST AUTHORISATION/RENEWAL OF THE AUTHORISATION

10.07.1995 / 09.02.2004

10. DATE OF REVISION OF THE TEXT

03/08/2009

Sinemet 62.5, 110, Plus and 275 Tablets

(Merck Sharp & Dohme Limited)

1. NAME OF THE MEDICINAL PRODUCT

SINEMET®-62.5 Tablets

SINEMET®-110 Tablets

SINEMET®-Plus Tablets

SINEMET®-275 Tablets

2. QUALITATIVE AND QUANTITATIVE COMPOSITION

Each tablet of 'Sinemet-62.5' contains 13.5 mg carbidopa (equivalent to 12.5 mg of anhydrous carbidopa) and 50 mg levodopa.

Each tablet of 'Sinemet-110' contains 10.8 mg carbidopa (equivalent to 10 mg of anhydrous carbidopa) and 100 mg levodopa.

Each tablet of 'Sinemet-Plus' contains 27.0 mg carbidopa (equivalent to 25 mg of anhydrous carbidopa) and 100 mg levodopa.

Each tablet of 'Sinemet-275' contains 27.0 mg carbidopa (equivalent to 25 mg of anhydrous carbidopa) and 250 mg levodopa.

3. PHARMACEUTICAL FORM

Tablets.

'Sinemet-62.5': yellow, oval-shaped tablets, one side scored and the other marked '520'.

'Sinemet-110': dapple blue, oval-shaped tablets, one side plain and the other scored and marked '647'.

'Sinemet-Plus': yellow, oval-shaped tablets, one side plain and the other scored and marked'650'.

'Sinemet-275': light dapple blue, oval-shaped tablets, one side plain and the other scored and marked '654'.

For excipients see 6.1.

4. CLINICAL PARTICULARS

4.1 Therapeutic indications

Antiparkinsonian agent.

For treatment of Parkinson's disease and syndrome.

4.2 Posology and method of administration

To be taken orally.

The optimum daily dosage of 'Sinemet' must be determined by careful titration in each patient.

'Sinemet' Tablets are available in a ratio of 1:4 or 1:10 of carbidopa to levodopa to provide facility for fine dosage titration for each patient.

General Considerations

Studies show that the peripheral dopa-decarboxylase is fully inhibited (saturated) by carbidopa at doses between 70 and 100 mg a day. Patients receiving less than this amount of carbidopa are more likely to experience nausea and vomiting.

Standard antiparkinsonian drugs, other than levodopa alone, may be continued while 'Sinemet' is being administered, although their dosage may have to be adjusted.

Because both therapeutic and adverse effects are seen more rapidly with 'Sinemet' than with levodopa, patients should be carefully monitored during the dosage adjustment period. Involuntary movements, particularly blepharospasm, are a useful early sign of excess dosage in some patients.

Patients not receiving levodopa

Dosage may be best initiated with one tablet of 'Sinemet-Plus' three times a day. This dosage schedule provides 75 mg of carbidopa per day. Dosage may be increased by one tablet of 'Sinemet-62.5' or 'Sinemet-Plus' every day or every other day, as necessary, until a dosage equivalent of eight tablets of 'Sinemet-Plus' a day is reached.

If 'Sinemet-110' or 'Sinemet-62.5' is used, dosage may be initiated with one tablet three or four times a day. Titration upward may be required in some patients to achieve optimum dosage of carbidopa. The dosage may be increased by one tablet every day or every other day until a total of eight tablets (two tablets q.d.s.) is reached.

For patients starting with 'Sinemet-275', the initial dose is one-half tablet taken once or twice daily. However, this may not provide the optimal amount of carbidopa needed by many patients. If necessary, add one-half tablet every day or every other day until optimal response is reached.

Response has been observed in one day, and sometimes after one dose. Fully effective doses usually are reached within seven days as compared to weeks or months with levodopa alone.

'Sinemet-62.5' or 'Sinemet-110' may be used to facilitate dosage titration according to the needs of the individual patient.

Patients receiving levodopa

Discontinue levodopa at least 12 hours (24 hours for slow-release preparations) before starting therapy with 'Sinemet'. The easiest way to do this is to give 'Sinemet' as the first morning dose after a night without any levodopa. The dose of 'Sinemet' should be approximately 20% of the previous daily dosage of levodopa.

Patients taking less than 1,500 mg levodopa a day should be started on one tablet of 'Sinemet-Plus' three or four times a day dependent on patient need. The suggested starting dose for most patients taking more than 1,500 mg levodopa a day is one tablet of 'Sinemet-275' three or four times a day.

Maintenance

Therapy with 'Sinemet' should be individualised and adjusted gradually according to response. When a greater proportion of carbidopa is required, each tablet of 'Sinemet-110' may be replaced with a tablet of 'Sinemet-Plus' or 'Sinemet-62.5'.

When more levodopa is required, 'Sinemet-275' should be substituted at a dosage of one tablet three or four times a day. If necessary, the dosage of 'Sinemet-275' may be increased by half to one tablet every other day to a maximum of eight tablets a day. Experience with a total daily dosage greater than 200 mg carbidopa is limited.

Patients receiving levodopa with another decarboxylase inhibitor

When transferring a patient to 'Sinemet' from levodopa combined with another decarboxylase inhibitor, discontinue dosage at least 12 hours before 'Sinemet' is started. Begin with a dosage of 'Sinemet' that will provide the same amount of levodopa as contained in the other levodopa/decarboxylase inhibitor combination.

Patients receiving other antiparkinsonian agents

Current evidence indicates that other antiparkinsonian agents may be continued when 'Sinemet' is introduced, although dosage may have to be adjusted in line with manufacturers recommendations.

Use in children

The safety of 'Sinemet' in patients under 18 years of age has not been established and its use in patients below the age of 18 is not recommended.

Use in the elderly

There is wide experience in the use of this product in elderly patients. The recommendations set out above reflect the clinical data derived from this experience.

4.3 Contraindications

Nonselective monoamine oxidase (MAO) inhibitors are contraindicated for use with 'Sinemet'. These inhibitors must be discontinued at least two weeks before starting 'Sinemet'. 'Sinemet' may be administered concomitantly with the manufacturer's recommended dose of an MAO inhibitor with selectivity for MAO type B (e.g. selegiline hydrochloride). (See 4.5 'Interaction with other medicinal products and other forms of interaction'.)

'Sinemet' is contraindicated in patients with narrow-angle glaucoma and in patients with known hypersensitivity to any component of this medication.

Since levodopa may activate a malignant melanoma, it should not be used in patients with suspicious undiagnosed skin lesions or a history of melanoma.

Use in patients with severe psychoses.

See also 4.6 'Pregnancy and lactation'.

4.4 Special warnings and precautions for use

'Sinemet' is not recommended for the treatment of drug-induced extrapyramidal reactions.

'Sinemet' should be administered cautiously to patients with severe cardiovascular or pulmonary disease, bronchial asthma, renal, hepatic or endocrine disease, or history of peptic ulcer disease (because of the possibility of upper gastro-intestinal haemorrhage).

Care should be exercised when 'Sinemet' is administered to patients with a history of myocardial infarction who have residual atrial nodal, or ventricular arrhythmias. Cardiac function should be monitored with particular care in such patients during the period of initial dosage adjustment.

Levodopa has been associated with somnolence and episodes of sudden sleep onset. Sudden onset of sleep during daily activities, in some cases without awareness or warning signs, has been reported very rarely. Patients must be informed of this and advised to exercise caution while driving or operating machines during treatment with levodopa. Patients who have experienced somnolence and/or an episode of sudden sleep onset must refrain from driving or operating machines. Furthermore a reduction of dosage or termination of therapy may be considered.

All patients should be monitored carefully for the development of mental changes, depression with suicidal tendencies, and other serious antisocial behaviour. Patients with current psychoses should be treated with caution.

Dyskinesias may occur in patients previously treated with levodopa alone because carbidopa permits more levodopa to reach the brain and, thus, more dopamine to be formed. The occurrence of dyskinesias may require dosage reduction.

As with levodopa, 'Sinemet' may cause involuntary movements and mental disturbances. Patients with a history of severe involuntary movements or psychotic episodes when treated with levodopa alone should be observed carefully when 'Sinemet' is substituted. These reactions are thought to be due to increased brain dopamine following administration of levodopa, and use of 'Sinemet' may cause a recurrence. A syndrome resembling the neuroleptic malignant syndrome including muscular rigidity, elevated body temperature, mental changes and increased serum creatine phosphokinase has been reported with the abrupt withdrawal of antiparkinsonian agents. Therefore, any abrupt dosage reduction or withdrawal of 'Sinemet' should be carefully observed, particularly in patients who are also receiving neuroleptics.

Pathological gambling, increased libido and hypersexuality have been reported in patients treated with dopamine agonists for Parkinson's disease.

Concomitant administration of psycho-active drugs such as phenothiazines or butyrophenones should be carried out with caution, and the patient carefully observed for loss of antiparkinsonian effect. Patients with a history of convulsions should be treated with caution.

As with levodopa, periodic evaluation of hepatic, haematopoetic, cardiovascular and renal function are recommended during extended therapy.

Patients with chronic wide-angle glaucoma may be treated cautiously with 'Sinemet', provided the intra-ocular pressure is well controlled and the patient monitored carefully for changes in intra-ocular pressure during therapy.

If general anaesthesia is required, therapy with 'Sinemet' may be continued for as long as the patient is permitted to take fluids and medication by mouth. If therapy has to be stopped temporarily, 'Sinemet' may be restarted as soon as oral medication can be taken at the same daily dosage as before.

Epidemiological studies have shown that patients with Parkinson's disease have a higher risk of developing melanoma than the general population (approximately 2-6 fold higher). It is unclear whether the increased risk observed was due to Parkinson's disease, or other factors such as drugs used to treat Parkinson's disease. Therefore patients and providers are advised to monitor for melanomas on a regular basis when using 'Sinemet' for any indication. Ideally, periodic skin examinations should be performed by appropriately qualified individuals (e.g., dermatologists).

Laboratory Tests

Commonly, levels of blood urea nitrogen, creatinine, and uric acid are lower during administration of 'Sinemet' than with levodopa. Transient abnormalities include elevated levels of blood urea, AST (SGOT), ALT (SGPT), LDH, bilirubin, and alkaline phosphatase.

Decreased haemoglobin, haematocrit, elevated serum glucose and white blood cells, bacteria and blood in the urine have been reported.

Positive Coombs' tests have been reported, both with 'Sinemet' and levodopa alone.

'Sinemet' may cause a false positive result when a dipstick is used to test for urinary ketone; and this reaction is not altered by boiling the urine. The use of glucose oxidase methods may give false negative results for glycosuria.

4.5 Interaction with other medicinal products and other forms of interaction

Caution should be exercised when the following drugs are administered concomitantly with 'Sinemet'.

Antihypertensive agents

Postural hypotension can occur when 'Sinemet' is added to the treatment of patients already receiving antihypertensive drugs. Dosage adjustment of the antihypertensive agent may be required.

Antidepressants

Rarely, reactions including hypertension and dyskinesia have been reported with the concomitant use of tricyclic antidepressants. (See first paragraph of 4.3 'Contraindication' for patients receiving MAOIs).

Anticholinergics

Anticholinergics may affect the absorption and thus the patient's response.

Iron

Studies demonstrate a decrease in the bioavailability of carbidopa and/or levodopa when it is ingested with ferrous sulphate or ferrous gluconate.

Other drugs

To date there has been no indication of interactions that would preclude concurrent use of standard antiparkinsonian drugs.

Dopamine D_2 receptor antagonists (e.g. phenothiazines, butyrophenones, and risperidone) and isoniazid, may reduce the therapeutic effects of levodopa. The beneficial effects of levodopa in Parkinson's disease have been reported to be reversed by phenytoin and papaverine. Patients taking these drugs with 'Sinemet' should be carefully observed for loss of therapeutic response.

Concomitant therapy with selegiline and carbidopa-levodopa may be associated with severe orthostatic hypotension not attributable to carbidopa-levodopa alone (See 4.3 'Contraindications')

Since levodopa competes with certain amino acids, the absorption of 'Sinemet' may be impaired in some patients on a high protein diet.

The effect of simultaneous administration of antacids with 'Sinemet' on the bioavailability of levodopa has not been studied.

'Sinemet' may be given to patients with Parkinson's disease and syndrome who are taking vitamin preparations that contain pyridoxine hydrochloride (Vitamin B6).

4.6 Pregnancy and lactation

Pregnancy

Although the effects of 'Sinemet' on human pregnancy are unknown, both levodopa and combinations of carbidopa and levodopa have caused visceral and skeletal malformations in rabbits. Therefore, the use of 'Sinemet' in women of childbearing potential requires that the anticipated benefits of the drug be weighed against possible hazards should pregnancy occur.

Breast-feeding mothers

It is not known whether carbidopa is excreted in human milk. In a study of one nursing mother with Parkinson's disease, excretion of levodopa in human breast milk was reported. Because many drugs are excreted in human milk and because of the potential for serious adverse reactions in infants, a decision should be made whether to discontinue breast-feeding or discontinue the use of 'Sinemet', taking into account the importance of the drug to the mother.

4.7 Effects on ability to drive and use machines

Individual responses to medication may vary and certain side effects that have been reported with 'Sinemet' may affect some patients' ability to drive or operate machinery. Patients treated with levodopa and presenting with somnolence and/or sudden sleep episodes must be informed to refrain from driving or engaging in activities where impaired alertness may put themselves or others at risk of serious injury or death (e.g. operating machines), until such recurrent episodes and somnolence have resolved (see also section 4.4 'Special warnings and precautions for use').

4.8 Undesirable effects

Side effects that occur frequently with 'Sinemet' are those due to the central neuropharmacological activity of dopamine. These reactions can usually be diminished by dosage reduction. The most common are dyskinesias including choreiform, dystonic and other involuntary movements and nausea. Muscle twitching and blepharospasm may be taken as early signs to consider dosage reduction.

Other side effects reported in clinical trials or in post-marketing experience include:

Body as a whole: syncope, chest pain, anorexia.

Cardiovascular: cardiac irregularities and/or palpitations, orthostatic effects including hypotensive episodes, hypertension, phlebitis.

Gastro-intestinal: vomiting, gastrointestinal bleeding, development of duodenal ulcer, diarrhoea, dark saliva.

Haemotologic: leucopenia, haemolytic and non-haemolytic anaemia, thrombocytopenia, agranulocytosis.

Hypersensitivity: angioedema, urticaria, pruritus, Henoch-Schonlein purpura.

Nervous System/Psychiatric: neuroleptic malignant syndrome (see 4.3 'Contraindications'), bradykinetic episodes (the "on-off" phenomenon), dizziness, paraesthesia, psychotic episodes including delusions, hallucinations and paranoid ideation, depression with or without development of suicidal tendencies, dementia, dream abnormalities, agitation, confusion, increased libido. Levodopa is associated with somnolence and has been associated very rarely with excessive daytime somnolence and sudden sleep onset episodes.

Respiratory: dyspnoea.

Skin: alopecia, rash, dark sweat.

Urogenital: dark urine.

Rarely convulsions have occurred; however, a causal relationship with 'Sinemet' has not been established.

Other side effects that have been reported with levodopa or levodopa/carbidopa combinations and may be potential side effects with 'Sinemet' include:

Gastro-intestinal: dyspepsia, dry mouth, bitter taste, sialorrhoea, dysphagia, bruxism, hiccups, abdominal pain and distress, constipation, flatulence, burning sensation of the tongue.

Metabolic: weight gain or loss, oedema.

Nervous System/Psychiatric: asthenia, decreased mental acuity, disorientation, ataxia, numbness, increased hand tremor, muscle cramp, trismus, activation of latent Horner's syndrome, insomnia, anxiety, euphoria, falling and gait abnormalities.

Patients treated with dopamine agonists for treatment of Parkinson's disease, especially at high doses, have been reported as exhibiting signs of pathological gambling, increased libido and hypersexuality, generally reversible upon reduction of the dose or treatment discontinuation.

Skin: flushing, increased sweating.

Special senses: diplopia, blurred vision, dilated pupils, oculogyric crises.

Urogenital: urinary retention, urinary incontinence, priapism.

Miscellaneous: weakness, faintness, fatigue, headache, hoarseness, malaise, hot flushes, sense of stimulation, bizarre breathing patterns, malignant melanoma (see 4.3 'Contraindications').

4.9 Overdose
Treatment

Management of acute overdosage with 'Sinemet' is basically the same as management of acute overdosage with levodopa; however pyridoxine is not effective in reversing the actions of 'Sinemet'. ECG monitoring should be instituted, and the patient carefully observed for the possible development of arrhythmias; if required, appropriate anti-arrhythmic therapy should be given. The possibility that the patient may have taken other drugs as well as 'Sinemet' should be taken into consideration. To date, no experience has been reported with dialysis, and hence its value in the treatment of overdosage is not known.

The terminal half-life of levodopa is about two hours in the presence of carbidopa.

5. PHARMACOLOGICAL PROPERTIES

5.1 Pharmacodynamic properties

Levodopa is a precursor of dopamine, and is given as replacement therapy in Parkinson's disease.

Carbidopa is a peripheral dopa decarboxylase inhibitor. It prevents metabolism of levodopa to dopamine in the peripheral circulation, ensuring that a higher proportion of the dose reaches the brain, where dopamine acts. A lower dose of levodopa can be used, reducing the incidence and severity of side effects.

'Sinemet' is useful in relieving many of the symptoms of parkinsonism, particularly rigidity and bradykinesia. It is frequently helpful in the management of tremor, dysphagia, sialorrhoea, and postural instability associated with Parkinson's disease and syndrome.

When response to levodopa alone is irregular, and signs and symptoms of Parkinson's disease are not controlled evenly throughout the day, substitution of 'Sinemet' usually reduces fluctuations in response. By reducing some of the adverse reactions produced by levodopa alone, 'Sinemet' permits more patients to obtain adequate relief from the symptoms of Parkinson's disease.

5.2 Pharmacokinetic properties

Following oral dosing levodopa, in the absence of decarboxylase inhibitor, is rapidly but variably absorbed from the gastro-intestinal tract. It has a plasma half life of about 1 hour and is mainly converted by decarboxylation to dopamine, a proportion of which is converted to noradrenaline. Up to 30 % is converted to 3-O-methyldopa which has a half life of 9 to 22 hours. About 80 % of levodopa is excreted in the urine within 24 hours mainly as homovanillic acid and dihydroxyphenylactic acid. Less than 1% is excreted unchanged.

Once in the circulation it competes with other neutral amino acids for transport across the blood brain barrier. Once it has entered the striatal neurones it is decarboxylated to dopamine, stored and released from presynaptic neurones. Because levodopa is so rapidly decarboxylated in the gastrointestinal tract and the liver, very little unchanged drug is available for transport into the brain. The peripheral decarboxylation reduces the therapeutic effectiveness of levodopa but is responsible for many of its side effects. For this reason levodopa is usually administered together with a peripheral decarboxylase inhibitor such as carbidopa, so that lower doses may be given to achieve the same therapeutic effect.

Carbidopa in the absence of levodopa, is rapidly but incompletely absorbed from the gastrointestinal tract following oral dosing. Following an oral dose approximately 50% is recorded in the urine, with about 3 % of this as unchanged drug. It does not cross the blood brain barrier but crosses the placenta and is excreted in breast milk. Turnover of the drug is rapid and virtually all unchanged drug appears in the urine within 7 hours.

Carbidopa inhibits the peripheral decarboxylation of levodopa to dopamine but as it does not cross the blood brain barrier, effective brain levels of dopamine get produced with lower levels of levodopa therapy reducing the peripheral side effects, noticeably nausea and vomiting and cardiac arrhythmias.

5.3 Preclinical safety data

'Sinemet' is well established in medical use. Preclinical data is broadly consistent with clinical experience. (For reproductive toxicity, see section 4.6 'Pregnancy and Lactation'.)

6. PHARMACEUTICAL PARTICULARS

6.1 List of excipients

'Sinemet-62.5' and 'Sinemet-Plus' tablets contain quinoline yellow (E104), maize starch, pregelatinised maize starch, microcrystalline cellulose, magnesium stearate.

'Sinemet-110' and 'Sinemet-275' tablets contain indigo carmine (E132), maize starch pregelatinised maize starch, microcrystalline cellulose, magnesium stearate.

6.2 Incompatibilities

Not applicable.

6.3 Shelf life

36 months

6.4 Special precautions for storage

Do not store above 25°C. Store in the original package in order to protect from light.

6.5 Nature and contents of container

PVC/AL blister packs of 30 or 90 tablets.

Amber glass bottles or HDPE bottles of 84 or 100 tablets

6.6 Special precautions for disposal and other handling

Not applicable.

7. MARKETING AUTHORISATION HOLDER

Merck Sharp & Dohme Limited
Hertford Road
Hoddesdon
Hertfordshire EN11 9BU, UK.

8. MARKETING AUTHORISATION NUMBER(S)

Sinemet-62.5 PL 0025/0226
Sinemet-110 PL 0025/0084
Sinemet-Plus PL 0025/0150
Sinemet-275 PL 0025/0085

9. DATE OF FIRST AUTHORISATION/RENEWAL OF THE AUTHORISATION

Sinemet-62.5 11 February 1988 / 16 April 2008
Sinemet-110 23 October 1973 / 16 April 2008
Sinemet-Plus 11 June 1981 / 16 April 2008
Sinemet-275 23 October 1973 / 16 April 2008

10. DATE OF REVISION OF THE TEXT

April 2009

LEGAL CATEGORY

POM

® Registered trademark of Merck & Co, Inc., Whitehouse Station, New Jersey, USA.

SPC.SEM.08.UK.2987

Sinemet CR and Half Sinemet CR

(Merck Sharp & Dohme Limited)

1. NAME OF THE MEDICINAL PRODUCT

SINEMET® CR 50/200 mg Prolonged-Release Tablets

HALF SINEMET® CR 25/100 mg Prolonged-Release Tablets

2. QUALITATIVE AND QUANTITATIVE COMPOSITION

Each tablet of 'Sinemet CR' contains carbidopa (equivalent to 50 mg of anhydrous carbidopa) and 200 mg levodopa.

Each tablet of 'Half Sinemet CR' contains carbidopa (equivalent to 25 mg of anhydrous carbidopa) and 100 mg levodopa.

3. PHARMACEUTICAL FORM

Modified-release tablets.

'Sinemet CR': peach-coloured, oval shaped, biconvex tablets, plain one side and the other scored and marked '521'.

'Half Sinemet CR': pink-coloured, oval-shaped, biconvex tablets, plain one side and the other marked '601'.

4. CLINICAL PARTICULARS

4.1 Therapeutic indications

Antiparkinson agent.

Idiopathic Parkinson's disease, in particular to reduce off-period in patients who previously have been treated with levodopa/decarboxylase inhibitors, or with levodopa alone and who have experienced motor fluctuations. The experience is limited with 'Sinemet CR' and 'Half Sinemet CR' in patients who have not been treated with levodopa before.

4.2 Posology and method of administration

'Sinemet CR' and 'Half Sinemet CR' tablets contain a 1:4 ratio of carbidopa to levodopa ('Sinemet CR': carbidopa 50 mg/levodopa 200 mg, 'Half Sinemet CR' 25mg/100mg per tablet). The daily dosage of 'Sinemet CR' must be determined by careful titration. Patients should be monitored closely during the dose adjustment period, particularly with regard to appearance or worsening of nausea or abnormal involuntary movements, including dyskinesias, chorea and dystonia.

Route of administration: oral

'Sinemet CR' and 'Half Sinemet CR' may only be administered as whole tablets. So that the controlled release properties of the product can be maintained, tablets should not be chewed, crushed, or halved.

Standard antiparkinson drugs, other than levodopa alone, may be continued while 'Sinemet CR' or 'Half Sinemet CR' are being administered, although their dosage may have to be adjusted. Since carbidopa prevents the reversal of levodopa effects caused by pyridoxine, 'Sinemet CR' or 'Half Sinemet CR' can be given to patients receiving supplemental pyridoxine (vitamin B6).

Initial Dose

Patients currently treated with conventional levodopa/decarboxylase inhibitor combinations

Dosage with 'Sinemet CR' should be substituted initially at an amount that provides no more than approximately 10% more levodopa per day when higher dosages are given (more than 900 mg per day). The dosing interval between doses should be prolonged by 30 to 50% at intervals ranging from 4 to 12 hours. It is recommended to give the smaller dose, if divided doses are not equal, at the end of the day. The dose needs to be titrated further depending on clinical response, as indicated below under 'Titration'. Dosages that provide up to 30% more levodopa per day may be necessary.

A guide for substitution of 'Sinemet CR' treatment for conventional levodopa/decarboxylase inhibitor combinations is shown in the table below:

Guideline for Conversion from 'Sinemet' to 'Sinemet CR'

'Sinemet' Daily Dosage Levodopa (mg)	'Sinemet CR' Daily Dosage Levodopa (mg)	Dosage Regimen
300 - 400	400	1 Tablet 2 × daily
500 - 600	600	1 Tablet 3 × daily
700 - 800	800	4 Tablets in 3 or more divided doses
900 - 1000	1000	5 Tablets in 3 or more divided doses
1100 - 1200	1200	6 Tablets in 3 or more divided doses
1300 - 1400	1400	7 Tablets in 3 or more divided doses
1500 - 1600	1600	8 Tablets in 3 or more divided doses

'Half Sinemet CR' is available to facilitate titration when 100 mg steps are required.

Patients currently treated with levodopa alone

Levodopa must be discontinued at least eight hours before therapy with 'Sinemet CR' is started. In patients with mild to moderate disease, the initial recommended dose is one tablet of 'Sinemet CR' twice daily.

Patients not receiving levodopa

In patients with mild to moderate disease, the initial recommended dose is one tablet of 'Sinemet CR' twice daily. Initial dosages should not exceed 600 mg per day of levodopa, nor be given at intervals of less than six hours.

Titration

Following initiation of therapy, doses and dosing intervals may be increased or decreased, depending upon therapeutic response. Most patients have been adequately treated with two to eight tablets per day of 'Sinemet CR' administered as divided doses at intervals ranging from four to twelve hours during the waking day. Higher doses (up to 12 tablets) and shorter intervals (less than four hours) have been used, but are not usually recommended.

When doses of 'Sinemet CR' are given at intervals of less than four hours, or if the divided doses are not equal, it is recommended that the smaller doses be given at the end of the day. In some patients the onset of effect of the first morning dose may be delayed for up to one hour compared with the response usually obtained from the first morning dose of 'Sinemet'.

An interval of at least three days between dosage adjustments is recommended.

Maintenance

Because Parkinson's disease is progressive, periodic clinical evaluations are recommended and adjustment of the dosage regimen of 'Sinemet CR' or 'Half Sinemet CR' may be required.

Addition of other antiparkinson medication

Anticholinergic agents, dopamine agonists and amantadine can be given with 'Sinemet CR' or 'Half Sinemet CR'. Dosage adjustment of 'Sinemet CR' or 'Half Sinemet CR' may be necessary when these agents are added to an existing treatment regimen for 'Sinemet CR' or 'Half Sinemet CR'.

Interruption of therapy

Patients should be observed carefully if abrupt reduction or discontinuation of 'Sinemet CR' or 'Half Sinemet CR' is required, especially if the patient is receiving antipsychotics (see 4.4 'Special warnings and precautions for use').

Use in Children

Safety and effectiveness of 'Sinemet CR' or 'Half Sinemet CR' in infants and children have not been established, and its use in patients below the age of 18 is not recommended.

4.3 Contraindications

'Sinemet CR' or 'Half Sinemet CR' should not be given when administration of a sympathomimetic amine is contraindicated.

Nonselective monoamine oxidase (MAO) inhibitors are contraindicated for use with 'Sinemet CR' or 'Half Sinemet CR'. These inhibitors must be discontinued at least two weeks prior to initiating therapy with 'Sinemet CR' or 'Half Sinemet CR'. 'Sinemet CR' or 'Half Sinemet CR' may be administered concomitantly with the manufacturer's recommended dose of an MAO inhibitor with selectivity for MAO type B (e.g. selegiline hydrochloride) (See 4.5 'Interactions with other medicinal products and other forms of interaction').

'Sinemet CR' or 'Half Sinemet CR' is contraindicated in patients with known hypersensitivity to any component of this medication, and in patients with narrow-angle glaucoma.

Because levodopa may activate a malignant melanoma, 'Sinemet CR' or 'Half Sinemet CR' should not be used in patients with suspicious undiagnosed skin lesions or a history of melanoma.

Use in patients with severe psychoses.

4.4 Special warnings and precautions for use

When patients are receiving levodopa monotherapy, levodopa must be discontinued at least eight hours before therapy with 'Sinemet CR' or 'Half Sinemet CR' is started (at least 12 hours if slow-release levodopa has been administered).

Dyskinesias may occur in patients previously treated with levodopa alone because carbidopa permits more levodopa to reach the brain and, thus, more dopamine to be formed. The occurrence of dyskinesias may require dosage reduction.

'Sinemet CR' and 'Half Sinemet CR' are not recommended for the treatment of drug-induced extrapyramidal reactions or for the treatment of Huntingdon's chorea.

Based on the pharmacokinetic profile of 'Sinemet CR' the onset of effect in patients with early morning dyskinesias may be slower than with conventional 'Sinemet'. The incidence of dyskinesias is slightly higher during treatment with 'Sinemet CR' than with conventional 'Sinemet' (16.5% vs 12.2%) in advanced patients with motor fluctuations.

'Sinemet CR' or 'Half Sinemet CR' should be administered cautiously to patients with severe cardiovascular or pulmonary disease, bronchial asthma, renal, hepatic or endocrine disease, or with a history of peptic ulcer disease or of convulsions.

Care should be exercised in administering 'Sinemet CR' or 'Half Sinemet CR' to patients with a history of recent myocardial infarction who have residual atrial, nodal, or ventricular arrhythmia. In such patients, cardiac function should be monitored with particular care during the period of initial dosage administration and titration.

Levodopa has been associated with somnolence and episodes of sudden sleep onset. Sudden onset of sleep during daily activities, in some cases without awareness or warning signs, has been reported very rarely. Patients must be informed of this and advised to exercise caution while driving or operating machines during treatment with Levodopa. Patients who have experienced somnolence and/or an episode of sudden sleep onset must refrain from driving or operating machines. Furthermore a reduction of dosage or termination of therapy may be considered.

As with levodopa, 'Sinemet CR' or 'Half Sinemet CR' may cause involuntary movements and mental disturbances. Patients with a history of severe involuntary movements or psychotic episodes when treated with levodopa alone or levodopa/decarboxylase inhibitor combination should be observed carefully when 'Sinemet CR' or 'Half Sinemet CR' is substituted. These reactions are thought to be due to increased brain dopamine following administration of levodopa and use of 'Sinemet CR' or 'Half Sinemet CR' may cause recurrence. Dosage reduction may be required. All patients should be observed carefully for the development of depression with concomitant suicidal tendencies. Patients with past or current psychoses should be treated with caution.

Pathological gambling, increased libido and hypersexuality have been reported in patients treated with dopamine agonists for Parkinson's disease.

A symptom complex resembling the neuroleptic malignant syndrome including muscular rigidity, elevated body temperature, mental changes, and increased serum creatine phosphokinase has been reported when antiparkinsonian agents were withdrawn abruptly. Therefore, patients should be observed carefully when the dosage of carbidopa-levodopa combinations is reduced abruptly or discontinued, especially if the patient is receiving antipsychotics.

Patients with chronic wide-angle glaucoma may be treated cautiously with 'Sinemet CR' or 'Half Sinemet CR', provided the intraocular pressure is well controlled and the patient monitored carefully for changes in intraocular pressure during therapy.

Periodic evaluations of hepatic, haematopoietic, cardiovascular and renal function are recommended during extended therapy.

If general anaesthesia is required, 'Sinemet CR' or 'Half Sinemet CR' may be continued as long as the patient is permitted to take oral medication. If therapy is interrupted temporarily, the usual dosage should be administered as soon as the patient is able to take oral medicine.

Epidemiological studies have shown that patients with Parkinson's disease have a higher risk of developing melanoma than the general population (approximately 2-6 fold higher). It is unclear whether the increased risk observed was due to Parkinson's disease, or other factors such as drugs used to treat Parkinson's disease. Therefore patients and providers are advised to monitor for melanomas on a regular basis when using 'Sinemet CR' for any indication. Ideally, periodic skin examinations should be performed by appropriately qualified individuals (e.g., dermatologists).

Laboratory Tests

Abnormalities in various laboratory tests have occurred with carbidopa-levodopa preparations and may occur with 'Sinemet CR' or 'Half Sinemet CR'. These include elevations of liver function tests such as alkaline phosphatase, SGOT (AST), SGPT (ALT), LDH, bilirubin, blood urea nitrogen, creatinine, uric acid and positive Coombs' test.

Carbidopa-levodopa preparations may cause a false-positive reaction for urinary ketone bodies when a test tape is used for determination of ketonuria. This reaction will not be altered by boiling the urine specimen. False-negative tests may result with the use of glucose-oxidase methods of testing for glycosuria.

Decreased haemoglobin and haematocrit, elevated serum glucose and white blood cells, bacteria and blood in the urine have been reported with standard 'Sinemet'.

4.5 Interaction with other medicinal products and other forms of interaction

Caution should be exercised when the following drugs are administered concomitantly with 'Sinemet CR' or 'Half Sinemet CR':

Antihypertensive agents

Symptomatic postural hypotension has occurred when levodopa/decarboxylase inhibitor combinations were added to the treatment of patients receiving some antihypertensive drugs. Therefore when therapy with 'Sinemet CR' or 'Half Sinemet CR' is started, dosage adjustment of the antihypertensive drug may be required.

Antidepressants

There have been rare reports of adverse reactions, including hypertension and dyskinesia, resulting from the concomitant use of tricyclic antidepressants and carbidopa-levodopa preparations. (For patients receiving monamine oxidase inhibitors, see 4.3 'Contraindications').

Anticholinergics

Anticholinergics may affect the absorption and thus the patient's response.

Iron

Studies demonstrate a decrease in the bioavailability of carbidopa and/or levodopa when it is ingested with ferrous sulphate or ferrous gluconate.

Other drugs

Dopamine D2 receptor antagonists (e.g. phenothiazines, butyrophenones and risperidone) and isoniazid may reduce the therapeutic effects of levodopa. The beneficial effects of levodopa in Parkinson's disease have been reported to be reversed by phenytoin and papaverine. Patients taking these drugs with 'Sinemet CR' or 'Half Sinemet CR' should be observed carefully for loss of therapeutic response.

Concomitant therapy with selegiline and carbidopa-levodopa may be associated with severe orthostatic hypotension not attributable to carbidopa-levodopa alone (See 4.3 'Contraindications').

Since levodopa competes with certain amino acids, the absorption of levodopa may be impaired in some patients on a high protein diet.

The effect of simultaneous administration of antacids with 'Sinemet CR' or 'Half Sinemet CR' on the bioavailability of levodopa has not been studied.

4.6 Pregnancy and lactation

There are insufficient data to evaluate the possible harmfulness of this substance when used in human pregnancy. (See 5.3 'Preclinical Safety Data'). It is not known whether carbidopa is excreted in human milk. In a study of one nursing mother with Parkinson's disease, excretion of levodopa in breast milk was reported. 'Sinemet CR' or 'Half Sinemet CR' should not be given during pregnancy and to nursing mothers.

4.7 Effects on ability to drive and use machines

Individual responses to medication may vary. Certain side effects that have been reported with 'Sinemet CR' may affect some patients' ability to drive or operate machinery. Patients treated with Levodopa and presenting with somnolence and/or sudden sleep episodes must be informed to refrain from driving or engaging in activities where impaired alertness may put themselves or other at risk of serious injury or death (e.g. operating machines) until such recurrent episodes and somnolence have resolved (see also section 4.4 'Special warnings and precautions for use').

4.8 Undesirable effects

In controlled clinical trials in patients with moderate to severe motor fluctuations 'Sinemet CR' did not produce side-effects which were unique to the modified-release formulation.

The side-effect reported most frequently was dyskinesia (a form of abnormal involuntary movements). A greater incidence of dyskinesias was seen with 'Sinemet CR' than with 'Sinemet'.

Other side-effects that also were reported frequently (above 2%) were: nausea, hallucinations, confusion, dizziness, chorea and dry mouth.

Side effects occurring less frequently (1-2%) were: dream abnormalities, dystonia, somnolence, insomnia, depression, asthenia, vomiting and anorexia.

Other side effects reported in clinical trials or in post-marketing experience include:

Body as a whole: chest pain, syncope.

Cardiovascular: palpitation, orthostatic effects including hypotensive episodes.

Gastrointestinal: constipation, diarrhoea, dyspepsia, gastrointestinal pain, dark saliva.

Hypersensitivity: angioedema, urticaria, pruritus.

Metabolic: weight loss.

Nervous System/Psychiatric: neuroleptic malignant syndrome (see 4.3 'Contraindications'), agitation, anxiety, decreased mental acuity, paraesthesia, disorientation, fatigue, headache, extrapyramidal and movement disorders, falling, gait abnormalities, muscle cramps, on-off phenomenon, increased libido, psychotic episodes including delusions and paranoid ideation. Levodopa is associated with somnolence and has been associated very rarely with excessive daytime somnolence and sudden sleep onset episodes.

Respiratory: dyspnoea

Skin: flushing, alopecia, rash, dark sweat.

Special Senses: blurred vision.

Urogenital: dark urine.

Other side effects that have been reported with levodopa or levodopa/carbidopa combinations and may be potential side-effects with 'Sinemet CR' are listed below:

Cardiovascular: cardiac irregularities, hypertension, phlebitis.

Gastrointestinal: bitter taste, sialorrhoea, dysphagia, bruxism, hiccups, gastrointestinal bleeding, flatulence, burning sensation of tongue, development of duodenal ulcer.

Haematologic: leucopenia, haemolytic and non-haemolytic anaemia, thrombocytopenia, agranulocytosis.

Nervous system/Psychiatric: ataxia, numbness, increased hand tremor, muscle twitching, blepharospasm, trismus, activation of latent Horner's syndrome, euphoria, and dementia, depression with suicidal tendencies.

Patients treated with dopamine agonists for treatment of Parkinson's disease, especially at high doses, have been reported as exhibiting signs of pathological gambling, increased libido and hypersexuality, generally reversible upon reduction of the dose or treatment discontinuation.

Skin: increased sweating.

Special senses: diplopia, dilated pupils, oculogyric crises.

Urogenital: urinary retention, urinary incontinence, priapism.

Miscellaneous: weight gain, oedema, weakness, faintness, hoarseness, malaise, hot flashes, sense of stimulation, bizarre breathing patterns, malignant melanoma (see 4.3 Contraindications), Henoch-Schonlein purpura.

Convulsions have occurred; however, a causal relationship with levodopa or levodopa/carbidopa combinations has not been established.

4.9 Overdose

Management of acute overdosage with 'Sinemet CR' or 'Half Sinemet CR' is basically the same as management of acute overdosage with levodopa; however, pyridoxine is not effective in reversing the actions of 'Sinemet CR' or 'Half Sinemet CR'.

Electrocardiographic monitoring should be instituted and the patient observed carefully for the development of arrhythmias; if required, appropriate antiarrhythmic therapy should be given. The possibility that the patient may have taken other drugs as well as 'Sinemet CR' or 'Half Sinemet CR' should be taken into consideration. To date, no experience has been reported with dialysis; hence, its value in overdosage is not known.

5. PHARMACOLOGICAL PROPERTIES

5.1 Pharmacodynamic properties

'Sinemet CR' and 'Half Sinemet CR' are a combination of carbidopa, an aromatic amino acid decarboxylase inhibitor, and levodopa, the metabolic precursor of dopamine, in a polymer-based controlled-release tablet formulation, for use in the treatment of Parkinson's disease. 'Sinemet CR' and 'Half Sinemet CR' are particularly useful to reduce 'off' time in patients treated previously with a conventional levodopa/decarboxylase inhibitor combination who have had dyskinesias and motor fluctuations.

Patients with Parkinson's disease treated with preparations containing levodopa may develop motor fluctuations characterised by end-of-dose failure, peak dose dyskinesia, and akinesia. The advanced form of motor fluctuations ('on-off' phenomenon) is characterised by unpredictable swings from mobility to immobility. Although the causes of the motor fluctuations are not completely understood, it has been demonstrated that they can be attenuated by treatment regimens that produce steady plasma levels of levodopa.

Levodopa relieves the symptoms of Parkinson's disease by being decarboxylated to dopamine in the brain. Carbidopa, which does not cross the blood-brain barrier, inhibits only the extracerebral decarboxylation of levodopa, making more levodopa available for transport to the brain and subsequent conversion to dopamine. This normally obviates the necessity for large doses of levodopa at frequent intervals. The lower dosage reduces or may help eliminate gastrointestinal and cardiovascular side-effects, especially those which are attributed to dopamine being formed in extracerebral tissues.

'Sinemet CR' and 'Half Sinemet CR' are designed to release their active ingredients over a four-six hour period. With this formulation there is less variation in plasma levodopa levels and the peak plasma level is 60% lower than with conventional 'Sinemet', as established in healthy volunteers.

In clinical trials, patients with motor fluctuations experienced reduced 'off'-time with 'Sinemet CR' when compared with 'Sinemet'. The reduction of the 'off'-time is rather small (about 10%) and the incidence of dyskinesias increases slightly after administration of 'Sinemet CR' compared to standard 'Sinemet'. Global ratings of improvement and activities of daily living in the 'on' and 'off' state, as assessed by both patient and physician, were better during therapy with 'Sinemet CR' than with 'Sinemet'. Patients considered 'Sinemet CR' to be more helpful for their clinical fluctuations, and preferred it over 'Sinemet'. In patients without motor fluctuations, 'Sinemet CR' under controlled conditions, provided the same therapeutic benefit with less frequent dosing than with 'Sinemet'. Generally, there was no further improvement of other symptoms of Parkinson's disease.

5.2 Pharmacokinetic properties

The pharmacokinetics of levodopa following administration of 'Sinemet CR' were studied in young and elderly healthy volunteers. The mean time to peak plasma levodopa level after 'Sinemet CR' was approximately two hours compared to 0.75 hours with 'Sinemet'. The mean peak plasma levodopa levels were 60% lower with 'Sinemet CR' than with 'Sinemet'. The in vivo absorption of levodopa following administration of 'Sinemet CR' was continuous for 4 to 6 hours. In these studies, as with patients, plasma levodopa concentrations fluctuated in a narrower range than with 'Sinemet'. Because the bioavailability of levodopa from 'Sinemet CR' relative to 'Sinemet' is approximately 70%, the daily dosage of levodopa in the controlled release formulation will usually be higher than with conventional formulations. There was no evidence that 'Sinemet CR' released its ingredients in a rapid or uncontrolled fashion.

The pharmacokinetics of levodopa following administration of 'Half Sinemet CR' were studied in patients with Parkinson's disease. Chronic three month, open-label, twice daily dosing with 'Half Sinemet CR' (range: 50 mg carbidopa, 200 mg levodopa up to 150 mg carbidopa, 600 mg levodopa per day) did not result in accumulation of plasma levodopa. The dose-adjusted bioavailability for one 'Half Sinemet CR' tablet was equivalent to that for one 'Sinemet CR' tablet. The mean peak concentration of levodopa following administration of one 'Half Sinemet CR' tablet was greater than 50% of that following one 'Sinemet CR' tablet. Mean time-to-peak plasma levels may be slightly less for 'Half Sinemet CR' than for 'Sinemet CR'.

It is not known whether or not to what extent the absorption is influenced by a protein rich diet. The bioavailability may be influenced by drugs which affect the gastrointestinal propulsion.

5.3 Preclinical safety data

The medicine has appeared harmful in animal trials (visceral and skeletal malformations in rabbits). For reproductive toxicity, see section 4.6 'Pregnancy and lactation'.

6. PHARMACEUTICAL PARTICULARS

6.1 List of excipients

Hydroxypropylcellulose

Magnesium Stearate

Poly (Vinyl Acetate-Crotonic Acid) Copolymer

Quinoline Yellow 10 Aluminium Lake E104 (Sinemet CR only)

Red Iron Oxide E172

6.2 Incompatibilities

Not applicable

6.3 Shelf life

36 months

6.4 Special precautions for storage

Do not store above 30°C. Store in the original package in order to protect from light.

6.5 Nature and contents of container

Amber glass bottles or HDPE bottles in packs of 100, 84, or 56 tablets.

All aluminium blister pack of 60 tablets.

6.6 Special precautions for disposal and other handling

Not applicable.

7. MARKETING AUTHORISATION HOLDER

Merck Sharp & Dohme Limited

Hertford Road, Hoddesdon, Hertfordshire, EN11 9BU, UK.

8. MARKETING AUTHORISATION NUMBER(S)

Sinemet CR 50/200 mg Prolonged-Release Tablets PL 0025/0269

Half Sinemet CR 25/100 mg Prolonged-Release Tablets PL 0025/0287

9. DATE OF FIRST AUTHORISATION/RENEWAL OF THE AUTHORISATION

Sinemet CR 50/200 mg Prolonged-Release Tablets 5 September 1991/Renewed 16 April 2008

Half Sinemet CR 25/100 mg Prolonged-Release Tablets 7 October 1992/Renewed 16 April 2008

10. DATE OF REVISION OF THE TEXT

April 2009

LEGAL CATEGORY

POM

® Registered trademark of Merck & Co., Inc., Whitehouse Station, New Jersey, USA

SPC.SEMCR.08.UK.2988

Singulair 10 mg Tablets

(Merck Sharp & Dohme Limited)

1. NAME OF THE MEDICINAL PRODUCT

SINGULAIR® 10 mg film-coated tablets

2. QUALITATIVE AND QUANTITATIVE COMPOSITION

One film-coated tablet contains montelukast sodium, which is equivalent to 10 mg montelukast.

Excipient: Lactose monohydrate 89.3 mg per tablet

For a full list of excipients, see section 6.1.

3. PHARMACEUTICAL FORM

Film-coated tablet.

Beige, rounded square, film-coated, size 7.9 mm × 7.9 mm with 'SINGULAIR' engraved on one side and 'MSD 117' on the other.

4. CLINICAL PARTICULARS

4.1 Therapeutic indications

SINGULAIR is indicated in the treatment of asthma as add-on therapy in those patients with mild to moderate persistent asthma who are inadequately controlled on inhaled corticosteroids and in whom "as-needed" short acting β-agonists provide inadequate clinical control of asthma. In those asthmatic patients in whom SINGULAIR is indicated in asthma, SINGULAIR can also provide symptomatic relief of seasonal allergic rhinitis.

SINGULAIR is also indicated in the prophylaxis of asthma in which the predominant component is exercise-induced bronchoconstriction.

4.2 Posology and method of administration

The dosage for adults 15 years of age and older with asthma, or with asthma and concomitant seasonal allergic rhinitis, is one 10 mg tablet daily to be taken in the evening.

General recommendations. The therapeutic effect of SINGULAIR on parameters of asthma control occurs within one day. SINGULAIR may be taken with or without food. Patients should be advised to continue taking SINGULAIR even if their asthma is under control, as well as during periods of worsening asthma. SINGULAIR should not be used concomitantly with other products containing the same active ingredient, montelukast.

No dosage adjustment is necessary for the elderly, or for patients with renal insufficiency, or mild to moderate hepatic impairment. There are no data on patients with severe hepatic impairment. The dosage is the same for both male and female patients.

Therapy with SINGULAIR in relation to other treatments for asthma.

SINGULAIR can be added to a patient's existing treatment regimen.

Inhaled corticosteroids: Treatment with SINGULAIR can be used as add-on therapy in patients when inhaled corticosteroids plus "as needed" short acting β-agonists provide inadequate clinical control. SINGULAIR should not be substituted for inhaled corticosteroids (see section 4.4).

5-mg chewable tablets are available for paediatric patients 6 to 14 years of age.

4.3 Contraindications

Hypersensitivity to the active substance or to any of the excipients.

4.4 Special warnings and precautions for use

Patients should be advised never to use oral montelukast to treat acute asthma attacks and to keep their usual appropriate rescue medication for this purpose readily available. If an acute attack occurs, a short-acting inhaled β-agonist should be used. Patients should seek their doctor's advice as soon as possible if they need more inhalations of short-acting β-agonists than usual.

Montelukast should not be substituted for inhaled or oral corticosteroids.

There are no data demonstrating that oral corticosteroids can be reduced when montelukast is given concomitantly.

In rare cases, patients on therapy with anti-asthma agents including montelukast may present with systemic eosinophilia, sometimes presenting with clinical features of vasculitis consistent with Churg-Strauss syndrome, a condition which is often treated with systemic corticosteroid therapy. These cases usually, but not always, have been associated with the reduction or withdrawal of oral corticosteroid therapy. The possibility that leukotriene receptor antagonists may be associated with emergence of Churg-Strauss syndrome can neither be excluded nor established. Physicians should be alert to eosinophilia, vasculitic rash, worsening pulmonary symptoms, cardiac complications, and/or neuropathy presenting in their patients. Patients who develop these symptoms should be reassessed and their treatment regimens evaluated.

Treatment with montelukast does not alter the need for patients with aspirin-sensitive asthma to avoid taking aspirin and other non-steroidal anti-inflammatory drugs.

Patients with rare hereditary problems of galactose intolerance, the Lapp lactase deficiency or glucose-galactose malabsorption should not take this medicine.

4.5 Interaction with other medicinal products and other forms of interaction

Montelukast may be administered with other therapies routinely used in the prophylaxis and chronic treatment of asthma. In drug-interactions studies, the recommended clinical dose of montelukast did not have clinically important effects on the pharmacokinetics of the following medicinal products: theophylline, prednisone, prednisolone, oral contraceptives (ethinyl estradiol/ norethindrone 35/1), terfenadine, digoxin and warfarin.

The area under the plasma concentration curve (AUC) for montelukast was decreased approximately 40% in subjects with co-administration of phenobarbital. Since montelukast is metabolised by CYP 3A4, caution should be exercised, particularly in children, when montelukast is co-administered with inducers of CYP 3A4, such as phenytoin, phenobarbital and rifampicin.

In vitro studies have shown that montelukast is a potent inhibitor of CYP 2C8. However, data from a clinical drug-drug interaction study involving montelukast and rosiglitazone (a probe substrate representative of medicinal products primarily metabolized by CYP 2C8) demonstrated that montelukast does not inhibit CYP 2C8 *in vivo*. Therefore, montelukast is not anticipated to markedly alter the metabolism of medicinal products metabolised by this enzyme (e.g., paclitaxel, rosiglitazone, and repaglinide.)

4.6 Pregnancy and lactation

Use during pregnancy

Animal studies do not indicate harmful effects with respect to effects on pregnancy or embryonal/foetal development.

Limited data from available pregnancy databases do not suggest a causal relationship between SINGULAIR and malformations (i.e. limb defects) that have been rarely reported in worldwide post marketing experience.

SINGULAIR may be used during pregnancy only if it is considered to be clearly essential.

Use during lactation

Studies in rats have shown that montelukast is excreted in milk (see section 5.3). It is not known if montelukast is excreted in human milk.

SINGULAIR may be used in breast-feeding only if it is considered to be clearly essential.

4.7 Effects on ability to drive and use machines

Montelukast is not expected to affect a patient's ability to drive a car or operate machinery. However, in very rare cases, individuals have reported drowsiness or dizziness.

4.8 Undesirable effects

Montelukast has been evaluated in clinical studies as follows:

- 10 mg film-coated tablets in approximately 4000 adult asthmatic patients 15 years of age and older.
- 10 mg film-coated tablets in approximately 400 adult asthmatic patients with seasonal allergic rhinitis 15 years of age and older.
- 5 mg chewable tablets in approximately 1750 paediatric asthmatic patients 6 to 14 years of age.

The following drug-related adverse reactions in clinical studies were reported commonly (≥1/100 to <1/10) in asthmatic patients treated with montelukast and at a greater incidence than in patients treated with placebo:

Body System Class	Adult Patients 15 years and older (two 12-week studies; n=795)	Paediatric Patients 6 to 14 years old (one 8-week study; n=201) (two 56-week studies; n=615)
Nervous system disorders	headache	headache
Gastro-intestinal disorders	abdominal pain	

With prolonged treatment in clinical trials with a limited number of patients for up to 2 years for adults, and up to 12 months for paediatric patients 6 to 14 years of age, the safety profile did not change.

The following adverse reactions have been reported in post-marketing use:

Blood and lymphatic system disorders: increased bleeding tendency.

Immune system disorders: hypersensitivity reactions including anaphylaxis, hepatic eosinophilic infiltration.

Psychiatric disorders: dream abnormalities including nightmares, hallucinations, insomnia, irritability, anxiety, restlessness, agitation including aggressive behaviour, tremor, depression, suicidal thinking and behaviour (suicidality) in very rare cases.

Nervous system disorders: dizziness drowsiness, paraesthesia/hypoesthesia, seizure.

Cardiac disorders: palpitations.

Respiratory, thoracic and mediastinal disorders: epistaxis

Gastro-intestinal disorders: diarrhoea, dry mouth, dyspepsia, nausea, vomiting.

Hepatobiliary disorders: elevated levels of serum transaminases (ALT, AST), cholestatic hepatitis

Skin and subcutaneous tissue disorders: angiooedema, bruising, urticaria, pruritus, rash, erythema nodosum.

Musculoskeletal and connective tissue disorders: arthralgia, myalgia including muscle cramps.

General disorders and administration site conditions: asthenia/fatigue, malaise, oedema, pyrexia.

Very rare cases of Churg-Strauss Syndrome (CSS) have been reported during montelukast treatment in asthmatic patients (see section 4.4).

4.9 Overdose

No specific information is available on the treatment of overdose with montelukast. In chronic asthma studies, montelukast has been administered at doses up to 200 mg/day to patients for 22 weeks and in short term studies, up to 900 mg/day to patients for approximately one week without clinically important adverse experiences.

There have been reports of acute overdose in post-marketing experience and clinical studies with montelukast. These include reports in adults and children with a dose as high as 1000 mg (approximately 61 mg/kg in a 42 month old child). The clinical and laboratory findings observed were consistent with the safety profile in adults and paediatric patients. There were no adverse experiences in the majority of overdose reports. The most frequently occurring adverse experiences were consistent with the safety profile of montelukast and included abdominal pain, somnolence, thirst, headache, vomiting, and psychomotor hyperactivity.

It is not known whether montelukast is dialysable by peritoneal- or haemo-dialysis.

5. PHARMACOLOGICAL PROPERTIES

5.1 Pharmacodynamic properties

Pharmacotherapeutic group: Leukotriene receptor antagonist

ATC-code: R03D C03

The cysteinyl leukotrienes (LTC_4, LTD_4, LTE_4) are potent inflammatory eicosanoids released from various cells including mast cells and eosinophils. These important pro-asthmatic mediators bind to cysteinyl leukotriene (CysLT) receptors. The CysLT type-1 ($CysLT_1$) receptor is found in the human airway (including airway smooth muscle cells and airway macrophages) and on other pro-inflammatory cells (including eosinophils and certain myeloid stem cells). CysLTs have been correlated with the pathophysiology of asthma and allergic rhinitis. In asthma, leukotriene-mediated effects include bronchoconstriction, mucous secretion, vascular permeability, and eosinophil recruitment. In allergic rhinitis, CysLTs are released from the nasal mucosa after allergen exposure during both early- and late-phase reactions and are associated with symptoms of allergic rhinitis. Intranasal challenge with CysLTs has been shown to increase nasal airway resistance and symptoms of nasal obstruction.

Montelukast is an orally active compound which binds with high affinity and selectivity to the $CysLT_1$ receptor. In clinical studies, montelukast inhibits bronchoconstriction due to inhaled LTD_4 at doses as low as 5 mg. Bronchodilation was observed within 2 hours of oral administration. The bronchodilation effect caused by a β-agonist was additive to that caused by montelukast. Treatment with montelukast inhibited both early- and late-phase bronchoconstriction due to antigen challenge. Montelukast, compared with placebo, decreased peripheral blood eosinophils in adult and paediatric patients. In a separate study, treatment with montelukast significantly decreased eosinophils in the airways (as measured in sputum) and in peripheral blood while improving clinical asthma control.

In studies in adults, montelukast, 10 mg once daily, compared with placebo, demonstrated significant improvements in morning FEV_1 (10.4% vs 2.7% change from baseline), AM peak expiratory flow rate (PEFR) (24.5 L/min vs 3.3 L/min change from baseline), and significant decrease in total β-agonist use (-26.1% vs -4.6% change from baseline). Improvement in patient-reported daytime and nighttime asthma symptoms scores was significantly better than placebo.

Studies in adults demonstrated the ability of montelukast to add to the clinical effect of inhaled corticosteroid (% change from baseline for inhaled beclometasone plus montelukast vs beclometasone, respectively for FEV_1: 5.43% vs 1.04%; β-agonist use: -8.70% vs 2.64%). Compared with inhaled beclometasone (200 μg twice daily with a spacer device), montelukast demonstrated a more rapid initial response, although over the 12-week study, beclometasone provided a greater average treatment effect (% change from baseline for montelukast vs beclometasone, respectively for FEV_1: 7.49% vs 13.3%; β-agonist use: -28.28% vs -43.89%). However, compared with beclometasone, a high percentage of patients treated with montelukast achieved similar clinical responses (e.g., 50% of patients treated with beclometasone achieved an improvement in FEV_1 of approximately 11% or more over baseline while approximately 42% of patients treated with montelukast achieved the same response).

A clinical study was conducted to evaluate montelukast for the symptomatic treatment of seasonal allergic rhinitis in adult asthmatic patients 15 years of age and older with concomitant seasonal allergic rhinitis. In this study, montelukast 10 mg tablets administered once daily demonstrated a statistically significant improvement in the Daily Rhinitis Symptoms score, compared with placebo. The Daily Rhinitis Symptoms score is the average of the Daytime Nasal Symptoms score (mean of nasal congestion, rhinorrhea, sneezing, nasal itching) and the Nighttime Symptoms score (mean of nasal congestion upon awakening, difficulty going to sleep, and nighttime awakenings scores). Global evaluations of allergic rhinitis by patients and physicians were significantly improved, compared with placebo. The evaluation of asthma efficacy was not a primary objective in this study.

In an 8-week study in paediatric patients 6 to 14 years of age, montelukast 5 mg once daily, compared with placebo, significantly improved respiratory function (FEV_1 8.71% vs 4.16% change from baseline; AM PEFR 27.9 L/min vs 17.8 L/min change from baseline) and decreased "as-needed" β-agonist use (-11.7% vs +8.2% change from baseline).

Significant reduction of exercise-induced bronchoconstriction (EIB) was demonstrated in a 12-week study in adults (maximal fall in FEV_1 22.33% for montelukast vs 32.40% for placebo; time to recovery to within 5% of baseline FEV_1 44.22 min vs 60.64 min). This effect was consistent throughout the 12-week study period. Reduction in EIB was also demonstrated in a short term study in paediatric patients (maximal fall in FEV_1 18.27% vs 26.11%; time to recovery to within 5% of baseline FEV_1 17.76 min vs 27.98 min). The effect in both studies was demonstrated at the end of the once-daily dosing interval.

In aspirin-sensitive asthmatic patients receiving concomitant inhaled and/or oral corticosteroids, treatment with montelukast, compared with placebo, resulted in significant improvement in asthma control (FEV_1 8.55% vs - 1.74% change from baseline and decrease in total β-agonist use -27.78% vs 2.09% change from baseline).

5.2 Pharmacokinetic properties

Absorption. Montelukast is rapidly absorbed following oral administration. For the 10 mg film-coated tablet, the mean peak plasma concentration (C_{max}) is achieved 3 hours (T_{max}) after administration in adults in the fasted state. The mean oral bioavailability is 64%. The oral bioavailability and C_{max} are not influenced by a standard meal. Safety and efficacy were demonstrated in clinical trials where the 10 mg film-coated tablet was administered without regard to the timing of food ingestion.

For the 5 mg chewable tablet, the C_{max} is achieved in 2 hours after administration in adults in the fasted state. The mean oral bioavailability is 73% and is decreased to 63% by a standard meal.

Distribution. Montelukast is more than 99% bound to plasma proteins. The steady-state volume of distribution of montelukast averages 8-11 litres. Studies in rats with radiolabelled montelukast indicate minimal distribution across the blood-brain barrier. In addition, concentrations of radiolabelled material at 24 hours post-dose were minimal in all other tissues.

Biotransformation. Montelukast is extensively metabolised. In studies with therapeutic doses, plasma concentrations of metabolites of montelukast are undetectable at steady state in adults and children.

In vitro studies using human liver microsomes indicate that cytochrome P450 3A4, 2A6 and 2C9 are involved in the metabolism of montelukast. Based on further *in vitro* results in human liver microsomes, therapeutic plasma concentrations of montelukast do not inhibit cytochromes P450 3A4, 2C9, 1A2, 2A6, 2C19, or 2D6. The contribution of metabolites to the therapeutic effect of montelukast is minimal.

Elimination. The plasma clearance of montelukast averages 45 ml/min in healthy adults. Following an oral dose of radiolabelled montelukast, 86% of the radioactivity was recovered in 5-day faecal collections and <0.2% was recovered in urine. Coupled with estimates of montelukast oral bioavailability, this indicates that montelukast and its metabolites are excreted almost exclusively via the bile.

Characteristics in patients. No dosage adjustment is necessary for the elderly or mild to moderate hepatic insufficiency. Studies in patients with renal impairment have not been undertaken. Because montelukast and its metabolites are eliminated by the biliary route, no dose adjustment is anticipated to be necessary in patients with renal impairment. There are no data on the pharmacokinetics of montelukast in patients with severe hepatic insufficiency (Child-Pugh score >9).

With high doses of montelukast (20- and 60-fold the recommended adult dose), decrease in plasma theophylline concentration was observed. This effect was not seen at the recommended dose of 10 mg once daily.

5.3 Preclinical safety data

In animal toxicity studies, minor serum biochemical alterations in ALT, glucose, phosphorus and triglycerides were observed which were transient in nature. The signs of toxicity in animals were increased excretion of saliva, gastro-intestinal symptoms, loose stools and ion imbalance. These occurred at dosages which provided >17-fold the systemic exposure seen at the clinical dosage. In monkeys, the adverse effects appeared at doses from 150 mg/kg/day (>232-fold the systemic exposure seen at the clinical dose). In animal studies, montelukast did not affect fertility or reproductive performance at systemic exposure exceeding the clinical systemic exposure by greater than 24-fold. A slight decrease in pup body weight was noted in the female fertility study in rats at 200 mg/kg/day >69-fold the clinical systemic exposure). In studies in rabbits, a higher incidence of incomplete ossification, compared with concurrent control animals, was seen at systemic exposure >24-fold the clinical systemic exposure seen at the clinical dose. No abnormalities were seen in rats. Montelukast has been shown to cross the placental barrier and is excreted in breast milk of animals.

No deaths occurred following a single oral administration of montelukast sodium at doses up to 5000 mg/kg in mice and rats (15,000 mg/m² and 30,000 mg/m² in mice and rats, respectively), the maximum dose tested. This dose is equivalent to 25,000 times the recommended daily adult human dose (based on an adult patient weight of 50 kg).

Montelukast was determined not to be phototoxic in mice for UVA, UVB or visible light spectra at doses up to 500 mg/kg/day (approximately >200-fold based on systemic exposure).

Montelukast was neither mutagenic in *in vitro* and *in vivo* tests nor tumorigenic in rodent species.

6. PHARMACEUTICAL PARTICULARS

6.1 List of excipients

Microcrystalline cellulose

Lactose monohydrate

Croscarmellose sodium

Hyprolose (E 463)

Magnesium stearate

Film coating:

Hypromellose

Hyprolose (E 463)

Titanium dioxide (E 171)

Red and yellow ferric oxide (E 172)

Carnauba wax

6.2 Incompatibilities

Not applicable.

6.3 Shelf life

3 years.

6.4 Special precautions for storage

Store in the original package in order to protect from light and moisture.

6.5 Nature and contents of container

Packaged in polyamide/PVC/aluminium blister package in:

Blisters in packages of: 7, 10, 14, 20, 28, 30, 50, 56, 84, 90, 98, 100, 140 and 200 tablets.

Blisters (unit doses), in packages of: 49, 50 and 56 tablets.

Not all pack sizes may be marketed.

6.6 Special precautions for disposal and other handling

Any unused product or waste material should be disposed of in accordance with local requirements.

7. MARKETING AUTHORISATION HOLDER

Merck Sharp & Dohme Limited

Hertford Road, Hoddesdon, Hertfordshire EN11 9BU, UK

8. MARKETING AUTHORISATION NUMBER(S)

PL 00025/0358

9. DATE OF FIRST AUTHORISATION/RENEWAL OF THE AUTHORISATION

15 January 1998/25 August 2007

10. DATE OF REVISION OF THE TEXT

14 August 2009

LEGAL CATEGORY

POM

SPC.SGA-10mg.09.UK.3032.II-049

SINGULAIR PAEDIATRIC 4 mg GRANULES

(Merck Sharp & Dohme Limited)

1. NAME OF THE MEDICINAL PRODUCT

SINGULAIR® Paediatric 4 mg Granules

2. QUALITATIVE AND QUANTITATIVE COMPOSITION

One sachet of granules contains montelukast sodium, which is equivalent to 4 mg montelukast. For a full list of excipients, see section 6.1.

3. PHARMACEUTICAL FORM

Granules

White granules

4. CLINICAL PARTICULARS

4.1 Therapeutic indications

SINGULAIR is indicated in the treatment of asthma as add-on therapy in those 6 months to 5 year old patients with mild to moderate persistent asthma who are inadequately controlled on inhaled corticosteroids and in whom "as-needed" short acting β-agonists provide inadequate clinical control of asthma.

SINGULAIR may also be an alternative treatment option to low-dose inhaled corticosteroids for 2 to 5 year old patients with mild persistent asthma who do not have a recent history of serious asthma attacks that required oral corticosteroid use, and who have demonstrated that they are not capable of using inhaled corticosteroids (see section 4.2).

SINGULAIR is also indicated in the prophylaxis of asthma from 2 years of age and older in which the predominant component is exercise-induced bronchoconstriction.

4.2 Posology and method of administration

This medicinal product is to be given to a child under adult supervision. The dosage for paediatric patients 6 months to 5 years of age is one sachet of 4-mg granules daily to be taken in the evening. No dosage adjustment within this age group is necessary. Efficacy data from clinical trials in paediatric patients 6 months to 2 years of age with persistent asthma are limited. Patients should be evaluated after 2 to 4 weeks for response to montelukast treatment. Treatment should be discontinued if a lack of response is observed. The SINGULAIR Paediatric 4 mg granules formulation is not recommended below 6 months of age.

Administration of SINGULAIR granules:

SINGULAIR granules can be administered either directly in the mouth, or mixed with a spoonful of cold or room temperature soft food (e.g., applesauce, ice cream, carrots and rice). The sachet should not be opened until ready to use. After opening the sachet, the full dose of SINGULAIR granules must be administered immediately (within 15 minutes). If mixed with food, SINGULAIR granules must not be stored for future use. SINGULAIR granules are not intended to be dissolved in liquid for administration. However, liquids may be taken subsequent to administration. SINGULAIR granules can be administered without regard to the timing of food ingestion.

General recommendations. The therapeutic effect of SINGULAIR on parameters of asthma control occurs within one day. Patients should be advised to continue taking SINGULAIR even if their asthma is under control, as well as during periods of worsening asthma.

No dosage adjustment is necessary for patients with renal insufficiency, or mild to moderate hepatic impairment. There are no data on patients with severe hepatic impairment. The dosage is the same for both male and female patients.

SINGULAIR as an alternative treatment option to low-dose inhaled corticosteroids for mild, persistent asthma:

Montelukast is not recommended as monotherapy in patients with moderate persistent asthma. The use of montelukast as an alternative treatment option to low-dose inhaled corticosteroids for children 2 to 5 years old with mild persistent asthma should only be considered for patients who do not have a recent history of serious asthma attacks that required oral corticosteroid use and who have demonstrated that they are not capable of using inhaled corticosteroids (see section 4.1). Mild persistent asthma is defined as asthma symptoms more than once a week but less than once a day, nocturnal symptoms more than twice a month but less than once a week, normal lung function between episodes. If satisfactory control of asthma is not achieved at follow-up (usually within one month), the need for an additional or different anti-inflammatory therapy based on the step system for asthma therapy should be evaluated. Patients should be periodically evaluated for their asthma control.

SINGULAIR as prophylaxis of asthma for 2 to 5 year old patients in whom the predominant component is exercise-induced bronchoconstriction.

In 2 to 5 year old patients, exercise-induced bronchoconstriction may be the predominant manifestation of persistent asthma that requires treatment with inhaled corticosteroids. Patients should be evaluated after 2 to 4 weeks of treatment with montelukast. If satisfactory response is not achieved, an additional or different therapy should be considered.

Therapy with SINGULAIR in relation to other treatments for asthma.

When treatment with SINGULAIR is used as add-on therapy to inhaled corticosteroids, SINGULAIR should not be abruptly substituted for inhaled corticosteroids (see section 4.4).

10-mg film-coated tablets are available for adults 15 years of age and older.

5-mg chewable tablets are available for paediatric patients 6 to 14 years of age.

4-mg chewable tablets are available as an alternative formulation for paediatric patients 2 to 5 years of age.

4.3 Contraindications

Hypersensitivity to the active substance or to any of the excipients.

4.4 Special warnings and precautions for use

The diagnosis of persistent asthma in very young children (6 months – 2 years) should be established by a paediatrician or pulmonologist.

Patients should be advised never to use oral montelukast to treat acute asthma attacks and to keep their usual appropriate rescue medication for this purpose readily available. If an acute attack occurs, a short-acting inhaled β-agonist should be used. Patients should seek their doctors' advice as soon as possible if they need more inhalations of short-acting β-agonists than usual.

Montelukast should not be abruptly substituted for inhaled or oral corticosteroids.

There are no data demonstrating that oral corticosteroids can be reduced when montelukast is given concomitantly.

In rare cases, patients on therapy with anti-asthma agents including montelukast may present with systemic eosinophilia, sometimes presenting with clinical features of vasculitis consistent with Churg-Strauss syndrome, a condition which is often treated with systemic corticosteroid therapy. These cases usually, but not always, have been associated with the reduction or withdrawal of oral corticosteroid therapy. The possibility that leukotriene receptor antagonists may be associated with emergence of Churg-Strauss syndrome can neither be excluded nor established. Physicians should be alert to eosinophilia, vasculitic rash, worsening pulmonary symptoms, cardiac complications, and/or neuropathy presenting in their patients. Patients who develop these symptoms should be reassessed and their treatment regimens evaluated.

4.5 Interaction with other medicinal products and other forms of interaction

Montelukast may be administered with other therapies routinely used in the prophylaxis and chronic treatment of asthma. In drug-interactions studies, the recommended clinical dose of montelukast did not have clinically important effects on the pharmacokinetics of the following medicinal products: theophylline, prednisone, prednisolone, oral contraceptives (ethinyl estradiol/norethindrone 35/1), terfenadine, digoxin and warfarin.

The area under the plasma concentration curve (AUC) for montelukast was decreased approximately 40% in subjects with co-administration of phenobarbital. Since montelukast is metabolised by CYP 3A4, caution should be exercised, particularly in children, when montelukast is co-administered with inducers of CYP 3A4, such as phenytoin, phenobarbital and rifampicin.

In vitro studies have shown that montelukast is a potent inhibitor of CYP 2C8. However, data from a clinical drug-drug interaction study involving montelukast and rosiglitazone (a probe substrate representative of medicinal products primarily metabolised by CYP 2C8) demonstrated that montelukast does not inhibit CYP 2C8 *in vivo*. Therefore, montelukast is not anticipated to markedly alter the metabolism of medicinal products metabolised by this enzyme (e.g., paclitaxel, rosiglitazone, and repaglinide.)

4.6 Pregnancy and lactation

Use during pregnancy

Animal studies do not indicate harmful effects with respect to effects on pregnancy or embryonal/foetal development.

Limited data from available pregnancy databases do not suggest a causal relationship between SINGULAIR and malformations (i.e. limb defects) that have been rarely reported in worldwide post marketing experience.

SINGULAIR may be used during pregnancy only if it is considered to be clearly essential.

Use during lactation

Studies in rats have shown that montelukast is excreted in milk (see section 5.3). It is not known if montelukast is excreted in human milk.

SINGULAIR may be used in breast-feeding mothers only if it is considered to be clearly essential.

4.7 Effects on ability to drive and use machines

Montelukast is not expected to affect a patient's ability to drive a car or operate machinery. However, in very rare cases, individuals have reported drowsiness or dizziness.

4.8 Undesirable effects

Montelukast has been evaluated in clinical studies as follows:

- 10-mg film-coated tablets in approximately 4000 adult patients 15 years of age and older
- 5-mg chewable tablets in approximately 1750 paediatric patients 6 to 14 years of age
- 4-mg chewable tablets in 851 paediatric patients 2 to 5 years of age, and
- 4-mg granules in 175 paediatric patients 6 months to 2 years of age.

The following drug-related adverse reactions in clinical studies were reported commonly (≥1/100 to <1/10) in patients treated with montelukast and at a greater incidence than in patients treated with placebo:

(see Table 1 on next page)

With prolonged treatment in clinical trials with a limited number of patients for up to 2 years for adults, and up to 12 months for paediatric patients 6 to 14 years of age, the safety profile did not change.

Cumulatively, 502 paediatric patients 2 to 5 years of age were treated with montelukast for at least 3 months, 338 for 6 months or longer, and 534 patients for 12 months or longer. With prolonged treatment, the safety profile did not change in these patients either.

The safety profile in paediatric patients 6 months to 2 years of age did not change with treatment up to 3 months.

The following adverse reactions have been reported in post-marketing use:

Blood and lymphatic system disorders: increased bleeding tendency.

Immune system disorders: hypersensitivity reactions including anaphylaxis, hepatic eosinophilic infiltration.

Psychiatric disorders: dream abnormalities including nightmares, hallucinations, insomnia, irritability, anxiety, restlessness, agitation including aggressive behaviour, tremor, depression, suicidal thinking and behaviour (suicidality) in very rare cases.

Nervous system disorders: dizziness drowsiness, paraesthesia/hypoesthesia, seizure.

Cardiac disorders: palpitations.

Respiratory, thoracic and mediastinal disorders: epistaxis.

Gastro-intestinal disorders: diarrhoea, dry mouth, dyspepsia, nausea, vomiting.

Table 1

Body System Class	Adult Patients 15 years and older (two 12-week studies; n=795)	Paediatric Patients 6 to 14 years old (one 8-week study; n=201) (two 56-week studies; n=615)	Paediatric Patients 2 to 5 years old (one 12-week study; n=461) (one 48-week study; n=278)	Paediatric Patients 6 months up to 2 years old (one 6-week study; n=175)
Nervous system disorders	headache	headache		hyperkinesia
Respiratory, thoracic, and mediastinal disorders				asthma
Gastro-intestinal disorders	abdominal pain		abdominal pain	diarrhoea
Skin and subcutaneous tissue disorders				eczematous dermatitis, rash
General disorders and administration site conditions			thirst	

Hepatobiliary disorders: elevated levels of serum transaminases (ALT, AST), cholestatic hepatitis

Skin and subcutaneous tissue disorders: angiooedema, bruising, urticaria, pruritus, rash, erythema nodosum.

Musculoskeletal and connective tissue disorders: arthralgia, myalgia including muscle cramps.

General disorders and administration site conditions: asthenia/fatigue, malaise, oedema, pyrexia.

Very rare cases of Churg-Strauss Syndrome (CSS) have been reported during montelukast treatment in asthmatic patients (see section 4.4).

4.9 Overdose

No specific information is available on the treatment of overdose with montelukast. In chronic asthma studies, montelukast has been administered at doses up to 200 mg/day to adult patients for 22 weeks and in short term studies, up to 900 mg/day to patients for approximately one week without clinically important adverse experiences.

There have been reports of acute overdose in post-marketing experience and clinical studies with montelukast. These include reports in adults and children with a dose as high as 1000 mg (approximately 61 mg/kg in a 42 month old child). The clinical and laboratory findings observed were consistent with the safety profile in adults and paediatric patients. There were no adverse experiences in the majority of overdose reports. The most frequently occurring adverse experiences were consistent with the safety profile of montelukast and included abdominal pain, somnolence, thirst, headache, vomiting, and psychomotor hyperactivity.

It is not known whether montelukast is dialysable by peritoneal- or haemo-dialysis.

5. PHARMACOLOGICAL PROPERTIES

5.1 Pharmacodynamic properties

Pharmacotherapeutic group: Leukotriene receptor antagonist

ATC-code: R03D C03

The cysteinyl leukotrienes (LTC_4, LTD_4, LTE_4) are potent inflammatory eicosanoids released from various cells including mast cells and eosinophils. These important pro-asthmatic mediators bind to cysteinyl leukotriene receptors (CysLT) found in the human airway and cause airway actions, including bronchoconstriction, mucous secretion, vascular permeability, and eosinophil recruitment.

Montelukast is an orally active compound which binds with high affinity and selectivity to the $CysLT_1$ receptor. In clinical studies, montelukast inhibits bronchoconstriction due to inhaled LTD_4 at doses as low as 5 mg. Bronchodilation was observed within 2 hours of oral administration. The bronchodilation effect caused by a β-agonist was additive to that caused by montelukast. Treatment with montelukast inhibited both early- and late-phase bronchoconstriction due to antigen challenge. Montelukast, compared with placebo, decreased peripheral blood eosinophils in adult and paediatric patients. In a separate study, treatment with montelukast significantly decreased eosinophils in the airways (as measured in sputum). In adult and paediatric patients 2 to 14 years of age, montelukast, compared with placebo, decreased peripheral blood eosinophils while improving clinical asthma control.

In studies in adults, montelukast, 10 mg once daily, compared with placebo, demonstrated significant improvements in morning FEV_1 (10.4% vs 2.7% change from baseline), AM peak expiratory flow rate (PEFR) (24.5 L/min vs 3.3 L/min change from baseline), and significant decrease in total β-agonist use (-26.1% vs -4.6% change from baseline). Improvement in patient-reported daytime and night-time asthma symptoms scores was significantly better than placebo.

Studies in adults demonstrated the ability of montelukast to add to the clinical effect of inhaled corticosteroid (% change from baseline for inhaled beclometasone plus montelukast vs beclometasone, respectively for FEV_1: 5.43% vs 1.04%; β-agonist use: -8.70% vs 2.64%). Compared with inhaled beclometasone (200 μg twice daily with a spacer device), montelukast demonstrated a more rapid initial response, although over the 12-week study, beclometasone provided a greater average treatment effect (% change from baseline for montelukast vs beclometasone, respectively for FEV_1: 7.49% vs 13.3%; β-agonist use: -28.28% vs -43.89%). However, compared with beclometasone, a high percentage of patients treated with montelukast achieved similar clinical responses (e.g., 50% of patients treated with beclometasone achieved an improvement in FEV_1 of approximately 11% or more over baseline while approximately 42% of patients treated with montelukast achieved the same response).

In an 8-week study in paediatric patients 6 to 14 years of age, montelukast 5 mg once daily, compared with placebo, significantly improved respiratory function (FEV_1 8.71% vs 4.16% change from baseline; AM PEFR 27.9 L/min vs 17.8 L/min change from baseline) and decreased "as-needed" β-agonist use (-11.7% vs +8.2% change from baseline).

In a 12-month study comparing the efficacy of montelukast to inhaled fluticasone on asthma control in paediatric patients 6 to 14 years of age with mild persistent asthma, montelukast was non-inferior to fluticasone in increasing the percentage of asthma rescue-free days (RFDs), the primary endpoint. Averaged over the 12-month treatment period, the percentage of asthma RFDs increased from 61.6 to 84.0 in the montelukast group and from 60.9 to 86.7 in the fluticasone group. The between group difference in LS mean increase in the percentage of asthma RFDs was statistically significant (-2.8 with a 95% CI of -4.7, -0.9), but within the limit pre-defined to be clinically not inferior. Both montelukast and fluticasone also improved asthma control on secondary variables assessed over the 12 month treatment period:

- FEV_1 increased from 1.83 L to 2.09 L in the montelukast group and from 1.85 L to 2.14 L in the fluticasone group. The between-group difference in LS mean increase in FEV_1 was -0.02 L with a 95% CI of (-0.06, 0.02. The mean increase from baseline in % predicted FEV_1 was 0.6% in the montelukast treatment group, and 2.7% in the fluticasone treatment group. The difference in LS means for the change from baseline in the % predicted FEV_1 was significant: -2.2% with a 95% CI of -3.6, -0.7.
- The percentage of days with β-agonist use decreased from 38.0 to 15.4 in the montelukast group, and from 38.5 to 12.8 in the fluticasone group. The between group difference in LS means for the percentage of days with β-agonist use was significant: 2.7 with a 95% CI of 0.9, 4.5.
- The percentage of patients with an asthma attack (an asthma attack being defined as a period of worsening asthma that required treatment with oral steroids, an unscheduled visit to the doctor's office, an emergency room visit, or hospitalisation) was 32.2 in the montelukast group and 25.6 in the fluticasone group; the odds ratio (95% CI) being significant: equal to 1.38 (1.04, 1.84).
- The percentage of patients with systemic (mainly oral) corticosteroid use during the study period was 17.8% in the montelukast group and 10.5% in the fluticasone group. The between group difference in LS means was significant: 7.3% with a 95%CI of 2.9; 11.7.

In a 12-week, placebo-controlled study in paediatric patients 2 to 5 years of age, montelukast 4 mg once daily improved parameters of asthma control compared with placebo irrespective of concomitant controller therapy (inhaled/nebulised corticosteroids or inhaled/nebulised sodium cromoglycate). Sixty percent of patients were not on any other controller therapy. Montelukast improved daytime symptoms (including coughing, wheezing, trouble breathing and activity limitation) and night-time symptoms compared with placebo. Montelukast also decreased "as-needed" β-agonist use and corticosteroid rescue for worsening asthma compared with placebo. Patients receiving montelukast had more days without asthma than those receiving placebo. A treatment effect was achieved after the first dose.

In a 12-month, placebo-controlled study in paediatric patients 2 to 5 years of age with mild asthma and episodic exacerbations, montelukast 4 mg once daily significantly ($p \leqslant 0.001$) reduced the yearly rate of asthma exacerbation episodes (EE) compared with placebo (1.60 EE vs. 2.34 EE, respectively), [EE defined as $\geqslant$ 3 consecutive days with daytime symptoms requiring β-agonist use, or corticosteroids (oral or inhaled), or hospitalisation for asthma]. The percentage reduction in yearly EE rate was 31.9%, with a 95% CI of 16.9, 44.1.

Efficacy of montelukast is supported in paediatric patients 6 months to 2 years of age by extrapolation from the demonstrated efficacy in patients 2 years of age and older with asthma, and is based on similar pharmacokinetic data, as well as the assumption that the disease course, pathophysiology and the medicinal product's effect are substantially similar among these populations.

Significant reduction of exercise-induced bronchoconstriction (EIB) was demonstrated in a 12-week study in adults (maximal fall in FEV_1 22.33% for montelukast vs 32.40% for placebo; time to recovery to within 5% of baseline FEV_1 44.22 min vs 60.64 min). This effect was consistent throughout the 12-week study period. Reduction in EIB was also demonstrated in a short term study in paediatric patients 6 to 14 years of age (maximal fall in FEV_1 18.27% vs 26.11%; time to recovery to within 5% of baseline FEV_1 17.76 min vs 27.98 min). The effect in both studies was demonstrated at the end of the once-daily dosing interval.

In aspirin-sensitive asthmatic patients receiving concomitant inhaled and/or oral corticosteroids, treatment with montelukast, compared with placebo, resulted in significant improvement in asthma control (FEV_1 8.55% vs -1.74% change from baseline and decrease in total β-agonist use -27.78% vs 2.09% change from baseline).

5.2 Pharmacokinetic properties

Absorption. Montelukast is rapidly absorbed following oral administration. For the 10-mg film-coated tablet, the mean peak plasma concentration (C_{max}) is achieved 3 hours (T_{max}) after administration in adults in the fasted state. The mean oral bioavailability is 64%. The oral bioavailability and C_{max} are not influenced by a standard meal. Safety and efficacy were demonstrated in clinical trials where the 10-mg film-coated tablet was administered without regard to the timing of food ingestion.

For the 5-mg chewable tablet, the C_{max} is achieved in 2 hours after administration in adults in the fasted state. The mean oral bioavailability is 73% and is decreased to 63% by a standard meal.

After administration of the 4-mg chewable tablet to paediatric patients 2 to 5 years of age in the fasted state, C_{max} is achieved 2 hours after administration. The mean C_{max} is 66% higher while mean C_{min} is lower than in adults receiving a 10-mg tablet.

The 4-mg granule formulation is bioequivalent to the 4-mg chewable tablet when administered to adults in the fasted state. In paediatric patients 6 months to 2 years of age, C_{max} is achieved 2 hours after administration of the 4-mg granules formulation. C_{max} is nearly 2-fold greater than in adults receiving a 10-mg tablet. The co-administration of applesauce or a high-fat standard meal with the granule formulation did not have a clinically meaningful effect on the pharmacokinetics of montelukast as determined by AUC (1225.7 vs 1223.1 ng·hr/mL with and without applesauce, respectively, and 1191.8 vs 1148.5 ng·hr/mL with and without a high-fat standard meal, respectively).

Distribution. Montelukast is more than 99% bound to plasma proteins. The steady-state volume of distribution of montelukast averages 8-11 litres. Studies in rats with radiolabelled montelukast indicate minimal distribution across the blood-brain barrier. In addition, concentrations of radiolabelled material at 24 hours post-dose were minimal in all other tissues.

Biotransformation. Montelukast is extensively metabolised. In studies with therapeutic doses, plasma concentrations of metabolites of montelukast are undetectable at steady state in adults and children.

In vitro studies using human liver microsomes indicate that cytochrome P450 3A4, 2A6 and 2C9 are involved in the metabolism of montelukast. Based on further *in vitro* results in human liver microsomes, therapeutic plasma concentrations of montelukast do not inhibit cytochromes P450 3A4, 2C9, 1A2, 2A6, 2C19, or 2D6. The contribution of metabolites to the therapeutic effect of montelukast is minimal.

Elimination. The plasma clearance of montelukast averages 45 ml/min in healthy adults. Following an oral dose of radiolabelled montelukast, 86% of the radioactivity was recovered in 5-day faecal collections and <0.2% was recovered in urine. Coupled with estimates of montelukast oral bioavailability, this indicates that montelukast and its metabolites are excreted almost exclusively via the bile.

Characteristics in patients. No dosage adjustment is necessary for the elderly or mild to moderate hepatic insufficiency. Studies in patients with renal impairment have not been undertaken. Because montelukast and its metabolites are eliminated by the biliary route, no dose adjustment is anticipated to be necessary in patients with renal impairment. There are no data on the pharmacokinetics of montelukast in patients with severe hepatic insufficiency (Child-Pugh score >9).

With high doses of montelukast (20- and 60-fold the recommended adult dose), a decrease in plasma theophylline concentration was observed. This effect was not seen at the recommended dose of 10 mg once daily.

5.3 Preclinical safety data
In animal toxicity studies, minor serum biochemical alterations in ALT, glucose, phosphorus and triglycerides were observed which were transient in nature. The signs of toxicity in animals were increased excretion of saliva, gastro-intestinal symptoms, loose stools and ion imbalance. These occurred at dosages which provided >17-fold the systemic exposure seen at the clinical dosage. In monkeys, the adverse effects appeared at doses from 150 mg/kg/day (>232-fold the systemic exposure seen at the clinical dose). In animal studies, montelukast did not affect fertility or reproductive performance at systemic exposure exceeding the clinical systemic exposure by greater than 24-fold. A slight decrease in pup body weight was noted in the female fertility study in rats at 200 mg/kg/day (>69-fold the clinical systemic exposure). In studies in rabbits, a higher incidence of incomplete ossification, compared with concurrent control animals, was seen at systemic exposure >24-fold the clinical systemic exposure seen at the clinical dose. No abnormalities were seen in rats. Montelukast has been shown to cross the placental barrier and is excreted in breast milk of animals.

No deaths occurred following a single oral administration of montelukast sodium at doses up to 5000 mg/kg in mice and rats (15,000 mg/m^2 and 30,000 mg/m^2 in mice and rats, respectively), the maximum dose tested. This dose is equivalent to 25,000 times the recommended daily adult human dose (based on an adult patient weight of 50 kg).

Montelukast was determined not to be phototoxic in mice for UVA, UVB or visible light spectra at doses up to 500 mg/kg/day (approximately >200-fold based on systemic exposure).

Montelukast was neither mutagenic in *in vitro* and *in vivo* tests nor tumorigenic in rodent species.

6. PHARMACEUTICAL PARTICULARS

6.1 List of excipients
Mannitol

Hyprolose (E 463)

Magnesium stearate

6.2 Incompatibilities
Not applicable.

6.3 Shelf life
2 years.

6.4 Special precautions for storage
Store in the original package in order to protect from light and moisture.

6.5 Nature and contents of container
Packaged in polyethylene/aluminum/polyester sachet in:

Cartons of 7, 20, 28 and 30 sachets.

Not all pack sizes may be marketed.

6.6 Special precautions for disposal and other handling
Any unused product or waste material should be disposed of in accordance with local requirements.

7. MARKETING AUTHORISATION HOLDER
Merck Sharp & Dohme Limited

Hertford Road, Hoddesdon, Hertfordshire EN11 9BU, UK

8. MARKETING AUTHORISATION NUMBER(S)
PL 0025/0440

9. DATE OF FIRST AUTHORISATION/RENEWAL OF THE AUTHORISATION
14 February 2003/ 25 August 2007

10. DATE OF REVISION OF THE TEXT
14 August 2009

LEGAL CATEGORY
POM

® denotes registered trademark of Merck & Co., Inc., Whitehouse Station, NJ, USA.

SPC.SGA-OG-4mg.09.UK.3021.II-049

Singulair Paediatric 4 mg tablets

(Merck Sharp & Dohme Limited)

1. NAME OF THE MEDICINAL PRODUCT
SINGULAIR® Paediatric 4 mg Chewable Tablets

2. QUALITATIVE AND QUANTITATIVE COMPOSITION
One chewable tablet contains montelukast sodium, which is equivalent to 4 mg montelukast.

Excipient: Aspartame (E 951) 1.2 mg per tablet

For a full list of excipients, see section 6.1.

3. PHARMACEUTICAL FORM
Chewable tablet.

Pink, oval, biconvex-shaped, 'SINGULAIR' engraved on one side and 'MSD 711' on the other.

4. CLINICAL PARTICULARS

4.1 Therapeutic indications
SINGULAIR is indicated in the treatment of asthma as add-on therapy in those 2 to 5 year old patients with mild to moderate persistent asthma who are inadequately controlled on inhaled corticosteroids and in whom 'as-needed' short-acting β-agonists provide inadequate clinical control of asthma.

SINGULAIR may also be an alternative treatment option to low-dose inhaled corticosteroids for 2 to 5 year old patients with mild persistent asthma who do not have a recent history of serious asthma attacks that required oral corticosteroid use, and who have demonstrated that they are not capable of using inhaled corticosteroids (see section 4.2).

SINGULAIR is also indicated in the prophylaxis of asthma from 2 years of age and older in which the predominant component is exercise-induced bronchoconstriction.

4.2 Posology and method of administration
This medicinal product is to be given to a child under adult supervision. For children who have problems consuming a chewable tablet, a granule formulation is available (See SINGULAIR® Paediatric 4 mg Granules SPC). The dosage for paediatric patients 2-5 years of age is one 4 mg chewable tablet daily to be taken in the evening. If taken in connection with food, SINGULAIR should be taken 1 hour before or 2 hours after food. No dosage adjustment within this age group is necessary. The SINGULAIR Paediatric 4 mg chewable tablet formulation is not recommended below 2 years of age.

General recommendations:

The therapeutic effect of SINGULAIR on parameters of asthma control occurs within one day. Patients should be advised to continue taking SINGULAIR even if their asthma is under control, as well as during periods of worsening asthma.

No dosage adjustment is necessary for patients with renal insufficiency, or mild to moderate hepatic impairment. There are no data on patients with severe hepatic impairment. The dosage is the same for both male and female patients.

SINGULAIR *as an alternative treatment option to low-dose inhaled corticosteroids for mild, persistent asthma:*

Montelukast is not recommended as monotherapy in patients with moderate persistent asthma. The use of montelukast as an alternative treatment option to low-dose inhaled corticosteroids for children with mild persistent asthma should only be considered for patients who do not have a recent history of serious asthma attacks that required oral corticosteroid use and who have demonstrated that they are not capable of using inhaled corticosteroids (see section 4.1). Mild persistent asthma is defined as asthma symptoms more than once a week but less than once a day, nocturnal symptoms more than twice a month but less than once a week, normal lung function between episodes. If satisfactory control of asthma is not achieved at follow-up (usually within one month), the need for an additional or different anti-inflammatory therapy based on the step system for asthma therapy should be evaluated. Patients should be periodically evaluated for their asthma control.

SINGULAIR as prophylaxis of asthma for 2 to 5 year old patients in whom the predominant component is exercise-induced bronchoconstriction.

In 2 to 5 year old patients, exercise-induced bronchoconstriction may be the predominant manifestation of persistent asthma that requires treatment with inhaled corticosteroids. Patients should be evaluated after 2 to 4 weeks of treatment with montelukast. If satisfactory response is not achieved, an additional or different therapy should be considered.

Therapy with SINGULAIR *in relation to other treatments for asthma.*

When treatment with SINGULAIR is used as add-on therapy to inhaled corticosteroids, SINGULAIR should not be abruptly substituted for inhaled corticosteroids (see section 4.4).

10 mg film-coated tablets are available for adults 15 years of age and older.

5 mg chewable tablets are available for paediatric patients 6 to 14 years of age.

4 mg granules are available for paediatric patients 6 months to 5 years of age.

4.3 Contraindications
Hypersensitivity to the active substance or to any of the excipients.

4.4 Special warnings and precautions for use
Patients should be advised never to use oral montelukast to treat acute asthma attacks and to keep their usual appropriate rescue medication for this purpose readily available. If an acute attack occurs, a short-acting inhaled β-agonist should be used. Patients should seek their doctor's advice as soon as possible if they need more inhalations of short-acting β-agonists than usual.

Montelukast should not be abruptly substituted for inhaled or oral corticosteroids.

There are no data demonstrating that oral corticosteroids can be reduced when montelukast is given concomitantly.

In rare cases, patients on therapy with anti-asthma agents including montelukast may present with systemic eosinophilia, sometimes presenting with clinical features of vasculitis consistent with Churg-Strauss syndrome, a condition which is often treated with systemic corticosteroid therapy. These cases usually, but not always, have been associated with the reduction or withdrawal of oral corticosteroid therapy. The possibility that leukotriene receptor antagonists may be associated with emergence of Churg-Strauss syndrome can neither be excluded nor established. Physicians should be alert to eosinophilia, vasculitic rash, worsening pulmonary symptoms, cardiac complications, and/or neuropathy presenting in their patients. Patients who develop these symptoms should be reassessed and their treatment regimens evaluated.

SINGULAIR contains aspartame, a source of phenylalanine. Patients with phenylketonuria should take into account that each 4 mg chewable tablet contains phenylalanine in an amount equivalent to 0.674 mg phenylalanine per dose.

4.5 Interaction with other medicinal products and other forms of interaction
Montelukast may be administered with other therapies routinely used in the prophylaxis and chronic treatment of asthma. In drug-interactions studies, the recommended clinical dose of montelukast did not have clinically important effects on the pharmacokinetics of the following medicinal products: theophylline, prednisone, prednisolone, oral contraceptives (ethinyl oestradiol/norethindrone 35/1), terfenadine, digoxin and warfarin.

The area under the plasma concentration curve (AUC) for montelukast was decreased approximately 40% in subjects with co-administration of phenobarbital. Since montelukast is metabolised by CYP 3A4, caution should be exercised, particularly in children, when montelukast is co-administered with inducers of CYP 3A4, such as phenytoin, phenobarbital and rifampicin.

In vitro studies have shown that montelukast is a potent inhibitor of CYP 2C8. However, data from a clinical drug-drug interaction study involving montelukast and rosiglitazone (a probe substrate representative of medicinal products primarily metabolised by CYP 2C8) demonstrated that montelukast does not inhibit CYP 2C8 *in vivo*. Therefore, montelukast is not anticipated to markedly alter the metabolism of medicinal products metabolised by this enzyme (eg., paclitaxel, rosiglitazone, and repaglinide).

4.6 Pregnancy and lactation
Use during pregnancy

Animal studies do not indicate harmful effects with respect to effects on pregnancy or embryonal/foetal development.

Limited data from available pregnancy databases do not suggest a causal relationship between SINGULAIR and malformations (i.e. limb defects) that have been rarely reported in worldwide post marketing experience.

SINGULAIR may be used during pregnancy only if it is considered to be clearly essential.

Use during lactation

Studies in rats have shown that montelukast is excreted in milk (see section 5.3). It is not known if montelukast is excreted in human milk.

SINGULAIR may be used in breast-feeding mothers only if it is considered to be clearly essential.

4.7 Effects on ability to drive and use machines
Montelukast is not expected to affect a patient's ability to drive a car or operate machinery. However, in very rare cases, individuals have reported drowsiness or dizziness.

4.8 Undesirable effects
Montelukast has been evaluated in clinical studies as follows:

- 10 mg film-coated tablets in approximately 4,000 adult patients 15 years of age and older
- 5 mg chewable tablets in approximately 1,750 paediatric patients 6 to 14 years of age, and
- 4 mg chewable tablets in 851 paediatric patients 2 to 5 years of age.

The following drug-related adverse reactions in clinical studies were reported commonly (≥1/100 to <1/10) in patients treated with montelukast and at a greater incidence than in patients treated with placebo:

(see Table 1 on next page)

With prolonged treatment in clinical trials with a limited number of patients for up to 2 years for adults, and up to 12 months for paediatric patients 6 to 14 years of age, the safety profile did not change.

Table 1

Body System Class	Adult Patients 15 years and older (two 12-week studies; n=795)	Paediatric Patients 6 to 14 years old (one 8-week study; n=201) (two 56-week studies; n=615)	Paediatric Patients 2 to 5 years old (one 12-week study; n=461) (one 48-week study; n=278)
Nervous system disorders	headache	headache	
Gastro-intestinal disorders	abdominal pain		abdominal pain
General disorders and administration site conditions			thirst

Cumulatively, 502 paediatric patients 2 to 5 years of age were treated with montelukast for at least 3 months, 338 for 6 months or longer, and 534 patients for 12 months or longer. With prolonged treatment, the safety profile did not change in these patients either.

The following adverse reactions have been reported in post-marketing use:

Blood and lymphatic system disorders: increased bleeding tendency.

Immune system disorders: hypersensitivity reactions including anaphylaxis, hepatic eosinophilic infiltration.

Psychiatric disorders: dream abnormalities including nightmares, hallucinations, insomnia, irritability, anxiety, restlessness, agitation including aggressive behaviour, tremor, depression, suicidal thinking and behaviour (suicidality) in very rare cases.

Nervous system disorders: dizziness, drowsiness, paraesthesia/hypoesthesia, seizure.

Cardiac disorders: palpitations.

Respiratory, thoracic and mediastinal disorders: epistaxis.

Gastro-intestinal disorders: diarrhoea, dry mouth, dyspepsia, nausea, vomiting.

Hepatobiliary disorders: elevated levels of serum transaminases (ALT, AST), cholestatic hepatitis.

Skin and subcutaneous tissue disorders: angiooedema, bruising, urticaria, pruritus, rash, erythema nodosum.

Musculoskeletal and connective tissue disorders: arthralgia, myalgia including muscle cramps.

General disorders and administration site conditions: asthenia/fatigue, malaise, oedema, pyrexia.

Very rare cases of Churg-Strauss Syndrome (CSS) have been reported during montelukast treatment in asthmatic patients (see section 4.4).

4.9 Overdose

No specific information is available on the treatment of overdose with montelukast. In chronic asthma studies, montelukast has been administered at doses up to 200 mg/day to adult patients for 22 weeks and in short-term studies, up to 900 mg/day to patients for approximately one week without clinically important adverse experiences.

There have been reports of acute overdose in post-marketing experience and clinical studies with montelukast. These include reports in adults and children with a dose as high as 1000 mg (approximately 61 mg/kg in a 42 month old child). The clinical and laboratory findings observed were consistent with the safety profile in adults and paediatric patients. There were no adverse experiences in the majority of overdose reports. The most frequently occurring adverse experiences were consistent with the safety profile of montelukast and included abdominal pain, somnolence, thirst, headache, vomiting, and psychomotor hyperactivity.

It is not known whether montelukast is dialysable by peritoneal- or haemo-dialysis.

5. PHARMACOLOGICAL PROPERTIES

5.1 Pharmacodynamic properties

Pharmacotherapeutic group: Leukotriene receptor antagonist

ATC Code: RO3D CO3

The cysteinyl leukotrienes (LTC_4, LTD_4, LTE_4) are potent inflammatory eicosanoids released from various cells including mast cells and eosinophils. These important pro-asthmatic mediators bind to cysteinyl leukotriene receptors (CysLT) found in the human airway and cause airway actions, including bronchoconstriction, mucous secretion, vascular permeability, and eosinophil recruitment.

Montelukast is an orally active compound which binds with high affinity and selectivity to the $CysLT_1$ receptor. In clinical studies, montelukast inhibits bronchoconstriction due to inhaled LTD_4 at doses as low as 5 mg. Bronchodilation was observed within two hours of oral administration. The bronchodilation effect caused by a β-agonist was additive to that caused by montelukast. Treatment with montelukast inhibited both early- and late-phase bronchoconstriction due to antigen challenge. Montelukast, compared with placebo, decreased peripheral blood eosinophils in adult and paediatric patients. In a separate study, treatment with montelukast significantly decreased eosinophils in the airways (as measured in sputum). In adult and paediatric patients 2 to 14 years of age, montelukast, compared with placebo, decreased peripheral blood eosinophils while improving clinical asthma control.

In studies in adults, montelukast 10 mg once daily, compared with placebo, demonstrated significant improvements in morning FEV_1 (10.4% vs 2.7% change from baseline), AM peak expiratory flow rate (PEFR) (24.5 L/min vs 3.3 L/min change from baseline), and significant decrease in total β-agonist use (-26.1% vs -4.6% change from baseline). Improvement in patient-reported daytime and night-time asthma symptoms scores was significantly better than placebo.

Studies in adults demonstrated the ability of montelukast to add to the clinical effect of inhaled corticosteroid (% change from baseline for inhaled beclometasone plus montelukast vs beclometasone, respectively for FEV_1 : 5.43% vs 1.04%; β-agonist use: -8.70% vs 2.64%). Compared with inhaled beclometasone (200 μg twice daily with a spacer device), montelukast demonstrated a more rapid initial response, although over the 12-week study, beclometasone provided a greater average treatment effect (% change from baseline for montelukast vs beclometasone, respectively for FEV_1 : 7.49% vs 13.3%; β-agonist use: -28.28% vs -43.89%). However, compared with beclometasone, a high percentage of patients treated with montelukast achieved similar clinical responses (e.g. 50% of patients treated with beclometasone achieved an improvement in FEV_1 of approximately 11% or more over baseline while approximately 42% of patients treated with montelukast achieved the same response).

In a 12-week, placebo-controlled study in paediatric patients 2 to 5 years of age, montelukast 4 mg once daily improved parameters of asthma control compared with placebo irrespective of concomitant controller therapy (inhaled/nebulised corticosteroids or inhaled/nebulised sodium cromoglycate). Sixty percent of patients were not on any other controller therapy. Montelukast improved daytime symptoms (including coughing, wheezing, trouble breathing and activity limitation) and night-time symptoms compared with placebo. Montelukast also decreased 'as needed' β-agonist use and corticosteroid rescue for worsening asthma compared with placebo. Patients receiving montelukast had more days without asthma than those receiving placebo. A treatment effect was achieved after the first dose.

In a 12-month, placebo-controlled study in paediatric patients 2 to 5 years of age with mild asthma and episodic exacerbations, montelukast 4 mg once daily significantly ($p \leqslant 0.001$) reduced the yearly rate of asthma exacerbation episodes (EE) compared with placebo (1.60 EE vs. 2.34 EE, respectively), [EE defined as $\geqslant$ 3 consecutive days with daytime symptoms requiring β-agonist use, or corticosteroids (oral or inhaled), or hospitalisation for asthma]. The percentage reduction in yearly EE rate was 31.9%, with a 95% CI of 16.9, 44.1.

In an 8-week study in paediatric patients 6 to 14 years of age, montelukast 5 mg once daily, compared with placebo, significantly improved respiratory function (FEV_1 8.71% vs 4.16% change from baseline; AM PEFR 27.9 L/min vs 17.8 L/min change from baseline) and decreased 'as-needed' β-agonist use (-11.7% vs +8.2% change from baseline).

In a 12-month study comparing the efficacy of montelukast to inhaled fluticasone on asthma control in paediatric patients 6 to 14 years of age with mild persistent asthma, montelukast was non-inferior to fluticasone in increasing the percentage of asthma rescue-free days (RFDs), the primary endpoint. Averaged over the 12-month treatment period, the percentage of asthma RFDs increased from 61.6 to 84.0 in the montelukast group and from 60.9 to 86.7 in the fluticasone group. The between group difference in LS mean increase in the percentage of asthma RFDs was statistically significant (-2.8 with a 95% CI of -4.7, -0.9), but within the limit pre-defined to be clinically not inferior. Both montelukast and fluticasone also improved asthma control on secondary variables assessed over the 12 month treatment period:

- FEV_1 increased from 1.83 L to 2.09 L in the montelukast group and from 1.85 L to 2.14 L in the fluticasone group. The between-group difference in LS mean increase in FEV_1 was -0.02 L with a 95% CI of -0.06, 0.02. The mean increase from baseline in % predicted FEV_1 was 0.6% in the montelukast treatment group, and 2.7% in the fluticasone treatment group. The difference in LS means for the change from baseline in the % predicted FEV_1 was significant: -2.2% with a 95% CI of -3.6, -0.7.
- The percentage of days with β-agonist use decreased from 38.0 to 15.4 in the montelukast group, and from 38.5 to 12.8 in the fluticasone group. The between group difference in LS means for the percentage of days with β-agonist use was significant: 2.7 with a 95% CI of 0.9, 4.5.
- The percentage of patients with an asthma attack (an asthma attack being defined as a period of worsening asthma that required treatment with oral steroids, an unscheduled visit to the doctor's office, an emergency room visit, or hospitalisation) was 32.2 in the montelukast group and 25.6 in the fluticasone group; the odds ratio (95% CI) being significant: equal to 1.38 (1.04, 1.84).
- The percentage of patients with systemic (mainly oral) corticosteroid use during the study period was 17.8% in the montelukast group and 10.5% in the fluticasone group. The between group difference in LS means was significant: 7.3% with a 95% CI of 2.9; 11.7.

Significant reduction of exercise-induced bronchoconstriction (EIB) was demonstrated in a 12-week study in adults (maximal fall in FEV_1 22.33% for montelukast vs 32.40% for placebo; time to recovery to within 5% of baseline FEV_1 44.22 min vs 60.64 min). This effect was consistent throughout the 12-week study period. Reduction in EIB was also demonstrated in a short term study in paediatric patients 6 to 14 years of age (maximal fall in FEV_1 18.27% vs 26.11%; time to recovery to within 5% of baseline FEV_1 17.76 min vs 27.98 min). The effect in both studies was demonstrated at the end of the once-daily dosing interval.

In aspirin-sensitive asthmatic patients receiving concomitant inhaled and/or oral corticosteroids, treatment with montelukast, compared with placebo, resulted in significant improvement in asthma control (FEV_1 8.55% vs -1.74% change from baseline and decrease in total β-agonist use -27.78% vs 2.09% change from baseline).

5.2 Pharmacokinetic properties

Absorption: Montelukast is rapidly absorbed following oral administration. For the 10 mg film-coated tablet, the mean peak plasma concentration (C_{max}) is achieved three hours (T_{max}) after administration in adults in the fasted state. The mean oral bioavailability is 64%. The oral bioavailability and C_{max} are not influenced by a standard meal. Safety and efficacy were demonstrated in clinical trials where the 10 mg film-coated tablet was administered without regard to the timing of food ingestion.

For the 5 mg chewable tablet, the C_{max} is achieved in two hours after administration in adults in the fasted state. The mean oral bioavailability is 73% and is decreased to 63% by a standard meal.

After administration of the 4 mg chewable tablet to paediatric patients 2 to 5 years of age in the fasted state, C_{max} is achieved 2 hours after administration. The mean C_{max} is 66% higher while mean C_{min} is lower than in adults receiving a 10 mg tablet.

Distribution: Montelukast is more than 99% bound to plasma proteins. The steady-state volume of distribution of montelukast averages 8-11 litres. Studies in rats with radiolabelled montelukast indicate minimal distribution across the blood-brain barrier. In addition, concentrations of radiolabelled material at 24 hours post-dose were minimal in all other tissues.

Biotransformation: Montelukast is extensively metabolised. In studies with therapeutic doses, plasma concentrations of metabolites of montelukast are undetectable at steady state in adults and children.

In vitro studies using human liver microsomes indicate that cytochromes P450 3A4, 2A6 and 2C9 are involved in the metabolism of montelukast. Based on further *in vitro* results in human liver microsomes, therapeutic plasma concentrations of montelukast do not inhibit cytochromes P450 3A4, 2C9, 1A2, 2A6, 2C19, or 2D6. The contribution of metabolites to the therapeutic effect of montelukast is minimal.

Elimination: The plasma clearance of montelukast averages 45 ml/min in healthy adults. Following an oral dose of radiolabelled montelukast, 86% of the radioactivity was recovered in 5-day faecal collections and <0.2% was recovered in urine. Coupled with estimates of montelukast oral bioavailability, this indicates that montelukast and its metabolites are excreted almost exclusively *via* the bile.

Characteristics in patients: No dosage adjustment is necessary for the elderly or mild to moderate hepatic insufficiency. Studies in patients with renal impairment have not been undertaken. Because montelukast and its metabolites are eliminated by the biliary route, no dose adjustment is anticipated to be necessary in patients with renal impairment. There are no data on the pharmacokinetics of montelukast in patients with severe hepatic insufficiency (Child-Pugh score >9).

With high doses of montelukast (20- and 60-fold the recommended adult dose), a decrease in plasma theophylline concentration was observed. This effect was not seen at the recommended dose of 10 mg once daily.

5.3 Preclinical safety data

In animal toxicity studies, minor serum biochemical alterations in ALT, glucose, phosphorus and triglycerides were observed which were transient in nature. The signs of toxicity in animals were increased excretion of saliva, gastro-intestinal symptoms, loose stools and ion imbalance. These occurred at dosages which provided >17-fold the systemic exposure seen at the clinical dosage. In monkeys, the adverse effects appeared at doses from 150 mg/kg/day (>232-fold the systemic exposure seen at the clinical dose). In animal studies, montelukast did not affect fertility or reproductive performance at systemic exposure exceeding the clinical systemic exposure by greater than 24-fold. A slight decrease in pup body weight was noted in the female fertility study in rats at 200 mg/kg/day (>69-fold the clinical systemic exposure). In studies in rabbits, a higher incidence of incomplete ossification, compared with concurrent control animals, was seen at systemic exposure >24-fold the clinical systemic exposure seen at the clinical dose. No abnormalities were seen in rats. Montelukast has been shown to cross the placental barrier and is excreted in breast milk of animals.

No deaths occurred following a single oral administration of montelukast sodium at doses up to 5000 mg/kg in mice and rats (15,000 mg/m^2 and 30,000 mg/m^2 in mice and rats, respectively) the maximum dose tested. This dose is equivalent to 25,000 times the recommended daily adult human dose (based on an adult patient weight of 50 kg).

Montelukast was determined not to be phototoxic in mice for UVA, UVB or visible light spectra at doses up to 500 mg/kg/day (approximately >200-fold based on systemic exposure).

Montelukast was neither mutagenic in *in vitro* and *in vivo* tests nor tumorigenic in rodent species.

6. PHARMACEUTICAL PARTICULARS

6.1 List of excipients

Mannitol

Microcrystalline cellulose

Hyprolose (E463)

Red ferric oxide (E172)

Croscarmellose sodium

Cherry flavour

Aspartame (E951)

Magnesium stearate.

6.2 Incompatibilities

Not applicable

6.3 Shelf life

2 years

6.4 Special precautions for storage

Store in the original package in order to protect from light and moisture.

6.5 Nature and contents of container

Packaged in polyamide/PVC/aluminium blister package in:

Blisters in packages of: 7, 10, 14, 20, 28, 30, 50, 56, 98, 100, 140 and 200 tablets.

Blisters (unit doses), in packages of: 49, 50 and 56 tablets.

Not all pack sizes may be marketed

6.6 Special precautions for disposal and other handling

Any unused product or waste material should be disposed of in accordance with local requirements.

7. MARKETING AUTHORISATION HOLDER

Merck Sharp & Dohme Limited

Hertford Road, Hoddesdon, Hertfordshire EN11 9BU, UK

8. MARKETING AUTHORISATION NUMBER(S)

4 mg Chewable tablets: PL 0025/0412

9. DATE OF FIRST AUTHORISATION/RENEWAL OF THE AUTHORISATION

4 mg Chewable tablets: 24 January 2001/25 August 2007

10. DATE OF REVISION OF THE TEXT

14 August 2009

LEGAL CATEGORY

POM

® denotes registered trademark of Merck & Co., Inc., Whitehouse Station, NJ, USA.

MSD (logo)

Merck Sharp & Dohme Limited

Hertford Road, Hoddesdon, Hertfordshire EN11 9BU, UK

SPC.SGA-4mg.09.UK.3020.II-049

Singulair Paediatric 5 mg Chewable Tablets

(Merck Sharp & Dohme Limited)

1. NAME OF THE MEDICINAL PRODUCT

SINGULAIR® Paediatric 5 mg Chewable Tablets

2. QUALITATIVE AND QUANTITATIVE COMPOSITION

One chewable tablet contains montelukast sodium, which is equivalent to 5 mg montelukast.

Excipient: Aspartame (E 951) 1.5 mg per tablet.

For a full list of excipients, see section 6.1.

3. PHARMACEUTICAL FORM

Chewable tablet.

Pink, round, biconvex, diameter 9.5 mm, with 'SINGULAIR' engraved on one side and 'MSD 275' on the other.

4. CLINICAL PARTICULARS

4.1 Therapeutic indications

SINGULAIR is indicated in the treatment of asthma as add-on therapy in those patients with mild to moderate persistent asthma who are inadequately controlled on inhaled corticosteroids and in whom "as-needed" short-acting β-agonists provide inadequate clinical control of asthma.

SINGULAIR may also be an alternative treatment option to low-dose inhaled corticosteroids for patients with mild persistent asthma who do not have a recent history of serious asthma attacks that required oral corticosteroid use, and who have demonstrated that they are not capable of using inhaled corticosteroids (see section 4.2).

SINGULAIR is also indicated in the prophylaxis of asthma in which the predominant component is exercise-induced bronchoconstriction.

4.2 Posology and method of administration

The dosage for paediatric patients 6-14 years of age is one 5 mg chewable tablet daily to be taken in the evening. If taken in connection with food, SINGULAIR should be taken 1 hour before or 2 hours after food. No dosage adjustment within this age group is necessary.

General recommendations:

The therapeutic effect of SINGULAIR on parameters of asthma control occurs within one day. Patients should be advised to continue taking SINGULAIR even if their asthma is under control, as well as during periods of worsening asthma.

No dosage adjustment is necessary for patients with renal insufficiency, or mild to moderate hepatic impairment. There are no data on patients with severe hepatic impairment. The dosage is the same for both male and female patients.

SINGULAIR *as an alternative treatment option to low-dose inhaled corticosteroids for mild persistent asthma:*

Montelukast is not recommended as monotherapy in patients with moderate persistent asthma. The use of montelukast as an alternative treatment option to low-dose inhaled corticosteroids for children with mild persistent asthma should only be considered for patients who do not have a recent history of serious asthma attacks that required oral corticosteroid use and who have demonstrated that they are not capable of using inhaled corticosteroids (see section 4.1). Mild persistent asthma is defined as asthma symptoms more than once a week but less than once a day, nocturnal symptoms more than twice a month but less than once a week, normal lung function between episodes. If satisfactory control of asthma is not achieved at follow-up (usually within one month), the need for an additional or different anti-inflammatory therapy based on the step system for asthma therapy should be evaluated. Patients should be periodically evaluated for their asthma control.

Therapy with SINGULAIR *in relation to other treatments for asthma.*

When treatment with SINGULAIR is used as add-on therapy to inhaled corticosteroids, SINGULAIR should not be abruptly substituted for inhaled corticosteroids (see section 4.4).

10 mg tablets are available for adults 15 years of age and older.

4.3 Contraindications

Hypersensitivity to the active substance or to any of the excipients.

4.4 Special warnings and precautions for use

Patients should be advised never to use oral montelukast to treat acute asthma attacks and to keep their usual appropriate rescue medication for this purpose readily available. If an acute attack occurs, a short-acting inhaled β-agonist should be used. Patients should seek their doctor's advice as soon as possible if they need more inhalations of short-acting β-agonists than usual.

Montelukast should not be abruptly substituted for inhaled or oral corticosteroids.

There are no data demonstrating that oral corticosteroids can be reduced when montelukast is given concomitantly.

In rare cases, patients on therapy with anti-asthma agents including montelukast may present with systemic eosinophilia, sometimes presenting with clinical features of vasculitis consistent with Churg-Strauss syndrome, a condition which is often treated with systemic corticosteroid therapy. These cases usually, but not always, have been associated with the reduction or withdrawal of oral corticosteroid therapy. The possibility that leukotriene receptor antagonists may be associated with emergence of Churg-Strauss syndrome can neither be excluded nor established. Physicians should be alert to eosinophilia, vasculitic rash, worsening pulmonary symptoms, cardiac complications, and/or neuropathy presenting in their patients. Patients who develop these symptoms should be reassessed and their treatment regimens evaluated.

SINGULAIR contains aspartame, a source of phenylalanine. Patients with phenylketonuria should take into account that each 5 mg chewable tablet contains phenylalanine in an amount equivalent to 0.842 mg phenylalanine per dose.

4.5 Interaction with other medicinal products and other forms of interaction

Montelukast may be administered with other therapies routinely used in the prophylaxis and chronic treatment of asthma. In drug-interactions studies, the recommended clinical dose of montelukast did not have clinically important effects on the pharmacokinetics of the following medicinal products: theophylline, prednisone, prednisolone, oral contraceptives (ethinyl oestradiol/norethindrone 35/1), terfenadine, digoxin and warfarin.

The area under the plasma concentration curve (AUC) for montelukast was decreased approximately 40% in subjects with co-administration of phenobarbital. Since montelukast is metabolised by CYP 3A4, caution should be exercised, particularly in children, when montelukast is co-administered with inducers of CYP 3A4, such as phenytoin, phenobarbital and rifampicin.

In vitro studies have shown that montelukast is a potent inhibitor of CYP 2C8. However, data from a clinical drug-drug interaction study involving montelukast and rosiglitazone (a probe substrate representative of medicinal products primarily metabolised by CYP 2C8) demonstrated that montelukast does not inhibit CYP 2C8 *in vivo*. Therefore, montelukast is not anticipated to markedly alter the metabolism of medicinal products metabolised by this enzyme (eg., paclitaxel, rosiglitazone, and repaglinide).

4.6 Pregnancy and lactation

Use during pregnancy

Animal studies do not indicate harmful effects with respect to effects on pregnancy or embryonal/foetal development.

Limited data from available pregnancy databases do not suggest a causal relationship between SINGULAIR and malformations (i.e. limb defects) that have been rarely reported in worldwide post marketing experience.

SINGULAIR may be used during pregnancy only if it is considered to be clearly essential.

Use during lactation

Studies in rats have shown that montelukast is excreted in milk (see section 5.3). It is not known if montelukast is excreted in human milk.

SINGULAIR may be used in breast-feeding mothers only if it is considered to be clearly essential.

4.7 Effects on ability to drive and use machines

Montelukast is not expected to affect a patient's ability to drive a car or operate machinery. However, in very rare cases, individuals have reported drowsiness or dizziness.

4.8 Undesirable effects

Montelukast has been evaluated in clinical studies as follows:

- 10 mg film-coated tablets in approximately 4,000 adult patients 15 years of age and older, and
- 5 mg chewable tablets in approximately 1,750 paediatric patients 6 to 14 years of age.

The following drug-related adverse reactions in clinical studies were reported commonly (≥1/100 to <1/10) in patients treated with montelukast and at a greater incidence than in patients treated with placebo:

Body System Class	Adult Patients 15 years and older (two 12-week studies; n=795)	Paediatric Patients 6 to 14 years old (one 8-week study; n=201) (two 56-week studies; n=615)
Nervous system disorders	headache	headache
Gastro-intestinal disorders	abdominal pain	

With prolonged treatment in clinical trials with a limited number of patients for up to 2 years for adults, and up to 12 months for paediatric patients 6 to 14 years of age, the safety profile did not change.

The following adverse reactions have been reported in post-marketing use:

Blood and lymphatic system disorders: increased bleeding tendency.

Immune system disorders: hypersensitivity reactions including anaphylaxis, hepatic eosinophilic infiltration.

Psychiatric disorders: dream abnormalities including nightmares, hallucinations, insomnia, irritability, anxiety, restlessness, agitation including aggressive behaviour, tremor, depression, suicidal thinking and behaviour (suicidality) in very rare cases.

Nervous system disorders: dizziness, drowsiness, paraesthesia/hypoesthesia, seizure.

Cardiac disorders: palpitations.

Respiratory, thoracic and mediastinal disorders: epistaxis.

Gastro-intestinal disorders: diarrhoea, dry mouth, dyspepsia, nausea, vomiting.

Hepatobiliary disorders: elevated levels of serum transaminases (ALT, AST), cholestatic hepatitis.

Skin and subcutaneous tissue disorders: angio-oedema, bruising, urticaria, pruritus, rash, erythema nodosum.

Musculoskeletal and connective tissue disorders: arthralgia, myalgia including muscle cramps.

General disorders and administration site conditions: asthenia/fatigue, malaise, oedema, pyrexia.

Very rare cases of Churg-Strauss Syndrome (CSS) have been reported during montelukast treatment in asthmatic patients (see section 4.4).

4.9 Overdose

No specific information is available on the treatment of overdose with montelukast. In chronic asthma studies, montelukast has been administered at doses up to 200 mg/day to patients for 22 weeks and in short-term studies, up to 900 mg/day to patients for approximately one week without clinically important adverse experiences.

There have been reports of acute overdose in post-marketing experience and clinical studies with montelukast. These include reports in adults and children with a dose as high as 1000 mg (approximately 61 mg/kg in a 42 month old child). The clinical and laboratory findings observed were consistent with the safety profile in adults and paediatric patients. There were no adverse experiences in the majority of overdose reports. The most frequently occurring adverse experiences were consistent with the safety profile of montelukast and included abdominal pain, somnolence, thirst, headache, vomiting, and psychomotor hyperactivity.

It is not known whether montelukast is dialysable by peritoneal- or haemo-dialysis.

5. PHARMACOLOGICAL PROPERTIES

5.1 Pharmacodynamic properties

Pharmacotherapeutic group: Leukotriene receptor antagonist

ATC Code: RO3D CO3

The cysteinyl leukotrienes (LTC_4, LTD_4, LTE_4) are potent inflammatory eicosanoids released from various cells including mast cells and eosinophils. These important pro-asthmatic mediators bind to cysteinyl leukotriene receptors (CysLT) found in the human airway and cause airway actions, including bronchoconstriction, mucous secretion, vascular permeability, and eosinophil recruitment.

Montelukast is an orally active compound which binds with high affinity and selectivity to the $CysLT_1$ receptor. In clinical studies, montelukast inhibits bronchoconstriction due to inhaled LTD_4 at doses as low as 5 mg. Bronchodilation was observed within two hours of oral administration. The bronchodilation effect caused by a β-agonist was additive to that caused by montelukast. Treatment with montelukast inhibited both early- and late-phase bronchoconstriction due to antigen challenge. Montelukast, compared with placebo, decreased peripheral blood eosinophils in adult and paediatric patients. In a separate study, treatment with montelukast significantly decreased eosinophils in the airways (as measured in sputum) and in peripheral blood while improving clinical asthma control.

In studies in adults, montelukast 10 mg once daily, compared with placebo, demonstrated significant improvements in morning FEV_1 (10.4% vs 2.7% change from baseline), AM peak expiratory flow rate (PEFR) (24.5 L/min vs 3.3 L/min change from baseline), and significant decrease in total β-agonist use (-26.1% vs -4.6% change from baseline). Improvement in patient-reported daytime and night-time asthma symptoms scores was significantly better than placebo.

Studies in adults demonstrated the ability of montelukast to add to the clinical effect of inhaled corticosteroid (% change from baseline for inhaled beclometasone plus montelukast vs beclometasone, respectively for FEV_1 : 5.43% vs 1.04%; β-agonist use: -8.70% vs 2.64%). Compared with inhaled beclometasone (200 μg twice daily with a spacer device), montelukast demonstrated a more rapid initial response, although over the 12-week study, beclometasone provided a greater average treatment effect (% change from baseline for montelukast vs beclometasone, respectively for FEV_1 : 7.49% vs 13.3%; β-agonist use: -28.28% vs -43.89%). However, compared with beclometasone, a high percentage of patients treated with montelukast achieved similar clinical responses (e.g. 50% of patients treated with beclometasone achieved an improvement in FEV_1 of approximately 11% or more over baseline while approximately 42% of patients treated with montelukast achieved the same response).

In an 8-week study in paediatric patients 6 to 14 years of age, montelukast 5 mg once daily, compared with placebo, significantly improved respiratory function (FEV_1 8.71% vs 4.16% change from baseline; AM PEFR 27.9 L/min vs 17.8 L/min change from baseline) and decreased 'as-needed' β-agonist use (-11.7% vs +8.2% change from baseline).

In a 12-month study comparing the efficacy of montelukast to inhaled fluticasone on asthma control in paediatric patients 6 to 14 years of age with mild persistent asthma, montelukast was non-inferior to fluticasone in increasing the percentage of asthma rescue-free days (RFDs), the primary endpoint. Averaged over the 12-month treatment period, the percentage of asthma RFDs increased from 61.6 to 84.0 in the montelukast group and from 60.9 to 86.7 in the fluticasone group. The between group difference in LS mean increase in the percentage of asthma RFDs was statistically significant (-2.8 with a 95% CI of -4.7, -0.9), but within the limit pre-defined to be clinically not inferior. Both montelukast and fluticasone also improved asthma control on secondary variables assessed over the 12 month treatment period:

- FEV_1 increased from 1.83 L to 2.09 L in the montelukast group and from 1.85 L to 2.14 L in the fluticasone group. The between-group difference in LS mean increase in FEV_1 was -0.02 L with a 95% CI of -0.06, 0.02. The mean increase from baseline in % predicted FEV_1 was 0.6% in the montelukast treatment group, and 2.7% in the fluticasone treatment group. The difference in LS means for the change from baseline in the % predicted FEV_1 was -2.2% with a 95% CI of -3.6, -0.7.
- The percentage of days with β-agonist use decreased from 38.0 to 15.4 in the montelukast group, and from 38.5 to 12.8 in the fluticasone group. The between group difference in LS means for the percentage of days with β-agonist use was 2.7 with a 95% CI of 0.9, 4.5.
- The percentage of patients with an asthma attack (an asthma attack being defined as a period of worsening asthma that required treatment with oral steroids, an unscheduled visit to the doctor's office, an emergency room visit, or hospitalisation) was 32.2 in the montelukast group and 25.6 in the fluticasone group; the odds ratio (95% CI) being significant: equal to 1.38 (1.04, 1.84).
- The percentage of patients with systemic (mainly oral) corticosteroid use during the study period was 17.8% in the montelukast group and 10.5% in the fluticasone group. The between group difference in LS means was significant: 7.3% with a 95% CI of 2.9; 11.7.

Significant reduction of exercise-induced bronchoconstriction (EIB) was demonstrated in a 12-week study in adults (maximal fall in FEV_1 22.33% for montelukast vs 32.40% for placebo; time to recovery to within 5% of baseline FEV_1 44.22 min vs 60.64 min). This effect was consistent throughout the 12-week study period. Reduction in EIB was also demonstrated in a short term study in paediatric patients (maximal fall in FEV_1 18.27% vs 26.11%; time to recovery to within 5% of baseline FEV_1 17.76 min vs 27.98 min). The effect in both studies was demonstrated at the end of the once-daily dosing interval.

In aspirin-sensitive asthmatic patients receiving concomitant inhaled and/or oral corticosteroids, treatment with montelukast, compared with placebo, resulted in significant improvement in asthma control (FEV_1 8.55% vs -1.74% change from baseline and decrease in total β-agonist use -27.78% vs 2.09% change from baseline).

5.2 Pharmacokinetic properties

Absorption: Montelukast is rapidly absorbed following oral administration. For the 10 mg film-coated tablet, the mean peak plasma concentration (C_{max}) is achieved three hours (T_{max}) after administration in adults in the fasted state. The mean oral bioavailability is 64%. The oral bioavailability and C_{max} are not influenced by a standard meal. Safety and efficacy were demonstrated in clinical trials where the 10 mg film-coated tablet was administered without regard to the timing of food ingestion.

For the 5 mg chewable tablet, the C_{max} is achieved in two hours after administration in adults in the fasted state. The mean oral bioavailability is 73% and is decreased to 63% by a standard meal.

Distribution: Montelukast is more than 99% bound to plasma proteins. The steady-state volume of distribution of montelukast averages 8-11 litres. Studies in rats with radiolabelled montelukast indicate minimal distribution across the blood-brain barrier. In addition, concentrations of radiolabelled material at 24 hours post-dose were minimal in all other tissues.

Biotransformation: Montelukast is extensively metabolised. In studies with therapeutic doses, plasma concentrations of metabolites of montelukast are undetectable at steady state in adults and children.

In vitro studies using human liver microsomes indicate that cytochromes P450 3A4, 2A6 and 2C9 are involved in the metabolism of montelukast. Based on further *in vitro* results in human liver microsomes, therapeutic plasma concentrations of montelukast do not inhibit cytochromes P450 3A4, 2C9, 1A2, 2A6, 2C19, or 2D6. The contribution of metabolites to the therapeutic effect of montelukast is minimal.

Elimination: The plasma clearance of montelukast averages 45 ml/min in healthy adults. Following an oral dose of radiolabelled montelukast, 86% of the radioactivity was recovered in 5-day faecal collections and <0.2% was recovered in urine. Coupled with estimates of montelukast oral bioavailability, this indicates that montelukast and its metabolites are excreted almost exclusively via the bile.

Characteristics in patients: No dosage adjustment is necessary for the elderly or mild to moderate hepatic insufficiency. Studies in patients with renal impairment have not been undertaken. Because montelukast and its metabolites are eliminated by the biliary route, no dose adjustment is anticipated to be necessary in patients with renal impairment. There are no data on the pharmacokinetics of montelukast in patients with severe hepatic insufficiency (Child-Pugh score >9).

With high doses of montelukast (20- and 60-fold the recommended adult dose), a decrease in plasma theophylline concentration was observed. This effect was not seen at the recommended dose of 10 mg once daily.

5.3 Preclinical safety data

In animal toxicity studies, minor serum biochemical alterations in ALT, glucose, phosphorus and triglycerides were observed which were transient in nature. The signs of toxicity in animals were increased excretion of saliva, gastro-intestinal symptoms, loose stools and ion imbalance. These occurred at dosages which provided >17-fold the systemic exposure seen at the clinical dosage. In monkeys, the adverse effects appeared at doses from 150 mg/kg/day (>232-fold the systemic exposure seen at the clinical dose). In animal studies, montelukast did not affect fertility or reproductive performance at systemic exposure exceeding the clinical systemic exposure by greater than 24-fold. A slight decrease in pup body weight was noted in the female fertility study in rats at 200 mg/kg/day (>69-fold the clinical systemic exposure). In studies in rabbits, a higher incidence of incomplete ossification, compared with concurrent control animals, was seen at systemic exposure >24-fold the clinical systemic exposure seen at the clinical dose. No abnormalities were seen in rats. Montelukast has been shown to cross the placental barrier and is excreted in breast milk of animals.

No deaths occurred following a single oral administration of montelukast sodium at doses up to 5000 mg/kg in mice and rats (15,000 mg/m^2 and 30,000 mg/m^2 in mice and rats, respectively) the maximum dose tested. This dose is equivalent to 25,000 times the recommended daily adult human dose (based on an adult patient weight of 50 kg).

Montelukast was determined not to be phototoxic in mice for UVA, UVB or visible light spectra at doses up to 500 mg/kg/day (approximately >200-fold based on systemic exposure).

Montelukast was neither mutagenic in *in vitro* and *in vivo* tests nor tumorigenic in rodent species.

6. PHARMACEUTICAL PARTICULARS

6.1 List of excipients

Mannitol

Microcrystalline cellulose

Hyprolose (E463)

Red ferric oxide (E172)

Croscarmellose sodium

Cherry flavour

Aspartame (E951)

Magnesium stearate.

6.2 Incompatibilities

Not applicable

6.3 Shelf life

2 years

6.4 Special precautions for storage

Store in the original package in order to protect from light and moisture.

6.5 Nature and contents of container

Packaged in polyamide/PVC/aluminium blister package in:

Blisters in packages of: 7, 10, 14, 20, 28, 30, 50, 56, 84, 90, 98, 100, 140 and 200 tablets.

Blisters (unit doses), in packages of: 49, 50 and 56 tablets.

Not all pack sizes may be marketed

6.6 Special precautions for disposal and other handling

Any unused product or waste material should be disposed of in accordance with local requirements.

7. MARKETING AUTHORISATION HOLDER

Merck Sharp & Dohme Limited

Hertford Road, Hoddesdon, Hertfordshire EN11 9BU, UK

8. MARKETING AUTHORISATION NUMBER(S)

PL 00025/0357

9. DATE OF FIRST AUTHORISATION/RENEWAL OF THE AUTHORISATION

15 January 1998/25 August 2007

10. DATE OF REVISION OF THE TEXT

14 August 2009

LEGAL CATEGORY

POM

MSD (logo)

Merck Sharp & Dohme Limited

Hertford Road, Hoddesdon, Hertfordshire EN11 9BU, UK

SPC.SGA-5mg.09.UK.3019.II-049

Sinthrome Tablets 1mg

(Alliance Pharmaceuticals)

1. NAME OF THE MEDICINAL PRODUCT
Sinthrome® Tablets 1mg.

2. QUALITATIVE AND QUANTITATIVE COMPOSITION
Acenocoumarol BP 1mg.

3. PHARMACEUTICAL FORM
White, round, flat tablets with slightly bevelled edges, with one side bearing the imprint "CG", and the other the imprint "AA".

4. CLINICAL PARTICULARS
4.1 Therapeutic indications
Treatment and prevention of thromboembolic diseases.

4.2 Posology and method of administration
Sensitivity to anticoagulants varies from patient to patient and may also fluctuate during the course of treatment. Therefore, it is essential to perform regular testing of prothrombin time (PT)/International Normalised Ratio (INT) and to adjust the patient's dosage accordingly. If this is not possible, Sinthrome should not be used.

Sinthrome should be given in a single oral dose at the same time every day.

Adults

Initial dosage: If the thromboplastin time is within the normal range before starting treatment, the following dosage schedule is recommended:

First day: Starting dose of 4 mg/day (lower doses may be required if patients are receiving heparin).

The administration of a loading dose may not be necessary if the PT/INR value before treatment is within the therapeutic range.

Second day: 4 to 8mg.

If the initial thromboplastin time is abnormal, treatment should be instituted with caution.

Elderly patients, patients with liver disease or severe heart failure with hepatic congestion or malnourished patients may require lower doses during treatment initiation and maintenance (see section 4.4 Special warnings and precautions for use).

Maintenance therapy: the maintenance dose of Sinthrome varies from patient to patient and must be determined on the basis of regular laboratory estimations of the patient's blood coagulation time.

Adjustment of the maintenance dose can only be made by monitoring the Quick value of international normalised ratio (INR) at regular intervals, ensuring that the dosage remains within the therapeutic range. Depending on the individual, the maintenance dose generally lies between 1 to 8mg daily.

Before the start of treatment, up to the time when the coagulation valency is stabilised within the optimum range, routine measurement of the thromboplastin time should be carried out daily in hospital. Blood samples for laboratory tests should always be taken at the same time of day.

The INR is the ratio of the patient's plasma thromboplastin time and the normal thromboplastin time raised to a power determined for a reference thromboplastin. As the Quick value decreases, the patient's thromboplastin time increases and the INR is greater. The therapeutic range generally lies between INR values of 2 to 4.5. Within this range, the majority of patients show no risk of severe haemorrhagic complications nor a recurrence of thrombosis.

Generally, after withdrawal of Sinthrome, there is usually no danger of reactive hypercoagulability and therefore it is not necessary to give gradually diminishing doses. However, in extremely rare cases, in some high risk patients (e.g. after myocardial infarction), withdrawal should be gradual.

Children: Not recommended.

Elderly: A dose lower than the recommended adult dose may be sufficient in elderly patients (see Section 4.4, " Special warnings and precautions for use").

4.3 Contraindications
Pregnancy. Known hypersensitivity to acenocoumarol and related coumarin derivatives or to the excipients of Sinthrome, and in patients unable to co-operate (e.g. unsupervised and senile patients, alcoholics and patients with psychiatric disorders).

All conditions where the risk of haemorrhage exceeds possible clinical benefit e.g. haemorrhagic diathesis and/or blood dyscrasia; immediately prior to, or after surgery on the central nervous system or eyes and traumatising surgery involving extensive exposure of the tissues; peptic ulceration or haemorrhage in the gastro-intestinal tract, urogenital tract or respiratory system; cerebrovascular haemorrhages; acute pericarditis; pericardial effusion; infective endocarditis; severe hypertension (due to occult risks); severe hepatic or renal disease; and in cases of increased fibrinolytic activity following operations on the lung, prostate or uterus.

4.4 Special warnings and precautions for use
Strict medical supervision should be given in cases where the disease or condition may reduce the protein binding of Sinthrome (e.g. thyrotoxicosis, tumours, renal disease, infections and inflammation).

Particular care should be taken in patients with hepatic dysfunction since the synthesis of blood coagulation factors may be impaired or there may be an underlying platelet dysfunction (see also Section 4.2 Posology and method of administration). Disorders affecting gastro-intestinal absorption may alter the anticoagulant activity of Sinthrome. In severe heart failure, a very cautious dosage schedule must be adopted, since hepatic congestion may reduce the activation of gamma-carboxylation of coagulation factors. However with reversal of the hepatic congestion, it may be necessary to raise the dosage.

In elderly patients, anticoagulant medication should be monitored with special care (see Sections 4.2 "Posology and method of administration" and 5.2 "Pharmacokinetic properties").

Caution should be exercised in patients with known or suspected (e.g. abnormal bleeding after injury) protein C or protein S deficiency (see Section 4.8 Undesirable effects).

Since acenocoumarol is extensively metabolised by the liver, impaired renal function will not greatly affect the elimination of the drug, although care should be taken due to the possibility of underlying platelet dysfunction.

During treatment with anticoagulants, intramuscular injections may cause haematomas and should be avoided. Subcutaneous and intravenous injections may be given without such complications.

Meticulous care should be taken where it is necessary to shorten the PT/INR (thromboplastin time) for diagnostic or therapeutic procedures (eg angiography, lumbar puncture, minor surgery, tooth extractions etc).

Patients with rare hereditary problems of galactose intolerance, the Lapp lactase deficiency or glucose-galactose malabsorption should not take this medicine.

4.5 Interaction with other medicinal products and other forms of interaction
There are many possible interactions between coumarins and other drugs; those of clinical relevance are given below. Many of these are isolated reports only or have been reported with warfarin rather than acenocoumarol; for completeness, all have been included. The mechanisms of these interactions include disturbances of absorption, inhibition or induction of the metabolising enzyme system (mainly CYP2C9), see section 5.2 Pharmacokinetic properties), and reduced availability of vitamin K_1, necessary for gamma-carboxylation of prothrombin–complex factors. It is important to note that some drugs may interact by more than one mechanism. Every form of therapy may involve the risk of an interaction, although not all will be significant. Thus careful surveillance is important and frequent coagulation tests (e.g. twice weekly) should be carried out when initially prescribing any drug in combination with Sinthrome, or when withdrawing a concomitantly administered drug.

The anticoagulant effect may be potentiated by concomitant administration of the following drugs:

- allopurinol;
- anabolic steroids;
- androgens;
- anti-arrhythmic agents (e.g. amiodarone, quinidine);
- antibiotics:

o broad spectrum antibiotics (e.g. amoxicillin, co-amoxiclav) macrolides (e.g. erythromycin, clarithromycin);

o cephalosporins second and third generation;

o metronidazole;

o quinolones (e.g. ciprofloxacin, norfloxacin, ofloxacin);

o tetracyclines;

o neomycin;

o chloramphenicol.

- Fibrates (e.g. clofibric acid), its derivatives and structural analogues (e.g. fenofibrate, gemfibrozil);
- disulfiram;
- etacrynic acid;
- glucagon;
- H_2 antagonists (e.g. cimetidine);
- Imidazole derivatives, including topical administration (e.g. econazole, fluconazole, ketoconazole, miconazole);
- paracetamol
- sulfonamides (including co-trimoxazole);
- oral antidiabetics (e.g. glibenclamide);
- thyroid hormones (including dextrothyroxine);
- sulfinpyrazone;
- sulphonylureas (such as tolbutamide and chlorpropamide)
- statins (e.g. atorvastatin, fluvastatin, simvastatin);
- selective serotonin re-uptake inhibitors (e.g. fluoxetine, paroxetine)
- tamoxifen;
- 5-fluorouracil and analogues;
- Tramadol.

Corticosteroids (e.g. methylprednisolone, prednisone) have also been reported to potentiate the anticoagulant effect of coumarin derivatives.

Inhibitors of CYP2C9 may potentiate the anticoagulant effect of acenocoumarol.

Drugs altering haemostasis may potentiate the anticoagulant activity of Sinthrome and thereby increase the risk of haemorrhage. Consequently, Sinthrome should not be prescribed with such drugs, which include:

- heparin (including low-molecular-weight heparin);
- platelet-aggregation inhibitors (e.g. dipyridamole, clopidogrel), salicyclic acid and its derivatives, acetylsalicylic acid, para-aminosalicylic acid;
- diflunisal, phenylbutazone or other pyrazolone derivatives (e.g. sulfinpyrazone), and other non-steroidal anti-inflammatory drugs (NSAIDs) including COX-2 inhibitors (e.g. celecoxib), high dose IV methylprednisolone.

The risk of gastrointestinal haemorrhage is increased if Sinthrome is prescribed in combination with NSAIDs, including selective COX-2 inhibitors. In the case of unavoidable concurrent use, coagulation tests should be performed more frequently.

The anticoagulant effect may be diminished by concomitant administration of the following drugs:

- aminoglutethimide;
- antineoplastic drugs (e.g. azathioprine, 6-mercaptopurine);
- barbiturates (e.g. Phenobarbital);
- carbamazepine;
- colestyramine (see Section 4.9 "Overdose");
- griseofulvin;
- oral contraceptives;
- rifampicin;
- thiazide diuretics;
- St. John's Wort/Hypericum perforatum;
- Inducers of CYP2C9, CYP2C19 or CYP3A4 may diminish the anticoagulant effect of acenocoumarol.

Unpredictable effect on anticoagulation, including both increase and decrease in anticoagulant activity have been reported with the following drugs:

- protease inhibitors (e.g. indinavir, nelfinavir, ritonavir, saquinavir).

Effects of acenocoumarol on other drugs:

During concomitant treatment with hydantoin derivatives (such as phenytoin), the serum hydantoin concentration may rise.

Sinthrome may potentiate the hypoglycaemic effect of sulphonylurea derivatives e.g. glibenclamide, glimepiride.

Patients being treated with Sinthrome (especially those suffering from hepatic dysfunction) should limit their alcohol intake, since it is not possible to predict the severity of any drug interactions, nor identify any early signs of such interactions.

Cranberry juice should be avoided in patients receiving Sinthrome due to a theoretical risk of enhanced anti-coagulation. Increased medical supervision and INR monitoring should be considered for any patient receiving Sinthrome and regularly drinking cranberry juice. It is not known whether other cranberry products, such as capsules or concentrates, might also interact with Sinthrome. Therefore similar caution should be observed with these products.

4.6 Pregnancy and lactation
Pregnancy

Sinthrome, like other coumarin derivatives, may be associated with congenital malformations of the embryo, therefore Sinthrome is contra-indicated for use in pregnancy. Women of child-bearing potential should take contraceptive measures during treatment with Sinthrome.

Lactation

Acenocoumarol passes into the breast milk of lactating mothers, but in quantities so small that no undesirable effects on the infant are to be expected. However, as a precaution, the infant should be given 1mg vitamin K_1 per week as a prophylactic measure.

The decision to breast-feed should be carefully considered and may include coagulation tests and vitamin K status evaluation in infants before advising women to breast-feed. Women who are breast-feeding and treated with Sinthrome should be carefully monitored to ensure that recommended PT/INR values are not exceeded.

4.7 Effects on ability to drive and use machines
None known.

4.8 Undesirable effects
Haemorrhage, in various organs, is the most common side-effect associated with Sinthrome; its occurrence is related to the dosage of the drug, the patient's age and the nature of the underlying disease (but not the duration of treatment). Fatalities have been reported. Possible sites of haemorrhage include the gastro-intestinal tract, brain, urogenital tract, uterus, liver, gall bladder and the eye. If haemorrhage occurs in a patient with a thromboplastin time within the therapeutic range, diagnosis of their condition must be clarified.

Rare effects noted with acenocoumarol and similar coumarin derivatives include gastro-intestinal disorders (loss of appetite, nausea, vomiting), allergic reactions (urticaria and other rashes, dermatitis and fever) and reversible alopecia. Isolated cases of haemorrhagic skin necrosis (usually associated with congenital protein C deficiency or its cofactor protein S), vasculitis and liver damage have also been reported.

Immune system disorders

Rare:	Allergic reactions (e.g. urticaria, rash)

Vascular disorders

Very rare:	Vasculitis

Gastrointestinal disorders

Rare	Loss of appetite, nausea, vomiting

Hepatobiliary disorders

Very rare:	Liver damage

Skin and subcutaneous tissue disorders

Rare:	Alopecia
Very rare:	Skin necrosis haemorrhagic (usually associated with congenital deficiency of protein C or its cofactor protein S)

4.9 Overdose

Clinical manifestations of overdosage are unlikely with large single doses, but more likely following prolonged use of daily doses exceeding those required therapeutically.

Hospital referral is recommended for any amount of Sinthrome taken above the therapeutic dose.

Symptoms:

The onset and severity of the symptoms are dependent on the individual's sensitivity to oral anticoagulants, the severity of the overdose and the duration of treatment.

Haemorrhage is the prominent feature of an overdose and may occur within 1 to 5 days after ingestion. Nose-bleeds, haematemesis, haemoptysis, gastro-intestinal haemorrhage, vaginal bleeding, haematuria (with renal colic), cutaneous haemorrhages, gingival bleeding, haematomata, and bleeding into the joints or menorrhagia may be experienced.

Further symptoms include tachycardia, hypotension, peripheral circulatory disorders due to loss of blood, nausea, vomiting, diarrhoea and abdominal pains.

Laboratory tests will show an extremely low Quick value (or high PT/INR value), pronounced prolongation of the recalcification time or thromboplastin time and disturbed gamma-carboxylation of factors II, VII, IX and X.

Treatment:

The necessity, or desirability of the treatment by gastric lavage in addition to the activated charcoal and cholestyramine administration is controversial. The benefits of these treatments should be balanced against the risk of bleeding in each patient.

For patients who have not previously received anticoagulants, arriving within 1 hour of ingestion, who are not obtunded, comatose or convulsing, and show no signs of bleeding from any source, then drug absorption may be reduced by gastric lavage. (However, note that gastric lavage may provoke bleeding). This may then be followed by the administration of activated charcoal. It should also be noted that vitamin-K mediated reversal of anticoagulation may be dangerous for patients who require constant anticoagulation such as those with prosthetic heart valves.

Colestyramine may markedly enhance the drug's elimination by inhibiting the enterohepatic circulation.

A temporary reduction of the dose of Sinthrome is often sufficient to control slight bleeding.

Emergency and supportive measures:

In emergency situations of severe haemorrhage, clotting factors can be returned to normal by administering fresh whole blood or fresh frozen plasma, complex concentrate or recombinant factor VIIa supplemented with vitamin K1.

Antidote:

Vitamin K_1 (phytomenadione) may antagonise the inhibitory effect of Sinthrome within 3 to 5 hours. In cases of moderate haemorrhage, 2 to 5 mg Vitamin K_1 should be given orally; in severe haemorrhage, 5 to 10mg Vitamin K_1 should be injected very slowly (at a rate less than 1mg/min) intravenously. Additional doses (up to a maximum dose of 40mg daily) should be given at 4-hour intervals. Vitamin K_1 should not be given by intramuscular injection.

Doses of Vitamin K_1 in excess of 5mg can cause resistance to further anticoagulant therapy for several days. If an anticoagulant is required, heparin may be used temporarily, although oral anticoagulant therapy should be resumed at the same time and heparin withdrawn once the therapeutic range has been reached.

In the case of life-threatening haemorrhage, intravenous transfusions of fresh frozen plasma or whole blood, complex concentrate or recombinant factor VIIa supplemented with vitamin K1 can abolish the effects of Sinthrome.

5. PHARMACOLOGICAL PROPERTIES

5.1 Pharmacodynamic properties

Pharmacotherapeutic group: Antithrombotic, vitamin K antagonists. ATC code: B01AA07

To initiate blood clotting, Vitamin K causes gamma-carboxylation of certain glutamic acid molecules on the coagulation factors II, VII, IX and X, and of protein C and its cofactor protein S. Coumarin derivatives, such as Sinthrome, prevent gamma-carboxylation of these proteins by Vitamin K, although the precise nature of this antagonism has yet to be established.

Depending on the initial dosage, Sinthrome prolongs the thromboplastin time within approximately 36 to 72 hours. Following withdrawal of Sinthrome, the thromboplastin time usually reverts to normal after a few days.

5.2 Pharmacokinetic properties

Absorption

Following oral administration, Sinthrome is rapidly absorbed; at least 60% of the administered dose is systemically available. Peak plasma concentrations are achieved within 1 to 3 hours after a single dose of 10mg and AUC values are proportional to the size of the dose over a dosage range of 8 to 16mg.

No correlation between plasma concentrations of acenocoumarol and the apparent prothombin levels can be established, due to the variation of plasma drug concentrations between patients.

Plasma drug concentrations are generally higher in patients of 70 years or over when compared with younger patients, after the same dose.

Distribution

Over 98% of acenocoumarol is protein-bound, mainly to albumin. The calculated apparent volume of distribution is 0.16-0.18 L/kg for the R(+) enantiomer and 0.22-0.34 L/kg for the S(-) enantiomer.

Metabolism

Acenocoumarol is extensively metabolised, although the metabolites appear to be pharmacologically inactive in man.

Elimination

The elimination half-life of acenocoumarol from the plasma is 8 to 11 hours. 29% is excreted in the faeces and 60% in the urine, with less than 0.2% of the dose renally excreted being unchanged.

5.3 Preclinical safety data

There are no other clinically relevant pre-clinical safety data in addition to those mentioned in other sections of the Summary of Product Characteristics.

6. PHARMACEUTICAL PARTICULARS

6.1 List of excipients

Aerosil 200 (silica aerogel), hypromellose, lactose, magnesium stearate, maize starch and talc.

6.2 Incompatibilities

None stated.

6.3 Shelf life

3 years.

6.4 Special precautions for storage

None stated.

6.5 Nature and contents of container

Blister packs of 100 tablets.

6.6 Special precautions for disposal and other handling

None stated

7. MARKETING AUTHORISATION HOLDER

Alliance Pharmaceuticals Ltd.

Avonbridge House

2 Bath Road

Chippenham

Wiltshire

SN15 2BB

8. MARKETING AUTHORISATION NUMBER(S)

PL16853/0013

9. DATE OF FIRST AUTHORISATION/RENEWAL OF THE AUTHORISATION

25 June 1998

10. DATE OF REVISION OF THE TEXT

March 2007

11 LEGAL STATUS

POM

Alliance, Alliance Pharmaceuticals and associated devices are registered Trademarks of Alliance Pharmaceuticals Ltd.

Skelid 200mg Tablet

(sanofi-aventis)

1. NAME OF THE MEDICINAL PRODUCT

SKELID 200mg Tablet

2. QUALITATIVE AND QUANTITATIVE COMPOSITION

Disodium tiludronate	240.00 mg
Quantity corresponding to tiludronic acid for one tablet	200.00 mg

For full list of excipients see section 6.1

3. PHARMACEUTICAL FORM

Tablet: Round, biconvex, white tablets with "SW" engraved on one side and "200" on the other.

4. CLINICAL PARTICULARS

4.1 Therapeutic indications

Treatment of Paget's disease

4.2 Posology and method of administration

Oral route

For adults only

Daily dosage: 400 mg (*i.e.* 2 tablets) as a single dose for three months (*i.e.* 12 weeks).

Most patients respond to treatment during the first three months regardless of whether or not they were previously treated with another bisphosphonate.

Serum alkaline phosphatase levels can continue to improve 18 months after withdrawal of treatment.

Treatment can be repeated if the biochemical markers (increase in serum alkaline phosphatase levels with or without elevated hydroxyprolinuria) or pain indicate a recurrence of the condition.

Allow a period of at least 6 months to elapse before administering a second course of treatment.

The tablets should be taken with the help of a glass of water on an empty stomach (at least two hours) before / after meals.

Foodstuffs, particularly those with a high calcium contents (e.g. milk and dairy products) and antacids providing gastric protection should be avoided for two hours pre and post-dose (see Interactions).

4.3 Contraindications

- History of allergy to bisphosphonates
- Severe kidney failure (creatinine clearance less than 30 ml/min)
- Juvenile Paget's disease
- Pregnancy and lactation (see 4.6 pregnancy and lactation)
- Hypersensitivity to any of the excipients
- Patients with rare hereditary problems of galactose intolerance, Lapp lactase deficiency or glucose-galactose malabsorption, should not take this medicine.

4.4 Special warnings and precautions for use

- Tiludronate is not metabolised and is excreted unchanged via the kidneys. Tiludronate must be administered with caution to patients suffering from mild (creatinine clearance ranging from 60 to 90 ml/min) and moderately severe kidney failure (creatinine clearance between 30 and 60 ml/min) (kidney function should be monitored on a regular basis).

- Patients must have an adequate calcium and vitamin D intake. calcium metabolism disorders (hypocalcaemia, vitamin D deficiency) must be controlled before instituting treatment.

- Osteonecrosis of the jaw, generally associated with tooth extraction and/or local infection (including osteomyelitis) has been reported in patients with cancer receiving treatment regimens including primarily intravenously administered bisphosphonates. Many of these patients were also receiving chemotherapy and corticosteroids. Osteonecrosis of the jaw has also been reported in patients with osteoporosis receiving oral bisphosphonates.

A dental examination with appropriate preventive dentistry should be considered prior to treatment with bisphophonates in patients with concomitant risk factors (e.g. cancer, chemotherapy, radiotherapy, corticosteroids, poor oral hygiene).

While on treatment, these patients should avoid invasive dental procedures if possible. For patients who develop osteonecrosis of the jaw while on bisphosphonate therapy, dental surgery may exacerbate the condition. For patients requiring dental procedures, there are no data available to suggest whether discontinuation of bisphosphonate treatment reduces the risk of osteonecrosis of the jaw.

Clinical judgement of the treating physician should guide the management plan of each patient based on individual benefit/risk assessment.

4.5 Interaction with other medicinal products and other forms of interaction

- Combination therapy warranting precautions in use:

Allow over two hours between administration of tiludronate and consumption of:

. calcium salts, topical gastro-intestinal agents, oral antacids (reduced gastro-intestinal absorption of bisphosphonates).

. indomethacin (increased bioavailability of tiludronic acid).

- The pharmacokinetic parameters of tiludronate are not significantly changed by concomitant administration of aspirin or diclofenac.

- The pharmacokinetic parameters of digoxin are not significantly changed by concurrent administration of tiludronate.

- Tiludronate should not be combined with products likely to induce mineralisation disorders.

4.6 Pregnancy and lactation

Pregnancy

Administration is contraindicated during pregnancy (lack of data).

Although there is no evidence of any deleterious effects with tiludronate in reproduction studies, delayed skeletal and bone development in the fetus has been reported in animals experiments conducted with other bisphosphonates. The passage of tiludronate through human placenta has not been documented.

Lactation

Administration is contraindicated during lactation (lack of data).

4.7 Effects on ability to drive and use machines

Drivers and machine operators are not required to take any specific precautions.

4.8 Undesirable effects

Adverse reactions are listed according the following categories:

"Very common (≥1/10); common (≥1/100 to ≤1/10); uncommon (≥1/1,000 to ≤1/100); rare (≥1/10,000 to ≤1/1,000); very rare (≤1/10,000), not known (can not be estimated from available data)"

- Gastro-intestinal disorders:

Common: abdominal pain, nausea, and diarrhoea. These events are of slight to moderate severity and their incidence is dose-related.

- Skin and subcutaneous tissue disorders:

Uncommon: rash

- Nervous system disorders:

Rare: dizziness, headache.

- General disorders and administration site conditions:

Rare: asthenia

- Musculo-skeletal disorders:

Not known: bone pain

4.9 Overdose

Some patients may present with hypocalcaemia and kidney failure following a massive overdose. Gastric lavage may prove useful in order to evacuate any as yet unabsorbed tiludronate.

Symptomatic treatment of hypocalcaemia (intravenous administration of calcium salts such as calcium gluconate) and/or kidney failure should be instituted.

5. PHARMACOLOGICAL PROPERTIES

5.1 Pharmacodynamic properties

Used in the treatment of bone diseases.

(M05 BA bisphosphonates).

Like other bisphosphonates, tiludronate inhibits the bone absorption of osteoclasts.

Tiludronate slows down the bone remodelling of lesions due to Paget's disease, as manifested by the fall in serum alkaline phosphatase levels. Preliminary studies of Paget's disease involving a small number of biopsies showed that tiludronate reduces excessive remodelling due to this disease.

No clinical data on potential long-term mineralisation disorders are available. However, long-term administration (6 months to 1 year) of high daily doses did not cause osteomalacia in rats or baboons.

5.2 Pharmacokinetic properties

The absolute bioavailability of tiludronate is low (averaging 6 %) and variable (2 to 11 %). Plasma concentration peaks following repeated dosing with 400 mg per day were extremely variable (generally between 1 and 5 mg/L occurring 1 to 2 hours post-dose). Bioavailability is decreased when the product is administered during or after a meal and falls considerably in the presence of calcium.

Plasma protein binding is of the order of 91 % and is constant within the therapeutic concentration range. Albumin is the protein responsible for this phenomenon. Less than 5 % binds to red blood cells. Approximately half of the dose absorbed is bound to bone.

Tiludronate is excreted unchanged via the kidneys. 3.5 ≠ 1.9 % of excreted unchanged tiludronate are detected 48 hours after single oral administration.

The decrease in tiludronate plasma levels following treatment withdrawal occurs in two stages, the second of which is much slower and difficult to assess accurately due to the very low plasma concentrations (half-life of over 100 hours). This last phase is due to bone remodelling and to the very slow absorption of tiludronate from the bones.

5.3 Preclinical safety data

- Single dose toxicity: Acute moderate toxicity (LD50 of about 550 mg/kg) and low toxicity (LD50 ≥ 1000 mg/kg) were observed in the rat and mouse respectively following oral administration. The principal target organs are the kidney, stomach and lungs.

- Repeated dose toxicity: gastritis and proximal renal tubulopathies were observed mainly in the rat and baboon following repeated oral dosing with ≥50mg/kg/day for up to a year. These dose levels are considerably higher than the pharmacologically active daily dose levels of 5 to 10 mg/kg which lead to inhibition of bone resorption and increase the bone density of trabecular bone.

- Genotoxicity and carcinogenicity: in-vitro and in-vivo studies of gene mutation, chromosomal aberration and DNA repair processes did not reveal any signs of toxicity.

No evidence of carcinogenicity was detected in mice given up to 50 mg/kg/day for 80 weeks or in rats receiving up to 25 mg/kg/day for 2 years.

- Reproduction toxicity: orally administered doses of up to 375 mg/kg/day did not induce any direct teratogenic or embryotoxic effect in rats, mice or rabbits.

Neither fertility nor peri- and post-natal development were affected in the rat following administration of up to 75 mg/kg/day.

However, given the retarded skeletal and bone maturation observed in animal foetuses during studies with other bisphosphonates, and since no data are available on the passage of tiludronate through human placenta, this product is contraindicated during pregnancy.

6. PHARMACEUTICAL PARTICULARS

6.1 List of excipients

Sodium laurilsulfate, Hypromellose, Crospovidone, Magnesium stearate, Lactose monohydrate

6.2 Incompatibilities

Not applicable

6.3 Shelf life

3 years

6.4 Special precautions for storage

No special precautions for storage.

6.5 Nature and contents of container

28 tablets in heat-formed blister packs (polyamide - aluminium - PVC/aluminium)

6.6 Special precautions for disposal and other handling

No special requirements

7. MARKETING AUTHORISATION HOLDER

Sanofi-aventis

One Onslow Street

Guildford

Surrey GU1 4YS

8. MARKETING AUTHORISATION NUMBER(S)

PL 11723/0207

9. DATE OF FIRST AUTHORISATION/RENEWAL OF THE AUTHORISATION

25th January 2006

10. DATE OF REVISION OF THE TEXT

24th November 2008

Legal category: POM

Slo-Phyllin 60mg, 125mg, 250mg, Capsules

(Merck Serono)

1. NAME OF THE MEDICINAL PRODUCT

Slo-Phyllin 60mg Capsules

Slo-Phyllin 125mg Capsules

Slo-Phyllin 250mg Capsules

2. QUALITATIVE AND QUANTITATIVE COMPOSITION

Slo-Phyllin 60mg capsules each contain theophylline (anhydrous) EP 60mg

Slo-Phyllin 125mg capsules each contain theophylline (anhydrous) EP 125mg

Slo-Phyllin 250mg capsules each contain theophylline (anhydrous) EP 250mg

3. PHARMACEUTICAL FORM

Prolonged release capsule

4. CLINICAL PARTICULARS

4.1 Therapeutic indications

As a bronchodilator in the symptomatic and prophylactic treatment of asthma and for reversible bronchoconstriction associated with chronic bronchitis and bronchial asthma.

4.2 Posology and method of administration

Method of administration

Oral

Dosage

Children:

2-6 years (10-20kg):	60-120mg twice daily
6-12 years (20-35kg)	125-250mg twice daily
over 12 years	250 - 500 mg twice daily

Adults: 250-500 mg twice daily

Elderly: There is a tendency for theophylline clearance to decrease with age leading to higher serum levels. A reduction of the adult dosage may therefore be necessary and close monitoring is advised.

Each patient should be titrated to a suitable dosage regimen by clinical assessment. It may also be necessary to measure plasma theophylline levels.

Initially the lowest dosage for each group is recommended. This may be increased gradually if optimal bronchodilator effects are not achieved. The total dosage should not normally exceed 24 mg/kg body weight for children and 13 mg/kg for adults. However the plasma theophylline level measured 4-8 hours after dosing and at least three days after any dosage adjustment, provides a more accurate assessment of the patients' dosage need, especially as significant variations in the rate of drug elimination can occur between individuals. The following table provides a guide:

Plasma level (mcg/ml)	Result	Directions (if clinically indicated)
Below 10	Too low	Increase dose by 25%
10-20	Correct	Maintain dose
20-25	Too high	Decrease dose by 10%
25-30	Too high	Miss next dose and decrease subsequent doses by 25%
Over 30	Too high	Miss next two doses and decrease subsequent doses by 50%

It is advisable to recheck the plasma level after dose adjustment and every 6-12 months.

It is not possible to ensure bioequivalence between different sustained release theophylline products. Once titrated to an effective dose, patients should not be changed from Slo-Phyllin to another sustained release xanthine preparation without re-titration and clinical assessment.

4.3 Contraindications

Hypersensitivity to theophylline or other xanthines. Concomitant use of theophylline and ephedrine in children.

4.4 Special warnings and precautions for use

Smoking and alcohol consumption can increase the clearance of theophylline and a higher dose may be necessary.

Careful monitoring is recommended for patients with congestive heart failure, chronic alcoholism, hepatic dysfunction, or viral infections, as they may have a lower clearance of theophylline, which could lead to higher than normal plasma levels.

Caution should be exercised in patients with peptic ulcers, cardiac arrhythmias, other cardiovascular diseases, hyperthyroidism or hypertension. Slo-Phyllin should not be used concurrently with other preparations containing xanthines derivatives. If it is necessary to administer aminophylline to a patient who is already receiving Slo-Phyllin, plasma theophylline concentration should be monitored.

The use of alternative treatments is advised in patients with a history of seizures, as these may be exacerbated by theophylline.

4.5 Interaction with other medicinal products and other forms of interaction

Theophylline has been reported to interact with a number of drugs. The following increase clearance and it may therefore be necessary to increase dosage to ensure therapeutic effect: barbiturates, carbamazepine, lithium, phenytoin, rifampicin and sulphinpyrazone.

The following reduce clearance and a reduced dosage may therefore be necessary to avoid side-effects: allopurinol, cimetidine, ciprofloxacin, corticosteroids, diltiazem, erythromycin, frusemide, isoprenaline, oral contraceptives, thiabendazole and verapamil. There is some evidence of an interaction between theophylline and influenza vaccine.

Xanthines can potentiate hypokalaemia resulting from $beta_2$ agonist therapy, steroids, diuretics and hypoxia. Particular caution is advised in severe asthma. It is recommended that serum potassium levels are monitored in such situations.

The concomitant use of theophylline and fluvoxamine should usually be avoided. Where this is not possible, patients should have their theophylline dose halved and plasma theophylline should be monitored closely.

Plasma concentrations of theophylline can be reduced by concomitant use of the herbal remedy St John's wort (Hypericum perforatum).

4.6 Pregnancy and lactation

Slo-Phyllin is not recommended since theophylline is known to cross the placenta and its safety in pregnancy has not been established.

Theophylline is distributed in breast milk and therefore Slo-Phyllin should be used with caution in nursing mothers.

4.7 Effects on ability to drive and use machines

None known

4.8 Undesirable effects

Side effects usually occur when theophylline blood levels exceed 20 micrograms/ml and include gastric irritation, nausea, vomiting, abdominal discomfort, palpitations, a fall in blood pressure, headache, occasional diarrhoea and insomnia. CNS stimulation and diuresis may also occur, especially in children.

4.9 Overdose

Over 3 g could be serious in an adult (40 mg/kg in a child). The fatal dose may be as little as 4.5 g in an adult (60 mg/kg in a child), but is generally higher.

Symptoms

Warning: Serious features may develop as long as 12 hours after overdosage with sustained release formulations.

Alimentary features: Nausea, vomiting (which is often severe), epigastric pain and haematemesis. Consider pancreatitis if abdominal pain persists.

Neurological features: Restlessness, hypertonia, exaggerated limb reflexes and convulsions. Coma may develop in very severe cases.

Cardiovascular features: Sinus tachycardia is common. Ectopic beats and supraventricular and ventricular tachycardia may follow.

Metabolic features: Hypokalaemia due to shift of potassium from plasma into cells is common, can develop rapidly and may be severe. Hyperglycaemia, hypomagnesaemia and metabolic acidosis may also occur. Rhabdomyolysis may also occur.

Management

Activated charcoal or gastric lavage should be considered if a significant overdose has been ingested within 1-2 hours. Repeated doses of activated charcoal given by mouth can enhance theophylline elimination. Measure the plasma potassium concentration urgently, repeat frequently and correct hypokalaemia. BEWARE! If large amounts of potassium have been given, serious hyperkalaemia may develop during recovery. If plasma potassium is low then the plasma magnesium concentration should be measured as soon as possible.

In the treatment of ventricular arrhythmias, proconvulsant antiarrhythmic agents such as lignocaine (lidocaine) should be avoided because of the risk of causing or exacerbating seizures.

Measure the plasma theophylline concentration regularly when severe poisoning is suspected, until concentrations are falling. Vomiting should be treated with an antiemetic such as metoclopramide or ondansetron.

Tachycardia with an adequate cardiac output is best left untreated. Beta-blockers may be given in extreme cases but not if the patient is asthmatic. Control isolated convulsions with intravenous diazepam. Exclude hypokalaemia as a cause.

5. PHARMACOLOGICAL PROPERTIES

5.1 Pharmacodynamic properties

The mechanism of action of theophylline is unclear although a number of pharmacological actions have been implicated. The principal of these are: -

1) Inhibition of the enzyme phosphodiesterase leading to raised cyclic AMP levels.

2) Antagonism of adenosine receptors.

3) Inhibition of the intracellular release of calcium.

4) Stimulation of catecholamine release

5) Anti-inflammatory action possible involving the inhibition of submucosal action.

5.2 Pharmacokinetic properties

Following administration of Slo-Phyllin capsules at an appropriate twice-daily dosage, peak levels occur 4-8 hours after dosing, and steady state is achieved in three days.

5.3 Preclinical safety data

No adverse effects can be predicted from animal toxicology studies other than those documented from human use of theophylline.

6. PHARMACEUTICAL PARTICULARS

6.1 List of excipients

The inactive ingredients are sucrose, maize starch, refined bleached lac, talc and ethanol. The gelatine capsules contain the following shell colours: Slo-Phyllin 60mg E171; Slo-Phyllin 125mg E171 and E172; Slo-Phyllin 250mg E171, E127 and E132.

Printing ink: black iron oxide (E172), shellac glaze, propylene glycol.

6.2 Incompatibilities

None stated.

6.3 Shelf life

Three years.

6.4 Special precautions for storage

Do not store above 25 degree C. Store in the original package.

6.5 Nature and contents of container

PVC/Foil blister packs of 56 tablets

Sample PVC/Foil blister packs of 8 tablets

Plastic container of 100 tablets.

6.6 Special precautions for disposal and other handling

Patients should be instructed not to chew or suck the capsules or pellets as this destroys the time-release properties. However, for those who experience difficulty in swallowing capsules, the contents of a capsule may be sprinkled on to a spoonful of soft food, e.g. yoghurt.

7. MARKETING AUTHORISATION HOLDER

Rona Laboratories Ltd, Bedfont Cross, Stanwell Road, Feltham, Middlesex, TW14 8NX, UK

8. MARKETING AUTHORISATION NUMBER(S)

Slo-Phyllin 60mg capsules PL 0161/0021

Slo-Phyllin 125mg capsules PL 0161/0019

Slo-Phyllin 250mg capsules PL 0161/0020

9. DATE OF FIRST AUTHORISATION/RENEWAL OF THE AUTHORISATION

Year granted - 1977

10. DATE OF REVISION OF THE TEXT

30 May 2008

Slow Sodium

(HK Pharma Limited)

1. NAME OF THE MEDICINAL PRODUCT

®Slow Sodium

2. QUALITATIVE AND QUANTITATIVE COMPOSITION

The active ingredient is Sodium Chloride Ph.Eur. Sodium Chloride contains not less than 99.0 per cent and not more than 100.5 per cent of NaCl.

One coated tablet contains 600 mg sodium chloride.

3. PHARMACEUTICAL FORM

Coated tablets.

4. CLINICAL PARTICULARS

4.1 Therapeutic indications

For the treatment and prophylaxis of sodium chloride deficiency.

4.2 Posology and method of administration

It is important that the tablets should be swallowed whole with water (approx. 70ml per tablet where kidney function is normal to avoid hypernatraemia), and not chewed.

Adults: For prophylaxis 4-8 tablets per day. For treatment dosage to be adjusted to individual needs up to a maximum of 20 tablets per day in cases of severe salt depletion.

For control of muscle cramps during routine maintenance haemodialysis usually 10-16 tablets per dialysis. In some cases of chronic renal salt-wasting up to 20 tablets per day may be required with appropriate fluid intake.

Children: Dosage should be adjusted to individual needs.

Elderly: No special dosage adjustment.

4.3 Contraindications

Slow Sodium is contra-indicated in any situation where salt retention is undesirable, such as oedema, heart disease, cardiac decompensation and primary or secondary aldosteronism; or where therapy is being given to produce salt and water loss.

4.4 Special warnings and precautions for use

Warnings

None

Precautions

Use of Slow Sodium without adequate water supplementation can produce hypernatraemia. The matrix (ghost) is often eliminated intact and owing to the risk of obstruction Slow Sodium should not be given to patients suffering from Crohn's disease or any other intestinal condition where strictures or diverticula may form.

4.5 Interaction with other medicinal products and other forms of interaction

In hypertensive patients with chronic renal failure Slow Sodium may tend to impair the efficacy of antihypertensive drugs.

4.6 Pregnancy and lactation

As with most medicines, consult your doctor first if you are pregnant or breastfeeding.

4.7 Effects on ability to drive and use machines

Nil

4.8 Undesirable effects

No side effects have been reported with Slow Sodium at the recommended dosage.

4.9 Overdose

Signs and symptoms

Excessive intake of sodium chloride can result in hypernatraemia. Symptoms of hypernatraemia include restlessness, weakness, thirst, reduced salivation and lachrymation, swollen tongue, flushing of the skin, pyrexia, dizziness, headache, oliguria, hypertension, tachycardia, delirium, hyperpnoea and respiratory arrest.

Treatment

Treatment requires the use of sodium-free liquids and the cessation of excessive sodium intake. In the event of a significant overdose serum sodium levels should be evaluated as soon as possible and appropriate steps taken to correct any abnormalities. The use of a loop diuretic eg frusemide (with potassium supplementation as required) may be appropriate in severe cases of hypernatraemia. Levels should be monitored until they return to normal.

5. PHARMACOLOGICAL PROPERTIES

5.1 Pharmacodynamic properties

Mode of action: Sodium chloride is the principle salt involved in maintaining the osmotic tension of blood and tissues, changes in osmotic tension influence the movement of fluids and diffusion of salts in cellular tissue.

Slow Sodium provides a source of sodium (in the form of sodium chloride) where a deficiency exists.

5.2 Pharmacokinetic properties

Sodium chloride is readily absorbed from the gastro-intestinal tract. It is present in all body fluids but specially in the extracellular fluid. The amount of sodium lost (as sweat) is normally small. Osmotic balance is maintained by excretion of surplus amounts in the urine.

5.3 Preclinical safety data

No information available.

6. PHARMACEUTICAL PARTICULARS

6.1 List of excipients

Cetostearyl alcohol

Gelatin

Magnesium stearate

Tablet coating

Acacia

Gelatin

Talc

Titanium dioxide (E171)

Polyethylene glycol

Printing ink

Shellac

Red Iron Oxide (E172)

Lecithin (E322)

Antifoam DC 1510-US

6.2 Incompatibilities

None known.

6.3 Shelf life

Five years.

6.4 Special precautions for storage

Protect from moisture and store below 30°C.

The tablets should be dispensed in moisture proof containers.

Medicines should be kept out of reach of children.

6.5 Nature and contents of container

The tablets are available in containers of 100 tablets.

6.6 Special precautions for disposal and other handling

None

Administrative Data

7. MARKETING AUTHORISATION HOLDER

HK Pharma Ltd

PO Box 105

Hitchin

SG5 2GG

8. MARKETING AUTHORISATION NUMBER(S)

PL 16784/0003

9. DATE OF FIRST AUTHORISATION/RENEWAL OF THE AUTHORISATION

28 April 1998

10. DATE OF REVISION OF THE TEXT

26th November 2008

Slow-K Tablets 600 mg

(Alliance Pharmaceuticals)

1. NAME OF THE MEDICINAL PRODUCT

Slow-K® Tablets 600mg

2. QUALITATIVE AND QUANTITATIVE COMPOSITION

Potassium chloride 600mg PhEur

Excipients: also includes sucrose.

For a full list of excipients see 6.1.

3. PHARMACEUTICAL FORM

Pale orange, round, biconvex, sugar-coated modified release tablets.

4. CLINICAL PARTICULARS

4.1 Therapeutic indications

The correction and/or prevention of hypokalaemia in those patients who cannot tolerate and/or refuse to take liquid or effervescent potassium chloride, or when there is a problem of compliance with these preparations.

4.2 Posology and method of administration

Slow-K is taken orally. It is important that the tablets should be swallowed whole, with fluid, during meals, whilst the patient is sitting upright.

Adults:

The dosage of Slow-K should be adapted to the cause, degree and duration of potassium depletion. 2 to 3 tablets daily are usually an adequate supplement. In states of severe potassium deficiency, a higher dose of 9 to 12 tablets daily may be needed.

If the dosage exceeds 16mmol K^+ (2 tablets) it should be taken in divided doses. Where intermittent diuretic therapy is being used, it is advisable to give Slow-K on intervening days between administration of the diuretic. The response to treatment should preferably be monitored by repeat determination of plasma potassium and Slow-K continued until the hypokalaemia has been corrected.

Children: Not recommended.

Elderly: No special dosage regime is usually necessary, but concurrent renal insufficiency should be taken into account (See Section 4.4 "Special warnings and precautions").

4.3 Contraindications

Hypersensitivity to potassium administration, eg hyperkalaemic periodic paralysis, congenital paramyotonia. Marked renal failure (even when not yet associated with manifest hyperkalaemia), untreated Addison's Disease, hyporeninaemic hypoaldosteronism, acute dehydration, hyperkalaemia and conditions involving extensive cell destruction (eg severe burns).

All solid forms of potassium medication are contra-indicated in the presence of obstructions in the digestive tract (eg resulting from compression of the oesophagus due to dilation of the left atrium or from stenosis of the gut).

In cases of metabolic acidosis, the hypokalaemia should be treated not with potassium chloride but with an alkaline potassium salt (eg potassium bicarbonate).

Concomitant treatment with potassium sparing diuretics (eg spironolactone, triamterene, amiloride).

4.4 Special warnings and precautions for use

If a patient under treatment with Slow-K develops severe vomiting, severe abdominal pains or flatulence, or gastro-intestinal haemorrhage, the preparation should be withdrawn at once, because in the presence of an obstruction it could conceivably give rise to ulceration or perforation.

Oral potassium preparations should be prescribed with particular caution in patients with a history of peptic ulcer.

Caution should be exercised when prescribing solid oral potassium preparations, particularly in high dosage, in patients concurrently receiving anticholinergics, because of their potential to slow gastro-intestinal motility.

Patients with ostomies may have altered intestinal transit times and are better treated with other forms of potassium salts.

In patients suffering from impaired renal function, special care should be exercised when prescribing potassium salts owing to the risk of their producing hyperkalaemia. Monitoring of the serum electrolytes is particularly necessary in patients with diseases of the heart or kidneys.

In some patients, diuretic-induced magnesium deficiency will prevent restoration of intracellular deficits of potassium, so that hypomagnesaemia should be corrected at the same time as hypokalaemia.

Patients with rare hereditary problems of fructose intolerance, glucose-galactose malabsorption or sucrase-isomaltase insufficiency should not take this medicine.

4.5 Interaction with other medicinal products and other forms of interaction

Combined treatment with the following increase the risk of hyperkalaemia: ACE inhibitors, ciclosporin, NSAIDs, β-blockers, heparin, digoxin, potassium sparing diuretics (see Section 4.3 "Contra-indications").

4.6 Pregnancy and lactation

Because of gastro-intestinal hypomotility associated with pregnancy, solid forms of oral potassium preparations should be given to pregnant women only if clearly needed.

The normal K^+ content of human milk is about 13mmol/litre. Since oral potassium becomes part of the body's potassium pool, provided this is not excessive, Slow-K can be expected to have little or no effect on the potassium level in human milk.

4.7 Effects on ability to drive and use machines

None known.

4.8 Undesirable effects

Side effects are rare with Slow-K, as any excess potassium is rapidly excreted in the urine.

Gastrointestinal tract: Rare: oral potassium preparations may provoke gastro-intestinal disturbances (nausea, vomiting, abdominal pains, diarrhoea) necessitating either a reduction in dosage or withdrawal of medication (see Section 4.4 "Special warnings and precautions for use"). Isolated cases: obstruction, bleeding and ulceration, with or without perforation of the upper or lower GIT, have been reported, usually associated with other factors known to predispose a patient to these effects (eg delayed GIT transit time, obstruction of GIT).

Skin: Rare: Pruritus and/or skin rash, urticaria.

Electrolytes: Hyperkalaemia may develop in patients having difficulty with either renal potassium excretion or potassium metabolism.

4.9 Overdose

Signs and symptoms: Mainly cardiovascular (hypotension, shock, ventricular arrhythmias, bundle-branch block, ventricular fibrillation leading possibly to cardiac arrest) and neuromuscular (paraesthesiae, convulsions, areflexia, flaccid paralysis of striated muscle leading possibly to respiratory paralysis). Beside elevation of serum potassium concentration, typical ECG changes are also encountered (increasing amplitude and peaking of T waves, disappearance of P wave, widening of QRS complex and S-T segment depression).

Treatment: Gastric lavage, administration of cation exchange agents, infusion of glucose and insulin, forced diuresis and possibly peritoneal dialysis or haemodialysis.

5. PHARMACOLOGICAL PROPERTIES

5.1 Pharmacodynamic properties

The potassium chloride in Slow-K is finely distributed in a neutral wax base, from which it is gradually released over a period of 3 to 6 hours during its passage through the digestive tract. This special form of potassium substitution therapy is designed to avoid high localised concentrations of potassium chloride which might irritate or damage the mucosa. The potassium chloride in Slow-K is completely absorbed in the intestinal tract.

5.2 Pharmacokinetic properties

The potassium chloride in Slow-K has been shown to be completely absorbed; occasionally patients may notice "ghost" tablet cores in the faeces, these do not contain any potassium.

Following a single dose of Slow-K, potassium chloride is released over a period of approximately 4 hours. Renal excretion of potassium chloride following ingestion of Slow-K occurs 30 to 60 minutes later than when the same dose is given in the form of a solution. In the presence of a normal potassium balance, 90% of the potassium supplied by Slow-K is excreted renally within 8 hours, and more than 98% by 24 hours.

5.3 Preclinical safety data

There are no pre-clinical data of relevance to the prescriber which are additional to those already included in other sections of the Summary of Product Characteristics.

6. PHARMACEUTICAL PARTICULARS

6.1 List of excipients

Cetostearyl alcohol

Gelatin

Magnesium stearate

Acacia

Titanium dioxide (E171)

Talc

Sucrose

Red iron oxide (E172)

Yellow iron oxide (E172)

Carnauba wax

6.2 Incompatibilities

None known.

6.3 Shelf life

5 years.

6.4 Special precautions for storage

Do not store above 30°C. Keep the container tightly closed.

6.5 Nature and contents of container

Polypropylene Securitainer with polyethylene cap containing 100 tablets.

6.6 Special precautions for disposal and other handling

None.

Administrative Data

7. MARKETING AUTHORISATION HOLDER

Alliance Pharmaceuticals Ltd

Avonbridge House

Bath Road

Chippenham

Wiltshire

SN15 2BB

8. MARKETING AUTHORISATION NUMBER(S)

PL16853/0014

9. DATE OF FIRST AUTHORISATION/RENEWAL OF THE AUTHORISATION

25 June 1998

10. DATE OF REVISION OF THE TEXT

January 2008

11. Legal Status

Pharmacy

Alliance, Alliance Pharmaceuticals and associated devices are registered Trademarks of Alliance Pharmaceuticals Ltd.

Slozem 120mg, 180mg, 240mg, 300mg Capsules

(Merck Serono)

1. NAME OF THE MEDICINAL PRODUCT

Slozem 120mg Capsules

Slozem 180mg Capsules

Slozem 240mg Capsules

Slozem 300mg Capsules

2. QUALITATIVE AND QUANTITATIVE COMPOSITION

Slozem 120mg Capsules each contain 120mg diltiazem hydrochloride

Slozem 180mg Capsules each contain 180mg diltiazem hydrochloride

Slozem 240mg Capsules each contain 240mg diltiazem hydrochloride

Slozem 300mg Capsules each contain 300mg diltiazem hydrochloride

For excipients, see 6.1.

3. PHARMACEUTICAL FORM

Prolonged release capsule, hard.

Slozem 120mg Capsules have a natural transparent cap with a pink transparent body and contain white-grey to light yellow approximately spherical pellets.

Slozem 180mg Capsules have a natural transparent cap with a pink opaque body and contain white-grey to light yellow approximately spherical pellets.

Slozem 240mg Capsules have a natural transparent cap with a scarlet opaque body and contain white-grey to light yellow approximately spherical pellets.

Slozem 300mg Capsules have an opaque white cap with an opaque scarlet body and contain white-grey to light yellow approximately spherical pellets.

4. CLINICAL PARTICULARS

4.1 Therapeutic indications

Mild to moderate hypertension. Angina pectoris.

4.2 Posology and method of administration

Adults

240mg once daily

Dosage titration in 60mg to 120mg steps at 2-weekly intervals may be required to obtain satisfactory clinical response (usually 240mg to 360mg daily will suffice). Dosage should be reduced in the presence of adverse reactions or if the pulse rate falls below 50 per minute.

Elderly and patients with impaired hepatic or renal function

Starting dose 120mg once daily.

Children

Not recommended.

4.3 Contraindications

In pregnancy and in women of childbearing potential. Slozem depresses atrioventricular node conduction and is therefore contraindicated in patients with marked bradycardia, sick sinus syndrome, uncontrolled heart failure or second or third degree AV block.

Hypersensitivity to diltiazem or any of the inactive ingredients.

As Slozem contains sucrose, patients with rare hereditary problems of fructose intolerance, glucose-galactose malabsorption or sucrase-isomaltase insufficiency should not take this medicine.

4.4 Special warnings and precautions for use

Slozem should be used with caution in patients with reduced left ventricular function. Patients with mild bradycardia, and/or having a prolonged PR interval, should be observed closely.

4.5 Interaction with other medicinal products and other forms of interaction

In common with other calcium antagonists, when Slozem is used with drugs which may induce bradycardia (eg amiodarone and beta-blockers) or with other antihypertensive drugs the possibility of an additive effect should be borne in mind.

Diltiazem has been used safely in combination with beta-blockers, diuretics, ACE inhibitors and other antihypertensive agents. It is recommended that patients receiving these combinations should be regularly monitored. Concomitant use with alpha blockers such as prazosin should be strictly monitored because of the possible marked synergistic hypotensive effect of this combination. Case reports have suggested that blood levels of carbamazepine, cyclosporin and theophylline may be increased when given concurrently with diltiazem hydrochloride. Care should be exercised in patients taking these drugs. In common with other calcium antagonists diltiazem may cause small increases in plasma levels of digoxin.

In patients taking H_2 receptor antagonists concurrently with diltiazem increased levels of diltiazem may be produced.

Diltiazem hydrochloride treatment has been continued without problem during anaesthesia, but the anaesthetist should be informed that the patient is receiving a calcium antagonist.

4.6 Pregnancy and lactation

Diltiazem hydrochloride is teratogenic in some animal species. In the absence of adequate evidence of safety in human pregnancy Slozem should not be used in pregnancy or in women of child-bearing potential.

Nursing mothers:

Diltiazem hydrochloride is excreted in breast milk. One report suggests that concentrations in breast milk reach similar levels to those in serum. If use of Slozem is considered essential, an alternative method of infant feeding should be instituted.

4.7 Effects on ability to drive and use machines

None known

4.8 Undesirable effects

The following have been reported: ankle oedema, malaise, headache, hot flushes, gastro-intestinal disturbances and very rarely symptomatic bradycardia, sino-atrial block and atrio-ventricular block. Rashes and other cutaneous reactions have been reported in association with diltiazem. These reactions are generally mild and resolve on cessation of therapy, however there have been occasional reports of severe vascular skin reactions, and of erythema multiforme. Isolated cases of moderate and transient elevation of liver transaminases have been observed at the start of treatment. Isolated cases of clinical hepatitis have been reported which resolved on cessation of therapy.

The current literature suggests that the effects of vasodilation, particularly ankle oedema, are dose dependent and are more frequent in the elderly.

4.9 Overdose

Signs and symptoms:

Acute intoxication can lead to severe hypotension, bradycardia, first to third degree atrioventricular block and, on occasions, to cardiac arrest. Hyperglycaemia may require treatment. Onset of symptoms may be delayed for several hours after ingestion and have been described after as little as 900mg diltiazem.

Treatment:

Observation in a coronary or intensive care unit is advisable if a substantial overdose has been ingested. Soon after ingestion, gastric lavage followed by activated charcoal may reduce absorption. Profound hypotension requires plasma expanders, I V calcium gluconate and inotropic agents (e.g. dopamine, dobutamine or isoprenaline). Symptomatic bradycardia and heart block may respond to atropine, isoprenaline or, if necessary, cardiac pacing. Slozem capsules are extended release capsules and effects may be slow in onset and prolonged.

5. PHARMACOLOGICAL PROPERTIES

5.1 Pharmacodynamic properties

Diltiazem hydrochloride is a calcium antagonist. It selectively reduces calcium entry through voltage-dependent calcium channels into vascular smooth muscle cells and myocardial cells. This lowers the concentration of intracellular calcium which is available to active contractile proteins. In vascular tissue, diltiazem relaxes arterial smooth muscle, reducing systemic peripheral resistance and dilating the coronary arteries. In cardiac muscle diltiazem reduces contractility and slows the heart rate through its negative chronotropic and inotropic actions. Cardiac work and oxygen demand can therefore be reduced and high blood pressure lowered without reflex tachycardia.

5.2 Pharmacokinetic properties

Diltiazem is well absorbed from the gastrointestinal tract and is subject to an extensive first-pass effect, giving an absolute bioavailability (compared to intravenous administration) of about 40%.

Diltiazem in plasma is 80-85% protein bound. Plasma levels above 40-50ng/ml are associated with pharmacological activity.

Diltiazem is extensively metabolised by the liver, the plasma elimination half-life being on average 3-4.5 hours.

The two major active circulating metabolites, desacetyl-diltiazem and N-monodesmethyl diltiazem possess coronary artery vasodilatory activity equivalent to about 50% of that of diltiazem. Only 0.2 to 4% diltiazem is found unchanged in the urine.

The prolonged release pellets in this presentation usually achieve maximum plasma diltiazem levels six to eight hours after dosing and have an apparent plasma half-life of approximately 7 hours, allowing once daily dosing

The bioavailability of diltiazem from the Slozem formulation given once a day is equivalent to that obtained from a conventional release tablet given three times a day, when the same total daily dose is administered.

Data from studies in patients and healthy volunteers have also demonstrated that trough plasma levels (i.e. 24 hours post dosing) can be maintained within the minimum therapeutic range by appropriate dose titration.

Plasma concentrations in elderly patients and in hepatic failure are in general higher than in young subjects, due to an increase in apparent bioavailability. In renal failure, a reduction in dosage is only necessary as a function of the clinical response

5.3 Preclinical safety data

There are no preclinical data of relevance to the prescriber which are additional to that already included in other sections of the SPC.

6. PHARMACEUTICAL PARTICULARS

6.1 List of excipients

Maize starch, sucrose, povidone, shellac, ethylcellulose, talc, gelatin, erythrosine (E127), indigo carmine (E132) and (180mg, 240mg and 300mg only), titanium dioxide (E171). Printing ink: black iron oxide (E172), shellac, propylene glycol.

6.2 Incompatibilities

Not applicable

6.3 Shelf life

3 years.

6.4 Special precautions for storage

Slozem 120mg, 180mg and 240mg Capsules:

Do not store above 30°C.

Slozem 300mg Capsules:

Do not store above 25°C.

6.5 Nature and contents of container

28 capsules in PVC/PVDC/Aluminium blisters enclosed in a cardboard carton.

6.6 Special precautions for disposal and other handling

None

7. MARKETING AUTHORISATION HOLDER

Merck Serono Ltd,

Bedfont Cross

Stanwell Road

Feltham

Middlesex

TW14 8NX

UK

8. MARKETING AUTHORISATION NUMBER(S)

Slozem 120mg Capsules PL 11648/0045

Slozem 180mg Capsules PL 11648/0046

Slozem 240mg Capsules PL 11648/0047

Slozem 300mg Capsules PL 11648/0042

9. DATE OF FIRST AUTHORISATION/RENEWAL OF THE AUTHORISATION

Slozem 120mg, 180mg and 240mg Capsules:

27 October 2004

Slozem 300mg Capsules:

15 January 2001

10. DATE OF REVISION OF THE TEXT

13 October 2008

LEGAL CATEGORY

POM

Sodiofolin 50 mg/ml, solution for injection

(medac GmbH)

1. NAME OF THE MEDICINAL PRODUCT

Sodiofolin 50 mg/ml, solution for injection

2. QUALITATIVE AND QUANTITATIVE COMPOSITION

Sodiofolin 50 mg/ml, solution for injection contains 54.65 mg/ml disodium folinate equivalent to 50 mg/ml folinic acid.

2 ml of solution contains 109.3 mg disodium folinate equivalent to 100 mg folinic acid.

4 ml of solution contains 218.6 mg disodium folinate equivalent to 200 mg folinic acid.

6 ml of solution contains 327.9 mg disodium folinate equivalent to 300 mg folinic acid.

7 ml of solution contains 382.55 mg disodium folinate equivalent to 350 mg folinic acid.

8 ml of solution contains 437.2 mg disodium folinate equivalent to 400 mg folinic acid.

10 ml of solution contains 546.5 mg disodium folinate equivalent to 500 mg folinic acid.

18 ml of solution contains 983.7 mg disodium folinate equivalent to 900 mg folinic acid.

For a full list of excipients, see section 6.1.

3. PHARMACEUTICAL FORM

Solution for injection or intravenous infusion

Slightly yellow, clear solution.

4. CLINICAL PARTICULARS

4.1 Therapeutic indications

Disodium folinate is indicated

- to diminish the toxicity and counteract the action of folic acid antagonists such as methotrexate in cytotoxic therapy and overdose in adults and children. In cytotoxic therapy, the procedure is commonly known as "Folinate Rescue";

in combination with 5-fluorouracil in cytotoxic therapy.

Note:

Persistently high serum methotrexate levels may also be expected in low-dose methotrexate therapy particularly in pleural effusions, ascites, renal insufficiency and inadequate fluid intake during methotrexate therapy.

4.2 Posology and method of administration

Sodiofolin 50 mg/ml, solution for injection or infusion is administered intravenously, either undiluted by injection or by infusion after dilution (for dilution see section 6.6). Disodium folinate should not be administered intrathecally.

Disodium folinate in combination with 5-fluorouracil in cytotoxic therapy

The combined use of disodium folinate and fluorouracil is reserved for physicians experienced in the combination of folinates with 5-fluorouracil in cytotoxic therapy.

Different regimes and different dosages are used, without any dosage having been proven to be the optimal one.

The following regimes have been used in adults and elderly in the treatment of advanced or metastatic colorectal cancer and are given as examples.

There are no data on the use of these combinations in children.

1. Weekly regime

1.1 Moderately high-dose fluorouracil

500 mg/m^2 folinic acid (= 546.5 mg/m^2 disodium folinate) as i.v. infusion over a period of 2 hours plus 600 mg/m^2 fluorouracil as i.v. bolus injection 1 hour after the start of the disodium folinate infusion.

Repeat once a week for a total of 6 weeks (= 1 cycle).

Repeat the cycle after a 2-week treatment interval. The number of cycles will depend on the response of the tumour.

Dose adjustment of fluorouracil

The fluorouracil dosage should be adjusted in accordance with the toxicity observed:

Gastrointestinal toxicity WHO ⩾ 1:	Reduction to 500 mg/m^2. Resumption of therapy only when findings have completely returned to normal.
Bone marrow toxicity WHO ⩾ 1:	Reduction to 500 mg/m^2. Resumption of therapy only when the findings are as follows: Leukocytes > 3,000/µl Thrombocytes > 100,000/µl

1.2 High-dose fluorouracil

500 mg/m^2 folinic acid (= 546.5 mg/m^2 disodium folinate) as i.v. infusion over a period of 1-2 hours and subsequently 2,600 mg/m^2 fluorouracil by continuous infusion over 24 hours.

Repeat once a week for a total of 6 weeks (= 1 cycle).

Repeat the cycle after a 2-week treatment interval. The number of cycles will depend on the response of the tumour.

Dose adjustment of fluorouracil

The fluorouracil dosage should be adjusted in accordance with the toxicity observed:

Life-threatening cardiotoxicity:	Termination of therapy
Bone marrow toxicity WHO ⩾ 3:	Reduction by 20% Resumption of therapy only when the findings are as follows: Leukocytes > 3,000/µl Thrombocytes > 100,000/µl
Gastrointestinal toxicity WHO ⩾ 3:	Reduction by 20%

2. Monthly regime

2.1 Moderately high-dosed disodium folinate

200 mg/m^2 folinic acid (= 218.6 mg/m^2 disodium folinate) daily, followed by 370 mg/m^2 fluorouracil daily, both given as i.v. bolus injection. Repeat on 5 successive days (= 1 cycle).

Repeat the cycle after 4 weeks, 8 weeks and every 5 weeks after that. The number of cycles will depend on the response of the tumour.

Dose adjustment of fluorouracil

The dosage of fluorouracil should be adjusted in each subsequent cycle in accordance with the toxicity (WHO) observed, as follows:

WHO toxicity 0:	Increase daily dose by 30 mg/m^2
WHO toxicity 1:	Daily dose unchanged
WHO toxicity ⩾ 2:	Reduce daily dose by 30 mg/m^2

2.2 Low-dose disodium folinate

20 mg/m^2 folinic acid (= 21.86 mg/m^2 disodium folinate) daily, followed by 425 mg/m^2 fluorouracil daily, both given as i.v. bolus injection. Repeat on 5 successive days (= 1 cycle).

Repeat the cycle after 4 weeks, 8 weeks and every 5 weeks after that. The number of cycles will depend on the response of the tumour.

Dose adjustment of fluorouracil

In the absence of toxicity (especially if no significant bone marrow toxicity and no non-haematological side-effects occur in the interval) it is recommended to increase the dosage of fluorouracil by 10% in each case.

Preventing the manifestations of intoxication in methotrexate therapy (folinate rescue):

Only physicians experienced in the use of high-dose methotrexate therapy should use prophylactic disodium folinate.

The prophylactic use of disodium folinate with methotrexate may start as mentioned below, without waiting for results of methotrexate serum level monitoring, and then posology may be further adapted according to results of methotrexate serum levels when available.

The use of a dose of methotrexate at $\geqslant$ 100 mg/m^2 (body surface) must be followed by the administration of disodium folinate. There are no uniform recommendations for the dosage and mode of use of disodium folinate as an antidote in high-dose methotrexate therapy. The following dosage recommendations are therefore given as examples:

Disodium folinate rescue following the intravenous administration of methotrexate (MTX):

MTX serum levels 24-30 hours after administration of MTX	Disodium folinate dose (mg/m^2 body surface) calculated as folinic acid and dosage interval (hours)	Duration of treatment
1.0 $\times$ 10^{-8} mol/l - 1.5 $\times$ 10^{-6} mol/l	10 to 15 mg/m^2 every 6 hours	48 hours
1.5 $\times$ 10^{-6} mol/l - 5.0 $\times$ 10^{-6} mol/l	30 mg/m^2 every 6 hours	up to MTX serum level < 5 $\times$ 10^{-8} mol/l
> 5.0 $\times$ 10^{-6} mol/l	60 to 100 mg/m^2 every 6 hours	up to MTX serum level < 5 $\times$ 10^{-8} mol/l

Start of rescue

Not later than 18 to 30 hours after the start of methotrexate intravenous administration.

End of rescue

72 hours after the start of methotrexate intravenous administration at the earliest. On completion of the rescue, the methotrexate level should be below 10^{-7} mol/l, preferably below 10^{-8} mol/l.

An "over-rescue" may impair the efficacy of methotrexate. With inadequate rescue, considerable toxic side-effects are likely with high-dosed methotrexate therapy.

4.3 Contraindications

Hypersensitivity to disodium folinate or any of the excipients

The combination of disodium folinate with fluorouracil is not indicated in:

- existing contraindications against fluorouracil, in particular pregnancy and lactation,
- severe diarrhoea.

Therapy with disodium folinate combined with fluorouracil must not be initiated or continued in patients who have symptoms of gastrointestinal toxicity of any severity until those symptoms have completely resolved. Patients with diarrhoea must be monitored with particular care until the diarrhoea has resolved, as rapid clinical deterioration leading to death can occur (see also sections 4.2, 4.4 and 4.5).

Disodium folinate is not suitable for the treatment of pernicious anaemia or other anaemias due to Vitamin B_{12} deficiency. Although haematological remissions may occur, the neurological manifestations remain progressive.

4.4 Special warnings and precautions for use

Disodium folinate should only be used under the direct supervision of a clinician experienced in the use of cancer chemotherapeutic agents.

Disodium folinate should not be given simultaneously with an antineoplastic folic acid antagonist (e.g. methotrexate) to modify or abort clinical toxicity, as the therapeutic effect of the antagonist may be nullified except in the case of folic acid antagonist overdose - see below.

Concomitant disodium folinate will not, however, inhibit the antibacterial activity of other folic acid antagonists such as trimethoprim and pyrimethamine.

In the combination regimen with fluorouracil, the toxicity profile of fluorouracil may be enhanced or shifted by disodium folinate. The commonest manifestations are leucopenia, mucositis, stomatitis and/or diarrhoea which may be dose limiting. When disodium folinate and fluorouracil are used in combination, the fluorouracil dosage must be reduced more in cases of toxicity than when fluorouracil is used alone. Toxicities observed in patients treated with the combination are qualitatively similar to those observed in patients treated with fluorouracil alone. Gastrointestinal toxicities are observed more commonly and may be more severe or even life threatening (particularly stomatitis and diarrhoea). In severe cases, treatment is withdrawal of fluorouracil and disodium folinate, and supportive intravenous therapy. Patients should be instructed to consult their treating physician immediately if stomatitis (mild to moderate ulcers) and/or diarrhoea (watery stools or bowel movements) two times per day occur (see also section 4.2).

Particular care should be taken in the treatment of elderly or debilitated patients, as these patients may be at increased risk of severe toxicity.

In the treatment of accidental overdosage of folic acid antagonists, disodium folinate should be administered as promptly as possible. With increasing time interval between antifolate administration (e.g. methotrexate) and disodium folinate rescue the effectiveness of disodium folinate in counteracting toxicity decreases. Monitoring of the serum methotrexate concentration is essential in determining the optimal dose and duration of treatment with disodium folinate. Delayed methotrexate excretion may be caused by third space fluid accumulation (i.e., ascites, pleural effusion), renal insufficiency, inadequate hydration or non steroidal anti inflammatory or salicylates drug administration. Under such circumstances, higher doses of disodium folinate or prolonged administration may be indicated.

Disodium folinate has no effect on non-haematological toxicities of methotrexate such as the nephrotoxicity resulting from drug and/or metabolite precipitation in the kidney.

In epileptic patients treated with phenobarbital, phenytoine, primidone, there is a risk to increase the frequency of seizures due to decrease of plasmatic concentrations of anti epileptic drugs. Clinical monitoring, possibly monitoring of the plasmatic concentrations and if necessary, dose adaptation of the anti-epileptic drug during disodium folinate administration and after discontinuation is recommended (see 4.5).

4.5 Interaction with other medicinal products and other forms of interaction

Disodium folinate is an antidote of folic acid antagonists - e.g. methotrexate. Following the use of methotrexate, disodium folinate overdosage may lead to a loss of the effect of methotrexate therapy ("over-rescue").

Concomitant use of disodium folinate counteracts the antineoplastic activity of methotrexate and increases the cytotoxic effects of fluorouracil.

The following side-effects for disodium folinate used in conjunction with fluorouracil were reported frequently: diarrhoea, dehydration, stomatitis and leucopenia. Less commonly infections, thrombocytopenia, nausea, vomiting, constipation, malaise, alopecia, dermatitis and anorexia have been observed.

Life threatening diarrhoeas have been observed if 600 mg/m^2 of fluorouracil (i.v. bolus once weekly) is given together with disodium folinate. When disodium folinate and fluorouracil are used in combination, the fluorouracil dosage must be reduced more than when fluorouracil is used alone.

Concomitant use requiring precautions for use: Phenobarbital, primidone, phenytoine: decreased plasma levels of enzymatic inductor anticonvulsivant drugs by increasing the hepatic metabolism for which folates are one of the cofactors (see 4.4).

4.6 Pregnancy and lactation

Methotrexate therapy is contra-indicated during pregnancy and lactation period. Therefore, prevention of consequences of a methotrexate therapy does not apply.

Combination therapy with disodium folinate and fluorouracil is contra-indicated during pregnancy and lactation period.

No information is available on the effects of folinic acid alone on fertility and general reproductive performance.

4.7 Effects on ability to drive and use machines

Disodium folinate is unlikely to affect the ability to drive or operate machines. The general condition of the patient is likely to be more significant than any drug-induced effects.

4.8 Undesirable effects

Adverse reactions to disodium folinate are rare but occasional pyrexial reactions have been reported following parenteral administration. Isolated case of allergic reactions - sensitisation, including anaphylactoid reactions and urticaria, can occur. At high dosage gastrointestinal disorders have been observed.

Disodium folinate enhances the toxicity of 5-fluorouracil (see section 4.5 Interactions).

4.9 Overdose

When using methotrexate, an overdosage of disodium folinate may result in a decrease of efficacy of methotrexate ("over-rescue").

Should overdosage of the combination of fluorouracil and Sodiofolin 50 mg/ml, solution for injection or infusion occur, overdosage instructions for fluorouracil should be followed.

5. PHARMACOLOGICAL PROPERTIES

5.1 Pharmacodynamic properties

Pharmacotherapeutic group: Antidote

ATC code: V 03 AF

Folinic acid is the formyl derivative of tetrahydrofolic acid resp. the active form of folic acid. It is involved in various metabolic processes including purine synthesis, pyrimidine nucleotide synthesis and amino acid metabolism.

Biochemical rationale for the combination of disodium folinate with fluorouracil:

Fluorouracil inhibits *inter alia* DNA synthesis by binding thymidilate synthetase. The combination of disodium folinate with fluorouracil results in the formation of a stable ternary complex consisting of thymidilate synthetase, 5-fluorodeoxy-uridinemonophosphate and 5,10-methylenetetrahydrofolate.

This leads to an extended blockade of thymidilate synthetase with enhanced inhibition of DNA biosynthesis, resulting in increased cytotoxicity as compared to fluorouracil monotherapy.

5.2 Pharmacokinetic properties

Bioequivalence

A pharmacokinetic study was performed to demonstrate the bioequivalence of disodium folinate in comparison with a licensed calcium folinate reference preparation. The bioequivalence criteria determined were fulfilled in respect of the pharmacokinetic parameters for D- and L-folinic acid and for the metabolite 5-methyltetrahydrofolic acid. Calcium folinate and disodium folinate solutions are bioequivalent.

Distribution

The distribution volume of folinic acid is not known. With i.v. application, peak serum levels of the parent substance (D/L-formyltetrahydrofolic acid, folinic acid) are obtained after 10 minutes.

Metabolism

The active isomeric form L-5-formyltetrahydrofolic acid is quickly metabolised to 5-methyltetrahydrofolic acid in the liver. It is assumed that this conversion is not linked to the presence of dihydrofolate reductase and occurs more quickly and more completely after oral application than after parenteral application.

Excretion

The inactive isomeric form D-5-formyltetrahydrofolic acid is excreted virtually completely unchanged via the kidneys. The active isomeric form L-5-formyltetra-hydrofolic acid is in part excreted unchanged via the kidneys, but is predominantly metabolised to folic acid.

5.3 Preclinical safety data

Toxicity tests on combined use with fluorouracil have not been carried out.

No further information is available of relevance to the prescriber which is not already included in other relevant sections of the SPC.

6. PHARMACEUTICAL PARTICULARS

6.1 List of excipients

Sodium hydroxide

Hydrochloric acid

Water for injection

6.2 Incompatibilities

This medicinal product should not be mixed with other medicinal products except those mentioned in section 6.6.

6.3 Shelf life

36 months

After dilution (see section 6.4 and 6.6): 72 hours.

6.4 Special precautions for storage

Store in a refrigerator (2 - 8 °C). Keep the container in the outer carton in order to protect from light.

After mixing with fluorouracil or dilution with 0.9 % sodium chloride solution (see section 6.6). Chemical and physical in use stability has been demonstrated for 72 hours at 20 - 25 °C. From a microbiological point of view the product should be used immediately. If not used immediately, in use storage times and conditions prior to use are the responsibility of the user and would normally not be longer than 24 hours at 2 - 8 °C unless dilution has taken place in controlled and validated aseptic conditions.

6.5 Nature and contents of container

Colourless glass vials type 1 of 5, 10 and 20 ml respectively

Closure: bromobutyl rubber stopper with aluminium flip-off cap as seal.

Vials with 2 ml, 4 ml, 6 ml, 7 ml, 8 ml, 10 ml or 18 ml solution for injection or infusion.

Packs containing 1 vial or 5 vials. Not all pack sizes may be marketed.

6.6 Special precautions for disposal and other handling

Sodiofolin 50 mg/ml, solution for injection or infusion is administered intravenously, either undiluted by injection or by infusion after dilution. Preparation of solution for infusion must take place in aseptic conditions. The solution for injection or infusion may be diluted with 0.9 % sodium chloride solution.

Sodiofolin 50 mg/ml is compatible with fluorouracil.

Only clear solutions without visible particles should be used.

For single use only. Any unused product must be discarded.

7. MARKETING AUTHORISATION HOLDER

medac

Gesellschaft für klinische

Spezialpräparate mbH

Fehlandtstraβe 3

D-20354 Hamburg

Germany

8. MARKETING AUTHORISATION NUMBER(S)

PL: 11587/0005

9. DATE OF FIRST AUTHORISATION/RENEWAL OF THE AUTHORISATION

2 August 2000 / 30 May 2006

10. DATE OF REVISION OF THE TEXT

09/2006

Sodium Bicarbonate Injection Bp Minijet 8.4% (International Medication Systems)

(International Medication Systems (UK) Ltd)

1. NAME OF THE MEDICINAL PRODUCT
Sodium Bicarbonate Injection BP Minijet 8.4% w/v

2. QUALITATIVE AND QUANTITATIVE COMPOSITION
Sodium Bicarbonate BP 8.4% w/v

3. PHARMACEUTICAL FORM
Sterile aqueous solution for parenteral administration to humans.

4. CLINICAL PARTICULARS

4.1 Therapeutic indications
For the correction of metabolic acidosis associated with cardiac arrest after other resuscitative measures such as cardiac compression, ventilation, adrenaline and antiarrhythmic agents have been used.

4.2 Posology and method of administration
For intravenous administration only.

Adults: the usual dose is 1mmol/kg (2ml/kg 4.2% solution or 1ml/kg 8.4% solution) followed by 0.5mmol/kg (1ml/kg 4.2% solution or 0.5ml/kg 8.4% solution) given at 10 minute intervals.

Children: the usual dose is 1mmol/kg by slow iv injection.

In premature infants and neonates, the 4.2% solution should be used or the 8.4% solution should be diluted 1:1 with 5% dextrose.

Elderly: as for adults.

4.3 Contraindications
Administration of sodium bicarbonate is contraindicated in patients with renal failure, metabolic or respiratory alkalosis, hypertension, oedema, congestive heart failure, a history of urinary calculi and coexistent potassium depletion or hypocalcaemia, hypoventilation, chloride depletion or hypernatraemia.

4.4 Special warnings and precautions for use
Whenever sodium bicarbonate is used intravenously, arterial blood gas analyses, in particular arterial/venous blood pH and carbon dioxide levels, should be performed before and during the course of treatment to minimise the possibility of overdosage and resultant alkalosis.

Accidental extravascular injection of hypertonic solutions may cause vascular irritation or sloughing. The use of scalp veins should be avoided.

Whenever respiratory acidosis is concomitant with metabolic acidosis, both pulmonary ventilation and perfusion must be adequately supported to get rid of excess CO_2.

4.5 Interaction with other medicinal products and other forms of interaction
Caution should be used when administering sodium ions to patients receiving corticosteroids or corticotrophin.

Urinary alkalisation will increase the renal clearance of tetracyclines, especially doxycycline but it will increase the half life and duration of action of basic drugs such as quinidine, amphetamines, ephedrine and pseudoephedrine.

Hypochloraemic alkalosis may occur if sodium bicarbonate is used in conjunction with potassium depleting diuretics such as bumetamide, ethacrynic acid, frusemide and thiazides. Concurrent use in patients taking potassium supplements may reduce serum potassium concentration by promoting an intracellular ion shift.

4.6 Pregnancy and lactation
Safe use in pregnancy has not been established. The use of any drug in pregnant or lactating women requires that the expected benefit be carefully weighed against the possible risk to the mother and child.

Patients requiring i.v. sodium bicarbonate are unlikely to be fit enough to breast feed.

4.7 Effects on ability to drive and use machines
Not applicable; this preparation is intended for use only in emergencies.

4.8 Undesirable effects
Alkalosis and/or hypokalaemia may ensue as a result of prolonged use or over-correction of the bicarbonate deficit.

Hyperirritability or tetany may occur caused by rapid shifts of free ionised calcium or due to serum protein alterations arising from pH changes.

4.9 Overdose
Symptoms: metabolic alkalosis accompanied by compensatory hyperventilation, paradoxical acidosis of the cerebrospinal fluid, severe hypokalaemia, hyperirritability and tetany.

Treatment: discontinue the administration of sodium bicarbonate, rebreathe expired air or, if more severe administer calcium gluconate especially if tetany is present. In severe alkalosis, an infusion of 2.14% ammonium chloride is recommended, except in patients with pe-existing hepatic disease. If hypokalaemia is present administer potassium chloride.

5. PHARMACOLOGICAL PROPERTIES

5.1 Pharmacodynamic properties
Sodium bicarbonate therapy increases plasma bicarbonate, buffers excess hydrogen ion concentration, raises blood pH and reverses clinical manifestations of metabolic acidosis.

5.2 Pharmacokinetic properties
Sodium bicarbonate is eliminated principally in the urine and effectively alkalises it.

5.3 Preclinical safety data
Not applicable since sodium bicarbonate has been used in clinical practice for many years and its effects in man are well known.

6. PHARMACEUTICAL PARTICULARS

6.1 List of excipients
Water for Injection USP

6.2 Incompatibilities
The addition of sodium bicarbonate to parenteral solutions containing calcium should be avoided except where compatibility has been previously established; precipitation or haze may result, should this occur, the solution should not be used.

6.3 Shelf life
36 months.

6.4 Special precautions for storage
Store below 25°C.

6.5 Nature and contents of container
The solution is contained in a USP type I glass vial with an elastomeric closure which meets all the relevant USP specifications.

The 8.4% w/v is available as 10 or 50ml.

6.6 Special precautions for disposal and other handling
The container is specially designed for use with the IMS Minijet injector.

Administrative Data

7. MARKETING AUTHORISATION HOLDER
International Medication Systems (UK) Limited

208 Bath Road

Slough

Berkshire

SL1 3WE

UK

8. MARKETING AUTHORISATION NUMBER(S)
PL 3265/0003R

9. DATE OF FIRST AUTHORISATION/RENEWAL OF THE AUTHORISATION
Date first granted: 28 February 1991

Date renewed: 29 November 1996

10. DATE OF REVISION OF THE TEXT
April 2001

POM

Sodium Bicarbonate Injection Minijet 4.2%

(International Medication Systems (UK) Ltd)

1. NAME OF THE MEDICINAL PRODUCT
Sodium Bicarbonate Injection BP Minijet 4.2% w/v

2. QUALITATIVE AND QUANTITATIVE COMPOSITION
Sodium Bicarbonate BP 4.2% w/v

3. PHARMACEUTICAL FORM
Sterile aqueous solution for parenteral administration to humans.

4. CLINICAL PARTICULARS

4.1 Therapeutic indications
For the correction of metabolic acidosis associated with cardiac arrest after other resuscitative measures such as cardiac compression, ventilation, adrenaline and antiarrhythmic agents have been used.

4.2 Posology and method of administration
For intravenous administration only.

Adults: the usual dose is 1mmol/kg (2ml/kg 4.2% solution or 1ml/kg 8.4% solution) followed by 0.5mmol/kg (1ml/kg 4.2% solution or 0.5ml/kg 8.4% solution) given at 10 minute intervals.

Children: the usual dose is 1mmol/kg by slow iv injection.

In premature infants and neonates, the 4.2% solution should be used or the 8.4% solution should be diluted 1:1 with 5% dextrose.

Elderly: as for adults.

4.3 Contraindications
Administration of sodium bicarbonate is contraindicated in patients with renal failure, metabolic or respiratory alkalosis, hypertension, oedema, congestive heart failure, a history of urinary calculi and coexistent potassium depletion or hypocalcaemia, hypoventilation, chloride depletion or hypernatraemia.

4.4 Special warnings and precautions for use
Whenever sodium bicarbonate is used intravenously, arterial blood gas analyses, in particular arterial/venous blood pH and carbon dioxide levels, should be performed before and during the course of treatment to minimise the possibility of overdosage and resultant alkalosis.

Accidental extravascular injection of hypertonic solutions may cause vascular irritation or sloughing. The use of scalp veins should be avoided.

Whenever respiratory acidosis is concomitant with metabolic acidosis, both pulmonary ventilation and perfusion must be adequately supported to get rid of excess CO_2.

4.5 Interaction with other medicinal products and other forms of interaction
Caution should be used when administering sodium ions to patients receiving corticosteroids or corticotrophin.

Urinary alkalisation will increase the renal clearance of tetracyclines, especially doxycycline but it will increase the half life and duration of action of basic drugs such as quinidine, amphetamines, ephedrine and pseudoephedrine.

Hypochloraemic alkalosis may occur if sodium bicarbonate is used in conjunction with potassium depleting diuretics such as bumetamide, ethacrynic acid, frusemide and thiazides. Concurrent use in patients taking potassium supplements may reduce serum potassium concentration by promoting an intracellular ion shift.

4.6 Pregnancy and lactation
Safe use in pregnancy has not been established. The use of any drug in pregnant or lactating women requires that the expected benefit be carefully weighed against the possible risk to the mother and child.

Patients requiring i.v. sodium bicarbonate are unlikely to be fit enough to breast feed.

4.7 Effects on ability to drive and use machines
Not applicable; this preparation is intended for use only in emergencies.

4.8 Undesirable effects
Alkalosis and/or hypokalaemia may ensue as a result of prolonged use or over-correction of the bicarbonate deficit.

Hyperirritability or tetany may occur caused by rapid shifts of free ionised calcium or due to serum protein alterations arising from pH changes.

4.9 Overdose
Symptoms: metabolic alkalosis accompanied by compensatory hyperventilation, paradoxical acidosis of the cerebrospinal fluid, severe hypokalaemia, hyperirritability and tetany.

Treatment: discontinue the administration of sodium bicarbonate, rebreathe expired air or, if more severe administer calcium gluconate especially if tetany is present. In severe alkalosis, an infusion of 2.14% ammonium chloride is recommended, except in patients with pe-existing hepatic disease. If hypokalaemia is present administer potassium chloride.

5. PHARMACOLOGICAL PROPERTIES

5.1 Pharmacodynamic properties
Sodium bicarbonate therapy increases plasma bicarbonate, buffers excess hydrogen ion concentration, raises blood pH and reverses clinical manifestations of metabolic acidosis.

5.2 Pharmacokinetic properties
Sodium bicarbonate is eliminated principally in the urine and effectively alkalises it.

5.3 Preclinical safety data
Not applicable since sodium bicarbonate has been used in clinical practice for many years and its effects in man are well known.

6. PHARMACEUTICAL PARTICULARS

6.1 List of excipients
Water for Injection USP

6.2 Incompatibilities
The addition of sodium bicarbonate to parenteral solutions containing calcium should be avoided except where compatibility has been previously established; precipitation or haze may result, should this occur, the solution should not be used.

6.3 Shelf life
36 months.

6.4 Special precautions for storage
Store below 25°C.

6.5 Nature and contents of container
The solution is contained in a USP type I glass vial with an elastomeric closure which meets all the relevant USP specifications.

The 4.2% w/v is available as 10ml.

6.6 Special precautions for disposal and other handling
The container is specially designed for use with the IMS Minijet injector.

Administrative Data

7. MARKETING AUTHORISATION HOLDER
International Medication Systems (UK) Limited
208 Bath Road
Slough
Berkshire
SL1 3WE
UK

8. MARKETING AUTHORISATION NUMBER(S)
PL 3265/0001R

9. DATE OF FIRST AUTHORISATION/RENEWAL OF THE AUTHORISATION
Date first granted: 28 February 1991

Date renewed: 29 November 1996

10. DATE OF REVISION OF THE TEXT
April 2001
POM

Sodium Fusidate 500mg for Intravenous Infusion

(Leo Laboratories Limited)

1. NAME OF THE MEDICINAL PRODUCT
Sodium Fusidate 500mg for Intravenous Infusion

2. QUALITATIVE AND QUANTITATIVE COMPOSITION
Sodium Fusidate Ph.Eur. 500mg (equivalent to 480mg fusidic acid) contained in one vial. (The second vial contains buffer solution).

3. PHARMACEUTICAL FORM
Powder for reconstitution and use as an intravenous infusion.

4. CLINICAL PARTICULARS

4.1 Therapeutic indications
This product is indicated in the treatment of all staphylococcal infections due to susceptible organisms such as: osteomyelitis, pneumonia, septicaemia, wound infections, endocarditis, superinfected cystic fibrosis, cutaneous infections.

It should be administered intravenously whenever oral therapy is inappropriate, which includes cases where absorption from the gastro-intestinal tract is unpredictable.

4.2 Posology and method of administration
Adults weighing more than 50 kg: 500 mg sodium fusidate three times daily.

Children and adults weighing less than 50 kg: 6-7 mg sodium fusidate per kg bodyweight three times daily.

Recommended procedure: To reconstitute, dissolve the contents of one vial containing 500 mg sodium fusidate powder (equivalent to 480 mg of fusidic acid) in the 10 ml buffer provided.

For adults weighing more than 50 kg: Add the 10 ml fusidate/buffer solution to 500 ml of infusion fluid.

For children and adults weighing less than 50 kg: Add the 10 ml fusidate/buffer solution to 500 ml of infusion fluid. Each dose corresponds to 6-7 ml of the resulting solution per kg bodyweight.

The diluted fluid should be infused via a central venous line over 2 hours. If a superficial vein is employed a more prolonged period of at least 6 hours is advisable.

This product should be administered intravenously into a wide bore vein with a good blood flow. Excessive doses may cause venospasm, thrombophlebitis and haemolysis of erythrocytes. Both oral and intravenous presentations have been given concurrently with other antibiotics, e.g. cloxacillin, flucloxacillin, ampicillin, methicillin and erythromycin.

Since it is excreted in the bile, no dosage modifications are needed in renal impairment.

The dosage in patients undergoing haemodialysis needs no adjustment as this product is not significantly dialysed.

Dosage in the elderly: No dosage alterations are necessary in the elderly.

If additional antibacterial therapy is to be employed, it is recommended that for parenteral administration, separate infusion fluids be used.

4.3 Contraindications
Contra-indicated in patients with known hypersensitivity to fusidic acid and its salts. This product should not be infused with amino acid solutions or in whole blood. Due to local tissue injury, this product should not be administered intramuscularly or subcutaneously.

4.4 Special warnings and precautions for use
Caution should be exercised with other antibiotics which have similar biliary excretion pathways e.g. lincomycin and rifampicin. Periodic liver function tests should be carried out when high oral doses are used, when the drug is given for prolonged periods and in patients with liver dysfunction.

This product displaces bilirubin from its albumin binding site *in vitro*. The clinical significance of this finding is uncertain and kernicterus has not been observed in neonates receiving Sodium Fusidate 500mg for Intravenous Infusion. However, this observation should be borne in mind when the drug is given to pre-term, jaundiced, acidotic or seriously ill neonates.

The use of this product in combination with drugs that are CYP-3A4 biotransformed should be avoided. See Section 4.5.

Patients given this product systemically in combination with HMG-CoA reductase inhibitors should be closely clinically monitored. See Section 4.5.

4.5 Interaction with other medicinal products and other forms of interaction
See 4.4.

In vitro compatibility studies of Sodium Fusidate 500mg for Intravenous Infusion with commonly used infusion solutions have been carried out.

The results showed that sodium fusidate reconstituted at 50 mg/ml in buffer solution is physically and chemically compatible for at least 24 hours at room temperature with the following infusion solutions (the figure in parenthesis shows the concentration of sodium fusidate in the final admixture):

Sodium Chloride Intravenous Infusion BP 0.9% (1-2 mg/ml)

Dextrose Intravenous Infusion BP 5% (1-2 mg/ml)

Compound Sodium Lactate Intravenous Infusion ("Ringer-Lactate Solution") (1 mg/ml)

Sodium Lactate Intravenous Infusion BP (1 mg/ml)

Sodium Chloride (0.18%) and Dextrose (4%) Intravenous Infusion BP (1 mg/ml)

Potassium Chloride (0.3%) and Dextrose (5%) Intravenous Infusion BP (1 mg/ml)

Specific pathways of metabolism of this product in the liver are not known, however, an interaction between this product and drugs being CYP-3A4 biotransformed can be suspected. The mechanism of this interaction is presumed to be a mutual inhibition of metabolism. There is insufficient data to characterise the effect of fusidic acid on CYPs *in-vitro*. The use of this product systemically should be avoided in patients treated with CYP-3A4 biotransformed drugs.

When this product is administered systemically and concomitantly with oral anticoagulants such as coumarin derivatives or anticoagulants with similar actions, the plasma concentration of these agents may increase enhancing the anticoagulant effect. Anticoagulation should be closely monitored and a decrease of the oral anticoagulant dose may be necessary in order to maintain the desired level of anticoagulation. Similarly, discontinuation of this product may require the maintenance dose of anticoagulant to be re-assessed. The mechanism of this suspected interaction remains unknown.

Systemic co-administration of this product with HMG-CoA reductase inhibitors such as statins may cause increased plasma concentrations of both agents and rare cases of rhabdomyolysis have been reported for this combination. Patients on this combination should be closely clinically monitored.

Co-administration of this product systemically with ciclosporin has been reported to cause increased plasma concentration of ciclosporin.

4.6 Pregnancy and lactation
There is inadequate evidence of safety in human pregnancy. Animal studies and many years of clinical experience suggest that fusidic acid is devoid of teratogenic effects. There is evidence to suggest that when given systemically, fusidic acid can cross the placental barrier. If the administration of the product to pregnant patients is considered essential, its use requires that the potential benefits be weighed against the possible hazards to the foetus.

Safety in nursing mothers has not been established. When fusidic acid (as the sodium salt) has been given systemically, levels have been detected in the breast milk. Caution is therefore required when the product is used in mothers who wish to breast feed.

4.7 Effects on ability to drive and use machines
None known.

4.8 Undesirable effects
In some patients, particularly in the young and elderly, a reversible jaundice has been reported. Jaundice has been seen most frequently in patients receiving this product in high dosage, or where the drug has been infused too rapidly or at too high a concentration in the infusion fluid. In some instances instituting oral therapy may be beneficial. If the jaundice persists this product should be withdrawn, following which the serum bilirubin will invariably return to normal. Reported reactions are thrombophlebitis and, rarely, skin rashes and other allergic reactions including anaphylaxis. Isolated cases of haematological abnormalities which can affect the 3 blood cell lines but mainly white blood cells e.g. bone marrow depression, neutropenia, granulocytopenia, agranulocytosis and pancytopenia have been reported. Reported less often is a depressive effect on the platelets and red blood cells with reports of thrombocytopenia and various anaemias. These abnormalities have been observed especially with treatment of more than 15 days. Acute renal failure has been described in patients with jaundice, particularly in the presence of other factors predisposing to renal failure.

4.9 Overdose
There has been no experience of overdosage. Treatment should be restricted to symptomatic and supportive measures. Dialysis is of no benefit, since the drug is not significantly dialysed.

5. PHARMACOLOGICAL PROPERTIES

5.1 Pharmacodynamic properties
Fusidic acid and its salts are potent anti-staphylococcal agents with unusual ability to penetrate tissue. Bactericidal levels have been assayed in bone and necrotic tissue.

Concentrations of 0.03 - 0.12 micrograms/ml inhibit nearly all strains of *Staphylococcus aureus*. Fusidic acid is active against *Staphylococcus epidermidis* and methicillin resistant staphylococci.

In severe or deep seated infections and when prolonged therapy may be required, systemic administration of this product should generally be given concurrently with other anti-staphylococcal antibiotic therapy.

5.2 Pharmacokinetic properties
500 mg of sodium fusidate given as a single infusion over 2 hours results in a Cmax of 52 micrograms/ml. Blood levels are cumulative, reaching concentrations of 60-120 micrograms/ml after repeated infusion of 500 mg sodium fusidate every 8 hours for 2-3 days.

The plasma half-life is approximately 10-15 hours.

This product is excreted mainly in the bile, little or none being excreted in the urine.

5.3 Preclinical safety data
There are no pre-clinical data of relevance to the prescriber which are additional to that already included in other sections of the SPC.

6. PHARMACEUTICAL PARTICULARS

6.1 List of excipients
The vial of 10 ml sterile phosphate-citrate buffer solution (pH 7.4 - 7.6) contains disodium hydrogen phosphate, citric acid, disodium edetate and water for injections. (When reconstituted with powder vial contains 3.1 mMol sodium and 1.1 mMol phosphate).

6.2 Incompatibilities
Sodium fusidate reconstituted at 50 mg/ml in buffer solution is physically incompatible with infusion fluids containing 20% or more of dextrose, lipid infusions and peritoneal dialysis fluids. Precipitation may occur at dilutions which result in a pH of less than 7.4.

6.3 Shelf life
3 years for the sodium fusidate dry powder.

After the sodium fusidate dry powder is dissolved in the buffer solution provided and added to 500ml of infusion fluid, the shelf-life of this solution is 24 hours.

6.4 Special precautions for storage
The sodium fusidate dry powder is stable for 3 years when stored at room temperature (below 25°C) and protected from light. When the buffer solution is transferred to the powder vial, this vial should be regarded as a unit dose. The required amount of the sodium fusidate/buffer solution should be used once only and any unused portion discarded.

6.5 Nature and contents of container
Pack containing a single pair of vials; one glass vial of sodium fusidate closed with a butyl rubber stopper secured with metal rings and one glass vial of sterile buffer solution 10ml closed with a bromobutyl rubber stopper secured with metal rings.

6.6 Special precautions for disposal and other handling
None

7. MARKETING AUTHORISATION HOLDER
LEO Laboratories Limited, Longwick Road, Princes Risborough, Bucks. HP27 9RR.

8. MARKETING AUTHORISATION NUMBER(S)
0043/0184

9. DATE OF FIRST AUTHORISATION/RENEWAL OF THE AUTHORISATION
14.10.1992

10. DATE OF REVISION OF THE TEXT
February 2006

LEGAL CATEGORY
POM

Sofradex Ear / Eye Drops

(sanofi-aventis)

1. NAME OF THE MEDICINAL PRODUCT
Sofradex Ear/Eye Drops.

2. QUALITATIVE AND QUANTITATIVE COMPOSITION
Each bottle contains 0.5% w/v of Framycetin Sulphate Ph.Eur., Dexamethasone Sodium Metasulphobenzoate (equivalent to 0.050% w/v of Dexamethasone) and 0.005% w/v of Gramicidin USP.

3. PHARMACEUTICAL FORM

Sterile clear colourless ear/eye drops.

4. CLINICAL PARTICULARS

4.1 Therapeutic indications

In the Eye: For the short term treatment of steroid responsive conditions of the eye when prophylactic antibiotic treatment is also required, after excluding the presence of fungal and viral disease.

In the Ear: Otitis Externa.

4.2 Posology and method of administration

DOSAGE

Adults (and the Elderly) and Children:

In the Eye: One or two drops applied to each affected eye up to six times daily or more frequently if required.

In the Ear: Two or three drops instilled into the ear three or four times daily.

ADMINISTRATION

Auricular and Ocular use.

4.3 Contraindications

Viral, fungal, tuberculous or purulent conditions of the eye. Use is contraindicated if glaucoma is present or herpetic keratitis (e.g. dendritic ulcer) is considered a possibility. Use of topical steroids in the latter condition can lead to extension of the ulcer and marked visual deterioration.

Otitis Externa should not be treated when the eardrum is perforated because of the risk of ototoxicity.

Hypersensitivity to the preparation.

4.4 Special warnings and precautions for use

Topical corticosteroids should never be given for an undiagnosed red eye as inappropriate use is potentially blinding.

Treatment with corticosteroid/antibiotic combinations should not be continued for more than 7 days in the absence of any clinical improvement, since prolonged use may lead to occult extension of infections due to the masking effect of the steroid. Prolonged use may also lead to skin sensitisation and the emergence of resistant organisms.

Prolonged use may lead to the risk of adrenal suppression in infants.

Treatment with corticosteroid preparations should not be repeated or prolonged without regular review to exclude raised intraocular, pressure, cataract formation or unsuspected infections.

Aminoglycosides antibiotics may cause irreversible, partial or total deafness when given systemically or when applied topically to open wounds or damaged skin. This effect is dose related and is enhanced by renal or hepatic impairment. Although this effect has not been reported following ocular use, the possibility should be considered when high dose topical is given to small children or infants.

4.5 Interaction with other medicinal products and other forms of interaction

None relevant to topical use

4.6 Pregnancy and lactation

Safety for use in pregnancy and lactation has not been established. There is inadequate evidence of safety in human pregnancy. Topical administration of corticosteroids to pregnant animals can cause abnormalities of foetal development including cleft palate and intrauterine growth retardation. There may therefore be a very small risk of such effects in the human foetus. There is a risk of foetal ototoxicity if aminoglycoside antibiotics preparations are administrated during pregnancy.

4.7 Effects on ability to drive and use machines

May cause transient blurring of vision on instillation. Warn patients not to drive or operate hazardous machinery unless vision is clear.

4.8 Undesirable effects

Hypersensitivity reactions, usually of the delayed type, may occur leading to irritation, burning, stinging, itching and dermatitis.

Topical steroid use may result in increased intraocular pressure leading to optic nerve damage, reduced visual acuity and visual field defects.

Intensive or prolonged use of topical corticosteroids may lead to formation of posterior subcapsular cataracts.

In those diseases causing thinning of the cornea or sclera, corticosteroid therapy may result in the thinning of the globe leading to perforation.

4.9 Overdose

Long-term intensive topical use may lead to systemic effects.

Oral ingestion of the contents of one bottle (up to 10ml) is unlikely to lead to any serious adverse effects.

5. PHARMACOLOGICAL PROPERTIES

5.1 Pharmacodynamic properties

Framycetin Sulphate is an aminoglycoside antibiotic with a spectrum of activity similar to that of neomycin, this includes *Staph. aureus* and most clinically significant gram negative organisms.

Gramicidin is an antimicrobial cyclic polypeptide active in vitro against many gram positive bacteria. It is used for the local treatment of susceptible infections, sometimes in combination with other antimicrobial agents and frequently with a corticosteroid.

Dexamethasone is a synthetic glucocorticoid and has the general properties as other corticosteroids.

5.2 Pharmacokinetic properties

Framycetin Sulphate absorption occurs from inflamed skin and wounds. Once absorbed it is rapidly excreted by the kidneys in active form. It has been reported to have a half life of 2-3 hours

Gramicidin has properties similar to those of Tyrothricin and is too toxic to be administered systemically.

Dexamethasone is readily absorbed from the gastro-intestinal tract. It has a biological half-life in plasma of about 190 minutes.

5.3 Preclinical safety data

Not applicable.

6. PHARMACEUTICAL PARTICULARS

6.1 List of excipients

The ear/eye drops contains Citric Acid BP, Sodium Citrate BP, Lithium Chloride, Phenylethyl Alcohol, Industrial Methylated Spirit BP, Polysorbate 80 BP, Purified Water BP.

6.2 Incompatibilities

None known.

6.3 Shelf life

24 Months.

Discard contents 28 days after opening.

6.4 Special precautions for storage

Store below 25°C, do not refrigerate.

6.5 Nature and contents of container

Glass bottle fitted with a special dropper attachment: Pack size of 8 or 10ml.

Plastic dropper bottle: Pack size of 10ml.

6.6 Special precautions for disposal and other handling

Not applicable.

7. MARKETING AUTHORISATION HOLDER

Sanofi-aventis

One Onslow Street

Guildford

Surrey

GU1 4YS

UK

8. MARKETING AUTHORISATION NUMBER(S)

PL 04425/0210

9. DATE OF FIRST AUTHORISATION/RENEWAL OF THE AUTHORISATION

4th June 2005

10. DATE OF REVISION OF THE TEXT

December 2006

Legal Category

POM

Solian

(sanofi-aventis)

1. NAME OF THE MEDICINAL PRODUCT

SOLIAN 50

SOLIAN 100

SOLIAN 200

SOLIAN 400

Solian® Solution, 100mg/ml

2. QUALITATIVE AND QUANTITATIVE COMPOSITION

Active ingredient: Amisulpride (INN) 50 mg, 100 mg, 200 mg or 400 mg per tablet; Solian Solution: Amisulpride (INN) 100 mg/ml.

For excipients, see 6.1.

3. PHARMACEUTICAL FORM

Solian 50: White to off-white, round, flat-faced tablet engraved with AMI 50 on one face.

Solian 100: White to off-white, round, flat-faced tablet engraved AMI 100 on one face and with a breakable bar on the other face

Solian 200: White to off-white, round, flat-faced tablet engraved AMI 200 on one face and with a breakable bar on the other face

Solian 400: Tablet

Solian Solution: Oral Solution: A clear yellow liquid in appearance.

4. CLINICAL PARTICULARS

4.1 Therapeutic indications

Solian is indicated for the treatment of acute and chronic schizophrenic disorders, in which positive symptoms (such as delusions, hallucinations, thought disorders) and/or negative symptoms (such as blunted affect, emotional and social withdrawal) are prominent, including patients characterised by predominant negative symptoms.

4.2 Posology and method of administration

For acute psychotic episodes, oral doses between 400 mg/d and 800 mg/d are recommended. In individual cases, the daily dose may be increased up to 1200 mg/d. Doses above 1200 mg/d have not been extensively evaluated for safety and therefore should not be used. No specific titration is required when initiating the treatment with Solian. Doses should be adjusted according to individual response.

For patients with mixed positive and negative symptoms, doses should be adjusted to obtain optimal control of positive symptoms ie between 400-800mg/day.

Maintenance treatment should be established individually with the minimally effective dose.

For patients characterised by predominant negative symptoms, oral doses between 50 mg/d and 300 mg/d are recommended. Doses should be adjusted individually.

Solian can be administered once daily at oral doses up to 300 mg, higher doses should be administered bid.

The minimum effective dose should be used.

Elderly: Solian should be used with particular caution because of a possible risk of hypotension or sedation.

Children: Solian is contra-indicated in children under 15 years of age as its safety has not yet been established.

Renal insufficiency: Solian is eliminated by the renal route. In renal insufficiency, the dose should be reduced to half in patients with creatinine clearance (CR_{CL}) between 30-60 ml/min and to a third in patients with CR_{CL} between 10-30 ml/min.

As there is no experience in patients with severe renal impairment ($CR_{CL} < 10$ ml/min) particular care is recommended in these patients (see 4.4 Special warning and precautions for use).

Hepatic insufficiency: since the drug is weakly metabolised a dosage reduction should not be necessary.

Method of administration (Solian Solution): The graduations on the dosage pipette measure the milligrams of active ingredient. After introducing the measuring syringe into the bottle, draw the plunger of the measuring syringe up to the graduation mark corresponding to the number of milligrams to be administered. The oral solution should be drunk with a liquid, which does not contain alcohol.

4.3 Contraindications

Hypersensitivity to the active ingredient or to other ingredients of the medicinal product.

Concomitant prolactin-dependent tumours e.g. pituitary gland prolactinomas and breast cancer.

Phaeochromocytoma.

Children under 15 years of age.

Lactation.

Combination with the following medications which could induce torsades de pointes:

- Class Ia antiarrhythmic agents such as quinidine, disopyramide, procainamide.

- Class III antiarrhythmic agents such as amiodarone, sotalol.

- Others medications such as bepridil, cisapride, sultopride, thioridazine, methadone, IV erythromycin, IV vincamine, halofantrine, pentamidine, sparfloxacin.

This list is not exhaustive.

Combination with levodopa (see 4.5 Interactions with other medical products and other forms of interaction)

4.4 Special warnings and precautions for use

As with other neuroleptics, Neuroleptic Malignant Syndrome, characterized by hyperthermia, muscle rigidity, autonomic instability, altered consciousness and elevated CPK, may occur. In the event of hyperthermia, particularly with high daily doses, all antipsychotic drugs including Solian should be discontinued.

Hyperglycaemia has been reported in patients treated with some atypical antipsychotic agents, including amisulpride, therefore patients with an established diagnosis of diabetes mellitus or with risk factors for diabetes who are started on amisulpride, should get appropriate glycaemic monitoring.

Solian is eliminated by the renal route. In cases of renal insufficiency, the dose should be decreased or intermittent treatment could be considered (see Section 4.2 Posology and method of administration).

Solian may lower the seizure threshold. Therefore patients with a history of epilepsy should be closely monitored during Solian therapy.

In elderly patients, Solian, like other neuroleptics, should be used with particular caution because of a possible risk of hypotension or sedation.

As with other antidopaminergic agents, caution should be also exercised when prescribing Solian to patients with Parkinson's disease since it may cause worsening of the disease. Solian should be used only if neuroleptic treatment cannot be avoided.

Acute withdrawal symptoms including nausea, vomiting and insomnia have very rarely been described after abrupt cessation of high doses of antipsychotic drugs.

Recurrence of psychotic symptoms may also occur, and the emergence of involuntary movement disorders (such as akathisia, dystonia and dyskinesia) has been reported. Therefore, gradual withdrawal is advisable.

Prolongation of the QT interval

Amisulpride induces a dose-dependent prolongation of the QT interval (see Section 4.8 Undesirable effects). This effect is known to potentiate the risk of serious ventricular arrhythmias such as torsades de pointes.

Before any administration, and if possible according to the patient's clinical status, it is recommended to monitor factors which could favour the occurrence of this rhythm disorder:

- bradycardia less than 55 bpm,
- cardiac disease or family history of sudden death or QT prolongation,
- electrolyte imbalance, in particular hypokalaemia,
- congenital prolongation of the QT interval,
- on-going treatment with a medication likely to produce pronounced bradycardia (< 55 bpm), hypokalaemia, decreased intracardiac conduction, or prolongation of the QT interval (see Section 4.5 Interaction with other medicinal products and other forms of interaction).

Baseline ECG is recommended prior to treatment in all patients especially in the elderly and patients with a positive personal or family history of cardiac disease or abnormal findings on cardiac clinical examination.

During therapy, the need for ECG monitoring (e.g. at dose escalation) should be assessed on an individual patient basis.

The dose of Solian should be reduced if QT is prolonged and discontinued if QTc is >500ms.

Periodic electrolyte monitoring is recommended particularly if the patient is taking diuretics or during inter-current illness.

Concomitant antipsychotics should be avoided.

Stroke

In randomized clinical trials versus placebo performed in a population of elderly patients with dementia and treated with certain atypical antipsychotic drugs, a 3-fold increase of the risk of cerebrovascular events has been observed. The mechanism of such risk increase is not known. An increase in the risk with other antipsychotic drugs, or other populations of patients cannot be excluded. Solian should be used with caution in patients with stroke risk factors.

4.5 Interaction with other medicinal products and other forms of interaction

COMBINATIONS WHICH ARE CONTRAINDICATED

Medications which could induce torsades de pointes:

- Class Ia antiarrhythmic agents such as quinidine, disopyramide, procainamide.
- Class III antiarrhythmic agents such as amiodarone, sotalol.
- Other medications such as bepridil, cisapride, sultopride, thioridazine, methadone, IV erythromycin, IV vincamine, halofantrine, pentamidine, sparfloxacin.

This list is not exhaustive.

Levodopa: reciprocal antagonism of effects between levodopa and neuroleptics.

COMBINATIONS WHICH ARE NOT RECOMMENDED

Solian may enhance the central effects of alcohol.

COMBINATIONS WHICH REQUIRE PRECAUTIONS FOR USE

Medications which enhance the risk of torsades de pointes or could prolong the QT interval:

- Bradycardia-inducing medications such as beta-blockers, bradycardia- inducing calcium channel blockers such as diltiazem and verapamil, clonidine, guanfacine; digitalis.
- Medications which induce hypokalaemia or electrolyte imbalance: hypokalemic diuretics, stimulant laxatives, IV amphotericin B, glucocorticoids, tetracosactides.
- Neuroleptics such as pimozide, haloperidol; imipramine antidepressants; lithium.

COMBINATIONS TO BE TAKEN INTO ACCOUNT

CNS depressants including narcotics, anaesthetics, analgesics, sedative H1 antihistamines, barbiturates, benzodiazepines and other anxiolytic drugs, clonidine and derivatives

Antihypertensive drugs and other hypotensive medications

Dopamine agonists (eg: levodopa) since it may attenuate their action

4.6 Pregnancy and lactation

Pregnancy

In animals, Solian did not show reproductive toxicity. A decrease in fertility linked to the pharmacological effects of the drug (prolactin mediated effect) was observed. No teratogenic effects of Solian were noted.

Very limited clinical data on exposed pregnancies are available. Therefore, the safety of Solian during human pregnancy has not been established.

Use of the drug is not recommended during pregnancy unless the benefits justify the potential risks. If amisulpride is used during pregnancy, neonates may show adverse effects of amisulpride and thus appropriate monitoring should be considered.

For women of childbearing potential, effective contraception should be fully discussed with the physician prior to treatment.

Lactation

It is not known whether Solian is excreted in breast milk, breast-feeding is therefore contra-indicated.

4.7 Effects on ability to drive and use machines

Even used as recommended, Solian may cause somnolence so that the ability to drive vehicles or operate machinery can be impaired (see Section 4.8 Undesirable effects).

4.8 Undesirable effects

Adverse effects have been ranked under headings of frequency using the following convention: very common (≥1/10); common (≥1/100; <1/10); uncommon (≥1/1,000; <1/100); rare (≥1/10,000; <1/1,000); very rare (<1/10,000); frequency not known (cannot be estimated from the available data).

Clinical trials data

The following adverse effects have been observed in controlled clinical trials. It should be noted that in some instances it can be difficult to differentiate adverse events from symptoms of the underlying disease.

- Nervous system disorders:

Very common: Extrapyramidal symptoms may occur: tremor, rigidity, hypokinesia, hypersalivation, akathisia, dyskinesia. These symptoms are generally mild at optimal dosages and partially reversible without discontinuation of amisulpride upon administration of antiparkinsonian medication. The incidence of extrapyramidal symptoms which is dose related, remains very low in the treatment of patients with predominantly negative symptoms with doses of 50-300 mg/day.

Common: Acute dystonia (spasm torticollis, oculogyric crisis, trismus) may appear. This is reversible without discontinuation of amisulpride upon treatment with an antiparkinsonian agent. Somnolence.

Uncommon: Tardive dyskinesia characterized by rhythmic, involuntary movements primarily of the tongue and/or face have been reported, usually after long term administration. Antiparkinsonian medication is ineffective or may induce aggravation of the symptoms. Seizures

- Psychiatric disorders:

Common: Insomnia, anxiety, agitation, orgasmic dysfunction

- Gastrointestinal disorders

Common: Constipation, nausea, vomiting, dry mouth

- Endocrine disorders:

Common: Amisulpride causes an increase in plasma prolactin levels which is reversible after drug discontinuation. This may result in galactorrhoea, amenorrhoea, gynaecomastia, breast pain, and erectile dysfunction.

- Metabolism and nutrition disorders

Uncommon: Hyperglycemia (see 4.4 Special warnings and precautions for use).

- Cardiovascular disorders

Common: Hypotension

Uncommon: Bradycardia

- Investigations:

Common: Weight gain

Uncommon: Elevations of hepatic enzymes, mainly transaminases

- Immune system disorders

Uncommon: Allergic reaction

Post Marketing data

In addition, cases of the following adverse reactions have been reported through spontaneous reporting only:

- Nervous system disorders:

Frequency not known: Neuroleptic Malignant Syndrome (see 4.4 Special warnings and precautions for use).

- Cardiac disorders:

Frequency not known: QT interval prolongation and ventricular arrhythmias such as torsade de pointes, ventricular tachycardia, which may result in ventricular fibrillation or cardiac arrest, sudden death (see 4.4 Special warnings and precautions for use).

4.9 Overdose

Experience with Solian in overdosage is limited. Exaggeration of the known pharmacological effects of the drug have been reported. These include drowsiness and sedation, coma, hypotension and extrapyramidal symptoms.

In cases of acute overdosage, the possibility of multiple drug intake should be considered.

Since Solian is weakly dialysed, haemodialysis is of no use to eliminate the drug.

There is no specific antidote to Solian.

Appropriate supportive measures should therefore be instituted with close supervision of vital functions including continuous cardiac monitoring due to the risk of prolongation of the QT interval.

If severe extrapyramidal symptoms occur, anticholinergic agents should be administered.

5. PHARMACOLOGICAL PROPERTIES

5.1 Pharmacodynamic properties

Pharmcotherapeutic group: Antipsychotics

ATC Code: NO5A LO5

Amisulpride binds selectively with a high affinity to human dopaminergic D_2/D_3 receptor subtypes whereas it is devoid of affinity for D_1, D_4 and D_5 receptor subtypes.

Unlike classical and atypical neuroleptics, amisulpride has no affinity for serotonin, α-adrenergic, histamine H_1 and cholinergic receptors. In addition, amisulpride does not bind to sigma sites.

In animal studies, at high doses, amisulpride blocks dopamine receptors located in the limbic structures in preference to those in the striatum.

At low doses it preferentially blocks pre-synaptic D_2/D_3 receptors, producing dopamine release responsible for its disinhibitory effects.

This pharmacological profile explains the clinical efficacy of Solian against both negative and positive symptoms of schizophrenia.

5.2 Pharmacokinetic properties

In man, amisulpride shows two absorption peaks: one which is attained rapidly, one hour post-dose and a second between 3 and 4 hours after administration. Corresponding plasma concentrations are 39 ± 3 and 54 ± 4 ng/ml after a 50 mg dose.

The volume of distribution is 5.8 l/kg, plasma protein binding is low (16%) and no drug interactions are suspected.

Absolute bioavailability is 48%. Amisulpride is weakly metabolised: two inactive metabolites, accounting for approximately 4% of the dose, have been identified. There is no accumulation of amisulpride and its pharmacokinetics remain unchanged after the administration of repeated doses. The elimination half-life of amisulpride is approximately 12 hours after an oral dose.

Amisulpride is eliminated unchanged in the urine. Fifty percent of an intravenous dose is excreted via the urine, of which 90% is eliminated in the first 24 hours. Renal clearance is in the order of 20 l/h or 330 ml/min.

A carbohydrate rich meal (containing 68% fluids) significantly decreases the AUCs, Tmax and Cmax of amisulpride but no changes were seen after a high fat meal. However, the significance of these findings in routine clinical use is not known.

Hepatic insufficiency: since the drug is weakly metabolised a dosage reduction should not be necessary in patients with hepatic insufficiency.

Renal insufficiency: The elimination half-life is unchanged in patients with renal insufficiency while systemic clearance is reduced by a factor of 2.5 to 3. The AUC of amisulpride in mild renal failure increased two fold and almost tenfold in moderate renal failure (see chapter 4.2). Experience is however limited and there is no data with doses greater than 50 mg.

Amisulpride is very weakly dialysed.

Limited pharmacokinetic data in elderly subjects (> 65 years) show that a 10-30 % rise occurs in Cmax, T1/2 and AUC after a single oral dose of 50 mg. No data are available after repeat dosing.

5.3 Preclinical safety data

An overall review of the completed safety studies indicates that Solian is devoid of any general, organ-specific, teratogenic, mutagenic or carcinogenic risk. Changes observed in rats and dogs at doses below the maximum tolerated dose are either pharmacological effects or are devoid of major toxicological significance under these conditions. Compared with the maximum recommended dosages in man, maximum tolerated doses are 2 and 7 times greater in the rat (200 mg/kg/d) and dog (120 mg/kg/d) respectively in terms of AUC. No carcinogenic risk, relevant to man, was identified in the rat at up to 1.5 to 4.5 times the expected human AUC.

A mouse carcinogenicity study (120 mg/kg/d) and reproductive studies (160, 300 and 500 mg/kg/d respectively in rat, rabbit and mouse) were performed. The exposure of the animals to amisulpride during these latter studies was not evaluated.

6. PHARMACEUTICAL PARTICULARS

6.1 List of excipients

Solian 50mg, 100mg & 200mg tablets

Sodium starch glycolate, lactose monohydrate, microcrystalline cellulose, hypromellose, magnesium stearate.

Solian 400mg tablets

Sodium starch glycollate, lactose monohydrate, microcrystalline cellulose, hypromellose, magnesium stearate, polyoxyl 40 stearate, titanium dioxide (E171).

Solian Solution

Saccharin sodium, sodium gluconate, glucono delta lactone, hydrochloric acid, methyl parahydroxybenzoate, propyl parahydroxybenzoate, potassium sorbate, caramel flavour (tonka beans extract, vanillin, benzaldehyde, acetyl methyl carbinol, gamma and delta decalactones, esters from acetic, butyric and 2 methyl butyric acid, esters from ethyl and cinnamyl alcohol, propylene glycol and ethyl alcohol), purified water.

6.2 Incompatibilities

None known.

6.3 Shelf life

Tablets		3 years
Solution	Shelf life of the medicinal product as packaged for sale:	3 years
	Shelf life after first opening the container:	2 months
	Dispose of within two months of opening.	

6.4 Special precautions for storage
No special precautions.

6.5 Nature and contents of container

Tablets	PVC/aluminium foil blister packs containing 60 tablets
Solution	60 ml brown glass bottle (type III) and child resistant cap with a PVDC/PE seal, with a 5ml graduated oral syringe.

6.6 Special precautions for disposal and other handling
No special precautions

7. MARKETING AUTHORISATION HOLDER
sanofi-aventis
One Onslow Street
Guildford
Surrey
GU1 4YS
United Kingdom

8. MARKETING AUTHORISATION NUMBER(S)

50mg tablets	PL 04425/0650
100mg tablets	PL 04425/0651
200mg tablets	PL 04425/0652
400mg tablets	PL 11723/0356
Solution	PL 04425/0654

9. DATE OF FIRST AUTHORISATION/RENEWAL OF THE AUTHORISATION

50 mg, 100mg, 200mg tablets	7 February 2009
400mg tablets	5 September 2000 / 4 April 2007
Solution	13 February 2009

10. DATE OF REVISION OF THE TEXT

50mg, 100mg, 200mg:	7 February 2009
400mg:	27 March 2008
Solution:	13 February 2009

Legal Category
POM

Solpadol Capsules, Solpadol Effervescent Tablets, Solpadol Caplets

(sanofi-aventis)

1. NAME OF THE MEDICINAL PRODUCT
Solpadol Caplets
Solpadol Capsules
Solpadol Effervescent Tablets

2. QUALITATIVE AND QUANTITATIVE COMPOSITION
Active Constituents
Paracetamol 500.0mg
Codeine Phosphate Hemihydrate 30.0mg
For excipients see 6.1.

3. PHARMACEUTICAL FORM
Tablet: Solpadol Caplets are white capsule shaped tablets, marked SOLPADOL on one side.

Capsule: Solpadol Capsules are grey and purple with SOLPADOL printed on them in black ink.

Effervescent Tablets: Solpadol Effervescent Tablets are white bevelled-edge tablets scored on one face.

4. CLINICAL PARTICULARS

4.1 Therapeutic indications
For the relief of severe pain.

4.2 Posology and method of administration
Adults: Two tablets not more frequently than every 4 hours, up to a maximum of 8 tablets in any 24 hour period.

Elderly: As adults, however a reduced dose may be required. See warnings.

Children: Not recommended for children under 12 years of age.

Solpadol Caplets, Capsules and Effervescent Tablets are for oral administration.

4.3 Contraindications
Hypersensitivity to paracetamol or codeine which is rare.

Hypersensitivity to any of the other constituents.

Conditions where morphine and opioids are contraindicated e.g:

- Acute asthma
- Respiratory depression
- Acute alcoholism
- Head injuries
- Raised intra-cranial pressure
- Following biliary tract surgery

Monoamine oxidase inhibitor therapy, concurrent or within 14 days.

4.4 Special warnings and precautions for use
Each tablet of the soluble formulation contains 388mg sodium (16.87m Equivalents). This sodium content should be taken into account when prescribing for patients in whom sodium restriction is indicated.

As the effervescent tablet contains sorbitol, patients with rare hereditary problems of fructose intolerance should not take this medicine.

Care should be observed in administering the product to any patient whose condition may be exacerbated by opioids, particularly the elderly, who may be sensitive to their central and gastro-intestinal effects, those on concurrent CNS depressant drugs, those with prostatic hypertrophy and those with inflammatory or obstructive bowel disorders. Care should also be observed if prolonged therapy is contemplated.

Care is advised in the administration of paracetamol to patients with severe renal or severe hepatic impairment. The hazards of overdose are greater in those with alcoholic liver disease.

Patients should be advised not to exceed the recommended dose and not take other paracetamol containing products concurrently.

Patients should be advised to consult a doctor should symptoms persist and to keep the product out of the reach and sight of children.

The risk-benefit of continued use should be assessed regularly by the prescriber.

The leaflet will state in a prominent position in the 'before taking' section:

Do not take for longer than directed by your prescriber.

Taking codeine regularly for a long time can lead to addiction, which might cause you to feel restless and irritable when you stop the tablets.

Taking a pain killer for headaches too often or for too long can make them worse.

The label will state (To be displayed prominently on outer pack (not boxed):

Do not take for longer than directed by your prescriber as taking codeine regularly for a long time can lead to addiction.

4.5 Interaction with other medicinal products and other forms of interaction
Paracetamol may increase the elimination half-life of chloramphenicol. Oral contraceptives may increase its rate of clearance. The speed of absorption of paracetamol may be increased by metoclopramide or domperidone and absorption reduced by colestyramine.

The anticoagulant effect of warfarin and other coumarins may be enhanced by prolonged regular use of paracetamol with increased risk of bleeding; occasional doses have no significant effect.

The effects of CNS depressants (including alcohol) may be potentiated by codeine.

4.6 Pregnancy and lactation
There is inadequate evidence of the safety of codeine in human pregnancy, but there is epidemiological evidence for the safety of paracetamol. Both substances have been used for many years without apparent ill consequences and animal studies have not shown any hazard. Nonetheless careful consideration should be given before prescribing the products for pregnant patients. Opioid analgesics may depress neonatal respiration and cause withdrawal effects in neonates of dependent mothers.

Paracetamol is excreted in breast milk but not in a clinically significant amount.

4.7 Effects on ability to drive and use machines
Patients should be advised not to drive or operate machinery if affected by dizziness or sedation.

4.8 Undesirable effects
Codeine can produce typical opioid effects including constipation, nausea, vomiting, dizziness, light-headedness, confusion, drowsiness and urinary retention. The frequency and severity are determined by dosage, duration of treatment and individual sensitivity. Tolerance and dependence can occur, especially with prolonged high dosage of codeine.

Adverse effects of paracetamol are rare but hypersensitivity including skin rash may occur. There have been reports of blood dyscrasias including thrombocytopenia and agranulocytosis, but these were not necessarily causally related to paracetamol.

- Regular prolonged use of codeine/DHC is known to lead to addiction and tolerance. Symptoms of restlessness and irritability may result when treatment is then stopped.
- Prolonged use of a painkiller for headaches can make them worse.

Very rare occurrence of pancreatitis.

4.9 Overdose

Codeine

The effects of Codeine overdosage will be potentiated by simultaneous ingestion of alcohol and psychotropic drugs.

Symptoms

Central nervous system depression, including respiratory depression, may develop but is unlikely to be severe unless other sedative agents have been co-ingested, including alcohol, or the overdose is very large. The pupils may be pin-point in size; nausea and vomiting are common. Hypotension and tachycardia are possible but unlikely.

Management

Management should include general symptomatic and supportive measures including a clear airway and monitoring of vital signs until stable. Consider activated charcoal if an adult presents within one hour of ingestion of more than 350 mg or a child more than 5 mg/kg.

Give naloxone if coma or respiratory depression is present. Naloxone is a competitive antagonist and has a short half-life so large and repeated doses may be required in a seriously poisoned patient. Observe for at least 4 hours after ingestion, or 8 hours if a sustained release preparation has been taken.

Paracetamol

Patients in whom oxidative liver enzymes have been induced, including alcoholics and those receiving barbiturates and patients who are chronically malnourished, may be particularly sensitive to the toxic effects of paracetamol in overdose.

Symptoms

Symptoms of paracetamol overdosage in the first 24 hours are pallor, nausea, vomiting, anorexia and abdominal pain. Liver damage may become apparent 12 to 48 hours after ingestion. Abnormalities of glucose metabolism and metabolic acidosis may occur. In severe poisoning, hepatic failure may progress to encephalopathy, coma and death. Acute renal failure with acute tubular necrosis may develop even in the absence of severe liver damage. Cardiac arrhythmias and pancreatitis have been reported.

Liver damage is likely in adults who have taken 10g or more of paracetamol. It is considered that excess quantities of a toxic metabolite (usually adequately detoxified by glutathione when normal doses of paracetamol are ingested), become irreversibly bound to liver tissue.

Management

Immediate treatment is essential in the management of paracetamol overdose. Despite a lack of significant early symptoms, patients should be referred to hospital urgently for immediate medical attention and any patient who has ingested around 7.5g or more of paracetamol in the preceding 4 hours should undergo gastric lavage. Administration of oral methionine or intravenous N-acetylcysteine which may have a beneficial effect up to at least 48 hours after the overdose, may be required. General supportive measures must be available.

5. PHARMACOLOGICAL PROPERTIES

5.1 Pharmacodynamic properties
Pharmacotherapeutic group: Anilides, Paracetamol combinations

ATC Code: NO2B E51

Paracetamol is an analgesic which acts peripherally, probably by blocking impulse generation at the bradykinin sensitive chemo-receptors which evoke pain. Although it is a prostaglandin synthetase inhibitor, the synthetase system in the CNS rather than the periphery appears to be more sensitive to it. This may explain paracetamol's lack of appreciable anti-inflammatory activity. Paracetamol also exhibits antipyretic activity.

Codeine is a centrally acting analgesic which produces its effect by its action at opioid-binding sites (m-receptors) within the CNS. It is a full agonist.

5.2 Pharmacokinetic properties
The bioavailabilities of paracetamol and codeine phosphate when given as the combination are similar to those when they are given separately.

Caplets

Following oral administration of two tablets (ie, a dose of paracetamol 1000mg and codeine 60mg) the mean maximum plasma concentrations of paracetamol and codeine were 15.96mg/ml and 212.4ng/ml respectively. The mean times to maximum plasma concentrations were 0.88 hours for paracetamol and 1.05 hours for codeine.

The mean AUC for the 9 hours following administration was 49.05mg.ml $^{-1}$.h for paracetamol and 885.0 ng/ml $^{-1}$.h for codeine.

Capsules

Following oral administration of two capsules (ie, a dose of paracetamol 1000mg and codeine phosphate 60mg) the mean maximum plasma concentrations of paracetamol and codeine phosphate were 17.5 µg/ml and 327ng/ml respectively. The mean times to maximum plasma concentrations were 1.03 hours for paracetamol and 1.10 hours for codeine phosphate.

The mean $AUC_{(0-10)}$ following administration was 48.0µg.ml $^{-1}$.h for paracetamol and 1301 ng/ml $^{-1}$.h for codeine.

Effervescent tablets

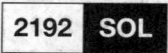

Following oral administration of two effervescent tablets (i.e., a dose of paracetamol 1000mg and codeine 60mg) the mean maximum plasma concentrations of paracetamol and codeine were 20.4µg/ml and 218.8ng/ml respectively. The mean times to maximum plasma concentrations were 0.34 hours for paracetamol and 0.42 hours for codeine phosphate.

The mean AUC for the 10 hours following administration was 50.0µg.ml^{-1}.h for paracetamol and 450.0 ng/ml^{-1}.h for codeine.

5.3 Preclinical safety data

Caplets & Effervescent Tablets: There are no preclinical data of relevance which are additional to that already included in other sections of the SPC.

Capsules: None stated

6. PHARMACEUTICAL PARTICULARS

6.1 List of excipients

Solpadol Caplets: Pregelatinised starch, Maize starch, Povidone, Potassium sorbate, Microcrystalline cellulose, Stearic acid, Talc, Magnesium stearate, Croscarmellose sodium (type A).

Solpadol Capsules: Maize starch, Magnesium stearate, Talc, Indigotine E132, Azorubine E122, Titanium dioxide E171, Gelatin, Black iron oxide E172, Shellac, Propylene glycol

Solpadol Effervescent: Sodium bicarbonate, Anhydrous citric acid, Anhydrous sodium carbonate, Sorbitol powder, Saccharin sodium, Povidone, Dimeticone,

Sodium lauril sulfate.

6.2 Incompatibilities

None known.

6.3 Shelf life

Caplets: 5 years.

Capsules: 3 years

Effervescent: 4 years

6.4 Special precautions for storage

Caplets and Capsules: Store in the original package. Do not store above 25°C.

Effervescent: Do not store above 25°C.

6.5 Nature and contents of container

Caplets: PVC/aluminium foil (250µm/20µm) / PVC (15µm) blister packs. Pack sizes: 30 and 100 tablets.

Capsules: White, opaque PVC (250µm)/aluminium foil (20µm)/ PVC (15µm) blister packs or White, opaque PVC (250µm)/ 35gsm Glassine (Pergamin) paper/9µm soft temper Aluminium foil contained in cardboard cartons. Pack sizes of 100 capsules.

Effervescent: PPFP strips in cardboard containers. Pack sizes: 32 and 100 tablets.

6.6 Special precautions for disposal and other handling

Capsules and caplets: no special requirements.

Solpadol Effervescent Tablets should be dissolved in half a tumberful of water before taking.

7. MARKETING AUTHORISATION HOLDER

Sanofi-aventis

One Onslow Street

Guildford

Surrey GU1 4YS

UK

8. MARKETING AUTHORISATION NUMBER(S)

Caplets: PL 04425/0637

Capsules: PL 04425/0635

Effervescent: PL 04425/0636

9. DATE OF FIRST AUTHORISATION/RENEWAL OF THE AUTHORISATION

4th December 2008

10. DATE OF REVISION OF THE TEXT

27 January 2009

Legal category: POM

Soltamox 10mg/5ml Oral Solution

(Rosemont Pharmaceuticals Limited)

1. NAME OF THE MEDICINAL PRODUCT

Soltamox 10mg/5ml Oral Solution

2. QUALITATIVE AND QUANTITATIVE COMPOSITION

Each 5ml dose of oral solution contains tamoxifen 10mg (as tamoxifen citrate)

Excipients:

Ethanol - 750mg per 5ml

Liquid sorbitol (non-crystallising) (E420) - 1g per 5ml

For a full list of excipients, see section 6.1.

3. PHARMACEUTICAL FORM

Oral Solution

A clear colourless liquid

4. CLINICAL PARTICULARS

4.1 Therapeutic indications

- Adjuvant treatment of oestrogen-receptor positive early breast cancer

- Treatment of oestrogen-receptor positive locally advanced or metastatic breast cancer

4.2 Posology and method of administration

Adjuvant treatment of breast cancer, Adults (including elderly):

The recommended dose is 20mg, given either in divided doses twice daily or as a single dose once daily. The current recommended treatment duration is five years; however the optimum duration has not been established.

Treatment of locally advanced or metastatic breast cancer:

The recommended dose is 20mg to 40mg, given either in divided doses twice daily or as a single dose once daily.

Children: Not applicable.

4.3 Contraindications

Pregnancy and lactation

Hypersensitivity to tamoxifen or to any of the excipients

Concurrent anastrozole therapy (see section 4.5)

4.4 Special warnings and precautions for use

Premenopausal patients must be carefully examined before treatment to exclude pregnancy.

Women should be informed of the potential risks to the foetus, should they become pregnant whilst taking tamoxifen; or within two months of cessation of therapy.

A number of secondary primary tumours, occurring at sites other than the endometrium and the opposite breast, have been reported in clinical trials, following the treatment of breast cancer patients with tamoxifen. No causal link has been established and the clinical significance of these observations remains unclear.

Menstruation is suppressed in a proportion of premenopausal women receiving tamoxifen for the treatment of breast cancer.

Any patients who have received tamoxifen therapy and have reported abnormal vaginal bleeding or patients presenting with menstrual irregularities, vaginal discharge and pelvic pressure or pain should undergo prompt investigation due to the increased incidence of endometrial changes including hyperplasia, polyps, cancer and uterine sarcoma (mostly malignant mixed Mullerian tumours) which has been reported in association with tamoxifen treatment. The underlying mechanism is unknown, but may be related to the oestrogenic-like effect of tamoxifen.

Before initiating tamoxifen a complete personal history should be taken. Physical examination (including pelvic examination) should be guided by the patients past medical history and by the 'contraindications' and 'special warnings and precautions for use' warnings for use for tamoxifen. During treatment periodic check-ups including gynaecological examination focussing on endometrial changes are recommended of a frequency and nature adapted to the individual woman and modified according to her clinical needs.

When starting tamoxifen therapy the patient should undergo an ophthalmological examination. If visual changes (cataracts and retinopathy) occur while on tamoxifen therapy it is urgent that an ophthalmological investigation be performed, because some of such changes may resolve after cessation of treatment if recognised at an early stage.

In cases of severe thrombocytopenia, leucocytopenia or hypercalcaemia, individual risk-benefit assessment and thorough medical supervision are necessary.

Venous thromboembolism:

- A 2-3-fold increase in the risk for VTE has been demonstrated in healthy tamoxifen-treated women (see section 4.8).
- Caution is advised regarding use of tamoxifen in patients who screen positive for thrombophilic factors; occasionally concomitant prophylactic anticoagulation may be justified (see section 4.5).
- VTE risk is further increased by severe obesity, increasing age and concomitant chemotherapy (see section 4.5). Long-term anti-coagulant prophylaxis may be justified for some patients with breast cancer who have multiple risk factors for VTE.
- Surgery and immobility: Tamoxifen treatment should only be stopped if the risk of tamoxifen-induced thrombosis clearly outweighs the risks associated with interrupting treatment. All patients should receive appropriate thrombosis prophylactic measures.
- Patients should be advised to seek immediate medical attention if they become aware of any symptoms of VTE; in such cases, tamoxifen therapy should be stopped and appropriate anti-thrombosis measures initiated.
- In the above all cases, the risks and benefits to the patient of tamoxifen therapy must be carefully considered.

The blood count including thrombocytes, liver function test and serum calcium should be controlled regularly.

Assessment of triglycerides in serum may be advisable because in most published cases of severe hypertriglyceridemia dyslipoproteinemia was the underlying disorder.

This product contains 19%v/v ethanol, i.e. 750mg per dose equivalent to 19ml of beer or 8ml of wine per dose. It is harmful for those suffering from alcoholism. It should be taken into account in high-risk groups such as patients with liver disease or epilepsy. It may modify or increase the effect of other medicines.

This product contains glycerol which may cause headache, stomach upset and diarrhoea.

This product also contains sorbitol. Patients with rare hereditary problems of fructose intolerance should not take this medicine.

Tamoxifen is not intended for use in children.

4.5 Interaction with other medicinal products and other forms of interaction

Coumarin-type anti-coagulants:

When used in combination with tamoxifen solution a significant increase in anticoagulant effect may occur. In the case of concomitant treatment particularly during the initial phase thorough monitoring of the coagulation status is mandatory.

Thrombocyte aggregation inhibitors:

In order to avoid bleeding during a possible thrombocytopenic interval thrombocyte aggregation inhibitors should not be combined with tamoxifen.

Cytotoxic agents:

When used in combination with tamoxifen solution there is increased risk of thromboembolic events occurring (see also Sections 4.4 and 4.8). Because of this increase in risk of VTE, thrombosis prophylaxis should be considered for these patients for the period of concomitant chemotherapy. Tamoxifen and its metabolites have been found to be inhibitors of hepatic cytochrome p-450 mixed function oxidases. The effect of tamoxifen on metabolism and excretion of other antineoplastic drugs, such as cyclophosphamide and other drugs that require mixed function oxidases of activation, is not known.

Anastrozole:

The use of tamoxifen in combination with anastrozole as adjuvant therapy has not shown improved efficacy compared with tamoxifen alone.

Bromocriptine:

Tamoxifen increases the dopaminergic effect of bromocriptine.

Hormone preparations:

Hormone preparations, particularly oestrogens (e.g. oral contraceptives) should not be combined with tamoxifen because a mutual decrease in effect is possible.

As tamoxifen is metabolised by cytochrome P450 34A, care is required when co-administered with drugs known to induce this enzyme, such as rifampicin, as tamoxifen levels may be reduced. The clinical relevance of this reduction is unknown.

Plasma concentrations of tamoxifen may be increased by concomitant treatment with CYP3A4 inhibitors.

Pharmacokinetic interaction with CYP2D6 inhibitors, showing a reduction in plasma level of an active tamoxifen metabolite, 4-hydroxy-N-desmethyltamoxifen (endoxifen), has been reported in the literature. The relevance of this to clinical practice is not known.

4.6 Pregnancy and lactation

Pregnancy:

There are only data from a small number of women who have been exposed to tamoxifen during pregnancy. Although no causal relationship has been established, only a small number of spontaneous abortions, birth defects and foetal deaths in women treated with tamoxifen during pregnancy have been reported.

Animal studies have shown reproduction toxicity (see section 5.3). Although the clinical relevance of the observed preclinical effects is unknown, some of them, especially vaginal adenosis, are similar to those seen in young women who were exposed to DES in utero and who have a 1 in 1000 risk of developing clear cell carcinoma of the vagina or cervix. Such exposure has not been reported to cause subsequent vaginal adenosis or clear cell carcinoma of the vagina or cervix in the small number of young women known to have been exposed in utero to tamoxifen.

Since the use of tamoxifen during pregnancy is contraindicated, women should be advised not to become pregnant whilst taking tamoxifen and within two months after stopping tamoxifen medication and should use barrier or other non hormonal contraceptive methods if sexually active.

Lactation:

It is not known whether tamoxifen is excreted into breast milk. Therefore, tamoxifen treatment is contraindicated during breast-feeding. Tamoxifen inhibits lactation in humans and no rebound lactation was observed after completion of therapy.

4.7 Effects on ability to drive and use machines

No studies on the effects of the ability to drive and use machines have been performed.

Since visual disturbances and light-headedness have been observed commonly with the use of tamoxifen, caution is advised when driving or using machines. The amount of alcohol in this product may impair the ability to drive or use machines.

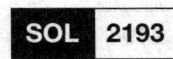

4.8 Undesirable effects
(see Table 1 below)

Cases of optic neuropathy and optic neuritis have been reported in patients receiving tamoxifen and, in a small number of cases, blindness has occurred.

Endometriosis has been reported.

Leucopenia has been observed following the administration of tamoxifen, sometimes in association with anaemia and/or thrombocytopenia.

When undesirable events are severe it may be possible to control them by a simple reduction of dosage without loss of control of the disease. If undesirable events do not respond to this measure, it may be necessary to cease treatment.

4.9 Overdose

At doses of 160mg/m^2 daily and higher, changes in ECG (QT-prolongation) and at doses of 300 mg/m^2 daily, neurotoxicity (tremor, hyperreflexia, gait disorders, and dizziness) occurred.

Overdosage of tamoxifen will increase the anti-oestrogenic effects. There is no specific antidote to overdosage and treatment should therefore be symptomatic.

5. PHARMACOLOGICAL PROPERTIES

5.1 Pharmacodynamic properties

Pharmacotherapeutic group: Hormone antagonists and related agents

ATC Code: L02B A01

Tamoxifen is a non-steroidal anti-oestrogen and inhibits the effects of endogenous oestrogen, probably by binding with oestrogen receptors. Tamoxifen competes for the binding sites with estradiol and by occupying the receptor reduces the amount of receptor available for endogenous estradiol. Tamoxifen also prevents the normal feedback inhibition of oestrogen synthesis in the hypothalamus and in the pituitary.

Tamoxifen decreases cell division in oestrogen-dependent tissues. In metastatic breast cancer, partial or complete remissions were observed in 50-60% of cases, particularly in bone and soft tissue metastases if oestrogen-receptors were found in the tumour. In cases of negative hormone-receptor status, particularly of the metastases only approx. 10% showed objective remissions. Women with oestrogen receptor-positive tumours or tumours with unknown receptor status who received adjuvant treatment with tamoxifen experienced significantly less tumour recurrences and had a higher 10-year survival rate. The effect was greater after 5 years of adjuvant treatment compared with 1-2 years of treatment. The benefit appears to be independent of age, menopausal status, daily tamoxifen dose and additional chemotherapy.

In postmenopausal women, tamoxifen has no effect on the plasma concentrations of oestrogens but reduces the concentrations of LH-, FSH-, and prolactin, however within the normal range. Additionally tamoxifen has been reported to lead to maintenance of bone mineral density in postmenopausal women.

In premenopausal women, tamoxifen can increase the concentrations of oestrogens and prostagens but they will return to predose levels after discontinuation of the treatment.

In the clinical situation, it is recognised that tamoxifen leads to reduction in levels of blood total cholesterol and low density lipoproteins in postmenopausal women of the order of 10 - 20%. Tamoxifen increases steroid- and thyroxine-binding proteins and can thus affect the concentrations of cortisol and thyroid hormones. Additionally, tamoxifen reduces the plasma concentrations of antithrombin III

5.2 Pharmacokinetic properties

Absorption:

After oral administration tamoxifen is well-absorbed achieving maximum serum concentrations within 4 - 7 hours and is extensively metabolised.

Distribution:

Tamoxifen concentrations have been observed in lung, liver, adrenals, kidney, pancreas, uterus and mammary tissues.

Metabolism:

Tamoxifen is highly protein bound to serum albumin (>99%). Metabolism is by hydroxylation, demethylation and conjugation, giving rise to several metabolites which have a similar pharmacological profile to the parent compound and thus contribute to the therapeutic effect. After four weeks of daily therapy, it was observed that steady state serum levels were achieved and an elimination half-life of seven days was calculated whereas that for N-desmethyltamoxifen, the principal circulating metabolite, is 14 days.

Excretion:

Elimination occurs, chiefly as conjugates with practically no unchanged drug, principally through the faeces and to a lesser extent through the kidneys.

5.3 Preclinical safety data

Although reproductive toxicology studies in rats, rabbits and monkeys have shown no teratogenic potential, tamoxifen was associated in rodent models of foetal reproductive tract development with changes similar to those caused by estradiol, ethynylestradiol, clomifene and diethylstilbestrol (DES). The clinical relevance of these changes is unknown. However some of them, especially vaginal adenosis, are

Table 1

	Very common (>1/10)	Common (>1/100, <1/10)	Uncommon (>1/1000, <1/100)	Rare (>1/10,000, <1/1000)	Very Rare (<1/10,000) including isolated reports.
Blood and lymphatic system disorders				Temporary reductions in blood count such as temporary anaemia, neutropenia and temporary thrombocytopenia (usually to 80,000 - 90,000 per cu mm but occasionally lower)	Severe neutropenia and pancytopenia.
Endocrine disorders			Patients with bony metastases have developed hypercalcaemia on initiation of therapy		
Metabolism disorders		Fluid retention. Increase in serum triglycerides.			Severe hypertriglyceridemia which may be partly combined with pancreatitis.
Nervous system disorders		Light-headedness and headache			
Eye disorders		Visual disturbances including corneal changes, cataracts and/or retinopathy that are only partly reversible. The risk for cataracts increases with the duration of tamoxifen treatment.			
Vascular disorders		Venous thromboembolic events. The risk including deep vein thrombosis and pulmonary embolism increases when tamoxifen is used in combination with cytotoxic agents.			
Respiratory disorders					Cases of interstitial pneumonitis have been reported.
Gastrointestinal disorders		Nausea	Vomiting		
Hepato-biliary disorders				Changes in liver enzyme levels and more severe liver abnormalities including fatty liver, cholestasis and hepatitis	A single case of agranulocytosis and liver cell necrosis was reported.
Skin and Subcutaneous tissue disorders		Alopecia		Hypersensitivity, including angioneurotic oedema, skin rash	Erythema multiforme, Stevens-Johnson-syndrome or bullous pemphigoid.
Reproductive system and breast disorders	Vaginal discharge, pruritus vulvae, vaginal bleeding			Endometrial changes, including hyperplasia and polyps, endometrial cancer and uterine sarcoma (mostly malignant mixed Mullerian tumours), suppression of menstruation, cystic ovarian swellings and uterine fibroids	
General	Hot flushes	Bone and tumour pain, leg cramps			

similar to those seen in young women who were exposed to DES in utero (see section 4.6).

Tamoxifen was not mutagenic in a range if in vitro and in vivo mutagenicity tests. Investigations in different in vivo and in vitro systems have shown that tamoxifen has a genotoxic potential following hepatic activation. Gonadal tumours in mice and liver tumours in rats receiving tamoxifen have been reported in long-term studies. The clinical relevance of these findings has not been established.

6. PHARMACEUTICAL PARTICULARS

6.1 List of excipients

Ethanol

Glycerol (E422)

Propylene glycol (E1520)

Sorbitol liquid (non-crystallising) (E420)

Natural aniseed flavouring A05 (flavouring preparations, isopropyl alcohol, water)

Liquorice flavouring L03 (flavouring preparations, natural flavouring substances, artificial flavouring substances, propylene glycol (E1520), isopropyl alcohol)

Purified water

6.2 Incompatibilities

Not applicable

6.3 Shelf life

Shelf life of the medicinal product as packaged for sale: 2 years

Shelf life after first opening the container: 3 months

6.4 Special precautions for storage

Do not store above 25°C. Do not refrigerate or freeze. Store in the original package in order to protect from light.

6.5 Nature and contents of container

Bottle: Amber (Type III) glass

Closure: a) Aluminium, polyethylene wadded, tamper evident screw cap

b) HDPE, polyethylene wadded, tamper evident screw cap

c) HDPE, polyethylene wadded, tamper evident, child resistant closure.

Pack: 1 bottle with 150ml or 250ml oral solution

4 bottles with 250ml oral solution

Not all pack sizes may be marketed.

6.6 Special precautions for disposal and other handling

No special requirements.

7. MARKETING AUTHORISATION HOLDER

Rosemont Pharmaceuticals Ltd

Rosemont House

Yorkdale Industrial Park

Braithwaite Street

Leeds

LS11 9XE

UK

8. MARKETING AUTHORISATION NUMBER(S)

PL 00427/0121

9. DATE OF FIRST AUTHORISATION/RENEWAL OF THE AUTHORISATION

Date of first authorisation: 16 August 1999

Date of last renewal: 5 December 2008

10. DATE OF REVISION OF THE TEXT

April 2009

Solu-Cortef

(Pharmacia Limited)

1. NAME OF THE MEDICINAL PRODUCT

Solu-Cortef® 100 mg or Hydrocortisone sodium succinate for injection BP 100 mg.

2. QUALITATIVE AND QUANTITATIVE COMPOSITION

Hydrocortisone sodium succinate 133.7 mg equivalent to hydrocortisone 100.0 mg.

3. PHARMACEUTICAL FORM

White, freeze dried powder for parenteral use.

4. CLINICAL PARTICULARS

4.1 Therapeutic indications

Anti-inflammatory agent.

Solu-Cortef is indicated for any condition in which rapid and intense corticosteroid effect is required such as:

1. Endocrine disorders

Primary or secondary adrenocortical insufficiency

2. Collagen diseases

Systemic lupus erythematosus

3. Dermatological diseases

Severe erythema multiforme (Stevens-Johnson syndrome)

4. Allergic states

Bronchial asthma, anaphylactic reactions

5. Gastro-intestinal diseases

Ulcerative colitis, Crohn's disease

6. Respiratory diseases

Aspiration of gastric contents

7. Medical emergencies

Solu-Cortef is indicated in the treatment of shock secondary to adrenocortical insufficiency or shock unresponsive to conventional therapy when adrenocortical insufficiency may be present.

4.2 Posology and method of administration

Solu-Cortef may be administered by intravenous injection, by intravenous infusion, or by intramuscular injection, the preferred method for initial emergency use being intravenous injection. Following the initial emergency period, consideration should be given to employing a longer-acting injectable preparation or an oral preparation.

Dosage usually ranges from 100 mg to 500 mg depending on the severity of the condition, administered by intravenous injection over a period of one to ten minutes. This dose may be repeated at intervals of 2, 4 or 6 hours as indicated by the patient's response and clinical condition.

In general high-dose corticosteroid therapy should be continued only until the patient's condition has stabilised - usually not beyond 48 to 72 hours. If hydrocortisone therapy must be continued beyond 48 to 72 hours hypernatraemia may occur, therefore it may be preferable to replace Solu-Cortef with a corticosteroid such as methylprednisolone sodium succinate as little or no sodium retention occurs. Although adverse effects associated with high dose, short-term corticoid therapy are uncommon, peptic ulceration may occur. Prophylactic antacid therapy may be indicated.

Patients subjected to severe stress following corticoid therapy should be observed closely for signs and symptoms of adrenocortical insufficiency.

Corticosteroid therapy is an adjunct to, and not a replacement for, conventional therapy.

Elderly patients: Solu-Cortef is primarily used in acute short-term conditions. There is no information to suggest that a change in dosage is warranted in the elderly. However, treatment of elderly patients should be planned bearing in mind the more serious consequences of the common side-effects of corticosteroids in old age and close clinical supervision is required (see Special warnings and special precautions for use).

Children: While the dose may be reduced for infants and children, it is governed more by the severity of the condition and response of the patient than by age or body weight but should not be less than 25 mg daily (see Special warnings and special precautions for use).

Preparation of solutions: For intravenous or intramuscular injection prepare the solution aseptically by adding not more than 2 ml of Sterile Water for Injections to the contents of one vial of Solu-Cortef 100 mg, shake and withdraw for use.

For intravenous infusion, first prepare the solution by adding not more than 2 ml of Sterile Water for Injections to the vial; this solution may then be added to 100 ml - 1000 ml (but not less than 100 ml) of 5% dextrose in water (or isotonic saline solution or 5% dextrose in isotonic saline solution if patient is not on sodium restriction).

When reconstituted as directed the pH of the solution will range from 7.0 to 8.0.

4.3 Contraindications

Solu-Cortef is contra-indicated where there is known hypersensitivity to components and in systemic fungal infection unless specific anti-infective therapy is employed.

Administration of live or live, attenuated vaccines is contra-indicated in patients receiving immunosuppressive doses of corticosteroids.

4.4 Special warnings and precautions for use

Warnings and Precautions:

1. A Patient Information Leaflet is provided in the pack by the manufacturer.

2. Undesirable effects may be minimised by using the lowest effective dose for the minimum period. Frequent patient review is required to appropriately titrate the dose against disease activity (see Posology and method of administration).

3. Adrenal cortical atrophy develops during prolonged therapy and may persist for months after stopping treatment. In patients who have received more than physiological doses of systemic corticosteroids (approximately 30 mg hydrocortisone) for greater than 3 weeks, withdrawal should not be abrupt. How dose reduction should be carried out depends largely on whether the disease is likely to relapse as the dose of systemic corticosteroids is reduced. Clinical assessment of disease activity may be needed during withdrawal. If the disease is unlikely to relapse on withdrawal of systemic corticosteroids, but there is uncertainty about HPA suppression, the dose of systemic corticosteroid may be reduced rapidly to physiological doses. Once a daily dose of 30 mg hydrocortisone is reached, dose reduction should be slower to allow the HPA-axis to recover.

Abrupt withdrawal of systemic corticosteroid treatment, which has continued up to 3 weeks is appropriate if it considered that the disease is unlikely to relapse. Abrupt withdrawal of doses up to 160 mg hydrocortisone for 3 weeks is unlikely to lead to clinically relevant HPA-axis suppression, in the majority of patients. In the following patient groups, gradual withdrawal of systemic corticosteroid therapy should be ***considered*** even after courses lasting 3 weeks or less:

- Patients who have had repeated courses of systemic corticosteroids, particularly if taken for greater than 3 weeks.
- When a short course has been prescribed within one year of cessation of long-term therapy (months or years).
- Patients who may have reasons for adrenocortical insufficiency other than exogenous corticosteroid therapy.
- Patients receiving doses of systemic corticosteroid greater than 160 mg hydrocortisone.
- Patients repeatedly taking doses in the evening.

4. Patients should carry 'Steroid Treatment' cards which give clear guidance on the precautions to be taken to minimise risk and which provide details of prescriber, drug, dosage and the duration of treatment.

5. Corticosteroids may mask some signs of infection, and new infections may appear during their use. Suppression of the inflammatory response and immune function increases the susceptibility to fungal, viral and bacterial infections and their severity. The clinical presentation may often be atypical and may reach an advanced stage before being recognised.

6. Chickenpox is of serious concern since this normally minor illness may be fatal in immunosuppressed patients. Patients (or parents of children) without a definite history of chickenpox should be advised to avoid close personal contact with chickenpox or herpes zoster and if exposed they should seek urgent medical attention. Passive immunization with varicella/zoster immunoglobin (VZIG) is needed by exposed non-immune patients who are receiving systemic corticosteroids or who have used them within the previous 3 months; this should be given within 10 days of exposure to chickenpox. If a diagnosis of chickenpox is confirmed, the illness warrants specialist care and urgent treatment. Corticosteroids should not be stopped and the dose may need to be increased.

7. Exposure to measles should be avoided. Medical advice should be sought immediately if exposure occurs. Prophylaxis with normal intramuscular immuneglobulin may be needed.

8. Live vaccines should not be given to individuals with impaired immune responsiveness. The antibody response to other vaccines may be diminished.

9 The use of Solu-Cortef in active tuberculosis should be restricted to those cases of fulminating or disseminated tuberculosis in which the corticosteroid is used for the management of the disease in conjunction with appropriate antituberculosis regimen. If corticosteroids are indicated in patients with latent tuberculosis or tuberculin reactivity, close observation is necessary as reactivation of the disease may occur. During prolonged corticosteroid therapy, these patients should receive chemoprophylaxis.

10. Rarely anaphylactoid reactions have been reported following parenteral Solu-Cortef therapy. Physicians using the drug should be prepared to deal with such a possibility. Appropriate precautionary measures should be taken prior to administration, especially when the patient has a history of drug allergy.

11. Care should be taken for patients receiving cardioactive drugs such as digoxin because of steroid induced electrolyte disturbance/potassium loss (see Undesirable effects).

Special precautions:

Particular care is required when considering the use of systemic corticosteroids in patients with the following conditions and frequent patient monitoring is necessary.

1. Osteoporosis (post-menopausal females are particularly at risk).
2. Hypertension or congestive heart failure.
3. Existing or previous history of severe affective disorders (especially previous steroid psychosis).
4. Diabetes mellitus (or a family history of diabetes).
5. History of tuberculosis.
6. Glaucoma (or a family history of glaucoma).
7. Previous corticosteroid-induced myopathy.
8. Liver failure or cirrhosis.
9. Renal insufficiency.
10. Epilepsy.
11. Peptic ulceration.
12. Fresh intestinal anastomoses.
13. Predisposition to thrombophlebitis.
14. Abscess or other pyogenic infections.
15. Ulcerative colitis.
16. Diverticulitis.
17. Myasthenia gravis.
18. Ocular herpes simplex, for fear of corneal perforation.
19. Hypothyroidism.

20. Recent myocardial infarction (myocardial rupture has been reported).

21. Kaposi's sarcoma has been reported to occur in patients receiving corticosteroid therapy. Discontinuation of corticosteroids may result in clinical remission.

22. Hydrocortisone can cause elevation of blood pressure, salt and water retention and increased excretion of potassium. Dietary salt restriction and potassium supplementation may be necessary. All corticosteroids increase calcium excretion.

23. Patients and/or carers should be warned that potentially severe psychiatric adverse reactions may occur with systemic steroids (see section 4.8). Symptoms typically emerge within a few days or weeks of starting treatment. Risks may be higher with high doses/systemic exposure (see also section 4.5 Interaction with Other Medicaments and Other Forms of Interaction that can increase the risk of side effects), although dose levels do not allow prediction of the onset, type, severity or duration of reactions. Most reactions recover after either dose reduction or withdrawal, although specific treatment may be necessary. Patients/carers should be encouraged to seek medical advice if worrying psychological symptoms develop, especially if depressed mood or suicidal ideation is suspected. Patients/carers should be alert to possible psychiatric disturbances that may occur either during or immediately after dose tapering/withdrawal of systemic steroids, although such reactions have been reported infrequently.

Particular care is required when considering the use of systemic corticosteroids in patients with existing or previous history of severe affective disorders in themselves or in their first degree relatives. These would include depressive or manic-depressive illness and previous steroid psychosis.

Use in children: Corticosteroids cause growth retardation in infancy, childhood and adolescence, which may be irreversible. Treatment should be limited to the minimum dosage for the shortest possible time. The use of steroids should be restricted to the most serious indications.

Use in the elderly: The common adverse effects of systemic corticosteroids may be associated with more serious consequences in old age, especially osteoporosis, hypertension, hypokalaemia, diabetes, susceptibility to infection and thinning of the skin. Close clinical supervision is required to avoid life-threatening reactions.

"Corticosteroids should not be used for the management of head injury or stroke because it is unlikely to be of benefit and may even be harmful."

4.5 Interaction with other medicinal products and other forms of interaction

1. Convulsions have been reported with concurrent use of corticosteroids and cyclosporin. Since concurrent administration of these agents results in a mutual inhibition of metabolism, it is possible that convulsions and other adverse effects associated with the individual use of either drug may be more apt to occur.

2. Drugs that induce hepatic enzymes, such as rifampicin, rifabutin, carbamazepine, phenobarbitone, phenytoin, primidone, and aminoglutethimide enhance the metabolism of corticosteroids and its therapeutic effects may be reduced.

3. Drugs which inhibit the CYP3A4 enzyme, such as cimetidine, erythromycin, ketoconazole, itraconazole, diltiazem and mibefradil, may decrease the rate of metabolism of corticosteroids and hence increase the serum concentration.

4. Steroids may reduce the effects of anticholinesterases in myasthenia gravis. The desired effects of hypoglycaemic agents (including insulin), anti-hypertensives and diuretics are antagonised by corticosteroids, and the hypokalaemic effects of acetazolamide, loop diuretics, thiazide diuretics and carbenoxolone are enhanced.

5. The efficacy of coumarin anticoagulants may be enhanced by concurrent corticosteroid therapy and close monitoring of the INR or prothrombin time is required to avoid spontaneous bleeding.

6. The renal clearance of salicylates is increased by corticosteroids and steroid withdrawal may result in salicylate intoxication. Salicylates and non-steroidal anti-inflammatory agents should be used cautiously in conjunction with corticosteroids in hypothrombinaemia.

7. Steroids have been reported to interact with neuromuscular blocking agents such as pancuronium with partial reversal of the neuromuscular block.

4.6 Pregnancy and lactation

Pregnancy

The ability of corticosteroids to cross the placenta varies between individual drugs, however, hydrocortisone readily crosses the placenta.

Administration of corticosteroids to pregnant animals can cause abnormalities of foetal development including cleft palate, intra-uterine growth retardation and affects on brain growth and development. There is no evidence that corticosteroids result in an increased incidence of congenital abnormalities, such as cleft palate in man, however, when administered for long periods or repeatedly during pregnancy, corticosteroids may increase the risk of intra-uterine growth retardation. Hypoadrenalism may, in theory, occur in the neonate following prenatal exposure to corticosteroids but usually resolves spontaneously following birth and is rarely clinically important. As with all drugs, corticosteroids should only be prescribed when the benefits to the mother and child outweigh the risks. When corticosteroids are essential, however, patients with normal pregnancies may be treated as though they were in the non-gravid state.

Lactation

Corticosteroids are excreted in breast milk, although no data are available for hydrocortisone. Doses up to 160 mg daily of hydrocortisone are unlikely to cause systemic effects in the infant. Infants of mothers taking higher doses than this may have a degree of adrenal suppression, but the benefits of breastfeeding are likely to outweigh any theoretical risk.

4.7 Effects on ability to drive and use machines

None stated.

4.8 Undesirable effects

Since Solu-Cortef is normally employed on a short-term basis it is unlikely that side-effects will occur; however, the possibility of side-effects attributable to corticosteroid therapy should be recognised (see Special warnings and special precautions for use). Such side-effects include:

PARENTERAL CORTICOSTEROID THERAPY - Anaphylactoid reaction e.g. bronchospasm, hypopigmentation or hyperpigmentation, subcutaneous and cutaneous atrophy, sterile abscess, laryngeal oedema and urticaria.

GASTRO-INTESTINAL - Dyspepsia, peptic ulceration with perforation and haemorrhage, abdominal distension, oesophageal ulceration, oesophageal candidiasis, acute pancreatitis, perforation of bowel, gastric haemorrhage.

Increases in alanine transaminase (ALT, SGPT) aspartate transaminase (AST, SGOT) and alkaline phosphatase have been observed following corticosteroid treatment. These changes are usually small, not associated with any clinical syndrome and are reversible upon discontinuation.

ANTI-INFLAMMATORY AND IMMUNOSUPPRESSIVE EFFECTS - Increased susceptibility and severity of infections with suppression of clinical symptoms and signs, opportunistic infections, may suppress reactions to skin tests, recurrence of dormant tuberculosis (see Special warnings and special precautions for use).

MUSCULOSKELETAL - Proximal myopathy, osteoporosis, vertebral and long bone fractures, avascular osteonecrosis, tendon rupture, aseptic necrosis, muscle weakness.

FLUID AND ELECTROLYTE DISTURBANCE - Sodium and water retention, potassium loss, hypertension, hypokalaemic alkalosis, congestive heart failure in susceptible patients.

DERMATOLOGICAL - Impaired healing, petechiae and ecchymosis, skin atrophy, bruising, striae, increased sweating, telangiectasia, acne. Kaposi's sarcoma has been reported to occur in patients receiving corticosteroid therapy. Discontinuation of corticosteroids may result in clinical remission.

ENDOCRINE/METABOLIC - Suppression of the hypothalamo-pituitary-adrenal axis; growth suppression in infancy, childhood and adolescence; menstrual irregularity and amenorrhoea, Cushingoid facies, hirsutism, weight gain, impaired carbohydrate tolerance with increased requirement for antidiabetic therapy, negative nitrogen and calcium balance. Increased appetite.

NEUROPSYCHIATRIC - A wide range of psychiatric reactions including affective disorders (such as irritable, euphoric, depressed and labile mood psychological dependence and suicidal thoughts), psychotic reactions (including mania, delusions, hallucinations and aggravation of schizophrenia), behavioural disturbances, irritability, anxiety, sleep disturbances, seizures and cognitive dysfunction including confusion and amnesia have been reported for all corticosteroids. Reactions are common and may occur in both adults and children. In adults, the frequency of severe reactions was estimated to be 5-6%. Psychological effects have been reported on withdrawal of corticosteroids; the frequency is unknown. Increased intra-cranial pressure with papilloedema in children (pseudotumour cerebri) has been reported, usually after treatment withdrawal of hydrocortisone.

OPHTHALMIC - Increased intra-ocular pressure, glaucoma, papilloedema with possible damage to the optic nerve, cataracts, corneal or scleral thinning, exacerbation of ophthalmic viral or fungal disease, exophthalmos.

CARDIOVASCULAR – Myocardial rupture following a myocardial infarction.

GENERAL - Leucocytosis, hypersensitivity reactions including anaphylaxis, thrombo-embolism, nausea, malaise, persistent hiccups with high doses of corticosteroids.

WITHDRAWAL SYMPTOMS - Too rapid a reduction of corticosteroid dosage following prolonged treatment can lead to acute adrenal insufficiency, hypotension and death. However, this is more applicable to corticosteroids with an indication where continuous therapy is given (see Special warnings and special precautions for use).

A 'withdrawal syndrome' may also occur including, fever, myalgia, arthralgia, rhinitis, conjunctivitis, painful itchy skin nodules and loss of weight.

4.9 Overdose

There is no clinical syndrome of acute overdosage with Solu-Cortef. Hydrocortisone is dialysable.

5. PHARMACOLOGICAL PROPERTIES

5.1 Pharmacodynamic properties

Hydrocortisone sodium succinate has the same metabolic and anti-inflammatory actions as hydrocortisone. It is a glucocorticosteroid. Used in pharmacological doses, its actions supress the clinical manifestations of disease in a wide range of disorders.

5.2 Pharmacokinetic properties

Twelve normal subjects received 100, 200 or 400 mg Solu-Cortef intravenously. Radio-immunoassay results were as follows:-

DOSE (mg)	CMAX (mcg/100 ml)	TMAX (hr)	12-HR AUC (mG/100 ml × hr)
100	132.3	0.35	418.0
200	231.8	0.25	680.0
400	629.8	0.37	1024.0

In another study, a 1 mg/kg i.m. dose of Solu-Cortef peaked in 30-60 minutes, with a plasma cmax of 80 mg/100 ml.

In analysing hydrocortisone metabolism, a 25 mg IV dose resulted in higher plasma concentrations in females than in males.

6. PHARMACEUTICAL PARTICULARS

6.1 List of excipients

Sodium biphosphate, sodium phosphate.

6.2 Incompatibilities

None stated.

6.3 Shelf life

Shelf-life of the medicinal product as packaged for sale: 60 months.

After reconstitution with Sterile Water for Injections, use immediately, discard any remainder.

6.4 Special precautions for storage

Store below 25°C.

Refer to Section 4.2 Dosage and Administration. No diluents other than those referred to are recommended. Parenteral drug products should be inspected visually for particulate matter and discoloration prior to administration.

6.5 Nature and contents of container

Type I flint glass vials with a butyl rubber plug and metal seal. Each vial of Solu-Cortef 100 mg contains the equivalent of 100 mg hydrocortisone as the sodium succinate for reconstitution with 2 ml of Sterile Water for Injections.

6.6 Special precautions for disposal and other handling

No special requirements.

7. MARKETING AUTHORISATION HOLDER

Pharmacia Limited
Ramsgate Road
Sandwich
Kent
CT13 9NJ
UK

8. MARKETING AUTHORISATION NUMBER(S)

PL 0032/5019

9. DATE OF FIRST AUTHORISATION/RENEWAL OF THE AUTHORISATION

PL 0032/5019 date of first authorisation: 18 May 1990

Last renewal date: 15 March 2005

10. DATE OF REVISION OF THE TEXT

3rd April 2008

Legal category

POM

Ref: SC 3_0 UK

Solu-Medrone 2 Gram

(Pharmacia Limited)

1. NAME OF THE MEDICINAL PRODUCT

Solu-Medrone™ 2 gram or methylprednisolone sodium succinate for injection.

2. QUALITATIVE AND QUANTITATIVE COMPOSITION

Methylprednisolone sodium succinate 2.652 grams equivalent to 2 grams of methylprednisolone.

3. PHARMACEUTICAL FORM

Powder for injection.

4. CLINICAL PARTICULARS

4.1 Therapeutic indications

Solu-Medrone is indicated to treat any condition in which rapid and intense corticosteroid effect is required such as:

1. Dermatological disease

Severe erythema multiforme (Stevens-Johnson syndrome)

2. Allergic states

Bronchial asthma

Severe seasonal and perennial allergic rhinitis

Angioneurotic oedema

Anaphylaxis

3. Gastro-intestinal diseases

Ulcerative colitis

Crohn's disease

4. Respiratory diseases

Aspiration of gastric contents

Fulminating or disseminated tuberculosis (with appropriate antituberculous chemotherapy)

5. Neurological disorders

Cerebral oedema secondary to cerebral tumour

6. Miscellaneous

TB meningitis (with appropriate antituberculous chemotherapy)

Transplantation

7. Acute spinal cord injury. The treatment should begin within eight hours of injury.

4.2 Posology and method of administration

Solu-Medrone may be administered intravenously or intramuscularly, the preferred method for emergency use being intravenous injection given over a suitable time interval. When administering Solu-Medrone in high doses intravenously it should be given over a period of at least 30 minutes. Doses up to 250 mg should be given intravenously over a period of at least five minutes.

For intravenous infusion the initially prepared solution may be diluted with 5% dextrose in water, isotonic saline solution, or 5% dextrose in isotonic saline solution. To avoid compatibility problems with other drugs Solu-Medrone should be administered separately, only in the solutions mentioned.

Undesirable effects may be minimised by using the lowest effective dose for the minimum period (see Special warnings and special precautions for use).

Parenteral drug products should wherever possible be visually inspected for particulate matter and discoloration prior to administration.

Adults: Dosage should be varied according to the severity of the condition, initial dosage will vary from 10 to 500 mg. In the treatment of graft rejection reactions following transplantation, a dose of up to 1 g/day may be required. Although doses and protocols have varied in studies using methylprednisolone sodium succinate in the treatment of graft rejection reactions, the published literature supports the use of doses of this level, with 500 mg to 1 g most commonly used for acute rejection. Treatment at these doses should be limited to a 48-72 hour period until the patient's condition has stabilised, as prolonged high dose corticosteroid therapy can cause serious corticosteroid induced side-effects (see Undesirable effects and Special warnings and special precautions for use).

Children: In the treatment of high dose indications, such as haematological, rheumatic, renal and dermatological conditions, a dosage of 30 mg/kg/day to a maximum of 1 g/day is recommended. This dosage may be repeated for three pulses either daily or on alternate days. In the treatment of graft rejection reactions following transplantation, a dosage of 10 to 20 mg/kg/day for up to 3 days, to a maximum of 1 g/day, is recommended. In the treatment of status asthmaticus, a dosage of 1 to 4 mg/kg/day for 1-3 days is recommended.

Solu-Medrone is not recommended for use in spinal cord injury in children.

Elderly patients: Solu-Medrone is primarily used in acute short-term conditions. There is no information to suggest that a change in dosage is warranted in the elderly. However, treatment of elderly patients should be planned bearing in mind the more serious consequences of the common side-effects of corticosteroids in old age and close clinical supervision is required (see Special warnings and special precautions for use).

Detailed recommendations for adult dosage are as follows:

In anaphylactic reactions adrenaline or noradrenaline should be administered first for an immediate haemodynamic effect, followed by intravenous injection of Solu-Medrone (methylprednisolone sodium succinate) with other accepted procedures. There is evidence that corticosteroids through their prolonged haemodynamic effect are of value in preventing recurrent attacks of acute anaphylactic reactions.

In sensitivity reactions Solu-Medrone is capable of providing relief within one half to two hours. In patients with status asthmaticus Solu-Medrone may be given at a dose of 40 mg intravenously, repeated as dictated by patient response. In some asthmatic patients it may be advantageous to administer by slow intravenous drip over a period of hours.

In graft rejection reactions following transplantation doses of up to 1 g per day have been used to suppress rejection crises, with doses of 500 mg to 1 g most commonly used for acute rejection. Treatment should be continued only until the patient's condition has stabilised; usually not beyond 48-72 hours.

In cerebral oedema corticosteroids are used to reduce or prevent the cerebral oedema associated with brain tumours (primary or metastatic).

In patients with oedema due to tumour, tapering the dose of corticosteroid appears to be important in order to avoid a rebound increase in intracranial pressure. If brain swelling does occur as the dose is reduced (intracranial bleeding having been ruled out), restart larger and more frequent doses parenterally. Patients with certain malignancies may need to remain on oral corticosteroid therapy for months or even life. Similar or higher doses may be helpful to control oedema during radiation therapy.

The following are suggested dosage schedules for oedemas due to brain tumour.

Schedule A (1)	Dose (mg)	Route	Interval in hours	Duration
Pre-operative:	20	IM	3-6	
During Surgery:	20 to 40	IV	hourly	
Post operative:	20	IM	3	24 hours
	16	IM	3	24 hours
	12	IM	3	24 hours
	8	IM	3	24 hours
	4	IM	3	24 hours
	4	IM	6	24 hours
	4	IM	12	24 hours

Schedule B (2)	Dose (mg)	Route	Interval in hours	Days Duration
Pre-operative:	40	IM	6	2-3
Post-operative:	40	IM	6	3-5
	20	Oral	6	1
	12	Oral	6	1
	8	Oral	8	1
	4	Oral	12	1
	4	Oral		1

Aim to discontinue therapy after a total of 10 days.

REFERENCES

1. Fox JL, MD. "Use of Methylprednisolone in Intracranial Surgery" Medical Annals of the District of Columbia, 34:261-265,1965.

2. Cantu RC, MD Harvard Neurological Service, Boston, Massachusetts. Letter on file, The Upjohn Company (February 1970).

For treatment of acute spinal cord injury, administer intravenously 30 mg methylprednisolone per kilogram of body weight in a bolus dose over a 15 minute period, followed by a 45 minute pause, and then a continuous infusion of 5.4 mg/kg per hour for 23 hours. There should be a separate intravenous site for the infusion pump. The treatment should begin within eight hours of injury.

In other indications, initial dosage will vary from 10 to 500 mg depending on the clinical problem being treated. Larger doses may be required for short-term management of severe, acute conditions. The initial dose, up to 250 mg, should be given intravenously over a period of at least 5 minutes, doses exceeding 250 mg should be given intravenously over a period of at least 30 minutes. Subsequent doses may be given intravenously or intramuscularly at intervals dictated by the patient's response and clinical condition. Corticosteroid therapy is an adjunct to, and not replacement for, conventional therapy.

4.3 Contraindications

Solu-Medrone is contra-indicated where there is known hypersensitivity to components, in systemic fungal infections unless specific anti-infective therapy is employed and in cerebral oedema in malaria.

4.4 Special warnings and precautions for use

Warnings and Precautions:

1. A Patient Information Leaflet is provided in the pack by the manufacturer.

2. Undesirable effects may be minimised by using the lowest effective dose for the minimum period. Frequent patient review is required to appropriately titrate the dose against disease activity (see Posology and method of administration).

3. Adrenal cortical atrophy develops during prolonged therapy and may persist for months after stopping treatment. In patients who have received more than physiological doses of systemic corticosteroids (approximately 6 mg methylprednisolone) for greater than 3 weeks, withdrawal should not be abrupt. How dose reduction should be carried out depends largely on whether the disease is likely to relapse as the dose of systemic corticosteroids is reduced. Clinical assessment of disease activity may be needed during withdrawal. If the disease is unlikely to relapse on withdrawal of systemic corticosteroids, but there is uncertainty about HPA suppression, the dose of systemic corticosteroid may be reduced rapidly to physiological doses. Once a daily dose of 6 mg methylprednisolone is reached, dose reduction should be slower to allow the HPA-axis to recover.

Abrupt withdrawal of systemic corticosteroid treatment, which has continued up to 3 weeks is appropriate if it considered that the disease is unlikely to relapse. Abrupt withdrawal of doses up to 32 mg daily of methylprednisolone for 3 weeks is unlikely to lead to clinically relevant HPA-axis suppression, in the majority of patients. In the following patient groups, gradual withdrawal of systemic corticosteroid therapy should be *considered* even after courses lasting 3 weeks or less:

- Patients who have had repeated courses of systemic corticosteroids, particularly if taken for greater than 3 weeks.
- When a short course has been prescribed within one year of cessation of long-term therapy (months or years).
- Patients who may have reasons for adrenocortical insufficiency other than exogenous corticosteroid therapy.
- Patients receiving doses of systemic corticosteroid greater than 32 mg daily of methylprednisolone.
- Patients repeatedly taking doses in the evening.

4. Patients should carry 'Steroid Treatment' cards which give clear guidance on the precautions to be taken to minimise risk and which provide details of prescriber, drug, dosage and the duration of treatment.

5. Although Solu-Medrone is not approved in the UK for use in any shock indication, the following warning statement should be adhered to. Data from a clinical study conducted to establish the efficacy of Solu-Medrone in septic shock, suggest that a higher mortality occurred in subsets of patients who entered the study with elevated serum creatinine levels or who developed a secondary infection after therapy began. Therefore this product should not be used in the treatment of septic syndrome or septic shock.

6. There have been a few reports of cardiac arrhythmias and/or circulatory collapse and/or cardiac arrest associated with the rapid intravenous administration of large doses of Solu-Medrone (greater than 500 mg administered over a period of less than 10 minutes). Bradycardia has been reported during or after the administration of large doses of methylprednisolone sodium succinate, and may be unrelated to the speed and duration of infusion.

7. Corticosteroids may mask some signs of infection, and new infections may appear during their use. Suppression of the inflammatory response and immune function increases the susceptibility to fungal, viral and bacterial infections and their severity. The clinical presentation may often be atypical and may reach an advanced stage before being recognised.

8. Chickenpox is of serious concern since this normally minor illness may be fatal in immunosuppressed patients. Patients (or parents of children) without a definite history of chickenpox should be advised to avoid close personal contact with chickenpox or herpes zoster and if exposed they should seek urgent medical attention. Passive immunisation with varicella/zoster immunoglobin (VZIG) is needed by exposed non-immune patients who are receiving systemic corticosteroids or who have used them within the previous 3 months; this should be given within 10 days of exposure to chickenpox. If a diagnosis of chickenpox is confirmed, the illness warrants specialist care and urgent treatment. Corticosteroids should not be stopped and the dose may need to be increased.

9. Exposure to measles should be avoided. Medical advice should be sought immediately if exposure occurs. Prophylaxis with normal intramuscular immuneglobulin may be needed.

10. Live vaccines should not be given to individuals with impaired immune responsiveness. The antibody response to other vaccines may be diminished.

11. The use of Solu-Medrone in active tuberculosis should be restricted to those cases of fulminating or disseminated tuberculosis in which the corticosteroid is used for the management of the disease in conjunction with an appropriate anti-tuberculous regimen. If corticosteroids are indicated in patients with latent tuberculosis or tuberculin reactivity, close observation is necessary as reactivation of the disease may occur. During prolonged corticosteroid therapy, these patients should receive chemoprophylaxis.

12. Rarely anaphylactoid reactions have been reported following parenteral Solu-Medrone therapy. Physicians using the drug should be prepared to deal with such a possibility. Appropriate precautionary measures should be taken prior to administration, especially when the patient has a history of drug allergy.

13. Care should be taken for patients receiving cardioactive drugs such as digoxin because of steroid induced electrolyte disturbance/potassium loss (see Undesirable effects).

14. Corticosteroids should not be used for the management of head injury or stroke because it is unlikely to be of benefit and may even be harmful.

Special precautions:

Particular care is required when considering the use of systemic corticosteroids in patients with the following conditions and frequent patient monitoring is necessary.

1. Osteoporosis (post-menopausal females are particularly at risk).
2. Hypertension or congestive heart failure.
3. Existing or previous history of severe affective disorders (especially previous steroid psychosis).
4. Diabetes mellitus (or a family history of diabetes).
5. History of tuberculosis.
6. Glaucoma (or a family history of glaucoma).

7. Previous corticosteroid-induced myopathy.
8. Liver failure or cirrhosis.
9. Renal insufficiency.
10. Epilepsy.
11. Peptic ulceration.
12. Fresh intestinal anastomoses.
13. Predisposition to thrombophlebitis.
14. Abscess or other pyogenic infections.
15. Ulcerative colitis.
16. Diverticulitis.
17. Myasthenia gravis.
18. Ocular herpes simplex, for fear of corneal perforation.
19. Hypothyroidism.
20. Recent myocardial infarction (myocardial rupture has been reported).
21. Kaposi's sarcoma has been reported to occur in patients receiving corticosteroid therapy. Discontinuation of corticosteroids may result in clinical remission.
22. Patients and/or carers should be warned that potentially severe psychiatric adverse reactions may occur with systemic steroids (see section 4.8). Symptoms typically emerge within a few days or weeks of starting treatment. Risks may be higher with high doses/systemic exposure (see also section 4.5 Interaction with Other Medicaments and Other Forms of Interaction that can increase the risk of side effects), although dose levels do not allow prediction of the onset, type, severity or duration of reactions. Most reactions recover after either dose reduction or withdrawal, although specific treatment may be necessary. Patients/carers should be encouraged to seek medical advice if worrying psychological symptoms develop, especially if depressed mood or suicidal ideation is suspected. Patients/carers should be alert to possible psychiatric disturbances that may occur either during or immediately after dose tapering/withdrawal of systemic steroids, although such reactions have been reported infrequently.

Particular care is required when considering the use of systemic corticosteroids in patients with existing or previous history of severe affective disorders in themselves or in their first degree relatives. These would include depressive or manic-depressive illness and previous steroid psychosis.

Use in children: Corticosteroids cause growth retardation in infancy, childhood and adolescence, which may be irreversible. Treatment should be limited to the minimum dosage for the shortest possible time. In order to minimise suppression of the hypothalamo-pituitary-adrenal axis and growth retardation, treatment should be administered where possible as a single dose on alternate days.

Use in the elderly: The common adverse effects of systemic corticosteroids may be associated with more serious consequences in old age, especially osteoporosis, hypertension, hypokalaemia, diabetes, susceptibility to infection and thinning of the skin. Close clinical supervision is required to avoid life-threatening reactions.

4.5 Interaction with other medicinal products and other forms of interaction

1. Convulsions have been reported with concurrent use of methylprednisolone and ciclosporin. Since concurrent administration of these agents results in a mutual inhibition of metabolism, it is possible that convulsions and other adverse events associated with the individual use of either drug may be more apt to occur.
2. Drugs that induce hepatic enzymes, such as rifampicin, rifabutin, carbamazepine, phenobarbitone, phenytoin, primidone, and aminoglutethimide enhance the metabolism of corticosteroids and its therapeutic effects may be reduced.
3. Drugs which inhibit the CYP3A4 enzyme, such as cimetidine, erythromycin, ketoconazole, itraconazole, diltiazem and mibefradil, may decrease the rate of metabolism of corticosteroids and hence increase the serum concentration.
4. Steroids may reduce the effects of anticholinesterases in myasthenia gravis. The desired effects of hypoglycaemic agents (including insulin), anti-hypertensives and diuretics are antagonised by corticosteroids, and the hypokalaemic effects of acetazolamide, loop diuretics, thiazide diuretics and carbenoxolone are enhanced.
5. The efficacy of coumarin anticoagulants may be enhanced by concurrent corticosteroid therapy and close monitoring of the INR or prothrombin time is required to avoid spontaneous bleeding.
6. The renal clearance of salicylates is increased by corticosteroids and steroid withdrawal may result in salicylate intoxication. Salicylates and non-steroidal anti-inflammatory agents should be used cautiously in conjunction with corticosteroids in hypothrombinaemia.
7. Steroids have been reported to interact with neuromuscular blocking agents such as pancuronium with partial reversal of the neuromuscular block.

4.6 Pregnancy and lactation

Pregnancy

The ability of corticosteroids to cross the placenta varies between individual drugs, however, methylprednisolone does cross the placenta.

Administration of corticosteroids to pregnant animals can cause abnormalities of foetal development including cleft palate, intra-uterine growth retardation and affects on brain growth and development. There is no evidence that corticosteroids result in an increased incidence of congenital abnormalities, such as cleft palate in man, however, when administered for long periods or repeatedly during pregnancy, corticosteroids may increase the risk of intra-uterine growth retardation. Hypoadrenalism may, in theory, occur in the neonate following prenatal exposure to corticosteroids but usually resolves spontaneously following birth and is rarely clinically important. As with all drugs, corticosteroids should only be prescribed when the benefits to the mother and child outweigh the risks. When corticosteroids are essential, however, patients with normal pregnancies may be treated as though they were in the non-gravid state.

Lactation

Corticosteroids are excreted in small amounts in breast milk, however, doses of up to 40 mg daily of methylprednisolone are unlikely to cause systemic effects in the infant. Infants of mothers taking higher doses than this may have a degree of adrenal suppression, but the benefits of breastfeeding are likely to outweigh any theoretical risk.

4.7 Effects on ability to drive and use machines

None stated.

4.8 Undesirable effects

Under normal circumstances Solu-Medrone therapy would be considered as short-term. However, the possibility of side-effects attributable to corticosteroid therapy should be recognised, particularly when high-dose therapy is being used (see Special warnings and special precautions for use). Such side-effects include:

PARENTERAL CORTICOSTEROID THERAPY - Anaphylactic reaction with or without circulatory collapse, cardiac arrest, bronchospasm, cardiac arrhythmias, hypotension or hypertension, hypopigmentation or hyperpigmentation.

GASTRO-INTESTINAL - Dyspepsia, peptic ulceration with perforation and haemorrhage, abdominal distension, oesophageal ulceration, oesophageal candidiasis, acute pancreatitis, perforation of the bowel, gastric haemorrhage. Nausea, vomiting and bad taste in mouth may occur especially with rapid administration.

Increases in alanine transaminase (ALT, SGPT) aspartate transaminase (AST, SGOT) and alkaline phosphatase have been observed following corticosteroid treatment. These changes are usually small, not associated with any clinical syndrome and are reversible upon discontinuation.

ANTI-INFLAMMATORY AND IMMUNOSUPPRESSIVE EFFECTS - Increased susceptibility and severity of infections with suppression of clinical symptoms and signs, opportunistic infections, may suppress reactions to skin tests, recurrence of dormant tuberculosis (see Special warnings and special precautions for use).

MUSCULOSKELETAL - Proximal myopathy, osteoporosis, vertebral and long bone fractures, avascular osteonecrosis, tendon rupture.

FLUID AND ELECTROLYTE DISTURBANCE - Sodium and water retention, potassium loss, hypertension, hypokalaemic alkalosis, congestive heart failure in susceptible patients.

DERMATOLOGICAL - Impaired healing, petechiae and ecchymosis, skin atrophy, bruising, striae, telangiectasia, acne. Kaposi's sarcoma has been reported to occur in patients receiving corticosteroid therapy. Discontinuation of corticosteroids may result in clinical remission.

ENDOCRINE/METABOLIC - Suppression of the hypothalamo-pituitary-adrenal axis; growth suppression in infancy, childhood and adolescence; menstrual irregularity and amenorrhoea. Cushingoid facies, hirsutism, weight gain, impaired carbohydrate tolerance with increased requirement for antidiabetic therapy, negative nitrogen and calcium balance. Increased appetite.

NEUROPSYCHIATRIC - A wide range of psychiatric reactions including affective disorders (such as irritable, euphoric, depressed and labile mood psychological dependence and suicidal thoughts), psychotic reactions (including mania, delusions, hallucinations and aggravation of schizophrenia), behavioural disturbances, irritability, anxiety, sleep disturbances, seizures and cognitive dysfunction including confusion and amnesia have been reported for all corticosteroids. Reactions are common and may occur in both adults and children. In adults, the frequency of severe reactions was estimated to be 5-6%. Psychological effects have been reported on withdrawal of corticosteroids; the frequency is unknown. Increased intra-cranial pressure with papilloedema in children (pseudotumour cerebri) has been reported, usually after treatment withdrawal of methylprednisolone.

OPHTHALMIC - Increased intra-ocular pressure, glaucoma, papilloedema with possible damage to the optic nerve, cataracts, corneal or scleral thinning, exacerbation of ophthalmic viral or fungal disease.

CARDIOVASCULAR – Myocardial rupture following a myocardial infarction.

GENERAL - Leucocytosis, hypersensitivity including anaphylaxis, thrombo-embolism, malaise, persistent hiccups with high doses of corticosteroids.

WITHDRAWAL SYMPTOMS - Too rapid a reduction of corticosteroid dosage following prolonged treatment can lead to acute adrenal insufficiency, hypotension and death. However, this is more applicable to corticosteroids with an indication where continuous therapy is given (see Special warnings and special precautions for use).

A 'withdrawal syndrome' may also occur including, fever, myalgia, arthralgia, rhinitis, conjunctivitis, painful itchy skin nodules and loss of weight.

4.9 Overdose

There is no clinical syndrome of acute overdosage with Solu-Medrone. Methylprednisolone is dialysable. Following chronic overdosage the possibility of adrenal suppression should be guarded against by gradual diminution of dose levels over a period of time. In such event the patient may require to be supported during any further stressful episode.

5. PHARMACOLOGICAL PROPERTIES

5.1 Pharmacodynamic properties

Medrone is a corticosteroid with an anti-inflammatory activity at least five times that of hydrocortisone. An enhanced separation of glucocorticoid and mineralocorticoid effect results in a reduced incidence of sodium and water retention.

5.2 Pharmacokinetic properties

Methylprednisolone is extensively bound to plasma proteins, mainly to globulin and less so to albumin. Only unbound corticosteroid has pharmacological effects or is metabolised. Metabolism occurs in the liver and to a lesser extent in the kidney. Metabolites are excreted in the urine.

Mean elimination half-life ranges from 2.4 to 3.5 hours in normal healthy adults and appears to be independent of the route of administration.

Total body clearance following intravenous or intramuscular injection of methylprednisolone to healthy adult volunteers is approximately 15-16l/hour. Peak methylprednisolone plasma levels of 33.67 micrograms/100 ml were achieved in 2 hours after a single 40 mg i.m. injection to 22 adult male volunteers.

6. PHARMACEUTICAL PARTICULARS

6.1 List of excipients

Sodium biphosphate and sodium phosphate.

6.2 Incompatibilities

None stated.

6.3 Shelf life

Shelf-life of the medicinal product as packaged for sale: 60 months.

After reconstitution with Sterile Water for Injections, use immediately, discard any remainder.

6.4 Special precautions for storage

Store below 25°C.

Refer to Section 4.2 Dosage and Administration. No diluents other than those referred to are recommended. Parenteral drug products should be inspected visually for particulate matter and discoloration prior to administration.

6.5 Nature and contents of container

Type I clear glass vial with butyl rubber plug and flip top seal. Each vial contains 2 grams of methylprednisolone as the sodium succinate for reconstitution with 31.2 ml of Sterile Water for Injections.

6.6 Special precautions for disposal and other handling

No special requirements.

7. MARKETING AUTHORISATION HOLDER

Pharmacia Limited
Ramsgate Road
Sandwich
Kent
CT13 9NJ
United Kingdom

8. MARKETING AUTHORISATION NUMBER(S)

PL 0032/0073

9. DATE OF FIRST AUTHORISATION/RENEWAL OF THE AUTHORISATION

6th January 2005

10. DATE OF REVISION OF THE TEXT

3rd April 2008

Legal category

POM

Ref: SMB 3_0 UK

Solu-Medrone 40mg, 125mg, 500mg and 1 gram

(Pharmacia Limited)

1. NAME OF THE MEDICINAL PRODUCT

Solu-Medrone 40 mg
Solu-Medrone 125mg
Solu-Medrone 500mg
Solu-Medrone 1gram

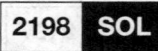

2. QUALITATIVE AND QUANTITATIVE COMPOSITION

Solu-Medrone 40 mg: Methylprednisolone sodium succinate 53.0 mg equivalent to 40 mg of methylprednisolone.

Solu-Medrone 125mg: Methylprednisolone sodium succinate 165.8 mg equivalent to 125 mg of methylprednisolone.

Solu-Medrone 500mg: Methylprednisolone sodium succinate 663.0 mg equivalent to 500 mg of methylprednisolone.

Solu-Medrone 1g: Methylprednisolone sodium succinate 1.326 gm equivalent to 1.0 g of methylprednisolone.

3. PHARMACEUTICAL FORM

Powder for injection.

4. CLINICAL PARTICULARS

4.1 Therapeutic indications

Solu-Medrone is indicated to treat any condition in which rapid and intense corticosteroid effect is required such as:

1. Dermatological disease

Severe erythema multiforme (Stevens-Johnson syndrome)

2. Allergic states

Bronchial asthma

Severe seasonal and perennial allergic rhinitis

Angioneurotic oedema

Anaphylaxis

3. Gastro-intestinal diseases

Ulcerative colitis

Crohn's disease

4. Respiratory diseases

Aspiration of gastric contents

Fulminating or disseminated tuberculosis (with appropriate antituberculous chemotherapy)

5. Neurological disorders

Cerebral oedema secondary to cerebral tumour

Acute exacerbations of multiple sclerosis superimposed on a relapsing-remitting background.

6. Miscellaneous

T.B. meningitis (with appropriate antituberculous chemotherapy)

Transplantation

4.2 Posology and method of administration

Solu-Medrone may be administered intravenously or intramuscularly, the preferred method for emergency use being intravenous injection given over a suitable time interval. When administering Solu-Medrone in high doses intravenously it should be given over a period of at least 30 minutes. Doses up to 250 mg should be given intravenously over a period of at least five minutes.

For intravenous infusion the initially prepared solution may be diluted with 5% dextrose in water, isotonic saline solution, or 5% dextrose in isotonic saline solution. To avoid compatibility problems with other drugs Solu-Medrone should be administered separately, only in the solutions mentioned.

Undesirable effects may be minimised by using the lowest effective dose for the minimum period (see Other special warnings and precautions).

Parenteral drug products should wherever possible be visually inspected for particulate matter and discoloration prior to administration.

Adults: Dosage should be varied according to the severity of the condition, initial dosage will vary from 10 to 500 mg. In the treatment of graft rejection reactions following transplantation, a dose of up to 1 g/day may be required. Although doses and protocols have varied in studies using methylprednisolone sodium succinate in the treatment of graft rejection reactions, the published literature supports the use of doses of this level, with 500 mg to 1 g most commonly used for acute rejection. Treatment at these doses should be limited to a 48-72 hour period until the patient's condition has stabilised, as prolonged high dose corticosteroid therapy can cause serious corticosteroid induced side-effects (see Undesirable effects and Special warnings and special precautions for use).

Children: In the treatment of high dose indications, such as haematological, rheumatic, renal and dermatological conditions, a dosage of 30 mg/kg/day to a maximum of 1 g/day is recommended. This dosage may be repeated for three pulses either daily or on alternate days. In the treatment of graft rejection reactions following transplantation, a dosage of 10 to 20 mg/kg/day for up to 3 days, to a maximum of 1 g/day, is recommended. In the treatment of status asthmaticus, a dosage of 1 to 4 mg/kg/day for 1-3 days is recommended.

Elderly patients: Solu-Medrone is primarily used in acute short-term conditions. There is no information to suggest that a change in dosage is warranted in the elderly. However, treatment of elderly patients should be planned bearing in mind the more serious consequences of the common side-effects of corticosteroids in old age and close clinical supervision is required (see Special warnings and special precautions for use).

Detailed recommendations for adult dosage are as follows:

In anaphylactic reactions adrenaline or noradrenaline should be administered first for an immediate haemodynamic effect, followed by intravenous injection of Solu-Medrone (methylprednisolone sodium succinate) with other accepted procedures. There is evidence that corticosteroids through their prolonged haemodynamic effect are of value in preventing recurrent attacks of acute anaphylactic reactions.

In sensitivity reactions Solu-Medrone is capable of providing relief within one half to two hours. In patients with status asthmaticus Solu-Medrone may be given at a dose of 40 mg intravenously, repeated as dictated by patient response. In some asthmatic patients it may be advantageous to administer by slow intravenous drip over a period of hours.

In graft rejection reactions following transplantation doses of up to 1 g per day have been used to suppress rejection crises, with doses of 500 mg to 1 g most commonly used for acute rejection. Treatment should be continued only until the patient's condition has stabilised; usually not beyond 48-72 hours.

In cerebral oedema corticosteroids are used to reduce or prevent the cerebral oedema associated with brain tumours (primary or metastatic).

In patients with oedema due to tumour, tapering the dose of corticosteroid appears to be important in order to avoid a rebound increase in intracranial pressure. If brain swelling does occur as the dose is reduced (intracranial bleeding having been ruled out), restart larger and more frequent doses parenterally. Patients with certain malignancies may need to remain on oral corticosteroid therapy for months or even life. Similar or higher doses may be helpful to control oedema during radiation therapy.

The following are suggested dosage schedules for oedemas due to brain tumour.

Schedule A (1)	Dose (mg)	Route	Interval in hours	Duration
Pre-operative:	20	IM	3-6	
During Surgery:	20 to 40	IV	hourly	
Post operative:	20	IM	3	24 hours
	16	IM	3	24 hours
	12	IM	3	24 hours
	8	IM	3	24 hours
	4	IM	3	24 hours
	4	IM	6	24 hours
	4	IM	12	24 hours

Schedule B (2)	Dose (mg)	Route	Interval in hours	Duration
Pre-operative:	40	IM	6	2-3
Post operative:	40	IM	6	3-5
	20	Oral	6	1
	12	Oral	6	1
	8	Oral	8	1
	4	Oral	12	1
	4	Oral		1

Aim to discontinue therapy after a total of 10 days.

REFERENCES

1. Fox JL, MD. "Use of Methylprednisolone in Intracranial Surgery" Medical Annals of the District of Columbia, 34:261-265,1965.

2. Cantu RC, MD Harvard Neurological Service, Boston, Massachusetts. Letter on file, The Upjohn Company (February 1970).

In the treatment of **acute exacerbations of multiple sclerosis** in adults, the recommended dose is 1 g daily for 3 days. Solu-Medrone should be given as an intravenous infusion over at least 30 minutes.

In other indications, initial dosage will vary from 10 to 500 mg depending on the clinical problem being treated. Larger doses may be required for short-term management of severe, acute conditions. The initial dose, up to 250 mg, should be given intravenously over a period of at least 5 minutes, doses exceeding 250 mg should be given intravenously over a period of at least 30 minutes. Subsequent doses may be given intravenously or intramuscularly at intervals dictated by the patient's response and clinical condition. Corticosteroid therapy is an adjunct to, and not replacement for, conventional therapy.

4.3 Contraindications

Solu-Medrone is contra-indicated where there is known hypersensitivity to components, in systemic infection unless specific anti-infective therapy is employed and in cerebral oedema in malaria.

4.4 Special warnings and precautions for use

Warnings and Precautions:

1. A Patient Information Leaflet is provided in the pack by the manufacturer.

2. Undesirable effects may be minimised by using the lowest effective dose for the minimum period. Frequent patient review is required to appropriately titrate the dose against disease activity (see Posology and method of administration).

3. Adrenal cortical atrophy develops during prolonged therapy and may persist for months after stopping treatment. In patients who have received more than physiological doses of systemic corticosteroids (approximately 6 mg methylprednisolone) for greater than 3 weeks, withdrawal should not be abrupt. How dose reduction should be carried out depends largely on whether the disease is likely to relapse as the dose of systemic corticosteroids is reduced. Clinical assessment of disease activity may be needed during withdrawal. If the disease is unlikely to relapse on withdrawal of systemic corticosteroids, but there is uncertainty about HPA suppression, the dose of systemic corticosteroid may be reduced rapidly to physiological doses. Once a daily dose of 6 mg methylprednisolone is reached, dose reduction should be slower to allow the HPA-axis to recover.

Abrupt withdrawal of systemic corticosteroid treatment, which has continued up to 3 weeks is appropriate if it considered that the disease is unlikely to relapse. Abrupt withdrawal of doses up to 32 mg daily of methylprednisolone for 3 weeks is unlikely to lead to clinically relevant HPA-axis suppression, in the majority of patients. In the following patient groups, gradual withdrawal of systemic corticosteroid therapy should be *considered* even after courses lasting 3 weeks or less:

- Patients who have had repeated courses of systemic corticosteroids, particularly if taken for greater than 3 weeks.
- When a short course has been prescribed within one year of cessation of long-term therapy (months or years).
- Patients who may have reasons for adrenocortical insufficiency other than exogenous corticosteroid therapy.
- Patients receiving doses of systemic corticosteroid greater than 32 mg daily of methylprednisolone.
- Patients repeatedly taking doses in the evening.

4. Patients should carry 'Steroid Treatment' cards which give clear guidance on the precautions to be taken to minimise risk and which provide details of prescriber, drug, dosage and the duration of treatment.

5. Although Solu-Medrone is not approved in the UK for use in any shock indication, the following warning statement should be adhered to. Data from a clinical study conducted to establish the efficacy of Solu-Medrone in septic shock, suggest that a higher mortality occurred in subsets of patients who entered the study with elevated serum creatinine levels or who developed a secondary infection after therapy began. Therefore this product should not be used in the treatment of septic syndrome or septic shock.

6. There have been a few reports of cardiac arrhythmias and/or circulatory collapse and/or cardiac arrest associated with the rapid intravenous administration of large doses of Solu-Medrone (greater than 500 mg administered over a period of less than 10 minutes). Bradycardia has been reported during or after the administration of large doses of methylprednisolone sodium succinate, and may be unrelated to the speed and duration of infusion.

7. Corticosteroids may mask some signs of infection, and new infections may appear during their use. Suppression of the inflammatory response and immune function increases the susceptibility to fungal, viral and bacterial infections and their severity. The clinical presentation may often be atypical and may reach an advanced stage before being recognised.

8. Chickenpox is of serious concern since this normally minor illness may be fatal in immunosuppressed patients. Patients (or parents of children) without a definite history of chickenpox should be advised to avoid close personal contact with chickenpox or herpes zoster and if exposed they should seek urgent medical attention. Passive immunization with varicella/zoster immunoglobin (VZIG) is needed by exposed non-immune patients who are receiving systemic corticosteroids or who have used them within the previous 3 months; this should be given within 10 days of exposure to chickenpox. If a diagnosis of chickenpox is confirmed, the illness warrants specialist care and urgent treatment. Corticosteroids should not be stopped and the dose may need to be increased.

9. Exposure to measles should be avoided. Medical advice should be sought immediately if exposure occurs. Prophylaxis with normal intramuscular immuneglobulin may be needed.

10. Live vaccines should not be given to individuals with impaired immune responsiveness. The antibody response to other vaccines may be diminished.

11. The use of Solu-Medrone in active tuberculosis should be restricted to those cases of fulminating or disseminated tuberculosis in which the corticosteroid is used for the management of the disease in conjunction with an appropriate anti-tuberculous regimen. If corticosteroids are indicated in patients with latent tuberculosis or tuberculin reactivity, close observation is necessary as reactivation of the disease may occur. During prolonged corticosteroid therapy, these patients should receive chemoprophylaxis.

12. Rarely anaphylactoid reactions have been reported following parenteral Solu-Medrone therapy. Physicians using the drug should be prepared to deal with such a possibility. Appropriate precautionary measures should be taken prior to administration, especially when the patient has a history of drug allergy.

13. Care should be taken for patients receiving cardioactive drugs such as digoxin because of steroid induced

electrolyte disturbance/potassium loss (see Undesirable effects).

14. Corticosteroids should not be used for the management of head injury or stroke because it is unlikely to be of benefit and may even be harmful.

Special precautions:

Particular care is required when considering the use of systemic corticosteroids in patients with the following conditions and frequent patient monitoring is necessary.

1. Osteoporosis (post-menopausal females are particularly at risk).
2. Hypertension or congestive heart failure.
3. Existing or previous history of severe affective disorders (especially previous steroid psychosis).
4. Diabetes mellitus (or a family history of diabetes).
5. History of tuberculosis.
6. Glaucoma (or a family history of glaucoma).
7. Previous corticosteroid-induced myopathy.
8. Liver failure or cirrhosis.
9. Renal insufficiency.
10. Epilepsy.
11. Peptic ulceration.
12. Fresh intestinal anastomoses.
13. Predisposition to thrombophlebitis.
14. Abscess or other pyogenic infections.
15. Ulcerative colitis.
16. Diverticulitis.
17. Myasthenia gravis.
18. Ocular herpes simplex, for fear of corneal perforation.
19. Hypothyroidism.
20. Recent myocardial infarction (myocardial rupture has been reported).
21. Kaposi's sarcoma has been reported to occur in patients receiving corticosteroid therapy. Discontinuation of corticosteroids may result in clinical remission.
22. Patients and/or carers should be warned that potentially severe psychiatric adverse reactions may occur with systemic steroids (see section 4.8). Symptoms typically emerge within a few days or weeks of starting treatment. Risks may be higher with high doses/systemic exposure (see also section 4.5 Interaction with Other Medicaments and Other Forms of Interaction that can increase the risk of side effects), although dose levels do not allow prediction of the onset, type, severity or duration of reactions. Most reactions recover after either dose reduction or withdrawal, although specific treatment may be necessary. Patients/carers should be encouraged to seek medical advice if worrying psychological symptoms develop, especially if depressed mood or suicidal ideation is suspected. Patients/carers should be alert to possible psychiatric disturbances that may occur either during or immediately after dose tapering/withdrawal of systemic steroids, although such reactions have been reported infrequently.

Particular care is required when considering the use of systemic corticosteroids in patients with existing or previous history of severe affective disorders in themselves or in their first degree relatives. These would include depressive or manic-depressive illness and previous steroid psychosis.

Use in children: Corticosteroids cause growth retardation in infancy, childhood and adolescence, which may be irreversible. Treatment should be limited to the minimum dosage for the shortest possible time. In order to minimise suppression of the hypothalamo-pituitary-adrenal axis and growth retardation, treatment should be administered where possible as a single dose on alternate days.

Use in the elderly: The common adverse effects of systemic corticosteroids may be associated with more serious consequences in old age, especially osteoporosis, hypertension, hypokalaemia, diabetes, susceptibility to infection and thinning of the skin. Close clinical supervision is required to avoid life-threatening reactions.

4.5 Interaction with other medicinal products and other forms of interaction

1. Convulsions have been reported with concurrent use of methylprednisolone and ciclosporin. Since concurrent administration of these agents results in a mutual inhibition of metabolism, it is possible that convulsions and other adverse events associated with the individual use of either drug may be more apt to occur.
2. Drugs that induce hepatic enzymes, such as rifampicin, rifabutin, carbamazepine, phenobarbitone, phenytoin, primidone, and aminoglutethimide enhance the metabolism of corticosteroids and its therapeutic effects may be reduced.
3. Drugs which inhibit the CYP3A4 enzyme, such as cimetidine, erythromycin, ketoconazole, itraconazole, diltiazem and mibefradil, may decrease the rate of metabolism of corticosteroids and hence increase the serum concentration.
4. Steroids may reduce the effects of anticholinesterases in myasthenia gravis. The desired effects of hypoglycaemic agents (including insulin), anti-hypertensives and diuretics are antagonised by corticosteroids, and the hypokalaemic effects of acetazolamide, loop diuretics, thiazide diuretics and carbenoxolone are enhanced.
5. The efficacy of coumarin anticoagulants may be enhanced by concurrent corticosteroid therapy and close monitoring of the INR or prothrombin time is required to avoid spontaneous bleeding.
6. The renal clearance of salicylates is increased by corticosteroids and steroid withdrawal may result in salicylate intoxication. Salicylates and non-steroidal anti-inflammatory agents should be used cautiously in conjunction with corticosteroids in hypothrombinaemia.
7. Steroids have been reported to interact with neuromuscular blocking agents such as pancuronium with partial reversal of the neuromuscular block.

4.6 Pregnancy and lactation

Pregnancy

The ability of corticosteroids to cross the placenta varies between individual drugs, however, methylprednisolone does cross the placenta.

Administration of corticosteroids to pregnant animals can cause abnormalities of foetal development including cleft palate, intra-uterine growth retardation and affects on brain growth and development. There is no evidence that corticosteroids result in an increased incidence of congenital abnormalities, such as cleft palate in man, however, when administered for long periods or repeatedly during pregnancy, corticosteroids may increase the risk of intra-uterine growth retardation. Hypoadrenalism may, in theory, occur in the neonate following prenatal exposure to corticosteroids but usually resolves spontaneously following birth and is rarely clinically important. As with all drugs, corticosteroids should only be prescribed when the benefits to the mother and child outweigh the risks. When corticosteroids are essential, however, patients with normal pregnancies may be treated as though they were in the non-gravid state.

Lactation

Corticosteroids are excreted in small amounts in breast milk, however, doses of up to 40 mg daily of methylprednisolone are unlikely to cause systemic effects in the infant. Infants of mothers taking higher doses than this may have a degree of adrenal suppression, but the benefits of breastfeeding are likely to outweigh any theoretical risk.

4.7 Effects on ability to drive and use machines

None stated.

4.8 Undesirable effects

Under normal circumstances Solu-Medrone therapy would be considered as short-term. However, the possibility of side-effects attributable to corticosteroid therapy should be recognised, particularly when high-dose therapy is being used (see Special warnings and special precautions for use). Such side-effects include:

PARENTERAL CORTICOSTEROID THERAPY - Anaphylactic reaction with or without circulatory collapse, cardiac arrest, bronchospasm, cardiac arrhythmias, hypotension or hypertension, hypopigmentation or hyperpigmentation.

GASTRO-INTESTINAL - Dyspepsia, peptic ulceration with perforation and haemorrhage, abdominal distension, oesophageal ulceration, oesophageal candidiasis, acute pancreatitis, perforation of the bowel, gastric haemorrhage. Nausea, vomiting and bad taste in mouth may occur especially with rapid administration.

Increases in alanine transaminase (ALT, SGPT) aspartate transaminase (AST, SGOT) and alkaline phosphatase have been observed following corticosteroid treatment. These changes are usually small, not associated with any clinical syndrome and are reversible upon discontinuation.

ANTI-INFLAMMATORY AND IMMUNOSUPPRESSIVE EFFECTS - Increased susceptibility and severity of infections with suppression of clinical symptoms and signs, opportunistic infections, may suppress reactions to skin tests, recurrence of dormant tuberculosis (see Special warnings and special precautions for use).

MUSCULOSKELETAL - Proximal myopathy, osteoporosis, vertebral and long bone fractures, avascular osteonecrosis, tendon rupture.

FLUID AND ELECTROLYTE DISTURBANCE - Sodium and water retention, potassium loss, hypertension, hypokalaemic alkalosis, congestive heart failure in susceptible patients.

DERMATOLOGICAL - Impaired healing, petechiae and ecchymosis, skin atrophy, bruising, striae, telangiectasia, acne. Kaposi's sarcoma has been reported to occur in patients receiving corticosteroid therapy. Discontinuation of corticosteroids may result in clinical remission.

ENDOCRINE/METABOLIC - Suppression of the hypothalamo-pituitary-adrenal axis, growth suppression in infancy, childhood and adolescence, menstrual irregularity and amenorrhoea. Cushingoid facies, hirsutism, weight gain, impaired carbohydrate tolerance with increased requirement for antidiabetic therapy, negative nitrogen and calcium balance. Increased appetite.

NEUROPSYCHIATRIC - A wide range of psychiatric reactions including affective disorders (such as irritable, euphoric, depressed and labile mood psychological dependence and suicidal thoughts), psychotic reactions (including mania, delusions, hallucinations and aggravation of schizophrenia), behavioural disturbances, irritability, anxiety, sleep disturbances, seizures and cognitive dysfunction including confusion and amnesia have been reported for all corticosteroids. Reactions are common and may occur in both adults and children. In adults, the frequency of severe reactions was estimated to be 5-6%. Psychological effects have been reported on withdrawal of corticosteroids; the frequency is unknown. Increased intra-cranial pressure with papilloedema in children (pseudotumour cerebri) has been reported, usually after treatment withdrawal of methylprednisolone.

OPHTHALMIC - Increased intra-ocular pressure, glaucoma, papilloedema with possible damage to the optic nerve, cataracts, corneal or scleral thinning, exacerbation of ophthalmic viral or fungal disease.

CARDIOVASCULAR – Myocardial rupture following a myocardial infarction.

GENERAL - Leucocytosis, hypersensitivity including anaphylaxis, thrombo-embolism, malaise, persistent hiccups with high doses of corticosteroids.

WITHDRAWAL SYMPTOMS - Too rapid a reduction of corticosteroid dosage following prolonged treatment can lead to acute adrenal insufficiency, hypotension and death. However, this is more applicable to corticosteroids with an indication where continuous therapy is given (see Special warnings and special precautions for use).

A 'withdrawal syndrome' may also occur including, fever, myalgia, arthralgia, rhinitis, conjunctivitis, painful itchy skin nodules and loss of weight.

4.9 Overdose

There is no clinical syndrome of acute overdosage with Solu-Medrone. Methylprednisolone is dialysable. Following chronic overdosage the possibility of adrenal suppression should be guarded against by gradual diminution of dose levels over a period of time. In such event the patient may require to be supported during any further stressful episode.

5. PHARMACOLOGICAL PROPERTIES

5.1 Pharmacodynamic properties

Medrone is a corticosteroid with an anti-inflammatory activity at least five times that of hydrocortisone. An enhanced separation of glucocorticoid and mineralocorticoid effect results in a reduced incidence of sodium and water retention.

5.2 Pharmacokinetic properties

Methylprednisolone is extensively bound to plasma proteins, mainly to globulin and less so to albumin. Only unbound corticosteroid has pharmacological effects or is metabolised. Metabolism occurs in the liver and to a lesser extent in the kidney. Metabolites are excreted in the urine.

Mean elimination half-life ranges from 2.4 to 3.5 hours in normal healthy adults and appears to be independent of the route of administration.

Total body clearance following intravenous or intramuscular injection of methylprednisolone to healthy adult volunteers is approximately 15-16l/hour. Peak methylprednisolone plasma levels of 33.67 mcg/100 ml were achieved in 2 hours after a single 40 mg i.m. injection to 22 adult male volunteers.

6. PHARMACEUTICAL PARTICULARS

6.1 List of excipients

Sodium biphosphate and sodium phosphate.

The 40 mg vial also contains lactose.

6.2 Incompatibilities

None stated.

6.3 Shelf life

Shelf-life of the medicinal product as packaged for sale: 60 months.

After reconstitution with Sterile Water for injections, use immediately, discard any remainder.

6.4 Special precautions for storage

Store below 25°C.

Refer to Section 4.2 Dosage and Administration. No diluents other than those referred to are recommended. Parenteral drug products should be inspected visually for particulate matter and discoloration prior to administration.

6.5 Nature and contents of container

Type I clear glass vial with butyl rubber plug and flip top seal.

Each vial of Solu-Medrone 40 mg contains the equivalent of 40 mg of methylprednisolone as the sodium succinate for reconstitution with 1 ml of Sterile Water for Injections.

Each vial of Solu-Medrone 125 mg contains the equivalent of 125 mg of methylprednisolone as the sodium succinate for reconstitution with 2 ml of Sterile Water for Injections.

Each vial of Solu-Medrone 500 mg contains the equivalent of 500 mg of methylprednisolone as the sodium succinate for reconstitution with 7.8 ml of Sterile Water for Injections.

Each vial of Solu-Medrone 1 g contains the equivalent of 1 g of methylprednisolone as the sodium succinate for reconstitution with 15.6 ml of Sterile Water for Injections.

6.6 Special precautions for disposal and other handling

No special requirements.

7. MARKETING AUTHORISATION HOLDER
Pharmacia Limited
Ramsgate Road
Sandwich
Kent
CT13 9NJ
United Kingdom

8. MARKETING AUTHORISATION NUMBER(S)
Solu-Medrone 40 mg PL 0032/0033
Solu-Medrone 125mg PL 0032/0034
Solu-Medrone 500mg PL 0032/0035
Solu-Medrone 1g PL 0032/0039

9. DATE OF FIRST AUTHORISATION/RENEWAL OF THE AUTHORISATION
2nd February 2005

10. DATE OF REVISION OF THE TEXT
3rd April 2008

Legal category: POM

SM 3_0 UK

Solvazinc

(Galen Limited)

1. NAME OF THE MEDICINAL PRODUCT
Solvazinc® Effervescent Tablets.

2. QUALITATIVE AND QUANTITATIVE COMPOSITION
Each Solvazinc® tablet contains the following active ingredient: Zinc sulphate monohydrate: 125mg (equivalent to 45mg elemental zinc).

3. PHARMACEUTICAL FORM
Effervescent tablet.

4. CLINICAL PARTICULARS

4.1 Therapeutic indications
Zinc sulphate is a source of zinc which is an essential trace element and involved in a number of body enzyme systems.

Indications: For the treatment of zinc deficiency.

4.2 Posology and method of administration
Method of Administration: oral after dissolution in water.

Adults: One tablet, dissolved in water, once to three times daily after meals.

Children: More than 30kg: One tablet, dissolved in water, once to three times daily after meals.

10-30kg: ½ tablet, dissolved in water, once to three times daily after meals.

Less than 10kg: ½ tablet, dissolved in water, once daily after meals.

4.3 Contraindications
None.

4.4 Special warnings and precautions for use
Accumulation of zinc may occur in cases of renal failure.

4.5 Interaction with other medicinal products and other forms of interaction
Zinc may inhibit the absorption of concurrently administered tetracyclines; when both are being given an interval of at least three hours should be allowed.

4.6 Pregnancy and lactation
The safety of this product in human pregnancy has not been established. Zinc crosses the placenta and is present in breast milk.

4.7 Effects on ability to drive and use machines
Solvazinc® is not expected to affect ability to drive and use machines.

4.8 Undesirable effects
Zinc salts may cause abdominal pain and dyspepsia.

4.9 Overdose
Zinc sulphate is corrosive in overdosage. Symptoms are corrosion and inflammation of the mucous membrane of the mouth and stomach; ulceration of the stomach followed by perforation may occur. Gastric lavage and emesis should be avoided. Demulcents such as milk should be given. Chelating agents such as sodium calcium edetate may be useful.

5. PHARMACOLOGICAL PROPERTIES

5.1 Pharmacodynamic properties
Zinc is an essential trace element involved in many enzyme systems. Severe deficiency causes skin lesion, alopecia, diarrhoea, increased susceptibility to infections and failure to thrive in children. Symptoms of less severe deficiency include distorted or absent perceptions of taste and smell and poor wound healing.

5.2 Pharmacokinetic properties
Zinc is absorbed from the gastrointestinal tract and distributed throughout the body. The highest concentrations occur in hair, eyes, male reproductive organs and bone. Lower levels are present in liver, kidney and muscle. In blood 80% is found in erythrocytes. Plasma zinc levels range from 70 to 110µg/dL and about 50% of this is loosely bound to albumin. About 7% is amino-acid bound and the rest is tightly bound to alpha 2-macroglobulins and other proteins.

5.3 Preclinical safety data
None stated.

6. PHARMACEUTICAL PARTICULARS

6.1 List of excipients
Solvazinc® contains the following excipients:

Sorbitol, mannitol, sodium hydrogen carbonate, citric acid, saccharin sodium, povidone K25, sodium citrate and sodium carbonate anhydrous.

6.2 Incompatibilities
None.

6.3 Shelf life
Three years.

6.4 Special precautions for storage
Store below 25°C, protect from moisture.

6.5 Nature and contents of container
Polypropylene containers with polyethylene caps and packed in cartons of three containers. Each tablet container contains 30 tablets. The tablet containers also contain a desiccant capsule.

6.6 Special precautions for disposal and other handling
None.

7. MARKETING AUTHORISATION HOLDER
Galen Limited
Seagoe Industrial Estate
Craigavon
BT63 5UA
UK

8. MARKETING AUTHORISATION NUMBER(S)
PL 27827/0003.

9. DATE OF FIRST AUTHORISATION/RENEWAL OF THE AUTHORISATION
01 November 1983.

10. DATE OF REVISION OF THE TEXT
01 April 2008.

Somatuline Autogel 60 mg, Somatuline Autogel 90 mg, Somatuline Autogel 120 mg

(Ipsen Ltd)

1. NAME OF THE MEDICINAL PRODUCT
SOMATULINE® Autogel® 60mg, solution for injection.
SOMATULINE® Autogel® 90mg, solution for injection.
SOMATULINE® Autogel® 120mg, solution for injection.

2. QUALITATIVE AND QUANTITATIVE COMPOSITION
Lanreotide (I.N.N.), 60mg, 90mg or 120mg (as acetate)

For excipients, see 6.1.

3. PHARMACEUTICAL FORM
Solution for injection.

White to off-white, translucent and viscous supersaturated solution in a pre-filled syringe, ready for use.

4. CLINICAL PARTICULARS

4.1 Therapeutic indications
SOMATULINE AUTOGEL is indicated for the treatment of individuals with acromegaly when the circulating levels of Growth Hormone (GH) and/or Insulin-like Growth Factor-1 (IGF-1) remain abnormal after surgery and/or radiotherapy, or in patients who otherwise require medical treatment. The goal of treatment in acromegaly is to reduce GH and IGF-1 levels and where possible to normalise these values.

SOMATULINE AUTOGEL is also indicated for the treatment of symptoms associated with neuroendocrine (particularly carcinoid) tumours.

4.2 Posology and method of administration
Posology

Acromegaly

In patients receiving a somatostatin analogue for the first time, the recommended starting dose is 60mg of Somatuline Autogel administered every 28 days.

In patients previously treated with Somatuline LA 30mg once every 14 days, the initial dose of SOMATULINE AUTOGEL should be 60mg every 28 days; in patients previously treated with Somatuline LA 30mg once every 10 days, the initial dose of SOMATULINE AUTOGEL should be 90mg every 28 days; and in patients treated with Somatuline LA 30mg once every 7 days, the initial dose of SOMATULINE AUTOGEL should be 120mg every 28 days.

Thereafter, for all patients, the dose should be individualised according to the response of the patient (as judged by a reduction in symptoms and/or a reduction in GH and/or IGF-1 levels).

For patients whose GH concentration are below 1ng/mL (approx 2mU/L), whose IGF-1 serum concentrations have normalised, and in whom most reversible signs of acromegaly have disappeared, the monthly dose should be decreased. If appropriate, this may be achieved by giving Somatuline Autogel 120mg at increased intervals of 42-56 days.

For patients on Somatuline Autogel 60mg or 90mg every 28 days who are well controlled (GH concentrations less than 2.5ng/mL (approx 5mU/L) but above 1ng/mL (approx 2mU/L) and normalised IGF-1 levels) the dose should be maintained, or alternatively Somatuline Autogel 120mg may be given at increased intervals of 56 or 42 days respectively.

For patients in whom clinical symptoms and biochemical parameters are not adequately controlled (GH concentrations still above 2.5ng/mL (approx 5mU/L) or IGF-1 greater than age matched normal) the dose of Somatuline Autogel may be increased to a maximum of 120mg at 28 day intervals.

Long term monitoring of symptoms, GH and IGF-1 levels should be routinely carried out in all patients.

Neuroendocrine tumours:

The recommended starting dose is 60 to 120mg administered every 28 days.

The dose should be adjusted according to the degree of symptomatic relief obtained.

Hepatic/renal impairment and the elderly.

Subjects with severe renal impairment show an approximately 2-fold decrease in total serum clearance of lanreotide, with a consequent increase in half-life and AUC. In hepatic impairment, an increase in volume of distribution and mean residence time are observed, but there is no difference in total clearance or AUC. Elderly subjects show an increase in half-life and mean residence time compared with healthy young subjects. Due to the wide therapeutic window of lanreotide, it is not necessary to alter the dose in these circumstances.

Children

Currently there is no experience of administration of Somatuline Autogel in children, therefore use of Somatuline Autogel in children cannot be recommended.

Method of administration

SOMATULINE AUTOGEL should be injected, via the deep subcutaneous route, into the superior, external quadrant of the buttock.

The injection may be given by a healthcare professional or, for patients considered by their healthcare professional to be stabilised on their treatment with Somatuline Autogel, by an appropriately trained friend or relative of the patient (see section 5.1) Alternatively, such patients may self-administer the product after appropriate training. In this case the injection should be given in the upper, outer thigh.

Regardless of the site of administration, the skin should be stretched prior to injection. The needle should be inserted rapidly to its full length, perpendicularly to the skin. The injection site should be alternated between the right and left sides.

4.3 Contraindications
Hypersensitivity to lanreotide or related peptides.

4.4 Special warnings and precautions for use
Pharmacological studies in animals and humans show that lanreotide, like somatostatin and its analogues, may produce a transient inhibition of the secretion of insulin and glucagon. Hence, diabetic patients treated by SOMATULINE AUTOGEL may experience a slight transient change in blood glucose levels. Blood glucose levels should be checked in order to determine whether anti-diabetic treatment needs to be adjusted.

Slight decreases in thyroid function have been seen during treatment with lanreotide in acromegalic patients, although clinical hypothyroidism is rare (<1%). Tests of thyroid function should be done where clinically indicated.

Lanreotide may reduce gall bladder motility and therefore, gall bladder echography may be advisable at the start of treatment and as clinically indicated thereafter. If gallstones do occur, they are generally asymptomatic. Symptomatic stones should be treated as medically indicated.

4.5 Interaction with other medicinal products and other forms of interaction
The gastrointestinal effects of SOMATULINE AUTOGEL may reduce the intestinal absorption of co-administered drugs.

Concomitant administration of lanreotide injection with cyclosporin may decrease blood levels of cyclosporin, hence blood levels of cyclosporin should be monitored.

Interactions with highly plasma bound drugs are unlikely in view of the moderate binding of lanreotide to serum proteins (78 % mean serum binding).

4.6 Pregnancy and lactation
Reproductive studies in rats and rabbits at doses up to 33 times the human dose have failed to demonstrate a risk to the foetus; however there are no adequate and well-controlled studies in pregnant women. Because animal reproductive studies are not always predictive of human response, this drug should be used during pregnancy only if clearly needed.

Six pregnancies and one suspected pregnancy have been reported in patients who were being treated with lanreotide. Four pregnancies resulted in healthy, full term infants. One acromegalic patient delivered prematurely due to maternal complications. One patient with acromegaly had a first trimester miscarriage. One additional patient with acromegaly had a suspected first trimester miscarriage.

There is no information available on the presence of lanreotide in human breast milk. SOMATULINE AUTOGEL should not be used during breast-feeding unless clearly necessary.

4.7 Effects on ability to drive and use machines
Therapy with SOMATULINE AUTOGEL is unlikely to impair patients' ability to drive or use machines.

4.8 Undesirable effects
Clinical tolerance

The adverse reactions related to SOMATULINE AUTOGEL during clinical trials are consistent with those seen with other prolonged release formulations of lanreotide, and are predominantly gastrointestinal. In clinical trials of SOMATULINE AUTOGEL in acromegalic patients, 80% of patients experienced at least 1 adverse event. More than 50% of these adverse events were classified as gastrointestinal system disorders. The most commonly reported adverse reactions are diarrhoea, abdominal pain and nausea. These reactions are usually mild and transient.

Very common adverse reactions: the following adverse reactions occurred in more than 10% of patients: diarrhoea, abdominal pain, nausea.

Common adverse reactions: the following adverse reactions occurred in greater than 5% but less than 10% of patients: constipation, flatulence, cholelithiasis, gall bladder sludge.

Less common adverse reactions: the following adverse reactions occurred in between 1 and 5% of patients: asthenia, fatigue, increased bilirubin.

Uncommon adverse reactions: the following adverse reactions occurred in less than 1% of patients: injection site pain, skin nodule, hot flushes, leg pain, malaise, headache, tenesmus, vomiting, abnormal glucose tolerance, hyperglycaemia, decreased libido, somnolence, pruritus, increased sweating, skin disorder (not specified).

In rare instances, acute pancreatitis has been reported within a short time after the first administration of lanreotide in prolonged release formulations other than SOMATULINE AUTOGEL.

Cardiovascular effects including sinus bradycardia, a myocardial infarction (ref Section 4.9 "Overdose"), high blood pressure episodes and ventricular tachycardia have also been reported in exceptional cases with other prolonged release formulations of lanreotide.

Local tolerance

Reactions at the injection site may occur after the deep subcutaneous injection of SOMATULINE AUTOGEL in the buttock. When specific enquiry was made, pain, redness, itching and induration were reported at the injection site 30 minutes after dosing in up to 8%, 5%, 5% and 19% of patients respectively. After 3 dosing intervals, these symptoms or signs were reduced to 6%, 2% 3% and 9% of patients or fewer. In all cases, the symptoms were described as mild.

4.9 Overdose
In clinical trials, lanreotide has been administered in doses up to 15mg per day without serious adverse events related to the treatment. Human experience of overdose of prolonged release forms of lanreotide is limited to one unconfirmed case report of overdose where a patient was reported to have taken one intramuscular injection of the 30mg prolonged release formulation daily for two months (instead of 1 injection every 7 to 14 days). One week after stopping therapy the 52 year-old man with a history of acromegaly, diabetes mellitus and arterial hypertension suffered a fatal cardiac infarction.

If overdosage occurs, symptomatic management is indicated.

5. PHARMACOLOGICAL PROPERTIES
5.1 Pharmacodynamic properties
Pharmacotherapeutic group: Antigrowth hormones, ATC code: H01C B03.

Lanreotide is an octapeptide analogue of natural somatostatin. Like somatostatin, lanreotide is an inhibitor of various endocrine, neuroendocrine, exocrine and paracrine functions. It shows high binding affinity for human somatostatin receptors (SSTR) 2, 3 and 5, and reduced affinity for human SSTR 1 and 4. Activity at SSTR 2 and 5 is the primary mechanism considered to be responsible for GH inhibition.

Lanreotide, like somatostatin, exhibits a general exocrine antisecretory action. It inhibits the basal secretion of motilin, gastric inhibitory peptide and pancreatic polypeptide, but has no significant effect on fasting secretin or gastrin secretion. Lanreotide markedly inhibits meal-induced increases in superior mesenteric artery blood flow and portal venous blood flow. Lanreotide significantly reduces prostaglandin E1-stimulated jejunal secretion of water, sodium, potassium and chloride. Lanreotide reduces prolactin levels in acromegalic patients treated long term.

During an open label, controlled study involving acromegalic patients treated with a stable dose of Somatuline Autogel for at least 4 months, 93% of the patients who received self or partner administered injections of Somatuline Autogel after appropriate training were considered competent to perform unsupervised injections (maintenance of GH and IGF-1 levels).

5.2 Pharmacokinetic properties
Pharmacokinetic parameters of lanreotide after intravenous administration in healthy volunteers indicated limited extravascular distribution, with a steady-state volume of distribution of 13L. Total clearance was 20L/h, terminal half-life was 2.5 hours and mean residence time was 0.68 hours.

After a single subcutaneous injection of SOMATULINE AUTOGEL 60mg in healthy volunteers, a maximum serum concentration (Cmax) of 5.8 ± 4ng/mL was reached after 6 hours, followed by a slow decrease (mean residence time: 30 ± 6 days, apparent half-life: 33 ± 14 days). The absolute bioavailability was 63 ± 10%.

After a single intramuscular injection of SOMATULINE AUTOGEL 60mg in healthy volunteers, a maximum serum concentration (Cmax) of 6.8 ± 3ng/mL was reached after 15 hours, followed by a slow decrease (mean residence time: 23 ± 11 days, apparent half-life: 23 ± 9 days). The absolute bioavailability was 79 ± 10%.

Therefore the route of administration (subcutaneous or intramuscular) does not show any marked influence on the lanreotide pharmacokinetic profile.

After a single intramuscular injection of SOMATULINE AUTOGEL 90mg in healthy volunteers, a maximum serum concentration (Cmax) of 9.8 ± 5ng/mL was reached after 10 hours, followed by a slow decrease (mean residence time: 26 ± 4 days, apparent half-life: 31 ± 16 days). The absolute bioavailability was 58 ± 10%.

After a single intramuscular injection of SOMATULINE AUTOGEL 120mg in healthy volunteers, a maximum serum concentration (Cmax) of 12.8 ± 7ng/mL was reached after 16 hours, followed by a slow decrease (mean residence time: 29 ± 3 days, apparent half-life: 28 ± 6 days). The absolute bioavailability was 55 ± 10%.

Therefore lanreotide serum concentration after intramuscular administration of SOMATULINE AUTOGEL 60, 90 and 120mg shows an almost log-linear first order lanreotide release profile.

Trough lanreotide serum levels obtained after three deep subcutaneous injections of SOMATULINE AUTOGEL 60, 90 or 120mg given every 28 days are similar to the steady-state trough lanreotide serum levels obtained in acromegalic patients previously treated with intramuscular administrations of lanreotide 30mg prolonged release microparticles (Somatuline LA) every 14, 10 or 7 days respectively.

Lanreotide serum levels of 1ng/mL are able to suppress GH to < 5ng/mL in more than 60% of patients studied. Lanreotide serum levels of 2.5ng/mL are able to suppress GH to < 5ng/mL in more than 90% of patients studied.

5.3 Preclinical safety data
In vitro and animal toxicology studies have not shown any specific toxic potential for lanreotide. The observed effects are related to the pharmacological properties of lanreotide on the endocrine system.

6. PHARMACEUTICAL PARTICULARS
6.1 List of excipients
Water for injections

6.2 Incompatibilities
Not applicable.

6.3 Shelf life
24 months.

6.4 Special precautions for storage
Store in refrigerator between +2°C and +8°C in its original package. Do not freeze

6.5 Nature and contents of container
SOMATULINE AUTOGEL is supplied in a clear polypropylene pre-filled syringe with a stainless steel needle and a plunger stopper made from bromobutyl rubber coated with silicone.

Each pre-filled syringe is packed in a nylon/polyethylene/aluminium laminated bag.

Box of one individual 60mg dose in a 0.3mL syringe with a needle (1.2 mm × 20mm).

Box of one individual 90mg dose in a 0.3mL syringe with a needle (1.2 mm × 20mm).

Box of one individual 120mg dose in a 0.5mL syringe with a needle (1.4 mm × 20mm).

6.6 Special precautions for disposal and other handling
The solution for injection in a pre-filled syringe is ready for use.

For immediate and single use following first opening.

7. MARKETING AUTHORISATION HOLDER
Ipsen Limited

190 Bath Road

Slough, Berkshire

SL1 3XE, UK

8. MARKETING AUTHORISATION NUMBER(S)
PL 06958/0013 (Somatuline® Autogel® 60mg)

PL 06958/0014 (Somatuline® Autogel® 90mg)

PL 06958/0015 (Somatuline® Autogel® 120mg)

9. DATE OF FIRST AUTHORISATION/RENEWAL OF THE AUTHORISATION
16th October 2001

10. DATE OF REVISION OF THE TEXT
August 2007

Somatuline LA

(Ipsen Ltd)

1. NAME OF THE MEDICINAL PRODUCT
Somatuline LA

2. QUALITATIVE AND QUANTITATIVE COMPOSITION
Lanreotide (I.N.N., B.A.N.) 0.030 g*

*Each vial is filled with a quantity of microparticles of lanreotide acetate and co-polymers corresponding to 40 mg of lanreotide base, which ensures the actual injection of 30 mg of lanreotide.

3. PHARMACEUTICAL FORM
Powder for suspension for injection.

4. CLINICAL PARTICULARS
4.1 Therapeutic indications
Acromegaly:

Somatuline LA is indicated for the treatment of acromegaly when the circulating levels of growth hormone remain abnormal after surgery and/or radiotherapy.

Thyrotrophic Adenomas:

Somatuline LA is indicated for the treatment of thyrotrophic adenomas when the circulating level of thyroid stimulating hormone remains inappropriately high after surgery and/or radiotherapy.

Neuroendocrine Tumours:

Somatuline LA is also indicated for the relief of symptoms associated with neuroendocrine (particularly carcinoid) tumours.

4.2 Posology and method of administration
Acromegaly and Neuroendocrine Tumours:

Initially, one intramuscular injection should be given every 14 days. The frequency of subsequent injections may be varied in accordance with the individual patient's response (as judged by a reduction in symptoms and/or a reduction in GH and/or IGF-1 levels) such that injections can be given every 7 to 10 days as necessary.

Thyroid tumours:

Treatment should only be initiated and maintained by physicians experienced in the management of this condition.

Initially, one intra-muscular injection should be given every 14 days. In the case of an insufficient response, as judged by the levels of thyroid hormone and TSH, the frequency of injection may be increased to 1 every 10 days. Continued treatment should be guided by periodic measurement of thyroid hormone and TSH.

Elderly:

No dose modification is required in elderly patients.

Children:

As there is no experience of the use of the product in children, the use of Somatuline LA in children cannot be advised.

4.3 Contraindications
Somatuline LA should not be prescribed during pregnancy and lactation, nor in patients presenting with hypersensitivity to the peptide or related peptides.

4.4 Special warnings and precautions for use
Pharmacological studies in animals and humans show that lanreotide, like somatostatin and its analogues, inhibit secretion of insulin and glucagon. Hence, patients treated with Somatuline LA may experience hypoglycaemia or hyperglycaemia. Blood glucose levels should be monitored when lanreotide treatment is initiated and treatment of diabetic patients should be accordingly adjusted (see Section 4.8).

Lanreotide may reduce gall bladder motility and therefore, gall bladder echography is advised at the start of treatment and every six months thereafter. If gallstones do occur, they are generally asymptomatic. Symptomatic stones should be treated as medically indicated.

Fat concentrations in stools may increase to levels high enough to result in steatorrhoea, requiring the use of appropriate corrective therapy.

In patients with hepatic/renal dysfunction, kidney and liver function should be regularly monitored and the dose interval adjusted if necessary.

4.5 Interaction with other medicinal products and other forms of interaction
The gastrointestinal effects of Somatuline LA may reduce the intestinal absorption of co-administered drugs. As with other somatostatin analogues, Somatuline LA may reduce the intestinal absorption of cyclosporin A. Interactions with highly plasma bound drugs are unlikely in view of the moderate binding of lanreotide to serum proteins (78 % mean serum binding).

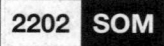

4.6 Pregnancy and lactation
Studies in animals showed transitory growth retardation of offspring prior to weaning. Although no teratogenic effects have been observed in animals, in the absence of clinical experience, lanreotide must not be administered to pregnant or lactating women.

4.7 Effects on ability to drive and use machines
Therapy with Somatuline LA is unlikely to impair a patient's ability to drive or use machinery.

4.8 Undesirable effects
Clinical tolerance

The side effects of Somatuline LA reported in the clinical trials are mainly local and gastrointestinal.

Local tolerance: moderate, transitory pain at the injection site is sometimes associated with local redness.

General tolerance: gastrointestinal side effects are the most common and include: diarrhoea or soft stools, abdominal pain, flatulence, anorexia, nausea and vomiting. In general, all these side effects are mild to moderate in intensity; in most cases the frequency and the intensity of such effects appear to diminish or to resolve with continued therapy.

Cases of asymptomatic and symptomatic gallbladder lithiasis have been reported in patients during prolonged treatment. A precautionary statement is included in section 4.4. In rare instances, acute pancreatitis has been reported within a short time after the first administration.

Biological tolerance

Altered glucose regulation has been reported in healthy volunteers. In non-diabetic patients both glucose intolerance and hyperglycaemia has been observed (See section 4.4).

4.9 Overdose
There is no human experience of overdosage. Animal data do not predict any effects other than those on insulin and glucagon secretion and the gastrointestinal system. If overdosage occurs, symptomatic management is indicated.

5. PHARMACOLOGICAL PROPERTIES
5.1 Pharmacodynamic properties
Like natural somatostatin, lanreotide is a peptide inhibitor of a number of endocrine, neuroendocrine, exocrine and paracrine functions. It shows good affinity for peripheral somatostatin receptors (anterior pituitary and pancreatic). In contrast, its affinity for central receptors is much lower. This profile confers a good specificity of action at the level of growth hormone and digestive hormone secretion.

Lanreotide shows a much longer duration of action than natural somatostatin. In addition, its marked selectivity for the secretion of growth hormone, compared to that of insulin, makes it a suitable candidate for the treatment of acromegaly. By inhibiting the synthesis of thyroid stimulating hormone (TSH), lanreotide also normalised thyroid function of patients with thyrotrophin secreting adenomas in 50% (8/16) of the per-protocol population treated for 6 months. There was no significant reduction in the size of the adenoma. Furthermore, the inhibitory action of lanreotide on intestinal exocrine secretion, digestive hormones and cellular proliferation mechanisms is suited to the symptomatic treatment of endocrine digestive tumours, especially carcinoids.

5.2 Pharmacokinetic properties
The plasma profile of lanreotide administered intramuscularly in healthy volunteers, is characterised by an initial rapid release phase (phase 1) followed by a prolonged slow release phase (phase 2). The first plasma peak (C_{max1}: 6.8 ± 3.8µg/l) occurs at 1.4 ± 0.8 hours and the second (C_{max2}: 2.5 ± 0.9µg/l) at 1.9 ± 1.8 days. The absolute bioavailability is 46.1 ± 16.7%. The mean residence time of 8.0 ± 1.0 days and the apparent half-life of 5.2 ± 2.5 days, confirm the prolonged release of the product.

After a single administration in acromegaly patients, a comparable pharmacokinetic profile is observed and the levels of growth hormone and IGF-1 are significantly reduced for a period of about 14 days. With repeated administration over several months, there is no evidence of accumulation of lanreotide.

5.3 Preclinical safety data
In vitro and animal toxicology studies have not shown any specific toxic potential for lanreotide. The observed effects are related to the pharmacological properties of lanreotide on the endocrine system. The resorption of Somatuline LA is complete in 45-60 days.

6. PHARMACEUTICAL PARTICULARS
6.1 List of excipients
Lactide-glycolide copolymer

Lactic-glycolic copolymer

Mannitol

Carmellose (Na)

Polysorbate 80

6.2 Incompatibilities
Somatuline LA must be made up immediately prior to use, using only the solution supplied in the package.

6.3 Shelf life
2 years

6.4 Special precautions for storage
Store at a temperature between +2°C and 8°C (in the refrigerator), do not freeze.

6.5 Nature and contents of container
Type I, clear, slightly tinted, glass vial containing sterile Somatuline LA.

Box of 1 vial, 1 ampoule (vehicle), 2 needles and 1 syringe.

Box of 2 vials, 2 ampoules (vehicle), 4 needles and 2 syringes.

Box of 6 vials, 6 ampoules (vehicle), 12 needles and 6 syringes.

6.6 Special precautions for disposal and other handling
Somatuline LA must be made up in the supplied solution immediately before injection, by shaking the vial, gently, 20 to 30 times, in order to obtain a homogenous suspension with a milky appearance. This must not be mixed with other medications.

NB: It is important that injection of this product is performed according to the instructions in the leaflet.

7. MARKETING AUTHORISATION HOLDER
IPSEN LIMITED

190 BATH ROAD

SLOUGH SL 1 3XE

8. MARKETING AUTHORISATION NUMBER(S)
Somatuline LA PL number: 06958 / 0018

9. DATE OF FIRST AUTHORISATION/RENEWAL OF THE AUTHORISATION
26 January 1998

10. DATE OF REVISION OF THE TEXT
4th August 2003

SOMAVERT 10mg, 15mg & 20mg powder and solvent for solution for injection

(Pfizer Limited)

1. NAME OF THE MEDICINAL PRODUCT
SOMAVERT▼ 10 mg powder and solvent for solution for injection.

SOMAVERT▼ 15 mg Powder and solvent for solution for injection.

SOMAVERT▼ 20 mg Powder and solvent for solution for injection.

2. QUALITATIVE AND QUANTITATIVE COMPOSITION

Presentations	
SOMAVERT 10mg	Each vial contains 10 mg of pegvisomant. After reconstitution, 1 ml of solution contains 10 mg pegvisomant.
SOMAVERT 15mg	Each vial contains 15 mg of pegvisomant. After reconstitution, 1 ml of solution contains 15 mg pegvisomant.
SOMAVERT 20mg	Each vial contains 20 mg of pegvisomant. After reconstitution, 1 ml of solution contains 20 mg pegvisomant.

Pegvisomant is produced in *E Coli* by recombinant DNA technology.

For a full list of excipients, see section 6.1.

3. PHARMACEUTICAL FORM
Powder and solvent for solution for injection.

The powder is white to slightly off-white.

4. CLINICAL PARTICULARS
4.1 Therapeutic indications
Treatment of patients with acromegaly who have had an inadequate response to surgery and/or radiation therapy and in whom an appropriate medical treatment with somatostatin analogues did not normalize IGF-I concentrations or was not tolerated.

4.2 Posology and method of administration
Treatment should be initiated under the supervision of a physician experienced in the treatment of acromegaly.

For the different dosage regimens the following strengths are available: SOMAVERT 10 mg, SOMAVERT 15 mg and SOMAVERT 20 mg.

For instructions on preparation see section 6.6

A loading dose of 80 mg pegvisomant should be administered subcutaneously under medical supervision. Following this, SOMAVERT 10 mg reconstituted in 1 ml of solvent should be administered once daily as a subcutaneous injection.

The site of injection should be rotated daily to help prevent lipohypertrophy.

Dose adjustments should be based on serum IGF-I levels. Serum IGF-I concentrations should be measured every four to six weeks and appropriate dose adjustments made in increments of 5 mg/day in order to maintain the serum IGF-I concentration within the age-adjusted normal range and to maintain an optimal therapeutic response.

The maximum dose should not exceed 30 mg/day.

Elderly patients

No dose adjustment is required.

Paediatric patients

There is no experience in children

Patients with impaired hepatic or renal function

The safety and effectiveness of SOMAVERT in patients with renal or hepatic insufficiency has not been established.

4.3 Contraindications
Hypersensitivity to the active substance or to any of the excipients.

4.4 Special warnings and precautions for use
Growth hormone-secreting pituitary tumours may sometimes expand, causing serious complications (for example, visual field defects). Treatment by SOMAVERT does not reduce tumour size. All patients with these tumours should be carefully monitored in order to avoid any eventual progression in tumour size under treatment.

SOMAVERT is a potent antagonist of growth hormone action. A growth hormone deficient state may result from SOMAVERT administration, despite the presence of elevated serum growth hormone levels. Serum IGF-I concentrations should be monitored and maintained within the age-adjusted normal range by adjustment of SOMAVERT dosing.

Serum concentrations of alanine aminotransferase (ALT) and aspartate transaminase (AST) should be monitored at four to six week intervals for the first six months of treatment with SOMAVERT, or at any time in patients exhibiting symptoms suggestive of hepatitis. Evidence of obstructive biliary tract disease should be ruled out in patients with elevations of ALT and AST or in patients with a prior history of treatment with any somatostatin analogue. Administration of SOMAVERT should be discontinued if signs of liver disease persist.

The study conducted with SOMAVERT in diabetic patients treated either by insulin or by oral hypoglycaemic medicinal products revealed the risk of hypoglycemia in this population. Therefore, in acromegalic patients with diabetes mellitus, doses of insulin or hypoglycaemic medicinal products may need to be decreased (see also section 4.5).

The therapeutic benefits of a reduction in IGF-I concentration which results in improvement of the patient's clinical condition could potentially increase fertility in female patients. Patients should be advised to use adequate contraception if necessary. SOMAVERT is not recommended during pregnancy (see also section 4.6).

4.5 Interaction with other medicinal products and other forms of interaction
No interaction studies have been performed. It should be considered whether to continue treatment with somatostatin analogues. The use of SOMAVERT in combination with other medicinal products for the treatment of acromegaly has not been extensively investigated.

Patients receiving insulin or oral hypoglycaemic medicinal products may require dose reduction of these active substances due to the effect of pegvisomant on insulin sensitivity (see section 4.4).

SOMAVERT has significant structural similarity to growth hormone which causes it to cross-react in commercially available growth hormone assays. Since serum concentrations of therapeutically-effective doses of SOMAVERT are generally 100 to 1000 times higher than the actual serum growth hormone concentrations seen in acromegalics, measurements of serum growth hormone concentrations will be spuriously reported in commercially available growth hormone assays. SOMAVERT treatment should therefore not be monitored or adjusted based on serum growth hormone concentrations reported from these assays.

4.6 Pregnancy and lactation
For pegvisomant no clinical data on exposed pregnancies are available.

Animal studies are insufficient with respect to effects on pregnancy, embryonal/foetal development, parturition or postnatal development (see section 5.3). The potential risk for humans is unknown.

SOMAVERT should not be used during pregnancy unless clearly necessary (see also section 4.4).

Use during lactation

The excretion of pegvisomant in breast milk has not been studied in animals. Clinical data are too limited (one reported case) to draw any conclusion on the excretion of pegvisomant in human breast milk. Therefore, SOMAVERT should not be used in breast-feeding women. However, breast-feeding may be continued if SOMAVERT is discontinued: this decision should take into account the benefit of SOMAVERT therapy to the mother and the benefit of breastfeeding to the child

4.7 Effects on ability to drive and use machines
No studies on the effect on the ability to drive and use machines have been performed.

4.8 Undesirable effects
The list below contains adverse reactions seen in clinical trials.

In clinical studies, for patients treated with pegvisomant (n=160), the majority of adverse reactions to pegvisomant were of mild to moderate intensity, of limited duration and did not require discontinuation of treatment.

The most commonly reported adverse reactions considered related to SOMAVERT occurring in ⩾ 5% of patients with acromegaly during the clinical trials were injection site reactions 11%, sweating 7%, headache 6% and asthenia 6%.

Adverse reactions are listed according to the following categories:

Very common: ⩾ 1/10
Common: ⩾1/100 to <1/10
Uncommon: ⩾1/1,000 to <1/100

Blood and lymphatic system disorders:
Uncommon: thrombocytopenia, leukopenia, leukocytosis, bleeding tendency

Nervous system disorders:
Common: headache, dizziness, somnolence, tremor
Uncommon: hypoesthesia, dysgeusia, migraine, narcolepsy

Eye disorders:
Uncommon: asthenopia, eye pain

Ear and labyrinth disorders:
Uncommon: Meniere's disease

Respiratory, thoracic and mediastinal disorders:
Uncommon: dyspnea

Gastrointestinal disorders:
Common: diarrhoea, constipation, nausea, vomiting, abdominal distension, dyspepsia, flatulence
Uncommon: dry mouth, hemorrhoids, salivary hypersecretion, tooth disorder

Renal and urinary disorders:
Uncommon: heamaturia, proteinuria, polyuria, renal impairment

Skin and subcutaneous tissue disorders:
Common: sweating, pruritis, rash
Uncommon: face oedema, dry skin, contusion, tendency to bruise, night sweats

Musculoskeletal and connective tissue disorders:
Common: arthralgia, myalgia, peripheral swelling
Uncommon: arthritis

Metabolism and nutrition disorders:
Common: hypercholesterolemia, weight gain, hyperglycemia, hunger
Uncommon: hypertriglyceridemia, hypoglycemia

Vascular disorders:
Common: hypertension

General disorders and administration site conditions
Common: influenza-like illness, fatigue, injection site bruising or bleeding, injection site reaction, (including injection site hypersensitivity), injection site hypertrophy, (e.g. lipohypertrophy)*
Uncommon: oedema lower limb, pyrexia, weakness, asthenia, feeling abnormal, impaired healing, peripheral oedema

Hepatobiliary disorders
Common abnormal liver function tests (e.g. transaminase elevation) (see section 4.4)

Psychiatric disorders:
Common: abnormal dreams, sleep disorder
Uncommon: anger, apathy, confusion, increased libido, panic attack, short term memory loss

*see Additional Information below.

Additional Information
Most injection site reactions characterised as localised erythemas and soreness, spontaneously resolved with local symptomatic treatment, while SOMAVERT therapy continued. Occurrence of injection site hypertrophies has been observed, including lipohypertrophy.

The development of isolated low-titre anti-growth hormone antibodies was observed in 16.9% of patients treated with SOMAVERT. The clinical significance of these antibodies is unknown.

4.9 Overdose
There is limited experience of overdosage with SOMAVERT. In the one reported incident of acute overdosage, where 80 mg/day was administered for 7 days, the patient experienced a slight increase in fatigue and dry mouth. In the week following discontinuation of treatment the adverse reactions noted were: insomnia, increased fatigue, a trace of foot oedema, fine tremor, and weight gain. Two weeks after stopping treatment, leukocytosis and moderate bleeding from injection and vein puncture sites was observed which were considered possibly related to SOMAVERT.

In cases of overdose, administration of SOMAVERT should be discontinued and not resumed until IGF-I levels return to within or above the normal range.

5. PHARMACOLOGICAL PROPERTIES
5.1 Pharmacodynamic properties
Pharmacotherapeutic group: Other anterior pituitary lobe hormones and analogues, ATC code: H01AX01.

Pegvisomant is an analogue of human growth hormone that has been genetically modified to be a growth hormone receptor antagonist. Pegvisomant binds to growth hormone receptors on cell surfaces, where it blocks growth hormone binding, and thus interferes with intracellular growth hormone signal transduction. Pegvisomant is highly selective for the GH receptor, and does not cross-react with other cytokine receptors, including prolactin. Inhibition of growth hormone action with pegvisomant leads to decreased serum concentrations of insulin-like growth factor-I (IGF-I), as well as other growth hormone-responsive serum proteins such as free IGF-I, the acid-labile subunit of IGF-I (ALS), and insulin-like growth factor binding protein-3 (IGFBP-3).

Acromegalic patients (n=112) have been treated in a 12-week, randomised, double-blind, multicentre study comparing placebo and pegvisomant. Dose-dependent, statistically significant reductions in mean IGF-I ($p<0.0001$), free IGF-I ($p<0.05$), IGFBP-3 ($p<0.05$) and ALS ($p<0.05$) were observed at all post-baseline visits in the pegvisomant treatment groups. The serum IGF-1 was normalised at the end of the study (week 12) in 9.7%, 38.5%, 75% and 82% of subjects treated with placebo, 10 mg/day, 15 mg/day or 20 mg/day SOMAVERT respectively.

Statistically significant differences from placebo ($p<0.05$) were observed for improvements in the total signs and symptoms score for all dose groups compared to placebo.

A cohort of 38 acromegalic subjects has been followed in a long-term, open-label, dose-titration study for at least 12 consecutive months of daily dosing with pegvisomant (mean = 55 weeks). The mean IGF-I concentration in this cohort fell from 917 ng/ml to 299 ng/ml on pegvisomant, with 92% achieving a normal (age-adjusted) IGF-I concentration.

5.2 Pharmacokinetic properties
Absorption of pegvisomant following subcutaneous administration is slow and prolonged, and peak serum pegvisomant concentrations are not generally attained until 33-77 hours after administration. The mean extent of absorption of a subcutaneous dose was 57% relative to an intravenous dose.

The apparent volume of distribution of pegvisomant is relatively small (7-12 l). The mean total body systemic clearance of pegvisomant following multiple doses is estimated to be 28 ml/h for subcutaneous doses ranging from 10 to 20 mg/day. Renal clearance of pegvisomant is negligible and accounts for less than 1% of total body clearance. Pegvisomant is slowly eliminated from serum, with mean estimates of half-life generally ranging from 74 to 172 hours following either single or multiple-doses. The metabolism of pegvisomant is not studied.

After single subcutaneous pegvisomant administration no linearity is observed with rising doses of 10, 15 or 20 mg. Approximately linear pharmacokinetics is observed at steady state in the population pharmacokinetic studies. The data from 145 patients in two long-term studies who received daily doses of 10, 15, or 20 mg, demonstrate pegvisomant mean serum concentrations (± SD) of approximately 8800 ± 6300, 13200 ± 8000 and 15600 ± 10300 ng/ml, respectively.

The pharmacokinetics of pegvisomant are similar in normal healthy volunteers and acromegaly patients, although heavier individuals tend to have a higher total body clearance of pegvisomant than lighter individuals, and may thus require greater doses of pegvisomant.

No pharmacokinetic data in special populations (children, populations with renal and hepatic impairment) are available.

5.3 Preclinical safety data
Non-clinical data revealed no special hazard for humans based on conventional studies of repeated dose toxicity in rat and monkey. However, due to the marked pharmacological response in monkey, systemic exposures higher than those achieved in patients at therapeutic doses have not been studied. Except for one segment II test in the rabbit, no other reproductive toxicity studies were conducted.

No data on carcinogenic potential are available.

6. PHARMACEUTICAL PARTICULARS
6.1 List of excipients
Powder:
Glycine
Mannitol (E421)
Sodium phosphate dibasic anhydrous
Sodium phosphate monobasic monohydrate
Solvent:
Water for Injections

6.2 Incompatibilities
This medicinal product must not be mixed with other medicinal products except those mentioned in section 6.6.

6.3 Shelf life
3 years
After reconstitution, the product should be used immediately.

6.4 Special precautions for storage
Store in a refrigerator (2°C – 8°C). Do not freeze. Keep the container in the outer carton in order to protect from light.
After reconstitution:
Use immediately.

6.5 Nature and contents of container
Powder in a vial (type I glass) with a rubber stopper (butyl) and 8 ml solvent in a vial (type I glass) with a (rubber butyl). Pack size: 30 vials of powder along with 30 vials of solvent. SOMAVERT 20 mg also available in pack size of 1 vial

6.6 Special precautions for disposal and other handling
Reconstitute using 1 ml solvent

Add solvent to vial with powder for injection. Gently dissolve the powder with a slow, swirling motion. Do not shake vigorously, as this might cause denaturation of the active ingredient.

After reconstitution, if the solution is cloudy or contains particulate matter, the product must be discarded.

For single use only. Any unused product or waste material should be disposed of in accordance with local requirements.

7. MARKETING AUTHORISATION HOLDER
Pfizer Limited
Sandwich
Kent CT13 9NJ
United Kingdom

8. MARKETING AUTHORISATION NUMBER(S)
EU/1/02/240/001 - SOMAVERT 10 mg; pack size 30 vials
EU/1/02/240/002 - SOMAVERT 15 mg; pack size 30 vials
EU/1/02/240/003 - SOMAVERT 20 mg; pack size 30 vials
EU/1/02/240/004 - SOMAVERT 20 mg; pack size 1 vial

9. DATE OF FIRST AUTHORISATION/RENEWAL OF THE AUTHORISATION
Date of first authorization: 13/11/2002
Date of last renewal: 20/09/2007

10. DATE OF REVISION OF THE TEXT
June 2008

11. LEGAL CATEGORY
POM

Ref: SV5_0

Sominex Tablets (Actavis UK Ltd)

(Actavis UK Ltd)

1. NAME OF THE MEDICINAL PRODUCT
Sominex

2. QUALITATIVE AND QUANTITATIVE COMPOSITION
Promethazine hydrochloride EP 20mg/tab

3. PHARMACEUTICAL FORM
Tablet

4. CLINICAL PARTICULARS
4.1 Therapeutic indications
As a night-time sleep aid, for the correction of temporary disturbances of sleep pattern where there is difficulty in going to sleep or staying asleep, caused for example by specific dislocation of normal routine.

4.2 Posology and method of administration
Oral

For bedtime use only.

Adults: one tablet at bedtime. May be taken up to one hour after going to bed when sleep is difficult to achieve.

Not to be given to children under the age of 16 years except on medical advice.

Elderly: the normal adult dose may be taken.

4.3 Contraindications
Known hypersensitivity to promethazine or phenothiazines. Patients taking MAOIs or within 14 days of taking MAOIs. Patients with any form of CNS depression.

4.4 Special warnings and precautions for use
Cause drowsiness. Do not drive or operate machinery.

Not to be used for more than 7 days without medical advice.

Concomitant use of alcohol should be avoided.

In patients with asthma or other respiratory disorders (eg bronchitis or bronchiectasis), glaucoma, epilepsy, urinary retention, prostatic hypertrophy, hepatic or renal impairment, cardiovascular problems or pyloroduodenal obstruction the product should only be taken after consulting a doctor.

Patients with rare hereditary problems of galactose intolerance, the Lapp lactase deficiency or glucose-galactose malabsorption should not take this medicine.

4.5 Interaction with other medicinal products and other forms of interaction
Promethazine hydrochloride may potentiate the action of alcohol and other centrally acting depressants, hypnotics

and anxiolytics. MAOIs may enhance the antimuscarinic effects of antihistamines.

Antihistamines have an added antimuscarinic effect with other antimuscarinic drugs such as atropine and tricyclic antidepressants. Promethazine may interfere with immunologic urine pregnancy tests to produce false positive or negative results.

4.6 Pregnancy and lactation

The advice of a doctor should be sought before use.

4.7 Effects on ability to drive and use machines

This product causes drowsiness. Do not drive or operate machinery.

4.8 Undesirable effects

Drowsiness, headache, psychomotor impairment, antimuscarinic effects (such as urinary retention, dry mouth, blurred vision), disorientation, restlessness and gastrointestinal disturbances, palpitations, arrhythmias, hypotension and anaphylaxis may occasionally occur.

Dizziness, tremor, extrapyramidal effects, angle closure glaucoma and hypersensitivity reactions (including bronchospasm, angioedema, anaphylaxis and rashes) are rare side effects of antihistamines.

Jaundice and blood dyscrasias occur rarely.

Photosensitivity reactions have been reported.

The elderly are particularly susceptible to the anticholinergic effects and confusion due to promethazine.

4.9 Overdose

In children, promethazine overdose can cause CNS stimulation, including ataxia, tremors and hallucinations, and antimuscarinic effects. In severe cases in both adults and children, CNS depression with coma and convulsions may occur. Cardiorespiratory depression is uncommon.

Gastric lavage or activated charcoal is only recommended if the patient presents within 1 hour of ingestion of a potentially toxic amount.

Treatment is otherwise supportive with attention to maintenance of adequate respiratory and circulatory status. Convulsions should be treated with diazepam or other suitable anticonvulsants.

Forced diuresis, haemodialysis and haemoperfusion are of no value

5. PHARMACOLOGICAL PROPERTIES

5.1 Pharmacodynamic properties

Promethazine hydrochloride – sedative. The drug is an antihistamine with anticholinergic activity.

5.2 Pharmacokinetic properties

Promethazine hydrochloride is readily absorbed from the gastrointestinal tract, but undergoes extensive first pass metabolism in the liver. With only 25% of the oral dose reaching the systemic circulation unchanged. After oral therapy therapeutic effects are identifiable at 15-30 minutes and peak plasma concentrations at 2 to 3 hours. Estimates of terminal half-life in blood plasma have been quoted as 4-6 hours. It is extensively plasma protein bound. It is eliminated mainly as metabolites, predominantly by the faecal (via biliary) route, with <1% of the parent compound and CA 10% as the sulphoxide metabolite being excreted in the urine over a 72 hour period.

5.3 Preclinical safety data

None stated.

6. PHARMACEUTICAL PARTICULARS

6.1 List of excipients

Lactose, maize starch, croscarmellose sodium, magnesium stearate.

6.2 Incompatibilities

None known.

6.3 Shelf life

60 months unopened.

6.4 Special precautions for storage

None.

6.5 Nature and contents of container

Opaque blister strip of polyvinylchloride/polyvinylidine chloride. Backed with aluminium foil. Each strip contains 8 tablets. One or two strips are packed into each cardboard carton.

6.6 Special precautions for disposal and other handling

None.

7. MARKETING AUTHORISATION HOLDER

Actavis Group PTC ehf

Reykjavíkurvegi 76-78

220 Hafnarfjordur

Iceland.

8. MARKETING AUTHORISATION NUMBER(S)

PL 30306/0080

9. DATE OF FIRST AUTHORISATION/RENEWAL OF THE AUTHORISATION

6th September 2002

10. DATE OF REVISION OF THE TEXT

11 DOSIMETRY (IF APPLICABLE)

Not Applicable

12 INSTRUCTIONS FOR PREPARATION OF RADIOPHARMACEUTICALS (IF APPLICABLE)

Not Applicable

SonoVue 8 microlitres/ml, powder and solvent for dispersion for injection

(Bracco UK Limited)

1. NAME OF THE MEDICINAL PRODUCT

SonoVue 8 microlitres / ml powder and solvent for dispersion for injection

2. QUALITATIVE AND QUANTITATIVE COMPOSITION

One ml contains 8μl of sulphur hexafluoride microbubbles

On reconstitution as directed, 1 ml of the resulting dispersion contains 8 μl sulphur hexafluoride in the microbubbles, equivalent to 45 microgrammes.

For a full list of excipients, see section 6.1

3. PHARMACEUTICAL FORM

Powder and solvent for dispersion for injection.

SonoVue is a kit including

1 vial containing 25 mg of lyophilised powder

1 pre-filled syringe containing 5 ml sodium chloride

1 Mini-Spike transfer system

Information on the appearance of the reconstituted solution is given in section 6.6.

4. CLINICAL PARTICULARS

4.1 Therapeutic indications

This medicinal product is for diagnostic use only.

SonoVue is for use with ultrasound imaging to enhance the echogenicity of the blood, which results in an improved signal to noise ratio.

SonoVue should only be used in patients where study without contrast enhancement is inconclusive.

Echocardiography

SonoVue is a transpulmonary echocardiographic contrast agent for use in patients with suspected or established cardiovascular disease to provide opacification of cardiac chambers and enhance left ventricular endocardial border delineation.

Doppler of macrovasculature

SonoVue increases the accuracy in detection or exclusion of abnormalities in cerebral arteries and extracranial carotid or peripheral arteriesby improving the Doppler signal to noise ratio.

SonoVue increases the quality of the Doppler flow image and the duration of clinically-useful signal enhancement in portal vein assessment.

Doppler of microvasculature

SonoVue improves display of the vascularity of liver and breast lesions during Doppler sonography, leading to more specific lesion characterisation.

4.2 Posology and method of administration

This product should only be used by physicians experienced in diagnostic ultrasound imaging.

The recommended doses of SonoVue are:

B-mode imaging of cardiac chambers, at rest or with stress: 2 ml.

Vascular Doppler imaging: 2.4 ml.

During a single examination, a second injection of the recommended dose can be made when deemed necessary by the physician.

Elderly Patients

The dosage recommendations also apply to elderly patients.

Paediatric Patients

The safety and effectiveness of SonoVue in patients under 18 years old has not been established and the product should not be used in these patients.

The microbubble dispersion is prepared before use by injecting through the septum 5 ml of sodium chloride 9 mg/ml (0.9%) solution for injection to the contents of the vial. The vial is then shaken vigorously for a few seconds until the lyophilisate is completely dissolved. The desired volume of the dispersion can be drawn into a syringe any time up to six hours after reconstitution. Just before drawing into the syringe, the vial should be agitated to re-suspend the microbubbles. SonoVue should be administered immediately after drawing into the syringe by injection into a peripheral vein. Every injection should be followed by a flush with 5 ml of sodium chloride 9 mg/ml (0.9%) solution for injection.

For instructions for preparation see section 6.6.

4.3 Contraindications

SonoVue should not be administered to patients with known hypersensitivity to sulphur hexafluoride or to any of the components of SonoVue.

SonoVue is contraindicated for use in patients with recent acute coronary syndrome or clinically unstable ischaemic cardiac disease, including: evolving or ongoing myocardial infarction, typical angina at rest within last 7 days, significant worsening of cardiac symptoms within last 7 days, recent coronary artery intervention or other factors suggesting clinical instability (for example, recent deterioration of ECG, laboratory or clinical findings), acute cardiac failure, Class III/IV cardiac failure, or severe rhythm disorders.

SonoVue is contraindicated in patients known to have right-to-left shunts, severe pulmonary hypertension (pulmonary artery pressure >90 mmHg), uncontrolled systemic hypertension, and in patients with adult respiratory distress syndrome.

The safety and efficacy of SonoVue have not been established in pregnant and lactating women therefore, SonoVue should not be administered during pregnancy and lactation (see Section 4.6).

4.4 Special warnings and precautions for use

ECG monitoring should be performed in high-risk patients as clinically indicated.

It should be emphasised that stress echocardiography, which can mimic an ischaemic episode, could potentially increase the risk of SonoVue utilisation. Therefore, if SonoVue is to be used in conjunction with stress echocardiography patients must have a stable condition verified by absence of chest pain or ECG modification during the two preceding days.

Moreover, ECG and blood pressure monitoring should be performed during SonoVue-enhanced echocardiography with a pharmacological stress (e.g. with dobutamine).

Care should be taken in patients with ischaemic cardiac disease because in these patients allergy-like and/or vasodilatory reactions may lead to life-threatening conditions.

Emergency equipment and personnel trained in its use must be readily available. Caution is advised when SonoVue is administered to patients with clinically significant pulmonary disease, including severe chronic obstructive pulmonary disease.

It is recommended to keep the patient under close medical supervision during and for at least 30 minutes following the administration of SonoVue.

Numbers of patients with the following conditions who were exposed to SonoVue in the clinical trials were limited, and therefore, caution is advisable when administering the product to patients with: acute endocarditis, prosthetic valves, acute systemic inflammation and/or sepsis, hyperactive coagulation states and/or recent thromboembolism, and end-stage renal or hepatic disease.

SonoVue is not suitable for use in ventilated patients, and those with unstable neurological diseases.

In animal studies, the application of echo-contrast agents revealed biological side effects (e.g. endothelial cell injury, capillary rupture) by interaction with the ultrasound beam. Although these biological side effects have not been reported in humans, the use of a low mechanical index is recommended.

4.5 Interaction with other medicinal products and other forms of interaction

No specific interaction studies have been performed. There was no apparent relationship with respect to occurrence of adverse events in the clinical studies for patients receiving various categories of the most common concomitant medications.

4.6 Pregnancy and lactation

No clinical data on exposed pregnancies are available. Animal studies do not indicate harmful effects with respect to pregnancy, embryonal/foetal development, parturition or postnatal development

(see section 5.3 Preclinical safety data). Caution should be exercised when prescribing to pregnant women. It is not known if sulphur hexafluoride is excreted in human milk. Therefore, caution should be exercised when SonoVue is administered to breast-feeding women.

4.7 Effects on ability to drive and use machines

On the basis of the pharmacokinetic and pharmacodynamic profiles, no or negligible influence is expected with the use of SonoVue on the ability to drive or use machines.

4.8 Undesirable effects

The undesirable effects reported with SonoVue were, in general, non-serious, transient and resolved spontaneously without residual effects.

In clinical trials, the most commonly reported adverse reactions are headache (2.3%), injection site reaction including bruising, burning and paraesthesia at the injection site (1.7%) and injection site pain (1.4%).

There were changes in ECG, blood pressure and in some laboratory parameters measured, but these were not deemed to be of clinical significance.

The adverse reactions reported among 1788 adult patients in clinical studies are:

Body system	Common >1/100, <1/10)	Uncommon >1/1,000 - <1/100)
Metabolism and nutrition disorders		Hyperglycaemia

Nervous system disorders	Headache	Paraesthesia, dizziness, insomnia, taste perversion
Eye disorders		Vision blurred
Vascular disorder		Vasodilatation
Respiratory, thoracic and mediastinal disorders		Pharyngitis, sinus pain
Gastrointestinal disorders	Nausea	Abdominal pain
Skin and subcutaneous tissue disorders		Pruritus, rash erythematous
Musculoskeletal, connective tissue and bone disorders		Back pain
General disorders and administration site conditions	Injection site pain, injection site reaction, including bruising, burning and paraesthesia at the injection site	Chest pain, pain no organ system, asthenia

One case of sensory-motor paresis was reported.

Post marketing

Rare cases suggestive of hypersensitivity, which could include skin erythema, bradycardia, hypotension or anaphylactic shock have been reported following the injection of SonoVue. In some of these cases, in patients with underlying coronary artery disease, bradycardia and hypotension were accompanied by myocardial ischemia and/or myocardial infarctions.

In very rare cases, fatal outcomes have been reported in temporal association with the use of SonoVue. In all these patients there was a high underlying risk for major cardiac complications, which could have led to the fatal outcome.

4.9 Overdose

Since there have been no cases of overdose reported to date, neither signs nor symptoms of overdose have been identified. In a Phase I study doses up to 56 ml of SonoVue were administered to normal volunteers without serious adverse events being reported. In the event of overdose occurring, the patient should be observed and treated symptomatically.

5. PHARMACOLOGICAL PROPERTIES

5.1 Pharmacodynamic properties

Pharmacotherapeutic group: Ultrasound contrast media

ATC code: VO8DA.

The addition of sodium chloride 9 mg/ml (0.9%) solution for injection to the lyophilised powder followed by vigorous shaking results in the production of the microbubbles of sulphur hexafluoride. The microbubbles have a mean diameter of about 2.5μm, with 90% having a diameter less than 6μm and 99% having a diameter less than 11μm. Each millilitre of SonoVue contains 8μl of the microbubbles.The interface between the sulphur hexafluoride bubble and the aqueous medium acts as a reflector of the ultrasound beam thus enhancing blood echogenicity and increasing contrast between the blood and the surrounding tissues.

The intensity of the reflected signal is dependent on concentration of the microbubbles and frequency of the ultrasound beam. At the proposed clinical doses, SonoVue has been shown to provide marked increase in signal intensity of more than 2 minutes for B-mode imaging in echocardiography and of 3 to 8 minutes for Doppler imaging of the macrovasculature and microvasculature.

Sulphur hexafluoride is an inert, innocuous gas, poorly soluble in aqueous solutions. There are literature reports of the use of the gas in the study of respiratory physiology and in pneumatic retinopexy.

5.2 Pharmacokinetic properties

The total amount of sulphur hexafluoride administered in a clinical dose is extremely small, (in a 2 ml dose the microbubbles contain 16 μl of gas). The sulphur hexafluoride dissolves in the blood and is subsequently exhaled.

After a single intravenous injection of 0.03 or 0.3 ml of SonoVue/kg (approximately 1 and 10 times the maximum clinical dose) to human volunteers, the sulphur hexafluoride was cleared rapidly. The mean terminal half-life was 12 minutes (range 2 to 33 minutes). More than 80% of the administered sulphur hexafluoride was recovered in exhaled air within 2 minutes after injection and almost 100% after 15 minutes.

In patients with diffuse interstitial pulmonary fibrosis, the percent of dose recovered in expired air averaged 100% and the terminal half-life was similar to that measured in healthy volunteers.

Figure 1 Presentation 02 (with separate MiniSpike transfer system)

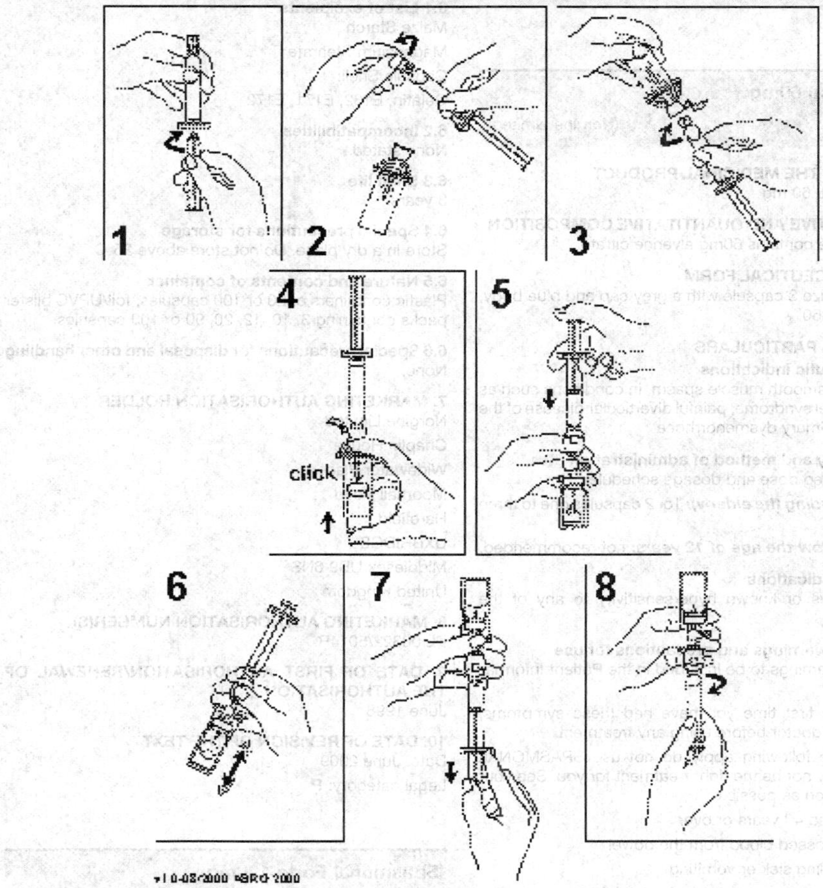

1. Connect the plunger rod by screwing it clockwise into the syringe.
2. Open the MiniSpike transfer system blister and remove syringe tip cap.
3. Open the transfer system cap and connect the syringe to the transfer system by screwing it in clockwise.
4. Remove Flipcap glass protective disk from the vial. Slide the vial into the transparent sleeve of the transfer system and press firmly to lock the vial in place.
5. Empty the contents of the syringe into the vial by pushing on the plunger rod.
6. Shake vigorously for 20 seconds to mix all the contents in the vial (white milky liquid).
7. Invert the system and carefully withdraw SonoVue into the syringe.
8. Unscrew the syringe from the transfer system.

5.3 Preclinical safety data

Non-clinical data reveal no special hazard for humans based on conventional studies of safety pharmacology, genotoxicity and toxicity to reproduction. Caecal lesions observed in some repeat- dose studies with rats, but not in monkeys, are not relevant for humans under normal conditions of administration.

6. PHARMACEUTICAL PARTICULARS

6.1 List of excipients

Powder:

Macrogol 4000

Distearoylphosphatidylcholine

Dipalmitoylphosphatidylglycerol Sodium

Palmitic acid

Solvent:

Sodium chloride 9 mg/ml (0.9%) solution for injection

6.2 Incompatibilities

In the absence of compatibility studies, SonoVue should not be admixed with any other medicinal product except the solvent provided.

6.3 Shelf life

2 years.

Once reconstituted, chemical and physical stability has been demonstrated for 6 hours. From a microbiological point of view, the product should be used immediately. If not used immediately, in use storage times and conditions prior to use are the responsibility of the user.

6.4 Special precautions for storage

The medicinal product does not require any special storage conditions.

For storage conditions of the reconstituted medicinal product, see section 6.3.

6.5 Nature and contents of container

Presentation 02 (with separate MiniSpike transfer system):-

25 mg of dry, lyophilised powder in an atmosphere of sulphur hexafluoride in a colourless

Type I glass vial, with elastomeric closure.

Separate transfer system.

Type I glass pre-filled syringe containing 5 ml sodium chloride 9 mg/ml (0.9%) solution for injection.

6.6 Special precautions for disposal and other handling

Before use examine the product to ensure that the container and closure have not been damaged.

SonoVue must be prepared before use by injecting through the septum 5 ml of sodium chloride 9 mg/ml (0.9%) solution for injection to the contents of the vial. The vial is then shaken vigorously for twenty seconds after which the desired volume of the dispersion can be drawn into a syringe as follows, depending on the presentation:

Presentation 02 (with separate MiniSpike transfer system)

(see Figure 1 above)

SonoVue should be administered immediately by injection into a peripheral vein.

After reconstitution, a homogeneous white milky liquid is obtained. If solid parts of the lyophilisate are seen or the suspension is not homogeneous, the product should be discarded. If SonoVue is not used immediately after reconstitution the microbubble dispersion should be shaken again before being drawn up into a syringe. Chemical and physical stability of the microbubble dispersion has been demonstrated for 6 hours.

The vial is for a single examination only. Any unused dispersion remaining at the end of an examination or waste material must be discarded in accordance with local requirements.

7. MARKETING AUTHORISATION HOLDER

Bracco International B.V.

Strawinskylaan 3051

NL - 1077 ZX Amsterdam

The Netherlands

8. MARKETING AUTHORISATION NUMBER(S)

EU/1/01/177/002

9. DATE OF FIRST AUTHORISATION/RENEWAL OF THE AUTHORISATION

26 March 2001/ 24 April 2006

10. DATE OF REVISION OF THE TEXT
24 April 2006

Spasmonal 60mg

(Norgine Limited)

1. NAME OF THE MEDICINAL PRODUCT
SPASMONAL 60 mg

2. QUALITATIVE AND QUANTITATIVE COMPOSITION
Each capsule contains 60mg alverine citrate.

3. PHARMACEUTICAL FORM
An opaque size 3 capsule with a grey cap and blue body, marked "SP 60".

4. CLINICAL PARTICULARS
4.1 Therapeutic indications
The relief of smooth muscle spasm, in conditions such as irritable bowel syndrome, painful diverticular disease of the colon and primary dysmenorrhoea

4.2 Posology and method of administration
Recommended dose and dosage schedules:

Adults (including the elderly): 1or 2 capsules one to three times daily.

Children below the age of 12 years: not recommended.

4.3 Contraindications
Paralytic ileus or known hypersensitivity to any of the ingredients.

4.4 Special warnings and precautions for use
Additional warnings to be included in the Patient Information Leaflet:

If this is the first time you have had these symptoms, consult your doctor before using any treatment.

If any of the following apply do not use SPASMONAL 60 mg; it may not be the right treatment for you. See your doctor as soon as possible if:

- you are aged 40 years or over
- you have passed blood from the bowel
- you are feeling sick or vomiting
- you have lost your appetite or lost weight
- you are looking pale and feeling tired
- you are suffering from severe constipation
- you have a fever
- you have recently travelled abroad
- you are or may be pregnant
- you have abnormal vaginal bleeding or discharge
- you have difficulty or pain passing urine.

Consult your doctor if you have developed new symptoms, or if your symptoms worsen, or if they do not improve after 2 weeks treatment.

4.5 Interaction with other medicinal products and other forms of interaction
None stated.

4.6 Pregnancy and lactation
Although no teratogenic effects have been reported, use during pregnancy or lactation is not recommended as evidence of safety in Preclinical studies is limited.

4.7 Effects on ability to drive and use machines
None.

4.8 Undesirable effects
Possible side effects may include nausea, headache, dizziness, itching, rash, and allergic reactions. There have been isolated reports of jaundice due to hepatitis, which may have been immune-mediated; but this adverse reaction resolved on cessation of alverine treatment.

4.9 Overdose
Can produce hypotension and atropine-like toxic effects. Management is as for atropine poisoning with supportive therapy for hypotension.

5. PHARMACOLOGICAL PROPERTIES
5.1 Pharmacodynamic properties
Alverine citrate is a spasmolytic, which has a specific action on the smooth muscle of the alimentary tract and uterus, without affecting the heart, blood vessels and tracheal muscle at therapeutic doses.

5.2 Pharmacokinetic properties
After oral administration, alverine is rapidly converted to its primary active metabolite, which is then further converted to two secondary metabolites. There is a high renal clearance of all metabolites indicating that they are eliminated by active renal secretion. The peak plasma level of the most active metabolite occurs between 1 and 1½ hours after oral dosing. The plasma half-life averages 0.8 hours for alverine and 5.7 hours for the active primary metabolite.

5.3 Preclinical safety data
Preclinical studies provide evidence that alverine citrate has no significant systemic toxicity potential at the proposed dosage.

6. PHARMACEUTICAL PARTICULARS
6.1 List of excipients
Maize Starch

Magnesium Stearate

Capsule Shell:

Gelatin, E132, E171, E172

6.2 Incompatibilities
None stated.

6.3 Shelf life
3 years.

6.4 Special precautions for storage
Store in a dry place. Do not store above 25°C.

6.5 Nature and contents of container
Plastic containers of 20 or 100 capsules; foil/UPVC blister packs containing 3, 10, 12, 20, 90 or 100 capsules.

6.6 Special precautions for disposal and other handling
None.

7. MARKETING AUTHORISATION HOLDER
Norgine Limited
Chaplin House
Widewater Place
Moorhall Road
Harefield
UXBRIDGE
Middlesex UB9 6NS
United Kingdom

8. MARKETING AUTHORISATION NUMBER(S)
PL 00322/5014R

9. DATE OF FIRST AUTHORISATION/RENEWAL OF THE AUTHORISATION
June 1998

10. DATE OF REVISION OF THE TEXT
Date: June 2009

Legal category: **P**

Spasmonal Forte 120mg

(Norgine Limited)

1. NAME OF THE MEDICINAL PRODUCT
SPASMONAL Forte 120 mg, Hard capsules.

2. QUALITATIVE AND QUANTITATIVE COMPOSITION
Each capsule contains 120 mg alverine citrate.

3. PHARMACEUTICAL FORM
An opaque, size 1 capsule with a grey cap and blue body, marked "SP120".

4. CLINICAL PARTICULARS
4.1 Therapeutic indications
The relief of smooth muscle spasm in conditions such as irritable bowel syndrome, painful diverticular disease of the colon and primary dysmenorrhoea.

4.2 Posology and method of administration
Recommended dose and dosage schedules:

Adults (including the elderly): 1 capsule one to three times daily.

Children below the age of 12 years: Not recommended.

4.3 Contraindications
Paralytic ileus or known hypersensitivity to any of the ingredients.

4.4 Special warnings and precautions for use
Additional warnings to be included in the Patient Information Leaflet:

If this is the first time you have had these symptoms, consult your doctor before using any treatment.

If any of the following apply do not use SPASMONAL Forte 120 mg, it may not be the right treatment for you. See your doctor as soon as possible if:

- you are aged 40 years or over
- you have passed blood from the bowel
- you are feeling sick or vomiting
- you have lost your appetite or lost weight
- you are looking pale and feeling tired
- you are suffering from severe constipation
- you have a fever
- you have recently travelled abroad
- you are or may be pregnant
- you have abnormal vaginal bleeding or discharge
- you have difficulty or pain passing urine.

Consult your doctor if you have developed new symptoms or if your symptoms worsen, or if they do not improve after 2 weeks treatment.

4.5 Interaction with other medicinal products and other forms of interaction
None stated.

4.6 Pregnancy and lactation
Although no teratogenic effects have been reported, use during pregnancy or lactation is not recommended as evidence of safety in preclinical studies is limited.

4.7 Effects on ability to drive and use machines
None.

4.8 Undesirable effects
Possible side effects may include nausea, headache, dizziness, itching, rash and allergic reactions including anaphylaxis.

There have been isolated reports of jaundice due to hepatitis which have been immune-mediated; but this adverse reaction resolved on cessation of alverine treatment.

4.9 Overdose
Can produce hypotension and atropine-like toxic effects. Management is as for atropine poisoning with supportive therapy for hypotension.

5. PHARMACOLOGICAL PROPERTIES
5.1 Pharmacodynamic properties
Alverine citrate is a spasmolytic which has a specific action on the smooth muscle of the alimentary tract and uterus without affecting the heart, blood vessels and tracheal muscle at therapeutic doses.

5.2 Pharmacokinetic properties
After oral administration, alverine is rapidly converted to its primary active metabolite, which is then further converted to two secondary metabolites. There is a high renal clearance of all metabolites indicating that they are eliminated by active renal secretion. The peak plasma level of the most active metabolite occurs between 1 and 1½ hours after oral dosing. The plasma half-life averages 0.8 hours for alverine and 5.7 hours for the active primary metabolite.

5.3 Preclinical safety data
Preclinical studies provide evidence that alverine citrate has no significant systemic toxicity potential at the proposed dosage.

6. PHARMACEUTICAL PARTICULARS
6.1 List of excipients
Maize starch

Magnesium stearate

Capsule shell: gelatine, E132, E171, E172

6.2 Incompatibilities
None stated.

6.3 Shelf life
3 years.

6.4 Special precautions for storage
Store in a dry place. Do not store above 25°C.

6.5 Nature and contents of container
A box of aluminium foil/UPVC blister strip packs containing 2, 10, 20, 30, 60 or 90 capsules, in strips of 10 capsules as appropriate.

6.6 Special precautions for disposal and other handling
None.

7. MARKETING AUTHORISATION HOLDER
Norgine Limited
Chaplin House
Widewater Place
Moorhall Road
Harefield
UXBRIDGE
Middlesex, UB9 6NS
United Kingdom

8. MARKETING AUTHORISATION NUMBER(S)
PL 00322/0075

9. DATE OF FIRST AUTHORISATION/RENEWAL OF THE AUTHORISATION
09 October 1997/ 04 April 2003

10. DATE OF REVISION OF THE TEXT
June 2009

Legal category: **P**

Spiriva 18 microgram inhalation powder, hard capsule

(Boehringer Ingelheim Limited)

1. NAME OF THE MEDICINAL PRODUCT
SPIRIVA® 18 microgram, inhalation powder, hard capsule

2. QUALITATIVE AND QUANTITATIVE COMPOSITION
Each capsule contains 22.5 microgram tiotropium bromide monohydrate equivalent to 18 microgram tiotropium.

The delivered dose (the dose that leaves the mouthpiece of the HandiHaler® device) is 10 microgram tiotropium.

Excipient: Lactose monohydrate

For a full list of excipients, see section 6.1.

3. PHARMACEUTICAL FORM
Inhalation powder, hard capsule.

Light green hard capsules with the product code TI 01 and company logo printed on the capsule.

4. CLINICAL PARTICULARS

4.1 Therapeutic indications

Tiotropium is indicated as a maintenance bronchodilator treatment to relieve symptoms of patients with chronic obstructive pulmonary disease (COPD).

4.2 Posology and method of administration

The recommended dosage of tiotropium bromide is inhalation of the contents of one capsule once daily with the HandiHaler device at the same time of day.

The recommended dose should not be exceeded.

Tiotropium bromide capsules must not be swallowed.

Tiotropium bromide should only be inhaled with the HandiHaler device.

Instructions for handling and use:

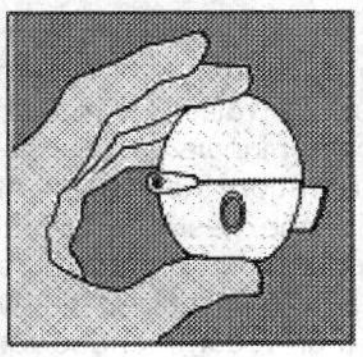

Remember to carefully follow your doctor's instructions for using SPIRIVA. The HandiHaler is especially designed for SPIRIVA. You must not use it to take any other medication. You can use your HandiHaler for up to one year to take your medication.

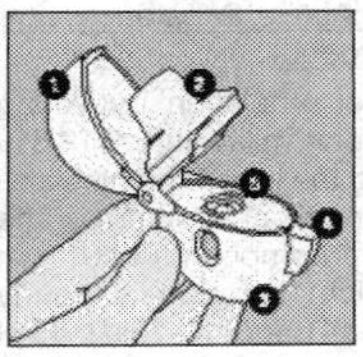

The HandiHaler
1 Dust cap
2 Mouthpiece
3 Base
4 Piercing button
5 Centre chamber

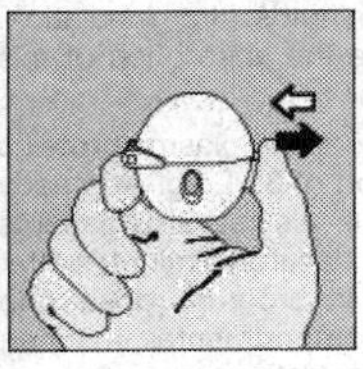

1. To release the dust cap press the piercing button completely in and let go.

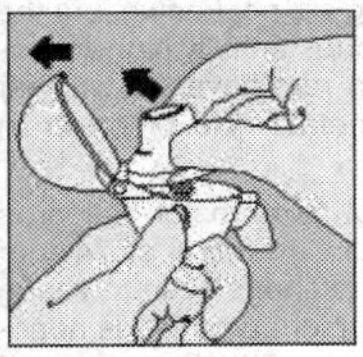

2. Open the dust cap completely by pulling it upwards. Then open the mouthpiece by pulling it upwards.

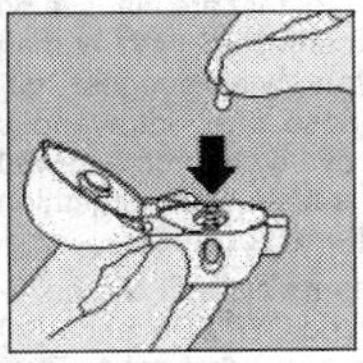

3. Remove a SPIRIVA capsule from the blister (only immediately before use) and place it in the centre chamber (5), as illustrated. It does not matter which way the capsule is placed in the chamber.

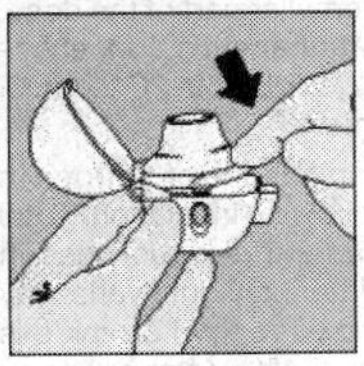

4. Close the mouthpiece firmly until you hear a click, leaving the dust cap open.

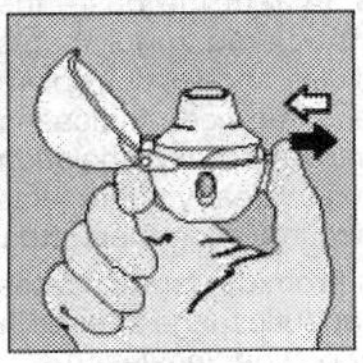

5. Hold the HandiHaler device with the mouthpiece upwards and press the piercing button completely in only once, and release. This makes holes in the capsule and allows the medication to be released when you breathe in.

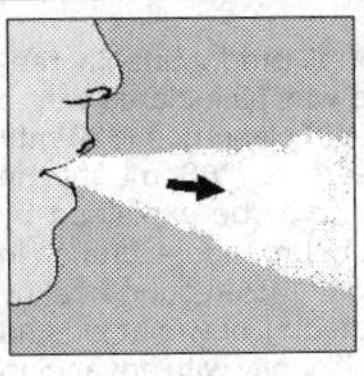

6. Breathe out completely. Important: Please avoid breathing into the mouthpiece at any time.

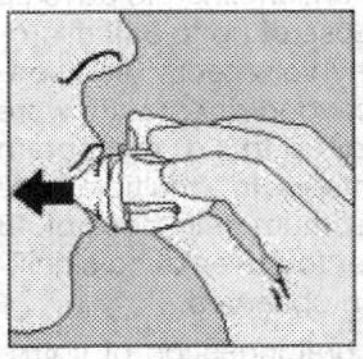

7. Raise the HandiHaler to your mouth and close your lips tightly around the mouthpiece. Keep your head in an upright position and breathe in slowly and deeply but at a rate sufficient to hear or feel the capsule vibrate. Breathe in until your lungs are full; then hold your breath as long as comfortable and at the same time take the HandiHaler out of your mouth. Resume normal breathing. Repeat steps 6 and 7 once, in order to empty the capsule completely.

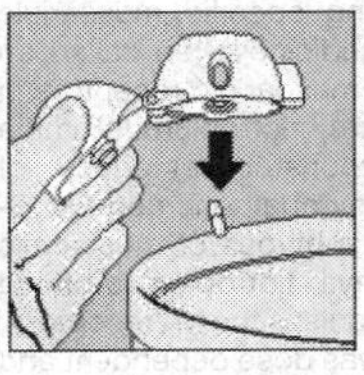

8. Open the mouthpiece again. Tip out the used capsule and dispose. Close the mouthpiece and dust cap for storage of your HandiHaler device.

Cleaning your HandiHaler

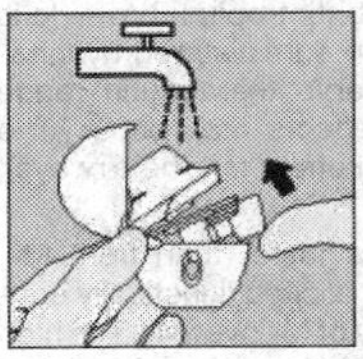

Clean the HandiHaler once a month. Open the dust cap and mouthpiece. Then open the base by lifting the piercing button. Rinse the complete inhaler with warm water to remove any powder. Dry the HandiHaler thoroughly by tipping excess of water out on a paper towel and air-dry afterwards, leaving the dust cap, mouthpiece and base open. It takes 24 hours to air dry, so clean it right after you used it and it will be ready for your next dose. If needed, the outside of the mouthpiece may be cleaned with a moist but not wet tissue.

Blister handling

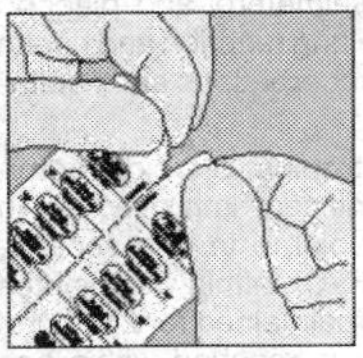

A. Separate the blister strips by tearing along the perforation.

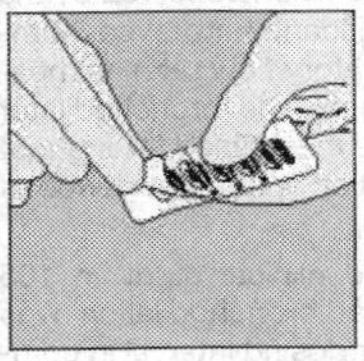

B. Peel back foil (only immediately before use) using the tab until one capsule is fully visible.
In case a second capsule is exposed to air inadvertently this capsule has to be discarded.

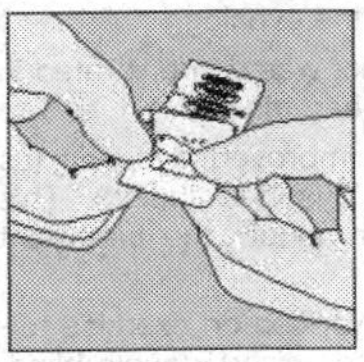

C. Remove capsule.

SPIRIVA® capsules contain only a small amount of powder so that the capsule is only partially filled.

Special Populations:

Geriatric patients can use tiotropium bromide at the recommended dose.

Renally impaired patients can use tiotropium bromide at the recommended dose. For patients with moderate to severe impairment (creatinine clearance ⩽ 50 ml/min) see 4.4 Special warnings and special precautions for use and 5.2 Pharmacokinetic properties.

Hepatically impaired patients can use tiotropium bromide at the recommended dose (see 5.2 Pharmacokinetic properties).

Paediatric patients: Safety and effectiveness of tiotropium bromide inhalation powder in paediatric patients have not been established and therefore it should not be used in patients under 18 years of age.

4.3 Contraindications

Tiotropium bromide inhalation powder is contraindicated in patients with a hypersensitivity to tiotropium bromide, atropine or its derivatives, e.g. ipratropium or oxitropium or to the excipient lactose monohydrate which contains milk protein.

4.4 Special warnings and precautions for use

Tiotropium bromide, as a once daily maintenance bronchodilator, should not be used for the initial treatment of acute episodes of bronchospasm, i.e. rescue therapy.

Immediate hypersensitivity reactions may occur after administration of tiotropium bromide inhalation powder.

Consistent with its anticholinergic activity, tiotropium bromide should be used with caution in patients with narrow-angle glaucoma, prostatic hyperplasia or bladder-neck obstruction. (see 4.8 undesirable effects)

Inhaled medicines may cause inhalation-induced bronchospasm.

As plasma concentration increases with decreased renal function in patients with moderate to severe renal impairment (creatinine clearance ⩽ 50 ml/min) tiotropium bromide should be used only if the expected benefit outweighs the potential risk. There is no long term experience in patients with severe renal impairment. (see 5.2 Pharmacokinetic properties).

Patients should be cautioned to avoid getting the drug powder into their eyes. They should be advised that this may result in precipitation or worsening of narrow-angle glaucoma, eye pain or discomfort, temporary blurring of vision, visual halos or coloured images in association with red eyes from conjunctival congestion and corneal oedema. Should any combination of these eye symptoms develop, patients should stop using tiotropium bromide and consult a specialist immediately.

Dry mouth, which has been observed with anti-cholinergic treatment, may in the long term be associated with dental caries.

Tiotropium bromide should not be used more frequently than once daily (see section 4.9 Overdose).

SPIRIVA capsules contain 5.5 mg lactose monohydrate.

4.5 Interaction with other medicinal products and other forms of interaction

Although no formal drug interaction studies have been performed, tiotropium bromide inhalation powder has been used concomitantly with other drugs without clinical evidence of drug interactions. These include sympathomimetic bronchodilators, methylxanthines, oral and inhaled steroids, commonly used in the treatment of COPD.

The co-administration of tiotropium bromide with other anticholinergic-containing drugs has not been studied and is therefore not recommended.

4.6 Pregnancy and lactation

For tiotropium bromide, no documented clinical data on exposed pregnancies are available. Studies in animals have shown reproductive toxicity associated with maternal toxicity (see section 5.3, Preclinical Safety Data). The potential risk for humans is unknown. SPIRIVA should therefore only be used during pregnancy when clearly indicated.

It is unknown whether tiotropium bromide is excreted in human breast milk. Despite studies in rodents which have demonstrated that excretion of tiotropium bromide in breast milk occurs only in small amounts, use of SPIRIVA is not recommended during breast-feeding. Tiotropium bromide is a long-acting compound. A decision on whether to continue/discontinue breast-feeding or to continue/discontinue therapy with SPIRIVA should be made taking into account the benefit of breast-feeding to the child and the benefit of SPIRIVA therapy to the woman.

4.7 Effects on ability to drive and use machines

No studies on the effects on the ability to drive and use machines have been performed. The occurrence of dizziness, blurred vision, or headache may influence the ability to drive and use machinery.

4.8 Undesirable effects

a) General Description

Many of the listed undesirable effects can be assigned to the anticholinergic properties of SPIRIVA. In controlled clinical studies, the most commonly observed undesirable effect was dry mouth which occurred in approximately 3% of patients.

b) Table of Undesirable Effects

The frequencies assigned to the undesirable effects listed below are based on crude incidence rates of adverse drug reactions (i.e. events attributed to tiotropium by study investigators) observed in the tiotropium group (5,437 patients) from 19 pooled placebo-controlled clinical trials with treatment periods ranging from four weeks to one year.

MedDRA Preferred Term	Frequency[1]
Nervous system disorders	
Dizziness	Uncommon
Headache	Uncommon
Taste disorders	Uncommon

Eye disorders	
Vision blurred	Rare
Intraocular pressure increased	Rare
Glaucoma	Not known*
Cardiac disorders	
Tachycardia	Rare
Palpitations	Rare
Supraventricular tachycardia	Not known*
Atrial fibrillation	Not known*
Respiratory, thoracic and mediastinal disorders	
Bronchospasm	Uncommon
Cough	Uncommon
Pharyngitis and other application site irritation	Uncommon
Dysphonia	Uncommon
Epistaxis	Rare
Sinusitis	Not known*
Gastrointestinal Disorders	
Dry Mouth	Common
Oral candidiasis	Uncommon
Nausea	Uncommon
Gastroesophageal reflux disease	Rare
Constipation	Rare
Dental caries	Not known*
Dysphagia	Not known*
Intestinal obstruction, including ileus paralytic	Not known*
Skin and subcutaneous tissue disorders, Immune system disorders:	
Rash	Rare
Urticaria	Rare
Pruritus	Rare
Other Hypersensitivity (including immediate reactions)	Rare
Angioneurotic oedema	Not known*
Renal and Urinary Disorders	
Dysuria	Rare
Urinary retention	Rare
Urinary tract infection	Rare

[1]very common > 1/10; common > 1/100, < 1/10; uncommon > 1/1,000, < 1/100, rare >1/10,000, < 1/1,000 according to frequency convention

*no events attributed to tiotropium by study investigators in 5,437 tiotropium treated patients; however, events are considered adverse drug reactions associated with tiotropium

c) Information Characterising Individual Serious and/or Frequently Occurring Undesirable Effects

The most common anticholinergic undesirable effect reported by COPD patients was dry mouth. Dry mouth was mild in the majority of cases. In general, dry mouth had an onset between 3 and 5 weeks. Dry mouth commonly resolved while patients continued to receive tiotropium bromide. Dry mouth led to discontinuation from the one-year studies by 3 of 906 patients (0.3% of the treated patients).

Serious undesirable effects consistent with anticholinergic effects include constipation and intestinal obstruction including ileus paralytic as well as urinary retention although none was attributed to tiotropium in the tiotropium group of 5,437 patients pooled from controlled clinical trials.

d) Pharmacological Class - Undesirable effects

Several organ systems and functions are under control of the parasympathetic nervous system and thus can be affected by anticholinergic agents. Possible adverse events attributable to systemic anticholinergic effects include dry mouth, dry throat, increased heart rate, blurred vision, increased intraocular pressure, glaucoma, urinary difficulty, urinary retention, and constipation. Urinary retention was usually observed in elderly men with predisposing factors, (e.g. prostatic hyperplasia).

In common with all inhaled medications, tiotropium may cause inhalation-induced bronchospasm. Local upper airway irritant phenomena have also been observed in patients receiving tiotropium bromide.

An increased incidence of dry mouth and constipation may occur with increasing age.

4.9 Overdose

High doses of tiotropium bromide may lead to anticholinergic signs and symptoms.

However, there were no systemic anticholinergic adverse effects following a single inhaled dose of up to 340 microgram tiotropium bromide in healthy volunteers. Additionally, no relevant adverse effects, beyond dry mouth, were observed following 7 day dosing of up to 170 microgram tiotropium bromide in healthy volunteers. In a multiple dose study in COPD patients with a maximum daily dose of 43 microgram tiotropium bromide over four weeks no significant undesirable effects have been observed.

Acute intoxication by inadvertent oral ingestion of tiotropium bromide capsules is unlikely due to low oral bioavailability.

5. PHARMACOLOGICAL PROPERTIES

5.1 Pharmacodynamic properties

Pharmacotherapeutic group: Anticholinergics

ATC code: R03B B04

Tiotropium bromide is a long-acting, specific, muscarinic receptor antagonist, in clinical medicine often called an anticholinergic. By binding to the muscarinic receptors in the bronchial smooth musculature, tiotropium bromide inhibits the cholinergic (bronchoconstrictive) effects of acetylcholine, released from parasympathetic nerve endings. It has similar affinity to the subtypes of muscarinic receptors, M_1 to M_5. In the airways, tiotropium bromide competitively and reversibly antagonises the M_3 receptors, resulting in relaxation. The effect was dose dependent and lasted longer than 24h. The long duration is probably due to the very slow dissociation from the M_3 receptor, exhibiting a significantly longer dissociation half-life than ipratropium. As an N-quaternary anticholinergic, tiotropium bromide is topically (broncho-) selective when administered by inhalation, demonstrating an acceptable therapeutic range before systemic anticholinergic effects may occur. The bronchodilation is primarily a local effect (on the airways), not a systemic one.

Dissociation from M_2-receptors is faster than from M_3, which in functional in vitro studies, elicited (kinetically controlled) receptor subtype selectivity of M_3 over M_2. The high potency and slow receptor dissociation found its clinical correlate in significant and long-acting bronchodilation in patients with COPD.

Electrophysiology: In a dedicated QT study involving 53 healthy volunteers, SPIRIVA 18 mcg and 54 mcg (i.e. three times the therapeutic dose) over 12 days did not significantly prolong QT intervals of the ECG.

The clinical development programme included four one-year and two six-month randomised, double-blind studies in 2663 patients (1308 receiving tiotropium bromide). The one-year programme consisted of two placebo-controlled trials and two trials with an active control (ipratropium). The two six-month trials were both, salmeterol and placebo controlled. These studies included lung function and health outcome measures of dyspnea, exacerbations and health-related quality of life.

In the aforementioned studies, tiotropium bromide, administered once daily, provided significant improvement in lung function (forced expiratory volume in one second, FEV_1 and forced vital capacity, FVC) within 30 minutes following the first dose which was maintained for 24 hours. Pharmacodynamic steady state was reached within one week with the majority of bronchodilation observed by the third day. Tiotropium bromide significantly improved morning and evening PEFR (peak expiratory flow rate) as measured by patient's daily recordings. The bronchodilator effects of tiotropium bromide were maintained throughout the one-year period of administration with no evidence of tolerance.

A randomised, placebo-controlled clinical study in 105 COPD patients demonstrated that bronchodilation was maintained throughout the 24 hour dosing interval in comparison to placebo regardless of whether the drug was administered in the morning or in the evening.

The following health outcome effect was demonstrated in the long term (6-month and one-year) trials:

Tiotropium bromide significantly improved dyspnea (as evaluated using the Transition Dyspnea Index.). This improvement was maintained throughout the treatment period.

The impact of improvements in dyspnea on exercise tolerance was investigated in two randomised, double-blind, placebo-controlled trials in 433 patients with moderate to severe COPD. In these trials, six weeks of treatment with SPIRIVA significantly improved symptom-limited exercise endurance time during cycle ergometry at 75% of maximal work capacity by 19.7% (Trial A: 640 seconds with SPIRIVA vs. 535 seconds with placebo, compared with a pre-treatment baseline of 492 seconds) and 28.3% (Trial B: 741 seconds with SPIRIVA vs. 577 seconds with placebo, compared with a pre-treatment baseline of 537 seconds).

In a randomized, double-blind, placebo controlled trial of 1,829 patients with moderate to very severe COPD, tiotropium bromide statistically significantly reduced the proportion of patients who experienced exacerbations of COPD (32.2% to 27.8%) and statistically significantly reduced the number of exacerbations by 19% (1.05 to 0.85 events per patient year of exposure). In addition, 7.0% of patients in the tiotropium bromide group and 9.5% of patients in the placebo group were hospitalized due to a COPD exacerbation (p=0.056). The number of hospitalizations due to COPD was reduced by 30% (0.25 to 0.18 events per patient year of exposure).

In a 9-month, randomized, double-blind, placebo-controlled clinical trial of 492 patients, SPIRIVA improved health-related quality of life as determined by the St. George's Respiratory Questionnaire (SGRQ) total score. The proportion of patients treated with SPIRIVA which achieved a meaningful improvement in the SGRQ total score (i.e. > 4 units) was 10.9% higher compared with placebo (59,1% in the SPIRIVA groups vs. 48.2% in the placebo group (p=0.029). The mean difference between the groups was 4.19 units (p=0.001; confidence interval: 1.69 – 6.68). While the SGRQ subdomains "activity" and "impact on daily life" were not improved significantly, the improvement on total score resulted from a marked improvement in the SGRQ subdomain disease related "symptoms".

5.2 Pharmacokinetic properties

a) General Introduction

Tiotropium bromide is a non-chiral quaternary ammonium compound and is sparingly soluble in water. Tiotropium bromide is administered by dry powder inhalation. Generally with the inhaled route of administration, the majority of the delivered dose is deposited in the gastro-intestinal tract, and to a lesser extent in the intended organ of the lung. Many of the pharmacokinetic data described below were obtained with higher doses than recommended for therapy.

b) General Characteristics of the Active Substance after Administration of the Medicinal Product

Absorption: Following dry powder inhalation by young healthy volunteers, the absolute bioavailability of 19.5% suggests that the fraction reaching the lung is highly bioavailable. It is expected from the chemical structure of the compound (quaternary ammonium compound) and from in-vitro experiments that tiotropium bromide is poorly absorbed from the gastrointestinal tract (10-15%). Oral solutions of tiotropium bromide have an absolute bioavailability of 2-3%. Maximum tiotropium bromide plasma concentrations were observed five minutes after inhalation. Food is not expected to influence the absorption of this quaternary ammonium compound.

Distribution: The drug is bound by 72% to plasma proteins and shows a volume of distribution of 32 L/kg. At steady state, tiotropium bromide plasma levels in COPD patients at peak were 17 – 19 pg/ml when measured 5 minutes after dry powder inhalation of a 18 microgram dose and decreased rapidly in a multi-compartmental manner. Steady state trough plasma concentrations were 3-4 pg/ml. Local concentrations in the lung are not known, but the mode of administration suggests substantially higher concentrations in the lung. Studies in rats have shown that tiotropium bromide does not penetrate the blood-brain barrier to any relevant extent.

Biotransformation: The extent of biotransformation is small. This is evident from a urinary excretion of 74% of unchanged substance after an intravenous dose to young healthy volunteers. The ester tiotropium bromide is nonenzymatically cleaved to the alcohol (N-methylscopine) and acid compound (dithienylglycolic acid) that are inactive on muscarinic receptors. In-vitro experiments with human liver microsomes and human hepatocytes suggest that some further drug (< 20% of dose after intravenous administration) is metabolised by cytochrome P450 (CYP) dependent oxidation and subsequent glutathion conjugation to a variety of Phase II-metabolites.

In vitro studies in liver microsomes reveal that the enzymatic pathway can be inhibited by the CYP 2D6 (and 3A4) inhibitors, quinidine, ketoconazole and gestodene. Thus CYP 2D6 and 3A4 are involved in metabolic pathway that is responsible for the elimination of a smaller part of the dose. Tiotropium bromide even in supra-therapeutic concentrations does not inhibit CYP 1A1, 1A2, 2B6, 2C9, 2C19, 2D6, 2E1 or 3A in human liver microsomes.

Elimination: The terminal elimination half-life of tiotropium bromide is between 5 and 6 days following inhalation. Total clearance was 880 ml/min after an intravenous dose in young healthy volunteers with an interindividual variability of 22%. Intravenously administered tiotropium bromide is mainly excreted unchanged in urine (74%). After dry powder inhalation urinary excretion is 14% of the dose, the remainder being mainly non-absorbed drug in gut that is eliminated via the faeces. The renal clearance of tiotropium bromide exceeds the creatinine clearance, indicating secretion into the urine. After chronic once daily inhalation by COPD patients, pharmacokinetic steady state was reached after 2-3 weeks with no accumulation thereafter.

Linearity / Nonlinearity: Tiotropium bromide demonstrates linear pharmacokinetics in the therapeutic range after both intravenous administration and dry powder inhalation.

c) Characteristics in Patients

Geriatric Patients: As expected for all predominantly renally excreted drugs, advanced age was associated with a decrease of tiotropium bromide renal clearance (326 mL/min in COPD patients < 58 years to 163 mL/min in COPD patients > 70 years) which may be explained by decreased renal function. Tiotropium bromide excretion in urine after inhalation decreased from 14% (young healthy volunteers) to about 7% (COPD patients), however plasma concentrations did not change significantly with advancing age within COPD patients if compared to inter- and intraindividual variability (43% increase in AUC_{0-4h} after dry powder inhalation.

Renally Impaired Patients: In common with all other drugs that undergo predominantly renal excretion, renal impairment was associated with increased plasma drug concentrations and reduced renal drug clearance after both intravenous infusion and dry powder inhalations. Mild renal impairment (CL_{CR} 50-80 ml/min) which is often seen in elderly patients increased tiotropium bromide plasma concentrations slightly (39% increase in AUC_{0-4h} after intravenous infusion). In COPD patients with moderate to severe renal impairment (CL_{CR} < 50 ml/min) the intravenous administration of tiotropium bromide resulted in doubling of the plasma concentrations (82% increase in AUC_{0-4h}), which was confirmed by plasma concentrations after dry powder inhalation.

Hepatically Impaired Patients: Liver insufficiency is not expected to have any relevant influence on tiotropium bromide pharmacokinetics. Tiotropium bromide is predominantly cleared by renal elimination (74% in young healthy volunteers) and simple non-enzymatic ester cleavage to pharmacologically inactive products.

Paediatric Patients: See 4.2 Posology and Method of Administration

d) Pharmacokinetic / Pharmacodynamic Relationship(s)

There is no direct relationship between pharmacokinetics and pharmacodynamics.

5.3 Preclinical safety data

Many effects observed in conventional studies of safety pharmacology, repeated dose toxicity, and reproductive toxicity could be explained by the anticholinergic properties of tiotropium bromide. Typically in animals reduced food consumption, inhibited body weight gain, dry mouth and nose, reduced lacrimation and salivation, mydriasis and increased heart rate were observed. Other relevant effects noted in repeated dose toxicity studies were: mild irritancy of the respiratory tract in rats and mice evinced by rhinitis and epithelial changes of the nasal cavity and larynx, and prostatitis along with proteinaceous deposits and lithiasis in the bladder in rats.

Harmful effects with respect to pregnancy, embryonal/foetal development, parturition or postnatal development could only be demonstrated at maternally toxic dose levels. Tiotropium bromide was not teratogenic in rats or rabbits. The respiratory (irritation) and urogenital (prostatitis) changes and reproductive toxicity were observed at local or systemic exposures more than five-fold the therapeutic exposure. Studies on genotoxicity and carcinogenic potential revealed no special hazard for humans.

6. PHARMACEUTICAL PARTICULARS

6.1 List of excipients

Lactose monohydrate (which contains milk protein)

6.2 Incompatibilities

Not applicable

6.3 Shelf life

2 years

After first opening of the blister: 9 days

Discard the HandiHaler device 12 months after first use.

6.4 Special precautions for storage

Do not store above 25°C

Do not freeze

6.5 Nature and contents of container

Aluminium / PVC / Aluminium blister strips containing 10 capsules

The HandiHaler is a single dose inhalation device made from plastic materials (ABS) and stainless steel.

Package sizes and devices supplied:

- Cardboard box containing 30 capsules (3 blister strips)
- Cardboard box containing 60 capsules (6 blister strips)
- Cardboard box containing 90 capsules (9 blister strips)
- Cardboard box containing HandiHaler device
- Cardboard box containing HandiHaler device and 10 capsules (1 blister strip)
- Cardboard box containing HandiHaler device and 30 capsules (3 blister strips)
- Hospital pack: Bundle pack containing 5 cardboard boxes of 30 capsules plus HandiHaler device
- Hospital pack: Bundle pack containing 5 cardboard boxes of 60 capsules

Not all pack sizes may be marketed

6.6 Special precautions for disposal and other handling

No special requirements.

7. MARKETING AUTHORISATION HOLDER

Boehringer Ingelheim International GmbH

Binger Straβe 173

D-55216 Ingelheim am Rhein

Germany

8. MARKETING AUTHORISATION NUMBER(S)

PL 14598/0062

9. DATE OF FIRST AUTHORISATION/RENEWAL OF THE AUTHORISATION

09/10/2006

10. DATE OF REVISION OF THE TEXT

June 2008

Legal Category

POM

Spiriva Respimat 2.5 micrograms solution for inhalation

(Boehringer Ingelheim Limited)

1. NAME OF THE MEDICINAL PRODUCT

Spiriva▼ Respimat 2.5 microgram, solution for inhalation

2. QUALITATIVE AND QUANTITATIVE COMPOSITION

The delivered dose is 2.5 microgram tiotropium per puff (2 puffs comprise one medicinal dose) and is equivalent to 3.124 microgram tiotropium bromide monohydrate.

The delivered dose is the dose which is available for the patient after passing the mouthpiece.

For a full list of excipients, see section 6.1.

3. PHARMACEUTICAL FORM

Solution for inhalation

Clear, colourless, solution for inhalation

4. CLINICAL PARTICULARS

4.1 Therapeutic indications

Tiotropium is indicated as a maintenance bronchodilator treatment to relieve symptoms of patients with chronic obstructive pulmonary disease (COPD).

4.2 Posology and method of administration

The medicinal product is intended for inhalation use only. The cartridge can only be inserted and used in the Respimat inhaler (see 4.2).

Two puffs from the Respimat inhaler comprise one medicinal dose.

The recommended dose for adults is 5 microgram tiotropium given as two puffs from the Respimat inhaler once daily, at the same time of the day.

The recommended dose should not be exceeded.

Special Populations:

Geriatric patients can use tiotropium bromide at the recommended dose.

Renally impaired patients can use tiotropium bromide at the recommended dose. For patients with moderate to severe impairment (creatinine clearance ⩽ 50 ml/min, see 4.4 and 5.2).

Hepatically impaired patients can use tiotropium bromide at the recommended dose (see 5.2).

Paediatric patients:

Spiriva Respimat is not recommended for use in children and adolescents below 18 years due to lack of data on safety and efficacy (see 5.1 and 5.2).

To ensure proper administration of the medicinal product, the patient should be shown how to use the inhaler by a physician or other health professionals.

Patient's instructions for use and handling

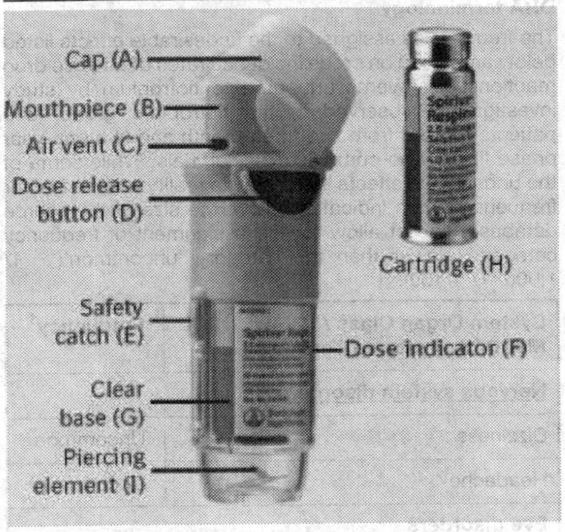

Spiriva Respimat inhaler and Spiriva Respimat cartridge

Inserting the cartridge and preparation for use

The following steps 1-6 are necessary before first use:

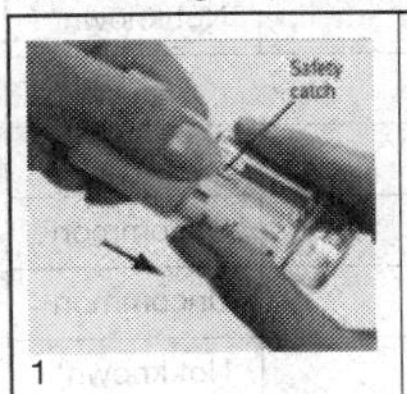

1

1

With the green cap (A) closed, press the safety catch (E) and pull off the clear base (G).

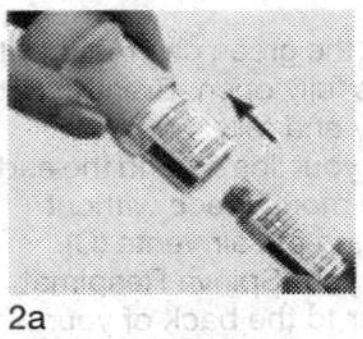

2a

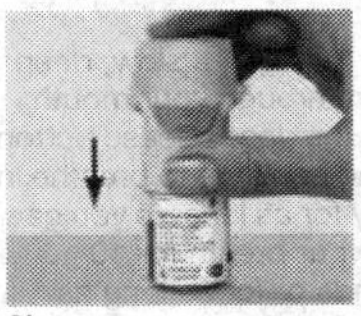

2b

2

Take the cartridge (H) out of the box. Push the **narrow** end of the cartridge into the inhaler until it clicks into place. The cartridge should be pushed **gently** against a firm surface to ensure that it has gone all the way in (2b).

Do not remove the cartridge once it has been inserted into the inhaler.

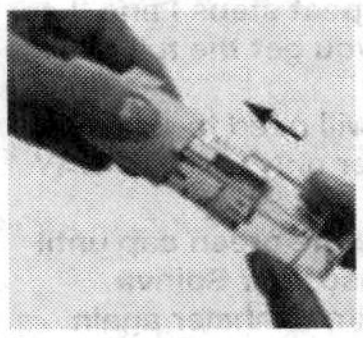

3

3

Replace the clear base (G).

Do not remove the clear base again.

To prepare the Spiriva Respimat inhaler for first-time use

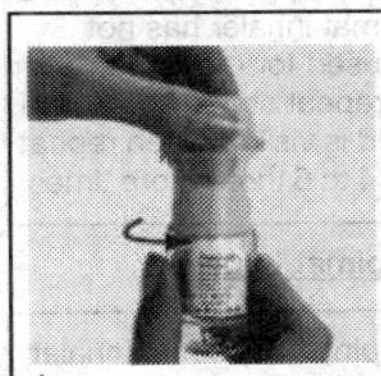

4

4

Hold the Spiriva Respimat inhaler upright, with the green cap (A) closed. Turn the base (G) in the direction of the red arrows on the label until it clicks (half a turn).

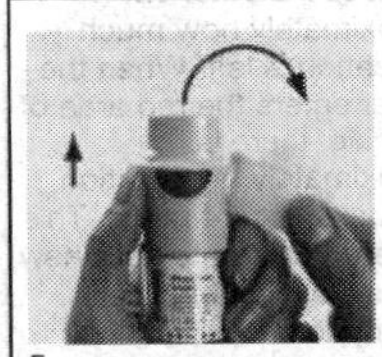

5

5

Open the green cap (A) until it snaps fully open.

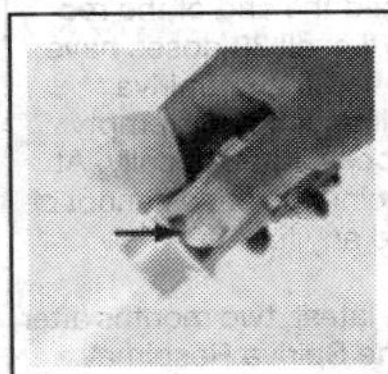

6

6

Point the Spiriva Respimat inhaler towards the ground. Press the dose release button (D). Close the green cap (A).

Repeat steps 4, 5 and 6 until a cloud is visible.

Then repeat steps 4, 5 and 6 three more times to ensure the inhaler is prepared for use.

Your Spiriva Respimat inhaler is now ready to use.

These steps will not affect the number of doses available. After preparation your Spiriva Respimat inhaler will be able to deliver your 60 puffs (30 medicinal doses).

Using the Spiriva Respimat inhaler

You will need to use this inhaler ONLY ONCE A DAY. Each time you use it take TWO PUFFS.

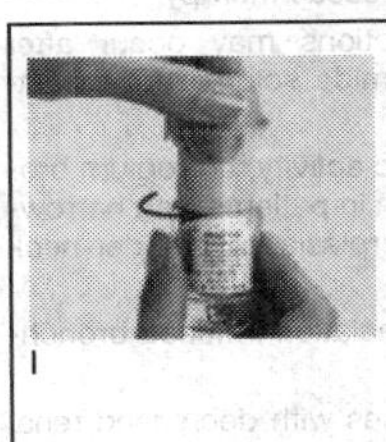

I

I

Hold the Spiriva Respimat inhaler upright, with the green cap (A) closed, to avoid accidental release of dose. Turn the base (G) in the direction of the red arrows on the label until it clicks (half a turn).

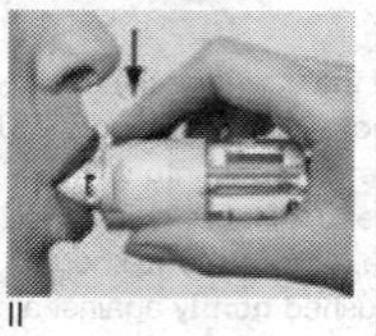

II

II
Open the green cap (A) until it snaps fully open. Breathe out slowly and fully, and then close your lips around the end of the mouthpiece without covering the air vents (C). Point your Spiriva Respimat inhaler to the back of your throat.

While taking in a slow, deep breath through your mouth, press the dose release button (D) and continue to breathe in slowly for as long as you can. Hold your breath for 10 seconds or for as long as comfortable.

III Repeat steps I and II so that you get the full dose.

You will need to use this inhaler only ONCE A DAY.

Close the green cap until you use your Spiriva Respimat inhaler again.

If Spiriva Respimat inhaler has not been used for more than 7 days release one puff towards the ground. If Spiriva Respimat inhaler has not been used for more than 21 days repeat steps 4 to 6 until a cloud is visible. Then repeat steps 4 to 6 three more times.

When to get a new Spiriva Respimat inhaler

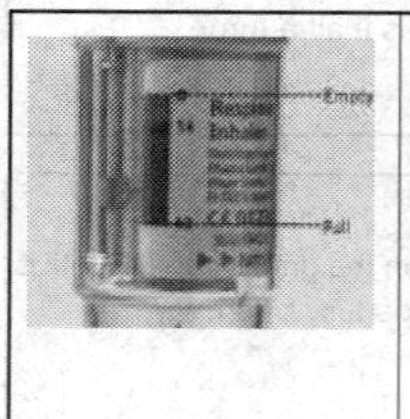

The Spiriva Respimat inhaler contains 60 puffs (30 medicinal doses).
The dose indicator shows approximately how much medication is left. When the pointer enters the red area of the scale, there is, approximately, medication for 7 days left (14 puffs). This is when you need to get a new Spiriva Respimat inhaler prescription.

Once the dose indicator has reached the end of the red scale (i.e. all 30 doses have been used), the Spiriva Respimat inhaler is empty and locks automatically. At this point, the base cannot be turned any further.

At the latest, two months after use the Spiriva Respimat inhaler should be discarded even if not all medication has been used.

How to care for your inhaler

Clean the mouthpiece including the metal part inside the mouthpiece with a damp cloth or tissue only, at least once a week.

Any minor discoloration in the mouthpiece does not affect your Spiriva Respimat inhaler performance.

If necessary, wipe the outside of your Spiriva Respimat inhaler with a damp cloth.

4.3 Contraindications

Spiriva Respimat is contraindicated in patients with hypersensitivity to tiotropium bromide, atropine or its derivatives, e.g. ipratropium or oxitropium or to any of the excipients (see 6.1).

4.4 Special warnings and precautions for use

Tiotropium bromide, as a once daily maintenance bronchodilator, should not be used for the initial treatment of acute episodes of bronchospasm, i.e. rescue therapy.

Immediate hypersensitivity reactions may occur after administration of tiotropium bromide solution for inhalation.

Consistent with its anticholinergic activity, tiotropium bromide should be used with caution in patients with narrow-angle glaucoma, prostatic hyperplasia or bladder-neck obstruction.

Inhaled medicines may cause inhalation-induced bronchospasm.

As plasma concentration increases with decreased renal function in patients with moderate to severe renal impairment (creatinine clearance ⩽ 50 ml/min) tiotropium bromide should be used only if the expected benefit outweighs the potential risk. There is no long term experience in patients with severe renal impairment (see 5.2).

Patients should be cautioned to avoid getting the spray into their eyes. They should be advised that this may result in precipitation or worsening of narrow-angle glaucoma, eye pain or discomfort, temporary blurring of vision, visual halos or coloured images in association with red eyes from conjunctival congestion and corneal oedema. Should any combination of these eye symptoms develop, patients should stop using tiotropium bromide and consult a specialist immediately

Dry mouth, which has been observed with anti-cholinergic treatment, may in the long term be associated with dental caries.

Tiotropium bromide should not be used more frequently than once daily (see 4.9).

4.5 Interaction with other medicinal products and other forms of interaction

Although no formal drug interaction studies have been performed, tiotropium bromide has been used concomitantly with other drugs commonly used in the treatment of COPD, including sympathomimetic bronchodilators, methylxanthines, oral and inhaled steroids without clinical evidence of drug interactions.

The co-administration of tiotropium bromide with other anticholinergic containing drugs has not been studied and therefore is not recommended.

4.6 Pregnancy and lactation

For tiotropium bromide, no clinical data on exposed pregnancies are available. Animal studies have shown reproductive toxicity associated with maternal toxicity (see 5.3).

The potential risk for humans is unknown. Spiriva Respimat should therefore only be used during pregnancy when clearly indicated.

It is unknown whether tiotropium bromide is excreted in human breast milk. Despite studies in rodents which have demonstrated that excretion of tiotropium bromide in breast milk occurs only in small amounts, use of Spiriva Respimat is not recommended during breast-feeding. Tiotropium bromide is a long-acting compound. A decision on whether to continue/discontinue breast-feeding or to continue/discontinue therapy with Spiriva Respimat should be made taking into account the benefit of breast-feeding to the child and the benefit of Spiriva Respimat therapy to the woman.

4.7 Effects on ability to drive and use machines

No studies on the effects on the ability to drive and use machines have been performed. The occurrence of dizziness or blurred vision may influence the ability to drive and use machinery.

4.8 Undesirable effects

a) General description

Many of the listed undesirable effects can be assigned to the anticholinergic properties of tiotropium bromide.

In combined one-year and three month studies of 849 patients receiving tiotropium bromide, the most commonly observed undesirable effect was dry mouth which occurred in approximately 6% of patients.

b) Table of Undesirable effects according to the MedDRA terminology

The frequencies assigned to the undesirable effects listed below are based on crude incidence rates of adverse drug reactions (i.e. events attributed to tiotropium by study investigators) observed in the tiotropium group (849 patients) pooled from two three-month and two one-year phase III placebo-controlled clinical trials. While some of the undesirable effects listed may in reality occur at lower frequencies than indicated below, the size of the source database did not allow for the assignment of frequency categories lower than the category 'uncommon'(⩾ 1/1,000, < 1/100).

System Organ Class / MedDRA Preferred Term	Frequency[1]
Nervous system disorders	
Dizziness	Uncommon
Headache	Uncommon
Eye disorders	
Vision blurred	Uncommon
Intraocular pressure increased	Not known*
Glaucoma	Not known*
Cardiac disorders	
Palpitations	Uncommon
Supraventricular tachycardia	Uncommon
Atrial fibrillation	Uncommon
Tachycardia	Not known*
Respiratory, thoracic and mediastinal disorders	
Cough	Uncommon
Pharyngitis and other application site irritation	Uncommon
Dysphonia	Uncommon
Bronchospasm	Not known*
Epistaxis	Not known*
Sinusitis	Not known*
Gastrointestinal Disorders	
Dry Mouth[2]	Common
Oral candidiasis	Uncommon
Gastrooesophageal reflux disease	Uncommon
Dysphagia	Uncommon
Dental caries	Not known*
Constipation[2]	Not known*
Intestinal obstruction, including ileus paralytic[2]	Not known*
Nausea	Not known*
Skin and subcutaneous tissue disorders, Immune system disorders	
Pruritus	Uncommon
Angioneurotic oedema	Not known*
Rash	Not known*
Urticaria	Not known*
Other Hypersensitivity (including immediate reactions)	Not known*
Renal and urinary Disorders	
Dysuria	Uncommon
Urinary retention[2]	Uncommon
Urinary tract infection	Not known*

[1] common ⩾ 1/100, < 1/10; uncommon ⩾ 1/1,000, < 1/100 according to frequency convention

[2] see section c)

* frequency not known, no adverse drug reaction observed in 849 patients

c) Information characterising individual serious and/or frequently occurring undesirable effects

The most common anticholinergic adverse reaction reported by COPD patients was dry mouth. Dry mouth was mild in the majority of cases. In general, dry mouth had an onset between 3 and 5 weeks. Dry mouth commonly resolved while patients continued to receive tiotropium bromide, but led to discontinuation from the combined one-year and 3-month trials by 2 of 849 (0.2%) patients in the active treatment group.

Serious undesirable effects consistent with anticholinergic effects include constipation, intestinal obstruction including ileus paralytic and urinary retention, though none were reported in the tiotropium Respimat development program.

d) Pharmacological class - undesirable effects

Several organ systems and functions are under control of the parasympathetic nervous system and thus can be affected by anticholinergic agents. Possible adverse events attributable to systemic anticholinergic effects include dry mouth, dry throat, tachycardia, blurred vision, increased intraocular pressure, glaucoma, urinary difficulty, urinary retention, and constipation. Urinary retention, when reported in the overall tiotropium data base, was usually observed in elderly men with predisposing factors, (e.g. prostatic hyperplasia). Increased incidences of dry mouth and constipation may occur with increasing age. In common with all inhaled medications, tiotropium bromide may cause inhalation-induced bronchospasm. Local upper airway irritant phenomena have also been observed in patients receiving tiotropium bromide.

4.9 Overdose

High doses of tiotropium bromide may lead to anticholinergic signs and symptoms.

However, there were no systemic anticholinergic adverse effects following a single inhaled dose of up to 340 microgram tiotropium bromide in healthy volunteers. Additionally, no relevant adverse effects, beyond dry mouth/throat and dry nasal mucosa, were observed following 14-day dosing of up to 40 microgram tiotropium solution for inhalation in healthy volunteers with the exception of pronounced reduction in salivary flow from day 7 onwards. No significant undesirable effects have been observed in four long term-studies in COPD patients with a daily dose of 10 microgram tiotropium solution for inhalation over 4-48 weeks.

Acute intoxication by inadvertent oral ingestion of tiotropium solution for inhalation from the cartridge is unlikely due to low oral bioavailability.

5. PHARMACOLOGICAL PROPERTIES

5.1 Pharmacodynamic properties

Pharmacotherapeutic group: Anticholinergics

ATC code: R03B B04

Tiotropium bromide is a long-acting, specific antagonist at muscarinic receptors. It has similar affinity to the subtypes, M_1 to M_5. In the airways, tiotropium bromide competitively and reversibly binds to the M_3 receptors in the bronchial smooth musculature, antagonising the cholinergic (bronchoconstrictive) effects of acetylcholine, resulting in bronchial smooth muscle relaxation. The effect was dose dependent and lasted longer than 24h. As an N-quaternary anticholinergic, tiotropium bromide is topically (broncho-) selective when administered by inhalation, demonstrating an acceptable therapeutic range before systemic anticholinergic effects may occur.

The dissociation of tiotropium from especially M_3-receptors is very slow, exhibiting a significantly longer dissociation half-life than ipratropium. Dissociation from M_2-receptors is faster than from M_3, which in functional in vitro studies, elicited (kinetically controlled) receptor subtype selectivity of M_3 over M_2. The high potency, very slow receptor dissociation and topical inhaled selectivity found its clinical correlate in significant and long-acting bronchodilation in patients with COPD.

The clinical Phase III development programme included two 1-year, two 12-weeks and two 4-weeks randomised, double-blind studies in 2901 COPD patients (1038 receiving the 5 µg tiotropium dose). The 1-year programme consisted of two placebo-controlled trials. The two 12-week trials were both active (ipratropium) - and placebo-controlled. All six studies included lung function measurements. In addition, the two 1-year studies included health outcome measures of dyspnoea, health-related quality of life and effect on exacerbations.

In the aforementioned studies, tiotropium solution for inhalation, administered once daily, provided significant improvement in lung function (forced expiratory volume in one second and forced vital capacity) within 30 minutes following the first dose, compared to placebo (FEV_1 mean improvement at 30 minutes: 0.113 litres; 95% confidence interval (CI): 0.102 to 0.125 litres, $p < 0.0001$). Improvement of lung function was maintained for 24 hours at steady state compared to placebo (FEV_1 mean improvement: 0.122 litres; 95% CI: 0.106 to 0.138 litres, $p < 0.0001$).

Pharmacodynamic steady state was reached within one week.

Spiriva Respimat significantly improved morning and evening PEFR (peak expiratory flow rate) as measured by patient's daily recordings compared to placebo (PEFR mean improvement: mean improvement in the morning 22 L/min; 95% CI: 18 to 55 L/min, $p < 0.0001$; evening 26 L/min; 95% CI: 23 to 30 L/min, $p < 0.0001$). The use of Spiriva Respimat resulted in a reduction of rescue bronchodilator use compared to placebo (mean reduction in rescue use 0.66 occasions per day, 95% CI: 0.51 to 0.81 occasions per day, $p < 0.0001$).

The bronchodilator effects of Spiriva Respimat were maintained throughout the 1-year period of administration with no evidence of tolerance.

The following health outcome effects were demonstrated in the long term 1-year studies:

(a) Spiriva Respimat significantly improved dyspnoea (as evaluated using the Transition Dyspnoea Index) compared to placebo (mean improvement 1.05 units; 95% CI: 0.73 to 1.38 units, $p < 0.0001$). An improvement was maintained throughout the treatment period.

(b) The improvement in mean total score of patient's evaluation of their Quality of Life (as measured using the St. George's Respiratory Questionnaire) between Spiriva Respimat versus placebo at the end of the two 1-year studies was 3.5 units (95% CI: 2.1 to 4.9, $p < 0.0001$). A 4-unit decrease is considered clinically relevant.

(c) Spiriva Respimat significantly reduced the number of COPD exacerbations (study A: mean reduction 21% per year, 95% CI; 1% to 37% reduction per year, p=0.04; study B: mean reduction 23% per year; 95% CI: 4% to 38% reduction per year, p=0.02; studies A and B pooled mean reduction 22% per year; 95% CI: 8% to 33% reduction per year, p=0.002) and delayed the time to first COPD exacerbation (study A: one in four placebo patients had an exacerbation by day 112, whereas for Spiriva Respimat one in four had an exacerbation by day 173, p=0.09; study B: one in four placebo patients had an exacerbation by day 74, whereas for Spiriva Respimat one in four had an exacerbation by day 149 ($p < 0.0001$); studies A and B pooled: one in four placebo patients had an exacerbation by day 86, whereas for Spiriva Respimat one in four had an exacerbation by day 160 ($p < 0.0001$)).

5.2 Pharmacokinetic properties

a) General Introduction

Tiotropium bromide is a non-chiral quaternary ammonium compound and is sparingly soluble in water. Tiotropium bromide is available as solution for inhalation administered by the Respimat inhaler. Approximately 40% of the inhaled dose is deposited in the lungs, the target organ, the remaining amount being deposited in the gastrointestinal tract. Some of the pharmacokinetic data described below were obtained with higher doses than recommended for therapy.

b) General Characteristics of the Active Substance after Administration of the Medicinal Product

Absorption: Following inhalation of the solution by young healthy volunteers, urinary excretion data suggest that approximately 33% of the inhaled dose reach the systemic circulation. It is expected from the chemical structure of the compound (quaternary ammonium compound) and from in-vitro experiments that tiotropium bromide is poorly absorbed from the gastrointestinal tract (10-15%). Oral solutions of tiotropium bromide have an absolute bioavailability of 2-3%. At steady state, tiotropium bromide plasma levels in COPD patients at peak were 10.5-11.7 pg/ml when measured 10 minutes after administration of a 5 microgram dose delivered by the Respimat inhaler and decreased rapidly in a multi-compartmental manner. Steady state trough plasma concentrations were 1.49-1.68 pg/ml. Food is not expected to influence the absorption of this quaternary ammonium compound.

Distribution: The drug is bound by 72% to plasma proteins and shows a volume of distribution of 32 l/kg. Local concentrations in the lung are not known, but the mode of administration suggests substantially higher concentrations in the lung. Studies in rats have shown that tiotropium bromide does not penetrate the blood-brain barrier to any relevant extent.

Biotransformation: The extent of biotransformation is small. This is evident from a urinary excretion of 74% of unchanged substance after an intravenous dose to young healthy volunteers. The ester tiotropium bromide is nonenzymatically cleaved to the alcohol (N-methylscopine) and acid compound (dithienylglycolic acid) that are inactive on muscarinic receptors. In-vitro experiments with human liver microsomes and human hepatocytes suggest that some further drug (< 20% of dose after intravenous administration) is metabolised by cytochrome P450 (CYP) dependent oxidation and subsequent glutathion conjugation to a variety of Phase II-metabolites.

In vitro studies in liver microsomes reveal that the enzymatic pathway can be inhibited by the CYP 2D6 (and 3A4) inhibitors, quinidine, ketoconazole and gestodene. Thus CYP 2D6 and 3A4 are involved in metabolic pathway that is responsible for the elimination of a smaller part of the dose.

Tiotropium bromide even in supra-therapeutic concentrations does not inhibit CYP 1A1, 1A2, 2B6, 2C9, 2C19, 2D6, 2E1 or 3A in human liver microsomes.

Elimination: The terminal elimination half-life of tiotropium bromide is between 5 and 6 days following inhalation. Total clearance was 880 ml/min after an intravenous dose in young healthy volunteers with an interindividual variability of 22%. Intravenously administered tiotropium bromide is mainly excreted unchanged in urine (74%). After inhalation of the solution urinary excretion is 20.1-29.4 % of the dose, the remainder being mainly non-absorbed drug in gut that is eliminated via the faeces. The renal clearance of tiotropium bromide exceeds the creatinine clearance, indicating secretion into the urine.

Linearity / Nonlinearity: Tiotropium bromide demonstrates linear pharmacokinetics in the therapeutic range after intravenous administration, dry powder inhalation and inhalation of the solution.

c) Characteristics in Patients

Geriatric Patients: As expected for all predominantly renally excreted drugs, advanced age was associated with a decrease of tiotropium bromide renal clearance (326 ml/min in COPD patients < 58 years to 163 ml/min in COPD patients > 70years) which may be explained by decreased renal function. Tiotropium bromide excretion in urine after inhalation decreased from 14 % (young healthy volunteers) to about 7 % (COPD patients); however plasma concentrations did not change significantly with advancing age within COPD patients if compared to inter- and intraindividual variability (43 % increase in AUC_{0-4} after dry powder inhalation).

Renally Impaired Patients: In common with all other drugs that undergo predominantly renal excretion, renal impairment was associated with increased plasma drug concentrations and reduced renal drug clearance after both intravenous infusion and dry powder inhalation. Mild renal impairment (CL_{CR} 50-80 ml/min) which is often seen in elderly patients increased tiotropium bromide plasma concentrations slightly (39% increase in AUC_{0-4h} after intravenous infusion). In COPD patients with moderate to severe renal impairment (CL_{CR} < 50 ml/min) the intravenous administration of tiotropium bromide resulted in doubling of the plasma concentrations (82% increase in AUC_{0-4h}), which was confirmed by plasma concentrations after dry powder inhalation and also by inhalation of the solution via the Respimat inhaler.

Hepatically Impaired Patients: Liver insufficiency is not expected to have any relevant influence on tiotropium bromide pharmacokinetics. Tiotropium bromide is predominantly cleared by renal elimination (74% in young healthy volunteers) and simple non-enzymatic ester cleavage to pharmacologically inactive products.

Paediatric Patients: See 4.2

d) Pharmacokinetic / Pharmacodynamic Relationship(s)

There is no direct relationship between pharmacokinetics and pharmacodynamics.

5.3 Preclinical safety data

Many effects observed in conventional studies of safety pharmacology, repeat-dose toxicity, and reproductive toxicity could be explained by the anticholinergic properties of tiotropium bromide. Typically in animals reduced food consumption, inhibited body weight gain, dry mouth and nose, reduced lacrimation and salivation, mydriasis and increased heart rate were observed. Other relevant effects noted in repeated dose toxicity studies were: mild irritancy of the respiratory tract in rats and mice evinced by rhinitis and epithelial changes of the nasal cavity and larynx, and prostatitis along with proteinaceous deposits and lithiasis in the bladder in rats.

Harmful effects with respect to pregnancy, embryonal/foetal development, parturition or postnatal development could only be demonstrated at maternally toxic dose levels. Tiotropium bromide was not teratogenic in rats or rabbits. The respiratory (irritation) and urogenital (prostatitis) changes and reproductive toxicity was observed at local or systemic exposures more than five-fold the therapeutic exposure. Studies on genotoxicity and carcinogenic potential revealed no special hazard for humans.

6. PHARMACEUTICAL PARTICULARS

6.1 List of excipients

Benzalkonium chloride

Disodium edetate

Water, purified

Hydrochloric acid 3.6 % (for pH adjustment)

6.2 Incompatibilities

Not applicable.

6.3 Shelf life

2 years

In-use shelf life: 2 months

6.4 Special precautions for storage

Do not freeze.

6.5 Nature and contents of container

Type and material of the container in contact with the medicinal product:

Solution filled into a polyethylene/polypropylene cartridge with a polypropylene cap with integrated silicone sealing ring. The cartridge is enclosed within an aluminium cylinder.

Pack sizes and devices supplied:

Single pack: 1 Respimat inhaler and 1 cartridge, providing 60 puffs (30 medicinal doses)

Double pack: 2 single packages, each containing 1 Respimat inhaler and 1 cartridge, providing 60 puffs (30 medicinal doses)

Triple pack: 3 single packages, each containing 1 Respimat inhaler and 1 cartridge, providing 60 puffs (30 medicinal doses)

Eight pack: 8 single packages, each containing 1 Respimat inhaler and 1 cartridge, providing 60 puffs (30 medicinal doses)

Not all pack sizes may be marketed.

6.6 Special precautions for disposal and other handling

Any unused product or waste material should be disposed of in accordance with local requirements.

7. MARKETING AUTHORISATION HOLDER

Boehringer Ingelheim International GmbH

Binger Strasse 173

D-55216 Ingelheim am Rhein

Germany

8. MARKETING AUTHORISATION NUMBER(S)

PL 14598/0084

9. DATE OF FIRST AUTHORISATION/RENEWAL OF THE AUTHORISATION

12/09/2007

10. DATE OF REVISION OF THE TEXT

12/9/2007

Legal Category

POM

Sporanox 10 mg/ml Oral Solution

(Janssen-Cilag Ltd)

1. NAME OF THE MEDICINAL PRODUCT

Sporanox® 10 mg/ml Oral Solution.

2. QUALITATIVE AND QUANTITATIVE COMPOSITION

1 ml Sporanox oral solution contains 10mg itraconazole.

Sorbitol E420 (190 microlitre per ml).

For a full list of excipients, see section 6.1.

3. PHARMACEUTICAL FORM

Oral solution.

Sporanox oral solution is clear, yellow to slightly amber solution with an odour of cherry.

4. CLINICAL PARTICULARS

4.1 Therapeutic indications

Sporanox oral solution is indicated:

– For the treatment of oral and/or oesophageal candidosis in HIV-positive or other immunocompromised patients.

– As prophylaxis of deep fungal infections anticipated to be susceptible to itraconazole, when standard therapy is considered inappropriate, in patients with haematological malignancy or undergoing bone marrow transplant, and who are expected to become neutropenic (ie < 500 cells/µl). At present there are insufficient clinical efficacy data in the prevention of aspergillosis.

Consideration should be given to national and/or local guidance regarding the appropriate use of antifungal agents.

4.2 Posology and method of administration

For optimal absorption, Sporanox oral solution should be taken without food (patients are advised to refrain from eating for at least 1 hour after intake).

For the treatment of oral and/or oesophageal candidosis, the liquid should be swished around the oral cavity (approx. 20 seconds) and swallowed. There should be no rinsing after swallowing.

Treatment of oral and/or oesophageal candidosis: 200 mg (2 measuring cups) per day in two intakes, or alternatively in one intake, for 1 week. If there is no response after 1 week, treatment should be continued for another week.

Treatment of fluconazole resistant oral and/or oesophageal candidosis: 100 to 200 mg (1-2 measuring cups) twice daily for 2 weeks. If there is no response after 2 weeks, treatment should be continued for another 2 weeks. The 400mg daily dose should not be used for longer than 14 days if there are no signs of improvement.

Prophylaxis of fungal infections: 5 mg/kg per day administered in two intakes. In clinical trials, prophylaxis treatment was started immediately prior to the cytostatic treatment and generally one week before transplant procedure. Almost all proven deep fungal infections occurred in patients reaching neutrophil counts below 100 cells/µl. Treatment was continued until recovery of neutrophils (ie > 1000 cells/µl).

Pharmacokinetic parameters from clinical studies in neutropenic patients demonstrate considerable intersubject variation. Blood level monitoring should be considered particularly in the presence of gastrointestinal damage, diarrhoea and during prolonged courses of Sporanox oral solution.

<u>Use in children:</u>

Since clinical data on the use of Sporanox oral solution in paediatric patients is limited, its use in children is not recommended unless the potential benefit outweighs the potential risks. See section 4.4 Special warnings and special precautions for use.

Prophylaxis of fungal infections: there are no efficacy data available in neutropenic children. Limited safety experience is available with a dose of 5 mg/kg per day administered in two intakes. The incidence of adverse events such as diarrhoea, abdominal pain, vomiting, fever, rash and mucositis was higher than in adults.

<u>Use in elderly:</u>

Since clinical data on the use of Sporanox oral solution in elderly patients is limited, it is advised to use Sporanox oral solution in these patients only if the potential benefit outweighs the potential risks. See section 4.4 Special warnings and special precautions for use.

<u>Use in patients with hepatic impairment</u>

Limited data are available on the use of oral itraconazole in patients with hepatic impairment. Caution should be exercised when this drug is administered in this patient population. (See 5.2 Pharmacokinetic properties, Special populations, Hepatic impairment)

<u>Use in patients with renal impairment</u>

Limited data are available on the use of oral itraconazole in patients with renal impairment. Caution should be exercised when this drug is administered in this patient population.

4.3 Contraindications

Sporanox oral solution is contraindicated in patients with a known hypersensitivity to itraconazole or to any of the excipients.

Co-administration of the following drugs is contraindicated with Sporanox oral solution (see also 4.5 Interaction with other medicinal products and other forms of interaction):

- CYP3A4 metabolised substrates that can prolong the QT-interval e.g., astemizole, bepridil, cisapride, dofetilide, levacetylmethadol (levomethadyl), mizolastine, pimozide, quinidine, sertindole and terfenadine are contraindicated with Sporanox oral solution. Co-administration may result in increased plasma concentrations of these substrates, which can lead to QT prolongation and rare occurrences of *torsade de pointes*.

- CYP3A4 metabolized HMG-CoA reductase inhibitors such as atorvastatin, lovastatin and simvastatin

- Triazolam and oral midazolam

- Ergot alkaloids such as dihydroergotamine, ergometrine (ergonovine), ergotamine and methylergometrine (methylergonovine).

- Eletriptan

- Nisoldipine

- Sporanox oral solution should not be administered to patients with evidence of ventricular dysfunction such as congestive heart failure (CHF) or a history of CHF except for the treatment of life-threatening or other serious infections. (see section 4.6 Pregnancy and lactation)

Sporanox oral solution should not be used during pregnancy for non life-threatening indications (see section 4.6 Pregnancy and lactation).

4.4 Special warnings and precautions for use

<u>Cardiac effects</u>

In a healthy volunteer study with Sporanox IV, a transient asymptomatic decrease of the left ventricular ejection fraction was observed.

Itraconazole has been shown to have a negative inotropic effect and Sporanox has been associated with reports of congestive heart failure. Heart failure was more frequently reported among spontaneous reports of 400mg total daily dose than among those of lower total daily doses, suggesting that the rsik of heart failure might increase with the total daily dose of itraconazole.

Sporanox oral solution should not be used in patients with congestive heart failure or with a history of congestive heart failure unless the benefit clearly outweighs the risk. This individual benefit/risk assessment should take into consideration factors such as the severity of the indication, the dose and duration of the treatment, and individual risk factors for congestive heart failure. Such patients should be informed of the signs and symptoms of congestive heart failure, should be treated with caution, and should be monitored for signs and symptoms of congestive heart failure during treatment; if such signs or symptoms do occur during treatment, Sporanox oral solution should be discontinued.

Caution should be exercised when co-administering itraconazole and calcium channel blockers (see section 4.5. Interaction with other medicinal products).

<u>Interaction potential</u>

Sporanox oral solution has a potential for clinically important drug interactions. (See section 4.5. Interaction with other medicinal products and other forms of interaction).

<u>Use in children</u>

Since clinical data on the use of Sporanox oral solution in paediatric patients is limited, its use in children is not recommended unless the potential benefit outweighs the potential risks.

<u>Use in elderly</u>

Since clinical data on the use of Sporanox oral solution in elderly patients is limited, it is advised to use Sporanox oral solution in these patients only if the potential benefit outweighs the potential risks.

<u>Hepatic effects</u>

Very rare cases of serious hepatotoxicity, including some cases of fatal acute liver failure, have occurred with the use of Sporanox. Some of these cases involved patients with no pre-existing liver disease. Some of these cases have been observed within the first month of treatment, including some within the first week. Liver function monitoring should be considered in patients receiving Sporanox treatment. Patients should be instructed to promptly report to their physician signs and symptoms suggestive of hepatitis such as anorexia, nausea, vomiting, fatigue, abdominal pain or dark urine. In these patients treatment should be stopped immediately and liver function testing should be conducted. Most cases of serious hepatotoxicity involved patients who had pre-existing liver disease, were treated for systemic indications, had significant other medical conditions and/or were taking other hepatotoxic drugs. In patients with raised liver enzymes or active liver disease, or who have experienced liver toxicity with other drugs, treatment should not be started unless the expected benefit exceeds the risk of hepatic injury. In patients with impaired hepatic function liver enzyme should be carefully monitored when taking itraconazole.

<u>Hepatic impairment</u>

Limited data are available on the use of oral itraconazole in patients with hepatic impairment. Caution should be exercised when the drug is administered in this patient population. (See 5.2 Pharmacokinetic properties, Special populations, Hepatic impairment)

<u>Renal impairment</u>

Limited data are available on the use of oral itraconazole in patients with renal impairment. Caution should be exercised when this drug is administered in this patient population.

<u>Prophylaxis in neutropenic patients</u>

In clinical trials diarrhoea was the most frequent adverse event. This disturbance of the gastrointestinal tract may result in impaired absorption and may alter the microbiological flora potentially favouring fungal colonisation. Consideration should be given to discontinuing Sporanox oral solution in these circumstances.

<u>Treatment of severely neutropenic patients</u>

Sporanox oral solution as treatment for oral and/or oesophageal candidosis was not investigated in severely neutropenic patients. Due to the pharmacokinetic properties (See 5.2 Pharmacokinetic properties), Sporanox oral solution is not recommended for initiation of treatment in patients at immediate risk of systemic candidosis.

<u>Neuropathy</u>

If neuropathy occurs that may be attributable to Sporanox oral solution, the treatment should be discontinued.

<u>Hearing Loss</u>

Transient or permanent hearing loss has been reported in patients receiving treatment with itraconazole. Several of these reports included concurrent administration of quinidine which is contraindicated (see sections 4.3 and 4.5). The hearing loss usually resolves when treatment is stopped, but can persist in some patients.

<u>Cross-hypersensitivity</u>

There is no information regarding cross hypersensitivity between itraconazole and other azole antifungal agents. Caution should be used in prescribing Sporanox oral solution to patients with hypersensitivity to other azoles.

Sporanox oral solution contains sorbitol and should not be given to patients with rare hereditary problems of fructose intolerance.

4.5 Interaction with other medicinal products and other forms of interaction

4.5.1. Drugs affecting the metabolism of itraconazole:

Itraconazole is mainly metabolised through the cytochrome CYP3A4. Interaction studies have been performed with rifampicin, rifabutin and phenytoin, which are potent enzyme inducers of CYP3A4. Since the bioavailability of itraconazole and hydroxy-itraconazole was decreased in these studies to such an extent that efficacy may be largely reduced, the combination of itraconazole with these potent enzyme inducers is not recommended. No formal study data are available for other enzyme inducers, such as carbamazepine, phenobarbital and isoniazid, but similar effects should be anticipated.

Potent inhibitors of this enzyme such as ritonavir, indinavir, clarithromycin and erythromycin may increase the bioavailability of itraconazole.

4.5.2. Effect of itraconazole on the metabolism of other drugs:

4.5.2.1 Itraconazole can inhibit the metabolism of drugs metabolised by the cytochrome 3A family. This can result in an increase and/or a prolongation of their effects, including side effects. When using concomitant medication, the corresponding label should be consulted for information on the route of metabolism. After stopping treatment, itraconazole plasma levels decline gradually, depending on the dose and duration of treatment (See Section 5.2. Pharmacokinetic Properties). This should be taken into account when the inhibitory effect of itraconazole on comedicated drugs is considered.

Examples are:

The following drugs are contraindicated with itraconazole:

- Astemizole, cisapride, dofetilide, levacetylmethadol (levomethadyl), mizolastine, pimozide, quinidine, sertindole and terfenadine are contraindicated with Sporanox oral solution since co-administration may result in increased plasma concentrations of these substrates, which can lead to QT prolongation and rare occurrences of *torsade de pointes*.

- CYP3A4 metabolized HMG-CoA reductase inhibitors such as atorvastatin, lovastatin and simvastatin.

- Triazolam and oral midazolam.

- Ergot alkaloids such as dihydroergotamine, ergometrine (ergonovine), ergotamine and methylergometrine (methylergonovine).

- Eletriptan

- Nisoldipine

Caution should be exercised when co-administering itraconazole with calcium channel blockers due to an increased risk of congestive heart failure. In addition to possible pharmacokinetic interactions involving the drug metabolising enzyme CYP3A4, calcium channel blockers can have negative inotropic effects which may be additive to those of itraconazole.

The following drugs should be used with caution, and their plasma concentrations, effects or side effects should be monitored. Their dosage, if co-administered with itraconazole, should be reduced if necessary:

- Oral anticoagulants;
- HIV protease inhibitors such as ritonavir, indinavir, saquinavir;
- Certain antineoplastic agents such as busulfan, docetaxel, trimetrexate and vinca alkaloids;
- CYP3A4 metabolised calcium channel blockers such as dihydropyridines and verapamil;
- Certain immunosuppressive agents: cyclosporine, tacrolimus, rapamycin (also known as sirolimus);
- Certain glucocorticosteroids such as budesonide, dexamethasone, fluticasone and methylprednisolone;
- Digoxin (via inhibiton of P-glycoprotein)

- Others: cilostazol, disopyramide, carbamazepine, buspirone, alfentanil, alprazolam, brotizolam, midazolam IV, rifabutin, ebastine, repaglinide, fentanyl, halofantrine, reboxetine and loperamide. The importance of the concentration increase and the clinical relevance of these changes during the co-administration with itraconazole remain to be established.

4.5.2.2

No interaction of itraconazole with zidovudine (AZT) and fluvastatin has been observed.

No inducing effects of itraconazole on the metabolism of ethinyloestradiol and norethisterone were observed.

4.5.3. Effect on protein binding:

In vitro studies have shown that there are no interactions on the plasma protein binding between itraconazole and imipramine, propranolol, diazepam, cimetidine, indometacin, tolbutamide and sulfamethazine.

4.6 Pregnancy and lactation

Pregnancy:

Sporanox oral solution must not be used during pregnancy except for life-threatening cases where the potential benefit to the mother outweighs the potential harm to the foetus (see 4.3 Contraindications).

In animal studies itraconazole has shown reproduction toxicity (see 5.3 Preclinical safety data).

Epidemiological data on exposure to Sporanox during the first trimester of pregnancy - mostly in patients receiving short-term treatment for vulvovaginal candidosis - did not show an increased risk for malformations as compared to control subjects not exposed to any known teratogens.

Women of child-bearing potential:

Women of childbearing potential taking Sporanox oral solution should use contraceptive precautions. Effective contraception should be continued until the next menstrual period following the end of Sporanox therapy.

Lactation:

A very small amount of itraconazole is excreted in human milk. Sporanox Oral Solution must not be used during lactation.

4.7 Effects on ability to drive and use machines

No studies on the effects on the ability to drive and use machines have been performed. When driving vehicles and operating machinery the possibility of adverse reactions such as dizziness (see Section 4.8 Undesirable effects), which may occur in some instances, must be taken into account.

4.8 Undesirable effects

Approximately 9% of patients can be expected to experience adverse reactions while taking itraconazole. In patients receiving prolonged (approximately 1 month) continuous treatment especially, the incidence of adverse events has been higher (about 15%). The most frequently reported adverse experiences have been of gastrointestinal, hepatic and dermatological origin.

The table below presents adverse drug reactions by System Organ Class. Within each System Organ Class, the adverse drug reactions are presented by incidence, using the following convention:

Very common (⩾ 1/10); Common (⩾ 1/100 to < 1/10); Uncommon (⩾ 1/1,000 to < 1/100); Rare (⩾ 1/10,000 to < 1/1,000); Very rare (< 1/10,000), Not known (cannot be estimated from the available data).

Adverse Drug Reactions	
Blood and lymphatic system disorders	
Uncommon	Leukopenia, Neutropenia, Thrombocytopenia
Immune system disorders	
Not Known	Serum Sickness, Angioneurotic Oedema, Anaphylactic Reaction, Anaphylactoid Reaction, Hypersensitivity
Metabolism and nutrition disorders	
Uncommon	Hypokalemia
Not Known	Hypertriglyceridemia
Nervous system disorders	
Common	Headache
Uncommon	Peripheral Neuropathy, Dizziness
Not Known	Paraesthesia, Hypoaesthesia
Eye disorders	
Uncommon	Visual Disorders, including Vision Blurred and Diplopia
Ear and labyrinth disorder	
Not Known	Tinnitus; Transient or permanent hearing loss
Cardiac disorders	
Not Known	Congestive Heart Failure
Respiratory, thoracic and mediastinal disorders	
Not Known	Pulmonary Oedema
Gastrointestinal disorders	
Common	Abdominal Pain, Vomiting, Nausea, Diarrhoea, Dysgeusia
Uncommon	Dyspepsia, Constipation
Hepato-biliary disorders	
Common	Hepatic enzyme increased
Uncommon	Hepatitis, Hyperbilirubinaemia
Not Known	Hepatotoxicity, Acute hepatic failure
Skin and subcutaneous tissue disorders	
Common	Rash
Uncommon	Pruritus
Not Known	Toxic epidermal necrolysis, Stevens-Johnson syndrome, erythema multiforme, exfoliative dermatitis, leukocytoclastic vasculitis, urticaria, alopecia, photosensitivity
Musculoskeletal and connective tissue disorders	
Not Known	Myalgia, arthralgia
Renal and urinary disorders	
Not Known	Pollakiuria, urinary incontinence
Reproductive system and breast disorders	
Not Known	Menstrual disorders, erectile dysfunction
General disorders and administration site conditions	
Uncommon	Oedema

4.9 Overdose

Symptoms:

There are limited data on the outcomes of patients ingesting high doses of itraconazole. In patients taking either 1000 mg of Sporanox oral solution or up to 3000 mg of Sporanox capsules, the adverse event profile was similar to that observed at recommended doses.

Treatment:

In the event of an overdose, supportive measures should be employed. Within the first hour after ingestion, gastric lavage may be performed. Activated charcoal may be given if considered appropriate. Itraconazole cannot be removed by haemodialysis. No specific antidote is available.

5. PHARMACOLOGICAL PROPERTIES

5.1 Pharmacodynamic properties

Pharmacotherapeutic group: Antimycotic for systemic use, triazole derivative.

ATC code: J02A C02

Mode of action

Itraconazole inhibits fungal 14α-demethylase, resulting in a depletion of ergosterol and disruption of membrane synthesis by fungi.

PK/PD relationship

The PK/PD relationship for itraconazole, and for triazoles in general, is poorly understood and is complicated by limited understanding of antifungal pharmacokinetics.

Mechanism(s) of resistance

Resistance of fungi to azoles appears to develop slowly and is often the result of several genetic mutations. Mechanisms that have been described are

- Over-expression of *ERG11*, the gene that encodes 14-alpha-demethylase (the target enzyme)
- Point mutations in *ERG11* that lead to decreased affinity of 14-alpha-demethylase for itraconazole
- Drug-transporter over-expression resulting in increased efflux of itraconazole from fungal cells (i.e., removal of itraconazole from its target)
- Cross-resistance. Cross-resistance amongst members of the azole class of drugs has been observed within *Candida* species though resistance to one member of the class does not necessarily confer resistance to other azoles.

Breakpoints

Breakpoints for itraconazole have not yet been established for fungi using EUCAST methods.

Using CLSI methods, breakpoints for itraconazole have only been established for *Candida* species from superficial mycotic infections. The CLSI breakpoints are: susceptible ≤0.125 mg/L and resistant ≥1 mg/L.

The prevalence of acquired resistance may vary geographically and with time for selected species, and local information on resistance is desirable, particularly when treating severe infections. As necessary, expert advice should be sought when the local prevalence of resistance is such that the utility of the agent in at least some types of infections is questionable.

The *in vitro* susceptibility of fungi to itraconazole depends on the inoculum size, incubation temperature, growth phase of the fungi, and the culture medium used. For these reasons, the minimum inhibitory concentration of itraconazole may vary widely. Susceptibility in the table below is based on MIC_{90} < 1 mg itraconazole/L. There is no correlation between *in vitro* susceptibility and clinical efficacy.

Commonly susceptible species
Aspergillus spp.[2]
Blastomyces dermatitidis[1]
Candida albicans
Candida parapsilosis
Cladosporium spp.
Coccidioides immitis[1]
Cryptococcus neoformans
Epidermophyton floccosum
Fonsecaea spp. [1]
Geotrichum spp.
Histoplasma spp.
Malassezia (formerly Pityrosporum) spp.
Microsporum spp.
Paracoccidioides brasiliensis[1]
Penicillium marneffei[1]
Pseudallescheria boydii
Sporothrix schenckii
Trichophyton spp.
Trichosporon spp.
Species for which acquired resistance may be a problem
Candida glabrata[3]
Candida krusei
Candida tropicalis[3]
Inherently resistant organisms
Absidia spp.
Fusarium spp.
Mucor spp.
Rhizomucor spp.
Rhizopus spp.
Scedosporium proliferans
Scopulariopsis spp.

[1] These organisms may be encountered in patients who have returned from travel outside Europe.

[2] Itraconazole-resistant strains of *Aspergillus fumigatus* have been reported.

[3] Natural intermediate susceptibility.

5.2 Pharmacokinetic properties

General pharmacokinetic characteristics

The pharmacokinetics of itraconazole has been investigated in healthy subjects, special populations and patients after single and multiple dosing.

Absorption

Itraconazole is rapidly absorbed after administration of the oral solution. Peak plasma concentrations of the unchanged drug are reached within 2.5 hours following an oral dose under fasting conditions. The observed absolute bioavailability of itraconazole under fed conditions is about 55% and increases by 30 % when the oral solution is taken in fasting conditions.

Distribution

Most of the itraconazole in plasma is bound to protein (99.8%) with albumin being the main binding component (99.6% for the hydroxy- metabolite). It has also a marked affinity for lipids. Only 0.2% of the itraconazole in plasma is present as free drug. Itraconazole is distributed in a large apparent volume in the body (> 700 L), suggesting its extensive distribution into tissues: Concentrations in lung, kidney, liver, bone, stomach, spleen and muscle were found to be two to three times higher than corresponding concentrations in plasma. Brain to plasma ratios were about 1 as measured in beagle dogs. The uptake into keratinous tissues, skin in particular, is up to four times higher than in plasma.

Biotransformation

Itraconazole is extensively metabolised by the liver into a large number of metabolites. One of the main metabolites is hydroxy-itraconazole, which has *in vitro* antifungal activity comparable to itraconazole. Plasma concentrations of the hydroxy-itraconazole are about twice those of itraconazole.

As shown in *in vitro* studies, CYP 3A4 is the major enzyme that is involved in the metabolism of itraconazole.

Elimination

Itraconazole is excreted as inactive metabolites to about 35% in urine within one week and to about 54% with feces. Renal excretion of the parent drug accounts for less than 0.03% of the dose, whereas fecal excretion of unchanged drug varies between 3 - 18% of the dose. Itraconazole clearance decreases at higher doses due to saturable hepatic metabolism.

Linearity/non-linearity

As a consequence of non-linear pharmacokinetics, itraconazole accumulates in plasma during multiple dosing. Steady-state concentrations are generally reached within about 15 days, with Cmax and AUC values 4 to 7-fold higher than those seen after a single dose. The mean elimination half-life of itraconazole is about 40 hours after repeated dosing.

Special Populations

Hepatic Insufficiency: A pharmacokinetic study using a single 100 mg dose of itraconazole (one 100 mg capsule) was conducted in 6 healthy and 12 cirrhotic subjects. No statistically significant differences in AUC_∞ were seen between these two groups. A statistically significant reduction in average C_{max} (47%) and a two fold increase in the elimination half-life (37 ± 17 versus 16 ±5 hours) of itraconazole were noted in cirrhotic subjects compared with healthy subjects.

Data are not available in cirrhotic patients during long-term use of itraconazole.

Renal Insufficiency: Limited data are available on the use of oral itraconazole in patients with renal impairment. Caution should be exercised when the drug is administered in this patient population.

5.3 Preclinical safety data

Nonclinical data on itraconazole revealed no indications for gene toxicity, primary carcinogenicity or impairment of fertility. At high doses, effects were observed in the adrenal cortex, liver and the mononuclear phagocyte system but appear to have a low relevance for the proposed clinical use. Itraconazole was found to cause a dose-related increase in maternal toxicity, embryotoxicity and teratogenicity in rats and mice at high doses. A global lower bone mineral density was observed in juvenile dogs after chronic itraconazole administration, and in rats, a decreased bone plate activity, thinning of the zona compacta of the large bones, and an increased bone fragility was observed.

6. PHARMACEUTICAL PARTICULARS

6.1 List of excipients

Hydroxypropyl-β-cyclodextrin, sorbitol E420, propylene glycol, cherry flavour 1 (contains 1,2-propylene glycol E1520 and acetic acid E260), cherry flavour 2 (contains 1,2-propylene glycol E1520 and lactic acid E270), caramel, sodium saccharin, hydrochloric acid and sodium hydroxide (for pH adjustment), purified water.

6.2 Incompatibilities

In the absence of compatibility studies this medicinal product must not be mixed with other medicinal products.

6.3 Shelf life

24months as packaged for sale.

1 month after first opening the container.

6.4 Special precautions for storage

Do not store above 25°C.

6.5 Nature and contents of container

150 ml amber glass bottle, with child resistant polypropylene screw cap and LDPE liner ring.

A measuring cup graduated to indicate 10 ml is provided.

6.6 Special precautions for disposal and other handling

Sporanox oral solution is supplied in bottles with a child-proof cap, and should be opened as follows: push the plastic screw cap down while turning it counter clockwise.

Administrative Data

7. MARKETING AUTHORISATION HOLDER

Janssen-Cilag Ltd
50-100 Holmers Farm Way
High Wycombe
Buckinghamshire
HP12 4EG
UK

8. MARKETING AUTHORISATION NUMBER(S)

00242/0307

9. DATE OF FIRST AUTHORISATION/RENEWAL OF THE AUTHORISATION

26 April 1996/26 April 2006

10. DATE OF REVISION OF THE TEXT

November 2008

Legal category POM.

Sporanox Capsules

(Janssen-Cilag Ltd)

1. NAME OF THE MEDICINAL PRODUCT

SPORANOX® 100 mg Capsules.

2. QUALITATIVE AND QUANTITATIVE COMPOSITION

Each capsule contains itraconazole 100 mg.

For excipients, see 6.1.

3. PHARMACEUTICAL FORM

Capsules, hard

Capsule (Size 0): opaque blue cap and pink transparent body containing coated beads.

4. CLINICAL PARTICULARS

4.1 Therapeutic indications

1. Vulvovaginal candidosis.

2. Pityriasis versicolor.

3. Dermatophytoses caused by organisms susceptible to itraconazole *(Trichophyton spp., Microsporum spp., Epidermophyton floccosum)* e.g. tinea pedis, tinea cruris, tinea corporis, tinea manuum.

4. Oropharyngeal candidosis.

5. Onychomycosis caused by dermatophytes and/or yeasts.

6. The treatment of histoplasmosis.

7. Sporanox is indicated in the following systemic fungal conditions when first-line systemic anti-fungal therapy is inappropriate or has proved ineffective. This may be due to underlying pathology, insensitivity of the pathogen or drug toxicity.

- Treatment of aspergillosis and candidosis

- Treatment of cryptococcosis (including cryptococcal meningitis): in immunocompromised patients with cryptococcosis and in all patients with cryptococcosis of the central nervous system.

- Maintenance therapy in AIDS patients to prevent relapse of underlying fungal infection.

Sporanox is also indicated in the prevention of fungal infection during prolonged neutropenia when standard therapy is considered inappropriate.

4.2 Posology and method of administration

Sporanox is for oral administration and must be taken immediately after a meal for maximal absorption.

Treatment schedules in adults for each indication are as follows:

Indication	*Dose*	*Remarks*
Vulvovaginal candidosis	200 mg twice daily for 1 day	
Pityriasis versicolor	200 mg once daily for 7 days	
Tinea corporis, tinea cruris	100 mg once daily for 15 days or 200 mg once daily for 7 days	
Tinea pedis, tinea manuum	100 mg once daily for 30 days	
Oropharyngeal candidosis	100 mg once daily for 15 days	Increase dose to 200 mg once daily for 15 days in AIDS or neutropenic patients because of impaired absorption in these groups.
Onychomycosis (toenails with or without fingernail involvement)	200 mg once daily for 3 months	

For skin, vulvovaginal and oropharyngeal infections, optimal clinical and mycological effects are reached 1 - 4 weeks after cessation of treatment and for nail infections, 6 - 9 months after the cessation of treatment. This is because elimination of itraconazole from skin, nails and mucous membranes is slower than from plasma.

The length of treatment for systemic fungal infections should be dictated by the mycological and clinical response to therapy:

Indication	*Dose*[1]	*Remarks*
Aspergillosis	200 mg once daily	Increase dose to 200 mg twice daily in case of invasive or disseminated disease
Candidosis	100-200 mg once daily	Increase dose to 200 mg twice daily in case of invasive or disseminated disease
Non-meningeal Cryptococcosis	200 mg once daily	
Cryptococcal meningitis	200 mg twice daily	See 4.4. Special warnings and special precautions for use.
Histoplasmosis	200 mg once daily - 200 mg twice daily	See note on impaired absorption below
Maintenance in AIDS	200 mg once daily	See note on impaired absorption below
Prophylaxis in neutropenia	200 mg once daily	

[1] The duration of treatment should be adjusted depending on the clinical response.

Impaired absorption in AIDS and neutropenic patients may lead to low itraconazole blood levels and lack of efficacy. In such cases, blood level monitoring and if necessary, an increase in itraconazole dose to 200 mg twice daily, is indicated.

Use in children

Not recommended. See 4.4 Special warnings and special precautions for use.

In Elderly

Not recommended. See 4.4 Special warnings and special precautions for use.

Use in patients with renal impairment

The oral bioavailability of itraconazole may be lower in patients with renal insufficiency, a dose adjustment may be considered. See 4.4 Special warnings and special precautions for use.

Use in patients with hepatic impairment

Itraconazole is predominantly metabolised by the liver. The terminal half-life of itraconazole in cirrhotic patients is somewhat prolonged. The oral bioavailability in cirrhotic patients is somewhat decreased. A dose adjustment may be considered. See 4.4 Special warnings and special precautions for use.

4.3 Contraindications

• Sporanox capsules are contra-indicated in patients who have shown hypersensitivity to the drug or its excipients.

• Coadministration of the following drugs is contraindicated with Sporanox capsules. (see also section 4.5 Interaction with other medicinal products and other forms of interaction):

- CYP3A4 metabolised substrates that can prolong the QT-interval e.g., astemizole, bepridil, cisapride, dofetilide, levacetylmethadol (levomethadyl), mizolastine, pimozide, quinidine, sertindole and terfenadine are contraindicated with Sporanox capsules. Coadministration may result in increased plasma concentrations of these substrates which can lead to QTc prolongation and rare occurrences of *torsades de pointes*.

- CYP3A4 metabolised HMG-CoA reductase inhibitors such as lovastatin and simvastatin

- Triazolam and oral midazolam

- Ergot alkaloids such as dihydroergotamine, ergometrine (ergonovine), ergotamine and methylergometrine (methylergonovine)

- Eletriptan

- Nisoldipine

- Sporanox capsules should not be administered for non-life threatening indications to patients receiving disopyramide or halofantrine.

Sporanox capsules should not be administered to patients with evidence of ventricular dysfunction such as congestive heart failure (CHF) or a history of CHF except for the treatment of life-threatening or other serious infections. See 4.4 Special warnings and precautions for use.

Sporanox capsules must not be used during pregnancy for non life-threatening indications (see section 4.6 Pregnancy and lactation).

4.4 Special warnings and precautions for use

Cardiac effects

In a healthy volunteer study with Sporanox® IV, a transient asymptomatic decrease of the left ventricular ejection fraction was observed.

Itraconazole has been shown to have a negative inotropic effect and Sporanox has been associated with reports of congestive heart failure. Heart failure was more frequently reported among spontaneous reports of 400 mg total daily dose than among those of lower total daily doses, suggesting that the risk of heart failure might increase with the total daily dose of itraconazole.

Sporanox should not be used in patients with congestive heart failure or with a history of congestive heart failure unless the benefit clearly outweighs the risk. This individual benefit/risk assessment should take into consideration factors such as the severity of the indication, the dose and duration of treatment (e.g. total daily dose), and individual risk factors for congestive heart failure. Such patients should be informed of the signs and symptoms of congestive heart failure, should be treated with caution, and should be monitored for signs and symptoms of congestive heart failure during treatment; if such signs or symptoms do occur during treatment, Sporanox should be discontinued.

Calcium channel blockers can have negative inotropic effects which may be additive to those of itraconazole. In addition, itraconazole can inhibit the metabolism of calcium channel blockers. Therefore, caution should be exercised when co-administering itraconazole and calcium channel blockers (see section 4.5, Interactions with other medicinal products and other forms of interaction) due to an increased risk of congestive heart failure.

Interaction Potential

Sporanox has a potential for clinically important drug interactions. (See 4.5: Interaction with other medicaments and other forms of interaction).

Reduced gastric acidity

Absorption of itraconazole is impaired when gastric acidity is reduced. In patients also receiving acid neutralising medicines (e.g. aluminium hydroxide), these should be administered at least 2 hours after the intake of Sporanox. In patients with achlorhydria, such as certain AIDS patients and patients on acid secretion suppressors (e.g. H_2 - antagonists, proton-pump inhibitors), it is advisable to administer Sporanox with a cola beverage.

Use in children

Clinical data on the use of Sporanox capsules in paediatric patients is limited. Sporanox capsules should not be used in paediatric patients unless the potential benefit outweighs the potential risks.

Use in elderly

Clinical data on the use of Sporanox-Pulse capsules in elderly patients is limited. Sporanox-Pulse capsules should not be used in these patients unless the potential benefit outweighs the potential risks.

Hepatic effects

Very rare cases of serious hepatotoxicity, including some cases of fatal acute liver failure, have occurred with the use of Sporanox. Some of these cases involved patients with no pre-existing liver disease. Some of these cases were observed within the first month of treatment, including some within the first week. Liver function monitoring should be considered in patients receiving Sporanox treatment. Patients should be instructed to promptly report to their physician signs and symptoms suggestive of hepatitis such as anorexia, nausea, vomiting, fatigue, abdominal pain or dark urine. In these patients treatment should be stopped immediately and liver function testing conducted. Most cases of serious hepatotoxicity involved patients who had pre-existing liver disease, were treated for systemic indications, had significant other medical conditions and/ or were taking other hepatotoxic drugs. In patients with raised liver enzymes or active liver disease, or who have experienced liver toxicity with other drugs, treatment should not be started unless the expected benefit exceeds the risk of hepatic injury. In such cases liver enzyme monitoring is necessary.

Hepatic impairment

Itraconazole is predominantly metabolised in the liver. A slight decrease in oral bioavailability in cirrhotic patients has been observed, although this was not of statistical significance. The terminal half-life was however significantly increased. The dose should be adapted if necessary.

Renal impairment

The oral bioavailability of itraconazole may be lower in patients with renal insufficiency. Dose adaptation may be considered.

Immunocompromised patients

In some immunocompromised patients (e.g., neutropenic, AIDS or organ transplant patients), the oral bioavailability of Sporanox capsules may be decreased.

Patients with immediately life-threatening systemic fungal infections

Due to the pharmacokinetic properties (See section 5.2), Sporanox capsules are not recommended for initiation of treatment in patients with immediately life-threatening systemic fungal infections.

Patients with AIDS

In patients with AIDS having received treatment for a systemic fungal infection such as sporotrichosis, blastomycosis, histoplasmosis or cryptococcosis (meningeal or non-meningeal) and who are considered at risk for relapse, the treating physician should evaluate the need for a maintenance treatment.

Neuropathy

If neuropathy occurs which may be attributable to Sporanox, treatment should be discontinued.

Cross-hypersensitivity

There is no information regarding cross hypersensitivity between itraconazole and other azole antifungal agents. Caution should be used in prescribing Sporanox to patients with hypersensitivity to other azoles.

Patients with rare hereditary problems of fructose intolerance, glucose-galactose malabsorption or sucrase-isomaltase insufficiency should not take this medicine.

• In systemic candidosis, if fluconazole-resistant strains of *Candida* species are suspected, it cannot be assumed that these are sensitive to itraconazole, hence their sensitivity should be tested before the start of Sporanox therapy.

4.5 Interaction with other medicinal products and other forms of interaction

1. Drugs affecting the absorption of itraconazole

Drugs that reduce the gastric acidity impair the absorption of itraconazole from Sporanox capsules (See 4.4 Special warnings and special precautions for use).

2. Drugs affecting the metabolism of itraconazole:

Itraconazole is mainly metabolised through the cytochrome CYP3A4. Interaction studies have been performed with rifampicin, rifabutin and phenytoin, which are potent inducers of CYP3A4. Since the bioavailability of itraconazole and hydroxy-itraconazole was decreased in these studies to such an extent that efficacy may be largely reduced, the combination of itraconazole with these potent enzyme inducers is not recommended. No formal study data are available for other enzyme inducers, such as carbamazepine, phenobarbital and isoniazid, but similar effects should be anticipated.

Potent inhibitors of this enzyme such as ritonavir, indinavir, clarithromycin and erythromycin may increase the bioavailability of itraconazole.

3. Effects of itraconazole on the metabolism of other drugs:

3.1 Itraconazole can inhibit the metabolism of drugs metabolised by the cytochrome 3A family. This can result in an increase and/or a prolongation of their effects, including side effects. When using concomitant medication, the corresponding label should be consulted for information on the route of administration. After stopping treatment, itraconazole plasma concentrations decline gradually, depending on the dose and duration of treatment (see 5.2 Pharmacokinetic Properties). This should be taken into account when the inhibitory effect of itraconazole on co-administered drugs is considered.

Examples are:

The following drugs are contraindicated with itraconazole:

Astemizole, bepridil, cisapride, dofetilide, levacetylmethadol (levomethadyl), mizolastine, pimozide, quinidine, sertindole or terfenadine are contraindicated with Sporanox since co-administration may result in increased plasma concentrations of these substrates, which can lead to QT prolongation and rare occurrences of torsades de pointes.

• CYP3A4 metabolised HMG-CoA reductase inhibitors such as lovastatin and simvastatin.

• Triazolam and oral midazolam.

• Ergot alkaloids such as dihydroergotamine, ergometrine (ergonovine), ergotamine and methylergometrine (methylergonovine).

• Eletriptan

• Nisoldipine

Caution should be exercised when co-administering itraconazole with calcium channel blockers due to an increased risk of congestive heart failure. In addition to possible pharmacokinetic interactions involving the drug metabolising enzyme CYP3A4, calcium channel blockers can have negative inotropic effects which may be additive to those of itraconazole.

The following drugs should be used with caution, and their plasma concentrations, effects or side effects should be monitored. Their dosage, when co-administered with itraconazole, should be reduced if necessary:

• Oral anticoagulants

• HIV protease inhibitors such as ritonavir, indinavir, saquinavir

• Certain antineoplastic agents such as vinca alkaloids, busulfan, docetaxel and trimetrexate

• CYP3A4 metabolised calcium channel blockers such as dihydropyridines and verapamil

• Certain immunosuppressive agents: ciclosporin, tacrolimus, rapamycin (also known as sirolimus)

• Certain CYP3A4 metabolised HMG-CoA reductase inhibitors such as atorvastatin

• Certain glucocorticoids such as budesonide, dexamethasone, fluticasone and methyl prednisolone

• Digoxin

• Others: carbamazepine, cilostazol, buspirone, disopyramide, alfentanil, alprazolam, brotizolam, midazolam IV, rifabutin, ebastine, fentanyl, halofantrine, repaglinide and reboxetine. The importance of the concentration increase and the clinical relevance of these changes during co-administration with itraconazole remain to be established.

3.2. No interaction of itraconazole with zidovudine (AZT) and fluvastatin has been observed.

No inducing effects of itraconazole on the metabolism of ethinyloestradiol and norethisterone were observed.

4. Effect on protein binding:

In vitro studies have shown that there are no interactions on the plasma protein binding between itraconazole and imipramine, propranolol, diazepam, cimetidine, indometacin, tolbutamide or sulphadimidine.

4.6 Pregnancy and lactation

Pregnancy

Sporanox capsules must not be used during pregnancy except for life-threatening cases where the potential benefit to the mother outweighs the potential harm to the foetus (see 4.3 Contraindications).

In animal studies itraconazole has shown reproduction toxicity (see 5.3 Preclinical safety data).

Epidemiological data on exposure to Sporanox during the first trimester of pregnancy-mostly in patients receiving short-term treatment for vulvovaginal candidosis-did not show an increased risk for malformations as compared to control subjects not exposed to any known teratogens.

Women of child bearing potential

Women of childbearing potential taking Sporanox capsules should use contraceptive precautions. Effective contraception should be continued until the next menstrual period following the end of Sporanox therapy.

Lactation

A very small amount of itraconazole is excreted in human milk. Sporanox capsules must not be used during lactation.

4.7 Effects on ability to drive and use machines

None known.

4.8 Undesirable effects

Approximately 9% of patients can be expected to experience adverse reactions while taking itraconazole. In patients receiving prolonged (approximately 1 month) continuous treatment, the incidence of adverse events was higher (about 15%). The most frequently reported adverse experiences were of gastrointestinal, hepatic and dermatological origin. Within each system organ class, the adverse reactions are ranked under the headings of frequency, using the following convention: Rare (>1/10,000, <1/1,000) and very rare (<1/10,000), including isolated reports. Based upon the post-marketing experience, the following adverse reactions have also been reported:

• Metabolism and Nutrition Disorders

• ***Very rare:*** *hypokalemia*

• Nervous System Disorders

• ***Very rare:*** *peripheral neuropathy, headache, and dizziness*

• Cardiac Disorders

• ***Very rare:*** *congestive heart failure*

• Respiratory, Thoracic and Mediastinal Disorders

• ***Very rare:*** *pulmonary oedema*

• Gastrointestinal Disorders

• ***Very rare:*** *abdominal pain, vomiting, dyspepsia, nausea, diarrhoea and constipation*

• Hepato-Biliary Disorders

• ***Very rare:*** *fatal acute liver failure, serious hepatotoxicity, hepatitis, and reversible increases in hepatic enzymes*

• Skin and Subcutaneous Tissue Disorders

• ***Very rare:*** *Stevens-Johnson syndrome, angio-oedema, urticaria, alopecia, rash, and pruritis*

• Reproductive System and Breast Disorders

• ***Very rare:*** *menstrual disorder*

• General Disorders and Administrative Site Conditions

• ***Very rare:*** *allergic reaction, and oedema*

4.9 Overdose

In the event of overdosage, patients should be treated symptomatically with supportive measures. Within the first hour after ingestion, gastric lavage may be performed. Activated charcoal may be given if considered appropriate. No specific antidote is available. Itraconazole cannot be removed by haemodialysis.

5. PHARMACOLOGICAL PROPERTIES

5.1 Pharmacodynamic properties

Pharmacotherapeutic classification: (Antimycotics for systemic use, triazole derivatives).

ATC code: J02A C02

Itraconazole, a triazole derivative, has a broad spectrum of activity.

In vitro studies have demonstrated that itraconazole impairs the synthesis of ergosterol in fungal cells. Ergosterol is a vital cell membrane component in fungi.

Impairment of its synthesis ultimately results in an antifungal effect.

For itraconazole, breakpoints have only been established for *Candida* spp. From superficial mycotic infections (CLSI M27-A2, breakpoints have not been established for EUCAST methodology). The CLSI breakpoints are as follows: susceptible ⩽0.125; susceptible, dose-dependent 0.25-0.5 and resistant ⩾ 1μg/mL. Interpretive breakpoints have not been established for the filamentous fungi.

In vitro studies demonstrate that itraconazole inhibits the growth of a broad range of fungi pathogenic for humans at concentrations usually ⩽ 1 μg/ml. These include:

dermatophytes (Trichophyton spp., Microsporum spp., *Epidermophyton floccosum*); yeasts (Candida spp., including *C. albicans*, *C. glabrata* and *C. krusei*, *Cryptococcus neoformans*, Pityrosporum spp., Trichosporon spp., Geotrichum spp.); Aspergillus spp.; Histoplasma spp.; *Paracoccidioides brasiliensis*; *Sporothrix schenckii*; Fonsecaea spp.; Cladosporium spp.; *Blastomyces dermatitidis*; *Coccidiodes immitis*; *Pseudallescheria boydii*; *Penicillium marneffei*; and various other yeasts and fungi.

Candida krusei, *Candida glabrata* and *Candida tropicalis* are generally the least susceptible Candida species, with some isolates showing unequivocal resistance to itraconazole *in vitro*.

The principal fungus types that are not inhibited by itraconazole are Zygomycetes (e.g. Rhizopus spp., Rhizomucor spp., Mucor spp. and Absidia spp.), Fusarium spp., *Scedosporium proliferans* and Scopulariopsis spp.

Azole resistance appears to develop slowly and is often the result of several genetic mutations. Mechanisms that have been described are overexpression of ERG11, which encodes the target enzyme 14α-demethylase, point mutations in ERG11 that lead to decreased target affinity and/or transporter overexpression resulting in increased efflux. Cross resistance between members of the azole class has been observed within Candida spp., although resistance to one member of the class does not necessarily confer resistance to other azoles. Itraconazole-resistant strains of *Aspergillus fumigatus* have been reported.

5.2 Pharmacokinetic properties

General pharmacokinetic characteristics

The pharmacokinetics of itraconazole has been investigated in healthy subjects, special populations and patients after single and multiple dosing.

Absorption

Itraconazole is rapidly absorbed after oral administration. Peak plasma concentrations of the unchanged drug are reached within 2 to 5 hours following an oral dose. The observed absolute bioavailability of itraconazole is about 55%. Oral bioavailability is maximal when the capsules are taken immediately after a full meal.

Distribution

Most of the itraconazole in plasma is bound to protein (99.8%) with albumin being the main binding component (99.6% for the hydroxy- metabolite). It has also a marked affinity for lipids. Only 0.2% of the itraconazole in plasma is present as free drug. Itraconazole is distributed in a large apparent volume in the body (> 700 L), suggesting its extensive distribution into tissues: Concentrations in lung, kidney, liver, bone, stomach, spleen and muscle were found to be two to three times higher than corresponding concentrations in plasma. Brain to plasma ratios were about 1 as measured in beagle dogs. The uptake into keratinous tissues, skin in particular, is up to four times higher than in plasma.

Biotransformation

Itraconazole is extensively metabolised by the liver into a large number of metabolites. One of the main metabolites is hydroxy-itraconazole, which has *in vitro* antifungal activity comparable to itraconazole. Plasma concentrations of the hydroxy-itraconazole are about twice those of itraconazole.

As shown in *in vitro* studies, CYP 3A4 is the major enzyme that is involved in the metabolism of itraconazole.

Elimination

Itraconazole is excreted as inactive metabolites to about 35% in urine within one week and to about 54% with feces. Renal excretion of the parent drug accounts for less than 0.03% of the dose, whereas fecal excretion of unchanged drug varies between 3 – 18% of the dose. Itraconazole clearance decreases at higher doses due to saturable hepatic metabolism.

Linearity/non-linearity

As a consequence of non-linear pharmacokinetics, itraconazole accumulates in plasma during multiple dosing. Steady-state concentrations are generally reached within about 15 days, with Cmax and AUC values 4 to 7-fold higher than those seen after a single dose. The mean elimination half-life of itraconazole is about 40 hours after repeated dosing.

Special Populations

Hepatic Insufficiency: A pharmacokinetic study using a single 100 mg dose of itraconazole (one 100 mg capsule) was conducted in 6 healthy and 12 cirrhotic subjects. No statistically significant differences in AUC_∞ were seen between these two groups. A statistically significant reduction in average C_{max} (47%) and a two fold increase in the elimination half-life (37 ± 17 versus 16 ±5 hours) of itraconazole were noted in cirrhotic subjects compared with healthy subjects.

Data are not available in cirrhotic patients during long-term use of itraconazole.

Renal Insufficiency: Limited data are available on the use of oral itraconazole in patients with renal impairment. Caution should be exercised when the drug is administered in this patient population.

5.3 Preclinical safety data

Nonclinical data on itraconazole revealed no indications for gene toxicity, primary carcinogenicity or impairment of fertility. At high doses, effects were observed in the adrenal cortex, liver and the mononuclear phagocyte system but appear to have a low relevance for the proposed clinical use. Itraconazole was found to cause a dose-related increase in maternal toxicity, embryotoxicity and teratogenicity in rats and mice at high doses. A global lower bone mineral density was observed in juvenile dogs after chronic itraconazole administration, and in rats, a decreased bone plate activity, thinning of the zona compacta of the large bones, and an increased bone fragility was observed.

6. PHARMACEUTICAL PARTICULARS

6.1 List of excipients

Sugar spheres

Hypromellose 2910 5mPa.s

Macrogol 20000

Capsule shell:

Titanium dioxide

Indigo carmine

Gelatin

Erythrosine

6.2 Incompatibilities

Not applicable.

6.3 Shelf life

3 years

6.4 Special precautions for storage

Do not store above 30°C.

Store in the original container.

6.5 Nature and contents of container

Perlalux tristar blister - plastic foil consisting of 3 layers

* Polyvinylchloride on the outside;

* Low density polyethylene in the middle;

* Polyvinylidene chloride on the inside;

Aluminium foil (thickness 20 μm) coated on the inner side with colourless heat-seal Lacquer: PVC mixed polymers with acrylates, 6 g/m^2.

or:

PVC blister consisting of -

Polyvinylchloride 'genotherm' glass clear, thickness 250 μm;

Aluminium foil (thickness 20μm) coated on the inner side with a colourless heat-seal Lacquer: PVC mixed polymers with acrylates, 6g/m^2.

Pack sizes: 4, **6*not marketed**, 15, 60 capsules.

6.6 Special precautions for disposal and other handling

No special requirements.

7. MARKETING AUTHORISATION HOLDER

Janssen-Cilag Ltd

50-100 Holmers Farm Way

High Wycombe

Buckinghamshire

HP12 4EG

UK

8. MARKETING AUTHORISATION NUMBER(S)

00242/0142

9. DATE OF FIRST AUTHORISATION/RENEWAL OF THE AUTHORISATION

18/01/89, 11/01/95

10. DATE OF REVISION OF THE TEXT

April 2009

Legal category POM.

Sporanox I.V. 10 mg/ml concentrate and solvent for solution for infusion

(Janssen-Cilag Ltd)

1. NAME OF THE MEDICINAL PRODUCT

Sporanox® I.V. 10 mg/ml concentrate and solvent for solution for infusion.

2. QUALITATIVE AND QUANTITATIVE COMPOSITION

Each ml of the concentrate contains 10 mg itraconazole.

One ampoule with 25 ml contains 250 mg itraconazole (itraconazole trihydrochloride salt formed *in situ*).

Each ml of the admixed solution contains 3.33 mg itraconazole.

One single dose of 200 mg itraconazole corresponds to 60 ml of the admixed solution.

For a full list of excipients, see 6.1.

3. PHARMACEUTICAL FORM

Concentrate and solvent for solution for infusion.

4. CLINICAL PARTICULARS

4.1 Therapeutic indications

Sporanox I.V. is indicated for the treatment of histoplasmosis.

Sporanox I.V. is indicated in the following systemic fungal conditions when first-line systemic anti-fungal therapy is inappropriate or has proved ineffective. (This may be due to underlying pathology, insensitivity of the pathogen or drug toxicity).

Treatment of aspergillosis, candidosis and cryptococcosis (including cryptococcal meningitis).

Consideration should be given to national and/or local guidance regarding the appropriate use of antifungal agents.

4.2 Posology and method of administration

Sporanox I.V. is given on the first two days in a loading dose twice daily, followed by once daily dosing.

Day 1 and 2 of the treatment: 1-hour infusion of 200 mg (60 ml of the admixed solution) Sporanox I.V. twice daily. See section 6.6.

From day 3 on: one 1-hour infusion of 200 mg (60 ml of the admixed solution) Sporanox I.V. each day. Safety for periods longer than 14 days has not been established.

Use in children: Since clinical data on the use of Sporanox I.V. in paediatric patients are unavailable, Sporanox I.V. should not be used in children unless the potential benefit outweighs the potential risk. See section 4.4. (Special warning and precautions for use).

Use in elderly: Since clinical data of the use of Sporanox I.V. in elderly patients are limited, it is advised to use Sporanox I.V. in these patients only if the potential benefit outweighs the potential risk. See section 4.4. (Special warning and precautions for use).

Use in patients with renal impairment: Limited data are available on the use of intravenous itraconazole in patients with renal impairment.

Hydroxypropyl-β-cyclodextrin, a required component of Sporanox intravenous formulation, is eliminated through glomerular filtration. Therefore, in patients with severe renal impairment defined as creatinine clearance below 30 ml/min the use of Sporanox I.V. is contraindicated. (See section 4.3 Contraindications).

In patients with mild and moderate renal impairment, Sporanox I.V. should be used with caution. Serum creatinine levels should be closely monitored and, if renal toxicity is suspected, consideration should be given to changing to the oral capsule formulation. See sections 4.4. Special warnings and special precautions for use and 5.2 Pharmacokinetic properties).

Use in patients with hepatic impairment: Limited data are available on the use of itraconazole in patients with hepatic impairment. Caution should be exercised when this drug is administered in this patient population. (See section 5.2 Pharmacokinetic properties).

4.3 Contraindications

– Sporanox I.V. is contraindicated in patients with a known hypersensitivity to itraconazole or to any of the excipients.

– Sporanox I.V. cannot be used when administration of Sodium Chloride Injection is contraindicated.

– The excipient hydroxypropyl-β-cyclodextrin is eliminated through glomerular filtration. Therefore, Sporanox I.V. is contraindicated in patients with severe renal impairment (defined as creatinine clearance below 30 ml/min). See section 4.4 Special warning and precautions for use and section 5.2 Pharmacokinetic Properties.

– Coadministration of the following drugs is contraindicated with Sporanox I.V. (see also section 4.5 Interaction with other medicinal products and other forms of interaction):

• CYP3A4 metabolised substrates that can prolong the QT-interval e.g., terfenadine, astemizole, bepridil, mizolastine, cisapride, dofetilide, quinidine, levacetylmethadol (levomethadyl), quinidine, sertindole or pimozide coadministration may result in increased plasma levels of these substrates which can lead to QTc prolongation and rare occurrences of torsades de pointes.

• CYP3A4 metabolised HMG-CoA reductase inhibitors such as simvastatin, lovastatin and atorvastatin

• Triazolam and oral midazolam

• Ergot alkaloids such as dihydroergotamine, ergometrine (ergonovine), ergotamine and methylergometrine (methylergonovine).

• Eletriptan

• Nisoldipine

– Sporanox I.V. must not be given during pregnancy for non life-threatening indications (see section 4.6 Pregnancy and lactation).

4.4 Special warnings and precautions for use

Interaction potential

Sporanox has a potential for clinically important drug interactions. (See 4.5: Interaction with other medicinal products and other forms of interaction).

Use in children

Since clinical data on the use of Sporanox I.V. in paediatric patients are unavailable, Sporanox I.V. should not be used in children unless the potential benefit outweighs the potential risk.

Use in elderly

Since clinical data of the use of Sporanox I.V. in elderly patients are limited, it is advised to use Sporanox I.V. in these patients only if the potential benefit outweighs the potential risk.

Hepatic effects

Very rare cases of serious hepatotoxicity, including some cases of fatal acute liver failure, have occurred with the use of Sporanox. Some of these cases involved patients with no pre-existing liver disease. Some of these cases have been observed within the first month of treatment, including some within the first week. Liver function monitoring should be considered in patients receiving Sporanox treatment. Patients should be instructed to promptly report to their physician signs and symptoms suggestive of hepatitis such as anorexia, nausea, vomiting, fatigue, abdominal pain or dark urine. In these patients treatment should be stopped immediately and liver function testing should be conducted. Most cases of serious hepatotoxicity involved patients who had pre-existing liver disease, were treated for systemic indications, had significant other medical conditions and/or were taking other hepatotoxic drugs. In patients with raised liver enzymes or active liver disease, or who have experienced liver toxicity with other drugs, treatment should not be started unless the expected benefit exceeds the risk of hepatic injury. In patients with impaired hepatic function liver enzyme should be carefully monitored when taking itraconazole.

Hepatic impairment

Studies have not been conducted with intravenous itraconazole in patients with hepatic impairment. Limited data are available on the use of oral itraconazole in patients with hepatic impairment. Caution should be exercised when the drug is administered to this patient population. (See Section 4.2 Posology and method of administration and 5.2 Pharmacokinetic properties)

Renal impairment

Hydroxypropyl-β-cyclodextrin, when administered intravenously, is eliminated through glomerular filtration. Therefore, patients with renal impairment defined as creatinine clearance below 30 ml/min Sporanox IV is contraindicated (see section 4.3 Contraindications and 5.2 Pharmacokinetic properties.)

Sporanox I.V. should be used with caution in patients with a lesser degree of renal failure. In patients with mild and moderate renal impairment, serum creatinine levels should be closely monitored and, if renal toxicity is suspected, consideration should be given to changing to the oral capsule formulation. See section 4.4. Special warning and precautions for use.

Neuropathy

If neuropathy occurs that may be attributable to Sporanox I.V., the treatment should be discontinued.

Cross hypersensitivity

There is no information regarding cross hypersensitivity between itraconazole and other azole antifungal agents. Caution should be used in prescribing Sporanox I.V. to patients with hypersensitivity to other azoles.

Cardiac effects

In a healthy volunteer study with Sporanox I.V., a transient asymptomatic decrease of the left ventricular ejection fraction was observed; this resolved before the next infusion. A similar investigation was not performed in the target patient population.

Itraconazole has been shown to have a negative inotropic effect and Sporanox has been associated with reports of congestive heart failure. Heart failure was more frequently reported among spontaneous reports of 400 mg total daily dose than among those of lower total daily doses, suggesting that the risk of heart failure might increase with the total daily dose of itraconazole.

Sporanox should not be used in patients with congestive heart failure or with a history of congestive heart failure unless the benefit clearly outweighs the risk.

Physicians should carefully review the risks and benefits of Sporanox therapy for patients with known risk factors for congestive heart failure. These risk factors include *cardiac disease, such as ischaemic and valvular disease; significant pulmonary disease, such as chronic obstructive pulmonary disease; and renal failure and other edematous disorders.* Such patients should be informed of the signs and symptoms of congestive heart failure, should be treated with caution, and should be monitored for signs and symptoms of congestive heart failure during treatment. If such signs or symptoms do occur during treatment, Sporanox should be discontinued.

Caution should be exercised when co-administering itraconazole and calcium channel blockers (see section 4.5, Interactions with other medicinal products).

Hearing Loss

Transient or permanent hearing loss has been reported in patients receiving treatment with itraconazole. Several of these reports included concurrent administration of quinidine which is contraindicated (see sections 4.3 and 4.5). The hearing loss usually resolves when treatment is stopped, but can persist in some patients.

4.5 Interaction with other medicinal products and other forms of interaction

1. Drugs affecting the metabolism of itraconazole:

Itraconazole is mainly metabolised through the cytochrome CYP3A4. Interaction studies have been performed with rifampicin, rifabutin and phenytoin, which are potent enzyme inducers of CYP3A4. Since the bioavailability of itraconazole and hydroxy-itraconazole was decreased in these studies to such an extent that efficacy may be largely reduced, the combination of itraconazole with these potent enzyme inducers is not recommended. No formal study data are available for other enzyme inducers, such as carbamazepine, *Hypericum perforatum* (St John's Wort), phenobarbital and isoniazid but similar effects should be anticipated.

Potent inhibitors of this enzyme such as ritonavir, indinavir, clarithromycin and erythromycin may increase the bioavailability of itraconazole.

2. Effect of itraconazole on the metabolism of other drugs:

Itraconazole can inhibit the metabolism of drugs metabolised by the cytochrome 3A family. This can result in an increase and/or a prolongation of their effects, including side effects. When using concomitant medication, the corresponding label should be consulted for information on the route of metabolism. After stopping treatment, itraconazole plasma concentrations decline gradually, depending on the dose and duration of treatment (see 5.2. Pharmacokinetic Properties). This should be taken into account when the inhibitory effect of itraconazole on co-medicated drugs is considered.

Drugs which are contraindicated with itraconazole:

- Terfenadine, astemizole, bepridil, mizolastine, levacetylmethadol (levomethadyl), cisapride, dofetilide, quinidine, sertindole or pimozide are contraindicated with Sporanox I.V. since coadministration may result in increased plasma levels of these substrates which can lead to QTc prolongation and rare occurrences of torsades de pointes (see section 4.3).
- CYP3A4 metabolised HMG-CoA reductase inhibitors such as simvastatin, lovastatin, and atorvastatin.
- Triazolam and oral midazolam.
- Ergot alkaloids such as dihydroergotamine, ergometrine (ergonovine), ergotamine and methylergometrine (methylergonovine).
- Eletriptan.
- Nisoldipine

Caution should be exercised when co-administering itraconazole with calcium channel blockers due to an increased risk of congestive heart failure. In addition to possible pharmacokinetic interactions involving the drug metabolising enzyme CYP3A4, calcium channel blockers can have negative inotropic effects which may be additive to those of itraconazole.

The following drugs should be used with caution and their plasma concentrations, effects or side effects should be monitored. Their dosage, if co-administered with itraconazole, should be reduced if necessary.

– Oral anticoagulants;

– HIV Protease Inhibitors such as ritonavir, indinavir, saquinavir;

– Certain antineoplastic agents such as vinca alkaloids, busulfan, docetaxel and trimetrexate;

– CYP3A4 metabolised calcium channel blockers such as dihydropyridines and verapamil;

– Certain CYP3A4 metabolised HMG-CoA reductase inhibitors such as cerivastatin (see also drugs which are contraindicated with itraconazole);

– Certain immunosuppressive agents: cyclosporine, tacrolimus, rapamycin (also known as sirolimus);

– Certain glucocorticosteroids such as budesonide, dexamethasone, fluticasone and methylprednisolone;

– Digoxin: (via inhibition of P-glycoprotein)

– Others: carbamazepine, cilostazol, buspirone, alfentanil, alprazolam, brotizolam, midazolam I.V., rifabutin, disopyramide ebastine, fentanyl, halofantrine, repaglinide and reboxetine. The importance of the concentration increase and clinical relevance of these changes during co-administration with itraconazole remain to be established.

No interaction of itraconazole with zidovudine (AZT) and fluvastatine has been observed.

No inducing effects of itraconazole on the metabolism of ethinyloestradiol and norethisterone were observed.

3. Effect on protein binding:

In vitro studies have shown that there are no interactions on the plasma protein binding between itraconazole and imipramine, propranolol, diazepam, cimetidine, indometacin, tolbutamide and sulfamethazine.

4.6 Pregnancy and lactation

Pregnancy

Sporanox IV must not be used during pregnancy except for life-threatening cases where the potential benefit to the mother outweighs the potential harm to the foetus (see section 4.3 Contraindications).

In animal studies itraconazole shows reproduction toxicity (see section 5.3 Preclinical safety data).

Epidemiological data on exposure to Sporanox during the first trimester of pregnancy – mostly in patients receiving short-term treatment for vulvovaginal candidosis – did not show an increased risk for malformations as compared to control subjects not exposed to any known teratogens.

Women of child bearing potential

Women of child-bearing potential receiving Sporanox IV should use contraceptive precautions. Effective contraception should be continued until the next menstrual period following the end of Sporanox IV therapy.

Lactation

A very small amount of itraconazole is excreted in human milk and must not be administered to lactating women. Breast-feeding is to be discontinued prior to taking itraconazole.

4.7 Effects on ability to drive and use machines

No effects have been observed.

4.8 Undesirable effects

In clinical trials with intravenous itraconazole, the most frequently reported adverse experiences were of gastrointestinal, metabolic and nutritional, and hepatobiliary origin.

The table below presents adverse drug reactions by System Organ Class. Within each System Organ Class, the adverse drug reactions are presented by incidence, using the following convention:

Very common (≥ 1/10); Common (≥ 1/100 to < 1/10); Uncommon (≥ 1/1,000 to < 1/100); Rare (≥ 1/10,000 to < 1/1,000); Very rare (< 1/10,000), Not known (cannot be estimated from the available data).

Adverse Drug Reactions	
Blood and lymphatic system disorders	
Not Known	Leukopenia, neutropenia, thrombocytopenia
Immune system disorders	
Not Known	Serum Sickness, Angioneurotic Oedema, Anaphylactic Reaction, Anaphylactoid Reaction, Hypersensitivity
Metabolism and nutrition disorders	
Common	Hypokalemia
Uncommon	Hyperglycaemia
Not Known	Hypertriglyceridemia
Nervous system disorders	
Common	Headache, Dizziness
Uncommon	Hypoaesthesia
Not Known	Peripheral Neuropathy, Paraesthesia
Eye disorders	
Uncommon	Visual Disorders, including Vision Blurred and Diplopia
Ear and labyrinth disorder	
Not Known	Tinnitus, Transient or permanent hearing loss
Cardiac disorders	
Not Known	Congestive Heart Failure, Hypertension
Respiratory, thoracic and mediastinal disorders	
Uncommon	Pulmonary Oedema
Gastrointestinal disorders	
Very Common	Nausea
Common	Abdominal Pain, Vomiting, Diarrhea, Constipation
Uncommon	Dysgeusia
Not Known	Dyspepsia
Hepato-biliary disorders	
Common	Hepatitis, Jaundice, Hyperbilirubinaemia, Hepatic Enzymes Increased
Not Known	Hepatotoxicity, Acute Hepatic Failure

Skin and subcutaneous tissue disorders	
Common	Rash, Pruritus
Not Known	Toxic Epidermal Necrolysis, Stevens-Johnson Syndrome, Erythema Multiforme, Exfoliative Dermatitis, Leukocytoclastic Vasculitis, Urticaria, Alopecia, Photosensitivity
Musculoskeletal and connective tissue disorders	
Uncommon	Myalgia
Not Known	Arthralgia
Renal and urinary disorders	
Not Known	Pollakiuria, urinary incontinence
Reproductive system and breast disorders	
Not Known	Menstrual Disorders, Erectile Dysfunction
General disorders and administration site conditions	
Common	Oedema

4.9 Overdose

In the event of overdose, supportive measures should be employed. Itraconazole cannot be removed by haemodialysis. No specific antidote is available.

5. PHARMACOLOGICAL PROPERTIES

5.1 Pharmacodynamic properties

Pharmacotherapeutic group: Antimycotic for systemic use, triazole derivatives

ATC code: J02A C02

Mode of action

Itraconazole inhibits fungal 14α-demethylase, resulting in a depletion of ergosterol and disruption of membrane synthesis by fungi.

PK/PD relationship

The PK/PD relationship for itraconazole, and for triazoles in general, is poorly understood and is complicated by limited understanding of antifungal pharmacokinetics.

Mechanism(s) of resistance

Resistance of fungi to azoles appears to develop slowly and is often the result of several genetic mutations. Mechanisms that have been described are:

- Over-expression of *ERG11*, the gene that encodes 14-alpha-demethylase (the target enzyme)
- Point mutations in *ERG11* that lead to decreased affinity of 14-alpha-demethylase for itraconazole
- Drug-transporter over-expression resulting in increased efflux of itraconazole from fungal cells (i.e., removal of itraconazole from its target)
- Cross-resistance. Cross-resistance amongst members of the azole class of drugs has been observed within *Candida* species though resistance to one member of the class does not necessarily conver resistance to other azoles.

Breakpoints

Breakpoints for itraconazole have not yet been established for fungi using EUCAST methods.

Using CLSI methods, breakpoints for itraconazole have only been established for *Candida* species from superficial mycotic infections. The CLSI breakpoints are: susceptible ⩽0.125 mg/L and resistant ⩾1 mg/L.

The prevalence of acquired resistance may vary geographically and with time for selected species, and local information on resistance is desirable, particularly when treating severe infections. As necessary, expert advice should be sought when the local prevalence of resistance is such that the utility of the agent in at least some types of infections is questionable.

The *in vitro* susceptibility of fungi to itraconazole depends on the inoculum size, incubation temperature, growth phase of the fungi, and the culture medium used. For these reasons, the minimum inhibitory concentration of itraconazole may vary widely. Susceptibility in the table below is based on MIC_{90} < 1 mg itraconazole/L. There is no correlation between *in vitro* susceptibility and clinical efficacy.

Commonly susceptible species
Aspergillus spp.[2]
Blastomyces dermatitidis[1]
Candida albicans
Candida parapsilosis
Cladosporium spp.
Coccidioides immitis[1]
Cryptococcus neoformans
Epidermophyton floccosum
Fonsecaea spp.[1]
Geotrichum spp.
Histoplasma spp.
Malassezia (formerly Pityrosporum) spp.
Microsporum spp.
Paracoccidioides brasiliensis[1]
Penicillium marneffei[1]
Pseudallescheria boydii
Sporothrix schenckii
Trichophyton spp.
Trichosporon spp.
Species for which acquired resistance may be a problem
Candida glabrata[3]
Candida krusei
Candida tropicalis[3]
Inherently resistant organisms
Absidia spp.
Fusarium spp.
Mucor spp.
Rhizomucor spp.
Rhizopus spp.
Scedosporium proliferans
Scopulariopsis spp.

[1] These organisms may be encountered in patients who have returned from travel outside Europe.

[2] Itraconazole-resistant strains of *Aspergillus fumigatus* have been reported.

[3] Natural intermediate susceptibility.

5.2 Pharmacokinetic properties

General pharmacokinetic characteristics

The pharmacokinetics of intravenously administered itraconazole has been investigated in healthy subjects, and patients after single and multiple dosing and in special populations after single doses.

Peak plasma concentrations of itraconazole are reached at the end of the intravenous infusion, declining thereafter. Peak plasma concentrations of hydroxyl-itraconazole (see Biotransformation below) are reached within 3 hours of beginning of a one-hour infusion, declining thereafter.

Each 200 mg intravenous dose of itraconazole contains 8g hydroxypropyl-β-cyclodextrin to increase the solubility of itraconazole. The pharmacokinetic profiles of each are described below. (See Itraconazole; see Special populations-Renal Impairment, Hydroxypropyl-β-cyclodextrin.)

Distribution

Most of the itraconazole in plasma is bound to protein (99.8%) with albumin being the main binding component (99.6% for the hydroxy-metabolite). It has also a marked affinity for lipids. Only 0.2% of the itraconazole in plasma is present as free drug. Itraconazole is distributed in a large apparent volume in the body (>700 L), suggesting its extensive distribution into tissues: Concentrations in lung, kidney, liver, bone, stomach, spleen and muscle were found to be two to three times higher than corresponding concentrations in plasma, and the uptake into keratinous tissues, skin in particular, up to four times higher. Brain to plasma ratios were about 1 as measured in beagle dogs.

Biotransformation

Itraconazole is extensively metabolised by the liver into a large number of metabolites. One of the main metabolites is hydroxy-itraconazole, which has *in vitro* antifungal activity comparable to itraconazole. Trough plasma concentrations of the hydroxy-metabolite are about twice those of itraconazole.

As shown in in-vitro studies, CYP3A4 is the major enzyme that is involved in the metabolism of itraconazole.

Elimination

Itraconazole total plasma clearance following intravenous administration is on average 381 ml/min. Itraconazole is excreted as inactive metabolites to about 35% in urine within one week and about 54% with feces. Renal excretion of the itraconazole and the active metabolite hydroxy-itraconazole account for less than 1%of an intravenous dose. Based on an oral dose, fecal excretion of unchanged drug ranges from 3% to 18% of the dose. Itraconazole is excreted mainly as inactive metabolites in urine (35%) and in feces (54%) within one week of an oral dose.

Linearity/non-linearity

As a consequence of non-linear pharmacokinetics, itraconazole accumulates in plasma during multiple dosing. In a multiple-dose pharmacokinetic study, itraconazole I.V. was administered as a 1-hour infusion of 200 mg itraconazole twice daily on days 1 and 2 of treatment, followed by a 1-hour infusion of 200 mg once daily from day 3 to 7. Steady-state concentrations were reached after the fourth dose of itraconazole I.V. and by the seventh dose for hydroxy-itraconazole. Mean C_{max} and C_{min} values after 4 doses of 200 mg itraconazole I.V. in healthy subjects were 3055 ng/ml and 687 ng/ml respectively, while mean values for hydroxy-itraconazole at the same time points were 1058 ng/ml and 1263 ng/ml respectively. Itraconazole mean total plasma clearance following intravenous administration is 278 ml/min. The mean elimination half-life of itraconazole is about 32.5 hours after repeated dosing.

Special Populations

Hepatic Impairment

Studies have not been conducted with intravenous itraconazole in patients with hepatic impairment. Itraconazole is predominantly metabolised in the liver. A single oral dose (100 mg capsule) was administered to 12 patients with cirrhosis and six healthy control subjects; Cmax, AUC and terminal half-life of itraconazole were measured and compared between groups. Mean itraconazole Cmax was reduced significantly (by 47%) in patients with cirrhosis. Mean elimination half-life was prolonged compared to that found in subjects without hepatic impairment (37 vs. 16 hours, respectively). Data are not available in cirrhotic patients during long-term use of itraconazole.

Renal Impairment

A small fraction (<1%) of an intravenous dose of itraconazole is excreted unchanged in urine.

After a single intravenous dose, the mean terminal half-lives of itraconazole in patients with mild (CrCl 50-79 ml/min), moderate (CrCl 20-49 ml/min), and severe renal impairment (CrCl <20 ml/min) were similar to that in healthy subjects, (range of means 42-49 hr vs 48 hr in renally impaired patients and healthy subjects, respectively.) Overall exposure to itraconazole, based on AUC, was decreased in patients with moderate and severe renal impairment by approximately 30% and 40%, respectively, as compared with subjects with normal renal function.

Data are not available in renally impaired patients during long-term use of itraconazole. Dialysis has no effect on the half-life or clearance of itraconazole or hydroxy-itraconazole.

Hydroxypropyl-β-Cyclodextrin

In patients with normal renal function, the pharmacokinetic profile of hydroxypropyl-β-cyclodextrin, an ingredient of Sporanox intravenous formulation, has a short half-life of 1 to 2 hours, and demonstrates no accumulation following successive daily doses. In healthy subjects and in patients with mild to severe renal insufficiency, the majority of an 8 g dose of hydroxypropyl-β-cyclodextrin is eliminated in the urine. Following a single intravenous dose of itraconazole 200 mg, clearance of hydroxypropyl-β-cyclodextrin was reduced in subjects with renal impairment, resulting in higher exposure to hydroxypropyl-β-cyclodextrin. In subjects with mild, moderate, and severe renal impairment, half-life values were increased over normal values by approximately two-, four-, and six-fold, respectively. In these patients, successive infusions may result in accumulation of hydroxypropyl-β-cyclodextrin until steady state is reached. Hydroxypropyl-β-cyclodextrin is removed by hemodialysis.

5.3 Preclinical safety data

Nonclinical data on itraconazole revealed no indications for gene toxicity, primary carcinogenicity or impairment of fertility. At high doses, effects were observed in the adrenal cortex, liver and the mononuclear phagocyte system but appear to have a low relevance for the proposed clinical use. Itraconazole was found to cause a dose-related increase in maternal toxicity, embryotoxicity and teratogenicity in rats and mice at high doses. A global lower bone mineral density was observed in juvenile dogs after chronic itraconazole administration, and in rats, a decreased bone plate activity, thinning of the zona compacta of the large bones, and an increased bone fragility was observed.

6. PHARMACEUTICAL PARTICULARS

6.1 List of excipients

Sporanox I.V.:	Hydroxypropyl-β-cyclodextrin, propylene glycol, hydrochloric acid, sodium hydroxide, water for injections.
0.9% Sodium Chloride Injection:	Sodium Chloride, water for Injection

6.2 Incompatibilities

Itraconazole has the potential to precipitate when Sporanox I.V. is diluted in solutions other than the 50ml 0.9% sodium chloride injection supplied.

6.3 Shelf life

Sporanox I.V.:

Shelf life as packaged:

2 years

0.9 % Sodium Chloride Injection:

24 months

Admixed Solution:

24 hours.

Figure 1 Breaking the ampoule

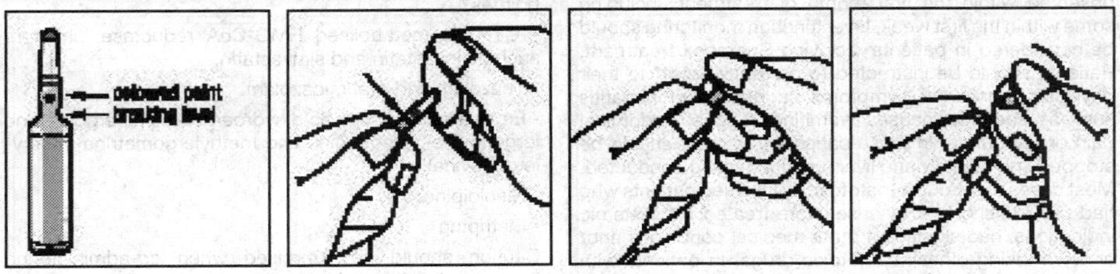

6.4 Special precautions for storage

Sporanox I.V.:

Do not store above 25°C. Store in the original container.

0.9 % Sodium Chloride Injection:

Do not store above 25°C. Do not freeze.

Admixed solution:

Protect from direct sunlight.

From a microbiological point of view, the product should be used immediately. If not used immediately, in-use storage times and conditions prior to use are the responsibility of the user and would not normally be longer than 24 hours at 2 to 8°C, unless the admixture has taken place in controlled and validated aseptic conditions.

6.5 Nature and contents of container

Sporanox I.V.:

25 ml siliconised type I glass ampoule with 25 ml containing 250 mg itraconazole.

0.9 % Sodium Chloride:

Flexible 75ml polypropylene infusion bag, equipped with a flexible inlet and outlet port, and containing 52 to 56ml of 0.9% Sodium Chloride Injection.

Extension Line:

Polyvinylchloride tubing with 2-way stopcock and in-line filter.

6.6 Special precautions for disposal and other handling

Sporanox I.V.:

Itraconazole has the potential to precipitate when 25 ml of Sporanox I.V. concentrate are diluted in solutions other than 50 ml 0.9% Sodium Chloride Injection. The full amount of 25 ml of Sporanox I.V. concentrate from the ampoule must be diluted into the Sodium Chloride Infusion Bag, which is intended to be used exclusively in combination with Sporanox I.V. No other bag should be used. Use the dedicated Sporanox extension line. Sporanox I.V. cannot be co-administered with other drugs or fluids. See section 6.2. Incompatabilities

The Sporanox I.V. concentrate, the solvent (Sodium Chloride) and the admixed solution for infusion are to be visually inspected prior to use. **Only clear solutions without particles should be used.**

Sporanox I.V. should be prepared for administration according to the following instructions:

Opening ampoule:

– Break the ampoule as shown:

(see Figure 1 above)

Opening sodium chloride bag:

Tear outer wrap at notch and remove infusion bag. Some opacity of the plastic due to moisture absorption during the sterilisation process may be observed. This is normal and does not affect the solution quality or safety. The opacity will diminish gradually.

Admixing Sporanox I.V. Concentrate and 0.9% Sodium Chloride Injection:

– Each component must be at room temperature.

– Admix only in the **infusion bag** provided.

– Using aseptic technique and an additive delivery needle of appropriate length (not supplied with the kit), draw up all the concentrate from the ampoule and subsequently add the Sporanox I.V. concentrate to the infusion bag by puncturing the resealable additive port and inject.

– Add the entire volume (25 ml) of **Sporanox I.V.** to the bag in a single action.

– Gently mix the bag once the Sporanox I.V. concentrate is completely transferred to the bag.

The admixture should be used immediately and should be protected from direct sunlight. During administration, exposure to normal room light is acceptable: see section 6.3. (Shelf life) and section 6.4 (Special precautions for storage).

Infusion:

– The admixed solution is intended for single-dose infusion only. No administration should occur unless the solution is clear and the infusion bag undamaged.

– The infusion bag should now contain 25 ml Sporanox I.V. concentrate and 50 ml 0.9% Sodium Chloride Injection.

– Note: An infusion line with drip chamber is not supplied with the kit. Close the flow control device (e.g. rotary clamp) on the infusion line. Using aseptic technique, push the pin of the infusion line in the flexible port of the infusion bag.

– Slowly release the flow control device and fill the drip chamber to half full by squeezing (pumping) it.

– Connect the infusion line to the two-way stop cock of the extension line.

– Open the flow control device until all the air has been expelled from the infusion and extension line.

– The Sporanox infusion is now ready for intravenous infusion to the patient.

– Connect the extension line to the indwelling line the patient (e.g. the catheter).

– Adjust the infusion rate to 1 ml/min (approximately 25 drops/min) by means of a flow control device (e.g. rotary clamp or infusion pump).

– Administer **60 ml** of the solution to the patient over approximately one hour.

– Stop the infusion when 60 ml is administered.

– Note that 200 mg of itraconazole has been administered.

– Flush the line as per the flushing procedure described below.

Figure 2

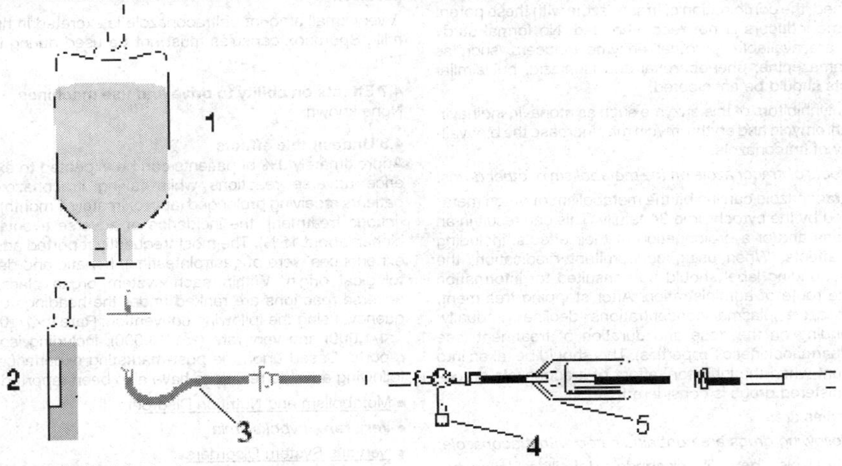

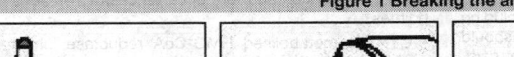

1. Sodium chloride infusion bag
2. Sporanox ampoule
3. Infusion line with drip chamber (not provided)
4. & 5. Extension line with 2-way stopcock and in-line filter.

Flush procedure post infusion:

– After the infusion a complete flush procedure must be started to clean the catheter. This is done to avoid compatibility problems between residual amounts of itraconazole and other drugs which later could be administered through the same catheter.

– Flush the extension line with 15 – 20 ml 0.9% sodium chloride solution at the two-way stop cock, just before the 0.2 µm in-line filter.

– Perform the flush in a continuous run of between 30 seconds to 15 minutes.

– After flushing, disconnect and discard the bag, the infusion line and the extension line.

– Discard the infusion set after use. Do not re-sterilise or re-use the Sporanox infusion set.

To avoid precipitation, other medicine should only be administered via the catheter after flushing.

If using a multi-lumen catheter, other medication may not be administered until the Sporanox I.V. infusion has been completed and the catheter has been flushed.

(see Figure 2 below)

Administrative Data

7. MARKETING AUTHORISATION HOLDER

Janssen-Cilag Ltd.
50-100 Holmers Farm Way
High Wycombe
Buckinghamshire
HP12 4EG
UK

8. MARKETING AUTHORISATION NUMBER(S)

PL 0242/0344

9. DATE OF FIRST AUTHORISATION/RENEWAL OF THE AUTHORISATION

22 July 1999 / 22nd July 2004

10. DATE OF REVISION OF THE TEXT

November 2008

Sporanox -Pulse

(Janssen-Cilag Ltd)

1. NAME OF THE MEDICINAL PRODUCT

SPORANOX®-Pulse.

2. QUALITATIVE AND QUANTITATIVE COMPOSITION

Itraconazole 100 mg.

For excipients, see 6.1.

3. PHARMACEUTICAL FORM

Capsule (Size 0): opaque blue cap and pink transparent body containing coated beads.

4. CLINICAL PARTICULARS

4.1 Therapeutic indications

Onychomycosis caused by dermatophytes and/or yeasts.

Tinea pedis and/or tinea manuum.

4.2 Posology and method of administration

Sporanox-Pulse is for oral administration and must be taken immediately after a meal for maximal absorption.

Treatment schedules in adults are as follows:

Indication	Dose	Remarks
Tinea pedis and/or tinea manuum	1 pulse treatment	A pulse treatment consists of 200 mg bd. for 7 days.
Onychomycosis – fingernails	2 pulse treatments	Pulse treatments are separated by a 3-week
Onychomycosis – toenails	3 pulse treatments	drug-free interval

Impaired absorption in AIDS and neutropenic patients may lead to low itraconazole blood levels and lack of efficacy. In such cases, blood level monitoring is indicated.

Use in children

Not recommended. See 4.4 Special warnings and special precautions for use.

In Elderly

Not recommended. See 4.4 Special warnings and special precautions for use.

Use in patients with renal impairment

The oral bioavailability of itraconazole may be lower in patients with renal insufficiency, a dose adjustment may be considered. See 4.4 Special warnings and special precautions for use.

Use in patients with hepatic impairment

Itraconazole is predominantly metabolised by the liver. The terminal half-life of itraconazole in cirrhotic patients is somewhat prolonged. The oral bioavailability in cirrhotic patients is somewhat decreased. A dose adjustment may be considered. See 4.4 Special warnings and special precautions for use.

4.3 Contraindications

Sporanox-Pulse is contra-indicated in patients who have shown hypersensitivity to the drug or its excipients.

Co-administration of the following drugs is contraindicated with Sporanox-Pulse capsules (see also section 4.5 Interaction with other medicinal products and other forms of interaction):

- CYP3A4 metabolised substrates that can prolong the QT-interval e.g., astemizole, bepridil, cisapride, dofetilide, levacetylmethadol (levomethadyl), mizolastine, pimozide, quinidine, sertindole and terfenadine are contraindicated with Sporanox-Pulse capsules. Co-administration may result in increased plasma concentrations of these substrates, which can lead to QTc prolongation and rare occurrences of *torsades de pointes*.

- CYP3A4 metabolised HMG-CoA reductase inhibitors such as lovastatin and simvastatin

- Triazolam and oral midazolam

- Ergot alkaloids such as dihydroergotamine, ergometrine (ergonovine), ergotamine and methylergometrine (methylergonovine)

- Eletriptan

- Nisoldipine

- Sporanox-Pulse capsules should not be administered to patients receiving disopyramide or halofantrine

Sporanox-Pulse capsules should not be administered to patients with evidence of ventricular dysfunction such as congestive heart failure (CHF) or a history of CHF except for the treatment of life-threatening or other serious infections. See 4.4 Special warnings and precautions for use.

Sporanox-Pulse must not be used during pregnancy. See section 4.6 Pregnancy and lactation.

4.4 Special warnings and precautions for use

Cardiac effects

In a healthy volunteer study with Sporanox® IV, a transient asymptomatic decrease of the left ventricular ejection fraction was observed.

Itraconazole has been shown to have a negative inotropic effect and Sporanox has been associated with reports of congestive heart failure. Heart failure was more frequently reported among spontaneous reports of 400 mg total daily dose than among those of lower total daily doses, suggesting that the risk of heart failure might increase with the total daily dose of itraconazole.

Sporanox-Pulse should not be used in patients with congestive heart failure or with a history of congestive heart failure unless the benefit clearly outweighs the risk. This individual benefit/risk assessment should take into consideration factors such as the severity of the indication, the dose and duration of treatment (e.g. total daily dose), and individual risk factors for congestive heart failure. Such patients should be informed of the signs and symptoms of congestive heart failure, should be treated with caution, and should be monitored for signs and symptoms of congestive heart failure during treatment; if such signs or symptoms do occur during treatment, Sporanox-Pulse should be discontinued.

Calcium channel blockers can have negative inotropic effects which may be additive to those of itraconazole. In addition, itraconazole can inhibit the metabolism of calcium channel blockers. Therefore, caution should be exercised when co-administering itraconazole and calcium channel blockers (see section 4.5, Interactions with other medicinal products and other forms of interaction) due to an increased risk of congestive heart failure.

Interaction potential

Sporanox-Pulse has a potential for clinically important drug interactions. (See section 4.5: Interactions with other medicinal products and other forms of interaction.)

Reduced gastric acidity

Absorption of itraconazole from Sporanox-Pulse is impaired when the gastric acidity is reduced. In patients also receiving acid neutralising medicines (eg aluminium hydroxide), these should be administered at least 2 hours after the intake of Sporanox-Pulse. In patients with achlorhydria such as certain AIDS patients and patients on secretion suppressors (eg H2-antagonists, proton-pump inhibitors), it is advisable to administer Sporanox-Pulse with a cola beverage.

Use in children

Clinical data on the use of Sporanox-Pulse capsules in paediatric patients is limited. Sporanox-Pulse capsules should not be used in paediatric patients unless the potential benefit outweighs the potential risks.

Use in elderly

Clinical data on the use of Sporanox-Pulse capsules in elderly patients is limited. Sporanox-Pulse capsules should not be used in these patients unless the potential benefit outweighs the potential risks.

Hepatic effects

Very rare cases of serious hepatotoxicity, including some cases of fatal acute liver failure, have occurred with the use of Sporanox. Some of these cases involved patients with no pre-existing liver disease. Some of these cases were observed within the first month of treatment, including some within the first week. Liver function monitoring should be considered in patients receiving Sporanox treatment. Patients should be instructed to promptly report to their physician signs and symptoms suggestive of hepatitis such as anorexia, nausea, vomiting, fatigue, abdominal pain or dark urine. In these patients treatment should be stopped immediately and liver function testing conducted. Most cases of serious hepatotoxicity involved patients who had pre-existing liver disease, were treated for systemic indications, had significant other medical conditions and/or were taking other hepatotoxic drugs. In patients with raised liver enzymes or active liver disease, or who have experienced liver toxicity with other drugs, treatment should not be started unless the expected benefit exceeds the risk of hepatic injury. In such cases liver enzyme monitoring is necessary.

Hepatic impairment

Itraconazole is predominantly metabolised in the liver. A slight decrease in oral bioavailability in cirrhotic patients has been observed, although this was not of statistical significance. The terminal half-life was however significantly increased. The dose should be adapted if necessary.

Renal impairment

The oral bioavailability of itraconazole may be lower in patients with renal insufficiency. Dose adaptation may be considered.

Immunocompromised patients

In some immunocompromised patients (e.g., neutropenic, AIDS or organ transplant patients), the oral bioavailability of Sporanox-Pulse capsules may be decreased.

Patients with immediately life-threatening systemic fungal infections

Due to the pharmacokinetic properties (See section 5.2), Sporanox-Pulse capsules are not recommended for initiation of treatment in patients with immediately life-threatening systemic fungal infections.

Patients with AIDS

In patients with AIDS having received treatment for a systemic fungal infection such as sporotrichosis, blastomycosis, histoplasmosis or cryptococcosis (meningeal or non-meningeal) and who are considered at risk for relapse, the treating physician should evaluate the need for a maintenance treatment.

Neuropathy

If neuropathy occurs which may be attributable to Sporanox-Pulse, treatment should be discontinued.

Cross-hypersensitivity

There is no information regarding cross hypersensitivity between itraconazole and other azole antifungal agents. Caution should be used in prescribing Sporanox to patients with hypersensitivity to other azoles.

Patients with rare hereditary problems of fructose intolerance, glucose-galactose malabsorption or sucrase-isomaltase insufficiency should not take this medicine.

4.5 Interaction with other medicinal products and other forms of interaction

1. Drugs affecting the absorption of itraconazole

Drugs that reduce the gastric acidity impair the absorption of itraconazole from Sporanox-Pulse capsules (See 4.4 Special warnings and special precautions for use).

2. Drugs affecting the metabolism of itraconazole:

Itraconazole is mainly metabolised through the cytochrome CYP3A4. Interaction studies have been performed with rifampicin, rifabutin and phenytoin, which are potent inducers of CYP3A4. Since the bioavailability of itraconazole and hydroxy-itraconazole was decreased in these studies to such an extent that efficacy may be largely reduced, the combination of itraconazole with these potent enzyme inducers is not recommended. No formal study data are available for other enzyme inducers, such as carbamazepine, phenobarbital and isoniazid, but similar effects should be anticipated.

Potent inhibitors of this enzyme such as ritonavir, indinavir, clarithromycin and erythromycin may increase the bioavailability of itraconazole.

3. Effects of itraconazole on the metabolism of other drugs:

3.1 Itraconazole can inhibit the metabolism of drugs metabolised by the cytochrome 3A family. This can result in an increase and/or a prolongation of their effects, including side effects. When using concomitant medication, the corresponding label should be consulted for information on the route of administration. After stopping treatment, itraconazole plasma concentrations decline gradually, depending on the dose and duration of treatment (see 5.2 Pharmacokinetic Properties). This should be taken into account when the inhibitory effect of itraconazole on co-administered drugs is considered.

Examples are:

The following drugs are contraindicated with itraconazole:

- Astemizole, bepridil, cisapride, dofetilide, levacetylmethadol (levomethadyl), mizolastine, pimozide, quinidine, sertindole or terfenadine are contraindicated with Sporanox-Pulse since co-administration may result in increased plasma concentrations of these substrates, which can lead to QT prolongation and rare occurrences of Torsades de pointes.

- CYP3A4 metabolised HMG-CoA reductase inhibitors such as lovastatin and simvastatin.

- Triazolam and oral midazolam.

- Ergot alkaloids such as dihydroergotamine, ergometrine (ergonovine), ergotamine and methylergometrine (methylergonovine).

- Nisoldipine

- Eletriptan

Caution should be exercised when co-administering itraconazole with calcium channel blockers due to an increased risk of congestive heart failure. In addition to possible pharmacokinetic interactions involving the drug metabolising enzyme CYP3A4, calcium channel blockers can have negative inotropic effects which may be additive to those of itraconazole.

The following drugs should be used with caution, and their plasma concentrations, effects or side effects should be monitored. Their dosage, when co-administered with itraconazole, should be reduced if necessary:

- Oral anticoagulants
- HIV protease inhibitors such as ritonavir, indinavir, saquinavir
- Certain antineoplastic agents such as vinca alkaloids, busulfan, docetaxel and trimetrexate
- CYP3A4 metabolised calcium channel blockers such as dihydropyridines and verapamil
- Certain immunosuppressive agents: ciclosporin, tacrolimus, rapamycin (also known as sirolimus)
- Certain CYP3A4 metabolised HMG-CoA reductase inhibitors such as atorvastatin
- Certain glucocorticoids such as budesonide, dexamethasone, fluticasone and methylprednisolone
- Digoxin
- Others: carbamazepine, cilostazol, buspirone, disopyramide, alfentanil, alprazolam, brotizolam, midazolam IV, rifabutin, ebastine, fentanyl, halofantrine, repaglinide and reboxetine. The importance of the concentration increase and the clinical relevance of these changes during co-administration remain to be established.

3.2. No interaction of itraconazole with zidovudine (AZT) and fluvastatin has been observed.

No inducing effects of itraconazole on the metabolism of ethinyloestradiol and norethisterone were observed.

4. Effect on protein binding:

In vitro studies have shown that there are no interactions on the plasma protein binding between itraconazole and imipramine, propranolol, diazepam, cimetidine, indometacin, tolbutamide or sulphadimidine.

4.6 Pregnancy and lactation

Pregnancy

Sporanox-Pulse is contra-indicated in pregnancy.

In animal studies itraconazole has shown reproduction toxicity (see 5.3 Preclinical safety data).

Epidemiological data on exposure to Sporanox-Pulse during the first trimester of pregnancy-mostly in patients receiving short-term treatment for vulvovaginal candidosis did not show an increased risk for malformations as compared to control subjects not exposed to any known teratogens.

Women of child bearing potential

Women of childbearing potential taking Sporanox capsules should use contraceptive precautions. Effective contraception should be continued until the next menstrual period following the end of Sporanox therapy.

Lactation

A very small amount of itraconazole is excreted in human milk. Sporanox capsules must not be used during lactation.

4.7 Effects on ability to drive and use machines

None known.

4.8 Undesirable effects

Approximately 9% of patients can be expected to experience adverse reactions while taking itraconazole. In patients receiving prolonged (approximately 1 month) continuous treatment, the incidence of adverse events was higher (about 15%). The most frequently reported adverse experiences were of gastrointestinal, hepatic and dermatological origin. Within each system organ class, the adverse reactions are ranked under the headings of frequency, using the following convention: Rare (>1/10,000, <1/1,000) and very rare (<1/10,000), including isolated reports. Based upon the post-marketing experience, the following adverse reactions have also been reported:

- Metabolism and Nutrition Disorders
- ***Very rare:*** *hypokalemia*
- Nervous System Disorders
- ***Very rare:*** *peripheral neuropathy, headache, and dizziness*
- Cardiac Disorders
- ***Very rare:*** *congestive heart failure*

• Respiratory, Thoracic and Mediastinal Disorders

• ***Very rare:*** *pulmonary oedema*

• Gastrointestinal Disorders

• ***Very rare:*** *abdominal pain, vomiting, dyspepsia, nausea, diarrhoea and constipation*

• Hepato-Biliary Disorders

• ***Very rare:*** *fatal acute liver failure, serious hepatotoxicity, hepatitis, and reversible increases in hepatic enzymes*

• Skin and Subcutaneous Tissue Disorders

• ***Very rare:*** *Stevens-Johnson syndrome, angio-oedema, urticaria, alopecia, rash, and pruritis*

• Reproductive System and Breast Disorders

• ***Very rare:*** *menstrual disorder*

• General Disorders and Administrative Site Conditions

• ***Very rare:*** *allergic reaction, and oedema*

4.9 Overdose

In the event of overdosage, patients should be treated symptomatically with supportive measures. Within the first hour after ingestion, gastric lavage may be performed. Activated charcoal may be given if considered appropriate. No specific antidote is available. Itraconazole cannot be removed by haemodialysis.

5. PHARMACOLOGICAL PROPERTIES

5.1 Pharmacodynamic properties

Pharmacotherapeutic classification: (Antimycotics for systemic use, triazole derivatives).

ATC code: J02A C02

Itraconazole, a triazole derivative, has a broad spectrum of activity.

In vitro studies have demonstrated that itraconazole impairs the synthesis of ergosterol in fungal cells. Ergosterol is a vital cell membrane component in fungi. Impairment of its synthesis ultimately results in an antifungal effect.

For itraconazole, breakpoints have only been established for Candida spp. From superficial mycotic infections (CLSI M27-A2, breakpoints have not been established for EUCAST methodology). The CLSI breakpoints are as follows: susceptible $\leqslant 0.125$; susceptible, dose-dependent 0.25-0.5 and resistant $\geqslant 1\mu g/mL$. Interpretive breakpoints have not been established for the filamentous fungi.

In vitro studies demonstrate that itraconazole inhibits the growth of a broad range of fungi pathogenic for humans at concentrations usually $\leqslant 1$ μg/ml. These include:

dermatophytes (Trichophyton spp., *Epidermophyton floccosum*); yeasts (Candida spp., including *C. albicans* and *C. glabrata*), Malassezia (formerly Pityrosporum) spp., Trichosporon spp., Geotrichum spp.); Aspergillus spp.; *Blastomyces dermatitidis*; and various other yeasts and fungi.

Candida glabrata and *Candida tropicalis* are generally the least susceptible Candida species, with some isolates showing unequivocal resistance to itraconazole *in vitro*.

The principal fungus types that are not inhibited by itraconazole are *Zygomycetes* (e.g. Rhizopus spp., Rhizomucor spp., Mucor spp. and Absidia spp.), Fusarium spp., *Scedosporium proliferans* and Scopulariopsis spp.

Azole resistance appears to develop slowly and is often the result of several genetic mutations. Mechanisms that have been described are overexpression of ERG11, which encodes the target enzyme 14α-demethylase, point mutations in ERG11 that lead to decreased target affinity and/or transporter overexpression resulting in increased efflux. Cross resistance between members of the azole class has been observed within Candida spp., although resistance to one member of the class does not necessarily confer resistance to other azoles. Itraconazole-resistant strains of *Aspergillus fumigatus* have been reported.

5.2 Pharmacokinetic properties

General pharmacokinetic characteristics

The pharmacokinetics of itraconazole has been investigated in healthy subjects, special populations and patients after single and multiple dosing.

Absorption

Itraconazole is rapidly absorbed after oral administration. Peak plasma concentrations of the unchanged drug are reached within 2 to 5 hours following an oral dose. The observed absolute bioavailability of itraconazole is about 55%. Oral bioavailability is maximal when the capsules are taken immediately after a full meal.

Distribution

Most of the itraconazole in plasma is bound to protein (99.8%) with albumin being the main binding component (99.6% for the hydroxy- metabolite). It has also a marked affinity for lipids. Only 0.2% of the itraconazole in plasma is present as free drug. Itraconazole is distributed in a large apparent volume in the body (> 700 L), suggesting its extensive distribution into tissues: Concentrations in lung, kidney, liver, bone, stomach, spleen and muscle were found to be two to three times higher than corresponding concentrations in plasma. Brain to plasma ratios were about 1 as measured in beagle dogs. The uptake into keratinous tissues, skin in particular, is up to four times higher than in plasma.

Biotransformation

Itraconazole is extensively metabolised by the liver into a large number of metabolites. One of the main metabolites is hydroxy-itraconazole, which has in vitro antifungal activity comparable to itraconazole. Plasma concentrations of the hydroxy-itraconazole are about twice those of itraconazole.

As shown in *in vitro* studies, CYP 3A4 is the major enzyme that is involved in the metabolism of itraconazole.

Elimination

Itraconazole is excreted as inactive metabolites to about 35% in urine within one week and to about 54% with feces. Renal excretion of the parent drug accounts for less than 0.03% of the dose, whereas fecal excretion of unchanged drug varies between 3 – 18% of the dose. Itraconazole clearance decreases at higher doses due to saturable hepatic metabolism.

Linearity/non-linearity

As a consequence of non-linear pharmacokinetics, itraconazole accumulates in plasma during multiple dosing. Steady-state concentrations are generally reached within about 15 days, with Cmax and AUC values 4 to 7-fold higher than those seen after a single dose. The mean elimination half-life of itraconazole is about 40 hours after repeated dosing.

Special Populations

Hepatic Insufficiency: A pharmacokinetic study using a single 100 mg dose of itraconazole (one 100 mg capsule) was conducted in 6 healthy and 12 cirrhotic subjects. No statistically significant differences in AUC_∞ were seen between these two groups. A statistically significant reduction in average C_{max} (47%) and a two fold increase in the elimination half-life (37 ± 17 versus 16 ±5 hours) of itraconazole were noted in cirrhotic subjects compared with healthy subjects.

Data are not available in cirrhotic patients during long-term use of itraconazole.

Renal Insufficiency: Limited data are available on the use of oral itraconazole in patients with renal impairment. Caution should be exercised when the drug is administered in this patient population.

5.3 Preclinical safety data

Nonclinical data on itraconazole revealed no indications for gene toxicity, primary carcinogenicity or impairment of fertility. At high doses, effects were observed in the adrenal cortex, liver and the mononuclear phagocyte system but appear to have a low relevance for the proposed clinical use. Itraconazole was found to cause a dose-related increase in maternal toxicity, embryotoxicity and teratogenicity in rats and mice at high doses. A global lower bone mineral density was observed in juvenile dogs after chronic itraconazole administration, and in rats, a decreased bone plate activity, thinning of the zona compacta of the large bones, and an increased bone fragility was observed.

6. PHARMACEUTICAL PARTICULARS

6.1 List of excipients

Sugar spheres Ph.Eur

Hypromellose 2910 5mPa.s PhEur.

Macrogol 20000 NF

Capsule shell:

Titanium dioxide E171

Indigotin carmine E132

Gelatin PhEur.

Erythrosine E127

6.2 Incompatibilities

None known.

6.3 Shelf life

36 months.

6.4 Special precautions for storage

Do not store above 30°C.

Store in the original container.

6.5 Nature and contents of container

Tristar blister - plastic foil consisting of 3 layers

• polyvinylchloride on the outside

• low density polyethylene in the middle

• polyvinylidene chloride on the inside

Aluminium foil (thickness 20 μm) coated on the inner side with colourless heatseal lacquer: PVC mixed polymers with acrylates 6 g/m²

or:

PVC blister consisting of:-

Polyvinylchloride "genotherm" glass clear, thickness 250 μm

Aluminium foil (thickness 20 μm) coated on the inner side with a colourless heatseal lacquer: PVC mixed polymers with acrylates 6 g/m²

Pack size: 28 capsules.

6.6 Special precautions for disposal and other handling

Not applicable.

7. MARKETING AUTHORISATION HOLDER

Janssen-Cilag Ltd

50-100 Holmers Farm Way

High Wycombe

Buckinghamshire

HP12 4EG

UK

8. MARKETING AUTHORISATION NUMBER(S)

00242/0334

9. DATE OF FIRST AUTHORISATION/RENEWAL OF THE AUTHORISATION

26 March 1997

10. DATE OF REVISION OF THE TEXT

April 2009

Legal category POM.

Stalevo 100/25/200mg

(Orion Pharma (UK) Limited)

1. NAME OF THE MEDICINAL PRODUCT

Stalevo 100 mg/25 mg/200 mg film-coated tablets

2. QUALITATIVE AND QUANTITATIVE COMPOSITION

Each tablet contains 100 mg of levodopa, 25 mg of carbidopa and 200 mg of entacapone.

Excipient: Each tablet contains 1.6 mg of sucrose.

For a full list of excipients, see section 6.1.

3. PHARMACEUTICAL FORM

Film-coated tablet

Brownish or greyish red, oval, unscored film-coated tablets marked with 'LCE 100' on one side.

4. CLINICAL PARTICULARS

4.1 Therapeutic indications

Stalevo is indicated for the treatment of adult patients with Parkinson's disease and end-of-dose motor fluctuations not stabilised on levodopa/dopa decarboxylase (DDC) inhibitor treatment.

4.2 Posology and method of administration

Each tablet is to be taken orally either with or without food (see section 5.2). One tablet contains one treatment dose and the tablet may only be administered as whole tablets.

The optimum daily dose must be determined by careful titration of levodopa in each patient. The daily dose should be preferably optimised using one of the six available tablet strengths (50 mg/12.5 mg/200 mg, 75 mg/18.75 mg/200 mg, 100 mg/25 mg/200 mg, 125 mg/31.25 mg/200 mg 150 mg/37.5 mg/200 mg or 200 mg/50 mg/200 mg levodopa/carbidopa/entacapone).

Patients should be instructed to take only one Stalevo tablet per dose administration. Patients receiving less than 70-100 mg carbidopa a day are more likely to experience nausea and vomiting. While the experience with total daily dose greater than 200 mg carbidopa is limited, the maximum recommended daily dose of entacapone is 2,000 mg and therefore the maximum dose is 10 tablets per day for the Stalevo strengths of 50 mg/12.5 mg/200 mg, 75 mg/18.75 mg/200 mg, 100 mg/25 mg/200 mg, 125 mg/31.25 mg/200 mg and 150 mg/37.5 mg/200 mg. Ten tablets of Stalevo 150 mg/37.5 mg/200 mg equals 375 mg of carbidopa a day. According to this daily carbidopa dose, the maximum recommended daily Stalevo 200 mg/50 mg/200 mg dose is 7 tablets per day.

Usually Stalevo is to be used in patients who are currently treated with corresponding doses of standard release levodopa/DDC inhibitor and entacapone.

How to transfer patients taking levodopa/DDC inhibitor (carbidopa or benserazide) preparations and entacapone tablets to Stalevo

a. Patients who are currently treated with entacapone and with standard release levodopa/carbidopa in doses equal to Stalevo tablet strengths can be directly transferred to corresponding Stalevo tablets.

For example, a patient taking one tablet of 100 mg/25 mg of levodopa/carbidopa with one tablet of entacapone 200 mg four times daily can take one 100 mg/25 mg/200 mg Stalevo tablet four times daily in place of their usual levodopa/carbidopa and entacapone doses.

b. When initiating Stalevo therapy for patients currently treated with entacapone and levodopa/carbidopa in doses not equal to Stalevo 100 mg/25 mg/200 mg, (or 50 mg/12.5 mg/200 mg or 75 mg/18.75 mg/200 mg or 125 mg/31.25 mg/200 mg or 150 mg/37.5 mg/200 mg or 200 mg/50 mg/200 mg) tablets, Stalevo dosing should be carefully titrated for optimal clinical response. At the initiation, Stalevo should be adjusted to correspond as closely as possible to the total daily dose of levodopa currently used.

c. When initiating Stalevo in patients currently treated with entacapone and levodopa/benserazide in a standard release formulation, discontinue dosing of levodopa/benserazide the previous night, and start Stalevo the next morning. Begin with a dose of Stalevo that will provide either the same amount of levodopa or slightly (5-10%) more.

How to transfer patients not currently treated with entacapone to Stalevo

Initiation of Stalevo may be considered at corresponding doses to current treatment in some patients with Parkinson's disease and end-of-dose motor fluctuations, who are not stabilised on their current standard release levodopa/DDC inhibitor treatment. However, a direct switch from levodopa/DDC inhibitor to Stalevo is not recommended for patients who have dyskinesias or whose daily levodopa dose is above 800 mg. In such patients it is advisable to introduce entacapone treatment as a separate treatment (entacapone tablets) and adjust the levodopa dose if necessary, before switching to Stalevo.

Entacapone enhances the effects of levodopa. It may therefore be necessary, particularly in patients with dyskinesia, to reduce levodopa dose by 10-30% within the first days to first weeks after initiating Stalevo treatment. The daily dose of levodopa can be reduced by extending the dosing intervals and/or by reducing the amount of levodopa per dose, according to the clinical condition of the patient.

Dose adjustment during the course of the treatment

When more levodopa is required, an increase in the frequency of doses and/or the use of an alternative strength of Stalevo should be considered, within the dose recommendations.

When less levodopa is required, the total daily dose of Stalevo should be reduced either by decreasing the frequency of administration by extending the time between doses, or by decreasing the strength of Stalevo at an administration.

If other levodopa products are used concomitantly with a Stalevo tablet, the maximum dose recommendations should be followed.

Discontinuation of Stalevo therapy: If Stalevo treatment (levodopa/carbidopa/entacapone) is discontinued and the patient is transferred to levodopa/DDC inhibitor therapy without entacapone, it is necessary to adjust the dosing of other antiparkinsonian treatments, especially levodopa, to achieve a sufficient level of control of the parkinsonian symptoms.

Children and adolescents: Stalevo is not recommended for use in children below 18 years due to a lack of data on safety and efficacy.

Elderly: No dose adjustment of Stalevo is required for elderly patients.

Hepatic impairment: It is advised that Stalevo should be administered cautiously to patients with mild to moderate hepatic impairment. Dose reduction may be needed (see section 5.2). For severe hepatic impairment see section 4.3

Renal impairment: Renal impairment does not affect the pharmacokinetics of entacapone. No particular studies are reported on the pharmacokinetics of levodopa and carbidopa in patients with renal insufficiency, therefore Stalevo therapy should be administered cautiously to patients in severe renal impairment including those receiving dialysis therapy (see section 5.2).

4.3 Contraindications

- Hypersensitivity to the active substances or to any of the excipients.
- Severe hepatic impairment.
- Narrow-angle glaucoma.
- Pheochromocytoma.
- Concomitant use of Stalevo with non-selective monoamine oxidase (MAO-A and MAO-B) inhibitors (e.g. phenelzine, tranylcypromine).
- Concomitant use of a selective MAO-A inhibitor and a selective MAO-B inhibitor (see section 4.5).
- A previous history of Neuroleptic Malignant Syndrome (NMS) and/or non-traumatic rhabdomyolysis.

4.4 Special warnings and precautions for use

- Stalevo is not recommended for the treatment of drug-induced extrapyramidal reactions
- Stalevo therapy should be administered cautiously to patients with severe cardiovascular or pulmonary disease, bronchial asthma, renal or endocrine disease, history of peptic ulcer disease or history of convulsions.
- In patients with a history of myocardial infarction who have residual atrial nodal or ventricular arrhythmias; cardiac function should be monitored with particular care during the period of initial dose adjustments.
- All patients treated with Stalevo should be monitored carefully for the development of mental changes, depression with suicidal tendencies, and other serious antisocial behaviour. Patients with past or current psychosis should be treated with caution.
- Concomitant administration of antipsychotics with dopamine receptor-blocking properties, particularly D_2 receptor antagonists should be carried out with caution, and the patient carefully observed for loss of antiparkinsonian effect or worsening of parkinsonian symptoms.
- Patients with chronic wide-angle glaucoma may be treated with Stalevo with caution, provided the intra-ocular pressure is well controlled and the patient is monitored carefully for changes in intra-ocular pressure.
- Stalevo may induce orthostatic hypotension. Therefore Stalevo should be given cautiously to patients who are taking other medicinal products which may cause orthostatic hypotension.
- Entacapone in association with levodopa has been associated with somnolence and episodes of sudden sleep onset in patients with Parkinson's disease and caution should therefore be exercised when driving or operating machines (see section 4.7).
- In clinical studies, dopaminergic adverse reactions, e.g. dyskinesia, were more common in patients who received entacapone and dopamine agonists (such as bromocriptine), selegiline or amantadine compared to those who received placebo with this combination. The doses of other antiparkinsonian medicinal products may need to be adjusted when Stalevo treatment is substituted for a patient currently not treated with entacapone.
- Rhabdomyolysis secondary to severe dyskinesias or neuroleptic malignant syndrome (NMS) has been observed rarely in patients with Parkinson's disease. Therefore, any abrupt dose reduction or withdrawal of levodopa should be carefully observed, particularly in patients who are also receiving neuroleptics. NMS, including rhabdomyolysis and hyperthermia, is characterised by motor symptoms (rigidity, myoclonus, tremor), mental status changes (e.g., agitation, confusion, coma), hyperthermia, autonomic dysfunction (tachycardia, labile blood pressure) and elevated serum creatine phosphokinase. In individual cases, only some of these symptoms and/or findings may be evident. The early diagnosis is important for the appropriate management of NMS. A syndrome resembling the neuroleptic malignant syndrome including muscular rigidity, elevated body temperature, mental changes and increased serum creatine phosphokinase has been reported with the abrupt withdrawal of antiparkinsonian agents. Neither NMS nor rhabdomyolysis have been reported in association with entacapone treatment from controlled trials in which entacapone was discontinued abruptly. Since the introduction of entacapone into the market, isolated cases of NMS have been reported, especially following abrupt reduction or discontinuation of entacapone and other concomitant dopaminergic medicinal products. When considered necessary, the replacement of Stalevo with levodopa and DDC inhibitor without entacapone or other dopaminergic treatment should proceed slowly and an increase in levodopa dose may be necessary.
- If general anaesthesia is required, therapy with Stalevo may be continued for as long as the patient is permitted to take fluids and medicinal products by mouth. If therapy has to be stopped temporarily, Stalevo may be restarted as soon as oral medicinal products can be taken at the same daily dose as before.
- Periodic evaluation of hepatic, haematopoietic, cardiovascular and renal function is recommended during extended therapy with Stalevo.
- For patients experiencing diarrhoea, a follow-up of weight is recommended in order to avoid potential excessive weight decrease.
- Pathological gambling, increased libido and hypersexuality have been reported in Parkinson's disease patients treated with dopamine agonists and other dopaminergic treatments such as Stalevo.
- For patients who experience progressive anorexia, asthenia and weight decrease within a relatively short period of time, a general medical evaluation including liver function should be considered.
- Stalevo contains sucrose, and therefore patients with rare hereditary problems of fructose intolerance, glucose-galactose malabsorption or sucrase-isomaltase insufficiency should not take this medicine.

4.5 Interaction with other medicinal products and other forms of interaction

Other antiparkinsonian medicinal products: To date there has been no indication of interactions that would preclude concurrent use of standard antiparkinsonian medicinal products with Stalevo therapy. Entacapone in high doses may affect the absorption of carbidopa. However, no interaction with carbidopa has been observed with the recommended treatment schedule (200 mg of entacapone up to 10 times daily). Interactions between entacapone and selegiline have been investigated in repeated dose studies in Parkinson's disease patients treated with levodopa/DDC inhibitor and no interaction was observed. When used with Stalevo, the daily dose of selegiline should not exceed 10 mg.

Caution should be exercised when the following active substances are administered concomitantly with levodopa therapy.

Antihypertensives: Symptomatic postural hypotension may occur when levodopa is added to the treatment of patients already receiving antihypertensives. Dose adjustment of the antihypertensive agent may be required.

Antidepressants: Rarely, reactions including hypertension and dyskinesia have been reported with the concomitant use of tricyclic antidepressants and levodopa/carbidopa. Interactions between entacapone and imipramine and between entacapone and moclobemide have been investigated in single dose studies in healthy volunteers. No pharmacodynamic interactions were observed. A significant number of Parkinson's disease patients have been treated with the combination of levodopa, carbidopa and entacapone with several active substances including MAO-A inhibitors, tricyclic antidepressants, noradrenaline reuptake inhibitors such as desipramine, maprotiline and venlafaxine and medicinal products that are metabolised by COMT (e.g. catechol-structured compounds, paroxetine). No pharmacodynamic interactions have been observed. However, caution should be exercised when these medicinal products are used concomitantly with Stalevo (see sections 4.3 and 4.4).

Other active substances: Dopamine receptor antagonists (e.g. some antipsychotics and antiemetics), phenytoin and papaverine may reduce the therapeutic effect of levodopa. Patients taking these medicinal products with Stalevo should be carefully observed for loss of therapeutic response.

Due to entacapone's affinity to cytochrome P450 2C9 *in vitro* (see section 5.2), Stalevo may potentially interfere with active substances whose metabolism is dependent on this isoenzyme, such as S-warfarin. However, in an interaction study with healthy volunteers, entacapone did not change the plasma levels of S-warfarin, while the AUC for R-warfarin increased on average by 18% [CI_{90} 11-26%]. The INR values increased on average by 13% [CI_{90} 6-19%]. Thus, a control of INR is recommended when Stalevo is initiated for patients receiving warfarin.

Other forms of interactions: Since levodopa competes with certain amino acids, the absorption of Stalevo may be impaired in some patients on high protein diet.

Levodopa and entacapone may form chelates with iron in the gastrointestinal tract. Therefore, Stalevo and iron preparations should be taken at least 2-3 hours apart (see section 4.8).

In vitro data: Entacapone binds to human albumin binding site II which also binds several other medicinal products, including diazepam and ibuprofen. According to *in vitro* studies, significant displacement is not anticipated at therapeutic concentrations of the medicinal products. Accordingly, to date there has been no indication of such interactions.

4.6 Pregnancy and lactation

There are no adequate data from the use of the combination of levodopa/carbidopa/entacapone in pregnant women. Studies in animals have shown reproductive toxicity of the separate compounds (see section 5.3). The potential risk for humans is unknown. Stalevo should not be used during pregnancy unless the benefits for the mother outweigh the possible risks to the foetus.

Levodopa is excreted in human breast milk. There is evidence that lactation is suppressed during treatment with levodopa. Carbidopa and entacapone were excreted in milk in animals but is not known whether they are excreted in human breast milk. The safety of levodopa, carbidopa or entacapone in the infant is not known. Women should not breast-feed during treatment with Stalevo.

4.7 Effects on ability to drive and use machines

Stalevo may have major influence on the ability to drive and use machines. Levodopa, carbidopa and entacapone together may cause dizziness and symptomatic orthostatism. Therefore, caution should be exercised when driving or using machines.

Patients being treated with Stalevo and presenting with somnolence and/or sudden sleep onset episodes must be instructed to refrain from driving or engaging in activities where impaired alertness may put themselves or others at risk of serious injury or death (e.g. operating machines) until such recurrent episodes have resolved (see section 4.4).

4.8 Undesirable effects

The following section describes the undesirable effects reported for levodopa/carbidopa and for entacapone used in combination with levodopa/DDC inhibitor.

Levodopa /carbidopa

Adverse reactions that occur frequently with levodopa/carbidopa are those due to central neuropharmacological activity of dopamine. These reactions can usually be diminished by levodopa dose reduction. The most common adverse reactions are dyskinesias including choreiform, dystonic and other involuntary movements. Muscle twitching and blepharospasm may be taken as early signs to consider levodopa dose reduction. Nausea, also related to enhanced central dopaminergic activity, is a common adverse reaction of levodopa/carbidopa.

Other adverse reactions associated with levodopa/carbidopa therapy are mental changes, including paranoid ideation and psychotic episodes; depression with or without development of suicidal tendencies; and cognitive dysfunction. Adding of entacapone to levodopa/DDC inhibitor therapy (carbidopa or benserazide), i.e. initiation of Stalevo treatment in an entacapone naive patient, may aggravate some of these mental changes.

Less frequent adverse reactions of levodopa/carbidopa therapy are irregular heart rhythm and/or palpitations, orthostatic hypotensive episodes, bradykinetic episodes (the 'on-off' phenomenon), anorexia, vomiting, dizziness, and somnolence.

Gastrointestinal bleeding, development of duodenal ulcer, hypertension, phlebitis, leucopenia, haemolytic and non-haemolytic anaemia, thrombocytopenia, agranulocytosis, chest pain, dyspnoea and paraesthesia have occurred rarely with levodopa/carbidopa.

Convulsions have occurred rarely with levodopa/carbidopa; however a causal relationship to levodopa/carbidopa therapy has not been established.

Parkinson's disease patients treated with dopamine agonists and other dopaminergic treatments such as Stalevo, especially at high doses, have been reported as exhibiting signs of pathological gambling, increased libido and hypersexuality, generally reversible upon reduction of the dose or treatment discontinuation.

Other adverse reactions that have been reported with levodopa and may, therefore, be potential adverse reactions of Stalevo as well, include:

Nervous system disorders: Ataxia, numbness, increased hand tremor, muscle twitching, muscle cramp, trismus, activation of latent Horner's syndrome. Also falling and gait abnormalities are potential undesirable effects.

Eye disorders: Diplopia, blurred vision, dilated pupils, oculogyric crises.

Gastrointestinal disorders: Dry mouth, bitter taste, sialorrhoea, dysphagia, bruxism, hiccups, abdominal pain and distress, constipation, diarrhoea, flatulence, burning sensation of the tongue.

Renal and urinary disorders: Urinary retention, urinary incontinence, dark urine, priapism.

Skin and subcutaneous tissue disorders: Flushing, increased sweating, dark sweat, rash, hair loss.

Metabolism and nutrition disorders: Weight gain or loss, oedema.

Psychiatric disorders: Confusion, insomnia, nightmares, hallucinations, delusions, agitation, anxiety, euphoria.

Miscellaneous: Weakness, faintness, fatigue, headache, hoarseness, malaise, hot flushes, sense of stimulation, bizarre breathing patterns, neuroleptic malignant syndrome, malignant melanoma.

Entacapone

The most frequent adverse reactions caused by entacapone relate to the increased dopaminergic activity and occur most commonly at the beginning of the treatment. Reduction of levodopa dose decreases the severity and frequency of the reactions. The other major class of adverse reactions are gastrointestinal symptoms, including nausea, vomiting, abdominal pain, constipations and diarrhoea. Urine may be discoloured reddish-brown by entacapone, but this is a harmless phenomenon.

The following adverse reactions, listed in Table 1, have been accumulated both from clinical studies with entacapone and since the introduction of entacapone into the market for the combination use of entacapone with levodopa/DDC inhibitor.

Table 1. Adverse reactions

Nervous system disorders

Very common: Dyskinesia, Parkinsonism aggravated.

Common: Dizziness, dystonia, hyperkinesia.

Gastrointestinal disorders

Very common: Nausea.

Common: Diarrhoea, abdominal pain, dry mouth, constipation, vomiting.

Very rare: Anorexia.

Not known: Colitis.

Renal and urinary disorders

Very common: Urine discolouration.

Skin and subcutaneous tissue disorders

Rare: Erythematous or maculopapular rash.

Very rare: Urticaria.

Not known: Skin, hair, beard and nail discolorations.

General disorders and administration site conditions

Common: Fatigue, sweating increased, fall.

Uncommon: Weight decrease.

Hepatobiliarydisorders

Rare: Hepatic function tests abnormal.

Not known: Hepatitis with mainly cholestatic features (see section 4.4).

Psychiatric disorders

Common: Insomnia, hallucinations, confusion, nightmares, agitation.

*Adverse reactions are ranked under headings of frequency, the most frequent first, using the following convention: Very common (≥1/10); common (1≥100 to <1/10); uncommon (≥1/1,000 to <1/100); rare (≥1/10,000 to <1/1,000), very rare (<1/10,000), not known (cannot be estimated from the available data), since no valid estimate can be derived from clinical trials or epidemiological studies).

Entacapone in association with levodopa has been associated with isolated cases of excessive daytime somnolence and sudden sleep onset episodes.

Isolated cases of NMS have been reported following the abrupt reduction or discontinuation of entacapone and other dopaminergic treatments.

Isolated cases of rhabdomyolysis have been reported.

Isolated cases of angioedema have been reported after the initiation of Stalevo.

Laboratory tests:

The following laboratory abnormalities have been reported with levodopa/carbidopa treatment and should, therefore, be acknowledged when treating patients with Stalevo:

Commonly, levels of blood urea nitrogen, creatinine, and uric acid are lower during administration of levodopa/carbidopa than with levodopa alone. Transient abnormalities include elevated values of blood urea, AST (SGOT), ALT (SGPT), LDH, bilirubin, and alkaline phosphatase.

Decreased haemoglobin, haematocrit, elevated serum glucose and white blood cells, bacteria and blood in the urine have been reported.

Positive Coombs' tests have been reported, both for levodopa/carbidopa and for levodopa alone, but haemolytic anaemia is extremely rare.

Levodopa/carbidopa may cause false positive result when a dipstick is used to test for urinary ketone and this reaction is not altered by boiling the urine sample. The use of glucose oxidase methods may give false negative results for glycosuria.

4.9 Overdose

The post-marketing data includes isolated cases of overdose in which the reported highest daily doses of levodopa and entacapone have been at least 10,000 mg and 40,000 mg, respectively. The acute symptoms and signs in these cases of overdose included agitation, confusional state, coma, bradycardia, ventricular tachycardia, Cheyne-Stokes respiration, discolourations of skin, tongue and conjunctiva, and chromaturia. Management of acute overdose with Stalevo therapy is similar to acute overdose with levodopa. Pyridoxine, however, is not effective in reversing the actions of Stalevo. Hospitalisation is advised and general supportive measures should be employed with immediate gastric lavage and repeated doses of charcoal over time. This may hasten the elimination of entacapone in particular by decreasing its absorption/reabsorption from the GI tract. The adequacy of the respiratory, circulatory and renal systems should be carefully monitored and appropriate supportive measures employed. ECG monitoring should be started and the patient carefully monitored for the possible development of arrhythmias. If required, appropriate anti-arrhythmic therapy should be given. The possibility that the patient has taken other active substances in addition to Stalevo should be taken into consideration. The value of dialysis in the treatment of overdose is not known.

5. PHARMACOLOGICAL PROPERTIES

5.1 Pharmacodynamic properties

Pharmacotherapeutic group: dopa and dopa derivatives, ATC code: N04BA03

According to the current understanding, the symptoms of Parkinson's disease are related to depletion of dopamine in the corpus striatum. Dopamine does not cross the blood-brain barrier. Levodopa, the precursor of dopamine, crosses the blood brain barrier and relieves the symptoms of the disease. As levodopa is extensively metabolised in the periphery, only a small portion of a given dose reaches the central nervous system when levodopa is administered without metabolic enzyme inhibitors.

Carbidopa and benserazide are peripheral DDC inhibitors which reduce the peripheral metabolism of levodopa to dopamine, and thus, more levodopa is available to the brain. When decarboxylation of levodopa is reduced with the co-administration of a DDC inhibitor, a lower dose of levodopa can be used and the incidence of undesirable effects such as nausea is reduced.

With inhibition of the decarboxylase by a DDC inhibitor, catechol-*O*-methyltransferase (COMT) becomes the major peripheral metabolic pathway catalyzing the conversion of levodopa to 3-O-methyldopa (3-OMD), a potentially harmful metabolite of levodopa. Entacapone is a reversible, specific and mainly peripherally acting COMT inhibitor designed for concomitant administration with levodopa. Entacapone slows the clearance of levodopa from the bloodstream resulting in an increased area under the curve (AUC) in the pharmacokinetic profile of levodopa. Consequently the clinical response to each dose of levodopa is enhanced and prolonged.

The evidence of the therapeutic effects of Stalevo is based on two phase III double-blind studies, in which 376 Parkinson's disease patients with end-of-dose motor fluctuations received either entacapone or placebo with each levodopa/DDC inhibitor dose. Daily ON time with and without entacapone was recorded in home-diaries by patients. In the first study, entacapone increased the mean daily ON time by 1 h 20 min ($CI_{95\%}$ 45 min, 1 h 56 min) from baseline. This corresponded to an 8.3% increase in the proportion of daily ON time. Correspondingly, the decrease in daily OFF time was 24% in the entacapone group and 0% in the placebo group. In the second study, the mean proportion of daily ON time increased by 4.5% ($CI_{95\%}$ 0.93%, 7.97%) from baseline. This is translated to a mean increase of 35 min in the daily ON time. Correspondingly, the daily OFF time decreased by 18% on entacapone and by 5% on placebo. Because the effects of Stalevo tablets are equivalent with entacapone 200 mg tablet administered concomitantly with the commercially available standard release carbidopa/levodopa preparations in corresponding doses these results are applicable to describe the effects of Stalevo as well.

5.2 Pharmacokinetic properties

General characteristics of the active substances

Absorption/Distribution: There are substantial inter- and intra-individual variations in the absorption of levodopa, carbidopa and entacapone. Both levodopa and entacapone are rapidly absorbed and eliminated. Carbidopa is absorbed and eliminated slightly slower compared with levodopa. When given separately without the two other active substances, the bioavailability for levodopa is 15-33%, for carbidopa 40-70% and for entacapone 35% after a 200 mg oral dose. Meals rich in large neutral amino acids may delay and reduce the absorption of levodopa. Food does not significantly affect the absorption of entacapone. The distribution volume of both levodopa (Vd 0.36-1.6 l/kg) and entacapone (Vd_{ss} 0.27 l/kg) is moderately small while no data for carbidopa are available.

Levodopa is bound to plasma protein only to a minor extent of about 10-30% and carbidopa is bound approximately 36%, while entacapone is extensively bound to plasma proteins (about 98%) –mainly to serum albumin. At therapeutic concentrations, entacapone does not displace other extensively bound active substances (e.g. warfarin, salicylic acid, phenylbutazone, or diazepam), nor is it displaced to any significant extent by any of these substances at therapeutic or higher concentrations.

Metabolism and Elimination: Levodopa is extensively metabolised to various metabolites: decarboxylation by dopa decarboxylase (DDC) and O-methylation by catechol-O-methyltransferase (COMT) being the most important pathways.

Carbidopa is metabolized to two main metabolites which are excreted in the urine as glucuronides and unconjugated compounds. Unchanged carbidopa accounts for 30% of the total urinary excretion.

Entacapone is almost completely metabolized prior to excretion via urine (10 to 20%) and bile/faeces (80 to 90%). The main metabolic pathway is glucuronidation of entacapone and its active metabolite, the cis-isomer, which accounts for about 5% of plasma total amount.

Total clearance for levodopa is in the range of 0.55-1.38 l/kg/h and for entacapone is in the range of 0.70 l/kg/h. The elimination-half life is ($t_{1/2}$) is 0.6-1.3 hours for levodopa, 2-3 hours for carbidopa and 0.4-0.7 hours for entacapone, each given separately.

Due to short elimination half-lives, no true accumulation of levodopa or entacapone occurs on repeated administration.

Data from *in vitro* studies using human liver microsomal preparations indicate that entacapone inhibits cytochrome P450 2C9 (IC50 ~ 4 μM). Entacapone showed little or no inhibition of other types of P450 isoenzymes (CYP1A2, CYP2A6, CYP2D6, CYP2E1, CYP3A and CYP2C19); see section 4.5.

Characteristics in patients

Elderly: When given without carbidopa and entacapone, the absorption of levodopa is greater and elimination is slower in elderly than in young subjects. However, after combination of carbidopa with levodopa, the absorption of levodopa is similar between the elderly and the young, but the AUC is still 1.5 fold greater in the elderly due to decreased DDC activity and lower clearance by aging. There are no significant differences in the AUC of carbidopa or entacapone between younger (45–64 years) and elderly subjects (65–75 years).

Gender: Bioavailability of levodopa is significantly higher in women than in men. In the pharmacokinetic studies with Stalevo the bioavailability of levodopa is higher in women than in men, primarily due to the difference in body weight, while there is no gender difference with carbidopa and entacapone.

Hepatic impairment: The metabolism of entacapone is slowed in patients with mild to moderate hepatic impairment (Child-Pugh Class A and B) leading to an increased plasma concentration of entacapone both in the absorption and elimination phases (see sections 4.2 and 4.3). No particular studies on the pharmacokinetics of carbidopa and levodopa in patients with hepatic impairment are reported, however, it is advised that Stalevo should be administered cautiously to patients with mild or moderate hepatic impairment.

Renal impairment: Renal impairment does not affect the pharmacokinetics of entacapone. No particular studies are reported on the pharmacokinetics of levodopa and carbidopa in patients with renal impairment. However, a longer dosing interval of Stalevo may be considered for patients who are receiving dialysis therapy (see section 4.2).

5.3 Preclinical safety data

Preclinical data of levodopa, carbidopa and entacapone, tested alone or in combination, revealed no special hazard for humans based on conventional studies of safety pharmacology, repeated dose toxicity, genotoxicity, and carcinogenic potential. In repeated dose toxicity studies with entacapone, anaemia most likely due to iron chelating properties of entacapone was observed. Regarding reproduction toxicity of entacapone, decreased foetal weight and a slightly delayed bone development were noticed in rabbits treated at systemic exposure levels in the therapeutic range. Both levodopa and combinations of carbidopa and levodopa have caused visceral and skeletal malformations in rabbits.

6. PHARMACEUTICAL PARTICULARS

6.1 List of excipients

Tablet core:

Croscarmellose sodium

Magnesium stearate

Maize starch

Mannitol (E421)

Povidone (E1201)

Film-coating:

Glycerol (85 per cent) (E422)

Hypromellose

Magnesium stearate

Polysorbate 80

Red iron oxide (E172)

Sucrose

Titanium dioxide (E171)

Yellow iron oxide (E172)

6.2 Incompatibilities

Not applicable.

6.3 Shelf life

3 years.

6.4 Special precautions for storage

This medicinal product does not require any special storage conditions.

6.5 Nature and contents of container

HDPE bottle with a child resistant PP-closure.

Pack sizes:

10, 30, 100, 130, 175 and 250 tablets.

Not all pack sizes may be marketed.

6.6 Special precautions for disposal and other handling

Any unused product or waste material should be disposed of in accordance with local requirements.

7. MARKETING AUTHORISATION HOLDER

Orion Corporation

Orionintie 1

FI-02200 Espoo

Finland

8. MARKETING AUTHORISATION NUMBER(S)

EU/1/03/260/005-008

EU/1/03/260/014

EU/1/03/260/017

9. DATE OF FIRST AUTHORISATION/RENEWAL OF THE AUTHORISATION

Date of first authorisation: 17 October 2003

Date of last renewal: 15 September 2008

10. DATE OF REVISION OF THE TEXT

27 March 2009

Detailed information on this medicine is available on the European Medicine's Agency (EMEA) web site: http://www.emea.europa.eu

Stalevo 125/31.25/200mg

(Orion Pharma (UK) Limited)

1. NAME OF THE MEDICINAL PRODUCT

Stalevo 125 mg/31.25 mg/200 mg film-coated tablets

2. QUALITATIVE AND QUANTITATIVE COMPOSITION

Each tablet contains 125 mg of levodopa, 31.25 mg of carbidopa and 200 mg of entacapone.

Excipient: Each tablet contains 1.6 mg of sucrose.

For a full list of excipients, see section 6.1.

3. PHARMACEUTICAL FORM

Film-coated tablet

Light brownish red, oval film-coated tablets marked with 'LCE 125' on one side.

4. CLINICAL PARTICULARS

4.1 Therapeutic indications

Stalevo is indicated for the treatment of adult patients with Parkinson's disease and end-of-dose motor fluctuations not stabilised on levodopa/dopa decarboxylase (DDC) inhibitor treatment.

4.2 Posology and method of administration

Each tablet is to be taken orally either with or without food (see section 5.2). One tablet contains one treatment dose and the tablet may only be administered as whole tablets.

The optimum daily dose must be determined by careful titration of levodopa in each patient. The daily dose should be preferably optimised using one of the six available tablet strengths (50 mg/12.5 mg/200 mg, 75 mg/18.75 mg/200 mg, 100 mg/25 mg/200 mg, 125 mg/31.25 mg/200 mg, 150 mg/37.5 mg/200 mg or 200 mg/50 mg/200 mg levodopa/carbidopa/entacapone).

Patients should be instructed to take only one Stalevo tablet per dose administration. Patients receiving less than 70-100 mg carbidopa a day are more likely to experience nausea and vomiting. While the experience with total daily dose greater than 200 mg carbidopa is limited, the maximum recommended daily dose of entacapone is 2,000 mg and therefore the maximum dose is 10 tablets per day for the Stalevo strengths of 50 mg/12.5 mg/200 mg, 75 mg/18.75 mg/200 mg, 100 mg/25 mg/200 mg, 125 mg/31.25 mg/200 mg and 150 mg/37.5 mg/200 mg. Ten tablets of Stalevo 150 mg/37.5 mg/200 mg equals 375 mg of carbidopa a day. According to this daily carbidopa dose, the maximum recommended daily Stalevo 200 mg/50 mg/200 mg dose is 7 tablets per day.

Usually Stalevo is to be used in patients who are currently treated with corresponding doses of standard release levodopa/DDC inhibitor and entacapone.

How to transfer patients taking levodopa/DDC inhibitor (carbidopa or benserazide) preparations and entacapone tablets to Stalevo

a. Patients who are currently treated with entacapone and with standard release levodopa/carbidopa in doses equal to Stalevo tablet strengths can be directly transferred to corresponding Stalevo tablets.

For example, a patient taking one tablet of 50 mg/12.5 mg of levodopa/carbidopa with one tablet of entacapone 200 mg four times daily can take one 50 mg/12.5 mg/200 mg Stalevo tablet four times daily in place of their usual levodopa/carbidopa and entacapone doses.

b. When initiating Stalevo therapy for patients currently treated with entacapone and levodopa/carbidopa in doses not equal to Stalevo, 125 mg/31.25 mg/200 mg (or 50 mg/12.5 mg/200 mg or 75 mg/18.75 mg/200 mg or 100 mg/25 mg/200 mg or 150 mg/37.5 mg/200 mg or 200 mg/50 mg/200 mg) tablets, Stalevo dosing should be carefully titrated for optimal clinical response. At the initiation, Stalevo should be adjusted to correspond as closely as possible to the total daily dose of levodopa currently used.

c. When initiating Stalevo in patients currently treated with entacapone and levodopa/benserazide in a standard release formulation, discontinue dosing of levodopa/benserazide the previous night, and start Stalevo the next morning. Begin with a dose of Stalevo that will provide either the same amount of levodopa or slightly (5-10%) more.

How to transfer patients not currently treated with entacapone to Stalevo

Initiation of Stalevo may be considered at corresponding doses to current treatment in some patients with Parkinson's disease and end-of-dose motor fluctuations, who are not stabilised on their current standard release levodopa/DDC inhibitor treatment. However, a direct switch from levodopa/DDC inhibitor to Stalevo is not recommended for patients who have dyskinesias or whose daily levodopa dose is above 800 mg. In such patients it is advisable to introduce entacapone treatment as a separate treatment (entacapone tablets) and adjust the levodopa dose if necessary, before switching to Stalevo.

Entacapone enhances the effects of levodopa. It may therefore be necessary, particularly in patients with dyskinesia, to reduce levodopa dose by 10-30% within the first days to first weeks after initiating Stalevo treatment. The daily dose of levodopa can be reduced by extending the dosing intervals and/or by reducing the amount of levodopa per dose, according to the clinical condition of the patient.

Dose adjustment during the course of the treatment

When more levodopa is required, an increase in the frequency of doses and/or the use of an alternative strength of Stalevo should be considered, within the dose recommendations.

When less levodopa is required, the total daily dose of Stalevo should be reduced either by decreasing the frequency of administration by extending the time between doses, or by decreasing the strength of Stalevo at an administration.

If other levodopa products are used concomitantly with a Stalevo tablet, the maximum dose recommendations should be followed.

Discontinuation of Stalevo therapy: If Stalevo treatment (levodopa/carbidopa/entacapone) is discontinued and the patient is transferred to levodopa/DDC inhibitor therapy without entacapone, it is necessary to adjust the dosing of other antiparkinsonian treatments, especially levodopa, to achieve a sufficient level of control of the parkinsonian symptoms.

Children and adolescents: Stalevo is not recommended for use in children below 18 years due to a lack of data on safety and efficacy.

Elderly: No dose adjustment of Stalevo is required for elderly patients.

Hepatic impairment: It is advised that Stalevo should be administered cautiously to patients with mild to moderate hepatic impairment. Dose reduction may be needed (see section 5.2). For severe hepatic impairment see section 4.3.

Renal impairment: Renal impairment does not affect the pharmacokinetics of entacapone. No particular studies are reported on the pharmacokinetics of levodopa and carbidopa in patients with renal insufficiency, therefore Stalevo therapy should be administered cautiously to patients in severe renal impairment including those receiving dialysis therapy (see section 5.2).

4.3 Contraindications

- Hypersensitivity to the active substances or to any of the excipients.
- Severe hepatic impairment.
- Narrow-angle glaucoma.
- Pheochromocytoma.
- Concomitant use of Stalevo with non-selective monoamine oxidase (MAO-A and MAO-B) inhibitors (e.g. phenelzine, tranylcypromine).
- Concomitant use of a selective MAO-A inhibitor and a selective MAO-B inhibitor (see section 4.5).
- A previous history of Neuroleptic Malignant Syndrome (NMS) and/or non-traumatic rhabdomyolysis.

4.4 Special warnings and precautions for use

- Stalevo is not recommended for the treatment of drug-induced extrapyramidal reactions
- Stalevo therapy should be administered cautiously to patients with severe cardiovascular or pulmonary disease, bronchial asthma, renal or endocrine disease, history of peptic ulcer disease or history of convulsions.
- In patients with a history of myocardial infarction who have residual atrial nodal or ventricular arrhythmias; cardiac function should be monitored with particular care during the period of initial dose adjustments.
- All patients treated with Stalevo should be monitored carefully for the development of mental changes, depression with suicidal tendencies, and other serious antisocial behaviour. Patients with past or current psychosis should be treated with caution.
- Concomitant administration of antipsychotics with dopamine receptor-blocking properties, particularly D_2 receptor antagonists should be carried out with caution, and the patient carefully observed for loss of antiparkinsonian effect or worsening of parkinsonian symptoms.
- Patients with chronic wide-angle glaucoma may be treated with Stalevo with caution, provided the intra-ocular pressure is well controlled and the patient is monitored carefully for changes in intra-ocular pressure.
- Stalevo may induce orthostatic hypotension. Therefore Stalevo should be given cautiously to patients who are taking other medicinal products which may cause orthostatic hypotension.
- Entacapone in association with levodopa has been associated with somnolence and episodes of sudden sleep onset in patients with Parkinson's disease and caution should therefore be exercised when driving or operating machines (see section 4.7).
- In clinical studies, undesirable dopaminergic adverse reactions, e.g. dyskinesia, were more common in patients who received entacapone and dopamine agonists (such as bromocriptine), selegiline or amantadine compared to those who received placebo with this combination. The doses of other antiparkinsonian medicinal products may need to be adjusted when Stalevo treatment is substituted for a patient currently not treated with entacapone.
- Rhabdomyolysis secondary to severe dyskinesias or neuroleptic malignant syndrome (NMS) has been observed rarely in patients with Parkinson's disease. Therefore, any abrupt dose reduction or withdrawal of levodopa should be carefully observed, particularly in patients who are also receiving neuroleptics. NMS, including rhabdomyolysis and hyperthermia, is characterised by motor symptoms (rigidity, myoclonus, tremor), mental status changes (e.g., agitation, confusion, coma), hyperthermia, autonomic dysfunction (tachycardia, labile blood pressure) and elevated serum creatine phosphokinase. In individual cases, only some of these symptoms and/or findings may be evident. The early diagnosis is important for the appropriate management of NMS. A syndrome resembling the neuroleptic malignant syndrome including muscular rigidity, elevated body temperature, mental changes and increased serum creatine phosphokinase has been reported with the abrupt withdrawal of antiparkinsonian agents. Neither NMS nor rhabdomyolysis have been reported in association with entacapone treatment from controlled trials in which entacapone was discontinued abruptly. Since the introduction of entacapone into the market, isolated cases of NMS have been reported, especially following abrupt reduction or discontinuation of entacapone and other concomitant dopaminergic medicinal products. When considered necessary, the replacement of Stalevo with levodopa and DDC inhibitor without entacapone or other dopaminergic treatment should proceed slowly and an increase in levodopa dose may be necessary.
- If general anaesthesia is required, therapy with Stalevo may be continued for as long as the patient is permitted to take fluids and medicinal products by mouth. If therapy has to be stopped temporarily, Stalevo may be restarted as soon as oral medicinal products can be taken at the same daily dose as before.
- Periodic evaluation of hepatic, haematopoietic, cardiovascular and renal function is recommended during extended therapy with Stalevo.
- For patients experiencing diarrhoea, a follow-up of weight is recommended in order to avoid potential excessive weight decrease.

- Pathological gambling, increased libido and hypersexuality have been reported in Parkinson's disease patients treated with dopamine agonists and other dopaminergic treatments such as Stalevo.

- For patients who experience progressive anorexia, asthenia and weight decrease within a relatively short period of time, a general medical evaluation including liver function should be considered.

- Stalevo contains sucrose, and therefore patients with rare hereditary problems of fructose intolerance, glucose-galactose malabsorption or sucrase-isomaltase insufficiency should not take this medicine.

4.5 Interaction with other medicinal products and other forms of interaction

Other antiparkinsonian medicinal products: To date there has been no indication of interactions that would preclude concurrent use of standard antiparkinsonian medicinal products with Stalevo therapy. Entacapone in high doses may affect the absorption of carbidopa. However, no interaction with carbidopa has been observed with the recommended treatment schedule (200 mg of entacapone up to 10 times daily). Interactions between entacapone and selegiline have been investigated in repeated dose studies in Parkinson's disease patients treated with levodopa/DDC inhibitor and no interaction was observed. When used with Stalevo, the daily dose of selegiline should not exceed 10 mg.

Caution should be exercised when the following active substances are administered concomitantly with levodopa therapy.

Antihypertensives: Symptomatic postural hypotension may occur when levodopa is added to the treatment of patients already receiving antihypertensives. Dose adjustment of the antihypertensive agent may be required.

Antidepressants: Rarely, reactions including hypertension and dyskinesia have been reported with the concomitant use of tricyclic antidepressants and levodopa/carbidopa. Interactions between entacapone and imipramine and between entacapone and moclobemide have been investigated in single dose studies in healthy volunteers. No pharmacodynamic interactions were observed. A significant number of Parkinson's disease patients have been treated with the combination of levodopa, carbidopa and entacapone with several active substances including MAO-A inhibitors, tricyclic antidepressants, noradrenaline reuptake inhibitors such as desipramine, maprotiline and venlafaxine and medicinal products that are metabolised by COMT (e.g. catechol-structured compounds, paroxetine). No pharmacodynamic interactions have been observed. However, caution should be exercised when these medicinal products are used concomitantly with Stalevo (see sections 4.3 and 4.4).

Other active substances: Dopamine receptor antagonists (e.g. some antipsychotics and antiemetics), phenytoin and papaverine may reduce the therapeutic effect of levodopa. Patients taking these medicinal products with Stalevo should be carefully observed for loss of therapeutic response.

Due to entacapone's affinity to cytochrome P450 2C9 *in vitro* (see section 5.2), Stalevo may potentially interfere with active substances whose metabolism is dependent on this isoenzyme, such as S-warfarin. However, in an interaction study with healthy volunteers, entacapone did not change the plasma levels of S-warfarin, while the AUC for R-warfarin increased on average by 18% [CI_{90} 11-26%]. The INR values increased on average by 13% [CI_{90} 6-19%]. Thus, a control of INR is recommended when Stalevo is initiated for patients receiving warfarin.

Other forms of interactions: Since levodopa competes with certain amino acids, the absorption of Stalevo may be impaired in some patients on high protein diet.

Levodopa and entacapone may form chelates with iron in the gastrointestinal tract. Therefore, Stalevo and iron preparations should be taken at least 2-3 hours apart (see section 4.8).

In vitro data: Entacapone binds to human albumin binding site II which also binds several other medicinal products, including diazepam and ibuprofen. According to *in vitro* studies, significant displacement is not anticipated at therapeutic concentrations of the medicinal products. Accordingly, to date there has been no indication of such interactions.

4.6 Pregnancy and lactation

There are no adequate data from the use of the combination of levodopa/carbidopa/entacapone in pregnant women. Studies in animals have shown reproductive toxicity of the separate compounds (see section 5.3). The potential risk for humans is unknown. Stalevo should not be used during pregnancy unless the benefits for the mother outweigh the possible risks to the foetus.

Levodopa is excreted in human breast milk. There is evidence that lactation is suppressed during treatment with levodopa. Carbidopa and entacapone were excreted in milk in animals but is not known whether they are excreted in human breast milk. The safety of levodopa, carbidopa or entacapone in the infant is not known. Women should not breast-feed during treatment with Stalevo.

4.7 Effects on ability to drive and use machines

Stalevo may have major influence on the ability to drive and use machines. Levodopa, carbidopa and entacapone together may cause dizziness and symptomatic orthostatism. Therefore, caution should be exercised when driving or using machines.

Patients being treated with Stalevo and presenting with somnolence and/or sudden sleep onset episodes must be instructed to refrain from driving or engaging in activities where impaired alertness may put themselves or others at risk of serious injury or death (e.g. operating machines) until such recurrent episodes have resolved (see section 4.4).

4.8 Undesirable effects

The following section describes the undesirable effects reported for levodopa/carbidopa and for entacapone used in combination with levodopa/DDC inhibitor.

<u>Levodopa /carbidopa</u>

Adverse reactions that occur frequently with levodopa/carbidopa are those due to central neuropharmacological activity of dopamine. These reactions can usually be diminished by levodopa dose reduction. The most common adverse reactions are dyskinesias including choreiform, dystonic and other involuntary movements. Muscle twitching and blepharospasm may be taken as early signs to consider levodopa dose reduction. Nausea, also related to enhanced central dopaminergic activity, is a common adverse reaction of levodopa/carbidopa.

Other adverse reactions associated with levodopa/carbidopa therapy are mental changes, including paranoid ideation and psychotic episodes; depression with or without development of suicidal tendencies; and cognitive dysfunction. Adding of entacapone to levodopa/DDC inhibitor therapy (carbidopa or benserazide), i.e. initiation of Stalevo treatment in an entacapone naive patient, may aggravate some of these mental changes.

Less frequent adverse reactions of levodopa/carbidopa therapy are irregular heart rhythm and/or palpitations, orthostatic hypotensive episodes, bradykinetic episodes (the 'on-off' phenomenon), anorexia, vomiting, dizziness, and somnolence.

Gastrointestinal bleeding, development of duodenal ulcer, hypertension, phlebitis, leucopenia, haemolytic and non-haemolytic anaemia, thrombocytopenia, agranulocytosis, chest pain, dyspnoea and paraesthesia have occurred rarely with levodopa/carbidopa.

Convulsions have occurred rarely with levodopa/carbidopa; however a causal relationship to levodopa/carbidopa therapy has not been established.

Parkinson's disease patients treated with dopamine agonists and other dopaminergic treatments such as Stalevo, especially at high doses, have been reported as exhibiting signs of pathological gambling, increased libido and hypersexuality, generally reversible upon reduction of the dose or treatment discontinuation.

Other adverse reactions that have been reported with levodopa and may, therefore, be potential adverse reactions of Stalevo as well, include:

Nervous system disorders: Ataxia, numbness, increased hand tremor, muscle twitching, muscle cramp, trismus, activation of latent Horner's syndrome. Also falling and gait abnormalities are potential undesirable effects.

Eye disorders: Diplopia, blurred vision, dilated pupils, oculogyric crises.

Gastrointestinal disorders: Dry mouth, bitter taste, sialorrhoea, dysphagia, bruxism, hiccups, abdominal pain and distress, constipation, diarrhoea, flatulence, burning sensation of the tongue.

Renal and urinary disorders: Urinary retention, urinary incontinence, dark urine, priapism.

Skin and subcutaneous tissue disorders: Flushing, increased sweating, dark sweat, rash, hair loss.

Metabolism and nutrition disorders: Weight gain or loss, oedema.

Psychiatric disorders: Confusion, insomnia, nightmares, hallucinations, delusions, agitation, anxiety, euphoria.

Miscellaneous: Weakness, faintness, fatigue, headache, hoarseness, malaise, hot flushes, sense of stimulation, bizarre breathing patterns, neuroleptic malignant syndrome, malignant melanoma.

<u>Entacapone</u>

The most frequent adverse reactions caused by entacapone relate to the increased dopaminergic activity and occur most commonly at the beginning of the treatment. Reduction of levodopa dose decreases the severity and frequency of the reactions. The other major class of adverse reactions are gastrointestinal symptoms, including nausea, vomiting, abdominal pain, constipations and diarrhoea. Urine may be discoloured reddish-brown by entacapone, but this is a harmless phenomenon.

The following adverse reactions, listed in Table 1, have been accumulated both from clinical studies with entacapone and since the introduction of entacapone into the market for the combination use of entacapone with levodopa/DDC inhibitor.

Table 1. Adverse reactions

Nervous system disorders

Very common: Dyskinesia, Parkinsonism aggravated.

Common: Dizziness, dystonia, hyperkinesia.

Gastrointestinal disorders

Very common: Nausea.

Common: Diarrhoea, abdominal pain, dry mouth, constipation, vomiting.

Very rare: Anorexia.

Not known: Colitis.

Renal and urinary disorders

Very common: Urine discolouration.

Skin and subcutaneous tissue disorders

Rare: Erythematous or maculopapular rash.

Very rare: Urticaria.

Not known: Skin, hair, beard and nail discolorations.

General disorders and administration site conditions

Common: Fatigue, sweating increased, fall.

Uncommon: Weight decrease.

Hepatobiliary disorders

Rare: Hepatic function tests abnormal.

Not known: Hepatitis with mainly cholestatic features (see section 4.4).

Psychiatric disorders

Common: Insomnia, hallucinations, confusion, nightmares, agitation.

*Adverse reactions are ranked under headings of frequency, the most frequent first, using the following convention: Very common (≥1/10); common (1≥100 to <1/10); uncommon (≥1/1,000 to <1/100); rare (≥1/10,000 to <1/1,000), very rare (<1/10,000), not known (cannot be estimated from the available data, since no valid estimate can be derived from clinical trials or epidemiological studies).

Entacapone in association with levodopa has been associated with isolated cases of excessive daytime somnolence and sudden sleep onset episodes.

Isolated cases of NMS have been reported following the abrupt reduction or discontinuation of entacapone and other dopaminergic treatments.

Isolated cases of rhabdomyolysis have been reported.

Isolated cases of angioedema have been reported after the initiation of Stalevo.

<u>Laboratory tests</u>:

The following laboratory abnormalities have been reported with levodopa/carbidopa treatment and should, therefore, be acknowledged when treating patients with Stalevo:

Commonly, levels of blood urea nitrogen, creatinine, and uric acid are lower during administration of levodopa/carbidopa than with levodopa alone. Transient abnormalities include elevated values of blood urea, AST (SGOT), ALT (SGPT), LDH, bilirubin, and alkaline phosphatase.

Decreased haemoglobin, haematocrit, elevated serum glucose and white blood cells, bacteria and blood in the urine have been reported.

Positive Coombs' tests have been reported, both for levodopa/carbidopa and for levodopa alone, but haemolytic anaemia is extremely rare.

Levodopa/carbidopa may cause false positive result when a dipstick is used to test for urinary ketone and this reaction is not altered by boiling the urine sample. The use of glucose oxidase methods may give false negative results for glycosuria.

4.9 Overdose

The post-marketing data includes isolated cases of overdose in which the reported highest daily doses of levodopa and entacapone have been at least 10,000 mg and 40,000 mg, respectively. The acute symptoms and signs in these cases of overdose included agitation, confusional state, coma, bradycardia, ventricular tachycardia, Cheyne-Stokes respiration, discolourations of skin, tongue and conjunctiva, and chromaturia. Management of acute overdose with Stalevo therapy is similar to acute overdose with levodopa. Pyridoxine, however, is not effective in reversing the actions of Stalevo. Hospitalisation is advised and general supportive measures should be employed with immediate gastric lavage and repeated doses of charcoal over time. This may hasten the elimination of entacapone in particular by decreasing its absorption/reabsorption from the GI tract. The adequacy of the respiratory, circulatory and renal systems should be carefully monitored and appropriate supportive measures employed. ECG monitoring should be started and the patient carefully monitored for the possible development of arrhythmias. If required, appropriate anti-arrhythmic therapy should be given. The possibility that the patient has taken other active substances in addition to Stalevo should be taken into consideration. The value of dialysis in the treatment of overdose is not known.

5. PHARMACOLOGICAL PROPERTIES

5.1 Pharmacodynamic properties

Pharmacotherapeutic group: dopa and dopa derivatives, ATC code: N04BA03

According to the current understanding, the symptoms of Parkinson's disease are related to depletion of dopamine in the corpus striatum. Dopamine does not cross the blood-brain barrier. Levodopa, the precursor of dopamine, crosses the blood brain barrier and relieves the symptoms of the disease. As levodopa is extensively metabolised in the periphery, only a small portion of a given dose reaches the central nervous system when levodopa is administered without metabolic enzyme inhibitors.

Carbidopa and benserazide are peripheral DDC inhibitors which reduce the peripheral metabolism of levodopa to dopamine, and thus, more levodopa is available to the brain. When decarboxylation of levodopa is reduced with the co-administration of a DDC inhibitor, a lower dose of levodopa can be used and the incidence of undesirable effects such as nausea is reduced.

With inhibition of the decarboxylase by a DDC inhibitor, catechol-O-methyltransferase (COMT) becomes the major peripheral metabolic pathway catalyzing the conversion of levodopa to 3-O-methyldopa (3-OMD), a potentially harmful metabolite of levodopa. Entacapone is a reversible, specific and mainly peripherally acting COMT inhibitor designed for concomitant administration with levodopa. Entacapone slows the clearance of levodopa from the bloodstream resulting in an increased area under the curve (AUC) in the pharmacokinetic profile of levodopa. Consequently the clinical response to each dose of levodopa is enhanced and prolonged.

The evidence of the therapeutic effects of Stalevo is based on two phase III double-blind studies, in which 376 Parkinson's disease patients with end-of-dose motor fluctuations received either entacapone or placebo with each levodopa/DDC inhibitor dose. Daily ON time with and without entacapone was recorded in home-diaries by patients. In the first study, entacapone increased the mean daily ON time by 1 h 20 min ($CI_{95\%}$ 45 min, 1 h 56 min) from baseline. This corresponded to an 8.3% increase in the proportion of daily ON time. Correspondingly, the decrease in daily OFF time was 24% in the entacapone group and 0% in the placebo group. In the second study, the mean proportion of daily ON time increased by 4.5% ($CI_{95\%}$ 0.93%, 7.97%) from baseline. This is translated to a mean increase of 35 min in the daily ON time. Correspondingly, the daily OFF time decreased by 18% on entacapone and by 5% on placebo. Because the effects of Stalevo tablets are equivalent with entacapone 200 mg tablet administered concomitantly with the commercially available standard release carbidopa/levodopa preparations in corresponding doses these results are applicable to describe the effects of Stalevo as well.

5.2 Pharmacokinetic properties

General characteristics of the active substances

Absorption/Distribution: There are substantial inter- and intra-individual variations in the absorption of levodopa, carbidopa and entacapone. Both levodopa and entacapone are rapidly absorbed and eliminated. Carbidopa is absorbed and eliminated slightly slower compared with levodopa. When given separately without the two other active substances, the bioavailability for levodopa is 15-33%, for carbidopa 40-70% and for entacapone 35% after a 200 mg oral dose. Meals rich in large neutral amino acids may delay and reduce the absorption of levodopa. Food does not significantly affect the absorption of entacapone. The distribution volume of both levodopa (Vd 0.36-1.6 l/kg) and entacapone (Vd_{ss} 0.27 l/kg) is moderately small while no data for carbidopa are available.

Levodopa is bound to plasma protein only to a minor extent of about 10-30% and carbidopa is bound approximately 36%, while entacapone is extensively bound to plasma proteins (about 98%) – mainly to serum albumin. At therapeutic concentrations, entacapone does not displace other extensively bound active substances (e.g. warfarin, salicylic acid, phenylbutazone, or diazepam), nor is it displaced to any significant extent by any of these substances at therapeutic or higher concentrations.

Metabolism and Elimination: Levodopa is extensively metabolised to various metabolites: decarboxylation by dopa decarboxylase (DDC) and O-methylation by catechol-O-methyltransferase (COMT) being the most important pathways.

Carbidopa is metabolized to two main metabolites which are excreted in the urine as glucuronides and unconjugated compounds. Unchanged carbidopa accounts for 30% of the total urinary excretion.

Entacapone is almost completely metabolized prior to excretion via urine (10 to 20%) and bile/faeces (80 to 90%). The main metabolic pathway is glucuronidation of entacapone and its active metabolite, the cis-isomer, which accounts for about 5% of plasma total amount.

Total clearance for levodopa is in the range of 0.55-1.38 l/kg/h and for entacapone is in the range of 0.70 l/kg/h. The elimination-half life is ($t_{1/2}$) is 0.6-1.3 hours for levodopa, 2-3 hours for carbidopa and 0.4-0.7 hours for entacapone, each given separately.

Due to short elimination half-lives, no true accumulation of levodopa or entacapone occurs on repeated administration.

Data from *in vitro* studies using human liver microsomal preparations indicate that entacapone inhibits cytochrome P450 2C9 (IC50 ~ 4 μM). Entacapone showed little or no inhibition of other types of P450 isoenzymes (CYP1A2, CYP2A6, CYP2D6, CYP2E1, CYP3A and CYP2C19); see section 4.5.

Characteristics in patients

Elderly: When given without carbidopa and entacapone, the absorption of levodopa is greater and elimination is slower in elderly than in young subjects. However, after combination of carbidopa with levodopa, the absorption of levodopa is similar between the elderly and the young, but the AUC is still 1.5 fold greater in the elderly due to decreased DDC activity and lower clearance by aging. There are no significant differences in the AUC of carbidopa or entacapone between younger (45–64 years) and elderly subjects (65–75 years).

Gender: Bioavailability of levodopa is significantly higher in women than in men. In the pharmacokinetic studies with Stalevo the bioavailability of levodopa is higher in women than in men, primarily due to the difference in body weight, while there is no gender difference with carbidopa and entacapone.

Hepatic impairment: The metabolism of entacapone is slowed in patients with mild to moderate hepatic impairment (Child-Pugh Class A and B) leading to an increased plasma concentration of entacapone both in the absorption and elimination phases (see sections 4.2 and 4.3). No particular studies on the pharmacokinetics of carbidopa and levodopa in patients with hepatic impairment are reported, however, it is advised that Stalevo should be administered cautiously to patients with mild or moderate hepatic impairment.

Renal impairment: Renal impairment does not affect the pharmacokinetics of entacapone. No particular studies are reported on the pharmacokinetics of levodopa and carbidopa in patients with renal impairment. However, a longer dosing interval of Stalevo may be considered for patients who are receiving dialysis therapy (see section 4.2).

5.3 Preclinical safety data

Preclinical data of levodopa, carbidopa and entacapone, tested alone or in combination, revealed no special hazard for humans based on conventional studies of safety pharmacology, repeated dose toxicity, genotoxicity, and carcinogenic potential. In repeated dose toxicity studies with entacapone, anaemia most likely due to iron chelating properties of entacapone was observed. Regarding reproduction toxicity of entacapone, decreased foetal weight and a slightly delayed bone development were noticed in rabbits treated at systemic exposure levels in the therapeutic range. Both levodopa and combinations of carbidopa and levodopa have caused visceral and skeletal malformations in rabbits.

6. PHARMACEUTICAL PARTICULARS

6.1 List of excipients

Tablet core:

Croscarmellose sodium

Magnesium stearate

Maize starch

Mannitol (E421)

Povidone (E1201)

Film-coating:

Glycerol (85 per cent) (E422)

Hypromellose

Magnesium stearate

Polysorbate 80

Red iron oxide (E172)

Sucrose

Titanium dioxide (E171)

Yellow iron oxide (E172)

6.2 Incompatibilities

Not applicable.

6.3 Shelf life

3 years.

6.4 Special precautions for storage

This medicinal product does not require any special storage conditions.

6.5 Nature and contents of container

HDPE bottle with a child resistant PP-closure.

Pack sizes:

10, 30, 100, 130 and 175 tablets.

Not all pack sizes may be marketed.

6.6 Special precautions for disposal and other handling

Any unused product or waste material should be disposed of in accordance with local requirements.

7. MARKETING AUTHORISATION HOLDER

Orion Corporation

Orionintie 1

FI-02200 Espoo

Finland

8. MARKETING AUTHORISATION NUMBER(S)

EU/1/03/260/029-033

9. DATE OF FIRST AUTHORISATION/RENEWAL OF THE AUTHORISATION

Date of first authorisation: 17 October 2003

Date of last renewal: 15 September 2008

10. DATE OF REVISION OF THE TEXT

27 March 2009

Detailed information on this medicine is available on the European Medicine's Agency (EMEA) web site: http://www.emea.europa.eu

Stalevo 150/37.5/200mg

(Orion Pharma (UK) Limited)

1. NAME OF THE MEDICINAL PRODUCT

Stalevo 150 mg/37.5 mg/200 mg film-coated tablets

2. QUALITATIVE AND QUANTITATIVE COMPOSITION

Each tablet contains 150 mg of levodopa, 37.5 mg of carbidopa and 200 mg of entacapone.

Excipient: Each tablet contains 1.9 mg of sucrose.

For a full list of excipients, see section 6.1.

3. PHARMACEUTICAL FORM

Film-coated tablet

Brownish or greyish red, elongated-ellipse shaped, unscored film-coated tablets marked with 'LCE 150' on one side.

4. CLINICAL PARTICULARS

4.1 Therapeutic indications

Stalevo is indicated for the treatment of adult patients with Parkinson's disease and end-of-dose motor fluctuations not stabilised on levodopa/dopa decarboxylase (DDC) inhibitor treatment.

4.2 Posology and method of administration

Each tablet is to be taken orally either with or without food (see section 5.2). One tablet contains one treatment dose and the tablet may only be administered as whole tablets.

The optimum daily dose must be determined by careful titration of levodopa in each patient. The daily dose should be preferably optimised using one of the six available tablet strengths (50 mg/12.5 mg/200 mg, 75 mg/18.75 mg/200 mg, 100 mg/25 mg/200 mg, 125 mg/31.25 mg/200 mg, 150 mg/37.5 mg/200 mg or 200 mg/50 mg/200 mg levodopa/carbidopa/entacapone).

Patients should be instructed to take only one Stalevo tablet per dose administration. Patients receiving less than 70-100 mg carbidopa a day are more likely to experience nausea and vomiting. While the experience with total daily dose greater than 200 mg carbidopa is limited, the maximum recommended daily dose of entacapone is 2,000 mg and therefore the maximum dose is 10 tablets per day for the Stalevo strengths of 50 mg/12.5 mg/200 mg, 75 mg/18.75 mg/200 mg, 100 mg/25 mg/200 mg, 125 mg/31.25 mg/200 mg and 150 mg/37.5 mg/200 mg. Ten tablets of Stalevo 150 mg/37.5 mg/200 mg equals 375 mg of carbidopa a day. According to this daily carbidopa dose, the maximum recommended daily Stalevo 200 mg/50 mg/200 mg dose is 7 tablets per day.

Usually Stalevo is to be used in patients who are currently treated with corresponding doses of standard release levodopa/DDC inhibitor and entacapone.

How to transfer patients taking levodopa/DDC inhibitor (carbidopa or benserazide) preparations and entacapone tablets to Stalevo

a. Patients who are currently treated with entacapone and with standard release levodopa/carbidopa in doses equal to Stalevo tablet strengths can be directly transferred to corresponding Stalevo tablets.

For example, a patient taking one tablet of 150 mg/37.5 mg of levodopa/carbidopa with one tablet of entacapone 200 mg four times daily can take one 150 mg/37.5 mg/200 mg Stalevo tablet four times daily in place of their usual levodopa/carbidopa and entacapone doses.

b. When initiating Stalevo therapy for patients currently treated with entacapone and levodopa/carbidopa in doses not equal to Stalevo 150 mg/37.5 mg/200 mg, (or 50 mg/12.5 mg/200 mg, or 75 mg/18.75 mg/200 mg or 100 mg/25 mg/200 mg or 125 mg/31.25 mg/200 mg or 200 mg/50 mg/200 mg) tablets, Stalevo dosing should be carefully titrated for optimal clinical response. At the initiation, Stalevo should be adjusted to correspond as closely as possible to the total daily dose of levodopa currently used.

c. When initiating Stalevo in patients currently treated with entacapone and levodopa/benserazide in a standard release formulation, discontinue dosing of levodopa/benserazide the previous night, and start Stalevo the next morning. Begin with a dose of Stalevo that will provide either the same amount of levodopa or slightly (5-10%) more.

How to transfer patients not currently treated with entacapone to Stalevo

Initiation of Stalevo may be considered at corresponding doses to current treatment in some patients with Parkinson's disease and end-of-dose motor fluctuations, who are not stabilised on their current standard release levodopa/DDC inhibitor treatment. However, a direct switch from levodopa/DDC inhibitor to Stalevo is not recommended for patients who have dyskinesias or whose daily levodopa dose is above 800 mg. In such patients it is advisable to introduce entacapone treatment as a separate treatment (entacapone tablets) and adjust the levodopa dose if necessary, before switching to Stalevo.

Entacapone enhances the effects of levodopa. It may therefore be necessary, particularly in patients with dyskinesia, to reduce levodopa dose by 10-30% within the first days to first weeks after initiating Stalevo treatment. The daily dose of levodopa can be reduced by extending the dosing intervals and/or by reducing the amount of levodopa per dose, according to the clinical condition of the patient.

Dose adjustment during the course of the treatment

When more levodopa is required, an increase in the frequency of doses and/or the use of an alternative strength of Stalevo should be considered, within the dose recommendations.

When less levodopa is required, the total daily dose of Stalevo should be reduced either by decreasing the frequency of administration by extending the time between doses, or by decreasing the strength of Stalevo at an administration.

If other levodopa products are used concomitantly with a Stalevo tablet, the maximum dose recommendations should be followed.

Discontinuation of Stalevo therapy: If Stalevo treatment (levodopa/carbidopa/entacapone) is discontinued and the patient is transferred to levodopa/DDC inhibitor therapy without entacapone, it is necessary to adjust the dosing of other antiparkinsonian treatments, especially levodopa, to achieve a sufficient level of control of the parkinsonian symptoms.

Children and adolescents: Stalevo is not recommended for use in children below 18 years due to a lack of data on safety and efficacy.

Elderly: No dose adjustment of Stalevo is required for elderly patients.

Hepatic impairment: It is advised that Stalevo should be administered cautiously to patients with mild to moderate hepatic impairment. Dose reduction may be needed (see section 5.2). For severe hepatic impairment see section 4.3.

Renal impairment: Renal impairment does not affect the pharmacokinetics of entacapone. No particular studies are reported on the pharmacokinetics of levodopa and carbidopa in patients with renal insufficiency, therefore Stalevo therapy should be administered cautiously to patients in severe renal impairment including those receiving dialysis therapy (see section 5.2).

4.3 Contraindications

- Hypersensitivity to the active substances or to any of the excipients.
- Severe hepatic impairment.
- Narrow-angle glaucoma.
- Pheochromocytoma.
- Concomitant use of Stalevo with non-selective monoamine oxidase (MAO-A and MAO-B) inhibitors (e.g. phenelzine, tranylcypromine).
- Concomitant use of a selective MAO-A inhibitor and a selective MAO-B inhibitor (see section 4.5).
- A previous history of Neuroleptic Malignant Syndrome (NMS) and/or non-traumatic rhabdomyolysis.

4.4 Special warnings and precautions for use

- Stalevo is not recommended for the treatment of drug-induced extrapyramidal reactions
- Stalevo therapy should be administered cautiously to patients with severe cardiovascular or pulmonary disease, bronchial asthma, renal or endocrine disease, history of peptic ulcer disease or history of convulsions.
- In patients with a history of myocardial infarction who have residual atrial nodal or ventricular arrhythmias; cardiac function should be monitored with particular care during the period of initial dose adjustments.
- All patients treated with Stalevo should be monitored carefully for the development of mental changes, depression with suicidal tendencies, and other serious antisocial behaviour. Patients with past or current psychosis should be treated with caution.
- Concomitant administration of antipsychotics with dopamine receptor-blocking properties, particularly D_2 receptor antagonists should be carried out with caution, and the patient carefully observed for loss of antiparkinsonian effect or worsening of parkinsonian symptoms.
- Patients with chronic wide-angle glaucoma may be treated with Stalevo with caution, provided the intra-ocular pressure is well controlled and the patient is monitored carefully for changes in intra-ocular pressure.
- Stalevo may induce orthostatic hypotension. Therefore Stalevo should be given cautiously to patients who are taking other medicinal products which may cause orthostatic hypotension.
- Entacapone in association with levodopa has been associated with somnolence and episodes of sudden sleep onset in patients with Parkinson's disease and caution should therefore be exercised when driving or operating machines (see section 4.7).
- In clinical studies, dopaminergic adverse reactions, e.g. dyskinesia, were more common in patients who received entacapone and dopamine agonists (such as bromocriptine), selegiline or amantadine compared to those who received placebo with this combination. The doses of other antiparkinsonian medicinal products may need to be adjusted when Stalevo treatment is substituted for a patient currently not treated with entacapone.
- Rhabdomyolysis secondary to severe dyskinesias or neuroleptic malignant syndrome (NMS) has been observed rarely in patients with Parkinson's disease. Therefore, any abrupt dose reduction or withdrawal of levodopa should be carefully observed, particularly in patients who are also receiving neuroleptics. NMS, including rhabdomyolysis and hyperthermia, is characterised by motor symptoms (rigidity, myoclonus, tremor), mental status changes (e.g., agitation, confusion, coma), hyperthermia, autonomic dysfunction (tachycardia, labile blood pressure) and elevated serum creatine phosphokinase. In individual cases, only some of these symptoms and/or findings may be evident. The early diagnosis is important for the appropriate management of NMS. A syndrome resembling the neuroleptic malignant syndrome including muscular rigidity, elevated body temperature, mental changes and increased serum creatine phosphokinase has been reported with the abrupt withdrawal of antiparkinsonian agents. Neither NMS nor rhabdomyolysis have been reported in association with entacapone treatment from controlled trials in which entacapone was discontinued abruptly. Since the introduction of entacapone into the market, isolated cases of NMS have been reported, especially following abrupt reduction or discontinuation of entacapone and other concomitant dopaminergicmedicinal products. When considered necessary, the replacement of Stalevo with levodopa and DDC inhibitor without entacapone or other dopaminergic treatment should proceed slowly and an increase in levodopa dose may be necessary.
- If general anaesthesia is required, therapy with Stalevo may be continued for as long as the patient is permitted to take fluids and medicinal products by mouth. If therapy has to be stopped temporarily, Stalevo may be restarted as soon as oral medicinal products can be taken at the same daily dose as before.
- Periodic evaluation of hepatic, haematopoietic, cardiovascular and renal function is recommended during extended therapy with Stalevo.
- For patients experiencing diarrhoea, a follow-up of weight is recommended in order to avoid potential excessive weight decrease.
- Pathological gambling, increased libido and hypersexuality have been reported in Parkinson's disease patients treated with dopamine agonists and other dopaminergic treatments such as Stalevo.
- For patients who experience progressive anorexia, asthenia and weight decrease within a relatively short period of time, a general medical evaluation including liver function should be considered.
- Stalevo contains sucrose, and therefore patients with rare hereditary problems of fructose intolerance, glucose-galactose malabsorption or sucrase-isomaltase insufficiency should not take this medicine.

4.5 Interaction with other medicinal products and other forms of interaction

Other antiparkinsonian medicinal products: To date there has been no indication of interactions that would preclude concurrent use of standard antiparkinsonian medicinal products with Stalevo therapy. Entacapone in high doses may affect the absorption of carbidopa. However, no interaction with carbidopa has been observed with the recommended treatment schedule (200 mg of entacapone up to 10 times daily). Interactions between entacapone and selegiline have been investigated in repeated dose studies in Parkinson's disease patients treated with levodopa/DDC inhibitor and no interaction was observed. When used with Stalevo, the daily dose of selegiline should not exceed 10 mg.

Caution should be exercised when the following active substances are administered concomitantly with levodopa therapy.

Antihypertensives: Symptomatic postural hypotension may occur when levodopa is added to the treatment of patients already receiving antihypertensives. Dose adjustment of the antihypertensive agent may be required.

Antidepressants: Rarely, reactions including hypertension and dyskinesia have been reported with the concomitant use of tricyclic antidepressants and levodopa/carbidopa. Interactions between entacapone and imipramine and between entacapone and moclobemide have been investigated in single dose studies in healthy volunteers. No pharmacodynamic interactions were observed. A significant number of Parkinson's disease patients have been treated with the combination of levodopa, carbidopa and entacapone with several active substances including MAO-A inhibitors, tricyclic antidepressants, noradrenaline reuptake inhibitors such as desipramine, maprotiline and venlafaxine and medicinal products that are metabolised by COMT (e.g. catechol-structured compounds, paroxetine). No pharmacodynamic interactions have been observed. However, caution should be exercised when these medicinal products are used concomitantly with Stalevo (see sections 4.3 and 4.4).

Other active substances: Dopamine receptor antagonists (e.g. some antipsychotics and antiemetics), phenytoin and papaverine may reduce the therapeutic effect of levodopa. Patients taking these medicinal products with Stalevo should be carefully observed for loss of therapeutic response.

Due to entacapone's affinity to cytochrome P450 2C9 *in vitro* (see section 5.2), Stalevo may potentially interfere with active substances whose metabolism is dependent on this isoenzyme, such as S-warfarin. However, in an interaction study with healthy volunteers, entacapone did not change the plasma levels of S-warfarin, while the AUC for R-warfarin increased on average by 18% [CI_{90} 11-26%]. The INR values increased on average by 13% [CI_{90} 6-19%]. Thus, a control of INR is recommended when Stalevo is initiated for patients receiving warfarin.

Other forms of interactions: Since levodopa competes with certain amino acids, the absorption of Stalevo may be impaired in some patients on high protein diet.

Levodopa and entacapone may form chelates with iron in the gastrointestinal tract. Therefore, Stalevo and iron preparations should be taken at least 2-3 hours apart (see section 4.8).

In vitro data: Entacapone binds to human albumin binding site II which also binds several other medicinal products, including diazepam and ibuprofen. According to *in vitro* studies, significant displacement is not anticipated at therapeutic concentrations of the medicinal products. Accordingly, to date there has been no indication of such interactions.

4.6 Pregnancy and lactation

There are no adequate data from the use of the combination of levodopa/carbidopa/entacapone in pregnant women. Studies in animals have shown reproductive toxicity of the separate compounds (see section 5.3). The potential risk for humans is unknown. Stalevo should not be used during pregnancy unless the benefits for the mother outweigh the possible risks to the foetus.

Levodopa is excreted in human breast milk. There is evidence that lactation is suppressed during treatment with levodopa. Carbidopa and entacapone were excreted in milk in animals but is not known whether they are excreted in human breast milk. The safety of levodopa, carbidopa or entacapone in the infant is not known. Women should not breast-feed during treatment with Stalevo.

4.7 Effects on ability to drive and use machines

Stalevo may have major influence on the ability to drive and use machines. Levodopa, carbidopa and entacapone together may cause dizziness and symptomatic orthostatism. Therefore, caution should be exercised when driving or using machines.

Patients being treated with Stalevo and presenting with somnolence and/or sudden sleep onset episodes must be instructed to refrain from driving or engaging in activities where impaired alertness may put themselves or others at risk of serious injury or death (e.g. operating machines) until such recurrent episodes have resolved (see section 4.4).

4.8 Undesirable effects

The following section describes the undesirable effects reported for levodopa/carbidopa and for entacapone used in combination with levodopa/DDC inhibitor.

Levodopa /carbidopa

Adverse reactions that occur frequently with levodopa/carbidopa are those due to central neuropharmacological activity of dopamine. These reactions can usually be diminished by levodopa dose reduction. The most common adverse reactions are dyskinesias including choreiform, dystonic and other involuntary movements. Muscle twitching and blepharospasm may be taken as early signs to consider levodopa dose reduction. Nausea, also related to enhanced central dopaminergic activity, is a common adverse reaction of levodopa/carbidopa.

Other adverse reactions associated with levodopa/carbidopa therapy are mental changes, including paranoid ideation and psychotic episodes; depression with or without development of suicidal tendencies; and cognitive dysfunction. Adding of entacapone to levodopa/DDC inhibitor therapy (carbidopa or benserazide), i.e. initiation of Stalevo treatment in an entacapone naive patient, may aggravate some of these mental changes.

Less frequent adverse reactions of levodopa/carbidopa therapy are irregular heart rhythm and/or palpitations, orthostatic hypotensive episodes, bradykinetic episodes (the 'on-off' phenomenon), anorexia, vomiting, dizziness, and somnolence.

Gastrointestinal bleeding, development of duodenal ulcer, hypertension, phlebitis, leucopenia, haemolytic and non-haemolytic anaemia, thrombocytopenia, agranulocytosis, chest pain, dyspnoea and paraesthesia have occurred rarely with levodopa/carbidopa.

Convulsions have occurred rarely with levodopa/carbidopa; however a causal relationship to levodopa/carbidopa therapy has not been established.

Parkinson's disease patients treated with dopamine agonists and other dopaminergic treatments such as Stalevo, especially at high doses, have been reported as exhibiting signs of pathological gambling, increased libido and hypersexuality, generally reversible upon reduction of the dose or treatment discontinuation.

Other adverse reactions that have been reported with levodopa and may, therefore, be potential adverse reactions of Stalevo as well, include:

Nervous system disorders: Ataxia, numbness, increased hand tremor, muscle twitching, muscle cramp, trismus, activation of latent Horner's syndrome. Also falling and gait abnormalities are potential undesirable effects.

Eye disorders: Diplopia, blurred vision, dilated pupils, oculogyric crises.

Gastrointestinal disorders: Dry mouth, bitter taste, sialorrhoea, dysphagia, bruxism, hiccups, abdominal pain and distress, constipation, diarrhoea, flatulence, burning sensation of the tongue.

Renal and urinary disorders: Urinary retention, urinary incontinence, dark urine, priapism.

Skin and subcutaneous tissue disorders: Flushing, increased sweating, dark sweat, rash, hair loss.

Metabolism and nutrition disorders: Weight gain or loss, oedema.

Psychiatric disorders: Confusion, insomnia, nightmares, hallucinations, delusions, agitation, anxiety, euphoria.

Miscellaneous: Weakness, faintness, fatigue, headache, hoarseness, malaise, hot flushes, sense of stimulation, bizarre breathing patterns, neuroleptic malignant syndrome, malignant melanoma.

Entacapone

The most frequent adverse reactions caused by entacapone relate to the increased dopaminergic activity and occur most commonly at the beginning of the treatment. Reduction of levodopa dose decreases the severity and frequency of the reactions. The other major class of adverse reactions are gastrointestinal symptoms, including nausea, vomiting, abdominal pain, constipations and diarrhoea. Urine may be discoloured reddish-brown by entacapone, but this is a harmless phenomenon.

The following adverse reactions, listed in Table 1, have been accumulated both from clinical studies with entacapone and since the introduction of entacapone into the market for the combination use of entacapone with levodopa/DDC inhibitor.

Table 1. Adverse reactions

Nervous system disorders

Very common: Dyskinesia, Parkinsonism aggravated.

Common: Dizziness, dystonia, hyperkinesia.

Gastrointestinal disorders

Very common: Nausea.

Common: Diarrhoea, abdominal pain, dry mouth, constipation, vomiting.

Very rare: Anorexia.

Not known: Colitis.

Renal and urinary disorders

Very common: Urine discolouration.

Skin and subcutaneous tissue disorders

Rare: Erythematous or maculopapular rash.

Very rare: Urticaria.

Not known: Skin, hair, beard, and nail discolorations.

General disorders and administration site conditions

Common: Fatigue, sweating increased, fall.

Uncommon: Weight decrease.

Hepatobiliary disorders

Rare: Hepatic function tests abnormal.

Not known: Hepatitis with mainly cholestatic features (see section 4.4).

Psychiatric disorders

Common: Insomnia, hallucinations, confusion, nightmares, agitation.

*Adverse reactions are ranked under headings of frequency, the most frequent first, using the following convention: Very common (≥1/10); common (≥1/100 to <1/10); uncommon (≥1/1,000 to <1/100); rare (≥1/10,000 to <1/1,000), very rare (<1/10,000), not known (cannot be estimated from the available data, since no valid estimate can be derived from clinical trials or epidemiological studies).

Entacapone in association with levodopa has been associated with isolated cases of excessive daytime somnolence and sudden sleep onset episodes.

Isolated cases of NMS have been reported following the abrupt reduction or discontinuation of entacapone and other dopaminergic treatments.

Isolated cases of rhabdomyolysis have been reported.

Isolated cases of angioedema have been reported after the initiation of Stalevo.

Laboratory tests:

The following laboratory abnormalities have been reported with levodopa/carbidopa treatment and should, therefore, be acknowledged when treating patients with Stalevo:

Commonly, levels of blood urea nitrogen, creatinine, and uric acid are lower during administration of levodopa/carbidopa than with levodopa alone. Transient abnormalities include elevated values of blood urea, AST (SGOT), ALT (SGPT), LDH, bilirubin, and alkaline phosphatase.

Decreased haemoglobin, haematocrit, elevated serum glucose and white blood cells, bacteria and blood in the urine have been reported.

Positive Coombs' tests have been reported, both for levodopa/carbidopa and for levodopa alone, but haemolytic anaemia is extremely rare.

Levodopa/carbidopa may cause false positive result when a dipstick is used to test for urinary ketone and this reaction is not altered by boiling the urine sample. The use of glucose oxidase methods may give false negative results for glycosuria.

4.9 Overdose

The post-marketing data includes isolated cases of overdose in which the reported highest daily doses of levodopa and entacapone have been at least 10,000 mg and 40,000 mg, respectively. The acute symptoms and signs in these cases of overdose included agitation, confusional state, coma, bradycardia, ventricular tachycardia, Cheyne-Stokes respiration, discolourations of skin, tongue and conjunctiva, and chromaturia. Management of acute overdose with Stalevo therapy is similar to acute overdose with levodopa. Pyridoxine, however, is not effective in reversing the actions of Stalevo. Hospitalisation is advised and general supportive measures should be employed with immediate gastric lavage and repeated doses of charcoal over time. This may hasten the elimination of entacapone in particular by decreasing its absorption/reabsorption from the GI tract. The adequacy of the respiratory, circulatory and renal systems should be carefully monitored and appropriate supportive measures employed. ECG monitoring should be started and the patient carefully monitored for the possible development of arrhythmias. If required, appropriate anti-arrhythmic therapy should be given. The possibility that the patient has taken other active substances in addition to Stalevo should be taken into consideration. The value of dialysis in the treatment of overdose is not known.

5. PHARMACOLOGICAL PROPERTIES

5.1 Pharmacodynamic properties

Pharmacotherapeutic group: dopa and dopa derivatives, ATC code: N04BA03

According to the current understanding, the symptoms of Parkinson's disease are related to depletion of dopamine in the corpus striatum. Dopamine does not cross the blood-brain barrier. Levodopa, the precursor of dopamine, crosses the blood brain barrier and relieves the symptoms of the disease. As levodopa is extensively metabolised in the periphery, only a small portion of a given dose reaches the central nervous system when levodopa is administered without metabolic enzyme inhibitors.

Carbidopa and benserazide are peripheral DDC inhibitors which reduce the peripheral metabolism of levodopa to dopamine, and thus, more levodopa is available to the brain. When decarboxylation of levodopa is reduced with the co-administration of a DDC inhibitor, a lower dose of levodopa can be used and the incidence of undesirable effects such as nausea is reduced.

With inhibition of the decarboxylase by a DDC inhibitor, catechol-*O*-methyltransferase (COMT) becomes the major peripheral metabolic pathway catalyzing the conversion of levodopa to 3-O-methyldopa (3-OMD), a potentially harmful metabolite of levodopa. Entacapone is a reversible, specific and mainly peripherally acting COMT inhibitor designed for concomitant administration with levodopa. Entacapone slows the clearance of levodopa from the bloodstream resulting in an increased area under the curve (AUC) in the pharmacokinetic profile of levodopa. Consequently the clinical response to each dose of levodopa is enhanced and prolonged.

The evidence of the therapeutic effects of Stalevo is based on two phase III double-blind studies, in which 376 Parkinson's disease patients with end-of-dose motor fluctuations received either entacapone or placebo with each levodopa/DDC inhibitor dose. Daily ON time with and without entacapone was recorded in home-diaries by patients. In the first study, entacapone increased the mean daily ON time by 1 h 20 min ($CI_{95\%}$ 45 min, 1 h 56 min) from baseline. This corresponded to an 8.3% increase in the proportion of daily ON time. Correspondingly, the decrease in daily OFF time was 24% in the entacapone group and 0% in the placebo group. In the second study, the mean proportion of daily ON time increased by 4.5% ($CI_{95\%}$ 0.93%, 7.97%) from baseline. This is translated to a mean increase of 35 min in the daily ON time. Correspondingly, the daily OFF time decreased by 18% on entacapone and by 5% on placebo. Because the effects of Stalevo tablets are equivalent with entacapone 200 mg tablet administered concomitantly with the commercially available standard release carbidopa/levodopa preparations in corresponding doses these results are applicable to describe the effects of Stalevo as well.

5.2 Pharmacokinetic properties

General characteristics of the active substances

Absorption/Distribution: There are substantial inter- and intra-individual variations in the absorption of levodopa, carbidopa and entacapone. Both levodopa and entacapone are rapidly absorbed and eliminated. Carbidopa is absorbed and eliminated slightly slower compared with levodopa. When given separately without the two other active substances, the bioavailability for levodopa is 15-33%, for carbidopa 40-70% and for entacapone 35% after a 200 mg oral dose. Meals rich in large neutral amino acids may delay and reduce the absorption of levodopa. Food does not significantly affect the absorption of entacapone. The distribution volume of both levodopa (Vd 0.36-1.6 l/kg) and entacapone (Vd_{ss} 0.27 l/kg) is moderately small while no data for carbidopa are available.

Levodopa is bound to plasma protein only to a minor extent of about 10-30% and carbidopa is bound approximately 36%, while entacapone is extensively bound to plasma proteins (about 98%) –mainly to serum albumin. At therapeutic concentrations, entacapone does not displace other extensively bound active substances (e.g. warfarin, salicylic acid, phenylbutazone, or diazepam), nor is it displaced to any significant extent by any of these substances at therapeutic or higher concentrations.

Metabolism and Elimination: Levodopa is extensively metabolised to various metabolites: decarboxylation by dopa decarboxylase (DDC) and O-methylation by catechol-O-methyltransferase (COMT) being the most important pathways.

Carbidopa is metabolized to two main metabolites which are excreted in the urine as glucuronides and unconjugated compounds. Unchanged carbidopa accounts for 30% of the total urinary excretion.

Entacapone is almost completely metabolized prior to excretion via urine (10 to 20%) and bile/faeces (80 to 90%). The main metabolic pathway is glucuronidation of entacapone and its active metabolite, the cis-isomer, which accounts for about 5% of plasma total amount.

Total clearance for levodopa is in the range of 0.55-1.38 l/kg/h and for entacapone is in the range of 0.70 l/kg/h. The elimination-half life is ($t_{1/2}$) is 0.6-1.3 hours for levodopa, 2-3 hours for carbidopa and 0.4-0.7 hours for entacapone, each given separately.

Due to short elimination half-lives, no true accumulation of levodopa or entacapone occurs on repeated administration.

Data from *in vitro* studies using human liver microsomal preparations indicate that entacapone inhibits cytochrome P450 2C9 (IC50 ~ 4 µM). Entacapone showed little or no inhibition of other types of P450 isoenzymes (CYP1A2, CYP2A6, CYP2D6, CYP2E1, CYP3A and CYP2C19); see section 4.5.

Characteristics in patients

Elderly: When given without carbidopa and entacapone, the absorption of levodopa is greater and elimination is slower in elderly than in young subjects. However, after combination of carbidopa with levodopa, the absorption of levodopa is similar between the elderly and the young, but the AUC is still 1.5 fold greater in the elderly due to decreased DDC activity and lower clearance by aging. There are no significant differences in the AUC of carbidopa or entacapone between younger (45–64 years) and elderly subjects (65–75 years).

Gender: Bioavailability of levodopa is significantly higher in women than in men. In the pharmacokinetic studies with Stalevo the bioavailability of levodopa is higher in women than in men, primarily due to the difference in body weight, while there is no gender difference with carbidopa and entacapone.

Hepatic impairment: The metabolism of entacapone is slowed in patients with mild to moderate hepatic impairment (Child-Pugh Class A and B) leading to an increased plasma concentration of entacapone both in the absorption and elimination phases (see sections 4.2 and 4.3). No particular studies on the pharmacokinetics of carbidopa and levodopa in patients with hepatic impairment are reported, however, it is advised that Stalevo should be administered cautiously to patients with mild or moderate hepatic impairment.

Renal impairment: Renal impairment does not affect the pharmacokinetics of entacapone. No particular studies are reported on the pharmacokinetics of levodopa and carbidopa in patients with renal impairment. However, a longer dosing interval of Stalevo may be considered for patients who are receiving dialysis therapy (see section 4.2).

5.3 Preclinical safety data

Preclinical data of levodopa, carbidopa and entacapone, tested alone or in combination, revealed no special hazard for humans based on conventional studies of safety pharmacology, repeated dose toxicity, genotoxicity, and carcinogenic potential. In repeated dose toxicity studies with entacapone, anaemia most likely due to iron chelating properties of entacapone was observed. Regarding reproduction toxicity of entacapone, decreased foetal weight and a slightly delayed bone development were noticed in rabbits treated at systemic exposure levels in the therapeutic range. Both levodopa and combinations of carbidopa and levodopa have caused visceral and skeletal malformations in rabbits.

6. PHARMACEUTICAL PARTICULARS

6.1 List of excipients

Tablet core:

Croscarmellose sodium

Magnesium stearate

Maize starch

Mannitol (E421)

Povidone (E1201)

Film-coating:

Glycerol (85 per cent) (E422)

Hypromellose

Magnesium stearate

Polysorbate 80

Red iron oxide (E172)

Sucrose

Titanium dioxide (E171)

Yellow iron oxide (E172)

6.2 Incompatibilities
Not applicable.

6.3 Shelf life
3 years.

6.4 Special precautions for storage
This medicinal product does not require any special storage conditions.

6.5 Nature and contents of container
HDPE bottle with a child resistant PP-closure.

Pack sizes:

10, 30, 100, 130, 175 and 250 tablets.

Not all pack sizes may be marketed.

6.6 Special precautions for disposal and other handling
Any unused product or waste material should be disposed of in accordance with local requirements.

7. MARKETING AUTHORISATION HOLDER
Orion Corporation

Orionintie 1

FI-02200 Espoo

Finland

8. MARKETING AUTHORISATION NUMBER(S)
EU/1/03/260/009-012

EU/1/03/260/015

EU/1/03/260/018

9. DATE OF FIRST AUTHORISATION/RENEWAL OF THE AUTHORISATION
Date of first authorisation: 17 October 2003

Date of last renewal: 15 September 2008

10. DATE OF REVISION OF THE TEXT
27 March 2009

Detailed information on this medicine is available on the European Medicine's Agency (EMEA) web site: http://www.emea.europa.eu

Stalevo 200/50/200mg

(Orion Pharma (UK) Limited)

1. NAME OF THE MEDICINAL PRODUCT
Stalevo 200 mg/50 mg/200 mg film-coated tablets

2. QUALITATIVE AND QUANTITATIVE COMPOSITION
Each tablet contains 200 mg of levodopa, 50 mg of carbidopa and 200 mg of entacapone.

Excipient: Each tablet contains 2.3 mg of sucrose.

For a full list of excipients, see section 6.1.

3. PHARMACEUTICAL FORM
Film-coated tablet

Dark brownish red, oval, unscored film-coated tablets marked with 'LCE 200' on one side.

4. CLINICAL PARTICULARS

4.1 Therapeutic indications
Stalevo is indicated for the treatment of adult patients with Parkinson's disease and end-of-dose motor fluctuations not stabilised on levodopa/dopa decarboxylase (DDC) inhibitor treatment.

4.2 Posology and method of administration
Each tablet is to be taken orally either with or without food (see section 5.2). One tablet contains one treatment dose and the tablet may only be administered as whole tablets.

The optimum daily dose must be determined by careful titration of levodopa in each patient. The daily dose should be preferably optimised using one of the six available tablet strengths (50 mg/12.5 mg/200 mg, 75 mg/18.75 mg/200 mg, 100 mg/25 mg/200 mg, 125 mg/31.25 mg/200 mg, 150 mg/37.5 mg/200 mg or 200 mg/50 mg/200 mg levodopa/carbidopa/entacapone).

Patients should be instructed to take only one Stalevo tablet per dose administration. Patients receiving less than 70-100 mg carbidopa a day are more likely to experience nausea and vomiting. While the experience with total daily dose greater than 200 mg carbidopa is limited, the maximum recommended daily dose of entacapone is 2,000 mg and therefore the maximum dose is 10 tablets per day for the Stalevo strengths of 50 mg/12.5 mg/200 mg, 75 mg/18.75 mg/200 mg, 100 mg/25 mg/200 mg, 125 mg/31.25 mg/200 mg and 150 mg/37.5 mg/200 mg. Ten tablets of Stalevo 150 mg/37.5 mg/200 mg equals 375 mg of carbidopa a day. According to this daily carbidopa dose, the maximum recommended daily Stalevo 200 mg/50 mg/200 mg dose is 7 tablets per day.

Usually Stalevo is to be used in patients who are currently treated with corresponding doses of standard release levodopa/DDC inhibitor and entacapone.

How to transfer patients taking levodopa/DDC inhibitor (carbidopa or benserazide) preparations and entacapone tablets to Stalevo

a. Patients who are currently treated with entacapone and with standard release levodopa/carbidopa in doses equal to Stalevo tablet strengths can be directly transferred to corresponding Stalevo tablets.

For example, a patient taking one tablet of 200 mg/50 mg of levodopa/carbidopa with one tablet of entacapone 200 mg four times daily can take one 200 mg/50 mg/200 mg Stalevo tablet four times daily in place of their usual levodopa/carbidopa and entacapone doses.

b. When initiating Stalevo therapy for patients currently treated with entacapone and levodopa/carbidopa in doses not equal to Stalevo 200 mg/50 mg/200 mg, (or 50 mg/12.5 mg/200 mg or 75 mg/18.75 mg/200 mg or 100 mg/25 mg200 mg 125 mg/31.25 mg/200 mg or 150 mg/37.5 mg/200 mg) tablets, Stalevo dosing should be carefully titrated for optimal clinical response. At the initiation, Stalevo should be adjusted to correspond as closely as possible to the total daily dose of levodopa currently used.

c. When initiating Stalevo in patients currently treated with entacapone and levodopa/benserazide in a standard release formulation, discontinue dosing of levodopa/benserazide the previous night, and start Stalevo the next morning. Begin with a dose of Stalevo that will provide either the same amount of levodopa or slightly (5-10%) more.

How to transfer patients not currently treated with entacapone to Stalevo

Initiation of Stalevo may be considered at corresponding doses to current treatment in some patients with Parkinson's disease and end-of-dose motor fluctuations, who are not stabilised on their current standard release levodopa/DDC inhibitor treatment. However, a direct switch from levodopa/DDC inhibitor to Stalevo is not recommended for patients who have dyskinesias or whose daily levodopa dose is above 800 mg. In such patients it is advisable to introduce entacapone treatment as a separate treatment (entacapone tablets) and adjust the levodopa dose if necessary, before switching to Stalevo.

Entacapone enhances the effects of levodopa. It may therefore be necessary, particularly in patients with dyskinesia, to reduce levodopa dose by 10-30% within the first days to first weeks after initiating Stalevo treatment. The daily dose of levodopa can be reduced by extending the dosing intervals and/or by reducing the amount of levodopa per dose, according to the clinical condition of the patient.

Dose adjustment during the course of the treatment

When more levodopa is required, an increase in the frequency of doses and/or the use of an alternative strength of Stalevo should be considered, within the dose recommendations.

When less levodopa is required, the total daily dose of Stalevo should be reduced either by decreasing the frequency of administration by extending the time between doses, or by decreasing the strength of Stalevo at an administration.

If other levodopa products are used concomitantly with a Stalevo tablet, the maximum dose recommendations should be followed.

Discontinuation of Stalevo therapy: If Stalevo treatment (levodopa/carbidopa/entacapone) is discontinued and the patient is transferred to levodopa/DDC inhibitor therapy without entacapone, it is necessary to adjust the dosing of other antiparkinsonian treatments, especially levodopa, to achieve a sufficient level of control of the parkinsonian symptoms.

Children and adolescents: Stalevo is not recommended for use in children below 18 years due to a lack of data on safety and efficacy.

Elderly: No dose adjustment of Stalevo is required for elderly patients.

Hepatic impairment: It is advised that Stalevo should be administered cautiously to patients with mild to moderate hepatic impairment. Dose reduction may be needed (see section 5.2). For severe hepatic impairment see section 4.3.

Renal impairment: Renal impairment does not affect the pharmacokinetics of entacapone. No particular studies are reported on the pharmacokinetics of levodopa and carbidopa in patients with renal insufficiency, therefore Stalevo therapy should be administered cautiously to patients in severe renal impairment including those receiving dialysis therapy (see section 5.2).

4.3 Contraindications
- Hypersensitivity to the active substances or to any of the excipients.
- Severe hepatic impairment.
- Narrow-angle glaucoma.
- Pheochromocytoma.
- Concomitant use of Stalevo with non-selective monoamine oxidase (MAO-A and MAO-B) inhibitors (e.g. phenelzine, tranylcypromine).
- Concomitant use of a selective MAO-A inhibitor and a selective MAO-B inhibitor (see section 4.5).
- A previous history of Neuroleptic Malignant Syndrome (NMS) and/or non-traumatic rhabdomyolysis.

4.4 Special warnings and precautions for use
- Stalevo is not recommended for the treatment of drug-induced extrapyramidal reactions
- Stalevo therapy should be administered cautiously to patients with severe cardiovascular or pulmonary disease, bronchial asthma, renal or endocrine disease, history of peptic ulcer disease or history of convulsions.
- In patients with a history of myocardial infarction who have residual atrial nodal or ventricular arrhythmias; cardiac function should be monitored with particular care during the period of initial dose adjustments.
- All patients treated with Stalevo should be monitored carefully for the development of mental changes, depression with suicidal tendencies, and other serious antisocial behaviour. Patients with past or current psychosis should be treated with caution.
- Concomitant administration of antipsychotics with dopamine receptor-blocking properties, particularly D_2 receptor antagonists should be carried out with caution, and the patient carefully observed for loss of antiparkinsonian effect or worsening of parkinsonian symptoms.
- Patients with chronic wide-angle glaucoma may be treated with Stalevo with caution, provided the intra-ocular pressure is well controlled and the patient is monitored carefully for changes in intra-ocular pressure.
- Stalevo may induce orthostatic hypotension. Therefore Stalevo should be given cautiously to patients who are taking other medicinal products which may cause orthostatic hypotension.
- Entacapone in association with levodopa has been associated with somnolence and episodes of sudden sleep onset in patients with Parkinson's disease and caution should therefore be exercised when driving or operating machines (see section 4.7).
- In clinical studies, dopaminergic adverse reactions, e.g. dyskinesia, were more common in patients who received entacapone and dopamine agonists (such as bromocriptine), selegiline or amantadine compared to those who received placebo with this combination. The doses of other antiparkinsonian medicinal products may need to be adjusted when Stalevo treatment is substituted for a patient currently not treated with entacapone.
- Rhabdomyolysis secondary to severe dyskinesias or neuroleptic malignant syndrome (NMS) has been observed rarely in patients with Parkinson's disease. Therefore, any abrupt dose reduction or withdrawal of levodopa should be carefully observed, particularly in patients who are also receiving neuroleptics. NMS, including rhabdomyolysis and hyperthermia, is characterised by motor symptoms (rigidity, myoclonus, tremor), mental status changes (e.g., agitation, confusion, coma), hyperthermia, autonomic dysfunction (tachycardia, labile blood pressure) and elevated serum creatine phosphokinase. In individual cases, only some of these symptoms and/or findings may be evident. The early diagnosis is important for the appropriate management of NMS. A syndrome resembling the neuroleptic malignant syndrome including muscular rigidity, elevated body temperature, mental changes and increased serum creatine phosphokinase has been reported with the abrupt withdrawal of antiparkinsonian agents. Neither NMS nor rhabdomyolysis have been reported in association with entacapone treatment from controlled trials in which entacapone was discontinued abruptly. Since the introduction of entacapone into the market, isolated cases of NMS have been reported, especially following abrupt reduction or discontinuation of entacapone and other concomitant dopaminergic medicinal products. When considered necessary, the replacement of Stalevo with levodopa and DDC inhibitor without entacapone or other dopaminergic treatment should proceed slowly and an increase in levodopa dose may be necessary.
- If general anaesthesia is required, therapy with Stalevo may be continued for as long as the patient is permitted to take fluids and medicinal products by mouth. If therapy has to be stopped temporarily, Stalevo may be restarted as soon as oral medicinal products can be taken at the same daily dose as before.
- Periodic evaluation of hepatic, haematopoietic, cardiovascular and renal function is recommended during extended therapy with Stalevo.
- For patients experiencing diarrhoea, a follow-up of weight is recommended in order to avoid potential excessive weight decrease.
- Pathological gambling, increased libido and hypersexuality have been reported in Parkinson's disease patients treated with dopamine agonists and other dopaminergic treatments such as Stalevo.
- For patients who experience progressive anorexia, asthenia and weight decrease within a relatively short period of time, a general medical evaluation including liver function should be considered.

- Stalevo contains sucrose, and therefore patients with rare hereditary problems of fructose intolerance, glucose-galactose malabsorption or sucrase-isomaltase insufficiency should not take this medicine.

4.5 Interaction with other medicinal products and other forms of interaction

Other antiparkinsonian medicinal products: To date there has been no indication of interactions that would preclude concurrent use of standard antiparkinsonian medicinal products with Stalevo therapy. Entacapone in high doses may affect the absorption of carbidopa. However, no interaction with carbidopa has been observed with the recommended treatment schedule (200 mg of entacapone up to 10 times daily). Interactions between entacapone and selegiline have been investigated in repeated dose studies in Parkinson's disease patients treated with levodopa/DDC inhibitor and no interaction was observed. When used with Stalevo, the daily dose of selegiline should not exceed 10 mg.

Caution should be exercised when the following active substances are administered concomitantly with levodopa therapy.

Antihypertensives: Symptomatic postural hypotension may occur when levodopa is added to the treatment of patients already receiving antihypertensives. Dose adjustment of the antihypertensive agent may be required.

Antidepressants: Rarely, reactions including hypertension and dyskinesia have been reported with the concomitant use of tricyclic antidepressants and levodopa/carbidopa. Interactions between entacapone and imipramine and between entacapone and moclobemide have been investigated in single dose studies in healthy volunteers. No pharmacodynamic interactions were observed. A significant number of Parkinson's disease patients have been treated with the combination of levodopa, carbidopa and entacapone with several active substances including MAO-A inhibitors, tricyclic antidepressants, noradrenaline reuptake inhibitors such as desipramine, maprotiline and venlafaxine and medicinal products that are metabolised by COMT (e.g. catechol-structured compounds, paroxetine). No pharmacodynamic interactions have been observed. However, caution should be exercised when these medicinal products are used concomitantly with Stalevo (see sections 4.3 and 4.4).

Other active substances: Dopamine receptor antagonists (e.g. some antipsychotics and antiemetics), phenytoin and papaverine may reduce the therapeutic effect of levodopa. Patients taking these medicinal products with Stalevo should be carefully observed for loss of therapeutic response.

Due to entacapone's affinity to cytochrome P450 2C9 *in vitro* (see section 5.2), Stalevo may potentially interfere with active substances whose metabolism is dependent on this isoenzyme, such as S-warfarin. However, in an interaction study with healthy volunteers, entacapone did not change the plasma levels of S-warfarin, while the AUC for R-warfarin increased on average by 18% [CI_{90} 11-26%]. The INR values increased on average by 13% [CI_{90} 6-19%]. Thus, a control of INR is recommended when Stalevo is initiated for patients receiving warfarin.

Other forms of interactions: Since levodopa competes with certain amino acids, the absorption of Stalevo may be impaired in some patients on high protein diet.

Levodopa and entacapone may form chelates with iron in the gastrointestinal tract. Therefore, Stalevo and iron preparations should be taken at least 2-3 hours apart (see section 4.8).

In vitro data: Entacapone binds to human albumin binding site II which also binds several other medicinal products, including diazepam and ibuprofen. According to *in vitro* studies, significant displacement is not anticipated at therapeutic concentrations of the medicinal products. Accordingly, to date there has been no indication of such interactions.

4.6 Pregnancy and lactation

There are no adequate data from the use of the combination of levodopa/carbidopa/entacapone in pregnant women. Studies in animals have shown reproductive toxicity of the separate compounds (see section 5.3). The potential risk for humans is unknown. Stalevo should not be used during pregnancy unless the benefits for the mother outweigh the possible risks to the foetus.

Levodopa is excreted in human breast milk. There is evidence that lactation is suppressed during treatment with levodopa. Carbidopa and entacapone were excreted in milk in animals but is not known whether they are excreted in human breast milk. The safety of levodopa, carbidopa or entacapone in the infant is not known. Women should not breast-feed during treatment with Stalevo.

4.7 Effects on ability to drive and use machines

Stalevo may have major influence on the ability to drive and use machines. Levodopa, carbidopa and entacapone together may cause dizziness and symptomatic orthostatism. Therefore, caution should be exercised when driving or using machines.

Patients being treated with Stalevo and presenting with somnolence and/or sudden sleep onset episodes must be instructed to refrain from driving or engaging in activities where impaired alertness may put themselves or others at risk of serious injury or death (e.g. operating machines) until such recurrent episodes have resolved (see section 4.4).

4.8 Undesirable effects

The following section describes the undesirable effects reported for levodopa/carbidopa and for entacapone used in combination with levodopa/DDC inhibitor.

Levodopa /carbidopa

Adverse reactions that occur frequently with levodopa/carbidopa are those due to central neuropharmacological activity of dopamine. These reactions can usually be diminished by levodopa dose reduction. The most common adverse reactions are dyskinesias including choreiform, dystonic and other involuntary movements. Muscle twitching and blepharospasm may be taken as early signs to consider levodopa dose reduction. Nausea, also related to enhanced central dopaminergic activity, is a common adverse reaction of levodopa/carbidopa.

Other adverse reactions associated with levodopa/carbidopa therapy are mental changes, including paranoid ideation and psychotic episodes; depression with or without development of suicidal tendencies; and cognitive dysfunction. Adding of entacapone to levodopa/DDC inhibitor therapy (carbidopa or benserazide), i.e. initiation of Stalevo treatment in an entacapone naive patient, may aggravate some of these mental changes.

Less frequent adverse reactions of levodopa/carbidopa therapy are irregular heart rhythm and/or palpitations, orthostatic hypotensive episodes, bradykinetic episodes (the 'on-off' phenomenon), anorexia, vomiting, dizziness, and somnolence.

Gastrointestinal bleeding, development of duodenal ulcer, hypertension, phlebitis, leucopenia, haemolytic and non-haemolytic anaemia, thrombocytopenia, agranulocytosis, chest pain, dyspnoea and paraesthesia have occurred rarely with levodopa/carbidopa.

Convulsions have occurred rarely with levodopa/carbidopa; however a causal relationship to levodopa/carbidopa therapy has not been established.

Parkinson's disease patients treated with dopamine agonists and other dopaminergic treatments such as Stalevo, especially at high doses, have been reported as exhibiting signs of pathological gambling, increased libido and hypersexuality, generally reversible upon reduction of the dose or treatment discontinuation.

Other adverse reactions that have been reported with levodopa and may, therefore, be potential adverse reactions of Stalevo as well, include:

Nervous system disorders: Ataxia, numbness, increased hand tremor, muscle twitching, muscle cramp, trismus, activation of latent Horner's syndrome. Also falling and gait abnormalities are potential undesirable effects.

Eye disorders: Diplopia, blurred vision, dilated pupils, oculogyric crises.

Gastrointestinal disorders: Dry mouth, bitter taste, sialorrhoea, dysphagia, bruxism, hiccups, abdominal pain and distress, constipation, diarrhoea, flatulence, burning sensation of the tongue.

Renal and urinary disorders: Urinary retention, urinary incontinence, dark urine, priapism.

Skin and subcutaneous tissue disorders: Flushing, increased sweating, dark sweat, rash, hair loss.

Metabolism and nutrition disorders: Weight gain or loss, oedema.

Psychiatric disorders: Confusion, insomnia, nightmares, hallucinations, delusions, agitation, anxiety, euphoria.

Miscellaneous: Weakness, faintness, fatigue, headache, hoarseness, malaise, hot flushes, sense of stimulation, bizarre breathing patterns, neuroleptic malignant syndrome, malignant melanoma.

Entacapone

The most frequent adverse reactions caused by entacapone relate to the increased dopaminergic activity and occur most commonly at the beginning of the treatment. Reduction of levodopa dose decreases the severity and frequency of the reactions. The other major class of adverse reactions are gastrointestinal symptoms, including nausea, vomiting, abdominal pain, constipations and diarrhoea. Urine may be discoloured reddish-brown by entacapone, but this is a harmless phenomenon.

The following adverse reactions, listed in Table 1, have been accumulated both from clinical studies with entacapone and since the introduction of entacapone into the market for the combination use of entacapone with levodopa/DDC inhibitor.

Table 1. Adverse reactions

Nervous system disorders

Very common: Dyskinesia, Parkinsonism aggravated.

Common: Dizziness, dystonia, hyperkinesia.

Gastrointestinal disorders

Very common: Nausea.

Common: Diarrhoea, abdominal pain, dry mouth, constipation, vomiting.

Very rare: Anorexia.

Not known: Colitis.

Renal and urinary disorders

Very common: Urine discolouration.

Skin and subcutaneous tissue disorders

Rare: Erythematous or maculopapular rash.

Very rare: Urticaria.

Not known: Skin, hair, beard and nail discolorations.

General disorders and administration site conditions

Common: Fatigue, sweating increased, fall.

Uncommon: Weight decrease.

Hepatobiliary disorders

Rare: Hepatic function tests abnormal.

Not known: Hepatitis with mainly cholestatic features (see section 4.4).

Psychiatric disorders

Common: Insomnia, hallucinations, confusion, nightmares, agitation.

*Adverse reactions are ranked under headings of frequency, the most frequent first, using the following convention: Very common (≥1/10); common (≥1/100 to <1/10); uncommon (≥1/1,000 to <1/100); rare (≥1/10,000 to <1/1,000), very rare (<1/10,000), not known (cannot be estimated from the available data, since no valid estimate can be derived from clinical trials or epidemiological studies).

Entacapone in association with levodopa has been associated with isolated cases of excessive daytime somnolence and sudden sleep onset episodes.

Isolated cases of NMS have been reported following the abrupt reduction or discontinuation of entacapone and other dopaminergic treatments.

Isolated cases of rhabdomyolysis have been reported.

Isolated cases of angioedema have been reported after the initiation of Stalevo.

Laboratory tests:

The following laboratory abnormalities have been reported with levodopa/carbidopa treatment and should, therefore, be acknowledged when treating patients with Stalevo:

Commonly, levels of blood urea nitrogen, creatinine, and uric acid are lower during administration of levodopa/carbidopa than with levodopa alone. Transient abnormalities include elevated values of blood urea, AST (SGOT), ALT (SGPT), LDH, bilirubin, and alkaline phosphatase.

Decreased haemoglobin, haematocrit, elevated serum glucose and white blood cells, bacteria and blood in the urine have been reported.

Positive Coombs' tests have been reported, both for levodopa/carbidopa and for levodopa alone, but haemolytic anaemia is extremely rare.

Levodopa/carbidopa may cause false positive result when a dipstick is used to test for urinary ketone and this reaction is not altered by boiling the urine sample. The use of glucose oxidase methods may give false negative results for glycosuria.

4.9 Overdose

The post-marketing data includes isolated cases of overdose in which the reported highest daily doses of levodopa and entacapone have been at least 10,000 mg and 40,000 mg, respectively. The acute symptoms and signs in these cases of overdose included agitation, confusional state, coma, bradycardia, ventricular tachycardia, Cheyne-Stokes respiration, discolourations of skin, tongue and conjunctiva, and chromaturia. Management of acute overdose with Stalevo therapy is similar to acute overdose with levodopa. Pyridoxine, however, is not effective in reversing the actions of Stalevo. Hospitalisation is advised and general supportive measures should be employed with immediate gastric lavage and repeated doses of charcoal over time. This may hasten the elimination of entacapone in particular by decreasing its absorption/reabsorption from the GI tract. The adequacy of the respiratory, circulatory and renal systems should be carefully monitored and appropriate supportive measures employed. ECG monitoring should be started and the patient carefully monitored for the possible development of arrhythmias. If required, appropriate anti-arrhythmic therapy should be given. The possibility that the patient has taken other active substances in addition to Stalevo should be taken into consideration. The value of dialysis in the treatment of overdose is not known.

5. PHARMACOLOGICAL PROPERTIES

5.1 Pharmacodynamic properties

Pharmacotherapeutic group: dopa and dopa derivatives, ATC code: N04BA03

According to the current understanding, the symptoms of Parkinson's disease are related to depletion of dopamine in the corpus striatum. Dopamine does not cross the blood-brain barrier. Levodopa, the precursor of dopamine, crosses the blood brain barrier and relieves the symptoms of the disease. As levodopa is extensively metabolised in the periphery, only a small portion of a given dose reaches the central nervous system when levodopa is administered without metabolic enzyme inhibitors.

Carbidopa and benserazide are peripheral DDC inhibitors which reduce the peripheral metabolism of levodopa to dopamine, and thus, more levodopa is available to the brain. When decarboxylation of levodopa is reduced with the co-administration of a DDC inhibitor, a lower dose of levodopa can be used and the incidence of undesirable effects such as nausea is reduced.

With inhibition of the decarboxylase by a DDC inhibitor, catechol-*O*-methyltransferase (COMT) becomes the major peripheral metabolic pathway catalyzing the conversion of levodopa to 3-O-methyldopa (3-OMD), a potentially harmful metabolite of levodopa. Entacapone is a reversible, specific and mainly peripherally acting COMT inhibitor designed for concomitant administration with levodopa. Entacapone slows the clearance of levodopa from the bloodstream resulting in an increased area under the curve (AUC) in the pharmacokinetic profile of levodopa. Consequently the clinical response to each dose of levodopa is enhanced and prolonged.

The evidence of the therapeutic effects of Stalevo is based on two phase III double-blind studies, in which 376 Parkinson's disease patients with end-of-dose motor fluctuations received either entacapone or placebo with each levodopa/DDC inhibitor dose. Daily ON time with and without entacapone was recorded in home-diaries by patients. In the first study, entacapone increased the mean daily ON time by 1 h 20 min ($CI_{95\%}$ 45 min, 1 h 56 min) from baseline. This corresponded to an 8.3% increase in the proportion of daily ON time. Correspondingly, the decrease in daily OFF time was 24% in the entacapone group and 0% in the placebo group. In the second study, the mean proportion of daily ON time increased by 4.5% ($CI_{95\%}$ 0.93%, 7.97%) from baseline. This is translated to a mean increase of 35 min in the daily ON time. Correspondingly, the daily OFF time decreased by 18% on entacapone and by 5% on placebo. Because the effects of Stalevo tablets are equivalent with entacapone 200 mg tablet administered concomitantly with the commercially available standard release carbidopa/levodopa preparations in corresponding doses these results are applicable to describe the effects of Stalevo as well.

5.2 Pharmacokinetic properties

General characteristics of the active substances

Absorption/Distribution: There are substantial inter- and intra-individual variations in the absorption of levodopa, carbidopa and entacapone. Both levodopa and entacapone are rapidly absorbed and eliminated. Carbidopa is absorbed and eliminated slightly slower compared with levodopa. When given separately without the two other active substances, the bioavailability for levodopa is 15-33%, for carbidopa 40-70% and for entacapone 35% after a 200 mg oral dose. Meals rich in large neutral amino acids may delay and reduce the absorption of levodopa. Food does not significantly affect the absorption of entacapone. The distribution volume of both levodopa (Vd 0.36-1.6 l/kg) and entacapone (Vd_{ss} 0.27 l/kg) is moderately small while no data for carbidopa are available.

Levodopa is bound to plasma protein only to a minor extent of about 10-30% and carbidopa is bound approximately 36%, while entacapone is extensively bound to plasma proteins (about 98%) –mainly to serum albumin. At therapeutic concentrations, entacapone does not displace other extensively bound active substances (e.g. warfarin, salicylic acid, phenylbutazone, or diazepam), nor is it displaced to any significant extent by any of these substances at therapeutic or higher concentrations.

Metabolism and Elimination: Levodopa is extensively metabolised to various metabolites: decarboxylation by dopa decarboxylase (DDC) and O-methylation by catechol-O-methyltransferase (COMT) being the most important pathways.

Carbidopa is metabolized to two main metabolites which are excreted in the urine as glucuronides and unconjugated compounds. Unchanged carbidopa accounts for 30% of the total urinary excretion.

Entacapone is almost completely metabolized prior to excretion via urine (10 to 20%) and bile/faeces (80 to 90%). The main metabolic pathway is glucuronidation of entacapone and its active metabolite, the cis-isomer, which accounts for about 5% of plasma total amount.

Total clearance for levodopa is in the range of 0.55-1.38 l/kg/h and for entacapone is in the range of 0.70 l/kg/h. The elimination-half life is ($t_{1/2}$) is 0.6-1.3 hours for levodopa, 2-3 hours for carbidopa and 0.4-0.7 hours for entacapone, each given separately.

Due to short elimination half-lives, no true accumulation of levodopa or entacapone occurs on repeated administration.

Data from *in vitro* studies using human liver microsomal preparations indicate that entacapone inhibits cytochrome P450 2C9 (IC50 ~ 4 μM). Entacapone showed little or no inhibition of other types of P450 isoenzymes (CYP1A2, CYP2A6, CYP2D6, CYP2E1, CYP3A and CYP2C19); see section 4.5.

Characteristics in patients

Elderly: When given without carbidopa and entacapone, the absorption of levodopa is greater and elimination is slower in elderly than in young subjects. However, after combination of carbidopa with levodopa, the absorption of levodopa is similar between the elderly and the young, but the AUC is still 1.5 fold greater in the elderly due to decreased DDC activity and lower clearance by aging. There are no significant differences in the AUC of carbidopa or entacapone between younger (45–64 years) and elderly subjects (65–75 years).

Gender: Bioavailability of levodopa is significantly higher in women than in men. In the pharmacokinetic studies with Stalevo the bioavailability of levodopa is higher in women than in men, primarily due to the difference in body weight, while there is no gender difference with carbidopa and entacapone.

Hepatic impairment: The metabolism of entacapone is slowed in patients with mild to moderate hepatic impairment (Child-Pugh Class A and B) leading to an increased plasma concentration of entacapone both in the absorption and elimination phases (see sections 4.2 and 4.3). No particular studies on the pharmacokinetics of carbidopa and levodopa in patients with hepatic impairment are reported, however, it is advised that Stalevo should be administered cautiously to patients with mild or moderate hepatic impairment.

Renal impairment: Renal impairment does not affect the pharmacokinetics of entacapone. No particular studies are reported on the pharmacokinetics of levodopa and carbidopa in patients with renal impairment. However, a longer dosing interval of Stalevo may be considered for patients who are receiving dialysis therapy (see section 4.2).

5.3 Preclinical safety data

Preclinical data of levodopa, carbidopa and entacapone, tested alone or in combination, revealed no special hazard for humans based on conventional studies of safety pharmacology, repeated dose toxicity, genotoxicity, and carcinogenic potential. In repeated dose toxicity studies with entacapone, anaemia most likely due to iron chelating properties of entacapone was observed. Regarding reproduction toxicity of entacapone, decreased foetal weight and a slightly delayed bone development were noticed in rabbits treated at systemic exposure levels in the therapeutic range. Both levodopa and combinations of carbidopa and levodopa have caused visceral and skeletal malformations in rabbits.

6. PHARMACEUTICAL PARTICULARS

6.1 List of excipients

Tablet core:

Croscarmellose sodium

Magnesium stearate

Maize starch

Mannitol (E421)

Povidone (E1201)

Film-coating:

Glycerol (85 per cent) (E422)

Hypromellose

Magnesium stearate

Polysorbate 80

Red iron oxide (E172)

Sucrose

Titanium dioxide (E171)

6.2 Incompatibilities

Not applicable.

6.3 Shelf life

3 years.

6.4 Special precautions for storage

This medicinal product does not require any special storage conditions.

6.5 Nature and contents of container

HDPE bottle with a child resistant PP-closure.

Pack sizes:

10, 30, 100, 130, and 175 tablets.

Not all pack sizes may be marketed.

6.6 Special precautions for disposal and other handling

Any unused product or waste material should be disposed of in accordance with local requirements.

7. MARKETING AUTHORISATION HOLDER

Orion Corporation

Orionintie 1

FI-02200 Espoo

Finland

8. MARKETING AUTHORISATION NUMBER(S)

EU/1/03/260/019-023

9. DATE OF FIRST AUTHORISATION/RENEWAL OF THE AUTHORISATION

Date of first authorisation: 17 October 2003

Date of last renewal: 15 September 2008

10. DATE OF REVISION OF THE TEXT

27 March 2009

Detailed information on this medicine is available on the European Medicine's Agency (EMEA) web site: http://www.emea.europa.eu

Stalevo 50/12.5/200mg

(Orion Pharma (UK) Limited)

1. NAME OF THE MEDICINAL PRODUCT

Stalevo 50 mg/12.5 mg/200 mg film-coated tablets

2. QUALITATIVE AND QUANTITATIVE COMPOSITION

Each tablet contains 50 mg of levodopa, 12.5 mg of carbidopa and 200 mg of entacapone.

Excipient: Each tablet contains 1.2 mg of sucrose.

For a full list of excipients, see section 6.1.

3. PHARMACEUTICAL FORM

Film-coated tablet

Brownish or greyish red, round, convex, unscored film-coated tablets marked with 'LCE 50' on one side.

4. CLINICAL PARTICULARS

4.1 Therapeutic indications

Stalevo is indicated for the treatment of adult patients with Parkinson's disease and end-of-dose motor fluctuations not stabilised on levodopa/dopa decarboxylase (DDC) inhibitor treatment.

4.2 Posology and method of administration

Each tablet is to be taken orally either with or without food (see section 5.2). One tablet contains one treatment dose and the tablet may only be administered as whole tablets.

The optimum daily dose must be determined by careful titration of levodopa in each patient. The daily dose should be preferably optimised using one of the six available tablet strengths (50 mg/12.5 mg/200 mg, 75 mg/18.75 mg/200 mg 100 mg/25 mg/200 mg, 125 mg/31.25 mg/200 mg 150 mg/37.5 mg/200 mg or 200 mg/50 mg/200 mg levodopa/carbidopa/entacapone).

Patients should be instructed to take only one Stalevo tablet per dose administration. Patients receiving less than 70-100 mg carbidopa a day are more likely to experience nausea and vomiting. While the experience with total daily dose greater than 200 mg carbidopa is limited, the maximum recommended daily dose of entacapone is 2,000 mg and therefore the maximum dose is 10 tablets per day for the Stalevo strengths of 50 mg/12.5 mg/200 mg, 75 mg/18.75 mg/200 mg 100 mg/25 mg/200 mg, 125 mg/31.25 mg/200 mg and 150 mg/37.5 mg/200 mg. Ten tablets of Stalevo 150 mg/37.5 mg/200 mg equals 375 mg of carbidopa a day. According to this daily carbidopa dose, the maximum recommended daily Stalevo 200 mg/50 mg/200 mg dose is 7 tablets per day.

Usually Stalevo is to be used in patients who are currently treated with corresponding doses of standard release levodopa/DDC inhibitor and entacapone.

How to transfer patients taking levodopa/DDC inhibitor (carbidopa or benserazide) preparations and entacapone tablets to Stalevo

a. Patients who are currently treated with entacapone and with standard release levodopa/carbidopa in doses equal to Stalevo tablet strengths can be directly transferred to corresponding Stalevo tablets.

For example, a patient taking one tablet of 50 mg/12.5 mg of levodopa/carbidopa with one tablet of entacapone 200 mg four times daily can take one 50 mg/12.5 mg/200 mg Stalevo tablet four times daily in place of their usual levodopa/carbidopa and entacapone doses.

b. When initiating Stalevo therapy for patients currently treated with entacapone and levodopa/carbidopa in doses not equal to Stalevo 50 mg/12.5 mg/200 mg, (or 75 mg/18.75 mg/200 mg or 100 mg/25 mg/200 mg or 125 mg/31.25 mg/200 mg or 150 mg/37.5 mg/200 mg or 200 mg/50 mg/200 mg) tablets, Stalevo dosing should be carefully titrated for optimal clinical response. At the initiation, Stalevo should be adjusted to correspond as closely as possible to the total daily dose of levodopa currently used.

c. When initiating Stalevo in patients currently treated with entacapone and levodopa/benserazide in a standard release formulation, discontinue dosing of levodopa/benserazide the previous night, and start Stalevo the next morning. Begin with a dose of Stalevo that will provide either the same amount of levodopa or slightly (5-10%) more.

How to transfer patients not currently treated with entacapone to Stalevo

Initiation of Stalevo may be considered at corresponding doses to current treatment in some patients with Parkinson's disease and end-of-dose motor fluctuations, who are not stabilised on their current standard release levodopa/DDC inhibitor treatment. However, a direct switch from levodopa/DDC inhibitor to Stalevo is not recommended for patients who have dyskinesias or whose daily levodopa dose is above 800 mg. In such patients it is advisable to introduce entacapone treatment as a separate treatment (entacapone tablets) and adjust the levodopa dose if necessary, before switching to Stalevo.

Entacapone enhances the effects of levodopa. It may therefore be necessary, particularly in patients with dyskinesia, to reduce levodopa dose by 10-30% within the first days to first weeks after initiating Stalevo treatment. The daily dose of levodopa can be reduced by extending the dosing intervals and/or by reducing the amount of levodopa per dose, according to the clinical condition of the patient.

Dose adjustment during the course of the treatment

When more levodopa is required, an increase in the frequency of doses and/or the use of an alternative strength of Stalevo should be considered, within the dose recommendations.

When less levodopa is required, the total daily dose of Stalevo should be reduced either by decreasing the frequency of administration by extending the time between doses, or by decreasing the strength of Stalevo at an administration.

If other levodopa products are used concomitantly with a Stalevo tablet, the maximum dose recommendations should be followed.

Discontinuation of Stalevo therapy: If Stalevo treatment (levodopa/carbidopa/entacapone) is discontinued and the patient is transferred to levodopa/DDC inhibitor therapy without entacapone, it is necessary to adjust the dosing of other antiparkinsonian treatments, especially levodopa, to achieve a sufficient level of control of the parkinsonian symptoms.

Children and adolescents: Stalevo is not recommended for use in children below 18 years due to a lack of data on safety and efficacy.

Elderly: No dose adjustment of Stalevo is required for elderly patients.

Hepatic impairment: It is advised that Stalevo should be administered cautiously to patients with mild to moderate hepatic impairment. Dose reduction may be needed (see section 5.2). For severe hepatic impairment see section 4.3.

Renal impairment: Renal impairment does not affect the pharmacokinetics of entacapone. No particular studies are reported on the pharmacokinetics of levodopa and carbidopa in patients with renal insufficiency, therefore Stalevo therapy should be administered cautiously to patients in severe renal impairment including those receiving dialysis therapy (see section 5.2).

4.3 Contraindications

- Hypersensitivity to the active substances or to any of the excipients.
- Severe hepatic impairment.
- Narrow-angle glaucoma.
- Pheochromocytoma.
- Concomitant use of Stalevo with non-selective monoamine oxidase (MAO-A and MAO-B) inhibitors (e.g. phenelzine, tranylcypromine).
- Concomitant use of a selective MAO-A inhibitor and a selective MAO-B inhibitor (see section 4.5).
- A previous history of Neuroleptic Malignant Syndrome (NMS) and/or non-traumatic rhabdomyolysis.

4.4 Special warnings and precautions for use

- Stalevo is not recommended for the treatment of drug-induced extrapyramidal reactions
- Stalevo therapy should be administered cautiously to patients with severe cardiovascular or pulmonary disease, bronchial asthma, renal or endocrine disease, history of peptic ulcer disease or history of convulsions.
- In patients with a history of myocardial infarction who have residual atrial nodal or ventricular arrhythmias; cardiac function should be monitored with particular care during the period of initial dose adjustments.
- All patients treated with Stalevo should be monitored carefully for the development of mental changes, depression with suicidal tendencies, and other serious antisocial behaviour. Patients with past or current psychosis should be treated with caution.
- Concomitant administration of antipsychotics with dopamine receptor-blocking properties, particularly D_2 receptor antagonists should be carried out with caution, and the patient carefully observed for loss of antiparkinsonian effect or worsening of parkinsonian symptoms.
- Patients with chronic wide-angle glaucoma may be treated with Stalevo with caution, provided the intra-ocular pressure is well controlled and the patient is monitored carefully for changes in intra-ocular pressure.
- Stalevo may induce orthostatic hypotension. Therefore Stalevo should be given cautiously to patients who are taking other medicinal products which may cause orthostatic hypotension.
- Entacapone in association with levodopa has been associated with somnolence and episodes of sudden sleep onset in patients with Parkinson's disease and caution should therefore be exercised when driving or operating machines (see section 4.7).
- In clinical studies, dopaminergic adverse reactions, e.g. dyskinesia, were more common in patients who received entacapone and dopamine agonists (such as bromocriptine), selegiline or amantadine compared to those who received placebo with this combination. The doses of other antiparkinsonian medicinal products may need to be adjusted when Stalevo treatment is substituted for a patient currently not treated with entacapone.
- Rhabdomyolysis secondary to severe dyskinesias or neuroleptic malignant syndrome (NMS) has been observed rarely in patients with Parkinson's disease. Therefore, any abrupt dose reduction or withdrawal of levodopa should be carefully observed, particularly in patients who are also receiving neuroleptics. NMS, including rhabdomyolysis and hyperthermia, is characterised by motor symptoms (rigidity, myoclonus, tremor), mental status changes (e.g., agitation, confusion, coma), hyperthermia, autonomic dysfunction (tachycardia, labile blood pressure) and elevated serum creatine phosphokinase. In individual cases, only some of these symptoms and/or findings may be evident. The early diagnosis is important for the appropriate management of NMS. A syndrome resembling the neuroleptic malignant syndrome including muscular rigidity, elevated body temperature, mental changes and increased serum creatine phosphokinase has been reported with the abrupt withdrawal of antiparkinsonian agents. Neither NMS nor rhabdomyolysis have been reported in association with entacapone treatment from controlled trials in which entacapone was discontinued abruptly. Since the introduction of entacapone into the market, isolated cases of NMS have been reported, especially following abrupt reduction or discontinuation of entacapone and other concomitant dopaminergic medicinal products. When considered necessary, the replacement of Stalevo with levodopa and DDC inhibitor without entacapone or other dopaminergic treatment should proceed slowly and an increase in levodopa dose may be necessary.
- If general anaesthesia is required, therapy with Stalevo may be continued for as long as the patient is permitted to take fluids and medicinal products by mouth. If therapy has to be stopped temporarily, Stalevo may be restarted as soon as oral medicinal products can be taken at the same daily dose as before.
- Periodic evaluation of hepatic, haematopoietic, cardiovascular and renal function is recommended during extended therapy with Stalevo.
- For patients experiencing diarrhoea, a follow-up of weight is recommended in order to avoid potential excessive weight decrease.
- Pathological gambling, increased libido and hypersexuality have been reported in Parkinson's disease patients treated with dopamine agonists and other dopaminergic treatments such as Stalevo.
- For patients who experience progressive anorexia, asthenia and weight decrease within a relatively short period of time, a general medical evaluation including liver function should be considered.
- Stalevo contains sucrose, and therefore patients with rare hereditary problems of fructose intolerance, glucose-galactose malabsorption or sucrase-isomaltase insufficiency should not take this medicine.

4.5 Interaction with other medicinal products and other forms of interaction

Other antiparkinsonian medicinal products: To date there has been no indication of interactions that would preclude concurrent use of standard antiparkinsonian medicinal products with Stalevo therapy. Entacapone in high doses may affect the absorption of carbidopa. However, no interaction with carbidopa has been observed with the recommended treatment schedule (200 mg of entacapone up to 10 times daily). Interactions between entacapone and selegiline have been investigated in repeated dose studies in Parkinson's disease patients treated with levodopa/DDC inhibitor and no interaction was observed. When used with Stalevo, the daily dose of selegiline should not exceed 10 mg.

Caution should be exercised when the following active substances are administered concomitantly with levodopa therapy.

Antihypertensives: Symptomatic postural hypotension may occur when levodopa is added to the treatment of patients already receiving antihypertensives. Dose adjustment of the antihypertensive agent may be required.

Antidepressants: Rarely, reactions including hypertension and dyskinesia have been reported with the concomitant use of tricyclic antidepressants and levodopa/carbidopa. Interactions between entacapone and imipramine and between entacapone and moclobemide have been investigated in single dose studies in healthy volunteers. No pharmacodynamic interactions were observed. A significant number of Parkinson's disease patients have been treated with the combination of levodopa, carbidopa and entacapone with several active substances including MAO-A inhibitors, tricyclic antidepressants, noradrenaline reuptake inhibitors such as desipramine, maprotiline and venlafaxine and medicinal products that are metabolised by COMT (e.g. catechol-structured compounds, paroxetine). No pharmacodynamic interactions have been observed. However, caution should be exercised when these medicinal products are used concomitantly with Stalevo (see sections 4.3 and 4.4).

Other active substances: Dopamine receptor antagonists (e.g. some antipsychotics and antiemetics), phenytoin and papaverine may reduce the therapeutic effect of levodopa. Patients taking these medicinal products with Stalevo should be carefully observed for loss of therapeutic response.

Due to entacapone's affinity to cytochrome P450 2C9 *in vitro* (see section 5.2), Stalevo may potentially interfere with active substances whose metabolism is dependent on this isoenzyme, such as S-warfarin. However, in an interaction study with healthy volunteers, entacapone did not change the plasma levels of S-warfarin, while the AUC for R-warfarin increased on average by 18% [CI_{90} 11-26%]. The INR values increased on average by 13% [CI_{90} 6-19%]. Thus, a control of INR is recommended when Stalevo is initiated for patients receiving warfarin.

Other forms of interactions: Since levodopa competes with certain amino acids, the absorption of Stalevo may be impaired in some patients on high protein diet.

Levodopa and entacapone may form chelates with iron in the gastrointestinal tract. Therefore, Stalevo and iron preparations should be taken at least 2-3 hours apart (see section 4.8).

In vitro data: Entacapone binds to human albumin binding site II which also binds several other medicinal products, including diazepam and ibuprofen. According to *in vitro* studies, significant displacement is not anticipated at therapeutic concentrations of the medicinal products. Accordingly, to date there has been no indication of such interactions.

4.6 Pregnancy and lactation

There are no adequate data from the use of the combination of levodopa/carbidopa/entacapone in pregnant women. Studies in animals have shown reproductive toxicity of the separate compounds (see section 5.3). The potential risk for humans is unknown. Stalevo should not be used during pregnancy unless the benefits for the mother outweigh the possible risks to the foetus.

Levodopa is excreted in human breast milk. There is evidence that lactation is suppressed during treatment with levodopa. Carbidopa and entacapone were excreted in milk in animals but is not known whether they are excreted in human breast milk. The safety of levodopa, carbidopa or entacapone in the infant is not known. Women should not breast-feed during treatment with Stalevo.

4.7 Effects on ability to drive and use machines

Stalevo may have major influence on the ability to drive and use machines. Levodopa, carbidopa and entacapone together may cause dizziness and symptomatic orthostatism. Therefore, caution should be exercised when driving or using machines.

Patients being treated with Stalevo and presenting with somnolence and/or sudden sleep onset episodes must be instructed to refrain from driving or engaging in activities where impaired alertness may put themselves or others at risk of serious injury or death (e.g. operating machines) until such recurrent episodes have resolved (see section 4.4).

4.8 Undesirable effects

The following section describes the undesirable effects reported for levodopa/carbidopa and for entacapone used in combination with levodopa/DDC inhibitor.

Levodopa /carbidopa

Adverse reactions that occur frequently with levodopa/carbidopa are those due to central neuropharmacological activity of dopamine. These reactions can usually be diminished by levodopa dose reduction. The most common adverse reactions are dyskinesias including choreiform, dystonic and other involuntary movements. Muscle twitching and blepharospasm may be taken as early signs to consider levodopa dose reduction. Nausea, also related to enhanced central dopaminergic activity, is a common adverse reaction of levodopa/carbidopa.

Other adverse reactions associated with levodopa/carbidopa therapy are mental changes, including paranoid ideation and psychotic episodes; depression with or without development of suicidal tendencies; and cognitive dysfunction. Adding of entacapone to levodopa/DDC inhibitor therapy (carbidopa or benserazide), i.e. initiation of Stalevo treatment in an entacapone naive patient, may aggravate some of these mental changes.

Less frequent adverse reactions of levodopa/carbidopa therapy are irregular heart rhythm and/or palpitations, orthostatic hypotensive episodes, bradykinetic episodes (the 'on-off' phenomenon), anorexia, vomiting, dizziness, and somnolence.

Gastrointestinal bleeding, development of duodenal ulcer, hypertension, phlebitis, leucopenia, haemolytic and non-haemolytic anaemia, thrombocytopenia, agranulocytosis, chest pain, dyspnoea and paraesthesia have occurred rarely with levodopa/carbidopa.

Convulsions have occurred rarely with levodopa/carbidopa; however a causal relationship to levodopa/carbidopa therapy has not been established.

Parkinson's disease patients treated with dopamine agonists and other dopaminergic treatments such as Stalevo, especially at high doses, have been reported as exhibiting signs of pathological gambling, increased libido and hypersexuality, generally reversible upon reduction of the dose or treatment discontinuation.

Other adverse reactions that have been reported with levodopa and may, therefore, be potential adverse reactions of Stalevo as well, include:

Nervous system disorders: Ataxia, numbness, increased hand tremor, muscle twitching, muscle cramp, trismus, activation of latent Horner's syndrome. Also falling and gait abnormalities are potential undesirable effects.

Eye disorders: Diplopia, blurred vision, dilated pupils, oculogyric crises.

Gastrointestinal disorders: Dry mouth, bitter taste, sialorrhoea, dysphagia, bruxism, hiccups, abdominal pain and distress, constipation, diarrhoea, flatulence, burning sensation of the tongue.

Renal and urinary disorders: Urinary retention, urinary incontinence, dark urine, priapism.

Skin and subcutaneous tissue disorders: Flushing, increased sweating, dark sweat, rash, hair loss.

Metabolism and nutrition disorders: Weight gain or loss, oedema.

Psychiatric disorders: Confusion, insomnia, nightmares, hallucinations, delusions, agitation, anxiety, euphoria.

Miscellaneous: Weakness, faintness, fatigue, headache, hoarseness, malaise, hot flushes, sense of stimulation, bizarre breathing patterns, neuroleptic malignant syndrome, malignant melanoma.

Entacapone

The most frequent adverse reactions caused by entacapone relate to the increased dopaminergic activity and occur most commonly at the beginning of the treatment. Reduction of levodopa dose decreases the severity and frequency of the reactions. The other major class of adverse reactions are gastrointestinal symptoms, including nausea, vomiting, abdominal pain, constipations and diarrhoea. Urine may be discoloured reddish-brown by entacapone, but this is a harmless phenomenon.

The following adverse reactions, listed in Table 1, have been accumulated both from clinical studies with entacapone and since the introduction of entacapone into the market for the combination use of entacapone with levodopa/DDC inhibitor.

Table 1. Adverse reactions

Nervous system disorders

Very common: Dyskinesia, Parkinsonism aggravated.

Common: Dizziness, dystonia, hyperkinesia.

Gastrointestinal disorders

Very common: Nausea.

Common: Diarrhoea, abdominal pain, dry mouth, constipation, vomiting.

Very rare: Anorexia.

Not known: Colitis.

Renal and urinary disorders

Very common: Urine discolouration.

Skin and subcutaneous tissue disorders

Rare: Erythematous or maculopapular rash.

Very rare: Urticaria.

Not known: Skin, hair, beard and nail discolorations.

General disorders and administration site conditions

Common: Fatigue, sweating increased, fall.

Uncommon: Weight decrease.

Hepatobiliary disorders

Rare: Hepatic function tests abnormal.

Not known: Hepatitis with mainly cholestatic features (see section 4.4).

Psychiatric disorders

Common: Insomnia, hallucinations, confusion, nightmares, agitation.

*Adverse reactions are ranked under headings of frequency, the most frequent first, using the following convention: Very common ($\geqslant$1/10); common (1$\geqslant$100 to $<$1/10); uncommon ($\geqslant$1/1,000 to $<$1/100); rare ($\geqslant$1/10,000 to $<$1/1,000), very rare ($<$1/10,000), not known (cannot be estimated from the available data, since no valid estimate can be derived from clinical trials or epidemiological studies).

Entacapone in association with levodopa has been associated with isolated cases of excessive daytime somnolence and sudden sleep onset episodes.

Isolated cases of NMS have been reported following the abrupt reduction or discontinuation of entacapone and other dopaminergic treatments.

Isolated cases of rhabdomyolysis have been reported.

Isolated cases of angioedema have been reported after the initiation of Stalevo.

Laboratory tests:

The following laboratory abnormalities have been reported with levodopa/carbidopa treatment and should, therefore, be acknowledged when treating patients with Stalevo:

Commonly, levels of blood urea nitrogen, creatinine, and uric acid are lower during administration of levodopa/carbidopa than with levodopa alone. Transient abnormalities include elevated values of blood urea, AST (SGOT), ALT (SGPT), LDH, bilirubin, and alkaline phosphatase.

Decreased haemoglobin, haematocrit, elevated serum glucose and white blood cells, bacteria and blood in the urine have been reported.

Positive Coombs' tests have been reported, both for levodopa/carbidopa and for levodopa alone, but haemolytic anaemia is extremely rare.

Levodopa/carbidopa may cause false positive result when a dipstick is used to test for urinary ketone and this reaction is not altered by boiling the urine sample. The use of glucose oxidase methods may give false negative results for glycosuria.

4.9 Overdose

The post-marketing data includes isolated cases of overdose in which the reported highest daily doses of levodopa and entacapone have been at least 10,000 mg and 40,000 mg, respectively. The acute symptoms and signs in these cases of overdose included agitation, confusional state, coma, bradycardia, ventricular tachycardia, Cheyne-Stokes respiration, discolourations of skin, tongue and conjunctiva, and chromaturia. Management of acute overdose with Stalevo therapy is similar to acute overdose with levodopa. Pyridoxine, however, is not effective in reversing the actions of Stalevo. Hospitalisation is advised and general supportive measures should be employed with immediate gastric lavage and repeated doses of charcoal over time. This may hasten the elimination of entacapone in particular by decreasing its absorption/reabsorption from the GI tract. The adequacy of the respiratory, circulatory and renal systems should be carefully monitored and appropriate supportive measures employed. ECG monitoring should be started and the patient carefully monitored for the possible development of arrhythmias. If required, appropriate anti-arrhythmic therapy should be given. The possibility that the patient has taken other active substances in addition to Stalevo should be taken into consideration. The value of dialysis in the treatment of overdose is not known.

5. PHARMACOLOGICAL PROPERTIES

5.1 Pharmacodynamic properties

Pharmacotherapeutic group: dopa and dopa derivatives, ATC code: N04BA03

According to the current understanding, the symptoms of Parkinson's disease are related to depletion of dopamine in the corpus striatum. Dopamine does not cross the blood-brain barrier. Levodopa, the precursor of dopamine, crosses the blood brain barrier and relieves the symptoms of the disease. As levodopa is extensively metabolised in the periphery, only a small portion of a given dose reaches the central nervous system when levodopa is administered without metabolic enzyme inhibitors.

Carbidopa and benserazide are peripheral DDC inhibitors which reduce the peripheral metabolism of levodopa to dopamine, and thus, more levodopa is available to the brain. When decarboxylation of levodopa is reduced with the co-administration of a DDC inhibitor, a lower dose of levodopa can be used and the incidence of undesirable effects such as nausea is reduced.

With inhibition of the decarboxylase by a DDC inhibitor, catechol-*O*-methyltransferase (COMT) becomes the major peripheral metabolic pathway catalyzing the conversion of levodopa to 3-O-methyldopa (3-OMD), a potentially harmful metabolite of levodopa. Entacapone is a reversible, specific and mainly peripherally acting COMT inhibitor designed for concomitant administration with levodopa. Entacapone slows the clearance of levodopa from the bloodstream resulting in an increased area under the curve (AUC) in the pharmacokinetic profile of levodopa. Consequently the clinical response to each dose of levodopa is enhanced and prolonged.

The evidence of the therapeutic effects of Stalevo is based on two phase III double-blind studies, in which 376 Parkinson's disease patients with end-of-dose motor fluctuations received either entacapone or placebo with each levodopa/DDC inhibitor dose. Daily ON time with and without entacapone was recorded in home-diaries by patients. In the first study, entacapone increased the mean daily ON time by 1 h 20 min ($CI_{95\%}$ 45 min, 1 h 56 min) from baseline. This corresponded to an 8.3% increase in the proportion of daily ON time. Correspondingly, the decrease in daily OFF time was 24% in the entacapone group and 0% in the placebo group. In the second study, the mean proportion of daily ON time increased by 4.5% ($CI_{95\%}$ 0.93%, 7.97%) from baseline. This is translated to a mean increase of 35 min in the daily ON time. Correspondingly, the daily OFF time decreased by 18% on entacapone and by 5% on placebo. Because the effects of Stalevo tablets are equivalent with entacapone 200 mg tablet administered concomitantly with the commercially available standard release carbidopa/levodopa preparations in corresponding doses these results are applicable to describe the effects of Stalevo as well.

5.2 Pharmacokinetic properties

General characteristics of the active substances

Absorption/Distribution: There are substantial inter- and intra-individual variations in the absorption of levodopa, carbidopa and entacapone. Both levodopa and entacapone are rapidly absorbed and eliminated. Carbidopa is absorbed and eliminated slightly slower compared with levodopa. When given separately without the two other active substances, the bioavailability for levodopa is 15-33%, for carbidopa 40-70% and for entacapone 35% after a 200 mg oral dose. Meals rich in large neutral amino acids may delay and reduce the absorption of levodopa. Food does not significantly affect the absorption of entacapone. The distribution volume of both levodopa (Vd 0.36-1.6 l/kg) and entacapone (Vd_{ss} 0.27 l/kg) is moderately small while no data for carbidopa are available.

Levodopa is bound to plasma protein only to a minor extent of about 10-30% and carbidopa is bound approximately 36%, while entacapone is extensively bound to plasma proteins (about 98%) –mainly to serum albumin. At therapeutic concentrations, entacapone does not displace other extensively bound active substances (e.g. warfarin, salicylic acid, phenylbutazone, or diazepam), nor is it displaced to any significant extent by any of these substances at therapeutic or higher concentrations.

Metabolism and Elimination: Levodopa is extensively metabolised to various metabolites: decarboxylation by dopa decarboxylase (DDC) and O-methylation by catechol-O-methyltransferase (COMT) being the most important pathways.

Carbidopa is metabolized to two main metabolites which are excreted in the urine as glucuronides and unconjugated compounds. Unchanged carbidopa accounts for 30% of the total urinary excretion.

Entacapone is almost completely metabolized prior to excretion via urine (10 to 20%) and bile/faeces (80 to 90%). The main metabolic pathway is glucuronidation of entacapone and its active metabolite, the cis-isomer, which accounts for about 5% of plasma total amount.

Total clearance for levodopa is in the range of 0.55-1.38 l/kg/h and for entacapone is in the range of 0.70 l/kg/h. The elimination-half life is ($t_{1/2}$) is 0.6-1.3 hours for levodopa, 2-3 hours for carbidopa and 0.4-0.7 hours for entacapone, each given separately.

Due to short elimination half-lives, no true accumulation of levodopa or entacapone occurs on repeated administration.

Data from *in vitro* studies using human liver microsomal preparations indicate that entacapone inhibits cytochrome P450 2C9 (IC50 ~ 4 μM). Entacapone showed little or no inhibition of other types of P450 isoenzymes (CYP1A2, CYP2A6, CYP2D6, CYP2E1, CYP3A and CYP2C19); see section 4.5.

Characteristics in patients

Elderly: When given without carbidopa and entacapone, the absorption of levodopa is greater and elimination is slower in elderly than in young subjects. However, after combination of carbidopa with levodopa, the absorption of levodopa is similar between the elderly and the young, but the AUC is still 1.5 fold greater in the elderly due to decreased DDC activity and lower clearance by aging. There are no significant differences in the AUC of carbidopa or entacapone between younger (45–64 years) and elderly subjects (65–75 years).

Gender: Bioavailability of levodopa is significantly higher in women than in men. In the pharmacokinetic studies with Stalevo the bioavailability of levodopa is higher in women than in men, primarily due to the difference in body weight, while there is no gender difference with carbidopa and entacapone.

Hepatic impairment: The metabolism of entacapone is slowed in patients with mild to moderate hepatic impairment (Child-Pugh Class A and B) leading to an increased plasma concentration of entacapone both in the absorption and elimination phases (see sections 4.2 and 4.3). No particular studies on the pharmacokinetics of carbidopa and levodopa in patients with hepatic impairment are reported, however, it is advised that Stalevo should be administered cautiously to patients with mild or moderate hepatic impairment.

Renal impairment: Renal impairment does not affect the pharmacokinetics of entacapone. No particular studies are reported on the pharmacokinetics of levodopa and carbidopa in patients with renal impairment. However, a longer dosing interval of Stalevo may be considered for patients who are receiving dialysis therapy (see section 4.2).

5.3 Preclinical safety data

Preclinical data of levodopa, carbidopa and entacapone, tested alone or in combination, revealed no special hazard for humans based on conventional studies of safety pharmacology, repeated dose toxicity, genotoxicity, and carcinogenic potential. In repeated dose toxicity studies with entacapone, anaemia most likely due to iron chelating properties of entacapone was observed. Regarding reproduction toxicity of entacapone, decreased foetal weight and a slightly delayed bone development were noticed in rabbits treated at systemic exposure levels in the therapeutic range. Both levodopa and combinations of carbidopa and levodopa have caused visceral and skeletal malformations in rabbits.

6. PHARMACEUTICAL PARTICULARS

6.1 List of excipients

Tablet core:

Croscarmellose sodium

Magnesium stearate

Maize starch

Mannitol (E421)

Povidone (E1201)

Film-coating:

Glycerol (85 per cent) (E422)

Hypromellose

Magnesium stearate

Polysorbate 80

Red iron oxide (E172)

Sucrose

Titanium dioxide (E171)

Yellow iron oxide (E172)

6.2 Incompatibilities

Not applicable.

6.3 Shelf life

3 years.

6.4 Special precautions for storage
This medicinal product does not require any special storage conditions.

6.5 Nature and contents of container
HDPE bottle with a child resistant PP-closure.

Pack sizes:

10, 30, 100, 130, 175 and 250 tablets.

Not all pack sizes may be marketed.

6.6 Special precautions for disposal and other handling
Any unused product or waste material should be disposed of in accordance with local requirements.

7. MARKETING AUTHORISATION HOLDER
Orion Corporation

Orionintie 1

FI-02200 Espoo

Finland

8. MARKETING AUTHORISATION NUMBER(S)
EU/1/03/260/001-004

EU/1/03/260/013

EU/1/03/260/016

9. DATE OF FIRST AUTHORISATION/RENEWAL OF THE AUTHORISATION
Date of first authorisation: 17 October 2003

Date of last renewal: 15 September 2008

10. DATE OF REVISION OF THE TEXT
27 March 2009

Detailed information on this medicine is available on the European Medicine's Agency (EMEA) web site: http://www.emea.europa.eu

Stalevo 75/18.75/200mg

(Orion Pharma (UK) Limited)

1. NAME OF THE MEDICINAL PRODUCT
Stalevo 75 mg/18.75 mg/200 mg film-coated tablets

2. QUALITATIVE AND QUANTITATIVE COMPOSITION
Each tablet contains 75 mg of levodopa, 18.75 mg of carbidopa and 200 mg of entacapone.

Excipient: Each tablet contains 1.4 mg of sucrose.

For a full list of excipients, see section 6.1.

3. PHARMACEUTICAL FORM
Film-coated tablet

Light brownish red, oval film-coated tablets marked with 'LCE 75' on one side.

4. CLINICAL PARTICULARS

4.1 Therapeutic indications
Stalevo is indicated for the treatment of adult patients with Parkinson's disease and end-of-dose motor fluctuations not stabilised on levodopa/dopa decarboxylase (DDC) inhibitor treatment.

4.2 Posology and method of administration
Each tablet is to be taken orally either with or without food (see section 5.2). One tablet contains one treatment dose and the tablet may only be administered as whole tablets.

The optimum daily dose must be determined by careful titration of levodopa in each patient. The daily dose should be preferably optimised using one of the six available tablet strengths (50 mg/12.5 mg/200 mg, 75 mg/18.75 mg/200 mg, 100 mg/25 mg/200 mg, 125 mg/31.25 mg/200 mg, 150 mg/37.5 mg/200 mg or 200 mg/50 mg/200 mg levodopa/carbidopa/entacapone).

Patients should be instructed to take only one Stalevo tablet per dose administration. Patients receiving less than 70-100 mg carbidopa a day are more likely to experience nausea and vomiting. While the experience with total daily dose greater than 200 mg carbidopa is limited, the maximum recommended daily dose of entacapone is 2,000 mg and therefore the maximum dose is 10 tablets per day for the Stalevo strengths of 50 mg/12.5 mg/200 mg, 75 mg/18.75 mg/200 mg, 100 mg/25 mg/200 mg, 125 mg/31.25 mg/200 mg and 150 mg/37.5 mg/200 mg. Ten tablets of Stalevo 150 mg/37.5 mg/200 mg equals 375 mg of carbidopa a day. According to this daily carbidopa dose, the maximum recommended daily Stalevo 200 mg/50 mg/200 mg dose is 7 tablets per day.

Usually Stalevo is to be used in patients who are currently treated with corresponding doses of standard release levodopa/DDC inhibitor and entacapone.

How to transfer patients taking levodopa/DDC inhibitor (carbidopa or benserazide) preparations and entacapone tablets to Stalevo

a. Patients who are currently treated with entacapone and with standard release levodopa/carbidopa in doses equal to Stalevo tablet strengths can be directly transferred to corresponding Stalevo tablets.

For example, a patient taking one tablet of 50 mg/12.5 mg of levodopa/carbidopa with one tablet of entacapone 200 mg four times daily can take one 50 mg/12.5 mg/200 mg Stalevo tablet four times daily in place of their usual levodopa/carbidopa and entacapone doses.

b. When initiating Stalevo therapy for patients currently treated with entacapone and levodopa/carbidopa in doses not equal to Stalevo, 75 mg/18.75 mg/200 mg (or 50 mg/12.5 mg/200 mg or 100 mg/25 mg/200 mg or 125 mg/31.25 mg/200 mg or 150 mg/37.5 mg/200 mg or 200 mg/50 mg/200 mg) tablets, Stalevo dosing should be carefully titrated for optimal clinical response. At the initiation, Stalevo should be adjusted to correspond as closely as possible to the total daily dose of levodopa currently used.

c. When initiating Stalevo in patients currently treated with entacapone and levodopa/benserazide in a standard release formulation, discontinue dosing of levodopa/benserazide the previous night, and start Stalevo the next morning. Begin with a dose of Stalevo that will provide either the same amount of levodopa or slightly (5-10%) more.

How to transfer patients not currently treated with entacapone to Stalevo

Initiation of Stalevo may be considered at corresponding doses to current treatment in some patients with Parkinson's disease and end-of-dose motor fluctuations, who are not stabilised on their current standard release levodopa/DDC inhibitor treatment. However, a direct switch from levodopa/DDC inhibitor to Stalevo is not recommended for patients who have dyskinesias or whose daily levodopa dose is above 800 mg. In such patients it is advisable to introduce entacapone treatment as a separate treatment (entacapone tablets) and adjust the levodopa dose if necessary, before switching to Stalevo.

Entacapone enhances the effects of levodopa. It may therefore be necessary, particularly in patients with dyskinesia, to reduce levodopa dose by 10-30% within the first days to first weeks after initiating Stalevo treatment. The daily dose of levodopa can be reduced by extending the dosing intervals and/or by reducing the amount of levodopa per dose, according to the clinical condition of the patient.

Dose adjustment during the course of the treatment

When more levodopa is required, an increase in the frequency of doses and/or the use of an alternative strength of Stalevo should be considered, within the dose recommendations.

When less levodopa is required, the total daily dose of Stalevo should be reduced either by decreasing the frequency of administration by extending the time between doses, or by decreasing the strength of Stalevo at an administration.

If other levodopa products are used concomitantly with a Stalevo tablet, the maximum dose recommendations should be followed.

Discontinuation of Stalevo therapy: If Stalevo treatment (levodopa/carbidopa/entacapone) is discontinued and the patient is transferred to levodopa/DDC inhibitor therapy without entacapone, it is necessary to adjust the dosing of other antiparkinsonian treatments, especially levodopa, to achieve a sufficient level of control of the parkinsonian symptoms.

Children and adolescents: Stalevo is not recommended for use in children below 18 years due to a lack of data on safety and efficacy.

Elderly: No dose adjustment of Stalevo is required for elderly patients.

Hepatic impairment: It is advised that Stalevo should be administered cautiously to patients with mild to moderate hepatic impairment. Dose reduction may be needed (see section 5.2). For severe hepatic impairment see section 4.3.

Renal impairment: Renal impairment does not affect the pharmacokinetics of entacapone. No particular studies are reported on the pharmacokinetics of levodopa and carbidopa in patients with renal insufficiency, therefore Stalevo therapy should be administered cautiously to patients in severe renal impairment including those receiving dialysis therapy (see section 5.2).

4.3 Contraindications
- Hypersensitivity to the active substances or to any of the excipients.

- Severe hepatic impairment.

- Narrow-angle glaucoma.

- Pheochromocytoma.

- Concomitant use of Stalevo with non-selective monoamine oxidase (MAO-A and MAO-B) inhibitors (e.g. phenelzine, tranylcypromine).

- Concomitant use of a selective MAO-A inhibitor and a selective MAO-B inhibitor (see section 4.5).

- A previous history of Neuroleptic Malignant Syndrome (NMS) and/or non-traumatic rhabdomyolysis.

4.4 Special warnings and precautions for use
- Stalevo is not recommended for the treatment of drug-induced extrapyramidal reactions

- Stalevo therapy should be administered cautiously to patients with severe cardiovascular or pulmonary disease, bronchial asthma, renal or endocrine disease, history of peptic ulcer disease or history of convulsions.

- In patients with a history of myocardial infarction who have residual atrial nodal or ventricular arrhythmias; cardiac function should be monitored with particular care during the period of initial dose adjustments.

- All patients treated with Stalevo should be monitored carefully for the development of mental changes, depression with suicidal tendencies, and other serious antisocial behaviour. Patients with past or current psychosis should be treated with caution.

- Concomitant administration of antipsychotics with dopamine receptor-blocking properties, particularly D_2 receptor antagonists should be carried out with caution, and the patient carefully observed for loss of antiparkinsonian effect or worsening of parkinsonian symptoms.

- Patients with chronic wide-angle glaucoma may be treated with Stalevo with caution, provided the intra-ocular pressure is well controlled and the patient is monitored carefully for changes in intra-ocular pressure.

- Stalevo may induce orthostatic hypotension. Therefore Stalevo should be given cautiously to patients who are taking other medicinal products which may cause orthostatic hypotension.

- Entacapone in association with levodopa has been associated with somnolence and episodes of sudden sleep onset in patients with Parkinson's disease and caution should therefore be exercised when driving or operating machines (see section 4.7).

- In clinical studies, dopaminergic adverse reactions, e.g. dyskinesia, were more common in patients who received entacapone and dopamine agonists (such as bromocriptine), selegiline or amantadine compared to those who received placebo with this combination. The doses of other antiparkinsonian medicinal products may need to be adjusted when Stalevo treatment is substituted for a patient currently not treated with entacapone.

- Rhabdomyolysis secondary to severe dyskinesias or neuroleptic malignant syndrome (NMS) has been observed rarely in patients with Parkinson's disease. Therefore, any abrupt dose reduction or withdrawal of levodopa should be carefully observed, particularly in patients who are also receiving neuroleptics. NMS, including rhabdomyolysis and hyperthermia, is characterised by motor symptoms (rigidity, myoclonus, tremor), mental status changes (e.g., agitation, confusion, coma), hyperthermia, autonomic dysfunction (tachycardia, labile blood pressure) and elevated serum creatine phosphokinase. In individual cases, only some of these symptoms and/or findings may be evident. The early diagnosis is important for the appropriate management of NMS. A syndrome resembling the neuroleptic malignant syndrome including muscular rigidity, elevated body temperature, mental changes and increased serum creatine phosphokinase has been reported with the abrupt withdrawal of antiparkinsonian agents. Neither NMS nor rhabdomyolysis have been reported in association with entacapone treatment from controlled trials in which entacapone was discontinued abruptly. Since the introduction of entacapone into the market, isolated cases of NMS have been reported, especially following abrupt reduction or discontinuation of entacapone and other concomitant dopaminergic medicinal products. When considered necessary, the replacement of Stalevo with levodopa and DDC inhibitor without entacapone or other dopaminergic treatment should proceed slowly and an increase in levodopa dose may be necessary.

- If general anaesthesia is required, therapy with Stalevo may be continued for as long as the patient is permitted to take fluids and medicinal products by mouth. If therapy has to be stopped temporarily, Stalevo may be restarted as soon as oral medicinal products can be taken at the same daily dose as before.

- Periodic evaluation of hepatic, haematopoietic, cardiovascular and renal function is recommended during extended therapy with Stalevo.

- For patients experiencing diarrhoea, a follow-up of weight is recommended in order to avoid potential excessive weight decrease.

- Pathological gambling, increased libido and hypersexuality have been reported in Parkinson's disease patients treated with dopamine agonists and other dopaminergic treatments such as Stalevo.

- For patients who experience progressive anorexia, asthenia and weight decrease within a relatively short period of time, a general medical evaluation including liver function should be considered.

- Stalevo contains sucrose, and therefore patients with rare hereditary problems of fructose intolerance, glucose-galactose malabsorption or sucrase-isomaltase insufficiency should not take this medicine.

4.5 Interaction with other medicinal products and other forms of interaction
Other antiparkinsonian medicinal products: To date there has been no indication of interactions that would preclude concurrent use of standard antiparkinsonian medicinal products with Stalevo therapy. Entacapone in high doses may affect the absorption of carbidopa. However, no interaction with carbidopa has been observed with the recommended treatment schedule (200 mg of entacapone up to 10 times daily). Interactions between entacapone and selegiline have been investigated in repeated dose studies in Parkinson's disease patients treated with levodopa/DDC

inhibitor and no interaction was observed. When used with Stalevo, the daily dose of selegiline should not exceed 10 mg.

Caution should be exercised when the following active substances are administered concomitantly with levodopa therapy.

Antihypertensives: Symptomatic postural hypotension may occur when levodopa is added to the treatment of patients already receiving antihypertensives. Dose adjustment of the antihypertensive agent may be required.

Antidepressants: Rarely, reactions including hypertension and dyskinesia have been reported with the concomitant use of tricyclic antidepressants and levodopa/carbidopa. Interactions between entacapone and imipramine and between entacapone and moclobemide have been investigated in single dose studies in healthy volunteers. No pharmacodynamic interactions were observed. A significant number of Parkinson's disease patients have been treated with the combination of levodopa, carbidopa and entacapone with several active substances including MAO-A inhibitors, tricyclic antidepressants, noradrenaline reuptake inhibitors such as desipramine, maprotiline and venlafaxine and medicinal products that are metabolised by COMT (e.g. catechol-structured compounds, paroxetine). No pharmacodynamic interactions have been observed. However, caution should be exercised when these medicinal products are used concomitantly with Stalevo (see sections 4.3 and 4.4).

Other active substances: Dopamine receptor antagonists (e.g. some antipsychotics and antiemetics), phenytoin and papaverine may reduce the therapeutic effect of levodopa. Patients taking these medicinal products with Stalevo should be carefully observed for loss of therapeutic response.

Due to entacapone's affinity to cytochrome P450 2C9 *in vitro* (see section 5.2), Stalevo may potentially interfere with active substances whose metabolism is dependent on this isoenzyme, such as S-warfarin. However, in an interaction study with healthy volunteers, entacapone did not change the plasma levels of S-warfarin, while the AUC for R-warfarin increased on average by 18% [CI_{90} 11-26%]. The INR values increased on average by 13% [CI_{90} 6-19%]. Thus, a control of INR is recommended when Stalevo is initiated for patients receiving warfarin.

Other forms of interactions: Since levodopa competes with certain amino acids, the absorption of Stalevo may be impaired in some patients on high protein diet.

Levodopa and entacapone may form chelates with iron in the gastrointestinal tract. Therefore, Stalevo and iron preparations should be taken at least 2-3 hours apart (see section 4.8).

In vitro data: Entacapone binds to human albumin binding site II which also binds several other medicinal products, including diazepam and ibuprofen. According to *in vitro* studies, significant displacement is not anticipated at therapeutic concentrations of the medicinal products. Accordingly, to date there has been no indication of such interactions.

4.6 Pregnancy and lactation

There are no adequate data from the use of the combination of levodopa/carbidopa/entacapone in pregnant women. Studies in animals have shown reproductive toxicity of the separate compounds (see section 5.3). The potential risk for humans is unknown. Stalevo should not be used during pregnancy unless the benefits for the mother outweigh the possible risks to the foetus.

Levodopa is excreted in human breast milk. There is evidence that lactation is suppressed during treatment with levodopa. Carbidopa and entacapone were excreted in milk in animals but is not known whether they are excreted in human breast milk. The safety of levodopa, carbidopa or entacapone in the infant is not known. Women should not breast-feed during treatment with Stalevo.

4.7 Effects on ability to drive and use machines

Stalevo may have major influence on the ability to drive and use machines. Levodopa, carbidopa and entacapone together may cause dizziness and symptomatic orthostatism. Therefore, caution should be exercised when driving or using machines.

Patients being treated with Stalevo and presenting with somnolence and/or sudden sleep onset episodes must be instructed to refrain from driving or engaging in activities where impaired alertness may put themselves or others at risk of serious injury or death (e.g. operating machines) until such recurrent episodes have resolved (see section 4.4).

4.8 Undesirable effects

The following section describes the undesirable effects reported for levodopa/carbidopa and for entacapone used in combination with levodopa/DDC inhibitor.

Levodopa /carbidopa

Adverse reactions that occur frequently with levodopa/carbidopa are those due to central neuropharmacological activity of dopamine. These reactions can usually be diminished by levodopa dose reduction. The most common adverse reactions are dyskinesias including choreiform, dystonic and other involuntary movements. Muscle twitching and blepharospasm may be taken as early signs to consider levodopa dose reduction. Nausea, also related to enhanced central dopaminergic activity, is a common adverse reaction of levodopa/carbidopa.

Other adverse reactions associated with levodopa/carbidopa therapy are mental changes, including paranoid ideation and psychotic episodes; depression with or without development of suicidal tendencies; and cognitive dysfunction. Adding of entacapone to levodopa/DDC inhibitor therapy (carbidopa or benserazide), i.e. initiation of Stalevo treatment in an entacapone naive patient, may aggravate some of these mental changes.

Less frequent adverse reactions of levodopa/carbidopa therapy are irregular heart rhythm and/or palpitations, orthostatic hypotensive episodes, bradykinetic episodes (the 'on-off' phenomenon), anorexia, vomiting, dizziness, and somnolence.

Gastrointestinal bleeding, development of duodenal ulcer, hypertension, phlebitis, leucopenia, haemolytic and non-haemolytic anaemia, thrombocytopenia, agranulocytosis, chest pain, dyspnoea and paraesthesia have occurred rarely with levodopa/carbidopa.

Convulsions have occurred rarely with levodopa/carbidopa; however a causal relationship to levodopa/carbidopa therapy has not been established.

Parkinson's disease patients treated with dopamine agonists and other dopaminergic treatments such as Stalevo, especially at high doses, have been reported as exhibiting signs of pathological gambling, increased libido and hypersexuality, generally reversible upon reduction of the dose or treatment discontinuation.

Other adverse reactions that have been reported with levodopa and may, therefore, be potential adverse reactions of Stalevo as well, include:

Nervous system disorders: Ataxia, numbness, increased hand tremor, muscle twitching, muscle cramp, trismus, activation of latent Horner's syndrome. Also falling and gait abnormalities are potential undesirable effects.

Eye disorders: Diplopia, blurred vision, dilated pupils, oculogyric crises.

Gastrointestinal disorders: Dry mouth, bitter taste, sialorrhoea, dysphagia, bruxism, hiccups, abdominal pain and distress, constipation, diarrhoea, flatulence, burning sensation of the tongue.

Renal and urinary disorders: Urinary retention, urinary incontinence, dark urine, priapism.

Skin and subcutaneous tissue disorders: Flushing, increased sweating, dark sweat, rash, hair loss.

Metabolism and nutrition disorders: Weight gain or loss, oedema.

Psychiatric disorders: Confusion, insomnia, nightmares, hallucinations, delusions, agitation, anxiety, euphoria.

Miscellaneous: Weakness, faintness, fatigue, headache, hoarseness, malaise, hot flushes, sense of stimulation, bizarre breathing patterns, neuroleptic malignant syndrome, malignant melanoma.

Entacapone

The most frequent adverse reactions caused by entacapone relate to the increased dopaminergic activity and occur most commonly at the beginning of the treatment. Reduction of levodopa dose decreases the severity and frequency of the reactions. The other major class of adverse reactions are gastrointestinal symptoms, including nausea, vomiting, abdominal pain, constipations and diarrhoea. Urine may be discoloured reddish-brown by entacapone, but this is a harmless phenomenon.

The following adverse reactions, listed in Table 1, have been accumulated both from clinical studies with entacapone and since the introduction of entacapone into the market for the combination use of entacapone with levodopa/DDC inhibitor.

Table 1. Adverse reactions

Nervous system disorders

Very common: Dyskinesia, Parkinsonism aggravated.

Common: Dizziness, dystonia, hyperkinesia.

Gastrointestinal disorders

Very common: Nausea.

Common: Diarrhoea, abdominal pain, dry mouth, constipation, vomiting.

Very rare: Anorexia.

Not known: Colitis.

Renal and urinary disorders

Very common: Urine discolouration.

Skin and subcutaneous tissue disorders

Rare: Erythematous or maculopapular rash.

Very rare: Urticaria.

Not known: Skin, hair, beard and nail discolorations.

General disorders and administration site conditions

Common: Fatigue, sweating increased, fall.

Uncommon: Weight decrease.

Hepatobiliary disorders

Rare: Hepatic function tests abnormal.

Not known: Hepatitis with mainly cholestatic features (see section 4.4).

Psychiatric disorders

Common: Insomnia, hallucinations, confusion, nightmares, agitation.

*Adverse reactions are ranked under headings of frequency, the most frequent first, using the following convention: Very common (≥1/10); common (≥100 to <1/10); uncommon (≥1/1,000 to <1/100); rare (≥1/10,000 to <1/1,000), very rare (<1/10,000), not known (cannot be estimated from the available data, since no valid estimate can be derived from clinical trials or epidemiological studies).

Entacapone in association with levodopa has been associated with isolated cases of excessive daytime somnolence and sudden sleep onset episodes.

Isolated cases of NMS have been reported following the abrupt reduction or discontinuation of entacapone and other dopaminergic treatments.

Isolated cases of rhabdomyolysis have been reported.

Isolated cases of angioedema have been reported after the initiation of Stalevo.

Laboratory tests:

The following laboratory abnormalities have been reported with levodopa/carbidopa treatment and should, therefore, be acknowledged when treating patients with Stalevo:

Commonly, levels of blood urea nitrogen, creatinine, and uric acid are lower during administration of levodopa/carbidopa than with levodopa alone. Transient abnormalities include elevated values of blood urea, AST (SGOT), ALT (SGPT), LDH, bilirubin, and alkaline phosphatase.

Decreased haemoglobin, haematocrit, elevated serum glucose and white blood cells, bacteria and blood in the urine have been reported.

Positive Coombs' tests have been reported, both for levodopa/carbidopa and for levodopa alone, but haemolytic anaemia is extremely rare.

Levodopa/carbidopa may cause false positive result when a dipstick is used to test for urinary ketone and this reaction is not altered by boiling the urine sample. The use of glucose oxidase methods may give false negative results for glycosuria.

4.9 Overdose

The post-marketing data includes isolated cases of overdose in which the reported highest daily doses of levodopa and entacapone have been at least 10,000 mg and 40,000 mg, respectively. The acute symptoms and signs in these cases of overdose included agitation, confusional state, coma, bradycardia, ventricular tachycardia, Cheyne-Stokes respiration, discolourations of skin, tongue and conjunctiva, and chromaturia. Management of acute overdose with Stalevo therapy is similar to acute overdose with levodopa. Pyridoxine, however, is not effective in reversing the actions of Stalevo. Hospitalisation is advised and general supportive measures should be employed with immediate gastric lavage and repeated doses of charcoal over time. This may hasten the elimination of entacapone in particular by decreasing its absorption/reabsorption from the GI tract. The adequacy of the respiratory, circulatory and renal systems should be carefully monitored and appropriate supportive measures employed. ECG monitoring should be started and the patient carefully monitored for the possible development of arrhythmias. If required, appropriate anti-arrhythmic therapy should be given. The possibility that the patient has taken other active substances in addition to Stalevo should be taken into consideration. The value of dialysis in the treatment of overdose is not known.

5. PHARMACOLOGICAL PROPERTIES

5.1 Pharmacodynamic properties

Pharmacotherapeutic group: dopa and dopa derivatives, ATC code: N04BA03

According to the current understanding, the symptoms of Parkinson's disease are related to depletion of dopamine in the corpus striatum. Dopamine does not cross the blood-brain barrier. Levodopa, the precursor of dopamine, crosses the blood brain barrier and relieves the symptoms of the disease. As levodopa is extensively metabolised in the periphery, only a small portion of a given dose reaches the central nervous system when levodopa is administered without metabolic enzyme inhibitors.

Carbidopa and benserazide are peripheral DDC inhibitors which reduce the peripheral metabolism of levodopa to dopamine, and thus, more levodopa is available to the brain. When decarboxylation of levodopa is reduced with the co-administration of a DDC inhibitor, a lower dose of levodopa can be used and the incidence of undesirable effects such as nausea is reduced.

With inhibition of the decarboxylase by a DDC inhibitor, catechol-*O*-methyltransferase (COMT) becomes the major peripheral metabolic pathway catalyzing the conversion of levodopa to 3-O-methyldopa (3-OMD), a potentially harmful metabolite of levodopa. Entacapone is a reversible, specific and mainly peripherally acting COMT inhibitor designed for concomitant administration with levodopa. Entacapone slows the clearance of levodopa from the bloodstream resulting in an increased area under the curve (AUC) in the pharmacokinetic profile of levodopa. Consequently the clinical response to each dose of levodopa is enhanced and prolonged.

The evidence of the therapeutic effects of Stalevo is based on two phase III double-blind studies, in which 376 Parkinson's disease patients with end-of-dose motor fluctuations received either entacapone or placebo with each levodopa/DDC inhibitor dose. Daily ON time with and without entacapone was recorded in home-diaries by patients. In the first study, entacapone increased the mean daily ON time by 1 h 20 min ($CI_{95\%}$ 45 min, 1 h 56 min) from baseline. This corresponded to an 8.3% increase in the proportion of daily ON time. Correspondingly, the decrease in daily OFF time was 24% in the entacapone group and 0% in the placebo group. In the second study, the mean proportion of daily ON time increased by 4.5% ($CI_{95\%}$ 0.93%, 7.97%) from baseline. This is translated to a mean increase of 35 min in the daily ON time. Correspondingly, the daily OFF time decreased by 18% on entacapone and by 5% on placebo. Because the effects of Stalevo tablets are equivalent with entacapone 200 mg tablet administered concomitantly with the commercially available standard release carbidopa/levodopa preparations in corresponding doses these results are applicable to describe the effects of Stalevo as well.

5.2 Pharmacokinetic properties

General characteristics of the active substances

Absorption/Distribution: There are substantial inter- and intra-individual variations in the absorption of levodopa, carbidopa and entacapone. Both levodopa and entacapone are rapidly absorbed and eliminated. Carbidopa is absorbed and eliminated slightly slower compared with levodopa. When given separately without the two other active substances, the bioavailability for levodopa is 15-33%, for carbidopa 40-70% and for entacapone 35% after a 200 mg oral dose. Meals rich in large neutral amino acids may delay and reduce the absorption of levodopa. Food does not significantly affect the absorption of entacapone. The distribution volume of both levodopa (Vd 0.36-1.6 l/kg) and entacapone (Vd_{ss} 0.27 l/kg) is moderately small while no data for carbidopa are available.

Levodopa is bound to plasma protein only to a minor extent of about 10-30% and carbidopa is bound approximately 36%, while entacapone is extensively bound to plasma proteins (about 98%) – mainly to serum albumin. At therapeutic concentrations, entacapone does not displace other extensively bound active substances (e.g. warfarin, salicylic acid, phenylbutazone, or diazepam), nor is it displaced to any significant extent by any of these substances at therapeutic or higher concentrations.

Metabolism and Elimination: Levodopa is extensively metabolised to various metabolites: decarboxylation by dopa decarboxylase (DDC) and O-methylation by catechol-O-methyltransferase (COMT) being the most important pathways.

Carbidopa is metabolized to two main metabolites which are excreted in the urine as glucuronides and unconjugated compounds. Unchanged carbidopa accounts for 30% of the total urinary excretion.

Entacapone is almost completely metabolized prior to excretion via urine (10 to 20%) and bile/faeces (80 to 90%). The main metabolic pathway is glucuronidation of entacapone and its active metabolite, the cis-isomer, which accounts for about 5% of plasma total amount.

Total clearance for levodopa is in the range of 0.55-1.38 l/kg/h and for entacapone is in the range of 0.70 l/kg/h. The elimination-half life is ($t_{1/2}$) is 0.6-1.3 hours for levodopa, 2-3 hours for carbidopa and 0.4-0.7 hours for entacapone, each given separately.

Due to short elimination half-lives, no true accumulation of levodopa or entacapone occurs on repeated administration.

Data from *in vitro* studies using human liver microsomal preparations indicate that entacapone inhibits cytochrome P450 2C9 (IC50 ~ 4 μM). Entacapone showed little or no inhibition of other types of P450 isoenzymes (CYP1A2, CYP2A6, CYP2D6, CYP2E1, CYP3A and CYP2C19); see section 4.5.

Characteristics in patients

Elderly: When given without carbidopa and entacapone, the absorption of levodopa is greater and elimination is slower in elderly than in young subjects. However, after combination of carbidopa with levodopa, the absorption of levodopa is similar between the elderly and the young, but the AUC is still 1.5 fold greater in the elderly due to decreased DDC activity and lower clearance by aging. There are no significant differences in the AUC of carbidopa or entacapone between younger (45–64 years) and elderly subjects (65–75 years).

Gender: Bioavailability of levodopa is significantly higher in women than in men. In the pharmacokinetic studies with Stalevo the bioavailability of levodopa is higher in women than in men, primarily due to the difference in body weight, while there is no gender difference with carbidopa and entacapone.

Hepatic impairment: The metabolism of entacapone is slowed in patients with mild to moderate hepatic impairment (Child-Pugh Class A and B) leading to an increased plasma concentration of entacapone both in the absorption and elimination phases (see sections 4.2 and 4.3). No particular studies on the pharmacokinetics of carbidopa and levodopa in patients with hepatic impairment are reported, however, it is advised that Stalevo should be administered cautiously to patients with mild or moderate hepatic impairment.

Renal impairment: Renal impairment does not affect the pharmacokinetics of entacapone. No particular studies are reported on the pharmacokinetics of levodopa and carbidopa in patients with renal impairment. However, a longer dosing interval of Stalevo may be considered for patients who are receiving dialysis therapy (see section 4.2).

5.3 Preclinical safety data

Preclinical data of levodopa, carbidopa and entacapone, tested alone or in combination, revealed no special hazard for humans based on conventional studies of safety pharmacology, repeated dose toxicity, genotoxicity, and carcinogenic potential. In repeated dose toxicity studies with entacapone, anaemia most likely due to iron chelating properties of entacapone was observed. Regarding reproduction toxicity of entacapone, decreased foetal weight and a slightly delayed bone development were noticed in rabbits treated at systemic exposure levels in the therapeutic range. Both levodopa and combinations of carbidopa and levodopa have caused visceral and skeletal malformations in rabbits.

6. PHARMACEUTICAL PARTICULARS

6.1 List of excipients

Tablet core:

Croscarmellose sodium

Magnesium stearate

Maize starch

Mannitol (E421)

Povidone (E1201)

Film-coating:

Glycerol (85 per cent) (E422)

Hypromellose

Magnesium stearate

Polysorbate 80

Red iron oxide (E172)

Sucrose

Titanium dioxide (E171)

Yellow iron oxide (E172)

6.2 Incompatibilities

Not applicable.

6.3 Shelf life

3 years.

6.4 Special precautions for storage

This medicinal product does not require any special storage conditions.

6.5 Nature and contents of container

HDPE bottle with a child resistant PP-closure.

Pack sizes:

10, 30, 100, 130 and 175 tablets.

Not all pack sizes may be marketed.

6.6 Special precautions for disposal and other handling

Any unused product or waste material should be disposed of in accordance with local requirements.

7. MARKETING AUTHORISATION HOLDER

Orion Corporation

Orionintie 1

FI-02200 Espoo

Finland

8. MARKETING AUTHORISATION NUMBER(S)

EU/1/03/260/024-028

9. DATE OF FIRST AUTHORISATION/RENEWAL OF THE AUTHORISATION

Date of first authorisation: 17 October 2003

Date of last renewal: 15 September 2008

10. DATE OF REVISION OF THE TEXT

27 March 2009

Detailed information on this medicine is available on the European Medicine's Agency (EMEA) web site: http://www.emea.europa.eu

Stelara 45 mg solution for injection

(Janssen-Cilag Ltd)

1. NAME OF THE MEDICINAL PRODUCT

STELARA▼45 mg solution for injection

2. QUALITATIVE AND QUANTITATIVE COMPOSITION

Each vial contains 45 mg ustekinumab in 0.5 ml.

Ustekinumab is a fully human IgG1κ monoclonal antibody to interleukin (IL)-12/23 produced in a murine myeloma cell line using recombinant DNA technology.

For a full list of excipients, see section 6.1.

3. PHARMACEUTICAL FORM

Solution for injection.

The solution is clear to slightly opalescent, colourless to light yellow.

4. CLINICAL PARTICULARS

4.1 Therapeutic indications

STELARA is indicated for the treatment of moderate to severe plaque psoriasis in adults who failed to respond to, or who have a contraindication to, or are intolerant to other systemic therapies including ciclosporin, methotrexate and PUVA (see section 5.1).

4.2 Posology and method of administration

STELARA is intended for use under the guidance and supervision of a physician experienced in the diagnosis and treatment of psoriasis.

Posology

The recommended posology of STELARA is an initial dose of 45 mg administered subcutaneously at week 0, followed by a 45 mg dose at week 4, then every 12 weeks thereafter.

Consideration should be given to discontinuing treatment in patients who have shown no response up to 28 weeks of treatment.

Patients with body weight > 100 kg

For patients with a body weight > 100 kg the dose is 90 mg administered subcutaneously at week 0, followed by a 90 mg dose at week 4, then every 12 weeks thereafter (see section 5.1). In patients weighing > 100 kg, 45 mg was also shown to be efficacious. However, 90 mg resulted in greater efficacy in these patients.

Elderly patients (≥ 65 years)

No dose adjustment is needed for elderly patients.

Children and adolescents (< 18 years)

STELARA is not recommended for use in children below age 18 due to a lack of data on safety and efficacy.

Renal and hepatic impairment

STELARA has not been studied in these patient populations. No dose recommendations can be made.

Method of administration

STELARA is for subcutaneous injection. If possible, areas of the skin that show psoriasis should be avoided as injection sites.

After proper training in subcutaneous injection technique, patients may self-inject STELARA if a physician determines that it is appropriate. However, the physician should ensure appropriate follow-up of patients. Patients should be instructed to inject the full amount of STELARA according to the directions provided in the package leaflet. Comprehensive instructions for administration are given in the package leaflet.

For further instructions on preparation and special precautions for handling, see section 6.6.

4.3 Contraindications

Hypersensitivity to the active substance or to any of the excipients (see section 6.1).

Clinically important, active infection.

4.4 Special warnings and precautions for use

Infections

Ustekinumab may have the potential to increase the risk of infections and reactivate latent infections. In clinial studies, serious bacterial, fungal, and viral infections have been observed in patients receiving STELARA (see section 4.8).

Caution should be exercised when considering the use of STELARA in patients with a chronic infection or a history of recurrent infection (see section 4.3).

Prior to initiating treatment with STELARA, patients should be evaluated for tuberculosis infection. STELARA must not be given to patients with active tuberculosis (see section 4.3). Treatment of latent tuberculosis infection should be initiated prior to administering STELARA. Anti-tuberculosis therapy should also be considered prior to initiation of STELARA in patients with a history of latent or active tuberculosis in whom an adequate course of treatment cannot be confirmed. Patients receiving STELARA should be monitored closely for signs and symptoms of active tuberculosis during and after treatment.

Patients should be instructed to seek medical advice if signs or symptoms suggestive of an infection occur. If a patient develops a serious infection, the patient should be closely monitored and STELARA should not be administered until the infection resolves.

Malignancies

Immunosuppressants like ustekinumab have the potential to increase the risk of malignancy. Some patients who received STELARA in clinical studies developed cutaneous and non-cutaneous malignancies (see section 4.8).

No studies have been conducted that include patients with a history of malignancy or that continue treatment in patients who develop malignancy while receiving STELARA. Thus, caution should be exercised when considering the use of STELARA in these patients.

Hypersensitivity reactions

If an anaphylactic or other serious allergic reaction occurs, administration of STELARA should be discontinued immediately and appropriate therapy instituted (see section 4.8).

Vaccinations

It is recommended that live viral or live bacterial vaccines (such as Bacillus of Calmette and Guérin (BCG)) should not be given concurrently with STELARA. Specific studies have not been conducted in patients who had recently received live viral or live bacterial vaccines. Before live viral or live bacterial vaccination, treatment with STELARA should be withheld for at least 15 weeks after the last dose and can be resumed at least 2 weeks after vaccination. Prescribers should consult the Summary of Product Characteristics for the specific vaccine for additional information and guidance on concomitant use of immunosuppressive agents post-vaccination.

Patients receiving STELARA may receive concurrent inactivated or non-live vaccinations.

Concomitant immunosuppressive therapy

The safety and efficacy of STELARA in combination with other immunosuppressants, including biologics, or phototherapy have not been evaluated. Caution should be exercised when considering concomitant use of other immunosuppressants and STELARA or when transitioning from other immunosuppressive biologics (see section 4.5).

Special populations

Children and adolescents (< 18 years)

STELARA is not recommended for use in children below age 18 due to a lack of data on safety and efficacy.

Elderly patients (⩾ 65 years)

No overall differences in efficacy or safety in patients age 65 and older who received STELARA were observed compared to younger patients. Because there is a higher incidence of infections in the elderly population in general, caution should be used in treating the elderly.

Hepatic and renal impairment

Specific studies have not been conducted in patients with hepatic and renal impairment (see section 4.2).

4.5 Interaction with other medicinal products and other forms of interaction

No interaction studies have been performed. In the population pharmacokinetic analysis of the phase III studies, the effect of the most frequently used concomitant medicinal products in patients with psoriasis (including paracetamol, ibuprofen, acetylsalicylic acid, metformin, atorvastatin, levothyroxine) on pharmacokinetics of ustekinumab was explored. There were no indications of an interaction with these concomitantly administered medicinal products. The basis for this analysis was that at least 100 patients (> 5% of the studied population) were treated concomitantly with these medicinal products for at least 90% of the study period.

Live vaccines should not be given concurrently with STELARA (see section 4.4).

The safety and efficacy of STELARA in combination with other immunosuppressants, including biologics, or phototherapy have not been evaluated (see section 4.4).

4.6 Pregnancy and lactation

Pregnancy

There are no adequate data from the use of ustekinumab in pregnant women. Animal studies do not indicate direct or indirect harmful effects with respect to pregnancy, embryonic/foetal development, parturition or postnatal development (see section 5.3). As a precautionary measure, it is preferable to avoid the use of STELARA in pregnancy. Women of childbearing potential should use effective methods of contraception during treatment and up to 15 weeks after treatment.

Lactation

It is unknown whether ustekinumab is excreted in human breast milk. Animal studies have shown excretion of ustekinumab at low levels in breast milk. It is not known if ustekinumab is absorbed systemically after ingestion. Because of the potential for adverse reactions in nursing infants from ustekinumab, a decision on whether to discontinue breast-feeding during treatment and up to 15 weeks after treatment or to discontinue therapy with STELARA must be made taking into account the benefit of breast-feeding to the child and the benefit of STELARA therapy to the woman.

4.7 Effects on ability to drive and use machines

No studies on the effects on the ability to drive and use of machines have been performed.

4.8 Undesirable effects

The safety data described below reflect exposure to ustekinumab in 3 studies of 2,266 patients, including 1,970 exposed for at least 6 months and 1,285 exposed for at least 1 year, and 373 for at least 18 months.

The following serious adverse reactions were reported:

- Serious infections
- Malignancies

The most common adverse reactions (> 10%) in controlled and uncontrolled portions of the psoriasis clinical studies with ustekinumab were nasopharyngitis and upper respiratory tract infection. Most were considered to be mild and did not necessitate discontinuation of study treatment.

Table 1 provides a summary of adverse reactions from psoriasis clinical studies. The adverse reactions are classified by System Organ Class and frequency, using the following convention: Very common (⩾ 1/10), Common (⩾ 1/100 to < 1/10), Uncommon (⩾ 1/1,000 to < 1/100), Rare (⩾ 1/10,000 to < 1/1,000), Very rare (< 1/10,000), not known (cannot be estimated from the available data).

Within each frequency grouping, adverse reactions are presented in order of decreasing seriousness.

Table 1 Summary of adverse reactions in psoriasis clinical studies

System Organ Class	Frequency: Adverse reaction
Infections and infestations	Very common: Upper respiratory tract infection, nasopharyngitis Common: Cellulitis, viral upper respiratory tract infection
Psychiatric disorders	Common: Depression
Nervous system disorders	Common: Dizziness, headache
Respiratory, thoracic and mediastinal disorders	Common: Pharyngolaryngeal pain, nasal congestion
Gastrointestinal disorders	Common: Diarrhoea
Skin and subcutaneous tissue disorders	Common: Pruritus
Musculoskeletal and connective tissue disorders	Common: Back pain, myalgia
General disorders and administration site conditions	Common: Fatigue, injection site erythema Uncommon: Injection site reactions (including pain, swelling, pruritus, induration, haemorrhage, bruising and irritation)

Infections

In controlled studies of psoriasis patients, the rates of infection or serious infection were similar between ustekinumab-treated patients and those treated with placebo. In the placebo-controlled period of clinical studies of psoriasis patients, the rate of infection was 1.39 per patient-year of follow-up in ustekinumab-treated patients, and 1.21 in placebo-treated patients. Serious infections occurred in 0.01 per patient-year of follow-up in ustekinumab-treated patients (5 serious infections in 407 patient-years of follow-up) and 0.02 in placebo-treated patients (3 serious infections in 177 patient-years of follow-up) (see section 4.4).

In the controlled and non-controlled portions of psoriasis clinical studies, the rate of infection was 1.24 per patient-year of follow-up in ustekinumab-treated patients, and the incidence of serious infections was 0.01 per patient-year of follow-up in ustekinumab-treated patients (24 serious infections in 2,251 patient-years of follow-up) and serious infections reported included cellulitis, diverticulitis, osteomyelitis, viral infections, gastroenteritis, pneumonia, and urinary tract infections.

In clinical studies, patients with latent tuberculosis who were concurrently treated with isoniazid did not develop tuberculosis.

Malignancies

In the placebo-controlled period of the psoriasis clinical studies, the incidence of malignancies excluding non-melanoma skin cancer was 0.25 per 100 patient-years of follow-up for ustekinumab-treated patients (1 patient in 406 patient-years of follow-up) compared with 0.57 for placebo-treated patients (1 patient in 177 patient-years of follow-up). The incidence of non-melanoma skin cancer was 0.74 per 100 patient-years of follow-up for ustekinumab-treated patients (3 patients in 406 patient-years of follow-up) compared to 1.13 for placebo-treated patients (2 patients in 176 patient-years of follow-up).

In the controlled and non-controlled portions of psoriasis clinical studies, the incidence of malignancies excluding non-melanoma skin cancers was 0.36 per 100 patient-years of follow-up for ustekinumab-treated patients (8 patients in 2,249 patient-years of follow-up) and malignancies reported included breast, colon, head and neck, kidney, prostate, and thyroid cancers. The rate of malignancies reported in ustekinumab-treated patients was comparable to the rate expected in the general population (standardised incidence ratio = 0.68 [95% confidence interval: 0.29, 1.34]). The incidence of non-melanoma skin cancer was 0.80 per 100 patient-years of follow-up for ustekinumab-treated patients (18 patients in 2,245 patient-years of follow-up) (see section 4.4).

Hypersensitivity reactions

In clinical studies of ustekinumab, rash and urticaria have each been observed in < 2% of patients.

Immunogenicity

Approximately 5% of ustekinumab-treated patients developed antibodies to ustekinumab, which were generally low-titer. No apparent correlation of antibody development to injection site reactions was seen. Efficacy tended to be lower in patients positive for antibodies to ustekinumab; however, antibody positivity does not preclude a clinical response.

4.9 Overdose

No cases of overdose have been reported.

Single doses up to 4.5 mg/kg have been administered intravenously in clinical studies without dose-limiting toxicity. In case of overdose, it is recommended that the patient be monitored for any signs or symptoms of adverse reactions and appropriate symptomatic treatment be instituted immediately.

5. PHARMACOLOGICAL PROPERTIES

5.1 Pharmacodynamic properties

Pharmacotherapeutic group: Interleukin inhibitors, ATC code: L04AC05.

Mechanism of action

Ustekinumab is a fully human IgG1κ monoclonal antibody that binds with high affinity and specificity to the p40 protein subunit of the human cytokines IL-12 and IL-23. Ustekinumab inhibits the activity of human IL-12 and IL-23 by preventing these cytokines from binding to their IL-12Rβ1 receptor protein expressed on the surface of immune cells. Ustekinumab cannot bind to IL-12 or IL-23 that is pre-bound to IL-12Rβ1 cell surface receptors. Thus, ustekinumab is not likely to contribute to complement- or antibody-mediated cytotoxicity of the receptor-bearing cell. IL-12 and IL-23 are heterodimeric cytokines secreted by activated antigen presenting cells, such as macrophages and dendritic cells. IL-12 and IL-23 participate in immune function by contributing to natural killer (NK) cell activation and CD4+ T-cell differentiation and activation. However, abnormal regulation of IL-12 and IL-23 has been associated with immune-mediated diseases, such as psoriasis. Ustekinumab prevents IL-12 and IL-23 contributions to immune cell activation, such as intracellular signaling and cytokine secretion. Thus, ustekinumab is believed to interrupt signaling and cytokine cascades that are relevant to psoriasis pathology.

Clinical efficacy and safety

The safety and efficacy of ustekinumabwas assessed in 1,996 patients in two randomised, double-blind, placebo-controlled studies in patients with moderate to severe plaque psoriasis and who were candidates for phototherapy or systemic therapy.

Psoriasis Study 1 (PHOENIX 1) evaluated 766 patients. 53% of these patients were either non-responsive, intolerant, or had a contraindication to other systemic therapy. Patients randomised to ustekinumab received 45 mg or 90 mg doses at Weeks 0 and 4 and followed by the same dose every 12 weeks. Patients randomised to receive placebo at Weeks 0 and 4 crossed over to receive ustekinumab (either 45 mg or 90 mg) at Weeks 12 and 16 followed by dosing every 12 weeks. Patients originally randomised to ustekinumab who achieved Psoriasis Area and Severity Index 75 response (PASI improvement of at least 75% relative to baseline) at both Weeks 28 and 40 were re-randomised to receive ustekinumab every 12 weeks or to placebo (i.e., withdrawal of therapy). Patients who were re-randomised to placebo at Week 40 reinitiated ustekinumab at their original dosing regimen when they experienced at least a 50% loss of their PASI improvement obtained at Week 40. All patients were followed for up to 76 weeks following first administration of study treatment.

Psoriasis Study 2 (PHOENIX 2) evaluated 1230 patients. 61% of these patients were either non-responsive, intolerant, or had a contraindication to other systemic therapy. Patients randomised to ustekinumab received 45 mg or 90 mg doses at Weeks 0 and 4 followed by an additional dose at 16 weeks. Patients randomised to receive placebo at Weeks 0 and 4 crossed over to receive ustekinumab (either 45 mg or 90 mg) at Weeks 12 and 16. All patients were followed for up to 52 weeks following first administration of study treatment.

In both studies, baseline disease characteristics were generally consistent across all treatment groups with a median baseline PASI score from 17 to 18 and median baseline Body Surface Area (BSA) ⩾ 20, median Dermatology Life Quality Index (DLQI) range from 10 to 12. Approximately one third (PHOENIX 1) and one quarter (PHOENIX 2) of subjects had Psoriatic Arthritis (PsA).

The primary endpoint in both studies was the proportion of patients who achieved PASI 75 response from baseline at Week 12 (see Table 2).

Table 2 Summary of clinical response in Psoriasis Study 1 (PHOENIX 1) and Psoriasis Study 2 (PHOENIX 2)

(see Table 2 on next page)

In Psoriasis Study 1 maintenance of PASI 75 was significantly superior with continuous treatment compared with treatment withdrawal ($p < 0.001$). Similar results were seen with each dose of ustekinumab. At Week 52, 89% of patients re-randomised to maintenance treatment were PASI 75 responders compared with 63% of patients re-randomised to placebo (treatment withdrawal) ($p < 0.001$). At week 76, 84% of patients re-randomised to maintenance treatment were PASI 75 responders compared with 19% of patients re-randomised to placebo (treatment withdrawal).

In patients re-randomised to placebo, and who reinitiated their original ustekinumab treatment regimen after loss of

Table 2 Summary of clinical response in Psoriasis Study 1 (PHOENIX 1) and Psoriasis Study 2 (PHOENIX 2)

	Week 12 (2 injections)			Week 28 (3 injections)	
	PBO	45 mg	90 mg	45 mg	90 mg
Psoriasis Study 1					
Number of patients randomised	255	255	256	250	243
PASI 50 response N (%)	26 (10%)	213 (84%) [a]	220 (86%) [a]	228 (91%)	234 (96%)
PASI 75 response N (%)	8 (3%)	171 (67%) [a]	170 (66%) [a]	178 (71%)	191 (79%)
PASI 90 response N (%)	5 (2%)	106 (42%) [a]	94 (37%) [a]	123 (49%)	135 (56%)
PGA[b] of cleared or minimal N (%)	10 (4%)	151 (59%) [a]	156 (61%) [a]	146 (58%)	160 (66%)
Psoriasis Study 2					
Number of patients randomised	410	409	411	397	400
PASI 50 response N (%)	41 (10%)	342 (84%) [a]	367 (89%) [a]	369 (93%)	380 (95%)
PASI 75 response N (%)	15 (4%)	273 (67%) [a]	311 (76%) [a]	276 (70%)	314 (79%)
PASI 90 response N (%)	3 (1%)	173 (42%) [a]	209 (51%) [a]	178 (45%)	217 (54%)
PGA[b] of cleared or minimal N (%)	18 (4%)	277 (68%) [a]	300 (73%) [a]	241 (61%)	279 (70%)

[a] $p < 0.001$ for 45 mg or 90 mg in comparison with placebo (PBO).
[b] PGA = Physician Global Assessment

≥ 50% of PASI improvement 85% regained PASI 75 response within 12 weeks after re-initiating therapy.

In Psoriasis Study 1, at Week 2 and Week 12, significantly greater improvements from baseline were demonstrated in the DLQI in each ustekinumab treatment group compared with placebo. The improvement was sustained through Week 28. Similarly, significant improvements were seen in Psoriasis Study 2 at Week 4 and 12, which were sustained through Week 24. In Psoriasis Study 1, improvements in nail psoriasis (Nail Psoriasis Severity Index), in the physical and mental component summary scores of the SF-36 and in the Itch Visual Analogue Scale (VAS) were also significant in each ustekinumab treatment group compared with placebo. In Psoriasis Study 2, the Hospital Anxiety and Depression Scale (HADS) and Work Limitations Questionnaire (WLQ) were also significantly improved in each ustekinumab treatment group compared with placebo.

5.2 Pharmacokinetic properties

Absorption

The median time to reach the maximum serum concentration (t_{max}) was 8.5 days after a single 90 mg subcutaneous administration in healthy subjects. The median t_{max} values of ustekinumab following a single subcutaneous administration of either 45 mg or 90 mg in patients with psoriasis were comparable to those observed in healthy subjects.

The absolute bioavailability of ustekinumab following a single subcutaneous administration was estimated to be 57.2% in patients with psoriasis.

Distribution

Median volume of distribution during the terminal phase (Vz) following a single intravenous administration to patients with psoriasis ranged from 57 to 83 ml/kg.

Metabolism

The exact metabolic pathway for ustekinumab is unknown.

Elimination

Median systemic clearance (CL) following a single intravenous administration to patients with psoriasis ranged from 1.99 to 2.34 ml/day/kg. Median half-life ($t_{1/2}$) of ustekinumab was approximately 3 weeks in patients with psoriasis, ranging from 15 to 32 days across all psoriasis studies. In a population pharmacokinetic analysis, the apparent clearance (CL/F) and apparent volume of distribution (V/F) were 0.465 l/day and 15.7 l, respectively, in patients with psoriasis. The CL/F of ustekinumab was not impacted by gender. Population pharmacokinetic analysis showed that there was a trend towards a higher clearance of ustekinumab in patients who tested positive for antibodies to ustekinumab.

Dose linearity

The systemic exposure of ustekinumab (C_{max} and AUC) increased in an approximately dose-proportional manner after a single intravenous administration at doses ranging from 0.09 mg/kg to 4.5 mg/kg or following a single subcutaneous administration at doses ranging from approximately 24 mg to 240 mg in patients with psoriasis.

Single dose vs. multiple doses

Serum concentration-time profiles of ustekinumab were generally predictable after single or multiple subcutaneous dose administrations. Steady-state serum concentrations of ustekinumab were achieved by Week 28 after initial subcutaneous doses at Weeks 0 and 4 followed by doses every 12 weeks. The median steady-state trough concentration ranged from 0.21 μg/ml to 0.26 μg/ml (45 mg) and from 0.47 μg/ml to 0.49 μg/ml (90 mg). There was no apparent accumulation in serum ustekinumab concentration over time when given subcutaneously every 12 weeks.

Impact of weight on pharmacokinetics

In a population pharmacokinetic analysis, body weight was found to be the most significant covariate affecting the clearance of ustekinumab. The median CL/F in patients with weight > 100 kg was approximately 55% higher compared to patients with weight ≤ 100 kg. The median V/F in patients with weight > 100 kg was approximately 37% higher as compared to patients with weight ≤ 100 kg. The median trough serum concentrations of ustekinumab in patients with higher weight (> 100 kg) in the 90 mg group were comparable to those in patients with lower weight (≤ 100 kg) in the 45 mg group.

Special populations

No pharmacokinetic data are available in patients with impaired renal or hepatic function.

No specific studies have been conducted in elderly patients.

In the population pharmacokinetic analysis, there were no indications of an effect of tobacco or alcohol on the pharmacokinetics of ustekinumab.

5.3 Preclinical safety data

Non-clinical data reveal no special hazard (e.g. organ toxicity) for humans based on studies of repeated-dose toxicity and developmental and reproductive toxicity, including safety pharmacology evaluations. In developmental and reproductive toxicity studies in cynomolgus monkeys, neither adverse effects on male fertility indices nor birth defects or developmental toxicity were observed. No adverse effects on female fertility indices were observed using an analogous antibody to IL-12/23 in mice.

Dose levels in animal studies were up to approximately 45-fold higher than the highest equivalent dose intended to be administered to psoriasis patients and resulted in peak serum concentrations in monkeys that were more than 100-fold higher than observed in humans.

Carcinogenicity studies were not performed with ustekinumab due to the lack of appropriate models for an antibody with no cross-reactivity to rodent IL-12/23 p40.

6. PHARMACEUTICAL PARTICULARS

6.1 List of excipients

Sucrose

L-histidine

L-histidine monohydrochloride monohydrate

Polysorbate 80

Water for injections

6.2 Incompatibilities

In the absence of compatibility studies, this medicinal product must not be mixed with other medicinal products.

6.3 Shelf life

12 months

6.4 Special precautions for storage

Store in a refrigerator (2°C - 8°C). Do not freeze.

Keep the vial in the outer carton in order to protect from light.

6.5 Nature and contents of container

STELARA is supplied as a sterile solution in a single-use type I glass 2 ml vial closed with a coated butyl rubber stopper. STELARA is available in a 1 vial pack.

6.6 Special precautions for disposal and other handling

The solution in the STELARA vial should not be shaken. The solution should be visually inspected for particulate matter or discoloration prior to subcutaneous administration. The solution is clear to slightly opalescent, colourless to light yellow and may contain a few small translucent or white particles of protein. This appearance is not unusual for proteinaceous solutions. The product should not be used if the solution is discoloured or cloudy, or if foreign particulate matter is present. Before administration, STELARA should be allowed to reach a comfortable temparature for injection (approximately half an hour). STELARA does not contain preservatives; therefore any unused product remaining in the vial and the syringe should not be used. Detailed instructions for use are provided in the package leaflet.

Any unused product or waste material should be disposed of in accordance with local requirements.

7. MARKETING AUTHORISATION HOLDER

Janssen-Cilag International NV
Turnhoutseweg 30
2340 Beerse
Belgium

8. MARKETING AUTHORISATION NUMBER(S)

EU/1/08/494/001

9. DATE OF FIRST AUTHORISATION/RENEWAL OF THE AUTHORISATION

16th January 2009

10. DATE OF REVISION OF THE TEXT

Detailed information on this medicinal product is available on the website of the European Medicines Agency (EMEA) http://www.emea.europa.eu/

Stemetil Injection

(sanofi-aventis)

1. NAME OF THE MEDICINAL PRODUCT

Stemetil injection 1.25% w/v

2. QUALITATIVE AND QUANTITATIVE COMPOSITION

Each 1 ml of Stemetil injection contains 12.5 mg prochlorperazine mesilate.

3. PHARMACEUTICAL FORM

Colourless sterile solution.

4. CLINICAL PARTICULARS

4.1 Therapeutic indications

Stemetil is a potent phenothiazine neuroleptic.

Uses: The treatment of nausea and vomiting and in schizophrenia (particularly the chronic stage) and acute mania.

4.2 Posology and method of administration

Adults

For deep intramuscular injection.

Indication	**Dosage**
Treatment of nausea and vomiting	12.5 mg by deep i.m. injection followed by oral medication 6 hours later if necessary.
Schizophrenia and other psychotic disorders	12.5 mg to 25 mg b.i.d. or t.d.s. by deep i.m. injection until oral treatment becomes possible.

Children

Intramuscular Stemetil should not be given to children.

Elderly

A lower dose is recommended. Please see Special Warnings and Precautions for Use.

4.3 Contraindications

Known hypersensitivity to prochlorperazine or to any of the other ingredients. The use of Stemetil injection is contraindicated in children as it has been associated with dystonic reactions after the cumulative dose of 0.5 mg/kg.

4.4 Special warnings and precautions for use

Stemetil should be avoided in patients with liver or renal dysfunction, Parkinson's disease, hypothyroidism, cardiac failure, phaeochromocytoma, myasthenia gravis, prostate hypertrophy. It should be avoided in patients known to be hypersensitive to phenothiazines or with a history of narrow angle glaucoma or agranulocytosis.

Close monitoring is required in patients with epilepsy or a history of seizures, as phenothiazines may lower the seizure threshold.

As agranulocytosis has been reported, regular monitoring of the complete blood count is recommended. The occurrence of unexplained infections or fever may be evidence of blood dyscrasia (see section 4.8 below), and requires immediate haematological investigation.

It is imperative that treatment be discontinued in the event of unexplained fever, as this may be a sign of neuroleptic malignant syndrome (pallor, hyperthermia, autonomic dysfunction, altered consciousness, muscle rigidity). Signs of autonomic dysfunction, such as sweating and arterial instability, may precede the onset of hyperthermia and serve as early warning signs. Although neuroleptic malignant syndrome may be idiosyncratic in origin, dehydration and organic brain disease are predisposing factors.

Acute withdrawal symptoms, including nausea, vomiting and insomnia, have very rarely been reported following the abrupt cessation of high doses of neuroleptics. Relapse may also occur, and the emergence of extrapyramidal reactions has been reported. Therefore, gradual withdrawal is advisable.

In schizophrenia, the response to neuroleptic treatment may be delayed. If treatment is withdrawn, the recurrence of symptoms may not become apparent for some time.

Neuroleptic phenothiazines may potentiate QT interval prolongation which increases the risk of onset of serious ventricular arrhythmias of the torsade de pointes type, which is potentially fatal (sudden death). QT prolongation is exacerbated, in particular, in the presence of bradycardia, hypokalaemia, and congenital or acquired (i.e. drug induced) QT prolongation. The risk-benefit should be fully assessed before Stemetil treatment is commenced. If the clinical situation permits, medical and laboratory evaluations (e.g. biochemical status and ECG) should be performed to rule out possible risk factors (e.g. cardiac disease; family history of QT prolongation; metabolic abnormalities such as hypokalaemia, hypocalcaemia or hypomagnesaemia; starvation; alcohol abuse; concomitant therapy with other drugs known to prolong the QT interval) before initiating treatment with Stemetil and during the initial phase of treatment, or as deemed necessary during the treatment (see also sections 4.5 and 4.8).

Avoid concomitant treatment with other neuroleptics (see section 4.5).

In randomised clinical trials versus placebo performed in a population with elderly patients with dementia and treated with certain atypical antipsychotic drugs, a 3-fold increase of the risk of cerebrovascular events has been observed. The mechanism of such risk increase is not known. An increase in the risk with other antipsychotic drugs or other populations of patients cannot be excluded. Stemetil should be used with caution with stroke risk factors.

As with all antipsychotic drugs, Stemetil should not be used alone where depression is predominant. However, it may be combined with antidepressant therapy to treat those conditions in which depression and psychosis coexist.

Because of the risk of photosensitisation, patients should be advised to avoid exposure to direct sunlight.

To prevent skin sensitisation in those frequently handling preparations of phenothiazines, the greatest care must be taken to avoid contact of the drug with the skin (see section 4.8, below).

Postural hypotension with tachycardia as well as local pain or nodule formation may occur after i.m. administration.

It should be used with caution in the elderly, particularly during very hot or very cold weather (risk of hyper-, hypothermia).

The elderly are particularly susceptible to postural hypotension.

Stemetil should be used cautiously in the elderly owing to their susceptibility to drugs acting on the central nervous system and a lower initial dosage is recommended. There is an increased risk of drug-induced Parkinsonism in the elderly particularly after prolonged use. Care should also be taken not to confuse the adverse effects of Stemetil, e.g. orthostatic hypotension, with the effects due to the underlying disorder.

4.5 Interaction with other medicinal products and other forms of interaction

Adrenaline must not be used in patients overdosed with Stemetil (see section 4.9, below).

The CNS depressant actions of neuroleptic agents may be intensified (additively) by alcohol, barbiturates and other sedatives. Respiratory depression may occur.

Anticholinergic agents may reduce the antipsychotic effect of neuroleptics and the mild anticholinergic effect of neuroleptics may be enhanced by other anticholinergic drugs, possibly leading to constipation, heat stroke, etc.

Some drugs interfere with absorption of neuroleptic agents: antacids, anti-Parkinson drugs and lithium.

Where treatment for neuroleptic-induced extrapyramidal symptoms is required, anticholinergic antiparkinsonian agents should be used in preference to levodopa, since neuroleptics antagonise the antiparkinsonian action of dopaminergics.

High doses of neuroleptics reduce the response to hypoglycaemic agents, the dosage of which might have to be raised.

The hypotensive effect of most antihypertensive drugs especially alpha adrenoceptor blocking agents may be exaggerated by neuroleptics.

The action of some drugs may be opposed by phenothiazine neuroleptics; these include amfetamine, levodopa, clonidine, guanethidine, adrenaline.

Increases or decreases in the plasma concentrations of a number of drugs, e.g. propranolol, phenobarbital have been observed but were not of clinical significance.

Simultaneous administration of desferrioxamine and prochlorperazine has been observed to induce transient metabolic encephalopathy characterised by loss of consciousness for 48-72 hours.

There is an increased risk of arrhythmias when antipsychotics are used with concomitant QT prolonging drugs (including certain antiarrhythmics, antidepressants and other antipsychotics) and drugs causing electrolyte imbalance.

There is an increased risk of agranulocytosis when neuroleptics are used concurrently with drugs with myelosuppressive potential, such as carbamazepine or certain antibiotics and cytotoxics.

In patients treated concurrently with neuroleptics and lithium, there have been rare reports of neurotoxicity.

4.6 Pregnancy and lactation

There is inadequate evidence of safety in pregnancy. There is evidence of harmful effects in animals. Stemetil should be avoided in pregnancy unless the physician considers it essential. Neuroleptics may occasionally prolong labour and at such time should be withheld until the cervix is dilated 3-4 cm. Possible adverse effects on the neonate include lethargy or paradoxical hyperexcitability, tremor and low apgar score.

Phenothiazines may be excreted in milk, therefore breast feeding should be suspended during treatment.

4.7 Effects on ability to drive and use machines

Patients should be warned about drowsiness during the early days of treatment and advised not to drive or operate machinery.

4.8 Undesirable effects

Generally, adverse reactions occur at a low frequency; the most common reported adverse reactions are nervous system disorders.

Adverse effects:

Blood and lymphatic system disorders: A mild leukopenia occurs in up to 30% of patients on prolonged high dosage. Agranulocytosis may occur rarely: it is not dose related (see section 4.4, above).

Endocrine: Hyperprolactinaemia which may result in galactorrhoea, gynaecomastia, amenorrhoea; impotence.

Nervous system disorders: Acute dystonia or dyskinesias, usually transitory are commoner in children and young adults, and usually occur within the first 4 days of treatment or after dosage increases.

Akathisia characteristically occurs after large initial doses.

Parkinsonism is more common in adults and the elderly. It usually develops after weeks or months of treatment. One or more of the following may be seen: tremor, rigidity, akinesia or other features of Parkinsonism. Commonly just tremor.

Tardive dyskinesia: If this occurs it is usually, but not necessarily, after prolonged or high dosage. It can even occur after treatment has been stopped. Dosage should therefore be kept low whenever possible.

Insomnia and agitation may occur.

Eye disorders: Ocular changes and the development of metallic greyish-mauve coloration of exposed skin have been noted in some individuals mainly females, who have received chlorpromazine continuously for long periods (four to eight years). This could possibly happen with Stemetil.

Cardiac disorders: ECG changes include QT prolongation (as with other neuroleptics), ST depression, U-Wave and T-Wave changes. Cardiac arrhythmias, including ventricular arrhythmias and atrial arrhythmias, a-v block, ventricular tachycardia, which may result in ventricular fibrillation or cardiac arrest have been reported during neuroleptic phenothiazine therapy, possibly related to dosage. Pre-existing cardiac disease, old age, hypokalaemia and concurrent tricyclic antidepressants may predispose.

There have been isolated reports of sudden death, with possible causes of cardiac origin (see section 4.4, above), as well as cases of unexplained sudden death, in patients receiving neuroleptic phenothiazines.

Vascular disorders: Hypotension, usually postural, commonly occurs. Elderly or volume depleted subjects are particularly susceptible; it is more likely to occur after intramuscular injection.

Gastrointestinal disorders: dry mouth may occur.

Respiratory, thoracic and mediastinal disorders: Respiratory depression is possible in susceptible patients. Nasal stuffiness may occur.

Hepato-biliary disorders: Jaundice, usually transient, occurs in a very small percentage of patients taking neuroleptics. A premonitory sign may be sudden onset of fever after one to three weeks of treatment followed by the development of jaundice. Neuroleptic jaundice has the biochemical and other characteristics of obstructive jaundice and is associated with obstruction of the canaliculi by bile thrombi; the frequent presence of an accompanying eosinphilia indicates the allergic nature of this phenomenon. Treatment should be withheld on the development of jaundice (see section 4.4, above).

Skin and subcutaneous tissue disorders: Contact skin sensitisation may occur rarely in those frequently handling preparations of certain phenothiazines (see section 4.4, above). Skin rashes of various kinds may also be seen in patients treated with the drug. Patients on high dosage should be warned that they may develop photosensitivity in sunny weather and should avoid exposure to direct sunlight.

General disorders and administration site conditions: Neuroleptic malignant syndrome (hyperthermia, rigidity, autonomic dysfunction and altered consciousness) may occur with any neuroleptic (see section 4.4, above).

4.9 Overdose

Symptoms of phenothiazine overdosage include drowsiness or loss of consciousness, hypotension, tachycardia, ECG changes, ventricular arrhythmias and hypothermia. Severe extrapyramidal dyskinesias may occur.

If the patient is seen sufficiently soon (up to 6 hours) after ingestion of a toxic dose, gastric lavage may be attempted. Pharmacological induction of emesis is unlikely to be of any use. Activated charcoal should be given. There is no specific antidote. Treatment is supportive.

Generalised vasodilatation may result in circulatory collapse; raising the patient's legs may suffice. In severe cases, volume expansion by intravenous fluids may be needed; infusion fluids should be warmed before administration in order not to aggravate hypothermia.

Positive inotropic agents such as dopamine may be tried if fluid replacement is insufficient to correct the circulatory collapse. Peripheral vasoconstrictor agents are not generally recommended. Avoid the use of adrenaline.

Ventricular or supraventricular tachy-arrhythmias usually respond to restoration of normal body temperature and correction of circulatory or metabolic disturbances. If persistent or life threatening, appropriate anti-arrhythmic therapy may be considered. Avoid lidocaine and, as far as possible, long acting anti-arrhythmic drugs.

Pronounced central nervous system depression requires airway maintenance or, in extreme circumstances, assisted respiration. Severe dystonic reactions usually respond to procyclidine (5-10 mg) or orphenadrine (20-40 mg) administered intramuscularly or intravenously. Convulsions should be treated with intravenous diazepam.

Neuroleptic malignant syndrome should be treated with cooling. Dantrolene sodium may be tried.

5. PHARMACOLOGICAL PROPERTIES

5.1 Pharmacodynamic properties

Stemetil is a potent phenothiazine neuroleptic.

5.2 Pharmacokinetic properties

There is little information about blood levels, distribution and excretion in humans. The rate of metabolism and excretion of phenothiazines decreases in old age.

5.3 Preclinical safety data

There are no preclinical data of relevance to the prescriber which are additional to that already included in other sections of the SPC.

6. PHARMACEUTICAL PARTICULARS

6.1 List of excipients

Stemetil injection also contains the following excipients: sodium sulphite anhydrous (E221), sodium metabisulphite powder (E223), sodium chloride, ethanolamine and water for injections (non-sterilised).

6.2 Incompatibilities

None stated.

6.3 Shelf life

60 months.

6.4 Special precautions for storage

Protect from light. Discoloured solutions should not be used.

6.5 Nature and contents of container

Stemetil injection is supplied in colourless glass ampoules in packs of 10 × 1ml.

6.6 Special precautions for disposal and other handling

None.

Administrative Data

7. MARKETING AUTHORISATION HOLDER

Sanofi-aventis

One Onslow Street

Guildford

Surrey

GU1 4YS

UK

8. MARKETING AUTHORISATION NUMBER(S)

PL 04425/0590

9. DATE OF FIRST AUTHORISATION/RENEWAL OF THE AUTHORISATION

2nd October 2006

10. DATE OF REVISION OF THE TEXT

22 June 2007

11. Legal Classification

POM

Stemetil Syrup

(sanofi-aventis)

1. NAME OF THE MEDICINAL PRODUCT
Stemetil Syrup

2. QUALITATIVE AND QUANTITATIVE COMPOSITION
The active component of the Stemetil syrup is prochlorperazine mesilate 5 mg per 5 ml.

3. PHARMACEUTICAL FORM
A dark straw coloured syrup.

4. CLINICAL PARTICULARS

4.1 Therapeutic indications
Vertigo due to Meniere's Syndrome, labyrinthitis and other causes, and for nausea and vomiting from whatever cause including that associated with migraine. It may also be used for schizophrenia (particularly in the chronic stage), acute mania and as an adjunct to the short-term management of anxiety.

4.2 Posology and method of administration
Adults

Indication	Dosage
Prevention of nausea and vomiting	5 to 10 mg b.d. or t.d.s.
Treatment of nausea and vomiting	20 mg stat, followed if necessary by 10 mg two hours later.
Vertigo and Meniere's syndrome	5 mg t.d.s. increasing if necessary to a total of 30 mg daily. After several weeks dosage may be reduced gradually to 5-10 mg daily.
Adjunct in the short term management of anxiety	15-20 mg daily in divided doses initially but this may be increased if necessary to a maximum of 40 mg daily in divided doses.
Schizophrenia and other psychotic disorders	Usual effective daily oral dosage is in the order of 75-100 mg daily. Patients vary widely in response. The following schedule is suggested: Initially 12.5 mg twice daily for 7 days, the daily amount being subsequently increased by 12.5 mg at 4 to 7 days interval until a satisfactory response is obtained. After some weeks at the effective dosage, an attempt should be made reduce this dosage. Total daily amounts as small as 50 mg or even 25 mg have sometimes been found to be effective.

Children

Indication	Dosage
Prevention and treatment of nausea and vomiting	If it is considered unavoidable to use Stemetil for a child, the dosage is 0.25 mg/kg bodyweight two or three times a day. Stemetil is not recommended for children weighing less than 10 kg or below 1 year of age.

Elderly

A lower dose is recommended - please see Special Warnings and Precautions for Use.

4.3 Contraindications
Known hypersensitivity to prochlorperazine or to any of the other ingredients.

4.4 Special warnings and precautions for use
Stemetil should be avoided in patients with liver or renal dysfunction, Parkinson's disease, hypothyroidism, cardiac failure, phaeochromocytoma, myasthenia gravis, prostate hypertrophy. It should be avoided in patients known to be hypersensitive to phenothiazines or with a history of narrow angle glaucoma or agranulocytosis.

Close monitoring is required in patients with epilepsy or a history of seizures, as phenothiazines may lower the seizure threshold.

As agranulocytosis has been reported, regular monitoring of the complete blood count is recommended. The occurrence of unexplained infections or fever may be evidence of blood dyscrasia (see section 4.8 below), and requires immediate haematological investigation.

It is imperative that treatment be discontinued in the event of unexplained fever, as this may be a sign of neuroleptic malignant syndrome (pallor, hyperthermia, autonomic dysfunction, altered consciousness, muscle rigidity). Signs of autonomic dysfunction, such as sweating and arterial instability, may precede the onset of hyperthermia and serve as early warning signs. Although neuroleptic malignant syndrome may be idiosyncratic in origin, dehydration and organic brain disease are predisposing factors.

Acute withdrawal symptoms, including nausea, vomiting and insomnia, have very rarely been reported following the abrupt cessation of high doses of neuroleptics. Relapse may also occur, and the emergence of extrapyramidal reactions has been reported. Therefore, gradual withdrawal is advisable.

In schizophrenia, the response to neuroleptic treatment may be delayed. If treatment is withdrawn, the recurrence of symptoms may not become apparent for some time.

Neuroleptic phenothiazines may potentiate QT interval prolongation which increases the risk of onset of serious ventricular arrhythmias of the torsade de pointes type, which is potentially fatal (sudden death). QT prolongation is exacerbated, in particular, in the presence of bradycardia, hypokalaemia, and congenital or acquired (i.e. drug induced) QT prolongation. The risk-benefit should be fully assessed before Stemetil treatment is commenced. If the clinical situation permits, medical and laboratory evaluations (e.g. biochemical status and ECG) should be performed to rule out possible risk factors (e.g. cardiac disease; family history of QT prolongation; metabolic abnormalities such as hypokalaemia, hypocalcaemia or hypomagnesaemia; starvation; alcohol abuse; concomitant therapy with other drugs known to prolong the QT interval) before initiating treatment with Stemetil and during the initial phase of treatment, or as deemed necessary during the treatment (see also sections 4.5 and 4.8).

Avoid concomitant treatment with other neuroleptics (see section 4.5).

In randomised clinical trials versus placebo performed in a population with elderly patients with dementia and treated with certain atypical antipsychotic drugs, a 3-fold increase of the risk of cerebrovascular events has been observed. The mechanism of such risk increase is not known. An increase in the risk with other antipsychotic drugs or other populations of patients cannot be excluded. Stemetil should be used with caution with stroke risk factors.

As with all antipsychotic drugs, Stemetil should not be used alone where depression is predominant. However, it may be combined with antidepressant therapy to treat those conditions in which depression and psychosis coexist.

Because of the risk of photosensitisation, patients should be advised to avoid exposure to direct sunlight.

To prevent skin sensitisation in those frequently handling preparations of phenothiazines, the greatest care must be taken to avoid contact of the drug with the skin (see section 4.8, below).

It should be used with caution in the elderly, particularly during very hot or very cold weather (risk of hyper-, hypothermia).

The elderly are particularly susceptible to postural hypotension.

Stemetil should be used cautiously in the elderly owing to their susceptibility to drugs acting on the central nervous system and a lower initial dosage is recommended. There is an increased risk of drug-induced Parkinsonism in the elderly particularly after prolonged use. Care should also be taken not to confuse the adverse effects of Stemetil, e.g. orthostatic hypotension, with the effects due to the underlying disorder.

Children: Stemetil has been associated with dystonic reactions particularly after a cumulative dosage of 0.5 mg/kg. It should therefore be used cautiously in children.

4.5 Interaction with other medicinal products and other forms of interaction
Adrenaline must not be used in patients overdosed with Stemetil (see section 4.9, below).

The CNS depressant actions of neuroleptic agents may be intensified (additively) by alcohol, barbiturates and other sedatives. Respiratory depression may occur.

Anticholinergic agents may reduce the antipsychotic effect of neuroleptics and the mild anticholinergic effect of neuroleptics may be enhanced by other anticholinergic drugs, possibly leading to constipation, heat stroke, etc.

Some drugs interfere with absorption of neuroleptic agents: antacids, anti-Parkinson drugs and lithium.

Where treatment for neuroleptic-induced extrapyramidal symptoms is required, anticholinergic antiparkinsonian agents should be used in preference to levodopa, since neuroleptics antagonise the antiparkinsonian action of dopaminergics.

High doses of neuroleptics reduce the response to hypoglycaemic agents, the dosage of which might have to be raised.

The hypotensive effect of most antihypertensive drugs especially alpha adrenoceptor blocking agents may be exaggerated by neuroleptics.

The action of some drugs may be opposed by phenothiazine neuroleptics; these include amfetamine, levodopa, clonidine, guanethidine, adrenaline.

Increases or decreases in the plasma concentrations of a number of drugs, e.g. propranolol, phenobarbital have been observed but were not of clinical significance.

Simultaneous administration of desferrioxamine and prochlorperazine has been observed to induce transient metabolic encephalopathy characterised by loss of consciousness for 48-72 hours.

There is an increased risk of arrhythmias when antipsychotics are used with concomitant QT prolonging drugs (including certain antiarrhythmics, antidepressants and other antipsychotics) and drugs causing electrolyte imbalance.

There is an increased risk of agranulocytosis when neuroleptics are used concurrently with drugs with myelosuppressive potential, such as carbamazepine or certain antibiotics and cytotoxics.

In patients treated concurrently with neuroleptics and lithium, there have been rare reports of neurotoxicity.

4.6 Pregnancy and lactation
There is inadequate evidence of safety in pregnancy. There is evidence of harmful effects in animals. Stemetil should be avoided in pregnancy unless the physician considers it essential. Neuroleptics may occasionally prolong labour and at such time should be withheld until the cervix is dilated 3-4 cm. Possible adverse effects on the neonate include lethargy or paradoxical hyperexcitability, tremor and low apgar score.

Phenothiazines may be excreted in milk, therefore breast feeding should be suspended during treatment.

4.7 Effects on ability to drive and use machines
Patients should be warned about drowsiness during the early days of treatment and advised not to drive or operate machinery.

4.8 Undesirable effects
Generally, adverse reactions occur at a low frequency; the most common reported adverse reactions are nervous system disorders.

Adverse effects:

Blood and lymphatic system disorders: A mild leukopenia occurs in up to 30% of patients on prolonged high dosage. Agranulocytosis may occur rarely: it is not dose related (see section 4.4, above).

Endocrine: Hyperprolactinaemia which may result in galactorrhoea, gynaecomastia, amenorrhoea; impotence.

Nervous system disorders: Acute dystonia or dyskinesias, usually transitory are commoner in children and young adults, and usually occur within the first 4 days of treatment or after dosage increases.

Akathisia characteristically occurs after large initial doses.

Parkinsonism is more common in adults and the elderly. It usually develops after weeks or months of treatment. One or more of the following may be seen: tremor, rigidity, akinesia or other features of Parkinsonism. Commonly just tremor.

Tardive dyskinesia: If this occurs it is usually, but not necessarily, after prolonged or high dosage. It can even occur after treatment has been stopped. Dosage should therefore be kept low whenever possible.

Insomnia and agitation may occur.

Eye disorders: Ocular changes and the development of metallic greyish-mauve coloration of exposed skin have been noted in some individuals mainly females, who have received chlorpromazine continuously for long periods (four to eight years). This could possibly happen with Stemetil.

Cardiac disorders: ECG changes include QT prolongation (as with other neuroleptics), ST depression, U-Wave and T-Wave changes. Cardiac arrhythmias, including ventricular arrhythmias and atrial arrhythmias, a-v block, ventricular tachycardia, which may result in ventricular fibrillation or cardiac arrest have been reported during neuroleptic phenothiazine therapy, possibly related to dosage. Pre-existing cardiac disease, old age, hypokalaemia and concurrent tricyclic antidepressants may predispose.

There have been isolated reports of sudden death, with possible causes of cardiac origin (see section 4.4, above), as well as cases of unexplained sudden death, in patients receiving neuroleptic phenothiazines.

Vascular disorders: Hypotension, usually postural, commonly occurs. Elderly or volume depleted subjects are particularly susceptible; it is more likely to occur after intramuscular injection.

Gastrointestinal disorders: dry mouth may occur.

Respiratory, thoracic and mediastinal disorders: Respiratory depression is possible in susceptible patients. Nasal stuffiness may occur.

Hepato-biliary disorders: Jaundice, usually transient, occurs in a very small percentage of patients taking neuroleptics. A premonitory sign may be sudden onset of fever after one to three weeks of treatment followed by the development of jaundice. Neuroleptic jaundice has the biochemical and other characteristics of obstructive jaundice and is associated with obstruction of the canaliculi by bile thrombi; the frequent presence of an accompanying eosinphilia indicates the allergic nature of this phenomenon. Treatment should be withheld on the development of jaundice (see section 4.4, above).

Skin and subcutaneous tissue disorders: Contact skin sensitisation may occur rarely in those frequently handling preparations of certain phenothiazines (see section 4.4, above). Skin rashes of various kinds may also be seen in patients treated with the drug. Patients on high dosage should be warned that they may develop photosensitivity in sunny weather and should avoid exposure to direct sunlight.

General disorders and administration site conditions: Neuroleptic malignant syndrome (hyperthermia, rigidity, autonomic dysfunction and altered consciousness) may occur with any neuroleptic (see section 4.4, above).

4.9 Overdose

Symptoms of phenothiazine overdosage include drowsiness or loss of consciousness, hypotension, tachycardia, ECG changes, ventricular arrhythmias and hypothermia. Severe extrapyramidal dyskinesias may occur.

If the patient is seen sufficiently soon (up to 6 hours) after ingestion of a toxic dose, gastric lavage may be attempted. Pharmacological induction of emesis is unlikely to be of any use. Activated charcoal should be given. There is no specific antidote. Treatment is supportive.

Generalised vasodilatation may result in circulatory collapse; raising the patient's legs may suffice. In severe cases, volume expansion by intravenous fluids may be needed; infusion fluids should be warmed before administration in order not to aggravate hypothermia.

Positive inotropic agents such as dopamine may be tried if fluid replacement is insufficient to correct the circulatory collapse. Peripheral vasoconstrictor agents are not generally recommended. Avoid the use of adrenaline.

Ventricular or supraventricular tachy-arrhythmias usually respond to restoration of normal body temperature and correction of circulatory or metabolic disturbances. If persistent or life threatening, appropriate anti-arrhythmic therapy may be considered. Avoid lidocaine and, as far as possible, long acting anti-arrhythmic drugs.

Pronounced central nervous system depression requires airway maintenance or, in extreme circumstances, assisted respiration. Severe dystonic reactions usually respond to procyclidine (5-10 mg) or orphenadrine (20-40 mg) administered intramuscularly or intravenously. Convulsions should be treated with intravenous diazepam.

Neuroleptic malignant syndrome should be treated with cooling. Dantrolene sodium may be tried.

5. PHARMACOLOGICAL PROPERTIES

5.1 Pharmacodynamic properties

Stemetil is a potent phenothiazine neuroleptic.

5.2 Pharmacokinetic properties

There is little information about blood levels, distribution and excretion in humans. The rate of metabolism and excretion of phenothiazines decreases in old age.

5.3 Preclinical safety data

There are no preclinical data of relevance to the prescriber which are additional to that already included in other sections of the SPC.

6. PHARMACEUTICAL PARTICULARS

6.1 List of excipients

Sucrose, Polysorbate 80 (E433), banana flavour, caramel (E150a), anhydrous citric acid (E330), sodium citrate (E331), sodium benzoate (E211), sodium sulphite anhydrous (E221), sodium metabisulphite (E223), ascorbic acid L(+) (E300) and purified water.

6.2 Incompatibilities

None stated.

6.3 Shelf life

36 months.

6.4 Special precautions for storage

Store protected from light.

6.5 Nature and contents of container

Stemetil Syrup is available in amber glass bottles containing 100ml. Rolled on pilfer proof aluminium cap and a PVDC emulsion coated wad or HDPE/ Polypropylene child resistant cap with a tamper evident band.

6.6 Special precautions for disposal and other handling

None.

7. MARKETING AUTHORISATION HOLDER

Sanofi-aventis

One Onslow Street

Guildford

Surrey

GU1 4YS

UK

8. MARKETING AUTHORISATION NUMBER(S)

PL 04425/0595

9. DATE OF FIRST AUTHORISATION/RENEWAL OF THE AUTHORISATION

1 August 2006

10. DATE OF REVISION OF THE TEXT

4 April 2008

Legal Category

POM

Stemetil Tablets 5mg

(sanofi-aventis)

1. NAME OF THE MEDICINAL PRODUCT

Stemetil tablets 5mg

2. QUALITATIVE AND QUANTITATIVE COMPOSITION

The active component of the Stemetil tablets is prochlorperazine maleate BP 5 mg

3. PHARMACEUTICAL FORM

Stemetil tablets 5 mg and prochlorperazine tablets BP 5mg (1000 tablet pack): Off-white to pale cream coloured circular tablets for oral use. The tablets are marked on one face 'STEMETIL' around a centrally impressed '5', reverse face plain.

Prochlorperazine tablets BP 5mg ('own label' supplier for 84 and 1000 tablets): Off-white to pale cream coloured circular tablets for oral use. The tablets are marked on one face '4L1'', reverse face plain.

4. CLINICAL PARTICULARS

4.1 Therapeutic indications

Vertigo due to Meniere's Syndrome, labyrinthis and other causes, and for nausea and vomiting from whatever cause including that associated with migraine. It may also be used for schizophrenia (particularly in the chronic stage), acute mania and as an adjunct to the short-term management of anxiety.

4.2 Posology and method of administration

__Adults__

Indication	Dosage
Prevention of nausea and vomiting	5 to 10 mg b.d. or t.d.s.
Treatment of nausea and vomiting	20 mg stat, followed if necessary by 10 mg two hours later.
Vertigo and Meniere's syndrome	5 mg t.d.s. increasing if necessary to a total of 30 mg daily. After several weeks dosage may be reduced gradually to 5-10 mg daily.
Adjunct in the short term management of anxiety	15-20 mg daily in divided doses initially but this may be increased if necessary to a maximum of 40 mg daily in divided doses.
Schizophrenia and other psychotic disorders	Usual effective daily oral dosage is in the order of 75-100 mg daily. Patients vary widely in response. The following schedule is suggested: Initially 12.5 mg twice daily for 7 days, the daily amount being subsequently increased 12.5 mg at 4 to 7 days interval until a satisfactory response is obtained. After some weeks at the effective dosage, an attempt should be made reduce this dosage. Total daily amounts as small as 50 mg or even 25 mg have sometimes been found to be effective.

__Children__

Indication	Dosage
Prevention and treatment of nausea and vomiting	If it is considered unavoidable to use Stemetil for a child, the dosage is 0.25 mg/kg bodyweight two or three a day. Stemetil is not recommended for children weighing less than 10 Kg or below 1 year of age.

__Elderly__

A lower dose is recommended. Please see Special Warnings and Special Precautions for Use.

4.3 Contraindications

Known hypersensitivity to prochlorperazine or to any of the other ingredients.

4.4 Special warnings and precautions for use

Stemetil should be avoided in patients with liver or renal dysfunction, Parkinson's disease, hypothyroidism, cardiac failure, phaeochromocytoma, myasthenia gravis, prostate hypertrophy. It should be avoided in patients known to be hypersensitive to phenothiazines or with a history of narrow angle glaucoma or agranulocytosis.

Close monitoring is required in patients with epilepsy or a history of seizures, as phenothiazines may lower the seizure threshold.

As agranulocytosis has been reported, regular monitoring of the complete blood count is recommended. The occurrence of unexplained infections or fever may be evidence of blood dyscrasia (see section 4.8 below), and requires immediate haematological investigation.

It is imperative that treatment be discontinued in the event of unexplained fever, as this may be a sign of neuroleptic malignant syndrome (pallor, hyperthermia, autonomic dysfunction, altered consciousness, muscle rigidity). Signs of autonomic dysfunction, such as sweating and arterial instability, may precede the onset of hyperthermia and serve as early warning signs. Although neuroleptic malignant syndrome may be idiosyncratic in origin, dehydration and organic brain disease are predisposing factors.

Acute withdrawal symptoms, including nausea, vomiting and insomnia, have very rarely been reported following the abrupt cessation of high doses of neuroleptics. Relapse may also occur, and the emergence of extrapyramidal reactions has been reported. Therefore, gradual withdrawal is advisable.

In schizophrenia, the response to neuroleptic treatment may be delayed. If treatment is withdrawn, the recurrence of symptoms may not become apparent for some time.

Neuroleptic phenothiazines may potentiate QT interval prolongation which increases the risk of onset of serious ventricular arrhythmias of the torsade de pointes type, which is potentially fatal (sudden death). QT prolongation is exacerbated, in particular, in the presence of bradycardia, hypokalaemia, and congenital or acquired (i.e. drug induced) QT prolongation. The risk-benefit should be fully assessed before Stemetil treatment is commenced. If the clinical situation permits, medical and laboratory evaluations (e.g. biochemical status and ECG) should be performed to rule out possible risk factors (e.g. cardiac disease; family history of QT prolongation; metabolic abnormalities such as hypokalaemia, hypocalcaemia or hypomagnesaemia; starvation; alcohol abuse; concomitant therapy with other drugs known to prolong the QT interval) before initiating treatment with Stemetil and during the initial phase of treatment, or as deemed necessary during the treatment (see also sections 4.5 and 4.8).

Avoid concomitant treatment with other neuroleptics (see section 4.5).

Stroke: In randomised clinical trials versus placebo performed in a population of elderly patients with dementia and treated with certain atypical antipsychotic drugs, a 3-fold increase of the risk of cerebrovascular events has been observed. The mechanism of such risk increase is not known. An increase in the risk with other antipsychotic drugs or other populations of patients cannot be excluded. Stemetil should be used with caution in patients with stroke risk factors.

As with all antipsychotic drugs, Stemetil should not be used alone where depression is predominant. However, it may be combined with antidepressant therapy to treat those conditions in which depression and psychosis coexist.

Because of the risk of photosensitisation, patients should be advised to avoid exposure to direct sunlight.

To prevent skin sensitisation in those frequently handling preparations of phenothiazines, the greatest care must be taken to avoid contact of the drug with the skin (see section 4.8, below).

It should be used with caution in the elderly, particularly during very hot or very cold weather (risk of hyper-, hypothermia).

The elderly are particularly susceptible to postural hypotension.

Stemetil should be used cautiously in the elderly owing to their susceptibility to drugs acting on the central nervous system and a lower initial dosage is recommended. There is an increased risk of drug-induced Parkinsonism in the elderly particularly after prolonged use. Care should also be taken not to confuse the adverse effects of Stemetil, e.g. orthostatic hypotension, with the effects due to the underlying disorder.

Children: Stemetil has been associated with dystonic reactions particularly after a cumulative dosage of 0.5 mg/kg. It should therefore be used cautiously in children.

4.5 Interaction with other medicinal products and other forms of interaction

Adrenaline must not be used in patients overdosed with Stemetil (see section 4.9, below).

The CNS depressant actions of neuroleptic agents may be intensified (additively) by alcohol, barbiturates and other sedatives. Respiratory depression may occur.

Anticholinergic agents may reduce the antipsychotic effect of neuroleptics and the mild anticholinergic effect of neuroleptics may be enhanced by other anticholinergic drugs, possibly leading to constipation, heat stroke, etc.

Some drugs interfere with absorption of neuroleptic agents: antacids, anti-Parkinson drugs and lithium.

Where treatment for neuroleptic-induced extrapyramidal symptoms is required, anticholinergic antiparkinsonian agents should be used in preference to levodopa, since neuroleptics antagonise the antiparkinsonian action of dopaminergics.

High doses of neuroleptics reduce the response to hypoglycaemic agents, the dosage of which might have to be raised.

The hypotensive effect of most antihypertensive drugs especially alpha adrenoceptor blocking agents may be exaggerated by neuroleptics.

The action of some drugs may be opposed by phenothiazine neuroleptics; these include amfetamine, levodopa, clonidine, guanethidine, adrenaline.

Increases or decreases in the plasma concentrations of a number of drugs, e.g. propranolol, phenobarbital have been observed but were not of clinical significance.

Simultaneous administration of desferrioxamine and prochlorperazine has been observed to induce transient metabolic encephalopathy characterised by loss of consciousness for 48-72 hours.

There is an increased risk of arrhythmias when neuroleptics are used with concomitant QT prolonging drugs (including certain antiarrhythmics, antidepressants and other antipsychotics) and drugs causing electrolyte imbalance.

There is an increased risk of agranulocytosis when neuroleptics are used concurrently with drugs with myelosuppressive potential, such as carbamazepine or certain antibiotics and cytotoxics.

In patients treated concurrently with neuroleptics and lithium, there have been rare reports of neurotoxicity.

4.6 Pregnancy and lactation
There is inadequate evidence of safety in pregnancy. There is evidence of harmful effects in animals. Stemetil should be avoided in pregnancy unless the physician considers it essential. Neuroleptics may occasionally prolong labour and at such time should be withheld until the cervix is dilated 3-4 cm. Possible adverse effects on the neonate include lethargy or paradoxical hyperexcitability, tremor and low apgar score.

Phenothiazines may be excreted in milk, therefore breast feeding should be suspended during treatment.

4.7 Effects on ability to drive and use machines
Patients should be warned about drowsiness during the early days of treatment and advised not to drive or operate machinery.

4.8 Undesirable effects
Generally, adverse reactions occur at a low frequency; the most common reported adverse reactions are nervous system disorders.

Adverse effects:

Blood and lymphatic system disorders: A mild leukopenia occurs in up to 30% of patients on prolonged high dosage. Agranulocytosis may occur rarely: it is not dose related (see section 4.4, above).

Endocrine: Hyperprolactinaemia which may result in galactorrhoea, gynaecomastia, amenorrhoea; impotence.

Nervous system disorders: Acute dystonia or dyskinesias, usually transitory are commoner in children and young adults, and usually occur within the first 4 days of treatment or after dosage increases.

Akathisia characteristically occurs after large initial doses.

Parkinsonism is more common in adults and the elderly. It usually develops after weeks or months of treatment. One or more of the following may be seen: tremor, rigidity, akinesia or other features of Parkinsonism. Commonly just tremor.

Tardive dyskinesia: If this occurs it is usually, but not necessarily, after prolonged or high dosage. It can even occur after treatment has been stopped. Dosage should therefore be kept low whenever possible.

Insomnia and agitation may occur.

Eye disorders: Ocular changes and the development of metallic greyish-mauve coloration of exposed skin have been noted in some individuals mainly females, who have received chlorpromazine continuously for long periods (four to eight years). This could possibly happen with Stemetil.

Cardiac disorders: ECG changes include QT prolongation (as with other neuroleptics), ST depression, U-Wave and T-Wave changes. Cardiac arrhythmias, including ventricular arrhythmias and atrial arrhythmias, a-v block, ventricular tachycardia, which may result in ventricular fibrillation or cardiac arrest have been reported during neuroleptic phenothiazine therapy, possibly related to dosage. Pre-existing cardiac disease, old age, hypokalaemia and concurrent tricyclic antidepressants may predispose.

There have been isolated reports of sudden death, with possible causes of cardiac origin (see section 4.4, above), as well as cases of unexplained sudden death, in patients receiving neuroleptic phenothiazines.

Vascular disorders: Hypotension, usually postural, commonly occurs. Elderly or volume depleted subjects are particularly susceptible; it is more likely to occur after intramuscular injection.

Gastrointestinal disorders: dry mouth may occur.

Respiratory, thoracic and mediastinal disorders: Respiratory depression is possible in susceptible patients. Nasal stuffiness may occur.

Hepato-biliary disorders: Jaundice, usually transient, occurs in a very small percentage of patients taking neuroleptics. A premonitory sign may be sudden onset of fever after one to three weeks of treatment followed by the development of jaundice. Neuroleptic jaundice has the biochemical and other characteristics of obstructive jaundice and is associated with obstruction of the canaliculi by bile thrombi; the frequent presence of an accompanying eosinphilia indicates the allergic nature of this phenomenon. Treatment should be withheld on the development of jaundice (see section 4.4, above).

Skin and subcutaneous tissue disorders: Contact skin sensitisation may occur rarely in those frequently handling preparations of certain phenothiazines (see section 4.4, above). Skin rashes of various kinds may also be seen in patients treated with the drug. Patients on high dosage should be warned that they may develop photosensitivity in sunny weather and should avoid exposure to direct sunlight.

General disorders and administration site conditions: Neuroleptic malignant syndrome (hyperthermia, rigidity, autonomic dysfunction and altered consciousness) may occur with any neuroleptic (see section 4.4, above).

4.9 Overdose
Symptoms of phenothiazine overdosage include drowsiness or loss of consciousness, hypotension, tachycardia, ECG changes, ventricular arrhythmias and hypothermia. Severe extrapyramidal dyskinesias may occur.

If the patient is seen sufficiently soon (up to 6 hours) after ingestion of a toxic dose, gastric lavage may be attempted. Pharmacological induction of emesis is unlikely to be of any use. Activated charcoal should be given. There is no specific antidote. Treatment is supportive.

Generalised vasodilatation may result in circulatory collapse; raising the patient's legs may suffice. In severe cases, volume expansion by intravenous fluids may be needed; infusion fluids should be warmed before administration in order not to aggravate hypothermia.

Positive inotropic agents such as dopamine may be tried if fluid replacement is insufficient to correct the circulatory collapse. Peripheral vasoconstrictor agents are not generally recommended. Avoid the use of adrenaline.

Ventricular or supraventricular tachy-arrhythmias usually respond to restoration of normal body temperature and correction of circulatory or metabolic disturbances. If persistent or life threatening, appropriate anti-arrhythmic therapy may be considered. Avoid lidocaine and, as far as possible, long acting anti-arrhythmic drugs.

Pronounced central nervous system depression requires airway maintenance or, in extreme circumstances, assisted respiration. Severe dystonic reactions usually respond to procyclidine (5-10 mg) or orphenadrine (20-40 mg) administered intramuscularly or intravenously. Convulsions should be treated with intravenous diazepam.

Neuroleptic malignant syndrome should be treated with cooling. Dantrolene sodium may be tried.

5. PHARMACOLOGICAL PROPERTIES

5.1 Pharmacodynamic properties
Stemetil is a potent phenothiazine neuroleptic

5.2 Pharmacokinetic properties
There is little information about blood levels, distribution and excretion in humans. The rate of metabolism and excretion of phenothiazines decreases in old age.

5.3 Preclinical safety data
There are no pre-clinical data of relevance to the prescriber which are additional to that already included in other sections of the SPC.

6. PHARMACEUTICAL PARTICULARS

6.1 List of excipients
Stemetil tablets also contain the following excipients: lactose BP, starch maize BP, aerosil (E551), and magnesium stearate BP.

6.2 Incompatibilities
None stated.

6.3 Shelf life
60 months.

6.4 Special precautions for storage
Store protected from light.

6.5 Nature and contents of container
Stemetil tablets 5mg are available in PVDC coated UPVC/aluminium foil blisters containing 84 tablets.

6.6 Special precautions for disposal and other handling
None

7. MARKETING AUTHORISATION HOLDER
Sanofi-aventis
One Onslow Street
Guildford
Surrey
GU1 4YS
UK

8. MARKETING AUTHORISATION NUMBER(S)
PL 04425/0593

9. DATE OF FIRST AUTHORISATION/RENEWAL OF THE AUTHORISATION
9 January 2007

10. DATE OF REVISION OF THE TEXT
15 August 2007

11. LEGAL CLASSIFICATION
POM

Sterile Dopamine Concentrate BP Selectajet (International Medication Systems)

(International Medication Systems (UK) Ltd)

1. NAME OF THE MEDICINAL PRODUCT
Sterile Dopamine Concentrate BP Selectajet

2. QUALITATIVE AND QUANTITATIVE COMPOSITION
Dopamine Hydrochloride 40 mg/ml

For full list of excipients, see section 6.1.

3. PHARMACEUTICAL FORM
Solution for injection.

4. CLINICAL PARTICULARS

4.1 Therapeutic indications
For the correction of haemodynamic imbalances present in the shock syndrome due to myocardial infarction, trauma, endotoxic septicaemia, cardiac surgery, renal failure and chronic cardiac decompensation as in congestive failure.

4.2 Posology and method of administration
Adults, elderly and children over 12 years old:

Begin infusion at between 1 - 5 mcg/kg/min. Increase dose by 1 - 5 mcg/kg/min, as required every 10 - 30 minutes, up to 20 - 50 mcg/kg/min. Most patients can be maintained at 20mcg/kg/min or less. Doses in excess of 50mcg/kg/min have been used in advanced states of circulatory decompensation.

Patients with severe refractory chronic congestive heart failure should be started on 0.5 - 2mcg/kg/min and the dose increased by 1 - 3 mcg/kg/min as urinary output increases.

ECG, blood pressure and urine output should be monitored. Cardiac output and pulmonary wedge pressure should be monitored if possible.

Children under 12 years:

The safety and efficacy of dopamine in children has not been established.

4.3 Contraindications
Dopamine should not be used in patients with phaeochromocytoma, uncorrected tachyarrhythmias, or ventricular fibrillation.

4.4 Special warnings and precautions for use
Correct hypovolaemia, before administering dopamine if possible.

Administer dilute solution through as large a vein as possible, to minimise the risk of extravasation. A metering chamber or device should be used to accurately control dosage in drops/minute.

Dopamine infusion should be withdrawn gradually, to avoid unnecessary hypotension.

Patients with a history of occlusive vascular disease (e.g. atherosclerosis, arterial embolism, Raynaud's disease, cold injury, diabetic endarteritis and Buerger's disease) should be closely monitored for any changes in colour or temperature of the skin in the extremities. If ischaemia occurs and is thought to be the result of vasoconstriction, the benefits of continued dopamine infusion should be weighed against the risk of possible necrosis. This condition may be reversed by either decreasing the rate or discontinuing the infusion. IV administration of phentolamine mesylate 5-10 mg may reverse the ischaemia.

If excessive vasoconstriction (as indicated by a disproportionate rise in diastolic pressure and a marked decrease in pulse pressure) is observed, the infusion rate should be decreased or suspended and the patient observed closely.

As the effect of dopamine on impaired renal and hepatic function is not known, close monitoring is advised.

4.5 Interaction with other medicinal products and other forms of interaction
The action of dopamine is potentiated by monoamine oxidase inhibitors (MAOI's). In patients who have received MAOI's within the previous 2-3 weeks, the initial dopamine dose should be no greater than 10% of the usual dose.

The concurrent administration of dopamine in patients with a chronic use of selegiline (given for Parkinson disease) should be avoided.

The concurrent administration of cyclopropane or halogenated hydrocarbon anaesthetics may cause ventricular arrhythmias.

The cardiac effects of dopamine are antagonised by beta-adrenergic blocking agents such as propranolol and metoprolol.

The ergot alkaloids should be avoided because of the possibility of excessive vasoconstriction. Tricyclic antidepressants and guanethidine may potentiate the pressor response to dopamine.

Hypotension and bradycardia have been observed in patients receiving phenytoin.

Dopamine may increase the effect of diuretic agents.

Peripheral vasoconstriction may be antagonised by alpha-adrenergic blocking agents, such as phentolamine. Other vasodilators may also be useful in patients with heart failure, allowing greater inotropic and renal effects without the associated vasoconstriction. Care must be taken to avoid hypotension.

4.6 Pregnancy and lactation
The use of any drug in pregnant women or women of child-bearing potential requires that the expected benefit be carefully weighed against the possible risk to mother and child. Animal studies have shown no evidence of teratogenic effect. It is not known whether dopamine crosses the placenta or enters breast milk.

4.7 Effects on ability to drive and use machines
This drug is intended for use in life threatening situations.

4.8 Undesirable effects

Extravasation of dopamine into the tissues may cause local necrosis. The area should be infiltrated with 5-10mg phentolamine in 10-15mL saline.

The most frequent adverse reactions include ectopic beats, nausea, vomiting, tachycardia, anginal pain, palpitations, dyspnoea, headache, hypotension, hypertension and vasoconstriction. Other less frequent adverse reactions are aberrant ventricular conduction, bradycardia, piloerection, mydriasis, widened QRS complex, azotaemia, elevated blood pressure and diabetes insipidus. Peripheral ischaemic gangrene in patients with pre-existing vascular disease. Fatal ventricular arrhythmias have been reported on rare occasions.

4.9 Overdose

In case of accidental overdosage, as evidenced by excessive blood pressure elevation, reduce the rate of administration or temporarily discontinue dopamine until the patients condition stabilises. Since the duration of action of dopamine is quite short, no additional measures are usually necessary. If these measures fail to stabilise the patient's condition, use of the short-acting alpha- adrenergic blocking agent such as phentolamine should be considered.

5. PHARMACOLOGICAL PROPERTIES

5.1 Pharmacodynamic properties

ATC code: C01CA 04; adrenergic and dopaminergic agents

Dopamine is a catecholamine. It is an agonist for specific dopamine receptors in the CNS, renal and other vascular beds (vasodilation) and for b_1 adrenoceptors in the heart (positive introprope). At high doses it activates a-adrenoceptors (vasoconstriction).

5.2 Pharmacokinetic properties

The half life of an iv bolus of dopamine is about 2 minutes, thus it is given by continuous infusion. Steady state is reached within 5 - 10 minutes. On termination of the infusion, dopamine is cleared from the plasma with a half life of about 9 minutes.

Dopamine is widely distributed throughout the body, but does not cross the blood/brain barrier. Dopamine like all catecholamines is metabolised by monoamine oxidase (MAO) and catechol-O-methyl transerase (COMT), in the liver, kidney and plasma. A small amount of unchanged drug plus its main metabolites, homovanillic acid (HVA) and 3,4-dihydroxyphenyl acetic acid (DOPAC) are excreted in the urine.

5.3 Preclinical safety data

The LD_{50} values for IV dopamine hydrochloride have been determined as 290 mg/kg in mice and 38.8 mg/kg in rats; the animals suffered massive internal bleeding and pulmonary congestion.

Subacute toxicity tests in rats revealed prostatic hypertrophy with associated bladder distension and hydronephrosis. In animals given higher doses (570 mg/kg daily) weights of heart, kidneys and lung were significantly higher than in controls, the weight of the spleen was significantly lower. Dogs given dopamine continuously for two weeks suffered intractable vomiting. Subsequent examination showed an increase in weight of the adrenal glands in all animals and an increase in weight of the prostate gland in dogs given the higher doses, some of which also had small areas of myocardial necrosis.

6. PHARMACEUTICAL PARTICULARS

6.1 List of excipients

Sodium bisulphite

Water for Injection

6.2 Incompatibilities

Do not add dopamine to any alkaline diluent solution e.g. sodium bicarbonate, since the drug is inactivated by these solutions.

6.3 Shelf life

36 months

6.4 Special precautions for storage

Do not store above 25°C. Keep vial in the outer carton.

6.5 Nature and contents of container

The solution is contained in a USP type I glass vial with an elastomeric closure which meets all the relevant USP specifications. The product is available as 5 ml, 10 ml and 20ml.

6.6 Special precautions for disposal and other handling

Dopamine must be diluted before use. Appropriate diluents include 5% dextrose, sodium chloride 0.9% or compound sodium lactate. Incompatible with sodium bicarbonate or any other alkali solution.

Dopamine is stable for about 24 hours in sodium chloride or dextrose. It should be used as soon as possible after mixing.

The container is specially designed for use with the IMS Select-A-Jet injector.

Any unused product should be disposed of in accordance with local requirements.

7. MARKETING AUTHORISATION HOLDER

International Medication Systems (UK) Ltd.

208 Bath Road

Slough

Berkshire

SL1 3WE

UK

8. MARKETING AUTHORISATION NUMBER(S)

PL 03265/0027

9. DATE OF FIRST AUTHORISATION/RENEWAL OF THE AUTHORISATION

16th July 1979 / 24th August 2001

10. DATE OF REVISION OF THE TEXT

Approved: March 2009

Sterile Saline Solution (0.9%)

(GlaxoSmithKline UK)

1. NAME OF THE MEDICINAL PRODUCT

Sterile Saline Solution (0.9%)

2. QUALITATIVE AND QUANTITATIVE COMPOSITION

None

3. PHARMACEUTICAL FORM

Diluent containing sterile solution for the reconstitution of lyophilised vaccine preparations.

4. CLINICAL PARTICULARS

4.1 Therapeutic indications

For reconstitution of lyophilised vaccines.

4.2 Posology and method of administration

Subcutaneous or intramuscular injection.

4.3 Contraindications

As for the product to be reconstituted.

4.4 Special warnings and precautions for use

As for the product to be reconstituted.

4.5 Interaction with other medicinal products and other forms of interaction

As for the product to be reconstituted.

4.6 Pregnancy and lactation

As for the product to be reconstituted.

4.7 Effects on ability to drive and use machines

As for the product to be reconstituted.

4.8 Undesirable effects

As for the product to be reconstituted.

4.9 Overdose

As for the product to be reconstituted.

5. PHARMACOLOGICAL PROPERTIES

5.1 Pharmacodynamic properties

Not applicable.

5.2 Pharmacokinetic properties

Not applicable.

5.3 Preclinical safety data

Not applicable.

6. PHARMACEUTICAL PARTICULARS

6.1 List of excipients

Sodium Chloride

Water for Injection

6.2 Incompatibilities

As for the product to be reconstituted.

6.3 Shelf life

60 months.

6.4 Special precautions for storage

Protect from light, store between 2°C and 8°C. Do not freeze.

6.5 Nature and contents of container

Type I, Ph Eur glass syringes with or without needles, fitted with rubber stoppers. The stoppers are attached to a polypropylene or polystyrene plunger.

This diluent is for use with the following vaccines:

Hiberix	PL 10592/0120
ACWY Vax	PL 10592/0014

6.6 Special precautions for disposal and other handling

As for the product to be reconstituted.

7. MARKETING AUTHORISATION HOLDER

Smith Kline & French Laboratories Limited

Great West Road, Brentford, Middlesex TW8 9GS

Trading as:

GlaxoSmithKline UK, Stockley Park West, Uxbridge, Middlesex, UB11 1BT

Or

SmithKline Beecham Pharmaceuticals*

**At the time of printing, only the marketed trading style will be printed*

8. MARKETING AUTHORISATION NUMBER(S)

PL 00002/0236

9. DATE OF FIRST AUTHORISATION/RENEWAL OF THE AUTHORISATION

15 May 1998 / 28/01/2009

10. DATE OF REVISION OF THE TEXT

07/05/2009

Stesolid Rectal Tubes 10mg

(Actavis UK Ltd)

1. NAME OF THE MEDICINAL PRODUCT

Stesolid® rectal tubes 10 mg.

2. QUALITATIVE AND QUANTITATIVE COMPOSITION

Diazepam 4 mg/ml.

3. PHARMACEUTICAL FORM

Enema.

4. CLINICAL PARTICULARS

4.1 Therapeutic indications

Diazepam has anticonvulsant, sedative, and muscle relaxant properties. It is used in the treatment of severe anxiety and tension states, as a sedative and premedication, in the control of muscle spasm, and in the management of alcohol withdrawal symptoms.

Stesolid rectal tubes 10 mg may be used in acute severe anxiety and agitation, epileptic and febrile convulsions, tetanus, as a sedative in minor surgical and dental procedures, or in other circumstances in which a rapid effect is required but where intravenous injection is impracticable or undesirable.

Stesolid rectal tubes 10 mg may be of particular value for the immediate treatment of convulsions in infants and children.

4.2 Posology and method of administration

Sensitivity to diazepam varies with age.

Children above 1 year of age: 0.5 mg/kg body weight

Adults: 0.5 mg/kg body weight

Elderly patients: 0.25 mg/kg body weight

A maximum dose of 30 mg diazepam is recommended, unless adequate medical supervision and monitoring are available.

4.3 Contraindications

Myasthenia gravis, hypersensitivity to benzodiazepines, severe respiratory insufficiency, sleep apnoea syndrome, severe hepatic insufficiency and porphyria.

4.4 Special warnings and precautions for use

Tolerance

Some loss of efficacy to the hypnotic effects of diazepam may develop after repeated use for a few weeks.

Dependence

Use of benzodiazepines may lead to development of physical and psychic dependence upon these products. The risk of dependence increases with dose and duration of treatment; it is also greater in patients with a history of alcohol or drug abuse.

Once physical dependence has developed, abrupt termination of treatment will be accompanied by withdrawal symptoms. These may consist of headaches, muscle pain, extreme anxiety, tension, restlessness, confusion and irritability. In severe cases the following symptoms may occur: derealisation, depersonalisation, hyperacusis, numbness and tingling of the extremities, hypersensitivity to light, noise and physical contact, hallucinations or epileptic seizures.

Rebound insomnia and anxiety: a transient syndrome whereby the symptoms that led to treatment with a benzodiazepine recur in an enhanced form may occur on withdrawal of treatment. It may be accompanied by other reactions including mood changes, anxiety or sleep disturbances and restlessness. Since the risk of withdrawal phenomena/rebound phenomena is greater after abrupt discontinuation of treatment, it is recommended that the dosage is decreased gradually.

Psychiatric and paradoxical reactions

Reactions like restlessness, agitation, irritability, aggressiveness, delusion, rages, nightmares, hallucinations, psychosis, inappropriate behaviour and other adverse behavioural effects are known to occur when using benzodiazepines. Should this occur, use of the medicinal product should be discontinued.

They are more likely to occur in children and the elderly.

Specific patient groups

Benzodiazepines should not be given to children without careful assessment of the need to do so; the duration of treatment must be kept to a minimum. Elderly should be given a reduced dose (see Posology). A lower dose is also recommended for patients with chronic respiratory insufficiency due to the risk of respiratory depression. Benzodiazepines are not indicated to treat patients with severe hepatic insufficiency as they may precipitate encephalopathy.

Benzodiazepines are not recommended for the primary treatment of psychotic illness.

Benzodiazepines should not be used alone to treat depression or anxiety associated with depression (suicide may be precipitated in such patients).

In common with other benzodiazepines, the use of diazepam may be associated with amnesia and should not be used in cases of loss or bereavement as psychological adjustment may be inhibited.

Stesolid rectal tubes 10 mg should not be used in phobic or obsessional states, as there is insufficient evidence of efficacy and safety in such conditions.

Benzodiazepines should be used with extreme caution in patients with a history of alcohol or drug abuse.

4.5 Interaction with other medicinal products and other forms of interaction

- Not recommended: concomitant intake with alcohol.

The sedative effects may be enhanced when the product is used in combination with alcohol. This affects the ability to drive or use machines.

- Take into account: combination with CNS depressants.

Enhancement of the central depressive effect may occur in cases of concomitant use with antipsychotics (neuroleptics), hypnotics, anxiolytics/sedatives, antidepressant agents, narcotic analgesics, anti-epileptic products, anaesthetics and sedative antihistamines.

In the case of narcotic analgesics enhancement of the euphoria may also occur leading to an increase in psychic dependence.

Compounds which inhibit certain hepatic enzymes (particularly cytochrome P450) may enhance the activity of benzodiazepines. To a lesser degree this also applies to benzodiazepines that are metabolised only by conjugation.

4.6 Pregnancy and lactation

In animal studies administration of benzodiazepines during gestation has lead to cleft palate, CNS malformation and permanent functional disturbances in the offspring.

There is no evidence as to the safety of diazepam in human pregnancy. It should not be used, especially during the first and last trimesters, unless the benefit is considered to outweigh the potential risk.

In labour, high single doses or repeated low doses have been reported to produce hypotonia, poor sucking, and hyperthermia in the neonate, and irregularities in the foetal heart.

If benzodiazepines are prescribed to a woman of child-bearing potential, she should be warned to contact her physician regarding discontinuance of the product if she intends to become or suspects that she is pregnant.

If, for compelling medical reasons, the product is administered during the late phase of pregnancy, or during labour at high doses, effects on neonate, such as hypothermia, hypotonia and moderate respiratory depression, can be expected, due to the pharmacological action of the compound.

Infants born to mothers who took benzodiazepines chronically during the later states of pregnancy may have developed physical dependence and may be at some risk for developing withdrawal symptoms in the postnatal period.

Since benzodiazepines are found in breast milk, benzodiazepines should not be given to breast feeding mothers.

4.7 Effects on ability to drive and use machines

Sedation, amnesia, impaired muscular function may adversely affect the ability to drive or use machines. If insufficient sleep occurs, the likelihood of impaired alertness may be increased (see also Interactions).

4.8 Undesirable effects

The side effects of diazepam are usually mild and infrequent.

The most common side effects are drowsiness, light-headedness, unsteadiness, and ataxia. Elderly patients are particularly susceptible to these effects.

Rare side effects include hypotension, apnoea, gastrointestinal and visual disturbances, skin rashes, urinary retention, headache, confusion, vertigo, changes in libido, blood dyscrasias, jaundice, and respiratory depression.

Paradoxical reactions to the benzodiazepines, provoking excitement instead of sedation, have been reported.

4.9 Overdose

As with other benzodiazepines, overdose should not present a threat to life unless combined with other CNS depressants (including alcohol).

In the management of overdose with any medical product, it should be borne in mind that multiple agents might have been taken.

Overdose of benzodiazepines is usually manifested by degrees of central nervous system depression ranging from drowsiness to coma. In mild cases, symptoms include drowsiness, mental confusion and lethargy, in more serious cases, symptoms may include ataxia, hypotonia, hypotension, respiratory depression, rarely coma and very rarely death.

Emergency procedure is to secure adequate airway maintenance. Otherwise, the treatment is symptomatic. Intravenous fluids may be administered and Flumazenil may be useful as an antidote.

5. PHARMACOLOGICAL PROPERTIES

5.1 Pharmacodynamic properties

Pharmacotherapeutic group: Diazepam has anticonvulsant, sedative, and muscle relaxant properties.

5.2 Pharmacokinetic properties

Absorption: Diazepam is quickly absorbed from the rectal mucosa. The maximum serum concentration is reached within 17 minutes. Absorption is 100% compared with that of intravenous injection of diazepam.

5.3 Preclinical safety data

Not applicable.

6. PHARMACEUTICAL PARTICULARS

6.1 List of excipients

Benzoic acid

Ethanol

Propylene glycol

Sodium benzoate

Benzyl alcohol

Purified water.

6.2 Incompatibilities

None known.

6.3 Shelf life

30 months at 25°C.

6.4 Special precautions for storage

The storage temperature must not exceed 25°C.

6.5 Nature and contents of container

Carton containing sealed low density polyethylene tubes, single packed in aluminium laminated bags.

Package size: 5 × 2.5 ml

6.6 Special precautions for disposal and other handling

Not applicable.

Administrative Data

7. MARKETING AUTHORISATION HOLDER

Actavis Group PTC ehf.

Reykjavikurvegi 76-78

220 Hafnarfjordur

Iceland

8. MARKETING AUTHORISATION NUMBER(S)

PL -30306/0041

9. DATE OF FIRST AUTHORISATION/RENEWAL OF THE AUTHORISATION

26/06/2006

10. DATE OF REVISION OF THE TEXT

31/07/2007

Stesolid Rectal Tubes 5mg

(Actavis UK Ltd)

1. NAME OF THE MEDICINAL PRODUCT

Stesolid® rectal tubes 5 mg.

2. QUALITATIVE AND QUANTITATIVE COMPOSITION

Diazepam 2 mg/ml.

3. PHARMACEUTICAL FORM

Enema.

4. CLINICAL PARTICULARS

4.1 Therapeutic indications

Diazepam has anticonvulsant, sedative, and muscle relaxant properties. It is used in the treatment of severe anxiety and tension states, as a sedative and premedication, in the control of muscle spasm, and in the management of alcohol withdrawal symptoms.

Stesolid rectal tubes 5 mg may be used in acute severe anxiety and agitation, epileptic and febrile convulsions, tetanus, as a sedative in minor surgical and dental procedures, or in other circumstances in which a rapid effect is required but where intravenous injection is impracticable or undesirable.

Stesolid rectal tubes 5 mg may be of particular value for the immediate treatment of convulsions in infants and children.

4.2 Posology and method of administration

Sensitivity to diazepam varies with age.

Children above 1 year of age: 0.5 mg/kg body weight

Adults: 0.5 mg/kg body weight

Elderly patients: 0.25 mg/kg body weight

A maximum dose of 30 mg diazepam is recommended, unless adequate medical supervision and monitoring are available.

4.3 Contraindications

Myasthenia gravis, hypersensitivity to benzodiazepines, severe respiratory insufficiency, sleep apnoea syndrome, severe hepatic insufficiency and porphyria.

4.4 Special warnings and precautions for use

Tolerance

Some loss of efficacy to the hypnotic effects of diazepam may develop after repeated use for a few weeks.

Dependence

Use of benzodiazepines may lead to development of physical and psychic dependence upon these products. The risk of dependence increases with dose and duration of treatment; it is also greater in patients with a history of alcohol or drug abuse.

Once physical dependence has developed, abrupt termination of treatment will be accompanied by withdrawal symptoms. These may consist of headaches, muscle pain, extreme anxiety, tension, restlessness, confusion and irritability. In severe cases the following symptoms may occur: derealisation, depersonalisation, hyperacusis, numbness and tingling of the extremities, hypersensitivity to light, noise and physical contact, hallucinations or epileptic seizures.

Rebound insomnia and anxiety: a transient syndrome whereby the symptoms that led to treatment with a benzodiazepine recur in an enhanced form may occur on withdrawal of treatment. It may be accompanied by other reactions including mood changes, anxiety or sleep disturbances and restlessness. Since the risk of withdrawal phenomena/rebound phenomena is greater after abrupt discontinuation of treatment, it is recommended that the dosage is decreased gradually.

Psychiatric and paradoxical reactions

Reactions like restlessness, agitation, irritability, aggressiveness, delusion, rages, nightmares, hallucinations, psychosis, inappropriate behaviour and other adverse behavioural effects are known to occur when using benzodiazepines. Should this occur, use of the medicinal product should be discontinued.

They are more likely to occur in children and the elderly.

Specific patient groups

Benzodiazepines should not be given to children without careful assessment of the need to do so; the duration of treatment must be kept to a minimum. Elderly should be given a reduced dose (see posology). A lower dose is also recommended for patients with chronic respiratory insufficiency due to the risk of respiratory depression. Benzodiazepines are not indicated to treat patients with severe hepatic insufficiency as they may precipitate encephalopathy.

Benzodiazepines are not recommended for the primary treatment of psychotic illness.

Benzodiazepines should not be used alone to treat depression or anxiety associated with depression (suicide may be precipitated in such patients).

In common with other benzodiazepines, the use of diazepam may be associated with amnesia and should not be used in cases of loss or bereavement as psychological adjustment may be inhibited.

Stesolid rectal tubes 5 mg should not be used in phobic or obsessional states, as there is insufficient evidence of efficacy and safety in such conditions.

Benzodiazepines should be used with extreme caution in patients with a history of alcohol or drug abuse.

4.5 Interaction with other medicinal products and other forms of interaction

- Not recommended: concomitant intake with alcohol.

The sedative effects may be enhanced when the product is used in combination with alcohol. This affects the ability to drive or use machines.

- Take into account: combination with CNS depressants.

Enhancement of the central depressive effect may occur in cases of concomitant use with antipsychotics (neuroleptics), hypnotics, anxiolytics/sedatives, antidepressant agents, narcotic analgesics, anti-epileptic products, anaesthetics and sedative antihistamines.

In the case of narcotic analgesics enhancement of the euphoria may also occur leading to an increase in psychic dependence.

Compounds which inhibit certain hepatic enzymes (particularly cytochrome P450) may enhance the activity of benzodiazepines. To a lesser degree this also applies to benzodiazepines that are metabolised only by conjugation.

4.6 Pregnancy and lactation

In animal studies administration of benzodiazepines during gestation has lead to cleft palate, CNS malformation and permanent functional disturbances in the offspring.

There is no evidence as to the safety of diazepam in human pregnancy. It should not be used, especially during the first and last trimesters, unless the benefit is considered to outweigh the potential risk.

In labour, high single doses or repeated low doses have been reported to produce hypotonia, poor sucking, and hyperthermia in the neonate, and irregularities in the foetal heart.

If benzodiazepines are prescribed to a woman of child-bearing potential, she should be warned to contact her physician regarding discontinuance of the product if she intends to become or suspects that she is pregnant.

If, for compelling medical reasons, the product is administered during the late phase of pregnancy, or during labour at high doses, effects on neonate, such as hypothermia, hypotonia and moderate respiratory depression, can be expected, due to the pharmacological action of the compound.

Infants born to mothers who took benzodiazepines chronically during the later states of pregnancy may have developed physical dependence and may be at some risk for developing withdrawal symptoms in the postnatal period.

Since benzodiazepines are found in breast milk, benzodiazepines should not be given to breast feeding mothers.

4.7 Effects on ability to drive and use machines
Sedation, amnesia, impaired muscular function may adversely affect the ability to drive or use machines. If insufficient sleep occurs, the likelihood of impaired alertness may be increased (see also Interactions).

4.8 Undesirable effects
The side effects of diazepam are usually mild and infrequent.

The most common side effects are drowsiness, light-headedness, unsteadiness, and ataxia. Elderly patients are particularly susceptible to these effects.

Rare side effects include hypotension, apnoea, gastrointestinal and visual disturbances, skin rashes, urinary retention, headache, confusion, vertigo, changes in libido, blood dyscrasias, jaundice and respiratory depression.

Paradoxical reactions to the benzodiazepines, provoking excitement instead of sedation, have been reported.

4.9 Overdose
As with other benzodiazepines, overdose should not present a threat to life unless combined with other CNS depressants (including alcohol).

In the management of overdose with any medical product, it should be borne in mind that multiple agents might have been taken.

Overdose of benzodiazepines is usually manifested by degrees of central nervous system depression ranging from drowsiness to coma. In mild cases, symptoms include drowsiness, mental confusion and lethargy, in more serious cases, symptoms may include ataxia, hypotonia, hypotension, respiratory depression, rarely coma and very rarely death.

Emergency procedure is to secure adequate airway maintenance. Otherwise, the treatment is symptomatic. Intravenous fluids may be administered and Flumazenil may be useful as an antidote.

5. PHARMACOLOGICAL PROPERTIES

5.1 Pharmacodynamic properties
Pharmacotherapeutic group: Diazepam has anticonvulsant, sedative, and muscle relaxant properties.

5.2 Pharmacokinetic properties
Absorption: Diazepam is quickly absorbed from the rectal mucosa. The maximum serum concentration is reached within 17 minutes. Absorption is 100% compared with that of intravenous injection of diazepam.

5.3 Preclinical safety data
Not applicable.

6. PHARMACEUTICAL PARTICULARS

6.1 List of excipients
Benzoic acid
Ethanol
Propylene glycol
Sodium benzoate
Benzyl alcohol
Purified water.

6.2 Incompatibilities
None known.

6.3 Shelf life
30 months at 25°C.

6.4 Special precautions for storage
The storage temperature must not exceed 25°C.

6.5 Nature and contents of container
Carton containing sealed low density polyethylene tubes, single packed in aluminium laminated bags.

Package size: 5 × 2.5 ml

6.6 Special precautions for disposal and other handling
Not applicable.

Administrative Data

7. MARKETING AUTHORISATION HOLDER
Actavis Group PTC ehf.
Reykjavikurvegi 76-78
220 Hafnarfjordur
Iceland

8. MARKETING AUTHORISATION NUMBER(S)
PL 30306/0040

9. DATE OF FIRST AUTHORISATION/RENEWAL OF THE AUTHORISATION
01/06/2007

10. DATE OF REVISION OF THE TEXT
31/07/2007

Stiemycin

(Stiefel Laboratories (UK) Limited)

1. NAME OF THE MEDICINAL PRODUCT
Stiemycin 2.0% w/w.

2. QUALITATIVE AND QUANTITATIVE COMPOSITION
Erythromycin Base EP 2.46 w/w.

3. PHARMACEUTICAL FORM
Solution for topical use.

4. CLINICAL PARTICULARS

4.1 Therapeutic indications
Stiemycin is indicated for use in the treatment of acne vulgaris.

4.2 Posology and method of administration
To be applied to the affected area twice daily after washing with soap and water.

4.3 Contraindications
Stiemycin is contraindicated in patients with known sensitivity to any of the ingredients.

4.4 Special warnings and precautions for use
Avoid contact with eyes and other mucous membranes. Concomitant topical acne therapy should be used with caution because a cumulative irritant effect may occur.

4.5 Interaction with other medicinal products and other forms of interaction
None known.

4.6 Pregnancy and lactation
There is no evidence of hazard from erythromycin in human pregnancy. It has been in wide use for many years without apparent ill consequence.

4.7 Effects on ability to drive and use machines
None.

4.8 Undesirable effects
None.

4.9 Overdose
Not applicable.

5. PHARMACOLOGICAL PROPERTIES

5.1 Pharmacodynamic properties
Erythromycin suppresses *propionibacterium acnes*, a resident bacterial of sebaceous follicles, and as a result of this organism's role in the hydrolysis of triglycerides to free fatty acids, administration decreases fatty acid formation. This is thought to be responsible for its effectiveness in reducing acne lesion counts and the fatty acid to fatty ester ratios in acne patients.

5.2 Pharmacokinetic properties
Not applicable.

5.3 Preclinical safety data
None.

6. PHARMACEUTICAL PARTICULARS

6.1 List of excipients
Propylene Glycol
Ethanol Absolute
Laureth 4 (BRIJ 30).

6.2 Incompatibilities
None

6.3 Shelf life
Store in a cool place

6.4 Special precautions for storage
Store in a cool place

6.5 Nature and contents of container
Amber glass screw capped bottle of 25ml and 50ml.

6.6 Special precautions for disposal and other handling
There are no special instructions for use or handling of Stiemycin.

7. MARKETING AUTHORISATION HOLDER
Stiefel Laboratories (UK) Ltd
Eurasia Headquarters
Concorde Road
Maidenhead
SL6 4BY
UK

8. MARKETING AUTHORISATION NUMBER(S)
PL 0174/0047

9. DATE OF FIRST AUTHORISATION/RENEWAL OF THE AUTHORISATION
21 June 1988 / 21 June 1993

10. DATE OF REVISION OF THE TEXT
August 2009

Stilnoct 5mg, Stilnoct 10mg

(sanofi-aventis)

1. NAME OF THE MEDICINAL PRODUCT
Stilnoct 5mg
Stilnoct 10mg

2. QUALITATIVE AND QUANTITATIVE COMPOSITION
Stilnoct 5mg Tablets: Round white film coated tablets containing 5mg zolpidem tartrate.

Stilnoct 10mg Tablets: White to off-white film-coated oblong tablet, scored and engraved SN 10 on one side, containing 10mg zolpidem tartrate.

3. PHARMACEUTICAL FORM
Coated tablets for oral administration.

4. CLINICAL PARTICULARS

4.1 Therapeutic indications
The short-term treatment of insomnia in situations where the insomnia is debilitating or is causing severe distress for the patient.

4.2 Posology and method of administration
Route of administration: Oral

Zolpidem tartrate acts rapidly and therefore should be taken immediately before retiring, or in bed.

The recommended daily dose for adults is 10 mg.

The duration of treatment should usually vary from a few days to two weeks with a maximum of four weeks including tapering off where clinically appropriate.

As with all hypnotics, long-term use is not recommended and a course of treatment should not exceed four weeks.

Special Populations

Children

Safety and effectiveness of zolpidem in paediatric patients under the age of 18 years have not been established. Therefore, zolpidem should not be prescribed in this population (see Section 4.4 Special warnings and precautions for use).

Elderly

Elderly or debilitated patients may be especially sensitive to the effects of zolpidem tartrate therefore a 5mg dose is recommended. These recommended doses should not be exceeded.

Hepatic impairment

As clearance and metabolism of zolpidem tartrate is reduced in hepatic impairment, dosage should begin at 5mg in these patients with particular caution being exercised in elderly patients. In adults (under 65 years) dosage may be increased to 10mg only where the clinical response is inadequate and the drug is well tolerated.

4.3 Contraindications
Zolpidem tartrate is contraindicated in patients with a hypersensitivity to zolpidem tartrate or any of the inactive ingredients, obstructive sleep apnoea, myasthenia gravis, severe hepatic insufficiency, acute and/or severe respiratory depression. In the absence of data, zolpidem tartrate should not be prescribed for children or patients with psychotic illness.

4.4 Special warnings and precautions for use
Respiratory Insufficiency

As hypnotics have the capacity to depress respiratory drive, precautions should be observed if zolpidem is prescribed to patients with compromised respiratory function.

Hepatic Insufficiency: See section 4.2.

The cause of insomnia should be identified wherever possible and the underlying factors treated before a hypnotic is prescribed. The failure of insomnia to remit after a 7-14 day course of treatment may indicate the presence of a primary psychiatric or physical disorder, and the patient should be carefully re-evaluated at regular intervals.

Elderly: See dose recommendations.

Paediatric Patients:

Safety and effectiveness of zolpidem have not been established in patients below the age of 18 years. In an 8-week study in paediatric patients (aged 6-17 years) with insomnia associated with attention-deficit/hyperactivity disorder (ADHD), psychiatric and nervous system disorders comprised the most frequent treatment emergent adverse events observed with zolpidem versus placebo and included dizziness (23.5% vs. 1.5%), headache (12.5% vs. 9.2%), and hallucinations (7.4% vs. 0%). (See Section 4.2 Posology and method of administration).

Depression:

As with other sedative/hypnotic drugs, zolpidem tartrate should be administered with caution in patients exhibiting symptoms of depression. Suicidal tendencies may be present therefore the least amount of zolpidem that is feasible should be supplied to these patients to avoid the possibility of intentional overdosage by the patient. Pre-existing depression may be unmasked during use of zolpidem. Since insomnia may be a symptom of depression, the patient should be re-evaluated if insomnia persists.

Use in patients with a history of drug or alcohol abuse: Extreme caution should be exercised when prescribing for patients with a history of drug or alcohol abuse. These patients should be under careful surveillance when receiving zolpidem tartrate or any other hypnotic, since they are at risk of habituation and psychological dependence.

General information relating to effects seen following administration of benzodiazepines and other hypnotic agents which should be taken into account by the prescribing physician are described below.

Tolerance: Some loss of efficacy to the hypnotic effects of short-acting benzodiazepines and benzodiazepine-like agents like zolpidem may develop after repeated use for a few weeks

Dependence

Use of benzodiazepines or benzodiazepine-like agents like zolpidem may lead to the development of physical and psychological dependence. The risk of dependence increases with dose and duration of treatment; it is also greater in patients with a history of psychiatric disorders and/or alcohol or drug abuse.

These patients should be under careful surveillance when receiving hypnotics.

Once physical dependence has developed, abrupt termination of treatment will be accompanied by withdrawal symptoms. These may consist of headaches or muscle pain, extreme anxiety and tension, restlessness, confusion and irritability. In severe cases the following symptoms may occur: derealisation, depersonalisation, hyperacusis, numbness and tingling of the extremities, hypersensitivity to light, noise and physical contact, hallucinations or epileptic seizures.

Rebound insomnia

A transient syndrome whereby the symptoms that led to treatment with a benzodiazepine or benzodiazepine-like agent recur in an enhanced form, may occur on withdrawal of hypnotic treatment. It may be accompanied by other reactions including mood changes, anxiety and restlessness.

It is important that the patient should be aware of the possibility of rebound phenomena, thereby minimising anxiety over such symptoms should they occur when the medicinal product is discontinued. Since the risk of withdrawal phenomena or rebound has been shown to be greater after abrupt discontinuation of treatment, it is recommended that the dosage is decreased gradually where clinically appropriate.

There are indications that, in the case of benzodiazepines and benzodiazepine-like agents with a short duration of action, withdrawal phenomena can become manifest within the dosage interval, especially when the dosage is high.

Amnesia

Benzodiazepines or benzodiazepine-like agents such as zolpidem may induce anterograde amnesia. The condition occurs most often several hours after ingesting the product and therefore to reduce the risk patients should ensure that they will be able to have an uninterrupted sleep of 7-8 hours.

Other psychiatric and "paradoxical" reactions

Other psychiatric and paradoxical reactions like restlessness, exacerbated insomnia, agitation, irritability, aggression, delusion, anger, nightmares, hallucinations, psychosis, abnormal behaviour and other adverse behavioural effects are known to occur when using benzodiazepines or benzodiazepine-like agents. Should this occur, use of the product should be discontinued. These reactions are more likely to occur in the elderly.

Somnambulism and associated behaviours:

Sleep walking and other associated behaviours such as "sleep driving", preparing and eating food, making phone calls or having sex, with amnesia for the event, have been reported in patients who had taken zolpidem and were not fully awake. The use of alcohol and other CNS-depressants with zolpidem appears to increase the risk of such behaviours, as does the use of zolpidem at doses exceeding the maximum recommended dose. Discontinuation of zolpidem should be strongly considered for patients who report such behaviours (See Section 4.5 Interactions with other medicinal products and other forms of interaction; and Section 4.8 Undesirable effects).

4.5 Interaction with other medicinal products and other forms of interaction

- **Not recommended**: Concomitant intake with alcohol.

The sedative effect may be enhanced when the product is used in combination with alcohol. This affects the ability to drive or use machines.

- **Take into account**: Combination with CNS depressants.

Enhancement of the central depressive effect may occur in cases of concomitant use with antipsychotics (neuroleptics), hypnotics, anxiolytics/sedatives, antidepressant agents, narcotic analgesics, antiepileptic drugs, anaesthetics and sedative antihistamines.

Zolpidem tartrate appears to interact with sertraline. This interaction may cause increased drowsiness. Also, isolated cases of visual hallucinations were reported

In the case of narcotic analgesics enhancement of euphoria may also occur leading to an increase in psychological dependence.

Compounds which inhibit certain hepatic enzymes (particularly cytochrome P450) may enhance the activity of benzodiazepines and benzodiazepine-like agents.

Zolpidem tartrate is metabolised via several hepatic cytochrome P450 enzymes, the main enzyme being CYP3A4 with the contribution of CYP1A2. The pharmacodynamic effect of zolpidem tartrate is decreased when it is administered with rifampicin (a CYP3A4 inducer).

However when zolpidem tartrate was administered with itraconazole (a CYP3A4 inhibitor) its pharmacokinetics and pharmacodynamics were not significantly modified. The clinical relevance of these results is unknown.

Since CYP3A4 plays an important role in zolpidem tartrate metabolism, possible interactions with drugs that are substrates or inducers of CYP3A4 should be considered.

Others: When zolpidem tartrate was administered with ranitidine or cimetidine, no significant pharmacokinetic interactions were observed.

4.6 Pregnancy and lactation

Although animal studies have shown no teratogenic or embryotoxic effects, safety in pregnancy has not been established. As with all drugs zolpidem tartrate should be avoided in pregnancy particularly during the first trimester.

If the product is prescribed to a woman of childbearing potential, she should be warned to contact her physician about stopping the product if she intends to become or suspects that she is pregnant.

If, for compelling medical reasons, zolpidem tartrate is administered during the late phase of pregnancy, or during labour, effects on the neonate, such as hypothermia, hypotonia and moderate respiratory depression, can be expected due to the pharmacological action of the product.

Infants born to mothers who took benzodiazepines or benzodiazepine-like agents chronically during the latter stages of pregnancy may have developed physical dependence and may be at some risk of developing withdrawal symptoms in the postnatal period.

Small quantities of zolpidem tartrate appear in breast milk. The use of zolpidem tartrate in nursing mothers is therefore not recommended.

4.7 Effects on ability to drive and use machines

Vehicle drivers and machine operators should be warned that, as with other hypnotics, there may be a possible risk of drowsiness the morning after therapy. In order to minimise this risk a resting period of 7 to 8 hours is recommended between taking zolpidem tartrate and driving.

4.8 Undesirable effects

The following CIOMS frequency rating is used, when applicable:

Very common ⩾10%

Common ⩾ 1 and < 10%

Uncommon ⩾ 0.1 and < 1%

Rare ⩾0.01 and < 0.1%

Very rare < 0.01%

Not known: cannot be estimated based on available data.

There is evidence of a dose-relationship for adverse effects associated with zolpidem tartrate use, particularly for certain CNS and gastrointestinal events. As recommended in section 4.2, they should in theory be less if zolpidem tartrate is taken immediately before retiring, or in bed. They occur most frequently in elderly patients.

Immune system disorders

Not known: angioneurotic oedema

Psychiatric disorders

Common: hallucination, agitation, nightmare

Uncommon: confusional state, irritability

Not known: restlessness, aggression, delusion, anger, psychosis, abnormal behaviour, sleep walking (See Section 4.4), dependence (withdrawal symptoms, or rebound effects may occur after treatment discontinuation), libido disorder

Most of these psychiatric undesirable effects are related to paradoxical reactions

Nervous system disorders:

Common: somnolence, headache, dizziness, exacerbated insomnia, anterograde amnesia: (amnestic effects may be associated with inappropriate behaviour)

Not known: depressed level of consciousness

Eye disorders

Uncommon: diplopia

Gastro-intestinal Disorders

Common: diarrhoea

Hepatobiliary disorders

Not known: Liver enzymes elevated

Skin and subcutaneous tissue disorders

Not known: rash, pruritus, urticaria

Musculoskeletal and connective tissue disorders

Not known: muscular weakness

General disorders and administration site conditions

Common: fatigue

Not known: gait disturbance, drug tolerance, fall (predominantly in elderly patients and when zolpidem was not taken in accordance with prescribing recommendation)

4.9 Overdose

Signs and Symptoms:

In cases of overdose involving zolpidem tartrate alone or with other CNS-depressant agents (including alcohol), impairment of consciousness ranging from somnolence to coma and including fatal outcomes have been reported.

Management:

General symptomatic and supportive measures should be used. If there is no advantage in emptying the stomach, activated charcoal should be given to reduce absorption. Sedating drugs should be withheld even if excitation occurs.

Use of flumazenil may be considered where serious symptoms are observed.

Flumazenil is reported to have an elimination half-life of about 40 to 80 minutes. Patients should be kept under close observation because of this short duration of action; further doses of flumazenil may be necessary. However, flumazenil administration may contribute to the appearance of neurological symptoms (convulsions).

The value of dialysis in the treatment of an overdose has not been determined. Dialysis in patients with renal failure receiving therapeutic doses of zolpidem have demonstrated no reduction in levels of zolpidem.

In the management of overdose with any medicinal product, it should be borne in mind that multiple agents may have been taken.

5. PHARMACOLOGICAL PROPERTIES

5.1 Pharmacodynamic properties

(GABA-A receptor modulator selective for omega-1 receptor subtype hypnotic agent).

Zolpidem tartrate is an imidazopyridine which preferentially binds the omega-1 receptor subtype (also known as the benzodiazepine-1 subtype) which corresponds to GABA-A receptors containing the alpha-1 sub-unit, whereas benzodiazepines non-selectively bind both omega-1 and omega-2 subtypes. The modulation of the chloride anion channel via this receptor leads to the specific sedative effects demonstrated by zolpidem tartrate. These effects are reversed by the benzodiazepine antagonist flumazenil.

In animals: The selective binding of zolpidem tartrate to omega-1 receptors may explain the virtual absence at hypnotic doses of myorelaxant and anti-convulsant effects in animals which are normally exhibited by benzodiazepines which are not selective for omega-1 sites.

In man: zolpidem tartrate decreases sleep latency and the number of awakenings, and increases sleep duration and sleep quality. These effects are associated with a characteristic EEG profile, different from that of the benzodiazepines. In studies that measured the percentage of time spent in each sleep stage, zolpidem tartrate has generally been shown to preserve sleep stages. At the recommended dose, zolpidem tartrate has no influence on the paradoxical sleep duration (REM). The preservation of deep sleep (stages 3 and 4 - slow-wave sleep) may be explained by the selective omega-1 binding by zolpidem tartrate. All identified effects of zolpidem tartrate are reversed by the benzodiazepine antagonist flumazenil.

5.2 Pharmacokinetic properties

Zolpidem tartrate has both a rapid absorption and onset of hypnotic action. Bioavailability is 70% following oral administration and demonstrates linear kinetics in the therapeutic dose range. Peak plasma concentration is reached at between 0.5 and 3 hours.

The elimination half-life is short, with a mean of 2.4 hours (± 0.2 h) and a duration of action of up to 6 hours.

Protein binding amounts to 92.5% ± 0.1%. First pass metabolism by the liver amounts to approximately 35%. Repeated administration has been shown not to modify protein binding indicating a lack of competition between zolpidem tartrate and its metabolites for binding sites.

The distribution volume in adults is 0.54 ± 0.02 L/kg and decreases to 0.34 ± 0.05 L/kg in the very elderly.

All metabolites are pharmacologically inactive and are eliminated in the urine (56%) and in the faeces (37%).

Zolpidem tartrate has been shown in trials to be non-dialysable.

Plasma concentrations in elderly subjects and those with hepatic impairment are increased. In patients with renal insufficiency, whether dialysed or not, there is a moderate reduction in clearance. The other pharmacokinetic parameters are unaffected.

Zolpidem tartrate is metabolised via several hepatic cytochrome P450 enzymes, the main enzyme being CYP3A4 with the contribution of CYP1A2. Since CYP3A4 plays an important role in zolpidem tartrate metabolism, possible interactions with drugs that are substrates or inducers of CYP3A4 should be considered.

5.3 Preclinical safety data

No data of therapeutic relevance.

6. PHARMACEUTICAL PARTICULARS

6.1 List of excipients

Tablet core: Lactose monohydrate, Microcrystalline cellulose, Hypromellose, Sodium starch glycollate, Magnesium stearate.

Film coating: Hypromellose, Titanium dioxide (E171), Macrogol 400 (Stilnoct 10mg only), Polyethylene glycol 400 (Stilnoct 5mg only).

6.2 Incompatibilities
None known

6.3 Shelf life
Stilnoct 5mg: 3 years
Stilnoct 10mg: 4 years

6.4 Special precautions for storage
Stilnoct 5mg: Store in a dry place below 30°C
Stilnoct 10mg: No special precautions

6.5 Nature and contents of container
Stilnoct 5mg: Cartons of 28 tablets in PVC/foil blister strips.
Stilnoct 10mg: Cartons of 28 tablets in PVC/foil blister strips.

6.6 Special precautions for disposal and other handling
Please consult the package insert before use. Do not use after the stated expiry date on the carton and blister.

KEEP OUT OF THE REACH OF CHILDREN

7. MARKETING AUTHORISATION HOLDER
sanofi-aventis
One Onslow Street
Guildford
Surrey
GU1 4YS
UK

8. MARKETING AUTHORISATION NUMBER(S)
Stilnoct 5mg: PL11723/0323
Stilnoct 10mg: PL 04425/0619

9. DATE OF FIRST AUTHORISATION/RENEWAL OF THE AUTHORISATION
Stilnoct 5mg: 1st February 2003
Stilnoct 10mg: 27 January 2009

10. DATE OF REVISION OF THE TEXT
Stilnoct 5mg: August 2008
Stilnoct 10mg 27 January 2009

Legal Category: POM

Strattera 10mg, 18mg, 25mg, 40mg, 60mg or 80mg hard capsules.

(Eli Lilly and Company Limited)

1. NAME OF THE MEDICINAL PRODUCT
STRATTERA* ▼ 10mg, 18mg, 25mg, 40mg, 60mg or 80mg hard capsules.

2. QUALITATIVE AND QUANTITATIVE COMPOSITION
The active substance is atomoxetine hydrochloride. Each STRATTERA 10mg, 18mg, 25mg, 40mg, 60mg or 80mg capsule contains atomoxetine hydrochloride equivalent to 10mg, 18mg, 25mg, 40mg, 60mg or 80mg of atomoxetine.

For a full list of excipients, see section 6.1.

3. PHARMACEUTICAL FORM
Capsule, hard.

STRATTERA 10mg capsules are opaque white, imprinted with 'Lilly 3227' on the cap and '10mg' on the body in black ink.

STRATTERA 18mg capsules are gold (cap) and opaque white (body), imprinted with 'Lilly 3238' on the cap and '18mg' on the body in black ink.

STRATTERA 25mg capsules are opaque blue (cap) and opaque white (body), imprinted with 'Lilly 3228' on the cap and '25mg' on the body in black ink.

STRATTERA 40mg capsules are opaque blue, imprinted with 'Lilly 3229' on the cap and '40mg' on the body in black ink.

STRATTERA 60mg capsules are opaque blue (cap) and gold (body), imprinted with 'Lilly 3239' on the cap and '60mg' on the body in black ink.

STRATTERA 80 mg capsules are opaque brown (cap) and opaque white (body), imprinted with 'Lilly 3250' and '80 mg' in black ink.

4. CLINICAL PARTICULARS

4.1 Therapeutic indications
STRATTERA is indicated for the treatment of Attention-Deficit/Hyperactivity Disorder (ADHD) in children of 6 years and older and in adolescents as part of a comprehensive treatment programme. Treatment must be initiated by a specialist in the treatment of ADHD. Diagnosis should be made according to DSM-IV criteria or the guidelines in ICD-10.

Additional information for the safe use of this product: A comprehensive treatment programme typically includes psychological, educational, and social measures and is aimed at stabilising children with a behavioural syndrome characterised by symptoms which may include chronic history of short attention span, distractibility, emotional lability, impulsivity, moderate to severe hyperactivity, minor neurological signs, and abnormal EEG. Learning may or may not be impaired.

Pharmacological treatment is not indicated in all children with this syndrome and the decision to use the drug must be based on a very thorough assessment of the severity of the child's symptoms in relation to the child's age and the persistence of symptoms.

4.2 Posology and method of administration
For oral use. STRATTERA can be administered as a single daily dose in the morning, with or without food. Patients who do not achieve a satisfactory clinical response (tolerability or efficacy) when taking STRATTERA as a single daily dose might benefit from taking it as twice daily evenly divided doses in the morning and late afternoon or early evening.

Dosing of children/adolescents up to 70 kg body weight: STRATTERA should be initiated at a total daily dose of approximately 0.5mg/kg. The initial dose should be maintained for a minimum of 7 days prior to upward dose titration according to clinical response and tolerability. The recommended maintenance dose is approximately 1.2mg/kg/day (depending on the patient's weight and available dosage strengths of atomoxetine). No additional benefit has been demonstrated for doses higher than 1.2mg/kg/day. The safety of single doses over 1.8mg/kg/day and total daily doses above 1.8mg/kg have not been systematically evaluated. In some cases it might be appropriate to continue treatment into adulthood.

Dosing of children/adolescents over 70 kg body weight: STRATTERA should be initiated at a total daily dose of 40mg. The initial dose should be maintained for a minimum of 7 days prior to upward dose titration according to clinical response and tolerability. The recommended maintenance dose is 80mg. No additional benefit has been demonstrated for doses higher than 80mg (see section 5.1). The maximum recommended total daily dose is 100mg. The safety of single doses over 120mg and total daily doses above 150mg have not been systematically evaluated. In some cases it might be appropriate to continue treatment into adulthood.

Additional information for the safe use of this product: Atomoxetine should be used in accordance with national clinical guidance on treatment of ADHD where available.

In the study programme, no distinct withdrawal symptoms have been described. In cases of significant adverse effects, atomoxetine may be stopped abruptly; otherwise the drug may be tapered off over a suitable time period.

Where patients are continuing treatment with atomoxetine beyond 1 year, re-evaluation of the need for therapy by a specialist in the treatment of ADHD is recommended.

In adolescents whose symptoms persist into adulthood and who have shown clear benefit from treatment, it may be appropriate to continue treatment into adulthood. However, start of treatment with STRATTERA in adults is not appropriate.

Special Populations

Hepatic insufficiency: For patients with moderate hepatic insufficiency (Child-Pugh class B), initial and target doses should be reduced to 50% of the usual dose. For patients with severe hepatic insufficiency (Child-Pugh class C), initial dose and target doses should be reduced to 25% of usual dose (see section 5.2).

Renal insufficiency: Subjects with end-stage renal disease had higher systemic exposure to atomoxetine than healthy subjects (about a 65% increase), but there was no difference when exposure was corrected for mg/kg dose. STRATTERA can therefore be administered to ADHD patients with end-stage renal disease or lesser degrees of renal insufficiency using the usual dosing regimen. Atomoxetine may exacerbate hypertension in patients with end-stage renal disease (see section 5.2).

Approximately 7% of Caucasians have a genotype corresponding to a non-functional CYP2D6 enzyme (called CYP2D6 poor metabolisers). Patients with this genotype have a several-fold higher exposure to atomoxetine when compared to patients with a functional enzyme. Poor metabolisers are therefore at higher risk of adverse events (see section 4.8 and section 5.2). For patients with a known poor metaboliser genotype, a lower starting dose and slower up titration of the dose may be considered.

Elderly patients: Not applicable.

Children under six years of age: The safety and efficacy of STRATTERA in children under 6 years of age have not been established. Therefore, STRATTERA should not be used in children under 6 years of age (see section 4.4).

4.3 Contraindications
Hypersensitivity to atomoxetine or to any of the excipients.

Atomoxetine should not be used in combination with monoamine oxidase inhibitors (MAOIs). Atomoxetine should not be used within a minimum of 2 weeks after discontinuing therapy with a MAOI. Treatment with a MAOI should not be initiated within 2 weeks after discontinuing atomoxetine.

Atomoxetine should not be used in patients with narrow-angle glaucoma, as in clinical trials the use of atomoxetine was associated with an increased incidence of mydriasis.

4.4 Special warnings and precautions for use
Possible allergic events: Although uncommon, allergic reactions, including rash, angioneurotic oedema, and urticaria, have been reported in patients taking atomoxetine.

Sudden death and pre-existing structural cardiac abnormalities or other serious heart problems: Sudden death has been reported in children and adolescents with structural cardiac abnormalities who were taking atomoxetine at usual doses. Although some serious structural cardiac abnormalities alone carry an increased risk of sudden death, atomoxetine should only be used with caution in children or adolescents with known serious structural cardiac abnormalities and in consultation with a cardiac specialist.

Cardiovascular effects: Many patients taking atomoxetine experience a modest increase in pulse (mean <10 bpm) and/or increase in blood pressure (mean <5 mmHg) (see section 4.8). For most patients, these changes are not clinically important. Atomoxetine should be used with caution in patients with hypertension, tachycardia, or cardiovascular or cerebrovascular disease. Pulse and blood pressure should be measured periodically while on therapy. Orthostatic hypotension has also been reported. Use with caution in any condition that may predispose patients to hypotension.

Atomoxetine should be used with caution in patients with congenital or acquired long QT or a family history of QT prolongation (see section 4.5 and section 4.8).

Hepatic effects: STRATTERA should be discontinued in patients with jaundice or laboratory evidence of liver injury, and should not be restarted. Very rarely, liver toxicity, manifested by elevated hepatic enzymes and bilirubin with jaundice, has been reported.

Growth and development: Growth and development should be monitored during treatment with atomoxetine. Patients requiring long-term therapy should be monitored and consideration should be given to dose reduction or interrupting therapy in patients who are not growing or gaining weight satisfactorily.

Clinical data do not suggest a deleterious effect of atomoxetine on cognition or sexual maturation; however, the amount of available long-term data is limited. Therefore, patients requiring long-term therapy should be carefully monitored.

Suicide-related behaviour: Suicide-related behaviour (suicide attempts and suicidal ideation) has been reported in patients treated with atomoxetine. In double-blind clinical trials, suicide-related behaviours were uncommon, but more frequently observed among children and adolescents treated with atomoxetine compared to those treated with placebo, where there were no events. Patients who are being treated for ADHD should be carefully monitored for the appearance or worsening of suicide-related behaviour.

Psychotic or manic symptoms: Treatment-emergent psychotic or manic symptoms, e.g., hallucinations, delusional thinking, mania or agitation in children and adolescents without a prior history of psychotic illness or mania can be caused by atomoxetine at usual doses. If such symptoms occur, consideration should be given to a possible causal role of atomoxetine, and discontinuation of treatment should be considered. The possibility that STRATTERA will cause the exacerbation of pre-existing psychotic or manic symptoms cannot be excluded.

Aggressive behaviour, hostility or emotional lability: Hostility (predominantly aggression, oppositional behaviour and anger) and emotional lability were more frequently observed in clinical trials among children and adolescents treated with STRATTERA compared to those treated with placebo. Patients should be closely monitored for the appearance or worsening of aggressive behaviour, hostility or emotional lability.

Seizures: Seizures are a potential risk with atomoxetine. Atomoxetine should be introduced with caution in patients with a history of seizure. Discontinuation of atomoxetine should be considered in any patient developing a seizure or if there is an increase in seizure frequency where no other cause is identified.

Children under six years of age: STRATTERA should not be used in patients less than six years of age as efficacy and safety have not been established in this age group.

Other indications: STRATTERA is not indicated for the treatment of major depressive episodes and/or anxiety, as the results of clinical trials that were conducted in adults did not show any effect compared to placebo and therefore were negative.

4.5 Interaction with other medicinal products and other forms of interaction
Effects of Other Drugs on Atomoxetine

MAOIs: Atomoxetine should not be used with MAOIs (see section 4.3).

CYP2D6 inhibitors (SSRIs [e.g., fluoxetine, paroxetine, quinidine, terbinafine]): Atomoxetine is primarily metabolised by the CYP2D6 pathway to 4-hydroxyatomoxetine. In CYP2D6 extensive metaboliser patients, potent inhibitors of CYP2D6 increase atomoxetine steady-state plasma concentrations to exposures similar to those observed in CYP2D6 poor metaboliser patients. In extensive metaboliser individuals treated with paroxetine or fluoxetine, the

AUC of atomoxetine is approximately 6- to 8-fold and $C_{ss,max}$ is about 3- to 4-fold greater than atomoxetine alone. Dose adjustment and slower titration of atomoxetine may be necessary in those patients who are also taking CYP2D6 inhibitor drugs. If a CYP2D6 inhibitor is prescribed or discontinued after titration to the appropriate atomoxetine dose has occurred, the clinical response and tolerability should be re-evaluated for that patient to determine if dose adjustment is needed.

Caution is advised when combining atomoxetine with potent inhibitors of cytochrome P450 enzymes other than CYP2D6 in patients who are poor CYP2D6 metabolisers as the risk of clinically relevant increases in atomoxetine exposure *in vivo* is unknown.

Salbutamol: Atomoxetine should be administered with caution to patients being treated with high dose nebulised or systemically administered (oral or intravenous) salbutamol (or other beta$_2$ agonists) because the action of salbutamol on the cardiovascular system can be potentiated. Systemically administered salbutamol (600 µg i.v. over 2 hrs) induced increases in heart rate and blood pressure. These effects were potentiated by atomoxetine (60 mg twice daily for 5 days) and were most marked after the initial co-administration of salbutamol and atomoxetine. In a study of healthy Asian adults who were extensive atomoxetine metabolisers, the effects on blood pressure and heart rate of a standard inhaled dose of salbutamol (200 µg) were not clinically significant compared to intravenous administration and not increased by the short-term co-administration of atomoxetine (80 mg once daily for 5 days). Heart rate after multiple inhalations of salbutamol (800 µg) was similar in the presence or absence of atomoxetine.

There is the potential for an increased risk of QT interval prolongation when atomoxetine is administered with other QT prolonging drugs (such as neuroleptics, class IA and III anti-arrhythmics, moxifloxacin, erythromycin, methadone, mefloquine, tricyclic antidepressants, lithium, or cisapride), drugs that cause electrolyte imbalance (such as thiazide diuretics), and drugs that inhibit CYP2D6.

Seizures are a potential risk with atomoxetine. Caution is advised with concomitant use of medicinal drugs which are known to lower the seizure threshold (such as antidepressants, neuroleptics, mefloquine, bupropion, or tramadol) (see section 4.4).

Pressor agents: Because of possible effects on blood pressure, atomoxetine should be used cautiously with pressor agents.

Drugs that affect noradrenaline: Drugs that affect noradrenaline should be used cautiously when co-administered with atomoxetine because of the potential for additive or synergistic pharmacological effects. Examples include antidepressants, such as imipramine, venlafaxine, and mirtazapine, or the decongestants pseudoephedrine or phenylephrine.

Drugs that affect gastric pH: Drugs that elevate gastric pH (magnesium hydroxide/aluminium hydroxide, omeprazole) had no effect on atomoxetine bioavailability.

Drugs highly bound to plasma protein: In vitro drug-displacement studies were conducted with atomoxetine and other highly-bound drugs at therapeutic concentrations. Warfarin, acetylsalicylic acid, phenytoin, or diazepam did not affect the binding of atomoxetine to human albumin. Similarly, atomoxetine did not affect the binding of these compounds to human albumin.

Effects of Atomoxetine on Other Drugs

Cytochrome P450 enzymes: Atomoxetine did not cause clinically significant inhibition or induction of cytochrome P450 enzymes, including CYP1A2, CYP3A, CYP2D6, and CYP2C9. *In vitro* studies indicate that atomoxetine does not cause clinically significant induction of CYP1A2 and CYP3A.

4.6 Pregnancy and lactation

For atomoxetine, no clinical data on exposed pregnancies are available.

Animal studies in general do not indicate direct harmful effects with respect to pregnancy, embryonal/foetal development, parturition, or postnatal development (see section 5.3).

Atomoxetine should not be used during pregnancy unless the potential benefit justifies the potential risk to the foetus.

Atomoxetine and/or its metabolites were excreted in the milk of rats. It is not known if atomoxetine is excreted in human milk. Because of the lack of data, atomoxetine should be avoided during breast-feeding.

4.7 Effects on ability to drive and use machines

No studies on the effects on the ability to drive and use machines have been performed. Atomoxetine was associated with increased rates of fatigue relative to placebo. In paediatric patients only, atomoxetine was associated with increased rates of somnolence relative to placebo. Patients should be advised to use caution when driving a car or operating hazardous machinery until they are reasonably certain that their performance is not affected by atomoxetine.

4.8 Undesirable effects

Children and adolescents: In paediatric placebo-controlled trials, headache, abdominal pain[1] and decreased appetite are the adverse events most commonly associated with atomoxetine, and are reported by about 19%, 18% and 16% of patients, respectively, but seldom lead to drug discontinuation (discontinuation rates are 0.1% for headache, 0.2 % for abdominal pain and 0.0% for decreased appetite). Abdominal pain and decreased appetite are usually transient.

Associated with decreased appetite, some patients lost weight early in therapy (average about 0.5 kg), and effects were greatest at the highest doses. After an initial decrease in weight, patients treated with atomoxetine showed a mean increase in weight during long-term treatment. Growth rates (weight and height) after 2 years of treatment are near normal (see section 4.4).

Nausea, vomiting and somnolence[2] can occur in about 10% to 11% of patients, particularly during the first month of therapy. However, these episodes were usually mild to moderate in severity and transient, and did not result in a significant number of discontinuations from therapy (discontinuation rates ⩽ 0.5%).

In paediatric placebo-controlled trials, patients taking atomoxetine experienced a mean increase in heart rate of about 6 beats/minute and mean increases in systolic and diastolic blood pressure of about 2 mmHg compared with placebo. In adult placebo-controlled trials, patients taking atomoxetine experienced a mean increase in heart rate of 5 beats/minute and mean increases in systolic (about 2 mmHg) and diastolic (about 1 mmHg) blood pressures compared with placebo.

Because of its effect on noradrenergic tone, orthostatic hypotension (0.2%) and syncope (0.8%) have been reported in patients taking atomoxetine. Atomoxetine should be used with caution in any condition that may predispose patients to hypotension.

The following table of undesirable effects is based on adverse event reporting and laboratory investigations from clinical trials in child and adolescent patients and spontaneous reporting from children/adolescents and adults post-marketing:

Table: **Adverse Reactions**

Frequency estimate: Very common (⩾1/10), common (⩾1/100 to <1/10), uncommon (⩾1/1,000 to <1/100), rare (⩾1/10,000 to <1/1,000), very rare (<1/10,000), data from spontaneous reports (frequency not known – cannot be estimated from the available data).

(see Table 1 below)

CYP2D6 poor metabolisers (PM): The following adverse events occurred in at least 2% of CYP2D6 poor metaboliser (PM) patients and were statistically significantly more frequent in PM patients compared with CYP2D6 extensive metaboliser (EM) patients: appetite decreased (24.1% of PMs, 17.0% of EMs); insomnia combined (including insomnia, middle insomnia and initial insomnia, 14.9% of PMs, 9.7% of EMs); depression combined (including depression, major depression, depressive symptom, depressed mood and dysphoria, 6.5% of PMs and 4.1% of EMs), weight decreased (7.3% of PMs, 4.4% of EMs), constipation 6.8% of PMs, 4.3% of EMs); tremor (4.5% of PMs, 0.9% of EMs); sedation (3.9% of PMs, 2.1% of EMs); excoriation (3.9% of PMs, 1.7% of EMs); enuresis (3.0% of PMs, 1.2% of EMs); conjunctivitis (2.5% of PMs, 1.2% of EMs); syncope (2.5% of PMs, 0.7% of EMs); early morning awakening (2.3% of PMs, 0.8% of EMs); mydriasis (2.0% of PMs, 0.6% of EMs). The following event did not meet the above criteria but is noteworthy: generalised anxiety disorder (0.8% of PMs and 0.1% of EMs). In addition, in trials lasting up to 10 weeks, weight loss was more pronounced in PM patients (mean of 0.6 kg in EM and 1.1kg in PM).

Adults: In adults, the adverse events reported most frequently with atomoxetine treatment were gastro-intestinal and insomnia. A complaint of urinary retention or urinary hesitancy in adults should be considered potentially related to atomoxetine. No serious safety concerns were observed during acute or long-term treatment.

The following table of undesirable effects is based on adverse event reporting and laboratory investigations from clinical trials in adults and spontaneous reporting from children/adolescents and adults post-marketing:

Table: **Adverse Reactions**

Frequency estimate: Very common (⩾1/10), common (⩾1/100 to <1/10), uncommon (⩾1/1,000 to <1/100), rare (⩾1/10,000 to <1/1,000), very rare (<1/10,000), data from spontaneous reports (frequency not known – cannot be estimated from the available data).

(see Table 2 on next page)

4.9 Overdose

Signs and symptoms: During post-marketing there have been reports of non-fatal acute and chronic overdoses of atomoxetine alone. The most commonly reported symptoms accompanying acute and chronic overdoses were somnolence, agitation, hyperactivity, abnormal behaviour, and gastro-intestinal symptoms. Most events were mild to moderate. Signs and symptoms consistent with mild to

Table 1 Adverse Reactions

System Organ Class	Very Common	Common	Uncommon	Post-Marketing Experience Spontaneous Reports*
Metabolism and Nutrition Disorders	Appetite decreased	Anorexia (loss of appetite)		
Psychiatric Disorders		Irritability, mood swings, insomnia[3]	Suicide-related events, aggression, hostility, emotional lability**, Early morning awakening	Psychosis (including hallucinations),** agitation**
Nervous System Disorders	Headache, somnolence[2]	Dizziness	Syncope, tremor, migraine	Seizure***
Eye Disorders			Mydriasis	
Cardiac Disorders			Palpitations, sinus tachycardia	QT interval prolongation***
Vascular Disorders				Raynaud's phenomenon
Gastro-intestinal Disorders	Abdominal pain[1], vomiting, nausea	Constipation, dyspepsia		
Hepato-biliary Disorders				Abnormal liver function tests, jaundice, hepatitis**
Skin and Subcutaneous Tissue Disorders		Dermatitis, rash	Pruritus, hyperhidrosis, Allergic reactions	
Renal and Urinary Disorders				Urinary hesitation, urinary retention
Reproductive System and Breast Disorders				Priapism, male genital pain
General Disorders and Administration Site Conditions		Fatigue, lethargy	Asthenia	
Investigations		Weight decreased, blood pressure increased		

[1] Also includes abdominal pain upper, stomach discomfort, abdominal discomfort and epigastric discomfort.
[2] Also includes sedation.
[3] Also includes initial insomnia and middle insomnia.
* These reports are derived from spontaneous event reporting and it is not possible to determine frequency accurately.
** See section 4.4.
*** See section 4.4 and section 4.6.

Table 2 Adverse Reactions

System Organ Class	Very Common	Common	Uncommon	Post-Marketing Experience Spontaneous Reports*
Metabolism and Nutrition Disorders	Appetite decreased			
Psychiatric Disorders	Insomnia[2]	Libido decreased, sleep disorder	Early morning awakening	Suicide-related events, aggression, hostility and emotional lability,** psychosis (including hallucinations),** agitation**
Nervous System Disorders		Dizziness, sinus headache, paraesthesia, tremor	Syncope, migraine	Seizure***
Cardiac Disorders		Palpitations, tachycardia		QT interval prolongation ***
Vascular Disorders		Hot flushes	Peripheral coldness	Raynaud's phenomenon
Gastro-intestinal Disorders	Dry mouth, nausea	Abdominal pain[1], constipation, dyspepsia, flatulence		
Hepato-biliary Disorders				Abnormal liver function tests, jaundice, hepatitis **
Skin and Subcutaneous Tissue Disorders		Dermatitis, hyperhidrosis, rash	Allergic reactions	
Renal and Urinary Disorders		Dysuria, urinary hesitation, urinary retention		
Reproductive System and Breast Disorders		Dysmenorrhoea, ejaculation disorder, erectile dysfunction, menstruation irregular, orgasm abnormal, prostatitis, male genital pain	Ejaculation failure	Priapism
General Disorders and Administration Site Conditions		Fatigue, lethargy, chills		
Investigations		Weight decreased	Blood pressure increased	

[1]Also includes abdominal pain upper, stomach discomfort, abdominal discomfort and epigastric discomfort.

[2] Also includes initial insomnia and middle insomnia.

* These reports are derived from spontaneous event reporting and it is not possible to determine frequency accurately.

** See section 4.4.

*** See section 4.4 and section 4.5.

moderate sympathetic nervous system activation (e.g., mydriasis, tachycardia, dry mouth) were also observed and reports of pruritus and rash have been received. All patients recovered from these events. In some cases of overdose involving atomoxetine, seizures have been reported and, very rarely, QT prolongation. There have also been reports of fatal, acute overdoses involving a mixed ingestion of atomoxetine and at least one other drug.

There is limited clinical trial experience with atomoxetine overdose. No fatal overdoses occurred in clinical trials.

Management of overdose: An airway should be established. Activated charcoal may be useful in limiting absorption if the patient presents within 1 hour of ingestion. Monitoring of cardiac and vital signs is recommended, along with appropriate symptomatic and supportive measures. The patient should be observed for a minimum of 6 hours. Because atomoxetine is highly protein-bound, dialysis is not likely to be useful in the treatment of overdose.

5. PHARMACOLOGICAL PROPERTIES

5.1 Pharmacodynamic properties

Pharmacotherapeutic group: Centrally acting sympathomimetics. *ATC code:* N06BA09.

Atomoxetine is a highly selective and potent inhibitor of the pre-synaptic noradrenaline transporter, its presumed mechanism of action, without directly affecting the serotonin or dopamine transporters. Atomoxetine has minimal affinity for other noradrenergic receptors or for other neurotransmitter transporters or receptors. Atomoxetine has two major oxidative metabolites: 4-hydroxyatomoxetine and N-desmethylatomoxetine. 4-hydroxyatomoxetine is equipotent to atomoxetine as an inhibitor of the noradrenaline transporter but, unlike atomoxetine, this metabolite also exerts some inhibitory activity at the serotonin transporter. However, any effect on this transporter is likely to be minimal, as the majority of 4-hydroxyatomoxetine is further metabolised such that it circulates in plasma at much lower concentrations (1% of atomoxetine concentration in extensive metabolisers and 0.1% of atomoxetine concentration in poor metabolisers). N-desmethylatomoxetine has substantially less pharmacological activity compared with atomoxetine. It circulates in plasma at lower concentrations in extensive metabolisers and at comparable concentrations to the parent drug in poor metabolisers at steady-state.

Atomoxetine is not a psychostimulant and is not an amphetamine derivative. In a randomised, double-blind, placebo-controlled, abuse-potential study in adults comparing effects of atomoxetine and placebo, atomoxetine was not associated with a pattern of response that suggested stimulant or euphoriant properties.

STRATTERA has been studied in trials in over 5000 children and adolescents with ADHD. The acute efficacy of STRATTERA in the treatment of ADHD was initially established in six randomised, double-blind, placebo-controlled trials of six to nine weeks duration. Signs and symptoms of ADHD were evaluated by a comparison of mean change from baseline to endpoint for STRATTERA-treated and placebo-treated patients. In each of the six trials, atomoxetine was statistically significantly superior to placebo in reducing ADHD signs and symptoms.

Additionally, the efficacy of atomoxetine in maintaining symptom response was demonstrated in a 1 year, placebo-controlled trial with over 400 patients, primarily conducted in Europe (approximately 3 months of open-label acute treatment followed by 9 months of double-blind, placebo-controlled maintenance treatment). The proportion of patients relapsing after 1 year was 18.7% and 31.4% (atomoxetine and placebo, respectively). After 1 year of atomoxetine treatment, patients who continued atomoxetine for 6 additional months were less likely to relapse or to experience partial symptom return compared with patients who discontinued active treatment and switched to placebo (2% versus 12%, respectively). For children and adolescents, periodic assessment of the value of ongoing treatment during long-term treatment should be performed.

STRATTERA was effective as a single daily dose and as a divided dose administered in the morning and late afternoon/early evening. STRATTERA administered once daily demonstrated statistically significantly greater reduction in severity of ADHD symptoms compared with placebo, as judged by teachers and parents.

Atomoxetine does not worsen tics in patients with ADHD and comorbid chronic motor tics or Tourette's Disorder.

536 adult patients with ADHD were enrolled in 2 randomised, double-blind, placebo-controlled clinical studies of 10 weeks duration.

Patients received STRATTERA twice daily titrated according to clinical response in a range of 60 to 120mg/day. The mean final dose of STRATTERA for both studies was approximately 95mg/day. In both studies, ADHD symptoms were statistically significantly improved on STRATTERA, as measured on the ADHD Symptom score from the CAARS scale. Magnitude of symptom improvement in adults was less than that observed in children. Long-term maintenance of effect in adults has not been shown.

5.2 Pharmacokinetic properties

The pharmacokinetics of atomoxetine in children and adolescents are similar to those in adults. The pharmacokinetics of atomoxetine have not been evaluated in children under 6 years of age.

Absorption: Atomoxetine is rapidly and almost completely absorbed after oral administration, reaching mean maximal observed plasma concentration (C_{max}) approximately 1 to 2 hours after dosing. The absolute bioavailability of atomoxetine following oral administration ranged from 63% to 94%, depending upon inter-individual differences in the modest first pass metabolism. Atomoxetine can be administered with or without food.

Distribution: Atomoxetine is widely distributed and is extensively (98%) bound to plasma proteins, primarily albumin.

Biotransformation: Atomoxetine undergoes biotransformation primarily through the cytochrome P450 2D6 (CYP2D6) enzymatic pathway. Individuals with reduced activity of this pathway (poor metabolisers) represent about 7% of the Caucasian population and have higher plasma concentrations of atomoxetine compared with people with normal activity (extensive metabolisers). For poor metabolisers, AUC of atomoxetine is approximately 10-fold greater and $C_{ss,max}$ is about 5-fold greater than extensive metabolisers. The major oxidative metabolite formed is 4-hydroxyatomoxetine that is rapidly glucuronidated. 4-hydroxyatomoxetine is equipotent to atomoxetine but circulates in plasma at much lower concentrations. Although 4-hydroxyatomoxetine is primarily formed by CYP2D6, in individuals that lack CYP2D6 activity, 4-hydroxyatomoxetine can be formed by several other cytochrome P450 enzymes, but at a slower rate. Atomoxetine does not inhibit or induce CYP2D6 at therapeutic doses.

Elimination: The mean elimination half-life of atomoxetine after oral administration is 3.6 hours in extensive metabolisers and 21 hours in poor metabolisers. Atomoxetine is excreted primarily as 4-hydroxyatomoxetine-*O*-glucuronide, mainly in the urine.

Linearity/non-linearity: Pharmacokinetics of atomoxetine are linear over the range of doses studied in both extensive and poor metabolisers.

Special populations: Hepatic impairment results in a reduced atomoxetine clearance, increased atomoxetine exposure (AUC increased 2-fold in moderate impairment and 4-fold in severe impairment), and a prolonged half-life of parent drug compared to healthy controls with the same CYP2D6 extensive metaboliser genotype. In patients with moderate to severe hepatic impairment (Child-Pugh class B and C) initial and target doses should be adjusted (see section 4.2).

Atomoxetine mean plasma concentrations for end-stage renal disease (ESRD) subjects were generally higher than the mean for healthy control subjects shown by C_{max} (7% difference) and $AUC_{0-\infty}$ (about 65% difference) increases. After adjustment for body weight, the differences between the two groups are minimised. Pharmacokinetics of atomoxetine and its metabolites in individuals with ESRD suggest that no dose adjustment would be necessary (see section 4.2).

5.3 Preclinical safety data

Preclinical data revealed no special hazard for humans based on conventional studies of safety pharmacology, repeated dose toxicity, genotoxicity, carcinogenicity, or reproduction and development. Due to the dose limitation imposed by the clinical (or exaggerated pharmacological) response of the animals to the drug combined with metabolic differences among species, maximum tolerated doses in animals used in non-clinical studies produced atomoxetine exposures similar to or slightly above those that are achieved in CYP2D6 poor metabolising patients at the maximum recommended daily dose.

A study was conducted in young rats to evaluate the effects of atomoxetine on growth and neurobehavioural and sexual development. Slight delays in onset of vaginal patency (all doses) and preputial separation (≥10mg/kg/day), and slight decreases in epididymal weight and sperm number (≥10mg/kg/day) were seen; however, there were no effects on fertility or reproductive performance. The significance of these findings to humans is unknown.

Pregnant rabbits were treated with up to 100mg/kg/day of atomoxetine by gavage throughout the period of organogenesis. At this dose, in 1 of 3 studies, decrease in live foetuses, increase in early resorption, slight increases in the incidences of atypical origin of carotid artery and absent subclavian artery were observed. These findings were observed at doses that caused slight maternal toxicity. The incidence of these findings is within historical control values. The no-effect dose for these findings was 30mg/kg/day. Exposure (AUC) to unbound atomoxetine in rabbits, at 100mg/kg/day, was approximately 3.3-times (CYP2D6 extensive metabolisers) and 0.4-times (CYP2D6 poor metabolisers) those in humans at the maximum daily dose of 1.4mg/kg/day. The findings in one of three rabbit studies were equivocal and the relevance to man is unknown.

6. PHARMACEUTICAL PARTICULARS

6.1 List of excipients

The capsules contain:

Starch, pregelatinised (Maize)

Dimeticone

Capsule shell:

Sodium laurilsulfate

Gelatin

Edible black ink SW-9008 or edible black ink SW-9010 (containing shellac and black iron oxide E172)

Capsule shell cap colourants:

10 mg: Titanium dioxide E171

18 mg: Yellow iron oxide E172

25 mg, 40mg, and 60mg: FD&C Blue 2 (indigo carmine) E132 and Titanium dioxide E171

80 mg: Yellow iron oxide E172, Red iron oxide E172, Titanium dioxide E171

Capsule shell body colourants:

10 mg, 18mg, 25mg and 80mg: Titanium dioxide E171

40 mg: FD&C Blue 2 (indigo carmine) E132 and Titanium dioxide E171

60 mg: Yellow iron oxide E172

6.2 Incompatibilities

Not applicable.

6.3 Shelf life

3 years.

6.4 Special precautions for storage

This medicinal product does not require any special storage conditions.

6.5 Nature and contents of container

Polyvinyl chloride (PVC)/polyethylene (PE)/polychlorotrifluoroethylene (PCTFE) blister sealed with aluminium foil lid.

Available in pack sizes of 7, 14, 28, and 56 capsules. Not all pack sizes may be marketed.

6.6 Special precautions for disposal and other handling

Atomoxetine capsules are not intended to be opened. Atomoxetine is an ocular irritant. In the event of capsules content coming in contact with the eye, the affected eye should be flushed immediately with water, and medical advice obtained. Hands and any potentially contaminated surfaces should be washed as soon as possible.

7. MARKETING AUTHORISATION HOLDER

Eli Lilly and Company Limited

Lilly House,

Priestley Road,

Basingstoke,

Hampshire RG24 9NL

United Kingdom

8. MARKETING AUTHORISATION NUMBER(S)

STRATTERA 10mg hard capsules: PL 00006/0375

STRATTERA 18mg hard capsules: PL 00006/0376

STRATTERA 25mg hard capsules: PL 00006/0377

STRATTERA 40mg hard capsules: PL 00006/0378

STRATTERA 60mg hard capsules: PL 00006/0379

STRATTERA 80mg hard capsules: PL 00006/0615

9. DATE OF FIRST AUTHORISATION/RENEWAL OF THE AUTHORISATION

27 May 2009

10. DATE OF REVISION OF THE TEXT

27 May 2009

LEGAL CATEGORY

POM

*STRATTERA (atomoxetine) is a trademark of Eli Lilly and Company. ST14M

Stronazon 400 micrograms MR Capsules

(Actavis UK Ltd)

1. NAME OF THE MEDICINAL PRODUCT

Stronazon 400 micrograms MR Capsules

2. QUALITATIVE AND QUANTITATIVE COMPOSITION

One capsule contains 0.4 mg of tamsulosin hydrochloride.

For excipients, see 6.1

3. PHARMACEUTICAL FORM

Modified-release capsule, hard

Orange/olive-green capsule, with the black printed mark TSL 0.4 and with a black stripe at both ends. The capsules contain white to off-white pellets.

4. CLINICAL PARTICULARS

4.1 Therapeutic indications

Lower urinary tract symptoms (LUTS) associated with benign prostatic hyperplasia (BPH).

4.2 Posology and method of administration

One capsule a day after breakfast or the first meal of the day. The capsule is swallowed whole with a glass of water while standing or sitting (not lying down). The capsule should not be broken or pulled apart as this may have an effect on the release of the long-acting active ingredient.

4.3 Contraindications

Hypersensitivity to tamsulosin, including drug-induced angio-oedema, or to any of the excipients.

Orthostatic hypotension observed earlier (history of orthostatic hypotension).

Severe hepatic insufficiency.

4.4 Special warnings and precautions for use

The use of tamsulosin may lower blood pressure, which in rare cases may cause fainting. If initial symptoms of orthostatic hypotension start to appear (dizziness, weakness), then the patient should sit or lie down until the symptoms have gone.

The patient should be examined before commencement of therapy with tamsulosin to exclude the presence of other conditions that can produce similar symptoms to those of BPH. The prostate should be examined via the rectum and, if necessary, the PSA count determined prior to commencement of treatment and again later at regular intervals.

The treatment of severely renally impaired patients (creatinine clearance of < 10 ml/min) should be approached with caution as these patients have not been studied.

Angio-oedema has been rarely reported after the use of tamsulosin. Treatment should be discontinued immediately, the patient should be monitored until disappearance of the oedema, and tamsulosin should not be re-administered.

The 'Intraoperative Floppy Iris Syndrome' (IFIS, a variant of small pupil syndrome) has been observed during cataract surgery in some patients on or previously treated with tamsulosin. IFIS may lead to increased procedural complications during the operation. The initiation of therapy with tamsulosin in patients for whom cataract surgery is scheduled is not recommended.

Discontinuing tamsulosin 1-2 weeks prior to cataract surgery is anecdotally considered helpful, but the benefit and duration of requirement of stopping the therapy prior to cataract surgery has not yet been established.

During pre-operative assessment, cataract surgeons and ophthalmic teams should consider whether patients scheduled for cataract surgery are being or have been treated with tamsulosin in order to ensure that appropriate measures will be in place to manage the IFIS during surgery.

4.5 Interaction with other medicinal products and other forms of interaction

No interactions have been observed when tamsulosin has been given concomitantly with atenolol, enalapril, nifedipine or theophylline. Concomitant cimetidine raises, and concomitant furosemide lowers, plasma concentrations of tamsulosin but, as the concentration of tamsulosin remains within the normal range, posology need not be altered.

Tamsulosin has not been found to interact with amitriptyline, salbutamol, glibenclamide or finasteride during *in vitro* studies with liver microsomal fractions (representing the cytochrome P450-linked metabolising enzyme system). Diclofenac and Warfarin may increase the elimination rate of tamsulosin.

Concurrent administration with another α_1-adrenoreceptor antagonist may lower blood pressure.

4.6 Pregnancy and lactation

Tamsulosin is intended for males only.

4.7 Effects on ability to drive and use machines

No studies on the effects on the ability to drive and use machines have been performed. However patients should be aware of the fact that dizziness can occur.

4.8 Undesirable effects

(see Table 1 below)

During cataract surgery a small pupil situation, known as Intraoperative Floppy Iris Syndrome (IFIS), has been associated with therapy of tamsulosin during post-marketing surveillance (See section 4.4).

4.9 Overdose

No cases of acute overdosage have been reported. However, acute hypotension could theoretically occur after overdosage in which case cardiovascular support should be given. Blood pressure can be restored and heart rate brought back to normal by lying the patient down. If this does not help then volume expanders and, when necessary, vasopressors could be employed. Renal function should be monitored and general supportive measures applied. Dialysis is unlikely to be of help as tamsulosin is very highly bound to plasma proteins.

If large quantities of the medicinal product are involved, gastric lavage may be performed and activated charcoal and an osmotic laxative, such as sodium sulphate, may be given.

5. PHARMACOLOGICAL PROPERTIES

5.1 Pharmacodynamic properties

Pharmacotherapeutic group

Tamsulosin is an α_{1A} adrenoreceptor antagonist. The medicinal product is only used for the treatment of prostatic conditions.

ATC code: G04CA02

Mechanism of action

Tamsulosin binds selectively and competitively to postsynaptic α_{1A} adrenoreceptors, which convey smooth muscle contraction, thereby relaxing prostatic and urethral smooth muscle.

Pharmacodynamic effects

Tamsulosin increases the maximum urinary flow rate by relaxing prostatic and urethral smooth muscle, thus relieving obstruction.

The medicinal product also improves the irritative and obstructive symptoms in which the contraction of smooth muscle in the lower urinary tract plays an important role.

Alpha-blockers can reduce blood pressure by lowering peripheral resistance. No reduction in blood pressure of any clinical significance was observed during studies with tamsulosin in normotensive patients.

The medicinal product's effect on storage and voiding symptoms are also maintained during long-term therapy, as a result of which the need for surgical treatment is significantly postponed.

5.2 Pharmacokinetic properties

Absorption

Tamsulosin is rapidly absorbed from the intestines and its bioavailability is almost complete. Absorption is slowed down if a meal has been eaten before taking the medicinal product. Uniformity of absorption can be assured by always taking tamsulosin after breakfast.

Tamsulosin shows linear kinetics.

Peak plasma levels are achieved at approximately six hours after a single dose of tamsulosin taken after a full meal. The steady state is reached by day five of multiple dosing, when C_{max} in patients is about two-thirds higher than that reached after a single dose. Although this has been demonstrated only in the elderly, the same result would also be expected in younger patients.

There are huge inter-patient variations in plasma levels of tamsulosin, both after single as well as multiple dosing.

Distribution

In humans, tamsulosin is more than 99% bound to plasma proteins and the volume of distribution is small (about 0.2 l/kg).

Table 1

	Common ($>1/100$, $<1/10$)	Uncommon ($>1/1\,000$, $<1/100$)	Rare ($>1/10\,000$, $<1/1\,000$)	Very rare ($<1/10\,000$)
Nervous system disorders	Dizziness	Headache	Syncope	
Cardiac disorders		Tachycardia		
Vascular disorders		Orthostatic hypotension		
Respiratory, thoracic and mediastinum-related disorders		Rhinitis		
Gastrointestinal disorders		Constipation, diarrhoea, nausea, vomiting		
Skin and subcutaneous tissue disorders		Rash, itching, urticaria	Angio-oedema	
Reproductive systems and breast disorders		Abnormal ejaculation		Priapism
General disorders and administration site conditions		Asthenia		

Biotransformation

Tamsulosin has a low first pass metabolic effect. Most tamsulosin is found unaltered in plasma. The substance is metabolised in the liver.

In studies on rats, tamsulosin was found to cause only a slight induction of microsomal liver enzymes.

The metabolites are not as effective and toxic as the active medicinal product itself.

Excretion

Tamsulosin and its metabolites are mainly excreted in the urine with about 9% of the dose being present in unchanged form.

The elimination half-life of tamsulosin in patients is approximately 10 hours (when taken after a meal) and 13 hours in the steady state.

5.3 Preclinical safety data

Toxicity after a single dose and multiple dosing has been investigated in mice, rats and dogs. Reproductive toxicity has also been investigated in rats, carcinogenicity in mice and rats, and genotoxicity *in vivo* and *in vitro*.

The common toxicity profile found with large doses of tamsulosin is equivalent to the pharmacological effect associated with alpha adrenergic antagonists.

Changes in ECG readings were found with very large doses in dogs. This is not, however, assumed to be of any clinical significance. Tamsulosin has not been found to have any significant genotoxic properties.

Greater proliferative changes in the mammary glands of female rats and mice have been discovered on exposure to tamsulosin. These findings, which are probably indirectly linked to hyperprolactinaemia and only occur as a result of large doses having been taken, are considered clinically insignificant.

6. PHARMACEUTICAL PARTICULARS

6.1 List of excipients

Content of capsule

Microcrystalline cellulose

Methacrylic acid-ethyl acrylate copolymer

Polysorbate 80

Sodium laurilsulfate

Triethyl citrate

Talc

Capsule body

Gelatine

Indigotine (E 132)

Titanium dioxide (E 171)

Yellow iron oxide (E 172)

Red iron oxide (E 172)

Black iron oxide (E 172)

Ink

Shellac

Black iron oxide (E 172)

Propylene glycol

6.2 Incompatibilities

Not applicable.

6.3 Shelf life

36 months.

6.4 Special precautions for storage

Blister packs: Store in the original package.

Tablet containers: Keep the container tightly closed.

6.5 Nature and contents of container

PVC/PE/PVDC/Aluminium blister packs in cardboard boxes and HDPE tablet containers with PP child-resistant closures containing 10, 14, 20, 28, 30, 50, 56, 60, 90, 100 or 200 modified-release capsules.

Not all pack sizes may be marketed.

6.6 Special precautions for disposal and other handling

No special requirements.

7. MARKETING AUTHORISATION HOLDER

Actavis UK Limited (Trading style: Actavis)

Whiddon Valley

BARNSTAPLE

N Devon EX32 8NS

8. MARKETING AUTHORISATION NUMBER(S)

PL 0142/0639

9. DATE OF FIRST AUTHORISATION/RENEWAL OF THE AUTHORISATION

20.01.06

10. DATE OF REVISION OF THE TEXT

June 2007

Stugeron 15mg

(Janssen-Cilag Ltd)

1. NAME OF THE MEDICINAL PRODUCT

Stugeron® 15 mg.

2. QUALITATIVE AND QUANTITATIVE COMPOSITION

Each tablet contains 15 mg cinnarizine.

3. PHARMACEUTICAL FORM

White circular tablet with S/15 on one side and Janssen on the other side.

4. CLINICAL PARTICULARS

4.1 Therapeutic indications

Stugeron is for the control of vestibular disorders such as vertigo, tinnitus, nausea and vomiting such as is seen in Meniere's Disease.

Stugeron is also effective in the control of motion sickness.

4.2 Posology and method of administration

Route of administration

Oral. The tablets may be chewed, sucked or swallowed whole.

Dosage

Stugeron should preferably be taken after meals.

Vestibular symptoms

Adults, elderly and children over 12 years: 2 tablets three times a day.

Children 5 to 12 years: One half the adult dose.

These doses should not be exceeded.

Motion sickness

Adults, elderly and children over 12 years: 2 tablets 2 hours before you travel and 1 tablet every 8 hours during your journey.

Children 5 to 12 years: One half the adult dose.

4.3 Contraindications

Stugeron should not be given to patients with known hypersensitivity to cinnarizine.

4.4 Special warnings and precautions for use

As with other antihistamines, Stugeron may cause epigastric discomfort; taking it after meals may diminish the gastric irritation.

In patients with Parkinson's Disease, Stugeron should only be given if the advantages outweigh the possible risk of aggravating this disease.

Because of its antihistamine effect, Stugeron may prevent an otherwise positive reaction to dermal reactivity indicators if used within 4 days prior to testing.

Use of cinnarizine should be avoided in porphyria.

There have been no specific studies in hepatic or renal dysfunction. Stugeron should be used with care in patients with hepatic or renal insufficiency.

Patients with rare hereditary problems of fructose or galactose intolerance, Lapp lactase deficiency, glucose-galactose malabsorption or sucrase-isomaltase insufficiency, should not take this medicine because it contains lactose and sucrose.

4.5 Interaction with other medicinal products and other forms of interaction

Concurrent use of alcohol, CNS depressants or tricyclic antidepressants may potentiate the sedative effects of either these drugs or of Stugeron.

4.6 Pregnancy and lactation

The safety of Stugeron in human pregnancy has not been established although studies in animals have not demonstrated teratogenic effects. As with other drugs it is not advisable to administer Stugeron in pregnancy.

There are no data on the excretion of Stugeron in human breast milk. Use of Stugeron is not recommended in nursing mothers.

4.7 Effects on ability to drive and use machines

Stugeron may cause drowsiness, especially at the start of treatment; patients affected in this way should not drive or operate machinery.

4.8 Undesirable effects

For all indications: Drowsiness and gastro-intestinal disturbances may occur. These are usually transient.

In rare cases, headache, dry mouth, perspiration or allergic reactions may occur.

For long term treatment, i.e. vestibular symptoms: Rare cases of weight gain and very rare cases of lichen planus, lupus-like skin reactions and cholestatic jaundice have been reported. Rare cases of aggravation or appearance of extrapyramidal symptoms (sometimes associated with depressive feelings) have been described, predominantly in elderly people during prolonged therapy. The treatment should be discontinued in such cases.

4.9 Overdose

Symptoms

The signs and symptoms are mainly due to the anticholinergic (atropine-like) activity of cinnarizine.

Acute cinnarizine overdoses have been reported with doses ranging from 90 to 2,250 mg. The most commonly reported signs and symptoms associated with overdose of cinnarizine include: alterations in consciousness ranging from somnolence to stupor and coma, vomiting, extrapyramidal symptoms, and hypotonia. In a small number of young children, seizures developed. Clinical consequences were not severe in most cases, but deaths have been reported after single and polydrug overdoses involving cinnarizine.

Treatment

There is no specific antidote. For any overdose, the treatment is symptomatic and supportive care.

Within the first hour after ingestion, gastric lavage may be performed provided that the airway is protected. However, the benefit of gastric lavage is uncertain.

Activated charcoal should only be considered in patients presenting within one hour of taking a potentially toxic overdose (ie more than 15mg/kg).

5. PHARMACOLOGICAL PROPERTIES

5.1 Pharmacodynamic properties

Cinnarizine has been shown to be a non-competitive antagonist of the smooth muscle contractions caused by various vasoactive agents including histamine.

Cinnarizine also acts on vascular smooth muscle by selectively inhibiting the calcium influx into depolarised cells, thereby reducing the availability of free Ca^{2+} ions for the induction and maintenance of contraction.

Vestibular eye reflexes induced by caloric stimulation of the labyrinth in guinea pigs are markedly depressed by cinnarizine.

Cinnarizine has been shown to inhibit nystagmus.

5.2 Pharmacokinetic properties

In animals, cinnarizine is extensively metabolised, N-dealkylation being the major pathway. Approx. two thirds of the metabolites are excreted with the faeces, the rest in the urine, mainly during the first five days after a single dose.

In man, after oral administration, absorption is relatively slow, peak serum concentrations occurring after 2.5 to 4 hours.

Cinnarizine undergoes extensive metabolism but there is considerable interindividual variation in the extent of metabolism. The drug is excreted in the urine unchanged as metabolites and glucuronide conjugates. The terminal elimination half life is about 3 hours.

5.3 Preclinical safety data

No relevant information additional to that contained elsewhere in the Summary of Product Characteristics.

6. PHARMACEUTICAL PARTICULARS

6.1 List of excipients

Lactose monohydrate

Maize starch

Sucrose

Talc

Magnesium stearate

0025Polyvidone K90

6.2 Incompatibilities

None known.

6.3 Shelf life

5 years

6.4 Special precautions for storage

None.

6.5 Nature and contents of container

PVC/Aluminium foil blisters

or

Polystyrene tubs with polyethylene caps

Each pack containing 15, 25, 100, 250 or 1000 tablets.

6.6 Special precautions for disposal and other handling

The tablets may be chewed, sucked or swallowed whole.

7. MARKETING AUTHORISATION HOLDER

Janssen-Cilag Limited

50-100 Holmers Farm Way

High Wycombe

Buckinghamshire

HP12 4EG

UK

8. MARKETING AUTHORISATION NUMBER(S)

PL 0242/5009R

9. DATE OF FIRST AUTHORISATION/RENEWAL OF THE AUTHORISATION

Date of First Authorisation: 14/09/89

Renewal of Authorisation: 23/03/95

10. DATE OF REVISION OF THE TEXT

28 April 2009

Sublimaze

(Janssen-Cilag Ltd)

1. NAME OF THE MEDICINAL PRODUCT

Sublimaze®

2. QUALITATIVE AND QUANTITATIVE COMPOSITION

Fentanyl citrate 78.5 micrograms equivalent to 50 micrograms per ml fentanyl base.

3. PHARMACEUTICAL FORM
Injection.

4. CLINICAL PARTICULARS

4.1 Therapeutic indications
Sublimaze is an opioid analgesic used:

a. In low doses to provide analgesia during short surgical procedures.

b. In high doses as an analgesic/respiratory depressant in patients requiring assisted ventilation.

c. In combination with a neuroleptic in the technique of neuroleptanalgesia.

d. In the treatment of severe pain, such as the pain of myocardial infarction

4.2 Posology and method of administration
Route of administration

Fentanyl should be given only in an environment where the airway can be controlled and by personnel who can control the airway (see section 4.4).

Intravenous administration either as a bolus or by infusion.

Intramuscular administration.

Sublimaze, by the intravenous route, can be administered to both adults and children. The dose of Sublimaze should be individualised according to age, body weight, physical status, underlying pathological condition, use of other drugs and type of surgery and anaesthesia.

Adults

The usual dosage regimen in adults is as follows:

	Initial	Supplemental
Spontaneous Respiration	50-200 mcg	50 mcg
Assisted Ventilation	300-3500 mcg	100-200 mcg

Doses in excess of 200 mcg are for use in anaesthesia only. As a premedicant, 1-2 ml Sublimaze may be given intramuscularly 45 minutes before induction of anaesthesia.

After intravenous administration in unpremedicated adult patients, 2 ml Sublimaze may be expected to provide sufficient analgesia for 10-20 minutes in surgical procedures involving low pain intensity. 10 ml Sublimaze injected as a bolus gives analgesia lasting about one hour. The analgesia produced is sufficient for surgery involving moderately painful procedures. Giving a dose of 50 mcg/kg Sublimaze will provide intense analgesia for some four to six hours, for intensely stimulating surgery.

Sublimaze may also be given as an infusion. In ventilated patients, a loading dose of Sublimaze may be given as a fast infusion of approximately 1 mcg/kg/min for the first 10 minutes followed by an infusion of approximately 0.1 mcg/kg/min. Alternatively the loading dose of Sublimaze may be given as a bolus. Infusion rates should be titrated to individual patient response; lower infusion rates may be adequate. Unless it is planned to ventilate post-operatively, the infusion should be terminated at about 40 minutes before the end of surgery.

Lower infusion rates, e.g. 0.05-0.08 mcg/kg/minute are necessary if spontaneous ventilation is to be maintained. Higher infusion rates (up to 3 mcg/kg/minute) have been used in cardiac surgery.

Sublimaze is chemically incompatible with the induction agents thiopentone and methohexitone because of wide differences in pH.

Children

The usual dosage regimen in children is as follows:

	Age	Initial	Supplemental
Spontaneous Respiration	2-12 yrs	2-3 mcg/kg	1 mcg/kg
Assisted Ventilation	2-12 yrs	2-3 mcg/kg	1 mcg/kg

Use in children:

Analgesia during operation, enhancement of anaesthesia with spontaneous respiration

Techniques that involve analgesia in a spontaneous breathing child should only be used as part of an anaesthetic technique, or given as part of a sedation/ analgesia technique with experienced personnel in an environment that can manage sudden chest wall rigidity requiring intubation, or apnoea requiring airway support (see section 4.4).

The usual dosage regimen is as follows:

Spontaneous respiration:

Child 2 years –12 years: initially 2–3 micrograms/kg, then 1 microgram/kg as required

Assisted ventilation:

Child 2 years –12 years: initially 2–3 micrograms/kg, then 1 microgram/kg as required

Use in elderly and debilitated patients: It is wise to reduce the dosage in the elderly and debilitated patients. The effect of the initial dose should be taken into account in determining supplemental doses.

4.3 Contraindications
Respiratory depression, obstructive airways disease. Concurrent administration with monoamine oxidase inhibitors, or within 2 weeks of their discontinuation. Known intolerance to fentanyl or other morphinomimetics.

4.4 Special warnings and precautions for use
Warnings:

Tolerance and dependence may occur. Following intravenous administration of fentanyl, a transient fall in blood pressure may occur, especially in hypovolaemic patients. Appropriate measures to maintain a stable arterial pressure should be taken.

Significant respiratory depression will occur following the administration of fentanyl in doses in excess of 200 mcg. This, and the other pharmacological effects of fentanyl, can be reversed by specific narcotic antagonists (e.g. naloxone). Additional doses of the latter may be necessary because the respiratory depression may last longer than the duration of action of the opioid antagonist.

Bradycardia and possibly cardiac arrest can occur in non-atropinised patients, and can be antagonised by atropine.

Muscular rigidity (morphine-like effect) may occur.

Rigidity, which may also involve the thoracic muscles, can be avoided by the following measures:

– slow IV injection (usually sufficient for lower doses);
– premedication with benzodiazepines;
– use of muscle relaxants.

Precautions:

Fentanyl should be given only in an environment where the airway can be controlled and by personnel who can control the airway.

Techniques that involve analgesia in a spontaneous breathing child should only be used as part of an anaesthetic technique, or given as part of a sedation/ analgesia technique with experienced personnel in an environment that can manage sudden chest wall rigidity requiring intubation, or apnoea requiring airway support.

As with all opioid analgesics, care should be observed when administering fentanyl to patients with myasthenia gravis.

It is wise to reduce dosage in the elderly and debilitated patients.

In hypothyroidism, pulmonary disease, decreased respiratory reserve, alcoholism and liver or renal impairment the dosage should be titrated with care and prolonged monitoring may be required.

Patients on chronic opioid therapy or with a history of opioid abuse may require higher doses.

Administration in labour may cause respiratory depression in the new born infant.

As with all potent opioids, profound analgesia is accompanied by marked respiratory depression, which may persist into or recur in the early postoperative period. Care should be taken after large doses or infusions of fentanyl to ensure that adequate spontaneous breathing has been established and maintained before discharging the patient from the recovery area.

Resuscitation equipment and opioid antagonists should be readily available. Hyperventilation during anaesthesia may alter the patient's response to CO_2, thus affecting respiration postoperatively.

The use of rapid bolus injections of opioids should be avoided in patients with compromised intracerebral compliance; in such patients the transient decrease in the mean arterial pressure has occasionally been accompanied by a transient reduction of the cerebral perfusion pressure.

4.5 Interaction with other medicinal products and other forms of interaction
Effect of other drugs on fentanyl

The use of opioid premedication, barbiturates, benzodiazepines, neuroleptics, halogenic gases and other non-selective CNS depressants (e.g. alcohol) may enhance or prolong the respiratory depression of fentanyl.

When patients have received other CNS-depressants, the dose of fentanyl required will be less than usual.

Fentanyl, a high clearance drug, is rapidly and extensively metabolised mainly by CYP3A4.

Itraconazole (a potent CYP3A4 inhibitor) at 200 mg/day given orally for 4 days had no significant effect on the pharmacokinetics of IV fentanyl.

Oral ritonavir (one of the most potent CYP3A4 inhibitors) reduced the clearance of IV fentanyl by two thirds; however, peak plasma concentrations after a single dose of IV fentanyl were not affected.

When fentanyl is used in a single dose, the concomitant use of potent CYP3A4 inhibitors such as ritonavir requires special patient care and observation.

Co-administration of fluconazole or voriconazole (moderate CYP3A4 inhibitors) and fentanyl may result in an increased exposure to fentanyl.

With continuous treatment of fentanyl and concomitant administration of CYP3A4 inhibitors, a dose reduction of fentanyl may be required to avoid accumulation, which may increase the risk of prolonged or delayed respiratory depression.

Bradycardia and possibly cardiac arrest can occur when fentanyl is combined with non-vagolytic muscle relaxants.

The concomitant use of droperidol can result in a higher incidence of hypotension.

Effect of fentanyl on other drugs

Following the administration of fentanyl, the dose of other CNS depressant drugs should be reduced.

The total plasma clearance and volume of distribution of etomidate is decreased by a factor 2 to 3 without a change in half-life when administered with fentanyl.

Simultaneous administration of fentanyl and intravenous midazolam results in an increase in the terminal plasma half-life and a reduction in the plasma clearance of midazolam. When these drugs are co-administered with fentanyl their dose may need to be reduced.

4.6 Pregnancy and lactation
There are no adequate data from the use of fentanyl in pregnant women. Fentanyl can cross the placenta in early pregnancy. Studies in animals have shown some reproductive toxicity (see Section 5.3, Preclinical safety data). The potential risk for humans is unknown.

Administration during childbirth (including Caesarean section) is not recommended because fentanyl crosses the placenta and the foetal respiratory centre is particularly sensitive to opioids. If fentanyl is nevertheless administered, an antidote for the child should always be at hand.

Fentanyl is excreted into human milk. It is therefore recommended that breast-feeding is not initiated within 24 hours of treatment. The risk/benefit of breast-feeding following fentanyl administration should be considered.

4.7 Effects on ability to drive and use machines
Where early discharge is envisaged, patients should be advised not to drive or operate machinery for 24 hours following administration.

4.8 Undesirable effects
The safety of fentanyl IV was evaluated in 376 subjects who participated in 20 clinical trials evaluating fentanyl IV as an anaesthetic. These subjects took at least 1 dose of fentanyl IV and provided safety data. Based on pooled safety data from these clinical trials, the most commonly reported (≥5% incidence) Adverse Drug Reactions (ADRs) were (with % incidence): nausea (26.1); vomiting (18.6); muscle rigidity (10.4); hypotension (8.8); hypertension (8.8); bradycardia (6.1); and sedation (5.3).

Including the above-mentioned ADRs, Table 1 displays ADRs that have been reported with the use of fentanyl IV from either clinical trials or postmarketing experience.

The displayed frequency categories use the following convention: Very common (≥1/10); common (≥1/100 to <1/10); uncommon (≥1/1,000 to <1/100); rare (≥1/10,000 to <1/1,000); very rare (<1/10,000); and not known (cannot be estimated from the available clinical trial data).

Table 1: Adverse Drug Reactions

(see Table 1 on next page)

When a neuroleptic is used with fentanyl, the following adverse reactions may be observed: chills and/or shivering, restlessness, postoperative hallucinatory episodes and extrapyramidal symptoms (see Section 4.4).

4.9 Overdose
Symptoms:

The manifestations of fentanyl overdosage are generally an extension of its pharmacological action. Depending on the individual sensitivity, the clinical picture is determined primarily by the degree of respiratory depression, which varies from bradypnoea to apnoea.

Treatment:

Hypoventilation or apnoea:	O_2 administration, assisted or controlled respiration.
Respiratory depression:	Specific narcotic antagonist (e.g. naloxone). This does not preclude the use of immediate countermeasures.
Muscular rigidity:	Intravenous neuromuscular blocking agent.

The patient should be carefully observed; body warmth and adequate fluid intake should be maintained. If hypotension is severe or if it persists, the possibility of hypovolaemia should be considered and, if present, it should be controlled with appropriate parenteral fluid administration.

5. PHARMACOLOGICAL PROPERTIES

5.1 Pharmacodynamic properties
Fentanyl is a synthetic opiate with a clinical potency of 50 to 100 times that of morphine. Its onset of action is rapid and its duration of action is short. In man, a single IV dose of 0.5-1 mg/70 kg body weight immediately produces a pronounced state of surgical analgesia, respiratory depression, bradycardia and other typical morphine-like effects. The duration of action of the peak effects is about 30 minutes. All potent morphine-like drugs produce relief from pain, ventilatory depression, emesis, constipation,

Table 3 Adverse Drug Reactions

System Organ Class	Adverse Drug Reactions			
	Frequency Category			
	Very Common (≥ 1/10)	Common (≥ 1/100 to < 1/10)	Uncommon (≥ 1/1,000 to < 1/100)	Not Known
Immune System Disorders				Hypersensitivity (such as anaphylactic shock, anaphylactic reaction, urticaria)
Psychiatric Disorders		Agitation	Euphoric mood	
Nervous System Disorders	Muscle rigidity (which may also involve the thoracic muscles)	Dyskinesia; Sedation; Dizziness	Headache	Convulsions; Loss of consciousness; Myoclonus
Eye Disorders		Visual disturbance		
Cardiac Disorders		Bradycardia; Tachycardia; Arrhythmia		Cardiac arrest
Vascular Disorders		Hypotension; Hypertension; Venous pain	Phlebitis; Blood pressure fluctuation	
Respiratory, Thoracic and Mediastinal Disorders		Laryngospasm; Bronchospasm; Apnoea	Hyperventilation; Hiccups	Respiratory depression
Gastrointestinal Disorders	Nausea; Vomiting			
Skin and Subcutaneous Tissue Disorders		Allergic dermatitis		Pruritus
General Disorders and Administration Site Conditions			Chills; Hypothermia	
Injury, Poisoning and Procedural Complications		Postoperative confusion	Airway complication of anaesthesia	

physical dependence, certain vagal effects and varying degrees of sedation. Fentanyl, however, differs from morphine not only by its short duration of action but also by its lack of emetic effect and minimal hypotensive activity in animals.

5.2 Pharmacokinetic properties

Some pharmacokinetic parameters for fentanyl are as follows:

Urinary excretion = 8%

Bound in plasma = 80%

Clearance (ml/min/kg) = 13±2

Volume of distribution (litres/kg) = 4.0±0.4

Estimates of terminal half-life range from 141 to 853 minutes.

5.3 Preclinical safety data

In vitro fentanyl showed, like other opioid analgesics, mutagenic effects in a mammalian cell culture assay, only at cytotoxic concentrations and along with metabolic activation. Fentanyl showed no evidence of mutagenicity when tested in *in vivo* rodent studies and bacterial assays. There are no long-term animal studies to investigate the tumor-forming potential of fentanyl.

Some tests on female rats showed reduced fertility as well as embryo mortality. These findings were related to maternal toxicity and not a direct effect of the drug on the developing embryo. There was no evidence of teratogenic effects.

6. PHARMACEUTICAL PARTICULARS

6.1 List of excipients

Sodium chloride

Water for injections

6.2 Incompatibilities

The product is chemically incompatible with the induction agents thiopentone and methohexitone because of the wide differences in pH.

6.3 Shelf life

36 months

6.4 Special precautions for storage

Protect from light.

Do not store above 30°C.

Keep container in the outer carton.

Keep out of reach and sight of children.

6.5 Nature and contents of container

Colourless glass ampoules (PhEur, USP Type I).

Pack size: packs of 10 **and 50*** of 2 ml and **5 ml*** ampoules; packs of 5 and **10*** of 10 ml ampoules.

*** not marketed**

6.6 Special precautions for disposal and other handling

Not applicable (store as a CD).

7. MARKETING AUTHORISATION HOLDER

Janssen-Cilag Ltd

50-100 Holmers Farm Way

High Wycombe

Buckinghamshire

HP12 4EG

UK

8. MARKETING AUTHORISATION NUMBER(S)

PL 00242/5001R

9. DATE OF FIRST AUTHORISATION/RENEWAL OF THE AUTHORISATION

26 February 1980 / 25 March 2002

10. DATE OF REVISION OF THE TEXT

04 September 2009

Legal category POM/CD

Sudocrem Antiseptic Healing Cream

(Forest Laboratories UK Limited)

1. NAME OF THE MEDICINAL PRODUCT

Sudocrem Antiseptic Healing Cream

2. QUALITATIVE AND QUANTITATIVE COMPOSITION

	% w/w
Zinc oxide, EP	15.25
Benzyl alcohol, BP	0.39
Benzyl benzoate, BP	1.01
Benzyl cinnamate	0.15
Lanolin (hypoallergenic)	4.00

3. PHARMACEUTICAL FORM

Emulsified water in oil cream

4. CLINICAL PARTICULARS

4.1 Therapeutic indications

In the treatment of:

1. Napkin rash
2. Eczema
3. Bedsores
4. Acne
5. Minor burns
6. Surface wounds
7. Sunburn
8. Chilblains

4.2 Posology and method of administration

Apply a thin layer with suitable covering where necessary. Renew application as required. No distinction is required between indications or between adults, children and the elderly.

Topical cream for external use only.

4.3 Contraindications

Hypersensitivity to any of the ingredients.

4.4 Special warnings and precautions for use

For external use only and should not be allowed to come into contact with the eyes and the mucous membranes.

4.5 Interaction with other medicinal products and other forms of interaction

None known

4.6 Pregnancy and lactation

There are no known contraindications.

4.7 Effects on ability to drive and use machines

Not applicable

4.8 Undesirable effects

Side effects include local hypersensitivity occasionally.

4.9 Overdose

No cases of overdose have been reported. If large amounts are swallowed accidentally, this may cause vomiting, diarrhoea, CNS stimulation and convulsions. Symptomatic treatment should be provided.

5. PHARMACOLOGICAL PROPERTIES

5.1 Pharmacodynamic properties

Zinc oxide:

A dermatological agent with astringent, soothing and protective properties.

Benzyl alcohol:

A local anaesthetic with disinfectant properties.

Benzyl benzoate:

An acaricide and has been used as a pediculicide, insect repellent and pharmaceutical solubilising agent. It is a constituent of many natural balsams and is one of the principal esters of Peru Balsam.

Benzyl cinnamate:

This is the other principal ester of Peru Balsam BPC 1973. It is synthesised from benzyl alcohol and cinnamic acid which has antibacterial and antifungal properties. Peru Balsam is categorised as having a mild antiseptic action because of cinnamic acid and its derivatives present.

Lanolin:

Resembles the sebaceous secretions of human skin. The grade (hypoallergenic) used is manufactured so as to exclude many sensitising substances present in the lanolin.

5.2 Pharmacokinetic properties

Not applicable.

5.3 Preclinical safety data

Not applicable

6. PHARMACEUTICAL PARTICULARS

6.1 List of excipients

Purified Water

Sodium Benzoate

Paraffin wax

Microcrystalline wax

Heavy Liquid Paraffin

Synthetic Beeswax

Sorbitan sesquioleate

Propylene glycol

Antioxidant (formulation consisting of butylated hydroxyanisole (BHA), citric acid and propylene glycol)

Linalyl acetate

Lavender

6.2 Incompatibilities

None known

6.3 Shelf life

Not exceeding 5 years from date of manufacture.

6.4 Special precautions for storage

No special precautions for storage.

6.5 Nature and contents of container

		Pack size (g)
a)	Polypropylene jars with polyethylene tamper-evident caps	(1) 60
		(2) 125
		(3) 250
		(4) 400
		(5) 750
		(6) 1000
b)	Polypropylene jars with polyethylene caps	(1) 15
		(2) 25
c)	Aluminium or laminated plastic aluminium tubes with aluminium membrane and plastic caps	(1) 30
		(2) 50

6.6 Special precautions for disposal and other handling

Not applicable

7. MARKETING AUTHORISATION HOLDER

Marketing Authorisation Holder	UK Distributor
Forest Tosara Limited	Forest Laboratories UK
Unit 146 Baldoyle Industrial	Limited
Estate	Bourne Road
Baldoyle	Bexley
Dublin 13	Kent DA5 1NX
Republic of Ireland	UK

8. MARKETING AUTHORISATION NUMBER(S)
PL 06166/0003

9. DATE OF FIRST AUTHORISATION/RENEWAL OF THE AUTHORISATION
5 March 2004

10. DATE OF REVISION OF THE TEXT

11. Legal Category
GSL

Sulpor 200mg/5ml Oral Solution.

(Rosemont Pharmaceuticals Limited)

1. NAME OF THE MEDICINAL PRODUCT
Sulpiride 200mg/5ml Oral Solution.

Sulpor

2. QUALITATIVE AND QUANTITATIVE COMPOSITION
Sulpiride 200mg/5ml.

3. PHARMACEUTICAL FORM
A colourless to slightly yellow oral solution.

4. CLINICAL PARTICULARS

4.1 Therapeutic indications
Acute and chronic schizophrenia.

4.2 Posology and method of administration
For oral administration only.

Adults:

A starting dose of 400mg to 800mg daily, given in two divided doses (morning and early evening) is recommended.

Predominantly positive symptoms (formal thought disorder, hallucinations, delusions, incongruity of affect) respond to higher doses, and a starting dose of at least 400mg twice daily is recommended, increasing if necessary up to a suggested maximum of 1200mg twice daily. Increasing the dose beyond this level has not been shown to produce further improvement. Predominantly negative symptoms (flattening of affect, poverty of speech, anergia, apathy), as well as depression, respond to doses below 800mg daily; therefore, a starting dose of 400mg twice daily is recommended. Reducing this dose towards 200mg twice daily will normally increase the alerting effect of sulpiride.

Patients with mixed positive and negative symptoms, with neither predominating, will normally respond to dosage of 400-600mg twice daily.

Children:

Clinical experience in children under the age of 14 years of age is insufficient to permit specific recommendations.

Elderly:

The same dose ranges may be required in the elderly, but should be reduced if there is evidence of renal impairment.

4.3 Contraindications
Phaeochromocytoma. Acute porphyria. Hypersensitivity to any of the ingredients in this product. Severe renal, haematological or hepatic disease. Alcoholic intoxication and other disorders which depress CNS function.

Concomitant prolactin-dependant tumours e.g. pituitary gland prolactinomas and breast cancer

Association with levodopa (See 4.5 Interactions with other medicinal products and other forms of interaction)

4.4 Special warnings and precautions for use
Increased motor agitation has been reported at high dosage in a small number of patients: in aggressive, agitated or excited phases of the disease process, low doses of sulpiride may aggravate symptoms. Care should be exercised where hypomania is present.

If extrapyramidal reactions occur, a reduction in dosage of sulpiride or initiation of anti-parkinsonian medication may be necessary.

As with all neuroleptic drugs, the presence of unexplained hyperthermia could indicate the neuroleptic malignant syndrome (NMS). In this event sulpiride and any associated neuroleptic treatment should be discontinued until the origin of the fever has been determined.

Although sulpiride only induces slight EEG modifications, caution is advised in prescribing it for patients with unstable epilepsy. Patients requiring sulpiride who are receiving anti-convulsant therapy should continue unchanged on the latter medication. Cases of convulsions, sometimes in patients with no previous history, have been reported.

Sulpiride has no significant anticholinergic or cardiovascular activity.

As with all drugs for which the kidney is the major elimination pathway, the usual precautions should be taken in cases of renal failure.

Patients should be warned against taking alcohol with sulpiride as reaction capacity may be impaired.

Abrupt cessation of treatment in some patients may produce a withdrawal response.

Elderly patients are more susceptible to postural hypotension, sedation and extrapyramidal effects. As with other neuroleptics, sulpiride should be used with particular caution (see section 4.2).

When neuroleptic treatment is absolutely necessary in a patient with Parkinson's disease, sulpiride can be used, although caution is in order.

Prolongation of the QT interval

Sulpiride may induce a prolongation of the QT interval. This effect, known to potentiate the risk of serious ventricular arrhythmias such as torsade de pointes is enhanced by the pre-existence of bradycardia or cardiovascular disease, hypokalaemia, congenital or acquired long QT interval, concomitant neuroleptic treatment, or a family history of QT prolongation (See section 4.5).

An approximately 3-fold increased risk of cerebrovascular adverse events have been seen in randomised placebo controlled clinical trials in the dementia population with some atypical antipsychotics. The mechanism for this increased risk cannot be excluded for other antipsychotics or other patient populations. Sulpiride should be used with caution in patients with risk factors for stroke.

Excipient Warnings

The product contains liquid maltitol. Patients with rare hereditary problems of fructose intolerance should not take this medicine.

This product also contains parahydroxybenzoates (preservatives) which may cause allergic reactions (possibly delayed).

4.5 Interaction with other medicinal products and other forms of interaction
While no drug interactions are known, unnecessary polypharmacy should be avoided. As with other psychotropic compounds, sulpiride may increase the effect of antihypertensives and CNS depressants or stimulants.

Sulpiride results in reciprocal antagonism of effects between levodopa and neuroleptics.

The bioavailability of sulpiride is reduced by concomitant administration with sucralfate and antacids and should not, therefore, be taken at the same time.

Also concurrent use with lithium may cause extrapyramidal symptoms to develop.

Sulpiride may reduce the effectiveness of ropinorole.

Combination with the following medications which could induce torsade de pointes:

- Bradycardia-inducing medications such as beta-blockers, bradycardia-inducing calcium channel blockers such as diltiazem and verapamil, clonidine; digitalics.
- Medications which induce hypokalaemia: Hypokalaemic diuretics, stimulant laxatives, IV amphotericin B, glucocorticoids, tetracosactides.
- Class Ia antiarrhythmic agents such as quinidine, disopyramide.
- Class III antiarrhythmic agents such as amiodarone, sotalol.
- Other medications such as pimozide, haloperidol; imipramine antidepressants; cisapride, thioridazine, IV erythromycin, pentamidine.

Use with concomitant QT prolonging drugs and with drugs causing electrolyte imbalance is not recommended. If the benefit is considered to outweigh the risk in the individual patient, co-administration should be undertaken with caution and ECG monitoring should be considered. (See section 4.4).

4.6 Pregnancy and lactation
Despite the negative results of teratogenicity studies in animals and the lack of teratogenic effects during widespread clinical use in other countries, sulpiride should not be considered an exception to the general principle of avoiding drug treatment in pregnancy, particularly during the first 16 weeks, with potential benefits being weighed against possible hazards.

Sulpiride has been found in low concentrations in breast milk. It is, therefore, recommended that the use of sulpiride be avoided in patients who are breast feeding.

4.7 Effects on ability to drive and use machines
Patients should be advised not to drive or operate machinery if they experience symptoms of slowing of reaction time, drowsiness or loss of concentration.

4.8 Undesirable effects
Sulpiride is very well tolerated and usually only minor side-effects occur, if at all, at the recommended doses.

Neuroleptic malignant syndrome. As with other neuroleptics, rare cases of neuroleptic malignant syndrome, characterised by hyperthermia, muscle rigidity, autonomic instability, altered consciousness and elevated CPK levels, have been reported. In such an event, all antipsychotic drugs, including Sulpor, Sulpiride 200mg/5ml Oral Solution, should be discontinued (section 4.4 Special warnings and precautions for use).

Very rare cases of convulsions have been reported, in particular in epileptic patients (see section 4.4 Special warnings and precautions for use).

Extrapyramidal symptoms and related disorders:

- parkinsonism and related symptoms (tremor, hypertonia, hypokinesia, hypersalivation)
- acute dyskinesia and dystonia (spasm torticollis, oculogyric crisis, trismus)
- akinesia.

These symptoms are generally reversible upon administration of antiparkinsonian medication.

- tardive dyskinesia (characterised by rhythmic, involuntary movements primarily of the tongue and/or the face) have been reported, as with all neuroleptics, after a neuroleptic administration of more than 3 months. Antiparkinsonian medication is ineffective or may induce aggravation of the symptoms.

Sedation or drowsiness. Insomnia has been reported.

Hepatic reactions including jaundice and hepatitis have been reported.

As is usual with neuroleptics and psychotic drugs, sulpiride raises serum prolactin levels, which may be associated with galactorrhoea, oligomenorrhoea and amenorrhoea, and less frequently with gynaecomastia. Sexual function may also be increased or decreased.

Postural hypotension, body weight gain (potentially significant in very rare cases) and very rare cases of hypersensitivity reactions such as skin reactions have been reported.

A mild laxative effect or diarrhoea may be caused by the liquid maltitol in the formulation.

Very rare cases of QT prolongation and very rare cases of torsade de pointes have been reported.

Ventricular arrhythmias such as VF, VT (rare), sudden unexplained death, cardiac arrest are class effects of neuroleptics.

4.9 Overdose
The range of single toxic doses is 1 to 16g but no death has occurred even at the 16g dose.

The clinical manifestations of poisoning vary depending upon the size of the dose taken. After single doses of 1 to 3g restlessness and clouding of consciousness have been reported and (rarely) extrapyramidal symptoms.

Doses of 3 to 7g may produce a degree of agitation, confusion and extrapyramidal symptoms; more than 7g can cause, in addition, coma and low blood pressure.

The duration of intoxication is generally short, the symptoms disappearing within a few hours. Comas which have occurred after large doses have lasted up to four days. There are no specific complications from overdose. In particular no haematological or hepatic toxicity has been reported.

Overdose may be treated with alkaline osmotic diuresis and, if necessary, anti-parkinsonian drugs. Coma needs appropriate nursing. Emetic drugs are unlikely to be effective in sulpiride overdosage.

5. PHARMACOLOGICAL PROPERTIES

5.1 Pharmacodynamic properties
One of the characteristics of sulpiride is its bimodal activity, as it has both antidepressant and neuroleptic properties. Schizophrenia characterised by a lack of social contact can benefit strikingly. Mood elevation is observed after a few days treatment, followed by disappearance of the florid schizophrenic symptoms. The sedation and lack of effect characteristically associated with classical neuroleptics of the phenothiazine or butyrophenone type are not features of sulpiride therapy.

Sulpiride is a member of the group of substituted benzamides, which are structurally distinct from the phenothiazines, butyrophenones and thioxanthenes. Current evidence suggests that the actions of sulpiride hint at an important distinction between different types of dopamine receptors or receptor mechanisms in the brain.

Behaviourally and biochemically, sulpiride shares with these classical neuroleptics a number of properties indicative of cerebral dopamine receptor antagonism. Essential and intriguing differences include lack of catalepsy at doses active in other behavioural tests, lack of effect in the dopamine sensitive adenylate cyclase systems, lack of effect upon noradrenaline or 5HT turnover, negligible anticholinesterase activity, no effect on muscarinic or GABA receptor binding, and a radical difference in the binding of tritiated sulpiride to striatal preparations in-vitro, compared to ^{3}H-spiperone and ^{3}H-haloperidol. These findings indicate a major differentiation between sulpiride and classical neuroleptics which lack such specificity.

5.2 Pharmacokinetic properties
Peak sulpiride serum levels are reached 3-6 hours after an oral dose. The plasma half-life in man is approximately 8 hours. Approximately 40% sulpiride is bound to plasma proteins. 95% of the compound is excreted in the urine and faeces as unchanged sulpiride.

5.3 Preclinical safety data
In long-term animal studies with neuroleptic drugs, including sulpiride, an increased incidence of various endocrine

tumours (some of which have occasionally been malignant) has been seen in some but not all strains of rats and mice studied. The significance of these findings to man is not known; there is no current evidence of any association between neuroleptic use and tumour risk in man. However, when prescribing neuroleptics to patients with existing mammary neoplasia or a history of this disease, possible risks should be weighed against benefits of therapy.

6. PHARMACEUTICAL PARTICULARS

6.1 List of excipients

Methyl parahydroxybenzoate, propyl parahydroxybenzoate, propylene glycol, citric acid monohydrate, liquid maltitol, lemon flavour, aniseed flavour and purified water.

6.2 Incompatibilities

None known.

6.3 Shelf life

36 months – unopened

3 months - opened

6.4 Special precautions for storage

Do not store above 25°C.

6.5 Nature and contents of container

Bottle: 150ml amber (Type III) glass.

Closure: a) Aluminium, EPE wadded, roll-on pilfer-proof screw cap.

b) HDPE, EPE wadded, tamper evident screw cap.

c) HDPE, EPE wadded, tamper evident, child resistant closure.

6.6 Special precautions for disposal and other handling

The date of opening should be entered on the label next to the "use within 3 months of opening" statement.

Administrative Data

7. MARKETING AUTHORISATION HOLDER

Rosemont Pharmaceuticals Ltd, Rosemont House, Yorkdale Industrial Park, Braithwaite Street, Leeds, LS11 9XE, UK.

8. MARKETING AUTHORISATION NUMBER(S)

PL 00427/0129

9. DATE OF FIRST AUTHORISATION/RENEWAL OF THE AUTHORISATION

08.08.01/07.04.09

10. DATE OF REVISION OF THE TEXT

07.04.09

Supralip 160mg

(Solvay Healthcare Limited)

1. NAME OF THE MEDICINAL PRODUCT

Supralip® 160 mg, film-coated tablet.

2. QUALITATIVE AND QUANTITATIVE COMPOSITION

Each tablet contains 160.0 mg fenofibrate.

For excipients, see 6.1.

3. PHARMACEUTICAL FORM

Film coated tablet.

White, oblong, film-coated tablets engraved "160" on one side and "Fournier logo" on the other side.

4. CLINICAL PARTICULARS

4.1 Therapeutic indications

Hypercholesterolaemia and hypertriglyceridaemia alone or combined (types IIa, IIb, IV dyslipidaemias, as well as types III and V dyslipidaemias although only a few patients have been treated during clinical trials) in patients unresponsive to dietary and other non-drug therapeutic measures (e.g. weight reduction or increased physical activity), particularly when there is evidence of associated risk factors.

The treatment of secondary hyperlipoproteinaemias is indicated if the hyperlipoproteinaemia persists despite effective treatment of the underlying disease (e.g. dyslipidaemia in diabetes mellitus).

Dietary measures initiated before therapy should be continued.

4.2 Posology and method of administration

Posology:

Adults: The recommended dose is one tablet containing 160 mg fenofibrate taken once daily. Patients currently taking one Lipantil Micro 200mg capsule can be changed to one Supralip 160 mg tablet without further dose adjustment.

Elderly patients: The usual adult dose is recommended.

Patients with renal impairment: Dosage reduction is required in patients with renal impairment. The use of dosage forms containing a lower dose of active ingredient (67 mg micronised fenofibrate capsules or 100 mg standard fenofibrate capsules) is recommended in these patients.

Children: The use of the 160 mg dosage form is contra-indicated in children.

Hepatic disease: Patients with hepatic disease have not been studied.

Dietary measures initiated before therapy should be continued.

If after several months of fenofibrate administration (e.g. 3 months) serum lipid levels have not been reduced satisfactorily, complementary or different therapeutic measures should be considered.

Method of administration: Tablet should be swallowed whole during a meal.

4.3 Contraindications

– hepatic insufficiency (including biliary cirrhosis),

– renal insufficiency,

– children,

– hypersensitivity to fenofibrate or any component of this medication,

– known photoallergy or phototoxic reaction during treatment with fibrates or ketoprofen,

– gallbladder disease.

Chronic or acute pancreatitis with the exception of acute pancreatitis due to severe hypertriglyceridemia.

Use during pregnancy and lactation: see section 4.6.

Supralip 160mg should not be taken in patients allergic to peanut or arachis oil or soya lecithin or related products due to the risk of hypersensitivity reactions.

4.4 Special warnings and precautions for use

Liver function

As with other lipid lowering agents, increases have been reported in transaminase levels in some patients. In the majority of cases these elevations were transient, minor and asymptomatic. It is recommended that transaminase levels be monitored every 3 months during the first 12 months of treatment. Attention should be paid to patients who develop increase in transaminase levels and therapy should be discontinued if ASAT and ALAT levels increase to more than 3 times the upper limit of the normal range or 100 IU.

Pancreatitis

Pancreatitis has been reported in patients taking fenofibrate (see sections 4.3 and 4.8). This occurrence may represent a failure of efficacy in patients with severe hypertriglyceridemia, a direct drug effect, or a secondary phenomenon mediated through biliary tract stone or sludge formation, resulting in the obstruction of the common bile duct.

Muscle

Muscle toxicity, including very rare cases of rhabdomyolysis, has been reported with administration of fibrates and other lipid-lowering agents. The incidence of this disorder increases in cases of hypoalbuminaemia and previous renal insufficiency. Muscle toxicity should be suspected in patients presenting diffuse myalgia, myositis, muscular cramps and weakness and/or marked increases in CPK (levels exceeding 5 times the normal range). In such cases treatment with fenofibrate should be stopped.

Patients with pre-disposing factors for myopathy and/or rhabdomyolysis, including age above 70 years old, personal or familial history of hereditary muscular disorders, renal impairment, hypothyroidism and high alcohol intake, may be at an increased risk of developing rhabdomyolysis. For these patients, the putative benefits and risks of fenofibrate therapy should be carefully weighed up.

The risk of muscle toxicity may be increased if the drug is administered with another fibrate or an HMG-CoA reductase inhibitor, especially in cases of pre-existing muscular disease. Consequently, the co-prescription of fenofibrate with a statin should be reserved to patients with severe combined dyslipidaemia and high cardiovascular risk without any history of muscular disease. This combination therapy should be used with caution and patients should be monitored closely for signs of muscle toxicity.

For hyperlipidaemic patients taking oestrogens or contraceptives containing oestrogens it should be ascertained whether the hyperlipidaemia is of primary or secondary nature (possible elevation of lipid values caused by oral oestrogen).

This medicinal product contains lactose. Therefore patients with rare hereditary problems of galactose intolerance, the Lapp lactase deficiency or glucose-galactose malabsorptionshould nottake this medicine.

Renal function:

Treatment should be interrupted in case of an increase in creatinine levels > 50% ULN (upper limit of normal).

It is recommended that creatinine measurement may be considered during the first three months after initiation of treatment.

4.5 Interaction with other medicinal products and other forms of interaction

Oral anticoagulants

Fenofibrate enhances oral anticoagulant effect and may increase risk of bleeding. It is recommended that the dose of anticoagulants is reduced by about one third at the start of treatment and then gradually adjusted if necessary according to INR (International Normalised Ratio) monitoring. Therefore, this combination is not recommended.

Cyclosporin

Some severe cases of reversible renal function impairment have been reported during concomitant administration of fenofibrate and cyclosporin. The renal function of these patients must therefore be closely monitored and the treatment with fenofibrate stopped in the case of severe alteration of laboratory parameters.

HMG-CoA reductase inhibitors and other fibrates

The risk of serious muscle toxicity is increased if fenofibrate is used concomitantly with HMG-CoA reductase inhibitors or other fibrates. Such combination therapy should be used with caution and patients monitored closely for signs of muscle toxicity (See section 4.4).

4.6 Pregnancy and lactation

There are no adequate data from the use of fenofibrate in pregnant women. Animal studies have not demonstrated any teratogenic effects. Embryotoxic effects have been shown at doses in the range of maternal toxicity (see section 5.3). The potential risk for humans is unknown. Therefore, Supralip 160mg film-coated tablet should only be used during pregnancy after a careful benefit/riskassessment.

There are no data on the excretion of fenofibrate and/or its metabolites into breast milk.

Consequently Supralip 160mg film-coated tablet should not be used in nursing mother.

4.7 Effects on ability to drive and use machines

No effect noted.

4.8 Undesirable effects

The frequencies of adverse events are ranked according to the following: Very common (>1/10); Common (>1/100, <1/10); Uncommon (>1/1,000, <1/100); Rare (>1/10,000, <1/1,000); Very rare (<1/10,000), including isolated reports.

Gastrointestinal disorders:

Common: Digestive, gastric or intestinal disorders (abdominal pain, nausea, vomiting, diarrhoea, and flatulence) moderate in severity

Uncommon: Pancreatitis *

Hepato-biliary disorders:

Common: Moderately elevated levels of serum transaminases (see Special precautions for use)

Uncommon: Development of gallstones

Very rare: episodes of hepatitis. When symptoms (e.g. jaundice, pruritus) indicative of hepatitis occur, laboratory tests are to be conducted for verification and fenofibrate discontinued, if applicable (see Special warnings)

Cardiovascular system

Uncommon: Thromboembolism (pulmonary embolism, deep vein thrombosis)*

Skin and subcutaneous tissue disorders:

Uncommon: rashes, pruritus, urticaria or photosensitivity reactions

Rare: alopecia

Very rare: cutaneous photosensitivity with erythema, vesiculation or nodulation on parts of the skin exposed to sunlight or artificial UV light (e.g. sunlamp) in individual cases (even after many months of uncomplicated use)

Musculoskeletal, connective tissue and bone disorders:

Rare: diffuse myalgia, myositis, muscular cramps and weakness

Very rare: rhabdomyolysis

Blood and lymphatic system disorders:

Rare: decrease in haemoglobin and leukocytes

Nervous system disorders:

Rare: sexual asthenia

Respiratory, thoracic and mediastinal disorders:

Very rare: interstitial pneumopathies

Investigation:

Uncommon: Increases in serum creatinine and urea.

* In the FIELD-study, a randomized placebo-controlled trial performed in 9795 patients with type 2 diabetes mellitus, a statistically significant increase in pancreatitis cases was observed in patients receiving fenofibrate versus patients receiving placebo (0.8% versus 0.5%; p = 0.031). In the same study, a statistically significant increase was reported in the incidence of pulmonary embolism (0.7% in the placebo group versus 1.1% in the fenofibrate group; p = 0.022) and a statistically non-significant increase in deep vein thromboses (placebo: 1.0 % [48/4900 patients] versus fenofibrate 1.4% [67/4895 patients]; p = 0.074).

4.9 Overdose

No case of overdosage has been reported. No specific antidote is known. If an overdose is suspected, treat symptomatically and institute appropriate supportive measures as required. Fenofibrate cannot be eliminated by haemodialysis.

5. PHARMACOLOGICAL PROPERTIES

5.1 Pharmacodynamic properties

Serum Lipid Reducing Agents / Cholesterol and Triglycerides Reducers / Fibrates.

ATC code: C10 AB 05

Fenofibrate is a fibric acid derivative whose lipid modifying effects reported in humans are mediated via activation of Peroxisome Proliferator Activated Receptor type alpha (PPARα).

Through activation of PPARα, fenofibrate increases the lipolysis and elimination of atherogenic triglyceride-rich particles from plasma by activating lipoprotein lipase and reducing production of apoprotein CIII. Activation of PPARα also induces an increase in the synthesis of apoproteins AI and AII.

The above stated effects of fenofibrate on lipoproteins lead to a reduction in very low- and low density fractions (VLDL and LDL) containing apoprotein B and an increase in the high density lipoprotein fraction (HDL) containing apoprotein AI and AII.

In addition, through modulation of the synthesis and the catabolism of VLDL fractions fenofibrate increases the LDL clearance and reduces small dense LDL, the levels of which are elevated in the atherogenic lipoprotein phenotype, a common disorder in patients at risk for coronary heart disease.

During clinical trials with fenofibrate, total cholesterol was reduced by 20 to 25%, triglycerides by 40 to 55% and HDL cholesterol was increased by 10 to 30%.

In hypercholesterolaemic patients, where LDL cholesterol levels are reduced by 20 to 35%, the overall effect on cholesterol results in a decrease in the ratios of total cholesterol to HDL cholesterol, LDL cholesterol to HDL cholesterol, or Apo B to Apo AI, all of which are markers of atherogenic risk.

Because of its significant effect on LDL cholesterol and triglycerides, treatment with fenofibrate should be beneficial in hypercholesterolaemic patients with or without hypertriglyceridaemia, including secondary hyperlipoproteinaemia such as type 2 diabetes mellitus.

At the present time, no results of long-term controlled clinical trials are available to demonstrate the efficacy of fenofibrate in the primary or secondary prevention of atherosclerotic complications.

Extravascular deposits of cholesterol (tendinous and tuberous xanthoma) may be markedly reduced or even entirely eliminated during fenofibrate therapy.

Patients with raised levels of fibrinogen treated with fenofibrate have shown significant reductions in this parameter, as have those with raised levels of Lp(a). Other inflammatory markers such as C Reactive Protein are reduced with fenofibrate treatment.

The uricosuric effect of fenofibrate leading to reduction in uric acid levels of approximately 25% should be of additional benefit in those dyslipidaemic patients with hyperuricaemia.

Fenofibrate has been shown to possess an anti-aggregatory effect on platelets in animals and in a clinical study, which showed a reduction in platelet aggregation induced by ADP, arachidonic acid and epinephrine.

5.2 Pharmacokinetic properties

Supralip 160 mg is a film-coated tablet containing 160 mg of micronised fenofibrate and is suprabioavailable (larger bioavailability) compared to the previous formulations.

Absorption: Maximum plasma concentrations (Cmax) occur within 4 to 5 hours after oral administration. Plasma concentrations are stable during continuous treatment in any given individual.

The absorption of fenofibrate is increased when administered with food.

Distribution: Fenofibric acid is strongly bound to plasma albumin (more than 99%).

Plasma half-life: The plasma elimination half-life of fenofibric acid is approximately 20 hours.

Metabolism and excretion: No unchanged fenofibrate can be detected in the plasma where the principal metabolite is fenofibric acid. The drug is excreted mainly in the urine. Practically all the drug is eliminated within 6 days. Fenofibrate is mainly excreted in the form of fenofibric acid and its glucuronide conjugate. In elderly patients, the fenofibric acid apparent total plasma clearance is not modified.

Kinetic studies following the administration of a single dose and continuous treatment have demonstrated that the drug does not accumulate. Fenofibric acid is not eliminated by haemodialysis.

5.3 Preclinical safety data

Chronic toxicity studies have yielded no relevant information about specific toxicity of fenofibrate.

Studies on mutagenicity of fenofibrate have been negative.

In rats and mice, liver tumours have been found at high dosages, which are attributable to peroxisome proliferation. These changes are specific to small rodents and have not been observed in other animal species. This is of no relevance to therapeutic use in man.

Studies in mice, rats and rabbits did not reveal any teratogenic effect. Embryotoxic effects were observed at doses in the range of maternal toxicity. Prolongation of the gestation period and difficulties during delivery were observed at high doses. No sign of any effect on fertility has been detected.

6. PHARMACEUTICAL PARTICULARS

6.1 List of excipients

Sodium laurilsulfate, lactose monohydrate, povidone, crospovidone, microcrystalline cellulose, silica colloidal anhydrous, sodium stearyl fumarate.

Composition of the coating

Opadry®: polyvinyl alcohol, titanium dioxide (E171), talc, soybean lecithin, xanthan gum.

6.2 Incompatibilities

Not applicable.

6.3 Shelf life

2 years.

6.4 Special precautions for storage

Store in the original package in order to protect from moisture.

Do not store above 30°C.

6.5 Nature and contents of container

Thermoformed blister strips (PVC/PE/PVDC) of 10 or 14 tablets each.

Boxes of 10, 20, 28, 30, 50, 84, 90, 98 and 100 tablets.

Hospital pack sizes: 280 (10 × 28) and 300 (10 × 30) tablets.

Not all pack sizes may be marketed.

6.6 Special precautions for disposal and other handling

No special requirements.

7. MARKETING AUTHORISATION HOLDER

Solvay Healthcare Ltd

Mansbridge Road

West End

Southampton

SO18 3JD

United Kingdom

8. MARKETING AUTHORISATION NUMBER(S)

PL 00512/0389

9. DATE OF FIRST AUTHORISATION/RENEWAL OF THE AUTHORISATION

Date of first authorisation: September 2000

Date of last renewal: 4 November 2004

10. DATE OF REVISION OF THE TEXT

July 2007

11. Legal category

POM

Suprax Powder for Paediatric Oral Suspension

(sanofi-aventis)

1. NAME OF THE MEDICINAL PRODUCT

Suprax Powder for Paediatric Oral Suspension

2. QUALITATIVE AND QUANTITATIVE COMPOSITION

Each 5mL of reconstituted suspension contains 100 mg cefixime (anhydrous).

3. PHARMACEUTICAL FORM

For oral administration.

Bottles of powder for the preparation of suspension. When reconstituted, each 5 ml volume contains 100 mg of cefixime. The suspension contains 2.5 g of sucrose in 5 ml.

4. CLINICAL PARTICULARS

4.1 Therapeutic indications

Suprax is an orally active cephalosporin antibiotic which has marked *in vitro* bactericidal activity against a wide variety of Gram-positive and Gram-negative organisms.

It is indicated for the treatment of the following acute infections when caused by susceptible micro-organisms:

Upper Respiratory Tract Infections (URTI): e.g. otitis media; and other URTI where the causative organism is known or suspected to be resistant to other commonly used antibiotics, or where treatment failure may carry significant risk.

Lower Respiratory Tract Infection: e.g. bronchitis.

Urinary Tract Infections: e.g. cystitis, cystourethritis, uncomplicated pyelonephritis.

Clinical efficacy has been demonstrated in infections caused by commonly occuring pathogens including *Streptococcus pneumoniae, Streptococcus pyogenes, Escherichia coli, Proteus mirabilis, Kliebsiella* species, *Haemophilus influenzae* (beta-lactamase positive and negative), *Branhamella catarrhalis* (beta-lactamase positive and negative) and *Enterobacter* species. Suprax is highly stable in the presence of beta-lactamase enzymes.

Most strains of enterococci (*Streptococcus faecalis*, group D Streptococci) and Staphylococci (including coagulase positive and negative strains and methicillin-resistant strains) are resistant to Suprax. In addition, most strains of *Pseudomonas, Bacteriodes fragalis, Listeria monocytogenes* and *Clostridia* are resistant to Suprax.

4.2 Posology and method of administration

Route of Administration: Oral

Absorption of Suprax is not significantly modified by the presence of food. The usual course of treatment is 7 days. This may be continued for up to 14 days if required.

Adults and Children over 10 Years: The recommended adult dosage is 200-400 mg daily according to the severity of infection, given either as a single dose or in two divided doses.

The Elderly: Elderly patients may be given the same dose as recommended for adults. Renal function should be assessed and dosage should be adjusted in severe renal impairment (See "Dosage in Renal Impairment").

Children (Use Paediatric Oral Suspension): The recommended dosage for children is 8 mg/kg/day administered as a single dose or in two divided doses. As a general guide for prescribing in children the following daily doses in terms of volume of Paediatric Oral Suspension are suggested:

6 months up to 1 year: 3.75 ml daily

Children 1-4 years: 5 ml daily

Children 5-10 years: 10 ml daily

(A spoon is supplied to aid correct dosing - see "Nature and Contents of Container").

Children weighing more than 50 kg or older than 10 years should be treated with the recommended adult dose (200 - 400 mg daily depending on the severity of infection).

The safety and efficacy of cefixime has not been established in children less than 6 months.

Dosage In Renal Impairment: Suprax may be administered in the presence of impaired renal function. Normal dose and schedule may be given in patients with creatinine clearances of 20 ml/min or greater. In patients whose creatinine clearance is less than 20 ml/min, it is recommended that a dose of 200 mg once daily should not be exceeded. The dose and regimen for patients who are maintained on chronic ambulatory peritoneal dialysis or haemodialysis should follow the same recommendation as that for patients with creatinine clearances of less than 20 ml/min.

4.3 Contraindications

Patients with known hypersensitivity to cephalosporin antibiotics.

4.4 Special warnings and precautions for use

Suprax should be given with caution to patients who have shown hypersensitivity to other drugs. Cephalosporins should be given with caution to penicillin-sensitive patients, as there is some evidence of partial cross-allergenicity between the penicillins and cephalosporins.

Patients have had severe reactions (including anaphylaxis) to both classes of drugs. If an allergic effect occurs with Suprax, the drug should be discontinued and the patient treated with appropriate agents if necessary.

Suprax should be administered with caution in patients with markedly impaired renal function (See "Dosage in Renal Impairment").

Treatment with broad spectrum antibiotics alters the normal flora of the colon and may permit overgrowth of clostridia. Studies indicate that a toxin produced by *Clostridium difficile* is a primary cause of antibiotic-associated diarrhoea. Pseudomembranous colitis is associated with the use of broad-spectrum antibiotics (including macrolides, semi-synthetic penicillins, lincosamides and cephalosporins); it is therefore important to consider its diagnosis in patients who develop diarrhoea in association with the use of antibiotics. Symptoms of pseudomembranous colitis may occur during or after antibiotic treatment.

Management of pseudomembranous colitis should include sigmoidoscopy, appropriate bacteriologic studies, fluids, electrolytes and protein supplementation. If the colitis does not improve after the drug has been discontinued, or if the symptoms are severe, oral vancomycin is the drug of choice for antibiotic-associated pseudomembranous colitis produced by *C. difficile*. Other causes of colitis should be excluded.

4.5 Interaction with other medicinal products and other forms of interaction

A false positive reaction for glucose in the urine may occur with Benedict's or Fehling's solutions or with copper sulphate test tablets, but not with tests based on enzymatic glucose oxidase reactions.

A false positive direct Coombs test has been reported during treatment with cephalosporin antibiotics, therefore it should be recognised that a positive Coombs test may be due to the drug.

In common with other cephalosporins, increases in prothrombin times have been noted in a few patients. Care should therefore be taken in patients receiving anticoagulation therapy.

4.6 Pregnancy and lactation

Reproduction studies have been performed in mice and rats at doses up to 400 times the human dose and have revealed no evidence of impaired fertility or harm to the foetus due to cefixime. In the rabbit, at doses up to 4 times the human dose, there was no evidence of a teratogenic effect; there was a high incidence of abortion and maternal death which is an expected consequence of the known sensitivity of rabbits to antibiotic-induced changes in the population of the microflora of the intestine. There are no adequate and well-controlled studies in pregnant women. Suprax should therefore not be used in pregnancy or in nursing mothers unless considered essential by the physician.

4.7 Effects on ability to drive and use machines
None.

4.8 Undesirable effects
Suprax is generally well tolerated. The majority of adverse reactions observed in clinical trials were mild and self-limiting in nature.

Gastrointestinal Disturbances: The most frequent side effects seen with Suprax are diarrhoea and stool changes; diarrhoea has been more commonly associated with higher doses. Some cases of moderate to severe diarrhoea have been reported; this has occasionally warranted cessation of therapy. Suprax should be discontinued if marked diarrhoea occurs. Other gastrointestinal side effects seen less frequently are nausea, abdominal pain, dyspepsia, vomiting and flatulence. Pseudomembranous colitis has been reported (see above).

Central Nervous System: Headache and dizziness.

Hypersensitivity Reactions: Allergies in the form of rash, pruritus, drug fever and arthralgia have been observed, including rare cases of urticaria or angioedema. These reactions usually subsided upon discontinuation of therapy. Rarely, erythema multiforme, Stevens-Johnson syndrome and toxic epidermal necrolysis have been reported.

Haematological and Clinical Chemistry: Thrombocytosis, thrombocytopenia, leucopenia, hypereosinophilia, neutropenia and agranulocytosis have been reported. These reactions were infrequent and reversible. Mild transient changes in liver and renal function tests have been observed.

Hepatic Disorders: Transient rises in liver transaminases, alkaline phosphatase and jaundice can also occur.

Miscellaneous: Other possible reactions include genital pruritus and vaginitis.

4.9 Overdose
There is no experience with overdoses with Suprax.

Adverse reactions seen at dose levels up to 2 g Suprax in normal subjects did not differ from the profile seen in patients treated at the recommended doses. Gastric lavage may be indicated in overdosage. No specific antidote exists. Cefixime is not removed from the circulation in significant quantities by dialysis.

5. PHARMACOLOGICAL PROPERTIES

5.1 Pharmacodynamic properties
Cefixime is an oral third generation cephalosporin which has marked *in vitro* bactericidal activity against a wide variety of Gram-positive and Gram-negative organisms.

Clinical efficacy has been demonstrated in infections caused by commonly occurring pathogens including *Streptococcus pneumoniae, Streptococcus pyogenes, Escherichia coli, Proteus mirabilis, Klebsiella* species, *Haemophilus influenzae* (beta-lactamase positive and negative), *Branhamella catarrhalis* (beta-lactamase positive and negative) and *Enterobacter* species. It is highly stable in the presence of beta-lactamase enzymes.

Most strains of enterococci (*Streptococcus faecalis*, group D Streptococci) and Staphylococci (including coagulase positive and negative strains and methicillin-resistant strains) are resistant to cefixime. In addition, most strains of *Pseudomonas, Bacteroides fragilis, Listeria monocytogenes* and *Clostridia* are resistant to cefixime.

5.2 Pharmacokinetic properties
The absolute oral bioavailability of cefixime is in the range of 22-54%. Absorption is not significantly modified by the presence of food. Cefixime may therefore be given without regard to meals.

From *in vitro* studies, serum or urine concentrations of 1 mcg/ml or greater were considered to be adequate for most common pathogens against which cefixime is active. Typically, the peak serum levels following the recommended adult or paediatric doses are between 1.5 and 3 mcg/ml. Little or no accumulation of cefixime occurs following multiple dosing.

The pharmacokinetics of cefixime in healthy elderly (age > 64 years) and young volunteers (11-35) compared the administration of 400 mg doses once daily for 5 days. Mean C_{max} and AUC values were slightly greater in the elderly. Elderly patients may be given the same dose as the general population.

Cefixime is predominantly eliminated as unchanged drug in the urine. Glomerular filtration is considered the predominant mechanism. Metabolites of cefixime have not been isolated from human serum or urine.

Serum protein binding is well characterised for human and animal sera; cefixime is almost exclusively bound to the albumin fraction, the mean free fraction being approximately 30%. Protein binding of cefixime is only concentration dependent in human serum at very high concentrations which are not seen following clinical dosing.

Transfer of ^{14}C-labelled cefixime from lactating rats to their nursing offspring through breast milk was quantitatively small (approximately 1.5% of the mothers' body content of cefixime in the pup). No data are available on secretion of cefixime in human breast milk. Placetal transfer of cefixime was small in pregnant rats dosed with labelled cefixime.

5.3 Preclinical safety data
There are no pre-clinical data of relevance to the prescriber which are additional to that already included in other sections of the Summary of Product Characteristics.

6. PHARMACEUTICAL PARTICULARS

6.1 List of excipients
Sucrose, xantham gum, sodium benzoate and strawberry flavour.

6.2 Incompatibilities
None.

6.3 Shelf life
2 years unopened.

2 weeks after reconstitution.

6.4 Special precautions for storage
Do not store unreconstituted product above 25°C.

Bottled product: To reconstitute, add 33 ml of water (50 ml bottle) or 66 ml of water (100 ml bottle) in two portions shaking after each addition. After reconstitution, the suspension may be stored at room temperature (below 25° C) for 14 days without significant loss of potency. Do not freeze. Keep bottles tightly closed and shake well before use. Discard any unused portion after 14 days. Dilution of the suspension is not recommended.

6.5 Nature and contents of container
Type III amber glass screw necked bottle with child resistant push/turn closure with white polyethylene cap with polyethylene film seal on expanded low density polyethylene. Bottles are supplied with a single ended transparent polypropylene (plastic) spoon capable of measuring 3.75 and 5.0ml of the suspension. Pack sizes of 50 and 100 ml.

6.6 Special precautions for disposal and other handling
None stated.

7. MARKETING AUTHORISATION HOLDER
sanofi-aventis
One Onslow Street
Guildford
Surrey
GU1 4YS
UK

8. MARKETING AUTHORISATION NUMBER(S)
PL 00012/0318

9. DATE OF FIRST AUTHORISATION/RENEWAL OF THE AUTHORISATION
14 October 1998

10. DATE OF REVISION OF THE TEXT
4th July 2008

11 LEGAL CLASSIFICATION
POM

Suprax Tablets 200 mg

(sanofi-aventis)

1. NAME OF THE MEDICINAL PRODUCT
Suprax Tablets 200mg

2. QUALITATIVE AND QUANTITATIVE COMPOSITION
Each tablet contains 200mg cefixime (anhydrous).

3. PHARMACEUTICAL FORM
Convex, off-white, film-coated tablets engraved with 'ORO' on one side.

For oral administration.

4. CLINICAL PARTICULARS

4.1 Therapeutic indications
Suprax is an orally active cephalosporin antibiotic which has marked *in vitro* bactericidal activity against a wide variety of Gram-positive and Gram-negative organisms.

It is indicated for the treatment of the following acute infections when caused by susceptible micro-organisms:

Upper Respiratory Tract Infections (URTI): e.g. otitis media; and other URTI where the causative organism is known or suspected to be resistant to other commonly used antibiotics, or where treatment failure may carry significant risk.

Lower Respiratory Tract Infection: e.g. bronchitis.

Urinary Tract Infections: e.g. cystitis, cystourethritis, uncomplicated pyelonephritis.

Clinical efficacy has been demonstrated in infections caused by commonly occuring pathogens including *Streptococcus pneumoniae, Streptococcus pyogenes, Escherichia coli, Proteus mirabilis, Kliebsiella* species, *Haemophilus influenzae* (beta-lactamase positive and negative), *Branhamella catarrhalis* (beta-lactamase positive and negative) and *Enterobacter* species. Suprax is highly stable in the presence of beta-lactamase enzymes.

Most strains of enterococci (*Streptococcus faecalis*, group D Streptococci) and Staphylococci (including coagulase positive and negative strains and meticillin-resistant strains) are resistant to Suprax. In addition, most strains of *Pseudomonas, Bacteriodes fragalis, Listeria monocytogenes* and *Clostridia* are resistant to Suprax.

4.2 Posology and method of administration
Absorption of Suprax is not significantly modified by the presence of food. The usual course of treatment is 7 days. This may be continued for up to 14 days if required.

Adults and Children over 10 Years: The recommended adult dosage is 200-400 mg daily according to the severity of infection, given either as a single dose or in two divided doses.

The Elderly: Elderly patients may be given the same dose as recommended for adults. Renal function should be assessed and dosage should be adjusted in severe renal impairment (See "Dosage in Renal Impairment").

Children (Use Paediatric Oral Suspension): The recommended dosage for children is 8 mg/kg/day administered as a single dose or in two divided doses. As a general guide for prescribing in children the following daily doses in terms of volume of Paediatric Oral Suspension are suggested:

6 months up to 1 year: 3.75 ml daily

Children 1-4 years: 5 ml daily

Children 5-10 years: 10 ml daily

Children weighing more than 50 kg or older than 10 years should be treated with the recommended adult dose (200 - 400 mg daily depending on the severity of infection).

The safety and efficacy of cefixime has not been established in children less than 6 months.

Dosage In Renal Impairment: Suprax may be administered in the presence of impaired renal function. Normal dose and schedule may be given in patients with creatinine clearances of 20 ml/min or greater. In patients whose creatinine clearance is less than 20 ml/min, it is recommended that a dose of 200 mg once daily should not be exceeded. The dose and regimen for patients who are maintained on chronic ambulatory peritoneal dialysis or haemodialysis should follow the same recommendation as that for patients with creatinine clearances of less than 20 ml/min.

4.3 Contraindications
Patients with known hypersensitivity to cephalosporin antibiotics.

4.4 Special warnings and precautions for use
Suprax should be given with caution to patients who have shown hypersensitivity to other drugs. Cephalosporins should be given with caution to penicillin-sensitive patients, as there is some evidence of partial cross-allergenicity between the penicillins and cephalosporins.

Patients have had severe reactions (including anaphylaxis) to both classes of drugs. If an allergic effect occurs with Suprax, the drug should be discontinued and the patient treated with appropriate agents if necessary.

Suprax should be administered with caution in patients with markedly impaired renal function (See "Dosage in Renal Impairment").

Treatment with broad spectrum antibiotics alters the normal flora of the colon and may permit overgrowth of clostridia. Studies indicate that a toxin produced by *Clostridium difficile* is a primary cause of antibiotic-associated diarrhoea. Pseudomembranous colitis is associated with the use of broad-spectrum antibiotics (including macrolides, semi-synthetic penicillins, lincosamides and cephalosporins); it is therefore important to consider its diagnosis in patients who develop diarrhoea in association with the use of antibiotics. Symptoms of pseudomembranous colitis may occur during or after antibiotic treatment.

Management of pseudomembranous colitis should include sigmoidoscopy, appropriate bacteriologic studies, fluids, electrolytes and protein supplementation. If the colitis does not improve after the drug has been discontinued, or if the symptoms are severe, oral vancomycin is the drug of choice for antibiotic-associated pseudomembranous colitis produced by *C. difficile*. Other causes of colitis should be excluded.

4.5 Interaction with other medicinal products and other forms of interaction
A false positive reaction for glucose in the urine may occur with Benedict's or Fehling's solutions or with copper sulphate test tablets, but not with tests based on enzymatic glucose oxidase reactions.

A false positive direct Coombs test has been reported during treatment with cephalosporin antibiotics, therefore it should be recognised that a positive Coombs test may be due to the drug.

In common with other cephalosporins, increases in prothrombin times have been noted in a few patients. Care should therefore be taken in patients receiving anticoagulation therapy.

4.6 Pregnancy and lactation
Reproduction studies have been performed in mice and rats at doses up to 400 times the human dose and have revealed no evidence of impaired fertility or harm to the foetus due to cefixime. In the rabbit, at doses up to 4 times the human dose, there was no evidence of a teratogenic effect; there was a high incidence of abortion and maternal death which is an expected consequence of the known sensitivity of rabbits to antibiotic-induced changes in the population of the microflora of the intestine. There are no

adequate and well-controlled studies in pregnant women. Suprax should therefore not be used in pregnancy or in nursing mothers unless considered essential by the physician.

4.7 Effects on ability to drive and use machines
None.

4.8 Undesirable effects
Suprax is generally well tolerated. The majority of adverse reactions observed in clinical trials were mild and self-limiting in nature.

Gastrointestinal Disturbances: The most frequent side effects seen with Suprax are diarrhoea and stool changes; diarrhoea has been more commonly associated with higher doses. Some cases of moderate to severe diarrhoea have been reported; this has occasionally warranted cessation of therapy. Suprax should be discontinued if marked diarrhoea occurs. Other gastrointestinal side effects seen less frequently are nausea, abdominal pain, dyspepsia, vomiting and flatulence. Pseudomembranous colitis has been reported (see above).

Central Nervous System: Headache and dizziness.

Hypersensitivity Reactions: Allergies in the form of rash, pruritus, drug fever and arthralgia have been observed, including rare cases of urticaria or angioedema. These reactions usually subsided upon discontinuation of therapy. Rarely, erythema multiforme, Stevens-Johnson syndrome and toxic epidermal necrolysis have been reported.

Haematological and Clinical Chemistry: Thrombocytosis, thrombocytopenia, leucopenia, hypereosinophilia, neutropenia and agranulocytosis have been reported. These reactions were infrequent and reversible. Mild transient changes in liver and renal function tests have been observed.

Hepatic Disorders: Transient rises in liver transaminases, alkaline phosphatase and jaundice can also occur.

Miscellaneous: Other possible reactions include genital pruritus and vaginitis.

4.9 Overdose
There is no experience with overdoses with Suprax.

Adverse reactions seen at dose levels up to 2 g Suprax in normal subjects did not differ from the profile seen in patients treated at the recommended doses. Gastric lavage may be indicated in overdosage. No specific antidote exists. Cefixime is not removed from the circulation in significant quantities by dialysis.

5. PHARMACOLOGICAL PROPERTIES

5.1 Pharmacodynamic properties
Cefixime is an oral third generation cephalosporin which has marked *in vitro* bactericidal activity against a wide variety of Gram-positive and Gram-negative organisms.

Clinical efficacy has been demonstrated in infections caused by commonly occurring pathogens including *Streptococcus pneumoniae, Streptococcus pyogenes, Escherichia coli, Proteus mirabilis, Klebsiella* species, *Haemophilus influenzae* (beta-lactamase positive and negative), *Branhamella catarrhalis* (beta-lactamase positive and negative) and *Enterobacter* species. It is highly stable in the presence of beta-lactamase enzymes.

Most strains of enterococci (*Streptococcus faecalis*, group D Streptococci) and Staphylococci (including coagulase positive and negative strains and meticillin-resistant strains) are resistant to cefixime. In addition, most strains of *Pseudomonas, Bacteroides fragilis, Listeria monocytogenes* and *Clostridia* are resistant to cefixime.

5.2 Pharmacokinetic properties
The absolute oral bioavailability of cefixime is in the range of 22-54%. Absorption is not significantly modified by the presence of food. Cefixime may therefore be given without regard to meals.

From *in vitro* studies, serum or urine concentrations of 1 mcg/mL or greater were considered to be adequate for most common pathogens against which cefixime is active. Typically, the peak serum levels following the recommended adult or paediatric doses are between 1.5 and 3 mcg/mL. Little or no accumulation of cefixime occurs following multiple dosing.

The pharmacokinetics of cefixime in healthy elderly (age > 64 years) and young volunteers (11-35) compared the administration of 400 mg doses once daily for 5 days. Mean C_{max} and AUC values were slightly greater in the elderly. Elderly patients may be given the same dose as the general population.

Cefixime is predominantly eliminated as unchanged drug in the urine. Glomerular filtration is considered the predominant mechanism. Metabolites of cefixime have not been isolated from human serum or urine.

Serum protein binding is well characterised for human and animal sera; cefixime is almost exclusively bound to the albumin fraction, the mean free fraction being approximately 30%. Protein binding of cefixime is only concentration dependent in human serum at very high concentrations which are not seen following clinical dosing.

Transfer of ^{14}C-labelled cefixime from lactating rats to their nursing offspring through breast milk was quantitatively small (approximately 1.5% of the mothers' body content of cefixime in the pup). No data are available on secretion of cefixime in human breast milk. Placetal transfer of cefixime was small in pregnant rats dosed with labelled cefixime.

5.3 Preclinical safety data
There are no pre-clinical data of relevance to the prescriber which are additional to that already included in other sections of the Summary of Product Characteristics.

6. PHARMACEUTICAL PARTICULARS

6.1 List of excipients
Tablet cores: microcrystalline cellulose, pregelatinised starch, calcium hydrogen phosphate dihydrate and magnesium stearate.

Tablet coating: hypromellose, Macrogol 6000 and titanium dioxide.

6.2 Incompatibilities
None.

6.3 Shelf life
2 Years

6.4 Special precautions for storage
Do not store above 25°C.

6.5 Nature and contents of container
PVC/aluminium foil blister packs - pack sizes of 7.

6.6 Special precautions for disposal and other handling
None.

7. MARKETING AUTHORISATION HOLDER
sanofi-aventis
One Onslow Street
Guildford
Surrey
GU1 4YS
UK

8. MARKETING AUTHORISATION NUMBER(S)
PL 00012/0316

9. DATE OF FIRST AUTHORISATION/RENEWAL OF THE AUTHORISATION
12 August 1998

10. DATE OF REVISION OF THE TEXT
4th July 2008

LEGAL CATEGORY
POM

Suprecur Injection

(sanofi-aventis)

1. NAME OF THE MEDICINAL PRODUCT
Suprecur Injection

2. QUALITATIVE AND QUANTITATIVE COMPOSITION
Suprecur injection contains 1.00 mg buserelin as buserelin acetate in 1 ml aqueous solution.

1.00 mg buserelin is equivalent to 1.05 mg buserelin acetate.

3. PHARMACEUTICAL FORM
Solution for Injection.

4. CLINICAL PARTICULARS

4.1 Therapeutic indications
Pituitary desensitisation in preparation for ovulation induction regimens using gonadotrophins

4.2 Posology and method of administration
The total daily dose is usually in the range 200 - 500 microgram (µg) given as a single injection by the subcutaneous route. Treatment should start in the early follicular phase (day 1) or, provided the existence of an early pregnancy has been excluded, in the midluteal phase (day 21). It should continue at least until down-regulation is achieved e.g. serum estradiol <180pmol/l and serum progesterone <3nmol/l. This will usually take about 1 - 3 weeks. Doses may have to be adjusted for individuals. Occasionally, patients may require up to 500 µg twice daily in order to achieve down-regulation. When down-regulation is achieved, stimulation with gonadotropin is commenced while the dosage of buserelin is maintained. At the appropriate stage of follicular development, gonadotropin and buserelin are stopped and hCG is given to induce ovulation.

Treatment monitoring, oocyte transfer and fertilisation techniques are performed according to the normal practice of the individual clinic.

Luteal support with hCG or progesterone should be given as appropriate.

4.3 Contraindications
Buserelin should not be used if the tumour is found to be insensitive to hormone manipulation or in cases of undiagnosed vaginal bleeding. It is contraindicated in cases of known hypersensitivity to benzalkonium chloride, LHRH or buserelin. It should not be used during pregnancy or lactation (see 4.6 Pregnancy and lactation).

4.4 Special warnings and precautions for use
Suprecur injection is for subcutaneous administration ONLY

Patients known to suffer from depression should be carefully monitored and treated if necessary during treatment with Suprecur.

In patients with hypertension, blood pressure must be monitored regularly.

In diabetic patients, blood glucose levels must be checked regularly.

Before treatment is started, it is recommended that a pregnancy test be performed

Whenever the treatment is self-administered, it is strongly recommended that initial doses should be administered under close medical supervision due to the possibility of hypersensitivity reactions. Patients should cease injections and seek medical attention should any adverse event occur which may represent an allergic reaction.

Treatment with Suprecur should be initiated only under the supervision of a specialist with experience of the indication.

Induction of ovulation should be carried out under close medical supervision. Risks specific to IVF/ET and related assisted reproduction procedures such as increase in miscarriages, ectopic and multiple pregnancies are unaltered under adjunctive use of buserelin. However, follicle recruitment may be increased especially in patients with polycystic ovarian disorder (PCOD).

Combined use of buserelin with gonadotrophins may bear a higher risk of ovarian hyperstimulation syndrome (OHSS) than the use of gonadotrophins alone. The stimulation cycle should be monitored carefully to identify patients at risk of developing OHSS. hCG should be withheld if necessary.

Possible clinical signs of ovarian hyperstimulation syndrome (OHSS) include: abdominal pain, feeling of abdominal tension, increased abdominal girth, occurrence of ovarian cysts, nausea, vomiting, as well as massive enlargement of the ovaries, dyspnoea, diarrhoea, oliguria, haemoconcentration, hypercoagulability. Pedicle tension or rupture of the ovary may lead to an acute abdomen. Severe thromboembolic events may also occur. Fatal outcome is possible.

Ovarian cysts have been observed in the initial phase of buserelin treatment. No impact on the stimulation cycle has been reported so far.

4.5 Interaction with other medicinal products and other forms of interaction
During treatment with Suprecur, the effect of antidiabetic agents may be attenuated.

In concomitant treatment with sexual hormones ("add back"), the dosage is to be selected so as to ensure that the overall therapeutic effect is not affected.

4.6 Pregnancy and lactation
Pregnancy must be excluded before starting buserelin and the medication should be stopped on the day of administration of hCG.

Buserelin passes into breast milk in small amounts. Although negative effects on the infant have not been observed, it is recommended that breast-feeding be avoided during treatment with Suprecur in order to prevent the infant from ingesting small quantities of buserelin with breast milk.

4.7 Effects on ability to drive and use machines
Certain adverse effects (e.g. dizziness) may impair the ability to concentrate and react, and therefore constitute a risk in situations where these abilities are of special importance (e.g. operating a vehicle or machinery).

4.8 Undesirable effects
After administration of the injection, pain or local reaction at the injection site is possible. Hypersensitivity reactions may also occur. These may become manifest for example as reddening of the skin, itching, skin rashes (including urticaria) and allergic asthma with dyspnoea as well as, in isolated cases, anaphylactic / anaphylactoid shock.

Treatment with buserelin inhibits oestrogen production. As evidence of the biological response to hormone deprivation, patients may experience menopausal-like symptoms and withdrawal bleeding, which are directly related to the pharmacological action of the drug. Symptoms such as hot flushes, increased sweating, dry vagina, dyspareunia and loss of libido generally occur some weeks after starting treatment and may be severe in some patients. Withdrawal bleeding may occur during the first few weeks of treatment. Breakthrough bleeding may occur during continuing treatment. **After several months' treatment, a decrease in bone mass may occur.**

Changes in bone density: a decrease in bone mineral, the magnitude of which relates to the duration of therapy, occurs during treatment with buserelin alone. The evidence available indicates that six months treatment is associated with a decrease in bone mineral density of the spine of 3.5 %. These changes are similar to those seen with other agonists. Increased levels of serum alkaline phosphatase may occur.

Other adverse effects may include:

Neoplasms benign and malignant - Very rare cases of pituitary adenomas were reported during treatment with LH-RH agonists, including buserelin.

Blood disorders - Very rare cases of thrombocytopenia or leucopenia.

Metabolism and nutrition disorders – Frequent increase or decrease in weight Occasional changes in appetite and increased thirst. Rarely increase or decrease in blood lipid levels. Very rarely, reduction in glucose tolerance which may lead to the worsening of metabolic control in diabetics.

Psychiatric disorders – Frequent nervousness, emotional instability. Occasional anxiety, depression or worsening of existing depression.

Nervous system disorders – Dizziness, headache (in women in rare cases migraine-like), sleep disturbances, tiredness, drowsiness. Occasional paraesthesia (especially in the arms and legs), disturbances of memory and concentration.

Eye disorders – Occassional dry eyes (possibly leading to eye irritations in people who wear contact lenses), impaired vision (eg blurred vision), feeling of pressure behind the eyes.

Ear and labyrinth disorders – Rare cases of tinnitus, hearing disorders found.

Cardiac disorders – Frequent palpitations.

Vascular disorders – Occassional oedema (of face and extremities) and hot flushes. Very rare cases of a deterioration of blood pressure levels in patients with hypertension.

Gastrointestinal disorders – Frequent lower abdominal pain, stomach ache, nausea, vomiting, diarrhoea, constipation.

Hepato-biliary disorders – Occasional, increase in serum liver enzyme levels (e.g. transaminases), increase in serum bilirubin.

Skin and subcutaneous tissue disorders – Frequent dry skin, acne, increase or decrease in scalp hair (alopecia, hirsutism). Occasional increase or decrease in body hair, splitting nails.

Musculoskeletal and bone disorders – Frequent musculoskeletal discomfort and pain (including shoulder pain/stiffness). The use of LHRH-agonists may be associated with decreased bone density and may lead to osteoporosis and an increased risk of bone fracture. The risk of skeletal fracture increases with the duration of therapy.

Reproductive system and breast disorders – Frequent Vaginal discharge, increase or decrease in breast size, breast tenderness. Occasional lactation.

In the initial phase of treatment with buserelin, ovarian cysts may develop (see also section 4.4).

Combined use of buserelin with gonadotrophins may bear a higher risk of ovarian hyperstimulation syndrome (OHSS) than the use of gonadotrophins alone (see section 4.4).

4.9 Overdose

Overdose may lead to signs and symptoms such as asthenia, headache, nervousness, hot flushes, dizziness, nausea, abdominal pain, oedemas of the lower extremities, and mastodynia as well as to local reactions at the injection site such as pain, haemorrhage and induration. Treatment should be symptomatic.

5. PHARMACOLOGICAL PROPERTIES

5.1 Pharmacodynamic properties

Buserelin is a synthetic peptide. It is a superactive analogue of natural gonadotrophin releasing hormone (gonadorelin, LHRH or GNRH). After an initial stimulation of gonadotrophin release, it down-regulates the hypothalamic-pituitary-gonadal (HPO) axis such that a decrease in ovarian steroid secretion into the post-menopausal range occurs. The time taken to achieve these levels varies between individuals and with the regimen of administration, so that close monitoring of circulating levels of estradiol and progesterone should be performed during treatment. This effect provides an appropriate setting for the administration of follicle-stimulating therapy and reduces the incidence of premature ovulation by inhibition of surges in LH.

5.2 Pharmacokinetic properties

The bioavailability of buserelin after subcutaneous injection is 100%. C_{max} occurs at about 1 hour post-injection. The half-life after injection is about 80 minutes.

Buserelin accumulates preferentially in the liver, kidneys and in the anterior pituitary lobe, the biological target organ. Buserelin circulates in serum predominantly in the intact, active form. Protein binding is about 15 %.

Buserelin is inactivated by peptidases (pyrogutamyl peptidase and chymotrypsin-like endopeptidases) in the liver and kidneys. In the pituitary gland, receptor-bound buserelin is inactivated by membrane-located enzymes. Buserelin and inactive buserelin metabolites are excreted via the renal and the biliary route.

5.3 Preclinical safety data

No signs of toxicity or histopathological changes were detected in long-term pharmacology and toxicology studies with buserelin in rats, dogs, and monkeys; the endocrine effects observed were restricted to the gonads. Pituitary adenoma occurred during long-term treatment in rats, this phenomenon has not been found in dogs and monkeys. There are no indications of a mutagenic or carcinogenic potential.

6. PHARMACEUTICAL PARTICULARS

6.1 List of excipients

sodium chloride Ph.Eur.

sodium dihydrogen phosphate BP.

sodium hydroxide BP.

benzyl alcohol BP.

Water for Injections Ph. Eur.

6.2 Incompatibilities

Not applicable.

6.3 Shelf life

Unopened: 36 months

(see section 6.6).

6.4 Special precautions for storage

Store between 2°C and 25°C. Do not freeze. Protect from light.

6.5 Nature and contents of container

Box of 2 × 5.5 ml multidose vials each containing 1.05 mg buserelin acetate per 1 ml, corresponding to 1.00 mg buserelin per 1 ml.

6.6 Special precautions for disposal and other handling

Each vial contains enough material for 10 doses. After finishing the course of treatment the vial should be disposed of and a new vial started for the next treatment. Do not use if the contents of the vial are cloudy or discoloured. Patients should be instructed on the correct handling of the vial (aseptic technique) by a doctor or nurse.

7. MARKETING AUTHORISATION HOLDER

Sanofi-aventis

One Onslow Street

Guildford

Surrey

GU1 4YS

UK

8. MARKETING AUTHORISATION NUMBER(S)

PL 04425/0278

9. DATE OF FIRST AUTHORISATION/RENEWAL OF THE AUTHORISATION

23 April 2002

10. DATE OF REVISION OF THE TEXT

17 July 2008

Legal category

POM

Suprecur Nasal Spray

(sanofi-aventis)

1. NAME OF THE MEDICINAL PRODUCT

Suprecur Nasal Spray

2. QUALITATIVE AND QUANTITATIVE COMPOSITION

Suprecur nasal spray contains 150 micrograms buserelin, as buserelin acetate, in one spray dose.

150 micrograms buserelin is equivalent to 157.5 micrograms buserelin acetate.

3. PHARMACEUTICAL FORM

Nasal Spray

4. CLINICAL PARTICULARS

4.1 Therapeutic indications

The treatment of endometriosis in cases that do not require surgery as primary therapy.

Pituitary desensitisation in preparation for ovulation induction regimens using gonadotrophins.

4.2 Posology and method of administration

Endometriosis: The total daily dose is 900 micrograms buserelin, administered as one spray dose in each nostril in the morning, at mid-day and in the evening. The product may be used before or after meals or at other times, provided that uniform intervals are maintained between doses.

The usual duration of treatment is six months and this should not be exceeded. Only a single course of treatment is recommended.

Repeated courses of treatment must only be administered after a careful review of the risk/benefit ratio by the attending physician since the possibility of additive effects on bone mass (reduction in bone mass) cannot be excluded (see also section 4.4).

Pituitary desensitisation prior to ovulation induction: The total daily intranasal dose for this indication is 600 micrograms buserelin, given in four divided dosages of 150 micrograms (one application in one nostril) spread over the waking hours. Treatment should start in the early follicular phase (day 1) or, provided the existence of an early pregnancy has been excluded in the midluteal phase (day 21). It should continue at least until down-regulation is achieved e.g. serum estradiol <50 ng/l and serum progesterone <1 microgram/l. This will usually take about 2-3 weeks. In some patients, dosages up to 4 × 300 micrograms may be required to achieve these levels. When down-regulation is achieved, stimulation with gonadotropin is commenced while the dosage of buserelin is maintained. At the appropriate stage of follicular development, gonadotropin and buserelin are stopped and hCG is given to induce ovulation.

Treatment monitoring, oocyte transfer and fertilisation techniques are performed according to the normal practice of the individual clinic.

Luteal support with hCG or progesterone should be given as appropriate.

If used correctly, reliable absorption of the active ingredient takes place via nasal mucous membranes. The drug is absorbed even if the patient has a cold; however, in such cases the nose should be blown thoroughly before administration.

If nasal decongestants are being used concurrently, they should be administered at least 30 minutes after the buserelin.

Children: Suprecur is not suitable for use in children.

Elderly: Suprecur is not suitable for use in post-menopausal women.

4.3 Contraindications

Buserelin should not be used if the tumour is found to be insensitive to hormone manipulation, after surgical removal of the testes or in cases of undiagnosed vaginal bleeding. It is contraindicated in cases of known hypersensitivity to benzalkonium chloride, LHRH or buserelin. It should not be used during pregnancy or lactation (see 4.6 Pregnancy and lactation).

4.4 Special warnings and precautions for use

Patients known to suffer from depression should be carefully monitored and treated if necessary during treatment with Suprecur.

In patients with hypertension, blood pressure must be checked regularly.

In diabetic patients blood glucose levels must be checked regularly.

Endometriosis: Patients should discontinue oral contraceptives before starting treatment. Where appropriate, alternative, non-hormonal methods of contraception should be used. If treatment is interrupted even for only a few days, ovulation may occur and there is a risk of pregnancy.

Suprecur treatment should be started on the first or second day of menstruation in order to exclude pre-existing pregnancy as far as possible. A pregnancy test is advisable if there is any doubt.

It is not expected that pregnancy will occur during the course of the treatment if the recommended doses are taken regularly. However, if treatment is interrupted for only a few days, ovulation and pregnancy may occur. If pregnancy does occur, treatment with buserelin must be discontinued immediately and a physician must me informed (see also section 4.6).

Repeated courses of treatment must only be administered after a careful review of the risk/benefit ratio by the attending physician since the possibility of additive effects on bone mass (reduction in bone mass) cannot be excluded (see also section 4.8).

A menstruation-like bleed usually occurs during the first few weeks of treatment. Breakthrough bleeding may also occur during continuing courses of treatment in some patients. Recovery of pituitary-gonadal function usually occurs within 8 weeks of discontinuing treatment.

In the initial treatment with buserelin, ovarian cysts may develop.

Pituitary desensitisation prior to ovulation induction:

Before treatment is started, it is recommended that a pregnancy test be performed.

Induction of ovulation should be carried out under close medical supervision. Risks specific to IVF/ET and related assisted reproduction procedures such as increase in miscarriages, ectopic and multiple pregnancies are unaltered under adjunctive use of buserelin. In addition, follicle recruitment may be increased especially in patients with PCOD.

Combined use of buserelin with gonadotrophins may bear a higher risk of ovarian hyperstimulation syndrome (OHSS) than the use of gonadotrophins alone. The stimulation cycle should be monitored carefully to identify patients at risk of developing OHSS. hCG should be withheld if necessary.

Possible clinical signs of ovarian hyperstimulation syndrome (OHSS) include: abdominal pain, feeling of abdominal tension, increased abdominal girth, occurrence of ovarian cysts, nausea, vomiting, as well as massive enlargement of the ovaries, dyspnoea, diarrhoea, oligurea, haemoconcentration, hypercoagulability. Pedicle tension or rupture of the ovary may lead to an acute abdomen. Severe thromboembolic events may also occur. Fatal outcome is possible.

Ovarian cysts have been observed in the initial phase of buserelin treatment. No impact on the stimulation cycle has been reported so far.

Treatment with Suprecur should be initiated only under the supervision of a specialist with experience of the indication.

4.5 Interaction with other medicinal products and other forms of interaction

During treatment with buserelin, the effect of antidiabetic agents may be attenuated.

In concomitant treatment with sexual hormones ("add back"), the dosage is to be selected so as to ensure that the overall therapeutic effect is not affected.

4.6 Pregnancy and lactation

Suprecur is contraindicated in pregnancy and lactation. In rats, fetal malformations have been seen after very high doses.

Buserelin passes into breast milk in small amounts. Although negative effects on the infant have not been observed, it is recommended that breast-feeding be avoided during treatment with Suprecur in order to prevent the infant from ingesting small quantities of buserelin with breast milk.

In endometriosis: It is unlikely that pregnancy will occur in the later stages of treatment if the recommended doses are taken regularly. However, if treatment is interrupted even for only a few days, ovulation may occur and the patient may become pregnant. In this event, Suprecur must be withdrawn immediately and a physician must be informed (see also section 4.4).

In pituitary desensitisation prior to ovulation induction: Pregnancy should be excluded before starting Suprecur, and the medication should be stopped on the day of administration of hCG.

4.7 Effects on ability to drive and use machines

Certain adverse effects (e.g. dizziness) may impair the patients ability to concentrate and react, and therefore, constitute a risk in those situations where these abilities are of special importance (e.g. operating a vehicle or machinery).

4.8 Undesirable effects

In isolated cases severe hypersensitivity reactions with shock can occur. These may become manifest as, e.g. reddening of the skin, itching, skin rashes (including urticaria) and allergic asthma with dyspnoea as well as, in isolated cases leading to anaphylactic/anaphylactoid shock.

The nasal spray may irritate the nasal mucosa, leading to nosebleeds and hoarseness as well as to disturbances of smell and taste.

Treatment with buserelin inhibits oestrogen production. As evidence of the biological response to hormone deprivation, patients may experience menopausal-like symptoms and withdrawal bleeding, which are directly related to the pharmacological action of the drug. Symptoms such as hot flushes, increased sweating, dry vagina, dyspareunia, loss of libido generally occur some weeks after starting treatment and may be severe in some patients. Withdrawal bleeding may occur during the first few weeks of treatment. Breakthrough bleeding may occur during continuing treatment. After several months' treatment, a decrease in bone mass may occur.

Changes in bone density: A decrease in bone mineral, the magnitude of which relates to the duration of therapy, occurs during treatment with buserelin alone. The evidence available indicates that six months' treatment is associated with a decrease in bone mineral density of the spine of 3.5%. These changes are similar to those seen with other agonists. Increased levels of serum alkaline phosphatase may occur. These are reversible on discontinuing treatment.

Buserelin treatment may also lead to:

Neoplasms benign and malignant - Very rare cases of pituitary adenomas were reported during treatment with LH-RH agonists, including buserelin.

Blood disorders - Very rare cases of thrombocytopenia or leucopenia.

Metabolism and nutrition disorders – Frequent increase or decrease in weight. Occasional changes in appetite and increased thirst. Rarely increase or decrease in blood lipid levels. Very rarely, reduction in glucose tolerance which may lead to the worsening of metabolic control in diabetics.

Psychiatric disorders – Frequent nervousness, emotional instability. Occasional anxiety, depression or worsening of existing depression.

Nervous system disorders – Dizziness, headache (in women in rare cases migraine-like), sleep disturbances, tiredness, drowsiness. Occasional paraesthesia (especially in the arms and legs), disturbances of memory and concentration.

Eye disorders – Occassional dry eyes (possibly leading to eye irritations in people who wear contact lenses), impaired vision (eg blurred vision), feeling of pressure behind the eyes.

Ear and labyrinth disorders – Rare cases of tinnitus, hearing disorders found.

Cardiac disorders – Frequent palpitations.

Vascular disorders – Occassional oedema (of face and extremities) and hot flushes. Very rare cases of a deterioration of blood pressure levels in patients with hypertension.

Gastrointestinal disorders – Frequent lower abdominal pain, stomach ache, nausea, vomiting, diarrhoea, constipation.

Hepato-biliary disorders – Occasional, increase in serum liver enzyme levels (e.g. transaminases), increase in serum bilirubin.

Skin and subcutaneous tissue disorders – Frequent dry skin, acne, increase or decrease in scalp hair (alopecia, hirsutism). Occasional increase or decrease in body hair, splitting nails.

Musculoskeletal and bone disorders – Frequent musculoskeletal discomfort and pain (including shoulder pain/stiffness). The use of LHRH-agonists may be associated with decreased bone density and may lead to osteoporosis and an increased risk of bone fracture. The risk of skeletal fracture increases with the duration of therapy.

Reproductive system and breast disorders – Frequent Vaginal discharge, increase or decrease in breast size, breast tenderness. Occasional lactation.

In the initial phase of treatment with buserelin, ovarian cysts may develop (see also section 4.4).

Combined use of buserelin with gonadotrophins may bear a higher risk of ovarian hyperstimulation syndrome (OHSS) than the use of gonadotrophins alone (see also section 4.4).

4.9 Overdose

Overdose may lead to signs and symptoms such as asthenia, headache, nervousness, hot flushes, dizziness, nausea, abdominal pain, oedema of the lower extremities and mastodynia. Treatment should be symptomatic.

5. PHARMACOLOGICAL PROPERTIES

5.1 Pharmacodynamic properties

Buserelin is a synthetic peptide. It is a superactive analogue of natural gonadotrophin releasing hormone (gonadorelin, LHRH or GNRH). After an initial stimulation of gonadotrophin release, it down-regulates the hypothalamic-pituitary-gonadal axis.

5.2 Pharmacokinetic properties

The intra-nasal absorption rate of buserelin is about 3%. Metabolic inactivation by peptides occurs in the liver and kidney. The drug is also inactivated by pituitary membrane enzymes. After intra-nasal administration to humans, buserelin is excreted for more than 8 hours in the urine. Virtually all the serum fraction, and half the urine fraction of buserelin, are present as the parent drug.

The bioavailability of buserelin after nasal administration is not adversely influenced by the presence of rhinitis.

5.3 Preclinical safety data

None of clinical relevance.

6. PHARMACEUTICAL PARTICULARS

6.1 List of excipients

The nasal spray also contains citric acid, sodium citrate, sodium chloride and benzalkonium chloride in aqueous solution.

6.2 Incompatibilities

None

6.3 Shelf life

3 years. 5 weeks after first opening.

6.4 Special precautions for storage

Store between 2 and 25°C. Do not freeze.

6.5 Nature and contents of container

Cartons containing two bottles and two metered-dose pumps (nebulisers). Each bottle contains 10g solution.

6.6 Special precautions for disposal and other handling

How to use the spray bottle:

1. Remove screw cap from bottle.
2. Remove metered-dose nebulizer from transparent plastic container and take off both protective caps.
3. Screw nebulizer on to bottle.
4. Before first application only, pump 5-8 times, holding bottle vertical, until the solution has filled the system and a uniform spray is emitted. The preliminary pumping is for the purpose of filling the system and testing the spray. It must not be repeated after the first use, in order to avoid wasting the contents.
5. Keeping bottle vertical and bending head over it slightly, spray solution into nose. If necessary, the nose should be cleaned before applying the solution.
6. After use leave nebulizer on bottle. After replacing protective cap, spray bottle is best stored in its transparent container in an upright position.

7. MARKETING AUTHORISATION HOLDER

Sanofi-aventis

One Onslow Street

Guildford, GU1 4YS

8. MARKETING AUTHORISATION NUMBER(S)

PL 04425/0277

9. DATE OF FIRST AUTHORISATION/RENEWAL OF THE AUTHORISATION

23 April 2002

10. DATE OF REVISION OF THE TEXT

15th September 2008

Legal category

POM

Suprefact Injection

(sanofi-aventis)

1. NAME OF THE MEDICINAL PRODUCT

Suprefact® Injection

2. QUALITATIVE AND QUANTITATIVE COMPOSITION

Suprefact injection contains 1.00 mg buserelin as buserelin acetate in 1ml aqueous solution.

1.00 mg buserelin is equivalent to 1.05 mg buserelin acetate.

3. PHARMACEUTICAL FORM

Injection

4. CLINICAL PARTICULARS

4.1 Therapeutic indications

For the treatment of advanced prostatic carcinoma (stage C or stage D according to the classification of Murphy *et al*, in Cancer 45, p1889-95, 1980) in which suppression of testosterone is indicated. Buserelin acts by blockade and subsequent down-regulation of pituitary LHRH receptor synthesis. Gonadotrophin release is consequently inhibited. As a result of this inhibition there is reduced stimulation of testosterone secretion and serum testosterone levels fall to castration range. Before inhibition occurs there is a brief stimulatory phase during which testosterone levels may rise.

4.2 Posology and method of administration

Initiation of therapy: is most conveniently carried out in hospital; 0.5ml Suprefact injection should be injected subcutaneously at 8 hourly intervals for 7 days.

Maintenance therapy: on the 8th day of treatment the patient is changed to intranasal administration of Suprefact. (see literature for dosage).

4.3 Contraindications

Buserelin should not be used if the tumour is found to be insensitive to hormone manipulation or after surgical removal of the testes. It is contraindicated in cases of known hypersensitivity to LHRH or buserelin. It should not be used during pregnancy or lactation (see 4.6 Pregnancy and lactation).

4.4 Special warnings and precautions for use

Patients known to suffer from depression should be carefully monitored and treated if necessary during treatment with Suprefact.

In patients with hypertension, blood pressure must be monitored regularly.

In diabetic patients blood glucose levels must be checked regularly.

Prostatic carcinoma: Monitoring of the effect of clinical effect of Suprefact is carried out by methods generally used in prostatic carcinoma. Initially serum testosterone levels rise and a clinical effect will not be seen until levels start to fall into therapeutic (castration) range. Disease flare (temporary deterioration of the patient's condition) has been reported at the beginning of the treatment. The incidence is variable, but of the order of the 10%. Symptoms are usually confined to transient increase in pain, but the exact nature depends on the site of the lesions.

Disease flare is prevented by the prophylactic use of an anti-androgen so it is strongly recommended that administration of an anti-androgen be started as adjunctive therapy (e.g. cyproterone acetate, 300 mg daily) about 5 days before starting treatment. This adjunctive therapy must be continued in parallel with buserelin therapy for 3 to 4 weeks.

Neurological sequelae have been reported where secondary deposits impinge upon the spinal cord or CNS. In patients with known metastases, e.g. of the spinal column, this adjunctive therapy with an anti-androgen is indispensable to prevent initial complications up to and including, for example, spinal compression and paralysis, arising from a transient activation of the tumour and metastases.

Once testosterone levels have started to fall below their baseline concentration clinical improvement should start to become apparent. If testosterone levels do not reach the therapeutic range within 4 weeks (6 weeks at the latest) the dose schedule should be checked to be sure that it is being followed exactly. It is unlikely that a patient who is taking the full dose will not show a suppression of testosterone to the therapeutic range. If this is the case, alternative therapy should be considered.

After the initial determination, testosterone levels should be monitored at 3-monthly intervals. A proportion of patients will have tumours that are not sensitive to hormone manipulation. Absence of clinical improvement in the face of adequate testosterone suppression is diagnostic of this condition, which will not benefit from further therapy with buserelin.

4.5 Interaction with other medicinal products and other forms of interaction

During treatment with Suprefact, the effect of antidiabetic agents may be attenuated.

4.6 Pregnancy and lactation

Suprefact is contraindicated in pregnancy. It is intended for the treatment of advanced prostatic carcinoma, it should not be used in pregnant or lactating women (see 4.3 Contraindications).

Buserelin passed into breast milk in small amounts. Although negative effects on the infant have not been observed, it is recommended that breast-feeding be avoided during treatment with Suprefact in order to prevent the infant from ingesting small quantities of buserelin with breast milk.

4.7 Effects on ability to drive and use machines

Certain adverse effects (eg.dizziness) may impair the ability to concentrate and react, and therefore constitute a risk in situations where these abilities are of special importance (eg. Operating a vehicle or machinery).

4.8 Undesirable effects

In isolated cases severe hypersensitivity reactions with shock can occur. These may become manifest as, eg. reddening of the skin, itching, skin rashes (including urticaria) and allergic asthma with dyspnoea as well as, in isolated cases leading to anaphylactic / anaphylactoid shock.

After administration of the injection, pain or local reaction at the injection site is possible.

At the beginning of treatment, a transient rise in the serum testosterone level usually develops and may lead to temporary activation of the tumour with secondary reactions such as:

- occurrence of exacerbation of bone pain in patients with metastases.
- signs of neurological deficit due to tumour compression with eg. muscle weakness in the legs.
- impaired micturition, hydronephrosis or lymphostasis.
- thrombosis with pulmonary embolism.

Such reactions can be largely avoided when an anti-androgen is given concomitantly in the initial phase of buserelin treatment (see Precautions and Warnings). However, even with concomitant anti-androgen therapy, a mild but transient increase in tumour pain as well as a deterioration in general well being may develop in some patients.

Suprefact treatment may also lead to:

Neoplasms bening and malignant - Very rare cases of pituitary adenomas were reported during treatment with LH-RH agonists, including buserelin.

Blood disorders - Very rare cases of thrombocytopenia or leucopenia.

Metabolism and nutrition disorders – Frequent increase or decrease in weight Occasional changes in appetite and increased thirst. Rarely increase or decrease in blood lipid levels. Very rarely, reduction in glucose tolerance which may lead to the worsening of metabolic control in diabetics.

Psychiatric disorders – Frequent nervousness, emotional instability. Occasional anxiety, depression or worsening of existing depression.

Nervous system disorders – Dizziness, headache, sleep disturbances, tiredness, drowsiness. Occasional paraesthesia (especially in the arms or legs), disturbances of memory and concentration.

Eye disorders – Occassional dry eyes (possibly leading to eye irritations in people who wear contact lenses), impaired vision (eg blurred vision), feeling of pressure behind the eyes.

Ear and labyrinth disorders – Rare cases of tinnitus, hearing disorders found.

Cardiac disorders – Frequent palpitations.

Vascular disorders – Occassional oedema (of face and extremities) and hot flushes. Very rare cases of a deterioration of blood pressure levels in patients with hypertension.

Gastrointestinal disorders – Frequent lower abdominal pain, stomach ache, nausea, vomiting, diarrhoea, constipation.

Hepato-biliary disorders – Occasional, increase in serum liver enzyme levels (e.g. transaminases), increase in serum bilirubin.

Skin and subcutaneous tissue disorders – Frequent dry skin, acne, increase or decrease in scalp hair (alopecia, hirsutism). Occasional increase or decrease in body hair, splitting nails.

Musculoskeletal and bone disorders – Frequent musculoskeletal discomfort and pain (including shoulder pain/stiffness). The use of LHRH-agonists may be associated with decreased bone density and may lead to osteoporosis and an increased risk of bone fracture. The risk of skeletal fracture increases with the duration of therapy.

Reproductive system and breast disorders – Ocassional gynaecomastia (increase in breast size), which is usually painless, decrease in libido and potency.

Most of the effects listed above are directly or indirectly related to the suppression of testosterone by buserelin (symptoms of androgen deficiency).

4.9 Overdose

Overdose may lead to signs and symptoms such as asthenia, headache, nervousness, hot flushes, dizziness, nausea, abdominal pain, oedemas of the lower extremities, and mastodynia as well as to local reactions at the injection site such as pain, haemorrhage and induration (see section 4.8). Treatment should be symptomatic.

5. PHARMACOLOGICAL PROPERTIES

5.1 Pharmacodynamic properties

Buserelin is a synthetic peptide. It is a superactive analogue of natural gonadotrophin releasing hormone (gonadorelin, LHRH or GNRH). After an initial stimulation of gonadotrophin release, it down-regulates the hypothalamic-pituitary-gonadal axis.

5.2 Pharmacokinetic properties

Metabolic inactivation by peptidases occurs in the liver and kidney. The drug is also inactivated by pituitary membrane enzymes.

5.3 Preclinical safety data

None stated

6. PHARMACEUTICAL PARTICULARS

6.1 List of excipients

Sodium Chloride

Sodium Dihydrogen Phosphate

Sodium Hydroxide

Benzyl Alcohol

Water for injections

6.2 Incompatibilities

Not applicable

6.3 Shelf life

3 years

6.4 Special precautions for storage

Store between 2° and 25°C. Protect from light.

6.5 Nature and contents of container

Box of 1 × 5.5 ml multidose vial containing 1.05 mg buserelin acetate per 1ml, corresponding to 1.00mg buserelin per 1 ml.

Pack size: 2 individual cardboard boxes are wrapped together in a clear plastic outer.

6.6 Special precautions for disposal and other handling

No special instructions

7. MARKETING AUTHORISATION HOLDER

Sanofi-aventis

One Onslow Street

Guildford

Surrey

GU1 4YS

UK

8. MARKETING AUTHORISATION NUMBER(S)

PL 04425/0268

9. DATE OF FIRST AUTHORISATION/RENEWAL OF THE AUTHORISATION

16 June 2006

10. DATE OF REVISION OF THE TEXT

17 July 2008

Legal Category

POM

Suprefact Nasal Spray

(sanofi-aventis)

1. NAME OF THE MEDICINAL PRODUCT

Suprefact Nasal Spray

2. QUALITATIVE AND QUANTITATIVE COMPOSITION

Suprefact nasal spray contains 100 micrograms buserelin as buserelin acetate in 1 spray dose of aqueous solution containing benzalkonium chloride as preservative.

100 micrograms buserelin is equivalent to 105 micrograms buserelin acetate.

3. PHARMACEUTICAL FORM

Nasal spray

4. CLINICAL PARTICULARS

4.1 Therapeutic indications

For the treatment of advanced prostatic carcinoma (stage C or stage D according to the classification of Murphy et al. in Cancer, 45, p 1889–95, 1980) in which suppression of testosterone is indicated. Buserelin acts by blockade and subsequent down-regulation of pituitary LHRH receptor synthesis. Gonadotrophin release is consequently inhibited. As a result of this inhibition there is reduced stimulation of testosterone secretion and serum testosterone levels fall to the castration range. Before inhibition occurs there is a brief stimulatory phase during which testosterone levels may rise.

4.2 Posology and method of administration

Initiation of therapy: is most conveniently carried out in hospital; 0.5 ml Suprefact injection should be injected subcutaneously at 8 hourly intervals for 7 days.

Maintenance therapy: on the 8th day of treatment the patient is changed to intranasal administration of Suprefact. One spray dose is introduced into each nostril 6 times a day according to the following schedule:

1st dose before breakfast

2nd dose after breakfast

3rd and 4th doses before and after midday meal

5th and 6th doses before and after evening meal.

This dosage regimen is to ensure adequate absorption of the material and to distribute the dose throughout the day.

If used correctly, reliable absorption of the active ingredient takes place via nasal mucous membranes. Suprefact nasal spray is absorbed even if the patient has a cold.

If nasal decongestants are being used concurrently, they should be administered at least 30 minutes after buserelin.

4.3 Contraindications

Buserelin should not be used if the tumour is found to be insensitive to hormone manipulation, after surgical removal of the testes. It is contraindicated in cases of known hypersensitivity to benzalkonium chloride, LHRH or buserelin. It should not be used during pregnancy or lactation (see 4.6 Pregnancy and lactation).

4.4 Special warnings and precautions for use

Patients known to suffer from depression should be carefully monitored and treated if necessary during treatment with Suprefact.

In patients with hypertension, blood pressure must be monitored regularly.

In diabetic patients blood glucose levels must be checked regularly.

Monitoring of the clinical effect of Suprefact is carried out by the methods generally used in prostatic carcinoma. Initially serum testosterone levels rise and a clinical effect will not be seen until levels start to fall into the therapeutic (castration) range. Disease flare (temporary deterioration of patient's condition) has been reported at the beginning of treatment. The incidence is variable, but of the order of 10%. Symptoms are usually confined to transient increase in pain, but the exact nature depends on the site of the lesions.

Disease flare is prevented by the prophylactic use of an anti-androgen so it is strongly recommended that administration of an anti-androgen be started as adjunctive therapy (e.g. cyproterone acetate, 300 mg daily) about 5 days before starting treatment. This adjunctive therapy must be continued in parallel with buserelin therapy for 3 to 4 weeks.

Neurological sequelae have been reported where secondary deposits impinge upon the spinal cord or CNS. In patients with known metastases, e.g. of the spinal column, this adjunctive therapy with an anti-androgen is indispensable to prevent initial complications up to and including, for example, spinal compression and paralysis, arising from a transient activation of the tumour and metastases.

Once testosterone levels have started to fall below their baseline concentration clinical improvement should start to become apparent. If testosterone levels do not reach the therapeutic range within 4 weeks (6 weeks at the latest) the dose schedule should be checked to be sure that it is being followed exactly. It is unlikely that a patient who is taking the full dose will not show a suppression of testosterone to the therapeutic range. If this is the case, alternative therapy should be considered.

After the initial determination, testosterone levels should be monitored at 3–monthly intervals. A proportion of patients will have tumours that are not sensitive to hormone manipulation. Absence of clinical improvement in the face of adequate testosterone suppression is diagnostic of this condition, which will not benefit from further therapy with buserelin.

4.5 Interaction with other medicinal products and other forms of interaction

During treatment with Suprefact, the effect of antidiabetic agents may be attenuated.

4.6 Pregnancy and lactation

Suprefact is contraindicated in pregnancy. It is intended for the treatment of advanced prostatic carcinoma, it should not be used in pregnant or lactating women (see 4.3 Contraindications).

Buserelin passed into breast milk in small amounts. Although negative effects on the infant have not been observed, it is recommended that breast-feeding be avoided during treatment with Suprefact in order to prevent the infant from ingesting small quantities of buserelin with breast milk.

4.7 Effects on ability to drive and use machines

Certain adverse effects (eg dizziness) may impair the ability to concentrate and react, and therefore constitute a risk in situations where these abilities are of special importance (eg operating a vehicle or machinery).

4.8 Undesirable effects

In isolated cases severe hypersensitivity reactions can occur. These may become manifest as, eg. reddening of the skin, itching, skin rashes (including urticaria) and allergic asthma with dyspnoea as well as, in isolated cases leading to anaphylactic / anaphylactoid shock.

Administration of the nasal spray, may irritate the mucosa in the nasopharynx. This may lead to nosebleeds and hoarseness as well as to disturbances of taste and smell.

At the beginning of treatment, a transient rise in the serum testosterone level usually develops and may lead to temporary activation of the tumour with secondary reactions such as:

– occurence or exacerbation of bone pain in patients with metastases.

– signs of neurological deficit due to tumour compression with eg. muscle weakness in the legs.

– impaired micturition, hydronephrosis or lymphostasis.

– thrombosis with pulmonary embolism.

Such reactions can be largely avoided when an anti-androgen is given concomitantly in the initial phase of buserelin treatment (see Precautions and Warnings). However, even with concomitant anti-androgen therapy, a mild but transient increase in tumour pain as well as a deterioration in general well-being may develop in some patients.

Suprefact treatment may also lead to:

Neoplasms benign and malignant - Very rare cases of pituitary adenomas were reported during treatment with LH-RH agonists, including buserelin.

Blood disorders - Very rare cases of thrombocytopenia or leucopenia.

Metabolism and nutrition disorders – Frequent increase or decrease in weight Occasional changes in appetite and increased thirst. Rarely increase or decrease in blood lipid levels. Very rarely, reduction in glucose tolerance which may lead to the worsening of metabolic control in diabetics.

Psychiatric disorders – Frequent nervousness, emotional instability. Occasional anxiety, depression or worsening of existing depression.

Nervous system disorders – Dizziness, headache, sleep disturbances, tiredness, drowsiness. Occasional paraesthesia (especially in the arms or legs), disturbances of memory and concentration.

Eye disorders – Occasional dry eyes (possibly leading to eye irritations in people who wear contact lenses), impaired vision (eg blurred vision), feeling of pressure behind the eyes.

Ear and labyrinth disorders – Rare cases of tinnitus, hearing disorders found.

Cardiac disorders – Frequent palpitations.

Vascular disorders –Very rare cases of a deterioration of blood pressure levels in patients with hypertension.

Gastrointestinal disorders – Frequent lower abdominal pain, stomach ache, nausea, vomiting, diarrhoea, constipation.

Hepato-biliary disorders – Occasional, increase in serum liver enzyme levels (e.g. transaminases), increase in serum bilirubin.

Skin and subcutaneous tissue disorders – Frequent dry skin, acne, increase or decrease in scalp hair (alopecia, hirsutism). Occasional increase or decrease in body hair, splitting nails.

Musculoskeletal and bone disorders – Frequent musculoskeletal discomfort and pain (including shoulder pain/stiffness). The use of LHRH-agonists may be associated with decreased bone density and may lead to osteoporosis and an increased risk of bone fracture. The risk of skeletal fracture increases with the duration of therapy.

Reproductive system and breast disorders – Occasional gynaecomastia (increase in breast size) which is usually painless, decrease in libido and potency.

Most of the effects listed above are directly or indirectly related to the suppression of testosterone by buserelin (symptoms of androgen deficiency).

4.9 Overdose
Overdose may lead to signs and symptoms such as asthenia, headache, nervousness, hot flushes, dizziness, nausea, abdominal pain, oedemas of the lower extremities, and mastodynia. Treatment should be symptomatic.

5. PHARMACOLOGICAL PROPERTIES

5.1 Pharmacodynamic properties
Buserelin is a synthetic peptide. It is a superactive analogue of natural gonadotrophin releasing hormone (gonadorelin, LHRH or GNRH). After an initial stimulation of gonadotrophin release, it down-regulates the hypothalamic-pituitary-gonadal axis.

5.2 Pharmacokinetic properties
The intra-nasal absorption rate of buserelin is about 3%. Metabolic inactivation by peptidases occurs in the liver and kidney. The drug is also inactivated by pituitary membrane enzymes. After intra-nasal administration to humans, buserelin is excreted for more than 8 hours in the urine. Virtually all the serum fraction, and half the urine fraction of buserelin, are present as the parent drug.

The bioavailability of buserelin after nasal administration is not adversely influenced by the presence of rhinitis.

5.3 Preclinical safety data
None stated

6. PHARMACEUTICAL PARTICULARS

6.1 List of excipients
Sodium Chloride

Citric Acid Monohydrate

Sodium Citrate Dihydrate

Benzalkonium Chloride

Water for Injections

6.2 Incompatibilities
Not applicable.

6.3 Shelf life
2½ years.

6.4 Special precautions for storage
Store below 25°C. The spray solution should last for 1 week of treatment. Any residual material after this time should be discarded.

6.5 Nature and contents of container
Box of 4 bottles each containing 10g solution and 4 spray pumps

6.6 Special precautions for disposal and other handling
How to use the spray bottle.

1. Remove spray cap from bottle.

2. Remove metered dose nebulizer from transparent plastic container and take off both protective caps.

3. Screw nebuliser on to bottle.

4. Before first application only, pump 5-8 times, holding bottle vertical, until the solution has filled the system and a uniform spray is emitted. The preliminary pumping is for the purpose of filling the system and testing the spray. It must not be repeated after the first use, in order to avoid wasting the contents.

5. Keeping the bottle vertical and bending head over it slightly, spray solution into nose. If necessary the nose should be cleaned before applying the solution.

6. After use leave nebulizer on bottle. After replacing protective cap, spray bottle is best stored in its transparent container in an upright position.

7. MARKETING AUTHORISATION HOLDER
Sanofi-aventis

One Onslow Street

Guildford

Surrey

GU1 4YS

UK

8. MARKETING AUTHORISATION NUMBER(S)
PL 04425/0279

9. DATE OF FIRST AUTHORISATION/RENEWAL OF THE AUTHORISATION
16 June 2006

10. DATE OF REVISION OF THE TEXT
17 July 2008

Legal Category
POM

Surgam 300mg

(sanofi-aventis)

1. NAME OF THE MEDICINAL PRODUCT
Surgam Tablets 300 mg.

2. QUALITATIVE AND QUANTITATIVE COMPOSITION
Each tablet contains 300 mg Tiaprofenic Acid.

3. PHARMACEUTICAL FORM
Tablets

4. CLINICAL PARTICULARS

4.1 Therapeutic indications
Rheumatoid arthritis, osteoarthritis, ankylosing spondylitis, low back pain, musculo-skeletal disorders such as fibrositis, capsulitis, epicondylitis and other soft-tissue inflammatory conditions, sprains and strains, post-operative inflammation and pain and other soft tissue injuries.

4.2 Posology and method of administration
For oral administration.

To be swallowed whole.

To be taken preferably with or after food.

Adults:

600 mg daily in divided doses

300mg twice a day

Alternatively 200mg three times a day

Elderly:

As for adults (see Section 4.4, Special Warnings and Precautions). NSAIDs should be used with particular caution in older patients who are at increased risk of the serious consequences of adverse reactions.

In cases of renal, cardiac or hepatic impairment, the dosage should be kept as low as possible. It is suggested that in such cases, the dosage be reduced to 200 mg twice daily.

If an NSAID is considered necessary, elderly patients should receive the lowest effective dose for the shortest possible duration and be monitored regularly for gastro-intestinal bleeding for following initiation of NSAID therapy

Children:

There are insufficient data to recommend use of Surgam in children.

Undesirable effects may be minimised by using the lowest effective dose for the shortest duration necessary to control symptoms (see section 4.4).

4.3 Contraindications
- Active or history of recurrent peptic ulcer/hemorrage (two or more distinct episodes of proven ulceration or bleeding).

- History of gastrointestinal bleeding or perforation, related to previous NSAIDs therapy.

- Active bladder or prostatic disease or symptoms.

- History of recurrent urinary tract disorders.

- Hypersensitivity to tiaprofenic acid or to any of the excipients.

- NSAIDs are contraindicated in patients who have previously shown hypersensitivity reactions (e.g. asthma, rhinitis, angioedema or urticaria) in response to ibuprofen, aspirin, or other non-steroidal anti-inflammatory drugs.

- During the last trimester of pregnancy (see Section 4.6)

- Severe heart failure, hepatic failure and renal failure (see section 4.4).

4.4 Special warnings and precautions for use
Undesirable effects may be minimised by using the lowest effective dose for the shortest duration necessary to control symptoms (see section 4.2, and GI and cardiovascular risks below). Patients treated with NSAIDs long-term should undergo regular medical supervision to monitor for adverse events.

The use of Surgam with concomitant NSAIDs including cyclooxygenase-2 selective inhibitors should be avoided (see section 4.5).

Tiaprofenic acid should be used with caution in:

- patients with chronic renal insufficiency (particularly careful monitoring of renal function is required)

- patients with arterial hypertension and/or heart failure

- elderly subjects as they have an increased frequency of adverse reactions to NSAIDs, particularly gastrointestinal bleeding and perforation, which may be fatal (see section 4.2)

- patients with a history of hepatic insufficiency

Respiratory disorders:

Caution is required if administered to patients suffering from, or with a previous history of, bronchial asthma since NSAIDs have been reported to precipitate bronchospasm in such patients.

Tiaprofenic acid may cause sodium and water retention with oedema. At the start of therapy, urine volume and renal function should be carefully monitored in patients with a history of hypertension, cardiac insufficiency, liver cirrhosis, or nephrotic syndrome, and in patients on diuretics.

Urinary symptoms and cystitis have been reported with tiaprofenic acid and other NSAIDs. Tiaprofenic acid appears to have a greater propensity than other NSAIDs to generate reports of cystitis. Tiaprofenic acid can cause cystitis which may become severe if the treatment is continued after the onset of urinary symptoms. Non-recognition has led to extensive investigations and even surgical intervention, in some patients. If urinary symptoms such as frequency, urgency, dysuria, nocturia or haematuria occur, tiaprofenic acid should be stopped immediately and urinalysis and urine culture performed and complete recovery is the rule. Before starting treatment with tiaprofenic acid, the patient should be asked to inform his/her physician of any urinary symptom, even if the physician is familiar with these symptoms from the patient's medical history (see Adverse Reactions). Patients should be warned about the onset of urinary symptoms which may suggest cystitis and are advised to stop taking the drug and seek medical advice if these occur.

Gastrointestinal bleeding, ulceration and perforation:

GI bleeding, ulceration or perforation, which can be fatal, has been reported with all NSAIDs at anytime during treatment, with or without warning symptoms or a previous history of serious GI events.

The risk of GI bleeding, ulceration or perforation is higher with increasing NSAID doses, in patients with a history of ulcer, particularly if complicated with haemorrhage or perforation (see section 4.3), and in the elderly. These patients should commence treatment on the lowest dose available. Combination therapy with protective agents (e.g. misoprostol or proton pump inhibitors) should be considered for these patients, and also for patients requiring concomitant low dose aspirin, or other drugs likely to increase gastrointestinal risk (see below and section 4.5).

Patients with a history of GI toxicity, particularly when elderly, should report any unusual abdominal symptoms (especially GI bleeding) particularly in the initial stages of treatment.

Caution should be advised in patients receiving concomitant medications which could increase the risk of ulceration or bleeding, such as oral corticosteroids, anticoagulants such as warfarin, selective serotonin-reuptake inhibitors or anti-platelet agents such as aspirin (see section 4.5).

When GI bleeding or ulceration occurs in patients receiving Surgam, the treatment should be withdrawn.

NSAIDs should be given with care to patients with a history of gastrointestinal disease (ulcerative colitis, Crohn's disease) as their condition may be exacerbated (see section 4.8).

Dermatological:

Serious skin reactions, some of them fatal, including exfoliative dermatitis, Stevens-Johnson syndrome, and toxic epidermal necrolysis, have been reported very rarely in association with the use of NSAIDSs. Patients appear to be at highest risk of these reactions early in the course of therapy, the onset of the reaction occurring in the majority of cases within the first month of treatment. Surgam should be discontinued at the first appearance of skin rash, mucosal lesions, or any other sign of hypersensitivity.

Impaired female fertility:

The use of Surgam may impair female fertility and is not recommended in women attempting to conceive. In women who have difficulties conceiving or who are undergoing investigation of infertility, withdrawal of Surgam should be considered.

There is a risk of cross-sensitivity among aspirin and NSAIDs, including the group to which tiaprofenic acid belongs. These pseudo-allergic reactions may include rash, urticaria and angioedema or more potentially severe manifestations (e.g. laryngeal oedema, bronchoconstriction and shock). The risk of pseudo-allergic reactions is greater in patients with recurrent rhino-sinusitis, nasal polyposis or chronic urticaria. Asthmatic patients are particularly at risk of dangerous reactions. Therefore tiaprofenic acid must not be administered to patients with a history of asthma.

As NSAIDs can interfere with platelet function, they should be used with caution in patients with intracranial haemorrhage and bleeding diathesis.

Cardiovascular, Renal and Hepatic Impairment:

The administration of an NSAID may cause a dose dependent reduction in prostaglandin formation and precipitate renal failure. Patients at greatest risk of this reaction are those with impaired renal function, cardiac impairment, liver dysfunction, those taking diuretics and the elderly. Renal function should be monitored in these patients (see also section 4.3).

Cardiovascular and cerebrovascular effects

Appropriate monitoring and advice are required for patients with a history of hypertension and/or mild to moderate congestive heart failure as fluid retention and oedema have been reported in association with NSAID therapy.

Clinical trial and epidemiological data suggest that use of some NSAIDs (particularly at high doses and in long term treatment) may be associated with a small increased risk of arterial thrombotic events (for example myocardial infarction or stroke). There are insufficient data to exclude such a risk for *tiaprofenic acid*.

Patients with uncontrolled hypertension, congestive heart failure, established ischaemic heart disease, peripheral arterial disease, and/or cerebrovascular disease should only be treated with *tiaprofenic acid* after careful consideration. Similar consideration should be made before initiating longer-term treatment of patients with risk factors for cardiovascular disease (e.g. hypertension, hyperlipidaemia, diabetes mellitus, smoking).

SLE and mixed connective tissue disease:

In patients with systemic lupus erythematosus (SLE) and mixed connective tissue disorders there may be an increased risk of aseptic meningitis (see section 4.8).

4.5 Interaction with other medicinal products and other forms of interaction

Heparin, Hypoglycaemic agents and Diuretics: Since Surgam is highly protein-bound, it is not recommended for co-administration with other highly protein-bound drugs such as heparin. Modification of the dosage may be necessary with hypoglycaemic agents, phenytoin and diuretics. With oral hypoglycaemic agents, an inhibition of metabolism of sulphonylurea drugs, prolonged half-life and increased risk of hypoglycaemia has been reported.

Anticoagulants and antiplatelet agents: It is considered unsafe to take NSAIDs in combination with anticoagulants (i.e. heparin, warfarin) and platelet aggregation inhibitors (i.e. ticlopidine, clopidogrel) due to increased risk of bleeding. If coadministration is unavoidable, patient should be closely monitored.

Other analgesics including cyclooxygenase-2 selective inhibitors: Concomitant use of Surgam with other NSAIDs (including cyclooxygenase-2 selective inhibitors) and high-dose salicylates should be avoided due to an increased risk of adverse effects, particulary upper gastrointestinal disorders.

Corticosteroids: Caution must be exercised when Surgam is administered with corticosteroids due to increased risk of gastrointestinal ulceration or bleeding.

Cardiac glycosides and sulphonamides: Caution should be exercised when Surgam is administered with cardiac glycosides and sulphonamides. With cardiac glycosides, NSAIDs may exacerbate cardiac failure, reduce GFR and increase plasma cardiac glycoside levels.

Methotrexate: Concomitant use of Surgam with methotrexate causes a decreased elimination of methotrexate. Concomitant use with high dose methotrexate should be avoided. Use with caution with low dose methotrexate.

Lithium: Decreased elimination of lithium

NSAIDs have been reported to increase steady state plasma levels of lithium and it is, therefore, recommended that these levels are monitored in patients receiving Surgam therapy.

Mifepristone: Aspirin and other NSAIDs should not be used for at least 8-12 days after mifepristone administration as NSAIDs can reduce the effect of mifepristone.

Diuretics: Caution must be exercised when Surgam is administered with diuretics: it reduces both the diuretic and antihypertensive effect of diuretics and increase risk of renal impairment and/or hyperkalemia.

Diuretics can increase the risk of nephrotoxicity of NSAIDs.

Tacrolimus: Possible increased risk of nephrotoxicity when NSAIDs are given with tacrolimus.

Zidovudine: Increased risk of haematological toxicity when NSAIDs are given with zidovudine. There is evidence of an increased risk of haemarthroses and haematoma in HIV(+) haemophiliacs receiving concurrent treatment with zidovudine and ibuprofen.

Caution must be exercised when Surgam is administered with ACE inhibitors and Angiotensin II Receptor Antagonists: Further deterioration of renal function, including possible acute renal failure, in patients with compromised renal function (e.g. dehydrated patients or elderly patients).

The possibility of interaction must be taken into account with:

- Thrombolytics: Increased risk of haemorrhage.
- anti-hypertensives agents (diuretics, beta-blockers, ACE-inhibitors, Angiotensin II Receptor Antagonists): Reduced activity of these drugs. This should be borne in mind in patients with incipient or actual congestive heart failure and/or hypertension.

Selective serotonin reuptake inhibitors (SSRIs): The possibility of interaction must be taken into account with selective serotonin reuptake inhibitors (SSRIs): increased risk of gastrointestinal bleeding.

Ciclosporin: The risk of nephrotoxicity may be increased if NSAIDs are given with ciclosporins.

Quinolone antibiotics: Animal data indicate that NSAIDs can increase the risk of convulsions associated with quinolone antibiotics. Patients taking NSAIDs and quinolones may have an increased risk of developing convulsions.

Aminoglycosides or probenecid: Care should also be taken if Surgam is concomitantly administered with aminoglycosides or probenecid. Aminoglycosides may interact with NSAIDs to cause a reduction in renal function in susceptible individuals, decreased elimination of aminoglycoside and increased plasma concentrations. A reduction in metabolism and elimination of NSAID and metabolites has been observed with probenecid.

4.6 Pregnancy and lactation

Pregnancy:

Congenital abnormalities have been reported in association with NSAID administration in man; however, these are low in frequency and do not appear to follow any discernible pattern. Tiaprofenic acid crosses the placental barrier. Although animal studies have not revealed evidence of teratogenicity, safety in human pregnancy and lactation cannot be assumed and, in common with other NSAIDs, Surgam should not be used during the first two trimesters of pregnancy or labour unless the potential benefit to the patient outweighs the potential risk to the foetus.

In view of the known effects of NSAIDs on the foetal cardiovascular system (a closure of ductus arteriosus), use in the last trimester of pregnancy is contraindicated. The onset of labour may be delayed and the duration increased with an increased bleeding tendency in both mother and child (see section 4.3).

Lactation: The level of Surgam in mother's milk has been studied and the total daily exposure is very small; approximately 0.2% of the administered dose and is unlikely to be of pharmacological significance. Breast feeding or treatment of the mother should be stopped as necessary.

See section 4.4 Special warnings and precautions for use, regarding female fertility.

4.7 Effects on ability to drive and use machines

Undesirable effects such as dizziness, drowsiness, fatigue and visual disturbances are possible after taking NSAIDs. If affected, patients should not drive or operate machinery.

4.8 Undesirable effects

Gastrointestinal disorders:

Reported reactions include dyspepsia, nausea, vomiting, abdominal / upper abdominal pain, melaena, haematemesis, anorexia, indigestion, heartburn, disorders of intestinal transit (flatulence, diarrhoea, constipation), gastritis, ulcerative stomatitis, exacerbation of colitis and Crohn's disease (See section 4.4). Pancreatitis has been reported very rarely.

Peptic ulcers, occult or active gastrointestinal haemorrhage and perforation have occasionally been reported, particularly in the elderly, and in exceptional case may have been associated with fatalities.

Skin and subcutaneous tissue disorders:

Rash, urticaria, pruritus, purpura, alopecia and erythema multiforme and dermatitis bullous (Stevens-Johnson Syndrome or toxic epidermal necrolysis), photosensitivity reactions have been reported.

Immune system disorders:

Hypersensitivity reactions have been reported following treatment with NSAIDs.

Non-specific allergic reactions, asthma, especially in subjects allergic to aspirin and other NSAIDs, bronchospasm, dyspnoea, angio-oedema, anaphylactic shock has also been reported.

Blood and lymphatic system disorders:

Thrombocytopenia, prolonged bleeding time anemia due to bleeding may occur.

Ear and labyrinth disorders:

Vertigo, dizziness, tinnitus and drowsiness.

Nervous system disorders:

Headaches

Renal and urinary disorders:

- bladder pain, dysuria, and pollakiuria
- hematuria or cystitis may occur
- after continuous, prolonged treatment with tiaprofenic acid in presence of urinary symptoms, inflammatory changes to the urinary tract, sometimes severe, have been observed.
- sodium and water retention (see Section 4.4, Special Warnings and Precautions).
- NSAIDs have been reported to cause nephrotoxicity in various forms. As with other NSAIDs, isolated cases of interstitial nephritis, nephrotic syndrome and renal failure have also been reported with tiaprofenic acid.

Hepatobiliary disorders:

Hepatitis, jaundice.

Investigations:

Abnormal liver function test

Other side-effects that have been reported with NSAIDS but not specifically with Surgam are:

- Nervous system disorders: – optic neuritis
- Eye disorders: visual disturbances
- Musculoskeletal and connective tissue disorders: paraesthesia
- Psychiatric disorders: depression, confusion, hallucinations
- General disorders and administration site conditions: fatigue, malaise
- Blood and lymphatic system disorders – Neutropenia, agranulocytosis, aplastic anaemia, haemolytic anaemia.
- Nervous disorders: reports of aseptic meningitis (especially in patients with existing auto-immune disorders, such as systemic lupus erythematosus, mixed connective tissue disease), with symptoms such as stiff neck, headache, nausea, vomiting, fever or disorientation (See section 4.4)

Vascular and cardiac disorders:

Oedema, hypertension, and cardiac failure, have been reported in association with NSAID treatment.

Clinical trial and epidemiological data suggest that use of some NSAIDs (particularly at high doses and in long term treatment) may be associated with an increased risk of arterial thrombotic events (for example myocardial infarction or stroke) (see section 4.4).

4.9 Overdose

In the event of overdosage with Surgam, supportive and symptomatic therapy is indicated.

a) Symptoms

- Symptoms include headache, nausea, vomiting, epigastric pain, gastrointestinal bleeding, rarely diarrhoea, disorientation, excitation, coma, drowsiness, dizziness, tinnitus, fainting, occasionally convulsions. In cases of significant poisoning acute renal failure and liver damage are possible.

b) Therapeutic measure

- Patients should be treated symptomatically as required.
- Within one hour of ingestion of a potentially toxic amount, activated charcoal should be considered. Alternatively, in adults, gastric lavage should be considered within one hour of ingestion of a potentially life-threatening overdose.
- Good urine output should be ensured.
- Renal and liver function should be closely monitored.
- Patients should be observed for at least four hours after ingestion of potentially toxic amounts.
- Frequent or prolonged convulsions should be treated with intravenous diazepam.
- Other measures may be indicated by the patient's clinical condition.

5. PHARMACOLOGICAL PROPERTIES

5.1 Pharmacodynamic properties

Non-steroidal anti-inflammatory drug.

Further Information:

The effects of tiaprofenic acid on articular cartilage have been investigated in in-vitro experiments and in ex-vivo studies using different animal models of arthritis. Ex-vivo experiments on human chondrocyte cultures have also been conducted. In these experiments, tiaprofenic acid, in concentrations equivalent to the therapeutic dose, did not depress the biosynthesis of proteoglycans and did not alter the differentiation of proteoglycans secreted. The degradation of proteoglycan aggregates was inhibited. These results suggest a neutral or possibly beneficial effect of tiaprofenic acid on joint cartilage under experimental conditions. The clinical significance of these findings has been studied in a long term double-blind controlled study, in which tiaprofenic acid did not significantly increase the rate of radiological deterioration of joint space in patients with osteoarthritis of the knee.

5.2 Pharmacokinetic properties

Single dose studies: Following oral administration (max. at 90mins). Plasma level zero at 24 hours. t½ = 1.5 to 2 hours.

Repeated dose studies: Surgam is rapidly eliminated and there is no accumulation after repeated doses of 600mg/day in divided doses. Steady state after first day. No impairment of absorption in patients with RA undergoing long term therapy. There is no evidence of different pharmacokinetics in the elderly.

Protein Binding = 97 - 98%

Plasma clearance = 6 litres/hour

Elimination = 60% of urine remainder in bile

Metabolites = there two main metabolites which account for about 10% of urinary excretion and have low pharmacological activity. The parent compound is excreted mostly in the form of acylglucuronide.

5.3 Preclinical safety data

Not applicable

6. PHARMACEUTICAL PARTICULARS

6.1 List of excipients

Maize starch, pluronic F68, magnesium stearate and talc.

6.2 Incompatibilities

None known

6.3 Shelf life

60 months

6.4 Special precautions for storage

Store below 25°C. Protect from light.

6.5 Nature and contents of container

Blister packs sealed with aluminium foil in a cardboard carton in packs of 56.

6.6 Special precautions for disposal and other handling

Not applicable.

7. MARKETING AUTHORISATION HOLDER

Sanofi-aventis

One Onslow Street

Guildford

Surrey,

GU1 4YS,

UK

8. MARKETING AUTHORISATION NUMBER(S)

04425/0318

9. DATE OF FIRST AUTHORISATION/RENEWAL OF THE AUTHORISATION

27 February 2009

10. DATE OF REVISION OF THE TEXT

16 July 2009

Legal category: POM

Surmontil 10mg and 25mg Tablets

(sanofi-aventis)

1. NAME OF THE MEDICINAL PRODUCT

Surmontil 10mg tablets

Surmontil 25mg tablets

2. QUALITATIVE AND QUANTITATIVE COMPOSITION

In terms of the active ingredient (BAN rINN if appropriate)

Trimipramine Maleate EP 14 mg equivalent to 10 mg trimipramine per tablet

Trimipramine Maleate EP 34.9mg equivalent to 25 mg trimipramine per tablet

3. PHARMACEUTICAL FORM

Film-coated tablet

4. CLINICAL PARTICULARS

4.1 Therapeutic indications

Surmontil has a potent antidepressant action similar to that of other tricyclic antidepressants. It also possesses pronounced sedative action. It is, therefore, indicated in the treatment of depressive illness, especially where sleep disturbance, anxiety or agitation are presenting symptoms. Sleep disturbance is controlled within 24 hours and true antidepressant action follows within 7 to 10 days.

4.2 Posology and method of administration

Adults

For depression 50-75 mg/day initially increasing to 150-300 mg/day in divided doses or one dose at night. The maintenance dose is 75-150 mg/day.

Elderly

10-25 mg three times a day initially. The initial dose should be increased with caution under close supervision. Half the normal maintenance dose may be sufficient to produce a satisfactory clinical response.

Children

Not recommended.

Route of administration is oral.

4.3 Contraindications

Recent myocardial infarction. Any degree of heart block or other cardiac arrhythmias. Mania. Severe liver disease. During breast feeding.

4.4 Special warnings and precautions for use

Suicide/suicidal thoughts or clinical worsening

Depression is associated with an increased risk of suicidal thoughts, self harm and suicide (suicide-related events). This risk persists until significant remission occurs. As improvement may not occur during the first few weeks or more of treatment, patients should be closely monitored until such improvement occurs. It is general clinical experience that the risk of suicide may increase in the early stages of recovery.

Other psychiatric conditions for which Surmontil is prescribed can also be associated with an increased risk of suicide-related events. In addition, these conditions may be co-morbid with major depressive disorder. The same precautions observed when treating patients with major depressive disorder should therefore be observed when treating patients with other psychiatric disorders.

Patients with a history of suicide-related events, or those exhibiting a significant degree of suicidal ideation prior to commencement of treatment are known to be at greater risk of suicidal thoughts or suicide attempts, and should receive careful monitoring during treatment. A meta-analysis of placebo-controlled clinical trials of antidepressant drugs in adult patients with psychiatric disorders showed an increased risk of suicidal behaviour with antidepressants compared to placebo in patients less than 25 years old.

Close supervision of patients and in particular those at high risk should accompany drug therapy especially in early treatment and following dose changes. Patients (and caregivers of patients) should be alerted about the need to monitor for any clinical worsening, suicidal behaviour or thoughts and unusual changes in behaviour and to seek medical advice immediately if these symptoms present.

The elderly are particularly liable to experience adverse reactions, especially agitation, confusion and postural hypotension.

Avoid if possible in patients with narrow angle glaucoma, symptoms suggestive of prostatic hypertrophy and a history of epilepsy.

Patients posing a high suicidal risk require close initial supervision. Tricyclic antidepressants potentiate the central nervous depressant action of alcohol.

Anaesthetics given during tri/tetracyclic antidepressant therapy may increase the risk of arrhythmias and hypotension. If surgery is necessary, the anaesthetist should be informed that a patient is being so treated.

It may be advisable to monitor liver function in patients on long term treatment with Surmontil.

Patients with rare hereditary problems of galactose intolerance, the Lapp lactase deficiency or glucose-galactose malabsorption should not take this medicine.

4.5 Interaction with other medicinal products and other forms of interaction

Trimipramine should not be given concurrently with, or within 2 weeks of cessation of, therapy with monoamine oxidase inhibitors. Trimipramine may decrease the antihypertensive effect of guanethidine, debrisoquine, betanidine and possibly clonidone. It would be advisable to review all antihypertensive therapy during treatment with tricyclic antidepressants.

Trimipramine should not be given with sympathomimetic agents such as adrenaline, ephedrine, isoprenaline, noradrenaline, phenylephrine and phenylpropanolamine.

Barbiturates may increase the rate of metabolism.

Surmontil should be administered with care in patients receiving therapy for hyperthyroidism.

4.6 Pregnancy and lactation

Do not use in pregnancy especially during the first and last trimesters unless there are compelling reasons. There is no evidence from animal work that it is free from hazard.

Trimipramine is contraindicated during lactation.

4.7 Effects on ability to drive and use machines

Trimipramine may initially impair alertness. Patients should be warned of the possible hazard when driving or operating machinery.

4.8 Undesirable effects

Cases of suicidal ideation and suicidal behaviours have been reported during trimipramine therapy or early after treatment discontinuation (see section 4.4).

Cardiac arrhythmias and severe hypotension are likely to occur with high dosage or in deliberate overdosage. They may also occur in patients with pre-existing heart disease taking normal dosage.

The following adverse effects, although not necessarily all reported with trimipramine, have occurred with other tricyclic antidepressants.

Atropine-like side effects including dry mouth, disturbance of accommodation, tachycardia, constipation and hesitancy of micturation are common early in treatment but usually lessen.

Other common adverse effects include drowsiness, sweating, postural hypotension, tremor and skin rashes. Interference with sexual function may occur.

Serious adverse effects are rare; the following have been reported: depression of bone marrow, including agranulocytosis, cholestatic jaundice, hypomania, convulsions and peripheral neuropathy. Psychotic manifestations including mania and paranoid delusions, may be excacerbated during treatment with tricyclic antidepressants. Withdrawal symptoms may occur on abrupt cessation of therapy and include insomnia, irritability and excessive perspiration.

Adverse effects such as withdrawal symptoms, respiratory depression and agitation have been reported in neonates whose mothers had taken trimipramine during the last trimester of pregnancy.

4.9 Overdose

Acute overdosage may be accompanied by hypotensive collapse, convulsions and coma. Provided coma is not present, gastric lavage should be carries out without delay even though some time may have passed since the drug was ingested. Patients in coma should have an endotracheal tube passed before gastric lavage is started. Absorption of trimipramine is slow but, as cardiac effects may appear soon after the drug is absorbed, a saline purge should be given. Electrocardiography monitoring is essential.

It is important to treat acidosis as soon as it appears with, for example, 20 ml per kg of M/6 sodium lactate injection by slow intravenous injection. Intubation is necessary and the patient should be ventilated before convulsions develop. Convulsions should be treated with diazepam administered intravenously.

Ventricular tachycardia or fibrillation should be treated by electrical defibrillation. If supraventricular tachycardia develops, pyridostigmine bromide 1 mg (adults) intravenously or propranolol 1mg (adults) should be administered at intervals as required.

Treatment should be continued for at least three days even if the patient appears to have recovered.

5. PHARMACOLOGICAL PROPERTIES

5.1 Pharmacodynamic properties

Trimipramine is a tricyclic antidepressant. It has marked sedative properties.

5.2 Pharmacokinetic properties

Trimipramine undergoes high first-pass hepatic clearance, with a mean value for bioavailability of about 41% after oral administration.

The absolute volume of distribution is 31 litres/kg and total metabolic clearance is 16 ml/min/kg.

Plasma protein binding of trimipramine is about 95%. The plasma elimination half-life is around 23 hours. Trimipramine is largely metabolised by demethylation prior to conjugation yielding a glucuronide.

5.3 Preclinical safety data

No additional pre-clinical data of relevance to the prescriber.

6. PHARMACEUTICAL PARTICULARS

6.1 List of excipients

Calcium Hydrogen Phosphate
Starch Potato
Magnesium Stearate
Talc
Coat
Opadry OY-L-28900 *

* Opadry OY-L-28900 contains: Lactose Monohydrate Hypromellose, Titanium Dioxide, Macrogol.

6.2 Incompatibilities

None known

6.3 Shelf life

60 months

6.4 Special precautions for storage

Protect from light

6.5 Nature and contents of container

Surmontil 10mg tablets; Cartons containing PVDC/coated UPVC/aluminium foil blister packs of 84 or 28 tablets.

Surmontil 25mg tablets; Cardboard cartons containing blisters of 84 or 28 tablets.

6.6 Special precautions for disposal and other handling

None stated.

7. MARKETING AUTHORISATION HOLDER

Sanofi-aventis

One Onslow Street

Guildford

Surrey

GU1 4YS

UK

8. MARKETING AUTHORISATION NUMBER(S)

Surmontil 10mg tablets: PL 04425/0266

Surmontil 25mg tablets: PL 04425/0267

9. DATE OF FIRST AUTHORISATION/RENEWAL OF THE AUTHORISATION

13th July, 2001

10. DATE OF REVISION OF THE TEXT

5 March 2008

LEGAL CATEGORY

POM

Surmontil Capsules 50mg

(sanofi-aventis)

1. NAME OF THE MEDICINAL PRODUCT

Surmontil Capsules 50mg

2. QUALITATIVE AND QUANTITATIVE COMPOSITION

In terms of the active ingredient (BAN rINN if appropriate)

Trimipramine Maleate EP 69.75 mg per capsule

3. PHARMACEUTICAL FORM

Capsule

4. CLINICAL PARTICULARS

4.1 Therapeutic indications

Surmontil has a potent antidepressant action similar to that of other tricyclic antidepressants. It also possesses pronounced sedative action. It is, therefore, indicated in the treatment of depressive illness, especially where sleep disturbance, anxiety or agitation are presenting symptoms. Sleep disturbance is controlled within 24 hours and true antidepressant action follows within 7 to 10 days.

4.2 Posology and method of administration

Adults

For depression 50-75 mg/day initially increasing to 150-300 mg/day in divided doses or one dose at night. The maintenance dose is 75-150 mg/day.

Elderly

10-25 mg three times a day initially. The initial dose should be increased with caution under close supervision. Half the normal maintenance dose may be sufficient to produce a satisfactory clinical response.

Children

Not recommended.

Route of administration is oral.

4.3 Contraindications

Recent myocardial infarction. Any degree of heart block or other cardiac arrhythmias. Mania. Severe liver disease. During breast feeding.

4.4 Special warnings and precautions for use

Suicide/suicidal thoughts or clinical worsening

Depression is associated with an increased risk of suicidal thoughts, self harm and suicide (suicide-related events). This risk persists until significant remission occurs. As improvement may not occur during the first few weeks or more of treatment, patients should be closely monitored until such improvement occurs. It is general clinical experience that the risk of suicide may increase in the early stages of recovery.

Other psychiatric conditions for which Surmontil is prescribed can also be associated with an increased risk of suicide-related events. In addition, these conditions may be co-morbid with major depressive disorder. The same precautions observed when treating patients with major depressive disorder should therefore be observed when treating patients with other psychiatric disorders.

Patients with a history of suicide-related events, or those exhibiting a significant degree of suicidal ideation prior to commencement of treatment are known to be at greater risk of suicidal thoughts or suicide attempts, and should receive careful monitoring during treatment. A meta-analysis of placebo-controlled clinical trials of antidepressant drugs in adult patients with psychiatric disorders showed an increased risk of suicidal behaviour with antidepressants compared to placebo in patients less than 25 years old.

Close supervision of patients and in particular those at high risk should accompany drug therapy especially in early treatment and following dose changes. Patients (and caregivers of patients) should be alerted about the need to monitor for any clinical worsening, suicidal behaviour or thoughts and unusual changes in behaviour and to seek medical advice immediately if these symptoms present.

The elderly are particularly liable to experience adverse reactions, especially agitation, confusion and postural hypotension.

Avoid if possible in patients with narrow angle glaucoma, symptoms suggestive of prostatic hypertrophy and a history of epilepsy.

Patients posing a high suicidal risk require close initial supervision. Tricyclic antidepressants potentiate the central nervous depressant action of alcohol.

Anaesthetics given during tri/tetracyclic antidepressant therapy may increase the risk of arrhythmias and hypotension. If surgery is necessary, the anaesthetist should be informed that a patient is being so treated.

It may be advisable to monitor liver function in patients on long term treatment with Surmontil.

4.5 Interaction with other medicinal products and other forms of interaction

Trimipramine should not be given concurrently with, or within 2 weeks of cessation of, therapy with monoamine oxidase inhibitors. Trimipramine may decrease the antihypertensive effect of guanethidine, debrisoquine, betanidine and possibly clonidone. It would be advisable to review all antihypertensive therapy during treatment with tricyclic antidepressants.

Trimipramine should not be given with sympathomimetic agents such as adrenaline, ephedrine, isoprenaline, noradrenaline, phenylephrine and phenylpropanolamine.

Barbiturates may increase the rate of metabolism.

Surmontil should be administered with care in patients receiving therapy for hyperthyrodism.

4.6 Pregnancy and lactation

Do not use in pregnancy especially during the first and last trimesters unless there are compelling reasons. There is no evidence from animal work that it is free from hazard.

Trimipramine is contraindicated during lactation.

4.7 Effects on ability to drive and use machines

Trimipramine may initially impair alertness. Patients should be warned of the possible hazard when driving or operating machinery.

4.8 Undesirable effects

Cases of suicidal ideation and suicidal behaviours have been reported during trimipramine therapy or early after treatment discontinuation (see section 4.4).

Cardiac arrhythmias and severe hypotension are likely to occur with high dosage or in deliberate overdosage. They may also occur in patients with pre-existing heart disease taking normal dosage.

The following adverse effects, although not necessarily all reported with trimipramine, have occurred with other tricyclic antidepressants.

Atropine-like side effects including dry mouth, disturbance of accommodation, tachycardia, constipation and hesitancy of micturation are common early in treatment but usually lessen.

Other common adverse effects include drowsiness, sweating, postural hypotension, tremor and skin rashes. Interference with sexual function may occur.

Serious adverse effects are rare. The following have been reported: depression of the bone marrow, including agranulocytosis, cholestatic jaundice, hypomania, convulsions and peripheral neuropathy. Psychotic manifestations including mania and paranoid delusions, may be exacerbated during treatment with tricyclic antidepressants.

Withdrawal symptoms may occur on abrupt cessation of therapy and include insomnia, irritability and excessive perspiration.

Adverse effects such as withdrawal symptoms, respiratory depression and agitation have been reported in neonates whose mothers had taken trimipramine during the last trimester of pregnancy.

4.9 Overdose

Acute overdosage may be accompanied by hypotensive collapse, convulsions and coma. Provided coma is not present, gastric lavage should be carries out without delay even though some time may have passed since the drug was ingested. Patients in coma should have an endotracheal tube passed before gastric lavage is started. Absorption of trimipramine is slow but, as cardiac effects may appear soon after the drug is absorbed, a saline purge should be given. Electrocardiography monitoring is essential.

It is important to treat acidosis as soon as it appears with, for example, 20 ml per kg of M/6 sodium lactate injection by slow intravenous injection. Intubation is necessary and the patient should be ventilated before convulsions develop. Convulsions should be treated with diazepam administered intravenously.

Ventricular tachycardia or fibrillation should be treated by electrical defibrillation. If supraventricular tachycardia develops, pyridostigmine bromide 1 mg (adults) intravenously or propranolol 1mg (adults) should be administered at intervals as required.

Treatment should be continued for at least three days even if the patient appears to have recovered.

5. PHARMACOLOGICAL PROPERTIES

5.1 Pharmacodynamic properties

Trimipramine is a tricyclic antidepressant. It has marked sedative properties.

5.2 Pharmacokinetic properties

Trimipramine undergoes high first-pass hepatic clearance, with a mean value for bioavailability of about 41% after oral administration.

The absolute volume of distribution is 31 litres/kg.

The metabolic clearance is 16 ml/min/kg.

Plasma protein binding of trimipramine is about 95%. The plasma elimination half-life is around 23 hours. Trimipramine is largely metabolised by demethylation prior to conjugation yielding a glucuronide.

5.3 Preclinical safety data

No additional pre-clinical data of relevance to the prescriber.

6. PHARMACEUTICAL PARTICULARS

6.1 List of excipients

Starch Maize

Microcrystalline cellulose E460

Magnesium stearate

Colloidal anhydrous silica

Capsule shell:

Titanium dioxide E171

Indigo Carmine E132

Iron Oxide Yellow E172

Gelatin

Ink – Iron Oxide Black E172

6.2 Incompatibilities

None known

6.3 Shelf life

36 months

6.4 Special precautions for storage

Store in a dry place below 25°C and protect from light.

6.5 Nature and contents of container

Cartons containing PVC/aluminium blisters of 28.

6.6 Special precautions for disposal and other handling

None stated.

7. MARKETING AUTHORISATION HOLDER

Sanofi-aventis

One Onslow Street

Guildford

Surrey

GU1 4YS

UK

8. MARKETING AUTHORISATION NUMBER(S)

PL 04425/0265

9. DATE OF FIRST AUTHORISATION/RENEWAL OF THE AUTHORISATION

13 July 2001

10. DATE OF REVISION OF THE TEXT

5 March 2008

Legal category

POM

Survanta

(Abbott Laboratories Limited)

1. NAME OF THE MEDICINAL PRODUCT

Survanta

2. QUALITATIVE AND QUANTITATIVE COMPOSITION

Each ml contains Beractant equivalent to:

Phospholipids 25 mg/ml

(including disaturated phosphatidylcholines 11.0 - 15.5 mg/ml)

Triglycerides 0.5 - 1.75 mg/ml

Free Fatty Acids 1.4 - 3.5 mg/ml

Protein 0.1 - 1.0 mg/ml

3. PHARMACEUTICAL FORM

Sterile suspension for intratracheal administration

4. CLINICAL PARTICULARS

4.1 Therapeutic indications

Survanta is indicated for treatment of Respiratory Distress Syndrome (RDS) (hyaline membrane disease) in new born premature infants with a birth weight of 700g or greater and who are intubated and are receiving mechanical ventilation.

Survanta is also indicated for the prophylactic treatment of premature infants <32 weeks gestational age at risk of developing RDS.

4.2 Posology and method of administration

Dosage In Infants

100 mg phospholipid/kg birth weight in a volume not exceeding 4ml/kg.

Treatment: Survanta should be administered early in the course of RDS, i.e. preferably less than 8 hours of age. Depending on clinical course, this dose may be repeated within 48 hours at intervals of at least six hours for up to 4 doses.

Prophylaxis: The first dose of Survanta should be administered as soon as possible after birth, preferably within 15 minutes. Depending on clinical course, this dose may be repeated within 48 hours at intervals of at least six hours for up to 4 doses.

Method of Administration:

Survanta should be administered by intratracheal administration (i.e. drug should be conducted into the lungs via an endotracheal tube) using a 5 Fr catheter. The tip of the catheter should lie at the end of the endotracheal tube. Infants should not be intubated solely for the administration of Survanta.

Survanta should be warmed to room temperature before administration (see Precautions).

Before administering Survanta to infants on mechanical ventilation, set the respiratory frequency at 60/minute - with inspiration time 0.5s and F_{i2} at 1.0. Inspiratory pressure needs no change at this point.

To ensure distribution of Survanta throughout the lungs, each dose is divided into fractional doses. Each dose can be administered as either two half-doses or four quarter-doses. Each fractional dose is administered with the infant in different positions as given below. Between each position the infant should be ventilated for 30 seconds.

For Four quarter-doses, the recommended positions are:

Right Lateral Position with the head lowered (i.e. head and body slanting down at an angle of approximately 15°).

Left Lateral Position with the head lowered (i.e. head and body slanting down at an angle of approximately 15°).

Right Lateral Position with head elevated (i.e. head and body slanting up at an angle of approximately 15°).

Left Lateral Position with head elevated (i.e. head and body slanting up at an angle of approximately 15°).

For administration of each quarter dose, the ventilator is disconnected, the catheter inserted, the dose administered then the ventilator reconnected. Between each quarter dose the infant is ventilated for 30 seconds.

For two half-doses, the recommended positions are:

With infant supine, the head and body turned approximately 45° to the right.

With infant supine, the head and body turned approximately 45° to the left.

When two half-doses of Survanta are being administered there are 2 alternative methods of administration:

Installation with disconnection from the ventilator

Each half dose is administered by disconnecting the endotracheal tube from the ventilator, inserting the catheter and administering the half dose. Between the half doses, the ventilator is reconnected for 30 seconds.

Alternatively,

Instillation without disconnection from the ventilator (through a suction port connector).

The first half dose is administered by inserting the catheter through a suction port connector without disconnection from the ventilator. There should be at least 30 seconds between the half doses during which time the catheter is retracted from the endotracheal tube but not removed from the connector. The catheter is then reinserted into the endotracheal tube and the second half dose administered. The catheter is then withdrawn completely.

Dosage in Adults

Not applicable.

Dosage in Elderly

Not applicable.

4.3 Contraindications

No specific contraindications for Survanta have been defined by the clinical studies.

4.4 Special warnings and precautions for use

Survanta should only be administered with adequate facilities for ventilation and monitoring of babies with RDS.

Marked improvements in oxygenation may occur within minutes of the administration of Survanta. Therefore, frequent and careful monitoring of systemic oxygenation is essential to avoid hyperoxia. Following Survanta administration, monitoring of the arterial blood gases, the fraction of inspired oxygen and ventilatory change is required to ensure appropriate adjustments.

During the dosing procedure, transient episodes of bradycardia and/or oxygen desaturation have been reported. If these occur, dosing should be stopped and appropriate measures to alleviate the condition should be initiated. After stabilisation, the dosing procedure should be resumed.

Survanta is stored refrigerated (2-8°C). Before administration, Survanta should be warmed by standing at room temperature for 20 minutes or warmed in the hand for 8 minutes. ARTIFICIAL WARMING METHODS SHOULD NOT BE USED. Discard each vial if not used within 8 hours of rewarming to room temperature. Vials should not be returned to the refrigerator once warmed.

Each vial of Survanta is for single use only. Used vials with residual drug should be discarded.

Survanta should be inspected visually for discolouration prior to administration. The colour of Survanta is off-white to light brown. Some settling may occur during storage. If this occurs, gently invert the vial several times (DO NOT SHAKE) to redisperse.

4.5 Interaction with other medicinal products and other forms of interaction

None known to date.

4.6 Pregnancy and lactation

Not applicable.

4.7 Effects on ability to drive and use machines

Not applicable.

4.8 Undesirable effects

Intracranial haemorrhage has been observed in patients who received either Survanta or placebo. The incidence of intracranial haemorrhage in all patients is similar to that reported in the literature in this patient population. Pulmonary haemorrhage has also been reported. No other serious adverse reactions have been reported. No antibody production to Survanta proteins has been observed. Blockage of the endotracheal tube by mucous secretions has been reported.

4.9 Overdose

If an excessively large dose of Survanta is given, observe the infant for signs of acute airway obstruction. Treatment should be symptomatic and supportive. Rales and moist breath sounds can transiently occur after Survanta is given, and do not indicate overdosage. Endotracheal suction or other remedial action is not required unless clear-cut signs of airway obstruction are present.

5. PHARMACOLOGICAL PROPERTIES

5.1 Pharmacodynamic properties

The mode of action of Survanta is biophysical rather than biochemical, i.e. it reduces surface tension and concomitantly increases lung compliance.

Intratracheally administered Survanta distributes rapidly to the alveolar surfaces and stabilises the alveoli against collapse during respiration thereby increasing alveolar ventilation.

In clinical studies of premature infants with Respiratory Distress Syndrome (RDS), a significant improvement in oxygenation was demonstrated after treatment with a single dose of Survanta.

These infants showed a decreased need for supplemental oxygen and an increase in the arterial/alveolar oxygen ratio (a/ApO_2). Significantly decreased need for respiratory support, as indicated by a lower mean airway pressure, was also observed. In most cases these effects were maintained for at least 72 hours after the administration of the single dose of Survanta.

5.2 Pharmacokinetic properties

In preclinical studies using radiolabelled phosphatidylcholine, the clearance rate of Survanta in the lung of three day old rabbits has been shown to be similar to that of natural calf and sheep surfactants (approximately 13% within 24 hours). In addition some re-uptake and secretion of Survanta was shown, implying its entry into a metabolically active surfactant pool.

Since an exogenous preparation of Survanta is delivered directly to the lung, classical clinical pharmocokinetic parameters (blood levels, plasma half-life etc.) have not been studied.

5.3 Preclinical safety data

There are no pre-clinical data of relevance to the prescriber which are additional to that already included in other sections of the SPC.

6. PHARMACEUTICAL PARTICULARS

6.1 List of excipients

Sodium chloride and water for injection.

6.2 Incompatibilities

None experienced to date, as product administration is unique.

6.3 Shelf life

18 months

6.4 Special precautions for storage

Store under refrigerated conditions (2-8°C) protected from light.

6.5 Nature and contents of container

21ml glass bottle with a 20mm rubber stopper and a 20mm aluminium seal finish containing 8ml of product.

Pack sizes: 1, 3 and 10

6.6 Special precautions for disposal and other handling

Do not freeze. Any inadvertently frozen product should be discarded.

Administrative Data

7. MARKETING AUTHORISATION HOLDER

Abbott Laboratories Limited

Queenborough

Kent

ME11 5EL

8. MARKETING AUTHORISATION NUMBER(S)

PL 0037 / 0218

MA 150 / 00501

9. DATE OF FIRST AUTHORISATION/RENEWAL OF THE AUTHORISATION

13th October 1998

10. DATE OF REVISION OF THE TEXT

March 2005

Suscard Buccal Tablets

(Forest Laboratories UK Limited)

1. NAME OF THE MEDICINAL PRODUCT

SUSCARD BUCCAL TABLETS 2MG

SUSCARD BUCCAL TABLETS 3MG

SUSCARD BUCCAL TABLETS 5MG

2. QUALITATIVE AND QUANTITATIVE COMPOSITION

Each tablet contains 2mg, 3mg or 5mg glyceryl trinitrate as Diluted Nitroglycerin USP.

3. PHARMACEUTICAL FORM

Prolonged release muco-adhesive buccal tablet.

4. CLINICAL PARTICULARS

4.1 Therapeutic indications

Management and treatment of angina pectoris. This product may also be of benefit in the in-patient management of unstable angina.

Acute and congestive cardiac failure.

4.2 Posology and method of administration

For buccal administration

Dosage

Adults and Elderly Patients:

Angina:

Administration of Suscard Tablets should start with the 2mg strength. If angina occurs while the tablet is in place, the dosage strength used should be increased to 3mg where necessary. The 5mg dosage strength should be reserved for patients with severe angina pectoris refractory to treatment with the lower dosage strengths.

Suggested dosage frequency in angina:

A) For patients suffering only occasional angina pectoris – the tablets may be administered on a p.r.n. basis to relieve the acute attack.

B) For patients suffering angina pectoris in response to known stimuli - the tablet may be administered a few minutes prior to encountering the angina-precipitating stimulus.

C) For patients in whom chronic therapy is indicated - the tablet should be administered on a thrice daily basis or as dictated by the dissolution rate of the tablet in an individual patient. If angina occurs during the period between the disappearance of one tablet and the time the next tablet is due to be put in place, dosage frequency should be increased.

Note that if an acute attack of angina pectoris is suffered while a tablet is in place, an additional tablet may be positioned on the opposite side of the mouth.

Unstable Angina:

Dosage should be rapidly titrated upwards in order to relieve and prevent symptoms. Suscard Tablets may be used in addition to pre-existing anti-anginal therapy, where considered appropriate.

As indicated in the above section the higher 5mg dosage strength may be required to achieve a satisfactory therapeutic response in patients exhibiting severe symptoms. Unstable angina is a serious condition managed under hospitalised conditions and involving continuous monitoring of ECG changes with frequent monitoring of appropriate haemodynamic variables. In common with other nitrate therapy a fall in systolic blood pressure, of 10-15mm hg may occur.

Acute heart failure:

Administer 5mg, repeated as indicated by the patient response until the symptoms abate.

Congestive cardiac failure:

Dosage should commence with the 5mg strength, administered three times daily. In moderately severe or severe cases, particularly where patients have not responded to standard therapy (digitalis/diuretics), the dosage may need to be increased to 10mg (2 × 5mg tablets) t.i.d. over a period of three or four days. In such instances one tablet should be placed between the upper lip and the gum, on each side of the front teeth.

Method of Administration

Suscard is for buccal administration. The Suscard tablet is placed high up between the upper lip and gum to either side of the front teeth

The onset of action of Suscard tablets is extremely rapid and the tablets may be substituted for sublingual glyceryl trinitrate tablets in the treatment of acute angina pectoris. The duration of action of the Suscard Tablet, once in place correlates with the dissolution time of the tablet. This is normally 3-5 hours. However, the first few doses may dissolve more rapidly until the patient is used to the presence of the tablet.

During the dissolution period the tablet will soften and adhere to the gum; in practice the presence of the tablet is not noticeable to the patient after a short time.

Patients should be instructed as to the correct placement of the tablet and should note the following points

A) The tablet should not be moved about the mouth with the tongue, as this will cause it to dissolve more rapidly.

B) A slight stinging sensation (as for sublingual glyceryl trinitrate) may be felt for a few minutes after placement of the tablet.

C) If a tablet is accidentally swallowed it may be replaced by a further tablet.

D) In patients who wear dentures, the tablet may be placed in any comfortable position between the lip and the gum.

E) The patient may alternate the placement of successive tablets on the right and left sides of the front teeth.

The tablets should not be placed under the tongue, chewed or intentionally swallowed.

4.3 Contraindications

As for glyceryl trinitrate. Suscard Tablets should not be used in patients with marked anaemia, head trauma, cerebral haemorrhage or close angle glaucoma.

Sildenafil has been shown to potentiate the hypotensive effects of nitrates, and its co-administration with nitrates or nitric oxide donors is therefore contraindicated.

4.4 Special warnings and precautions for use

Rarely, prolonged use in susceptible individuals with poor dental hygiene and associated plaque may lead to an increased risk of dental caries. Patients should, therefore be instructed to alternate the site of application and careful attention should be paid to dental hygiene, particularly in those areas where the tablet is applied. In conditions where xerostomia (dry mouth) may occur, e.g. during concomitant medication with drugs having anticholinergic effects, patients should be instructed to moisten the buccal mucosa with the tongue, or with a little water, prior to insertion of Suscard.

Prescribe with caution to patients with; hypothyroidism, malnutrition, hepatic impairment, renal impairment, hypothermia, hypoxaemia or other ventilation and perfusion abnormalities.

4.5 Interaction with other medicinal products and other forms of interaction

The hypotensive effects of nitrates are potentiated by concurrent administration of sildenafil.

4.6 Pregnancy and lactation

There is no information on the safety of nitrates in pregnancy and lactation. Nitrates should not be administered to pregnant women and nursing mothers unless considered essential by the physician.

4.7 Effects on ability to drive and use machines

None known

4.8 Undesirable effects

Side effects are predominantly headache, dizziness, facial flushing and postural hypotension. In the unlikely event of severe side effects, the tablet may simply be removed from the mouth. Blisters of the tongue and oral mucosa have been associated with glyceryl trinitrate treatment.

4.9 Overdose

Toxic effects of glyceryl trinitrate include vomiting, restlessness, cyanosis, methaemoglobinaemia and syncope. Overdosage (i.e. if large numbers of tablets have been swallowed) should be treated with gastric aspiration and lavage plus attention to the respiratory and circulatory systems.

5. PHARMACOLOGICAL PROPERTIES

5.1 Pharmacodynamic properties

The principal action of glyceryl trinitrate is relaxation of vascular smooth muscle producing a vasodilator effect on both peripheral arteries and veins. Dilation of the postcapillary vessels, including large veins, promotes peripheral pooling of blood and decreases venous return to the heart, thereby reducing left ventricular end-diastolic pressure (preload). Arteriolar relaxation reduces systemic vascular resistance and arterial pressure (afterload). Myocardial oxygen consumption or demand for a given level of exercise is decreased by both the arterial and venous effects of nitroglycerin. Dilatation of the large epicardial coronary arteries by nitroglycerin contributes to the relief of exertional angina.

5.2 Pharmacokinetic properties

Bioavailability:

relative to sublingual GTN 107%.

Mean plasma levels:

0.7ng/ml obtained with 5mg Buccal Tablet over 5 hours compared with 0.4ng/ml over 30 minutes with 0.4mg sublingual GTN.

Maximum plasma concentration:

1.7ng/ml following 5mg Buccal compared with 0.9ng/ml following 0.4mg sublingual GTN.

Time to maximum plasma concentration:

1.52 hours following Buccal GTN compared with 6 minutes following sublingual GTN.

Apparent elimination half-life:

1.30 hours for Buccal GTN compared with an elimination half-life of 5 minutes following sublingual GTN.

Pharmacodynamic studies have shown a dose-related response with a rapid onset equivalent to sublingual GTN together with a prolonged duration of activity of 4-5 hours.

5.3 Preclinical safety data

There are no preclinical data of relevance to the prescriber which are additional to that already included in other sections of the SPC.

6. PHARMACEUTICAL PARTICULARS

6.1 List of excipients

Lactose hydrous

Hypromellose

Purified Water

Peppermint flavour

Spearmint flavour

Stearic acid

Silica gel

6.2 Incompatibilities

None stated

6.3 Shelf life

3 years

6.4 Special precautions for storage

Do not store above 25°C

6.5 Nature and contents of container

Aluminium foil blister strips in cartons of 30, 50, 60, 90 and 100 tablets.

Professional sample pack size of 10 tablets.

6.6 Special precautions for disposal and other handling

None stated.

7. MARKETING AUTHORISATION HOLDER

Forest Laboratories UK Limited

Bourne Road

Bexley

Kent DA5 1NX

8. MARKETING AUTHORISATION NUMBER(S)

Suscard Buccal Tablets 2mg: 0108/0069

Suscard Buccal Tablets 3mg: 0108/0073

Suscard Buccal Tablets 5mg: 0108/0071

9. DATE OF FIRST AUTHORISATION/RENEWAL OF THE AUTHORISATION

Suscard Buccal Tablets 2mg, 5mg: 15 March 1982 / 20 March 2003

Suscard Buccal Tablets 3mg: 7 October 1982 / 20 March 2003

10. DATE OF REVISION OF THE TEXT

May 2009

11. Legal Category

P

SUTENT 12.5mg, 25mg, 37.5mg and 50mg Hard Capsules

(Pfizer Limited)

1. NAME OF THE MEDICINAL PRODUCT

SUTENT® 12.5 mg hard capsules

SUTENT® 25 mg hard capsules

SUTENT® 37.5 mg hard capsules

SUTENT® 50 mg hard capsules

2. QUALITATIVE AND QUANTITATIVE COMPOSITION

SUTENT® 12.5 mg hard capsules

Each capsule contains sunitinib malate, equivalent to 12.5 mg of sunitinib.

SUTENT® 25 mg hard capsules

Each capsule contains sunitinib malate, equivalent to 25.0 mg of sunitinib

SUTENT® 37.5 mg hard capsules

Each capsule contains sunitinib malate, equivalent to 37.5 mg of sunitinib

SUTENT® 50 mg hard capsules

Each capsule contains sunitinib malate equivalent to 50 mg of sunitinib

For a full list of excipients, see section 6.1.

3. PHARMACEUTICAL FORM

SUTENT® 12.5 mg

Hard capsule

Gelatin capsules with orange cap and orange body, printed with white ink "Pfizer" on the cap, "STN 12.5 mg" on the body, and containing yellow to orange granules.

SUTENT® 25 mg

Hard Capsule

Gelatin capsule with caramel cap and orange body, printed with white ink "Pfizer" on the cap and "STN 25 mg" on the body and containing yellow to orange granules.

SUTENT® 37.5 mg

Hard Capsule

Gelatin capsules with yellow cap and yellow body, printed with black ink "Pfizer" on the cap and "STN 37.5 mg" on the body and containing yellow to orange granules.

SUTENT® 50 mg

Hard capsule

Gelatin capsules with caramel cap and caramel body, printed with white ink "Pfizer" on the cap and "STN 50 mg" on the body and containing yellow to orange granules.

4. CLINICAL PARTICULARS

4.1 Therapeutic indications

Gastrointestinal stromal tumour (GIST)

SUTENT is indicated for the treatment of unresectable and/or metastatic malignantgastrointestinal stromal tumour (GIST) after failure of imatinib mesilate treatment due to resistance or intolerance.

Metastatic renal cell carcinoma (MRCC)

SUTENT is indicated for the treatment of advanced/metastatic renal cell carcinoma (MRCC).

4.2 Posology and method of administration

Therapy with sunitinib should be initiated by a physician experienced in the treatment of MRCC or GIST.

The recommended dose of SUTENT is 50 mg once daily, taken orally for 4 consecutive weeks, followed by a 2-week rest period (schedule 4/2) to comprise a complete cycle of 6 weeks.

Dose adjustments

Safety and tolerability

Dose modifications in 12.5-mg steps may be applied based on individual safety and tolerability. Daily dose should not exceed 75 mg nor be decreased below 25 mg.

CYP3A4 inhibitors/inducers

Co-administration of SUTENT with potent CYP3A4 inducers such as rifampicin, should be avoided (see sections 4.4 and 4.5). If this is not possible, the dose of SUTENT may need to be increased in 12.5 mg increments (up to 87.5 mg per day) based on careful monitoring of tolerability.

Co-administration of SUTENT with potent CYP3A4 inhibitors, such as ketoconazole, should be avoided (see sections 4.4 and 4.5). If this is not possible, the doses of SUTENT may need to be reduced to a minimum of 37.5 mg daily, based on careful monitoring of the tolerability.

Selection of an alternative concomitant medicinal product with no, or minimal potential to induce or inhibit CYP3A4 should be considered.

Special populations

Children and adolescents (< 18 years old)

The safety and efficacy of SUTENT in paediatric patients below 18 years of age have not been established.

SUTENT should not be used in paediatric population until further data become available.

Elderly patients *(≥ 65 years old)*

Approximately 34% of the subjects in clinical studies of sunitinib were 65 or over. No significant differences in safety or effectiveness were observed between younger and older patients.

Hepatic Insufficiency

No starting dose adjustment is recommended when administering sunitinib to patients with mild or moderate (Child-Pugh Class A and B) hepatic impairment. Sunitinib has not been studied in subjects with severe (Child-Pugh Class C) hepatic impairment (see section 5.2).

Renal Insufficiency

No clinical studies have been performed in patients with impaired renal function.(see section 5.2).

Method of administration

SUTENT is for oral administration. It may be taken with or without food.

If a dose is missed the patient should not be given an additional dose. The patient should take the usual prescribed dose on the following day.

4.3 Contraindications

Hypersensitivity to the active substance or to any of the excipients.

4.4 Special warnings and precautions for use

Co-administration with potent CYP3A4 inducers should be avoided because it may decrease sunitinib plasma concentration (see sections 4.2 and 4.5).

Co-administration with potent CYP3A4 inhibitors should be avoided because it may increase the plasma concentration of sunitinib (see sections 4.2 and 4.5).

Skin and tissues disorders

Skin discolouration, possibly due to the active substance colour (yellow) is a common adverse reaction occurring in approximately 30% of patients. Patients should be advised that depigmentation of the hair or skin may also occur during treatment with sunitinib. Other possible dermatologic effects may include dryness, thickness or cracking of the skin, blisters or occasional rash on the palms of the hands and soles of the feet.

Mouth pain/irritation was reported in approximately 14% of patients. The above events were not cumulative, were typically reversible and generally did not result in treatment discontinuation.

Haemorrhage and tumour bleeding

Haemorrhagic events, some of which were fatal, reported through post-marketing experience, have included gastro-intestinal, respiratory, tumour, urinary tract and brain haemorrhages. In clinical trials treatment-related tumour haemorrhage occurred in approximately 2% of patients with GIST. These events may occur suddenly, and in the case of pulmonary tumours, may present as severe and life-threatening haemoptysis or pulmonary haemorrhage. Fatal pulmonary haemorrhage occurred in 2 patients (~ 1.8%) receiving SUTENT on a phase 2 clinical trial of patients with metastatic non-small cell lung cancer (NSCLC). Both patients had squamous cell histology. SUTENT is not approved for use in patients with NSCLC. Bleeding events occurred in 18% of patients receiving SUTENT in a phase 3 GIST Study compared to 17% of patients receiving placebo. In patients receiving SUTENT for treatment-naïve MRCC, 28% had bleeding events compared to 7% of patients receiving IFN- α. Seven (1.9%) patients on sunitinib malate versus 0% of patients on IFN-α experienced Grade 3 or greater treatment-related bleeding events. Of patients receiving sunitinib malate for cytokine-refractory MRCC, 26% experienced bleeding. Routine assessment of this event should include complete blood counts and physical examination.

Epistaxis was the most common haemorrhagic adverse reactions, having been reported for approximately half of the patients with solid tumours who experienced haemorrhagic events. Some of the epistaxis events were severe, but very rarely fatal.

Gastrointestinal disorders

Nausea, diarrhoea, stomatitis, dyspepsia and vomiting were the most commonly reported treatment-related gastrointestinal adverse reactions (see section 4.8).

Supportive care for gastrointestinal adverse reactions requiring treatment may include medicinal products with an anti-emetic or anti-diarrhoeal properties.

Serious, sometimes fatal gastrointestinal complications including gastrointestinal perforation have occurred rarely in patients with intra-abdominal malignancies treated with sunitinib. Treatment-related fatal gastrointestinal bleeding occurred in 0.5% of patients receiving placebo in the GIST Phase 3 study.

Hypertension

Treatment-related hypertension was reported in approximately 16% of patients with solid tumours. The dose of sunitinib was reduced or its administration temporarily suspended in approximately 2.7% of the patients who experienced hypertension. In none of these patients sunitinib was permanently discontinued. Severe hypertension (>200 mmHg systolic or 110 mmHg diastolic) occurred in 4.7% of patients with solid tumours. Treatment-related hypertension was reported in approximately 24% of patients receiving sunitinib for treatment-naïve MRCC compared to 1% of patients receiving IFN-α. Severe hypertension occurred in 5% of treatment-naïve patients on sunitinib and 1% of patients on IFN-α. Patients should be screened for hypertension and controlled as appropriate. Temporary suspension is recommended in patients with severe hypertension that is not controlled with medical management. Treatment may be resumed once hypertension is appropriately controlled.

Haematological disorders

Decreased absolute neutrophil counts of grade 3 and 4 severity were reported in 10% and 1.7% of patients on the phase 3 GIST study, respectively, and in 16% and 1.6% of patients on the phase 3 MRCC study, respectively. Decreased platelet counts of grade 3 and 4 severity were reported in 3.7% and 0.4% of patients on the phase 3 GIST study, respectively, and in 8.2% and 1.1% of patients on the phase 3 MRCC study, respectively. The above events were not cumulative, were typically reversible and generally did not result in treatment discontinuation. None of these events in the phase 3 studies were fatal, but rare fatal haematological events have been reported through post-marketing experience.

Complete blood counts should be performed at the beginning of each treatment cycle for patients receiving treatment with sunitinib.

Cardiac disorders

Cardiovascular events, some of which were fatal, reported through post-marketing experience, have included left ventricular ejection fraction (LVEF) decreased and cardiac failure. In clinical trials, decreases in LVEF of ⩾ 20% and below the lower limit of normal occurred in approximately 2% of SUTENT-treated GIST patients, 4% of cytokine-refractory MRCC patients, and 2% of placebo-treated GIST patients. These LVEF declines do not appear to have been progressive and often improved as treatment continued. In the treatment-naïve MRCC study, 21% patients on SUTENT and 12% of patients on IFN-α, had an LVEF value below the lower limit of normal. One (<1%) patient who received sunitinib was diagnosed with congestive heart failure (CHF).

In GIST patients treatment-related 'cardiac failure', 'cardiac failure congestive' or 'left ventricular failure' were reported in 0.7% of patients treated with SUTENT and 1% of patients treated with placebo. In the pivotal phase 3 GIST study (n=312), treatment-related fatal cardiac reactions occurred in 1% of patients on each arm of the study (i.e. sunitinib and placebo arms). In a phase 2 study in cytokine-refractory MRCC patients, 0.9% of patients experienced treatment-related fatal myocardial infarction and in the phase 3 study in treatment-naïve MRCC patients, 0.6% of patients on the IFN-αarm and 0% patients on the sunitinib arm experienced fatal cardiac events. The relationship, if any, between receptor tyrosine kinase (RTK) inhibition and cardiac function remains unclear.

Patients who presented with cardiac events within 12 months prior to sunitinib administration, such as myocardial infarction (including severe/unstable angina), coronary/peripheral artery bypass graft, symptomatic CHF, cerebrovascular accident or transient ischemic attack, or pulmonary embolism were excluded from SUTENT clinical studies.

Close monitoring for clinical signs and symptoms of CHF should be performed, especially in patients with cardiac risk factors and/or history of coronary artery disease.

Physicians are advised to weigh this risk against the potential benefits of SUTENT. These patients should be carefully monitored for clinical signs and symptoms of CHF while receiving sunitinib. Baseline and periodic evaluations of LVEF should also be considered while the patient is receiving sunitinib. In patients without cardiac risk factors, a baseline evaluation of ejection fraction should be considered.

In the presence of clinical manifestations of CHF, discontinuation of SUTENT is recommended. The administration of SUTENT should be interrupted and/or the dose reduced in patients without clinical evidence of CHF but with an ejection fraction <50% and >20% below baseline.

QT Interval prolongation

Data from non-clinical (*in vitro* and *in vivo*) studies, at doses higher than the recommended human dose, indicate that sunitinib has the potential to inhibit the cardiac action potential repolarisation process (e.g. prolongation of QT interval).

Increases in the QTc interval to over 500 msec occurred in 0.5% and changes from baseline in excess of 60 msec occurred in 1.1% of the 450 solid tumours patients; both of these parameters are recognized as potentially significant changes. At approximately twice therapeutic concentrations, sunitinib has been shown to prolong the QTcF Inteval (Frederica's Correction).

QTc interval prolongation was investigated in a trial in 24 patients, ages 20-87 years, with advanced malignancies. The results of this study demonstrated that sunitinib had an effect on QTc (defined as a mean placebo-adjusted change of > 10 msec with a 90% CI upper limit > 15 msec) at therapeutic concentration (day 3) using the within-day baseline correction method, and at greater than therapeutic concentration (Day 9) using both baseline correction methods. No patients had a QTc value >500 msec. Although an effect on QTcF interval was observed on Day 3 at 24 hours post-dose (i.e. at therapeutic plasma concentration expected after the recommended starting dose of 50 mg) with the within-day baseline correction method, the clinical significance of this finding is unclear.

Using comprehensive serial ECG assessments at times corresponding to either therapeutic or greater than therapeutic exposures, none of the patients in the evaluable or ITT populations were observed to develop QTc interval prolongation considered as "severe" (i.e. equal to or greater than Grade 3 by CTCAE version 3.0).

At therapeutic plasma concentrations, the maximum QTcF interval (Frederica's correction) mean change from baseline was 9.6 msec (90% CI 15.1msec). At approximately twice therapeutic concentrations, the maximum QTcF interval change from baseline was 15.4 msec (90% CI 22.4 msec). Moxifloxacin (400 mg) used as a positive control showed a 5.6 msec maximum mean QTcF interval change from baseline. No subjects experienced an effect on the QTc interval greater than Grade 2 (CTCAE version 3.0). No patient presented with a cardiac arrhythmia.

QT interval prolongation may lead to an increased risk of ventricular arrhythmias including *Torsade de pointes*. *Torsade de pointes* has been observed in <0.1% of sunitinib-exposed patients. Sunitinib should be used with caution in patients with a known history of QT interval prolongation, patients who are taking antiarrhythmics, or patients with relevant pre-existing cardiac disease, bradycardia, or electrolyte disturbances. Concomitant administration of sunitinib with potent CYP3A4 inhibitors should be limited because of the possible increase in sunitinib plasma concentrations, (see section 4.2 and 4.5).

Venous thromboembolic events

Treatment-related venous thromboembolic events were reported in approximately 1.0% of patients with solid tumours who received SUTENT on clinical trials, including GIST and MRCC.

Seven patients (3%) on SUTENT and none on placebo in a phase 3 GIST study experienced venous thromboembolic events; five of the seven were Grade 3 deep venous thromboses (DVT), and two were Grade 1 or 2. Four of these seven GIST patients discontinued treatment following first observation of DVT.

Seven patients (1.9%) receiving SUTENT in the phase 3 for treatment-naïve MRCC study and four patients (2%) on the two cytokine-refractory MRCC studies had treatment-related venous thromboembolic events reported. Six of these patients had pulmonary embolisms, one was Grade 3 and five were Grade 4, and five of these patients had DVT, one each with Grade 1 and 2, and three with Grade 3.

In treatment-naïve MRCC patients receiving IFN-α, six (2%) venous thromboembolic events occurred; one patient (<1%) experienced a Grade 3 DVT and five patients (1%) had pulmonary embolism, one Grade 1 and four with Grade 4.

No cases with fatal outcome were reported in GIST and MRCC registrational studies. Cases with fatal out-come had been observed in post-marketing setting (see pulmonary events and section 4.8).

Respiratory events

Patients who presented with pulmonary embolism within the previous 12 months were excluded from SUTENT clinical studies.

In patients who received SUTENT in Phase 3 registrational studies, treatment-related pulmonary events (i.e. dyspnoea, pleural effusion, pulmonary embolism or pulmonary oedema) were reported in approximately 5% of patients with GIST and in approximately 14% of patients with MRCC. Rare cases with fatal outcome were reported.

Approximately 8% of patients with solid tumours, including GIST and MRCC, who received SUTENT in clinical trials experienced treatment-related pulmonary events.

Cases of Pulmonary embolism were observed in approximately 1.3% of patients with GIST and in approximately 0.8% of patients with MRCC, who received Sutent in Phase 3 studies (see section 4.4 - Venous thromboembolic events)

Thyroid Dysfunction

Baseline laboratory measurement of thyroid function is recommended and patients with hypothyroidism or hyperthyroidism should be treated as per standard medical practice prior to the start of sunitinib treatment. All patients should be observed closely for signs and symptoms of thyroid dysfunction on sunitinib treatment. Patients with signs and/or symptoms suggestive of thyroid dysfunction should have laboratory monitoring of thyroid function performed and be treated as per standard medical practice.

Hypothyroidism was reported as an adverse event in 7 patients (4%) receiving SUTENT across the two cytokine-refractory MRCC studies; in nine patients (2%) on SUTENT and one patient (<1%) in the IFN-α arm in the treatment-naïve MRCC study. Additionally, TSH elevations were reported in 4 cytokine-refractory MRCC patients (2%). Overall, 7% of the MRCC population had either clinical or laboratory evidence of treatment-emergent hypothyroidism. Treatment-emergent acquired hypothyroidism was noted in 8 GIST patients (4%) on SUTENT *versus* 1 (1%) on placebo.

Rare cases of hyperthyroidism, some followed by hypothyroidism, have been reported in clinical trials and through post-marketing experience.

Pancreatitis

Increases in serum lipase and amylase activities were observed in patients with various solid tumours who received sunitinib. Increases in lipase activities were transient and were generally not accompanied by signs or symptoms of pancreatitis in subjects with various solid tumours. Pancreatitis has been observed uncommonly (<1%) in patients receiving SUTENT for GIST or MRCC.

Cases of serious pancreatic events, some with fatal outcome, have been reported. If symptoms of pancreatitis are present, patients should have sunitinib discontinued and be provided with appropriate supportive care.

Hepatic Function

Serious cases of sunitinib-related hepatobiliary events have been reported in patients with solid tumours; hepatic failure was observed in <1% of these patients. Cases of hepatobiliary events some with fatal outcome, have been reported. If signs or symptoms of hepatic failure are present, SUTENT should be discontinued and appropriate supportive care should be provided.

Renal function

The safety of continued SUTENT treatment in patients with moderate to severe proteinuria has not been systematically evaluated.

Cases of proteinuria and rare cases of nephrotic syndrome have been reported. Baseline urinalysis is recommended, and patients should be monitored for the development or worsening of proteinuria. Discontinue SUTENT in patients with nephrotic syndrome.

Fistula

If fistula formation occurs, sunitinib treatment should be interrupted. Limited information is available on the continued use of sunitinib in patients with fistulae.

Hypersensitivity/Angioedema

If angioedema due to hypersensitivity occurs, sunitinib treatment should be interrupted and standard medical care provided.

Nervous system disorders

Taste disturbance

Dysgeusia was reported in approximately 28% of patients receiving SUTENT in clinical trials.

Seizures

In clinical studies of SUTENT and from post-marketing experience, seizures have been observed in subjects with or without radiological evidence of brain metastases. In addition, there have been few reports (<1%) of subjects presenting with seizures and radiological evidence of reversible posterior leukoencephalopathy syndrome (RPLS). Patients with seizures and signs/symptoms consistent with RPLS, such as hypertension, headache, decreased alertness, altered mental functioning and visual loss, including cortical blindness should be controlled with medical management including control of hypertension. Temporary suspension of SUTENT is recommended; following resolution, treatment may be resumed at the discretion of the treating physician.

4.5 Interaction with other medicinal products and other forms of interaction

Medicinal products that may ***increase*** *sunitinib plasma concentrations*

In healthy volunteers, concomitant administration of a single dose of sunitinib with the potent CYP3A4 inhibitor, ketoconazole, resulted in an increase of the combined [sunitinib + primary metabolite] C_{max} and $AUC_{0-\infty}$ values of 49% and 51%, respectively.

Administration of sunitinib with potent CYP3A4 inhibitors (e.g. ritonavir, itraconazole, erythromycin, clarithromycin, grapefruit juice) may increase sunitinib concentrations.

Combination with CYP3A4 inhibitors should therefore be avoided, or the selection of an alternate concomitant medicinal product with no, or minimal potential to inhibit CYP3A4 should be considered.

If this is not possible, the dose of SUTENT may need to be reduced to a minimum of 37.5 mg daily, based on careful monitoring of tolerability (see section 4.2).

Medicinal products that may ***decrease*** *sunitinib plasma concentrations:*

In healthy volunteers, concomitant administration of a single dose of sunitinib with the CYP3A4 inducer, rifampin, resulted in a reduction of the combined [sunitinib + primary metabolite] C_{max} and $AUC_{0-\infty}$ values of 23% and 46%, respectively.

Administration of sunitinib with potent CYP3A4 inducers (e.g., dexamethasone, phenytoin, carbamazepine, rifampin, phenobarbital or herbal preparations containing St. John's Wort/ *Hypericum perforatum* may decrease sunitinib concentrations. Combination with CYP3A4 inducers should therefore be avoided, or selection of an alternate concomitant medicinal product with no, or minimal potential to induce CYP3A4 should be considered. If this is not possible, the dosage of SUTENT may need to be increased in 12.5 mg increments (up to 87.5 mg per day) based on careful monitoring of tolerability (see section 4.2).

Anticoagulants

Haemorrhage has been observed rarely in patients treated with sunitinib (see section 4.4 and 4.8). Patients receiving concomitant treatment with anti-coagulants (e.g. warfarin; acenocumarole) may be periodically monitored by complete blood counts (platelets), coagulation factors (PT/INR), and physical examination

4.6 Pregnancy and lactation

Pregnancy

There are no studies in pregnant women using SUTENT. Studies in animals have shown reproductive toxicity including foetal malformations (see section 5.3). SUTENT should not be used during pregnancy or in any women not using effective contraception, unless the potential benefit justifies the potential risk to the foetus. If SUTENT is used during pregnancy or if the patient becomes pregnant while on treatment with SUTENT, the patient should be apprised of the potential hazard to the foetus.

Women of childbearing potential should be advised to use affective contraception and avoid becoming pregnant while receiving treatment with SUTENT.

Lactation

Sunitinib and/or its metabolites are excreted in rat milk. It is not known whether sunitinib or its primary active metabolite is excreted in human milk. Because active substances are commonly excreted in human milk and because of the potential for serious adverse reactions in nursing infants, women should not breast feed while taking SUTENT.

Table 1 Adverse reactions reported in GIST studies with SUTENT

System Organ Class	Frequency	Adverse reactions	All Grades n (%)	Grade 3 n (%)	Grade 4 n (%)
Blood and the lymphatic system disorders	Very common	Anaemia	86 (19.5%)	24 (5.5%)	3 (0.7%)
	Very common	Neutropoenia	81 (18.4%)	39 (8.9%)	5 (1.1%)
	Very common	Thrombocytopoenia	67 (15.2%)	19 (4.3%)	6 (1.4%)
	Common	Leukopoenia	26 (5.9%)	9 (2.0%)	1 (0.2%)
	Common	Lymphopoenia	10 (2.3%)	3 (0.7%)	1 (0.2%)
Endocrine disorders	Very common	Hypothyroidism	59 (13.4%)	5 (1.1%)	1 (0.2%)
Metabolism and nutrition disorders	Very common	Decreased appetite [a]	117 (26.6%)	8 (1.8%)	0 (0.0%)
Psychiatric disorders	Common	Insomnia	14 (3.2%)	0 (0.0%)	0 (0.0%)
Nervous system disorders	Very common	Taste disturbance [b]	105 (23.9%)	1 (0.2%)	0 (0.0%)
	Very common	Headache	76 (17.3%)	5 (1.1%)	0 (0.0%)
	Common	Paraesthesia	27 (6.1%)	1 (0.2%)	0 (0.0%)
	Common	Dizziness	18 (4.1%)	1 (0.2%)	0 (0.0%)
	Common	Neuropathy peripheral	11 (2.5%)	0 (0.0%)	0 (0.0%)
	Common	Hypoaesthesia	10 (2.3%)	0 (0.0%)	0 (0.0%)
Vascular disorders	Very common	Hypertension	101 (23.0%)	43 (9.8%)	0 (0.0%)
Respiratory, thoracic and mediastinal disorders	Common	Epistaxis	28 (6.4%)	1 (0.2%)	0 (0.0%)
	Common	Dyspnoea	16 (3.6%)	2 (0.5%)	0 (0.0%)
Renal and urinary disorders	Common	Chromaturia	18 (4.1%)	0 (0.0%)	0 (0.0%)
Gastrointestinal disorders	Very common	Diarrhoea	187 (42.5%)	24 (5.5%)	0 (0.0%)
	Very common	Nausea	161 (36.6%)	15 (3.4%)	0 (0.0%)
	Very common	Vomiting	98 (22.2%)	7 (1.6%)	0 (0.0%)
	Very common	Stomatitis	90 (20.5%)	7 (1.6%)	0 (0.0%)
	Very common	Dyspepsia	80 (18.2%)	4 (0.9%)	0 (0.0%)
	Very common	Abdominal pain [c] / distension	77 (17.5%)	15 (3.4%)	2 (0.5%)
	Very common	Flatulence	46 (10.5%)	0 (0.0%)	0 (0.0%)
	Very common	Oral pain	44 (10.0%)	2 (0.5%)	0 (0.0%)
	Common	Constipation	37 (8.4%)	2 (0.5%)	0 (0.0%)
	Common	Glossodynia	37 (8.4%)	0 (0.0%)	0 (0.0%)
	Common	Dry mouth	31 (7.0%)	0 (0.0%)	0 (0.0%)
	Common	Gastro-oesophageal reflux disease	12 (2.7%)	1 (0.2%)	0 (0.0%)
	Common	Mouth ulceration	11 (2.5%)	0 (0.0%)	0 (0.0%)
	Common	Oral discomfort	11 (2.5%)	0 (0.0%)	0 (0.0%)
Skin and subcutaneous tissue disorders	Very common	Yellow skin/ Skin discolouration	146 (33.2%)	0 (0.0%)	0 (0.0%)
	Very common	Palmar-plantar erythrodysaesthesia syndrome	106 (24.1%)	27 (6.1%)	0 (0.0%)
	Very common	Hair colour changes	67 (15.2%)	0 (0.0%)	0 (0.0%)
	Very common	Rash	64 (14.5%)	3 (0.7%)	0 (0.0%)
	Common	Dry skin	41 (9.3%)	0 (0.0%)	0 (0.0%)
	Common	Alopecia	33 (7.5%)	0 (0.0%)	0 (0.0%)
	Common	Dermatitis	29 (6.6%)	1 (0.2%)	0 (0.0%)
	Common	Periorbital oedema	20 (4.5%)	0 (0.0%)	0 (0.0%)
	Common	Skin Reaction	20 (4.5%)	3 (0.7%)	0 (0.0%)
	Common	Erythema	18 (4.1%)	0 (0.0%)	0 (0.0%)
	Common	Eczema	16 (3.6%)	1 (0.2%)	0 (0.0%)
	Common	Pruritus	16 (3.6%)	0 (0.0%)	0 (0.0%)
	Common	Skin hyperpigmentation	15 (3.4%)	0 (0.0%)	0 (0.0%)
	Common	Skin exfoliation	12 (2.7%)	0 (0.0%)	0 (0.0%)
	Common	Blister	10 (2.3%)	1 (0.2%)	0 (0.0%)
	Common	Skin lesion	10 (2.3%)	1 (0.2%)	0 (0.0%)
Musculoskeletal and connective tissue and bone disorders	Very Common	Pain in extremity/limb	54 (12.3%)	5 (1.1%)	0 (0.0%)
	Common	Arthralgia	39 (8.9%)	3 (0.7%)	0 (0.0%)
	Common	Myalgia	29 (6.6%)	0 (0.0%)	0 (0.0%)
	Common	Muscle spasm	21 (4.8%)	1 (0.2%)	0 (0.0%)
	Common	Back pain	11 (2.5%)	2 (0.5%)	0 (0.0%)
	Common	Muscular weakness	10 (2.3%)	1 (0.2%)	0 (0.0%)
General disorders and administration site conditions	Very common	Fatigue/Asthenia	287 (65.2%)	64 (14.5%)	5 (1.1%)
	Very common	Mucosal inflammation	70 (15.9%)	6 (1.4%)	1 (0.2%)
	Very common	Oedema [d]	59 (13.4%)	1 (0.2%)	0 (0.0%)
	Common	Pyrexia	26 (5.9%)	2 (0.5%)	0 (0.0%)
Investigations	Common	Lipase increase	35 (8.0%)	12 (2.7%)	7 (1.6%)
	Common	White blood cell count decreased [e]	33 (7.5%)	15 (3.4%)	0 (0.0%)
	Common	Ejection fraction decreased	27 (6.1%)	5 (1.2%)	0 (0.0%)
	Common	Haemoglobin decreased	27 (6.1%)	6 (1.4%)	0 (0.0%)
	Common	Blood creatinine phosphokinase increased	22 (5.0%)	1 (0.2%)	1 (0.2%)
	Common	Platelet count decrease	25 (5.7%)	4 (0.9%)	1 (0.2%)
	Common	Weight decreased	23 (5.2%)	1 (0.2%)	0 (0.0%)
	Common	Amylase increased	21 (4.8%)	8 (1.8%)	0 (0.0%)
	Common	Aspartate aminotransferase increased	18 (4.1%)	2 (0.5%)	1 (0.2%)
	Common	Alanine aminotransferase increased	12 (2.7%)	1 (0.2%)	0 (0.0%)
		Any adverse event	414 (94.1%)	204 (46.4%)	53 (12.0%)

The following terms have been combined:

[a] Anorexia and decreased appetite

[b] Dysgeusia, ageusia and taste disturbance

[c] Abdominal pain and abdominal pain upper

[d] Oedema, oedema peripheral and oedema face

[e] White blood cell count decreased, neutrophil count decreased, and leukocyte count decreased

Table 2 Adverse reactions reported in cytokine-refractory and treatment-naïve MRCC studies with SUTENT

System Organ Class	*Frequency*	*Adverse reactions*	*All Grades n (%)*	*Grade 3 n (%)*	*Grade 4 n (%)*
Blood and lymphatic system disorders	Very common	Neutropoenia	89 (16.4%)	46 (8.5%)	5 (0.9%)
	Very common	Thrombocytopoenia	86 (15.8%)	37 (6.8%)	5 (0.9%)
	Very common	Anaemia	67 (12.3%)	20 (3.7%)	3 (0.6%)
	Common	Leukopoenia	45 (8.3%)	16 (2.9%)	0 (0%)
	Common	Lymphopenia	21 (3.9%)	12 (2.2%)	1 (0.2%)
Endocrine disorders	Very common	Hypothyroidism	67 (12.3%)	7 (1.3%)	0 (0%)
Metabolism and nutrition disorders	Very Common	Decreased appetite [a]	205 (37.7%)	9 (1.7%)	0 (0%)
	Common	Dehydration	33 (6.1%)	7 (1.3%)	1 (0.2%)
Psychiatric disorders	Common	Insomnia	22 (4.0%)	0 (0%)	0 (0%)
	Common	Depression	15 (2.8%)	1 (0.2%)	0 (0%)
Nervous system disorders	Very common	Taste disturbance [b]	250 (46.0%)	1 (0.2%)	0 (0%)
	Very common	Headache	82 (15.1%)	3 (0.6%)	0 (0%)
	Common	Dizziness	38 (7.0%)	2 (0.4%)	0 (0%)
	Common	Paraesthesia	36 (5.9%)	0 (0%)	0 (0%)
	Common	Neuropathy peripheral	33 (6.1%)	1 (0.2%)	0 (0%)
	Common	Hypoaesthesia	20 (3.7%)	0 (0%)	0 (0%)
	Common	Hyperaesthesia	17 (3.1%)	0 (0%)	0 (0%)
Eye disorders	Common	Lacrimation increased	39 (7.2%)	0 (0%)	0 (0%)
	Common	Eyelid oedema	12 (2.2%)	0 (0%)	0 (0%)
Vascular disorders	Very common	Hypertension	143 (26.3%)	55 (10.1%)	0 (0%)
	Common	Flushing	17 (3.1%)	0 (0%)	0 (0%)
	Common	Hot flush	12 (2.2%)	0 (0%)	0 (0%)
Respiratory, thoracic and mediastinal disorders	Very common	Epistaxis	86 (15.8%)	3 (0.6%)	0 (0%)
	Common	Dyspnoea	45 (8.3%)	6 (1.1%)	0 (0%)
	Common	Pharyngolaryngeal pain	29 (5.3%)	2 (0.4%)	0 (0%)
	Common	Cough	23 (4.2%)	0 (0%)	0 (0%)
	Common	Dysphonia	16 (2.9%)	0 (0%)	0 (0%)
	Common	Nasal dryness	14 (2.6%)	0 (0%)	0 (0%)
	Common	Dyspnoea exertional	12 (2.2%)	0 (0%)	0 (0%)
	Common	Nasal congestion	12 (2.2%)	0 (0%)	0 (0%)
	Common	Pleural effusion	12 (2.2%)	3 (0.6%)	0 (0%)
Gastrointestinal disorders	Very common	Diarrhoea	326 (59.9%)	38 (7.0%)	0 (0%)
	Very common	Nausea	290 (53.3%)	19 (3.5%)	0 (0%)
	Very common	Dyspepsia	189 (34.7%)	8 (1.5%)	0 (0%)
	Very common	Stomatitis	185 (34.0%)	13 (2.4%)	0 (0%)
	Very common	Vomiting	178 (32.7%)	17 (3.1%)	0 (0%)
	Very common	Abdominal pain [c] / distension	106 (19.5%)	10 (1.8%)	0 (0%)
	Very common	Constipation	83 (15.3%)	1 (0.2%)	0 (0%)
	Very common	Glossodynia	63 (11.6%)	0 (0%)	0 (0%)
	Very common	Flatulence	60 (11.0%)	0 (0%)	0 (0%)
	Very common	Oral pain	60 (11.0%)	2 (0.4%)	0 (0%)
	Very common	Dry mouth	56 (10.3%)	0 (0%)	0 (0%)
	Common	Gastroesophageal reflux disease	50 (9.2%)	2 (0.4%)	0 (0%)
	Common	Dysphagia	20 (3.7%)	2 (0.4%)	1 (0.2%)
	Common	Cheilitis	19 (3.5%)	1 (0.2%)	1 (0.2%)
	Common	Gingival bleeding	18 (3.3%)	0 (0%)	0 (0%)
	Common	Haemorrhoids	18 (3.3%)	0 (0%)	0 (0%)
	Common	Proctalgia	17 (3.1%)	1 (0.2%)	0 (0%)
	Common	Mouth ulceration	16 (2.9%)	0 (0%)	1 (0.2%)
	Common	Stomach discomfort	15 (2.8%)	0 (0%)	0 (0%)
	Common	Rectal haemorrhage	13 (2.4%)	0 (0%)	0 (0%)
Skin and subcutaneous tissue disorders	Very common	Palmar-plantar erythrodysaesthesia syndrome	144 (26.5%)	46 (8.5%)	0 (0%)
	Very common	Yellow discolouration/ Skin discolouration	144 (26.5%)	1 (0.2%)	0 (0%)
	Very common	Rash	121 (22.2%)	2 (0.4%)	1 (0.2%)
	Very common	Dry skin	108 (19.9%)	1 (0.2%)	0 (0%)
	Very common	Hair colour changes	103 (18.9%)	0 (0%)	0 (0%)
	Very common	Alopecia	64 (11.8%)	0 (0%)	0 (0%)
	Common	Erythema	51 (9.4%)	2 (0.4%)	0 (0%)
	Common	Skin exfoliation	47 (8.6%)	4 (0.7%)	0 (0%)
	Common	Pruritus	40 (7.4%)	1 (0.2%)	0 (0%)
	Common	Periorbital oedema	31 (5.7%)	1 (0.2%)	0 (0%)
	Common	Dermatitis	27 (5.0%)	4 (0.7%)	0 (0%)
	Common	Skin lesion	26 (4.8%)	1 (0.2%)	0 (0%)
	Common	Nail disorder/ discolouration	25 (4.6%)	0 (0%)	0 (0%)
	Common	Blister	23 (4.2%)	1 (0.2%)	0 (0%)
	Common	Skin reaction	23 (4.2%)	6 (1.1%)	0 (0%)
	Common	Hyperkeratosis	22 (4.0%)	4 (0.7%)	0 (0%)
	Common	Acne	19 (3.5%)	0 (0%)	0 (0%)
Musculoskeletal and connective tissue disorders	Very common	Pain in extremity	96 (17.6%)	6 (1.1%)	0 (0%)
	Common	Arthralgia	49 (9.0%)	1 (0.2%)	0 (0%)
	Common	Myalgia	48 (8.8%)	2 (0.4%)	0 (0%)
	Common	Muscle Spasm	26 (4.8%)	0 (0%)	0 (0%)
	Common	Back pain	17 (3.1%)	2 (0.4%)	0 (0%)

System Organ Class	*Frequency*	*Adverse reactions*	*All Grades n (%)*	*Grade 3 n (%)*	*Grade 4 n (%)*
General disorders and administration site conditions	Very common	Fatigue/asthenia	397 (73.0%)	95 (17.5%)	1 (0.2%)
	Very common	Mucosal inflammation	127 (23.3%)	8 (1.5%)	0 (0%)
	Very common	Oedema [d]	99 (18.2%)	5 (0.9%)	0 (0%)
	Common	Pyrexia	37 (6.8%)	3 (0.6%)	0 (0%)
	Common	Chills	35 (6.4%)	2 (0.4%)	0 (0%)
	Common	Pain	20 (3.7%)	0 (0%)	0 (0%)
	Common	Chest pain	13 (2.4%)	2 (0.4%)	0 (0%)
Investigations	Very common	Ejection fraction decreased	84 (15.4%)	16 (2.9%)	0 (0%)
	Very common	Weight decreased	57 (10.5%)	1 (0.2%)	0 (0%)
	Common	Platelet count decreased	41 (7.5%)	15 (2.8%)	2 (0.4%)
	Common	White blood cell count decreased [e]	37 (6.8%)	16 (2.9%)	0 (0%)
	Common	Lipase increased	36 (6.6%)	19 (3.5%)	11 (2%)
	Common	Haemoglobin decreased	25 (4.6%)	8 (1.5%)	0 (0%)
	Common	Blood creatine phosphokinase increased	19 (3.5%)	7 (1.3%)	2 (0.4%)
	Common	Aspartate aminotransferase increased	18 (3.3%)	7 (1.3%)	0 (0%)
	Common	Blood amylase increased	18 (3.3%)	11 (2.0%)	2 (0.4%)
	Common	Blood creatinine increased	15 (2.8%)	2 (0.4%)	0 (0%)
	Common	Blood pressure increased	15 (2.8%)	2 (0.4%)	0 (0%)
	Common	Alanine aminotransferase increased	14 (2.6%)	7 (1.3%)	2 (0.4%)
		Any adverse event	524 (96.3%)	296 (54.4%)	57 (10.5%)

The following terms have been combined:

[a] Anorexia and decreased appetite

[b] Dysgeusia, ageusia and taste disturbance

[c] Abdominal pain and abdominal pain upper

[d] Oedema, oedema peripheral and oedema face

[e] White blood cell count decreased, neutrophil count decreased, and leukocyte count decreased

Fertility

Based on nonclinical findings, male and female fertility may be compromised by treatment with SUTENT (see section 5.3).

4.7 Effects on ability to drive and use machines

No studies on the effects on the ability to drive and use machines have been performed. Patients should be advised that they may experience dizziness during treatment with sunitinib.

4.8 Undesirable effects

The most important serious adverse reactions associated with SUTENT in patients with solid tumours were pulmonary embolism (1%), thrombocytopoenia (1%), tumour haemorrhage (0.9%), febrile neutropoenia (0.4%), and hypertension (0.4%). The most common adverse reactions (experienced by at least 20% of the patients) of any grade included: fatigue; gastrointestinal disorders, such as diarrhoea, nausea, stomatitis, dyspepsia and vomiting; skin discolouration; dysgeusia and anorexia. Fatigue, hypertension and neutropoenia were the most common Grade 3 adverse reactions and increased lipase was the most frequent Grade 4 adverse reaction in patients with solid tumours. Hepatitis and hepatic failure occurred in <1% of patients and prolonged QT interval in < 0.1% (see section 4.4).

Fatal events other than those listed in section 4.4 above or in section 4.8 below that were considered possibly related to sunitinib included multi-system organ failure, disseminated intravascular coagulation, peritoneal haemorrhage, rhabdomyolysis, cerebrovascular accident, dehydration, adrenal insufficiency, renal failure, respiratory failure, pleural effusion, pneumothorax, shock, and sudden death.

Adverse reactions that were reported in >2% of solid tumour patients are listed below, by system organ class, frequency and grade of severity (NCI-CTCAE). Within each frequency grouping, undesirable effects are presented in order of decreasing seriousness.

Frequencies are defined as: Very common (⩾1/10); common (⩾1/100 to <1/10); uncommon (⩾1/1,000 to <1/100); rare (⩾1/10,000 to <1/1,000); very rare (<1/10,000), not known (cannot be estimated from the available data).

Table 1 - Adverse reactions reported in GIST studies with SUTENT

(see Table 1 on page 2269)

Table 2 - Adverse reactions reported in cytokine-refractory and treatment-naïve MRCC studies with SUTENT

(see Table 2 on previous page)

Table 3 - Adverse reactions reported through post-marketing experience

The following adverse reactions have been identified during post-approval use of SUTENT. This includes spontaneous case reports as well as serious adverse events from ongoing studies, the expanded access programmes, clinical pharmacology studies and exploratory studies in unapproved indications.

Infections and infestations [a]	
Non known	Infections (with or without neutropoenia)
Blood and lymphatic system disorder[b]	
Non known	Thrombotic microangiopathy
Immune system disorders[c]	
Non known	Angioedema, hypersensitivity reaction
Endocrine disorderse[d]	
Non known	Hyperthyroidism
Cardiac disorders:	
Uncommon:	Cardiac failure, cardiac failure congestive, left ventricular failure
Rare:	Prolonged QT interval, Torsade de pointes
Gastrointestinal disorders:	
Uncommon:	Pancreatitis
Rare:	Gastrointestinal perforation
Hepatobiliary disorders:	
Uncommon:	Hepatic failure
Musculoskeletal and connective tissue disorders[e]	
Not known	Myopathy and/or rhabdomyolysis
Not known	Fistula formation
Renal and urinary disorders[f]	
Not known	Proteinuria, Nephrotic syndrome
Pulmonary disorders[g]	
Not known:	Pleural effusion
Not known:	Pulmonary embolism and respiratory failure
Investigations:	
Common:	Elevated thyroid stimulating hormone (TSH)

[a] ***Infection and infestations***: Cases of serious infection (with or without neutropoenia), including pneumonia, have been reported. Few cases had a fatal outcome.

[b] ***Blood and lymphatic system disorders:*** Rare cases of thrombotic microangiopathy have been reported. Temporary suspension of SUTENT is recommended; following resolution, treatment may be resumed at the discretion of the treating physician.

[c] ***Immune system disorders:*** Hypersensitivity reactions, including angioedema, have been reported.

[d] ***Endocrine Disorders:*** Rare cases of hyperthyroidism, some followed by hypothyroidism, have been reported in clinical trials and through post-marketing experience (See also section 4.4).

[e] ***Musculoskeletal and connective tissue disorders***: Rare cases of myopathy and/or rhabdomyolysis, some with acute renal failure, have been reported. Patients with signs or symptoms of muscle toxicity should be managed as per standard medical practice.

Cases of fistula formation, sometimes associated with tumour necrosis and regression, in some cases with fatal outcomes, have been reported.

[f] ***Renal and urinary disorders:*** Cases of proteinuria and rare cases of nephrotic syndrome have been reported. The safety of continued SUTENT treatment in patients with moderate to severe proteinuria has not been systematically evaluated. Discontinue SUTENT in patients with nephrotic syndrome (see also section 4.4).

[g] ***Pulmonary disorders:*** Cases of pulmonary embolism, in some cases with fatal outcome, have been reported.

4.9 Overdose

There is no experience of acute overdose with SUTENT. There is no specific antidote for overdose with sunitinib and treatment of overdose should consist of general supportive measures. If indicated, elimination of unabsorbed active substance may be achieved by emesis or gastric lavage.

5. PHARMACOLOGICAL PROPERTIES

5.1 Pharmacodynamic properties

Pharmacotherapeutic group: – Protein kinase inhibitors, ATC Code: LO1XE04

Mechanism of action

Sunitinib inhibits multiple receptor tyrosine kinases (RTKs) that are implicated in tumour growth, neoangiogenesis, and metastatic progression of cancer. Sunitinib was identified as an inhibitor of platelet-derived growth factor receptors (PDGFRα and PDGFRβ), vascular endothelial growth factor receptors (VEGFR1, VEGFR2 and VEGFR3), stem cell factor receptor (KIT), Fms-like tyrosine kinase-3 (FLT3), colony stimulating factor receptor (CSF-1R), and the glial cell-line derived neurotrophic factor receptor (RET). The primary metabolite exhibits similar potency compared to sunitinib in biochemical and cellular assays.

Clinical studies

The clinical safety and efficacy of SUTENT has been studied in the treatment of patients with GIST who were resistant to imatinib (i.e. those who experienced disease progression during or following treatment with imatinib) or intolerant to imatinib (i.e. those who experienced significant toxicity during treatment with imatinib that precluded further treatment) and the treatment of patients with MRCC.

Efficacy is based on time to tumour progression and an increase in survival in GIST and on progression free survival and objective response rates for treatment-naïve and cytokine-refractory MRCC respectively.

Gastrointestinal stromal tumours (GIST)

An initial open-label, dose-escalation study was conducted in patients with GIST after failure of imatinib (median maximum daily dose 800 mg) due to resistance or intolerance. Ninety-seven patients were enrolled at various doses and schedules; 55 patients received 50 mg SUTENT at the recommended treatment schedule 4 weeks on /2 weeks off ("schedule 4/2").

In this study the median Time to Progression (TTP) was 34.0 weeks (95% CI = 22.0 – 46.0 weeks).

A phase 3, randomized, double-blind, placebo-controlled study of SUTENT was conducted in patients with GIST who were intolerant to, or had experienced disease progression during or following treatment with, imatinib (Median maximum daily dose 800 mg). In this study, 312 patients were randomized (2:1) to receive either 50 mg SUTENT or placebo, orally once daily on Schedule 4/2 until disease progression or withdrawal from the study for another reason (207 patients received SUTENT and 105 patients received placebo). The primary efficacy endpoint of the study was TTP, defined as the time from randomization to first documentation of objective tumour progression.

The median TTP on SUTENT was 28.9 weeks (95% CI = 21.3-34.1 weeks) and was statistically significantly longer than the TTP of 5.1 weeks (95% CI = 4.4-10.1 weeks, $p<0.001$) on placebo. The difference in overall survival was statistically in favour of SUTENT [hazard ratio: 0.491 (95% C.I. 0.290- 0.831)]; the risk of death was 2 times higher in patients in the placebo arm compared to the SUTENT arm. The percentages of deaths were 14% for SUTENT *vs* 25% for placebo. Median overall survival had not yet been reached in either treatment arm at the time of analysis.

Treatment-naïve metastatic renal cell carcinoma (MRCC)

A phase 3 randomized, multicentre, international, study evaluating the efficacy and safety of sunitinib compared with interferon IFN-α in treatment-naïve MRCC patients was conducted. Seven hundred and fifty patients were randomized 1:1 to the treatment arms; they received treatment with either sunitinib in repeated 6-week cycles, consisting of 4 weeks of 50 mg daily oral administration followed by 2 weeks of rest (Schedule 4/2), or IFN-α, administered as a subcutaneous injection of 3 million units (MU) the first week, 6 MU the second week, and 9 MU the third week and thereafter on 3 non-consecutive days each week.

The primary efficacy endpoint was progression free survival (PFS). In this study the median PFS for the sunitinib-treated group was 47.3 weeks compared with 22.0 weeks for the IFN-α-treated group; the hazard ratio was 0.415 (95% CI: 0.320-0.539, p-value <0.001).

Cytokine-Refractory metastatic renal cell carcinoma (MRCC).

A phase 2 study of SUTENT was conducted in patients who were refractory to prior cytokine therapy with interleukin-2 or IFN-α. Sixty three patients received a starting dose of 50 mg of sunitinib orally, once daily for 4 consecutive weeks followed by a 2-week rest period, to comprise a complete cycle of 6 weeks (schedule 4/2). The primary efficacy endpoint was objective response rate (ORR) based on Response Evaluation Criteria in Solid Tumours (RECIST).

In this study the objective response rate was 36.5% (95% C.I. 24.7% - 49.6%) and the median time to progression (TTP) was 37.7 weeks (95% C.I. 24.0 - 46.4 weeks).

A confirmatory, open-label, single-arm, multi-centre study evaluating the efficacy and safety of SUTENT was conducted in patients with MRCC who were refractory to prior cytokine therapy. One hundred and six patients received at least one 50 mg dose of SUTENT on schedule 4/2.

The primary efficacy endpoint of this study was Objective Response Rate (ORR). Secondary endpoints included TTP, duration of response (DR) and overall survival (OS).

In this study the ORR was 35.8% (95% C.I. 26.8% – 47.5 %) The median DR and OS had not yet been reached.

5.2 Pharmacokinetic properties

The pharmacokinetics of sunitinib has been evaluated in 135 healthy volunteers and 266 patients with solid tumours. The pharmacokinetics were similar in all solid tumours populations tested and in healthy volunteers.

In the dosing ranges of 25 to 100 mg, the area under the plasma concentration-time curve (AUC) and Cmax increase proportionally with dose. With repeated daily administration, sunitinib accumulates 3- to 4-fold and its primary active metabolite accumulates 7- to 10-fold. Steady-state concentrations of sunitinib and its primary active metabolite are achieved within 10 to 14 days. By day 14, combined plasma concentrations of sunitinib and is active metabolite are 62.9 - 101 ng/ml which are target concentrations predicted from preclinical data to inhibit receptor phosphorylation in vitro and result in tumour stasis/growth reduction in vivo. The primary active metabolite comprises 23 to 37% of the total exposure. No significant changes in the pharmacokinetics of sunitinib or the primary, active metabolite are observed with repeated daily administration or with repeated cycles in the dosing schedules tested.

Absorption

After oral administration of sunitinib, maximum concentrations (C_{max}) are generally observed from 6 to 12 hours (T_{max}) post-administration.

Food has no effect on the bioavailability of sunitinib.

Distribution

In vitro binding of sunitinib and its primary active metabolite to human plasma protein in *in vitro* assays was 95% and 90%, respectively, with no apparent concentration dependence. The apparent volume of distribution (V_d) for sunitinib was large - 2230 l -, indicating distribution into the tissues.

Metabolic interactions

The calculated *invitro* Ki values for all cytochrome (CYP) isoforms tested (CYP1A2, CYP2A6, CYP2B6, CYP2C8, CYP2C9, CYP2C19, CYP2D6, CYP2E1, CYP3A4/5 and CYP4A9/11) indicated that sunitinib and its primary active metabolite are unlikely to induce metabolism, to any clinically relevant extent, of other active substances that may be metabolized by these enzymes.

Biotransformation

Sunitinib is metabolized primarily by CYP3A4, the cytochrome P450 isoform, which produces its primary active metabolite, desethyl sunitinib, which is then further metabolized by the same isoenzyme.

Co-administration of SUTENT with potent CYP3A4 inducers or inhibitors should be avoided because the plasma levels of sunitinib may be altered (see sections 4.4 and 4.5)

Elimination

Excretion is primarily via faeces (61%) with renal elimination of unchanged active substance and metabolites accounting for 16% of the administered dose. Sunitinib and its primary active metabolite were the major compounds identified in plasma, urine and faeces, representing 91.5%, 86.4% and 73.8% of radioactivity in pooled samples, respectively. Minor metabolites were identified in urine and faeces, but generally were not found in plasma. Total oral clearance (CL/F) was 34-62 l/hr. Following oral administration in healthy volunteers, the elimination half-lives of sunitinib and its primary active desethyl metabolite are approximately 40 – 60 hours, and 80 – 110 hours, respectively.

Special Populations

Hepatic impairment: Sunitinib and its primary metabolite are mainly metabolized by the liver. Systemic exposures after a single dose of sunitinib were similar in subjects with mild or moderate (Child-Pugh Class A and B) hepatic impairment compared to subjects with normal hepatic function. SUTENT was not studied in subjects with severe (Child-Pugh class C) hepatic impairment.

Studies in cancer patients have excluded patients with ALT or AST$>2.5 \times$ ULN (Upper Limit of Normal) or, if due to liver metastasis $> 5.0 \times$ ULN.

Renal impairment: No clinical studies have been completed in patients with impaired renal function

Studies excluded patients with serum creatinine $> 2.0 \times$ ULN. Population pharmacokinetic analyses indicated that sunitinib apparent clearance (CL/F) was not affected by creatinine clearance within the range evaluated (42-347 ml/min).

Weight, performance status: Population pharmacokinetic analyses of demographic data indicate that no starting dose adjustments are necessary for weight or Eastern Cooperative Oncology Group (ECOG) performance status.

Gender: Available data indicate that females could have about 30% lower apparent clearance (CL/F) of sunitinib than males: this difference, however, does not necessitate starting dose adjustments.

5.3 Preclinical safety data

In rat and monkey repeated-dose toxicity studies up to 9-months duration, the primary target organ effects were identified in the gastrointestinal tract (emesis and diarrhoea in monkeys), adrenal gland (cortical congestion and/or haemorrhage in rats and monkeys, with necrosis followed by fibrosis in rats), haemolymphopoietic system (bone morrow hypocelularity, and lymphoid depletion of thymus, spleen, and lymph node), exocrine pancreas (acinar cell degranulation with single cell necrosis), salivary gland (acinar hypertrophy), bone joint (growth plate thickening), uterus (atrophy) and ovaries (decreased follicular development). All findings occurred at clinically relevant sunitinib plasma exposure levels. Additional effects, observed in other studies included QTc interval prolongation, LVEF reduction, pituitary hypertrophy, and testicular tubular atrophy, increased mesangial cells in kidney, haemorrhage in gastro-intestinal tract and oral mucosa, and hypertrophy of anterior pituitary cells. Changes in the uterus (endometrial atrophy) and bone growth plate (physeal thickening or dysplasia of cartilage) are thought to be related to the pharmacological action of sunitinib. Most of these findings were reversible after 2 to 6 weeks without treatment.

Genotoxicity

The genotoxic potential of sunitinib was assessed *in vitro* and *in vivo*. Sunitinib was not mutagenic in bacteria using metabolic activation provided by rat liver. Sunitinib did not induce structural chromosome aberrations in human peripheral blood lymphocyte cells *in vitro*. Polyploidy (numerical chromosome aberrations) was observed in human peripheral blood lymphocytes *in vitro*, both in the presence and absence of metabolic activation. Sunitinib was not clastogenic in rat bone marrow *in vivo*. The major active metabolite was not evaluated for genotoxic potential.

Carcinogenicity

Carcinogenicity studies with sunitinib have not been performed.

Reproductive and Developmental toxicity.

No effects on male or female fertility were observed in reproductive toxicity studies. However, in repeated-dose toxicity studies performed in rats and monkeys, effects on female fertility were observed in the form of follicular atresia, degeneration of corpora lutea, endometrial changes in the uterus and decreased uterine and ovarian weights at clinically relevant systemic exposure levels. Effects on male fertility in rat were observed in the form of tubular atrophy in the testes, reduction of spermatozoa in epididimes and colloid depletion in prostate and seminal vesicles at plasma exposure levels 18-fold higher than is observed in clinic.

In rats, embryo-foetal mortality was evident as significant reductions in the number of live foetuses, increased numbers of resorptions increased postimplantation loss, and total litter loss in 8 of 28 pregnant females at plasma exposure levels 5.5-fold higher than observed in clinic. In rabbits, reductions in gravid uterine weights and number of live foetuses were due to increases in the number of resorptions, increases in post-implantation loss and complete litter loss in 4 of 6 pregnant females at plasma exposure levels 3-fold higher than observed in clinic.

Sunitinib treatment in rats during organogenesis resulted in developmental effects at ⩾5 mg/kg/day consisting of increased incidence of foetal skeletal malformations, predominantly characterized as retarded ossification of thoracic/lumbar vertebrae and occurred at plasma exposure levels 6-fold higher than is observed in clinic. In rabbits, developmental effects consisted of increased incidence of cleft lip at plasma exposure levels approximately equal to that observed in clinic, and cleft lip and cleft palate at plasma exposure levels 2.7-fold higher than observed in clinic.

6. PHARMACEUTICAL PARTICULARS

6.1 List of excipients

SUTENT® 12.5 mg, 25 mg, 37.5 mg, 50 mg hard capsules
Capsule content
Mannitol (E421)
Croscarmellose Sodium
Povidone (K-25)
Magnesium Stearate
SUTENT® 12.5 mg, 25 mg hard capsules
Orange Capsule Shell
Gelatin
Red Iron Oxide (E172)
Titanium dioxide (E171)
SUTENT® 25 mg, 50 mg hard capsules
Caramel Capsule Shell
Gelatin
Titanium dioxide (E171)
Yellow Iron Oxide (E172)
Red Iron Oxide (E172)
Black Iron Oxide (E172)
SUTENT® 37.5 mg hard capsules
Yellow Capsule Shell
Gelatin
Titanium dioxide (E171)
Yellow Iron Oxide (E172)
SUTENT® 12.5 mg, 25 mg, 50 mg hard capsules
Printing ink.
Shellac
Propylene glycol
Sodium hydroxide
Povidone
Titanium dioxide (E171)
SUTENT® 37.5 mg hard capsules
Printing ink.
Shellac
Propylene glycol
Potassium hydroxide
Black Iron Oxide (E172)

6.2 Incompatibilities

Not applicable.

6.3 Shelf life

2 years.

6.4 Special precautions for storage

This medicinal product does not require any special storage conditions.

6.5 Nature and contents of container

High-density polyethylene (HDPE) bottle with a polypropylene closure containing 30 hard capsules.

Aclar/PVC transparent blister with aluminium foil coated with heat seal lacquer containing 28 (4×7) hard capsules

Not all pack sizes may be marketed.

6.6 Special precautions for disposal and other handling

No special requirements.

7. MARKETING AUTHORISATION HOLDER
Pfizer Ltd
Ramsgate Road
Sandwich, Kent CT13 9NJ
United Kingdom

8. MARKETING AUTHORISATION NUMBER(S)
EU/1/06/347/001-008

9. DATE OF FIRST AUTHORISATION/RENEWAL OF THE AUTHORISATION
Date of first authorisation: July 19, 2006
Due-date for next renewal: July 19, 2011

10. DATE OF REVISION OF THE TEXT
20 August 2009

LEGAL CATEGORY
POM
ST 9_0

Symbicort Turbohaler 100/6, Inhalation powder.

(AstraZeneca UK Limited)

1. NAME OF THE MEDICINAL PRODUCT
Symbicort® Turbohaler® 100 micrograms/6 micrograms/inhalation, inhalation powder.

2. QUALITATIVE AND QUANTITATIVE COMPOSITION
Each delivered dose (the dose that leaves the mouthpiece) contains: budesonide 80 micrograms/inhalation and formoterol fumarate dihydrate 4.5 micrograms/inhalation.

Symbicort Turbohaler® 100 micrograms/6 micrograms/inhalation delivers the same amount of budesonide and formoterol as the corresponding Turbohaler monoproducts, i.e. budesonide 100 micrograms/inhalation (metered dose) and formoterol 6 micrograms/inhalation (metered dose) alternatively labelled as 4.5 micrograms/inhalation (delivered dose).

Excipient: lactose monohydrate 810 micrograms per dose.
For a full list of excipients, see section 6.1.

3. PHARMACEUTICAL FORM
Inhalation powder.
White powder.

4. CLINICAL PARTICULARS
4.1 Therapeutic indications
Symbicort Turbohaler is indicated in the regular treatment of asthma where use of a combination (inhaled corticosteroid and long-acting beta$_2$-agonist) is appropriate:

- patients not adequately controlled with inhaled corticosteroids and "as needed" inhaled short-acting beta$_2$-agonists.

or

- patients already adequately controlled on both inhaled corticosteroids and long-acting beta$_2$-agonists.

Note: Symbicort Turbohaler (100 micrograms/6 micrograms/inhalation) is not appropriate in patients with severe asthma.

4.2 Posology and method of administration
Symbicort Turbohaler is not intended for the initial management of asthma. The dosage of the components of Symbicort is individual and should be adjusted to the severity of the disease. This should be considered not only when treatment with combination products is initiated but also when the maintenance dose is adjusted. If an individual patient should require a combination of doses other than those available in the combination inhaler, appropriate doses of beta$_2$-agonists and/or corticosteroids by individual inhalers should be prescribed.

The dose should be titrated to the lowest dose at which effective control of symptoms is maintained. Patients should be regularly reassessed by their prescriber/health care provider so that the dosage of Symbicort remains optimal. When long-term control of symptoms is maintained with the lowest recommended dosage, then the next step could include a test of inhaled corticosteroid alone.

For Symbicort there are two treatment approaches:

A. Symbicort maintenance therapy: Symbicort is taken as regular maintenance treatment with a separate rapid-acting bronchodilator as rescue.

B. Symbicort maintenance and reliever therapy: Symbicort is taken as regular maintenance treatment and as needed in response to symptoms.

A. Symbicort maintenance therapy

Patients should be advised to have their separate rapid-acting bronchodilator available for rescue use at all times.

Recommended doses:

Adults (18 years and older): 1-2 inhalations twice daily. Some patients may require up to a maximum of 4 inhalations twice daily.

Adolescents (12 - 17 years): 1-2 inhalations twice daily.

Children (6 years and older): 2 inhalations twice daily.

In usual practice when control of symptoms is achieved with the twice daily regimen, titration to the lowest effective dose could include Symbicort given once daily, when in the opinion of the prescriber, a long-acting bronchodilator would be required to maintain control.

Increasing use of a separate rapid acting bronchodilator indicates a worsening of the underlying condition and warrants a reassessment of the asthma therapy.

Children under 6 years: Symbicort is not recommended for children under 6 years of age.

B. Symbicort maintenance and reliever therapy

Patients take a daily maintenance dose of Symbicort and in addition take Symbicort as needed in response to symptoms. Patients should be advised to always have Symbicort available for rescue use.

Symbicort maintenance and reliever therapy should especially be considered for patients with:

- inadequate asthma control and in frequent need of reliever medication
- asthma exacerbations in the past requiring medical intervention

Close monitoring for dose-related adverse effects is needed in patients who frequently take high numbers of Symbicort as-needed inhalations.

Recommended doses:

Adults (18 years and older): The recommended maintenance dose is 2 inhalations per day, given either as one inhalation in the morning and evening or as 2 inhalations in either the morning or evening. Patients should take 1 additional inhalation as needed in response to symptoms. If symptoms persist after a few minutes, an additional inhalation should be taken. Not more than 6 inhalations should be taken on any single occasion.

A total daily dose of more than 8 inhalations is not normally needed; however, a total daily dose of up to 12 inhalations could be used for a limited period. Patients using more than 8 inhalations daily should be strongly recommended to seek medical advice. They should be reassessed and their maintenance therapy should be reconsidered.

Children and adolescents under 18 years: Symbicort maintenance and reliever therapy is not recommended for children and adolescents.

General information

Special patient groups:

There are no special dosing requirements for elderly patients. There are no data available for use of Symbicort in patients with hepatic or renal impairment. As budesonide and formoterol are primarily eliminated via hepatic metabolism, an increased exposure can be expected in patients with severe liver cirrhosis.

Instructions for correct use of Turbohaler:

Turbohaler is inspiratory flow-driven, which means that when the patient inhales through the mouthpiece, the substance will follow the inspired air into the airways.

Note: It is important to instruct the patient

- to carefully read the instructions for use in the patient information leaflet which is packed together with each inhaler
- to breathe in forcefully and deeply through the mouthpiece to ensure that an optimal dose is delivered to the lungs
- never to breathe out through the mouthpiece
- to replace the cover of the Symbicort Turbohaler after use
- to rinse their mouth out with water after inhaling the maintenance dose to minimise the risk of oropharyngeal thrush. If oropharyngeal thrush occurs, patients should also rinse their mouth with water after the as-needed inhalations.

The patient may not taste or feel any medication when using Symbicort Turbohaler due to the small amount of drug dispensed.

4.3 Contraindications
Hypersensitivity (allergy) to budesonide, formoterol or lactose (which contains small amounts of milk proteins).

4.4 Special warnings and precautions for use
It is recommended that the dose is tapered when the treatment is discontinued and should not be stopped abruptly.

If patients find the treatment ineffective, or exceed the highest recommended dose of Symbicort, medical attention must be sought (see section 4.2 Posology and method of administration). Sudden and progressive deterioration in control of asthma is potentially life threatening and the patient should undergo urgent medical assessment. In this situation consideration should be given to the need for increased therapy with corticosteroids e.g. a course of oral corticosteroids, or antibiotic treatment if an infection is present.

Patients should be advised to have their rescue inhaler available at all times, either Symbicort (for patients using Symbicort as maintenance and reliever therapy) or a separate rapid-acting bronchodilator (for patients using Symbicort as maintenance therapy only).

Patients should be reminded to take their Symbicort maintenance dose as prescribed, even when asymptomatic. The prophylactic use of Symbicort, e.g. before exercise, has not been studied. The reliever inhalations of Symbicort should be taken in response to asthma symptoms but are not intended for regular prophylactic use, e.g. before exercise. For such use, a separate rapid-acting bronchodilator should be considered.

Once asthma symptoms are controlled, consideration may be given to gradually reducing the dose of Symbicort. Regular review of patients as treatment is stepped down is important. The lowest effective dose of Symbicort should be used (see section 4.2 Posology and method of administration).

Patients should not be initiated on Symbicort during an exacerbation, or if they have significantly worsening or acutely deteriorating asthma.

Serious asthma-related adverse events and exacerbations may occur during treatment with Symbicort. Patients should be asked to continue treatment but to seek medical advice if asthma symptoms remain uncontrolled or worsen after initiation with Symbicort.

As with other inhalation therapy, paradoxical bronchospasm may occur, with an immediate increase in wheezing after dosing. Symbicort should then be discontinued; treatment should be re-assessed and alternative therapy instituted if necessary.

Systemic effects may occur with any inhaled corticosteroid, particularly at high doses prescribed for long periods. These effects are much less likely to occur with inhalation treatment than with oral corticosteroids. Possible systemic effects include adrenal suppression, growth retardation in children and adolescents, decrease in bone mineral density, cataract and glaucoma.

It is recommended that the height of children receiving prolonged treatment with inhaled corticosteroids is regularly monitored. If growth is slowed, therapy should be re-evaluated with the aim of reducing the dose of inhaled corticosteroid. The benefits of the corticosteroid therapy and the possible risks of growth suppression must be carefully weighed. In addition consideration should be given to referring the patient to a paediatric respiratory specialist.

Limited data from long-term studies suggest that most children and adolescents treated with inhaled budesonide will ultimately achieve their adult target height. However, an initial small but transient reduction in growth (approximately 1 cm) has been observed. This generally occurs within the first year of treatment.

Long-term studies with inhaled budesonide in children at mean daily doses of 400 micrograms (metered dose) or in adults at daily doses of 800 micrograms (metered dose) have not shown any significant effects on bone mineral density. No information regarding the effect of Symbicort at higher doses is available.

If there is any reason to suppose that adrenal function is impaired from previous systemic steroid therapy, care should be taken when transferring patients to Symbicort therapy.

The benefits of inhaled budesonide therapy would normally minimise the need for oral steroids, but patients transferring from oral steroids may remain at risk of impaired adrenal reserve for a considerable time. Patients who have required high dose emergency corticosteroid therapy in the past or prolonged treatment with high doses of inhaled corticosteroids, may also be at risk. Additional systemic corticosteriod cover should be considered during periods of stress or elective surgery.

To minimise the risk of oropharyngeal candida infection, the patient should be instructed to rinse their mouth out with water after inhaling the maintenance dose. If oropharyngeal thrush occurs, patients should also rinse their mouth with water after the as-needed inhalations.

Concomitant treatment with itraconazole, ritonavir or other potent CYP3A4 inhibitors should be avoided (see section 4.5 Interaction with other medicinal products and other forms of interaction). If this is not possible the time interval between administration of the interacting drugs should be as long as possible. In patients using potent CYP3A4 inhibitors, Symbicort maintenance and reliever therapy is not recommended.

Symbicort should be administered with caution in patients with thyrotoxicosis, phaeochromocytoma, diabetes mellitus, untreated hypokalaemia, hypertrophic obstructive cardiomyopathy, idiopathic subvalvular aortic stenosis, severe hypertension, aneurysm or other severe cardiovascular disorders, such as ischaemic heart disease, tachyarrhythmias or severe heart failure.

Caution should be observed when treating patients with prolongation of the QTc-interval. Formoterol itself may induce prolongation of the QTc-interval.

The need for, and dose of inhaled corticosteroids should be re-evaluated in patients with active or quiescent pulmonary tuberculosis, fungal and viral infections in the airways.

Potentially serious hypokalaemia may result from high doses of beta$_2$-agonists. Concomitant treatment of beta$_2$-agonists with drugs which can induce hypokalaemia or potentiate a hypokalaemic effect, e.g. xanthine-derivatives, steroids and diuretics, may add to a possible hypokalaemic effect of the beta$_2$-agonist. Particular caution is recommended in unstable asthma with variable use of rescue bronchodilators, in acute severe asthma as the associated risk may be augmented by hypoxia and in other conditions when the likelihood for hypokalaemia adverse effects is increased. It is recommended that serum potassium levels are monitored during these circumstances.

As for all beta$_2$-agonists, additional blood glucose controls should be considered in diabetic patients.

Symbicort Turbohaler contains lactose (<1 mg/inhalation). This amount does not normally cause problems in lactose intolerant people. The excipient lactose contains small amounts of milk proteins, which may cause allergic reactions.

4.5 Interaction with other medicinal products and other forms of interaction

Pharmacokinetic interactions

The metabolic conversion of budesonide is impeded by substances metabolized by CYP P450 3A4 (e.g. itraconazole, ritonavir). The concomitant administration of these potent inhibitors of CYP P450 3A4 may increase plasma levels of budesonide. The concomitant use of these drugs should be avoided unless the benefit outweighs the increased risk of systemic side-effects. In patients using potent CYP3A4 inhibitors, Symbicort maintenance and reliever therapy is not recommended.

Pharmacodynamic interactions

Beta-adrenergic blockers can weaken or inhibit the effect of formoterol. Symbicort should therefore not be given together with beta-adrenergic blockers (including eye drops) unless there are compelling reasons.

Concomitant treatment with quinidine, disopyramide, procainamide, phenothiazines, antihistamines (terfenadine), monoamine oxidase inhibitors and tricyclic antidepressants can prolong the QTc-interval and increase the risk of ventricular arrhythmias.

In addition L-Dopa, L-thyroxine, oxytocin and alcohol can impair cardiac tolerance towards beta$_2$-sympathomimetics.

Concomitant treatment with monoamine oxidase inhibitors including agents with similar properties such as furazolidone and procarbazine may precipitate hypertensive reactions.

There is an elevated risk of arrhythmias in patients receiving concomitant anaesthesia with halogenated hydrocarbons.

Concomitant use of other beta-adrenergic drugs can have a potentially additive effect.

Hypokalaemia may increase the disposition towards arrhythmias in patients who are treated with digitalis glycosides.

Budesonide and formoterol have not been observed to interact with any other drugs used in the treatment of asthma.

4.6 Pregnancy and lactation

For Symbicort or the concomitant treatment with formoterol and budesonide, no clinical data on exposed pregnancies are available. Data from an embryo-fetal development study in the rat, showed no evidence of any additional effect from the combination.

There are no adequate data from use of formoterol in pregnant women. In animal studies formoterol has caused adverse effects in reproduction studies at very high systemic exposure levels (see section 5.3 Preclinical safety data).

Data on approximately 2000 exposed pregnancies indicate no increased teratogenic risk associated with the use of inhaled budesonide. In animal studies glucocorticosteroids have been shown to induce malformations (see section 5.3 Preclinical safety data). This is not likely to be relevant for humans given recommended doses.

Animal studies have also identified an involvement of excess prenatal glucocorticoids in increased risks for intrauterine growth retardation, adult cardiovascular disease and permanent changes in glucocorticoid receptor density, neurotransmitter turnover and behaviour at exposures below the teratogenic dose range.

During pregnancy, Symbicort should only be used when the benefits outweigh the potential risks. The lowest effective dose of budesonide needed to maintain adequate asthma control should be used.

Budesonide is excreted in breast milk. However, at therapeutic doses no effects on the suckling child are anticipated. It is not known whether formoterol passes into human breast milk. In rats, small amounts of formoterol have been detected in maternal milk. Administration of Symbicort to women who are breastfeeding should only be considered if the expected benefit to the mother is greater than any possible risk to the child.

4.7 Effects on ability to drive and use machines

Symbicort has no or negligible influence on the ability to drive and use machines.

4.8 Undesirable effects

Since Symbicort Turbohaler contains both budesonide and formoterol, the same pattern of undesirable effects as reported for these substances may occur. No increased incidence of adverse reactions has been seen following concurrent administration of the two compounds. The most common drug related adverse reactions are pharmacologically predictable side-effects of beta$_2$-agonist therapy, such as tremor and palpitations. These tend to be mild and usually disappear within a few days of treatment.

Adverse reactions, which have been associated with budesonide or formoterol, are given below, listed by system organ class and frequency. Frequency are defined as: very common (≥1/10), common (≥1/100 and <1/10), uncommon (≥1/1000 and <1/100), rare (≥1/10 000 and <1/1000) and very rare (<1/10 000).

Cardiac disorders	Common	Palpitations
	Uncommon	Tachycardia
	Rare	Cardiac arrhythmias, e.g. atrial fibrillation, supraventricular tachycardia, extrasystoles
	Very rare	Angina pectoris
Endocrine disorders	Very rare	Signs or symptoms of systemic glucocorticosteroid effects e.g. adrenal suppression, growth retardation, decrease in bone mineral density, cataract and glaucoma
Gastrointestinal disorders	Uncommon	Nausea
Immune system disorders	Rare	Immediate and delayed hypersensitivity reactions, e.g. exanthema, urticaria, pruritus, dermatitis, angioedema and anaphylactic reaction
Infections and infestations	Common	Candida infections in the oropharynx
Metabolic and nutrition disorders	Rare	Hypokalemia
	Very rare	Hyperglycemia
Musculoskeletal, connective tissue and bone disorders	Uncommon	Muscle cramps
Nervous system disorders	Common	Headache, tremor
	Uncommon	Dizziness
	Very rare	Taste disturbances
Psychiatric disorders	Uncommon	Agitation, restlessness, nervousness, sleep disturbances
	Very rare	Depression, behavioural disturbances (mainly in children)
Respiratory, thoracic and mediastinal disorders	Common	Mild irritation in the throat, coughing, hoarseness
	Rare	Bronchospasm
Skin and subcutaneous tissue disorders	Uncommon	Bruises
Vascular disorders	Very rare	Variations in blood pressure

As with other inhalation therapy, paradoxical bronchospasm may occur in very rare cases (see section 4.4 Special warning and precautions for use).

Treatment with beta$_2$-agonists may result in an increase in blood levels of insulin, free fatty acids, glycerol and ketone bodies.

4.9 Overdose

An overdose of formoterol would likely lead to effects that are typical for beta$_2$-adrenergic agonists: tremor, headache, palpitations. Symptoms reported from isolated cases are tachycardia, hyperglycaemia, hypokalaemia, prolonged QTc-interval, arrhythmia, nausea and vomiting. Supportive and symptomatic treatment may be indicated. A dose of 90 micrograms administered during three hours in patients with acute bronchial obstruction raised no safety concerns.

Acute overdosage with budesonide, even in excessive doses, is not expected to be a clinical problem. When used chronically in excessive doses, systemic glucocorticosteroid effects, such as hypercorticism and adrenal suppression, may appear.

If Symbicort therapy has to be withdrawn due to overdose of the formoterol component of the drug, provision of appropriate inhaled corticosteroid therapy must be considered.

5. PHARMACOLOGICAL PROPERTIES

5.1 Pharmacodynamic properties

Pharmacotherapeutic group: Adrenergics and other drugs for obstructive airway diseases.

ATC-code: R03AK07

Mechanisms of action and pharmacodynamic effects

Symbicort contains formoterol and budesonide, which have different modes of action and show additive effects in terms of reduction of asthma exacerbations. The specific properties of budesonide and formoterol allow the combination to be used both as maintenance and reliever therapy, or as maintenance treatment of asthma.

Budesonide

Budesonide is a glucocorticosteroid which when inhaled has a dose-dependent anti-inflammatory action in the airways, resulting in reduced symptoms and fewer asthma exacerbations. Inhaled budesonide has less severe adverse effects than systemic corticosteroids. The exact mechanism responsible for the anti-inflammatory effect of glucocorticosteroids is unknown.

Formoterol

Formoterol is a selective beta$_2$-adrenergic agonist that when inhaled results in rapid and long-acting relaxation of bronchial smooth muscle in patients with reversible airways obstruction. The bronchodilating effect is dose-dependent, with an onset of effect within 1-3 minutes. The duration of effect is at least 12 hours after a single dose.

Symbicort Turbohaler

Clinical efficacy for Symbicort maintenance therapy

Clinical studies in adults have shown that the addition of formoterol to budesonide improved asthma symptoms and lung function, and reduced exacerbations.

In two 12-week studies the effect on lung function of Symbicort was equal to that of the free combination of budesonide and formoterol, and exceeded that of budesonide alone. All treatment arms used a short-acting beta$_2$-agonist as needed. There was no sign of attenuation of the anti-asthmatic effect over time.

In a 12-week paediatric study, 85 children aged 6-11 years were treated with a maintenance dose of Symbicort Turbohaler (2 inhalations of 80 micrograms/4.5 micrograms/inhalation twice daily), and a short-acting beta$_2$-agonist as needed. Lung function was improved, and the treatment was well tolerated compared to the corresponding dose of budesonide Turbohaler.

Clinical efficacy for Symbicort maintenance and reliever therapy

A total of 12076 asthma patients were included in 5 double-blind efficacy and safety studies (4447 were randomised to Symbicort maintenance and reliever therapy) for 6 or 12 months. Patients were required to be symptomatic despite use of inhaled glucocorticosteroids.

Symbicort maintenance and reliever therapy provided statistically significant and clinically meaningful reductions in severe exacerbations for all comparisons in all 5 studies. This included a comparison with Symbicort at a higher maintenance dose with terbutaline as reliever (study 735) and Symbicort at the same maintenance dose with either formoterol or terbutaline as reliever (study 734) (Table 1). In Study 735, lung function, symptom control, and reliever use were similar in all treatment groups. In Study 734, symptoms and reliever use were reduced and lung function improved, compared with both comparator treatments. In the 5 studies combined, patients receiving Symbicort maintenance and reliever therapy used, on average, no reliever inhalations on 57% of treatment days. There was no sign of development of tolerance over time.

Table 1 Overview of severe exacerbations in clinical studies

(see Table 1 on next page)

In 2 other studies with patients seeking medical attention due to acute asthma symptoms, Symbicort provided rapid and effective relief of bronchoconstriction similar to salbutamol and formoterol.

5.2 Pharmacokinetic properties

Absorption

Symbicort Turbohaler and the corresponding monoproducts have been shown to be bioequivalent with regard to systemic exposure of budesonide and formoterol, respectively. In spite of this, a small increase in cortisol suppression was seen after administration of Symbicort Turbohaler compared to the monoproducts. The difference is considered not to have an impact on clinical safety.

There was no evidence of pharmacokinetic interactions between budesonide and formoterol.

Pharmacokinetic parameters for the respective substances were comparable after the administration of budesonide and formoterol as monoproducts or as Symbicort Turbohaler. For budesonide, AUC was slightly higher, rate of absorption more rapid and maximal plasma concentration higher after administration of the fixed combination. For formoterol, maximal plasma concentration was similar after administration of the fixed combination. Inhaled budesonide is rapidly absorbed and the maximum plasma concentration is reached within 30 minutes after inhalation. In studies, mean lung deposition of budesonide after inhalation via Turbohaler ranged from 32% to 44% of the

Table 2 Overview of severe exacerbations in clinical studies

Study No. Duration	Treatment groups	N	Severe exacerbations[a]	
			Events	Events/ patient-year
Study 735 6 months	**Symbicort 160/4.5 μg bd + as needed**	**1103**	**125**	**0.23[b]**
	Symbicort 320/9 μg bd + terbutaline 0.4 mg as needed	1099	173	0.32
	Salmeterol/fluticasone 2 × 25/125 μg bd + terbutaline 0.4 mg as needed	1119	208	0.38
Study 734 12 months	**Symbicort 160/4.5 μg bd + as needed**	**1107**	**194**	**0.19[b]**
	Symbicort 160/4.5 μg bd + formoterol 4.5 μg as needed	1137	296	0.29
	Symbicort 160/4.5 μg bd + terbutaline 0.4 mg as needed	1138	377	0.37

[a] Hospitalisation/emergency room treatment or treatment with oral steroids

[b] Reduction in exacerbation rate is statistically significant (P value <0.01) for both comparisons

delivered dose. The systemic bioavailability is approximately 49% of the delivered dose. In children 6-16 years the lung deposition fall in the same range as in adults for the same given dose, the resulting plasma concentrations were not determined.

Inhaled formoterol is rapidly absorbed and the maximum plasma concentration is reached within 10 minutes after inhalation. In studies the mean lung deposition of formoterol after inhalation via Turbohaler ranged from 28% to 49% of the delivered dose. The systemic bioavailability is about 61% of the delivered dose.

Distribution and metabolism

Plasma protein binding is approximately 50% for formoterol and 90% for budesonide. Volume of distribution is about 4 L/kg for formoterol and 3 L/kg for budesonide. Formoterol is inactivated via conjugation reactions (active O-demethylated and deformylated metabolites are formed, but they are seen mainly as inactivated conjugates). Budesonide undergoes an extensive degree (approximately 90%) of biotransformation on first passage through the liver to metabolites of low glucocorticosteroid activity. The glucocorticosteroid activity of the major metabolites, 6-beta-hydroxy-budesonide and 16-alfa-hydroxy-prednisolone, is less than 1% of that of budesonide. There are no indications of any metabolic interactions or any displacement reactions between formoterol and budesonide.

Elimination

The major part of a dose of formoterol is transformed by liver metabolism followed by renal elimination. After inhalation, 8% to 13% of the delivered dose of formoterol is excreted unmetabolised in the urine. Formoterol has a high systemic clearance (approximately 1.4 L/min) and the terminal elimination half-life averages 17 hours.

Budesonide is eliminated via metabolism mainly catalysed by the enzyme CYP3A4. The metabolites of budesonide are eliminated in urine as such or in conjugated form. Only negligible amounts of unchanged budesonide have been detected in the urine. Budesonide has a high systemic clearance (approximately 1.2 L/min) and the plasma elimination half-life after i.v. dosing averages 4 hours.

The pharmacokinetics of formoterol in children have not been studied. The pharmacokinetics of budesonide and formoterol in patients with renal failure are unknown. The exposure of budesonide and formoterol may be increased in patients with liver disease.

5.3 Preclinical safety data

The toxicity observed in animal studies with budesonide and formoterol, given in combination or separately, were effects associated with exaggerated pharmacological activity.

In animal reproduction studies, corticosteroids such as budesonide have been shown to induce malformations (cleft palate, skeletal malformations). However, these animal experimental results do not seem to be relevant in humans at the recommended doses. Animal reproduction studies with formoterol have shown a somewhat reduced fertility in male rats at high systemic exposure and implantation losses as well as decreased early postnatal survival and birth weight at considerably higher systemic exposures than those reached during clinical use. However, these animal experimental results do not seem to be relevant in humans.

6. PHARMACEUTICAL PARTICULARS

6.1 List of excipients

Lactose monohydrate (which contains milk proteins).

6.2 Incompatibilities

Not applicable.

6.3 Shelf life

2 years.

6.4 Special precautions for storage

Do not store above 30°C. Keep the container tightly closed.

6.5 Nature and contents of container

Symbicort Turbohaler is an inspiratory flow-driven, multi-dose powder inhaler. The inhaler is white with a red turning grip. The inhaler is made of different plastic materials (PP, PC, HDPE, LDPE, LLDPE, PBT). Each inhaler contains 60 doses or 120 doses. In each secondary package there are 1, 2, 3, 10 or 18 inhalers. Not all pack-sizes may be marketed.

6.6 Special precautions for disposal and other handling

No special requirements.

7. MARKETING AUTHORISATION HOLDER

AstraZeneca UK Limited,

600 Capability Green,

Luton, LU1 3LU, UK.

8. MARKETING AUTHORISATION NUMBER(S)

PL 17901/0091

9. DATE OF FIRST AUTHORISATION/RENEWAL OF THE AUTHORISATION

Date of first authorisation: 15th May 2001

Date of last renewal: 25th August 2005

10. DATE OF REVISION OF THE TEXT

10th December 2008

Symbicort Turbohaler 200/6 Inhalation powder

(AstraZeneca UK Limited)

1. NAME OF THE MEDICINAL PRODUCT

Symbicort® Turbohaler® 200 micrograms/6 micrograms/ inhalation, inhalation powder.

2. QUALITATIVE AND QUANTITATIVE COMPOSITION

Each delivered dose (the dose that leaves the mouthpiece) contains: budesonide 160 micrograms/inhalation and formoterol fumarate dihydrate 4.5 micrograms/inhalation.

Symbicort Turbohaler 200 micrograms/6 micrograms/ inhalation delivers the same amount of budesonide and formoterol as the corresponding Turbohaler monoproducts, i.e. budesonide 200 micrograms/inhalation (metered dose) and formoterol 6 micrograms/inhalation (metered dose) alternatively labelled as 4.5 micrograms/ inhalation (delivered dose).

Excipient: lactose monohydrate 730 micrograms per dose.

For a full list of excipients, see section 6.1.

3. PHARMACEUTICAL FORM

Inhalation powder.

White powder.

4. CLINICAL PARTICULARS

4.1 Therapeutic indications

Asthma

Symbicort Turbohaler is indicated in the regular treatment of asthma where use of a combination (inhaled corticosteroid and long-acting beta$_2$-agonist) is appropriate:

- patients not adequately controlled with inhaled corticosteroids and "as needed" inhaled short-acting beta$_2$-agonists.

or

- patients already adequately controlled on both inhaled corticosteroids and long-acting beta$_2$-agonists.

COPD

Symptomatic treatment of patients with severe COPD (FEV$_1$ < 50% predicted normal) and a history of repeated exacerbations, who have significant symptoms despite regular therapy with long-acting bronchodilators.

4.2 Posology and method of administration

Asthma

Symbicort Turbohaler is not intended for the initial management of asthma. The dosage of the components of Symbicort is individual and should be adjusted to the severity of the disease. This should be considered not only when treatment with combination products is initiated but also when the maintenance dose is adjusted. If an individual patient should require a combination of doses other than those available in the combination inhaler, appropriate doses of beta$_2$-agonists and/or corticosteroids by individual inhalers should be prescribed.

The dose should be titrated to the lowest dose at which effective control of symptoms is maintained. Patients should be regularly reassessed by their prescriber/health care provider so that the dosage of Symbicort remains optimal. When long-term control of symptoms is maintained with the lowest recommended dosage, then the next step could include a test of inhaled corticosteroid alone.

For Symbicort there are two treatment approaches:

A. Symbicort maintenance therapy: Symbicort is taken as regular maintenance treatment with a separate rapid-acting bronchodilator as rescue.

B. Symbicort maintenance and reliever therapy: Symbicort is taken as regular maintenance treatment and as needed in response to symptoms.

A. Symbicort maintenance therapy

Patients should be advised to have their separate rapid-acting bronchodilator available for rescue use at all times.

Recommended doses:

Adults (18 years and older): 1-2 inhalation twice daily. Some patients may require up to a maximum of 4 inhalations twice daily.

Adolescents (12 – 17 years): 1-2 inhalations twice daily.

In usual practice when control of symptoms is achieved with the twice daily regimen, titration to the lowest effective dose could include Symbicort given once daily, when in the opinion of the prescriber, a long-acting bronchodilator would be required to maintain control.

Increasing use of a separate rapid-acting bronchodilator indicates a worsening of the underlying condition and warrants a reassessment of the asthma therapy.

Children (6 years and older): A lower strength is available for children 6-11 years.

B. Symbicort maintenance and reliever therapy

Patients take a daily maintenance dose of Symbicort and in addition take Symbicort as needed in response to symptoms. Patients should be advised to always have Symbicort available for rescue use.

Symbicort maintenance and reliever therapy should especially be considered for patients with:

- inadequate asthma control and in frequent need of reliever medication
- asthma exacerbations in the past requiring medical intervention

Close monitoring for dose-related adverse effects is needed in patients who frequently take high numbers of Symbicort as-needed inhalations.

Recommended doses:

Adults (18 years and older): The recommended maintenance dose is 2 inhalations per day, given either as one inhalation in the morning and evening or as 2 inhalations in either the morning or evening. For some patients a maintenance dose of 2 inhalations twice daily may be appropriate. Patients should take 1 additional inhalation as needed in response to symptoms. If symptoms persist after a few minutes, an additional inhalation should be taken. Not more than 6 inhalations should be taken on any single occasion.

A total daily dose of more than 8 inhalations is not normally needed; however, a total daily dose of up to 12 inhalations could be used for a limited period. Patients using more than 8 inhalations daily should be strongly recommended to seek medical advice. They should be reassessed and their maintenance therapy should be reconsidered.

Children and adolescents under 18 years: Symbicort maintenance and reliever therapy is not recommended for children and adolescents.

COPD

Recommended doses:

Adults: 2 inhalations twice daily

General information

Special patient groups:

There are no special dosing requirements for elderly patients. There are no data available for use of Symbicort in patients with hepatic or renal impairment. As budesonide and formoterol are primarily eliminated via hepatic metabolism, an increased exposure can be expected in patients with severe liver cirrhosis.

Instructions for correct use of Turbohaler:

Turbohaler is inspiratory flow-driven, which means that when the patient inhales through the mouthpiece, the substance will follow the inspired air into the airways.

Note: It is important to instruct the patient

- to carefully read the instructions for use in the patient information leaflet which is packed together with each inhaler
- to breathe in forcefully and deeply through the mouthpiece to ensure that an optimal dose is delivered to the lungs
- never to breathe out through the mouthpiece
- to replace the cover of the Symbicort Turbohaler after use
- to rinse their mouth out with water after inhaling the maintenance dose to minimise the risk of oropharyngeal thrush. If oropharyngeal thrush occurs, patients should also rinse their mouth with water after the as-needed inhalations.

The patient may not taste or feel any medication when using Symbicort Turbohaler due to the small amount of drug dispensed.

4.3 Contraindications

Hypersensitivity (allergy) to budesonide, formoterol or lactose (which contains small amounts of milk proteins).

4.4 Special warnings and precautions for use

It is recommended that the dose is tapered when the treatment is discontinued and should not be stopped abruptly.

If patients find the treatment ineffective, or exceed the highest recommended dose of Symbicort, medical attention must be sought (see section 4.2 Posology and method of administration). Sudden and progressive deterioration in control of asthma or COPD is potentially life threatening and the patient should undergo urgent medical assessment. In this situation, consideration should be given to the need for increased therapy with corticosteroids e.g. a course of oral corticosteroids, or antibiotic treatment if an infection is present.

Patients should be advised to have their rescue inhaler available at all times, either Symbicort (for asthma patients using Symbicort as maintenance and reliever therapy) or a separate rapid-acting bronchodilator (for all patients using Symbicort as maintenance therapy only).

Patients should be reminded to take their Symbicort maintenance dose as prescribed, even when asymptomatic. The prophylactic use of Symbicort, e.g. before exercise, has not been studied. The reliever inhalations of Symbicort should be taken in response to symptoms but are not intended for regular prophylactic use, e.g. before exercise. For such use, a separate rapid-acting bronchodilator should be considered.

Once asthma symptoms are controlled, consideration may be given to gradually reducing the dose of Symbicort. Regular review of patients as treatment is stepped down is important. The lowest effective dose of Symbicort should be used (see section 4.2 Posology and method of administration).

Patients should not be initiated on Symbicort during an exacerbation, or if they have significantly worsening or acutely deteriorating asthma.

Serious asthma-related adverse events and exacerbations may occur during treatment with Symbicort. Patients should be asked to continue treatment but to seek medical advice if asthma symptoms remain uncontrolled or worsen after initiation with Symbicort. As with other inhalation therapy, paradoxical bronchospasm may occur, with an immediate increase in wheezing after dosing. Symbicort should then be discontinued; treatment should be re-assessed and alternative therapy instituted if necessary.

Systemic effects may occur with any inhaled corticosteroid, particularly at high doses prescribed for long periods. These effects are much less likely to occur with inhalation treatment than with oral corticosteroids. Possible systemic effects include adrenal suppression, growth retardation in children and adolescents, decrease in bone mineral density, cataract and glaucoma.

It is recommended that the height of children receiving prolonged treatment with inhaled corticosteroids is regularly monitored. If growth is slowed, therapy should be re-evaluated with the aim of reducing the dose of inhaled corticosteroid. The benefits of the corticosteroid therapy and the possible risks of growth suppression must be carefully weighed. In addition consideration should be given to referring the patient to a paediatric respiratory specialist.

Limited data from long-term studies suggest that most children and adolescents treated with inhaled budesonide will ultimately achieve their adult target height. However, an initial small but transient reduction in growth (approximately 1 cm) has been observed. This generally occurs within the first year of treatment.

Potential effects on bone density should be considered particularly in patients on high doses for prolonged periods that have co-existing risk factors for osteoporosis. Long-term studies with inhaled budesonide in children at mean daily doses of 400 micrograms (metered dose) or in adults at daily doses of 800 micrograms (metered dose) have not shown any significant effects on bone mineral density. No information regarding the effect of Symbicort at higher doses is available.

If there is any reason to suppose that adrenal function is impaired from previous systemic steroid therapy, care should be taken when transferring patients to Symbicort therapy.

The benefits of inhaled budesonide therapy would normally minimise the need for oral steroids, but patients transferring from oral steroids may remain at risk of impaired adrenal reserve for a considerable time. Patients who have required high dose emergency corticosteroid therapy in the past or prolonged treatment with high doses of inhaled corticosteroids, may also be at risk. Additional systemic corticosteriod cover should be considered during periods of stress or elective surgery.

To minimise the risk of oropharyngeal candida infection, the patient should be instructed to rinse their mouth out with water after inhaling the maintenance dose. If oropharyngeal thrush occurs, patients should also rinse their mouth with water after the as-needed inhalations.

Concomitant treatment with itraconazole, ritonavir or other potent CYP3A4 inhibitors should be avoided (see section 4.5 Interaction with other medicinal products and other forms of interaction). If this is not possible the time interval between administration of the interacting drugs should be as long as possible. In patients using potent CYP3A4 inhibitors, Symbicort maintenance and reliever therapy is not recommended.

Symbicort should be administered with caution in patients with thyrotoxicosis, phaeochromocytoma, diabetes mellitus, untreated hypokalaemia, hypertrophic obstructive cardiomyopathy, idiopathic subvalvular aortic stenosis, severe hypertension, aneurysm or other severe cardiovascular disorders, such as ischaemic heart disease, tachyarrhythmias or severe heart failure.

Caution should be observed when treating patients with prolongation of the QTc-interval. Formoterol itself may induce prolongation of the QTc-interval.

The need for, and dose of inhaled corticosteroids should be re-evaluated in patients with active or quiescent pulmonary tuberculosis, fungal and viral infections in the airways.

Potentially serious hypokalaemia may result from high doses of beta$_2$-agonists. Concomitant treatment of beta$_2$-agonists with drugs which can induce hypokalaemia or potentiate a hypokalaemic effect, e.g. xanthine-derivatives, steroids and diuretics, may add to a possible hypokalaemic effect of the beta$_2$-agonist. Particular caution is recommended in unstable asthma with variable use of rescue bronchodilators, in acute severe asthma as the associated risk may be augmented by hypoxia and in other conditions when the likelihood for hypokalaemia adverse effects is increased. It is recommended that serum potassium levels are monitored during these circumstances.

As for all beta$_2$-agonists, additional blood glucose controls should be considered in diabetic patients.

Symbicort Turbohaler contains lactose (< 1 mg/inhalation). This amount does not normally cause problems in lactose intolerant people. The excipient lactose contains small amounts of milk proteins, which may cause allergic reactions.

4.5 Interaction with other medicinal products and other forms of interaction

Pharmacokinetic interactions

The metabolic conversion of budesonide is impeded by substances metabolized by CYP P450 3A4 (e.g. itraconazole, ritonavir). The concomitant administration of these potent inhibitors of CYP P450 3A4 may increase plasma levels of budesonide. The concomitant use of these drugs should be avoided unless the benefit outweighs the increased risk of systemic side-effects. In patients using potent CYP3A4 inhibitors, Symbicort maintenance and reliever therapy is not recommended.

Pharmacodynamic interactions

Beta-adrenergic blockers can weaken or inhibit the effect of formoterol. Symbicort should therefore not be given together with beta-adrenergic blockers (including eye drops) unless there are compelling reasons.

Concomitant treatment with quinidine, disopyramide, procainamide, phenothiazines, antihistamines (terfenadine), monoamine oxidase inhibitors and tricyclic antidepressants can prolong the QTc-interval and increase the risk of ventricular arrhythmias.

In addition L-Dopa, L-thyroxine, oxytocin and alcohol can impair cardiac tolerance towards beta$_2$-sympathomimetics.

Concomitant treatment with monoamine oxidase inhibitors, including agents with similar properties such as furazolidone and procarbazine, may precipitate hypertensive reactions.

There is an elevated risk of arrhythmias in patients receiving concomitant anaesthesia with halogenated hydrocarbons.

Concomitant use of other beta-adrenergic drugs can have a potentially additive effect.

Hypokalaemia may increase the disposition towards arrhythmias in patients who are treated with digitalis glycosides.

Budesonide and formoterol have not been observed to interact with any other drugs used in the treatment of asthma.

4.6 Pregnancy and lactation

For Symbicort or the concomitant treatment with formoterol and budesonide, no clinical data on exposed pregnancies are available. Data from an embryo-fetal development study in the rat, showed no evidence of any additional effect from the combination.

There are no adequate data from use of formoterol in pregnant women. In animal studies formoterol has caused adverse effects in reproduction studies at very high systemic exposure levels (see section 5.3 Preclinical safety data).

Data on approximately 2000 exposed pregnancies indicate no increased teratogenic risk associated with the use of inhaled budesonide. In animal studies glucocorticosteroids have been shown to induce malformations (see section 5.3 Preclinical safety data). This is not likely to be relevant for humans given recommended doses.

Animal studies have also identified an involvement of excess prenatal glucocorticoids in increased risks for intrauterine growth retardation, adult cardiovascular disease and permanent changes in glucocorticoid receptor density, neurotransmitter turnover and behaviour at exposures below the teratogenic dose range.

During pregnancy, Symbicort should only be used when the benefits outweigh the potential risks. The lowest effective dose of budesonide needed to maintain adequate asthma control should be used.

Budesonide is excreted in breast milk. However, at therapeutic doses no effects on the suckling child are anticipated. It is not known whether formoterol passes into human breast milk. In rats, small amounts of formoterol have been detected in maternal milk. Administration of Symbicort to women who are breastfeeding should only be considered if the expected benefit to the mother is greater than any possible risk to the child.

4.7 Effects on ability to drive and use machines

Symbicort has no or negligible influence on the ability to drive and use machines.

4.8 Undesirable effects

Since Symbicort contains both budesonide and formoterol, the same pattern of undesirable effects as reported for these substances may occur. No increased incidence of adverse reactions has been seen following concurrent administration of the two compounds. The most common drug related adverse reactions are pharmacologically predictable side-effects of beta$_2$-agonist therapy, such as tremor and palpitations. These tend to be mild and usually disappear within a few days of treatment. In a 3-year clinical trial with budesonide in COPD, skin bruises and pneumonia occurred at a frequency of 10% and 6%, respectively, compared with 4% and 3% in the placebo group ($p < 0.001$ and $p < 0.01$, respectively).

Adverse reactions, which have been associated with budesonide or formoterol, are given below, listed by system organ class and frequency. Frequency are defined as: very common (≥ 1/10), common (≥ 1/100 and < 1/10), uncommon (≥ 1/1000 and < 1/100), rare (≥ 1/10 000 and < 1/1000) and very rare (< 1/10 000).

Cardiac disorders	Common	Palpitations
	Uncommon	Tachycardia
	Rare	Cardiac arrhythmias, e.g. atrial fibrillation, supraventricular tachycardia, extrasystoles
	Very rare	Angina pectoris
Endocrine disorders	Very rare	Signs or symptoms of systemic glucocorticosteroid effects e.g. adrenal suppression, growth retardation, decrease in bone mineral density, cataract and glaucoma
Gastrointestinal disorders	Uncommon	Nausea
Immune system disorders	Rare	Immediate and delayed hypersensitivity reactions, e.g. exanthema, urticaria, pruritus, dermatitis, angioedema and anaphylactic reaction
Infections and infestations	Common	Candida infections in the oropharynx
Metabolic and nutrition disorders	Rare	Hypokalemia
	Very rare	Hyperglycemia
Musculoskeletal, connective tissue and bone disorders	Uncommon	Muscle cramps
Nervous system disorders	Common	Headache, tremor
	Uncommon	Dizziness
	Very rare	Taste disturbances

Psychiatric disorders	Uncommon	Agitation, restlessness, nervousness, sleep disturbances
	Very rare	Depression, behavioural disturbances (mainly in children)
Respiratory, thoracic and mediastinal disorders	Common	Mild irritation in the throat, coughing, hoarseness
	Rare	Bronchospasm
Skin and subcutaneous tissue disorders	Uncommon	Bruises
Vascular disorders	Very rare	Variations in blood pressure

As with other inhalation therapy, paradoxical bronchospasm may occur in very rare cases (see section 4.4 Special warning and precautions for use).

Treatment with beta$_2$-agonists may result in an increase in blood levels of insulin, free fatty acids, glycerol and ketone bodies.

4.9 Overdose

An overdose of formoterol would likely lead to effects that are typical for beta$_2$-adrenergic agonists: tremor, headache, palpitations. Symptoms reported from isolated cases are tachycardia, hyperglycaemia, hypokalaemia, prolonged QTc-interval, arrhythmia, nausea and vomiting. Supportive and symptomatic treatment may be indicated. A dose of 90 micrograms administered during three hours in patients with acute bronchial obstruction raised no safety concerns.

Acute overdosage with budesonide, even in excessive doses, is not expected to be a clinical problem. When used chronically in excessive doses, systemic glucocorticosteroid effects, such as hypercorticism and adrenal suppression, may appear.

If Symbicort therapy has to be withdrawn due to overdose of the formoterol component of the drug, provision of appropriate inhaled corticosteroid therapy must be considered.

5. PHARMACOLOGICAL PROPERTIES

5.1 Pharmacodynamic properties

Pharmacotherapeutic group: Adrenergics and other drugs for obstructive airway diseases.

ATC-code: R03AK07

Mechanisms of action and pharmacodynamic effects

Symbicort contains formoterol and budesonide, which have different modes of action and show additive effects in terms of reduction of asthma exacerbations. The specific properties of budesonide and formoterol allow the combination to be used both as maintenance and reliever therapy, or as maintenance treatment of asthma.

Budesonide

Budesonide is a glucocorticosteroid which when inhaled has a dose-dependent anti-inflammatory action in the airways, resulting in reduced symptoms and fewer asthma exacerbations. Inhaled budesonide has less severe adverse effects than systemic corticosteroids. The exact mechanism responsible for the anti-inflammatory effect of glucocorticosteroids is unknown.

Formoterol

Formoterol is a selective beta$_2$-adrenergic agonist that when inhaled results in rapid and long-acting relaxation of bronchial smooth muscle in patients with reversible airways obstruction. The bronchodilating effect is dose-dependent, with an onset of effect within 1-3 minutes. The duration of effect is at least 12 hours after a single dose.

Symbicort Turbohaler

Asthma

Clinical efficacy for Symbicort maintenance therapy

Clinical studies in adults have shown that the addition of formoterol to budesonide improved asthma symptoms and lung function, and reduced exacerbations.

In two 12-week studies the effect on lung function of Symbicort was equal to that of the free combination of budesonide and formoterol, and exceeded that of budesonide alone. All treatment arms used a short-acting beta$_2$-agonist as needed. There was no sign of attenuation of the anti-asthmatic effect over time.

In a 12-week paediatric study 85 children aged 6-11 years were treated with a maintenance dose of Symbicort Turbohaler (2 inhalations of 80 micrograms/4.5 micrograms/inhalation twice daily), and a short-acting beta$_2$-agonist as needed. Lung function was improved and the treatment was well tolerated compared to the corresponding dose of budesonide Turbohaler.

Clinical efficacy for Symbicort maintenance and reliever therapy

A total of 12076 asthma patients were included in 5 double-blind clinical studies (4447 were randomised to Symbicort maintenance and reliever therapy) for 6 or 12 months. Patients were required to be symptomatic despite use of inhaled glucocorticosteroids.

Symbicort maintenance and reliever therapy provided statistically significant and clinically meaningful reductions in severe exacerbations for all comparisons in all 5 studies. This included a comparison with Symbicort at a higher maintenance dose with terbutaline as reliever (study 735) and Symbicort at the same maintenance dose with either formoterol or terbutaline as reliever (study 734) (Table 2). In Study 735, lung function, symptom control, and reliever use were similar in all treatment groups. In Study 734, symptoms and reliever use were reduced and lung function improved, compared with both comparator treatments. In the 5 studies combined, patients receiving Symbicort maintenance and reliever therapy used, on average, no reliever inhalations on 57% of treatment days. There was no sign of development of tolerance over time.

Table 2 Overview of severe exacerbations in clinical studies

(see Table 2 below)

In 2 other studies with patients seeking medical attention due to acute asthma symptoms, Symbicort provided rapid and effective relief of bronchoconstriction similar to salbutamol and formoterol.

COPD

In two 12-month studies, the effects on lung function and the rate of exacerbation (defined as courses of oral steroids and/or course of antibiotics and/or hospitalisations) in patients with severe COPD was evaluated. Median FEV$_1$ at inclusion in the trials was 36% of predicted normal. The mean number of exacerbations per year (as defined above) was significantly reduced with Symbicort as compared with treatment with formoterol alone or placebo (mean rate 1.4 compared with 1.8-1.9 in the placebo/formoterol group). The mean number of days on oral corticosteroids/patient during the 12 months was slightly reduced in the Symbicort group (7-8 days/patient/year compared with 11-12 and 9-12 days in the placebo and formoterol groups, respectively). For changes in lung-function parameters, such as FEV$_1$, Symbicort was not superior to treatment with formoterol alone.

5.2 Pharmacokinetic properties

Absorption

Symbicort Turbohaler and the corresponding monoproducts have been shown to be bioequivalent with regard to systemic exposure of budesonide and formoterol, respectively. In spite of this, a small increase in cortisol suppression was seen after administration of Symbicort Turbohaler compared to the monoproducts. The difference is considered not to have an impact on clinical safety.

There was no evidence of pharmacokinetic interactions between budesonide and formoterol.

Pharmacokinetic parameters for the respective substances were comparable after the administration of budesonide and formoterol as monoproducts or as Symbicort Turbohaler. For budesonide, AUC was slightly higher, rate of absorption more rapid and maximal plasma concentration higher after administration of the fixed combination. For formoterol, maximal plasma concentration was similar after administration of the fixed combination. Inhaled budesonide is rapidly absorbed and the maximum plasma concentration is reached within 30 minutes after inhalation. In studies, mean lung deposition of budesonide after inhalation via Turbohaler ranged from 32% to 44% of the delivered dose. The systemic bioavailability is approximately 49% of the delivered dose.

Inhaled formoterol is rapidly absorbed and the maximum plasma concentration is reached within 10 minutes after inhalation. In studies the mean lung deposition of formoterol after inhalation via Turbohaler ranged from 28% to 49% of the delivered dose. The systemic bioavailability is about 61% of the delivered dose.

Distribution and metabolism

Plasma protein binding is approximately 50% for formoterol and 90% for budesonide. Volume of distribution is about 4 L/kg for formoterol and 3 L/kg for budesonide. Formoterol is inactivated via conjugation reactions (active O-demethylated and deformylated metabolites are formed, but they are seen mainly as inactivated conjugates). Budesonide undergoes an extensive degree (approximately 90%) of biotransformation on first passage through the liver to metabolites of low glucocorticosteroid activity. The glucocorticosteroid activity of the major metabolites, 6-beta-hydroxy-budesonide and 16-alfa-hydroxy-prednisolone, is less than 1% of that of budesonide. There are no indications of any metabolic interactions or any displacement reactions between formoterol and budesonide.

Elimination

The major part of a dose of formoterol is transformed by liver metabolism followed by renal elimination. After inhalation, 8% to 13% of the delivered dose of formoterol is excreted unmetabolised in the urine. Formoterol has a high systemic clearance (approximately 1.4 L/min) and the terminal elimination half-life averages 17 hours.

Budesonide is eliminated via metabolism mainly catalysed by the enzyme CYP3A4. The metabolites of budesonide are eliminated in urine as such or in conjugated form. Only negligible amounts of unchanged budesonide have been detected in the urine. Budesonide has a high systemic clearance (approximately 1.2 L/min) and the plasma elimination half-life after i.v. dosing averages 4 hours.

The pharmacokinetics of budesonide or formoterol in patients with renal failure is unknown. The exposure of budesonide and formoterol may be increased in patients with liver disease.

5.3 Preclinical safety data

The toxicity observed in animal studies with budesonide and formoterol, given in combination or separately, were effects associated with exaggerated pharmacological activity.

In animal reproduction studies, corticosteroids such as budesonide have been shown to induce malformations (cleft palate, skeletal malformations). However, these animal experimental results do not seem to be relevant in humans at the recommended doses. Animal reproduction studies with formoterol have shown a somewhat reduced fertility in male rats at high systemic exposure and implantation losses as well as decreased early postnatal survival and birth weight at considerably higher systemic exposures than those reached during clinical use. However, these animal experimental results do not seem to be relevant in humans.

6. PHARMACEUTICAL PARTICULARS

6.1 List of excipients

Lactose monohydrate (which contains milk proteins).

6.2 Incompatibilities

Not applicable.

6.3 Shelf life

2 years.

6.4 Special precautions for storage

Do not store above 30°C. Keep the container tightly closed.

6.5 Nature and contents of container

Symbicort Turbohaler is an inspiratory flow-driven, multi-dose powder inhaler. The inhaler is white with a red turning grip. The inhaler is made of different plastic materials (PP, PC, HDPE, LDPE, LLDPE, PBT). Each inhaler contains 60 doses or 120 doses. In each secondary package there are 1, 2, 3, 10 or 18 inhalers. Not all pack-sizes may be marketed.

6.6 Special precautions for disposal and other handling

No special requirements.

7. MARKETING AUTHORISATION HOLDER

AstraZeneca UK Limited,
600 Capability Green,
Luton, LU1 3LU, UK.

Table 2 Overview of severe exacerbations in clinical studies

Study No. Duration	Treatment groups	N	Severe exacerbations[a]	
			Events	Events/ patient-year
Study 735 6 months	**Symbicort 160/4.5 μg bd + as needed**	**1103**	**125**	**0.23[b]**
	Symbicort 320/9 μg bd + terbutaline 0.4 mg as needed	1099	173	0.32
	Salmeterol/fluticasone 2 × 25/125 μg bd + terbutaline 0.4 mg as needed	1119	208	0.38
Study 734 12 months	**Symbicort 160/4.5 μg bd + as needed**	**1107**	**194**	**0.19[b]**
	Symbicort 160/4.5 μg bd + formoterol 4.5 μg as needed	1137	296	0.29
	Symbicort 160/4.5 μg bd + terbutaline 0.4 mg as needed	1138	377	0.37

[a] Hospitalisation/emergency room treatment or treatment with oral steroids

[b] Reduction in exacerbation rate is statistically significant (P value <0.01) for both comparisons

8. MARKETING AUTHORISATION NUMBER(S)
PL 17901/0092

9. DATE OF FIRST AUTHORISATION/RENEWAL OF THE AUTHORISATION
Date of first authorisation: 15 May 2001

Date of last renewal: 25 August 2005

10. DATE OF REVISION OF THE TEXT
10th December 2008

Symbicort Turbohaler 400/12, Inhalation powder.

(AstraZeneca UK Limited)

1. NAME OF THE MEDICINAL PRODUCT
Symbicort® Turbohaler® 400 micrograms/12 micrograms, inhalation powder.

2. QUALITATIVE AND QUANTITATIVE COMPOSITION
Each delivered dose (the dose that leaves the mouthpiece) contains: budesonide 320 micrograms/inhalation and formoterol fumarate dihydrate 9 micrograms/inhalation.

Symbicort Turbohaler 400 micrograms/12 micrograms/ inhalation delivers the same amount of budesonide and formoterol as the corresponding Turbohaler monoproducts, i.e. budesonide 400 micrograms/inhalation (metered dose) and formoterol 12 micrograms/inhalation (metered dose) alternatively labelled as 9 micrograms/ inhalation (delivered dose).

Excipient: lactose monohydrate 491 micrograms per dose.

For a full list of excipients, see section 6.1.

3. PHARMACEUTICAL FORM
Inhalation powder.

White powder.

4. CLINICAL PARTICULARS
4.1 Therapeutic indications
Asthma
Symbicort Turbohaler is indicated in the regular treatment of asthma where use of a combination (inhaled corticosteroid and long-acting beta$_2$-agonist) is appropriate:

- patients not adequately controlled with inhaled corticosteroids and "as needed" inhaled short-acting beta$_2$-agonists.

or

- patients already adequately controlled on both inhaled corticosteroids and long-acting beta$_2$-agonists.

COPD
Symptomatic treatment of patients with severe COPD (FEV_1 < 50% predicted normal) and a history of repeated exacerbations, who have significant symptoms despite regular therapy with long-acting bronchodilators.

4.2 Posology and method of administration
Asthma
Symbicort Turbohaler is not intended for the initial management of asthma. The dosage of the components of Symbicort is individual and should be adjusted to the severity of the disease. This should be considered not only when treatment with combination products is initiated but also when the maintenance dose is adjusted. If an individual patient should require a combination of doses other than those available in the combination inhaler, appropriate doses of beta$_2$-agonists and/or corticosteroids by individual inhalers should be prescribed.

Recommended doses:

Adults (18 years and older): 1 inhalation twice daily. Some patients may require up to a maximum of 2 inhalations twice daily.

Adolescents (12-17 years): 1 inhalation twice daily.

Patients should be regularly reassessed by their prescriber/health care provider, so that the dosage of Symbicort remains optimal. The dose should be titrated to the lowest dose at which effective control of symptoms is maintained. When long-term control of symptoms is maintained with the lowest recommended dosage, then the next step could include a test of inhaled corticosteroid alone.

In usual practice when control of symptoms is achieved with the twice daily regimen, titration to the lowest effective dose could include Symbicort given once daily, when in the opinion of the prescriber, a long-acting bronchodilator would be required to maintain control.

Children (6 years and older): A lower strength is available for children 6-11 years.

Symbicort 400/12 should be used as Symbicort maintenance therapy only. Lower strengths are available for the Symbicort maintenance and reliever therapy regimen.

COPD
Recommended doses:

Adults: 1 inhalation twice daily.

General information
Special patient groups: There are no special dosing requirements for elderly patients. There are no data available for use of Symbicort in patients with hepatic or renal impairment. As budesonide and formoterol are primarily eliminated via hepatic metabolism, an increased exposure can be expected in patients with severe liver cirrhosis.

Instructions for correct use of Turbohaler:
Turbohaler is inspiratory flow-driven, which means that when the patient inhales through the mouthpiece, the substance will follow the inspired air into the airways.

Note: It is important to instruct the patient

- to carefully read the instructions for use in the patient information leaflet which is packed together with each inhaler
- to breathe in forcefully and deeply through the mouthpiece to ensure that an optimal dose is delivered to the lungs
- never to breathe out through the mouthpiece
- to replace the cover of the Symbicort Turbohaler after use
- to rinse their mouth out with water after inhaling the maintenance dose to minimise the risk of oropharyngeal thrush.

The patient may not taste or feel any medication when using Symbicort Turbohaler due to the small amount of drug dispensed.

4.3 Contraindications
Hypersensitivity (allergy) to budesonide, formoterol or lactose (which contains small amounts of milk protein).

4.4 Special warnings and precautions for use
It is recommended that the dose is tapered when the treatment is discontinued and should not be stopped abruptly.

If patients find the treatment ineffective, or exceed the highest recommended dose of Symbicort, medical attention must be sought. Increasing use of rescue bronchodilators indicates a worsening of the underlying condition and warrants a reassessment of the asthma therapy. Sudden and progressive deterioration in control of asthma or COPD is potentially life threatening and the patient should undergo urgent medical assessment. In this situation consideration should be given to the need for increased therapy with corticosteroids e.g. a course of oral corticosteroids, or antibiotic treatment if an infection is present.

Patients should be advised to have their rescue inhaler available at all times.

Patients should be reminded to take their Symbicort maintenance dose as prescribed, even when asymptomatic.

Once asthma symptoms are controlled, consideration may be given to gradually reducing the dose of Symbicort. Regular review of patients as treatment is stepped down is important. The lowest effective dose of Symbicort should be used (see section 4.2 Posology and method of administration).

Patients should not be initiated on Symbicort during an exacerbation, or if they have significantly worsening or acutely deteriorating asthma.

Serious asthma-related adverse events and exacerbations may occur during treatment with Symbicort. Patients should be asked to continue treatment but to seek medical advice if asthma symptoms remain uncontrolled or worsen after initiation with Symbicort.

As with other inhalation therapy, paradoxical bronchospasm may occur, with an immediate increase in wheezing after dosing. Symbicort should then be discontinued; treatment should be re-assessed and alternative therapy instituted if necessary.

Systemic effects may occur with any inhaled corticosteroid, particularly at high doses prescribed for long periods. These effects are much less likely to occur with inhalation treatment than with oral corticosteroids. Possible systemic effects include adrenal suppression, growth retardation in children and adolescents, decrease in bone mineral density, cataract and glaucoma.

It is recommended that the height of children receiving prolonged treatment with inhaled corticosteroids is regularly monitored. If growth is slowed, therapy should be re-evaluated with the aim of reducing the dose of inhaled corticosteroid. The benefits of the corticosteroid therapy and the possible risks of growth suppression must be carefully weighed. In addition consideration should be given to referring the patient to a paediatric respiratory specialist.

Limited data from long-term studies suggest that most children and adolescents treated with inhaled budesonide will ultimately achieve their adult target height. However, an initial small but transient reduction in growth (approximately 1 cm) has been observed. This generally occurs within the first year of treatment.

Potential effects on bone should be considered, particularly in patients on high doses for prolonged periods that have co-existing risk factors for osteoporosis. Long-term studies with inhaled budesonide in children at mean daily doses of 400 micrograms (metered dose) or in adults at daily doses of 800 micrograms (metered dose) have not shown any significant effects on bone mineral density. No information regarding the effect of Symbicort at higher doses is available.

If there is any reason to suppose that adrenal function is impaired from previous systemic steroid therapy, care should be taken when transferring patients to Symbicort therapy.

The benefits of inhaled budesonide therapy would normally minimise the need for oral steroids, but patients transferring from oral steroids may remain at risk of impaired adrenal reserve for a considerable time. Patients who have required high dose emergency corticosteroid therapy in the past or prolonged treatment with high doses of inhaled corticosteroids, may also be at risk. Additional systemic corticosteriod cover should be considered during periods of stress or elective surgery.

To minimise the risk of oropharyngeal candida infection, the patient should be instructed to rinse their mouth out with water after inhaling the maintenance dose.

Concomitant treatment with itraconazole, ritonavir or other potent CYP3A4 inhibitors should be avoided (see section 4.5 Interaction with other medicinal products and other forms of interaction). If this is not possible, the time interval between administration of the interacting drugs should be as long as possible.

Symbicort should be administered with caution in patients with thyrotoxicosis, phaeochromocytoma, diabetes mellitus, untreated hypokalaemia, hypertrophic obstructive cardiomyopathy, idiopathic subvalvular aortic stenosis, severe hypertension, aneurysm or other severe cardiovascular disorders, such as ischaemic heart disease, tachyarrhythmias or severe heart failure.

Caution should be observed when treating patients with prolongation of the QTc-interval. Formoterol itself may induce prolongation of the QTc-interval.

The need for, and dose of inhaled corticosteroids should be re-evaluated in patients with active or quiescent pulmonary tuberculosis, fungal and viral infections in the airways.

Potentially serious hypokalaemia may result from high doses of beta$_2$-agonists. Concomitant treatment of beta$_2$-agonists with drugs which can induce hypokalaemia or potentiate a hypokalaemic effect, e.g. xanthine-derivatives, steroids and diuretics, may add to a possible hypokalaemic effect of the beta$_2$-agonist. Particular caution is recommended in unstable asthma with variable use of rescue bronchodilators, in acute severe asthma as the associated risk may be augmented by hypoxia and in other conditions when the likelihood for hypokalaemia adverse effects is increased. It is recommended that serum potassium levels are monitored during these circumstances.

As for all beta$_2$-agonists, additional blood glucose controls should be considered in diabetic patients.

Symbicort Turbohaler contains lactose (< 1 mg/inhalation). This amount does not normally cause problems in lactose intolerant people. The excipient lactose contains small amounts of milk proteins, which may cause allergic reactions.

4.5 Interaction with other medicinal products and other forms of interaction
Pharmacokinetic interactions
The metabolic conversion of budesonide is impeded by substances metabolized by CYP P450 3A4 (e.g. itraconazole, ritonavir). The concomitant administration of these potent inhibitors of CYP P450 3A4 may increase plasma levels of budesonide. The concomitant use of these drugs should be avoided unless the benefit outweighs the increased risk of systemic side-effects.

Pharmacodynamic interactions
Beta-adrenergic blockers can weaken or inhibit the effect of formoterol. Symbicort should therefore not be given together with beta-adrenergic blockers (including eye drops) unless there are compelling reasons.

Concomitant treatment with quinidine, disopyramide, procainamide, phenothiazines, antihistamines (terfenadine), monoamine oxidase inhibitors and tricyclic antidepressants can prolong the QTc-interval and increase the risk of ventricular arrhythmias.

In addition L-Dopa, L-thyroxine, oxytocin and alcohol can impair cardiac tolerance towards beta$_2$-sympathomimetics.

Concomitant treatment with monoamine oxidase inhibitors, including agents with similar properties such as furazolidone and procarbazine, may precipitate hypertensive reactions.

There is an elevated risk of arrhythmias in patients receiving concomitant anaesthesia with halogenated hydrocarbons.

Concomitant use of other beta-adrenergic drugs can have a potentially additive effect.

Hypokalaemia may increase the disposition towards arrhythmias in patients who are treated with digitalis glycosides.

Budesonide and formoterol have not been observed to interact with any other drugs used in the treatment of asthma.

4.6 Pregnancy and lactation
For Symbicort or the concomitant treatment with formoterol and budesonide, no clinical data on exposed pregnancies are available. Data from an embryo-fetal development study in the rat, showed no evidence of any additional effect from the combination.

There are no adequate data from use of formoterol in pregnant women. In animal studies formoterol has caused adverse effects in reproduction studies at very high systemic exposure levels (see section 5.3 Preclinical safety data).

Data on approximately 2000 exposed pregnancies indicate no increased teratogenic risk associated with the use of inhaled budesonide. In animal studies glucocorticosteroids have been shown to induce malformations (see section 5.3 Preclinical safety data). This is not likely to be relevant for humans given recommended doses.

Animal studies have also identified an involvement of excess prenatal glucocorticoids in increased risks for intrauterine growth retardation, adult cardiovascular disease and permanent changes in glucocorticoid receptor density, neurotransmitter turnover and behaviour at exposures below the teratogenic dose range.

During pregnancy, Symbicort should only be used when the benefits outweigh the potential risks. The lowest effective dose of budesonide needed to maintain adequate asthma control should be used.

Budesonide is excreted in breast milk. However, at therapeutic doses no effects on the suckling child are anticipated. It is not known whether formoterol passes into human breast milk. In rats, small amounts of formoterol have been detected in maternal milk. Administration of Symbicort to women who are breast-feeding should only be considered if the expected benefit to the mother is greater than any possible risk to the child.

4.7 Effects on ability to drive and use machines

Symbicort has no or negligible influence on the ability to drive and use machines.

4.8 Undesirable effects

Since Symbicort contains both budesonide and formoterol, the same pattern of undesirable effects as reported for these substances may occur. No increased incidence of adverse reactions has been seen following concurrent administration of the two compounds. The most common drug related adverse reactions are pharmacologically predictable side-effects of beta$_2$-agonist therapy, such as tremor and palpitations. These tend to be mild and usually disappear within a few days of treatment. In a 3-year clinical trial with budesonide in COPD, skin bruises and pneumonia occurred at a frequency of 10% and 6%, respectively, compared with 4% and 3% in the placebo group ($p < 0.001$ and $p < 0.01$, respectively).

Adverse reactions, which have been associated with budesonide or formoterol, are given below, listed by system organ class and frequency. Frequency are defined as: very common (≥1/10), common (≥1/100 and <1/10), uncommon (≥1/1000 and <1/100), rare (≥1/10 000 and <1/1000) and very rare (<1/10 000).

Cardiac disorders	Common	Palpitations
	Uncommon	Tachycardia
	Rare	Cardiac arrhythmias, e.g. atrial fibrillation, supraventricular tachycardia, extrasystoles
	Very rare	Angina pectoris
Endocrine disorders	Very rare	Signs or symptoms of systemic glucocorticosteroid effects e.g. adrenal suppression, growth retardation, decrease in bone mineral density, cataract and glaucoma
Gastrointestinal disorders	Uncommon	Nausea
Immune system disorders	Rare	Immediate and delayed hypersensitivity reactions, e.g. exanthema, urticaria, pruritus, dermatitis, angioedema and anaphylactic reaction
Infections and infestations	Common	Candida infections in the oropharynx
Metabolic and nutrition disorders	Rare	Hypokalemia
	Very rare	Hyperglycemia
Musculoskeletal, connective tissue and bone disorders	Uncommon	Muscle cramps
Nervous system disorders	Common	Headache, tremor
	Uncommon	Dizziness
	Very rare	Taste disturbances
Psychiatric disorders	Uncommon	Agitation, restlessness, nervousness, sleep disturbances
	Very rare	Depression, behavioural disturbances (mainly in children)
Respiratory, thoracic and mediastinal disorders	Common	Mild irritation in the throat, coughing, hoarseness
	Rare	Bronchospasm
Skin and subcutaneous tissue disorders	Uncommon	Bruises
Vascular disorders	Very rare	Variations in blood pressure

As with other inhalation therapy, paradoxical bronchospasm may occur in very rare cases (see section 4.4 Special warning and precautions for use).

Treatment with beta$_2$-agonists may result in an increase in blood levels of insulin, free fatty acids, glycerol and ketone bodies.

4.9 Overdose

An overdose of formoterol would likely lead to effects that are typical for beta$_2$-adrenergic agonists: tremor, headache, palpitations. Symptoms reported from isolated cases are tachycardia, hyperglycaemia, hypokalaemia, prolonged QTc-interval, arrhythmia, nausea and vomiting. Supportive and symptomatic treatment may be indicated. A dose of 90 micrograms administered during three hours in patients with acute bronchial obstruction raised no safety concerns.

Acute overdosage with budesonide, even in excessive doses, is not expected to be a clinical problem. When used chronically in excessive doses, systemic glucocorticosteroid effects, such as hypercorticism and adrenal suppression, may appear.

If Symbicort therapy has to be withdrawn due to overdose of the formoterol component of the drug, provision of appropriate inhaled corticosteroid therapy must be considered.

5. PHARMACOLOGICAL PROPERTIES

5.1 Pharmacodynamic properties

Pharmacotherapeutic group: Adrenergics and other drugs for obstructive airway diseases.

ATC-code: R03AK07

Mechanisms of action and pharmacodynamic effects

Symbicort contains formoterol and budesonide, which have different modes of action and show additive effects in terms of reduction of asthma exacerbations. The mechanisms of action of the two substances, respectively are discussed below.

Budesonide

Budesonide is a glucocorticosteroid which when inhaled has a dose-dependent anti-inflammatory action in the airways, resulting in reduced symptoms and fewer asthma exacerbations. Inhaled budesonide has less severe adverse effects than systemic corticosteroids. The exact mechanism responsible for the anti-inflammatory effect of glucocorticosteroids is unknown.

Formoterol

Formoterol is a selective beta$_2$-adrenergic agonist that when inhaled results in rapid and long-acting relaxation of bronchial smooth muscle in patients with reversible airways obstruction. The bronchodilating effect is dose-dependent, with an onset of effect within 1-3 minutes. The duration of effect is at least 12 hours after a single dose.

Symbicort Turbohaler

Asthma

Clinical studies in adults have shown that the addition of formoterol to budesonide improved asthma symptoms and lung function, and reduced exacerbations.

In two12-week studies, the effect on lung function of Symbicort was equal to that of the free combination of budesonide and formoterol, and exceeded that of budesonide alone. All treatment arms used a short-acting beta$_2$-agonist as needed. There was no sign of attenuation of the anti-asthmatic effect over time.

In a 12-week paediatric study 85 children aged 6-11 years were treated with a maintenance dose of Symbicort Turbohaler (2 inhalations of 80 micrograms/4.5 micrograms/inhalation twice daily), and a short-acting beta$_2$-agonist as needed. Lung function was improved and the treatment was well tolerated compared to the corresponding dose of budesonide Turbohaler.

COPD

In two 12-month studies, the effect on lung function and the rate of exacerbation (defined as courses of oral steroids and/or course of antibiotics and/or hospitalisations) in patients with severe COPD was evaluated. Median FEV$_1$ at inclusion in the trials was 36% of predicted normal. The mean number of exacerbations per year (as defined above) was significantly reduced with Symbicort as compared with treatment with formoterol alone or placebo (mean rate 1.4 compared with 1.8-1.9 in the placebo/formoterol group). The mean number of days on oral corticosteroids/patient during the 12 months was slightly reduced in the Symbicort group (7-8 days/patient/year compared with 11-12 and 9-12 days in the placebo and formoterol groups, respectively). For changes in lung-function parameters, such as FEV$_1$, Symbicort was not superior to treatment with formoterol alone.

5.2 Pharmacokinetic properties

Absorption

Symbicort Turbohaler and the corresponding monoproducts have been shown to be bioequivalent with regard to systemic exposure of budesonide and formoterol, respectively. In spite of this, a small increase in cortisol suppression was seen after administration of Symbicort Turbohaler compared with the monoproducts. The difference is considered not to have an impact on clinical safety.

There was no evidence of pharmacokinetic interactions between budesonide and formoterol.

Pharmacokinetic parameters for the respective substances were comparable after the administration of budesonide and formoterol as monoproducts or as Symbicort Turbohaler. For budesonide, AUC was slightly higher, rate of absorption more rapid and maximal plasma concentration higher after administration of the fixed combination. For formoterol, maximal plasma concentration was similar after administration of the fixed combination. Inhaled budesonide is rapidly absorbed and the maximum plasma concentration is reached within 30 minutes after inhalation. In studies, mean lung deposition of budesonide after inhalation via Turbohaler ranged from 32% to 44% of the delivered dose. The systemic bioavailability is approximately 49% of the delivered dose.

Inhaled formoterol is rapidly absorbed and the maximum plasma concentration is reached within 10 minutes after inhalation. In studies the mean lung deposition of formoterol after inhalation via Turbohaler ranged from 28% to 49% of the delivered dose. The systemic bioavailability is about 61% of the delivered dose.

Distribution and metabolism

Plasma protein binding is approximately 50% for formoterol and 90% for budesonide. Volume of distribution is about 4 L/kg for formoterol and 3 L/kg for budesonide. Formoterol is inactivated via conjugation reactions (active O-demethylated and deformylated metabolites are formed, but they are seen mainly as inactivated conjugates). Budesonide undergoes an extensive degree (approximately 90%) of biotransformation on first passage through the liver to metabolites of low glucocorticosteroid activity. The glucocorticosteroid activity of the major metabolites, 6-beta-hydroxy-budesonide and 16-alfa-hydroxy-prednisolone, is less than 1% of that of budesonide. There are no indications of any metabolic interactions or any displacement reactions between formoterol and budesonide.

Elimination

The major part of a dose of formoterol is transformed by liver metabolism followed by renal elimination. After inhalation, 8% to 13% of the delivered dose of formoterol is excreted unmetabolised in the urine. Formoterol has a high systemic clearance (approximately 1.4 L/min) and the terminal elimination half-life averages 17 hours.

Budesonide is eliminated via metabolism mainly catalysed by the enzyme CYP3A4. The metabolites of budesonide are eliminated in urine as such or in conjugated form. Only negligible amounts of unchanged budesonide have been detected in the urine. Budesonide has a high systemic clearance (approximately 1.2 L/min) and the plasma elimination half-life after i.v. dosing averages 4 hours.

The pharmacokinetics of budesonide or formoterol in children and patients with renal failure is unknown. The exposure of budesonide and formoterol may be increased in patients with liver disease.

5.3 Preclinical safety data

The toxicity observed in animal studies with budesonide and formoterol, given in combination or separately, were effects associated with exaggerated pharmacological activity.

In animal reproduction studies, corticosteroids such as budesonide have been shown to induce malformations (cleft palate, skeletal malformations). However, these animal experimental results do not seem to be relevant in humans at the recommended doses. Animal reproduction studies with formoterol have shown a somewhat reduced fertility in male rats at high systemic exposure and implantation losses as well as decreased early postnatal survival and birth weight at considerably higher systemic exposures than those reached during clinical use. However, these animal experimental results do not seem to be relevant in humans.

6. PHARMACEUTICAL PARTICULARS

6.1 List of excipients

Lactose monohydrate (which contains milk proteins).

6.2 Incompatibilities

Not applicable.

6.3 Shelf life

2 years.

6.4 Special precautions for storage

Do not store above 30°C. Keep the container tightly closed.

6.5 Nature and contents of container

Symbicort Turbohaler is an inspiratory flow-driven, multi-dose powder inhaler. The inhaler is white with a red turning grip. The inhaler is made of different plastic materials (PP, PC, HDPE, LDPE, LLDPE, PBT). Each inhaler contains

60 doses. In each secondary package there are 1, 2, 3, 10 or 18 inhalers. Not all pack sizes may be marketed.

6.6 Special precautions for disposal and other handling
No special requirements.

7. MARKETING AUTHORISATION HOLDER
AstraZeneca UK Limited
600 Capability Green
Luton
LU1 3LU, UK

8. MARKETING AUTHORISATION NUMBER(S)
PL 17901/0200

9. DATE OF FIRST AUTHORISATION/RENEWAL OF THE AUTHORISATION
Date of first authorisation: 20 March 2003
Date of last renewal: 25 August 2005

10. DATE OF REVISION OF THE TEXT
10th December 2008

Symmetrel Capsules

(Alliance Pharmaceuticals)

1. NAME OF THE MEDICINAL PRODUCT
Symmetrel® capsules 100mg

2. QUALITATIVE AND QUANTITATIVE COMPOSITION
Amantadine hydrochloride PhEur 100mg.

3. PHARMACEUTICAL FORM
Brownish-red, hard gelatin capsules imprinted SYMM in white on both cap and body.

4. CLINICAL PARTICULARS

4.1 Therapeutic indications
Parkinson's disease.

Herpes zoster. It is recommended that Symmetrel be given to elderly or debilitated patients in whom the physician suspects that a severe and painful rash could occur. Symmetrel can significantly reduce the proportion of patients experiencing pain of long duration.

4.2 Posology and method of administration
Parkinson's disease: Initially 100mg daily for the first week, increasing to 100mg twice daily. The dose can be titrated against signs and symptoms. Doses exceeding 200mg daily may provide some additional relief, but may also be associated with increasing toxicity. A dose of 400mg/day should not be exceeded. The dose should be increased gradually, at intervals of not less than 1 week. Since patients over 65 years of age tend to show lower renal clearance and consequently higher plasma concentrations, the lowest effective dose should be used.

Amantadine acts within a few days, but may appear to lose efficacy within a few months of continuous treatment. Its effectiveness may be prolonged by withdrawal for three to four weeks, which seems to restore activity. During this time, existing concomitant antiparkinsonian therapy should be continued, or low dose L-dopa treatment initiated if clinically necessary.

Symmetrel withdrawal should be gradual, e.g. half the dose at weekly intervals. Abrupt discontinuation may exacerbate Parkinsonism, regardless of the patient's response to therapy (see Section 4.4, "Special warnings and precautions for use"). *Combined treatment:* any antiparkinson drug already in use should be continued during initial Symmetrel treatment. It may then be possible to reduce the other drug gradually. If increased side effects occur, the dosage should be reduced more quickly. In patients receiving large doses of anticholinergic agents or L-dopa, the initial phase of Symmetrel treatment should be extended to 15 days.

Herpes zoster: 100mg twice daily for 14 days. Treatment should be started as soon as possible after diagnosis. If post-herpetic pain persists treatment can be continued for a further 14 days.

In patients with **renal impairment**: the dose of amantadine should be reduced. This can be achieved by either reducing the total daily dose, or by increasing the dosage interval in accordance with the creatinine clearance. For example,

Creatinine clearance ml/(min)	Dose
< 15	Symmetrel contra-indicated.
15 – 35	100mg every 2 to 3 days.
> 35	100mg every day

The above recommendations are for guidance only and physicians should continue to monitor their patients for signs of unwanted effects.

4.3 Contraindications
Known hypersensitivity to amantadine or any of the excipients. Individuals subject to convulsions. A history of gastric ulceration. Severe renal disease. Pregnancy.

4.4 Special warnings and precautions for use
Symmetrel should be used with caution in patients with confusional or hallucinatory states or underlying psychiatric disorders, in patients with liver or kidney disorders, and those suffering from, or who have a history of, cardiovascular disorders. Caution should be applied when prescribing amantadine with other medications having an effect on the CNS (See section 4.5, Interactions with other medicaments and other forms of interaction).

Abrupt discontinuation of amantadine may result in worsening of Parkinsonism. Symmetrel should not be stopped abruptly in patients who are treated concurrently with neuroleptics. There have been isolated reports of precipitation or aggravation of neuroleptic malignant syndrome or neuroleptic-induced catatonia following the withdrawal of amantadine in patients taking neuroleptic agents. A similar syndrome has also been reported rarely following withdrawal of amantadine and other anti-parkinson agents in patients who were not taking concurrent psychoactive medication.

As some individuals have attempted suicide with amantadine, prescriptions should be written for the smallest quantity consistent with good patient management.

Peripheral oedema (thought to be due to an alteration in the responsiveness of peripheral vessels) may occur in some patients during chronic treatment (not usually before four weeks) with Symmetrel. This should be taken into account in patients with congestive heart failure.

4.5 Interaction with other medicinal products and other forms of interaction
Concurrent administration of amantadine and anticholinergic agents or levodopa may increase confusion, hallucinations, nightmares, gastro-intestinal disturbances, or other atropine-like side effects (see Section 4.9 "Overdose"). Psychotic reactions have been observed in patients receiving amantadine and levodopa.

In isolated cases, worsening of psychotic symptoms has been reported in patients receiving amantadine and concomitant neuroleptic medication.

Concurrent administration of amantadine and drugs or substances (e.g. alcohol) acting on the CNS may result in additive CNS toxicity. Close observation is recommended (see Section 4.9 "Overdose").

There have been isolated reports of a suspected interaction between amantadine and combination diuretics (hydrochlorothiazide + potassium sparing diuretics). One or both of the components apparently reduce the clearance of amantadine, leading to higher plasma concentrations and toxic effects (confusion, hallucinations, ataxia, myoclonus).

4.6 Pregnancy and lactation
Amantadine-related complications during pregnancy have been reported. Symmetrel is contra-indicated during pregnancy and in women trying to become pregnant. Amantadine passes into breast milk. Undesirable effects have been reported in breast-fed infants. Nursing mothers should not take Symmetrel.

4.7 Effects on ability to drive and use machines
Patients should be warned of the potential hazards of driving or operating machinery if they experience side effects such as dizziness or blurred vision.

4.8 Undesirable effects
Amantadine's undesirable effects are often mild and transient, usually appearing within the first 2 to 4 days of treatment and promptly disappearing 24 to 48 hours after discontinuation. A direct relationship between dose and incidence of side effects has not been demonstrated, although there seems to be a tendency towards more frequent undesirable effects (particularly affecting the CNS) with increasing doses.

Side effects reported include:

Frequency estimates: frequent > 10%, occasional 1%-10%, rare 0.001%-1%, isolated cases < 0.001%.

Central nervous system: Occasional: anxiety, elevation of mood, lightheadedness, headache, lethargy, hallucinations, nightmares, ataxia, slurred speech, blurred vision, loss of concentration, nervousness, depression, insomnia, myalgia. Hallucinations, confusion and nightmares are more common when amantadine is administered concurrently with anticholinergic agents or when the patient has an underlying psychiatric disorder. Rare: confusion, disorientation, psychosis, tremor, dyskinesia, convulsions, neuroleptic malignant-like syndrome. Delirium, hypomanic state and mania have been reported but their incidence cannot be readily deduced from the literature. *Cardiovascular system:* Frequent: oedema of ankles, livedo reticularis (usually after very high doses or use over many months). Occasional: palpitations, orthostatic hypotension. Isolated cases: heart insufficiency/failure. *Blood:* Isolated cases: leucopenia, reversible elevation of liver enzymes. *Gastrointestinal tract:* Occasional: dry mouth, anorexia, nausea, vomiting, constipation. Rare: diarrhoea. *Skin and appendages:* Occasional: diaphoresis. Rare: exanthema. Isolated cases: photosensitisation. *Sense organs*: Rare: corneal lesions, e.g. punctate subepithelial opacities which might be associated with superficial punctate keratitis, corneal epithelial oedema, and markedly reduced visual acuity. *Urogenital tract:* Rare: urinary retention, urinary incontinence.

4.9 Overdose
Signs and symptoms: *Neuromuscular* disturbances and symptoms of acute psychosis are prominent. *Central nervous system:* Hyperreflexia, motor restlessness, convulsions, extrapyramidal signs, torsion spasms, dystonic posturing, dilated pupils, confusion, disorientation, delirium, visual hallucinations. *Respiratory system*: hyperventilation, pulmonary oedema, respiratory distress, including adult respiratory distress syndrome. *Cardiovascular system*: sinus tachycardia, arrhythmia. *Gastrointestinal system*: nausea, vomiting, dry mouth. *Renal function*: urine retention, renal dysfunction, including increase in BUN and decreased creatinine clearance.

Overdose from combined drug treatment: the effects of anticholinergic drugs are increased by amantadine. Acute psychotic reactions (which may be identical to those of atropine poisoning) may occur when large doses of anticholinergic agents are used. Where alcohol or central nervous stimulants have been taken at the same time, the signs and symptoms of acute poisoning with amantadine may be aggravated and/or modified.

Management: There is no specific antidote. Induction of vomiting and/or gastric aspiration (and lavage if patient is conscious), activated charcoal or saline cathartic may be used if judged appropriate. Since amantadine is excreted mainly unchanged in the urine, maintenance of renal function and copious diuresis (forced diuresis if necessary) are effective ways to remove it from the blood stream. Acidification of the urine favours its excretion. Haemodialysis does not remove significant amounts of amantadine.

Monitor the blood pressure, heart rate, ECG, respiration and body temperature, and treat for possible hypotension and cardiac arhythmias, as necessary. *Convulsions and excessive motor restlessness*: administer anticonvulsants such as diazepam iv, paraldehyde im or per rectum, or phenobarbital im. *Acute psychotic symptoms, delirium, dystonic posturing, myoclonic manifestations*: physostigmine by slow iv infusion (1mg doses in adults, 0.5mg in children) repeated administration according to the initial response and the subsequent need, has been reported. *Retention of urine*: bladder should be catheterised; an indwelling catheter can be left in place for the time required.

5. PHARMACOLOGICAL PROPERTIES

5.1 Pharmacodynamic properties
Parkinson's disease: Symmetrel has been shown to be a low affinity antagonist at the N-methyl-D-aspartate (NMDA) subtype of glutamate receptors. Overactivity of glutamatergic neurotransmission has been implicated in the generation of parkinsonian symptoms. The clinical efficacy of amantadine is thought to be mediated through its antagonism at the NMDA subtype of glutamate receptors. In addition, amantadine may also exert some anticholinergic activity.

Herpes Zoster: The mechanism of action of Symmetrel in herpes zoster has not been fully characterised.

5.2 Pharmacokinetic properties
Absorption: Amantadine is absorbed slowly but almost completely. Peak plasma concentrations of approximately 250ng/ml and 500ng/ml are seen 3 to 4 hours after single oral administration of 100mg and 200mg amantadine, respectively. Following repeated administration of 200mg daily, the steady-state plasma concentration settles at 300ng/ml within 3 days.

Distribution: Amantadine accumulates after several hours in nasal secretions and crosses the blood-brain barrier (this has not been quantified). *In vitro*, 67% is bound to plasma proteins, with a substantial amount bound to red blood cells. The concentration in erythrocytes in normal healthy volunteers is 2.66 times the plasma concentration. The apparent volume of distribution is 5 to 10L/kg, suggesting extensive tissue binding. This declines with increasing doses. The concentrations in the lung, heart, kidney, liver and spleen are higher than in the blood.

Biotransformation: Amantadine is metabolised to a minor extent, principally by N-acetylation.

Elimination: The drug is eliminated in healthy young adults with a mean plasma elimination half-life of 15 hours (10 to 31 hours). The total plasma clearance is about the same as renal clearance (250ml/min). The renal amantadine clearance is much higher than the creatinine clearance, suggesting renal tubular secretion. After 4 to 5 days, 90% of the dose appears unchanged in urine. The rate is considerably influenced by urinary pH: a rise in pH brings about a fall in excretion.

Characteristics in special patient populations:

Elderly patients: compared with healthy young adults, the half-life may be doubled and renal clearance diminished. Tubular secretion diminishes more than glomerular filtration in the elderly. In elderly patients with renal impairment, repeated administration of 100mg daily for 14 days raised the plasma concentration into the toxic range.

Renal impairment: amantadine may accumulate in renal failure, causing severe side effects. The rate of elimination from plasma correlates to creatinine clearance divided by body surface area, although total renal elimination exceeds this value (possibly due to tubular secretion). The effects of reduced kidney function are dramatic: a reduction of creatinine clearance to 40ml/min may result in a five-fold increase in elimination half-life. The urine is the almost exclusive route of excretion, even with renal failure, and amantadine may persist in the plasma for several days. Haemodialysis does not remove significant amounts of amantadine, possibly due to extensive tissue binding.

5.3 Preclinical safety data

Reproductive toxicity studies were performed in rats and rabbits. In rat oral doses of 50 and 100 mg/kg proved to be teratogenic. The maximum recommended dose of 400mg is less than 6mg/kg.

There are no other pre-clinical data of relevance to the prescriber which are additional to those already included in other sections of the Summary of Product Characteristics.

6. PHARMACEUTICAL PARTICULARS

6.1 List of excipients

Lactose, polyvinylpyrrolidone, magnesium stearate, red iron oxide (E172), titanium dioxide (E171), gelatin and white printer's ink.

6.2 Incompatibilities

None known.

6.3 Shelf life

Five years.

6.4 Special precautions for storage

Protect from moisture. Medicines should be kept out of reach of children.

6.5 Nature and contents of container

Aluminium/PVdC blister packs of 56 capsules.

6.6 Special precautions for disposal and other handling

None.

7. MARKETING AUTHORISATION HOLDER

Alliance Pharmaceuticals Ltd
Avonbridge House
Bath Road
Chippenham
Wiltshire
SN15 2BB

8. MARKETING AUTHORISATION NUMBER(S)

PL16853/0015

9. DATE OF FIRST AUTHORISATION/RENEWAL OF THE AUTHORISATION

26 June 1998

10. DATE OF REVISION OF THE TEXT

January 2008

11. Legal Status

POM

Alliance, Alliance Pharmaceuticals and associated devices are registered Trademarks of Alliance Pharmaceuticals Ltd.

Symmetrel syrup

(Alliance Pharmaceuticals)

1. NAME OF THE MEDICINAL PRODUCT

Symmetrel® syrup 50mg/5ml

2. QUALITATIVE AND QUANTITATIVE COMPOSITION

Amantadine hydrochloride PhEur 50mg/5 mL.

3. PHARMACEUTICAL FORM

Clear, citrus flavoured syrup with a lemon odour.

4. CLINICAL PARTICULARS

4.1 Therapeutic indications

Prophylaxis and treatment of signs and symptoms of infection caused by influenza A virus. It is suggested that Symmetrel be given to patients suffering from clinical influenza in which complications might be expected to occur. In addition, Symmetrel is recommended prophylactically in cases particularly at risk. This can include those with chronic respiratory disease or debilitating conditions, the elderly and those living in crowded conditions. It can also be used for individuals in families where influenza has already been diagnosed, for control of institutional outbreaks or for those in essential services who are unvaccinated or when vaccination is unavailable or contra-indicated.

Symmetrel does not completely prevent the host immune response to influenza A infection, so individuals who take this drug still develop immune responses to the natural disease or vaccination and may be protected when later exposed to antigenically related viruses. Symmetrel may also be used in post-exposure prophylaxis in conjunction with inactivated vaccine during an outbreak until protective antibodies develop, or in patients who are not expected to have a substantial antibody response (immunosuppression).

Parkinson's disease.

Herpes zoster. It is recommended that Symmetrel be given to elderly or debilitated patients in whom the physician suspects that a severe and painful rash could occur. Symmetrel can significantly reduce the proportion of patients experiencing pain of long duration.

4.2 Posology and method of administration

Influenza A: Treatment: It is advisable to start treating influenza as early as possible and to continue for 4 to 5 days. When amantadine is started within 48 hours of symptoms appearing, the duration of fever and other effects is reduced by one or two days and the inflammatory reaction of the bronchial tree that usually accompanies influenza resolves more quickly. ***Prophylaxis:*** Treat daily for as long as protection from infection is required. In most instances this is expected to be for 6 weeks. When used with inactivated influenza A vaccine, amantadine is continued for 2 to 3 weeks following inoculation.

Adults: 100mg daily for the recommended period.

Children aged 10-15 years: 100mg daily for the recommended period.

Children under 10 years of age: Dosage not established.

Adults over 65 years of age: Plasma amantadine concentrations are influenced by renal function. In elderly patients, the elimination half-life is longer and renal clearance of the compound is diminished in comparison to young people. Therefore a daily dose of less than 100mg, or 100mg given at intervals of greater than one day, may be appropriate.

Parkinson's disease: Initially 100mg daily for the first week, increasing to 100mg twice daily. The dose can be titrated against signs and symptoms. Doses exceeding 200mg daily may provide some additional relief, but may also be associated with increasing toxicity. A dose of 400mg/day should not be exceeded. The dose should be increased gradually, at intervals of not less than 1 week. Since patients over 65 years of age tend to show lower renal clearance and consequently higher plasma concentrations, the lowest effective dose should be used.

Amantadine acts within a few days, but may appear to lose efficacy within a few months of continuous treatment. Its effectiveness may be prolonged by withdrawal for three to four weeks, which seems to restore activity. During this time, existing concomitant antiparkinsonian therapy should be continued, or low dose L-dopa treatment initiated if clinically necessary.

Symmetrel withdrawal should be gradual, e.g. half the dose at weekly intervals. Abrupt discontinuation may exacerbate Parkinsonism, regardless of the patient's response to therapy (see Section 4.4, "Special warnings and precautions for use"). *Combined treatment:* any antiparkinson drug already in use should be continued during initial Symmetrel treatment. It may then be possible to reduce the other drug gradually. If increased side effects occur, the dosage should be reduced more quickly. In patients receiving large doses of anticholinergic agents or L-dopa, the initial phase of Symmetrel treatment should be extended to 15 days.

Herpes zoster: 100mg twice daily for 14 days. Treatment should be started as soon as possible after diagnosis. If post-herpetic pain persists treatment can be continued for a further 14 days.

In patients with **renal impairment**: the dose of amantadine should be reduced. This can be achieved by either reducing the total daily dose, or by increasing the dosage interval in accordance with the creatinine clearance. For example,

Creatinine clearance ml/(min)	Dose
< 15	Symmetrel contra-indicated.
15 – 35	100mg every 2 to 3 days.
> 35	100mg every day

The above recommendations are for guidance only and physicians should continue to monitor their patients for signs of unwanted effects.

4.3 Contraindications

Known hypersensitivity to amantadine or any of the excipients. Individuals subject to convulsions. A history of gastric ulceration. Severe renal disease. Pregnancy.

4.4 Special warnings and precautions for use

Symmetrel should be used with caution in patients with confusional or hallucinatory states or underlying psychiatric disorders, in patients with liver or kidney disorders, and those suffering from, or who have a history of, cardiovascular disorders. Caution should be applied when prescribing amantadine with other medications having an effect on the CNS (See section 4.5, Interactions with other medicaments and other forms of interaction).

Abrupt discontinuation of amantadine may result in worsening of Parkinsonism. Symmetrel should not be stopped abruptly in patients who are treated concurrently with neuroleptics. There have been isolated reports of precipitation or aggravation of neuroleptic malignant syndrome or neuroleptic-induced catatonia following the withdrawal of amantadine in patients taking neuroleptic agents. A similar syndrome has also been reported rarely following withdrawal of amantadine and other anti-parkinson agents in patients who were not taking concurrent psychoactive medication.

Resistance to amantadine occurs during serial passage of influenza virus strains in vitro or in vivo in the presence of the drug. Apparent transmission of drug-resistant viruses may have been the cause of failure of prophylaxis and treatment in household contacts and in nursing-home patients. However, there is no evidence to date that the resistant virus produces a disease that is in any way different from that produced by sensitive viruses.

As some individuals have attempted suicide with amantadine, prescriptions should be written for the smallest quantity consistent with good patient management.

Peripheral oedema (thought to be due to an alteration in the responsiveness of peripheral vessels) may occur in some patients during chronic treatment (not usually before 4 weeks) with Symmetrel. This should be taken into account in patients with congestive heart failure.

4.5 Interaction with other medicinal products and other forms of interaction

Concurrent administration of amantadine and anticholinergic agents or levodopa may increase confusion, hallucinations, nightmares, gastro-intestinal disturbances, or other atropine-like side effects (see Section 4.9 "Overdose"). Psychotic reactions have been observed in patients receiving amantadine and levodopa.

In isolated cases, worsening of psychotic symptoms has been reported in patients receiving amantadine and concomitant neuroleptic medication.

Concurrent administration of amantadine and drugs or substances (e.g. alcohol) acting on the CNS may result in additive CNS toxicity. Close observation is recommended (see Section 4.9 "Overdose").

There have been isolated reports of a suspected interaction between amantadine and combination diuretics (hydrochlorothiazide + potassium sparing diuretics). One or both of the components apparently reduce the clearance of amantadine, leading to higher plasma concentrations and toxic effects (confusion, hallucinations, ataxia, myoclonus).

4.6 Pregnancy and lactation

Amantadine-related complications during pregnancy have been reported. Symmetrel is contra-indicated during pregnancy and in women wishing to become pregnant. Amantadine passes into breast milk. Undesirable effects have been reported in breast-fed infants. Nursing mothers should not take Symmetrel.

4.7 Effects on ability to drive and use machines

Patients should be warned of the potential hazards of driving or operating machinery if they experience side effects such as dizziness or blurred vision.

4.8 Undesirable effects

Amantadine's undesirable effects are often mild and transient, usually appearing within the first 2 to 4 days of treatment and promptly disappearing 24 to 48 hours after discontinuation. A direct relationship between dose and incidence of side effects has not been demonstrated, although there seems to be a tendency towards more frequent undesirable effects (particularly affecting the CNS) with increasing doses.

The side effects reported after the pivotal clinical studies in influenza in over 1200 patients receiving amantadine at 100mg daily were mostly mild, transient, and equivalent to placebo. Only 7% of subjects reported adverse events, many being similar to the effects of influenza itself. The most commonly reported effects were gastro-intestinal disturbances (anorexia, nausea), CNS effects (loss of concentration, dizziness, agitation, nervousness, depression, insomnia, fatigue, weakness), or myalgia.

Side effects reported after higher doses or chronic use, in addition to those already stated, include:

Frequency estimates: frequent > 10%, occasional 1%-10%, rare 0.001%-1%, isolated cases < 0.001%.

Central nervous system: Occasional: anxiety, elevation of mood, lightheadedness, headache, lethargy, hallucinations, nightmares, ataxia, slurred speech, blurred vision. Hallucinations, confusion and nightmares are more common when amantadine is administered concurrently with anticholinergic agents or when the patient has an underlying psychiatric disorder. Rare: confusion, disorientation, psychosis, tremor, dyskinesia, convulsions and neuroleptic malignant-like syndrome. Delirium, hypomanic state and mania have been reported but their incidence cannot be readily deduced from the literature. *Cardiovascular system:* Frequent: oedema of ankles, livedo reticularis (usually after very high doses or use over many months). Occasional: palpitations, orthostatic hypotension. Isolated cases: heart insufficiency/failure. *Blood:* Isolated cases: leucopenia, reversible elevation of liver enzymes. *Gastro-intestinal tract:* Occasional: dry mouth, anorexia, nausea, vomiting, constipation. Rare: diarrhoea. *Skin and appendages:* Occasional: diaphoresis. Rare: exanthema. Isolated cases: photosensitisation. *Sense organs:* Rare: corneal lesions, e.g. punctate subepithelial opacities which might be associated with superficial punctate keratitis, corneal epithelial oedema, and markedly reduced visual acuity. *Urogenital tract:* Rare: urinary retention, urinary incontinence.

4.9 Overdose

Signs and symptoms: *Neuromuscular* disturbances and symptoms of acute psychosis are prominent. *Central nervous system:* Hyperreflexia, motor restlessness, convulsions, extrapyramidal signs, torsion spasms, dystonic posturing, dilated pupils, confusion, disorientation, delirium, visual hallucinations. *Respiratory system*: hyperventilation, pulmonary oedema, respiratory distress, including adult respiratory distress syndrome. *Cardiovascular system*: sinus tachycardia, arrhythmia. *Gastrointestinal system*: nausea, vomiting, dry mouth. *Renal function*: urine retention, renal dysfunction, including increase in BUN and decreased creatinine clearance.

Overdose from combined drug treatment: the effects of anticholinergic drugs are increased by amantadine. Acute psychotic reactions (which may be identical to those of atropine poisoning) may occur when large doses of anticholinergic agents are used. Where alcohol or central nervous stimulants have been taken at the same time, the signs and symptoms of acute poisoning with amantadine may be aggravated and/or modified.

Management: There is no specific antidote. Induction of vomiting and/or gastric aspiration (and lavage if patient is conscious), activated charcoal or saline cathartic may be used if judged appropriate. Since amantadine is excreted mainly unchanged in the urine, maintenance of renal function and copious diuresis (forced diuresis if necessary) are effective ways to remove it from the blood stream. Acidification of the urine favours its excretion. Haemodialysis does not remove significant amounts of amantadine.

Monitor the blood pressure, heart rate, ECG, respiration and body temperature, and treat for possible hypotension and cardiac arrhythmias, as necessary. *Convulsions and excessive motor restlessness*: administer anticonvulsants such as diazepam iv, paraldehyde im or per rectum, or phenobarbital im. *Acute psychotic symptoms, delirium, dystonic posturing, myoclonic manifestations*: physostigmine by slow iv infusion (1mg doses in adults, 0.5mg in children) repeated administration according to the initial response and the subsequent need, has been reported. *Retention of urine*: bladder should be catheterised; an indwelling catheter can be left in place for the time required.

5. PHARMACOLOGICAL PROPERTIES

5.1 Pharmacodynamic properties

Influenza: Amantadine specifically inhibits the replication of influenza A viruses at low concentrations. If using a sensitive plaque-reduction assay, human influenza viruses, including H_1N_1, H_2N_2 and H_3N_2 subtypes, are inhibited by $\leqslant 0.4\ \mu$ g/ml of amantadine. Amantadine inhibits an early stage in viral replication by blocking the proton pump of the M_2 protein in the virus. This has two actions; it stops the virus uncoating and inactivates newly synthesised viral haemagglutinin. Effects on late replicative steps have been found for representative avian influenza viruses.

Data from tests with representative strains of influenza A virus indicate that Symmetrel is likely to be active against previously unknown strains, and could be used in the early stages of an epidemic, before a vaccine against the causative strain is generally available.

Herpes Zoster: The mechanism of action of Symmetrel in herpes zoster has not been fully characterised.

Parkinson's disease: Symmetrel has been shown to be a low affinity antagonist at the N-methyl-D-aspartate (NDMA) subtype of glutamate receptors. Overactivity of glutamatergic neurotransmission has been implicated in the generation of parkinsonian symptoms. The clinical efficacy of amantadine is thought to be mediated through its antagonism at the NDMA subtype of glutamate receptors. In addition, amantadine may also exert some anticholinergic activity.

5.2 Pharmacokinetic properties

Absorption: Amantadine is absorbed slowly but almost completely. Peak plasma concentrations of approximately 250ng/ml and 500ng/ml are seen 3 to 4 hours after single oral administration of 100mg and 200mg amantadine, respectively. Following repeated administration of 200mg daily, the steady-state plasma concentration settles at 300ng/ml within 3 days.

Distribution: Amantadine accumulates after several hours in nasal secretions and crosses the blood-brain barrier (this has not been quantified). *In vitro*, 67% is bound to plasma proteins, with a substantial amount bound to red blood cells. The concentration in erythrocytes in normal healthy volunteers is 2.66 times the plasma concentration. The apparent volume of distribution is 5 to 10L/kg, suggesting extensive tissue binding. This declines with increasing doses. The concentrations in the lung, heart, kidney, liver and spleen are higher than in the blood.

Biotransformation: Amantadine is metabolised to a minor extent, principally by N-acetylation.

Elimination: The drug is eliminated in healthy young adults with a mean plasma elimination half-life of 15 hours (10 to 31 hours). The total plasma clearance is about the same as renal clearance (250ml/min). The renal amantadine clearance is much higher than the creatinine clearance, suggesting renal tubular secretion. After 4 to 5 days, 90% of the dose appears unchanged in urine. The rate is considerably influenced by urinary pH: a rise in pH brings about a fall in excretion.

Characteristics in special patient populations:

Elderly patients: compared with healthy young adults, the half-life may be doubled and renal clearance diminished. Tubular secretion diminishes more than glomerular filtration in the elderly. In elderly patients with renal impairment, repeated administration of 100mg daily for 14 days raised the plasma concentration into the toxic range.

Renal impairment: amantadine may accumulate in renal failure, causing severe side effects. The rate of elimination from plasma correlates to creatinine clearance divided by body surface area, although total renal elimination exceeds this value (possibly due to tubular secretion). The effects of reduced kidney function are dramatic: a reduction of creatinine clearance to 40ml/min may result in a five-fold increase in elimination half-life. The urine is the almost exclusive route of excretion, even with renal failure, and amantadine may persist in the plasma for several days. Haemodialysis does not remove significant amounts of amantadine, possibly due to extensive tissue binding.

5.3 Preclinical safety data

Reproductive toxicity studies were performed in rats and rabbits. In rat oral doses of 50 and 100 mg/kg proved to be teratogenic. This is 33-fold the recommended dose of 100mg for influenza. The maximum recommended dose, of 400mg in Parkinson's disease, is less than 6mg/kg.

There are no other pre-clinical data of relevance to the prescriber which are additional to those already included in other sections of the Summary of Product Characteristics.

6. PHARMACEUTICAL PARTICULARS

6.1 List of excipients

Methyl hydroxybenzoate, propyl hydroxybenzoate, sorbitol, disodium hydrogen citrate, lemon flavouring, strawberry flavouring and water.

6.2 Incompatibilities

None known.

6.3 Shelf life

Five years.

6.4 Special precautions for storage

Protect from heat and light. Keep container closed.

6.5 Nature and contents of container

150ml amber glass bottles with child proof closures.

6.6 Special precautions for disposal and other handling

None

Administrative Data

7. MARKETING AUTHORISATION HOLDER

Alliance Pharmaceuticals Ltd

Avonbridge House

Bath Road

Chippenham

Wiltshire

SN15 2BB

8. MARKETING AUTHORISATION NUMBER(S)

PL16853/0016.

9. DATE OF FIRST AUTHORISATION/RENEWAL OF THE AUTHORISATION

25 June 1998

10. DATE OF REVISION OF THE TEXT

6 April 2009

11. Legal Status

POM

Alliance, Alliance Pharmaceuticals and associated devices are registered Trademarks of Alliance Pharmaceuticals Ltd.

Synacthen Ampoules 250mcg

(Alliance Pharmaceuticals)

1. NAME OF THE MEDICINAL PRODUCT

Synacthen® Ampoules 250mcg

2. QUALITATIVE AND QUANTITATIVE COMPOSITION

Tetracosactide acetate PhEur 250micrograms per ampoule.

3. PHARMACEUTICAL FORM

A clear colourless sterile solution in a clear glass ampoule.

4. CLINICAL PARTICULARS

4.1 Therapeutic indications

Diagnostic test for the investigation of adrenocortical insufficiency.

4.2 Posology and method of administration

Adults: This preparation of Synacthen is intended for administration for diagnostic purposes only as a single intramuscular or intravenous dose; it is not to be used for repeated therapeutic administration.

The 30-minute Synacthen diagnostic test: This test is based on measurement of the plasma cortisol concentration immediately before and exactly 30 minutes after an intramuscular or intravenous injection of 250micrograms (1ml) Synacthen. Adrenocortical function can be regarded as normal if the post-injection rise in plasma cortisol concentration amounts to at least 200nmol/litre (70micrograms/litre).

Where the 30-minute test has yielded inconclusive results, or where it is desired to determine the functional reserve of the adrenal cortex, a 5-hour test can be performed with Synacthen Depot (see separate Summary of Product Characteristics). Furthermore, a 3-day test with Synacthen Depot may be used to differentiate between primary and secondary adrenocortical insufficiency.

Children: An intravenous dose of 250micrograms/1.73m^2 body surface area has been suggested. Thus for children aged 5 to 7 years, approximately half the adult dose will be adequate. For more accurate dosing of other ages, standard body surface area tables should be consulted.

Elderly: There is no evidence to suggest that dosage should be different in the elderly.

4.3 Contraindications

History of hypersensitivity to ACTH, Synachen or Synacthen Depot. Synacthen is contra-indicated in patients with allergic disorders (e.g. asthma).

4.4 Special warnings and precautions for use

Before using Synacthen, the doctor should make every effort to find out whether the patient is suffering from, or has a history of, allergic disorders (see Section 4.3 "Contra-indications"). In particular, he should enquire whether the patient has previously experienced adverse reactions to ACTH, Synacthen or other drugs.

Synacthen should only be administered under the supervision of appropriate senior hospital medical staff (e.g. consultants).

If local or systemic hypersensitivity reactions occur after the injection (for example, marked redness and pain at the injection site, urticaria, pruritus, flushing, faintness or dyspnoea), Synacthen or other ACTH preparations should be avoided in the future. Hypersensitivity reactions tend to occur within 30 minutes of an injection. The patient should therefore be kept under observation during this time.

Preparation should be made in advance to combat any anaphylactic reaction that may occur after an injection of Synacthen. In the event of a serious anaphylactic reaction occurring, the following measures must be taken immediately: administer adrenaline (0.4 to 1ml of a 0.1% solution intramuscularly or 0.1 to 0.2ml of a 0.1% solution in 10ml physiological saline slowly intravenously) as well as a large intravenous dose of a corticosteroid (for example 100mg to 500mg hydrocortisone, three or four times in 24 hours), repeating the dose if necessary.

The hydrocortisone product information prepared by the manufacturer should also be consulted.

4.5 Interaction with other medicinal products and other forms of interaction

None known.

4.6 Pregnancy and lactation

The Synacthen test should not be utilised during pregnancy and lactation unless there are compelling reasons for doing so.

4.7 Effects on ability to drive and use machines

Patients should be warned of the potential hazards of driving or operating machinery if they experience side effects such as dizziness.

4.8 Undesirable effects

Hypersensitivity reactions:

Synacthen may provoke hypersensitivity reactions. In patients suffering from, or susceptible to, allergic disorders (especially asthma) this may take the form of anaphylactic shock (see Section 4.3 "Contra-indications").

Hypersensitivity may be manifested as skin reactions at the injection site, dizziness, nausea, vomiting, urticaria, pruritus, flushing, malaise, dyspnoea, angioneurotic oedema and Quinke's oedema.

Other side effects are unlikely to be observed with short-term use of Synacthen as a diagnostic tool. Should information be required on the side effects reported with therapeutic use of tetracosactide acetate, see Synacthen Depot Summary of Product Characteristics.

4.9 Overdose

Overdosage is unlikely to be a problem when the product is used as a single dose for diagnostic purposes.

5. PHARMACOLOGICAL PROPERTIES

5.1 Pharmacodynamic properties

Tetracosactide acetate consists of the first 24 amino acids occurring in the natural corticotropic hormone (ACTH) sequence and displays the same physiological properties as ACTH. In the adrenal cortex, it stimulates the biosynthesis of glucocorticoids, mineralocorticoids, and, to a lesser extent androgens.

The site of action of ACTH is the plasma membrane of the adrenocortical cells, where it binds to a specific receptor. The hormone-receptor complex activates adenylate cyclase, stimulating the production of cyclic AMP (adenosine monophosphate) and so promoting the synthesis of pregnenolone from cholesterol. From pregnenolone the various corticosteroids are produced via different enzymatic pathways.

5.2 Pharmacokinetic properties

Following an intravenous injection, elimination of tetracosactide acetate from the plasma consists of 3 phases. The half-lives of these phases are approximately 7 minutes (0 to 1 hour), 37 minutes (1 to 2 hours) and 3 hours thereafter.

Tetracosactide acetate has an apparent volume of distribution of approximately 0.4L/kg.

In the serum, tetracosactide acetate is broken down by serum endopeptidases into inactive oligopeptides and then by aminopeptidases into free amino acids. The rapid elimination from plasma is probably not attributable to this relatively slow cleavage process, but rather to the rapid concentration of the active substance in the adrenal glands and kidneys.

Following an iv dose of ^{131}I-labelled tetracosactide acetate, 95 to 100% of the radioactivity is excreted in the urine within 24 hours.

5.3 Preclinical safety data
There are no pre-clinical data of relevance to the prescriber, which are additional to those already included in other sections of the Summary of Product Characteristics.

6. PHARMACEUTICAL PARTICULARS
6.1 List of excipients
Acetic acid, sodium acetate, sodium chloride and water.

6.2 Incompatibilities
None known.

6.3 Shelf life
5 years.

6.4 Special precautions for storage
Synacthen should be protected from light and stored in a refrigerator (2 - 8°C).

6.5 Nature and contents of container
The ampoules are colourless glass PhEur type I. Five ampoules are packed in a cardboard box.

6.6 Special precautions for disposal and other handling
Shake well before use.

Administrative Data
7. MARKETING AUTHORISATION HOLDER
Alliance Pharmaceuticals Ltd

Avonbridge House

Bath Road

Chippenham

Wiltshire

SN15 2BB

8. MARKETING AUTHORISATION NUMBER(S)
PL 16853/0017

9. DATE OF FIRST AUTHORISATION/RENEWAL OF THE AUTHORISATION
25 June 1998

10. DATE OF REVISION OF THE TEXT
February 2005

11. Legal Status
POM

Alliance, Alliance Pharmaceuticals and associated devices are registered Trademarks of Alliance Pharmaceuticals Ltd.

Synacthen Depot

(Alliance Pharmaceuticals)

1. NAME OF THE MEDICINAL PRODUCT
Synacthen Depot® Ampoules 1mg/ml

2. QUALITATIVE AND QUANTITATIVE COMPOSITION
Tetracosactide acetate PhEur 1mg/ml

Contains benzyl alcohol (50mg/5ml), for a full list of excipients, see sections 6.1

3. PHARMACEUTICAL FORM
Tetracosactide acetate is absorbed on to zinc phosphate. A sterile, milky white suspension, which settles on standing, in a clear glass ampoule.

4. CLINICAL PARTICULARS
4.1 Therapeutic indications
Therapeutic use: Synacthen Depot should normally only be used for short-term therapy in conditions for which glucocorticoids are indicated in principle, for example, in ulcerative colitis and Crohn's disease, juvenile rheumatoid arthritis, or as adjunct therapy in patients with rheumatoid arthritis and osteoarthrosis. Synacthen Depot may be particularly useful in patients unable to tolerate oral glucocorticoid therapy or in patients where normal therapeutic doses of glucocorticoids have been ineffective.

Diagnostic use: As a diagnostic aid for the investigation of adrenocortical insufficiency.

4.2 Posology and method of administration
Synacthen Depot is intended for intramuscular injection. The ampoule should be shaken before use.

Therapeutic use: Initially, daily doses of Synacthen Depot should be given but after approximately 3 days, intermittent doses may be given.

Adults: Initially 1mg intramuscularly daily or 1mg every 12 hours in acute cases. After the acute symptoms of the disease have disappeared, treatment may be continued at a dose of 1mg every 2 to 3 days; in patients who respond well, the dosage may be reduced to 0.5mg every 2 to 3 days or 1mg per week.

Infants and children under 3 years: Not recommended due to the presence of benzyl alcohol in the formulation.

Children aged 3 to 5 years: Initially 0.25 to 0.5mg intramuscularly daily; the maintenance dose is 0.25 to 0.5mg every 2 to 8 days.

Children aged 5 to 12 years: Initially 0.25 to 1mg intramuscularly daily; the maintenance dose is 0.25 to 1mg every 2 to 8 days.

Elderly: There is no evidence to suggest that dosage should be different in the elderly.

Diagnostic use: In cases of suspected adrenocortical insufficiency, where the 30-minute diagnostic test with Synacthen ampoules (see Synacthen Summary of Product Characteristics) has yielded inconclusive results or where it is desired to determine the functional reserve of the adrenal cortex, a 5-hour test with Synacthen Depot may be performed.

Adults: This test is based on measurement of the plasma cortisol concentration before and exactly 30 minutes, 1, 2, 3, 4 and 5 hours after an intramuscular injection of 1mg Synacthen Depot. Adrenocortical function can be regarded as normal if the post-injection rise in plasma cortisol concentration increases 2-fold in the first hour, and continues to rise steadily. The values expected would be 600 to 1,250nmol/l in the first hour increasing slowly up to 1,000 to 1,800nmol/l by the fifth hour. Lower concentrations of plasma cortisol may be attributable to Addison's disease, secondary adrenocortical insufficiency due to a disorder of hypothalamo-pituitary function, or overdosage of corticosteroids.

A 3-day test with Synacthen Depot may be used to differentiate between primary and secondary adrenocortical insufficiency.

Children: No paediatric dosage has been established. Synacthen Depot is not recommended for children under 3 years of age due to the presence of benzyl alcohol in the formulation.

Elderly: There is no evidence to suggest that dosage should be different in the elderly.

4.3 Contraindications
History of hypersensitivity to ACTH, Synacthen or Synacthen Depot. Acute psychoses, infectious diseases, Cushing's syndrome, peptic ulcer, refractory heart failure, adrenogenital syndrome and for therapeutic use in adrenocortical insufficiency.

In view of the increased risk of anaphylactic reactions, Synacthen Depot should not be used in patients known to have asthma and/or other forms of allergy.

Synacthen Depot is contra-indicated for use in children under 3 years of age as it contains benzyl alcohol, which can cause severe poisoning and hypersensitivity reactions.

Therapeutic use is contra-indicated during pregnancy or lactation. Diagnostic use should only occur during pregnancy or lactation if there are compelling reasons.

Synacthen Depot must not be administered intravenously.

4.4 Special warnings and precautions for use
Before using Synacthen Depot, the doctor should make every effort to find out whether the patient is suffering from, or has a history of, allergic disorders. In particular, he should enquire whether the patient has previously experienced adverse reactions to ACTH, Synacthen Depot or other drugs.

Synacthen Depot should only be administered under medical supervision.

If local or systemic hypersensitivity reactions occur during or after an injection (for example, marked redness and pain at the injection site, urticaria, pruritus, flushing, faintness or dyspnoea), Synacthen Depot or other ACTH preparations should be avoided in the future. Hypersensitivity reactions tend to occur within 30 minutes of the injection. The patient should therefore be kept under observation during this time.

In the event of a serious anaphylactic reaction occurring despite these precautions, the following measures must be taken immediately: administer adrenaline (0.4 to 1ml of a 0.1% solution intramuscularly or 0.1 to 0.2ml of a 0.1% solution in 10ml physiological saline slowly intravenously) as well as a large intravenous dose of a corticosteroid (for example 100 to 500mg hydrocortisone, three or four times in 24 hours) repeating the dose if necessary.

The hydrocortisone product information prepared by the manufacturer should also be consulted.

Synacthen Depot should not be used in the presence of active infectious or systemic diseases, when the use of live vaccine is contemplated or in the presence of a reduced immune response, unless adequate disease specific therapy is being given.

Use with care in patients with non-specific ulcerative colitis, diverticulitis, recent intestinal anastomosis, renal insufficiency, hypertension, thromboembolic tendencies, osteoporosis and myasthenia gravis.

The increased production of adrenal steroids may result in corticosteroid type effects:

- Salt and water retention can occur and may respond to a low salt diet. Potassium supplementation may be necessary during long term treatment.

- Psychological disturbances may be triggered or aggravated.

- Latent infections (e.g. amoebiasis, tuberculosis) may become activated.

- Ocular effects may be produced (e.g. glaucoma, cataracts).

- Provided the dose is chosen to meet the individual's needs, Synacthen Depot is unlikely to inhibit growth in children. Nevertheless, growth should be monitored in children undergoing long-term treatment. In infants and children aged up to 5 years, reversible myocardial hypertrophy may occur in very rare cases following long-term treatment with high doses. Therefore echocardiographic recordings should be made regularly.

- Dosage adjustments may be necessary in patients being treated for diabetes or hypertension.

An enhanced effect of tetracosactide acetate therapy may occur in patients with hypothyroidism and in those with cirrhosis of the liver.

4.5 Interaction with other medicinal products and other forms of interaction
Interactions are likely with drugs whose actions are affected by adrenal steroids (see Section 4.4 "Special warnings and precautions for use").

4.6 Pregnancy and lactation
Synacthen Depot is contra-indicated for therapeutic use during pregnancy and lactation. It should not be used as a diagnostic tool unless there are compelling reasons for doing so.

4.7 Effects on ability to drive and use machines
Patients should be warned of the potential hazards of driving or operating machinery if they experience side effects such as dizziness.

4.8 Undesirable effects
Since Synacthen Depot stimulates the adrenal cortex to increase the output of glucocorticoids and mineralocorticoids, side effects associated with excessive adrenocorticotropic activity may be encountered, as well as those related to tetracosactide and to the presence of benzyl alcohol in the formulation.

Undesirable effects related to tetracosactide

Immune system disorders: Synacthen Depot may provoke hypersensitivity reactions. In patients suffering from, or susceptible to, allergic disorders (especially asthma) this may take the form of anaphylactic shock (see Section 4.3 Contraindications).

Hypersensitivity may be manifested as skin reactions at the injection site, dizziness, nausea, vomiting, urticaria, pruritus, flushing, malaise, dyspnoea, angioneurotic oedema and Quincke's oedema.

Endocrine disorders: Adrenal haemorrhage (very rare)

Undesirable effects related to benzyl alcohol

The benzyl alcohol contained as an excipient in Synacthen Depot may provoke toxic and anaphylactoid reactions in children aged under 3 years (see Section 4.3 Contraindications, Section 4.4 Special warnings and special precautions for use).

Immune system disorders: Hypersensitivity reactions

Undesirable effects related to glucocorticoid and mineralocorticoid effects

The undesirable effects related to glucocorticoid and mineralocorticoid effects are unlikely to be observed with short-tem use of Synacthen Depot as a diagnostic tool, but may be reported when Synacthen Depot is used for therapeutic indications.

Infections and infestations: Increased susceptibility to infection, abscess.

Blood and lymphatic system disorders: Leucocytosis.

Endocrine disorders: Menstrual irregularities, Cushing's syndrome, secondary adrenocortical and pituitary insufficiency, particularly in times of stress, as in trauma, surgery or illness, decreased carbohydrate tolerance, hyperglycaemia, manifestations of latent diabetes mellitus, hirsutism.

Metabolism and nutrition disorders: Sodium retention, fluid retention, hypokalaemia, hypokalaemic alkalosis, calcium loss, increased appetite.

Psychiatric disorders: Mental disorder.

Nervous system disorders: Headache, convulsions, increased intracranial pressure with papilloedema (benign intracranial hypertension) usually after treatment.

Eye disorders: Posterior subcapsular cataracts, increased intraocular pressure, glaucoma, exophthalmos.

Ear and labyrinth disorders: Vertigo.

Cardiac disorders: Blood pressure increased, congestive heart failure. There have been very rare reports of reversible myocardial hypertrophy in infants and small children treated over a prolonged period with high doses.

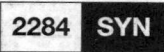

Vascular disorders: Thromboembolism, necrotising vasculitis.

Gastrointestinal disorders: Peptic ulceration with possible perforation and haemorrhage, pancreatitis, abdominal distension, ulcerative oesophagitis.

Skin and subcutaneous tissue disorders: Skin atrophy, petechia, ecchymosis, facial erythema, hyperhidrosis, acne, skin hyperpigmentation.

Musculoskeletal, connective tissue and bone disorders: Osteoporosis, muscle weakness, steroid myopathy, loss of muscle mass, vertebral compression fractures, aseptic necrosis of femoral and humeral heads, pathologic fracture of long bones, tendon rupture.

General disorders and administration site conditions: Impaired wound healing, growth retardation in children.

Investigations: Weight increase, suppression of skin test reactions, negative nitrogen balance due to protein catabolism.

4.9 Overdose

Relating to therapeutic usage of Synacthen Depot:

Overdosage may lead to fluid retention and signs of excessive adrenocorticotropic activity (Cushing's Syndrome). In such cases, Synacthen Depot should either be withdrawn temporarily, given in lower doses or the interval between injections should be prolonged (e.g. 5 to 7 days).

Treatment: There is no known antidote. Treatment should be symptomatic.

5. PHARMACOLOGICAL PROPERTIES

5.1 Pharmacodynamic properties

Tetracosactide acetate consists of the first 24 amino acids occurring in the natural corticotropic hormone (ACTH) sequence and displays the same physiological properties as ACTH. In the adrenal cortex, it stimulates the biosynthesis of glucocorticoids, mineralocorticoids, and, to a lesser extent, androgens, which explains its therapeutic effect in conditions responsive to glucocorticoid treatment.

However, its pharmacological activity is not comparable to that of corticosteroids, because under ACTH treatment (in contrast to treatment with a single glucocorticoid) the tissues are exposed to a physiological spectrum of corticosteroids.

The site of action of ACTH is the plasma membrane of the adrenocortical cells, where it binds to a specific receptor. The hormone-receptor complex activates adenylate cyclase, stimulating the production of cyclic AMP (adenosine monophosphate) and so promoting the synthesis of pregnenolone from cholesterol. From pregnenolone the various corticosteroids are produced via different enzymatic pathways.

5.2 Pharmacokinetic properties

Tetracosactide acetate is absorbed on to a zinc phosphate complex which ensures the sustained release of the active substance from the intramuscular injection site. After an intramuscular injection of 1mg Synacthen Depot, the radioimmunologically determined plasma concentrations of tetracosactide acetate range between 200 to 300pg/ml and are maintained for 12 hours.

Tetracosactide acetate has an apparent volume of distribution of approximately 0.4litres/kg.

In the serum, tetracosactide acetate is broken down by serum endopeptidases into inactive oligopeptides and then by aminopeptidases into free amino acids.

Following an intravenous dose of ^{131}I-labelled tetracosactide acetate, 95 to 100% of the radioactivity is excreted in the urine within 24 hours.

5.3 Preclinical safety data

There are no pre-clinical data of relevance to the prescriber which are additional to those already included in other sections of the Summary of Product Characteristics.

6. PHARMACEUTICAL PARTICULARS

6.1 List of excipients

Zinc chloride, disodium phosphate dodecahydrate, benzyl alcohol, sodium chloride, sodium hydroxide and water for injections.

6.2 Incompatibilities

None known

6.3 Shelf life

3 years

6.4 Special precautions for storage

Protect from light. Store in a refrigerator (2 to 8C).

6.5 Nature and contents of container

1ml ampoules packed in boxes of 10.

6.6 Special precautions for disposal and other handling

None

7. MARKETING AUTHORISATION HOLDER

Alliance Pharmaceuticals Ltd
Avonbridge House
Bath Road
Chippenham
Wiltshire
SN15 2BB

8. MARKETING AUTHORISATION NUMBER(S)

PL16853/0018

9. DATE OF FIRST AUTHORISATION/RENEWAL OF THE AUTHORISATION

25 June 1998

10. DATE OF REVISION OF THE TEXT

February 2007

Synagis

(Abbott Laboratories Limited)

1. NAME OF THE MEDICINAL PRODUCT

SYNAGIS ▼ 50 mg or 100 mg powder and solvent for solution for injection

2. QUALITATIVE AND QUANTITATIVE COMPOSITION

Each vial contains 50 mg or 100 mg palivizumab*, providing 100 mg/ml of palivizumab when reconstituted as recommended.

*recombinant humanised monoclonal antibody produced by DNA technology in mouse myeloma host cells.

For a full list of excipients, see section 6.1.

3. PHARMACEUTICAL FORM

Powder and solvent for solution for injection.

The powder is a white to off-white cake.

4. CLINICAL PARTICULARS

4.1 Therapeutic indications

SYNAGIS is indicated for the prevention of serious lower respiratory tract disease requiring hospitalisation caused by respiratory syncytial virus (RSV) in children at high risk for RSV disease:

- Children born at 35 weeks of gestation or less and less than 6 months of age at the onset of the RSV season.
- Children less than 2 years of age and requiring treatment for bronchopulmonary dysplasia within the last 6 months.
- Children less than 2 years of age and with haemodynamically significant congenital heart disease.

4.2 Posology and method of administration

Recommended dose

The recommended dose of palivizumab is 15 mg/kg of body weight, given once a month during anticipated periods of RSV risk in the community. Where possible, the first dose should be administered prior to commencement of the RSV season. Subsequent doses should be administered monthly throughout the RSV season.

The majority of experience including the pivotal phase III clinical trials with palivizumab has been gained with 5 injections during one season (see section 5.1). Data, although limited, are available on greater than 5 doses (see sections 4.8 and 5.1), therefore the benefit in terms of protection beyond 5 doses has not been established.

To reduce risk of rehospitalisation, it is recommended that children receiving palivizumab who are hospitalised with RSV continue to receive monthly doses of palivizumab for the duration of the RSV season.

For children undergoing cardiac bypass, it is recommended that a 15 mg/kg of body weight injection of palivizumab be administered as soon as stable after surgery to ensure adequate palivizumab serum levels. Subsequent doses should resume monthly through the remainder of the RSV season for children that continue to be at high risk of RSV disease (see section 5.2).

Method of administration

Palivizumab is administered in a dose of 15 mg/kg of body weight once a month intramuscularly, preferably in the anterolateral aspect of the thigh. The gluteal muscle should not be used routinely as an injection site because of the risk of damage to the sciatic nerve. The injection should be given using standard aseptic technique. Injection volumes over 1 ml should be given as a divided dose.

For information on reconstituting SYNAGIS, see section 6.6.

4.3 Contraindications

Known hypersensitivity to the active substance or to any of the excipients (see section 6.1), or other humanised monoclonal antibodies.

4.4 Special warnings and precautions for use

Allergic reactions including very rare cases of anaphylaxis have been reported following palivizumab administration (see section 4.8).

Medicinal products for the treatment of severe hypersensitivity reactions, including anaphylaxis, should be available for immediate use following administration of palivizumab.

A moderate to severe acute infection or febrile illness may warrant delaying the use of palivizumab, unless, in the opinion of the physician, withholding palivizumab entails a greater risk. A mild febrile illness, such as mild upper respiratory infection, is not usually reason to defer administration of palivizumab.

As with any intramuscular injection, palivizumab should be given with caution to patients with thrombocytopaenia or any coagulation disorder.

The efficacy of palivizumab when administered to patients as a second course of treatment during an ensuing RSV season has not been formally investigated in a study performed with this objective. The possible risk of enhanced RSV infection in the season following the season in which the patients were treated with palivizumab has not been conclusively ruled out by studies performed aiming at this particular point.

4.5 Interaction with other medicinal products and other forms of interaction

No formal interactions studies with other medicinal products were conducted, however no interactions have been described to date. In the phase III IMpact-RSV study in the premature and bronchopulmonary dysplasia paediatric populations, the proportions of patients in the placebo and palivizumab groups who received routine childhood vaccines, influenza vaccine, bronchodilators or corticosteroids were similar and no incremental increase in adverse reactions was observed among patients receiving these agents.

Since the monoclonal antibody is specific for RSV, palivizumab is not expected to interfere with the immune response to vaccines.

4.6 Pregnancy and lactation

Not relevant. SYNAGIS is not indicated for use in adults. Data on pregnancy and lactation are not available.

4.7 Effects on ability to drive and use machines

Not relevant.

4.8 Undesirable effects

Adverse drug reactions (ADRs) reported in the prophylactic paediatric studies were similar in the placebo and palivizumab groups. The majority of ADRs were transient and mild to moderate in severity.

Adverse events at least possibly causally-related to palivizumab, both clinical and laboratory, are displayed by system organ class and frequency (common $\geq$1/100 to $<$ 1/10; uncommon $\geq$1/1,000 to $<$ 1/100) in studies conducted in premature and bronchopulmonary dysplasia paediatric patients, and congenital heart disease patients (Tables 1 and 2, respectively).

Within each frequency grouping, adverse reactions have been presented in order of decreasing seriousness.

Table 1
Undesirable effects in prophylactic clinical studies with premature and bronchopulmonary dysplasia paediatric populations

Infections and infestations	Uncommon	Viral infection Upper respiratory infection
Blood and lymphatic system disorders	Uncommon	Leucopaenia
Psychiatric disorders	Common	Nervousness
Respiratory, thoracic and mediastinal disorders	Uncommon	Wheeze Rhinitis Cough
Gastrointestinal disorders	Common Uncommon	Diarrhoea Vomiting
Skin and subcutaneous tissue disorders	Uncommon	Rash
General disorders and administration site conditions	Common Uncommon	Fever Injection site reaction Pain
Investigations	Uncommon	AST increase ALT increase Abnormal liver function test

No medically important differences were observed during the prophylactic studies carried out in the premature and bronchopulmonary dysplasia paediatric populations in ADRs by body system or when evaluated in subgroups of children by clinical category, gender, age, gestational age, country, race/ethnicity or quartile serum palivizumab concentration. No significant difference in safety profile was observed between children without active RSV infection and those hospitalised for RSV. Permanent discontinuation of palivizumab due to ADRs was rare (0.2%). Deaths were balanced between the integrated placebo and palivizumab groups and were not drug-related.

Table 2
Undesirable effects in the prophylactic paediatric congenital heart disease clinical study

Infections and infestations	Uncommon	Gastroenteritis Upper respiratory infection

Psychiatric disorders	Uncommon	Nervousness
Nervous system disorders	Uncommon	Somnolence Hyperkinesia
Vascular disorders	Uncommon	Haemorrhage
Respiratory, thoracic and mediastinal disorders	Uncommon	Rhinitis
Gastrointestinal disorders	Uncommon	Vomiting Diarrhoea Constipation
Skin and subcutaneous tissue disorders	Uncommon	Rash Eczema
General disorders and administration site conditions	Common	Fever Injection site reaction
	Uncommon	Asthenia

In the congenital heart disease study no medically important differences were observed in ADRs by body system or when evaluated in subgroups of children by clinical category. The incidence of serious adverse events was significantly lower in the palivizumab group compared to the placebo group. No serious adverse events related to palivizumab were reported. The incidences of cardiac surgeries classified as planned, earlier than planned or urgent were balanced between the groups. Deaths associated with RSV infection occurred in 2 patients in the palivizumab group and 4 patients in the placebo group and were not drug-related.

Post-marketing experience:

The following events were reported during post-marketing experience of palivizumab:

Rare ADRs (> 1/10,000, < 1/1,000): apnoea

Very rare ADRs (< 1/10,000): anaphylaxis, urticaria

Post-marketing serious spontaneous adverse events reported during palivizumab treatment between 1998 and 2002 covering four RSV seasons were evaluated. A total of 1,291 serious reports were received where palivizumab had been administered as indicated and the duration of therapy was within one season. The onset of the adverse event occurred after the sixth or greater dose in only 22 of these reports (15 after the sixth dose, 6 after the seventh doses and 1 after the eight dose). These events are similar in character to those after the initial five doses.

Palivizumab treatment schedule and adverse events were monitored in a group of nearly 20,000 infants tracked through a patient compliance registry between 1998 and 2000. Of this group 1,250 enrolled infants had 6 injections, 183 infants had 7 injections, and 27 infants had either 8 or 9 injections. Adverse events observed in patients after a sixth or greater dose were similar in character and frequency to those after the initial 5 doses.

Human anti-human antibody (HAHA) response:

Antibody to palivizumab was observed in approximately 1% of patients in the IMpact-RSV during the first course of therapy. This was transient, low titre, resolved despite continued use (first and second season), and could not be detected in 55/56 infants during the second season (including 2 with titres during the first season). Therefore, HAHA responses appear to be of no clinical relevance.

Immunogenicity was not studied in the congenital heart disease study.

4.9 Overdose

In clinical studies, three children received an overdose of more than 15 mg/kg. These doses were 20.25 mg/kg, 21.1 mg/kg and 22.27 mg/kg. No medical consequences were identified in these instances.

5. PHARMACOLOGICAL PROPERTIES

5.1 Pharmacodynamic properties

Pharmacotherapeutic group: specific immunoglobulins; ATC Code: J06BB16

Palivizumab is a humanised $IgG_{1\kappa}$ monoclonal antibody directed to an epitope in the A antigenic site of the fusion protein of respiratory syncytial virus (RSV). This humanised monoclonal antibody is composed of human (95%) and murine (5%) antibody sequences. It has potent neutralising and fusion-inhibitory activity against both RSV subtype A and B strains.

Palivizumab serum concentrations of approximately 30 µg/ml have been shown to produce a 99% reduction in pulmonary RSV replication in the cotton rat model.

Clinical studies

In a placebo-controlled trial of RSV disease prophylaxis in (IMpact-RSV trial) 1502 high-risk children (1002 SYNAGIS; 500 placebo), 5 monthly doses of 15 mg/kg reduced the incidence of RSV related hospitalisation by 55% (p = < 0.001). The RSV hospitalisation rate was 10.6% in the placebo group. On this basis, the absolute risk reduction is 5.8% which means the number needed to treat is 17 to prevent one hospitalisation. The severity of RSV disease in children hospitalised despite prophylaxis with palivizumab in terms of days in ICU stay per 100 children and days of mechanical ventilation per 100 children was not affected.

A total of 222 children were enrolled in two separate studies to examine the safety of palivizumab when it is administered for a second RSV season. One hundred and three (103) children received monthly palivizumab injections for the first time, and 119 children received palivizumab for two consecutive seasons. No difference between groups regarding immunogenicity was observed in either study. However, as the efficacy of palivizumab when administered to patients as a second course of treatment during an ensuing RSV season has not been formally investigated in a study performed with this objective, the relevance of these data in terms of efficacy is unknown.

In an open label prospective trial designed to evaluate pharmacokinetics, safety and immunogenicity after administration of 7 doses of palivizumab within a single RSV season, pharmacokinetic data indicated that adequate mean palivizumab levels were achieved in all 18 children enrolled. Transient, low levels of antipalivizumab antibody were observed in one child after the second dose of palivizumab that dropped to undetectable levels at the fifth and seventh dose.

In a placebo-controlled trial in 1,287 patients ≤ 24 months of age with haemodynamically significant congenital heart disease (639 SYNAGIS; 648 placebo), 5 monthly doses of 15 mg/kg SYNAGIS reduced the incidence of RSV hospitalisations by 45% (p = 0.003) (congenital heart disease study). Groups were equally balanced between cyanotic and acyanotic patients. The RSV hospitalisation rate was 9.7% in the placebo group and 5.3% in the SYNAGIS group. Secondary efficacy endpoints showed significant reductions in the SYNAGIS group compared to placebo in total days of RSV hospitalisation (56% reduction, p = 0.003) and total RSV days with increased supplemental oxygen (73% reduction, p = 0.014) per 100 children.

5.2 Pharmacokinetic properties

In studies in adult volunteers, palivizumab had a pharmacokinetic profile similar to a human IgG_1 antibody with regard to volume of distribution (mean 57 ml/kg) and half-life (mean 18 days). In prophylactic studies in premature and bronchopulmonary dysplasia paediatric populations, the mean half-life of palivizumab was 20 days and monthly intramuscular doses of 15 mg/kg achieved mean 30 day trough serum active substance concentrations of approximately 40 µg/ml after the first injection, approximately 60 µg/ml after the second injection, approximately 70 µg/ml after the third injection and fourth injection. In the congenital heart disease study, monthly intramuscular doses of 15 mg/kg achieved mean 30 day trough serum active substance concentrations of approximately 55 µg/ml after the first injection and approximately 90 µg/ml after the fourth injection.

Among 139 children in the congenital heart disease study receiving palivizumab who had cardio-pulmonary bypass and for whom paired serum samples were available, the mean serum palivizumab concentration was approximately 100 µg/ml pre-cardiac bypass and declined to approximately 40 µg/ml after bypass.

5.3 Preclinical safety data

Single dose toxicology studies have been conducted in cynomolgus monkeys (maximum dose 30 mg/kg), rabbits (maximum dose 50 mg/kg) and rats (maximum dose 840 mg/kg). No significant findings were observed.

Studies carried out in rodents gave no indication of enhancement of RSV replication, or RSV-induced pathology or generation of virus escape mutants in the presence of palivizumab under the chosen experimental conditions.

6. PHARMACEUTICAL PARTICULARS

6.1 List of excipients

Powder:

Histidine

Glycine

Mannitol (E421)

Solvent:

Water for injections

6.2 Incompatibilities

Palivizumab should not be mixed with any medicinal products or diluents other than water for injections.

6.3 Shelf life

3 years.

After reconstitution, the product should be used immediately. However in-use stability has been demonstrated for 3 hours at 20 - 24°C.

6.4 Special precautions for storage

Store in a refrigerator (2°C to 8°C).

Do not freeze.

Store in the original container.

For storage conditions of the reconstituted medicinal product, see section 6.3.

6.5 Nature and contents of container

50 mg of powder in a 4 ml vial (Type I glass) with a stopper (bromobutyl rubber) and a flip-off seal (aluminium).

100 mg of powder in a 10 ml vial (Type I glass) with a stopper (bromobutyl rubber) and a flip-off seal (aluminium).

1ml of water for injections in an ampoule (type I glass).

Pack size of 1.

6.6 Special precautions for disposal and other handling

SLOWLY add 0.6 ml of water for injections for the 50 mg vial or 1.0 ml of water for injections for the 100 mg vial along the inside wall of the vial to minimise foaming. After the water is added, tilt the vial slightly and gently rotate the vial for 30 seconds. DO NOT SHAKE THE VIAL. Palivizumab solution should stand at room temperature for a minimum of 20 minutes until the solution clarifies. Palivizumab solution does not contain a preservative and should be administered within 3 hours of preparation.

When reconstituted as recommended, the final concentration is 100 mg/ml.

The appearance of the reconstituted solution is clear to slightly opalescent.

Any unused product or waste material should be disposed of in accordance with local requirements.

7. MARKETING AUTHORISATION HOLDER

Abbott Laboratories Limited

Queenborough

Kent ME11 5EL

United Kingdom

8. MARKETING AUTHORISATION NUMBER(S)

50 mg vial: EU/1/99/117/001

100 mg vial: EU/1/99/117/002

9. DATE OF FIRST AUTHORISATION/RENEWAL OF THE AUTHORISATION

Date of first authorisation: 13 August 1999

Date of latest renewal: 27 July 2009

10. DATE OF REVISION OF THE TEXT

27 July 2009

Synarel Nasal Spray

(Pharmacia Limited)

1. NAME OF THE MEDICINAL PRODUCT

SYNAREL®

2. QUALITATIVE AND QUANTITATIVE COMPOSITION

Solution containing 2mg/ml of nafarelin (as acetate) supplied in bottles fitted with a metered spray pump that delivers 200 micrograms of nafarelin base per spray.

3. PHARMACEUTICAL FORM

Nasal spray

4. CLINICAL PARTICULARS

4.1 Therapeutic indications

The hormonal management of endometriosis, including pain relief and reduction of endometriotic lesions.

Use in controlled ovarian stimulation programmes prior to in-vitro fertilisation, under the supervision of an infertility specialist.

4.2 Posology and method of administration

Adult: Synarel is for administration by the intranasal route only.

Experience with the treatment of endometriosis has been limited to women 18 years of age and older.

Endometriosis: In the use of Synarel in endometriosis, the aim is to induce chronic pituitary desensitisation, which gives a menopause-like state maintained over many months.

The recommended daily dose of Synarel is 200 mcg taken twice daily as one spray (200 mcg of nafarelin) to one nostril in the morning and one spray into the other nostril in the evening (400 mcg/day). Treatment should be started between days 2 and 4 of the menstrual cycle. The recommended duration of therapy is six months; only one 6-month course is advised. In clinical studies the majority of women have only received up to six-months treatment with Synarel.

Controlled ovarian stimulation prior to in vitro fertilisation: In the use of Synarel associated with controlled ovarian stimulation prior to *in vitro* fertilisation, the long protocol should be employed, whereby Synarel is continued through a period of transient gonadotrophin stimulation lasting 10-15 days (the 'flare effect') through to pituitary desensitisation (down-regulation). Down-regulation may be defined as serum oestradiol ≤50pg/ml and serum progesterone ≤1ng/ml, and the majority of patients down-regulate within 4 weeks.

The recommended daily dose of Synarel is 400 mcg taken twice daily as one spray to each nostril in the morning, and one spray to each nostril in the evening (800 mcg/day).

Once down-regulation is achieved, controlled ovarian stimulation with gonadotrophins, e.g. hMG, is commenced, and the Synarel dosage maintained until the administration of hCG at follicular maturity (usually a further 8-12 days).

If patients do not down-regulate within 12 weeks of starting Synarel, it is recommended that Synarel therapy be discontinued and the cycle cancelled.

Treatment may begin in either the early follicular phase (day 2) or the mid-luteal phase (usually day 21).

If the use of a nasal decongestant is required at the time of nafarelin administration, it is recommended that the nasal decongestant be used at least 30 minutes after nafarelin dosing.

Sneezing during or immediately after dosing may impair absorption of Synarel. If sneezing occurs upon administration, repeating the dose may be advisable.

Bottles contain either 30 or 60 doses and should not be used for a greater number of doses. The 60 dose-unit bottle is sufficient for 30 days' treatment at 400mcg (2 sprays) per day, and 15 days treatment at 800mcg (4 sprays) per day.

The 30 dose-unit bottle is sufficient for 15 days' treatment at 400mcg (2 sprays) per day, and 7 days' treatment at 800mcg (4 sprays) per day. Patients should therefore be advised that continued use after this time may result in delivery of an insufficient amount of nafarelin.

4.3 Contraindications

A small loss of trabecula bone mineral content occurs during 6 months treatment with nafarelin. Although this is mostly reversible within 6 months of stopping treatment, there are no data on the effects of repeat courses on bone loss. Retreatment with Synarel or use for longer than 6 months is, therefore, not recommended. (See Side-effects section on 'Changes in bone density').

Synarel should not be administered to patients who:

1. are hypersensitive to GnRH, GnRH agonist analogues or any of the excipients in Synarel;

2. have undiagnosed vaginal bleeding;

3. are pregnant or may become pregnant whilst taking Synarel (see 'use in pregnancy and lactation');

4. are breast-feeding.

4.4 Special warnings and precautions for use

When regularly used at the recommended dose, nafarelin inhibits ovulation. Patients should be advised to use non-hormonal, barrier methods of contraception. In the event of missed doses there may be breakthrough ovulation and a potential for conception. If a patient becomes pregnant during treatment, administration of the drug must be discontinued and the patient must be informed of a potential risk to fetal development. NB Synarel treatment will be stopped at least 3 days before fertilised embryos are placed in the uterine cavity.

As with other drugs in this class ovarian cysts have been reported to occur in the first two months of therapy with Synarel. Many, but not all, of these events occurred in patients with polycystic ovarian disease. These cystic enlargements may resolve spontaneously, generally by about four to six weeks of therapy, but in some cases may require discontinuation of drug and/or surgical intervention.

Controlled ovarian stimulation prior to in vitro fertilisation; Transient ovarian cyst formation is a recognised complication of GnRH agonist use. These cysts tend to regress spontaneously over a number of weeks and are more common when GnRH agonists are commenced in the follicular phase of the cycle.

There are no clinical data available on the use of Synarel in ovulation induction regimens involving patients with polycystic ovarian syndrome. Caution is advised in this patient group as they are at greater risk of excessive follicular recruitment when undergoing ovulation induction regimes.

Administration of nafarelin in therapeutic doses results in suppression of the pituitary-gonadal system. Normal function is usually restored within 8 weeks after treatment is discontinued. Diagnostic tests of pituitary-gonadal function conducted during the treatment and up to 8 weeks after discontinuation of nafarelin therapy may therefore be misleading.

4.5 Interaction with other medicinal products and other forms of interaction

Nafarelin would not be expected to participate in pharmacokinetic-based drug-drug interactions because degradation of the compound is primarily by the action of peptidases not cytochrome P-450 enzymes. Additionally, because nafarelin is only about 80% bound to plasma proteins (albumin), drug interactions at the protein-binding level would not be expected to occur.

Rhinitis does not impair nasal absorption of nafarelin. Nasal decongestants used 30 minutes before nafarelin administration decrease absorption.

4.6 Pregnancy and lactation

When administered intramuscularly to rats on days 6-15 of pregnancy at doses of 0.4, 1.6 and 6.4 mcg/kg/day (0.6, 2.5 and 10.0 times the intranasal human dose of 400mcg per day), 4/80 fetuses in the highest dose group had major fetal abnormalities that were not seen in a repeat study in rats. Moreover, studies in mice and rabbits failed to demonstrate an increase in fetal abnormalities. In rats, there was a dose-related increase in fetal mortality, and a decrease in fetal weight with the highest dose. These effects on rat fetal mortality are logical consequences of the alterations in hormonal levels brought about by nafarelin in this species.

Use of nafarelin in human pregnancy has not been studied.

Synarel should not therefore be used during pregnancy or suspected pregnancy. Before starting treatment with Synarel pregnancy must be excluded. If a patient becomes pregnant during treatment, administration of the drug must be discontinued and the patient must be informed of a potential risk to fetal development.

Controlled ovarian stimulation prior to in vitro fertilisation: Pregnancy should be excluded before starting treatment with Synarel, and the medication should be stopped on the day of administration of hCG. Barrier methods of contraception should be employed whilst Synarel is being taken.

It is not known whether or to what extent nafarelin is excreted into human breast milk. The effects, if any on the breast-fed child have not been determined and therefore Synarel should not be used by breast-feeding women.

4.7 Effects on ability to drive and use machines

Not applicable.

4.8 Undesirable effects

In approximately 0.2% of adult patients, symptoms suggestive of drug sensitivity, such as shortness of breath, chest pain, urticaria, rash and pruritus have occurred.

As would be expected with a drug which lowers serum oestradiol levels to menopausal concentrations the most frequently reported adverse reactions are those related to hypo-oestrogenism.

In controlled studies of nafarelin 400mcg/day, adverse reactions that were most frequently reported are listed in order of decreasing frequency; hot flushes, changes in libido, vaginal dryness, headaches, emotional lability, acne, myalgia, decreased breast size and irritation of the nasal mucosa.

During post-marketing surveillance, depression, paraesthesia, alopecia, migraine, palpitations, blurred vision have been reported. Emotional lability and depression would be expected with a drug that towers serum oestradiol to post-menopausal levels.

Changes in bone density: After six months of Synarel treatment there was a reduction in vertebral trabecular bone density and total vertebral mass, averaging about 9% and 4%, respectively. There was very little, if any, decrease in the mineral content of compact bone of the distal radius and second metacarpal. Substantial recovery of bone occurred during the post-treatment period. Total vertebral bone mass, measured by dual photon absorptiometry (DPA), decreased by a mean of about 6% at the end of treatment. Mean total vertebral mass, re-examined by DPA six months after completion of treatment, was 1.4% below pretreatment levels. These changes are similar to those which occur during treatment with other GnRH agonists.

Carcinogenesis/mutagenesis: As seen with other GnRH agonists, nafarelin given parenterally in high doses to laboratory rodents for prolonged periods induced hyperplasia and neoplasia of endocrine organs, including the anterior pituitary (adenoma/carcinoma) of both mice and rats; tumours of the pancreatic islets, adrenal medulla, testes and ovaries occurred only in long-term studies in rats. No metastases of these tumours were observed. Monkeys treated with high doses of nafarelin for one year did not develop any tumours or proliferative changes. Experience in humans is limited but there is no evidence for tumorigenesis of GnRH analogues in human beings.

In vitro studies conducted in bacterial and mammalian systems provided no indication of a mutagenic potential for nafarelin.

Impairment of fertility: Reproduction studies in rats of both sexes have shown full reversibility of fertility suppression when drug treatment was discontinued after continuous administration for up to six months.

Laboratory values: Increased levels of SGOT/SGPT and serum alkaline phosphatase may rarely occur which are reversible on discontinuing treatment.

4.9 Overdose

In animals, subcutaneous administration of up to 60 times the recommended human dose (expressed on a mcg/kg basis) had no adverse effects. Orally-administered nafarelin is subject to enzymatic degradation in the gastro-intestinal tract and is therefore inactive. At present there is no clinical experience with overdosage of nafarelin.

Based on studies in monkeys, nafarelin is not absorbed after oral administration.

5. PHARMACOLOGICAL PROPERTIES

5.1 Pharmacodynamic properties

Nafarelin is a potent agonistic analogue of gonadotrophin releasing hormone (GnRH). Given as a single dose, nafarelin stimulates release of the pituitary gonadotrophins, LH and FSH, with consequent increase of ovarian and testicular steroidogenesis. During repeated dosing this response to stimulation gradually diminishes. Within three to four weeks, daily administration leads to decreased pituitary gonadotrophin secretion and/or the secretion of gonadotrophin secretion and/or the secretion of gonadotrophins with lowered biological activity. There is a consequent suppression of gonadal steroidogenesis and inhibition of functions in tissues that depend on gonadal steroids for their maintenance.

5.2 Pharmacokinetic properties

Nafarelin is rapidly absorbed into the circulation after intranasal administration. Maximum plasma concentration is achieved 20 minutes after dosing and the plasma half-life is approximately 4 hours. Bioavailability of the intranasal dose averages 2.8% (range 1.2-5.6%).

5.3 Preclinical safety data

This is discussed in Section 4.8 undesirable effects.

6. PHARMACEUTICAL PARTICULARS

6.1 List of excipients

Synarel contains:

Sorbitol, benzalkonium chloride, glacial acetic acid and water.

Sodium hydroxide or hydrochloric acid to adjust pH.

6.2 Incompatibilities

None stated.

6.3 Shelf life

The shelf life of Synarel is 2 years.

6.4 Special precautions for storage

Store upright below 25°C. Avoid heat above 30°C. Protect from light and freezing.

6.5 Nature and contents of container

White, high density polyethylene bottles with a 0.1ml metered spray pump, containing 6.5ml or 10ml.

PVC-coated glass bottles with an internal conical reservoir in the base and a valois pump, with either an aluminium crimp-on cap or a polypropylene snap-on cap, containing 4ml or 8ml.

6.6 Special precautions for disposal and other handling

None.

7. MARKETING AUTHORISATION HOLDER

Pharmacia Limited

Ransgate Road

Sandwich

Kent CT13 9NJ

UK

8. MARKETING AUTHORISATION NUMBER(S)

PL 00032/0421

9. DATE OF FIRST AUTHORISATION/RENEWAL OF THE AUTHORISATION

13 August 2003

10. DATE OF REVISION OF THE TEXT

July 2007

11. LEGAL CATEGORY

POM

Company Ref: SL2_0

Syndol Caplets

(SSL International plc)

1. NAME OF THE MEDICINAL PRODUCT

Syndol Caplets.

2. QUALITATIVE AND QUANTITATIVE COMPOSITION

Paracetamol BP 450.0mg, Codeine Phosphate BP 10.0mg, Doxylamine Succinate NF 5.0mg, Caffeine BP 30.0mg.

3. PHARMACEUTICAL FORM

Tablets.

4. CLINICAL PARTICULARS

4.1 Therapeutic indications

For the treatment of mild to moderate pain and as an antipyretic. Syndol Caplets are recommended for the symptomatic relief of headache, including muscle contraction or tension headache, migraine, neuralgia, toothache, sore throat, dysmenorrhoea, muscular and rheumatic aches and pains and for post-operative analgesia following surgical or dental procedures.

4.2 Posology and method of administration

For oral administration. Adults and children over 12 years: 1 or 2 tablets every four to six hours as needed for relief. Total dosage over a 24 hour period should not normally exceed 8 tablets. Do not take for more than three days continuously without medical review.

Codeine should be used with caution in the elderly and debilitated patients, as they may be more susceptible to the respiratory depressant effects.

4.3 Contraindications

Hypersensitivity to paracetamol, codeine or other opioid analgesics, or any of the other constituents.

4.4 Special warnings and precautions for use

Do not exceed the stated dose. Do not take concurrently with any other paracetamol or codeine containing compounds. Keep out of the reach of children. Care is advised in the administration of this preparation to patients with impaired kidney or liver function and in those with hypertension, hypothyroidism, adrenocortical insufficiency, prostatic hypertrophy, shock, obstructive bowel disorders, acute abdominal conditions, recent gastrointestinal surgery, gallstones, myasthenia gravis, a history of cardiac arrhythmias or convulsions and in patients with a history of drug abuse or emotional instability.

Codeine may induce faecal impaction, producing incontinence, spurious diarrhoea, abdominal pain and rarely colonic obstruction. Elderly patients may metabolise or eliminate opioid analgesics more slowly than younger adults.

The leaflet will state in a prominent position in the before taking section:

If you need to use this medicine for more than three days at a time, see your doctor, pharmacist or healthcare professional. Taking codeine regularly for a long time can lead to addiction, which might cause you to feel restless and irritable when you stop taking the tablets. Taking a painkiller for headaches too often or for too long can make them worse.

The label will state (to be displayed prominently on outer pack, not boxed):

If you need to use this medicine for more than three days at a time, see your doctor or pharmacist. Taking codeine regularly for a long time can lead to addiction. Taking a painkiller for headaches too often or for too long can make them worse.

4.5 Interaction with other medicinal products and other forms of interaction

The speed of absorption of paracetamol may be increased by metoclopramide or domperidone and absorption reduced by cholestyramine. The anticoagulant effect of warfarin and other coumarins may be enhanced by prolonged regular daily use of paracetamol with increased risk of bleeding; occasional doses have no significant effect.

The depressant effects of codeine are enhanced by depressants of the central nervous system such as alcohol, anaesthetics, hypnotics, sedatives, tricyclic antidepressants and phenothiazines. The hypotensive actions of diuretics and anti hypertensive agents may be potentiated when used concurrently with opioid analgesics. Concurrent use of hydroxyzine with codeine may result in increased analgesia as well as increased CNS depressant and hypotensive effects. Concurrent use of codeine with antidiarrhoeal and antiperistaltic agents such as loperamide and kaolin may increase the risk of severe constipation. Concomitant use of antimuscarinics or medications with antimuscarinic action may result in an increased risk of severe constipation that may lead to paralytic ileus and/or urinary retention. The respiratory depressant effect caused by neuromuscular blocking agents may be additive to the central respiratory depressant effects of opioid analgesics. CNS depression or excitation may occur if codeine is given to patients receiving monoamine oxidase inhibitors, or within two weeks of stopping treatment with them. Quinidine can inhibit the analgesic effect of codeine. Codeine may delay the absorption of mexiletine and thus reduce the antiarrhythmic effect of the latter. Codeine may antagonise the gastrointestinal effects of metoclopramide, cisapride and domperidone. Cimetidine inhibits the metabolism of opioid analgesics resulting in increased plasma concentrations. Naloxone antagonises the analgesic, CNS and respiratory depressant effects of opioid analgesics. Naltrexone also blocks the therapeutic effect of opioids.

Incompatibilities: Codeine has been reported to be incompatible with phenobarbitone sodium forming a codeine-phenobarbitone complex, and with potassium iodide, forming crystals of codeine periodide. Acetylation of codeine phosphate by aspirin has occurred in solid dosage forms containing the two drugs, even at low moisture levels.

Interference with laboratory tests: Opioid analgesics interfere with a number of laboratory tests including plasma amylase, lipase, bilirubin, alkaline phosphatase, lactate dehydrogenase, alanine aminotransferase and aspartate aminotransferase. Opioids may also interfere with gastric emptying studies as they delay gastric emptying and with hepatobiliary imaging-using technetium Tc 99m disofenin as opioid treatment may cause constriction of the sphincter of Oddi and increase biliary tract pressure.

4.6 Pregnancy and lactation

Epidemiological studies in human pregnancy have shown no ill effects due to paracetamol used in the recommended dosage, but patients should follow the advice of their doctor regarding its use. Codeine crosses the placenta. There is no adequate evidence of safety in human pregnancy and a possible association with respiratory and cardiac malformations has been reported. Regular use during pregnancy may cause physical dependence in the foetus leading to withdrawal symptoms in the neonate. Use during pregnancy should be avoided if possible.

Use of opioid analgesia during labour may cause respiratory depression in the neonate, especially the premature neonate. These agents should not be given during the delivery of a premature baby.

Codeine passes into breast milk in very small amounts that are considered to be compatible with breast feeding.

4.7 Effects on ability to drive and use machines

Not applicable.

4.8 Undesirable effects

Doxylamine succinate may cause drowsiness or dizziness in some patients.

Adverse effects of paracetamol are rare but hypersensitivity including skin rash may occur. There have been a few reports of blood dyscrasias including thrombocytopenia and agranulocytosis but these were not necessarily causally related to paracetamol.

The most frequent undesirable effects of codeine are constipation and drowsiness. Less frequent effects are nausea, vomiting, sweating, facial flushing, dry mouth, blurred or double vision, dizziness, orthostatic hypotension, malaise, tiredness, headache, anorexia, vertigo, bradycardia, palpitations, respiratory depression, dyspnoea, allergic reactions (itch, skin rash, facial oedema) and difficulties in micturition (dysuria, increased frequency, decrease in amount). Side effects that occur rarely include convulsions, hallucinations, nightmares, uncontrolled muscle movements, muscle rigidity, mental depression and stomach cramps.

Regular prolonged use of codeine is known to lead to addiction and symptoms of restlessness and irritability may result when treatment is stopped. Prolonged use of a painkiller for headaches can make them worse.

4.9 Overdose

Symptoms of overdose in the first 24 hours are pallor, nausea, vomiting, anorexia, and abdominal pain. Liver damage may become apparent 12 to 48 hours after ingestion. Abnormalities of glucose metabolism and metabolic acidosis may occur. In severe poisoning, hepatic failure may progress to encephalopathy, coma and death. Acute renal failure with acute tubular necrosis may develop even in the absence of severe liver damage. Cardiac arrhythmias and pancreatitis have been reported. Liver damage is possible in adults who have taken 10g or more of paracetamol. It is considered that excess quantities of a toxic metabolite (usually adequately detoxified by glutathione when normal doses of paracetamol are ingested) become irreversibly bound to liver tissue. Immediate treatment is essential in the management of a paracetamol overdose. Despite a lack of significant early symptoms, patients should be referred to hospital urgently for immediate medical attention and any patient who has ingested around 7.5g or more of paracetamol in the preceding 4 hours should undergo gastric lavage. Administration of oral methionine or intravenous N-acetylcysteine which may have a beneficial effect up to at least 48 hours after the overdose, may be required. General supportive measures must be available.

While the dose of codeine phosphate in this preparation is relatively small and therefore less likely to prove a problem, symptoms of overdose include cold clammy skin, confusion, convulsions, dizziness, drowsiness, nervousness or restlessness, miosis, bradycardia, dyspnoea, unconsciousness and weakness. Codeine in large doses may produce respiratory depression, hypotension, circulatory failure and deepening coma. Death may occur from respiratory failure.

Initial treatment includes emptying the stomach by aspiration and lavage. Intensive support therapy may be required to correct respiratory failure and shock. In addition the specific narcotic antagonist, naloxone hydrochloride, may be used rapidly to counteract the severe respiratory depression and coma. A dose of 0.4-2 mg is given intravenously or intramuscularly to adults, this is repeated at intervals of 2-3 minutes; if necessary up to 10mg of naloxone may be given. In children doses of 5-10μg/kg body weight may be given intravenously or intramuscularly. Codeine is not dialysable.

5. PHARMACOLOGICAL PROPERTIES

5.1 Pharmacodynamic properties

Paracetamol - antipyretic, analgesic; codeine phosphate - analgesic; doxylamine succinate - antihistamine; caffeine - mild stimulant.

5.2 Pharmacokinetic properties

The pharmacokinetics of paracetamol, codeine phosphate and caffeine are widely published (see Goodman & Gilman's The Pharmacological Basis of Therapeutics, Seventh Edition, pp 693, 505 and 596 respectively). Doxylamine succinate is readily absorbed from the gastrointestinal tract. Following oral administration, the effects start within 15 to 30 minutes and peak within one hour. In humans, 60-80% of doxylamine given has been recovered in urine at 24 hours post-dose.

5.3 Preclinical safety data

None stated.

6. PHARMACEUTICAL PARTICULARS

6.1 List of excipients

Tablet Core: Povidone; Croscarmellose Sodium; Corn Starch; Magnesium Stearate; Talc; Purified water.

Coating: Opadry II Yellow (Lactose Monohydrate; Hydroxypropyl Methyl Cellulose (Methocel E15); Polyethylene Glycol 4000; Quinoline Yellow Aluminium Lake (E104); Sunset Yellow Aluminium Lake (E110); Titanium Dioxide)

6.2 Incompatibilities

Not applicable.

6.3 Shelf life

60 months.

6.4 Special precautions for storage

None stated.

6.5 Nature and contents of container

Blister strips: 250 micron PVC and aluminium foil 20 micron coated with a 15 micron PVC layer.

Blister strips are presented in cardboard cartons.

Pack sizes are 10,20 or 30 tablets.

6.6 Special precautions for disposal and other handling

None.

7. MARKETING AUTHORISATION HOLDER

Seton Products Limited, Tubiton House, Oldham, OL1 3HS

8. MARKETING AUTHORISATION NUMBER(S)

PL 11314/0122.

9. DATE OF FIRST AUTHORISATION/RENEWAL OF THE AUTHORISATION

16th January 1999.

10. DATE OF REVISION OF THE TEXT

October 2006

Syner-KINASE 10,000 IU, 25,000 IU, 100,000 IU, 250,000 IU, 500,000 IU, 1,000,000 IU

(Syner-Med (Pharmaceutical Products) Ltd)

1. NAME OF THE MEDICINAL PRODUCT

Syner-KINASE® 10,000 IU

Syner-KINASE® 25,000 IU

Syner-KINASE® 100,000 IU

Syner-KINASE® 250,000 IU

Syner-KINASE®500,000 IU

Syner-KINASE® 1,000,000 IU

Powder for solution for injection or infusion

2. QUALITATIVE AND QUANTITATIVE COMPOSITION

Each vial contains 10,000, 25,000, 100,000, 250,000, 500,000 or 1,000,000 IU of human urokinase.

For excipients, see 6.1.

3. PHARMACEUTICAL FORM

White powder for solution for injection or infusion.

4. CLINICAL PARTICULARS

4.1 Therapeutic indications

Syner-KINASE® is indicated for the lysis of blood clots in these conditions:

a) thrombosed intravascular catheters and cannulae that are blocked by fibrin clots.

b) thromboembolic occlusive vascular disease such as deep vein thrombosis, pulmonary embolism and peripheral vascular occlusion.

4.2 Posology and method of administration

Syner-KINASE® must be reconstituted before use with the correct volume of sterile physiological saline (not provided).

The route of administration is by direct intravenous injection or infusion. It must not be given as a subcutaneous or intramuscular injection.

Adults:

a) Thrombosed intravascular catheters and cannula

5,000 to 25,000 IU Syner-KINASE® should be dissolved in the volume of sterile physiological saline required to completely fill the lumen of the catheter or cannula and locked for a duration of 20 to 60 minutes. The lysate is then aspirated and the procedure repeated if necessary.

Alternatively, an infusion of up to 250,000 IU Syner-KINASE® can be administered into the catheter or cannula over a period of 90 to 180 minutes using a solution of 1,000 to 2,500 IU/ml in sterile physiological saline.

b) Thromboembolic occlusive vascular disease

Deep vein thrombosis: an initial loading dose of 4,400 IU/kg body weight dissolved in 15 ml sterile physiological saline infused over 10 minutes followed by 4,400 IU/kg/hour for 12-24 hours.

Pulmonary embolism: an initial loading dose of 4,400 IU/kg body weight dissolved in 15 ml sterile physiological saline infused over 10 minutes followed by 4,400 IU/kg/hour for 12 hours. Alternatively a bolus injection into the pulmonary artery repeated for up to 3 times in 24 hours may be used. An initial dosage of 15,000 IU/kg body weight may be adjusted if necessary for subsequent injections depending on the plasma fibrinogen concentration produced by the previous injection.

Peripheral vascular occlusion: infusion of a solution of 2,000 IU/ml (500,000 IU Syner-KINASE® dissolved in 250 ml sterile physiological saline) into the clot with angiographic monitoring of progress of treatment. It is recommended that the rate of infusion should be 4,000 IU/minute for 2 hours when angiography should be repeated. Following this, the catheter should be advanced into the occluded segment of vessel and Syner-KINASE® infused at the same rate of 4,000 IU/minute for another 2 hours. The process can be repeated up to 4 times if flow has not been achieved. Once a channel has been created through the blocked segment, the catheter may be withdrawn until it lies proximal to the remaining thrombus. Infusion should continue at the rate of 1,000 IU/minute until the clot has completely lysed. Usually, a dose of 500,000 IU over 8 hours should be sufficient. If the length of the clot has not been reduced by more than 25% after the initial dose of 500,000 IU and further reductions of 10% by subsequent infusions of 500,000 IU, discontinuation of treatment should be considered.

After fibrinolytic therapy has been completed, suitable anticoagulant therapy should be considered.

Elderly:

The initial dosage as in adults should be used but the dosage may be adjusted depending on response.

4.3 Contraindications

Hypersensitivity to urokinase or to any of the excipients. The risk of haemorrhage should be balanced against the dangers of untreated occlusion particularly in the situation of recent bleeding such as following: surgery, cerebrovascular bleeding, severe hypertension, pregnancy and the immediate post-partum period, severe hepatic or renal insufficiency unless the patient is receiving renal replacement therapy.

4.4 Special warnings and precautions for use

If bleeding occurs following systemic treatment with Syner-KINASE®, infusion should be stopped immediately. However, the risks of haemorrhage must be balanced against the risk of stopping treatment.

Care should be taken in patients known to have peptic ulcer disease or at risk of other gastrointestinal bleeding. Also due caution should be exercised in patients who have had recent repeated intravascular or intracardiac puncture as in those who have undergone recent cardio-pulmonary resuscitation.

4.5 Interaction with other medicinal products and other forms of interaction

Loss of activity of urokinase has been noted when dissolved in 5% glucose at a concentration of 1,500 IU/ml and stored in PVC containers. No information is available regarding other dilutions of urokinase.

4.6 Pregnancy and lactation

Syner-KINASE® should not be given during pregnancy or in the immediate post-partum period. Breast feeding should be avoided.

4.7 Effects on ability to drive and use machines

Not relevant.

4.8 Undesirable effects

Local sensations of warmth, dull ache or pain may be felt locally in the vessel being treated. Overt bleeding and haemorrhagic complications may occur. Pyrexia and haematuria have been reported.

Embolic episodes have been noted after fragments of clot have been released. Cholesterol embolism may occur.

Allergic reactions have been reported.

4.9 Overdose

Haemorrhage that occurs during treatment with Syner-KINASE® may be controlled with local pressure and treatment continued. If severe bleeding occurs, treatment with Syner-KINASE® must be stopped and inhibitors such as aprotinin, epsilon-amino caproic acid, p-aminoethylbenzoic acid or tranexamic acid can be given. In serious cases, human fibrinogen, Factor XII, packed red cells or whole blood should be given as appropriate. For correction of volume deficiency, dextrans should be avoided.

5. PHARMACOLOGICAL PROPERTIES

5.1 Pharmacodynamic properties

ATC code: B01A D04, antithrombotic agent.

Syner-KINASE® is a highly purified form of naturally occurring human urokinase extracted from urine. It is a thrombolytic agent which converts plasminogen into plasmin (fibrinolysin) a proteolytic enzyme that breaks down fibrin. As it is of human origin, it is not antigenic although allergic reactions have been reported following the use of urokinase.

5.2 Pharmacokinetic properties

Syner-KINASE® is eliminated rapidly from the circulation by the liver with a half-life of up to 20 minutes. Elimination is delayed in patients with liver disease and impaired kidney function.

5.3 Preclinical safety data

There is no pre-clinical safety data of additional value to the prescribing physician.

6. PHARMACEUTICAL PARTICULARS

6.1 List of excipients

Mannitol

Disodium edetate

Disodium phosphate dodecahydrate

Sodium hydroxide

6.2 Incompatibilities

Syner-KINASE® should be reconstituted before use with sterile physiological saline. It has been reported to lose 15-20% of its activity in solutions of 5% glucose containing 1,500 units/ml in PVC containers. No information is available regarding other dilutions of urokinase.

Patel J P, *et al.* Activity of urokinase diluted in 0.9% sodium chloride injection or 5% dextrose injection and stored in glass or plastic syringes. *Am. J. Hosp. Pharm.* 1991; 48:1511-1514

6.3 Shelf life

10,000IU, 25,000IU, 100,000IU, 250,000IU and 500,000IU strengths – 3 Years

1,000,000IU strength – 2 Years

Use reconstituted material immediately

6.4 Special precautions for storage

Do not store above 25°C.

Keep the vial in the outer container to protect from light.

6.5 Nature and contents of container

All presentations are contained in borosilicate clear type 1 glass vials closed with chlorobutyl rubber stoppers and sealed with an aluminium flip-off cap.

6.6 Special precautions for disposal and other handling

No special requirements.

7. MARKETING AUTHORISATION HOLDER

Syner-Medica Ltd
2nd Floor, Beech House
840 Brighton Road
Purley
Surrey
CR8 2BH
Telephone No. 0845 634 2100
Fax No. 0845 634 2101

8. MARKETING AUTHORISATION NUMBER(S)

Syner-KINASE®	10,000 IU	MA20675/0006
Syner-KINASE®	25,000 IU	MA20675/0001
Syner-KINASE®	100,000 IU	MA20675/0002
Syner-KINASE®	250,000 IU	MA20675/0003
Syner-KINASE®	500,000 IU	MA20675/0004
Syner-KINASE®	1,000,000 IU	MA20675/0005

9. DATE OF FIRST AUTHORISATION/RENEWAL OF THE AUTHORISATION

Syner-KINASE® 25,000 IU, 100,000 IU, 250,000 IU, 500,000 IU and 1,000,000 IU: 21st September 2006

Syner-KINASE® 10,000 IU: 15th August 2008

10. DATE OF REVISION OF THE TEXT

June 2009

Marketing and Distribution

Syner-Med Pharmaceutical Products Ltd
2nd Floor, Beech House
840 Brighton Road
Purley
Surrey
CR8 2BH
United Kingdom
Tel: 0845 634 2100
Fax: 0845 634 2101
Email: mail@syner-medica.com

Syner-KINASE® is a registered trademark

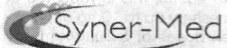

Syner-Med

Synflex 275mg Tablets

(Roche Products Limited)

1. NAME OF THE MEDICINAL PRODUCT

Synflex 275mg Tablets

2. QUALITATIVE AND QUANTITATIVE COMPOSITION

Each tablet contains 275mg naproxen sodium (equivalent to naproxen 250mg).

For excipients, see 6.1.

3. PHARMACEUTICAL FORM

Film-coated Tablet.

Oval, pale blue, opaque film-coated tablet, imprinted with 'NPS-275' on one side.

4. CLINICAL PARTICULARS

4.1 Therapeutic indications

Synflex is indicated for the treatment of musculoskeletal disorders (including sprains and strains, direct trauma, lumbo-sacral pain, cervical spondylitis, fibrositis, bursitis and tendinitis); uterine pain following IUCD insertion, post-operative (including orthopaedic) pain; post-partum pain, rheumatoid arthritis, osteoarthrosis, ankylosing spondylitis, acute gout and dysmenorrhoea.

Synflex is also indicated for the relief of migraine.

4.2 Posology and method of administration

For oral administration.

To be taken preferably with or after food.

Therapy should be started at the lowest recommended dose, especially in the elderly.

Undesirable effects may be minimised by using the lowest effective dose for the shortest duration necessary to control symptoms (see section 4.4).

Adults

For musculoskeletal disorders and post-operative pain, post IUCD insertion, rheumatoid arthritis, osteoarthrosis and ankylosing spondylitis the recommended dosage is 550mg twice daily, not more than 1100mg being taken per day.

For post-partum pain a single dose of 550mg is recommended.

For dysmenorrhoea and acute gout the recommended dosage is 550mg initially, followed by 275mg at 6 - 8 hour intervals as needed. This represents a maximum dose on the first day of 1375mg and 1100mg per day thereafter.

For the relief of migraine, the recommended dose is 825mg at the first symptom of an impending attack. 275 - 550mg can be taken in addition throughout the day, if necessary, but not before half an hour after the initial dose. A total dose of 1375mg per day should not be exceeded.

Elderly

Studies indicate that although the total plasma concentration of naproxen is unchanged, the unbound plasma fraction of naproxen is increased in the elderly. The implication of this finding for Synflex dosing is unknown. As with other drugs used in the elderly it is prudent to use the lowest effective dose and for the shortest possible duration as elderly patients are more prone to adverse events. The patient should be monitored regularly for GI bleeding during NSAID therapy. For the effect of reduced elimination in the elderly, refer to section 4.4.

Children

Synflex is not recommended for use in children under sixteen years of age.

Renal/hepatic impairment

A lower dose should be considered in patients with renal or hepatic impairment. Synflex is contraindicated in patients with baseline creatinine clearance less than 30 ml/minute because accumulation of naproxen metabolites has been seen in patients with severe renal failure or those on dialysis (see section 4.3).

Treatment should be reviewed at regular intervals and discontinued if no benefit is seen.

4.3 Contraindications

Active or history of peptic ulceration or active gastrointestinal bleeding (two or more distinct episodes of proven ulceration or bleeding). History of gastrointestinal bleeding or perforation, related to previous NSAIDs therapy.

Hypersensitivity to naproxen, naproxen sodium, or any of the excipients. Since the potential exists for cross-sensitivity reactions, Synflex should not be given to patients in whom aspirin or other non-steroidal anti-inflammatory/analgesic drugs induce asthma, rhinitis, nasal polyps or urticaria. These reactions have the potential of being fatal. Severe anaphylactic-like reactions to naproxen have been reported in such patients.

Severe renal, hepatic or heart failure.

Synflex is contraindicated during the last trimester of pregnancy (see Section 4.6).

4.4 Special warnings and precautions for use

Undesirable effects may be minimised by using the lowest effective dose for the shortest duration necessary to control symptoms (see section 4.2 and GI and cardiovascular risks below). Patients treated with non-steroidal drugs long-term should undergo regular supervision to monitor for adverse events.

Elderly and/or debilitated patients are particularly susceptible to the adverse events of NSAIDS, especially gastro-intestinal bleeding and perforation, which may be fatal. Prolonged use of NSAIDs in these patients is not recommended. Where prolonged therapy is required, patients should be reviewed regularly.

The antipyretic and anti-inflammatory activities of Synflex may reduce fever and inflammation, thereby diminishing their usefulness as diagnostic signs.

Bronchospasm may be precipitated in patients suffering from, or with a history of, bronchial asthma or allergic disease.

As with other non-steroidal anti-inflammatory drugs, elevations of one or more liver function tests may occur. Hepatic abnormalities may be the result of hypersensitivity rather than direct toxicity. Severe hepatic reactions, including jaundice and hepatitis (some cases of hepatitis have been fatal) have been reported with this drug as with other non-steroidal anti-inflammatory drugs. Cross reactivity has been reported.

Naproxen decreases platelet aggregation and prolongs bleeding time. This effect should be kept in mind when bleeding times are determined.

Although sodium retention has not been reported in metabolic studies, it is possible that patients with questionable or compromised cardiac function may be at a greater risk when taking Synflex.

Each Synflex tablet contains approximately 25mg of sodium (about 1m Eq), so the total amount of sodium ingested with the maximum recommended daily dose is 125mg, about 16% of the 800mg of sodium permitted on a severely sodium-restricted diet. This should be considered in patients whose overall intake of sodium must be markedly restricted.

Gastrointestinal bleeding, ulceration and perforation

GI bleeding, ulceration or perforation, which can be fatal, has been reported with all NSAIDs at anytime during treatment, with or without warning symptoms or a previous history of serious GI events.

The risk of GI bleeding, ulceration or perforation is higher with increasing NSAID doses, in patients with a history of ulcer, particularly if complicated with haemorrhage or perforation (see section 4.3), and in the elderly. These patients should commence treatment on the lowest dose available. Combination therapy with protective agents (e.g. misoprostol or proton pump inhibitors) should be considered for these patients, and also for patients requiring concomitant low dose aspirin, or other drugs likely to increase gastrointestinal risk (see section 4.5).

Patients with a history of GI toxicity, particularly when elderly, should report any unusual abdominal symptoms (especially GI bleeding) particularly in the initial stages of treatment.

Caution should be advised in patients receiving concomitant medications which could increase the risk of ulceration or bleeding, such as oral corticosteroid, anticoagulants such as warfarin, selective serotonin-reuptake inhibitors or anti-platelet agents such as aspirin (see Section 4.5).

When GI bleeding or ulceration occurs in patients receiving Synflex, the treatment should be withdrawn.

NSAIDs should be given with care to patients with a history of gastrointestinal disease (ulcerative colitis, Crohn's disease) as these conditions may be exacerbated (see section 4.8)

Renal Effects

There have been reports of impaired renal function, renal failure, acute interstitial nephritis, haematuria, proteinuria, renal papillary necrosis and occasionally nephrotic syndrome associated with Synflex.

Renal failure linked to reduced prostaglandin production

The administration of an NSAID may cause a dose dependent reduction in prostaglandin formation and precipitate renal failure. Patients at greatest risk of this reaction are those with impaired renal function, cardiac impairment, liver dysfunction, those taking diuretics and the elderly. Renal function should be monitored in these patients (see also section 4.3).

Use in patients with impaired renal function

As naproxen is eliminated to a large extent (95%) by urinary excretion via glomerular filtration, it should be used with great caution in patients with impaired renal function and the monitoring of serum creatinine and/or creatinine clearance is advised in these patients. Synflex is contraindicated in patients having baseline creatinine clearance of less than 30 ml/minute.

Haemodialysis does not decrease the plasma concentration of naproxen because of the high degree of protein binding.

Certain patients, specifically those whose renal blood flow is compromised, such as in extracellular volume depletion, cirrhosis of the liver, sodium restriction, congestive heart failure, and pre-existing renal disease, should have renal function assessed before and during Synflex therapy. Some elderly patients in whom impaired renal function may be expected, as well as patients using diuretics, may also fall within this category. A reduction in daily dosage should be considered to avoid the possibility of excessive accumulation of naproxen metabolites in these patients.

Use in patients with impaired liver function

Chronic alcoholic liver disease and probably also other forms of cirrhosis reduce the total plasma concentration of naproxen, but the plasma concentration of unbound naproxen is increased. The implication of this finding for Synflex dosing is unknown but it is prudent to use the lowest effective dose.

Haematological

Patients who have coagulation disorders or are receiving drug therapy that interferes with haemostasis should be carefully observed if naproxen-containing products are administered.

Patients at high risk of bleeding or those on full anticoagulation therapy (e.g. dicoumarol derivatives) may be at increased risk of bleeding if given naproxen-containing products concurrently.

Anaphylactic (anaphylactoid) reactions

Hypersensitivity reactions may occur in susceptible individuals. Anaphylactic (anaphylactoid) reactions may occur both in patients with and without a history of hypersensitivity or exposure to aspirin, other non-steroidal anti-inflammatory drugs or naproxen-containing products. They may also occur in individuals with a history of angio-oedema, bronchospastic reactivity (e.g. asthma), rhinitis and nasal polyps.

Anaphylactoid reactions, like anaphylaxis, may have a fatal outcome.

Steroids

If steroid dosage is reduced or eliminated during therapy, the steroid dosage should be reduced slowly and the patients must be observed closely for any evidence of adverse effects, including adrenal insufficiency and exacerbation of symptoms of arthritis.

Ocular effects

Studies have not shown changes in the eye attributable to naproxen administration. In rare cases, adverse ocular disorders including papillitis, retrobulbar optic neuritis and papilloedema, have been reported in users of NSAIDs including naproxen, although a cause-and-effect relationship cannot be established; accordingly, patients who develop visual disturbances during treatment with naproxen-containing products should have an ophthalmological examination.

Cardiovascular and cerebrovascular effects

Appropriate monitoring and advice are required for patients with a history of hypertension and/or mild to moderate congestive heart failure as fluid retention and oedema have been reported in association with NSAID therapy.

Clinical trial and epidemiological data suggest that use of coxibs and some NSAIDs (particularly at high doses and in long term treatment) may be associated with a small increased risk of arterial thrombotic events (for example myocardial infarction or stroke). Although data suggest that the use of naproxen (1000mg daily) may be associated with a lower risk, some risk cannot be excluded.

Patients with uncontrolled hypertension, congestive heart failure, established ischaemic heart disease, peripheral arterial disease, and/or cerebrovascular disease should only be treated with naproxen after careful consideration. Similar consideration should be made before initiating longer-term treatment of patients with risk factors for cardiovascular events (e.g. hypertension, hyperlipidaemia, diabetes mellitus, smoking).

SLE and mixed connective tissue disease

In patients with systemic lupus erythematosus (SLE) and mixed connective tissue disorders there may be an increased risk of aseptic meningitis (see section 4.8).

Dermatological

Serious skin reactions, some of them fatal, including exfoliative dermatitis, Stevens-Johnson syndrome, and toxic epidermal necrolysis, have been reported very rarely in association with the use of NSAIDs (see 4.8). Patients appear to be at highest risk for these reactions early in the course of therapy: the onset of the reactions occurring in the majority of cases within the first month of treatment. Synflex should be discontinued at the first appearance of skin rash, mucosal lesions, or any other sign of hypersensitivity.

Precautions related to fertility

The use of naproxen, as with any drug known to inhibit cyclooxygenase/prostaglandin synthesis, may impair fertility and is not recommended in women attempting to conceive. In women who have difficulty conceiving or are undergoing investigation of infertility, withdrawal of naproxen should be considered.

Combination with other NSAIDs

The combination of naproxen-containing products and other NSAIDs, including cyclooxygenase-2 selective inhibitors, is not recommended, because of the cumulative risks of inducing serious NSAID-related adverse events.

4.5 Interaction with other medicinal products and other forms of interaction

It is considered unsafe to take NSAIDs in combination with anti-coagulants such as warfarin or heparin unless under direct medical supervision, as NSAIDs may enhance the effects of anti-coagulants (see section 4.4).

Other analgesics including cyclooxygenase-2 selective inhibitors: Avoid concomitant use of two or more NSAIDs (including aspirin) as this may increase the risk of adverse effects (see section 4.4).

Concomitant administration of antacid or colestyramine can delay the absorption of naproxen but does not affect its extent. Concomitant administration of food can delay the absorption of naproxen, but does not affect its extent.

Due to the high plasma protein binding of naproxen, patients simultaneously receiving hydantoins, anti-coagulants, other NSAIDS, aspirin or a highly protein-bound sulfonamide should be observed for signs of overdosage of these drugs. Patients simultaneously receiving Synflex and a hydantoin, sulphonamide or sulphonylurea should be observed for adjustment of dose if required. No interactions have been observed in clinical studies with naproxen sodium or naproxen and anti-coagulants or sulfonylureas, but caution is nevertheless advised since interaction has been seen with other non-steroidal agents of this class.

Caution is advised when Synflex is co-administered with diuretics as there can be a decreased diuretic effect. The natriuretic effect of furosemide has been reported to be inhibited by some drugs of this class. Diuretics can increase the risk of nephrotoxicity of NSAIDs

Inhibition of renal lithium clearance leading to increases in plasma lithium concentrations has also been reported.

Naproxen and other non-steroidal anti-inflammatory drugs can reduce the anti-hypertensive effect of anti-hypertensives and may increase the risk of renal impairment associated with the use of ACE-inhibitors.

Probenecid given concurrently increases naproxen plasma levels and extends its half-life considerably.

Caution is advised where methotrexate is given concurrently because of possible enhancement of its toxicity since naproxen, among other non-steroidal anti-inflammatory drugs, has been reported to reduce the tubular secretion of methotrexate in an animal model.

NSAIDs may exacerbate cardiac failure, reduce GFR and increase plasma cardiac glycoside levels when co-administered with cardiac glycosides.

As with all NSAIDs caution is advised when ciclosporin is co-administered because of the increased risk of nephrotoxicity.

NSAIDs should not be used for 8 - 12 days after mifepristone administration as NSAIDs can reduce the effects of mifepristone.

As with all NSAIDs, caution should be taken when co-administering with corticosteroids because of the increased risk of gastrointestinal ulceration or bleeding.

Animal data indicate that NSAIDs can increase the risk of convulsions associated with quinolone antibiotics. Patients taking quinolones may have an increased risk of developing convulsions.

There is an increased risk of gastrointestinal bleeding (see section 4.4) when anti-platelet agents and selective serotonin reuptake inhibitors (SSRIs) are combined with NSAIDs.

There is a possible risk of nephrotoxicity when NSAIDs are given with tacrolimus.

There is an increased risk of haematological toxicity when NSAIDs are given with zidovudine. There is evidence of an increased risk of haemarthroses and haematoma in HIV(+) haemophiliacs receiving concurrent treatment with zidovudine and ibuprofen.

It is suggested that Synflex therapy be temporarily discontinued 48 hours before adrenal function tests are performed because naproxen may artifactually interfere with some tests for 17-ketogenic steroids. Similarly, naproxen may interfere with some assays of urinary 5-hydroxyindoleacetic acid.

4.6 Pregnancy and lactation

Pregnancy

Congenital abnormalities have been reported in association with NSAID administration in man; however, these are low in frequency and do not appear to follow any discernible pattern. As with other drugs of this type, naproxen produces delay in parturition in animals and also affects the human foetal cardiovascular system (closure of ductus arteriosus). Use of Synflex in the last trimester of pregnancy is contraindicated (see section 4.3). NSAIDS should not be used during the first two trimesters of pregnancy, unless the potential benefit to the patient outweighs the potential risk to the foetus.

Labour and delivery

Naproxen containing products are not recommended in labour and delivery because, through its prostaglandin synthesis inhibitory effect, naproxen may adversely affect foetal circulation and inhibit contractions, with an increased bleeding tendency in both mother and child.

Nursing mothers

Naproxen has been found in the milk of lactating women. The use of Synflex should be avoided in patients who are breast-feeding.

See section 4.4 regarding female fertility.

4.7 Effects on ability to drive and use machines

Some patients may experience drowsiness, dizziness, vertigo, insomnia, fatigue, visual disturbances or depression with the use of Synflex. If patients experience these or similar undesirable effects, they should not drive or operate machinery.

4.8 Undesirable effects

The following adverse events have been reported with NSAIDs and with naproxen.

Gastrointestinal disorders: The most commonly observed adverse events are gastrointestinal in nature. Heartburn, nausea, vomiting, constipation, diarrhoea, flatulence, dyspepsia, abdominal discomfort and epigastric distress. More serious reactions which may occur are gastro-intestinal bleeding, which is sometimes fatal, particularly in the elderly (see section 4.4), peptic ulceration, perforation, non-peptic gastro-intestinal ulceration, melaena, haematemesis, stomatitis, ulcerative stomatitis, exacerbation of ulcerative colitis and Crohn's disease (see section 4.4), oesophagitis, gastritis and pancreatitis.

Blood and lymphatic system disorders: Neutropenia, thrombocytopenia, granulocytopenia including agranulocytosis, eosinophilia, leucopenia, aplastic anaemia and haemolytic anaemia.

Immune system disorders: Hypersensitivity reactions have been reported following treatment with NSAIDs in patients with, or without, a history of previous hypersensitivity reactions to NSAIDs. These may consist of (a) non-specific allergic reactions and anaphylaxis (b) respiratory tract reactivity comprising asthma, aggravated asthma, bronchospasm or dyspnoea, or (c) assorted skin disorders, including rashes of various types, pruritus, urticaria, purpura, angio-oedema and more rarely exfoliative and bullous dermatoses (including epidermal necrolysis and erythema multiforme).

Table 1

Parameter	2 × 275mg Naproxen-Na tablet	2 × 250mg Naproxen tablet	p. value
Biol T1/2 (hrs)	13.41	13.43	0.993
T max (min)	56.67	110.0	0.036
Cp max (mcg/ml)	74.67	65.58	0.007
AUC Total (mcg/ml × hr)	1050.9	1006.1	0.478

Metabolic and nutrition disorders: hyperkalaemia.

Psychiatric disorders: Insomnia, dream abnormalities, depression, confusion and hallucinations.

Nervous system disorders: Convulsions, dizziness, headache, lightheadedness, drowsiness, paraesthesia, retrobulbar optic neuritis, inability to concentrate and cognitive dysfunction have been reported. Aseptic meningitis (especially in patients with existing auto-immune disorders, such as systemic lupus erythematosus, mixed connective tissue disease), with symptoms such as stiff neck, headache, nausea, vomiting, fever or disorientation (see section 4.4).

Eye Disorders: Visual disturbances, corneal opacity, papillitis and papilloedema.

Ear and Labyrinth disorders: Tinnitus, hearing disturbances including impairment and vertigo.

Cardiac disorders: Oedema, palpitations, cardiac failure and congestive heart failure have been reported.

Clinical trial and epidemiological data suggest that use of coxibs and some NSAIDs (particularly at high doses and in long term treatment) may be associated with a small increased risk of arterial thrombotic events (for example myocardial infarction or stroke) (see section 4.4).

Vascular disorders: Hypertension, vasculitis.

Respiratory, thoracic and mediastinal disorders: Dyspnoea, asthma, eosinophilic pneumonitis and pulmonary oedema.

Hepatobiliary disorders: Jaundice, fatal hepatitis and abnormal liver function tests.

Skin and subcutaneous tissue disorders: Skin rashes including fixed drug eruption, itching (pruritus), urticaria, ecchymoses, purpura, sweating. Alopecia, erythema multiforme, Stevens Johnson syndrome, erythema nodosum, lichen planus, pustular reaction, SLE, epidermal necrolysis, very rarely toxic epidermal necrolysis, photosensitivity reactions (including cases in which skin resembles porphyria cutanea tarda "pseudoporphyria") or epidermolysis bullosa-like reactions which may occur rarely.

If skin fragility, blistering or other symptoms suggestive of pseudoporphyria occur, treatment should be discontinued and the patient monitored.

Musculoskeletal and connective tissue disorders: Myalgia and muscle weakness.

Renal and urinary disorders: Including, but not limited to, glomerular nephritis, interstitial nephritis, nephrotic syndrome, haematuria, raised serum creatinine, renal papillary necrosis and renal failure.

Reproductive system and breast disorders: Female infertility.

General disorders and administration site conditions: Thirst, pyrexia, fatigue and malaise.

4.9 Overdose

Symptoms include headache, heartburn, nausea, vomiting, epigastric pain, gastrointestinal bleeding, rarely diarrhoea, disorientation, excitation, drowsiness, dizziness, tinnitus, fainting. In cases of significant poisoning acute renal failure and liver damage are possible.

Respiratory depression and coma may occur after the ingestion of NSAIDs but are rare.

In one case of naproxen overdose, transient prolongation of the prothrombin time due to hypothrombinaemia may have been due to selective inhibition of the synthesis of vitamin-K dependent clotting factors.

A few patients have experienced seizures, but it is not clear whether these were naproxen-related or not. It is not known what dose of the drug would be life-threatening.

Patients should be treated symptomatically as required. Within one hour of ingestion of a potentially toxic amount activated charcoal should be considered. Alternatively in adults gastric lavage should be considered within one hour of ingestion of a potentially life-threatening overdose.

Good urine output should be ensured.

Renal and liver function should be closely monitored.

Patients should be observed for at least four hours after ingestion of potentially toxic amounts.

Frequent or prolonged convulsions should be treated with intravenous diazepam.

Other measures may be indicated by the patient's clinical condition.

Haemodialysis does not decrease the plasma concentration of naproxen because of the high degree of protein binding. However, haemodialysis may still be appropriate in a patient with renal failure who has taken Synflex.

5. PHARMACOLOGICAL PROPERTIES

5.1 Pharmacodynamic properties

Synflex is a non-steroidal, anti-inflammatory agent. It has analgesic, anti-inflammatory and antipyretic properties.

5.2 Pharmacokinetic properties

The sodium salt of naproxen is absorbed more rapidly than naproxen leading to earlier and higher plasma levels of naproxen. This is particularly useful for analgesia, where early availability of the drug in circulation is advantageous.

Typical pharmacokinetic values for naproxen sodium and naproxen are as follows:

(see Table 1 above)

See also *Special warnings and special precautions for use* for certain patients, i.e. the elderly and those with impaired renal or liver function.

5.3 Preclinical safety data

Carcinogenicity

Naproxen was administered with food to Sprague-Dawley rats for 24 months at doses of 8, 16 and 24mg/kg/day. Naproxen was not carcinogenic in rats.

Mutagenicity

Mutagenicity was not seet in *Salmonella typhimurium* (5 cell lines), *Sachharomyces cerevisisae* (1 cell line), and mouse lymphoma tests.

Fertility

Naproxen did not affect the fertility of rats when administered orally at doses of 30mg/kg/day to males and 20mg/kg/day to females.

Teratogenicity

Naproxen was not teratogenic when administered orally at does of 20mg/kg/day during organogenesis to rats and rabbits.

Perinatal/Postnatal Reproduction

Oral administration of naproxen to pregnant rats at doses of 2, 10 and 20mg/kg/day during the third trimester of pregnancy resulted in difficult labour. These are know effects of this class of compounds and were demonstrated in pregnant rats with aspirin and indometacin.

6. PHARMACEUTICAL PARTICULARS

6.1 List of excipients

Tablet core

Povidone

Magnesium stearate

Microcrystalline cellulose

Talc,

Printing ink

Hypromellose

Titanium dioxide (E171)

Macrogol

FD&C blue no. 2 - aluminium lake (E132)

6.2 Incompatibilities

None stated.

6.3 Shelf life

5 years.

6.4 Special precautions for storage

Containers: Keep the container tightly closed.
Store in the original package.

Blisters: Store in the original package.
Keep blister in the outer carton.

6.5 Nature and contents of container

a. Opaque high density polyethylene container containing 100 tablets.

b. PVC/foil blister pack containing 60 tablets.

c. Polypropylene securitainers with high density polyethylene lid containing 2 or 4 tablets.

6.6 Special precautions for disposal and other handling

None stated.

Administrative Data

7. MARKETING AUTHORISATION HOLDER

Roche Products Limited
6 Falcon Way
Shire Park
Welwyn Garden City
AL7 1TW
United Kingdom

8. MARKETING AUTHORISATION NUMBER(S)

PL 00031/0478

9. DATE OF FIRST AUTHORISATION/RENEWAL OF THE AUTHORISATION

09 February 2009

10. DATE OF REVISION OF THE TEXT

February 2009

LEGAL STATUS

POM

Synflex is a registered trade mark Item Code

Synphase Tablets

(Pharmacia Limited)

1. NAME OF THE MEDICINAL PRODUCT

Synphase.

2. QUALITATIVE AND QUANTITATIVE COMPOSITION

Synphase consists of 7 blue tablets containing norethisterone 500 micrograms and ethinylestradiol 35 micrograms, marked 'BX' on one side and 'SEARLE' on the other; 9 white tablets containing norethisterone 1.0 milligram and ethinylestradiol 35 micrograms inscribed 'SEARLE' on one face and 'BX' on the other; 5 blue tablets containing norethisterone 500 micrograms and ethinylestradiol 35 micrograms, marked 'BX' on one side and 'SEARLE' on the other.

3. PHARMACEUTICAL FORM

Tablets for oral administration.

4. CLINICAL PARTICULARS

4.1 Therapeutic indications

Synphase is indicated for oral contraception, with the benefit of a low intake of oestrogen.

4.2 Posology and method of administration

Oral Administration: The dosage of Synphase for the initial cycle of therapy is 1 tablet taken at the same time each day from the first day of the menstrual cycle. For subsequent cycles, no tablets are taken for 7 days, then a new course is started of 1 tablet daily for the next 21 days. This sequence of 21 days on treatment, seven days off treatment is repeated for as long as contraception is required.

Patients unable to start taking Synphase tablets on the first day of the menstrual cycle may start treatment on any day up to and including the 5th day of the menstrual cycle.

Patients starting on day 1 of their period will be protected at once. Those patients delaying therapy up to day 5 may not be protected immediately and it is recommended that another method of contraception is used for the first 7 days of tablet-taking. Suitable methods are condoms, caps plus spermicides and intra-uterine devices.

The rhythm, temperature and cervical-mucus methods should not be relied upon.

Tablet omissions

Tablets must be taken daily in order to maintain adequate hormone levels and contraceptive efficacy.

If a tablet is missed within 12 hours of the correct dosage time then the missed tablet should be taken as soon as possible, even if this means taking 2 tablets on the same day, this will ensure that contraceptive protection is maintained. If one or more tablets are missed for more than 12 hours from the correct dosage time it is recommended that the patient takes the last missed tablet as soon as possible and then continues to take the rest of the tablets in the normal manner. In addition, it is recommended that extra contraceptive protection, such as a condom, is used for the next 7 days.

Patients who have missed one or more of the last 7 tablets in a pack should be advised to start the next pack of tablets as soon as the present one has finished (i.e. without the normal seven day gap between treatments). This reduces the risk of contraceptive failure resulting from tablets being missed close to a 7 day tablet free period.

Changing from another oral contraceptive

In order to ensure that contraception is maintained it is advised that the first dose of Synphase tablets is taken on the day immediately after the patient has finished the previous pack of tablets.

Use after childbirth, miscarriage or abortion

Providing the patient is not breast feeding the first dose of Synphase tablets should be taken on the 21st day after childbirth. This will ensure the patient is protected immediately. If there is any delay in taking the first dose, contraception may not be established until 7 days after the first tablet has been taken. In these circumstances patients should be advised that extra contraceptive methods will be necessary.

After a miscarriage or abortion patients can take the first dose of Synphase tablets on the next day; in this way they will be protected immediately.

Figure 1 Estimated cumulative numbers of breast cancers per 10,000 women diagnosed in 5 years of use and up to 10 years after stopping COCs, compared with numbers of breast cancers diagnosed in 10,000 women who had never used COCs.

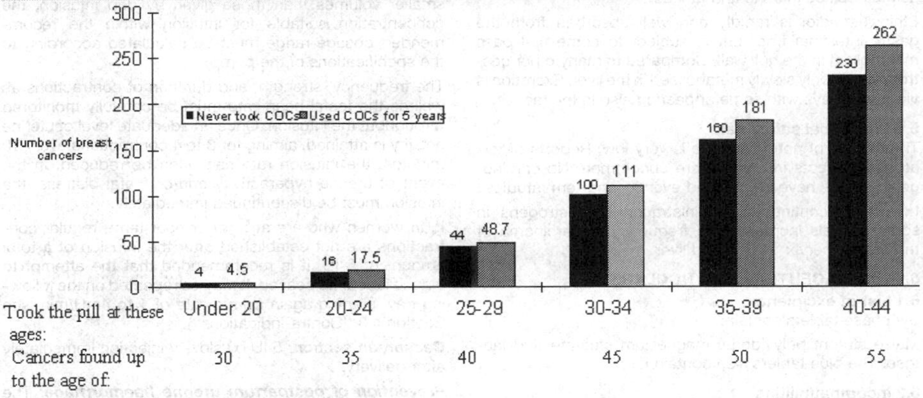

4.3 Contraindications

As with all combined progestogen/oestrogen oral contraceptives, the following conditions should be regarded as contra-indications:

i. History of confirmed venous thromboembolic disease (VTE), family history of idiopathic VTE and other known risk factors of VTE

ii. Thrombophlebitis, cerebrovascular disorders, coronary artery disease, myocardial infarction, angina, hyperlipidaemia or a history of these conditions.

iii. Acute or severe chronic liver disease, including liver tumours, Dubin-Johnson or Rotor syndrome.

iv. History during pregnancy of idiopathic jaundice, severe pruritus or pemphigoid gestationis.

v. Known or suspected breast or genital cancer.

vi. Known or suspected oestrogen-dependent neoplasia.

vii. Undiagnosed abnormal vaginal bleeding.

viii. A history of migraines classified as classical, focal or crescendo.

ix. Pregnancy.

4.4 Special warnings and precautions for use

Assessment of women prior to starting oral contraceptives (and at regular intervals thereafter) should include a personal and family medical history of each woman. Physical examination should be guided by this and by the contraindications (section 4.3) and warnings (section 4.4) for this product. The frequency and nature of these assessments should be based upon relevant guidelines and should be adapted to the individual woman, but should include measurement of blood pressure and, if judged appropriate by the clinician, breast, abdominal and pelvic examination including cervical cytology.

Women taking oral contraceptives require careful observation if they have or have had any of the following conditions: breast nodules; fibrocystic disease of the breast or an abnormal mammogram; uterine fibroids; a history of severe depressive states; varicose veins; sickle-cell anaemia; diabetes; hypertension; cardiovascular disease; migraine; epilepsy; asthma; otosclerosis; multiple sclerosis; porphyria; tetany; disturbed liver functions; gallstones; kidney disease; chloasma; any condition that is likely to worsen during pregnancy. The worsening or first appearance of any of these conditions may indicate that the oral contraceptive should be stopped. Discontinue treatment if there is a gradual or sudden, partial or complete loss of vision or any evidence of ocular changes, onset or aggravation of migraine or development of headache of a new kind which is recurrent, persistent or severe.

Gastro-intestinal upsets, such as vomiting and diarrhoea, may interfere with the absorption of the tablets leading to a reduction in contraceptive efficacy. Patients should continue to take Synphase, but they should also be encouraged to use another contraceptive method during the period of gastro-intestinal upset and for the next 7 days.

Progestogen oestrogen preparations should be used with caution in patients with a history of hepatic dysfunction or hypertension.

An increased risk of venous thromboembolic disease (VTE) associated with the use of oral contraceptives is well established but is smaller than that associated with pregnancy, which has been estimated at 60 cases per 100,000 pregnancies. Some epidemiological studies have reported a greater risk of VTE for women using combined oral contraceptives containing desogestrel or gestodene (the so-called 'third generation' pills) than for women using pills containing levonorgestrel or norethisterone (the so-called 'second generation' pills)

The spontaneous incidence of VTE in healthy non-pregnant women (not taking any oral contraceptive) is about 5 cases per 100,000 per year. The incidence in users of second generation pills is about 15 per 100,000 women per year of use. The incidence in users of third generation pills is about 25 cases per 100,000 women per year of use; this excess incidence has not been satisfactorily explained by bias or confounding. The level of all of these risks of VTE increases with age and is likely to be further increased in women with other known risk factors for VTE such as obesity. The excess risk of VTE is highest during the first year a woman ever uses a combined oral contraceptive.

Patients receiving oral contraceptives should be kept under regular surveillance, in view of the possibility of development of conditions such as thromboembolism.

The risk of coronary artery disease in women taking oral contraceptives is increased by the presence of other predisposing factors such as cigarette smoking, hypercholesterolaemia, obesity, diabetes, history of pre-eclamptic toxaemia and increasing age. After the age of thirty-five years, the patient and physician should carefully re-assess the risk/benefit ratio of using combined oral contraceptives as opposed to alternative methods of contraception.

Synphase should be discontinued at least four weeks before, and for two weeks following, elective operations and during immobilisation. Patients undergoing injection treatment for varicose veins should not resume taking Synphase until 3 months after the last injection.

Benign and malignant liver tumours have been associated with oral contraceptive use. The relationship between occurrence of liver tumours and use of female sex hormones is not known at present. These tumours may rupture causing intra-abdominal bleeding. If the patient presents with a mass or tenderness in the right upper quadrant or an acute abdomen, the possible presence of a tumour should be considered.

An increased risk of congenital abnormalities, including heart defects and limb defects, has been reported following the use of sex hormones, including oral contraceptives, in pregnancy. If the patient does not adhere to the prescribed schedule, the possibility of pregnancy should be considered at the time of the first missed period and further use of oral contraceptives should be withheld until pregnancy has been ruled out. It is recommended that for any patient who has missed two consecutive periods, pregnancy should be ruled out before continuing the contraceptive regimen. If pregnancy is confirmed the patient should be advised of the potential risks to the foetus and the advisability of continuing the pregnancy should be discussed in the light of these risks. It is advisable to discontinue Synphase three months before a planned pregnancy.

The risk of arterial thrombosis associated with combined oral contraceptives increases with age, and this risk is aggravated by cigarette smoking. The use of combined oral contraceptives by women in the older age group, especially those who are cigarette smokers, should therefore be discouraged and alternative methods advised.

The use of this product in patients suffering from epilepsy, migraine, asthma or cardiac dysfunction may result in exacerbation of these disorders because of fluid retention. Caution should also be observed in patients who wear contact lenses.

Decreased glucose tolerance may occur in diabetic patients on this treatment, and their control must be carefully supervised.

The use of oral contraceptives has also been associated with a possible increased incidence of gall bladder disease.

Women with a history of oligomenorrhoea or secondary amenorrhoea or young women without regular cycles may have a tendency to remain anovulatory or to become amenorrhoeic after discontinuation of oral contraceptives. Women with these pre-existing problems should be advised of this possibility and encouraged to use other contraceptive methods.

Numerous epidemiological studies have been reported on the risks of ovarian, endometrial, cervical and breast cancer in women using combined oral contraceptives. The evidence is clear that combined oral contraceptives offer substantial protection against both ovarian and endometrial cancer.

An increased risk of cervical cancer in long-term users of combined oral contraceptives has been reported in some studies, but there continues to be controversy about the extent to which this is attributable to the confounding effects of sexual behaviour and other factors.

A meta-analysis from 54 epidemiological studies reported that there is a slightly increased relative risk (RR = 1.24) of having breast cancer diagnosed in women who are currently using combined oral contraceptives (COCs). The observed pattern of increased risk may be due to an earlier diagnosis of breast cancer in COC users, the biological effects of COCs or a combination of both. The additional breast cancers diagnosed in current users of COCs or in women who have used COCs in the last ten years are more likely to be localised to the breast than those in women who never used COCs.

Breast cancer is rare among women under 40 years of age whether or not they take COCs. Whilst this background risk increases with age, the excess number of breast cancer diagnoses in current and recent COC users is small in relation to the overall risk of breast cancer (see bar chart).

The most important risk factor for breast cancer in COC users is the age women discontinue the COC; the older the age at stopping, the more breast cancers are diagnosed. Duration of use is less important and the excess risk gradually disappears during the course of the 10 years after stopping COC use such that by 10 years there appears to be no excess.

The possible increase in risk of breast cancer should be discussed with the user and weighed against the benefits of COCs taking into account the evidence that they offer substantial protection against the risk of developing certain other cancers (e.g. ovarian and endometrial cancer).

(see Figure 1 above)

4.5 Interaction with other medicinal products and other forms of interaction

The herbal remedy St John's wort (*Hypericum perforatum*) should not be taken concomitantly with this medicine as this could potentially lead to a loss of contraceptive effect.

Some drugs may modify the metabolism of Synphase reducing its effectiveness; these include certain sedatives, antibiotics, anti-epileptic and anti-arthritic drugs. During the time such agents are used concurrently, it is advised that mechanical contraceptives also be used.

The results of a large number of laboratory tests have been shown to be influenced by the use of oestrogen containing oral contraceptives, which may limit their diagnostic value. Among these are: biochemical markers of thyroid and liver function; plasma levels of carrier proteins, triglycerides, coagulation and fibrinolysis factors.

4.6 Pregnancy and lactation

Contra-indicated in pregnancy.

Patients who are fully breast-feeding should not take Synphase tablets since, in common with other combined oral contraceptives, the oestrogen component may reduce the amount of milk produced. In addition, active ingredients or their metabolites have been detected in the milk of mothers taking oral contraceptives. The effect of Synphase on breast-fed infants has not been determined.

4.7 Effects on ability to drive and use machines

Not applicable.

4.8 Undesirable effects

As with all oral contraceptives, there may be slight nausea at first, weight gain or breast discomfort, which soon disappear.

Other side-effects known or suspected to occur with oral contraceptives include gastro-intestinal symptoms, changes in libido and appetite, headache, exacerbation of existing uterine fibroid disease, depression, and changes in carbohydrate, lipid and vitamin metabolism.

Spotting or bleeding may occur during the first few cycles. Usually menstrual bleeding becomes light and occasionally there may be no bleeding during the tablet-free days.

Hypertension, which is usually reversible on discontinuing treatment, has occurred in a small percentage of women taking oral contraceptives.

4.9 Overdose

Overdosage may be manifested by nausea, vomiting, breast enlargement and vaginal bleeding. There is no specific antidote and treatment should be symptomatic. Gastric lavage may be employed if the overdose is large and the patient is seen sufficiently early (within four hours).

5. PHARMACOLOGICAL PROPERTIES

5.1 Pharmacodynamic properties

The mode of action of Synphase is similar to that of other progestogen/oestrogen oral contraceptives and includes the inhibition of ovulation, the thickening of cervical mucus so as to constitute a barrier to sperm and the rendering of the endometrium unreceptive to implantation. Such activity is exerted through a combined effect on one or more of the following: hypothalamus, anterior pituitary, ovary, endometrium and cervical mucus.

5.2 Pharmacokinetic properties

Norethisterone is rapidly and completely absorbed after oral administration, peak plasma concentrations occurring in the majority of subjects between 1 and 3 hours. Due to first-pass metabolism, blood levels after oral administration are 60% of those after i.v. administration. The half life of elimination varies from 5 to 12 hours, with a mean of 7.6 hours. Norethisterone is metabolised mainly in the liver. Approximately 60% of the administered dose is excreted as metabolites in urine and faeces.

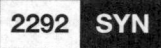

Ethinylestradiol is rapidly and well absorbed from the gastro-intestinal tract but is subject to some first-pass metabolism in the gut-wall. Compared to many other oestrogens it is only slowly metabolised in the liver. Excretion is via the kidneys with some appearing also in the faeces.

5.3 Preclinical safety data

The toxicity of norethisterone is very low. Reports of teratogenic effects in animals are uncommon. No carcinogenic effects have been found even in long-term studies.

Long-term continuous administration of oestrogens in some animals increases the frequency of carcinoma of the breast, cervix, vagina and liver.

6. PHARMACEUTICAL PARTICULARS

6.1 List of excipients

Synphase tablets contain:

Maize starch, polyvidone, magnesium stearate and lactose. The blue tablets also contain E132.

6.2 Incompatibilities

None stated.

6.3 Shelf life

The shelf life of Synphase tablets is 5 years.

6.4 Special precautions for storage

Store in a dry place below 25°C away from direct sunlight.

6.5 Nature and contents of container

Synphase tablets are supplied in pvc/foil blister packs of 21 and 63 tablets.

6.6 Special precautions for disposal and other handling

None.

7. MARKETING AUTHORISATION HOLDER

Pharmacia Limited
Ramsgate Road
Sandwich
Kent
CT13 9JN

8. MARKETING AUTHORISATION NUMBER(S)

PL 0032/0422

9. DATE OF FIRST AUTHORISATION/RENEWAL OF THE AUTHORISATION

May 10th 1996 / 25/02/2009

10. DATE OF REVISION OF THE TEXT

February 2009

Company Ref: SY3_0

Syntocinon Ampoules 10 IU/ml

(Alliance Pharmaceuticals)

1. NAME OF THE MEDICINAL PRODUCT

Syntocinon® Ampoules 10 IU/ml

2. QUALITATIVE AND QUANTITATIVE COMPOSITION

Oxytocin PhEur 10 units in 1ml.

For excipients, see section 6.1.

3. PHARMACEUTICAL FORM

A clear, colourless, sterile solution in 1ml clear glass ampoules.

4. CLINICAL PARTICULARS

4.1 Therapeutic indications

Induction of labour for medical reasons; stimulation of labour in hypotonic uterine inertia; during caesarean section, following delivery of the child; prevention and treatment of postpartum uterine atony and haemorrhage.

Early stages of pregnancy as a adjunctive therapy for the management of incomplete, inevitable, or missed abortion.

4.2 Posology and method of administration

Induction or enhancement of labour: Oxytocin should not be started for 6 hours following administration of vaginal prostaglandins. Syntocinon should be administered as an iv drip infusion or, preferably, by means of a variable-speed infusion pump. For drip infusion it is recommended that 5 IU of Syntocinon be added to 500ml of a physiological electrolyte solution. For patients in whom infusion of sodium chloride must be avoided, 5% dextrose solution may be used as the diluent (see Section 4.4 "Special warnings and precautions for use"). To ensure even mixing, the bottle or bag must be turned upside down several times before use.

The initial infusion rate should be set at 1 to 4mU/min (2 to 8 drops/min). It may be gradually increased at intervals not shorter than 20 min, until a contraction pattern similar to that of normal labour is established. In pregnancy near term this can often be achieved with an infusion of less than 10mU/min (20 drops/min), and the recommended maximum rate is 20mU/min (40 drops/min). In the unusual event that higher rates are required, as may occur in the management of foetal death *in utero* or for induction of labour at an earlier stage of pregnancy, when the uterus is less sensitive to oxytocin, it is advisable to use a more concentrated Syntocinon solution, e.g., 10 IU in 500ml.

When using a motor-driven infusion pump which delivers smaller volumes than those given by drip infusion, the concentration suitable for infusion within the recommended dosage range must be calculated according to the specifications of the pump.

The frequency, strength, and duration of contractions as well as the foetal heart rate must be carefully monitored throughout the infusion. Once an adequate level of uterine activity is attained, aiming for 3 to 4 contractions every 10 minutes, the infusion rate can often be reduced. In the event of uterine hyperactivity and/or foetal distress, the infusion must be discontinued immediately.

If, in women who are at term or near term, regular contractions are not established after the infusion of a total amount of 5 IU, it is recommended that the attempt to induce labour be ceased; it may be repeated on the following day, starting again from a rate of 1 to 4mU/min (see Section 4.3 "Contra-indications").

Caesarean section: 5 IU by slow iv injection immediately after delivery.

Prevention of postpartum uterine haemorrhage: The usual dose is 5 IU slowly iv after delivery of the placenta. In women given Syntocinon for induction or enhancement of labour, the infusion should be continued at an increased rate during the third stage of labour and for the next few hours thereafter.

Treatment of postpartum uterine haemorrhage: 5 IU slowly iv, followed in severe cases by iv infusion of a solution containing 5 to 20 IU of oxytocin in 500ml of a non-hydrating diluent, run at the rate necessary to control uterine atony.

Incomplete, inevitable, or missed abortion: 5 IU slowly iv, if necessary followed by iv infusion at a rate of 20 to 40mU/min or higher.

Children: Not applicable.

Elderly: Not applicable.

Route of administration: Intravenous infusion or intravenous injection.

4.3 Contraindications

Known hypersensitivity to oxytocin or to any of the excipients of Syntocinon. Hypertonic uterine contractions, mechanical obstruction to delivery, foetal distress. Any condition in which, for foetal or maternal reasons, spontaneous labour is inadvisable and/or vaginal delivery is contra-indicated: e.g., significant cephalopelvic disproportion; foetal malpresentation; placenta praevia and vasa praevia; placental abruption; cord presentation or prolapse; overdistension or impaired resistance of the uterus to rupture as in multiple pregnancy; polyhydramnios; grand multiparity and in the presence of a uterine scar resulting from major surgery including classical caesarean section.

Syntocinon should not be used for prolonged periods in patients with oxytocin-resistant uterine inertia, severe pre-eclamptic toxaemia or severe cardiovascular disorders.

4.4 Special warnings and precautions for use

The induction of labour by means of oxytocin should be attempted only when strictly indicated for medical reasons. Administration should only be under hospital conditions and qualified medical supervision. When given for induction and enhancement of labour, Syntocinon must only be administered as an iv infusion and never by iv bolus injection. Administration of oxytocin at excessive doses results in uterine overstimulation which may cause foetal distress, asphyxia and death, or may lead to hypertonicity, titanic contractions or rupture of the uterus. Careful monitoring of foetal heart rate and uterine motility (frequency, strength, and duration of contractions) is essential, so that the dosage may be adjusted to individual response.

When Syntocinon is given for induction or enhancement of labour, particular caution is required in the presence of borderline cephalopelvic disproportion, secondary uterine inertia, mild or moderate degrees of pregnancy-induced hypertension or cardiac disease, and in patients above 35 years of age or with a history of lower-uterine-segment caesarean section.

In rare circumstances, the pharmacological induction of labour using uterotonic agents increases the risk of post patum disseminated intravascular coagulation (DIC). The pharmacological induction itself and not a particular agent is linked to such risk. This risk is increased in particular if the woman has additional risk factors for DIC such as being 35 years of age or over, complications during pregnancy and gestational age more than 40 weeks. In these women, oxytocin or any other alternative drug should be used with care, and the practitioner should be alerted by signs of DIC.

In the case of foetal death *in utero*, and/or in the presence of meconium-stained amniotic fluid, tumultous labour must be avoided, as it may cause amniotic fluid embolism.

Because oxytocin possesses slight antidiuretic activity, its prolonged iv administration at high doses in conjunction with large volumes of fluid, as may be the case in the treatment of inevitable or missed abortion or in the management of postpartum haemorrhage, may cause water intoxication associated with hyponatraemia. To avoid this rare complication, the following precautions must be observed whenever high doses of oxytocin are administered over a long time: an electrolyte-containing diluent must be used (not dextrose); the volume of infused fluid should be kept low (by infusing oxytocin at a higher concentration than recommended for the induction or enhancement of labour at term); fluid intake by mouth must be restricted; a fluid balance chart should be kept, and serum electrolytes should be measured when electrolyte imbalance is suspected.

When Syntocinon is used for prevention or treatment of uterine haemorrhage, rapid iv injection should be avoided, as it may cause an acute short-lasting drop in blood pressure accompanied with flushing and reflex tachycardia.

4.5 Interaction with other medicinal products and other forms of interaction

Since it has been found that prostaglandins potentiate the effect of oxytocin, it is not recommended that these drugs are used together. If used in sequence, the patient's uterine activity should be carefully monitored.

Some inhalation anaesthetics, e.g., cyclopropane or halothane, may enhance the hypotensive effect of oxytocin and reduce its oxytocic action. Their concurrent use with oxytocin has also been reported to cause cardiac rhythm disturbances.

When given during or after caudal block anaesthesia, oxytocin may potentiate the pressor effect of sympathomimetic vasoconstrictor agents.

4.6 Pregnancy and lactation

Animal reproduction studies have not been conducted with oxytocin. Based on the wide experience with this drug and its chemical structure and pharmacological properties, it is not expected to present a risk of foetal abnormalities when used as indicated.

Oxytocin may be found in small quantities in mother's breast milk. However, oxytocin is not expected to cause harmful effects in the newborn because It passes into the alimentary tract where it undergoes rapid inactivation.

4.7 Effects on ability to drive and use machines

Syntocinon can induce labour, therefore caution should be exercised when driving or operating machines. Women with uterine contractions should not drive or use machines.

4.8 Undesirable effects

As there is a wide variation in uterine sensitivity, uterine spasm may be caused in some instances by what are normally considered to be low doses. When oxytocin is used by iv infusion for the induction or enhancement of labour, administration at too high doses results in uterine overstimulation which may cause foetal distress, asphyxia, and death, or may lead to hypertonicity, tetanic contractions, soft tissue damage or rupture of the uterus.

Water intoxication associated with maternal and neonatal hyponatraemia has been reported in cases where high doses of oxytocin together with large amounts of electrolyte-free fluid have been administered over a prolonged period of time (see Section 4.4 "Special warnings and precautions for use"). Symptoms of water intoxication include:

1. Headache, anorexia, nausea, vomiting and abdominal pain.

2. Lethargy, drowsiness, unconsciousness and grand-mal type seizures.

3. Low blood electrolyte concentration.

Rapid iv bolus injection of oxytocin at doses amounting to several IU may result in acute short-lasting hypotension accompanied with flushing and reflex tachycardia.

In rare circumstances the pharmacological induction of labour using uterotonic agents increases the risk of postpartum disseminated intravascular coagulation (see section 4.4 Special warnings and special precautions for use).

Oxytocin may occasionally cause nausea, vomiting, haemorrhageor cardiac arrhythmias. In a few cases, skin rashes and anaphylactoid reactions associated with dyspnoea, hypotension, or shock have been reported.

Immune System disorders	
Rare:	Anaphylactoid reaction associated with dyspnoea, hypotension or shock
Nervous system disorders	
Common:	Headache
Cardiac disorders	
Common:	Tachycardia, bradycardia
Uncommon:	Arrhythmia
Gastrointestinal disorders	
Common:	Nausea, vomiting
Skin and subcutaneous tissue disorders	
Rare:	Rash

4.9 Overdose

The fatal dose of Syntocinon has not been established. Syntocinon is subject to inactivation by proteolytic enzymes of the alimentary tract. Hence it is not absorbed from the intestine and is not likely to have toxic effects when ingested.

The symptoms and consequences of overdosage are those mentioned under Section 4.8 "Undesirable effects". In addition, as a result of uterine overstimulation, placental abruption and/or amniotic fluid embolism have been reported.

Treatment: When signs or symptoms of overdosage occur during continuous iv administration of Syntocinon, the infusion must be discontinued at once and oxygen should be given to the mother. In cases of water intoxication it is essential to restrict fluid intake, promote diuresis, correct electrolyte imbalance, and control convulsions that may eventually occur, by judicious use of diazepam. In the case of coma, a free airway should be maintained with routine measures normally employed in the nursing of the unconscious patient.

5. PHARMACOLOGICAL PROPERTIES

5.1 Pharmacodynamic properties

The active principle of Syntocinon is a synthetic nonapeptide identical with oxytocin, a hormone released by the posterior lobe of the pituitary. It exerts a stimulatory effect on the smooth musculature of the uterus, particularly towards the end of pregnancy, during labour, after delivery, and in the puerperium, i.e., at times when the number of specific oxytocin receptors in the myometrium is increased.

When given by low-dose iv infusion, Syntocinon elicits rhythmic uterine contractions that are indistinguishable in frequency, force, and duration from those observed during spontaneous labour. At higher infusion dosages, or when given by single injection, the drug is capable of causing sustained uterine contractions.

Being synthetic, Syntocinon does not contain vasopressin, but even in its pure form oxytocin possesses some weak intrinsic vasopressin-like antidiuretic activity.

Another pharmacological effect observed with high doses of oxytocin, particularly when administered by rapid iv bolus injection, consists of a transient direct relaxing effect on vascular smooth muscle, resulting in brief hypotension, flushing and reflex tachycardia.

5.2 Pharmacokinetic properties

The plasma half-life of oxytocin is of the order of five minutes, hence the need for continuous iv infusion. Elimination is via the liver, kidney, functional mammary gland and oxytocinase.

5.3 Preclinical safety data

There are no pre-clinical data of relevance to the prescriber which are additional to those already included in other sections of the Summary of Product Characteristics.

6. PHARMACEUTICAL PARTICULARS

6.1 List of excipients

Sodium acetate tri-hydrate, acetic acid, chlorobutanol, ethanol and water for injections.

6.2 Incompatibilities

Syntocinon should not be infused via the same apparatus as blood or plasma, because the peptide linkages are rapidly inactivated by oxytocin-inactivating enzymes. Syntocinon is incompatible with solutions containing sodium metabisulphite as a stabiliser.

6.3 Shelf life

Five years

6.4 Special precautions for storage

Store between 2°C and 8°C. May be stored up to 30°C for 3 months, but must then be discarded.

6.5 Nature and contents of container

Clear glass 1ml ampoules. Boxes of 5 ampoules.

6.6 Special precautions for disposal and other handling

Snap ampoules: no file required.

Syntocinon is compatible with the following infusion fluids, but due attention should be paid to the advisability of using electrolyte fluids in individual patients: sodium/potassium chloride (103mmol Na^+ and 51mmol K^+), sodium bicarbonate 1.39%, sodium chloride 0.9%, sodium lactate 1.72%, dextrose 5%, laevulose 20%, macrodex 6%, rheomacrodex 10%, Ringer's solution.

7. MARKETING AUTHORISATION HOLDER

Alliance Pharmaceuticals Ltd

Avonbridge House

Bath Road

Chippenham

Wiltshire

SN15 2BB

8. MARKETING AUTHORISATION NUMBER(S)

PL 16853/0020

9. DATE OF FIRST AUTHORISATION/RENEWAL OF THE AUTHORISATION

25 June 1998

10. DATE OF REVISION OF THE TEXT

February 2007

11. Legal Status

POM

Syntocinon Ampoules 5 IU/ml

(Alliance Pharmaceuticals)

1. NAME OF THE MEDICINAL PRODUCT

Syntocinon® Ampoules 5 IU/ml

2. QUALITATIVE AND QUANTITATIVE COMPOSITION

Oxytocin PhEur 5 units in 1ml.

For excipients, see section 6.1.

3. PHARMACEUTICAL FORM

A clear, colourless, sterile solution in 1ml clear glass ampoules.

4. CLINICAL PARTICULARS

4.1 Therapeutic indications

Induction of labour for medical reasons; stimulation of labour in hypotonic uterine inertia; during caesarean section, following delivery of the child; prevention and treatment of postpartum uterine atony and haemorrhage.

Early stages of pregnancy as a adjunctive therapy for the management of incomplete, inevitable, or missed abortion.

4.2 Posology and method of administration

Induction or enhancement of labour: Oxytocin should not be started for 6 hours following administration of vaginal prostaglandins. Syntocinon should be administered as an iv drip infusion or, preferably, by means of a variable-speed infusion pump. For drip infusion it is recommended that 5 IU of Syntocinon be added to 500ml of a physiological electrolyte solution. For patients in whom infusion of sodium chloride must be avoided, 5% dextrose solution may be used as the diluent (see Section 4.4 "Special warnings and precautions for use"). To ensure even mixing, the bottle or bag must be turned upside down several times before use.

The initial infusion rate should be set at 1 to 4mU/min (2 to 8 drops/min). It may be gradually increased at intervals not shorter than 20 min, until a contraction pattern similar to that of normal labour is established. In pregnancy near term this can often be achieved with an infusion of less than 10mU/min (20 drops/min), and the recommended maximum rate is 20mU/min (40 drops/min). In the unusual event that higher rates are required, as may occur in the management of foetal death *in utero* or for induction of labour at an earlier stage of pregnancy, when the uterus is less sensitive to oxytocin, it is advisable to use a more concentrated Syntocinon solution, e.g., 10 IU in 500ml.

When using a motor-driven infusion pump which delivers smaller volumes than those given by drip infusion, the concentration suitable for infusion within the recommended dosage range must be calculated according to the specifications of the pump.

The frequency, strength, and duration of contractions as well as the foetal heart rate must be carefully monitored throughout the infusion. Once an adequate level of uterine activity is attained, aiming for 3 to 4 contractions every 10 minutes, the infusion rate can often be reduced. In the event of uterine hyperactivity and/or foetal distress, the infusion must be discontinued immediately.

If, in women who are at term or near term, regular contractions are not established after the infusion of a total amount of 5 IU, it is recommended that the attempt to induce labour be ceased; it may be repeated on the following day, starting again from a rate of 1 to 4mU/min (see Section 4.3 "Contra-indications").

Caesarean section: 5 IU by slow iv injection immediately after delivery.

Prevention of postpartum uterine haemorrhage: The usual dose is 5 IU slowly iv after delivery of the placenta. In women given Syntocinon for induction or enhancement of labour, the infusion should be continued at an increased rate during the third stage of labour and for the next few hours thereafter.

Treatment of postpartum uterine haemorrhage: 5 IU slowly iv, followed in severe cases by iv infusion of a solution containing 5 to 20 IU of oxytocin in 500ml of a non-hydrating diluent, run at the rate necessary to control uterine atony.

Incomplete, inevitable, or missed abortion: 5 IU slowly iv, if necessary followed by iv infusion at a rate of 20 to 40mU/min or higher.

Children: Not applicable.

Elderly: Not applicable.

Route of administration: Intravenous infusion or intravenous injection.

4.3 Contraindications

Known hypersensitivity to oxytocin or to any of the excipients of Syntocinon. Hypertonic uterine contractions, mechanical obstruction to delivery, foetal distress. Any condition in which, for foetal or maternal reasons, spontaneous labour is inadvisable and/or vaginal delivery is contra-indicated: e.g., significant cephalopelvic disproportion; foetal malpresentation; placenta praevia and vasa praevia; placental abruption; cord presentation or prolapse; overdistension or impaired resistance of the uterus to rupture as in multiple pregnancy; polyhydramnios; grand multiparity and in the presence of a uterine scar resulting from major surgery including classical caesarean section.

Syntocinon should not be used for prolonged periods in patients with oxytocin-resistant uterine inertia, severe pre-eclamptic toxaemia or severe cardiovascular disorders.

4.4 Special warnings and precautions for use

The induction of labour by means of oxytocin should be attempted only when strictly indicated for medical reasons. Administration should only be under hospital conditions and qualified medical supervision. When given for induction and enhancement of labour, Syntocinon must only be administered as an iv infusion and never by iv bolus injection. Administration of oxytocin at excessive doses results in uterine overstimulation which may cause foetal distress, asphyxia and death, or may lead to hypertonicity, titanic contractions or rupture of the uterus. Careful monitoring of foetal heart rate and uterine motility (frequency, strength, and duration of contractions) is essential, so that the dosage may be adjusted to individual response.

When Syntocinon is given for induction or enhancement of labour, particular caution is required in the presence of borderline cephalopelvic disproportion, secondary uterine inertia, mild or moderate degrees of pregnancy-induced hypertension or cardiac disease, and in patients above 35 years of age or with a history of lower-uterine-segment caesarean section.

In rare circumstances, the pharmacological induction of labour using uterotonic agents increases the risk of post patum disseminated intravascular coagulation (DIC). The pharmacological induction itself and not a particular agent is linked to such risk. This risk is increased in particular if the woman has additional risk factors for DIC such as being 35 years of age or over, complications during pregnancy and gestational age more than 40 weeks. In these women, oxytocin or any other alternative drug should be used with care, and the practitioner should be alerted by signs of DIC.

In the case of foetal death *in utero*, and/or in the presence of meconium-stained amniotic fluid, tumultous labour must be avoided, as it may cause amniotic fluid embolism.

Because oxytocin possesses slight antidiuretic activity, its prolonged iv administration at high doses in conjunction with large volumes of fluid, as may be the case in the treatment of inevitable or missed abortion or in the management of postpartum haemorrhage, may cause water intoxication associated with hyponatraemia. To avoid this rare complication, the following precautions must be observed whenever high doses of oxytocin are administered over a long time: an electrolyte-containing diluent must be used (not dextrose); the volume of infused fluid should be kept low (by infusing oxytocin at a higher concentration than recommended for the induction or enhancement of labour at term); fluid intake by mouth must be restricted; a fluid balance chart should be kept, and serum electrolytes should be measured when electrolyte imbalance is suspected.

When Syntocinon is used for prevention or treatment of uterine haemorrhage, rapid iv injection should be avoided, as it may cause an acute short-lasting drop in blood pressure accompanied with flushing and reflex tachycardia.

4.5 Interaction with other medicinal products and other forms of interaction

Since it has been found that prostaglandins potentiate the effect of oxytocin, it is not recommended that these drugs are used together. If used in sequence, the patient's uterine activity should be carefully monitored.

Some inhalation anaesthetics, e.g., cyclopropane or halothane, may enhance the hypotensive effect of oxytocin and reduce its oxytocic action. Their concurrent use with oxytocin has also been reported to cause cardiac rhythm disturbances.

When given during or after caudal block anaesthesia, oxytocin may potentiate the pressor effect of sympathomimetic vasoconstrictor agents.

4.6 Pregnancy and lactation

Animal reproduction studies have not been conducted with oxytocin. Based on the wide experience with this drug and its chemical structure and pharmacological properties, it is not expected to present a risk of foetal abnormalities when used as indicated.

Oxytocin may be found in small quantities in mother's breast milk. However, oxytocin is not expected to cause harmful effects in the newborn because It passes into the alimentary tract where it undergoes rapid inactivation.

4.7 Effects on ability to drive and use machines

Syntocinon can induce labour, therefore caution should be exercised when driving or operating machines. Women with uterine contractions should not drive or use machines.

4.8 Undesirable effects

As there is a wide variation in uterine sensitivity, uterine spasm may be caused in some instances by what are normally considered to be low doses. When oxytocin is used by iv infusion for the induction or enhancement of labour, administration at too high doses results in uterine overstimulation which may cause foetal distress, asphyxia, and death, or may lead to hypertonicity, tetanic contractions, soft tissue damage or rupture of the uterus.

Water intoxication associated with maternal and neonatal hyponatraemia has been reported in cases where high doses of oxytocin together with large amounts of electrolyte-free fluid have been administered over a prolonged period of time (see Section 4.4 "Special warnings and precautions for use"). Symptoms of water intoxication include:

1. Headache, anorexia, nausea, vomiting and abdominal pain.

2. Lethargy, drowsiness, unconsciousness and grand-mal type seizures.

3. Low blood electrolyte concentration.

Rapid iv bolus injection of oxytocin at doses amounting to several IU may result in acute short-lasting hypotension accompanied with flushing and reflex tachycardia.

In rare circumstances the pharmacological induction of labour using uterotonic agents increases the risk of postpartum disseminated intravascular coagulation (see section 4.4 Special warnings and special precautions for use).

Oxytocin may occasionally cause nausea, vomiting, haemorrhage or cardiac arrhythmias. In a few cases, skin rashes and anaphylactoid reactions associated with dyspnoea, hypotension, or shock have been reported.

Immune System disorders	
Rare:	Anaphylactoid reaction associated with dyspnoea, hypotension or shock
Nervous system disorders	
Common:	Headache
Cardiac disorders	
Common:	Tachycardia, bradycardia
Uncommon:	Arrhythmia
Gastrointestinal disorders	
Common:	Nausea, vomiting
Skin and subcutaneous tissue disorders	
Rare:	Rash

4.9 Overdose

The fatal dose of Syntocinon has not been established. Syntocinon is subject to inactivation by proteolytic enzymes of the alimentary tract. Hence it is not absorbed from the intestine and is not likely to have toxic effects when ingested.

The symptoms and consequences of overdosage are those mentioned under Section 4.8 "Undesirable effects". In addition, as a result of uterine overstimulation, placental abruption and/or amniotic fluid embolism have been reported.

Treatment: When signs or symptoms of overdosage occur during continuous iv administration of Syntocinon, the infusion must be discontinued at once and oxygen should be given to the mother. In cases of water intoxication it is essential to restrict fluid intake, promote diuresis, correct electrolyte imbalance, and control convulsions that may eventually occur, by judicious use of diazepam. In the case of coma, a free airway should be maintained with routine measures normally employed in the nursing of the unconscious patient.

5. PHARMACOLOGICAL PROPERTIES

5.1 Pharmacodynamic properties

The active principle of Syntocinon is a synthetic nonapeptide identical with oxytocin, a hormone released by the posterior lobe of the pituitary. It exerts a stimulatory effect on the smooth musculature of the uterus, particularly towards the end of pregnancy, during labour, after delivery, and in the puerperium, i.e., at times when the number of specific oxytocin receptors in the myometrium is increased.

When given by low-dose iv infusion, Syntocinon elicits rhythmic uterine contractions that are indistinguishable in frequency, force, and duration from those observed during spontaneous labour. At higher infusion dosages, or when given by single injection, the drug is capable of causing sustained uterine contractions.

Being synthetic, Syntocinon does not contain vasopressin, but even in its pure form oxytocin possesses some weak intrinsic vasopressin-like antidiuretic activity.

Another pharmacological effect observed with high doses of oxytocin, particularly when administered by rapid iv bolus injection, consists of a transient direct relaxing effect on vascular smooth muscle, resulting in brief hypotension, flushing and reflex tachycardia.

5.2 Pharmacokinetic properties

The plasma half-life of oxytocin is of the order of five minutes, hence the need for continuous iv infusion. Elimination is via the liver, kidney, functional mammary gland and oxytocinase.

5.3 Preclinical safety data

There are no pre-clinical data of relevance to the prescriber which are additional to those already included in other sections of the Summary of Product Characteristics.

6. PHARMACEUTICAL PARTICULARS

6.1 List of excipients

Sodium acetate tri-hydrate, acetic acid, chlorobutanol, ethanol and water for injections.

6.2 Incompatibilities

Syntocinon should not be infused via the same apparatus as blood or plasma, because the peptide linkages are rapidly inactivated by oxytocin-inactivating enzymes. Syntocinon is incompatible with solutions containing sodium metabisulphite as a stabiliser.

6.3 Shelf life

Five years

6.4 Special precautions for storage

Store between 2°C and 8°C. May be stored up to 30°C for 3 months, but must then be discarded.

6.5 Nature and contents of container

Clear glass 1ml ampoules. Boxes of 5 ampoules.

6.6 Special precautions for disposal and other handling

Snap ampoules: no file required.

Syntocinon is compatible with the following infusion fluids, but due attention should be paid to the advisability of using electrolyte fluids in individual patients: sodium/potassium chloride (103mmol Na^+ and 51mmol K^+), sodium bicarbonate 1.39%, sodium chloride 0.9%, sodium lactate 1.72%, dextrose 5%, laevulose 20%, macrodex 6%, rheomacrodex 10%, Ringer's solution.

7. MARKETING AUTHORISATION HOLDER

Alliance Pharmaceuticals Ltd
Avonbridge House
Bath Road
Chippenham
Wiltshire
SN15 2BB

8. MARKETING AUTHORISATION NUMBER(S)

PL 16853/0019

9. DATE OF FIRST AUTHORISATION/RENEWAL OF THE AUTHORISATION

25 June 1998

10. DATE OF REVISION OF THE TEXT

February 2007

11. Legal Status

POM

Syntometrine Ampoules

(Alliance Pharmaceuticals)

1. NAME OF THE MEDICINAL PRODUCT

Syntometrine® Ampoules

2. QUALITATIVE AND QUANTITATIVE COMPOSITION

Each 1ml ampoule contains 5IU oxytocin PhEur and 0.5mg ergometrine maleate PhEur.

3. PHARMACEUTICAL FORM

A clear colourless sterile liquid in a 1ml clear colourless glass ampoule.

4. CLINICAL PARTICULARS

4.1 Therapeutic indications

The active management of the third stage of labour, or routinely, following the birth of the placenta, to prevent or treat postpartum haemorrhage.

4.2 Posology and method of administration

Syntometrine is usually administered by intramuscular injection.

Adults:

Active management of third stage of labour: Intramuscular injection of 1ml after delivery of the anterior shoulder, or at the latest, immediately after delivery of the child. Expulsion of the placenta, which is normally separated by the first strong uterine contraction, should be assisted by gentle suprapubic pressure and controlled cord traction.

Prevention and treatment of postpartum haemorrhage: Intramuscular injection of 1ml following expulsion of the placenta, or when bleeding occurs.

Third stage of labour and postpartum haemorrhage: Syntometrine may also be administered by a slow intravenous injection in a dose of 0.5 to 1ml. This route of administration is not generally recommended.

Children: Not applicable.

Elderly: Not applicable.

4.3 Contraindications

Hypersensitivity to any of the components.

Pregnancy, first stage of labour, primary or secondary uterine inertia. Second stage of labour before crowning of the head.

Severe disorders of cardiac, liver or kidney functions; occlusive vascular disease, sepsis, severe hypertension, pre-eclampsia, eclampsia.

4.4 Special warnings and precautions for use

When the intravenous route is employed, care should be exercised in patients of doubtful cardiac status.

In breech presentations and other abnormal presentations, Syntometrine should not be given until after delivery of the child, and in multiple births not until the last child has been delivered. In postpartum haemorrhage, if bleeding is not arrested by the injection of Syntometrine, the possibility of retained placental fragments, of soft tissue injury (cervical or vaginal laceration), or of a clotting defect, should be excluded before a further injection is given. Caution should be exercised in the presence of mild or moderate hypertension, or with mild or moderate degrees of cardiac, liver or kidney disease.

4.5 Interaction with other medicinal products and other forms of interaction

Halothane anaesthesia may diminish the uterotonic effect of Syntometrine. Syntometrine may enhance the effects of vasoconstrictors and of prostaglandins.

4.6 Pregnancy and lactation

See Section 4.1 "Therapeutic Indications".

4.7 Effects on ability to drive and use machines

None known.

4.8 Undesirable effects

Nausea, vomiting, abdominal pain, headache, dizziness and skin rashes. On rare occasions hypertension, bradycardia, cardiac arrhythmias, chest pain or anaphylactoid reactions associated with dyspnoea, hypotension, collapse or shock.

4.9 Overdose

No case of maternal intoxication with Syntometrine has been reported to the company. If such a case were to occur the most likely symptoms would be those of ergometrine intoxication: nausea, vomiting, hypertension or hypotension, vasospastic reactions, respiratory depression, convulsions, coma. Treatment would have to be symptomatic.

Accidental administration to the newborn infant has been reported and has proved fatal. In these accidental neonatal overdosage cases, symptoms such as respiratory depression, convulsions and hypertonia, heart arrhythmia have been reported. In treatment has been symptomatic in most cases; respiratory and cardiovascular support have been required.

5. PHARMACOLOGICAL PROPERTIES

5.1 Pharmacodynamic properties

Syntometrine combines the known sustained oxytocic action of ergometrine with the more rapid action of oxytocin on the uterus.

5.2 Pharmacokinetic properties

Ergometrine is reported to be rapidly and completely absorbed after an intramuscular injection. Uterine stimulation occurs within 7 minutes of im injection and immediately after iv injection. Oxytocin is also rapidly absorbed and is rapidly metabolised by the liver and the kidneys.

5.3 Preclinical safety data

There are no pre-clinical data of relevance to the prescriber which are additional to those already included in other sections of the Summary of Product Characteristics.

6. PHARMACEUTICAL PARTICULARS

6.1 List of excipients

Sodium chloride, maleic acid, water for injections.

6.2 Incompatibilities

None.

6.3 Shelf life

3 years.

6.4 Special precautions for storage

For prolonged periods store between 2° and 8°C. Protect from light. Syntometrine may be stored up to 25°C for 2 months when protected from light, but must then be discarded.

6.5 Nature and contents of container

Uncoloured borosilicate glass Type I snap ampoule. Packs of 5 ampoules.

6.6 Special precautions for disposal and other handling

None

Administrative Data

7. MARKETING AUTHORISATION HOLDER

Alliance Pharmaceuticals Ltd
Avonbridge House
Bath Road
Chippenham
Wiltshire
SN15 2BB

8. MARKETING AUTHORISATION NUMBER(S)

PL16853/0021

9. DATE OF FIRST AUTHORISATION/RENEWAL OF THE AUTHORISATION

25 June 1998

10. DATE OF REVISION OF THE TEXT

January 1999

11. Legal Status
POM

Alliance, Alliance Pharmaceuticals and associated devices are registered Trademarks of Alliance Pharmaceuticals Ltd.

Syprol 40mg/5ml Oral Solution

(Rosemont Pharmaceuticals Limited)

1. NAME OF THE MEDICINAL PRODUCT
Syprol 40mg/5ml Oral Solution

2. QUALITATIVE AND QUANTITATIVE COMPOSITION
Propranolol Hydrochloride 40mg/5ml

For excipients see Section 6.1.

3. PHARMACEUTICAL FORM
Oral Solution

A clear bright orange liquid with odour of orange/tangerine

4. CLINICAL PARTICULARS
4.1 Therapeutic indications
Propranolol is indicated in:

- the control of hypertension
- the management of angina pectoris
- the long term prophylaxis against reinfarction after recovery from acute myocardial infarction
- the control of most forms of cardiac arrhythmia
- the prophylaxis of migraine
- the management of essential tremor
- relief of situational anxiety and generalised anxiety symptoms, particularly those of the somatic type
- prophylaxis of upper gastro-intestinal bleeding in patients with portal hypertension and oesophageal varices
- the adjunctive management of thyrotoxicosis and thyrotoxic crisis
- management of hypertrophic obstructive cardiomyopathy
- management of phaeochromocytoma perioperatively (with an alpha-adrenoceptor blocking drug).

4.2 Posology and method of administration
For oral administration only.

Adults:

Hypertension – A starting dose of 80mg twice a day may be increased at weekly intervals according to response. The usual dose range is 160 – 320mg per day. With concurrent diuretic or other antihypertensive drugs a further reduction of blood pressure is obtained.

Angina, migraine and essential tremor – A starting dose of 40mg two or three times daily may be increased by the same amount at weekly intervals according to patient response. An adequate response in migraine and essential tremor is usually seen in the range 80-160mg/day and in angina in the range 120-240mg/day.

Situational and generalised anxiety – A dose of 40mg daily may provide short term relief of acute situational anxiety. Generalised anxiety, requiring longer term therapy, usually responds adequately to 40mg twice daily which, in individual cases, may be increased to 40mg three times daily. Treatment should be continued according to response. Patients should be reviewed after six to twelve months treatment.

Arrhythmias, anxiety, tachycardia, hypertrophic obstructive cardiomyopathy and thyrotoxicosis – A dosage range of 10-40mg three or four times a day usually achieves the required response.

Post myocardial infarction - Treatment should start between days 5 and 21 after myocardial infarction with an initial dose of 40mg four times a day for 2 or 3 days. In order to improve compliance the total daily dosage may thereafter be given as 80mg twice daily.

Portal hypertension:

Dosage should be titrated to achieve approximately 25% reduction in resting heart rate. Dosage should begin with 40mg twice daily, increasing to 80mg twice daily depending on heart rate response. If necessary, the dose may be increased incrementally to a maximum of 160mg twice daily.

Phaeochromocytoma (Used only with an alpha-receptor blocking drug)- Preoperative: 60mg daily for three days is recommended.

Non-operable malignant cases: 30mg daily.

Children

Arrhythmias, phaeochromocytoma, thyrotoxicosis – Dosage should be individually determined and the following is only a guide: 250 – 500 micrograms per Kilogram three or four times daily as required.

Migraine – Under the age of 12: 20mg two or three times daily

Over the age of 12: the adult dose

Fallots' tetralogy – The value of propranolol in this condition is confined mainly to the relief of right-ventricular outflow tract shut-down. It is also useful for treatment of associated arrhythmias and angina. Dosage should be individually determined and the following is only a guide: Up to 1mg/Kg repeated three or four times a day as required.

Elderly

With regard to the elderly the optimum dose should be individually determined according to the clinical response.

4.3 Contraindications
Propranolol must not be used if there is a history of bronchial asthma or bronchospasm.

The product label states the following warning: "Do not take propranolol if you have a history of asthma or wheezing". A similar warning appears in the patient information leaflet.

Bronchospasm can usually be reversed by beta2-agonist bronchodilators such as salbutamol. Large doses of the beta2-agonist bronchodilator may be required to overcome the beta-blockade produced by propranolol and the dose should be titrated according to the clinical response; both intravenous and inhalational administration should be considered. The use of intravenous aminophylline and/or the use of ipratropium (given by nebuliser) may also be considered. Glucagon (1 to 2mg given intravenously) has also been reported to produce a bronchodilator effect in asthmatic patients. Oxygen or artificial ventilation may be required in severe cases.

Propranolol as with other beta-adrenoceptor blocking drugs must not be used in patients with any of the following:

Hypersensitivity to propranolol hydrochloride or any of the ingredients; the presence of second or third degree heart block; in cardiogenic shock; metabolic acidosis; after prolonged fasting; bradycardia; hypotension; severe peripheral arterial circulatory disturbances; sick sinus syndrome; untreated phaeochromocytoma; uncontrolled heart failure or Prinzmetal's angina.

Propranolol must not be used in patients prone to hypoglycaemia, i.e. patients after prolonged fasting or patients with restricted counter-regulatory reserves. Patients with restricted counter-regulatory reserves may have reduced autonomic and hormonal responses to hypoglycaemia which includes glycogenolysis, gluconeogenesis and/or impaired modulation of insulin secretion. Patients at risk for an inadequate response to hypoglycaemia includes individuals with malnutrition, prolonged fasting, starvation, chronic liver disease, diabetes and concomitant use of drugs which block the full response to catecholamines.

4.4 Special warnings and precautions for use
Although contra-indicated in uncontrolled heart failure, propranolol may be used where the signs of heart failure have been controlled by the use of appropriate concomitant medication. Propranolol should be used with caution in patients whose cardiac reserve is poor.

Treatment should not be discontinued abruptly in patients with ischaemic heart disease. Either the equivalent dose of another beta-adrenoceptor blocking drug may be substituted or the withdrawal of propranolol should be gradual.

Propranolol should not be used in combination with calcium channel blockers with negative inotropic effects (e.g. verapamil, diltiazem), as it can lead to an exaggeration of these effects particularly in patients with impaired ventricular function and/or SA or AV conduction abnormalities. This may result in severe hypotension, bradycardia and cardiac failure. Neither the beta-blocker nor the calcium channel blocker should be administered intravenously within 48 hours of discontinuing the other.

Propranolol may block/modify the signs and symptoms of hypoglycaemia (especially tachycardia). Propranolol occasionally causes hypoglycaemia, even in non-diabetic patients, e.g. neonates, infants, children, elderly patients, patients on haemodialysis or patients suffering from chronic liver disease and patients suffering from overdose. Severe hypoglycaemia associated with propranolol has rarely presented with seizures and/or coma in isolated patients. Caution must be exercised in the concurrent use of propranolol and hypoglycaemic therapy in diabetic patients. Propranolol may prolong the hypoglycaemic response to insulin (see section 4.3).

When a patient is scheduled for surgery and a decision is made to discontinue betablocker therapy, this should be done at least 24 hours prior to the procedure. The risk/benefit of stopping beta blockade should be made for each patient.

Propranolol should not be used in untreated phaeochromocytoma. However, in patients with phaeochromocytoma, an alpha-blocker may be given concomitantly.

Although contra-indicated in severe peripheral arterial circulatory disturbances, propranolol may also aggravate less severe peripheral arterial circulatory disturbances.

One of the pharmacological actions of propranolol is to reduce the heart rate. Therefore the dosage should be reduced in those rare cases where symptoms are attributable to a slow heart rate.

Due to propranolol having a negative effect on conduction time, caution must be exercised if it is given to patients with first degree heart block.

Since the half life may be increased in patients with significant hepatic or renal impairment, caution must be exercised when starting treatment and selecting the initial dose.

In patients with portal hypertension, liver function may deteriorate and hepatic encephalopathy may develop. There have been reports suggesting that treatment with propranolol may increase the risk of developing hepatic encephalopathy.

Propranolol may cause a more severe reaction to a variety of allergens, when given to patients with a history of anaphylactic reaction to such allergens. Such patients may be unresponsive to the usual doses of adrenaline used to treat the allergic reactions.

Propranolol may mask the signs of thyrotoxicosis.

Propranolol must be used with caution in patients with decompensated cirrhosis.

Laboratory Tests: Propranolol has been reported to interfere with the estimation of serum bilirubin by the diazo method and with the determination of catecholamines by methods using fluorescence.

Excipient Warnings

This product contains parahydroxybenzoates which may cause allergic reactions (possibly delayed).

This product also contains liquid maltitol. Patients with rare hereditary problems of fructose intolerance should not take this medicine.

In addition, this product contains Sunset Yellow (E110) which may cause allergic reactions.

medicine.

4.5 Interaction with other medicinal products and other forms of interaction
Hypoglycaemic agents: Tachycardia associated with hypoglycaemia may be modified by propranolol. Use of propranolol alongside hypoglycaemic therapy in diabetic patients should be with caution since it may prolong the hypoglycaemic response to insulin.

Clonidine: Caution should be exercised when transferring patients from clonidine to beta-adrenoceptor blocking drugs. If propranolol and clonidine are given concurrently, clonidine should not be discontinued until several days after the withdrawal of the beta blocker. If replacing clonidine by beta-adrenoceptor blocking drug therapy, the introduction of the beta-adrenoceptor blocking drugs should be delayed for several days after clonidine administration has stopped.

Anti-arrhythmics: Care should be taken when prescribing a beta-adrenergic blocking drug with Class 1 anti-arrhythmic agents such as disopyramide. Flecainaide may have additive cardiac depressant effects.

Calcium Channel Blockers: Combined use of beta-adrenoceptor blocking drugs and calcium channel blockers with negative inotropic effects (eg, verapamil, diltiazem) can lead to an exaggeration of these effects particularly in patients with impaired ventricular function and/or SA or AV conduction abnormalities. This may result in severe hypotension, bradycardia and cardiac failure. Neither drug should be administered intravenously within 48 hours of discontinuing the other.

Concomitant therapy with dihydropyridine calcium channel blockers eg, nifedipine, may increase the risk of hypotension, and cardiac failure may occur in patients with latent cardiac insufficiency.

Drugs with hypotensive effects: Dynamic interactions between propranolol and other drugs with hypotensive effects are to be expected. Reactions are sometimes severe and careful monitoring is advised in co-administration of propranolol with other drugs including ACE inhibitors, diuretics, angiotensin II receptor antagonists, vasodilator antihypertensives, diazoxide, adrenergic neurone blockers, alpha blockers, moxisylyte, moxonidine, nitrates and methyldopa.

Anaesthesia: Caution must be exercised when using anaesthetic agents with propranolol. The anaesthetist should be informed and the choice of anaesthetic should be the agent with as little negative inotropic activity as possible. Use of beta-adrenoceptor blocking drugs with anaesthetic drugs may result in attenuation of the reflex tachycardia and increase the risk of hypotension. Anaesthetic agents causing myocardial depression are best avoided.

Neostigmine and other anticholinesterases: Propranolol reduces the efficacy of these compounds in treatment of myasthenia gravis.

Sympathomimetic Agents and Parenteral Adrenaline: Concomitant use of sympathomimetic agents e.g. adrenaline, may counteract the effect of beta-adrenoceptor blocking drugs. Caution should be taken in the parenteral administration of preparations containing adrenaline to people taking beta-adrenoceptor blocking drugs as, in rare cases, vasoconstriction, hypertension and bradycardia may result.

Muscle relaxants (e.g. balcofen): Concomitant use may result in a fall in blood pressure. Tizanidine may also result in bradycardia.

Antidepressants, anxiolytics and hypnotics: Plasma levels of propranolol can be increased by fluvoxamine. Anxiolytics, hypnotics and MAOIs when given with propranolol may have an enhanced hypotensive effect. Propranolol may increase plasma concentration of imipramine. Barbiturates may reduce the plasma concentration of propranolol.

Corticosteroids: Can antagonise the effects of beta-blockers.

Dihydropyridines: Concomitant therapy with dihydropyridines e.g. nifedipine, may increase the risk of hypotension, and cardiac failure may occur in patients with latent cardiac insufficiency.

Digitalis Glycosides: These preparations in association with beta-adrenoceptor blocking drugs, may increase atrio-ventricular conduction time.

Lignocaine: Administration of propranolol during infusion of lignocaine may increase the plasma concentration of lignocaine by approximately 30%. Patients already receiving propranolol tend to have higher lignocaine levels than controls. The combination should be avoided.

Ergotamine: Caution should be exercised if ergotamine, dihydroergotamine or related compounds are given in combination with propranolol since vasospastic reactions have been reported in a few patients.

Prostaglandin Synthetase Inhibiting Drugs: Concomitant use of these e.g. ibuprofen or indomethacin, may decrease the hypotensive effects of propranolol.

Chlorpromazine: Concomitant administration with propranolol may result in an increase in plasma levels of both drugs. This may lead to an enhanced antipsychotic effect for chlorpromazine and an increased antihypertensive effect for propranolol.

Mefolquine: May lead to an increased risk of bradycardia.

Cimetidine, hydralazine, alcohol: Concomitant use of cimetidine and hydralazine will increase, whereas concomitant use of alcohol will decrease, the plasma level of propranolol.

Dopaminergics (e.g. Levodopa), Aldesleukin, Prostaglandins (alprostadil): May have an enhanced hypotensive effect when used concomitantly with propranolol.

Oestrogens: May antagonise the hypotensive effect of propranolol.

5HT$_1$ agonists: Propranolol may increase plasma concentrations of rizatriptan.

Pharmacokinetic studies have shown that the following agents may interact with propranolol due to effects on enzyme systems in the liver which metabolise propranolol and these agents: quinidine, propafenone, rifampicin, theophylline, warfarin, thioridazine and dihydropyridine calcium channel blockers such as nifedipine, nisoldipine, nicardipine, isradipine and lacidipine. Owing to the fact that blood concentrations of either agent may be affected, dosage adjustments may be needed according to clinical judgement. (See also the interaction above concerning the concomitant therapy with dihydropyridine calcium channel blockers).

4.6 Pregnancy and lactation

As with all drugs, propranolol should not be given in pregnancy unless absolutely essential. There is no evidence of teratogenicity with propranolol. However, beta adrenoceptor blocking agents reduce placenta perfusion, which may result in intrauterine foetal death, immature and premature deliveries. In addition, adverse effects (especially hypoglycaemia and bradycardia in the neonate and bradycardia in the foetus) may occur. There is an increased risk of cardiac and pulmonary complications in the neonate in the post-natal period.

Most beta-adrenoceptor blocking drugs particularly lipophilic compounds, will pass into breast milk although to a variable extent. Breast feeding is therefore not recommended following administration of these compounds.

4.7 Effects on ability to drive and use machines

Use is unlikely to result in any impairment of the ability of patients to drive or operate machinery. However, it should be taken into account that occasionally dizziness or fatigue may occur.

4.8 Undesirable effects

Propranolol is usually well tolerated, however, listed below are the side effects that may occur:-

Cardiovascular: Bradycardia, heart failure deterioration, postural hypotension which may be associated with syncope, heart block and congestive cardiac failure, exacerbation of claudication, cold extremities, Raynaud's phenomenon.

Respiratory: Bronchospasm (especially in patients with a history of asthma), sometimes with fatal outcome (see Section 4.3)

Neurological and CNS: Confusion, dizziness, mood changes, nightmares, psychoses and hallucinations, sleep disturbances, paraesthesia especially of the hands.

Haematological: Purpura, thrombocytopenia.

Endocrine: Hypoglycaemia in neonates, infants, children, elderly patients, patients on haemodialysis, patients on concomitant antidiabetic therapy, patients with prolonged fasting and patients with chronic liver disease has been reported (see Section 4.3, 4.4 and 4.5).

Gastro-intestinal: Gastro-intestinal disturbance, nausea, diarrhoea.

Integumentary: Alopecia, dry eyes, psoriasiform skin reactions and exacerbation of psoriasis, skin rashes.

Senses: Visual disturbances.

Others: Muscle fatigue, lassitude, insomnia, an increase in ANA (antinuclear antibodies) although the clinical relevance of this has not been established. Isolated reports of myasthenia gravis have been reported in patients administered propranolol.

If these effects occur, thought should be given to withdrawing the drug. However, it should be withdrawn gradually.

Bradycardia and hypotension are usually a sign of overdosage but may be rarely linked to intolerance. If this occurs the drug should be withdrawn and overdosage treatment initiated.

4.9 Overdose

The symptoms of overdosage may include bradycardia, hypotension, acute cardiac insufficiency and bronchospasm.

General treatment should include: close supervision, treatment in an intensive care ward, the use of gastric lavage, activated charcoal and a laxative to prevent absorption of any drug still present in the gastrointestinal tract, the use of plasma or plasma substitutes to treat hypotension and shock.

Excessive bradycardia can be countered with atropine 1-2mg intravenously and/or a cardiac pacemaker. If necessary, this may be followed by a bolus dose of glucagons 10mg intravenously. If required, this may be repeated or followed by an intravenous infusion of glucagon 1-10mg/hour depending on response. If no response to glucagons occurs or if glucagon is unavailable, a beta-adrenoceptor stimulant such as dobutamine 2.5 to 10 micrograms/Kg/minute by intravenous infusion may be given. Dobutamine, because of its positive inotropic effect could also be used to treat hypotension and acute cardiac insufficiency. It is likely that these doses would be inadequate to reverse the cardiac effects of beta-blockade if a large overdose has been taken. The dose of dobutamine should therefore be increased if necessary to achieve the required response according to the clinical condition of the patient.

5. PHARMACOLOGICAL PROPERTIES

5.1 Pharmacodynamic properties

Pharmacotherapeutic group: Beta blocking agents, non-selective.

ATC Code: C07A A05

Propranolol is a competitive antagonist at both beta1 and beta2-adrenoceptors.

It has no agonist activity at the beta-adrenoceptor, but has membrane stabilising activity at concentrations exceeding 1-3mg/litre, though such concentrations are rarely achieved during oral therapy. Competitive beta-adrenoceptor blockade has been demonstrated in man by a parallel shift to the right in the dose-heart rate response curve to beta-agonists such as isoprenaline.

Propranolol, as with other beta-adrenoceptor blocking drugs, has negative inotropic effects, and is therefore contra-indicated in uncontrolled heart failure.

Propranolol is a racemic mixture and the active form is the S(-) isomer. With the exception of inhibition of the conversion of thyroxine to triiodothyronine it is unlikely that any additional ancillary properties possessed by R(+) propranolol, in comparison with the racemic mixture will give rise to different therapeutic effects.

Propranolol is effective and well tolerated in most ethnic populations, although the response may be less in black patients.

5.2 Pharmacokinetic properties

Following intravenous administration, the plasma half-life of propranolol is about 2 hours and the ratio of metabolites to parent drug in the blood is lower than after oral administration. In particular, 4-hydroxypropranolol is not present after intravenous administration.

Propranolol is completely absorbed after oral administration and peak plasma concentrations occur 1-2 hours after dosing in fasting patients. The liver removes up to 90% of an oral dose with an elimination half-life of 3 to 6 hours. Propranolol is widely and rapidly distributed throughout the body with highest levels occurring in the lungs, liver, kidney, brain and heart.

Propranolol is highly protein bound (80-95%).

5.3 Preclinical safety data

Propranolol is a drug on which extensive clinical experience has been obtained.

Relevant information for the prescriber is provided elsewhere in the Summary of Product Characteristics.

6. PHARMACEUTICAL PARTICULARS

6.1 List of excipients

Citric acid monohydrate (E330), methyl parahydroxybenzoate (E218), propyl parahydroxybenzoate (E216), propylene glycol (E1520), liquid maltitol (E965), sunset yellow E110, orange/tangerine flavour (including ethanol (0.12%v/v) and butylhydroxyanisole E320) and purified water.

6.2 Incompatibilities

None known

6.3 Shelf life

24 months unopened

3 months opened

6.4 Special precautions for storage

Do not store above 25°C. Do not refrigerate or freeze.

6.5 Nature and contents of container

Amber (Type III) glass bottles

Closures: - a) Aluminium, EPE wadded, roll-on pilfer-proof screw cap.

b) HDPE, EPE wadded, tamper evident screw cap.

c) HDPE, EPE wadded, tamper evident, child resistant closure.

Pack Size: 150ml

6.6 Special precautions for disposal and other handling

Not applicable.

Administrative Data

7. MARKETING AUTHORISATION HOLDER

Rosemont Pharmaceuticals Ltd Rosemont House, Yorkdale Industrial Park, Braithwaite Street, Leeds, LS11 9XE, UK.

8. MARKETING AUTHORISATION NUMBER(S)

PL 00427/0135

9. DATE OF FIRST AUTHORISATION/RENEWAL OF THE AUTHORISATION

29/05/2008

10. DATE OF REVISION OF THE TEXT

10/08/2009

Syprol Oral Solution 10mg/5ml

(Rosemont Pharmaceuticals Limited)

1. NAME OF THE MEDICINAL PRODUCT

Propranolol Hydrochloride 10mg/5ml Oral Solution

Syprol 10mg/5ml

2. QUALITATIVE AND QUANTITATIVE COMPOSITION

Propranolol Hydrochloride 10mg/5ml.

3. PHARMACEUTICAL FORM

Oral Solution

Clear colourless liquid with odour of orange/tangerine.

4. CLINICAL PARTICULARS

4.1 Therapeutic indications

Propranolol is indicated in:

- the control of hypertension
- the management of angina pectoris
- the long term prophylaxis against reinfarction after recovery from acute myocardial infarction
- the control of most forms of cardiac arrhythmia
- the prophylaxis of migraine
- the management of essential tremor
- relief of situational anxiety and generalised anxiety symptoms, particularly those of the somatic type.
- prophylaxis of upper gastro-intestinal bleeding in patients with portal hypertension and oesophageal varices.
- the adjunctive management of thyrotoxicosis and thyrotoxic crisis
- management of hypertrophic obstructive cardiomyopathy
- management of phaeochromocytoma perioperatively (with an alpha-adrenoceptor blocking drug).

4.2 Posology and method of administration

For oral administration only.

Adults:

Hypertension– A starting dose of 80mg twice a day may be increased at weekly intervals according to response. The usual dose range is 160 – 320mg per day. With concurrent diuretic or other antihypertensive drugs a further reduction of blood pressure is obtained.

Angina, migraine and essential tremor– A starting dose of 40mg two or three times daily may be increased by the same amount at weekly intervals according to patient response. An adequate response in migraine and essential tremor is usually seen in the range 80-160mg/day and in angina in the range 120-240mg/day.

Situational and generalised anxiety– A dose of 40mg daily may provide short term relief of acute situational anxiety. Generalised anxiety, requiring longer term therapy, usually responds adequately to 40mg twice daily which, in individual cases, may be increased to 40mg three times daily. Treatment should be continued according to response. Patients should be reviewed after six to twelve months treatment.

Arrhythmias, anxiety, tachycardia, hypertrophic obstructive cardiomyopathy and thyrotoxicosis– A dosage range of 10-40mg three or four times a day usually achieves the required response.

Post myocardial infarction - Treatment should start between days 5 and 21 after myocardial infarction with an initial dose of 40mg four times a day for 2 or 3 days. In order to improve compliance the total daily dosage may thereafter be given as 80mg twice daily.

Portal hypertension:

Dosage should be titrated to achieve approximately 25% reduction in resting heart rate. Dosage should begin with 40mg twice daily, increasing to 80mg twice daily depending on heart rate response. If necessary, the dose may be increased incrementally to a maximum of 160mg twice daily.

Phaeochromocytoma (Used only with an alpha-receptor blocking drug)- Pre-operative: 60mg daily for three days is recommended. Non-operable malignant cases: 30mg daily.

Children

Arrhythmias, phaeochromocytoma, thyrotoxicosis– Dosage should be individually determined and the following is only a guide: 250 – 500 micrograms per Kilogram three or four times daily as required.

Migraine– Under the age of 12: 20mg two or three times daily

Over the age of 12: the adult dose

Fallot's tetralogy– The value of propranolol in this condition is confined mainly to the relief of right-ventricular outflow tract shut-down. It is also useful for treatment of associated arrhythmias and angina. Dosage should be individually determined and the following is only a guide: Up to 1mg/Kg repeated three or four times a day as required.

Elderly

With regard to the elderly the optimum dose should be individually determined according to the clinical response.

4.3 Contraindications

Propranolol must not be used if there is a history of bronchial asthma or bronchospasm.

The product label states the following warning: "Do not take propranolol if you have a history of asthma or wheezing". A similar warning appears in the patient information leaflet.

Bronchospasm can usually be reversed by beta$_2$-agonist bronchodilators such as salbutamol. Large doses of the beta$_2$-agonist bronchodilator may be required to overcome the beta-blockade produced by propranolol and the dose should be titrated according to the clinical response; both intravenous and inhalational administration should be considered. The use of intravenous aminophylline and/or the use of ipratropium (given by nebuliser) may also be considered. Glucagon (1 to 2mg given intravenously) has also been reported to produce a bronchodilator effect in asthmatic patients. Oxygen or artificial ventilation may be required in severe cases.

Propranolol as with other beta-adrenoceptor blocking drugs must not be used in patients with any of the following:

hypersensitivity to propranolol hydrochloride or any of the ingredients; the presence of second or third degree heart block; in cardiogenic shock; metabolic acidosis; after prolonged fasting; bradycardia; hypotension; severe peripheral arterial circulatory disturbances; sick sinus syndrome; untreated phaeochromocytoma; uncontrolled heart failure or Prinzmetal's angina.

Propranolol must not be used in patients prone to hypoglycaemia, i.e., patients after prolonged fasting or patients with restricted counter-regulatory reserves. Patients with restricted counter-regulatory reserves may have reduced autonomic and hormonal responses to hypoglycaemia which includes glycogenolysis, gluconeogenesis and /or impaired modulation of insulin secretion. Patients at risk for an inadequate response to hypoglycaemia includes individuals with malnutrition, prolonged fasting, starvation, chronic liver disease, diabetes and concomitant use of drugs which block the full response to catecholamines.

4.4 Special warnings and precautions for use

Although contra-indicated in uncontrolled heart failure, propranolol may be used where the signs of heart failure have been controlled by the use of appropriate concomitant medication. Propranolol should be used with caution in patients whose cardiac reserve is poor.

Treatment should not be discontinued abruptly in patients with ischaemic heart disease. Either the equivalent dose of another beta-adrenoceptor blocking drug may be substituted or the withdrawal of propranolol should be gradual.

Propranolol should not be used in combination with calcium channel blockers with negative inotropic effects (e.g. verapamil, diltiazem), as it can lead to an exaggeration of these effects particularly in patients with impaired ventricular function and/or SA or AV conduction abnormalities. This may result in severe hypotension, bradycardia and cardiac failure. Neither the beta-blocker nor the calcium channel blocker should be administered intravenously within 48 hours of discontinuing the other.

Propranolol may block/modify the signs and symptoms of hypoglycaemia (especially tachycardia). Propranolol occasionally causes hypoglycaemia, even in non-diabetic patients, e.g., neonates, infants, children, elderly patients, patients on haemodialysis or patients suffering from chronic liver disease and patients suffering from overdose. Severe hypoglycaemia associated with propranolol has rarely presented with seizures and/or coma in isolated patients. Caution must be exercised in the concurrent use of propranolol and hypoglycaemic therapy in diabetic patients. Propranolol may prolong the hypoglycaemic response to insulin (see section 4.3).

When a patient is scheduled for surgery and a decision is made to discontinue beta-blocker therapy, this should be done at least 24 hours prior to the procedure. The risk/benefit of stopping beta blockade should be made for each patient

Propranolol should not be used in untreated phaeochromocytoma. However, in patients with phaeochromocytoma, an alpha-blocker may be given concomitantly.

Although contra-indicated in severe peripheral arterial circulatory disturbances, propranolol may also aggravate less severe peripheral arterial circulatory disturbances.

One of the pharmacological actions of propranolol is to reduce the heart rate. Therefore the dosage should be reduced in those rare cases where symptoms are attributable to a slow heart rate.

Due to propranolol having a negative effect on conduction time, caution must be exercised if it is given to patients with first degree heart block.

Since the half life may be increased in patients with significant hepatic or renal impairment, caution must be exercised when starting treatment and selecting the initial dose.

In patients with portal hypertension, liver function may deteriorate and hepatic encephalopathy may develop. There have been reports suggesting that treatment with propranolol may increase the risk of developing hepatic encephalopathy.

Propranolol may cause a more severe reaction to a variety of allergens, when given to patients with a history of anaphylactic reaction to such allergens. Such patients may be unresponsive to the usual doses of adrenaline used to treat the allergic reactions.

Propranolol may mask the signs of thyrotoxicosis.

Propranolol must be used with caution in patients with decompensated cirrhosis.

Laboratory Tests: Propranolol has been reported to interfere with the estimation of serum bilirubin by the diazo method and with the determination of catecholamines by methods using fluorescence.

Excipient Warnings

This product contains parahydroxybenzoates which may cause allergic reactions (possibly delayed)

This product also contains liquid maltitol. Patients with rare hereditary problems of fructose intolerance should not take this medicine.

4.5 Interaction with other medicinal products and other forms of interaction

Hypoglycaemic agents: Tachycardia associated with hypoglycaemia may be modified by propranolol. Use of propranolol alongside hypoglycaemic therapy in diabetic patients should be with caution since it may prolong the hypoglycaemic response to insulin.

Clonidine: Caution should be exercised when transferring patients from clonidine to beta-adrenoceptor blocking drugs. If propranolol and clonidine are given concurrently, clonidine should not be discontinued until several days after the withdrawal of the beta blocker. If replacing clonidine by beta-adrenoceptor blocking drug therapy, the introduction of the beta-adrenoceptor blocking drugs should be delayed for several days after clonidine administration has stopped.

Anti-arrhythmics: Care should be taken when prescribing a beta-adrenergic blocking drug with Class 1 anti-arrhythmic agents such as disopyramide. Flecainaide may have additive cardiac depressant effects.

Calcium Channel Blockers: Combined use of beta-adrenoceptor blocking drugs and calcium channel blockers with negative inotropic effects (eg, verapamil, diltiazem) can lead to an exaggeration of these effects particularly in patients with impaired ventricular function and/or SA or AV conduction abnormalities. This may result in severe hypotension, bradycardia and cardiac failure. Neither drug should be administered intravenously within 48 hours of discontinuing the other.

Concomitant therapy with dihydropyridine calcium channel blockers eg, nifedipine, may increase the risk of hypotension, and cardiac failure may occur in patients with latent cardiac insufficiency.

Drugs with hypotensive effects: Dynamic interactions between propranolol and other drugs with hypotensive effects are to be expected. Reactions are sometimes severe and careful monitoring is advised in co-administration of propranolol with other drugs including ACE inhibitors, diuretics, angiotensin II receptor antagonists, vasodilator antihypertensives, diazoxide, adrenergic neurone blockers, alpha blockers, moxisylyte, moxonidine, nitrates and methyldopa.

Anaesthesia: Caution must be exercised when using anaesthetic agents with propranolol. The anaesthetist should be informed and the choice of anaesthetic should be the agent with as little negative inotropic activity as possible. Use of beta-adrenoceptor blocking drugs with anaesthetic drugs may result in attenuation of the reflex tachycardia and increase the risk of hypotension. Anaesthetic agents causing myocardial depression are best avoided.

Neostigmine and other anticholinesterases: Propranolol reduces the efficacy of these compounds in treatment of myasthenia gravis.

Sympathomimetic Agents and Parenteral Adrenaline: Concomitant use of sympathomimetic agents e.g. adrenaline, may counteract the effect of beta-adrenoceptor blocking drugs. Caution should be taken in the parenteral administration of preparations containing adrenaline to people taking beta-adrenoceptor blocking drugs as, in rare cases, vasoconstriction, hypertension and bradycardia may result.

Muscle relaxants (e.g. balcofen): Concomitant use may result in a fall in blood pressure. Tizanidine may also result in bradycardia.

Antidepressants, anxiolytics and hypnotics: Plasma levels of propranolol can be increased by fluvoxamine. Anxiolytics, hypnotics and MAOIs when given with propranolol may have an enhanced hypotensive effect. Propranolol may increase plasma concentration of imipramine. Barbiturates may reduce the plasma concentration of propranolol.

Corticosteroids: Can antagonise the effects of beta-blockers.

Dihydropyridines: Concomitant therapy with dihydropyridines e.g. nifedipine, may increase the risk of hypotension, and cardiac failure may occur in patients with latent cardiac insufficiency.

Digitalis Glycosides: These preparations in association with beta-adrenoceptor blocking drugs, may increase atrio-ventricular conduction time.

Lignocaine: Administration of propranolol during infusion of lignocaine may increase the plasma concentration of lignocaine by approximately 30%. Patients already receiving propranolol tend to have higher lignocaine levels than controls. The combination should be avoided.

Ergotamine: Caution should be exercised if ergotamine, dihydroergotamine or related compounds are given in combination with propranolol since vasospastic reactions have been reported in a few patients.

Prostaglandin Synthetase Inhibiting Drugs: Concomitant use of these e.g. ibuprofen or indomethacin, may decrease the hypotensive effects of propranolol.

Chlorpromazine: Concomitant administration with propranolol may result in an increase in plasma levels of both drugs. This may lead to an enhanced antipsychotic effect for chlorpromazine and an increased antihypertensive effect for propranolol.

Mefolquine: May lead to an increased risk of bradycardia.

Cimetidine, hydralazine, alcohol: Concomitant use of cimetidine and hydralazine will increase, whereas concomitant use of alcohol will decrease, the plasma level of propranolol.

Dopaminergics (e.g. Levodopa), Aldesleukin, Prostaglandins (alprostadil): May have an enhanced hypotensive effect when used concomitantly with propranolol.

Oestrogens: May antagonise the hypotensive effect of propranolol.

5 HT$_1$ agonists: Propranolol may increase plasma concentrations of rizatriptan.

Pharmacokinetic studies have shown that the following agents may interact with propranolol due to effects on enzyme systems in the liver which metabolise propranolol and these agents: quinidine, propafenone, rifampicin, theophylline, warfarin, thioridazine and dihydropyridine calcium channel blockers such as nifedipine, nisoldipine, nicardipine, isradipine and lacidipine. Owing to the fact that blood concentrations of either agent may be affected, dosage adjustments may be needed according to clinical judgement. (See also the interaction above concerning the concomitant therapy with dihydropyridine calcium channel blockers).

4.6 Pregnancy and lactation

As with all drugs, propranolol should not be given in pregnancy unless absolutely essential. There is no evidence of teratogenicity with propranolol. However, beta adrenoceptor blocking agents reduce placenta perfusion, which may result in intra-uterine foetal death, immature and premature deliveries. In addition, adverse effects (especially hypoglycaemia and bradycardia in the neonate and bradycardia in the foetus) may occur. There is an increased risk of cardiac and pulmonary complications in the neonate in the post-natal period.

Most beta-adrenoceptor blocking drugs particularly lipophilic compounds, will pass into breast milk although to a variable extent. Breast feeding is therefore not recommended following administration of these compounds.

4.7 Effects on ability to drive and use machines

Use is unlikely to result in any impairment of the ability of patients to drive or operate machinery. However, it should be taken into account that occasionally dizziness or fatigue may occur.

4.8 Undesirable effects

Propranolol is usually well tolerated, however, listed below are the side effects that may occur:-

Cardiovascular: Bradycardia, heart failure deterioration, postural hypotension which may be associated with syncope, heart block and congestive cardiac failure, exacerbation of claudication, cold extremities, Raynaud's phenomenon.

Respiratory: Bronchospasm (especially in patients with a history of asthma), sometimes with fatal outcome (see Section 4.3).

Neurological and CNS: Confusion, dizziness, mood changes, nightmares, psychoses and hallucinations, sleep disturbances, paraesthesia especially of the hands.

Haematological: Purpura, thrombocytopenia.

Endocrine: Hypoglycaemia in neonates, infants, children, elderly patients, patients on haemodialysis, patients on concomitant antidiabetic therapy, patients with prolonged fasting and patients with chronic liver disease has been reported (see section 4.3, 4.4 and 4.5).

Gastro-intestinal: Gastro-intestinal disturbance, nausea, diarrhoea.

Integumentary: Alopecia, dry eyes, psoriasiform skin reactions and exacerbation of psoriasis, skin rashes.

Senses: Visual disturbances.

Others: Muscle fatigue, lassitude, insomnia, an increase in ANA (antinuclear antibodies) although the clinical relevance of this has not been established. Isolated reports of myasthenia gravis like syndrome or exacerbation of myasthenia gravis have been reported in patients administered propranolol.

If these effects occur, thought should be given to withdrawing the drug. However, it should be withdrawn gradually.

Bradycardia and hypotension are usually a sign of overdosage but may be rarely linked to intolerance. If this occurs the drug should be withdrawn and overdosage treatment initiated.

4.9 Overdose

The symptoms of overdosage may include bradycardia, hypotension, acute cardiac insufficiency and bronchospasm.

General treatment should include: close supervision, treatment in an intensive care ward, the use of gastric lavage, activated charcoal and a laxative to prevent absorption of any drug still present in the gastrointestinal tract, the use of plasma or plasma substitutes to treat hypotension and shock.

Excessive bradycardia can be countered with atropine 1-2mg intravenously and/or a cardiac pacemaker. If necessary, this may be followed by a bolus dose of glucagon 10mg intravenously. If required, this may be repeated or followed by an intravenous infusion of glucagon 1-10mg/hour depending on response. If no response to glucagon occurs or if glucagon is unavailable, a beta-adrenoceptor stimulant such as dobutamine 2.5 to 10 micrograms/Kg/minute by intravenous infusion may be given. Dobutamine, because of its positive inotropic effect could also be used to treat hypotension and acute cardiac insufficiency. It is likely that these doses would be inadequate to reverse the cardiac effects of beta-blockade if a large overdose has been taken. The dose of dobutamine should therefore be increased if necessary to achieve the required response according to the clinical condition of the patient.

5. PHARMACOLOGICAL PROPERTIES

5.1 Pharmacodynamic properties

Propranolol is a competitive antagonist at both $beta_1$ and $beta_2$-adrenoceptors.

It has no agonist activity at the beta-adrenoceptor, but has membrane stabilising activity at concentrations exceeding 1-3mg/litre, though such concentrations are rarely achieved during oral therapy. Competitive beta-adrenoceptor blockade has been demonstrated in man by a parallel shift to the right in the dose-heart rate response curve to beta-agonists such as isoprenaline.

Propranolol, as with other beta-adrenoceptor blocking drugs, has negative inotropic effects, and is therefore contra-indicated in uncontrolled heart failure.

Propranolol is a racemic mixture and the active form is the S(-) isomer. With the exception of inhibition of the conversion of thyroxine to triiodothyronine it is unlikely that any additional ancillary properties possessed by R(+) propranolol, in comparison with the racemic mixture will give rise to different therapeutic effects.

Propranolol is effective and well tolerated in most ethnic populations, although the response may be less in black patients.

5.2 Pharmacokinetic properties

Following intravenous administration, the plasma half-life of propranolol is about 2 hours and the ratio of metabolites to parent drug in the blood is lower than after oral administration. In particular, 4-hydroxypropranolol is not present after intravenous administration.

Propranolol is completely absorbed after oral administration and peak plasma concentrations occur 1-2 hours after dosing in fasting patients. The liver removes up to 90% of an oral dose with an elimination half-life of 3 to 6 hours. Propranolol is widely and rapidly distributed throughout the body with highest levels occurring in the lungs, liver, kidney, brain and heart.

Propranolol is highly protein bound (80-95%).

5.3 Preclinical safety data

Propranolol is a drug on which extensive clinical experience has been obtained. Relevant information for the prescriber is provided elsewhere in the Summary of Product Characteristics.

6. PHARMACEUTICAL PARTICULARS

6.1 List of excipients

Citric acid monohydrate, methyl parahydroxybenzoate (E218), propyl parahydroxybenzoate (E216), propylene glycol, liquid maltitol, orange/tangerine flavour (including ethanol (0.12%v/v) and butylhydroxyanisol E320) and purified water.

6.2 Incompatibilities

None known.

6.3 Shelf life

24 months unopened

3 months opened.

6.4 Special precautions for storage

Do not store above 25°C. Do not refrigerate or freeze.

6.5 Nature and contents of container

Amber (Type III) glass bottles

Closures: - a) Aluminium, EPE wadded, roll-on pilfer-proof screw cap.

b) HDPE, EPE wadded, tamper evident screw cap.

c) HDPE, EPE wadded, tamper evident, child resistant closure.

Pack Size: 150ml

6.6 Special precautions for disposal and other handling

Not applicable.

Administrative Data

7. MARKETING AUTHORISATION HOLDER

Rosemont Pharmaceuticals Ltd, Rosemont House, Yorkdale Industrial Park, Braithwaite Street, Leeds, LS11 9XE, UK.

8. MARKETING AUTHORISATION NUMBER(S)

PL 00427/0123

9. DATE OF FIRST AUTHORISATION/RENEWAL OF THE AUTHORISATION

11th December 2000, Renewal: 30th August 2006

10. DATE OF REVISION OF THE TEXT

10th August 2009

11. Legal Category

POM

Syprol Oral Solution 50mg/5ml

(Rosemont Pharmaceuticals Limited)

1. NAME OF THE MEDICINAL PRODUCT

Propranolol Hydrochloride 50mg/5ml Oral Solution

Syprol 50mg/5ml

2. QUALITATIVE AND QUANTITATIVE COMPOSITION

Propranolol Hydrochloride 50mg/5ml.

3. PHARMACEUTICAL FORM

Oral Solution

A clear bright orange liquid with odour of orange/tangerine.

4. CLINICAL PARTICULARS

4.1 Therapeutic indications

Propranolol is indicated in:

- the control of hypertension
- the management of angina pectoris
- the long term prophylaxis against reinfarction after recovery from acute myocardial infarction
- the control of most forms of cardiac arrhythmia
- the prophylaxis of migraine
- the management of essential tremor
- relief of situational anxiety and generalised anxiety symptoms, particularly those of the somatic type.
- prophylaxis of upper gastro-intestinal bleeding in patients with portal hypertension and oesophageal varices.
- the adjunctive management of thyrotoxicosis and thyrotoxic crisis
- management of hypertrophic obstructive cardiomyopathy
- management of phaeochromocytoma perioperatively (with an alpha-adrenoceptor blocking drug).

4.2 Posology and method of administration

For oral administration only.

Adults:

Hypertension– A starting dose of 80mg twice a day may be increased at weekly intervals according to response. The usual dose range is 160 – 320mg per day. With concurrent diuretic or other antihypertensive drugs a further reduction of blood pressure is obtained.

Angina, migraine and essential tremor– A starting dose of 40mg two or three times daily may be increased by the same amount at weekly intervals according to patient response. An adequate response in migraine and essential tremor is usually seen in the range 80-160mg/day and in angina in the range 120-240mg/day.

Situational and generalised anxiety– A dose of 40mg daily may provide short term relief of acute situational anxiety. Generalised anxiety, requiring longer term therapy, usually responds adequately to 40mg twice daily which, in individual cases, may be increased to 40mg three times daily. Treatment should be continued according to response. Patients should be reviewed after six to twelve months treatment.

Arrhythmias, anxiety, tachycardia, hypertrophic obstructive cardiomyopathy and thyrotoxicosis– A dosage range of 10-40mg three or four times a day usually achieves the required response.

Post myocardial infarction - Treatment should start between days 5 and 21 after myocardial infarction with an initial dose of 40mg four times a day for 2 or 3 days. In order to improve compliance the total daily dosage may thereafter be given as 80mg twice daily.

Portal hypertension:

Dosage should be titrated to achieve approximately 25% reduction in resting heart rate. Dosage should begin with 40mg twice daily, increasing to 80mg twice daily depending on heart rate response. If necessary, the dose may be increased incrementally to a maximum of 160mg twice daily.

Phaeochromocytoma (Used only with an alpha-receptor blocking drug)- Pre-operative: 60mg daily for three days is recommended. Non-operable malignant cases: 30mg daily.

Children

Arrhythmias, phaeochromocytoma, thyrotoxicosis– Dosage should be individually determined and the following is only a guide: 250 – 500 micrograms per Kilogram three or four times daily as required.

Migraine– Under the age of 12: 20mg two or three times daily

Over the age of 12: the adult dose

Fallot's tetralogy– The value of propranolol in this condition is confined mainly to the relief of right-ventricular outflow tract shut-down. It is also useful for treatment of associated arrhythmias and angina. Dosage should be individually determined and the following is only a guide: Up to 1mg/Kg repeated three or four times a day as required.

Elderly

With regard to the elderly the optimum dose should be individually determined according to the clinical response.

4.3 Contraindications

Propranolol must not be used if there is a history of bronchial asthma or bronchospasm.

The product label states the following warning: "Do not take propranolol if you have a history of asthma or wheezing". A similar warning appears in the patient information leaflet.

Bronchospasm can usually be reversed by $beta_2$-agonist bronchodilators such as salbutamol. Large doses of the $beta_2$-agonist bronchodilator may be required to overcome the beta-blockade produced by propranolol and the dose should be titrated according to the clinical response; both intravenous and inhalational administration should be considered. The use of intravenous aminophylline and/or the use of ipratropium (given by nebuliser) may also be considered. Glucagon (1 to 2mg given intravenously) has also been reported to produce a bronchodilator effect in asthmatic patients. Oxygen or artificial ventilation may be required in severe cases.

Propranolol as with other beta-adrenoceptor blocking drugs must not be used in patients with any of the following:

hypersensitivity to propranolol hydrochloride or any of the ingredients; the presence of second or third degree heart block; in cardiogenic shock; metabolic acidosis; after prolonged fasting; bradycardia; hypotension; severe peripheral arterial circulatory disturbances; sick sinus syndrome; untreated phaeochromocytoma; uncontrolled heart failure or Prinzmetal's angina.

Propranolol must not be used in patients prone to hypoglycaemia, i.e., patients after prolonged fasting or patients with restricted counter-regulatory reserves. Patients with restricted counter-regulatory reserves may have reduced autonomic and hormonal responses to hypoglycaemia which includes glycogenolysis, gluconeogenesis and /or impaired modulation of insulin secretion. Patients at risk for an inadequate response to hypoglycaemia includes individuals with malnutrition, prolonged fasting, starvation, chronic liver disease, diabetes and concomitant use of drugs which block the full response to catecholamines.

4.4 Special warnings and precautions for use

Although contra-indicated in uncontrolled heart failure, propranolol may be used where the signs of heart failure have been controlled by the use of appropriate concomitant medication. Propranolol should be used with caution in patients whose cardiac reserve is poor.

Treatment should not be discontinued abruptly in patients with ischaemic heart disease. Either the equivalent dose of another beta-adrenoceptor blocking drug may be substituted or the withdrawal of propranolol should be gradual.

Propranolol should not be used in combination with calcium channel blockers with negative inotropic effects (e.g. verapamil, diltiazem), as it can lead to an exaggeration of these effects particularly in patients with impaired ventricular function and/or SA or AV conduction abnormalities. This may result in severe hypotension, bradycardia and cardiac failure. Neither the beta-blocker nor the calcium channel blocker should be administered intravenously within 48 hours of discontinuing the other.

Propranolol may block/modify the signs and symptoms of hypoglycaemia (especially tachycardia). Propranolol occasionally causes hypoglycaemia, even in non-diabetic patients, e.g., neonates, infants, children, elderly patients, patients on haemodialysis or patients suffering from chronic liver disease and patients suffering from overdose. Severe hypoglycaemia associated with propranolol has rarely presented with seizures and/or coma in isolated patients. Caution must be exercised in the concurrent use of propranolol and hypoglycaemic therapy in diabetic patients. Propranolol may prolong the hypoglycaemic response to insulin (see section 4.3).

When a patient is scheduled for surgery and a decision is made to discontinue beta-blocker therapy, this should be done at least 24 hours prior to the procedure. The risk/benefit of stopping beta blockade should be made for each patient

Propranolol should not be used in untreated phaeochromocytoma. However, in patients with phaeochromocytoma, an alpha-blocker may be given concomitantly.

Although contra-indicated in severe peripheral arterial circulatory disturbances, propranolol may also aggravate less severe peripheral arterial circulatory disturbances.

One of the pharmacological actions of propranolol is to reduce the heart rate. Therefore the dosage should be reduced in those rare cases where symptoms are attributable to a slow heart rate.

Due to propranolol having a negative effect on conduction time, caution must be exercised if it is given to patients with first degree heart block.

Since the half life may be increased in patients with significant hepatic or renal impairment, caution must be exercised when starting treatment and selecting the initial dose.

In patients with portal hypertension, liver function may deteriorate and hepatic encephalopathy may develop. There have been reports suggesting that treatment with propranolol may increase the risk of developing hepatic encephalopathy.

Propranolol may cause a more severe reaction to a variety of allergens, when given to patients with a history of anaphylactic reaction to such allergens. Such patients may be unresponsive to the usual doses of adrenaline used to treat the allergic reactions.

Propranolol may mask the signs of thyrotoxicosis.

Propranolol must be used with caution in patients with decompensated cirrhosis.

Laboratory Tests: Propranolol has been reported to interfere with the estimation of serum bilirubin by the diazo method and with the determination of catecholamines by methods using fluorescence.

Excipient Warnings

This product contains parahydroxybenzoates which may cause allergic reactions (possibly delayed)

This product also contains liquid maltitol. Patients with rare hereditary problems of fructose intolerance should not take this medicine.

In addition, this product contains Sunset Yellow (E110) which may cause allergic reactions.

4.5 Interaction with other medicinal products and other forms of interaction

Hypoglycaemic agents: Tachycardia associated with hypoglycaemia may be modified by propranolol. Use of propranolol alongside hypoglycaemic therapy in diabetic patients should be with caution since it may prolong the hypoglycaemic response to insulin.

Clonidine: Caution should be exercised when transferring patients from clonidine to beta-adrenoceptor blocking drugs. If propranolol and clonidine are given concurrently, clonidine should not be discontinued until several days after the withdrawal of the beta blocker. If replacing clonidine by beta-adrenoceptor blocking drug therapy, the introduction of the beta-adrenoceptor blocking drugs should be delayed for several days after clonidine administration has stopped.

Anti-arrhythmics: Care should be taken when prescribing a beta-adrenergic blocking drug with Class 1 anti-arrhythmic agents such as disopyramide. Flecainaide may have additive cardiac depressant effects.

Calcium Channel Blockers: Combined use of beta-adrenoceptor blocking drugs and calcium channel blockers with negative inotropic effects (eg, verapamil, diltiazem) can lead to an exaggeration of these effects particularly in patients with impaired ventricular function and/or SA or AV conduction abnormalities. This may result in severe hypotension, bradycardia and cardiac failure. Neither drug should be administered intravenously within 48 hours of discontinuing the other.

Concomitant therapy with dihydropyridine calcium channel blockers eg, nifedipine, may increase the risk of hypotension, and cardiac failure may occur in patients with latent cardiac insufficiency.

Drugs with hypotensive effects: Dynamic interactions between propranolol and other drugs with hypotensive effects are to be expected. Reactions are sometimes severe and careful monitoring is advised in co-administration of propranolol with other drugs including ACE inhibitors, diuretics, angiotensin II receptor antagonists, vasodilator antihypertensives, diazoxide, adrenergic neurone blockers, alpha blockers, moxisylyte, moxonidine, nitrates and methyldopa.

Anaesthesia: Caution must be exercised when using anaesthetic agents with propranolol. The anaesthetist should be informed and the choice of anaesthetic should be the agent with as little negative inotropic activity as possible. Use of beta-adrenoceptor blocking drugs with anaesthetic drugs may result in attenuation of the reflex tachycardia and increase the risk of hypotension. Anaesthetic agents causing myocardial depression are best avoided.

Neostigmine and other anticholinesterases: Propranolol reduces the efficacy of these compounds in treatment of myasthenia gravis.

Sympathomimetic Agents and Parenteral Adrenaline: Concomitant use of sympathomimetic agents e.g. adrenaline, may counteract the effect of beta-adrenoceptor blocking drugs. Caution should be taken in the parenteral administration of preparations containing adrenaline to people taking beta-adrenoceptor blocking drugs as, in rare cases, vasoconstriction, hypertension and bradycardia may result.

Muscle relaxants (e.g. balcofen): Concomitant use may result in a fall in blood pressure. Tizanidine may also result in bradycardia.

Antidepressants, anxiolytics and hypnotics: Plasma levels of propranolol can be increased by fluvoxamine. Anxiolytics, hypnotics and MAOIs when given with propranolol may have an enhanced hypotensive effect. Propranolol may increase plasma concentration of imipramine. Barbiturates may reduce the plasma concentration of propranolol.

Corticosteroids: Can antagonise the effects of beta-blockers.

Dihydropyridines: Concomitant therapy with dihydropyridines e.g. nifedipine, may increase the risk of hypctension, and cardiac failure may occur in patients with latent cardiac insufficiency.

Digitalis Glycosides: These preparations in association with beta-adrenoceptor blocking drugs, may increase atrio-ventricular conduction time.

Lignocaine: Administration of propranolol during infusion of lignocaine may increase the plasma concentration of lignocaine by approximately 30%. Patients already receiving propranolol tend to have higher lignocaine levels than controls. The combination should be avoided.

Ergotamine: Caution should be exercised if ergotamine, dihydroergotamine or related compounds are given in combination with propranolol since vasospastic reactions have been reported in a few patients.

Prostaglandin Synthetase Inhibiting Drugs: Concomitant use of these e.g. ibuprofen or indomethacin, may decrease the hypotensive effects of propranolol.

Chlorpromazine: Concomitant administration with propranolol may result in an increase in plasma levels of both drugs. This may lead to an enhanced antipsychotic effect for chlorpromazine and an increased antihypertensive effect for propranolol.

Mefolquine: May lead to an increased risk of bradycardia.

Cimetidine, hydralazine, alcohol: Concomitant use of cimetidine and hydralazine will increase, whereas concomitant use of alcohol will decrease, the plasma level of propranolol.

Dopaminergics (e.g. Levodopa), Aldesleukin, Prostaglandins (alprostadil): May have an enhanced hypotensive effect when used concomitantly with propranolol.

Oestrogens: May antagonise the hypotensive effect of propranolol.

$5HT_1$ agonists: Propranolol may increase plasma concentrations of rizatriptan.

Pharmacokinetic studies have shown that the following agents may interact with propranolol due to effects on enzyme systems in the liver which metabolise propranolol and these agents: quinidine, propafenone, rifampicin, theophylline, warfarin, thioridazine and dihydropyridine calcium channel blockers such as nifedipine, nisoldipine, nicardipine, isradipine and lacidipine. Owing to the fact that blood concentrations of either agent may be affected, dosage adjustments may be needed according to clinical judgement. (See also the interaction above concerning the concomitant therapy with dihydropyridine calcium channel blockers).

4.6 Pregnancy and lactation

As with all drugs, propranolol should not be given in pregnancy unless absolutely essential. There is no evidence of teratogenicity with propranolol. However, beta adrenoceptor blocking agents reduce placenta perfusion, which may result in intra-uterine foetal death, immature and premature deliveries. In addition, adverse effects (especially hypoglycaemia and bradycardia in the neonate and bradycardia in the foetus) may occur. There is an increased risk of cardiac and pulmonary complications in the neonate in the post-natal period.

Most beta-adrenoceptor blocking drugs particularly lipophilic compounds, will pass into breast milk although to a variable extent. Breast feeding is therefore not recommended following administration of these compounds.

4.7 Effects on ability to drive and use machines

Use is unlikely to result in any impairment of the ability of patients to drive or operate machinery. However, it should be taken into account that occasionally dizziness or fatigue may occur.

4.8 Undesirable effects

Propranolol is usually well tolerated, however, listed below are the side effects that may occur:-

Cardiovascular: Bradycardia, heart failure deterioration, postural hypotension which may be associated with syncope, heart block and congestive cardiac failure, exacerbation of claudication, cold extremities, Raynaud's phenomenon.

Respiratory: Bronchospasm (especially in patients with a history of asthma), sometimes with fatal outcome (see Section 4.3).

Neurological and CNS: Confusion, dizziness, mood changes, nightmares, psychoses and hallucinations, sleep disturbances, paraesthesia especially of the hands.

Haematological: Purpura, thrombocytopenia.

Endocrine: Hypoglycaemia in neonates, infants, children, elderly patients, patients on haemodialysis, patients on concomitant antidiabetic therapy, patients with prolonged fasting and patients with chronic liver disease has been reported (see section 4.3, 4.4 and 4.5).

Gastro-intestinal: Gastro-intestinal disturbance, nausea, diarrhoea.

Integumentary: Alopecia, dry eyes, psoriasiform skin reactions and exacerbation of psoriasis, skin rashes.

Senses: Visual disturbances.

Others: Muscle fatigue, lassitude, insomnia, an increase in ANA (antinuclear antibodies) although the clinical relevance of this has not been established. Isolated reports of myasthenia gravis like syndrome or exacerbation of myasthenia gravis have been reported in patients administered propranolol.

If these effects occur, thought should be given to withdrawing the drug. However, it should be withdrawn gradually.

Bradycardia and hypotension are usually a sign of overdosage but may be rarely linked to intolerance. If this occurs the drug should be withdrawn and overdosage treatment initiated.

4.9 Overdose

The symptoms of overdosage may include bradycardia, hypotension, acute cardiac insufficiency and bronchospasm.

General treatment should include: close supervision, treatment in an intensive care ward, the use of gastric lavage, activated charcoal and a laxative to prevent absorption of any drug still present in the gastrointestinal tract, the use of plasma or plasma substitutes to treat hypotension and shock.

Excessive bradycardia can be countered with atropine 1-2mg intravenously and/or a cardiac pacemaker. If necessary, this may be followed by a bolus dose of glucagon 10mg intravenously. If required, this may be repeated or followed by an intravenous infusion of glucagon 1-10mg/hour depending on response. If no response to glucagon occurs or if glucagon is unavailable, a beta-adrenoceptor stimulant such as dobutamine 2.5 to 10 micrograms/Kg/minute by intravenous infusion may be given. Dobutamine, because of its positive inotropic effect could also be used to treat hypotension and acute cardiac insufficiency. It is likely that these doses would be inadequate to reverse the cardiac effects of beta-blockade if a large overdose has been taken. The dose of dobutamine should therefore be increased if necessary to achieve the required response according to the clinical condition of the patient.

5. PHARMACOLOGICAL PROPERTIES

5.1 Pharmacodynamic properties

Propranolol is a competitive antagonist at both $beta_1$ and $beta_2$-adrenoceptors.

It has no agonist activity at the beta-adrenoceptor, but has membrane stabilising activity at concentrations exceeding 1-3mg/litre, though such concentrations are rarely achieved during oral therapy. Competitive beta-adrenoceptor blockade has been demonstrated in man by a parallel shift to the right in the dose-heart rate response curve to beta-agonists such as isoprenaline.

Propranolol, as with other beta-adrenoceptor blocking drugs, has negative inotropic effects, and is therefore contra-indicated in uncontrolled heart failure.

Propranolol is a racemic mixture and the active form is the S(-) isomer. With the exception of inhibition of the conversion of thyroxine to triiodothyronine it is unlikely that any additional ancillary properties possessed by R(+) propranolol, in comparison with the racemic mixture will give rise to different therapeutic effects.

Propranolol is effective and well tolerated in most ethnic populations, although the response may be less in black patients.

5.2 Pharmacokinetic properties
Following intravenous administration, the plasma half-life of propranolol is about 2 hours and the ratio of metabolites to parent drug in the blood is lower than after oral administration. In particular, 4-hydroxypropranolol is not present after intravenous administration.

Propranolol is completely absorbed after oral administration and peak plasma concentrations occur 1-2 hours after dosing in fasting patients. The liver removes up to 90% of an oral dose with an elimination half-life of 3 to 6 hours. Propranolol is widely and rapidly distributed throughout the body with highest levels occurring in the lungs, liver, kidney, brain and heart.

Propranolol is highly protein bound (80-95%).

5.3 Preclinical safety data
Propranolol is a drug on which extensive clinical experience has been obtained. Relevant information for the prescriber is provided elsewhere in the Summary of Product Characteristics.

6. PHARMACEUTICAL PARTICULARS
6.1 List of excipients
Citric acid monohydrate, methyl parahydroxybenzoate (E218), propyl parahydroxybenzoate (E216), propylene glycol, liquid maltitol, sunset yellow E110, orange/tangerine flavour (including ethanol (0.12%v/v) and butylhydroxyanisol E320) and purified water.

6.2 Incompatibilities
None known.

6.3 Shelf life
24 months unopened

3 months opened.

6.4 Special precautions for storage
Do not store above 25°C. Do not refrigerate or freeze.

6.5 Nature and contents of container
Amber (Type III) glass bottles

Closures: - a) Aluminium, EPE wadded, roll-on pilfer-proof screw cap.

b) HDPE, EPE wadded, tamper evident screw cap.

c) HDPE, EPE wadded, tamper evident, child resistant closure.

Pack Size: 150ml

6.6 Special precautions for disposal and other handling
Not applicable.

Administrative Data
7. MARKETING AUTHORISATION HOLDER
Rosemont Pharmaceuticals Ltd, Rosemont House, Yorkdale Industrial Park, Braithwaite Street, Leeds, LS11 9XE, UK.

8. MARKETING AUTHORISATION NUMBER(S)
PL 00427/0124

9. DATE OF FIRST AUTHORISATION/RENEWAL OF THE AUTHORISATION
11th December 2000, Renewal 30th August 2006

10. DATE OF REVISION OF THE TEXT
10th August 2009

11. Legal Category
POM

Syprol Oral Solution 5mg/5ml
(Rosemont Pharmaceuticals Limited)

1. NAME OF THE MEDICINAL PRODUCT
Propranolol Hydrochloride 5mg/5ml Oral Solution
Syprol 5mg/5ml

2. QUALITATIVE AND QUANTITATIVE COMPOSITION
Propranolol Hydrochloride 5mg/5ml.

3. PHARMACEUTICAL FORM
Oral Solutions

Clear colourless liquid with odour of orange/tangerine.

4. CLINICAL PARTICULARS
4.1 Therapeutic indications
Propranolol is indicated in:
- the control of hypertension
- the management of angina pectoris
- the long term prophylaxis against reinfarction after recovery from acute myocardial infarction
- the control of most forms of cardiac arrhythmia
- the prophylaxis of migraine
- the management of essential tremor
- relief of situational anxiety and generalised anxiety symptoms, particularly those of the somatic type.
- prophylaxis of upper gastro-intestinal bleeding in patients with portal hypertension and oesophageal varices.
- the adjunctive management of thyrotoxicosis and thyrotoxic crisis
- management of hypertrophic obstructive cardiomyopathy
- management of phaeochromocytoma perioperatively (with an alpha-adrenoceptor blocking drug).

4.2 Posology and method of administration
For oral administration only.

Adults:
Hypertension – A starting dose of 80mg twice a day may be increased at weekly intervals according to response. The usual dose range is 160 – 320mg per day. With concurrent diuretic or other antihypertensive drugs a further reduction of blood pressure is obtained.

Angina, migraine and essential tremor – A starting dose of 40mg two or three times daily may be increased by the same amount at weekly intervals according to patient response. An adequate response in migraine and essential tremor is usually seen in the range 80-160mg/day and in angina in the range 120-240mg/day.

Situational and generalised anxiety – A dose of 40mg daily may provide short term relief of acute situational anxiety. Generalised anxiety, requiring longer term therapy, usually responds adequately to 40mg twice daily which, in individual cases, may be increased to 40mg three times daily. Treatment should be continued according to response. Patients should be reviewed after six to twelve months treatment.

Arrhythmias, anxiety, tachycardia, hypertrophic obstructive cardiomyopathy and thyrotoxicosis – A dosage range of 10-40mg three or four times a day usually achieves the required response.

Post myocardial infarction - Treatment should start between days 5 and 21 after myocardial infarction with an initial dose of 40mg four times a day for 2 or 3 days. In order to improve compliance the total daily dosage may thereafter be given as 80mg twice daily.

Portal hypertension:

Dosage should be titrated to achieve approximately 25% reduction in resting heart rate. Dosage should begin with 40mg twice daily, increasing to 80mg twice daily depending on heart rate response. If necessary, the dose may be increased incrementally to a maximum of 160mg twice daily.

Phaeochromocytoma (Used only with an alpha-receptor blocking drug)- Pre-operative: 60mg daily for three days is recommended. Non-operable malignant cases: 30mg daily.

Children
Arrhythmias, phaeochromocytoma, thyrotoxicosis– Dosage should be individually determined and the following is only a guide: 250 – 500 micrograms per Kilogram three or four times daily as required.

Migraine– Under the age of 12: 20mg two or three times daily

Over the age of 12: the adult dose

Fallot's tetralogy– The value of propranolol in this condition is confined mainly to the relief of right-ventricular outflow tract shut-down. It is also useful for treatment of associated arrhythmias and angina. Dosage should be individually determined and the following is only a guide: Up to 1mg/Kg repeated three or four times a day as required.

Elderly
With regard to the elderly the optimum dose should be individually determined according to the clinical response.

4.3 Contraindications
Propranolol must not be used if there is a history of bronchial asthma or bronchospasm.

The product label states the following warning: "Do not take propranolol if you have a history of asthma or wheezing". A similar warning appears in the patient information leaflet.

Bronchospasm can usually be reversed by $beta_2$-agonist bronchodilators such as salbutamol. Large doses of the $beta_2$-agonist bronchodilator may be required to overcome the beta-blockade produced by propranolol and the dose should be titrated according to the clinical response; both intravenous and inhalational administration should be considered. The use of intravenous aminophylline and/or the use of ipratropium (given by nebuliser) may also be considered. Glucagon (1 to 2mg given intravenously) has also been reported to produce a bronchodilator effect in asthmatic patients. Oxygen or artificial ventilation may be required in severe cases.

Propranolol as with other beta-adrenoceptor blocking drugs must not be used in patients with any of the following:

hypersensitivity to propranolol hydrochloride or any of the ingredients; the presence of second or third degree heart block; in cardiogenic shock; metabolic acidosis; after prolonged fasting; bradycardia; hypotension; severe peripheral arterial circulatory disturbances; sick sinus syndrome; untreated phaeochromocytoma; uncontrolled heart failure or Prinzmetal's angina.

Propranolol must not be used in patients prone to hypoglycaemia, i.e., patients after prolonged fasting or patients with restricted counter-regulatory reserves. Patients with restricted counter-regulatory reserves may have reduced autonomic and hormonal responses to hypoglycaemia which includes glycogenolysis, gluconeogenesis and /or impaired modulation of insulin secretion. Patients at risk for an inadequate response to hypoglycaemia includes individuals with malnutrition, prolonged fasting, starvation, chronic liver disease, diabetes and concomitant use of drugs which block the full response to catecholamines.

4.4 Special warnings and precautions for use
Although contra-indicated in uncontrolled heart failure, propranolol may be used where the signs of heart failure have been controlled by the use of appropriate concomitant medication. Propranolol should be used with caution in patients whose cardiac reserve is poor.

Treatment should not be discontinued abruptly in patients with ischaemic heart disease. Either the equivalent dose of another beta-adrenoceptor blocking drug may be substituted or the withdrawal of propranolol should be gradual.

Propranolol should not be used in combination with calcium channel blockers with negative inotropic effects (e.g. verapamil, diltiazem), as it can lead to an exaggeration of these effects particularly in patients with impaired ventricular function and/or SA or AV conduction abnormalities. This may result in severe hypotension, bradycardia and cardiac failure. Neither the beta-blocker nor the calcium channel blocker should be administered intravenously within 48 hours of discontinuing the other.

Propranolol may block/modify the signs and symptoms of hypoglycaemia (especially tachycardia). Propranolol occasionally causes hypoglycaemia, even in non-diabetic patients, e.g., neonates, infants, children, elderly patients, patients on haemodialysis or patients suffering from chronic liver disease and patients suffering from overdose. Severe hypoglycaemia associated with propranolol has rarely presented with seizures and/or coma in isolated patients.

Caution must be exercised in the concurrent use of propranolol and hypoglycaemic therapy in diabetic patients. Propranolol may prolong the hypoglycaemic response to insulin (see section 4.3).

When a patient is scheduled for surgery and a decision is made to discontinue beta-blocker therapy, this should be done at least 24 hours prior to the procedure. The risk/benefit of stopping beta blockade should be made for each patient

Propranolol should not be used in untreated phaeochromocytoma. However, in patients with phaeochromocytoma, an alpha-blocker may be given concomitantly.

Although contra-indicated in severe peripheral arterial circulatory disturbances, propranolol may also aggravate less severe peripheral arterial circulatory disturbances.

One of the pharmacological actions of propranolol is to reduce the heart rate. Therefore the dosage should be reduced in those rare cases where symptoms are attributable to a slow heart rate.

Due to propranolol having a negative effect on conduction time, caution must be exercised if it is given to patients with first degree heart block.

Since the half life may be increased in patients with significant hepatic or renal impairment, caution must be exercised when starting treatment and selecting the initial dose.

In patients with portal hypertension, liver function may deteriorate and hepatic encephalopathy may develop. There have been reports suggesting that treatment with propranolol may increase the risk of developing hepatic encephalopathy.

Propranolol may cause a more severe reaction to a variety of allergens, when given to patients with a history of anaphylactic reaction to such allergens. Such patients may be unresponsive to the usual doses of adrenaline used to treat the allergic reactions.

Propranolol may mask the signs of thyrotoxicosis.

Propranolol must be used with caution in patients with decompensated cirrhosis.

Laboratory Tests: Propranolol has been reported to interfere with the estimation of serum bilirubin by the diazo method and with the determination of catecholamines by methods using fluorescence.

Excipient Warnings

This product contains parahydroxybenzoates which may cause allergic reactions (possibly delayed)

This product also contains liquid maltitol. Patients with rare hereditary problems of fructose intolerance should not take this medicine.

4.5 Interaction with other medicinal products and other forms of interaction
Hypoglycaemic agents: Tachycardia associated with hypoglycaemia may be modified by propranolol. Use of propranolol alongside hypoglycaemic therapy in diabetic patients should be with caution since it may prolong the hypoglycaemic response to insulin.

Clonidine: Caution should be exercised when transferring patients from clonidine to beta-adrenoceptor blocking drugs. If propranolol and clonidine are given concurrently, clonidine should not be discontinued until several days after the withdrawal of the beta blocker. If replacing clonidine by beta-adrenoceptor blocking drug therapy, the introduction of the beta-adrenoceptor blocking drugs should be delayed for several days after clonidine administration has stopped.

Anti-arrhythmics: Care should be taken when prescribing a beta-adrenergic blocking drug with Class 1 anti-arrhythmic agents such as disopyramide. Flecainaide may have additive cardiac depressant effects.

Calcium Channel Blockers: Combined use of beta-adrenoceptor blocking drugs and calcium channel blockers with negative inotropic effects (eg, verapamil, diltiazem) can lead to an exaggeration of these effects particularly in patients with impaired ventricular function and/or SA or AV conduction abnormalities. This may result in severe hypotension, bradycardia and cardiac failure. Neither drug should be administered intravenously within 48 hours of discontinuing the other.

Concomitant therapy with dihydropyridine calcium channel blockers eg, nifedipine, may increase the risk of hypotension, and cardiac failure may occur in patients with latent cardiac insufficiency.

Drugs with hypotensive effects: Dynamic interactions between propranolol and other drugs with hypotensive effects are to be expected. Reactions are sometimes severe and careful monitoring is advised in co-administration of propranolol with other drugs including ACE inhibitors, diuretics, angiotensin II receptor antagonists, vasodilator antihypertensives, diazoxide, adrenergic neurone blockers, alpha blockers, moxisylyte, moxonidine, nitrates and methyldopa.

Anaesthesia: Caution must be exercised when using anaesthetic agents with propranolol. The anaesthetist should be informed and the choice of anaesthetic should be the agent with as little negative inotropic activity as possible. Use of beta-adrenoceptor blocking drugs with anaesthetic drugs may result in attenuation of the reflex tachycardia and increase the risk of hypotension. Anaesthetic agents causing myocardial depression are best avoided.

Neostigmine and other anticholinesterases: Propranolol reduces the efficacy of these compounds in treatment of myasthenia gravis.

Sympathomimetic Agents and Parenteral Adrenaline: Concomitant use of sympathomimetic agents e.g. adrenaline, may counteract the effect of beta-adrenoceptor blocking drugs. Caution should be taken in the parenteral administration of preparations containing adrenaline to people taking beta-adrenoceptor blocking drugs as, in rare cases, vasoconstriction, hypertension and bradycardia may result.

Muscle relaxants (e.g. balcofen): Concomitant use may result in a fall in blood pressure. Tizanidine may also result in bradycardia.

Antidepressants, anxiolytics and hypnotics: Plasma levels of propranolol can be increased by fluvoxamine. Anxiolytics, hypnotics and MAOIs when given with propranolol may have an enhanced hypotensive effect. Propranolol may increase plasma concentration of imipramine. Barbiturates may reduce the plasma concentration of propranolol.

Corticosteroids: Can antagonise the effects of beta-blockers.

Dihydropyridines: Concomitant therapy with dihydropyridines e.g. nifedipine, may increase the risk of hypotension, and cardiac failure may occur in patients with latent cardiac insufficiency.

Digitalis Glycosides: These preparations in association with beta-adrenoceptor blocking drugs, may increase atrio-ventricular conduction time.

Lignocaine: Administration of propranolol during infusion of lignocaine may increase the plasma concentration of lignocaine by approximately 30%. Patients already receiving propranolol tend to have higher lignocaine levels than controls. The combination should be avoided.

Ergotamine: Caution should be exercised if ergotamine, dihydroergotamine or related compounds are given in combination with propranolol since vasospastic reactions have been reported in a few patients.

Prostaglandin Synthetase Inhibiting Drugs: Concomitant use of these e.g. ibuprofen or indomethacin, may decrease the hypotensive effects of propranolol.

Chlorpromazine: Concomitant administration with propranolol may result in an increase in plasma levels of both drugs. This may lead to an enhanced antipsychotic effect for chlorpromazine and an increased antihypertensive effect for propranolol.

Mefolquine: May lead to an increased risk of bradycardia.

Cimetidine, hydralazine, alcohol: Concomitant use of cimetidine and hydralazine will increase, whereas concomitant use of alcohol will decrease, the plasma level of propranolol.

Dopaminergics (e.g. Levodopa), Aldesleukin, Prostaglandins (alprostadil): May have an enhanced hypotensive effect when used concomitantly with propranolol.

Oestrogens: May antagonise the hypotensive effect of propranolol.

5 HT_1 agonists: Propranolol may increase plasma concentrations of rizatriptan.

Pharmacokinetic studies have shown that the following agents may interact with propranolol due to effects on enzyme systems in the liver which metabolise propranolol and these agents: quinidine, propafenone, rifampicin, theophylline, warfarin, thioridazine and dihydropyridine calcium channel blockers such as nifedipine, nisoldipine, nicardipine, isradipine and lacidipine. Owing to the fact that blood concentrations of either agent may be affected, dosage adjustments may be needed according to clinical judgement. (See also the interaction above concerning the concomitant therapy with dihydropyridine calcium channel blockers).

4.6 Pregnancy and lactation

As with all drugs, propranolol should not be given in pregnancy unless absolutely essential. There is no evidence of teratogenicity with propranolol. However, beta adrenoceptor blocking agents reduce placenta perfusion, which may result in intra-uterine foetal death, immature and premature deliveries. In addition, adverse effects (especially hypoglycaemia and bradycardia in the neonate and bradycardia in the foetus) may occur. There is an increased risk of cardiac and pulmonary complications in the neonate in the postnatal period.

Most beta-adrenoceptor blocking drugs particularly lipophilic compounds, will pass into breast milk although to a variable extent. Breast feeding is therefore not recommended following administration of these compounds.

4.7 Effects on ability to drive and use machines

Use is unlikely to result in any impairment of the ability of patients to drive or operate machinery. However, it should be taken into account that occasionally dizziness or fatigue may occur.

4.8 Undesirable effects

Propranolol is usually well tolerated, however, listed below are the side effects that may occur:-

Cardiovascular: Bradycardia, heart failure deterioration, postural hypotension which may be associated with syncope, heart block and congestive cardiac failure, exacerbation of claudication, cold extremities, Raynaud's phenomenon.

Respiratory: Bronchospasm (especially in patients with a history of asthma), sometimes with fatal outcome (see Section 4.3).

Neurological and CNS: Confusion, dizziness, mood changes, nightmares, psychoses and hallucinations, sleep disturbances, paraesthesia especially of the hands.

Haematological: Purpura, thrombocytopenia.

Endocrine: Hypoglycaemia in neonates, infants, children, elderly patients, patients on haemodialysis, patients on concomitant antidiabetic therapy, patients with prolonged fasting and patients with chronic liver disease has been reported (see section 4.3, 4.4 and 4.5).

Gastro-intestinal: Gastro-intestinal disturbance, nausea, diarrhoea.

Integumentary: Alopecia, dry eyes, psoriasiform skin reactions and exacerbation of psoriasis, skin rashes.

Senses: Visual disturbances.

Others: Muscle fatigue, lassitude, insomnia, an increase in ANA (antinuclear antibodies) although the clinical relevance of this has not been established. Isolated reports of myasthenia gravis like syndrome or exacerbation of myasthenia gravis have been reported in patients administered propranolol.

If these effects occur, thought should be given to withdrawing the drug. However, it should be withdrawn gradually.

Bradycardia and hypotension are usually a sign of overdosage but may be rarely linked to intolerance. If this occurs the drug should be withdrawn and overdosage treatment initiated.

4.9 Overdose

The symptoms of overdosage may include bradycardia, hypotension, acute cardiac insufficiency and bronchospasm.

General treatment should include: close supervision, treatment in an intensive care ward, the use of gastric lavage, activated charcoal and a laxative to prevent absorption of any drug still present in the gastrointestinal tract, the use of plasma or plasma substitutes to treat hypotension and shock.

Excessive bradycardia can be countered with atropine 1-2mg intravenously and/or a cardiac pacemaker. If necessary, this may be followed by a bolus dose of glucagon 10mg intravenously. If required, this may be repeated or followed by an intravenous infusion of glucagon 1-10mg/hour depending on response. If no response to glucagon occurs or if glucagon is unavailable, a beta-adrenoceptor stimulant such as dobutamine 2.5 to 10 micrograms/Kg/minute by intravenous infusion may be given. Dobutamine, because of its positive inotropic effect could also be used to treat hypotension and acute cardiac insufficiency. It is likely that these doses would be inadequate to reverse the cardiac effects of beta-blockade if a large overdose has been taken. The dose of dobutamine should therefore be increased if necessary to achieve the required response according to the clinical condition of the patient.

5. PHARMACOLOGICAL PROPERTIES

5.1 Pharmacodynamic properties

Propranolol is a competitive antagonist at both $beta_1$ and $beta_2$-adrenoceptors.

It has no agonist activity at the beta-adrenoceptor, but has membrane stabilising activity at concentrations exceeding 1-3mg/litre, though such concentrations are rarely achieved during oral therapy. Competitive beta-adrenoceptor blockade has been demonstrated in man by a parallel shift to the right in the dose-heart rate response curve to beta-agonists such as isoprenaline.

Propranolol, as with other beta-adrenoceptor blocking drugs, has negative inotropic effects, and is therefore contra-indicated in uncontrolled heart failure.

Propranolol is a racemic mixture and the active form is the S(-) isomer. With the exception of inhibition of the conversion of thyroxine to triiodothyronine it is unlikely that any additional ancillary properties possessed by R(+) propranolol, in comparison with the racemic mixture will give rise to different therapeutic effects.

Propranolol is effective and well tolerated in most ethnic populations, although the response may be less in black patients.

5.2 Pharmacokinetic properties

Following intravenous administration, the plasma half-life of propranolol is about 2 hours and the ratio of metabolites to parent drug in the blood is lower than after oral administration. In particular, 4-hydroxypropranolol is not present after intravenous administration.

Propranolol is completely absorbed after oral administration and peak plasma concentrations occur 1-2 hours after dosing in fasting patients. The liver removes up to 90% of an oral dose with an elimination half-life of 3 to 6 hours. Propranolol is widely and rapidly distributed throughout the body with highest levels occurring in the lungs, liver, kidney, brain and heart.

Propranolol is highly protein bound (80-95%).

5.3 Preclinical safety data

Propranolol is a drug on which extensive clinical experience has been obtained. Relevant information for the prescriber is provided elsewhere in the Summary of Product Characteristics.

6. PHARMACEUTICAL PARTICULARS

6.1 List of excipients

Citric acid monohydrate, methyl parahydroxybenzoate (E218), propyl parahydroxybenzoate (E216), propylene glycol, liquid maltitol, orange/tangerine flavour (including ethanol (0.12%v/v) and butylhydroxyanisol E320) and purified water.

6.2 Incompatibilities

None known.

6.3 Shelf life

24 months unopened

3 months opened.

6.4 Special precautions for storage

Do not store above 25°C. Do not refrigerate or freeze.

6.5 Nature and contents of container

Amber (Type III) glass bottles

Closures: - a) Aluminium, EPE wadded, roll-on pilfer-proof screw cap.

b) HDPE, EPE wadded, tamper evident screw cap.

c) HDPE, EPE wadded, tamper evident, child resistant closure.

Pack Size: 150ml

6.6 Special precautions for disposal and other handling

Not applicable.

Administrative Data

7. MARKETING AUTHORISATION HOLDER

Rosemont Pharmaceuticals Ltd, Rosemont House, Yorkdale Industrial Park, Braithwaite Street, Leeds, LS11 9XE, UK.

8. MARKETING AUTHORISATION NUMBER(S)

PL 00427/0122

9. DATE OF FIRST AUTHORISATION/RENEWAL OF THE AUTHORISATION

11th December 2000, Renewal 30th August 2006

10. DATE OF REVISION OF THE TEXT

10th August 2009

11. Legal Category

POM

Tabphyn MR

(ProStrakan)

1. NAME OF THE MEDICINAL PRODUCT
Tabphyn™ MR 400 microgram

2. QUALITATIVE AND QUANTITATIVE COMPOSITION
One capsule contains 400 micrograms tamsulosin hydrochloride, equivalent to 367 micrograms tamsulosin.

For excipients, see 6.1.

3. PHARMACEUTICAL FORM
Modified-release capsule, hard.

Orange/olive-green capsule, with the black printed mark TSL 0.4 and with a black stripe at both ends. The capsules contain white to off-white pellets.

4. CLINICAL PARTICULARS

4.1 Therapeutic indications
Lower urinary tract symptoms (LUTS) associated with benign prostatic hyperplasia (BPH).

4.2 Posology and method of administration
One capsule a day after breakfast or the first meal of the day. The capsule is swallowed whole with a glass of water while standing or sitting (not lying down). The capsule should not be broken or pulled apart as this may have an effect on the release of the long-acting active ingredient.

4.3 Contraindications
Hypersensitivity to tamsulosin, including drug-induced angio-oedema, or to any of the excipients.

Orthostatic hypotension observed earlier (history of orthostatic hypotension).

Severe hepatic insufficiency.

4.4 Special warnings and precautions for use
The use of tamsulosin may lower blood pressure, which in rare cases may cause fainting. If initial symptoms of orthostatic hypotension start to appear (dizziness, weakness), then the patient should sit or lie down until the symptoms have gone.

The patient should be examined before commencement of therapy with tamsulosin to exclude the presence of other conditions that can produce similar symptoms to those of BPH. The prostate should be examined via the rectum and, if necessary, the PSA count determined prior to commencement of treatment and again later at regular intervals.

The treatment of severely renally impaired patients (creatinine clearance of < 10 ml/min) should be approached with caution as these patients have not been studied.

Angio-oedema has been rarely reported after the use of tamsulosin. Treatment should be discontinued immediately, the patient should be monitored until disappearance of the oedema, and tamsulosin should not be re-administered.

The 'Intraoperative Floppy Iris Syndrome' (IFIS, a variant of small pupil syndrome) has been observed during cataract surgery in some patients on or previously treated with tamsulosin. IFIS may lead to increased procedural complications during the operation. The initiation of therapy with tamsulosin in patients for whom cataract surgery is scheduled is not recommended.

Discontinuing tamsulosin 1-2 weeks prior to cataract surgery is anecdotally considered helpful, but the benefit and duration of requirement of stopping the therapy prior to cataract surgery has not yet been established.

During pre-operative assessment, cataract surgeons and ophthalmic teams should consider whether patients scheduled for cataract surgery are being or have been treated with tamsulosin in order to ensure that appropriate measures will be in place to manage the IFIS during surgery.

4.5 Interaction with other medicinal products and other forms of interaction
No interactions have been observed when tamsulosin has been given concomitantly with atenolol, enalapril, nifedipine or theophylline. Concomitant cimetidine raises, and concomitant furosemide lowers, plasma concentrations of tamsulosin but, as the concentration of tamsulosin remains within the normal range, posology need not be altered.

Tamsulosin has not been found to interact with amitriptyline, salbutamol, glibenclamide or finasteride during *in vitro* studies with liver microsomal fractions (representing the cytochrome P450-linked metabolising enzyme system). Diclofenac and Warfarin may increase the elimination rate of tamsulosin.

Concurrent administration with another α1-adrenoreceptor antagonist may lower blood pressure.

4.6 Pregnancy and lactation
Tamsulosin is intended for males only.

4.7 Effects on ability to drive and use machines
No studies on the effects on the ability to drive and use machines have been performed. However patients should be aware of the fact that dizziness can occur.

4.8 Undesirable effects
(see Table 1 below)

During cataract surgery a small pupil situation, known as Intraoperative Floppy Iris Syndrome (IFIS), has been associated with therapy of tamsulosin during post-marketing surveillance (See also Section 4.4).

4.9 Overdose
No cases of acute overdosage have been reported. However, acute hypotension could theoretically occur after overdosage in which case cardiovascular support should be given. Blood pressure can be restored and heart rate brought back to normal by lying the patient down. If this does not help then volume expanders and, when necessary, vasopressors could be employed. Renal function should be monitored and general supportive measures applied. Dialysis is unlikely to be of help as tamsulosin is very highly bound to plasma proteins.

If large quantities of the medicinal product are involved, gastric lavage may be performed and activated charcoal and an osmotic laxative, such as sodium sulphate, may be given.

5. PHARMACOLOGICAL PROPERTIES

5.1 Pharmacodynamic properties
Pharmacotherapeutic group:
Tamsulosin is an α_{1A} adrenoreceptor antagonist. The medicinal product is only used for the treatment of prostatic conditions.

ATC code: G04CA02

Mechanism of action:
Tamsulosin binds selectively and competitively to postsynaptic α1A adrenoreceptors, which convey smooth muscle contraction, thereby relaxing prostatic and urethral smooth muscle.

Pharmacodynamic effects:
Tamsulosin increases the maximum urinary flow rate by relaxing prostatic and urethral smooth muscle, thus relieving obstruction.

The medicinal product also improves the irritative and obstructive symptoms in which the contraction of smooth muscle in the lower urinary tract plays an important role.

Alpha-blockers can reduce blood pressure by lowering peripheral resistance. No reduction in blood pressure of any clinical significance was observed during studies with tamsulosin in normotensive patients.

The medicinal product's effect on storage and voiding symptoms are also maintained during long-term therapy, as a result of which the need for surgical treatment is significantly postponed.

5.2 Pharmacokinetic properties

Absorption

Tamsulosin is rapidly absorbed from the intestines and its bioavailability is almost complete. Absorption is slowed down if a meal has been eaten before taking the medicinal product. Uniformity of absorption can be assured by always taking tamsulosin after breakfast. Tamsulosin shows linear kinetics.

Peak plasma levels are achieved at approximately six hours after a single dose of tamsulosin taken after a full meal. The steady state is reached by day five of multiple dosing, when C_{max} in patients is about two-thirds higher than that reached after a single dose. Although this has been demonstrated only in the elderly, the same result would also be expected in younger patients.

There are huge inter-patient variations in plasma levels of tamsulosin, both after single as well as multiple dosing.

Distribution

In humans, tamsulosin is more than 99% bound to plasma proteins and the volume of distribution is small (about 0.2 l/kg).

Biotransformation

Tamsulosin has a low first pass metabolic effect. Most tamsulosin is found unaltered in plasma. The substance is metabolised in the liver.

In studies on rats, tamsulosin was found to cause only a slight induction of microsomal liver enzymes.

The metabolites are not as effective and toxic as the active medicinal product itself.

Excretion

Tamsulosin and its metabolites are mainly excreted in the urine with about 9% of the dose being present in unchanged form.

The elimination half-life of tamsulosin in patients is approximately 10 hours (when taken after a meal) and 13 hours in the steady state.

5.3 Preclinical safety data
Toxicity after a single dose and multiple dosing has been investigated in mice, rats and dogs. Reproductive toxicity has also been investigated in rats, carcinogenicity in mice and rats, and genotoxicity *in vivo* and *in vitro*.

The common toxicity profile found with large doses of tamsulosin is equivalent to the pharmacological effect associated with alpha adrenergic antagonists.

Changes in ECG readings were found with very large doses in dogs. This is not, however, assumed to be of any clinical significance. Tamsulosin has not been found to have any significant genotoxic properties.

Greater proliferative changes in the mammary glands of female rats and mice have been discovered on exposure to tamsulosin. These findings, which are probably indirectly linked to hyperprolactinaemia and only occur as a result of large doses having been taken, are considered clinically insignificant.

6. PHARMACEUTICAL PARTICULARS

6.1 List of excipients

Content of capsule:

Microcrystalline cellulose
Methacrylic acid-ethyl acrylate copolymer
Polysorbate 80
Sodium laurilsulfate
Triethyl citrate
Talc

Capsule body:

Gelatine
Indigotine (E 132)
Titanium dioxide (E 171)
Yellow iron oxide (E 172)
Red iron oxide (E 172)
Black iron oxide (E 172)

Table 1

	Common (>1/100, <1/10)	Uncommon (>1/1 000, <1/100)	Rare (>1/10 000, <1/1 000)	Very rare (<1/10 000)
Nervous system disorders	Dizziness	Headache	Syncope	
Cardiac disorders		Tachycardia		
Vascular disorders		Orthostatic hypotension		
Respiratory, thoracic and mediastinum-related disorders		Rhinitis		
Gastrointestinal disorders		Constipation, diarrhoea, nausea, vomiting		
Skin and subcutaneous tissue disorders		Rash, itching, urticaria	Angio-oedema	
Reproductive systems and breast disorders		Abnormal ejaculation		Priapism
General disorders and administration site conditions		Asthenia		

Ink:

Shellac

Black iron oxide (E 172)

Propylene glycol

6.2 Incompatibilities
Not applicable.

6.3 Shelf life
36 months.

6.4 Special precautions for storage
Blister packs: Store in the original package.

Tablet container: Keep the container tightly closed.

6.5 Nature and contents of container
PVC/PE/PVDC/Aluminium blister packs in cardboard boxes containing 10, 14, 15, 20, 28, 30, 50, 56, 60, 90 or 100 modified-release capsules.

HDPE tablet containers with PP child-resistant closures containing 60 or 250 modified-release capsules.

Not all pack sizes may be marketed.

6.6 Special precautions for disposal and other handling
No special requirements.

7. MARKETING AUTHORISATION HOLDER
Genus Pharmaceuticals Ltd

T/A Genus Pharmaceuticals

Park View House

65 London Road

Newbury

Berkshire

RG14 1JN UK

8. MARKETING AUTHORISATION NUMBER(S)
PL 06831/0157

9. DATE OF FIRST AUTHORISATION/RENEWAL OF THE AUTHORISATION
23/02/2006

10. DATE OF REVISION OF THE TEXT
15/08/2008

11. LEGAL CATEGORY
POM

TachoSil medicated sponge

(Nycomed UK Ltd)

1. NAME OF THE MEDICINAL PRODUCT
TachoSil medicated sponge

2. QUALITATIVE AND QUANTITATIVE COMPOSITION
TachoSil contains per cm^2:

Human Fibrinogen 5.5 mg

Human Thrombin 2.0 IU

For a full list of excipients, see section 6.1.

3. PHARMACEUTICAL FORM
Medicated sponge

TachoSil is an off-white sponge. The active side of the sponge, which is coated with fibrinogen and thrombin, is marked by a yellow colour.

4. CLINICAL PARTICULARS

4.1 Therapeutic indications
TachoSil is indicated for supportive treatment in surgery for improvement of haemostasis, to promote tissue sealing, and for suture support in vascular surgery where standard techniques are insufficient (see section 5.1).

4.2 Posology and method of administration

Posology

The use of TachoSil is restricted to experienced surgeons.

There is insufficient information for use in paediatric patients.

The number of TachoSil sponges to be applied should always be oriented towards the underlying clinical need for the patient. The number of TachoSil sponges to be applied is governed by the size of the wound area.

Application of TachoSil must be individualised by the treating surgeon. In clinical trials, the individual dosages have typically ranged from 1-3 sponges (9.5 cm × 4.8 cm); application of up to 7 sponges has been reported. For smaller wounds, e.g. in minimal invasive surgery the smaller size sponges (4.8 cm × 4.8 cm or 3.0 cm × 2.5 cm) are recommended.

Method and route of administration

For local use only.

See section 6.6 for more detailed instructions.

4.3 Contraindications
Hypersensitivity to the active substances or to any of the excipients.

4.4 Special warnings and precautions for use
For local use only. Do not use intravascularly.

Specific data have not been obtained on the use of this product in neurosurgery or in gastrointestinal anastomoses surgery.

Life threatening thromboembolic complications may occur if the preparation is unintentionally applied intravascularly.

As with any protein product, allergic type hypersensitivity reactions are possible. Signs of hypersensitivity reactions include hives, generalised urticaria, tightness of the chest, wheezing, hypotension and anaphylaxis. If these symptoms occur, the administration has to be discontinued immediately.

In case of shock, the current medical standards for shock treatment should be observed.

Standard measures to prevent infections resulting from the use of medicinal products prepared from human blood or plasma include selection of donors, screening of individual donations and plasma pools for specific markers of infection and the inclusion of effective manufacturing steps for the inactivation/removal of viruses. Despite this, when medicinal products prepared from human blood or plasma are administered, the possibility of transmitting infective agents cannot be totally excluded. This also applies to unknown or emerging viruses and other pathogens.

The measures taken are considered effective for enveloped viruses such as HIV, HBV and HCV and for the non-enveloped virus HAV. The measures taken may be of limited value against non-enveloped viruses such as parvovirus B19. Parvovirus B19 infection may be serious for pregnant women (fetal infection) and for individuals with immunodeficiency or increased erythropoiesis (e.g. haemolytic anaemia).

It is strongly recommended that every time that TachoSil is administered to a patient, the name and batch number of the product are recorded in order to maintain a link between the patient and the batch of the product.

4.5 Interaction with other medicinal products and other forms of interaction
No formal interaction studies have been performed.

Similar to comparable products or thrombin solutions, the sealant may be denaturated after exposure to solutions containing alcohol, iodine or heavy metals (e.g. antiseptic solutions). Such substances should be removed to the greatest possible extent before applying the sealant.

4.6 Pregnancy and lactation
The safety of TachoSil for use in human pregnancy or breastfeeding has not been established in controlled clinical trials. Experimental animal studies are insufficient to assess the safety with respect to reproduction, development of the embryo or foetus, the course of gestation and peri- and postnatal development.

Therefore, TachoSil should be administered to pregnant and lactating women only if clearly needed.

4.7 Effects on ability to drive and use machines
Not relevant.

4.8 Undesirable effects
Hypersensitivity or allergic reactions (which may include angioedema, burning and stinging at the application site, bronchospasm, chills, flushing, generalised urticaria, headache, hives, hypotension, lethargy, nausea, restlessness, tachycardia, tightness of the chest, tingling, vomiting, wheezing) may occur in rare cases in patients treated with fibrin sealants/haemostatics. In isolated cases, these reactions may progress to severe anaphylaxis. Such reactions may especially be seen, if the preparation is applied repeatedly, or administered to patients known to be hypersensitive to constituents of the product.

Antibodies against components of fibrin sealant/haemostatic products may occur rarely.

Thromboembolic complications may occur if the preparation is unintentionally applied intravascularly (see section 4.4).

For viral safety see section 4.4

Frequency of undesirable effects for TachoSil based on all adverse event data from six clinical trials, two post-authorisation safety studies and spontaneous reporting.

Summary of the safety profile

The safety data of TachoSil generally reflect the type of post-operative complications related to the surgical settings in which the trials were conducted and the underlying disease of the patients.

Tabulated summary of adverse reactions

Data from the six controlled clinical trials conducted by the MAH has been pooled into an integrated dataset and the frequencies of occurrence in this SmPC originate from this integrated dataset. In the integrated analyses, 521 patients were treated with TachoSil and 511 patients were treated with comparator treatment. Due to practical reasons (comparison to standard surgical and standard haemostatic treatment), blinding was not possible in the TachoSil trials. Therefore the studies were performed as open-label studies.

The following categories are used to rank the undesirable effects by frequency of occurrence: very common (≥1/10); common (≥1/100 to <1/10); uncommon (≥1/1,000 to <1/100); rare (≥1/10,000 to <1/1,000); and very rare (<1/10,000), not known (cannot be estimated from the available data).

(see Table 1 below)

4.9 Overdose
No case of overdose has been reported.

5. PHARMACOLOGICAL PROPERTIES

5.1 Pharmacodynamic properties
Pharmaco-therapeutic group:

Local haemostatics, ATC code: B02BC30

TachoSil contains fibrinogen and thrombin as a dried coating on the surface of a collagen sponge. At contact with physiological fluids, e.g. blood, lymph or physiological saline solution the components of the coating dissolve and partly diffuse into the wound surface. This is followed by the fibrinogen-thrombin reaction which initiates the last phase of physiological blood coagulation. Fibrinogen is converted into fibrin monomers which spontaneously polymerise to a fibrin clot, which holds the collagen sponge tightly to the wound surface. The fibrin is then cross linked by endogenous factor XIII, creating a firm, mechanically stable network with good adhesive properties and provides sealing as well.

Clinical studies demonstrating haemostasis were conducted in a total of 240 patients (118 TachoSil, 122 argon beamer) undergoing partial liver resection surgery and 185 patients (95 TachoSil, 93 standard surgical treatment) undergoing surgical resection of superficial renal tumour. A further controlled study in 119 patients (59 TachoSil, 60 haemostatic fleece) demonstrated sealing, haemostasis and suture support in patients undergoing cardiovascular surgery. Tissue sealing in lung surgery was investigated in two controlled trials in patients undergoing lung surgery. The first controlled clinical trial investigating tissue sealing in lung surgery failed to document superiority over standard treatment measured by air leakage due to the inclusion of a large group of patients (53%) without air leakage. However, the second study investigating tissue sealing in 299 patients (148 TachoSil, 151 standard surgical treatment) with demonstrated intraoperative air leakage showed the superiority of TachoSil compared to standard treatment.

5.2 Pharmacokinetic properties
TachoSil is intended for local application only. Intravascular administration is not possible.

As a consequence, intravascular pharmacokinetic studies were not performed in man.

In animal studies TachoSil shows a progressive biodegradation. The fibrin clot is metabolised in the same way as endogenous fibrin by fibrinolysis and phagocytosis. The collagen sponge is degraded by resorptive granulation tissue. Approximately 24 weeks after application only a few remnants were present without any signs of local irritation.

5.3 Preclinical safety data
Single dose toxicity studies in different species of animals have shown no signs of acute toxic effect.

6. PHARMACEUTICAL PARTICULARS

6.1 List of excipients
Equine collagen

Human albumin

Riboflavine (E 101)

Sodium chloride

Sodium citrate

L-arginin-hydrochloride.

Table 1

Frequency / Organ class	Common (≥1/100 to <1/10)	Uncommon (≥1/1,000 to <1/100)	Very rare (<1/10,000), not known (cannot be estimated from the available data)
Vascular disorders			Thromboembolism (if applied intravascularly)
General disorders and administration site conditions	Pyrexia*		
Immune system disorders		Hypersensitivity	

*Pyrexia occurred in 6.3% of the patients treated with TachoSil and in 5.9% of the patients treated with comparator treatment.

6.2 Incompatibilities
Not applicable.

6.3 Shelf life
3 years.

Once the foil sachet is opened, TachoSil must be used immediately.

6.4 Special precautions for storage
Do not store above 25°C.

6.5 Nature and contents of container
TachoSil is packed in a double packaging:

- An outer container consisting of an aluminium-bonded foil sachet

- An inner container (sterile) consisting of a polystyrene blister sealed with a peel lacquer-laminate paper

- A desiccant bag is included in the outer container

Each sponge is packed individually.

Pack sizes:

Package with 1 sponge of 9.5 cm × 4.8 cm

Package with 2 sponges of 4.8 cm × 4.8 cm

Package with 1 sponge of 3.0 cm × 2.5 cm

Package with 5 sponges of 3.0 cm × 2.5 cm

Not all pack sizes may be marketed.

6.6 Special precautions for disposal and other handling
TachoSil comes ready to use in sterile packages and must be handled accordingly. Use only undamaged packages. Once the package is opened post-sterilisation is not possible. The outer aluminium foil sachet may be opened in a non-sterile operating area. The inner sterile blister must be opened in a sterile operating room area. TachoSil should be used immediately after opening the inner sterile cover.

TachoSil is used under sterile conditions. Prior to application the wound area should be cleansed, e.g. from blood, disinfectants and other fluids. After removal of TachoSil from the sterile package the sponge should be pre-moistened in saline solution and then applied immediately. The yellow, active side of the sponge is applied to the bleeding/leaking surface and held against it with a gentle pressure for 3-5 minutes. This procedure enables an easy adhesion of TachoSil to the wound surface.

Pressure is applied with moistened gloves or a moist pad. Due to the strong affinity of collagen to blood, TachoSil may also stick to surgical instruments or gloves covered with blood. This can be avoided by pre-moistening surgical instruments and gloves with physiological saline solution. After pressing TachoSil to the wound, the glove or the pad must be removed carefully. To avoid the sponge from being pulled loose it may be held in place at one end, e.g. with a pair of forceps.

Alternatively, e.g. in case of stronger bleeding, TachoSil may be applied without pre-moistening, while also pressing gently to the wound for 3-5 minutes.

The TachoSil sponge should be applied so that it extends 1-2 cm beyond the margins of the wound. If more than one sponge is used the sponges should overlap. The sponge can be cut to the correct size and shaped if too large.

Any unused product or waste material should be disposed of in accordance with local requirements.

7. MARKETING AUTHORISATION HOLDER
Nycomed Austria GmbH

St. Peter Strasse 25

A-4020 Linz

Austria

8. MARKETING AUTHORISATION NUMBER(S)
EU/1/04/277/001-004

9. DATE OF FIRST AUTHORISATION/RENEWAL OF THE AUTHORISATION
08.06.2004

10. DATE OF REVISION OF THE TEXT
February 2009

Tagamet Injection

(GlaxoSmithKline UK)

1. NAME OF THE MEDICINAL PRODUCT
Tagamet® Injection

2. QUALITATIVE AND QUANTITATIVE COMPOSITION
Tagamet Injection contains 200 mg cimetidine in 2 ml.

3. PHARMACEUTICAL FORM
Ampoules containing 200 mg cimetidine in 2 ml solution.

4. CLINICAL PARTICULARS

4.1 Therapeutic indications
Tagamet is a histamine H_2-receptor antagonist which rapidly inhibits both basal and stimulated gastric secretion of acid and reduces pepsin output.

Tagamet is indicated in the treatment of duodenal and benign gastric ulceration, including that associated with non-steroidal anti-inflammatory agents, recurrent and stomal ulceration, oesophageal reflux disease and other conditions where reduction of gastric acid by Tagamet has been shown to be beneficial: persistent dyspeptic symptoms with or without ulceration, particularly meal-related upper abdominal pain, including such symptoms associated with non-steroidal anti-inflammatory agents; the prophylaxis of gastrointestinal haemorrhage from stress ulceration in seriously ill patients; before general anaesthesia in patients thought to be at risk of acid aspiration (Mendelson's) syndrome, particularly obstetric patients during labour; to reduce malabsorption and fluid loss in the short bowel syndrome; and in pancreatic insufficiency to reduce degradation of enzyme supplements. Tagamet is also recommended in the management of the Zollinger-Ellison syndrome.

4.2 Posology and method of administration
Tagamet is usually given orally, but parenteral dosing may be substituted for all or part of the recommended oral dose in cases where oral dosing is impracticable or considered inappropriate.

The total daily dose by any route should not normally exceed 2.4 g. Dosage should be reduced in patients with impaired renal function (see *Section 4.4*).

ADULTS

Tagamet may be given intramuscularly or intravenously.

The dose by intramuscular injection is normally 200 mg, which may be repeated at four- to six-hourly intervals.

The usual dosage for intravenous administration is 200 - 400 mg, which may be repeated four to six-hourly.

If direct intravenous injection cannot be avoided, 200 mg should be given *slowly* over at least five minutes, and may be repeated four to six-hourly. Rapid intravenous injection has been associated with cardiac arrest and arrhythmias. For critically ill patients and patients with cardiovascular impairment, or if a larger dose is needed, the dose should be diluted and given over at least 10 minutes. In such cases infusion is preferable.

For intermittent intravenous infusion, Tagamet may be given at a dosage of 200 mg to 400 mg every 4 to 6 hours.

If continuous intravenous infusion is required, Tagamet may be given at an average rate of 50 to 100 mg/hour over 24 hours.

In the prophylaxis of haemorrhage from stress ulceration in seriously ill patients, doses of 200 - 400 mg can be given every four to six hours by oral, nasogastric or parenteral routes. By direct intravenous injection a dose of 200 mg should not be exceeded: see above.

In patients thought to be at risk of acid aspiration syndrome an oral dose of 400 mg can be given 90 - 120 minutes before induction of general anaesthesia or, in obstetric practice, at the start of labour. While such a risk persists, a dose of up to 400 mg may be repeated (parenterally if appropriate) at four-hourly intervals as required up to the usual daily maximum of 2.4 g. The usual precautions to avoid acid aspiration should be taken.

To reduce degradation of pancreatic enzyme supplements, 800 - 1600 mg a day may be given according to response in four divided doses, one to one and a half hours before meals.

ELDERLY

The normal adult dosage may be used unless renal function is markedly impaired (see *Section 4.4*).

CHILDREN

Experience in children is less than that in adults. In children more than one year old, Tagamet 25 - 30 mg/kg body weight per day in divided doses may be administered.

The use of Tagamet in infants under one year old is not fully evaluated; 20 mg/kg body weight per day in divided doses has been used.

4.3 Contraindications
Hypersensitivity to cimetidine.

4.4 Special warnings and precautions for use
Rapid intravenous injection of cimetidine (less than 5 minutes) should be avoided as there have been rare associations with cardiac arrest and arrhythmias. Transient hypotension has also been observed, particularly in critically ill patients (see *Section 4.2*).

Dosage should be reduced in patients with impaired renal function according to creatinine clearance. The following dosages are suggested: creatinine clearance of 0 to 15 ml per minute, 200 mg twice a day; 15 to 30 ml per minute, 200 mg three times a day; 30 to 50 ml per minute, 200 mg four times a day; over 50 ml per minute, normal dosage.

Clinical trials of over six years' continuous treatment and more than 15 years' widespread use have not revealed unexpected adverse reactions related to long-term therapy. The safety of prolonged use is not, however, fully established and care should be taken to observe periodically patients given prolonged treatment.

Tagamet treatment can mask the symptoms and allow transient healing of gastric cancer. The potential delay in diagnosis should particularly be borne in mind in patients of middle age and over with new or recently changed dyspeptic symptoms.

Care should be taken that patients with a history of peptic ulcer, particularly the elderly, being treated with Tagamet and a non-steroidal anti-inflammatory agent are observed regularly.

In patients such as the elderly, persons with chronic lung disease, diabetes or the immunocompromised, there may be an increased risk of developing community acquired pneumonia. A large epidemiological study showed an increased risk of developing community acquired pneumonia in current users of H_2 receptor antagonists versus those who had stopped treatment, with an observed adjusted relative risk increase of 1.63 (95% CI, 1.07-2.48).

Due to the possible interaction with coumarins, close monitoring of prothrombin time is recommended when cimetidine is concurrently used.

Coadministration of therapeutic agents with a narrow therapeutic index, such as phenytoin or theophylline, may require dosage adjustment when starting or stopping concomitantly administered cimetidine (*see Section 4.5*).

4.5 Interaction with other medicinal products and other forms of interaction
Tagamet can prolong the elimination of drugs metabolised by oxidation in the liver. Although pharmacological interactions with a number of drugs (e.g. diazepam, propranolol) have been demonstrated, only those with oral anticoagulants, phenytoin, theophylline and intravenous lidocaine appear, to date, to be of clinical significance. Close monitoring of patients on Tagamet receiving oral anticoagulants or phenytoin is recommended and a reduction in the dosage of these drugs may be necessary.

In patients on drug treatment or with illnesses that could cause falls in blood cell count, the possibility that H_2-receptor antagonism could potentiate this effect should be borne in mind.

Cimetidine has the potential to affect the absorption, metabolism or renal excretion of other drugs which is particularly important when drugs with a narrow therapeutic index are administered concurrently. The altered pharmacokinetics may necessitate dosage adjustment of the affected drug or discontinuation of treatment (see *Section 4.4*).

Interactions may occur by several mechanisms including:

1) Inhibition of certain cytochrome P450 enzymes (including CYP1A2, CYP2C9, CYP2D6 and CYP3A3/A4, and CYP2C18); Inhibition of these enzymes may result in increased plasma levels of certain drugs including warfarin-type coumarin anticoagulants (e.g. warfarin), tricyclic antidepressants (e.g. amitriptyline), class I antiarrhythmics (e.g. lidocaine, quinidine), calcium channel blockers (e.g. nifedipine, diltiazem), oral sulfonylureas (e.g. glipizide), phenytoin, theophylline and metoprolol.

2) Competition for renal tubular secretion; This may result in increased plasma levels of certain drugs including procainamide, quinidine, metformin, ciclosporin and tacrolimus.

3)Alteration of gastric pH; The bioavailability of certain drugs may be affected. This can result in either an increase in absorption (e.g. atazanavir) or a decrease in absorption (e.g. some azole antifungals such as ketoconazole, itraconazole or posaconazole).

4) Unknown mechanisms; Cimetidine may potentiate the myelosuppressive effects (e.g. neutropenia, agranulocytosis) of chemotherapeutic agents such as carmustine, fluorouracil, epirubicin, or therapies such as radiation. Isolated cases of clinically relevant interactions have been documented with narcotic analgesics (e.g. morphine).

4.6 Pregnancy and lactation
Although tests in animals and clinical evidence have not revealed any hazards from the administration of Tagamet during pregnancy or lactation, both animal and human studies have shown that it does cross the placental barrier and is excreted in milk. As with most drugs, the use of Tagamet should be avoided during pregnancy and lactation unless essential.

4.7 Effects on ability to drive and use machines
Not applicable.

4.8 Undesirable effects
Adverse experiences with cimetidine are listed below by system organ class and frequency. Frequencies are defined as: very common (>1/10), common (>1/100, <1/10), uncommon (>1/1000, <1/100), rare (>1/10000, <1/1000), very rare (<1/10000)

Blood and lymphatic system disorders

Uncommon: Leukopenia

Rare: Thrombocytopenia, aplastic anaemia

Very rare: Pancytopenia, agranulocytosis

Immune system disorders

Very rare: Anaphylaxis

Anaphylaxis is usually cleared on withdrawal of the drug.

Psychiatric disorders

Uncommon: Depression, confusional states, hallucinations

Confusional states, reversible within a few days of withdrawing cimetidine, have been reported, usually in elderly or ill patients.

Nervous system disorders

Common: Headache, dizziness

Cardiac disorders

Uncommon: Tachycardia

Rare: Sinus bradycardia

Very rare: Heart block

Gastrointestinal disorders
Common: Diarrhoea
Very rare: Pancreatitis
Pancreatitis cleared on withdrawal of the drug.
Hepatobiliary disorders
Uncommon: Hepatitis
Rare: Increases in serum transaminase levels
Hepatitis and increases in serum tranaminase levels cleared on withdrawal of the drug.
Skin and subcutaneous tissue disorders
Common: Skin rashes
Very rare: Reversible alopecia and hypersensitivity vasculitis
Hypersensitivity vasculitis usually cleared on withdrawal of the drug.
Musculoskeletal and connective tissue disorders
Common: Myalgia
Very rare: Arthralgia
Renal and urinary disorders
Uncommon: Increases in plasma creatinine
Rare: Interstitial nephritis
Interstitial nephritis cleared on withdrawal of the drug.
Small increases in plasma creatinine have been reported, unassociated with changes in glomerular filtration rate. The increases do not progress with continued therapy and disappear at the end of therapy.
Reproductive system and breast disorders
Uncommon: Gynaecomastia and reversible impotence
Gynaecomastia is usually reversible upon discontinuation of cimetidine therapy.
Reversible impotence has been reported particularly in patients receiving high doses (e.g. in Zollinger-Ellison Syndrome). However, at regular dosage, the incidence is similar to that in the general population.
Very rare: Galactorrhoea
General disorders and administration site conditions
Common: Tiredness
Very rare: Fever
Fever cleared on withdrawal of the drug.

4.9 Overdose
Acute over-dosage of up to 20 grams has been reported several times with no significant ill effects. Induction of vomiting and/or gastric lavage may be employed together with symptomatic and supportive therapy.

5. PHARMACOLOGICAL PROPERTIES
5.1 Pharmacodynamic properties
Cimetidine is a histamine H_2-receptor antagonist which rapidly inhibits both basal and stimulated gastric secretion of acid and reduces pepsin output.

5.2 Pharmacokinetic properties
Cimetidine is metabolised in the liver and excreted mainly through the kidney with a half-life of about two hours. The effects on acid secretion are of longer duration.

5.3 Preclinical safety data
Not applicable.

6. PHARMACEUTICAL PARTICULARS
6.1 List of excipients
The injection contains hydrochloric acid (E507) and water for injections.

6.2 Incompatibilities
Not applicable.

6.3 Shelf life
Five years.

6.4 Special precautions for storage
Store ampoules below 30°C, protected from light.

6.5 Nature and contents of container
2 ml clear glass ampoules in boxes of 20.

6.6 Special precautions for disposal and other handling
Tagamet is compatible with electrolyte and dextrose solutions commonly used for intravenous infusion.

Administrative Data
7. MARKETING AUTHORISATION HOLDER
Smith Kline & French Laboratories Ltd
Great West Road, Brentford, Middlesex TW8 9GS.
trading as:
GlaxoSmithKline UK,
Stockley Park West,
Uxbridge, Middlesex, UB11 1BT

8. MARKETING AUTHORISATION NUMBER(S)
PL 0002/0059R

9. DATE OF FIRST AUTHORISATION/RENEWAL OF THE AUTHORISATION
4 September 2002

10. DATE OF REVISION OF THE TEXT
14 August 2008

11. Legal Status
POM.

Tamiflu 12 mg/ml powder for oral suspension
(Roche Products Limited)

1. NAME OF THE MEDICINAL PRODUCT
Tamiflu▼
(Oseltamivir phosphate)
Tamiflu 12 mg/ml powder for oral suspension.

2. QUALITATIVE AND QUANTITATIVE COMPOSITION
1 g of powder for oral suspension contains oseltamivir phosphate equivalent to 30 mg of oseltamivir.
After reconstitution, each ml of suspension contains 12 mg oseltamivir.
One bottle of reconstituted suspension (75 ml) contains 900 mg of active substance (oseltamivir).
A bottle of 30 g Tamiflu powder for oral suspension contains 25.713 g of sorbitol. One dose of 45 mg oseltamivir administered twice daily delivers 2.6 g of sorbitol.
For a full list of excipients, see section 6.1.

3. PHARMACEUTICAL FORM
Powder for oral suspension
The powder is a granulate or clumped granulate with a white to light yellow colour.

4. CLINICAL PARTICULARS
4.1 Therapeutic indications
Treatment of influenza
In patients one year of age and older who present with symptoms typical of influenza, when influenza virus is circulating in the community. Efficacy has been demonstrated when treatment is initiated within two days of first onset of symptoms. This indication is based on clinical studies of naturally occurring influenza in which the predominant infection was influenza A (see section 5.1).
Tamiflu is indicated for the treatment of children 6 to 12 months of age during a pandemic influenza outbreak.
Prevention of influenza
- Post-exposure prevention in individuals one year of age or older following contact with a clinically diagnosed influenza case when influenza virus is circulating in the community.
- The appropriate use of Tamiflu for prevention of influenza should be determined on a case by case basis by the circumstances and the population requiring protection. In exceptional situations (e.g., in case of a mismatch between the circulating and vaccine virus strains, and a pandemic situation) seasonal prevention could be considered in individuals one year of age or older.
Tamiflu is not a substitute for influenza vaccination.
The use of antivirals for the treatment and prevention of influenza should be determined on the basis of official recommendations. Decisions regarding the use of antivirals for treatment and prophylaxis should take into consideration what is known about the characteristics of the circulating influenza viruses and the impact of the disease in different geographical areas and patient populations.
Based on limited pharmacokinetic and safety data, Tamiflu can be used in children 6 to 12 months of age for treatment during a pandemic influenza outbreak. The treating physician should take into account the pathogenicity of the circulating strain and the underlying condition of the patient to ensure there is a potential benefit to the child.

4.2 Posology and method of administration
Tamiflu suspension and Tamiflu capsules are bioequivalent formulations. 75 mg doses can be administered as either
- one 75 mg capsule or
- one 30 mg capsule plus one 45 mg capsule or
- by administering one 30 mg dose plus one 45 mg dose of suspension.
Adults, adolescents or children (> 40 kg) who are able to swallow capsules may receive appropriate doses of Tamiflu capsules.
Treatment of influenza
Treatment should be initiated as soon as possible within the first two days of onset of symptoms of influenza.
For adolescents (13 to 17 years of age) and adults: The recommended oral dose is 75 mg oseltamivir twice daily for 5 days.
For infants older than 1 year of age and for children 2 to 12 years of age: The recommended dose of Tamiflu oral suspension is indicated in the table below. Tamiflu 30 mg and 45 mg capsules are available as an alternative to the recommended dose of Tamiflu suspension.
The following weight-adjusted dosing regimens are recommended for children 1 year of age and older:

Body Weight	Recommended dose for 5 days
≤ 15 kg	30 mg twice daily
> 15 kg to 23 kg	45 mg twice daily
> 23 kg to 40 kg	60 mg twice daily
> 40 kg	75 mg twice daily

For dosing, an oral dispenser with 30 mg, 45 mg and 60 mg graduations is provided in the box. For accurate dosing, the oral dispenser supplied should be used exclusively.
Children weighing > 40 kg and who are able to swallow capsules may receive treatment with the adult dosage of 75 mg capsules twice daily for 5 days as an alternative to the recommended dose of Tamiflu suspension.
For children 6 to 12 months of age: Depending on the pathogenicity of the circulating influenza virus strain, children between 6 and 12 months of age can be treated with Tamiflu during a pandemic influenza outbreak, although the available data are limited. Pharmacokinetic data indicate that a dosage of 3 mg/kg twice daily in children 6 to 12 months of age provides plasma drug exposures in the majority of patients similar to those shown to be clinically efficacious in children age one or older and adults (see section 5.2).
The recommended dose for treatment of children 6 to 12 months of age is 3 mg per kg body weight twice daily for 5 days for treatment
Prevention of influenza
Post-exposure prevention
For adolescents (13 to 17 years of age) and adults: The recommended dose for prevention of influenza following close contact with an infected individual is 75 mg oseltamivir once daily for 10 days. Therapy should begin as soon as possible within two days of exposure to an infected individual.
For infants older than 1 year of age and for children 2 to 12 years of age: Tamiflu 30 mg and 45 mg capsules are available as an alternative to the recommended dose of Tamiflu suspension.
The recommended post-exposure prevention dose of Tamiflu is:

Body Weight	Recommended dose for 10 days
≤ 15 kg	30 mg once daily
> 15 kg to 23 kg	45 mg once daily
> 23 kg to 40 kg	60 mg once daily
> 40 kg	75 mg once daily

For dosing, an oral dispenser with 30 mg, 45 mg and 60 mg graduations is provided in the box. For accurate dosing, the oral dispenser supplied should be used exclusively.
It is recommended that Tamiflu powder for oral suspension be constituted by a pharmacist prior to dispensing to the patient (see section 6.6).
Children weighing > 40 kg and who are able to swallow capsules may receive prophylaxis with a 75 mg capsule once daily for 10 days as an alternative to the recommended dose of Tamiflu suspension.
Prevention during an influenza epidemic in the community
The recommended dose for prevention of influenza during a community outbreak is 75 mg oseltamivir once daily for up to 6 weeks.
Special populations
Hepatic impairment
No dose adjustment is required either for treatment or for prevention in patients with hepatic dysfunction. No studies have been carried out in paediatric patients with hepatic disorder.
Renal impairment
Treatment of influenza: Dose adjustment is recommended for adults with severe renal impairment. Recommended doses are detailed in the table below.

Creatinine clearance	Recommended dose for treatment
> 30 (ml/min)	75 mg twice daily
> 10 to ≤ 30 (ml/min)	75 mg once daily, or 30 mg suspension twice daily, or 30 mg capsules twice daily
≤ 10 (ml/min)	Not recommended
dialysis patients	Not recommended

Prevention of influenza: Dose adjustment is recommended for adults with severe renal impairment as detailed in the table below.

Creatinine clearance	Recommended dose for prevention
> 30 (ml/min)	75 mg once daily

> 10 to ⩽ 30 (ml/min)	75 mg every second day, or 30 mg suspension once daily, or 30 mg capsules once daily
⩽ 10 (ml/min)	Not recommended
dialysis patients	Not recommended

Elderly

No dose adjustment is required, unless there is evidence of severe renal impairment.

Children

There is insufficient clinical data available in children with renal impairment to be able to make any dosing recommendation.

4.3 Contraindications

Hypersensitivity to the active substance or to any of the excipients.

4.4 Special warnings and precautions for use

Oseltamivir is effective only against illness caused by influenza viruses. There is no evidence for efficacy of oseltamivir in any illness caused by agents other than influenza viruses.

No information is available regarding the safety and efficacy of oseltamivir in patients with any medical condition sufficiently severe or unstable to be considered at imminent risk of requiring hospitalisation.

The safety and efficacy of oseltamivir in either treatment or prevention of influenza in immunocompromised patients have not been established.

Efficacy of oseltamivir in the treatment of subjects with chronic cardiac disease and/or respiratory disease has not been established. No difference in the incidence of complications was observed between the treatment and placebo groups in this population (see section 5.1).

Tamiflu is not a substitute for influenza vaccination. Use of Tamiflu must not affect the evaluation of individuals for annual influenza vaccination. The protection against influenza lasts only as long as Tamiflu is administered. Tamiflu should be used for the treatment and prevention of influenza only when reliable epidemiological data indicate that influenza virus is circulating in the community.

Severe renal impairment

Dose adjustment is recommended for both treatment and prevention in adults with severe renal insufficiency. There is insufficient clinical data available in children with renal impairment to be able to make any dosing recommendation (see sections 4.2 and 5.2).

This medicinal product contains sorbitol. Patients with rare hereditary problems of fructose intolerance should not take this medicine.

4.5 Interaction with other medicinal products and other forms of interaction

Pharmacokinetic properties of oseltamivir, such as low protein binding and metabolism independent of the CYP450 and glucuronidase systems (see section 5.2), suggest that clinically significant drug interactions via these mechanisms are unlikely.

No dose adjustment is required when co-administering with probenecid in patients with normal renal function. Co-administration of probenecid, a potent inhibitor of the anionic pathway of renal tubular secretion, results in an approximate 2-fold increase in exposure to the active metabolite of oseltamivir.

Oseltamivir has no kinetic interaction with amoxicillin, which is eliminated via the same pathway, suggesting that oseltamivir interaction with this pathway is weak.

Clinically important drug interactions involving competition for renal tubular secretion are unlikely, due to the known safety margin for most of these substances, the elimination characteristics of the active metabolite (glomerular filtration and anionic tubular secretion) and the excretion capacity of these pathways. However, care should be taken when prescribing oseltamivir in subjects when taking co-excreted agents with a narrow therapeutic margin (e.g., chlorpropamide, methotrexate, phenylbutazone).

No pharmacokinetic interactions between oseltamivir or its major metabolite have been observed when co-administering oseltamivir with paracetamol, acetyl-salicylic acid, cimetidine or with antacids (magnesium and aluminium hydroxides and calcium carbonates).

4.6 Pregnancy and lactation

While no controlled clinical trials have been conducted on the use of oseltamivir in pregnant women, there is limited data available from post-marketing and retrospective observational surveillance reports. These data in conjunction with animal studies do not indicate direct or indirect harmful effects with respect to pregnancy, embryonal/foetal or postnatal development (see section 5.3). Pregnant women may receive Tamiflu, after considering the available safety information, the pathogenicity of the circulating influenza virus strain and the underlying condition of the pregnant woman.

In lactating rats, oseltamivir and the active metabolite are excreted in milk. Very limited information is available on children breast-fed by mothers taking oseltamivir and on excretion of oseltamivir in breast milk. Limited data demonstrated that oseltamivir and the active metabolite were detected in breast milk, however the levels were low, which would result in a subtherapeutic dose to the infant. Considering this information, the pathogenicity of the circulating influenza virus strain and the underlying condition of the lactating woman, administration of oseltamivir may be considered, where there are clear potential benefits to lactating mothers.

4.7 Effects on ability to drive and use machines

Tamiflu has no influence on the ability to drive and use machines.

4.8 Undesirable effects

The overall safety profile of Tamiflu is based on data from 2107 adult and 1032 paediatric patients treated for influenza, and on data from 2914 adult and 99 paediatric patients receiving Tamiflu for the prophylaxis of influenza in clinical trials.

In adults, the most commonly reported adverse drug reactions (ADRs) were vomiting and nausea in the treatment studies, and nausea and headache in the prevention studies. The majority of these ADRs were reported on a single occasion on either the first or second treatment day and resolved spontaneously within 1-2 days. In children, the most commonly reported adverse drug reaction was vomiting.

The ADRs listed in the tables below fall into the following categories: Very Common (⩾ *1/10*), Common (⩾ *1/100* to < *1/10*), Uncommon (⩾ *1/1,000* to < *1/100*), Rare (⩾ *1/10,000* to < *1/1,000*), Very rare (< *1/10,000*) and not known (cannot be estimated from the available data). ADRs are added to the appropriate category in the tables according to the pooled analysis from clinical trials. Within each

Table 1

System Organ Class (SOC) *Frequency Category* Adverse Drug Reaction	Percentage of Patients Experiencing the ADR: Treatment – Oseltamivir 75 mg bid (n = 1057)	Treatment – Placebo (n = 1050)	Prevention – Oseltamivir 75 mg od (n = 1480)	Prevention – Placebo (n = 1434)
Infections and infestations				
Common:				
Bronchitis	4 %	5 %	1 %	1 %
Bronchitis acute	1 %	1 %	0 %	< 1 %
Upper respiratory tract infections	0 %	0 %	8 %	8 %
Psychiatric disorders				
Uncommon:				
Hallucination[a]	< 1 %	0 %	< 1 %	0 %
Nervous system disorders				
Very Common:				
Headache	2 %	2 %	20 %	18 %
Common:				
Insomnia	1 %	1 %	1 %	1 %
Uncommon:				
Convulsion[a]	< 1 %	0 %	0 %	0 %
Disorders of the ear and labyrinth				
Common:				
Vertigo	1 %	1 %	< 1 %	< 1 %
Respiratory, thoracic and mediastinal disorders				
Common:				
Cough	1 %	1 %	6 %	6 %
Rhinorrhoea	< 1 %	0 %	2 %	1 %
Gastrointestinal disorders				
Very Common:				
Nausea[b,c]	11 %	7 %	8 %	4 %
Common:				
Vomiting[c]	8 %	3 %	2 %	1 %
Abdominal pain	2 %	2 %	2 %	2 %
Diarrhoea	6 %	8 %	3 %	3 %
Dyspepsia	1 %	1 %	2 %	2 %
Skin and subcutaneous tissue disorders				
Uncommon:				
Dermatitis[a]	< 1 %	< 1 %	1 %	1 %
Rash[a]	< 1 %	< 1 %	< 1 %	< 1 %
Urticaria[a]	< 1 %	< 1 %	< 1 %	< 1 %
Eczema[a]	< 1 %	0 %	< 1 %	< 1 %
General disorders				
Common:				
Dizziness	2 %	3 %	2 %	2 %
Fatigue	1 %	1 %	8 %	8 %
Pain	< 1 %	< 1 %	4 %	3 %

[a] These are events identified during post-marketing surveillance. They were also reported in the pooled clinical studies the incidence presented in the table above.

[b] Subjects who experienced nausea alone; excludes subjects who experienced nausea in association with vomiting.

[c] The difference between the placebo and oseltamivir groups was statistically significant.

Table 2

System Organ Class (SOC) *Frequency Category* Adverse Drug Reaction	Percentage of Patients Experiencing the ADR			
	Treatment		Treatment	Prevention[a]
	Oseltamivir 2 mg/kg bid (n=515)	Placebo (n=517)	Oseltamivir 30 to 75 mg[b] (n=158)	Oseltamivir 30 to 75 mg[b] (n=99)
Infections and infestations				
Common:				
Pneumonia	2 %	3 %	0 %	0 %
Sinusitis	2 %	3 %	0 %	0 %
Bronchitis	2 %	2 %	2 %	0 %
Otitis media	9 %	11 %	1 %	2 %
Disorders of the blood and lymphatic system				
Common:				
Lymphadenopathy	1 %	2 %	< 1 %	0 %
Respiratory, thoracic and mediastinal disorders				
Common:				
Asthma (incl. aggravated)	4 %	4 %	0 %	1 %
Epistaxis	3 %	3 %	1 %	1 %
Gastrointestinal disorder				
Very Common:				
Vomiting	15 %	9 %	20 %	10 %
Diarrhoea	10 %	11 %	3 %	1 %
Common:				
Nausea	3 %	4 %	6 %	4 %
Abdominal pain	5 %	4 %	2 %	1 %
Disorders of the eye				
Common:				
Conjunctivitis	1 %	< 1 %	0 %	0 %
Disorders of the ear and labyrinth				
Common:				
Ear disorder[c]	2 %	1 %	0 %	0 %
Tympanic membrane disorder	1 %	1 %	0 %	0 %
Skin and subcutaneous tissue disorders				
Common:				
Dermatitis	1 %	2 %	< 1 %	0 %

[a] The prevention study did not contain a placebo arm, i.e. was an uncontrolled study.
[b] Unit dose = weight-based dosing (see section 4.2).
[c] Patients experienced ear ache and ear pain.

frequency grouping ADRs are presented in the order of decreasing seriousness.

Treatment and prevention of influenza in adults and adolescents:

Most Frequent Adverse Drug Reactions (⩾ 1 % in the oseltamivir group) in Studies Investigating Tamiflu for Treatment and Prevention of Influenza in Adults and Adolescents or Through Post-Marketing Surveillance

(see Table 1 on previous page)

Treatment and prevention of influenza in children:

The table below shows the most frequently reported ADRs from paediatric clinical trials.

Most Frequent Adverse Drug Reactions (⩾ 1 % in the oseltamivir group in the treatment studies and ⩾ 10 % in the oseltamivir group in the prophylaxis study) in Children

(see Table 2 above)

In general, the adverse event profile in children with pre-existing bronchial asthma was qualitatively similar to that of otherwise healthy children.

Further post marketing surveillance data on selected serious adverse drug reactions:

Immune system disorders

Frequency not known: hypersensitivity reactions, including anaphylactic/anaphylactoid reactions.

Psychiatric disorders and nervous system disorders

Frequency not known: influenza can be associated with a variety of neurologic and behavioural symptoms which can include events such as hallucinations, delirium, and abnormal behaviour, in some cases resulting in fatal outcomes. These events may occur in the setting of encephalitis or encephalopathy but can occur without obvious severe disease.

In patients with influenza who were receiving Tamiflu, there have been postmarketing reports of convulsions and delirium (including symptoms such as altered level of consciousness, confusion, abnormal behaviour, delusions, hallucinations, agitation, anxiety, nightmares), in a very few cases resulting in accidental injury or fatal outcomes. These events were reported primarily among paediatric and adolescent patients and often had an abrupt onset and rapid resolution. The contribution of Tamiflu to those events is unknown. Such neuropsychiatric events have also been reported in patients with influenza who were not taking Tamiflu.

Eye disorders

Frequency not known: visual disturbance.

Cardiac disorders

Frequency not known: cardiac arrhythmia.

Gastrointestinal disorders

Frequency not known: gastrointestinal bleedings and haemorrhagic colitis.

Hepato-biliary disorders

Frequency not known: hepato-biliary system disorders, including hepatitis and elevated liver enzymes in patients with influenza-like illness. These cases include fatal fulminant hepatitis/hepatic failure.

Skin and subcutaneous tissue disorders

Frequency not known: severe skin reactions, including Stevens-Johnson syndrome, toxic epidermal necrolysis, erythema multiforme and angioneurotic oedema.

Additional information on special populations:

There were no clinically relevant differences in the safety population of the elderly subjects who received oseltamivir or placebo compared with the adult population aged up to 65 years.

The adverse event profile in adolescents and patients with chronic cardiac and/or respiratory disease was qualitatively similar to those of healthy young adults.

Safety information available on oseltamivir administered for treatment of influenza in children less than one year of age from prospective and retrospective observational trials (comprising together more than 2400 children of that age class), epidemiological databases research and postmarketing reports suggest that the safety profile in children less than one year of age is similar to the established safety profile of children aged one year and older.

4.9 Overdose

There is no experience with overdose. However, the anticipated manifestations of acute overdose would be nausea, with or without accompanying vomiting, and dizziness. Patients should discontinue the treatment in the event of overdose. No specific antidote is known.

5. PHARMACOLOGICAL PROPERTIES

5.1 Pharmacodynamic properties

Pharmacotherapeutic group: Antiviral ATC code: J05AH02

Oseltamivir phosphate is a pro-drug of the active metabolite (oseltamivir carboxylate). The active metabolite is a selective inhibitor of influenza virus neuraminidase enzymes, which are glycoproteins found on the virion surface. Viral neuraminidase enzyme activity is important both for viral entry into uninfected cells and for the release of recently formed virus particles from infected cells, and for the further spread of infectious virus in the body.

Oseltamivir carboxylate inhibits influenza A and B neuraminidases *in vitro*. Oseltamivir phosphate inhibits influenza virus infection and replication *in vitro*. Oseltamivir given orally inhibits influenza A and B virus replication and pathogenicity *in vivo* in animal models of influenza infection at antiviral exposures similar to that achieved in man with 75 mg twice daily.

Antiviral activity of oseltamivir was supported for influenza A and B by experimental challenge studies in healthy volunteers.

Neuraminidase enzyme IC50 values for oseltamivir for clinically isolated influenza A ranged from 0.1 nM to 1.3 nM, and for influenza B was 2.6 nM. Higher IC50 values for influenza B, up to a median of 8.5 nM, have been observed in published trials.

Reduced sensitivity of viral neuraminidase

There has been no evidence for emergence of drug resistance associated with the use of Tamiflu in clinical studies conducted to date in post-exposure (7 days), post-exposure within household groups (10 days) and seasonal (42 days) prevention of influenza.

The risk of emergence of influenza viruses with reduced susceptibility or frank resistance to oseltamivir has been examined during Roche-sponsored clinical studies. All patients who were found to carry oseltamivir-resistant virus did so transiently, cleared the virus normally and showed no clinical deterioration.

Patient Population	Patients with Resistance Mutations (%)	
	Phenotyping*	Geno- and Phenotyping*
Adults and adolescents	4/1245 (0.32%)	5/1245 (0.4%)
Children (1-12 years)	19/464 (4.1%)	25/464 (5.4%)

* Full genotyping was not performed in all studies.

The rate of emergence of resistance may be higher in the youngest age groups, and in immunosupressed patients. Oseltamivir-resistant viruses isolated from oseltamivir-treated patients and oseltamivir-resistant laboratory strains of influenza viruses have been found to contain mutations in N1 and N2 neuraminidases. Resistance mutations tend to be viral sub-type specific (including those found in H5N1 variants).

Naturally occurring mutations in influenza A/H1N1 virus associated with reduced susceptibility to oseltamivir *in vitro* have been detected in patients who, based on the reported information, have not been exposed to oseltamivir. The extent of reduction in susceptibility to oseltamivir and the prevalence of such viruses appears to vary seasonally and geographically.

Treatment of influenza infection

Oseltamivir is effective only against illnesses caused by influenza virus. Statistical analyses are therefore presented only for influenza-infected subjects. In the pooled treatment study population, which included both influenza-positive and -negative subjects (ITT), primary efficacy was reduced proportional to the number of influenza-negative individuals. In the overall treatment population, influenza infection was confirmed in 67 % (range 46 % to 74 %) of the recruited patients. Of the elderly subjects, 64 % were influenza-positive and of those with chronic cardiac and/or respiratory disease 62 % were influenza-positive. In all phase III treatment studies, patients were recruited only during the period in which influenza was circulating in the local community.

Adults and adolescents 13 years of age and older: Patients were eligible if they reported within 36 hours of onset of symptoms, had fever ⩾ 37.8 °C, accompanied by at least one respiratory symptom (cough, nasal symptoms or sore throat) and at least one systemic symptom (myalgia, chills/ sweats, malaise, fatigue or headache). In a pooled analysis of all influenza-positive adults and adolescents (N = 2413) enrolled into treatment studies, oseltamivir 75 mg twice daily for 5 days reduced the median duration of influenza illness by approximately one day from 5.2 days (95 % CI 4.9 – 5.5 days) in the placebo group to 4.2 days (95 % CI 4.0 – 4.4 days; p ⩽ 0.0001).

The proportion of subjects who developed specified lower respiratory tract complications (mainly bronchitis) treated with antibiotics was reduced from 12.7 % (135/1063) in the placebo group to 8.6 % (116/1350) in the oseltamivir treated population (p = 0.0012).

Treatment of influenza in high risk populations: The median duration of influenza illness in elderly subjects (⩾ 65 years) and in subjects with chronic cardiac and/or respiratory disease receiving oseltamivir 75 mg twice daily for 5 days was not reduced significantly. The total duration of fever was reduced by one day in the groups treated with oseltamivir. In the influenza-positive elderly, oseltamivir significantly reduced the incidence of specified lower respiratory tract complications (mainly bronchitis) treated with antibiotics from 19 % (52/268) in the placebo group to 12 % (29/250) in the oseltamivir treated population (p = 0.0156).

In influenza-positive patients with chronic cardiac and/or respiratory disease, the combined incidence of lower respiratory tract complications (mainly bronchitis) treated with antibiotics was 17 % (22/133) in the placebo group and 14 % (16/118) in the oseltamivir treated population (p = 0.5976).

Treatment of influenza in children: In a study of otherwise healthy children (65 % influenza-positive) aged 1 to 12 years (mean age 5.3 years) who had fever (⩾ 37.8 °C) plus either cough or coryza, 67 % of influenza-positive patients were infected with influenza A and 33 % with influenza B. Oseltamivir treatment, started within 48 hours of onset of symptoms, significantly reduced the duration of time to freedom from illness (defined as the simultaneous return to normal health and activity and alleviation of fever, cough and coryza) by 1.5 days (95 % CI 0.6 – 2.2 days; p < 0.0001) compared to placebo. Oseltamivir reduced the incidence of acute otitis media from 26.5 % (53/200) in the placebo group to 16 % (29/183) in the oseltamivir treated children (p = 0.013).

A second study was completed in 334 asthmatic children aged 6 to 12 years old of which 53.6 % were influenza-positive. In the oseltamivir treated group, the median duration of illness was not reduced significantly. By day 6 (the last day of treatment) FEV_1 had increased by 10.8 % in the oseltamivir treated group compared to 4.7 % on placebo (p = 0.0148) in this population.

Treatment of influenza B infection: Overall, 15 % of the influenza-positive population were infected by influenza B, proportions ranging from 1 to 33 % in individual studies. The median duration of illness in influenza B infected subjects did not differ significantly between the treatment groups in individual studies. Data from 504 influenza B infected subjects were pooled across all studies for analysis. Oseltamivir reduced the time to alleviation of all symptoms by 0.7 days (95 % CI 0.1 – 1.6 days; p = 0.022) and the duration of fever (⩾ 37.8 °C), cough and coryza by one day (95 % CI 0.4 – 1.7 days; p < 0.001) compared to placebo.

Prevention of influenza

The efficacy of oseltamivir in preventing naturally occurring influenza illness has been demonstrated in a post-exposure prevention study in households and two seasonal prevention studies. The primary efficacy parameter for all of these studies was the incidence of laboratory-confirmed influenza. The virulence of influenza epidemics is not predictable and varies within a region and from season to season, therefore the number needed to treat (NNT) in order to prevent one case of influenza illness varies.

Post-exposure prevention: In a study in contacts (12.6 % vaccinated against influenza) of an index case of influenza, oseltamivir 75 mg once daily was started within 2 days of onset of symptoms in the index case and continued for seven days. Influenza was confirmed in 163 out of 377 index cases. Oseltamivir significantly reduced the incidence of clinical influenza illness occurring in the contacts of confirmed influenza cases from 24/200 (12 %) in the placebo group to 2/205 (1 %) in the oseltamivir group (92 % reduction [95 % CI 6 – 16; p ⩽ 0.0001]). The number needed to treat (NNT) in contacts of true influenza cases was 10 (95 % CI 9 – 12) and was 16 (95 % CI 15 – 19) in the whole population (ITT) regardless of infection status in the index case.

The efficacy of oseltamivir in preventing naturally occurring influenza illness has been demonstrated in a post-exposure prevention study in households that included adults, adolescents, and children aged 1 to 12 years, both as index cases and as family contacts. The primary efficacy parameter for this study was the incidence of laboratory-confirmed clinical influenza in the households. Oseltamivir prophylaxis lasted for 10 days. In the total population, there was a reduction in the incidence of laboratory-confirmed clinical influenza in households from 20 % (27/136) in the group not receiving prevention to 7 % (10/135) in the group receiving prevention (62.7 % reduction [95 % CI 26.0 – 81.2; p = 0.0042]). In households of influenza-infected index cases, there was a reduction in the incidence of influenza from 26 % (23/89) in the group not receiving prevention to 11 % (9/84) in the group receiving prevention (58.5 % reduction [95 % CI 15.6 – 79.6; p = 0.0114]).

According to subgroup analysis in children at 1 to 12 years of age, the incidence of laboratory-confirmed clinical influenza among children was significantly reduced from 19 % (21/111) in the group not receiving prevention to 7 % (7/104) in the group receiving prevention (64.4 % reduction [95 % CI 15.8 – 85.0; p = 0.0188]). Among children who were not already shedding virus at baseline, the incidence of laboratory-confirmed clinical influenza was reduced from 21 % (15/70) in the group not receiving prevention to 4 % (2/47) in the group receiving prevention (80.1 % reduction [95 % CI 22.0 – 94.9; p = 0.0206]). The NNT for the total paediatric population was 9 (95 % CI 7 – 24) and 8 (95 % CI 6, upper limit not estimable) in the whole population (ITT) and in paediatric contacts of infected index cases (ITTII), respectively.

Prevention during an influenza epidemic in the community: In a pooled analysis of two other studies conducted in unvaccinated otherwise healthy adults, oseltamivir 75 mg once daily given for 6 weeks significantly reduced the incidence of clinical influenza illness from 25/519 (4.8 %) in the placebo group to 6/520 (1.2 %) in the oseltamivir group (76 % reduction [95 % CI 1.6 – 5.7; p = 0.0006]) during a community outbreak of influenza. The NNT in this study was 28 (95 % CI 24 – 50).

A study in elderly residents of nursing homes, where 80 % of participants received vaccine in the season of the study, oseltamivir 75 mg once daily given for 6 weeks significantly reduced the incidence of clinical influenza illness from 12/272 (4.4 %) in the placebo group to 1/276 (0.4 %) in the oseltamivir group (92 % reduction [95 % CI 1.5 – 6.6; p = 0.0015]). The NNT in this study was 25 (95 % CI 23 – 62).

Specific studies have not been conducted to assess of the reduction in the risk of complications.

5.2 Pharmacokinetic properties

Absorption

Oseltamivir is readily absorbed from the gastrointestinal tract after oral administration of oseltamivir phosphate (pro-drug) and is extensively converted by predominantly hepatic esterases to the active metabolite (oseltamivir carboxylate). At least 75 % of an oral dose reaches the systemic circulation as the active metabolite. Exposure to the pro-drug is less than 5 % relative to the active metabolite. Plasma concentrations of both pro-drug and active metabolite are proportional to dose and are unaffected by co-administration with food.

Distribution

The mean volume of distribution at steady state of the oseltamivir carboxylate is approximately 23 litres in humans, a volume equivalent to extracellular body fluid. Since neuraminidase activity is extracellular, oseltamivir carboxylate distributes to all sites of influenza virus spread.

The binding of the oseltamivir carboxylate to human plasma protein is negligible (approximately 3 %).

Metabolism

Oseltamivir is extensively converted to oseltamivir carboxylate by esterases located predominantly in the liver. *In vitro* studies demonstrated that neither oseltamivir nor the active metabolite is a substrate for, or an inhibitor of, the major cytochrome P450 isoforms. No phase 2 conjugates of either compound have been identified *in vivo*.

Elimination

Absorbed oseltamivir is primarily (> 90 %) eliminated by conversion to oseltamivir carboxylate. It is not further metabolised and is eliminated in the urine. Peak plasma concentrations of oseltamivir carboxylate decline with a half-life of 6 to 10 hours in most subjects. The active metabolite is eliminated entirely by renal excretion. Renal clearance (18.8 l/h) exceeds glomerular filtration rate (7.5 l/h) indicating that tubular secretion occurs in addition to glomerular filtration. Less than 20 % of an oral radiolabelled dose is eliminated in faeces.

Renal impairment

Administration of 100 mg oseltamivir phosphate twice daily for 5 days to patients with various degrees of renal impairment showed that exposure to oseltamivir carboxylate is inversely proportional to declining renal function. For dosing, see section 4.2.

Hepatic impairment

In vitro studies have concluded that exposure to oseltamivir is not expected to be increased significantly nor is exposure to the active metabolite expected to be significantly decreased in patients with hepatic impairment (see section 4.2).

Elderly

Exposure to the active metabolite at steady state was 25 to 35 % higher in elderly (age 65 to 78 years) compared to adults less than 65 years of age given comparable doses of oseltamivir. Half-lives observed in the elderly were similar to those seen in young adults. On the basis of drug exposure and tolerability, dosage adjustments are not required for elderly patients unless there is evidence of severe renal impairment (creatinine clearance below 30 ml/min) (see section 4.2).

Children

Children 1 year of age and older: The pharmacokinetics of oseltamivir have been evaluated in single-dose pharmacokinetic studies in children aged 1 to 16 years. Multiple-dose pharmacokinetics were studied in a small number of children enrolled in a clinical efficacy study. Younger children cleared both the pro-drug and its active metabolite faster than adults, resulting in a lower exposure for a given mg/kg dose. Doses of 2 mg/kg give oseltamivir carboxylate exposures comparable to those achieved in adults receiving a single 75 mg dose (approximately 1 mg/kg). The pharmacokinetics of oseltamivir in children over 12 years of age are similar to those in adults.

Children 6 to 12 months of age: Limited exposure data from children 6 to 12 months of age from a pharmacodynamic, pharmacokinetic and safety study in influenza-infected children less than 2 years of age, suggest that for most children 6 to 12 months of age, the exposure following 3 mg/kg dosing is similar to the exposures seen in older children and adults using the approved dose.

5.3 Preclinical safety data

Preclinical data reveal no special hazard for humans based on conventional studies of safety pharmacology, repeated-dose toxicity and genotoxicity. Results of the conventional rodent carcinogenicity studies showed a trend towards a dose-dependent increase in the incidence of some tumours that are typical for the rodent strains used. Considering the margins of exposure in relation to the expected exposure in the human use, these findings do not change the benefit-risk of Tamiflu in its adopted therapeutic indications.

Teratology studies have been conducted in rats and rabbits at doses of up to 1500 mg/kg/day and 500 mg/kg/day, respectively. No effects on foetal development were observed. A rat fertility study up to a dose of 1500 mg/kg/day demonstrated no adverse effects on either sex. In pre- and post-natal rat studies, prolonged parturition was noted at 1500 mg/kg/day: the safety margin between human exposure and the highest no-effect dose (500 mg/kg/day) in rats is 480-fold for oseltamivir and 44-fold for the active metabolite, respectively. Foetal exposure in the rats and rabbits was approximately 15 to 20 % of that of the mother.

In lactating rats, oseltamivir and the active metabolite are excreted in the milk. Limited data indicate that oseltamivir and the active metabolite are excreted in human milk. Extrapolation of the animal data provides estimates of 0.01 mg/day and 0.3 mg/day for the respective compounds.

A potential for skin sensitisation to oseltamivir was observed in a "maximisation" test in guinea pigs. Approximately 50 % of the animals treated with the unformulated active ingredient showed erythema after challenging the induced animals. Reversible irritancy of rabbits' eyes was detected.

Whereas very high oral single doses of oseltamivir phosphate had no effect in adult rats, such doses resulted in toxicity in juvenile 7-day-old rat pups, including death. These effects were seen at doses of 657 mg/kg and higher. At 500 mg/kg, no adverse effects were seen, including upon chronic treatment (500 mg/kg/day administered from 7 to 21 days post partum).

6. PHARMACEUTICAL PARTICULARS

6.1 List of excipients

Powder for oral suspension:

Sorbitol (E420),

Sodium dihydrogen citrate (E331[a])

Xanthan gum (E415)

Sodium benzoate (E211)

Saccharin sodium (E954)

Titanium dioxide (E171)

Tutti frutti flavour (including maltodextrins [maize], propylene glycol, arabic gum E414 and natural identical flavouring substances [mainly consisting of banana, pineapple and peach flavour]).

6.2 Incompatibilities

Not applicable.

6.3 Shelf life

2 years for powder for oral suspension.

6.4 Special precautions for storage

Powder: Do not store above 30°C.

After reconstitution, the suspension can be stored either at room temperature (not above 25°C) for 10 days or in a refrigerator (2°C - 8°C) for 17 days.

6.5 Nature and contents of container

Carton containing a 100 ml amber glass bottle (with child-resistant plastic screw cap) with 30 g of powder for oral suspension, a plastic adapter, a plastic oral dispenser and a plastic measuring cup. After reconstitution with 52 ml of water, the usable volume of oral suspension allows for the retrieval of a total of 10 doses of 75 mg oseltamivir.

6.6 Special precautions for disposal and other handling
It is recommended that Tamiflu oral suspension should be reconstituted by the pharmacist prior to its dispensing to the patient.

Preparation of Oral Suspension

1. Tap the closed bottle gently several times to loosen the powder.

2. Measure 52 ml of water by filling the measuring cup to the indicated level (measuring cup included in the box).

3. Add all 52 ml of water into the bottle, recap the bottle and shake the closed bottle well for 15 seconds.

4. Remove the cap and push the bottle adapter into the neck of the bottle.

5. Close the bottle tightly with the cap (on the top of the bottle adapter). This will make sure that the bottle adapter fits in the bottle in the right position.

Tamiflu powder for suspension will appear as an opaque and white to light yellow suspension after reconstitution.

Any unused product or waste material should be disposed of in accordance with local requirements.

7. MARKETING AUTHORISATION HOLDER
Roche Registration Limited

6 Falcon Way

Shire Park

Welwyn Garden City

AL7 1TW

United Kingdom

8. MARKETING AUTHORISATION NUMBER(S)
EU/1/02/222/002

9. DATE OF FIRST AUTHORISATION/RENEWAL OF THE AUTHORISATION
Date of first authorisation: 20 June 2002

Date of last renewal: 20 June 2007

10. DATE OF REVISION OF THE TEXT
9 September 2009

LEGAL STATUS
POM

Detailed information on this medicinal product is available on the website of the European Medicines Agency (EMEA) http://www.emea.europa.eu/.

Tamiflu 30 mg and 45 mg Hard Capsules

(Roche Products Limited)

1. NAME OF THE MEDICINAL PRODUCT
Tamiflu▼ 30 mg hard capsule.

Tamiflu▼ 45 mg hard capsule.

2. QUALITATIVE AND QUANTITATIVE COMPOSITION
Tamiflu 30 mg hard capsule: Each hard capsule contains oseltamivir phosphate equivalent to 30 mg of oseltamivir.

Tamiflu 45 mg hard capsule: Each hard capsule contains oseltamivir phosphate equivalent to 45 mg of oseltamivir.

For a full list of excipients, see section 6.1.

3. PHARMACEUTICAL FORM
Hard capsule

Tamiflu 30 mg hard capsule: The hard capsule consists of a light yellow opaque body bearing the imprint "ROCHE" and a light yellow opaque cap bearing the imprint "30 mg". Imprints are blue.

Tamiflu 45 mg hard capsule: The hard capsule consists of a grey opaque body bearing the imprint "ROCHE" and a grey opaque cap bearing the imprint "45 mg". Imprints are blue.

4. CLINICAL PARTICULARS
4.1 Therapeutic indications
Treatment of influenza
In patients one year of age and older who present with symptoms typical of influenza, when influenza virus is circulating in the community. Efficacy has been demonstrated when treatment is initiated within two days of first onset of symptoms. This indication is based on clinical studies of naturally occurring influenza in which the predominant infection was influenza A (see section 5.1).

Tamiflu is indicated for the treatment of children 6 to 12 months of age during a pandemic influenza outbreak.

Prevention of influenza

- Post-exposure prevention in individuals one year of age or older following contact with a clinically diagnosed influenza case when influenza virus is circulating in the community.
- The appropriate use of Tamiflu for prevention of influenza should be determined on a case by case basis by the circumstances and the population requiring protection. In exceptional situations (e.g., in case of a mismatch between the circulating and vaccine virus strains, and a pandemic situation) seasonal prevention could be considered in individuals one year of age or older.

Tamiflu is not a substitute for influenza vaccination.

The use of antivirals for the treatment and prevention of influenza should be determined on the basis of official recommendations. Decisions regarding the use of antivirals for treatment and prophylaxis should take into consideration what is known about the characteristics of the circulating influenza viruses and the impact of the disease in different geographical areas and patient populations.

Based on limited pharmacokinetic and safety data, Tamiflu can be used in children 6 to 12 months of age for treatment during a pandemic influenza outbreak. The treating physician should take into account the pathogenicity of the circulating strain and the underlying condition of the patient to ensure there is a potential benefit to the child.

4.2 Posology and method of administration
Tamiflu capsules and Tamiflu suspension are bioequivalent formulations. 75 mg doses can be administered as either

- one 75 mg capsule or
- one 30 mg capsule plus one 45 mg capsule or
- by administering one 30 mg dose plus one 45 mg dose of suspension.

Adults, adolescents or children (> 40 kg) who are unable to swallow capsules may receive appropriate doses of Tamiflu suspension.

During situations when commercially manufactured Tamiflu oral suspension is not readily available, adults, adolescents or children who are unable to swallow capsules may receive appropriate doses of Tamiflu (see section 3 in Package Leaflet) by opening capsules and pouring the contents of capsules into a suitable, small amount (1 teaspoon maximum) of sweetened food product such as regular or sugar-free chocolate syrup, honey (only for children two years or older), light brown or table sugar dissolved in water, dessert toppings, sweetened condensed milk, apple sauce or yogurt to mask the bitter taste. The mixture should be stirred and the entire contents given to the patient. The mixture must be swallowed immediately after its preparation.

Treatment of influenza

Treatment should be initiated as soon as possible within the first two days of onset of symptoms of influenza.

For adolescents (13 to 17 years of age) and adults: The recommended oral dose is 75 mg oseltamivir twice daily for 5 days.

For infants older than 1 year of age and for children 2 to 12 years of age: Tamiflu 30 mg and 45 mg capsules and oral suspension are available.

The following weight-adjusted dosing regimens are recommended for children 1 year of age and older:

Body Weight	Recommended dose for 5 days
⩽ 15 kg	30 mg twice daily
> 15 kg to 23 kg	45 mg twice daily
> 23 kg to 40 kg	60 mg twice daily
> 40 kg	75 mg twice daily

Children weighing > 40 kg and who are able to swallow capsules may receive treatment with the adult dosage of 75 mg capsules twice daily for 5 days as an alternative to the recommended dose of Tamiflu suspension.

For children 6 to 12 months of age: Depending on the pathogenicity of the circulating influenza virus strain, children between 6 and 12 months of age can be treated with Tamiflu during a pandemic influenza outbreak, although the available data are limited. Pharmacokinetic data indicate that a dosage of 3 mg/kg twice daily in children 6 to 12 months of age provides plasma drug exposures in the majority of patients similar to those shown to be clinically efficacious in children age one or older and adults (see section 5.2).

The recommended dose for treatment of children 6 to 12 months of age is 3 mg per kg body weight twice daily for 5 days for treatment

Prevention of influenza

Post-exposure prevention

For adolescents (13 to 17 years of age) and adults: The recommended dose for prevention of influenza following close contact with an infected individual is 75 mg oseltamivir once daily for 10 days. Therapy should begin as soon as possible within two days of exposure to an infected individual.

For infants older than 1 year of age and for children 2 to 12 years of age: Tamiflu 30 mg and 45 mg capsules and oral suspension are available.

The recommended post-exposure prevention dose of Tamiflu is:

Body Weight	Recommended dose for 10 days
⩽ 15 kg	30 mg once daily
> 15 kg to 23 kg	45 mg once daily
> 23 kg to 40 kg	60 mg once daily
> 40 kg	75 mg once daily

Children weighing > 40 kg and who are able to swallow capsules may receive prevention with a 75 mg capsule once daily for 10 days as an alternative to the recommended dose of Tamiflu suspension.

Prevention during an influenza epidemic in the community
The recommended dose for prevention of influenza during a community outbreak is 75 mg oseltamivir once daily for up to 6 weeks.

Special populations

Hepatic impairment
No dose adjustment is required either for treatment or for prevention in patients with hepatic dysfunction. No studies have been carried out in paediatric patients with hepatic disorder.

Renal impairment
Treatment of influenza: Dose adjustment is recommended for adults with severe renal impairment. Recommended doses are detailed in the table below.

Creatinine clearance	Recommended dose for treatment
> 30 (ml/min)	75 mg twice daily
> 10 to ⩽ 30 (ml/min)	75 mg once daily, or 30 mg suspension twice daily, or 30 mg capsules twice daily
⩽ 10 (ml/min)	Not recommended
dialysis patients	Not recommended

Prevention of influenza: Dose adjustment is recommended for adults with severe renal impairment as detailed in the table below.

Creatinine clearance	Recommended dose for prevention
> 30 (ml/min)	75 mg once daily
> 10 to ⩽ 30 (ml/min)	75 mg every second day, or 30 mg suspension once daily, or 30 mg capsules once daily
⩽ 10 (ml/min)	Not recommended
dialysis patients	Not recommended

Elderly
No dose adjustment is required, unless there is evidence of severe renal impairment.

Children
There is insufficient clinical data available in children with renal impairment to be able to make any dosing recommendation.

4.3 Contraindications
Hypersensitivity to the active substance or to any of the excipients.

4.4 Special warnings and precautions for use
Oseltamivir is effective only against illness caused by influenza viruses. There is no evidence for efficacy of oseltamivir in any illness caused by agents other than influenza viruses.

No information is available regarding the safety and efficacy of oseltamivir in patients with any medical condition sufficiently severe or unstable to be considered at imminent risk of requiring hospitalisation.

The safety and efficacy of oseltamivir in either treatment or prevention of influenza in immunocompromised patients have not been established.

Efficacy of oseltamivir in the treatment of subjects with chronic cardiac disease and/or respiratory disease has not been established. No difference in the incidence of complications was observed between the treatment and placebo groups in this population (see section 5.1).

Tamiflu is not a substitute for influenza vaccination. Use of Tamiflu must not affect the evaluation of individuals for annual influenza vaccination. The protection against influenza lasts only as long as Tamiflu is administered. Tamiflu should be used for the treatment and prevention of influenza only when reliable epidemiological data indicate that influenza virus is circulating in the community.

Severe renal impairment
Dose adjustment is recommended for both treatment and prevention in adults with severe renal insufficiency. There is insufficient clinical data available in children with renal impairment to be able to make any dosing recommendation.(see sections 4.2 and 5.2).

4.5 Interaction with other medicinal products and other forms of interaction
Pharmacokinetic properties of oseltamivir, such as low protein binding and metabolism independent of the CYP450 and glucuronidase systems (see section 5.2), suggest that clinically significant drug interactions via these mechanisms are unlikely.

No dose adjustment is required when co-administering with probenecid in patients with normal renal function. Co-administration of probenecid, a potent inhibitor of the anionic pathway of renal tubular secretion, results in an approximate 2-fold increase in exposure to the active metabolite of oseltamivir.

Oseltamivir has no kinetic interaction with amoxicillin, which is eliminated via the same pathway, suggesting that oseltamivir interaction with this pathway is weak.

Clinically important drug interactions involving competition for renal tubular secretion are unlikely, due to the known safety margin for most of these substances, the elimination characteristics of the active metabolite (glomerular filtration and anionic tubular secretion) and the excretion capacity of these pathways. However, care should be taken when prescribing oseltamivir in subjects when taking co-excreted agents with a narrow therapeutic margin (e.g., chlorpropamide, methotrexate, phenylbutazone).

No pharmacokinetic interactions between oseltamivir or its major metabolite have been observed when co-administering oseltamivir with paracetamol, acetyl-salicylic acid, cimetidine or with antacids (magnesium and aluminium hydroxides and calcium carbonates).

4.6 Pregnancy and lactation

While no controlled clinical trials have been conducted on the use of oseltamivir in pregnant women, there is limited data available from post-marketing and retrospective observational surveillance reports. These data in conjunction with animal studies do not indicate direct or indirect harmful effects with respect to pregnancy, embryonal/foetal or postnatal development (see section 5.3). Pregnant women may receive Tamiflu, after considering the available safety information, the pathogenicity of the circulating influenza virus strain and the underlying condition of the pregnant woman.

In lactating rats, oseltamivir and the active metabolite are excreted in milk. Very limited information is available on children breast-fed by mothers taking oseltamivir and on excretion of oseltamivir in breast milk. Limited data demonstrated that oseltamivir and the active metabolite were detected in breast milk, however the levels were low, which would result in a subtherapeutic dose to the infant. Considering this information, the pathogenicity of the circulating influenza virus strain and the underlying condition of the lactating woman, administration of oseltamivir may be considered, where there are clear potential benefits to lactating mothers.

4.7 Effects on ability to drive and use machines

Tamiflu has no influence on the ability to drive and use machines.

4.8 Undesirable effects

The overall safety profile of Tamiflu is based on data from 2107 adult and 1032 paediatric patients treated for influenza, and on data from 2914 adult and 99 paediatric patients receiving Tamiflu for the prophylaxis of influenza in clinical trials.

In adults, the most commonly reported adverse drug reactions (ADRs) were vomiting and nausea in the treatment studies, and nausea and headache in the prevention studies. The majority of these ADRs were reported on a single occasion on either the first or second treatment day and resolved spontaneously within 1-2 days. In children, the most commonly reported adverse drug reaction was vomiting.

The ADRs listed in the tables below fall into the following categories: Very Common (≥ *1/10*), Common (≥ *1/100* to < *1/10*), Uncommon (≥ *1/1,000* to < *1/100*), Rare (≥ *1/10,000* to < *1/1,000*), Very rare (< *1/10,000*) and not known (cannot be estimated from the available data). ADRs are added to the appropriate category in the tables according to the pooled analysis from clinical trials. Within each frequency grouping ADRs are presented in the order of decreasing seriousness.

Treatment and prevention of influenza in adults and adolescents:

Most Frequent Adverse Drug Reactions (≥ 1 % in the oseltamivir group) in Studies Investigating Tamiflu for Treatment and Prevention of Influenza in Adults and Adolescents or Through Post-Marketing Surveillance

(see Table 1 opposite)

Treatment and prevention of influenza in children:

The table below shows the most frequently reported ADRs from paediatric clinical trials.

Most Frequent Adverse Drug Reactions (≥ 1 % in the oseltamivir group in the treatment studies and ≥ 10 % in the oseltamivir group in the prophylaxis study) in Children

(see Table 2 on next page)

In general, the adverse event profile in children with pre-existing bronchial asthma was qualitatively similar to that of otherwise healthy children.

Further post marketing surveillance data on selected serious adverse drug reactions:

Immune system disorder

Frequency not known: hypersensitivity reactions, including anaphylactic/anaphylactoid reactions.

Table 1

System Organ Class (SOC) *Frequency Category* Adverse Drug Reaction	Percentage of Patients Experiencing the ADR			
	Treatment		Prevention	
	Oseltamivir 75 mg bid (n = 1057)	Placebo (n = 1050)	Oseltamivir 75 mg od (n = 1480)	Placebo (n = 1434)
Infections and infestations				
Common:				
Bronchitis	4 %	5 %	1 %	1 %
Bronchitis acute	1 %	1 %	0 %	< 1 %
Upper respiratory tract infections	0 %	0 %	8 %	8 %
Psychiatric disorders				
Uncommon:				
Hallucination[a]	< 1 %	0 %	< 1 %	0 %
Nervous system disorders				
Very Common:				
Headache	2 %	2 %	20 %	18 %
Common:				
Insomnia	1 %	1 %	1 %	1 %
Uncommon:				
Convulsion[a]	< 1 %	0 %	0 %	0 %
Disorders of the ear and labyrinth				
Common:				
Vertigo	1 %	1 %	< 1 %	< 1 %
Respiratory, thoracic and mediastinal disorders				
Common:				
Cough	1 %	1 %	6 %	6 %
Rhinorrhoea	< 1 %	0 %	2 %	1 %
Gastrointestinal disorders				
Very Common:				
Nausea[b,c]	11 %	7 %	8 %	4 %
Common:				
Vomiting[c]	8 %	3 %	2 %	1 %
Abdominal pain	2 %	2 %	2 %	2 %
Diarrhoea	6 %	8 %	3 %	3 %
Dyspepsia	1 %	1 %	2 %	2 %
Skin and subcutaneous tissue disorders				
Uncommon:				
Dermatitis[a]	< 1 %	< 1 %	1 %	1 %
Rash[a]	< 1 %	< 1 %	< 1 %	< 1 %
Urticaria[a]	< 1 %	< 1 %	< 1 %	< 1 %
Eczema[a]	< 1 %	0 %	< 1 %	< 1 %
General disorders				
Common:				
Dizziness	2 %	3 %	2 %	2 %
Fatigue	1 %	1 %	8 %	8 %
Pain	< 1 %	< 1 %	4 %	3 %

[a] These are events identified during post-marketing surveillance. They were also reported in the pooled clinical studies at the incidence presented in the table above.

[b] Subjects who experienced nausea alone; excludes subjects who experienced nausea in association with vomiting.

[c] The difference between the placebo and oseltamivir groups was statistically significant.

Psychiatric disorders and nervous system disorders

Frequency not known: influenza can be associated with a variety of neurologic and behavioural symptoms which can include events such as hallucinations, delirium, and abnormal behaviour, in some cases resulting in fatal outcomes. These events may occur in the setting of encephalitis or encephalopathy but can occur without obvious severe disease.

In patients with influenza who were receiving Tamiflu, there have been postmarketing reports of convulsions and delirium (including symptoms such as altered level of consciousness, confusion, abnormal behaviour, delusions, hallucinations, agitation, anxiety, nightmares), in a very few cases resulting in accidental injury or fatal outcomes. These events were reported primarily among paediatric and adolescent patients and often had an abrupt onset and rapid resolution. The contribution of Tamiflu to those events is unknown. Such neuropsychiatric events have also been reported in patients with influenza who were not taking Tamiflu.

Eye disorders

Frequency not known: visual disturbance.

Cardiac disorders

Frequency not known: cardiac arrhythmia.

Gastrointestinal disorders

Frequency not known: gastrointestinal bleedings and hemorrhagic colitis.

Hepato-biliary disorders

Frequency not known: hepato-biliary system disorders, including hepatitis and elevated liver enzymes in patients with influenza-like illness. These cases include fatal fulminant hepatitis/hepatic failure.

Table 2

System Organ Class (SOC) *Frequency Category* Adverse Drug Reaction	Percentage of Patients Experiencing the ADR			
	Treatment		Treatment	Prevention[a]
	Oseltamivir 2 mg/kg bid (n = 515)	Placebo (n = 517)	Oseltamivir 30 to 75 mg[b] (n = 158)	Oseltamivir 30 to 75 mg[b] (n = 99)
Infections and infestations				
Common:				
Pneumonia	2 %	3 %	0 %	0 %
Sinusitis	2 %	3 %	0 %	0 %
Bronchitis	2 %	2 %	2 %	0 %
Otitis media	9 %	11 %	1 %	2 %
Disorders of the blood and lymphatic system				
Common:				
Lymphadenopathy	1 %	2 %	< 1 %	0 %
Respiratory, thoracic and mediastinal disorders				
Common:				
Asthma (incl. aggravated)	4 %	4 %	0 %	1 %
Epistaxis	3 %	3 %	1 %	1 %
Gastrointestinal disorder				
Very Common:				
Vomiting	15 %	9 %	20 %	10 %
Diarrhoea	10 %	11 %	3 %	1 %
Common:				
Nausea	3 %	4 %	6 %	4 %
Abdominal pain	5 %	4 %	2 %	1 %
Disorders of the eye				
Common:				
Conjunctivitis	1 %	< 1 %	0 %	0 %
Disorders of the ear and labyrinth				
Common:				
Ear disorder[c]	2 %	1 %	0 %	0 %
Tympanic membrane disorder	1 %	1 %	0 %	0 %
Skin and subcutaneous tissue disorders				
Common:				
Dermatitis	1 %	2 %	< 1 %	0 %

[a] The prevention study did not contain a placebo arm, i.e. was an uncontrolled study.
[b] Unit dose = weight-based dosing (see section 4.2).
[c] Patients experienced ear ache and ear pain.

Skin and subcutaneous tissue disorders

Frequency not known: severe skin reactions, including Stevens-Johnson syndrome, toxic epidermal necrolysis, erythema multiforme and angioneurotic oedema.

Additional information on special populations:

There were no clinically relevant differences in the safety population of the elderly subjects who received oseltamivir or placebo compared with the adult population aged up to 65 years.

The adverse event profile in adolescents and patients with chronic cardiac and/or respiratory disease was qualitatively similar to those of healthy young adults.

Safety information available on oseltamivir administered for treatment of influenza in children less than one year of age from prospective and retrospective observational trials (comprising together more than 2400 children of that age class), epidemiological databases research and postmarketing reports suggest that the safety profile in children less than one year of age is similar to the established safety profile of children aged one year and older.

4.9 Overdose

There is no experience with overdose. However, the anticipated manifestations of acute overdose would be nausea, with or without accompanying vomiting, and dizziness. Patients should discontinue the treatment in the event of overdose. No specific antidote is known.

5. PHARMACOLOGICAL PROPERTIES

5.1 Pharmacodynamic properties

Pharmacotherapeutic group: Antiviral ATC code: J05AH02

Oseltamivir phosphate is a pro-drug of the active metabolite (oseltamivir carboxylate). The active metabolite is a selective inhibitor of influenza virus neuraminidase enzymes, which are glycoproteins found on the virion surface. Viral neuraminidase enzyme activity is important both for viral entry into uninfected cells and for the release of recently formed virus particles from infected cells, and for the further spread of infectious virus in the body.

Oseltamivir carboxylate inhibits influenza A and B neuraminidases *in vitro*. Oseltamivir phosphate inhibits influenza virus infection and replication *in vitro*. Oseltamivir given orally inhibits influenza A and B virus replication and pathogenicity *in vivo* in animal models of influenza infection at antiviral exposures similar to that achieved in man with 75 mg twice daily.

Antiviral activity of oseltamivir was supported for influenza A and B by experimental challenge studies in healthy volunteers.

Neuraminidase enzyme IC50 values for oseltamivir for clinically isolated influenza A ranged from 0.1 nM to 1.3 nM, and for influenza B was 2.6 nM. Higher IC50 values for influenza B, up to a median of 8.5 nM, have been observed in published trials.

Reduced sensitivity of viral neuraminidase

There has been no evidence for emergence of drug resistance associated with the use of Tamiflu in clinical studies conducted to date in post-exposure (7 days), post-exposure within household groups (10 days) and seasonal (42 days) prevention of influenza.

The risk of emergence of influenza viruses with reduced susceptibility or frank resistance to oseltamivir has been examined during Roche-sponsored clinical studies. All patients who were found to carry oseltamivir-resistant virus did so transiently, cleared the virus normally and showed no clinical deterioration.

Patient Population	Patients with Resistance Mutations (%)	
	Phenotyping*	Geno- and Phenotyping*
Adults and adolescents	4/1245 (0.32%)	5/1245 (0.4%)
Children (1-12 years)	19/464 (4.1%)	25/464 (5.4%)

* Full genotyping was not performed in all studies.

The rate of emergence of resistance may be higher in the youngest age groups, and in immunosupressed patients. Oseltamivir-resistant viruses isolated from oseltamivir-treated patients and oseltamivir-resistant laboratory strains of influenza viruses have been found to contain mutations in N1 and N2 neuraminidases. Resistance mutations tend to be viral sub-type specific (including those found in H5N1 variants).

Naturally occurring mutations in influenza A/H1N1 virus associated with reduced susceptibility to oseltamivir *in vitro* have been detected in patients who, based on the reported information, have not been exposed to oseltamivir. The extent of reduction in susceptibility to oseltamivir and the prevalence of such viruses appears to vary seasonally and geographically.

Treatment of influenza infection

Oseltamivir is effective only against illnesses caused by influenza virus. Statistical analyses are therefore presented only for influenza-infected subjects. In the pooled treatment study population, which included both influenza-positive and -negative subjects (ITT), primary efficacy was reduced proportional to the number of influenza-negative individuals. In the overall treatment population, influenza infection was confirmed in 67 % (range 46 % to 74 %) of the recruited patients. Of the elderly subjects, 64 % were influenza-positive and of those with chronic cardiac and/or respiratory disease 62 % were influenza-positive. In all phase III treatment studies, patients were recruited only during the period in which influenza was circulating in the local community.

Adults and adolescents 13 years of age and older: Patients were eligible if they reported within 36 hours of onset of symptoms, had fever $\geq$ 37.8 °C, accompanied by at least one respiratory symptom (cough, nasal symptoms or sore throat) and at least one systemic symptom (myalgia, chills/sweats, malaise, fatigue or headache). In a pooled analysis of all influenza-positive adults and adolescents (N = 2413) enrolled into treatment studies, oseltamivir 75 mg twice daily for 5 days reduced the median duration of influenza illness by approximately one day from 5.2 days (95 % CI 4.9 – 5.5 days) in the placebo group to 4.2 days (95 % CI 4.0 – 4.4 days; p $\leq$ 0.0001).

The proportion of subjects who developed specified lower respiratory tract complications (mainly bronchitis) treated with antibiotics was reduced from 12.7 % (135/1063) in the placebo group to 8.6 % (116/1350) in the oseltamivir treated population (p = 0.0012).

Treatment of influenza in high risk populations: The median duration of influenza illness in elderly subjects ($\geq$ 65 years) and in subjects with chronic cardiac and/or respiratory disease receiving oseltamivir 75 mg twice daily for 5 days was not reduced significantly. The total duration of fever was reduced by one day in the groups treated with oseltamivir. In the influenza-positive elderly, oseltamivir significantly reduced the incidence of specified lower respiratory tract complications (mainly bronchitis) treated with antibiotics from 19 % (52/268) in the placebo group to 12 % (29/250) in the oseltamivir treated population (p = 0.0156).

In influenza-positive patients with chronic cardiac and/or respiratory disease, the combined incidence of lower respiratory tract complications (mainly bronchitis) treated with antibiotics was 17 % (22/133) in the placebo group and 14 % (16/118) in the oseltamivir treated population (p = 0.5976).

Treatment of influenza in children: In a study of otherwise healthy children (65 % influenza-positive) aged 1 to 12 years (mean age 5.3 years) who had fever ($\geq$ 37.8 °C) plus either cough or coryza, 67 % of influenza-positive patients were infected with influenza A and 33 % with influenza B. Oseltamivir treatment, started within 48 hours of onset of symptoms, significantly reduced the time to freedom from illness (defined as the simultaneous return to normal health and activity and alleviation of fever, cough and coryza) by 1.5 days (95 % CI 0.6 – 2.2 days; p < 0.0001) compared to placebo. Oseltamivir reduced the incidence of acute otitis media from 26.5 % (53/200) in the placebo group to 16 % (29/183) in the oseltamivir treated children (p = 0.013).

A second study was completed in 334 asthmatic children aged 6 to 12 years old of which 53.6 % were influenza-positive. In the oseltamivir treated group, the median duration of illness was not reduced significantly. By day 6 (the last day of treatment) FEV_1 had increased by 10.8 % in the oseltamivir treated group compared to 4.7 % on placebo (p = 0.0148) in this population.

Treatment of influenza B infection: Overall, 15 % of the influenza-positive population were infected by influenza B, proportions ranging from 1 to 33 % in individual studies.

The median duration of illness in influenza B infected subjects did not differ significantly between the treatment groups in individual studies. Data from 504 influenza B infected subjects were pooled across all studies for analysis. Oseltamivir reduced the time to alleviation of all symptoms by 0.7 days (95 % CI 0.1 – 1.6 days; p = 0.022) and the duration of fever (≥ 37.8 °C), cough and coryza by one day (95 % CI 0.4 – 1.7 days; p < 0.001) compared to placebo.

Prevention of influenza

The efficacy of oseltamivir in preventing naturally occurring influenza illness has been demonstrated in a post-exposure prevention study in households and two seasonal prevention studies. The primary efficacy parameter for all of these studies was the incidence of laboratory-confirmed influenza. The virulence of influenza epidemics is not predictable and varies within a region and from season to season, therefore the number needed to treat (NNT) in order to prevent one case of influenza illness varies.

Post-exposure prevention: In a study in contacts (12.6 % vaccinated against influenza) of an index case of influenza, oseltamivir 75 mg once daily was started within 2 days of onset of symptoms in the index case and continued for seven days. Influenza was confirmed in 163 out of 377 index cases. Oseltamivir significantly reduced the incidence of clinical influenza illness occurring in the contacts of confirmed influenza cases from 24/200 (12 %) in the placebo group to 2/205 (1 %) in the oseltamivir group (92 % reduction [95 % CI 6 – 16; p ≤ 0.0001]). The number needed to treat (NNT) in contacts of true influenza cases was 10 (95 % CI 9 – 12) and was 16 (95 % CI 15 – 19) in the whole population (ITT) regardless of infection status in the index case.

The efficacy of oseltamivir in preventing naturally occurring influenza illness has been demonstrated in a post-exposure prevention study in households that included adults, adolescents, and children aged 1 to 12 years, both as index cases and as family contacts. The primary efficacy parameter for this study was the incidence of laboratory-confirmed clinical influenza in the households. Oseltamivir prophylaxis lasted for 10 days. In the total population, there was a reduction in the incidence of laboratory-confirmed clinical influenza in households from 20 % (27/136) in the group not receiving prevention to 7 % (10/135) in the group receiving prevention (62.7 % reduction [95 % CI 26.0 – 81.2; p = 0.0042]). In households of influenza-infected index cases, there was a reduction in the incidence of influenza from 26 % (23/89) in the group not receiving prevention to 11 % (9/84) in the group receiving prevention (58.5 % reduction [95 % CI 15.6 – 79.6; p = 0.0114]).

According to subgroup analysis in children at 1 to 12 years of age, the incidence of laboratory-confirmed clinical influenza among children was significantly reduced from 19 % (21/111) in the group not receiving prevention to 7 % (7/104) in the group receiving prevention (64.4 % reduction [95 % CI 15.8 – 85.0; p = 0.0188]). Among children who were not already shedding virus at baseline, the incidence of laboratory-confirmed clinical influenza was reduced from 21 % (15/70) in the group not receiving prevention to 4 % (2/47) in the group receiving prevention (80.1 % reduction [95 % CI 22.0 – 94.9; p = 0.0206]). The NNT for the total paediatric population was 9 (95 % CI 7 – 24) and 8 (95 % CI 6, upper limit not estimable) in the whole population (ITT) and in paediatric contacts of infected index cases (ITTII), respectively.

Prevention during an influenza epidemic in the community: In a pooled analysis of two other studies conducted in unvaccinated otherwise healthy adults, oseltamivir 75 mg once daily given for 6 weeks significantly reduced the incidence of clinical influenza illness from 25/519 (4.8 %) in the placebo group to 6/520 (1.2 %) in the oseltamivir group (76 % reduction [95 % CI 1.6 – 5.7; p = 0.0006]) during a community outbreak of influenza. The NNT in this study was 28 (95 % CI 24 – 50).

A study in elderly residents of nursing homes, where 80 % of participants received vaccine in the season of the study, oseltamivir 75 mg once daily given for 6 weeks significantly reduced the incidence of clinical influenza illness from 12/272 (4.4 %) in the placebo group to 1/276 (0.4 %) in the oseltamivir group (92 % reduction [95 % CI 1.5 – 6.6; p = 0.0015]). The NNT in this study was 25 (95 % CI 23 – 62).

Specific studies have not been conducted to assess of the reduction in the risk of complications.

5.2 Pharmacokinetic properties

Absorption

Oseltamivir is readily absorbed from the gastrointestinal tract after oral administration of oseltamivir phosphate (pro-drug) and is extensively converted by predominantly hepatic esterases to the active metabolite (oseltamivir carboxylate). At least 75 % of an oral dose reaches the systemic circulation as the active metabolite. Exposure to the pro-drug is less than 5 % relative to the active metabolite. Plasma concentrations of both pro-drug and active metabolite are proportional to dose and are unaffected by co-administration with food.

Distribution

The mean volume of distribution at steady state of the oseltamivir carboxylate is approximately 23 litres in humans, a volume equivalent to extracellular body fluid. Since neuraminidase activity is extracellular, oseltamivir carboxylate distributes to all sites of influenza virus spread.

The binding of the oseltamivir carboxylate to human plasma protein is negligible (approximately 3 %).

Metabolism

Oseltamivir is extensively converted to oseltamivir carboxylate by esterases located predominantly in the liver. *In vitro* studies demonstrated that neither oseltamivir nor the active metabolite is a substrate for, or an inhibitor of, the major cytochrome P450 isoforms. No phase 2 conjugates of either compound have been identified *in vivo*.

Elimination

Absorbed oseltamivir is primarily (> 90 %) eliminated by conversion to oseltamivir carboxylate. It is not further metabolised and is eliminated in the urine. Peak plasma concentrations of oseltamivir carboxylate decline with a half-life of 6 to 10 hours in most subjects. The active metabolite is eliminated entirely by renal excretion. Renal clearance (18.8 l/h) exceeds glomerular filtration rate (7.5 l/h) indicating that tubular secretion occurs in addition to glomerular filtration. Less than 20 % of an oral radiolabelled dose is eliminated in faeces.

Renal impairment

Administration of 100 mg oseltamivir phosphate twice daily for 5 days to patients with various degrees of renal impairment showed that exposure to oseltamivir carboxylate is inversely proportional to declining renal function. For dosing, see section 4.2.

Hepatic impairment

In vitro studies have concluded that exposure to oseltamivir is not expected to be increased significantly nor is exposure to the active metabolite expected to be significantly decreased in patients with hepatic impairment (see section 4.2).

Elderly

Exposure to the active metabolite at steady state was 25 to 35 % higher in elderly (age 65 to 78 years) compared to adults less than 65 years of age given comparable doses of oseltamivir. Half-lives observed in the elderly were similar to those seen in young adults. On the basis of drug exposure and tolerability, dosage adjustments are not required for elderly patients unless there is evidence of severe renal impairment (creatinine clearance below 30 ml/min) (see section 4.2).

Children

Children 1 year of age and older: The pharmacokinetics of oseltamivir have been evaluated in single-dose pharmacokinetic studies in children aged 1 to 16 years. Multiple-dose pharmacokinetics were studied in a small number of children enrolled in a clinical efficacy study. Younger children cleared both the pro-drug and its active metabolite faster than adults, resulting in a lower exposure for a given mg/kg dose. Doses of 2 mg/kg give oseltamivir carboxylate exposures comparable to those achieved in adults receiving a single 75 mg dose (approximately 1 mg/kg). The pharmacokinetics of oseltamivir in children over 12 years of age are similar to those in adults.

Children 6 to 12 months of age: Limited exposure data from children 6 to 12 months of age from a pharmacodynamic, pharmacokinetic and safety study in influenza-infected children less than 2 years of age, suggest that for most children 6 to 12 months of age, the exposure following 3 mg/kg dosing is similar to the exposures seen in older children and adults using the approved dose.

5.3 Preclinical safety data

Preclinical data reveal no special hazard for humans based on conventional studies of safety pharmacology, repeated-dose toxicity and genotoxicity. Results of the conventional rodent carcinogenicity studies showed a trend towards a dose-dependent increase in the incidence of some tumours that are typical for the rodent strains used. Considering the margins of exposure in relation to the expected exposure in the human use, these findings do not change the benefit-risk of Tamiflu in its adopted therapeutic indications.

Teratology studies have been conducted in rats and rabbits at doses of up to 1500 mg/kg/day and 500 mg/kg/day, respectively. No effects on foetal development were observed. A rat fertility study up to a dose of 1500 mg/kg/day demonstrated no adverse effects on either sex. In pre- and post-natal rat studies, prolonged parturition was noted at 1500 mg/kg/day: the safety margin between human exposure and the highest no-effect dose (500 mg/kg/day) in rats is 480-fold for oseltamivir and 44-fold for the active metabolite, respectively. Foetal exposure in the rats and rabbits was approximately 15 to 20 % of that of the mother.

In lactating rats, oseltamivir and the active metabolite are excreted in the milk. Limited data indicate that oseltamivir and the active metabolite are excreted in human milk. Extrapolation of the animal data provides estimates of 0.01 mg/day and 0.3 mg/day for the respective compounds.

A potential for skin sensitisation to oseltamivir was observed in a "maximisation" test in guinea pigs. Approximately 50 % of the animals treated with the unformulated active ingredient showed erythema after challenging the induced animals. Reversible irritancy of rabbits' eyes was detected.

Whereas very high oral single doses of oseltamivir phosphate had no effect in adult rats, such doses resulted in toxicity in juvenile 7-day-old rat pups, including death. These effects were seen at doses of 657 mg/kg and higher. At 500 mg/kg, no adverse effects were seen, including upon chronic treatment (500 mg/kg/day administered from 7 to 21 days post partum).

6. PHARMACEUTICAL PARTICULARS

6.1 List of excipients

Tamiflu 30 mg hard capsule.	Tamiflu 45 mg hard capsule.
Capsule core: Pregelatinised starch (derived from maize starch) Talc Povidone Croscarmellose sodium Sodium stearyl fumarate	*Capsule core:* Pregelatinised starch (derived from maize starch) Talc Povidone Croscarmellose sodium Sodium stearyl fumarate
Capsule shell: Gelatin Yellow iron oxide (E172) Red iron oxide (E172) Titanium dioxide (E171)	*Capsule shell:* Gelatin Black iron oxide (E172) Titanium dioxide (E171)
Printing ink: Shellac Titanium dioxide (E171) FD and C Blue 2 (indigo carmine, E132)	*Printing ink:* Shellac Titanium dioxide (E171) FD and C Blue 2 (indigo carmine, E132)

6.2 Incompatibilities

Not applicable.

6.3 Shelf life

7 years

6.4 Special precautions for storage

Do not store above 25 °C.

6.5 Nature and contents of container

One box contains 10 capsules in a triplex blister pack (PVC/PE/PVDC, sealed with aluminium foil).

6.6 Special precautions for disposal and other handling

No special requirements.

Any unused product or waste material should be disposed of in accordance with local requirements.

7. MARKETING AUTHORISATION HOLDER

Roche Registration Limited

6 Falcon Way

Shire Park

Welwyn Garden City

AL7 1TW

United Kingdom

8. MARKETING AUTHORISATION NUMBER(S)

EU/1/02/222/003 – Tamiflu 30 mg hard capsule.

EU/1/02/222/004 – Tamiflu 45 mg hard capsule.

9. DATE OF FIRST AUTHORISATION/RENEWAL OF THE AUTHORISATION

Date of first authorisation: 20 June 2002

Date of last renewal: 20 June 2007

10. DATE OF REVISION OF THE TEXT

9 September 2009

LEGAL STATUS

POM

Detailed information on this medicinal product is available on the website of the European Medicines Agency (EMEA) http://www.emea.europa.eu/.

Tamiflu▼ 75mg hard capsule

(Roche Products Limited)

1. NAME OF THE MEDICINAL PRODUCT

Tamiflu▼ 75 mg hard capsule.

2. QUALITATIVE AND QUANTITATIVE COMPOSITION

Each hard capsule contains oseltamivir phosphate equivalent to 75 mg of oseltamivir.

For a full list of excipients, see section 6.1.

3. PHARMACEUTICAL FORM

Hard capsule

The hard capsule consists of a grey opaque body bearing the imprint "ROCHE" and a light yellow opaque cap bearing the imprint "75 mg". Imprints are blue.

4. CLINICAL PARTICULARS

4.1 Therapeutic indications

Treatment of influenza

In patients one year of age and older who present with symptoms typical of influenza, when influenza virus is circulating in the community. Efficacy has been demonstrated when treatment is initiated within two days of first onset of symptoms. This indication is based on clinical studies of naturally occurring influenza in which the predominant infection was influenza A (see section 5.1).

Tamiflu is indicated for the treatment of children 6 to 12 months of age during a pandemic influenza outbreak.

Prevention of influenza

- Post-exposure prevention in individuals one year of age or older following contact with a clinically diagnosed influenza case when influenza virus is circulating in the community.

- The appropriate use of Tamiflu for prevention of influenza should be determined on a case by case basis by the circumstances and the population requiring protection. In exceptional situations (e.g., in case of a mismatch between the circulating and vaccine virus strains, and a pandemic situation) seasonal prevention could be considered in individuals one year of age or older.

Tamiflu is not a substitute for influenza vaccination.

The use of antivirals for the treatment and prevention of influenza should be determined on the basis of official recommendations. Decisions regarding the use of antivirals for treatment and prophylaxis should take into consideration what is known about the characteristics of the circulating influenza viruses and the impact of the disease in different geographical areas and patient populations.

Based on limited pharmacokinetic and safety data, Tamiflu can be used in children 6 to 12 months of age for treatment during a pandemic influenza outbreak. The treating physician should take into account the pathogenicity of the circulating strain and the underlying condition of the patient to ensure there is a potential benefit to the child.

4.2 Posology and method of administration

Tamiflu capsules and Tamiflu suspension are bioequivalent formulations. 75 mg doses can be administered as either

- one 75 mg capsule or
- one 30 mg capsule plus one 45 mg capsule or
- by administering one 30 mg dose plus one 45 mg dose of suspension.

Adults, adolescents or children (> 40 kg) who are unable to swallow capsules may receive appropriate doses of Tamiflu suspension.

During situations when commercially manufactured Tamiflu oral suspension is not readily available, adults, adolescents or children who are unable to swallow capsules may receive appropriate doses of Tamiflu (see section 3 in Package Leaflet) by opening capsules and pouring the contents of capsules into a suitable, small amount (1 teaspoon maximum) of sweetened food product such as regular or sugar-free chocolate syrup, honey (only for children two years or older), light brown or table sugar dissolved in water, dessert toppings, sweetened condensed milk, apple sauce or yogurt to mask the bitter taste. The mixture should be stirred and the entire contents given to the patient. The mixture must be swallowed immediately after its preparation. It is not necessary to administer any undissolved white powder as this is inert material.

Treatment of influenza

Treatment should be initiated as soon as possible within the first two days of onset of symptoms of influenza.

For adolescents (13 to 17 years of age) and adults: The recommended oral dose is 75 mg oseltamivir twice daily for 5 days.

For infants older than 1 year of age and for children 2 to 12 years of age: Tamiflu 30 mg and 45 mg capsules and oral suspension are available.

For recommended treatment dose of Tamiflu for infants older than 1 year of age and for children 2 to 12 years of age, see SmPC of Tamiflu suspension and Tamiflu 30 and 45 mg capsules.

Children weighing > 40 kg and who are able to swallow capsules may receive treatment with the adult dosage of 75 mg capsules twice daily for 5 days as an alternative to the recommended dose of Tamiflu suspension or Tamiflu 30 mg and 45 mg capsules.

For children 6 to 12 months of age: Depending on the pathogenicity of the circulating influenza virus strain, children between 6 and 12 months of age can be treated with Tamiflu during a pandemic influenza outbreak, although the available data are limited. Pharmacokinetic data indicate that a dosage of 3 mg/kg twice daily in children 6 to 12 months of age provides plasma drug exposures in the majority of patients similar to those shown to be clinically efficacious in children age one or older and adults (see section 5.2).

The recommended dose for treatment of children 6 to 12 months of age is 3 mg per kg body weight twice daily for 5 days for treatment

Prevention of influenza

Post-exposure prevention

For adolescents (13 to 17 years of age) and adults: The recommended dose for prevention of influenza following close contact with an infected individual is 75 mg oseltamivir once daily for 10 days. Therapy should begin as soon as possible within two days of exposure to an infected individual.

For infants older than 1 year of age and for children 2 to 12 years of age: Tamiflu 30 mg and 45 mg capsules and oral suspension are available.

Table 1

System Organ Class (SOC) *Frequency Category* Adverse Drug Reaction	Percentage of Patients Experiencing the ADR			
	Treatment		Prevention	
	Oseltamivir 75 mg bid (n = 1057)	Placebo (n = 1050)	Oseltamivir 75 mg od (n = 1480)	Placebo (n = 1434)
Infections and infestations				
Common:				
Bronchitis	4 %	5 %	1 %	1 %
Bronchitis acute	1 %	1 %	0 %	< 1 %
Upper respiratory tract infections	0 %	0 %	8 %	8 %
Psychiatric disorders				
Uncommon:				
Hallucination[a]	< 1 %	0 %	< 1 %	0 %
Nervous system disorders				
Very Common:				
Headache	2 %	2 %	20 %	18 %
Common:				
Insomnia	1 %	1 %	1 %	1 %
Uncommon:				
Convulsion[a]	< 1 %	0 %	0 %	0 %
Disorders of the ear and labyrinth				
Common:				
Vertigo	1 %	1 %	< 1 %	< 1 %
Respiratory, thoracic and mediastinal disorders				
Common:				
Cough	1 %	1 %	6 %	6 %
Rhinorrhoea	< 1 %	0 %	2 %	1 %
Gastrointestinal disorders				
Very Common:				
Nausea[b,c]	11 %	7 %	8 %	4 %
Common:				
Vomiting[c]	8 %	3 %	2 %	1 %
Abdominal pain	2 %	2 %	2 %	2 %
Diarrhoea	6 %	8 %	3 %	3 %
Dyspepsia	1 %	1 %	2 %	2 %
Skin and subcutaneous tissue disorders				
Uncommon:				
Dermatitis[a]	< 1 %	< 1 %	1 %	1 %
Rash[a]	< 1 %	< 1 %	< 1 %	< 1 %
Urticaria[a]	< 1 %	< 1 %	< 1 %	< 1 %
Eczema[a]	< 1 %	0 %	< 1 %	< 1 %
General disorders				
Common:				
Dizziness	2 %	3 %	2 %	2 %
Fatigue	1 %	1 %	8 %	8 %
Pain	< 1 %	< 1 %	4 %	3 %

[a] These are events identified during post-marketing surveillance. They were also reported in the pooled clinical studies at the incidence presented in the table above.

[b] Subjects who experienced nausea alone; excludes subjects who experienced nausea in association with vomiting.

[c] The difference between the placebo and oseltamivir groups was statistically significant.

For recommended post-exposure prevention dose of Tamiflu for infants older than 1 year of age and for children of 2 to 12 years of age, see SmPC of Tamiflu suspension and Tamiflu 30 mg and 45 mg capsules.

Children weighing > 40 kg and who are able to swallow capsules may receive prevention with a 75 mg capsule once daily for 10 days as an alternative to the recommended dose of Tamiflu suspension or Tamiflu 30 mg and 45 mg capsules.

Prevention during an influenza epidemic in the community

The recommended dose for prevention of influenza during a community outbreak is 75 mg oseltamivir once daily for up to 6 weeks.

Special populations

Hepatic impairment

No dose adjustment is required either for treatment or for prevention in patients with hepatic dysfunction. No studies have been carried out in paediatric patients with hepatic disorder.

Renal impairment

Treatment of influenza: Dose adjustment is recommended for adults with severe renal impairment. Recommended doses are detailed in the table below.

Creatinine clearance	Recommended dose for treatment
> 30 (ml/min)	75 mg twice daily
> 10 to ⩽ 30 (ml/min)	75 mg once daily, or 30 mg suspension twice daily, or 30 mg capsules twice daily
⩽ 10 (ml/min)	Not recommended
dialysis patients	Not recommended

Prevention of influenza: Dose adjustment is recommended for adults with severe renal impairment as detailed in the table below.

Creatinine clearance	Recommended dose for prevention
> 30 (ml/min)	75 mg once daily
> 10 to ⩽ 30 (ml/min)	75 mg every second day, or 30 mg suspension once daily, or 30 mg capsules once daily
⩽ 10 (ml/min)	Not recommended
dialysis patients	Not recommended

Elderly

No dose adjustment is required, unless there is evidence of severe renal impairment.

Children

There is insufficient clinical data available in children with renal impairment to be able to make any dosing recommendation.

4.3 Contraindications

Hypersensitivity to the active substance or to any of the excipients.

4.4 Special warnings and precautions for use

Oseltamivir is effective only against illness caused by influenza viruses. There is no evidence for efficacy of oseltamivir in any illness caused by agents other than influenza viruses.

No information is available regarding the safety and efficacy of oseltamivir in patients with any medical condition sufficiently severe or unstable to be considered at imminent risk of requiring hospitalisation.

The safety and efficacy of oseltamivir in either treatment or prevention of influenza in immunocompromised patients have not been established.

Efficacy of oseltamivir in the treatment of subjects with chronic cardiac disease and/or respiratory disease has not been established. No difference in the incidence of complications was observed between the treatment and placebo groups in this population (see section 5.1).

Tamiflu is not a substitute for influenza vaccination. Use of Tamiflu must not affect the evaluation of individuals for annual influenza vaccination. The protection against influenza lasts only as long as Tamiflu is administered. Tamiflu should be used for the treatment and prevention of influenza only when reliable epidemiological data indicate that influenza virus is circulating in the community.

Severe renal impairment

Dose adjustment is recommended for both treatment and prevention in adults with severe renal insufficiency. There is insufficient clinical data available in children with renal impairment to be able to make any dosing recommendation.(see sections 4.2 and 5.2).

4.5 Interaction with other medicinal products and other forms of interaction

Pharmacokinetic properties of oseltamivir, such as low protein binding and metabolism independent of the CYP450 and glucuronidase systems (see section 5.2), suggest that clinically significant drug interactions via these mechanisms are unlikely.

No dose adjustment is required when co-administering with probenecid in patients with normal renal function. Co-administration of probenecid, a potent inhibitor of the anionic pathway of renal tubular secretion, results in an approximate 2-fold increase in exposure to the active metabolite of oseltamivir.

Oseltamivir has no kinetic interaction with amoxicillin, which is eliminated via the same pathway, suggesting that oseltamivir interaction with this pathway is weak.

Clinically important drug interactions involving competition for renal tubular secretion are unlikely, due to the known safety margin for most of these substances, the elimination characteristics of the active metabolite (glomerular filtration and anionic tubular secretion) and the excretion capacity of these pathways. However, care should be taken when prescribing oseltamivir in subjects when taking co-excreted agents with a narrow therapeutic margin (e.g., chlorpropamide, methotrexate, phenylbutazone).

No pharmacokinetic interactions between oseltamivir or its major metabolite have been observed when co-administering oseltamivir with paracetamol, acetyl-salicylic acid, cimetidine or with antacids (magnesium and aluminium hydroxides and calcium carbonates).

4.6 Pregnancy and lactation

While no controlled clinical trials have been conducted on the use of oseltamivir in pregnant women, there is limited data available from post-marketing and retrospective observational surveillance reports. These data in conjunction with animal studies do not indicate direct or indirect harmful effects with respect to pregnancy, embryonal/foetal or postnatal development (see section 5.3). Pregnant women may receive Tamiflu, after considering the available safety information, the pathogenicity of the circulating influenza virus strain and the underlying condition of the pregnant woman.

In lactating rats, oseltamivir and the active metabolite are excreted in milk. Very limited information is available on children breast-fed by mothers taking oseltamivir and on excretion of oseltamivir in breast milk. Limited data demonstrated that oseltamivir and the active metabolite were detected in breast milk, however the levels were low, which would result in a subtherapeutic dose to the infant. Considering this information, the pathogenicity of the circulating influenza virus strain and the underlying condition of the lactating woman, administration of oseltamivir may be considered, where there are clear potential benefits to lactating mothers.

4.7 Effects on ability to drive and use machines

Tamiflu has no influence on the ability to drive and use machines.

4.8 Undesirable effects

The overall safety profile of Tamiflu is based on data from 2107 adult and 1032 paediatric patients treated for influenza, and on data from 2914 adult and 99 paediatric patients receiving Tamiflu for the prophylaxis of influenza in clinical trials.

In adults, the most commonly reported adverse drug reactions (ADRs) were vomiting and nausea in the treatment studies, and nausea and headache in the prevention studies. The majority of these ADRs were reported on a single occasion on either the first or second treatment day and resolved spontaneously within 1-2 days. In children, the most commonly reported adverse drug reaction was vomiting.

The ADRs listed in the tables below fall into the following categories: Very Common (⩾ *1/10*), Common (⩾ *1/100* to < *1/10*), Uncommon (⩾ *1/1,000* to < *1/100*), Rare (⩾ *1/10,000* to < *1/1,000*), Very rare (< *1/10,000*) and not known (cannot be estimated from the available data). ADRs are added to the appropriate category in the tables according to the pooled analysis from clinical trials. Within each frequency grouping ADRs are presented in the order of decreasing seriousness.

Treatment and prevention of influenza in adults and adolescents:

Most Frequent Adverse Drug Reactions (⩾ 1 % in the oseltamivir group) in Studies Investigating Tamiflu for Treatment and Prevention of Influenza in Adults and Adolescents or Through Post-Marketing Surveillance

(see Table 1 on previous page)

Treatment and prevention of influenza in children:

The table below shows the most frequently reported ADRs from paediatric clinical trials.

Most Frequent Adverse Drug Reactions (⩾ 1 % in the treatment studies and ⩾ 10 % in the oseltamivir group in the prophylaxis study) in Children

(see Table 2 on next page)

In general, the adverse event profile in children with pre-existing bronchial asthma was qualitatively similar to that of otherwise healthy children.

Further post marketing surveillance data on selected serious adverse drug reactions:

Immune system disorders

Frequency not known: hypersensitivity reactions, including anaphylactic/anaphylactoid reactions.

Psychiatric disorders and nervous system disorders

Frequency not known: influenza can be associated with a variety of neurologic and behavioural symptoms which can include events such as hallucinations, delirium, and abnormal behaviour, in some cases resulting in fatal outcomes. These events may occur in the setting of encephalitis or encephalopathy but can occur without obvious severe disease.

In patients with influenza who were receiving Tamiflu, there have been postmarketing reports of convulsions and delirium (including symptoms such as altered level of consciousness, confusion, abnormal behaviour, delusions, hallucinations, agitation, anxiety, nightmares), in a very few cases resulting in accidental injury or fatal outcomes. These events were reported primarily among paediatric and adolescent patients and often had an abrupt onset and rapid resolution. The contribution of Tamiflu to those events is unknown. Such neuropsychiatric events have also been reported in patients with influenza who were not taking Tamiflu.

Eye disorders

Frequency not known: visual disturbance.

Cardiac disorders

Frequency not known: cardiac arrhythmia.

Gastrointestinal disorders

Frequency not known: gastrointestinal bleedings and hemorrhagic colitis.

Hepato-biliary disorders

Frequency not known: hepato-biliary system disorders, including hepatitis and elevated liver enzymes in patients with influenza-like illness. These cases include fatal fulminant hepatitis/hepatic failure.

Skin and subcutaneous tissue disorders

Frequency not known: severe skin reactions, including Stevens-Johnson syndrome, toxic epidermal necrolysis, erythema multiforme and angioneurotic oedema.

Additional information on special populations:

There were no clinically relevant differences in the safety population of the elderly subjects who received oseltamivir or placebo compared with the adult population aged up to 65 years.

The adverse event profile in adolescents and patients with chronic cardiac and/or respiratory disease was qualitatively similar to those of healthy young adults.

Safety information available on oseltamivir administered for treatment of influenza in children less than one year of age from prospective and retrospective observational trials (comprising together more than 2400 children of that age class), epidemiological databases research and postmarketing reports suggest that the safety profile in children less than one year of age is similar to the established safety profile of children aged one year and older.

4.9 Overdose

There is no experience with overdose. However, the anticipated manifestations of acute overdose would be nausea, with or without accompanying vomiting, and dizziness. Patients should discontinue the treatment in the event of overdose. No specific antidote is known.

5. PHARMACOLOGICAL PROPERTIES

5.1 Pharmacodynamic properties

Pharmacotherapeutic group: Antiviral ATC code: J05AH02

Oseltamivir phosphate is a pro-drug of the active metabolite (oseltamivir carboxylate). The active metabolite is a selective inhibitor of influenza virus neuraminidase enzymes, which are glycoproteins found on the virion surface. Viral neuraminidase enzyme activity is important both for viral entry into uninfected cells and for the release of recently formed virus particles from infected cells, and for the further spread of infectious virus in the body.

Oseltamivir carboxylate inhibits influenza A and B neuraminidases *in vitro*. Oseltamivir phosphate inhibits influenza virus infection and replication *in vitro*. Oseltamivir given orally inhibits influenza A and B virus replication and pathogenicity *in vivo* in animal models of influenza infection at antiviral exposures similar to that achieved in man with 75 mg twice daily.

Antiviral activity of oseltamivir was supported for influenza A and B by experimental challenge studies in healthy volunteers.

Neuraminidase enzyme IC50 values for oseltamivir for clinically isolated influenza A ranged from 0.1 nM to 1.3 nM, and for influenza B was 2.6 nM. Higher IC50 values for influenza B, up to a median of 8.5 nM, have been observed in published trials.

Reduced sensitivity of viral neuraminidase

There has been no evidence for emergence of drug resistance associated with the use of Tamiflu in clinical studies conducted to date in post-exposure (7 days), post-exposure within household groups (10 days) and seasonal (42 days) prevention of influenza.

The risk of emergence of influenza viruses with reduced susceptibility or frank resistance to oseltamivir has been examined during Roche-sponsored clinical studies. All patients who were found to carry oseltamivir-resistant virus did so transiently, cleared the virus normally and showed no clinical deterioration.

Patient Population	Patients with Resistance Mutations (%)	
	Phenotyping*	Geno- and Phenotyping*
Adults and adolescents	4/1245 (0.32%)	5/1245 (0.4%)
Children (1-12 years)	19/464 (4.1%)	25/464 (5.4%)

* Full genotyping was not performed in all studies.

The rate of emergence of resistance may be higher in the youngest age groups, and in immunosupressed patients. Oseltamivir-resistant viruses isolated from oseltamivir-treated patients and oseltamivir-resistant laboratory

Table 2

System Organ Class (SOC) *Frequency Category* Adverse Drug Reaction	Percentage of Patients Experiencing the ADR			
	Treatment		Treatment	Prevention[a]
	Oseltamivir 2 mg/kg bid (n=515)	Placebo (n=517)	Oseltamivir 30 to 75 mg[b] (n=158)	Oseltamivir 30 to 75 mg[b] (n=99)
Infections and infestations				
Common:				
Pneumonia	2 %	3 %	0 %	0 %
Sinusitis	2 %	3 %	0 %	0 %
Bronchitis	2 %	2 %	2 %	0 %
Otitis media	9 %	11 %	1 %	2 %
Disorders of the blood and lymphatic system				
Common:				
Lymphadenopathy	1 %	2 %	< 1 %	0 %
Respiratory, thoracic and mediastinal disorders				
Common:				
Asthma (incl. aggravated)	4 %	4 %	0 %	1 %
Epistaxis	3 %	3 %	1 %	1 %
Gastrointestinal disorder				
Very Common:				
Vomiting	15 %	9 %	20 %	10 %
Diarrhoea	10 %	11 %	3 %	1 %
Common:				
Nausea	3 %	4 %	6 %	4 %
Abdominal pain	5 %	4 %	2 %	1 %
Disorders of the eye				
Common:				
Conjunctivitis	1 %	< 1 %	0 %	0 %
Disorders of the ear and labyrinth				
Common:				
Ear disorder[c]	2 %	1 %	0 %	0 %
Tympanic membrane disorder	1 %	1 %	0 %	0 %
Skin and subcutaneous tissue disorders				
Common:				
Dermatitis	1 %	2 %	< 1 %	0 %

[a] The prevention study did not contain a placebo arm, i.e. was an uncontrolled study.
[b] Unit dose = weight-based dosing (see section 4.2).
[c] Patients experienced ear ache and ear pain.

strains of influenza viruses have been found to contain mutations in N1 and N2 neuraminidases. Resistance mutations tend to be viral sub-type specific (including those found in H5N1 variants).

Naturally occurring mutations in influenza A/H1N1 virus associated with reduced susceptibility to oseltamivir *in vitro* have been detected in patients who, based on the reported information, have not been exposed to oseltamivir. The extent of reduction in susceptibility to oseltamivir and the prevalence of such viruses appears to vary seasonally and geographically.

Treatment of influenza infection

Oseltamivir is effective only against illnesses caused by influenza virus. Statistical analyses are therefore presented only for influenza-infected subjects. In the pooled treatment study population, which included both influenza-positive and -negative subjects (ITT), primary efficacy was reduced proportional to the number of influenza-negative individuals. In the overall treatment population, influenza infection was confirmed in 67 % (range 46 % to 74 %) of the recruited patients. Of the elderly subjects, 64 % were influenza-positive and of those with chronic cardiac and/or respiratory disease 62 % were influenza-positive. In all phase III treatment studies, patients were recruited only during the period in which influenza was circulating in the local community.

Adults and adolescents 13 years of age and older: Patients were eligible if they reported within 36 hours of onset of symptoms, had fever $\geqslant$ 37.8 °C, accompanied by at least one respiratory symptom (cough, nasal symptoms or sore throat) and at least one systemic symptom (myalgia, chills/sweats, malaise, fatigue or headache). In a pooled analysis of all influenza-positive adults and adolescents (N = 2413) enrolled into treatment studies, oseltamivir 75 mg twice daily for 5 days reduced the median duration of influenza illness by approximately one day from 5.2 days (95 % CI 4.9 – 5.5 days) in the placebo group to 4.2 days (95 % CI 4.0 – 4.4 days; $p \leqslant 0.0001$).

The proportion of subjects who developed specified lower respiratory tract complications (mainly bronchitis) treated with antibiotics was reduced from 12.7 % (135/1063) in the placebo group to 8.6 % (116/1350) in the oseltamivir treated population (p = 0.0012).

Treatment of influenza in high risk populations: The median duration of influenza illness in elderly subjects ($\geqslant$ 65 years) and in subjects with chronic cardiac and/or respiratory disease receiving oseltamivir 75 mg twice daily for 5 days was not reduced significantly. The total duration of fever was reduced by one day in the groups treated with oseltamivir. In the influenza-positive elderly, oseltamivir significantly reduced the incidence of specified lower respiratory tract complications (mainly bronchitis) treated with antibiotics from 19 % (52/268) in the placebo group to 12 % (29/250) in the oseltamivir treated population (p = 0.0156).

In influenza-positive patients with chronic cardiac and/or respiratory disease, the combined incidence of lower respiratory tract complications (mainly bronchitis) treated with antibiotics was 17 % (22/133) in the placebo group and 14 % (16/118) in the oseltamivir treated population (p = 0.5976).

Treatment of influenza in children: In a study of otherwise healthy children (65 % influenza-positive) aged 1 to 12 years (mean age 5.3 years) who had fever ($\geqslant$ 37.8 °C) plus either cough or coryza, 67 % of influenza-positive patients were infected with influenza A and 33 % with influenza B. Oseltamivir treatment, started within 48 hours of onset of symptoms, significantly reduced the time to freedom from illness (defined as the simultaneous return to normal health and activity and alleviation of fever, cough and coryza) by 1.5 days (95 % CI 0.6 – 2.2 days; $p < 0.0001$) compared to placebo. Oseltamivir reduced the incidence of acute otitis media from 26.5 % (53/200) in the placebo group to 16 % (29/183) in the oseltamivir treated children (p = 0.013).

A second study was completed in 334 asthmatic children aged 6 to 12 years old of which 53.6 % were influenza-positive. In the oseltamivir treated group, the median duration of illness was not reduced significantly. By day 6 (the last day of treatment) FEV_1 had increased by 10.8 % in the oseltamivir treated group compared to 4.7 % on placebo (p = 0.0148) in this population.

Treatment of influenza B infection: Overall, 15 % of the influenza-positive population were infected by influenza B, proportions ranging from 1 to 33 % in individual studies. The median duration of illness in influenza B infected subjects did not differ significantly between the treatment groups in individual studies. Data from 504 influenza B infected subjects were pooled across all studies for analysis. Oseltamivir reduced the time to alleviation of all symptoms by 0.7 days (95 % CI 0.1 – 1.6 days; p = 0.022) and the duration of fever ($\geqslant$ 37.8 °C), cough and coryza by one day (95 % CI 0.4 – 1.7 days; $p < 0.001$) compared to placebo.

Prevention of influenza

The efficacy of oseltamivir in preventing naturally occurring influenza illness has been demonstrated in a post-exposure prevention study in households and two seasonal prevention studies. The primary efficacy parameter for all of these studies was the incidence of laboratory-confirmed influenza. The virulence of influenza epidemics is not predictable and varies within a region and from season to season, therefore the number needed to treat (NNT) in order to prevent one case of influenza illness varies.

Post-exposure prevention: In a study in contacts (12.6 % vaccinated against influenza) of an index case of influenza, oseltamivir 75 mg once daily was started within 2 days of onset of symptoms in the index case and continued for seven days. Influenza was confirmed in 163 out of 377 index cases. Oseltamivir significantly reduced the incidence of clinical influenza illness occurring in the contacts of confirmed influenza cases from 24/200 (12 %) in the placebo group to 2/205 (1 %) in the oseltamivir group (92 % reduction [95 % CI 6 – 16; $p \leqslant 0.0001$]). The number needed to treat (NNT) in contacts of true influenza cases was 10 (95 % CI 9 – 12) and was 16 (95 % CI 15 – 19) in the whole population (ITT) regardless of infection status in the index case.

The efficacy of oseltamivir in preventing naturally occurring influenza illness has been demonstrated in a post-exposure prevention study in households that included adults, adolescents, and children aged 1 to 12 years, both as index cases and as family contacts. The primary efficacy parameter for this study was the incidence of laboratory-confirmed clinical influenza in the households. Oseltamivir prophylaxis lasted for 10 days. In the total population, there was a reduction in the incidence of laboratory-confirmed clinical influenza in households from 20 % (27/136) in the group not receiving prevention to 7 % (10/135) in the group receiving prevention (62.7 % reduction [95 % CI 26.0 – 81.2; p = 0.0042]). In households of influenza-infected index cases, there was a reduction in the incidence of influenza from 26 % (23/89) in the group not receiving prevention to 11 % (9/84) in the group receiving prevention (58.5 % reduction [95 % CI 15.6 – 79.6; p = 0.0114]).

According to subgroup analysis in children at 1 to 12 years of age, the incidence of laboratory-confirmed clinical influenza among children was significantly reduced from 19 % (21/111) in the group not receiving prevention to 7 % (7/104) in the group receiving prevention (64.4 % reduction [95 % CI 15.8 – 85.0; p = 0.0188]). Among children who were not already shedding virus at baseline, the incidence of laboratory-confirmed clinical influenza was reduced from 21 % (15/70) in the group not receiving prevention to 4 % (2/47) in the group receiving prevention (80.1 % reduction [95 % CI 22.0 – 94.9; p = 0.0206]). The NNT for the total paediatric population was 9 (95 % CI 7 – 24) and 8 (95 % CI 6, upper limit not estimable) in the whole population (ITT) and in paediatric contacts of infected index cases (ITTII), respectively.

Prevention during an influenza epidemic in the community: In a pooled analysis of two other studies conducted in unvaccinated otherwise healthy adults, oseltamivir 75 mg once daily given for 6 weeks significantly reduced the incidence of clinical influenza illness from 25/519 (4.8 %) in the placebo group to 6/520 (1.2 %) in the oseltamivir group (76 % reduction [95 % CI 1.6 – 5.7; p = 0.0006]) during a community outbreak of influenza. The NNT in this study was 28 (95 % CI 24 – 50).

A study in elderly residents of nursing homes, where 80 % of participants received vaccine in the season of the study, oseltamivir 75 mg once daily given for 6 weeks significantly reduced the incidence of clinical influenza illness from 12/272 (4.4 %) in the placebo group to 1/276 (0.4 %) in the oseltamivir group (92 % reduction [95 % CI 1.5 – 6.6; p = 0.0015]). The NNT in this study was 25 (95 % CI 23 – 62).

Specific studies have not been conducted to assess of the reduction in the risk of complications.

5.2 Pharmacokinetic properties

Absorption

Oseltamivir is readily absorbed from the gastrointestinal tract after oral administration of oseltamivir phosphate (pro-drug) and is extensively converted by predominantly hepatic esterases to the active metabolite (oseltamivir carboxylate). At least 75 % of an oral dose reaches the systemic circulation as the active metabolite. Exposure to the pro-drug is less than 5 % relative to the active metabolite. Plasma concentrations of both pro-drug and active metabolite are proportional to dose and are unaffected by co-administration with food.

Distribution

The mean volume of distribution at steady state of the oseltamivir carboxylate is approximately 23 litres in humans, a volume equivalent to extracellular body fluid. Since neuraminidase activity is extracellular, oseltamivir carboxylate distributes to all sites of influenza virus spread.

The binding of the oseltamivir carboxylate to human plasma protein is negligible (approximately 3 %).

Metabolism

Oseltamivir is extensively converted to oseltamivir carboxylate by esterases located predominantly in the liver. *In vitro* studies demonstrated that neither oseltamivir nor the active metabolite is a substrate for, or an inhibitor of, the major cytochrome P450 isoforms. No phase 2 conjugates of either compound have been identified *in vivo*.

Elimination

Absorbed oseltamivir is primarily (> 90 %) eliminated by conversion to oseltamivir carboxylate. It is not further metabolised and is eliminated in the urine. Peak plasma concentrations of oseltamivir carboxylate decline with a half-life of 6 to 10 hours in most subjects. The active metabolite is eliminated entirely by renal excretion. Renal clearance (18.8 l/h) exceeds glomerular filtration rate (7.5 l/h) indicating that tubular secretion occurs in addition to glomerular filtration. Less than 20 % of an oral radiolabelled dose is eliminated in faeces.

Renal impairment

Administration of 100 mg oseltamivir phosphate twice daily for 5 days to patients with various degrees of renal impairment showed that exposure to oseltamivir carboxylate is inversely proportional to declining renal function. For dosing, see section 4.2.

Hepatic impairment

In vitro studies have concluded that exposure to oseltamivir is not expected to be increased significantly nor is exposure to the active metabolite expected to be significantly decreased in patients with hepatic impairment (see section 4.2).

Elderly

Exposure to the active metabolite at steady state was 25 to 35 % higher in elderly (age 65 to 78 years) compared to adults less than 65 years of age given comparable doses of oseltamivir. Half-lives observed in the elderly were similar to those seen in young adults. On the basis of drug exposure and tolerability, dosage adjustments are not required for elderly patients unless there is evidence of severe renal impairment (creatinine clearance below 30 ml/min) (see section 4.2).

Children

Children 1 year of age and older: The pharmacokinetics of oseltamivir have been evaluated in single-dose pharmacokinetic studies in children aged 1 to 16 years. Multiple-dose pharmacokinetics were studied in a small number of children enrolled in a clinical efficacy study. Younger children cleared both the pro-drug and its active metabolite faster than adults, resulting in a lower exposure for a given mg/kg dose. Doses of 2 mg/kg give oseltamivir carboxylate exposures comparable to those achieved in adults receiving a single 75 mg dose (approximately 1 mg/kg). The pharmacokinetics of oseltamivir in children over 12 years of age are similar to those in adults.

Children 6 to 12 months of age: Limited exposure data from children 6 to 12 months of age from a pharmacodynamic, pharmacokinetic and safety study in influenza-infected children less than 2 years of age, suggest that for most children 6 to 12 months of age, the exposure following 3 mg/kg dosing is similar to the exposures seen in older children and adults using the approved dose.

5.3 Preclinical safety data

Preclinical data reveal no special hazard for humans based on conventional studies of safety pharmacology, repeated-dose toxicity and genotoxicity. Results of the conventional rodent carcinogenicity studies showed a trend towards a dose-dependent increase in the incidence of some tumours that are typical for the rodent strains used. Considering the margins of exposure in relation to the expected exposure in the human use, these findings do not change the benefit-risk of Tamiflu in its adopted therapeutic indications.

Teratology studies have been conducted in rats and rabbits at doses of up to 1500 mg/kg/day and 500 mg/kg/day, respectively. No effects on foetal development were observed. A rat fertility study up to a dose of 1500 mg/kg/day demonstrated no adverse effects on either sex. In pre- and post-natal rat studies, prolonged parturition was noted at 1500 mg/kg/day: the safety margin between human exposure and the highest no-effect dose (500 mg/kg/day) in rats is 480-fold for oseltamivir and 44-fold for the active metabolite, respectively. Foetal exposure in the rats and rabbits was approximately 15 to 20 % of that of the mother.

In lactating rats, oseltamivir and the active metabolite are excreted in the milk. Limited data indicate that oseltamivir and the active metabolite are excreted in human milk. Extrapolation of the animal data provides estimates of 0.01 mg/day and 0.3 mg/day for the respective compounds.

A potential for skin sensitisation to oseltamivir was observed in a "maximisation" test in guinea pigs. Approximately 50 % of the animals treated with the unformulated active ingredient showed erythema after challenging the induced animals. Reversible irritancy of rabbits' eyes was detected.

Whereas very high oral single doses of oseltamivir phosphate had no effect in adult rats, such doses resulted in toxicity in juvenile 7-day-old rat pups, including death. These effects were seen at doses of 657 mg/kg and higher. At 500 mg/kg, no adverse effects were seen, including upon chronic treatment (500 mg/kg/day administered from 7 to 21 days post partum).

6. PHARMACEUTICAL PARTICULARS

6.1 List of excipients

Capsule core:

Pregelatinised starch (derived from maize starch)

Talc

Povidone

Croscarmellose sodium

Sodium stearyl fumarate

Capsule shell:

Gelatin

Yellow iron oxide (E172)

Red iron oxide (E172)

Black iron oxide (E172)

Titanium dioxide (E171)

Printing ink:

Shellac

Titanium dioxide (E171)

FD and C Blue 2 (indigo carmine, E132)

6.2 Incompatibilities

Not applicable.

6.3 Shelf life

7 years

6.4 Special precautions for storage

Do not store above 25°C.

6.5 Nature and contents of container

One box contains 10 capsules in a triplex blister pack (PVC/PE/PVDC, sealed with aluminium foil).

6.6 Special precautions for disposal and other handling

No special requirements.

Any unused product or waste material should be disposed of in accordance with local requirements.

7. MARKETING AUTHORISATION HOLDER

Roche Registration Limited
6 Falcon Way
Shire Park
Welwyn Garden City
AL7 1TW
United Kingdom

8. MARKETING AUTHORISATION NUMBER(S)

EU/1/02/222/001

9. DATE OF FIRST AUTHORISATION/RENEWAL OF THE AUTHORISATION

Date of first authorisation: 20 June 2002

Date of last renewal: 20 June 2007

10. DATE OF REVISION OF THE TEXT

9 September 2009

LEGAL STATUS

POM

Detailed information on this medicinal product is available on the website of the European Medicines Agency (EMEA) http://www.emea.europa.eu/.

Tarceva 25mg, 100mg and 150mg Film-Coated Tablets

(Roche Products Limited)

1. NAME OF THE MEDICINAL PRODUCT

Tarceva▼ 25 mg, 100 mg, and 150 mg film-coated tablets

2. QUALITATIVE AND QUANTITATIVE COMPOSITION

Tarceva 25 mg

One film-coated tablet contains 25 mg erlotinib (as erlotinib hydrochloride).

Tarceva 100 mg

One film-coated tablet contains 100 mg erlotinib (as erlotinib hydrochloride).

Tarceva 150 mg

One film-coated tablet contains 150 mg erlotinib (as erlotinib hydrochloride).

For a full list of excipients, see section 6.1.

3. PHARMACEUTICAL FORM

Film-coated tablet

White to yellowish, round, biconvex tablets with 'Tarceva 25' and logo printed in brownish yellow on one side.

White to yellowish, round, biconvex tablets with 'Tarceva 100' and logo printed in grey on one side.

White to yellowish, round, biconvex tablets with 'Tarceva 150' and logo printed in brown on one side.

4. CLINICAL PARTICULARS

4.1 Therapeutic indications

Non-small cell lung cancer (NSCLC):

Tarceva is indicated for the treatment of patients with locally advanced or metastatic non-small cell lung cancer after failure of at least one prior chemotherapy regimen.

When prescribing Tarceva, factors associated with prolonged survival should be taken into account.

No survival benefit or other clinically relevant effects of the treatment have been demonstrated in patients with EGFR-negative tumours (see section 5.1).

Pancreatic cancer:

Tarceva in combination with gemcitabine is indicated for the treatment of patients with metastatic pancreatic cancer.

When prescribing Tarceva, factors associated with prolonged survival should be taken into account (see section 4.2 and 5.1).

No survival advantage could be shown for patients with locally advanced disease.

4.2 Posology and method of administration

Tarceva treatment should be supervised by a physician experienced in the use of anticancer therapies.

Non-small cell lung cancer:

The recommended daily dose of Tarceva is 150 mg taken at least one hour before or two hours after the ingestion of food.

Pancreatic cancer:

The recommended daily dose of Tarceva is 100 mg taken at least one hour before or two hours after the ingestion of food, in combination with gemcitabine (see the summary of product characteristics of gemcitabine for the pancreatic cancer indication).

In patients who do not develop rash within the first 4 – 8 weeks of treatment, further Tarceva treatment should be re-assessed (see section 5.1).

When dose adjustment is necessary, reduce in 50 mg steps (see section 4.4).

Tarceva is available in strengths of 25 mg, 100 mg and 150 mg.

Concomitant use of CYP3A4 substrates and modulators may require dose adjustment (see section 4.5).

Hepatic impairment: Erlotinib is eliminated by hepatic metabolism and biliary excretion. Although erlotinib exposure was similar in patients with moderately impaired hepatic function (Child-Pugh score 7-9) compared with patients with adequate hepatic function, caution should be used when administering Tarceva to patients with hepatic impairment. Dose reduction or interruption of Tarceva should be considered if severe adverse reactions occur. The safety and efficacy of erlotinib has not been studied in patients with severe hepatic impairment. Use of Tarceva in patients with severe hepatic impairment is not recommended (see section 5.2).

Renal impairment: The safety and efficacy of erlotinib has not been studied in patients with renal impairment (serum creatinine concentration >1.5 times the upper normal limit). Based on pharmacokinetic data no dose adjustments appear necessary in patients with mild or moderate renal impairment (see section 5.2). Use of Tarceva in patients with severe renal impairment is not recommended.

Paediatric use: The safety and efficacy of erlotinib has not been studied in patients under the age of 18 years. Use of Tarceva in paediatric patients is not recommended.

Smokers: Cigarette smoking has been shown to reduce erlotinib exposure by 50-60%. The maximum tolerated dose of Tarceva in NSCLC patients who currently smoke cigarettes was 300 mg. Efficacy and long term safety of a dose higher than the recommended starting doses have not been established in patients who continue to smoke cigarettes (see sections 4.5 and 5.2). Therefore, current smokers should be advised to stop smoking, as plasma concentrations of erlotinib in smokers as compared to non-smokers are reduced.

4.3 Contraindications

Severe hypersensitivity to erlotinib or to any of the excipients.

4.4 Special warnings and precautions for use

Potent inducers of CYP3A4 may reduce the efficacy of erlotinib whereas potent inhibitors of CYP3A4 may lead to increased toxicity. Concomitant treatment with these types of agents should be avoided (see section 4.5).

Current smokers should be advised to stop smoking, as plasma concentrations of erlotinib in smokers as compared to non-smokers are reduced. The degree of reduction is likely to be clinically significant (see section 4.5).

Cases of interstitial lung disease (ILD)-like events, including fatalities, have been reported uncommonly in patients receiving Tarceva for treatment of non-small cell lung cancer (NSCLC), pancreatic cancer or other advanced solid tumours. In the pivotal study BR.21 in NSCLC, the incidence of ILD (0.8 %) was the same in both the placebo and Tarceva groups. In the pancreatic cancer study in combination with gemcitabine, the incidence of ILD-like events was 2.5 % in the Tarceva plus gemcitabine group versus 0.4 % in the placebo plus gemcitabine treated group. The overall incidence in Tarceva-treated patients from all studies (including uncontrolled studies and studies with concurrent chemotherapy) is approximately 0.6 % compared to 0.2 % in patients on placebo. Reported diagnoses in patients suspected of having ILD-like events included pneumonitis, radiation pneumonitis, hypersensitivity pneumonitis, interstitial pneumonia, interstitial lung disease, obliterative bronchiolitis, pulmonary fibrosis, Acute Respiratory Distress Syndrome (ARDS), alveolitis, and lung infiltration. Symptoms started from a few days to several months after initiating Tarceva therapy. Confounding or contributing factors such as concomitant or prior chemotherapy, prior radiotherapy, pre-existing parenchymal lung disease, metastatic lung disease, or pulmonary infections were frequent.

In patients who develop acute onset of new and/or progressive unexplained pulmonary symptoms such as dyspnoea, cough and fever, Tarceva therapy should be interrupted pending diagnostic evaluation. Patients treated concurrently with erlotinib and gemcitabine should be monitored carefully for the possibility to develop ILD-like toxicity. If ILD is diagnosed, Tarceva should be discontinued and appropriate treatment initiated as necessary (see section 4.8).

Diarrhoea has occurred in approximately 50 % of patients on Tarceva and moderate or severe diarrhoea should be treated with e.g. loperamide. In some cases dose reduction may be necessary. In the clinical studies doses were reduced by 50 mg steps. Dose reductions by 25 mg steps have not been investigated. In the event of severe or persistent diarrhoea, nausea, anorexia, or vomiting associated with dehydration, Tarceva therapy should be interrupted and appropriate measures should be taken to treat the dehydration (see section 4.8). There have been rare reports of hypokalaemia and renal failure (including fatalities). Some cases were secondary to severe dehydration due to diarrhoea, vomiting and/or anorexia, while others were confounded by concomitant chemotherapy. In more severe or persistent cases of diarrhoea, or cases leading to dehydration, particularly in groups of patients with aggravating risk factors (concomitant medications, symptoms or diseases or other predisposing conditions including advanced age), Tarceva therapy should be interrupted and appropriate measures should be taken to intensively rehydrate the patients intravenously. In addition, renal function and serum electrolytes including potassium should be monitored in patients at risk of dehydration.

Rare cases of hepatic failure (including fatalities) have been reported during use of Tarceva. Confounding factors have included pre-existing liver disease or concomitant hepatotoxic medications. Therefore, in such patients, periodic liver function testing should be considered. Tarceva dosing should be interrupted if changes in liver function are severe (see section 4.8).

Patients receiving Tarceva are at increased risk of developing gastrointestinal perforation, which was observed uncommonly. Patients receiving concomitant anti-angiogenic agents, corticosteroids, NSAIDs, and/or taxane based chemotherapy, or who have prior history of peptic ulceration or diverticular disease are at increased risk. Tarceva should be permanently discontinued in patients who develop gastrointestinal perforation (see section 4.8).

Bullous, blistering and exfoliative skin conditions have been reported, including very rare cases suggestive of Stevens-Johnson syndrome/Toxic epidermal necrolysis, which in some cases were fatal (see section 4.8). Tarceva treatment should be interrupted or discontinued if the patient develops severe bullous, blistering or exfoliating conditions.

Very rare cases of corneal perforation or ulceration have been reported during use of Tarceva. Other ocular disorders including abnormal eyelash growth, keratoconjunctivitis sicca or keratitis have been observed with Tarceva treatment which are also risk factors for corneal perforation/ulceration. Tarceva therapy should be interrupted or discontinued if patients present with acute/worsening ocular disorders such as eye pain (see section 4.8).

The tablets contain lactose and should not be administered to patients with rare hereditary problems of galactose intolerance, Lapp lactase deficiency or glucose-galactose malabsorption.

Erlotinib is characterised by a decrease in solubility at pH above 5. Drugs that alter the pH of the upper GI tract, like proton pump inhibitors, H2 antagonists and antacids, may alter the solubility of erlotinib and hence its bioavailability. Increasing the dose of Tarceva when coadministered with such agents is not likely to compensate for the loss of exposure. Combination of erlotinib with proton pump inhibitors should be avoided. The effects of concomitant administration of erlotinib with H2 antagonists and antacids are unknown; however, reduced bioavailability is likely. Therefore, concomitant administration of these combinations should be avoided (see section 4.5). If the use of antacids is considered necessary during treatment with Tarceva, they should be taken at least 4 hours before or 2 hours after the daily dose of Tarceva.

4.5 Interaction with other medicinal products and other forms of interaction

Interaction studies have only been performed in adults.

Erlotinib is a potent inhibitor of CYP1A1, and a moderate inhibitor of CYP3A4 and CYP2C8, as well as a strong inhibitor of glucuronidation by UGT1A1 *in vitro*.

The physiological relevance of the strong inhibition of CYP1A1 is unknown due to the very limited expression of CYP1A1 in human tissues.

When erlotinib was co-administered with ciprofloxacin, a moderate CYP1A2 inhibitor, the erlotinib exposure [AUC] increased significantly by 39 %, while no statistically significant change in C_{max} was found. Similarly, the exposure to the active metabolite increased by about 60% and 48% for AUC and C_{max}, respectively. The clinical relevance of this increase has not been established. Caution should be exercised when ciprofloxacin or potent CYP1A2 inhibitors (e.g. fluvoxamine) are combined with erlotinib. If adverse events related to erlotinib are observed, the dose of erlotinib may be reduced.

Pretreatment or coadministration of Tarceva did not alter the clearance of the prototypical CYP3A4 substrates, midazolam and erythromycin, but did appear to decrease the oral bioavailability of midazolam by up to 24%. In another clinical study, erlotinib was shown not to affect pharmacokinetics of the concomitantly administered CYP3A4/2C8 substrate paclitaxel. Significant interactions with the clearance of other CYP3A4 substrates are therefore unlikely.

The inhibition of glucuronidation may cause interactions with medicinal products which are substrates of UGT1A1 and exclusively cleared by this pathway. Patients with low expression levels of UGT1A1 or genetic glucuronidation disorders (e.g. Gilbert's disease) may exhibit increased serum concentrations of bilirubin and must be treated with caution.

Erlotinib is metabolised in the liver by the hepatic cytochromes in humans, primarily CYP3A4 and to a lesser extent by CYP1A2. Extrahepatic metabolism by CYP3A4 in intestine, CYP1A1 in lung, and CYP1B1 in tumour tissue also potentially contribute to the metabolic clearance of erlotinib. Potential interactions may occur with active substances which are metabolised by, or are inhibitors or inducers of, these enzymes.

Potent inhibitors of CYP3A4 activity decrease erlotinib metabolism and increase erlotinib plasma concentrations. In a clinical study, the concomitant use of erlotinib with ketoconazole (200 mg orally twice daily for 5 days), a potent CYP3A4 inhibitor, resulted in an increase of erlotinib exposure (86 % of AUC and 69 % of C_{max}). Therefore, caution should be used when erlotinib is combined with a potent CYP3A4 inhibitor, e.g. azole antifungals (i.e. ketoconazole, itraconazole, voriconazole), protease inhibitors, erythromycin or clarithromycin. If necessary the dose of erlotinib should be reduced, particularly if toxicity is observed.

Potent inducers of CYP3A4 activity increase erlotinib metabolism and significantly decrease erlotinib plasma concentrations. In a clinical study, the concomitant use of erlotinib and rifampicin (600 mg orally once daily for 7 days), a potent CYP3A4 inducer, resulted in a 69 % decrease in the median erlotinib AUC. Co-administration of rifampicin with a single 450 mg dose of Tarceva resulted in a mean erlotinib exposure (AUC) of 57.5% of that after a single 150 mg Tarceva dose in the absence of rifampicin treatment. Co-administration of Tarceva with CYP3A4 inducers should therefore be avoided. For patients who require concomitant treatment with Tarceva and a potent CYP3A4 inducer such as rifampicin an increase in dose to 300 mg should be considered while their safety (including renal and liver functions and serum electrolytes) is closely monitored, and if well tolerated for more than 2 weeks, further increase to 450 mg could be considered with close safety monitoring. Reduced exposure may also occur with other inducers e.g. phenytoin, carbamazepine, barbiturates or St. Johns Wort (*hypericum perforatum*). Caution should be observed when these active substances are combined with erlotinib. Alternate treatments lacking potent CYP3A4 inducing activity should be considered when possible.

International Normalized Ratio (INR) elevations, and bleeding events including gastrointestinal bleeding have been reported in clinical studies, some associated with concomitant warfarin administration (see section 4.8) and some with concomitant NSAID administration. Patients taking warfarin or other coumarin-derivative anticoagulants should be monitored regularly for changes in prothrombin time or INR.

Results of a pharmacokinetic interaction study indicated a significant 2.8-, 1.5- and 9-fold reduced AUC_{inf}, C_{max} and plasma concentration at 24 hours, respectively, after administration of Tarceva in smokers as compared to non-smokers (see section 5.2). Therefore, patients who are still smoking should be encouraged to stop smoking as early as possible before initiation of treatment with Tarceva, as plasma erlotinib concentrations are reduced otherwise. The clinical effect of the decreased exposure has not been formally assessed but it is likely to be clinically significant.

Erlotinib is a substrate for the P-glycoprotein active substance transporter. Concomitant administration of inhibitors of Pgp, e.g. cyclosporine and verapamil, may lead to altered distribution and/or altered elimination of erlotinib. The consequences of this interaction for e.g. CNS toxicity has not been established. Caution should be exercised in such situations.

Erlotinib is characterised by a decrease in solubility at pH above 5. Drugs that alter the pH of the upper GI tract may alter the solubility of erlotinib and hence its bioavailability. Co-administration of erlotinib with omeprazole, a proton pump inhibitor (PPI), decreased the erlotinib exposure [AUC] and maximum concentration [C_{max}] by 46 % and 61 %, respectively. There was no change to T_{max} or half-life. Concomitant administration of Tarceva with 300 mg ranitidine, an H2-receptor antagonist, decreased erlotinib exposure [AUC] and maximum concentrations [C_{max}] by 33% and 54%, respectively. Increasing the dose of Tarceva when co-administered with such agents is not likely to compensate for this loss of exposure. However, when Tarceva was dosed in a staggered manner 2 hours before or 10 hours after ranitidine 150 mg b.i.d., erlotinib exposure [AUC] and maximum concentrations [C_{max}] decreased only by 15% and 17%, respectively. The effect of antacids on the absorption of erlotinib have not been investigated but absorption may be impaired, leading to lower plasma levels. In summary, the combination of erlotinib with proton pump inhibitors should be avoided. If the use of antacids is considered necessary during treatment with Tarceva, they should be taken at least 4 hours before or 2 hours after the daily dose of Tarceva. If the use of ranitidine is considered, it should be used in a staggered manner; i.e. Tarceva must be taken at least 2 hours before or 10 hours after ranitidine dosing.

In a Phase Ib study, there were no significant effects of gemcitabine on the pharmacokinetics of erlotinib nor were there significant effects of erlotinib on the pharmacokinetics of gemcitabine.

Erlotinib increases platinum concentrations. In a clinical study, the concomitant use of erlotinib with carboplatin and paclitaxel led to an increase of total platinum AUC_{0-48} of 10.6%. Although statistically significant, the magnitude of this difference is not considered to be clinically relevant. In clinical practice, there may be other co-factors leading to an increased exposure to carboplatin like renal impairment. There were no significant effects of carboplatin or paclitaxel on the pharmacokinetics of erlotinib.

Capecitabine may increase erlotinib concentrations. When erlotinib was given in combination with capecitabine, there was a statistically significant increase in erlotinib AUC and a borderline increase in C_{max} when compared with values observed in another study in which erlotinib was given as single agent. There were no significant effects of erlotinib on the pharmacokinetics of capecitabine.

4.6 Pregnancy and lactation

There are no studies in pregnant women using erlotinib. Studies in animals have shown some reproductive toxicity (see section 5.3). The potential risk for humans is unknown. Women of childbearing potential must be advised to avoid pregnancy while on Tarceva. Adequate contraceptive methods should be used during therapy, and for at least 2 weeks after completing therapy. Treatment should only be continued in pregnant women if the potential benefit to the mother outweighs the risk to the foetus.

It is not known whether erlotinib is excreted in human milk. Because of the potential harm to the infant, mothers should be advised against breastfeeding while receiving Tarceva.

4.7 Effects on ability to drive and use machines

No studies on the effects on the ability to drive and use machines have been performed; however erlotinib is not associated with impairment of mental ability.

4.8 Undesirable effects

Non-small cell lung cancer (Tarceva administered as single agent in study BR.21):

Rash (75 %) and diarrhoea (54 %) were the most commonly reported adverse drug reactions (ADRs). Most were Grade 1/2 in severity and manageable without intervention. Grade 3/4 rash and diarrhoea occurred in 9 % and 6 %, respectively in Tarceva-treated patients and each resulted in study discontinuation in 1 % of patients. Dose reduction for rash and diarrhoea was needed in 6 % and 1 % of patients, respectively. In study BR.21, the median time to onset of rash was 8 days, and the median time to onset of diarrhoea was 12 days.

In general, rash manifests as a mild or moderate erythematous and papulopustular rash, which may occur or worsen in sun exposed areas. For patients who are exposed to sun, protective clothing, and/or use of sun screen (e.g. mineral-containing) may be advisable.

Adverse events occurring more frequently (≥3 %) in Tarceva-treated patients than in the placebo group in the pivotal study BR.21, and in at least 10 % of patients in the Tarceva group, are summarised by National Cancer Institute-Common Toxicity Criteria (NCI-CTC) Grade in Table 1.

Table 1: Very common ADRs in study BR.21

(see Table 1 opposite)

(see Table 1 opposite)

Pancreatic cancer (Tarceva administered concurrently with gemcitabine in study PA.3):

The most common adverse reactions in pivotal study PA.3 in pancreatic cancer patients receiving Tarceva 100 mg plus gemcitabine were fatigue, rash and diarrhoea. In the Tarceva plus gemcitabine arm, Grade 3/4 rash and diarrhoea were each reported in 5 % of patients. The median time to onset of rash and diarrhoea was 10 days and 15 days, respectively. Rash and diarrhoea each resulted in dose reductions in 2 % of patients, and resulted in study discontinuation in up to 1 % of patients receiving Tarceva plus gemcitabine.

Adverse events occurring more frequently (≥3 %) in Tarceva 100 mg plus gemcitabine-treated patients than in the placebo plus gemcitabine group in the pivotal study PA.3, and in at least 10 % of patients in the Tarceva 100 mg plus gemcitabine group, are summarised by National Cancer Institute-Common Toxicity Criteria (NCI-CTC) Grade in Table 2.

Table 2: Very common ADRs in study PA.3 (100 mg cohort)

(see Table 2 on next page)

Other Observations:

Safety evaluation of Tarceva is based on the data from 759 patients treated with at least one 150 mg dose of Tarceva monotherapy during Phase III NSCLC study BR.21, Phase II NSCLC study A248-1007, and three Phase II studies in populations other than NSCLC: 248-101 (ovarian cancer), A248-1003 (head and neck cancer), and OSI2288g (metastatic breast cancer) and the 285 patients who received Tarceva 100 or 150 mg plus gemcitabine in the phase III pancreatic cancer study PA.3.

The following terms are used to rank the undesirable effects by frequency: very common (>1/10); common (>1/100, <1/10); uncommon (>1/1,000, <1/100); rare (>1/10,000, <1/1000); very rare (<1/10,000) including isolated reports.

The following adverse reactions have been observed in patients who received Tarceva administered as single agent and patients who received Tarceva concurrently with chemotherapy.

Very common ADR's are presented in Tables 1 and 2, ADR's in other frequency categories are summarized below.

Gastrointestinal disorders:

Common: Gastrointestinal bleeding. In clinical studies, some cases have been associated with concomitant warfarin administration (see section 4.5) and some with concomitant NSAID administration.

Uncommon: Gastrointestinal perforations.

Skin and subcutaneous tissue disorders:

Common: Alopecia.

Common (in PA.3): Dry skin.

Common: Paronychia.

Uncommon Hirsutism, eyebrow changes and brittle and loose nails.

Uncommon Mild skin reactions such as hyperpigmentation.

Very rare: Cases suggestive of Stevens-Johnson syndrome/Toxic epidermal necrolysis, which in some cases were fatal.

Hepato-biliary disorders:

Very common (in PA.3)

Common (in BR.21): Liver function test abnormalities (including increased alanine aminotransferase [ALT], aspartate aminotransferase [AST], bilirubin). These were mainly mild or moderate in severity, transient in nature or associated with liver metastases.

Rare: Rare cases of hepatic failure (including fatalities) have been reported during use of Tarceva. Confounding factors have included pre-existing liver disease or concomitant hepatotoxic medications (see section 4.4).

Eye disorders:

Common: Keratitis.

Common: Conjunctivitis in study PA.3.

Uncommon: Eyelash changes (including in-growing eyelashes, excessive growth and thickening of the eyelashes).

Very rare: Corneal ulcerations and perforations.

Respiratory, thoracic and mediastinal disorders:

Common: Epistaxis.

Uncommon: Serious interstitial lung disease (ILD), including fatalities, in patients receiving Tarceva for treatment of NSCLC or other advanced solid tumours (see section 4.4).

Table 1 Very common ADRs in study BR.21

	Erlotinib N = 485			Placebo N = 242		
NCI-CTC Grade	**Any Grade**	**3**	**4**	**Any Grade**	**3**	**4**
MedDRA Preferred Term	%	%	%	%	%	%
Total patients with any AE	99	40	22	96	36	22
Infections and infestations						
Infection*	24	4	0	15	2	0
Metabolism and nutrition disorders						
Anorexia	52	8	1	38	5	<1
Eye disorders						
Conjunctivitis	12	<1	0	2	<1	0
Keratoconjunctivitis sicca	12	0	0	3	0	0
Respiratory, thoracic and mediastinal disorders						
Dyspnoea	41	17	11	35	15	11
Cough	33	4	0	29	2	0
Gastrointestinal disorders						
Diarrhoea**	54	6	<1	18	<1	0
Nausea	33	3	0	24	2	0
Vomiting	23	2	<1	19	2	0
Stomatitis	17	<1	0	3	0	0
Abdominal pain	11	2	<1	7	1	<1
Skin and subcutaneous tissue disorders						
Rash***	75	8	<1	17	0	0
Pruritus	13	<1	0	5	0	0
Dry skin	12	0	0	4	0	0
General disorders and administration site conditions						
Fatigue	52	14	4	45	16	4

* Severe infections, with or without neutropenia, have included pneumonia, sepsis, and cellulitis.

** Can lead to dehydration, hypokalemia and renal failure.

*** Rash included dermatitis acneiform.

4.9 Overdose

Single oral doses of Tarceva up to 1000 mg erlotinib in healthy subjects, and up to 1600 mg in cancer patients have been tolerated. Repeated twice daily doses of 200 mg in healthy subjects were poorly tolerated after only a few days of dosing. Based on the data from these studies, severe adverse events such as diarrhoea, rash and possibly increased activity of liver aminotransferases may occur above the recommended dose. In case of suspected overdose, Tarceva should be withheld and symptomatic treatment initiated.

5. PHARMACOLOGICAL PROPERTIES

5.1 Pharmacodynamic properties

Pharmacotherapeutic group: antineoplastic agent, ATC code: L01XE03

Erlotinib is an epidermal growth factor receptor/human epidermal growth factor receptor type 1 (EGFR also known as HER1) tyrosine kinase inhibitor. Erlotinib potently inhibits the intracellular phosphorylation of EGFR. EGFR is expressed on the cell surface of normal cells and cancer cells. In non-clinical models, inhibition of EGFR phosphotyrosine results in cell stasis and/or death.

Non-small cell lung cancer (Tarceva administered as single agent in study BR.21):

The efficacy and safety of Tarceva was demonstrated in a randomised, double-blind, placebo-controlled trial (BR.21), in 731 patients with locally advanced or metastatic NSCLC after failure of at least one chemotherapy regimen. Patients were randomised 2:1 to receive Tarceva 150 mg or placebo orally once daily. Study endpoints included overall survival, progression-free survival (PFS), response rate, duration of response, time to deterioration of lung cancer-related symptoms (cough, dyspnoea and pain), and safety. The primary endpoint was survival.

Demographic characteristics were well balanced between the two treatment groups. About two-thirds of the patients were male and approximately one-third had a baseline ECOG performance status (PS) of 2, and 9 % had a baseline ECOG PS of 3. Ninety-three percent and 92 % of all patients in the Tarceva and placebo groups, respectively, had received a prior platinum-containing regimen and 36 % and 37 % of all patients, respectively, had received a prior taxane therapy.

The adjusted hazard ratio (HR) for death in the Tarceva group relative to the placebo group was 0.73 (95 % CI, 0.60 to 0.87) (p = 0.001). The percent of patients alive at 12 months was 31.2 % and 21.5 %, for the Tarceva and placebo groups, respectively. The median overall survival was 6.7 months in the Tarceva group (95 % CI, 5.5 to 7.8 months) compared with 4.7 months in the placebo group (95 % CI, 4.1 to 6.3 months).

The effect on overall survival was explored across different patient subsets. The effect of Tarceva on overall survival was similar in patients with a baseline performance status (ECOG) of 2-3 (HR = 0.77, CI 0.6-1.0) or 0-1 (HR = 0.73, 0.6-0.9), male (HR = 0.76, CI 0.6-0.9) or female patients (HR = 0.80, CI 0.6-1.1), patients < 65 years of age (HR = 0.75, CI 0.6-0.9) or older patients (HR = 0.79, CI 0.6-1.0), patients with one prior regimen (HR = 0.76, CI 0.6-1.0) or more than one prior regimen (HR = 0.75, CI 0.6-1.0), Caucasian (HR = 0.79, CI 0.6-1.0) or Asian patients (HR = 0.61, 0.4-1.0), patients with adenocarcinoma (HR = 0.71, CI 0.6-0.9) or squamous cell carcinoma (HR = 0.67, CI 0.5-0.9), but not in patients with other histologies (HR 1.04, CI 0.7-1.5), patients with stage IV disease at diagnosis (HR = 0.92, CI 0.7-1.2) or < stage IV disease at diagnosis (HR = 0.65, 0.5-0.8). Patients who never smoked had a much greater benefit from erlotinib (survival HR = 0.42, CI 0.28-0.64) compared with current or ex-smokers (HR = 0.87, CI 0.71-1.05).

In the 45 % of patients with known EGFR-expression status, the hazard ratio was 0.68 (CI 0.49-0.94) for patients with EGFR-positive tumours and 0.93 (CI 0.63-1.36) for patients with EGFR-negative tumours (defined by IHC using EGFR pharmDx kit and defining EGFR-negative as less than 10 % tumour cells staining). In the remaining 55 % of patients with unknown EGFR-expression status, the hazard ratio was 0.77 (CI 0.61-0.98).

The median PFS was 9.7 weeks in the Tarceva group (95 % CI, 8.4 to 12.4 weeks) compared with 8.0 weeks in the placebo group (95 % CI, 7.9 to 8.1 weeks).

The objective response rate by RECIST in the Tarceva group was 8.9 % (95 % CI, 6.4 to 12.0).

The first 330 patients were centrally assessed (response rate 6.2 %); 401 patients were investigator-assessed (response rate 11.2 %).

The median duration of response was 34.3 weeks, ranging from 9.7 to 57.6+ weeks. The proportion of patients who experienced complete response, partial response or stable disease was 44.0 % and 27.5 %, respectively, for the Tarceva and placebo groups (p = 0.004).

A survival benefit of Tarceva was also observed in patients who did not achieve an objective tumour response (by RECIST). This was evidenced by a hazard ratio for death

Table 2 Very common ADRs in study PA.3 (100 mg cohort)

	Erlotinib N = 259			Placebo N = 256		
NCI-CTC Grade	**Any Grade**	**3**	**4**	**Any Grade**	**3**	**4**
MedDRA Preferred Term	**%**	**%**	**%**	**%**	**%**	**%**
Total patients with any AE	99	48	22	97	48	16
Infections and infestations						
Infection*	31	3	<1	24	6	<1
Metabolism and nutrition disorders						
Weight decreased	39	2	0	29	<1	0
Psychiatric disorders						
Depression	19	2	0	14	<1	0
Nervous system disorders						
Headache	15	<1	0	10	0	0
Neuropathy	13	1	<1	10	<1	0
Respiratory, thoracic and mediastinal disorders						
Cough	16	0	0	11	0	0
Gastrointestinal disorders						
Diarrhoea**	48	5	<1	36	2	0
Stomatitis	22	<1	0	12	0	0
Dyspepsia	17	<1	0	13	<1	0
Flatulence	13	0	0	9	<1	0
Skin and subcutaneous tissue disorders						
Rash***	69	5	0	30	1	0
Alopecia	14	0	0	11	0	0
General disorders and administration site conditions						
Pyrexia	36	3	0	30	4	0
Fatigue	73	14	2	70	13	2
Rigors	12	0	0	9	0	0

* Severe infections, with or without neutropenia, have included pneumonia, sepsis, and cellulitis.

** Can lead to dehydration, hypokalemia and renal failure.

*** Rash included dermatitis acneiform.

Table 3

Outcome	Tarceva (months)	Placebo (months)	Δ (months)	CI of Δ	HR	CI of HR	P- value
Overall Population							
Median overall survival	6.4	6.0	0.41	-0.54-1.64	0.82	0.69-0.98	0.028
Mean overall survival	8.8	7.6	1.16	-0.05-2.34			
Metastatic Population							
Median overall survival	5.9	5.1	0.87	-0.26-1.56	0.80	0.66-0.98	0.029
Mean overall survival	8.1	6.7	1.43	0.17-2.66			
Locally Advanced Population							
Median overall survival	8.5	8.2	0.36	-2.43-2.96	0.93	0.65-1.35	0.713
Mean overall survival	10.7	10.5	0.19	-2.43-2.69			

of 0.82 (95 % CI, 0.68 to 0.99) among patients whose best response was stable disease or progressive disease.

Tarceva resulted in symptom benefits by significantly prolonging time to deterioration in cough, dyspnoea and pain, versus placebo.

Pancreatic cancer (Tarceva administered concurrently with gemcitabine in study PA.3):

The efficacy and safety of Tarceva in combination with gemcitabine as a first-line treatment was assessed in a randomised, double-blind, placebo-controlled trial in patients with locally advanced, unresectable or metastatic pancreatic cancer. Patients were randomised to receive Tarceva or placebo once daily on a continuous schedule plus gemcitabine IV (1000 mg/m^2, Cycle 1 - Days 1, 8, 15, 22, 29, 36 and 43 of an 8 week cycle; Cycle 2 and subsequent cycles - Days 1, 8 and 15 of a 4 week cycle [approved dose and schedule for pancreatic cancer, see the gemcitabine SPC]). Tarceva or placebo was taken orally once daily until disease progression or unacceptable toxicity. The primary endpoint was overall survival.

Baseline demographic and disease characteristics of the patients were similar between the 2 treatment groups, 100 mg Tarceva plus gemcitabine or placebo plus gemcitabine, except for a slightly larger proportion of females in the erlotinib/gemcitabine arm compared with the placebo/gemcitabine arm:

Baseline	Tarceva	Placebo
Females	51%	44%
Baseline ECOG performance status (PS) = 0	31%	32%
Baseline ECOG performance status (PS) = 1	51%	51%
Baseline ECOG performance status (PS) = 2	17%	17%
Metastatic disease at baseline	77%	76%

Survival was evaluated in the intent-to-treat population based on follow-up survival data. Results are shown in the table below (results for the group of metastatic and locally advanced patients are derived from exploratory subgroup analysis).

(see Table 3 below)

(see Figure 1 on next page)

(see Figure 2 on next page)

In a post-hoc analysis, patients with favourable clinical status at baseline (low pain intensity, good QoL and good PS) may derive more benefit from Tarceva. The benefit is mostly driven by the presence of a low pain intensity score.

In a post-hoc analysis, patients on Tarceva who developed a rash had a longer overall survival compared to patients who did not develop rash (median OS 7.2 months vs 5 months, HR:0.61).

90% of patients on Tarceva developed rash within the first 44 days. The median time to onset of rash was 10 days.

5.2 Pharmacokinetic properties

Absorption: After oral administration, erlotinib peak plasma levels are obtained in approximately 4 hours after oral dosing. A study in normal healthy volunteers provided an estimate of the absolute bioavailability of 59 %. The exposure after an oral dose may be increased by food.

Distribution: Erlotinib has a mean apparent volume of distribution of 232 l and distributes into tumour tissue of humans. In a study of 4 patients (3 with non-small cell lung cancer [NSCLC], and 1 with laryngeal cancer) receiving 150 mg daily oral doses of Tarceva, tumour samples from surgical excisions on Day 9 of treatment revealed tumour concentrations of erlotinib that averaged 1,185 ng/g of tissue. This corresponded to an overall average of 63 % (range 5-161 %) of the steady state observed peak plasma concentrations. The primary active metabolites were present in tumour at concentrations averaging 160 ng/g tissue, which corresponded to an overall average of 113 % (range 88-130 %) of the observed steady state peak plasma concentrations. Plasma protein binding is approximately 95 %. Erlotinib binds to serum albumin and alpha-1 acid glycoprotein (AAG).

Metabolism: Erlotinib is metabolised in the liver by the hepatic cytochromes in humans, primarily CYP3A4 and to a lesser extent by CYP1A2. Extrahepatic metabolism by CYP3A4 in intestine, CYP1A1 in lung, and 1B1 in tumour tissue potentially contribute to the metabolic clearance of erlotinib.

There are three main metabolic pathways identified: 1) O-demethylation of either side chain or both, followed by oxidation to the carboxylic acids; 2) oxidation of the acetylene moiety followed by hydrolysis to the aryl carboxylic acid; and 3) aromatic hydroxylation of the phenyl-acetylene moiety. The primary metabolites OSI-420 and OSI-413 of erlotinib produced by O-demethylation of either side chain have comparable potency to erlotinib in non-clinical *in vitro* assays and *in vivo* tumour models. They are present in plasma at levels that are <10 % of erlotinib and display similar pharmacokinetics as erlotinib.

Elimination: Erlotinib is excreted predominantly as metabolites via the faeces (>90 %) with renal elimination accounting for only a small amount (approximately 9 %) of an oral dose. Less than 2 % of the orally administered dose is excreted as parent substance. A population pharmacokinetic analysis in 591 patients receiving single agent Tarceva shows a mean apparent clearance of 4.47 l/hour with a median half-life of 36.2 hours. Therefore, the time to reach steady state plasma concentration would be expected to occur in approximately 7-8 days.

Pharmacokinetics in special populations:

Based on population pharmacokinetic analysis, no clinically significant relationship between predicted apparent clearance and patient age, bodyweight, gender and ethnicity were observed. Patient factors, which correlated with erlotinib pharmacokinetics, were serum total bilirubin, AAG and current smoking. Increased serum concentrations of total bilirubin and AAG concentrations were associated with a reduced erlotinib clearance. The clinical relevance of these differences is unclear. However, smokers had an increased rate of erlotinib clearance. This was confirmed in a pharmacokinetic study in non-smoking and currently cigarette smoking healthy subjects receiving a single oral dose of 150 mg erlotinib. The geometric mean of the C_{max} was 1056 ng/mL in the non-smokers and 689 ng/mL in the smokers with a mean ratio for smokers to non-smokers of 65.2 % (95 % CI: 44.3 to 95.9, p = 0.031). The geometric mean of the AUC_{0-inf} was 18726 ng•h/mL in the non-smokers and 6718 ng•h/mL in the smokers with a mean ratio of 35.9 % (95 % CI: 23.7 to 54.3, p < 0.0001). The geometric mean of the C_{24h} was 288 ng/mL in the non-smokers and 34.8 ng/mL in the smokers with a mean ratio of 12.1 % (95 % CI: 4.82 to 30.2, p = 0.0001).

In the pivotal Phase III NSCLC trial, current smokers achieved erlotinib steady state trough plasma concentration of 0.65 µg/mL (n=16) which was approximately 2-fold less than the former smokers or patients who had never smoked (1.28 µg/mL, n=108). This effect was accompanied by a 24% increase in apparent erlotinib plasma clearance. In a phase I dose escalation study in NSCLC patients who were current smokers, pharmacokinetic analyses at steady-state indicated a dose proportional increase in erlotinib exposure when the Tarceva dose was increased from 150 mg to the maximum tolerated dose of 300 mg. Steady-state trough plasma concentrations at a 300 mg

Figure 1

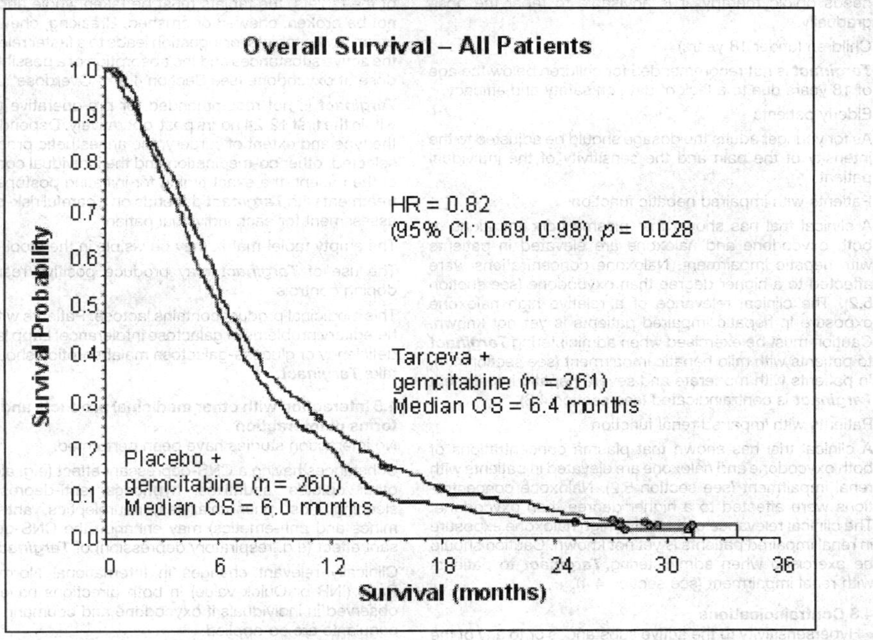

Figure 2

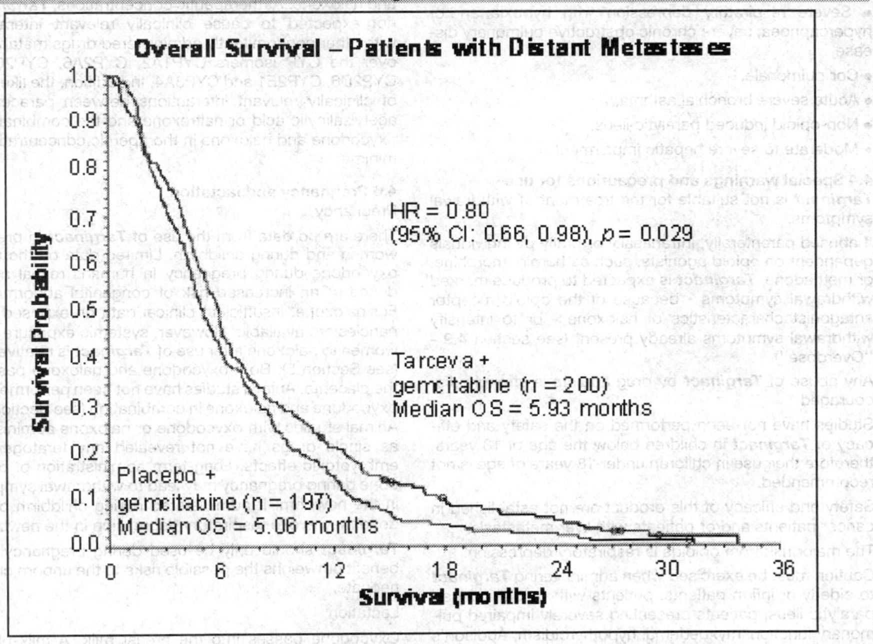

dose in current smokers in this study was 1.22 μg/mL (n=17).

Based on the results of pharmacokinetic studies, current smokers should be advised to stop smoking while taking Tarceva, as plasma concentrations could be reduced otherwise.

Based on population pharmacokinetic analysis, the presence of an opioid appeared to increase exposure by about 11 %.

A second population pharmacokinetic analysis was conducted that incorporated erlotinib data from 204 pancreatic cancer patients who received erlotinib plus gemcitabine. This analysis demonstrated that covariants affecting erlotinib clearance in patients from the pancreatic study were very similar to those seen in the prior single agent pharmacokinetic analysis. No new covariate effects were identified. Co-administration of gemcitabine had no effect on erlotinib plasma clearance.

There have been no specific studies in paediatric or elderly patients.

Hepatic impairment: Erlotinib is primarily cleared by the liver. In patients with solid tumours and with moderately impaired hepatic function (Child-Pugh score 7-9), geometric mean erlotinib AUC_{0-t} and C_{max} was 27000 ng•h/mL and 805 ng/mL, respectively, as compared to 29300 ng•h/mL and 1090 ng/mL in patients with adequate hepatic function including patients with primary liver cancer or hepatic metastases. Although the C_{max} was statistically significant lower in moderately hepatic impaired patients, this difference is not considered clinically relevant. No data are available regarding the influence of severe hepatic dysfunction on the pharmacokinetics of erlotinib. In population pharmacokinetic analysis, increased serum concentrations of total bilirubin were associated with a slower rate of erlotinib clearance.

Renal impairment: Erlotinib and its metabolites are not significantly excreted by the kidney, as less than 9 % of a single dose is excreted in the urine. In population pharmacokinetic analysis, no clinically significant relationship was observed between erlotinib clearance and creatinine clearance, but there are no data available for patients with creatinine clearance < 15 ml/min.

5.3 Preclinical safety data

Chronic dosing effects observed in at least one animal species or study included effects on the cornea (atrophy, ulceration), skin (follicular degeneration and inflammation, redness, and alopecia), ovary (atrophy), liver (liver necrosis), kidney (renal papillary necrosis and tubular dilatation), and gastrointestinal tract (delayed gastric emptying and diarrhoea). Red blood cell parameters were decreased and white blood cells, primarily neutrophils, were increased. There were treatment-related increases in ALT, AST and bilirubin. These findings were observed at exposures well below clinically relevant exposures.

Based on the mode of action, erlotinib, has the potential to be a teratogen. Data from reproductive toxicology tests in rats and rabbits at doses near the maximum tolerated dose and/or maternally toxic doses showed reproductive (embryotoxicity in rats, embryo resorption and foetotoxicity in rabbits) and developmental (decrease in pup growth and survival in rats) toxicity, but was not teratogenic and did not impair fertility. These findings were observed at clinically relevant exposures.

Erlotinib tested negative in conventional genotoxicity studies. Carcinogenicity studies have not been performed.

A mild phototoxic skin reaction was observed in rats after UV irradiation.

6. PHARMACEUTICAL PARTICULARS

6.1 List of excipients

Tablet core:

Lactose monohydrate

Cellulose, microcrystalline (E460)

Sodium starch glycolate Type A

Sodium laurilsulfate

Magnesium stearate (E470 b)

Tablet coat:

Hydroxypropyl cellulose (E463)

Titanium dioxide (E171)

Macrogol

Hypromellose (E464)

Printing ink yellow: 25 mg film-coated tablet

Shellac (E904)

Iron oxide yellow (E172)

Printing ink grey:100 mg film-coated tablet

Shellac (E904)

Iron oxide yellow (E172)

Iron oxide black (E172)

Titanium dioxide (E171)

Printing ink brown:150 mg film-coated tablet

Shellac (E904)

Iron oxide red (E172)

6.2 Incompatibilities

Not applicable.

6.3 Shelf life

3 years.

6.4 Special precautions for storage

This medicinal product does not require any special storage conditions.

6.5 Nature and contents of container

PVC blister sealed with aluminium foil containing 30 tablets.

6.6 Special precautions for disposal and other handling

No special requirements.

7. MARKETING AUTHORISATION HOLDER

Roche Registration Limited
6 Falcon Way
Shire Park
Welwyn Garden City
AL7 1TW
United Kingdom

8. MARKETING AUTHORISATION NUMBER(S)

EU/1/05/311/001 – 25 mg film-coated tablet
EU/1/05/311/002 – 100 mg film-coated tablet
EU/1/05/311/003 – 150 mg film-coated tablet

9. DATE OF FIRST AUTHORISATION/RENEWAL OF THE AUTHORISATION

19 September 2005

10. DATE OF REVISION OF THE TEXT

28 May 2009

Not all strengths may be marketed.

LEGAL STATUS

POM

Targinact 10mg/5mg and 20mg/10mg prolonged-release tablets

(Napp Pharmaceuticals Limited)

1. NAME OF THE MEDICINAL PRODUCT

Targinact▼® 10 mg/5 mg prolonged-release tablets

Targinact▼® 20 mg/10 mg prolonged-release tablets

2. QUALITATIVE AND QUANTITATIVE COMPOSITION

Targinact 10 mg/5 mg

Each prolonged-release tablet contains:

10 mg of oxycodone hydrochloride equivalent to 9.0 mg oxycodone

5.45 mg of naloxone hydrochloride dihydrate equivalent to 5.0 mg naloxone hydrochloride and 4.5 mg naloxone.

Targinact 20 mg/10 mg

Each prolonged-release tablet contains:

20 mg of oxycodone hydrochloride equivalent to 18.0 mg oxycodone,

10.9 mg of naloxone hydrochloride dihydrate equivalent to 10.0 mg naloxone hydrochloride and 9.0 mg naloxone

Excipients:

Targinact 10 mg/5 mg

Each prolonged-release tablet contains 64.25 mg lactose monohydrate

Targinact 20 mg/10 mg

Each prolonged-release tablet contains 54.50 mg lactose monohydrate

For a full list of excipients, see section 6.1.

3. PHARMACEUTICAL FORM

Prolonged-release tablet

Targinact 10 mg/5 mg prolonged-release tablets are oblong, white film-coated tablets, unscored and marked "OXN" on one side and "10" on the other side

Targinact 20 mg/10 mg prolonged-release tablets are oblong, pink film-coated tablets, unscored and marked "OXN" on one side and "20" on the other side.

4. CLINICAL PARTICULARS

4.1 Therapeutic indications

Severe pain, which can be adequately managed only with opioid analgesics

The opioid antagonist naloxone is added to counteract opioid-induced constipation by blocking the action of oxycodone at opioid receptors locally in the gut.

4.2 Posology and method of administration

Targinact is for oral administration.

The dosage should be adjusted to the intensity of pain and the sensitivity of the individual patient. Unless otherwise prescribed, ***Targinact*** should be administered as follows:

Adults

The usual starting dose for an opioid naïve patient is 10 mg/5 mg of oxycodone hydrochloride/ naloxone hydrochloride at 12 hourly intervals. ***Targinact*** 10 mg/5 mg prolonged-release tablets are available for these patients. Patients requiring higher doses are recommended ***Targinact*** 20 mg/10 mg prolonged-release tablets.

Patients already receiving opioids may be started on higher doses of ***Targinact***, depending on their previous opioid experience.

In clinical studies, only patients who had previously been dosed on oxycodone were switched to ***Targinact***. To date there is no clinical experience to refer to for switching from other analgesics to ***Targinact*** pursuant to steps II or III of the WHO analgesic ladder.

The analgesic efficacy of ***Targinact*** is equivalent to oxycodone prolonged-release formulations.

The maximum daily dose of ***Targinact*** is limited to 40 mg/20 mg (corresponding to 40 mg oxycodone hydrochloride and 20 mg naloxone hydrochloride, or e.g. twice daily administration of ***Targinact*** 20 mg/10 mg prolonged-release tablets). Patients requiring higher doses should be administered supplemental prolonged-release oxycodone at the same time intervals, taking into account the maximum daily dose of 400 mg prolonged-release oxycodone. In the case of supplemental oxycodone dosing, the beneficial effect of naloxone on bowel function may be impaired.

Some patients taking ***Targinact*** according to a regular time schedule require immediate release analgesics as "rescue" medication for breakthrough pain. ***Targinact*** is not intended for the treatment of breakthrough pain. For the treatment of breakthrough pain, a single dose of "rescue medication" should amount to one sixth of the equivalent daily dose of oxycodone hydrochloride. The need for more than two "rescues" per day is usually an indication that the dose of ***Targinact*** requires upward adjustment. This adjustment should be made every 1-2 days in steps of 2 × daily 10 mg/5 mg oxycodone hydrochloride/naloxone hydrochloride until a stable dose is reached. The aim is to establish a patient-specific 2 × daily dose that will maintain adequate analgesia and make use of as little rescue medication as possible for as long as pain therapy is necessary.

Targinact is taken at the determined dosage twice daily according to a fixed time schedule. While symmetric administration (the same dose mornings and evenings) subject to a fixed time schedule (every 12 hours) is appropriate for the majority of patients, some patients, depending on the individual pain situation, may benefit from asymmetric dosing tailored to their pain pattern. In general, the lowest effective analgesic dose should be selected.

In non-malignant pain therapy, daily doses of up to 40 mg/20 mg oxycodone hydrochloride/naloxone hydrochloride (corresponding to 40 mg oxycodone hydrochloride and 20 mg naloxone hydrochloride, the twice daily administration of ***Targinact*** 20 mg/10mg prolonged-release tablets) are usually sufficient, but higher doses of prolonged-release oxycodone hydrochloride may be needed.

The prolonged-release tablets can be taken with or without food with sufficient liquid. ***Targinact*** must be swallowed whole, and not broken or chewed.

Targinact should not be administered for longer than absolutely necessary. If long-term pain treatment is necessary given the nature and severity of the illness, careful and regular monitoring is required to establish to what extent further treatment is necessary. When the patient no longer needs opioid therapy, it is advisable to taper the dose gradually.

Children (under 18 years)

Targinact is not recommended for children below the age of 18 years due to a lack of data on safety and efficacy.

Elderly patients

As for younger adults the dosage should be adjusted to the intensity of the pain and the sensitivity of the individual patient.

Patients with impaired hepatic function

A clinical trial has shown that plasma concentrations of both oxycodone and naloxone are elevated in patients with hepatic impairment. Naloxone concentrations were affected to a higher degree than oxycodone (see section 5.2). The clinical relevance of a relative high naloxone exposure in hepatic impaired patients is yet not known. Caution must be exercised when administering ***Targinact*** to patients with mild hepatic impairment (see section 4.4). In patients with moderate and severe hepatic impairment ***Targinact*** is contraindicated (see section 4.3).

Patients with impaired renal function

A clinical trial has shown that plasma concentrations of both oxycodone and naloxone are elevated in patients with renal impairment (see section 5.2). Naloxone concentrations were affected to a higher degree than oxycodone. The clinical relevance of a relative high naloxone exposure in renal impaired patients is yet not known. Caution should be exercised when administering ***Targinact*** to patients with renal impairment (see section 4.4).

4.3 Contraindications

- Hypersensitivity to the active substances or to any of the excipients;
- Any situation where opioids are contraindicated;
- Severe respiratory depression with hypoxia and/or hypercapnoea; severe chronic obstructive pulmonary disease,
- Cor pulmonale,
- Acute severe bronchial asthma,
- Non-opioid induced paralytic ileus,
- Moderate to severe hepatic impairment.

4.4 Special warnings and precautions for use

Targinact is not suitable for the treatment of withdrawal symptoms.

If abused parenterally, intranasally or orally by individuals dependent on opioid agonists, such as heroin, morphine, or methadone, ***Targinact*** is expected to produce marked withdrawal symptoms - because of the opioid receptor antagonist characteristics of naloxone - or to intensify withdrawal symptoms already present (see section 4.9 - "Overdose").

Any abuse of ***Targinact*** by drug addicts is strongly discouraged.

Studies have not been performed on the safety and efficacy of ***Targinact*** in children below the age of 18 years, therefore their use in children under 18 years of age is not recommended.

Safety and efficacy of this product are not established in cancer patients and/or patients with liver metastasis.

The major risk from opioids is respiratory depression.

Caution must be exercised when administering ***Targinact*** to elderly or infirm patients, patients with opioid-induced paralytic ileus, patients presenting severely impaired pulmonary function, myxoedema, hypothyroidism, Addison's disease (adrenal cortical insufficiency), toxic psychosis, cholelithiasis, prostate hypertrophy, alcoholism, delirium tremens, pancreatitis, hypotension, hypertension, pre-existing cardiovascular diseases, head injury (due to the risk of increased intracranial pressure), epileptic disorder or predisposition to convulsions, or patients taking MAO inhibitors.

Caution must also be exercised when administering ***Targinact*** to patients with mild hepatic or renal impairment. A careful medical monitoring is particularly necessary for patients with severe renal impairment.

The occurrence of diarrhoea should be considered as a possible effect of naloxone.

In patients under long-term opioid treatment with higher doses of opioids, the switch to ***Targinact*** can initially provoke withdrawal symptoms. Such patients may require specific attention.

During long-term administration, the patient may develop tolerance to the drug and require higher doses to maintain the desired analgesic effect. Chronic administration of ***Targinact*** may lead to physical dependence. Withdrawal symptoms may occur upon the abrupt cessation of therapy. If therapy with ***Targinact*** is no longer required, it may be advisable to reduce the daily dose gradually.

Targinact consists of a dual-polymer matrix, intended for oral use only. Abusive parenteral injections of the tablet constituents (especially talc) can be expected to result in local tissue necrosis and pulmonary granulomas or may lead to other serious, potentially fatal undesirable effects. In opioid addicts who abuse ***Targinact***, acute withdrawal symptoms will be induced or already existing symptoms will be intensified.

In order not to impair the prolonged-release characteristic of the tablets, the tablets must be taken whole and must not be broken, chewed or crushed. Breaking, chewing or crushing the tablets for ingestion leads to a faster release of the active substances and the absorption of a possibly fatal dose of oxycodone (see Section 4.9 - "Overdose").

Targinact is not recommended for pre-operative use or within the first 12-24 hours post-operatively. Depending on the type and extent of surgery, the anaesthetic procedure selected, other co-medication and the individual condition of the patient, the exact timing for initiating postoperative treatment with ***Targinact*** depends on a careful risk-benefit assessment for each individual patient.

The empty tablet matrix may be visible in the stool.

The use of ***Targinact*** may produce positive results in doping controls

This medicinal product contains lactose. Patients with rare hereditary problems of galactose intolerance, Lapp lactase deficiency or glucose-galactose malabsorption should not take ***Targinact***.

4.5 Interaction with other medicinal products and other forms of interaction

No interaction studies have been performed.

Substances having a CNS-depressant effect (e.g. alcohol, other opioids, sedatives, hypnotics, anti-depressants, sleeping aids, phenothiazines, neuroleptics, anti-histamines and anti-emetics) may enhance the CNS-depressant effect (e.g. respiratory depression) of ***Targinact***.

Clinically relevant changes in International Normalized Ratio (INR or Quick-value) in both directions have been observed in individuals if oxycodone and coumarin anticoagulants are co-applied.

In vitro metabolism studies indicate that no clinically relevant interactions are to be expected between oxycodone and naloxone. At therapeutic concentrations, ***Targinact*** is not expected to cause clinically relevant interactions with other concomitantly administered drugs metabolised over the CYP isomers CYP1A2, CYP2A6, CYP2C9/19, CYP2D6, CYP2E1 and CYP3A4. In addition, the likelihood of clinically relevant interactions between paracetamol, acetylsalicylic acid or naltrexone and the combination of oxycodone and naloxone in therapeutic concentrations is minimal.

4.6 Pregnancy and lactation

Pregnancy

There are no data from the use of ***Targinact*** in pregnant women and during childbirth. Limited data on the use of oxycodone during pregnancy in humans reveal no evidence of an increased risk of congenital abnormalities. For naloxone, insufficient clinical data on exposed pregnancies are available. However, systemic exposure of the women to naloxone after use of ***Targinact*** is relatively low (see Section 5). Both oxycodone and naloxone pass into the placenta. Animal studies have not been performed with oxycodone and naloxone in combination (see Section 5.3). Animal studies with oxycodone or naloxone administered as single drugs have not revealed any teratogenic or embryotoxic effects. Long-term administration of oxycodone during pregnancy may lead to withdrawal symptoms in the newborn. If administered during childbirth oxycodone may evoke respiratory depression in the newborn.

Targinact should only be used during pregnancy if the benefit outweighs the possible risks to the unborn child or neonate.

Lactation

Oxycodone passes into the breast milk. A milk-plasma concentration ratio of 3.4:1 was measured and oxycodone effects in the suckling infant are therefore conceivable. It is not known whether naloxone also passes into the breast milk. However, after use of ***Targinact*** systemic naloxone levels are very low (see Section 5).

Breast-feeding should be discontinued during treatment with ***Targinact***.

4.7 Effects on ability to drive and use machines

Targinact may impair the ability to drive and use machines. This is particularly likely at the beginning of treatment with ***Targinact***, after dose increase or product rotation and if ***Targinact*** is combined with alcohol or other CNS depressant agents. Patients stabilised on a specific dosage will not necessarily be restricted. Therefore, patients should consult with their physician as to whether driving or the use of machinery is permitted.

4.8 Undesirable effects

The following frequencies are the basis for assessing undesirable effects:

Very common (≥ 1/10)

Common (≥ 1/100 to < 1/10)

Uncommon (≥ 1/1,000 to < 1/100)

Rare (≥ 1/10,000 to < 1/1,000)

Very rare (<1/10,000), not known (cannot be estimated from the available data)

Within each frequency grouping, undesirable effects are presented in order of decreasing seriousness.

Immune system disorders

Uncommon: Hypersensitivity

Metabolism and nutrition disorders

Common: Decreased appetite up to loss of appetite

Psychiatric disorders

Common: Anxiety, restlessness

Uncommon: Abnormal thinking, confusion, depression, hallucination

Nervous system disorders

Common: Headache, sedation, tremor

Uncommon: Disturbance in attention, paraesthesia, speech disorder

Rare: Convulsions (particularly in persons with epileptic disorder or predisposition to convulsions)

Unknown: Syncope

Eye disorders

Uncommon: Visual disturbances

Ear and labyrinth disorders

Common: Vertigo

Cardiac disorders

Uncommon: Angina pectoris in particular in patients with history of coronary artery disease, palpitations

Vascular disorders

Common: Decrease in blood pressure

Uncommon: Increase in blood pressure

Respiratory, thoracic and mediastinal disorders

Common: Rhinorrhoea, yawning

Uncommon: Dyspnoea

Gastrointestinal disorders

Common: Abdominal pain, diarrhoea, dry mouth, flatulence, vomiting, nausea

Unknown: Constipation

Hepatobiliary disorders

Unknown: Biliary colic

Reproductive system and breast disorders

Uncommon: Erectile dysfunction

Skin and subcutaneous tissue disorders

Common: Pruritus, skin reactions, hyperhidrosis

Musculoskeletal and connective tissue disorders

Common: Muscle spasms, muscle twitching, myalgia

General disorders and application site conditions

Common: Drug withdrawal syndrome, feeling hot and cold, chills, asthenic conditions

Uncommon: Chest pain, insomnia, malaise, peripheral oedema

Injury, poisoning and procedural complications

Uncommon: Injuries from accidents

For the active substance oxycodone, the following additional undesirable effects are known:

Due to its pharmacological properties, oxycodone may cause respiratory depression, miosis, bronchial spasm and spasms of nonstriated muscles as well as suppress the cough reflex.

Infections and infestations

Rare: Herpes simplex

Immune system disorders

Very rare: Anaphylactic reaction

Metabolism and nutrition disorders

Rare: Dehydration, increased appetite

Psychiatric disorders

Common: Altered mood and personality change (e.g. depression, euphoric mood), decreased activity, psychomotor hyperactivity, agitation, nervousness, insomnia, abnormal thinking, confusion

Uncommon: Perception disturbances (e.g. hallucination, derealisation), reduced libido

The development of psychological dependence on opioid analgesics in properly managed patients with pain has been reported to be rare. However, there are no data to establish the true incidence of psychological dependence in chronic pain patients.

Nervous system disorders

Very common: Sedation (somnolence up to a depressed level of consciousness), dizziness, headache

Common: Syncope, paraesthesia

Uncommon: Migraine, dysgeusia, hypertonia, involuntary muscle contractions, hypoaesthesia, abnormal coordination

Ear and labyrinth disorders

Uncommon: Hearing impaired

Cardiac disorders

Uncommon: Tachycardia

Vascular disorders

Uncommon: Vasodilatation

Respiratory, thoracic and mediastinal disorders

Common: Dyspnoea

Uncommon: Dysphonia, cough

Gastrointestinal disorders

Very common: Constipation, vomiting, nausea

Common: Hiccups, dyspepsia

Uncommon: Mouth ulceration, stomatitis

Rare: Melaena, tooth disorder, gingival bleeding, dysphagia

Very rare: Ileus

Hepatobiliary disorders

Uncommon: Biliary colic

Very rare: Hepatic enzymes increased

Skin and subcutaneous tissue disorders

Very common: Pruritus

Rare: Dry skin

Very rare: Urticaria

Renal and urinary disorders

Common: Urinary retention, dysuria, micturition urgency

Reproductive system and breast disorders

Rare: Amenorrhoea

General disorders and administration site conditions

Uncommon: Pain, oedema

Rare: Weight increase, weight decrease, thirst

Unknown: Drug tolerance

4.9 Overdose

Symptoms and intoxication:

Depending on the history of the patient, an overdose of ***Targinact*** may be manifested by symptoms that are either triggered by oxycodone (opioid receptor agonist) or by naloxone (opioid receptor antagonist).

Symptoms of oxycodone overdose include miosis, respiratory depression, somnolence progressing to stupor, skeletal muscle flaccidity, bradycardia as well as hypotension. Coma, non-cardiogenic pulmonary oedema and circulatory failure may occur in more severe cases and may lead to a fatal outcome.

Symptoms of a naloxone overdose alone are unlikely.

Therapy of intoxications:

Withdrawal symptoms due to an overdose of naloxone should be treated symptomatically in a closely-supervised environment.

Clinical symptoms suggestive of an oxycodone overdose may be treated by the administration of opioid antagonists (e.g. naloxone 0.4-2 mg intravenously). Administration should be repeated at 2-3 minute intervals, as clinically necessary. It is also possible to apply an infusion of 2 mg naloxone in 500 ml of 0.9% sodium chloride or 5% dextrose (0.004 mg/ml naloxone). The infusion should run at a rate aligned to the previously administered bolus doses and to the patient's response.

Consideration may be given to gastric lavage.

Supportive measures (artificial ventilation, oxygen, vasopressors and infusions) should be employed, as necessary, to manage the circulatory shock accompanying an overdose. Cardiac arrest or arrhythmias may require cardiac massage or defibrillation. Artificial ventilation should be applied if necessary. Fluid and electrolyte metabolism should be maintained.

5. PHARMACOLOGICAL PROPERTIES

5.1 Pharmacodynamic properties

Oxycodone hydrochloride:

Pharmacotherapeutic group: Natural opium alkaloids

Naloxone hydrochloride:

Pharmacotherapeutic group: Opioid receptor antagonists

Oxycodone and naloxone have an affinity for kappa, mu and delta opiate receptors in the brain, spinal cord and peripheral organs (e.g. intestine). Oxycodone acts as opioid-receptor agonist at these receptors and affects pain relief by binding to the endogenous opioid receptors in the CNS. By contrast, naloxone is a pure antagonist acting on all types of opioid receptors.

Because of the pronounced first-pass metabolism, the bioavailability of naloxone upon oral administration is <3%, therefore a clinically relevant systemic effect is unlikely. Due to the local competitive antagonism of the opioid receptor mediated oxycodone effect by naloxone in the gut, naloxone reduces the bowel function disorders that are typical for opioid treatment.

In a 12 weeks parallel controlled, blinded study in 322 patients with opioid-induced constipation, patients who were treated with oxycodone-naloxone had on average one extra spontaneous bowel movement in the last week of treatment, compared to patients who continued using similar doses of oxycodone prolonged release tablets ($p<0.0001$). The use of laxatives in the first four weeks was significantly lower in the oxycodone-naloxone group compared to the oxycodone monotherapy group (31% versus 55%, respectively, $p<0.0001$).

Compared to immediate release oxycodone preparations, ***Targinact*** tablets relieve pain for a considerably longer period of time.

Opioids can influence the hypothalamic-pituitary-adrenal or gonadal axes. Among the changes observed are an increase of prolactin in the serum and a reduced level of cortisol and testosterone in the plasma. Clinical symptoms may occur because of these hormone changes.

Preclinical studies show differing effects of natural opioids on components of the immune system. The clinical significance of these findings is not known. It is not known whether oxycodone, a semi-synthetic opioid, has similar effects on the immune system to natural opioids.

5.2 Pharmacokinetic properties

Oxycodone hydrochloride

Absorption

Oxycodone has a high absolute bioavailability of up to 87% following oral administration.

Distribution

Following absorption, oxycodone is distributed throughout the entire body. Plasma protein binding is approximately 45%. Oxycodone also crosses the placenta and may be detected in breast milk.

Metabolism

Oxycodone is metabolised in the liver, via the cytochrome P450-dependent enzyme system, to noroxycodone, oxymorphone, noroxymorphone and various glucuronides. Oxycodone is metabolised to noroxycodone primarily via CYP3A4 enzymes and to oxymorphone via CYP2D6. Both metabolites are further converted to Noroxymorphone. The formation of noroxymorphone is catalysed by recombinant CYP2D6 and CYP3A4 from noroxycodone and oxymorphone, respectively. CYP3A4 is the major CYP isoform responsible for noroxycodone formation, followed by CYP2B6, CYP2C9, CYP2C19, and CYP2D6. CYP2D6 is the major CYP isoform responsible for oxymorphone formation followed by CYP2C19. The analgesic effects of these metabolites are thought to be clinically insignificant. Noroxymorphone, with its high receptor potency and relative abundance in plasma may contribute to the pharmacodynamics of oxycodone. However, due to its low lipophilicity and its low ability to cross the blood-brain barrier, its prevalence in the brain is minimal.

Elimination

Oxycodone and its metabolites are excreted in both urine and faeces.

The plasma concentrations of oxycodone are only nominally affected by age, i.e. 15% higher concentrations in elderly patients than in young subjects. Female subjects have, on average, plasma oxycodone concentrations up to 25% higher than males on a bodyweight-adjusted basis.

When compared to healthy subjects, patients with mild to severe hepatic dysfunction may demonstrate higher plasma concentrations of oxycodone and noroxycodone, and lower concentrations of oxymorphone. There may be an increase in the elimination half-life of oxycodone that could be accompanied by enhanced efficacy.

When compared to healthy subjects, patients with mild to severe renal dysfunction (creatinine clearance < 60 ml/min) may show higher plasma concentrations of oxycodone and its metabolites. There may be an increase in the elimination half-life of oxycodone that could be accompanied by enhanced efficacy.

Naloxone hydrochloride

Absorption

Following oral administration, naloxone has a very low systemic availability of <3%.

Distribution

Naloxone passes into the placenta. It is not known, whether naloxone also passes into breast milk.

Metabolism & Elimination

After parenteral administration, the plasma half-life is approximately one hour. The duration of action depends upon the dose and route of administration, intramuscular injection producing a more prolonged effect than intravenous doses. It is metabolised in the liver and excreted in the urine. The principal metabolites are naloxone glucuronide, 6β-Naloxol and its glucuronide.

Oxycodone hydrochloride/ naloxone hydrochloride combination (***Targinact***)

Pharmacokinetics of the combination

The pharmacokinetic characteristics of oxycodone from ***Targinact*** is equivalent to those of prolonged-release oxycodone tablets (***OxyContin®***) administered together with prolonged-release naloxone tablets.

The interchangeability of the two strengths (***Targinact*** 10 mg/5mg and ***Targinact*** 20 mg/10mg prolonged-release tablets) has been demonstrated.

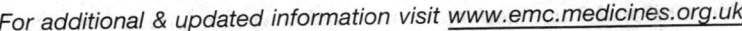

After the oral administration of ***Targinact*** in maximum dose, the plasma concentrations of naloxone are so low that it is not feasible to carry out a pharmacokinetic analysis. However, it is possible to conduct a pharmacokinetic

analysis of naloxone-3-glucuronide as surrogate marker, since the plasma concentration is high enough to measure.

The maximum plasma concentration and bioavailability of oxycodone after ingestion of ***Targinact*** following a high-fat breakfast was approximately 15-20% higher compared to administration in the fasting state. This was evaluated as clinically not relevant, therefore ***Targinact*** may be taken with or without food (see section 4.2 Posology and method of administration).

Drug interactions

In vitro drug metabolism studies have indicated that the occurrence of clinically relevant interactions involving ***Targinact*** is unlikely.

Patients with impaired hepatic function

Oxycodone:

For AUCINF of oxycodone, on average there was an increase to 143% (90% C.I.: 111, 184), 319% (90% C.I.: 248, 411) and 310% (90% C.I.: 241, 398) for mild, moderate and severe hepatically impaired subjects, respectively, compared with healthy volunteers. For Cmax of oxycodone, on average there was an increase to 120% (90% C.I.: 99, 144), 201% (90% C.I.: 166, 242) and 191% (90% C.I.: 158, 231) for mild, moderate and severe hepatically impaired subjects, respectively, compared with healthy volunteers. For t1/2Z of oxycodone, on average there was an increase to 108% (90% C.I.: 70, 146), 176% (90% C.I.: 138, 215) and 183% (90% C.I.: 145, 221) for mild, moderate and severe hepatically impaired subjects, respectively, compared with healthy volunteers.

Naloxone:

For AUCt of naloxone, on average there was an increase to 411% (90% C.I.: 152, 1112), 11518% (90% C.I.: 4259, 31149) and 10666% (90% C.I.: 3944, 28847) for mild, moderate and severe hepatically impaired subjects, respectively, compared with healthy volunteers. For Cmax of naloxone, on average there was an increase to 193% (90% C.I.: 115, 324), 5292% (90% C.I: 3148, 8896) and 5252% (90% C.I.: 3124, 8830) for mild, moderate and severe hepatically impaired subjects, respectively, compared with healthy volunteers. Due to insufficient amount of data available t1/2Z and the corresponding AUCINF of naloxone were not calculated. The bioavailability comparisons for naloxone were therefore based on AUCt values.

Naloxone-3-glucuronide:

For AUCINF of naloxone-3-glucuronide, on average there was an increase to 157% (90% C.I.: 89, 279), 128% (90% C.I.: 72, 227) and 125% (90% C.I.: 71, 222) for mild, moderate and severe hepatically impaired subjects, respectively, compared with healthy volunteers. For Cmax of naloxone-3-glucuronide, on average there was an increase to 141% (90% C.I.: 100, 197), 118% (90% C.I.: 84, 166) and a decrease to 98% (90% C.I.: 70, 137) for mild, moderate and severe hepatically impaired subjects, respectively, compared with healthy volunteers. For t1/2Z of naloxone-3-glucuronide, on average there was an increase to 117% (90% C.I.: 72, 161), a decrease to 77% (90% C.I.: 32, 121) and a decrease to 94% (90% C.I.: 49, 139) for mild, moderate and severe hepatically impaired subjects, respectively, compared with healthy volunteers.

Patients with impaired renal function

Oxycodone:

For AUCINF of oxycodone, on average there was an increase to 153% (90% C.I.: 130, 182), 166% (90% C.I.: 140, 196) and 224% (90% C.I.: 190, 266) for mild, moderate and severe renally impaired subjects, respectively, compared with healthy volunteers. For Cmax of oxycodone, on average there was an increase to 110% (90% C.I.: 94, 129), 135% (90% C.I.: 115, 159) and 167% (90% C.I.: 142, 196) for mild, moderate and severe renally impaired subjects, respectively, compared with healthy volunteers. For t1/2Z of oxycodone, on average there was an increase to 149%, 123% and 142% for mild, moderate and severe renally impaired subjects, respectively, compared with healthy volunteers.

Naloxone:

For AUCt of naloxone, on average there was an increase to 2850% (90% C.I.: 369, 22042), 3910% (90% C.I.: 506, 30243) and 7612% (90% C.I.: 984, 58871) for mild, moderate and severe renally impaired subjects, respectively, compared with healthy volunteers. For Cmax of naloxone, on average there was an increase to 1076% (90% C.I.: 154, 7502), 858% (90% C.I.: 123, 5981) and 1675% (90% C.I.: 240, 11676) for mild, moderate and severe renally impaired subjects, respectively, compared with healthy volunteers. Due to insufficient amount of data available t1/2Z and the corresponding AUCINF of naloxone were not calculated. The bioavailability comparisons for naloxone were therefore based on AUCt values. The ratios may have been influenced by the inability to fully characterize the naloxone plasma profiles for the healthy subjects.

Naloxone-3-glucuronide:

For AUCINF of naloxone-3-glucuronide, on average there was an increase to 220% (90% C.I.: 148, 327), 370% (90% C.I.: 249, 550) and 525% (90% C.I.: 354, 781) for mild, moderate and severe renally impaired subjects, respectively, compared with healthy subjects. For Cmax of naloxone-3-glucuronide, on average there was an increase to 148% (90% C.I.: 110, 197), 202% (90% C.I.: 151, 271) and 239% (90% C.I.: 179, 320) for mild, moderate and severe renally impaired subjects, respectively, compared with healthy subjects. For t1/2Z of naloxone-3-glucuronide, on average there was no significant change between the renally impaired subjects and the healthy subjects.

Abuse

To avoid damage to the prolonged-release properties of the tablets, ***Targinact*** must not be broken, crushed or chewed, as this leads to a faster release of the active substances. In addition, following intra-nasal administration, naloxone has significant systemic bioavailability and a slow elimination rate when administered intranasally. These properties mean that abuse of ***Targinact*** will not have the effect intended. In oxycodone-dependent rats, the intravenous administration of oxycodone/ naloxone at a ratio of 2:1 resulted in withdrawal symptoms.

5.3 Preclinical safety data

There are no data from studies on reproductive toxicity of the combination of oxycodone and naloxone. Studies with the single components showed that oxycodone had no effect on fertility and early embryonic development in male and female rats in doses of up to 8 mg/kg body weight and induced no malformations in rats in doses of up to 8 mg/kg and in rabbits in doses of 125 mg/kg bodyweight. However, in rabbits, when individual foetuses were used in statistical evaluation, a dose related increase in developmental variations was observed (increased incidences of 27 presacral vertebrae, extra pairs of ribs). When these parameters were statistically evaluated using litters, only the incidence of 27 presacral vertebrae was increased and only in the 125 mg/kg group, a dose level that produced severe pharmacotoxic effects in the pregnant animals. In a study on pre- and postnatal development in rats F1 body weights were lower at 6 mg/kg/d when compared to body weights of the control group at doses which reduced maternal weight and food intake (NOAEL 2 mg/kg body weight). There were neither effects on physical, reflexological, and sensory developmental parameters nor on behavioural and reproductive indices. The standard oral reproduction toxicity studies with naloxone show that at high oral doses naloxone was not teratogenic and/or embryo/foetotoxic, and does not affect perinatal/postnatal development. At very high doses (800 mg/kg/day) naloxone produced increased pup deaths in the immediate post-partum period at dosages that produced significant toxicity in maternal rats (e.g., body weight loss, convulsions). However, in surviving pups, no effects on development or behaviour were observed.

Long-term carcinogenicity studies with oxycodone/naloxone in combination or oxycodone as single entity were not performed. Naloxone was not carcinogenic in a long-term study in rats.

Oxycodone and naloxone as single entities show a clastogenic potential in *in vitro* assays. No similar effects were observed, however, under *in vivo* conditions, even at toxic doses. The results indicate that the mutagenic risk of ***Targinact*** to humans at therapeutic concentrations may be ruled out with adequate certainty.

For naloxone, a 24-months oral carcinogenicity study was performed in rats with naloxone doses up to 100 mg/kg/day. The results indicate that naloxone is not carcinogenic under these conditions.

6. PHARMACEUTICAL PARTICULARS

6.1 List of excipients

Tablet core:

Povidone K30,

Ethylcellulose N45,

Stearyl alcohol,

Lactose monohydrate,

Talc,

Magnesium stearate

Targinact 10 mg/5 mg

Tablet coat

Poly(vinylalcohol),

Titanium dioxide (E171),

Macrogol 3350,

Talc

Targinact 20 mg/10 mg

Tablet coat:

Poly(vinylalcohol),

Titanium dioxide (E171),

Macrogol 3350,

Talc

Iron (III) oxide red (E172)

6.2 Incompatibilities

Not applicable.

6.3 Shelf life

3 years

6.4 Special precautions for storage

Do not store above 25°C.

6.5 Nature and contents of container

Polyvinylchloride/aluminium foil blisters containing 56 prolonged-release tablets

6.6 Special precautions for disposal and other handling

None

7. MARKETING AUTHORISATION HOLDER

Napp Pharmaceuticals Ltd

Cambridge Science Park

Milton Road

Cambridge CB4 0GW

8. MARKETING AUTHORISATION NUMBER(S)

PL16950/0157-8

9. DATE OF FIRST AUTHORISATION/RENEWAL OF THE AUTHORISATION

29/12/2008

10. DATE OF REVISION OF THE TEXT

29/12/2008

11 LEGAL CATEGORY

CD (Sch 2) POM

Targinact 5mg/2.5mg and 40mg/20mg prolonged release tablets

(Napp Pharmaceuticals Limited)

1. NAME OF THE MEDICINAL PRODUCT

Targinact®▼ 5 mg/2.5 mg prolonged-release tablets

Targinact®▼ 40 mg/20 mg prolonged-release tablets

2. QUALITATIVE AND QUANTITATIVE COMPOSITION

Targinact 5 mg/2.5 mg

Each prolonged-release tablet contains 5 mg of oxycodone hydrochloride equivalent to 4.5 mg oxycodone,

2.73 mg of naloxone hydrochloride dihydrate equivalent to 2.5 mg naloxone hydrochloride and 2.25 mg naloxone.

Excipients: Each prolonged-release tablet contains 68.17 mg lactose anhydrous

Targinact 40 mg/20 mg

Each prolonged-release tablet contains 40 mg of oxycodone hydrochloride equivalent to 36.0 mg oxycodone,

21.8 mg of naloxone hydrochloride dihydrate equivalent to 20.0 mg naloxone hydrochloride and 18.0 mg naloxone

Excipients: Each prolonged-release tablet contains 103.55 mg lactose anhydrous

For a full list of excipients, see section 6.1.

3. PHARMACEUTICAL FORM

Prolonged-release tablet

Targinact 5 mg/2.5 mg

Oblong, blue film-coated tablets, marked "OXN" on one side and "5" on the other side.

Targinact 40 mg/20 mg

Oblong, yellow film-coated tablets, marked "OXN" on one side and "40" on the other side.

4. CLINICAL PARTICULARS

4.1 Therapeutic indications

Severe pain, which can be adequately managed only with opioid analgesics

The opioid antagonist naloxone is added to counteract opioid-induced constipation by blocking the action of oxycodone at opioid receptors locally in the gut.

4.2 Posology and method of administration

Targinact is for oral use.

Posology

The analgesic efficacy of ***Targinact*** is equivalent to oxycodone hydrochloride prolonged-release formulations.

The dosage should be adjusted to the intensity of pain and the sensitivity of the individual patient. Unless otherwise prescribed, ***Targinact*** should be administered as follows:

Adults

The usual starting dose for an opioid naïve patient is 10 mg/ 5 mg of oxycodone hydrochloride/naloxone hydrochloride at 12 hourly intervals.

Patients already receiving opioids may be started on higher doses of ***Targinact*** depending on their previous opioid experience.

Targinact 5 mg/2.5 mg is intended for dose titration when initiating opioid therapy and individual dose adjustment.

The maximum daily dose of ***Targinact*** is 80 mg oxycodone hydrochloride and 40 mg naloxone hydrochloride. For patients requiring higher doses of ***Targinact***, administration of supplemental oxycodone hydrochloride prolonged-release at the same time intervals should be considered, taking into account the maximum daily dose of 400 mg prolonged-release oxycodone hydrochloride. In the case of supplemental oxycodone hydrochloride dosing, the beneficial effect of naloxone hydrochloride on bowel function may be impaired.

After complete discontinuation of therapy with ***Targinact*** with a subsequent switch to another opioid a worsening of the bowel function can be expected.

Some patients taking ***Targinact*** according to a regular time schedule require immediate-release analgesics as "rescue" medication for breakthrough pain. ***Targinact*** is a prolonged-release formulation and therefore not intended for the treatment of breakthrough pain. For the treatment of breakthrough pain, a single dose of "rescue medication" should approximate one sixth of the equivalent daily dose of oxycodone hydrochloride. The need for more than two"rescues" per day is usually an indication that the dose of **Targinact** requires upward adjustment. This adjustment should be made every 1-2 days in steps of twice daily 5 mg/2.5 mg, or where demanded 10 mg/5 mg, oxycodone hydrochloride/naloxone hydrochoride until a stable dose is reached. The aim is to establish a patient-specific twice daily dose that will maintain adequate analgesia and make use of as little rescue medication as possible for as long as pain therapy is necessary.

Targinact is taken at the determined dosage twice daily according to a fixed time schedule. While symmetric administration (the same dose mornings and evenings) subject to a fixed time schedule (every 12 hours) is appropriate for the majority of patients, some patients, depending on the individual pain situation, may benefit from asymmetric dosing tailored to their pain pattern. In general, the lowest effective analgesic dose should be selected.

In non-malignant pain therapy, daily doses of up to 40 mg/ 20 mg oxycodone hydrochloride/naloxone hydrochloride are usually sufficient, but higher doses may be needed.

For doses not realisable/practicable with this strength other strengths of this medicinal product are available.

Children and adolescents (under 18 years)

Targinact is not recommended for use in children and adolescents below the age of 18 years due to a lack of data on safety and efficacy.

Elderly patients

As for younger adults the dosage should be adjusted to the intensity of the pain and the sensitivity of the individual patient.

Patients with impaired hepatic function

A clinical trial has shown that plasma concentrations of both oxycodone and naloxone are elevated in patients with hepatic impairment. Naloxone concentrations were affected to a higher degree than oxycodone (see section 5.2). The clinical relevance of a relative high naloxone exposure in hepatic impaired patients is yet not known. Caution must be exercised when administering **Targinact** to patients with mild hepatic impairment (see section 4.4). In patients with moderate and severe hepatic impairment **Targinact** is contraindicated (see section 4.3).

Patients with impaired renal function

A clinical trial has shown that plasma concentrations of both oxycodone and naloxone are elevated in patients with renal impairment (see section 5.2). Naloxone concentrations were affected to a higher degree than oxycodone. The clinical relevance of a relative high naloxone exposure in renal impaired patients is yet not known. Caution should be exercised when administering **Targinact** to patients with renal impairment (see section 4.4).

Method of administration

Targinact is taken in the determined dosage twice daily in a fixed time schedule.

The prolonged-release tablets may be taken with or without food with sufficient liquid. **Targinact** must be swallowed whole, and not broken or chewed.

Duration of use

Targinact should not be administered for longer than absolutely necessary. If long-term pain treatment is necessary in view the nature and severity of the illness, careful and regular monitoring is required to establish whether and to what extent further treatment is necessary. When the patient no longer requires opioid therapy, it may be advisable to taper the dose gradually (see section 4.4).

4.3 Contraindications

- Hypersensitivity to the active substances or to any of the excipients,
- Any situation where opioids are contraindicated,
- Severe respiratory depression with hypoxia and/or hypercapnia,
- Severe chronic obstructive pulmonary disease,
- Cor pulmonale,
- Severe bronchial asthma,
- Non-opioid induced paralytic ileus,
- Moderate to severe hepatic impairment.

4.4 Special warnings and precautions for use

The major risk from opioids is respiratory depression.

Caution must be exercised when administering **Targinact** to elderly or infirm patients, patients with opioid-induced paralytic ileus, patients presenting severely impaired pulmonary function, myxoedema, hypothyroidism, Addison's disease (adrenal cortical insufficiency), toxic psychosis, cholelithiasis, prostate hypertrophy, alcoholism, delirium tremens, pancreatitis, hypotension, hypertension, pre-existing cardiovascular diseases, head injury (due to the risk of increased intracranial pressure), epileptic disorder or predisposition to convulsions, or patients taking MAO inhibitors.

Caution must also be exercised when administering **Targinact** to patients with mild hepatic or renal impairment. A careful medical monitoring is particularly necessary for patients with severe renal impairment.

Diarrhoea may be considered as a possible effect of naloxone.

In patients under long-term opioid treatment with higher doses of opioids, the switch to **Targinact** can initially provoke withdrawal symptoms. Such patients may require specific attention.

Targinact is not suitable for the treatment of withdrawal symptoms.

During long-term administration, the patient may develop tolerance to the medicinal product and require higher doses to maintain the desired analgesic effect. Chronic administration of **Targinact** may lead to physical dependence. Withdrawal symptoms may occur upon the abrupt cessation of therapy. If therapy with **Targinact** is no longer required, it may be advisable to reduce the daily dose gradually in order to avoid the occurrence of withdrawal syndrome.

There is potential for development of psychological dependence (addiction) to opioid analgesics, including **Targinact. Targinact** should be used with particular care in patients with a history of alcohol and drug abuse. Oxycodone alone has an abuse profile similar to other strong agonist opioids.

In order not to impair the prolonged-release characteristic of the prolonged-release tablets, the prolonged-release tablets must be taken whole and must not be broken, chewed or crushed. Breaking, chewing or crushing the prolonged-release tablets for ingestion leads to a faster release of the active substances and the absorption of a possibly fatal dose of oxycodone (see section 4.9).

Studies have not been performed on the safety and efficacy of **Targinact** in children and adolescents below the age of 18 years. Therefore, their use in children and adolescents under 18 years of age is not recommended.

There is no clinical experience in patients with cancer associated to peritoneal carcinomatosis or with sub-occlusive syndrome in advanced stages of digestive and pelvic cancers. Therefore, the use of **Targinact** in this population is not recommended.

Targinact is not recommended for pre-operative use or within the first 12-24 hours post-operatively. Depending on the type and extent of surgery, the anaesthetic procedure selected, other co-medication and the individual condition of the patient, the exact timing for initiating postoperative treatment with **Targinact** depends on a careful risk-benefit assessment for each individual patient.

Any abuse of **Targinact** by drug addicts is strongly discouraged.

If abused parenterally, intranasally or orally by individuals dependent on opioid agonists, such as heroin, morphine, or methadone, **Targinact** is expected to produce marked withdrawal symptoms - because of the opioid receptor antagonist characteristics of naloxone - or to intensify withdrawal symptoms already present (see section 4.9).

Targinact consists of a dual-polymer matrix, intended for oral use only. Abusive parenteral injections of the prolonged-release tablet constituents (especially talc) can be expected to result in local tissue necrosis and pulmonary granulomas or may lead to other serious, potentially fatal undesirable effects.

The empty prolonged-release tablet matrix may be visible in the stool.

The use of **Targinact** may produce positive results in doping controls.

The use of **Targinact** as a doping agent may become a health hazard.

This medicinal product contains lactose. Patients with rare hereditary problems of galactose intolerance, Lapp lactase deficiency or glucose-galactose malabsorption should not take **Targinact.**

4.5 Interaction with other medicinal products and other forms of interaction

No interaction studies have been performed in adults.

Substances having a CNS-depressant effect (e.g. alcohol, other opioids, sedatives, hypnotics, anti-depressants, sleeping aids, phenothiazines, neuroleptics, anti-histamines and anti-emetics) may enhance the CNS-depressant effect (e.g. respiratory depression) of **Targinact.**

Clinically relevant changes in International Normalized Ratio (INR or Quick-value) in both directions have been observed in individuals if oxycodone and coumarin anticoagulants are co-applied.

In vitro metabolism studies indicate that no clinically relevant interactions are to be expected between oxycodone and naloxone. At therapeutic concentrations, **Targinact** is not expected to cause clinically relevant interactions with other concomitantly administered active substances metabolised over the CYP isomers CYP1A2, CYP2A6, CYP2C9/19, CYP2D6, CYP2E1 and CYP3A4. In addition, the likelihood of clinically relevant interactions between paracetamol, acetylsalicylic acid or naltrexone and the combination of oxycodone and naloxone in therapeutic concentrations is minimal.

4.6 Pregnancy and lactation

Pregnancy

There are no data from the use of **Targinact** in pregnant women and during childbirth. Limited data on the use of oxycodone during pregnancy in humans reveal no evidence of an increased risk of congenital abnormalities. For naloxone, insufficient clinical data on exposed pregnancies are available. However, systemic exposure of the women to naloxone after use of **Targinact** is relatively low (see section 5.2). Both oxycodone and naloxone pass into the placenta. Animal studies have not been performed with oxycodone and naloxone in combination (see section 5.3). Animal studies with oxycodone or naloxone administered as single drugs have not revealed any teratogenic or embryotoxic effects.

Long-term administration of oxycodone during pregnancy may lead to withdrawal symptoms in the newborn. If administered during childbirth, oxycodone may evoke respiratory depression in the newborn.

Targinact should only be used during pregnancy if the benefit outweighs the possible risks to the unborn child or neonate.

Lactation

Oxycodone passes into the breast milk. A milk-plasma concentration ratio of 3.4:1 was measured and oxycodone effects in the suckling infant are therefore conceivable. It is not known whether naloxone also passes into the breast milk. However, after use of **Targinact** systemic naloxone levels are very low (see section 5.2).

A risk to the suckling child cannot be excluded in particular following intake of multiple doses of **Targinact** by the breast-feeding mother.

Breast-feeding should be discontinued during treatment with **Targinact.**

4.7 Effects on ability to drive and use machines

Targinact may impair the ability to drive and use machines. This is particularly likely at the beginning of treatment with **Targinact**, after dose increase or product rotation and if **Targinact** is combined with alcohol or other CNS depressant agents. Patients stabilised on a specific dosage will not necessarily be restricted. Therefore, patients should consult with their physician as to whether driving or the use of machinery is permitted.

4.8 Undesirable effects

The following frequencies are the basis for assessing undesirable effects:

Very common ($\geqslant$ 1/10)

Common ($\geqslant$ 1/100 to $<$ 1/10)

Uncommon ($\geqslant$ 1/1,000 to $<$ 1/100)

Rare ($\geq$ 1/10,000 to $<$ 1/1,000)

Very rare ($<$1/10,000)

Not known (cannot be estimated from the available data)

Within each frequency grouping, undesirable effects are presented in order of decreasing seriousness.

Immune system disorders

Uncommon: Hypersensitivity

Metabolism and nutrition disorders

Common: Decreased appetite up to loss of appetite

Psychiatric disorders

Common: Restlessness

Uncommon: Abnormal thinking, anxiety, confusion, depression, euphoric mood, hallucination, insomnia, nervousness

Rare: Nightmares

Nervous system disorders

Common: Dizziness, headache,

Uncommon: Disturbance in attention, paraesthesia, somnolence, speech disorder, tremor

Rare: Convulsions (particularly in persons with epileptic disorder or predisposition to convulsions), sedation, syncope

Eye disorders

Uncommon: Visual disturbances

Ear and labyrinth disorders

Common: Vertigo

Cardiac disorders

Uncommon: Angina pectoris in particular in patients with history of coronary artery disease, palpitations

Rare: Tachycardia

Vascular disorders

Common: Decrease in blood pressure

Uncommon: Increase in blood pressure

Respiratory, thoracic and mediastinal disorders

Uncommon: Dyspnoea, rhinorrhoe, cough

Rare: Yawning

Very rare: Respiratory depression

Gastrointestinal disorders

Common: Abdominal pain, constipation, diarrhoea, dry mouth, dyspepsia, vomiting, nausea, flatulence

Uncommon: Abdominal distension, eructation

Rare: Tooth disorder

Hepatobiliary disorders

Common: Hepatic enzymes increased

Uncommon: Biliary colic

Reproductive system and breast disorders

Uncommon: Erectile dysfunction

Skin and subcutaneous tissue disorders

Common: Pruritus, skin reactions, hyperhidrosis

Musculoskeletal and connective tissue disorders

Uncommon: Muscle spasms, muscle twitching, myalgia

Renal and urinary disorders

Uncommon: Micturition urgency

Rare: Urinary retention

General disorders and application site conditions

Common: Drug withdrawal syndrome, feeling hot and cold, chills, asthenic conditions

Uncommon: Chest pain, malaise, pain, peripheral oedema, weight decrease

Rare: Weight increase

Injury, poisoning and procedural complications

Uncommon: Injuries from accidents

For the active substance oxycodone hydrochloride, the following additional undesirable effects are known:

Due to its pharmacological properties, oxycodone hydrochloride may cause respiratory depression, miosis, bronchial spasm and spasms of nonstriated muscles as well as suppress the cough reflex.

Infections and infestations

Rare: Herpes simplex

Immune system disorders

Very rare: Anaphylactic responses

Metabolism and nutrition disorders

Rare: Dehydration, increased appetite

Psychiatric disorders

Common: Altered mood and personality change, decreased activity, psychomotor hyperactivity, agitation

Uncommon: Perception disturbances (e.g. derealisation), reduced libido

Not known: Drug dependence.

Nervous system disorders

Uncommon: Concentration impaired, migraine, dysgeusia, hypertonia, involuntary muscle contractions, hypoaesthesia, abnormal coordination

Ear and labyrinth disorders

Uncommon: Hearing impaired

Vascular disorders

Uncommon: Vasodilatation

Respiratory, thoracic and mediastinal disorders

Uncommon: Dysphonia

Gastrointestinal disorders

Common: Hiccups

Uncommon: Mouth ulceration, stomatitis

Rare: Melaena, gingival bleeding, dysphagia

Very rare: Ileus

Skin and subcutaneous tissue disorders

Rare: Dry skin

Very rare: Urticaria

Renal and urinary disorders

Common: Dysuria

Reproductive system and breast disorders

Rare: Amenorrhoea

General disorders and administration site conditions

Uncommon: Oedema

Rare: Thirst

Not known: Drug tolerance.

4.9 Overdose

Symptoms of intoxication

Depending on the history of the patient, an overdose of ***Targinact*** may be manifested by symptoms that are either triggered by oxycodone (opioid receptor agonist) or by naloxone (opioid receptor antagonist).

Symptoms of oxycodone overdose include miosis, respiratory depression, somnolence progressing to stupor, skeletal muscle flaccidity, bradycardia as well as hypotension. Coma, non-cardiogenic pulmonary oedema and circulatory failure may occur in more severe cases and may lead to a fatal outcome.

Symptoms of a naloxone overdose alone are unlikely.

Therapy of intoxication

Withdrawal symptoms due to an overdose of naloxone should be treated symptomatically in a closely-supervised environment.

Clinical symptoms suggestive of an oxycodone overdose may be treated by the administration of opioid antagonists (e.g. naloxone hydrochloride 0.4-2 mg intravenously). Administration should be repeated at 2-3 minute intervals, as clinically necessary. It is also possible to apply an infusion of 2 mg naloxone hydrochloride in 500 ml of 0.9% sodium chloride or 5% dextrose (0.004 mg/ml naloxone). The infusion should be run at a rate aligned to the previously administered bolus doses and to the patient's response.

Consideration may be given to gastric lavage.

Supportive measures (artificial ventilation, oxygen, vasopressors and fluid infusions) should be employed, as necessary, to manage the circulatory shock accompanying an overdose. Cardiac arrest or arrhythmias may require cardiac massage or defibrillation. Artificial ventilation should be applied if necessary. Fluid and electrolyte metabolism should be maintained.

5. PHARMACOLOGICAL PROPERTIES

5.1 Pharmacodynamic properties

Oxycodone:

Pharmacotherapeutic group: Natural opium alkaloids

ATC code: N02AA05

Naloxone:

Pharmacotherapeutic group: Antidotes

ATC code: V03AB15

Oxycodone and naloxone have an affinity for kappa, mu and delta opiate receptors in the brain, spinal cord and peripheral organs (e.g. intestine). Oxycodone acts as opioid-receptor agonist at these receptors and affects pain relief by binding to the endogenous opioid receptors in the CNS. By contrast, naloxone is a pure antagonist acting on all types of opioid receptors.

Because of the pronounced first-pass metabolism, the bioavailability of naloxone upon oral administration is $< 3\%$, therefore a clinically relevant systemic effect is unlikely. Due to the local competitive antagonism of the opioid receptor mediated oxycodone effect by naloxone in the gut, naloxone reduces the bowel function disorders that are typical for opioid treatment.

In a 12 weeks parallel group double-blinded study in 322 patients with opioid-induced constipation, patients who were treated with oxycodone hydrochloride - naloxone hydrochloride had on average one extra complete spontaneous (without laxatives) bowel movement in the last week of treatment, compared to patients who continued using similar doses of oxycodone hydrochloride prolonged release tablets ($p < 0.0001$). The use of laxatives in the first four weeks was significantly lower in the oxycodone-naloxone group compared to the oxycodone monotherapy group (31% versus 55%, respectively, $p < 0.0001$). Similar results were shown in a study with 265 non-cancer patients comparing daily doses of oxycodone hydrochloride/naloxone hydrochloride of 60 mg/30 mg to up to 80 mg/40 mg with oxycodone hydrochloride monotherapy in the same dose range.

Opioids can influence the hypothalamic-pituitary-adrenal or gonadal axes. Among the changes observed are an increase of prolactin in the serum and a reduced level of cortisol and testosterone in the plasma. Clinical symptoms may occur because of these hormone changes.

Preclinical studies show differing effects of natural opioids on components of the immune system. The clinical significance of these findings is not known. It is not known whether oxycodone, a semi-synthetic opioid, has similar effects on the immune system to natural opioids.

5.2 Pharmacokinetic properties

Oxycodone hydrochloride

Absorption

Oxycodone has a high absolute bioavailability of up to 87% following oral administration.

Distribution

Following absorption, oxycodone is distributed throughout the entire body. Approximately 45% is bound to plasma protein.

Oxycodone crosses the placenta and may be detected in breast milk.

Metabolism

Oxycodone is metabolized in the gut and the liver to noroxycodone and oxymorphone and to various glucuronide conjugates. Noroxycodone, oxymorphone and noroxymorphone are produced via the cytochrome P450 system. *In vitro* studies suggest that therapeutic doses of cimetidine are not likely to significantly influence the production of noroxycodone. Quinidine reduces the production of oxymorphone in man without substantially influencing the pharmacodynamics of oxycodone. The contribution of the metabolites to overall pharmacodynamic effect is insignificant.

Elimination

Oxycodone and its metabolites are excreted in both urine and faeces.

Naloxone hydrochloride

Absorption

Following oral administration, naloxone has a very low systemic availability of $<3\%$.

Distribution

Naloxone passes into the placenta. It is not known, whether naloxone also passes into breast milk.

Metabolism and Elimination

After parenteral administration, the plasma half-life is approximately one hour. The duration of action depends upon the dose and route of administration, intramuscular injection producing a more prolonged effect than intravenous doses. It is metabolised in the liver and excreted in the urine. The principal metabolites are naloxone glucuronide, 6β-Naloxol and its glucuronide.

Oxycodone hydrochloride/ naloxone hydrochloride combination *Targinact*

The pharmacokinetic characteristics of oxycodone from ***Targinact*** is equivalent to those of prolonged-release oxycodone hydrochloride tablets administered together with prolonged-release naloxone hydrochloride tablets.

All dosage strengths of ***Targinact*** are interchangeable.

After the oral administration of ***Targinact*** in maximum dose to healthy subjects, the plasma concentrations of naloxone are so low that it is not feasible to carry out a pharmacokinetic analysis. To conduct a pharmacokinetic analysis naloxone-3-glucuronide as surrogate marker is used, since its plasma concentration is high enough to measure.

Overall, following ingestion of a high-fat breakfast, the bioavailability and peak plasma concentration (C_{max}) of oxycodone were increased by an average of 16% and 30% respectively compared to administration in the fasting state. This was evaluated as clinically not relevant, therefore ***Targinact*** prolonged-release tablets may be taken with or without food (see section 4.2).

In vitro drug metabolism studies have indicated that the occurrence of clinically relevant interactions involving ***Targinact*** is unlikely.

Elderly patients

Oxycodone:

For AUC_τ of oxycodone, on average there was an increase to 118% (90% C.I.: 103, 135), for elderly compared with younger volunteers. For C_{max} of oxycodone, on average there was an increase to 114% (90% C.I.: 102, 127). For C_{min} of oxycodone, on average there was an increase to 128% (90% C.I.: 107, 152).

Naloxone:

For AUC_τ of naloxone, on average there was an increase to 182% (90% C.I.: 123, 270), for elderly compared with younger volunteers. For C_{max} of naloxone, on average there was an increase to 173% (90% C.I.: 107, 280). For C_{min} of naloxone, on average there was an increase to 317% (90% C.I.: 142, 708).

Naloxone-3-glucuronide:

For AUC_τ of naloxone-3-glucuronide, on average there was an increase to 128% (90% C.I.: 113, 147), for elderly compared with younger volunteers. For C_{max} of naloxone-3-glucuronide, on average there was an increase to 127% (90% C.I.: 112, 144). For C_{min} of naloxone-3-glucuronide, on average there was an increase to 125% (90% C.I.: 105, 148).

Patients with impaired hepatic function

Oxycodone:

For AUC_{INF} of oxycodone, on average there was an increase to 143% (90% C.I.: 111, 184), 319% (90% C.I.: 248, 411) and 310% (90% C.I.: 241, 398) for mild, moderate and severe hepatically impaired subjects, respectively, compared with healthy volunteers. For C_{max} of oxycodone, on average there was an increase to 120% (90% C.I.: 99, 144), 201% (90% C.I.: 166, 242) and 191% (90% C.I.: 158, 231) for mild, moderate and severe hepatically impaired subjects, respectively, compared with healthy volunteers. For $t_{1/2Z}$ of oxycodone, on average there was an increase to 108% (90% C.I.: 70, 146), 176% (90% C.I.: 138, 215) and 183% (90% C.I.: 145, 221) for mild, moderate and severe hepatically impaired subjects, respectively, compared with healthy volunteers.

Naloxone:

For AUC_t of naloxone, on average there was an increase to 411% (90% C.I.: 152, 1112), 11518% (90% C.I.: 4259, 31149) and 10666% (90% C.I.: 3944, 28847) for mild, moderate and severe hepatically impaired subjects, respectively, compared with healthy volunteers. For C_{max} of naloxone, on average there was an increase to 193% (90% C.I.: 115, 324), 5292% (90% C.I: 3148, 8896) and 5252% (90% C.I.: 3124, 8830) for mild, moderate and severe hepatically impaired subjects, respectively, compared with healthy volunteers. Due to insufficient amount of data available $t_{1/2Z}$ and the corresponding AUC_{INF} of naloxone were not calculated. The bioavailability comparisons for naloxone were therefore based on AUC_t values.

Naloxone-3-glucuronide:

For AUC_{INF} of naloxone-3-glucuronide, on average there was an increase to 157% (90% C.I.: 89, 279), 128% (90% C.I.: 72, 227) and 125% (90% C.I.: 71, 222) for mild, moderate and severe hepatically impaired subjects, respectively, compared with healthy volunteers. For C_{max} of naloxone-3-glucuronide, on average there was an increase to 141% (90% C.I.: 100, 197), 118% (90% C.I.: 84, 166) and a decrease to 98% (90% C.I.: 70, 137) for mild, moderate and severe hepatically impaired subjects, respectively, compared with healthy volunteers. For $t_{1/2Z}$ of naloxone-3-glucuronide, on average there was an increase to 117% (90% C.I.: 72, 161), a decrease to 77% (90% C.I.: 32, 121) and a decrease to 94% (90% C.I.: 49, 139) for mild, moderate and severe hepatically impaired subjects, respectively, compared with healthy volunteers.

Patients with impaired renal function

Oxycodone:

For AUC_{INF} of oxycodone, on average there was an increase to 153% (90% C.I.: 130, 182), 166% (90% C.I.: 140, 196) and 224% (90% C.I.: 190, 266) for mild, moderate and severe renally impaired subjects, respectively, compared with healthy volunteers. For C_{max} of oxycodone, on average there was an increase to 110% (90% C.I.: 94, 129), 135% (90% C.I.: 115, 159) and 167% (90% C.I.: 142, 196) for mild, moderate and severe renally impaired subjects, respectively, compared with healthy volunteers. For $t_{1/2Z}$ of oxycodone, on average there was an increase to 149%, 123% and 142% for mild, moderate and severe renally impaired subjects, respectively, compared with healthy volunteers.

Naloxone:

For AUC_t of naloxone, on average there was an increase to 2850% (90% C.I.: 369, 22042), 3910% (90% C.I.: 506, 30243) and 7612% (90% C.I.: 984, 58871) for mild, moderate and severe renally impaired subjects, respectively, compared with healthy volunteers. For C_{max} of naloxone, on average there was an increase to 1076% (90% C.I.: 154, 7502), 858% (90% C.I.: 123, 5981) and 1675% (90% C.I.: 240, 11676) for mild, moderate and severe renally impaired subjects, respectively, compared with healthy volunteers. Due to insufficient amount of data available $t_{1/2Z}$ and the corresponding AUC_{INF} of naloxone were not calculated. The bioavailability comparisons for naloxone were therefore based on AUC_t values. The ratios may have been influenced by the inability to fully characterize the naloxone plasma profiles for the healthy subjects.

Naloxone-3-glucuronide:

For AUC_{INF} of naloxone-3-glucuronide, on average there was an increase to 220% (90% C.I.: 148, 327), 370% (90% C.I.: 249, 550) and 525% (90% C.I.: 354, 781) for mild, moderate and severe renally impaired subjects, respectively, compared with healthy subjects. For C_{max} of naloxone-3-glucuronide, on average there was an increase to 148% (90% C.I.: 110, 197), 202% (90% C.I.: 151, 271) and 239% (90% C.I.: 179, 320) for mild, moderate and severe renally impaired subjects, respectively, compared with healthy subjects. For $t_{1/2Z}$ of naloxone-3-glucuronide, on average there was no significant change between the renally impaired subjects and the healthy subjects.

Abuse

To avoid damage to the prolonged-release properties of the tablets, ***Targinact*** must not be broken, crushed or chewed, as this leads to a rapid release of the active substances. In addition, naloxone has a slower elimination rate when administered intranasally. Both properties mean that abuse of ***Targinact*** will not have the effect intended. In oxycodone-dependent rats, the intravenous administration of oxycodone hydrochloride / naloxone hydrochloride at a ratio of 2:1 resulted in withdrawal symptoms.

5.3 Preclinical safety data

There are no data from studies on reproductive toxicity of the combination of oxycodone and naloxone.

Studies with the single components showed that oxycodone had no effect on fertility and early embryonic development in male and female rats in doses of up to 8 mg/kg body weight and induced no malformations in rats in doses of up to 8 mg/kg and in rabbits in doses of 125 mg/kg bodyweight. However, in rabbits, when individual fetuses were used in statistical evaluation, a dose related increase in developmental variations was observed (increased incidences of 27 presacral vertebrae, extra pairs of ribs). When these parameters were statistically evaluated using litters, only the incidence of 27 presacral vertebrae was increased and only in the 125 mg/kg group, a dose level that produced severe pharmacotoxic effects in the pregnant animals. In a study on pre- and postnatal development in rats F1 body weights were lower at 6 mg/kg/d when compared to body weights of the control group at doses which reduced maternal weight and food intake (NOAEL 2 mg/kg body weight). There were neither effects on physical, reflexological, and sensory developmental parameters nor on behavioural and reproductive indices. The standard oral reproduction toxicity studies with naloxone show that at high oral doses naloxone was not teratogenic and/or embryo/fetotoxic, and does not affect perinatal/postnatal development. At very high doses (800 mg/kg/day) naloxone produced increased pup deaths in the immediate post-partum period at dosages that produced significant toxicity in maternal rats (e.g., body weight loss, convulsions). However, in surviving pups, no effects on development or behaviour were observed.

Long-term carcinogenicity studies with oxycodone/naloxone in combination or oxycodone as a single entity have not been performed. For naloxone, a 24-months oral carcinogenicity study was performed in rats with naloxone doses up to 100 mg/kg/day. The results indicate that naloxone is not carcinogenic under these conditions.

Oxycodone and naloxone as single entities show a clastogenic potential in *in vitro* assays. No similar effects were observed, however, under in vivo conditions, even at toxic doses. The results indicate that the mutagenic risk of ***Targinact*** to humans at therapeutic concentrations may be ruled out with adequate certainty.

6. PHARMACEUTICAL PARTICULARS

6.1 List of excipients

Tablet core:

Ethylcellulose,

Stearyl alcohol,

Lactose monohydrate,

Talc,

Magnesium stearate

Targinact 5 mg/2.5 mg: Hydroxylpropylcellulose

Targinact 40 mg/20 mg: Povidone K30

Tablet coat:

Poly(vinylalcohol),

Titanium dioxide (E171),

Macrogol 3350,

Talc

Targinact 5 mg/2.5 mg: Brilliant Blue FCF aluminium lake (E133)

Targinact 40 mg/20 mg: Iron oxide yellow (E172)

6.2 Incompatibilities

Not applicable.

6.3 Shelf life

Targinact 5 mg/2.5 mg

2 years

Targinact 40 mg/20 mg

3 years

6.4 Special precautions for storage

Do not store above 25°C.

Targinact 5 mg/2.5 mg

Store in the original package in order to protect from light

6.5 Nature and contents of container

Polyvinylchloride/aluminium foil blisters

10 prolonged-release tablets

14 prolonged-release tablets

20 prolonged-release tablets

28 prolonged-release tablets

30 prolonged-release tablets

50 prolonged-release tablets

56 prolonged-release tablets

60 prolonged-release tablets

98 prolonged-release tablets

100 prolonged-release tablets.

Hospital pack of 100 (10 × 10) prolonged-release tablets

Not all pack sizes may be marketed.

6.6 Special precautions for disposal and other handling

Any unused product or waste material should be disposed of in accordance with local requirements.

7. MARKETING AUTHORISATION HOLDER

Napp Pharmaceuticals Limited

Cambridge Science Park

Milton Road

Cambridge

CB4 OGW

UK

8. MARKETING AUTHORISATION NUMBER(S)

PL16950/0161-0162

9. DATE OF FIRST AUTHORISATION/RENEWAL OF THE AUTHORISATION

23 July 2009

10. DATE OF REVISION OF THE TEXT

Targocid 200mg & 400mg

(sanofi-aventis)

1. NAME OF THE MEDICINAL PRODUCT

Targocid 200mg

Teicoplanin 200mg Powder for Injection

Targocid 400mg

Teicoplanin 400mg Powder for Injection

2. QUALITATIVE AND QUANTITATIVE COMPOSITION

Teicoplanin 200mg

Teicoplanin 400mg

3. PHARMACEUTICAL FORM

Powder for Injection

4. CLINICAL PARTICULARS

4.1 Therapeutic indications

Targocid is indicated in potentially serious Gram-positive infections including those which cannot be treated with other antimicrobial drugs, eg. penicillins and cephalosporins.

Targocid is useful in the therapy of serious staphylococcal infections in patients who cannot receive or who have failed to respond to the penicillins and cephalosporins, or who have infections with staphylococci resistant to other antibiotics.

The effectiveness of teicoplanin has been documented in the following infections:-

Skin and soft tissue infections, urinary tract infections, lower respiratory tract infections, joint and bone infections, septicaemia, endocarditis and peritonitis related to continuous ambulatory peritoneal dialysis.

Targocid may be used for antimicrobial prophylaxis in orthopaedic surgery at risk of Gram-positive infection.

4.2 Posology and method of administration

Administration

The reconstituted Targocid injection may be administered directly either intravenously or intramuscularly. The intravenous injection may be administered either as a bolus or as a 30 minute infusion. Dosage is usually once daily but, in cases of severe infection, a second injection should be administered on the first day in order to reach more rapidly the required serum concentrations.

The majority of patients with infections caused by organisms sensitive to the antibiotic show a therapeutic response within 48-72 hours. The total duration of therapy is determined by the type and severity of the infection and the clinical response of the patient. In endocarditis and osteomyelitis, treatment for three weeks or longer is recommended.

Determination of teicoplanin serum concentrations may optimise therapy. In severe infections, trough serum concentrations should not be less than 10mg/l. Peak concentrations measured one hour after a 400mg intravenous dose are usually in the range of 20-50mg/l; peak serum concentrations of up to 250mg/l have been reported after intravenous doses of 25mg/kg. A relationship between serum concentration and toxicity has not been established.

Therapeutic dosage:

Adult or elderly patients with normal renal function

Prophylaxis: 400mg intravenously as a single dose at induction of anaesthesia

Moderate infections: Skin and soft tissue infection, urinary tract infection, lower respiratory tract infection

Loading dose: One single i.v. or i.m. injection of 400mg on the first day maintenance dose: A single i.v. or i.m. injection of 200mg daily

Severe infections: Joint and bone infection, septicaemia, endocarditis

Loading dose: Three 400mg i.v. injections, administered 12 hours apart

Maintenance dose: A single i.v. or i.m. injection of 400mg daily

1. Standard doses of 200 and 400mg equate respectively to mean doses of 3 and 6mg/kg. In patients weighing more than 85kg it is recommended to adapt the dosage to the weight following the same therapeutic schedule: moderate infection 3mg/kg, severe infection 6mg/kg.

2. In some clinical situations, such as infected, severely burned patients or Staphylococcus aureus endocarditis, unit maintenance doses of up to 12mg/kg have been administered (intravenously).

Children

Teicoplanin can be used to treat Gram-positive infections in children from the age of 2 months. For severe infections and neutropenic patients the recommended dose is 10mg/kg every 12 hours for the first three doses; thereafter a dose of 10mg/kg should be administered by either intravenous or intramuscular injection as a single dose each day.

For moderate infections the recommended dose is 10mg/kg every twelve hours for the first three doses; thereafter a dose of 6mg/kg should be administered by either intravenous or intramuscular injection as a single dose each day.

The recommended dosage regimen for neonates is a loading dose of 16mg/kg followed by a daily dose of 8mg/kg.

In continuous ambulatory periotoneal dialysis

After a single loading IV dose of 400mg if the patient is febrile, the recommended dosage is 20mg/l per bag in the first week, 20mg/l in alternate bags in the second week and 20mg/l in the overnight dwell bag only during the third week.

Adults and elderly patients with renal insufficiency

For patients with impaired renal function, reduction of dosage is not required until the fourth day of Targocid treatment. Measurement of the serum concentration of teicoplanin may optimise therapy (see section 'Administration').

From the fourth day of treatment

In mild renal insufficiency

Creatinine clearance between 40 and 60ml/min, Targocid dose should be halved, either by administering the initial unit dose every two days, or by administering half of this dose once a day.

In severe renal insufficiency

Creatinine clearance less than 40ml/min and in haemodialysed patients, Targocid dose should be one third of the normal either by administering the initial unit dose every third day, or by administering one third of this dose once a day. Teicoplanin is not removed by dialysis.

4.3 Contraindications

Teicoplanin is contra-indicated in patients who have exhibited previous hypersensitivity to the drug.

4.4 Special warnings and precautions for use

Warnings:

Targocid should be administered with caution in patients known to be hypersensitive to vancomycin since cross hypersensitivity may occur. However, a history of the "Red Man Syndrome" that can occur with vancomycin is not a contra-indication to Targocid.

Thrombocytopenia has been reported with teicoplanin, especially at higher doses than those usually recommended. It is advisable for periodic haematological studies to be performed during treatment. Liver and renal function tests are advised during treatment.

Serial renal and auditory function tests should be undertaken in the following circumstances:

Prolonged treatment in patients with renal insufficiency.

Concurrent and sequential use of other drugs which may have neurotoxic and/or nephrotoxic properties. These include aminoglycosides, colistin, amphotericin B, ciclosporin, cisplatin, furosemide and etacrynic acid.

However, there is no evidence of synergistic toxicity with combinations with Targocid.

Dosage must be adapted in patients with renal impairment (see 'Dosage').

Precautions:

Superinfection: as with other antibiotics, the use of teicoplanin, especially if prolonged, may result in overgrowth of non-susceptible organisms. Repeated evaluation of the patients condition is essential. If superinfection occurs during therapy, appropriate measures should be taken.

4.5 Interaction with other medicinal products and other forms of interaction

Targocid should be used with care in conjunction with or sequentially with other drugs with known nephrotoxic or ototoxic potential. Of particular concern are streptomycin, neomycin, kanamycin, gentamicin, amikacin, tobramycin, cephaloridine, colistin.

In clinical trials teicoplanin has been administered to many patients already receiving various medications including other antibiotics, antihypertensives, anaesthetic agents, cardiac drugs and antidiabetic agents without evidence of adverse interaction.

Animal studies have shown lack of interaction with diazepam, thiopental, morphine, neuromuscular blocking agents or halothane.

4.6 Pregnancy and lactation

Animal reproduction studies have not shown evidence of impairment of fertility or teratogenic effect. At high doses in rats there was an increased incidence of stillbirths and neonatal mortality. It is recommended that Targocid should not be used during confirmed or presumed pregnancy or during lactation unless a physician considers that the potential benefits outweigh a possible risk. There is no information about the excretion of teicoplanin in milk or placental transfer of the drug.

4.7 Effects on ability to drive and use machines

There is no indication to suggest an effect of teicoplanin on a patient's ability to drive or use machinery.

4.8 Undesirable effects

Targocid is generally well tolerated. Side-effects rarely require cessation of therapy and are generally mild and transient: serious side-effects are rare. The following adverse events have been reported:

Local reactions: erythema, local pain, thrombophlebitis, injection site abscess.

Hypersensitivity: rash, pruritis, fever, bronchospasm, anaphylactic reactions, anaphylactic shock, rigors, urticaria, angioedema, rare reports of exfolative dermatitis, toxic epidermal necrolysis, rare cases of erythema multiforme including Stevens-Johnson Syndrome. In addition, infusion-related events, such as erythema or flushing of the upper body, have been rarely reported in which the events occurred without a history of previous teicoplanin exposure and did not recur on re-exposure when the infusion rate was slowed and/or concentration decreased. These events were not specific to any concentration or rate of infusion.

Gastric-intestinal: nausea, vomiting, diarrhoea.

Blood: eosinophilia, leucopenia, thrombocytopenia, thrombocytosis, neutropenia, rare cases of reversible agranulocytosis.

Liver function: increases in serum transaminases and/or serum alkaline phosphatase.

Renal function: transient elevations of serum creatinine, renal failure.

Central nervous system: dizziness, headache.

Auditory/vestibular: mild hearing loss, tinnitus and vestibular disorder.

Other: Superinfection (overgrowth of non-susceptible organisms).

4.9 Overdose

Teicoplanin is not removed by haemodialysis. Treatment of overdosage should be symptomatic. Several overdoses of 100mg/kg/day have been administered in error to two neutropenic patients aged 4 and 8 years. Despite high plasma concentrations of teicoplanin up to 300mg/ml there were no symptoms or laboratory abnormalities.

5. PHARMACOLOGICAL PROPERTIES

5.1 Pharmacodynamic properties

Teicoplanin is a bactericidial, glycopeptide antibiotic, produced by fermentation of *Actinoplanes teichomyceticus*. It is active against both aerobic and anaerobic Gram-positive bacteria.

Species usually sensitive (MIC less than or equal to 16mg/l):

Staphylococcus aureus and coagulase negative staphylococci (sensitive or resistant to meticillin), streptococci, enterococci, *Listeria monocytogenes*, micrococci, *Eikenella corrodens*, group *JK corynebacteria* and Gram-positive anaerobes including *Clostridium difficile*, and peptococci.

Species usually resistant (MIC superior to 16mg/l):

Nocardia asteroides, Lactobacillus spp, Leuconostoc and all Gram-negative bacteria.

Bactericidal synergy has been demonstrated *in vitro* with aminoglycosides against group D streptococci and staphylococci. *In vitro* combinations of teicoplanin with rifampicin or fluorinated quinolones show primarily additive effects and sometimes synergy.

One-step resistance to teicoplanin could not be obtained *in vitro* and multi-step resistance was only reached *in vitro* after 11-14 passages.

Teicoplanin does not show cross-resistance with other classes of antibiotics.

The use of teicoplanin may result in overgrowth of non-susceptible organisms. If new infections due to bacteria or fungi appear during treatment appropriate measures should be taken.

Susceptibility testing:

Sensidiscs are charged with 30 micrograms of teicoplanin. Strains showing an inhibition zone diameter of 14mm or more are susceptible and those of 10mm or less are resistant.

5.2 Pharmacokinetic properties

Following injection teicoplanin rapidly penetrates into tissues, including skin, fat and bones and reaches the highest concentrations in the kidney, trachea, lungs and adrenals. Teicoplanin does not readily penetrate into the cerebrospinal fluid (CSF).

In man the plasma level profile after intravenous administration indicates a biphasic distribution (with a rapid distribution phase having a half-life of about 0.3 hours, followed by a more prolonged distribution phase having a half-life of about 3 hours), followed by slow elimination (with a terminal elimination half-life of about 150 hours). At 6mg/kg administered intravenously at 0, 12, 24 hours and every 24 hours thereafter as a 30 minute infusion, a predicted trough serum concentration of 10mg/l would be reached by Day 4. The steady state volume of distribution after 3 to 6mg/kg intravenously ranges from 0.94 l/kg to 1.4 l/kg. The volume of distribution in children is not substantially different from that in adults.

Approximately 90-95% teicoplanin is bound with weak affinity to plasma proteins. Teicoplanin penetrates readily into blister exudates and into joint fluid; it penetrates neutrophils and enhances their bactericidal activity; it does not penetrate red blood cells.

No metabolites of teicoplanin have been identified; more than 97% of the administered teicoplanin is excreted unchanged. The elimination of teicoplanin from the plasma is prolonged with a terminal half-life of elimination in man of about 150 hours. Teicoplanin is excreted mainly in the urine.

5.3 Preclinical safety data

Not Applicable

6. PHARMACEUTICAL PARTICULARS

6.1 List of excipients

Sodium chloride

6.2 Incompatibilities

Solutions of teicoplanin and aminoglycosides are incompatible when mixed directly and should not be mixed before injection.

6.3 Shelf life

3 years unopened.

24 hours after reconstitution.

6.4 Special precautions for storage

Finished Product:

Vials of dry Targocid should not be stored above 25°C.

Reconstituted Product:

In keeping with good clinical pharmaceutical practise reconstituted vials of Targocid should be used immediately and any unused portion discarded. On the few occasions when changing circumstances make this impractical reconstituted solutions should be kept at 2 - 8°C and discarded within 24 hours.

Do not store in a syringe.

6.5 Nature and contents of container

Colourless, BP, Type I glass vials, closed with a butyl rubber plug and combination aluminium/plastic "flip-off cap" (200mg colour coded yellow, 400mg colour coded green).

Pack size: 1 vial

6.6 Special precautions for disposal and other handling

Preparation of Injection

The entire contents of the water ampoule should be slowly added to the vial of Targocid and the vial rolled gently until the powder is completely dissolved, taking care to avoid formation of foam. If the solution does become foamy then allow to stand for about 15 minutes for the foam to subside.

A calculated excess is included in each vial of Targocid so that, when prepared as described above, a full dose of 100mg, 200mg or 400mg (depending on the strength of the vial) will be obtained if all the reconstituted solution is withdrawn from the vial by a syringe. The concentration of teicoplanin in these injections will be 100mg in 1.5ml (from the 100mg and 200mg vials) and 400mg in 3ml (from the 400mg vial).

The reconstituted solution may be injected directly, or alternatively diluted with:

- 0.9% Sodium Chloride Injection
- Compound Sodium Lactate Injection (Ringer-Lactate Solution, Hartmanns Solution)
- 5% Dextrose Injection
- 0.18% Sodium Chloride and 4% Dextrose Injection
- Peritoneal dialysis solution containing 1.36% or 3.86% Dextrose.

7. MARKETING AUTHORISATION HOLDER

Sanofi-aventis

One Onslow Street

Guildford

Surrey

GU1 4YS

8. MARKETING AUTHORISATION NUMBER(S)

200 mg: PL 04425/0088

400 mg: PL 04425/0089

9. DATE OF FIRST AUTHORISATION/RENEWAL OF THE AUTHORISATION

2 August 1989/7 March 2001

10. DATE OF REVISION OF THE TEXT

29 November 2006

LEGAL CATEGORY:

POM

TARGRETIN CAPSULES

(Cephalon Limited)

1. NAME OF THE MEDICINAL PRODUCT

Targretin 75 mg soft capsules

2. QUALITATIVE AND QUANTITATIVE COMPOSITION

Each capsule contains 75 mg of bexarotene.

For a full list of excipients, see section 6.1.

3. PHARMACEUTICAL FORM

Soft capsule.

Off-white capsule, containing a liquid suspension and imprinted with "Targretin".

4. CLINICAL PARTICULARS

4.1 Therapeutic indications

Targretin capsules are indicated for the treatment of skin manifestations of advanced stage cutaneous T-cell lymphoma (CTCL) patients refractory to at least one systemic treatment.

4.2 Posology and method of administration

Bexarotene therapy should only be initiated and maintained by physicians experienced in the treatment of patients with CTCL.

The recommended initial dose is 300 mg/m^2/day. Targretin capsules should be taken as a single oral daily dose with a meal (see section 4.5). Initial dose calculations according to body surface area are as follows:

Initial dose level (300 mg/m^2/day)		Number of 75 mg Targretin capsules
Body Surface Area (m^2)	Total daily dose (mg/day)	
0.88 – 1.12	300	4
1.13 - 1.37	375	5
1.38 - 1.62	450	6
1.63 - 1.87	525	7
1.88 - 2.12	600	8
2.13 - 2.37	675	9
2.38 - 2.62	750	10

Dose modification guidelines: the 300 mg/m^2/day dose level may be adjusted to 200 mg/m^2/day then to 100 mg/m^2/day, or temporarily suspended, if necessitated by toxicity. When toxicity is controlled, doses may be carefully readjusted upward. With appropriate clinical monitoring, individual patients may benefit from doses above 300 mg/m^2/day. Doses greater than 650 mg/m^2/day have not been evaluated in patients with CTCL. In clinical trials, bexarotene was administered for up to 118 weeks to patients with CTCL. Treatment should be continued as long as the patient is deriving benefit.

Use in children and adolescents: the clinical safety and effectiveness of bexarotene in the paediatric population (below 18 years of age) have not been studied and this product should not be used in a paediatric population until further data become available.

Use in the elderly: of the total number of patients with CTCL in clinical studies, 61% were 60 years or older, while 30% were 70 years or older. No overall differences in safety were observed between patients 70 years or older and younger patients, but greater sensitivity of some older individuals to bexarotene cannot be ruled out. The standard dose should be used in the elderly.

Renal insufficiency: no formal studies have been conducted in patients with renal insufficiency. Clinical pharmacokinetic data indicate that urinary elimination of bexarotene and its metabolites is a minor excretory pathway for bexarotene. In all evaluated patients, the estimated renal clearance of bexarotene was less than 1 ml/minute. In view of the limited data, patients with renal insufficiency should be monitored carefully while on bexarotene therapy.

4.3 Contraindications

Known hypersensitivity to bexarotene or to any of the excipients of the product.

Pregnancy and lactation.

Women of child-bearing potential without effective birth-control measures.

History of pancreatitis.

Uncontrolled hypercholesterolaemia.

Uncontrolled hypertriglyceridaemia.

Hypervitaminosis A.

Uncontrolled thyroid disease.

Hepatic insufficiency.

Ongoing systemic infection.

4.4 Special warnings and precautions for use

General: Targretin capsules should be used with caution in patients with a known hypersensitivity to retinoids. No clinical instances of cross-reactivity have been noted. Patients receiving bexarotene should not donate blood for transfusion. Butylated hydroxyanisole, an ingredient in Targretin, may cause irritation to the mucous membranes, therefore the capsules must be swallowed intact and not chewed.

Lipids: hyperlipidaemia has been identified as an effect associated with the use of bexarotene in clinical studies. Fasting blood lipid determinations (triglycerides and cholesterol) should be performed before bexarotene therapy is initiated and at weekly intervals until the lipid response to bexarotene is established, which usually occurs within two to four weeks, and then at intervals no less than monthly thereafter. Fasting triglycerides should be normal or normalised with appropriate intervention prior to bexarotene therapy. Every attempt should be made to maintain triglyceride levels below 4.52 mmol/l in order to reduce the risk of clinical sequelae. If fasting triglycerides are elevated or become elevated during treatment, institution of antilipaemic therapy is recommended, and if necessary, dose reductions (from 300 mg/m^2/day of bexarotene to 200 mg/m^2/day, and if necessary to 100 mg/m^2/day) or treatment discontinuation. Data from clinical studies indicate that bexarotene concentrations were not affected by concomitant administration of atorvastatin. However, concomitant administration of gemfibrozil resulted in substantial increases in plasma concentrations of bexarotene and therefore, concomitant administration of gemfibrozil with bexarotene is not recommended (see section 4.5). Elevations of serum cholesterol should be managed according to current medical practice.

Pancreatitis: acute pancreatitis associated with elevations of fasting serum triglycerides has been reported in clinical studies. Patients with CTCL having risk factors for pancreatitis (e.g., prior episodes of pancreatitis, uncontrolled hyperlipidaemia, excessive alcohol consumption, uncontrolled diabetes mellitus, biliary tract disease, and medications known to increase triglyceride levels or to be associated with pancreatic toxicity) should not be treated with bexarotene, unless the potential benefit outweighs the risk.

Liver Function Test (LFT) abnormalities: LFT elevations associated with the use of bexarotene have been reported. Based on data from ongoing clinical trials, elevation of LFTs resolved within one month in 80% of patients following a decrease in dose or discontinuation of therapy. Baseline LFTs should be obtained, and LFTs should be carefully monitored weekly during the first month and then monthly thereafter. Consideration should be given to a suspension or discontinuation of bexarotene if test results reach greater than three times the upper limit of normal values for SGOT/AST, SGPT/ALT, or bilirubin.

Thyroid function test alterations: changes in thyroid function tests have been observed in patients receiving bexarotene, most often noted as a reversible reduction in thyroid hormone (total thyroxine [total T_4]) and thyroid-stimulating hormone (TSH) levels. Baseline thyroid function tests should be obtained and then monitored at least monthly during treatment and as indicated by the emergence of symptoms consistent with hypothyroidism. Patients with symptomatic hypothyroidism on bexarotene therapy have been treated with thyroid hormone supplements with resolution of symptoms.

Leucopenia: leucopenia associated with bexarotene therapy has been reported in clinical studies. The majority of cases resolved after dose reduction or discontinuation of treatment. Determination of white blood cell count with differential count should be obtained at baseline, weekly during the first month and then monthly thereafter.

Anaemia: anaemia associated with bexarotene therapy has been reported in clinical studies. Determination of haemoglobin should be obtained at baseline, weekly during the first month and then monthly thereafter. Decreases of haemoglobin should be managed according to current medical practice.

Lens opacities: following bexarotene treatment, some patients were observed to have previously undetected lens opacities or a change in pre-existing lens opacities unrelated to treatment duration or dose level of exposure. Given the high prevalence and natural rate of cataract formation in the older patient population represented in the clinical studies, there was no apparent association between the incidence of lens opacity formation and bexarotene administration. However, an adverse effect of long-term bexarotene treatment on lens opacity formation in humans has not been excluded. Any patient treated with bexarotene who experiences visual difficulties should have an appropriate ophthalmologic examination.

Vitamin A supplementation: because of the relationship of bexarotene to vitamin A, patients should be advised to limit vitamin A supplements to ⩽15,000 IU/day to avoid potential additive toxic effects.

Patients with diabetes mellitus: caution should be exercised when administering bexarotene in patients using insulin, agents enhancing insulin secretion (e.g. sulfonylureas), or insulin-sensitisers (e.g. thiazolidinediones). Based on the known mechanism of action, bexarotene may potentially enhance the action of these agents, resulting in hypoglycaemia. No cases of hypoglycaemia associated with the use of bexarotene as monotherapy have been reported.

Photosensitivity: the use of some retinoids has been associated with photosensitivity. Patients should be advised to minimise exposure to sunlight and avoid sun lamps during therapy with bexarotene, as *in vitro* data indicate that bexarotene may potentially have a photosensitising effect.

Oral contraceptives: bexarotene can potentially induce metabolic enzymes and thereby theoretically reduce the efficacy of oestroprogestive contraceptives. Thus, if treatment with bexarotene is intended in a woman of child-bearing potential, a reliable, non-hormonal form of contraception is also required, because bexarotene belongs to a therapeutic class for which the human malformative risk is high.

4.5 Interaction with other medicinal products and other forms of interaction

Effects of other substances on bexarotene: no formal studies to evaluate interactions with bexarotene have been conducted. On the basis of the oxidative metabolism of bexarotene by cytochrome P450 3A4 (CYP3A4), coadministration with other CYP3A4 substrates such as ketoconazole, itraconazole, protease inhibitors, clarithromycin and erythromycin may theoretically lead to an increase in plasma bexarotene concentrations. Furthermore, co-administration with CYP3A4 inducers such as rifampicin, phenytoin, dexamethasone or phenobarbital may theoretically cause a reduction in plasma bexarotene concentrations.

A population analysis of plasma bexarotene concentrations in patients with CTCL indicated that concomitant administration of gemfibrozil resulted in substantial increases in plasma concentrations of bexarotene. The mechanism of this interaction is unknown. Under similar conditions, bexarotene concentrations were not affected by concomitant administration of atorvastatin or levothyroxine. Concomitant administration of gemfibrozil with bexarotene is not recommended.

Effects of bexarotene on other substances: there are indications that bexarotene may induce CYP3A4. Therefore, repeated administration of bexarotene may result in an auto-induction of its own metabolism and, particularly at dose levels greater than 300 mg/m^2/day, may increase the rate of metabolism and reduce plasma concentrations of other substances metabolised by cytochrome P450 3A4, such as tamoxifen. For example bexarotene may reduce the efficacy of oral contraceptives (see sections 4.4 and 4.6).

Laboratory test interactions: CA125 assay values in patients with ovarian cancer may be accentuated with bexarotene therapy.

Food interactions: in all clinical trials, patients were instructed to take Targretin capsules with or immediately following a meal. In one clinical study, plasma bexarotene AUC and C_{max} values were substantially higher following the administration of a fat-containing meal versus those following the administration of a glucose solution. Because safety and efficacy data from clinical trials are based upon administration with food, it is recommended that Targretin capsules be administered with food.

On the basis of the oxidative metabolism of bexarotene by cytochrome P450 3A4, grapefruit juice may theoretically lead to an increase in plasma bexarotene concentrations.

4.6 Pregnancy and lactation

Pregnancy: there are no adequate data from the use of bexarotene in pregnant women. Studies in animals have shown reproductive toxicity. Based on the comparison of animal and patient exposures to bexarotene, a margin of safety for human teratogenicity has not been demonstrated (see section 5.3). Bexarotene is contraindicated in pregnancy (see section 4.3).

If this medicinal product is used inadvertently during pregnancy, or if the patient becomes pregnant while taking this medicinal product, the patient should be informed of the potential hazard to the foetus.

Women of childbearing potential must use adequate birth-control measures when bexarotene is used. A negative, sensitive, pregnancy test (e.g. serum beta-human chorionic gonadotropin, beta-HCG) should be obtained within one week prior to bexarotene therapy. Effective contraception must be used from the time of the negative pregnancy test through the initiation of therapy, during therapy and for at least one month following discontinuation of therapy. Whenever contraception is required, it is recommended that two reliable forms of contraception be used simultaneously. Bexarotene can potentially induce metabolic enzymes and thereby theoretically reduce the efficacy of oestroprogestative contraceptives (see section 4.5). Thus, if treatment with bexarotene is intended in a woman with childbearing potential, a reliable, non-hormonal contraceptive method is also recommended. Male patients with sexual partners who are pregnant, possibly pregnant, or may potentially become pregnant must use condoms during sexual intercourse while taking bexarotene and for at least one month after the last dose.

Lactation: it is not known whether bexarotene is excreted in human milk. Bexarotene should not be used in breast-feeding mothers.

4.7 Effects on ability to drive and use machines

No studies on the effects on the ability to drive and use machines have been performed. However, dizziness and visual difficulties have been reported in patients taking Targretin. Patients who experience dizziness or visual difficulties during therapy must not drive or operate machinery.

4.8 Undesirable effects

The safety of bexarotene has been examined in clinical studies of 193 patients with CTCL who received bexarotene for up to 118 weeks and in 420 non-CTCL cancer patients in other studies.

In 109 patients with CTCL treated at the recommended initial dose of 300 mg/m^2/day, the most commonly reported adverse reactions to Targretin were hyperlipaemia ((primarily elevated triglycerides) 74%), hypothyroidism (29%), hypercholesterolaemia (28%), headache (27%), leucopenia (20%), pruritus (20%), asthenia (19%), rash (16%), exfoliative dermatitis (15%), and pain (12%).

The following Targretin-related adverse reactions were reported during clinical studies in patients with CTCL (N=109) treated at the recommended initial dose of 300 mg/m^2/day. The frequencies of adverse reactions are classified as very common >1/10), common >1/100, <1/10), uncommon >1/1,000, <1/100), rare >1/10,000, <1/1,000), and very rare (<1/10,000).

Within each frequency grouping, undesirable effects are presented in order of decreasing seriousness.

Blood and lymphatic system disorders

Very common: Leucopenia

Common: Lymphoma Like Reaction, Lymphadenopathy, Hypochromic Anaemia[1,2,3]

Uncommon: Blood Dyscrasia, Purpura, Coagulation Disorder, Coagulation Time Increased[2,3], Anaemia[1], Thrombocytopenia[3], Thrombocythemia, Eosinophilia[1], Leukocytosis[2], Lymphocytosis

Endocrine disorders

Very common: Hypothyroidism

Common: Thyroid Disorder

Uncommon: Hyperthyroidism

Metabolism and nutrition disorders

Very common: Hyperlipaemia, Hypercholesterolaemia

Common: Weight Gain, SGOT Increased, SGPT Increased, Lactic Dehydrogenase Increased, Creatinine Increased, Hypoproteinaemia,

Uncommon: Gout, Bilirubinemia[1,3], BUN Increased[1], High Density Lipoprotein Decreased

Nervous system disorders

Common: Dizziness, Hypesthesia, Insomnia

Uncommon: Ataxia, Neuropathy, Vertigo, Hyperaesthesia, Depression[1,2,3], Agitation

Eye disorders

Common: Dry Eyes, Eye Disorder

Uncommon: Cataract Specified[1,2,3], Amblyopia[3], Visual Field Defect, Corneal Lesion, Abnormal Vision[1,2,3], Blepharitis, Conjunctivitis[3]

Ear and labyrinth disorders

Common: Deafness

Uncommon: Ear disorder

Cardiac disorders

Uncommon: Tachycardia

Vascular disorders

Common: Peripheral Oedema

Uncommon: Haemorrhage, Hypertension, Oedema[3], Vasodilatation[1,2,3], Varicose Vein

Gastrointestinal disorders

Common: Vomiting, Diarrhoea[1,3], Nausea[3], Anorexia[1], Liver Function Tests Abnormal, Cheilitis[2], Dry Mouth[2,3], Constipation, Flatulence,

Uncommon: Pancreatitis[1,3], Hepatic Failure, Gastrointestinal Disorder[1]

Skin and subcutaneous tissue disorders

Very common: Exfoliative Dermatitis, Pruritus, Rash

Common: Skin Ulcer, Alopecia[1], Skin Hypertrophy, Skin Nodule, Acne, Sweating, Dry Skin[2,3], Skin Disorder

Uncommon: Serous Drainage[1], Herpes Simplex, Pustular Rash, Skin Discoloration[3] Hair Disorder[1], Nail Disorder[1,3]

Musculoskeletal and connective tissue disorders

Common: Bone Pain, Arthralgia, Myalgia

Uncommon: Myasthaenia[1]

Renal and urinary disorders

Uncommon: Albuminuria[1,3], Kidney Function Abnormal

General Disorders and administration site conditions

Very common: Pain, Headache, Asthaenia

Common: Allergic Reaction, Infection, Chills[1], Abdominal Pain, Hormone Level Altered[1]

Uncommon: Neoplasm, Fever[1,2,3], Cellulitis, Infection Parasitic, Mucous Membrane Disorder[3], Back Pain[1,2,3], Lab Test Abnormal

1: adverse reactions noted with increased frequency when bexarotene was administered at a dose $>$300mg/m^2/day.

2: adverse reactions noted with increased frequency when bexarotene was administered at a dose of 300 mg/m^2/day in non-CTCL cancer patients.

3: adverse reactions noted with increased frequency when bexarotene was administered at a dose of $>$300 mg/m^2/day (compared to administration to CTCL patients at 300 mg/m^2/day) in non-CTCL cancer patients.

Additional adverse reactions observed when used outside of the recommended dose and indication (i.e. used in CTCL at an initial dose $>$300mg/m ^{2} /day or in non-CTCL cancer indications):

Newly observed adverse reactions: ecchymosis, petechia, abnormal white blood cells, thromboplastin decreased, abnormal erythrocytes, dehydration, increased gonadotrophic luteinizing hormone, weight loss, increased alkaline phosphatase, increased creatinine phosphokinase, lipase increased, hypercalcaemia, migraine, peripheral neuritis, paraesthesia, hypertonia, confusion, anxiety, emotional lability, somnolence, decreased libido, nervousness, night blindness, nystagmus, lacrimation disorder, tinnitus, taste perversion, chest pain, arrhythmia, peripheral vascular disorder, generalized oedema, haemoptysis, dyspnoea, increased cough, sinusitis, pharyngitis, dysphagia, mouth ulceration, oral moniliasis, stomatitis, dyspepsia, thirst, abnormal stools, eructation, vesicobullous rash, maculopapular rash, leg cramps, haematuria, flu syndrome, pelvic pain, and body odour.

Single observations of the following were also reported: bone marrow depression, decreased prothrombin, decreased gonadotrophic luteinizing hormone, increased amylase, hyponatraemia, hypokalaemia, hyperuricaemia, hypocholesterolaemia, hypolipaemia, hypomagnesaemia, abnormal gait, stupor, circumoral paraesthesia, abnormal thinking, eye pain, hypovolaemia, subdural haematoma, congestive heart failure, palpitation, epistaxis, vascular anomaly, vascular disorder, pallor, pneumonia, respiratory disorder, lung disorder, pleural disorder, cholecystitis, liver damage, jaundice, cholestatic jaundice, melaena, vomiting, laryngismus, tenesmus, rhinitis, increased appetite, gingivitis, herpes zoster, psoriasis, furunculosis, contact dermatitis, seborrhoea, lichenoid dermatitis, arthritis, joint disorder, urinary retention, impaired urination, polyuria, nocturia, impotence, urine abnormality, breast enlargement, carcinoma, photosensitivity reaction, face oedema, malaise, viral infection, enlarged abdomen.

The majority of adverse reactions were noted at a higher incidence at doses greater than 300 mg/m^2/day. Generally, these resolved without sequelae on dose reduction or withdrawal of treatment. However, among a total of 810 patients, including those without malignancy, treated with bexarotene, there were three serious adverse reactions with fatal outcome (acute pancreatitis, subdural haematoma and liver failure). Of these, liver failure, subsequently determined to be not related to bexarotene, was the only one to occur in a CTCL patient.

Hypothyroidism generally occurs 4-8 weeks after commencement of therapy. It may be asymptomatic and responds to treatment with thyroxine and resolves upon withdrawal of treatment.

Bexarotene has a different adverse reaction profile to other oral, non-retinoid X receptor (RXR) -selective retinoids. Owing to its primarily RXR-binding activity, bexarotene is less likely to cause mucocutaneous, nail, and hair toxicities; arthralgia; and myalgia; which are frequently reported with retinoic acid receptor (RAR) -binding agents.

4.9 Overdose

No clinical experience with an overdose of Targretin has been reported. Any overdose should be treated with supportive care for the signs and symptoms exhibited by the patient.

Doses up to 1000 mg/m^2/day of bexarotene have been administered in clinical studies with no acute toxic effects. Single doses of 1500 mg/kg (9000 mg/m^2) and 720 mg/kg (14,400 mg/m^2) were tolerated without significant toxicity in rats and dogs, respectively.

5. PHARMACOLOGICAL PROPERTIES

5.1 Pharmacodynamic properties

Pharmacotherapeutic Group: other antineoplastic agents, ATC code: L01XX25

Bexarotene is a synthetic compound that exerts its biological action through selective binding and activation of the three RXRs: α, β, and γ. Once activated, these receptors function as transcription factors that regulate processes such as cellular differentiation and proliferation, apoptosis, and insulin sensitisation. The ability of the RXRs to form heterodimers with various receptor partners that are important in cellular function and in physiology indicates that the biological activities of bexarotene are more diverse than those of compounds that activate the RARs. *In vitro*, bexarotene inhibits the growth of tumour cell lines of haematopoietic and squamous cell origin. *In vivo*, bexarotene causes tumour regression in some animal models and prevents tumour induction in others. However, the exact mechanism of action of bexarotene in the treatment of cutaneous T-cell lymphoma (CTCL) is unknown.

Bexarotene capsules were evaluated in clinical trials of 193 patients with CTCL of whom 93 had advanced stage disease refractory to prior systemic therapy. Among the 61 patients treated at an initial dose of 300 mg/m^2/day, the overall response rate, according to a global assessment by the physician, was 51% (31/61) with a clinical complete response rate of 3%. Responses were also determined by a composite score of five clinical signs (surface area, erythema, plaque elevation, scaling and hypo/hyperpigmentation) which also considered all extracutaneous CTCL manifestations. The overall response rate according to this composite assessment was 31% (19/61) with a clinical complete response rate of 7% (4/61).

5.2 Pharmacokinetic properties

Absorption/dose proportionality: pharmacokinetics were linear up to a dose of 650 mg/m^2. Terminal elimination half-life values were generally between one and three hours. Following repeat once daily dose administration at dose levels $\geq$ 230 mg/m^2, C_{max} and AUC in some patients were less than respective single dose values. No evidence of prolonged accumulation was observed. At the recommended initial daily-dose level (300 mg/m^2), single-dose and repeated daily-dose bexarotene pharmacokinetic parameters were similar.

Protein binding/distribution: bexarotene is highly bound $>$99%) to plasma proteins. The uptake of bexarotene by organs or tissues has not been evaluated.

Metabolism: bexarotene metabolites in plasma include 6- and 7-hydroxy-bexarotene and 6- and 7-oxo-bexarotene. *In vitro* studies suggest glucuronidation as a metabolic pathway, and that cytochrome P450 3A4 is the major cytochrome P450 isozyme responsible for formation of the oxidative metabolites. Based on the *in vitro* binding and the retinoid receptor activation profile of the metabolites, and on the relative amounts of individual metabolites in plasma, the metabolites have little impact on the pharmacological profile of retinoid receptor activation by bexarotene.

Excretion: neither bexarotene nor its metabolites are excreted in urine in any appreciable amounts. The estimated renal clearance of bexarotene is less than 1 ml/minute. Renal excretion is not a significant elimination pathway for bexarotene.

5.3 Preclinical safety data

Carcinogenesis, mutagenesis, impairment of fertility: bexarotene is not genotoxic. Carcinogenicity studies have not been conducted. Fertility studies have not been conducted; however, in sexually immature male dogs, reversible aspermatogenesis (28-day study) and testicular degeneration (91-day study) were seen. When bexarotene was administered for six months to sexually mature dogs, no testicular effects were seen. Effects on fertility cannot be excluded. Bexarotene, in common with the majority of retinoids, was teratogenic and embryotoxic in an animal test species at systemic exposures that are achievable clinically in humans. Irreversible cataracts involving the posterior area of the lens occurred in rats and dogs treated with bexarotene at systemic exposures that are achievable clinically in humans. The aetiology of this finding is unknown. An adverse effect of long-term bexarotene treatment on cataract formation in humans has not been excluded.

6. PHARMACEUTICAL PARTICULARS

6.1 List of excipients

Capsule content:

macrogol

polysorbate

povidone

butylated hydroxyanisole

Capsule shell:

gelatin

sorbitol special-glycerin blend (glycerin, sorbitol, sorbitol anhydrides (1,4-sorbitan), mannitol and water)

titanium dioxide (E171)

printing ink (shellac glaze-45% (20% esterified) in SD-45 alcohol, indigo carmine lake (E132) and simethicone)

6.2 Incompatibilities

Not applicable.

6.3 Shelf life

3 years

6.4 Special precautions for storage

Do not store above 30°C.

Keep the bottle tightly closed.

6.5 Nature and contents of container

High-density polyethylene bottles with child-resistant closures containing 100 capsules.

6.6 Special precautions for disposal and other handling

No special requirements.

7. MARKETING AUTHORISATION HOLDER

Eisai Ltd.

3 Shortlands

London

W6 8EE

United Kingdom

8. MARKETING AUTHORISATION NUMBER(S)

EU/1/01/178/001

9. DATE OF FIRST AUTHORISATION/RENEWAL OF THE AUTHORISATION

Date of first authorisation: 29 March 2001.

Date of last renewal: 24 April 2006.

10. DATE OF REVISION OF THE TEXT

30 April 2007

Tarivid 200mg & 400mg Tablets

(sanofi-aventis)

1. NAME OF THE MEDICINAL PRODUCT

Tarivid 200 mg Tablets

Tarivid 400 mg Tablets

2. QUALITATIVE AND QUANTITATIVE COMPOSITION

Tarivid Tablets 200mg contain 200mg of ofloxacin

Tarivid Tablets 400mg contain 400mg of ofloxacin

For a full list of excipients, see section 6.1.

3. PHARMACEUTICAL FORM

Film coated tablets

4. CLINICAL PARTICULARS

4.1 Therapeutic indications

Ofloxacin is a synthetic 4-fluoroquinolone antibacterial agent with bactericidal activity against a wide range of Gram-negative and Gram-positive organisms. It is indicated for the treatment of the following infections when caused by sensitive organisms: Upper and lower urinary tract infections; lower respiratory tract infections; uncomplicated urethral and cervical gonorrhoea; non-gonococcal urethritis and cervicitis, skin and soft tissue infections.

4.2 Posology and method of administration

General dosage recommendations: The dose of ofloxacin is determined by the type and severity of the infection. The dosage range for adults is 200mg to 800mg daily. Up to 400mg may be given as a single dose, preferably in the morning, larger doses should be given as two divided doses. Generally, individual doses are to be given at approximately equal intervals. Tarivid tablets should be swallowed with liquid; they should not be taken within two hours of magnesium/aluminium containing antacids, sucralfate, zinc or iron preparations since reduction of absorption of ofloxacin can occur.

Lower urinary tract infection: 200-400 mg daily.

Upper urinary tract infection: 200-400 mg daily increasing, if necessary, to 400 mg twice a day.

Lower respiratory tract infection: 400 mg daily increasing, if necessary, to 400 mg twice daily.

Uncomplicated urethral and cervical gonorrhoea: A single dose of 400 mg.

Non-gonococcal urethritis and cervicitis: 400 mg daily in single or divided doses.

Skin and soft tissue infections: 400 mg twice daily.

Impaired renal function: Following a normal initial dose, dosage should be reduced in patients with impairment of renal function. When creatinine clearance is 20-50 ml/minute (serum creatinine 1.5-5.0 mg/dl) the dosage should be reduced by half (100-200 mg daily). If creatinine clearance is less than 20 ml/minute (serum creatinine greater than 5 mg/dl) 100 mg should be given every 24 hours. In patients undergoing haemodialysis or peritoneal dialysis, 100 mg should be given every 24 hours.

Impaired liver function: The excretion of ofloxacin may be reduced in patients with severe hepatic dysfunction.

Elderly: No adjustment of dosage is required in the elderly, other than that imposed by consideration of renal or hepatic function. (See section 4.4 QT interval prolongation).

Children: Ofloxacin is not indicated for use in children or growing adolescents.

Duration of treatment: Duration of treatment is dependent on the severity of the infection and the response to treatment. The usual treatment period is 5-10 days except in uncomplicated gonorrhoea, where a single dose is recommended.

Treatment should not exceed 2 months duration.

4.3 Contraindications

Ofloxacin should not be used in patients with known hypersensitivity to 4-quinolone antibacterials or any of the tablet excipients.

Ofloxacin should not be used in patients with a past history of tendonitis.

Ofloxacin, like other 4-quinolones, is contra-indicated in patients with a history of epilepsy or with a lowered seizure threshold. Ofloxacin is contra-indicated in children or growing adolescents, and in pregnant or breast-feeding women, since animal experiments do not entirely exclude the risk of damage to the cartilage of joints in the growing subject.

Patients with latent or actual defects in glucose-6-phosphate dehydrogenese activity may be prone to haemolytic reactions when treated with quinolone antibacterial agents.

4.4 Special warnings and precautions for use

QT interval prolongation

Very rare cases of QT interval prolongation have been reported in patients taking fluoroquinolones. Caution should be taken when using fluoroquinolones, including ofloxacin, in patients with known risk factors for prolongation of the QT interval such as, for example:

- elderly
- uncorrected electrolyte imbalance (e.g. hypokalemia, hypomagnesemia)
- congenital long QT syndrome
- acquired QT prolongation
- cardiac disease (e.g. heart failure, myocardial infarction, bradycardia)
- concomitant use of drugs that are known to prolong the QT interval (e.g. Class IA and III antiarrrhythmics, tricyclic antidepressants, macrolides).

See also section 4.2 Elderly and section 4.5.

Patients being treated with ofloxacin should not expose themselves unnecessarily to strong sunlight and should avoid UV rays (sun lamps, solaria). Caution is recommended if the drug is to be used in psychotic patients or in patients with a history of psychiatric disease.

Administration of antibiotics, especially of prolonged, may lead to proliferation of resistant micro-organisms. The patient's condition must therefore be checked at regular intervals. If a secondary infection occurs, appropriate measures must be taken.

Peripheral neuropathy

Sensory or sensorimotor peripheral neuropathy has been reported in patients receiving fluoroquinolones, including ofloxacin. Ofloxacin should be discontinued if the patient experiences symptoms of neuropathy in order to prevent the development of an irreversible condition.

4.5 Interaction with other medicinal products and other forms of interaction

Drugs known to prolong QT interval

Ofloxacin, like other fluoroquinolones, should be used with caution in patients receiving drugs known to prolong the QT interval (e.g. Class IA and III antiarrhythmics, tricyclic antidepressants, macrolides).(See Section 4.4 QT interval prolongation).

Antacids, Sucralfate, Metal Cations

Co-administered magnesium/aluminium antacids, sucralfate, zinc or iron preparations can reduce absorption. Therefore, ofloxacin should be taken 2 hours before such preparations. Prolongation of bleeding time has been reported during concomitant administration of Tarivid and anticoagulants.

There may be a further lowering of the cerebral seizure threshold when quinolones are given concurrently with other drugs which lower the seizure threshold, e.g. theophylline. However ofloxacin is not thought to cause a pharmacokinetic interaction with theophylline, unlike some other fluoroquinolones.

Further lowering of the cerebral seizure threshold may also occur with certain nonsteroidal anti-inflammatory drugs.

Ofloxacin may cause a slight increase in serum concentrations of glibenclamide administered concurrently; patients treated with this combination should be closely monitored.

With high doses of quinolones, impairment of excretion and an increase in serum levels may occur when co-administered with other drugs that undergo renal tubular secretion (e.g. probenecid, cimetidine, frusemide and methotrexate).

Interaction with laboratory tests: Determination of opiates or porphyrins in urine may give false-positive results during treatment with ofloxacin. It may be necessary to confirm positive opiate or porphyrin screens by more specific methods.

4.6 Pregnancy and lactation

The safety of this medicinal product for use in human pregnancy has not been established. Reproduction studies performed in rats and rabbits did not reveal any evidence of teratogenicity, impairment of fertility or impairment of peri- and post-natal development. However, as with other quinolones, ofloxacin has been shown to cause arthropathy in immature animals and therefore its use during pregnancy is not recommended. Studies in rats have indicated that ofloxacin is secreted in milk. It should therefore not be used during lactation.

4.7 Effects on ability to drive and use machines

Since there have been occasional reports of somnolence, impairment of skills, dizziness and visual disturbances, patients should know how they react to Tarivid before they drive or operate machinery. These effects may be enhanced by alcohol.

4.8 Undesirable effects

The overall frequency of adverse reactions from the clinical trial data base is about 7%. The commonest events involved the gastrointestinal system (about 5.0%) and the nervous system (about 2.0%).

The following provides a tabulation based on post marketing experience where occasional represents a frequency of 0.1 - 1.0%, rare <0.1%, very rare <0.01% and isolated cases <0.01%:

Digestive and Liver side effects:

Occasional: Nausea and vomiting, diarrhoea, abdominal pain, gastric symptoms. (Diarrhoea may sometimes be a symptom of enterocolitis which may, in some cases, be haemorrhagic).

Rare: Loss of appetite, increase in liver enzymes and/or bilirubin.

Very rare: cholestatic jaundice; hepatitis or severe liver damage may develop. A particular form of enterocolitis that can occur with antibiotics is pseudomembranous colitis (in most cases due to Clostridium difficile). Even if Clostridium difficile is only suspected, administration of ofloxacin should be discontinued immediately, and appropriate treatment given. Drugs that inhibit peristalsis should not be administered in such cases.

Central nervous system:

Occasional: Headache, dizziness, sleep disorders, restlessness.

Rare: Confusion, nightmares, anxiety, depression, hallucinations and psychotic reactions, drowsiness, unsteady gait and tremor (due to disorders of muscular co-ordination), neuropathy, numbness and paraesthesia, sensory or sensorimotor peripheral neuropathy (see Section 4.4 Special Warnings and Precautions for Use), visual disturbances, disturbances of taste and smell (including, in exceptional cases, loss of function), extrapyramidal symptoms.

Very rare: Convulsions, hearing disorders (including, in exceptional cases, loss of hearing).

These reactions have occurred in some patients after the first dose of ofloxacin. In such cases, discontinue treatment immediately.

Isolated cases: Psychotic reactions and depression with self-endangering behaviour including suicidal ideation or acts.

Cardiovascular system:

Tachycardia and a temporary decrease in blood pressure have been reported.

Rare: circulatory collapse (due to pronounced drop in blood pressure).

Haematological side effects:

Very rare: anaemia, leucopenia (including agranulocytosis), thrombocytopenia, pancytopenia.

Only in some cases are these due to bone marrow depression. In very rare cases, haemolytic anaemia may develop.

Renal side effects:

Rare: Disturbances of kidney function.

Isolated cases: Acute interstitial nephritis, or an increase in serum creatinine, which may progress to acute renal failure.

Allergic and skin side effects:

Occasional: Skin rash, itching.

Very rare: Rash on exposure to strong sunlight, other severe skin reactions. Hypersensitivity reactions, immediate or delayed, usually involving the skin (e.g. erythema multiforme, Stevens-Johnson syndrome, Lyell's syndrome, and vasculitis) may occur. In exceptional circumstances, vasculitis can lead to skin lesions including necrosis and may also involve internal organs. There are rarely other signs of anaphylaxis such as tachycardia, fever, dyspnoea, shock, angioneurotic oedema, vasculitic reactions, eosinophilia. In these cases treatment should be discontinued immediately and where appropriate, supportive treatment given.

Isolated cases: Pneumonitis.

Other side effects:

Rare: Malaise.

Very rare: Excessive rise or fall in blood-sugar levels. Weakness, joint and muscle pains (in isolated cases these may be symptoms of rhabdomyolysis).

Isolated cases: Tendon discomfort including inflammation and rupture of tendons (e.g. the Achilles tendon) particularly in patients treated concurrently with corticosteroids. In the event of signs of inflammation of a tendon, treatment with Tarivid must be halted immediately and appropriate treatment must be initiated for the affected tendon.

The possibility cannot be ruled out that ofloxacin may trigger an attack of porphyria in predisposed patients.

Except in very rare instances (e.g. isolated cases of smell, taste and hearing disorders) the adverse effects observed subsided after discontinuation of ofloxacin.

4.9 Overdose

The most important signs to be expected following acute overdosage are CNS symptoms such as confusion, dizziness, impairment of consciousness and convulsive seizures as well as gastrointestinal reactions such as nausea and mucosal erosions.

In the case of overdose steps to remove any unabsorbed ofloxacin eg gastric lavage, administration of adsorbants and sodium sulphate, if possible during the first 30 minutes, are recommended; antacids are recommended for protection of the gastric mucosa.

Elimination of ofloxacin may be increased by forced diuresis.

5. PHARMACOLOGICAL PROPERTIES

5.1 Pharmacodynamic properties

Pharmacotherapeutic group: Quinolone antibacterials, Fluoroquinolones. ATC code J01M A01

Ofloxacin is a quinolone-carboxylic acid derivative with a wide range of antibacterial activity against both gram negative and gram positive organisms. It is active after oral administration. It inhibits bacterial DNA replication by blocking DNA topo-isomerases, in particular DNA gyrase.

Therapeutic doses of ofloxacin are devoid of pharmacological effects on the voluntary or autonomic nervous systems.

Microbiological results indicate that the following pathogens may be regarded as sensitive: *Staphylococcus aureus* (including methicillin resistant staphylococci), *Staphylococcus epidermidis*, Neisseria species, *Escherichia coli*, Citrobacter, Klebsiella, Enterobacter, Hafnia, Proteus (indole-negative and indole-positive strains), *Haemophilus influenzae*, Chlamydiae, Legionella, Gardnerella.

Variable sensitivity is shown by Streptococci, *Serratia marcescens*, *Pseudomonas aeruginosa* and Mycoplasmas.

Anaerobic bacteria (e.g. Fusobacterium species, Bacteroides species, Eubacterium species, Peptococci, Peptostreptococci) are normally resistant.

Tarivid is not active against *Treponema pallidum*.

5.2 Pharmacokinetic properties

Ofloxacin is almost completely absorbed after oral administration. Maximal blood levels occur 1-3 hours after dosing and the elimination half-life is 4-6 hours. Ofloxacin is primarily excreted unchanged in the urine.

In renal insufficiency the dose should be reduced.

No clinically relevant interactions were seen with food and no interaction was found between ofloxacin and theophylline.

5.3 Preclinical safety data

Not Applicable

6. PHARMACEUTICAL PARTICULARS

6.1 List of excipients

Tarivid 200mg: Maize starch, lactose, hyprolose, carmellose NS300, magnesium stearate, hypromellose (2910), titanium dioxide (E171) talc, macrogol 8000.

Tarivid 400mg: Lactose, maize starch, sodium starch glycolate, hyprolose, magnesium stearate, hypromellose, macrogol 8000, talc, titanium dioxide (E171), yellow ferric oxide (E172), purified water.

6.2 Incompatibilities

Not applicable.

6.3 Shelf life

Tarivid 200mg: 5 years

Tarivid 400mg: 3 years

6.4 Special precautions for storage

Tarivid 200mg: This medicinal product does not require any special storage conditions.

Tarivid 400mg: Store in the original package.

6.5 Nature and contents of container
Tarivid 200mg: Blister packs of 10, 20 and 100 tablets

Tarivid 400mg: Aluminium/PVC blister pack with aluminium foil 20µg and PVC (bluish clear) 250µg. Pack sizes: 5, 10 and 50 tablets

6.6 Special precautions for disposal and other handling
No special requirements.

7. MARKETING AUTHORISATION HOLDER
Sanofi-aventis

One Onslow Street

Guildford

Surrey,

GU1 4YS,

UK

8. MARKETING AUTHORISATION NUMBER(S)
Tarivid 200mg: PL 04425/0216

Tarivid 400mg: PL 04425/0217

9. DATE OF FIRST AUTHORISATION/RENEWAL OF THE AUTHORISATION
Tarivid 200mg: April 2002

Tarivid 400mg: 1st January 2002

10. DATE OF REVISION OF THE TEXT
January 2008

11. LEGAL CLASSIFICATION
POM

Tarivid IV Infusion Solution

(sanofi-aventis)

1. NAME OF THE MEDICINAL PRODUCT
Tarivid™ IV Infusion Solution.

2. QUALITATIVE AND QUANTITATIVE COMPOSITION
Ofloxacin, 2 mg/ml.

For a full list of excipients, see section 6.1.

3. PHARMACEUTICAL FORM
Solution for Infusion.

4. CLINICAL PARTICULARS

4.1 Therapeutic indications
Ofloxacin is a synthetic 4-fluoroquinolone antibacterial agent with bactericidal activity against a wide range of Gram-negative and Gram-positive organisms. It is indicated for the treatment of the following infections when caused by sensitive organisms:

Lower Respiratory Tract: Acute and chronic infections.

Upper and Lower Urinary Tract: Acute and chronic lower urinary tract infections; acute and chronic upper urinary tract infections (pyelonephritis). Septicaemia.

Skin and soft tissue infections.

Microbiological results indicate that the following pathogens may be regarded as sensitive: *Staphylococcus aureus* (including methicillin resistant staphylococci), *Staphylococcus epidermidis*, Neisseria species, *Escherichia coli*, Citrobacter, Klebsiella, Enterobacter, Hafnia, Proteus (indole-negative and indole-positive strains), Salmonella, Shigella, Acinetobacter, *Yersinia enterocolitica*, *Campylobacter jejuni*, Aeromonas, Plesiomonas, *Vibrio cholerae*, *Vibrio parahaemolyticus*, *Haemophilus influenzae*, Chlamydiae, Legionella, Gardenerella.

Variable sensitivity is shown by Streptococci, *Serratia marcescens*, *Pseudomonas aeruginosa*, Clostridium species and Mycoplasmas.

Anaerobic bacteria (e.g. Fusobacterium species, Bacteroides species, Eubacterium species, Peptococci, Peptostreptococci) are normally resistant.

Tarivid is not active against *Treponema pallidum*.

4.2 Posology and method of administration
General dosage recommendations: The dose of ofloxacin is determined by the type and severity of the infection.

Adults: The usual intravenous dosages in adults are:

Complicated urinary tract infection: 200 mg daily.

Lower respiratory tract infection: 200 mg twice daily.

Septicaemia: 200 mg twice daily.

Skin and soft tissue infections: 400 mg twice daily.

The infusion time for Tarivid IV should not be less than 30 minutes for 200 mg. Generally, individual doses are to be given at approximately equal intervals.

The dose may be increased to 400 mg twice daily in severe or complicated infections.

Impaired renal function: Following a normal initial dose, dosage should be reduced in patients with impairment of renal function. When creatinine clearance is 20-50 ml/minute (serum creatinine 1.5-5.0 mg/dl) the dosage should be reduced by half (100-200 mg daily). If creatinine clearance is less than 20 ml/minute (serum creatinine greater than 5 mg/dl) 100 mg should be given every 24 hours. In patients undergoing haemodialysis or peritoneal dialysis, 100 mg should be given every 24 hours.

Impaired liver function: The excretion of ofloxacin may be reduced in patients with severe hepatic dysfunction.

Children: Ofloxacin is not indicated for use in children or growing adolescents.

Elderly: No adjustment of dosage is required in the elderly, other than that imposed by consideration of renal or hepatic function. (See section 4.4 QT interval prolongation).

Duration of treatment: The duration of treatment is determined according to the response of the causative organisms and the clinical picture. As with all antibacterial agents, treatment with Tarivid should be continued for at least 3 days after the body temperature has returned to normal and the symptoms have subsided.

In most cases of acute infection, a course of treatment lasting 7 to 10 days is sufficient. Once the patient's condition has improved, the mode of administration should be changed from parenteral to oral, normally at the same total daily dose.

Treatment should not exceed 2 months duration.

4.3 Contraindications
Hypersensitivity to the active substance or to any of the excipients.

Ofloxacin should not be used in patients with a past history of tendinitis.

Ofloxacin, like other 4-quinolones, is contra-indicated in patients with a history of epilepsy or with a lowered seizure threshold. Ofloxacin is contra-indicated in children or growing adolescents, and in pregnant or breast-feeding women, since animal experiments do not entirely exclude the risk of damage to the cartilage of joints in the growing subject.

Patients with latent or actual defects in glucose-6-phosphate dehydrogenase activity may be prone to haemolytic reactions when treated with quinolone antibacterial agents.

4.4 Special warnings and precautions for use

QT interval prolongation

Very rare cases of QT interval prolongation have been reported in patients taking fluoroquinolones. Caution should be taken when using fluoroquinolones, including ofloxacin, in patients with known risk factors for prolongation of the QT interval such as, for example:

- Elderly
- uncorrected electrolyte imbalance (e.g. hypokalemia, hypomagnesemia)
- congenital long QT syndrome
- acquired QT prolongation
- cardiac disease (e.g. heart failure, myocardial infarction, bradycardia)
- concomitant use of drugs that are known to prolong the QT interval (e.g. Class IA and III antiarrhythmics, tricyclic antidepressants, macrolides).

See also section 4.2 Elderly and section 4.5.

Patients being treated with ofloxacin should not expose themselves unnecessarily to strong sunlight and should avoid UV rays (sunlamps, solaria). Caution is recommended if the drug is to be used in psychotic patients or in patients with a history of psychiatric disease.

Sudden reductions in blood pressure may occur when Tarivid IV is administered with hypotensive agents. In such cases, or if the drug is given concomitantly with barbiturate anaesthetics, cardiovascular function should be monitored.

Administration of antibiotics, especially if prolonged, may lead to proliferation of resistant micro-organisms. The patient's condition must therefore be checked at regular intervals. If a secondary infection occurs, appropriate measures must be taken.

Peripheral neuropathy

Sensory or sensorimotor peripheral neuropathy has been reported in patients receiving fluoroquinolones, including ofloxacin. Ofloxacin should be discontinued if the patient experiences symptoms of neuropathy in order to prevent the development of an irreversible condition.

4.5 Interaction with other medicinal products and other forms of interaction

Drugs known to prolong QT interval

Ofloxacin, like other fluoroquinolones, should be used with caution in patients receiving drugs known to prolong the QT interval (e.g. Class IA and III antiarrhythmics, tricyclic antidepressants, macrolides).(See Section 4.4 QT interval prolongation).

Prolongation of bleeding time has been reported during concomitant administration of Tarivid and anticoagulants.

There may be a further lowering of the cerebral seizure threshold when quinolones are given concurrently with other drugs which lower the seizure threshold, e.g. theophylline. However ofloxacin is not thought to cause a pharmacokinetic interaction with theophylline, unlike some other fluoroquinolones.

Further lowering of the cerebral seizure threshold may also occur with certain nonsteroidal anti-inflammatory drugs.

Ofloxacin may cause a slight increase in serum concentrations of glibenclamide administered concurrently; patients treated with this combination should be closely monitored.

With high doses of quinolones, impairment of excretion and an increase in serum levels may occur when co-administered with other drugs that undergo renal tubular secretion (e.g. probenecid, cimetidine, frusemide and methotrexate).

Interaction with laboratory tests: Determination of opiates or porphyrins in urine may give false-positive results during treatment with ofloxacin. It may be necessary to confirm positive opiate or porphyrin screens by more specific methods.

4.6 Pregnancy and lactation
The safety of this medicinal product for use in human pregnancy has not been established. Reproduction studies performed in rats and rabbits did not reveal any evidence of teratogenicity, impairment of fertility or impairment of peri- and post-natal development. However, as with other quinolones, ofloxacin has been shown to cause arthropathy in immature animals and therefore its use during pregnancy is not recommended. Studies in rats have indicated that ofloxacin is secreted in milk. It should therefore not be used during lactation.

4.7 Effects on ability to drive and use machines
Since there have been occasional reports of somnolence, impairment of skills, dizziness and visual disturbances, patients should know how they react to Tarivid before they drive or operate machinery. These effects may be enhanced by alcohol.

4.8 Undesirable effects
In rare cases after i.v. infusion, a reduction in blood pressure may occur. If this effect is marked, the infusion should be stopped. Pain, reddening of the infusion site and thrombophlebitis have been reported in rare cases.

The overall frequency of adverse reactions from the clinical trial data base is about 7%. The commonest events involved the gastrointestinal system (about 5.0%) and the nervous system (about 2.0%).

The following provides a tabulation based on post marketing experience where occasional represents a frequency of 0.1-1.0%, rare <0.1%, very rare <0.01% and isolated cases <0.01%.

Digestive and liver side effects:

Occasional: Nausea and vomiting, diarrhoea, abdominal pain, gastric symptoms. (Diarrhoea may sometimes be a symptom of enterocolitis which may, in some cases, be haemorrhagic).

Rare: Loss of appetite, increase in liver enzymes and/or bilirubin.

Very rare: cholestatic jaundice, hepatitis or severe liver damage may develop. A particular form of enterocolitis that can occur with antibiotics is pseudomembranous colitis (in most cases due to *Clostridium difficile*). Even if *Clostridium difficile* is only suspected, administration of ofloxacin should be discontinued immediately, and appropriate treatment given. Drugs that inhibit peristalsis should not be administered in such cases.

Central nervous system:

Occasional: Headache, dizziness, sleep disorders, restlessness.

Rare: Confusion, nightmares, anxiety, depression, hallucinations and psychotic reactions, drowsiness, unsteady gait and tremor (due to disorders of muscular co-ordination), neuropathy, numbness and paraesthesia, sensory or sensorimotor peripheral neuropathy (see Section 4.4 Special Warnings and Precautions for Use), visual disturbances, disturbances of taste and smell (including, in exceptional cases, loss of function), extrapyramidal symptoms.

Very rare: Convulsions, hearing disorders (including, in exceptional cases, loss of hearing).

Isolated cases: Psychotic reactions and depression with self-endangering behaviour including suicidal ideation or acts.

These reactions have occurred in some patients after the first dose of ofloxacin. In such cases, discontinue treatment immediately.

Cardiovascular system:

Tachycardia and a temporary decrease in blood pressure have been reported.

Rare: circulatory collapse (due to pronounced drop in blood pressure).

Haematological side effects:

Very rare: anaemia, leucopenia (including agranulocytosis), thrombocytopenia, pancytopenia. Only in some cases are these due to bone marrow depression. In very rare cases, haemolytic anaemia may develop.

Renal side effects:

Rare: Disturbances of kidney function.

Isolated cases: Acute interstitial nephritis, or an increase in serum creatinine, which may progress to acute renal failure.

Allergic and skin side effects:

Occasional: Skin rash, itching.

Very rare: Rash on exposure to strong sunlight, other severe skin reactions. Hypersensitivity reactions, immediate or delayed, usually involving the skin (e.g. erythema multiforme, Stevens-Johnson syndrome, Lyell's syndrome and vasculitis) may occur. In exceptional circumstances, vasculitis can lead to skin lesions including necrosis and may also involve internal organs. There are rarely other signs of anaphylaxis such as tachycardia, fever, dyspnoea, shock, angioneurotic oedema, vasculitic reactions, eosinophilia. In these cases treatment should be discontinued immediately and where appropriate, supportive treatment given.

Isolated cases: Pneumonitis.

Other side effects:

Rare: Malaise.

Very rare: Excessive rise or fall in blood-sugar levels. Weakness, joint and muscle pains (in isolated cases these may be symptoms of rhabdomyolysis).

Isolated cases: Tendon discomfort, including inflammation and rupture of tendons (e.g. the Achilles tendon) particularly in patients treated concurrently with corticosteroids. In the event of signs of inflammation of a tendon, treatment with Tarivid must be halted immediately and appropriate treatment must be initiated for the affected tendon.

The possibility cannot be ruled out that ofloxacin may trigger an attack of porphyria in predisposed patients.

Except in very rare instances (e.g. isolated cases of smell, taste and hearing disorders) the adverse effects observed subsided after discontinuation of ofloxacin.

4.9 Overdose

The most important signs to be expected following acute overdosage are CNS symptoms such as confusion, dizziness, impairment of consciousness and convulsive seizures, as well as gastrointestinal reactions such as nausea and mucosal erosions.

Elimination of ofloxacin may be increased by forced diuresis.

5. PHARMACOLOGICAL PROPERTIES

5.1 Pharmacodynamic properties

Pharmacotherapeutic group: Quinolone antibacterials, Fluoroquinolones. ATC code J01M A01

Ofloxacin is a quinolone-carboxylic acid derivative with a wide range of antibacterial activity against both Gram-negative and Gram-positive organisms. It inhibits bacterial DNA replication by blocking DNA topo-isomerases, in particular DNA gyrase.

Therapeutic doses of ofloxacin are devoid of pharmacological effects on the voluntary or autonomic nervous systems.

5.2 Pharmacokinetic properties

Maximum plasma concentrations occur within five minutes of the end of the infusion. The plasma half life is about five hours. Ofloxacin is primarily excreted unchanged in the urine.

Urinary clearance is reduced in renal insufficiency.

5.3 Preclinical safety data

None stated.

6. PHARMACEUTICAL PARTICULARS

6.1 List of excipients

Sodium chloride, hydrochloric acid and water for injections.

6.2 Incompatibilities

Tarivid IV should be administered alone unless compatibility with other infusion fluids has been demonstrated. Compatible infusion solutions include isotonic sodium chloride, Ringer's solution and 5 % glucose solution. Heparin and ofloxacin are incompatible.

6.3 Shelf life

3 years.

6.4 Special precautions for storage

Tarivid IV presented in glass infusion bottles should be protected from light.

6.5 Nature and contents of container

Clear, colourless Type I glass vials with grey chlorobutyl rubber closures and aluminium caps containing 100ml infusion solution.

6.6 Special precautions for disposal and other handling

No special requirements.

7. MARKETING AUTHORISATION HOLDER

Sanofi-aventis

One Onslow Street

Guildford

Surrey,

GU1 4YS,

UK

8. MARKETING AUTHORISATION NUMBER(S)

PL 04425/0215

9. DATE OF FIRST AUTHORISATION/RENEWAL OF THE AUTHORISATION

28/06/2002

10. DATE OF REVISION OF THE TEXT

January 2008

11 LEGAL CLASSIFICATION

POM

Tarka 180/2 mg Capsules

(Abbott Laboratories Limited)

1. NAME OF THE MEDICINAL PRODUCT

Tarka 180 mg/2 mg modified-release capsule

2. QUALITATIVE AND QUANTITATIVE COMPOSITION

Each modified-release capsule contains 180 mg of verapamil hydrochloride and 2 mg of trandolapril.

Excipient: 54.50 mg lactose monohydrate/modified-release capsule

For a full list of excipients see section 6.1.

3. PHARMACEUTICAL FORM

Modified-release capsule

Pale pink opaque

4. CLINICAL PARTICULARS

4.1 Therapeutic indications

Essential hypertension in patients whose blood pressure has been normalised with the individual components in the same proportion of doses.

Refer to section 4.4 (special warnings and precautions for use).

4.2 Posology and method of administration

The usual dosage is one capsule once daily, taken in the morning before, with or after breakfast. The capsules should be swallowed whole.

Children and adolescents: Tarka is contraindicated in children and adolescents (<18 years) (see also section 4.3).

Elderly: As systemic availability is higher in elderly patients compared to younger hypertensives, some elderly patients might experience a more pronounced blood pressure lowering effect (see section 4.4).

Renal insufficiency: Tarka is contraindicated in severe renal impairment (see section 4.3).

Hepatic insufficiency: the use of Tarka is not recommended in patients with severe hepatic impairment; Tarka is contraindicated in patients with liver cirrhosis with ascites (see sections 4.3 and 4.4)

4.3 Contraindications

- Hypersensitivity to trandolapril or any other ACE inhibitor and/or verapamil or to any of the excipients
- History of angioneurotic oedema associated with previous ACE inhibitor therapy
- Hereditary/idiopathic angioneurotic oedema
- Cardiogenic shock
- Recent myocardial infarction with complications
- Second- or third-degree AV block without a functioning pacemaker
- SA block
- Sick sinus syndrome in patients without a functioning pacemaker
- Congestive heart failure
- Atrial flutter/fibrillation in association with an accessory pathway (e.g. WPW-syndrome)
- Severe renal impairment (creatinine clearance < 30 ml/min)
- Dialysis
- Liver cirrhosis with ascites
- Aortic or mitral stenosis, obstructive hypertrophic cardiomyopathy
- Primary aldosteronism
- 2nd and 3rd trimester of pregnancy (see section 4.4 and 4.6)
- Use in children and adolescents (< 18 years)
- Is contraindicated in patients concomitantly treated with i.v. β-adrenoreceptor antagonists (exception: intensive care unit).

4.4 Special warnings and precautions for use

Symptomatic hypotension:

Under certain circumstances, Tarka may occasionally produce symptomatic hypotension. This risk is elevated in patients with a stimulated renin-angiotensin-aldosterone system (e.g., volume or salt depletion, due to the use of diuretics, a low-sodium diet, dialysis, dehydration, diarrhoea or vomiting; decreased left ventricular function, renovascular hypertension)

Such patients should have their volume or salt depletion corrected beforehand and therapy should preferably be initiated in a hospital setting. Patients experiencing hypotension during titration should lie down and may require volume expansion by oral fluid supply or intravenous administration of normal saline. Tarka therapy can usually be continued once blood volume and pressure have been effectively corrected.

Close monitoring during initiation of therapy and dose adjustment is also needed in patients with ischaemic heart or cerebrovascular disease in whom an excessive fall in blood pressure could result in a myocardial infarction or cerebrovascular accident.

Kidney function impairment (see also section 4.3):

Patients with moderate renal impairment should have their kidney function monitored.

Tarka may produce hyperkalaemia in patients with renal dysfunction.

Acute deterioration of kidney function (acute renal failure) may occur especially in patients with pre-existing kidney function impairment, or congestive heart failure.

There is insufficient experience with Tarka in secondary hypertension and particularly in renal vascular hypertension. Hence, Tarka should not be administered to these patients, especially since patients with bilateral renal artery stenosis or unilateral renal artery stenosis in individuals with a single functioning kidney (e.g., renal transplant patients) are endangered to suffer an acute loss of kidney function.

Proteinuria:

Proteinuria may occur particularly in patients with existing renal function impairment or on relatively high doses of ACE inhibitors.

Diabetic Patients:

In diabetic patients treated with oral antidiabetic agents or insulin, glycaemic control should be closely monitored during the first month of treatment with an ACE inhibitor (see section 4.5).

Severe hepatic impairment:

Since there is insufficient therapeutic experience in patients with severe hepatic impairment, the use of Tarka cannot be recommended. Tarka is contraindicated in patients with severe liver cirrhosis with ascites (see also section 4.3). Very rarely, ACE inhibitor therapy has been associated with a syndrome that starts with cholestatic jaundice or hepatitis and progresses to fulminant necrosis and sometimes death. The mechanism of this syndrome is not understood. Patients receiving Tarka who develop jaundice or marked elevations of hepatic enzymes should discontinue Tarka and receive medical follow-up.

Angioneurotic oedema:

Rarely, ACE inhibitors (such as trandolapril) may cause angioneurotic oedema that includes swelling of the face, extremities, tongue, glottis, and/or larynx. Patients experiencing angioneurotic oedema must immediately discontinue trandolapril therapy and be monitored until oedema resolution.

Angioneurotic oedema confined to the face will usually resolve spontaneously. Oedema involving not only the face but also the glottis may be life-threatening because of the risk of airway obstruction.

Compared to non-black patients a higher incidence of angioedema has been reported in black patients treated with ACE inhibitors.

Angioneurotic oedema involving the tongue, glottis or larynx requires immediate subcutaneous administration of 0.3-0.5 ml of epinephrine solution (1:1000) along with other therapeutic measures as appropriate.

Caution must be exercised in patients with a history of idiopathic angioneurotic oedema, and Tarka is contraindicated if angioneurotic oedema was an adverse reaction to an ACE inhibitor (see also section 4.3)

Neutropenia/agranulocytosis:

The risk of neutropenia appears to be dose-and type-related and is dependent on the patient's clinical status. It is rarely seen in uncomplicated patients but may occur in patients with some degree of renal impairment especially when it is associated with collagen vascular disease e.g. systemic lupus erythematosus, scleroderma and therapy with immunosuppressive medicinal products. It is reversible after discontinuation of the ACE inhibitor.

Cough:

During treatment with an ACE inhibitor a dry and non-productive cough may occur which disappears after discontinuation.

Hyperkalaemia:

Hyperkalaemia may occur during treatment with an ACE inhibitor, especially in the presence of renal insufficiency and/or heart failure. Potassium supplements or potassium sparing diuretics are generally not recommended, since they may lead to significant increases in plasma potassium. If concomitant use of the above mentioned medicinal products is deemed appropriate, they should be used with frequent monitoring of serum potassium.

Elderly:

Tarka has been studied in a limited number of elderly hypertensive patients only. Pharmacokinetic data show that the systemic availability of Tarka is higher in elderly compared to younger hypertensives. Some elderly patients might experience a more pronounced blood pressure lowering effect than others. Evaluation of the renal function at the beginning of treatment is recommended.

Surgical patients:

In patients undergoing major surgery requiring general anaesthesia, ACE inhibitors may produce hypotension, which can be corrected by plasma volume expanders.

Conduction disturbances:

Treatments should be used with caution in patients with first degree atrioventricular block. (see also section 4.3).

Bradycardia:

Tarka should be used with caution in patients with bradycardia (see also section 4.3).

Diseases in which neuromuscular transmission is affected:

Tarka should be used with caution in patients with diseases in which neuromuscular transmission is affected (myasthenia gravis, Lambert-Eaton syndrome, advanced Duchenne muscular dystrophy).

Desensitisation:

Anaphylactoid reactions (in some cases life threatening) may develop in patients receiving ACE inhibitor therapy and concomitant desensitisation against animal venoms.

LDL-aphaeresis:

Life threatening anaphylactoid reactions have been noted when patients on LDL-aphaeresis take ACE inhibitors at the same time.

Evaluation of the patients should include assessment of renal function prior to initiation of therapy and during treatment.

Blood pressure readings for evaluation of therapeutic response to Tarka should always be taken before the next dose.

Lactose:

Tarka capsules contain lactose. Each modified-release capsule contains 54.50 mg of lactose monohydrate. Patients with rare hereditary problems of galactose intolerance, the Lapp lactase deficiency or glucose-galactose malabsorption should not take this medicinal product.

Sodium:

This medicinal product contains 1.12 mmol (or 25.71 mg) sodium per dose. To be taken into consideration by patients on a controlled sodium diet.

Lithium:

The combination of lithium and Tarka is not recommended (see section 4.5).

Pregnancy

ACE inhibitors should not be initiated during pregnancy. Unless continued ACE inhibitor therapy is considered essential, patients planning pregnancy should be changed to alternative anti-hypertensive treatments which have an established safety profile for use in pregnancy. When pregnancy is diagnosed, treatment with ACE inhibitors should be stopped immediately, and, if appropriate, alternative therapy should be started (see sections 4.3 and 4.6).

Lactation:

The use of Tarka is not recommended in women whom are breastfeeding (see section 4.6).

4.5 Interaction with other medicinal products and other forms of interaction

Not recommended association

- *Potassium sparing diuretics or potassium supplements*: ACE inhibitors attenuate diuretic induced potassium loss. Potassium sparing diuretics e.g. spironolactone, triamterene, or amiloride, potassium supplements, or potassium containing salt substitutes may lead to significant increases in serum potassium, particularly in the presence of renal function impairment. If concomitant use is indicated because of demonstrated hypokalaemia they should be used with caution and with frequent monitoring of serum potassium.

- *Dantrolene:* The simultaneous use of verapamil with dantrolene is not recommended.

Precaution for use

- *Antihypertensive medicinal products*: increase of the hypotensive effect of Tarka.

- *Diuretics*: patients on diuretics and especially those who are volume-and / or salt depleted may experience an excessive reduction of blood pressure after initiation of therapy with an ACE inhibitor. The possibility of hypotensive effects can be reduced by discontinuation of the diuretic, by increasing volume or salt intake prior to intake and by initiation of therapy with low doses. Further increases in dosage should be performed with caution.

- *Lithium:* there have been reports of both an increase and a reduction in the effects of lithium used concurrently with verapamil. The concomitant administration of ACE inhibitors with lithium may reduce the excretion of lithium. Serum lithium levels should be monitored frequently (see section 4.4).

- *Anaesthetics*: Tarka may enhance the hypotensive effects of certain anaesthetic medicinal products.

- *Narcotics/antipsychotics:* postural hypotension may occur.

- *Allopurinol, cytostatic or immunosuppressive medicinal products, systemic corticosteroids or procainamide*: concomitant administration with ACE inhibitors may lead to an increased risk for leucopenia.

- *Cardiodepressive medicinal products:* the concurrent use of verapamil and cardiodepressives, i.e., medicinal products that inhibit cardiac impulse generation and conduction (e.g., beta-adrenergic blockers, antiarrhythmics, inhalation anaesthetics), may produce undesirable additive effects.

- *Quinidine:* the concomitant use of quinidine and oral verapamil in patients with hypertrophic (obstructive) cardiomyopathy has resulted in hypotension and pulmonary oedema in a small number of cases.

- *Digoxin*: concurrent use of digoxin and verapamil has been reported to result in 50-75% higher digoxin plasma concentrations, requiring reduction of the digoxin dosage.

- *Muscle relaxants:* the effect of muscle relaxants (such as neuromuscular blockers) may be enhanced.

- *Tranquillisers/antidepressants*: as with all antihypertensives, there is an elevated risk of orthostatic hypotension when combining Tarka with major tranquillisers or antidepressant medicinal products containing imipramine.

Take into account

- *Non-steroidal anti-inflammatory drugs (NSAIDs)*: the administration of a non-steroidal anti-inflammatory drug may reduce the antihypertensive effect of an ACE inhibitor. Furthermore it has been described that NSAIDs and ACE inhibitors exert an additive effect on the increase in serum potassium, whereas renal function may decrease. These effects are in principle reversible, and occur especially in patients with compromised renal function.

- *Antacids:* induce decreased bioavailability of ACE inhibitors.

- *Sympathomimetics:* may reduce the antihypertensive effects of ACE inhibitors; patient should be carefully monitored to confirm that the desired effect is being obtained.

- *Alcohol:* enhances the hypotensive effect.

In-vitro metabolic studies indicate that verapamil is metabolised by cytochrome P450 CYP3A4, CYP1A2, CYP2C8, CYP2C9 and CYP2C18. Verapamil is a known inhibitor of CYP3A4 enzymes. Clinically significant interactions have been reported with inhibitors of CYP3A4 causing elevation of plasma levels of verapamil, while inducers of CYP3A4 have caused lowering of plasma levels of verapamil, therefore patients should be monitored for drug interactions. Examples of such interactions are:

- Verapamil may increase the plasma concentrations of *carbamazepine, cyclosporin,* and *theophylline* thus increasing risk of toxicity from these compounds.

- *Rifampin, phenytoin,* and *phenobarbital* reduce the plasma concentrations of verapamil, whereas *cimetidine* may increase the plasma concentrations of verapamil.

- Verapamil may increase plasma concentrations of *prazosin*.

- HMG-CoA Reductase Inhibitors: An increase in serum exposure has been reported for simvastatin (metabolised by CYP3A4) when concomitantly administered with verapamil. The concomitant administration of verapamil and high doses of simvastatin has been reported to increase the risk of myopathia/rabdomyolysis. The dose of simvastatin (and other statins metabolised by CYP3A4 such as atorvastatin and lovastatin) should be adapted accordingly

- *Antidiabetics:* a dose adjustment of antidiabetics or of Tarka may be necessary in individual cases especially at the start of therapy due to increased reduction of blood glucose (see section 4.4).

- *Acetylsalicylic Acid (Aspirin):* The concomitant use of acetylsalicylic acid can increase the side effect profile of acetylsalicylic acid (may increase the risk of bleeding).

- *Grapefruit juice* has been shown to increase the plasma levels of verapamil, which is a component of Tarka. Grapefruit juice should therefore not be ingested with Tarka.

4.6 Pregnancy and lactation

The use of ACE inhibitors is not recommended during the first trimester of pregnancy (see section 4.4). The use of ACE inhibitors is contra-indicated during the 2nd and 3rd trimester of pregnancy (see section 4.3 and 4.4).

Epidemiological evidence regarding the risk of teratogenicity following exposure to ACE inhibitors during the first trimester of pregnancy has not been conclusive; however a small increase in risk cannot be excluded. Unless continued ACE inhibitor therapy is considered essential, patients planning pregnancy should be changed to alternative antihypertensive treatments which have an established safety profile for use in pregnancy. When pregnancy is diagnosed, treatment with ACE inhibitors should be stopped immediately, and, if appropriate, alternative therapy should be started.

ACE inhibitor therapy exposure during the second and third trimesters is known to induce human fetotoxicity (decreased renal function, oligohydramnios, skull ossification retardation) and neonatal toxicity (renal failure, hypotension, hyperkalaemia) (see also 5.3 'Preclinical safety data'). Should exposure to ACE inhibitor have occurred from the second trimester of pregnancy, ultrasound check of renal function and skull is recommended. Infants whose mothers have taken ACE inhibitors should be closely observed for hypotension (see also section 4.3 and 4.4).

Verapamil may inhibit contractions if used at the end of the pregnancy. Also, foetal bradycardia and hypotension cannot be excluded, based on the pharmacological properties.

It is not known whether trandolapril is excreted into human breast milk.

Verapamil is excreted in low amounts into human breast milk.

The use of Tarka is not recommended in women who are breastfeeding (see section 4.4)

4.7 Effects on ability to drive and use machines

No studies on the effects on the ability to drive and use machines have been performed.

There are no data available, but an effect cannot be ruled out, since the undesirable effects such as dizziness and fatigue can occur.

4.8 Undesirable effects

The adverse drug reactions for Tarka are consistent with those known for its components or the respective class of medicinal products. The most commonly reported adverse drug reactions are cough, headache, constipation, vertigo, dizziness and hot flushes (see table below). Adverse events either reported spontaneously or observed in clinical trials are depicted in the following table. Within each system organ class, the adverse drug reactions are ranked under headings of frequency, using the following convention: common (>1/100, <1/10), uncommon (>1/1,000, <1/100), rare (>1/10,000, <1/1,000), very rare (<1/10,000), including isolated reports.

System Organ Class	Frequency	Undesirable Effects
Blood and lymphatic system disorders		
	very rare	- leucopenia - pancytopenia - thrombocytopenia
Immune system disorders		
	uncommon	- allergic reaction, unspecified
	very rare	- increase in gammaglobulin - hypersensitivity, unspecified
Metabolism and nutritional disorders		
	uncommon	- hyperlipidaemia
	rare	- anorexia
Psychiatric disorders		
	uncommon	- somnolence
	very rare	- aggression - anxiety - depression - nervousness
Nervous system disorders		
	common	- dizziness - vertigo
	uncommon	- tremor
	rare	- collapse
	very rare	- impaired balance - insomnia - paresthesia or hyperesthesia - syncope or acute circulatory failures with loss of consciousness - taste aberration - weakness
Eye disorders		
	very rare	- abnormal/blurred vision
Cardiac disorders/ vascular disorders		
	common	- hot flushes
	uncommon	- AV block, first degree - palpitation
	very rare	- angina pectoris - atrial fibrillation - AV block, complete - AV block, unspecified - bradycardia - cardiac arrest - cerebral haemorrhage - oedema, peripheral - oedema, unspecified - flushing - heart failure - hypotension events including orthostasis or fluctuation of blood pressure (see also section 4.4) - tachycardia

Respiratory, thoracic and mediastinal disorders		
	common	- cough
	very rare	- asthma - bronchitis - dyspnoea - sinus congestion
Gastrointestinal disorders		
	common	- constipation
	uncommon	- abdominal pain - diarrhoea - gastrointestinal disorders unspecified - nausea
	very rare	- dry mouth/throat - pancreatitis - vomiting
Hepatobiliary disorders		
	very rare	- cholestasis - hepatitis - increase in γGT - increase in LDH - increase in lipase - jaundice
Skin and subcutaneous tissue disorders		
	uncommon	- facial oedema - pruritus - rash - sweating increased
	rare	- alopecia - herpes simplex - skin disorders, unspecified
	very rare	- angioneurotic oedema (see also section 4.4) - erythema multiforme - exanthema or dermatitis - psoriasis - urticaria
Musculoskeletal, connective tissue and bone disorders		
	very rare	- arthralgia - myalgia - myasthenia
Renal and urinary disorders		
	uncommon	- polyuria
	very rare	- acute renal failure (see also - section 4.4)
Reproductive system and breast disorders		
	very rare	- gynaecomastia - impotence
General disorders and administration site conditions		
	common	- headache
	uncommon	- chest pain
	very rare	- fatigue or asthenia
Investigations		
	uncommon	- liver function test, abnormal
	rare	- hyperbilirubinemia
	very rare	- increase in alkaline phosphatase - increase in serum potassium - increase in transaminases

The following adverse reactions have not yet been reported in relation to Tarka, but are generally accepted as being attributable to ACE inhibitors:

- *Blood and lymphatic system disorders*: decreases in haemoglobin and haematocrit, and in individual cases agranulocytosis. Isolated cases of haemolytic anaemia have been reported in patients with congenital G-6-PDH deficiency.

- *Psychiatric disorders*: occasionally confusion.

- *Nervous system disorders*: rarely, sleep disorders.

- *Ear and labyrinth disorders*: rarely, problems with balance, tinnitus.

- *Cardiac disorders/vascular disorders*: Individual cases of arrhythmia, myocardial infarction and transient ischemic attacks have been reported for ACE inhibitors in association with hypotension.

- *Respiratory, thoracic and mediastinal disorders*: Rarely, sinusitis, rhinitis, glossitis, and bronchospasm.

- *Gastrointestinal disorders*: occasionally indigestion. Individual cases of ileus.

- *Hepatobiliary disorders*: individual cases of cholestatic icterus.

- *Skin and subcutaneous tissue disorders*: occasionally allergic and hypersensitivity reactions such as Stevens-Johnson syndrome, toxic epidermic necrolysis. This can be accompanied by fever, myalgia, arthralgia, eosinophilia and / or increased ANA - titers.

- *Investigations*: increases in blood urea and plasma creatinine may occur especially in the presence of renal insufficiency, severe heart failure and renovascular hypertension. These increases are however reversible on discontinuation.

Symptomatic or severe hypotension has occasionally occurred after initiation of therapy with ACE inhibitors. This occurs especially in certain risk groups, such as patients with a stimulated renin-angiotensin-aldosterone system.

The following adverse reactions have not yet been reported in relation to Tarka, but are generally accepted as being attributable to phenylalkylamine calcium-channel blockers:

- *Nervous system disorders*: in some cases, there may be extrapyramidal symptoms (Parkinson's disease, choreoathetosis, dystonic syndrome). Experience so far has shown that these symptoms resolve once the medicinal product is discontinued. There have been isolated reports of exacerbation of myasthenia gravis, Lambert-Eaton syndrome and advanced cases of Duchenne's muscular dystrophy.

- *Gastrointestinal disorders*: gingival hyperplasia following long-term treatment is extremely rare and reversible after discontinuation of therapy.

- *Skin and subcutaneous tissue disorders*: Stevens-Johnson syndrome and erythromelalgia have been described. In isolated cases allergic skin reactions like erythema.

- *Reproductive system and breast disorders*: Hyperprolactinemia and galactorrhea have been described.

Excessive hypotension in patients with angina pectoris or cerebrovascular disease treated with Verapamil may result in myocardial infarction or cerebrovascular accident.

4.9 Overdose

The highest dose used in clinical trials was 16 mg of trandolapril. This dose produced no signs or symptoms of intolerance.

During overdose with Tarka, the following signs and symptoms may occur due to the verapamil component: hypotension, bradycardia, AV block, asytole and negative inotropy. Fatalities have occurred as a result of overdose.

During overdose with Tarka, the following signs and symptoms may occur due to the ACE inhibitor component: severe hypotension, shock, stupor, bradycardia, electrolyte disturbance, renal failure, hyperventilation, tachycardia, palpitations, dizziness, anxiety, and cough.

Treatment:

After ingestion of an overdose of Tarka Tablets total intestinal lavage should be considered. Further absorption of verapamil present in the gastrointestinal tract should be prevented by gastric lavage, administration of an absorbent (activated charcoal) and a laxative.

Except for general measures (maintenance of an adequate circulation volume with plasma or plasma replacements) against severe hypotension (e.g. shock), inotropic support with dopamine dobutamine or isoprenaline can also be administered.

Treatment of overdose with Tarka should be supportive. Treatment of the overdose of the verapamil hydrochloride component has included the administration of parenteral calcium, beta adrenergic stimulation and gastrointestinal irrigation. Due to the potential for delayed absorption of the sustained release verapamil portion of Tarka, patients may require observation and hospitalisation for up to 48 hours. Verapamil hydrochloride can not be removed by haemodialysis.

The recommended treatment of trandolapril overdose is intravenous infusion of normal saline solution. If hypotension occurs, the patient should be placed in the shock position. If available, treatment with angiotensin II infusion and/or intravenous catecholamines may also be considered. If ingestion is recent, take measures to eliminate trandolapril (e.g. emesis, gastric lavage, administration of absorbents and sodium sulphate). It is not known whether trandolapril (or the active metabolite, trandolaprilat) can be removed via haemodialysis. Pacemaker therapy is indicated for therapy-resistant bradycardia. Vital signs, serum electrolytes and creatinine concentrations should be monitored frequently.

5. PHARMACOLOGICAL PROPERTIES

5.1 Pharmacodynamic properties

Pharmacotherapeutic group: Verapamil, combinations

ATC code: C08DA51

Tarka is a fixed combination of the heart-rate lowering calcium antagonist verapamil and the ACE inhibitor trandolapril.

Verapamil

The pharmacologic action of verapamil is due to inhibition of the influx of calcium ions through the slow channels of the cell membrane of vascular smooth muscle cells and of the conductile and contractile cells in the heart.

The mechanism of action of verapamil produces the following effects:

1. Arterial vasodilation.

In general, verapamil reduces arterial pressure both at rest and at a given level of exercise by dilating peripheral arterioles.

This reduction in total peripheral resistance (afterload) reduces myo-cardial oxygen require-ments and energy consumption.

2. Reduction of myocardial contractility.

The negative inotropic activity of verapamil can be compensated by the reduction in total peripheral resistance.

The cardiac index will not be decreased unless in patients with preexisting left ventricular dysfunction.

Verapamil does not interfere with sympathetic regulation of the heart because it does not block the beta-adrenergic receptors.

Spastic bronchitis and similar conditions, therefore, are not contraindications to verapamil.

Trandolapril

Trandolapril suppresses the plasma renin-angiotensin-aldosterone system (RAS). Renin is an endogenous enzyme synthesized by the kidneys and released into the circulation where it converts angiotensinogen to angiotensin I a relatively inactive decapeptide. Angiotensin I is then converted by angiotensin converting enzyme, a peptidyldipeptidase, to angiotensin II. Angiotensin II is a potent vasoconstrictor responsible for arterial vasoconstriction and increased blood pressure, as well as for stimulation of the adrenal gland to secrete aldosterone. Inhibition of ACE results in decreased plasma angiotensin II, which leads to decreased vasopressor activity and to reduced aldosterone secretion. Although the latter decrease is small, small increase in serum potassium concentrations may occur, along with sodium and fluid loss. The cessation of the negative feedback of angiotensin II on the renin secretion results in an increase of the plasma renin activity.

Another function of the converting enzyme is to degrade the potent vasodilating kinin peptide bradykinin to inactive metabolites. Therefore inhibition of ACE results in an increased activity of circulating and local kallikrein-kinin system which contributes to peripheral vasodilation by activating the prostaglandin system. It is possible that this mechanism is involved in the hypotensive effects of ACE inhibitors and is responsible for certain adverse reactions.

In patients with hypertension administration of ACE inhibitors results in a reduction of supine and standing blood pressure to about the same extent with no compensatory increase of the heart rate. Peripheral arterial resistance is reduced with either no change or an increase in cardiac output.

There is an increase in renal blood flow and glomerular filtration rate is usually unchanged. Achievement of optimal blood pressure reduction may require several weeks of therapy in some patients. The antihypertensive effects are maintained during long term therapy. Abrupt withdrawal of therapy has not been associated with a rapid increase in blood pressure.

The antihypertensive effect of trandolapril sets in one hour post-dose and lasts for at least 24 hours, but trandolapril does not interfere with the circadian blood pressure pattern.

Tarka

Neither animal studies nor healthy volunteer studies could demonstrate pharmacokinetic or RAS interactions between verapamil and trandolapril. The observed synergistic activity of these two active substances must therefore be due to their complementary pharmacodynamic actions.

In clinical trials Tarka was more effective in reducing high blood pressure than either active substance alone.

5.2 Pharmacokinetic properties

The capsules contain verapamil hydrochloride in a sustained-release form and trandolapril in an immediate release form.

Verapamil

Absorption:

About 90% of orally administered verapamil is absorbed. The mean bioavailability is as low as 22% because of extensive hepatic first-pass extraction, and shows great variation (10-35%). The mean bioavailability following repeated administration may increase to 30%.

The presence of food has no effect on the bioavailability of verapamil.

Distribution and biotransformation:

The mean time to peak plasma concentration is 4 hours. The peak plasma concentration of norverapamil is attained about 6 hours post-dose.

Steady state after multiple once daily dosing is reached after 3-4 days.

Plasma protein binding of verapamil is about 90%.

Elimination:

The mean elimination half-life after repeated administration is 8 hours. 3-4% of a dose is excreted renally as unchanged drug. Metabolite excretion is in the urine (70%) and in the faeces (16%). Norverapamil is one of 12 metabolites identified in urine, has 10-20% of the pharmacologic activity of verapamil, and accounts for 6% of excreted drug. The steady-state plasma concentrations of norverapamil and verapamil are similar. Verapamil kinetics is not altered by renal function impairment.

The bioavailability and elimination half-life of verapamil are increased in patients with liver cirrhosis. Verapamil kinetics is, however, unchanged in patients with compensated hepatic dysfunction. Kidney function has no effect on verapamil elimination.

Trandolapril

Absorption:

Orally administered trandolapril is absorbed rapidly. Absorption is 40-60% and independent of the presence of food.

The time to peak plasma concentration is about 30 minutes.

Distribution and biotransformation:

Trandolapril disappears very rapidly from plasma, and its half-life is less than one hour.

Trandolapril is hydrolysed in plasma to form trandolaprilat, a specific angiotensin converting enzyme (ACE) inhibitor. The amount of trandolaprilat formed is independent of food intake.

The time to peak plasma concentration of trandolaprilat is 4-6 hours.

Plasma protein binding of trandolaprilat is greater than 80%. Trandolaprilat binds with great affinity to ACE, and this is a saturable process. Most of circulating trandolaprilat binds to albumin in a non saturable process. Steady state after multiple once daily dosing is reached after about 4 days in healthy volunteers as well as in younger and elderly hypertensive patients.

The effective half-life calculated from accumulation is 16-24 hours.

Elimination:

10-15% of an administered trandolapril dose is excreted as unchanged trandolaprilat in urine. Following oral administration of radioactively labelled trandolapril, one third of radioactivity is recovered in urine and two thirds in faeces.

The renal clearance of trandolaprilat shows a linear correlation with creatinine clearance. The trandolaprilat plasma concentration is significantly higher in patients whose creatinine clearance is ≤ 30 ml/min. Following repeated administration to patients with chronic renal dysfunction, steady state is, however, also reached after four days, independently of the extent of kidney function impairment.

The trandolapril plasma concentration may be 10 times higher in patients with liver cirrhosis than in healthy volunteers. The plasma concentration and renal excretion of trandolaprilat are also increased in cirrhotic patients, albeit to a lesser extent.

Trandolapril(at) kinetics are unchanged in patients with compensated hepatic dysfunction.

Tarka

As there are no known kinetic interactions between verapamil and trandolapril or trandolaprilat, the single active substance kinetic parameters of these two active substances apply to the combination product as well.

5.3 Preclinical safety data

General toxicity effects were observed in animals only at exposures that were sufficiently in excess of the maximum human exposure to make any concern for human safety negligible. Genotoxicity assays revealed no special hazard for humans.

Animal studies have shown that ACE inhibitors tend to have an adverse effect on late foetal development, resulting in foetal death and congenital abnormalities of the skull in particular. Foetoxicity, intrauterine growth retardation and patent ductus arteriosus have also been reported. These abnormalities are thought to be partly due to the pharmacologic activity of these active substances and may be related to ACE inhibitor-induced oligo-hydramnios. The abnormalities may also be partly due to ischaemia resulting from maternal hypotension and decreases in foetal-placental blood flow and oxygen/nutrients delivery to the foetus.

There is no evidence of tumorigenic potential with either trandolapril or verapamil.

6. PHARMACEUTICAL PARTICULARS

6.1 List of excipients

Ingredients of the verapamil film-coated tablet:

- Microcrystalline cellulose
- Povidone
- Sodium alginate
- Magnesium stearate
- Hypromellose
- Hyprolose
- Macrogol 400
- Macrogol 6000
- Talc
- Silica, colloidal anhydrous
- Docusate sodium
- Titanium dioxide, E171

Ingredients of the trandolapril granule:

- Maize starch
- Lactose monohydrate
- Povidone
- Sodium stearyl fumarate

Ingredients of the hard gelatin capsule:

- Titanium dioxide, E171
- Iron oxide red, E172
- Gelatin
- Sodium lauryl sulphate

6.2 Incompatibilities

Not applicable.

6.3 Shelf life

3 years

6.4 Special precautions for storage

Do not store above 25°C.

6.5 Nature and contents of container

Transparent colourless PVC/PVDC-aluminium blisters

Calender packs of 14, 28, 56, 98, 280 capsules in blisters

Packs of 20, 30, 50, 100 and 300 capsules in blisters

Not all pack sizes may be marketed.

6.6 Special precautions for disposal and other handling

No special requirements.

7. MARKETING AUTHORISATION HOLDER

Abbott Laboratories Limited

Queenborough

Kent

ME11 5EL

United Kingdom

8. MARKETING AUTHORISATION NUMBER(S)

PL 00037/0371

9. DATE OF FIRST AUTHORISATION/RENEWAL OF THE AUTHORISATION

Date of last renewal: 26 June 2006.

10. DATE OF REVISION OF THE TEXT

30 March 2009

Tavanic 250mg tablets

(sanofi-aventis)

1. NAME OF THE MEDICINAL PRODUCT

Tavanic 250 mg film-coated tablet

2. QUALITATIVE AND QUANTITATIVE COMPOSITION

Each film-coated tablet of Tavanic contains 250 mg of levofloxacin as active substance corresponding to 256.23 mg of levofloxacin hemihydrate.

For excipients, see 6.1

3. PHARMACEUTICAL FORM

Film-coated tablet.

Score line pale yellowish-white to reddish-white film-coated tablets

4. CLINICAL PARTICULARS

4.1 Therapeutic indications

In adults with infections of mild or moderate severity, Tavanic tablets are indicated for the treatment of the following infections when due to levofloxacin-susceptible microorganisms:

- Acute bacterial sinusitis (adequately diagnosed according to national and/or local guidelines on the treatment of respiratory tract infections)
- Acute bacterial exacerbations of chronic bronchitis (adequately diagnosed according to national and/or local guidelines on the treatment of respiratory tract infections)
- Community-acquired pneumonia
- Uncomplicated urinary tract infections
- Complicated urinary tract infections including pyelonephritis
- Chronic bacterial prostatitis.
- Skin and soft tissue infections.

Before prescribing Tavanic, consideration should be given to national and/or local guidance on the appropriate use of fluoroquinolones.

4.2 Posology and method of administration

Tavanic tablets are administered once or twice daily. The dosage depends on the type and severity of the infection and the sensitivity of the presumed causative pathogen.

Duration of treatment

The duration of treatment varies according to the course of the disease (see table below). As with antibiotic therapy in general, administration of Tavanic tablets should be continued for a minimum of 48 to 72 hours after the patient has become afebrile or evidence of bacterial eradication has been obtained.

Method of administration

Tavanic tablets should be swallowed without crushing and with sufficient amount of liquid. They may be divided at the score line to adapt the dosage. The tablets may be taken during meals or between meals. Tavanic tablets should be taken at least two hours before or after iron salts, antacids and sucralfate administration since reduction of absorption can occur (see section 4.5).

Posology

The following dose recommendations can be given for Tavanic:

Dosage in patients with normal renal function (creatinine clearance > 50 ml/min)

Indication	Daily dose regimen *(according to severity)*	Duration of treatment
Acute sinusitis	500 mg once daily	10 - 14 days
Acute exacerbations of chronic bronchitis	250 to 500 mg once daily	7 - 10 days
Community-acquired pneumonia	500 mg once or twice daily	7 - 14 days
Uncomplicated urinary tract infections	250 mg once daily	3 days
Complicated urinary tract infections including pyelonephritis	250 mg once daily	7 - 10 days
Chronic bacterial prostatitis.	500 mg once daily	28 days
Skin and soft tissue infections	250 mg once daily or 500 mg once or twice daily	7 - 14 days

Special populations

Impaired renal function (creatinine clearance ≤ 50ml/min)

(see Table 1 on next page)

Impaired liver function

No adjustment of dosage is required since levofloxacin is not metabolised to any relevant extent by the liver and is mainly excreted by the kidneys.

In the elderly

No adjustment of dosage is required in the elderly, other than that imposed by consideration of renal function. (See section 4.4 QT interval prolongation).

In children

Tavanic is contraindicated in children and growing adolescents (see section 4.3).

4.3 Contraindications

Tavanic tablets must not be used:

- in patients hypersensitive to levofloxacin or other quinolones or any of the excipients,
- in patients with epilepsy,
- in patients with history of tendon disorders related to fluoroquinolone administration,
- in children or growing adolescents,
- during pregnancy,
- in breast-feeding women.

4.4 Special warnings and precautions for use

In the most severe cases of pneumococcal pneumonia Tavanic may not be the optimal therapy.

Nosocomial infections due to *P. aeruginosa* may require combination therapy.

Tendinitis and tendon rupture

Tendinitis may rarely occur. It most frequently involves the Achilles tendon and may lead to tendon rupture. The risk of tendinitis and tendon rupture is increased in the elderly and in patients using corticosteroids. Close monitoring of these patients is therefore necessary if they are prescribed Tavanic. All patients should consult their physician if they experience symptoms of tendinitis. If tendinitis is

Table 1

	Dose regimen		
	250 mg/24 h	500 mg/24 h	500 mg/12 h
Creatinine clearance	*first dose:* 250 mg	*first dose:* 500 mg	*first dose:* 500 mg
50-20 ml/min	*then:* 125 mg/24 h	*then:* 250 mg/24 h	*then:* 250 mg/12 h
19-10 ml/min	*then:* 125 mg/48 h	*then:* 125 mg/24 h	*then:* 125 mg/12 h
< 10 ml/min (including haemodialysis and CAPD) [1]	*then:* 125 mg/48 h	*then:* 125 mg/24 h	*then:* 125 mg/24 h

[1] No additional doses are required after haemodialysis or continuous ambulatory peritoneal dialysis (CAPD).

suspected, treatment with Tavanic must be halted immediately, and appropriate treatment (e.g. immobilisation) must be initiated for the affected tendon.

Clostridium difficile-associated disease

Diarrhoea, particularly if severe, persistent and/or bloody, during or after treatment with Tavanic tablets, may be symptomatic of *Clostridium difficile*-associated disease, the most severe form of which is pseudomembranous colitis. If pseudomembranous colitis is suspected, Tavanic tablets must be stopped immediately and patients should be treated with supportive measures ± specific therapy without delay (e.g. oral vancomycin). Products inhibiting the peristalsis are contraindicated in this clinical situation.

Patients predisposed to seizures

Tavanic tablets are contraindicated in patients with a history of epilepsy and, as with other quinolones, should be used with extreme caution in patients predisposed to seizures, such as patients with pre-existing central nervous system lesions, concomitant treatment with fenbufen and similar non-steroidal anti-inflammatory drugs or with drugs which lower the cerebral seizure threshold, such as theophylline (see section 4.5). In case of convulsive seizures, treatment with levofloxacin should be discontinued.

Patients with G-6- phosphate dehydrogenase deficiency

Patients with latent or actual defects in glucose-6-phosphate dehydrogenase activity may be prone to haemolytic reactions when treated with quinolone antibacterial agents, and so levofloxacin should be used with caution.

Patients with renal impairment

Since levofloxacin is excreted mainly by the kidneys, the dose of Tavanic should be adjusted in patients with renal impairment (see section 4.2).

Hypersensitivity reactions

Levofloxacin can cause serious, potentially fatal hypersensitivity reactions (e.g. angioedema up to anaphylactic shock), occasionally following the initial dose (see section 4.8). Patients should discontinue treatment immediately and contact their physician or an emergency physician, who will initiate appropriate emergency measures.

Hypoglycemia

As with all quinolones, hypoglycemia has been reported, usually in diabetic patients receiving concomitant treatment with an oral hypoglycemic agent (e.g., glibenclamide) or with insulin. In these diabetic patients, careful monitoring of blood glucose is recommended. (See section 4.8).

Prevention of photosensitisation

Although photosensitisation is very rare with levofloxacin, it is recommended that patients should not expose themselves unnecessarily to strong sunlight or to artificial UV rays (e.g. sunray lamp, solarium), in order to prevent photosensitisation.

Patients treated with Vitamin K antagonists

Due to possible increase in coagulation tests (PT/INR) and/or bleeding in patients treated with Tavanic in combination with a vitamin K antagonist (e.g. warfarin), coagulation tests should be monitored when these drugs are given concomittantly (see section 4.5).

Psychotic reactions

Psychotic reactions have been reported in patients receiving quinolones, including levofloxacin. In very rare cases these have progressed to suicidal thoughts and self-endangering behaviour- sometimes after only a single dose of levofloxacin (see section 4.8). In the event that the patient develops these reactions, levofloxacin should be discontinued and appropriate measures instituted. Caution is recommended if levofloxacin is to be used in psychotic patients or in patients with history of psychiatric disease.

QT interval prolongation

Caution should be taken when using fluoroquinolones, including levofloxacin, in patients with known risk factors for prolongation of the QT interval such as, for example:

- congenital long QT syndrome
- concomitant use of drugs that are known to prolong the QT interval (e.g. Class IA and III antiarrhythmics, tricyclic antidepressants, macrolides).
- uncorrected electrolyte imbalance (e.g. hypokalemia, hypomagnesemia)
- elderly
- cardiac disease (e.g. heart failure, myocardial infarction, bradycardia)

(See section 4.2 *Elderly*, section 4.5, section 4.8, section 4.9).

Peripheral neuropathy

Sensory or sensorimotor peripheral neuropathy has been reported in patients receiving fluoroquinolones, including levofloxacin, which can be rapid in its onset. Levofloxacin should be discontinued if the patient experiences symptoms of neuropathy in order to prevent the development of an irreversible condition.

Opiates

In patients treated with levofloxacin, determination of opiates in urine may give false-positive results. It may be necessary to confirm positive opiate screens by more specific method.

Hepatobiliary disorders

Cases of hepatic necrosis up to life threatening hepatic failure have been reported with levofloxacin, primarily in patients with severe underlying diseases, e.g. sepsis (see section 4.8). Patients should be advised to stop treatment and contact their doctor if signs and symptoms of hepatic disease develop such as anorexia, jaundice, dark urine, pruritus or tender abdomen.

4.5 Interaction with other medicinal products and other forms of interaction

Effect of other medicinal products on Tavanic

Iron salts, magnesium- or aluminium-containing antacids

Levofloxacin absorption is significantly reduced when iron salts, or magnesium- or aluminium-containing antacids are administered concomitantly with Tavanic tablets. It is recommended that preparations containing divalent or trivalent cations such as iron salts, or magnesium- or aluminium-containing antacids should not be taken 2 hours before or after Tavanic tablet administration (see section 4.2). No interaction was found with calcium carbonate.

Sucralfate

The bioavailability of Tavanic tablets is significantly reduced when administered together with sucralfate. If the patient is to receive both sucralfate and Tavanic, it is best to administer sucralfate 2 hours after the Tavanic tablet administration (see section 4.2).

Theophylline, fenbufen or similar non-steroidal anti-inflammatory drugs

No pharmacokinetic interactions of levofloxacin were found with theophylline in a clinical study. However a pronounced lowering of the cerebral seizure threshold may occur when quinolones are given concurrently with theophylline, non-steroidal anti-inflammatory drugs, or other agents which lower the seizure threshold.

Levofloxacin concentrations were about 13% higher in the presence of fenbufen than when administered alone.

Probenecid and cimetidine

Probenecid and cimetidine had a statistically significant effect on the elimination of levofloxacin. The renal clearance of levofloxacin was reduced by cimetidine (24%) and probenecid (34%). This is because both drugs are capable of blocking the renal tubular secretion of levofloxacin. However, at the tested doses in the study, the statistically significant kinetic differences are unlikely to be of clinical relevance.

Caution should be exercised when levofloxacin is coadministered with drugs that affect the tubular renal secretion such as probenecid and cimetidine, especially in renally impaired patients.

Other relevant information

Clinical pharmacology studies have shown that the pharmacokinetics of levofloxacin were not affected to any clinically relevant extent when levofloxacin was administered together with the following drugs: calcium carbonate, digoxin, glibenclamide, ranitidine.

Effect of Tavanic on other medicinal products

Ciclosporin

The half-life of ciclosporin was increased by 33% when coadministered with levofloxacin.

Vitamin K antagonists

Increased coagulation tests (PT/INR) and/or bleeding, which may be severe, have been reported in patients treated with levofloxacin in combination with a vitamin K antagonist (e.g. warfarin). Coagulation tests, therefore, should be monitored in patients treated with vitamin K antagonists (see section 4.4).

Drugs known to prolong QT interval

Levofloxacin, like other fluoroquinolones, should be used with caution in patients receiving drugs known to prolong the QT interval (e.g. Class IA and III antiarrhythmics, tricyclic antidepressants, macrolides). (See section 4.4 QT interval prolongation).

Other forms of interactions

Meals

There is no clinically relevant interaction with food. Tavanic tablets may therefore be administered regardless of food intake.

4.6 Pregnancy and lactation

Pregnancy

Reproductive studies in animals did not raise specific concern. However in the absence of human data and due to the experimental risk of damage by fluoroquinolones to the weight-bearing cartilage of the growing organism, Tavanic tablets must not be used in pregnant women. (see sections 4.3 and 5.3)

Lactation

In the absence of human data and due to the experimental risk of damage by fluoroquinolones to the weight-bearing cartilage of the growing organism, Tavanic tablets must not be used in breast-feeding women. (see sections 4.3 and 5.3)

4.7 Effects on ability to drive and use machines

Some undesirable effects (e.g. dizziness/vertigo, drowsiness, visual disturbances) may impair the patient's ability to concentrate and react, and therefore may constitute a risk in situations where these abilities are of special importance (e.g. driving a car or operating machinery).

4.8 Undesirable effects

The information given below is based on data from clinical studies in more than 5000 patients and on extensive post marketing experience.

The adverse reactions are described according to the MedDRA system organ class below.

Frequencies are defined using the following convention: very common (≥1/10), common (≥1/100, <1/10), uncommon (≥1/1000, ≤1/100), rare (≥1/10000, ≤1/1000), very rare (≤1/10000), not known (cannot be estimated from the available data).

Within each frequency grouping, undesirable effects are presented in order of decreasing seriousness.

Infections and infestations

Uncommon: Fungal infection (and proliferation of other resistant microorganisms)

Blood and lymphatic system disorders

Uncommon: Leukopenia, eosinophilia

Rare: Thrombocytopenia, neutropenia

Very rare: Agranulocytosis

Not Known: Pancytopenia, haemolytic anaemia

Immune system disorders

Very rare: Anaphylactic shock (see section 4.4)

Anaphylactic and anaphylactoid reactions may sometimes occur even after the first dose

Not known: Hypersensitivity (see section 4.4)

Metabolism and nutrition disorders

Uncommon: Anorexia

Very rare: Hypoglycemia, particularly in diabetic patients (see section 4.4)

Psychiatric disorders

Uncommon: Insomnia, nervousness

Rare: Psychotic disorder, Depression, confusional state, agitation, anxiety

Very rare: Psychotic reactions with self-endangering behaviour including suicidal ideation or acts (see section 4.4), hallucination

Nervous system disorders

Uncommon: Dizziness, headache, somnolence

Rare: Convulsion, tremor, paraesthesia,

Very rare: sensory or sensorimotor peripheral neuropathy, dysgeusia including ageusia, parosmia including anosmia

Eye disorders

Very rare: Visual disturbance

Ear and Labyrinth disorders

Uncommon: Vertigo

Very rare: Hearing impaired

Not known: Tinnitus

Cardiac disorders

Rare: Tachycardia

Not Known: Electrocardiogram QT prolonged (see section 4.4 QT interval prolongation and section 4.9)

Vascular disorders

Rare: Hypotension

Respiratory, thoracic and mediastinal disorders

Rare: Bronchospasm, dyspnoea

Very rare: Pneumonitis allergic

Gastrointestinal disorders

Common: Diarrhoea, nausea

Uncommon: Vomiting, abdominal pain, dyspepsia, flatulence, constipation

Rare: Diarrhoea –haemorrhagic which in very rare cases may be indicative of enterocolitis, including pseudomembranous colitis

Hepatobiliary disorders

Common: Hepatic enzyme increased (ALT/AST, alkaline phosphatase, GGT)

Uncommon: Blood bilirubin increased

Very rare: Hepatitis

Not known: Jaundice and severe liver injury, including cases with acute liver failure, have been reported with levofloxacin, primarily in patients with severe underlying diseases (see section 4.4).

Skin and subcutaneous tissue disorders

Uncommon: Rash, pruritus

Rare: Urticaria

Very rare: Angioneurotic oedema, photosensitivity reaction

Not Known: Toxic epidermal necrolysis, Stevens-Johnson syndrome, erythema multiforme, hyperhidrosis

Mucocutaneous reactions may sometimes occur even after the first dose

Musculoskeletal and Connective tissue disorders

Rare: Tendon disorder (see section 4.4) including tendinitis (e.g. Achilles tendon), arthralgia, myalgia

Very rare: Tendon rupture (see section 4.4). This undesirable effect may occur within 48 hours of starting treatment and may be bilateral, muscular weakness which may be of special importance in patients with myasthenia gravis

Not Known: Rhabdomyolysis

Renal and urinary disorders

Uncommon: Blood creatinine increased

Very rare: Renal failure acute (e.g. due to nephritis interstitial)

General disorders and administration site conditions

Uncommon: Asthenia

Very rare: Pyrexia

Not known: Pain (including pain in back, chest, and extremities)

Other undesirable effects which have been associated with fluoroquinolone administration include:

- extrapyramidal symptoms and other disorders of muscular coordination,
- hypersensitivity vasculitis,
- attacks of porphyria in patients with porphyria.

4.9 Overdose

According to toxicity studies in animals or clinical pharmacology studies performed with supra-therapeutic doses, the most important signs to be expected following acute overdosage of Tavanic tablets are central nervous system symptoms such as confusion, dizziness, impairment of consciousness, and convulsive seizures, increases in QT interval as well as gastro-intestinal reactions such as nausea and mucosal erosions.

In the event of overdose, symptomatic treatment should be implemented. ECG monitoring should be undertaken, because of the possibility of QT interval prolongation. Antacids may be used for protection of gastric mucosa. Haemodialysis, including peritoneal dialysis and CAPD, are not effective in removing levofloxacin from the body. No specific antidote exists.

5. PHARMACOLOGICAL PROPERTIES

5.1 Pharmacodynamic properties

Pharmacotherapeutic group: quinolone antibacterials, fluoroquinolones

ATC code: J01MA12

Levofloxacin is a synthetic antibacterial agent of the fluoroquinolone class and is the S (-) enantiomer of the racemic drug substance ofloxacin.

Mechanism of action

As a fluoroquinolone antibacterial agent, levofloxacin acts on the DNA-DNA-gyrase complex and topoisomerase IV.

PK/PD relationship

The degree of the bactericidal activity of levofloxacin depends on the ratio of the maximum concentration in serum (Cmax) or the area under the curve (AUC) and the minimal inhibitory concentration (MIC).

Mechanism of resistance

The main mechanism of resistance is due to a *gyr-A* mutation. *In vitro* there is a cross-resistance between levofloxacin and other fluoroquinolones.

Due to the mechanism of action, there is generally no cross-resistance between levofloxacin and other classes of antibacterial agents.

Breakpoints

The EUCAST recommended MIC breakpoints for levofloxacin, separating susceptible from intermediately susceptible organisms and intermediately susceptible from resistant organisms are presented in the below table for MIC testing (mg/L).

EUCAST clinical MIC breakpoints for levofloxacin (2006-06-20):

Pathogen	Susceptible	Resistant
Enterobacteriacae	≤1 mg/L	>2 mg/L
Pseudomonas spp.	≤1 mg/L	>2 mg/L
Acinetobacter spp.	≤1 mg/L	>2 mg/L
Staphylococcus spp.	≤1 mg/L	>2 mg/L
S.pneumoniae [1]	≤2 mg/L	>2 mg/L
Streptococcus A,B,C,G	≤1 mg/L	>2 mg/L
H. influenzae *M. catarrhalis* [2]	≤1 mg/L	>1 mg/L
Non-species related breakpoints[3]	≤1 mg/L	>2 mg/L

[1] the S/I-breakpoint was increased from 1.0 to 2.0 to avoid dividing the wild type MIC distribution. The breakpoints relate to high dose therapy.

[2] Strains with MIC values above the S/I breakpoint are very rare or not yet reported. The identification and antimicrobial susceptibility tests on any such isolate must be repeated and if the result is confirmed the isolate sent to a reference laboratory.

[3] Non-species related breakpoints have been determined mainly on the basis of pharmacokinetic/pharmacodynamic data and are independent of MIC distributions of specific species. They are for use only for species that have not been given a species-specific breakpoint and are not for use with species where susceptibility testing is not recommended or for which there is insufficient evidence that the species in question is a good target (Enterococcus, Neisseria, Gram negative anaerobes)

The CLSI (Clinical And Laboratory Standards Institute, formerly NCCLS) recommended MIC breakpoints for levofloxacin, separating susceptible from intermediately susceptible organisms and intermediately susceptible from resistant organisms are presented in the below table for MIC testing (μg/mL) or disc diffusion testing (zone diameter [mm] using a 5 μg levofloxacin disc).

CLSI recommended MIC and disc diffusion breakpoints for levofloxacin (M100-S17, 2007):

Pathogen	Susceptible	Resistant
Enterobacteriaceae	≤2 μg/mL ≥17 mm	≥8 μg/mL ≤13 mm
Non Enterobacteriaceae.	≤2 μg/mL ≥17 mm	≥8 μg/mL ≤13 mm
Acinetobacter spp.	≤2 μg/mL ≥17 mm	≥8 μg/mL ≤13 mm
Stenotrophomonas maltophilia	≤2 μg/mL ≥17 mm	≥8 μg/mL ≤13 mm
Staphylococcus spp.	≤1 μg/mL ≥19 mm	≥4 μg/mL ≤15 mm
Enterococcus spp.	≤2 μg/mL ≥17 mm	≥8 μg/mL ≤13 mm
H. influenzae *M. catarrhalis* [1]	≤2 μg/mL ≥17 mm	
Streptococcus pneumoniae	≤2 μg/mL ≥17 mm	≥8 μg/mL ≤13 mm
beta-hemolytic Streptococcus	≤2 μg/mL ≥17 mm	≥8 μg/mL ≤13 mm

[1] The absence or rare occurrence of resistant strains precludes defining any results categories other than « susceptible ». for strains yielding results suggestive of a « nonsusceptible » category, organism identification and antimicrobial susceptibility test results should be confirmed by a reference laboratory using CLSI reference dilution method.

Antibacterial spectrum

The prevalence of resistance may vary geographically and with time for selected species and local information on resistance is desirable, particularly when treating severe infections. As necessary, expert advice should be sought when the local prevalence of resistance is such that the utility of the agent in at least some types of infections is questionable

Commonly susceptible species

Aerobic Gram-positive bacteria

*Staphylococcus aureus** methicillin-susceptible
Staphylococcus saprophyticus
Streptococci, group C and G
Streptococcus agalactiae
Streptococcus pneumoniae *
Streptococcus pyogenes *

Aerobic Gram-negative bacteria

Burkholderia cepacia$
Eikenella corrodens
Haemophilus influenzae *
Haemophilus para-influenzae *
Klebsiella oxytoca
Klebsiella pneumoniae *
Moraxella catarrhalis *
Pasteurella multocida
Proteus vulgaris
Providencia rettgeri

Anaerobic bacteria

Peptostreptococcus

Other

Chlamydophila *pneumoniae* *
Chlamydophila *psittaci*
Chlamydia trachomatis
*Legionella pneumophila**
Mycoplasma pneumoniae *
Mycoplasma hominis
Ureaplasma urealyticum

Species for which acquired resistance may be a problem

Aerobic Gram-positive bacteria

*Enterococcus faecalis**
Staphylococcus aureus methicillin-resistant
Staphylococcus coagulase *spp*

Aerobic Gram-negative bacteria

Acinetobacter baumannii *
Citrobacter freundii *
Enterobacter aerogenes
Enterobacter agglomerans
Enterobacter cloacae *
Escherichia coli *
Morganella morganii *
Proteus mirabilis *
Providencia stuartii
*Pseudomonas aeruginosa**
Serratia marcescens *

Anaerobic bacteria

Bacteroides fragilis
Bacteroides ovatus$
Bacteroides thetaiotamicron$
Bacteroides vulgatus$
Clostridium difficile$

* Clinical efficacy has been demonstrated for susceptible isolates in the approved clinical indications.

$ natural intermediate susceptibility

Other information

Nosocomial infections due to *P. aeruginosa* may require combination therapy.

5.2 Pharmacokinetic properties

Absorption

Orally administered levofloxacin is rapidly and almost completely absorbed with peak plasma concentrations being obtained within 1h. The absolute bioavailability is approximately 100 %.

Food has little effect on the absorption of levofloxacin.

Distribution

Approximately 30 - 40 % of levofloxacin is bound to serum protein. 500 mg once daily multiple dosing with levofloxacin showed negligible accumulation. There is modest but predictable accumulation of levofloxacin after doses of 500 mg twice daily. Steady-state is achieved within 3 days.

Penetration into tissues and body fluids:

Penetration into Bronchial Mucosa, Epithelial Lining Fluid (ELF)

Maximum levofloxacin concentrations in bronchial mucosa and epithelial lining fluid after 500 mg p.o. were 8.3 μg/g and 10.8 μg/ml respectively. These were reached approximately one hour after administration.

Penetration into Lung Tissue

Maximum levofloxacin concentrations in lung tissue after 500 mg p.o. were approximately 11.3 μg/g and were reached between 4 and 6 hours after administration. The concentrations in the lungs consistently exceeded those in plasma.

Penetration into Blister Fluid

Maximum levofloxacin concentrations of about 4.0 and 6.7 μg/ml in the blister fluid were reached 2 - 4 hours after administration following 3 days dosing at 500 mg once or twice daily, respectively.

Penetration into Cerebro-Spinal Fluid

Levofloxacin has poor penetration into cerebro-spinal fluid.

Penetration into prostatic tissue

After administration of oral 500mg levofloxacin once a day for three days, the mean concentrations in prostatic tissue were 8.7 μg/g, 8.2 μg/g and 2.0 μg/g respectively after 2 hours, 6 hours and 24 hours; the mean prostate/plasma concentration ratio was 1.84.

Concentration in urine

The mean urine concentrations 8 -12 hours after a single oral dose of 150 mg, 300 mg or 500 mg levofloxacin were 44 mg/L, 91 mg/L and 200 mg/L, respectively.

Biotransformation

Levofloxacin is metabolised to a very small extent, the metabolites being desmethyl-levofloxacin and levofloxacin N-oxide. These metabolites account for < 5 % of the dose excreted in urine. Levofloxacin is stereochemically stable and does not undergo chiral inversion.

Elimination

Following oral and intravenous administration of levofloxacin, it is eliminated relatively slowly from the plasma ($t_{½}$: 6 - 8 h). Excretion is primarily by the renal route (> 85 % of the administered dose).

There are no major differences in the pharmacokinetics of levofloxacin following intravenous and oral administration, suggesting that the oral and intravenous routes are interchangeable.

Linearity

Levofloxacin obeys linear pharmacokinetics over a range of 50 to 600 mg.

Subjects with renal insufficiency

The pharmacokinetics of levofloxacin are affected by renal impairment. With decreasing renal function renal elimination and clearance are decreased, and elimination half-lives increased as shown in the table below:

Cl_{cr} [ml/min]	< 20	20 - 40	50 - 80
Cl_R [ml/min]	13	26	57
$t_{1/2}$ [h]	35	27	9

Elderly subjects

There are no significant differences in levofloxacin pharmacokinetics between young and elderly subjects, except those associated with differences in creatinine clearance.

Gender differences

Separate analysis for male and female subjects showed small to marginal gender differences in levofloxacin pharmacokinetics. There is no evidence that these gender differences are of clinical relevance.

5.3 Preclinical safety data

Acute toxicity

The median lethal dose (LD_{50}) values obtained in mice and rats after oral administration of levofloxacin were in the range 1500-2000 mg/kg.

Administration of 500 mg/kg p.o. to monkeys induced little effect apart from vomiting.

Repeated dose toxicity

Studies of one and six months duration by gavage have been carried out in the rat and monkey. Doses were 50, 200, 800 mg/kg/day and 20, 80, 320 mg/kg/day for 1 and 6 months in the rat and 10, 30, 100 mg/kg/day and 10, 25, 62.5 mg/kg/day for 1 and 6 months in the monkey.

Signs of reaction to treatment were minor in the rat with slight effects principally at 200 mg/kg/day and above in reducing food consumption and slightly altering haematological and biochemical parameters. The No Observed Adverse Effect Levels (NOELs) in these studies were concluded to be 200 and 20 mg/kg/day after 1 and 6 months respectively.

Toxicity after oral dosing in the monkey was minimal with reduced body weight at 100 mg/kg/day together with salivation, diarrhoea and decreased urinary pH in some animals at this dose. No toxicity was seen in the 6-month study. The NOELs were concluded to be 30 and 62.5 mg/kg/day after 1 and 6 months respectively.

The NOELs in the six-month studies were concluded to be 20 and 62.5 mg/kg/day in the rat and monkey respectively.

Reproductive toxicity

Levofloxacin caused no impairment of fertility or reproductive performance in rats at oral doses as high as 360 mg/kg/day or intravenous doses up to 100 mg/kg/day.

Levofloxacin was not teratogenic in rats at oral doses as high as 810 mg/kg/day, or at intravenous doses as high as 160 mg/kg/day. No teratogenicity was observed when rabbits were dosed orally with up to 50 mg/kg/day or intravenously with up to 25 mg/kg/day.

Levofloxacin had no effect on fertility and its only effect on foetuses was delayed maturation as a result of maternal toxicity.

Genotoxicity

Levofloxacin did not induce gene mutations in bacterial or mammalian cells but did induce chromosome aberrations in Chinese hamster lung cells *in vitro* at or above 100 µg/ml, in the absence of metabolic activation. *In vivo* tests (micronucleus, sister chromatid exchange, unscheduled DNA synthesis, dominant lethal tests) did not show any genotoxic potential.

Phototoxic potential

Studies in the mouse after both oral and intravenous dosing showed levofloxacin to have phototoxic activity only at very high doses. Levofloxacin did not show any genotoxic potential in a photomutagenicity assay, and it reduced tumour development in a photocarcinogenicity assay.

Carcinogenic potential

No indication of carcinogenic potential was seen in a two year study in the rat with dietary administration (0, 10, 30 and 100 mg/kg/day).

Toxicity to joints

In common with other fluoroquinolones, levofloxacin showed effects on cartilage (blistering and cavities) in rats and dogs. These findings were more marked in young animals.

6. PHARMACEUTICAL PARTICULARS

6.1 List of excipients

Tavanic 250 mg film-coated tablets contain the following excipients for a weight of 315 mg:

Tablet core:

Crospovidone, hypromellose, microcrystalline cellulose and sodium stearyl fumarate.

Tablet coating:

Hypromellose, titanium dioxide (E 171), talc, macrogol, yellow ferric oxide (E 172) and red ferric oxide (E 172).

6.2 Incompatibilities

Not applicable.

6.3 Shelf life

5 years.

6.4 Special precautions for storage

This medicine does not require any special conditions for storage.

6.5 Nature and contents of container

PVC aluminium blisters containing film-coated tablets.

Pack sizes for 250 mg tablets: 5 or 10.

6.6 Special precautions for disposal and other handling

A score line allows adaptation of the dose in patients with impaired renal function.

As for all medicines, any unused medicinal product should be disposed of accordingly and in compliance with local environmental regulations.

7. MARKETING AUTHORISATION HOLDER

Sanofi-aventis
One Onslow Street
Guildford
Surrey
GU1 4YS
UK

8. MARKETING AUTHORISATION NUMBER(S)

PL 13042/0011

9. DATE OF FIRST AUTHORISATION/RENEWAL OF THE AUTHORISATION

Date of first authorisation: 6 June 1997

Date of last renewal: 5 June 2007

10. DATE OF REVISION OF THE TEXT

14 September 2007

Legal category: POM

Tavanic 500mg tablets

(sanofi-aventis)

1. NAME OF THE MEDICINAL PRODUCT

Tavanic 500 mg film-coated tablet

2. QUALITATIVE AND QUANTITATIVE COMPOSITION

Each film-coated tablet of Tavanic contains 500 mg of levofloxacin as active substance corresponding to 512.46 mg of levofloxacin hemihydrate.

For excipients, see 6.1

3. PHARMACEUTICAL FORM

Film-coated tablet.

Score line pale yellowish-white to reddish-white film-coated tablets

4. CLINICAL PARTICULARS

4.1 Therapeutic indications

In adults with infections of mild or moderate severity, Tavanic tablets are indicated for the treatment of the following infections when due to levofloxacin-susceptible microorganisms:

- Acute bacterial sinusitis (adequately diagnosed according to national and/or local guidelines on the treatment of respiratory tract infections)
- Acute bacterial exacerbations of chronic bronchitis (adequately diagnosed according to national and/or local guidelines on the treatment of respiratory tract infections)
- Community-acquired pneumonia
- Uncomplicated urinary tract infections
- Complicated urinary tract infections including pyelonephritis
- Chronic bacterial prostatitis.
- Skin and soft tissue infections.

Before prescribing Tavanic, consideration should be given to national and/or local guidance on the appropriate use of fluoroquinolones.

4.2 Posology and method of administration

Tavanic tablets are administered once or twice daily. The dosage depends on the type and severity of the infection and the sensitivity of the presumed causative pathogen.

Duration of treatment

The duration of treatment varies according to the course of the disease (see table below). As with antibiotic therapy in general, administration of Tavanic tablets should be continued for a minimum of 48 to 72 hours after the patient has become afebrile or evidence of bacterial eradication has been obtained.

Method of administration

Tavanic tablets should be swallowed without crushing and with sufficient amount of liquid. They may be divided at the score line to adapt the dosage. The tablets may be taken during meals or between meals. Tavanic tablets should be taken at least two hours before or after iron salts, antacids and sucralfate administration since reduction of absorption can occur (see section 4.5).

Posology

The following dose recommendations can be given for Tavanic:

Dosage in patients with normal renal function (creatinine clearance > 50 ml/min)

Indication	**Daily dose regimen** *(according to severity)*	**Duration of treatment**
Acute sinusitis	500 mg once daily	10 - 14 days
Acute exacerbations of chronic bronchitis	250 to 500 mg once daily	7 - 10 days
Community-acquired pneumonia	500 mg once or twice daily	7 - 14 days
Complicated urinary tract infections including pyelonephritis	250 mg once daily	7 - 10 days
Chronic bacterial prostatitis.	500 mg once daily	28 days
Skin and soft tissue infections	250 mg once daily or 500 mg once or twice daily	7 - 14 days

Special populations

Impaired renal function (creatinine clearance ≤ 50ml/min)

(see Table 1 on next page)

Impaired liver function

No adjustment of dosage is required since levofloxacin is not metabolised to any relevant extent by the liver and is mainly excreted by the kidneys.

In the elderly

No adjustment of dosage is required in the elderly, other than that imposed by consideration of renal function.(See section 4.4 QT interval prolongation).

In children

Tavanic is contraindicated in children and growing adolescents (see section 4.3).

4.3 Contraindications

Tavanic tablets must not be used:

- in patients hypersensitive to levofloxacin or other quinolones or any of the excipients,
- in patients with epilepsy,
- in patients with history of tendon disorders related to fluoroquinolone administration,
- in children or growing adolescents,
- during pregnancy,
- in breast-feeding women.

4.4 Special warnings and precautions for use

In the most severe cases of pneumococcal pneumonia Tavanic may not be the optimal therapy.

Nosocomial infections due to *P. aeruginosa* may require combination therapy.

Tendinitis and tendon rupture

Tendinitis may rarely occur. It most frequently involves the Achilles tendon and may lead to tendon rupture. The risk of tendinitis and tendon rupture is increased in the elderly and in patients using corticosteroids. Close monitoring of these patients is therefore necessary if they are prescribed Tavanic. All patients should consult their physician if they experience symptoms of tendinitis. If tendinitis is suspected, treatment with Tavanic must be halted immediately, and appropriate treatment (e.g. immobilisation) must be initiated for the affected tendon.

Table 1

Creatinine clearance	Dose regimen		
	250 mg/24 h	**500 mg/24 h**	**500 mg/12 h**
	first dose: 250 mg	*first dose:* 500 mg	*first dose:* 500 mg
50-20 ml/min	*then:* 125 mg/24 h	*then:* 250 mg/24 h	*then:* 250 mg/12 h
19-10 ml/min	*then:* 125 mg/48 h	*then:* 125 mg/24 h	*then:* 125 mg/12 h
< 10 ml/min (including haemodialysis and CAPD) [1]	*then:* 125 mg/48 h	*then:* 125 mg/24 h	*then:* 125 mg/24 h

[1] No additional doses are required after haemodialysis or continuous ambulatory peritoneal dialysis (CAPD).

Clostridium difficile-associated disease

Diarrhoea, particularly if severe, persistent and/or bloody, during or after treatment with Tavanic tablets, may be symptomatic of *Clostridium difficile*-associated disease, the most severe form of which is pseudomembranous colitis. If pseudomembranous colitis is suspected, Tavanic tablets must be stopped immediately and patients should be treated with supportive measures ± specific therapy without delay (e.g. oral vancomycin). Products inhibiting the peristalsis are contraindicated in this clinical situation.

Patients predisposed to seizures

Tavanic tablets are contraindicated in patients with a history of epilepsy and, as with other quinolones, should be used with extreme caution in patients predisposed to seizures, such as patients with pre-existing central nervous system lesions, concomitant treatment with fenbufen and similar non-steroidal anti-inflammatory drugs or with drugs which lower the cerebral seizure threshold, such as theophylline (see section 4.5). In case of convulsive seizures, treatment with levofloxacin should be discontinued.

Patients with G-6- phosphate dehydrogenase deficiency

Patients with latent or actual defects in glucose-6-phosphate dehydrogenase activity may be prone to haemolytic reactions when treated with quinolone antibacterial agents, and so levofloxacin should be used with caution.

Patients with renal impairment

Since levofloxacin is excreted mainly by the kidneys, the dose of Tavanic should be adjusted in patients with renal impairment (see section 4.2).

Hypersensitivity reactions

Levofloxacin can cause serious, potentially fatal hypersensitivity reactions (e.g. angioedema up to anaphylactic shock), occasionally following the initial dose (see section 4.8). Patients should discontinue treatment immediately and contact their physician or an emergency physician, who will initiate appropriate emergency measures.

Hypoglycemia

As with all quinolones, hypoglycemia has been reported, usually in diabetic patients receiving concomitant treatment with an oral hypoglycemic agent (e.g., glibenclamide) or with insulin. In these diabetic patients, careful monitoring of blood glucose is recommended. (See section 4.8).

Prevention of photosensitisation

Although photosensitisation is very rare with levofloxacin, it is recommended that patients should not expose themselves unnecessarily to strong sunlight or to artificial UV rays (e.g. sunray lamp, solarium), in order to prevent photosensitisation.

Patients treated with Vitamin K antagonists

Due to possible increase in coagulation tests (PT/INR) and/or bleeding in patients treated with Tavanic in combination with a vitamin K antagonist (e.g. warfarin), coagulation tests should be monitored when these drugs are given concomittantly (see section 4.5).

Psychotic reactions

Psychotic reactions have been reported in patients receiving quinolones, including levofloxacin. In very rare cases these have progressed to suicidal thoughts and self-endangering behaviour- sometimes after only a single dose of levofloxacin (see section 4.8). In the event that the patient develops these reactions, levofloxacin should be discontinued and appropriate measures instituted. Caution is recommended if levofloxacin is to be used in psychotic patients or in patients with history of psychiatric disease.

QT interval prolongation

Caution should be taken when using fluoroquinolones, including levofloxacin, in patients with known risk factors for prolongation of the QT interval such as, for example:

- congenital long QT syndrome
- concomitant use of drugs that are known to prolong the QT interval (e.g. Class IA and III antiarrhythmics, tricyclic antidepressants, macrolides).
- uncorrected electrolyte imbalance (e.g. hypokalemia, hypomagnesemia)
- elderly
- cardiac disease (e.g. heart failure, myocardial infarction, bradycardia)

(See section 4.2 *Elderly*, section 4.5, section 4.8, section 4.9).

Peripheral neuropathy

Sensory or sensorimotor peripheral neuropathy has been reported in patients receiving fluoroquinolones, including levofloxacin, which can be rapid in its onset. Levofloxacin should be discontinued if the patient experiences symptoms of neuropathy in order to prevent the development of an irreversible condition.

Opiates

In patients treated with levofloxacin, determination of opiates in urine may give false-positive results. It may be necessary to confirm positive opiate screens by more specific method.

Hepatobiliary disorders

Cases of hepatic necrosis up to life threatening hepatic failure have been reported with levofloxacin, primarily in patients with severe underlying diseases, e.g. sepsis (see section 4.8). Patients should be advised to stop treatment and contact their doctor if signs and symptoms of hepatic disease develop such as anorexia, jaundice, dark urine, pruritus or tender abdomen.

4.5 Interaction with other medicinal products and other forms of interaction

Effect of other medicinal products on Tavanic

Iron salts, magnesium- or aluminium-containing antacids

Levofloxacin absorption is significantly reduced when iron salts, or magnesium- or aluminium-containing antacids are administered concomitantly with Tavanic tablets. It is recommended that preparations containing divalent or trivalent cations such as iron salts, or magnesium- or aluminium-containing antacids should not be taken 2 hours before or after Tavanic tablet administration (see section 4.2). No interaction was found with calcium carbonate.

Sucralfate

The bioavailability of Tavanic tablets is significantly reduced when administered together with sucralfate. If the patient is to receive both sucralfate and Tavanic, it is best to administer sucralfate 2 hours after the Tavanic tablet administration (see section 4.2).

Theophylline, fenbufen or similar non-steroidal anti-inflammatory drugs

No pharmacokinetic interactions of levofloxacin were found with theophylline in a clinical study. However a pronounced lowering of the cerebral seizure threshold may occur when quinolones are given concurrently with theophylline, non-steroidal anti-inflammatory drugs, or other agents which lower the seizure threshold.

Levofloxacin concentrations were about 13% higher in the presence of fenbufen than when administered alone.

Probenecid and cimetidine

Probenecid and cimetidine had a statistically significant effect on the elimination of levofloxacin. The renal clearance of levofloxacin was reduced by cimetidine (24%) and probenecid (34%). This is because both drugs are capable of blocking the renal tubular secretion of levofloxacin. However, at the tested doses in the study, the statistically significant kinetic differences are unlikely to be of clinical relevance.

Caution should be exercised when levofloxacin is coadministered with drugs that affect the tubular renal secretion such as probenecid and cimetidine, especially in renally impaired patients.

Other relevant information

Clinical pharmacology studies have shown that the pharmacokinetics of levofloxacin were not affected to any clinically relevant extent when levofloxacin was administered together with the following drugs: calcium carbonate, digoxin, glibenclamide, ranitidine.

Effect of Tavanic on other medicinal products

Ciclosporin

The half-life of ciclosporin was increased by 33% when coadministered with levofloxacin.

Vitamin K antagonists

Increased coagulation tests (PT/INR) and/or bleeding, which may be severe, have been reported in patients treated with levofloxacin in combination with a vitamin K antagonist (e.g. warfarin). Coagulation tests, therefore, should be monitored in patients treated with vitamin K antagonists (see section 4.4).

Drugs known to prolong QT interval

Levofloxacin, like other fluoroquinolones, should be used with caution in patients receiving drugs known to prolong the QT interval (e.g. Class IA and III antiarrhythmics, tricyclic antidepressants, macrolides). (See section 4.4 QT interval prolongation).

Other forms of interactions

Meals

There is no clinically relevant interaction with food. Tavanic tablets may therefore be administered regardless of food intake.

4.6 Pregnancy and lactation

Pregnancy

Reproductive studies in animals did not raise specific concern. However in the absence of human data and due to the experimental risk of damage by fluoroquinolones to the weight-bearing cartilage of the growing organism, Tavanic tablets must not be used in pregnant women. (see sections 4.3 and 5.3)

Lactation

In the absence of human data and due to the experimental risk of damage by fluoroquinolones to the weight-bearing cartilage of the growing organism, Tavanic tablets must not be used in breast-feeding women. (see sections 4.3 and 5.3)

4.7 Effects on ability to drive and use machines

Some undesirable effects (e.g. dizziness/vertigo, drowsiness, visual disturbances) may impair the patient's ability to concentrate and react, and therefore may constitute a risk in situations where these abilities are of special importance (e.g. driving a car or operating machinery).

4.8 Undesirable effects

The information given below is based on data from clinical studies in more than 5000 patients and on extensive post marketing experience.

The adverse reactions are described according to the MedDRA system organ class below.

Frequencies are defined using the following convention: very common (≥ 1/10), common (≥ 1/100, < 1/10), uncommon (≥ 1/1000, ≤ 1/100), rare (≥ 1/10000, ≤ 1/1000), very rare (≤ 1/10000), not known (cannot be estimated from the available data).

Within each frequency grouping, undesirable effects are presented in order of decreasing seriousness.

Infections and infestations

Uncommon: Fungal infection (and proliferation of other resistant microorganisms)

Blood and lymphatic system disorders

Uncommon: Leukopenia, eosinophilia

Rare: Thrombocytopenia, neutropenia

Very rare: Agranulocytosis

Not Known: Pancytopenia, haemolytic anaemia

Immune system disorders

Very rare: Anaphylactic shock (see section 4.4)

Anaphylactic and anaphylactoid reactions may sometimes occur even after the first dose

Not known: Hypersensitivity (see section 4.4)

Metabolism and nutrition disorders

Uncommon: Anorexia

Very rare: Hypoglycemia, particularly in diabetic patients (see section 4.4)

Psychiatric disorders

Uncommon: Insomnia, nervousness

Rare: Psychotic disorder, depression, confusional state, agitation, anxiety

Very rare: Psychotic reactions with self-endangering behaviour including suicidal ideation or acts (see section 4.4), hallucination

Nervous system disorders

Uncommon: Dizziness, headache, somnolence

Rare: Convulsion, tremor, paraesthesia

Very rare: sensory or sensorimotor peripheral neuropathy, dysgeusia including ageusia, parosmia including anosmia

Eye disorders

Very rare: Visual disturbance

Ear and Labyrinth disorders

Uncommon: Vertigo

Very rare: Hearing impaired

Not known: Tinnitus

Cardiac disorders

Rare: Tachycardia

Not Known: Electrocardiogram QT prolonged (see section 4.4 QT interval prolongation and section 4.9)

Vascular disorders

Rare: Hypotension

Respiratory, thoracic and mediastinal disorders

Rare: Bronchospasm, dyspnoea

Very rare: Pneumonitis allergic

Gastrointestinal disorders

Common: Diarrhoea, nausea

Uncommon: Vomiting, abdominal pain, dyspepsia, flatulence, constipation.

Rare: Diarrhoea –haemorrhagic which in very rare cases may be indicative of enterocolitis, including pseudomembranous colitis

Hepatobiliary disorders

Common: Hepatic enzyme increased (ALT/AST, alkaline phosphatase, GGT)

Uncommon: Blood bilirubin increased

Very rare: Hepatitis

Not known: Jaundice and severe liver injury, including cases with acute liver failure, have been reported with levofloxacin, primarily in patients with severe underlying diseases (see section 4.4).

Skin and subcutaneous tissue disorders

Uncommon: Rash, pruritus

Rare: Urticaria

Very rare: Angioneurotic oedema, photosensitivity reaction

Not Known: Toxic epidermal necrolysis, Stevens-Johnson syndrome, erythema multiforme, hyperhidrosis

Mucocutaneous reactions may sometimes occur even after the first dose

Musculoskeletal and Connective tissue disorders

Rare: Tendon disorder (see section 4.4) including tendinitis (e.g. Achilles tendon), Arthralgia, Myalgia

Very rare: Tendon rupture (see section 4.4). This undesirable effect may occur within 48 hours of starting treatment and may be bilateral, muscular weakness which may be of special importance in patients with myasthenia gravis

Not Known: Rhabdomyolysis

Renal and urinary disorders

Uncommon: Blood creatinine increased

Very rare: Renal failure acute (e.g. due to nephritis interstitial)

General disorders and administration site conditions

Uncommon: Asthenia

Very rare: Pyrexia

Not known: Pain (including pain in back, chest, and extremities)

Other undesirable effects which have been associated with fluoroquinolone administration include:

- extrapyramidal symptoms and other disorders of muscular coordination,
- hypersensitivity vasculitis,
- attacks of porphyria in patients with porphyria

4.9 Overdose

According to toxicity studies in animals or clinical pharmacology studies performed with supra-therapeutic doses, the most important signs to be expected following acute overdosage of Tavanic tablets are central nervous system symptoms such as confusion, dizziness, impairment of consciousness, and convulsive seizures, increases in QT interval as well as gastro-intestinal reactions such as nausea and mucosal erosions.

In the event of overdose, symptomatic treatment should be implemented. ECG monitoring should be undertaken, because of the possibility of QT interval prolongation. Antacids may be used for protection of gastric mucosa. Haemodialysis, including peritoneal dialysis and CAPD, are not effective in removing levofloxacin from the body. No specific antidote exists.

5. PHARMACOLOGICAL PROPERTIES

5.1 Pharmacodynamic properties

Pharmacotherapeutic group: quinolone antibacterials, fluoroquinolones

ATC code: J01MA12

Levofloxacin is a synthetic antibacterial agent of the fluoroquinolone class and is the S (-) enantiomer of the racemic drug substance ofloxacin.

Mechanism of action

As a fluoroquinolone antibacterial agent, levofloxacin acts on the DNA-DNA-gyrase complex and topoisomerase IV.

PK/PD relationship

The degree of the bactericidal activity of levofloxacin depends on the ratio of the maximum concentration in serum (Cmax) or the area under the curve (AUC) and the minimal inhibitory concentration (MIC).

Mechanism of resistance

The main mechanism of resistance is due to a *gyr-A* mutation. *In vitro* there is a cross-resistance between levofloxacin and other fluoroquinolones.

Due to the mechanism of action, there is generally no cross-resistance between levofloxacin and other classes of antibacterial agents.

Breakpoints

The EUCAST recommended MIC breakpoints for levofloxacin, separating susceptible from intermediately susceptible organisms and intermediately susceptible from resistant organisms are presented in the below table for MIC testing (mg/L).

EUCAST clinical MIC breakpoints for levofloxacin (2006-06-20):

Pathogen	Susceptible	Resistant
Enterobacteriacae	⩽1 mg/L	>2 mg/L
Pseudomonas spp.	⩽1 mg/L	>2 mg/L
Acinetobacter spp.	⩽1 mg/L	>2 mg/L
Staphylococcus spp.	⩽1 mg/L	>2 mg/L
S.pneumoniae [1]	⩽2 mg/L	>2 mg/L
Streptococcus A,B,C,G	⩽1 mg/L	>2 mg/L
H. influenzae *M. catarrhalis* [2]	⩽1 mg/L	>1 mg/L
Non-species related breakpoints[3]	⩽1 mg/L	>2 mg/L

[1] the S/I-breakpoint was increased from 1.0 to 2.0 to avoid dividing the wild type MIC distribution. The breakpoints relate to high dose therapy.

[2] Strains with MIC values above the S/I breakpoint are very rare or not yet reported. The identification and antimicrobial susceptibility tests on any such isolate must be repeated and if the result is confirmed the isolate sent to a reference laboratory.

[3] Non-species related breakpoints have been determined mainly on the basis of pharmacokinetic/pharmacodynamic data and are independent of MIC distributions of specific species. They are for use only for species that have not been given a species-specific breakpoint and are not for use with species where susceptibility testing is not recommended or for which there is insufficient evidence that the species in question is a good target (Enterococcus, Neisseria, Gram negative anaerobes).

The CLSI (Clinical And Laboratory Standards Institute, formerly NCCLS) recommended MIC breakpoints for levofloxacin, separating susceptible from intermediately susceptible organisms and intermediately susceptible from resistant organisms are presented in the below table for MIC testing (μg/mL) or disc diffusion testing (zone diameter [mm] using a 5 μg levofloxacin disc).

CLSI recommended MIC and disc diffusion breakpoints for levofloxacin (M100-S17, 2007):

Pathogen	Susceptible	Resistant
Enterobacteriaceae	⩽2 μg/mL ⩾17 mm	⩾8 μg/mL ⩽13 mm
Non Enterobacteriaceae.	⩽2 μg/mL ⩾17 mm	⩾8 μg/mL ⩽13 mm
Acinetobacter spp.	⩽2 μg/mL ⩾17 mm	⩾8 μg/mL ⩽13 mm
Stenotrophomonas maltophilia	⩽2 μg/mL ⩾17 mm	⩾8 μg/mL ⩽13 mm
Staphylococcus spp.	⩽1 μg/mL ⩾19 mm	⩾4 μg/mL ⩽15 mm
Enterococcus spp.	⩽2 μg/mL ⩾17 mm	⩾8 μg/mL ⩽13 mm
H. influenzae *M. catarrhalis* [1]	⩽2 μg/mL ⩾17 mm	
Streptococcus pneumoniae	⩽2 μg/mL ⩾17 mm	⩾8 μg/mL ⩽13 mm
beta-hemolytic Streptococcus	⩽2 μg/mL ⩾17 mm	⩾8 μg/mL ⩽13 mm

[1] The absence or rare occurrence of resistant strains precludes defining any results categories other than « susceptible ». for strains yielding results suggestive of a « nonsusceptible » category, organism identification and antimicrobial susceptibility test results should be confirmed by a reference laboratory using CLSI reference dilution method.

Antibacterial spectrum

The prevalence of resistance may vary geographically and with time for selected species and local information on resistance is desirable, particularly when treating severe infections. As necessary, expert advice should be sought when the local prevalence of resistance is such that the utility of the agent in at least some types of infections is questionable

Commonly susceptible species

Aerobic Gram-positive bacteria

*Staphylococcus aureus**
methicillin-susceptible
Staphylococcus saprophyticus
Streptococci, group C and G
Streptococcus agalactiae
*Streptococcus pneumoniae**
*Streptococcus pyogenes**

Aerobic Gram-negative bacteria

Burkholderia cepacia$
Eikenella corrodens
*Haemophilus influenzae**
*Haemophilus para-influenzae**
Klebsiella oxytoca
*Klebsiella pneumoniae**
*Moraxella catarrhalis**
Pasteurella multocida
Proteus vulgaris
Providencia rettgeri

Anaerobic bacteria

Peptostreptococcus

Other

Chlamydophila *pneumoniae**
Chlamydophila *psittaci*
Chlamydia trachomatis
*Legionella pneumophila**
*Mycoplasma pneumoniae**
Mycoplasma hominis
Ureaplasma urealyticum

Species for which acquired resistance may be a problem

Aerobic Gram-positive bacteria

*Enterococcus faecalis**
Staphylococcus aureus
methicillin-resistant
Staphylococcus coagulase *spp*

Aerobic Gram-negative bacteria

*Acinetobacter baumannii**
*Citrobacter freundii**
Enterobacter aerogenes
Enterobacter agglomerans
*Enterobacter cloacae**
*Escherichia coli**
*Morganella morganii**
*Proteus mirabilis**
Providencia stuartii
*Pseudomonas aeruginosa**
*Serratia marcescens**

Anaerobic bacteria

Bacteroides fragilis
Bacteroides ovatus$
Bacteroides thetaiotamicron$
Bacteroides vulgatus$
Clostridium difficile$

* Clinical efficacy has been demonstrated for susceptible isolates in the approved clinical indications.

$ natural intermediate susceptibility

Other information

Nosocomial infections due to *P. aeruginosa* may require combination therapy.

5.2 Pharmacokinetic properties

Absorption

Orally administered levofloxacin is rapidly and almost completely absorbed with peak plasma concentrations being obtained within 1h. The absolute bioavailability is approximately 100 %.

Food has little effect on the absorption of levofloxacin.

Distribution

Approximately 30 - 40 % of levofloxacin is bound to serum protein. 500 mg once daily multiple dosing with levofloxacin showed negligible accumulation. There is modest but predictable accumulation of levofloxacin after doses of 500 mg twice daily. Steady-state is achieved within 3 days.

Penetration into tissues and body fluids:

Penetration into Bronchial Mucosa, Epithelial Lining Fluid (ELF)

Maximum levofloxacin concentrations in bronchial mucosa and epithelial lining fluid after 500 mg p.o. were 8.3 μg/g and 10.8 μg/ml respectively. These were reached approximately one hour after administration.

Penetration into Lung Tissue

Maximum levofloxacin concentrations in lung tissue after 500 mg p.o. were approximately 11.3 μg/g and were reached between 4 and 6 hours after administration. The concentrations in the lungs consistently exceeded those in plasma.

Penetration into Blister Fluid

Maximum levofloxacin concentrations of about 4.0 and 6.7 μg/ml in the blister fluid were reached 2 - 4 hours after administration following 3 days dosing at 500 mg once or twice daily, respectively.

Penetration into Cerebro-Spinal Fluid

Levofloxacin has poor penetration into cerebro-spinal fluid.

Penetration into prostatic tissue

After administration of oral 500mg levofloxacin once a day for three days, the mean concentrations in prostatic tissue were 8.7 μg/g, 8.2 μg/g and 2.0 μg/g respectively after 2 hours, 6 hours and 24 hours; the mean prostate/plasma concentration ratio was 1.84.

Concentration in urine

The mean urine concentrations 8 -12 hours after a single oral dose of 150 mg, 300 mg or 500 mg levofloxacin were 44 mg/L, 91 mg/L and 200 mg/L, respectively.

Biotransformation

Levofloxacin is metabolised to a very small extent, the metabolites being desmethyl-levofloxacin and levofloxacin N-oxide. These metabolites account for < 5 % of the dose excreted in urine. Levofloxacin is stereochemically stable and does not undergo chiral inversion.

Elimination

Following oral and intravenous administration of levofloxacin, it is eliminated relatively slowly from the plasma ($t_{½}$: 6 - 8 h). Excretion is primarily by the renal route (> 85 % of the administered dose).

There are no major differences in the pharmacokinetics of levofloxacin following intravenous and oral administration, suggesting that the oral and intravenous routes are interchangeable.

Linearity

Levofloxacin obeys linear pharmacokinetics over a range of 50 to 600 mg.

Subjects with renal insufficiency

The pharmacokinetics of levofloxacin are affected by renal impairment. With decreasing renal function renal elimination and clearance are decreased, and elimination half-lives increased as shown in the table below:

Cl_{cr} [ml/min]	< 20	20 - 40	50 - 80
Cl_R [ml/min]	13	26	57
$t_{1/2}$ [h]	35	27	9

Elderly subjects

There are no significant differences in levofloxacin pharmacokinetics between young and elderly subjects, except those associated with differences in creatinine clearance.

Gender differences

Separate analysis for male and female subjects showed small to marginal gender differences in levofloxacin pharmacokinetics. There is no evidence that these gender differences are of clinical relevance.

5.3 Preclinical safety data

Acute toxicity

The median lethal dose (LD_{50}) values obtained in mice and rats after oral administration of levofloxacin were in the range 1500-2000 mg/kg.

Administration of 500 mg/kg p.o. to monkeys induced little effect apart from vomiting.

Repeated dose toxicity

Studies of one and six months duration by gavage have been carried out in the rat and monkey. Doses were 50, 200, 800 mg/kg/day and 20, 80, 320 mg/kg/day for 1 and 6 months in the rat and 10, 30, 100 mg/kg/day and 10, 25, 62.5 mg/kg/day for 1 and 6 months in the monkey.

Signs of reaction to treatment were minor in the rat with slight effects principally at 200 mg/kg/day and above in reducing food consumption and slightly altering haematological and biochemical parameters. The No Observed Adverse Effect Levels (NOELs) in these studies were concluded to be 200 and 20 mg/kg/day after 1 and 6 months respectively.

Toxicity after oral dosing in the monkey was minimal with reduced body weight at 100 mg/kg/day together with salivation, diarrhoea and decreased urinary pH in some animals at this dose. No toxicity was seen in the 6-month study. The NOELs were concluded to be 30 and 62.5 mg/kg/day after 1 and 6 months respectively.

The NOELs in the six-month studies were concluded to be 20 and 62.5 mg/kg/day in the rat and monkey respectively.

Reproductive toxicity

Levofloxacin caused no impairment of fertility or reproductive performance in rats at oral doses as high as 360 mg/kg/day or intravenous doses up to 100 mg/kg/day.

Levofloxacin was not teratogenic in rats at oral doses as high as 810 mg/kg/day, or at intravenous doses as high as 160 mg/kg/day. No teratogenicity was observed when rabbits were dosed orally with up to 50 mg/kg/day or intravenously with up to 25 mg/kg/day.

Levofloxacin had no effect on fertility and its only effect on foetuses was delayed maturation as a result of maternal toxicity.

Genotoxicity

Levofloxacin did not induce gene mutations in bacterial or mammalian cells but did induce chromosome aberrations in Chinese hamster lung cells *in vitro* at or above 100 µg/ml, in the absence of metabolic activation. *In vivo* tests (micronucleus, sister chromatid exchange, unscheduled DNA synthesis, dominant lethal tests) did not show any genotoxic potential.

Phototoxic potential

Studies in the mouse after both oral and intravenous dosing showed levofloxacin to have phototoxic activity only at very high doses. Levofloxacin did not show any genotoxic potential in a photomutagenicity assay, and it reduced tumour development in a photocarcinogenicity assay.

Carcinogenic potential

No indication of carcinogenic potential was seen in a two year study in the rat with dietary administration (0, 10, 30 and 100 mg/kg/day).

Toxicity to joints

In common with other fluoroquinolones, levofloxacin showed effects on cartilage (blistering and cavities) in rats and dogs. These findings were more marked in young animals.

6. PHARMACEUTICAL PARTICULARS

6.1 List of excipients

Tavanic 500 mg film-coated tablets contain the following excipients for a weight of 630 mg:

Tablet core:

Crospovidone, hypromellose, microcrystalline cellulose and sodium stearyl fumarate.

Tablet coating:

Hypromellose, titanium dioxide (E 171), talc, macrogol, yellow ferric oxide (E 172) and red ferric oxide (E 172).

6.2 Incompatibilities

Not applicable.

6.3 Shelf life

5 years.

6.4 Special precautions for storage

This medicine does not require any special conditions for storage.

6.5 Nature and contents of container

PVC aluminium blisters containing film-coated tablets.

Pack sizes for 500 mg tablets: 1, 5 or 10.

6.6 Special precautions for disposal and other handling

A score line allows adaptation of the dose in patients with impaired renal function.

As for all medicines, any unused medicinal product should be disposed of accordingly and in compliance with local environmental regulations.

7. MARKETING AUTHORISATION HOLDER

Sanofi-aventis
One Onslow Street
Guildford
Surrey
GU1 4YS
UK

8. MARKETING AUTHORISATION NUMBER(S)

PL 13402/0012

9. DATE OF FIRST AUTHORISATION/RENEWAL OF THE AUTHORISATION

Date of first authorisation: 6 June 1997

Date of last renewal: 5 June 2007

10. DATE OF REVISION OF THE TEXT

14 September 2007

Legal category: POM

Tavanic i.v.

(sanofi-aventis)

1. NAME OF THE MEDICINAL PRODUCT

Tavanic. 5 mg/ml solution for infusion

2. QUALITATIVE AND QUANTITATIVE COMPOSITION

500 mg of levofloxacin in a 100 ml glass bottle

One ml of solution for infusion contains 5 mg of levofloxacin

For a full list of excipients, see section 6.1

3. PHARMACEUTICAL FORM

Solution for infusion.

Clear greenish-yellow solution

4. CLINICAL PARTICULARS

4.1 Therapeutic indications

In adults for whom intravenous therapy is considered to be appropriate, Tavanic solution for infusion is indicated for the treatment of the following infections when due to levofloxacin-susceptible microorganisms:

- Community-acquired pneumonia.
- Complicated urinary tract infections including pyelonephritis.
- Chronic bacterial prostatitis.
- Skin and soft tissue infections.

Before prescribing Tavanic, consideration should be given to national and/or local guidance on the appropriate use of fluoroquinolones.

4.2 Posology and method of administration

Tavanic solution for infusion is administered by slow intravenous infusion once or twice daily. The dosage depends on the type and severity of the infection and the sensitivity of the presumed causative pathogen. It is usually possible to switch from initial intravenous treatment to the oral route after a few days (Tavanic 250 or 500 mg tablets), according to the condition of the patient. Given the bioequivalence of the parenteral and oral forms, the same dosage can be used.

Duration of treatment

The duration of treatment varies according to the course of the disease. As with antibiotic therapy in general, administration of Tavanic (solution for infusion or tablets) should be continued for a minimum of 48 to 72 hours after the patient has become afebrile or evidence of bacterial eradication has been obtained.

Method of administration

Tavanic solution for infusion is only intended for slow intravenous infusion; it is administered once or twice daily. The infusion time must be at least 30 minutes for 250 mg or 60 minutes for 500 mg Tavanic solution for infusion (see section 4.4). It is possible to switch from an initial intravenous application to the oral route at the same dosage after a few days, according to the condition of the patient.

For incompatibilities see section 6.2 and compatibility with other infusion solutions see section 6.6.

Posology

The following dose recommendations can be given for Tavanic:

Dosage in patients with normal renal function (creatinine clearance > 50 ml/min)

Indication	Daily dose regimen (according to severity)
Community-acquired pneumonia	500 mg once or twice daily
Complicated urinary tract infections including pyelonephritis	250 mg[1] once daily
Chronic bacterial prostatitis.	500mg once daily
Skin and soft tissue infections	500 mg twice daily

[1]Consideration should be given to increasing the dose in cases of severe infection.

Special populations

Impaired renal function (creatinine clearance ≤ 50ml/min)

(see Table 1 on next page)

Impaired liver function

No adjustment of dosage is required since levofloxacin is not metabolised to any relevant extent by the liver and is mainly excreted by the kidneys.

In the elderly

No adjustment of dosage is required in the elderly, other than that imposed by consideration of renal function (See section 4.4 QT interval prolongation).

In children

Tavanic is contraindicated in children and growing adolescents (see section 4.3).

4.3 Contraindications

Tavanic solution for infusion must not be used:

- in patients hypersensitive to levofloxacin or any other quinolone and any of the excipients,
- in patients with epilepsy,
- in patients with history of tendon disorders related to fluoroquinolone administration,
- in children or growing adolescents,
- during pregnancy,
- in breast-feeding women.

4.4 Special warnings and precautions for use

In the most severe cases of pneumococcal pneumonia Tavanic may not be the optimal therapy.

Nosocomial infections due to *P. aeruginosa* may require combination therapy.

Infusion Time

The recommended infusion time of at least 30 minutes for 250 mg or 60 minutes for 500mg Tavanic solution for infusion should be observed. It is known for ofloxacin, that during infusion tachycardia and a temporary decrease in blood pressure may develop. In rare cases, as a consequence of a profound drop in blood pressure, circulatory collapse may occur. Should a conspicuous drop in blood pressure occur during infusion of levofloxacin, (*l*-isomer of ofloxacin) the infusion must be halted immediately.

Tendinitis and tendon rupture

Tendinitis may rarely occur. It most frequently involves the Achilles tendon and may lead to tendon rupture. The risk of tendinitis and tendon rupture is increased in the elderly and in patients using corticosteroids. Close monitoring of these patients is therefore necessary if they are prescribed Tavanic. All patients should consult their physician if they experience symptoms of tendinitis. If tendinitis is suspected, treatment with Tavanic must be halted immediately, and appropriate treatment (e.g. immobilisation) must be initiated for the affected tendon.

Clostridium difficile-associated disease

Diarrhoea, particularly if severe, persistent and/or bloody, during or after treatment with Tavanic solution for infusion, may be symptomatic of *Clostridium difficile*-associated disease, the most severe form of which is pseudomembranous colitis. If pseudomembranous colitis is suspected, Tavanic solution for infusion must be stopped immediately and patients should be treated with supportive measures ± specific therapy without delay (e.g. oral vancomycin). Products inhibiting the peristalsis are contraindicated in this clinical situation.

Patients predisposed to seizures

Tavanic solution for infusion is contraindicated in patients with a history of epilepsy and, as with other quinolones,

Table 1

	Dose regimen		
	250 mg/24 h	500 mg/24 h	500 mg/12 h
Creatinine clearance	*first dose*: 250 mg	*first dose*: 500 mg	*first dose*: 500 mg
50 - 20 ml/min	*then*: 125 mg/24 h	*then*: 250 mg/24 h	*then*: 250 mg/12 h
19-10 ml/min	*then*: 125 mg/48 h	*then*: 125 mg/24 h	*then*: 125 mg/12 h
< 10 ml/mi (including haemodialysis and CAPD) [1]	*then*: 125 mg/48 h	*then*: 125 mg/24 h	*then*: 125 mg/24 h

[1]No additional doses are required after haemodialysis or continuous ambulatory peritoneal dialysis (CAPD).

should be used with extreme caution in patients predisposed to seizures, such as patients with pre-existing central nervous system lesions, concomitant treatment with fenbufen and similar non-steroidal anti-inflammatory drugs or with drugs which lower the cerebral seizure threshold, such as theophylline (see section 4.5). In case of convulsive seizures, treatment with levofloxacin should be discontinued.

Patients with G-6- phosphate dehydrogenase deficiency

Patients with latent or actual defects in glucose-6-phosphate dehydrogenase activity may be prone to haemolytic reactions when treated with quinolone antibacterial agents, and so levofloxacin should be used with caution.

Patients with renal impairment

Since levofloxacin is excreted mainly by the kidneys, the dose of Tavanic should be adjusted in patients with renal impairment (see section 4.2).

Hypersensitivity reactions

Levofloxacin can cause serious, potentially fatal hypersensitivity reactions (e.g. angioedema up to anaphylactic shock), occasionally following the initial dose (see section 4.8). Patients should discontinue treatment immediately and contact their physician or an emergency physician, who will initiate appropriate emergency measures.

Hypoglycemia

As with all quinolones, hypoglycemia has been reported, usually in diabetic patients receiving concomitant treatment with an oral hypoglycemic agent (e.g., glibenclamide) or with insulin. In these diabetic patients, careful monitoring of blood glucose is recommended. (See section 4.8).

Prevention of photosensitisation

Although photosensitisation is very rare with levofloxacin, it is recommended that patients should not expose themselves unnecessarily to strong sunlight or to artificial UV rays (e.g. sunray lamp, solarium), in order to prevent photosensitisation.

Patients treated with Vitamin K antagonists

Due to possible increase in coagulation tests (PT/INR) and/or bleeding in patients treated with Tavanic in combination with a vitamin K antagonist (e.g. warfarin), coagulation tests should be monitored when these drugs are given concomittantly (see section 4.5).

Psychotic reactions

Psychotic reactions have been reported in patients receiving quinolones, including levofloxacin. In very rare cases these have progressed to suicidal thoughts and self-endangering behaviour- sometimes after only a single dose of levofloxacin (see section 4.8). In the event that the patient develops these reactions, levofloxacin should be discontinued and appropriate measures instituted. Caution is recommended if levofloxacin is to be used in psychotic patients or in patients with history of psychiatric disease.

QT interval prolongation

Caution should be taken when using fluoroquinolones, including levofloxacin, in patients with known risk factors for prolongation of the QT interval such as, for example:

- congenital long QT syndrome
- concomitant use of drugs that are known to prolong the QT interval (e.g. Class IA and III antiarrhythmics, tricyclic antidepressants, macrolides).
- uncorrected electrolyte imbalance (e.g. hypokalemia, hypomagnesemia)
- elderly
- cardiac disease (e.g. heart failure, myocardial infarction, bradycardia)

(See section 4.2 *Elderly*, section 4.5, section 4.8, section 4.9).

Peripheral neuropathy

Sensory or sensorimotor peripheral neuropathy has been reported in patients receiving fluoroquinolones, including levofloxacin, which can be rapid in its onset. Levofloxacin should be discontinued if the patient experiences symptoms of neuropathy in order to prevent the development of an irreversible condition.

Opiates

In patients treated with levofloxacin, determination of opiates in urine may give false-positive results. It may be necessary to confirm positive opiate screens by more specific method.

Hepatobiliary disorders

Cases of hepatic necrosis up to life threatening hepatic failure have been reported with levofloxacin, primarily in patients with severe underlying diseases, e.g. sepsis (see section 4.8). Patients should be advised to stop treatment and contact their doctor if signs and symptoms of hepatic disease develop such as anorexia, jaundice, dark urine, pruritus or tender abdomen.

4.5 Interaction with other medicinal products and other forms of interaction

Effect of other medicinal products on Tavanic

Theophylline, fenbufen or similar non-steroidal anti-inflammatory drugs

No pharmacokinetic interactions of levofloxacin were found with theophylline in a clinical study. However a pronounced lowering of the cerebral seizure threshold may occur when quinolones are given concurrently with theophylline, non-steroidal anti-inflammatory drugs, or other agents which lower the seizure threshold.

Levofloxacin concentrations were about 13% higher in the presence of fenbufen than when administered alone.

Probenecid and cimetidine

Probenecid and cimetidine had a statistically significant effect on the elimination of levofloxacin. The renal clearance of levofloxacin was reduced by cimetidine (24%) and probenecid (34%). This is because both drugs are capable of blocking the renal tubular secretion of levofloxacin. However, at the tested doses in the study, the statistically significant kinetic differences are unlikely to be of clinical relevance.

Caution should be exercised when levofloxacin is coadministered with drugs that affect the tubular renal secretion such as probenecid and cimetidine, especially in renally impaired patients.

Other relevant information

Clinical pharmacology studies have shown that the pharmacokinetics of levofloxacin were not affected to any clinically relevant extent when levofloxacin was administered together with the following drugs: calcium carbonate, digoxin, glibenclamide, ranitidine.

Effect of Tavanic on other medicinal products

Ciclosporin

The half-life of ciclosporin was increased by 33% when coadministered with levofloxacin.

Vitamin K antagonists

Increased coagulation tests (PT/INR) and/or bleeding, which may be severe, have been reported in patients treated with levofloxacin in combination with a vitamin K antagonist (e.g. warfarin). Coagulation tests, therefore, should be monitored in patients treated with vitamin K antagonists (see section 4.4)

Drugs known to prolong QT interval

Levofloxacin, like other fluoroquinolones, should be used with caution in patients receiving drugs known to prolong the QT interval (e.g. Class IA and III antiarrhythmics, tricyclic antidepressants, macrolides). (See section 4.4 QT interval prolongation).

4.6 Pregnancy and lactation

Pregnancy

Reproductive studies in animals did not raise specific concern. However in the absence of human data and due to the experimental risk of damage by fluoroquinolones to the weight-bearing cartilage of the growing organism, Tavanic must not be used in pregnant women (see sections 4.3 and 5.3).

Lactation

In the absence of human data and due to the experimental risk of damage by fluoroquinolones to the weight-bearing cartilage of the growing organism, Tavanic solution for infusion must not be used in breast-feeding women (see sections 4.3 and 5.3).

4.7 Effects on ability to drive and use machines

Some undesirable effects (e.g. dizziness/vertigo, drowsiness, visual disturbances) may impair the patient's ability to concentrate and react, and therefore may constitute a risk in situations where these abilities are of special importance (e.g. driving a car or operating machinery).

4.8 Undesirable effects

The information given below is based on data from clinical studies in more than 5000 patients and on extensive post marketing experience.

The adverse reactions are described according to the MedDRA system organ class in the table below.

Frequencies in this table are defined using the following convention: very common (≥1/10), common (≥1/100, <1/10), uncommon (≥1/1000, ≤1/100), rare (≥1/10000, ≤1/1000), very rare (≤1/10000), not known (cannot be estimated from the available data).

Within each frequency grouping, undesirable effects are presented in order of decreasing seriousness.

Infections and infestations

Uncommon: Fungal infection (and proliferation of other resistant microorganisms)

Blood and lymphatic system disorders

Uncommon: Leukopenia, eosinophilia

Rare: Thrombocytopenia, neutropenia

Very rare: Agranulocytosis

Not Known: Pancytopenia, haemolytic anaemia

Immune system disorders

Very rare: Anaphylactic shock (see section 4.4)

Anaphylactic and anaphylactoid reactions may sometimes occur even after the first dose

Not known: Hypersensitivity (see section 4.4)

Metabolism and nutrition disorders

Uncommon: Anorexia

Very rare: Hypoglycemia, particularly in diabetic patients (see section 4.4)

Psychiatric disorders

Uncommon: Insomnia, nervousness

Rare: Psychotic disorder, depression, confusional state, agitation, anxiety

Very rare: Psychotic reactions with self-endangering behaviour including suicidal ideation or acts (see section 4.4), hallucination

Nervous system disorders

Uncommon: Dizziness, headache, somnolence

Rare: Convulsion, tremor, paraesthesia

Very rare: sensory or sensorimotor peripheral neuropathy, dysgeusia including ageusia, parosmia including anosmia

Eye disorders

Very rare: Visual disturbance

Ear and Labyrinth disorders

Uncommon: Vertigo

Very rare: Hearing impaired

Not known: Tinnitus

Cardiac disorders

Rare: Tachycardia

Not Known: Electrocardiogram QT prolonged (see section 4.4 QT interval prolongation and section 4.9)

Vascular disorders

Common: Phlebitis

Rare: Hypotension

Respiratory, thoracic and mediastinal disorders

Rare: Bronchospasm, dyspnoea

Very rare: Pneumonitis allergic

Gastrointestinal disorders

Common: Diarrhoea, nausea

Uncommon: Vomiting, abdominal pain, dyspepsia, flatulence, constipation

Rare: Diarrhoea –haemorrhagic which in very rare cases may be indicative of enterocolitis, including pseudomembranous colitis

Hepatobiliary disorders

Common: Hepatic enzyme increased (ALT/AST, alkaline phosphatase, GGT)

Uncommon: Blood bilirubin increased

Very rare: Hepatitis

Not known: Jaundice and severe liver injury, including cases with acute liver failure, have been reported with levofloxacin, primarily in patients with severe underlying diseases (see section 4.4).

Skin and subcutaneous tissue disorders

Uncommon: Rash, pruritus

Rare: Urticaria

Very rare: Angioneurotic oedema, photosensitivity reaction

Not Known: Toxic epidermal necrolysis, Stevens-Johnson syndrome, erythema multiforme, hyperhidrosis

Mucocutaneous reactions may sometimes occur even after the first dose

Musculoskeletal and Connective tissue disorders

Rare: Tendon disorder (see section 4.4) including tendinitis (e.g. Achilles tendon), arthralgia, myalgia

Very rare: Tendon rupture (see section 4.4). This undesirable effect may occur within 48 hours of starting treatment and may be bilateral, muscular weakness which may be of special importance in patients with myasthenia gravis

Not Known: Rhabdomyolysis

Renal and urinary disorders

Uncommon: Blood creatinine increased

Very rare: Renal failure acute (e.g. due to nephritis interstitial)

General disorders and administration site conditions

Common: Infusion site reaction

Uncommon: Asthenia

Very rare: Pyrexia

Not known: Pain (including pain in back, chest, and extremities)

Other undesirable effects which have been associated with fluoroquinolone administration include:

- extrapyramidal symptoms and other disorders of muscular coordination,
- hypersensitivity vasculitis,
- attacks of porphyria in patients with porphyria

4.9 Overdose

According to toxicity studies in animals or clinical pharmacology studies performed with supra-therapeutic doses, the most important signs to be expected following acute overdosage of Tavanic solution for infusion are central nervous system symptoms such as confusion, dizziness, impairment of consciousness, and convulsive seizures, increases in QT interval.

In the event of overdose, symptomatic treatment should be implemented. ECG monitoring should be undertaken, because of the possibility of QT interval prolongation. Haemodialysis, including peritoneal dialysis and CAPD, are not effective in removing levofloxacin from the body. No specific antidote exists.

5. PHARMACOLOGICAL PROPERTIES

5.1 Pharmacodynamic properties

Pharmacotherapeutic group: quinolone antibacterials, fluoroquinolones

ATC code: J01MA12

Levofloxacin is a synthetic antibacterial agent of the fluoroquinolone class and is the S (-) enantiomer of the racemic drug substance ofloxacin.

Mechanism of action

As a fluoroquinolone antibacterial agent, levofloxacin acts on the DNA-DNA-gyrase complex and topoisomerase IV.

PK/PD relationship

The degree of the bactericidal activity of levofloxacin depends on the ratio of the maximum concentration in serum (Cmax) or the area under the curve (AUC) and the minimal inhibitory concentration (MIC).

Mechanism of resistance

The main mechanism of resistance is due to a *gyr-A* mutation. *In vitro* there is a cross-resistance between levofloxacin and other fluoroquinolones.

Due to the mechanism of action, there is generally no cross-resistance between levofloxacin and other classes of antibacterial agents.

Breakpoints

The EUCAST recommended MIC breakpoints for levofloxacin, separating susceptible from intermediately susceptible organisms and intermediately susceptible from resistant organisms are presented in the below table for MIC testing (mg/L).

EUCAST clinical MIC breakpoints for levofloxacin (2006-06-20):

Pathogen	Susceptible	Resistant
Enterobacteriacae	≤1 mg/L	>2 mg/L
Pseudomonas spp.	≤1 mg/L	>2 mg/L
Acinetobacter spp.	≤1 mg/L	>2 mg/L
Staphylococcus spp.	≤1 mg/L	>2 mg/L
S.pneumoniae [1]	≤2 mg/L	>2 mg/L
Streptococcus A,B,C,G	≤1 mg/L	>2 mg/L
H. influenzae *M. catarrhalis* [2]	≤1 mg/L	>1 mg/L
Non-species related breakpoints[3]	≤1 mg/L	>2 mg/L

[1] the S/I-breakpoint was increased from 1.0 to 2.0 to avoid dividing the wild type MIC distribution. The breakpoints relate to high dose therapy.

[2] Strains with MIC values above the S/I breakpoint are very rare or not yet reported. The identification and antimicrobial susceptibility tests on any such isolate must be repeated and if the result is confirmed the isolate sent to a reference laboratory.

[3] Non-species related breakpoints have been determined mainly on the basis of pharmacokinetic/pharmacodynamic data and are independent of MIC distributions of specific species. They are for use only for species that have not been given a species-specific breakpoint and are not for use with species where susceptibility testing is not recommended or for which there is insufficient evidence that the species in question is a good target (Enterococcus, Neisseria, Gram negative anaerobes)

The CLSI (Clinical And Laboratory Standards Institute, formerly NCCLS)recommended MIC breakpoints for levofloxacin, separating susceptible from intermediately susceptible organisms and intermediately susceptible from resistant organisms are presented in the below table for MIC testing (µg/mL) or disc diffusion testing (zone diameter [mm] using a 5 µg levofloxacin disc).

CLSI recommended MIC and disc diffusion breakpoints for levofloxacin (M100-S17, 2007):

Pathogen	Susceptible	Resistant
Enterobacteriaceae	≤2 µg/mL ≥17 mm	≥8 µg/mL ≤13 mm
Non Enterobacteriaceae.	≤2 µg/mL ≥17 mm	≥8 µg/mL ≤13 mm
Acinetobacter spp.	≤2 µg/mL ≥17 mm	≥8 µg/mL ≤13 mm
Stenotrophomonas maltophilia	≤2 µg/mL ≥17 mm	≥8 µg/mL ≤13 mm
Staphylococcus spp.	≤1 µg/mL ≥19 mm	≥4 µg/mL ≤15 mm
Enterococcus spp.	≤2 µg/mL ≥17 mm	≥8 µg/mL ≤13 mm
H. influenzae *M. catarrhalis* [1]	≤2 µg/mL ≥17 mm	
Streptococcus pneumoniae	≤2 µg/mL ≥17 mm	≥8 µg/mL ≤13 mm
beta-hemolytic Streptococcus	≤2 µg/mL ≥17 mm	≥8 µg/mL ≤13 mm

[1] The absence or rare occurrence of resistant strains precludes defining any results categories other than « susceptible ». for strains yielding results suggestive of a « nonsusceptible » category, organism identification and antimicrobial susceptibility test results should be confirmed by a reference laboratory using CLSI reference dilution method.

Antibacterial spectrum

The prevalence of resistance may vary geographically and with time for selected species and local information on resistance is desirable, particularly when treating severe infections. As necessary, expert advice should be sought when the local prevalence of resistance is such that the utility of the agent in at least some types of infections is questionable

Commonly susceptible species

Aerobic Gram-positive bacteria

*Staphylococcus aureus**
methicillin-susceptible
Staphylococcus saprophyticus
Streptococci, group C and G
Streptococcus agalactiae
*Streptococcus pneumoniae**
*Streptococcus pyogenes**

Aerobic Gram-negative bacteria

Burkholderia cepacia$
Eikenella corrodens
*Haemophilus influenzae**
*Haemophilus para-influenzae**
Klebsiella oxytoca
*Klebsiella pneumoniae**
*Moraxella catarrhalis**
Pasteurella multocida
Proteus vulgaris
Providencia rettgeri

Anaerobic bacteria

Peptostreptococcus

Other

*Chlamydophila pneumoniae**
Chlamydophila psittaci
Chlamydia trachomatis
*Legionella pneumophila**
*Mycoplasma pneumoniae**
Mycoplasma hominis
Ureaplasma urealyticum

Species for which acquired resistance may be a problem

Aerobic Gram-positive bacteria

*Enterococcus faecalis**
Staphylococcus aureus
methicillin-resistant
Coagulase negative *Staphylococcus spp*

Aerobic Gram-negative bacteria

*Acinetobacter baumannii**
*Citrobacter freundii**
Enterobacter aerogenes
Enterobacter agglomerans
*Enterobacter cloacae**
*Escherichia coli**
*Morganella morganii**
*Proteus mirabilis**
Providencia stuartii
*Pseudomonas aeruginosa**
*Serratia marcescens**

Anaerobic bacteria

Bacteroides fragilis
Bacteroides ovatus$
Bacteroides thetaiotamicron$
Bacteroides vulgatus$
Clostridium difficile$

* Clinical efficacy has been demonstrated for susceptible isolates in the approved clinical indications.

$ natural intermediate susceptibility

Other information

Nosocomial infections due to *P. aeruginosa* may require combination therapy.

5.2 Pharmacokinetic properties

Absorption

Orally administered levofloxacin is rapidly and almost completely absorbed with peak plasma concentrations being obtained within 1h. The absolute bioavailability is approximately 100 %.

Food has little effect on the absorption of levofloxacin.

Distribution

Approximately 30 - 40 % of levofloxacin is bound to serum protein. 500 mg once daily multiple dosing with levofloxacin showed negligible accumulation. There is modest but predictable accumulation of levofloxacin after doses of 500 mg twice daily. Steady-state is achieved within 3 days.

Penetration into tissues and body fluids:

Penetration into Bronchial Mucosa, Epithelial Lining Fluid (ELF)

Maximum levofloxacin concentrations in bronchial mucosa and epithelial lining fluid after 500 mg po were 8.3 µg/g and 10.8 µg/ml respectively. These were reached approximately one hour after administration.

Penetration into Lung Tissue

Maximum levofloxacin concentrations in lung tissue after 500 mg po were approximately 11.3 µg/g and were reached between 4 and 6 hours after administration. The concentrations in the lungs consistently exceeded those in plasma.

Penetration into Blister Fluid

Maximum levofloxacin concentrations of about 4.0 and 6.7 µg/ml in the blister fluid were reached 2 - 4 hours after administration following 3 days dosing at 500 mg once or twice daily respectively.

Penetration into Cerebro-Spinal Fluid

Levofloxacin has poor penetration into cerebro-spinal fluid.

Penetration into prostatic tissue

After administration of oral 500mg levofloxacin once a day for three days, the mean concentrations in prostatic tissue were 8.7 µg/g, 8.2 µg/g and 2.0 µg/g respectively after 2 hours, 6 hours and 24 hours; the mean prostate/plasma concentration ratio was 1.84.

Concentration in urine

The mean urine concentrations 8 -12 hours after a single oral dose of 150 mg, 300 mg or 500 mg levofloxacin were 44 mg/L, 91 mg/L and 200 mg/L, respectively.

Biotransformation

Levofloxacin is metabolised to a very small extent, the metabolites being desmethyl-levofloxacin and levofloxacin N-oxide. These metabolites account for < 5 % of the dose excreted in urine. Levofloxacin is stereochemically stable and does not undergo chiral inversion.

Elimination

Following oral and intravenous administration of levofloxacin, it is eliminated relatively slowly from the plasma ($t_{½}$: 6 - 8 h). Excretion is primarily by the renal route (> 85 % of the administered dose).

There are no major differences in the pharmacokinetics of levofloxacin following intravenous and oral administration, suggesting that the oral and intravenous routes are interchangeable.

Linearity

Levofloxacin obeys linear pharmacokinetics over a range of 50 to 600 mg.

Subjects with renal insufficiency

The pharmacokinetics of levofloxacin are affected by renal impairment. With decreasing renal function renal elimination and clearance are decreased, and elimination half-lives increased as shown in the table below:

Cl_{cr} [ml/min]	< 20	20 - 40	50 - 80
Cl_R [ml/min]	13	26	57
$t_{1/2}$ [h]	35	27	9

Elderly subjects

There are no significant differences in levofloxacin pharmacokinetics between young and elderly subjects, except those associated with differences in creatinine clearance.

Gender differences

Separate analysis for male and female subjects showed small to marginal gender differences in levofloxacin pharmacokinetics. There is no evidence that these gender differences are of clinical relevance.

5.3 Preclinical safety data

Acute toxicity

The median lethal dose (LD_{50}) values obtained in mice and rats after intravenous administration of levofloxacin were in the range 250-400 mg/kg; in dogs the LD_{50} value was approximately 200 mg/kg with one of two animals which received this dose dying.

Repeated dose toxicity

Studies of one month duration with intravenous administration have been carried out in the rat (20, 60, 180 mg/kg/day) and monkey (10, 25, 63 mg/kg/day) and a three-month study has also been carried in the rat (10, 30, 90 mg/kg/day).

The "No Observed Adverse Effect Levels" (NOEL) in the rat studies were concluded to be 20 and 30 mg/kg/day in the one-month and three-month studies respectively. Crystal deposits in urine were seen in both studies at doses of 20 mg/kg/day and above. High doses (180 mg/kg/day for 1 month or 30 mg/kg/day and above for 3 months) slightly decreased food consumption and body weight gain. Haematological examination showed reduced erythrocytes and increased leucocytes and reticulocytes at the end of the 1 month, but not the 3 months study.

The NOEL in the monkey study was concluded to be 63 mg/kg/day with only minor reduction in food and water consumption at this dose.

Reproductive toxicity

Levofloxacin caused no impairment of fertility or reproductive performance in rats at oral doses as high as 360 mg/kg/day or intravenous doses up to 100 mg/kg/day.

Levofloxacin was not teratogenic in rats at oral doses as high as 810 mg/kg/day, or at intravenous doses as high as 160 mg/kg/day. No teratogenicity was observed when rabbits were dosed orally with up to 50 mg/kg/day or intravenously with up to 25 mg/kg/day.

Levofloxacin had no effect on fertility and its only effect on fetuses was delayed maturation as a result of maternal toxicity.

Genotoxicity

Levofloxacin did not induce gene mutations in bacterial or mammalian cells but did induce chromosome aberrations in Chinese hamster lung (CHL) cells *in vitro* at or above 100 μg/ml, in the absence of metabolic activation. *In vivo* tests (micronucleus, sister chromatid exchange, unscheduled DNA synthesis, dominant lethal tests) did not show any genotoxic potential.

Phototoxic potential

Studies in the mouse after both intravenous and oral dosing showed levofloxacin to have phototoxic activity only at very high doses. Levofloxacin did not show any genotoxic potential in a photomutagenicity assay, and it reduced tumour development in a photocarcinogenicity assay.

Carcinogenic potential

No indication of carcinogenic potential was seen in a two-year study in the rat with dietary administration (0, 10, 30 and 100 mg/kg/day).

Toxicity to joints

In common with other fluoroquinolones, levofloxacin showed effects on cartilage (blistering and cavities) in rats and dogs. These findings were more marked in young animals.

6. PHARMACEUTICAL PARTICULARS

6.1 List of excipients

Sodium chloride, sodium hydroxide, hydrochloric acid *(qs: pH 4.8)* and water for injection. (Na^+ concentration: 154 mmol / L).

6.2 Incompatibilities

Tavanic 5 mg/ml solution for infusion should not be mixed with heparin or alkaline solutions (e.g. sodium hydrogen carbonate). This medicinal product must not be mixed with other medicinal products except those mentioned in section 6.6.

6.3 Shelf life

3 years

Shelf life after removal of the outer packaging: 3 days (under indoor light conditions).

Shelf life after perforation of the rubber stopper: (see 6.6).

From a microbiological point of view, the solution for infusion should be used immediately. If not used immediately, in-use storage times and conditions are the responsibility of the user.

6.4 Special precautions for storage

Keep the bottle in the outer carton in order to protect from light (see section 6.3). Inspect visually prior to use. Only clear solutions without particles should be used.

6.5 Nature and contents of container

100ml, type 1 glass bottle with flanged aluminium cap, chlorobutyl rubber stopper and tear-off polypropylene lid. Each bottle contains 100 ml solution. Packs of 1 bottle are available.

6.6 Special precautions for disposal and other handling

Tavanic solution for infusion should be used immediately (within 3 hours) after perforation of the rubber stopper in order to prevent any bacterial contamination. No protection from light is necessary during infusion.

As for all medicines, any unused medicinal product should be disposed of accordingly and in compliance with local environmental regulations.

Mixture with other solutions for infusion:

Tavanic solution for infusion is compatible with the following solutions for infusion:

0.9 % sodium chloride solution USP.

5 % dextrose injection USP.

2.5 % dextrose in Ringer solution.

Combination solutions for parenteral nutrition (amino acids, carbohydrates, electrolytes).

See section 6.2 for incompatibilities.

7. MARKETING AUTHORISATION HOLDER

Sanofi-aventis

One Onslow Street

Guildford

Surrey

GU1 4YS

UK

8. MARKETING AUTHORISATION NUMBER(S)

PL 13402/0013

9. DATE OF FIRST AUTHORISATION/RENEWAL OF THE AUTHORISATION

Date of first authorisation: 6 June 1997

Date of last renewal: 5 June 2007

10. DATE OF REVISION OF THE TEXT

May 2009

LEGAL CATEGORY

POM

Taxotere 20mg and 80mg concentrate and solvent for infusion

(sanofi-aventis)

1. NAME OF THE MEDICINAL PRODUCT

TAXOTERE 20 mg concentrate and solvent for solution for infusion

TAXOTERE 80 mg concentrate and solvent for solution for infusion

2. QUALITATIVE AND QUANTITATIVE COMPOSITION

Each single-dose vial of TAXOTERE 20 mg concentrate contains docetaxel which is a trihydrate corresponding to 20 mg of docetaxel (anhydrous). The viscous solution contains 40 mg/ml docetaxel (anhydrous).

Each single-dose vial of TAXOTERE 80 mg concentrate contains docetaxel which is a trihydrate corresponding to 80 mg of docetaxel (anhydrous). The viscous solution contains 40 mg/ml docetaxel (anhydrous).

Excipient: Each single-dose vial of solvent contains 13% (w/w) ethanol 95% in water for injection.

For a full list of excipients, see section 6.1.

3. PHARMACEUTICAL FORM

Concentrate and solvent for solution for infusion.

The concentrate is a clear viscous, yellow to brown-yellow solution.

The solvent is a colourless solution.

4. CLINICAL PARTICULARS

4.1 Therapeutic indications

<u>Breast cancer</u>

TAXOTERE in combination with doxorubicin and cyclophosphamide is indicated for the adjuvant treatment of patients with operable node- positive breast cancer.

TAXOTERE in combination with doxorubicin is indicated for the treatment of patients with locally advanced or metastatic breast cancer who have not previously received cytotoxic therapy for this condition.

TAXOTERE monotherapy is indicated for the treatment of patients with locally advanced or metastatic breast cancer after failure of cytotoxic therapy. Previous chemotherapy should have included an anthracycline or an alkylating agent.

TAXOTERE in combination with trastuzumab is indicated for the treatment of patients with metastatic breast cancer whose tumors overexpress HER2 and who previously have not received chemotherapy for metastatic disease.

TAXOTERE in combination with capecitabine is indicated for the treatment of patients with locally advanced or metastatic breast cancer after failure of cytotoxic chemotherapy. Previous therapy should have included an anthracycline.

<u>Non-small cell lung cancer</u>

TAXOTERE is indicated for the treatment of patients with locally advanced or metastatic non-small cell lung cancer after failure of prior chemotherapy.

TAXOTERE in combination with cisplatin is indicated for the treatment of patients with unresectable, locally advanced or metastatic non-small cell lung cancer, in patients who have not previously received chemotherapy for this condition.

<u>Prostate cancer</u>

TAXOTERE in combination with prednisone or prednisolone is indicated for the treatment of patients with hormone refractory metastatic prostate cancer.

<u>Gastric adenocarcinoma</u>

TAXOTERE in combination with cisplatin and 5-fluorouracil is indicated for the treatment of patients with metastatic gastric adenocarcinoma, including adenocarcinoma of the gastroesophageal junction, who have not received prior chemotherapy for metastatic disease.

<u>Head and neck cancer</u>

TAXOTERE in combination with cisplatin and 5-fluorouracil is indicated for the induction treatment of patients with locally advanced squamous cell carcinoma of the head and neck.

4.2 Posology and method of administration

The use of docetaxel should be confined to units specialised in the administration of cytotoxic chemotherapy and it should only be administered under the supervision of a physician qualified in the use of anticancer chemotherapy (see section 6.6).

<u>Recommended dose</u>

For breast, non-small cell lung, gastric, and head and neck cancers, premedication consisting of an oral corticosteroid, such as dexamethasone 16 mg per day (e.g. 8 mg BID) for 3 days starting 1 day prior to docetaxel administration, unless contraindicated, can be used (see section 4.4). Prophylactic G-CSF may be used to mitigate the risk of hematological toxicities.

For prostate cancer, given the concurrent use of prednisone or prednisolone the recommended premedication regimen is oral dexamethasone 8 mg, 12 hours, 3 hours and 1 hour before the docetaxel infusion (see section 4.4).

Docetaxel is administered as a one-hour infusion every three weeks.

<u>Breast cancer</u>

In the adjuvant treatment of operable node-positive breast cancer, the recommended dose of docetaxel is 75 mg/m^2 administered 1-hour after doxorubicin 50 mg/m^2 and cyclophosphamide 500 mg/m^2 every 3 weeks for 6 cycles (see also Dose adjustments during treatment).

For the treatment of patients with locally advanced or metastatic breast cancer, the recommended dose of docetaxel is 100 mg/m^2 in monotherapy. In first-line treatment, docetaxel 75 mg/m^2 is given in combination therapy with doxorubicin (50 mg/m^2).

In combination with trastuzumab the recommended dose of docetaxel is 100 mg/m^2 every three weeks, with trastuzumab administered weekly. In the pivotal trial the initial docetaxel infusion was started the day following the first dose of trastuzumab. The subsequent docetaxel doses were administered immediately after completion of the trastuzumab infusion, if the preceding dose of trastuzumab was well tolerated. For trastuzumab dose and administration, see trastuzumab summary of product characteristics.

In combination with capecitabine, the recommended dose of docetaxel is 75 mg/m^2 every three weeks, combined with capecitabine at 1250 mg/m^2 twice daily (within 30 minutes after a meal) for 2 weeks followed by 1-week rest period. For capecitabine dose calculation according to body surface area, see capecitabine summary of product characteristics.

<u>Non-small cell lung cancer</u>

In chemotherapy naïve patients treated for non-small cell lung cancer, the recommended dose regimen is docetaxel 75 mg/m^2 immediately followed by cisplatin 75 mg/m^2 over 30-60 minutes. For treatment after failure of prior platinum-based chemotherapy, the recommended dose is 75 mg/m^2 as a single agent.

<u>Prostate cancer</u>

The recommended dose of docetaxel is 75 mg/m^2. Prednisone or prednisolone 5 mg orally twice daily is administered continuously (see section 5.1).

<u>Gastric adenocarcinoma</u>

The recommended dose of docetaxel is 75 mg/m^2 as a 1 hour infusion, followed by cisplatin 75 mg/m^2, as a 1 to 3 hour infusion (both on day 1 only), followed by 5-fluorouracil 750 mg/m^2 per day given as a 24-hour continuous infusion for 5 days, starting at the end of the cisplatin infusion. Treatment is repeated every three weeks. Patients must receive premedication with antiemetics and appropriate hydration for cisplatin administration. Prophylactic G-CSF should be used to mitigate the risk of hematological toxicities (see also Dose adjustments during treatment).

Head and neck cancer

Patients must receive premedication with antiemetics and appropriate hydration (prior to and after cisplatin administration). Prophylactic G-CSF may be used to mitigate the risk of hematological toxicities. All patients on the docetaxel-containing arm of the TAX 323 and TAX 324 studies, received prophylactic antibiotics.

• Induction chemotherapy followed by radiotherapy (TAX 323)

For the induction treatment of inoperable locally advanced squamous cell carcinoma of the head and neck (SCCHN), the recommended dose of docetaxel is 75 mg/m^2 as a 1 hour infusion followed by cisplatin 75 mg/m^2 over 1 hour, on day one, followed by 5-fluorouracil as a continuous infusion at 750 mg/m^2 per day for five days. This regimen is administered every 3 weeks for 4 cycles. Following chemotherapy, patients should receive radiotherapy.

• Induction chemotherapy followed by chemoradiotherapy (TAX 324)

For the induction treatment of patients with locally advanced (technically unresectable, low probability of surgical cure, and aiming at organ preservation) squamous cell carcinoma of the head and neck (SCCHN), the recommended dose of docetaxel is 75 mg/m^2 as a 1 hour intravenous infusion on day 1, followed by cisplatin 100 mg/m^2 administered as a 30-minute to 3 hour infusion, followed by 5-fluorouracil 1000 mg/m^2/day as a continuous infusion from day 1 to day 4. This regimen is administered every 3 weeks for 3 cycles. Following chemotherapy, patients should receive chemoradiotherapy.

For cisplatin and 5-fluorouracil dose modifications, see the corresponding summary of product characteristics.

Dose adjustments during treatment

General

Docetaxel should be administered when the neutrophil count is ≥1,500 cells/mm^3.

In patients who experienced either febrile neutropenia, neutrophil < 500 cells/mm^3 for more than one week, severe or cumulative cutaneous reactions or severe peripheral neuropathy during docetaxel therapy, the dose of docetaxel should be reduced from 100 mg/m^2 to 75 mg/m^2 and/or from 75 to 60 mg/m^2. If the patient continues to experience these reactions at 60 mg/m^2, the treatment should be discontinued.

Adjuvant therapy for breast cancer

In the pivotal trial in patients who received adjuvant therapy for breast cancer and who experienced complicated neutropenia (including prolonged neutropenia, febrile neutropenia, or infection), it was recommended to use G-CSF to provide prophylactic coverage (eg, day 4 to 11) in all subsequent cycles. Patients who continued to experience this reaction should remain on G-CSF and have their docetaxel dose reduced to 60 mg/m^2.

However, in clinical practice neutropenia could occur earlier. Thus the use of G-CSF should be considered function of the neutropenic risk of the patient and current recommendations. Patients who experience Grade 3 or 4 stomatitis should have their dose decreased to 60 mg/m^2.

In combination with cisplatin

For patients who are dosed initially at docetaxel 75 mg/m^2 in combination with cisplatin and whose nadir of platelet count during the previous course of therapy is < 25,000 cells/mm^3, or in patients who experience febrile neutropenia, or in patients with serious non-hematologic toxicities, the docetaxel dose in subsequent cycles should be reduced to 65 mg/m^2. For cisplatin dose adjustments, see the corresponding summary of product characteristics.

In combination with capecitabine

• For capecitabine dose modifications, see capecitabine summary of product characteristics.

• For patients developing the first appearance of a Grade 2 toxicity, which persists at the time of the next docetaxel/capecitabine treatment, delay treatment until resolved to Grade 0-1, and resume at 100% of the original dose.

• For patients developing the second appearance of a Grade 2 toxicity, or the first appearance of a Grade 3 toxicity, at any time during the treatment cycle, delay treatment until resolved to Grade 0-1, then resume treatment with docetaxel 55 mg/m^2.

• For any subsequent appearances of toxicities, or any Grade 4 toxicities, discontinue the docetaxel dose.

For trastuzumab dose modifications, see trastuzumab summary of product characteristics.

In combination with cisplatin and 5-fluorouracil

If an episode of febrile neutropenia, prolonged neutropenia or neutropenic infection occurs despite G-CSF use, the docetaxel dose should be reduced from 75 to 60 mg/m^2. If subsequent episodes of complicated neutropenia occur the docetaxel dose should be reduced from 60 to 45 mg/m^2. In case of Grade 4 thrombocytopenia the docetaxel dose should be reduced from 75 to 60 mg/m^2. Patients should not be retreated with subsequent cycles of docetaxel until neutrophils recover to a level > 1,500 cells/mm^3 and platelets recover to a level > 100,000 cells/mm^3. Discontinue treatment if these toxicities persist. (See section 4.4).

Recommended dose modifications for toxicities in patients treated with docetaxel in combination with cisplatin and 5-fluorouracil (5-FU):

Toxicity	Dose adjustment
Diarrhea grade 3	First episode: reduce 5-FU dose by 20%. Second episode: then reduce docetaxel dose by 20%.
Diarrhea grade 4	First episode: reduce docetaxel and 5-FU doses by 20%. Second episode: discontinue treatment.
Stomatitis/ mucositis grade 3	First episode: reduce 5-FU dose by 20%. Second episode: stop 5-FU only, at all subsequent cycles. Third episode: reduce docetaxel dose by 20%.
Stomatitis/ mucositis grade 4	First episode: stop 5-FU only, at all subsequent cycles. Second episode: reduce docetaxel dose by 20%.

For cisplatin and 5-fluorouracil dose adjustments, see the corresponding summary of product characteristics.

In the pivotal SCCHN trials patients who experienced complicated neutropenia (including prolonged neutropenia, febrile neutropenia, or infection), it was recommended to use G-CSF to provide prophylactic coverage (eg, day 6-15) in all subsequent cycles.

Special populations:

Patients with hepatic impairment

Based on pharmacokinetic data with docetaxel at 100 mg/m^2 as single agent, patients who have both elevations of transaminase (ALT and/or AST) greater than 1.5 times the upper limit of the normal range (ULN) and alkaline phosphatase greater than 2.5 times the ULN, the recommended dose of docetaxel is 75 mg/m^2 (see sections 4.4 and 5.2). For those patients with serum bilirubin > ULN and/or ALT and AST > 3.5 times the ULN associated with alkaline phosphatase 6 times the ULN, no dose-reduction can be recommended and docetaxel should not be used unless strictly indicated.

In combination with cisplatin and 5-fluorouracil for the treatment of patients with gastric adenocarcinoma, the pivotal clinical trial excluded patients with ALT and/or AST > 1.5 × ULN associated with alkaline phosphatase > 2.5 × ULN, and bilirubin >1 × ULN; for these patients, no dose-reductions can be recommended and docetaxel should not be used unless strictly indicated. No data are available in patients with hepatic impairment treated by docetaxel in combination in the other indications.

Children and adolescents

The experience in children is limited.

Elderly

Based on a population pharmacokinetic analysis, there are no special instructions for use in the elderly.

In combination with capecitabine, for patients 60 years of age or more, a starting dose reduction of capecitabine to 75% is recommended (see capecitabine summary of product characteristics).

4.3 Contraindications

Hypersensitivity to the active substance or to any of the excipients.

Docetaxel must not be used in patients with baseline neutrophil count of < 1,500 cells/mm^3.

Docetaxel must not be used in pregnant or breast-feeding women.

Docetaxel must not be used in patients with severe liver impairment since there is no data available (see sections 4.2 and 4.4).

Contraindications for other medicinal products also apply, when combined with docetaxel.

4.4 Special warnings and precautions for use

For breast and non-small cell lung cancers, premedication consisting of an oral corticosteroid, such as dexamethasone 16 mg per day (e.g. 8 mg BID) for 3 days starting 1 day prior to docetaxel administration, unless contraindicated, can reduce the incidence and severity of fluid retention as well as the severity of hypersensitivity reactions. For prostate cancer, the premedication is oral dexamethasone 8 mg, 12 hours, 3 hours and 1 hour before the docetaxel infusion (see section 4.2).

Haematology

Neutropenia is the most frequent adverse reaction of docetaxel. Neutrophil nadirs occurred at a median of 7 days but this interval may be shorter in heavily pre-treated patients. Frequent monitoring of complete blood counts should be conducted on all patients receiving docetaxel. Patients should be retreated with docetaxel when neutrophils recover to a level ≥ 1,500 cells/mm^3 (see section 4.2).

In the case of severe neutropenia (< 500 cells/mm^3 for seven days or more) during a course of docetaxel therapy, a reduction in dose for subsequent courses of therapy or the use of appropriate symptomatic measures are recommended (see section 4.2).

In patients treated with docetaxel in combination with cisplatin and 5-fluorouracil (TCF), febrile neutropenia and neutropenic infection occurred at lower rates when patients received prophylactic G-CSF. Patients treated with TCF should receive prophylactic G-CSF to mitigate the risk of complicated neutropenia (febrile neutropenia, prolonged neutropenia or neutropenic infection). Patients receiving TCF should be closely monitored (see sections 4.2 and 4.8).

Hypersensitivity reactions

Patients should be observed closely for hypersensitivity reactions especially during the first and second infusions. Hypersensitivity reactions may occur within a few minutes following the initiation of the infusion of docetaxel, thus facilities for the treatment of hypotension and bronchospasm should be available. If hypersensitivity reactions occur, minor symptoms such as flushing or localised cutaneous reactions do not require interruption of therapy. However, severe reactions, such as severe hypotension, bronchospasm or generalised rash/erythema require immediate discontinuation of docetaxel and appropriate therapy. Patients who have developed severe hypersensitivity reactions should not be re-challenged with docetaxel.

Cutaneous reactions

Localised skin erythema of the extremities (palms of the hands and soles of the feet) with oedema followed by desquamation has been observed. Severe symptoms such as eruptions followed by desquamation which lead to interruption or discontinuation of docetaxel treatment were reported (see section 4.2).

Fluid retention

Patients with severe fluid retention such as pleural effusion, pericardial effusion and ascites should be monitored closely.

Patients with liver impairment

In patients treated with docetaxel at 100 mg/m^2 as single agent who have serum transaminase levels (ALT and/or AST) greater than 1.5 times the ULN concurrent with serum alkaline phosphatase levels greater than 2.5 times the ULN, there is a higher risk of developing severe adverse reactions such as toxic deaths including sepsis and gastrointestinal haemorrhage which can be fatal, febrile neutropenia, infections, thrombocytopenia, stomatitis and asthenia. Therefore, the recommended dose of docetaxel in those patients with elevated liver function test (LFTs) is 75 mg/m^2 and LFTs should be measured at baseline and before each cycle (see section 4.2).

For patients with serum bilirubin levels > ULN and/or ALT and AST > 3.5 times the ULN concurrent with serum alkaline phosphatase levels > 6 times the ULN, no dose-reduction can be recommended and docetaxel should not be used unless strictly indicated.

In combination with cisplatin and 5-fluorouracil for the treatment of patients with gastric adenocarcinoma, the pivotal clinical trial excluded patients with ALT and/or AST > 1.5 × ULN associated with alkaline phosphatase > 2.5 × ULN, and bilirubin > 1 × ULN; for these patients, no dose-reductions can be recommended and docetaxel should not be used unless strictly indicated. No data are available in patients with hepatic impairment treated by docetaxel in combination in the other indications.

Patients with renal impairment

There are no data available in patients with severely impaired renal function treated with docetaxel.

Nervous system

The development of severe peripheral neurotoxicity requires a reduction of dose (see section 4.2).

Cardiac toxicity

Heart failure has been observed in patients receiving docetaxel in combination with trastuzumab, particularly following anthracycline (doxorubicin or epirubicin)-containing chemotherapy. This may be moderate to severe and has been associated with death (see section 4.8).

When patients are candidates for treatment with docetaxel in combination with trastuzumab, they should undergo baseline cardiac assessment. Cardiac function should be further monitored during treatment (e.g. every three months) to help identify patients who may develop cardiac dysfunction. For more details see summary of product characteristics of trastuzumab.

Others

Contraceptive measures must be taken during and for at least three months after cessation of therapy.

Additional cautions for use in adjuvant treatment of breast cancer

Complicated neutropenia

For patients who experience complicated neutropenia (prolonged neutropenia, febrile neutropenia or infection), G-CSF and dose reduction should be considered (see section 4.2).

Gastrointestinal reactions

Symptoms such as early abdominal pain and tenderness, fever, diarrhea, with or without neutropenia, may be early manifestations of serious gastrointestinal toxicity and should be evaluated and treated promptly.

Congestive heart failure

Patients should be monitored for symptoms of congestive heart failure during therapy and during the follow up period.

Leukemia

In the docetaxel, doxorubicin and cyclophosphamide (TAC) treated patients, the risk of delayed myelodysplasia or myeloid leukemia requires haematological follow-up.

Patients with 4+ nodes

The benefit/risk ratio for TAC in patients with 4+ nodes was not defined fully at the interim analysis (see section 5.1).

Elderly

There are no data available in patients > 70 years of age on docetaxel use in combination with doxorubicin and cyclophosphamide.

Of the 333 patients treated with docetaxel every three weeks in a prostate cancer study, 209 patients were 65 years of age or greater and 68 patients were older than 75 years. In patients treated with docetaxel every three weeks, the incidence of related nail changes occurred at a rate ⩾ 10% higher in patients who were 65 years of age or greater compared to younger patients. The incidence of related fever, diarrhea, anorexia, and peripheral edema occurred at rates ⩾ 10% higher in patients who were 75 years of age or greater versus less than 65 years.

Among the 300 (221 patients in the phase III part of the study and 79 patients in the phase II part) patients treated with docetaxel in combination with cisplatin and 5-fluorouracil in the gastric cancer study, 74 were 65 years of age or older and 4 patients were 75 years of age or older. The incidence of serious adverse events was higher in the elderly patients compared to younger patients. The incidence of the following adverse events (all grades): lethargy, stomatitis, neutropenic infection occurred at rates ⩾ 10% higher in patients who were 65 years of age or older compared to younger patients.

Elderly patients treated with TCF should be closely monitored.

4.5 Interaction with other medicinal products and other forms of interaction

In vitro studies have shown that the metabolism of docetaxel may be modified by the concomitant administration of compounds which induce, inhibit or are metabolised by (and thus may inhibit the enzyme competitively) cytochrome P450-3A such as ciclosporine, terfenadine, ketoconazole, erythromycin and troleandomycin. As a result, caution should be exercised when treating patients with these medicinal products as concomitant therapy since there is a potential for a significant interaction.

Docetaxel is highly protein bound (> 95%). Although the possible *in vivo* interaction of docetaxel with concomitantly administered medication has not been investigated formally, *in vitro* interactions with tightly protein-bound agents such as erythromycin, diphenhydramine, propranolol, propafenone, phenytoin, salicylate, sulfamethoxazole and sodium valproate did not affect protein binding of docetaxel. In addition, dexamethasone did not affect protein binding of docetaxel. Docetaxel did not influence the binding of digitoxin.

The pharmacokinetics of docetaxel, doxorubicin and cyclophosphamide were not influenced by their coadministration. Limited data from a single uncontrolled study were suggestive of an interaction between docetaxel and carboplatin. When combined to docetaxel, the clearance of carboplatin was about 50% higher than values previously reported for carboplatin monotherapy.

Docetaxel pharmacokinetics in the presence of prednisone was studied in patients with metastatic prostate cancer. Docetaxel is metabolised by CYP3A4 and prednisone is known to induce CYP3A4. No statistically significant effect of prednisone on the pharmacokinetics of docetaxel was observed.

Docetaxel should be administered with caution in patients concomitantly receiving potent CYP3A4 inhibitors (e.g. protease inhibitors like ritonavir, azole antifungals like ketoconazole or itraconazole). A drug interaction study performed in patients receiving ketoconazole and docetaxel showed that the clearance of docetaxel was reduced by half by ketoconazole, probably because the metabolism of docetaxel involves CYP3A4 as a major (single) metabolic pathway. Reduced tolerance of docetaxel may occur, even at lower doses.

4.6 Pregnancy and lactation

There is no information on the use of docetaxel in pregnant women. Docetaxel has been shown to be both embryotoxic and foetotoxic in rabbits and rats, and to reduce fertility in rats. As with other cytotoxic medicinal products, docetaxel may cause foetal harm when administered to pregnant women. Therefore, docetaxel must not be used during pregnancy. Women of childbearing age receiving docetaxel should be advised to avoid becoming pregnant, and to inform the treating physician immediately should this occur.

Docetaxel is a lipophilic substance but it is not known whether it is excreted in human milk. Consequently, because of the potential for adverse reactions in nursing infants, breast feeding must be discontinued for the duration of docetaxel therapy.

Table 1 TAXOTERE 100 mg/m² single agent

MedDRA System Organ classes	Very common adverse reactions ⩾ 10% of patients	Common adverse reactions ⩾ 1 to < 10% of patients	Uncommon adverse reactions ⩾ 0.1 to < 1% of patients
Investigations		G3/4 Blood bilirubin increased (< 5%); G3/4 Blood alkaline phosphatase increased (< 4%); G3/4 AST increased (< 3%); G3/4 ALT increased (< 2%)	
Cardiac disorders		Arrhythmia (G3/4: 0.7%)	Cardiac failure
Blood and lymphatic system disorders	Neutropenia (G4: 76.4%); Anaemia (G3/4: 8.9%); Febrile neutropenia	Thrombocytopenia (G4: 0.2%)	
Nervous system disorders	Peripheral sensory neuropathy (G3: 4.1%); Peripheral motor neuropathy (G3/4: 4%); Dysgeusia (severe: 0.07%)		
Respiratory, thoracic and mediastinal disorders	Dyspnoea (severe: 2.7%)		
Gastrointestinal disorders	Stomatitis (G3/4: 5.3%); Diarrhoea (G3/4: 4%); Nausea (G3/4: 4%); Vomiting (G3/4: 3%)	Constipation (severe: 0.2%); Abdominal pain (severe: 1%); Gastrointestinal haemorrhage (severe: 0.3%)	Oesophagitis (severe: 0.4%)
Skin and subcutaneous tissue disorders	Alopecia; Skin reaction (G3/4: 5.9%); Nail disorders (severe: 2.6%)		
Musculoskeletal and connective tissue disorders	Myalgia (severe: 1.4%)	Arthralgia	
Metabolism and nutrition disorders	Anorexia		
Infections and infestations	Infections (G3/4: 5.7%; including sepsis and pneumonia, fatal in 1.7%)	Infection associated with G4 neutropenia (G3/4: 4.6%)	
Vascular disorders		Hypotension; Hypertension; Haemorrhage	
General disorders and administration site conditions	Fluid retention (severe: 6.5%); Asthenia (severe: 11.2%); Pain	Infusion site reaction; Non-cardiac chest pain (severe: 0.4%)	
Immune system disorders	Hypersensitivity (G3/4: 5.3%)		

4.7 Effects on ability to drive and use machines

No studies on the effects on the ability to drive and use machines have been performed.

4.8 Undesirable effects

The adverse reactions considered to be possibly or probably related to the administration of docetaxel have been obtained in:

- 1312 and 121 patients who received 100 mg/m² and 75 mg/m² of docetaxel as a single agent respectively.
- 258 patients who received docetaxel in combination with doxorubicin.
- 406 patients who received docetaxel in combination with cisplatin.
- 92 patients treated with docetaxel in combination with trastuzumab.
- 255 patients who received docetaxel in combination with capecitabine.
- 332 patients who received docetaxel in combination with prednisone or prednisolone (clinically important treatment related adverse events are presented).
- 744 patients who received docetaxel in combination with doxorubicin and cyclophosphamide (clinically important treatment related adverse events are presented).
- 300 gastric adenocarcinoma patients (221 patients in the phase III part of the study and 79 patients in the phase II part) who received docetaxel in combination with cisplatin and 5-fluorouracil (clinically important treatment related adverse events are presented).
- 174 and 251 head and neck cancer patients who received docetaxel in combination with cisplatin and 5-fluorouracil (clinically important treatment related adverse events are presented).

These reactions were described using the NCI Common Toxicity Criteria (grade 3 = G3; grade 3-4 = G3/4; grade 4 = G4) and the COSTART terms. Frequencies are defined as: very common (⩾ 1/10), common (⩾ 1/100, < 1/10); uncommon (⩾ 1/1,000, < 1/100); rare (⩾ 1/10,000, < 1/1,000); very rare (< 1/10,000).

Within each frequency grouping, undesirable effects are presented in order of decreasing seriousness.

The most commonly reported adverse reactions of docetaxel alone are: neutropenia (which was reversible and not cumulative; the median day to nadir was 7 days and the median duration of severe neutropenia (< 500 cells/mm³) was 7 days), anemia, alopecia, nausea, vomiting, stomatitis, diarrhea and asthenia. The severity of adverse events of docetaxel may be increased when docetaxel is given in combination with other chemotherapeutic agents.

For combination with trastuzumab, adverse events (all grades) reported in ⩾ 10% are displayed. There was an increased incidence of SAEs (40% vs. 31%) and Grade 4 AEs (34% vs. 23%) in the trastuzumab combination arm compared to docetaxel monotherapy.

For combination with capecitabine, the most frequent treatment-related undesirable effects (⩾ 5%) reported in a phase III trial in breast cancer patients failing anthracycline treatment are presented (see capecitabine summary of product characteristics).

The following adverse reactions are frequently observed with docetaxel:

Nervous system disorders

The development of severe peripheral neurotoxicity requires a reduction of dose (see sections 4.2 and 4.4). Mild to moderate neuro-sensory signs are characterised by paresthesia, dysesthesia or pain including burning. Neuromotor events are mainly characterised by weakness.

Skin and subcutaneous tissue disorders

Reversible cutaneous reactions have been observed and were generally considered as mild to moderate. Reactions were characterised by a rash including localised eruptions mainly on the feet and hands (including severe hand and foot syndrome), but also on the arms, face or thorax, and frequently associated with pruritus. Eruptions generally occurred within one week after the docetaxel infusion. Less frequently, severe symptoms such as eruptions followed by desquamation which rarely lead to interruption or discontinuation of docetaxel treatment were reported (see

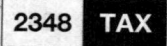

Table 2 TAXOTERE 75 mg/m² in combination with doxorubicin

MedDRA System Organ classes	Very common adverse reactions ⩾ 10% of patients	Common adverse reactions ⩾ 1 to < 10% of patients	Uncommon adverse reactions ⩾ 0.1 to < 1% of patients
Investigations		G3/4 Blood bilirubin increased (< 2.5%); G3/4 Blood alkaline phosphatase increased (< 2.5%)	G3/4 AST increased (< 1%); G3/4 ALT increased (< 1%)
Cardiac disorders		Cardiac failure; Arrhythmia (no severe)	
Blood and lymphatic system disorders	Neutropenia (G4: 91.7%); Anaemia (G3/4: 9.4%); Febrile neutropenia; Thrombocytopenia (G4: 0.8%)		
Nervous system disorders	Peripheral sensory neuropathy (G3: 0.4%)	Peripheral motor neuropathy (G3/4: 0.4%)	
Gastrointestinal disorders	Nausea (G3/4: 5%); Stomatitis (G3/4: 7.8%); Diarrhoea (G3/4: 6.2%); Vomiting (G3/4: 5%); Constipation		
Skin and subcutaneous tissue disorders	Alopecia; Nail disorders (severe: 0.4%); Skin reaction (no severe)		
Musculoskeletal and connective tissue disorders		Myalgia	
Metabolism and nutrition disorders		Anorexia	
Infections and infestations	Infection (G3/4: 7.8%)		
Vascular disorders			Hypotension
General disorders and administration site conditions	Asthenia (severe: 8.1%); Fluid retention (severe: 1.2%); Pain	Infusion site reaction	
Immune system disorders		Hypersensitivity (G3/4: 1.2%)	

Table 3 TAXOTERE 75 mg/m² in combination with cisplatin

MedDRA System Organ classes	Very common adverse reactions ⩾ 10% of patients	Common adverse reactions ⩾ 1 to <10% of patients	Uncommon adverse reactions ⩾ 0.1 to <1% of patients
Investigations		G3/4 Blood bilirubin increased (2.1%); G3/4 ALT increased (1.3%)	G3/4 AST increased (0.5%); G3/4 Blood alkaline phosphatase increased (0.3%)
Cardiac disorders		Arrhythmia (G3/4: 0.7%)	Cardiac failure
Blood and lymphatic system disorders	Neutropenia (G4: 51.5%); Anaemia (G3/4: 6.9%); Thrombocytopenia (G4: 0.5%)	Febrile neutropenia	
Nervous system disorders	Peripheral sensory neuropathy (G3: 3.7%); Peripheral motor neuropathy (G3/4: 2%)		
Gastrointestinal disorders	Nausea (G3/4: 9.6%); Vomiting (G3/4: 7.6%); Diarrhoea (G3/4: 6.4%); Stomatitis (G3/4: 2%)	Constipation	
Skin and subcutaneous tissue disorders	Alopecia; Nail disorders (severe: 0.7%); Skin reaction (G3/4: 0.2%)		
Musculoskeletal and connective tissue disorders	Myalgia (severe: 0.5%)		
Metabolism and nutrition disorders	Anorexia		
Infections and infestations	Infection (G3/4: 5.7%)		
Vascular disorders		Hypotension (G3/4: 0.7%)	
General disorders and administration site conditions	Asthenia (severe: 9.9%); Fluid retention (severe: 0.7%); Fever (G3/4: 1.2%)	Infusion site reaction; Pain	
Immune system disorders	Hypersensitivity (G3/4: 2.5%)		

sections 4.2 and 4.4). Severe nail disorders are characterised by hypo- or hyperpigmentation and sometimes pain and onycholysis.

General disorders and administration site conditions

Infusion site reactions were generally mild and consisted of hyper pigmentation, inflammation, redness or dryness of the skin, phlebitis or extravasation and swelling of the vein.

Fluid retention includes events such as peripheral oedema and less frequently pleural effusion, pericardial effusion, ascites and weight gain. The peripheral oedema usually starts at the lower extremities and may become generalised with a weight gain of 3 kg or more. Fluid retention is cumulative in incidence and severity (see section 4.4).

Immune system disorders

Hypersensitivity reactions have generally occurred within a few minutes following the start of the infusion of docetaxel and were usually mild to moderate. The most frequently reported symptoms were flushing, rash with or without pruritus, chest tightness, back pain, dyspnoea and fever or chills. Severe reactions were characterised by hypotension and/or bronchospasm or generalized rash/erythema (see section 4.4).

TAXOTERE 100 mg/m² single agent

(see Table 1 on previous page)

Blood and lymphatic system disorders

Rare: bleeding episodes associated with grade 3/4 thrombocytopenia.

Nervous system disorders

Reversibility data are available among 35.3% of patients who developed neurotoxicity following docetaxel treatment at 100 mg/m² as single agent. The events were spontaneously reversible within 3 months.

Skin and subcutaneous tissue disorders

Very rare: one case of alopecia non-reversible at the end of the study. 73% of the cutaneous reactions were reversible within 21 days.

General disorders and administration site conditions

The median cumulative dose to treatment discontinuation was more than 1,000 mg/m² and the median time to fluid retention reversibility was 16.4 weeks (range 0 to 42 weeks). The onset of moderate and severe retention is delayed (median cumulative dose: 818.9 mg/m²) in patients with premedication compared with patients without premedication (median cumulative dose: 489.7 mg/m²); however, it has been reported in some patients during the early courses of therapy.

TAXOTERE 75 mg/m² single agent

MedDRA System Organ classes	Very common adverse reactions ⩾ 10% of patients	Common adverse reactions ⩾ 1 to <10% of patients
Investigations		G3/4 Blood bilirubin increased (<2%)
Cardiac disorders		Arrhythmia (no severe)
Blood and lymphatic system disorders	Neutropenia (G4: 54.2%); Anaemia (G3/4: 10.8%); Thrombocytopenia (G4: 1.7%)	Febrile neutropenia
Nervous system disorders	Peripheral sensory neuropathy (G3/4: 0.8%)	Peripheral motor neuropathy (G3/4: 2.5%)
Gastrointestinal disorders	Nausea (G3/4: 3.3%); Stomatitis (G3/4: 1.7%); Vomiting (G3/4: 0.8%); Diarrhea (G3/4: 1.7%)	Constipation
Skin and subcutaneous tissue disorders	Alopecia; Skin reaction (G3/4: 0.8%)	Nail disorders (severe: 0.8%)
Musculoskeletal and connective tissue disorders		Myalgia
Metabolism and nutrition disorders	Anorexia	
Infections and infestations	Infections (G3/4: 5%)	
Vascular disorders		Hypotension
General disorders and administration site conditions	Asthenia (severe: 12.4%); Fluid retention (severe: 0.8%); Pain	
Immune system disorders		Hypersensitivity (no severe)

TAXOTERE 75 mg/m² in combination with doxorubicin

(see Table 2 above)

TAXOTERE 75 mg/m² in combination with cisplatin

(see Table 3 on previous page)

TAXOTERE 100 mg/m² in combination with trastuzumab

MedDRA System Organ classes	Very common adverse reactions ≥ 10% of patients	Common adverse reactions ≥ 1 to < 10% of patients
Investigations	Weight increased	
Cardiac disorders		Cardiac failure
Blood and lymphatic system disorders	Neutropenia (G3/4: 32%); Febrile neutropenia (includes neutropenia associated with fever and antibiotic use) or neutropenic sepsis	
Nervous system disorders	Paresthesia; Headache; Dysgeusia; Hypoaesthesia	
Eye disorders	Lacrimation increased; Conjunctivitis	
Respiratory, thoracic and mediastinal disorders	Epistaxis; Pharyngolaryngeal pain; Nasopharyngitis; Dyspnoea; Cough; Rhinorrhoea	
Gastrointestinal disorders	Nausea; Diarrhoea; Vomiting; Constipation; Stomatitis; Dyspepsia; Abdominal pain	
Skin and subcutaneous tissue disorders	Alopecia; Erythema; Rash; Nail disorders	
Musculoskeletal and connective tissue disorders	Myalgia; Arthralgia; Pain in extremity; Bone pain; Back pain	
Metabolism and nutrition disorders	Anorexia	
Vascular disorders	Lymphoedema	
General disorders and administration site conditions	Asthenia; Oedema peripheral; Pyrexia; Fatigue; Mucosal inflammation; Pain; Influenza like illness; Chest pain; Chills	Lethargy
Psychiatric disorders	Insomnia	

Cardiac disorders

Symptomatic cardiac failure was reported in 2.2% of the patients who received docetaxel plus trastuzumab compared to 0% of patients given docetaxel alone. In the docetaxel plus trastuzumab arm, 64% had received a prior anthracycline as adjuvant therapy compared with 55% in the docetaxel arm alone.

Blood and lymphatic system disorders

Very common: Haematological toxicity was increased in patients receiving trastuzumab and docetaxel, compared with docetaxel alone (32% grade 3/4 neutropenia versus 22%, using NCI-CTC criteria). Note that this is likely to be an underestimate since docetaxel alone at a dose of 100 mg/m² is known to result in neutropenia in 97% of patients, 76% grade 4, based on nadir blood counts. The incidence of febrile neutropenia/neutropenic sepsis was also increased in patients treated with Herceptin plus docetaxel (23% versus 17% for patients treated with docetaxel alone).

TAXOTERE 75 mg/m² in combination with capecitabine

MedDRA System Organ classes	Very common adverse reactions ≥ 10% of patients	Common adverse reactions ≥ 1 to < 10% of patients
Investigations		Weight decreased; G3/4 Blood bilirubin increased (9%)
Blood and lymphatic system disorders	Neutropenia (G3/4: 63%); Anaemia (G3/4: 10%)	Thrombocytopenia (G3/4: 3%)
Nervous system disorders	Dysgeusia (G3/4: <1%); Paraesthesia (G3/4: <1%)	Dizziness; Headache (G3/4: <1%); Neuropathy peripheral
Eye disorders	Lacrimation increased	
Respiratory, thoracic and mediastinal disorders	Pharyngolaryngeal pain (G3/4: 2%)	Dyspnoea (G3/4: 1%); Cough (G3/4: <1%); Epistaxis (G3/4: <1%)
Gastrointestinal disorders	Stomatitis (G3/4: 18%); Diarrhoea (G3/4: 14%); Nausea (G3/4: 6%); Vomiting (G3/4: 4%); Constipation (G3/4: 1%); Abdominal pain (G3/4: 2%); Dyspepsia	Abdominal pain upper; Dry mouth
Skin and subcutaneous tissue disorders	Hand-foot syndrome (G3/4: 24%); Alopecia (G3/4: 6%); Nail disorders (G3/4: 2%)	Dermatitis; Rash erythematous (G3/4: <1%); Nail discolouration; Onycholysis (G3/4: 1%)
Musculoskeletal and connective tissue disorders	Myalgia (G3/4: 2%); Arthralgia (G3/4: 1%)	Pain in extremity (G3/4: <1%); Back pain (G3/4: 1%)
Metabolism and nutrition disorders	Anorexia (G3/4: 1%); Decreased appetite	Dehydration (G3/4: 2%)
Infections and infestations		Oral candidiasis (G3/4: < 1%)
General disorders and administration site conditions	Asthenia (G3/4: 3%); Pyrexia (G3/4: 1%); Fatigue/weakness (G3/4: 5%); Oedema peripheral (G3/4: 1%)	Lethargy; Pain

TAXOTERE 75 mg/m² in combination with prednisone or prednisolone

MedDRA System Organ classes	Very common adverse reactions ≥ 10% of patients	Common adverse reactions ≥1 to < 10% of patients
Cardiac disorders		Cardiac left ventricular function decrease (G3/4: 0.3%)
Blood and lymphatic system disorders	Neutropenia (G3/4: 32%); Anaemia (G3/4: 4.9%)	Thrombocytopenia (G3/4: 0.6%); Febrile neutropenia
Nervous system disorders	Peripheral sensory neuropathy (G3/4: 1.2%); Dysgeusia (G3/4: 0%)	Peripheral motor neuropathy (G3/4: 0%)
Eye disorders		Lacrimation increased (G3/4: 0.6%)
Respiratory, thoracic and mediastinal disorders		Epistaxis (G3/4: 0%); Dyspnoea (G3/4: 0.6%); Cough (G3/4: 0%)
Gastrointestinal disorders	Nausea (G3/4: 2.4%); Diarrhoea (G3/4: 1.2%); Stomatitis/ Pharyngitis (G3/4: 0.9%); Vomiting (G3/4: 1.2%)	
Skin and subcutaneous tissue disorders	Alopecia; Nail disorders (no severe)	Exfoliative rash (G3/4: 0.3%)
Musculoskeletal and connective bone disorders		Arthralgia (G3/4: 0.3%); Myalgia (G3/4: 0.3%)
Metabolism and nutrition disorders	Anorexia (G3/4: 0.6%)	
Infections and infestations	Infection (G3/4: 3.3%)	
General disorders and administration site conditions	Fatigue (G3/4: 3.9%); Fluid retention (severe: 0.6%)	
Immune system disorders		Hypersensitivity (G3/4: 0.6%)

TAXOTERE 75 mg/m² in combination with doxorubicin and cyclophosphamide

(see Table 4 on next page)

Cardiac disorders

Congestive Heart Failure (CHF) (2.3% at 70 months median follow-up) has also been reported. One patient in each treatment arm died due to cardiac failure.

Nervous system disorders

Peripheral sensory neuropathy was observed to be ongoing at the median follow-up time of 55 months in 9 patients out of the 73 patients with peripheral sensory neuropathy at the end of the chemotherapy.

Skin and subcutaneous tissue disorders

Alopecia was observed to be ongoing at the median follow-up time of 55 months in 22 patients out of the 687 patients with alopecia at the end of the chemotherapy.

General disorders and administration site conditions

Oedema peripheral was observed to be ongoing at the median follow-up time of 55 months in 18 patients out of the 112 patients with oedema peripheral at the end of the chemotherapy.

Reproductive system and breast disorders

Amenorrhoea was observed to be ongoing at the median follow-up time of 55 months in 133 patients out of the 233 patients with amenorrhoea at the end of the chemotherapy.

TAXOTERE 75 mg/m² in combination with cisplatin and 5-fluorouracil for gastric adenocarcinoma cancer

MedDRA System Organ classes	Very common adverse reactions ≥ 10% of patients	Common adverse reactions ≥ 1 to <10% of patients
Cardiac disorders		Arrhythmia (G3/4: 1.0%)
Blood and lymphatic system disorders	Anaemia (G3/4: 20.9%); Neutropenia (G3/4: 83.2%); Thrombocytopenia (G3/4: 8.8%); Febrile neutropenia	
Nervous system disorders	Peripheral sensory neuropathy (G3/4: 8.7%)	Dizziness (G3/4: 2.3%); Peripheral motor neuropathy (G3/4: 1.3%)
Eye disorders		Lacrimation increased (G3/4: 0%)
Ear and labyrinth disorders		Hearing impaired (G3/4: 0%)
Gastrointestinal disorders	Diarrhoea (G3/4: 19.7%); Nausea (G3/4: 16%); Stomatitis (G3/4: 23.7%); Vomiting (G3/4: 14.3%)	Constipation (G3/4: 1.0%); Gastrointestinal pain (G3/4: 1.0%); Oesophagitis/ dysphagia/ odynophagia (G3/4: 0.7%)
Skin and subcutaneous tissue disorders	Alopecia (G3/4: 4.0%)	Rash pruritus (G3/4: 0.7%); Nail disorders (G3/4: 0.7%); Skin exfoliation (G3/4: 0%)
Metabolism and nutrition disorders	Anorexia (G3/4: 11.7%)	
Infections and infestations	Neutropenic infection; Infection (G3/4: 11.7%)	
General disorders and administration site conditions	Lethargy (G3/4: 19.0%); Fever (G3/4: 2.3%); Fluid retention (severe/life-threatening: 1%)	
Immune system disorders	Hypersensitivity (G3/4: 1.7%)	

Blood and lymphatic system disorders

Febrile neutropenia and neutropenic infection occurred in 17.2% and 13.5% of patients respectively, regardless of G-CSF use. G-CSF was used for secondary prophylaxis in 19.3% of patients (10.7% of the cycles). Febrile neutropenia and neutropenic infection occurred respectively in 12.1% and 3.4% of patients when patients received prophylactic G-CSF, in 15.6% and 12.9% of patients without prophylactic G-CSF (see section 4.2).

TAXOTERE 75 mg/m² in combination with cisplatin and 5-fluorouracil for Head and Neck cancer

- Induction chemotherapy followed by radiotherapy (TAX 323)

(see Table 5 on page 4932351)

- Induction chemotherapy followed by chemoradiotherapy (TAX 324)

Table 4 TAXOTERE 75 mg/m² in combination with doxorubicin and cyclophosphamide

MedDRA System Organ classes	Very common adverse reactions ⩾ 10% of patients	Common adverse reactions ⩾ 1 to < 10% of patients	Uncommon adverse reactions ⩾ 0.1 to < 1% of patients
Investigations	Weight increased or decreased (G3/4: 0.3%)		
Cardiac disorders		Arrhythmia (G3/4: 0.1%); Congestive heart failure	
Blood and lymphatic system disorders	Anaemia (G3/4: 4.3%); Neutropenia (G3/4: 65.5%); Thrombocytopenia (G3/4: 2.0%); Febrile neutropenia		
Nervous system disorders	Dysgeusia (G3/4: 0.7%); Peripheral sensory neuropathy (G3/4: 0%)	Peripheral motor neuropathy (G3/4: 0%); Neurocortical (G3/4: 0.3%); Neurocerebellar (G3/4: 0.1%)	Syncope (G3/4: 0%)
Eye disorders		Lacrimation disorder (G3/4: 0.1%); Conjunctivitis (G3/4: 0.3%)	
Respiratory, thoracic and mediastinal disorders		Cough (G3/4: 0%)	
Gastrointestinal disorders	Nausea (G3/4: 5.1%); Stomatitis (G3/4: 7.1%); Vomiting (G3/4: 4.3%); Diarrhoea (G3/4: 3.2%); Constipation (G3/4: 0.4%)	Abdominal pain (G3/4: 0.5%)	Colitis/enteritis/large intestine perforation
Skin and subcutaneous tissue disorders	Alopecia; Skin toxicity (G3/4: 0.7%); Nail disorders (G3/4: 0.4%)		
Musculoskeletal and connective tissue disorders	Myalgia (G3/4: 0.8%); Arthralgia (G3/4: 0.4%)		
Metabolism and nutrition disorders	Anorexia (G3/4: 2.2%)		
Infections and infestations	Infection (G3/4: 3.2%); Neutropenic infection. There were no septic deaths.		
Vascular disorders	Vasodilatation (G3/4: 0.9%)	Hypotension (G3/4: 0%)	Phlebitis (G3/4: 0%); Lymphoedema (G3/4: 0%)
General disorders and administration site conditions	Asthenia (G3/4: 11%); Fever (G3/4: 1.2%); Oedema peripheral (G3/4: 0.4%)		
Immune system disorders	Hypersensitivity (G3/4: 1.1%)		
Reproductive system and breast disorders	Amenorrhoea		

(see Table 6 on page 4932352)

Post-marketing experience

Cardiac disorders

Rare cases of myocardial infarction have been reported.

Blood and lymphatic system disorders

Bone marrow suppression and other hematologic adverse reactions have been reported. Disseminated intravascular coagulation (DIC), often in association with sepsis or multi-organ failure, has been reported.

Nervous system disorders

Rare cases of convulsion or transient loss of consciousness have been observed with docetaxel administration. These reactions sometimes appear during the infusion of the medicinal product.

Eye disorders

Very rare cases of transient visual disturbances (flashes, flashing lights, scotomata) typically occurring during infusion of the medicinal product and in association with hypersensitivity reactions have been reported. These were reversible upon discontinuation of the infusion. Cases of lacrimation with or without conjunctivitis, as cases of lacrimal duct obstruction resulting in excessive tearing have been rarely reported.

Ear and labyrinth disorders

Rare cases of ototoxicity, hearing impaired and/or hearing loss have been reported.

Respiratory, thoracic and mediastinal disorders

Acute respiratory distress syndrome, interstitial pneumonia and pulmonary fibrosis have rarely been reported. Rare cases of radiation pneumonitis have been reported in patients receiving concomitant radiotherapy.

Gastrointestinal disorders

Rare occurrences of dehydration as a consequence of gastrointestinal events, gastrointestinal perforation, colitis ischaemic, colitis and neutropenic enterocolitis have been reported. Rare cases of ileus and intestinal obstruction have been reported.

Skin and subcutaneous tissue disorders

Very rare cases of cutaneous lupus erythematosus and bullous eruptions such as erythema multiforme, Stevens-Johnson syndrome, toxic epidermal necrolysis, have been reported with docetaxel. In some cases concomitant factors may have contributed to the development of these effects. Sclerodermal-like changes usually preceded by peripheral lymphedema have been reported with docetaxel.

Neoplasms benign, malignant and unspecified (incl cysts and polyps)

Very rare cases of acute myeloid leukaemia and myelodysplastic syndrome have been reported in association with docetaxel when used in combination with other chemotherapy agents and/or radiotherapy.

Vascular disorders

Venous thromboembolic events have rarely been reported.

General disorders and administration site conditions

Radiation recall phenomena have rarely been reported.

Fluid retention has not been accompanied by acute episodes of oliguria or hypotension. Dehydration and pulmonary oedema have rarely been reported.

Immune system disorders

Some cases of anaphylactic shock, sometimes fatal, have been reported.

Hepatobiliary disorders

Very rare cases of hepatitis, sometimes fatal primarily in patients with pre-existing liver disorders, have been reported.

4.9 Overdose

There were a few reports of overdose. There is no known antidote for docetaxel overdose. In case of overdose, the patient should be kept in a specialised unit and vital functions closely monitored. In cases of overdose, exacerbation of adverse events may be expected. The primary anticipated complications of overdose would consist of bone marrow suppression, peripheral neurotoxicity and mucositis. Patients should receive therapeutic G-CSF as soon as possible after discovery of overdose. Other appropriate symptomatic measures should be taken, as needed.

5. PHARMACOLOGICAL PROPERTIES

5.1 Pharmacodynamic properties

Pharmacotherapeutic group: Antineoplastic agents, ATC Code: L01CD 02

Preclinical data

Docetaxel is an antineoplastic agent which acts by promoting the assembly of tubulin into stable microtubules and inhibits their disassembly which leads to a marked decrease of free tubulin. The binding of docetaxel to microtubules does not alter the number of protofilaments.

Docetaxel has been shown *in vitro* to disrupt the microtubular network in cells which is essential for vital mitotic and interphase cellular functions.

Docetaxel was found to be cytotoxic *in vitro* against various murine and human tumour cell lines and against freshly excised human tumour cells in clonogenic assays. Docetaxel achieves high intracellular concentrations with a long cell residence time. In addition, docetaxel was found to be active on some but not all cell lines over expressing the p-glycoprotein which is encoded by the multidrug resistance gene. *In vivo*, docetaxel is schedule independent and has a broad spectrum of experimental antitumour activity against advanced murine and human grafted tumours.

Clinical data

Breast cancer

TAXOTERE in combination with doxorubicin and cyclophosphamide: adjuvant therapy

Data from a multicenter open label randomized trial support the use of docetaxel for the adjuvant treatment of patients with operable node-positive breast cancer and KPS ⩾ 80%, between 18 and 70 years of age. After stratification according to the number of positive lymph nodes (1-3, 4+), 1491 patients were randomized to receive either docetaxel 75 mg/m² administered 1-hour after doxorubicin 50 mg/m² and cyclophosphamide 500 mg/m² (TAC arm), or doxorubicin 50 mg/m² followed by fluorouracil 500 mg/m² and cyclosphosphamide 500 mg/m² (FAC arm). Both regimens were administered once every 3 weeks for 6 cycles. Docetaxel was administered as a 1-hour infusion, all other medicinal products were given as intravenous bolus on day one. G-CSF was administered as secondary prophylaxis to patients who experienced complicated neutropenia (febrile neutropenia, prolonged neutropenia, or infection). Patients on the TAC arm received antibiotic prophylaxis with ciprofloxacin 500 mg orally twice daily for 10 days starting on day 5 of each cycle, or equivalent. In both arms, after the last cycle of chemotherapy, patients with positive estrogen and/or progesterone receptors received tamoxifen 20 mg daily for up to 5 years. Adjuvant radiation therapy was prescribed according to guidelines in place at participating institutions and was given to 69% of patients who received TAC and 72% of patients who received FAC.

An interim analysis was performed with a median follow up of 55 months. Significantly longer disease-free survival for the TAC arm compared to the FAC arm was demonstrated. Incidence of relapses at 5 years was reduced in patients receiving TAC compared to those who received FAC (25% versus 32%, respectively) i.e. an absolute risk reduction by 7% ($p = 0.001$). Overall survival at 5 years was also significantly increased with TAC compared to FAC (87% versus 81%, respectively) i.e. an absolute reduction of the risk of death by 6% ($p = 0.008$). TAC-treated patient subsets according to prospectively defined major prognostic factors were analyzed:

(see Table 7 on page 4932352)

The beneficial effect of TAC was not proven in patients with 4 and more positive nodes (37% of the population) at the interim analysis stage. The effect appears to be less pronounced than in patients with 1-3 positive nodes. The benefit/risk ratio was not defined fully in patients with 4 and more positive nodes at this analysis stage.

TAXOTERE as single agent

Two randomised phase III comparative studies, involving a total of 326 alkylating or 392 anthracycline failure metastatic breast cancer patients, have been performed with docetaxel at the recommended dose and regimen of 100 mg/m² every 3 weeks.

Table 5 TAXOTERE 75 mg/m² in combination with cisplatin and 5-fluorouracil for Head and Neck cancer

MedDRA System Organ classes	Very common adverse reactions $\geq$ 10% of patients	Common adverse reactions $\geq$ 1 to $<$10% of patients	Uncommon adverse reactions $\geq$ 0.1 to $<$ 1% of patients
Investigations		Weight increased	
Cardiac disorders		Myocardial ischemia (G3/4:1.7%)	Arrhythmia (G3/4: 0.6%)
Blood and lymphatic system disorders	Neutropenia (G3/4: 76.3%); Anemia (G3/4: 9.2%); Thrombocytopenia (G3/4: 5.2%)	Febrile neutropenia	
Nervous system disorders	Dysgeusia/Parosmia; Peripheral sensory neuropathy (G3/4: 0.6%)	Dizziness	
Eye disorders		Lacrimation increased; Conjunctivitis	
Ear and labyrinth disorders		Hearing impaired	
Gastrointestinal disorders	Nausea (G3/4: 0.6%); Stomatitis (G3/4: 4.0%); Diarrhea (G3/4: 2.9%); Vomiting (G3/4: 0.6%)	Constipation; Esophagitis/dysphagia/ odynophagia (G3/4: 0.6%); Abdominal pain; Dyspepsia; Gastrointestinal haemorrhage (G3/4: 0.6%)	
Skin and subcutaneous tissue disorders	Alopecia (G3/4: 10.9%)	Rash pruritic; Dry skin; Skin exfoliative (G3/4: 0.6%)	
Musculoskeletal and connective tissue disorders		Myalgia (G3/4: 0.6%)	
Metabolism and nutrition disorders	Anorexia (G3/4: 0.6%)		
Infections and infestations	Infection (G3/4: 6.3%); Neutropenic infection		
Neoplasms benign, malignant and unspecified (incl cysts and polyps)		Cancer pain (G3/4: 0.6%)	
Vascular disorders		Venous disorder (G3/4: 0.6%)	
General disorders and administration site conditions	Lethargy (G3/4: 3.4%); Pyrexia (G3/4: 0.6%); Fluid retention; Oedema		
Immune system disorders		Hypersensitivity (no severe)	

In alkylating-failure patients, docetaxel was compared to doxorubicin (75 mg/m² every 3 weeks). Without affecting overall survival time (docetaxel 15 months vs. doxorubicin 14 months, p = 0.38) or time to progression (docetaxel 27 weeks vs. doxorubicin 23 weeks, p = 0.54), docetaxel increased response rate (52% vs. 37%, p = 0.01) and shortened time to response (12 weeks vs. 23 weeks, p = 0.007). Three docetaxel patients (2%) discontinued the treatment due to fluid retention, whereas 15 doxorubicin patients (9%) discontinued due to cardiac toxicity (three cases of fatal congestive heart failure).

In anthracycline-failure patients, docetaxel was compared to the combination of mitomycin C and vinblastine (12 mg/m² every 6 weeks and 6 mg/m² every 3 weeks). Docetaxel increased response rate (33% vs. 12%, p < 0.0001), prolonged time to progression (19 weeks vs. 11 weeks, p = 0.0004) and prolonged overall survival (11 months vs. 9 months, p = 0.01).

During these two phase III studies, the safety profile of docetaxel was consistent with the safety profile observed in phase II studies (see section 4.8).

An open-label, multicenter, randomized phase III study was conducted to compare docetaxel monotherapy and paclitaxel in the treatment of advanced breast cancer in patients whose previous therapy should have included an anthracycline. A total of 449 patients were randomized to receive either docetaxel monotherapy 100 mg/m² as a 1 hour infusion or paclitaxel 175 mg/m² as a 3 hour infusion. Both regimens were administered every 3 weeks.

Without affecting the primary endpoint, overall response rate (32% vs 25%, p = 0.10), docetaxel prolonged median time to progression (24.6 weeks vs 15.6 weeks; p < 0.01) and median survival (15.3 months vs 12.7 months; p = 0.03).

More grade 3/4 adverse events were observed for docetaxel monotherapy (55.4%) compared to paclitaxel (23.0%).

TAXOTERE in combination with doxorubicin

One large randomized phase III study, involving 429 previously untreated patients with metastatic disease, has been performed with doxorubicin (50 mg/m²) in combination with docetaxel (75 mg/m²) (AT arm) versus doxorubicin (60 mg/m²) in combination with cyclophosphamide (600 mg/m²) (AC arm). Both regimens were administered on day 1 every 3 weeks.

- Time to progression (TTP) was significantly longer in the AT arm versus AC arm, p = 0.0138. The median TTP was 37.3 weeks (95% CI: 33.4 - 42.1) in AT arm and 31.9 weeks (95% CI: 27.4 - 36.0) in AC arm.
- Overall response rate (ORR) was significantly higher in the AT arm versus AC arm, p = 0.009. The ORR was 59.3% (95% CI: 52.8 - 65.9) in AT arm versus 46.5% (95% CI: 39.8 - 53.2) in AC arm.

In this trial, AT arm showed a higher incidence of severe neutropenia (90% versus 68.6%), febrile neutropenia (33.3% versus 10%), infection (8% versus 2.4%), diarrhea (7.5% versus 1.4%), asthenia (8.5% versus 2.4%), and pain (2.8% versus 0%) than AC arm. On the other hand, AC arm showed a higher incidence of severe anemia (15.8% versus 8.5%) than AT arm, and, in addition, a higher incidence of severe cardiac toxicity: congestive heart failure (3.8% versus 2.8%), absolute LVEF decrease $\geq$ 20% (13.1% versus 6.1%), absolute LVEF decrease ³ 30% (6.2% versus 1.1%). Toxic deaths occurred in 1 patient in the AT arm (congestive heart failure) and in 4 patients in the AC arm (1 due to septic shock and 3 due to congestive heart failure).

In both arms, quality of life measured by the EORTC questionnaire was comparable and stable during treatment and follow-up.

TAXOTERE in combination with trastuzumab

Docetaxel in combination with trastuzumab was studied for the treatment of patients with metastatic breast cancer whose tumors overexpress HER2, and who previously had not received chemotherapy for metastatic disease. One hundred eighty six patients were randomized to receive docetaxel (100 mg/m²) with or without trastuzumab; 60% of patients received prior anthracycline-based adjuvant chemotherapy. Docetaxel plus trastuzumab was efficacious in patients whether or not they had received prior adjuvant anthracyclines. The main test method used to determine HER2 positivity in this pivotal trial was immunohistochemistry (IHC). A minority of patients were tested using fluorescence in-situ hybridization (FISH). In this trial, 87% of patients had disease that was IHC 3+, and 95% of patients entered had disease that was IHC 3+ and/or FISH positive. Efficacy results are summarized in the following table:

Parameter	Docetaxel plus trastuzumab[1] n = 92	Docetaxel[1] n = 94
Response rate (95% CI)	61% (50-71)	34% (25-45)
Median Duration of response (months) (95% CI)	11.4 (9.2-15.0)	5.1 (4.4-6.2)
Median TTP (months) (95% CI)	10.6 (7.6-12.9)	5.7 (5.0-6.5)
Median Survival (months) (95% CI)	30.5[2] (26.8-ne)	22.1[2] (17.6-28.9)

TTP = time to progression; "ne" indicates that it could not be estimated or it was not yet reached.

[1] Full analysis set (intent-to-treat)

[2] Estimated median survival

TAXOTERE in combination with capecitabine

Data from one multicenter, randomised, controlled phase III clinical trial support the use of docetaxel in combination with capecitabine for treatment of patients with locally advanced or metastatic breast cancer after failure of cytotoxic chemotherapy, including an anthracycline. In this trial, 255 patients were randomised to treatment with docetaxel (75 mg/m² as a 1 hour intravenous infusion every 3 weeks) and capecitabine (1250 mg/m² twice daily for 2 weeks followed by 1-week rest period). 256 patients were randomised to treatment with docetaxel alone (100 mg/m² as a 1 hour intravenous infusion every 3 weeks). Survival was superior in the docetaxel + capecitabine combination arm (p = 0.0126). Median survival was 442 days (docetaxel + capecitabine) vs. 352 days (docetaxel alone). The overall objective response rates in the all-randomised population (investigator assessment) were 41.6% (docetaxel + capecitabine) vs. 29.7% (docetaxel alone); p = 0.0058. Time to progressive disease was superior in the docetaxel + capecitabine combination arm (p < 0.0001). The median time to progression was 186 days (docetaxel + capecitabine) vs. 128 days (docetaxel alone).

<u>Non-small cell lung cancer</u>

Patients previously treated with chemotherapy with or without radiotherapy

In a phase III study, in previously treated patients, time to progression (12.3 weeks versus 7 weeks) and overall survival were significantly longer for docetaxel at 75 mg/m² compared to Best Supportive Care. The 1-year survival rate was also significantly longer in docetaxel (40%) versus BSC (16%).

There was less use of morphinic analgesic (p < 0.01), non-morphinic analgesics (p < 0.01), other disease-related medications (p = 0.06) and radiotherapy (p < 0.01) in patients treated with docetaxel at 75 mg/m² compared to those with BSC.

The overall response rate was 6.8% in the evaluable patients, and the median duration of response was 26.1 weeks.

TAXOTERE in combination with platinum agents in chemotherapy-naïve patients

In a phase III trial, 1218 patients with unresectable stage IIIB or IV NSCLC, with KPS of 70% or greater, and who did not receive previous chemotherapy for this condition, were randomised to either docetaxel (T) 75 mg/m² as a 1 hour infusion immediately followed by cisplatin (Cis) 75 mg/m² over 30-60 minutes every 3 weeks, docetaxel 75 mg/m² as a 1 hour infusion in combination with carboplatin (AUC 6 mg/ml.min) over 30-60 minutes every 3 weeks, or vinorelbine (V) 25 mg/m² administered over 6-10 minutes on days 1, 8, 15, 22 followed by cisplatin 100 mg/m² administered on day 1 of cycles repeated every 4 weeks.

Survival data, median time to progression and response rates for two arms of the study are illustrated in the following table:

(see Table 8 on page 4932353)

Secondary end-points included change of pain, global rating of quality of life by EuroQoL-5D, Lung Cancer Symptom Scale, and changes in Karnosfky performance status. Results on these end-points were supportive of the primary end-points results.

For docetaxel/carboplatin combination, neither equivalent nor non-inferior efficacy could be proven compared to the reference treatment combination VCis.

<u>Prostate cancer</u>

The safety and efficacy of docetaxel in combination with prednisone or prednisolone in patients with hormone refractory metastatic prostate cancer were evaluated in a randomized multicenter phase III trial. A total of 1006 patients with KPS $\geq$ 60 were randomized to the following treatment groups:

- Docetaxel 75 mg/m² every 3 weeks for 10 cycles.

Table 6

MedDRA System Organ classes	Very common adverse reactions ≥ 10% of patients	Common adverse reactions ≥ 1 to < 10% of patients	Uncommon adverse reactions ≥ 0.1 to < 1% of patients
Investigations	Weight decreased		Weight increased
Cardiac disorders		Arrhythmia (G3/4: 2.0%)	Ischemia myocardial
Blood and lymphatic system disorders	Neutropenia (G3/4: 83.5%); Anemia (G3/4: 12.4%); Thrombocytopenia (G3/4: 4.0%); Febrile neutropenia		
Nervous system disorders	Dysgeusia/Parosmia (G3/4: 0.4%); Peripheral sensory neuropathy (G3/4: 1.2%)	Dizziness (G3/4: 2.0%); Peripheral motor neuropathy (G3/4: 0.4%)	
Eye disorders		Lacrimation increased	Conjunctivitis
Ear and labyrinth disorders	Hearing impaired (G3/4: 1.2%)		
Gastrointestinal disorders	Nausea (G3/4: 13.9%); Stomatitis (G3/4: 20.7%); Vomiting (G3/4: 8.4%); Diarrhea (G3/4: 6.8%); Esophagitis/dysphagia/odynophagia (G3/4: 12.0%); Constipation (G3/4: 0.4%)	Dyspepsia (G3/4: 0.8%); Gastrointestinal pain (G3/4: 1.2%); Gastrointestinal haemorrhage (G3/4: 0.4%)	
Skin and subcutaneous tissue disorders	Alopecia (G3/4: 4.0%); Rash pruritic	Dry skin; Desquamation	
Musculoskeletal, connective tissue bone disorders		Myalgia (G3/4: 0.4%)	
Metabolism and nutrition disorders	Anorexia (G3/4: 12.0%)		
Infections and infestations	Infection (G3/4: 3.6%)	Neutropenic infection	
Neoplasms benign, malignant and unspecified (incl cysts and polyps)		Cancer pain (G3/4: 1.2%)	
Vascular disorders			Venous disorder
General disorders and administration site conditions	Lethargy (G3/4: 4.0%); Pyrexia (G3/4: 3.6%); Fluid retention (G3/4: 1.2); Oedema (G3/4: 1.2%)		
Immune system disorders			Hypersensitivity

Table 7

Patient subset	Number of patients	Disease Free Survival			Overall Survival		
		Hazard ratio*	95% CI	p =	Hazard ratio*	95% CI	p =
No of positive nodes							
Overall	745	0.72	0.59-0.88	0.001	0.70	0.53-0.91	0.008
1-3	467	0.61	0.46-0.82	0.0009	0.45	0.29-0.70	0.0002
4+	278	0.83	0.63-1.08	0.17	0.94	0.66-1.33	0.72

*a hazard ratio of less than 1 indicates that TAC is associated with a longer disease-free survival and overall survival compared to FAC

- Docetaxel 30 mg/m^2 administered weekly for the first 5 weeks in a 6 week cycle for 5 cycles.
- Mitoxantrone 12 mg/m^2 every 3 weeks for 10 cycles.

All 3 regimens were administered in combination with prednisone or prednisolone 5 mg twice daily, continuously.

Patients who received docetaxel every three weeks demonstrated significantly longer overall survival compared to those treated with mitoxantrone. The increase in survival seen in the docetaxel weekly arm was not statistically significant compared to the mitoxantrone control arm. Efficacy endpoints for the docetaxel arms versus the control arm are summarized in the following table:

(see Table 9 on next page)

Given the fact that docetaxel every week presented a slightly better safety profile than docetaxel every 3 weeks, it is possible that certain patients may benefit from docetaxel every week.

No statistical differences were observed between treatment groups for Global Quality of Life.

Gastric adenocarcinoma

A multicenter, open-label, randomized trial, was conducted to evaluate the safety and efficacy of docetaxel for the treatment of patients with metastatic gastric adenocarcinoma, including adenocarcinoma of the gastroesophageal junction, who had not received prior chemotherapy for metastatic disease. A total of 445 patients with KPS > 70 were treated with either docetaxel (T) (75 mg/m^2 on day 1) in combination with cisplatin (C) (75 mg/m^2 on day 1) and 5-fluorouracil (F) (750 mg/m^2 per day for 5 days) or cisplatin (100 mg/m^2 on day 1) and 5-fluorouracil (1000 mg/m^2 per day for 5 days). The length of a treatment cycle was 3 weeks for the TCF arm and 4 weeks for the CF arm. The median number of cycles administered per patient was 6 (with a range of 1-16) for the TCF arm compared to 4 (with a range of 1-12) for the CF arm. Time to progression (TTP) was the primary endpoint. The risk reduction of progression was 32.1% and was associated with a significantly longer TTP (p = 0.0004) in favor of the TCF arm. Overall survival was also significantly longer (p = 0.0201) in favor of the TCF arm with a risk reduction of mortality of 22.7%. Efficacy results are summarized in the following table:

<u>Efficacy of docetaxel in the treatment of patients with gastric adenocarcinoma</u>

Endpoint	TCF n = 221	CF n = 224
Median TTP (months)	5.6	3.7
(95% CI)	(4.86-5.91)	(3.45-4.47)
Hazard ratio	1.473	
(95% CI)	(1.189-1.825)	
*p-value	0.0004	
Median survival (months)	9.2	8.6
(95% CI)	(8.38-10.58)	(7.16-9.46)
2-year estimate (%)	18.4	8.8
Hazard ratio	1.293	
(95% CI)	(1.041-1.606)	
*p-value	0.0201	
Overall Response Rate (CR+PR) (%)	36.7	25.4
p-value	0.0106	
Progressive Disease as Best Overall Response (%)	16.7	25.9

*Unstratified logrank test

Subgroup analyses across age, gender and race consistently favored the TCF arm compared to the CF arm.

A survival update analysis conducted with a median follow-up time of 41.6 months no longer showed a statistically significant difference although always in favour of the TCF regimen and showed that the benefit of TCF over CF is clearly observed between 18 and 30 months of follow up.

Overall, quality of life (QoL) and clinical benefit results consistently indicated improvement in favor of the TCF arm. Patients treated with TCF had a longer time to 5% definitive deterioration of global health status on the QLQ-C30 questionnaire (p = 0.0121) and a longer time to definitive worsening of Karnofsky performance status (p = 0.0088) compared to patients treated with CF.

Head and neck cancer

- Induction chemotherapy followed by radiotherapy (TAX323)

The safety and efficacy of docetaxel in the induction treatment of patients with squamous cell carcinoma of the head and neck (SCCHN) was evaluated in a phase III, multicenter, open-label, randomized trial (TAX323). In this study, 358 patients with inoperable locally advanced SCCHN, and WHO perfomance status 0 or 1, were randomized to one of two treatment arms. Patients on the docetaxel arm received docetaxel (T) 75 mg/m^2 followed by cisplatin (P) 75 mg/m^2 followed by 5-fluorouracil (F) 750 mg/m^2 per day as a continuous infusion for 5 days. This regimen was administered every three weeks for 4 cycles in case at least a minor response (≥ 25% reduction in bidimensionally measured tumour size) was observed after 2 cycles. At the end of chemotherapy, with a minimal interval of 4 weeks and a maximal interval of 7 weeks, patients whose disease did not progress received radiotherapy (RT) according to institutional guidelines for 7 weeks (TPF/RT). Patients on the comparator arm received cisplatin (P) 100 mg/m^2 followed by 5-fluorouracil (F) 1000 mg/m^2 per day for 5 days. This regimen was administered every three weeks for 4 cycles in case at least a minor response (≥ 25% reduction in bidimensionally measured tumour size) was observed after 2 cycles. At the end of chemotherapy, with a minimal interval of 4 weeks and a maximal interval of 7 weeks, patients whose disease did not progress received radiotherapy (RT) according to institutional guidelines for 7 weeks (PF/RT). Locoregional therapy with radiation was delivered either with a conventional fraction (1.8 Gy - 2.0 Gy once a day, 5 days per week for a total dose of 66 to 70 Gy), or accelerated/hyperfractionated regimens of radiation therapy (twice a day, with a minimum interfraction interval of 6 hours, 5 days per week). A total of 70 Gy was recommended for accelerated regimens and 74 Gy for hyperfractionated schemes. Surgical resection was allowed following chemotherapy, before or after radiotherapy. Patients on the TPF arm received antibiotic prophylaxis with ciprofloxacin 500 mg orally twice daily for 10 days starting on day 5 of each cycle, or equivalent. The primary endpoint in this study, progression-free survival (PFS), was significantly longer in the TPF arm compared to the PF arm, p = 0.0042 (median PFS: 11.4 vs. 8.3 months respectively) with an overall median follow up time of 33.7 months. Median overall survival was also significantly longer in favor of the TPF arm compared to the PF arm (median OS: 18.6 vs. 14.5 months respectively) with a 28% risk reduction of mortality, p = 0.0128. Efficacy results are presented in the table below:

<u>Efficacy of docetaxel in the induction treatment of patients with inoperable locally advanced SCCHN (Intent-to-Treat Analysis)</u>

Endpoint	Docetaxel + Cis + 5-FU n = 177	Cis + 5-FU n = 181
Median progression free survival (months) (95% CI)	11.4 (10.1-14.0)	8.3 (7.4-9.1)
Adjusted Hazard ratio (95% CI) *p-value	0.70 (0.55-0.89) 0.0042	
Median survival (months) (95% CI)	18.6 (15.7-24.0)	14.5 (11.6-18.7)
Hazard ratio (95% CI) **p-value	0.72 (0.56-0.93) 0.0128	

Best overall response to chemotherapy (%) (95% CI)	67.8 (60.4-74.6)	53.6 (46.0-61.0)
***p-value	0.006	
Best overall response to study treatment [chemotherapy +/- radiotherapy] (%) (95% CI)	72.3 (65.1-78.8)	58.6 (51.0-65.8)
***p-value	0.006	
Median duration of response to chemotherapy ± radiotherapy (months) (95% CI)	n = 128 15.7 (13.4-24.6)	n = 106 11.7 (10.2-17.4)
Hazard ratio (95% CI) **p-value	0.72 (0.52-0.99) 0.0457	

A Hazard ratio of less than 1 favors docetaxel + cisplatin + 5-FU

*Cox model (adjustment for Primary tumor site, T and N clinical stages and PSWHO)

**Logrank test

*** Chi-square test

Quality of life parameters

Patients treated with TPF experienced significantly less deterioration of their Global health score compared to those treated with PF (p = 0.01, using the EORTC QLQ-C30 scale).

Clinical benefit parameters

The performance status scale, for head and neck (PSS-HN) subscales designed to measure understandability of speech, ability to eat in public, and normalcy of diet, was significantly in favor of TPF as compared to PF.

Median time to first deterioration of WHO performance status was significantly longer in the TPF arm compared to PF. Pain intensity score improved during treatment in both groups indicating adequate pain management.

• Induction chemotherapy followed by chemoradiotherapy (TAX324)

The safety and efficacy of docetaxel in the induction treatment of patients with locally advanced squamous cell carcinoma of the head and neck (SCCHN) was evaluated in a randomized, multicenter open-label, phase III, trial (TAX324). In this study, 501 patients, with locally advanced SCCHN, and a WHO performance status of 0 or 1, were randomized to one of two arms. The study population comprised patients with technically unresectable disease, patients with low probability of surgical cure and patients aiming at organ preservation. The efficacy and safety evaluation solely addressed survival endpoints and the success of organ preservation was not formally addressed. Patients on the docetaxel arm received docetaxel (T) 75 mg/m^2 by intravenous infusion on day 1 followed by cisplatin (P) 100 mg/m^2 administered as a 30-minute to three-hour intravenous infusion, followed by the continuous intravenous infusion of 5-fluorouracil (F) 1000 mg/m^2/day from day 1 to day 4. The cycles were repeated every 3 weeks for 3 cycles. All patients who did not have progressive disease were to receive chemoradiotherapy (CRT) as per protocol (TPF/CRT). Patients on the comparator arm received cisplatin (P) 100 mg/m^2 as a 30-minute to three-hour intravenous infusion on day 1 followed by the continuous intravenous infusion of 5-fluorouracil (F) 1000 mg/m^2/day from day 1 to day 5. The cycles were repeated every 3 weeks for 3 cycles. All patients who did not have progressive disease were to receive CRT as per protocol (PF/CRT).

Patients in both treatment arms were to receive 7 weeks of CRT following induction chemotherapy with a minimum interval of 3 weeks and no later than 8 weeks after start of the last cycle (day 22 to day 56 of last cycle). During radiotherapy, carboplatin (AUC 1.5) was given weekly as a one-hour intravenous infusion for a maximum of 7 doses. Radiation was delivered with megavoltage equipment using once daily fractionation (2 Gy per day, 5 days per week for 7 weeks, for a total dose of 70-72 Gy). Surgery on the primary site of disease and/or neck could be considered at anytime following completion of CRT. All patients on the docetaxel-containing arm of the study received prophylactic antibiotics. The primary efficacy endpoint in this study, overall survival (OS) was significantly longer (log-rank test, p = 0.0058) with the docetaxel-containing regimen compared to PF (median OS: 70.6 versus 30.1 months respectively), with a 30% risk reduction in mortality compared to PF (hazard ratio (HR) = 0.70, 95% confidence interval (CI) = 0.54-0.90) with an overall median follow up time of 41.9 months. The secondary endpoint, PFS, demonstrated a 29% risk reduction of progression or death and a 22 month improvement in median PFS (35.5 months for TPF and 13.1 for PF). This was also statistically significant with an HR of 0.71; 95% CI 0.56-0.90; log-rank test p = 0.004. Efficacy results are presented in the table below:

Efficacy of docetaxel in the induction treatment of patients with locally advanced SCCHN (Intent-to-Treat Analysis)

Endpoint	**Docetaxel + Cis + 5-FU n = 255**	**Cis + 5-FU n = 246**
Median overall survival (months) (95% CI)	70.6 (49.0-NA)	30.1 (20.9-51.5)
Hazard ratio: (95% CI) *p-value	0.70 (0.54-0.90) 0.0058	
Median PFS (months) (95% CI)	35.5 (19.3-NA)	13.1 (10.6 - 20.2)
Hazard ratio: (95% CI) **p-value	0.71 (0.56 - 0.90) 0.004	
Best overall response (CR + PR) to chemotherapy (%) (95% CI)	71.8 (65.8-77.2)	64.2 (57.9-70.2)
***p-value	0.070	
Best overall response (CR + PR) to study treatment [chemotherapy +/- chemoradiotherapy] (%) (95%CI)	76.5 (70.8-81.5)	71.5 (65.5-77.1)
***p-value	0.209	

A Hazard ratio of less than 1 favors docetaxel + cisplatin + fluorouracil

*un-adjusted log-rank test

**un-adjusted log-rank test, not adjusted for multiple comparisons

***Chi square test, not adjusted for multiple comparisons

NA-not applicable

Table 8

	TCis n = 408	VCis n = 404	Statistical Analysis
Overall Survival (Primary end-point):			
Median Survival (months)	11.3	10.1	Hazard Ratio: 1.122 [97.2% CI: 0.937; 1.342]*
1-year Survival (%)	46	41	Treatment difference: 5.4% [95% CI: -1.1; 12.0]
2-year Survival (%)	21	14	Treatment difference: 6.2% [95% CI: 0.2; 12.3]
Median Time to Progression (weeks):	22.0	23.0	Hazard Ratio: 1.032 [95% CI: 0.876; 1.216]
Overall Response Rate (%):	31.6	24.5	Treatment difference: 7.1% [95% CI: 0.7; 13.5]

*: Corrected for multiple comparisons and adjusted for stratification factors (stage of disease and region of treatment), based on evaluable patient population.

Table 9

Endpoint	Docetaxel every 3 weeks	Docetaxel every week	Mitoxantrone every 3 weeks
Number of patients Median survival (months) 95% CI Hazard ratio 95% CI p-value†*	335 18.9 (17.0-21.2) 0.761 (0.619-0.936) 0.0094	334 17.4 (15.7-19.0) 0.912 (0.747-1.113) 0.3624	337 16.5 (14.4-18.6) – – –
Number of patients PSA** response rate (%) 95% CI p-value*	291 45.4 (39.5-51.3) 0.0005	282 47.9 (41.9-53.9) <0.0001	300 31.7 (26.4-37.3) –
Number of patients Pain response rate (%) 95% CI p-value*	153 34.6 (27.1-42.7) 0.0107	154 31.2 (24.0-39.1) 0.0798	157 21.7 (15.5-28.9) –
Number of patients Tumor response rate (%) 95% CI p-value*	141 12.1 (7.2-18.6) 0.1112	134 8.2 (4.2-14.2) 0.5853	137 6.6 (3.0-12.1) –

†Stratified log rank test

*Threshold for statistical significance = 0.0175

**PSA: Prostate-Specific Antigen

5.2 Pharmacokinetic properties

The pharmacokinetics of docetaxel have been evaluated in cancer patients after administration of 20-115 mg/m^2 in phase I studies. The kinetic profile of docetaxel is dose independent and consistent with a three-compartment pharmacokinetic model with half lives for the α, β and γ phases of 4 min, 36 min and 11.1 h, respectively. The late phase is due, in part, to a relatively slow efflux of docetaxel from the peripheral compartment. Following the administration of a 100 mg/m^2 dose given as a one-hour infusion a mean peak plasma level of 3.7 μg/ml was obtained with a corresponding AUC of 4.6 h.μg/ml. Mean values for total body clearance and steady-state volume of distribution were 21 l/h/m^2 and 113 l, respectively. Inter individual variation in total body clearance was approximately 50%. Docetaxel is more than 95% bound to plasma proteins.

A study of ^{14}C-docetaxel has been conducted in three cancer patients. Docetaxel was eliminated in both the urine and faeces following cytochrome P450-mediated oxidative metabolism of the tert-butyl ester group, within seven days, the urinary and faecal excretion accounted for about 6% and 75% of the administered radioactivity, respectively. About 80% of the radioactivity recovered in faeces is excreted during the first 48 hours as one major inactive metabolite and 3 minor inactive metabolites and very low amounts of unchanged medicinal product.

A population pharmacokinetic analysis has been performed with docetaxel in 577 patients. Pharmacokinetic parameters estimated by the model were very close to those estimated from phase I studies. The pharmacokinetics of docetaxel were not altered by the age or sex of the patient. In a small number of patients (n = 23) with clinical chemistry data suggestive of mild to moderate liver function impairment (ALT, AST ⩾ 1.5 times the ULN associated with alkaline phosphatase ⩾ 2.5 times the ULN), total clearance was lowered by 27% on average (see section 4.2). Docetaxel clearance was not modified in patients with mild to moderate fluid retention and there are no data available in patients with severe fluid retention.

When used in combination, docetaxel does not influence the clearance of doxorubicin and the plasma levels of doxorubicinol (a doxorubicin metabolite). The pharmacokinetics of docetaxel, doxorubicin and cyclophosphamide were not influenced by their coadministration.

Phase I study evaluating the effect of capecitabine on the pharmacokinetics of docetaxel and vice versa showed no effect by capecitabine on the pharmacokinetics of docetaxel (Cmax and AUC) and no effect by docetaxel on the pharmacokinetics of a relevant capecitabine metabolite 5'-DFUR.

Clearance of docetaxel in combination therapy with cisplatin was similar to that observed following monotherapy. The pharmacokinetic profile of cisplatin administered shortly after docetaxel infusion is similar to that observed with cisplatin alone.

The combined administration of docetaxel, cisplatin and 5-fluorouracil in 12 patients with solid tumors had no influence on the pharmacokinetics of each individual medicinal product.

The effect of prednisone on the pharmacokinetics of docetaxel administered with standard dexamethasone premedication has been studied in 42 patients. No effect of prednisone on the pharmacokinetics of docetaxel was observed.

5.3 Preclinical safety data

The carcinogenic potential of docetaxel has not been studied.

Docetaxel has been shown to be mutagenic in the *in vitro* micronucleus and chromosome aberration test in CHO-K1 cells and in the *in vivo* micronucleus test in the mouse. However, it did not induce mutagenicity in the Ames test or the CHO/HGPRT gene mutation assay. These results are consistent with the pharmacological activity of docetaxel.

Undesirable effects on the testis observed in rodent toxicity studies suggest that docetaxel may impair male fertility.

6. PHARMACEUTICAL PARTICULARS

6.1 List of excipients

Concentrate vial:

polysorbate 80.

Solvent vial:

ethanol 95%

water for injections.

6.2 Incompatibilities

This medicinal product must not be mixed with other medicinal products except those mentioned in section 6.6.

6.3 Shelf life

TAXOTERE 20mg vials: 24 months

TAXOTERE 80mg vials: 36 months

• Premix solution: The premix solution contains 10 mg/ml docetaxel and should be used immediately after preparation. However the chemical and physical stability of the premix solution has been demonstrated for 8 hours when stored either between 2°C and 8°C or at room temperature (below 25°C).

• Infusion solution: the infusion solution should be used within 4 hours at room temperature (below 25°C).

6.4 Special precautions for storage

Do not store above 25°C or below 2°C.

Store in the original package in order to protect from light.

For storage conditions of the diluted medicinal product, see section 6.3.

6.5 Nature and contents of container

Each blister pack contains:

• one single-dose vial of concentrate and,

• one single-dose vial of solvent.

<u>TAXOTERE 20 mg concentrate for solution for infusion vial</u>

7 ml clear glass Type I vial with a green flip-off cap.

This vial contains 0.5 ml of a 40 mg/ml solution of docetaxel in polysorbate 80 (fill volume: 24.4 mg/0.61 ml). This fill volume has been established during the development of TAXOTERE to compensate for liquid loss during preparation of the premix due to foaming, adhesion to the walls of the vial and "dead-volume". This overfill ensures that after dilution with the entire contents of the accompanying solvent for TAXOTERE vial, there is a minimal extractable premix volume of 2 ml containing 10 mg/ml docetaxel which corresponds to the labelled amount of 20 mg per vial.

<u>Solvent vial</u>

7 ml clear glass Type I vial with a transparent colourless flip-off cap.

Solvent vial contains 1.5 ml of a 13% w/w solution of ethanol 95% in water for injections (fill volume: 1.98 ml). The addition of the entire contents of the solvent vial to the contents of the TAXOTERE 20 mg concentrate for solution for infusion vial ensures a premix concentration of 10 mg/ml docetaxel.

<u>TAXOTERE 80 mg concentrate for solution for infusion vial</u>

15 ml clear glass Type I vial with a red flip-off cap.

This vial contains 2 ml of a 40 mg/ml solution of docetaxel in polysorbate 80 (fill volume: 94.4 mg/2.36 ml). This fill volume has been established during the development of TAXOTERE to compensate for liquid loss during preparation of the premix due to foaming, adhesion to the walls of the vial and "dead-volume". This overfill ensures that after dilution with the entire contents of the accompanying solvent for TAXOTERE vial, there is a minimal extractable premix volume of 8 ml containing 10 mg/ml docetaxel which corresponds to the labelled amount of 80 mg per vial.

<u>Solvent vial</u>

15 ml clear glass Type I vial with a transparent colourless flip-off cap.

Solvent vial contains 6 ml of a 13% w/w solution of ethanol 95% in water for injections (fill volume: 7.33 ml). The addition of the entire contents of the solvent vial to the contents of the TAXOTERE 80 mg concentrate for solution for infusion vial ensures a premix concentration of 10 mg/ml docetaxel.

6.6 Special precautions for disposal and other handling

TAXOTERE is an antineoplastic agent and, as with other potentially toxic compounds, caution should be exercised when handling it and preparing TAXOTERE solutions. The use of gloves is recommended.

If TAXOTERE concentrate, premix solution or infusion solution should come into contact with skin, wash immediately and thoroughly with soap and water. If TAXOTERE concentrate, premix solution or infusion solution should come into contact with mucous membranes, wash immediately and thoroughly with water.

<u>Preparation for the intravenous administration</u>

<u>*a) Preparation of the TAXOTERE premix solution (10 mg docetaxel/ml)*</u>

If the vials are stored under refrigeration, allow the required number of TAXOTERE boxes to stand at room temperature (below 25 °C) for 5 minutes.

Using a syringe fitted with a needle, aseptically withdraw the entire contents of the solvent for TAXOTERE vial by partially inverting the vial.

Inject the entire contents of the syringe into the corresponding TAXOTERE vial.

Remove the syringe and needle and mix manually by repeated inversions for at least 45 seconds. Do not shake.

Allow the premix vial to stand for 5 minutes at room temperature (below 25 °C) and then check that the solution is homogenous and clear (foaming is normal even after 5 minutes due to the presence of polysorbate 80 in the formulation).

The premix solution contains 10 mg/ml docetaxel and should be used immediately after preparation. However the chemical and physical stability of the premix solution has been demonstrated for 8 hours when stored either between 2°C and 8°C or at room temperature (below 25°C).

<u>*b) Preparation of the infusion solution*</u>

More than one premix vial may be necessary to obtain the required dose for the patient. Based on the required dose for the patient expressed in mg, aseptically withdraw the corresponding premix volume containing 10 mg/ml docetaxel from the appropriate number of premix vials using graduated syringes fitted with a needle. For example, a dose of 140 mg docetaxel would require 14 ml docetaxel premix solution.

Inject the required premix volume into a 250 ml infusion bag or bottle containing either 5% glucose solution or 0.9% sodium chloride solution.

If a dose greater than 200 mg of docetaxel is required, use a larger volume of the infusion vehicle so that a concentration of 0.74 mg/ml docetaxel is not exceeded.

Mix the infusion bag or bottle manually using a rocking motion.

The TAXOTERE infusion solution should be used within 4 hours and should be aseptically administered as a 1-hour infusion under room temperature (below 25 °C) and normal lighting conditions.

As with all parenteral products, TAXOTERE premix solution and infusion solution should be visually inspected prior to use, solutions containing a precipitate should be discarded.

Any unused product or waste material should be disposed of in accordance with local requirements.

7. MARKETING AUTHORISATION HOLDER

Aventis Pharma S.A., 20 avenue Raymond Aron, 92165 Antony Cedex, France

8. MARKETING AUTHORISATION NUMBER(S)

TAXOTERE 80 mg concentrate and solvent for solution for infusion: EU/1/95/002/001

TAXOTERE 80 mg concentrate and solvent for solution for infusion: EU/1/95/002/002

9. DATE OF FIRST AUTHORISATION/RENEWAL OF THE AUTHORISATION

Date of first authorisation: 27 November 1995

Date of latest renewal: 27 November 2005

10. DATE OF REVISION OF THE TEXT

December 2008

Legal Category:
POM

Tazocin 2g/0.25g and 4g/0.5g Powder for Solution for Injection or Infusion

(Wyeth Pharmaceuticals)

1. NAME OF THE MEDICINAL PRODUCT

TAZOCIN 2g/0.25g Powder for Solution for Injection or Infusion

TAZOCIN 4g/0.5g Powder for Solution for Injection or Infusion

2. QUALITATIVE AND QUANTITATIVE COMPOSITION

Piperacillin sodium/tazobactam sodium (INN)

TAZOCIN 2g/0.25g contains 2 active ingredients; piperacillin 2g and tazobactam 250mg both present as sodium salts.

This medicinal product contains 128mg of sodium per vial.

The product also contains 0.5 mg of disodium edetate (dihydrate) (EDTA) per vial.

TAZOCIN 4g/0.5g contains 2 active ingredients; piperacillin 4g and tazobactam 500mg both present as sodium salts.

This medicinal product contains 256 mg of sodium per vial.

The product also contains 1 mg of disodium edetate (dihydrate) (EDTA) per vial.

Each vial of piperacillin / tazobactam reformulation contains a total of 2.79 mmol (64mg) of sodium per gram of piperacillin.

For a full list of excipients, see section 6.1.

3. PHARMACEUTICAL FORM

TAZOCIN, an injectable antibacterial combination for intravenous administration is available as a white to off-white sterile, lyophilised powder for solution for injection or infusion packaged in glass vials.

4. CLINICAL PARTICULARS

4.1 Therapeutic indications

TAZOCIN is indicated for treatment of the following systemic and/or local bacterial infections in which susceptible organisms have been detected or are suspected:

Adults and the Elderly

Lower respiratory tract infections

Urinary tract infections (complicated and uncomplicated)

Intra-abdominal infections

Skin and skin structure infections

Bacterial septicaemia

Bacterial infections in neutropenic adults in combination with an aminoglycoside

Children

Appendicitis complicated by rupture with peritonitis and/or abscess formation in children aged 2-12 years.

Bacterial infections in neutropenic children in combination with an aminoglycoside.

TAZOCIN is indicated for the treatment of polymicrobic infections including those where gram-positive and gram-negative aerobic and/or anaerobic organisms are suspected (intra-abdominal, skin and skin structure, lower respiratory tract) see Section 5.1. As such, TAZOCIN is particularly useful in the treatment of polymicrobial infections and in presumptive therapy prior to the availability of the results of sensitivity tests because of its broad spectrum of activity.

4.2 Posology and method of administration

TAZOCIN may be given by slow intravenous injection (over at least 3-5 minutes) or by slow intravenous infusion (over 20-30 minutes).

Neutropenic patients with signs of infection (e.g. fever) should receive immediate empirical antibiotic therapy before laboratory results are available.

<u>Adults and Children Over 12 Years, Each with Normal Renal Function</u>

The usual dosage for adults and children over 12 years is 4.5g TAZOCIN (4g piperacillin / 0.5g tazobactam) given every 8 hours.

The total daily dose of TAZOCIN depends on the severity and localisation of the infection and can vary from 2g/0.25g (2g piperacillin / 0.25g tazobactam) to 4.5g (4g piperacillin / 0.5g tazobactam) administered every 6 or 8 hours.

In neutropenia the recommended dose is 4.5g TAZOCIN (4g piperacillin / 0.5g tazobactam) given every 6 hours in combination with an aminoglycoside.

<u>Elderly with Normal Renal Function</u>

TAZOCIN may be used at the same dose levels as adults except in cases of renal impairment (see below):

<u>Renal Insufficiency in Adults, the Elderly and Children Receiving the Adult Dose</u>

In patients with renal insufficiency, the intravenous dose should be adjusted to the degree of actual renal impairment. The suggested daily doses are as follows:

Creatinine Clearance (ml/min)	Recommended Piperacillin/Tazobactam Dosage
20 - 80	12g/1.5g/day Divided Doses 4g/0.5g q 8H
< 20	8g/1g/day Divided Doses 4g/0.5g q 12H

For patients on haemodialysis, the maximum daily dose is 8g/1g piperacillin/tazobactam. In addition, because haemodialysis removes 30%-50% of piperacillin in 4 hours, one additional dose of 2g/0.25g piperacillin/tazobactam should be administered following each dialysis period. For patients with renal failure and hepatic insufficiency, measurement of serum levels of TAZOCIN will provide additional guidance for adjusting dosage.

Children Aged 12 Years and Under with Normal Renal Function

TAZOCIN is only recommended for the treatment of children with neutropenia or complicated appendicitis.

Neutropenia

For children the dose should be adjusted to 90mg/kg (80mg piperacillin / 10mg tazobactam) administered every 6 hours, in combination with an aminoglycoside, not exceeding 4.5g (4g piperacillin / 0.5g tazobactam) every 6 hours.

Complicated Appendicitis.

For children aged 2 - 12 years the dose should be adjusted to 112.5mg/kg (100mg piperacillin / 12.5mg tazobactam) administered every 8 hours, not exceeding 4.5g (4g piperacillin / 0.5g tazobactam) every 8 hours.

Until further experience is available, TAZOCIN should not be used in children who do not have neutropenia or complicated appendicitis.

Renal Insufficiency in Children Aged 12 Years and Under

In children with renal insufficiency the intravenous dosage should be adjusted to the degree of actual renal impairment as follows:

Creatinine Clearance (ml/min)	Recommended Piperacillin / Tazobactam Dosage
⩾ 40	No adjustment
20-39	90mg (80mg piperacillin / 10mg tazobactam) /kg q 8H, not exceeding 13.5g/day
< 20	90mg (80mg piperacillin / 10mg tazobactam) /kg q 12H, not exceeding 9g/day

For children weighing < 50kg on haemodialysis the recommended dose is 45mg (40mg piperacillin /5mg tazobactam) /kg every 8 hours.

The above dosage modifications are only an approximation. Each patient must be monitored closely for signs of drug toxicity. Drug dose and interval should be adjusted accordingly.

Hepatic Impairment

No dose adjustment is necessary.

Duration of Therapy

The duration of therapy should be guided by the severity of the infection and the patient's clinical and bacteriological progress.

In acute infections, treatment with TAZOCIN should be continued for 48 hours beyond the resolution of clinical symptoms or the fever.

In paediatric complicated appendicitis treatment is recommended for a minimum of 5 days and a maximum of 14 days.

4.3 Contraindications

Hypersensitivity to any of the beta-lactams (including penicillins and cephalosporins) or to beta-lactamase inhibitors.

4.4 Special warnings and precautions for use

Warnings

Serious and occasionally fatal hypersensitivity (anaphylactic / anaphylactoid [including shock]) reactions have been reported in patients receiving therapy with penicillins including TAZOCIN. These reactions are more likely to occur in persons with a history of sensitivity to multiple allergens.

There have been reports of patients with a history of penicillin hypersensitivity who have experienced severe reactions when treated with a cephalosporin.

If an allergic reaction occurs during therapy with TAZOCIN, the antibiotic should be discontinued. Serious hypersensitivity reactions may require adrenaline and other emergency measures.

Before initiating therapy with TAZOCIN, careful inquiry should be made concerning previous hypersensitivity reactions to penicillins, cephalosporins, and other allergens.

In case of severe, persistent diarrhoea, the possibility of antibiotic-induced, life threatening pseudomembranous colitis must be taken into consideration. The onset of pseudomembranous colitis symptoms may occur during or after antibacterial treatment. Therefore, Tazocin must be discontinued immediately in such cases, and suitable therapy be initiated (e.g. oral metronidazole or oral vancomycin). Preparations which inhibit peristalsis are contraindicated.

Precautions

Leukopenia and neutropenia may occur, especially during prolonged therapy. Therefore, periodic assessment of hematopoietic function should be performed.

Table 1

PROPOSED MINIMUM INHIBITORY CONCENTRATION (MIC) BREAKPOINTS			
Pathogens	Susceptible	Intermediate	Resistant
Enterobacteriaceae	⩽ 16 mg/L	32 - 64 mg/L	⩾ 128 mg/L
Pseudomonas	⩽ 64 mg/L	-	⩾ 128 mg/L
Staphylococcus	⩽ 8 mg/L	-	⩾ 16 mg/L
Streptococcus	⩽ 1 mg/L	-	⩾ 2 mg/L
Anaerobes	⩽ 32 mg/L	64 mg/L	⩾ 128 mg/L

As with treatment with other penicillins, neurological complications in the form of convulsions may occur when high doses are administered, especially in patients with impaired renal function.

Periodic assessment of organ system functions including renal and hepatic during prolonged therapy is advisable.

Bleeding manifestations have occurred in some patients receiving β-lactam antibiotics. These reactions have sometimes been associated with abnormalities of coagulation tests such as clotting time, platelet aggregation and prothrombin time, and are more likely to occur in patients with renal failure. If bleeding manifestations occur, the antibiotic should be discontinued and appropriate therapy instituted.

As with other antibiotics, the possibility of the emergence of resistant organisms which might cause superinfections should be kept in mind, particularly during prolonged treatment. Microbiological follow-up may be required to detect any important superinfection. If this occurs, appropriate measures should be taken.

As with other penicillins, patients may experience neuromuscular excitability or convulsions if higher than recommended doses are given intravenously.

This product contains 2.79 mmol (64 mg) of sodium per gram of piperacillin which may increase a patient's overall sodium intake. This may be harmful to people on a low sodium diet.

Hypokalaemia may occur in patients with low potassium reserves or who are receiving concomitant medications that may lower potassium levels; periodic electrolyte determinations should be performed in such patients. Modest elevation of indices of liver function may be observed.

Antimicrobials used in high doses for short periods to treat gonorrhoea may mask or delay the symptoms of incubating syphilis. Therefore, prior to treatment, patients with gonorrhoea should also be evaluated for syphilis. Specimens for darkfield examination should be obtained from patients with any suspect primary lesion, and serologic tests should be made for a minimum of 4 months.

4.5 Interaction with other medicinal products and other forms of interaction

Concurrent administration of probenecid and piperacillin/tazobactam produced a longer half-life and lower renal clearance for both piperacillin and tazobactam. However, peak plasma concentrations of either drug are unaffected.

Piperacillin either alone or with tazobactam did not cause clinically important alterations to the pharmacokinetics of tobramycin in subjects with normal renal function and with mild or moderate renal impairment. The pharmacokinetics of piperacillin, tazobactam, and the M1 metabolite were not significantly altered by tobramycin administration. No clinically important pharmacokinetic interactions have been noted between TAZOCIN and vancomycin in healthy adults with normal renal function.

Due to the in vitro physical incompatibility of the aminoglycoside with beta-lactam antibiotics, reformulated TAZOCIN and the aminoglycoside should not be mixed and are recommended for separate administration. Reformulated TAZOCIN and the aminoglycoside should be reconstituted and diluted separately when concomitant therapy with aminoglycosides is indicated.

In circumstances where co-administration is thought essential, the reformulated TAZOCIN containing EDTA in vials has been shown to be compatible for simultaneous co-administration via **Y-site infusion only** with the aminoglycosides; amikacin and gentamicin under certain conditions:

Please see section 6.6 for instructions on dilution and administration.

Hartmann's solution is compatible with reformulated TAZOCIN containing EDTA (see section 6.6).

During simultaneous administration of heparin, oral anticoagulants and other drugs which may affect the blood coagulation system including thrombocyte function, appropriate coagulation tests should be performed more frequently and monitored regularly.

Piperacillin when used concomitantly with vecuronium has been implicated in the prolongation of the neuromuscular blockade of vecuronium. Due to their similar mechanism of action, it is expected that the neuromuscular blockade produced by any of the non-polarizing muscle relaxants could be prolonged in the presence of piperacillin.

Piperacillin may reduce the excretion of methotrexate. Serum levels of methotrexate should be monitored in patients on methotrexate therapy.

As with other penicillins, the administration of TAZOCIN may result in a false-positive reaction for glucose in the urine using a copper-reduction method. It is recommended that glucose tests based on enzymatic glucose oxidase reactions be used.

There have been reports of positive test results using the Bio-Rad Laboratories Platelia *Aspergillus* EIA test in patients receiving piperacillin-tazobactam injection who were subsequently found to be free of *Aspergillus* infection. Cross-reactions with non-*Aspergillus* polysaccharides and polyfuranoses with Bio-Rad Laboratories Platelia *Aspergillus* EIA test have been reported. Therefore, positive test results in patients receiving piperacillin-tazobactam should be interpreted cautiously and confirmed by other diagnostic methods.

4.6 Pregnancy and lactation

Studies in mice and rats have not demonstrated any embryotoxic or teratogenic effects of the piperacillin-tazobactam combination Tazocin. There are no adequate and well-controlled studies with piperacillin-tazobactam combination Tazocin or with piperacillin or tazobactam alone in pregnant women. Piperacillin and tazobactam cross the placenta. Pregnant women should be treated only if the expected benefit outweighs the possible risks to the pregnant woman and foetus.

Piperacillin is excreted in low concentrations in human milk; tazobactam concentrations in human milk have not been studied. Women who are breast-feeding should be treated only if the expected benefit outweighs the possible risks to the nursing woman and child.

4.7 Effects on ability to drive and use machines

TAZOCIN is not known to affect ability to drive or operate machines.

4.8 Undesirable effects

The most commonly reported adverse reactions are diarrhoea, nausea, vomiting, and rash, each having a frequency of ⩾ 1% but ⩽ 10%.

Body System	Adverse Reaction
Infections and infestations	
Uncommon:	Candidal superinfection
Blood and lymphatic system disorders	
Uncommon:	Leucopenia, neutropenia, thrombocytopenia
Rare:	Anaemia, bleeding manifestations (including purpura, epistaxis, bleeding time prolonged), eosinophilia, haemolytic anaemia
Very rare:	Agranulocytosis, Coombs direct test positive, pancytopenia, prolonged partial thromboplastin time, prothrombin time prolonged, thrombocytosis
Immune system disorders	
Uncommon:	Hypersensitivity reaction
Rare:	Anaphylactic/anaphylactoid reaction (including shock)
Metabolism and nutritional disorders	
Very rare:	Hypoalbuminaemia, hypoglycaemia, hypoproteinaemia, hypokalaemia
Nervous system disorders	
Uncommon:	Headache, insomnia
Rare:	Muscular weakness, hallucination, convulsion, dry mouth
Vascular disorders	
Uncommon:	Hypotension, phlebitis, thrombophlebitis
Rare:	Flushing
Gastrointestinal disorders	
Common:	Diarrhoea, nausea, vomiting
Uncommon:	Constipation, dyspepsia, jaundice, stomatitis
Rare:	Abdominal pain, pseudomembranous colitis, hepatitis

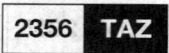

Hepatobiliary disorders

Uncommon:	Alanine aminotransferase increased, aspartate aminotransferase increased
Rare:	Bilirubin increased, blood alkaline phosphatase increased, gamma-glutamyltransferase increased, hepatitis

Skin and subcutaneous tissue disorders

Common:	Rash
Uncommon:	Pruritus, urticaria, erythema
Rare:	Bullous dermatitis, erythema multiforme, increased sweating, eczema, exanthema
Very rare:	Stevens-Johnson Syndrome, toxic epidermal necrolysis

Musculoskeletal, connective tissue and bone disorders

Rare:	Arthralgia, myalgia

Renal and urinary disorders

Uncommon:	Blood creatinine increased
Rare:	Interstitial nephritis, renal failure
Very rare:	Blood urea nitrogen increased

General disorders and administration site conditions

Uncommon:	Fever, injection site reaction
Rare:	Rigors, tiredness, oedema

Piperacillin therapy has been associated with an increased incidence of fever and rash in cystic fibrosis patients.

4.9 Overdose

There have been post-marketing reports of overdose with TAZOCIN. The majority of those events experienced including nausea, vomiting, and diarrhoea have also been reported with the usual recommended dosages. Patients may experience neuromuscular excitability or convulsions if higher than recommended doses are given intravenously (particularly in the presence of renal failure).

Treatment of Intoxication

No specific antidote is known.

Treatment should be supportive and symptomatic according to the patient's clinical presentation. In the event of an emergency, all required intensive medical measures are indicated as in the case of piperacillin.

Excessive serum concentrations of either piperacillin or tazobactam may be reduced by haemodialysis.

In case of motor excitability or convulsions, anticonvulsive agents (e.g. diazepam or barbiturates) may be indicated.

In case of severe, anaphylactic reactions, the usual counter-measures are to be initiated.

5. PHARMACOLOGICAL PROPERTIES

5.1 Pharmacodynamic properties

ATC Code: J01CR05

Pharmacotherapeutic group: Beta-lactam antibacterials, penicillins

Piperacillin, a broad spectrum, semisynthetic penicillin active against many gram-positive and gram-negative aerobic and anaerobic bacteria, exerts bactericidal activity by inhibition of both septum and cell wall synthesis. Tazobactam, a triazolylmethyl penicillanic acid sulphone, is a potent inhibitor of many β-lactamases, in particular the plasmid mediated enzymes which commonly cause resistance to penicillins and cephalosporins including third-generation cephalosporins. The presence of tazobactam in the TAZOCIN formulation enhances and extends the antibiotic spectrum of piperacillin to include many β-lactamase producing bacteria normally resistant to it and other β-lactam antibiotics. Thus, TAZOCIN combines the properties of a broad spectrum antibiotic and a β-lactamase inhibitor.

TAZOCIN is highly active against piperacillin-sensitive micro-organisms as well as many β-lactamase producing, piperacillin-resistant micro-organisms. TAZOCIN also acts synergistically with aminoglycosides against certain strains of *Pseudomonas aeruginosa*.

The prevalence of acquired resistance may vary geographically and with time for selected species. Local information of resistance is desirable, particularly when treating severe infections. Please refer to local guidelines for antibiotic sensitivity testing as appropriate.

The minimum inhibitory concentration (MIC) breakpoints separating susceptible from intermediately susceptible and intermediately susceptible from resistant organisms are suggested as follows:

(see Table 1 on previous page)

Resistance has been mainly observed for *Staphylococcus epidermidis*, *Burkholderia cepacia*, *Citrobacter freundii*, *Enterobacter cloacae*, *Pseudomonas* and *Serratia* species, *Enterococcus avium*, *Enterococcus faecium*, *Propionibacterium acnes*, *Acinetobacter* species, *Enterobacter aerogenes*, *Stenotrophomonas maltophilia*, *Corynebacterium jeikeium*, *Staphylococcus aureus* (methicillin resistant), and *Staphylococcus* coagulase negative (methicillin resistant).

Organism susceptibility to TAZOCIN observed in the European clinical studies conducted in adults or children with various infections published from 1997 to 1999 have been summarised in the following table.

It must be noted that this information gives only an approximate guidance on the probability that a micro-organism will be susceptible to TAZOCIN.

ESTIMATED EUROPEAN RANGE OF MICROBIOLOGIC RESISTANCE TO TAZOCIN (PIPERACILLIN/ TAZOBACTAM)

Susceptibility (classification) ***Pathogen***	**Resistance rate[a]**
Susceptible (Gram-Positive Aerobes)	
*Brevibacterium species**	
*Corynebacterium xerosis**	
Corynebacterium species	
Enterococcus durans	
*Enterococcus faecalis**	0 - 8 %
*Enterococcus species**	0 - 4 %
*Gemella haemolysans**	
*Gemella morbillorum**	
*Lactococcus lactis cremoris**	
*Propionibacterium granulosum**	
Propionibacterium species	
*Staphylococcus aureus, methicillin-susceptible**	0 - 12 %
*Staphylococcus epidermidis**	0 - 25 %
*Staphylococcus haemolyticus**	
*Staphylococcus hominis**	
*Staphylococcus saprophyticus**	
*Staphylococcus sciuri**	
*Staphylococcus xylosus**	
*Staphylococcus species, coagulase negative**	
Streptococcus agalactiae	2 %
*Streptococcus anginosus**	
*Streptococcus beta hemolysans non group A**	
*Streptococcus beta hemolysans group D**	
*Streptococcus constellatus**	
*Streptococcus gordonii**	
*Streptococcus intermedius**	
*Streptococcus milleri**	
*Streptococcus milleri-group**	
*Streptococcus mitis**	
*Streptococcus morbillorum**	
*Streptococcus oralis**	
*Streptococcus pneumoniae**	0 - 2 %
*Streptococcus pyogenes**	0 - 3 %
*Streptococcus sanguis**	
*Streptococcus viridans**	
*Streptococcus viridans group**	0 - 17 %
*Streptococcus species**	
Susceptible (Gram-Negative Aerobes)	
Acinetobacter anitratus	0 - 25 %
*Acinetobacter lwoffii**	0 - 4 %
*Aeromonas sobria**	
*Alcaligenens species**	
Branhamella catarrhalis	
Burkholderia cepacia	0 - 30 %
Citrobacter diversus	9 %
*Citrobacter farmeri**	
*Citrobacter freundii**	0 - 25 %
Citrobacter koseri	
*Citrobacter species**	
*Eikenella corrodens**	
Enterobacter agglomerans	17 %
*Enterobacter cloacae**	0 - 25 %
Enterobacter species	11 - 17 %
*Escherichia coli**	0 - 15 %
*Escherichia hermannii**	0 - 3 %
Escherichia vulneris	
*Haemophilus influenzae**	0 - 3 %
Haemophilus parainfluenzae	0 - 2 %
Haemophilus species	
*Klebsiella ornithinolytica**	
*Klebsiella oxytoca**	3 - 19 %
*Klebsiella pneumoniae**	3 - 17 %
Klebsiella species	0 - 18 %
Morganella morganii	0 - 5 %
*Pasteurella multocida**	
Proteus, indole positive	0 - 4 %
*Proteus mirabilis**	0 - 4 %
*Proteus vulgaris**	0 - 8 %
*Proteus species**	
Providencia stuartii	11 %
Providencia species	2 %
*Pseudomonas aeruginosa**	0 - 29 %
Pseudomonas fluorescens	22 %
Pseudomonas putida	20 %
Pseudomonas species	2 - 30 %
Salmonella arizonae	
Salmonella species	0 - 3 %
Serratia liquefaciens	12 - 22 %
*Serratia marcescens**	0 - 38 %
*Serratia odorifera**	
*Serratia species**	0 - 48 %
Shigella boydii	
Shigella dysenteriae	
Shigella flexneri	
Shigella sonnei	
Susceptible (Gram-Positive Anaerobes)	
*Bifidobacterium species**	
*Clostridium bifermentans**	
*Clostridium butyricum**	
*Clostridium cadaveris**	
*Clostridium clostridiforme**	
*Clostridium difficile**	
*Clostridium hastiforme**	
*Clostridium limosum**	
*Clostridium perfringens**	
*Clostridium ramosum**	
*Clostridium tertium**	
*Clostridium species**	
Eubacterium aerofaciens	
*Eubacterium lentum**	
Eubacterium species	
*Peptococcus asaccharolyticus**	
Peptococcus species	
*Peptostreptococcus anaerobius**	
*Peptostreptococcus magnus**	
*Peptostreptococcus micros**	
*Peptostreptococcus prevotii**	
*Peptostreptococcus species**	

Susceptible (Gram-Negative Anaerobes)	
*Bacteroides caccae**	0 - 2 %
*Bacteroides capillosus**	
*Bacteroides distasonis**	
*Bacteroides fragilis**	0 - 3 %
Bacteroides fragilis group	
*Bacteroides ovatus**	0 - 15 %
*Bacteroides putredinis**	
*Bacteroides stercoris**	
*Bacteroides thetaiotaomicron**	
*Bacteroides uniformis**	
*Bacteroides ureolyticus**	
*Bacteroides vulgatus**	
*Bacteroides species**	0 - 4 %
*Fusobacterium necrophorum**	
*Fusobacterium nucleatum**	
*Fusobacterium varium**	
*Fusobacterium species**	
*Porphyromonas asaccharolytica**	
*Porphyromonas gingivalis**	
*Porphyromonas species**	
Prevotella bivia	
*Prevotella disiens**	
*Prevotella intermedia**	
*Prevotella melaninogenica**	
*Prevotella oralis**	
*Prevotella species**	
Intermediate Susceptible (Gram-Positive Aerobes)	
*Enterococcus avium**	15 - 45 %
*Enterococcus faecium**	15 - 93 %
*Propionibacterium acnes**	50 %
Intermediate Susceptible (Gram-Negative Aerobes)	
*Acinetobacter baumannii**	16 - 63 %
Acinetobacter calcoaceticus	30 - 58 %
*Acinetobacter species**	0 - 75 %
Enterobacter aerogenes	7 - 79 %
*Pseudomonas stutzeri**	50 %
Stenotrophomonas maltophilia	1 - 53 %
Resistant (Gram-Positive Aerobes)	
Corynebacterium jeikeium	100 %
Staphylococcus aureus (methicillin resistant)	100 %
Staphylococcus coagulase negative (methicillin resistant)	100 %

[a] When no range is given this indicates that all isolates are susceptible; one percentage number (without any range) means that the organism was cited in one study.

* Clinical efficacy has been demonstrated for susceptible isolates in paediatric appendicitis complicated by rupture with peritonitis and/or abscess formation.

5.2 Pharmacokinetic properties

Distribution

Peak piperacillin and tazobactam plasma concentrations are attained immediately after completion of an intravenous infusion or injection. Piperacillin plasma levels produced when given with tazobactam are similar to those attained when equivalent doses of piperacillin are administered alone.

There is a greater proportional (approximately 28%) increase in plasma levels of piperacillin and tazobactam with increasing dose over the dosage range of 0.25g tazobactam/2g piperacillin to 0.5g tazobactam/4g piperacillin.

Both piperacillin and tazobactam are approximately 20 to 30% bound to plasma proteins. The protein binding of either piperacillin or tazobactam is unaffected by the presence of the other compound. Protein binding of the tazobactam metabolite is negligible.

TAZOCIN is widely distributed in tissue and body fluids including intestinal mucosa, gallbladder, lung, bile and bone.

Biotransformation

Piperacillin is metabolised to a minor microbiologically active desethyl metabolite. Tazobactam is metabolised to a single metabolite which has been found to be microbiologically inactive.

Elimination

Piperacillin and tazobactam are eliminated by the kidney via glomerular filtration and tubular secretion.

Piperacillin is excreted rapidly as unchanged drug with 68% of the administered dose appearing in the urine. Tazobactam and its metabolite are eliminated primarily by renal excretion with 80% of the administered dose appearing as unchanged drug and the remainder as the single metabolite. Piperacillin, tazobactam, and desethyl piperacillin are also secreted into the bile.

Following single or multiple doses of TAZOCIN to healthy subjects, the plasma half-life of piperacillin and tazobactam ranged from 0.7 to 1.2 hours and was unaffected by dose or duration of infusion. The elimination half-lives of both piperacillin and tazobactam are increased with decreasing renal clearance.

There are no significant changes in piperacillin pharmacokinetics due to tazobactam. Piperacillin appears to reduce the rate of elimination of tazobactam.

Impaired Renal Function

The half-lives of piperacillin and tazobactam increase with decreasing creatinine clearance. The increase is two-fold and four-fold for piperacillin and tazobactam, respectively, at creatinine clearance of below 20ml/min compared to patients with normal function.

Haemodialysis removes 30% to 50% of TAZOCIN with an additional 5% of the tazobactam dose removed as the tazobactam metabolite. Peritoneal dialysis removes approximately 6% and 21% of the piperacillin and tazobactam doses, respectively, with up to 18% of the tazobactam dose removed as the tazobactam metabolite.

Impaired Liver Function

Plasma concentrations of piperacillin and tazobactam are prolonged in hepatically impaired patients. The half-life of piperacillin and of tazobactam increases by approximately 25% and 18%, respectively, in patients with hepatic cirrhosis compared to healthy subjects. However, dosage adjustments in patients with hepatic impairment are not necessary.

5.3 Preclinical safety data

Preclinical mutagenicity and reproduction studies reveal no special hazards for humans.

Carcinogenicity studies have not been conducted with piperacillin, tazobactam, or the combination.

6. PHARMACEUTICAL PARTICULARS

6.1 List of excipients

Citric Acid

Disodium Edetate (dihydrate) (EDTA)

6.2 Incompatibilities

The mixing of beta-lactam antibiotics with aminoglycosides in vitro can result in physical incompatibility of the aminoglycoside. However, amikacin and gentamicin were determined to be compatible with TAZOCIN containing EDTA in vitro in certain diluents at specific concentrations. (See Section 4.5 and 6.6)

TAZOCIN should not be mixed with other drugs in a syringe or infusion bottle since compatibility has not been established.

TAZOCIN should be administered through an infusion set separately from any other drugs unless compatibility is proven.

Because of chemical instability, TAZOCIN should not be used with solutions containing only sodium bicarbonate.

TAZOCIN should not be added to blood products or albumin hydrolysates.

6.3 Shelf life

Vials containing sterile powder for injection: 36 months.

6.4 Special precautions for storage

Do not store above 25°C. Store in the original container.

To reduce the risk of microbial contamination TAZOCIN should be used immediately. However, when prepared under aseptic conditions, reconstituted and/or diluted TAZOCIN in vials, syringes or I.V. bags has demonstrated chemical and physical stability for 24 hours when stored in a refrigerator at 2-8°C.

If not used immediately, in use storage times and conditions prior to administration are the responsibility of the user. Unused solution should be discarded.

6.5 Nature and contents of container

Type I glass vial with butyl rubber stopper and aluminium/plastic seal containing TAZOCIN 2g/0.25g or TAZOCIN 4g/0.5g, boxed singly.

Infusion pack containing: One vial made of type I glass with a butyl rubber stopper and violet aluminium/plastic seal containing 4g/0.5g TAZOCIN; a 50ml type I glass bottle with a butyl rubber stopper and blue aluminium plastic seal containing Water For Injections BP; and a transfer needle.

6.6 Special precautions for disposal and other handling

Reconstitution Directions

Intravenous Injection

Each vial of TAZOCIN 2g/0.25g should be reconstituted with 10ml of one of the following diluents. Each vial of TAZOCIN 4g/0.5g should be reconstituted with 20ml of one of the following diluents:

- Sterile Water for Injection
- 0.9% Sodium Chloride for Injection

Swirl until dissolved. When swirled constantly, reconstitution should occur within 10 minutes. Intravenous injection should be given over at least 3-5 minutes.

Intravenous Infusion

Each vial of TAZOCIN 2g/0.25g should be reconstituted with 10ml of one of the above diluents. Each vial of TAZOCIN 4g/0.5g should be reconstituted with 20ml of one of the above diluents.

The reconstituted solution should be further diluted to the desired volume (a minimum of 50ml and a maximum of 150ml) with one of the following reconstitution diluents:

- 0.9% Sodium Cholride for Injection
- Dextrose 5% in Water
- Hartmann's solution (compatible only with TAZOCIN containing EDTA)
- Sterile Water for Injection (maximum recommend volume per dose is 50ml).

Displacement Volume

Each gram of TAZOCIN lyophilised powder has a displacement volume of 0.7ml.

2g/0.25g TAZOCIN will displace 1.58ml

(see Table 2 below)

4g/0.5g TAZOCIN will displace 3.15ml

(see Table 3 below)

Co-administration with aminoglycosides

In circumstances where co-administration is thought essential, the reformulated TAZOCIN containing EDTA in vials has been shown to be compatible for simultaneous co-administration via **Y-site infusion only** with the following aminoglycosides under certain conditions.

Tazocin can be co- administered via Y-site with either of the following aminoglycosides, please refer to the

Table 2 2g/0.25g TAZOCIN will displace 1.58ml

Tazocin Product Strength	**Tazocin 2g/0.25g Initial Reconstitution**	Tazocin Final Infusion Volume (0.9% Sodium Chloride)	**Tazocin Final Infusion Concentration**
2g/0.25g	10 ml of Water for Injection or 0.9%	100 ml	23 mg/mL
	Sodium Chloride for Injection	150 ml	15 mg/mL
INFUSION TIME: 20 – 30 MINUTES			

Table 2 4g/0.5g TAZOCIN will displace 3.15ml

Tazocin Product Strength	**Tazocin 4g/0.5g Initial Reconstitution**	Tazocin Final Infusion Volume (0.9% Sodium Chloride)	**Tazocin Final Infusion Concentration**
4g/0.5g	20 ml of Water for Injection or 0.9%	100 ml	45 mg/mL
	Sodium Chloride for Injection	150 ml	30 mg/mL
INFUSION TIME: 20 – 30 MINUTES			

Summary of Product Characteristics (SPC) of each respective product for full prescribing information:

AMIKACIN‡		
Final Infusion Concentration Range *(mg/ml)*	Product Strength *(mg/ml)*	Required Diluent Volume*
1.75 - 7.5	250	143 – 33 ml
INFUSION TIME: Please refer to the SPC for Amikacin		

GENTAMICIN‡		
Final Infusion Concentration Range *(mg/ml)*	Product Strength *(mg/ml)*	Required Diluent Volume*
0.7 - 3.32	40	57 – 12 ml
INFUSION TIME: Please refer to the SPC for Gentamicin		

* (0.9% Sodium Chloride)

‡ The dose of aminoglycoside should be based on patient weight, status of infection (serious or life threatening) and renal function (creatinine clearance).

Simultaneous co-administration of an aminoglycoside and beta lactam is not recommended due to physical incompatibility. However when necessary simultaneous co-administration of Tazocin containing EDTA and the specific aminoglycoside, amikacin and gentamicin, in the manner described above is acceptable.

Guidance on checks that need to be performed by the Health Professionals when co-administering infusions:

1. **Strict asepsis** should be maintained throughout and in general the giving set should not be used for more than 24 hours.

2. The infusion container should be labelled with the patient's name, the name and quantity of additives, and the date and time of addition (including the new expiry date or time if applicable).

3. The intravenous infusion should be examined from time to time. If **cloudiness, crystallisation, change of colour,** or **any other sign of interaction** or **contamination** is observed the infusion should be discontinued.

Tazocin diluents are to be used post reconstitution.

7. MARKETING AUTHORISATION HOLDER

John Wyeth & Brother Limited
Trading as Wyeth Pharmaceuticals
Huntercombe Lane South
Taplow
Maidenhead
Berkshire SL6 0PH
United Kingdom

8. MARKETING AUTHORISATION NUMBER(S)

TAZOCIN 2g/0.25g	PL 00011/0292
TAZOCIN 4g/0.5g	PL 00011/0293

9. DATE OF FIRST AUTHORISATION/RENEWAL OF THE AUTHORISATION

Tazocin 2g/0.25g:	30 January 2004
Tazocin 4g/0.5g:	30 January 2004

10. DATE OF REVISION OF THE TEXT

18 June 2009

* Trade marks

Telfast 120mg film-coated tablets

(sanofi-aventis)

1. NAME OF THE MEDICINAL PRODUCT

Telfast 120 mg film-coated tablets.

2. QUALITATIVE AND QUANTITATIVE COMPOSITION

Each tablet contains 120 mg of fexofenadine hydrochloride, which is equivalent to 112 mg of fexofenadine.

For a full list of excipients, see section 6.1.

3. PHARMACEUTICAL FORM

Film coated tablets.

Peach, modified capsule-shaped, debossed, film-coated tablet.

4. CLINICAL PARTICULARS

4.1 Therapeutic indications

Relief of symptoms associated with seasonal allergic rhinitis.

4.2 Posology and method of administration

Adults and children aged 12 years and over

The recommended dose of fexofenadine hydrochloride for adults and children aged 12 years and over is 120 mg once daily taken before a meal.

Fexofenadine is a pharmacologically active metabolite of terfenadine.

Children under 12 years of age

The efficacy and safety of fexofenadine hydrochloride has not been studied in children under 12.

Special risk groups

Studies in special risk groups (elderly, renally or hepatically impaired patients) indicate that it is not necessary to adjust the dose of fexofenadine hydrochloride in these patients.

4.3 Contraindications

Hypersensitivity to the active substance or to any of the excipients.

4.4 Special warnings and precautions for use

As with most new drugs there is only limited data in the elderly and renally or hepatically impaired patients. Fexofenadine hydrochloride should be administered with care in these special groups.

Patients with a history of or ongoing cardiovascular disease should be warned that, antihistamines as a drug class, have been associated with the adverse events, tachycardia and palpitations (see section 4.8).

4.5 Interaction with other medicinal products and other forms of interaction

Fexofenadine does not undergo hepatic biotransformation and therefore will not interact with other drugs through hepatic mechanisms. Coadministration of fexofenadine hydrochloride with erythromycin or ketoconazole has been found to result in a 2-3 times increase in the level of fexofenadine in plasma. The changes were not accompanied by any effects on the QT interval and were not associated with any increase in adverse events compared to the drugs given singly.

Animal studies have shown that the increase in plasma levels of fexofenadine observed after coadministration of erythromycin or ketoconazole, appears to be due to an increase in gastrointestinal absorption and either a decrease in biliary excretion or gastrointestinal secretion, respectively.

No interaction between fexofenadine and omeprazole was observed. However, the administration of an antacid containing aluminium and magnesium hydroxide gels 15 minutes prior to fexofenadine hydrochloride caused a reduction in bioavailability, most likely due to binding in the gastrointestinal tract. It is advisable to leave 2 hours between administration of fexofenadine hydrochloride and aluminium and magnesium hydroxide containing antacids.

4.6 Pregnancy and lactation

Pregnancy

There are no adequate data from the use of fexofenadine hydrochloride in pregnant women.

Limited animal studies do not indicate direct or indirect harmful effects with respect to effects on pregnancy, embryonal/foetal development, parturition or postnatal development (see section 5.3). Fexofenadine hydrochloride should not be used during pregnancy unless clearly necessary.

Lactation

There are no data on the content of human milk after administering fexofenadine hydrochloride. However, when terfenadine was administered to nursing mothers fexofenadine was found to cross into human breast milk. Therefore fexofenadine hydrochloride is not recommended for mothers breast feeding their babies.

4.7 Effects on ability to drive and use machines

On the basis of the pharmacodynamic profile and reported adverse events it is unlikely that fexofenadine hydrochloride tablets will produce an effect on the ability to drive or use machines. In objective tests, Telfast has been shown to have no significant effects on central nervous system function. This means that patients may drive or perform tasks that require concentration. However, in order to identify sensitive people who have an unusual reaction to drugs, it is advisable to check the individual response before driving or performing complicated tasks.

4.8 Undesirable effects

In controlled clinical trials the most commonly reported adverse events were headache (7.3%), drowsiness (2.3%), nausea (1.5%) and dizziness (1.5%). The incidence of these events observed with fexofenadine was similar to that observed with placebo.

Events that have been reported with incidences less than 1% and similar to placebo in controlled trials and have also been reported rarely during postmarketing surveillance include: fatigue, insomnia, nervousness and sleep disorders or paroniria, such as nightmares, and tachycardia, palpitations, diarrhoea. In rare cases, rash, urticaria, pruritus, and hypersensitivity reactions with manifestations such as angioedema, chest tightness, dyspnea, flushing and systemic anaphylaxis have also been reported.

4.9 Overdose

Dizziness, drowsiness, fatigue and dry mouth have been reported with overdose of fexofenadine hydrochloride. Single doses up to 800 mg and doses up to 690 mg twice daily for 1 month or 240 mg once daily for 1 year have been administered to healthy subjects without the development of clinically significant adverse events as compared with placebo. The maximum tolerated dose of fexofenadine hydrochloride has not been established.

Standard measures should be considered to remove any unabsorbed drug. Symptomatic and supportive treatment is recommended. Haemodialysis does not effectively remove fexofenadine hydrochloride from blood.

5. PHARMACOLOGICAL PROPERTIES

5.1 Pharmacodynamic properties

Pharmacotherapeutic group: Antihistamines for systemic use, ATC code: R06A X26

Fexofenadine hydrochloride is a non-sedating H_1 antihistamine. Fexofenadine is a pharmacologically active metabolite of terfenadine.

Human histamine wheal and flare studies following single and twice daily doses of fexofenadine hydrochloride demonstrate that the drug exhibits an antihistaminic effect beginning within one hour, achieving maximum at 6 hours and lasting 24 hours. There was no evidence of tolerance to these effects after 28 days of dosing. A positive dose-response relationship between doses of 10 mg to 130 mg taken orally was found to exist. In this model of antihistaminic activity, it was found that doses of at least 130 mg were required to achieve a consistent effect that was maintained over a 24 hour period. Maximum inhibition in skin wheal and flare areas were greater than 80%. Clinical studies conducted in seasonal allergic rhinitis have shown that a dose of 120 mg is sufficient for 24 hour efficacy.

No significant differences in QT_c intervals were observed in seasonal allergic rhinitis patients given fexofenadine hydrochloride up to 240 mg twice daily for 2 weeks when compared to placebo. Also, no significant change in QT_c intervals was observed in healthy subjects given fexofenadine hydrochloride up to 60 mg twice daily for 6 months, 400 mg twice daily for 6.5 days and 240 mg once daily for 1 year, when compared to placebo. Fexofenadine at concentrations 32 times greater than the therapeutic concentration in man had no effect on the delayed rectifier K+ channel cloned from human heart.

Fexofenadine hydrochloride (5-10 mg/kg po) inhibited antigen induced bronchospasm in sensitised guinea pigs and inhibited histamine release at supratherapeutic concentrations (10-100 μM) from peritoneal mast cells.

5.2 Pharmacokinetic properties

Fexofenadine hydrochloride is rapidly absorbed into the body following oral administration, with T_{max} occurring at approximately 1-3 hours post dose. The mean C_{max} value was approximately 427 ng/ml following the administration of a 120 mg dose once daily.

Fexofenadine is 60-70% plasma protein bound. Fexofenadine undergoes negligible metabolism (hepatic or non-hepatic), as it was the only major compound identified in urine and faeces of animals and man. The plasma concentration profiles of fexofenadine follow a bi-exponential decline with a terminal elimination half-life ranging from 11 to 15 hours after multiple dosing. The single and multiple dose pharmacokinetics of fexofenadine are linear for oral doses up to 120 mg BID. A dose of 240 mg BID produced slightly greater than proportional increase (8.8%) in steady state area under the curve, indicating that fexofenadine pharmacokinetics are practically linear at these doses between 40 mg and 240 mg taken daily. The major route of elimination is believed to be via biliary excretion while up to 10% of ingested dose is excreted unchanged through the urine.

5.3 Preclinical safety data

Dogs tolerated 450 mg/kg administered twice daily for 6 months and showed no toxicity other than occasional emesis. Also, in single dose dog and rodent studies, no treatment-related gross findings were observed following necropsy.

Radiolabelled fexofenadine hydrochloride in tissue distribution studies of the rat indicated that fexofenadine did not cross the blood brain barrier.

Fexofenadine hydrochloride was found to be non-mutagenic in various *in vitro* and *in vivo* mutagenicity tests.

The carcinogenic potential of fexofenadine hydrochloride was assessed using terfenadine studies with supporting pharmacokinetic studies showing fexofenadine hydrochloride exposure (via plasma AUC values). No evidence of carcinogenicity was observed in rats and mice given terfenadine (up to 150 mg/kg/day).

In a reproductive toxicity study in mice, fexofenadine hydrochloride did not impair fertility, was not teratogenic and did not impair pre- or postnatal development.

6. PHARMACEUTICAL PARTICULARS

6.1 List of excipients

Tablet core:

Microcrystalline Cellulose
Pregelatinised Maize Starch
Croscarmellose Sodium
Magnesium Stearate

Film coat:

Hypromellose
Povidone
Titanium Dioxide (E171)
Colloidal Anhydrous Silica
Macrogol 400
Iron oxide (E172)

6.2 Incompatibilities
Not applicable

6.3 Shelf life
3 years

6.4 Special precautions for storage
This medicinal product does not require any special storage conditions.

6.5 Nature and contents of container
PVC/PE/PVDC/Al blisters, packaged into cardboard boxes. 30tablets per package.

6.6 Special precautions for disposal and other handling
No special requirements.

7. MARKETING AUTHORISATION HOLDER
Sanofi-aventis

One Onslow Street

Guildford

Surrey

GU1 4YS

8. MARKETING AUTHORISATION NUMBER(S)
PL 4425/0157

9. DATE OF FIRST AUTHORISATION/RENEWAL OF THE AUTHORISATION
28/06/2006

10. DATE OF REVISION OF THE TEXT
20 February 2007

LEGAL CLASSIFICATION: POM

Telfast 180mg film-coated tablets

(sanofi-aventis)

1. NAME OF THE MEDICINAL PRODUCT
Telfast 180 mg film-coated tablets

2. QUALITATIVE AND QUANTITATIVE COMPOSITION
Each tablet contains 180 mg of fexofenadine hydrochloride, which is equivalent to 168 mg of fexofenadine.

For a full list of excipients, see section 6.1.

3. PHARMACEUTICAL FORM
Film coated tablets.

Peach, capsule-shaped, debossed, film-coated tablet.

4. CLINICAL PARTICULARS

4.1 Therapeutic indications
Relief of symptoms associated with chronic idiopathic urticaria.

4.2 Posology and method of administration
Adults and children aged 12 years and over

The recommended dose of fexofenadine hydrochloride for adults and children aged 12 years and over is 180 mg once daily taken before a meal.

Fexofenadine is a pharmacologically active metabolite of terfenadine.

Children under 12 years of age

The efficacy and safety of fexofenadine hydrochloride has not been studied in children under 12.

Special risk groups

Studies in special risk groups (elderly, renally or hepatically impaired patients) indicate that it is not necessary to adjust the dose of fexofenadine hydrochloride in these patients.

4.3 Contraindications
Hypersensitivity to the active substance or to any of the excipients.

4.4 Special warnings and precautions for use
As with most new drugs there is only limited data in the elderly and renally or hepatically impaired patients. Fexofenadine hydrochloride should be administered with care in these special groups.

Patients with a history of or ongoing cardiovascular disease should be warned that, antihistamines as a drug class, have been associated with the adverse events, tachycardia and palpitations (see section 4.8).

4.5 Interaction with other medicinal products and other forms of interaction
Fexofenadine does not undergo hepatic biotransformation and therefore will not interact with other drugs through hepatic mechanisms. Coadministration of fexofenadine hydrochloride with erythromycin or ketoconazole has been found to result in a 2-3 times increase in the level of fexofenadine in plasma. The changes were not accompanied by any effects on the QT interval and were not associated with any increase in adverse events compared to the drugs given singly.

Animal studies have shown that the increase in plasma levels of fexofenadine observed after coadministration of erythromycin or ketoconazole, appears to be due to an increase in gastrointestinal absorption and either a decrease in biliary excretion or gastrointestinal secretion, respectively.

No interaction between fexofenadine and omeprazole was observed. However, the administration of an antacid containing aluminium and magnesium hydroxide gels 15 minutes prior to fexofenadine hydrochloride caused a reduction in bioavailability, most likely due to binding in the gastrointestinal tract. It is advisable to leave 2 hours between administration of fexofenadine hydrochloride and aluminium and magnesium hydroxide containing antacids.

4.6 Pregnancy and lactation
Pregnancy
There are no adequate data from the use of fexofenadine hydrochloride in pregnant women.

Limited animal studies do not indicate direct or indirect harmful effects with respect to effects on pregnancy, embryonal/foetal development, parturition or postnatal development (see section 5.3). Fexofenadine hydrochloride should not be used during pregnancy unless clearly necessary.

Lactation
There are no data on the content of human milk after administering fexofenadine hydrochloride. However, when terfenadine was administered to nursing mothers fexofenadine was found to cross into human breast milk. Therefore fexofenadine hydrochloride is not recommended for mothers breast feeding their babies.

4.7 Effects on ability to drive and use machines
On the basis of the pharmacodynamic profile and reported adverse events it is unlikely that fexofenadine hydrochloride tablets will produce an effect on the ability to drive or use machines. In objective tests, Telfast has been shown to have no significant effects on central nervous system function. This means that patients may drive or perform tasks that require concentration. However, in order to identify sensitive people who have an unusual reaction to drugs, it is advisable to check the individual response before driving or performing complicated tasks.

4.8 Undesirable effects
In controlled clinical trials the most commonly reported adverse events were headache (7.3%), drowsiness (2.3%), nausea (1.5%) and dizziness (1.5%). The incidence of these events observed with fexofenadine was similar to that observed with placebo.

Events that have been reported with incidences less than 1% and similar to placebo in controlled trials and have also been reported rarely during postmarketing surveillance include: fatigue, insomnia, nervousness and sleep disorders or paroniria, such as nightmares, and tachycardia, palpitations, diarrhoea. In rare cases, rash, urticaria, pruritus, and hypersensitivity reactions with manifestations such as angioedema, chest tightness, dyspnea, flushing and systemic anaphylaxis have also been reported.

4.9 Overdose
Dizziness, drowsiness, fatigue and dry mouth have been reported with overdose of fexofenadine hydrochloride. Single doses up to 800 mg and doses up to 690 mg twice daily for 1 month or 240 mg once daily for 1 year have been administered to healthy subjects without the development of clinically significant adverse events as compared with placebo. The maximum tolerated dose of fexofenadine hydrochloride has not been established.

Standard measures should be considered to remove any unabsorbed drug. Symptomatic and supportive treatment is recommended. Haemodialysis does not effectively remove fexofenadine hydrochloride from blood.

5. PHARMACOLOGICAL PROPERTIES

5.1 Pharmacodynamic properties
Pharmacotherapeutic group: Antihistamines for systemic use, ATC code: R06A X26

Fexofenadine hydrochloride is a non-sedating H_1 antihistamine. Fexofenadine is a pharmacologically active metabolite of terfenadine.

Human histamine wheal and flare studies following single and twice daily doses of fexofenadine hydrochloride demonstrate that the drug exhibits an antihistaminic effect beginning within one hour, achieving maximum at 6 hours and lasting 24 hours. There was no evidence of tolerance to these effects after 28 days of dosing. A positive dose-response relationship between doses of 10 mg to 130 mg taken orally was found to exist. In this model of antihistaminic activity, it was found that doses of at least 130 mg were required to achieve a consistent effect that was maintained over a 24 hour period. Maximum inhibition in skin wheal and flare areas were greater than 80%.

No significant differences in QT_c intervals were observed in seasonal allergic rhinitis patients given fexofenadine hydrochloride up to 240 mg twice daily for 2 weeks when compared to placebo. Also, no significant change in QT_c intervals was observed in healthy subjects given fexofenadine hydrochloride up to 60 mg twice daily for 6 months, 400 mg twice daily for 6.5 days and 240 mg once daily for 1 year, when compared to placebo. Fexofenadine at concentrations 32 times greater than the therapeutic concentration in man had no effect on the delayed rectifier K+ channel cloned from human heart.

Fexofenadine hydrochloride (5-10 mg/kg po) inhibited antigen induced bronchospasm in sensitised guinea pigs and inhibited histamine release at supratherapeutic concentrations (10-100 μM) from peritoneal mast cells.

5.2 Pharmacokinetic properties
Fexofenadine hydrochloride is rapidly absorbed into the body following oral administration, with T_{max} occurring at approximately 1-3 hours post dose. The mean C_{max} value was approximately 494 ng/ml following the administration of a 180 mg dose once daily.

Fexofenadine is 60-70% plasma protein bound. Fexofenadine undergoes negligible metabolism (hepatic or non-hepatic), as it was the only major compound identified in urine and faeces of animals and man. The plasma concentration profiles of fexofenadine follow a bi-exponential decline with a terminal elimination half-life ranging from 11 to 15 hours after multiple dosing. The single and multiple dose pharmacokinetics of fexofenadine are linear for oral doses up to 120 mg BID. A dose of 240 mg BID produced slightly greater than proportional increase (8.8%) in steady state area under the curve, indicating that fexofenadine pharmacokinetics are practically linear at these doses between 40 mg and 240 mg taken daily. The major route of elimination is believed to be via biliary excretion while up to 10% of ingested dose is excreted unchanged through the urine.

5.3 Preclinical safety data
Dogs tolerated 450 mg/kg administered twice daily for 6 months and showed no toxicity other than occasional emesis. Also, in single dose dog and rodent studies, no treatment-related gross findings were observed following necropsy.

Radiolabelled fexofenadine hydrochloride in tissue distribution studies of the rat indicated that fexofenadine did not cross the blood brain barrier.

Fexofenadine hydrochloride was found to be non-mutagenic in various *in vitro* and *in vivo* mutagenicity tests.

The carcinogenic potential of fexofenadine hydrochloride was assessed using terfenadine studies with supporting pharmacokinetic studies showing fexofenadine hydrochloride exposure (via plasma AUC values). No evidence of carcinogenicity was observed in rats and mice given terfenadine (up to 150 mg/kg/day).

In a reproductive toxicity study in mice, fexofenadine hydrochloride did not impair fertility, was not teratogenic and did not impair pre- or postnatal development.

6. PHARMACEUTICAL PARTICULARS

6.1 List of excipients
Tablet core:

Microcrystalline Cellulose

Pregelatinised Maize Starch

Croscarmellose Sodium

Magnesium Stearate

Film coat:

Hypromellose

Povidone

Titanium Dioxide (E171)

Colloidal Anhydrous Silica

Macrogol 400

Iron oxide (E172)

6.2 Incompatibilities
Not applicable

6.3 Shelf life
3 years

6.4 Special precautions for storage
This medicinal product does not require any special storage conditions.

6.5 Nature and contents of container
PVC/PE/PVDC/Al blisters, packaged into cardboard boxes. 30 tablets per package.

6.6 Special precautions for disposal and other handling
No special requirements.

7. MARKETING AUTHORISATION HOLDER
Sanofi-aventis

One Onslow Street

Guildford

Surrey

GU1 4YS

8. MARKETING AUTHORISATION NUMBER(S)
PL 4425/0158

9. DATE OF FIRST AUTHORISATION/RENEWAL OF THE AUTHORISATION
28/06/2006

10. DATE OF REVISION OF THE TEXT
20 February 2007

LEGAL CLASSIFICATION: POM

Telfast 30mg tablets

(sanofi-aventis)

1. NAME OF THE MEDICINAL PRODUCT
Telfast 30 mg film-coated tablets

2. QUALITATIVE AND QUANTITATIVE COMPOSITION

Each tablet contains 30 mg of fexofenadine hydrochloride, which is equivalent to 28 mg of fexofenadine.

For a full list of excipients, see section 6.1.

3. PHARMACEUTICAL FORM

Film-coated tablet.

Peach round film-coated tablet marked with "03" on one side and "e" on the other side.

4. CLINICAL PARTICULARS

4.1 Therapeutic indications

Relief of symptoms associated with seasonal allergic rhinitis.

4.2 Posology and method of administration

Children 6 to 11 years of age

The recommended dose of Fexofenadine hydrochloride in children aged 6 to 11 years is 30 mg twice daily.

Children under 6 years of age

The efficacy of Fexofenadine hydrochloride has not been established in children under 6 years of age.

Special risk groups

The safety and efficacy of Fexofenadine hydrochloride in renally or hepatically impaired children have not been established (see section 4.4). Studies conducted in adults in special risk groups (renally or hepatically impaired patients) indicate that it is not necessary to adjust the dose of Fexofenadine hydrochloride in adults.

4.3 Contraindications

Hypersensitivity to the active substance or to any of the excipients.

4.4 Special warnings and precautions for use

The safety and efficacy of fexofenadine hydrochloride in renally or hepatically impaired children have not been established (see section 4.2). Fexofenadine hydrochloride should be administered with caution in these patients.

Patients with a history of or ongoing cardiovascular disease should be warned that, antihistamines as a drug class, have been associated with the adverse events, tachycardia and palpitations (see section 4.8).

4.5 Interaction with other medicinal products and other forms of interaction

Interaction studies have only been performed in adults.

Fexofenadine does not undergo hepatic biotransformation and therefore will not interact with other medicinal products through hepatic mechanisms.

Co administration of Fexofenadine hydrochloride with erythromycin or ketoconazole has been found to result in a 2-3 times increase in the level of Fexofenadine in plasma. The changes were not accompanied by any effects on the QT interval and were not associated with any increase in adverse events compared to the medicinal products given singly.

Animal studies have shown that the increase in plasma levels of Fexofenadine observed after co administration of erythromycin or ketoconazole, appears to be due to an increase in gastrointestinal absorption and either a decrease in biliary excretion or gastrointestinal secretion, respectively.

No interaction between Fexofenadine hydrochloride and omeprazole was observed. However, the administration of an antacid containing aluminium and magnesium hydroxide gels 15 minutes prior to Fexofenadine hydrochloride caused a reduction in bioavailability, most likely due to binding in the gastrointestinal tract. It is advisable to leave 2 hours between administration of Fexofenadine hydrochloride and aluminium and magnesium hydroxide containing antacids.

4.6 Pregnancy and lactation

There are no adequate data from the use of Fexofenadine hydrochloride in pregnant women. Limited animal studies do not indicate direct or indirect harmful effects with respect to effects on pregnancy, embryonal/foetal development, parturition or postnatal development (see section 5.3). Fexofenadine hydrochloride should not be used during pregnancy unless clearly necessary.

There are no data on the content of human milk after administering Fexofenadine hydrochloride. However, when terfenadine was administered to nursing mothers Fexofenadine was found to cross into human breast milk. Therefore Fexofenadine hydrochloride is not recommended for mothers breast-feeding their babies.

4.7 Effects on ability to drive and use machines

On the basis of the pharmacodynamic profile and reported adverse events it is unlikely that Fexofenadine hydrochloride tablets will produce an effect on the ability to drive or use machines.

In objective tests, Telfast has been shown to have no significant effects on central nervous system function. This means that patients may drive or perform tasks that require concentration. However, in order to identify sensitive people who have an unusual reaction to drugs, it is advisable to check the individual response before driving or performing complicated tasks

4.8 Undesirable effects

In controlled clinical trials in children aged 6 to 11 years, the most commonly reported adverse reaction considered at least possibly related to fexofenadine hydrochloride by the investigator was headache. The incidence of headache in pooled data from clinical trials was 1.0% for patients taking fexofenadine hydrochloride 30 mg (673 children) and for patients taking placebo (700 children). There are no clinical safety data in children treated with fexofenadine hydrochloride for periods longer than two weeks

In controlled clinical trials in 845 children aged 6 months to 5 years with allergic rhinitis, 415 children were administered 15 mg or 30 mg of fexofenadine hydrochloride (capsule content sprinkled onto dosing vehicle) and 430 children were administered placebo. There were no unexpected adverse events in the children treated with fexofenadine and the adverse event profile was similar to that of older children and adults (see section 4.2).

In adults, the following undesirable effects have been reported in clinical trials, with an incidence similar to that observed with placebo:

Nervous system disorders

Common ($\geq$1/100, $<$1/10): headache, drowsiness, dizziness

Gastrointestinal disorders

Common ($\geq$1/100, $<$1/10): nausea

General disorders and administration site conditions

Uncommon ($\geq$1/1000, $<$1/100): fatigue

In adults, the following undesirable effects have been rarely ($\geq$1/10 000, $<$1/1 000) reported in post-marketing surveillance:

Immune system disorders

hypersensitivity reactions with manifestations such as angioedema, chest tightness, dyspnoea, flushing and systemic anaphylaxis

Psychiatric disorders

insomnia, nervousness, sleep disorders or paroniria, such as nightmares

Cardiac disorders

tachycardia, palpitations

Gastrointestinal disorders

diarrhoea

Skin and subcutaneous tissue disorders

rash, urticaria, pruritus

4.9 Overdose

Dizziness, drowsiness, fatigue and dry mouth have been reported with overdose of Fexofenadine hydrochloride. Doses up to 60 mg twice daily for two weeks have been administered to children, and single doses up to 800 mg and doses up to 690 mg twice daily for 1 month or 240 mg once daily for 1 year have been administered to healthy adult subjects without the development of clinically significant adverse events as compared with placebo. The maximum tolerated dose of Fexofenadine hydrochloride has not been established.

Standard measures should be considered to remove any unabsorbed drug. Symptomatic and supportive treatment is recommended. Haemodialysis does not effectively remove Fexofenadine hydrochloride from blood.

5. PHARMACOLOGICAL PROPERTIES

5.1 Pharmacodynamic properties

Pharmacotherapeutic group: Antihistamines for systemic use, ATC code: R06A X26

Fexofenadine hydrochloride is a non-sedating H_1 antihistamine. Fexofenadine is a pharmacologically active metabolite of terfenadine.

In children aged 6 to 11 years, the suppressive effects of Fexofenadine hydrochloride on histamine – induced wheal and flare were comparable to that in adults at similar exposure. Inhibition of histamine-induced wheal and flare was observed at one hour post dose following single doses of 30 and 60 mg Fexofenadine hydrochloride. Peak inhibitory effects of Fexofenadine generally occurred at 3-6 hours post dose.

In a pooled analysis of three placebo-controlled double-blind phase III studies, involving 1369 children with seasonal allergic rhinitis aged 6 to 11 years, Fexofenadine hydrochloride at 30 mg twice daily was significantly better than placebo in reducing total symptom score (p=0.0001). All individual component symptoms including rhinorrhea (p=0.0058), sneezing (p=0.0001), itchy/ watery/red eyes (p=0.0001), itchy nose/ palate and throat (p=0.0001), and nasal congestion (p=0.0334) were significantly improved by fexofenadine hydrochloride.

In children aged 6 to 11 years, no significant differences in QT_c were observed following up to 60 mg Fexofenadine hydrochloride twice daily for two weeks compared with placebo. No significant differences in QT_c intervals were observed in adult and adolescent patients with seasonal allergic rhinitis, when given Fexofenadine hydrochloride up to 240 mg twice daily for 2 weeks when compared with placebo. Also, no significant change in QT_c intervals was observed in healthy adult subjects given Fexofenadine hydrochloride up to 60 mg twice daily for 6 months, 400 mg twice daily for 6.5 days and 240 mg once daily for 1 year, when compared with placebo. Fexofenadine at concentrations 32 times greater than the therapeutic concentration in man had no effect on the delayed rectifier K+ channel cloned from human heart.

5.2 Pharmacokinetic properties

Fexofenadine hydrochloride is rapidly absorbed into the body following oral administration, with T_{max} occurring at approximately 1-3 hours post dose. In children, the mean C_{max} value was approximately 128 ng/ml following a single dose oral administration of 30 mg Fexofenadine hydrochloride.

A dose of 30 mg BID was determined to provide plasma levels (AUC) in paediatric patients which are comparable to those achieved in adults with the approved adult regimen of 120 mg once daily.

After oral administration in adults, Fexofenadine is 60-70% plasma protein bound. Fexofenadine undergoes negligible metabolism (hepatic or non-hepatic), as it was the only major compound identified in urine and faeces of animals and man. The plasma concentration profiles of Fexofenadine follow a bi-exponential decline with a terminal elimination half-life ranging from 11 to 15 hours after multiple dosing. The single and multiple dose pharmacokinetics of Fexofenadine are linear for oral doses up to 120 mg BID. A dose of 240 mg BID produced slightly greater than proportional increase (8.8%) in steady state area under the curve, indicating that Fexofenadine pharmacokinetics are practically linear at these doses between 40 mg and 240 mg taken daily. The major route of elimination is believed to be via biliary excretion while up to 10% of ingested dose is excreted unchanged through the urine.

5.3 Preclinical safety data

Dogs tolerated 450 mg/kg administered twice daily for 6 months and showed no toxicity other than occasional emesis. Also, in single dose dog and rodent studies, no treatment-related gross findings were observed following necropsy.

Radiolabelled Fexofenadine hydrochloride in tissue distribution studies of the rat indicated that Fexofenadine did not cross the blood brain barrier.

Fexofenadine hydrochloride was found to be non-mutagenic in various in vitro and in vivo mutagenicity tests.

The carcinogenic potential of Fexofenadine hydrochloride was assessed using terfenadine studies with supporting pharmacokinetic studies showing Fexofenadine hydrochloride exposure (via plasma AUC values). No evidence of carcinogenicity was observed in rats and mice given terfenadine (up to 150 mg/kg/day).

In a reproductive toxicity study in mice, Fexofenadine hydrochloride did not impair fertility, was not teratogenic and did not impair pre- or postnatal development.

6. PHARMACEUTICAL PARTICULARS

6.1 List of excipients

Tablet core:

Microcrystalline Cellulose

Pregelatinised Starch

Croscarmellose Sodium

Magnesium Stearate

Film coat:

Hypromellose

Povidone

Titanium Dioxide (E171)

Colloidal Anhydrous Silica

Macrogol

Pink Iron oxide (E172) blend

Yellow Iron oxide (E172) blend

6.2 Incompatibilities

Not applicable.

6.3 Shelf life

3 years

6.4 Special precautions for storage

This medicinal product does not require any special storage condition

6.5 Nature and contents of container

PVC/PE/PVDC/Al blisters, packaged into cardboard boxes, 60 tablets per package.

6.6 Special precautions for disposal and other handling

No special requirements

7. MARKETING AUTHORISATION HOLDER

sanofi-aventis

One Onslow Street

Guildford

Surrey

GU1 4YS

8. MARKETING AUTHORISATION NUMBER(S)

PL 04425/0162

9. DATE OF FIRST AUTHORISATION/RENEWAL OF THE AUTHORISATION

1st April 2003

10. DATE OF REVISION OF THE TEXT

9 June 2008.

Legal category

POM

Telzir 700 mg film-coated tablets

(GlaxoSmithKline UK)

1. NAME OF THE MEDICINAL PRODUCT

Telzir 700 mg film-coated tablets

2. QUALITATIVE AND QUANTITATIVE COMPOSITION

Each film-coated tablet contains 700 mg of fosamprenavir as fosamprenavir calcium (equivalent to approximately 600 mg of amprenavir).

For a full list of excipients, see section 6.1.

3. PHARMACEUTICAL FORM

Film-coated tablet

Pink film coated, capsule shaped, biconvex tablets, marked with GXLL7 on one side.

4. CLINICAL PARTICULARS

4.1 Therapeutic indications

Telzir in combination with low dose ritonavir is indicated for the treatment of Human Immunodeficiency Virus Type 1 (HIV-1) infected adults, adolescents and children of 6 years and above in combination with other antiretroviral medicinal products.

In moderately antiretroviral experienced adults, Telzir in combination with low dose ritonavir has not been shown to be as effective as lopinavir / ritonavir. No comparative studies have been undertaken in children or adolescents.

In heavily pretreated patients the use of Telzir in combination with low dose ritonavir has not been sufficiently studied.

In protease inhibitor (PI) experienced patients the choice of Telzir should be based on individual viral resistance testing and treatment history (see section 5.1).

4.2 Posology and method of administration

Telzir must only be given with low dose ritonavir as a pharmacokinetic enhancer of amprenavir and in combination with other antiretroviral medicinal products. The Summary of Product Characteristics of ritonavir must therefore be consulted prior to initiation of therapy with Telzir.

Therapy should be initiated by a physician experienced in the management of HIV infection.

Fosamprenavir is a pro-drug of amprenavir and must not be administered concomitantly with other medicinal products containing amprenavir.

The importance of complying with the full recommended dosing regimen should be stressed to all patients.

Caution is advised if the recommended doses of Telzir with ritonavir detailed below are exceeded (see section 4.4).

Telzir tablet is administered orally.

Telzir tablet can be taken with or without food.

Telzir is also available as an oral suspension for use in patients unable to swallow tablets, and in paediatric patients less than 39 kg (please refer to the Summary of Product Characteristics for Telzir oral suspension).

Adults

The recommended dose is 700 mg fosamprenavir twice daily with 100 mg ritonavir twice daily.

Paediatric patients from 6 years of age

The adult dose of Telzir tablet 700 mg twice daily with ritonavir 100 mg twice daily may be used in children weighing at least 39 kg and able to swallow tablets.

For children weighing less than 39 kg, Telzir oral suspension is the recommended option for the most accurate dosing in children based on body weight (please refer to the Summary of Product Characteristics for Telzir oral suspension).

Children less than 6 years of age: Telzir with ritonavir is not recommended in children below 6 years due to insufficient data on pharmacokinetics, safety and antiviral response (see section 5.2).

Elderly (over 65 years of age)

The pharmacokinetics of fosamprenavir have not been studied in this patient population (see section 5.2). Therefore, no recommendations can be made in this patient population.

Renal impairment

No dose adjustment is considered necessary in patients with renal impairment (see section 5.2).

Hepatic impairment

For adults with mild hepatic impairment (Child-Pugh score: 5-6) the recommended dose is 700 mg fosamprenavir twice daily with 100 mg ritonavir **once** daily.

For adults with moderate hepatic impairment (Child-Pugh score: 7-9) the recommended dose is 450 mg fosamprenavir twice daily with 100 mg ritonavir **once** daily. As it is not possible to achieve this fosamprenavir dose using the tablet formulation, these patients should be treated with fosamprenavir oral suspension.

For adults with severe hepatic impairment (Child-Pugh score: 10-15): fosamprenavir should be used with caution and at a reduced dose of 300 mg fosamprenavir twice daily with 100 mg ritonavir **once** daily. As it is not possible to achieve this fosamprenavir dose using the tablet formulation, these patients should be treated with fosamprenavir oral suspension.

Even with these dose adjustments for adults, some patients with hepatic impairment may have higher or lower than anticipated amprenavir and/or ritonavir plasma concentrations as compared to patients with normal hepatic function, due to increased inter-patient variability (see section 5.2), therefore a close monitoring of safety and virologic response is warranted.

No dose recommendation can be made for children and adolescents with hepatic impairment as no studies have been conducted in these age groups.

4.3 Contraindications

Hypersensitivity to fosamprenavir, amprenavir, or ritonavir, or to any of the excipients.

Telzir must not be administered concurrently with medicinal products with narrow therapeutic windows that are substrates of cytochrome P450 3A4 (CYP3A4), e.g. amiodarone, astemizole, bepridil, cisapride, dihydroergotamine, ergotamine, pimozide, quinidine, terfenadine, oral midazolam (for caution on parenterally administered midazolam, see section 4.5), oral triazolam.

Telzir with ritonavir must not be co-administered with medicinal products with narrow therapeutic windows that are highly dependent on CYP2D6 metabolism, e.g. flecainide and propafenone (see section 4.5).

Combination of rifampicin with Telzir with concomitant low-dose ritonavir is contraindicated (see section 4.5).

Herbal preparations containing St John's wort (*Hypericum perforatum*) must not be used while taking Telzir due to the risk of decreased plasma concentrations and reduced clinical effects of amprenavir (see section 4.5).

4.4 Special warnings and precautions for use

Patients should be advised that treatment with Telzir, or any other current antiretroviral therapy, does not cure HIV and that they may still develop opportunistic infections and other complications of HIV infection. Current antiretroviral therapies, including Telzir, have not been proven to prevent the risk of transmission of HIV to others through sexual contact or blood contamination. Appropriate precautions should continue to be taken.

Fosamprenavir contains a sulphonamide moiety. The potential for cross-sensitivity between medicinal products in the sulphonamide class and fosamprenavir is unknown. In the pivotal studies of Telzir, in patients receiving fosamprenavir with ritonavir there was no evidence of an increased risk of rashes in patients with a history of sulphonamide allergy versus those who did not have a sulphonamide allergy. Yet, Telzir should be used with caution in patients with a known sulphonamide allergy.

Co-administration of Telzir 700 mg twice daily with ritonavir in doses greater than 100 mg twice daily has not been clinically evaluated. The use of higher ritonavir doses might alter the safety profile of the combination and therefore is not recommended.

Liver disease

Telzir with ritonavir should be used with caution and at reduced doses in adults with mild, moderate, or severe hepatic impairment (see section 4.2).

Patients with chronic hepatitis B or C and treated with combination antiretroviral therapy are at an increased risk of severe and potentially fatal hepatic adverse reactions. In case of concomitant antiviral therapy for hepatitis B or C, please refer also to the relevant Summary of Product Characteristics for these medicinal products.

Patients with pre-existing liver dysfunction, including chronic active hepatitis, have an increased frequency of liver function abnormalities during combination antiretroviral therapy and should be monitored according to standard practice. If there is evidence of worsening liver disease in such patients, interruption or discontinuation of treatment must be considered.

Medicinal products – interactions

The use of Telzir concomitantly with halofantrine or lidocaine (systemic) is not recommended (see section 4.5).

The use of Telzir concomitantly with PDE5 inhibitors (e.g. sildenafil and vardenafil) is not recommended (see section 4.5).

Concomitant use of Telzir with simvastatin or lovastatin is not recommended due to an increased risk of myopathy, including rhabdomyolysis (see section 4.5).

A reduction in the rifabutin dosage by at least 75 % is recommended when administered with Telzir with ritonavir. Further dose reduction may be necessary (see section 4.5).

Because there may be an increased risk of hepatic transaminase elevations and hormonal levels may be altered with co-administration of fosamprenavir, ritonavir and oral contraceptives, alternative non-hormonal methods of contraception are recommended for women of childbearing potential (see section 4.5).

No data are available on the co-administration of fosamprenavir and ritonavir with oestrogens and/or progestogens when used as hormonal replacement therapies. The efficacy and safety of these therapies with fosamprenavir and ritonavir has not been established.

Anticonvulsants (carbamazepine, phenobarbital) should be used with caution. Telzir may be less effective due to decreased amprenavir plasma concentrations in patients taking these medicinal products concomitantly (see section 4.5).

Therapeutic concentration monitoring is recommended for immunosuppressant medicinal products (cyclosporine, tacrolimus, rapamycin) when co-administered with Telzir (see section 4.5).

Therapeutic concentration monitoring is recommended for tricyclic antidepressants (e.g. desipramine and nortriptyline) when coadministered with Telzir (see section 4.5).

When warfarin or other oral anticoagulants are coadministered with Telzir a reinforced monitoring of INR (International Normalised Ratio) is recommended (see section 4.5).

Concomitant use of Telzir with ritonavir and fluticasone or other glucocorticoids that are metabolised by CYP3A4 is not recommended unless the potential benefit of treatment outweighs the risk of systemic corticosteroid effects, including Cushing's syndrome and adrenal suppression (see section 4.5).

Rash / cutaneous reactions

Most patients with mild or moderate rash can continue Telzir. Appropriate antihistamines (e.g. cetirizine dihydrochloride) may reduce pruritus and hasten the resolution of rash. Severe and life-threatening skin reactions, including Stevens-Johnson syndrome, were reported in less than 1 % of patients included in the clinical development programme. Telzir should be permanently discontinued in case of severe rash, or in case of rash of moderate intensity with systemic or mucosal symptoms (see section 4.8).

Haemophiliac patients

There have been reports of increased bleeding including spontaneous skin haematomas and haemarthroses in haemophiliac patients type A and B treated with protease inhibitors (PIs). In some patients administration of factor VIII was necessary. In more than half of the reported cases, treatment with protease inhibitors was continued, or reintroduced if treatment had been discontinued. A causal relationship has been evoked, although the mechanism of action has not been elucidated. Haemophiliac patients should therefore be informed of the possibility of increased bleeding.

Hyperglycaemia

New onset of diabetes mellitus, hyperglycaemia or exacerbations of existing diabetes mellitus have been reported in patients receiving antiretroviral therapy, including protease inhibitors. In some of these, the hyperglycaemia was severe and in some cases also associated with ketoacidosis. Many of the patients had confounding medical conditions, some of which required therapy with medicinal products that have been associated with the development of diabetes mellitus or hyperglycaemia.

Lipodystrophy

Combination antiretroviral therapy has been associated with the redistribution of body fat (lipodystrophy) in HIV patients. The long-term consequences of these events are currently unknown. Knowledge about the mechanism is incomplete. A connection between visceral lipomatosis and protease inhibitors and lipoatrophy and nucleoside reverse transcriptase inhibitors has been hypothesised. A higher risk of lipodystrophy has been associated with individual factors such as older age, and with drug related factors such as longer duration of antiretroviral treatment and associated metabolic disturbances. Clinical examination should include evaluation for physical signs of fat redistribution. Consideration should be given to the measurement of fasting serum lipids and blood glucose. Lipid disorders should be managed as clinically appropriate (see section 4.8).

Immune Reactivation Syndrome

In HIV-infected patients with severe immune deficiency at the time of institution of combination antiretroviral therapy (CART), an inflammatory reaction to asymptomatic or residual opportunistic pathogens may arise and cause serious clinical conditions, or aggravation of symptoms. Typically, such reactions have been observed within the first few weeks or months of initiation of CART. Relevant examples are cytomegalovirus retinitis, generalised and/or focal mycobacterium infections, and *Pneumocystis carinii* pneumonia. Any inflammatory symptoms should be evaluated and treatment instituted when necessary.

Osteonecrosis:

Although the aetiology is considered to be multifactorial (including corticosteroid use, alcohol consumption, severe immunosuppression, higher body mass index), cases of osteonecrosis have been reported particularly in patients with advanced HIV-disease and/or long-term exposure to combination antiretroviral therapy (CART). Patients should be advised to seek medical advice if they experience joint aches and pain, joint stiffness or difficulty in movement.

4.5 Interaction with other medicinal products and other forms of interaction

When fosamprenavir and ritonavir are co-administered, the ritonavir metabolic drug interaction profile may predominate because ritonavir is a more potent CYP3A4 inhibitor. The full prescribing information for ritonavir must therefore be consulted prior to initiation of therapy with Telzir with ritonavir. Ritonavir also inhibits CYP2D6 but to a lesser extent than CYP3A4. Ritonavir induces CYP3A4, CYP1A2, CYP2C9 and glucuronosyl transferase.

Additionally, both amprenavir, the active metabolite of fosamprenavir, and ritonavir are primarily metabolised in the liver by CYP3A4. Therefore, any medicinal products that either share this metabolic pathway or modify CYP3A4 activity may modify the pharmacokinetics of amprenavir and ritonavir. Similarly administration of fosamprenavir with ritonavir may modify the pharmacokinetics of other active substances that share this metabolic pathway.

Interaction studies have only been performed in adults.

• Associations contraindicated (see section 4.3)

CYP3A4 substrates with narrow therapeutic index

Telzir must not be administered concurrently with medicinal products with narrow therapeutic windows containing active substances that are substrates of cytochrome P450 3A4 (CYP3A4). Co-administration may result in competitive inhibition of the metabolism of these active substances thus increasing their plasma level and leading to serious and / or life-threatening adverse reactions such as cardiac arrhythmia (e.g. amiodarone, astemizole, bepridil, cisapride, pimozide, quinidine, terfenadine) or peripheral vasospasm or ischaemia (e.g. ergotamine, dihydroergotamine).

CYP2D6 substrates with narrow therapeutic index

Telzir with ritonavir must not be co-administered with medicinal products containing active substances that are highly dependent on CYP2D6 metabolism and for which elevated plasma concentrations are associated with serious and / or life-threatening adverse reactions. These active substances include flecainide and propafenone.

Rifampicin

Rifampicin is a strong CYP3A4 inducer and has been shown to cause an 82% decrease in amprenavir AUC, which can result in virological failure and resistance development. During attempts to overcome the decreased exposure by increasing the dose of other protease inhibitors with ritonavir, a high frequency of liver reactions was seen. The combination of rifampicin and Telzir with concomitant low-dose ritonavir is contraindicated (see section 4.3).

St John's wort (*Hypericum perforatum*)

Serum levels of amprenavir and ritonavir can be reduced by concomitant use of the herbal preparation St John's wort (*Hypericum perforatum*). This is due to induction of drug metabolising enzymes by St John's wort. Herbal preparations containing St John's wort should therefore not be combined with Telzir with ritonavir. If a patient is already taking St John's wort, check amprenavir, ritonavir and if possible viral levels and stop St John's wort. Amprenavir and ritonavir levels may increase on stopping St John's wort. The inducing effect may persist for at least 2 weeks after cessation of treatment with St John's wort.

• Other combinations

Antiretroviral medicinal products

Non-nucleoside reverse transcriptase inhibitors

Efavirenz: there was no clinically relevant interaction when fosamprenavir 700 mg twice daily and ritonavir 100 mg twice daily was used concurrently with efavirenz (600 mg once daily).

Nevirapine: there was no clinically relevant interaction when fosamprenavir 700 mg twice daily and ritonavir 100 mg twice daily was used concurrently with nevirapine (200 mg twice daily).

Nucleoside / Nucleotide reverse transcriptase inhibitors

Interaction studies with abacavir, lamivudine and zidovudine have been performed with amprenavir without ritonavir. Based on data derived from these studies and because ritonavir is not expected to have a significant impact on the pharmacokinetics of NRTIs, the co-administration of fosamprenavir and ritonavir with these medicinal products is not expected to significantly alter the exposure of the co-administered active substances.

Didanosine chewable tablet: no pharmacokinetic study has been performed with fosamprenavir in combination with didanosine. Clinically significant interaction resulting from an increase in the stomach pH due to the didanosine antacid component is unlikely and no dose separation or adjustment is considered necessary when fosamprenavir and didanosine are administered concomitantly (see chapter, Antacids). No significant interaction is expected with didanosine gastro-resistant capsule.

Tenofovir: no recommendations can be drawn at this stage on the co-administration of fosamprenavir with ritonavir with tenofovir.

Protease Inhibitors

Lopinavir / ritonavir: Co-administration of standard doses of lopinavir/ritonavir with fosamprenavir results in a significant reduction in amprenavir concentrations. Co-administration of increased doses of fosamprenavir 1400 mg twice daily with lopinavir/ritonavir 533/133 mg twice daily to PI-experienced patients resulted in a higher incidence of gastrointestinal adverse reactions and elevations in triglycerides with the combination regimen without increases in virological efficacy, when compared with standard doses of fosamprenavir/ritonavir.

Therefore, concomitant administration of these medicinal products is not recommended.

No interaction studies have been undertaken between fosamprenavir with ritonavir and the protease inhibitors: indinavir, saquinavir, nelfinavir and atazanavir.

Antibiotics / Antifungals

Clarithromycin: a reduction in the clarithromycin dose should be considered when co-administered with Telzir with ritonavir in patients with renal impairment as moderate increases in clarithromycin concentrations are expected when co-administered with Telzir with ritonavir.

Erythromycin: no pharmacokinetic study has been performed with fosamprenavir with ritonavir in combination with erythromycin, however, plasma levels of erythromycin may be increased when co-administered.

Ketoconazole / Itraconazole: co-administration of fosamprenavir 700 mg with ritonavir 100 mg twice daily and ketoconazole 200 mg once daily increased plasma ketoconazole C_{max} by 25 % and increased AUC(0-τ) to values 2.69-fold those observed on administration of ketoconazole 200 mg once daily without concurrent fosamprenavir with ritonavir. The C_{max}, AUC and C_{min} of amprenavir were unchanged. When used with Telzir with ritonavir, high doses (> 200 mg/day) of ketoconazole or itraconazole are not recommended.

Rifabutin: compared to rifabutin administered alone (300 mg once daily), plasma rifabutin AUC (0-48) was unchanged and C_{max} was decreased 14 % following co-administration of reduced doses of rifabutin (150 mg every other day) with fosamprenavir 700 mg twice daily with ritonavir 100 mg twice daily. However, 25-O-desacetylrifabutin AUC (0-48) and C_{max} were increased 11-fold and 6-fold respectively, which could potentially lead to an increase of rifabutin related adverse events, notably uveitis. Based on historical comparison, rifabutin did not appear to reduce amprenavir exposure. On the basis of these data, a 75 % reduction of the standard rifabutin dose (i.e. to 150 mg every other day) is recommended when administered with Telzir with ritonavir. Further dose reduction may be necessary.

Other medicinal products

Medicinal products that may reduce plasma amprenavir concentrations when co-administered with Telzir

Antacids, Histamine H_2 receptor antagonist and Proton-Pump inhibitors: no dose adjustment for any of the respective medicinal products is considered necessary when antacids, proton-pump inhibitors or histamine H_2 receptor antagonists are administered concomitantly with fosamprenavir. The AUC and C_{max} of amprenavir were decreased by 18 % and 35 % respectively, whilst the C_{min} (C12h) was comparable, when a single 1400 mg dose of fosamprenavir was co-administered with a single 30 ml dose of antacid suspension (equivalent to 3.6 grams aluminium hydroxide and 1.8 grams magnesium hydroxide).

Serum levels of amprenavir can be reduced by concomitant use of histamine H_2 receptor antagonists (for example ranitidine and cimetidine). Concurrent administration of ranitidine (300 mg single dose) with fosamprenavir (1400 mg single dose) decreased plasma amprenavir AUC by 30 % and C_{max} by 51 %. There was, however, no change observed in the amprenavir C_{min}(C12h).

Anticonvulsant active substances: The AUC and C_{min} of amprenavir were increased by 20 % and 19 % respectively, with C_{max} unchanged when fosamprenavir (700 mg twice daily) plus ritonavir (100 mg twice daily) was given concomitantly with phenytoin (300 mg once daily). The AUC, C_{max} and C_{min} of phenytoin were decreased by 22 %, 20 % and 29 % respectively. Therefore, if fosamprenavir plus ritonavir is given in combination with phenytoin, no change to the fosamprenavir plus ritonavir dosage regimen is required. However, it is recommended that phenytoin plasma concentrations be monitored and phenytoin dose increased as appropriate.

Concomitant administration of other anticonvulsant agents known to be enzymatic inducers (e.g. phenobarbital, carbamazepine) has not been studied but may lead to a decrease in the plasma concentrations of amprenavir. These combinations should be used with caution.

Medicinal products whose plasma levels may be increased when co-administered with Telzir

Other medicinal products with a narrow therapeutic window: some substances (e.g. lidocaine (by systemic route) and halofantrine) given with Telzir may cause serious adverse reactions. Concomitant use is not recommended.

Erectile dysfunction medicinal products: concomitant use is not recommended. Based on data for ritonavir and other protease inhibitors, plasma concentrations of PDE5 inhibitors (e.g. sildenafil and vardenafil) are expected to substantially increase when co-administered with Telzir with ritonavir and may result in an increase in PDE5 inhibitor associated adverse reactions, including hypotension, visual changes and priapism.

Fluticasone propionate (interaction with ritonavir): in a clinical study where ritonavir 100 mg capsules bid were co-administered with 50 µg intranasal fluticasone propionate (4 times daily) for 7 days in healthy subjects, the fluticasone propionate plasma levels increased significantly, whereas the intrinsic cortisol levels decreased by approximately 86 % (90 % confidence interval 82-89 %). Greater effects may be expected when fluticasone propionate is inhaled. Systemic corticosteroid effects including Cushing's syndrome and adrenal suppression have been reported in patients receiving ritonavir and inhaled or intranasally administered fluticasone propionate; this could also occur with other corticosteroids metabolised via the P450 3A pathway e.g. budesonide. Consequently, concomitant administration of Telzir with ritonavir and these glucocorticoids is not recommended unless the potential benefit of treatment outweighs the risk of systemic corticosteroid effects (see section 4.4). A dose reduction of the glucocorticoid should be considered with close monitoring of local and systemic effects or a switch to a glucocorticoid, which is not a substrate for CYP3A4 (e.g. beclomethasone). Moreover, in case of withdrawal of glucocorticoids progressive dose reduction may have to be performed over a longer period. The effects of high fluticasone systemic exposure on ritonavir plasma levels is yet unknown.

HMG-CoA reductase inhibitors: if treatment with a HMG-CoA reductase inhibitor is indicated, pravastatin or fluvastatin is recommended because their metabolism is not dependent on CYP 3A4 and interactions are not expected with protease inhibitors. HMG-CoA reductase inhibitors which are highly dependent on CYP3A4 for metabolism, such as lovastatin and simvastatin, are expected to have markedly increased plasma concentrations when co-administered with Telzir with ritonavir. Since increased concentrations of HMG-CoA reductase inhibitors may cause myopathy, including rhabdomyolysis, the combination of lovastatin or simvastatin with Telzir with ritonavir is not recommended. No adjustment of the fosamprenavir or ritonavir dose is required when co-administered with atorvastatin.

The C_{max}, AUC and C_{min} of atorvastatin were increased by 184 %, 153 % and 73 % respectively when atorvastatin (10 mg once daily for 4 days) was given with fosamprenavir 700 mg twice daily with ritonavir 100 mg twice daily for two weeks. The C_{max}, AUC and C_{min} of amprenavir were unchanged. When used with Telzir with ritonavir, doses of atorvastatin no greater than 20 mg / day should be administered, with careful monitoring for atorvastatin toxicity.

Immunosuppressants: frequent therapeutic concentration monitoring of immunosuppresant levels is recommended until levels have stabilised as plasma concentrations of cyclosporin, rapamycin and tacrolimus may be increased when co-administered with fosamprenavir with ritonavir.

Midazolam: midazolam is extensively metabolized by CYP3A4. Coadministration with Telzir/ritonavir may cause a large increase in the concentration of this benzodiazepine. No drug interaction study has been performed for the co-administration of Telzir/ritonavir with benzodiazepines. Based on data for other CYP3A4 inhibitors, plasma concentrations of midazolam are expected to be significantly higher when midazolam is given orally. Therefore Telzir/ritonavir should not be co-administered with orally administered midazolam (see section 4.3), whereas caution should be used with co-administration of Telzir/ritonavir and parenteral midazolam. Data from concomitant use of parenteral midazolam with other protease inhibitors suggest a possible 3-4 fold increase in midazolam plasma levels. If Telzir/ritonavir is co-administered with parenteral midazolam, it should be done in an intensive care unit (ICU) or similar setting which ensures close clinical monitoring and appropriate medical management in case of respiratory depression and/or prolonged sedation. Dosage adjustment for midazolam should be considered, especially if more than a single dose of midazolam is administered.

Tricyclic antidepressants: careful monitoring of the therapeutic and adverse reactions of tricyclic antidepressants is recommended when they (for example desipramine and nortriptyline) are concomitantly administered with Telzir.

Medicinal products whose plasma levels may be decreased when co-administered with Telzir

Methadone: co-administration of fosamprenavir 700 mg and ritonavir 100 mg twice daily with methadone once daily (≤ 200 mg) for 14 days decreased the active (R-) methadone enantiomer AUC(0-τ) and C_{max} by 18 % and 21 % respectively. This limited impact is not expected to be clinically significant. However, as a precaution, patients should be monitored for withdrawal syndrome.

Based on historical comparisons, methadone did not appear to alter plasma amprenavir pharmacokinetic parameters.

Oral anticoagulants: a reinforced monitoring of the International Normalised Ratio is recommended in case of administration of Telzir with ritonavir with warfarin or other oral anticoagulants, due to a possible decrease or increase of their antithrombotic effect.

Steroids: Co-administration of fosamprenavir 700 mg twice daily + ritonavir 100 mg twice daily with an oral contraceptive containing ethinyl estradiol (EE) 0.035 mg/ norethisterone (NE) 0.5 mg once daily decreased plasma EE AUC(0-τ) and C_{max} by 37% and 28%, respectively, and decreased plasma NE AUC(0-τ), C_{max}, and Cτ by 34%, 38%, and 26%, respectively. Steady state plasma amprenavir pharmacokinetic (PK) parameters were not significantly affected by co-administration with this oral contraceptive; however, ritonavir AUC(0-τ) and C_{max} were 45% and 63% higher, respectively, compared to historical data in female subjects dosed with fosamprenavir / ritonavir alone. In addition to the decreased hormonal contraceptive exposures, co-administration of fosamprenavir with ritonavir and this oral contraceptive resulted in clinically significant hepatic transaminase elevations in some healthy subjects. Therefore alternative non-hormonal methods of contraception are recommended for women of childbearing potential (see section 4.4).

Paroxetine: The C_{max} and AUC of paroxetine were decreased by 51% and 55% respectively when paroxetine 20 mg once daily was given with fosamprenavir 700 mg and ritonavir 100 mg twice daily for 10 days in healthy volunteers. The mechanism of this interaction remains unknown. Based on historical comparison, amprenavir pharmacokinetic parameters were not altered by paroxetine. Therefore, if paroxetine is co-administered with Telzir and ritonavir, the recommended approach is a dose titration of paroxetine based on a clinical assessment of antidepressant response. In addition, patients on stable dose of paroxetine who start treatment with Telzir and ritonavir should be monitored for antidepressant response.

4.6 Pregnancy and lactation

Pregnancy

There is no clinical experience with fosamprenavir in pregnant women. In animal studies at systemic plasma exposures (AUC) to amprenavir lower than therapeutic exposure in patients treated with Telzir, some developmental toxicity was observed (see section 5.3). In view of the low exposure in reproductive toxicity studies, the potential developmental toxicity of Telzir has not been fully determined.

Telzir should be used during pregnancy only if the potential benefit justifies the potential risk to the foetus.

Lactation

Amprenavir-related material was found in rat milk, but it is not known whether amprenavir is excreted in human milk. Rat pups exposed pre and post-natally to amprenavir and fosamprenavir showed developmental toxicity (see section 5.3).

It is therefore recommended that mothers treated with Telzir do not breast-feed their infants. As a general rule, it is recommended that HIV-infected women must not breast-feed under any circumstances to avoid transmission of HIV.

4.7 Effects on ability to drive and use machines

No studies on the effects of Telzir in combination with ritonavir on the ability to drive and use machines have been performed. The adverse reaction profile of Telzir should be borne in mind when considering the patient's ability to drive or operate machinery (see section 4.8).

4.8 Undesirable effects

The safety of fosamprenavir has been studied in 755 adult patients in Phase II and III controlled clinical trials. The safety of the co-administration of fosamprenavir with low dose ritonavir was established in two pivotal Phase III trials: APV30002 (n = 322) in antiretroviral naïve patients, fosamprenavir (1400 mg) given once daily in combination with ritonavir (200 mg) as part of a triple regimen including abacavir and lamivudine. APV30003 in protease inhibitor experienced patients, fosamprenavir given in combination with low dose ritonavir either once daily (1400 mg / 200 mg) (n = 106) or twice daily (700 mg / 100 mg) (n = 106) in combination with two active reverse transcriptase inhibitors (RTIs).

The most frequently > 5% of adult subjects treated) reported adverse reactions were gastrointestinal reactions (nausea, diarrhoea, abdominal pain and vomiting) and headache. Most adverse reactions associated with fosamprenavir/ritonavir combination therapies were mild to moderate in severity, early in onset and rarely treatment limiting.

The adverse reaction profile was similar across all the respective adult studies: antiretroviral naïve (APV30002) and protease inhibitor experienced (twice daily dosing, APV30003) patient populations.

Adverse reactions are listed by MedDRA system organ class and absolute frequency. Frequencies are defined as: Very common (≥ 1/10), Common (≥ 1/100 to < 1/10), Uncommon (≥ 1/1,000 to < 1/100), Rare (≥ 1/10,000 to < 1/1,000) or Very rare (< 1/10,000).

Frequency categories for the reactions below have been based on clinical trials and postmarketing data.

Most of the adverse reactions below were reported from two large clinical studies in adults, where the adverse events were of at least moderate intensity (Grade 2 or more) occurring in at least 1% of patients and reported by investigators as being attributable to the medicinal products used in the studies.

Body System	Adverse reaction	Frequency
Nervous system disorders	Headache, dizziness, oral paraesthesia	Common
Gastrointestinal disorders	Diarrhoea	Very common
	Loose stools, nausea, vomiting, abdominal pain	Common
Skin and subcutaneous tissue disorders	Stevens Johnson syndrome	Rare
	Angioedema	Uncommon
	Rash (see text below "rash/ cutaneous reactions")	Common
General disorders and administration site conditions	Fatigue	Common
Investigations	Alanine aminotransferase increased	Common
	Aspartate aminotransferase increased	Common
	Lipase increased	Common
	Blood triglycerides increased	Very Common
	Blood cholesterol increased	Uncommon

Children and adolescents: The adverse reaction profile in children and adolescents is based on integrated safety data from two studies (APV29005 and APV20003) in which 126 HIV-1 infected subjects 2 to 18 years of age received fosamprenavir with ritonavir with background nucleoside reverse transcriptase inhibitor therapy (see section 5.1 for information on dosing regimens applied for each age group). 70 % of subjects received greater than 48 weeks of exposure.

Overall the safety profile in these 126 children and adolescents was similar to that observed in the adult population. Drug-related adverse reactions were more common in APV20003 (55%) where subjects received once daily fosamprenavir / ritonavir when compared to APV29005 (39%) where subjects received twice daily fosamprenavir / ritonavir.

Rash / cutaneous reactions: erythematous or maculopapular cutaneous eruptions, with or without pruritus, may occur during therapy. The rash generally will resolve spontaneously without the necessity of discontinuing treatment with the fosamprenavir with ritonavir.

Severe or life-threatening cases of rash, including Stevens-Johnson syndrome are rare. Fosamprenavir with ritonavir therapy should be definitively stopped in case of severe rash or in case of rash of mild or moderate intensity associated with systemic or mucosal signs (see section 4.4).

Clinical chemistry abnormalities: clinical chemistry abnormalities (Grade 3 or 4) potentially related to treatment with fosamprenavir with ritonavir and reported in greater than or equal to 1 % of adult patients, included: increased ALT (*common*), AST (*common*), serum lipase (*common*) and triglycerides (*very common*). Grade 3 or 4 elevations in total cholesterol values were observed in less than 1 % of adult patients (< 1 % APV30002; 0 % APV 30003).

Lipodystrophy: combination antiretroviral therapy has been associated with redistribution of body fat (lipodystrophy) in HIV patients including the loss of peripheral and facial subcutaneous fat, increased intra-abdominal and visceral fat, breast hypertrophy and dorsocervical fat accumulation (buffalo hump) (see section 4.4).

Metabolic abnormalities: combination antiretroviral therapy has been associated with metabolic abnormalities such as hypertriglyceridaemia, hypercholesterolaemia, insulin resistance, hyperglycaemia and hyperlactataemia (see section 4.4).

Hyperglycaemia: new onset of diabetes mellitus, hyperglycaemia or exacerbations of existing diabetes mellitus have been reported in patients receiving antiretroviral protease inhibitors (see section 4.4).

Rhabdomyolysis: an increase in CPK, myalgia, myositis, and rarely, rhabdomyolysis, have been reported with protease inhibitors, more specifically in association with nucleoside analogues.

Haemophiliac patients: there have been reports of increased spontaneous bleeding in haemophiliac patients receiving antiretroviral protease inhibitors (see section 4.4).

Immune Reactivation Syndrome: in HIV-infected patients with severe immune deficiency at the time of initiation of combination antiretroviral therapy (CART), an inflammatory reaction to asymptomatic or residual opportunistic infections may arise (see section 4.4).

Osteonecrosis: cases of osteonecrosis have been reported, particularly in patients with generally acknowledged risk factors, advanced HIV disease or long-term exposure to combination antiretroviral therapy (CART). The frequency of this is unknown (see section 4.4).

4.9 Overdose

There is no known antidote for Telzir. It is not known whether amprenavir can be removed by peritoneal dialysis or haemodialysis. If overdose occurs, the patient should be monitored for evidence of toxicity (see section 4.8) and standard supportive treatment applied as necessary.

5. PHARMACOLOGICAL PROPERTIES

5.1 Pharmacodynamic properties

Pharmacotherapeutic group: Antivirals for systemic use, protease inhibitor, ATC Code: J05AE07

Mechanism of action

The *in vitro* antiviral activity observed with fosamprenavir is due to the presence of trace amounts of amprenavir. Amprenavir is a competitive inhibitor of the HIV-1 protease. Amprenavir binds to the active site of HIV-1 protease and thereby prevents the processing of viral gag and gag-pol polyprotein precursors, resulting in the formation of immature non-infectious viral particles.

Co-administration of ritonavir with fosamprenavir increase plasma amprenavir AUC by approximately 2-fold and plasma $C_{\tau,ss}$ by 4- to 6-fold, compared to values obtained when fosamprenavir is administered alone. Administration of fosamprenavir 700 mg twice daily with ritonavir 100 mg twice daily results in plasma amprenavir concentrations (data from study APV30003 in antiretroviral experienced patients) which results in protein adjusted median ratios of C_{min}/IC_{50} and C_{min}/IC_{95} of 21.7 (range 1.19-240) and 3.21 (range 0.26-30.0), respectively.

Antiviral activity *in vitro*

The *in vitro* antiviral activity of amprenavir was evaluated against HIV-1 IIIB in both acutely and chronically infected lymphoblastic cell lines (MT-4, CEM-CCRF, H9) and in peripheral blood lymphocytes. The 50% inhibitory concentration (IC_{50}) of amprenavir ranged from 0.012 to 0.08 μM in acutely infected cells and was 0.41 μM in chronically infected cells (1 μM = 0.50 μg/ml). The relationship between *in vitro* anti-HIV-1 activity of amprenavir and the inhibition of HIV-1 replication in humans has not been defined.

Resistance

In vitro

HIV-1 isolates with decreased susceptibility to amprenavir have been selected during *in vitro* serial passage experiments. Reduced susceptibility to amprenavir was associated with virus that had developed I50V or I84V or V32I+I47V or I54M mutations.

In vivo

a) ART-naïve or PI-naïve patients

Various regimens have been assessed in the amprenavir/ fosamprenavir development programs with and without co-administration of ritonavir. Analysis of the virological failure samples across these regimens defined four main resistance pathways: V32I+I47V, I50V, I54L/M and I84V. Additional mutations observed which may contribute to resistance were: L10V/F/R, I13V, K20R/T, L33F/V, M36I, M46I/L, I47V/L Q58E, I62V, L63P, V77I, I85V, and I93L.

When ART naïve patients were treated with the currently approved doses of fosamprenavir/ritonavir, as for other ritonavir boosted PI regimens, the mutations described were infrequently observed. Sixteen of 434 ART-naïve patients who received fosamprenavir 700mg/ritonavir 100mg twice daily in ESS100732 experienced virological failure by Week 48 with 14 isolates genotyped. Three of 14 isolates had protease resistance mutations. One resistance mutation was observed in each of 3 isolates: K20K/R, I54I/L and I93I/L respectively

Genotypic analysis of isolates from 13 of 14 paediatric patients exhibiting virological failure among the 59 PI-naïve patients enrolled, demonstrated resistance patterns similar to those observed in adults.

b) PI-experienced patients

Amprenavir

In the studies of PI-experienced patients, PRO30017 (amprenavir 600 mg / ritonavir 100 mg twice daily in sub-study A and B with 80 and 37 patients respectively), the following mutations emerged in patients with virological failure: L10F/I/V, V11I, I13V, K20R, V32I, L33F, E34Q, M36I, M46I/L, I47V, G48V, I50V, I54L/M/T/V, Q58E, D60E, I62V, A71V, V77I, V82A/I, I84V, I85V, L90M and I93L/M.

Fosamprenavir

In the studies of PI-experienced patients, APV30003 and its extension, APV30005 (fosamprenavir 700 mg / ritonavir 100 mg twice daily: n=107), the following mutations emerged in patients experiencing virological failure through 96 weeks: L10F/I, L24I, V32I, L33F, M36I, M46I/L, I47V, I50V, I54L/M/S, A71I/T/V, G73S, V82A, I84V, and L90M.

In the paediatric studies APV20003 and APV29005, 67 PI-experienced patients were treated with fosamprenavir / ritonavir and of 22 virological failure isolates genotyped, nine patients were found with treatment-emergent protease mutations. The mutational profiles were similar to those described for PI-experienced adults treated with fosamprenavir / ritonavir.

Analyses based on genotypic resistance testing.

Genotypic interpretation systems may be used to estimate the activity of amprenavir / ritonavir or fosamprenavir / ritonavir in subjects with PI-resistant isolates. The current (July 2006) ANRS AC-11 algorithm for fosamprenavir / ritonavir defines resistance as the presence of the mutations V32I+I47A/V, or I50V, or at least four mutations among: L10F/I/V, L33F, M36I, I54A/L/M/S/T/V, I62V, V82A/C/F/G, I84V and L90M and is associated with increased phenotypic resistance to fosamprenavir with ritonavir as well as reduced likelihood of virological response (resistance). Conclusions regarding the relevance of particular mutations or mutational patterns are subject to change with additional data, and it is recommended to always consult current interpretation systems for analysing resistance test results.

Analyses based on phenotypic resistance testing.

Clinically validated phenotypic interpretation systems may be used in association with the genotypic data to estimate the activity of amprenavir / ritonavir or fosamprenavir / ritonavir in patients with PI-resistant isolates. Resistance testing diagnostic companies have developed clinical phenotypic cut-offs for FPV/RTV that can be used to interpret resistance test results.

Cross-Resistance

HIV-1 isolates with a decreased susceptibility to amprenavir have been selected during *in vitro* serial passage experiments. Reduced susceptibility to amprenavir was associated with virus that had developed I50V or I84V or V32I+I47Vor I54M mutations. Each of these four genetic patterns associated with reduced susceptibility to amprenavir produces some cross-resistance to ritonavir but susceptibility to indinavir, nelfinavir and saquinavir is generally retained. There are currently data on cross-resistance between amprenavir and other protease inhibitors for all 4 fosamprenavir resistance pathways, either alone or in combination with other mutations. Based on data from twenty-five antiretroviral naïve patients failing a fosamprenavir containing regimen (one of whom showed Baseline resistance to lopinavir and saquinavir and another to tipranavir the resistance pathways associated with amprenavir produce limited cross-resistance to atazanavir/ritonavir (three of 25 isolates), darunavir/ritonavir (four of 25 isolates), indinavir/ritonavir (one of 25 isolates), lopinavir/ritonavir (three of 24 isolates, saquinavir (three of 24 isolates) and tipranavir/ritonavir (four of 24 isolates). Conversely amprenavir retains activity against some isolates with resistance to other PIs and this retained activity would depend on the number and type of protease resistance mutations present in the isolates.

The number of key PI-resistance mutations increases markedly the longer a failing PI-containing regimen is continued. Early discontinuation of failing therapies is recommended in order to limit the accumulation of multiple mutations, which may be detrimental to a subsequent rescue regimen.

Cross-resistance between amprenavir and reverse transcriptase inhibitors is unlikely to occur because the enzyme targets are different.

Telzir is not recommended for use as monotherapy, due to the rapid emergence of resistant virus.

Clinical experience

Clinical experience with fosamprenavir boosted with ritonavir is mainly based on three open label studies. Two studies performed in antiretroviral naïve patients, one in comparison to nelfinavir (study APV30002) and one in comparison to lopinavir / ritonavir (study ESS100732), and one study in antiretroviral experienced patients, in comparison to lopinavir / ritonavir (study APV30003).

Antiretroviral Naïve Adult Patients

In antiretroviral naïve patients in APV30002, fosamprenavir (1400 mg) given once daily in combination with low dose ritonavir (200 mg) as part of a triple regimen including abacavir (300 mg twice daily) and lamivudine (150 mg twice daily) showed similar efficacy over 48 weeks compared to nelfinavir (1250 mg) given twice daily in combination with abacavir with lamivudine (300 and 150 mg twice daily).

Non-inferiority was demonstrated between fosamprenavir with ritonavir and nelfinavir based on the proportions of patients achieving plasma HIV-1 RNA levels < 400 copies/ml at 48 weeks (primary endpoint). In the ITT (Rebound or Discontinuation = Failure) analysis, 69 % (221 / 322) of patients receiving fosamprenavir with ritonavir achieved < 400 copies/ml compared to 68 % (221 / 327) of patients receiving nelfinavir.

The median plasma HIV-1 RNA had decreased by 3.1 $\log_{10}$ copies/ml and 3.0 $\log_{10}$ copies/ml at Week 48 in the fosamprenavir with ritonavir and nelfinavir arms respectively.

The median baseline CD4 cell count was low (170 cells/ mm^3 overall) in both groups. CD4 + cell counts increased in both the fosamprenavir with ritonavir and nelfinavir groups, with median increases above baseline being similar in magnitude at Week 48 (+ 203 and + 207 cells/mm^3, respectively).

The data presented above demonstrates that the once daily regimen of fosamprenavir with ritonavir (1400 / 200 mg OD) in antiretroviral naïve patients showed similar efficacy compared to nelfinavir given twice daily. This study in view of its design (open label versus nelfinavir) did not provide a sufficiently robust efficacy demonstration in antiretroviral naïve patients to support the once daily regimen of fosamprenavir with ritonavir. As a conservative approach, based on enhanced amprenavir C_{trough} levels, the twice daily dosing regimen of fosamprenavir with ritonavir was recommended for optimal therapeutic management of this population (see section 4.2).

In a subsequent randomised open-label study (ESS100732) in antiretroviral naïve patients, fosamprenavir (700 mg) co-administered with low dose ritonavir (100 mg) in a twice daily regimen including abacavir / lamivudine (600 mg / 300 mg) fixed dose combination tablet once daily showed comparable efficacy over 48 weeks to lopinavir / ritonavir (400 mg / 100 mg) given twice daily in combination with abacavir / lamivudine (600 mg / 300 mg once daily).

Non-inferiority was demonstrated between fosamprenavir co-administered with ritonavir and lopinavir / ritonavir based on the proportions of patients achieving plasma HIV-1 RNA levels < 400 copies/ml at 48 weeks (primary endpoint). In the Time to loss of virological response (TLOVR) analysis for the ITT(E) population, the proportion of patients achieving <400 copies/ml was 73 % (315 / 434) in the fosamprenavir with ritonavir group compared to 71 % (317 / 444) of patients receiving lopinavir / ritonavir, with a 95 % confidence interval of the difference of [-4,84%; 7;05%].

The median plasma HIV-1 RNA had decreased by 3.34 $\log_{10}$ copies/ml and 3.33 $\log_{10}$ copies/ml at Week 48 in the fosamprenavir with ritonavir and lopinavir / ritonavir arms respectively.

Median increase in CD4 cell count was 176 cells/mm^3 in the fosamprenavir with ritonavir arm and 191 cells/mm^3 in the lopinavir / ritonavir arm respectively by Week 48.

Antiretroviral Experienced Adult Patients

In a randomised open-label study (APV30003) in protease inhibitor experienced patients with virological failure (less than or equal to two PIs) the fosamprenavir with ritonavir combination (700 / 100 mg twice daily or 1400 / 200 mg once daily) did not demonstrate non-inferiority to lopinavir / ritonavir with regard to viral suppression as measured by the average area under the curve minus baseline (AAUCMB) for plasma HIV-1 RNA over 48 weeks (the primary end point). Results were in favour of the lopinavir / ritonavir arm as detailed below.

All patients in this study had failed treatment with a previous protease inhibitor regimen (defined as plasma HIV-1 RNA that never went below 1,000 copies/ml after at least 12 consecutive weeks of therapy, or initial suppression of HIV-1 RNA which subsequently rebounded to ≥ 1,000 copies/ml). However, only 65 % of patients were receiving a PI based regimen at study entry.

The population enrolled mainly consisted of moderately antiretroviral experienced patients. The median durations of prior exposure to NRTIs were 257 weeks for patients receiving fosamprenavir with ritonavir twice daily (79 % had ≥ 3 prior NRTIs) and 210 weeks for patients receiving lopinavir/ritonavir (64 % had ≥ 3 prior NRTIs). The median durations of prior exposure to protease inhibitors were 149 weeks for patients receiving fosamprenavir with ritonavir twice daily (49 % received ≥ 2 prior PIs) and 130 weeks for patients receiving lopinavir/ritonavir (40 % received ≥ 2 prior PIs).

The mean AAUCMBs ($\log_{10}$ c/ml) in the ITT (E) population (Observed analysis) at 48 weeks are described in the table below:

Plasma HIV-1 RNA Average Area Under the Curve Minus Baseline (AAUCMB) Values ($\log_{10}$ copies/ml) at week 48 by Randomisation Strata in APV30003 ITT (E) Population (Observed Analysis)

(see Table 1 below)

When considering the proportion of patients with undetectable viral load in the fosamprenavir with ritonavir twice daily dosing regimens and lopinavir / ritonavir arms respectively, results showed a trend in favour of the lopinavir / ritonavir arms: 58 % versus 61 % (plasma HIV-1 RNA < 400 copies/ml) or 46 % versus 50 % (plasma HIV-1 RNA < 50 copies/ml) at Week 48 (secondary efficacy endpoint) in the intent to treat (RD=F) analysis.

In patients with high viral load at baseline (> 100,000 copies/ml) 7/14 (50 %) patients in the lopinavir / ritonavir group and 6/19 (32 %) patients in the fosamprenavir with ritonavir group had plasma HIV-1 RNA < 400 copies/ml.

The fosamprenavir with ritonavir twice daily regimen and the lopinavir / ritonavir twice daily regimen showed similar immunological improvements through 48 weeks of treatment as measured by median change from baseline in CD4 + cell count (fosamprenavir with ritonavir twice daily: 81 cells/mm^3: lopinavir / ritonavir twice daily: 91 cells/mm^3).

There are insufficient data to recommend the use of fosamprenavir with ritonavir in heavily pre-treated patients.

Children and adolescent patients above the age of six

Fosamprenavir tablets and oral suspension with ritonavir in combination with NRTIs have been evaluated in protease inhibitor naïve and experienced children and adolescent patients. The benefit in this age group has mainly been derived from the ongoing study, APV29005, an open label 48 week study evaluating the pharmacokinetic profiles, safety, and antiviral activity of fosamprenavir with ritonavir administered twice daily to HIV 1 protease inhibitor experienced and naive patients 2 to 18 years of age. Results through 24 weeks of treatment are provided below.

APV29005 enrolled 25 patients aged 6 to 11 (the majority of whom were treated with fosamprenavir / ritonavir 18/3 mg/kg twice daily or with the adult tablet regimen), and 29 patients aged 12 to 18 (the majority of whom were treated with the adult tablet regimen). Overall, 27 (50 %) were PI-naïve, 9 of whom were ART naïve, and 27 (50 %) were PI-experienced. Prior NRTI exposure was extensive, with median durations of 421 and 389 weeks for the PI naïve and experienced patients respectively. The median duration of prior PI exposure was 239 weeks. Overall, patients enrolled with a median 4.6 HIV-1 RNA log10 copies/ml (33 % of whom had > 100,000 copies/ml at baseline) and a median % CD4+ cell of 18 % (37 % of whom had % CD4+ of < 15% at baseline).

Through 24 weeks of therapy, 70 % (19/27) of protease inhibitor naive and 56 % (15/27) of protease inhibitor experienced patients achieved and maintained a plasma HIV 1 RNA <400 copies/ml (ITT(E), TLOVR). In the ITT(E) population (Observed analysis) at Week 24 the median % CD4+ cell counts increased by 8 % in the PI-naïve subjects and 4 % in the PI-experienced subjects.

These data were further substantiated by the supportive study APV20003; however, a different dosage regimen than that of study APV29005 was used.

5.2 Pharmacokinetic properties

After oral administration, fosamprenavir is rapidly and almost completely hydrolysed to amprenavir and inorganic phosphate prior to reaching the systemic circulation. The conversion of fosamprenavir to amprenavir appears to primarily occur in the gut epithelium.

The pharmacokinetic properties of amprenavir following co-administration of Telzir with ritonavir have been evaluated in healthy adult subjects and HIV-infected patients and no substantial differences were observed between these two groups.

Telzir tablet and oral suspension formulations, both given fasted, delivered equivalent plasma amprenavir AUC_∞ values and the Telzir oral suspension formulation delivered a 14 % higher plasma amprenavir C_{max} as compared to the oral tablet formulation.

Absorption

After single dose administration of fosamprenavir, amprenavir peak plasma concentrations are observed approximately 2 hours after administration. Fosamprenavir AUC values are, in general, less than 1 % of those observed for amprenavir. The absolute bioavailability of fosamprenavir in humans has not been established.

After multiple dose oral administration of equivalent fosamprenavir and amprenavir doses, comparable amprenavir AUC values were observed; however, C_{max} values were approximately 30 % lower and C_{min} values were approximately 28 % higher with fosamprenavir.

After multiple dose oral administration of fosamprenavir 700 mg with ritonavir 100 mg twice daily, amprenavir was rapidly absorbed with a geometric mean (95 % CI) steady state peak plasma amprenavir concentration (C_{max}) of 6.08 (5.38-6.86) µg/ml occurring approximately 1.5 (0.75-5.0) hours after dosing (t_{max}). The mean steady state plasma amprenavir trough concentration (C_{min}) was 2.12 (1.77-2.54) µg/ml and AUC_{0-tau} was 39.6 (34.5–45.3) h*µg/ml.

Table 1

Plasma HIV-1 RNA stratum	Observed analysis FPV/RTV BID N=107 Mean (n)	Observed analysis LPV/RTV BID N=103 Mean (n)	Observed analysis Mean Diff. (97.5% CI) FPV/RTV BID vs LPV/RTV BID
1000 – 10,000 copies/ml	-1.53 (41)	-1.43 (43)	-0.104 (-0.550, 0.342)
>10,000 – 100,000 copies/ml	-1.59 (45)	-1.81 (46)	0.216 (-0.213, 0.664)
>100,000 copies/ml	-1.38 (19)	-2.61 (14)	1.232 (0.512, 1.952)
Total population	-1.53 (105)	-1.76 (103)	0.244 (-0.047, 0.536)

Key: FPV/RTV BID – Fosamprenavir with ritonavir twice daily, LPV/RTV BID – Lopinavir / ritonavir twice daily

Administration of the fosamprenavir tablet formulation in the fed state (standardised high fat meal: 967 kcal, 67 grams fat, 33 grams protein, 58 grams carbohydrate) did not alter plasma amprenavir pharmacokinetics (C_{max}, t_{max} or $AUC_{0-\infty}$) compared to the administration of this formulation in the fasted state. Telzir tablets may be taken without regard to food intake.

Co-administration of amprenavir with grapefruit juice was not associated with clinically significant changes in plasma amprenavir pharmacokinetics.

Distribution

The apparent volume of distribution of amprenavir following administration of Telzir is approximately 430 l (6 l/kg assuming a 70 kg body weight), suggesting a large volume of distribution, with penetration of amprenavir freely into tissues beyond the systemic circulation. This value is decreased by approximately 40 % when Telzir is co-administered with ritonavir, most likely due to an increase in amprenavir bioavailability.

In *in vitro* studies, the protein binding of amprenavir is approximately 90 %. It is bound to the alpha-1-acid glycoprotein (AAG) and albumin, but has a higher affinity for AAG. Concentrations of AAG have been shown to decrease during the course of antiretroviral therapy. This change will decrease the total active substance concentration in the plasma, however the amount of unbound amprenavir, which is the active moiety, is likely to be unchanged.

CSF penetration of amprenavir is negligible in humans. Amprenavir appears to penetrate into semen, though semen concentrations are lower than plasma concentrations.

Metabolism

Fosamprenavir is rapidly and almost completely hydrolysed to amprenavir and inorganic phosphate as it is absorbed through the gut epithelium, following oral administration. Amprenavir is primarily metabolised by the liver with less than 1 % excreted unchanged in the urine. The primary route of metabolism is via the cytochrome P450 3A4 enzyme. Amprenavir metabolism is inhibited by ritonavir, via inhibition of CYP3A4, resulting in increased plasma concentrations of amprenavir. Amprenavir in addition is also an inhibitor of the CYP3A4 enzyme, although to a lesser extent than ritonavir. Therefore medicinal products that are inducers, inhibitors or substrates of CYP3A4 must be used with caution when administered concurrently with Telzir with ritonavir (see sections 4.3 and 4.5).

Elimination

Following administration of Telzir, the half-life of amprenavir is 7.7 hours. When Telzir is co-administered with ritonavir, the half-life of amprenavir is increased to 15 – 23 hours.

The primary route of elimination of amprenavir is via hepatic metabolism with less than 1 % excreted unchanged in the urine and no detectable amprenavir in faeces. Metabolites account for approximately 14 % of the administered amprenavir dose in the urine, and approximately 75 % in the faeces.

Special populations

Paediatrics

In a clinical study on pharmacokinetics of fosamprenavir in paediatric patients, eight subjects 12 to 18 years of age received the standard fosamprenavir adult tablet dose of 700 mg twice daily (with ritonavir 100 mg twice daily). Compared to the historical adult population receiving fosamprenavir / ritonavir 700 / 100 mg twice daily, 12 to 18 year old subjects had 20 % lower plasma APV AUC(0-24), 23 % lower C_{max}, and 20 % lower C_{min} values. Children 6 to 11 years of age (n=9) receiving fosamprenavir / ritonavir 18 / 3 mg/kg twice daily had 26 % higher AUC(0-24) and similar C_{max} and C_{min} values when compared to the historical adult population receiving fosamprenavir / ritonavir 700 / 100 mg twice daily.

APV20002 is a 48 week, Phase II, open label study designed to evaluate the pharmacokinetics, safety, tolerability and antiviral activity of fosamprenavir with and without ritonavir in paediatric subjects 4 weeks to < 2 years of age. Compared to the historical adult population receiving fosamprenavir with ritonavir 700 mg / 100 mg twice daily, a subset of five pediatric subjects ages 6 to < 24-months receiving fosamprenavir / ritonavir 45/7 mg/kg twice daily demonstrated that despite an approximately 5-fold increase in fosamprenavir and ritonavir doses on a mg/kg basis, plasma amprenavir AUC(0-τ) was approximately 48 % lower, C_{max} 26 % lower, and Cτ 29 % lower in the paediatric subjects. No dosing recommendations can be made for the very young (children < 2 years of age) and Telzir with ritonavir is not recommended for this patient population (see section 4.2).

Elderly

The pharmacokinetics of fosamprenavir in combination with ritonavir has not been studied in patients over 65 years of age.

Renal impairment

Patients with renal impairment have not been specifically studied. Less than 1 % of the therapeutic dose of amprenavir is excreted unchanged in the urine. Renal clearance of ritonavir is also negligible, therefore the impact of renal impairment on amprenavir and ritonavir elimination should be minimal.

Hepatic impairment

Fosamprenavir is converted in man to amprenavir. The principal route of amprenavir and ritonavir elimination is hepatic metabolism.

The plasma amprenavir pharmacokinetics were evaluated in a 14 day repeat-dose study in HIV-1 infected adult subjects with mild, moderate, or severe hepatic impairment receiving fosamprenavir with ritonavir compared to matched control subjects with normal hepatic function.

In subjects with mild hepatic impairment (Child-Pugh score of 5-6), the dosage regimen of fosamprenavir 700 mg twice daily with a reduced dosing frequency of ritonavir 100 mg once daily provided slightly higher plasma amprenavir C_{max} (17 %), slightly higher plasma amprenavir AUC(0-12) (22 %), similar plasma total amprenavir C12 values and approximately 117 % higher plasma unbound amprenavir C12 values compared to subjects with normal hepatic function receiving the standard fosamprenavir / ritonavir 700 mg /100 mg twice daily regimen.

In subjects with moderate hepatic impairment (Child-Pugh score of 7-9), a reduced dose of fosamprenavir 450 mg twice daily with a reduced dosing frequency of ritonavir 100 mg once daily is predicted to deliver similar plasma amprenavir C_{max} and AUC(0-12), but approximately 35 % lower plasma total amprenavir C12 values and approximately 88 % higher plasma unbound amprenavir C12 values than achieved in subjects with normal hepatic function receiving the standard fosamprenavir with ritonavir 700 mg / 100 mg twice daily regimen.

In subjects with severe hepatic impairment (Child-Pugh score of 10-13), a reduced dose of fosamprenavir 300 mg twice daily with a reduced dosing frequency of ritonavir 100 mg once daily delivered 19% lower plasma amprenavir Cmax, 23% lower AUC(0-12), and 38% lower C12 values, but similar unbound plasma amprenavir C12 values than achieved in subjects with normal hepatic function receiving the standard fosamprenavir with ritonavir 700 mg / 100 mg twice daily regimen. Despite reducing the dosing frequency of ritonavir, subjects with severe hepatic impairment had 64% higher ritonavir Cmax, 40% higher ritonavir AUC(0-24), and 38% higher ritonavir C12 than achieved in subjects with normal hepatic function receiving the standard fosamprenavir with ritonavir 700 mg / 100 mg twice daily regimen.

Fosamprenavir with ritonavir was generally well-tolerated in subjects with mild, moderate, or severe hepatic impairment, and these regimens had similar adverse event and clinical laboratory profiles as previous studies of HIV-1 infected subjects with normal hepatic function.

5.3 Preclinical safety data

Toxicity was similar to that of amprenavir and occurred at amprenavir plasma exposure levels below human exposure after treatment with fosamprenavir in combination with ritonavir at the recommended dose.

In repeated dose toxicity studies in adult rats and dogs, fosamprenavir produced evidence of gastrointestinal disturbances (salivation, vomiting and soft to liquid faeces), and hepatic changes (increased liver weights, raised serum liver enzyme activities and microscopic changes, including hepatocyte necrosis). Toxicity was not aggravated when juvenile animals were treated as compared with adult animals, but the data did indicate a steeper dose response.

In reproductive toxicity studies with fosamprenavir in rats, male fertility was not affected, but in females gravid uterine weights, numbers of ovarian corpora lutea and uterine implantation sites were reduced. In pregnant rats and rabbits there were no major effects on embryo-foetal development. However, the number of abortions increased. In rabbits, systemic exposure at the high dose level was only 0.3 times human exposure at the maximum clinical dose and thus the developmental toxicity of fosamprenavir has not been fully determined. In rats exposed pre- and post-natally to fosamprenavir, pups showed impaired physical and functional development and reduced growth. Pup survival was decreased. In addition, decreased number of implantation sites per litter and a prolongation of gestation were seen when pups were mated after reaching maturity.

Fosamprenavir was not mutagenic or genotoxic in a standard battery of *in vitro* and *in vivo* assays. In long-term carcinogenicity studies with fosamprenavir in mice and rats, there were increases in hepatocellular adenomas and hepatocellular carcinomas in mice at exposure levels equivalent to 0.1 to 0.3-fold those in humans given 700 mg of fosamprenavir plus 100mg ritonavir twice daily, and increases in hepatocellular adenomas and thyroid follicular cell adenomas in rats at exposure levels equivalent to 0.3 to 0.6-fold those in humans given 700 mg of fosamprenavir plus 100mg ritonavir twice daily. The relevance of the hepatocellular findings in the rodents for humans is uncertain; however, there is no evidence from clinical trials or marketed use to suggest that these findings are of clinical significance. Repeat dose studies with fosamprenavir in rats produced effects consistent with hepatic enzyme induction, which predisposes rats to thyroid neoplasms. The thyroid tumorigenic potential is regarded to be species-specific. The clinical relevance of these findings is unknown. In rats only there was an increase in interstitial cell hyperplasia in males at exposure levels equivalent to 0.5-fold those in humans, and an increase in uterine endometrial adenocarcinoma in females at an exposure level equivalent to 1.1-fold those in humans. The incidence of endometrial findings was slightly increased over concurrent controls, but within background range for female rats. The relevance of the uterine endometrial adenocarcinomas for humans is uncertain; however there is no evidence from clinical trials or marketed use to suggest that these findings are of clinical significance.

6. PHARMACEUTICAL PARTICULARS

6.1 List of excipients

Tablet core:

Microcrystalline cellulose

Croscarmellose sodium

Povidone K30

Magnesium stearate

Colloidal anhydrous silica

Tablet film-coat:

Hypromellose

Titanium dioxide (E171)

Glycerol triacetate

Iron oxide red (E172)

6.2 Incompatibilities

Not applicable.

6.3 Shelf life

3 years.

6.4 Special precautions for storage

This medicinal product does not require any special storage conditions.

6.5 Nature and contents of container

HDPE bottles with a child resistant polypropylene closure containing 60 tablets.

6.6 Special precautions for disposal and other handling

Any unused product should be disposed of in accordance with local requirements.

7. MARKETING AUTHORISATION HOLDER

Glaxo Group Ltd

Greenford Road

Greenford

Middlesex UB6 0NN

United Kingdom

8. MARKETING AUTHORISATION NUMBER(S)

EU/1/04/282/001

9. DATE OF FIRST AUTHORISATION/RENEWAL OF THE AUTHORISATION

Date of first authorisation: 12 July 2004

10. DATE OF REVISION OF THE TEXT

15 May 2009

Detailed information on this medicinal product is available on the website of the European Medicines Agency (EMEA) http://www.emea.europa.eu

Telzir Oral Suspension

(GlaxoSmithKline UK)

1. NAME OF THE MEDICINAL PRODUCT

Telzir 50 mg/ml oral suspension

2. QUALITATIVE AND QUANTITATIVE COMPOSITION

Each ml of oral suspension contains 50 mg fosamprenavir as fosamprenavir calcium (equivalent to approximately 43 mg amprenavir).

Excipients:

Methyl parahydroxybenzoate (E218) 1.5 mg/ml

Propyl parahydroxybenzoate (E216) 0.2 mg/ml

For a full list of excipients, see section 6.1.

3. PHARMACEUTICAL FORM

Oral suspension.

The suspension is white to off-white in colour.

4. CLINICAL PARTICULARS

4.1 Therapeutic indications

Telzir in combination with low dose ritonavir is indicated for the treatment of Human Immunodeficiency Virus Type 1 (HIV-1) infected adults, adolescents and children of 6 years and above in combination with other antiretroviral medicinal products.

In moderately antiretroviral experienced adults, Telzir in combination with low dose ritonavir has not been shown to be as effective as lopinavir / ritonavir. No comparative studies have been undertaken in children or adolescents.

In heavily pretreated patients the use of Telzir in combination with low dose ritonavir has not been sufficiently studied.

In protease inhibitor (PI) experienced patients, the choice of Telzir should be based on individual viral resistance testing and treatment history (see section 5.1).

4.2 Posology and method of administration

Telzir must only be given with low dose ritonavir as a pharmacokinetic enhancer of amprenavir and in combination with other antiretroviral medicinal products. The Summary of Product Characteristics of ritonavir must therefore be consulted prior to initiation of therapy with Telzir.

Therapy should be initiated by a physician experienced in the management of HIV infection.

Fosamprenavir is a pro-drug of amprenavir and must not be administered concomitantly with other medicinal products containing amprenavir.

The importance of complying with the full recommended dosing regimen should be stressed to all patients.

Caution is advised if the recommended dose of fosamprenavir with ritonavir detailed below are exceeded (see section 4.4).

Telzir suspension is administered orally.

Shake the bottle vigorously for 20 seconds before first dose is removed and 5 seconds before each subsequent dose.

Telzir is also available as 700 mg film-coated tablets.

Adults

In adults, the oral suspension **should** be taken **without** food and on an empty stomach.

Please refer to the table below for the dosing recommendations in adults.

Paediatric patients (from 6 years of age)

In paediatric patients, the oral suspension **should** be taken **with** food in order to aid palatability and assist compliance (see section 5.2).

Telzir oral suspension is the recommended option for the most accurate dosing in children based on body weight.

Please refer to the table below for the dosing recommendations in paediatric patients.

No dosing recommendations can be made for children weighing less than 25 kg.

Children less than 6 years of age: Telzir with ritonavir is not recommended in children below 6 years due to insufficient data on pharmacokinetics, safety and antiviral response (see section 5.2).

Dosing recommendations for Telzir with ritonavir

(see Table 1 below)

Elderly (over 65 years of age)

The pharmacokinetics of fosamprenavir have not been studied in this patient population (see section 5.2). Therefore, no recommendations can be made in this patient population.

Renal impairment

No dose adjustment is considered necessary in patients with renal impairment (see section 5.2).

Hepatic impairment

For adults with mild hepatic impairment (Child-Pugh score: 5-6) the recommended dose is 700 mg fosamprenavir twice daily with 100 mg ritonavir **once** daily.

For adults with moderate hepatic impairment (Child-Pugh score: 7-9) the recommended dose is 450 mg fosamprenavir (i.e. 9 ml Telzir oral suspension) twice daily with 100 mg ritonavir **once** daily.

For adults with severe hepatic impairment (Child-Pugh score: 10-15): fosamprenavir should be used with caution and at a reduced dose of 300 mg fosamprenavir twice daily with 100 mg ritonavir **once** daily.

Even with these dose adjustments for adults, some patients with hepatic impairment may have higher or lower than anticipated amprenavir and/or ritonavir plasma concentrations as compared to patients with normal hepatic function, due to increased inter-patient variability (see section 5.2), therefore a close monitoring of safety and virologic response is warranted.

In this patient population, the oral suspension **should** be taken **without** food and on an empty stomach.

No dose recommendation can be made for children and adolescents with hepatic impairment as no studies have been conducted in these age groups.

4.3 Contraindications

Hypersensitivity to fosamprenavir, amprenavir, or ritonavir, or to any of the excipients.

Telzir must not be administered concurrently with medicinal products with narrow therapeutic windows that are substrates of cytochrome P450 3A4 (CYP3A4), e.g. amiodarone, astemizole, bepridil, cisapride, dihydroergotamine, ergotamine, pimozide, quinidine, terfenadine, oral midazolam (for caution on parenterally administered midazolam, see section 4.5), oral triazolam.

Telzir with ritonavir must not be co-administered with medicinal products with narrow therapeutic windows that are highly dependent on CYP2D6 metabolism e.g. flecainide and propafenone (see section 4.5).

Combination of rifampicin with Telzir with concomitant low-dose ritonavir is contraindicated (see section 4.5).

Herbal preparations containing St John's wort (*Hypericum perforatum*) must not be used while taking Telzir due to the risk of decreased plasma concentrations and reduced clinical effects of amprenavir (see section 4.5).

4.4 Special warnings and precautions for use

Patients should be advised that treatment with the Telzir, or any other current antiretroviral therapy, does not cure HIV and that they may still develop opportunistic infections and other complications of HIV infection. Current antiretroviral therapies, including Telzir, have not been proven to prevent the risk of transmission of HIV to others through sexual contact or blood contamination. Appropriate precautions should continue to be taken.

Fosamprenavir contains a sulphonamide moiety. The potential for cross-sensitivity between medicinal products in the sulphonamide class and fosamprenavir is unknown. In the pivotal studies of Telzir, in patients receiving fosamprenavir with ritonavir there was no evidence of an increased risk of rashes in patients with a history of sulphonamide allergy versus those who did not have a sulphonamide allergy. Yet, Telzir should be used with caution in patients with a known sulphonamide allergy.

The Telzir oral suspension contains propyl and methyl parahydroxybenzoate. These products may cause an allergic reaction in some individuals. This reaction may be delayed.

Co-administration of Telzir 700 mg twice daily with ritonavir in doses greater than 100 mg twice daily has not been clinically evaluated. The use of higher ritonavir doses might alter the safety profile of the combination and therefore is not recommended.

Liver disease

Telzir with ritonavir should be used with caution and at reduced doses in adults with mild, moderate or severe hepatic impairment (see section 4.2).

Patients with chronic hepatitis B or C and treated with combination antiretroviral therapy are at an increased risk of severe and potentially fatal hepatic adverse reactions. In case of concomitant antiviral therapy for hepatitis B or C, please refer also to the relevant Summary of Product Characteristics for these medicinal products.

Patients with pre-existing liver dysfunction, including chronic active hepatitis, have an increased frequency of liver function abnormalities during combination antiretroviral therapy and should be monitored according to standard practice. If there is evidence of worsening liver disease in such patients, interruption or discontinuation of treatment must be considered.

Medicinal products – interactions

The use of Telzir concomitantly with halofantrine or lidocaine (systemic) is not recommended.

The use of Telzir concomitantly with PDE5 inhibitors (e.g. sildenafil and vardenafil) is not recommended (see section 4.5).

Concomitant use of Telzir with simvastatin or lovastatin is not recommended due to an increased risk of myopathy, including rhabdomyolysis (see section 4.5).

A reduction in the rifabutin dosage by at least 75 % is recommended when administered with Telzir with ritonavir. Further dose reduction may be necessary (see section 4.5).

Because there may be an increased risk of hepatic transaminase elevations and hormonal levels may be altered with co-administration of fosamprenavir, ritonavir and oral contraceptives, alternative non-hormonal methods of contraception are recommended for women of childbearing potential (see section 4.5).

No data are available on the co-administration of fosamprenavir and ritonavir with oestrogens and/or progestogens when used as hormonal replacement therapies. The efficacy and safety of these therapies with fosamprenavir and ritonavir has not been established.

Anticonvulsants (carbamazepine, phenobarbital) should be used with caution. Telzir may be less effective due to decreased amprenavir plasma concentrations in patients taking these medicinal products concomitantly (see section 4.5).

Therapeutic concentration monitoring is recommended for immunosuppressant medicinal products (cyclosporine, tacrolimus, rapamycin) when co-administered with Telzir (see section 4.5).

Therapeutic concentration monitoring is recommended for tricyclic antidepressants (e.g. desipramine and nortriptyline) when co-administered with Telzir (see section 4.5).

When warfarin or other oral anticoagulants are co-administered with Telzir a reinforced monitoring of INR (International normalised ratio) is recommended (see section 4.5).

Concomitant use of Telzir with ritonavir and fluticasone or other glucocorticoids that are metabolised by CYP3A4 is not recommended unless the potential benefit of treatment outweighs the risk of systemic corticosteroid effects, including Cushing's syndrome and adrenal suppression (see section 4.5).

Rash / cutaneous reactions

Most patients with mild or moderate rash can continue Telzir. Appropriate antihistamines (e.g. cetirizine dihydrochloride) may reduce pruritus and hasten the resolution of rash. Severe and life-threatening skin reactions, including Stevens-Johnson syndrome, were reported in less than 1 % of patients included in the clinical development programme. Telzir should be permanently discontinued in case of severe rash, or in case of rash of moderate intensity with systemic or mucosal symptoms (see section 4.8).

Haemophiliac patients

There have been reports of increased bleeding including spontaneous skin haematomas and haemarthroses in haemophiliac patients type A and B treated with protease inhibitors (PIs). In some patients administration of factor VIII was necessary. In more than half of the reported cases, treatment with protease inhibitors was continued, or reintroduced if treatment had been discontinued. A causal relationship has been evoked, although the mechanism of action has not been elucidated. Haemophiliac patients should therefore be informed of the possibility of increased bleeding.

Hyperglycaemia

New onset of diabetes mellitus, hyperglycaemia or exacerbations of existing diabetes mellitus have been reported in patients receiving antiretroviral therapy, including protease inhibitors. In some of these, the hyperglycaemia was severe and in some cases also associated with ketoacidosis. Many of the patients had confounding medical conditions, some of which required therapy with medicinal products that have been associated with the development of diabetes mellitus or hyperglycaemia.

Lipodystrophy

Combination antiretroviral therapy has been associated with the redistribution of body fat (lipodystrophy) in HIV patients. The long-term consequences of these events are currently unknown. Knowledge about the mechanism is incomplete. A connection between visceral lipomatosis and protease inhibitors and lipoatrophy and nucleoside reverse transcriptase inhibitors has been hypothesised. A higher risk of lipodystrophy has been associated with individual factors such as older age, and with drug related factors such as longer duration of antiretroviral treatment and associated metabolic disturbances. Clinical examination should include

Table 1 Dosing recommendations for Telzir with ritonavir

Age	Body weight	Telzir dose (TWICE DAILY)	Ritonavir dose (TWICE DAILY)
Adult (≥18 years)		Tablet or Oral suspension 700 mg (1 tablet or 14 ml suspension) Oral suspension should be taken **without** food	Capsule or Solution 100 mg
6-17 years	≥39 kg	Tablet or Oral suspension 700 mg (1 tablet or 14 ml suspension) Oral suspension should be taken **with** food	Capsule or Solution 100 mg
	33-38 kg	Oral suspension 18 mg/kg (0.36 ml/kg); maximum 700 mg or 14 ml Oral suspension should be taken **with** food	Capsule or Solution 100 mg
	25-32 kg	Oral suspension 18 mg/kg (0.36 ml/kg) Oral suspension should be taken **with** food	Solution 3 mg/kg
	<25 kg	No dosing recommendations	
<6 years		Not recommended	

evaluation for physical signs of fat redistribution. Consideration should be given to the measurement of fasting serum lipids and blood glucose. Lipid disorders should be managed as clinically appropriate (see section 4.8).

Immune Reactivation Syndrome

In HIV-infected patients with severe immune deficiency at the time of institution of combination antiretroviral therapy (CART), an inflammatory reaction to asymptomatic or residual opportunistic pathogens may arise and cause serious clinical conditions, or aggravation of symptoms. Typically, such reactions have been observed within the first few weeks or months of initiation of CART. Relevant examples are cytomegalovirus retinitis, generalised and/or focal mycobacterium infections, and *Pneumocystis carinii* pneumonia. Any inflammatory symptoms should be evaluated and treatment instituted when necessary.

Osteonecrosis:

Although the aetiology is considered to be multifactorial (including corticosteroid use, alcohol consumption, severe immunosuppression, higher body mass index), cases of osteonecrosis have been reported particularly in patients with advanced HIV-disease and/or long-term exposure to combination antiretroviral therapy (CART). Patients should be advised to seek medical advice if they experience joint aches and pain, joint stiffness or difficulty in movement.

4.5 Interaction with other medicinal products and other forms of interaction

When fosamprenavir and ritonavir are co-administered, the ritonavir metabolic drug interaction profile may predominate because ritonavir is a more potent CYP3A4 inhibitor. The full prescribing information for ritonavir must therefore be consulted prior to initiation of therapy with Telzir with ritonavir. Ritonavir also inhibits CYP2D6 but to a lesser extent than CYP3A4. Ritonavir induces CYP3A4, CYP1A2, CYP2C9 and glucuronosyl transferase. Additionally, both amprenavir, the active metabolite of fosamprenavir, and ritonavir are primarily metabolised in the liver by CYP3A4. Therefore, any medicinal products that either share this metabolic pathway or modify CYP3A4 activity may modify the pharmacokinetics of amprenavir and ritonavir. Similarily, administration of fosamprenavir with ritonavir may modify the pharmacokinetics of other active substances that share this metabolic pathway.

Interaction studies have only been performed in adults.

• Associations contraindicated (see section 4.3)

CYP3A4 substrates with narrow therapeutic index

Telzir must not be administered concurrently with medicinal products with narrow therapeutic windows containing active substances that are substrates of cytochrome P450 3A4 (CYP3A4). Co-administration may result in competitive inhibition of the metabolism of these active substances thus increasing their plasma levels and leading to serious and / or life-threatening adverse reactions such as cardiac arrhythmia (e.g. amiodarone, astemizole, bepridil, cisapride, pimozide, quinidine, terfenadine) or peripheral vasospasm or ischaemia (e.g. ergotamine, dihydroergotamine).

CYP2D6 substrates with narrow therapeutic index

Telzir with ritonavir must not be co-administered with medicinal products containing active substances that are highly dependent on CYP2D6 metabolism and for which elevated plasma concentrations are associated with serious and / or life-threatening adverse reactions. These active substances include flecainide and propafenone.

Rifampicin

Rifampicin is a strong CYP3A4 inducer and has been shown to cause an 82% decrease in amprenavir AUC, which can result in virological failure and resistance development. During attempts to overcome the decreased exposure by increasing the dose of other protease inhibitors with ritonavir, a high frequency of liver reactions was seen. The combination of rifampicin and Telzir with concomitant low-dose ritonavir is contraindicated (see section 4.3).

St John's wort (*Hypericum perforatum*)

Serum levels of amprenavir and ritonavir can be reduced by concomitant use of the herbal preparation St John's wort (*Hypericum perforatum*). This is due to induction of drug metabolising enzymes by St John's wort. Herbal preparations containing St John's wort should therefore not be combined with Telzir with ritonavir. If a patient is already taking St John's wort, check amprenavir, ritonavir and if possible viral levels and stop St John's wort. Amprenavir and ritonavir levels may increase on stopping St John's wort. The inducing effect may persist for at least 2 weeks after cessation of treatment with St John's wort.

• Other combinations

Antiretroviral medicinal products

Non-nucleoside reverse transcriptase inhibitors

Efavirenz: there was no clinically relevant interaction when fosamprenavir 700 mg twice daily and ritonavir 100 mg twice daily was used concurrently with efavirenz (600 mg once daily).

Nevirapine: there was no clinically relevant interaction when fosamprenavir 700 mg twice daily and ritonavir 100 mg twice daily was used concurrently with nevirapine (200 mg twice daily).

Nucleoside / Nucleotide reverse transcriptase inhibitors

Interaction studies with abacavir, lamivudine and zidovudine have been performed with amprenavir without ritonavir. Based on data derived from these studies and because ritonavir is not expected to have a significant impact on the pharmacokinetics of NRTIs, the co-administration of fosamprenavir and ritonavir with these medicinal products is not expected to significantly alter the exposure of the co-administered active substances.

Didanosine chewable tablet: no pharmacokinetic study has been performed with fosamprenavir in combination with didanosine. Clinically significant interaction resulting from an increase in the stomach pH due to the didanosine antacid component is unlikely and no dose separation or adjustment is considered necessary when fosamprenavir and didanosine are administered concomitantly (see chapter, Antacids). No significant interaction is expected with didanosine gastro-resistent capsule

Tenofovir: no recommendations can be drawn at this stage on the co-administration of fosamprenavir with ritonavir with tenofovir.

Protease Inhibitors

Lopinavir / ritonavir: Co-administration of standard doses of lopinavir/ritonavir with fosamprenavir results in a significant reduction in amprenavir concentrations. Co-administration of increased doses of fosamprenavir 1400 mg twice daily with lopinavir/ritonavir 533/133 mg twice daily to PI-experienced patients resulted in a higher incidence of gastrointestinal adverse reactions and elevations in triglycerides with the combination regimen without increases in virological efficacy, when compared with standard doses of fosamprenavir/ritonavir.

Therefore, concomitant administration of these medicinal products is not recommended.

No interaction studies have been undertaken between fosamprenavir with ritonavir and the following protease inhibitors: indinavir, saquinavir, nelfinavir and atazanavir.

Antibiotics / Antifungals

Clarithromycin: a reduction in the clarithromycin dose should be considered when co-administered with Telzir with ritonavir in patients with renal impairment as moderate increases in clarithromycin concentrations are expected when coadministered with Telzir with ritonavir.

Erythromycin: no pharmacokinetic study has been performed with fosamprenavir with ritonavir in combination with erythromycin, however, plasma levels of erythromycin may be increased when co-administered.

Ketoconazole / Itraconazole: co-administration of fosamprenavir 700 mg with ritonavir 100 mg twice daily and ketoconazole 200 mg once daily increased plasma ketoconazole C_{max} by 25 % and increased AUC(0-τ) to values 2.69-fold those observed on administration of ketoconazole 200 mg once daily without concurrent fosamprenavir with ritonavir. The C_{max}, AUC and C_{min} of amprenavir were unchanged. When used with Telzir with ritonavir, high doses (> 200 mg/day) of ketoconazole or itraconazole are not recommended.

Rifabutin: compared to rifabutin administered alone (300 mg once daily), plasma rifabutin AUC (0-48) was unchanged and C_{max} was decreased 14 % following co-administration of reduced doses of rifabutin (150 mg every other day) with fosamprenavir 700 mg twice daily with ritonavir 100 mg twice daily. However, 25-O-desacetylrifabutin AUC (0-48) and C_{max} were increased 11-fold and 6-fold respectively, which could potentially lead to an increase of rifabutin related adverse events, notably uveitis. Based on historical comparison, rifabutin did not appear to reduce amprenavir exposure. On the basis of these data, a 75 % reduction of the standard rifabutin dose (i.e. to 150 mg every other day) is recommended when administered with Telzir with ritonavir. Further dose reduction may be necessary.

Other medicinal products

Medicinal products that may reduce plasma amprenavir concentrations when co-administered with Telzir

Antacids, Histamine H_2 receptor antagonist and Proton-Pump inhibitors*:* no dose adjustment for any of the respective medicinal products is considered necessary when antacids, proton-pump inhibitors or histamine H_2 receptor antagonists are administered concomitantly with fosamprenavir. The AUC and C_{max} of amprenavir were decreased by 18 % and 35 % respectively, whilst the C_{min} (C12h) was comparable, when a single 1400 mg dose of fosamprenavir was co-administered with a single 30 ml dose of antacid suspension (equivalent to 3.6 grams aluminium hydroxide and 1.8 grams magnesium hydroxide).

Serum levels of amprenavir can be reduced by concomitant use of histamine H_2 receptor antagonists (for example ranitidine and cimetidine). Concurrent administration of ranitidine (300 mg single dose) with fosamprenavir (1400 mg single dose) decreased plasma amprenavir AUC by 30 % and C_{max} by 51 %. There was, however, no change observed in the amprenavir C_{min} (C12h).

Anticonvulsant active substances*:* The AUC and C_{min} of amprenavir were increased by 20 % and 19 % respectively, with C_{max} unchanged when fosamprenavir (700 mg twice daily) plus ritonavir (100 mg twice daily) was given concomitantly with phenytoin (300 mg once daily). The AUC, C_{max} and C_{min} of phenytoin were decreased by 22 %, 20 % and 29 % respectively. Therefore, if fosamprenavir plus ritonavir is given in combination with phenytoin, no change to the fosamprenavir plus ritonavir dosage regimen is required. However, it is recommended that phenytoin plasma concentrations be monitored and phenytoin dose increased as appropriate.

Concomitant administration of other anticonvulsant agents known to be enzymatic inducers (e.g. phenobarbital, carbamazepine) has not been studied but may lead to a decrease in the plasma concentrations of amprenavir. These combinations should be used with caution.

Medicinal products whose plasma levels may be increased when co-administered with Telzir

Other medicinal products with a narrow therapeutic window*:* some substances (e.g. lidocaine (by systemic route) and halofantrine) given with Telzir may cause serious adverse reactions. Concomitant use is not recommended.

Erectile dysfunction medicinal products*:* concomitant use is not recommended. Based on data for ritonavir and other protease inhibitors, plasma concentrations of PDE5 inhibitors (e.g. sildenafil and vardenafil) are expected to substantially increase when co-administered with Telzir with ritonavir and may result in an increase in PDE5 inhibitor associated adverse reactions, including hypotension, visual changes and priapism.

Fluticasone propionate (interaction with ritonavir)*:* in a clinical study where ritonavir 100 mg capsules bid were co-administered with 50 μg intranasal fluticasone propionate (4 times daily) for 7 days in healthy subjects, the fluticasone propionate plasma levels increased significantly, whereas the intrinsic cortisol levels decreased by approximately 86 % (90 % confidence interval 82-89 %). Greater effects may be expected when fluticasone propionate is inhaled. Systemic corticosteroid effects including Cushing's syndrome and adrenal suppression have been reported in patients receiving ritonavir and inhaled or intranasally administered fluticasone propionate; this could also occur with other corticosteroids metabolised via the P450 3A pathway e.g. budesonide. Consequently, concomitant administration of Telzir with ritonavir and these glucocorticoids is not recommended unless the potential benefit of treatment outweighs the risk of systemic corticosteroid effects (see section 4.4). A dose reduction of the glucocorticoid should be considered with close monitoring of local and systemic effects or a switch to a glucocorticoid, which is not a substrate for CYP3A4 (e.g. beclomethasone). Moreover, in case of withdrawal of glucocorticoids progressive dose reduction may have to be performed over a longer period. The effects of high fluticasone systemic exposure on ritonavir plasma levels is yet unknown.

HMG-CoA reductase inhibitors*:* if treatment with a HMG-CoA reductase inhibitor is indicated, pravastatin or fluvastatin is recommended because their metabolism is not dependent on CYP3A4 and interactions are not expected with protease inhibitors. HMG-CoA reductase inhibitors which are highly dependent on CYP3A4 for metabolism, such as lovastatin and simvastatin, are expected to have markedly increased plasma concentrations when co-administered with Telzir with ritonavir. Since increased concentrations of HMG-CoA reductase inhibitors may cause myopathy, including rhabdomyolysis, the combination of lovastatin or simvastatin with Telzir with ritonavir is not recommended. No adjustment of the fosamprenavir or ritonavir dose is required when co-administered with atorvastatin.

The C_{max}, AUC and C_{min} of atorvastatin were increased by 184 %, 153 % and 73 % respectively when atorvastatin (10 mg once daily for 4 days) was given with fosamprenavir 700 mg twice daily with ritonavir 100 mg twice daily for two weeks. The C_{max}, AUC and C_{min} of amprenavir were unchanged. When used with Telzir with ritonavir, doses of atorvastatin no greater than 20 mg/day should be administered, with careful monitoring for atorvastatin toxicity.

Immunosuppressants*:* frequent therapeutic concentration monitoring of immunosuppresant levels is recommended until levels have stabilised as plasma concentrations of cyclosporin, rapamycin and tacrolimus may be increased when co-administered with fosamprenavir with ritonavir.

Midazolam: midazolam is extensively metabolized by CYP3A4. Coadministration with Telzir/ritonavir may cause a large increase in the concentration of this benzodiazepine. No drug interaction study has been performed for the co-administration of Telzir/ritonavir with benzodiazepines. Based on data for other CYP3A4 inhibitors, plasma concentrations of midazolam are expected to be significantly higher when midazolam is given orally. Therefore Telzir/ritonavir should not be co-administered with orally administered midazolam (see section 4.3), whereas caution should be used with co-administration of Telzir/ritonavir and parenteral midazolam. Data from concomitant use of parenteral midazolam with other protease inhibitors suggest a possible 3-4 fold increase in midazolam plasma levels. If Telzir/ritonavir is co-administered with parenteral midazolam, it should be done in an intensive care unit (ICU) or similar setting which ensures close clinical monitoring and appropriate medical management in case of respiratory depression and/or prolonged sedation. Dosage adjustment for midazolam should be considered, especially if more than a single dose of midazolam is administered.

Tricyclic antidepressants: careful monitoring of the therapeutic and adverse reactions of tricyclic antidepressants is recommended when they (for example desipramine and nortriptyline) are concomitantly administered with Telzir.

Medicinal products whose plasma levels may be decreased when co-administered with Telzir

Methadone: co-administration of fosamprenavir 700 mg and ritonavir 100 mg twice daily with methadone once daily (≤ 200 mg) for 14 days decreased the active (R-) methadone enantiomer AUC(0-τ) and C_{max} by 18 % and 21 % respectively. This limited impact is not expected to be clinically significant. However, as a precaution, patients should be monitored for withdrawal syndrome.

Based on historical comparisons, methadone did not appear to alter plasma amprenavir pharmacokinetic parameters.

Oral anticoagulants: a reinforced monitoring of the International Normalised Ratio is recommended in case of administration of Telzir with ritonavir with warfarin or other oral anticoagulants, due to a possible decrease or increase of their antithrombotic effect.

Steroids: Co-administration of fosamprenavir 700 mg twice daily + ritonavir 100 mg twice daily with an oral contraceptive containing ethinyl estradiol (EE) 0.035 mg/ norethisterone (NE) 0.5 mg once daily decreased plasma EE AUC(0-τ) and C_{max} by 37% and 28%, respectively, and decreased plasma NE AUC(0-τ), C_{max}, and Cτ by 34%, 38%, and 26%, respectively. Steady state plasma amprenavir pharmacokinetic (PK) parameters were not significantly affected by co-administration with this oral contraceptive; however, ritonavir AUC(0-τ) and C_{max} were 45% and 63% higher, respectively, compared to historical data in female subjects dosed with fosamprenavir / ritonavir alone. In addition to the decreased hormonal contraceptive exposures, co-administration of fosamprenavir with ritonavir and this oral contraceptive resulted in clinically significant hepatic transaminase elevations in some healthy subjects. Therefore alternative non-hormonal methods of contraception are recommended for women of childbearing potential (see section 4.4).

Paroxetine: The C_{max} and AUC of paroxetine were decreased by 51% and 55% respectively when paroxetine 20 mg once daily was given with fosamprenavir 700 mg and ritonavir 100 mg twice daily for 10 days in healthy volunteers. The mechanism of this interaction remains unknown. Based on historical comparison, amprenavir pharmacokinetic parameters were not altered by paroxetine. Therefore, if paroxetine is co-administered with Telzir and ritonavir, the recommended approach is a dose titration of paroxetine based on a clinical assessment of antidepressant response. In addition, patients on stable dose of paroxetine who start treatment with Telzir and ritonavir should be monitored for antidepressant response.

4.6 Pregnancy and lactation

Pregnancy

There is no clinical experience with fosamprenavir in pregnant women. In animal studies at systemic plasma exposures (AUC) to amprenavir lower than therapeutic exposure in patients treated with Telzir, some developmental toxicity was observed (see section 5.3). In view of the low exposure in reproductive toxicity studies, the potential developmental toxicity of Telzir has not been fully determined.

Telzir should be used during pregnancy only if the potential benefit justifies the potential risk to the foetus.

Lactation

Amprenavir-related material was found in rat milk, but it is not known whether amprenavir is excreted in human milk. Rat pups exposed pre and post-natally to amprenavir and fosamprenavir showed developmental toxicity (see section 5.3).

It is therefore recommended that mothers treated with Telzir do not breast-feed their infants. As a general rule, it is recommended that HIV-infected women must not breast-feed under any circumstances to avoid transmission of HIV.

4.7 Effects on ability to drive and use machines

No studies on the effects of Telzir in combination with ritonavir on the ability to drive and use machines have been performed. The adverse reaction profile of Telzir should be borne in mind when considering the patient's ability to drive or operate machinery (see section 4.8).

4.8 Undesirable effects

It should be noted that the Telzir oral suspension has not been evaluated clinically in adults and that the adverse reaction profile detailed in this section is based on the experience in adults with the Telzir film coated tablets.

The safety of fosamprenavir has been studied in 755 adult patients in Phase II and III controlled clinical trials. The safety of the co-administration of fosamprenavir with low dose ritonavir was established in two pivotal Phase III trials: APV30002 (n = 322) in antiretroviral naïve patients, fosamprenavir (1400 mg) given once daily in combination with ritonavir (200 mg) as part of a triple regimen including abacavir and lamivudine. APV30003 in protease inhibitor experienced patients, fosamprenavir given in combination with low dose ritonavir either once daily (1400 mg / 200 mg) (n = 106) or twice daily (700 mg / 100 mg) (n = 106) in combination with two active reverse transcriptase inhibitors (RTIs).

The most frequently (> 5% of adult subjects treated) reported adverse reactions were gastrointestinal reactions (nausea, diarrhoea, abdominal pain and vomiting) and headache. Most adverse reactions associated with fosamprenavir/ritonavir combination therapies were mild to moderate in severity, early in onset and rarely treatment limiting.

The adverse reaction profile was similar across all the respective adult studies: antiretroviral naïve (APV30002) and protease inhibitor experienced (twice daily dosing, APV30003) patient populations.

Adverse reactions are listed by MedDRA system organ class and absolute frequency. Frequencies are defined as: Very common (≥ 1/10), Common (≥ 1/100 to < 1/10), Uncommon (≥ 1/1,000 to < 1/100), Rare (≥ 1/10,000 to < 1/1,000) or Very rare (< 1/10,000).

Frequency categories for the reactions below have been based on clinical trials and postmarketing data.

Most of the adverse reactions below were reported from two large clinical studies in adults, where the adverse events were of at least moderate intensity (Grade 2 or more) occurring in at least 1% of patients and reported by investigators as being attributable to the medicinal products used in the studies.

Body System	Adverse reaction	Frequency
Nervous system disorders	Headache, dizziness, oral paraesthesia	Common
Gastrointestinal disorders	Diarrhoea	Very common
	Loose stools, nausea, vomiting, abdominal pain	Common
Skin and subcutaneous tissue disorders	Stevens Johnson syndrome	Rare
	Angioedema	Uncommon
	Rash (see text below "rash/ cutaneous reactions")	Common
General disorders and administration site conditions	Fatigue	Common
Investigations	Alanine aminotransferase increased	Common
	Aspartate aminotransferase increased	Common
	Lipase increased	Common
	Blood triglycerides increased	Very Common
	Blood cholesterol increased	Uncommon

Children and adolescents: The adverse reaction profile in children and adolescents is based on integrated safety data from two studies (APV29005 and APV20003) in which 126 HIV-1 infected subjects 2 to 18 years of age received fosamprenavir with ritonavir with background nucleoside reverse transcriptase inhibitor therapy (see section 5.1 for information on dosing regimens applied for each age group). 70 % of subjects received greater than 48 weeks of exposure.

Overall the safety profile in these 126 children and adolescents was similar to that observed in the adult population. Drug-related adverse reactions were more common in APV20003 (55%) where subjects received once daily fosamprenavir / ritonavir when compared to APV29005 (39%) where subjects received twice daily fosamprenavir / ritonavir.

Rash / cutaneous reactions: erythematous or maculopapular cutaneous eruptions, with or without pruritus, may occur during therapy. The rash generally will resolve spontaneously without the necessity of discontinuing treatment with the fosamprenavir with ritonavir.

Severe or life-threatening cases of rash, including Stevens-Johnson syndrome are rare. Fosamprenavir with ritonavir therapy should be definitively stopped in case of severe rash or in case of rash of mild or moderate intensity associated with systemic or mucosal signs (see section 4.4).

Clinical chemistry abnormalities: clinical chemistry abnormalities (Grade 3 or 4) potentially related to treatment with fosamprenavir with ritonavir and reported in greater than or equal to 1 % of adult patients, included:

increased ALT (*common*), AST (*common*), serum lipase (*common*) and triglycerides (*very common*). Grade 3 or 4 elevations in total cholesterol values were observed in less than 1 % of adult patients (< 1 % APV30002; 0 % APV 30003).

Lipodystrophy: combination antiretroviral therapy has been associated with redistribution of body fat (lipodystrophy) in HIV patients including the loss of peripheral and facial subcutaneous fat, increased intra-abdominal and visceral fat, breast hypertrophy and dorsocervical fat accumulation (buffalo hump) (see section 4.4).

Metabolic abnormalities: combination antiretroviral therapy has been associated with metabolic abnormalities such as hypertriglyceridaemia, hypercholesterolaemia, insulin resistance, hyperglycaemia and hyperlactataemia (see section 4.4).

Hyperglycaemia: new onset of diabetes mellitus, hyperglycaemia or exacerbations of existing diabetes mellitus have been reported in patients receiving antiretroviral protease inhibitors (see section 4.4).

Rhabdomyolysis: an increase in CPK, myalgia, myositis, and rarely, rhabdomyolysis, have been reported with protease inhibitors, more specifically in association with nucleoside analogues.

Haemophiliac patients: there have been reports of increased spontaneous bleeding in haemophiliac patients receiving antiretroviral protease inhibitors (see section 4.4).

Immune Reactivation Syndrome: in HIV-infected patients with severe immune deficiency at the time of initiation of combination antiretroviral therapy (CART), an inflammatory reaction to asymptomatic or residual opportunistic infections may arise (see section 4.4).

Osteonecrosis: cases of osteonecrosis have been reported, particularly in patients with generally acknowledged risk factors, advanced HIV disease or long-term exposure to combination antiretroviral therapy (CART). The frequency of this is unknown (see section 4.4).

4.9 Overdose

There is no known antidote for Telzir. It is not known whether amprenavir can be removed by peritoneal dialysis or haemodialysis. If overdose occurs, the patient should be monitored for evidence of toxicity (see section 4.8) and standard supportive treatment applied as necessary.

5. PHARMACOLOGICAL PROPERTIES

5.1 Pharmacodynamic properties

Pharmacotherapeutic group: Antivirals for systemic use, protease inhibitor, ATC Code: J05AE07

Mechanism of action

The *in vitro* antiviral activity observed with fosamprenavir is due to the presence of trace amounts of amprenavir. Amprenavir is a competitive inhibitor of the HIV-1 protease. Amprenavir binds to the active site of HIV-1 protease and thereby prevents the processing of viral gag and gag-pol polyprotein precursors, resulting in the formation of immature non-infectious viral particles.

Co-administration of ritonavir with fosamprenavir increase plasma amprenavir AUC by approximately 2-fold and plasma $C_{\tau,ss}$ by 4- to 6-fold, compared to values obtained when fosamprenavir is administered alone. Administration of fosamprenavir 700 mg twice daily with ritonavir 100 mg twice daily results in plasma amprenavir concentrations (data from study APV30003 in antiretroviral experienced patients) which results in protein adjusted median ratios of C_{min}/IC_{50} and C_{min}/IC_{95} of 21.7 (range 1.19-240) and 3.21 (range 0.26-30.0), respectively.

Antiviral activity *in vitro*

The *in vitro* antiviral activity of amprenavir was evaluated against HIV-1 IIIB in both acutely and chronically infected lymphoblastic cell lines (MT-4, CEM-CCRF, H9) and in peripheral blood lymphocytes. The 50% inhibitory concentration (IC_{50}) of amprenavir ranged from 0.012 to 0.08 μM in acutely infected cells and was 0.41 μM in chronically infected cells (1 μM = 0.50 μg/ml). The relationship between *in vitro* anti-HIV-1 activity of amprenavir and the inhibition of HIV-1 replication in humans has not been defined.

Resistance

In vitro

HIV-1 isolates with decreased susceptibility to amprenavir have been selected during *in vitro* serial passage experiments. Reduced susceptibility to amprenavir was associated with virus that had developed I50V or I84V or V32I+I47V or I54M mutations.

In vivo

a) ART-naïve or PI-naïve patients

Various regimens have been assessed in the amprenavir/ fosamprenavir development programs with and without co-administration of ritonavir. Analysis of the virological failure samples across these regimens defined four main resistance pathways: V32I+I47V, I50V, I54L/M and I84V. Additional mutations observed which may contribute to resistance were: L10V/F/R, I13V, K20R/T, L33F/V, M36I, M46I/L, I47V/L Q58E, I62V, L63P, V77I, I85V, and I93L.

When ART naïve patients were treated with the currently approved doses of fosamprenavir/ritonavir, as for other ritonavir boosted PI regimens, the mutations described were infrequently observed. Sixteen of 434 ART-naïve patients who received fosamprenavir 700mg/ritonavir 100mg twice daily in ESS100732 experienced virological failure by Week 48 with 14 isolates genotyped. Three of 14 isolates had protease resistance mutations. One resistance mutation was observed in each of 3 isolates: K20K/R, I54I/L and I93I/L respectively

Genotypic analysis of isolates from 13 of 14 paediatric patients exhibiting virological failure among the 59 PI-naïve patients enrolled, demonstrated resistance patterns similar to those observed in adults.

b) PI-experienced patients

Amprenavir

In the studies of PI-experienced patients, PRO30017 (amprenavir 600 mg / ritonavir 100 mg twice daily in sub-study A and B with 80 and 37 patients respectively), the following mutations emerged in patients with virological failure: L10F/I/V, V11I, I13V, K20R, V32I, L33F, E34Q, M36I, M46I/L, I47V, G48V, I50V, I54L/M/T/V, Q58E, D60E, I62V, A71V, V77I, V82A/I, I84V, I85V, L90M and I93L/M.

Fosamprenavir

In the studies of PI-experienced patients, APV30003 and its extension, APV30005 (fosamprenavir 700 mg / ritonavir 100 mg twice daily: n=107), the following mutations emerged in patients experiencing virological failure through 96 weeks: L10F/I, L24I, V32I, L33F, M36I, M46I/L, I47V, I50V, I54L/M/S, A71I/T/V, G73S, V82A, I84V, and L90M.

In the paediatric studies APV20003 and APV29005, 67 PI-experienced patients were treated with fosamprenavir / ritonavir and of 22 virological failure isolates genotyped, nine patients were found with treatment-emergent protease mutations. The mutational profiles were similar to those described for PI-experienced adults treated with fosamprenavir / ritonavir.

Analyses based on genotypic resistance testing.

Genotypic interpretation systems may be used to estimate the activity of amprenavir / ritonavir or fosamprenavir / ritonavir in subjects with PI-resistant isolates. The current (July 2006) ANRS AC-11 algorithm for fosamprenavir / ritonavir defines resistance as the presence of the mutations V32I+I47A/V, or I50V, or at least four mutations among: L10F/I/V, L33F, M36I, I54A/L/M/S/T/V, I62V, V82A/C/F/G, I84V and L90M and is associated with increased phenotypic resistance to fosamprenavir with ritonavir as well as reduced likelihood of virological response (resistance). Conclusions regarding the relevance of particular mutations or mutational patterns are subject to change with additional data, and it is recommended to always consult current interpretation systems for analysing resistance test results.

Analyses based on phenotypic resistance testing.

Clinically validated phenotypic interpretation systems may be used in association with the genotypic data to estimate the activity of amprenavir / ritonavir or fosamprenavir / ritonavir in patients with PI-resistant isolates. Resistance testing diagnostic companies have developed clinical phenotypic cut-offs for FPV/RTV that can be used to interpret resistance test results.

Cross-Resistance

HIV-1 isolates with a decreased susceptibility to amprenavir have been selected during *in vitro* serial passage experiments. Reduced susceptibility to amprenavir was associated with virus that had developed I50V or I84V or V32I+I47Vor I54M mutations. Each of these four genetic patterns associated with reduced susceptibility to amprenavir produces some cross-resistance to ritonavir but susceptibility to indinavir, nelfinavir and saquinavir is generally retained. There are currently data on cross-resistance between amprenavir and other protease inhibitors for all 4 fosamprenavir resistance pathways, either alone or in combination with other mutations. Based on data from twenty-five antiretroviral naïve patients failing a fosamprenavir containing regimen (one of whom showed Baseline resistance to lopinavir and saquinavir and another to tipranavir) the resistance pathways associated with amprenavir produce limited cross-resistance to atazanavir/ritonavir (three of 25 isolates), darunavir/ritonavir (four of 25 isolates), indinavir/ritonavir (one of 25 isolates), lopinavir/ritonavir (three of 24 isolates, saquinavir (three of 24 isolates) and tipranavir/ritonavir (four of 24 isolates). Conversely amprenavir retains activity against some isolates with resistance to other PIs and this retained activity would depend on the number and type of protease resistance mutations present in the isolates.

The number of key PI-resistance mutations increases markedly the longer a failing PI-containing regimen is continued. Early discontinuation of failing therapies is recommended in order to limit the accumulation of multiple mutations, which may be detrimental to a subsequent rescue regimen.

Cross-resistance between amprenavir and reverse transcriptase inhibitors is unlikely to occur because the enzyme targets are different.

Telzir is not recommended for use as monotherapy, due to the rapid emergence of resistant virus.

Clinical experience

Clinical experience with fosamprenavir boosted with ritonavir is mainly based on three open label studies. Two studies performed in antiretroviral naïve patients, one in comparison to nelfinavir (study APV30002) and one in comparison to lopinavir / ritonavir (study ESS100732), and one study in antiretroviral experienced patients, in comparison to lopinavir / ritonavir (study APV30003).

Antiretroviral Naïve Adult Patients

In antiretroviral naïve patients in APV30002, fosamprenavir (1400 mg) given once daily in combination with low dose ritonavir (200 mg) as part of a triple regimen including abacavir (300 mg twice daily) and lamivudine (150 mg twice daily) showed similar efficacy over 48 weeks compared to nelfinavir (1250 mg) given twice daily in combination with abacavir plus lamivudine (300 and 150 mg twice daily).

Non-inferiority was demonstrated between fosamprenavir with ritonavir and nelfinavir based on the proportions of patients achieving plasma HIV-1 RNA levels < 400 copies/ml at 48 weeks (primary endpoint). In the ITT (Rebound or Discontinuation = Failure) analysis, 69 % (221 / 322) of patients receiving fosamprenavir with ritonavir achieved < 400 copies/ml compared to 68 % (221 / 327) of patients receiving nelfinavir.

The median plasma HIV-1 RNA had decreased by 3.1 $\log_{10}$ copies/ml and 3.0 $\log_{10}$ copies/ml at Week 48 in the fosamprenavir with ritonavir and nelfinavir arms respectively.

The median baseline CD4 cell count was low (170 cells/mm^3 overall) in both groups. CD4+ cell counts increased in both the fosamprenavir with ritonavir and nelfinavir groups, with median increases above baseline being similar in magnitude at Week 48 (+203 and +207 cells/mm^3, respectively).

The data presented above demonstrates that the once daily regimen of fosamprenavir with ritonavir (1400/200 mg OD) in antiretroviral naïve patients showed similar efficacy compared to nelfinavir given twice daily. This study in view of its design (open label versus nelfinavir) did not provide a sufficiently robust efficacy demonstration in antiretroviral naïve patients to support the once daily regimen of fosamprenavir with ritonavir. As a conservative approach, based on enhanced amprenavir C_{trough} levels, the twice daily dosing regimen of fosamprenavir with ritonavir was recommended for optimal therapeutic management of this population (see section 4.2).

In a subsequent randomised open-label study (ESS100732) in antiretroviral naïve patients, fosamprenavir (700 mg) co-administered with low dose ritonavir (100 mg) in a twice daily regimen including abacavir / lamivudine (600 mg / 300 mg) fixed dose combination tablet once daily showed comparable efficacy over 48 weeks to lopinavir / ritonavir (400 mg / 100 mg) given twice daily in combination with abacavir / lamivudine (600 mg / 300 mg once daily).

Non-inferiority was demonstrated between fosamprenavir co-administered with ritonavir and lopinavir / ritonavir based on the proportions of patients achieving plasma HIV-1 RNA levels < 400 copies/ml at 48 weeks (primary endpoint). In the Time to loss of virological response (TLOVR) analysis for the ITT(E) population, the proportion of patients achieving <400 copies/ml was 73 % (315 / 434) in the fosamprenavir with ritonavir group compared to 71 % (317 / 444) of patients receiving lopinavir / ritonavir, with a 95 % confidence interval of the difference of [-4,84%; 7;05%].

The median plasma HIV-1 RNA had decreased by 3.34 $\log_{10}$ copies/ml and 3.33 $\log_{10}$ copies/ml at Week 48 in the fosamprenavir with ritonavir and lopinavir / ritonavir arms respectively.

Median increase in CD4 cell count was 176 cells/mm^3 in the fosamprenavir with ritonavir arm and 191 cells/mm^3 in the lopinavir / ritonavir arm respectively by Week 48.

Antiretroviral Experienced Adult Patients

In a randomised open-label study (APV30003) in protease inhibitor experienced patients with virological failure (less than or equal to two PIs) the fosamprenavir with ritonavir (700 / 100 mg twice daily or 1400 / 200 mg once daily) did not demonstrate non-inferiority to lopinavir / ritonavir with regard to viral suppression as measured by the average area under the curve minus baseline (AAUCMB) for plasma HIV-1 RNA over 48 weeks (the primary end point). Results were in favour of the lopinavir / ritonavir arm as detailed below.

All patients in this study had failed treatment with a previous protease inhibitor regimen (defined as plasma HIV-1 RNA that never went below 1,000 copies/ml after at least 12 consecutive weeks of therapy, or initial suppression of HIV-1 RNA which subsequently rebounded to ⩾ 1,000 copies/ml). However, only 65 % of patients were receiving a PI based regimen at study entry.

The population enrolled mainly consisted of moderately antiretroviral experienced patients. The median durations of prior exposure to NRTIs were 257 weeks for patients receiving fosamprenavir with ritonavir twice daily (79 % had ⩾ 3 prior NRTIs) and 210 weeks for patients receiving lopinavir/ritonavir (64 % had ⩾ 3 prior NRTIs). The median durations of prior exposure to protease inhibitors were 149 weeks for patients receiving fosamprenavir with ritonavir twice daily (49 % received ⩾ 2 prior PIs) and 130 weeks for patients receiving lopinavir/ritonavir (40 % received ⩾2 prior PIs).

The mean AAUCMBs ($\log_{10}$ c/ml) in the ITT (E) population (Observed analysis) at 48 weeks are described in the table below:

Plasma HIV-1 RNA Average Area Under the Curve Minus Baseline (AAUCMB) Values ($\log_{10}$ copies/ml) at week 48 by Randomisation Strata in APV30003 ITT (E) Population (Observed Analysis)

(see Table 2 below)

When considering the proportion of patients with undetectable viral load in the fosamprenavir with ritonavir twice daily dosing regimens and lopinavir / ritonavir arms respectively, results showed a trend in favour of the lopinavir / ritonavir arms: 58 % versus 61 % (plasma HIV-1 RNA < 400 copies/ml) or 46 % versus 50 % (plasma HIV-1 RNA < 50 copies/ml) at Week 48 (secondary efficacy endpoint) in the intent to treat (RD=F) analysis.

In patients with high viral load at baseline (> 100,000 copies/ml) 7/14 (50 %) patients in the lopinavir / ritonavir group and 6/19 (32 %) patients in the fosamprenavir with ritonavir group had plasma HIV-1 RNA < 400 copies/ml.

The fosamprenavir with ritonavir twice daily regimen and the lopinavir / ritonavir twice daily regimen showed similar immunological improvements through 48 weeks of treatment as measured by median change from baseline in CD4+ cell count (fosamprenavir with ritonavir twice daily: 81 cells/mm^3: lopinavir / ritonavir twice daily: 91 cells/mm^3).

There are insufficient data to recommend the use of fosamprenavir with ritonavir in heavily pre-treated patients.

Children and adolescent patients above the age of six

Fosamprenavir tablets and oral suspension with ritonavir in combination with NRTIs have been evaluated in protease inhibitor naïve and experienced children and adolescent patients. The benefit in this age group has mainly been derived from the ongoing study, APV29005, an open label 48 week study evaluating the pharmacokinetic profiles, safety, and antiviral activity of fosamprenavir with ritonavir administered twice daily to HIV 1 protease inhibitor experienced and naive patients 2 to 18 years of age. Results through 24 weeks of treatment are provided below.

APV29005 enrolled 25 patients aged 6 to 11 (the majority of whom were treated with fosamprenavir / ritonavir 18/3 mg/kg twice daily or the adult tablet regimen) and 29 patients aged 12 to 18 (the majority of whom were treated with the adult tablet regimen). Overall, 27 (50 %) were PI-naïve, 9 of whom were ART naïve, and 27 (50 %) were PI-experienced. Prior NRTI exposure was extensive, with median durations of 421 and 389 weeks for the PI naïve and experienced patients respectively. The median duration of prior PI exposure was 239 weeks. Overall, patients enrolled with a median 4.6 HIV-1 RNA log10 copies/ml (33 % of whom had > 100,000 copies/ml at baseline) and a median % CD4+ cell of 18 % (39 % of whom had % CD4+ of < 15% at baseline).

Through 24 weeks of therapy, 70 % (19/27) of protease inhibitor naive and 56 % (15/27) of protease inhibitor experienced patients achieved and maintained a plasma HIV 1 RNA <400 copies/ml (ITT(E), TLOVR). In the ITT(E) population (Observed analysis) at Week 24 the median % CD4+ cell counts increased by 8 % in the PI-naïve subjects and 4 % in the PI-experienced subjects.

These data were further substantiated by the supportive study APV20003; however, a different dosage regimen than that of study APV29005 was used.

5.2 Pharmacokinetic properties

After oral administration, fosamprenavir is rapidly and almost completely hydrolysed to amprenavir and inorganic phosphate prior to reaching the systemic circulation. The

Table 2

Plasma HIV-1 RNA stratum	Observed analysis FPV/RTV BID N=107 Mean (n)	Observed analysis LPV/RTV BID N=103 Mean (n)	Observed analysis Mean Diff. (97.5% CI) FPV/RTV BID vs LPV/RTV BID
1000 – 10,000 copies/ml	-1.53 (41)	-1.43 (43)	-0.104 (-0.550, 0.342)
>10.000 – 100,000 copies/ml	-1.59 (45)	-1.81 (46)	0.216 (-0.213, 0.664)
>100,000 copies/ml	-1.38 (19)	-2.61 (14)	1.232 (0.512, 1.952)
Total population	-1.53 (105)	-1.76 (103)	0.244 (-0.047, 0.536)

Key: FPV/RTV BID – Fosamprenavir with ritonavir twice daily, LPV/RTV BID – Lopinavir / ritonavir twice daily conversion of fosamprenavir to amprenavir appears to primarily occur in the gut epithelium.

The pharmacokinetic properties of amprenavir following co-administration of Telzir with ritonavir have been evaluated in healthy adult subjects and HIV-infected patients and no substantial differences were observed between these two groups.

Telzir tablet and oral suspension formulations, both given fasted, delivered equivalent plasma amprenavir AUC_{∞} values and the Telzir oral suspension formulation delivered a 14 % higher plasma amprenavir C_{max} as compared to the oral tablet formulation. However, the bioequivalence could not be demonstrated when the oral suspension was given with food. Therefore for adult patients the Telzir oral suspension should be taken **without** food and on an empty stomach (see section 4.2).

Absorption

After single dose administration of fosamprenavir, amprenavir peak plasma concentrations are observed approximately 2 hours after administration. Fosamprenavir AUC values are, in general, less than 1 % of those observed for amprenavir. The absolute bioavailability of fosamprenavir in humans has not been established.

After multiple dose oral administration of equivalent fosamprenavir and amprenavir doses, comparable amprenavir AUC values were observed; however, C_{max} values were approximately 30 % lower and C_{min} values were approximately 28 % higher with fosamprenavir.

After multiple dose oral administration of fosamprenavir 700 mg with ritonavir 100 mg twice daily, amprenavir was rapidly absorbed with a geometric mean (95 % CI) steady state peak plasma amprenavir concentration (C_{max}) of 6.08 (5.38-6.86) μg/ml occurring approximately 1.5 (0.75-5.0) hours after dosing (t_{max}). The mean steady state plasma amprenavir trough concentration (C_{min}) was 2.12 (1.77-2.54) μg/ml and $AUC_{0\text{-}tau}$ was 39.6 (34.5–45.3) h*μg/ml.

Administration of the fosamprenavir oral suspension formulation with a high fat meal (967 kcal, 67 grams fat, 33 grams protein, 58 grams carbohydrate) reduced plasma amprenavir AUC(0-∞) by 28% and C_{max} by 46% and delayed T_{max} by 0.72 hours. For adult patients the fosamprenavir oral suspension should be taken **without** food and on an empty stomach. In children and adolescents the fosamprenavir oral suspension should be taken **with food**. The dose recommendations for this population therefore take into account the observed food effect (see section 4.2).

Co-administration of amprenavir with grapefruit juice was not associated with clinically significant changes in plasma amprenavir pharmacokinetics.

Distribution

The apparent volume of distribution of amprenavir following administration of Telzir is approximately 430 l (6 l/kg assuming a 70 kg body weight), suggesting a large volume of distribution, with penetration of amprenavir freely into tissues beyond the systemic circulation. This value is decreased by approximately 40 % when Telzir is co-administered with ritonavir, most likely due to an increase in amprenavir bioavailability.

In *in vitro* studies, the protein binding of amprenavir is approximately 90 %. It is bound to the alpha-1-acid glycoprotein (AAG) and albumin, but has a higher affinity for AAG. Concentrations of AAG have been shown to decrease during the course of antiretroviral therapy. This change will decrease the total active substance concentration in the plasma, however the amount of unbound amprenavir, which is the active moiety, is likely to be unchanged.

CSF penetration of amprenavir is negligible in humans. Amprenavir appears to penetrate into semen, though semen concentrations are lower than plasma concentrations.

Metabolism

Fosamprenavir is rapidly and almost completely hydrolysed to amprenavir and inorganic phosphate as it is absorbed through the gut epithelium, following oral administration. Amprenavir is primarily metabolised by the liver with less than 1 % excreted unchanged in the urine. The primary route of metabolism is via the cytochrome P450 3A4 enzyme. Amprenavir metabolism is inhibited by ritonavir, via inhibition of CYP3A4, resulting in increased plasma concentrations of amprenavir. Amprenavir in addition is also an inhibitor of the CYP3A4 enzyme, although to a lesser extent than ritonavir. Therefore medicinal products that are inducers, inhibitors or substrates of CYP3A4 must be used with caution when administered concurrently with Telzir with ritonavir (see sections 4.3 and 4.5).

Elimination

Following administration of Telzir, the half-life of amprenavir is 7.7 hours. When Telzir is co-administered with ritonavir, the half-life of amprenavir is increased to 15 – 23 hours.

The primary route of elimination of amprenavir is via hepatic metabolism with less than 1 % excreted unchanged in the urine and no detectable amprenavir in faeces. Metabolites account for approximately 14 % of the administered amprenavir dose in the urine, and approximately 75 % in the faeces.

Special populations

Paediatrics

In a clinical study on pharmacokinetics of fosamprenavir in paediatric patients, eight subjects 12 to 18 years of age received the standard fosamprenavir adult tablet dose of 700 mg twice daily (with ritonavir 100 mg twice daily). Compared to the historical adult population receiving fosamprenavir / ritonavir 700 / 100 mg twice daily, 12 to 18 year old subjects had 20 % lower plasma APV AUC(0-24), 23 % lower C_{max}, and 20 % lower C_{min} values. Children 6 to 11 years of age (n=9) receiving fosamprenavir / ritonavir 18 / 3 mg/kg twice daily had 26 % higher AUC(0-24) and similar C_{max} and C_{min} values when compared to the historical adult population receiving fosamprenavir / ritonavir 700 / 100 mg twice daily.

APV20002 is a 48 week, Phase II, open label study designed to evaluate the pharmacokinetics, safety, tolerability and antiviral activity of fosamprenavir with and without ritonavir in paediatric subjects 4 weeks to < 2 years of age. Compared to the historical adult population receiving fosamprenavir with ritonavir 700 mg / 100 mg twice daily, a subset of five pediatric subjects ages 6 to < 24-months receiving fosamprenavir / ritonavir 45/7 mg/kg twice daily demonstrated that despite an approximate 5-fold increase in fosamprenavir and ritonavir doses on a mg/kg basis, plasma amprenavir AUC(0-τ) was approximately 48 % lower, C_{max} 26 % lower, and Cτ 29 % lower in the paediatric subjects. No dosing recommendations can be made for the very young (children < 2 years of age) and Telzir with ritonavir is not recommended for this patient population (see section 4.2).

Elderly

The pharmacokinetics of fosamprenavir in combination with ritonavir has not been studied in patients over 65 years of age.

Renal impairment

Patients with renal impairment have not been specifically studied. Less than 1 % of the therapeutic dose of amprenavir is excreted unchanged in the urine. Renal clearance of ritonavir is also negligible, therefore the impact of renal impairment on amprenavir and ritonavir elimination should be minimal.

Hepatic impairment

Fosamprenavir is converted in man to amprenavir. The principal route of amprenavir and ritonavir elimination is hepatic metabolism.

The plasma amprenavir pharmacokinetics were evaluated in a 14 day repeat-dose study in HIV-1 infected adult subjects with mild, moderate, or severe hepatic impairment receiving fosamprenavir with ritonavir compared to matched control subjects with normal hepatic function.

In subjects with mild hepatic impairment (Child-Pugh score of 5-6), the dosage regimen of fosamprenavir 700 mg twice daily with a reduced dosing frequency of ritonavir 100 mg once daily provided slightly higher plasma amprenavir C_{max} (17 %), slightly higher plasma amprenavir AUC(0-12) (22 %), similar plasma total amprenavir C12 values and approximately 117 % higher plasma unbound amprenavir C12 values compared to subjects with normal hepatic function receiving the standard fosamprenavir / ritonavir 700 mg /100 mg twice daily regimen.

In subjects with moderate hepatic impairment (Child-Pugh score of 7-9), a reduced dose of fosamprenavir 450 mg twice daily with a reduced dosing frequency of ritonavir 100 mg once daily is predicted to deliver similar plasma amprenavir C_{max} and AUC(0-12), but approximately 35 % lower plasma total amprenavir C12 values and approximately 88 % higher plasma unbound amprenavir C12 values than achieved in subjects with normal hepatic function receiving the standard fosamprenavir with ritonavir 700 mg / 100 mg twice daily regimen.

In subjects with severe hepatic impairment (Child-Pugh score of 10-13), a reduced dose of fosamprenavir 300 mg twice daily with a reduced dosing frequency of ritonavir 100 mg once daily delivered 19% lower plasma amprenavir Cmax, 23% lower AUC(0-12), and 38% lower C12 values, but similar unbound plasma amprenavir C12 values than achieved in subjects with normal hepatic function receiving the standard fosamprenavir with ritonavir 700 mg / 100 mg twice daily regimen. Despite reducing the dosing frequency of ritonavir, subjects with severe hepatic impairment had 64% higher ritonavir Cmax, 40% higher ritonavir AUC(0-24), and 38% higher ritonavir C12 than achieved in subjects with normal hepatic function receiving the standard fosamprenavir with ritonavir 700 mg / 100 mg twice daily regimen.

Fosamprenavir with ritonavir was generally well-tolerated in subjects with mild, moderate, or severe hepatic impairment, and these regimens had similar adverse event and clinical laboratory profiles as previous studies of HIV-1 infected subjects with normal hepatic function.

5.3 Preclinical safety data

Toxicity was similar to that of amprenavir and occurred at amprenavir plasma exposure levels below human exposure after treatment with fosamprenavir in combination with ritonavir at the recommended dose.

In repeated dose toxicity studies in adult rats and dogs, fosamprenavir produced evidence of gastrointestinal disturbances (salivation, vomiting and soft to liquid faeces), and hepatic changes (increased liver weights, raised serum liver enzyme activities and microscopic changes, including hepatocyte necrosis). Toxicity was not aggravated when juvenile animals were treated as compared with adult animals, but the data did indicate a steeper dose response.

In reproductive toxicity studies with fosamprenavir in rats, male fertility was not affected, but in females gravid uterine weights, numbers of ovarian corpora lutea and uterine implantation sites were reduced. In pregnant rats and rabbits there were no major effects on embryo-foetal development. However, the number of abortions increased. In rabbits, systemic exposure at the high dose level was only 0.3 times human exposure at the maximum clinical dose and thus the development toxicity of fosamprenavir has not been fully determined. In rats exposed pre- and post-natally to fosamprenavir, pups showed impaired physical and functional development and reduced growth. Pup survival was decreased. In addition, decreased number of implantation sites per litter and a prolongation of gestation were seen when pups were mated after reaching maturity.

Fosamprenavir was not mutagenic or genotoxic in a standard battery of *in vitro* and *in vivo* assays. In long-term carcinogenicity studies with fosamprenavir in mice and rats, there were increases in hepatocellular adenomas and hepatocellular carcinomas in mice at exposure levels equivalent to 0.1 to 0.3-fold those in humans given 700 mg of fosamprenavir plus 100mg ritonavir twice daily, and increases in hepatocellular adenomas and thyroid follicular cell adenomas in rats at exposure levels equivalent to 0.3 to 0.6-fold those in humans given 700 mg of fosamprenavir plus 100mg ritonavir twice daily. The relevance of the hepatocellular findings in the rodents for humans is uncertain; however, there is no evidence from clinical trials or marketed use to suggest that these findings are of clinical significance. Repeat dose studies with fosamprenavir in rats produced effects consistent with hepatic enzyme induction, which predisposes rats to thyroid neoplasms. The thyroid tumorigenic potential is regarded to be species-specific. The clinical relevance of these findings is unknown. In rats only there was an increase in interstitial cell hyperplasia in males at exposure levels equivalent to 0.5-fold those in humans, and an increase in uterine endometrial adenocarcinoma in females at an exposure level equivalent to 1.1-fold those in humans. The incidence of endometrial findings was slightly increased over concurrent controls, but within background range for female rats. The relevance of the uterine endometrial adenocarcinomas for humans is uncertain; however there is no evidence from clinical trials or marketed use to suggest that these findings are of clinical significance.

6. PHARMACEUTICAL PARTICULARS

6.1 List of excipients

Hypromellose

Sucralose

Propylene glycol

Methyl parahydroxybenzoate (E218)

Propyl parahydroxybenzoate (E216)

Polysorbate 80

Calcium chloride dihydrate

Artificial grape bubblegum flavour

Natural peppermint flavour

Purified water

6.2 Incompatibilities

In the absence of compatibility studies, this medicinal product must not be mixed with other medicinal products.

6.3 Shelf life

2 years.

Discard 28 days after first opening.

6.4 Special precautions for storage

Do not freeze.

6.5 Nature and contents of container

HDPE bottle with a child resistant polypropylene closure containing 225 millilitres oral suspension.

A 10 ml graduated polypropylene dosing syringe and polyethylene adapter are provided in the pack.

6.6 Special precautions for disposal and other handling

Any unused product should be disposed of in accordance with local requirements.

7. MARKETING AUTHORISATION HOLDER

Glaxo Group Ltd

Greenford Road

Greenford

Middlesex UB6 0NN

United Kingdom

8. MARKETING AUTHORISATION NUMBER(S)

EU/1/04/282/002

9. DATE OF FIRST AUTHORISATION/RENEWAL OF THE AUTHORISATION

Date of first authorisation: 12 July 2004

10. DATE OF REVISION OF THE TEXT

15 May 2009

Detailed information on this medicinal product is available on the website of the European Medicines Agency (EMEA) http://www.emea.europa.eu

Tenif

(AstraZeneca UK Limited)

1. NAME OF THE MEDICINAL PRODUCT
Tenif

2. QUALITATIVE AND QUANTITATIVE COMPOSITION
Atenolol 50 mg
Nifedipine 20 mg
For excipients, see Section 6.1

3. PHARMACEUTICAL FORM
Capsules

Reddish brown capsules containing atenolol and a slow release formulation of nifedipine.

4. CLINICAL PARTICULARS

4.1 Therapeutic indications
Management of hypertension where therapy with either a calcium channel blocker or a beta-blocking drug proves inadequate.

Management of chronic stable angina pectoris where therapy with a calcium channel blocker or a beta-adrenoceptor blocking drug proves inadequate.

4.2 Posology and method of administration
For administration by the oral route.

Adults

Hypertension: One capsule daily swallowed with water. If necessary, the dosage may be increased to 1 capsule dosed every 12 hours. Patients can be transferred to the combination from other antihypertensive treatments with the *exception of clonidine* (see Section 4.4).

Angina: One capsule every 12 hours swallowed with water. Where additional efficacy is necessary, prophylactic nitrate therapy or additional nifedipine may be of benefit.

Elderly

Dosage should not exceed 1 capsule daily in hypertension or 1 capsule twice daily in angina.

The pharmacokinetics of nifedipine are altered in the elderly so that lower maintenance doses of nifedipine may be required compared to younger patients.

Children

There is no paediatric experience with Tenif and therefore Tenif should not be used in children.

Renal Impairment

Tenif should not be used in patients with marked renal impairment (see Section 4.3)

4.3 Contraindications
Tenif should not be used in patients with any of the following conditions:

- known hypersensitivity to either active component, or any other excipient or other dihydropyridines because of the theoretical risk of cross-reactivity;
- bradycardia;
- cardiogenic shock;
- hypotension;
- metabolic acidosis;
- severe peripheral arterial circulatory disturbances;
- second or third degree heart block;
- sick sinus syndrome;
- untreated phaeochromocytoma;
- uncontrolled heart failure;
- women capable of childbearing or during pregnancy or during lactation;
- patients with clinically significant aortic stenosis;
- patients with marked renal impairment (i.e. creatinine clearance below 15 ml/min/1.73 m^2; serum creatinine greater than 600 micromol/litre);
- patients receiving calcium channel blockers with negative inotropic effects eg.
verapamil and diltiazem; unstable angina;
- during or within one month of a myocardial infarction.

Tenif should not be used for the treatment of acute attacks of angina.

The safety of Tenif in malignant hypertension has not been established.

Tenif should not be used for secondary prevention of myocardial infarction.

Due to the nifedipine component, Tenif should not be administered in combination with rifampicin because plasma levels of nifedipine, predictive of efficacy, may not be attained due to enzyme induction. (see Section 4.5).

4.4 Special warnings and precautions for use
Due to its beta-blocker component, Tenif:

• Although contraindicated in uncontrolled heart failure (see section 4.3), may be substituted with care in patients already treated with a beta-blocking drug, and/or whose signs of heart failure have been controlled. Caution must be exercised in patients with conduction defects or whose cardiac reserve is poor, especially as nifedipine also has negative inotropic effects. However, in patients already treated with a beta-blocker and/or where signs of cardiac failure have been controlled, Tenif may be substituted with care if necessary.

• May increase the number and duration of angina attacks in patients with Prinzmetal's angina due to unopposed alpha-receptor mediated coronary artery vasoconstriction. Atenolol is a beta$_1$-selective beta-blocking drug; consequently, the use of Tenif may be considered although utmost caution must be exercised.

• Although contra-indicated in severe peripheral arterial circulatory disturbances (see section 4.3), may also aggravate less severe peripheral arterial circulatory disturbances.

• Due to its negative effect on conduction time, caution must be exercised if it is given to patients with first-degree heart block.

• May modify the tachycardia of hypoglycaemia.

• May mask the signs of thyrotoxicosis.

• Will reduce heart rate, as a result of its pharmacological action. In the rare instances when a treated patient develops symptoms, which may be attributable to a slow heart rate, the dose may be reduced.

• Should not be discontinued abruptly in patients suffering from ischaemic heart disease.

• May cause a more severe reaction to a variety of allergens, when given to patients with a history of anaphylactic reaction to such allergens. Such patients may be unresponsive to the usual doses of adrenaline (epinephrine) used to treat the allergic reactions.

• May cause a hypersensitivity reaction including angioedema and urticaria.

Obstructive airways disease

Tenif contains the cardioselective beta-blocking drug atenolol. Although cardioselective (beta$_1$) beta-blocking drugs may have less effect on lung function than non-selective beta-blocking drugs, as with all beta-blocking drugs, these should be avoided in patients with reversible obstructive airways disease, unless there are compelling clinical reasons for their use. Where such reasons exist, Tenif may be used with caution. Occasionally, some increase in airways resistance may occur in asthmatic patients, however, and this may usually be reversed by commonly used dosage of bronchodilators such as salbutamol or isoprenaline.

The label and patient information leaflet for this product state the following warning: "If you have ever had asthma or wheezing, you should not take this medicine unless you have discussed these symptoms with the prescribing doctor".

Due to its nifedipine component it should be noted that:

• In rare cases, a transient increase in blood glucose has been observed with nifedipine in acute studies. This should be considered in patients suffering from diabetes mellitus. Nifedipine has no diabetogenic effect.

• Ischaemic pain occurs in a small proportion of patients following introduction of nifedipine monotherapy. Although a "steal" effect has not been demonstrated, patients experiencing this effect should discontinue nifedipine therapy.

• In single cases of *in vitro* fertilisation, calcium antagonists like nifedipine have been associated with reversible biochemical changes in the spermatozoa's head section that may result in impaired sperm function. In those men who are repeatedly unsuccessful in fathering a child by *in vitro* fertilisation and where no other explanation can be found, calcium antagonists like nifedipine should be considered as possible causes.

Hypertensive or anginal patients with clinically significant liver disease have not been studied and no dosage adjustment is suggested from the systemic availability of the monocomponents in patients with cirrhosis. However nifedipine is metabolised primarily by the liver and therefore patients with liver dysfunction should be carefully monitored. As a precaution, it is recommended that the dose should not exceed one capsule daily.

4.5 Interaction with other medicinal products and other forms of interaction
Tenif must not be used in conjunction with calcium channel blockers with negative inotropic effects e.g. verapamil, diltiazem since this can lead to an exaggeration of these effects particularly in patients with impaired ventricular function and/or sino-atrial or atrioventricular conduction abnormalities. This may result in severe hypotension, bradycardia and cardiac failure (see section 4.3).

Concomitant therapy with additional dihydropyridines e.g. nifedipine, may increase the risk of hypotension, and cardiac failure may occur in patients with latent cardiac insufficiency.

Atenolol monotherapy:

Digitalis glycosides, in association with beta-blocking drugs, may increase atrioventricular conduction time.

Beta-blocking drugs may exacerbate the rebound hypertension, which can follow the withdrawal of clonidine. If the two drugs are co-administered, the beta-blocking drug should be withdrawn several days before discontinuing clonidine. If replacing clonidine by beta-blocking drug therapy, the introduction of beta-blocking drugs should be delayed for several days after clonidine administration has stopped.

Class I anti-arrhythmic drugs (eg, disopyramide) and amiodarone may have a potentiating effect on atrial-conduction time and induce negative inotropic effect.

Concomitant use of sympathomimetic agents, e.g. adrenaline (epinephrine), may counteract the effect of beta-blocking drugs.

Concomitant use with insulin and oral antidiabetic drugs may lead to the intensification of the blood sugar-lowering effects of these drugs.

Concomitant use of prostaglandin synthetase-inhibiting drugs, e.g. ibuprofen or indometacin, may decrease the hypotensive effects of beta-blocking drugs.

Caution must be exercised when using anaesthetic agents with Tenif. The anaesthetist should be informed and the choice of anaesthetic should be the agent with as little negative inotropic activity as possible. Use of beta-blocking drugs with anaesthetic drugs may result in attenuation of the reflex tachycardia and increase the risk of hypotension. Anaesthetic agents causing myocardial depression are best avoided.

Nifedipine monotherapy:

The antihypertensive effect of nifedipine can be potentiated by simultaneous administration of cimetidine.

The simultaneous administration of nifedipine and quinidine may lead to serum quinidine levels being suppressed regardless of dosage of quinidine.

The simultaneous administration of nifedipine and digoxin may lead to reduced digoxin clearance and hence an increase in the plasma digoxin level. Patients' plasma digoxin levels should be monitored and, if necessary, the digoxin dose reduced.

As with other dihydropyridines, nifedipine should not be taken with grapefruit juice because bioavailability is increased.

Due to enzyme induction, rifampicin has been shown to decrease the nifedipine AUC and C_{max} by 95% 288 ng l/ml to 8 ng l/ml and 154 ng/ml to 7.5 ng/ml respectively. This may result in reduced efficacy, therefore **co-administration of nifedipine is contraindicated** (see section 4.3).

Nifedipine may cause falsely increased spectrophotometric values of urinary vanillylmandelic acid. However, measurement with HPLC is unaffected.

4.6 Pregnancy and lactation
Tenif is contraindicated in women capable of childbearing or during pregnancy or during lactation (see Section 4.3).

4.7 Effects on ability to drive and use machines
The use of Tenif is unlikely to result in any impairment of the ability of patients to drive or operate machinery. However, it should be taken into account that occasionally dizziness or fatigue may occur.

4.8 Undesirable effects
Tenif is well tolerated. In clinical studies, the undesired events reported are usually attributed to the pharmacological actions of its components.

The following undesired events, listed by body system, have been reported:

Tenif

Cardiovascular: flushing, oedema

CNS: dizziness, headache

Gastrointestinal: gastrointestinal disturbance

Haematological: purpura

Reproductive: impotence

Others: fatigue

Atenolol monotherapy

Cardiovascular: bradycardia, heart failure deterioration, postural hypotension which may be associated with syncope, cold extremities. In susceptible patients: precipitation of heart block, intermittent claudication, Raynaud's phenomenon.

CNS: confusion, dizziness, headache, mood changes, nightmares, psychoses and hallucinations, sleep disturbances of the type noted with other beta-blockers.

Gastrointestinal: dry mouth, gastrointestinal disturbances, elevations of transaminase levels have been seen infrequently, rare cases of hepatic toxicity including intrahepatic cholestasis have been reported.

Haematological: purpura, thrombocytopenia.

Integumentary: alopecia, dry eyes, psoriasiform skin reactions, exacerbation of psoriasis, skin rashes.

Neurological: paraesthesia.

Respiratory: bronchospasm may occur in patients with bronchial asthma or a history of asthmatic complaints.

Reproductive: impotence

Special senses: visual disturbances.

Others: hypersensitivity reaction, including angioedema and urticaria, an increase in ANA (antinuclear antibodies) has been observed, however the clinical relevance of this is not clear. Fatigue.

Nifedipine monotherapy

Cardiovascular: palpitations, tachycardia, gravitational oedema, marked reduction in blood pressure in dialysis patients with malignant hypertension and hypovolaemia.

Neurological: paraesthesia.

Respiratory: dyspnoea.

Gastrointestinal: gingival hyperplasia, hypersensitivity type jaundice and disturbances of liver function such as increased transaminase or intrahepatic cholestasis which regress after discontinuing therapy.

Haematological: agranulocytosis.

Integumentary: skin reactions such as pruritus, urticaria, photosensitive dermatitis, exanthema and exfoliative dermatitis, erythromelalgia and systemic allergic reactions.

Musculoskeletal: myalgia, tremor (both after high doses).

Urogenital: increased frequency of micturition, gynaecomastia (in older men on long term therapy, which usually regresses on withdrawal of therapy).

As with other sustained release dihydropyridines, exacerbation of angina pectoris may occur rarely at the start of treatment with sustained release formulations of nifedipine. The occurrence of myocardial infarction has been described although it is not possible to distinguish such an event from the natural course of ischaemic heart disease.

Discontinuance of Tenif should be considered if, according to clinical judgement, the well-being of the patient is adversely affected by any of the above reactions.

4.9 Overdose

Symptoms

The symptoms of overdosage may include bradycardia, hypotension, acute cardiac insufficiency and bronchospasm.

Treatment

General treatment should include: close supervision, treatment in an intensive care ward, the use of gastric lavage, activated charcoal and a laxative to prevent absorption of any drug still present in the gastrointestinal tract, the use of plasma or plasma substitutes to treat hypotension and shock. The possible use of haemodialysis or haemoperfusion may be considered.

Excessive bradycardia can be countered with atropine 1 to 2 mg intravenously and/or a cardiac pacemaker. If necessary, this may be followed by a bolus dose of glucagon 10 mg intravenously. If required, this may be repeated or followed by an intravenous infusion of glucagon 1 to 10 mg/hour depending on response. Intravenous calcium gluconate combined with metaraminol may be beneficial for hypotension induced by nifedipine. If no response to glucagon occurs or if glucagon is unavailable, a beta-adrenoceptor stimulant such as dobutamine 2.5 to 10 micrograms/kg/minute by intravenous infusion may be given. Dobutamine, because of its positive inotropic effect could also be used to treat hypotension and acute cardiac insufficiency. It is likely that these doses would be inadequate to reverse the cardiac effects of beta-blockade if a large overdose has been taken. The dose of dobutamine should therefore be increased if necessary to achieve the required response according to the clinical condition of the patient. In severe cases of hypotension cardiac pacing with appropriate cardiorespiratory support may be necessary.

Bronchospasm can usually be reversed by bronchodilators.

5. PHARMACOLOGICAL PROPERTIES

5.1 Pharmacodynamic properties

CO7 FB

Beta-blocking agents, selective and other antihypertensives.

Atenolol is a beta-blocking drug which is beta$_1$selective (i.e. acts preferentially on beta$_1$-adrenergic receptors in the heart). Selectivity decreases with increasing dose.

Atenolol is without intrinsic sympathomimetic and membrane stabilising activities and as with other beta-blocking drugs, atenolol has negative inotropic effects (and is therefore contraindicated in uncontrolled heart failure).

As with other beta-blocking drugs, its mode of action in the treatment of hypertension is unclear.

It is probably the action of atenolol in reducing cardiac rate and contractility which makes it effective in eliminating or reducing the symptoms of patients with angina.

Atenolol is effective and well-tolerated in most ethnic populations although the response may be less in black patients.

It is unlikely that any additional ancillary properties possessed by S (-) atenolol, in comparison with the racemic mixture, will give rise to different therapeutic effects.

Nifedipine is a calcium channel blocker. It is a powerful coronary and peripheral vasodilator which increases myocardial oxygen supply and reduces blood pressure (afterload) and peripheral resistance. Concomitant use of atenolol, therefore, ameliorates the reflex sympathetic response to nifedipine monotherapy by blocking the rise in heart rate, while the tendency of atenolol to increase peripheral resistance is balanced by the vasodilation and increased sympathetic tone induced by the calcium antagonist.

Consequently, greater antihypertensive or antianginal efficacy is achieved by the concomitant use of nifedipine and atenolol than either drug alone. This beneficial pharmacodynamic interaction also results in fewer side effects when lower dosages of the two drugs are used in combination.

5.2 Pharmacokinetic properties

Absorption of atenolol following oral dosing is consistent but incomplete (approximately 40 to 50%) with peak plasma concentrations occurring 2 to 4 hours after dosing. The atenolol blood levels are consistent and subject to little variability. There is no significant hepatic metabolism of atenolol and more than 90% of that absorbed reaches the systemic circulation unaltered. The plasma half-life is about 6 hours but this may rise in severe renal impairment since the kidney is the major route of elimination. Atenolol penetrates tissues poorly due to its low lipid solubility and its concentration in brain tissue is low. Plasma protein binding is low (approximately 3%). Absorption of nifedipine following oral dosing is complete with peak plasma concentrations occurring about 3 hours after dosing. Nifedipine is >90% plasma protein bound. There is significant hepatic metabolism of nifedipine. The plasma half-life is between 6 and 11 hours for the sustained formulation of nifedipine.

Co-administration of atenolol and nifedipine has little effect on the pharmacokinetics of either. In the elderly, the systemic bioavailability and elimination half-life of both components are increased.

Tenif is effective when given either once or twice daily. This simplicity of dosing facilitates compliance by its acceptability to patients.

5.3 Preclinical safety data

Atenolol and nifedipine are drugs on which extensive clinical experience has been obtained. Relevant information for the prescriber is provided elsewhere in the Prescribing Information.

6. PHARMACEUTICAL PARTICULARS

6.1 List of excipients

Gelatin

Iron Oxide Red (E172)

Lactose

Macrogol

Maize starch

Magnesium carbonate

Magnesium stearate

Methylhydroxypropylcellulose

Microcrystalline cellulose

Polysorbate

Sodium Laurilsulfate

Titanium dioxide (E171)

6.2 Incompatibilities

Not applicable

6.3 Shelf life

48 months

6.4 Special precautions for storage

Do not store above 30°C. Protect from light and moisture Store in original package. Keep the container in the outer carton.

6.5 Nature and contents of container

PVC/PVDC/AL Blister strips of 28 capsules.

6.6 Special precautions for disposal and other handling

None

7. MARKETING AUTHORISATION HOLDER

AstraZeneca UK Limited,

600 Capability Green,

Luton, LU1 3LU, UK.

8. MARKETING AUTHORISATION NUMBER(S)

PL 17901/0047

9. DATE OF FIRST AUTHORISATION/RENEWAL OF THE AUTHORISATION

1st June 2000 / 7th December 2004

10. DATE OF REVISION OF THE TEXT

18th December 2007

Tenoret 50

(AstraZeneca UK Limited)

1. NAME OF THE MEDICINAL PRODUCT

Tenoret 50 Film-coated Tablets

2. QUALITATIVE AND QUANTITATIVE COMPOSITION

Atenolol. 50mg

Chlortalidone 12.5 mg

For excipients, see Section 6.1

3. PHARMACEUTICAL FORM

Film-coated tablets.

Brown, biconvex, film-coated tablet imprinted with the name Tenoret 50 on one face, and an 'S' logo on the reverse.

4. CLINICAL PARTICULARS

4.1 Therapeutic indications

The management of hypertension, particularly suited to older patients.

4.2 Posology and method of administration

Tenoret 50 Film-coated Tablets are administered orally.

Adults

One tablet daily.

Elderly

One tablet daily. Older patients with hypertension who do not respond to low dose therapy with a single agent should have a satisfactory response to a single tablet daily of Tenoret 50 Film-coated Tablets. Where hypertensive control is not achieved, addition of a small dose of a third agent e.g. as a vasodilator, may be appropriate.

Children

There is no paediatric experience with Tenoret 50 Film-coated Tablets, therefore this preparation is not recommended for children.

Renal Impairment

In patients with renal impairment a reduction in daily dose or in frequency of administration may be necessary. (See Section 4.4).

4.3 Contraindications

Tenoret 50 Film-coated Tablets should not be used in patients with any of the following:

- known hypersensitivity to either active component or any of the excipients;
- bradycardia;
- cardiogenic shock;
- hypotension;
- metabolic acidosis;
- severe peripheral arterial circulatory disturbances;
- second- or third-degree heart block;
- sick sinus syndrome;
- untreated phaeochromocytoma;
- uncontrolled heart failure.

Tenoret 50 Film-coated Tablets must not be given during pregnancy or lactation.

4.4 Special warnings and precautions for use

Due to its beta-blocker component Tenoret 50 Film-coated Tablets:

- although contraindicated in uncontrolled heart failure (See Section 4.3), may be used in patients whose signs of heart failure have been controlled. Caution must be exercised in patients whose cardiac reserve is poor.
- may increase the number and duration of angina attacks in patients with Prinzmetal's angina due to unopposed alpha receptor mediated coronary artery vasoconstriction. Atenolol is a beta$_1$-selective beta-blocker; consequently the use of Tenoret 50 Film-Coated Tablets may be considered although utmost caution must be exercised.
- although contraindicated in severe peripheral arterial circulatory disturbances (See Section 4.3), may also aggravate less severe peripheral arterial circulatory disturbances.
- due to its negative effect on conduction time, caution must be exercised if it is given to patients with first-degree heart block.
- may modify the tachycardia of hypoglycaemia.
- may mask the signs of thyrotoxicosis.
- will reduce heart rate, as a result of its pharmacological action. In the rare instances when a treated patient develops symptoms which may be attributable to a slow heart rate, the dose may be reduced.
- should not be discontinued abruptly in patients suffering from ischaemic heart disease.
- may cause a more severe reaction to a variety of allergens, when given to patients with a history of anaphylactic reactions to such allergens. Such patients may be unresponsive to the usual doses of adrenaline used to treat the allergic reactions.
- may cause a hypersensitivity reaction including angioedema and urticaria.

Tenoret 50 Film-coated Tablets contain the cardioselective beta-blocker atenolol. Although cardioselective (beta$_1$) beta-blockers may have less effect on lung function than non-selective beta-blockers, as with all beta-blockers, these should be avoided in patients with reversible obstructive airways disease, unless there are compelling clinical reasons for their use. Where such reasons exist, Tenoret 50 Film-coated Tablets may be used with caution. Occasionally, some increase in airways resistance may occur in asthmatic patients, however, and this may usually be reversed by commonly used dosage of bronchodilators such as salbutamol or isoprenaline.

The label and patient information leaflet for this product state the following warning: "If you have ever had asthma or wheezing, you should not take this medicine unless you have discussed these symptoms with the prescribing doctor".

Due to its chlortalidone component:

- hypokalaemia may occur. Measurement of potassium levels is appropriate, especially in the older patient, those receiving digitalis preparations for cardiac failure, those taking an abnormal (low in potassium) diet or those suffering from gastrointestinal complaints. Hypokalaemia may predispose to arrhythmias in patients receiving digitalis;
- caution must be exercised in patients with severe renal failure (See Section 4.2);

- impaired glucose tolerance may occur and caution must be exercised if chlortalidone is administered to patients with a known pre-disposition to diabetes mellitus;

- hyperuricaemia may occur. Only a minor increase in serum uric acid usually occurs but in cases of prolonged elevation, the concurrent use of a uricosuric agent will reverse the hyperuricaemia.

4.5 Interaction with other medicinal products and other forms of interaction

Combined use of beta-blockers and calcium channel blockers with negative inotropic effects, e.g. verapamil, diltiazem, can lead to an exaggeration of these effects particularly in patients with impaired ventricular function and/or sino-atrial or atrio-ventricular conduction abnormalities. This may result in severe hypotension, bradycardia and cardiac failure. Neither the beta-blocker nor the calcium channel blocker should be administered intravenously within 48 hours of discontinuing the other.

Concomitant therapy with dihydropyridines e.g. nifedipine, may increase the risk of hypotension, and cardiac failure may occur in patients with latent cardiac insufficiency.

Digitalis glycosides, in association with beta-blockers, may increase atrio-ventricular conduction time.

Beta-blockers may exacerbate the rebound hypertension which can follow the withdrawal of clonidine. If the two drugs are co-administered, the beta-blocker should be withdrawn several days before discontinuing clonidine. If replacing clonidine by beta-blocker therapy, the introduction of -blockers should be delayed for several days after clonidine administration has stopped.

Class I anti-arrhythmic drugs (e.g. disopyramide) and amiodarone may have a potentiating effect on atrial-conduction time and induce negative inotropic effect.

Concomitant use of sympathomimetic agents, e.g. adrenaline (epinephrine), may counteract the effect of beta-blockers.

Concomitant use with insulin and oral antidiabetic drugs may lead to the intensification of the blood sugar lowering effects of these drugs.

Concomitant use of prostaglandin synthetase-inhibiting drugs e.g. ibuprofen and indometacin, may decrease the hypotensive effects beta-blockers.

Preparations containing lithium should not be given with diuretics because they may reduce its renal clearance.

Caution must be exercised when using anaesthetic agents with Tenoret 50 Film-coated Tablets. The anaesthetist should be informed and the choice of anaesthetic should be an agent with as little negative inotropic activity as possible. Use of beta-blockers with anaesthetic drugs may result in attenuation of the reflex tachycardia and increase the risk of hypotension. Anaesthetic agents causing myocardial depression are best avoided.

4.6 Pregnancy and lactation

Pregnancy:

Tenoret 50 Film-coated Tablets must not be given during pregnancy

Lactation:

Tenoret 50 Film-coated Tablets must not be given during lactation.

4.7 Effects on ability to drive and use machines

Use is unlikely to result in any impairment of the ability of patients to drive or operate machinery. However, it should be taken into account that occasionally dizziness or fatigue may occur.

4.8 Undesirable effects

Tenoret 50 Film-Coated Tablets were well tolerated in clinical studies, the undesired events reported are usually attributable to the pharmacological actions of its components.

The following undesirable effects, listed by body system, have been reported with the following frequencies: Very common ($\geqslant$10%), common (1-9.9%), uncommon (0.1-0.9%), rare (0.01-0.09%), very rare ($<$0.01%), not known (cannot be estimated from the available data):

Blood and lymphatic system disorders:

Rare: Purpura, thrombocytopenia, leucopenia (related to chlortalidone).

Psychiatric disorders:

Uncommon: Sleep disturbances of the type noted with other beta blockers.

Rare: Mood changes, nightmares, confusion, psychoses and hallucinations.

Nervous system disorders:

Rare: Dizziness, headache, paraesthesia.

Eye disorders:

Rare: Dry eyes, visual disturbances.

Cardiac disorders:

Common: Bradycardia

Rare: Heart failure deterioration, precipitation of heart block.

Vascular disorders:

Common: Cold extremities.

Rare: Postural hypotension which may be associated with syncope, intermittent claudication may be increased if already present, in susceptible patients Raynaud's phenomenon.

Respiratory, thoracic and mediastinal disorders:

Rare: Bronchospasm may occur in patients with bronchial asthma or a history of asthmatic complaints.

Gastrointestinal disorders:

Common: Gastrointestinal disturbances (including nausea related to chlortalidone).

Rare: Dry mouth.

Hepatobiliary disorders:

Rare: Hepatic toxicity including intrahepatic cholestasis, pancreatitis (related to chlortalidone).

Skin and subcutaneous tissue disorders:

Rare: Alopecia, psoriasiform skin reaction, exacerbation of psoriasis, skin rashes.

Not known: Hypersensitivity reactions, including angioedema and urticaria.

Reproductive system and breast disorders:

Rare: Impotence.

General disorders and administration site conditions:

Common: Fatigue.

Investigations:

Common: Related to chlortalidone: Hyperuricaemia, hyponatraemia, hypokalaemia, impaired glucose tolerance.

Uncommon: Elevations of transaminase levels.

Very rare: An increase in ANA (Antinuclear Antibodies) has been observed, however the clinical relevance of this is not clear.

Discontinuance of Tenoret 50 Film-coated Tablets should be considered if, according to clinical judgement, the well-being of the patient is adversely affected by any of the above reactions.

4.9 Overdose

The symptoms of overdosage may include bradycardia, hypotension, acute cardiac insufficiency and bronchospasm.

General treatment should include: close supervision, treatment in an intensive care ward, the use of gastric lavage, activated charcoal and a laxative to prevent absorption of any drug still present in the gastrointestinal tract, the use of plasma or plasma substitutes to treat hypotension and shock. The possible use of haemodialysis or haemoperfusion may be considered.

Excessive bradycardia can be countered with atropine 1-2 mg intravenously and/or a cardiac pacemaker. If necessary, this may be followed by a bolus dose of glucagon 10 mg intravenously. If required, this may be repeated or followed by an intravenous infusion of glucagon 1-10 mg/hour depending on response. If no response to glucagon occurs or if glucagon is unavailable, a beta-adrenoceptor stimulant such as dobutamine 2.5 to 10 micrograms/kg/minute by intravenous infusion may be given.

Dobutamine, because of its positive inotropic effect, could also be used to treat hypotension and acute cardiac insufficiency. It is likely that these doses would be inadequate to reverse the cardiac effects of beta-blocker blockade if a large overdose has been taken. The dose of dobutamine should therefore be increased if necessary to achieve the required response according to the clinical condition of the patient.

Bronchospasm can usually be reversed by bronchodilators.

Excessive diuresis should be countered by maintaining normal fluid and electrolyte balance.

5. PHARMACOLOGICAL PROPERTIES

5.1 Pharmacodynamic properties

Beta-blocking agents, selective, and other diuretics.

C07C B03

Tenoret 50 Film-coated Tablets combines the antihypertensive activity of two agents, a beta-blocker (atenolol) and a diuretic (chlortalidone).

Atenolol

Atenolol is beta$_1$-selective (i.e. acts preferentially on beta$_1$-adrenergic receptors in the heart). Selectivity decreases with increasing dose.

Atenolol is without intrinsic sympathomimetic and membrane-stabilising activities and, as with other beta-blockers, has negative inotropic effects (and is therefore contraindicated in uncontrolled heart failure).

As with other beta-blockers, the mode of action in the treatment of hypertension is unclear.

It is unlikely that any additional ancillary properties possessed by S (-) atenolol, in comparison with the racemic mixture, will give rise to different therapeutic effects.

Atenolol is effective and well-tolerated in most ethnic populations. Black patients respond better to the combination of atenolol and chlortalidone, than to atenolol alone.

The combination of atenolol with thiazide-like diuretics has been shown to be compatible and generally more effective than either drug used alone.

Chlortalidone

Chlortalidone, a monosulfonamyl diuretic, increases excretion of sodium and chloride. Natriuresis is accompanied by some loss of potassium. The mechanism by which chlortalidone reduces blood pressure is not fully known but may be related to the excretion and redistribution of body sodium.

5.2 Pharmacokinetic properties

Atenolol

Absorption of atenolol following oral dosing is consistent but incomplete (approximately 40-50%) with peak plasma concentrations occurring 2-4 hours after dosing. The atenolol blood levels are consistent and subject to little variability. There is no significant hepatic metabolism of atenolol and more than 90% of that absorbed reaches the systemic circulation unaltered. The plasma half-life is about 6 hours but this may rise in severe renal impairment since the kidney is the major route of elimination. Atenolol penetrates tissues poorly due to its low lipid solubility and its concentration in brain tissue is low. Plasma protein binding is low (approximately 3%).

Chlortalidone

Absorption of chlortalidone following oral dosing is consistent but incomplete (approximately 60%) with peak plasma concentrations occurring about 12 hours after dosing. The chlortalidone blood levels are consistent and subject to little variability. The plasma half-life is about 50 hours and the kidney is the major route of elimination. Plasma protein binding is high (approximately 75%).

Coadministration of chlortalidone and atenolol has little effect on the pharmacokinetics of either.

Tenoret 50 Film-coated Tablets is effective for at least 24 hours after a single oral daily dose. This simplicity of dosing facilitates compliance by its acceptability to patients.

5.3 Preclinical safety data

Atenolol and chlortalidone are drugs on which extensive clinical experience has been obtained. Relevant information for the prescriber is provided elsewhere in the Summary of Product Characteristics.

6. PHARMACEUTICAL PARTICULARS

6.1 List of excipients

Magnesium Carbonate

Maize Starch

Sodium laurilsulfate

Gelatin

Magnesium Stearate

Methylhydroxypropylcellulose

Macrogol 300

Iron Oxide (E172)

6.2 Incompatibilities

Not applicable.

6.3 Shelf life

36 months.

6.4 Special precautions for storage

Do not store above 25°C.

Store in the original package. Keep the container in the outer carton

6.5 Nature and contents of container

Blister packs of 28 tablets contained in a carton.

6.6 Special precautions for disposal and other handling

Not applicable.

7. MARKETING AUTHORISATION HOLDER

AstraZeneca UK Limited.,

600 Capability Green,

Luton, LU1 3LU, UK.

8. MARKETING AUTHORISATION NUMBER(S)

PL 17901/0048

9. DATE OF FIRST AUTHORISATION/RENEWAL OF THE AUTHORISATION

01 June 2000/09 February 2005

10. DATE OF REVISION OF THE TEXT

28th April 2008

Tenoretic

(AstraZeneca UK Limited)

1. NAME OF THE MEDICINAL PRODUCT

Tenoretic Film-coated Tablets

2. QUALITATIVE AND QUANTITATIVE COMPOSITION

Atenolol 100 mg

Chlortalidone 25 mg

For excipients, see Section 6.1

3. PHARMACEUTICAL FORM

Film-coated tablets.

Brown

4. CLINICAL PARTICULARS

4.1 Therapeutic indications

Management of hypertension.

4.2 Posology and method of administration

Tenoretic Film-coated Tablets are administered orally.

Adults

One tablet daily. Most patients with hypertension will give a satisfactory response to a single tablet daily of Tenoretic Film-coated Tablets. There is little or no further fall in blood pressure with increased dosage and, where necessary, another antihypertensive drug, such as a vasodilator, can be added.

Elderly

Dosage requirements are often lower in this age group.

Children

There is no paediatric experience with Tenoretic Film-coated Tablets, therefore this preparation is not recommended for children.

Renal Impairment

In patients with severe renal impairment, a reduction in the daily dose or in frequency of administration may be necessary. (See Section 4.4).

4.3 Contraindications

Tenoretic Film-coated Tablets should not be used in patients with any of the following:

- known hypersensitivity to either active component or any of the excipients;
- bradycardia;
- cardiogenic shock;
- hypotension;
- metabolic acidosis;
- severe peripheral arterial circulatory disturbances;
- second- or third-degree heart block;
- sick sinus syndrome;
- untreated phaeochromocytoma;
- uncontrolled heart failure.

Tenoretic Film-coated Tablets must not be given during pregnancy or lactation.

4.4 Special warnings and precautions for use

Due to its beta-blocker component Tenoretic Film-coated Tablets:

- although contraindicated in uncontrolled heart failure (See section 4.3) may be used in patients whose signs of heart failure have been controlled. Caution must be exercised in patients whose cardiac reserve is poor.
- may increase the number and duration of angina attacks in patients with Prinzmetal's angina due to unopposed alpha receptor mediated coronary artery vasoconstriction. Atenolol is a $beta_1$-selective beta-blocker; consequently the use of Tenoretic Film-coated Tablets may be considered although utmost caution must be exercised.
- although contraindicated in severe peripheral arterial circulatory disturbances (See section 4.3) may also aggravate less severe peripheral arterial circulatory disturbances.
- due to its negative effect on conduction time, caution must be exercised if it is given to patients with first-degree heart block.
- may modify the tachycardia of hypoglycaemia.
- may mask the signs of thyrotoxicosis.
- will reduce heart rate, as a result of its pharmacological action. In the rare instances when a treated patient develops symptoms which may be attributable to a slow heart rate, the dose may be reduced.
- should not be discontinued abruptly in patients suffering from ischaemic heart disease.
- may cause a more severe reaction to a variety of allergens, when given to patients with a history of anaphylactic reaction to such allergens. Such patients may be unresponsive to the usual doses of adrenaline used to treat the allergic reactions.
- may cause a hypersensitivity reaction including angioedema and urticaria.

Tenoretic Film-coated Tablets contain the cardioselective beta-blocker atenolol. Although cardioselective ($beta_1$) beta-blockers may have less effect on lung function than non-selective beta-blockers, as with all beta-blockers, these should be avoided in patients with reversible obstructive airways disease, unless there are compelling clinical reasons for their use. Where such reasons exist, Tenoretic Film-coated Tablets may be used with caution. Occasionally, some increase in airways resistance may occur in asthmatic patients, however, and this may usually be reversed by commonly used dosage of bronchodilators such as salbutamol or isoprenaline.

The label and patient information leaflet for this product state the following warning:

"If you have ever had asthma or wheezing, you should not take this medicine unless you have discussed these symptoms with the prescribing doctor".

Due to its chlortalidone component:

- hypokalaemia may occur. Measurement of potassium levels is appropriate, especially in the older patient, those receiving digitalis preparations for cardiac failure, those taking an abnormal (low in potassium) diet or those suffering from gastrointestinal complaints. Hypokalaemia may predispose to arrhythmias in patients receiving digitalis;
- caution must be exercised in patients with severe renal failure (See Section 4.2);
- Impaired glucose tolerance may occur and caution must be exercised if chlortalidone is administered to patients with a known pre-disposition to diabetes mellitus;
- hyperuricaemia may occur. Only a minor increase in serum uric acid usually occurs but in cases of prolonged elevation, the concurrent use of a uricosuric agent will reverse the hyperuricaemia.

4.5 Interaction with other medicinal products and other forms of interaction

Combined use of beta-blockers and calcium channel blockers with negative inotropic effects e.g. verapamil, diltiazem, can lead to an exaggeration of these effects particularly in patients with impaired ventricular function and/or sino-atrial or atrio-ventricular conduction abnormalities. This may result in severe hypotension, bradycardia and cardiac failure. Neither the beta-blocker nor the calcium channel blocker should be administered intravenously within 48 hours of discontinuing the other.

Concomitant therapy with dihydropyridines e.g. nifedipine, may increase the risk of hypotension, and cardiac failure may occur in patients with latent cardiac insufficiency.

Digitalis glycosides, in association with beta-blockers, may increase atrio-ventricular conduction time.

Beta-blockers may exacerbate the rebound hypertension which can follow the withdrawal of clonidine. If the two drugs are co-administered, the beta-blocker should be withdrawn several days before discontinuing clonidine. If replacing clonidine by beta-blocker therapy, the introduction of beta-blockers should be delayed for several days after clonidine administration has stopped.

Class I anti-arrhythmic drugs (e.g. disopyramide) and amiodarone may have a potentiating effect on atrial-conduction time and induce negative inotropic effect.

Concomitant use of sympathomimetic agents, e.g. adrenaline (epinephrine), may counteract the effect of beta-blockers.

Concomitant use with insulin and oral antidiabetic drugs may lead to the intensification of the blood sugar lowering effects of these drugs.

Concomitant use of prostaglandin synthetase inhibiting drugs (e.g. ibuprofen, indometacin) may decrease the hypotensive effects of beta-blockers

Preparations containing lithium should not be given with diuretics because they may reduce its renal clearance.

Caution must be exercised when using anaesthetic agents with Tenoretic Film-coated Tablets. The anaesthetist should be informed and the choice of anaesthetic should be an agent with as little negative inotropic activity as possible. Use of beta-blockers with anaesthetic drugs may result in attenuation of the reflex tachycardia and increase the risk of hypotension. Anaesthetic agents causing myocardial depression are best avoided.

4.6 Pregnancy and lactation

Pregnancy:

Tenoretic Film-coated Tablets must not be given during pregnancy.

Lactation:

Tenoretic Film-coated Tablets must not be given during lactation.

4.7 Effects on ability to drive and use machines

Use is unlikely to result in any impairment of the ability of patients to drive or operate machinery. However, it should be taken into account that occasionally dizziness or fatigue may occur.

4.8 Undesirable effects

Tenoretic Film-coated Tablets are well tolerated. In clinical studies, the undesired events reported are usually attributable to the pharmacological actions of its components.

The following undesirable effects, listed by body system, have been reported with the following frequencies: Very common (≥10%), common (1-9.9%), uncommon (0.1-0.9%), rare (0.01-0.09%), very rare (<0.01%), not known (cannot be estimated from the available data):

Blood and lymphatic system disorders:

Rare: Purpura, thrombocytopenia, leucopenia (related to chlortalidone).

Psychiatric disorders:

Uncommon: Sleep disturbances of the type noted with other beta blockers.

Rare: Mood changes, nightmares, confusion, psychoses and hallucinations.

Nervous system disorders:

Rare: Dizziness, headache, paraesthesia.

Eye disorders:

Rare: Dry eyes, visual disturbances.

Cardiac disorders:

Common: Bradycardia

Rare: Heart failure deterioration, precipitation of heart block.

Vascular disorders:

Common: Cold extremities.

Rare: Postural hypotension which may be associated with syncope, intermittent claudication may be increased if already present, in susceptible patients Raynaud's phenomenon.

Respiratory, thoracic and mediastinal disorders:

Rare: Bronchospasm may occur in patients with bronchial asthma or a history of asthmatic complaints.

Gastrointestinal disorders:

Common: Gastrointestinal disturbances (including nausea related to chlortalidone).

Rare: Dry mouth.

Hepatobiliary disorders:

Rare: Hepatic toxicity including intrahepatic cholestasis, pancreatitis (related to chlortalidone).

Skin and subcutaneous tissue disorders:

Rare: Alopecia, psoriasiform skin reaction, exacerbation of psoriasis, skin rashes.

Not known: Hypersensitivity reactions, including angioedema and urticaria.

Reproductive system and breast disorders:

Rare: Impotence.

General disorders and administration site conditions:

Common: Fatigue.

Investigations:

Common: Related to chlortalidone: Hyperuricaemia, hyponatraemia, hypokalaemia, impaired glucose tolerance.

Uncommon: Elevations of transaminase levels.

Very rare: An increase in ANA (Antinuclear Antibodies) has been observed, however the clinical relevance of this is not clear.

Discontinuance of Tenoretic Film-coated Tablets should be considered if, according to clinical judgement, the well-being of the patient is adversely affected by any of the above reactions.

4.9 Overdose

The symptoms of overdosage may include bradycardia, hypotension, acute cardiac insufficiency and bronchospasm.

General treatment should include: close supervision, treatment in an intensive care ward, the use of gastric lavage, activated charcoal and a laxative to prevent absorption of any drug still present in the gastrointestinal tract, the use of plasma or plasma substitutes to treat hypotension and shock. The possible use of haemodialysis or haemoperfusion may be considered.

Excessive bradycardia may be countered with atropine 1-2 mg intravenously and/or a cardiac pacemaker. If necessary, this may be followed by a bolus dose of glucagon 10 mg intravenously. If required, this may be repeated or followed by an intravenous infusion of glucagon 1-10 mg/hour depending on response. If no response to glucagon occurs or if glucagon is unavailable, a beta-adrenoceptor stimulant such as dobutamine 2.5 to 10 micrograms/kg/minute by intravenous infusion may be given. Dobutamine, because of its positive inotropic effects could be used to treat hypotension and acute cardiac insufficiency. It is likely that these doses would be inadequate to reverse the cardiac effects of beta-blocker blockade if a large overdose has been taken. The dose of dobutamine should therefore be increased if necessary to achieve the required response according to the clinical condition of the patient.

Bronchospasm can usually be reversed by bronchodilators.

Excessive diuresis should be countered by maintaining normal fluid and electrolyte balance.

5. PHARMACOLOGICAL PROPERTIES

5.1 Pharmacodynamic properties

Beta-blocking agents, selective, and other diuretics.

C07C B03

Tenoretic Film-coated Tablets combines the antihypertensive activity of two agents, a beta-blocker (atenolol) and a diuretic (chlortalidone).

Atenolol

Atenolol is $beta_1$-selective (i.e. acts preferentially on $beta_1$-adrenergic receptors in the heart). Selectivity decreases with increasing dose.

Atenolol is without intrinsic sympathomimetic and membrane-stabilising activities and, as with other beta-adrenoceptor blocking drugs, has negative inotropic effects (and is therefore contraindicated in uncontrolled heart failure).

As with other beta-blockers, the mode of action in the treatment of hypertension is unclear.

It is unlikely that any additional ancillary properties possessed by S (-) atenolol, in comparison with the racemic mixture, will give rise to different therapeutic effects.

Atenolol is effective and well-tolerated in most ethnic populations. Black patients respond better to the combination of atenolol and chlortalidone, than to atenolol alone.

The combination of atenolol with thiazide-like diuretics has been shown to be compatible and generally more effective than either drug used alone.

Chlortalidone

Chlortalidone, a monosulfonamyl diuretic, increases excretion of sodium and chloride. Natriuresis is accompanied by some loss of potassium. The mechanism by which chlortalidone reduces blood pressure is not fully known but may be related to the excretion and redistribution of body sodium.

5.2 Pharmacokinetic properties

Atenolol

Absorption of atenolol following oral dosing is consistent but incomplete (approximately 40-50%) with peak plasma concentrations occurring 2-4 hours after dosing. The atenolol blood levels are consistent and subject to little variability. There is no significant hepatic metabolism of atenolol and more than 90% of that absorbed reaches the systemic circulation unaltered. The plasma half-life is about 6 hours but this may rise in severe renal impairment since the kidney is the major route of elimination. Atenolol penetrates tissues poorly due to its low lipid solubility and its concentration in brain tissue is low. Plasma protein binding is low (approximately 3%).

Chlortalidone

Absorption of chlortalidone following oral dosing is consistent but incomplete (approximately 60%) with peak plasma concentrations occurring about 12 hours after dosing. The chlortalidone blood levels are consistent and subject to little variability. The plasma half-life is about 50 hours and the kidney is the major route of elimination. Plasma protein binding is high (approximately 75%).

Coadministration of chlortalidone and atenolol has little effect on the pharmacokinetics of either.

Tenoretic Film-coated Tablets is effective for at least 24 hours after a single oral daily dose. This simplicity of dosing facilitates compliance by its acceptability to patients.

5.3 Preclinical safety data

Atenolol and chlortalidone are drugs on which extensive clinical experience has been obtained. Relevant information for the prescriber is provided elsewhere in the Summary of Product Characteristics.

6. PHARMACEUTICAL PARTICULARS

6.1 List of excipients

Heavy Magnesium Carbonate

Maize Starch.

Sodium laurilsulfate

Gelatin

Magnesium Stearate

Methylhydroxypropylcellulose.

Macrogol 300 BP

Iron Oxide yellow (E172)

Iron Oxide red (E172)

Magnesium Carbonate.

6.2 Incompatibilities

Not applicable.

6.3 Shelf life

4 years.

6.4 Special precautions for storage

Do not store above 25°C.

Store in the original package. Keep the container in the outer carton

6.5 Nature and contents of container

Blister packs of 28 tablets contained in a carton.

6.6 Special precautions for disposal and other handling

Not applicable.

7. MARKETING AUTHORISATION HOLDER

AstraZeneca UK Limited

600 Capability Green,

Luton, LU1 3LU, UK.

8. MARKETING AUTHORISATION NUMBER(S)

17901/0049

9. DATE OF FIRST AUTHORISATION/RENEWAL OF THE AUTHORISATION

1st June 2000/9th February 2005

10. DATE OF REVISION OF THE TEXT

28th April 2008

Tenormin 100mg Tablets

(AstraZeneca UK Limited)

1. NAME OF THE MEDICINAL PRODUCT

Tenormin 100 mg Tablets

2. QUALITATIVE AND QUANTITATIVE COMPOSITION

Atenolol 100 mg.

For excipients, see section 6.1.

3. PHARMACEUTICAL FORM

Film-coated tablet.

Orange film-coated tablets.

4. CLINICAL PARTICULARS

4.1 Therapeutic indications

i. Management of hypertension.

ii. Management of angina pectoris.

iii. Management of cardiac arrhythmias.

iv. Management of myocardial infarction. Early intervention in the acute phase.

4.2 Posology and method of administration

Oral administration.

The dose must always be adjusted to individual requirements of the patients, with the lowest possible starting dosage. The following are guidelines:

Adults

Hypertension

One tablet daily. Most patients respond to 100 mg daily given orally as a single dose. Some patients, however, will respond to 50 mg given as a single daily dose. The effect will be fully established after one to two weeks. A further reduction in blood pressure may be achieved by combining Tenormin with other antihypertensive agents. For example co-administration of Tenormin with a diuretic, as in Tenoretic, provides a highly effective and convenient antihypertensive therapy.

Angina

Most patients with angina pectoris will respond to 100 mg given orally once daily or 50 mg given twice daily. It is unlikely that additional benefit will be gained by increasing the dose.

Cardiac arrhythmias

A suitable initial dose of Tenormin is 2.5 mg (5 ml) injected intravenously over a 2.5 minute period (i.e. 1 mg/minute). (See also prescribing information for Tenormin Injection.) This may be repeated at 5 minute intervals, until a response is observed up to a maximum dosage of 10 mg. If Tenormin is given by infusion, 0.15 mg/kg bodyweight may be administered over a 20 minute period. If required, the injection or infusion may be repeated every 12 hours. Having controlled the arrhythmias with intravenous Tenormin, a suitable oral maintenance dosage is 50–100 mg daily, given as a single dose.

Myocardial infarction

For patients suitable for treatment with intravenous beta-blockade and presenting within 12 hours of the onset of chest pain, Tenormin 5–10 mg should be given by slow intravenous injection (1 mg/minute) followed by Tenormin 50 mg orally about 15 minutes later, provided no untoward effects have occurred from the intravenous dose. This should be followed by a further 50 mg orally 12 hours after the intravenous dose, and then 12 hours later by 100 mg orally, once daily. If bradycardia and/or hypotension requiring treatment, or any other untoward effects occur, Tenormin should be discontinued.

Elderly

Dosage requirements may be reduced, especially in patients with impaired renal function.

Children

There is no paediatric experience with Tenormin and for this reason it is not recommended for use in children.

Renal failure

Since Tenormin is excreted via the kidneys, the dosage should be adjusted in cases of severe impairment of renal function.

No significant accumulation of Tenormin occurs in patients who have a creatinine clearance greater than 35 ml/min/1.73 m^2 (normal range is 100–150 ml/min/1.73 m^2).

For patients with a creatinine clearance of 15–35 ml/min/1.73 m^2 (equivalent to serum creatinine of 300–600 micromol/litre), the oral dose should be 50 mg daily and the intravenous dose should be 10 mg once every two days.

For patients with a creatinine clearance of less than 15 ml/min/1.73 m^2 (equivalent to serum creatinine of greater than 600 micromol/litre), the oral dose should be 25 mg daily or 50 mg on alternate days and the intravenous dose should be 10 mg once every four days.

Patients on haemodialysis should be given 50 mg orally after each dialysis; this should be done under hospital supervision as marked falls in blood pressure can occur.

4.3 Contraindications

Tenormin, as with other beta-blockers, should not be used in patients with any of the following:

cardiogenic shock

uncontrolled heart failure

sick sinus syndrome

second-or third-degree heart block

untreated phaeochromocytoma

metabolic acidosis

bradycardia (<45 bpm)

hypotension

known hypersensitivity to the active substance, or any of the excipients

severe peripheral arterial circulatory disturbances.

4.4 Special warnings and precautions for use

Tenormin as with other beta-blockers:

- Should not be withdrawn abruptly. The dosage should be withdrawn gradually over a period of 7–14 days, to facilitate a reduction in beta-blocker dosage. Patients should be followed during withdrawal, especially those with ischaemic heart disease.
- When a patient is scheduled for surgery, and a decision is made to discontinue beta-blocker therapy, this should be done at least 24 hours prior to the procedure. The risk-benefit assessment of stopping beta-blockade should be made for each patient. If treatment is continued, an anaesthetic with little negative inotropic activity should be selected to minimise the risk of myocardial depression. The patient may be protected against vagal reactions by intravenous administration of atropine.
- Although contraindicated in uncontrolled heart failure (see section 4.3), may be used in patients whose signs of heart failure have been controlled. Caution must be exercised in patients whose cardiac reserve is poor.
- May increase the number and duration of angina attacks in patients with Prinzmetal's angina due to unopposed alpha-receptor mediated coronary artery vasoconstriction. Tenormin is a $beta_1$-selective beta-blocker; consequently, its use may be considered although utmost caution must be exercised.
- Although contraindicated in severe peripheral arterial circulatory disturbances (see section 4.3), may also aggravate less severe peripheral arterial circulatory disturbances.
- Due to its negative effect on conduction time, caution must be exercised if it is given to patients with first-degree heart block.
- May mask the symptoms of hypoglycaemia, in particular, tachycardia.
- May mask the signs of thyrotoxicosis.
- Will reduce heart rate as a result of its pharmacological action. In the rare instances when a treated patient develops symptoms which may be attributable to a slow heart rate and the pulse rate drops to less than 50–55 bpm at rest, the dose should be reduced.
- May cause a more severe reaction to a variety of allergens when given to patients with a history of anaphylactic reaction to such allergens. Such patients may be unresponsive to the usual doses of adrenaline (epinephrine) used to treat the allergic reactions.
- May cause a hypersensitivity reaction including angioedema and urticaria.
- Should be used with caution in the elderly, starting with a lesser dose (see Section 4.2).

Since Tenormin is excreted via the kidneys, dosage should be reduced in patients with a creatinine clearance of below 35 ml/min/1.73 m^2.

Although cardioselective ($beta_1$) beta-blockers may have less effect on lung function than non-selective beta-blockers, as with all beta-blockers, these should be avoided in patients with reversible obstructive airways disease, unless there are compelling clinical reasons for their use. Where such reasons exist, Tenormin may be used with caution. Occasionally, some increase in airways resistance may occur in asthmatic patients however, and this may usually be reversed by commonly used dosage of bronchodilators such as salbutamol or isoprenaline. The label and patient information leaflet for this product state the following warning: "If you have ever had asthma or wheezing, you should not take this medicine unless you have discussed these symptoms with the prescribing doctor".

As with other beta-blockers, in patients with a phaeochromocytoma, an alpha-blocker should be given concomitantly.

4.5 Interaction with other medicinal products and other forms of interaction

Combined use of beta-blockers and calcium channel blockers with negative inotropic effects, e.g. verapamil and diltiazem, can lead to an exaggeration of these effects particularly in patients with impaired ventricular function and/or sinoatrial or atrioventricular conduction abnormalities. This may result in severe hypotension, bradycardia and cardiac failure. Neither the beta-blocker nor the calcium channel blocker should be administered intravenously within 48 hours of discontinuing the other.

Concomitant therapy with dihydropyridines, e.g. nifedipine, may increase the risk of hypotension, and cardiac failure may occur in patients with latent cardiac insufficiency.

Digitalis glycosides, in association with beta-blockers, may increase atrioventricular conduction time.

Beta-blockers may exacerbate the rebound hypertension which can follow the withdrawal of clonidine. If the two drugs are co-administered, the beta-blocker should be withdrawn several days before discontinuing clonidine. If replacing clonidine by beta-blocker therapy, the introduction of beta-blockers should be delayed for several days after clonidine administration has stopped. (See also prescribing information for clonidine.)

Class I anti-arrhythmic drugs (e.g. disopyramide) and amiodarone may have a potentiating effect on atrial-conduction time and induce negative inotropic effect.

Concomitant use of sympathomimetic agents, e.g. adrenaline (epinephrine), may counteract the effect of beta-blockers.

Concomitant use with insulin and oral antidiabetic drugs may lead to the intensification of the blood sugar lowering effects of these drugs. Symptoms of hypoglycaemia, particularly tachycardia, may be masked (see section 4.4).

Concomitant use of prostaglandin synthetase-inhibiting drugs, e.g. ibuprofen and indometacin, may decrease the hypotensive effects of beta-blockers.

Caution must be exercised when using anaesthetic agents with Tenormin. The anaesthetist should be informed and the choice of anaesthetic should be an agent with as little negative inotropic activity as possible. Use of beta-blockers with anaesthetic drugs may result in attenuation of the reflex tachycardia and increase the risk of hypotension. Anaesthetic agents causing myocardial depression are best avoided.

4.6 Pregnancy and lactation

Tenormin crosses the placental barrier and appears in the cord blood. No studies have been performed on the use of Tenormin in the first trimester and the possibility of foetal injury cannot be excluded. Tenormin has been used under close supervision for the treatment of hypertension in the third trimester. Administration of Tenormin to pregnant women in the management of mild to moderate hypertension has been associated with intra-uterine growth retardation.

The use of Tenormin in women who are, or may become, pregnant requires that the anticipated benefit be weighed against the possible risks, particularly in the first and second trimesters, since beta-blockers, in general, have been associated with a decrease in placental perfusion which may result in intra-uterine deaths, immature and premature deliveries.

There is significant accumulation of Tenormin in breast milk.

Neonates born to mothers who are receiving Tenormin at parturition or breast-feeding may be at risk of hypoglycaemia and bradycardia.

Caution should be exercised when Tenormin is administered during pregnancy or to a woman who is breast-feeding.

4.7 Effects on ability to drive and use machines

Use is unlikely to result in any impairment of the ability of patients to drive or operate machinery. However, it should be taken into account that occasionally dizziness or fatigue may occur.

4.8 Undesirable effects

Tenormin is well tolerated. In clinical studies, the undesired events reported are usually attributable to the pharmacological actions of atenolol.

The following undesired events, listed by body system, have been reported with the following frequencies: very common ($\geqslant$10%), common (1–9.9%), uncommon (0.1–0.9%), rare (0.01–0.09%), very rare (<0.01%) including isolated reports, not known (cannot be estimated from the available data).

Blood and lymphatic system disorders:

Rare: Purpura, thrombocytopenia.

Psychiatric disorders:

Uncommon: Sleep disturbances of the type noted with other beta-blockers.

Rare: Mood changes, nightmares, confusion, psychoses and hallucinations.

Nervous system disorders:

Rare: Dizziness, headache, paraesthesia.

Eye disorders:

Rare: Dry eyes, visual disturbances.

Cardiac disorders:

Common: Bradycardia.

Rare: Heart failure deterioration, precipitation of heart block.

Vascular disorders:

Common: Cold extremities.

Rare: Postural hypotension which may be associated with syncope, intermittent claudication may be increased if already present, in susceptible patients Raynaud's phenomenon.

Respiratory, thoracic and mediastinal disorders:

Rare: Bronchospasm may occur in patients with bronchial asthma or a history of asthmatic complaints.

Gastrointestinal disorders:

Common: Gastrointestinal disturbances.

Rare: Dry mouth.

Hepato-biliary disorders:

Uncommon: Elevations of transaminase levels.

Rare: Hepatic toxicity including intrahepatic cholestasis.

Skin and subcutaneous tissue disorders:

Rare: Alopecia, psoriasiform skin reactions, exacerbation of psoriasis, skin rashes.

Not known: Hypersensitivity reactions, including angioedema and urticaria.

Reproductive system and breast disorders:

Rare: Impotence.

General disorders and administration site conditions:

Common: Fatigue.

Investigations:

Very rare: An increase in ANA (Antinuclear Antibodies) has been observed, however the clinical relevance of this is not clear.

Discontinuance of the drug should be considered if, according to clinical judgement, the well-being of the patient is adversely affected by any of the above reactions.

4.9 Overdose

The symptoms of overdosage may include bradycardia, hypotension, acute cardiac insufficiency and bronchospasm.

General treatment should include: close supervision; treatment in an intensive care ward; the use of gastric lavage; activated charcoal and a laxative to prevent absorption of any drug still present in the gastrointestinal tract; the use of plasma or plasma substitutes to treat hypotension and shock. The possible uses of haemodialysis or haemoperfusion may be considered.

Excessive bradycardia can be countered with atropine 1–2 mg intravenously and/or a cardiac pacemaker. If necessary, this may be followed by a bolus dose of glucagon 10 mg intravenously. If required, this may be repeated or followed by an intravenous infusion of glucagon 1–10 mg/hour depending on response. If no response to glucagon occurs or if glucagon is unavailable, a beta-adrenoceptor stimulant such as dobutamine 2.5 to 10 micrograms/kg/minute by intravenous infusion may be given. Dobutamine, because of its positive inotropic effect could also be used to treat hypotension and acute cardiac insufficiency. It is likely that these doses would be inadequate to reverse the cardiac effects of beta-blocker blockade if a large overdose has been taken. The dose of dobutamine should therefore be increased if necessary to achieve the required response according to the clinical condition of the patient.

Bronchospasm can usually be reversed by bronchodilators.

5. PHARMACOLOGICAL PROPERTIES

5.1 Pharmacodynamic properties

Beta-blocking agents, plain, selective.

CO7A B03.

Atenolol is a beta-blocker which is $beta_1$-selective, (i.e. acts preferentially on $beta_1$-adrenergic receptors in the heart). Selectivity decreases with increasing dose.

Atenolol is without intrinsic sympathomimetic and membrane-stabilising activities and as with other beta-blockers, has negative inotropic effects (and is therefore contraindicated in uncontrolled heart failure).

As with other beta-blockers, the mode of action of atenolol in the treatment of hypertension is unclear.

It is probably the action of atenolol in reducing cardiac rate and contractility which makes it effective in eliminating or reducing the symptoms of patients with angina.

It is unlikely that any additional ancillary properties possessed by S (-) atenolol, in comparison with the racemic mixture, will give rise to different therapeutic effects.

Tenormin is effective and well-tolerated in most ethnic populations although the response may be less in black patients.

Tenormin is effective for at least 24 hours after a single oral dose. The drug facilitates compliance by its acceptability to patients and simplicity of dosing. The narrow dose range and early patient response ensure that the effect of the drug in individual patients is quickly demonstrated. Tenormin is compatible with diuretics, other hypotensive agents and antianginals (see section 4.5). Since it acts preferentially on beta-receptors in the heart, Tenormin may, with care, be used successfully in the treatment of patients with respiratory disease, who cannot tolerate non-selective beta-blockers.

Early intervention with Tenormin in acute myocardial infarction reduces infarct size and decreases morbidity and mortality. Fewer patients with a threatened infarction progress to frank infarction; the incidence of ventricular arrhythmias is decreased and marked pain relief may result in reduced need of opiate analgesics. Early mortality is decreased. Tenormin is an additional treatment to standard coronary care.

5.2 Pharmacokinetic properties

Absorption of atenolol following oral dosing is consistent but incomplete (approximately 40–50%) with peak plasma concentrations occurring 2–4 hours after dosing. The atenolol blood levels are consistent and subject to little variability. There is no significant hepatic metabolism of atenolol and more than 90% of that absorbed reaches the systemic circulation unaltered. The plasma half-life is about 6 hours but this may rise in severe renal impairment since the kidney is the major route of elimination. Atenolol penetrates tissues poorly due to its low lipid solubility and its concentration in brain tissue is low. Plasma protein binding is low (approximately 3%).

5.3 Preclinical safety data

Atenolol is a drug on which extensive clinical experience has been obtained. Relevant information for the prescriber is provided elsewhere in the Prescribing Information.

6. PHARMACEUTICAL PARTICULARS

6.1 List of excipients

Gelatin

Magnesium Carbonate

Macrogol

Magnesium Stearate

Maize Starch

Methylhydroxypropylcellulose

Sodium Laurilsulfate

Sunset Yellow Lake (E110)

Talc

Titanium Dioxide (E171)

6.2 Incompatibilities

Not applicable.

6.3 Shelf life

60 months.

6.4 Special precautions for storage

Do not store above 25°C.

Store in the original package. Keep the container in the outer carton.

6.5 Nature and contents of container

Aluminium PVC/PVDC blister strips of 14 tablets in cartons: 28 Tablets

Aluminium PVC/PVDC blister strips of 7 tablets: 504 Tablets (for Hospital Use) (pack is subdivided into 6 cartons each containing 12 blister strips i.e. 84 tablets)

6.6 Special precautions for disposal and other handling

Not applicable.

7. MARKETING AUTHORISATION HOLDER

AstraZeneca UK Limited,

600 Capability Green,

Luton, LU1 3LU, UK.

8. MARKETING AUTHORISATION NUMBER(S)

PL 17901/0054

9. DATE OF FIRST AUTHORISATION/RENEWAL OF THE AUTHORISATION

01st June 2000 / 5th November 2003

10. DATE OF REVISION OF THE TEXT

18th Decmber 2007

Tenormin 25mg Tablets

(AstraZeneca UK Limited)

1. NAME OF THE MEDICINAL PRODUCT

Tenormin 25 mg Tablets

2. QUALITATIVE AND QUANTITATIVE COMPOSITION

Atenolol 25 mg.

For excipients, see Section 6.1.

3. PHARMACEUTICAL FORM

Film-coated tablet.

White film-coated tablets.

4. CLINICAL PARTICULARS

4.1 Therapeutic indications

i Management of hypertension.

ii Management of angina pectoris.

iii Management of cardiac arrhythmias.

iv Management of myocardial infarction. Early intervention in the acute phase.

4.2 Posology and method of administration

Oral administration.

The dose must always be adjusted to individual requirements of the patients, with the lowest possible starting dosage. The following are guidelines:

Adults

Hypertension

One tablet daily. Most patients respond to 100 mg daily given orally as a single dose. Some patients, however, will respond to 50 mg given as a single daily dose. The effect will be fully established after one to two weeks. A further reduction in blood pressure may be achieved by combining Tenormin with other antihypertensive agents. For example, co-administration of Tenormin with a diuretic, as in Tenoretic provides a highly effective and convenient antihypertensive therapy.

Angina

Most patients with angina pectoris will respond to 100 mg given orally once daily or 50 mg given twice daily. It is unlikely that additional benefit will be gained by increasing the dose.

Cardiac arrhythmias

A suitable initial dose of Tenormin is 2.5 mg (5 ml) injected intravenously over a 2.5 minute period (i.e. 1 mg/minute). (See also prescribing information for Tenormin Injection.) This may be repeated at 5 minute intervals, until a response is observed up to a maximum dosage of 10 mg. If Tenormin is given by infusion, 0.15 mg/kg bodyweight may be administered over a 20 minute period. If required, the injection or infusion may be repeated every 12 hours. Having controlled the arrhythmias with intravenous Tenormin, a suitable oral maintenance dosage is 50–100 mg daily, given as a single dose.

Myocardial infarction

For patients suitable for treatment with intravenous beta-blockade and presenting within 12 hours of the onset of chest pain, Tenormin 5–10 mg should be given by slow intravenous injection (1 mg/minute) followed by Tenormin 50 mg orally about 15 minutes later, provided no untoward effects have occurred from the intravenous dose. This should be followed by a further 50 mg orally 12 hours after the intravenous dose, and then 12 hours later by 100 mg orally, once daily. If bradycardia and/or hypotension requiring treatment, or any other untoward effects occur, Tenormin should be discontinued.

Elderly

Dosage requirements may be reduced, especially in patients with impaired renal function.

Children

There is no paediatric experience with Tenormin and for this reason it is not recommended for use in children.

Renal failure

Since Tenormin is excreted via the kidneys, the dosage should be adjusted in cases of severe impairment of renal function.

No significant accumulation of Tenormin occurs in patients who have a creatinine clearance greater than 35 ml/min/1.73 m^2 (normal range is 100–150 ml/min/1.73 m^2).

For patients with a creatinine clearance of 15–35 ml/min/1.73 m^2 (equivalent to serum creatinine of 300–600 micromol/litre), the oral dose should be 50 mg daily and the intravenous dose should be 10 mg once every two days.

For patients with a creatinine clearance of less than 15 ml/min/1.73 m^2 (equivalent to serum creatinine of greater than 600 micromol/litre), the oral dose should be 25 mg daily or 50 mg on alternate days and the intravenous dose should be 10 mg once every four days.

Patients on haemodialysis should be given 50 mg orally after each dialysis; this should be done under hospital supervision as marked falls in blood pressure can occur.

4.3 Contraindications

Tenormin, as with other beta-blockers, should not be used in patients with any of the following:

cardiogenic shock

uncontrolled heart failure

sick sinus syndrome

second-or third-degree heart block

untreated phaeochromocytoma

metabolic acidosis

bradycardia (<45 bpm)

hypotension

known hypersensitivity to the active substance, or any of the excipients

severe peripheral arterial circulatory disturbances.

4.4 Special warnings and precautions for use

Tenormin as with other beta-blockers:

- Should not be withdrawn abruptly. The dosage should be withdrawn gradually over a period of 7–14 days, to facilitate a reduction in beta-blocker dosage. Patients should be followed during withdrawal, especially those with ischaemic heart disease.
- When a patient is scheduled for surgery, and a decision is made to discontinue beta-blocker therapy, this should be done at least 24 hours prior to the procedure. The risk-benefit assessment of stopping beta-blockade should be made for each patient. If treatment is continued, an anaesthetic with little negative inotropic activity should be selected to minimise the risk of myocardial depression. The patient may be protected against vagal reactions by intravenous administration of atropine.
- Although contraindicated in uncontrolled heart failure (see section 4.3), may be used in patients whose signs of heart failure have been controlled. Caution must be exercised in patients whose cardiac reserve is poor.
- May increase the number and duration of angina attacks in patients with Prinzmetal's angina due to unopposed alpha-receptor mediated coronary artery vasoconstriction. Tenormin is a beta$_1$-selective beta-blocker; consequently, its use may be considered although utmost caution must be exercised.
- Although contraindicated in severe peripheral arterial circulatory disturbances (see section 4.3), may also aggravate less severe peripheral arterial circulatory disturbances.
- Due to its negative effect on conduction time, caution must be exercised if it is given to patients with first-degree heart block.
- May mask the symptoms of hypoglycaemia, in particular, tachycardia.
- May mask the signs of thyrotoxicosis.
- Will reduce heart rate as a result of its pharmacological action. In the rare instances when a treated patient develops symptoms which may be attributable to a slow heart rate and the pulse rate drops to less than 50–55 bpm at rest, the dose should be reduced.
- May cause a more severe reaction to a variety of allergens when given to patients with a history of anaphylactic reaction to such allergens. Such patients may be unresponsive to the usual doses of adrenaline (epinephrine) used to treat the allergic reactions.
- May cause a hypersensitivity reaction including angioedema and urticaria.
- Should be used with caution in the elderly, starting with a lesser dose (see Section 4.2).

Since Tenormin is excreted via the kidneys, dosage should be reduced in patients with a creatinine clearance of below 35 ml/min/1.73 m^2.

Although cardioselective (beta$_1$) beta-blockers may have less effect on lung function than non-selective beta-blockers, as with all beta-blockers, these should be avoided in patients with reversible obstructive airways disease, unless there are compelling clinical reasons for their use. Where such reasons exist, Tenormin may be used with caution. Occasionally, some increase in airways resistance may occur in asthmatic patients however, and this may usually be reversed by commonly used dosage of bronchodilators such as salbutamol or isoprenaline. The label and patient information leaflet for this product state the following warning: "If you have ever had asthma or wheezing, you should not take this medicine unless you have discussed these symptoms with the prescribing doctor".

As with other beta-blockers, in patients with a phaeochromocytoma, an alpha-blocker should be given concomitantly.

4.5 Interaction with other medicinal products and other forms of interaction

Combined use of beta-blockers and calcium channel blockers with negative inotropic effects, e.g. verapamil and diltiazem, can lead to an exaggeration of these effects particularly in patients with impaired ventricular function and/or sinoatrial or atrioventricular conduction abnormalities. This may result in severe hypotension, bradycardia and cardiac failure. Neither the beta-blocker nor the calcium channel blocker should be administered intravenously within 48 hours of discontinuing the other.

Concomitant therapy with dihydropyridines, e.g. nifedipine, may increase the risk of hypotension, and cardiac failure may occur in patients with latent cardiac insufficiency.

Digitalis glycosides, in association with beta-blockers, may increase atrioventricular conduction time.

Beta-blockers may exacerbate the rebound hypertension which can follow the withdrawal of clonidine. If the two drugs are co-administered, the beta-blocker should be withdrawn several days before discontinuing clonidine. If replacing clonidine by beta-blocker therapy, the introduction of beta-blockers should be delayed for several days after clonidine administration has stopped. (See also prescribing information for clonidine.)

Class I anti-arrhythmic drugs (e.g. disopyramide) and amiodarone may have a potentiating effect on atrial-conduction time and induce negative inotropic effect.

Concomitant use of sympathomimetic agents, e.g. adrenaline (epinephrine), may counteract the effect of beta-blockers.

Concomitant use with insulin and oral antidiabetic drugs may lead to the intensification of the blood sugar lowering effects of these drugs. Symptoms of hypoglycaemia, particularly tachycardia, may be masked (see section 4.4).

Concomitant use of prostaglandin synthetase-inhibiting drugs, e.g. ibuprofen and indometacin, may decrease the hypotensive effects of beta-blockers.

Caution must be exercised when using anaesthetic agents with Tenormin. The anaesthetist should be informed and the choice of anaesthetic should be an agent with as little negative inotropic activity as possible. Use of beta-blockers with anaesthetic drugs may result in attenuation of the reflex tachycardia and increase the risk of hypotension. Anaesthetic agents causing myocardial depression are best avoided.

4.6 Pregnancy and lactation

Tenormin crosses the placental barrier and appears in the cord blood. No studies have been performed on the use of Tenormin in the first trimester and the possibility of foetal injury cannot be excluded. Tenormin has been used under close supervision for the treatment of hypertension in the third trimester. Administration of Tenormin to pregnant women in the management of mild to moderate hypertension has been associated with intra-uterine growth retardation.

The use of Tenormin in women who are, or may become, pregnant requires that the anticipated benefit be weighed against the possible risks, particularly in the first and second trimesters, since beta-blockers, in general, have been associated with a decrease in placental perfusion which may result in intra-uterine deaths, immature and premature deliveries.

There is significant accumulation of Tenormin in breast milk.

Neonates born to mothers who are receiving Tenormin at parturition or breast-feeding may be at risk of hypoglycaemia and bradycardia.

Caution should be exercised when Tenormin is administered during pregnancy or to a woman who is breast-feeding.

4.7 Effects on ability to drive and use machines

Use is unlikely to result in any impairment of the ability of patients to drive or operate machinery. However, it should be taken into account that occasionally dizziness or fatigue may occur.

4.8 Undesirable effects

Tenormin is well tolerated. In clinical studies, the undesired events reported are usually attributable to the pharmacological actions of atenolol.

The following undesired events, listed by body system, have been reported with the following frequencies: very common (≥10%), common (1–9.9%), uncommon (0.1–0.9%), rare (0.01–0.09%), very rare (<0.01%) including isolated reports, not known (cannot be estimated from the available data).

Blood and lymphatic system disorders:

Rare: Purpura, thrombocytopenia.

Psychiatric disorders:

Uncommon: Sleep disturbances of the type noted with other beta-blockers.

Rare: Mood changes, nightmares, confusion, psychoses and hallucinations.

Nervous system disorders:

Rare: Dizziness, headache, paraesthesia.

Eye disorders:

Rare: Dry eyes, visual disturbances.

Cardiac disorders:

Common: Bradycardia.

Rare: Heart failure deterioration, precipitation of heart block.

Vascular disorders:

Common: Cold extremities.

Rare: Postural hypotension which may be associated with syncope, intermittent claudication may be increased if already present, in susceptible patients Raynaud's phenomenon.

Respiratory, thoracic and mediastinal disorders:

Rare: Bronchospasm may occur in patients with bronchial asthma or a history of asthmatic complaints.

Gastrointestinal disorders:

Common: Gastrointestinal disturbances.

Rare: Dry mouth.

Hepato-biliary disorders:

Uncommon: Elevations of transaminase levels.

Rare: Hepatic toxicity including intrahepatic cholestasis.

Skin and subcutaneous tissue disorders:

Rare: Alopecia, psoriasiform skin reactions, exacerbation of psoriasis, skin rashes.

Not known: Hypersensitivity reactions, including angioedema and urticaria.

Reproductive system and breast disorders:

Rare: Impotence.

General disorders and administration site conditions:

Common: Fatigue.

Investigations:

Very rare: An increase in ANA (Antinuclear Antibodies) has been observed, however the clinical relevance of this is not clear.

Discontinuance of the drug should be considered if, according to clinical judgement, the well-being of the patient is adversely affected by any of the above reactions.

4.9 Overdose

The symptoms of overdosage may include bradycardia, hypotension, acute cardiac insufficiency and bronchospasm.

General treatment should include: close supervision; treatment in an intensive care ward; the use of gastric lavage; activated charcoal and a laxative to prevent absorption of any drug still present in the gastrointestinal tract; the use of plasma or plasma substitutes to treat hypotension and shock. The possible uses of haemodialysis or haemoperfusion may be considered.

Excessive bradycardia can be countered with atropine 1–2 mg intravenously and/or a cardiac pacemaker. If necessary, this may be followed by a bolus dose of glucagon 10 mg intravenously. If required, this may be repeated or followed by an intravenous infusion of glucagon 1–10 mg/hour depending on response. If no response to glucagon occurs or if glucagon is unavailable, a beta-adrenoceptor stimulant such as dobutamine 2.5 to 10 micrograms/kg/minute by intravenous infusion may be given. Dobutamine, because of its positive inotropic effect could also be used to treat hypotension and acute cardiac insufficiency. It is likely that these doses would be inadequate to reverse the cardiac effects of beta-blocker blockade if a large overdose has been taken. The dose of dobutamine should therefore be increased if necessary to achieve the required response according to the clinical condition of the patient.

Bronchospasm can usually be reversed by bronchodilators.

5. PHARMACOLOGICAL PROPERTIES

5.1 Pharmacodynamic properties

Beta-blocking agents, plain, selective.

CO7A B03.

Atenolol is a beta-blocker which is $beta_1$-selective, (i.e. acts preferentially on $beta_1$-adrenergic receptors in the heart). Selectivity decreases with increasing dose.

Atenolol is without intrinsic sympathomimetic and membrane-stabilising activities and as with other beta-blockers, has negative inotropic effects (and is therefore contraindicated in uncontrolled heart failure).

As with other beta-blockers, the mode of action of atenolol in the treatment of hypertension is unclear.

It is probably the action of atenolol in reducing cardiac rate and contractility which makes it effective in eliminating or reducing the symptoms of patients with angina.

It is unlikely that any additional ancillary properties possessed by S (-) atenolol, in comparison with the racemic mixture, will give rise to different therapeutic effects.

Tenormin is effective and well-tolerated in most ethnic populations although the response may be less in black patients.

Tenormin is effective for at least 24 hours after a single oral dose. The drug facilitates compliance by its acceptability to patients and simplicity of dosing. The narrow dose range and early patient response ensure that the effect of the drug in individual patients is quickly demonstrated. Tenormin is compatible with diuretics, other hypotensive agents and antianginals (see section 4.5). Since it acts preferentially on beta-receptors in the heart, Tenormin may, with care, be used successfully in the treatment of patients with respiratory disease, who cannot tolerate non-selective beta-blockers.

Early intervention with Tenormin in acute myocardial infarction reduces infarct size and decreases morbidity and mortality. Fewer patients with a threatened infarction progress to frank infarction; the incidence of ventricular arrhythmias is decreased and marked pain relief may result in reduced need of opiate analgesics. Early mortality is decreased. Tenormin is an additional treatment to standard coronary care.

5.2 Pharmacokinetic properties

Absorption of atenolol following oral dosing is consistent but incomplete (approximately 40–50%) with peak plasma concentrations occurring 2–4 hours after dosing. The atenolol blood levels are consistent and subject to little variability. There is no significant hepatic metabolism of atenolol and more than 90% of that absorbed reaches the systemic circulation unaltered. The plasma half-life is about 6 hours but this may rise in severe renal impairment since the kidney is the major route of elimination. Atenolol penetrates tissues poorly due to its low lipid solubility and its concentration in brain tissue is low. Plasma protein binding is low (approximately 3%).

5.3 Preclinical safety data

Atenolol is a drug on which extensive clinical experience has been obtained. Relevant information for the prescriber is provided elsewhere in the Prescribing Information.

6. PHARMACEUTICAL PARTICULARS

6.1 List of excipients

Gelatin

Glycerol

Magnesium Carbonate

Magnesium Stearate

Maize Starch

Methylhydroxypropylcellulose

Sodium Laurilsulfate

Titanium Dioxide (E171)

6.2 Incompatibilities

Not applicable.

6.3 Shelf life

60 months.

6.4 Special precautions for storage

Do not store above 25°C.

Store in the original package. Keep the container in the outer carton.

6.5 Nature and contents of container

Aluminium PVC/PVDC blister strips: 28 tablets.

6.6 Special precautions for disposal and other handling

Not applicable.

7. MARKETING AUTHORISATION HOLDER

AstraZeneca UK Limited,

600 Capability Green,

Luton, LU1 3LU, UK.

8. MARKETING AUTHORISATION NUMBER(S)

PL 17901/0052

9. DATE OF FIRST AUTHORISATION/RENEWAL OF THE AUTHORISATION

1st June 2000 / 5th November 2003

10. DATE OF REVISION OF THE TEXT

18th December 2007

Tenormin Injection 0.5mg/ml

(AstraZeneca UK Limited)

1. NAME OF THE MEDICINAL PRODUCT

Tenormin Injection 0.5 mg/ml

2. QUALITATIVE AND QUANTITATIVE COMPOSITION

Atenolol 0.5 mg/ml (5 mg in 10 ml).

For excipients, see section 6.1.

3. PHARMACEUTICAL FORM

Solution for injection or infusion.

Type I clear glass ampoules containing a clear, colourless, sterile solution.

4. CLINICAL PARTICULARS

4.1 Therapeutic indications

Management of arrhythmias and for the early intervention treatment of acute myocardial infarction.

4.2 Posology and method of administration

Administered by the intravenous route.

The dose must always be adjusted to individual requirements of the patients, with the lowest possible starting dosage. The following are guidelines:

Adults

Cardiac arrhythmias

A suitable initial dose of Tenormin is 2.5 mg (5 ml) injected intravenously over a 2.5 minute period (i.e.1 mg/minute). This may be repeated at 5 minute intervals until a response is observed up to a maximum dosage of 10 mg. If Tenormin is given by infusion, 0.15 mg/kg bodyweight may be administered over a 20 minute period. If required, the injection or infusion may be repeated every 12 hours. Having controlled the arrhythmias with intravenous Tenormin, a suitable oral maintenance dosage is 50 to 100 mg daily (see prescribing information for Tenormin and Tenormin LS tablets).

Myocardial infarction

For patients suitable for treatment with intravenous beta-blockade and presenting within 12 hours of the onset of chest pain, Tenormin 5–10 mg should be given by slow intravenous injection (1 mg/minute) followed by Tenormin 50 mg orally about 15 minutes later, provided no untoward effects have occurred from the intravenous dose. This should be followed by a further 50 mg orally 12 hours after the intravenous dose, and then 12 hours later by 100 mg orally, once daily. If bradycardia and/or hypotension requiring treatment, or any other untoward effects occur, Tenormin should be discontinued

Elderly

Dosage requirements may be reduced, especially in patients with impaired renal function.

Children

There is no paediatric experience with Tenormin and for this reason it is not recommended for use in children.

Renal failure

Since Tenormin is excreted via the kidneys, the dosage should be adjusted in cases of severe impairment of renal function.

No significant accumulation of Tenormin occurs in patients who have a creatinine clearance greater than 35 ml/min/1.73 m^2 (normal range is 100–150 ml/min/1.73 m^2).

For patients with a creatinine clearance of 15–35 ml/min/1.73 m^2 (equivalent to serum creatinine of 300–600 micromol/litre), the oral dose should be 50 mg daily and the intravenous dose should be 10 mg once every two days.

For patients with a creatinine clearance of less than 15 ml/min/1.73 m^2 (equivalent to serum creatinine of greater than 600 micromol/litre), the oral dose should be 25 mg daily or 50 mg on alternate days and the intravenous dose should be 10 mg once every four days.

Patients on haemodialysis should be given 50 mg orally after each dialysis; this should be done under hospital supervision as marked falls in blood pressure can occur.

4.3 Contraindications

Tenormin, as with other beta-blockers, should not be used in patients with any of the following:

cardiogenic shock

uncontrolled heart failure

sick sinus syndrome

second- or third-degree heart block

untreated phaeochromocytoma

metabolic acidosis

bradycardia (<45 bpm)

hypotension

known hypersensitivity to the active substance, or any of the excipients

severe peripheral arterial circulatory disturbances.

4.4 Special warnings and precautions for use

Tenormin as with other beta-blockers:

• Should not be withdrawn abruptly. The dosage should be withdrawn gradually over a period of 7–14 days, to facilitate a reduction in beta-blocker dosage. Patients should be followed during withdrawal, especially those with ischaemic heart disease.

• When a patient is scheduled for surgery, and a decision is made to discontinue beta-blocker therapy, this should be done at least 24 hours prior to the procedure. The risk-benefit assessment of stopping beta-blockade should be made for each patient. If treatment is continued, an anaesthetic with little negative inotropic activity should be selected to minimise the risk of myocardial depression. The patient may be protected against vagal reactions by intravenous administration of atropine.

• Although contraindicated in uncontrolled heart failure (see section 4.3), may be used in patients whose signs of heart failure have been controlled. Caution must be exercised in patients whose cardiac reserve is poor.

• May increase the number and duration of angina attacks in patients with Prinzmetal's angina due to unopposed alpha-receptor mediated coronary artery vasoconstriction. Tenormin is a $beta_1$-selective beta-blocker; consequently, its use may be considered although utmost caution must be exercised.

• Although contraindicated in severe peripheral arterial circulatory disturbances (see section 4.3), may also aggravate less severe peripheral arterial circulatory disturbances.

• Due to its negative effect on conduction time, caution must be exercised if it is given to patients with first-degree heart block.

• May mask the symptoms of hypoglycaemia, in particular, tachycardia.

• May mask the signs of thyrotoxicosis.

• Will reduce heart rate as a result of its pharmacological action. In the rare instances when a treated patient develops symptoms which may be attributable to a slow heart rate and the pulse rate drops to less than 50–55 bpm at rest, the dose should be reduced.

• May cause a more severe reaction to a variety of allergens when given to patients with a history of anaphylactic reaction to such allergens. Such patients may be unresponsive to the usual doses of adrenaline (epinephrine) used to treat the allergic reactions.

• May cause a hypersensitivity reaction including angioedema and urticaria.

• Should be used with caution in the elderly, starting with a lesser dose (see Section 4.2).

Since Tenormin is excreted via the kidneys, dosage should be reduced in patients with a creatinine clearance of below 35 ml/min/1.73 m^2.

Although cardioselective ($beta_1$) beta-blockers may have less effect on lung function than non-selective beta-blockers, as with all beta-blockers, these should be avoided in patients with reversible obstructive airways disease, unless there are compelling clinical reasons for their use. Where such reasons exist, Tenormin may be used with caution. Occasionally, some increase in airways resistance may occur in asthmatic patients however, and this may usually be reversed by commonly used dosage of bronchodilators such as salbutamol or isoprenaline. The label and patient information leaflet for this product state the following warning: "If you have ever had asthma or wheezing, you should not take this medicine unless you have discussed these symptoms with the prescribing doctor".

As with other beta-blockers, in patients with a phaeochromocytoma, an alpha-blocker should be given concomitantly.

4.5 Interaction with other medicinal products and other forms of interaction

Combined use of beta-blockers and calcium channel blockers with negative inotropic effects, e.g. verapamil and diltiazem, can lead to an exaggeration of these effects particularly in patients with impaired ventricular function and/or sinoatrial or atrioventricular conduction abnormalities. This may result in severe hypotension, bradycardia and cardiac failure. Neither the beta-blocker nor the calcium channel blocker should be administered intravenously within 48 hours of discontinuing the other.

Concomitant therapy with dihydropyridines, e.g. nifedipine, may increase the risk of hypotension, and cardiac failure may occur in patients with latent cardiac insufficiency.

Digitalis glycosides, in association with beta-blockers, may increase atrioventricular conduction time.

Beta-blockers may exacerbate the rebound hypertension which can follow the withdrawal of clonidine. If the two drugs are co-administered, the beta-blocker should be withdrawn several days before discontinuing clonidine. If replacing clonidine by beta-blocker therapy, the introduction of beta-blockers should be delayed for several days after clonidine administration has stopped. (See also prescribing information for clonidine.)

Class I anti-arrhythmic drugs (e.g. disopyramide) and amiodarone may have a potentiating effect on atrial-conduction time and induce negative inotropic effect.

Concomitant use of sympathomimetic agents, e.g. adrenaline (epinephrine), may counteract the effect of beta-blockers.

Concomitant use with insulin and oral antidiabetic drugs may lead to the intensification of the blood sugar lowering effects of these drugs. Symptoms of hypoglycaemia, particularly tachycardia, may be masked (see section 4.4).

Concomitant use of prostaglandin synthetase-inhibiting drugs, e.g. ibuprofen and indometacin, may decrease the hypotensive effects of beta-blockers.

Caution must be exercised when using anaesthetic agents with Tenormin. The anaesthetist should be informed and the choice of anaesthetic should be an agent with as little negative inotropic activity as possible. Use of beta-blockers with anaesthetic drugs may result in attenuation of the reflex tachycardia and increase the risk of hypotension. Anaesthetic agents causing myocardial depression are best avoided.

4.6 Pregnancy and lactation

Tenormin crosses the placental barrier and appears in the cord blood. No studies have been performed on the use of Tenormin in the first trimester and the possibility of foetal injury cannot be excluded. Tenormin has been used under close supervision for the treatment of hypertension in the third trimester. Administration of Tenormin to pregnant women in the management of mild to moderate hypertension has been associated with intra-uterine growth retardation.

The use of Tenormin in women who are, or may become, pregnant requires that the anticipated benefit be weighed against the possible risks, particularly in the first and second trimesters, since beta-blockers, in general, have been associated with a decrease in placental perfusion which may result in intra-uterine deaths, immature and premature deliveries.

There is significant accumulation of Tenormin in breast milk.

Neonates born to mothers who are receiving Tenormin at parturition or breast-feeding may be at risk of hypoglycaemia and bradycardia.

Caution should be exercised when Tenormin is administered during pregnancy or to a woman who is breast-feeding.

4.7 Effects on ability to drive and use machines

The use of Tenormin is unlikely to result in any impairment of the ability of patients to drive or operate machinery. However, it should be taken into account that occasionally dizziness or fatigue may occur.

4.8 Undesirable effects

Tenormin is well tolerated. In clinical studies, the undesired events reported are usually attributable to the pharmacological actions of atenolol.

The following undesired events, listed by body system, have been reported with the following frequencies: very common (≥10%), common (1–9.9%), uncommon (0.1–0.9%), rare (0.01–0.09%), very rare (<0.01%) including isolated reports, not known (cannot be estimated from the available data).

Blood and lymphatic system disorders:

Rare: Purpura, thrombocytopenia.

Psychiatric disorders:

Uncommon: Sleep disturbances of the type noted with other beta-blockers.

Rare: Mood changes, nightmares, confusion, psychoses and hallucinations.

Nervous system disorders:

Rare: Dizziness, headache, paraesthesia.

Eye disorders:

Rare: Dry eyes, visual disturbances.

Cardiac disorders:

Common: Bradycardia.

Rare: Heart failure deterioration, precipitation of heart block.

Vascular disorders:

Common: Cold extremities.

Rare: Postural hypotension which may be associated with syncope, intermittent claudication may be increased if already present, in susceptible patients Raynaud's phenomenon.

Respiratory, thoracic and mediastinal disorders:

Rare: Bronchospasm may occur in patients with bronchial asthma or a history of asthmatic complaints.

Gastrointestinal disorders:

Common: Gastrointestinal disturbances.

Rare: Dry mouth.

Hepato-biliary disorders:

Uncommon: Elevations of transaminase levels.

Rare: Hepatic toxicity including intrahepatic cholestasis.

Skin and subcutaneous tissue disorders:

Rare: Alopecia, psoriasiform skin reactions, exacerbation of psoriasis, skin rashes.

Not known: Hypersensitivity reactions, including angioedema and urticaria.

Reproductive system and breast disorders:

Rare: Impotence.

General disorders and administration site conditions:

Common: Fatigue.

Investigations:

Very rare: An increase in ANA (Antinuclear Antibodies) has been observed, however the clinical relevance of this is not clear.

Discontinuance of the drug should be considered if, according to clinical judgement, the well-being of the patient is adversely affected by any of the above reactions.

4.9 Overdose

The symptoms of overdosage may include bradycardia, hypotension, acute cardiac insufficiency and bronchospasm.

General treatment should include: close supervision; treatment in an intensive care ward; the use of gastric lavage; activated charcoal and a laxative to prevent absorption of any drug still present in the gastrointestinal tract; the use of plasma or plasma substitutes to treat hypotension and shock. The possible uses of haemodialysis or haemoperfusion may be considered.

Excessive bradycardia can be countered with atropine 1–2 mg intravenously and/or a cardiac pacemaker. If necessary, this may be followed by a bolus dose of glucagon 10 mg intravenously. If required, this may be repeated or followed by an intravenous infusion of glucagon 1–10 mg/hour depending on response. If no response to glucagon occurs or if glucagon is unavailable, a beta-adrenoceptor stimulant such as dobutamine 2.5 to 10 micrograms/kg/minute by intravenous infusion may be given. Dobutamine, because of its positive inotropic effect could also be used to treat hypotension and acute cardiac insufficiency. It is likely that these doses would be inadequate to reverse the cardiac effects of beta-blocker blockade if a large overdose has been taken. The dose of dobutamine should therefore be increased if necessary to achieve the required response according to the clinical condition of the patient.

Bronchospasm can usually be reversed by bronchodilators.

5. PHARMACOLOGICAL PROPERTIES

5.1 Pharmacodynamic properties

Beta-blocking agents, plain, selective.

CO7A B03.

Atenolol is a beta-blocker which is $beta_1$-selective, (i.e. acts preferentially on $beta_1$-adrenergic receptors in the heart). Selectivity decreases with increasing dose.

Atenolol is without intrinsic sympathomimetic and membrane-stabilising activities and as with other beta-blockers, has negative inotropic effects (and is therefore contraindicated in uncontrolled heart failure).

As with other beta-blockers, the mode of action of atenolol in the treatment of hypertension is unclear.

It is probably the action of atenolol in reducing cardiac rate and contractility which makes it effective in eliminating or reducing the symptoms of patients with angina.

It is unlikely that any additional ancillary properties possessed by S (-) atenolol, in comparison with the racemic mixture, will give rise to different therapeutic effects.

Tenormin is effective and well-tolerated in most ethnic populations although the response may be less in black patients.

The narrow dose range and early patient response to Tenormin ensure that the effect of the drug in individual patients is quickly demonstrated. Tenormin is compatible with diuretics, other hypotensive agents and antianginals (see section 4.5). Since it acts preferentially on beta-adrenergic receptors in the heart, Tenormin may, with care be used successfully in the treatment of patients with respiratory disease who cannot tolerate non-selective beta-adrenoceptor blocking drugs.

Early intervention with Tenormin in acute myocardial infarction reduces infarct size and decreases morbidity and mortality. Fewer patients with a threatened infarction progress to frank infarction; the incidence of ventricular arrhythmias is decreased and marked pain relief may result in reduced need of opiate analgesics. Early mortality is decreased. Tenormin is an additional treatment to standard coronary care.

5.2 Pharmacokinetic properties

Following intravenous administration, the blood levels of atenolol decay tri-exponentially with an elimination half-life of about 6 hours. Throughout the intravenous dose range of 5 to 10 mg the blood level profile obeys linear pharmacokinetics and beta-adrenoceptor blockade is still measurable 24 hours after a 10 mg intravenous dose.

Absorption of atenolol following oral dosing is consistent but incomplete (approximately 40–50%) with peak plasma concentrations occurring 2–4 hours after dosing. The atenolol blood levels are consistent and subject to little variability. There is no significant hepatic metabolism of atenolol and more than 90% of that absorbed reaches the systemic circulation unaltered. The plasma half-life is about 6 hours but this may rise in severe renal impairment since the kidney is the major route of elimination. Atenolol penetrates tissues poorly due to its low lipid solubility and its concentration in brain tissue is low. Plasma protein binding is low (approximately 3%).

5.3 Preclinical safety data

Atenolol is a drug on which extensive clinical experience has been obtained. Relevant information for the prescriber is provided elsewhere in the Prescribing Information.

6. PHARMACEUTICAL PARTICULARS

6.1 List of excipients

Citric acid

Sodium chloride

Sodium hydroxide

Water for Injection

6.2 Incompatibilities

None known.

6.3 Shelf life

36 months.

6.4 Special precautions for storage

Do not store above 25°C. Keep the container in the outer carton.

6.5 Nature and contents of container

Glass ampoules.

10 ml ampoules are packed in boxes of 10.

6.6 Special precautions for disposal and other handling

Use as instructed by the prescriber.

Tenormin Injection is compatible with sodium chloride intravenous infusion (0.9 %w/v) and Glucose Intravenous Infusion BP (5 % w/v).

7. MARKETING AUTHORISATION HOLDER

AstraZeneca UK Limited,

600 Capability Green,

Luton, LU1 3LU, UK.

8. MARKETING AUTHORISATION NUMBER(S)

17901/0050

9. DATE OF FIRST AUTHORISATION/RENEWAL OF THE AUTHORISATION

01 June 2000/18th February 2004

10. DATE OF REVISION OF THE TEXT

18th December 2007

Tenormin LS 50mg Tablets

(AstraZeneca UK Limited)

1. NAME OF THE MEDICINAL PRODUCT

Tenormin LS 50 mg Tablets

2. QUALITATIVE AND QUANTITATIVE COMPOSITION

Atenolol 50 mg.

For excipients, see section 6.1.

3. PHARMACEUTICAL FORM

Film-coated tablet.

Orange film-coated tablets which are intagliated on one face and bisected on the other. Intagliations are highlighted in white.

4. CLINICAL PARTICULARS

4.1 Therapeutic indications

i. Management of hypertension.

ii. Management of angina pectoris.

iii. Management of cardiac arrhythmias.

iv. Management of myocardial infarction. Early intervention in the acute phase.

4.2 Posology and method of administration

Oral administration.

The dose must always be adjusted to individual requirements of the patients, with the lowest possible starting dosage. The following are guidelines:

Adults

Hypertension

One tablet daily. Most patients respond to 100 mg daily given orally as a single dose. Some patients, however, will respond to 50 mg given as a single daily dose. The effect will be fully established after one to two weeks. A further reduction in blood pressure may be achieved by combining Tenormin with other antihypertensive agents. For example, co-administration of Tenormin with a diuretic, as in Tenoretic provides a highly effective and convenient antihypertensive therapy.

Angina

Most patients with angina pectoris will respond to 100 mg given orally once daily or 50 mg given twice daily. It is unlikely that additional benefit will be gained by increasing the dose.

Cardiac arrhythmias

A suitable initial dose of Tenormin is 2.5 mg (5 ml) injected intravenously over a 2.5 minute period (i.e. 1 mg/minute). (See also prescribing information for Tenormin Injection.) This may be repeated at 5 minute intervals, until a response is observed up to a maximum dosage of 10 mg. If Tenormin is given by infusion, 0.15 mg/kg bodyweight may be administered over a 20 minute period. If required, the injection or infusion may be repeated every 12 hours. Having controlled the arrhythmias with intravenous Tenormin, a suitable oral maintenance dosage is 50–100 mg daily, given as a single dose.

Myocardial infarction

For patients suitable for treatment with intravenous beta-blockade and presenting within 12 hours of the onset of chest pain, Tenormin 5–10 mg should be given by slow intravenous injection (1 mg/minute) followed by Tenormin 50 mg orally about 15 minutes later, provided no untoward effects have occurred from the intravenous dose. This should be followed by a further 50 mg orally 12 hours after the intravenous dose, and then 12 hours later by 100 mg orally, once daily. If bradycardia and/or hypotension requiring treatment, or any other untoward effects occur, Tenormin should be discontinued.

Elderly

Dosage requirements may be reduced, especially in patients with impaired renal function.

Children

There is no paediatric experience with Tenormin and for this reason it is not recommended for use in children.

Renal failure

Since Tenormin is excreted via the kidneys, the dosage should be adjusted in cases of severe impairment of renal function.

No significant accumulation of Tenormin occurs in patients who have a creatinine clearance greater than 35 ml/min/1.73 m^2 (normal range is 100–150 ml/min/1.73 m^2).

For patients with a creatinine clearance of 15–35 ml/min/1.73 m^2 (equivalent to serum creatinine of 300–600 micromol/litre), the oral dose should be 50 mg daily and the intravenous dose should be 10 mg once every two days.

For patients with a creatinine clearance of less than 15 ml/min/1.73 m^2 (equivalent to serum creatinine of greater than 600 micromol/litre), the oral dose should be 25 mg daily or 50 mg on alternate days and the intravenous dose should be 10 mg once every four days.

Patients on haemodialysis should be given 50 mg orally after each dialysis; this should be done under hospital supervision as marked falls in blood pressure can occur.

4.3 Contraindications

Tenormin, as with other beta-blockers, should not be used in patients with any of the following:

cardiogenic shock

uncontrolled heart failure

sick sinus syndrome

second-or third-degree heart block

untreated phaeochromocytoma

metabolic acidosis

bradycardia (<45 bpm)

hypotension

known hypersensitivity to the active substance, or any of the excipients

severe peripheral arterial circulatory disturbances.

4.4 Special warnings and precautions for use

Tenormin as with other beta-blockers:

• Should not be withdrawn abruptly. The dosage should be withdrawn gradually over a period of 7–14 days, to facilitate a reduction in beta-blocker dosage. Patients should be followed during withdrawal, especially those with ischaemic heart disease.

• When a patient is scheduled for surgery, and a decision is made to discontinue beta-blocker therapy, this should be done at least 24 hours prior to the procedure. The risk-benefit assessment of stopping beta-blockade should be made for each patient. If treatment is continued, an anaesthetic with little negative inotropic activity should be selected to minimise the risk of myocardial depression. The patient may be protected against vagal reactions by intravenous administration of atropine.

• Although contraindicated in uncontrolled heart failure (see section 4.3), may be used in patients whose signs of heart failure have been controlled. Caution must be exercised in patients whose cardiac reserve is poor.

• May increase the number and duration of angina attacks in patients with Prinzmetal's angina due to unopposed alpha-receptor mediated coronary artery vasoconstriction. Tenormin is a beta$_1$-selective beta-blocker; consequently, its use may be considered although utmost caution must be exercised.

• Although contraindicated in severe peripheral arterial circulatory disturbances (see section 4.3), may also aggravate less severe peripheral arterial circulatory disturbances.

• Due to its negative effect on conduction time, caution must be exercised if it is given to patients with first-degree heart block.

• May mask the symptoms of hypoglycaemia, in particular, tachycardia.

• May mask the signs of thyrotoxicosis.

• Will reduce heart rate as a result of its pharmacological action. In the rare instances when a treated patient develops symptoms which may be attributable to a slow heart rate and the pulse rate drops to less than 50–55 bpm at rest, the dose should be reduced.

• May cause a more severe reaction to a variety of allergens when given to patients with a history of anaphylactic reaction to such allergens. Such patients may be unresponsive to the usual doses of adrenaline (epinephrine) used to treat the allergic reactions.

• May cause a hypersensitivity reaction including angioedema and urticaria.

• Should be used with caution in the elderly, starting with a lesser dose (see Section 4.2).

Since Tenormin is excreted via the kidneys, dosage should be reduced in patients with a creatinine clearance of below 35 ml/min/1.73 m^2.

Although cardioselective (beta$_1$) beta-blockers may have less effect on lung function than non-selective beta-blockers, as with all beta-blockers, these should be avoided in patients with reversible obstructive airways disease, unless there are compelling clinical reasons for their use. Where such reasons exist, Tenormin may be used with caution. Occasionally, some increase in airways resistance may occur in asthmatic patients however, and this may usually be reversed by commonly used dosage of bronchodilators such as salbutamol or isoprenaline. The label and patient information leaflet for this product state the following warning: "If you have ever had asthma or wheezing, you should not take this medicine unless you have discussed these symptoms with the prescribing doctor".

As with other beta-blockers, in patients with a phaeochromocytoma, an alpha-blocker should be given concomitantly.

4.5 Interaction with other medicinal products and other forms of interaction

Combined use of beta-blockers and calcium channel blockers with negative inotropic effects, e.g. verapamil and diltiazem, can lead to an exaggeration of these effects particularly in patients with impaired ventricular function and/or sinoatrial or atrioventricular conduction abnormalities. This may result in severe hypotension, bradycardia and cardiac failure. Neither the beta-blocker nor the calcium channel blocker should be administered intravenously within 48 hours of discontinuing the other.

Concomitant therapy with dihydropyridines, e.g. nifedipine, may increase the risk of hypotension, and cardiac failure may occur in patients with latent cardiac insufficiency.

Digitalis glycosides, in association with beta-blockers, may increase atrioventricular conduction time.

Beta-blockers may exacerbate the rebound hypertension which can follow the withdrawal of clonidine. If the two drugs are co-administered, the beta-blocker should be withdrawn several days before discontinuing clonidine. If replacing clonidine by beta-blocker therapy, the introduction of beta-blockers should be delayed for several days after clonidine administration has stopped. (See also prescribing information for clonidine.)

Class I anti-arrhythmic drugs (e.g. disopyramide) and amiodarone may have a potentiating effect on atrial-conduction time and induce negative inotropic effect.

Concomitant use of sympathomimetic agents, e.g. adrenaline (epinephrine), may counteract the effect of beta-blockers.

Concomitant use with insulin and oral antidiabetic drugs may lead to the intensification of the blood sugar lowering effects of these drugs. Symptoms of hypoglycaemia, particularly tachycardia, may be masked (see section 4.4).

Concomitant use of prostaglandin synthetase-inhibiting drugs, e.g. ibuprofen and indometacin, may decrease the hypotensive effects of beta-blockers.

Caution must be exercised when using anaesthetic agents with Tenormin. The anaesthetist should be informed and the choice of anaesthetic should be an agent with as little negative inotropic activity as possible. Use of beta-blockers with anaesthetic drugs may result in attenuation of the reflex tachycardia and increase the risk of hypotension. Anaesthetic agents causing myocardial depression are best avoided.

4.6 Pregnancy and lactation

Tenormin crosses the placental barrier and appears in the cord blood. No studies have been performed on the use of Tenormin in the first trimester and the possibility of foetal injury cannot be excluded. Tenormin has been used under close supervision for the treatment of hypertension in the third trimester. Administration of Tenormin to pregnant women in the management of mild to moderate hypertension has been associated with intra-uterine growth retardation.

The use of Tenormin in women who are, or may become, pregnant requires that the anticipated benefit be weighed against the possible risks, particularly in the first and second trimesters, since beta-blockers, in general, have been associated with a decrease in placental perfusion which may result in intra-uterine deaths, immature and premature deliveries.

There is significant accumulation of Tenormin in breast milk.

Neonates born to mothers who are receiving Tenormin at parturition or breast-feeding may be at risk of hypoglycaemia and bradycardia.

Caution should be exercised when Tenormin is administered during pregnancy or to a woman who is breast-feeding.

4.7 Effects on ability to drive and use machines

Use is unlikely to result in any impairment of the ability of patients to drive or operate machinery. However, it should be taken into account that occasionally dizziness or fatigue may occur.

4.8 Undesirable effects

Tenormin is well tolerated. In clinical studies, the undesired events reported are usually attributable to the pharmacological actions of atenolol.

The following undesired events, listed by body system, have been reported with the following frequencies: very common (⩾10%), common (1–9.9%), uncommon (0.1–0.9%), rare (0.01–0.09%), very rare (<0.01%) including isolated reports, not known (cannot be estimated from the available data).

Blood and lymphatic system disorders:

Rare: Purpura, thrombocytopenia.

Psychiatric disorders:

Uncommon: Sleep disturbances of the type noted with other beta-blockers.

Rare: Mood changes, nightmares, confusion, psychoses and hallucinations.

Nervous system disorders:

Rare: Dizziness, headache, paraesthesia.

Eye disorders:

Rare: Dry eyes, visual disturbances.

Cardiac disorders:

Common: Bradycardia.

Rare: Heart failure deterioration, precipitation of heart block.

Vascular disorders:

Common: Cold extremities.

Rare: Postural hypotension which may be associated with syncope, intermittent claudication may be increased if already present, in susceptible patients Raynaud's phenomenon.

Respiratory, thoracic and mediastinal disorders:

Rare: Bronchospasm may occur in patients with bronchial asthma or a history of asthmatic complaints.

Gastrointestinal disorders:

Common: Gastrointestinal disturbances.

Rare: Dry mouth.

Hepato-biliary disorders:

Uncommon: Elevations of transaminase levels.

Rare: Hepatic toxicity including intrahepatic cholestasis.

Skin and subcutaneous tissue disorders:

Rare: Alopecia, psoriasiform skin reactions, exacerbation of psoriasis, skin rashes.

Not known: Hypersensitivity reactions, including angioedema and urticaria.

Reproductive system and breast disorders:

Rare: Impotence.

General disorders and administration site conditions:

Common: Fatigue.

Investigations:

Very rare: An increase in ANA (Antinuclear Antibodies) has been observed, however the clinical relevance of this is not clear.

Discontinuance of the drug should be considered if, according to clinical judgement, the well-being of the patient is adversely affected by any of the above reactions.

4.9 Overdose

The symptoms of overdosage may include bradycardia, hypotension, acute cardiac insufficiency and bronchospasm.

General treatment should include: close supervision; treatment in an intensive care ward; the use of gastric lavage; activated charcoal and a laxative to prevent absorption of any drug still present in the gastrointestinal tract; the use of plasma or plasma substitutes to treat hypotension and shock. The possible uses of haemodialysis or haemoperfusion may be considered.

Excessive bradycardia can be countered with atropine 1–2 mg intravenously and/or a cardiac pacemaker. If necessary, this may be followed by a bolus dose of glucagon 10 mg intravenously. If required, this may be repeated or followed by an intravenous infusion of glucagon 1–10 mg/hour depending on response. If no response to glucagon occurs or if glucagon is unavailable, a beta-adrenoceptor stimulant such as dobutamine 2.5 to 10 micrograms/kg/minute by intravenous infusion may be given. Dobutamine, because of its positive inotropic effect could also be used to treat hypotension and acute cardiac insufficiency. It is likely that these doses would be inadequate to reverse the cardiac effects of beta-blocker blockade if a large overdose has been taken. The dose of dobutamine should therefore be increased if necessary to achieve the required response according to the clinical condition of the patient.

Bronchospasm can usually be reversed by bronchodilators.

5. PHARMACOLOGICAL PROPERTIES

5.1 Pharmacodynamic properties

Beta-blocking agents, plain, selective.

CO7A B03.

Atenolol is a beta-blocker which is beta$_1$-selective, (i.e. acts preferentially on beta$_1$-adrenergic receptors in the heart). Selectivity decreases with increasing dose.

Atenolol is without intrinsic sympathomimetic and membrane-stabilising activities and as with other beta-blockers, has negative inotropic effects (and is therefore contraindicated in uncontrolled heart failure).

As with other beta-blockers, the mode of action of atenolol in the treatment of hypertension is unclear.

It is probably the action of atenolol in reducing cardiac rate and contractility which makes it effective in eliminating or reducing the symptoms of patients with angina.

It is unlikely that any additional ancillary properties possessed by S (-) atenolol, in comparison with the racemic mixture, will give rise to different therapeutic effects.

Tenormin is effective and well-tolerated in most ethnic populations although the response may be less in black patients.

Tenormin is effective for at least 24 hours after a single oral dose. The drug facilitates compliance by its acceptability to patients and simplicity of dosing. The narrow dose range and early patient response ensure that the effect of the drug in individual patients is quickly demonstrated. Tenormin is compatible with diuretics, other hypotensive agents and antianginals (see section 4.5). Since it acts preferentially on beta-receptors in the heart, Tenormin may, with care, be used successfully in the treatment of patients with respiratory disease, who cannot tolerate non-selective beta-blockers.

Early intervention with Tenormin in acute myocardial infarction reduces infarct size and decreases morbidity and mortality. Fewer patients with a threatened infarction progress to frank infarction; the incidence of ventricular arrhythmias is decreased and marked pain relief may result in reduced need of opiate analgesics. Early mortality is decreased. Tenormin is an additional treatment to standard coronary care.

5.2 Pharmacokinetic properties

Absorption of atenolol following oral dosing is consistent but incomplete (approximately 40–50%) with peak plasma concentrations occurring 2–4 hours after dosing. The atenolol blood levels are consistent and subject to little variability. There is no significant hepatic metabolism of atenolol and more than 90% of that absorbed reaches the systemic circulation unaltered. The plasma half-life is about 6 hours but this may rise in severe renal impairment since the kidney is the major route of elimination. Atenolol penetrates tissues poorly due to its low lipid solubility and its concentration in brain tissue is low. Plasma protein binding is low (approximately 3%).

5.3 Preclinical safety data

Atenolol is a drug on which extensive clinical experience has been obtained. Relevant information for the prescriber is provided elsewhere in the Prescribing Information.

6. PHARMACEUTICAL PARTICULARS

6.1 List of excipients

Gelatin

Macrogol 300

Magnesium Carbonate

Magnesium Stearate

Maize Starch

Methylhydoxypropylcellulose

Sodium Laurilsulfate

Sunset Yellow Lake (E110)

Talc

Titanium Dioxide (E171)

6.2 Incompatibilities

Not applicable.

6.3 Shelf life

60 months.

6.4 Special precautions for storage

Do not store above 25°C.

Store in the original package. Keep the container in the outer carton.

6.5 Nature and contents of container

Aluminium PVC/PVDC blister strips of 14 tablets: 28 Tablets

Aluminium PVC/PVDC blister strips of 7 tablets: 504 Tablets (for Hospital Use) (pack is subdivided into 6 cartons each containing 12 blister strips i.e. 84 tablets)

6.6 Special precautions for disposal and other handling

Not applicable.

7. MARKETING AUTHORISATION HOLDER

AstraZeneca UK Limited,

600 Capability Green,

Luton, LU1 3LU, UK.

8. MARKETING AUTHORISATION NUMBER(S)

PL 17901/0053

9. DATE OF FIRST AUTHORISATION/RENEWAL OF THE AUTHORISATION

1st June 2000 / 5th November 2003

10. DATE OF REVISION OF THE TEXT

18th December 2007

Tenormin Syrup

(AstraZeneca UK Limited)

1. NAME OF THE MEDICINAL PRODUCT

Tenormin 5 mg/ml Syrup

2. QUALITATIVE AND QUANTITATIVE COMPOSITION

Atenolol 0.5 % w/v.

For excipients, see section 6.1.

3. PHARMACEUTICAL FORM

Syrup.

4. CLINICAL PARTICULARS

4.1 Therapeutic indications

i. Management of hypertension.

ii. Management of angina.

iii. Management of cardiac arrhythmias.

iv. Myocardial infarction. Early intervention in the acute phase.

4.2 Posology and method of administration

Oral administration.

Tenormin 5 mg/ml Syrup is intended for patients unable to swallow Tenormin tablets.

The dose must always be adjusted to individual requirements of the patients, with the lowest possible starting dosage. The following are guidelines:

Adults

Hypertension

Two or four 5 ml spoonfuls daily i.e. 50 mg or 100 mg in patients unable to take 50 mg or 100 mg tablets.

Most patients respond to 100 mg once daily. Some patients, however, will respond to 50 mg given as a single daily dose. The effect will be fully established after one to two weeks. A further reduction in blood pressure may be achieved by combining Tenormin with other antihypertensive agents.

Angina

Most patients with angina pectoris will respond to 100 mg (four 5 ml spoonfuls) given orally once a day, or 50 mg (two 5 ml spoonfuls) given twice daily. It is unlikely that additional benefit will be gained by increasing the dose.

Cardiac arrhythmias

A suitable initial dose of Tenormin Injection is 2.5 mg (5 ml) injected intravenously over a 2.5 minute period (i.e. 1 mg/minute). (See also prescribing information for Tenormin Injection.) This may be repeated at 5 minute intervals, until a response is observed up to a maximum dosage of 10 mg. If Tenormin Injection is given by infusion, 0.15 mg/kg bodyweight may be administered over a 20 minute period. If required, the injection or infusion may be repeated every 12 hours. Having controlled the arrhythmias with intravenous Tenormin, a suitable oral maintenance dosage is

50–100 mg (two to four 5 ml spoonfuls of Tenormin 5 mg/ml Syrup) daily, given as a single dose.

Myocardial infarction

For patients suitable for treatment with intravenous beta-blockade and presenting within 12 hours of the onset of chest pain, Tenormin 5–10 mg should be given by slow intravenous injection (1 mg/minute) followed by Tenormin 50 mg orally about 15 minutes later, provided no untoward effects have occurred from the intravenous dose. This should be followed by a further 50 mg orally 12 hours after the intravenous dose, and then 12 hours later by 100 mg orally, once daily. If bradycardia and/or hypotension requiring treatment, or any other untoward effects occur, Tenormin should be discontinued.

Elderly

Dosage requirements may be reduced, especially in patients with impaired renal function.

Children

There is no paediatric experience with Tenormin and for this reason it is not recommended for use in children.

Renal failure

Since Tenormin is excreted via the kidneys, the dosage should be adjusted in cases of severe impairment of renal function.

No significant accumulation of Tenormin occurs in patients who have a creatinine clearance greater than 35 ml/min/1.73 m^2 (normal range is 100–150 ml/min/1.73 m^2).

For patients with a creatinine clearance of 15–35 ml/min/1.73 m^2 (equivalent to serum creatinine of 300–600 micromol/litre), the oral dose should be 50 mg daily and the intravenous dose should be 10 mg once every two days.

For patients with a creatinine clearance of less than 15 ml/min/1.73 m^2 (equivalent to serum creatinine of greater than 600 micromol/litre), the oral dose should be 25 mg daily or 50 mg on alternate days and the intravenous dose should be 10 mg once every four days.

Patients on haemodialysis should be given 50 mg orally after each dialysis; this should be done under hospital supervision as marked falls in blood pressure can occur.

4.3 Contraindications

Tenormin, as with other beta-blockers, should not be used in patients with any of the following:

cardiogenic shock

uncontrolled heart failure

sick sinus syndrome

second-or third-degree heart block

untreated phaeochromocytoma

metabolic acidosis

bradycardia (<45 bpm)

hypotension

known hypersensitivity to the active substance, or any of the excipients

severe peripheral arterial circulatory disturbances.

4.4 Special warnings and precautions for use

Tenormin as with other beta-blockers:

- Should not be withdrawn abruptly. The dosage should be withdrawn gradually over a period of 7–14 days, to facilitate a reduction in beta-blocker dosage. Patients should be followed during withdrawal, especially those with ischaemic heart disease.
- When a patient is scheduled for surgery, and a decision is made to discontinue beta-blocker therapy, this should be done at least 24 hours prior to the procedure. The risk-benefit assessment of stopping beta-blockade should be made for each patient. If treatment is continued, an anaesthetic with little negative inotropic activity should be selected to minimise the risk of myocardial depression. The patient may be protected against vagal reactions by intravenous administration of atropine.
- Although contraindicated in uncontrolled heart failure (see section 4.3), may be used in patients whose signs of heart failure have been controlled. Caution must be exercised in patients whose cardiac reserve is poor.
- May increase the number and duration of angina attacks in patients with Prinzmetal's angina due to unopposed alpha-receptor mediated coronary artery vasoconstriction. Tenormin is a beta$_1$-selective beta-blocker; consequently, its use may be considered although utmost caution must be exercised.
- Although contraindicated in severe peripheral arterial circulatory disturbances (see section 4.3), may also aggravate less severe peripheral arterial circulatory disturbances.
- Due to its negative effect on conduction time, caution must be exercised if it is given to patients with first-degree heart block.
- May mask the symptoms of hypoglycaemia, in particular, tachycardia.
- May mask the signs of thyrotoxicosis.
- Will reduce heart rate as a result of its pharmacological action. In the rare instances when a treated patient develops symptoms which may be attributable to a slow heart rate and the pulse rate drops to less than 50–55 bpm at rest, the dose should be reduced.
- May cause a more severe reaction to a variety of allergens when given to patients with a history of anaphylactic reaction to such allergens. Such patients may be unresponsive to the usual doses of adrenaline (epinephrine) used to treat the allergic reactions.
- May cause a hypersensitivity reaction including angioedema and urticaria.
- Should be used with caution in the elderly, starting with a lesser dose (see Section 4.2).

Since Tenormin is excreted via the kidneys, dosage should be reduced in patients with a creatinine clearance of below 35 ml/min/1.73 m^2.

Although cardioselective (beta$_1$) beta-blockers may have less effect on lung function than non-selective beta-blockers, as with all beta-blockers, these should be avoided in patients with reversible obstructive airways disease, unless there are compelling clinical reasons for their use. Where such reasons exist, Tenormin may be used with caution. Occasionally, some increase in airways resistance may occur in asthmatic patients however, and this may usually be reversed by commonly used dosage of bronchodilators such as salbutamol or isoprenaline. The label and patient information leaflet for this product state the following warning: "If you have ever had asthma or wheezing, you should not take this medicine unless you have discussed these symptoms with the prescribing doctor".

As with other beta-blockers, in patients with a phaeochromocytoma, an alpha-blocker should be given concomitantly.

4.5 Interaction with other medicinal products and other forms of interaction

Combined use of beta-blockers and calcium channel blockers with negative inotropic effects, e.g. verapamil and diltiazem, can lead to an exaggeration of these effects particularly in patients with impaired ventricular function and/or sinoatrial or atrioventricular conduction abnormalities. This may result in severe hypotension, bradycardia and cardiac failure. Neither the beta-blocker nor the calcium channel blocker should be administered intravenously within 48 hours of discontinuing the other.

Concomitant therapy with dihydropyridines, e.g. nifedipine, may increase the risk of hypotension, and cardiac failure may occur in patients with latent cardiac insufficiency.

Digitalis glycosides, in association with beta-blockers, may increase atrioventricular conduction time.

Beta-blockers may exacerbate the rebound hypertension which can follow the withdrawal of clonidine. If the two drugs are co-administered, the beta-blocker should be withdrawn several days before discontinuing clonidine. If replacing clonidine by beta-blocker therapy, the introduction of beta-blockers should be delayed for several days after clonidine administration has stopped. (See also prescribing information for clonidine.)

Class I anti-arrhythmic drugs (e.g. disopyramide) and amiodarone may have a potentiating effect on atrial-conduction time and induce negative inotropic effect.

Concomitant use of sympathomimetic agents, e.g. adrenaline (epinephrine), may counteract the effect of beta-blockers.

Concomitant use with insulin and oral antidiabetic drugs may lead to the intensification of the blood sugar lowering effects of these drugs. Symptoms of hypoglycaemia, particularly tachycardia, may be masked (see section 4.4).

Concomitant use of prostaglandin synthetase-inhibiting drugs, e.g. ibuprofen and indometacin, may decrease the hypotensive effects of beta-blockers.

Caution must be exercised when using anaesthetic agents with Tenormin. The anaesthetist should be informed and the choice of anaesthetic should be an agent with as little negative inotropic activity as possible. Use of beta-blockers with anaesthetic drugs may result in attenuation of the reflex tachycardia and increase the risk of hypotension. Anaesthetic agents causing myocardial depression are best avoided.

4.6 Pregnancy and lactation

Tenormin crosses the placental barrier and appears in the cord blood. No studies have been performed on the use of Tenormin in the first trimester and the possibility of foetal injury cannot be excluded. Tenormin has been used under close supervision for the treatment of hypertension in the third trimester. Administration of Tenormin to pregnant women in the management of mild to moderate hypertension has been associated with intra-uterine growth retardation.

The use of Tenormin in women who are, or may become, pregnant requires that the anticipated benefit be weighed against the possible risks, particularly in the first and second trimesters, since beta-blockers, in general, have been associated with a decrease in placental perfusion which may result in intra-uterine deaths, immature and premature deliveries.

There is significant accumulation of Tenormin in breast milk.

Neonates born to mothers who are receiving Tenormin at parturition or breast-feeding may be at risk of hypoglycaemia and bradycardia.

Caution should be exercised when Tenormin is administered during pregnancy or to a woman who is breast-feeding.

4.7 Effects on ability to drive and use machines

Use is unlikely to result in any impairment of the ability of patients to drive or operate machinery. However, it should be taken into account that occasionally dizziness or fatigue may occur.

4.8 Undesirable effects

Tenormin is well tolerated. In clinical studies, the undesired events reported are usually attributable to the pharmacological actions of atenolol.

The following undesired events, listed by body system, have been reported with the following frequencies: very common (≥10%), common (1–9.9%), uncommon (0.1–0.9%), rare (0.01–0.09%), very rare (<0.01%) including isolated reports, not known (cannot be estimated from the available data).

Blood and lymphatic system disorders:

Rare: Purpura, thrombocytopenia.

Psychiatric disorders:

Uncommon: Sleep disturbances of the type noted with other beta-blockers.

Rare: Mood changes, nightmares, confusion, psychoses and hallucinations.

Nervous system disorders:

Rare: Dizziness, headache, paraesthesia.

Eye disorders:

Rare: Dry eyes, visual disturbances.

Cardiac disorders:

Common: Bradycardia.

Rare: Heart failure deterioration, precipitation of heart block.

Vascular disorders:

Common: Cold extremities.

Rare: Postural hypotension which may be associated with syncope, intermittent claudication may be increased if already present, in susceptible patients Raynaud's phenomenon.

Respiratory, thoracic and mediastinal disorders:

Rare: Bronchospasm may occur in patients with bronchial asthma or a history of asthmatic complaints.

Gastrointestinal disorders:

Common: Gastrointestinal disturbances.

Rare: Dry mouth.

Hepato-biliary disorders:

Uncommon: Elevations of transaminase levels.

Rare: Hepatic toxicity including intrahepatic cholestasis.

Skin and subcutaneous tissue disorders:

Rare: Alopecia, psoriasiform skin reactions, exacerbation of psoriasis, skin rashes.

Not known: Hypersensitivity reactions, including angioedema and urticaria.

Reproductive system and breast disorders:

Rare: Impotence.

General disorders and administration site conditions:

Common: Fatigue.

Investigations:

Very rare: An increase in ANA (Antinuclear Antibodies) has been observed, however the clinical relevance of this is not clear.

Discontinuance of the drug should be considered if, according to clinical judgement, the well-being of the patient is adversely affected by any of the above reactions.

4.9 Overdose

The symptoms of overdosage may include bradycardia, hypotension, acute cardiac insufficiency and bronchospasm.

General treatment should include: close supervision; treatment in an intensive care ward; the use of gastric lavage; activated charcoal and a laxative to prevent absorption of any drug still present in the gastrointestinal tract; the use of plasma or plasma substitutes to treat hypotension and shock. The possible uses of haemodialysis or haemoperfusion may be considered.

Excessive bradycardia can be countered with atropine 1–2 mg intravenously and/or a cardiac pacemaker. If necessary, this may be followed by a bolus dose of glucagon 10 mg intravenously. If required, this may be repeated or followed by an intravenous infusion of glucagon 1–10 mg/hour depending on response. If no response to glucagon occurs or if glucagon is unavailable, a beta-adrenoceptor stimulant such as dobutamine 2.5 to 10 micrograms/kg/minute by intravenous infusion may be given. Dobutamine, because of its positive inotropic effect could also be used to treat hypotension and acute cardiac insufficiency. It is likely that these doses would be inadequate to reverse the cardiac effects of beta-blocker blockade if a large overdose has been taken. The dose of dobutamine should therefore be increased if necessary to achieve the required response according to the clinical condition of the patient.

Bronchospasm can usually be reversed by bronchodilators.

5. PHARMACOLOGICAL PROPERTIES

5.1 Pharmacodynamic properties

Beta-blocking agents, plain, selective.

CO7 B03.

Atenolol is a beta-blocker which is $beta_1$-selective, (i.e. acts preferentially on $beta_1$-adrenergic receptors in the heart). Selectivity decreases with increasing dose.

Atenolol is without intrinsic sympathomimetic and membrane-stabilising activities and as with other beta-blockers, has negative inotropic effects (and is therefore contraindicated in uncontrolled heart failure).

As with other beta-blockers, the mode of action of atenolol in the treatment of hypertension is unclear.

It is probably the action of atenolol in reducing cardiac rate and contractility which makes it effective in eliminating or reducing the symptoms of patients with angina.

It is unlikely that any additional ancillary properties possessed by S (-) atenolol, in comparison with the racemic mixture, will give rise to different therapeutic effects.

Tenormin is effective and well-tolerated in most ethnic populations although the response may be less in black patients.

Tenormin is effective for at least 24 hours after once daily dosing with 10 ml or 20 ml Tenormin 5 mg/ml Syrup. Tenormin 5 mg/ml Syrup facilitates compliance by its acceptability to patients and the once daily dosing regimen. The narrow dose range and early patient response ensure that the effect of the drug in individual patients is quickly demonstrated. Tenormin is compatible with diuretics, other hypotensive agents and antianginals (see section 4.5). Since it acts preferentially on beta-adrenergic receptors in the heart, Tenormin may, with care, be used successfully in the treatment of patients with respiratory disease, who cannot tolerate non-selective beta-blockers.

Early intervention with Tenormin in acute myocardial infarction reduces infarct size and decreases morbidity and mortality. Fewer patients with a threatened infarction progress to frank infarction; the incidence of ventricular arrhythmias is decreased and marked pain relief may result in reduced need of opiate analgesics. Early mortality is decreased. Tenormin is an additional treatment to standard coronary care.

5.2 Pharmacokinetic properties

Absorption of atenolol following oral dosing is consistent but incomplete (approximately 40–50%) with peak plasma concentrations occurring 2–4 hours after dosing. The atenolol blood levels are consistent and subject to little variability. There is no significant hepatic metabolism of atenolol and more than 90% of that absorbed reaches the systemic circulation unaltered. The plasma half-life is about 6 hours but this may rise in severe renal impairment since the kidney is the major route of elimination. Atenolol penetrates tissues poorly due to its low lipid solubility and its concentration in brain tissue is low. Plasma protein binding is low (approximately 3%).

5.3 Preclinical safety data

Atenolol is a drug on which extensive clinical experience has been obtained. Relevant information for the prescriber is provided elsewhere in the Summary of Product Characteristics.

6. PHARMACEUTICAL PARTICULARS

6.1 List of excipients

Citric acid

Lemon and lime flavour

Methyl hydroxybenzoate

Propyl hydroxybenzoate

Purified water

Saccharin sodium

Sodium citrate

Sorbitol solution

6.2 Incompatibilities

Not applicable.

6.3 Shelf life

36 months.

6.4 Special precautions for storage

Do not store above 25°C.

Store in the original container.

6.5 Nature and contents of container

Amber-coloured PET bottles with white polypropylene screw caps containing 300 ml.

6.6 Special precautions for disposal and other handling

Not applicable.

7. MARKETING AUTHORISATION HOLDER

AstraZeneca UK Limited,

600 Capability Green,

Luton, LU1 3LU, UK.

8. MARKETING AUTHORISATION NUMBER(S)

PL 17901/0051

9. DATE OF FIRST AUTHORISATION/RENEWAL OF THE AUTHORISATION

01 June 2000 / 31 October 2003

10. DATE OF REVISION OF THE TEXT

22nd August 2008

Tensipine MR 10

(Genus Pharmaceuticals)

1. NAME OF THE MEDICINAL PRODUCT

Tensipine MR 10

2. QUALITATIVE AND QUANTITATIVE COMPOSITION

Tensipine MR 10 tablets: Pink-grey lacquered modified release tablets each containing 10mg nifedipine, one side marked TMR and the reverse side marked 10.

3. PHARMACEUTICAL FORM

Modified release tablets for oral administration.

4. CLINICAL PARTICULARS

4.1 Therapeutic indications

For the prophylaxis of chronic stable angina pectoris and the treatment of hypertension.

4.2 Posology and method of administration

Adults

The recommended starting dose of Tensipine MR is 10mg every 12 hours swallowed with water with subsequent titration of dosage according to response. The dose may be adjusted to 40mg every 12 hours.

Tensipine MR 10 permits titration of initial dosage. The recommended dose is one Tensipine MR 10 tablet (10mg) every 12 hours.

Nifedipine is metabolised primarily by the liver and therefore patients with liver dysfunction should be carefully monitored.

Patients with renal impairment should not require adjustment of dosage.

Elderly patients

The pharmacokinetics of nifedipine are altered in the elderly so that lower maintenance doses of nifedipine may be required compared to younger patients.

Children

Nifedipine is not recommended for use in children.

Treatment may be continued indefinitely.

4.3 Contraindications

Tensipine MR should not be administered to patients with known hypersensitivity to nifedipine or other dihydropyridines because of the theoretical risk of cross-reaction, to women capable of child-bearing or to nursing mothers.

Tensipine MR should not be used in cardiogenic shock, clinically significant aortic stenosis, unstable angina, or during or within one month of a myocardial infarction.

Tensipine MR should not be used for the treatment of acute attacks of angina.

The safety of Tensipine MR in malignant hypertension has not been established.

Tensipine MR should not be used for secondary prevention of myocardial infarction.

Tensipine MR should not be administered concomitantly with rifampicin since effective plasma levels of nifedipine may not be achieved owing to enzyme induction.

4.4 Special warnings and precautions for use

Tensipine MR is not a beta-blocker and therefore gives no protection against the dangers of abrupt beta-blocker withdrawal; any such withdrawal should be by gradual reduction of the dose of beta-blocker preferably over 8 - 10 days.

Tensipine MR may be used in combination with beta-blocking drugs and other antihypertensive agents but the possibility of an additive effect resulting in postural hypotension should be borne in mind. Tensipine MR will not prevent possible rebound effects after cessation of other antihypertensive therapy.

Tensipine MR should be used with caution in patients whose cardiac reserve is poor. Deterioration of heart failure has occasionally been observed with nifedipine.

Caution should be exercised in patients with severe hypotension.

Diabetic patients taking Tensipine MR may require adjustment of their control.

In dialysis patients with malignant hypertension and hypovolaemia, a marked decrease in blood pressure can occur.

4.5 Interaction with other medicinal products and other forms of interaction

The antihypertensive effect of Tensipine MR may be potentiated by simultaneous administration of cimetidine.

When used in combination with nifedipine, serum quinidine levels have been shown to be suppressed regardless of dosage of quinidine.

The simultaneous administration of nifedipine and digoxin may lead to reduced digoxin clearance and hence an increase in the plasma digoxin level. Plasma digoxin levels should be monitored and, if necessary, the digoxin dose reduced.

Diltiazem decreases the clearance of nifedipine and hence increases plasma nifedipine levels. Therefore, caution should be taken when both drugs are used in combination and a reduction of the nifedipine dose may be necessary.

Nifedipine may increase the spectrophotometric values of urinary vanillylmandelic acid falsely. However, HPLC measurements are unaffected.

Rifampicin interacts with nifedipine (see Contra-indications).

As with other dihydropyridines, nifedipine should not be taken with grapefruit juice because bioavailability is increased.

4.6 Pregnancy and lactation

Tensipine MR is contra-indicated in women capable of child-bearing and nursing mothers.

4.7 Effects on ability to drive and use machines

None known.

4.8 Undesirable effects

Ischaemic pain has been reported in a small proportion of patients within one to four hours of the introduction of Tensipine MR therapy. Although a "steal" effect has not been demonstrated, patients experiencing this effect should discontinue Tensipine MR.

Most side-effects are consequences of the vasodilatory effects of nifedipine. Headache, flushing, tachycardia and palpitations may occur, most commonly in the early stages of treatment with nifedipine. Gravitational oedema not associated with heart failure or weight gain may also occur.

Paraesthesia, dizziness, lethargy and gastro-intestinal symptoms such as nausea and altered bowel habit occur occasionally.

There are reports of skin reactions such as rash, pruritus and urticaria.

Other less frequently reported side-effects include myalgia, tremor and visual disturbances.

Impotence may occur rarely.

Increased frequency of micturition may occur.

There are reports of gingival hyperplasia and, in older men on long-term therapy, gynaecomastia, which usually regress upon withdrawal of therapy.

Mood changes may occur rarely.

Side-effects which may occur in isolated cases are photosensitivity, exfoliative dermatitis, systemic allergic reactions and purpura. Usually, these regress after discontinuation of the drug.

Rare cases of hypersensitivity-type jaundice have been reported. In addition, disturbances of liver function such as intra-hepatic cholestasis may occur. These regress after discontinuation of therapy.

As with other sustained release dihydropyridines, exacerbation of angina pectoris may occur rarely at the start of treatment. The occurrence of myocardial infarction has been described although it is not possible to distinguish such an event from the natural course of ischaemic heart disease.

4.9 Overdose

Clinical effects

Reports of nifedipine overdosage are limited and symptoms are not necessarily dose-related. Severe hypotension due to vasodilatation, and tachycardia or bradycardia are the most likely manifestations of overdose.

Metabolic disturbances include hyperglycaemia, metabolic acidosis and hypo- or hyperkalaemia.

Cardiac effects may include heart block, AV dissociation and asystole, and cardiogenic shock with pulmonary oedema.

Other toxic effects include nausea, vomiting, drowsiness, dizziness, confusion, lethargy, flushing, hypoxia and unconsciousness to the point of coma.

Treatment

As far as treatment is concerned, elimination of nifedipine and the restoration of stable cardiovascular conditions have priority.

After oral ingestion, gastric lavage is indicated, if necessary in combination with irrigation of the small intestine. Ipecacuanha should be given to children.

Elimination must be as complete as possible, including the small intestine, to prevent the otherwise inevitable subsequent absorption of the active substance. Activated charcoal should be given in 4-hourly doses of 25g for adults, 10g for children.

Blood pressure, ECG, central arterial pressure, pulmonary wedge pressure, urea and electrolytes should be monitored.

Hypotension as a result of cardiogenic shock and arterial vasodilatation should be treated with elevation of the feet and plasma expanders. If these measures are ineffective, hypotension may be treated with 10% calcium gluconate 10 - 20ml intravenously over 5 - 10 minutes. If the effects are inadequate, the treatment can be continued, with ECG monitoring. In addition, beta-sympathomimetics may be given, e.g. isoprenaline 0.2mg slowly i.v. or as a continuous infusion of 5µg/min. If an insufficient increase in blood pressure is achieved with calcium and isoprenaline, vasoconstricting sympathomimetics such as dopamine or noradrenaline should be administered. The dosage of these drugs should be determined by the patient's response.

Bradycardia may be treated with atropine, beta-sympathomimetics or a temporary cardiac pacemaker, as required.

Additional fluids should be administered with caution to avoid cardiac overload.

5. PHARMACOLOGICAL PROPERTIES

5.1 Pharmacodynamic properties

Mode of action

Nifedipine is a specific and potent calcium antagonist. In hypertension, the main action of Tensipine MR is to cause peripheral vasodilatation and thus reduce peripheral resistance.

In angina, Tensipine MR reduces peripheral and coronary vascular resistance, leading to an increase in coronary blood flow, cardiac output and stroke volume, whilst decreasing after-load.

Additionally, nifedipine dilates submaximally both clear and atherosclerotic coronary arteries, thus protecting the heart against coronary artery spasm and improving perfusion to the ischaemic myocardium.

Nifedipine reduces the frequency of painful attacks and the ischaemic ECG changes irrespective of the relative contribution from coronary artery spasm or atherosclerosis.

Tensipine MR administered twice-daily provides 24-hour control of raised blood pressure. Tensipine MR causes reduction in blood pressure such that the percentage lowering is directly related to its initial level. In normotensive individuals, Tensipine MR has little or no effect on blood pressure.

5.2 Pharmacokinetic properties

Nifedipine is absorbed almost completely from the gastro-intestinal tract regardless of the oral formulation used and undergoes extensive metabolism in the liver to inactive metabolites, with less than 1% of the parent drug appearing unchanged in the urine. The rate of absorption determines the drug's apparent elimination. The terminal elimination half-life of the modified release formulation is 6 - 11 hours.

After enteral or intravenous doses, 70 - 80% of activity is eliminated (primarily as metabolites) via the urine. Remaining excretion is via the faeces.

After 24 hours, 90% of the administered dose is eliminated.

Protein binding of nifedipine exceeds 90% in human serum.

5.3 Preclinical safety data

Reproduction toxicology

Nifedipine administration has been associated with a variety of embryotoxic, placentotoxic and fetotoxic effects in rats, mice and rabbits. All of the doses associated with the teratogenic, embryotoxic or fetotoxic effects in animals were maternally toxic and several times the recommended maximum dose for humans.

6. PHARMACEUTICAL PARTICULARS

6.1 List of excipients

Tensipine MR tablets contain the following excipients:

Microcrystalline cellulose, maize starch, lactose, polysorbate 80, magnesium stearate, hydroxypropyl methylcellulose, polyethylene glycol 4000, iron oxide red and titanium dioxide.

6.2 Incompatibilities

Not applicable.

6.3 Shelf life

PVC blister strips: 48 months

PP blister strips: 30 months

6.4 Special precautions for storage

The tablets should be protected from strong light and stored in the manufacturer's original container.

6.5 Nature and contents of container

Tensipine MR 10 tablets: blister strips of 14 tablets in a cardboard outer container, packs of 56 tablets.

Blister strips are composed of red polypropylene foil (0.3mm) with aluminium backing foil (0.02mm) or red PVC foil (0.3mm) with aluminium backing foil (0.02mm).

6.6 Special precautions for disposal and other handling

No additional information.

7. MARKETING AUTHORISATION HOLDER

Genus Pharmaceuticals Limited

T/A Genus Pharmaceuticals

Benham Valence

Newbury

Berkshire RG20 8LU

8. MARKETING AUTHORISATION NUMBER(S)

PL 06831/0048

9. DATE OF FIRST AUTHORISATION/RENEWAL OF THE AUTHORISATION

22 April 1996

10. DATE OF REVISION OF THE TEXT

19 February 2009

Tensipine MR 20

(Genus Pharmaceuticals)

1. NAME OF THE MEDICINAL PRODUCT

Tensipine MR 20

2. QUALITATIVE AND QUANTITATIVE COMPOSITION

Tensipine MR 20 tablets: Pink-grey lacquered modified release tablets each containing 20mg nifedipine, one side marked TMR and the reverse side marked 20.

3. PHARMACEUTICAL FORM

Modified release tablets for oral administration.

4. CLINICAL PARTICULARS

4.1 Therapeutic indications

For the prophylaxis of chronic stable angina pectoris and the treatment of hypertension.

4.2 Posology and method of administration

Adults

The recommended starting dose of Tensipine MR is 10mg every 12 hours swallowed with water with subsequent titration of dosage according to response. The dose may be adjusted to 40mg every 12 hours.

Tensipine MR 10 permits titration of initial dosage. The recommended dose is one Tensipine MR 10 tablet (10mg) every 12 hours.

Nifedipine is metabolised primarily by the liver and therefore patients with liver dysfunction should be carefully monitored.

Patients with renal impairment should not require adjustment of dosage.

Elderly patients

The pharmacokinetics of nifedipine are altered in the elderly so that lower maintenance doses of nifedipine may be required compared to younger patients.

Children

Nifedipine is not recommended for use in children.

Treatment may be continued indefinitely.

4.3 Contraindications

Tensipine MR should not be administered to patients with known hypersensitivity to nifedipine or other dihydropyridines because of the theoretical risk of cross-reaction, to women capable of child-bearing or to nursing mothers.

Tensipine MR should not be used in cardiogenic shock, clinically significant aortic stenosis, unstable angina, or during or within one month of a myocardial infarction.

Tensipine MR should not be used for the treatment of acute attacks of angina.

The safety of Tensipine MR in malignant hypertension has not been established.

Tensipine MR should not be used for secondary prevention of myocardial infarction.

Tensipine MR should not be administered concomitantly with rifampicin since effective plasma levels of nifedipine may not be achieved owing to enzyme induction.

4.4 Special warnings and precautions for use

Tensipine MR is not a beta-blocker and therefore gives no protection against the dangers of abrupt beta-blocker withdrawal; any such withdrawal should be by gradual reduction of the dose of beta-blocker preferably over 8 - 10 days.

Tensipine MR may be used in combination with beta-blocking drugs and other antihypertensive agents but the possibility of an additive effect resulting in postural hypotension should be borne in mind. Tensipine MR will not prevent possible rebound effects after cessation of other antihypertensive therapy.

Tensipine MR should be used with caution in patients whose cardiac reserve is poor. Deterioration of heart failure has occasionally been observed with nifedipine.

Caution should be exercised in patients with severe hypotension.

Diabetic patients taking Tensipine MR may require adjustment of their control.

In dialysis patients with malignant hypertension and hypovolaemia, a marked decrease in blood pressure can occur.

4.5 Interaction with other medicinal products and other forms of interaction

The antihypertensive effect of Tensipine MR may be potentiated by simultaneous administration of cimetidine.

When used in combination with nifedipine, serum quinidine levels have been shown to be suppressed regardless of dosage of quinidine.

The simultaneous administration of nifedipine and digoxin may lead to reduced digoxin clearance and hence an increase in the plasma digoxin level. Plasma digoxin levels should be monitored and, if necessary, the digoxin dose reduced.

Diltiazem decreases the clearance of nifedipine and hence increases plasma nifedipine levels. Therefore, caution should be taken when both drugs are used in combination and a reduction of the nifedipine dose may be necessary.

Nifedipine may increase the spectrophotometric values of urinary vanillylmandelic acid falsely. However, HPLC measurements are unaffected.

Rifampicin interacts with nifedipine (see Contra-indications).

As with other dihydropyridines, nifedipine should not be taken with grapefruit juice because bioavailability is increased.

4.6 Pregnancy and lactation

Tensipine MR is contra-indicated in women capable of child-bearing and nursing mothers.

4.7 Effects on ability to drive and use machines

None known.

4.8 Undesirable effects

Ischaemic pain has been reported in a small proportion of patients within one to four hours of the introduction of Tensipine MR therapy. Although a "steal" effect has not been demonstrated, patients experiencing this effect should discontinue Tensipine MR.

Most side-effects are consequences of the vasodilatory effects of nifedipine. Headache, flushing, tachycardia and palpitations may occur, most commonly in the early stages of treatment with nifedipine. Gravitational oedema not associated with heart failure or weight gain may also occur.

Paraesthesia, dizziness, lethargy and gastro-intestinal symptoms such as nausea and altered bowel habit occur occasionally.

There are reports of skin reactions such as rash, pruritus and urticaria.

Other less frequently reported side-effects include myalgia, tremor and visual disturbances.

Impotence may occur rarely.

Increased frequency of micturition may occur.

There are reports of gingival hyperplasia and, in older men on long-term therapy, gynaecomastia, which usually regress upon withdrawal of therapy.

Mood changes may occur rarely.

Side-effects which may occur in isolated cases are photosensitivity, exfoliative dermatitis, systemic allergic reactions and purpura. Usually, these regress after discontinuation of the drug.

Rare cases of hypersensitivity-type jaundice have been reported. In addition, disturbances of liver function such as intra-hepatic cholestasis may occur. These regress after discontinuation of therapy.

As with other sustained release dihydropyridines, exacerbation of angina pectoris may occur rarely at the start of treatment. The occurrence of myocardial infarction has been described although it is not possible to distinguish such an event from the natural course of ischaemic heart disease.

4.9 Overdose

Clinical effects

Reports of nifedipine overdosage are limited and symptoms are not necessarily dose-related. Severe hypotension due to vasodilatation, and tachycardia or bradycardia are the most likely manifestations of overdose.

Metabolic disturbances include hyperglycaemia, metabolic acidosis and hypo- or hyperkalaemia.

Cardiac effects may include heart block, AV dissociation and asystole, and cardiogenic shock with pulmonary oedema.

Other toxic effects include nausea, vomiting, drowsiness, dizziness, confusion, lethargy, flushing, hypoxia and unconsciousness to the point of coma.

Treatment

As far as treatment is concerned, elimination of nifedipine and the restoration of stable cardiovascular conditions have priority.

After oral ingestion, gastric lavage is indicated, if necessary in combination with irrigation of the small intestine. Ipecacuanha should be given to children.

Elimination must be as complete as possible, including the small intestine, to prevent the otherwise inevitable subsequent absorption of the active substance. Activated charcoal should be given in 4-hourly doses of 25g for adults, 10g for children.

Blood pressure, ECG, central arterial pressure, pulmonary wedge pressure, urea and electrolytes should be monitored.

Hypotension as a result of cardiogenic shock and arterial vasodilatation should be treated with elevation of the feet and plasma expanders. If these measures are ineffective, hypotension may be treated with 10% calcium gluconate 10 - 20ml intravenously over 5 - 10 minutes. If the effects are inadequate, the treatment can be continued, with ECG monitoring. In addition, beta-sympathomimetics may be given, e.g. isoprenaline 0.2mg slowly i.v. or as a continuous infusion of 5μg/min. If an insufficient increase in blood pressure is achieved with calcium and isoprenaline, vasoconstricting sympathomimetics such as dopamine or noradrenaline should be administered. The dosage of these drugs should be determined by the patient's response.

Bradycardia may be treated with atropine, beta-sympathomimetics or a temporary cardiac pacemaker, as required.

Additional fluids should be administered with caution to avoid cardiac overload.

5. PHARMACOLOGICAL PROPERTIES

5.1 Pharmacodynamic properties

Mode of action

Nifedipine is a specific and potent calcium antagonist. In hypertension, the main action of Tensipine MR is to cause peripheral vasodilatation and thus reduce peripheral resistance.

In angina, Tensipine MR reduces peripheral and coronary vascular resistance, leading to an increase in coronary blood flow, cardiac output and stroke volume, whilst decreasing after-load.

Additionally, nifedipine dilates submaximally both clear and atherosclerotic coronary arteries, thus protecting the heart against coronary artery spasm and improving perfusion to the ischaemic myocardium.

Nifedipine reduces the frequency of painful attacks and the ischaemic ECG changes irrespective of the relative contribution from coronary artery spasm or atherosclerosis.

Tensipine MR administered twice-daily provides 24-hour control of raised blood pressure. Tensipine MR causes reduction in blood pressure such that the percentage lowering is directly related to its initial level. In normotensive individuals, Tensipine MR has little or no effect on blood pressure.

5.2 Pharmacokinetic properties

Nifedipine is absorbed almost completely from the gastro-intestinal tract regardless of the oral formulation used and undergoes extensive metabolism in the liver to inactive metabolites, with less than 1% of the parent drug appearing unchanged in the urine. The rate of absorption determines the drug's apparent elimination. The terminal elimination half-life of the modified release formulation is 6 - 11 hours.

After enteral or intravenous doses, 70 - 80% of activity is eliminated (primarily as metabolites) via the urine. Remaining excretion is via the faeces.

After 24 hours, 90% of the administered dose is eliminated.

Protein binding of nifedipine exceeds 90% in human serum.

5.3 Preclinical safety data

Reproduction toxicology

Nifedipine administration has been associated with a variety of embryotoxic, placentotoxic and fetotoxic effects in rats, mice and rabbits. All of the doses associated with the teratogenic, embryotoxic or fetotoxic effects in animals were maternally toxic and several times the recommended maximum dose for humans.

6. PHARMACEUTICAL PARTICULARS

6.1 List of excipients

Tensipine MR tablets contain the following excipients:

Microcrystalline cellulose, maize starch, lactose, polysorbate 80, magnesium stearate, hydroxypropyl methylcellulose, polyethylene glycol 4000, iron oxide red and titanium dioxide.

6.2 Incompatibilities

Not applicable.

6.3 Shelf life

PVC blister strips: 48 months

PP blister strips: 30 months

6.4 Special precautions for storage

The tablets should be protected from strong light and stored in the manufacturer's original container.

6.5 Nature and contents of container

Tensipine MR 20 tablets: blister strips of 14 tablets in a cardboard outer container, packs of 56 tablets.

Blister strips are composed of red polypropylene foil (0.3mm) with aluminium backing foil (0.02mm) or red PVC foil (0.3mm) with aluminium backing foil (0.02mm).

6.6 Special precautions for disposal and other handling

No additional information.

7. MARKETING AUTHORISATION HOLDER

Genus Pharmaceuticals Limited

T/A Genus Pharmaceuticals

Benham Valence

Newbury

Berkshire RG20 8LU

8. MARKETING AUTHORISATION NUMBER(S)

PL 06831/0049

9. DATE OF FIRST AUTHORISATION/RENEWAL OF THE AUTHORISATION

22 April 1996/23 February 2009

10. DATE OF REVISION OF THE TEXT

23 February 2009

Testim Gel

(Ferring Pharmaceuticals Ltd)

1. NAME OF THE MEDICINAL PRODUCT

Testim 50mg Gel

2. QUALITATIVE AND QUANTITATIVE COMPOSITION

One tube of 5g contains 50mg testosterone.

Excipients: contains propylene glycol, see section 4.4.

For a full list of excipients, see section 6.1.

3. PHARMACEUTICAL FORM

Gel.

A clear to translucent gel.

4. CLINICAL PARTICULARS

4.1 Therapeutic indications

Testosterone replacement therapy for male hypogonadism when testosterone deficiency has been confirmed by clinical features and biochemical tests (see 4.4 Special warnings and precautions for use).

4.2 Posology and method of administration

Adults and the Elderly: The recommended starting dose of Testim is testosterone 50mg (1 tube).

Dose titration should be based on serum testosterone levels or the persistence of clinical signs and symptoms related to testosterone deficiency. To ensure proper serum testosterone levels are achieved, early morning serum testosterone should be measured before applying the next dose, approximately 7-14 days after initiation of therapy. Currently there is no consensus about age specific testosterone levels. The normal serum testosterone level for young eugonadal men is generally accepted to be approximately 300 – 1000 ng/dL (10.4 – 34.6 nmol/L). However, it should be taken into account that physiologically testosterone levels are lower with increasing age. If serum testosterone concentrations are below the normal range, the daily testosterone dose may be increased from 50mg (one tube) to 100mg (two tubes) once a day. The duration of treatment and frequency of subsequent testosterone measurements should be determined by the physician. Non-virilised patients may require treatment with one tube for a longer period of time before the dose is increased, as needed. At any time during treatment, after initial titration, the dose may need to be reduced if serum testosterone levels are raised above the upper limit of the normal range. If morning serum testosterone levels are above the normal range while applying 50mg (1 tube) of Testim, the use of Testim should be discontinued. If serum testosterone levels are below the normal limit, the dose may be increased, not exceeding 100mg per day.

Because of the variability in analytical values amongst diagnostic laboratories, all testosterone measurements should be performed at the same laboratory.

The gel should be applied once a day, at about the same time each day, to clean, dry, intact, skin of the shoulders and/or upper arms. It is preferable that the gel is applied in the morning. For patients who wash in the morning, Testim should be applied after washing, bathing or showering.

To apply the gel, patients should open one tube and squeeze the entire contents into the palm of one hand. They should then apply the gel immediately to their shoulders and/or upper arms. The gel should be spread on the skin gently as a thin layer. The gel should then be rubbed until no gel is left on the skin. This process should then be repeated with a second tube of Testim by patients who have been prescribed a daily dose of testosterone 100mg. It is suggested that patients who require two tubes of gel each day use both shoulders (one tube per shoulder) and/or upper arms as application sites. Patients should thoroughly wash their hands immediately with soap and water after Testim has been applied. After application of the gel, patients should allow the application sites to dry for a few minutes and then dress with clothing that covers the application sites.

Patients should be advised not to apply Testim to the genitals.

Children and women:

Testim is not indicated in children and has not been clinically evaluated in males under 18 years of age. For use in women, see Section 4.4 Special Warnings and Precautions for Use.

4.3 Contraindications

Androgens are contraindicated in men with carcinoma of the breast or known or suspected carcinoma of the prostate.

Testim should not be used in patients with known hypersensitivity to the active substance, which is chemically synthesized from soy, or to any of the excipients.

4.4 Special warnings and precautions for use

Prior to testosterone initiation, all patients must undergo a detailed examination in order to exclude the risk of pre-existing prostate cancer. Careful and regular monitoring of the breast and prostate gland must be performed in accordance with recommended methods (digital rectal examination and estimation of serum PSA) in patients receiving testosterone therapy at least once yearly and twice yearly in elderly patients and at risk patients (those with clinical or familial factors).

Androgens may accelerate the progression of sub-clinical prostate cancer and benign prostatic hyperplasia.

Care should be taken in patients with skeletal metastases due to the risk of hypercalcaemia/hypercalciuria developing from androgen therapy. In these patients, serum calcium levels should be determined regularly.

Testosterone may cause an increase in blood pressure and Testim should be used with caution in patients with hypertension.

In patients suffering from severe cardiac, hepatic or renal insufficiency, treatment with testosterone may cause severe complications characterised by oedema with or without congestive cardiac failure. In this case, treatment must be stopped immediately. In addition diuretic therapy may be required.

Testosterone should be used with caution in patients with ischaemic heart disease.

Testosterone should be used with caution in patients with epilepsy and migraine as these conditions may be aggravated.

There are published reports of increased risk of sleep apnoea in hypogonadal subjects treated with testosterone esters, especially in those with risk factors such as obesity or chronic respiratory disease.

Improved insulin sensitivity may occur in patients treated with androgens who achieve normal testosterone plasma concentrations following replacement therapy.

Certain clinical signs: irritability, nervousness, weight gain, prolonged or frequent erections may indicate excessive androgen exposure requiring dosage adjustment.

If the patient develops a severe application site reaction, treatment should be reviewed and discontinued if necessary.

The following checks should be carried out periodically; full blood count, lipid profile and liver function tests.

To ensure proper dosing, serum testosterone concentrations should be measured (see section 4.2: Posology and Method of Administration).

Testim should not be used to treat non-specific symptoms suggestive of hypogonadism if testosterone deficiency has not been demonstrated and if other aetiologies responsible for the symptoms have not been excluded. Testosterone deficiency should be clearly demonstrated by clinical features and confirmed by 2 separate blood testosterone measurements before initiating therapy with any testosterone replacement, including Testim treatment.

Testim is not a treatment for male infertility or sexual dysfunction/impotence in patients without demonstrated testosterone deficiency. For the restoration of fertility in patients with hypogonadotrophic hypogonadism, therapeutic measures in addition to treatment with Testim are required.

Athletes treated for testosterone replacement in primary and secondary male hypogonadism should be advised that the product contains an active substance which may produce a positive reaction in anti-doping tests. Androgens are not suitable for enhancing muscular development in healthy individuals or for increasing physical ability.

Testim should not be used in women due to possible virilising effects.

As washing after Testim administration reduces testosterone levels, patients are advised not to wash or shower for at least 6 hours after applying Testim. When washing occurs up to six hours after the gel application, the absorption of testosterone may be reduced.

Testim contains propylene glycol, which may cause skin irritation.

The contents of each tube are flammable.

Potential for Transfer

If no precaution is taken, testosterone gel can be transferred to other persons by close skin to skin contact, resulting in increased testosterone serum levels and possibly adverse effects (e.g. growth of facial and/or body hair, ***acne,*** deepening of the voice, irregularities of the menstrual cycle) in case of repeat contact (inadvertent androgenisation).

The physician should inform the patient carefully about the risk of testosterone transfer and about safety instructions (see below). Testim should not be prescribed in patients with a major risk of non-compliance with safety instructions (e.g. severe alcoholism, drug abuse, severe psychiatric disorders).

This transfer is avoided by wearing clothes covering the application area or showering prior to contact.

As a result, the following precautions are recommended:

For the patient:

- wash hands thoroughly with soap and water after applying the gel,
- cover the application area with clothing once the gel has dried,
- shower before any situation in which this type of contact is foreseen.

For people not being treated with Testim:

- in the event of contact with an application area which has not been washed or is not covered with clothing, wash the area of skin onto which testosterone may have been transferred as soon as possible, using soap and water.
- Report the development of signs of excessive androgen exposure such as acne or hair modification.

To guarantee partner safety, the patient should be advised for example to observe a long interval between Testim application and sexual intercourse, to wear a T-shirt covering the application site during contact period, or to shower before sexual intercourse.

Furthermore, it is recommended to wear a T-shirt covering the application site during contact periods with children in order to avoid a contamination risk of children's skin.

Pregnant women must avoid any contact with Testim application sites. In case of pregnancy of the partner, the patient must reinforce his attention to the precautions for use (see section 4.6).

4.5 Interaction with other medicinal products and other forms of interaction

When androgens are used simultaneously with anti-coagulants, the anti-coagulant effects may be increased. Patients receiving oral anticoagulants require close monitoring, especially when androgen therapy is started or stopped.

In a published pharmacokinetic study of an injectable testosterone product, administration of testosterone cypionate led to an increased clearance of propranolol in the majority of men tested.

The concurrent administration of testosterone with ACTH or corticosteroids may enhance oedema formation; thus these drugs should be administered cautiously, particularly in patients with cardiac or hepatic disease.

Laboratory Test Interactions: Androgens may decrease levels of thyroxine-binding globulin resulting in decreased total T4 serum levels and increased resin uptake of T3 and T4. Free thyroid hormone levels remain unchanged, however, and there is no clinical evidence of thyroid dysfunction.

4.6 Pregnancy and lactation

Testim is not indicated for women and must not be used in pregnant or breastfeeding women.

Testosterone may induce virilising effects on the female foetus.

Pregnant women should avoid skin contact with Testim application sites.

In the event that unwashed or unclothed skin to which Testim has been applied does come into direct contact with the skin of a pregnant woman, the general area of contact on the woman should be washed with soap and water immediately.

4.7 Effects on ability to drive and use machines

No studies on the effects on the ability to drive and use machines have been performed.

4.8 Undesirable effects

a. Summary of the safety profile

In double-blind clinical trials comparing Testim to placebo, the most frequently observed adverse drug reactions in Testim treated patients were application site erythema and increased PSA, both occurring in approximately 4% of patients.

b. Tabulated summary of adverse events

Adverse Drug Reactions terminology used for the classification of incidence: Very common ⩾10% - Common ⩾1% to <10% - Uncommon ⩾0.1% to <1% - Rare ⩾0.01% to <0.1% - Very rare <0.01% - Not known (can not be estimated from the available data).

The cumulative safety experience of testosterone is derived from Phase I to Phase III clinical trials and post-marketing experience.

The adverse reactions listed in the table below have been observed in clinical studies with testosterone and/or post-marketing experience.

System Organ Class	Adverse Reaction	Frequency
Nervous disorders	Headache	Common
Vascular disorders	Hypertension worsened	Common
	Hot flushes/flushing	Uncommon
Skin and subcutaneous tissue disorders	Acne	Common
	Pruritus	Uncommon
Reproductive system and breast disorders	Azoospermia	Very rare
General disorders and administration site disorders	Application site reaction (including erythema, rash and pruritus)	Common
	Peripheral oedema	Uncommon
Investigations	PSA increased, haematocrit increased, haemoglobin increased, red blood cell count increased	Common

Uncommonly, gynaecomastia may develop and persist in patients being treated for hypogonadism with Testim.

c. Additional information

Other known adverse drug reactions that may be associated with testosterone treatments are listed in the following table:

System Organ Class	Adverse reactions
Neoplasms benign and malignant (including cysts and polyps)	Prostate Cancer (Data on prostate cancer risk in association with testosterone therapy are inconclusive)
Metabolism and nutrition disorders	Electrolyte changes (retention of sodium, chloride, potassium, calcium, inorganic phosphate and water) during high dose and/or prolonged treatment,
Psychiatric disorders	Decreased libido, anxiety, emotional lability
Nervous system	Paresthesia generalised
Gastrointestinal disorders	Nausea
Hepatobiliary disorders	In very rare cases jaundice and liver function test abnormalities
Skin and subcutaneous tissue disorders	Various skin reactions may occur including hirsutism, alopecia and seborrhoea
Musculoskeletal and connective tissue disorders	Muscle cramps
Reproductive system and breast disorders	Increased frequency of erections; testosterone replacement therapy of hypogonadism can in rare cases cause persistent, painful erections (priapism), and prostate abnormalities
Investigations	Altered blood lipid levels including a reduction in HDL cholesterol and weight gain

Patients should be instructed to report any of the following to a physician; too frequent or persistent erections of the penis; any changes in skin colour, ankle swelling or unexplained nausea or vomiting; any breathing disturbances including those associated with sleep.

4.9 Overdose

Reports describing overdose have included doses up to Testim 150 mg. No dose limiting toxicity has been reported from these spontaneous cases.

5. PHARMACOLOGICAL PROPERTIES

5.1 Pharmacodynamic properties

Pharmacotherapeutic group: Androgens. ATC code: G03B A03.

Testosterone and dihydrotestosterone (DHT), endogenous androgens, are responsible for the normal growth and development of the male sex organs and for the maintenance of secondary sex characteristics. These effects include the growth and maturation of the prostate, seminal vesicles, penis and scrotum; the development of male hair distribution on the face, chest, axillae and pubis; laryngeal enlargement, vocal chord thickening, alterations in body musculature and fat distribution.

Insufficient secretion of testosterone due to testicular failure, pituitary pathology or gonadotropin or luteinising hormone-releasing hormone deficiency results in male hypogonadism and low serum testosterone concentration. Symptoms associated with low testosterone include decreased sexual desire with or without impotence, fatigue, loss of muscle mass, mood depression and regression of secondary sexual characteristics. Restoring testosterone levels to within the normal range can result in improvements over time in muscle mass, mood, sexual desire, libido and sexual function including sexual performance and number of spontaneous erections.

During exogenous administration of testosterone to normal males, endogenous testosterone release may be decreased through feedback inhibition of pituitary luteinising hormone (LH). With large doses of exogenous androgens, spermatogenesis may also be suppressed through inhibition of pituitary follicle stimulating hormone (FSH).

Androgen administration causes retention of sodium, nitrogen, potassium, phosphorus and decreased urinary excretion of calcium. Androgens have been reported to increase protein anabolism and decrease protein catabolism. Nitrogen balance is improved only when there is sufficient intake of calories and protein. Androgens have been reported to stimulate production of red blood cells by enhancing the production of erythropoietin.

5.2 Pharmacokinetic properties

Testim dries very quickly when applied to the skin surface. The skin acts as a reservoir for the sustained release of testosterone into the systemic circulation.

With once daily application of Testim 50mg or 100mg to adult males with early morning serum testosterone levels $\leqslant$ 300 ng/dL, follow up measurements at 30, 60 and 90 days after starting treatment have confirmed that serum testosterone concentrations are generally maintained within the normal range.

Following 50 mg Testim daily in hypogonadal men, the C_{avg} was shown to be 365±187 ng/dL (12.7±6.5 nmol/L), C_{max} was 538±371 ng/dL (18.7±12.9 nmol/L) and C_{min} was 223±126 ng/dl (7.7± 4.4 nmol/L), measured at steady-state. The corresponding concentrations following 100 mg Testim daily were C_{avg} = 612±286 ng/dL (21.3±9.9 nmol/L), C_{max} = 897±566 ng/dL (31.1± 19.6 nmol/L) and C_{min} = 394±189 ng/dL (13.7±6.6 nmol/L).

In the young eugonadal man, normal levels of serum testosterone are in the range of 300 – 1000 ng/dL (10.4 – 34.6 nmol/L).

The measurement of serum testosterone levels can be variable depending on the laboratory and method of assay used (see 4.2 Posology and method of administration).

Distribution:

Circulating testosterone is chiefly bound in the serum to sex hormone-binding globulin (SHBG) and albumin. The albumin-bound fraction of testosterone easily dissociates from albumin and is presumed to be bioactive. The portion of testosterone bound to SHBG is not considered biologically active. Approximately 40% of testosterone in plasma is bound to SHBG, 2% remains unbound (free) and the rest is bound to albumin and other proteins.

Metabolism:

There is considerable variation in the half-life of testosterone as reported in the literature, ranging from ten to 100 minutes.

Testosterone is metabolised to various 17-keto steroids through two different pathways. The major active metabolites of testosterone are oestradiol and dihydrotestosterone (DHT). Testosterone is metabolised to DHT by steroid 5α reductase located in the skin, liver and the urogenital tract of the male. DHT binds with greater affinity to SHBG than does testosterone. In many tissues, the activity of testosterone depends on its reduction to DHT, which binds to cytosol receptor proteins. The steroid-receptor complex is transported to the nucleus where it initiates transcription and cellular changes related to androgen action. In reproductive tissues, DHT is further metabolised to 3-α and 3-β androstanediol.

Inactivation of testosterone occurs primarily in the liver.

DHT concentrations increased during Testim treatment. After 90 days of treatment, mean DHT concentrations remained within the normal range for Testim treated subjects.

Excretion:

About 90% of testosterone given intramuscularly is excreted in the urine as glucuronic and sulphuric acid conjugates of testosterone and its metabolites; about 6% of a dose is excreted in the faeces, mostly in the unconjugated form.

Special patient groups:

In patients treated with Testim no differences in the average daily serum testosterone concentration at steady state were observed based on age or cause of hypogonadism.

5.3 Preclinical safety data

Toxicological studies have not revealed effects other than those which can be explained based on the hormonal profile of Testim.

6. PHARMACEUTICAL PARTICULARS

6.1 List of excipients

Purified water

Pentadecalactone

Carbomer 980

Carbomer 1342

Propylene glycol

Glycerol

Macrogol 1000

Ethanol

Trometamol

6.2 Incompatibilities

Not applicable.

6.3 Shelf life

2 years.

6.4 Special precautions for storage

Do not store above 25°C.

6.5 Nature and contents of container

Testim is supplied in unit dose aluminium tubes with epoxy phenolic liners and screw caps, each containing 5g gel. The tubes are packed in cartons containing 7, 14, 30 and 90 tubes.

Not all pack sizes may be marketed.

6.6 Special precautions for disposal and other handling

No special requirements.

7. MARKETING AUTHORISATION HOLDER

Ferring Pharmaceuticals Ltd

The Courtyard

Waterside Drive

Langley

Berkshire

SL3 6EZ

United Kingdom

8. MARKETING AUTHORISATION NUMBER(S)

PL 03194/0105

9. DATE OF FIRST AUTHORISATION/RENEWAL OF THE AUTHORISATION

31/07/2009

10. DATE OF REVISION OF THE TEXT

31/07/2009

Testosterone Enanthate Ampoules

(Cambridge Laboratories)

1. NAME OF THE MEDICINAL PRODUCT

Testosterone Enanthate Ampoules

2. QUALITATIVE AND QUANTITATIVE COMPOSITION

Each ampoule contains 250mg Testosterone Enanthate Ph.Eur in oily solution.

3. PHARMACEUTICAL FORM

Solution for injection.

4. CLINICAL PARTICULARS

4.1 Therapeutic indications

Mammary carcinoma in the female.

Androgen deficiency in the male.

4.2 Posology and method of administration

Females - mammary carcinoma: 250mg every two weeks by intramuscular injection.

Males - Hypogonadism: To stimulate development of underdeveloped androgen-dependent organs and for initial treatment of deficiency symptoms, 250mg Testosterone Enanthate intramuscularly every two to three weeks.

For maintenance treatment: 250mg Testosterone Enanthate intramuscularly every three to six weeks, according to individual requirement.

4.3 Contraindications

Prostatic carcinoma, mammary carcinoma in males and pregnancy. Previous or existing liver tumours (in advanced mammary carcinoma in the female only) if these are not due to metastases.

4.4 Special warnings and precautions for use

Androgens should not be used for enhancing muscular development in healthy individuals or for increasing physical ability.

High dose or long term administration of testosterone occasionally increases the tendency to water retention and oedema. Caution should therefore be exercised in patients predisposed to oedema.

In rare cases benign and in even rarer cases malignant liver tumours leading in isolated cases to life-threatening intra-abdominal haemorrhage have been observed after the use of hormonal substances such as Testosterone Enanthate. If severe upper abdominal complaints, liver enlargement or signs of intra-abdominal haemorrhage occur, a liver tumour should be included in the differential diagnosis and, if necessary, the preparation should be withdrawn. Regular examination of the prostate is advisable for men receiving androgen therapy.

If, in individual cases, frequent or persistent erections occur, the dose should be reduced or the treatment discontinued in order to avoid injury to the penis.

In women: If hypercalcaemia develops, therapy must be discontinued.

4.5 Interaction with other medicinal products and other forms of interaction

Phenobarbitone increases the break-down of steroid hormones in the liver (possible impairment of efficacy).

The clotting status should be monitored particularly closely when Testosterone Enanthate is administered together with coumarin derivatives.

4.6 Pregnancy and lactation

Contra-indicated in pregnancy.

4.7 Effects on ability to drive and use machines

None known.

4.8 Undesirable effects

Women treated with Testosterone Enanthate may develop signs of virilization, (e.g. acne, hirsutism, voice changes). Particular care is therefore necessary in women whose occupations involve singing or speaking.

Spermatogenesis is inhibited by long-term and high-dose treatment with Testosterone Enanthate.

In rare cases, coughing, dyspnoea and circulatory irregularities may occur during or immediately after the injection. Experience has shown that these reactions can be avoided by injecting very slowly.

4.9 Overdose

Acute toxicity data show that Testosterone Enanthate can be classified as non-toxic following a single intake. Even in the case of an inadvertent administration of a multiple of the dose required for therapy, no acute toxicity risk is expected.

5. PHARMACOLOGICAL PROPERTIES

5.1 Pharmacodynamic properties

Testosterone Enanthate is an ester of the natural male sex hormone testosterone and exhibits all the pharmacological effects of the natural hormone. It differs in that it has a depot effect, due to the fact that Testosterone Enanthate is only slowly degraded to testosterone in the body.

5.2 Pharmacokinetic properties

Following intramuscular administration of 200mg of Testosterone Enanthate to 6 hypogonadal males:-

- Peak serum testosterone levels of 1233 ± 484 ng/dl were achieved at 24 hours.
- Physiological levels of testosterone (approx. 500 ng/dl) were maintained for 11 days.

Half-life in blood was 2-3 days (healthy male volunteers).

5.3 Preclinical safety data

Studies in animals showed that the formulation has minimal potential for causing sensitisation or local irritation following intramuscular injection. Long-term systemic studies showed no evidence of testicular toxicity although a temporary inhibition of spermatogenesis may occur. No fertility studies with Testosterone Enanthate have been carried out. Administration of Testosterone Enanthate is contra-indicated during pregnancy due to the possibility of virilisation of the female foetus. However, investigations into embryotoxic, in particular teratogenic, effects gave no indication that further impairment of organ development may occur.

In vitro investigations of mutagenicity gave negative results.

6. PHARMACEUTICAL PARTICULARS

6.1 List of excipients

Benzyl benzoate

Castor oil for injection

6.2 Incompatibilities

None so far known.

6.3 Shelf life

5 years.

6.4 Special precautions for storage
Protect from light.

6.5 Nature and contents of container
Clear glass ampoules of 1 ml in packs of 3.

6.6 Special precautions for disposal and other handling
Not applicable.

7. MARKETING AUTHORISATION HOLDER
Cambridge Laboratories Limited
Deltic House
Kingfisher Way
Silverlink Business Park
Wallsend
Tyne & Wear
NE28 9NX

8. MARKETING AUTHORISATION NUMBER(S)
PL 12070/0015

9. DATE OF FIRST AUTHORISATION/RENEWAL OF THE AUTHORISATION
19 September 1996

10. DATE OF REVISION OF THE TEXT
September 2003

Tetralysal 300

(Galderma (U.K) Ltd)

1. NAME OF THE MEDICINAL PRODUCT
Tetralysal 300

2. QUALITATIVE AND QUANTITATIVE COMPOSITION
Lymecycline 408mg equivalent to 300mg tetracycline base

3. PHARMACEUTICAL FORM
Hard gelatin capsule, red cap and yellow body

4. CLINICAL PARTICULARS

4.1 Therapeutic indications
Tetralysal 300 is for the treatment of acne

As Tetralysal 300 contains a broad spectrum antibiotic, it is also recommended for the treatment of infections caused by tetracycline-sensitive organisms and may be utilised in all conditions where tetracycline is indicated, including use in penicillin-sensitive patients for the treatment of staphylococcal infections. Typical indications include: ear, nose and throat infections; acute and chronic bronchitis (including prophylaxis); infections of the gastro-intestinal and urinary tracts; non-gonococcal urethritis of chlamydial origin and other chlamydial infections such as trachoma; rickettsial fevers; soft tissue infections.

4.2 Posology and method of administration
Adults:

The usual dosage for the chronic treatment of acne is 1 capsule daily: treatment should be continued for at least 8 weeks.

For other infections, the usual dosage is 1 capsule b.d. If higher doses are required, 3-4 capsules may be given over 24 hours. Lower doses may be given for prophylaxis.

In the management of sexually transmitted disease both partners should be treated.

Elderly:

As for other tetracyclines, no specific dose adjustment is required.

Children:

Not recommended for children under the age of 12 years. For children over the age of 12 years the adult dosage may be given.

4.3 Contraindications
As lymecycline is mainly excreted by the kidneys, Tetralysal 300 should not be administered to patients with overt renal insufficiency. Its use is also contra-indicated in patients hypersensitive to tetracyclines.

Children under 12 years

Pregnancy and lactation (see section 4.6)

4.4 Special warnings and precautions for use
Prolonged use of broad spectrum antibiotics may result in the appearance of resistant organisms and superinfection.

Care should be exercised in administering tetracyclines to patients with hepatic impairment. Tetracyclines may cause photosensitivity reactions; however, very rare cases have been reported with lymecycline.

May cause exacerbation of systemic lupus erythematosus. Can cause weak neuromuscular blockade so should be used with caution in Myasthenia Gravis.

4.5 Interaction with other medicinal products and other forms of interaction
The absorption of tetracyclines may be affected by the simultaneous administration of calcium, aluminium, magnesium, bismuth and zinc salts, antacids, Bismuth containing ulcer-healing drugs, iron preparations and quinapril. These products should not be taken within two hours before or after taking Tetralysal 300.

Unlike earlier tetracyclines, absorption of Tetralysal 300 is not significantly impaired by moderate amounts of milk.

Concomitant use of oral retinoids should be avoided as this may increase the risk of benign intracranial hypertension. An increase in the effects of anticoagulants may occur with tetracyclines. Concomitant use of diuretics should be avoided.

Although not reported for Tetralysal 300, a few cases of pregnancy or breakthrough bleeding have been attributed to the concurrent use of tetracycline or oxytetracycline with oral contraceptives.

4.6 Pregnancy and lactation
Tetracyclines are selectively absorbed by developing bones and teeth and may cause dental staining and enamel hypoplasia. In addition these compounds readily cross the placental barrier and therefore Tetralysal 300 should not be given to pregnant or lactating women.

4.7 Effects on ability to drive and use machines
None known

4.8 Undesirable effects

- Rarely anaphylaxis
- Nausea, vomiting, diarrhoea
- Rarely dysphagia
- A few cases of oesophagitis and oesophageal ulceration have been reported, usually when taken before bed or with inadequate fluids.
- A few cases of pancreatitis have been reported.
- As with all antibiotics overgrowth of nonsusceptible organisms may cause candidiasis, pseudomembranous colitis (Clostridium difficile overgrowth), glossitis, stomatitis, vaginitis, or staphylococcal enterocolitis.
- Transient increases in liver function tests, hepatitis, jaundice and hepatic failure have been reported rarely.
- Bulging fontanelles in infants and benign intracranial hypertension in juveniles and adults have been reported. Presenting features were headache and visual disturbances including blurring of vision, scotomata and diplopia. Permanent visual loss has been reported.
- Skin rashes, photosensitivity, erythematous, and maculo-papular rashes, pruritis, bullous dermatoses, exfoliative dermatitis.
- Teeth discoloration – usually only obvious after repeated doses.

4.9 Overdose
There is no specific treatment, but gastric lavage should be performed as soon as possible. Supportive measure should be instituted as required and a high fluid intake maintained.

5. PHARMACOLOGICAL PROPERTIES

5.1 Pharmacodynamic properties
Lymecycline has antimicrobial activity and uses similar to those of tetracycline hydrochloride. It acts by interfering with bacterial protein synthesis and is active against a large number of Gram-positive and Gram-negative pathogenic bacteria including some which are resistant to penicillin.

5.2 Pharmacokinetic properties
Lymecycline is more readily absorbed from the gastro-intestinal tract than tetracycline, with a peak serum concentration of approximately 2mg/L after 3 hours following a 300 mg dose. In addition, similar blood concentrations are achieved with small doses. When the dose is doubled an almost correspondingly higher blood concentration has been reported to occur.

The serum half-life of lymecycline is approximately 10 hours.

5.3 Preclinical safety data
No specific information is presented given the vast experience gained with the use of tetracyclines in humans over the last forty years.

6. PHARMACEUTICAL PARTICULARS

6.1 List of excipients
Magnesium stearate
Colloidal hydrated silica
The capsule shells contain
gelatin
titanium dioxide (E171)
erythrosine (E127)
quinoline yellow (E104)
indigotine (E132)

6.2 Incompatibilities
None known

6.3 Shelf life
Thirty-six (36) months (unopened)

6.4 Special precautions for storage
Aluminium and polyethylene strips: Do not store above 25°C.

Store in the original container.

Aluminium-PVC/PVDC calendar blister strips: Do not store above 25°C.

Keep container in the outer carton.

As with all medicines, Tetralysal 300 should be kept out of the sight and reach of children.

6.5 Nature and contents of container
Aluminium-PVC/PVDC calendar blister strips of 14 capsules; two strips per carton, pack size = 28 capsules or Aluminium and polyethylene strips 28 or 56 capsule pack size.

6.6 Special precautions for disposal and other handling
No special instructions

7. MARKETING AUTHORISATION HOLDER
Galderma (UK) Limited
Meridien House
69-71 Clarendon Road
Watford
Herts.
WD17 1DS
UK

8. MARKETING AUTHORISATION NUMBER(S)
PL 10590/0019

9. DATE OF FIRST AUTHORISATION/RENEWAL OF THE AUTHORISATION
29th September 1995

10. DATE OF REVISION OF THE TEXT
February 2006

11 Legal category
POM

Teveten 300 mg Film-coated Tablets

(Solvay Healthcare Limited)

1. NAME OF THE MEDICINAL PRODUCT
Teveten 300 mg film-coated tablets

2. QUALITATIVE AND QUANTITATIVE COMPOSITION
Eprosartan mesylate equivalent to 300 mg eprosartan free base.

For excipients, see section 6.1

3. PHARMACEUTICAL FORM
Film-coated tablet.

Oval, biconvex, white film-coated tablets with inscriptions 'SOLVAY and '5043'.

4. CLINICAL PARTICULARS

4.1 Therapeutic indications
Eprosartan is indicated for the treatment of essential hypertension.

4.2 Posology and method of administration
The recommended dose is 600 mg eprosartan once daily.

The dose may be increased to 800 mg eprosartan once daily if further response is required. Achievement of maximal blood pressure reduction in most patients may take 2 to 3 weeks of treatment.

Eprosartan may be used alone or in combination with other anti-hypertensives, e.g. thiazide-type diuretics, calcium channel blockers, if a greater blood pressure lowering effect is required.

Eprosartan should be taken with food.

Elderly (>75 years): As clinical experience is limited in patients over 75 years, a starting dose of 300 mg once daily is recommended.

Dosage in hepatically impaired patients: There is limited experience in patients with hepatic impairment (see sections 4.3 and 5.2). In patients with mild to moderate hepatic impairment, a starting dose of 300 mg once daily is recommended.

Dosage in renally impaired patients: No dose adjustment is required in patients with creatinine clearance 60-80 ml/min. As clinical experience is limited in patients with creatinine clearance <60 ml/min, a starting dose of 300mg once daily is recommended (see section 4.4).

Children: As safety and efficacy in children have not been established, treatment of children is not recommended.

4.3 Contraindications
Known hypersensitivity to components of the product.

Pregnancy and lactation.

Severe hepatic impairment.

4.4 Special warnings and precautions for use
Risk of renal impairment

As a consequence of inhibiting the renin-angiotensin-aldosterone system, changes in renal function including renal failure have been reported with angiotensin converting enzyme (ACE) inhibitors and angiotensin receptor antagonists in susceptible individuals. Such changes in renal function may be reversible upon discontinuation of therapy.

As clinical experience is limited in patients with creatinine clearance <60 ml/min and in patients undergoing dialysis, caution is recommended.

As with other angiotensin II antagonists, pre-treatment and periodic monitoring of serum potassium and creatinine levels is recommended in patients with impaired renal function.

Sodium and/or volume depletion

At the start of therapy, symptomatic hypotension may occur in patients with severe sodium depletion and/or volume depletion (e.g. high dose diuretic therapy). Sodium and/or volume depletion should be corrected before commencing therapy or existing diuretic therapy should be reduced.

Hyperkalaemia

Although eprosartan has no significant effect on serum potassium there is no experience of concomitant administration with K-sparing diuretics or K-supplements. Consequently, as with other angiotensin II antagonists, the risk of hyperkalaemia when taken with K-sparing diuretics or K-supplements cannot be excluded. Regular monitoring for serum potassium levels is recommended when drugs that may increase potassium are administered with eprosartan in patients with renal impairment.

4.5 Interaction with other medicinal products and other forms of interaction

No clinically significant drug interactions have been observed. No effect on the pharmacokinetics of digoxin and the pharmacodynamics of warfarin or glyburide (glibenclamide) has been shown with eprosartan. Similarly no effect on eprosartan pharmacokinetics has been shown with ranitidine, ketoconazole or fluconazole.

Eprosartan has been safely used concomitantly with thiazide diuretics (e.g. hydrochlorothiazide) and calcium channel blockers (e.g. sustained-release nifedipine) without evidence of clinically significant adverse interactions. It has been safely co-administered with hypolipidaemic agents (e.g. lovastatin, simvastatin, pravastatin, fenofibrate, gemfibrozil, niacin).

Reversible increases in serum lithium concentrations and toxicity have been reported during concomitant administration of lithium with ACE inhibitors. While this is not documented with eprosartan, the possibility of a similar effect can not be excluded and careful monitoring of serum lithium levels is recommended during concomitant use.

Eprosartan has been shown not to inhibit human cytochrome P450 enzymes CYP1A, 2A6, 2C9/8, 2C19, 2D6, 2E and 3A *in vitro*.

Combination with NSAIDs: When Angiotensin II antagonists are administered simultaneously with non-steroidal anti-inflammatory drugs (i.e. selective COX-2 inhibitors, acetylsalicylic acid (> 3g/day) and non-selective NSAIDs), attenuation of the antihypertensive effect may occur.

As with ACE inhibitors, concomitant use of Angiotensin II antagonists and NSAIDs may lead to an increased risk of worsening of renal function, including possible acute renal failure, and an increase in serum potassium, especially in patients with poor pre-existing renal function. The combination should be administered with caution, especially in the elderly. Patients should be adequately hydrated and consideration should be given to monitoring renal function after initiation of concomitant therapy, and periodically thereafter.

4.6 Pregnancy and lactation

Pregnancy: There is little experience with the use of eprosartan during pregnancy. Drugs that act directly on the renin-angiotensin-aldosterone system can cause foetal and neonatal morbidity and death when administered to pregnant women during the second and third trimester. As with other drugs affecting the renin- angiotensin-aldosterone system, eprosartan should not be used in pregnancy, and if pregnancy is detected, eprosartan should be discontinued as soon as possible.

Lactation: Breast feeding women should not be treated with eprosartan (see Contraindications).

4.7 Effects on ability to drive and use machines

The effect of eprosartan on the ability to drive and use machines has not been studied, but based on its pharmacodynamic properties, eprosartan is unlikely to affect this ability. When driving vehicles or operating machines, it should be taken into account, that occasionally dizziness or weariness may occur during treatment of hypertension.

4.8 Undesirable effects

Clinical Trials

In placebo-controlled clinical trials, the overall incidence of adverse experiences reported with eprosartan was comparable to placebo. Adverse experiences have usually been mild and transient in nature and have only required discontinuation of therapy in 4.1% of patients treated with eprosartan in placebo-controlled studies (6.5% for placebo).

The following table shows the adverse experiences, regardless of causality, reported by patients with hypertension in placebo controlled studies of up to 13 weeks duration. It includes all adverse experiences occurring on eprosartan 600 - 800 mg once daily with an incidence at least 1% higher than placebo.

	Eprosartan 600/800mg O.D.	Placebo
Total Number of Patients	326	280
	%	%
Dizziness	4.6	2.9
Arthralgia	1.8	0.7
Rhinitis	1.5	0.4
Flatulence	1.5	0
Hypertriglyceridaemia	1.2	0

Angioedema has been infrequently reported.

Market Experience

The following adverse reactions have been reported during post-marketing experience with the following frequencies: very common (> 1/10); common (> 1/100, < 1/10); uncommon (> 1/1000, < 1/100); rare (> 1/10,000, < 1/1000); very rare (< 1/10,000)

Body as a whole:

Rare: Headache, asthenia

Nervous disorders:

Rare: Dizziness

Cardiovascular disorders:

Very rare: Hypotension (including postural hypotension)

Gastrointestinal disorders:

Very rare: Nausea

Skin disorders:

Rare: Rash, pruritus, urticaria

Very rare: Facial swelling, angioedema

Laboratory Findings

In placebo-controlled clinical studies, significantly elevated serum potassium concentrations were observed in 0.9% of patients treated with eprosartan and 0.3% of patients who received placebo.

Significantly low values of haemoglobin were observed in 0.1% and 0% patients treated with eprosartan and placebo respectively.

In rare cases elevations of BUN values were reported in patients treated with eprosartan. In rare cases increases in liver function values were also observed but were not considered to be causally related to eprosartan treatment.

4.9 Overdose

Limited data are available with regard to overdosage in humans. Eprosartan was well tolerated after oral dosing (maximum unit dose taken to date in humans 1200 mg) with no mortality in rats and mice up to 3000 mg/kg and in dogs up to 1000 mg/kg. The most likely manifestation of overdosage would be hypotension. If symptomatic hypotension occurs, supportive treatment should be instituted.

5. PHARMACOLOGICAL PROPERTIES

5.1 Pharmacodynamic properties

Eprosartan is a potent, synthetic, orally active non-biphenyl non-tetrazole angiotensin II receptor antagonist, which binds selectively to the AT_1 receptor. Angiotensin II is a potent vasoconstrictor and the primary active hormone of the renin-angiotensin-aldosterone system, playing a major part in the pathophysiology of hypertension. Angiotensin II binds to the AT_1 receptor in many tissues (e.g. smooth vascular musculature, suprarenals, kidney, heart) and produces important biological effects such as vasoconstriction, sodium retention and release of aldosterone. More recently, angiotensin II has been implicated in the genesis of cardiac and vascular hypertrophy through its effect on cardiac and smooth muscle cell growth.

Eprosartan antagonised the effect of angiotensin II on blood pressure, renal blood flow and aldosterone secretion in normal volunteers. In hypertensive patients, comparable blood pressure control is achieved when eprosartan is administered as a single dose or in two divided doses. In placebo-controlled studies, in 299 patients treated receiving 600-800 mg once daily, there was no evidence of first dose postural hypotension. Discontinuation of treatment with eprosartan does not lead to a rapid rebound increase in blood pressure.

Eprosartan was evaluated in mild to moderate hypertensive patients (sitting DBP ⩾95 mmHg and < 115 mmHg) and severe hypertensive patients (sitting DBP ⩾ 115 mmHg and ⩽125 mmHg).

A dose of 1200 mg once daily, for 8 weeks, has been shown in 72 patients in clinical trials to be effective. In placebo-controlled studies using doses up to 1200 mg once daily, there is no apparent dose relationship in the incidence of adverse experiences reported.

In patients with hypertension, blood pressure reduction did not produce a change in heart rate.

In hypertensive patients eprosartan does not affect fasting triglycerides, total cholesterol, or LDL (low density lipoprotein) cholesterol levels. In addition, eprosartan has no effect on fasting blood sugar levels.

Eprosartan does not compromise renal autoregulatory mechanisms. In normal adult males eprosartan has been shown to increase mean effective renal plasma flow. Effective renal plasma flow is not altered in patients with essential hypertension and patients with renal insufficiency treated with eprosartan. Eprosartan does not reduce glomerular filtration rate in normal males, in patients with hypertension or in patients with varying degrees of renal insufficiency. Eprosartan has a natriuretic effect in normal subjects on a salt restricted diet.

Eprosartan does not significantly affect the excretion of urinary uric acid.

Eprosartan does not potentiate effects relating to bradykinin (ACE-mediated), e.g. cough. In a study specifically designed to compare the incidence of cough in patients treated with eprosartan and an angiotensin converting enzyme inhibitor, the incidence of dry persistent cough in patients treated with eprosartan (1.5%) was significantly lower ($p < 0.05$) than that observed in patients treated with an angiotensin converting enzyme inhibitor (5.4%). In a further study investigating the incidence of cough in patients who had previously coughed while taking an angiotensin converting enzyme inhibitor, the incidence of dry, persistent cough was 2.6% on eprosartan, 2.7% on placebo, and 25.0% on an angiotensin converting enzyme inhibitor ($p < 0.01$, eprosartan versus angiotensin converting enzyme inhibitor).

5.2 Pharmacokinetic properties

Absolute bioavailability following a single 300 mg oral dose of eprosartan is about 13%, due to limited oral absorption. Eprosartan plasma concentrations peak at one to two hours after an oral dose in the fasted state. Plasma concentrations are dose proportional from 100 to 200 mg, but less than proportional for 400 and 800 mg doses. The terminal elimination half-life of eprosartan following oral administration is typically five to nine hours. A slight accumulation (14%) is seen with chronic use of eprosartan. Administration of eprosartan with food delays absorption with minor increases (<25%) observed in C_{max} and AUC.

Plasma protein binding of eprosartan is high (approximately 98%) and constant over the concentration range achieved with therapeutic doses. The extent of plasma protein binding is not influenced by gender, age, hepatic dysfunction or mild-moderate renal impairment but has shown to be decreased in a small number of patients with severe renal impairment.

Following oral and intravenous dosing with [^{14}C]eprosartan in human subjects, eprosartan was the only drug-related compound found in the plasma and faeces. In the urine, approximately 20% of the radioactivity excreted was an acyl glucuronide of eprosartan with the remaining 80% being unchanged eprosartan.

The volume of distribution of eprosartan is about 13 litres. Total plasma clearance is about 130 ml/min. Biliary and renal excretion contribute to the elimination of eprosartan. Following intravenous [^{14}C]eprosartan, about 61% of radioactivity is recovered in the faeces and about 37% in the urine. Following an oral dose of [^{14}C]eprosartan, about 90% of radioactivity is recovered in the faeces and about 7% in the urine.

Both AUC and C_{max} values of eprosartan are increased in the elderly (on average, approximately two-fold).

Following administration of a single 100 mg dose of eprosartan, AUC values of eprosartan (but not C_{max}) are increased, on average, by approximately 40% in patients with hepatic impairment. Since an intravenous dose of eprosartan was not administered to patients with hepatic impairment, the plasma clearance of eprosartan could not be measured.

Compared to subjects with normal renal function (n=7), mean AUC and C_{max} values were approximately 30% higher in patients with creatinine clearance 30-59 ml/min (n=11) and approximately 50% higher in patients with creatinine clearance 5-29 ml/min (n=3).

In a separate investigation, mean AUC was approximately 60% higher in patients undergoing dialysis (n=9) compared to subjects with normal renal function (n=10).

There is no difference in the pharmacokinetics of eprosartan between males and females.

5.3 Preclinical safety data

General toxicology

Eprosartan given orally at dosages up to 1000 mg/kg per day for up to six months in rat and up to one year in dogs did not result in any significant drug-related toxicity.

Reprotoxicity

In pregnant rabbits, eprosartan has been shown to produce maternal and foetal mortality at 10 mg/kg per day during late pregnancy only. This is most likely due to effects on the renin angiotensin aldosterone system. Maternal toxicity but no foetal effects were observed at 3 mg/kg per day.

Genotoxicity

Genotoxicity was not observed in a battery of *in vitro* and *in vivo* tests.

Carcinogenicity

Carcinogenicity was not observed in rats and mice given up to 600 or 2000 mg/kg per day respectively for two years.

6. PHARMACEUTICAL PARTICULARS

6.1 List of excipients

Tablet cores:

Lactose

Microcrystalline cellulose

Pregelatinised starch

Croscarmellose sodium

Magnesium stearate

Film-coat:

Hypromellose

Titanium dioxide (E171)

Macrogol 400

Polysorbate 80

6.2 Incompatibilities

None known.

6.3 Shelf life

PVC/Aclar blister packs: 36 months

HDPE bottles: 36 months

6.4 Special precautions for storage

Do not store above 25°C.

Keep container in the outer carton.

6.5 Nature and contents of container

Opaque PVC/Aclar blister packs containing 28 tablets or 56 tablets.

HDPE bottles containing 100 tablets.

6.6 Special precautions for disposal and other handling

No special instructions.

7. MARKETING AUTHORISATION HOLDER

Solvay Healthcare Limited

Mansbridge Road

West End

Southampton

SO18 3JD

8. MARKETING AUTHORISATION NUMBER(S)

PL 00512/0163

9. DATE OF FIRST AUTHORISATION/RENEWAL OF THE AUTHORISATION

23 August 1999/17 April 2003

10. DATE OF REVISION OF THE TEXT

June 2006

LEGAL CATEGORY

POM

Teveten 400 mg film-coated Tablets

(Solvay Healthcare Limited)

1. NAME OF THE MEDICINAL PRODUCT

Teveten 400 mg film-coated tablets

2. QUALITATIVE AND QUANTITATIVE COMPOSITION

Eprosartan mesylate equivalent to 400 mg eprosartan free base.

For excipients, see section 6.1

3. PHARMACEUTICAL FORM

Film-coated tablet.

Oval, biconvex, pink film-coated tablets with inscriptions 'SOLVAY' and '5044'.

4. CLINICAL PARTICULARS

4.1 Therapeutic indications

Eprosartan is indicated for the treatment of essential hypertension.

4.2 Posology and method of administration

The recommended dose is 600 mg eprosartan once daily.

The dose may be increased to 800 mg eprosartan once daily if further response is required. Achievement of maximal blood pressure reduction in most patients may take 2 to 3 weeks of treatment.

Eprosartan may be used alone or in combination with other anti-hypertensives, e.g. thiazide-type diuretics, calcium channel blockers, if a greater blood pressure lowering effect is required.

Eprosartan should be taken with food.

Elderly (>75 years): As clinical experience is limited in patients over 75 years, a starting dose of 300 mg once daily is recommended.

Dosage in hepatically impaired patients: There is limited experience in patients with hepatic impairment (see sections 4.3 and 5.2). In patients with mild to moderate hepatic impairment, a starting dose of 300 mg once daily is recommended.

Dosage in renally impaired patients: No dose adjustment is required in patients with creatinine clearance 60-80 ml/min. As clinical experience is limited in patients with creatinine clearance <60 ml/min, a starting dose of 300mg once daily is recommended (see section 4.4).

Children: As safety and efficacy in children have not been established, treatment of children is not recommended.

4.3 Contraindications

Known hypersensitivity to components of the product.

Pregnancy and lactation.

Severe hepatic impairment.

4.4 Special warnings and precautions for use

Risk of renal impairment

As a consequence of inhibiting the renin-angiotensin-aldosterone system, changes in renal function including renal failure have been reported with angiotensin converting enzyme (ACE) inhibitors and angiotensin receptor antagonists in susceptible individuals. Such changes in renal function may be reversible upon discontinuation of therapy.

As clinical experience is limited in patients with creatinine clearance <60 ml/min and in patients undergoing dialysis, caution is recommended.

As with other angiotensin II antagonists, pre-treatment and periodic monitoring of serum potassium and creatinine levels is recommended in patients with impaired renal function.

Sodium and/or volume depletion

At the start of therapy, symptomatic hypotension may occur in patients with severe sodium depletion and/or volume depletion (e.g. high dose diuretic therapy). Sodium and/or volume depletion should be corrected before commencing therapy or existing diuretic therapy should be reduced.

Hyperkalaemia

Although eprosartan has no significant effect on serum potassium there is no experience of concomitant administration with K-sparing diuretics or K-supplements. Consequently, as with other angiotensin II antagonists, the risk of hyperkalaemia when taken with K-sparing diuretics or K-supplements cannot be excluded. Regular monitoring for serum potassium levels is recommended when drugs that may increase potassium are administered with eprosartan in patients with renal impairment.

4.5 Interaction with other medicinal products and other forms of interaction

No clinically significant drug interactions have been observed. No effect on the pharmacokinetics of digoxin and the pharmacodynamics of warfarin or glyburide (glibenclamide) has been shown with eprosartan. Similarly no effect on eprosartan pharmacokinetics has been shown with ranitidine, ketoconazole or fluconazole.

Eprosartan has been safely used concomitantly with thiazide diuretics (e.g. hydrochlorothiazide) and calcium channel blockers (e.g. sustained-release nifedipine) without evidence of clinically significant adverse interactions. It has been safely co-administered with hypolipidaemic agents (e.g. lovastatin, simvastatin, pravastatin, fenofibrate, gemfibrozil, niacin).

Reversible increases in serum lithium concentrations and toxicity have been reported during concomitant administration of lithium with ACE inhibitors. While this is not documented with eprosartan, the possibility of a similar effect can not be excluded and careful monitoring of serum lithium levels is recommended during concomitant use.

Eprosartan has been shown not to inhibit human cytochrome P450 enzymes CYP1A, 2A6, 2C9/8, 2C19, 2D6, 2E and 3A *in vitro*.

Combination with NSAIDs: When Angiotensin II antagonists are administered simultaneously with non-steroidal anti-inflammatory drugs (i.e. selective COX-2 inhibitors, acetylsalicylic acid (> 3g/day) and non-selective NSAIDs), attenuation of the antihypertensive effect may occur.

As with ACE inhibitors, concomitant use of Angiotensin II antagonists and NSAIDs may lead to an increased risk of worsening of renal function, including possible acute renal failure, and an increase in serum potassium, especially in patients with poor pre-existing renal function. The combination should be administered with caution, especially in the elderly. Patients should be adequately hydrated and consideration should be given to monitoring renal function after initiation of concomitant therapy, and periodically thereafter.

4.6 Pregnancy and lactation

Pregnancy: There is little experience with the use of eprosartan during pregnancy. Drugs that act directly on the renin-angiotensin-aldosterone system can cause foetal and neonatal morbidity and death when administered to pregnant women during the second and third trimester. As with other drugs affecting the renin- angiotensin-aldosterone system, eprosartan should not be used in pregnancy, and if pregnancy is detected, eprosartan should be discontinued as soon as possible.

Lactation: Breast feeding women should not be treated with eprosartan (see Contraindications).

4.7 Effects on ability to drive and use machines

The effect of eprosartan on the ability to drive and use machines has not been studied, but based on its pharmacodynamic properties, eprosartan is unlikely to affect this ability. When driving vehicles or operating machines, it should be taken into account, that occasionally dizziness or weariness may occur during treatment of hypertension.

4.8 Undesirable effects

Clinical Trials

In placebo-controlled clinical trials, the overall incidence of adverse experiences reported with eprosartan was comparable to placebo. Adverse experiences have usually been mild and transient in nature and have only required discontinuation of therapy in 4.1% of patients treated with eprosartan in placebo-controlled studies (6.5% for placebo).

The following table shows the adverse experiences, regardless of causality, reported by patients with hypertension in placebo controlled studies of up to 13 weeks duration. It includes all adverse experiences occurring on eprosartan 600 - 800 mg once daily with an incidence at least 1% higher than placebo.

	Eprosartan 600/800mg O.D.	Placebo
Total Number of Patients	326	280
	%	%
Dizziness	4.6	2.9
Arthralgia	1.8	0.7
Rhinitis	1.5	0.4
Flatulence	1.5	0
Hypertriglyceridaemia	1.2	0

Angioedema has been infrequently reported.

Market Experience

The following adverse reactions have been reported during post-marketing experience with the following frequencies: very common (>1/10); common (>1/100, <1/10); uncommon (>1/1000, <1/100); rare (>1/10,000, <1/1000); very rare (<1/10,000)

Body as a whole:

Rare: Headache, asthenia

Nervous disorders:

Rare: Dizziness

Cardiovascular disorders:

Very rare: Hypotension (including postural hypotension)

Gastrointestinal disorders:

Very rare: Nausea

Skin disorders:

Rare: Rash, pruritus, urticaria

Very rare: Facial swelling, angioedema

Laboratory Findings

In placebo-controlled clinical studies, significantly elevated serum potassium concentrations were observed in 0.9% of patients treated with eprosartan and 0.3% of patients who received placebo.

Significantly low values of haemoglobin were observed in 0.1% and 0% patients treated with eprosartan and placebo respectively.

In rare cases elevations of BUN values were reported in patients treated with eprosartan. In rare cases increases in liver function values were also observed but were not considered to be causally related to eprosartan treatment.

4.9 Overdose

Limited data are available with regard to overdosage in humans. Eprosartan was well tolerated after oral dosing (maximum unit dose taken to date in humans 1200 mg) with no mortality in rats and mice up to 3000 mg/kg and in dogs up to 1000 mg/kg. The most likely manifestation of overdosage would be hypotension. If symptomatic hypotension occurs, supportive treatment should be instituted.

5. PHARMACOLOGICAL PROPERTIES

5.1 Pharmacodynamic properties

Eprosartan is a potent, synthetic, orally active non-biphenyl non-tetrazole angiotensin II receptor antagonist, which binds selectively to the AT_1 receptor. Angiotensin II is a potent vasoconstrictor and the primary active hormone of the renin-angiotensin-aldosterone system, playing a major part in the pathophysiology of hypertension. Angiotensin II binds to the AT_1 receptor in many tissues (e.g. smooth vascular musculature, suprarenals, kidney, heart) and produces important biological effects such as vasoconstriction, sodium retention and release of aldosterone. More recently, angiotensin II has been implicated in the genesis of cardiac and vascular hypertrophy through its effect on cardiac and smooth muscle cell growth.

Eprosartan antagonised the effect of angiotensin II on blood pressure, renal blood flow and aldosterone secretion in normal volunteers. In hypertensive patients, comparable blood pressure control is achieved when eprosartan is administered as a single dose or in two divided doses. In placebo-controlled studies, in 299 patients treated receiving 600-800 mg once daily, there was no evidence of first dose postural hypotension. Discontinuation of treatment with eprosartan does not lead to a rapid rebound increase in blood pressure.

Eprosartan was evaluated in mild to moderate hypertensive patients (sitting DBP ⩾95 mmHg and <115 mmHg) and severe hypertensive patients (sitting DBP ⩾115 mmHg and ⩽125 mmHg).

A dose of 1200 mg once daily, for 8 weeks, has been shown in 72 patients in clinical trials to be effective. In placebo-controlled studies using doses up to 1200 mg once daily, there is no apparent dose relationship in the incidence of adverse experiences reported.

In patients with hypertension, blood pressure reduction did not produce a change in heart rate.

In hypertensive patients eprosartan does not affect fasting triglycerides, total cholesterol, or LDL (low density lipoprotein) cholesterol levels. In addition, eprosartan has no effect on fasting blood sugar levels.

Eprosartan does not compromise renal autoregulatory mechanisms. In normal adult males eprosartan has been shown to increase mean effective renal plasma flow. Effective renal plasma flow is not altered in patients with essential hypertension and patients with renal insufficiency treated with eprosartan. Eprosartan does not reduce glomerular filtration rate in normal males, in patients with hypertension or in patients with varying degrees of renal insufficiency. Eprosartan has a natriuretic effect in normal subjects on a salt restricted diet.

Eprosartan does not significantly affect the excretion of urinary uric acid.

Eprosartan does not potentiate effects relating to bradykinin (ACE-mediated), e.g. cough. In a study specifically designed to compare the incidence of cough in patients treated with eprosartan and an angiotensin converting enzyme inhibitor, the incidence of dry persistent cough in patients treated with eprosartan (1.5%) was significantly lower ($p<0.05$) than that observed in patients treated with an angiotensin converting enzyme inhibitor (5.4%). In a further study investigating the incidence of cough in patients who had previously coughed while taking an angiotensin converting enzyme inhibitor, the incidence of dry, persistent cough was 2.6% on eprosartan, 2.7% on placebo, and 25.0% on an angiotensin converting enzyme inhibitor ($p<0.01$, eprosartan versus angiotensin converting enzyme inhibitor).

5.2 Pharmacokinetic properties

Absolute bioavailability following a single 300 mg oral dose of eprosartan is about 13%, due to limited oral absorption. Eprosartan plasma concentrations peak at one to two hours after an oral dose in the fasted state. Plasma concentrations are dose proportional from 100 to 200 mg, but less than proportional for 400 and 800 mg doses. The terminal elimination half-life of eprosartan following oral administration is typically five to nine hours. A slight accumulation (14%) is seen with chronic use of eprosartan. Administration of eprosartan with food delays absorption with minor increases (<25%) observed in C_{max} and AUC.

Plasma protein binding of eprosartan is high (approximately 98%) and constant over the concentration range achieved with therapeutic doses. The extent of plasma protein binding is not influenced by gender, age, hepatic dysfunction or mild-moderate renal impairment but has shown to be decreased in a small number of patients with severe renal impairment.

Following oral and intravenous dosing with [^{14}C]eprosartan in human subjects, eprosartan was the only drug-related compound found in the plasma and faeces. In the urine, approximately 20% of the radioactivity excreted was an acyl glucuronide of eprosartan with the remaining 80% being unchanged eprosartan.

The volume of distribution of eprosartan is about 13 litres. Total plasma clearance is about 130 ml/min. Biliary and renal excretion contribute to the elimination of eprosartan. Following intravenous [^{14}C]eprosartan, about 61% of radioactivity is recovered in the faeces and about 37% in the urine. Following an oral dose of [^{14}C]eprosartan, about 90% of radioactivity is recovered in the faeces and about 7% in the urine.

Both AUC and C_{max} values of eprosartan are increased in the elderly (on average, approximately two-fold).

Following administration of a single 100 mg dose of eprosartan, AUC values of eprosartan (but not C_{max}) are increased, on average, by approximately 40% in patients with hepatic impairment. Since an intravenous dose of eprosartan was not administered to patients with hepatic impairment, the plasma clearance of eprosartan could not be measured.

Compared to subjects with normal renal function (n=7), mean AUC and C_{max} values were approximately 30% higher in patients with creatinine clearance 30-59 ml/min (n=11) and approximately 50% higher in patients with creatinine clearance 5-29 ml/min (n=3).

In a separate investigation, mean AUC was approximately 60% higher in patients undergoing dialysis (n=9) compared to subjects with normal renal function (n=10).

There is no difference in the pharmacokinetics of eprosartan between males and females.

5.3 Preclinical safety data

General toxicology

Eprosartan given orally at dosages up to 1000 mg/kg per day for up to six months in rat and up to one year in dogs did not result in any significant drug-related toxicity.

Reprotoxicity

In pregnant rabbits, eprosartan has been shown to produce maternal and foetal mortality at 10 mg/kg per day during late pregnancy only. This is most likely due to effects on the renin angiotensin aldosterone system. Maternal toxicity but no foetal effects were observed at 3 mg/kg per day.

Genotoxicity

Genotoxicity was not observed in a battery of *in vitro* and *in vivo* tests.

Carcinogenicity

Carcinogenicity was not observed in rats and mice given up to 600 or 2000 mg/kg per day respectively for two years.

6. PHARMACEUTICAL PARTICULARS

6.1 List of excipients

Tablet core

Lactose

Microcrystalline cellulose

Pregelatinised starch

Croscarmellose sodium

Magnesium stearate

Film-coat

Hypromellose

Titanium dioxide (E171)

Macrogol 400

Polysorbate 80

Red iron oxide (E172)

Yellow iron oxide (E172)

6.2 Incompatibilities

None known.

6.3 Shelf life

PVC/Aclar blister packs: 2 years

HDPE bottles: 36 months

6.4 Special precautions for storage

Do not store above 25°C.

Keep container in the outer carton.

6.5 Nature and contents of container

White PVC/PCTFE blister packs containing 28 tablets or 56 tablets.

HDPE bottles containing 100 tablets.

6.6 Special precautions for disposal and other handling

No special instructions.

7. MARKETING AUTHORISATION HOLDER

Solvay Healthcare Limited

Mansbridge Road

West End

Southampton

SO18 3JD

8. MARKETING AUTHORISATION NUMBER(S)

PL 00512/0164

9. DATE OF FIRST AUTHORISATION/RENEWAL OF THE AUTHORISATION

23 August 1999/ 17 April 2003

10. DATE OF REVISION OF THE TEXT

October 2008

LEGAL CATEGORY

POM

Teveten 600mg Film-coated Tablets

(Solvay Healthcare Limited)

1. NAME OF THE MEDICINAL PRODUCT

Teveten 600 mg film-coated tablets

2. QUALITATIVE AND QUANTITATIVE COMPOSITION

Eprosartan mesylate equivalent to 600 mg eprosartan free base.

For excipients, see section 6.1.

3. PHARMACEUTICAL FORM

Film-coated tablet.

Capsule-shaped, biconvex, white film-coated tablets with the inscription '5046'.

4. CLINICAL PARTICULARS

4.1 Therapeutic indications

Eprosartan is indicated for the treatment of essential hypertension.

4.2 Posology and method of administration

The recommended dose is 600 mg eprosartan once daily.

The dose may be increased to 800 mg eprosartan once daily if further response is required. Achievement of maximal blood pressure reduction in most patients may take 2 to 3 weeks of treatment.

Eprosartan may be used alone or in combination with other anti-hypertensives, e.g. thiazide-type diuretics, calcium channel blockers, if a greater blood pressure lowering effect is required.

Eprosartan should be taken with food.

Elderly (>75 years): As clinical experience is limited in patients over 75 years, a starting dose of 300 mg once daily is recommended.

Dosage in hepatically impaired patients: There is limited experience in patients with hepatic impairment (see sections 4.3 and 5.2). In patients with mild to moderate hepatic impairment, a starting dose of 300 mg once daily is recommended.

Dosage in renally impaired patients: No dose adjustment is required in patients with creatinine clearance 60-80 ml/min. As clinical experience is limited in patients with creatinine clearance <60 ml/min, a starting dose of 300mg once daily is recommended (see section 4.4).

Children: As safety and efficacy in children have not been established, treatment of children is not recommended.

4.3 Contraindications

Known hypersensitivity to components of the product.

Pregnancy and lactation.

Severe hepatic impairment.

4.4 Special warnings and precautions for use

Risk of renal impairment

As a consequence of inhibiting the renin-angiotensin-aldosterone system, changes in renal function including renal failure have been reported with angiotensin converting enzyme (ACE) inhibitors and angiotensin receptor antagonists in susceptible individuals. Such changes in renal function may be reversible upon discontinuation of therapy.

As clinical experience is limited in patients with creatinine clearance <60 ml/min and in patients undergoing dialysis, caution is recommended.

As with other angiotensin II antagonists, pre-treatment and periodic monitoring of serum potassium and creatinine levels is recommended in patients with impaired renal function.

Sodium and/or volume depletion

At the start of therapy, symptomatic hypotension may occur in patients with severe sodium depletion and/or volume depletion (e.g. high dose diuretic therapy). Sodium and/or volume depletion should be corrected before commencing therapy or existing diuretic therapy should be reduced.

Hyperkalaemia

Although eprosartan has no significant effect on serum potassium there is no experience of concomitant administration with K-sparing diuretics or K-supplements. Consequently, as with other angiotensin II antagonists, the risk of hyperkalaemia when taken with K-sparing diuretics or K-supplements cannot be excluded. Regular monitoring for serum potassium levels is recommended when drugs that may increase potassium are administered with eprosartan in patients with renal impairment.

4.5 Interaction with other medicinal products and other forms of interaction

No clinically significant drug interactions have been observed. No effect on the pharmacokinetics of digoxin and the pharmacodynamics of warfarin or glyburide (glibenclamide) has been shown with eprosartan. Similarly no effect on eprosartan pharmacokinetics has been shown with ranitidine, ketoconazole or fluconazole.

Eprosartan has been safely used concomitantly with thiazide diuretics (e.g. hydrochlorothiazide) and calcium channel blockers (e.g. sustained-release nifedipine) without evidence of clinically significant adverse interactions. It has been safely co-administered with hypolipidaemic agents (e.g. lovastatin, simvastatin, pravastatin, fenofibrate, gemfibrozil, niacin).

Reversible increases in serum lithium concentrations and toxicity have been reported during concomitant administration of lithium with ACE inhibitors. While this is not documented with eprosartan, the possibility of a similar effect can not be excluded and careful monitoring of serum lithium levels is recommended during concomitant use.

Eprosartan has been shown not to inhibit human cytochrome P450 enzymes CYP1A, 2A6, 2C9/8, 2C19, 2D6, 2E and 3A *in vitro*.

Combination with NSAIDs: When Angiotensin II antagonists are administered simultaneously with non-steroidal anti-inflammatory drugs (i.e. selective COX-2 inhibitors, acetylsalicylic acid (> 3g/day) and non-selective NSAIDs), attenuation of the antihypertensive effect may occur.

As with ACE inhibitors, concomitant use of Angiotensin II antagonists and NSAIDs may lead to an increased risk of worsening of renal function, including possible acute renal failure, and an increase in serum potassium, especially in patients with poor pre-existing renal function. The combination should be administered with caution, especially in the elderly. Patients should be adequately hydrated and consideration should be given to monitoring renal function after initiation of concomitant therapy, and periodically thereafter.

4.6 Pregnancy and lactation

Pregnancy: There is little experience with the use of eprosartan during pregnancy. Drugs that act directly on the renin-angiotensin-aldosterone system can cause foetal and neonatal morbidity and death when administered to pregnant women during the second and third trimester. As with other drugs affecting the renin- angiotensin-aldosterone system, eprosartan should not be used in pregnancy, and if pregnancy is detected, eprosartan should be discontinued as soon as possible.

Lactation: It is not known whether eprosartan is excreted in human milk but it is in rat milk. Because of potential adverse effects on the nursing infant, eprosartan should be used in women who are breast feeding only if the benefits clearly outweigh the risks.

4.7 Effects on ability to drive and use machines

The effect of eprosartan on the ability to drive and use machines has not been studied, but based on its pharmacodynamic properties, eprosartan is unlikely to effect this ability. When driving vehicles or operating machines, it should be taken into account, that occasionally dizziness or weariness may occur during treatment of hypertension.

4.8 Undesirable effects

Clinical Trials

In placebo-controlled clinical trials, the overall incidence of adverse experiences reported with eprosartan was comparable to placebo. Adverse experiences have usually been mild and transient in nature and have only required discontinuation of therapy in 4.1% of patients treated with eprosartan in placebo-controlled studies (6.5% for placebo).

The following table shows the adverse experiences, regardless of causality, reported by patients with hypertension in placebo controlled studies of up to 13 weeks duration. It includes all adverse experiences occurring on eprosartan 600 - 800 mg once daily with an incidence at least 1% higher than placebo.

	Eprosartan 600/800mg O.D.	Placebo
Total Number of Patients	326	280
	%	%
Dizziness	4.6	2.9
Arthralgia	1.8	0.7
Rhinitis	1.5	0.4
Flatulence	1.5	0
Hypertriglyceridaemia	1.2	0

Angioedema has been infrequently reported.

Market Experience

The following adverse reactions have been reported during post-marketing experience with the following frequencies: very common (>1/10); common (>1/100, <1/10); uncommon (>1/1000, <1/100); rare (>1/10,000, <1/1000); very rare (<1/10,000).

Body as a whole:

Rare: Headache, asthenia

Nervous disorders:

Rare: Dizziness

Cardiovascular disorders:

Very rare: Hypotension (including postural hypotension)

Gastrointestinal disorders:

Very rare: Nausea

Skin disorders:

Rare: Rash, pruritus, urticaria

Very rare: Facial swelling, angioedema

Laboratory Findings

In placebo-controlled clinical studies, significantly elevated serum potassium concentrations were observed in 0.9% of patients treated with eprosartan and 0.3% of patients who received placebo.

Significantly low values of haemoglobin were observed in 0.1% and 0% patients treated with eprosartan and placebo respectively.

In rare cases elevations of BUN values were reported in patients treated with eprosartan. In rare cases increases in liver function values were also observed but were not considered to be causally related to eprosartan treatment.

4.9 Overdose

Limited data are available in regard to overdosage in humans. Eprosartan was well tolerated after oral dosing (maximum unit dose taken to date in humans 1200 mg) with no mortality in rats and mice up to 3000 mg/kg and in dogs up to 1000 mg/kg. The most likely manifestation of overdosage would be hypotension. If symptomatic hypotension occurs, supportive treatment should be instituted.

5. PHARMACOLOGICAL PROPERTIES

5.1 Pharmacodynamic properties

Eprosartan is a potent, synthetic, orally active non-biphenyl non-tetrazole angiotensin II receptor antagonist, which binds selectively to the AT_1 receptor. Angiotensin II is a potent vasoconstrictor and the primary active hormone of the renin-angiotensin-aldosterone system, playing a major part in the pathophysiology of hypertension. Angiotensin II binds to the AT_1 receptor in many tissues (e.g. smooth vascular musculature, suprarenals, kidney, heart) and produces important biological effects such as vasoconstriction, sodium retention and release of aldosterone. More recently, angiotensin II has been implicated in the genesis of cardiac and vascular hypertrophy through its effect on cardiac and smooth muscle cell growth.

Eprosartan antagonised the effect of angiotensin II on blood pressure, renal blood flow and aldosterone secretion in normal volunteers. In hypertensive patients, comparable blood pressure control is achieved when eprosartan is administered as a single dose or in two divided doses. In placebo-controlled studies, in 299 patients treated receiving 600-800 mg once daily, there was no evidence of first dose postural hypotension. Discontinuation of treatment with eprosartan does not lead to a rapid rebound increase in blood pressure.

Eprosartan was evaluated in mild to moderate hypertensive patients (sitting DBP ≥95 mmHg and <115 mmHg) and severe hypertensive patients (sitting DBP ≥115 mmHg and ≤125 mmHg).

A dose of 1200 mg once daily, for 8 weeks, has been shown in 72 patients in clinical trials to be effective. In placebo-controlled studies using doses up to 1200 mg once daily, there is no apparent dose relationship in the incidence of adverse experiences reported.

In patients with hypertension, blood pressure reduction did not produce a change in heart rate.

In hypertensive patients eprosartan does not affect fasting triglycerides, total cholesterol, or LDL (low density lipoprotein) cholesterol levels. In addition, eprosartan has no effect on fasting blood sugar levels.

Eprosartan does not compromise renal autoregulatory mechanisms. In normal adult males eprosartan has been shown to increase mean effective renal plasma flow. Effective renal plasma flow is not altered in patients with essential hypertension and patients with renal insufficiency treated with eprosartan. Eprosartan does not reduce glomerular filtration rate in normal males, in patients with hypertension or in patients with varying degrees of renal insufficiency. Eprosartan has a natriuretic effect in normal subjects on a salt restricted diet.

Eprosartan does not significantly affect the excretion of urinary uric acid.

Eprosartan does not potentiate effects relating to bradykinin (ACE-mediated), e.g. cough. In a study specifically designed to compare the incidence of cough in patients treated with eprosartan and an angiotensin converting enzyme inhibitor, the incidence of dry persistent cough in patients treated with eprosartan (1.5%) was significantly lower ($p<0.05$) than that observed in patients treated with an angiotensin converting enzyme inhibitor (5.4%). In a further study investigating the incidence of cough in patients who had previously coughed while taking an angiotensin converting enzyme inhibitor, the incidence of dry, persistent cough was 2.6% on eprosartan, 2.7% on placebo, and 25.0% on an angiotensin converting enzyme inhibitor ($p<0.01$, eprosartan versus angiotensin converting enzyme inhibitor).

5.2 Pharmacokinetic properties

Absolute bioavailability following a single 300 mg oral dose of eprosartan is about 13%, due to limited oral absorption. Eprosartan plasma concentrations peak at one to two hours after an oral dose in the fasted state. Plasma concentrations are dose proportional from 100 to 200 mg, but less than proportional for 400 and 800 mg doses. The terminal elimination half-life of eprosartan following oral administration is typically five to nine hours. A slight accumulation (14%) is seen with chronic use of eprosartan. Administration of eprosartan with food delays absorption with minor increases (<25%) observed in C_{max} and AUC.

Plasma protein binding of eprosartan is high (approximately 98%) and constant over the concentration range achieved with therapeutic doses. The extent of plasma protein binding is not influenced by gender, age, hepatic dysfunction or mild-moderate renal impairment but has shown to be decreased in a small number of patients with severe renal impairment.

Following oral and intravenous dosing with [^{14}C]eprosartan in human subjects, eprosartan was the only drug-related compound found in the plasma and faeces. In the urine, approximately 20% of the radioactivity excreted was an acyl glucuronide of eprosartan with the remaining 80% being unchanged eprosartan.

The volume of distribution of eprosartan is about 13 litres. Total plasma clearance is about 130 ml/min. Biliary and renal excretion contribute to the elimination of eprosartan. Following intravenous [^{14}C]eprosartan, about 61% of radioactivity is recovered in the faeces and about 37% in the urine. Following an oral dose of [^{14}C]eprosartan, about 90% of radioactivity is recovered in the faeces and about 7% in the urine.

Both AUC and C_{max} values of eprosartan are increased in the elderly (on average, approximately two-fold).

Following administration of a single 100 mg dose of eprosartan, AUC values of eprosartan (but not C_{max}) are increased, on average, by approximately 40% in patients with hepatic impairment. Since an intravenous dose of eprosartan was not administered to patients with hepatic impairment, the plasma clearance of eprosartan could not be measured.

Compared to subjects with normal renal function (n=7), mean AUC and C_{max} values were approximately 30% higher in patients with creatinine clearance 30-59 ml/min (n=11) and approximately 50% higher in patients with creatinine clearance 5-29 ml/min (n=3).

In a separate investigation, mean AUC was approximately 60% higher in patients undergoing dialysis (n=9) compared to subjects with normal renal function (n=10).

There is no difference in the pharmacokinetics of eprosartan between males and females.

5.3 Preclinical safety data

General toxicology

Eprosartan given orally at dosages up to 1000 mg/kg per day for up to six months in rat and up to one year in dogs did not result in any significant drug-related toxicity.

Reprotoxicity

In pregnant rabbits, eprosartan has been shown to produce maternal and foetal mortality at 10 mg/kg per day during late pregnancy only. This is most likely due to effects on the renin angiotensin aldosterone system. Maternal toxicity but no foetal effects were observed at 3 mg/kg per day.

Genotoxicity

Genotoxicity was not observed in a battery of *in vitro* and *in vivo* tests.

Carcinogenicity

Carcinogenicity was not observed in rats and mice given up to 600 or 2000 mg/kg per day respectively for two years.

6. PHARMACEUTICAL PARTICULARS

6.1 List of excipients

Tablet core

Lactose

Microcrystalline cellulose

Pregelatinised starch

Magnesium stearate

Crospovidone

Film-coat

Hypromellose

Titanium dioxide (E171)

Macrogol 400

Polysorbate 80

6.2 Incompatibilities

None known.

6.3 Shelf life

36 months.

6.4 Special precautions for storage

Do not store above 25°C. Keep container in the outer carton.

6.5 Nature and contents of container

White PVC/PCTFE/Alu blister packs or,

White PVC/PVDC/Alu blister packs containing 28 tablets or 56 tablets.

6.6 Special precautions for disposal and other handling

No special instructions.

7. MARKETING AUTHORISATION HOLDER

Solvay Healthcare Limited

Mansbridge Road

West End

Southampton

SO18 3JD

United Kingdom

8. MARKETING AUTHORISATION NUMBER(S)

PL 00512/0165

9. DATE OF FIRST AUTHORISATION/RENEWAL OF THE AUTHORISATION

29 November 1999/ 17 April 2003

10. DATE OF REVISION OF THE TEXT

July 2009

LEGAL CATEGORY

POM

Tilade CFC-Free Inhaler

(sanofi-aventis)

1. NAME OF THE MEDICINAL PRODUCT

Tilade CFC-Free Inhaler 2mg per actuation pressurised inhalation suspension ▼

2. QUALITATIVE AND QUANTITATIVE COMPOSITION

One metered dose (ex-valve) contains 2 mg nedocromil sodium.

For excipients, see 6.1.

3. PHARMACEUTICAL FORM

Pressurised inhalation suspension.

Tilade CFC-Free Inhaler contains a new propellant, HFA-227, and does not contain any chlorofluorocarbons (CFCs).

4. CLINICAL PARTICULARS

4.1 Therapeutic indications

Tilade CFC-Free is recommended for the treatment of bronchial asthma where regular preventative anti-inflammatory therapy is indicated and, in particular, in patients whose asthma is not adequately controlled by bronchodilators alone. Tilade CFC-Free may be given in addition to all existing therapies and in many cases will provide added therapeutic benefit.

4.2 Posology and method of administration
For inhalation use.

Adults, including the elderly and children over 6 years of age.

The initial dose is 4 mg (2 actuations) four times daily. Once control of symptoms has been achieved it may be possible to reduce the dose to a maintenance dose of 4mg (2 actuations) twice daily.

Tilade CFC-Free is intended for regular daily use and should not be used for the relief of symptoms in an acute attack.

Tilade CFC-Free is not recommended for use in children 6 years of age and younger.

Concomitant Bronchodilator Therapy

Where a concomitant inhaled bronchodilator is prescribed it is recommended that this be administered prior to Tilade CFC-Free.

Concomitant Steroid Therapy

In patients currently treated with steroids, the addition of Tilade CFC-Free to the regimen may make it possible to reduce the maintenance dose of steroids, or discontinue steroid therapy completely. The patient must be carefully supervised while the steroid dose is reduced; a rate of 10% weekly is suggested.

If a reduction of a steroid dose has been possible, Tilade CFC-Free should not be withdrawn until steroid cover has been re-instituted.

Method of Administration

If the inhaler is new, it should be primed by actuating 4 times prior to inhalation. If not used for more than 3 days, additional priming with 1-2 actuations is advised.

The inhaler should be well shaken and the dustcap removed. The mouthpiece of the inhaler should be placed in the mouth and the lips closed around it prior to the patient beginning to breathe in. The patient should then be instructed to breathe in slowly and deeply through the mouth and as inhalation begins the aerosol should be actuated by pressing the can down firmly with the first finger whilst continuing to breathe in. The breath should then be held for 10 seconds before exhaling into the air. To avoid condensation of moisture in the inhaler and blocking of the spray, exhalation through the inhaler should be avoided. If the patient needs two actuations they should be instructed to wait for about one minute before repeating the inhalation procedure. The dustcap should be replaced following use. To prevent excessive accumulation of powder the plastic body and mouthpiece cover should be rinsed in hand hot water twice a week and then thoroughly dried. If the Fisonair holding chamber is used this also should be washed in hand hot water twice a week and thoroughly dried.

Children and patients with difficulty in coordinating actuation of the inhaler with inhalation of the aerosol cloud, may benefit from using a holding chamber to assist inhalation of the medication. When using a holding chamber the procedure for inhalation is different from that through the standard mouthpiece. The medication is first released into the holding chamber from which it is subsequently inhaled (in one or more breaths) until the chamber is empty. Thus, there is no need to co-ordinate actuation of the inhaler with simultaneous breathing. However medication must still be inhaled slowly and deeply from the holding chamber. The standard mouthpiece, is suitable for use with large volume holding chambers such as Fisonair.

Detailed instructions for the inhalation of Tilade CFC-Free from each of the three devices are provided in the respective Patient Information Leaflet supplied with each pack.

4.3 Contraindications
TILADE CFC-Free is contraindicated in patients with known hypersensitivity to nedocromil sodium or to any of the other constituents.

4.4 Special warnings and precautions for use
TILADE CFC-Free must not be used for the relief of an acute attack of bronchospasm.

Since therapy is prophylactic, it is important that Tilade CFC-Free be used regularly, every day, in those patients who benefit, even if they become asymptomatic. The patient should also be advised that because several doses may be needed to establish benefit, relief may not be apparent immediately, but may take some weeks to develop.

Patients should be advised to have relief medication available (such as an inhaled short-acting bronchodilator) to relieve symptoms of acute asthma, and must be instructed to seek medical attention if their relief medication becomes less effective, or if more inhalations than usual are required to control symptoms.

In those cases where corticosteroid therapy has been reduced or discontinued, such therapy may need to be increased or be re-instated if symptoms of asthma worsen - particularly during periods of stress, such as infection, illness, trauma, severe antigen challenge. Alternative therapeutic management may also need to be considered.

Withdrawal of TILADE CFC-Free therapy

If it is necessary to withdraw this treatment, it should be done progressively over a period of one week. Symptoms of asthma may reoccur.

4.5 Interaction with other medicinal products and other forms of interaction
None known.

4.6 Pregnancy and lactation
Administration of drugs during pregnancy should only be considered if the expected benefit to the mother is greater than any possible risk to the fetus. As with all medications caution should be exercised especially during the first trimester of pregnancy.

There is no information on the use of nedocromil sodium formulated with propellant HFA-227 or with propellant HFA-227 alone in human pregnancy. However studies of HFA-227 administered to pregnant and lactating animals have not revealed any special risk and cumulative clinical experience with nedocromil sodium formulated with CFC propellants would suggest that nedocromil sodium has no adverse effects on fetal development. Nedocromil sodium formulated with propellant HFA-227 (in Tilade CFC-Free) should only be used in pregnancy where there is a clear need.

On the basis of animal studies and its physicochemical properties it is considered that only negligible amounts of nedocromil sodium may pass into human breast milk. There is no evidence to suggest that the use of nedocromil sodium during breast-feeding has any undesirable effects on the baby. However there is no experience to date with nedocromil sodium formulated with propellant HFA-227 or with propellant HFA-227 alone during lactation in female patients with asthma. Nedocromil sodium formulated with propellant HFA-227 (as in Tilade CFC-Free) should only be used in lactation where there is a clear need and its use should be restricted to those situations where it is felt that the expected benefit to the mother is likely to outweigh any potential risk to the neonate.

4.7 Effects on ability to drive and use machines
TILADE CFC- Free has no known effect on ability to drive or operate machinery.

4.8 Undesirable effects
The principal side effects reported are headache and upper gastrointestinal tract symptoms (nausea, vomiting, dyspepsia and abdominal pain). Throat irritation and pharyngitis may also occur. These are usually mild and transient. Rare occurrences of unusual or unpleasant taste have been reported. In common with other inhaled medications Tilade CFC- Free may produce cough or bronchospasm.

As with other inhalation therapy, paradoxical bronchospasm may occur with an immediate increase in wheezing, dyspnoea and/or tightness in the chest following administration. This requires immediate treatment with a fast-acting inhaled bronchodilator and immediate medical attention must be sought straightaway. Therapy with Tilade CFC-Free should be discontinued immediately and alternative treatment instituted.

4.9 Overdose
Animal studies have not shown evidence of toxic effects of nedocromil sodium even at high dosage, nor have extended human studies revealed any safety hazard with the drug. Overdosage is therefore unlikely to cause problems, but if suspected, treatment should be supportive and directed to the control of the relevant symptoms.

5. PHARMACOLOGICAL PROPERTIES

5.1 Pharmacodynamic properties
Tilade CFC-Free contains nedocromil sodium, a non-steroidal agent, which has anti-inflammatory properties when administered topically in the lung. In-vivo, ex-vivo and in-vitro studies have shown that nedocromil sodium has beneficial effects on cellular, humoral and neuronal mechanisms thought to be involved in the inflammation of bronchial asthma. In the treatment of bronchial asthma, nedocromil sodium reduces bronchospasm, cough and bronchial hyperreactivity and improves objective measurements of lung function.

5.2 Pharmacokinetic properties
After inhalation of nedocromil sodium (in common with other drugs inhaled using an MDI) a small fraction (generally 10%) reaches the lungs, while a major portion of the dose is deposited in the mouth or oropharynx and swallowed. The oral absorption of nedocromil sodium from the gastrointestinal tract is low, being approximately 2% of an orally administered dose. Hence, nedocromil sodium measured in plasma following inhalation is considered to represent mainly the drug absorbed by the airways. After inhalation, plasma concentrations of nedocromil sodium reach a maximum within one hour post-dosing and decline with a half-life of 1-2 hours.

Nedocromil sodium is moderately (80%) and reversibly bound to human plasma proteins, and is not metabolised in man or animals. In man nedocromil sodium is excreted unchanged in the urine (approximately 70%) and in faeces (approximately 30%). The plasma profiles of nedocromil sodium are similar following inhalation of TILADE®, TILADE Mint®, or TILADE CFC-Free, and are also similar in healthy volunteers and in asthmatic patients.

5.3 Preclinical safety data
Preclinical data reveal no special hazard for humans based on studies of safety pharmacology, repeated dose toxicity, genotoxicity, carcinogenic potential and toxicity to reproduction.

6. PHARMACEUTICAL PARTICULARS

6.1 List of excipients
1,1,1,2,3,3,3 - heptafluoropropane (HFA-227)

povidone K30

polyethylene glycol (PEG) 600

levomenthol

6.2 Incompatibilities
Not applicable.

6.3 Shelf life
2 years

6.4 Special precautions for storage
Do not store in a refrigerator or freezer. Protect from direct sunlight.

The canister contains a pressurised liquid. Do not expose to temperatures higher than 50°C. Do not pierce the canister.

6.5 Nature and contents of container
The aluminium can is fitted with a metering valve which delivers actuations each containing 2 mg of nedocromil sodium. Each canister contains 112 actuations.

Tilade CFC-Free Inhaler: The cartoned pack consists of an aerosol canister and two plastic adaptors with dustcaps

6.6 Special precautions for disposal and other handling
Not applicable.

7. MARKETING AUTHORISATION HOLDER
Sanofi-aventis

One Onslow Street

Guildford

Surrey

GU1 4YS

UK

8. MARKETING AUTHORISATION NUMBER(S)
PL 04425/0342

9. DATE OF FIRST AUTHORISATION/RENEWAL OF THE AUTHORISATION
11 October 2005

10. DATE OF REVISION OF THE TEXT
December 2006

11 Legal Category
POM

Tildiem LA 200, Tildiem LA 300

(sanofi-aventis)

1. NAME OF THE MEDICINAL PRODUCT
Tildiem LA 200

Tildiem LA 300

2. QUALITATIVE AND QUANTITATIVE COMPOSITION
Each capsule contains a combination of immediate-release and coated sustained-release pellets with 200mg or 300mg diltiazem hydrochloride as the active ingredient.

For a full list of excipients, see Section 6.1

3. PHARMACEUTICAL FORM
Sustained-release oral capsules

Tildiem LA 200: Opaque capsules with a grey body and pink cap, containing white to off-white pellets.

Tildiem LA 300: Opaque capsules with a white body and yellow cap, containing white to off-white pellets.

4. CLINICAL PARTICULARS

4.1 Therapeutic indications
Mild to moderate hypertension and angina pectoris.

4.2 Posology and method of administration
Tildiem LA 200 and Tildiem LA 300 are sustained release products for once daily dosing. The capsules should not be chewed but swallowed whole with water, ideally before or during a meal. The dosage requirements may differ in patients with angina or hypertension.

Tildiem (diltiazem hydrochloride) is available in a range of presentations to enable dosage to be adjusted to meet the individual requirements of the patient. Careful titration of the dose should be considered where appropriate, as individual patient response may vary. When changing from one type of Tildiem formulation to another it may be necessary to adjust the dosage until a satisfactory response is obtained. To ensure consistency of response once established, particularly in the sustained release formulations, Tildiem LA 200 should continue to be prescribed by brand name.

Adults:

Angina and hypertension: The usual starting dose is Tildiem LA 200 once daily. This dose may be increased to Tildiem LA 300 once daily, or 2 capsules of Tildiem LA 200 daily (400 mg), and if clinically indicated a higher dose of one Tildiem LA 300 plus one Tildiem LA 200 capsule (total 500 mg) may be considered.

Elderly and patients with impaired hepatic or renal function:

Heart rate should be monitored and if it falls below 50 beats per minute the dose should not be increased. Plasma levels of diltiazem can be increased in this group of patients.

Angina and hypertension: the initial dose should be one Tildiem LA 200 capsule daily. This dose may be increased to one capsule of Tildiem LA 300 daily if clinically indicated.

Children:

Safety and efficacy in children have not been established. Therefore diltiazem is not recommended for use in children.

4.3 Contraindications

Sick sinus syndrome, 2nd or 3rd degree AV block in patients without a functioning pacemaker.

Severe bradycardia (less than 50 beats per minute).

Left ventricular failure with pulmonary stasis.

Lactation.

Concurrent use with dantrolene infusion (see section 4.5 Interactions with other medicinal products and other forms of interaction).

Hypersensitivity to diltiazem or to any of the excipients

4.4 Special warnings and precautions for use

Close observation is necessary in patients with reduced left ventricular function, bradycardia (risk of exacerbation) or with a 1st degree AV block or prolonged PR interval detected on the electrocardiogram (risk of exacerbation and rarely, of complete block).

Plasma diltiazem concentrations can be increased in the elderly and patients with renal or hepatic insufficiency. The contraindications and precautions should be carefully observed and close monitoring, particularly of heart rate, should be carried out at the beginning of treatment.

In the case of general anaesthesia, the anaesthetist must be informed that the patient is taking diltiazem. The depression of cardiac contractility, conductivity and automaticity as well as the vascular dilatation associated with anaesthetics may be potentiated by calcium channel blockers.

4.5 Interaction with other medicinal products and other forms of interaction

COMBINATION CONTRAINDICATED FOR SAFETY REASONS:

Dantrolene (infusion)

Lethal ventricular fibrillation is regularly observed in animals when intravenous verapamil and dantrolene are administered concomitantly.

The combination of a calcium antagonist and dantrolene is therefore potentially dangerous *(see section 4.3 Contra-indications)*.

COMBINATIONS REQUIRING CAUTION:

Alpha-antagonists

Increased anti-hypertensive effects. Concomitant treatment with alpha-antagonists may produce or aggravate hypotension. The combination of diltiazem with an alpha antagonist should be considered only with strict monitoring of blood pressure.

Beta-blockers

Possibility of rhythm disturbances (pronounced bradycardia, sinus arrest), sino-atrial and atrio-ventricular conduction disturbances and heart failure (synergistic effect).

Such a combination must only be used under close clinical and ECG monitoring, particularly at the beginning of treatment.

Amiodarone, Digoxin

Increased risk of bradycardia; caution is required when these are combined with diltiazem, particularly in elderly subjects and when high doses are used.

Antiarrhythmic agents

Since diltiazem has antiarrhythmic properties, its concomitant prescription with other antiarrhythmic agents is not recommended due to the risk of increased cardiac adverse effects due to an additive effect. This combination should only be used under close clinical and ECG monitoring.

Nitrate derivatives:

Increased hypotensive effects and faintness (additive vasodilating effects).

In all patients treated with calcium antagonists, the prescription of nitrate derivatives should only be carried out at gradually increasing doses.

Ciclosporin

Increase in circulating ciclosporin levels. It is recommended that the ciclosporin dose be reduced, renal function be monitored, circulating ciclosporin levels be assayed and that the dose should be adjusted during combined therapy and after its discontinuation.

Carbamazepine

Increase in circulating carbamazepine levels. It is recommended that the plasma carbamazepine concentrations be assayed and that the dose should be adjusted if necessary.

Theophylline

Increase in circulating theophylline levels.

Anti-H_2 agents (cimetidine and ranitidine)

Increase in plasma diltiazem concentrations. Patients currently receiving diltiazem therapy should be carefully monitored when initiating or discontinuing therapy with anti-H_2 agents. An adjustment in diltiazem daily dose may be necessary.

Rifampicin

Risk of decrease of diltiazem plasma levels after initiating therapy with rifampicin. The patient should be carefully monitored when initiating or discontinuing rifampicin treatment.

Lithium

Risk of increase in lithium-induced neurotoxicity.

COMBINATIONS TO BE TAKEN INTO ACCOUNT:

Oral administration of diltiazem can raise the plasma concentration of drugs exclusively metabolised by CYP450 3A4. The concomitant therapy of diltiazem and such drugs may increase the risk of adverse reactions (e.g. muscular disorders with statins such as simvastatin (refer to manufacturer's prescribing information for simvastatin)).

4.6 Pregnancy and lactation

Pregnancy: There is very limited data from the use of diltiazem in pregnant patients. Diltiazem has been shown to have reproductive toxicity (see section 5.3) in certain animal species (rat, mice, rabbit). Diltiazem is therefore not recommended during pregnancy, as well as in women of child-bearing potential not using effective contraception.

Breast feeding: as this drug is excreted in breast milk, breast feeding whilst taking diltiazem is contraindicated.

4.7 Effects on ability to drive and use machines

No studies on the effects on the ability to drive and use machines have been performed.

4.8 Undesirable effects

Immune system disorders

More rarely, cases of angioneurotic oedema have been reported.

Psychiatric disorders

Nervousness, insomnia.

Cardiac disorders:

Rare cases of symptomatic bradycardia and sino-atrial block and atrioventricular block, palpitations.

Development or aggravation of congestive heart failure.

Vascular disorders

The manifestations of vasodilatation (headache, flushing and in particular oedema of the lower limbs) are dose-dependent and appear more frequent in elderly subjects and related to the pharmacological activity of the product.

Vasculitis, including leukocytoclastic vasculitis.

Orthostatic hypotension.

Gastrointestinal disorders:

Digestive disturbances such as dyspepsia, gastric pain, nausea, constipation, vomiting, dry mouth, diarrhoea.

Gingival hyperplasia

Hepatobiliary disorders:

Isolated cases of moderate and transient elevation of liver transaminases have been observed at the start of treatment. Isolated cases of clinical hepatitis have been reported which resolved on cessation of diltiazem therapy.

Skin and subcutaneous tissue disorders:

Muco-cutaneous reactions such as simple erythema, urticaria, or occasionally desquamative erythema, with or without fever and photosensitivity have been reported, recovering when the treatment is discontinued.

More rarely, cases of erythema multiforme (including rare cases of Steven-Johnson's syndrome) and/or exfoliative dermatitis and acute generalised exanthematous pustular dermatitis have been reported. Very rare cases of Toxic Epidermal Necrolysis have also been reported.

Others:

Malaise, dizziness, asthenia/fatigue.

As with some other calcium channel blockers, exceptional cases of extrapyramidal symptoms and gynaecomastia have been reported, reversible after discontinuation of calcium antagonists.

4.9 Overdose

The clinical effects of acute overdose can involve pronounced hypotension leading to collapse, sinus bradycardia with or without isorhythmic dissociation, and atrio-ventricular conduction disturbances.

Treatment, under hospital supervision, will include gastric lavage, osmotic diuresis. Conduction disturbances may be managed by temporary cardiac pacing.

Proposed corrective treatments: atropine, vasopressors, inotropic agents, glucagon and calcium gluconate infusion.

5. PHARMACOLOGICAL PROPERTIES

5.1 Pharmacodynamic properties

Pharmacotherapeutic group: Calcium channel blocker ATC code: C08DB01

Calcium antagonist, antihypertensive agent.

Diltiazem restricts calcium entry into the slow calcium channel of vascular smooth muscle and myocardial muscle fibres in a voltage-dependent manner. By this mechanism, diltiazem reduces the concentration of intracellular calcium in contractile protein.

In animals: diltiazem increases coronary blood flow without inducing any coronary steal phenomena. It acts both on small, large and collateral arteries. This vasodilator effect, which is moderate on peripheral systemic arterial territories, can be seen at doses that are not negatively inotropic.

The two major active circulating metabolites, i.e. desacetyl diltiazem and N-monodesmethyl diltiazem, possess pharmacological activity in angina corresponding to 10 and 20% respectively of that of the parent compound.

In humans: diltiazem increases coronary blood flow by reducing coronary resistance.

Due to its moderate bradycardia-inducing activity and the reduction in systemic arterial resistance, diltiazem reduces cardiac workload.

Tildiem LA does not have a significant myocardial depressant action in man.

5.2 Pharmacokinetic properties

Diltiazem is well absorbed (90%) in healthy volunteers following oral administration.

The sustained release capsule provides prolonged absorption of the active constituent, producing steady state plasma concentrations between 2 and 14 hours post-dose, during which time peak plasma levels occur.

Bioavailability of Tildiem LA relative to the Tildiem 60mg formulation is approximately 80%. The mean apparent plasma half-life is 8 hours.

Diltiazem in plasma is 80 to 85% protein bound and is poorly dialysed. It is extensively metabolised by the liver.

The major circulating metabolite, N-monodesmethyl diltiazem accounts for approximately 35% of the circulating diltiazem.

Less than 5% of diltiazem is excreted unchanged in the urine.

Twenty four hours after intake, plasma concentrations remain, even after the 200 mg dose administration, at the level of 50 ng/ml, in patients. During long term administration in any one patient, plasma concentrations of diltiazem remained constant.

Mean plasma concentrations in the elderly and patients with renal and hepatic insufficiency are higher than in young subjects.

Food intake does not significantly affect the kinetics of Tildiem LA, however, when administered with food, absorption was observed to be higher in the first few hours post-dose.

Diltiazem and its metabolites are poorly dialysed.

Once daily formulations of diltiazem have been shown to have different pharmacokinetic profiles and therefore it is not advised to substitute different brands for one another.

5.3 Preclinical safety data

Pregnancy: Reproduction studies have been conducted in mice, rats, and rabbits. Administration of doses ranging from 4 to 6 times (depending on species) the upper limit of the optimum dosage range in clinical trials (480 mg q.d. or 8 mg/kg q.d. for a 60-kg patient) resulted in embryo and fetal lethality. These studies revealed, in one species or another, a propensity to cause fetal abnormalities of the skeleton, heart, retina, and tongue. Also observed were reductions in early individual pup weights, pup survival, as well as prolonged delivery times and an increased incidence of stillbirths.

6. PHARMACEUTICAL PARTICULARS

6.1 List of excipients

Tildiem LA 200: Microcrystalline cellulose, Acrylic and methacrylic esters co-polymer, Ethylcellulose, sodium carboxymethylcellulose, Diacetylated monoglycerides, Magnesium stearate.

In the capsule: Gelatin, Black iron oxide (E172), Titanium dioxide (E171), Red iron oxide (E172).

Tildiem LA 300: Microcrystalline cellulose, Acrylic and methacrylic esters copolymer, Ethylcellulose, Carmellose sodium, Diacetylated monoglycerides

Magnesium stearate.

In the capsule: Gelatin, Titanium dioxide (E171), Yellow iron oxide (E172)

6.2 Incompatibilities

Not applicable

6.3 Shelf life

Tildiem LA 200: 3 years

Tildiem LA 300: 2 years

6.4 Special precautions for storage

Store below 25 C.

6.5 Nature and contents of container

Tildiem LA 200: 28 capsules, in a PVC/foil blister strip.

Tildiem LA 300: 28 capsules, in a PVC/foil blister strip.

6.6 Special precautions for disposal and other handling

No special requirements

7. MARKETING AUTHORISATION HOLDER

Sanofi-aventis

One Onslow Street

Guildford

Surrey

GU1 4YS

UK

8. MARKETING AUTHORISATION NUMBER(S)

Tildiem LA 200: PL 04425/0639

Tildiem LA 300: PL 04425/0638

9. DATE OF FIRST AUTHORISATION/RENEWAL OF THE AUTHORISATION

27th January 2009

10. DATE OF REVISION OF THE TEXT

January 2009

LEGAL CATEGORY

POM

Tildiem Retard 90mg, Tildiem Retard 120mg

(sanofi-aventis)

1. NAME OF THE MEDICINAL PRODUCT

Tildiem Retard 90mg.

Tildiem Retard 120mg

2. QUALITATIVE AND QUANTITATIVE COMPOSITION

Each 90mg tablet contains 90mg diltiazem hydrochloride as the active ingredient.

Each 120mg tablet contains 120mg diltiazem hydrochloride as the active ingredient.

For excipients see 6.1

3. PHARMACEUTICAL FORM

Sustained release tablet.

Off-white biconvex tablet.

4. CLINICAL PARTICULARS

4.1 Therapeutic indications

Mild to moderate hypertension and angina pectoris.

4.2 Posology and method of administration

Tildiem Retard tablets should be swallowed whole with a little water and not crushed or chewed.

Patients should be advised that the tablet membrane may pass through the gastro-intestinal tract unchanged.

Tildiem (diltiazem hydrochloride) is available in a range of presentations to enable dosage to be adjusted to meet the individual requirements of the patient. Careful titration of the dose should be considered where appropriate, as individual patient response may vary. When changing from one type of Tildiem formulation to another it may be necessary to adjust the dosage until a satisfactory response is obtained. To ensure consistency of response once established, particularly in the sustained release formulations, Tildiem Retard 90mg and 120mg should continue to be prescribed by brand name.

Adults:

Angina and hypertension:

The usual starting dose is one tablet (90mg or 120mg) twice daily. Patient responses may vary and dosage requirements can differ significantly between individual patients. Higher divided doses up to 480mg/day have been used with benefit in some angina patients especially in unstable angina. Doses of 360mg/day may be required to provide adequate BP control in hypertensive patients.

Elderly and patients with impaired hepatic or renal function:

Heart rate should be monitored in these patients and if it falls below 50 beats per minute the dose should not be increased.

Angina:

The recommended starting dose is one Tildiem 60mg tablet twice daily. This dose may be increased to one 90mg or 120mg Tildiem Retard tablet twice daily.

Hypertension:

The starting dose should be one 120mg Tildiem Retard tablet daily. Dose adjustment to one 90mg or one 120mg Tildiem Retard tablet twice daily may be required.

Children:

Safety and efficacy in children have not been established. Therefore diltiazem is not recommended for use in children.

4.3 Contraindications

Sick sinus syndrome, 2nd or 3rd degree AV block in patients without a functioning pacemaker.

Severe bradycardia (less than 50 beats per minute).

Left ventricular failure with pulmonary stasis.

Lactation.

Concurrent use with dantrolene infusion *(see section 4.5 Interactions with other medicinal products and other forms of interaction)*.

Hypersensitivity to diltiazem or to any of the excipients.

4.4 Special warnings and precautions for use

Close observation is necessary in patients with reduced left ventricular function, bradycardia (risk of exacerbation) or with a 1st degree AV block detected on the electrocardiogram (risk of exacerbation and rarely of complete block) or prolonged PR interval.

Plasma diltiazem concentrations can be increased in the elderly and patients with renal or hepatic insufficiency. The contraindications and precautions should be carefully observed and close monitoring, particularly of heart rate, should be carried out at the beginning of treatment.

In the case of general anaesthesia, the anaesthetist must be informed that the patient is taking diltiazem. The depression of cardiac contractility, conductivity and automaticity as well as the vascular dilatation associated with anaesthetics may be potentiated by calcium channel blockers.

Diltiazem does not affect the glucose or endogenous insulin responses to hypoglycaemia.

4.5 Interaction with other medicinal products and other forms of interaction

COMBINATION CONTRAINDICATED FOR SAFETY REASONS:

Dantrolene (infusion)

Lethal ventricular fibrillation is regularly observed in animals when intravenous verapamil and dantrolene are administered concomitantly.

The combination of a calcium antagonist and dantrolene is therefore potentially dangerous *(see section 4.3 Contraindications)*.

COMBINATIONS REQUIRING CAUTION:

Alpha-antagonists:

Increased anti-hypertensive effects.

Concomitant treatment with alpha-antagonists may produce or aggravate hypotension. The combination of diltiazem with an alpha antagonist should be considered only with strict monitoring of blood pressure.

Beta-blockers:

Possibility of rhythm disturbances (pronounced bradycardia, sinus arrest), sino-atrial and atrio-ventricular conduction disturbances and heart failure (synergistic effect).

Such a combination must only be used under close clinical and ECG monitoring, particularly at the beginning of treatment.

Amiodarone, Digoxin:

Increased risk of bradycardia; caution is required when these are combined with diltiazem, particularly in elderly subjects and when high doses are used.

Antiarrhythmic agents:

Since diltiazem has antiarrhythmic properties, its concomitant prescription with other antiarrhythmic agents is not recommended due to the risk of increased cardiac adverse effects due to an additive effect. This combination should only be used under close clinical and ECG monitoring.

Nitrate derivatives:

Increased hypotensive effects and faintness (additive vasodilating effects).

In all patients treated with calcium antagonists, the prescription of nitrate derivatives should only be carried out at gradually increasing doses.

Cyclosporin:

Increase in circulating cyclosporin levels. It is recommended that the cyclosporin dose be reduced, renal function be monitored, circulating cyclosporin levels be assayed and that the dose should be adjusted during combined therapy and after its discontinuation.

Carbamazepine:

Increase in circulating carbamazepine levels.

It is recommended that the plasma carbamazepine concentrations be assayed and that the dose should be adjusted if necessary.

Theophylline:

Increase in circulating theophylline levels.

Anti-H_2 agents (cimetidine and ranitidine):

Increase in plasma diltiazem concentrations.

Patients currently receiving diltiazem therapy should be carefully monitored when initiating or discontinuing therapy with anti-H_2 agents. An adjustment in diltiazem daily dose may be necessary.

Rifampicin

Risk of decrease of diltiazem plasma levels after initiating therapy with rifampicin. The patient should be carefully monitored when initiating or discontinuing rifampicin treatment.

Lithium

Risk of increase in lithium-induced neurotoxicity.

COMBINATIONS TO BE TAKEN INTO ACCOUNT:

Oral administration of diltiazem can raise the plasma concentration of drugs exclusively metabolised by CYP3A4. The concomitant therapy of diltiazem and such drugs may increase the risk of adverse reactions (e.g. muscular disorders with statins such as simvastatin (refer to manufacturer's prescribing information for simvastatin)).

4.6 Pregnancy and lactation

Pregnancy: There is very limited data from the use of diltiazem in pregnant patients. Diltiazem has been shown to have reproductive toxicity (see section 5.3) in certain animal species (rat, mice, rabbit). Diltiazem is therefore not recommended during pregnancy, as well as in women of child-bearing potential not using effective contraception.

Breast feeding: as this drug is excreted in breast milk, breast feeding whilst taking diltiazem is contraindicated.

4.7 Effects on ability to drive and use machines

No studies on the effects on the ability to drive and use machines have been performed

4.8 Undesirable effects

Immune system disorders

More rarely, cases of angioneurotic oedema have been reported.

Psychiatric disorders

Nervousness, insomnia.

Cardiac disorders:

Rare cases of symptomatic bradycardia and sino-atrial block and atrioventricular block, palpitations.

Development or aggravation of congestive heart failure.

Vascular disorders

The manifestations of vasodilatation (headache, flushing and in particular oedema of the lower limbs) are dose-dpendent and appear more frequent in elderly subjects and related to the pharmacological activity of the product.

Vasculitis, including leukocytoclastic vasculitis.

Orthostatic hypotension.

Gastrointestinal disorders:

Digestive disturbances such as dyspepsia, gastric pain, nausea, vomiting, constipation, dry mouth, diarrhoea.

Gingival hyperplasia

Hepatobiliary disorders:

Isolated cases of moderate and transient elevation of liver transaminases have been observed at the start of treatment. Isolated cases of clinical hepatitis have been reported which resolved on cessation of diltiazem therapy.

Skin and subcutaneous tissue disorders:

Muco-cutaneous reactions such as simple erythema, urticaria, or occasionally desquamative erythema, with or without fever and photosensitivity have been reported, recovering when the treatment is discontinued.

More rarely, cases of erythema multiforme (including rare cases of Steven-Johnson's syndrome) and/or exfoliative dermatitis and acute generalised exanthematous pustular dermatitis have been reported. Very rare cases of toxic epidermal necrolysis have also been reported.

Others:

Malaise, dizziness, asthenia/fatigue.

As with some other calcium channel blockers, exceptional cases of extrapyramidal symptoms and gynaecomastia have been reported, reversible after discontinuation of calcium antagonists.

4.9 Overdose

The clinical effects of acute overdose can involve pronounced hypotension leading to collapse, sinus bradycardia with or without isorhythmic dissociation, and atrio-ventricular conduction disturbances.

Treatment, under hospital supervision, will include gastric lavage, osmotic diuresis. Conduction disturbances may be managed by temporary cardiac pacing.

Proposed corrective treatments: atropine, vasopressors, inotropic agents, glucagon and calcium gluconate infusion.

5. PHARMACOLOGICAL PROPERTIES

5.1 Pharmacodynamic properties

Pharmacotherapeutic group: Calcium Channel Blocker, ATC code: C08D B01

Tildiem is a calcium antagonist. It restricts the slow channel entry of calcium into the cell and so reduces the liberation of calcium from stores in the sarcoplasmic reticulum. This results in a reduction of the amount of available intracellular calcium reducing myocardial oxygen consumption. It increases exercise capacity and improves all indices of myocardial ischaemia in the angina patient. Tildiem relaxes large and small coronary arteries and relieves the spasm of vasospastic (Prinzmetal's) angina and the response to catecholamines but has little effect on the peripheral vasculature. There is therefore no possibility of reflex tachycardia. A small reduction in heart rate occurs which is accompanied by an increase in cardiac output, improved myocardial perfusion and reduction of ventricular work. In animal studies, Tildiem protects the myocardium against the effects of ischaemia and reduces the damage produced by excessive entry of calcium into the myocardial cell during reperfusion.

5.2 Pharmacokinetic properties

Diltiazem is well absorbed (90%) in healthy volunteers following oral administration.

These formulations of diltiazem hydrochloride provide prolonged absorption of the active ingredient. Peak plasma concentrations occur between 4 and 8 hours post-dose.

Bioavailability of this formulation of diltiazem is approximately 90% of that of the conventional tablet. The mean apparent plasma half-life is 7 - 8 hours.

Diltiazem is 80 to 85% bound to plasma proteins. It is extensively metabolised by the liver.

The major circulating metabolite, N-monodesmethyl diltiazem accounts for approximately 35% of the circulating diltiazem.

Less than 5% of diltiazem is excreted unchanged in the urine.

During long term administration to any one patient, plasma concentrations of diltiazem remain constant.

Mean plasma concentrations in elderly subjects and patients with renal and hepatic insufficiency are higher than in young subjects.

Diltiazem and its metabolites are poorly dialysed.

Twice daily formulations of diltiazem have been shown to have different pharmacokinetic profiles and therefore it is not advised to substitute different brands for one another.

5.3 Preclinical safety data

Pregnancy: Reproduction studies have been conducted in mice, rats, and rabbits. Administration of doses ranging from 4 to 6 times (depending on species) the upper limit of the optimum dosage range in clinical trials (480 mg q.d. or 8 mg/kg q.d. for a 60-kg patient) resulted in embryo and fetal lethality. These studies revealed, in one species or another, a propensity to cause fetal abnormalities of the skeleton, heart, retina, and tongue. Also observed were reductions in early individual pup weights, pup survival, as well as prolonged delivery times and an increased incidence of stillbirths.

6. PHARMACEUTICAL PARTICULARS

6.1 List of excipients

Tablet core: Sodium dihydrogen citrate, sucrose, povidone, magnesium stearate, macrogol 6000.

Coating: Sucrose, coating polymer, acetyl tributyl citrate, castor oil polymerised, sodium hydrogen carbonate, ethyl vanillin, titanium dioxide (E171).

6.2 Incompatibilities

Not applicable

6.3 Shelf life

Two years.

6.4 Special precautions for storage

Do not store above 30°C. Store in the original package.

Tildiem Retard tablets are coated with a porous polymer membrane which enables the diltiazem to diffuse out of the tablet at a gradual rate. This membrane may pass through the gastro-intestinal tract unchanged. This has no bearing on the efficacy of the product.

6.5 Nature and contents of container

56 tablets in PVC/foil strips

6.6 Special precautions for disposal and other handling

No special requirements.

7. MARKETING AUTHORISATION HOLDER

Sanofi-aventis

One Onslow Street

Guildford

Surrey

GU1 4YS

8. MARKETING AUTHORISATION NUMBER(S)

Tildiem Retard 90mg 04425/0641

Tildiem Retard 120mg 04425/0642

9. DATE OF FIRST AUTHORISATION/RENEWAL OF THE AUTHORISATION

27th January 2009

10. DATE OF REVISION OF THE TEXT

January 2009

Legal Category: POM

Tildiem Tablets 60mg

(sanofi-aventis)

1. NAME OF THE MEDICINAL PRODUCT

Tildiem tablets 60mg

2. QUALITATIVE AND QUANTITATIVE COMPOSITION

Each modified release tablet contains diltiazem hydrochloride 60mg

For a full list of excipients, see section 6.1.

3. PHARMACEUTICAL FORM

Modified release tablet

Almost white, round, convex tablets, 8mm in diameter, engraved, 'Tildiem 60' <u>or</u> 'Dilt 60' <u>or</u> 'DTZ 60'

4. CLINICAL PARTICULARS

4.1 Therapeutic indications

Prophylaxis and treatment of Angina Pectoris

4.2 Posology and method of administration

<u>Adults:</u>The usual dose is one tablet (60mg) three times daily. However, patient responses may vary and dosage requirements can differ significantly between individual patients. If necessary the divided dose may be increased to 360mg/day. Higher doses up to 480mg/day have been used with benefit in some patients especially in unstable angina. There is no evidence of any decrease in efficacy at these high doses.

<u>Elderly and patients with impaired hepatic or renal function:</u> The recommended starting dose is one tablet (60mg) twice daily. The heart rate should be measured regularly in these groups of patients and the dose should not be increased if the heart rate falls below 50 beats per minute.

<u>Children:</u> Safety and efficacy in children have not been established. Therefore diltiazem is not recommended for use in children

4.3 Contraindications

Sick sinus syndrome, 2nd or 3rd degree AV block in patients without a functioning pacemaker.

Severe bradycardia (less than 50 beats per minute).

Left ventricular failure with pulmonary stasis.

Lactation.

Concurrent use with dantrolene infusion (see section 4.5 Interactions with other medicinal products and other forms of interactions).

Hypersensitivity to diltiazem or to any of the excipients.

4.4 Special warnings and precautions for use

Patients with rare hereditary problems of galactose intolerance, the Lapp lactase deficiency or glucose-galactose malabsorption should not take this medicine.

Close observation is necessary in patients with reduced left ventricular function, bradycardia (risk of exacerbation) or with a 1st degree AV block detected on the electrocardiogram (risk of exacerbation and rarely of complete block) or prolonged PR interval.

Plasma diltiazem concentrations can be increased in the elderly and patients with renal or hepatic insufficiency. The contraindications and precautions should be carefully observed and close monitoring, particularly of heart rate, should be carried out at the beginning of treatment.

In the case of general anaesthesia, the anaesthetist must be informed that the patient is taking diltiazem. The depression of cardiac contractility, conductivity and automaticity as well as the vascular dilatation associated with anaesthetics may be potentiated by calcium channel blockers.

4.5 Interaction with other medicinal products and other forms of interaction

<u>COMBINATION CONTRAINDICATED FOR SAFETY REASONS:</u>

<u>Dantrolene (infusion)</u>

Lethal ventricular fibrillation is regularly observed in animals when intravenous verapamil and dantrolene are administered concomitantly.

The combination of a calcium antagonist and dantrolene is therefore potentially dangerous *(see section 4.3 Contraindications)*.

<u>COMBINATIONS REQUIRING CAUTION:</u>

<u>Alpha-antagonists</u>

Increased anti-hypertensive effects. Concomitant treatment with alpha-antagonists may produce or aggravate hypotension. The combination of diltiazem with an alpha antagonist should be considered only with strict monitoring of blood pressure.

<u>Beta-blockers</u>

Possibility of rhythm disturbances (pronounced bradycardia, sinus arrest), sino-atrial and atrio-ventricular conduction disturbances and heart failure (synergistic effect).

Such a combination must only be used under close clinical and ECG monitoring, particularly at the beginning of treatment.

<u>Amiodarone, Digoxin</u>

Increased risk of bradycardia; caution is required when these are combined with diltiazem, particularly in elderly subjects and when high doses are used.

<u>Antiarrhythmic agents</u>

Since diltiazem has antiarrhythmic properties, its concomitant prescription with other antiarrhythmic agents is not recommended due to the risk of increased cardiac adverse effects due to an additive effect. This combination should only be used under close clinical and ECG monitoring.

<u>Nitrate derivatives:</u>

Increased hypotensive effects and faintness (additive vasodilating effects).

In all patients treated with calcium antagonists, the prescription of nitrate derivatives should only be carried out at gradually increasing doses.

<u>Cyclosporin</u>

Increase in circulating cyclosporin levels. It is recommended that the cyclosporin dose be reduced, renal function be monitored, circulating cyclosporin levels be assayed and that the dose should be adjusted during combined therapy and after its discontinuation.

<u>Carbamazepine</u>

Increase in circulating carbamazepine levels. It is recommended that the plasma carbamazepine concentrations be assayed and that the dose should be adjusted if necessary.

<u>Theophylline</u>

Increase in circulating theophylline levels.

<u>Anti-H_2 agents (cimetidine and ranitidine)</u>

Increase in plasma diltiazem concentrations. Patients currently receiving diltiazem therapy should be carefully monitored when initiating or discontinuing therapy with anti-H_2 agents. An adjustment in diltiazem daily dose may be necessary.

<u>Rifampicin</u>

Risk of decrease of diltiazem plasma levels after initiating therapy with rifampicin. The patient should be carefully monitored when initiating or discontinuing rifampicin treatment.

<u>Lithium</u>

Risk of increase in lithium-induced neurotoxicity.

<u>COMBINATIONS TO BE TAKEN INTO ACCOUNT:</u>

Oral administration of diltiazem can raise the plasma concentration of drugs exclusively metabolised by CYP3A4. The concomitant therapy of diltiazem and such drugs may increase the risk of adverse reactions (e.g. muscular disorders with statins such as simvastatin (refer to manufacturer's prescribing information for simvastatin)).

4.6 Pregnancy and lactation

Pregnancy: There is very limited data from the use of diltiazem in pregnant patients. Diltiazem has been shown to have reproductive toxicity (see section 5.3) in certain animal species (rat, mice, rabbit). Diltiazem is therefore not recommended during pregnancy, as well as in women of child-bearing potential not using effective contraception.

Breast feeding: as this drug is excreted in breast milk, breast feeding whilst taking diltiazem is contraindicated.

4.7 Effects on ability to drive and use machines

No studies on the effects on the ability to drive and use machines have been performed

4.8 Undesirable effects

Immune system disorders

<u>More rarely cases of angioneurotic oedema have been reported.</u>

<u>Psychiatric disorders</u>

Nervousness, insomnia.

<u>Cardiac disorders:</u>

Rare cases of symptomatic bradycardia and sino-atrial block and atrioventricular block, palpitations.

Development or aggravation of congestive heart failure.

<u>Vascular disorders</u>

The manifestations of vasodilatation (headache, flushing and in particular oedema of the lower limbs) are dosedpendent and appear more frequent in elderly subjects and related to the pharmacological activity of the product.

Vasculitis, including leukocytoclastic vasculitis.

Orthostatic hypotension.

<u>Gastrointestinal disorders:</u>

Digestive disturbances such as dyspepsia, gastric pain, nausea, vomiting dry mouth, constipation, diarrhoea.

Gingival hyperplasia

<u>Hepatobiliary disorders:</u>

Isolated cases of moderate and transient elevation of liver transaminases have been observed at the start of treatment. Isolated cases of clinical hepatitis have been reported which resolved on cessation of diltiazem therapy.

<u>Skin and subcutaneous tissue disorders:</u>

Muco-cutaneous reactions such as simple erythema, urticaria, or occasionally desquamative erythema, with or without fever and photosensitivity have been reported, recovering when the treatment is discontinued.

More rarely, cases of erythema multiforme (including rare cases of Steven-Johnson's syndrome) and/or exfoliative dermatitis and acute generalised exanthematous pustular dermatitis have been reported. Very rare cases of toxic epidermal necrolysis have also been reported.

<u>Others:</u>

Malaise, dizziness, asthenia/fatigue.

As with some other calcium channel blockers, exceptional cases of extrapyramidal symptoms and gynaecomastia have been reported, reversible after discontinuation of calcium antagonists.

4.9 Overdose

The clinical effects of acute overdose can involve pronounced hypotension leading to collapse, sinus bradycardia with or without isorhythmic dissociation, and atrioventricular conduction disturbances.

Treatment, under hospital supervision, will include gastric lavage, osmotic diuresis. Conduction disturbances may be managed by temporary cardiac pacing.

Proposed corrective treatments: atropine, vasopressors, inotropic agents, glucagon and calcium gluconate infusion.

5. PHARMACOLOGICAL PROPERTIES

5.1 Pharmacodynamic properties

Pharmacotherapeutic group: Calcium channel blocker ATC code: C08DB01

Tildiem is a calcium antagonist. It restricts the slow channel entry of calcium into the cell and so reduces the liberation of calcium from stores in the sarcoplasmic reticulum. This results in a reduction of the amount of available intracellular calcium reducing myocardial oxygen consumption. It increases exercise capacity and improves all indices of myocardial ischaemia in the angina patient. Tildiem relaxes large and small coronary arteries and relieves the spasm of vasospastic (prinzmetals) angina and the response to catecholamines but has little effect on the peripheral vasculature. There is therefore no possibility of reflex tachycardia. A small reduction in heart rate occurs which is accompanied by an increase in cardiac output, improved myocardial perfusion and reduction of ventricular work. In animal studies, Tildiem protects the myocardium against the effects of ischaemia and reduces the damage produced by excessive entry of calcium into the myocardial cell during reperfusion.

5.2 Pharmacokinetic properties

Diltiazem hydrochloride is effective in angina, protecting the heart against ischaemia, vasodilating coronary arteries and reducing myocardial oxygen requirements. It is well tolerated and does not generally give rise to side effects associated with peripheral vasodilators, nor cause significant myocardial depression.

Diltiazem is well absorbed (90%) in healthy volunteers following oral administration.

Peak plasma concentrations occur 3 to 4 hours after dosing.

Due to a first pass effect, the bioavailability of the 60 mg tablet is about 40 %.

The mean apparent plasma half-life is 4 - 8 hours.

Diltiazem is 80 to 85% bound to plasma proteins. It is extensively metabolised by the liver.

The major circulating metabolite, N-monodesmethyl diltiazem accounts for approximately 35% of the circulating diltiazem.

Less than 5% of diltiazem is excreted unchanged in the urine.

There is a linear relationship between dose and plasma concentration. During long term administration to any one patient, plasma concentrations of diltiazem remain constant.

Mean plasma concentrations in elderly subjects and patients with renal and hepatic insufficiency are higher than in young subjects.

Diltiazem and its metabolites are poorly dialysed.

5.3 Preclinical safety data

Pregnancy: Reproduction studies have been conducted in mice, rats, and rabbits. Administration of doses ranging from 4 to 6 times (depending on species) the upper limit of the optimum dosage range in clinical trials (480 mg q.d. or 8 mg/kg q.d. for a 60-kg patient) resulted in embryo and fetal lethality. These studies revealed, in one species or another, a propensity to cause fetal abnormalities of the skeleton, heart, retina, and tongue. Also observed were reductions in early individual pup weights, pup survival, as well as prolonged delivery times and an increased incidence of stillbirths.

6. PHARMACEUTICAL PARTICULARS

6.1 List of excipients

Lactose

Macrogol 6000

Hydrogenated caster oil

Magnesium stearate

6.2 Incompatibilities

Not applicable

6.3 Shelf life

3 years

6.4 Special precautions for storage

Store below 25°C. Store in the original package.

6.5 Nature and contents of container

PVC/ foil blister packs of 90 tablets

6.6 Special precautions for disposal and other handling

No special requirements

7. MARKETING AUTHORISATION HOLDER

Sanofi-aventis

One Onslow Street

Guildford

Surrey

GU1 4YS

UK

8. MARKETING AUTHORISATION NUMBER(S)

PL 04425/0640

9. DATE OF FIRST AUTHORISATION/RENEWAL OF THE AUTHORISATION

27th January 2009

10. DATE OF REVISION OF THE TEXT

January 2009

Legal category: POM

Timentin 0.8 G, 1.6 G, 3.2 G

(GlaxoSmithKline UK)

1. NAME OF THE MEDICINAL PRODUCT

Timentin® 0.8 G, 1.6 G, 3.2 G

2. QUALITATIVE AND QUANTITATIVE COMPOSITION

Timentin 0.8 g: Contains 50 mg clavulanic acid with 750 mg ticarcillin.

Timentin 1.6 g: Contains 100 mg clavulanic acid with 1.5 g ticarcillin.

Timentin 3.2 g: Contains 200 mg clavulanic acid with 3.0 g ticarcillin.

The clavulanic acid is present as Potassium Clavulanate BP and the ticarcillin as ticarcillin sodium.

3. PHARMACEUTICAL FORM

Powder for solution for infusion.

Vials containing sterile powder for reconstitution.

4. CLINICAL PARTICULARS

4.1 Therapeutic indications

Timentin is an injectable antibiotic agent with a broad spectrum of bactericidal activity against a wide range of Gram-positive and Gram-negative aerobic and anaerobic bacteria. The presence of clavulanate in the formulation extends the spectrum of activity of ticarcillin to include many β-lactamase-producing bacteria normally resistant to ticarcillin and other β-lactam antibiotics.

Timentin is indicated for the treatment of infections in which susceptible organisms have been detected or are suspected.

Typical indications include:

Severe infections in hospitalised patients and proven or suspected infections in patients with impaired or suppressed host defences including: septicaemia, bacteraemia, peritonitis, intra-abdominal sepsis, post-surgical infections, bone and joint infections, skin and soft tissue infections, respiratory tract infections, serious or complicated renal infections (e.g. pyelonephritis), ear, nose and throat infections.

A comprehensive list of sensitive and resistant organisms is provided in Section 5.1. Consideration should be given to official guidance regarding bacterial resistance and the appropriate use of antibacterial agents.

4.2 Posology and method of administration

Adult dosage (including elderly patients):

The usual dosage is 3.2 g Timentin given six to eight hourly. The maximum recommended dosage is 3.2 g four hourly.

Children's dosage (including infants, neonates and premature infants >2 kg in weight):

The usual dosage for children is 80 mg Timentin/kg body weight given every eight hours. The maximum dosage for children is 80 mg Timentin/kg body weight given every six hours. This should not exceed the maximum recommended adult dosage.

For premature infants <2 kg in weight, the dosage is 80 mg Timentin/kg body weight every 12 hours.

Dosage in renal impairment:

Mild impairment	Moderate impairment	Severe impairment
(Creatinine Clearance >30 ml/min)	(Creatinine Clearance 10-30 ml/min)	(Creatinine Clearance <10 ml/min)
3.2 g 8 hourly	1.6 g 8 hourly	1.6 g 12 hourly

Similar reductions in dosage should be made for children.

Administration:

Intravenous infusion

4.3 Contraindications

Timentin contains ticarcillin which is a penicillin, and should not be given to patients with a history of hypersensitivity to beta-lactam antibiotics (e.g. penicillins and cephalosporins).

4.4 Special warnings and precautions for use

Before initiating therapy with Timentin, careful inquiry should be made concerning previous hypersensitivity reactions to beta-lactams (e.g. penicillins and cephalosporins). Serious and occasionally fatal hypersensitivity reactions (anaphylaxis) have been reported in patients receiving beta-lactam antibiotics. These reactions are more likely to occur in individuals with a history of beta-lactam hypersensitivity.

Changes in liver function tests have been observed in some patients receiving Timentin. The clinical significance of these changes is uncertain but Timentin should be used with care in patients with evidence of severe hepatic dysfunction.

In patients with renal impairment, dosage should be adjusted according to the degree of impairment (see Section 4.2).

It should be noted that each gram of ticarcillin contains 5.3 mmol of sodium (approx.). This should be included in the daily allowance of patients on sodium restricted diets.

Timentin has only rarely been reported to cause hypokalemia; however, the possibility of this occurring should be kept in mind particularly when treating patients with fluid and electrolyte imbalance. Periodic monitoring of serum potassium may be advisable in patients receiving prolonged therapy.

Bleeding manifestations have occurred in some patients receiving beta-lactam antibiotics. These reactions have been associated with abnormalities of coagulation tests such as clotting time, platelet aggregation and prothrombin time and are more likely to occur in patients with renal impairment. If bleeding manifestations appear, Timentin treatment should be discontinued and appropriate therapy instituted.

The presence of clavulanic acid in Timentin may cause a non-specific binding of IgG and albumin by red cell membranes leading to a false positive Coombs test.

Prolonged use may occasionally result in overgrowth of non-susceptible organisms.

4.5 Interaction with other medicinal products and other forms of interaction

Timentin acts synergistically with aminoglycosides against a number of organisms including *Pseudomonas*. Timentin prescribed concurrently with an aminoglycoside, may therefore be preferred in the treatment of life-threatening infections, particularly in patients with impaired host defences. In such instances the two products should be administered separately, at the recommended dosages.

Co-administration of probenecid cannot be recommended. Probenecid decreases the renal tubular secretion of ticarcillin. Concurrent administration of probenecid delays ticarcillin renal excretion but does not delay the excretion of clavulanic acid.

The presence of clavulanic acid in Timentin may cause a non-specific binding of IgG and albumin by red cell membranes leading to a false positive Coombs test.

In common with other antibiotics, Timentin may affect the gut flora, leading to lower oestrogen reabsorption and reduced efficacy of combined oral contraceptives. Therefore, alternative non-hormonal methods of contraception are recommended.

Penicillins reduce the excretion of methotrexate (potential increase in toxicity).

4.6 Pregnancy and lactation

Pregnancy:

Animal studies with Timentin have shown no teratogenic effects. Penicillins are generally considered safe for use in pregnancy. Limited information is available concerning the results of the use of Timentin in human pregnancy. The decision to administer any drug during pregnancy should be taken with the utmost care. Therefore Timentin should only be used in pregnancy when the potential benefits outweigh the potential risks associated with treatment.

Lactation:

Trace quantities of Timentin are excreted in breast milk.

Timentin may be administered during the period of lactation. With the exception of the risk of sensitization, there are no detrimental effects for the breast-fed infant.

4.7 Effects on ability to drive and use machines

Adverse effects on the ability to drive or operate machinery have not been observed.

4.8 Undesirable effects

Hypersensitivity reactions:

Hypersensitivity effects, including skin rashes:

Skin rashes, pruritus, urticaria, and anaphylactic reactions.

Bullous reactions (including erythema multiforme, Stevens-Johnson syndrome and toxic epidermal necrolysis) have been reported very rarely.

Gastrointestinal effects:

Nausea, vomiting and diarrhea have been reported. Pseudomembranous colitis has been reported rarely.

Hepatic effects:

A moderate rise in AST and/or ALT has been noted in patients receiving ampicillin class antibiotics. Hepatitis and cholestatic jaundice have been reported very rarely. These events have been noted with other penicillins and cephalosporins.

Renal and urinary effects:

Hypokalaemia has been reported rarely. Haemorrhagic cystitis has been reported very rarely.

Central Nervous System effects:

Convulsions may occur rarely, particularly in patients with impaired renal function or in those receiving high doses.

Haematological effects:

Thrombocytopenia, leukopenia, eosinophilia and reduction of haemoglobin have been reported rarely. Haemolytic anaemia has been reported very rarely. Prolongation of prothrombin time and bleeding time. Bleeding manifestations have occurred.

Local effects:

Pain, burning, swelling and induration at the injection site and thrombophlebitis with intravenous administration.

4.9 Overdose

Gastrointestinal effects such as nausea, vomiting and diarrhoea may be evident and should be treated symptomatically.

Disturbances of the fluid and electrolyte balances may be evident and may be treated symptomatically.

Ticarcillin and clavulanic acid may be removed from circulation by haemodialysis.

As with other penicillins, Timentin overdosage has the potential to cause neuromuscular hyperirritability or convulsive seizures.

5. PHARMACOLOGICAL PROPERTIES

5.1 Pharmacodynamic properties

Timentin is an injectable antibiotic, active against a wide range of both Gram-positive and Gram-negative bacteria, including β-lactamase-producing strains.

Resistance to many antibiotics is caused by bacterial enzymes which destroy the antibiotic before it can act on the pathogen. The clavulanate in Timentin anticipates this defence mechanism by blocking the β-lactamase enzymes, thus rendering the organisms sensitive to ticarcillin's rapid bactericidal effect at concentrations readily attainable in the body.

Clavulanate, by itself, has little antibacterial effect; however, in association with ticarcillin, as Timentin it produces an antibiotic agent with a breadth of spectrum suitable for empiric use in a wide range of infections treated parenterally in hospital.

Gram-Positive

Aerobes: *Staphylococcus* species including *Staphylococcus aureus* and *Staphylococcus epidermidis, Streptococcus* species including *Enterococcus faecalis.*

Anaerobes: *Peptococcus* species, *Peptostreptococcus* species, *Clostridium* species, *Eubacterium* species.

Gram-Negative

Aerobes: *Escherichia coli, Haemophilus* species including *Haemophilus influenzae, Moraxella catarrhalis, Klebsiella* species including *Klebsiella pneumoniae, Enterobacter* species, *Proteus* species including indole-positive strains, *Providentia stuartii, Pseudomonas* species including *Pseudomonas aeruginosa, Serratia* species including *Serratia marcescens, Citrobacter* species, *Acinetobacter* species, *Yersinia enterocolitica*

Anaerobes: *Bacteroides* species *including Bacteroides fragilis, Fusobacterium* species, *Veillonella* species.

Breakpoints

The breakpoints listed below have been obtained from the National Committee for Clinical Laboratory Standards (NCCLS) (Performance Standards for Antimicrobial Disk Susceptibility Tests; Approved Standard - Seventh Edition).

Enterobacteriaceae	S ≤ 16/2 μg/mL	R ≥ 128/2 μg/mL
Pseudomonas aeruginosa	S ≤ 64/2 μg/mL	R ≥ 128/2 μg/mL
Other non-Enterobacteriaceae	S ≤ 16/2 μg/mL	R ≥ 128/2 μg/mL
Staphylococcus spp.	S ≤ 8/2 μg/mL	R ≥ 16/2 μg/mL

S = susceptible, R = resistant

There are no NCCLS breakpoints for other organisms listed in this document.

Table 1

Susceptible
Aerobic Gram-positive micro-organisms
Staphylococcus aureus
Aerobic Gram-negative micro-organisms
Acinetobacter species
Escherichia coli
Haemophilus influenzae
Klebsiella pneumoniae
Proteus species
Serratia species
Anaerobic micro-organisms
Bacteroides fragilis
Intermediate
Aerobic Gram-negative micro-organisms
Serratia marcescens
Insusceptible
Aerobic Gram-positive micro-organisms
Enterococcus
Aerobic Gram-negative micro-organisms
Citrobacter species
Enterobacter species
Pseudomonas aeruginosa

The prevalence of resistance may vary geographically and with time for selected species. Where possible, local information on resistance is included. This information gives only an approximate guidance on probabilities whether micro-organisms will be susceptible to ticarcillin disodium clavulanate potassium (commonly known as Timentin) or not.

5.2 Pharmacokinetic properties

The pharmacokinetics of the two components are closely matched and both components are well distributed in body fluids and tissues. Both clavulanate and ticarcillin have low levels of serum binding; about 20% and 45% respectively.

As with other penicillins the major route of elimination for ticarcillin is via the kidney; clavulanate is also excreted by this route.

5.3 Preclinical safety data

Not applicable.

6. PHARMACEUTICAL PARTICULARS

6.1 List of excipients

None

6.2 Incompatibilities

Timentin is not compatible with the following:

Proteinaceous fluids (e.g. protein hydrolysates); blood and plasma; intravenous lipids.

If Timentin is prescribed concurrently with an aminoglycoside the antibiotics should not be mixed in the syringe, intravenous fluid container or giving set because loss of activity of the aminoglycoside can occur under these conditions.

6.3 Shelf life

24 months.

6.4 Special precautions for storage

Timentin should be stored in a dry place at temperatures below 25°C.

6.5 Nature and contents of container

Clear Type I glass vials fitted with a chlorobutyl rubber bung and an aluminium seal. Supplied in packs of four vials.

6.6 Special precautions for disposal and other handling

The sterile powder should be dissolved in approximately 5 ml/10 ml (1.6 g/3.2 g vial) prior to dilution into the infusion container (e.g. mini-bag) or in-line burette.

The following approximate infusion volumes are suggested:

	Water for Injections BP	Glucose Intravenous Infusion BP (5% w/v)
3.2 g	100 ml	100-150 ml
1.6 g	50 ml	100 ml

Detailed instructions are given in the Package Enclosure Leaflet.

Each dose of Timentin should be infused intravenously over a period of 30-40 minutes; avoid continuous infusion over longer periods as this may result in subtherapeutic concentrations.

800 mg Timentin has a displacement value of 0.55 ml.

Heat is generated when Timentin dissolves. Reconstituted solutions are normally a pale straw colour.

Timentin presentations are not for multi-dose use or for direct IV or IM injection. Any residual antibiotic solution should be discarded if less than the fully made up vial is used.

Administrative Data

7. MARKETING AUTHORISATION HOLDER

Beecham Group plc, Great West Road

Brentford, Middlesex TW8 9GS

Trading as:

GlaxoSmithKline UK,

Stockley Park West,

Uxbridge,

Middlesex UB11 1BT

8. MARKETING AUTHORISATION NUMBER(S)

00038/0329

9. DATE OF FIRST AUTHORISATION/RENEWAL OF THE AUTHORISATION

15 April 2003

10. DATE OF REVISION OF THE TEXT

17 February 2009

11. Legal Status

POM

Timoptol 0.25% and 0.5% w/v Eye Drops Solution

(Merck Sharp & Dohme Limited)

1. NAME OF THE MEDICINAL PRODUCT

TIMOPTOL® 0.25% w/v Eye Drops Solution

TIMOPTOL® 0.5% w/v Eye Drops Solution

2. QUALITATIVE AND QUANTITATIVE COMPOSITION

'Timoptol' 0.25% w/v Eye Drops Solution contains timolol maleate equivalent to 0.25% w/v solution of timolol with preservative.

'Timoptol' 0.5% w/v Eye Drops Solution contains timolol maleate equivalent to 0.5% w/v solution of timolol with preservative.

3. PHARMACEUTICAL FORM

Eye drops solution.

Clear, colourless to light yellow, sterile eye drops solution.

4. CLINICAL PARTICULARS

4.1 Therapeutic indications

'Timoptol' Eye Drops Solution is a beta-adrenoreceptor blocking agent used topically in the reduction of elevated intra-ocular pressure in various conditions including the following: patients with ocular hypertension; patients with chronic open-angle glaucoma including aphakic patients; some patients with secondary glaucoma.

4.2 Posology and method of administration

Recommended therapy is one drop 0.25% solution in the affected eye twice a day.

If clinical response is not adequate, dosage may be changed to one drop 0.5% solution in each affected eye twice a day. If needed, 'Timoptol' may be used with other agent(s) for lowering intra-ocular pressure. The use of two topical beta-adrenergic blocking agents is not recommended (see 4.4 'Special warnings and precautions for use').

Intra-ocular pressure should be reassessed approximately four weeks after starting treatment because response to 'Timoptol' may take a few weeks to stabilise.

Provided that the intra-ocular pressure is maintained at satisfactory levels, many patients can than be placed on once-a-day therapy.

Transfer from other agents

When another topical beta-blocking agent is being used, discontinue its use after a full day of therapy and start treatment with 'Timoptol' the next day with one drop of 0.25% 'Timoptol' in each affected eye twice a day. The dosage may be increased to one drop of 0.5% solution in each affected eye twice a day, if the response is not adequate.

When transferring a patient from a single anti-glaucoma agent other than a topical beta-blocking agent, continue the agent and add one drop of 0.25% 'Timoptol' in each affected eye twice a day. On the following day, discontinue the previous agent completely, and continue with 'Timoptol'. If a higher dosage of 'Timoptol' is required, substitute one drop of 0.5% solution in each affected eye twice a day.

'Timoptol' Eye Drops Solution is also available as 'Timoptol' Unit dose: The Unit-dose Dispenser of 'Timoptol' is free from preservative and should be used for patients who may be sensitive to the preservative benzalkonium chloride, or when use of a preservative-free topical medication is advisable.

Paediatric use: is not currently recommended.

Use in the elderly: there has been wide experience with the use of timolol maleate in elderly patients. The dosage recommendations given above reflect the clinical data derived from this experience.

4.3 Contraindications

Bronchial asthma, history of bronchial asthma or severe chronic obstructive pulmonary disease; sinus bradycardia, second- and third-degree AV block, overt cardiac failure, cardiogenic shock; and hypersensitivity to this product or other beta-blocking agents.

4.4 Special warnings and precautions for use

Like other topically applied ophthalmic drugs, 'Timoptol' may be absorbed systemically and adverse reactions seen with oral beta-blockers may occur.

Cardiac failure should be adequately controlled before beginning therapy with 'Timoptol'. Patients with a history of severe cardiac disease should be watched for signs of cardiac failure and have their pulse rates checked.

Respiratory and cardiac reactions, including death due to bronchospasm in patients with asthma and, rarely, death associated with cardiac failure have been reported.

The effect on intra-ocular pressure or the known effects of systemic beta-blockade may be exaggerated when 'Timoptol' is given to the patients already receiving a systemic beta-blocking agent. The response of these patients should be closely observed. The use of two topical beta-adrenergic blocking agents is not recommended.

There have been reports of skin rashes and/or dry eyes associated with the use of beta-adrenoreceptor blocking drugs. The reported incidence is small and in most cases the symptoms have cleared when treatment was withdrawn. Discontinuation of the drug should be considered if any such reaction is not otherwise explicable. Cessation of therapy involving beta-blockade should be gradual.

Choroidal detachment has been reported with administration of aqueous suppressant therapy (e.g. timolol, acetazolamide) after filtration procedures.

'Timoptol' has been generally well tolerated in glaucoma patients wearing conventional hard contact lenses. 'Timoptol' has not been studied in patients wearing lenses made with material other than polymethylmethacrylate (PMMA), which is used to make hard contact lenses.

The Ocumeter® Dispenser of 'Timoptol' contains benzalkonium chloride as a preservative which may be deposited in soft contact lenses; therefore 'Timoptol' should not be used while wearing these lenses. The lenses should be removed before application of the drops and not reinserted earlier than 15 minutes after use.

In patients with angle-closure glaucoma, the immediate objective of treatment is to reopen the angle. This requires constricting the pupil with a miotic. 'Timoptol' has little or no effect on the pupil. When 'Timoptol' is used to reduce elevated intra-ocular pressure in angle-closure glaucoma it should be used with a miotic and not alone.

Patients should be advised that if they develop an intercurrent ocular condition (e.g. trauma, ocular surgery or infection), they should immediately seek their physician's advice concerning the continued use of the present multidose container (see 6.6 'Special precautions for disposal and other handling').

There have been reports of bacterial keratitis associated with the use of multiple dose containers of topical ophthalmic products. These containers had been inadvertently contaminated by patients who, in most cases, had a concurrent corneal disease or a disruption of the ocular epithelial surface.

Risk from anaphylactic reaction: While taking beta-blockers, patients with a history of atopy or a history of severe anaphylactic reaction to a variety of allergens may be more reactive to repeated challenge with such allergens, either accidental, diagnostic, or therapeutic. Such patients may be unresponsive to the usual doses of epinephrine (adrenaline) used to treat anaphylactic reactions.

4.5 Interaction with other medicinal products and other forms of interaction

Although 'Timoptol' alone has little or no effect on pupil size, mydriasis has occasionally been reported when 'Timoptol' is given with epinephrine (adrenaline).

Potentiated systemic beta-blockade (e.g. decreased heart rate, depression) has been reported during combined treatment with CYP2D6 inhibitors (e.g.quinidine, SSRIs) and timolol.

Oral β-adrenergic blocking agents may exacerbate the rebound hypertension which can follow the withdrawal of clonidine.

'Timoptol' may potentially add to the effects of oral calcium antagonists, rauwolfia alkaloids or beta-blockers, to induce hypotension and/or marked bradycardia.

Close observation of the patient is recommended when a beta-blocker is administered to patients receiving catecholamine-depleting drugs such as reserpine, because of possible additive effects and the production of hypotension and/or marked bradycardia, which may produce vertigo, syncope, or postural hypotension.

Oral calcium antagonists may be used in combination with beta-adrenergic blocking agents when heart function is normal, but should be avoided in patients with impaired cardiac function.

The potential exists for hypotension, AV conduction disturbances and left ventricular failure to occur in patients receiving a beta-blocking agent when an oral calcium entry blocker is added to the treatment regimen. The nature of any cardiovascular adverse effect tends to depend on the type of calcium blocker used. Dihydropyridine derivatives, such as nifedipine, may lead to hypotension, whereas verapamil or diltiazem have a greater propensity to lead to AV conduction disturbances or left ventricular failure when used with a beta-blocker.

Intravenous calcium channel blockers should be used with caution in patients receiving beta-adrenergic blocking agents.

The concomitant use of beta-adrenergic blocking agents and digitalis with either diltiazem or verapamil may have additive effects in prolonging AV conduction time.

4.6 Pregnancy and lactation

Use in pregnancy: 'Timoptol' has not been studied in human pregnancy. The use of 'Timoptol' requires that the anticipated benefit be weighed against possible hazards.

Breast-feeding mothers: Timolol is detectable in human milk. A decision for breast-feeding mothers, either to stop taking 'Timoptol' or stop nursing, should be based on the importance of the drug to the mother.

4.7 Effects on ability to drive and use machines

Possible side effects such as dizziness and visual disturbances may affect some patients' ability to drive or operate machinery.

4.8 Undesirable effects

Side effects

'Timoptol' is usually well tolerated. The following adverse reactions have been reported with *ocular* administration of this or other timolol maleate formulations, either in clinical trials or since the drug has been marketed. Additional side effects have been reported in clinical experiences with *systemic* timolol maleate, and may be considered potential effects of ophthalmic timolol maleate:

Special senses:

ocular: signs and symptoms of ocular irritation, including burning and stinging, conjunctivitis, blepharitis, keratitis, dry eyes and decreased corneal sensitivity. Tinnitus, visual disturbances, including refractive changes (due to withdrawal of miotic therapy in some cases), diplopia, ptosis and choroidal detachment following filtration surgery (see 4.4 'Special warnings and precautions for use').

Cardiovascular:

ocular: bradycardia, arrhythmia, hypotension, syncope, heart block, cerebrovascular accident, cerebral ischaemia, congestive heart failure, palpitation, cardiac arrest, oedema, claudication, Raynaud's phenomenon, cold hands and feet.

systemic: AV block (second- or third-degree), sino-atrial block, pulmonary oedema, worsening of arterial insufficiency, worsening of angina pectoris, vasodilatation.

Respiratory:

ocular: bronchospasm (predominantly in patients with pre-existing bronchospastic disease), respiratory failure, dyspnoea, cough.

systemic: rales

Body as a whole:

ocular: headache, asthenia, fatigue, chest pain.

systemic: extremity pain, decreased exercise tolerance.

Integumentary:

ocular: alopecia, psoriasiform rash or exacerbation of psoriasis.

systemic: pruritus, sweating, exfoliative dermatitis.

Hypersensitivity:

ocular: signs and symptoms of allergic reactions including anaphylaxis, angioedema, urticaria, localised and generalised rash.

Nervous system/psychiatric:

ocular: dizziness, depression, insomnia, nightmares, memory loss, increase in signs and symptoms of myasthenia gravis, paresthesia.

systemic: vertigo, local weakness, diminished concentration, increased dreaming.

Digestive:

ocular: nausea, diarrhoea, dyspepsia, dry mouth.

systemic: vomiting

Urogenital:

ocular: decreased libido, Peyronie's disease.

systemic: impotence, micturition difficulties.

Immunologic:

ocular: systemic lupus erythematosus

Endocrine:

systemic: hyperglycaemia, hypoglycaemia.

Musculoskeletal:

systemic: arthralgia.

Haematologic:

systemic: non-thrombocytopenic purpura.

4.9 Overdose

There have been reports of inadvertent overdosage with 'Timoptol' resulting in systemic effects similar to those seen with systemic beta-adrenergic blocking agents such as dizziness, headache, shortness of breath, bradycardia, bronchospasm, and cardiac arrest (see 'Side effects').

If overdosage occurs, the following measures should be considered:

1. Gastric lavage, if ingested. Studies have shown that timolol does not dialyse readily.

2. Symptomatic bradycardia: atropine sulphate, 0.25 to 2 mg intravenously, should be used to induce vagal blockade. If bradycardia persists, intravenous isoprenaline hydrochloride should be administered cautiously. In refractory cases, the use of a cardiac pacemaker may be considered.

3. Hypotension: a sympathomimetic pressor agent such as dopamine, dobutamine or noradrenaline should be used. In refractory cases, the use of glucagon has been reported to be useful.

4. Bronchospasm: isoprenaline hydrochloride should be used. Additional therapy with aminophylline may be considered.

5. Acute cardiac failure: conventional therapy with digitalis, diuretics, and oxygen should be instituted immediately. In refractory cases, the use of intravenous aminophylline is suggested. This may be followed, if necessary, by glucagon, which has been reported useful.

6. Heart block (second- or third-degree): isoprenaline hydrochloride or a pacemaker should be used.

5. PHARMACOLOGICAL PROPERTIES

5.1 Pharmacodynamic properties

Timolol maleate is a non-selective beta-adrenergic receptor blocking agent that does not have significant intrinsic sympathomimetic, direct myocardial depressant, or local anaesthetic activity. Timolol maleate combines reversibly with the beta-adrenergic receptor, and this inhibits the usual biologic response that would occur with stimulation of that receptor. This specific competitive antagonism blocks stimulation of the beta-adrenergic stimulating (agonist) activity, whether these originate from an endogenous or exogenous source. Reversal of this blockade can be accomplished by increasing the concentration of the agonist which will restore the usual biological response.

Unlike miotics, 'Timoptol' reduces IOP with little or no effect on accommodation or pupil size. In patients with cataracts, the inability to see around lenticular opacities when the pupil is constricted is avoided. When changing patients from miotics to 'Timoptol' a refraction might be necessary when the effects of the miotic have passed.

Diminished response after prolonged therapy with 'Timoptol' has been reported in some patients.

5.2 Pharmacokinetic properties

The onset of reduction in intra-ocular pressure can be detected within one-half hour after a single dose. The maximum effect occurs in one or two hours; significant lowering of IOP can be maintained for as long as 24 hours with a single dose.

5.3 Preclinical safety data

No adverse ocular effects were observed in rabbits and dogs administered 'Timoptol' topically in studies lasting one and two years, respectively. The oral LD_{50} of the drug is 1,190 and 900 mg/kg in female mice and female rats, respectively.

Carcinogenesis, mutagenesis, impairment of fertility

In a two-year oral study of timolol maleate in rats there was a statistically significant ($p \leqslant 0.05$) increase in the incidence of adrenal phaeochromocytomas in male rats administered 300 mg/kg/day (300 times the maximum recommended human oral dose). Similar differences were not observed in rats administered oral doses equivalent to 25 or 100 times the maximum recommended human oral dose.

In a lifetime oral study in mice, there were statistically significant ($p \leqslant 0.05$) increases in the incidence of benign and malignant pulmonary tumours, benign uterine polyps and mammary adenocarcinoma in female mice at 500 mg/kg/day (500 times the maximum recommended human dose), but not at 5 or 50 mg/kg/day. In a subsequent study in female mice, in which post-mortem examinations were limited to uterus and lungs, a statistically significant increase in the incidence of pulmonary tumours was again observed at 500 mg/kg/day.

The increased occurrence of mammary adenocarcinoma was associated with elevations in serum prolactin which occurred in female mice administered timolol at 500 mg/kg/day, but not at doses of 5 or 50 mg/kg/day. An increased incidence of mammary adenocarcinomas in rodents has been associated with administration of several other therapeutic agents which elevate serum prolactin, but no correlation between serum prolactin levels and mammary tumours has been established in man. Furthermore, in adult human female subjects who received oral dosages of up to 60 mg of timolol maleate, the maximum recommended human oral dosage, there were no clinically meaningful changes in serum prolactin.

Timolol maleate was devoid of mutagenic potential when evaluated *in vivo* (mouse) in the micronucleus test and cytogenetic assay (doses up to 800 mg/kg) and *in vitro* in a neoplastic cell transformation assay (up to 100 mcg/ml). In Ames tests the highest concentrations of timolol employed, 5,000 or 10,000 mcg/plate, were associated with statistically significant ($p \leqslant 0.05$) elevations of revertants observed with tester strain TA100 (in seven replicate assays) but not in the remaining three strains. In the assays with tester strain TA100, no consistent dose-response relationship was observed, nor did the ratio of test to control revertants reach 2. A ratio of 2 is usually considered the criterion for a positive Ames test.

Reproduction and fertility studies in rats showed no adverse effect on male or female fertility at doses up to 150 times the maximum recommended human oral dose.

6. PHARMACEUTICAL PARTICULARS

6.1 List of excipients

Disodium phosphate dodecahydrate (may be replaced by equivalent amounts of the dihydrate or anhydrous)

Sodium dihydrogen phosphate dihydrate (may be replaced by equivalent amounts of monohydrate)

Sodium hydroxide

Benzalkonium chloride

Water for injections

6.2 Incompatibilities

None known.

6.3 Shelf life

24 months

Discard 'Timoptol' Eye Drops Solution 28 days after opening the bottle.

6.4 Special precautions for storage

Do not store above 25°C. Store the bottle in the outer carton.

6.5 Nature and contents of container

The OCUMETER Plus ophthalmic dispenser consists of a translucent high-density polyethylene container with a sealed dropper tip, a flexible fluted side area, which is depressed to dispense the drops, and a two-piece cap assembly. The two-piece cap mechanism punctures the sealed dropper tip upon initial use, then locks together to provide a single cap during the usage period. Tamper evidence is provided by two perforated tabs on the container label extending on to the cap. The OCUMETER Plus ophthalmic dispenser contains 5 ml of solution.

6.6 Special precautions for disposal and other handling
Patients should be instructed to avoid allowing the tip of the dispensing container to contact the eye or surrounding structures.

Patients should also be instructed that ocular solutions, if handled improperly, can become contaminated by common bacteria known to cause ocular infections. Serious damage to the eye and subsequent loss of vision may result from using contaminated solutions.

7. MARKETING AUTHORISATION HOLDER
Merck Sharp & Dohme Limited

Hertford Road, Hoddesdon, Hertfordshire EN11 9BU, UK

8. MARKETING AUTHORISATION NUMBER(S)
0.25% w/v Eye Drops Solution PL0025/0134

0.5% w/v Eye Drops Solution PL0025/0135

9. DATE OF FIRST AUTHORISATION/RENEWAL OF THE AUTHORISATION
Granted: 5 January 1979

Last renewed: 12 February 2002

10. DATE OF REVISION OF THE TEXT
February 2008

LEGAL CATEGORY
POM

® denotes registered trademark of Merck & Co., Inc., Whitehouse Station, NJ, USA.

SPC.TOTOS.06.UK.2345 F.T. 020608

Timoptol Unit Dose 0.25% and 0.5% w/v Eye Drops Solution

(Merck Sharp & Dohme Limited)

1. NAME OF THE MEDICINAL PRODUCT
TIMOPTOL® Unit Dose 0.25% w/v Eye Drops Solution

TIMOPTOL® Unit Dose 0.5% w/v Eye Drops Solution

2. QUALITATIVE AND QUANTITATIVE COMPOSITION
'Timoptol' Unit Dose 0.25% w/v Eye Drops Solution contains timolol maleate equivalent to 0.25% w/v solution of timolol without preservative.

'Timoptol' Unit Dose 0.5% w/v Eye Drops Solution contains timolol maleate equivalent to 0.5% w/v solution of timolol without preservative.

3. PHARMACEUTICAL FORM
Eye drops solution.

Clear, colourless to light yellow, sterile eye drops.

4. CLINICAL PARTICULARS

4.1 Therapeutic indications
'Timoptol' Eye Drops Solution is a beta-adrenoreceptor blocking agent used topically in the reduction of elevated intra-ocular pressure in various conditions including the following: patients with ocular hypertension; patients with chronic open-angle glaucoma including aphakic patients; some patients with secondary glaucoma.

4.2 Posology and method of administration
Recommended therapy is one drop 0.25% solution in the affected eye twice a day.

If clinical response is not adequate, dosage may be changed to one drop 0.5% solution in each affected eye twice a day. If needed, 'Timoptol' may be used with other agent(s) for lowering intra-ocular pressure. The use of two topical beta-adrenergic blocking agents is not recommended (see 4.4 'Special warnings and precautions for use').

Intra-ocular pressure should be reassessed approximately four weeks after starting treatment because response to 'Timoptol' may take a few weeks to stabilise.

Provided that the intra-ocular pressure is maintained at satisfactory levels, many patients can than be placed on once-a-day therapy.

Transfer from other agents

When another topical beta-blocking agent is being used, discontinue its use after a full day of therapy and start treatment with 'Timoptol' the next day with one drop of 0.25% 'Timoptol' in each affected eye twice a day. The dosage may be increased to one drop of 0.5% solution in each affected eye twice a day if the response is not adequate.

When transferring a patient from a single anti-glaucoma agent other than a topical beta-blocking agent, continue the agent and add one drop of 0.25% 'Timoptol' in each affected eye twice a day. On the following day, discontinue the previous agent completely, and continue with 'Timoptol'. If a higher dosage of 'Timoptol' is required, substitute one drop of 0.5% solution in each affected eye twice a day.

'Timoptol' Unit dose: The Unit-dose Dispenser of 'Timoptol' is free from preservative and should be used for patients who may be sensitive to the preservative benzalkonium chloride, or when use of a preservative-free topical medication is advisable.

'Timoptol' Unit-dose is a sterile solution. The solution from one individual unit is to be used immediately after opening for administration to one or both eyes. Since sterility cannot be maintained after the individual unit is opened, the remaining contents should be discarded immediately after administration.

Paediatric use: is not currently recommended.

Use in the elderly: there has been wide experience with the use of timolol maleate in elderly patients. The dosage recommendations given above reflect the clinical data derived from this experience.

4.3 Contraindications
Bronchial asthma, history of bronchial asthma or severe chronic obstructive pulmonary disease; sinus bradycardia, second- and third-degree AV block, overt cardiac failure, cardiogenic shock; and hypersensitivity to this product or other beta-blocking agents.

4.4 Special warnings and precautions for use
Like other topically applied ophthalmic drugs, 'Timoptol' may be absorbed systemically and adverse reactions seen with oral beta-blockers may occur.

Cardiac failure should be adequately controlled before beginning therapy with 'Timoptol'. Patients with a history of severe cardiac disease should be watched for signs of cardiac failure and have their pulse rates checked.

Respiratory and cardiac reactions, including death due to bronchospasm in patients with asthma and, rarely, death associated with cardiac failure have been reported.

The effect on intra-ocular pressure or the known effects of systemic beta-blockade may be exaggerated when 'Timoptol' is given to patients already receiving a systemic beta-blocking agent. The response of these patients should be closely observed. The use of two topical beta-adrenergic blocking agents is not recommended.

There have been reports of skin rashes and/or dry eyes associated with the use of beta-adrenoreceptor blocking drugs. The reported incidence is small and in most cases the symptoms have cleared when treatment was withdrawn. Discontinuation of the drug should be considered if any such reaction is not otherwise explicable. Cessation of therapy involving beta-blockade should be gradual.

Choroidal detachment has been reported with administration of aqueous suppressant therapy (e.g. timolol, acetazolamide) after filtration procedures.

'Timoptol' has been generally well tolerated in glaucoma patients wearing conventional hard contact lenses. 'Timoptol' has not been studied in patients wearing lenses made with material other than polymethylmethacrylate (PMMA), which is used to make hard contact lenses.

The Unit-dose Dispenser of 'Timoptol' is free from preservative and should, therefore, be discarded after single use to one or both eyes.

In patients with angle-closure glaucoma, the immediate objective of treatment is to reopen the angle. This requires constricting the pupil with a miotic. 'Timoptol' has little or no effect on the pupil. When 'Timoptol' is used to reduce elevated intra-ocular pressure in angle-closure glaucoma it should be used with a miotic and not alone.

Patients should be advised that if they develop an intercurrent ocular condition (e.g. trauma, ocular surgery or infection), they should immediately seek their physician's advice concerning the continued use of the present multidose container (see 6.6 'Special precautions for disposal and other handling')

There have been reports of bacterial keratitis associated with the use of multiple dose containers of topical ophthalmic products. These containers had been inadvertently contaminated by patients who, in most cases, had a concurrent corneal disease or a disruption of the ocular epithelial surface.

Risk from anaphylactic reaction: While taking beta-blockers, patients with a history of atopy or a history of severe anaphylactic reaction to a variety of allergens may be more reactive to repeated challenge with such allergens, either accidental, diagnostic, or therapeutic. Such patients may be unresponsive to the usual doses of epinephrine (adrenaline) used to treat anaphylactic reactions.

4.5 Interaction with other medicinal products and other forms of interaction
Although 'Timoptol' alone has little or no effect on pupil size, mydriasis has occasionally been reported when 'Timoptol' is given with epinephrine (adrenaline).

Potentiated systemic beta-blockade (e.g. decreased heart rate, depression) has been reported during combined treatment with CYP2D6 inhibitors (e.g.quinidine, SSRIs) and timolol.

Oral β-adrenergic blocking agents may exacerbate the rebound hypertension which can follow the withdrawal of clonidine.

'Timoptol' may potentially add to the effects of oral calcium antagonists, rauwolfia alkaloids or beta-blockers, to induce hypotension and/or marked bradycardia.

Close observation of the patient is recommended when a beta-blocker is administered to patients receiving catecholamine-depleting drugs such as reserpine, because of possible additive effects and the production of hypotension and/or marked bradycardia, which may produce vertigo, syncope, or postural hypotension.

Oral calcium antagonists may be used in combination with beta-adrenergic blocking agents when heart function is normal, but should be avoided in patients with impaired cardiac function.

The potential exists for hypotension, AV conduction disturbances and left ventricular failure to occur in patients receiving a beta-blocking agent when an oral calcium entry blocker is added to the treatment regimen. The nature of any cardiovascular adverse effect tends to depend on the type of calcium blocker used. Dihydropyridine derivatives, such as nifedipine, may lead to hypotension, whereas verapamil or diltiazem have a greater propensity to lead to AV conduction disturbances or left ventricular failure when used with a beta-blocker.

Intravenous calcium channel blockers should be used with caution in patients receiving beta-adrenergic blocking agents.

The concomitant use of beta-adrenergic blocking agents and digitalis with either diltiazem or verapamil may have additive effects in prolonging AV conduction time.

4.6 Pregnancy and lactation
Use in pregnancy: 'Timoptol' has not been studied in human pregnancy. The use of 'Timoptol' requires that the anticipated benefit be weighed against possible hazards.

Breast-feeding mothers: Timolol is detectable in human milk. A decision for breast-feeding mothers, either to stop taking 'Timoptol' or stop nursing, should be based on the importance of the drug to the mother.

4.7 Effects on ability to drive and use machines
Possible side effects such as dizziness and visual disturbances may affect some patients' ability to drive or operate machinery.

4.8 Undesirable effects
Side effects

'Timoptol' is usually well tolerated. The following adverse reactions have been reported with *ocular* administration of this or other timolol maleate formulations, either in clinical trials or since the drug has been marketed. Additional side effects have been reported in clinical experiences with *systemic* timolol maleate, and may be considered potential effects of ophthalmic timolol maleate:

Special senses:

ocular: signs and symptoms of ocular irritation, including burning and stinging, conjunctivitis, blepharitis, keratitis, dry eyes, and decreased corneal sensitivity. Tinnitus, visual disturbances, including refractive changes (due to withdrawal of miotic therapy in some cases), diplopia, ptosis and choroidal detachment following filtration surgery (see 4.4 'Special warnings and precautions for use').

Cardiovascular:

ocular: bradycardia, arrhythmia, hypotension, syncope, heart block, cerebrovascular accident, cerebral ischaemia, congestive heart failure, palpitation, cardiac arrest, oedema, claudication, Raynaud's phenomenon, cold hands and feet.

systemic: AV block (second- or third-degree), sino-atrial block, pulmonary oedema, worsening of arterial insufficiency, worsening of angina pectoris, vasodilation.

Respiratory:

ocular: bronchospasm (predominantly in patients with pre-existing bronchospastic disease), respiratory failure, dyspnoea, cough.

systemic: rales

Body as a whole:

ocular: headache, asthenia, fatigue, chest pain.

systemic: extremity pain, decreased exercise tolerance.

Integumentary:

ocular: alopecia, psoriasiform rash or exacerbation of psoriasis.

systemic: pruritus, sweating, exfoliative dermatitis.

Hypersensitivity:

ocular: signs and symptoms of allergic reactions including anaphylaxis, angioedema, urticaria, localised and generalised rash.

Nervous system/psychiatric:

ocular: dizziness, depression, insomnia, nightmares, memory loss, increase in signs and symptoms of myasthenia gravis, paraesthesia.

systemic: vertigo, local weakness, diminished concentration, increased dreaming.

Digestive:

ocular: nausea, diarrhoea, dyspepsia, dry mouth.

systemic: vomiting.

Urogenital:

ocular: decreased libido, Peyronie's disease.

systemic: impotence, micturition difficulties.

Immunologic:

ocular: systemic lupus erythematosus.

Endocrine:

systemic: hyperglycaemia, hypoglycaemia.

Musculoskeletal:

systemic: arthralgia.

Haematologic:

systemic: non-thrombocytopenic purpura.

4.9 Overdose
There have been reports of inadvertent overdosage with 'Timoptol' resulting in systemic effects similar to those seen with systemic beta-adrenergic blocking agents such as dizziness, headache, shortness of breath, bradycardia, bronchospasm, and cardiac arrest (see 4.8 'Undesirable effects').

If overdosage occurs, the following measures should be considered:

1. Gastric lavage, if ingested. Studies have shown that timolol does not dialyse readily.

2. Symptomatic bradycardia: atropine sulphate, 0.25 to 2 mg intravenously, should be used to induce vagal blockade. If bradycardia persists, intravenous isoprenaline hydrochloride should be administered cautiously. In refractory cases, the use of a cardiac pacemaker may be considered.

3. Hypotension: a sympathomimetic pressor agent such as dopamine, dobutamine or noradrenaline should be used. In refractory cases, the use of glucagon has been reported to be useful.

4. Bronchospasm: isoprenaline hydrochloride should be used. Additional therapy with aminophylline may be considered.

5. Acute cardiac failure: conventional therapy with digitalis, diuretics, and oxygen should be instituted immediately. In refractory cases, the use of intravenous aminophylline is suggested. This may be followed, if necessary, by glucagon, which has been reported useful.

6. Heart block (second- or third-degree): isoprenaline hydrochloride or a pacemaker should be used.

5. PHARMACOLOGICAL PROPERTIES

5.1 Pharmacodynamic properties
Timolol maleate is a non-selective beta-adrenergic receptor blocking agent that does not have significant intrinsic sympathomimetic, direct myocardial depressant, or local anaesthetic activity. Timolol maleate combines reversibly with the beta-adrenergic receptor, and this inhibits the usual biologic response that would occur with stimulation of that receptor. This specific competitive antagonism blocks stimulation of the beta-adrenergic stimulating (agonist) activity, whether these originate from an endogenous or exogenous source. Reversal of this blockade can be accomplished by increasing the concentration of the agonist which will restore the usual biological response.

Unlike miotics, 'Timoptol' reduces IOP with little or no effect on accommodation or pupil size. In patients with cataracts, the inability to see around lenticular opacities when the pupil is constricted is avoided. When changing patients from miotics to 'Timoptol' a refraction might be necessary when the effects of the miotic have passed.

Diminished response after prolonged therapy with 'Timoptol' has been reported in some patients.

5.2 Pharmacokinetic properties
The onset of reduction in intra-ocular pressure can be detected within one-half hour after a single dose. The maximum effect occurs in one or two hours; significant lowering of IOP can be maintained for as long as 24 hours with a single dose.

5.3 Preclinical safety data
No adverse ocular effects were observed in rabbits and dogs administered 'Timoptol' topically in studies lasting one and two years, respectively. The oral LD_{50} of the drug is 1,190 and 900 mg/kg in female mice and female rats, respectively.

Carcinogenesis, mutagenesis, impairment of fertility

In a two-year oral study of timolol maleate in rats there was a statistically significant ($p \leqslant 0.05$) increase in the incidence of adrenal phaeochromocytomas in male rats administered 300 mg/kg/day (300 times the maximum recommended human oral dose). Similar differences were not observed in rats administered oral doses equivalent to 25 or 100 times the maximum recommended human oral dose.

In a lifetime oral study in mice, there were statistically significant ($p \leqslant 0.05$) increases in the incidence of benign and malignant pulmonary tumours, benign uterine polyps and mammary adenocarcinoma in female mice at 500 mg/kg/day (500 times the maximum recommended human dose), but not at 5 or 50 mg/kg/day. In a subsequent study in female mice, in which post-mortem examinations were limited to uterus and lungs, a statistically significant increase in the incidence of pulmonary tumours was again observed at 500 mg/kg/day.

The increased occurrence of mammary adenocarcinoma was associated with elevations in serum prolactin which occurred in female mice administered timolol at 500 mg/kg/day, but not at doses of 5 or 50 mg/kg/day. An increased incidence of mammary adenocarcinomas in rodents has been associated with administration of several other therapeutic agents which elevate serum prolactin, but no correlation between serum prolactin levels and mammary tumors has been established in man. Furthermore, in adult human female subjects who received oral dosages of up to 60 mg of timolol maleate, the maximum recommended human oral dosage, there were no clinically meaningful changes in serum prolactin.

Timolol maleate was devoid of mutagenic potential when evaluated *in vivo* (mouse) in the micronucleus test and cytogenetic assay (doses up to 800 mg/kg) and *in vitro* in a neoplastic cell transformation assay (up to 100 mcg/ml). In Ames tests the highest concentrations of timolol employed, 5,000 or 10,000 mcg/plate, were associated with statistically significant ($p \leqslant 0.05$) elevations of revertants observed with tester strain TA100 (in seven replicate assays) but not in the remaining three strains. In the assays with tester strain TA100, no consistent dose-response relationship was observed, nor did the ratio of test to control revertants reach 2. A ratio of 2 is usually considered the criterion for a positive Ames test.

Reproduction and fertility studies in rats showed no adverse effect on male or female fertility at doses up to 150 times the maximum recommended human oral dose.

6. PHARMACEUTICAL PARTICULARS

6.1 List of excipients
'Timoptol' Unit Dose Eye Drops Solution contains the following inactive ingredients:

Disodium phosphate dodecahydrate

(may be replaced by equivalent amounts of the dihydrate or anhydrous form)

Sodium dihydrogen phosphate dihydrate

(may be replaced by equivalent amounts of the monohydrate)

Sodium hydroxide

Water for injection

6.2 Incompatibilities
None known.

6.3 Shelf life
3 Years

'Timoptol' Unit Dose Eye Drops Solution should be used immediately after opening and any remaining contents should be discarded immediately after administration.

6.4 Special precautions for storage
Do not store above 25°C and keep in outer carton.

6.5 Nature and contents of container
Both the 0.25% and the 0.5% w/v solutions are presented in:

Unit-dose Dispensers, available in cartons of 30 unit doses.

6.6 Special precautions for disposal and other handling
Patients should be instructed to avoid allowing the tip of the dispensing container to contact the eye or surrounding structures.

Patients should also be instructed that ocular solutions, if handled improperly, can become contaminated by common bacteria known to cause ocular infections. Serious damage to the eye and subsequent loss of vision may result from using contaminated solutions.

7. MARKETING AUTHORISATION HOLDER
Merck Sharp & Dohme Limited
Hertford Road, Hoddesdon, Hertfordshire EN11 9BU, UK

8. MARKETING AUTHORISATION NUMBER(S)
0.25% w/v Eye Drops Solution, PL0025/0210

0.5% w/v Eye Drops Solution, PL0025/0211

9. DATE OF FIRST AUTHORISATION/RENEWAL OF THE AUTHORISATION
Granted: 17 March 1992

Last renewed: 21 March 2002

10. DATE OF REVISION OF THE TEXT
February 2008

LEGAL CATEGORY
POM.

® denotes registered trademark of Merck & Co., Inc., Whitehouse Station, NJ, USA.

SPC.TOTUD.06.UK.2347 F.T. 080608

Timoptol-LA 0.25 and 0.5% w/v Gel-Forming Eye Drops Solution

(Merck Sharp & Dohme Limited)

1. NAME OF THE MEDICINAL PRODUCT
TIMOPTOL®-LA 0.25% w/v Gel-Forming Eye Drops Solution

TIMOPTOL®-LA 0.5% w/v Gel-Forming Eye Drops Solution

2. QUALITATIVE AND QUANTITATIVE COMPOSITION
Each millilitre of 0.25% w/v solution contains an amount of timolol maleate equivalent to 2.5 mg/ml timolol.

Each millilitre of 0.5% w/v solution contains an amount of timolol maleate equivalent to 5 mg/ml timolol.

3. PHARMACEUTICAL FORM
Sterile gel-forming eye drops solution.

4. CLINICAL PARTICULARS

4.1 Therapeutic indications
A beta-adrenoreceptor blocker used topically in the reduction of elevated intra-ocular pressure in various conditions including the following: patients with ocular hypertension; patients with chronic open-angle glaucoma including aphakic patients; some patients with secondary glaucoma.

4.2 Posology and method of administration
Invert the closed container and shake once before each use. It is not necessary to shake the container more than once.

Recommended therapy is one drop 0.25% solution in each affected eye once a day.

If clinical response is not adequate, dosage may be changed to one drop 0.5% solution in each affected eye once a day.

If needed, 'Timoptol'-LA may be used with other agent(s) for lowering intra-ocular pressure. Other topically applied medication should be administered not less than 10 minutes before 'Timoptol'-LA. The use of two topical beta-adrenergic blocking agents is not recommended (see section 4.4 'Special warnings and precautions for use').

Intra-ocular pressure should be reassessed approximately four weeks after starting treatment because response to 'Timoptol'-LA may take a few weeks to stabilise.

Transfer from other agents: When transferring a patient from 'Timoptol' to 'Timoptol'-LA, discontinue 'Timoptol' after a full day of therapy, starting treatment with the same concentration of 'Timoptol'-LA on the following day.

When another topical beta-blocking agent is being used, discontinue its use after a full day of therapy and start treatment with 'Timoptol'-LA the next day with one drop of 0.25% 'Timoptol'-LA in each affected eye once a day. The dosage may be increased to one drop of 0.5% solution in each affected eye once a day if the response is not adequate.

When transferring a patient from a single anti-glaucoma agent other than a topical beta-blocking agent, continue the agent and add one drop of 0.25% 'Timoptol'-LA in each affected eye once a day. On the following day, discontinue the previous agent completely, and continue with 'Timoptol'-LA. If a higher dosage of 'Timoptol'-LA is required, substitute one drop of 0.5% solution in each affected eye once a day (see section 5.1 'Pharmacodynamic properties').

Paediatric use: is not currently indicated.

Use in the elderly: there has been wide-experience with the use of timolol maleate in elderly patients. The dosage recommendations given above reflect the clinical data derived from this experience.

4.3 Contraindications
Bronchial asthma, history of bronchial asthma or severe chronic obstructive pulmonary disease; sinus bradycardia, second- or third-degree AV block, overt cardiac failure, cardiogenic shock; and hypersensitivity to any component of this product or other beta-blocking agents. 'Timoptol'-LA should not be used in patients wearing contact lenses as it has not been studied in these patients.

4.4 Special warnings and precautions for use
Like other topically applied ophthalmic drugs, this drug may be absorbed systemically and adverse reactions seen with oral beta-blockers may occur.

Cardiac failure should be adequately controlled before beginning therapy with 'Timoptol'-LA. Patients with a history of severe cardiac disease should be watched for signs of cardiac failure and have their pulse rates monitored.

Respiratory and cardiac reactions, including death due to bronchospasm in patients with asthma and, rarely, death associated with cardiac failure, are potential complications of therapy with 'Timoptol'-LA.

The effect on intra-ocular pressure or the known effects of systemic beta-blockade may be exaggerated when 'Timoptol'-LA is given to patients already receiving a systemic beta-blocking agent. The response of these patients should be closely observed. The use of two topical beta-adrenergic blocking agents is not recommended.

There have been reports of skin rashes and/or dry eyes associated with the use of beta-adrenoreceptor blocking drugs. The reported incidence is small and in most cases the symptoms have cleared when treatment was withdrawn. Discontinuation of the drug should be considered if any such reaction is not otherwise explicable. Cessation of therapy involving beta-blockade should be gradual.

The dispenser of 'Timoptol'-LA contains benzododecinium bromide as a preservative. In a clinical study, the time required to eliminate 50% of the gellan solution from the eye was up to 30 minutes.

In patients with angle-closure glaucoma, the immediate objective of treatment is to reopen the angle. This requires constricting the pupil with a miotic. 'Timoptol'-LA has little or no effect on the pupil. When 'Timoptol'-LA is used to reduce elevated intra-ocular pressure in angle-closure glaucoma it should be used with a miotic and not alone.

Choroidal detachment has been reported with administration of aqueous suppressant therapy (e.g. timolol, acetazolamide) after filtration procedures.

Transient blurred vision following instillation may occur, generally lasting from 30 seconds to 5 minutes, and in rare cases up to 30 minutes or longer. Blurred vision and potential visual disturbances may impair the ability to perform hazardous tasks such as operating machinery or driving a motor vehicle.

Patients should be advised that if they develop an intercurrent ocular condition (e.g. trauma, ocular surgery or infection), they should immediately seek their physician's advice concerning the continued use of the present multidose container (see section 6.6 'Special precautions for disposal and other handling').

There have been reports of bacterial keratitis associated with the use of multiple dose containers of topical ophthalmic products. These containers had been inadvertently contaminated by patients who, in most cases, had a concurrent corneal disease or a disruption of the ocular epithelial surface.

Risk from anaphylactic reactions: While taking beta-blockers, patients with a history of atopy or a history of severe anaphylactic reaction to a variety of allergens may be more reactive to repeated challenge with such allergens, either accidental, diagnostic, or therapeutic. Such patients may be unresponsive to the usual doses of epinephrine (adrenaline) used to treat anaphylactic reactions.

4.5 Interaction with other medicinal products and other forms of interaction

Although 'Timoptol' alone has little or no effect on pupil size, mydriasis has occasionally been reported when 'Timoptol' is given with epinephrine (adrenaline). The potential for mydriasis exists from concomitant therapy with 'Timoptol'-LA and epinephrine.

Close observation of the patient is recommended when a beta-blocker is administered to patients receiving catecholamine-depleting drugs such as reserpine, because of possible additive effects and the production of hypotension and/or marked bradycardia, which may produce vertigo, syncope, or postural hypotension.

The potential exists for hypotension, atrioventricular (AV) conduction disturbances and left ventricular failure to occur in patients receiving a beta-blocking agent when an oral calcium-channel blocker is added to the treatment regimen. The nature of any cardiovascular adverse effect tends to depend on the type of calcium-channel blocker used. Dihydropyridine derivatives, such as nifedipine, may lead to hypotension, whereas verapamil or diltiazem have a greater propensity to lead to AV conduction disturbances or left ventricular failure when used with a beta-blocker.

The concomitant use of beta-adrenergic blocking agents and digitalis with either diltiazem or verapamil may have additive effects in prolonging AV conduction time.

Oral calcium-channel antagonists may be used in combination with beta-adrenergic blocking agents when heart function is normal, but should be avoided in patients with impaired cardiac function.

Intravenous calcium-channel blockers should be used with caution in patients receiving beta-adrenergic blocking agents.

Potentiated systemic beta-blockade (e.g. decreased heart rate, depression) has been reported during combined treatment with CYP2D6 inhibitors (e.g.quinidine, SSRIs) and timolol.

Oral-β-adrenergic blocking agents may exacerbate the rebound hypertension which can follow the withdrawal of clonidine.

4.6 Pregnancy and lactation

Use in pregnancy: 'Timoptol'-LA has not been studied in human pregnancy. The use of 'Timoptol'-LA requires that the anticipated benefit be weighed against possible hazards.

Breast-feeding mothers: Timolol is detectable in human milk. Because of the potential for adverse reactions to 'Timoptol'-LA in infants, a decision should be made whether to discontinue nursing or to discontinue the drug, taking into account the importance of the drug to the mother.

4.7 Effects on ability to drive and use machines

Transient blurred vision following instillation may occur, generally lasting from 30 seconds to 5 minutes, and in rare cases, up to 30 minutes or longer. Blurred vision and potential visual disturbances may impair the ability to perform hazardous tasks such as operating machinery or driving a motor vehicle.

4.8 Undesirable effects
Side effects

'Timoptol'-LA is usually well tolerated. The most frequent drug-related complaint in clinical studies was transient blurred vision (6.0%), lasting from 30 seconds to 5 minutes following instillation.

The following possibly, probably, or definitely drug-related adverse reactions occurred with frequency of at least 1% in parallel active treatment controlled clinical trials:

Ocular: burning and stinging, discharge, foreign body sensation, itching.

The following side effects reported with 'Timoptol', either in clinical trials or since the drug has been marketed, are potential side effects of 'Timoptol'-LA. Additional side effects have been reported in clinical experiences with *systemic* timolol maleate, and may be considered potential effects of ophthalmic timolol maleate

Special senses:

ocular: signs and symptoms of ocular irritation, including conjunctivitis, blepharitis, keratitis, decreased corneal sensitivity and dry eyes. Tinnitus, visual disturbances, including refractive changes (due to withdrawal of miotic therapy in some cases), diplopia, and ptosis. Choroidal detachment following filtration surgery (see section 4.4 'Special warnings and precautions for use').

Cardiovascular:

ocular: bradycardia, arrhythmia, hypotension, syncope, heart block, cerebrovascular accident, cerebral ischaemia, congestive heart failure, palpitation, cardiac arrest, oedema, claudication, Raynaud's phenomenon, cold hands and feet.

systemic: AV block (second- or third-degree), sino-atrial block, pulmonary oedema, worsening of arterial insufficiency, worsening of angina pectoris, vasodilation.

Respiratory:

ocular: bronchospasm (predominantly in patients with pre-existing bronchospastic disease), respiratory failure, dyspnoea, cough.

systemic: rales

Body as a whole:

ocular: headache, asthenia, fatigue, chest pain.

systemic: extremity pain, decreased exercise tolerance.

Integumentary:

ocular: alopecia, psoriasiform rash or exacerbation of psoriasis.

systemic: pruritis, sweating, exfoliative dermatitis.

Hypersensitivity:

ocular: signs and symptoms of allergic reactions including anaphylaxis, angioedema, urticaria, localised and generalised rash.

Nervous system/psychiatric:

ocular: dizziness, depression, insomnia, nightmares, memory loss, paraesthesia.

systemic: vertigo, local weakness, diminished concentration, increased dreaming.

Neuromuscular:

ocular: increase in signs and symptoms of myasthenia gravis.

Digestive:

ocular: nausea, diarrhoea, dyspepsia, dry mouth.

systemic: vomiting.

Urogenital:

ocular: decreased libido, Peyronie's disease.

systemic: impotence, micturition difficulties.

Immunologic:

ocular: systemic lupus erythematosus.

Endocrine:

systemic: hyperglycaemia, hypoglycaemia.

Musculoskeletal:

systemic: arthralgia.

Haematological:

systemic: non-thrombocytopenic purpura.

4.9 Overdose

There have been reports of inadvertent overdosage with 'Timoptol' resulting in systemic effects similar to those seen with systemic beta-adrenergic blocking agents such as dizziness, headache, shortness of breath, bradycardia, bronchospasm, and cardiac arrest (see section 4.8 'Undesirable effects' - Side effects).

If overdosage occurs, the following measures should be considered:

1. Symptomatic bradycardia: atropine sulphate, 0.25 to 2 mg intravenously, should be used to induce vagal blockade. If bradycardia persists, intravenous isoprenaline hydrochloride should be administered cautiously. In refractory cases, the use of a cardiac pacemaker may be considered.

2. Hypotension: a sympathomimetic pressor agent such as dopamine, dobutamine or norepinephrine (noradrenaline) should be used. In refractory cases, the use of glucagon has been reported to be useful.

3. Bronchospasm: isoprenaline hydrochloride should be used. Additional therapy with aminophylline may be considered.

4. Acute cardiac failure: conventional therapy with digitalis, diuretics, and oxygen should be instituted immediately. In refractory cases, the use of intravenous aminophylline is suggested. This may be followed, if necessary, by glucagon, which has been reported useful.

5. Heart block (second- or third-degree): isoprenaline hydrochloride or a pacemaker should be used.

Timolol does not dialyse readily.

5. PHARMACOLOGICAL PROPERTIES

5.1 Pharmacodynamic properties

Pharmacotherapeutic group

Beta-adrenergic receptor blocking agent.

Mechanism of action

The precise mechanism of action of timolol maleate in lowering intra-ocular pressure is not clearly established. A fluorescein study and tonography studies indicate that the predominant action may be related to reduced aqueous formation. However, in some studies a slight increase in outflow facility was also observed.

'Timoptol'-LA is an ophthalmic formulation comprising timolol maleate, which reduces intra-ocular pressure, whether or not associated with glaucoma, and a new delivery vehicle. Gellan solution contains a highly purified anionic heteropolysaccharide derived from gellan gum. Aqueous solutions of gellan gum form a clear transparent gel at low polymer concentrations in the presence of cations. When 'Timoptol'-LA contacts the precorneal tear film, it becomes a gel. Gellan gum increases the contact time of the drug with the eye.

Pharmacodynamics

In parallel active treatment controlled, double-masked, multiclinic studies in patients with untreated elevated intra-ocular pressure of greater than 22 mmHg in one or both eyes, 0.25% and 0.5% 'Timoptol'-LA administered once daily had an intra-ocular pressure-lowering effect equivalent to the same concentration of 'Timoptol' administered twice daily (see table below).

For the five independent comparative studies listed in the table below, the entrance criterion was an intra-ocular pressure of greater than 22 mmHg in one or both eyes after a washout period of one week for most antiglaucoma medications and up to three weeks for ophthalmic beta-adrenergic antagonists. The dosage used was one drop of 'Timoptol'-LA in each affected eye once daily versus one drop of 'Timoptol' in each affected eye twice daily.

Mean change in intra-ocular pressure (mmHg) from baseline at trough (immediately before the morning dose) for the final week of the double-masked study

Concentration	'Timoptol'-LA (n)	'Timoptol' (n)	Week
0.25%	-5.8 (94)	-5.9 (96)	12
0.25%	-6.0 (74)	-5.9 (73)	12
0.50%	-8.3 (110)*	-8.2 (111)*	12
0.50%	-5.6 (189)	-6.3 (94)	24
0.50%	-6.4 (212)	-6.1 (109)	24

*The baseline intra-ocular pressure was elevated in comparison to the other studies due to the higher intra-ocular pressure of patients with pseudoexfoliative glaucoma.

Onset of action of timolol maleate is usually rapid, occurring approximately 20 minutes after topical application to the eye.

Maximum reduction of intra-ocular pressure occurs in two to four hours with 'Timoptol'-LA. Significant lowering of intra-ocular pressure has been maintained for 24 hours with both 0.25% and 0.5% 'Timoptol'-LA.

As compared with 0.5% 'Timoptol' administered twice daily, in three clinical studies 0.5% 'Timoptol'-LA administered once daily reduced mean heart rate less and produced bradycardia less frequently (see section 4.4 'Special warnings and specialprecautions for use'). At trough (24 hours post-dose 'Timoptol'-LA, 12 hours post-dose 'Timoptol'), the mean reduction in heart rate was 0.8 beats/minute for 'Timoptol'-LA and 3.6 beats/minute for 'Timoptol'; whereas at two hours post-dose, the mean reduction was comparable (3.8 beats/minute for 'Timoptol'-LA and 5 beats/minute for 'Timoptol').

Timolol maleate is a non-selective beta-adrenergic receptor blocking agent that does not have significant intrinsic sympathomimetic, direct myocardial depressant, or local anaesthetic (membrane-stabilising) activity.

Unlike miotics, timolol maleate reduces intra-ocular pressure with little or no effect on accommodation or pupil size. Thus, changes in visual acuity due to increased accommodation are uncommon, and the dim or blurred vision and night blindness produced by miotics are not evident. In addition, in patients with cataracts the inability to see around lenticular opacities when the pupil is constricted by miotics is avoided. When changing patients from miotics to 'Timoptol'-LA, refraction may be necessary after the effects of the miotic have passed.

As with other antiglaucoma drugs, diminished responsiveness to timolol maleate after prolonged therapy has been reported in some patients. However, in clinical studies of 'Timoptol' in which 164 patients were followed for at least three years, no significant difference in mean intra-ocular pressure was observed after initial stabilisation. This indicates that the intra-ocular pressure-lowering effects of timolol maleate is well maintained.

5.2 Pharmacokinetic properties

Onset of action of timolol maleate is usually rapid, occurring approximately 20 minutes after topical application to the eye.

Maximum reduction of intra-ocular pressure occurs in two to four hours with 'Timoptol'-LA. Significant lowering of intra-ocular pressure has been maintained for 24 hours with both 0.25% and 0.5% 'Timoptol'-LA. In a study of plasma timolol concentrations, the systemic exposure to timolol was less when normal healthy volunteers received 0.5% 'Timoptol'-LA once daily than when they received 0.5% 'Timoptol' twice daily.

5.3 Preclinical safety data

No adverse ocular effects were observed in monkeys and rabbits administered 'Timoptol'-LA topically in studies lasting 12 months and one month, respectively. The oral

LD_{50} of timolol is 1,190 and 900 mg/kg in female mice and female rats, respectively. The oral LD_{50} of gellan gum is greater than 5,000 mg/kg in rats.

In a two-year oral study of timolol maleate in rats there was a statistically significant ($p \leq 0.05$) increase in the incidence of adrenal phaeochromocytomas in male rats administered 300 mg/kg/day (300 times the maximum recommended human oral dose*). Similar differences were not observed in rats administered oral doses equivalent to 25 or 100 times the maximum recommended human oral dose.

In a lifetime oral study in mice, there were statistically significant ($p \leq 0.05$) increases in the incidence of benign and malignant pulmonary tumours, benign uterine polyps and mammary adenocarcinoma in female mice at 500 mg/kg/day (500 times the maximum recommended human dose), but not at 5 or 50 mg/kg/day. In a subsequent study in female mice, in which post-mortem examinations were limited to uterus and lungs, a statistically significant increase in the incidence of pulmonary tumours was again observed at 500 mg/kg/day.

The increased occurrence of mammary adenocarcinoma was associated with elevations in serum prolactin which occurred in female mice administered timolol at 500 mg/kg/day, but not at doses of 5 or 50 mg/kg/day. An increased incidence of mammary adenocarcinomas in rodents has been associated with administration of several other therapeutic agents which elevate serum prolactin, but no correlation between serum prolactin levels and mammary tumours has been established in man. Furthermore, in adult human female subjects who received oral dosages of up to 60 mg of timolol maleate, the maximum recommended human oral dosage, there were no clinically meaningful changes in serum prolactin.

In oral studies of gellan gum administered to rats for up to 105 weeks at concentrations up to 5% of their diet and to mice for 96-98 weeks at concentrations up to 3% of their diet, no overt signs of toxicity and no increase in the incidence of tumours was observed.

Timolol maleate was devoid of mutagenic potential when evaluated *in vivo* (mouse) in the micronucleus test and cytogenetic assay (doses up to 800 mg/kg) and *in vitro* in a neoplastic cell-transformation assay (up to 100 mcg/ml). In Ames tests the highest concentrations of timolol employed, 5,000 or 10,000 mcg/plate, were associated with statistically significant ($p \leq 0.05$) elevations of revertants observed with tester strain TA100 (in seven replicate assays), but not in the remaining three strains. In the assays with tester strain TA100, no consistent dose-response relationship was observed, nor did the ratio of test to control revertants reach 2. A ratio of 2 is usually considered the criterion for a positive Ames test.

Gellan gum was devoid of mutagenic potential when evaluated *in vivo* (mouse) in micronucleus assay using doses up to 450 mg/kg. In addition, gellan gum in concentrations up to 20 mg/ml was not detectably mutagenic in the following *in-vitro* assays:

(1) unscheduled DNA synthesis in rat hepatocytes assay, (2) V-79 mammalian cell mutagenesis assay, and (3) chromosomal aberrations in Chinese hamster ovary cells assay.

In Ames tests, gellan gum (in concentrations up to 1,000 mcg/plate, which is its limit of solubility) did not induce a twofold or greater increase in revertants relative to the solvent control. It is therefore not detectably mutagenic.

*The maximum recommended daily oral dose of timolol is 60 mg. One drop of 0.5% 'Timoptol'-LA contains about 1/300 of this dose, which is about 0.2 mg.

6. PHARMACEUTICAL PARTICULARS

6.1 List of excipients

Gellan gum, trometamol, mannitol E421, and water for injection. Benzododecinium bromide (0.012%) is added as preservative.

6.2 Incompatibilities

None known.

6.3 Shelf life

The shelf life is 24 months. After opening the shelf life is 28 days.

6.4 Special precautions for storage

Do not store above 25°C. Do not freeze. Store bottle in the outer carton.

6.5 Nature and contents of container

The OCUMETER Plus ophthalmic dispenser consists of a translucent high-density polyethylene container with a sealed dropper tip, a flexible fluted side area, which is depressed to dispense the drops, and a two-piece assembly. The two-piece cap mechanism punctures the sealed dropper tip upon initial use, then locks together to provide a single cap during the usage period. Tamper evidence is provided by a safety strip on the container label. The OCUMETER Plus ophthalmic dispenser contains 2.5 ml of solution.

'Timoptol'-LA Gel-Forming Eye Drops Solution is available in single bottles containing 2.5 ml of solution.

6.6 Special precautions for disposal and other handling

Invert the container and shake once before each use. It is not necessary to shake the container more than once.

Discard 28 days after opening.

Patients should be instructed to avoid allowing the tip of the dispensing container to contact the eye or surrounding structures.

Patients should also be instructed that ocular solutions, if handled improperly, can become contaminated by common bacteria known to cause ocular infections. Serious damage to the eye and subsequent loss of vision may result from using contaminated solutions.

7. MARKETING AUTHORISATION HOLDER

Merck Sharp & Dohme Limited

Hertford Road, Hoddesdon, Hertfordshire EN11 9BU, UK.

8. MARKETING AUTHORISATION NUMBER(S)

0.25% PL 0025/0310

0.5% PL 0025/0311

9. DATE OF FIRST AUTHORISATION/RENEWAL OF THE AUTHORISATION

Granted: 2 April 1996/Renewed: 2 April 2001

10. DATE OF REVISION OF THE TEXT

February 2008

LEGAL CATEGORY

POM.

® denotes registered trademark of Merck & Co., Inc., Whitehouse Station, NJ, USA.

SPC.TOTX.06.UK.2343 F.T. 060608

Toctino 10mg and 30mg soft capsules

(Basilea Pharmaceuticals Ltd)

1. NAME OF THE MEDICINAL PRODUCT

Toctino®▼ 10mg soft capsules.

Toctino®▼ 30mg soft capsules.

2. QUALITATIVE AND QUANTITATIVE COMPOSITION

Each soft capsule contains 10mg or 30mg of alitretinoin.

This medicinal product contains the excipients soya-bean oil and sorbitol.

For a full list of excipients, see section 6.1 "List of excipients".

3. PHARMACEUTICAL FORM

Soft capsule

The Toctino 10mg capsule is an opaque brown soft capsule imprinted with "A1" in white.

The Toctino 30mg capsule is an opaque red-brown soft capsule imprinted with "A3" in white.

4. CLINICAL PARTICULARS

4.1 Therapeutic indications

Toctino is indicated for use in adults who have severe chronic hand eczema that is unresponsive to treatment with potent topical corticosteroids.

Patients in whom the eczema has predominantly hyperkeratotic features are more likely to respond to treatment than in those in whom the eczema predominantly presents as pompholyx (See section 5.1 "Pharmacodynamic properties").

4.2 Posology and method of administration

Toctino should only be prescribed by dermatologists, or physicians with experience in the use of systemic retinoids who have full understanding of the risks of systemic retinoid therapy and monitoring requirements. Prescriptions of Toctino for women of childbearing potential should be limited to 30 days of treatment and continuation of treatment requires a new prescription. Ideally, pregnancy testing, issuing a prescription and dispensing of Toctino should occur on the same day. Dispensing of Toctino should occur within a maximum of 7 days of the prescription.

The recommended dose range for Toctino is 10mg-30mg once daily.

The recommended start dose for Toctino is 30mg once daily. A dose reduction to 10mg once daily may be considered in patients with unacceptable adverse reactions to the higher dose. In studies investigating 10mg and 30mg daily doses, both doses resulted in clearing of the disease. The 30mg dose provided a more rapid response and a higher response rate. The 10mg daily dose was associated with fewer adverse events (see section 4.4 "Special warnings and precautions for use" and section 5.1 "Pharmacodynamic Properties").

A treatment course of Toctino may be given for 12 to 24 weeks depending on response. Discontinuation of therapy should be considered for patients who still have severe disease after the initial 12 weeks of treatment. In the event of relapse, patients may benefit from further treatment courses of Toctino.

The capsules should be taken with a meal once daily.

Toctino should not be prescribed if the patient's eczema can be adequately controlled by standard measures, including skin protection, avoidance of allergens and irritants, and treatment with potent topical corticosteroids.

Children

Toctino is not recommended for use in patients under 18 years of age.

4.3 Contraindications

Pregnancy is an absolute contraindication to treatment with Toctino (see section 4.6 "Pregnancy and lactation").

Toctino is contraindicated in woman of childbearing potential unless all of the conditions of the Pregnancy Prevention Programme are met (see section 4.4 "Special warnings and special precautions for use").

Toctino contains soya oil. Patients who are allergic to peanut, soya or with rare hereditary fructose intolerance should not take this medicine.

Toctino is contraindicated in breastfeeding.

Toctino is also contraindicated in patients

- With hepatic insufficiency
- With severe renal insufficiency
- With uncontrolled hypercholesterolaemia
- With uncontrolled hypertriglyceridaemia
- With uncontrolled hypothyroidism
- With hypervitaminosis A
- With hypersensitivity either to alitretinoin, to other retinoids or to any of the excipients, in particular in case of allergies to peanut or soya
- Receiving concomitant treatment with tetracyclines (see section 4.5 "Interactions with other medicinal products and other forms of interactions")

4.4 Special warnings and precautions for use

Pregnancy Prevention Programme

This medicinal product is **TERATOGENIC.**

Toctino is contraindicated in women of childbearing potential unless all of the following conditions of the Pregnancy Prevention Programme are met:

- She understands the teratogenic risk
- She understands the need for rigorous follow-up, on a monthly basis
- She understands and accepts the need for effective contraception, without interruption, 1 month before starting treatment, throughout the duration of treatment and 1 month after the end of treatment. At least one and preferably two complementary forms of contraception including a barrier method should be used
- Even if she has amenorrhoea she must follow all of the advice on effective contraception
- She should be capable of complying with effective contraceptive measures
- She is informed and understands the potential consequences of pregnancy and the need to rapidly consult if there is a risk of pregnancy
- She understands the need and accepts to undergo pregnancy testing before, during and 5 weeks after the end of treatment
- She has acknowledged that she has understood the hazards and necessary precautions associated with the use of Toctino

These conditions also concern women who are not currently sexually active unless the prescriber considers that there are compelling reasons to indicate that there is no risk of pregnancy.

The prescriber must ensure that:

- The patient complies with the conditions for pregnancy prevention as listed above, including confirmation that she has an adequate level of understanding
- The patient has acknowledged the aforementioned conditions
- The patient has used at least one and preferably two methods of effective contraception including a barrier method for at least 1 month prior to starting treatment and is continuing to use effective contraception throughout the treatment period and for at least 1 month after cessation of treatment
- Negative pregnancy test results have been obtained before, during and 5 weeks after the end of treatment. The dates and results of pregnancy tests should be documented

Contraception

Female patients must be provided with comprehensive information on pregnancy prevention and should be referred for contraceptive advice if they are not using effective contraception.

As a minimum requirement, female patients at potential risk of pregnancy must use at least one effective method of contraception. Preferably the patient should use two complementary forms of contraception including a barrier method. Contraception should be continued for at least 1 month after stopping treatment with Toctino, even in patients with amenorrhea.

Pregnancy testing

According to local practice, medically supervised pregnancy tests with a minimum sensitivity of 25mIU/mL are recommended to be performed in the first 3 days of the menstrual cycle, as follows:

One month prior to starting therapy

In order to exclude the possibility of pregnancy prior to starting contraception, it is recommended that an initial medically supervised pregnancy test should be performed and its date and result recorded. In patients without regular menses, the timing of this pregnancy test should reflect the sexual activity of the patient and should be undertaken approximately 3 weeks after the patient last had unprotected sexual intercourse. The prescriber should educate the patient about contraception.

At the start of therapy

A medically supervised pregnancy test should also be performed during the consultation when Toctino is prescribed or in the 3 days prior to the visit to the prescriber, and should have been delayed until the patient had been using effective contraception for at least 1 month. This test should ensure the patient is not pregnant when she starts treatment with Toctino.

Follow-up visits

Follow-up visits should be arranged at 28 day intervals. The need for repeated medically supervised pregnancy tests every month should be determined in consideration amongst other of the patient's sexual activity and recent menstrual history (abnormal menses, missed periods or amenorrhea). Where indicated, follow-up pregnancy tests should be performed on the day of the prescribing visit or in the 3 days prior to the visit to the prescriber.

End of treatment

Five weeks after stopping treatment, women should undergo a final pregnancy test to exclude pregnancy.

Prescribing and dispensing restrictions

Prescriptions of Toctino for women of childbearing potential should be limited to 30 days of treatment and continuation of treatment requires a new prescription. Ideally, pregnancy testing, issuing a prescription and dispensing of Toctino should occur on the same day. Dispensing of Toctino should be completed within a maximum of 7 days of the prescription.

Male patients

Small amounts of alitretinoin have been detected in the semen of healthy volunteers receiving 40 mg of alitretinoin and there is no indication of drug accumulation in semen. Assuming complete vaginal absorption of these amounts would have a negligible effect on the endogenous plasma levels of the female partner and therefore does not appear to pose a risk to the foetus if the partner is pregnant. Based on non-clinical findings, male fertility may be compromised by treatment with Toctino (see section 5.3 "Preclinical safety data").

Male patients should be reminded that they must not share their medication with anyone, particularly not females.

Additional precautions

Patients should be instructed never to give this medicinal product to another person and to return any unused capsules to their pharmacist at the end of treatment.

Patients should not donate blood during therapy and for 1 month following discontinuation of Toctino because of the potential risk to the foetus of a pregnant transfusion recipient.

Educational material

In order to assist prescribers, pharmacists and patients in avoiding foetal exposure to alitretinoin, the Marketing Authorisation Holder will provide educational material to reinforce the warnings about the teratogenicity of Toctino, to provide advice on contraception before therapy is started and to provide guidance on the need for pregnancy testing. Full patient information about the teratogenic risk and the strict pregnancy prevention measures as specified in the Pregnancy Prevention Programme should be given by the physician to all patients, both male and female.

Psychiatric disorders

Depression, aggravated depression, anxiety, aggressive tendencies, mood alterations, psychotic symptoms, and very rarely, suicidal ideation, suicide attempts and suicide have been reported in patients treated with systemic retinoids. Particular care needs to be taken in patients with a history of depression and patients on alitretinoin treatment should therefore be observed for signs of depression and referred for appropriate treatment if necessary. However, discontinuation of alitretinoin may be insufficient to alleviate symptoms and therefore further psychiatric or psychological evaluation may be necessary.

UV light

The effects of UV light are enhanced by retinoid therapy, therefore patients should avoid excessive exposure to sunlight and the unsupervised use of sun lamps. Where necessary a sun-protection product with a high protection factor of at least SPF 15 should be used.

Patients who experience dryness of the skin and lips should be advised to use a skin moisturising ointment or cream and a lip balm.

Musculo-skeletal and connective tissue disorders

Treatment with other systemic retinoids has been associated with bone changes including premature epiphyseal closure, hyperostosis, and calcification of tendons and ligaments.

Myalgia, arthralgia and increased serum creatinine phosphokinase values have been observed in patients treated with alitretinoin.

Eye disorders

Treatment with alitretinoin has been associated with dry eyes. The symptoms usually resolve after discontinuation of therapy. Dry eyes can be helped by the application of a lubricating eye ointment or by the application of tear replacement therapy. Intolerance to contact lenses may occur which may necessitate the patient wearing glasses during treatment.

Treatment with systemic retinoids has been associated with corneal opacities and keratitis. Decreased night vision has been observed in patients treated with alitretinoin. These effects usually resolve after discontinuation of therapy.

Patients experiencing visual difficulties should be referred to an ophthalmologist. Withdrawal of alitretinoin may be necessary.

Benign intracranial hypertension

Treatment with systemic retinoids, including alitretinoin, has been associated with the occurrence of benign intracranial hypertension, some of which involved concomitant use of tetracyclines (see section 4.3 "Contraindications" and section 4.5 "Interaction with other medicinal products and other forms of interaction"). Signs and symptoms of benign intracranial hypertension include headache, nausea and vomiting, visual disturbances and papilloedema. Patients who develop signs of benign intracranial hypertension should discontinue alitretinoin immediately.

Lipid Metabolism

Alitretinoin has been associated with an increase in plasma cholesterol and triglyceride levels. Serum cholesterol and triglycerides (fasting values) should be monitored.

Alitretinoin should be discontinued if hypertriglyceridaemia cannot be controlled at an acceptable level or if symptoms of pancreatitis occur (see section 4.8 "Undesirable effects"). Triglyceride levels in excess of 800mg/dL (9mmol/L) are sometimes associated with acute pancreatitis, which may be fatal.

Thyroid function

Changes in thyroid function tests have been observed in patients receiving alitretinoin, most often noted as a reversible reduction in thyroid stimulating hormone (TSH) levels and T4 (free thyroxine).

Hepatobiliary disorders

Treatment with other systemic retinoids has been associated with transient and reversible increases in liver transaminases. In the event of persistent clinically relevant elevation of transaminase levels, reduction of the dose or discontinuation of treatment should be considered.

Gastrointestinal disorders

Systemic retinoids have been associated with IBD (inflammatory bowel disease, including regional ileitis) in patients without a history of intestinal disorders. If severe diarrhoea is observed, diagnosis of IBD should be considered and alitretinoin should be discontinued immediately.

Allergic reactions

Anaphylactic reactions have been rarely reported in systemic retinoids, in some cases after previous topical exposure to retinoids. Allergic cutaneous reactions are reported infrequently. Serious cases of allergic vasculitis, often with purpura (bruises and red patches) of the extremities and extracutaneous involvement have been reported. Severe allergic reactions necessitate interruption of therapy and careful monitoring.

High risk patients

In patients with diabetes, obesity, cardiovascular risk factors or a lipid metabolism disorder undergoing treatment with alitretinoin, more frequent checks of serum values for lipids may be necessary. It is recommended that these patients are started with 10mg once daily and titrated up to the maximum dose of 30mg if necessary.

4.5 Interaction with other medicinal products and other forms of interaction

Pharmacokinetic interaction

Alitretinoin is metabolised by cytochrome P450 3A4 (CYP3A4).

Patients should be prospectively cautioned not to self-medicate with the herbal supplement St. John's Wort because a possible interaction has been suggested with hormonal contraceptives based on reports of breakthrough bleeding on oral contraceptives shortly after starting St. John's Wort. Pregnancies have been reported by users of combined hormonal contraceptives who also used some form of St. John's Wort.

Co-administration with CYP3A4 inhibitors such as ketoconazole increases the plasma level of alitretinoin and dose reduction may be required. The effects of other inhibitors of CYP3A4 have not been studied. Alitretinoin did not affect the pharmacokinetics of ketoconazole.

A 16% reduction of simvastatin plasma levels was observed when co-administered with alitretinoin.

The effects on other similar medicinal products have not been studied. Simvastatin did not affect the pharmacokinetics of alitretinoin.

No pharmacokinetic interactions were observed when alitretinoin was co-administered with ciclosporin or the oral contraceptive ethinyl estradiol and norgestimate.

Pharmacodynamic interactions

Patients should not take vitamin A or other retinoids as concurrent medication due to the risk of hypervitaminosis A.

Cases of benign intracranial hypertension (pseudotumour cerebri) have been reported with concomitant use of retinoids and tetracyclines. Therefore, concomitant treatment with tetracyclines must be avoided (see sections 4.3 "Contraindications" and section 4.4 "Special warnings and precautions for use").

4.6 Pregnancy and lactation

Pregnancy is an absolute contraindication to treatment with Toctino (see section 4.3, "Contraindications"). If pregnancy does occur in spite of the pregnancy prevention precautions during treatment with Toctino or in the month following discontinuation of therapy, there is a great risk of very severe and serious malformation of the foetus.

Alitretinoin is a retinoid and therefore is a potent teratogen. The foetal malformations associated with exposure to retinoids include central nervous system abnormalities (hydrocephalus, cerebellar malformation/ abnormalities, microcephaly), facial dysmorphia, cleft palate, external ear abnormalities (absence of external ear, small or absent external auditory canals), eye abnormalities (microphthalmia), cardiovascular abnormalities (conotruncal malformations such as tetralogy of Fallot, transposition of great vessels, septal defects), thymus gland abnormality and parathyroid gland abnormalities. There is also an increased incidence of spontaneous abortion.

If pregnancy occurs in a woman treated with Toctino, treatment must be stopped and the patient should be referred to a physician specialised or experienced in teratology for evaluation and advice.

Lactation

Alitretinoin is highly lipophilic, therefore the passage of alitretinoin into human milk is very likely. Due to the potential risk for the exposed child, the use of alitretinoin is contraindicated during breastfeeding.

Fertility

Small amounts of alitretinoin have been detected in the semen of healthy volunteers receiving 40mg of alitretinoin and there is no indication of drug accumulation in semen. In the event of complete vaginal absorption of these amounts, this would have a negligible effect on the endogenous plasma levels of the female partner and therefore does not appear to pose a risk to the foetus if the partner is pregnant. Based on non-clinical findings, male fertility may be compromised by treatment with Toctino (see section 5.3 "Preclinical safety data").

4.7 Effects on ability to drive and use machines

Decreased night vision has been reported in patients treated with alitretinoin and other retinoids. Patients should be advised of this potential problem and warned to be cautious when driving or operating machines.

4.8 Undesirable effects

The most frequent adverse drug reactions (ADRs) observed under alitretinoin therapy are headache (30mg: 21%; 10mg: 11%), flushing (30mg: 5.9%; 10mg: 1.6%), and laboratory changes consisting of increased levels of triglycerides (30mg: 35.4%; 10mg: 17.0%), increased cholesterol (30mg: 27.8%; 10mg: 16.7%), decreased levels of thyroid stimulating hormone (TSH, 30mg: 8.4%; 10mg: 6.0%) and decreased levels of free T4 (30mg: 10.5%; 10mg: 2.9%). These reversible ADRs are dose dependent and may therefore be alleviated by dose reduction.

(see Table 1 on next page)

Psychiatric effects, in particular depression, and mood changes and suicidal ideation, have been associated with retinoids. In clinical studies, where patients with a history or active psychiatric disorders were excluded patients have been monitored for depression using the CES-D (Center for Epidemiological Studies - Depression) score. Treatment with alitretinoin was not associated with changes in the CES-D score.

The following adverse events have not been observed in clinical trials with alitretinoin, but have been observed with other retinoids: inflammatory bowel disease, diabetes mellitus, colour blindness (colour vision deficiencies), and contact lens intolerance (see section 4.4 "Special warnings and precautions for use").

Changes in bone mineralisation and extra-osseous calcifications have been associated with systemic retinoid treatment. In clinical studies with alitretinoin, degenerative changes of the spine and ligamentous calcifications were frequent findings in patients with chronic hand eczema before treatment (baseline), with minor progression in a small number of patients during treatment. These observations were consistent with age dependent degenerative changes. Assessments of bone density (DXA) did not indicate a dose dependent effect on bone mineralisation.

4.9 Overdose

Alitretinoin is a derivative of vitamin A. Alitretinoin has been administered in oncological clinical studies at dosages of more than 10 times the therapeutic dosage given for chronic hand eczema. The adverse effects observed were consistent with retinoid toxicity, and included severe headache, diarrhoea, facial flushing, hypertriglyceridaemia. These effects were reversible.

Table 1

	Very common (≥ 1/10)	Common (≥ 1/100 < 1/10)	Uncommon (≥ 1/1000, < 1/100)	Rare (≥ 1/10.000 < 1/1000)
Blood and lymphatic system disorders		Anaemia, increased iron binding capacity, monocytes decreased; thrombocytes increased		
Endocrine Disorders		TSH decreased, free T4 decreased		
Nervous system disorders	Headache			Benign intracranial hypertension
Eye disorders		Conjunctivitis, dry eye, eye irritation	Blurred vision, cataract	
Vascular disorders		Flushing		Vasculitis
Respiratory, thoracic and mediastinal disorders			Epistaxis	
Hepatobiliary disorders		Transaminase increased[1)]		
Skin and subcutaneous tissues disorders		Dry skin, dry lips, cheilitis, eczema[1)], dermatitis[1)], erythema, alopecia	Pruritus, rash, skin exfoliation, asteatotic eczema	
Musculo-skeletal and connective tissue disorders		Arthralgia[1)], myalgia[1]	Exostosis, (hyperostosis), ankylosing spondylitis	
Investigations	Hypertriglyceridemia, high density lipoprotein decreased, hypercholesterolemia	Blood creatinine phosphokinase increased		

[1)] The incidence of adverse events was not higher than those observed in the corresponding placebo group.

5. PHARMACOLOGICAL PROPERTIES

5.1 Pharmacodynamic properties

ATC code: D11AX19

Mechanism of action

The pharmacological action of retinoids may be explained by their effects on cell proliferation, cell differentiation, apoptosis, angiogenesis, keratinisation, sebum secretion and immunomodulation. Unlike other retinoids, which are specific agonists of either RAR or RXR receptors, alitretinoin binds to members of both receptor families. The mechanism of action of alitretinoin in chronic hand eczema is unknown. Alitretinoin has demonstrated immunomodulatory and anti-inflammatory effects that are relevant to skin inflammation. CXCR3 ligands and CCL20 chemokines, expressed in eczematous skin lesions, are down-regulated by alitretinoin in cytokine-stimulated keratinocytes and dermal endothelial cells. In addition, alitretinoin suppresses the expansion of cytokine-activated leucocyte subsets and antigen presenting cells.

It has been observed that in humans alitretinoin only minimally affects sebum secretion.

Clinical efficacy

The safety and efficacy of Toctino in patients with severe chronic hand eczema (CHE) refractory to topical corticosteroids has been established in two randomised, double blind, placebo-controlled Phase 3 studies.

The primary endpoint in these studies was the proportion of patients achieving Physicians Global Assessment (PGA) ratings of clear or almost clear hands at the end of therapy. The treatment duration was 12 to 24 weeks.

The BACH (Benefit of Alitretinoin in Chronic Hand Dermatitis Study) included 1032 severe CHE patients who had no response or a transient response (initial improvement and worsening of disease despite continued treatment) to potent topical corticosteroids or who were intolerant of potent topical corticosteroids. All phenotypes of CHE were included: hyperkeratosis (87%), pompholyx (27%), fingertip dermatitis (43%), and other (15%). Essentially all patients had signs of skin inflammation, comprising of erythema and/or vesicles. Treatment with alitretinoin led to a significantly higher proportion of patients with clear/almost clear hands, compared to placebo. The response was dose dependent (see Table 2). Response rates for different CHE subtypes were also dose dependent, except for patients with pompholyx (see Table 3).

Table 2: Primary Efficacy Parameter - Results
(see Table 2 below)

Table 3: Response rate by CHE subtype
(see Table 3 below)

Secondary endpoints included the proportion of patients achieving at least mild disease, time to achieving clear to almost clear hands, reduction in total lesion symptom score, patient global assessment (PaGA) of disease severity, reduction in extent of disease (see Table 4). Patients with clear/almost clear hands at end of treatment were followed up for 24 weeks. During that period no active drug treatment for CHE was allowed. Relapse was defined as 75% of the initial total lesion symptom score.

Table 4: Secondary Efficacy Parameters - Results
(see Table 4 on next page)

The numbers of responding patients without observed relapse at the end of the 24-weeks follow-up period is given in Table 5 below. In this analysis, the majority of responders given 10mg and 30mg alitretinoin did not relapse by the end of the follow-up period.

Table 5: Relapse Rates* at the End of Follow-up

	Alitretinoin		Placebo
	10 mg N=418	**30 mg N=409**	**N=205**
Responders	115 (100%)	195 (100%)	34 (100%)
No Relapse	81 (70.4%)	122 (62.6%)	19 (55.9%)

* Corresponds to a last-observation-carried-forward (LOCF) computation

A follow-up study (the second Phase 3 study) investigated the efficacy and safety of a second course of treatment both in patients who previously responded (Cohort A) and in patients who did not (Cohort B). Cohort A patients who responded in the previous study but who relapsed were randomised to the same dose they received in their initial treatment (10 or 30mg) or to placebo in a 2:1 ratio. 80% of relapsing patients who again received the 30 mg dose achieved clear/almost clear hands vs. 8% of the corresponding placebo group ($p<0.001$). 48% of relapsing patients who again received the 10 mg dose achieved clear/almost clear hands vs. 10% of the corresponding placebo group ($p=0.1$). Patients who responded to treatment with placebo in the previous study also received placebo in this follow-up study. Many of these patients responded again to treatment with placebo (69.2%).

5.2 Pharmacokinetic properties

Absorption

The absorption of alitretinoin from the gastro-intestinal tract is variable and dose-proportional over the therapeutic range from 10-30mg. The absolute bioavailability of alitretinoin has not been determined. When alitretinoin is taken with food, the systemic exposure is enhanced by a factor of 4 and the variability of exposure is decreased. Therefore, alitretinoin should be taken with a meal.

Distribution

Alitretinoin strongly binds to plasma proteins. The volume of distribution of alitretinoin in man has not been determined, but animal studies indicate a volume of distribution greater than the extracellular volume.

Metabolism

Alitretinoin is metabolised by oxidation in the liver by CYP3A4 isoenzymes into 4-oxo-alitretinoin. Both compounds undergo isomerisation into all-trans retinoic acid and 4-oxo-all-trans retinoic acid. After oral administration, the contribution of the metabolites in plasma to the systemic exposure of alitretinoin is approximately 35% to 80% for 4-oxo-alitretinoin. The major metabolite 4-oxo-alitretinoin is further glucuronidated and eliminated in urine. Alitretinoin is degraded similarly to vitamin A by sequential cleavage of the carbon-side chain.

During a 12-to 24-week treatment period with 10 or 30mg, the exposure to alitretinoin remained stable.

Elimination

Alitretinoin is an endogenous retinoid. Alitretinoin concentrations return to normal range within 1 to 3 days after treatment cessation.

Excretion of radio-labelled alitretinoin was complete with approximately 94% of the dose recovered. Radio-labelled material was eliminated mainly in urine and a smaller fraction (approx. 30%) in faeces. The most abundant excretion compound is the glucuronide of 4-oxo-alitretinoin amounting to 6.5% of the dose in urine.

Elimination half-life of unchanged alitretinoin ranges between 2 to 10 hours. Alitretinoin and its 4-oxo-metabolite do not accumulate.

Pharmacokinetic in special populations

In a pharmacokinetic study in patients, gender, weight and age did not affect the pharmacokinetics of alitretinoin.

The pharmacokinetics of alitretinoin in CHE patients was similar to that in healthy volunteers.

Alitretinoin kinetics have not been studied in patients with hepatic or with severe renal insufficiency or in patients below 18 years (see section 4.3).

5.3 Preclinical safety data

Acute toxicity

As with other retinoids, the acute toxicity of alitretinoin was low in mice and rats. The LD_{50} after intraperitoneal administration was >4000 mg/kg after 24 hours and 1400 mg/kg after 10 days. The approximate LD_{50} after oral administration in rats was 3000 mg/kg.

Chronic toxicity

Alitretinoin was tested in long-term studies up to 9 months in dogs and 6 months in rats. Signs of toxicity were dose-related and occurred at exposures similar to the human

Table 2 Primary Efficacy Parameter - Results

	Alitretinoin		
Primary Endpoint	**10 mg**	**30 mg**	**Placebo**
ITT Population	**N=418**	**N=409**	**N=205**
PGA at end of study			
Total Response Rate	115 (27.5%)	195 (47.7%)	34 (16.6%)
Clear	39 (9.3%)	90 (22.0%)	6 (2.9%)
Almost clear	76 (18.2%)	105 (25.7%)	28 (13.7%)
Comparison to placebo	P=0.004	P=<0.001	N/A

Table 3 Response rate by CHE subtype

CHE subtype (% of ITT population)	Hyperkeratotic (64%)	Hyperkeratotic / Pompholyx (22%)	Pompholyx (5%)
Response rate (PGA)	30mg: 54% 10 mg: 30% Placebo: 12%	30mg: 33% 10 mg: 23% Placebo: 12%	30mg: 33% 10 mg: 22% Placebo: 30%

Table 4 Secondary Efficacy Parameters - Results

	Alitretinoin		
Efficacy Variable	**10 mg**	**30 mg**	**Placebo**
ITT Population	**N=418**	**N=409**	**N=205**
Partial Response Rate (clear, almost clear or mild disease)	207 (49.5%)	254 (62.1%)	74 (36.1%)
PaGA (clear or almost clear)	101 (24.2%)	163 (39.9%)	31 (15.1%)
mTLSS (mean % change from baseline)	-50.79 (n=411)	-60.80 (n=408)	-37.30 (n=204)
Extent of disease (mean % change from baseline)	-40.01 (n=402)	-54.15 (n=391)	-31.93 (n=197)

therapeutic exposure based on AUC. Effects were characteristic for retinoids (consistent with hypervitaminosis A), and were generally spontaneously reversible.

Teratogenicity

Like other retinoids, alitretinoin has been shown to be teratogenic *in vitro* and *in vivo*.

Due to the teratogenic potential of alitretinoin, women of childbearing potential must adhere to strict pregnancy prevention measurers during and 1 month following alitretinoin therapy (see section 4.3 "Contraindications", section 4.4 "Special warnings and special precautions for use" and section 4.6 "Pregnancy and lactation").

Fertility

Alitretinoin was tested in a study of fertility and early embryonic development in rats. No effects on male or female reproductive parameters were observed at the highest dose tested. However, systemic exposure in this study did not reach the level observed in patients.

As with other retinoids reversible effects on male reproductive organs were observed in experimental animals in the form of disturbed spermatogenesis and associated degenerative lesions of the testes. The safety margin in dogs with regard to the no-effect level of toxicity to male reproductive organs was 1-6 for a human dose of 30mg.

Mutagenicity

In *in vitro* or *in vivo* tests, alitretinoin has been shown not to be mutagenic.

Carcinogenicity

Alitretinoin was tested in 2-year carcinogenicity studies in rats and mice. Dose-related retinoid-specific toxicity was seen at higher doses, but no carcinogenic potential was noted.

Phototoxicity

Alitretinoin was found to be phototoxic *in vitro* and *in vivo*.

6. PHARMACEUTICAL PARTICULARS

6.1 List of excipients

Capsule content:

Soya-bean oil, refined

Partially hydrogenated soya-bean oil

Triglycerides, medium chain

Beeswax, yellow

All-rac-α-tocopherol

Capsule shell:

Gelatin

Glycerol

Sorbitol, liquid (non-crystallising)

Water purified

Iron oxide (E 172)

6.2 Incompatibilities

Not applicable

6.3 Shelf life

3 years

6.4 Special precautions for storage

Store in the original package. Keep the blister in the outer carton to protect from light.

6.5 Nature and contents of container

PVC/PE/PVDC/Aluminum or COC (cycloolefin copolymer)/ Aluminum blisters. Pack sizes of 30 capsules

6.6 Special precautions for disposal and other handling

Any unused product or waste material should be disposed in accordance with local requirements.

7. MARKETING AUTHORISATION HOLDER

Basilea Medical Ltd, 14/16 Frederick Sanger Road, The Surrey Research Park, Guildford, Surrey GU2 7YD

8. MARKETING AUTHORISATION NUMBER(S)

10mg, 30 capsules PL 32205/0001

30mg, 30 capsules PL 32205/0002

9. DATE OF FIRST AUTHORISATION/RENEWAL OF THE AUTHORISATION

5 SEPTEMBER 2008

10. DATE OF REVISION OF THE TEXT

5 SEPTEMBER 2008

Topamax 25 mg, 50mg, 100mg, 200mg Tablets and Sprinkle Capsules 15, 25 or 50 mg.

(Janssen-Cilag Ltd)

1. NAME OF THE MEDICINAL PRODUCT

TOPAMAX®▼ 25 mg Tablets

TOPAMAX®▼ 50 mg Tablets

TOPAMAX®▼ 100 mg Tablets

TOPAMAX®▼ 200 mg Tablets

TOPAMAX®▼ Sprinkle Capsules 15, 25 or 50 mg.

2. QUALITATIVE AND QUANTITATIVE COMPOSITION

Each tablet contains 25, 50, 100 and 200 mg of topiramate.

Topamax Sprinkle Capsules contain topiramate 15, 25 or 50 mg.

For excipients see Section 6.1.

3. PHARMACEUTICAL FORM

Topamax Tablets are available as engraved, round, film-coated tablets in the following strengths and colours: 25 mg - white, 50 mg – light - yellow, 100 mg - yellow, 200 mg - salmon. The tablets are engraved as follows:

25 mg "TOP" on one side; "25" on the other

50 mg "TOP" on one side; "50" on the other

100 mg "TOP" on one side; "100" on the other

200 mg "TOP" on one side; "200" on the other

Topamax Sprinkle Capsules are available as hard gelatin capsules containing topiramate in coated beads.

4. CLINICAL PARTICULARS

4.1 Therapeutic indications

Epilepsy

Topamax is indicated as monotherapy in adults and children aged 6 years and above with newly diagnosed epilepsy who have generalised tonic-clonic seizures or partial seizures with or without secondarily generalised seizures.

Topamax is indicated as adjunctive therapy for adults and children over 2 years of age who are inadequately controlled on conventional first line antiepileptic drugs for: partial seizures with or without secondarily generalised seizures; seizures associated with Lennox Gastaut Syndrome and primary generalised tonic-clonic seizures.

The efficacy and safety of conversion from adjunctive therapy to Topamax monotherapy has not been demonstrated.

Migraine

Topamax is indicated in adults for the prophylaxis of migraine headache. Initiation of treatment with topiramate should be restricted to specialist care and treatment should be managed under specialist supervision or shared care arrangements.

Prophylactic treatment of migraine may be considered in situations such as: Adults experiencing three or more migraine attacks per month; frequent migraine attacks that significantly interfere with the patient's daily routine.

Continuing therapy should be reviewed every six months.

The usefulness of Topamax in the acute treatment of migraine has not been studied.

4.2 Posology and method of administration

4.2.1 General

For optimal seizure control in both adults and children, it is recommended that therapy be initiated at a low dose followed by titration to an effective dose.

Tablets should not be broken. Topamax can be taken without regard to meals.

Topamax Sprinkle Capsules may be swallowed whole or may be administered by carefully opening the capsule and sprinkling the entire contents on a small amount (teaspoon) of soft food e.g. apple sauce, mashed banana, ice cream or yoghurts. This drug/food mixture should be swallowed immediately and not chewed. It should not be stored for future use.

It is not necessary to monitor topiramate plasma concentrations to optimise Topamax therapy.

The dosing recommendations apply to children and to all adults, including the elderly, in the absence of underlying renal disease. (See 4.4 Special warnings and special precautions for use.)

Since Topamax is removed from plasma by haemodialysis, a supplemental dose of Topamax equal to approximately one-half the daily dose should be administered on haemodialysis days. The supplemental dose should be administered in divided doses at the beginning and completion of the haemodialysis procedure. The supplemental dose may differ based on the characteristics of the dialysis equipment being used.

4.2.2 Epilepsy

a) Monotherapy

Adults and children over 16 years

Titration should begin at 25 mg nightly for 1 week. The dosage should then be increased at 1- or 2-week intervals by increments of 25 or 50 mg/day, administered in two divided doses. If the patient is unable to tolerate the titration regimen, smaller increments or longer intervals between increments can be used. Dose and titration rate should be guided by clinical outcome.

The recommended initial target dose for topiramate monotherapy in adults with newly diagnosed epilepsy is 100 mg/day and the maximum recommended daily dose is 400 mg. These dosing recommendations apply to all adults including the elderly in the absence of underlying renal disease.

Children aged 6-16 years

Treatment of children aged 6 years and above should begin at 0.5 to 1 mg/kg nightly for the first week. The dosage should then be increased at 1- or 2-week intervals by increments of 0.5 to 1 mg/kg/day, administered in two divided doses. If the child is unable to tolerate the titration regimen, smaller increments or longer intervals between dose increments can be used. Dose and dose titration rate should be guided by clinical outcome.

The recommended initial target dose range for topiramate monotherapy in children with newly diagnosed epilepsy aged 6 years and above is 3 to 6 mg/kg/day. Higher doses have been tolerated and rarely doses up to 16 mg/kg/day have been given.

The tablet formulations are not appropriate for children requiring doses of less than 25 mg/day. A suitable formulation (eg Topamax Sprinkle Capsules) should be prescribed.

b) Adjunctive Therapy

Adults and children over 16 years

The minimal effective dose as adjunctive therapy is 200 mg per day. The usual total daily dose is 200 mg to 400 mg in two divided doses. Some patients may require doses up to 800 mg per day, which is the maximum recommended dose. It is recommended that therapy be initiated at a low dose, followed by titration to an effective dose.

Titration should begin at 25 mg daily for one week. The total daily dose should then be increased by 25-50 mg increments at one to two weekly intervals and should be taken in two divided doses. If the patient is unable to tolerate the titration regimen then lower increments or longer intervals between increments may be used. Dose titration should be guided by clinical outcome.

Children aged 2 - 16 years

The recommended total daily dose of Topamax (topiramate) as adjunctive therapy is approximately 5 to 9 mg/kg/day in two divided doses. Titration should begin at 25 mg nightly for the first week. The dosage should then be increased at 1- or 2-week intervals by increments of 1 to 3 mg/kg/day (administered in two divided doses), to achieve optimal clinical response. Dose titration should be guided by clinical outcome.

Daily doses up to 30 mg/kg/day have been studied and were generally well tolerated.

4.2.3 Migraine

Adults and children over 16 years

Titration should begin at 25 mg nightly for 1 week. The dosage should then be increased in increments of 25 mg/day administered at 1-week intervals. If the patient is unable to tolerate the titration regimen, longer intervals between dose adjustments can be used.

The recommended total daily dose of topiramate as treatment for the prophylaxis of migraine headache is 100 mg/day administered in two divided doses. Some patients may experience a benefit at a total daily dose of 50 mg/day. No extra benefit has been demonstrated from the administration of doses higher than 100 mg/day. Dose and titration rate should be guided by clinical outcome.

Children

Topamax in migraine prophylaxis has not been studied in children under 16 years.

4.3 Contraindications

Hypersensitivity to any component of this product.

4.4 Special warnings and precautions for use

4.4.1 General

In patients with or without a history of seizures or epilepsy, antiepileptic drugs, including Topamax, should be gradually withdrawn to minimise the potential for seizures or increased seizure frequency. In clinical trials, daily dosages were decreased in weekly intervals by 50-100 mg in adults with epilepsy and by 25-50 mg in adults receiving Topamax at doses up to 100 mg/day for migraine prophylaxis. In clinical trials of children, Topamax was gradually withdrawn over a 2-8 week period. In situations where rapid withdrawal of Topamax is medically required, appropriate monitoring is recommended.

The major route of elimination of unchanged topiramate and its metabolites is via the kidney. Renal elimination is dependent on renal function and is independent of age. Patients with moderate or severe renal impairment may take 10 to 15 days to reach steady-state plasma concentrations as compared to 4 to 8 days in patients with normal renal function.

As with all patients, the titration schedule should be guided by clinical outcome (e.g. seizure control, avoidance of side effects, prophylaxis of migraine headache) with the knowledge that subjects with known renal impairment may require a longer time to reach steady state at each dose.

Some patients, especially those with a predisposition to nephrolithiasis, may be at increased risk for renal stone formation and associated signs and symptoms such as renal colic, renal pain or flank pain. Adequate hydration whilst using topiramate is very important as it can reduce the risk of developing renal stones. In addition, it may reduce the risk of heat-related adverse events during exercise and exposure to particularly warm environments (see section 4.8).

Risk factors for nephrolithiasis include prior stone formation, a family history of nephrolithiasis and hypercalciuria. None of these risk factors can reliably predict stone formation during topiramate treatment. In addition, patients taking other medication associated with nephrolithiasis may be at increased risk.

In hepatically impaired patients, topiramate should be administered with caution as the clearance of topiramate may be decreased.

Depression and mood alterations have been reported in patients treated with topiramate.

Suicidal ideation and behaviour have been reported in patients treated with anti-epileptic agents in several indications. A meta-analysis of randomised placebo controlled trials of anti-epileptic drugs has also shown a small increased risk of suicidal ideation and behaviour. The mechanism of this risk is not known and the available data do not exclude the possibility of an increased risk for topiramate.

In double blind clinical trials, suicide related events (SREs) (suicidal ideation, suicide attempts and suicide) occurred at a frequency of 0.5% in topiramate treated patients (43 out of 7,999 patients treated) and at a 3 fold higher incidence than in those treated with placebo (0.15%; 5 out of 3,150 patients treated).

Therefore patients should be monitored for signs of suicidal ideation and behaviours and appropriate treatment should be considered. Patients (and caregivers of patients) should be advised to seek medical advice should signs of suicidal ideation or behaviour emerge.

In accordance with good clinical practice, patients with a history of depression and/or suicidal behaviour, adolescents and young adults may be at a greater risk of suicidal thoughts or suicide attempts, and should receive careful monitoring during treatment.

Acute myopia with secondary angle-closure glaucoma has been reported rarely in both children and adults receiving Topamax. Symptoms typically occur within 1 month of the start of treatment and include decreased visual acuity and/or ocular pain. Ophthalmological findings include bilateral myopia, anterior chamber shallowing, hyperaemia and increased intra-ocular pressure with or without mydriasis. There may be supraciliary effusion resulting in anterior displacement of the lens and iris. Treatment includes discontinuation of Topamax as rapidly as is clinically feasible and appropriate measures to reduce intraocular pressure. These measures generally result in a decrease in intraocular pressure. If increased intraocular pressure is suspected, immediate specialist advice should be sought.

Metabolic Acidosis: Hyperchloraemic, non-anion gap, metabolic acidosis (ie decreased serum bicarbonate below the normal reference range in the absence of respiratory alkalosis) is associated with topiramate treatment. This decrease in serum bicarbonate is due to the inhibitory effect of topiramate on renal carbonic anhydrase. Generally, the decrease in bicarbonate occurs early in treatment although it can occur at any time during treatment. These decreases are usually mild to moderate (average decrease of 4 mmol/L at doses of 100 mg/day or above in adults and at approximately 6 mg/kg/day in paediatric patients). Rarely, patients have experienced decreases to values below 10 mmol/L. Conditions or therapies that predispose to acidosis (such as renal disease, severe respiratory disorders, status epilepticus, diarrhoea, surgery, ketogenic diet, or certain drugs) may be additive to the bicarbonate lowering effects of topiramate.

Chronic metabolic acidosis in paediatric patients can reduce growth rates. The effect of topiramate on growth and bone-related sequelae has not been systematically investigated in paediatric or adult populations.

Depending on underlying conditions, appropriate evaluation including serum bicarbonate levels is recommended with topiramate therapy. If metabolic acidosis develops and persists, consideration should be given to reducing the dose or discontinuing topiramate (using dose tapering).

A dietary supplement or increased food intake may be considered if the patient is losing weight or has inadequate weight gain while on this medication.

Patients with rare hereditary problems of galactose intolerance, the Lapp lactase deficiency or glucose-galactose malabsorption should not take this medicine.

4.4.2 Migraine Prophylaxis

In migraine prophylaxis, before discontinuation of treatment, dosage should be gradually reduced over at least 2 weeks to minimise the possibility of rebound migraine headaches.

Weight loss

During the double-blind treatment with topiramate 100 mg/day, the mean change from baseline to the final visit in body weight was -2.5 kg, compared to -0.1 kg in the placebo group. Overall, 68% of patients treated with topiramate 100 mg/day lost weight during the trials, compared to 33% of patients receiving placebo. Weight decrease was reported as an adverse event in 1% of all placebo-treated patients and in 9% of all patients receiving topiramate 100 mg/day.

Significant weight loss may occur during long-term topiramate treatment for migraine prophylaxis. In clinical studies of topiramate 100 mg in migraine prophylaxis, a continuing weight decrease was observed with a mean weight decrease of 5.5 kg over 20 months. Twenty-five per cent of patients treated with topiramate for migraine prophylaxis had a weight loss of ⩾ 10% of their body weight.

It is recommended that patients on long term topiramate for migraine prophylaxis should be regularly weighed and monitored for continuing weight loss.

4.5 Interaction with other medicinal products and other forms of interaction

For purposes of this section, a no effect dose is defined as a ⩽ 15% change.

Effects of Topamax on Other Antiepileptic Drugs

The addition of Topamax to other antiepileptic drugs (phenytoin, carbamazepine, valproic acid, phenobarbital, primidone) has no clinically significant effect on their steady-state plasma concentrations, except in some patients where the addition of Topamax to phenytoin may result in an increase of plasma concentrations of phenytoin. Consequently, it is advised that any patient on phenytoin should have phenytoin levels monitored.

A pharmacokinetic interaction study of patients with epilepsy indicated the addition of topiramate to lamotrigine had no effect on steady state plasma concentration of lamotrigine at topiramate doses of 100 to 400 mg/day. In addition, there was no change in steady state plasma concentration of topiramate during or after removal of lamotrigine treatment (mean dose of 327 mg/day).

Effects of Other Antiepileptic Drugs on Topamax

Phenytoin and carbamazepine decrease the plasma concentration of topiramate. The addition or withdrawal of phenytoin or carbamazepine to Topamax therapy may require an adjustment in dosage of the latter. This should be done by titrating to clinical effect.

The addition or withdrawal of valproic acid does not produce clinically significant changes in plasma concentrations of topiramate and, therefore, does not warrant dosage adjustment of Topamax.

The results of these interactions are summarised in the following table:

AED Coadministered	AED Concentration	Topiramate Concentration
Phenytoin	↔**	↓
Carbamazepine (CBZ)	↔	↓
Valproic Acid	↔	↔
Lamotrigine	↔	↔
Phenobarbital	↔	NS
Primidone	↔	NS

↔ = No effect on plasma concentration (⩽ 15% change)

** = Plasma concentrations increase in some patients

↓ = Plasma concentrations decrease

NS = Not studied

AED = antiepileptic drug

Other Drug Interactions

Digoxin: In a single-dose study, serum digoxin area under plasma concentration curve (AUC) decreased 12% due to concomitant administration of Topamax. The clinical relevance of this observation has not been established. When Topamax is added or withdrawn in patients on digoxin therapy, careful attention should be given to the routine monitoring of serum digoxin.

CNS Depressants: Concomitant administration of Topamax and alcohol or other CNS depressant drugs has not been evaluated in clinical studies. Because of the potential of topiramate to cause CNS depression, as well as other cognitive and/or neuropsychiatric adverse events, topiramate should be used with caution if used in combination with alcohol and other CNS depressants.

Oral Contraceptives: In an interaction study with a combined oral contraceptive, Topamax increased plasma clearance of the oestrogenic component significantly. Consequently, and bearing in mind the potential risk of teratogenicity, patients should receive a preparation containing not less than 50 μg of oestrogen or use some alternative non-hormonal method of contraception. Patients taking oral contraceptives should be asked to report any change in their bleeding patterns.

Lithium: In healthy volunteers, there was an observed reduction (18% for AUC) in systemic exposure for lithium during concomitant administration with topiramate 200 mg/day. In patients with bipolar disorder, the pharmacokinetics of lithium were unaffected during treatment with topiramate at doses of 200 mg/day; however, there was an observed increase in systemic exposure (26% for AUC) following topiramate doses of up to 600 mg/day. Lithium levels should be monitored when co-administered with topiramate.

Hydrochlorothiazide (HCTZ): A drug-drug interaction study conducted in healthy volunteers evaluated the steady-state pharmacokinetics of HCTZ (25 mg q24h) and topiramate (96 mg q12h) when administered alone and concomitantly. The results of this study indicate that topiramate C_{max} increased by 27% and AUC increased by 29% when HCTZ was added to topiramate. The clinical significance of this change is unknown. The addition of HCTZ to topiramate therapy may require an adjustment of the topiramate dose. The steady-state pharmacokinetics of HCTZ were not significantly influenced by the concomitant administration of topiramate. Clinical laboratory results indicated decreases in serum potassium after topiramate or HCTZ administration, which were greater when HCTZ and topiramate were administered in combination.

Metformin: A drug-drug interaction study conducted in healthy volunteers evaluated the steady-state pharmacokinetics of metformin 500mg bd and topiramate 100mg bd in plasma when metformin was given alone and when metformin and topiramate were given simultaneously. The results of this study indicated that metformin mean C_{max} and mean $AUC_{0\text{-}12h}$ increased by 18% and 25%, respectively, while mean CL/F decreased 20% when metformin was co-administered with topiramate. Topiramate did not affect metformin t_{max}. The clinical significance of the effect of topiramate on metformin pharmacokinetics is unclear. Oral plasma clearance of topiramate appears to be reduced when administered with metformin. The extent of change in the clearance is unknown. The clinical significance of the effect of metformin on topiramate pharmacokinetics is unclear. When Topamax is added or withdrawn in patients on metformin therapy, careful attention should be given to the routine monitoring for adequate control of their diabetic disease state.

Pioglitazone: A drug-drug interaction study conducted in healthy volunteers evaluated the steady-state pharmacokinetics of topiramate and pioglitazone when administered alone and concomitantly. A 15% decrease in the $AUC_{\tau,ss}$ of pioglitazone with no alteration in $C_{max,ss}$ was observed. This finding was not statistically significant. In addition, a 13% and 16% decrease in $C_{max,ss}$ and $AUC_{\tau,ss}$ respectively, of the active hydroxy-metabolite was noted as well as a 60% decrease in $C_{max,ss}$ and $AUC_{\tau,ss}$ of the active keto-metabolite. The clinical significance of these findings is not known. When Topamax is added to pioglitazone therapy or pioglitazone is added to Topamax therapy, careful attention should be given to the routine monitoring of patients for adequate control of their diabetic disease state.

Glibenclamide: A drug-drug interaction study conducted in patients with type 2 diabetes evaluated the steady-state pharmacokinetics of glibenclamide (5mg/day) alone and concomitantly with topiramate (150 mg/day). There was a 25% reduction in glibenclamide AUC_{24} during topiramate administration. Systemic exposure of the active metabolites, 4-*trans*-hydroxy-glibenclamide (M1) and 3-*cis*-hydroxyglibenclamide (M2), were also reduced by 13% and 15%, respectively. The steady-state pharmacokinetics of topiramate were unaffected by concomitant administration of glibenclamide. When topiramate is added to glibenclamide therapy or glibenclamide is added to topiramate therapy, careful attention should be given to the routine monitoring of patients for adequate control of their diabetic disease state.

Other forms of interactions:

Agents predisposing to nephrolithiasis

Topamax, when used concomitantly with other agents predisposing to nephrolithiasis, may increase the risk of nephrolithiasis. While using Topamax, agents like these should be avoided since they may create a physiological environment that increases the risk of renal stone formation. The interaction with benzodiazepines has not been studied.

Valproic Acid: Concomitant administration of topiramate and valproic acid has been associated with hyperammonemia with or without encephalopathy in patients who have tolerated either drug alone. In most cases, symptoms and signs abated with discontinuation of either drug. This adverse event is not due to a pharmacokinetic interaction.

An association of hyperammonemia with topiramate monotherapy or concomitant treatment with other antiepileptics has not been established.

Additional Pharmacokinetic Drug Interaction Studies: Clinical studies have been conducted to assess the potential pharmacokinetic drug interaction between topiramate and other agents. The changes in C_{max} or AUC as a result of the interactions are summarized below. The second column (concomitant drug concentration) describes what happens to the concentration of the concomitant drug listed in the first column when topiramate is added. The third column (topiramate concentration) describes how the coadministration of a drug listed in the first column modifies the concentration of topiramate.

Summary of Results from Additional Clinical Pharmacokinetic Drug Interaction Studies

Concomitant Drug	Concomitant Drug Concentration[a]	Topiramate Concentration[a]
Amitriptyline	↔ 20% increase in C_{max} and AUC of nortriptyline metabolite	NS
Dihydroergotamine (Oral and Subcutaneous)	↔	↔
Haloperidol	↔ 31% increase in AUC of the reduced metabolite	NS
Propranolol	↔ 17% increase in C_{max} for 4-OH propranolol (TPM 50 mg q12h)	16% increase in C_{max}, 17% increase in AUC (80 mg propranolol q12h)
Sumatriptan (Oral and Subcutaneous)	↔	NS
Pizotifen	↔	↔

[a] % values are the changes in treatment mean C_{max} or AUC with respect to monotherapy

↔ = No effect on C_{max} and AUC (≤ 15% change) of the parent compound

NS = Not studied

Interaction studies showed that Topamax did not significantly alter the serum levels of amitriptyline, propranolol or dihydroergotamine mesylate. The combination of Topamax with each of these drugs was well tolerated and no dose adjustments were necessary.

Laboratory Tests:

Clinical trial data indicates that topiramate has been associated with an average decrease of 4 mmol/L in the serum bicarbonate level (see Section 4.4 Special warnings and special precautions for use Metabolic Acidosis).

4.6 Pregnancy and lactation

Topiramate was teratogenic in mice, rats and rabbits. In rats, topiramate crosses the placental barrier.

There are no studies using Topamax in pregnant women. However, Topamax should not be used during pregnancy unless, in the opinion of the physician, the potential benefit outweighs the potential risk to the foetus.

Before starting Topamax, women of childbearing potential should be fully informed of the possible effects of Topamax on the unborn foetus and the risks should be discussed with the patient in relation to the benefits of Topamax treatment in migraine prophylaxis.

In post-marketing experience, hypospadias has been reported in male infants exposed in-utero to topiramate, with or without other anticonvulsants; however, a causal relationship with topiramate has not been established.

It is recommended that women of child bearing potential use adequate contraception.

Topiramate is excreted in the milk of lactating rats. The excretion of topiramate in human milk has not been evaluated in controlled studies. Limited observations in patients suggests an extensive excretion of topiramate into breast milk. Topamax should not be used during breast feeding.

4.7 Effects on ability to drive and use machines

Topamax can produce central nervous system related adverse events and may be more sedative than other antiepileptic drugs. Drowsiness is a likelihood. In addition, there have been reports of visual disturbances/blurred vision. Patients should be warned of these and advised that if affected, they should not drive, operate machinery and/or take part in activities where such reactions could put themselves or others at risk.

4.8 Undesirable effects

Reported adverse events were classified using a modified WHO-ART dictionary. The majority of the most common adverse events in clinical trials were mild-moderate in severity and dose-related. These dose-related adverse events typically began in the titration phase and often persisted into the maintenance phase but infrequently began in the maintenance phase. Rapid titration rate and higher initial dose were associated with higher incidences of adverse events leading to discontinuation.

4.8.1 Epilepsy

a) Monotherapy

Qualitatively, the types of adverse events observed in monotherapy trials were generally similar to those observed during adjunctive therapy trials (see below). With the exception of paraesthesia and fatigue in adults, these adverse events were reported at similar or lower incidence rates in monotherapy trials.

Adults:

In double-blind monotherapy clinical trials, the most common adverse events, i.e., those occurring in 10% or more of the topiramate-treated adult patients were paraesthesia, headache, fatigue, dizziness, somnolence, weight decrease, nausea and anorexia.

Adverse events occurring at 5% or more but less than 10% included: insomnia, difficulty with memory, depression, difficulty with concentration/attention, abdominal pain, nervousness, hypoaesthesia, mood problems and anxiety.

Children:

In double-blind monotherapy clinical trials, the most common adverse events, i.e., those occurring in 10% or more of the topiramate-treated children were headache, anorexia and somnolence.

Adverse events occurring at 5% or more but less than 10% included: difficulty with concentration/attention, fatigue, weight decrease, dizziness, paraesthesia, insomnia and nervousness.

b) Adjunctive Therapy

Adults:

Since Topamax has most frequently been co-administered with other antiepileptic agents, it is not possible to determine which agents, if any, are associated with adverse effects. In double blind clinical trials, some of which included a rapid titration period, adverse events which occurred with a frequency greater than or equal to 5% and with a higher incidence in the topiramate-treated adult patients than in placebo included: abdominal pain, ataxia, anorexia, asthenia, confusion, difficulty with concentration/attention, difficulty with memory, diplopia, dizziness, fatigue, language problems, nausea, nystagmus, paraesthesia, psychomotor slowing, somnolence, speech disorders/related speech problems, abnormal vision and weight decrease. Topamax may cause agitation and emotional lability (which may manifest mood problems and nervousness) and depression. Other less common adverse effects include, gait abnormal, aggressive reaction, apathy, cognitive problems, co-ordination problems, leucopenia, psychotic symptoms (such as hallucinations) and taste perversion.

Isolated cases of venous thromboembolic events have been reported. A causal association with the drug has not been established.

Reports of increases in liver enzymes in patients taking Topamax with and without other medications have been received. Isolated reports have been received of hepatitis and hepatic failure occurring in patients taking multiple medications while being treated with Topamax.

Children

In double blind clinical trials, some of which included a rapid titration period, adverse events which occurred with a frequency greater than or equal to 5% and with a higher incidence in the topiramate-treated children than in placebo included: somnolence, anorexia, fatigue, insomnia, nervousness, personality disorder (behaviour problems), difficulty with concentration/attention, aggressive reaction, weight decrease, gait abnormal, mood problems, ataxia, saliva increased, nausea, difficulty with memory, hyperkinesia, dizziness, speech disorders/related speech problems and paraesthesia.

Adverse events that occurred less frequently but were considered potentially medically relevant included: emotional lability, agitation, apathy, cognitive problems, psychomotor slowing, confusion, hallucination, depression and leucopenia.

4.8.2 Migraine prophylaxis

In double-blind clinical trials, clinically relevant adverse events which occurred at a frequency of 5% or more and seen at a higher incidence in topiramate-treated patients than placebo-treated patients included: fatigue, paraesthesia, dizziness, hypoaesthesia, language problems, nausea, diarrhoea, dyspepsia, dry mouth, weight decrease, anorexia, somnolence, difficulty with memory, difficulty with concentration/attention, insomnia, anxiety, mood problems, depression, taste perversion, abnormal vision. Fifty per cent of patients in these trials experienced paraesthesia.

During 6-month double-blind treatment with topiramate 100 mg/day for migraine prophylaxis, weight decrease was reported as an adverse event in 1% of all placebo-treated patients and in 9% of all patients receiving topiramate 100 mg/day. Weight loss continued with long-term topiramate treatment (see Section 4.4 Special warnings and special precautions for use).

Children

The effect of Topamax in children less than 16 years old with migraine has not been studied.

4.8.3 Post-marketing and Other Experience

Adverse drug reactions from spontaneous reports during the worldwide post-marketing experience with TOPAMAX are included in Table below. The adverse drug reactions are ranked by frequency, using the following convention (all calculated per patient-years of estimated exposure):

Very common ≥ 1/10

Common ≥ 1/100 and < 1/10

Uncommon ≥ 1/1,000 and < 1/100

Rare ≥ 1/10,000 and < 1/1000

Very rare < 1/10,000

The frequencies provided below reflect reporting rates for adverse drug reactions from spontaneous reports, and do not represent more precise estimates that might be obtained in clinical or experimental studies.

Topamax increases the risk of nephrolithiasis especially in those with a predisposition (see 4.4 Special warnings and special precautions for use). In the initial clinical trials none of the calculi required open surgery and three-quarters were passed spontaneously. Most of the patients opted to continue treatment despite nephrolithiasis.

Reduced sweating has been rarely reported. The majority of cases have been in children and some have been associated with flushing and raised temperature.

Very rarely, reports have been received for bullous skin and mucosal reactions (including erythema multiforme, pemphigus, Stevens-Johnson syndrome and toxic epidermal necrolysis). The majority of these reports have occurred in patients taking other medications also associated with bullous skin and mucosal reactions.

Post marketing reports of adverse drug reactions	
Blood and Lymphatic System Disorders	Very rare: leucopenia and neutropenia, thrombocytopenia
Metabolism and Nutrition Disorders	Rare: anorexia Very rare: metabolic acidosis (see section 4.4. Special warnings and Special precautions); decreased appetite, hyperammonemia (see section 4.5 Interactions with Other Medicinal Products and Other Forms of Interaction)
Psychiatric Disorders	Uncommon: suicidal ideation, attempts, and suicide (see section 4.4. Special warnings and Special precautions) Rare: depression (see section 4.4. Special warnings and Special precautions); agitation; somnolence
	Very rare: insomnia, confusional state, psychotic disorder, aggression, hallucination, expressive language disorder
Nervous System Disorders	Rare: paresthesia, convulsion, headache
	Very rare: speech disorder, dysgeusia, amnesia, memory impairment, drug withdrawal convulsion (see section 4.4. Special warnings and Special precautions)
Eye Disorders	Rare: visual disturbance, vision blurred Very rare: myopia, angle closure glaucoma (see section 4.4. Special warnings and Special precautions), eye pain
Gastrointestinal Disorders	Rare: nausea
	Very rare: diarrhoea, abdominal pain, vomiting
Skin and Subcutaneous Tissue Disorders	Rare: alopecia Very rare: rash
Renal and Urinary Disorders	Rare: nephrolithiasis (see section 4.4. Special warnings and Special precautions)
General Disorders and Administration Site Conditions	Rare: fatigue
	Very rare: pyrexia, feeling abnormal, asthenia
Investigations	Rare: weight decreased

4.9 Overdose

Signs and Symptoms

Overdoses of topiramate have been reported. Signs and symptoms included: convulsions, drowsiness, speech disturbances, blurred vision, diplopia, mentation impaired, lethargy, abnormal co-ordination, stupor, hypotension, abdominal pain, agitation, dizziness and depression. The clinical consequences were not severe in most cases, but deaths have been reported after polydrug overdoses involving topiramate.

Topiramate overdose can result in severe metabolic acidosis.

A patient who ingested a dose calculated to be between 96 and 110 g topiramate was admitted to hospital with coma lasting 20-24 hours followed by full recovery after 3 to 4 days.

Treatment

In acute topiramate overdose, if the ingestion is recent, the stomach should be emptied immediately by lavage or by induction of emesis. Activated charcoal has been shown to adsorb topiramate *in vitro*. Treatment should be appropriately supportive. Haemodialysis has been shown to be an effective means of removing topiramate from the body. The patient should be well hydrated.

5. PHARMACOLOGICAL PROPERTIES

5.1 Pharmacodynamic properties

Topiramate is classified as a sulphamate-substituted monosaccharide. Three pharmacological properties of topiramate have been identified that may contribute to its anticonvulsant activity:

Topiramate reduces the frequency at which action potentials are generated when neurones are subjected to a sustained depolarisation indicative of a state-dependent blockade of voltage-sensitive sodium channels.

Topiramate markedly enhances the activity of GABA at some types of GABA receptors but has no apparent effect on the activity of N-methyl-D-aspartate (NMDA) at the NMDA receptor subtype.

Topiramate weakly antagonises the excitatory activity of kainate/AMPA subtype of glutamate receptor.

In addition, topiramate inhibits some isoenzymes of carbonic anhydrase. This pharmacologic effect is much weaker than that of acetazolamide, a known carbonic anhydrase inhibitor, and is not thought to be a major component of topiramate's antiepileptic activity.

5.2 Pharmacokinetic properties

Topiramate is rapidly and well absorbed. Based on recovery of radioactivity from the urine, the mean extent of absorption of a 100 mg dose of ^{14}C topiramate was at least 81%. There is no clinically significant effect of food on topiramate. Generally 13-17% of topiramate is bound to plasma proteins. The mean apparent volume of distribution has been measured as 0.55-0.8 L/kg for single doses up to 1200 mg. There is an effect of gender on the volume of distribution. Values for females are circa 50% of those for males.

Topiramate is not extensively metabolised (≈20%) in healthy volunteers. Topiramate is metabolised up to 50% in patients receiving concomitant antiepileptic therapy with known inducers of drug metabolising enzymes. Six metabolites have been isolated, characterised and identified from plasma, urine and faeces of humans. Two metabolites, which retained most of the structure of topiramate, were tested and found to have little or no anticonvulsant activity.

In humans, the major route of elimination of unchanged topiramate and its metabolites is via the kidney. Overall, plasma clearance is approximately 20 to 30 mL/min in humans following oral administration.

Topiramate exhibits low intersubject variability in plasma concentrations and, therefore, has predictable pharmacokinetics. The pharmacokinetics of topiramate are linear with plasma clearance remaining constant and area under the plasma concentration curve increasing in a dose-proportional manner over a 100 to 400 mg single oral dose range in healthy subjects. Patients with normal renal function may take 4 to 8 days to reach steady-state plasma concentrations. The mean C_{max} following multiple, twice a day oral doses of 100 mg to healthy subjects was 6.76 μg/mL. Following administration of multiple doses of 50 mg and 100 mg of topiramate twice a day, the mean plasma elimination half-life was approximately 21 hours.

The plasma and renal clearance of topiramate are decreased in patients with impaired renal function ($CL_{CR} \leq 60$ mL/min), and the plasma clearance is decreased in patients with end-stage renal disease.

Plasma clearance of topiramate is unchanged in elderly subjects in the absence of underlying renal disease.

Plasma clearance of topiramate is decreased in patients with moderate to severe hepatic impairment.

The pharmacokinetics of topiramate in children, as in adults receiving add-on therapy, are linear, with clearance independent of dose and steady-state plasma concentrations increasing in proportion to dose. Children, however, have a higher clearance and shorter elimination half-life. Consequently, the plasma concentrations of topiramate for the same mg/kg dose may be lower in children compared to adults. As in adults, hepatic enzyme inducing anti-epileptic drugs decrease the steady-state plasma concentrations.

Topiramate modestly reduces the bioavailability of risperidone, but not that of the active antipsychotic fraction. Therefore, this interaction is unlikely to be of clinical significance.

Topiramate modestly reduces the bioavailability of diltiazem and one of its active metabolites. This is unlikely to be of clinical significance.

5.3 Preclinical safety data

Preclinical data reveal no special hazard for humans based on conventional studies of repeated dose toxicity and genotoxicity.

As with other antiepileptic drugs, topiramate was teratogenic in mice, rats and rabbits. Overall numbers of foetal malformations in mice were increased for all drug-treated groups, but no significant differences or dosage-response relationships were observed for overall or specific malformations, suggesting that other factors such as maternal toxicity may be involved.

6. PHARMACEUTICAL PARTICULARS

6.1 List of excipients

Topamax contains the following inactive ingredients:

Lactose monohydrate

Pregelatinized starch

Carnauba wax

Microcrystalline cellulose

Sodium starch glycolate

Magnesium stearate

OPADRY White, Yellow, Pink, Red depending on the colour

Contains:

hypromellose

titanium dioxide (E171)

macrogol 400

synthetic iron oxide

polysorbate 80.

Topamax Sprinkle Capsules contain the following inactive ingredients:

Sugar spheres

Povidone

Cellulose Acetate

Capsule Composition

Gelatin

Titanium dioxide (E171)

Silicon dioxide

Sodium lauryl sulphate

Ink Composition

OPACODE contains synthetic iron oxide, pharmaceutical glaze, n-butyl alcohol, alcohol, hypromellose, propylene glycol, ammonium hydroxide, simethicone and distilled water.

6.2 Incompatibilities

None known

6.3 Shelf life

Topamax Tablets: 36 months.

Topamax Sprinkle Capsules: 24 months.

6.4 Special precautions for storage

Topamax Tablets: Do not store above 25°C. Keep container tightly closed.

Topamax Sprinkle Capsules: Do not store above 25°C. Keep container tightly closed.

6.5 Nature and contents of container

Topamax Tablets: Available in high density polyethylene (HDPE) bottles with polypropylene (PP) child resistant closure, with a desiccant inserted into the cap. Each bottle contains 60 tablets.

Topamax Sprinkle Capsules: Available in opaque HDPE containers with tamper-evident closures containing 60 capsules. The closures consist of either an HDPE outer shell and polypropylene inner shell or polypropylene outer shell and LDPE inner shell.

6.6 Special precautions for disposal and other handling

Not applicable.

7. MARKETING AUTHORISATION HOLDER

Janssen–Cilag Ltd

50-100 Holmers Farm Way

High Wycombe

Buckinghamshire

HP12 4EG

UK

8. MARKETING AUTHORISATION NUMBER(S)

Topamax 25 mg Tablets PL 00242/0301

Topamax 50 mg Tablets PL 00242/0302

Topamax 100 mg Tablets PL 00242/0303

Topamax 200 mg Tablets PL 00242/0304

Topamax Sprinkle Capsules 15 mg PL 00242/0348

Topamax Sprinkle Capsules 25 mg PL 00242/0349

Topamax Sprinkle Capsules 50 mg PL 00242/0350

9. DATE OF FIRST AUTHORISATION/RENEWAL OF THE AUTHORISATION

Topamax Tablets: 18 July 1995 / 30 March 2005

Topamax Sprinkle Capsules: 17 February 1999 / 30 March 2005

10. DATE OF REVISION OF THE TEXT

Topamax Tablets: 10 December 2008

Topamax Sprinkle Capsules: 10 December 2008

Legal Category: POM

Toradol Injection

(Roche Products Limited)

1. NAME OF THE MEDICINAL PRODUCT

Toradol

2. QUALITATIVE AND QUANTITATIVE COMPOSITION

Toradol contains ketorolac trometamol 10mg or 30mg in ampoules of 1ml. It also contains ethanol, sodium chloride and water.

3. PHARMACEUTICAL FORM

Toradol is a clear, slightly yellow solution for intramuscular or bolus intravenous injection.

4. CLINICAL PARTICULARS

4.1 Therapeutic indications

Toradol is indicated for the short-term management of moderate to severe acute post-operative pain.

Treatment should only be initiated in hospitals. The maximum duration of treatment is two days.

4.2 Posology and method of administration

Toradol is for administration by intramuscular or bolus intravenous injection. Bolus intravenous doses should be given over no less than 15 seconds. Toradol should not be used for epidural or spinal administration.

The time to onset of analgesic effect following both IV and IM administration is similar and is approximately 30 minutes, with maximum analgesia occurring within one to two hours. The median duration of analgesia is generally four to six hours.

Dosage should be adjusted according to the severity of the pain and the patient response.

The administration of continuous multiple daily doses of ketorolac intramuscularly or intravenously should not exceed two days because adverse events may increase with prolonged usage. There has been limited experience with dosing for longer periods since the vast majority of patients have transferred to oral medication, or no longer require analgesic therapy after this time.

Undesirable effects may be minimised by using the lowest effective dose for the shortest duration necessary to control symptoms (see section 4.4).

Adults

The recommended initial dose of Toradol is 10mg, followed by 10 to 30mg every four to six hours as required. In the initial post-operative period, Toradol may be given as often as every two hours if needed. The lowest effective dose should be given. A total daily dose of 90mg for non-elderly and 60mg for the elderly, renally-impaired patients and patients less than 50kg should not be exceeded. The maximum duration of treatment should not exceed two days.

Reduce dosage in patients under 50kg.

Opioid analgesics (e.g. morphine, pethidine) may be used concomitantly, and may be required for optimal analgesic effect in the early post-operative period when pain is most severe. Ketorolac does not interfere with opioid binding and does not exacerbate opioid-related respiratory depression or sedation. When used in association with Toradol IM/IV, the daily dose of opioid is usually less than that normally required. However, opioid side-effects should still be considered, especially in day-case surgery.

For patients receiving parenteral Toradol, and who are converted to Toradol oral tablets, the total combined daily dose should not exceed 90mg (60mg for the elderly, renally-impaired patients and patients less than 50kg) and the oral component should not exceed 40mg on the day the change of formulation is made. Patients should be converted to oral treatment as soon as possible.

Elderly

The elderly are at increased risk of the serious consequences of adverse reactions. If an NSAID is considered necessary, the lowest effective dose should be used and for the shortest possible duration. The patient should be monitored regularly for GI bleeding during NSAID therapy.

A total daily dose of 60mg should not be exceeded (see section 4.4).

Children

Safety and efficacy in children have not been established. Therefore, Toradol is not recommended for use in children under 16 years of age.

Renal impairment

Contra-indicated in moderate to severe renal impairment; reduce dosage in lesser impairment (not exceeding 60mg/day IV or IM) (see section 4.3).

4.3 Contraindications

- active peptic ulcer or any history of gastrointestinal bleeding, ulceration or perforation

- severe heart failure, hepatic failure and renal failure (see section 4.4)
– suspected or confirmed cerebrovascular bleeding
– haemorrhagic diatheses, including coagulation disorders
– hypersensitivity to ketorolac trometamol or any of its ingredients, or other NSAIDs
– patients in whom ibuprofen, aspirin or other prostaglandin synthesis inhibitors induce allergic reactions e.g. asthma, rhinitis, angioedema, or urticaria (severe anaphylactic-like reactions have been observed in such patients)
– the complete or partial syndrome of nasal polyps, angioedema or bronchospasm
– concurrent treatment with other NSAIDs, (including cyclooxygenase-2 selective inhibitors), oxpentifylline, probenecid or lithium salts
– hypovolaemia from any cause or dehydration
– moderate or severe renal impairment (serum creatinine > 160 micromol/l)
– a history of asthma
– patients who have had operations with a high risk of haemorrhage or incomplete haemostasis
– patients on anti-coagulants including warfarin and low dose heparin (2500 - 5000 units twelve hourly)
– during pregnancy, labour, delivery or lactation (see section 4.6)
– children under 16 years of age
– Toradol is contra-indicated as prophylactic analgesia before surgery due to inhibition of platelet aggregation and is contra-indicated intra-operatively because of the increased risk of bleeding
– Toradol is contra-indicated in patients currently receiving aspirin.

4.4 Special warnings and precautions for use

Physicians should be aware that in some patients pain relief may not occur until upwards of 30 minutes after IV or IM administration.

Undesirable effects may be minimised by using the lowest effective dose for the shortest duration necessary to control symptoms (see section 4.2 and GI and cardiovascular risks below).

Use in the elderly: The elderly have an increased frequency of adverse reactions to NSAIDs especially gastrointestinal bleeding and perforation which may be fatal. This age-related risk is common to all NSAIDs. Compared to young adults, the elderly have an increased plasma half-life and reduced plasma clearance of ketorolac. With Toradol IM/IV, a total daily dose greater than 60mg is not recommended. With Toradol tablets, a longer dosing interval is advisable (see section 4.2).

Effects on fertility: The use of Toradol, as with any drug known to inhibit cyclo-oxygenase/prostaglandin synthesis may impair fertility and is not recommended in women attempting to conceive. In women who have difficulty conceiving or are undergoing investigation for fertility, withdrawal of Toradol should be considered.

Gastrointestinal bleeding, ulceration and perforation:

GI bleeding, ulceration or perforation, which can be fatal, has been reported with all NSAIDs at anytime during treatment, with or without warning symptoms or a previous history of serious GI events.

The risk of clinically serious gastro-intestinal bleeding is dose-dependent. This is particularly true in elderly patients who receive an average daily dose greater than 60mg/day of Toradol.

In a non-randomised, in-hospital post-marketing surveillance study, increased rates of clinically serious GI bleeding were seen in patients < 65 years of age who received an average daily dose of > 90mg ketorolac IM as compared to those patients receiving parenteral opioids.

Epidemiological evidence suggests that Ketorolac may be associated with a high risk of serious gastrointestinal toxicity, relative to some other NSAIDs, especially when used outside the licensed indications and/or for prolonged periods (see also section 4.1, 4.2 and 4.3).

The risk of GI bleeding, ulceration or perforation is higher with increasing NSAID doses, in patients with a history of ulcer, particularly if complicated with haemorrhage or perforation (see section 4.3), and in the elderly. These patients should commence treatment on the lowest dose available. Combination therapy with protective agents (e.g. misoprostol or proton pump inhibitors) should be considered for these patients, and also for patients requiring concomitant low dose aspirin, or other drugs likely to increase gastrointestinal risk (see below and section 4.5).

Patients with a history of GI toxicity, particularly when elderly, should report any unusual abdominal symptoms (especially GI bleeding) particularly in the initial stages of treatment.

Caution should be advised in patients receiving concomitant medications which could increase the risk of ulceration or bleeding, such as oral corticosteroids, selective serotonin-reuptake inhibitors or anti-platelet agents such as aspirin (see section 4.5).

Use in patients taking anticoagulants such as warfarin is contraindicated (see section 4.3).

When GI bleeding or ulceration occurs in patients receiving Ketorolac Trometamol, the treatment should be withdrawn.

NSAIDs should be given with care to patients with a history of gastrointestinal disease (ulcerative colitis, Crohn's disease) as these conditions may be exacerbated (see section 4.8).

Respiratory disorders: Caution is required if administered to patients suffering from, or with a previous history of, bronchial asthma since NSAIDs have been reported to precipitate bronchospasm in such patients.

Renal effects: Drugs that inhibit prostaglandin biosynthesis (including non-steroidal anti-inflammatory drugs) have been reported to cause nephrotoxicity, including but not limited to glomerular nephritis, interstitial nephritis, renal papillary necrosis, nephrotic syndrome and acute renal failure. In patients with renal, cardiac or hepatic impairment, caution is required since the use of NSAIDs may result in deterioration of renal function.

As with other drugs that inhibit prostaglandin synthesis, elevations of serum urea, creatinine and potassium have been reported with ketorolac trometamol and may occur after one dose.

Patients with impaired renal function: Since ketorolac trometamol and its metabolites are excreted primarily by the kidney, patients with moderate to severe impairment of renal function (serum creatinine greater than 160 micromol/l) should not receive Toradol. Patients with lesser renal impairment should receive a reduced dose of ketorolac (not exceeding 60mg/day IM or IV) and their renal status should be closely monitored.

Cardiovascular, Renal and Hepatic Impairment: Caution should be observed in patients with conditions leading to a reduction in blood volume and/or renal blood flow, where renal prostaglandins have a supportive role in the maintenance of renal perfusion. In these patients, administration of an NSAID may cause a dose-dependent reduction in renal prostaglandin formation and may precipitate overt renal failure. Patients at greatest risk of this reaction are those who are volume depleted because of blood loss or severe dehydration, patients with impaired renal function, heart failure, liver dysfunction, the elderly and those taking diuretics. Renal function should be monitored in these patients. Discontinuation of NSAID therapy is typically followed by recovery to the pre-treatment state. Inadequate fluid/blood replacement during surgery, leading to hypovolaemia, may lead to renal dysfunction which could be exacerbated when Toradol is administered. Therefore, volume depletion should be corrected and close monitoring of serum urea and creatinine and urine output is recommended until the patient is normovolaemic. In patients on renal dialysis, ketorolac clearance was reduced to approximately half the normal rate and terminal half-life increased approximately three-fold (see section 4.3).

Fluid retention and oedema: Fluid retention and oedema have been reported with the use of Toradol and it should therefore be used with caution in patients with cardiac decompensation, hypertension or similar conditions.

Cardiovascular and cerebrovascular effects

Appropriate monitoring and advice are required for patients with a history of hypertension and/or mild to moderate congestive heart failure as fluid retention and oedema have been reported in association with NSAID therapy.

Clinical trial and epidemiological data suggest that use of some NSAIDs (particularly at high doses and in long term treatment) may be associated with a small increased risk of arterial thrombotic events (for example myocardial infarction or stroke). There are insufficient data to exclude such a risk for Ketorolac Trometamol.

Patients with uncontrolled hypertension, congestive heart failure, established ischaemic heart disease, peripheral arterial disease, and/or cerebrovascular disease should only be treated with Ketorolac Trometamol after careful consideration. Similar consideration should be made before initiating longer-term treatment of patients with risk factors for cardiovascular disease (e.g. hypertension, hyperlipidaemia, diabetes mellitus, smoking).

SLE and mixed connective tissue disease:

In patients with systemic lupus erythematosus (SLE) and mixed connective tissue disorders there may be an increased risk of aseptic meningitis (see section 4.8).

Dermatological:

Serious skin reactions, some of them fatal, including exfoliative dermatitis, Stevens-Johnson syndrome, and toxic epidermal necrolysis, have been reported very rarely in association with the use of NSAIDs (see section 4.8). Patients appear to be at highest risk for these reactions early in the course of therapy: the onset of the reactions occurring in the majority of cases within the first month of treatment. Toradol should be discontinued at the first appearance of skin rash, mucosal lesions, or any other sign of hypersensitivity.

Use in patients with impaired liver function: Patients with impaired hepatic function from cirrhosis do not have any clinically important changes in ketorolac clearance or terminal half-life.

Borderline elevations of one or more liver function tests may occur. These abnormalities may be transient, may remain unchanged, or may progress with continued therapy. Meaningful elevations (greater than three times normal) of serum glutamate pyruvate transaminase (SGPT/ALT) or serum glutamate oxaloacetate transaminase (SGOT/AST) occurred in controlled clinical trials in less than 1% of patients. If clinical signs and symptoms consistent with liver disease develop, or if systemic manifestations occur, Toradol should be discontinued.

Haematological effects: Patients with coagulation disorders should not receive Toradol. Patients on anti-coagulation therapy may be at increased risk of bleeding if given Toradol concurrently. The concomitant use of ketorolac and prophylactic low-dose heparin (2500 - 5000 units twelve hourly) has not been studied extensively and may also be associated with an increased risk of bleeding. Patients already on anti-coagulants or who require low-dose heparin should not receive ketorolac. Patients who are receiving other drug therapy that interferes with haemostasis should be carefully observed if Toradol is administered. In controlled clinical studies, the incidence of clinically significant post-operative bleeding was less than 1%.

Ketorolac inhibits platelet aggregation and prolongs bleeding time. In patients with normal bleeding function, bleeding times were raised, but not outside the normal range of two to eleven minutes. Unlike the prolonged effects from aspirin, platelet function returns to normal within 24 to 48 hours after ketorolac is discontinued.

In post-marketing experience, post-operative wound haemorrhage has been reported in association with the immediate peri-operative use of Toradol IM/IV. Therefore, ketorolac should not be used in patients who have had operations with a high risk of haemorrhage or incomplete haemostasis. Caution should be used where strict haemostasis is critical, e.g. in cosmetic or day-case surgery. Haematomata and other signs of wound haemorrhage and epistaxis have been reported with the use of Toradol. Physicians should be aware of the pharmacological similarity of ketorolac to other non-steroidal anti-inflammatory drugs that inhibit cyclo-oxygenase and the risk of bleeding, particularly in the elderly.

Toradol is not an anaesthetic agent and possesses no sedative or anxiolytic properties; therefore it is not recommended as a pre-operative medication for the support of anaesthesia when these effects are required.

4.5 Interaction with other medicinal products and other forms of interaction

Ketorolac is highly bound to human plasma protein (mean 99.2%) and binding is concentration-independent.

The following medicinal products are NOT to be co-administered with Toradol:

Toradol should not be used with other NSAIDs including cyclooxygenase-2 selective inhibitors or in patients receiving aspirin because of the potential for adverse effects (see section 4.3).

Toradol is contraindicated in combination with anti-coagulants, such as warfarin since co-administration may cause an enhanced anti-coagulant effect (see section 4.3).

In patients receiving lithium, there is a possible inhibition of renal lithium clearance, increased plasma lithium concentration, and potential lithium toxicity (see section 4.3).

Probenecid should not be administered concurrently with ketorolac because of increases in ketorolac plasma level and half-life.

NSAIDs should not be used for eight to twelve days after mifepristone administration as NSAIDs can reduce the effects of mifepristone.

The following medicinal products in combination with Toradol, are to be co-administered with caution:

In normovolaemic healthy subjects, ketorolac reduces the diuretic response to furosemide by approximately 20%, so particular care should be taken in patients with cardiac decompensation.

NSAIDs may exacerbate cardiac failure, reduce GFR and increase plasma cardiac glycoside levels when co-administered with cardiac glycosides.

Toradol and other non-steroidal anti-inflammatory drugs can reduce the anti-hypertensive effect of beta-blockers and may increase the risk of renal impairment when administered concurrently with ACE inhibitors, particularly in volume depleted patients.

As with all NSAIDs caution is advised when ciclosporin is co-administered because of the increased risk of nephrotoxicity.

There is a possible risk of nephrotoxicity when NSAIDs are given with tacrolimus.

Co-administration with diuretics can lead to a reduced diuretic effect, and increase the risk of nephrotoxicity of NSAIDs.

As with all NSAIDs, caution should be taken when co-administering with corticosteroids because of the increased risk of gastro-intestinal ulceration or bleeding (see section 4.4).

There is an increased risk of gastrointestinal bleeding (see section 4.4) when anti-platelet agents and selective serotonin reuptake inhibitors (SSRIs) are combined with NSAIDs.

Because of an increased tendency to bleeding when oxpentifylline is administered concurrently, this combination should be avoided.

Caution is advised when methotrexate is administered concurrently, since some prostaglandin synthesis inhibiting drugs have been reported to reduce the clearance of methotrexate, and thus possibly enhance its toxicity.

Animal data indicate that NSAIDs can increase the risk of convulsions associated with quinolone antibiotics. Patients taking NSAIDs and quinolones may have an increased risk of developing convulsions.

NSAIDs given with zidovudine increase the risk of haematological toxicity. There is evidence of an increased risk of of haemarthroses and haematoma in HIV (+) haemophiliacs receiving concurrent treatment with zidovudine and ibuprofen.

The following medicinal products are unlikely to have an interaction with Toradol:

Ketorolac did not alter digoxin protein binding. *In vitro* studies indicated that at therapeutic concentrations of salicylate (300μg/ml) and above, the binding of ketorolac was reduced from approximately 99.2% to 97.5%. Therapeutic concentrations of digoxin, warfarin, paracetamol, phenytoin and tolbutamide did not alter ketorolac protein binding. Because ketorolac is a highly potent drug and present in low concentrations in plasma, it would not be expected to displace other protein-bound drugs significantly.

There is no evidence in animal or human studies that ketorolac trometamol induces or inhibits the hepatic enzymes capable of metabolising itself or other drugs. Hence Toradol would not be expected to alter the pharmacokinetics of other drugs due to enzyme induction or inhibition mechanisms.

4.6 Pregnancy and lactation

Pregnancy

The safety of Toradol during human pregnancy has not been established. There was no evidence of teratogenicity in rats or rabbits studied at maternally-toxic doses of ketorolac. Prolongation of the gestation period and/or delayed parturition were seen in the rat. Congenital abnormalities have been reported in association with NSAID administration in man, however these are low in frequency and do not follow any discernible pattern. In view of the known effects of NSAIDs on the foetal cardiovascular system (risk of closure of the ductus arteriosus) ketorolac is contra-indicated during pregnancy, labour or delivery. The onset of labour may be delayed and the duration increased with an increased bleeding tendency in both mother and child (see section 4.3).

See section 4.4 regarding female fertility.

Lactation

Ketorolac and its metabolites have been shown to pass into the foetus and milk of animals. Ketorolac has been detected in human milk at low levels therefore, ketorolac is contra-indicated in mothers who are breast-feeding.

4.7 Effects on ability to drive and use machines

Some patients may experience dizziness, drowsiness, fatigue, visual disturbances, headaches, vertigo, insomnia or depression with the use of Toradol. If patients experience these, or other similar undesirable effects, patients should not drive or operate machinery.

4.8 Undesirable effects

The following side-effects have been reported with Toradol.

Gastro-intestinal: The most commonly observed adverse events are gastrointestinal in nature.

Peptic ulcers, perforation or GI bleeding, sometimes fatal, particularly in the elderly, may occur (see section 4.4). Nausea, dyspepsia, gastro-intestinal pain, abdominal discomfort, haematemesis, gastritis, oesophagitis, diarrhoea, eructation, constipation, flatulence, fullness, melaena, non-peptic gastro-intestinal ulceration, rectal bleeding, ulcerative stomatitis, vomiting, haemorrhage, perforation, pancreatitis, exacerbation of colitis and Crohn's disease (see section 4.4) have been reported following administration.

Central nervous/musculoskeletal systems: Anxiety, visual disturbances, drowsiness, dizziness, headaches, sweating, dry mouth, nervousness, paraesthesia, functional disorders, abnormal thinking, depression, euphoria, convulsions, excessive thirst, inability to concentrate, insomnia, malaise, fatigue, stimulation, vertigo, abnormal taste and vision, optic neuritis, myalgia, abnormal dreams, confusion, hallucinations, hyperkinesia, hearing loss, tinnitus, aseptic meningitis (especially in patients with existing auto-immune disorders, such as systemic lupus erythematosus, mixed connective tissue disease), with symptoms such as stiff neck, headache, nausea, vomiting, fever or disorientation (see section 4.4), psychotic reactions.

Renal: Nephrotoxicity including increased urinary frequency, oliguria, acute renal failure, hyponatraemia, hyperkalaemia, haemolytic uraemic syndrome, flank pain (with or without haematuria), raised serum urea and creatinine, interstitial nephritis, urinary retention, nephrotic syndrome, renal failure.

Hepatic: abnormal liver function, hepatitis, jaundice and liver failure.

Cardiovascular: Flushing, bradycardia, pallor, hypertension, palpitations, chest pain.

Oedema, hypertension and cardiac failure have been reported in association with NSAID treatment. Clinical trial and epidemiological data suggest that use of some NSAIDs (particularly at high doses and in long term treatment) may be associated with an increased risk of arterial thrombotic events (for example myocardial infarction or stroke) (see section 4.4).

Reproductive, female: Infertility.

Respiratory: Dyspnoea, asthma, pulmonary oedema.

Haematological: Purpura, thrombocytopenia, neutropenia, agranulocytosis, aplastic anaemia and haemolytic anaemia.

Dermatological: Pruritus, urticaria, skin photosensitivity, Lyell's syndrome, bullous reactions including Stevens-Johnson syndrome and Toxic Epidermal Necrolysis (very rare), exfoliative dermatitis, maculopapular rash.

Hypersensitivity reactions: Hypersensitivity reactions have been reported following treatment with NSAIDs. These may consist of (a) non-specific allergic reactions and anaphylaxis (b) respiratory tract reactivity comprising asthma, aggravated asthma, bronchospasm, laryngeal oedema or dyspnoea, or (c) assorted skin disorders, including rashes of various types, pruritus, urticaria, purpura, angio-oedema and more rarely exfoliative and bullous dermatoses (including epidermal necrolysis and erythema multiforme). Other reactions include hypotension and flushing. Such reactions may occur in patients with or without known sensitivity to Toradol or other non-steroidal anti-inflammatory drugs.

These may also occur in individuals with a history of angioedema, bronchospastic reactivity (e.g. asthma and nasal polyps). Anaphylactoid reactions, like anaphylaxis, may have a fatal outcome (see section 4.3).

Bleeding: Post-operative wound haemorrhage, haematomata, epistaxis, increased bleeding time.

Other: Asthenia, oedema, weight gain, fever. Injection site pain has been reported in some patients.

4.9 Overdose

a) Symptoms

Symptoms include headache, nausea, vomiting, epigastric pain, gastrointestinal bleeding, rarely diarrhoea, disorientation, excitation, coma, drowsiness, dizziness, tinnitus, fainting, occasionally convulsions. In cases of significant poisoning acute renal failure and liver damage are possible.

b) Therapeutic measure

Patients should be treated symptomatically as required. Within one hour of ingestion of a potentially toxic amount, activated charcoal should be considered. Alternatively, in adults, gastric lavage should be considered within one hour of ingestion of a potentially life-threatening overdose.

Good urine output should be ensured. Renal and liver function should be closely monitored. Patients should be observed for at least four hours after ingestion of potentially toxic amounts. Frequent or prolonged convulsions should be treated with intravenous diazepam. Other measures may be indicated by the patient's clinical condition.

Doses of 360mg given intramuscularly over an eight hour interval for five consecutive days have caused abdominal pain and peptic ulcers which have healed after discontinuation of dosing. Two patients recovered from unsuccessful suicide attempts. One patient experienced nausea after 210mg ketorolac, and the other hyperventilation after 300mg ketorolac.

5. PHARMACOLOGICAL PROPERTIES

5.1 Pharmacodynamic properties

Toradol is a potent analgesic agent of the non-steroidal, anti-inflammatory class (NSAID). It is not an opioid and has no known effects on opioid receptors. Its mode of action is to inhibit the cyclo-oxygenase enzyme system and hence prostaglandin synthesis, and it demonstrates a minimal anti-inflammatory effect at its analgesic dose.

5.2 Pharmacokinetic properties

IM: Following intramuscular administration, ketorolac trometamol was rapidly and completely absorbed, a mean peak plasma concentration of 2.2μg/ml occurring an average of 50 minutes after a single 30mg dose. The influences of age, kidney and liver function on terminal plasma half-life and mean total clearance are outlined in the table below (estimated from a single 30mg IM dose of ketorolac).

Type of subjects	Total clearance (l/hr/kg) mean (range)	Terminal half-life (hrs) mean (range)
Normal subjects (n = 54)	0.023 (0.010 - 0.046)	5.3 (3.5 - 9.2)
Patients with hepatic dysfunction (n = 7)	0.029 (0.013 - 0.066)	5.4 (2.2 - 6.9)
Patients with renal impairment (n = 25) (serum creatinine 160 - 430 micromol/l)	0.016 (0.005 - 0.043)	10.3 (5.9 - 19.2)
Renal dialysis patients (n = 9)	0.016 (0.003 - 0.036)	13.6 (8.0 - 39.1)
Healthy elderly subjects (n = 13) (mean age 72)	0.019 (0.013 - 0.034)	7.0 (4.7 - 8.6)

IV: Intravenous administration of a single 10mg dose of ketorolac trometamol resulted in a mean peak plasma concentration of 2.4μg/ml occurring an average of 5.4 minutes after dosing, with a terminal plasma elimination half-life of 5.1 hours, an average volume of distribution of 0.15 l/kg, and a total plasma clearance of 0.35ml/min/kg.

The pharmacokinetics of ketorolac in man following single or multiple doses are linear. Steady-state plasma levels are achieved after dosing every six hours for one day. No changes in clearance occurred with chronic dosing. The primary route of excretion of ketorolac and its metabolites is renal: 91.4% (mean) of a given dose being found in the urine and 6.1% (mean) in the faeces.

More than 99% of the ketorolac in plasma is protein-bound over a wide concentration range.

5.3 Preclinical safety data

An 18-month study in mice with oral doses of ketorolac trometamol at 2mg/kg/day (0.9 times human systemic exposure at the recommended IM or IV dose of 30mg qid, based on area-under-the-plasma-concentration curve [AUC]), and a 24-month study in rats at 5mg/kg/day (0.5 times the human AUC), showed no evidence of tumourigenicity.

Ketorolac trometamol was not mutagenic in the Ames test, unscheduled DNA synthesis and repair, and in forward mutation assays. Ketorolac trometamol did not cause chromosome breakage in the *in vivo* mouse micronucleus assay. At 1590μg/ml and at higher concentrations, ketorolac trometamol increased the incidence of chromosomal aberrations in Chinese hamster ovarian cells.

Impairment of fertility did not occur in male or female rats at oral doses of 9mg/kg (0.9 times the human AUC) and 16mg/kg (1.6 times the human AUC) of ketorolac trometamol, respectively.

6. PHARMACEUTICAL PARTICULARS

6.1 List of excipients

Ethanol

Sodium Chloride

Water

6.2 Incompatibilities

Toradol should not be mixed in a small volume (e.g. in a syringe) with morphine sulphate, pethidine hydrochloride, promethazine hydrochloride or hydroxyzine hydrochloride as precipitation of ketorolac will occur.

It is compatible with normal saline, 5% dextrose, Ringer's, lactated Ringer's or Plasmacyte solutions. Compatibility of Toradol with other drugs is unknown.

6.3 Shelf life

3 years.

6.4 Special precautions for storage

Keep Toradol ampoules in the outer carton. Do not refrigerate or freeze. Do not use if particulate matter is present.

6.5 Nature and contents of container

Toradol 10mg and 30mg is available in single-dose ampoules containing 1ml of solution in cartons of 1, 5 or 10.

6.6 Special precautions for disposal and other handling

No special instructions applicable.

7. MARKETING AUTHORISATION HOLDER

Roche Products Limited, 6 Falcon Way, Shire Park, Welwyn Garden City, AL7 1TW, United Kingdom.

8. MARKETING AUTHORISATION NUMBER(S)

PL 0031/0480 (ampoules 10mg/ml)

PL 0031/0481 (ampoules 30mg/ml)

9. DATE OF FIRST AUTHORISATION/RENEWAL OF THE AUTHORISATION

31 May 1996/30 October 2000

10. DATE OF REVISION OF THE TEXT

25/02/2009

Toradol is a registered trade mark

Toradol Tablets

(Roche Products Limited)

1. NAME OF THE MEDICINAL PRODUCT

Toradol

2. QUALITATIVE AND QUANTITATIVE COMPOSITION

Ketorolac Trometamol 10mg.

3. PHARMACEUTICAL FORM

White to creamy white film coated, round tablet, marked "KET 10" on one face, the other face blank.

4. CLINICAL PARTICULARS

4.1 Therapeutic indications

Toradol tablets are indicated for the short-term management of moderate postoperative pain.

Treatment should only be initiated in hospitals. The maximum duration of treatment is seven days.

4.2 Posology and method of administration

For oral administration.

To be taken preferably with or after food.

Toradol tablets are recommended for short-term use only (up to 7 days) and are not recommended for chronic use.

Undesirable effects may be minimised by using the lowest effective dose for the shortest duration necessary to control symptoms (see section 4.4).

Adults

10mg every 4 to 6 hours as required. Doses exceeding 40mg per day are not recommended.

Opioid analgesics (e.g. morphine, pethidine) may be used concomitantly, and may be required for optimal analgesic effect in the early postoperative period when pain is most severe. Ketorolac does not interfere with opioid binding and does not exacerbate opioid-related respiratory depression or sedation.

For patients receiving parenteral Toradol, and who are converted to Toradol oral tablets, the total combined daily dose should not exceed 90mg (60mg for the elderly, renally-impaired patients and patients less than 50kg) and the oral component should not exceed 40mg on the day the change of formulation is made. Patients should be converted to oral treatment as soon as possible.

Elderly

The elderly are at increased risk of the serious consequences of adverse reactions. If an NSAID is considered necessary, the lowest effective dose should be used and for the shortest possible duration. The patient should be monitored regularly for GI bleeding during NSAID therapy.

A longer dosing interval, e.g. 6 - 8 hourly, is advisable in the elderly.

Children

Toradol is not recommended for use in children under 16 years of age.

4.3 Contraindications

– active peptic ulcer, or any history of gastrointestinal bleeding, ulceration or perforation

– severe heart failure, hepatic failure and renal failure (see section 4.4)

– suspected or confirmed cerebrovascular bleeding

– haemorrhagic diatheses, including coagulation disorders

– hypersensitivity to ketorolac trometamol or any of the excipients or other NSAIDs

– patients in whom ibuprofen, aspirin or other prostaglandin synthesis inhibitors induce allergic reactions e.g. asthma, rhinitis, angioedema, or urticaria (severe anaphylactic-like reactions have been observed in such patients)

– the complete or partial syndrome of nasal polyps, angioedema or bronchospasm

– concurrent treatment with other NSAIDs, (including cyclooxygenase-2 selective inhibitors), oxpentifylline, probenecid or lithium salts

– hypovolaemia from any cause or dehydration

– moderate or severe renal impairment (serum creatinine > 160 micromol/l)

– a history of asthma

– patients who have had operations with a high risk of haemorrhage or incomplete haemostasis

– patients on anticoagulants including low dose heparin (2500 - 5000 units 12 hourly)

– during pregnancy, labour, delivery or lactation (see section 4.6)

– children under 16 years of age

– Toradol is contra-indicated as prophylactic analgesia before surgery due to inhibition of platelet aggregation and is contra-indicated intraoperatively because of the increased risk of bleeding

– Toradol is contra-indicated in patients currently receiving aspirin.

4.4 Special warnings and precautions for use

Undesirable effects may be minimised by using the lowest effective dose for the shortest duration necessary to control symptoms (see section 4.2 and GI and cardiovascular risks below).

Use in the elderly: The elderly have an increased frequency of adverse reactions to NSAIDs especially gastrointestinal bleeding and perforation which may be fatal. This age-related risk is common to all NSAIDs. Compared to young adults, the elderly have an increased plasma half-life and reduced plasma clearance of ketorolac. A longer dosing interval is advisable (see section 4.2).

Effects on fertility: The use of Toradol, as with any drug known to inhibit cyclooxygenase/prostaglandin synthesis, may impair fertility and is not recommended in women attempting to conceive. In women who have difficulty conceiving or are undergoing investigation of fertility, withdrawal of Toradol should be considered.

Gastrointestinal bleeding, ulceration and perforation:

GI bleeding, ulceration or perforation, which can be fatal, has been reported with all NSAIDs at anytime during treatment, with or without warning symptoms or a previous history of serious GI events.

The risk of clinically serious gastro-intestinal bleeding is dose-dependent. This is particularly true in elderly patients who receive an average daily dose greater than 60mg/day of Toradol.

In a non-randomised, in-hospital post-marketing surveillance study, increased rates of clinically serious GI bleeding were seen in patients ⩽ 65 years of age who received an average daily dose of > 90mg ketorolac IM as compared to those patients receiving parenteral opioids.

Epidemiological evidence suggests that Ketorolac may be associated with a high risk of serious gastrointestinal toxicity, relative to some other NSAIDs, especially when used outside the licensed indications and/or for prolonged periods (see also section 4.1, 4.2 and 4.3).

The risk of GI bleeding, ulceration or perforation is higher with increasing NSAID doses, in patients with a history of ulcer, particularly if complicated with haemorrhage or perforation (see section 4.3), and in the elderly. These patients should commence treatment on the lowest dose available. Combination therapy with protective agents (e.g. misoprostol or proton pump inhibitors) should be considered for these patients, and also for patients requiring concomitant low dose aspirin, or other drugs likely to increase gastrointestinal risk (see below and section 4.5).

Patients with a history of GI toxicity, particularly when elderly, should report any unusual abdominal symptoms (especially GI bleeding) particularly in the initial stages of treatment.

Caution should be advised in patients receiving concomitant medications which could increase the risk of ulceration or bleeding, such as oral corticosteroids, selective serotonin-reuptake inhibitors or anti-platelet agents such as aspirin (see section 4.5).

Use in patients taking anticoagulants such as warfarin is contraindicated (see section 4.3).

When GI bleeding or ulceration occurs in patients receiving Ketorolac Trometamol, the treatment should be withdrawn.

NSAIDs should be given with care to patients with a history of gastrointestinal disease (ulcerative colitis, Crohn's disease) as these conditions may be exacerbated (see section 4.8).

Respiratory disorders: Caution is required if administered to patients suffering from, or with a previous history of, bronchial asthma since NSAIDs have been reported to precipitate bronchospasm in such patients.

Renal effects: Drugs that inhibit prostaglandin biosynthesis (including non-steroidal anti-inflammatory drugs) have been reported to cause nephrotoxicity, including but not limited to glomerular nephritis, interstitial nephritis, renal papillary necrosis, nephrotic syndrome and acute renal failure. In patients with renal, cardiac or hepatic impairment, caution is required since the use of NSAIDs may result in deterioration of renal function.

As with other drugs that inhibit prostaglandin synthesis, elevations of serum urea, creatinine and potassium have been reported with ketorolac trometamol and may occur after one dose.

Patients with impaired renal function: Since ketorolac trometamol and its metabolites are excreted primarily by the kidney, patients with moderate to severe impairment of renal function (serum creatinine greater than 160 micromol/l) should not receive Toradol. Patients with lesser renal impairment should receive a reduced dose of ketorolac (not exceeding 60mg/day IM or IV) and their renal status should be closely monitored.

Cardiovascular, Renal and Hepatic Impairment: Caution should be observed in patients with conditions leading to a reduction in blood volume and/or renal blood flow, where renal prostaglandins have a supportive role in the maintenance of renal perfusion. In these patients, administration of an NSAID may cause a dose-dependent reduction in renal prostaglandin formation and may precipitate overt renal failure. Patients at greatest risk of this reaction are those who are volume depleted because of blood loss or severe dehydration, patients with impaired renal function, heart failure, liver dysfunction, the elderly and those taking diuretics. Renal function should be monitored in these patients. Discontinuation of NSAID therapy is typically followed by recovery to the pre-treatment state. Inadequate fluid/blood replacement during surgery, leading to hypovolaemia, may lead to renal dysfunction which could be exacerbated when Toradol is administered. Therefore, volume depletion should be corrected and close monitoring of serum urea and creatinine and urine output is recommended until the patient is normovolaemic. In patients on renal dialysis, ketorolac clearance was reduced to approximately half the normal rate and terminal half-life increased approximately three-fold (see section 4.3).

Fluid retention and oedema: Fluid retention and oedema have been reported with the use of Toradol and it should therefore be used with caution in patients with cardiac decompensation, hypertension or similar conditions.

Cardiovascular and cerebrovascular effects

Appropriate monitoring and advice are required for patients with a history of hypertension and/or mild to moderate congestive heart failure as fluid retention and oedema have been reported in association with NSAID therapy.

Clinical trial and epidemiological data suggest that use of some NSAIDs (particularly at high doses and in long term treatment) may be associated with a small increased risk of arterial thrombotic events (for example myocardial infarction or stroke). There are insufficient data to exclude such a risk for Ketorolac Trometamol.

Patients with uncontrolled hypertension, congestive heart failure, established ischaemic heart disease, peripheral arterial disease, and/or cerebrovascular disease should only be treated with Ketorolac Trometamol after careful consideration. Similar consideration should be made before initiating longer-term treatment of patients with risk factors for cardiovascular disease (e.g. hypertension, hyperlipidaemia, diabetes mellitus, smoking).

SLE and mixed connective tissue disease:

In patients with systemic lupus erythematosus (SLE) and mixed connective tissue disorders there may be an increased risk of aseptic meningitis (see section 4.8).

Dermatological:

Serious skin reactions, some of them fatal, including exfoliative dermatitis, Stevens-Johnson syndrome, and toxic epidermal necrolysis, have been reported very rarely in association with the use of NSAIDs (see section 4.8). Patients appear to be at highest risk for these reactions early in the course of therapy: the onset of the reactions occurring in the majority of cases within the first month of treatment. Toradol should be discontinued at the first appearance of skin rash, mucosal lesions, or any other sign of hypersensitivity.

Use in patients with impaired liver function: Patients with impaired hepatic function from cirrhosis do not have any clinically important changes in ketorolac clearance or terminal half-life.

Borderline elevations of one or more liver function tests may occur. These abnormalities may be transient, may remain unchanged, or may progress with continued therapy. Meaningful elevations (greater than 3 times normal) of serum glutamate pyruvate transaminase (SGPT/ALT) or serum glutamate oxaloacetate transaminase (SGOT/AST) occurred in controlled clinical trials in less than 1% of patients. If clinical signs and symptoms consistent with liver disease develop, or if systemic manifestations occur, Toradol should be discontinued.

Haematological effects: Patients with coagulation disorders should not receive Toradol. Patients on anticoagulation therapy may be at increased risk of bleeding if given Toradol concurrently. The concomitant use of ketorolac and prophylactic low dose heparin (2500 - 5000 units 12-hourly) has not been studied extensively and may also be associated with an increased risk of bleeding. Patients already on anticoagulants or who require low-dose heparin should not receive ketorolac. Patients who are receiving other drug therapy that interferes with haemostasis should be carefully observed if Toradol is administered. In controlled clinical studies, the incidence of clinically significant postoperative bleeding was less than 1%.

Ketorolac inhibits platelet aggregation and prolongs bleeding time. In patients with normal bleeding function, bleeding times were raised, but not outside the normal range of 2 - 11 minutes. Unlike the prolonged effects from aspirin, platelet function returns to normal within 24 to 48 hours after ketorolac is discontinued.

In post-marketing experience, postoperative wound haemorrhage has been reported in association with the immediate peri-operative use of Toradol IM/IV. Therefore, ketorolac should not be used in patients who have had operations with a high risk of haemorrhage or incomplete haemostasis. Caution should be used where strict haemostasis is critical, e.g. in cosmetic or day-case surgery. Haematomata and other signs of wound haemorrhage and epistaxis have been reported with the use of Toradol. Physicians should be aware of the pharmacological similarity of ketorolac to other non-steroidal anti-inflammatory drugs that inhibit cyclo-oxygenase and the risk of bleeding, particularly in the elderly.

Toradol is not an anaesthetic agent and possesses no sedative or anxiolytic properties; therefore it is not recommended as a pre-operative medication for the support of anaesthesia when these effects are required.

4.5 Interaction with other medicinal products and other forms of interaction

Ketorolac is highly bound to human plasma protein (mean 99.2%) and binding is concentration-independent.

The following medicinal products are NOT to be co-administered with Toradol:

Toradol should not be used with other NSAIDs including cyclooxygenase-2 selective inhibitors or in patients receiving aspirin because of the potential for adverse effects (see section 4.3).

Toradol is contraindicated in combination with anti-coagulants, such as warfarin since co-administration may cause an enhanced anti-coagulant effect (see section 4.3).

In patients receiving lithium, there is a possible inhibition of renal lithium clearance, increased plasma lithium concentration, and potential lithium toxicity. (see section 4.3)

Probenecid should not be administered concurrently with ketorolac because of increases in ketorolac plasma level and half-life.

NSAIDs should not be used for 8 to 12 days after mifepristone administration as NSAIDs can reduce the effects of mifepristone.

The following medicinal products, in combination with Toradol, are to be co-administered with caution:

In normovolaemic healthy subjects, ketorolac reduces the diuretic response to furosemide by approximately 20%, so particular care should be taken in patients with cardiac decompensation.

NSAIDs may exacerbate cardiac failure, reduce GFR and increase plasma cardiac glycoside levels when co-administered with cardiac glycosides.

Toradol and other non-steroidal anti-inflammatory drugs can reduce the antihypertensive effect of anti-hypertensives.

There is an increased risk of renal impairment when ketorolac is administered concurrently with ACE inhibitors, particularly in volume depleted patients.

As with all NSAIDs caution is advised when ciclosporin is co-administered because of the increased risk of nephrotoxicity.

There is a possible risk of nephrotoxicity when NSAIDs are given with tacrolimus.

Co-administration with diuretics can lead to a reduced diuretic effect, and increase the risk of nephrotoxicity of NSAIDs.

As with all NSAIDs, caution should be taken when co-administering with corticosteroids because of the increased risk of gastro-intestinal ulceration or bleeding (see section 4.4).

There is an increased risk of gastrointestinal bleeding (see section 4.4) when antiplatelet agents and selective serotonin reuptake inhibitors (SSRIs) are combined with NSAIDs.

Because of an increased tendency to bleeding when oxpentifylline is administered concurrently, this combination should be avoided.

Caution is advised when methotrexate is administered concurrently, since some prostaglandin synthesis inhibiting drugs have been reported to reduce the clearance of methotrexate, and thus possibly enhance its toxicity.

Animal data indicate that NSAIDs can increase the risk of convulsions associated with quinolone antibiotics. Patients taking NSAIDs and quinolones may have an increased risk of developing convulsions.

NSAIDs given with zidovudine increase the risk of haematological toxicity. There is evidence of an increased risk of haemarthroses and haematoma in HIV (+) haemophiliacs receiving concurrent treatment with zidovudine and ibuprofen.

The following medicinal products are unlikely to have an interaction with Toradol:

Ketorolac did not alter digoxin protein binding. *In vitro* studies indicated that at therapeutic concentrations of salicylate (300mcg/ml) and above, the binding of ketorolac was reduced from approximately 99.2% to 97.5%. Therapeutic concentrations of digoxin, warfarin, paracetamol, phenytoin and tolbutamide did not alter ketorolac protein binding. Because ketorolac is a highly potent drug and present in low concentrations in plasma, it would not be expected to displace other protein-bound drugs significantly.

There is no evidence in animal or human studies that ketorolac trometamol induces or inhibits the hepatic enzymes capable of metabolising itself or other drugs. Hence Toradol would not be expected to alter the pharmacokinetics of other drugs due to enzyme induction or inhibition mechanisms.

4.6 Pregnancy and lactation

Pregnancy

The safety of Toradol during human pregnancy has not been established. There was no evidence of teratogenicity in rats or rabbits studied at maternally-toxic doses of ketorolac. Prolongation of the gestation period and/or delayed parturition were seen in the rat. Congenital abnormalities have been reported in association with NSAID administration in man; however, these are low in frequency and do not appear to follow any discernible pattern. In view of the known effects of NSAIDs on the foetal cardiovascular system (risk of closure of the ductus arteriosus) ketorolac is contraindicated during pregnancy, labour or delivery. The onset of labour may be delayed and the duration increased with an increased bleeding tendency in both mother and child (see section 4.3).

See section 4.4 regarding female fertility.

Lactation

Ketorolac and its metabolites have been shown to pass into the foetus and milk of animals. Ketorolac has been detected in human milk at low levels therefore, ketorolac is contra-indicated in mothers who are breast-feeding.

4.7 Effects on ability to drive and use machines

Some patients may experience drowsiness, dizziness, vertigo, insomnia, fatigue, visual disturbances or depression with the use of Toradol. If patients experience these, or other similar undesirable effects, they should not drive or operate machinery.

4.8 Undesirable effects

The following side-effects have been reported with Toradol.

Gastro-intestinal: The most commonly observed adverse events are gastrointestinal in nature. Peptic ulcers, perforation or GI bleeding, sometimes fatal, particularly in the elderly, may occur (see section 4.4). Nausea, dyspepsia, gastro-intestinal pain, abdominal discomfort, haematemesis, gastritis, oesophagitis, diarrhoea, eructation, constipation, flatulence, fullness, melaena, rectal bleeding, ulcerative stomatitis, vomiting, haemorrhage, perforation, pancreatitis, exacerbation of colitis and Crohn's disease (see section 4.4) have been reported following administration.

Central nervous/musculoskeletal systems: Anxiety, visual disturbances, optic neuritis, drowsiness, dizziness, headaches, sweating, dry mouth, nervousness, paraesthesia, functional disorders, abnormal thinking, depression, euphoria, convulsions, excessive thirst, inability to concentrate, insomnia, malaise, fatigue, stimulation, vertigo, abnormal taste and vision, myalgia, abnormal dreams, confusion, hallucinations, hyperkinesia, hearing loss, tinnitus, aseptic meningitis (especially in patients with existing auto-immune disorders, such as systemic lupus erythematosus, mixed connective tissue disease), with symptoms such as stiff neck, headache, nausea, vomiting, fever or disorientation (see section 4.4), psychotic reactions.

Renal: increased urinary frequency, oliguria, acute renal failure, hyponatraemia, hyperkalaemia, haemolytic uraemic syndrome, flank pain (with or without haematuria), raised serum urea and creatinine, interstitial nephritis, urinary retention, nephrotic syndrome, renal failure.

Hepatic: abnormal liver function, hepatitis, jaundice and liver failure.

Cardiovascular: Flushing, bradycardia, pallor, hypertension, palpitations, chest pain.

Oedema, hypertension and cardiac failure have been reported in association with NSAID treatment. Clinical trial and epidemiological data suggest that use of some NSAIDs (particularly at high doses and in long term treatment) may be associated with an increased risk of arterial thrombotic events (for example myocardial infarction or stroke) (see section 4.4).

Reproductive, female: Infertility.

Respiratory: Dyspnoea, asthma, pulmonary oedema.

Haematological: Purpura, thrombocytopenia, neutropenia, agranulocytosis, aplastic anaemia and haemolytic anaemia.

Dermatological: Pruritus, urticaria, skin photosensitivity, Lyell's syndrome, bullous reactions including Stevens-Johnson syndrome and Toxic Epidermal Necrolysis (very rare), exfoliative dermatitis, maculopapular rash.

Hypersensitivity: Hypersensitivity reactions have been reported following treatment with NSAIDs. These may consist of (a) non-specific allergic reactions and anaphylaxis (b) respiratory tract reactivity comprising asthma, aggravated asthma, bronchospasm, laryngeal oedema or dyspnoea, or (c) assorted skin disorders, including rashes of various types, pruritus, urticaria, purpura, angio-oedema and more rarely exfoliative and bullous dermatoses (including epidermal necrolysis and erythema multiforme). Other reactions include hypotension and flushing. Such reactions may occur in patients with or without known sensitivity to Toradol or other non-steroidal anti-inflammatory drugs. These may also occur in individuals with a history of angioedema, bronchospastic reactivity (e.g. asthma and nasal polyps). Anaphylactoid reactions, like anaphylaxis, may have a fatal outcome (see section 4.3).

Bleeding: Postoperative wound haemorrhage, haematomata, epistaxis, increased bleeding time.

Other: Asthenia, oedema, weight gain, fever.

4.9 Overdose

a) Symptoms

Symptoms include headache, nausea, vomiting, epigastric pain, gastrointestinal bleeding, rarely diarrhoea, disorientation, excitation, coma, drowsiness, dizziness, tinnitus, fainting, occasionally convulsions. In cases of significant poisoning acute renal failure and liver damage are possible.

b) Therapeutic measure

Patients should be treated symptomatically as required. Within one hour of ingestion of a potentially toxic amount, activated charcoal should be considered. Alternatively, in adults, gastric lavage should be considered with one hour of ingestion of a potentially life-threatening overdose.

Good urine output should be ensured. Renal and liver function should be closely monitored. Patients should be observed for at least four hours after ingestion of potentially toxic amounts. Frequent or prolonged convulsions should be treated with intravenous diazepam. Other measures may be indicated by the patient's clinical condition.

Doses of 360mg given intramuscularly over an 8-hour interval for five consecutive days have caused abdominal pain and peptic ulcers which have healed after discontinuation of dosing. Two patients recovered from unsuccessful suicide attempts. One patient experienced nausea after 210mg ketorolac, and the other hyperventilation after 300mg ketorolac.

5. PHARMACOLOGICAL PROPERTIES

5.1 Pharmacodynamic properties

Ketorolac trometamol is a non-narcotic analgesic. It is a nonsteroidal anti-inflammatory agent that exhibits anti-inflammatory and weak antipyretic activity.

Ketorolac trometamol inhibits the synthesis of prostaglandins and is considered a peripherally acting analgesic. It does not have known effects on opiate receptors.

No evidence of respiratory depression has been observed after administration of ketorolac trometamol in controlled clinical trials. Ketorolac trometamol does not cause pupil constriction.

5.2 Pharmacokinetic properties

Ketorolac trometamol is rapidly and completely absorbed following oral administration with a peak plasma concentration of 0.87mcg/ml occurring 50 minutes after a single 10mg dose. The terminal plasma elimination half-life averages 5.4 hours (S.D = 1.0) in healthy subjects. In elderly subjects (mean age 72) it is 6.2 hours (S.D = 1.0). More than 99% of the ketorolac in plasma is protein bound.

The pharmacokinetics of ketorolac in man following single or multiple doses are linear. Steady state plasma levels are achieved after 1 day of Q.I.D. dosing. No changes occurred with chronic dosing. Following a single intravenous dose, the volume of distribution is 0.25 l/kg, the half-life is 5 hours and the clearance 0.55ml/min/kg. The primary route of excretion of ketorolac and its metabolites (conjugates and the p-hydroxymetabolite) is in the urine (91.4%) and the remainder is excreted in the faeces.

A high fat diet decreased the rate, but not the extent of absorption, while antacid had no effect on ketorolac absorption.

5.3 Preclinical safety data

None stated.

6. PHARMACEUTICAL PARTICULARS

6.1 List of excipients

Tablet core:

Microcrystalline cellulose (E460) Lactose monohydrate

Magnesium stearate

Film-coating mixture:

Opadry white YS-1R-7002 containing:

Hypromellose,

Titanium dioxide (E171)

Macrogol

Printing ink:

Opacode Black-S-1-27794 containing:

Shellac, modified

Iron oxide black (E172)

Propylene glycol

Purified water

6.2 Incompatibilities

None known.

6.3 Shelf life

3 years.

6.4 Special precautions for storage

Toradol tablets should be kept in their original packaging to protect them from moisture and light.

6.5 Nature and contents of container

White HDPE bottles with polypropylene screw containers containing 50, 56, 100, 250 or 500 tablets.

Polypropylene securitainers containing 50, 56, 100, 250 or 500 tablets.

Amber or white OPA/PVC/aluminium foil blister packs in outer cardboard carton containing 4, 20, 28, 50, 56, 100, 250 or 500 tablets.

6.6 Special precautions for disposal and other handling

None stated.

7. MARKETING AUTHORISATION HOLDER

Roche Products Limited

6 Falcon Way

Shire Park

Welwyn Garden City

AL7 1TW

United Kingdom

8. MARKETING AUTHORISATION NUMBER(S)

PL 0031/0482

9. DATE OF FIRST AUTHORISATION/RENEWAL OF THE AUTHORISATION

24/02/2009

10. DATE OF REVISION OF THE TEXT

13 July 2009

LEGAL STATUS

POM

TORISEL 25 mg/ml concentrate and diluent for solution for infusion

(Wyeth Pharmaceuticals)

1. NAME OF THE MEDICINAL PRODUCT

TORISEL ▼ 25 mg/ml concentrate and diluent for solution for infusion.

2. QUALITATIVE AND QUANTITATIVE COMPOSITION

1 vial TORISEL 25 mg/ml concentrate contains:

30 mg temsirolimus dissolved in a total volume of 1.2 ml

Therefore, 1 ml of TORISEL concentrate contains 25 mg temsirolimus.

After dilution of TORISEL 25 mg/ml concentrate with 1.8 ml of withdrawn diluent, the concentration of temsirolimus is 10 mg/ml.

Excipients:

1 vial TORISEL 25 mg/ml concentrate contains 474 mg anhydrous ethanol.

1 vial of the diluent, provided contains 358 mg anhydrous ethanol.

For a full list of excipients, see section 6.1.

3. PHARMACEUTICAL FORM

Concentrate and diluent for solution for infusion.

The concentrate is a clear, colourless to light-yellow solution, essentially free from visible particulates.

The diluent is a clear to slightly turbid, light-yellow to yellow solution, essentially free from visible particulates.

4. CLINICAL PARTICULARS

4.1 Therapeutic indications

Renal cell carcinoma

TORISEL is indicated for the first-line treatment of patients with advanced renal cell carcinoma (RCC) who have at least three of six prognostic risk factors (see section 5.1).

Mantle cell lymphoma

TORISEL is indicated for the treatment of adult patients with relapsed and/or refractory mantle cell lymphoma [MCL], (see section 5.1).

4.2 Posology and method of administration

TORISEL must be administered under the supervision of a physician experienced in the use of antineoplastic medicinal products.

The total volume (1.2 ml) of 1 vial TORISEL 25 mg/ml concentrate must be diluted with 1.8 ml of withdrawn diluent to achieve a concentration of temsirolimus of 10 mg/ml. Withdraw the required amount of the temsirolimus 10 mg/ml mixture and then inject rapidly into sodium chloride 9 mg/ml (0.9%) solution for injection.

For instructions on preparation, see section 6.6.

Patients should be given intravenous diphenhydramine 25 to 50 mg (or similar antihistamine) approximately 30 minutes before the start of each dose of temsirolimus.

Treatment with TORISEL should continue until the patient is no longer clinically benefiting from therapy or until unacceptable toxicity occurs. No special dose modification is required for any of the populations that have been studied (gender, elderly).

Renal cell carcinoma

The recommended dose of temsirolimus for advanced renal cell carcinoma administered intravenously is 25 mg infused over a 30- to 60-minute period once weekly (see section 6.6 for instructions on dilution, administration and disposal).

Management of suspected adverse reactions may require temporary interruption and/or dose reduction of temsirolimus therapy. If a suspected reaction is not manageable with dose delays, then temsirolimus may be reduced by 5 mg/week decrements.

Mantle cell lymphoma

The recommended dosing regimen of temsirolimus for mantle cell lymphoma is 175 mg, infused over a 30-60 minute period once weekly for 3 weeks followed by weekly doses of 75 mg, infused over a 30-60 minute period. The starting dose of 175 mg was associated with a significant incidence of adverse events and required dose reductions/delays in the majority of patients. The contribution of the initial 175 mg doses to the efficacy outcome is currently not known.

Management of suspected adverse reactions may require temporary interruption and/or dose reduction of temsirolimus therapy according to the guidelines in the following tables. If a suspected reaction is not manageable with dose delays and/or optimal medical therapy, then the dose of temsirolimus should be reduced according to the dose reduction table below.

Dose Reduction Levels

Dose Reduction Level	Starting Dose 175 mg	Continuing Dose[a] 75 mg
-1	75 mg	50 mg
-2	50 mg	25 mg

[a] In the MCL Clinical Trial, up to two dose level reductions were allowed per patient.

Temsirolimus Dose Modifications Based on Weekly ANC and Platelet Counts

ANC	Platelets	Dose of Temsirolimus
$\geqslant 1.0 \times 10^9$/l	$\geqslant 50 \times 10^9$/l	100% of planned dose
$<1.0 \times 10^9$/l	$<50 \times 10^9$/l	Hold[a]

[a] Upon recovery to ANC $\geqslant 1.0 \times 10^9$/l (1000 cells/mm^3) and platelets to $\geqslant 50 \times 10^9$/l (50,000 cells/mm^3), the doses should be modified to the next lower dose level according to the table above. If the patient cannot maintain ANC $>1.0 \times 10^9$/l and platelets $>50 \times 10^9$/l on the new dose reduction level, then the next lower dose should be given once the counts have recovered.

Abbreviation: ANC = absolute neutrophil count.

Paediatric patients

Experience in paediatric patients is limited. The safety and effectiveness in paediatric patients have not been established. Therefore, the use of TORISEL in the paediatric population is not recommended until further information on effectiveness and safety is available.

Elderly patients

No specific dose adjustment is necessary.

Renal impairment

No dose adjustment of temsirolimus is recommended in patients with renal impairment. Temsirolimus should be used with caution in patients with severe renal impairment (see section 4.4).

Hepatic impairment

Temsirolimus should be used with caution in patients with hepatic impairment. Use of temsirolimus in patients with moderate (total bilirubin greater than 1.5-3 times upper limit of normal [ULN] and any AST greater than ULN) or severe (total bilirubin greater than 3 times ULN and any AST greater than ULN) hepatic impairment is not recommended (see section 4.4).

4.3 Contraindications

Hypersensitivity to temsirolimus, its metabolites (including sirolimus), polysorbate 80, or to any of the excipients of TORISEL.

Use of temsirolimus in patients with mantle cell lymphoma with moderate or severe hepatic impairment is not recommended (see section 4.4).

4.4 Special warnings and precautions for use

The incidence and severity of adverse events is dose-dependent. Patients receiving the starting dose of 175 mg weekly for the treatment of MCL must be followed closely to decide on dose reductions/delays.

Paediatric patients

Temsirolimus is not recommended for use in paediatric patients due to insufficient data on safety.

Elderly patients

Based on the results of a phase 3 study in renal cell carcinoma, elderly patients ($\geqslant$ 65 years of age) may be more likely to experience certain adverse reactions, including oedema, diarrhoea, and pneumonia. Based on the results of a phase 3 study in mantle cell lymphoma, elderly patients ($\geqslant$ 65 years of age) may be more likely to experience certain adverse reactions, including pleural effusion, anxiety, depression, insomnia, dyspnoea, leukopaenia, lymphopaenia, myalgia, arthralgia, taste loss, dizziness, upper respiratory infection, mucositis, and rhinitis.

Renal impairment

Temsirolimus elimination by the kidneys is negligible; studies in patients with varying renal impairment have not been conducted (see sections 4.2 and 5.2). TORISEL has not been studied in patients undergoing haemodialysis.

Renal failure

Renal failure (including fatal outcomes) has been observed in patients receiving TORISEL for advanced renal cell cancer and/or with pre-existing renal insufficiency (see section 4.8).

Hepatic impairment

Temsirolimus is cleared predominantly by the liver. No data are currently available regarding the influence of hepatic dysfunction and/or hepatic metastases on temsirolimus disposition. Use of temsirolimus 25 mg IV in patients with severe (total bilirubin >3 times ULN and any AST greater than ULN) hepatic impairment is not recommended. Use of temsirolimus doses >25 mg IV in patients who have moderate (total bilirubin >1.5-3 times upper limit of normal [ULN] and any AST $>$ ULN) or severe (total bilirubin >3 times ULN and any AST $>>$ ULN) hepatic impairment is not recommended (see section 4.2).

Intracerebral bleeding

Patients with central nervous system (CNS) tumours (primary CNS tumours or metastases) and/or receiving anticoagulation therapy may be at an increased risk of developing intracerebral bleeding (including fatal outcomes) while receiving therapy with temsirolimus.

Thrombocytopaenia and neutropaenia

Grades 3 and 4 thrombocytopaenia and/or neutropaenia have been observed in the MCL Clinical Trial (see section 4.8). Patients on temsirolimus who develop thrombocytopaenia may be at increased risk of bleeding events, including epistaxis (see section 4.8). Patients on temsirolimus with baseline neutropaenia may be at risk of developing febrile neutropaenia.

Infections

Patients may be immunosuppressed and should be carefully observed for the occurrence of infections, including opportunistic infections. Among patients receiving 175 mg/week for the treatment of MCL, infections (including grade 3 and 4 infections) were substantially increased compared to lower doses and compared to conventional chemotherapy.

Cataracts

Cataracts have been observed in some patients who received the combination of temsirolimus and interferon-α.

Hypersensitivity/infusion reactions

Hypersensitivity/infusion reactions (including some life-threatening and rare fatal reactions), including and not limited to flushing, chest pain, dyspnoea, hypotension, apnoea, loss of consciousness, hypersensitivity and anaphylaxis, have been associated with the administration of temsirolimus (see section 4.8). These reactions can occur very early in the first infusion, but may also occur with subsequent infusions. Patients should be monitored early during the infusion and appropriate supportive care should be available. Temsirolimus infusion should be interrupted in all patients with severe infusion reactions and appropriate medical therapy administered. A benefit-risk assessment should be done prior to the continuation of temsirolimus therapy in patients with severe or life-threatening reactions.

If a patient develops a hypersensitivity reaction during the TORISEL infusion, despite the premedication, the infusion must be stopped and the patient observed for at least 30 to 60 minutes (depending on the severity of the reaction). At the discretion of the physician, treatment may be resumed after the administration of an H_1-receptor antagonist (diphenhydramine or similar antihistamine) and a H_2-receptor antagonist (intravenous famotidine 20 mg or intravenous ranitidine 50 mg) approximately 30 minutes before restarting the TORISEL infusion. Administration of corticosteroids may be considered; however, the efficacy of corticosteroid treatment in this setting has not been established. The infusion may then be resumed at a slower rate (up to 60 minutes) and should be completed within six hours from the time that TORISEL is first added to sodium chloride 9 mg/ml (0.9%) solution for injection.

Because it is recommended that an H_1 antihistamine be administered to patients before the start of the intravenous temsirolimus infusion, temsirolimus should be used with caution in patients with known hypersensitivity to the antihistamine or in patients who cannot receive the antihistamine for other medical reasons.

Hypersensitivity reactions, including anaphylactic/anaphylactoid reactions, angioedema, exfoliative dermatitis and hypersensitivity vasculitis, have been associated with the oral administration of sirolimus.

Hyperglycaemia/glucose intolerance/diabetes mellitus

Patients should be advised that treatment with TORISEL may be associated with an increase in blood glucose levels in diabetic and non-diabetic patients. In the RCC Clinical Trial, a phase 3 clinical trial for renal cell carcinoma, 26% of patients reported hyperglycaemia as an adverse event. In the MCL Clinical Trial, a phase 3 clinical trial for mantle cell lymphoma, 11% of patients reported hyperglycaemia as an adverse event. This may result in the need for an increase in the dose of, or initiation of, insulin and/or hypoglycaemic agent therapy. Patients should be advised to report excessive thirst or any increase in the volume or frequency of urination.

Interstitial lung disease

There have been cases of non-specific interstitial pneumonitis, including rare fatal reports, occurring in patients who received weekly intravenous TORISEL. Some patients were asymptomatic with pneumonitis detected on computed tomography scan or chest radiograph. Others presented with symptoms such as dyspnoea, cough, and fever. Some patients required discontinuation of TORISEL or treatment with corticosteroids and/or antibiotics, while some patients continued treatment without additional intervention. Patients should be followed for clinical respiratory symptoms.

Hyperlipaemia

The use of TORISEL was associated with increases in serum triglycerides and cholesterol. In the RCC Clinical Trial 1, hyperlipaemia was reported as an adverse event in 27% of patients. In the MCL Clinical Trial, hyperlipaemia was reported as an adverse event in 9.3% of patients. This may require initiation, or increase, in the dose of lipid-lowering agents. Serum cholesterol and triglycerides should be tested before and during treatment with TORISEL.

Wound healing complications

The use of TORISEL has been associated with abnormal wound healing; therefore, caution should be exercised with the use of TORISEL in the peri-surgical period.

Concomitant use of temsirolimus with sunitinib

The combination of temsirolimus and sunitinib resulted in dose-limiting toxicity. Dose-limiting toxicities (grade 3/4 erythematous maculopapular rash, gout/cellulitis requiring hospitalisation) were observed in two out of three patients treated in the first cohort of a phase 1 study at doses of temsirolimus 15 mg intravenous per week and sunitinib 25 mg oral per day (days 1-28 followed by a 2-week rest).

Concomitant use of angiotensin-converting enzyme (ACE) inhibitors

Angioneurotic oedema-type reactions (including delayed reactions occurring two months following initiation of therapy) have been observed in some patients who received temsirolimus and ACE inhibitors concomitantly (see section 4.5).

Agents inducing CYP3A metabolism

Agents such as carbamazepine, phenobarbital, phenytoin, rifampicin, and St. John's Wort are strong inducers of CYP3A4/5 and may decrease composite exposure of the active moieties, temsirolimus and its metabolite, sirolimus. Therefore, for patients with renal cell carcinoma, continuous administration beyond 5-7 days with agents that have CYP3A4/5 induction potential should be avoided. For patients with mantle cell lymphoma, it is recommended that coadministration of CYP3A4/5 inducers should be avoided due to the higher dose of temsirolimus (see section 4.5).

Agents inhibiting CYP3A metabolism

Agents such as protease inhibitors (nelfinavir, ritonavir), antifungals (e.g., itraconazole, ketoconazole, voriconazole), and nefazodone are strong CYP3A4 inhibitors and may increase blood concentrations of the active moieties, temsirolimus and its metabolite, sirolimus. Therefore, concomitant treatment with agents that have strong CYP3A4 inhibition potential should be avoided. Concomitant treatment with moderate CYP3A4 inhibitors (e.g., aprepitant, erythromycin, fluconazole, verapamil, grapefruit juice) should only be administered with caution in patients receiving 25 mg and should be avoided in patients receiving temsirolimus doses higher than 25 mg (see section 4.5). Alternative treatments with agents that do not have CYP3A4 inhibition potential should be considered (see section 4.5).

Vaccinations

Immunosuppressants may affect responses to vaccination. During treatment with TORISEL, vaccination may be less effective. The use of live vaccines should be avoided during treatment with TORISEL. Examples of live vaccines are: measles, mumps, rubella, oral polio, BCG, yellow fever, varicella, and TY21a typhoid vaccines.

Excipients

This medicinal product (concentrate-diluent mixture) contains 35% volume ethanol (alcohol); i.e., up to 693.5 mg per dose, equivalent to 17.6 ml beer, 7.3 ml wine per dose.

Harmful for those suffering from alcoholism.

To be taken into account in pregnant or breast-feeding women, children and high-risk groups, such as patients with liver disease or epilepsy.

4.5 Interaction with other medicinal products and other forms of interaction

Interaction studies have only been performed in adults.

Concomitant use of angiotensin-converting enzyme (ACE) inhibitors

Angioneurotic oedema-type reactions (including delayed reactions occurring two months following initiation of therapy) have been observed in some patients who received temsirolimus and ACE inhibitors concomitantly (see section 4.4).

Agents inducing CYP3A metabolism

Co-administration of TORISEL with rifampicin, a potent CYP3A4/5 inducer, had no significant effect on temsirolimus C_{max} (maximum concentration) and AUC (area under the concentration vs. time curve) after intravenous administration, but decreased sirolimus C_{max} by 65% and AUC by 56%, compared to TORISEL treatment alone. Therefore, concomitant treatment with agents that have CYP3A4/5 induction potential should be avoided [e.g., carbamazepine, phenobarbital, phenytoin, rifampicin, and St. John's Wort] (see section 4.4).

Agents inhibiting CYP3A metabolism

Co-administration of TORISEL 5 mg with ketoconazole, a potent CYP3A4 inhibitor, had no significant effect on temsirolimus C_{max} or AUC; however, sirolimus AUC increased 3.1-fold, and AUC_{sum} (temsirolimus + sirolimus) increased 2.3-fold compared to TORISEL alone. The effect on the unbound concentrations of sirolimus has not been determined, but is expected to be larger than the effect on whole-blood concentrations due to the saturable binding to red blood cells. The effect may also be more pronounced at a 25 mg dose. Therefore, substances that are potent inhibitors of CYP3A4 activity (e.g., nelfinavir, ritonavir, itraconazole, ketoconazole, voriconazole, nefazodone) increase sirolimus blood concentrations. Concomitant treatment of TORISEL with these agents should be avoided (see section 4.4).

Concomitant treatment with moderate CYP3A4 inhibitors (e.g., diltiazem, verapamil, clarithromycin, erythromycin, aprepitant, amiodarone) should only be administered with caution in patients receiving 25 mg and should be avoided in patients receiving temsirolimus doses higher than 25 mg.

Interaction with medicinal products metabolised by CYP2D6

In 23 healthy subjects, the concentration of desipramine, a CYP2D6 substrate, was unaffected when 25 mg of temsirolimus was co-administered. No clinically significant effect is anticipated when TORISEL is co-administered with agents that are metabolised by CYP2D6 in patients with renal cell carcinoma. For patients with mantle cell lymphoma, the effect of a 175 or 75 mg temsirolimus dose on CYP2D6 or 3A4 substrates has not been studied.

Interactions with drugs that are P-glycoprotein substrates

In an *in vitro* study, temsirolimus inhibited the transport of P-glycoprotein substrates with an IC_{50} value of 2 μM. The clinical relevance of this finding is not known.

Table 1

Adverse Reactions in RCC Clinical Trial 1

System Organ Class	Frequency	Adverse Reactions	All Grades n (%)	Grade 3 & 4 n (%)
Infections and infestations	Very common	Bacterial and viral infections (including infection, cellulitis, herpes zoster, herpes simplex, bronchitis, sinusitis, abscess)*	42 (20)	6 (3)
	Very common	Urinary tract infection (including dysuria, haematuria, cystitis, urinary frequency, urinary tract infection)*	31 (15)	4 (2)
	Very common	Pharyngitis	25 (12)	0 (0)
	Very common	Rhinitis	20 (10)	0 (0)
	Common	Pneumonia	17 (8)	5 (2)
	Common	Upper respiratory tract infection	14 (7)	0 (0)
	Common	Folliculitis	4 (2)	0 (0)
Blood and lymphatic system disorders	Very common	Thrombocytopaenia	28 (14)	3 (1)
	Very common	Anaemia	94 (45)	41 (20)
	Common	Neutropaenia	15 (7)	6 (3)
	Common	Leukopoenia	13 (6)	1 (1)
	Common	Lymphopaenia	11 (5)	9 (4)
Immune system disorders	Common	Allergic/hypersensitivity reactions	18 (9)	0 (0)
Metabolism and nutrition disorders	Very common	Hypokalaemia	20 (10)	7 (3)
	Very common	Anorexia	66 (32)	6 (3)
	Very common	Hyperglycaemia/diabetes mellitus**	53 (26)	22 (11)
	Very common	Hypercholesterolaemia	51 (24)	1 (1)
	Very common	Hyperlipaemia	57 (27)	8 (4)
	Common	Hypophosphataemia	17 (8)	11 (5)
Psychiatric disorders	Very common	Insomnia	24 (12)	1 (1)
	Common	Anxiety	16 (8)	0 (0)
	Common	Depression	9 (4)	0 (0)
Nervous system disorders	Very common	Dysgeusia	31 (15)	0 (0)
	Common	Somnolence	14 (7)	3 (1)
	Common	Paresthaesia	13 (6)	1 (1)
	Common	Dizziness	19 (9)	1 (1)
	Common	Ageusia	11 (5)	0 (0)
	Uncommon	Intracerebral bleeding	1 (0.5)	1 (0.5)
Eye disorders	Common	Conjunctivitis (including conjunctivitis, lacrimation disorders)*	15 (7)	1 (1)
Cardiac disorders	Uncommon	Pericardial effusion (including haemodynamically significant pericardial effusions requiring intervention)	2 (1)	1 (1)
Vascular disorders	Common	Venous thromboembolism (including deep vein thrombosis, pulmonary embolus, thrombosis)*	6 (3)	3 (1)
	Common	Hypertension	14 (7)	3 (1)
	Common	Thrombophlebitis	2 (1)	0 (0)
Respiratory, thoracic and mediastinal disorders	Very common	Dyspnoea	58 (28)	18 (9)
	Very common	Epistaxis	25 (12)	0 (0)
	Very common	Cough	54 (26)	2 (1)
	Common	Pneumonitis [including fatal pneumonitis] (see section 4.4)	4 (2)	1 (1)
	Common	Pleural effusion	8 (4)	5 (2)
Gastrointestinal disorders	Very common	Abdominal pain	44 (21)	9 (4)
	Very common	Vomiting	40 (19)	4 (2)
	Very common	Stomatitis*	42 (20)	3 (1)
	Very common	Diarrhoea	57 (27)	3 (1)
	Very common	Nausea	77 (37)	5 (2)
	Common	Abdominal distension	9 (4)	1 (1)
	Common	Oral pain	5 (2)	0 (0)
	Common	Gingivitis	5 (2)	0 (0)
	Common	Aphthous stomatitis	8 (4)	1 (0)
	Uncommon	Bowel perforation	1 (0.5)	1 (0.5)
Skin and subcutaneous tissue disorders	Very common	Rash (including rash, pruritic rash, maculopapular rash, pustular rash)*	88 (42)	10 (5)
	Very common	Pruritus	40 (19)	1 (1)
	Very common	Acne	21 (10)	0 (0)
	Very common	Nail disorder	28 (14)	0 (0)
	Very common	Dry skin	22 (11)	1 (1)
	Common	Exfoliative dermatitis	16 (8)	0 (0)
Musculoskeletal and connective ti ssue disorders	Very common	Back pain	41 (20)	6 (3)
	Very common	Arthralgia	37 (18)	2 (1)
	Common	Myalgia (including myalgia, leg cramps)*	17 (8)	1 (1)
Renal and urinary disorders	Common	Renal failure [including fatal outcomes] (see section 4.4)	4 (2)	2 (1)

Adverse Reactions in RCC Clinical Trial 1				
System Organ Class	**Frequency**	**Adverse Reactions**	**All Grades n (%)**	**Grade 3 & 4 n (%)**
General disorders and administration site conditions	Very common	Oedema (including oedema, facial oedema, peripheral oedema)*	72 (35)	7 (3)
	Very common	Asthenia	106 (51)	23 (11)
	Very common	Pain	59 (28)	11 (5)
	Very common	Pyrexia	51 (24)	1 (1)
	Very common	Mucositis	39 (19)	2 (1)
	Very common	Chest pain	34 (16)	2 (1)
	Common	Chills	17 (8)	1 (1)
	Common	Impaired wound healing	3 (1)	0 (0)
Investigations	Very common	Blood creatinine increased	30 (14)	6 (3)
	Common	Increased aspartate aminotransferase	17 (8)	3 (1)
	Common	Increased alanine aminotransferase	12 (6)	1 (1)

*Body system totals are not necessarily the sum of the individual adverse events, since a subject may report two or more different adverse events in the same body system.

**Patients should be advised that treatment with TORISEL may be associated with an increase in blood glucose levels in diabetic and non-diabetic patients.

Amphiphilic agents

Temsirolimus has been associated with phospholipidosis in rats. Phospholipidosis has not been observed in mice or monkeys treated with temsirolimus, nor has it been documented in patients treated with temsirolimus. Although phospholipidosis has not been shown to be a risk for patients administered temsirolimus, it is possible that combined administration of temsirolimus with other amphiphilic agents such as amiodarone or statins could result in an increased risk of amphiphilic pulmonary toxicity.

4.6 Pregnancy and lactation

There are no adequate data from the use of temsirolimus in pregnant women. Studies in animals have shown reproductive toxicity. In reproduction studies in animals, temsirolimus caused embryo/foetotoxicity that was manifested as mortality and reduced foetal weights (with associated delays in skeletal ossification) in rats and rabbits. Teratogenic effects (omphalocele) were seen in rabbits. In male rats, decreased fertility and partly reversible reductions in sperm counts were reported (see section 5.3).

The potential risk for humans is unknown. TORISEL must not be used during pregnancy, unless the risk for the embryo is justified by the expected benefit for the mother.

Due to the unknown risk related to potential exposure during early pregnancy, women of childbearing potential must be advised not to become pregnant while using TORISEL.

Men with partners of childbearing potential should use medically acceptable contraception while receiving TORISEL (see section 5.3).

It is unknown whether temsirolimus is excreted in human breast milk. The excretion of temsirolimus in milk has not been studied in animals. However, sirolimus, the main metabolite of temsirolimus, is excreted in milk of lactating rats. Because of the potential for adverse reactions in breast-fed infants from temsirolimus, breast-feeding should be discontinued during therapy.

4.7 Effects on ability to drive and use machines

No studies on the effects on the ability to drive and use machines have been performed.

4.8 Undesirable effects

Due to the different approved posology for RCC and MCL and the dose-dependency of the frequency and severity of undesirable effects, adverse drug reactions are listed separately.

Renal cell carcinoma

A total of 626 patients were randomly assigned in a phase 3, three-arm, randomised, open-label study of Interferon alfa (IFN-α) alone, TORISEL alone, and TORISEL and IFN-α. A total of 616 patients received treatment: 200 patients received IFN-α weekly; 208 received TORISEL 25 mg weekly, and 208 patients received a combination of IFN-α and TORISEL weekly. Based on the results of the phase 3 study, elderly patients may be more likely to experience certain adverse reactions, including face oedema and pneumonia.

The most serious reactions observed with TORISEL are hypersensitivity/infusion reactions (including some life-threatening and rare fatal reactions), hyperglycaemia/glucose intolerance, infections, interstitial lung disease (pneumonitis), hyperlipaemia, intracerebral bleeding, renal failure, bowel perforation, and wound healing complication.

The most common (≥30%) adverse reactions (all grades) observed with TORISEL include anaemia, nausea, rash (including rash, pruritic rash, maculopapular rash, pustular rash), anorexia, oedema (including facial oedema and peripheral oedema), and asthenia.

Cataracts have been observed in some patients who received the combination of temsirolimus and interferon-α.

See section 4.4 for additional information concerning serious adverse reactions, including appropriate actions to be taken if specific reactions occur.

The following list contains adverse reactions seen in RCC Clinical Trial 1. Only events for which there is at least reasonable suspicion of a causal relationship to intravenous treatment with TORISEL are listed.

Within each frequency grouping, undesirable effects are presented in order of decreasing seriousness.

Adverse reactions are listed according to the following categories:

Very common: ≥1/10

Common: ≥1/100 to <1/10

Uncommon: ≥1/1,000 to <1/100

(see Table 1 on previous page)

Mantle cell lymphoma

A total of 54 patients were treated with 175/75 mg TORISEL in the MCL Clinical Trial, a phase 3, three-arm, randomised, open-label study of TORISEL comparing 2 different dosing regimens of temsirolimus with an investigator's choice of therapy in patients with relapsed and/or refractory mantle cell lymphoma. Based on the results of the phase 3 study, elderly patients (≥65 years) may be more likely to experience certain adverse reactions, including pleural effusion, anxiety, depression, insomnia, dyspnoea, leukopaenia, lymphopaenia, myalgia, arthralgia, taste loss, dizziness, upper respiratory infection, mucositis, and rhinitis.

The most serious reactions observed with TORISEL are thrombocytopaenia, neutropaenia, infections, interstitial lung disease (pneumonitis), bowel perforation, hypersensitivity reactions, and hyperglycaemia/glucose intolerance.

The most common (≥30%) adverse reactions (all grades) observed with TORISEL include thrombocytopaenia, asthenia, anaemia, diarrhoea, bacterial and viral infections*, rash*, pyrexia, anorexia, epistaxis, mucositis, oedema*, and stomatitis*.

The occurrence of undesirable effects following the dose of 175 mg TORISEL/week for MCL, e.g. grade 3 or 4 infections or thrombocytopaenia, is associated with a higher incidence than that observed with either 75 mg TORISEL/week or conventional chemotherapy.

*See table below for additional terms included with these adverse reactions.

See section 4.4 for additional information concerning serious adverse reactions, including appropriate actions to be taken if specific reactions occur.

The following list contains adverse reactions seen in the MCL Clinical Trial. Only events for which there is at least reasonable suspicion of a causal relationship to intravenous treatment with TORISEL are listed.

Within each frequency grouping, undesirable effects are presented in order of decreasing seriousness.

Adverse reactions are listed according to the following categories:

Very common: ≥1/10

Common: ≥1/100 to <1/10

(see Table 2 on next page)

Serious adverse reactions observed in clinical trials of temsirolimus for advanced renal cell carcinoma, but not in clinical trials of temsirolimus for mantle cell lymphoma include: anaphylaxis, impaired wound healing, renal failure with fatal outcomes, and pulmonary embolus.

Adverse reactions for which frequency is undetermined

Angioneurotic oedema-type reactions in some patients who received temsirolimus and ACE-inhibitors concomitantly.

4.9 Overdose

There is no specific treatment for TORISEL intravenous overdose. While TORISEL has been safely administered to patients with renal cancer with repeated intravenous doses of temsirolimus as high as 220 mg/m^2, in MCL, two administrations of 330 mg TORISEL/week in one patient resulted in grade 3 rectal bleeding and grade 2 diarrhoea.

5. PHARMACOLOGICAL PROPERTIES

5.1 Pharmacodynamic properties

Pharmacotherapeutic group: Protein Kinase Inhibitors; ATC code: L01X E09

Temsirolimus is a selective inhibitor of mTOR (mammalian target of rapamycin). Temsirolimus binds to an intracellular protein (FKBP-12), and the protein/temsirolimus complex binds and inhibits the activity of mTOR that controls cell division. *In vitro*, at high concentrations (10-20 μM), temsirolimus can bind and inhibit mTOR in the absence of FKBP-12. Biphasic dose response of cell growth inhibition was observed. High concentrations resulted in complete cell growth inhibition *in vitro*, whereas inhibition mediated by FKBP-12/temsirolimus complex alone resulted in approximately 50% decrease in cell proliferation. Inhibition of mTOR activity results in a G1 growth delay at nanomolar concentrations and growth arrest at micromolar concentrations in treated tumour cells resulting from selective disruption of translation of cell cycle regulatory proteins, such as D-type cyclins, c-myc, and ornithine decarboxylase. When mTOR activity is inhibited, its ability to phosphorylate, and thereby control the activity of protein translation factors (4E-BP1 and S6K, both downstream of mTOR in the P13 kinase/AKT pathway) that control cell division, is blocked.

In addition to regulating cell cycle proteins, mTOR can regulate translation of the hypoxia-inducible factors, HIF-1 and HIF-2 alpha. These transcription factors regulate the ability of tumours to adapt to hypoxic microenvironments and to produce the angiogenic factor vascular endothelial growth factor (VEGF). The anti-tumour effect of temsirolimus, therefore, may also in part stem from its ability to depress levels of HIF and VEGF in the tumour or tumour microenvironment, thereby impairing vessel development.

Clinical Efficacy

Renal cell carcinoma

The safety and efficacy of TORISEL in the treatment of advanced renal cell carcinoma were studied in the following two randomised clinical trials:

RCC Clinical Trial 1

RCC Clinical Trial 1 was a phase 3, multi-centre, three-arm, randomised, open-label study in previously untreated patients with advanced renal cell carcinoma and with 3 or more of 6 pre-selected prognostic risk factors (less than one year from time of initial renal cell carcinoma diagnosis to randomisation, Karnofsky performance status of 60 or 70, haemoglobin less than the lower limit of normal, corrected calcium of greater than 10 mg/dl, lactate dehydrogenase >1.5 times the upper limit of normal, more than one metastatic organ site). The primary study endpoint was overall survival (OS). Secondary endpoints included progression-free survival (PFS), objective response rate (ORR), clinical benefit rate, time to treatment failure (TTF), and quality adjusted survival measurement. Patients were stratified for prior nephrectomy status within three geographic regions and were randomly assigned (1:1:1) to receive IFN-α alone (n = 207), TORISEL alone (25 mg weekly; n = 209), or the combination of IFN-α and TORISEL (n = 210).

In RCC Clinical Trial 1, TORISEL 25 mg was associated with a statistically significant advantage over IFN-α in the primary endpoint of OS at the 2nd pre-specified interim analysis (n = 446 events, p = 0.0078). The TORISEL arm showed a 49% increase in median OS compared with the IFN-α arm. TORISEL also was associated with statistically significant advantages over IFN-α in the secondary endpoints of PFS, TTF, and clinical benefit rate.

The combination of TORISEL 15 mg and IFN-α did not result in a significant increase in overall survival when compared with IFN-α alone at either the interim analysis (median 8.4 vs. 7.3 months, hazard ratio = 0.96, p = 0.6965) or final analysis (median 8.4 vs. 7.3 months, hazard ratio = 0.93, p = 0.4902). Treatment with the combination of TORISEL and IFN-α resulted in a statistically significant increase in the incidence of certain grade 3-4 adverse events (weight loss, anaemia, neutropaenia, thrombocytopaenia and mucosal inflammation) when compared with the adverse events observed in the IFN-α or TORISEL-alone arms.

(see Table 3 on page 4932417)

In RCC Clinical Trial 1, 31% of patients treated with TORISEL were 65 or older. In patients younger than 65, median overall survival was 12 months (95% CI 9.9, 14.2) with a hazard ratio of 0.67 (95% CI 0.52, 0.87) compared with those treated with IFN-α. In patients 65 or older, median overall survival was 8.6 months (95% CI 6.4, 11.5) with a hazard ratio of 1.15 (95% CI 0.78, 1.68) compared with those treated with IFN-α.

RCC Clinical Trial 2

RCC Clinical Trial 2 was a randomised, double-blind, multi-centre, outpatient trial to evaluate the efficacy, safety, and pharmacokinetics of three dose levels of TORISEL when

Table 2

Adverse Reactions in MCL Clinical Trial

System Organ Class	Frequency	Adverse Reactions	All Grades n (%)	Grade 3 & 4 n (%)
Infections and infestations	Very common	Bacterial and viral infections (including infection, cellulitis, bronchitis, sinusitis, herpes zoster, herpes simplex)*	23 (43)	8 (15)
	Very common	Pneumonia (including interstitial pneumonia)**	8 (15)	6 (11)
	Very common	Urinary tract infection (including dysuria, urinary frequency, urinary tract infection, urinary urgency)*	8 (15)	0 (0)
	Very common	Pharyngitis	4 (7)	0 (0)
	Very common	Upper respiratory tract infection	8 (15)	0 (0)
	Common	Sepsis (including sepsis, septic shock)*	3 (6)	3 (6)
	Common	Rhinitis	5 (9)	0 (0)
	Common	Folliculitis	1 (2)	0 (0)
Blood and lymphatic system disorders	Very common	Thrombocytopaenia**	39 (72)	32 (59)
	Very common	Anaemia	28 (52)	11 (20)
	Very common	Neutropaenia**	13 (24)	8 (15)
	Very common	Leukopaenia	8 (15)	4 (7)
	Very common	Lymphopaenia	6 (11)	4 (7)
Immune system disorders	Common	Allergic/hypersensitivity reactions	1 (2)	0 (0)
Metabolism and nutrition disorders	Very common	Hypokalaemia	10 (19)	4 (7)
	Very common	Anorexia	20 (37)	1 (2)
	Very common	Hyperglycaemia***	6 (11)	6 (11)
	Very common	Hypercholesterolaemia	7 (13)	0 (0)
	Common	Dehydration	3 (6)	2 (4)
	Common	Hypophosphataemia	3 (6)	0 (0)
	Common	Hyperlipaemia	5 (9)	1 (2)
	Common	Hypocalcaemia	5 (9)	1 (2)
Psychiatric disorders	Very common	Insomnia	11 (20)	0 (0)
	Very common	Anxiety	8 (15)	0 (0)
	Common	Depression	5 (9)	0 (0)
Nervous system disorders	Very common	Dysgeusia	8 (15)	0 (0)
	Common	Paresthaesia	4 (7)	0 (0)
	Common	Dizziness	3 (6)	0 (0)
	Common	Ageusia	5 (9)	0 (0)
Eye disorders	Common	Conjunctivitis	4 (7)	0 (0)
	Common	Eye haemorrhage	2 (4)	0 (0)
Vascular disorders	Common	Thrombosis (including deep venous thrombosis, thrombosis)*	3 (6)	1 (2)
	Common	Hypertension	2 (4)	0 (0)
Respiratory, thoracic and mediastinal disorders	Very common	Dyspnoea	10 (19)	4 (7)
	Very common	Epistaxis	19 (35)	0 (0)
	Very common	Cough	14 (26)	0 (0)
	Common	Pneumonitis****	2 (4)	0 (0)
Gastrointestinal disorders	Very common	Abdominal pain	11 (20)	1 (2)
	Very common	Vomiting	9 (17)	0 (0)
	Very common	Stomatitis (including aphthous stomatitis, mouth ulceration, stomatitis, glossitis, oral pain)*	16 (30)	1 (2)
	Very common	Diarrhoea	24 (44)	4 (7)
	Very common	Nausea	14 (26)	0 (0)
	Common	Bowel perforation	1 (2)	1 (2)
	Common	Gastrointestinal haemorrhage (including gastrointestinal haemorrhage, rectal haemorrhage)*	6 (11)	2 (4)
	Common	Gingivitis	2 (4)	0 (0)
	Common	Gastritis	3 (6)	1 (2)
	Common	Dysphagia	4 (7)	0 (0)
Skin and subcutaneous tissue disorders	Very common	Rash (including rash, pruritic rash, maculopapular rash, pustular rash, eczema)*	22 (41)	4 (7)
	Very common	Pruritus	14 (26)	2 (4)
	Very common	Nail disorder	8 (15)	0 (0)
	Very common	Dry skin	7 (13)	0 (0)
	Common	Acne	4 (7)	0 (0)
	Common	Moniliasis (including moniliasis, oral moniliasis)*	2 (4)	0 (0)
	Common	Fungal dermatitis	1 (2)	0 (0)
	Common	Ecchymosis	4 (7)	0 (0)
Musculoskeletal, connective tissue and bone disorders	Very common	Back pain	7 (13)	0 (0)
	Very common	Arthralgia	11 (20)	1 (2)
	Very common	Myalgia (including muscle cramps, leg cramps, myalgia)*	9 (17)	0 (0)
General disorders and administration site conditions	Very common	Oedema (including oedema, facial oedema, peripheral oedema, scrotal oedema, genital oedema, generalised oedema)*	19 (35)	1 (2)
	Very common	Asthenia	34 (63)	7 (13)
	Very common	Pain	15 (28)	1 (2)
	Very common	Pyrexia	21 (39)	3 (6)
	Very common	Mucositis	19 (35)	3 (6)
	Very common	Chills	14 (26)	1 (2)
	Common	Chest pain	4 (7)	0 (0)

administered to previously treated patients with advanced renal cell carcinoma. The primary efficacy endpoint was ORR, and OS was also evaluated. One hundred eleven (111) patients were randomly assigned in a 1:1:1 ratio to receive 25 mg, 75 mg, or 250 mg temsirolimus intravenous weekly. In the 25 mg arm (n = 36), all patients had metastatic disease; 4 (11%) had no prior chemo- or immunotherapy; 17 (47%) had one prior treatment, and 15 (42%) had 2 or more prior treatments for renal cell carcinoma. Twenty-seven (27, 75%) had undergone a nephrectomy. Twenty-four (24, 67%) were Eastern Cooperative Oncology Group (ECOG) performance status (PS) = 1, and 12 (33%) were ECOG PS = 0.

For patients treated weekly with 25 mg temsirolimus OS was 13.8 months (95% CI: 9.0, 18.7 months); ORR was 5.6% (95% CI: 0.7, 18.7%).

Mantle cell lymphoma

The safety and efficacy of intravenous (IV) temsirolimus for the treatment of relapsed and/or refractory mantle cell lymphoma were studied in the following phase 3 clinical study.

MCL Clinical Trial

MCL Clinical Trial is a controlled, randomised, open-label, multicenter, outpatient study comparing 2 different dosing regimens of temsirolimus with an investigator's choice of therapy in patients with relapsed and/or refractory mantle cell lymphoma. Subjects with mantle cell lymphoma (that was confirmed by histology, immunophenotype, and cyclin D1 analysis) who had received 2 to 7 prior therapies that included anthracyclines and alkylating agents, and rituximab (and could include haematopoietic stem cell transplant) and whose disease was relapsed and/or refractory were eligible for the study. Subjects were randomly assigned in a 1:1:1 ratio to receive temsirolimus IV 175 mg (3 successive weekly doses) followed by 75 mg weekly (n = 54), temsirolimus IV 175 mg (3 successive weekly doses) followed by 25 mg weekly (n=54), or the investigator's choice of single-agent treatment (as specified in the protocol; n = 54). Investigator's choice therapies included: gemcitabine (IV: 22 [41.5%]), fludarabine (IV: 12 [22.6%] or oral: 2 [3.8%]), chlorambucil (oral: 3 [5.7%]), cladribine (IV: 3 [5.7%]), etoposide (IV: 3 [5.7%]), cyclophosphamide (oral: 2 [3.8%]), thalidomide (oral: 2 [3.8%]), vinblastine (IV: 2 [3.8%]), alemtuzumab (IV: 1 [1.9%]), and lenalidomide (oral: 1 [1.9%]). The primary endpoint of the study was progression-free survival (PFS), as assessed by an independent radiologist and oncology review. Secondary efficacy endpoints included overall survival (OS) and objective response rate (ORR).

The results for the MCL Clinical Trial are summarized in the following table. Temsirolimus 175/75 (temsirolimus 175 mg weekly for 3 weeks followed by 75 mg weekly) led to an improvement in PFS compared with investigator's choice in patients with relapsed and/or refractory mantle cell lymphoma that was statistically significant (hazard ratio = 0.44; p-value = 0.0009). Median PFS of the temsirolimus 175/75 mg group (4.8 months) was prolonged by 2.9 months compared to the investigator's choice group (1.9 months). Overall survival was similar.

Temsirolimus also was associated with statistically significant advantages over investigator's choice in the secondary endpoint of overall response rate (ORR). The evaluations of PFS and ORR were based on blinded independent radiologic assessment of tumour response using the International Workshop Criteria.

(see Table 4 on next page)

The temsirolimus 175 mg (3 successive weekly doses) followed by 25 mg weekly treatment arm did not result in a significant increase in PFS when compared with investigator's choice (median 3.4 vs. 1.9 months, hazard ratio = 0.65, CI = 0.39, 1.10, p = 0.0618).

In the MCL Clinical Trial, there was no difference in efficacy in patients with respect to age, sex, race, geographic region, or baseline disease characteristics.

5.2 Pharmacokinetic properties

Absorption

Following administration of a single 25 mg intravenous dose of temsirolimus in patients with cancer, mean C_{max} in whole blood was 585 ng/ml (coefficient of variation, CV = 14%), and mean AUC in blood was 1627 ng•h/ml (CV = 26%). For patients receiving 175 mg weekly for 3 weeks followed by 75 mg weekly, estimated C_{max} in whole blood at end of infusion was 2457 ng/ml during week 1, and 2574 ng/ml during week 3.

Distribution

Temsirolimus exhibits a polyexponential decline in whole blood concentrations, and distribution is attributable to preferential binding to FKBP-12 in blood cells. The mean (standard deviation, SD) dissociation constant (K_d) of binding was 5.1 (3.0) ng/ml, denoting the concentration at which 50% of binding sites in blood cells were occupied. Temsirolimus distribution is dose-dependent with mean (10th, 90th percentiles) maximal specific binding in blood cells of 1.4 mg (0.47 to 2.5 mg). Following a single 25 mg temsirolimus intravenous dose, mean steady-state volume of distribution in whole blood of patients with cancer was 172 liters.

Metabolism

Sirolimus, an equally potent metabolite to temsirolimus, was observed as the principal metabolite in humans

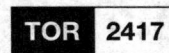

Adverse Reactions in MCL Clinical Trial				
System Organ Class	**Frequency**	**Adverse Reactions**	**All Grades n (%)**	**Grade 3 & 4 n (%)**
Investigations	Common	Blood creatinine increased	4 (7)	0 (0)
	Common	Increased aspartate aminotransferase	2 (4)	1 (2)
	Common	Increased alanine aminotransferase	1 (2)	1 (2)

*Body system totals are not necessarily the sum of the individual adverse events since a subject may report two or more different adverse events in the same body system.

**Grades 3 and 4 (thrombocytopaenia) are defined as 50,000-25,000 platelets/mm^3 and <25,000 platelets/mm^3, respectively. Grades 3 and 4 (neutropaenia) are defined as 1000-500 neutrophils/mm^3 and <500 neutrophils/mm^3, respectively.

***Patients should be advised that treatment with TORISEL may be associated with an increase in blood glucose levels in diabetic and non-diabetic patients.

****One case of fatal pneumonitis was reported in a mantle cell lymphoma patient receiving 175/25 mg/week that is not included in this table.

Table 3

Summary of Efficacy Results in TORISEL RCC Clinical Trial 1				
Parameter	**TORISEL** n = 209	**IFN-α** n = 207	**P-value**[a]	**Hazard ratio (95% CI)**[b]
Pre-specified interim analysis				
Median overall survival, Months (95% CI)	10.9 (8.6, 12.7)	7.3 (6.1, 8.8)	0.0078	0.73 (0.58, 0.92)
Final analysis				
Median overall survival, Months (95% CI)	10.9 (8.6, 12.7)	7.3 (6.1, 8.8)	0.0252	0.78 (0.63, 0.97)
Median progression-free survival by independent assessment Months (95% CI)	5.6 (3.9, 7.2)	3.2 (2.2, 4.0)	0.0042	0.74 (0.60, 0.91)
Median progression-free survival by investigator assessment Months (95% CI)	3.8 (3.6, 5.2)	1.9 (1.9, 2.2)	0.0028	0.74 (0.60, 0.90)
Overall response rate by independent assessment % (95% CI)	9.1 (5.2, 13.0)	5.3 (2.3, 8.4)	0.1361[c]	NA

CI = confidence interval; NA = not applicable.

[a] Based on log-rank test stratified by prior nephrectomy and region.

[b] Based on Cox proportional hazard model stratified by prior nephrectomy and region (95% CI are descriptive only).

[c] Based on Cochran-Mantel-Hansel test stratified by prior nephrectomy and region.

Table 4

Summary of Efficacy Results in TORISEL MCL Clinical Trial				
Parameter	**Temsirolimus Concentrate for Injection** 175/75 mg n = 54	**Investigator's Choice** n = 54	**P-value**	**Hazard Ratio (97.5% CI)**[a]
Median progression-free survival[b] Months (97.5% CI)	4.8 (3.1, 8.1)	1.9 (1.6, 2.5)	0.0009[c]	0.44 (0.25, 0.78)
Objective response rate[b] % (95% CI)	22.2 (11.1, 33.3)	1.9 (0.0, 5.4)	0.0019[d]	NA
Overall survival Months (95% CI)	11.1 (8.2, 18.0)	9.5 (5.3, 15.1)	0.3053[c]	0.77 (0.46, 1.28)
One-year survival rate % (97.5% CI)	0.47 (0.31, 0.61)	0.46 (0.30, 0.60)		

[a] Compared with INV CHOICE based on Cox proportional hazard model.

[b] Disease assessment is based on radiographic review by independent radiologists and review of clinical data by independent oncologists.

[c] Compared with INV CHOICE based on log-rank test.

[d] Compared with INV CHOICE alone based on Fisher's exact test.

Abbreviations: CI = confidence interval; NA = not applicable.

following intravenous treatment. During *in vitro* temsirolimus metabolism studies, sirolimus, seco-temsirolimus and seco-sirolimus were observed; additional metabolic pathways were hydroxylation, reduction and demethylation. Following a single 25 mg intravenous dose in patients with cancer, sirolimus AUC was 2.7-fold that of temsirolimus AUC, due principally to the longer half-life of sirolimus.

Elimination

Following a single 25 mg intravenous dose of temsirolimus, temsirolimus mean ± SD systemic clearance from whole blood was 11.4 ± 2.4 l/h. Mean half-lives of temsirolimus and sirolimus were 17.7 hr and 73.3 hr, respectively. Following administration of [^{14}C] temsirolimus, excretion was predominantly via the faeces (78%), with renal elimination of active substance and metabolites accounting for 4.6% of the administered dose. Model-predicted values for clearance from plasma, after applying a 175 mg dose for 3 weeks, and subsequently 75 mg for 3 weeks, indicate temsirolimus and sirolimus metabolite trough concentrations of approximately 1.2 ng/ml and 10.7 ng/ml, respectively.

Temsirolimus and sirolimus were demonstrated to be substrates for P-gp *in vitro*. Possible effects of inhibition of P-gp on elimination of temsirolimus and sirolimus *in vivo* have not been investigated.

Special Populations

Hepatic impairment

Temsirolimus and sirolimus pharmacokinetics have not been investigated in patients with hepatic impairment (see sections 4.2 and 4.4).

Gender, weight, race, age

Temsirolimus and sirolimus pharmacokinetics are not significantly affected by gender. No relevant differences in exposure were apparent when data from the Caucasian population was compared with either the Japanese or Black population.

In population pharmacokinetic-based data analysis, increased body weight (between 38.6 and 158.9 kg) was associated with a two-fold range of trough concentration of sirolimus in whole blood.

Pharmacokinetic data on temsirolimus and sirolimus are available in patients up to age 79 years. Age does not appear to affect temsirolimus and sirolimus pharmacokinetics significantly.

Paediatric population

Temsirolimus and sirolimus pharmacokinetics in the paediatric population have not been investigated.

5.3 Preclinical safety data

Adverse reactions not observed in clinical studies, but seen in animals at exposure levels similar to or even lower than clinical exposure levels and with possible relevance to clinical use, were as follows: pancreatic islet cell vacuolation (rat), testicular tubular degeneration (mouse, rat and monkey), lymphoid atrophy (mouse, rat and monkey), mixed cell inflammation of the colon/caecum (monkey), and pulmonary phospholipidosis (rat).

Diarrhoea with mixed cell inflammation of the caecum or colon was observed in monkeys and was associated with an inflammatory response, and may have been due to a disruption of the normal intestinal flora.

General inflammatory responses, as indicated by increased fibrinogen and neutrophils, and/or changes in serum protein, were observed in mice, rats, and monkeys, although in some cases these clinical pathology changes were attributed to skin or intestinal inflammation as noted above. For some animals, there were no specific clinical observations or histological changes that suggested inflammation.

Temsirolimus was not genotoxic in a battery of *in vitro* (bacterial reverse mutation in *Salmonella typhimurium* and *Escherichia coli*, forward mutation in mouse lymphoma cells, and chromosome aberrations in Chinese hamster ovary cells) and *in vivo* (mouse micronucleus) assays.

Carcinogenicity studies have not been conducted with temsirolimus; however, sirolimus, the major metabolite of temsirolimus in humans, was carcinogenic in mice and rats. The following effects were reported in mice and/or rats in the carcinogenicity studies conducted: granulocytic leukaemia, lymphoma, hepatocellular adenoma and carcinoma, and testicular adenoma.

Reductions in testicular weights and/or histological lesions (e.g., tubular atrophy and tubular giant cells) were observed in mice, rats, and monkeys. In rats, these changes were accompanied by a decreased weight of accessory sex organs (epididymides, prostate, seminal vesicles). In reproduction toxicity studies in animals, decreased fertility and partly reversible reductions in sperm counts were reported in male rats. Exposures in animals were lower than those seen in humans receiving clinically relevant doses of temsirolimus.

6. PHARMACEUTICAL PARTICULARS

6.1 List of excipients

Concentrate:

Anhydrous ethanol

all-*rac*-α-Tocopherol (E 307)

Propylene glycol

Anhydrous citric acid (E 330)

Diluent:

Polysorbate 80 (E 433)

Macrogol 400

Anhydrous ethanol

6.2 Incompatibilities

This medicinal product must not be mixed with other medicinal products, except those mentioned in section 6.6.

TORISEL 25 mg/ml concentrate for solution for infusion must not be added directly to aqueous infusion solutions. Direct addition of TORISEL 25 mg/ml concentrate to aqueous solutions will result in precipitation of medicinal product.

Always dilute TORISEL 25 mg/ml concentrate for solution for infusion with the supplied diluent before adding to infusion solutions. TORISEL may only be administered in sodium chloride 9 mg/ml (0.9%) solution for injection after the initial dilution of TORISEL 25 mg/ml concentrate with 1.8 ml of withdrawn diluent.

TORISEL, when diluted, contains polysorbate 80, which is known to increase the rate of di-(2-ethylhexyl) phthalate extraction (DEHP) from polyvinyl chloride (PVC). This incompatibility has to be considered during the preparation and administration of TORISEL. It is important that the recommendations in sections 4.2 and 6.6 be followed closely.

PVC bags and medical devices must not be used for the administration of preparations containing polysorbate 80, because polysorbate 80 leaches DEHP from PVC.

6.3 Shelf life

2 years.

After first dilution of TORISEL 25 mg/ml concentrate with 1.8 ml of withdrawn diluent: 24 hours when stored below 25°C and protected from light.

After further dilution of the concentrate-diluent mixture with sodium chloride 9 mg/ml (0.9%) solution for injection: 6 hours when stored below 25°C and protected from light.

6.4 Special precautions for storage
Store in a refrigerator (2°C-8°C).

Do not freeze.

Keep the vials in the outer carton in order to protect from light.

For storage conditions of the diluted medicinal product, see section 6.3.

6.5 Nature and contents of container
TORISEL 25 mg/ml concentrate:

Clear glass vial (type 1 glass) with butyl rubber stopper and a plastic flip-top closure sealed with aluminum.

Diluent:

Clear glass vial (type 1 glass) with butyl rubber stopper and a plastic flip-top closure sealed with aluminum.

Pack size: 1 vial of 1.2 ml of TORISEL 25 mg/ml concentrate and 1 vial of 2.2 ml of diluent.

6.6 Special precautions for disposal and other handling
During handling and preparation of admixtures, TORISEL should be protected from excessive room light and sunlight.

TORISEL, when diluted, contains polysorbate 80, which is known to increase the rate of di-(2-ethylhexyl) phthalate (DEHP) extraction from polyvinyl chloride (PVC).

Therefore, PVC bags and medical devices must not be used for the preparation, storage and administration of TORISEL solutions for infusions.

Bags/containers that come in contact with TORISEL must be made of glass, polyolefin, or polyethylene.

Dilution

TORISEL 25 mg/ml concentrate must be diluted with the supplied diluent before administration in sodium chloride infusion.

Note: For mantle cell lymphoma, multiple vials will be required for each dose over 25 mg. Each vial of TORISEL must be diluted according to the instructions below. The required amount of concentrate-diluent mixture from each vial must be combined in one syringe for rapid injection into 250 ml of sodium chloride 9 mg/ml (0.9%) solution for injection (see section 4.2).

In preparing the solution, the following two-step process must be carried out in an aseptic manner according to local standards for handling cytotoxic/cytostatic drugs:

STEP 1: DILUTION OF TORISEL 25 MG/ML CONCENTRATE WITH THE SUPPLIED DILUENT

• Withdraw 1.8 ml of the supplied diluent.

• Inject the 1.8 ml of diluent into the vial of Torisel 25 mg/ml concentrate, which contains 30 mg of temsirolimus (1.2 ml of concentrate).

• Mix the diluent and the concentrate well by inversion of the vial. Sufficient time should be allowed for air bubbles to subside. The solution should be a clear to slightly turbid, colourless to light-yellow to yellow solution, essentially free from visual particulates.

One vial of 1.2 ml of TORISEL 25 mg/ml concentrate contains 30 mg of temsirolimus: when the 1.2 ml concentrate is combined with 1.8 ml of withdrawn diluent, a total volume of 3.0 ml is obtained, and the concentration of temsirolimus will be 10 mg/ml. The concentrate-diluent mixture is stable below 25°C for up to 24 hours.

STEP 2: ADMINISTRATION OF CONCENTRATE-DILUENT MIXTURE IN SODIUM CHLORIDE INFUSION

• Withdraw the required amount of concentrate-diluent mixture (containing temsirolimus 10 mg/ml) from the vial; i.e., 2.5 ml for a temsirolimus dose of 25 mg.

• Inject the withdrawn volume rapidly into 250 ml of sodium chloride 9 mg/ml (0.9%) solution for injection to ensure adequate mixing.

The admixture should be mixed by inversion of the bag or bottle, avoiding excessive shaking, as this may cause foaming.

The resulting solution should be inspected visually for particulate matter and discolouration prior to administration, whenever solution and container permit. The admixture of TORISEL in sodium chloride 9 mg/ml (0.9%) solution for injection should be protected from excessive room light and sunlight.

Administration

• Administration of the final diluted solution should be completed within six hours from the time that the TORISEL is first added to sodium chloride 9 mg/ml (0.9%) solution for injection.

• TORISEL is infused over a 30- to 60-minute period once weekly. The use of an infusion pump is the preferred method of administration to ensure accurate delivery of the medicinal product.

• Appropriate administration materials must be composed of glass, polyolefin, or polyethylene to avoid excessive loss of medicinal product and to decrease the rate of DEHP extraction. The administration materials must consist of non-DEHP, non-PVC tubing with appropriate filter. An in-line polyethersulfone filter with a pore size of not greater than 5 microns is recommended for administration to avoid the possibility of particles bigger than 5 microns being infused. If the administration set available does not have an in-line filter incorporated, a filter should be added at the end of the set (i.e., an end-filter) before the admixture reaches the vein of the patient. Different end-filters can be used ranging in filter pore size from 0.2 microns up to 5 microns. The use of both an in-line and end-filter is not recommended.

• TORISEL, when diluted, contains polysorbate 80, which is known to increase the rate of DEHP extraction from PVC. This should be considered during the preparation and administration of TORISEL following constitution. It is important that the recommendations in section 4.2 be followed closely.

Disposal

Any unused product or waste material should be disposed of in accordance with local requirements.

7. MARKETING AUTHORISATION HOLDER
Wyeth Europa Ltd
Huntercombe Lane South
Taplow, Maidenhead
Berkshire SL6 0PH
United Kingdom

8. MARKETING AUTHORISATION NUMBER(S)
EU/1/07/424/001

9. DATE OF FIRST AUTHORISATION/RENEWAL OF THE AUTHORISATION
Date of first authorisation: 19 November 2007

10. DATE OF REVISION OF THE TEXT
21 August 2009

Detailed information on this medicinal product is available on the website of the European Medicines Agency (EMEA): http://www.emea.europa.eu/

Tostran 2% Gel

(ProStrakan)

1. NAME OF THE MEDICINAL PRODUCT
Tostran 2% Gel.

2. QUALITATIVE AND QUANTITATIVE COMPOSITION
One gram of gel contains 20 mg testosterone. One press of the canister piston delivers 0.5 g of gel containing 10 mg testosterone.

One gram of gel contains 1 mg butylhydroxytoluene.

One gram of gel contains 350 mg propylene glycol.

For a full list of excipients, see Section 6.1.

3. PHARMACEUTICAL FORM
Gel.

Clear, colourless gel.

4. CLINICAL PARTICULARS

4.1 Therapeutic indications
Replacement therapy with testosterone for male hypogonadism when testosterone deficiency has been confirmed by clinical symptoms and laboratory analyses (see Section 4.4).

4.2 Posology and method of administration
For cutaneous use

Adults and Elderly Men
The recommended starting dose of Tostran is 3 g gel (60 mg of testosterone) applied once daily at approximately the same time each morning. Dose titration should be based on both serum testosterone levels and the existence of clinical signs and symptoms related to androgen deficiency. It should be taken into account that physiological testosterone levels decline with increasing age.

The daily dose should not exceed 4 g of gel (80 mg testosterone).

The dose can be applied to the abdomen (entire dose over an area of at least 10 by 30 cm), or to **both** inner thighs (one half of the dose over an area of at least 10 by 15 cm for each inner thigh). Daily rotation between the abdomen and inner thighs is recommended to minimise application site reactions.

The gel should be applied to clean, dry, intact skin. It should be rubbed in gently with one finger until dry, then the application site should be covered, preferably with loose clothing. Hands should then be washed with soap and water.

Each full depression of the canister piston delivers one half gram of gel (10 mg testosterone). To obtain a full first dose, it is necessary to prime the canister pump. To do so, with the canister in the upright position, slowly and fully depress the actuator twice. The first depression may result in no discharge of gel. Discard the gel from the two depressions. It is only necessary to prime the pump before the first dose.

In Table 1 below the amount of gel dispensed and the amount of testosterone which would be applied to the skin from a number of piston depressions are shown.

TABLE 1: Dose of Tostran

No of Depressions	Amount of Gel (g)	Amount of Testosterone Applied to the Skin (mg)
1	0.5	10
2	1	20
4	2	40
6	3	60
8	4	80

Patients who wash in the morning should apply Tostran after washing, bathing or showering.

Tostran must not be applied to the genitals.

Treatment Control
Serum testosterone concentration should be measured approximately 14 days after initiation of therapy to ensure proper dosing. The blood sample for measurement of serum testosterone level should be obtained 2 hours after application of Tostran. If the serum testosterone concentration is between 5.0 and 15.0 μg/l, the dose should not be changed from 3 g/day. If the serum testosterone concentration is below 5.0 μg/l, the dose should be increased to 4 g/day (80 mg testosterone). If the testosterone concentration is above 15.0 μg/l, the dose should be reduced to 2 g/day (40 mg testosterone). Smaller 0.5 g gel (10 mg testosterone) dosage adjustment may be made if necessary.

Because of the variability in analytical values amongst diagnostic laboratories, all testosterone measurements should be performed in the same laboratory.

There is limited experience of treating men older than 65 years of age with Tostran.

No formal studies have been conducted with the product in patients with renal or hepatic impairment (see also Section 4.4).

Children
Tostran is not indicated for use in children and has not been clinically evaluated in males under 18 years of age.

4.3 Contraindications
Tostran 2% Gel is contraindicated in patients with:

• known or suspected carcinoma of the breast or the prostate

• known hypersensitivity to testosterone or any of the excipients

4.4 Special warnings and precautions for use
Tostran should not be used to treat non-specific symptoms suggestive of hypogonadism if testosterone deficiency has not been demonstrated and if other aetiologies responsible for the symptoms have not been excluded. Testosterone deficiency should be clearly demonstrated by clinical features and confirmed by two separate blood testosterone measurements before initiating therapy with any testosterone replacement, including Tostran treatment. For the time being there is no consensus concerning age specific reference values for testosterone. However it should be taken into consideration that the physiological serum levels of testosterone decrease with age.

To ensure proper dosing, serum testosterone concentrations should be measured (see Section 4.2).

Tostran is not indicated for treatment of male sterility or sexual impotence.

Prior to initiation of testosterone replacement therapy, all patients must undergo a detailed examination in order to exclude a risk of pre-existing prostatic cancer. Careful and regular monitoring of the prostate gland and breast must be performed in accordance with recommended methods (digital rectal examination and estimation of serum prostate specific antigen (PSA)) in patients receiving testosterone therapy at least annually and twice yearly in elderly patients and at risk patients (those with clinical or familial factors).

Androgens may accelerate the progression of sub-clinical prostatic cancer and benign prostatic hyperplasia.

Oedema with or without congestive heart failure may be a serious complication in patients with pre-existing cardiac, renal or hepatic disease. The treatment must be discontinued immediately if such complications occur. In addition, diuretic therapy may be required.

There are no studies undertaken to demonstrate the efficacy and safety of this medicinal product in patients with renal or hepatic impairment. Therefore, testosterone replacement therapy should be used with caution in these patients.

The treatment of hypogonadal men with testosterone may potentiate sleep apnoea in some patients, especially those with risk factors such as obesity or chronic lung disease.

The following checks should be carried out periodically: Full blood count (including haemoglobin and haematocrit to detect polycythaemia), lipid profile and liver function tests.

Care should be taken in patients with skeletal metastases due to the risk of hypercalcaemia/hypercalcuria developing from androgen therapy. Regular monitoring of the serum levels of calcium in these patients is recommended.

Testosterone may cause a rise in blood pressure and Tostran should be used with caution in men with hypertension.

Tostran should be used with caution in patients with ischemic heart disease, epilepsy and migraine as these conditions may be aggravated.

Improved insulin sensitivity may occur in patients treated with androgens who achieve normal testosterone plasma concentrations following replacement therapy.

General: Certain clinical signs may indicate excessive androgen exposure requiring dosage adjustment. The physician should instruct patients to report any of the following:

- Irritability, nervousness, weight gain.
- Too frequent or persistent erections of the penis.
- Any nausea, vomiting, changes in skin colour or ankle swelling.
- Breathing disturbances, including those associated with sleep.

If the patient develops a severe application site reaction, treatment should be reviewed and discontinued if necessary.

Athletes should be informed that Tostran contains an active substance (testosterone), which may give positive results in a doping test. Androgens are not suitable for enhancing muscular development in healthy individuals or for increasing physical ability.

Tostran should not be used in women due to possible virilising effects.

Potential for transfer

If no precautions are taken, testosterone gel can be transferred to other persons by close skin to skin contact, resulting in increased testosterone serum levels and possibly adverse effects (e.g. growth of facial and/or body hair, deepening of the voice, irregularities of the menstrual cycle) in case of repeat contact (inadvertent androgenisation).

The physician should inform the patient carefully about the risk of testosterone transfer and about safety instructions (see below). Tostran should not be prescribed in patients with a major risk of non-compliance with safety instructions (e.g. severe alcoholism, drug abuse, severe psychiatric disorders).

This transfer is avoided by wearing clothes covering the application area or bathing or showering prior to contact.

As a result, the following precautions are recommended:

For the patient:

- wash hands with soap and water after applying the gel,
- cover the application area with clothing once the gel has dried,
- bathe or shower before any situation in which this type of contact is foreseen.

For people not being treated with Tostran:

- in the event of contact with an application area which has not been washed or is not covered with clothing, wash the area of skin onto which testosterone may have been transferred as soon as possible, using soap and water,
- report the development of signs of excessive androgen exposure such as acne or hair modification.

To guarantee partner safety the patient should be advised for example to observe a minimum of four hours between Tostran application and sexual intercourse, to wear clothing covering the application site, during contact period or to bathe or shower before sexual intercourse.

Furthermore, it is recommended to wear clothing covering the application site during contact periods with children, in order to avoid a risk of contamination to children's skin.

Pregnant women must avoid contact with Tostran application sites. In case of pregnancy of a partner, the patient must take extra care with the precautions for use described above (see also Section 4.6).

Absorption studies of testosterone conducted in patients treated with Tostran indicate that patients should wait at least two hours between gel application and bathing or showering.

Tostran contains butylhydroxytoluene (E321) which may cause local skin reactions (eg contact dermatitis) or irritation of the eyes and mucous membranes. Tostran contains propylene glycol which may cause skin irritation.

4.5 Interaction with other medicinal products and other forms of interaction

When androgens are given simultaneously with anticoagulants, the anticoagulant effect can increase. Patients receiving oral anticoagulants require close monitoring of their INR especially when the androgen treatment is started, stopped or the dose of Tostran changed.

The concurrent administration of testosterone with ACTH or corticosteroids may increase the likelihood of oedema; thus these drugs should be administered with caution, particularly in patients with cardiac, renal or hepatic disease.

Laboratory test interactions: Androgens may decrease concentrations of thyroxin-binding globulin, resulting in decreased total T4 serum concentrations and increased resin uptake of T3 and T4. Free thyroid hormone concentrations remain unchanged, however and there is no clinical evidence of thyroid dysfunction.

4.6 Pregnancy and lactation

Tostran is only intended to be used by men.

Tostran is not indicated for pregnant or breastfeeding women. No studies on women have been carried out. Pregnant women should avoid all contact with skin treated with Tostran (see Section 4.4). Tostran can give rise to adverse, virilising effects on the foetus. In the event of contact with treated skin, the area should be washed with soap and water as soon as possible.

4.7 Effects on ability to drive and use machines

No studies on the effects on the ability to drive and use machines have been performed

4.8 Undesirable effects

The most commonly reported adverse reactions in a controlled clinical study (up to 4 g Tostran) were application site reactions (ASR; 26%) including; paresthesia, xerosis, pruritus and rash or erythema. The majority of these reactions were mild to moderate in severity and diminished or cleared, despite continued application.

All adverse reactions reported with a suspected relationship are listed by class and frequency (very common (> 1/10), common (> 1/100, < 1/10), uncommon (> 1/1000, < 1/100) and rare (< 1/1000)).

Organ System	Very Common > 1/10)	Common > 1/100, < 1/10)
General disorders and application site conditions	Application site reactions	Peripheral oedema
Vascular disorders		Hypertension
Blood and lymphatic system disorders		Increase in haemoglobin and haematocrit
Investigations		Increased PSA
Endocrine disorders		Increase in male pattern hair distribution
Reproductive system and breast disorders		Gynaecomastia

Hyperglycaemia was reported as an adverse event in two patients with a history of diabetes mellitus.

Gynecomastia develops in 1.5% of patients being treated with testosterone for hypogonadism and occasionally persists.

According to the literature, other known undesirable effects have been reported following testosterone treatment and are listed in the following table:

Organ System	Adverse reactions
Metabolism and nutrition disorders	Weight gain, electrolyte changes (retention of sodium, chloride, potassium, calcium, inorganic phosphate and water) during high dose and/or prolonged treatment.
Musculoskeletal system	Muscle cramps, muscle pain
Nervous system	Nervousness, hostility, depression.
Respiratory system	Sleep apnoea
Hepatobiliary disorders	In very rare cases jaundice and liver function test abnormalities.
Skin and appendages	Various skin reactions may occur including acne, seborrhoea and balding (alopecia).
Reproductive system and breast disorders	Libido changes, increased frequency of erections; therapy with high doses of testosterone preparations commonly reversibly interrupts or reduces spermatogenesis, thereby reducing the size of the testicles; testosterone replacement therapy of hypogonadism can in rare cases cause persistent, painful erections (priapism), prostate abnormalities, prostate cancer*, urinary obstruction.
General disorders and administration site conditions	High dose or long-term administration of testosterone occasionally increases the occurrences of water retention and oedema; hypersensitivity reactions may occur.
Digestive system	Nausea

* Data on prostate cancer risk in association with testosterone therapy are inconclusive.

Other rare known undesirable effects associated with excessive dosages of testosterone treatments include hepatic neoplasms.

Because of the excipients (butylhydroxytoluene and propylene glycol) contained in the product, applications to the skin may cause irritation and dry skin which usually reduce over time.

4.9 Overdose

There is a single case of acute overdosage after parenteral administration of testosterone enanthate reported in the literature. This resulted in testosterone concentrations of up to 114.0 µg/l, which was implicated in a cerebrovascular accident. Oral ingestion of Tostran will not result in clinically significant testosterone concentrations due to extensive first-pass metabolism. It is unlikely that such serum testosterone levels could be achieved using the transdermal route of administration.

Treatment of transdermal overdosage is by washing the site of application with soap and water as soon as possible, discontinuing application of Tostran and treatment of any symptoms.

5. PHARMACOLOGICAL PROPERTIES

5.1 Pharmacodynamic properties

Pharmacotherapeutic group: Androgens; ATC-code G03BA03

Endogenous androgens, which are excreted by the testicles, mainly testosterone and its main metabolite dihydrotestosterone (DHT) are responsible for the development of the external and internal male sex organs and for maintaining secondary sex characteristics (stimulation of the hair growth, voice breaking and development of libido). They have a general effect on the protein anabolism, affect the development of the skeletal muscles and the distribution of body fat, reduce the excretion in the urine of nitrogen, sodium, potassium, chloride, phosphates and water.

Testosterone does not affect the development of the testicles but reduces the excretion of gonadotrophin from the pituitary gland.

The effect of testosterone on certain target organs occurs after a peripheral transformation of testosterone to oestradiol which then binds to the oestradiol receptors in the nuclei of the target cell e.g in the pituitary gland, fat tissue, brain, bone tissue and the Leydig cells in the testicle.

5.2 Pharmacokinetic properties

Absorption

Tostran is a hydroalcoholic formulation that dries quickly when rubbed into the skin. The skin acts as a reservoir for the sustained release of testosterone into the systemic circulation. Testosterone absorption into the blood continues throughout the entire 24 hour dosing interval, with concentrations significantly above the base level the whole time. Varying application areas between 200 and 800 cm^2 in size has not been shown to have any clinically relevant effect on serum testosterone concentrations.

Application on the inside of the thighs and the abdomen results in comparable serum testosterone concentrations.

The bioavailability of Tostran is estimated to be 12%. Administration of 3 g gel daily over 6 months results in time-averaged serum testosterone concentrations of 5.0 ± 2.0 µg/l and individual minimal concentrations of 3.0 ± 1.0 µg/l and maximum concentrations of 12.0 ± 7.0 µg/l.

Distribution

About 40% of the testosterone in plasma is bound to sex hormone binding globulin (SHBG), 2% remains unbound (free) and the rest is loosely bound to albumin and other proteins. Albumin bound testosterone easily dissociates and is considered to be biologically active. However the binding to SHBG is strong. Thus, the concentration of serum bioactive testosterone is the unbound fraction plus that bound to albumin.

Metabolism

The major active metabolites of testosterone are oestradiol and DHT. DHT binds with greater affinity to SHBG than does testosterone. DHT is further metabolised to 3-α and 2-β androstanediol.

Excretion

About 90% of a dose of testosterone given intramuscularly is excreted in the urine as glucuronic acid and sulphate conjugates of testosterone and its metabolites; about 6% of a dose is excreted in the faeces, mostly in the unconjugated form.

5.3 Preclinical safety data

Toxicological studies have not revealed other effects than those which can be explained based on the hormone profile of Tostran.

Testosterone has been found to be non-mutagenic *in vitro* using the reverse mutation model (Ames test) or hamster ovary cells. A relationship between androgen treatment and certain cancers has been found in laboratory animals. Experimental data in rats have shown increased incidences of prostate cancer after treatment with testosterone. Sex hormones are known to facilitate the development of certain tumours induced by known carcinogenic agents. The clinical relevance of this observation is not known.

Fertility studies in rodents and primates have shown that treatment with testosterone can impair fertility by suppressing spermatogenesis in a dose dependent manner.

6. PHARMACEUTICAL PARTICULARS

6.1 List of excipients

Propylene glycol

Ethanol, dehydrated

Isopropyl alcohol

Oleic acid

Carbomer 1382

Trolamine

Butylhydroxytoluene (E321)

Purified water

6.2 Incompatibilities

Not applicable

6.3 Shelf life

2 years.

6.4 Special precautions for storage

Do not store above 25°C.

Do not refrigerate.

6.5 Nature and contents of container

60 g multi-dose container (comprised of an epoxy phenolic lined aluminium canister) with a fixed volume metering pump.

Pack sizes: 60 g, 2 × 60 g or 3 × 60 g

Not all pack sizes may be marketed.

6.6 Special precautions for disposal and other handling

No special requirements.

7. MARKETING AUTHORISATION HOLDER

ProStrakan Ltd

Galabank Business Park

Galashiels

TD1 1QH

United Kingdom

8. MARKETING AUTHORISATION NUMBER(S)

PL 16508/0025

9. DATE OF FIRST AUTHORISATION/RENEWAL OF THE AUTHORISATION

October 2006

10. DATE OF REVISION OF THE TEXT

TOVIAZ 4 mg prolonged-release tablets & TOVIAZ 8 mg prolonged-release tablets

(Pfizer Limited)

1. NAME OF THE MEDICINAL PRODUCT

TOVIAZ▼ 4 mg prolonged-release tablets

TOVIAZ▼ 8 mg prolonged-release tablets

2. QUALITATIVE AND QUANTITATIVE COMPOSITION

Each 4mg prolonged-release tablet contains fesoterodine fumarate 4 mg corresponding to 3.1 mg of fesoterodine.

Each 8mg prolonged-release tablet contains fesoterodine fumarate 8 mg corresponding to 6.2 mg of fesoterodine.

Excipients

Each 4 mg prolonged-release tablet contains 0.525 mg of soya lecithin and 91.125 mg lactose monohydrate.

Each 8 mg prolonged-release tablet contains 0.525 mg of soya lecithin and 58.125 mg lactose monohydrate.

For a full list of excipients, see section 6.1.

3. PHARMACEUTICAL FORM

Prolonged-release tablets

The 4 mg tablets are light blue, oval, biconvex, film-coated, and engraved on one side with the letters 'FS'.

The 8 mg tablets are blue, oval, biconvex, film-coated, and engraved on one side with the letters 'FT'.

4. CLINICAL PARTICULARS

4.1 Therapeutic indications

Treatment of the symptoms (increased urinary frequency and/or urgency and/or urgency incontinence) that may occur in patients with overactive bladder syndrome.

4.2 Posology and method of administration

Adults (including elderly)

The recommended starting dose is 4 mg once daily. Based upon individual response, the dose may be increased to 8 mg once daily. The maximum daily dose is 8 mg.

Full treatment effect was observed between 2 and 8 weeks. Hence, it is recommended to re-evaluate the efficacy for the individual patient after 8 weeks of treatment.

Tablets are to be taken once daily with liquid and swallowed whole. TOVIAZ can be administered with or without food.

In subjects with normal renal and hepatic function receiving concomitant administration of potent CYP3A4 inhibitors, the maximum daily dose of TOVIAZ should be 4 mg once daily (see section 4.5). During concomitant administration of a moderate CYP3A4 inhibitor, a dose increase to 8 mg should be preceded by an evaluation of the individual response and tolerability (see sections 4.4 and 4.5).

Renal and hepatic impairment

The following table provides the daily dosing recommendations for subjects with renal or hepatic impairment in the absence and presence of moderate and potent CYP3A4 inhibitors (see sections 4.3, 4.4, 4.5 and 5.2).

(see Table 1 below)

TOVIAZ is contraindicated in subjects with severe hepatic impairment (see section 4.3).

Paediatric population

TOVIAZ is not recommended for use in children and adolescents below 18 years of age due to lack of data on safety and efficacy (see section 5.2).

4.3 Contraindications

- Hypersensitivity to the active substance or to peanut or soya or any of the excipients
- Urinary retention
- Gastric retention
- Uncontrolled narrow angle glaucoma
- Myasthenia gravis
- Severe hepatic impairment (Child Pugh C)
- Concomitant use of potent CYP3A4 inhibitors in subjects with moderate to severe hepatic or renal impairment
- Severe ulcerative colitis
- Toxic megacolon.

4.4 Special warnings and precautions for use

TOVIAZ should be used with caution in patients with:

- Clinically significant bladder outflow obstruction at risk of urinary retention (see section 4.3)
- Gastrointestinal obstructive disorders (e.g. pyloric stenosis)
- Gastro-oesophageal reflux and/or who are concurrently taking medicinal products (such as oral bisphosphonates) that can cause or exacerbate oesophagitis
- Decreased gastrointestinal motility
- Autonomic neuropathy
- Controlled narrow-angle glaucoma

Caution should be exercised when prescribing or uptitrating fesoterodine to patients in whom an increased exposure to the active metabolite (see section 5.1) is expected:

- Hepatic impairment (see sections 4.2, 4.3 and 5.2)
- Renal impairment (see section 4.2, 4.3 and 5.2)
- Concomitant administration of potent or moderate CYP3A4 inhibitors (see sections 4.2 and 4.5)
- Concomitant administration of a potent CYP2D6 inhibitor (see sections 4.5 and 5.2).

In patients with a combination of these factors, additional exposure increases are expected. Dose dependent antimuscarinic side effects are likely to occur. In populations where the dose may be increased to 8 mg once daily, the dose increase should be preceded by an evaluation of the individual response and tolerability.

As with all medicinal products indicated for the treatment of overactive bladder, organic causes must be excluded before any treatment with antimuscarinics is considered. Safety and efficacy have not yet been established in patients with a neurogenic cause for detrusor overactivity.

Other causes of frequent urination (treatment of heart failure or renal disease) should be assessed before treatment with fesoterodine. If urinary tract infection is present, an appropriate medical approach should be taken/antibacterial therapy should be started.

The concomitant use of fesoterodine with a potent CYP3A4 inducer (i.e. carbamazepine, rifampicin, phenobarbital, phenytoin, St John's Wort) is not recommended (see section 4.5).

As with other antimuscarinics, fesoterodine should be used with caution in patients with risk for QT-prolongation (e.g. hypokalaemia, bradycardia and concomitant administration of medicines known to prolong QT interval) and relevant pre-existing cardiac diseases (e.g. myocardial ischaemia, arrhythmia, congestive heart failure), (see section 4.8). This especially holds true when taking potent CYP3A4 inhibitors (see sections 4.2, 4.5 and 5.1).

Lactose

TOVIAZ prolonged-release tablets contain lactose. Patients with rare hereditary problems of galactose intolerance, the Lapp lactase deficiency or glucose-galactose malabsorption should not take this medicinal product.

4.5 Interaction with other medicinal products and other forms of interaction

Pharmacological interactions

Caution should be exercised in coadministration of fesoterodine with other antimuscarinic agents and medicinal products with anticholinergic properties (e.g. amantadine, tri-cyclic antidepressants, certain neuroleptics) as this may lead to more pronounced therapeutic- and side-effects (e.g. constipation, dry mouth, drowsiness, urinary retention).

Fesoterodine may reduce the effect of medicinal products that stimulate the motility of the gastro-intestinal tract, such as metoclopromide.

Pharmacokinetic interactions

In vitro data demonstrate that the active metabolite of fesoterodine does not inhibit CYP1A2, 2B6, 2C8, 2C9, 2C19, 2D6, 2E1, or 3A4, or induce CYP1A2, 2B6, 2C9, 2C19, or 3A4 at clinically relevant plasma concentrations. Thus fesoterodine is unlikely to alter the clearance of medicinal products that are metabolised by these enzymes.

CYP3A4 Inhibitors

Potent CYP3A4 Inhibitors

Following inhibition of CYP3A4 by co-administration of ketoconazole 200 mg twice daily, C_{max} and AUC of the active metabolite of fesoterodine increased 2.0 and 2.3-fold in CYP2D6 extensive metabolisers and 2.1 and 2.5-fold in CYP2D6 poor metabolisers, respectively. Therefore, the maximum dose of fesoterodine should be restricted to 4 mg when used concomitantly with potent CYP3A4 inhibitors (e.g. atazanavir, clarithromycin, indinavir, itraconazole, ketoconazole, nefazodone, nelfinavir, ritonavir (and all ritonavir boosted PI-regimens), saquinavir and telithromycin (see sections 4.2 and 4.4)).

Moderate CYP3A4 Inhibitors

No study has been performed evaluating the effect of a moderate CYP3A4 inhibitor (e.g. amprenavir, aprepitant, diltiazem, erythromycin, fluconazole, fosamprenavir, grapefruit juice, verapamil) on the pharmacokinetics of fesoterodine. However, an increase in the exposure of the active metabolite of fesoterodine is expected, although a smaller increase than observed with a potent CYP3A4 inhibitor (see sections 4.2 and 4.4).

CYP3A4 Inducers

Following induction of CYP3A4 by coadministration of rifampicin 600 mg once a day, C_{max} and AUC of the active metabolite of fesoterodine decreased by approximately 70% and 75%, respectively, after oral administration of fesoterodine 8 mg.

Induction of CYP3A4 may lead to subtherapeutic plasma levels. Concomitant use with CYP3A4 inducers (e.g. carbamazepine, rifampicin, phenobarbital, phenytoin, St John's Wort) is not recommended (see section 4.4).

CYP2D6 Inhibitors

The interaction with CYP2D6 inhibitors was not tested clinically. Mean C_{max} and AUC of the active metabolite are 1.7 and 2-fold higher, respectively, in CYP2D6 poor metabolisers as compared to extensive metabolisers. Co-administration of a potent CYP2D6 inhibitor may result in increased exposure and adverse events. A dose reduction to 4 mg may be needed (see section 4.4).

Oral contraceptives

Fesoterodine does not impair the suppression of ovulation by oral hormonal contraception. In the presence of fesoterodine there are no changes in the plasma concentrations of combined oral contraceptives containing ethinylestradiol and levonorgestrel.

4.6 Pregnancy and lactation

Pregnancy

There are no adequate data from the use of fesoterodine in pregnant women. Reproductive toxicity studies with

Table 1

		Moderate(3) or potent(4) CYP3A4 inhibitors		
		None	Moderate	Potent
Renal impairment(1)	Mild	4→8 mg(2)	4 mg	Should be avoided
	Moderate	4→8 mg(2)	4 mg	Contraindicated
	Severe	4 mg	Should be avoided	Contraindicated
Hepatic impairment	Mild	4→8 mg(2)	4 mg	Should be avoided
	Moderate	4 mg	Should be avoided	Contraindicated

(1) Mild GFR = 50-80 ml/min; Moderate GFR = 30-50 ml/min; Severe GFR = <30 ml/min

(2) Cautious dose increase. See sections 4.4, 4.5 and 5.2

(3) Studies with moderate CYP3A4 inhibitors have not been conducted. See section 4.5

(4) Potent CYP3A4 inhibitors. See sections 4.3, 4.4 and 4.5

Table 2

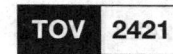

System Organ Class	Very common	Common	Uncommon*
Cardiac disorders			Tachycardia
Nervous system disorders		Dizziness; Headache	Dysgeusia; Somnolence
Eye disorders		Dry eye	
Ear and labyrinth disorders			Vertigo
Respiratory, thoracic and mediastinal disorders		Dry throat	Pharyngolaryngeal pain; Cough; Nasal dryness
Gastrointestinal disorders	Dry mouth	Abdominal pain; Diarrhoea; Dyspepsia; Constipation; Nausea	Abdominal discomfort; Flatulence
Renal and urinary disorders		Dysuria	Urinary retention (including feeling of residual urine; micturition disorder); Urinary hesitation
Skin and subcutaneous tissue disorders			Rash; Dry skin
Infections and infestations			Urinary tract infection
General disorders and administration site conditions			Fatigue
Hepatobiliary disorders			ALT increased; GGT increased
Psychiatric disorders		Insomnia	

***5 or more cases**

fesoterodine in animals show minor embryotoxicity (see section 5.3). The potential risk for humans is unknown. TOVIAZ is not recommended during pregnancy.

Lactation

It is not known whether fesoterodine is excreted into human milk; therefore, breast-feeding is not recommended during treatment with TOVIAZ.

4.7 Effects on ability to drive and use machines

No studies on the effects on the ability to drive and use machines have been performed. As with other antimuscarinic agents, caution should be exercised when driving or using machines due to possible occurrence of side effects such as blurred vision, dizziness, and somnolence (see section 4.8).

4.8 Undesirable effects

The safety of fesoterodine was evaluated in placebo-controlled clinical studies in a total of 2859 patients with overactive bladder, of which 780 received placebo.

Due to the pharmacological properties of fesoterodine, treatment may cause mild to moderate antimuscarinic effects like dry mouth, dry eye, dyspepsia and constipation.

Dry mouth, the only very common event, occurred with a frequency of 28.8% in the fesoterodine group compared to 8.5% in the placebo group. The majority of ADRs occurred during the first month of treatment with the exception of cases classified as urinary retention or post void residual urine greater than 200 ml, which could occur after long term treatment and was more common in male than female subjects.

The table below gives the frequency of treatment emergent adverse reactions from placebo-controlled clinical trials. The adverse reactions reported in this table are those events that were very common (≥1/10), common (≥1/100 to <1/10) or uncommon (≥1/1,000 to <1/100).

Within each frequency grouping, undesirable effects are presented in order of decreasing seriousness.

(see Table 2 opposite)

In clinical trials of fesoterodine, cases of markedly elevated liver enzymes were reported with the occurrence frequency no different from the placebo group. The relation to fesoterodine treatment is unclear.

Electrocardiograms were obtained from 782 patients treated with 4 mg, 785 treated with 8 mg, 222 treated with 12 mg fesoterodine and 780 with placebo. The heart rate corrected QT interval in fesoterodine treated patients did not differ from that seen in placebo treated patients. The incidence rates of QTc ≥ 500 ms post baseline or QTc increase of ≥60 ms is 1.9%, 1.3%, 1.4% and 1.5%, for fesoterodine 4 mg, 8 mg, 12 mg and placebo, respectively. The clinical relevance of these findings will depend on individual patient risk factors and susceptibilities present (see section 4.4).

4.9 Overdose

Overdose with antimuscarinic agents, including fesoterodine can result in severe anticholinergic effects. Treatment should be symptomatic and supportive. In the event of overdose, ECG monitoring is recommended; standard supportive measures for managing QT prolongation should be adopted. Fesoterodine has been safely administered in clinical studies at doses up to 28 mg/day.

In the event of fesoterodine overdose, treat with gastric lavage and give activated charcoal. Treat symptoms as follows:

– Severe central anticholinergic effects (e.g. hallucinations, severe excitation): treat with physostigmine

– Convulsions or pronounced excitation: treat with benzodiazepines

– Respiratory insufficiency: treat with artificial respiration

– Tachycardia: treat with beta-blockers

– Urinary retention: treat with catheterisation

Table 3 Mean changes from Baseline to end of treatment for primary and selected secondary endpoints

	Study 1				Study 2		
Parameter	**Placebo**	**Fesoterodine 4 mg**	**Fesoterodine 8 mg**	**Active comparator**	**Placebo**	**Fesoterodine 4 mg**	**Fesoterodine 8 mg**
Number of micturitions per 24 hours#							
	N=279	N=265	N=276	N=283	N=266	N=267	N=267
Baseline	12.0	11.6	11.9	11.5	12.2	12.9	12.0
Change from baseline	-1.02	-1.74	-1.94	-1.69	-1.02	-1.86	-1.94
p-value		<0.001	<0.001			0.032	<0.001
Responder rate (treatment response)#							
	N=279	N=265	N=276	N=283	N=266	N=267	N=267
Responder rate	53.4%	74.7%	79.0%	72.4%	45.1%	63.7%	74.2%
p-value		<0.001	<0.001			<0.001	<0.001
Number of urge incontinence episodes per 24 hours							
	N=211	N=199	N=223	N=223	N=205	N=228	N=218
Baseline	3.7	3.8	3.7	3.8	3.7	3.9	3.9
Change from baseline	-1.20	-2.06	-2.27	-1.83	-1.00	-1.77	-2.42
p-value		0.001	<0.001			0.003	<0.001
Number of continent days per week							
	N=211	N=199	N=223	N=223	N=205	N=228	N=218
Baseline	0.8	0.8	0.6	0.6	0.6	0.7	0.7
Change from baseline	2.1	2.8	3.4	2.5	1.4	2.4	2.8
p-value		0.007	<0.001			<0.001	<0.001
Voided volume per micturition (ml)							
	N=279	N=265	N=276	N=283	N=266	N=267	N=267
Baseline	150	160	154	154	159	152	156
Change from baseline	10	27	33	24	8	17	33
p-value		<0.001	<0.001			0.150	<0.001

primary end points

– Mydriasis: treat with pilocarpine eye drops and/or place patient in dark room.

5. PHARMACOLOGICAL PROPERTIES

5.1 Pharmacodynamic properties

Pharmacotherapeutic group: Urinary antispasmodics, ATC code: G04B D11.

Fesoterodine is a competitive, specific muscarinic receptor antagonist. It is rapidly and extensively hydrolysed by non-specific plasma esterases to the 5-hydroxymethyl derivative, its primary active metabolite, which is the main active pharmacological principle of fesoterodine.

The efficacy of fixed doses of fesoterodine 4 mg and 8 mg was evaluated in two Phase 3 randomised, double-blind, placebo-controlled, 12-week studies. Female (79%) and male (21%) patients with a mean age of 58 years (range 19-91 years) were included. A total of 33% of patients were ⩾65 years of age and 11% were ⩾75 years of age.

Fesoterodine treated patients had statistically significant mean reductions in the number of micturitions per 24 hours and in the number of urge incontinence episodes per 24 hours at the end of treatment compared to placebo. Likewise, the response rate (% of patients reporting that their condition has been "greatly improved" or "improved" using a 4-point Treatment Benefit Scale) was significantly greater with fesoterodine compared to placebo. Furthermore, fesoterodine improved the mean change in the voided volume per micturition, and the mean change in the number of continent days per week (see Table 3 on previous page).

Table 3: Mean changes from Baseline to end of treatment for primary and selected secondary endpoints

(see Table 3 on previous page)

Cardiac electrophysiology: The effect of fesoterodine 4 mg and 28 mg on the QT interval was thoroughly evaluated in a double-blind, randomised, placebo- and positive-controlled (moxifloxacin 400 mg) parallel group study with once-daily treatment over a period of 3 days in 261 male and female subjects aged 45 to 65 years. Change from baseline in QTc based on the Fridericia correction method did not show any differences between the active treatment and placebo group.

5.2 Pharmacokinetic properties

Absorption

After oral administration, due to rapid and extensive hydrolysis by non-specific plasma esterases, fesoterodine was not detected in plasma.

Bioavailability of the active metabolite is 52%. After single or multiple-dose oral administration of fesoterodine in doses from 4 mg to 28 mg, plasma concentrations of the active metabolite are proportional to the dose. Maximum plasma levels are reached after approximately 5 hours. Therapeutic plasma levels are achieved after the first administration of fesoterodine. No accumulation occurs after multiple-dose administration.

Distribution

Plasma protein binding of the active metabolite is low with approximately 50% bound to albumin and alpha-1-acid glycoprotein. The mean steady-state volume of distribution following intravenous infusion of the active metabolite is 169 l.

Metabolism

After oral administration, fesoterodine is rapidly and extensively hydrolysed to its active metabolite. The active metabolite is further metabolised in the liver to its carboxy, carboxy-N-desisopropyl, and N-desisopropyl metabolite with involvement of CYP2D6 and CYP3A4. None of these metabolites contribute significantly to the antimuscarinic activity of fesoterodine. Mean C_{max} and AUC of the active metabolite are 1.7 and 2-fold higher, respectively, in CYP2D6 poor metabolisers as compared to extensive metabolisers.

Elimination

Hepatic metabolism and renal excretion contribute significantly to the elimination of the active metabolite. After oral administration of fesoterodine, approximately 70% of the administered dose was recovered in urine as the active metabolite (16%), carboxy metabolite (34%), carboxy-N-desisopropyl metabolite (18%), or N-desisopropyl metabolite (1%), and a smaller amount (7%) was recovered in faeces. The terminal half-life of the active metabolite following oral administration is approximately 7 hours and is absorption rate-limited.

Age and gender

No dose adjustment is recommended in these subpopulations. The pharmacokinetics of fesoterodine are not significantly influenced by age and gender.

Paediatric patients

The pharmacokinetics of fesoterodine have not been evaluated in paediatric patients.

Renal impairment

In patients with mild or moderate renal impairment (GFR 30 – 80 ml/min), C_{max} and AUC of the active metabolite increased up to 1.5 and 1.8-fold, respectively, as compared to healthy subjects. In patients with severe renal impairment (GFR < 30 ml/min), C_{max} and AUC are increased 2.0 and 2.3-fold, respectively.

Hepatic impairment

In patients with moderate hepatic impairment (Child Pugh B), C_{max} and AUC of the active metabolite increased 1.4 and 2.1-fold, respectively, as compared to healthy subjects. Pharmacokinetics of fesoterodine in patients with severe hepatic impairment have not been studied.

5.3 Preclinical safety data

In non-clinical safety pharmacology, general toxicity, genotoxicity and carcinogenicity studies no clinically relevant effects have been observed, except those related to the pharmacological effect of the active substance.

Reproduction studies have shown minor embryotoxicity at doses close to maternally toxic ones (increased number of resorptions, pre-implantation and post-implantation losses).

Supratherapeutic concentrations of the active metabolite of fesoterodine, have been shown to inhibit K^+ current in cloned human ether-à-go-go-related gene (hERG) channels and prolong action potential duration (70% and 90% repolarisation) in canine isolated Purkinje fibres. However in conscious dogs, the active metabolite had no effect on the QT interval and QTc interval at plasma exposures at least 33-fold higher than mean peak free plasma concentration in human subjects who are extensive metabolisers and 21-fold higher than measured in subjects who are poor CYP2D6 metabolisers after fesoterodine 8 mg once daily.

6. PHARMACEUTICAL PARTICULARS

6.1 List of excipients

Tablet core

Xylitol

Lactose monohydrate

Microcrystalline cellulose

Hypromellose

Glycerol dibehenate

Talc

Film-coat

Polyvinyl alcohol

Titanium dioxide (E171)

Macrogol (3350)

Talc

Soya lecithin

Indigo carmine aluminium lake (E132)

6.2 Incompatibilities

Not applicable.

6.3 Shelf life

2 years

6.4 Special precautions for storage

Do not store above 25°C.

Store in the original package to protect from moisture.

6.5 Nature and contents of container

TOVIAZ 4 mg tablets and TOVIAZ 8 mg tablets are packed in aluminium-aluminium blisters in cartons containing 7, 14, 28, 56, 84, 98 or 100 tablets. In addition, TOVIAZ 4 mg and 8mg tablets are also packed in HDPE bottles containing 30 or 90 tablets.

Not all pack sizes may be marketed.

6.6 Special precautions for disposal and other handling

Any unused product or waste material should be disposed of in accordance with local requirements.

7. MARKETING AUTHORISATION HOLDER

Pfizer Limited

Ramsgate Road

Sandwich

Kent CT13 9NJ

United Kingdom

8. MARKETING AUTHORISATION NUMBER(S)

EU/1/07/386/001-018

9. DATE OF FIRST AUTHORISATION/RENEWAL OF THE AUTHORISATION

20/04/2007

10. DATE OF REVISION OF THE TEXT

July 2009

Tracrium Injection

(GlaxoSmithKline UK)

1. NAME OF THE MEDICINAL PRODUCT

Tracrium Injection

2. QUALITATIVE AND QUANTITATIVE COMPOSITION

Atracurium Besilate HSE 10mg/ml

3. PHARMACEUTICAL FORM

Injection

4. CLINICAL PARTICULARS

4.1 Therapeutic indications

Tracrium is a highly selective, competitive or non-depolarising neuromuscular blocking agent. It is used as an adjunct to general anaesthesia or sedation in the intensive care unit (ICU), to relax skeletal muscles, and to facilitate tracheal intubation and mechanical ventilation.

4.2 Posology and method of administration

Route of administration: Intravenous injection or continuous infusion.

Used by injection in adults: Tracrium is administered by intravenous injection.

The dosage range recommended for adults is 0.3 to 0.6 mg/kg (depending on the duration of full block required) and will provide adequate relaxation for about 15 to 35 minutes.

Endotracheal intubation can usually be accomplished within 90 seconds from the intravenous injection of 0.5 to 0.6 mg/kg.

Full block can be prolonged with supplementary doses of 0.1 to 0.2 mg/kg as required. Successive supplementary dosing does not give rise to accumulation of neuromuscular blocking effect.

Spontaneous recovery from the end of full block occurs in about 35 minutes as measured by the restoration of the tetanic response to 95% of normal neuromuscular function.

The neuromuscular block produced by Tracrium can be rapidly reversed by standard doses of anticholinesterase agents, such as neostigmine and edrophonium, accompanied or preceded by atropine, with no evidence of recurarisation.

Use as an infusion in adults: After an initial bolus dose of 0.2 to 0.6mg/kg, Tracrium can be used to maintain neuromuscular block during long surgical procedures by administration as a continuous infusion at rates of 0.3 to 0.6mg/kg/hour.

Tracrium can be administered by infusion during cardiopulmonary bypass surgery at the recommended infusion rates. Induced hypothermia to a body temperature of 25° to 26°C reduces the rate of inactivation of atracurium, therefore full neuromuscular block may be maintained by approximately half the original infusion rate at these low temperatures.

Tracrium is compatible with the following infusion solutions for the times stated below:

Infusion solution stability	*Period of*
Sodium Chloride Intravenous Infusion BP (0.9% w/v)	24 hours
Glucose Intravenous Infusion BP (5% w/v)	8 hours
Ringer's Injection USP	8 hours
Sodium Chloride (0.18%w/v) and Glucose (4% w/v) Intravenous Infusion BP	8 hours
Compound Sodium Lactate Intravenous Infusion BP (Hartmann's Solution for Injection)	4 hours

When diluted in these solutions to give atracurium besilate concentrations of 0.5 mg/ml and above, the resultant solutions will be stable in daylight for the stated periods at temperatures of up to 30°C.

Use in Children: The dosage in children over the age of one month is similar to that in adults on a bodyweight basis.

Use in Neonates: The use of Tracrium is not recommended in neonates since there are insufficient data available.

Use in the elderly: Tracrium may be used at standard dosage in elderly patients. It is recommended, however, that the initial dose be at the lower end of the range and that it be administered slowly.

Use in patients with reduced renal and/or hepatic function: Tracrium may be used at standard dosage at all levels of renal or hepatic function, including end stage failure.

Use in patients with cardiovascular disease: In patients with clinically significant cardiovascular disease, the initial dose of Tracrium should be administered over a period of 60 seconds.

Use in intensive care unit (ICU) patients: After an optional initial bolus dose of Tracrium of 0.3 to 0.6 mg/kg, Tracrium can be used to maintain neuromuscular block by administering a continuous infusion at rates of between 11 and 13 microgram/kg/min (0.65 to 0.78 mg/kg/hr). There may be wide inter-patient variability in dosage requirements and these may increase or decrease with time. Infusion rates as low as 4.5 microgram/kg/min (0.27 mg/kg/hr) or as high as 29.5 microgram/kg/min (1.77 mg/kg/hr) are required in some patients.

The rate of spontaneous recovery from neuromuscular block after infusion of Tracrium in ICU patients is independent of the duration of administration.

Spontaneous recovery to a train-of-four ratio > 0.75 (the ratio of the height of the fourth to the first twitch in a train-of-four) can be expected to occur in approximately 60 minutes. A range of 32 to 108 minutes has been observed in clinical trials.

Monitoring: In common with all neuromuscular blocking agents, monitoring of neuromuscular function is recommended during the use of Tracrium in order to individualise dosage requirements.

4.3 Contraindications
Atracurium is contraindicated in patients known to be hypersensitive to atracurium, cisatracurium or benzenesulfonic acid (see section 4.4, Special Warnings and Precautions for Use).

4.4 Special warnings and precautions for use
Precautions: In common with all the other neuromuscular blocking agents, Tracrium paralyses the respiratory muscles as well as other skeletal muscles but has no effect on consciousness. Tracrium should be administered only with adequate general anaesthesia and only by or under the close supervision of an experienced anaesthetist with adequate facilities for endotracheal intubation and artificial ventilation.

The potential for histamine release exists in susceptible patients during Tracrium administration. Caution should be exercised in administering Tracrium to patients with a history suggestive of an increased sensitivity to the effects of histamine.

High rates of cross-sensitivity (greater than 50%) between neuromuscular blocking agents have been reported. Therefore, where possible, before administering atracurium, hypersensitivity to other neuromuscular blocking agents should be excluded (see section 4.3, Contra-indications). Atracurium should only be used when absolutely essential in susceptible patients. Patients who experience a hypersensitivity reaction under general anaesthesia should be tested subsequently for hypersensitivity to other neuromuscular blockers.

Monitoring of serial creatinine phosphate (cpk) values should be considered in asthmatic patients receiving high dose corticosteroids and neuromuscular blocking agents in ICU.

Tracrium does not have significant vagal or ganglionic blocking properties in the recommended dosage range. Consequently, Tracrium has no clinically significant effects on heart rate in the recommended dosage range and it will not counteract the bradycardia produced by many anaesthetic agents or by vagal stimulation during surgery.

In common with other non-depolarising neuromuscular blocking agents, increased sensitivity to atracurium may be expected in patients with myasthenia gravis and other forms of neuromuscular disease.

As with other neuromuscular blocking agents severe acid-base and/or serum electrolyte abnormalities may increase or decrease the sensitivity of patients to atracrium.

As with other non-depolarising neuromuscular blockers hypophosphataemia may prolong recovery. Recovery may be hastened by correcting this condition.

Tracrium should be administered over a period of 60 seconds to patients who may be unusually sensitive to falls in arterial blood pressure, for example those who are hypovolaemic.

Tracrium is inactivated by high pH and so must not be mixed in the same syringe with thiopental or any alkaline agent.

When a small vein is selected as the injection site, Tracrium should be flushed through the vein with physiological saline after injection. When other anaesthetic drugs are administered through the same in-dwelling needle or cannula as Tracrium it is important that each drug is flushed through with an adequate volume of physiological saline. Atracurium besilate is hypotonic and must not be administered into the infusion line of a blood transfusion.

Studies in malignant hyperthermia in susceptible animals (swine), and clinical studies in patients susceptible to malignant hypothermia indicate that Tracrium does not trigger this syndrome.

In common with other non-depolarising neuromuscular blocking agents, resistance may develop in patients suffering from burns. Such patients may require increased doses, dependent on the time elapsed since the burn injury and the extent of the burn.

Intensive Care Unit (ICU) patients: When administered to laboratory animals in high doses, Laudanosine, a metabolite of atracrium has been associated with transient hypotension and, in some species, cerebral excitatory effects. Although seizures have been seen in ICU patients receiving atracurium, a causal relationship to laudanosine has not been established (see Undesirable Effects).

Carcinogenicity: Carcinogenicity studies have not been performed.

Teratogenicity: Animal studies have indicated that Tracrium has no significant effects on foetal development.

Fertility: Fertility studies have not been performed.

4.5 Interaction with other medicinal products and other forms of interaction
The neuromuscular block produced by Tracrium may be increased by the concomitant use of inhalational anaesthetics such as halothane, isoflurane and enflurane.

In common with all non-depolarising neuromuscular blocking agents the magnitude and/or duration of a non-depolarising neuromuscular block may be increased as a result of interaction with: antibiotics, including the aminoglycosides, polymyxins, spectinomycin, tetracyclines, lincomycin and clindamycin; antiarrhythmic drugs, propranolol, calcium channel blockers, lidocaine, procainamide and quinidine; diuretics: furosemide and possibly mannitol, thiazide diuretics and acetazolamide; magnesium sulphate, ketamine, lithium salts, ganglion blocking agents, trimetaphan, hexamethonium.

Rarely certain drugs may aggravate or unmask latent myasthenia gravis or actually induce a myasthenic syndrome; increased sensitivity to Tracrium would be consequent on such a development. Such drugs include various antibiotics, β-blockers (propranolol, oxprenolol), antiarrhythmic drugs (procainamide, quinidine), antirheumatic drugs (chloroquine, D-penicillamine), trimetaphan, chlorpromazine, steroids, phenytoin and lithium.

The onset of non-depolarising neuromuscular block is likely to be lengthened and the duration of block shortened in patients receiving chronic anticonvulsant therapy.

The administration of combinations of non-depolarising neuromuscular blocking agents in conjunction with Tracrium may produce a degree of neuromuscular blockage in excess of that which might be expected were an equipotent total dose of Tracrium administered. Any synergistic effect may vary between different drug combinations.

A depolarising muscle relaxant such as suxamethonium chloride should not be administered to prolong the neuromuscular blocking effects of non-depolarising blocking agents such as atracurium, as this may result in a prolonged and complex block which can be difficult to reverse with anticholinesterase drugs.

Treatment with anticholinesterases, commonly used in the treatment of Alzheimer's disease e.g. donepezil, may shorten the duration and diminish the magnitude of neuromuscular blockade with atracurium.

4.6 Pregnancy and lactation
In common with all neuromuscular blocking agents, Tracrium should be used during pregnancy only if the potential benefit to the mother outweighs any potential risk to the foetus.

Tracrium is suitable for maintenance of muscle relaxation during Caesarean section as it does not cross the placenta in clinically significant amounts following recommended doses. It is not known whether Tracrium is excreted in human milk.

4.7 Effects on ability to drive and use machines
This precaution is not relevant to the use of atracurium. Atracurium will always be used in combination with a general anaesthetic and therefore the usual precautions relating to performance of tasks following general anaesthesia apply.

4.8 Undesirable effects
Associated with the use of Tracrium there have been reports of skin flushing and mild transient hypotension or bronchospasm, which have been attributed to histamine release. Very rarely, severe anaphylactoid or anaphylactic reactions have been reported in patients receiving Tracrium in conjunction with one or more anaesthetic agents.

There have been rare reports of seizures in ICU patients who have been receiving atracurium concurrently with several other agents. These patients usually had one or more medical conditions predisposing to seizures (e.g. cranial trauma, cerebral oedema, viral encephalitis, hypoxic encephalopathy, uraemia). A causal relationship to laudanosine has not been established. In clinical trials, there appears to be no correlation between plasma laudanosine concentration and the occurrence of seizures.

There have been some reports of muscle weakness and/or myopathy following prolonged use of muscle relaxants in severely ill patients in the ICU. Most patients were receiving concomitant corticosteroids. These events have been seen infrequently in association with Tracrium. A causal relationship has not been established.

4.9 Overdose
Prolonged muscle paralysis and its consequences are the main signs of overdosage.

Treatment: It is essential to maintain a patient airway together with assisted positive pressure ventilation until spontaneous respiration is adequate. Full sedation will be required since consciousness is not impaired. Recovery may be hastened by the administration of anticholinesterase agents accompanied by atropine or glycopyrrolate, once evidence of spontaneous recovery is present.

5. PHARMACOLOGICAL PROPERTIES
5.1 Pharmacodynamic properties
Atracurium is a highly selective competitive (non-depolarising) neuromuscular blocking agent with an intermediate duration of action. Non-depolarising agents antagonise the neurotransmitter action of acetylcholine by binding with receptor sites on the motor-end-plate. Atracurium can be used in a wide range of surgical procedures and to facilitate controlled ventilation.

5.2 Pharmacokinetic properties
The pharmacokinetics of Atracurium in man are essentially linear with the 0.3-0.6 mg/kg dose range. The elimination half-life is approximately 20 minutes, and the volume of distribution is 0.16 L/kg. Atracurium is 82% bound to plasma proteins.

Atracurium is degraded spontaneously mainly by a non-enzymatic decomposition process (Hofmann elimination) which occurs at plasma pH and at body temperature and produces breakdown products which are inactive. Degradation also occurs by ester hydrolysis catalysed by non-specific esterases. Elimination of atracurium is not dependent on kidney or liver function.

The main breakdown products are laudanosine and a monoquaternary alcohol which have no neuromuscular blocking activity. The monoquaternary alcohol is degraded spontaneously by hofmann elimination and excreted by the kidney. Laudanosine is excreted by the kidney and metabolised by the liver. The half-life of laudanosine ranges from 3-6h in patients with normal kidney and liver function. It is about 15h in renal failure and is about 40h in renal and hepatic failure. Peak plasma levels of laudanosine are highest in patients without kidney or liver function and average 4 μg/ml with wide variation.

Concentration of metabolites are higher in ICU patients with abnormal renal and/or hepatic function (see Special Warnings and Special Precautions for Use). These metabolites do not contribute to neuromuscular block.

5.3 Preclinical safety data
There are no pre-clinical data of relevance to the prescriber which are additional to that already included in other sections of the SMPC.

6. PHARMACEUTICAL PARTICULARS
6.1 List of excipients
Benzene Sulphonic acid
Water for Injections

6.2 Incompatibilities
None

6.3 Shelf life
24 months

6.4 Special precautions for storage
Store between 2 and 8°C. Do not freeze. Keep container in the outer carton.

Any unused Tracrium from opened ampoules or vials should be discarded.

6.5 Nature and contents of container
Neutral glass ampoules or vials. Vials are closed with a rubber stopper, sealed with an aluminium collar and fitted with a plastic flip-off top. Pack sizes: Boxes of 5 × 2.5ml ampoules, 5 × 5ml ampoules and 2 × 25ml vials.

6.6 Special precautions for disposal and other handling
None

Administrative Data
7. MARKETING AUTHORISATION HOLDER
The Wellcome Foundation Ltd trading as:
GlaxoSmithKline UK
Stockley Park West
Uxbridge
Middlesex UB11 1BT
Glaxo Wellcome House
Berkeley Avenue
Greenford
Middlesex UB6 ONN

8. MARKETING AUTHORISATION NUMBER(S)
PL0003/0166

9. DATE OF FIRST AUTHORISATION/RENEWAL OF THE AUTHORISATION
12th January 1999

10. DATE OF REVISION OF THE TEXT
15/7/09

11. Legal Status
POM

Tractocile 7.5 mg/ml Concentrate for Solution for Infusion

(Ferring Pharmaceuticals Ltd)

1. NAME OF THE MEDICINAL PRODUCT
TRACTOCILE 7.5 mg/ml concentrate for solution for infusion

2. QUALITATIVE AND QUANTITATIVE COMPOSITION
One ml solution contains 7.5 mg atosiban free-base in the form of atosiban acetate.

After dilution, the concentration of atosiban is 0.75 mg/ml.

For excipients, see section 6.1.

3. PHARMACEUTICAL FORM
Concentrate for solution for infusion

Visual appearance: clear, colourless solution without particles.

4. CLINICAL PARTICULARS
4.1 Therapeutic indications
TRACTOCILE is indicated to delay imminent pre-term birth in pregnant women with:

– regular uterine contractions of at least 30 seconds duration at a rate of ⩾ 4 per 30 minutes

– a cervical dilation of 1 to 3 cm (0-3 for nulliparas) and effacement of ⩾ 50%

– age ⩾ 18 years

– a gestational age from 24 until 33 completed weeks

– a normal fetal heart rate

4.2 Posology and method of administration

Treatment with TRACTOCILE should be initiated and maintained by a physician experienced in the treatment of pre-term labour.

TRACTOCILE is administered intravenously in three successive stages: an initial bolus dose (6.75 mg), performed with TRACTOCILE 7.5 mg/ml solution for injection, immediately followed by a continuous high dose infusion (loading infusion 300 micrograms/min) of TRACTOCILE 7.5 mg/ml concentrate for solution for infusion during three hours, followed by a lower dose of TRACTOCILE 7.5 mg/ml concentrate for solution for infusion (subsequent infusion 100 micrograms/min) up to 45 hours. The duration of the treatment should not exceed 48 hours. The total dose given during a full course of TRACTOCILE therapy should preferably not exceed 330 mg of the active substance.

Intravenous therapy using the initial bolus injection of TRACTOCILE 7.5 mg/ml, solution for injection (see Summary of Product Characteristics of this product) should be started as soon as possible after diagnosis of pre-term labour. Once the bolus has been injected, proceed with the infusion. In the case of persistence of uterine contractions during treatment with TRACTOCILE, alternative therapy should be considered.

There is no data available regarding the need for dose adjustments in patients with renal or liver insufficiency.

The following table shows the full posology of the bolus injection followed by the infusion:

(see Table 1 below)

Re-treatment

In case a re-treatment with atosiban is needed, it should also commence with a bolus injection of TRACTOCILE 7.5 mg/ml, solution for injection followed by infusion with TRACTOCILE 7.5 mg/ml, concentrate for solution for infusion.

4.3 Contraindications

TRACTOCILE should not be used in the following conditions:

– Gestational age below 24 or over 33 completed weeks

– Premature rupture of the membranes >30 weeks of gestation

– Intrauterine growth retardation and abnormal fetal heart rate

– Antepartum uterine haemorrhage requiring immediate delivery

– Eclampsia and severe pre-eclampsia requiring delivery

– Intrauterine fetal death

– Suspected intrauterine infection

– Placenta praevia

– Abruptio placenta

– Any other conditions of the mother or fetus, in which continuation of pregnancy is hazardous

– Known hypersensitivity to the active substance or any of the excipients.

4.4 Special warnings and precautions for use

When atosiban is used in patients in whom premature rupture of membranes cannot be excluded, the benefits of delaying delivery should be balanced against the potential risk of chorioamnionitis.

There is no experience with atosiban treatment in patients with impaired function of the liver or kidneys (see sections 4.2 and 5.2).

Atosiban has not been used in patients with an abnormal placental site.

There is only limited clinical experience in the use of atosiban in multiple pregnancies or the gestational age group between 24 and 27 weeks, because of the small number of patients treated. The benefit of atosiban in these subgroups is therefore uncertain.

Re-treatment with TRACTOCILE is possible, but there is only limited clinical experience available with multiple re-treatments, up to 3 re-treatments (see section 4.2).

In case of intrauterine growth retardation, the decision to continue or reinitiate the administration of TRACTOCILE depends on the assessment of fetal maturity.

Monitoring of uterine contractions and fetal heart rate during administration of atosiban and in case of persistent uterine contractions should be considered.

As an antagonist of oxytocin, atosiban may theoretically facilitate uterine relaxation and postpartum bleeding therefore blood loss after delivery should be monitored. However, inadequate uterus contraction postpartum was not observed during the clinical trials.

4.5 Interaction with other medicinal products and other forms of interaction

It is unlikely that atosiban is involved in cytochrome P450 mediated drug-drug interactions as *in vitro* investigations have shown that atosiban is not a substrate for the cytochrome P450 system, and does not inhibit the drug metabolising cytochrome P450 enzymes.

Interaction studies were performed in healthy, female volunteers with betamethasone and labetalol. No clinically relevant interaction was observed between atosiban and betamethasone. When atosiban and labetalol were co-administrated, C_{max} of labetalol was decreased by 36% and T_{max} increased by 45 minutes. However, the extent of labetalol bioavailability in terms of AUC did not change. The interaction observed has no clinical relevance. Labetalol had no effect on atosiban pharmacokinetics.

No interaction study has been performed with antibiotics, ergot alkaloids, and anti-hypertensive agents other than labetalol.

4.6 Pregnancy and lactation

Atosiban should only be used when pre-term labour has been diagnosed between 24 and 33 completed weeks of gestation.

In atosiban clinical trials no effects were observed on lactation. Small amounts of atosiban have been shown to pass from plasma into the breast milk of lactating women.

Embryo-fetal toxicity studies have not shown toxic effects of atosiban. No studies were performed that covered fertility and early embryonic development (see section 5.3).

4.7 Effects on ability to drive and use machines

Not applicable.

4.8 Undesirable effects

Possible undesirable effects of atosiban were described for the mother during the use of atosiban in clinical trials. The observed undesirable effects were generally of a mild severity. In total 48% of the patients treated with atosiban experienced undesirable effects.

For the newborn, the clinical trials did not reveal any specific undesirable effects of atosiban. The infant adverse events were in the range of normal variation and were comparable with both placebo and beta-mimetic group incidences.

The undesirable effects in the women were the following:

Very common (>1/10)	*Gastrointestinal disorders:* nausea.
Common (>1/100, <1/10)	*Metabolism and nutrition disorders:* hyperglycaemia *Nervous system disorders:* headache, dizziness *Cardiac disorders:* tachycardia *Vascular disorders:* hot flush, hypotension *Gastrointestinal disorders:* vomiting *General disorders and administration site conditions:* injection site reaction
Uncommon (>1/1,000, <1/100)	*Psychiatric disorders:* insomnia *Skin and subcutaneous tissue disorders:* pruritis, rash *General disorders and administration site conditions:* pyrexia
Rare (>1/10,000, <1/1,000)	Incidental cases of uterine haemorrhage/uterine atony were reported. The frequency did not exceed that of the control groups in clinical trials. One case of allergic reaction was reported, which was considered to be probably related to atosiban.

4.9 Overdose

Few cases of atosiban overdosing were reported, they occurred without any specific signs or symptoms. There is no known specific treatment in case of an overdose.

5. PHARMACOLOGICAL PROPERTIES

5.1 Pharmacodynamic properties

Pharmacotherapeutic group: Other gynecologicals, ATC code: G02CX01

TRACTOCILE contains atosiban (INN), a synthetic peptide ([Mpa^1,D-Tyr(Et)^2,Thr^4,Orn^8]-oxytocin) which is a competitive antagonist of human oxytocin at receptor level. In rats and guinea pigs, atosiban was shown to bind to oxytocin receptors, to decrease the frequency of contractions and the tone of the uterine musculature, resulting in a suppression of uterine contractions. Atosiban was also shown to bind to the vasopressin receptor, thus inhibiting the effect of vasopressin. In animals atosiban did not exhibit cardiovascular effects.

In human pre-term labour, atosiban at the recommended dosage antagonises uterine contractions and induces uterine quiescence. The onset of uterus relaxation following atosiban is rapid, uterine contractions being significantly reduced within 10 minutes to achieve stable uterine quiescence ($\leqslant$ 4 contractions/hour) for 12 hours.

Phase III clinical trials (CAP-001 studies) include data from 742 women who were diagnosed with pre-term labour at 23–33 weeks of gestation and were randomised to receive either atosiban (according to this labelling) or β-agonist (dose-titrated).

Primary endpoint: the primary efficacy outcome was the proportion of women remaining undelivered and not requiring alternative tocolysis within 7 days of treatment initiation. The data show that 59.6% (n=201) and 47.7% (n=163) of atosiban- and β-agonist-treated women (p=0.0004), respectively, were undelivered and did not require alternative tocolysis within 7 days of starting treatment. Most of the treatment failures in CAP-001 were caused by poor tolerability. Treatment failures caused by insufficient efficacy were significantly (p=0.0003) more frequent in atosiban (n=48, 14.2%) than in the β-agonist-treated women (n=20, 5.8%).

In the CAP-001 studies the probability of remaining undelivered and not requiring alternative tocolytics within 7 days of treatment initiation was similar for atosiban and beta-mimetics treated women at gestational age of 24-28 weeks. However, this finding is based on a very small sample (n=129 patients).

Secondary endpoints: secondary efficacy parameters included the proportion of women remaining undelivered within 48 h of treatment initiation. There was no difference between the atosiban and beta-mimetic groups with regard to this parameter.

Mean (SD) gestational age at delivery was the same in the two groups: 35.6 (3.9) and 35.3 (4.2) weeks for the atosiban and β-agonist groups, respectively (p=0.37). Admission to a neonatal intensive care unit (NICU) was similar for both treatment groups (approximately 30%), as was length of stay and ventilation therapy. Mean (SD) birth weight was 2491 (813) grams in the atosiban group and 2461 (831) grams in the β-agonist group (p=0.58).

Fetal and maternal outcome did apparently not differ between the atosiban and the β-agonist group, but the clinical studies were not powered enough to rule out a possible difference.

Of the 361 women who received atosiban treatment in the phase III studies, 73 received at least one re-treatment, 8 received at least 2 re-treatments and 2 received 3 re-treatments (see section 4.4).

As the safety and efficacy of atosiban in women with a gestational age of less than 24 completed weeks has not been established in controlled randomised studies, the treatment of this patient group with atosiban is not recommended (see section 4.3).

In a placebo-controlled study, fetal/infant deaths were 5/295 (1.7%) in the placebo group and 15/288 (5.2%) in the atosiban group, of which two occurred at five and eight months of age. Eleven out of the 15 deaths in the atosiban group occurred in pregnancies with a gestational age of 20 to 24 weeks, although in this subgroup patient distribution was unequal (19 women on atosiban, 4 on placebo). For women with a gestational age greater than 24 weeks there was no difference in mortality rate (1.7% in the placebo group and 1.5% in the atosiban group).

5.2 Pharmacokinetic properties

In healthy non-pregnant subjects receiving atosiban infusions (10 to 300 micrograms/min over 12 hours), the steady state plasma concentrations increased proportionally to the dose.

The clearance, volume of distribution and half-life were found to be independent of the dose.

In women in pre-term labour receiving atosiban by infusion (300 micrograms/min for 6 to 12 hours), steady state plasma concentrations were reached within one hour following the start of the infusion (mean 442 ± 73 ng/ml, range 298 to 533 ng/ml).

Following completion of the infusion, plasma concentration rapidly declined with an initial (t_α) and terminal (t_β) half-life of 0.21 ± 0.01 and 1.7 ± 0.3 hours, respectively. Mean value for clearance was 41.8 ± 8.2 litres/h. Mean value of volume of distribution was 18.3 ± 6.8 litres.

Plasma protein binding of atosiban is 46 to 48% in pregnant women. It is not known whether the free fraction in the maternal and fetal compartments differs substantially. Atosiban does not partition into red blood cells.

Atosiban passes the placenta. Following an infusion of 300 micrograms/min in healthy pregnant women at term, the fetal/maternal atosiban concentration ratio was 0.12.

Two metabolites were identified in the plasma and urine from human subjects. The ratios of the main metabolite M1

Table 1

Step	Regimen	Injection/infusion rate	Atosiban dose
1	0.9 ml intravenous bolus	over 1 minute	6.75 mg
2	3 hours intravenous loading infusion	24 ml/hour	18 mg/hour
3	subsequent intravenous infusion	8 ml/hour	6 mg/hour

(des-(Orn[8], Gly-NH_2[9])-[Mpa[1], D-Tyr(Et)[2], Thr[4]]-oxytocin) to atosiban concentrations in plasma were 1.4 and 2.8 at the second hour and at the end of the infusion respectively. It is not known whether M1 accumulates in tissues. Atosiban is found in only small quantities in urine, its urinary concentration is about 50 times lower than that of M1. The proportion of atosiban eliminated in faeces is not known. Main metabolite M1 is apparently as potent as the parent compound in inhibiting oxytocin-induced uterine contractions *in vitro*. Metabolite M1 is excreted in milk (see section 4.6).

There is no experience with atosiban treatment in patients with impaired function of the liver or kidneys (see sections 4.2 and 4.4).

It is unlikely that atosiban inhibits hepatic cytochrome P450 isoforms in humans (see section 4.5).

5.3 Preclinical safety data

No systemic toxic effects were observed during the two-week intravenous toxicity studies (in rats and dogs) at doses which are approximately 10 times higher than the human therapeutic dose, and during the three-months toxicity studies in rats and dogs (up to 20 mg/kg/day s.c.). The highest atosiban subcutaneous dose not producing any adverse effects was approximately two times the therapeutic human dose.

No studies were performed that covered fertility and early embryonic development. Reproduction toxicity studies, with dosing from implantation up to late stage pregnancy, showed no effects on mothers and fetuses. The exposure of the rat fetus was approximately four times that received by the human fetus during intravenous infusions in women. Animal studies have shown inhibition of lactation as expected from the inhibition of action of oxytocin.

Atosiban was neither oncogenic nor mutagenic in *in vitro* and *in vivo* tests.

6. PHARMACEUTICAL PARTICULARS

6.1 List of excipients

Mannitol

Hydrochloric acid 1M

Water for injections

6.2 Incompatibilities

In the absence of compatibility studies, this medicinal product must not be mixed with other medicinal products except those mentioned in section 6.6.

6.3 Shelf life

2 years.

Once the vial has been opened, the dilution must be performed immediately.

Diluted solution for intravenous administration should be used within 24 hours after preparation.

6.4 Special precautions for storage

Store in a refrigerator (2°C - 8°C).

Store in the original package.

6.5 Nature and contents of container

One vial of concentrate for solution for infusion contains 5 ml solution, corresponding to 37.5 mg atosiban.

Colourless glass vials, clear borosilicated (type I) sealed with grey siliconised bromo-butyl rubber stopper, type I, and flip-off cap of polypropylene and aluminium.

6.6 Special precautions for disposal and other handling

The vials should be inspected visually for particulate matter and discoloration prior to administration.

Preparation of the intravenous infusion solution:

For intravenous infusion, following the bolus dose, TRACTOCILE 7.5 mg/ml, concentrate for solution for infusion should be diluted in one of the following solutions:

- 0.9% w/v NaCl
- Ringer's lactate solution
- 5% w/v glucose solution.

Withdraw 10 ml solution from a 100 ml infusion bag and discard. Replace it by 10 ml TRACTOCILE 7.5 mg/ml concentrate for solution for infusion from two 5 ml vials to obtain a concentration of 75 mg atosiban in 100 ml.

The reconstituted product is a clear, colourless solution without particles.

The loading infusion is given by infusing 24 ml/hour (i.e. 18 mg/h) of the above prepared solution over the 3 hour period under adequate medical supervision in an obstetric unit. After three hours the infusion rate is reduced to 8 ml/hour.

Prepare new 100 ml bags in the same way as described to allow the infusion to be continued.

If an infusion bag with a different volume is used, a proportional calculation should be made for the preparation.

To achieve accurate dosing, a controlled infusion device is recommended to adjust the rate of flow in drops/min. An intravenous microdrip chamber can provide a convenient range of infusion rates within the recommended dose levels for TRACTOCILE.

In the absence of compatibility studies, this medicinal product must not be mixed with other medicinal products (see section 6.2). If other medicinal products need to be given intravenously at the same time, the intravenous cannula can be shared or another site of intravenous administration can be used. This permits the continued independent control of the rate of infusion.

7. MARKETING AUTHORISATION HOLDER

Ferring AB
Soldattorpsvägen 5
Box 30 047
SE - 20061 - Limhamn
Sweden.

8. MARKETING AUTHORISATION NUMBER(S)

EU/1/99/124/002.

9. DATE OF FIRST AUTHORISATION/RENEWAL OF THE AUTHORISATION

20 January 2005.

10. DATE OF REVISION OF THE TEXT

January 2005.

11. LEGAL CATEGORY

POM.

Tractocile 7.5 mg/ml Solution for Injection

(Ferring Pharmaceuticals Ltd)

1. NAME OF THE MEDICINAL PRODUCT

TRACTOCILE 7.5 mg/ml solution for injection

2. QUALITATIVE AND QUANTITATIVE COMPOSITION

One ml solution contains 7.5 mg atosiban free-base in the form of atosiban acetate.

For excipients, see section 6.1.

3. PHARMACEUTICAL FORM

Solution for injection

Visual appearance: clear, colourless solution without particles.

4. CLINICAL PARTICULARS

4.1 Therapeutic indications

TRACTOCILE is indicated to delay imminent pre-term birth in pregnant women with:

- regular uterine contractions of at least 30 seconds duration at a rate of ⩾ 4 per 30 minutes
- a cervical dilation of 1 to 3 cm (0-3 for nulliparas) and effacement of ⩾ 50%
- age ⩾ 18 years
- a gestational age from 24 until 33 completed weeks
- a normal fetal heart rate

4.2 Posology and method of administration

Treatment with TRACTOCILE should be initiated and maintained by a physician experienced in the treatment of pre-term labour.

TRACTOCILE is administered intravenously in three successive stages: an initial bolus dose (6.75 mg), performed with TRACTOCILE 7.5 mg/ml solution for injection, immediately followed by a continuous high dose infusion (loading infusion 300 micrograms/min) of TRACTOCILE 7.5 mg/ml concentrate for solution for infusion during three hours, followed by a lower dose of TRACTOCILE 7.5 mg/ml concentrate for solution for infusion (subsequent infusion 100 micrograms/min) up to 45 hours. The duration of the treatment should not exceed 48 hours. The total dose given during a full course of TRACTOCILE therapy should preferably not exceed 330 mg of the active substance.

Intravenous therapy using the initial bolus injection should be started as soon as possible after diagnosis of pre-term labour. Once the bolus has been injected, proceed with the infusion (See Summary of Product Characteristics of TRACTOCILE 7.5 mg/ml, concentrate for solution for infusion). In the case of persistence of uterine contractions during treatment with TRACTOCILE, alternative therapy should be considered.

There is no data available regarding the need for dose adjustments in patients with renal or liver insufficiency.

The following table shows the full posology of the bolus injection followed by the infusion:

(see Table 1 below)

Re-treatment

In case a re-treatment with atosiban is needed, it should also commence with a bolus injection of TRACTOCILE 7.5 mg/ml, solution for injection followed by infusion with TRACTOCILE 7.5 mg/ml, concentrate for solution for infusion.

4.3 Contraindications

TRACTOCILE should not be used in the following conditions:

- Gestational age below 24 or over 33 completed weeks
- Premature rupture of the membranes >30 weeks of gestation
- Intrauterine growth retardation and abnormal fetal heart rate
- Antepartum uterine haemorrhage requiring immediate delivery
- Eclampsia and severe pre-eclampsia requiring delivery
- Intrauterine fetal death
- Suspected intrauterine infection
- Placenta praevia
- Abruptio placenta
- Any other conditions of the mother or fetus, in which continuation of pregnancy is hazardous
- Known hypersensitivity to the active substance or any of the excipients.

4.4 Special warnings and precautions for use

When atosiban is used in patients in whom premature rupture of membranes cannot be excluded, the benefits of delaying delivery should be balanced against the potential risk of chorioamnionitis.

There is no experience with atosiban treatment in patients with impaired function of the liver or kidneys (see sections 4.2 and 5.2).

Atosiban has not been used in patients with an abnormal placental site.

There is only limited clinical experience in the use of atosiban in multiple pregnancies or the gestational age group between 24 and 27 weeks, because of the small number of patients treated. The benefit of atosiban in these subgroups is therefore uncertain.

Re-treatment with TRACTOCILE is possible, but there is only limited clinical experience available with multiple re-treatments, up to 3 re-treatments (see section 4.2).

In case of intrauterine growth retardation, the decision to continue or reinitiate the administration of TRACTOCILE depends on the assessment of fetal maturity.

Monitoring of uterine contractions and fetal heart rate during administration of atosiban and in case of persistent uterine contractions should be considered.

As an antagonist of oxytocin, atosiban may theoretically facilitate uterine relaxation and postpartum bleeding therefore blood loss after delivery should be monitored. However, inadequate uterus contraction postpartum was not observed during the clinical trials.

4.5 Interaction with other medicinal products and other forms of interaction

It is unlikely that atosiban is involved in cytochrome P450 mediated drug-drug interactions as *in vitro* investigations have shown that atosiban is not a substrate for the cytochrome P450 system, and does not inhibit the drug metabolising cytochrome P450 enzymes.

Interaction studies were performed in healthy, female volunteers with betamethasone and labetalol. No clinically relevant interaction was observed between atosiban and betamethasone. When atosiban and labetalol were co-administrated, C_{max} of labetalol was decreased by 36% and T_{max} increased by 45 minutes. However, the extent of labetalol bioavailability in terms of AUC did not change. The interaction observed has no clinical relevance. Labetalol had no effect on atosiban pharmacokinetics.

No interaction study has been performed with antibiotics, ergot alkaloids, and anti-hypertensive agents other than labetalol.

4.6 Pregnancy and lactation

Atosiban should only be used when pre-term labour has been diagnosed between 24 and 33 completed weeks of gestation.

In atosiban clinical trials no effects were observed on lactation. Small amounts of atosiban have been shown to pass from plasma into the breast milk of lactating women.

Embryo-fetal toxicity studies have not shown toxic effects of atosiban. No studies were performed that covered fertility and early embryonic development (see section 5.3).

4.7 Effects on ability to drive and use machines

Not applicable.

4.8 Undesirable effects

Possible undesirable effects of atosiban were described for the mother during the use of atosiban in clinical trials.

Table 1

Step	Regimen	Injection/infusion rate	Atosiban dose
1	0.9 ml intravenous bolus	over 1 minute	6.75 mg
2	3 hours intravenous loading infusion	24 ml/hour	18 mg/hour
3	subsequent intravenous infusion	8 ml/hour	6 mg/hour

The observed undesirable effects were generally of a mild severity. In total 48% of the patients treated with atosiban experienced undesirable effects.

For the newborn, the clinical trials did not reveal any specific undesirable effects of atosiban. The infant adverse events were in the range of normal variation and were comparable with both placebo and beta-mimetic group incidences.

The undesirable effects in the women were the following:

Very common (>1/10)	*Gastrointestinal disorders:* nausea.
Common (>1/100, <1/10)	*Metabolism and nutrition disorders:* hyperglycaemia
	Nervous system disorders: headache, dizziness
	Cardiac disorders: tachycardia
	Vascular disorders: hot flush, hypotension
	Gastrointestinal disorders: vomiting
	General disorders and administration site conditions: injection site reaction
Uncommon (>1/1,000, <1/100)	*Psychiatric disorders:* insomnia
	Skin and subcutaneous tissue disorders: pruritis, rash
	General disorders and administration site conditions: pyrexia
Rare (>1/10,000, <1/1,000)	Incidental cases of uterine haemorrhage/ uterine atony were reported. The frequency did not exceed that of the control groups in clinical trials. One case of allergic reaction was reported, which was considered to be probably related to atosiban.

4.9 Overdose

Few cases of atosiban overdosing were reported, they occurred without any specific signs or symptoms. There is no known specific treatment in case of an overdose.

5. PHARMACOLOGICAL PROPERTIES

5.1 Pharmacodynamic properties

Pharmacotherapeutic group: Other gynecologicals, ATC code: G02CX01

TRACTOCILE contains atosiban (INN), a synthetic peptide ([Mpa^1,D-Tyr(Et)^2,Thr^4,Orn^8]-oxytocin) which is a competitive antagonist of human oxytocin at receptor level. In rats and guinea pigs, atosiban was shown to bind to oxytocin receptors, to decrease the frequency of contractions and the tone of the uterine musculature, resulting in a suppression of uterine contractions. Atosiban was also shown to bind to the vasopressin receptor, thus inhibiting the effect of vasopressin. In animals atosiban did not exhibit cardiovascular effects.

In human pre-term labour, atosiban at the recommended dosage antagonises uterine contractions and induces uterine quiescence. The onset of uterus relaxation following atosiban is rapid, uterine contractions being significantly reduced within 10 minutes to achieve stable uterine quiescence (≤ 4 contractions/hour) for 12 hours.

Phase III clinical trials (CAP-001 studies) include data from 742 women who were diagnosed with pre-term labour at 23–33 weeks of gestation and were randomised to receive either atosiban (according to this labelling) or β-agonist (dose-titrated).

Primary endpoint: the primary efficacy outcome was the proportion of women remaining undelivered and not requiring alternative tocolysis within 7 days of treatment initiation. The data show that 59.6% (n=201) and 47.7% (n=163) of atosiban- and β-agonist-treated women (p=0.0004), respectively, were undelivered and did not require alternative tocolysis within 7 days of starting treatment. Most of the treatment failures in CAP-001 were caused by poor tolerability. Treatment failures caused by insufficient efficacy were significantly (p=0.0003) more frequent in atosiban (n=48, 14.2%) than in the β-agonist-treated women (n=20, 5.8%).

In the CAP-001 studies the probability of remaining undelivered and not requiring alternative tocolytics within 7 days of treatment initiation was similar for atosiban and beta-mimetics treated women at gestational age of 24-28 weeks. However, this finding is based on a very small sample (n=129 patients).

Secondary endpoints: secondary efficacy parameters included the proportion of women remaining undelivered within 48 h of treatment initiation. There was no difference between the atosiban and beta-mimetic groups with regard to this parameter.

Mean (SD) gestational age at delivery was the same in the two groups: 35.6 (3.9) and 35.3 (4.2) weeks for the atosiban and β-agonist groups, respectively (p=0.37). Admission to a neonatal intensive care unit (NICU) was similar for both treatment groups (approximately 30%), as was length of stay and ventilation therapy. Mean (SD) birth weight was 2491 (813) grams in the atosiban group and 2461 (831) grams in the β-agonist group (p=0.58).

Fetal and maternal outcome did apparently not differ between the atosiban and the β-agonist group, but the clinical studies were not powered enough to rule out a possible difference.

Of the 361 women who received atosiban treatment in the phase III studies, 73 received at least one re-treatment, 8 received at least 2 re-treatments and 2 received 3 re-treatments (see section 4.4).

As the safety and efficacy of atosiban in women with a gestational age of less than 24 completed weeks has not been established in controlled randomised studies, the treatment of this patient group with atosiban is not recommended (see section 4.3).

In a placebo-controlled study, fetal/infant deaths were 5/295 (1.7%) in the placebo group and 15/288 (5.2%) in the atosiban group, of which two occurred at five and eight months of age. Eleven out of the 15 deaths in the atosiban group occurred in pregnancies with a gestational age of 20 to 24 weeks, although in this subgroup patient distribution was unequal (19 women on atosiban, 4 on placebo). For women with a gestational age greater than 24 weeks there was no difference in mortality rate (1.7% in the placebo group and 1.5% in the atosiban group).

5.2 Pharmacokinetic properties

In healthy non-pregnant subjects receiving atosiban infusions (10 to 300 micrograms/min over 12 hours), the steady state plasma concentrations increased proportionally to the dose.

The clearance, volume of distribution and half-life were found to be independent of the dose.

In women in pre-term labour receiving atosiban by infusion (300 micrograms/min for 6 to 12 hours), steady state plasma concentrations were reached within one hour following the start of the infusion (mean 442 ± 73 ng/ml, range 298 to 533 ng/ml).

Following completion of the infusion, plasma concentration rapidly declined with an initial (t_α) and terminal (t_β) half-life of 0.21 ± 0.01 and 1.7 ± 0.3 hours, respectively. Mean value for clearance was 41.8 ± 8.2 litres/h. Mean value of volume of distribution was 18.3 ± 6.8 litres.

Plasma protein binding of atosiban is 46 to 48% in pregnant women. It is not known whether the free fraction in the maternal and fetal compartments differs substantially. Atosiban does not partition into red blood cells.

Atosiban passes the placenta. Following an infusion of 300 micrograms/min in healthy pregnant women at term, the fetal/maternal atosiban concentration ratio was 0.12.

Two metabolites were identified in the plasma and urine from human subjects. The ratios of the main metabolite M1 (des-(Orn^8, Gly-NH$_2$^{9})-[Mpa^1, D-Tyr(Et)^2, Thr^4]-oxytocin) to atosiban concentrations in plasma were 1.4 and 2.8 at the second hour and at the end of the infusion respectively. It is not known whether M1 accumulates in tissues. Atosiban is found in only small quantities in urine, its urinary concentration is about 50 times lower than that of M1. The proportion of atosiban eliminated in faeces is not known. Main metabolite M1 is apparently as potent as the parent compound in inhibiting oxytocin-induced uterine contractions *in vitro*. Metabolite M1 is excreted in milk (see section 4.6).

There is no experience with atosiban treatment in patients with impaired function of the liver or kidneys (see sections 4.2 and 4.4).

It is unlikely that atosiban inhibits hepatic cytochrome P450 isoforms in humans (see section 4.5).

5.3 Preclinical safety data

No systemic toxic effects were observed during the two-week intravenous toxicity studies (in rats and dogs) at doses which are approximately 10 times higher than the human therapeutic dose, and during the three-months toxicity studies in rats and dogs (up to 20 mg/kg/day s.c.). The highest atosiban subcutaneous dose not producing any adverse effects was approximately two times the therapeutic human dose.

No studies were performed that covered fertility and early embryonic development. Reproduction toxicity studies, with dosing from implantation up to late stage pregnancy, showed no effects on mothers and fetuses. The exposure of the rat fetus was approximately four times that received by the human fetus during intravenous infusions in women. Animal studies have shown inhibition of lactation as expected from the inhibition of action of oxytocin.

Atosiban was neither oncogenic nor mutagenic in *in vitro* and *in vivo* tests.

6. PHARMACEUTICAL PARTICULARS

6.1 List of excipients

Mannitol

Hydrochloric acid 1M

Water for injections

6.2 Incompatibilities

In the absence of compatibility studies, this medicinal product must not be mixed with other medicinal products.

6.3 Shelf life

2 years.

Once the vial has been opened, the product must be used immediately.

6.4 Special precautions for storage

Store in a refrigerator (2°C - 8°C).

Store in the original package.

6.5 Nature and contents of container

One vial of solution for injection contains 0.9 ml solution, corresponding to 6.75 mg atosiban.

Colourless glass vials, clear borosilicated (type I) sealed with grey siliconised bromo-butyl rubber stopper, type I, and flip-off cap of polypropylene and aluminium.

6.6 Special precautions for disposal and other handling

The vials should be inspected visually for particulate matter and discoloration prior to administration.

Preparation of the initial intravenous injection:

Withdraw 0.9 ml of a 0.9 ml labelled vial of TRACTOCILE 7.5 mg/ml, solution for injection and administer slowly as an intravenous bolus dose over one minute, under adequate medical supervision in an obstetric unit. The TRACTOCILE 7.5 mg/ml, solution for injection should be used immediately.

In the absence of compatibility studies, this medicinal product must not be mixed with other medicinal products (see section 6.2).

7. MARKETING AUTHORISATION HOLDER

Ferring AB

Soldattorpsvägen 5

Box 30 047

SE - 20061 - Limhamn

Sweden.

8. MARKETING AUTHORISATION NUMBER(S)

EU/1/99/124/001.

9. DATE OF FIRST AUTHORISATION/RENEWAL OF THE AUTHORISATION

20 January 2005.

10. DATE OF REVISION OF THE TEXT

January 2005.

11. LEGAL CATEGORY

POM.

Tramacet 37.5 mg/ 325 mg film-coated tablets

(Grunenthal Ltd)

1. NAME OF THE MEDICINAL PRODUCT

TRAMACET 37.5 mg/325 mg, film coated-tablets

2. QUALITATIVE AND QUANTITATIVE COMPOSITION

One film-coated tablet contains 37.5 mg tramadol hydrochloride and 325 mg paracetamol

For a full list of excipients, see section 6.1.

3. PHARMACEUTICAL FORM

Film-coated tablet

Pale yellow film-coated tablet

4. CLINICAL PARTICULARS

4.1 Therapeutic indications

TRAMACET tablets are indicated for the symptomatic treatment of moderate to severe pain.

The use of TRAMACET should be restricted to patients whose moderate to severe pain is considered to require a combination of tramadol and paracetamol (see also Section 5.1).

4.2 Posology and method of administration

Posology

ADULTS AND ADOLESCENTS (12 years and older)

The use of TRAMACET should be restricted to patients whose moderate to severe pain is considered to require a combination of tramadol and paracetamol.

The dose should be individually adjusted according to intensity of pain and response of the patient.

An initial dose of two tablets of TRAMACET is recommended. Additional doses can be taken as needed, not exceeding 8 tablets (equivalent to 300 mg tramadol and 2600 mg paracetamol) per day.

The dosing interval should not be less than six hours.

TRAMACET should under no circumstances be administered for longer than is strictly necessary (see also section 4.4 - Special warnings and precautions for use). If repeated use or long term treatment with TRAMACET is required as a result of the nature and severity of the illness, then careful, regular monitoring should take place (with breaks in the treatment, where possible), to assess whether continuation of the treatment is necessary.

Children

The effective and safe use of TRAMACET has not been established in children below the age of 12 years. Treatment is therefore not recommended in this population.

Elderly patients

The usual dosages may be used although it should be noted that in volunteers aged over 75 years the elimination half life of tramadol was increased by 17% following oral administration. In patients over 75 years old, it is recommended that the minimum interval between doses should be not less than 6 hours, due to the presence of tramadol.

Renal insufficiency

Because of the presence of tramadol, the use of TRAMACET is not recommended in patients with severe renal insufficiency (creatinine clearance < 10 ml/min). In cases of moderate renal insufficiency (creatinine clearance between 10 and 30 ml/min), the dosing should be increased to 12-hourly intervals. As tramadol is removed only very slowly by haemodialysis or by haemofiltration, post dialysis administration to maintain analgesia is not usually required.

Hepatic insufficiency

In patients with severe hepatic impairment TRAMACET should not be used (see Section 4.3). In moderate cases prolongation of the dosage interval should be carefully considered (see Section 4.4).

Method of administration

Oral use

Tablets must be swallowed whole, with a sufficient quantity of liquid. They must not be broken or chewed.

4.3 Contraindications

- Hypersensitivity to tramadol, paracetamol or to any of the excipients (see 6.1. List of excipients) of the medicinal product,
- acute intoxication with alcohol, hypnotic drugs, centrally-acting analgesics, opioids or psychotropic drugs,
- TRAMACET should not be administered to patients who are receiving monoamine oxidase inhibitors or within two weeks of their withdrawal (see 4.5. Interactions with other medicinal products and other forms of interaction),
- severe hepatic impairment,
- epilepsy not controlled by treatment (see. 4.4. Special Warnings).

4.4 Special warnings and precautions for use

Warnings:

- In adults and adolescents 12 years and older. The maximum dose of 8 tablets of TRAMACET should not be exceeded. In order to avoid inadvertent overdose, patients should be advised not to exceed the recommended dose and not to use any other paracetamol (including over the counter) or tramadol hydrochloride containing products concurrently without the advice of a physician.
- In severe renal insufficiency (creatinine clearance <10 ml/mm), TRAMACET is not recommended.
- In patients with severe hepatic impairment TRAMACET should not be used (See Section 4.3). The hazards of paracetamol overdose are greater in patients with non-cirrhotic alcoholic liver disease. In moderate cases prolongation of dosage interval should be carefully considered.
- In severe respiratory insufficiency, TRAMACET is not recommended.
- Tramadol is not suitable as a substitute in opioid-dependent patients. Although it is an opioid agonist, tramadol cannot suppress morphine withdrawal symptoms.
- Convulsions have been reported in tramadol-treated patients susceptible to seizures or taking other medications that lower the seizure threshold, especially selective serotonin re-uptake inhibitors, tricyclic antidepressants, antipsychotics, centrally acting analgesics or local anaesthesia. Epileptic patients controlled by a treatment or patients susceptible to seizures should be treated with TRAMACET only if there are compelling circumstances. Convulsions have been reported in patients receiving tramadol at the recommended dose levels. The risk may be increased when doses of tramadol exceed the recommended upper dose limit
- Concomitant use of opioid agonists-antagonists (nalbuphine, buprenorphine, pentazocine) is not recommended (see 4.5 Interactions with other medicinal products and other forms of interaction).

Precautions for use

TRAMACET should be used with caution in opioid dependent patients, or in patients with cranial trauma, in patients prone to convulsive disorder, biliary tract disorders, in a state of shock, in an altered state of consciousness for unknown reasons, with problems affecting the respiratory center or the respiratory function, or with an increased intracranial pressure.

Paracetamol in overdosage may cause hepatic toxicity in some patients.

At therapeutic doses, tramadol has the potential to cause withdrawal symptoms. Rarely, cases of dependence and abuse have been reported (see section 4.8).

Symptoms of withdrawal reactions, similar to those occurring during opiate withdrawal may occur (see section 4.8).

In one study, use of tramadol during general anaesthesia with enflurane and nitrous oxide was reported to enhance intra-operative recall. Until further information is available, use of tramadol during light planes of anaesthesia should be avoided.

4.5 Interaction with other medicinal products and other forms of interaction

Concomitant use is contraindicated with:

• Non-selective MAO Inhibitors

Risk of serotoninergic syndrome: diarrhoea, tachycardia, sweating, trembling, confusion, even coma.

• Selective-A MAO Inhibitors

Extrapolation from non-selective MAO inhibitors

Risk of serotoninergic syndrome: diarrhoea, tachycardia, sweating, trembling, confusion, even coma.

• Selective-B MAO Inhibitors

Central excitation symptoms evocative of a serotoninergic syndrome: diarrhoea, tachycardia, sweating, trembling, confusion, even coma.

In case of recent treatment with MAO inhibitors, a delay of two weeks should occur before treatment with tramadol

Concomitant use is not recommended with:

• Alcohol

Alcohol increases the sedative effect of opioid analgesics.

The effect on alertness can make driving of vehicles and the use of machines dangerous.

Avoid intake of alcoholic drinks and of medicinal products containing alcohol.

• Carbamazepine and other enzyme inducers

Risk of reduced efficacy and shorter duration due to decreased plasma concentrations of tramadol.

• Opioid agonists-antagonists (buprenorphine, nalbuphine, pentazocine)

Decrease of the analgesic effect by competitive blocking effect at the receptors, with the risk of occurrence of withdrawal syndrome.

Concomitant use which needs to be taken into consideration:

• In isolated cases there have been reports of Serotonin Syndrome in a temporal connection with the therapeutic use of tramadol in combination with other serotoninergic medicines such as selective serotonin re-uptake inhibitors (SSRIs) and triptans. Signs of Serotonin Syndrome may be for example, confusion, agitation, fever, sweating, ataxia, hyperreflexia, myoclonus and diarrhoea.

• Other opioid derivatives (including antitussive drugs and substitutive treatments), benzodiazepines and barbiturates

Increased risk of respiratory depression which can be fatal in cases of overdose.

• Other central nervous system depressants, such as other opioid derivatives (including antitussive drugs and substitutive treatments), barbiturates, benzodiazepines, other anxiolytics, hypnotics, sedative antidepressants, sedative antihistamines, neuroleptics, centrally-acting antihypertensive drugs, thalidomide and baclofen.

These drugs can cause increased central depression. The effect on alertness can make driving of vehicles and the use of machines dangerous.

• As medically appropriate, periodic evaluation of prothrombin time should be performed when TRAMACET and warfarin like compounds are administered concurrently due to reports of increased INR.

• Other drugs known to inhibit CYP3A4, such as ketoconazole and erythromycin, might inhibit the metabolism of tramadol (N-demethylation) probably also the metabolism of the active O-demethylated metabolite. The clinical importance of such an interaction has not been studied.

• Medicinal products reducing the seizure threshold, such as bupropion, serotonin reuptake inhibitor antidepressants, tricyclic antidepressants and neuroleptics. Concomitant use of tramadol with these drugs can increase the risk of convulsions. The speed of absorption of paracetamol may be increased by metoclopramide or domperidone and absorption reduced by cholestyramine.

• In a limited number of studies the pre- or postoperative application of the antiemetic 5-HT3 antagonist ondansetron increased the requirement of tramadol in patients with postoperative pain.

4.6 Pregnancy and lactation

Pregnancy

Since TRAMACET is a fixed combination of active ingredients including tramadol, it should not be used during pregnancy.

• Data regarding paracetamol:

Epidemiological studies in human pregnancy have shown no ill effects due to paracetamol used in the recommended dosages.

• Data regarding tramadol:

Tramadol should not be used during pregnancy as there is inadequate evidence available to assess the safety of tramadol in pregnant women. Tramadol administered before or during birth does not affect uterine contractility. In neonates it may induce changes in the respiratory rate which are usually not clinically relevant. Long-term treatment during pregnancy may lead to withdrawal symptoms in the newborn after birth, as a consequence of habituation.

Lactation:

Since TRAMACET is a fixed combination of active ingredients including tramadol, it should not be ingested during breast feeding.

• Data regarding paracetamol:

Paracetamol is excreted in breast milk but not in a clinically significant amount. Available published data do not contraindicate breast feeding by women using single ingredient medicinal products containing only paracetamol.

• Data regarding tramadol:

Tramadol and its metabolites are found in small amounts in human breast milk. An infant could ingest about 0.1% of the dose given to the mother. Tramadol should not be ingested during breast feeding.

4.7 Effects on ability to drive and use machines

Tramadol may cause drowsiness or dizziness, which may be enhanced by alcohol or other CNS depressants. If affected, the patient should not drive or operate machinery.

4.8 Undesirable effects

The most commonly reported undesirable effects during the clinical trials performed with the paracetamol/tramadol combination were nausea, dizziness and somnolence, observed in more than 10 % of the patients.

Cardiovascular system disorders:

• Uncommon (≥ 1/1000 to < 1/100): hypertension, palpitations, tachycardia, arrythmia.

Central and peripheral nervous system disorders:

• Very common (≥ 1/10): dizziness, somnolence

• Common (≥ 1/100 to < 1/10): headache trembling

• Uncommon (≥ 1/1000 to < 1/100): involuntary muscular contractions, paraesthesia, tinnitus

• Rare (≥ 1/10000 to < 1/1000): ataxia, convulsions.

Psychiatric disorders:

• Common (≥ 1/100 to < 1/10): confusion, mood changes (anxiety, nervousness, euphoria), sleep disorders

• Uncommon (≥ 1/1000 to < 1/100): depression, hallucinations, nightmares, amnesia

• Rare (≥ 1/10000 to < 1/1000): drug dependence.

Post marketing surveillance

very rare (< 1/10000): abuse.

Vision disorders:

• Rare (≥ 1/10000 to < 1/1000): blurred vision

Respiratory system disorders:

• Uncommon (≥ 1/1000 to < 1/100): dyspnoea

Gastro-intestinal disorders:

• Very common (≥ 1/10): nausea

• Common (≥ 1/100 to < 1/10): vomiting, constipation, dry mouth, diarrhoea abdominal pain, dyspepsia, flatulence

• Uncommon (≥ 1/1000 to < 1/100): dysphagia, melaena.

Liver and biliary system disorders:

• Uncommon (≥ 1/1000 to < 1/100): hepatic transaminases increase.

Skin and appendages disorders:

• Common (≥ 1/100 to < 1/10): sweating, pruritus

• Uncommon (≥ 1/1000 to < 1/100): dermal reactions (e.g.rash, urticaria).

Urinary system disorders:

• Uncommon (≥ 1/1000 to < 1/100): albuminuria, micturition disorders (dysuria and urinary retention).

Body as a whole:

• Uncommon (≥ 1/1000 to < 1/100): shivers, hot flushes, thoracic pain.

Although not observed during clinical trials, the occurrence of the following undesirable effects known to be related to the administration of tramadol or paracetamol cannot be excluded:

Tramadol

• Postural hypotension, bradycardia, collapse (tramadol).

• Post-marketing surveillance of tramadol has revealed rare alterations of warfarin effect, including elevation of prothrombin times.

• Rare cases (≥ 1/10000 to < 1/1000): allergic reactions with respiratory symptoms (e.g. dyspnoea, bronchospasm, wheezing, angioneurotic oedema) and anaphylaxis

• Rare cases (≥ 1/10000 to < 1/1000): changes in appetite, motor weakness, and respiratory depression

• Psychic side-effects may occur following administration of tramadol which vary individually in intensity and nature (depending on personality and duration of medication). These include changes in mood, (usually elation occasionally dysphoria), changes in activity (usually suppression occasionally increase) and changes in cognitive and sensorial capacity (e.g. decision behaviour perception disorders).

• Worsening of asthma has been reported though a causal relationship has not been established.

• Symptoms of withdrawal reactions, similar to those occurring during opiate withdrawal may occur as follows: agitation, anxiety, nervousness, insomnia, hyperkinesia, tremor and gastrointestinal symptoms. Other symptoms that have very rarely been seen if tramadol hydrochloride is discontinued abruptly include: panic attacks, severe anxiety, hallucinations, paraesthesia, tinnitus and unusual CNS symptoms.

Paracetamol

• Adverse effects of paracetamol are rare but hypersensitivity including skin rash may occur. There have been reports of blood dyscrasias including thrombocytopenia and agranulocytosis, but these were not necessarily causally related to paracetamol.

- There have been several reports that suggest that paracetamol may produce hypoprothrombinemia when administered with warfarin-like compounds. In other studies, prothrombin time did not change.

4.9 Overdose
TRAMACET is a fixed combination of active ingredients. In case of overdose, the symptoms may include the signs and symptoms of toxicity of tramadol or paracetamol or of both these active ingredients.

Symptoms of overdose from tramadol:

In principle, on intoxication with tramadol, symptoms similar to those of other centrally acting analgesics (opioids) are to be expected. These include in particular, miosis, vomiting, cardiovascular collapse, consciousness disorders up to coma, convulsions and respiratory depression up to respiratory arrest.

Symptoms of overdose from paracetamol:

An overdose is of particular concern in young children. Symptoms of paracetamol overdosage in the first 24 hours are pallor, nausea, vomiting, anorexia and abdominal pain. Liver damage may become apparent 12 to 48 hours after ingestion. Abnormalities of glucose metabolism and metabolic acidosis may occur. In severe poisoning, hepatic failure may progress to encephalophathy, coma and death. Acute renal failure with acute tubular necrosis may develop even in the absence of severe liver damage. Cardiac arrhythmias and pancreatitis have been reported.

Liver damage is possible in adults who have taken 7.5-10 g or more of paracetamol. It is considered that excess quantities of a toxic metabolite (usually adequately detoxified by glutathione when normal doses of paracetamol are ingested), become irreversibly bound to liver tissue.

Emergency treatment:

- Transfer immediately to a specialised unit.
- Maintain respiratory and circulatory functions
- Prior to starting treatment, a blood sample should be taken as soon as possible after overdose in order to measure the plasma concentration of paracetamol and tramadol and in order to perform hepatic tests.
- Perform hepatic tests at the start (of overdose) and repeat every 24 hours. An increase in hepatic enzymes (ASAT, ALAT) is usually observed, which normalizes after one or two weeks.
- Empty the stomach by causing the patient to vomit (when the patient is conscious) by irritation or gastric lavage.
- Supportive measures such as maintaining the patency of the airway and maintaining cardiovascular function should be instituted; naloxone should be used to reverse respiratory depression; fits can be controlled with diazepam.
- Tramadol is minimally eliminated from the serum by haemodialysis or haemofiltration. Therefore treatment of acute intoxication with TRAMACET with haemodialysis or haemofiltration alone is not suitable for detoxification.

Immediate treatment is essential in the management of paracetamol overdose. Despite a lack of significant early symptoms, patients should be referred to hospital urgently for immediate medical attention and any adult or adolescent who had ingested around 7.5 g or more of paracetamol in the preceding 4 hours or any child who has ingested ≥150 mg/kg of paracetamol in the preceding 4 hours should undergo gastric lavage. Paracetamol concentrations in blood should be measured later than 4 hours after overdose in order to be able to assess the risk of developing liver damage (via the paracetamol overdose nomogram). Administration of oral methionine or intravenous N-acetylcysteine (NAC) which may have a beneficial effect up to at least 48 hours after the overdose, may be required. Administration of intravenous NAC is most beneficial when initiated within 8 hours of overdose ingestion. However, NAC should still be given if the time to presentation is greater than 8 hours after overdose and continued for a full course of therapy. NAC treatment should be started immediately when massive overdose is suspected. General supportive measures must be available.

Irrespective of the reported quantity of paracetamol ingested, the antidote for paracetamol, NAC, should be administered orally or intravenously, as quickly as possible, if possible, within 8 hours following the overdose.

5. PHARMACOLOGICAL PROPERTIES

5.1 Pharmacodynamic properties
Pharmacotherapeutic group: Tramadol, combinations

ATC code: N02A X 52

ANALGESICS

Tramadol is an opioid analgesic that acts on the central nervous system. Tramadol is a pure non selective agonists of the μ, δ, and κ opioid receptors with a higher affinity for the μ receptors. Other mechanisms which contribute to its analgesic effect are inhibition of neuronal reuptake of noradrenaline and enhancement of serotonin release. Tramadol has an antitussive effect. Unlike morphine, a broad range of analgesic doses of tramadol has no respiratory depressant effect. Similarly, the gastro-intestinal motility is not modified. The cardiovascular effects are generally slight. The potency of tramadol is considered to be one-tenth to one-sixth that of morphine.

The precise mechanism of the analgesic properties of paracetamol is unknown and may involve central and peripheral effects.

TRAMACET is positioned as a step II analgesic in the WHO pain ladder and should be utilised accordingly by the physician.

5.2 Pharmacokinetic properties
Tramadol is administered in racemic form and the [-] and [+] forms of tramadol and its metabolite M1, are detected in the blood. Although tramadol is rapidly absorbed after administration, its absorption is slower (and its half-life longer) than that of paracetamol.

After a single oral administration of a tramadol/paracetamol (37.5 mg/325 mg) tablet, peak plasma concentrations of 64.3/55.5 ng/ml [(+)-tramadol/(-)-tramadol] and 4.2 μg/ml (paracetamol) are reached after 1.8 h [(+)-tramadol/(-)-tramadol] and 0.9 h (paracetamol) respectively. The mean elimination half-lives $t_{1/2}$ are 5.1/4.7 h [(+)-tramadol/(-)-tramadol] and 2,5 h (paracetamol).

During pharmacokinetic studies in healthy volunteers after single and repeated oral administration of TRAMACET, no clinical significant change was observed in the kinetic parameters of each active ingredient compared to the parameters of the active ingredients used alone.

Absorption:

Racemic tramadol is rapidly and almost completely absorbed after oral administration. The mean absolute bioavailability of a single 100 mg dose is approximately 75 %. After repeated administration, the bioavailability is increased and reaches approximately 90 %.

After administration of TRAMACET, the oral absorption of paracetamol is rapid and nearly complete and takes place mainly in the small intestine. Peak plasma concentrations of paracetamol are reached in one hour and are not modified by concomitant administration of tramadol.

The oral administration of TRAMACET with food has no significant effect on the peak plasma concentration or extent of absorption of either tramadol or paracetamol so that TRAMACET can be taken independently of meal times.

Distribution:

Tramadol has a high tissue affinity ($V_{d,\beta}$=203 ± 40 l). It has a plasma protein binding of about 20%.

Paracetamol appears to be widely distributed throughout most body tissues except fat. Its apparent volume of distribution is about 0.9 l/kg. A relative small portion (~20%) of paracetamol is bound to plasma proteins.

Metabolism:

Tramadol is extensively metabolized after oral administration. About 30 % of the dose is excreted in urine as unchanged drug, whereas 60% of the dose is excreted as metabolites.

Tramadol is metabolised through O-demethylation (catalysed by the enzyme CYP2D6) to the metabolite M1, and through N-demethylation (catalysed by CYP3A) to the metabolite M2. M1 is further metabolised through N-demethylation and by conjugation with glucuronic acid. The plasma elimination half-life of M1 is 7 hours. The metabolite M1 has analgesic properties and is more potent than the parent drug. The plasma concentrations of M1 are several-fold lower than those of tramadol and the contribution to the clinical effect is unlikely to change on multiple dosing.

Paracetamol is principally metabolized in the liver through two major hepatic routes: glucuronidation and sulphation. The latter route can be rapidly saturated at doses above the therapeutic doses. A small fraction (less than 4%) is metabolized by cytochrome P 450 to an active intermediate (the N-acetyl benzoquinoneimine) which, under normal conditions of use, is rapidly detoxified by reduced glutathione and excreted in urine after conjugation to cysteine and mercapturic acid. However, during massive overdose, the quantity of this metabolite is increased.

Elimination:

Tramadol and its metabolites are eliminated mainly by the kidneys. The half-life of paracetamol is approximately 2 to 3 hours in adults. It is shorter in children and slightly longer in the newborn and in cirrhotic patients. Paracetamol is mainly eliminated by dose-dependent formation of glucuro- and sulpho-conjugate derivatives. Less than 9 % of paracetamol is excreted unchanged in urine. In renal insufficiency, the half-life of both compounds is prolonged.

5.3 Preclinical safety data
No preclinical study has been performed with the fixed combination (tramadol and paracetamol) to evaluate its carcinogenic or mutagenic effects or its effects on fertility.

No teratogenic effect that can be attributed to the medicine has been observed in the progeny of rats treated orally with the combination tramadol/paracetamol.

The combination tramadol/paracetamol has proven to be embryotoxic and foetotoxic in the rat at materno-toxic dose (50/434 mg/kg tramadol/paracetamol), i.e., 8.3 times the maximum therapeutic dose in man. No teratogenic effect has been observed at this dose. The toxicity to the embryo and the foetus results in a decreased foetal weight and an increase in supernumerary ribs. Lower doses, causing less severe materno-toxic effect (10/87 and 25/217 mg/kg tramadol/paracetamol) did not result in toxic effects in the embryo or the foetus.

Results of standard mutagenicity tests did not reveal a potential genotoxic risk for tramadol in man.

Results of carcinogenicity tests do not suggest a potential risk of tramadol for man.

Animal studies with tramadol revealed, at very high doses, effects on organ development, ossification and neonatal mortality, associated with maternotoxicity. Fertility reproductive performance and development of offspring were unaffected. Tramadol crosses the placenta. No effect on fertility has been observed after oral administration of tramadol up to doses of 50 mg/kg in the male rat and 75 mg/kg in the female rat.

Extensive investigations showed no evidence of a relevant genotoxic risk of paracetamol at therapeutic (i.e. non-toxic) doses.

Long-term studies in rats and mice yielded no evidence of relevant tumorigenic effects at non-hepatotoxic dosages of paracetamol.

Animal studies and extensive human experience to date yield no evidence of reproductive toxicity.

6. PHARMACEUTICAL PARTICULARS

6.1 List of excipients
Tablet core:

powdered cellulose

pregelatinised starch

sodium starch glycolate (Type A)

maize starch

magnesium stearate

Film-coating:

OPADRY yellow YS-1-6382 G (hypromellose, titanium dioxide (E171), macrogol 400, yellow iron oxide (E172), polysorbate 80),

carnauba wax

6.2 Incompatibilities
Not applicable.

6.3 Shelf life
3 years in thermoformed blister packs of (polypropylene / aluminium)

3 years in thermoformed blister packs of (PVC/aluminium)

6.4 Special precautions for storage
This medicinal product does not require any special storage conditions.

6.5 Nature and contents of container
TRAMACET tablets are packed in white opaque PVC/aluminium foil or white opaque polypropylene/aluminium.

Box of 2 tablets, of 10, 20, 30, 40, 50, 60, 70, 80, 90 and 100 tablets

Not all packaging sizes may be marketed.

6.6 Special precautions for disposal and other handling
No special requirements.

7. MARKETING AUTHORISATION HOLDER
Grünenthal Ltd

Regus Lakeside House

1 Furzeground Way

Stockley Park East

Uxbridge

Middlesex UB11 1BD

United Kingdom

8. MARKETING AUTHORISATION NUMBER(S)
PL 21727/0039

9. DATE OF FIRST AUTHORISATION/RENEWAL OF THE AUTHORISATION
Date of first authorisation: 25 September 2003

Date of last renewal: 22/06/07

10. DATE OF REVISION OF THE TEXT
01/04/2009

Tramacet 37.5 mg/325 mg film-coated tablets

(Janssen-Cilag Ltd)

1. NAME OF THE MEDICINAL PRODUCT
TRAMACET 37.5 mg/325 mg, film coated-tablets

2. QUALITATIVE AND QUANTITATIVE COMPOSITION
One film-coated tablet contains 37.5 mg tramadol hydrochloride and 325 mg paracetamol

For a full list of excipients, see section 6.1

3. PHARMACEUTICAL FORM
Film-coated tablet

Pale yellow film-coated tablet

4. CLINICAL PARTICULARS

4.1 Therapeutic indications
TRAMACET tablets are indicated for the symptomatic treatment of moderate to severe pain.

The use of TRAMACET should be restricted to patients whose moderate to severe pain is considered to require a combination of tramadol and paracetamol (see also Section 5.1).

4.2 Posology and method of administration

Posology

ADULTS AND ADOLESCENTS (12 years and older)

The use of TRAMACET should be restricted to patients whose moderate to severe pain is considered to require a combination of tramadol and paracetamol.

The dose should be individually adjusted according to intensity of pain and response of the patient.

An initial dose of two tablets of TRAMACET is recommended. Additional doses can be taken as needed, not exceeding 8 tablets (equivalent to 300 mg tramadol and 2600 mg paracetamol) per day.

The dosing interval should not be less than six hours.

TRAMACET should under no circumstances be administered for longer than is strictly necessary (see also section 4.4 - Special warnings and precautions for use). If repeated use or long term treatment with TRAMACET is required as a result of the nature and severity of the illness, then careful, regular monitoring should take place (with breaks in the treatment, where possible), to assess whether continuation of the treatment is necessary.

Children

The effective and safe use of TRAMACET has not been established in children below the age of 12 years. Treatment is therefore not recommended in this population.

Elderly Patients

The usual dosages may be used although it should be noted that in volunteers aged over 75 years the elimination half life of tramadol was increased by 17% following oral administration. In patients over 75 years old, it is recommended that the minimum interval between doses should be not less than 6 hours, due to the presence of tramadol.

Renal insufficiency

Because of the presence of tramadol, the use of TRAMACET is not recommended in patients with severe renal insufficiency (creatinine clearance < 10 ml/min). In cases of moderate renal insufficiency (creatinine clearance between 10 and 30 ml/min), the dosing should be increased to 12-hourly intervals. As tramadol is removed only very slowly by haemodialysis or by haemofiltration, post dialysis administration to maintain analgesia is not usually required.

Hapatic insufficiency

In patients with severe hepatic impairment TRAMACET should not be used (see Section 4.3). In moderate cases prolongation of the dosage interval should be carefully considered (see Section 4.4).

Method of administration

Oral use

Tablets must be swallowed whole, with a sufficient quantity of liquid. They must not be broken or chewed.

4.3 Contraindications

- Hypersensitivity to tramadol, paracetamol or to any of the excipients (see 6.1. List of excipients) of the medicinal product,
- acute intoxication with alcohol, hypnotic drugs, centrally-acting analgesics, opioids or psychotropic drugs,
- TRAMACET should not be administered to patients who are receiving monoamine oxidase inhibitors or within two weeks of their withdrawal (see 4.5. Interactions with other medicinal products and other forms of interaction),
- severe hepatic impairment,
- epilepsy not controlled by treatment (see. 4.4. Special Warnings)

4.4 Special warnings and precautions for use

Warnings:

- In adults and adolescents 12 years and older. The maximum dose of 8 tablets of TRAMACET should not be exceeded. In order to avoid inadvertent overdose, patients should be advised not to exceed the recommended dose and not to use any other paracetamol (including over the counter) or tramadol hydrochloride containing products concurrently without the advice of a physician.
- In severe renal insufficiency (creatinine clearance <10 ml/mm), TRAMACET is not recommended.
- In patients with severe hepatic impairment TRAMACET should not be used (See Section 4.3). The hazards of paracetamol overdose are greater in patients with non-cirrhotic alcoholic liver disease. In moderate cases prolongation of dosage interval should be carefully considered.
- In severe respiratory insufficiency, TRAMACET is not recommended.
- Tramadol is not suitable as a substitute in opioid-dependent patients. Although it is an opioid agonist, tramadol cannot suppress morphine withdrawal symptoms.
- Convulsions have been reported in tramadol-treated patients susceptible to seizures or taking other medications that lower the seizure threshold, especially selective serotonin re-uptake inhibitors, tricyclic antidepressants, antipsychotics, centrally acting analgesics or local anaesthesia. Epileptic patients controlled by a treatment or patients susceptible to seizures should be treated with TRAMACET only if there are compelling circumstances. Convulsions have been reported in patients receiving tramadol at the recommended dose levels. The risk may be increased when doses of tramadol exceed the recommended upper dose limit
- Concomitant use of opioid agonists-antagonists (nalbuphine, buprenorphine, pentazocine) is not recommended (see 4.5 Interactions with other medicinal products and other forms of interaction).

Precautions for use

TRAMACET should be used with caution in opioid dependent patients, or in patients with cranial trauma, in patients prone to convulsive disorder, biliary tract disorders, in a state of shock, in an altered state of consciousness for unknown reasons, with problems affecting the respiratory center or the respiratory function, or with an increased intracranial pressure.

Paracetamol in overdosage may cause hepatic toxicity in some patients.

At therapeutic doses, tramadol has the potential to cause withdrawal symptoms. Rarely, cases of dependence and abuse have been reported (see section 4.8).

Symptoms of withdrawal reactions, similar to those occurring during opiate withdrawal may occur (see section 4.8).

In one study, use of tramadol during general anaesthesia with enflurane and nitrous oxide was reported to enhance intra-operative recall. Until further information is available, use of tramadol during light planes of anaesthesia should be avoided.

4.5 Interaction with other medicinal products and other forms of interaction

Concomitant use is contraindicated with:

- Non-selective MAO Inhibitors

Risk of serotoninergic syndrome: diarrhoea, tachycardia, sweating, trembling, confusion, even coma.

- Selective-A MAO Inhibitors

Extrapolation from non-selective MAO inhibitors

Risk of serotoninergic syndrome: diarrhoea, tachycardia, sweating, trembling, confusion, even coma.

- Selective-B MAO Inhibitors

Central excitation symptoms evocative of a serotoninergic syndrome: diarrhoea, tachycardia, sweating, trembling, confusion, even coma.

In case of recent treatment with MAO inhibitors, a delay of two weeks should occur before treatment with tramadol

Concomitant use is not recommended with:

- Alcohol

Alcohol increases the sedative effect of opioid analgesics.

The effect on alertness can make driving of vehicles and the use of machines dangerous.

Avoid intake of alcoholic drinks and of medicinal products containing alcohol.

- Carbamazepine and other enzyme inducers

Risk of reduced efficacy and shorter duration due to decreased plasma concentrations of tramadol.

- Opioid agonists-antagonists (buprenorphine, nalbuphine, pentazocine)

Decrease of the analgesic effect by competitive blocking effect at the receptors, with the risk of occurrence of withdrawal syndrome.

Concomitant use which needs to be taken into consideration:

- In isolated cases there have been reports of Serotonin Syndrome in a temporal connection with the therapeutic use of tramadol in combination with other serotoninergic medicines such as selective serotonin re-uptake inhibitors (SSRIs) and triptans. Signs of Serotonin Syndrome may be for example, confusion, agitation, fever, sweating, ataxia, hyperreflexia, myoclonus and diarrhoea.
- Other opioid derivatives (including antitussive drugs and substitutive treatments), benzodiazepines and barbiturates

Increased risk of respiratory depression which can be fatal in cases of overdose.

- Other central nervous system depressants, such as other opioid derivatives (including antitussive drugs and substitutive treatments), barbiturates, benzodiazepines, other anxiolytics, hypnotics, sedative antidepressants, sedative antihistamines, neuroleptics, centrally-acting antihypertensive drugs, thalidomide and baclofen.

These drugs can cause increased central depression. The effect on alertness can make driving of vehicles and the use of machines dangerous.

- As medically appropriate, periodic evaluation of prothrombin time should be performed when TRAMACET and warfarin like compounds are administered concurrently due to reports of increased INR.
- Other drugs known to inhibit CYP3A4, such as ketoconazole and erythromycin, might inhibit the metabolism of tramadol (N-demethylation) probably also the metabolism of the active O-demethylated metabolite. The clinical importance of such an interaction has not been studied.
- Medicinal products reducing the seizure threshold, such as bupropion, serotonin reuptake inhibitor antidepressants, tricyclic antidepressants and neuroleptics. Concomitant use of tramadol with these drugs can increase the risk of convulsions. The speed of absorption of paracetamol may be increased by metoclopramide or domperidone and absorption reduced by cholestyramine.
- In a limited number of studies the pre- or postoperative application of the antiemetic 5-HT3 antagonist ondansetron increased the requirement of tramadol in patients with postoperative pain.

4.6 Pregnancy and lactation

Pregnancy

Since TRAMACET is a fixed combination of active ingredients including tramadol, it should not be used during pregnancy.

- Data regarding paracetamol:

Epidemiological studies in human pregnancy have shown no ill effects due to paracetamol used in the recommended dosages.

- Data regarding tramadol:

Tramadol should not be used during pregnancy as there is inadequate evidence available to assess the safety of tramadol in pregnant women. Tramadol administered before or during birth does not affect uterine contractility. In neonates it may induce changes in the respiratory rate which are usually not clinically relevant. Long-term treatment during pregnancy may lead to withdrawal symptoms in the newborn after birth, as a consequence of habituation.

Lactation:

Since TRAMACET is a fixed combination of active ingredients including tramadol, it should not be ingested during breast feeding.

- Data regarding paracetamol:

Paracetamol is excreted in breast milk but not in a clinically significant amount. Available published data do not contraindicate breast feeding by women using single ingredient medicinal products containing only paracetamol.

- Data regarding tramadol:

Tramadol and its metabolites are found in small amounts in human breast milk. An infant could ingest about 0.1% of the dose given to the mother. Tramadol should not be ingested during breast feeding.

4.7 Effects on ability to drive and use machines

Tramadol may cause drowsiness or dizziness, which may be enhanced by alcohol or other CNS depressants. If affected, the patient should not drive or operate machinery.

4.8 Undesirable effects

The most commonly reported undesirable effects during the clinical trials performed with the paracetamol/tramadol combination were nausea, dizziness and somnolence, observed in more than 10 % of the patients.

Cardiovascular system disorders:

- Uncommon (≥ 1/1000 to < 1/100): hypertension, palpitations, tachycardia, arrythmia.

Central and peripheral nervous system disorders:

- Very common (≥ 1/10): dizziness, somnolence
- Common (≥ 1/100 to < 1/10): headache trembling
- Uncommon (≥ 1/1000 to < 1/100): involuntary muscular contractions, paraesthesia, tinnitus
- Rare (≥ 1/10000 to < 1/1000): ataxia, convulsions.

Psychiatric disorders:

- Common (≥ 1/100 to < 1/10): confusion, mood changes (anxiety, nervousness, euphoria), sleep disorders
- Uncommon (≥ 1/1000 to < 1/100): depression, hallucinations, nightmares, amnesia
- Rare (≥ 1/10000 to < 1/1000): drug dependence.

Post marketing surveillance

very rare (< 1/10000): abuse.

Vision disorders:

- Rare (≥ 1/10000 to < 1/1000): blurred vision

Respiratory system disorders:

- Uncommon (≥ 1/1000 to < 1/100): dyspnoea

Gastro-intestinal disorders:

- Very common (≥ 1/10): nausea
- Common (≥ 1/100 to < 1/10): vomiting, constipation, dry mouth, diarrhoea abdominal pain, dyspepsia, flatulence
- Uncommon (≥ 1/1000 to < 1/100): dysphagia, melaena.

Liver and biliary system disorders:

- Uncommon (≥ 1/1000 to < 1/100): hepatic transaminases increase.

Skin and appendages disorders:

- Common (≥ 1/100 to < 1/10): sweating, pruritus
- Uncommon (≥ 1/1000 to < 1/100): dermal reactions (e.g.rash, urticaria).

Urinary system disorders:

- Uncommon (≥ 1/1000 to < 1/100): albuminuria, micturition disorders (dysuria and urinary retention).

Body as a whole:

- Uncommon (≥ 1/1000 to < 1/100): shivers, hot flushes, thoracic pain.

Although not observed during clinical trials, the occurrence of the following undesirable effects known to be related to the administration of tramadol or paracetamol cannot be excluded:

Tramadol

- Postural hypotension, bradycardia, collapse (tramadol).
- Post-marketing surveillance of tramadol has revealed rare alterations of warfarin effect, including elevation of prothrombin times.
- Rare cases (≥ 1/10000 to < 1/1000): allergic reactions with respiratory symptoms (e.g. dyspnoea, bronchospasm, wheezing, angioneurotic oedema) and anaphylaxis
- Rare cases (≥ 1/10000 to < 1/1000): changes in appetite, motor weakness, and respiratory depression
- Psychic side-effects may occur following administration of tramadol which vary individually in intensity and nature (depending on personality and duration of medication). These include changes in mood, (usually elation occasionally dysphoria), changes in activity (usually suppression occasionally increase) and changes in cognitive and sensorial capacity (e.g. decision behaviour perception disorders).
- Worsening of asthma has been reported though a causal relationship has not been established.
- Symptoms of withdrawal reactions, similar to those occurring during opiate withdrawal may occur as follows: agitation, anxiety, nervousness, insomnia, hyperkinesia, tremor and gastrointestinal symptoms. Other symptoms that have very rarely been seen if tramadol hydrochloride is discontinued abruptly include: panic attacks, severe anxiety, hallucinations, paraesthesia, tinnitus and unusual CNS symptoms.

Paracetamol

- Adverse effects of paracetamol are rare but hypersensitivity including skin rash may occur. There have been reports of blood dyscrasias including thrombocytopenia and agranulocytosis, but these were not necessarily causally related to paracetamol.
- There have been several reports that suggest that paracetamol may produce hypoprothrombinemia when administered with warfarin-like compounds. In other studies, prothrombin time did not change

4.9 Overdose

TRAMACET is a fixed combination of active ingredients. In case of overdose, the symptoms may include the signs and symptoms of toxicity of tramadol or paracetamol or of both these active ingredients.

Symptoms of overdose from tramadol:

In principle, on intoxication with tramadol, symptoms similar to those of other centrally acting analgesics (opioids) are to be expected. These include in particular, miosis, vomiting, cardiovascular collapse, consciousness disorders up to coma, convulsions and respiratory depression up to respiratory arrest.

Symptoms of overdose from paracetamol:

An overdose is of particular concern in young children. Symptoms of paracetamol overdosage in the first 24 hours are pallor, nausea, vomiting, anorexia and abdominal pain. Liver damage may become apparent 12 to 48 hours after ingestion. Abnormalities of glucose metabolism and metabolic acidosis may occur. In severe poisoning, hepatic failure may progress to encephalophathy, coma and death. Acute renal failure with acute tubular necrosis may develop even in the absence of severe liver damage. Cardiac arrhythmias and pancreatitis have been reported.

Liver damage is possible in adults who have taken 7.5-10 g or more of paracetamol. It is considered that excess quantities of a toxic metabolite (usually adequately detoxified by glutathione when normal doses of paracetamol are ingested), become irreversibly bound to liver tissue.

Emergency treatment:

- Transfer immediately to a specialised unit.
- Maintain respiratory and circulatory functions
- Prior to starting treatment, a blood sample should be taken as soon as possible after overdose in order to measure the plasma concentration of paracetamol and tramadol and in order to perform hepatic tests.
- Perform hepatic tests at the start (of overdose) and repeat every 24 hours. An increase in hepatic enzymes (ASAT, ALAT) is usually observed, which normalizes after one or two weeks.
- Empty the stomach by causing the patient to vomit (when the patient is conscious) by irritation or gastric lavage.
- Supportive measures such as maintaining the patency of the airway and maintaining cardiovascular function should be instituted; naloxone should be used to reverse respiratory depression; fits can be controlled with diazepam.
- Tramadol is minimally eliminated from the serum by haemodialysis or haemofiltration. Therefore treatment of acute intoxication with TRAMACET with haemodialysis or haemofiltration alone is not suitable for detoxification.
- Immediate treatment is essential in the management of paracetamol overdose. Despite a lack of significant early symptoms, patients should be referred to hospital urgently for immediate medical attention and any adult or adolescent who had ingested around 7.5 g or more of paracetamol in the preceding 4 hours or any child who has ingested ≥150 mg/kg of paracetamol in the preceding 4 hours should undergo gastric lavage. Paracetamol concentrations in blood should be measured later than 4 hours after overdose in order to be able to assess the risk of developing liver damage (via the paracetamol overdose nomogram). Administration of oral methionine or intravenous N-acetylcysteine (NAC) which may have a beneficial effect up to at least 48 hours after the overdose, may be required. Administration of intravenous NAC is most beneficial when initiated within 8 hours of overdose ingestion. However, NAC should still be given if the time to presentation is greater than 8 hours after overdose and continued for a full course of therapy. NAC treatment should be started immediately when massive overdose is suspected. General supportive measures must be available.
- Irrespective of the reported quantity of paracetamol ingested, the antidote for paracetamol, NAC, should be administered orally or intravenously, as quickly as possible, if possible, within 8 hours following the overdose.

5. PHARMACOLOGICAL PROPERTIES

5.1 Pharmacodynamic properties

Pharmacotherapeutic group: Tramadol, combinations

ATC code: N02A X 52

ANALGESICS

Tramadol is an opioid analgesic that acts on the central nervous system. Tramadol is a pure non selective agonists of the μ, δ, and κ opioid receptors with a higher affinity for the μ receptors. Other mechanisms which contribute to its analgesic effect are inhibition of neuronal reuptake of noradrenaline and enhancement of serotonin release. Tramadol has an antitussive effect. Unlike morphine, a broad range of analgesic doses of tramadol has no respiratory depressant effect. Similarly, the gastro-intestinal motility is not modified. The cardiovascular effects are generally slight. The potency of tramadol is considered to be one-tenth to one-sixth that of morphine.

The precise mechanism of the analgesic properties of paracetamol is unknown and may involve central and peripheral effects.

TRAMACET is positioned as a step II analgesic in the WHO pain ladder and should be utilised accordingly by the physician.

5.2 Pharmacokinetic properties

Tramadol is administered in racemic form and the [-] and [+] forms of tramadol and its metabolite M1, are detected in the blood. Although tramadol is rapidly absorbed after administration, its absorption is slower (and its half-life longer) than that of paracetamol.

After a single oral administration of a tramadol/paracetamol (37.5 mg/325 mg) tablet, peak plasma concentrations of 64.3/55.5 ng/ml [(+)-tramadol/(-)-tramadol] and 4.2 μg/ml (paracetamol) are reached after 1.8 h [(+)-tramadol/(-)-tramadol] and 0.9 h (paracetamol) respectively. The mean elimination half-lives $t_{1/2}$ are 5.1/4.7 h [(+)-tramadol/(-)-tramadol] and 2,5 h (paracetamol).

During pharmacokinetic studies in healthy volunteers after single and repeated oral administration of TRAMACET, no clinical significant change was observed in the kinetic parameters of each active ingredient compared to the parameters of the active ingredients used alone.

Absorption:

Racemic tramadol is rapidly and almost completely absorbed after oral administration. The mean absolute bioavailability of a single 100 mg dose is approximately 75 %. After repeated administration, the bioavailability is increased and reaches approximately 90 %.

After administration of TRAMACET, the oral absorption of paracetamol is rapid and nearly complete and takes place mainly in the small intestine. Peak plasma concentrations of paracetamol are reached in one hour and are not modified by concomitant administration of tramadol.

The oral administration of TRAMACET with food has no significant effect on the peak plasma concentration or extent of absorption of either tramadol or paracetamol so that TRAMACET can be taken independently of meal times.

Distribution:

Tramadol has a high tissue affinity ($V_{d,\beta}$=203 ± 40 l). It has a plasma protein binding of about 20%.

Paracetamol appears to be widely distributed throughout most body tissues except fat. Its apparent volume of distribution is about 0.9 l/kg. A relative small portion (~20%) of paracetamol is bound to plasma proteins.

Metabolism:

Tramadol is extensively metabolized after oral administration. About 30 % of the dose is excreted in urine as unchanged drug, whereas 60% of the dose is excreted as metabolites.

Tramadol is metabolised through *O*-demethylation (catalysed by the enzyme CYP2D6) to the metabolite M1, and through *N*-demethylation (catalysed by CYP3A) to the metabolite M2. M1 is further metabolised through N-demethylation and by conjugation with glucuronic acid. The plasma elimination half-life of M1 is 7 hours. The metabolite M1 has analgesic properties and is more potent than the parent drug. The plasma concentrations of M1 are several-fold lower than those of tramadol and the contribution to the clinical effect is unlikely to change on multiple dosing.

Paracetamol is principally metabolized in the liver through two major hepatic routes: glucuronidation and sulphation. The latter route can be rapidly saturated at doses above the therapeutic doses. A small fraction (less than 4%) is metabolized by cytochrome P 450 to an active intermediate (the N-acetyl benzoquinoneimine) which, under normal conditions of use, is rapidly detoxified by reduced glutathione and excreted in urine after conjugation to cysteine and mercapturic acid. However, during massive overdose, the quantity of this metabolite is increased.

Elimination:

Tramadol and its metabolites are eliminated mainly by the kidneys. The half-life of paracetamol is approximately 2 to 3 hours in adults. It is shorter in children and slightly longer in the newborn and in cirrhotic patients. Paracetamol is mainly eliminated by dose-dependent formation of gluco- and sulpho-conjugate derivatives. Less than 9 % of paracetamol is excreted unchanged in urine. In renal insufficiency, the half-life of both compounds is prolonged.

5.3 Preclinical safety data

No preclinical study has been performed with the fixed combination (tramadol and paracetamol) to evaluate its carcinogenic or mutagenic effects or its effects on fertility.

No teratogenic effect that can be attributed to the medicine has been observed in the progeny of rats treated orally with the combination tramadol/paracetamol.

The combination tramadol/paracetamol has proven to be embryotoxic and foetotoxic in the rat at materno-toxic dose (50/434 mg/kg tramadol/paracetamol), i.e., 8.3 times the maximum therapeutic dose in man. No teratogenic effect has been observed at this dose. The toxicity to the embryo and the foetus results in a decreased foetal weight and an increase in supernumerary ribs. Lower doses, causing less severe materno-toxic effect (10/87 and 25/217 mg/kg tramadol/paracetamol) did not result in toxic effects in the embryo or the foetus.

Results of standard mutagenicity tests did not reveal a potential genotoxic risk for tramadol in man.

Results of carcinogenicity tests do not suggest a potential risk of tramadol for man.

Animal studies with tramadol revealed, at very high doses, effects on organ development, ossification and neonatal mortality, associated with maternotoxicity. Fertility reproductive performance and development of offspring were unaffected. Tramadol crosses the placenta. No effect on fertility has been observed after oral administration of tramadol up to doses of 50 mg/kg in the male rat and 75 mg/kg in the female rat.

Extensive investigations showed no evidence of a relevant genotoxic risk of paracetamol at therapeutic (i.e. non-toxic) doses.

Long-term studies in rats and mice yielded no evidence of relevant tumorigenic effects at non-hepatotoxic dosages of paracetamol.

Animal studies and extensive human experience to date yield no evidence of reproductive toxicity.

6. PHARMACEUTICAL PARTICULARS

6.1 List of excipients

Tablet core:

powdered cellulose

pregelatinised starch

sodium starch glycolate (Type A)

maize starch

magnesium stearate

Film-coating:

OPADRY yellow YS-1-6382 G (hypromellose, titanium dioxide (E171),

macrogol 400, yellow iron oxide (E172), polysorbate 80),

carnauba wax

6.2 Incompatibilities

Not applicable.

6.3 Shelf life

3 years in thermoformed blister packs of (polypropylene / aluminium)

3 years in thermoformed blister packs of (PVC/aluminium)

6.4 Special precautions for storage

This medicinal product does not require any special storage conditions.

6.5 Nature and contents of container

TRAMACET tablets are packed in white opaque PVC/aluminium foil or white opaque polypropylene/aluminium.

Box of 2 tablets, of 10, 20, 30, 40, 50, 60, 70, 80, 90 and 100 tablets

Not all packaging sizes may be marketed.

6.6 Special precautions for disposal and other handling

No special requirements.

7. MARKETING AUTHORISATION HOLDER

Janssen-Cilag Ltd

Saunderton

High Wycombe

Buckinghamshire

HP14 4HJ

United Kingdom

8. MARKETING AUTHORISATION NUMBER(S)
PL 0242/0384

9. DATE OF FIRST AUTHORISATION/RENEWAL OF THE AUTHORISATION
Date of first authorisation: 25 September 2003

Date of last renewal: 22/06/07

10. DATE OF REVISION OF THE TEXT
22/06/07

Trandate Injection

(UCB Pharma Limited)

1. NAME OF THE MEDICINAL PRODUCT
Trandate Injection

2. QUALITATIVE AND QUANTITATIVE COMPOSITION
Labetalol hydrochloride 5mg/ml.

3. PHARMACEUTICAL FORM
Solution for Injection

4. CLINICAL PARTICULARS

4.1 Therapeutic indications
Trandate Injection is indicated for the treatment of:-

1. Severe hypertension, including severe hypertension of pregnancy, when rapid control of blood pressure is essential.

2. Anaesthesia when a hypotensive technique is indicated.

3. Hypertensive episodes following acute myocardial infarction.

4.2 Posology and method of administration

Adults:

Trandate Injection is intended for intravenous use in hospitalised patients. The plasma concentrations achieved after intravenous dose of Trandate in severe hypertension are substantially greater than those following oral administration of the drug and provide a greater degree of blockade of alpha-adrenoceptors necessary to control the more severe disease. Patients should, therefore, always receive the drug whilst in the supine or left lateral position. Raising the patient into the upright position, within three hours of intravenous Trandate administration, should be avoided since excessive postural hypotension may occur.

Bolus injection

If it is essential to reduce blood pressure quickly, as for example, in hypertensive encephalopathy, a dose of 50mg of Trandate should be given by intravenous injection over a period of at least one minute. If necessary, doses of 50mg may be repeated at five minute intervals until a satisfactory response occurs. The total dose should not exceed 200mg. After bolus injection, the maximum effect usually occurs within five minutes and the effective duration of action is usually about six hours but may be as long as eighteen hours.

Intravenous infusion

An alternative method of administering Trandate is intravenous infusion of a solution made by diluting the contents of two ampoules (200mg) to 200ml with Sodium Chloride and Dextrose Injection BP or 5% Dextrose Intravenous Infusion BP. The resultant infusion solution contains 1mg/ml of Trandate. It should be administered using a paediatric giving set fitted with a 50ml graduated burette to facilitate dosage.

In the hypertension of pregnancy: The infusion can be started at the rate of 20mg per hour and this dose may be doubled every thirty minutes until a satisfactory reduction in blood pressure has been obtained or a dosage of 160mg per hour is reached. Occasionally, higher doses may be necessary.

In hypertensive episodes following acute myocardial infarction: The infusion should be commenced at 15mg per hour and gradually increased to a maximum of 120mg per hour depending on the control of blood pressure.

In hypertension due to other causes: The rate of infusion of Trandate should be about 2mg (2ml of infusion solution) per minute, until a satisfactory response is obtained; the infusion should then be stopped. The effective dose is usually in the range of 50-200mg depending on the severity of the hypertension. For most patients it is unnecessary to administer more than 200mg but larger doses may be required especially in patients with phaeochromocytoma. The rate of infusion may be adjusted according to the response, at the discretion of the physician. The blood pressure and pulse rate should be monitored throughout the infusion.

It is desirable to monitor the heart rate after injection and during infusion. In most patients, there is a small decrease in the heart rate; severe bradycardia is unusual but may be controlled by injecting atropine 1-2 mg intravenously. Respiratory function should be observed particularly in patients with any known impairment.

Once the blood pressure has been adequately reduced, maintenance therapy with Trandate tablets should be instituted with a starting dose of one 100mg tablet twice daily (see Trandate tablets SmPC for further details). Trandate Injection has been administered to patients with uncontrolled hypertension already receiving other hypotensive agents, including beta-blocking drugs, without adverse effects.

In hypotensive anaesthesia: Induction should be with standard agents (e.g. sodium thiopentone) and anaesthesia maintained with nitrous oxide and oxygen with or without halothane. The recommended starting dose of Trandate Injection is 10-20mg intravenously depending on the age and condition of the patient. Patients for whom halothane is contra-indicated usually require a higher initial dose of Trandate (25-30mg). If satisfactory hypotension is not achieved after five minutes, increments of 5-10mg should be given until the desired level of blood pressure is attained.

Halothane and Trandate act synergistically therefore the halothane concentration should not exceed 1-1.5% as profound falls in blood pressure may be precipitated.

Following Trandate Injection the blood pressure can be quickly and easily adjusted by altering the halothane concentration and / or adjusting table tilt. The mean duration of hypotension following 20-25mg of Trandate is fifty minutes.

Hypotension induced by Trandate Injection is readily reversed by atropine 0.6mg and discontinuation of halothane.

Tubocurarine and pancuronium may be used when assisted or controlled ventilation is required. Intermittent Positive Pressure Ventilation (IPPV) may further increase the hypotension resulting from Trandate Injection and / or halothane.

Children:

Safety and efficacy have not been established.

4.3 Contraindications

- Cardiogenic shock.
- Uncontrolled, incipient or digitalis refractory heart failure.
- Sick sinus syndrome (including sino-atrial block).
- Second or third degree heart block.
- Prinzmetal's angina.
- History of wheezing or asthma.
- Untreated phaeochromocytoma.
- Metabolic acidosis.
- Bradycardia (<45-50 bpm).
- Hypotension.
- Hypersensitivity to labetalol.
- Severe peripheral circulatory disturbances.
- Where peripheral vasoconstriction suggests low cardiac output, the use of Trandate Injection to control hypertensive episodes following acute myocardial infarction is contra-indicated.

4.4 Special warnings and precautions for use
There have been reports of skin rashes and/ or dry eyes associated with the use of beta-adrenoceptor blocking drugs. The reported incidence is small and in most cases the symptoms have cleared when the treatment was withdrawn. Gradual discontinuance of the drug should be considered if any such reaction is not otherwise explicable.

There have been rare reports of severe hepatocellular injury with labetalol therapy. The hepatic injury is usually reversible and has occurred after both short and long term treatment. Appropriate laboratory testing should be done at the first sign or symptom of liver dysfunction. If there is laboratory evidence of liver injury or the patient is jaundiced, labetalol therapy should be stopped and not re-started.

Due to negative inotropic effects, special care should be taken with patients whose cardiac reserve is poor and heart failure should be controlled before starting Trandate therapy.

Patients particularly those with ischemic heart disease, should not interrupt/ discontinue abruptly Trandate therapy. The dosage should gradually be reduced, ie. over 1-2 weeks, if necessary at the same time initiating replacement therapy, to prevent exacerbation of angina pectoris. In addition, hypertension and arrhythmias may develop.

It is not necessary to discontinue Trandate therapy in patients requiring anaesthesia, but the anaesthetist must be informed and the patient should be given intravenous atropine prior to induction. During anaesthesia Trandate may mask the compensatory physiological responses to sudden haemorrhage (tachycardia and vasoconstriction). Close attention must therefore be paid to blood loss and the blood volume maintained. If beta-blockade is interrupted in preparation for surgery, therapy should be discontinued for at least 24 hours. Anaesthetic agents causing myocardial depression (eg. cyclopropane, trichloroethylene) should be avoided. Trandate may enhance the hypotensive effects of halothane.

In patients with peripheral circulatory disorders (Raynaud's disease or syndrome, intermittent claudication), beta-blockers should be used with great caution as aggravation of these disorders may occur.

Beta-blockers may induce bradycardia. If the pulse rate decreases to less than 50-55 beats per minute at rest and the patient experiences symptoms related to the bradycardia, the dosage should be reduced.

Beta-blockers, even those with apparent cardioselectivity, should not be used in patients with asthma or a history of obstructive airways disease unless no alternative treatment is available. In such cases the risk of inducing bronchospasm should be appreciated and appropriate precautions taken. If bronchospasm should occur after the use of Trandate it can be treated with a beta$_2$-agonist by inhalation, e.g. salbutamol (the dose of which may need to be greater than the usual in asthma) and, if necessary, intravenous atropine 1mg

Due to a negative effect on conduction time, beta-blockers should only be given with caution to patients with first degree heart block. Patients with liver or kidney insufficiency may need a lower dosage, depending on the pharmacokinetic profile of the compound. The elderly should be treated with caution, starting with a lower dosage but tolerance is usually good in the elderly.

Patients with a history of psoriasis should take beta-blockers only after careful consideration.

Risk of anaphylactic reaction: While taking beta-blockers, patients with a history of severe anaphylactic reaction to a variety of allergens may be more reactive to repeated challenge, either accidental, diagnostic or therapeutic. Such patients may be unresponsive to the usual doses of epinephrine use to treat allergic reaction.

The label will state "Do not take Trandate if you have a history of wheezing or asthma as it can make your breathing worse."

4.5 Interaction with other medicinal products and other forms of interaction
Concomitant use not recommended:

- Calcium antagonists such as verapamil and to a lesser extent diltiazem have a negative influence on contractility and atrio-ventricular conduction.
- Digitalis glycosides used in association with beta-blockers may increase atrio-ventricular conduction time.
- Clonidine: Beta-blockers increase the risk of rebound hypertension. When clonidine is used in conjunction with non-selective beta-blockers, such as propranolol, treatment with clonidine should be continued for some time after treatment with the beta-blocker has been discontinued.
- Monoamineoxidase inhibitors (except MOA-B inhibitors).

Use with caution:

- Class I antiarrhythmic agents (eg. disopyramide, quinidine) and amiodarone may have potentiating effects on atrial conduction time and induce negative inotropic effect.
- Insulin and oral antidiabetic drugs may intensify the blood sugar lowering effect, especially of non-selective beta-blockers. Beta- blockade may prevent the appearance of signs of hypoglycaemia (tachycardia).
- Anaesthetic drugs may cause attenuation of reflex tachycardia and increase the risk of hypotension. Continuation of beta-blockade reduces the risk of arrhythmia during induction and intubation. The anaesthesiologist should be informed when the patient is receiving a beta-blocking agent. Anaesthetic agents causing myocardial depression, such as cyclopropane and trichlorethylene, are best avoided.
- Cimetidine, hydralazine and alcohol may increase the bioavailability of labetalol.

Take into account:

- Calcium antagonists: dihydropyridine derivates such as nifedipine. The risk of hypotension may be increased. In patients with latent cardiac insufficiency, treatment with beta-blockers may lead to cardiac failure.
- Prostaglandin synthetase inhibiting drugs may decrease the hypotensive effect of beta-blockers.
- Sympathicomimetic agents may counteract the effect of beta-adrenergic blocking agents.
- Concomitant use of tricyclic antidepressants, barbiturates, phenothiazines or other antihypertensive agents may increase the blood pressure lowering effect of labetalol. Concomitant use of tricyclic antidepressants may increase the incidence of tremor.
- Labetalol has been shown to reduce the uptake of radioisotopes of metaiodobenzylguanidine (MIBG), and may increase the likelihood of a false negative study. Care should therefore be taken in interpreting results from MIBG scintigraphy. Consideration should be given to withdrawing labetalol for several days at least before MIBG scintigraphy, and substituting other beta or alpha-blocking drugs.

4.6 Pregnancy and lactation
Although no teratogenic effects have been demonstrated in animals, Trandate should only be used during the first trimester of pregnancy if the potential benefit outweighs the potential risk.

Trandate crosses the placental barrier and the possibility of the consequences of alpha- and beta- adrenoceptor blockade in the foetus and neonate should be borne in mind. Perinatal and neonatal distress (bradycardia, hypotension, respiratory depression, hypoglycaemia, hypothermia) has been rarely reported. Sometimes these symptoms have developed a day or two after birth. Response to supportive measures (e.g. intravenous fluids and glucose) is usually prompt but with severe pre-eclampsia, particularly after prolonged intravenous labetalol, recovery may be slower. This may be related to diminished liver metabolism in premature babies.

Beta-blockers reduce placental perfusion, which may result in intrauterine foetal death, immature and premature deliveries. There is an increased risk of cardiac and pulmonary complications in the neonate in the post-natal period. Intra-uterine and neonatal deaths have been reported with Trandate but other drugs (e.g. vasodilators, respiratory depressants) and the effects of pre-eclampsia, intra-uterine growth retardation and prematurity were implicated. Such clinical experience warns against unduly prolonging high dose labetalol and delaying delivery and against co-administration of hydralazine.

Trandate is excreted in breast milk. Breast-feeding is therefore not recommended.

4.7 Effects on ability to drive and use machines

There are no studies on the effect of this medicine on the ability to drive. When driving vehicles or operating machines it should be taken into account that occasionally dizziness or fatigue may occur.

4.8 Undesirable effects

Trandate Injection is usually well tolerated. Excessive postural hypotension may occur if patients are allowed to assume an upright position within three hours of receiving Trandate Injection.

Most side-effects are transient and occur during the first few weeks of treatment with Trandate. They include headache, tiredness, dizziness, depressed mood and lethargy, nasal congestion, sweating, and rarely, ankle oedema. A tingling sensation in the scalp, usually transient, also may occur in a few patients early in treatment. Tremor has been reported in the treatment of hypertension of pregnancy. Acute retention of urine, difficulty in micturition, ejaculatory failure, epigastric pain, nausea and vomiting have been reported.

There have been rare reports of positive anti-nuclear antibodies unassociated with disease, cases of systemic lupus erythematosus, drug fever, toxic myopathy, hypersensitivity (rash, pruritus, angioedema and dyspnoea), reversible lichenoid rash, impaired vision, dry eyes, cramps, raised liver function tests, jaundice (both hepatocellular and cholestatic), hepatitis and hepatic necrosis, bradycardia and heart block.

Other possible side effects of beta-blockers are: heart failure, cold or cyanotic extremities, Raynaud's phenomenon, paraesthesia of the extremities, increase of an existing intermittent claudication, hallucinations, psychoses, confusion, sleep disturbances, nightmares, diarrhoea, bronchospasm (in patients with asthma or a history of asthma), masking of the symptoms of thyrotoxicosis or hypoglycaemia.

4.9 Overdose

Symptoms of overdosage are bradycardia, hypotension, bronchospasm and acute cardiac insufficiency.

After an overdose or in case of hypersensitivity, the patient should be kept under close supervision and be treated in an intensive-care ward. Artificial respiration may be required. Bradycardia or extensive vagal reactions should be treated by administering atropine or methylatropine. Hypotension and shock should be treated with plasma/ plasma substitutes and, if necessary, catecholamines. The beta-blocking effect can be counteracted by slow intravenous administration of isoprenaline hydrochloride, starting with a dose of approximately 5mcg/min, or dobutamine, starting with a dose of approximately 2.5mcg/min, until the required effect has been obtained. If this does not produce the desired effect, intravenous administration of 8-10 mg glucagon may be considered. If required the injection should be repeated within one hour, to be followed, if necessary, by an iv infusion of glucagon at 1-3mg/hour. Administration of calcium ions, or the use of a cardiac pacemaker, may also be considered.

Oliguric renal failure has been reported after massive overdosage of labetalol orally. In one case, the use of dopamine to increase the blood pressure may have aggravated the renal failure.

Labetalol does have membrane stabilising activity which may have clinical significance in overdosage.

Haemodialysis removes less than 1% labetalol hydrochloride from the circulation.

5. PHARMACOLOGICAL PROPERTIES

5.1 Pharmacodynamic properties

Labetalol lowers the blood pressure primarily by blocking peripheral arteriolar alpha-adrenoceptors thus reducing peripheral resistance and, by concurrent beta-blockade, protects the heart from reflex sympathetic drive that would otherwise occur. Cardiac output is not significantly reduced at rest or after moderate exercise. Increases in systolic blood pressure during exercise are reduced but corresponding changes in diastolic pressure are essentially normal.

In patients with angina pectoris co-existing with hypertension, the reduced peripheral resistance decreases myocardial afterload and oxygen demand. All these effects would be expected to benefit hypertensive patients and those with co-existing angina.

5.2 Pharmacokinetic properties

The plasma half-life of labetalol is about 4 hours. About 50% of labetalol in the blood is protein bound. Labetalol is metabolised mainly through conjugation to inactive glucuronide metabolites. These are excreted both in urine and via the bile into the faeces.

Only negligible amounts of the drug cross the blood brain barrier in animal studies.

5.3 Preclinical safety data

Not applicable since Trandate Injection has been used in clinical practice for many years and its effects in man are well known.

6. PHARMACEUTICAL PARTICULARS

6.1 List of excipients

Hydrochloric acid dilute

Sodium hydroxide

Water for Injection

6.2 Incompatibilities

Trandate injection has been shown to be incompatible with sodium bicarbonate injection BP 4.2% w/v

6.3 Shelf life

24 months

6.4 Special precautions for storage

Protect from light. Store below 30°C

6.5 Nature and contents of container

Type I Glass ampoules: 5 ampoules per pack. Pack size 20.

6.6 Special precautions for disposal and other handling

None

7. MARKETING AUTHORISATION HOLDER

UCB Pharma Limited

208 Bath Road

Slough

Berkshire

SL1 3WE

UK

8. MARKETING AUTHORISATION NUMBER(S)

PL 0039/0492

9. DATE OF FIRST AUTHORISATION/RENEWAL OF THE AUTHORISATION

1 November 1996/ 3 October 1999

10. DATE OF REVISION OF THE TEXT

June 2005

POM

Trandate Tablets 50mg, 100mg, 200mg or 400mg

(UCB Pharma Limited)

1. NAME OF THE MEDICINAL PRODUCT

Trandate Tablets 50 mg

Trandate Tablets 100 mg

Trandate Tablets 200 mg

Trandate Tablets 400 mg

2. QUALITATIVE AND QUANTITATIVE COMPOSITION

Each tablet contains 50 mg, 100 mg, 200 mg or 400 mg labetalol hydrochloride

3. PHARMACEUTICAL FORM

Orange coloured, circular, biconvex film-coated tablets engraved Trandate 50, or 100, 200 or 400 on one face

4. CLINICAL PARTICULARS

4.1 Therapeutic indications

Trandate Tablets are indicated for the treatment of:-

1. Mild, moderate or severe hypertension
2. Hypertension in pregnancy
3. Angina pectoris with existing hypertension

4.2 Posology and method of administration

Trandate tablets should be taken orally with food.

Adults:

Hypertension

Treatment should start with 100mg twice daily. In patients already being treated with antihypertensives and in those of low body weight this may be sufficient to control blood pressure. In others, increases in dose of 100mg twice daily should be made at fortnightly intervals. Many patients' blood pressure is controlled by 200mg twice daily and up to 800mg daily may be given as a twice daily regimen. In severe, refractory hypertension, daily doses up to 2400mg have been given. Such doses should be divided into a three or four times a day regimen.

Elderly

In elderly patients, an initial dose of 50mg twice daily is recommended. This has provided satisfactory control in some cases.

In the hypertension of pregnancy

The initial dose of 100mg twice daily may be increased, if necessary, at weekly intervals by 100mg twice daily. During the second and third trimester, the severity of the hypertension may require further dose titration to a three times daily regimen, ranging from 100mg tds to 400mg tds. A total daily dose of 2400mg should not be exceeded.

Hospital in-patients with severe hypertension, particularly of pregnancy, may have daily increases in dosage.

General

If rapid reduction of blood pressure is necessary, see the SPC for Trandate Injection. If long-term control of hypertension following the use of Trandate Injection is required, oral therapy with Trandate tablets should start with 100mg twice daily.

Additive hypotensive effects may be expected if Trandate tablets are administered together with other antihypertensives e.g. diuretics, methyldopa etc. When transferring patients from such agents, Trandate tablets should be introduced with a dosage of 100mg twice daily and the previous therapy gradually decreased. Abrupt withdrawal of clonidine or beta-blocking agents is undesirable.

Angina co-existing with hypertension

In patients with angina pectoris co-existing with hypertension, the dose of Trandate will be that required to control the hypertension.

Children:

Safety and efficacy in children have not been established.

4.3 Contraindications

- Cardiogenic shock.
- Uncontrolled, incipient or digitalis-refractory heart failure.
- Sick sinus syndrome (including sino-atrial block).
- Second or third degree heart block.
- Prinzmetal's angina.
- History of wheezing or asthma.
- Untreated phaeochromocytoma.
- Metabolic acidosis.
- Bradycardia (<45-50 bpm).
- Hypotension.
- Hypersensitivity to labetalol.
- Severe peripheral circulatory disturbances.

4.4 Special warnings and precautions for use

There have been reports of skin rashes and/ or dry eyes associated with the use of beta-adrenoceptor blocking drugs. The reported incidence is small and in most cases the symptoms have cleared when the treatment was withdrawn. Gradual discontinuance of the drug should be considered if any such reaction is not otherwise explicable.

There have been rare reports of severe hepatocellular injury with labetalol therapy. The hepatic injury is usually reversible and has occurred after both short and long term treatment. Appropriate laboratory testing should be done at the first sign or symptom of liver dysfunction. If there is laboratory evidence of liver injury or the patient is jaundiced, labetalol therapy should be stopped and not restarted.

Due to negative inotropic effects, special care should be taken with patients whose cardiac reserve is poor and heart failure should be controlled before starting Trandate therapy.

Patients particularly those with ischemic heart disease, should not interrupt/ discontinue abruptly Trandate therapy. The dosage should gradually be reduced, ie. over 1-2 weeks, if necessary at the same time initiating replacement therapy, to prevent exacerbation of angina pectoris. In addition, hypertension and arrhythmias may develop.

It is not necessary to discontinue Trandate therapy in patients requiring anaesthesia but the anaesthetist must be informed and the patient should be given intravenous atropine prior to induction. If beta-blockade is interrupted in preparation for surgery, therapy should be discontinued for at least 24 hours. Anaesthetic agents causing myocardial depression (eg. cyclopropane, trichloroethylene) should be avoided. Trandate may enhance the hypotensive effects of halothane.

In patients with peripheral circulatory disorders (Raynaud's disease or syndrome, intermittent claudication), beta-blockers should be used with great caution as aggravation of these disorders may occur.

Beta-blockers may induce bradycardia. If the pulse rate decreases to less than 50-55 beats per minute at rest and the patient experiences symptoms related to the bradycardia, the dosage should be reduced.

Beta-blockers, even those with apparent cardioselectivity, should not be used in patients with asthma or a history of obstructive airways disease unless no alternative treatment is available. In such cases the risk of inducing bronchospasm should be appreciated and appropriate precautions taken. If bronchospasm should occur after the use of Trandate it can be treated with a beta2-agonist by inhalation, e.g. salbutamol (the dose of which may need to be greater than the usual in asthma) and, if necessary, intravenous atropine 1mg.

Due to a negative effect on conduction time, beta-blockers should only be given with caution to patients with first degree heart block. Patients with liver or kidney insufficiency may need a lower dosage, depending on the pharmacokinetic profile of the compound. The elderly should be treated with caution, starting with a lower dosage but tolerance is usually good in the elderly.

Patients with a history of psoriasis should take beta-blockers only after careful consideration.

Risk of anaphylactic reaction: While taking beta-blockers, patients with a history of severe anaphylactic reaction to a variety of allergens may be more reactive to repeated challenge, either accidental, diagnostic or therapeutic. Such patients may be unresponsive to the usual doses of epinephrine used to treat allergic reaction.

The label will state "Do not take Trandate if you have a history of wheezing or asthma as it can make your breathing worse."

Trandate Tablets contain sodium benzoate which is a mild irritant to the eyes, nose and mucous membranes. It may increase the risk of jaundice in newborn babies.

4.5 Interaction with other medicinal products and other forms of interaction

Concomitant use not recommended:

- Calcium antagonists such as verapamil and to a lesser extent diltiazem have a negative influence on contractility and atrio-ventricular conduction.
- Digitalis glycosides used in association with beta-blockers may increase atrio-ventricular conduction time.
- Clonidine: Beta-blockers increase the risk of rebound hypertension. When clonidine is used in conjunction with non-selective beta-blockers, such as propranolol, treatment with clonidine should be continued for some time after treatment with the beta-blocker has been discontinued.
- Monoamineoxidase inhibitors (except MOA-B inhibitors).

Use with caution:

- Class I antiarrhythmic agents (eg. disopyramide, quinidine) and amiodarone may have potentiating effects on atrial conduction time and induce negative inotropic effect.
- Insulin and oral antidiabetic drugs may intensify the blood sugar lowering effect, especially of non-selective beta-blockers. Beta- blockade may prevent the appearance of signs of hypoglycaemia (tachycardia).
- Anaesthetic drugs may cause attenuation of reflex tachycardia and increase the risk of hypotension. Continuation of beta-blockade reduces the risk of arrhythmia during induction and intubation. The anaesthesiologist should be informed when the patient is receiving a beta-blocking agent. Anaesthetic agents causing myocardial depression, such as cyclopropane and trichlorethylene, are best avoided.
- Cimetidine, hydralazine and alcohol may increase the bioavailability of labetalol.

Take into account:

- Calcium antagonists: dihydropyridine derivates such as nifedipine. The risk of hypotension may be increased. In patients with latent cardiac insufficiency, treatment with beta-blockers may lead to cardiac failure.
- Prostaglandin synthetase inhibiting drugs may decrease the hypotensive effect of beta-blockers.
- Sympathicomimetic agents may counteract the effect of beta-adrenergic blocking agents.
- Concomitant use of tricyclic antidepressants, barbiturates, phenothiazines or other antihypertensive agents may increase the blood pressure lowering effect of labetalol. Concomitant use of tricyclic antidepressants may increase the incidence of tremor.
- Labetalol has been shown to reduce the uptake of radioisotopes of metaiodobenzylguanidine (MIBG), and may increase the likelihood of a false negative study. Care should therefore be taken in interpreting results from MIBG scintigraphy. Consideration should be given to withdrawing labetalol for several days at least before MIBG scintigraphy, and substituting other beta or alpha-blocking drugs.

4.6 Pregnancy and lactation

Although no teratogenic effects have been demonstrated in animals, Trandate should only be used during the first trimester of pregnancy if the potential benefit outweighs the potential risk.

Trandate crosses the placental barrier and the possible consequences of alpha- and beta-adrenoceptor blockade in the foetus and neonate should be borne in mind. Perinatal and neonatal distress (bradycardia, hypotension, respiratory depression, hypoglycaemia, hypothermia) has been rarely reported. Sometimes these symptoms have developed a day or two after birth. Response to supportive measures (e.g. intravenous fluids and glucose) is usually prompt but with severe pre-eclampsia, particularly after prolonged intravenous labetalol, recovery may be slower. This may be related to diminished liver metabolism in premature babies.

Beta-blockers reduce placental perfusion, which may result in intrauterine foetal death, immature and premature deliveries. There is an increased risk of cardiac and pulmonary complications in the neonate in the post-natal period. Intra-uterine and neonatal deaths have been reported with Trandate but other drugs (e.g. vasodilators, respiratory depressants) and the effects of pre-eclampsia, intra-uterine growth retardation and prematurity were implicated. Such clinical experience warns against unduly prolonging high dose labetalol and delaying delivery and against co-administration of hydralazine.

Trandate is excreted in breast milk. Breast-feeding is therefore not recommended.

4.7 Effects on ability to drive and use machines

There are no studies on the effect of this medicine on the ability to drive. When driving vehicles or operating machines it should be taken into account that occasionally dizziness or fatigue may occur.

4.8 Undesirable effects

Most side-effects are transient and occur during the first few weeks of treatment with Trandate. They include headache, tiredness, dizziness, depressed mood and lethargy, nasal congestion, sweating, and rarely, ankle oedema. Postural hypotension is uncommon except at very high doses or if the initial dose is too high or doses are increased too rapidly. A tingling sensation in the scalp, usually transient, also may occur in a few patients early in treatment. Tremor has been reported in the treatment of hypertension of pregnancy. Acute retention of urine, difficulty in micturition, ejaculatory failure, epigastric pain, nausea and vomiting have been reported.

There have been rare reports of positive anti-nuclear antibodies unassociated with disease, cases of systemic lupus erythematosus, drug fever, toxic myopathy, hypersensitivity (rash, pruritus, angioedema and dyspnoea), reversible lichenoid rash, impaired vision, dry eyes, cramps, raised liver function tests, jaundice (both hepatocellular and cholestatic), hepatitis and hepatic necrosis, bradycardia and heart block.

Other possible side effects of beta-blockers are: heart failure, cold or cyanotic extremities, Raynaud's phenomenon, paraesthesia of the extremities, increase of an existing intermittent claudication, hallucinations, psychoses, confusion, sleep disturbances, nightmares, diarrhoea, bronchospasm (in patients with asthma or a history of asthma), masking of the symptoms of thyrotoxicosis or hypoglycaemia.

4.9 Overdose

Symptoms of overdosage are bradycardia, hypotension, bronchopasm and acute cardiac insufficency.

After ingestion of an overdose or in case of hypersensitivity, the patient should be kept under close supervision and be treated in an intensive-care ward. Absorption of any drug material still present in the gastro-intestinal tract can be prevented by gastric lavage, administration of activated charcoal and a laxative. Artificial respiration may be required. Bradycardia or extensive vagal reactions should be treated by administering atropine or methylatropine. Hypotension and shock should be treated with plasma/plasma substitutes and, if necessary, catecholamines. The beta-blocking effect can be counteracted by slow intravenous administration of isoprenaline hydrochloride, starting with a dose of approximately 5mcg/min, or dobutamine, starting with a dose of approximately 2.5mcg/min, until the required effect has been obtained. If this does not produce the desired effect, intravenous administration of 8-10 mg glucagon may be considered. If required the injection should be repeated within one hour, to be followed, if necessary, by an iv infusion of glucagon at 1-3mg/hour. Administration of calcium ions, or the use of a cardiac pacemaker, may also be considered.

Oliguric renal failure has been reported after massive overdosage of labetalol orally. In one case, the use of dopamine to increase the blood pressure may have aggravated the renal failure.

Labetalol does have membrane stabilising activity which may have clinical significance in overdosage.

Haemodialysis removes less than 1% labetalol hydrochloride from the circulation.

5. PHARMACOLOGICAL PROPERTIES

5.1 Pharmacodynamic properties

Labetalol lowers the blood pressure by blocking peripheral arteriolar alpha-adrenoceptors thus reducing peripheral resistance, and by concurrent beta-blockade, protects the heart from reflex sympathetic drive that would otherwise occur. Cardiac output is not significantly reduced at rest or after moderate exercise. Increases in systolic blood pressure during exercise are reduced but corresponding changes in diastolic pressure are essentially normal.

In patients with angina pectoris co-existing with hypertension, the reduced peripheral resistance decreases myocardial afterload and oxygen demand. All these effects would be expected to benefit hypertensive patients and those with co-existing angina.

5.2 Pharmacokinetic properties

The plasma half-life of labetalol is about 4 hours. About 50% of labetalol in the blood is protein bound. Labetalol is metabolised mainly through conjugation to inactive glucuronide metabolites. These are excreted both in urine and via the bile into the faeces.

Only negligible amounts of the drug cross the blood brain barrier in animal studies.

5.3 Preclinical safety data

Not applicable since Trandate Tablets have been used in clinical practice for many years and its effects in man are well known.

6. PHARMACEUTICAL PARTICULARS

6.1 List of excipients

Tablet Core:

Lactose BP

Magnesium stearate

Starch maize special

Starch maize pregelatinised

Film coating suspension:

Hydroxypropylmethylcellulose

Sodium benzoate

Titanium dioxide

Sunset yellow

Methyl hydroxybenzoate

Propyl hydroxybenzoate

IMS 740P

Purified Water

6.2 Incompatibilities

None stated

6.3 Shelf life

60 months

6.4 Special precautions for storage

No special storage conditions are necessary

6.5 Nature and contents of container

Calendar blister pack containing 56 tablets; composed of hard tempered aluminium foil and opaque PVC blister.

Polypropylene container with tamper-evident polyethylene lid containing 250 tablets.

6.6 Special precautions for disposal and other handling

None

7. MARKETING AUTHORISATION HOLDER

UCB Pharma Limited

208 Bath Road

Slough

Berkshire

SL1 3WE

UK

8. MARKETING AUTHORISATION NUMBER(S)

50 mg: PL 00039/0493

100 mg: PL 00039/0494

200 mg: PL 00039/0495

400 mg: PL 00039/0496

9. DATE OF FIRST AUTHORISATION/RENEWAL OF THE AUTHORISATION

1 November 1996/ 17 February 1999/17 March 2009

10. DATE OF REVISION OF THE TEXT

17 March 2009

POM

Transtec 35, 52.5 and 70 micrograms transdermal patch

(Napp Pharmaceuticals Limited)

1. NAME OF THE MEDICINAL PRODUCT

TRANSTEC 35® micrograms/h transdermal patch

TRANSTEC 52.5® micrograms/h transdermal patch

TRANSTEC 70® micrograms/h transdermal patch

2. QUALITATIVE AND QUANTITATIVE COMPOSITION

TRANSTEC 35 micrograms/h transdermal patch:

One transdermal patch contains 20 mg buprenorphine.

Area containing the active substance: 25 cm^2

Nominal release rate: 35 micrograms of buprenorphine per hour (over a period of 96 hours).

TRANSTEC 52.5 micrograms/h transdermal patch:

One transdermal patch contains 30 mg buprenorphine.

Area containing the active substance: 37.5 cm^2

Nominal release rate: 52.5 micrograms of buprenorphine per hour (over a period of 96 hours).

TRANSTEC 70 micrograms/h transdermal patch:

One transdermal patch contains 40 mg buprenorphine.

Area containing the active substance: 50 cm^2

Nominal release rate: 70 micrograms of buprenorphine per hour (over a period of 96 hours).

For a full list of excipients, see section 6.1.

3. PHARMACEUTICAL FORM

Transdermal patch

Skin coloured transdermal patch with rounded corners marked:

TRANSTEC 35 µg/h, buprenorphinum 20 mg

TRANSTEC 52.5 µg/h, buprenorphinum 30 mg

TRANSTEC 70 µg/h, buprenorphinum 40 mg

4. CLINICAL PARTICULARS

4.1 Therapeutic indications

Moderate to severe cancer pain and severe pain which does not respond to non-opioid analgesics.

TRANSTEC is not suitable for the treatment of acute pain.

4.2 Posology and method of administration

Posology Patients over 18 years of age

The TRANSTEC dosage should be adapted to the condition of the individual patient (pain intensity, suffering, individual reaction). The lowest possible dosage providing adequate pain relief should be given. Three transdermal patch strengths are available to provide such adaptive treatment: TRANSTEC 35 micrograms/h, TRANSTEC 52.5 micrograms/h and TRANSTEC 70 micrograms/h.

Initial dose selection: patients who have previously not received any analgesics should start with the lowest transdermal patch strength (TRANSTEC 35 micrograms/h). Patients previously given a WHO step-I analgesic (non-opioid) or a step-II analgesic (weak opioid) should also begin with TRANSTEC 35 micrograms/h. According to the WHO recommendations, the administration of a non-opioid analgesic can be continued, depending on the patient's overall medical condition.

When switching from a step-III analgesic (strong opioid) to TRANSTEC and choosing the initial transdermal patch strength, the nature of the previous medication, administration and the mean daily dose should be taken into account in order to avoid the recurrence of pain. In general it is advisable to titrate the dose individually, starting with the lowest transdermal patch strength (TRANSTEC 35 micrograms/h). Clinical experience has shown that patients who were previously treated with higher daily dosages of a strong opioid (in the dimension of approximately 120 mg oral morphine) may start the therapy with the next higher transdermal patch strength (see also section 5.1).

To allow for individual dose adaptation in an adequate time period sufficient supplementary immediate release analgesics should be made available during dose titration.

The necessary strength of TRANSTEC must be adapted to the requirements of the individual patient and checked at regular intervals.

After application of the first TRANSTEC transdermal patch the buprenorphine serum concentrations rise slowly both in patients who have been treated previously with analgesics and in those who have not. Therefore initially, there is unlikely to be a rapid onset of effect. Consequently, a first evaluation of the analgesic effect should only be made after 24 hours.

The previous analgesic medication (with the exception of transdermal opioids) should be given in the same dose during the first 12 hours after switching to TRANSTEC and appropriate rescue medication on demand in the following 12 hours.

Dose titration and maintenance therapy

TRANSTEC should be replaced after 96 hours (4 days) at the latest. For convenience of use, the transdermal patch can be changed twice a week at regular intervals, e.g. always on Monday morning and Thursday evening. The dose should be titrated individually until analgesic efficacy is attained. If analgesia is insufficient at the end of the initial application period, the dose may be increased, either by applying more than one transdermal patch of the same strength or by switching to the next transdermal patch strength. At the same time no more than two transdermal patches regardless of the strength should be applied.

Before application of the next TRANSTEC strength the amount of total opioids administered in addition to the previous transdermal patch should be taken into consideration, i.e. the total amount of opioids required, and the dosage adjusted accordingly. Patients requiring a supplementary analgesic (e.g. for breakthrough pain) during maintenance therapy may take for example one to two 0.2 mg buprenorphine sublingual tablets every 24 hours in addition to the transdermal patch. If the regular addition of 0.4 – 0.6 mg sublingual buprenorphine is necessary, the next strength should be used.

Patients under 18 years of age

As TRANSTEC has not been studied in patients under 18 years of age, the use of the medicinal product in patients below this age is not recommended.

Elderly patients

No dosage adjustment of TRANSTEC is required for elderly patients.

Patients with renal insufficiency

Since the pharmacokinetics of buprenorphine is not altered during the course of renal failure, its use in patients with renal insufficiency, including dialysis patients, is possible.

Patients with hepatic insufficiency

Buprenorphine is metabolised in the liver. The intensity and duration of its action may be affected in patients with impaired liver function. Therefore patients with liver insufficiency should be carefully monitored during treatment with TRANSTEC.

Method of application

TRANSTEC should be applied to non-irritated, clean skin on a non-hairy flat surface, but not to any parts of the skin with large scars. Preferable sites on the upper body are: upper back or below the collar-bone on the chest. Any remaining hairs should be cut off with a pair of scissors (not shaved). If the site of application requires cleansing, this should be done with water. Soap or any other cleansing agents should not be used. Skin preparations that might affect adhesion of the transdermal patch to the area selected for application of TRANSTEC should be avoided.

The skin must be completely dry before application. TRANSTEC is to be applied immediately after removal from the sachet. Following removal of the release liner, the transdermal patch should be pressed firmly in place with the palm of the hand for approximately 30 seconds. The transdermal patch will not be affected when bathing, showering or swimming. However, it should not be exposed to excessive heat (e.g. sauna, infrared-radiation).

TRANSTEC should be worn continuously for up to 4 days. After removal of the previous transdermal patch a new TRANSTEC transdermal patch should be applied to a different skin site. At least one week should elapse before a new transdermal patch is applied to the same area of skin.

Duration of administration

TRANSTEC should under no circumstances be administered for longer than absolutely necessary. If long-term pain treatment with TRANSTEC is necessary in view of the nature and severity of the illness, then careful and regular monitoring should be carried out (if necessary with breaks in treatment) to establish whether and to what extent further treatment is necessary.

Discontinuation of TRANSTEC

After removal of TRANSTEC buprenorphine serum concentrations decrease gradually and thus the analgesic effect is maintained for a certain amount of time. This should be considered when therapy with TRANSTEC is to be followed by other opioids. As a general rule, a subsequent opioid should not be administered within 24 hours after removal of TRANSTEC. For the time being only limited information is available on the starting dose of other opioids administered after discontinuation of TRANSTEC.

4.3 Contraindications

TRANSTEC is contraindicated in:

- hypersensitivity to the active substance buprenorphine or to any of the excipients (for the excipients, see section 6.1)
- in opioid-dependent patients and for narcotic withdrawal treatment
- conditions in which the respiratory centre and function are severely impaired or may become so
- patients who are receiving MAO inhibitors or have taken them within the last two weeks (see section 4.5)
- patients suffering from myasthenia gravis
- patients suffering from delirium tremens.
- pregnancy (see section 4.6)

4.4 Special warnings and precautions for use

TRANSTEC must only be used with particular caution in acute alcohol intoxication, convulsive disorders, in patients with head injury, shock, a reduced level of consciousness of uncertain origin, increased intracranial pressure without the possibility of ventilation.

Buprenorphine occasionally causes respiratory depression. Therefore care should be taken when treating patients with impaired respiratory function or patients receiving medicinal products which can cause respiratory depression.

Buprenorphine has a substantially lower dependence liability than pure opioid agonists. In healthy volunteer and patient studies with TRANSTEC, withdrawal reactions have not been observed. However, after long-term use of TRANSTEC withdrawal symptoms, similar to those occurring during opiate withdrawal, cannot be entirely excluded (see section 4.8). These symptoms are: agitation, anxiety, nervousness, insomnia, hyperkinesia, tremor and gastrointestinal disorders.

In patients abusing opioids, substitution with buprenorphine may prevent withdrawal symptoms. This has resulted in some abuse of buprenorphine and caution should be exercised when prescribing it to patients suspected of having drug abuse problems.

Buprenorphine is metabolised in the liver. The intensity and duration of effect may be altered in patients with liver function disorders. Therefore such patients should be carefully monitored during TRANSTEC treatment.

As TRANSTEC has not been studied in patients under 18 years of age, the use of the medicinal product in patients below this age is not recommended.

Patients with fever / external heat

Fever and the presence of heat may increase the permeability of the skin. Theoretically in such situations buprenorphine serum concentrations may be raised during TRANSTEC treatment. Therefore on treatment with TRANSTEC, attention should be paid to the increased possibility of opioid reactions in febrile patients or those with increased skin temperature due to other causes.

4.5 Interaction with other medicinal products and other forms of interaction

On administration of MAO inhibitors in the last 14 days prior to the administration of the opioid pethidine life-threatening interactions have been observed affecting the central nervous system and respiratory and cardiovascular function. The same interactions between MAO inhibitors and TRANSTEC cannot be ruled out (see section 4.3).

When TRANSTEC is applied together with other opioids, anaesthetics, hypnotics, sedatives, antidepressants, neuroleptics, and in general, medicinal products that depress respiration and the central nervous system, the CNS effects may be intensified. This applies also to alcohol.

Administered together with inhibitors or inducers of CYP 3A4 the efficacy of TRANSTEC may be intensified (inhibitors) or weakened (inducers).

4.6 Pregnancy and lactation

Pregnancy

There are no adequate data from the use of TRANSTEC in pregnant women. Studies in animals have shown reproductive toxicity (see section 5.3). The potential risk for humans is unknown.

Towards the end of pregnancy high doses of buprenorphine may induce respiratory depression in the neonate even after a short period of administration. Long-term administration of buprenorphine during the last three months of pregnancy may cause a withdrawal syndrome in the neonate.

Therefore TRANSTEC is contraindicated during pregnancy.

Lactation

Buprenorphine is excreted in human milk. In rats, buprenorphine has been found to inhibit lactation.

TRANSTEC should not be used during lactation.

4.7 Effects on ability to drive and use machines

TRANSTEC® has major influence on the ability to drive and use machines.

Even when used according to instructions, TRANSTEC® may affect the patient's reactions to such an extent that road safety and the ability to operate machinery may be impaired.

This applies particularly at the beginning of treatment, at any change of dosage and when TRANSTEC® is used in conjunction with other centrally acting substances including alcohol, tranquillisers, sedatives and hypnotics.

Patients who are affected (e.g. feeling dizzy or drowsy or experience blurred or double vision) should not drive or use machines while using TRANSTEC® and for at least 24 hours after the patch has been removed.

Patients stabilized on a specific dosage will not necessarily be restricted if the above mentioned symptoms are not present.

4.8 Undesirable effects

The following adverse reactions were reported after administration of TRANSTEC in clinical studies and from post-marketing surveillance.

The frequencies are given as follows:

Very common ($\geqslant$1/10)

Common ($\geqslant$1/100, <1/10)

Uncommon ($\geqslant$1/1,000, <1/100)

Rare ($\geqslant$1/10,000, <1/1,000)

Very rare ($\leqslant$1/10,000)

Not known (cannot be estimated from the available data)

a) The most commonly reported systemic adverse reactions were nausea and vomiting.

The most commonly reported local adverse reactions were erythema and pruritus.

b) **Immune system disorders**

Very rare: serious allergic reactions*

Metabolism and nutrition disorders

Rare: appetite lost

Psychiatric disorders

Uncommon: confusion, sleep disorder, restlessness

Rare: psychotomimetic effects (e.g. hallucinations, anxiety, nightmares), decreased libido

Very rare: dependence, mood swings

Nervous system disorders

Common: dizziness, headache

Uncommon: sedation, somnolence

Rare: concentration impaired, speech disorder, numbness, dysequilibrium, paraesthesia (e.g. pricking or burning skin sensation)

Very rare: muscle fasciculation, parageusia

Eye disorders

Rare: visual disturbance, blurring of vision, eyelid oedema

Very rare: miosis

Ear and labyrinth disorders

Very rare: ear pain

Cardiac/Vascular disorders

Uncommon: circulatory disorders (such as hypotension or, rarely, even circulatory collapse)

Rare: hot flushes

Respiratory, thoracic and mediastinal disorders

Common: dyspnoea

Rare: respiratory depression

Very rare: hyperventilation, hiccups

Gastrointestinal disorders

Very common: nausea

Common: vomiting, constipation

Uncommon: dry mouth

Rare: pyrosis

Very rare: retching

Skin and subcutaneous tissue disorders

Very common: erythema, pruritus

Common: exanthema, diaphoresis

Uncommon: rash

Rare: urticaria

Very rare: pustules, vesicles

Renal and urinary disorders

Uncommon: urinary retention, micturition disorders

Reproductive system and breast disorders

Rare: decreased erection

General disorders and administration site conditions

Common: oedema, tiredness

Uncommon: weariness

Rare: withdrawal symptoms*, administration site reactions

Very rare: thoracic pain

* see section c)

c) In some cases delayed allergic reactions occurred with marked signs of inflammation. In such cases treatment with TRANSTEC should be terminated.

Buprenorphine has a low risk of dependence. After discontinuation of TRANSTEC, withdrawal symptoms are unlikely. This is due to the very slow dissociation of buprenorphine from the opiate receptors and to the gradual decrease of buprenorphine serum concentrations (usually over a period of 30 hours after removal of the last transdermal patch). However, after long-term use of TRANSTEC withdrawal symptoms, similar to those occurring during opiate withdrawal, cannot be entirely excluded. These symptoms include: agitation, anxiety, nervousness, insomnia, hyperkinesia, tremor and gastro-intestinal disorders.

4.9 Overdose

Buprenorphine has a wide safety margin. Due to the rate-controlled delivery of small amounts of buprenorphine into the blood circulation high or toxic buprenorphine concentrations in the blood are unlikely. The maximum serum concentration of buprenorphine after the application of the TRANSTEC 70 micrograms/h transdermal patch is about six times less than after the intravenous administration of the therapeutic dose of 0.3 mg buprenorphine.

Symptoms

In principal, on overdose with buprenorphine, symptoms similar to those of other centrally acting analgesics (opioids) are to be expected. These are: respiratory depression, sedation, somnolence, nausea, vomiting, cardiovascular collapse, and marked miosis.

Treatment

General emergency measures apply. Keep the airway open (aspiration!), maintain respiration and circulation depending on the symptoms. Naloxone has a limited impact on the respiratory depressant effect of buprenorphine. High doses are needed given either as repeated boluses or infusion (for example starting with a bolus administration of 1-2 mg intravenously. Having attained an adequate antagonistic effect, administration by infusion is recommended to maintain constant naloxone plasma levels). Therefore, adequate ventilation should be established.

5. PHARMACOLOGICAL PROPERTIES

5.1 Pharmacodynamic properties

Pharmacotherapeutic group: Opioids, Oripavine derivatives. ATC code: N02AE01.

Buprenorphine is a strong opioid with agonistic activity at the mu-opioid receptor and antagonistic activity at the kappa-opioid receptor. Buprenorphine appears to have the general characteristics of morphine, but has its own specific pharmacology and clinical attributes.

In addition, numerous factors, e.g. indication and clinical setting, route of administration and the interindividual variability, have an impact on analgesia and therefore have to be considered when comparing analgesics.

In daily clinical practice different opioids are ranked by a relative potency, although this is to be considered a simplification.

The relative potency of buprenorphine in different application forms and in different clinical settings has been described in literature as follows:

- Morphine p.o.: BUP i.m. as 1: 67 - 150 (single dose; acute pain model)
- Morphine p.o.: BUP s.l. as 1: 60 - 100 (single dose, acute pain model; multiple dose, chronic pain, cancer pain)
- Morphine p.o.: BUP TTS as 1: 75 - 115 (multiple dose, chronic pain)

Abbreviations:

p.o = oral; i.m. = intramuscular; s.l. = sublingual; TTS = transdermal; BUP = buprenorphine

Adverse reactions are similar to those of other strong opioid analgesics. Buprenorphine appears to have a lower dependence liability than morphine.

5.2 Pharmacokinetic properties

a) General characteristics of the active substance

Buprenorphine has a plasma protein binding of about 96%.

Buprenorphine is metabolised in the liver to *N*-dealkylbuprenorphine (norbupren-orphine) and to glucuronide conjugated metabolites. $^{2}/_{3}$ of the active substance is eliminated unchanged in the faeces and $^{1}/_{3}$ eliminated as conjugates of unchanged or dealkylated buprenorphine via the urinary system. There is evidence of enterohepatic recirculation.

Studies in non-pregnant and pregnant rats have shown that buprenorphine passes the blood-brain and placental barriers. Concentrations in the brain (which contained only unchanged buprenorphine) after parenteral administration were 2-3 times higher than after oral administration. After intramuscular or oral administration buprenorphine apparently accumulates in the foetal gastrointestinal lumen – presumably due to biliary excretion, as enterohepatic circulation has not fully developed.

b) Characteristics of TRANSTEC in healthy volunteers

After the application of TRANSTEC, buprenorphine is absorbed through the skin. The continuous delivery of buprenorphine into the systemic circulation is by controlled release from the adhesive polymer-based matrix system.

After the initial application of TRANSTEC the plasma concentrations of buprenorphine gradually increase, and after 12-24 h the plasma concentrations reach the minimum effective concentration of 100 pg/ml. From the studies performed with the TRANSTEC 35 micrograms/h in healthy volunteers, an average C_{max} of 200 to 300 pg/ml and an average t_{max} of 60-80 h were determined. In one volunteer study, TRANSTEC 35 micrograms/h and TRANSTEC 70 micrograms/h were applied in a cross-over design. From this study, dose proportionality for the different strengths was demonstrated.

After removal of TRANSTEC the plasma concentrations of buprenorphine steadily decrease and are eliminated with a half-life of approx. 30 hours (range 22 - 36). Due to the continuous absorption of buprenorphine from the depot in the skin elimination is slower than after intravenous administration.

5.3 Preclinical safety data

Standard toxicological studies have not shown evidence of any particular potential risks for humans. In tests with repeated doses of buprenorphine in rats the increase in body weight was reduced.

Studies on fertility and general reproductive capacity of rats showed no detrimental effects. Studies in rats and rabbits revealed signs of fetotoxicity and increased post-implantation loss.

Studies in rats showed diminished intra-uterine growth, delays in the development of certain neurological functions and high peri/post natal mortality in the neonates after treatment of the dams during gestation or lactation. There is evidence that complicated delivery and reduced lactation contributed to these effects. There was no evidence of embryotoxicity including teratogenicity in rats or rabbits.

In vitro and *in vivo* examinations on the mutagenic potential of buprenorphine did not indicate any clinically relevant effects.

In long-term studies in rats and mice there was no evidence of any carcinogenic potential relevant for humans.

Toxicological data available did not indicate a sensitising potential of the additives of the transdermal patches.

6. PHARMACEUTICAL PARTICULARS

6.1 List of excipients

Adhesive matrix (containing buprenorphine): [(Z)-octadec-9-en-1-yl] oleate, povidone K90, 4-oxopentanic acid, poly[acrylic acid-co-butylacrylate-co-(2-ethylhexyl)acrylate-co-vinylacetate] (5:15:75:5), cross-linked

Adhesive matrix (without buprenorphine): poly[acrylic acid-co-butylacrylate-co-(2-ethylhexyl)acrylate-co-vinylacetate] (5:15:75:5), not cross-linked

Separating foil between the adhesive matrices with and without buprenorphine: poly(ethyleneterephthalate) - foil

Backing layer: poly(ethyleneterephthalate) – tissue

Release liner (on the front covering the adhesive matrix containing buprenorphine): poly(ethyleneterephthalate) – foil, siliconised, coated on one side with aluminium

6.2 Incompatibilities

Not applicable.

6.3 Shelf life

3 years.

6.4 Special precautions for storage

This medicinal product does not require any special storage conditions.

6.5 Nature and contents of container

Type of container:

Sealed sachet, composed of identical top and bottom layers of heat-sealable laminate, comprising (from outside to inside) paper, low density polyethylene, aluminium and poly-(acrylic acid-co-ethylene) (= surlyn).

Pack sizes:

Packs containing 4 individually sealed transdermal patches.

6.6 Special precautions for disposal and other handling

Any unused product or waste material should be disposed of in accordance with local requirements.

7. MARKETING AUTHORISATION HOLDER

Grünenthal GmbH, Zieglerstrasse 6, 52078 Aachen, Germany

8. MARKETING AUTHORISATION NUMBER(S)

PL 04539/0014-16

9. DATE OF FIRST AUTHORISATION/RENEWAL OF THE AUTHORISATION

27 FEBRUARY 2002

10. DATE OF REVISION OF THE TEXT

January 2009

TREDAPTIVE® 1000 mg/20 mg modified release tablets

(Merck Sharp & Dohme Limited)

1. NAME OF THE MEDICINAL PRODUCT

TREDAPTIVE®▼ 1000 mg/20 mg modified-release tablets.

2. QUALITATIVE AND QUANTITATIVE COMPOSITION

Each modified-release tablet contains 1000 mg of nicotinic acid and 20 mg of laropiprant.

Excipient

Each modified-release tablet contains 128.4 mg of lactose monohydrate.

For a full list of excipients, see section 6.1.

3. PHARMACEUTICAL FORM

Modified-release tablet.

Capsule-shaped, white to off-white tablet, with "552" debossed on one side.

4. CLINICAL PARTICULARS

4.1 Therapeutic indications

'Tredaptive' is indicated for the treatment of dyslipidaemia, particularly in patients with combined mixed dyslipidaemia (characterised by elevated levels of LDL-cholesterol and triglycerides and low HDL-cholesterol) and in patients with primary hypercholesterolaemia (heterozygous familial and non-familial).

'Tredaptive' should be used in patients in combination with HMG-CoA reductase inhibitors (statins), when the cholesterol lowering effect of HMG-CoA reductase inhibitor monotherapy is inadequate. It can be used as monotherapy only in patients in whom HMG-CoA reductase inhibitors are considered inappropriate or not tolerated. Diet and other non-pharmacological treatments (e.g. exercise, weight reduction) should be continued during therapy with 'Tredaptive'.

4.2 Posology and method of administration

Posology

The starting dose is one modified-release tablet (1000 mg nicotinic acid/20 mg laropiprant) once a day. After four weeks, it is recommended that patients be advanced to the maintenance dose of 2000 mg/40 mg taken as two modified-release tablets (1000 mg/20 mg each) once daily. Daily doses greater than 2000 mg/40 mg have not been studied and therefore are not recommended.

If 'Tredaptive' is missed for less than 7 consecutive days, patients can resume therapy at the last administered dose. If 'Tredaptive' is missed for 7 or more consecutive days, therapy should be resumed at the 1000 mg/20 mg dose for 1 week, before advancing to the maintenance dose of 2000 mg/40 mg.

Those patients switching from 2000 mg or more of prolonged-release nicotinic acid can initiate 'Tredaptive' at the 2000 mg/40 mg dose. Patients switching from less than 2000 mg of prolonged-release nicotinic acid should initiate therapy at the starting dose of 1000 mg/20 mg and advance to the 2000 mg/40 mg maintenance dose after four weeks. For patients switching from immediate-release nicotinic acid to 'Tredaptive', therapy should be initiated at the 1000 mg/20 mg dose and advanced to the 2000 mg/40 mg maintenance dose after four weeks.

Method of administration

The tablets should be taken whole, with food, in the evening or at bedtime. To preserve the modified-release properties, the tablets must not be split, broken, crushed, or chewed before swallowing. To reduce the possibility of flushing, alcohol or hot drinks should be avoided at the time of ingestion of the medicinal product.

Use in the elderly

No dose adjustment is required for elderly patients.

Use in paediatric patients

Safety and effectiveness of 'Tredaptive' in paediatric patients have not been established. Therefore, treatment is not recommended in this age group.

Use in patients with hepatic or renal insufficiency

Use of 'Tredaptive' in patients with hepatic or renal insufficiency has not been studied. Like other nicotinic acid medicinal products, 'Tredaptive' is contraindicated in patients with significant or unexplained hepatic dysfunction. It should be used with caution in patients with renal insufficiency, because nicotinic acid and its metabolites are primarily excreted by the kidneys (see sections 4.3, 4.4 and 5.2).

Concomitant therapy

Acetylsalicylic acid provides no additional reduction of flushing beyond that achieved by 'Tredaptive'. Therefore, treatment with acetylsalicylic acid to alleviate flushing symptoms is not necessary (see section 5.1).

Because co-administration of bile acid sequestrants may reduce the bioavailability of acidic medicinal products such as nicotinic acid, it is recommended that 'Tredaptive' be administered > 1 hour before or > 4 hours after administration of a bile acid sequestrant (see section 4.5).

4.3 Contraindications

- Hypersensitivity to the active substances or to any of the excipients.
- Significant or unexplained hepatic dysfunction.
- Active peptic ulcer disease.
- Arterial bleeding.

4.4 Special warnings and precautions for use

When 'Tredaptive' is co-administered with a statin, please refer to the Summary of Product Characteristics for that particular medicinal product.

Hepatic effects

Switching from immediate-release (crystalline) nicotinic acid to 'Tredaptive' has not been studied. However, cases of severe hepatic toxicity, including fulminant hepatic necrosis, have occurred in patients who have switched from immediate-release nicotinic acid to long-acting nicotinic acid at equivalent doses. Therefore, patients switching from immediate-release nicotinic acid to 'Tredaptive' should be initiated at the 1000 mg/20 mg dose.

'Tredaptive' should be used with caution in patients who consume substantial quantities of alcohol and/or have a past history of liver disease.

Like other lipid-lowering therapies, nicotinic acid medicinal products have been associated with abnormal liver function tests (see section 4.8). Transaminase elevations were reversible upon discontinuation of therapy.

Liver function tests are recommended before initiation, every 6 to 12 weeks for the first year, and periodically (e.g. semi-annually) thereafter. Patients who develop increased transaminase levels should be monitored until the abnormalities have resolved. Should an increase in alanine aminotransferase (ALT) or aspartate aminotransferase (AST) of ⩾ 3 X ULN persist, reduction of dose or withdrawal of 'Tredaptive' is recommended.

Effect on skeletal muscle

Rare cases of rhabdomyolysis have been associated with concomitant administration of lipid-altering doses (⩾ 1000 mg/day) of nicotinic acid and HMG-CoA reductase inhibitors (statins) (see section 4.8).

Physicians contemplating combined therapy with statins and 'Tredaptive' should carefully weigh the potential benefits and risks and should carefully monitor patients for any signs and symptoms of muscle pain, tenderness, or weakness, particularly during the initial months of therapy and when the dose of either medicinal product is increased. Periodic serum creatine kinase (CK) should be considered in such situations, but there is no assurance that such monitoring will prevent the occurrence of severe myopathy.

Caution should be exercised in patients with pre-disposing factors for rhabdomyolysis.

- Age > 70 years
- Renal impairment
- Uncontrolled hypothyroidism
- Personal or familial history of hereditary muscular disorders
- Previous history of muscular toxicity with a statin or fibrate
- Alcohol abuse.

If muscle pain, weakness or cramps occur while a patient is receiving 'Tredaptive' with a statin, their CK levels should be measured. If these levels are found, in the absence of strenuous exercise, to be significantly elevated (> 5 × ULN), treatment should be stopped.

Renal dysfunction

Because nicotinic acid and its metabolites are excreted through the kidneys, 'Tredaptive' should be used with caution in patients with renal dysfunction.

Effect on glucose

Nicotinic acid medicinal products have been associated with increases of fasting blood glucose levels (see section 4.8). Diabetic or potentially diabetic patients should be observed closely. Adjustment of diet and/or hypoglycaemic therapy may be necessary.

Acute coronary syndrome

As with other nicotinic acid medicinal products, caution should be used when 'Tredaptive' is used in patients with unstable angina or in the acute phase of an MI, particularly when such patients are also receiving vasoactive medicinal products such as nitrates, calcium channel blockers, or adrenergic blocking agents.

Haematologic effects

As with other nicotinic acid medicinal products, 'Tredaptive' (2000 mg/40 mg) was associated with small reductions in platelet count (see section 4.8). Therefore, patients undergoing surgery should be carefully evaluated.

Effect on uric acid

As with other nicotinic acid medicinal products, 'Tredaptive' (2000 mg/40 mg) was associated with small increases in uric acid levels (see section 4.8). Therefore, 'Tredaptive' should be used with caution in patients with or predisposed to gout.

Hypophosphataemia

As with other nicotinic acid medicinal products, 'Tredaptive' was associated with small decreases in phosphorus levels. Therefore, patients with a risk for hypophosphataemia should be closely followed.

Further Information

As with other nicotinic acid medicinal products, patients with a history of jaundice, hepato-biliary disorder or peptic ulcer should be observed closely (see sections 4.2 and 4.3).

Excipient

'Tredaptive' contains lactose. Patients with rare hereditary problems of galactose intolerance, the Lapp lactase deficiency or glucose-galactose malabsorption should not take this medicine.

4.5 Interaction with other medicinal products and other forms of interaction

Simultaneous use of alcohol or hot drinks can enhance the effects of flushing and should therefore be avoided around the time of ingestion of 'Tredaptive'.

Nicotinic acid

Effects of nicotinic acid on other medicinal products

Antihypertensive therapy: Nicotinic acid may potentiate the effects of ganglionic blocking agents and vasoactive medicinal products such as nitrates, calcium channel blockers, and adrenergic receptor blocking agents, resulting in postural hypotension.

HMG-CoA reductase inhibitors: When simvastatin is combined with nicotinic acid, a modest increase in AUC and C_{max} of simvastatin acid (the active form of simvastatin) was observed, which may be devoid of clinical relevance. The pharmacokinetic interaction of 'Tredaptive' with statins has been studied only with simvastatin (see section 4.4).

Effects of other medicinal products on nicotinic acid

Bile acid sequestrants: Because co-administration of bile acid sequestrants may reduce the bioavailability of acidic medicinal products such as nicotinic acid, it is recommended that 'Tredaptive' be administered > 1 hour before or > 4 hours after administration of a bile acid sequestrant.

Supplements containing nicotinic acid: Vitamins or other nutritional supplements containing (⩾ 50 mg/day) of nicotinic acid (or nicotinamide) have not been studied with 'Tredaptive'. Physicians should consider the nicotinic acid intake from vitamins and nutritional supplements when prescribing 'Tredaptive'.

Medicinal product /laboratory test interactions: In urine glucose tests, nicotinic acid may also give false-positive reactions with cupric sulphate solution (Benedict's reagent).

Laropiprant

Effects of laropiprant on other medicinal products

Midazolam: Multiple doses of laropiprant 40 mg did not affect the pharmacokinetics of midazolam, a sensitive CYP3A4 substrate. Therefore, laropiprant is not an inducer or inhibitor of CYP3A4. However, the plasma concentration of a metabolite of midazolam, 1'-hydroxymidazolam, was increased approximately 2-fold with multiple doses of laropiprant. Because 1'-hydroxymidazolam is an active metabolite, the sedative effect of midazolam may be increased and caution should be used when laropiprant is co-administered with midazolam.

Other medicinal products: Co-administration of laropiprant 40 mg with midazolam increased the $AUC_{0-\infty}$ and C_{max} of 1'-hydroxymidazolam, a midazolam metabolite, by 98 % and 59 %, respectively. 1'-hydroxymidazolam is metabolised predominantly by uridine diphosphate-glucuronosyltransferases (UGT) 2B4 and 2B7. Clinical and *in vitro* studies support the conclusion that laropiprant is a mild to moderate inhibitor of UGT2B4/UGT2B7. Very few medicinal products are known to be metabolised predominantly by UGT2B4 or UGT2B7. Caution should be used when 'Tredaptive' is co-administered with medicinal products metabolised predominantly by UGT2B4 or UGT2B7, for instance zidovudine.

In interaction studies, laropiprant did not have clinically significant effects on the pharmacokinetics of the following medicinal products: simvastatin, warfarin, oral contraceptives, rosiglitazone and digoxin. Based on these data, laropiprant is not expected to cause interactions with substrates of CYP isozymes 3A4, 2C9, 2C8 and human P-glycoprotein (P-gp). In *in vitro* studies, laropiprant did not inhibit CYP1A2, CYP2B6, CYP2C19, CYP2D6, or CYP2E1-mediated reactions.

Clopidogrel: In a clinical study, there was no meaningful effect of laropiprant on the inhibition of ADP-induced platelet aggregation by clopidogrel, but there was a modest increase in the inhibition of collagen-induced platelet aggregation by clopidogrel. This effect is unlikely to be clinically important as laropiprant did not increase bleeding time when co-administered with clopidogrel throughout the dosing interval.

Acetylsalicylic acid: In a clinical study, concomitant administration of laropiprant with acetylsalicylic acid did not have an effect on collagen-induced platelet aggregation or on bleeding time compared to treatment with acetylsalicylic acid alone (see section 5.1).

Acetylsalicylic acid and clopidogrel: A clinical study to evaluate the effect of laropiprant on platelet function in patients concomitantly receiving both acetylsalicylic acid and clopidogel was inconclusive. Because this study did not rule out the potential for prolongation of bleeding time patients receiving Tredaptive concomitantly with acetylsalicylic acid and clopidogel should be closely monitored.

Effects of other medicinal products on laropiprant

CYP3A4 inhibitor: Clarithromycin (a potent inhibitor of CYP3A4 and P-gp) did not have a clinically meaningful effect on the pharmacokinetics of laropiprant. Laropiprant is not a substrate of human P-gp, and therefore other inhibitors of CYP3A4 and/or P-gp are also not expected to have a clinically meaningful impact on the pharmacokinetics of laropiprant.

4.6 Pregnancy and lactation

Pregnancy

'Tredaptive'

There are no data from the combined use of nicotinic acid and laropiprant in pregnant women. The combination has not been tested in reproductive toxicity studies. The potential risk for humans is unknown. Therefore, 'Tredaptive' should not be used during pregnancy unless clearly necessary.

Nicotinic acid

There are no adequate data from the use of high dose nicotinic acid in pregnant women. Animal studies are insufficient with respect to reproductive toxicity (see section 5.3).

Laropiprant

There are no data from the use of laropiprant in pregnant women. Studies in animals have shown reproductive toxicity at high doses of laropiprant (see section 5.3).

Lactation

'Tredaptive'

No studies in lactating animals have been conducted with 'Tredaptive'. A decision on whether to continue/discontinue breast-feeding or to continue/discontinue therapy should be made taking into account the benefit of breast-feeding to the child and the benefit of 'Tredaptive' to the woman.

Nicotinic acid

Nicotinic acid is excreted in human breast milk.

Laropiprant

It is unknown whether laropiprant is excreted in human breast milk. Animal studies have shown excretion of laropiprant in milk.

4.7 Effects on ability to drive and use machines

No studies on the effects on the ability to drive and use machines have been performed. However, when driving vehicles or operating machines, it should be taken into account that dizziness has been reported (see section 4.8).

4.8 Undesirable effects

In clinical trials, over 2,500 patients received 'Tredaptive' alone or with an HMG-CoA reductase inhibitor. Adverse reactions have usually been mild and transient.

Flushing

Flushing is the most common adverse reaction of 'Tredaptive'. Flushing is most prominent in the head, neck, and upper torso. In a pool of four active- or placebo-controlled clinical trials (N=2,548), flushing was reported by the investigator as a possibly, probably, or definitely treatment-related adverse reaction in 12.3 % of patients taking 'Tredaptive'. In these studies, the percentage of patients taking 'Tredaptive', nicotinic acid (pooled prolonged-release formulations) or pooled placebo/simvastatin who discontinued due to any flushing-related symptom (redness, warmth, itching and tingling) was 7.2 %, 16.6 %, and 0.4 %, respectively. Discontinuations due to other specific adverse reactions among patients taking 'Tredaptive' were infrequent (< 1 %).

Overall adverse reactions with 'Tredaptive'

In addition to flushing, clinical adverse reactions reported by the investigators as possibly, probably, or definitely related to 'Tredaptive' in ⩾ 1 % of patients treated with 'Tredaptive' alone (n=947) or co-administered with statin (n=1,601) and clinically meaningful adverse reactions (< 1 %), for up to one year are listed below.

The frequencies of adverse reactions are ranked according to the following: Very common (⩾ 1/10), Common

($\geqslant$ 1/100 to < 1/10), Uncommon ($\geqslant$ 1/1,000 to < 1/100), Rare ($\geqslant$ 1/10,000 to < 1/1,000), Very rare (< 1/10,000).

System organ class	Adverse reaction	Frequency
Investigations	elevations in ALT and/or AST (consecutive, $\geqslant$ 3 X ULN), fasting glucose, uric acid (see below)	Common
	elevations in CK ($\geqslant$ 10 X ULN), total bilirubin, reductions in phosphorus and platelet counts (see below)	Uncommon
Nervous system disorders	dizziness, headache, paraesthesia	Common
Gastro-intestinal disorders	diarrhoea, dyspepsia, nausea, vomiting	Common
Skin and subcutaneous tissue disorders	erythema, pruritus, rash, urticaria	Common
Vascular disorders	flushing	Very common
General disorders and administration site conditions	feeling hot	Common
Immune system disorders	Hypersensitivity reaction (see below)	Uncommon

Hypersensitivity reactions

An apparent hypersensitivity reaction has been reported (< 1 %) This is characterised by multiple symptoms that may include: angio-oedema, pruritus, erythema, paraesthesia, loss of consciousness, vomiting, urticaria, flushing, dyspnoea, nausea, incontinence of urine and stool, cold sweats, shivering, chills, increased blood pressure, lip swelling, burning sensation, drug eruption, arthralgia, leg swelling, and tachycardia.

Investigations

Marked and persistent increases of serum transaminases have been reported infrequently (see section 4.4). In controlled clinical studies, the incidence of clinically important elevations in serum transaminases (ALT and/or AST $\geqslant$ 3 X ULN, consecutive) was 1.0 % for patients treated with 'Tredaptive' with or without a statin. These elevations were generally asymptomatic and returned to baseline after discontinuation of therapy or with continued treatment.

Clinically important elevations of CK ($\geqslant$ 10 X ULN) were seen in 0.3 % of the patients treated with 'Tredaptive' with or without a statin (see section 4.4).

Other abnormal laboratory values reported were elevations in LDH, fasting glucose, uric acid, total bilirubin, and amylase, and reductions in phosphorus and platelet counts (see section 4.4).

As with other nicotinic acid medicinal products, elevations in fasting glucose (a median increase of approximately 4 mg/dl), and uric acid (mean change from baseline of +14.7 %), and reductions in platelet counts (a mean change from baseline of -14.0 %) were reported in controlled clinical studies with 'Tredaptive' (2000 mg/40 mg) (see section 4.4). In diabetic patients a median increase in HbA_1c of 0.2 % was observed (where modification of hypoglycaemic therapy was allowed).

Nicotinic acid-related adverse reactions

The following nicotinic acid-related adverse reactions have been seen in clinical trials or post-marketing experience with other nicotinic acid medicinal products at unknown frequency or in clinical trials with 'Tredaptive' (or the nicotinic acid component of 'Tredaptive') in < 1 % of the patients treated:

Cardiac disorders: Atrial fibrillation and other cardiac arrhythmias, palpitations, tachycardia.

Nervous system disorders: Migraine, syncope.

Eye disorders: Cystoid macular oedema, toxic amblyopia.

Respiratory, thoracic, and mediastinal disorders: Dyspnoea.

Gastrointestinal disorders: Abdominal pain, mouth oedema, eructation, peptic ulcer.

Skin and subcutaneous tissue disorders: Acanthosis nigricans, dry skin, hyperpigmentation, macular rash, sweating (night or cold sweat), vesicular rash.

Musculoskeletal and connective tissue disorders: Muscular weakness, myalgia.

Metabolism and nutrition disorders: Impaired glucose tolerance, gout.

Infections and infestations: Rhinitis.

Vascular disorders: Hypotension, orthostatic hypotension.

General disorders and administration site conditions: Asthaenia, chills, face oedema, generalised oedema, pain, peripheral oedema.

Immune system disorders: Angio-oedema, type I hypersensitivity.

Hepatobiliary disorders: Jaundice.

Psychiatric disorders: Anxiety, insomnia.

4.9 Overdose

'Tredaptive'

In the event of an overdose, it is reasonable to employ the usual symptomatic and supportive measures. Cases of overdose have been reported; the maximum dose of 'Tredaptive' taken was 5000 mg/100 mg. All patients recovered without sequelae. The most commonly reported adverse reactions from the subjects who received this higher dose were consistent with a high dose of nicotinic acid and included: flushing, headache, pruritus, nausea, dizziness, vomiting, diarrhoea, epigastric and abdominal pain/discomfort, and back pain. Laboratory abnormalities included increased amylase and lipase, decreased haematocrit and occult blood in the stool.

Nicotinic acid

For an overdose of nicotinic acid, supportive measures should be employed.

Laropiprant

During controlled clinical trials in healthy subjects, single doses of up to 900 mg laropiprant and multiple doses up to 450 mg once daily for 10 days were generally well tolerated. There is no experience with doses of laropiprant above 900 mg in humans. Prolongation of collagen-induced platelet aggregation was observed in subjects taking multiple doses of 300 mg or greater (see section 5.1).

5. PHARMACOLOGICAL PROPERTIES

5.1 Pharmacodynamic properties

Pharmacotherapeutic group: nicotinic acid and derivatives, ATC code: C10AD52.

'Tredaptive' contains nicotinic acid, which at therapeutic doses is a lipid-modifying agent, and laropiprant, a potent, selective antagonist of the prostaglandin D_2 (PGD_2) receptor subtype 1 (DP_1). Nicotinic acid lowers the levels of low-density lipoprotein cholesterol (LDL-C), total cholesterol (TC), very low density lipoprotein cholesterol (VLDL-C), apolipoprotein B (apo B, the major LDL protein), triglycerides (TG), and lipoprotein(a) (Lp(a), a modified LDL particle) and elevates the levels of high-density lipoprotein cholesterol (HDL-C) and apolipoprotein A-I (apo A-I, the major protein component of HDL). Laropiprant suppresses PGD_2 mediated flushing associated with administration of nicotinic acid. Laropiprant has no effect on lipid levels nor does it interfere with the effects of nicotinic acid on lipids.

Nicotinic acid

Mechanism of action

The mechanisms by which nicotinic acid modifies the plasma lipid profile are not fully understood. Nicotinic acid inhibits release of free fatty acids (FFA) from adipose tissue, which may contribute to the reduced plasma LDL-C, TC, VLDL-C, apo B, TG, and Lp(a), as well as elevated HDL-C, and apo A-I, all of which are associated with lower cardiovascular risk. Additional explanations that do not invoke plasma FFA reduction as the central driver of lipid profile modification include nicotinic acid-mediated inhibition of *de novo* lipogenesis or esterification of fatty acids into TG in the liver.

Pharmacodynamic effects

Nicotinic acid causes a relative shift in the distribution of LDL subclasses from small, dense (most atherogenic) LDL particles to larger LDL particles. Nicotinic acid also elevates the HDL_2 subfraction to a greater extent than the HDL_3 subfraction, thereby increasing the HDL_2:HDL_3 ratio, which is associated with decreased cardiovascular disease risk. HDL is hypothesised to participate in the transport of cholesterol from tissues back to the liver, to suppress vascular inflammation associated with atherosclerosis, and to have anti-oxidative and anti-thrombotic effects.

Like LDL, cholesterol-enriched triglyceride-rich lipoproteins, including VLDL, intermediate-density lipoproteins (IDL), and remnants, can also promote atherosclerosis. Elevated plasma TG levels are frequently found in a triad with low HDL-C levels and small LDL particles, as well as in association with non-lipid metabolic risk factors for coronary heart disease (CHD).

Treatment with nicotinic acid reduces the risk of death and cardiovascular events, and slows progression or promotes regression of atherosclerotic lesions. The Coronary Drug Project, a five year study completed in 1975, showed that nicotinic acid had a statistically significant benefit in decreasing nonfatal, recurrent myocardial infarctions (MI) in men 30 to 64 years old with a history of MI. Though total mortality was similar in the two groups at five years, in a fifteen-year cumulative follow-up there were 11 % fewer deaths in the nicotinic acid group compared to the placebo cohort.

Laropiprant

Mechanism of action

Nicotinic acid-induced flushing is mediated primarily by release of prostaglandin D_2 (PGD_2) in the skin. Genetic and pharmacologic studies in animal models have provided evidence that PGD_2, acting through DP_1, one of the two receptors for PGD_2, plays a key role in nicotinic acid-induced flushing. Laropiprant is a potent and selective antagonist of DP_1. Laropiprant is not expected to inhibit the production of prostaglandins.

Pharmacodynamic effects

Laropiprant has been shown to be effective in reducing flushing symptoms induced by nicotinic acid. The reduction in flushing symptoms (assessed by patient questionnaires) was correlated with a reduction in nicotinic acid-induced vasodilatation (assessed by measurements of skin blood flow). In healthy subjects receiving 'Tredaptive', pretreatment with acetylsalicylic acid 325 mg had no additional beneficial effects in reducing nicotinic acid-induced flushing symptoms compared to 'Tredaptive' alone (see section 4.8).

Laropiprant also has affinity for the thromboxane A_2 receptor (TP) (although it is substantially less potent at TP as compared to DP_1). TP plays a role in platelet function; however, therapeutic doses of laropiprant had no clinically relevant effect on bleeding time and collagen-induced platelet aggregation (see section 4.5).

Clinical studies

Effect on lipids

'Tredaptive' was consistently efficacious across all pre-specified patient subpopulations defined by race, gender, baseline LDL-C, HDL-C and TG levels, age and diabetes status.

Patients taking 'Tredaptive' (2000 mg/40 mg) with or without a statin, versus placebo, had significantly decreased LDL-C (-18.9 % vs. -0.5 %), TG (-21.7 % vs. 3.6 %), LDL-C:HDL-C (-28.9 % vs. 2.3 %), non-HDL-C (-19.0 % vs. 0.8 %), apo B (-16.4 % vs. 2.5 %), TC (-9.2 % vs. -0.6 %), Lp(a) (-17.6 % vs. 1.1 %), and TC:HDL-C (-21.2 % vs. 1.9 %) and also had significantly increased HDL-C (18.8 % vs. -1.2 %), and apo A-I (11.2 % vs. 4.3 %) as measured by percent change from baseline. In general, the between-group treatment effects on all lipid parameters were consistent across all patient subgroups examined. Patients receiving 'Tredaptive', nicotinic acid (prolonged-released formulation), or placebo were also taking statins (29 % atorvastatin [5-80 mg], 54 % simvastatin [10-80 mg], 17 % other statins [2.5-180 mg] [pravastatin, fluvastatin, rosuvastatin, lovastatin]), of which 9 % were also taking ezetimibe (10 mg). The effect on lipids was similar whether 'Tredaptive' was given as monotherapy or was added to ongoing statin therapy with or without ezetimibe.

The placebo-adjusted LDL-C, HDL-C and TG responses appeared greater among women compared to men and appeared greater among elderly patients ($\geqslant$ 65 years) compared to younger patients (< 65 years).

In a multicentre, double-blind, 12-week factorial study, 'Tredaptive' 1000 mg/20 mg co-administered with simvastatin, when compared with simvastatin alone or 'Tredaptive' 1000 mg/20 mg alone, for 4 weeks, significantly lowered LDL-C (-44.2 %, -37.4 %, -8.2 % respectively), TG (-25.8 %, -15.7 %, -18.7 % respectively), TC (-27.9 %, -25.8 %, -4.9 % respectively) and significantly increased HDL-C (19.2 %, 4.2 %, 12.5 % respectively). 'Tredaptive' (2000 mg/40 mg) co-administered with simvastatin when compared with simvastatin alone or 'Tredaptive' (2000 mg/40 mg) alone for 12 weeks, significantly lowered LDL-C (-47.9 %, -37.0 %, -17.0 % respectively), TG (-33.3 %, -14.7 %, -21.6 % respectively), apo B (-41.0 %, -28.8 %, -17.1 % respectively), and TC (-29.6 %, -24.9 %, -9.1 % respectively), as well as LDL-C:HDL-C (-57.1 %, -39.8 %, -31.2 % respectively), non-HDL-C (-45.8 %, -33.4 %, -18.1 % respectively), and TC:HDL-C (-43.0 %, -28.0 %, -24.9 % respectively), and significantly increased HDL-C (27.5 %, 6.0 %, 23.4 % respectively). Further analysis showed 'Tredaptive' (2000 mg/40 mg) co-administered with simvastatin when compared with simvastatin alone significantly increased apo A-I (8.6 %, 2.3 % respectively) and significantly decreased Lp(a) (-19.8 %, 0.0 % respectively). Efficacy and safety of 'Tredaptive' in combination with simvastatin > 40 mg were not included in this study.

Flushing

In two large clinical trials measuring patient-reported flushing symptoms, patients taking 'Tredaptive' experienced less flushing than those taking nicotinic acid (prolonged-release formulations). In patients continuing in the first study (24 weeks), the frequency of moderate or greater flushing in patients treated with 'Tredaptive' declined and approached that of patients receiving placebo (see Figure 1), whereas in patients treated with nicotinic acid (prolonged-release formulation) the flushing frequency remained constant (after Week 6).

Flushing efficacy of laropiprant has not been established past 24 weeks.

Figure 1. Average number of days per week with moderate or greater* flushing symptoms across weeks 1-24

(see Figure 1 on next page)

In the second study (16 weeks) where acetylsalicylic acid was allowed, patients taking 'Tredaptive' experienced significantly fewer days per week with moderate or greater flushing compared to nicotinic acid (prolonged-release formulation taken as a 12-week multi-step 500 mg to 2000 mg titration) (p< 0.001).

Figure 1 Average number of days per week with moderate or greater* flushing symptoms across weeks 1-24

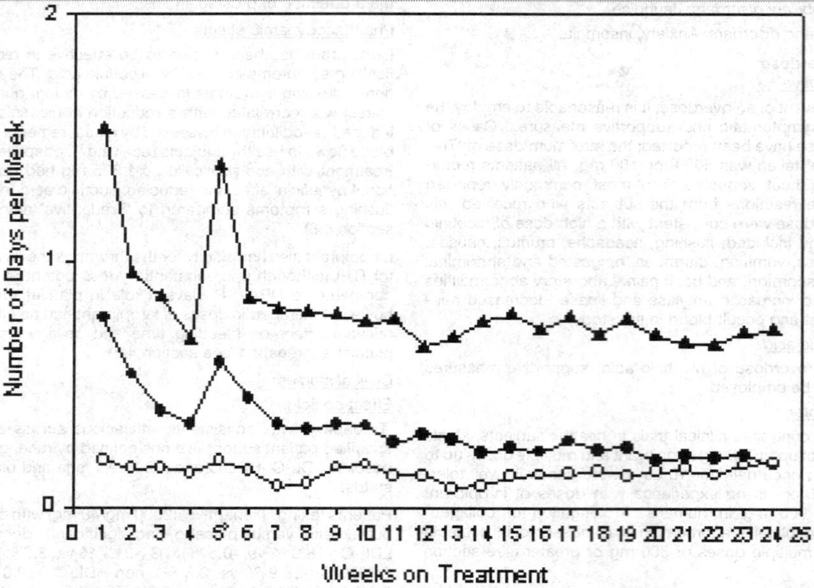

• 'Tredaptive' (1000 mg/20 mg to 2000 mg/40 mg at week 5)

▲ Nicotinic acid (prolonged-release 1000 mg to 2000 mg at week 5)

o Placebo

* Includes patients with moderate, severe, or extreme flushing symptoms

† Dose advancement at Week 5

5.2 Pharmacokinetic properties

Absorption

Nicotinic acid

Following a 2000 mg dose of nicotinic acid administered orally as two modified-release tablets of nicotinic acid/laropiprant with food, nicotinic acid was absorbed with a median time to peak plasma concentration (T_{max}) of 4 hours, a mean area under the plasma concentration-time curve ($AUC_{0\text{-}last}$) of approximately 58.0 μM·hr and a mean peak plasma concentration (C_{max}) of approximately 20.2 μM. Bioavailability with or without food is at least 72 % based on the recovery of the nicotinic acid dose in the urine. The oral bioavailability of nicotinic acid is not altered when it is taken with a high-fat meal.

Laropiprant

Following a 40 mg dose of laropiprant administered orally as two modified-release tablets of nicotinic acid/laropiprant with food, laropiprant is rapidly absorbed with a median T_{max} of 1 hour, a mean $AUC_{0\text{-}\infty}$ of approximately 13 μM·hr, and a mean C_{max} of approximately 1.6 μM. The rate and extent of absorption are not altered with a high-fat meal. The pharmacokinetics of laropiprant are linear, displaying approximately dose-proportional increases in AUC and C_{max} and no evidence of time-dependent clearance.

The mean absolute bioavailability of laropiprant is approximately 71 % following a 40 mg dose when administered as two modified-release tablets of nicotinic acid/laropiprant after an overnight fast.

Distribution

Nicotinic acid

Nicotinic acid is less than 20 % bound to serum proteins.

Laropiprant

The mean volume of distribution at steady state following a single 40 mg intravenous dose of laropiprant to healthy subjects is approximately 70 litres. Laropiprant is highly bound (> 99 %) to plasma proteins, and its binding is independent of concentration. Laropiprant crosses the placenta in rats and rabbits.

Metabolism

Nicotinic acid

Nicotinic acid undergoes extensive first-pass metabolism through two pathways that are dose and dose-rate dependent. The first pathway results in the formation of nicotinamide adenine dinucleotide (NAD) and nicotinamide. In humans, nicotinamide is further predominantly metabolised to N-methylnicotinamide (MNA) and to N-methyl-2-pyridone-5-carboxamide (2PY). In the second pathway, glycine is conjugated with nicotinic acid to form nicotinuric acid (NUA). With low doses of nicotinic acid or lower rates of absorption, the first pathway predominates. At higher doses or higher rates of absorption, the NAD pathway is saturable, and an increasing fraction of the oral dose reaches the bloodstream unchanged as nicotinic acid. The glycine conjugation pathway is not saturated across the clinically relevant dose range, based on the dose-proportional increase in the plasma concentrations of NUA from 1000 mg to 2000 mg.

In *in vitro* studies, nicotinic acid and its metabolites did not inhibit CYP1A2, CYP2B6, CYP2C9, CYP2C19, CYP2D6, CYP2E1, or CYP3A4-mediated reactions or UGT1A1-mediated 3-glucuronidation of estradiol.

Laropiprant

Laropiprant is metabolised primarily via acyl glucuronidation, with a smaller component of oxidative metabolism, followed by excretion of the glucuronide into faeces (via bile) and urine. Laropiprant and its acyl glucuronide conjugate are the major circulating components in human plasma. *In vitro* studies have shown that the acyl glucuronide conjugate of laropiprant had at least a 65-fold reduced affinity for DP_1 as compared to laropiprant; thus, it is not expected to contribute to the overall DP_1 activity of laropiprant. The major component (73 % of radioactivity) in faeces is laropiprant (comprising unabsorbed active substance and/or hydrolysed glucuronic acid conjugate). In urine, the primary component is the acyl glucuronide conjugate (64 % of radioactivity) with smaller contributions from the parent compound (5 %). The oxidative metabolism of laropiprant is catalysed primarily by CYP3A4, whereas several UGT isoforms (1A1, 1A3, 1A9 and 2B7) catalysed the acyl glucuronidation.

Elimination

Nicotinic acid

Nicotinic acid is predominantly excreted in the urine as metabolites.

Laropiprant

Laropiprant is eliminated primarily via acyl glucuronidation, followed by excretion of the glucuronide in faeces (via bile) and urine. Following oral administration of ^{14}C-laropiprant in humans, approximately 68 % of the dose was recovered in faeces (primarily as parent compound, comprising unabsorbed active substance and/or hydrolysed glucuronic acid conjugate) and 22 % was recovered in urine (primarily as metabolites). The majority of the dose was excreted within 96 hours. The apparent terminal half-life ($t_{1/2}$) following a 40 mg dose of laropiprant administered as two modified-release tablets of nicotinic acid/laropiprant with food was approximately 17 hours. Pharmacokinetic steady state is achieved within 2 days of once-daily dosing of laropiprant, with minimal accumulation in AUC (approximately 1.3-fold) and C_{max} (approximately 1.1-fold).

Characteristics in patients

Renal insufficiency

'Tredaptive': Use in patients with renal insufficiency has not been studied.

Nicotinic acid: see section 4.4.

Laropiprant: Administration of laropiprant 40 mg in non-dialysed patients with severe renal insufficiency resulted in no clinically meaningful change in the AUC and C_{max} of laropiprant, compared to healthy control subjects. As no effect was observed in severe renal insufficiency, no effect is expected in patients with mild and moderate renal insufficiency; however, the effects of end-stage renal failure and dialysis on laropiprant pharmacokinetics cannot be inferred from this study.

Hepatic insufficiency

'Tredaptive': Use in patients with hepatic insufficiency has not been studied.

Nicotinic acid: see sections 4.3 and 4.4.

Laropiprant: Consistent with the characteristics of a medicinal product that is primarily cleared by metabolism, moderate hepatic disease has a significant impact on laropiprant pharmacokinetics, with an increase in AUC and C_{max} of approximately 2.8- and 2.2-fold respectively.

Gender

Nicotinic acid: No dose adjustment is necessary based on gender. Gender has no clinically meaningful effect on pharmacokinetics of nicotinic acid (prolonged-release formulation). There is no difference in the oral bioavailability of nicotinic acid in men and women receiving 'Tredaptive'. Women have a modest increase in plasma concentrations of nicotinuric acid and nicotinic acid compared to men.

Laropiprant: No dose adjustment is necessary based on gender. Gender had no clinically meaningful effect on the pharmacokinetics of laropiprant.

Elderly

Nicotinic acid: There is no pharmacokinetic data in the elderly (⩾ 65 years). Age has no clinically meaningful effect on pharmacokinetics of nicotinic acid (prolonged-release formulation) based on a composite analysis of subjects ages 18-65 years. There is no change in the oral bioavailability of nicotinic acid with age.

Laropiprant: No dose adjustment is necessary in the elderly. Age had no clinically meaningful effect on the pharmacokinetics of laropiprant.

Paediatric

'Tredaptive': No studies have been performed in paediatric patients.

Race

Nicotinic acid: No dose adjustment is necessary based on race. Race has no clinically meaningful effect on the pharmacokinetics of nicotinic acid (prolonged-release formulation) based on pharmacokinetic data including subjects of Hispanic, White, Black, and Native American racial groups.

Laropiprant: No dose adjustment is necessary based on race. Race had no clinically meaningful effect on the pharmacokinetics of laropiprant based on a composite analysis of pharmacokinetic data including subjects of White, Hispanic, Black, Asian, and Native American racial groups.

5.3 Preclinical safety data

'Tredaptive'

Effects in non-clinical studies were observed only at exposures considered sufficiently in excess of the maximum human exposure, indicating little relevance to human use.

The safety of concomitant administration of nicotinic acid and laropiprant was assessed in dogs and rats. Toxicologic findings in these co-administration studies were consistent with those seen with nicotinic acid and laropiprant administered individually.

Nicotinic acid

Degeneration in the stomach and hepatocyte vacuolation were observed in rats following 6 months of dosing at systemic exposure values at least 179 times the human exposure based on the AUC of the recommended daily human dose. Retinopathy and/or corneal lesions were observed in dogs following 6 months of dosing at systemic exposure values at least 240 times the human exposure based on the AUC of the recommended daily human dose.

Nicotinic acid was not carcinogenic in mice when administered for the duration of their life. Mice in this study received approximately 9 to 13 times a human nicotinic acid dose of 2000 mg/day as determined on a mg/m^2 basis. Nicotinic acid showed no mutagenic effects in the *in vitro* assays.

No studies are available on possible effects of high dose nicotinic acid on fertility or on postnatal development after *in utero* exposure. Nicotinic acid induced reproduction toxic effects in rats when dosed at 1000 mg/kg/day during days 5-16 of gestation. Decreased placental and foetal weights were observed.

Laropiprant

Ketonuria and hepatocellular centrilobular hypertrophy were observed in rats in repeated dose toxicity studies for up to 6 months dosing. The hepatocellular centrilobular hypertrophy was consistent with rodent specific enzyme induction. The no-observed-adverse-effect level (NOAEL) was at least 118 times the human exposure based on the AUC of the recommended daily human dose.

Increases in serum alanine aminotransferase (ALT) levels were observed in all dog studies, at systemic exposure levels at least 14 times the human exposure based on the AUC of the recommended daily human dose. No other effects were observed in dog studies with exposures at least 100 times the human exposure based on the AUC of the recommended daily human dose.

Laropiprant was not carcinogenic in 2 year studies in mice and rats at the highest doses tested, which represents at least 218 to 289 times the human exposure based on the AUC of the recommended daily human dose.

Laropiprant was not mutagenic or clastogenic in a series of genetic toxicology studies.

No adverse effects on fertility were observed in male or female rats given laropiprant prior to mating and throughout mating, at systemic exposure levels at least 289 times the human exposure based on the AUC of the recommended daily human dose.

Laropiprant was not teratogenic in rats or in rabbits at least 153 and 438 times the human exposure based on the AUC of the recommended daily human dose. Reproduction toxicity studies showed slight treatment-related decreases in mean maternal weight gain and foetal body weight, slight increases in pup mortality, and increased incidence of supernumerary rib and incomplete ossification of the sternebra in the foetus were observed in rats at systemic exposure levels at least 513 times the human exposure based on the AUC of the recommended daily human dose.

6. PHARMACEUTICAL PARTICULARS

6.1 List of excipients

Hypromellose (E464)

Colloidal anhydrous silica (E551)

Sodium stearyl fumarate

Hydroxypropylcellulose (E463)

Microcrystalline cellulose (E460)

Croscarmellose sodium

Lactose monohydrate

Magnesium stearate

6.2 Incompatibilities

Not applicable.

6.3 Shelf life

2 years.

6.4 Special precautions for storage

PVC/Aclar blisters: Store in the original package in order to protect from light and moisture.

Aluminium/Aluminium blisters: Do not store above 30°C. Store in the original package in order to protect from light and moisture.

6.5 Nature and contents of container

Opaque PVC/Aclar blister with push-through aluminium lidding containing 14 modified-release tablets. Pack sizes of 14, 28, 56, 84, 98, 168 or 196 modified-release tablets, multi-packs containing 196 (2 packs of 98) modified-release tablets and 49 × 1 modified-release tablets in a perforated unit dose blister.

Aluminium/Aluminium blister with push-through lidding containing 7 modified-release tablets. Pack sizes of 14, 28, 56, 168 modified-release tablets, and 32x1 modified-release tablets in a perforated unit dose blister.

Not all pack sizes may be marketed.

6.6 Special precautions for disposal and other handling

No special requirements.

7. MARKETING AUTHORISATION HOLDER

Merck Sharp & Dohme Ltd.

Hertford Road, Hoddesdon

Hertfordshire EN11 9BU

United Kingdom

8. MARKETING AUTHORISATION NUMBER(S)

EU/1/08/459/002: Blister (Aclar/PVC)-28 tablets

EU/1/08/459/003: Blister (Aclar/PVC)-56 tablets

9. DATE OF FIRST AUTHORISATION/RENEWAL OF THE AUTHORISATION

03 July 2008

10. DATE OF REVISION OF THE TEXT

31 August 2009

Detailed information on this product is available on the website of the European Medicines Agency (EMEA) http://www.emea.europa.eu/.

® denotes registered trademark of Merck & Co., Inc., Whitehouse Station, NJ, USA.

SPC.TRE.09.UK.3096 II-008

Trental 400

(sanofi-aventis)

1. NAME OF THE MEDICINAL PRODUCT

TRENTAL 400.

2. QUALITATIVE AND QUANTITATIVE COMPOSITION

Pentoxifylline 400MG.

3. PHARMACEUTICAL FORM

Modified release tablet.

4. CLINICAL PARTICULARS

4.1 Therapeutic indications

Trental 400 is indicated in the treatment of peripheral vascular disease, including intermittent claudication and rest pain.

4.2 Posology and method of administration

The recommended initial dose is 1 tablet (400 mg) three times daily; two tablets daily may prove sufficient in some patients, particularly for maintenance therapy. Tablets should be taken with or immediately after meals, and swallowed whole with plenty of water.

Elderly: No special dosage requirements.

Children: Trental 400 is not suitable for use in children.

Special Cases: In patients with impairment of renal function (creatinine clearance below 30ml/min) a dose reduction by approximately 30% to 50% may be necessary guided by individual tolerance.

4.3 Contraindications

Trental 400 is contra-indicated in cases where there is known hypersensitivity to the active constituent, pentoxifylline other methyl xanthines or any of the excipients. Also in patients with cerebral haemorrhage, extensive retinal haemorrhage, acute myocardial infarction and severe cardiac arrhythmias.

4.4 Special warnings and precautions for use

In patients with hypotension or severe coronary artery disease, Trental 400 should be used with caution, as a transient hypotensive effect is possible and, in isolated cases, might result in a reduction in coronary artery perfusion.

Particularly careful monitoring is required in patients with impaired renal function. In patients with a creatinine clearance of less than 30 ml/min it may be necessary to reduce the daily dose of Trental 400 to one or two tablets to avoid accumulation. In patients with severely impaired liver function the dosage may need to be reduced.

4.5 Interaction with other medicinal products and other forms of interaction

High doses of Trental injection have been shown, in rare cases, to intensify the hypoglycaemic action of insulin and oral hypoglycaemic agents. However, no effect on insulin release has been observed with Trental following oral administration.

Trental 400 may potentiate the effect of anti-hypertensive agents and the dosage of the latter may need to be reduced.

Trental 400 should not be given concomitantly with ketorolac as there is increased risk of bleeding and/or prolongation of prothrombin time.

Concomitant administration of pentoxifylline and theophylline may increase theophylline levels in some patients. Therefore there may be an increase in and intensification of adverse effects of theophylline.

4.6 Pregnancy and lactation

There is no information on the use of Trental in pregnancy but no untoward effects have been found in animal studies. Trental 400 should not be administered during pregnancy.

Pentoxifylline passes into breast milk in minute quantities. Because insufficient experience has been gained, the possible risks and benefits must be weighed before administration of Trental 400 to breast feeding mothers.

4.7 Effects on ability to drive and use machines

No effect known.

4.8 Undesirable effects

Gastrointestinal side-effects (e.g. nausea, vomiting, diarrhoea), may occur which, in individual cases, could necessitate discontinuation of treatment. Headache, dizziness, agitation and sleep disorders may occasionally occur as well as, in isolated cases intrahepatic cholestasis and transaminase elevation.

There have been reports of flushing, occasionally tachycardia and rarely angina pectoris and hypotension, particularly if using high doses of pentoxifylline. In such cases a discontinuation of the medication or a reduction of the daily dosage is required.

Hypersensitivity reactions such as pruritus, rash, urticaria, anaphylactic or anaphylactoid reactions with angioneurotic edema or bronchospasm may occur in isolated cases and usually disappear rapidly after discontinuation of the drug treatment.

A few very rare events of bleeding (e.g. skin, mucosa) have been reported in patients treated with Trental with and without anticoagulants or platelet aggregation inhibitors. The serious cases are predominantly concentrated in the gastrointestinal, genitourinary, multiple site and surgical wound areas and are associated with bleeding risk factors. A causal relationship between Trental therapy and bleeding has not been established. Thrombocytopenia has occurred in isolated cases.

4.9 Overdose

The treatment of overdosage should be symptomatic with particular attention to supporting the cardiovascular system.

5. PHARMACOLOGICAL PROPERTIES

5.1 Pharmacodynamic properties

Leukocyte properties of haemorrheologic importance have been modified in animal and in vitro human studies. Pentoxifylline has been shown to increase leukocyte deformability and to inhibit neutrophil adhesion and activation.

5.2 Pharmacokinetic properties

The half life of absorption of Trental 400 is 4-6 hours. Pentoxifylline is extensively metabolised, mainly in the liver. Sixty percent of a single dose of Trental 400 is eliminated via the kidney over 24 hours.

5.3 Preclinical safety data

Nothing of clinical relevance.

6. PHARMACEUTICAL PARTICULARS

6.1 List of excipients

Hydroxyethyl cellulose, povidone, talc, magnesium stearate, hypromellose, macrogol 8000, erythrosine (E127). titanium dioxide (E171).

6.2 Incompatibilities

None known.

6.3 Shelf life

5 years.

6.4 Special precautions for storage

Do not store above 25°C. Store in the original package.

6.5 Nature and contents of container

Blister Pack (Alu/PVC): 90 tablets.

6.6 Special precautions for disposal and other handling

None.

Administrative Data

7. MARKETING AUTHORISATION HOLDER

Sanofi-aventis

One Onslow Street

Guildford

Surrey, GU1 4YS, UK

8. MARKETING AUTHORISATION NUMBER(S)

PL 04425/0213

9. DATE OF FIRST AUTHORISATION/RENEWAL OF THE AUTHORISATION

15th April 2002

10. DATE OF REVISION OF THE TEXT

October 2006

Legal category: POM

Treosulfan Capsules 250 mg (Medac UK)

(medac GmbH)

1. NAME OF THE MEDICINAL PRODUCT

Treosulfan Capsules 250 mg

2. QUALITATIVE AND QUANTITATIVE COMPOSITION

Capsules each containing 250 mg treosulfan as active substance.

For a full list of excipients see section 6.1.

3. PHARMACEUTICAL FORM

White opaque capsules.

4. CLINICAL PARTICULARS

4.1 Therapeutic indications

For the treatment of all types of ovarian cancer, either supplementary to surgery or palliatively. Some uncontrolled studies have suggested activity in a wider range of neoplasms.

Because of a lack of cross-resistance reported between Treosulfan and other cytotoxic agents Treosulfan may be useful in any neoplasm refractive to conventional therapy.

Treosulfan has been used in combination regimens in conjunction with vincristine, methotrexate, 5-FU and procarbazine.

4.2 Posology and method of administration

The following dosage regimens have been indicated. All regimens indicate that a total dose of 21-28 g of treosulfan should be given in the initial 8 weeks of treatment.

Regimen A: 1 g daily, given in four divided doses for four weeks, followed by four weeks off therapy.

Regimen B: 1 g daily, given in four divided doses for two weeks, followed by two weeks off therapy.

Regimen C: 1.5 g daily, given in three divided doses for one week only, followed by three weeks off therapy. If no evidence of haematological toxicity at this dose in Regimen C, increase to 2 g daily in four divided doses for one week for the second and subsequent courses.

These cycles should be repeated with the dose being adjusted if necessary, as outlined below, according to the effect on the peripheral blood counts. The capsules should be swallowed whole and not allowed to disintegrate within the mouth.

Dose modification (all regimens):

For excessive haematological toxicity (white blood cell count less than 3.000/microlitre or thrombocyte count less than 100.000/microlitre, a repeat blood count should be made after 1-2 weeks interval and treatment restarted if haematological parameters are satisfactory, reducing dose as follows:

Regimen A: 1 g daily × 28 to 0.75 g daily × 28 (and to 0.5 g daily × 28 if necessary).

Regimen B: 1 g daily × 14 to 0.75 g daily × 14 (and to 0.5 g daily × 14 if necessary).

Regimen C: 2 g daily × 7 to 1.5 g daily × 7 (and to 1 g daily × 7 if necessary).

Present evidence, whilst not definitive, suggests that Regimens B and C are less myelosuppressive than Regimen A, whilst retaining maximum cytotoxic efficacy.

Dosage in the elderly

Treosulfan is renally excreted. Blood counts should be carefully monitored in the elderly and the dosage adjusted accordingly.

Children

Treosulfan Capsules are not recommended for use in children.

4.3 Contraindications

Hypersensitivity to the active substance or to any of the excipients.

Severe and lasting bone marrow depression.

4.4 Special warnings and precautions for use

Risk of infections

The risk of infections (mycotic, viral, bacterial) is increased.

Haematological effects and monitoring of blood count

The dose limiting side effect of treosulfan is a myelosuppression, which is usually reversible. It is manifested by a reduction in leukocytes and platelets and a decrease in haemoglobin. The leukocytes and platelets usually reach their baseline level after 28 days.

Because the inhibition of bone marrow function is cumulative, the blood count should be monitored at shorter intervals starting with the third course of treatment.

This is especially important if combined with other forms of therapy that suppress bone marrow function such as radiotherapy.

Risk of malignancy

During a long term therapy with oral treosulfan doses eight patients (1.4 % of 553 patients) developed an acute non-lymphocytic leukaemia. The risk was depending on the cumulative dose of treosulfan. Single cases of myeloma, myeloproliferative disorder and myelodysplastic syndrome have additionally been reported.

Cardiac toxicity

It cannot be totally ruled out that one case of cardiomyopathy was related to treosulfan.

Pulmonary toxicity

If allergic alveolitis or pulmonary fibrosis develop treosulfan should be permanently discontinued.

Risk of stomatitis

Stomatitis may occur if the patients chew the capsule. Therefore the capsules should be swallowed whole.

Risk of cystitis

Because of the possible development of a haemorrhagic cystitis patients are advised to drink more fluids during the course of medication.

Use with vaccines

Cytostatic therapy may increase the risk of generalised infection after immunisation using live vaccines. Therefore live vaccines should not be used in patients receiving treosulfan.

4.5 Interaction with other medicinal products and other forms of interaction

In one patient the effect of ibuprofen/chloroquine was reduced with concomitant administration of treosulfan.

4.6 Pregnancy and lactation

Warning: This product should not normally be administered to patients who are pregnant or to mothers who are breast feeding.

Woman of childbearing age should take adequate contraceptive precautions.

4.7 Effects on ability to drive and use machines

Because of nausea and vomiting the ability to drive or operate machines may be influenced.

4.8 Undesirable effects

The most commonly reported adverse drug reactions are myelosuppression and gastrointestinal complaints. They are usually mild and resolve after therapy with treosulfan.

Frequency

Very common (≥1/10)

Common (≥1/100 to <1/10)

Uncommon (≥1/1,000 to <1/100)

Rare (≥1/10,000 to <1/1,000)

Very rare (<1/10,000)

Not known (cannot be estimated from the available data)

Within each frequency grouping, undesirable effects are presented in order of decreasing seriousness.

Frequency	
Very common ≥1/10	*Blood and lymphatic system disorders* Leucocytopenia, thrombocytopenia, anaemia, myelosuppression *Gastrointestinal disorders* Vomiting, nausea *Skin and subcutaneous tissue disorders* Alopecia (usually mild), bronze skin pigmentation
Uncommon (≥1/1,000 to <1/100	*Neoplasms benign, malignant and unspecified (incl cysts and polyps)* Treatment related secondary malignancies (acute non-lymphocytic leukaemia, myeloma, myeloproliferative disorder, myelodysplastic syndrome)
Not known	*Immune system disorders* Allergic reactions *Blood and lymphatic system disorders* Pancytopenia

The following undesirable effects have also been reported:

Addinson's disease, hypoglycaemia, paraesthesia, cardiomyopathy, stomatitis, alveolitis, pneumonia, pulmonary fibrosis, urticaria, erythema, scleroderma, triggering of psoriasis, haemorrhagic cystitis, flu-like complaints.

4.9 Overdose

Although there is no experience of acute overdosage with treosulfan, nausea, vomiting and gastritis may occur. Prolonged or excessive therapeutic doses may result in bone marrow depression which has occasionally been irreversible. The drug should be withdrawn, a blood transfusion given and general supportive measures given.

5. PHARMACOLOGICAL PROPERTIES

5.1 Pharmacodynamic properties

Pharmacotherapeutic group: Antineoplastic agents, ATC code: L 01 AB 02

Treosulfan is a bifunctional alkylating agent which has been shown to possess antineoplastic activity in the animal tumor screen and in clinical trials. The activity of treosulfan is due to the formation of epoxide compounds in vivo.

Treosulfan is converted in vitro under physiological conditions (pH 7.4; 37 °C) non-enzymatically via a monoepoxide to the diepoxide (diepoxybutane) with a half-life of 2.2 hours.

The epoxides formed react with nucleophilic centres of the DNA and are responsible via secondary biological mechanisms for the antineoplastic effect. It is important that in vivo the monoepoxide first formed can already alkylate a nucleophilic centre of the DNA. This fixes the compound to this centre by chemical reaction before the second epoxide ring is formed.

5.2 Pharmacokinetic properties

Oral absorption from treosulfan is excellent with the bioavailability approaching 100 %.

5.3 Preclinical safety data

Acute toxicity

In mice the oral LD_{50} is 3360 mg treosulfan/kg body weight and the intravenous LD_{50} >2500 mg treosulfan/kg body weight.

In rats the oral LD_{50} is 2575 mg treosulfan/kg body weight and the intraperitoneal LD_{50} > 2860 mg treosulfan/kg body weight.

Subacute toxicity

In monkeys receiving a subacute dose (56-111 mg/kg/day) the haematopoietic system was damaged. At higher doses (222-445 mg/kg/day) diarrhoea, anorexia and marked weight loss were also noted.

Chronic toxicity

Administration of treosulfan to rats for seven months led to a reduction in spermiogenesis in males and cycle disturbances in females. All other organs were unchanged.

Tumorogenic and mutagenic potential

In long-term therapy with oral treosulfan doses an acute non-lymphatic leukaemia was observed in 1.4 % of the patients.

Treosulfan, like other cytostatic agents with alkylating properties, has a mutagenic potential. Therefore, patients of child-bearing age should practice contraception while receiving treosulfan.

Reproductive toxicity

Treosulfan has not been tested for reproductive toxicity in animal experiments. However, during chronic toxicity testing in rats, a delayed spermiogenesis and the absence of corpora lutea and follicles was determined.

6. PHARMACEUTICAL PARTICULARS

6.1 List of excipients

Capsule content: maize starch, hydroxypropyl methylcellulose, magnesium stearate

Capsule shell: titanium dioxide E171, gelatine

6.2 Incompatibilities

None known

6.3 Shelf life

5 years

6.4 Special precautions for storage

This medicinal product does not require any special storage conditions.

6.5 Nature and contents of container

Amber glass bottles of 100 capsules.

6.6 Special precautions for disposal and other handling

The capsules should be swallowed whole and not allowed to disintegrate within the mouth.

7. MARKETING AUTHORISATION HOLDER

medac

Gesellschaft fuer klinische Spezialpraeparate

Fehlandtstraβe 3 · D-20354 Hamburg

Germany

Full information is available on request from

medac

Gesellschaft für klinische Spezialpräparate

Scion House

Stirling University Innovation Park

Stirling FK9 4NF

Tel.: 01786/ 458 086

Fax: 01786/ 458 032

8. MARKETING AUTHORISATION NUMBER(S)

11587/0001

9. DATE OF FIRST AUTHORISATION/RENEWAL OF THE AUTHORISATION

20/01/1992

10. DATE OF REVISION OF THE TEXT

24/06/2008

Treosulfan Injection (medac UK)

(medac GmbH)

1. NAME OF THE MEDICINAL PRODUCT

Treosulfan Injection

2. QUALITATIVE AND QUANTITATIVE COMPOSITION

Vials containing 1 g or 5 g Treosulfan.

3. PHARMACEUTICAL FORM

Powder for solution for injection or infusion.

A white crystalline powder.

4. CLINICAL PARTICULARS

4.1 Therapeutic indications

For the treatment of all types of ovarian cancer, either supplementary to surgery or palliatively. Some uncontrolled studies have suggested activity in a wider range of neoplasms.

Because of a lack of cross-resistance reported between treosulfan and other cytotoxic agents treosulfan may be useful in any neoplasm refractive to conventional therapy.

Treosulfan has been used in combination regimens in conjunction with vincristine, methotrexate, 5-FU and procarbazine.

4.2 Posology and method of administration

3 - 8 g/m^2 i.v. every 1-3 weeks depending on blood count and concurrent chemotherapy. Single injections of up to 8 g/m^2 have been given with no serious adverse effects. Doses up to 1.5 g/m^2 have been given intraperitoneally. Doses up to 3 g/m^2 treosulfan may be given as a bolus injection. Larger doses should be administered as an i.v. infusion at a rate of 3 g/m^2 every 5-10 minutes (8 g/m^2 as a 30 minutes infusion).

Treatment should not be given if the white blood cell count is less than 3.000/microlitre or the thrombocyte count less than 100.000/microlitre. A repeat blood count should be made after a weeks interval, when treatment may be restarted if haematological parameters are satisfactory. Lower doses of treosulfan should be used if other cytotoxic drugs or radiotherapy are being given concurrently. Treatment is initiated as soon as possible after diagnosis.

Care should be taken in administration of the injection to avoid extravasation into tissues since this will cause local pain and tissue damage. If extravasation occurs, the injection should be discontinued immediately and any remaining portion of the dose should be introduced into another vein.

Dosage in the elderly

Treosulfan is renally excreted. Blood counts should be carefully monitored in the elderly and the dosage adjusted accordingly.

Children

Treosulfan Injection is not recommended for use in children.

4.3 Contraindications

Hypersensitivity to the active substance.

Severe and lasting bone marrow depression.

4.4 Special warnings and precautions for use

Risk of infections

The risk of infections (mycotic, viral, bacterial) is increased.

Haematological effects and monitoring of blood count

The dose limiting side effect of treosulfan is a myelosuppression, which is usually reversible. It is manifested by a reduction in leukocytes and platelets and a decrease in haemoglobin. The leukocytes and platelets usually reach their baseline level after 28 days.

Because the inhibition of bone marrow function is cumulative, the blood count should be monitored at shorter intervals starting with the third course of treatment.

This is especially important if combined with other forms of therapy that suppress bone marrow function such as radiotherapy.

Risk of malignancy

During long term therapy with oral treosulfan doses eight patients (1.4% of 553 patients) developed an acute non-lymphocytic leukaemia. The risk was depending on the cumulative dose of treosulfan. Single cases of myeloma, myeloproliferative disorder and myelodysplastic syndrome have additionally been reported.

Cardiac toxicity

It cannot be totally ruled out that one case of cardiomyopathy was related to treosulfan.

Pulmonary toxicity

If allergic alveolitis or pulmonary fibrosis develop treosulfan should be permanently discontinued.

Risk of cystitis

Because of the possible development of a haemorrhagic cystitis patients are advised to drink more fluids for up to 24 hours after infusion.

Use with live vaccines

Cytostatic therapy may increase the risk of generalised infection after immunisation using live vaccines. Therefore live vaccines should not be used in patients receiving treosulfan.

Extravasation

During infusion, care must be taken to use a flawless technique, since painful inflammatory reactions may occur as a result of extravasation of treosulfan solution into surrounding tissue.

4.5 Interaction with other medicinal products and other forms of interaction

In one patient the effect of ibuprofen/chloroquine was reduced with concomitant administration of treosulfan.

4.6 Pregnancy and lactation

Warning: This product should not normally be administered to patients who are pregnant or to mothers who are breast feeding.

Woman of childbearing age should take adequate contraceptive precautions.

4.7 Effects on ability to drive and use machines

Because of nausea and vomiting the ability to drive or operate machines may be influenced.

4.8 Undesirable effects

The most commonly reported adverse drug reactions are myelosuppression and gastrointestinal complaints. They are usually mild and resolve after therapy with treosulfan.

Frequency

Very common (≥1/10)

Common (≥1/100 to <1/10)

Uncommon (≥1/1,000 to <1/100)

Rare (≥1/10,000 to <1/1,000)

Very rare (<1/10,000)

Within each frequency grouping, undesirable effects are presented in order of decreasing seriousness.

Frequency	
Very common ≥ 1/10	*Blood and lymphatic system disorders* Leucocytopenia, thrombocytopenia, anaemia, myelosuppression *Gastrointestinal disorders* Vomiting, nausea *Skin and subcutaneous tissue disorders* Alopecia (usually mild), bronze skin pigmentation
Uncommon (≥1/1,000 to <1/100	*Neoplasms benign, malignant and unspecified (incl cysts and polyps)* Treatment related secondary malignancies (acute non-lymphocytic leukaemia, myeloma, myeloproliferative disorder, myelodysplastic syndrome)
Not known	*Immune system disorders* Allergic reactions *Blood and lymphatic system disorders* Pancytopenia

The following undesirable effects have also been reported:

Addison's disease, hypoglycaemia, paraesthesia, cardiomyopathy, alveolitis, pneumonia, pulmonary fibrosis, urticaria, erythema, scleroderma, triggering of psoriasis, haemorrhagic cystitis, flu-like complaints, local painful inflammatory reactions (in cases of extravasation).

4.9 Overdose

Although there is no experience of acute overdosage with treosulfan, nausea, vomiting and gastritis may occur. Prolonged or excessive therapeutic doses may result in bone marrow depression which has occasionally been irreversible. The drug should be withdrawn, a blood transfusion given and general supportive measures given.

5. PHARMACOLOGICAL PROPERTIES

5.1 Pharmacodynamic properties

Pharmacotherapeutic group: Antineoplastic agents, ATC code: L 01 AB 02

Treosulfan is a bifunctional alkylating agent which has been shown to possess antineoplastic activity in the animal tumor screen and in clinical trials. The activity of treosulfan is due to the formation of epoxide compounds in vivo.

Treosulfan is converted in vitro under physiological conditions (pH 7.4; 37 °C) non-enzymatically via a monoepoxide to the diepoxide (diepoxybutane) with a half-life of 2.2 hours.

The epoxides formed react with nucleophilic centres of the DNA and are responsible via secondary biological mechanisms for the antineoplastic effect. It is important that in vivo the monoepoxide first formed can already alkylate a nucleophilic centre of the DNA. This fixes the compound to this centre by chemical reaction before the second epoxide ring is formed.

5.2 Pharmacokinetic properties

After intravenous administration treosulfan is rapidly distributed in the body.

Elimination follows a 1st order kinetics with a half-life of 1.6 h. Approximately 30 % of the substance are excreted unchanged with the urine within 24 hours, nearly 90 % of which within the first 6 hours after administration.

5.3 Preclinical safety data

Acute toxicity

In mice the oral LD_{50} is 3360 mg treosulfan/kg body weight and the intravenous LD_{50} >2500 mg treosulfan/kg body weight.

In rats the oral LD_{50} is 2575 mg treosulfan/kg body weight and the intraperitoneal LD_{50} > 2860 mg treosulfan/kg body weight.

Subacute toxicity

In monkeys receiving a subacute dose (56-111 mg/kg/day) the haematopoietic system was damaged. At higher doses (222-445 mg/kg/day) diarrhoea, anorexia and marked weight loss were also noted.

Chronic toxicity

Administration of treosulfan to rats for seven months led to a reduction in spermiogenesis in males and cycle disturbances in females. All other organs were unchanged.

Tumorogenic and mutagenic potential

In long-term therapy with oral treosulfan doses an acute non-lymphatic leukaemia was observed in 1.4 % of the patients.

Treosulfan, like other cytostatic agents with alkylating properties, has a mutagenic potential. Therefore, patients of child-bearing age should practice contraception while receiving treosulfan.

Reproductive toxicity

Treosulfan has not been tested for reproductive toxicity in animal experiments. However, during chronic toxicity testing in rats, a delayed spermiogenesis and the absence of corpora lutea and follicles was determined.

6. PHARMACEUTICAL PARTICULARS

6.1 List of excipients

None.

6.2 Incompatibilities

No incompatibilities are as yet known.

6.3 Shelf life

5 years when stored at room temperature.

The drug product should not be used after the expiration date.

Once brought into solution the injection should be used immediately.

6.4 Special precautions for storage

This medicinal product does not require any special storage conditions.

6.5 Nature and contents of container

100 ml colourless infusion glass vial (glass type I or II) with butyl rubber stopper and cap of aluminium completed with labels with integrated hanger.

100 ml colourless injection glass vial (glass type III) with butyl rubber stopper and cap of aluminium completed with labels with integrated hanger.

Each vial contains 1 g or 5 g treosulfan.

The vials are packed in boxes of 5.

6.6 Special precautions for disposal and other handling

Route of administration

Treosulfan Injection 1 g or 5 g is used for intravenous infusion after being dissolved in 20 or 100 ml of water for injection.

As with all cytotoxic substances, appropriate precautions should be taken when handling treosulfan.

Guidelines for the safe handling of antineoplastic agents:

1. Trained personnel should reconstitute the drug.

2. This should be performed in a designated area.

3. Adequate protective gloves, masks and clothing should be worn.

4. Precautions should be taken to avoid the drug accidentally coming into contact with the eyes.

5. Cytotoxic preparations should not be handled by staff who may be pregnant.

6. Adequate care and precautions should be taken in the disposal of items (syringes, needles, etc.) used to reconstitute cytotoxic drugs.

7. The work surface should be covered with disposable plastic-backed absorbent paper.

8. Use Luer-lock fittings on all syringes and sets. Large bore needles are recommended to minimise pressure and the possible formation of aerosols. The latter may also be reduced by the use of a venting needle.

Instructions for reconstitution of Treosulfan Injection

To avoid solubility problems during reconstitution the following aspects should be regarded.

1. The solvent, water for injection, is warmed to 25 - 30 °C (not higher !) by using a water bath.

2. The treosulfan is carefully removed from the inner surface of the infusion bottle by shaking.

This procedure is very important, because moistening of powder that sticks to the surface results in caking. In case caking occurs the bottle has to be shaken long and vigorously.

3. One side of the double sided cannula is put into the rubber stopper of the water bottle. The treosulfan bottle is then put on the other end of the cannula with the bottom on top. The whole construction is converted and the water let run into the lower bottle while the bottle is shaken gently.

Following these instructions, the whole reconstitution procedure should take not longer than 2 minutes.

7. MARKETING AUTHORISATION HOLDER

medac

Gesellschaft fuer klinische Spezialpraeparate

Fehlandtstrasse 3 · D-20354 Hamburg

Germany

8. MARKETING AUTHORISATION NUMBER(S)

11587/0002

9. DATE OF FIRST AUTHORISATION/RENEWAL OF THE AUTHORISATION

20/01/1992

10. DATE OF REVISION OF THE TEXT

24th June 2008

Full information is available on request from

medac

Gesellschaft für klinische Spezialpräparate

Scion House

Stirling University Innovation Park

Stirling FK9 4NF

Tel.: 01786/ 458 086

Fax: 01786/ 458 032

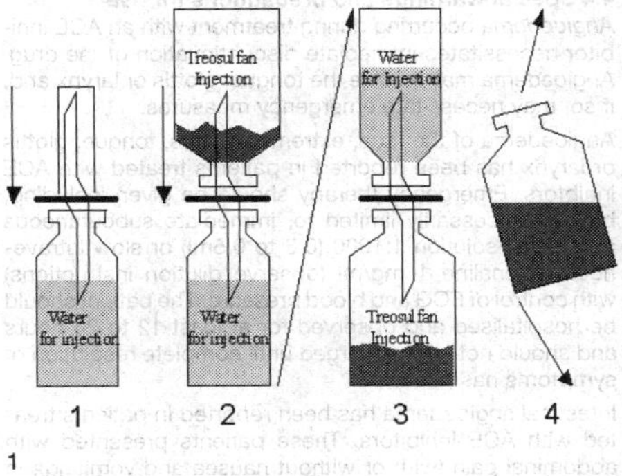

1

Triapin & Triapin Mite

(sanofi-aventis)

1. NAME OF THE MEDICINAL PRODUCT

Triapin mite 2.5mg/2.5mg prolonged release tablet

Triapin 5mg/5mg prolonged release tablet

2. QUALITATIVE AND QUANTITATIVE COMPOSITION

Triapin Mite: Each tablet contains 2.5 mg of felodipine and 2.5 mg of ramipril.

Each tablet contains 52 mg lactose anhydrous.

Triapin: Each tablet contains 5 mg of felodipine and 5 mg of ramipril.

Each tablet contains 51.5 mg lactose anhydrous.

For a full list of excipients, see section 6.1

3. PHARMACEUTICAL FORM

Triapin Mite 2.5mg/2.5mg tablets are circular (diameter approx 9 mm), apricot coloured, biconvex and engraved $\frac{H}{OD}$ on one side and marked 2.5 on the other side.

Triapin 5mg/5mg tablets are circular (diameter approx 9 mm), reddish-brown coloured, biconvex and engraved $\frac{H}{OE}$ on one side and marked 5 on the other side.

4. CLINICAL PARTICULARS

4.1 Therapeutic indications

Treatment of essential hypertension. Triapin mite/Triapin fixed dose combination is indicated in patients whose blood pressure is not adequately controlled on felodipine or ramipril alone.

4.2 Posology and method of administration

Use in adults, including elderly:

Triapin Mite: One tablet Triapin mite daily. The maximum dose is two tablets Triapin mite once daily.

Triapin: One tablet Triapin once daily, which is also the maximum dose.

Use in patients with impaired liver function:

See sections 4.3 and 4.4.

Use in patients with impaired renal function or patients already on diuretic treatment:

See sections 4.3 and 4.4.

Individual dose titration with the components can be recommended and when clinically appropriate, direct change from monotherapy to the fixed combination may be considered.

Use in children:

Triapin Mite is not recommended for use in children due to a lack of data.

Administration

The tablets should be swallowed whole with a sufficient amount of liquid. The tablets must not be divided, crushed or chewed.

The tablet can be administered without food or following a light meal not rich in fat or carbohydrate.

4.3 Contraindications

Triapin Mite/Triapin must not be used:

• in patients with hypersensitivity to felodipine (or other dihydropyridines), ramipril, other angiotensin converting enzyme (ACE) inhibitors or any of the excipients of Triapin mite/Triapin.

• in patients with a history of angioedema.

• in unstable haemodynamic conditions: cardiovascular shock, untreated heart failure, acute myocardial infarction, unstable angina pectoris, stroke.

• in patients with AV block II or III.

• in patients with severely impaired hepatic function.

• in patients with severely impaired renal function (creatinine clearance less than 20 ml/min) and in patients on dialysis.

• during pregnancy.

• during lactation.

4.4 Special warnings and precautions for use

Angioedema occurring during treatment with an ACE inhibitor necessitates immediate discontinuation of the drug. Angioedema may involve the tongue, glottis or larynx and, if so, may necessitate emergency measures.

Angioedema of the face, extremeties, lips, tongue, glottis or larynx has been reported in patients treated with ACE inhbitors. Emergency therapy should be given including, but not necessarily limited to, immediate subcutaneous adrenaline solution 1:1000 (0.3 to 0.5ml) or slow intravenous adrenaline 1 mg/ml (observe dilution instructions) with control of ECG and blood pressure. The patient should be hospitalised and observed for at least 12 to 24 hours and should not be discharged until complete resolution of symptoms has occurred.

Intestinal angioedema has been reported in patients treated with ACE inhibitors. These patients presented with abdominal pain (with or without nausea and vomiting); in some cases there was no prior history of facial angioedema and C1-esterase levels were normal. The angioedema was diagnosed by procedures including abdominal CT scan or ultrasound, or at surgery, and symptoms resolved after stopping the ACE inhibitor. Intestinal angioedema should be included in the differential diagnosis of patients on ACE inhibitors presenting with abdominal pain.

Compared with non-black patients, a higher incidence of angioedema has been reported in black patients treated with ACE inhibitors.

Renal function should be monitored, particularly in the initial weeks of treatment with ACE inhibitors. Caution should be observed in patients with an activated renin-angiotensin system.

Patients with mild to moderately impaired renal function (creatinine clearance 20-60 ml/min) and patients already on diuretic treatment. For dosage see the respective monoproducts

Hyperkalaemia. Elevations in serum potassium have been observed in some patients treated with ACE inhibitors, including ramipril. Patients at risk for the development of hyperkalaemia include those with renal insufficiency, diabetes mellitus, or those using concomitant potassium-sparing diuretics, potassium supplements or potassium-containing salt substitutes; or those patients taking other drugs associated with increases in serum potassium (e.g. heparin). If concomitant use of the above mentioned agents is deemed appropriate, regular monitoring of serum potassium is recommended

Proteinuria: It may occur particularly in patients with existing renal function impairment or on relatively high doses of ACE inhibitors.

Renovascular hypertension/renal artery stenosis: There is an increased risk of severe hypotension and renal insufficiency when patients with renovascular hypertension and pre-existing bilateral renal artery stenosis or stenosis of the artery to a solitary kidney are treated with ACE inhibitors. Loss of renal function may occur with only mild changes in serum creatinine even in patients with unilateral renal artery stenosis.

There is no experience regarding the administration of Triapin mite/Triapin in patients with a recent kidney transplantation.

Hepatic failure: Rarely, ACE inhibitors have been associated with a syndrome that starts with cholestatic jaundice and progress to fulminant hepatic necrosis and (sometimes) death. The mechanism of this syndrome is not understood. Patients receiving ACE inhibitors who develop jaundice or marked elevations of hepatic enzymes should discontinue the ACE inhibitor and receive appropriate medical follow up.

Patients with mild to moderately impaired liver function: For dosage see respective monoproducts

Surgery/Anaesthesia: Hypotension may occur in patients undergoing major surgery or during treatment with anaesthetic agents that are known to lower blood pressure. If hypotension occurs, it may be corrected by volume expansion.

Aortic stenosis/Hypertrophic cardiomyopathy: ACE inhibitors should be used with caution in patients with haemodynamically relevant left-ventricular inflow or outflow impediment (e.g. stenosis of the aortic or mitral valve, obstructive cardiomyopathy). The initial phase of treatment requires special medical supervision.

Symptomatic hypotension: In some patients, symptomatic hypotension may be observed after the initial dose, mainly in patients with heart failure (with or without renal insufficiency) treated with high doses of loop diuretics, in hyponatraemia or in reduced renal function. Therefore, Triapin mite/Triapin should only be given to such patients after special consideration and after the doses of the individual components have been carefully titrated. Triapin mite/Triapin should only be given if the patient is in a stable circulatory condition (see Section 4.3). In hypertensive patients without cardiac and renal insufficiency, hypotension may occur especially in patients with decreased blood volume due to diuretic therapy, salt restriction, diarrhoea or vomiting.

Patients who would be at particular risk from an undesirably pronounced reduction in blood pressure (e.g. patients with coronary or cerebrovascular insufficiency) should be treated with ramipril and felodipine in a free combination. If satisfactory and stable blood pressure control is achieved with the doses of ramipril and felodipine included in Triapin mite/Triapin, the patient can be switched to this combination. In some cases, felodipine may cause hypotension with tachycardia, which may aggravate angina pectoris.

Neutropenia/Agranulocytosis: Triapin mite/Triapin may cause agranulocytosis and neutropenia. These undesirable effects have also been shown with other ACE inhibitors, rarely in uncomplicated patients but more frequently in patients with some degree of renal impairment, especially when it is associated with collagen vascular disease (e.g. systemic lupus erythematodes, scleroderma) and therapy with immunosuppressive agents. Monitoring of white blood cell counts should be considered for patients who have collagen vascular disease, especially if the disease is associated with impaired renal function. Neutropenia and agranulocytosis are reversible after discontinuation of the ACE inhibitor. Should symptoms such as fever, swelling of the lymph nodes, and/or inflammation of the throat occur in the course of therapy with Triapin mite/Triapin, the treating physician must be consulted and the white blood picture investigated immediately.

Cough: During treatment with an ACE inhibitor a dry cough may occur which disappears after discontinuation.

Concomitant treatment with ACE inhibitors and antidiabetics (insulin and oral antidiabetics) may lead to an enhanced hypoglycaemic effect with the risk of hypoglycaemia. This effect may be most pronounced at the beginning of treatment and in patients with impaired renal function.

Felodipine is metabolised by CYP3A4. Therefore, combination with medicinal products which are potent CYP3A4 inhibitors or inducers should be avoided. For the same reason, the concomitant intake of grapefruit juice should be avoided (see Section 4.5).

Lithium: The combination of lithium and ACE inhibitor is not recommended. (see Section 4.5).

LDL-apheresis: Concomitant use of ACE inhibitors and extracorporeal treatments leading to contact of blood with negatively charged surfaces should be avoided since it may lead to severe anaphylactoid reactions. Such extracorporeal treatments include dialysis or haemofiltration with certain high-flux (e.g. polyacrylonitrile) membranes and low-density lipoprotein apheresis with dextran sulphate.

Desensitisation therapy: Increased likelihood and greater severity of anaphylactic and anaphylactoid reactions to insect venom (e.g. bee and wasp) as for other ACE inhibitors.

Ethnic differences: As with other angiotensin converting enzyme inhibitors, ramipril is apparently less effective in lowering blood pressure in black people than in non-blacks, possibly because of a higher prevalence of low-renin states in the black hypertensive population.

Children, patients with creatinine clearance under 20 ml/min and dialysis-treated patients: No experience is available. Triapin mite/Triapin should not be given to these patient groups.

This product contains lactose. Patients with rare hereditary problems of galactose intolerance, the Lapp lactase deficiency or glucose-galactose malabsorption should not take this medicine.

4.5 Interaction with other medicinal products and other forms of interaction

Not recommended associations

Potassium salts, potassium-retaining diuretics: Rise in serum potassium concentration is to be anticipated. Concomitant treatment with potassium-retaining diuretics (e.g. spironolactone, triamterene, or amiloride) or with potassium salts requires close monitoring of serum potassium.

Felodipine is a CYP3A4 substrate. Drugs that induce or inhibit CYP3A4 will have large influence on felodipine plasma concentrations.

Drugs that increase the metabolism of felodipine through induction of cytochrome P450 3A4 include carbamazepine, phenytoin, phenobarbital and rifampin as well as St John's wort (Hypericum perforatum). During concomitant administration of felodipine with carbamazepine, phenytoin, phenobarbital, AUC decreased by 93% and C_{max} by 82%. A similar effect is expected with St John's wort. Combination with CYP3A4 inducers should be avoided.

Potent inhibitors of cytochrome P450 3A4 include azole antifungals, macrolide antibiotics, telithomycin and HIV protease inhibitors. During concomitant administration of felodipine with itraconazole, C_{max} increased 8-fold and AUC 6-fold. During concomitant administration of felodipine with erythromycin, C_{max} and AUC increased approximately 2.5-fold. Combination with potent CYP3A4 inhibitors should be avoided.

Grapefruit juice inhibits cytochrome P450 3A4. Concomitant administration of felodipine with grapefruit juice increased felodipine C_{max} and AUC approximately 2-fold. The combination should be avoided.

Caution is recommended with concomitant use

Lithium: Excretion of lithium may be reduced by ACE inhibitors, leading to lithium toxicity. Lithium levels must, therefore, be monitored.

Antihypertensive agents and other substances with blood pressure lowering potential (e.g. nitrates, antipsychotics, narcotics, anaesthetics): Potentiation of the antihypertensive effect of Triapin mite/Triapin is to be anticipated.

Allopurinol, immunosuppressants, corticosteroids, procainamide, cytostatics and other substances that may change the blood picture: Increased likelihood of haematological reactions.

Nonsteroidal anti-inflammatory drugs (NSAIDS): Attenuation of the effect of ramipril is to be expected. Furthermore, concomitant treatment with ACE inhibitors and such drugs may lead to an increased risk of worsening of the renal function and an increase in serum potassium.

Vasopressor sympathomimetics: These may reduce the antihypertensive effect of Triapin mite/Triapin. Particularly close blood pressure monitoring is recommended.

Insulin, metformin, sulphonylureas: Concomitant treatment with ACE inhibitors and antidiabetic agents may cause a pronounced hypoglycaemic effect with the risk of hypoglycaemia. This effect is most pronounced at the beginning of treatment.

Theophylline: Concomitant administration of felodipine and oral theophylline reduces theophylline absorption by approximately 20%. This is probably of minor clinical importance.

Tacrolimus: Felodipine may increase the concentration of tacrolimus. When used together, the tacrolimus serum concentration should be followed and the tacrolimus dose may need to be adjusted.

Heparin: Rise in serum potassium concentration possible.

Salt: Increased dietary salt intake may attenuate the antihypertensive effect of Triapin mite.

Alcohol: Increased vasodilatation. The antihypertensive effect of Triapin mite/Triapin may increase.

4.6 Pregnancy and lactation

Use in pregnancy

Triapin mite/Triapin is contraindicated (see Section 4.3) in pregnancy.

Calcium antagonists may inhibit contractions of the uterus during labour. Definite evidence that labour is prolonged in full-term pregnancy is lacking. Risk of foetal hypoxia may occur if the mother is hypotensive and perfusion of the uterus is reduced due to redistribution of the blood-flow through peripheral vasodilatation. In animal experiments, calcium antagonists have caused embryotoxic and/or teratogenic effects, especially in the form of distal skeletal malformations in several species.

Appropriate and well-controlled studies with ramipril have not been done in humans. ACE inhibitors cross the placenta and can cause foetal and neonatal morbidity and mortality when administered to pregnant women.

Foetal exposure to ACE inhibitors during the second and third trimesters has been associated with neonatal hypotension, renal failure, face or skull deformities and/or death. Maternal oligohydramnios have also been reported reflecting decreasing renal function in the foetus. Limb contractures, craniofacial deformities, hypoplastic lung development and intrauterine growth retardation have been reported in association with oligohydramnios. Intrauterine growth retardation, prematurity, persistent ductus arteriosus and foetal death have also been reported, but it is not clear whether they are related to the ACE inhibitor or to the underlying maternal disease. Whether exposure limited to the first trimester can adversely effect foetal outcome is not known.

Use in lactation

In animals, ramipril is excreted in milk. No information is available on whether or not ramipril is excreted in human breast-milk. Felodipine is excreted in human breast-milk.

Women must not breast-feed during treatment with Triapin mite/Triapin (see Section 4.3).

4.7 Effects on ability to drive and use machines

Some undesirable effects (e.g. some symptoms of reduction in blood pressure such as dizziness) may be accompanied by an impairment of the ability to concentrate and react. This may constitute a risk in situations where these abilities are of special importance, e.g., when driving a car or operating machinery.

4.8 Undesirable effects

The frequencies used in the tables throughout this section are: very common (⩾ 1/10), common (⩾ 1/100, <1/10), uncommon (>1/1000, <1/100), rare (>1/10 000, <1/1000) and very rare (<1/10 000),

The following undesirable effects may occur in connection with felodipine treatment

(see Table 1 below)

The following undesirable effects may occur in connection with ramipril treatment

(see Table 2 on next page)

4.9 Overdose

Symptoms

Overdosage may cause excessive peripheral vasodilatation with marked hypotension, bradycardia, shock, electrolyte disturbances and renal failure.

Management

Primary detoxification by, for example, gastric lavage, administration of adsorbents and/or sodium sulphate (if possible during the first 30 minutes). In case of hypotension, administration of α_1-adrenergic sympathomimetics and angiotensin II must be considered in addition to volume and salt substitution. Bradycardia or extensive vagal reactions should be treated by administering atropine.

No experience is available concerning the efficacy of forced diuresis, alteration in urine pH, haemofiltration, or dialysis in speeding up the elimination of ramipril or ramiprilat. If dialysis or haemofiltration is nevertheless considered, see also under 4.4 Special Warnings and Special Precautions for use.

5. PHARMACOLOGICAL PROPERTIES

5.1 Pharmacodynamic properties

Pharmacotherapeutic group: Antihypertensive drugs. ATC code: C09B B05

Both the calcium antagonist felodipine and the ACE inhibitor ramipril reduce blood pressure by dilation of the peripheral blood vessels. Calcium antagonists dilate the arterial beds while ACE inhibitors dilate both arterial and venous beds. Vasodilatation and thereby reduction of blood pressure may lead to activation of the sympathetic nervous system and the renin-angiotensin system. Inhibition of ACE results in decreased plasma angiotensin II.

The onset of the antihypertensive effect of a single dose of Triapin mite/Triapin is 1 to 2 hours. The maximum antihypertensive effect is achieved within 2 to 4 weeks and is maintained during long-term therapy. The blood pressure reduction is maintained throughout the 24-hour dosage interval. Morbidity and mortality data are not available.

Felodipine is a vascular selective calcium antagonist, which lowers arterial blood pressure by decreasing peripheral vascular resistance via a direct relaxant action on vascular smooth muscles. Due to its selectivity for smooth muscle in the arterioles, felodipine, in therapeutic doses, has no direct effect on cardiac contractility or conduction. The renal vascular resistance is decreased by felodipine. The normal glomerular filtration rate is not influenced. In patients with impaired renal function, the glomerular filtration rate may increase. Felodipine possesses a mild natriuretic/diuretic effect and fluid retention does not occur.

Ramipril is a prodrug which hydrolyses to the active metabolite ramiprilat, a potent and long-acting ACE (angiotensin converting enzyme) inhibitor. In plasma and tissue, ACE catalyses the conversion of angiotensin I to the vasoconstrictor angiotensin II and also the breakdown of the vasodilator bradykinin. The vasodilatation induced by the ACE inhibitor reduces blood pressure pre-load and after-load. Since angiotensin II also stimulates the release of aldosterone, ramiprilat reduces secretion of aldosterone. Ramipril reduces peripheral arterial resistance without major changes in renal plasma flow or glomerular filtration rate. In hypertensive patients, ramipril leads to a reduction in supine and standing blood pressure without a compensatory rise in heart rate.

5.2 Pharmacokinetic properties

General characteristics of the active substances

Felodipine ER (extended-release formulation): The bioavailability is approximately 15% and is not influenced by concomitant intake of food. The peak plasma concentration is reached after 3 to 5 hours. Binding to plasma proteins is more than 99%. The distribution volume at steady state is 10 l/kg. The half-life for felodipine in the elimination phase is approximately 25 hours and steady state is reached after 5 days. There is no risk of accumulation during long-term treatment. Mean clearance is 1200 ml/min. Decreased clearance in elderly patients leads to higher plasma concentrations of felodipine. Age only partly explains the inter-individual variation in plasma concentration, however. Felodipine is metabolised in the liver and all identified metabolites are devoid of vasodilating properties. Approximately 70% of a given dose is excreted as metabolites in the urine and about 10% with the faeces. Less than 0.5% of the dose is excreted unchanged in the urine. Impaired renal function does not influence the plasma concentration of felodipine.

Ramipril: The pharmacokinetic parameters of ramiprilat are calculated after intravenous administration of ramipril. Ramipril is metabolised in the liver, and aside from the active metabolite ramiprilat, pharmacologically inactive metabolites have been identified. The formation of active ramiprilat may be decreased in patients with impaired liver function. The metabolites are excreted mainly via the kidneys. The bioavailability of ramiprilat is approximately 28% after oral administration of ramipril. After intravenous administration of 2.5 mg ramipril, approximately 53% of the dose is converted to ramiprilat. A maximum serum concentration of ramiprilat is achieved after 2 to 4 hours. Absorption and bioavailability are not influenced by concomitant intake of food. The protein binding of ramiprilat is approximately 55%. The distribution volume is approximately 500 litres. The effective half-life, after repeated daily dosage of 5 to 10 mg, is 13 to 17 hours. Steady-state is achieved after approximately 4 days. Renal clearance is 70 to 100 ml/min and total clearance is approximately 380 ml/min. Impaired renal function delays the elimination of ramiprilat and excretion in the urine is reduced.

Characteristics of the combination product

In Triapin mite/Triapin the pharmacokinetics of ramipril, ramiprilat and felodipine are essentially unaltered compared to the monoproducts, felodipine ER tablets and ramipril tablets. Felodipine does not influence the ACE inhibition caused by ramiprilat. The fixed combination tablets are thus regarded as bioequivalent to the free combination.

5.3 Preclinical safety data

Repeated-dose toxicity studies performed with the combination in rats and monkeys did not demonstrate any synergistic effects.

Non-clinical data for felodipine and ramipril reveal no special hazard for humans based on conventional studies of genotoxicity and carcinogenic potential.

Reproduction toxicity

Felodipine: In investigations on fertility and general reproductive performance in rats, a prolongation of parturition resulting in difficult labour/increased foetal deaths and early postnatal deaths was observed. Reproduction toxicity studies in rabbits have shown a dose-related reversible enlargement of the mammary glands of the parent animals and dose-related digital anomalies in the foetuses.

Ramipril: Studies in rats, rabbits and monkeys did not disclose any teratogenic properties. Daily doses during pregnancy and lactation in rats produced irreversible renal pelvis dilatation in the offspring.

6. PHARMACEUTICAL PARTICULARS

6.1 List of excipients

Cellulose microcrystalline

Hyprolose

Hypromellose

Iron oxides E172

Lactose anhydrous

Macrogol 6000

Macrogolglycerol hydroxystearate

Maize starch

Paraffin

Propyl gallate

Sodium aluminium silicate

Sodium stearyl fumarate

Titanium dioxide E 171

6.2 Incompatibilities

Not applicable.

6.3 Shelf life

Triapin mite: 2 years

Triapin: 30 months

6.4 Special precautions for storage

Do not store above 30°C.

6.5 Nature and contents of container

PVC/PVDC blisters: 28 tablets

6.6 Special precautions for disposal and other handling

No special requirements.

Table 1

Frequencies/ Organ System	Common (⩾ 1/100)	Uncommon (>1/1000, <1/100)	Rare (>1/10 000, <1/1000)	Very rare (<1/10 000)
Cardiac Disorders		Tachycardia, palpitations		
Nervous System Disorders	Headache	Dizziness, paraesthesiae	Syncope	
Gastrointestinal Disorders		Nausea, abdominal pain	Vomiting	Gingival hyperplasia, gingivitis
Renal and Urinary Disorders				Pollakisuria
Skin and Subcutaneous Tissue Disorders		Rash, pruritus	Urticaria	Photosensitivity reactions, angioedema
Musculoskeletal and Connective Tissue Disorders			Arthralgia, myalgia	
Metabolism and nutrition disorders				Hyperglycaemia
Vascular Disorders	Flush, peripheral oedema			Leucocytoclastic vasculitis
General Disorders and Administration Site conditions		Fatigue		Fever
Immune System Disorder				Hypersensitivity reactions
Hepatobiliary Disorders				Increased liver enzymes
Psychiatric Disorders			Impotence/ sexual dysfunction	

Table 2

Frequencies/ Organ System	Common (≥ 1/100)	Uncommon (>1/1000, <1/100)	Rare (>1/10 000, <1/1000)	Very rare (<1/10 000)
Investigation and Electrolyte Balance		Increase in serum urea and serum creatinine	Increase in serum potassium, increased levels of pancreatic enzymes	Decrease in serum sodium, raised titers of antinuclear antibodies
Cardiac Disorders			Severe hypotension, palpitations, disturbed orthostatic regulation, angina pectoris, cardiac arrhythmias	Myocardial ischemia, myocardial infarction, cardiovascular shock, coronary insufficiency
Blood and Lymphatic System Disorders			Reduction in the red blood cell count and haemoglobin content, white blood cell or blood platelet	Agranulocytosis, pancytopenia, bone marrow depression, haemolytical anaemia, eosinophilia, SR-elevation, leucocytosis
Nervous System Disorders		Headache, disorders of balance, impaired reactions	Dizziness, syncope, tremor, smell and taste disturbances, loss of taste	Paraesthesia
Eye Disorders		Conjunctivitis	Visual disturbances	
Ear and Labyrinth Disorders			Tinnitus, disturbed hearing	
Respiratory, Thoracic and mediastinal Disorders	Dry tickling cough		Sinusitis, bronchitis, bronchospasm, dyspnoea, aggravation of asthma, rhinitis	
Gastrointestinal Disorders		Nausea	Dryness of the mouth, glossitis, inflammatory reactions of the oral cavity and gastrointestinal tract, abdominal discomfort, gastric pain, digestive disturbances, constipation, diarrhea, vomiting	Ileus, Intestinal angioedema
Skin and Subcutaneous Tissue Disorders		Angioedema, pruritus, rash, urticaria		Maculopapular rash, pemphigus, exacerbation of psoriasis, psoriasiform, pemphigoid or lichenoid exanthema, enanthema, erythema multiforme, Steven-Johnson syndrome, toxic epidermal necrolysis, alopecia, onycholysis, photosensitivity, serositis
Musculoskeletal and Connective Tissue Disorders			Muscle cramps	Myalgia, arthralgia, myositis
Endocrine Disorders				Gynaecomastia
Metabolism and Nutrition Disorders			Loss of appetite	
Vascular Disorders		Tachycardia	Peripheral oedema, flushing	Exacerbation of perfusion disturbances due to vascular stenosis, precipitation or intensification of Raynaud's phenomenon, vasculitis, transient ischemic attack, ischemic stroke, cerebral ischemia
General Disorders and Administration Site conditions		Weakness, drowsiness, lightheadedness	Fatigue, sweating	Fever
Immune System Disorders			Anaphylactic or anaphylactoid reactions	
Hepatobiliary Disorders		Increases in serum levels of hepatic enzymes and/or bilirubin, cholestatic jaundice		Pancreatitis, liver failure, hepatocellular or cholestatic hepatitis
Reproductive System and Breast Disorders			Transient erectile impotence	
Psychiatric Disorders			Nervousness, depressed mood, restlessness, confusion, sleep disturbances, feeling of anxiety, somnolence, reduced libido	

7. MARKETING AUTHORISATION HOLDER
Sanofi-aventis
One Onslow Street
Guildford
Surrey
GU1 4YS
UK

8. MARKETING AUTHORISATION NUMBER(S)
Triapin Mite: PL 04425/0321
Triapin: PL 04425/0320

9. DATE OF FIRST AUTHORISATION/RENEWAL OF THE AUTHORISATION
15th April 2002/January 2008

10. DATE OF REVISION OF THE TEXT
January 2008

Legal Category: POM

Triclofos Elixir BP (UCB Pharma Ltd)

(UCB Pharma Limited)

1. NAME OF THE MEDICINAL PRODUCT
Triclofos Elixir BP

2. QUALITATIVE AND QUANTITATIVE COMPOSITION
Triclofos Sodium BP 10%w/v

For excipients, see 6.1

3. PHARMACEUTICAL FORM
An elixir for oral administration

4. CLINICAL PARTICULARS

4.1 Therapeutic indications
For the short-term treatment of severe insomnia which is interfering with normal daily life and where other therapies have failed.

Triclofos should be used as an adjunct to non-pharmacological therapies.

4.2 Posology and method of administration
As directed by a medical practitioner.

The following doses of Triclofos Elixir should be administered 15 to 30 minutes before bedtime:

Adults
1-2g (10-20ml)

Elderly and debilitated
Reduce dose (also see Special Warnings and Precautions for Use)

Children
The safety and efficacy of Triclofos Elixir has yet to be established in children

4.3 Contraindications
The use of Triclofos Elixir is contraindicated in:

cardiac disease, hepatic impairment, hypersensitivity (or previous idiosyncrasy) to Triclofos (or chloral hydrate), nursing mothers, pregnancy, renal impairment.

The use of Triclofos Elixir is not recommended in patients with gastritis, or in those with a history of acute attacks of porphyria.

4.4 Special warnings and precautions for use
There is a danger of misuse with Triclofos and habituation may develop. Tolerance to Triclofos may develop with high or prolonged dosage and dependence may occur. Sudden withdrawal after long term use may result in delirium. Other withdrawal symptoms which may occur include: apprehension, weakness, anxiety, headache, dizziness, irritability, tremors, nausea, vomiting, abdominal cramps, insomnia, visual distortions, muscle twitches, convulsions and hallucinations. Potential sequelae of such misuse are gastritis and parenchymatous renal injury. Delirium may occur, especially in the elderly, and particularly when Triclofos is used in conjunction with psychotropic or anticholinergic agents. Reduce dose in the elderly or debilitated. Caution should be taken in patients with respiratory disease, history of drug or alcohol abuse and marked personality disorder.

4.5 Interaction with other medicinal products and other forms of interaction
Patients established on anticoagulant therapy should be monitored for changes in prothrombin time when Triclofos is added or removed from the treatment regimen. Triclofos is known to potentiate the effects of alcohol. Administration of intravenous frusemide following administration of Triclofos may provoke a hypermetabolic state characterised by sweating, hot flushes, and variable blood pressure.

Coadministration of barbiturates and other sedatives may potentiate the drowsiness that can be caused by Triclofos.

4.6 Pregnancy and lactation
Contra-indicated

4.7 Effects on ability to drive and use machines
Patients should be warned that their ability to drive or use machines may be impaired by drowsiness.

4.8 Undesirable effects

Abdominal distension and flatulence; malaise; gastric irritation (gastro-intestinal upset, nausea and vomiting); eosinophilia, ketonuria, reduction in total white cell count; CNS type reactions (ataxia, drowsiness, headache, light-headedness, staggering gait, vertigo, confusion, sometimes with paranoia, excitement, hangover, nightmares); hypersensitivity reactions including skin reactions (angioedema, purpura, bullous lesions (erythema multiforme, Stevens Johnson syndrome), rashes and urticaria, have all been reported in patients following administration of Triclofos.

4.9 Overdose

Symptoms of overdose may include respiratory depression, arrhythmias, hypothermia, pin-point pupils, hypotension, coma, gastric irritation, areflexia, muscle flaccidity, oesophageal stricture, gastric perforation, gastro-intestinal haemorrhage and vomiting. Gastric necrosis, icterus, hepatic damage, albuminuria and renal damage may also occur. Serious problems have arisen in adults with doses as little as 4g and 10g can be fatal in adults.

Treatment: provided that the patient is conscious and a patent airway can be maintained, it may be appropriate to empty the stomach contents by gastric lavage. Activated charcoal should then be administered. General supportive measures, including ECG monitoring, should be employed. It may be necessary to consider haemodialysis or haemoperfusion in patients who deteriorate despite general supportive measures.

5. PHARMACOLOGICAL PROPERTIES

5.1 Pharmacodynamic properties

Triclofos sodium has hypnotic and sedative actions similar to those of chloral hydrate. It is hydrolysed in the body to trichloroethanol which is probably the active metabolite.

5.2 Pharmacokinetic properties

Following oral administration, triclofos is rapidly and completely hydrolysed in the gastro-intestinal tract to trichloroethanol. Peak serum levels of trichloroethanol are achieved within about one hour. Trichloroethanol is subject to conjugation with glucuronic acid and further metabolism to trichloroacetic acid. Trichloroethanol and trichloroacetic acid are approximately 35% and 95% protein bound respectively. Their half lives are estimated as between 8 and 11 hours and between 67 and 75 hours respectively. Approximately 12% of a dose is excreted in the urine within 24 hours. In infants the half lives are longer. The value for trichloroethanol is 35 hours, whilst for trichloroacetic acid the half life exceeds six days, with significant plasma concentrations present at 14 days.

5.3 Preclinical safety data

Triclofos Sodium has the same major metabolites as chloral hydrate, which has been shown to induce liver tumours in male mice, with no tumourigenic effects in rats. The mechanism of tumour induction is not known, but in the absence of clear evidence of mutagenic and clastogenic potential it is unlikely to be relevant to man. No data are available on the genotoxic or carcinogenic potential of triclofos sodium.

6. PHARMACEUTICAL PARTICULARS

6.1 List of excipients

Sugar Granulated

Vanillin

Nipastat GL75 containing: methyl-, ethyl-, propyl- and butyl-4- hydroxybenzoates

Disodium Edetate

Sodium Bicarbonate Powder

Sunset Yellow Ariavit 311831

Flavour IFF 1211

Purified Water

Activated Charcoal

6.2 Incompatibilities

None stated

6.3 Shelf life

24 months unopened - all bottles.

6 months once opened - 100ml and 300ml bottles.

6.4 Special precautions for storage

Store below 25°C. Keep well closed.

6.5 Nature and contents of container

Amber glass bottles (100ml) with screw on white pigmented polypropylene closure with saran faced expanded polyethylene wad.

Amber glass bottles (300ml) with screw on white pigmented polypropylene child resistant closure with natural expanded polyethylene wad

2 litre amber glass bottles with screw on white pigmented polypropylene closure with natural expanded polyethylene wad.

6.6 Special precautions for disposal and other handling

Discard elixir 6 months after first opening.

7. MARKETING AUTHORISATION HOLDER

UCB Pharma Ltd

208 Bath Road

Slough

Berkshire

SL1 3WE

8. MARKETING AUTHORISATION NUMBER(S)

PL 00039/0555

9. DATE OF FIRST AUTHORISATION/RENEWAL OF THE AUTHORISATION

April 2007

10. DATE OF REVISION OF THE TEXT

Approved: April 2009

Tridestra

(Orion Pharma (UK) Limited)

1. NAME OF THE MEDICINAL PRODUCT

Tridestra

2. QUALITATIVE AND QUANTITATIVE COMPOSITION

Tridestra tablet (white):

Estradiol valerate 2 mg

Tridestra tablet (blue):

Estradiol valerate 2 mg

Medroxyprogesterone acetate 20 mg

Tridestra tablet (yellow):

Placebo

For excipients, see 6.1

3. PHARMACEUTICAL FORM

Tablets, oral.

4. CLINICAL PARTICULARS

4.1 Therapeutic indications

i) Hormone replacement therapy (HRT) for estrogen deficiency symptoms in peri- and post-menopausal women.

ii) Prevention of osteoporosis in postmenopausal women at high risk of future fractures who are intolerant of, or contraindicated for, other medicinal products approved for the prevention of osteoporosis.

Please also refer to section 4.4

The experience of treating women older than 65 years is limited.

4.2 Posology and method of administration

Tridestra is a cyclic HRT that produces a vaginal bleed every 3 months. The bleeding occurs during treatment when the yellow (placebo) tablets are taken and is similar to the monthly bleed experienced during the normal menstrual cycle.

Tridestra consists of 91 tablets in a blister pack bearing calendar markings. Dosage is according to the calendar pack. One tablet should be taken daily without a break between packs.

The dosage during days 1 to 70 (inclusive) of the cycle is 2 mg estradiol valerate (white tablets). From day 71 to day 84 (inclusive) it is 2 mg of estradiol valerate and 20 mg of medroxyprogesterone acetate (blue tablets). From day 85 to day 91 (inclusive) a placebo preparation (yellow tablets) is taken when a menstrual like bleed occurs.

For initiation and continuation of treatment of postmenopausal symptoms, the lowest effective dose for the shortest duration (see also Section 4.4) should be used.

Women with amenorrhoea who are not taking HRT or who are switching to Tridestra from continuous combined HRT product, may start treatment on any day.

Women who are still having periods may start treatment 5 days after the start of the period.

Women who are switching from a cyclic or sequential HRT product to Tridestra treatment may start one week after completion of the cycle (28 days) ie at the end of a withdrawal bleed.

If the patient has forgotten to take one tablet, it should be taken within 12 hours otherwise the forgotten tablet should be discarded and the usual tablet taken the following day. Missing a dose may increase the likelihood of breakthrough bleeding and spotting.

4.3 Contraindications

- Known, past or suspected breast cancer
- Known or suspected estrogen-dependent malignant tumours (e.g. endometrial cancer)
- Undiagnosed genital bleeding
- Untreated endometrial hyperplasia
- Previous idiopathic or current venous thromboembolism [deep venous thrombosis (DVT), pulmonary embolism]
- Active or recent arterial thromboembolic disease (e.g. angina, myocardial infarction)
- Acute liver disease or a history of liver disease as long as liver function tests have failed to return to normal
- Known hypersensitivity to the active substances or to any of the excipients
- Porphyria
- Patients with rare hereditary problems of galactose intolerance, the Lapp lactase deficiency or glucose-galactose malabsorption should not take this medicine.

4.4 Special warnings and precautions for use

For the treatment of postmenopausal symptoms, HRT should only be initiated for symptoms that adversely affect quality of life. In all cases, a careful appraisal of the risks and benefits should be undertaken at least annually and HRT should only be continued as long as the benefit outweighs the risk.

Medical examination/follow-up

Before initiating or reinstituting HRT, a complete personal and family medical history should be taken. Physical (including pelvic and breast) examination should be guided by this and by the contraindications and warnings for use. During treatment, periodic check-ups are recommended of a frequency and nature adapted to the individual woman. Women should be advised what changes in their breasts should be reported to their doctor or nurse (see 'Breast Cancer' below). Investigations, including mammography, should be carried out in accordance with currently accepted screening practices, modified to the clinical needs of the individual.

Conditions which need supervision

If any of the following conditions are present, have occurred previously and/or have been aggravated during pregnancy or previous hormone treatment, the patient should be closely supervised. It should be taken into account that these conditions may recur or be aggravated during treatment with Tridestra, in particular:

- Leiomyoma (uterine fibroids) or endometriosis
- A history of or risk factors for thromboembolic disorders (see below)
- Risk factors for estrogen dependent tumours, e.g. 1st degree heredity for breast cancer
- Hypertension
- Liver disorders (e.g. liver adenoma)
- Diabetes mellitus with or without vascular involvement
- Cholelithiasis
- Migraine or (severe) headache
- Systemic lupus erythematosus
- A history of endometrial hyperplasia (see below)
- Epilepsy
- Asthma
- Otosclerosis

Reasons for immediate withdrawal of therapy

Therapy should be discontinued in case a contra-indication is discovered and in the following situations:

- Jaundice or deterioration of liver function
- Significant increase in blood pressure
- New onset of migraine-type headache
- Pregnancy

Endometrial hyperplasia

- The risk of endometrial hyperplasia and carcinoma is increased when estrogens are administered alone for prolonged periods (see Section 4.8). The addition of a progestagen for at least 12 days per cycle in non-hysterectomised women greatly reduces this risk.
- Breakthrough bleeding and spotting may occur during the first months of treatment. If breakthrough bleeding or spotting appears after some time of therapy, or continues after treatment has been discontinued, the reason should be investigated, which may include endometrial biopsy to excluded endometrial malignancy.

Breast cancer

A randomised placebo-controlled trial, the Women's Health Initiative study (WHI) and epidemiological studies including the Million Women Study (MWS), have reported an increased risk of breast cancer in women taking estrogens, estrogen-progestagen combinations or tibolone for HRT for several years (see Section 4.8). For all HRT, an excess risk becomes apparent within a few years of use and increase with duration of intake but returns to baseline within a few (at most 5 years) after stopping treatment.

In the MWS, the relative risk of breast cancer with conjugated equine estrogens (CEE) or estradiol (E2) was greater when a progestagen was added, either sequentially or continuously, and regardless of type of progestagen. There was no evidence of a difference in risk between the different routes of administration.

In the WHI study, the continuous combined conjugated equine estrogen and medroxyprogesterone acetate (CEE + MPA) product used was associated with breast cancers that were slightly larger in size and more frequently had local lymph node metastases compared to placebo.

HRT, especially estrogen-progestagen combined treatment, increases the density of mammographic images which may adversely affect the radiological detection of breast cancer.

Venous thromboembolism

- HRT is associated with a higher relative risk of developing venous thromboembolism (VTE), i.e. deep vein thrombosis or pulmonary embolism. One randomised controlled trial and epidemiological studies found a two- to threefold higher risk for users compared with non-users, For non-users it is estimated that the number of cases of VTE that will occur over a 5 year period is about 3 per 1000 women aged 50-59 years and 8 per 1000 women aged between 60-69 years. It is estimated that in healthy women who use HRT for 5 years, the number of additional cases of VTE over a 5 year period will be between 2 and 6 (best estimate = 4) per 1000 women aged 50-59 years and between 5 and 15 (best estimate = 9) per 1000 women aged 60-69 years. The occurrence of such an event is more likely in the first year of HRT than later.

• Generally recognised risk factors for VTE include a personal history or family history, severe obesity (BMI > 30 kg/m^2) and systemic lupus erythematosus (SLE). There is no consensus about the possible role of varicose veins in VTE.

• Patients with a history of VTE or known thrombophilic states have an increased risk of VTE. HRT may add to this risk. Personal or strong family history of thromboembolism or recurrent spontaneous abortion should be investigated in order to exclude a thrombophilic predisposition. Until a thorough evaluation of thrombophilic factors has been made or anticoagulant treatment initiated, use of HRT in such patients should be viewed as contraindicated. Those women already on anticoagulant treatment require careful consideration of the benefit-risk of use of HRT.

• The risk of VTE may be temporarily increased with prolonged immobilisation, major trauma or major surgery. As in all postoperative patients, scrupulous attention should be given to prophylactic measures to prevent VTE following surgery. Where prolonged immobilisation is liable to follow elective surgery, particularly abdominal or orthopaedic surgery to the lower limbs, consideration should be given to temporarily stopping HRT 4 to 6 weeks earlier, if possible. Treatment should not be restarted until the woman is completely mobilised.

• If VTE develops after initiating therapy, the drug should be discontinued. Patients should be told to contact their doctors immediately when they are aware of a potential thromboembolic symptom (eg, painful swelling of a leg, sudden pain in the chest, dyspnea).

Coronary artery disease (CAD)

• There is no evidence from randomised controlled trials of cardiovascular benefit with continuous combined conjugated estrogens and medroxyprogesterone acetate (MPA). Two large clinical trials (WHI and HERS i.e. Heart and Estrogen/progestin Replacement Study) showed a possible increased risk of cardiovascular morbidity in the first year of use and no overall benefit. For other HRT products there are only limited data from randomised controlled trials examining effects in cardiovascular morbidity and mortality. Therefore, it is uncertain whether these findings also extend to other HRT products.

Stroke

• One large randomised clinical trial (WHI-trial) found, as a secondary outcome, an increased risk of ischaemic stroke in healthy women during treatment with continuous combined conjugated estrogens and MPA. For women who do not use HRT, it is estimated that the number of cases of stroke that will occur over a 5 year period is about 3 per 1000 women aged 50-59 years and 11 per 1000 women aged 60-69 years. It is estimated that for women who use conjugated estrogens and MPA for 5 years, the number of additional cases will be between 0 and 3 (best estimate = 1) per 1000 users aged 50-59 years and between 1 and 9 (best estimate = 4) per 1000 users aged 60-69 years. It is unknown whether the increased risk also extends to other HRT products.

Ovarian cancer

• Long-term (at least 5-10 years) use of estrogen-only HRT products in hysterectomised women has been associated with an increased risk of ovarian cancer in some epidemiological studies. It is uncertain whether long-term use of combined HRT confers a different risk than estrogen-only products.

Other conditions

• Estrogens may cause fluid retention and, therefore, patients with cardiac or renal dysfunction should be carefully observed. Patients with terminal renal insufficiency should be closely observed, since it is expected that the level of circulating active ingredients of Tridestra is increased.

• Women with pre-existing hypertriglyceridaemia should be followed closely during estrogen replacement or HRT, since rare cases of large increases of plasma triglycerides leading to pancreatitis have been reported with estrogen therapy in this condition.

• Estrogens increase thyroid binding globulin (TBG), leading to increased circulating total thyroid hormone, as measured by protein-bound iodine (PBI), T4 levels (by column or by radio-immunoassay) or T3 levels (by radio-immunoassay). T3 resin uptake is decreased, reflecting the elevated TBG. Free T4 and free T3 concentrations are unaltered. Other binding proteins may be elevated in serum, i.e. corticoid binding globulin (CBG), sex-hormone-binding globulin (SHBG) leading to increased circulating corticosteroids and sex steroids, respectively. Free or biological active hormone concentrations are unchanged. Other plasma proteins may be increased (angiotensinogen/renin substrate, alpha-1-antitrypsin, ceruloplasmin).

• There is no conclusive evidence for improvement of cognitive function. There is some evidence from the WHI trial of increased risk of probable dementia in women who start using continuous combined CEE and MPA after the age of 65. It is unknown whether the findings apply to younger post-menopausal women or other HRT products.

4.5 Interaction with other medicinal products and other forms of interaction

The metabolism of estrogens and progestogens may be increased by concomitant use of substances known to induce drug-metabolising enzymes, specifically cytochrome P450 enzymes, such as anticonvulsants (e.g. phenobarbital, phenytoin, carbamazepine) and anti-infectives (e.g. rifampicin, rifabutin, nevirapine, efavirenz).

Ritonavir and nelfinavir, although known as strong inhibitors, by contrast exhibit inducing properties when used concomitantly with steroid hormones. Herbal preparations containing St John's wort (*Hypericum perforatum*) may induce the metabolism of estrogens and progestogens.

Clinically, an increased metabolism of estrogens and progestogens may lead to decreased effect and changes in the uterine bleeding profile.

4.6 Pregnancy and lactation

Tridestra is not indicated during pregnancy. If pregnancy occurs during medication with Tridestra treatment should be withdrawn immediately.

Clinically, data on a limited number of exposed pregnancies indicate no adverse effects of medroxyprogesterone acetate on the foetus.

The results of most epidemiological studies to date relevant to inadvertent foetal exposure to combinations of estrogens and progestogens indicate no teratogenic or foetotoxic effect.

Lactation

Tridestra is not indicated during lactation.

4.7 Effects on ability to drive and use machines

No effects on ability to drive and use machines have been observed

4.8 Undesirable effects

Adverse drug reactions occur most commonly in the first months of the treatment. The most common adverse effect is breakthrough bleeding and spotting appearing in 22% of patients. The overall percentage of treated patients experiencing at least 1 adverse reaction is 47%.

(see Table 1 below)

Breast Cancer

According to evidence from a large number of epidemiological studies and one randomised placebo-controlled trial, the Women's Health Initiative (WHI), the overall risk of breast cancer increases with increasing duration of HRT use in current or recent HRT users.

For estrogen only HRT, estimates of relative risk (RR) from a reanalysis of original data from 51 epidemiological studies (in which > 80% of HRT use was estrogen only HRT) and from the epidemiological Million Women Study (MWS) are similar at 1.35 (95% CI 1.21-1.49) and 1.30 (95% CI 1.21-1.40), respectively.

For estrogen plus progestagen combined HRT, several epidemiological studies have reported an overall higher risk for breast cancer than with estrogens alone.

The MWS reported that, compared to never users, the use of various types of estrogen-progestagen combined HRT was associated with a higher risk of breast cancer (RR = 2.00, 95%CI: 1.88-2.12) than use of estrogens alone (RR = 1.30, 95%CI: 1.21 – 1.40) or use of tibolone (RR=1.45; 95%CI 1.25-1.68).

The WHI trial reported a risk estimate of 1.24 (95% CI: 1.01-1.54) after 5.6 years of use of estrogen-progestagen combined HRT (CEE + MPA) in all users compared with placebo.

The absolute risks calculated from the MWS and the WHI trials are presented below:

The MWS has estimated, from the known average incidence of breast cancer in developed countries, that:

• For women not using HRT, about 32 in every 1000 are expected to have breast cancer diagnosed between the ages of 50 and 64 years.

• For 1000 current or recent users of HRT, the number of additional cases during the corresponding period will be

• For users of estrogen only replacement therapy,

  • between 0 and 3 (best estimate = 1.5) for 5 years' use
  • between 3 and 7 (best estimate = 5) for 10 years' use.

• For users of estrogen plus progestagen combined HRT,

  • between 5 and 7 (best estimate = 6) for 5 years' use
  • between 18 and 20 (best estimate = 19) for 10 years' use.

The WHI trial estimated that after 5.6 years of follow-up of women between the ages of 50 and 79 years, an additional 8 cases of invasive breast cancer would be due to estrogen-progestagen combined HRT (CEE + MPA) per 10,000 women years.

According to calculations from the trial data, it is estimated that:

• For 1000 women in the placebo group,

  • about 16 cases of invasive breast cancer would be diagnosed in 5 years.

• For 1000 women who used estrogen + progestagen combined HRT (CEE + MPA), the number of additional cases would be

  • between 0 and 9 (best estimate = 4) for 5 years' use.

The number of additional cases of breast cancer in women who use HRT is broadly similar for women who start HRT irrespective of age at start of use (between the ages of 45-65) (see section 4.4).'

Endometrial cancer

In women with an intact uterus, the risk of endometrial hyperplasia and endometrial cancer increases with increasing duration of use of unopposed estrogens. According to data from epidemiological studies, the best estimate of the risk is that for women not using HRT, about 5 in every 1000 are expected to have endometrial cancer diagnosed between the ages of 50 and 65. Depending on the duration of treatment and estrogen dose, the reported increase in endometrial cancer risk among unopposed estrogen users varies from 2-to 12-fold greater compared with non-users. Adding a progestagen to estrogen-only therapy greatly reduces this increased risk.

Other adverse reactions have been reported in association with estrogen/progestagen treatment:

• Estrogen-dependent neoplasms benign and malignant, e.g. endometrial cancer.

• Venous thromboembolism, i.e. deep leg or pelvic venous thrombosis and pulmonary embolism, is more frequent among HRT users than among non-users. For further information see sections 4.3. Contraindications and 4.4. Special warnings and precautions for use.

• Myocardial infarction and stroke.

• Gall bladder disease.

• Skin and subcutaneous disorders: chloasma, erythema multiforme, erythema nodosum, vascular purpura.

• Probable dementia (see section 4.4)

4.9 Overdose

Overdosage of estrogen may cause nausea, headache and withdrawal bleeding. Serious ill effects have not been reported following acute ingestion of large doses of estrogens and progestogens in contraceptive formulations by young children. When needed, therapy is symptomatic.

5. PHARMACOLOGICAL PROPERTIES

5.1 Pharmacodynamic properties

Pharmacotherapeutic group: Progestogens and Estrogens in Combination

ATC code: G03FB 06

•Estradiol / Estradiol valerate: the active ingredient, synthetic 17β-estradiol, is chemically and biologically identical to endogenous human estradiol. It substitutes for the loss of estrogen production in menopausal women, and

Table 1

Organ group	Common (>1/100)	Uncommon >1/1,000, <1/100	Rare >1/10,000; <1/1,000
Gastrointestinal disorders	Nausea, abdominal pain	vomiting	
Skin and subcutaneous tissue disorders			
Nervous System disorders	Headache, migraine		
Vision disorders	Visual disturbances		
Cardiac and vascular disorders			
Reproductive disorders and breast disorders	Dysmenorrhoea, breast tenderness, breast enlargement, breakthrough bleeding.	Uterine fibroids	Endometrial hyperplasia, menorrhagia
Miscellaneous	Oedema, tiredness, weight increase, changes in mood, changes in libido		

alleviates menopausal symptoms. Estrogens prevent bone loss following menopause or ovariectomy.

Progestagen: Medroxyprogesterone acetate (MPA) is a synthetic derivative of natural progesterone, a 17-α-hydroxy-6-methylprogesterone acetate. It has a similar effect to progesterone with slight androgenic activity. As estrogens promote the growth of the endometrium, unopposed estrogens increase the risk of endometrial hyperplasia and cancer. The addition of a progestagen greatly reduces the estrogen-induced risk of endometrial hyperplasia in non-hysterectomised women.

• Relief of estrogen-deficiency symptoms and bleeding patterns

- Relief of menopausal symptoms was achieved during the first few weeks of treatment.

- Tridestra causes a withdrawal bleed at the end of a 3 monthly cycle

- Regular withdrawal bleeding occurred in 77% of women with a mean duration of 5 days. Withdrawal bleeding usually started 2-3 days after the last tablet is taken of the 14 days of the estrogen/progestagen phase (2 mg E_2V + 20 mg MPA). Break through bleeding and/or spotting appeared in 15% of the women during the first three months of therapy and in 27% during months 10-12 of treatment. Amenorrhoea (no bleeding or spotting) occurred in 0% of the cycles during the first year of treatment (for cyclic or sequential products).

• Prevention of osteoporosis

- Estrogen deficiency at menopause is associated with an increasing bone turnover and decline in bone mass. The effect of estrogens on bone mineral density (BMD) is dose dependent. Protection appears to be effective for as long as treatment is continued. After discontinuation of HRT, bone mass is lost at a rate similar to that in untreated women.

- Evidence from the WHI trial and meta-analysed trials shows that current use of HRT, alone or in combination with a progestagen – given to predominantly healthy women – reduces the risk of hip, vertebral and other osteoporotic fractures. HRT may also prevent fractures in women with low bone density and/or established osteoporosis, but evidence for that is limited.

- After 1 year of treatment with Tridestra, the increase in lumbar spine bone mineral density (BMD) was 3.3 ± 3.6 % (mean ± SD). The percentage of women who maintained or gained BMD in lumbar zone during treatment was 72.7%. After 2 years of treatment with Tridestra, the increase in BMD was 5.9 ± 3.0 % (mean ± SD). The percentage of women who maintained or gained BMD in lumber zone during treatment was 95.2%.

- Tridestra also had an effect on hip BMD. The increase after 1 year was 2.3% ± 3.4% (mean ± SD) at the femoral neck. The percentage of women who maintained or gained BMD in the hip zone during treatment was 72.7%. The increase after 2 years was 0.6% ± 3.6% (mean ± SD) at femoral neck. The percentage of women who maintained or gained BMD in the hip zone during treatment was 52.4%.

5.2 Pharmacokinetic properties

Maximum plasma levels (C_{max}) of estradiol (about 250 pmol/l) are reached in about 5-7 hours. The trough concentration (C_{min}) of estradiol was about 142 pmol/l and the average concentration ($C_{average}$) about 185 pmol/l. In circulation, natural estrogens are bound to sex hormone binding globulin and albumin. Free estradiol is metabolised in the liver and partly converted to less active estrogens like estrone.

Maximum plasma levels (C_{max}) of estrone (about 1790 pmol/l) are reached in 5–7 hours after intake of the tablet. C_{min} of estrone was about 864 pmol/l, $C_{average}$ about 1160 pmol/l. Estrone is subjected to an enterohepatic cycle and its half-life is 15–20 hours. The majority of estrogens are excreted via kidneys as conjugates (sulphates or glucuronides).

MPA is well absorbed from the gastrointestinal tract and rapidly distributed from circulation to extravascular tissues. After the intake of the Tridestra combination tablet, the maximum plasma level (C_{max}) of MPA (about 5 μg/L) is reached in about 2 hours. $C_{average}$ (after a single dose) was about 1.3 μg/L. The elimination half-life is 40-50 hours. MPA is metabolised in the liver and excreted as glucuronides both in urine and bile. The extent of absorption from the combination tablet is comparable to MPA given alone.

5.3 Preclinical safety data

Data from animal toxicity studies with estradiol and medroxyprogesterone acetate have shown expected estrogenic and gestagenic effects, and do not reveal any particular risk for humans in the therapeutic dose-range.

6. PHARMACEUTICAL PARTICULARS

6.1 List of excipients

Tridestra tablet (white):

Lactose

Maize starch

Gelatine

Purified water

Magnesium stearate

Talc

Tridestra tablet (blue):

Lactose

Maize starch

Gelatine

Purified water

Magnesium stearate

Indigo carmine (E132)

Tridestra tablet (yellow):

Lactose

Maize starch

Gelatine

Purified water

Magnesium stearate

Yellow iron oxide (E172)

6.2 Incompatibilities

Not applicable

6.3 Shelf life

3 years

6.4 Special precautions for storage

Do not store above 25°C

Store in a dry place

6.5 Nature and contents of container

A PVC/PVDC/AL thermofoiled blister pack.

Quantity: 91

6.6 Special precautions for disposal and other handling

No special requirements

7. MARKETING AUTHORISATION HOLDER

Orion Corporation

P.O. Box 65,

FIN-02101 Espoo

Finland

8. MARKETING AUTHORISATION NUMBER(S)

PL 27925/0014

9. DATE OF FIRST AUTHORISATION/RENEWAL OF THE AUTHORISATION

11/01/2006

10. DATE OF REVISION OF THE TEXT

11/01/2006

Trimovate

(GlaxoSmithKline UK)

1. NAME OF THE MEDICINAL PRODUCT

Trimovate Cream

Trimovate

Clobetasone Butyrate

2. QUALITATIVE AND QUANTITATIVE COMPOSITION

Trimovate Cream is a yellow water-miscible cream containing clobetasone butyrate 0.05% w/w, oxytetracycline 3.0% w/w as calcium oxytetracycline and nystatin 100,000 units per gram.

3. PHARMACEUTICAL FORM

Cream for topical administration.

4. CLINICAL PARTICULARS

4.1 Therapeutic indications

Clobetasone butyrate is a topically active corticosteroid which provides an exceptional combination of activity and safety. Topical formulations have been shown to be more effective in the treatment of eczemas than 1% hydrocortisone, yet to have little effect on hypothalamic-pituitary-adrenal function.

The combination of the topically active antibiotics, nystatin and oxytetracycline, provides a broad spectrum of antibacterial and anticandidal activity against many of the organisms associated with infected dermatoses. Trimovate is indicated for the treatment and management of steroid responsive dermatoses where candidal or bacterial infection is present, suspected or likely to occur and the use of a more potent topical corticosteroid is not required. These include infected eczemas, intertrigo, napkin rash, anogenital pruritius and seborrhoeic dermatitis.

4.2 Posology and method of administration

Apply to the affected area up to four times a day.

Suitable for treating infants, children and adults.

4.3 Contraindications

Primary cutaneous infections caused by viruses (e.g. herpes simplex, chickenpox) fungi and bacteria. Secondary infections due to dermatophytes, Pseudomonas or Proteus species.

Hypersensitivity to the preparation.

4.4 Special warnings and precautions for use

Although generally regarded as safe, even for long term administration in adults, there is a potential for overdosage, and in children this may result in adrenal suppression. Extreme caution is required in dermatoses in such patients and treatment should not normally exceed seven days. In infants, the napkin may act as an occlusive dressing, and increase absorption.

If infection persists, systemic chemotherapy is likely to be required: Any spread of infection requires withdrawal of topical corticosteroid therapy. Bacterial infection is encouraged by the warm, moist conditions induced by occlusive dressings, and the skin should be cleansed before a fresh dressing is applied. Do not continue for more than seven days in the absence of clinical improvement, since occult extension of infection may occur due to the masking effect of the steroid.

As with all corticosteroids, prolonged application to the face is undesirable. If applied to the eyelids, care is needed to ensure that the preparation does not enter the eye, as glaucoma might result.

Trimovate may cause slight staining of hair, skin or fabric, but this can be removed by washing. The application may be covered with a non-occlusive dressing to protect clothing.

Extended or recurrent application may increase the risk of contact sensitisation.

Products which contain antimicrobial agents should not be diluted.

4.5 Interaction with other medicinal products and other forms of interaction

None reported.

4.6 Pregnancy and lactation

There is inadequate evidence of safety in human pregnancy. Topical administration of corticosteroids to pregnant animals can cause abnormalities of fetal development including cleft palate and intra-uterine growth retardation. There may therefore be a very small risk of such effects in the human fetus.

4.7 Effects on ability to drive and use machines

None stated.

4.8 Undesirable effects

Local hypersensitivity reactions such as erythema, rash, pruritus, urticaria, local skin burning and allergic contact dermatitis may occur at the site of application and may resemble symptoms of the condition under treatment.

In the unlikely event of signs of hypersensitivity appearing, application should be stopped immediately.

If large areas of the body were to be treated with Trimovate, it is possible that some patients would absorb sufficient steroid to cause transient adrenal suppression despite the low degree of systemic activity associated with clobetasone butyrate.

Local atrophic changes could possibly occur in situations where moisture increases absorption of clobetasone butyrate, but only after prolonged use.

There are reports of pigmentation changes and hypertrichosis with topical steroids. Exacerbation of underlying symptoms may occur with extensive use.

4.9 Overdose

Acute overdosage is very unlikely to occur, however, in the case of chronic overdosage or misuse the features of hypercortisolism may appear.

In this situation topical steroids should be reduced or discontinued gradually under medical supervision because of the risk of adrenal insufficiency

5. PHARMACOLOGICAL PROPERTIES

5.1 Pharmacodynamic properties

Clobetasone butyrate is a topically active corticosteroid.

Clobetasone butyrate is less potent than other available corticosteroid preparations and has been shown not to suppress the hypothalamo-pituitary-adrenal axis in patients treated for psoriasis or eczema. Pharmacological studies in man and animals have shown that clobetasone butyrate has a relatively high level of topical activity accompanied by a low level of systemic activity.

The use of nystatin in the local treatment of candidal infections of the skin and of the tetracyclines in localised bacterial infections is well known. Nystatin is included in Trimovate at the standard concentration recommended by the British Pharmaceutical codex for the topical preparation nystatin ointment (100,000 units/g) and oxytetracycline calcium is included at a concentration to give approximately the same level of activity as recommended for Oxytetracycline Ointment BPC (3.0% w/w).

The principle action of the preparation is based on the anti-inflammatory activity of the corticosteroid. The broad spectrum antibacterial and anti-candidal activity provided by the combination of oxytetracycline and nystatin allow this effect to be utilised in the treatment of conditions which are or are likely to become infected.

5.2 Pharmacokinetic properties

Trimovate has been shown to have a satisfactory pharmacokinetic profile by many years of successful clinical experience.

5.3 Preclinical safety data

No additional data of relevance.

6. PHARMACEUTICAL PARTICULARS

6.1 List of excipients

Titanium dioxide, glyceryl monostearate, cetostearyl alcohol, soft paraffin white, polyoxyl 40 stearate, dimeticone

20, glycerol, chlorocresol, sodium metabisulphite, sodium acid phosphate, disodium hydrogen phosphate anhydrous, purified water.

6.2 Incompatibilities
None reported.

6.3 Shelf life
18 months.

6.4 Special precautions for storage
Store below 25C.

6.5 Nature and contents of container
Collapsible latex banded aluminium tube, internally coated with epoxy resin based lacquer with polypropylene cap.

6.6 Special precautions for disposal and other handling
None stated.

Administrative Data

7. MARKETING AUTHORISATION HOLDER
Glaxo Wellcome UK Ltd trading as GlaxoSmithKline UK,
Stockley Park West,
Uxbridge, Middlesex.
UB11 1BT.

8. MARKETING AUTHORISATION NUMBER(S)
PL 10949/0040

9. DATE OF FIRST AUTHORISATION/RENEWAL OF THE AUTHORISATION
29 May 2002

10. DATE OF REVISION OF THE TEXT
14 February 2007

11. Legal Category
POM.

Trinovum

(Janssen-Cilag Ltd)

1. NAME OF THE MEDICINAL PRODUCT
Trinovum Oral Contraceptive Tablets

2. QUALITATIVE AND QUANTITATIVE COMPOSITION

7 white tablets	Norethisterone 0.5 mg Enthinylestradiol 0.035 mg
7 light peach coloured tablets	Norethisterone 0.75 mg Enthinylestradiol 0.035 mg
7 peach coloured tablets	Norethisterone 1.0 mg Enthinylestradiol 0.035 mg

3. PHARMACEUTICAL FORM
Tablets

4. CLINICAL PARTICULARS

4.1 Therapeutic indications
Oral contraception and the recognised indications for such oestrogen/progestogen combinations. Route of administration: Oral.

4.2 Posology and method of administration
Adults

It is preferable that tablet intake from the first pack is started on the first day of menstruation in which case no extra contraceptive precautions are necessary.

If menstruation has already begun (that is 2, 3 or 4 days previously). Tablet taking should commence on day 5 of the menstrual period. In this case additional contraceptive precautions must be taken for the first 7 days of tablet taking.

If menstruation began more than 5 days previously then the patient should be advised to wait until her next menstrual period before starting to take Trinovum.

How to take Trinovum

One tablet is taken daily at the same time (preferably in the evening) without interruption for 21 days, followed by a break of 7 tablet-free days. (A white tablet is taken every day for 7 days, then a light peach coloured tablet is taken every day for 7 days, then a peach coloured tablet every day for 7 days, then 7 tablet-free days.

Each subsequent pack is started after the 7 tablet-free days have elapsed. Additional contraceptive precautions are not then required.

Elderly

Not applicable.

Children

Not recommended.

4.3 Contraindications
Absolute contraindications

Pregnancy or suspected pregnancy (that cannot yet be excluded).

Circulatory disorders (cardiovascular or cerebrovascular) such as thrombophlebitis and thromboembolic processes or a history of these conditions (including history of confirmed venous thrombo-embolism (VTE), family history of idiopathic VTE and other known risk factors for VTE), moderate to severe hypertension, hyperlipoproteinaemia. In addition the presence of more than one of the risk factors for arterial disease.

Severe liver disease, cholestatic jaundice or hepatitis (viral or non-viral) or a history of these conditions if the results of liver function tests have failed to return to normal, and for 3 months after liver function tests have been found to be normal; a history of jaundice of pregnancy or jaundice due to the use of steroids, Rotor syndrome and Dubin-Johnson syndrome, hepatic cell tumours and porphyria.

Cholelithiasis.

Known or suspected oestrogen-dependent tumours; endometrial hyperplasia; undiagnosed vaginal bleeding.

Systemic lupus erythematosus or a history of this condition.

A history during pregnancy or previous use of steroids of:

Severe pruritus

Herpes gestationis

A manifestation or deterioration of otosclerosis.

Relative Contraindications

If any relative contraindications listed below is present, the benefits of oestrogen/progestogen containing preparations must be weighed against the possible risk for each individual case and the patient kept under close supervision. In case of aggravation or appearance of any of these conditions whilst the patient is taking the pill, its use should be discontinued.

Conditions implicating an increasing risk of developing venous thromboembolic complications, e.g. severe varicose veins or prolonged immobilisation or major surgery.

Disorders of coagulation.

Presence of any risk factor for arterial disease e.g. smoking, hyperlipidaemia or hypertension.

Other conditions associated with an increased risk of circulatory disease such as latent or overt cardiac failure, renal dysfunction, or a history of these conditions.

Epilepsy or a history of this condition.

Migraine or a history of this condition.

A history of cholelithiasis.

Presence of any risk factor for oestrogen-dependent tumours; oestrogen-sensitive gynaecological disorders such as uterine fibromyomata and endometriosis.

Diabetes mellitus.

Severe depression or a history of this condition. If this is accompanied by a disturbance in tryptophan metabolism, administration of vitamin B6 might be of therapeutic value.

Sickle cell haemoglobinopathy, since under certain circumstances, e.g. during infections or anoxia, oestrogen containing preparations may induce thromboembolic process in patients with this condition.

If the results of liver function tests become abnormal, use should be discontinued.

4.4 Special warnings and precautions for use
Post partum administration

Following a vaginal delivery, oral contraceptive administration to non-breast feeding mothers can be started 21 days post-partum provided the patient is fully ambulant and there are no puerperal complications. No additional contraceptive precautions are required. If post-partum administration begins more than 21 days after delivery, additional contraceptive precautions are required for the first 7 days of pill - taking. If intercourse has taken place post-partum, oral contraceptive use should be delayed until the first day of the first menstrual period.

After miscarriage or abortion administration should start immediately in which case no additional contraceptive precautions are required.

Changing from a 21 day pill or another 22 day pill to Trinovum

All tablets in the old pack should be finished. The first Trinovum Tablet is taken the next day i.e. no gap is left between taking tablets nor does the patient need to wait for her period to begin. Tablets should be taken as instructed in 'how to take Trinovum' (see 4.2). Additional contraceptive precautions are not required. The patient will not have a period until the end of the first Trinovum pack, but this is not harmful, nor does it matter if she experiences some bleeding on tablet-taking days.

Changing from a combined every day pill (28 day tablet) to Trinovum

Trinovum should be started after taking the last active tablet from the 'everyday pill' pack (i.e. after taking 21 or 22 tablets). The first Trinovum tablet is taken the next day i.e. no gap is left between taking tablets nor does the patient need to wait for her period to begin. Tablets should be taken as instructed in 'how to take Trinovum' (see 4.2). Additional contraceptive precautions are not required. Remaining tablets from the every day (ED) pack should be discarded.

The patient will not have a period until the end of the first Trinovum pack, but this is not harmful, nor does it matter if she experiences some bleeding on tablet-taking days.

Changing from a progestogen-only pill (POP or mini pill) to Trinovum

The first Trinovum tablet should be taken on the first day of the period, even if the patient has already taken a mini pill on that day. Tablets should be taken as instructed in 'how to take Trinovum' (see 4.2). Additional contraceptive precautions are not required. All the remaining progestogen-only pills in the mini pill pack should be discarded.

If the patient is taking a (mini) pill, then she may not always have a period, especially when she is breast feeding. The first Trinovum tablet should be taken on the day after stopping the mini pill. All remaining pills in the mini pill packet must be discarded. Additional contraceptive precautions must be taken for the first 7 days.

To skip a period

To skip a period, an new pack of Trinovum should be started on the day after finishing the current pack (the patient skips the tablet-free days). Tablet-taking should be continued in the usual way.

During the use of the second pack she may experience slight spotting or break-through bleeding but contraceptive protection will not be diminished provided there are no tablet omissions.

The next pack of Trinovum is started after the usual 7 tablet-free days, regardless of whether the period has completely finished or not.

Reduced reliability

When Trinovum is taken according to the directions for use the occurrence of pregnancy is highly unlikely. However the reliability of oral contraceptives may be reduced under the following circumstances:

Forgotten tablets

If the patient forgets to take a tablet, she should take it as soon as she remembers and take the next one at the normal tine. This may mean that two tablets are taken in one day. Provided she is less than 12 hours late in taking her tablet, Trinovum will still give contraceptive protection during this cycle and the rest of the pack should be taken as usual.

If she is more than 12 hours late in taking one or more tablets then she should take the last missed pill as soon as she remembers but leave the other missed pills in the pack. She should continue to take the rest of the pack as usual but must use extra precautions (e.g. sheath, diaphragm, plus spermicide) and follow the 7 day rules (see further information for 7 day rule).

If there are 7 or more pills left in the pack after the missed and delayed pills then the usual 7-day break can be left before starting the next pack. If there are less than 7 pills left in the pack after the missed and delayed pills then when the pack is finished the next pack should be started the next day. If withdrawal bleeding does not occur at the end of the second pack then a pregnancy test should be performed.

Vomiting or diarrhoea

If after tablet intake vomiting or diarrhoea occurs, a tablet may not be absorbed properly by the body. If the symptoms disappear within 12 hours of tablet-taking, the patient should take an extra tablet from a spare pack and continue with the rest of the pack as usual.

However, if the symptoms continue beyond the 12 hours, additional contraceptive precautions are necessary for any sexual intercourse during the stomach or bowel upset and for the following 7 days (the patient must be advised to follow '7-day rule').

Change in bleeding pattern

If after taking Trinovum for several months there is a sudden occurrence of spotting or breakthrough bleeding (not observed in previous cycles) or the absence of withdrawal bleeding, contraceptive effectiveness may be reduced. If withdrawal bleeding fails to occur and none of the above mentioned events has taken place, pregnancy is highly unlikely and oral contraceptive use can be continued until the end of the next pack.

(If withdrawal bleeding fails to occur at the end of the second cycle, tablet intake should be discontinued and pregnancy excluded before oral contraceptive use can be resumed). However, if withdrawal bleeding is absent and any of the above mentioned events has occurred, tablet intake should be discontinued and pregnancy excluded before oral contraceptive use can be resumed.

Medical examination/consultation

Assessment of women prior to starting oral contraceptives (and at regular intervals thereafter) should include a personal and family medical history of each woman. Physical examination should be guided by this and by the contra-indications (section 4.3) and warnings (section 4.4) for this product. The frequency and nature of these assessments should be based upon relevant guidelines and should be adapted to the individual woman, but should include measurement of blood pressure and, if judged appropriate by the clinician, breast, abdominal and pelvic examination including cervical cytology.

Caution should be observed when prescribing oral contraceptives to young women whose cycles are not yet stabilised.

Venous thrombo-embolic disease

An increased risk of venous thrombo-embolic disease (VTE) associated with the use of oral contraceptives is well established but is smaller than that associated with pregnancy, which has been estimated at 60 cases per 100,000 pregnancies. Some epidemiological studies have reported a greater risk of VTE for women using combined oral contraceptives containing desogestrel or gestodene (the so-called 'third generation' pills) than for women using pills containing levonorgestrel or norethisterone (the so-called 'second generation' pills).

The spontaneous incidence of VTE in healthy non-pregnant women (not taking any oral contraceptive) is about 5 cases per 100,000 per year. The incidence in users of second generation pills is about 15 per 100,000 women per year of use. The incidence in users of third generation pills is about 25 cases per 100,000 women per years of use; this excess incidence has not been satisfactorily explained by bias or confounding. The level of all of these risks of VTE increases with age and is likely to be further increased in women with other known risk factors for VTE such as obesity. The excess risk of VTE is highest during the first year a woman ever uses a combined oral contraceptive.

Surgery, varicose veins or immobilisation

In patients using oestrogen-containing preparations the risk of deep vein thrombosis may be temporarily increased when undergoing a major operation(e.g. abdominal, orthopaedic), any surgery to the legs, medical treatment for varicose veins or prolonged immobilisation. Therefore, it is advisable to discontinue oral contraceptive use at least 4 to 6 weeks prior to these procedures if performed electively and to (re) star not less than 2 weeks after full ambulation. The latter is also valid with regard to immobilisation after an accident or emergency surgery. In case of emergency surgery, thrombotic prophylaxis is usually indicated e.g. with subcutaneous heparin.

Chloasma

Chloasma may occasionally occur, especially in women with a history of chloasma gravidarum. Women with a tendency to chloasma should avoid exposure to the sun or ultraviolet radiation whilst taking this preparation. Chloasma is often not fully reversible.

Laboratory tests

The use of steroids may influence the results of certain laboratory tests. In the literature, at least a hundred different parameters have been reported to possibly be influenced by oral contraceptive use, predominantly by the oestrogenic component. Among these are: biochemical parameters of the liver, thyroid, adrenal and renal function, plasma levels of (carrier) proteins and lipid/lipoprotein fractions and parameters of coagulation and fibrinolysis.

Further information

Additional contraceptive precautions

When additional contraceptive precautions are required the patient should be advised either not to have sex, or to use a cap plus spermicide or for her partner to use a condom. Rhythm methods should not be advised as the pill disrupts the usual cyclical changes associated with the natural menstrual cycle e.g. changes in temperature and cervical mucus.

The 7 day rule

If any one tablet is forgotten for more than 12 hours:

If the patient has vomiting or diarrhoea for more than 12 hours:

If the patient is taking any of the drugs listed under interactions:

The patient should continue to take her tablets as usual and:

Additional contraceptive precautions must be taken for the next 7 days.

But - if these 7 days run beyond the end of the current pack, the next pack must be started as soon as the current one is finished, i.e. no gap should be left between packs. (This prevents an extended break in tablet taking which may increase the risk of the ovaries releasing an egg and thus reducing contraceptive protection). The patient will not have a period until the end of 2 packs but this is not harmful nor does it matter if she experiences some bleeding on tablet taking days.

4.5 Interaction with other medicinal products and other forms of interaction

Irregular cycles and reduced reliability of oral contraceptives may occur when these preparations are used concomitantly with drugs such as anticonvulsants, barbiturates, antibiotics, (e.g. tetracyclines, ampicillin, rifampicin, etc). griseofulvin, activated charcoal and certain laxatives. Special consideration should be given to patients being treated with antibiotics for acne. They should be advised to use a non-hormonal method of contraception, or to use an oral contraceptive containing a progestogen showing minimal androgenicity, which have been reported as helping to improve acne without using an antibiotic. Oral contraceptives may diminish glucose tolerance and increase the need for insulin or other antidiabetic drug in diabetics.

The herbal remedy St John's wort (*Hypericum perforatum*) should not be taken concomitantly with this medicine as this could potentially lead to a loss of contraceptive effect.

4.6 Pregnancy and lactation

Trinovum is contraindicated for use during pregnancy or suspected pregnancy, since it has been suggested that combined oral contraceptives, in common with many other substances, might be capable of affecting the normal development of the child in the early stages of pregnancy.

Figure 1

Estimated cumulative numbers of breast cancers per 10,000 women diagnosed in 5 years of use and up to 10 years after stopping COCs, compared with numbers of breast cancers diagnosed in 10,000 women who had never used COCs

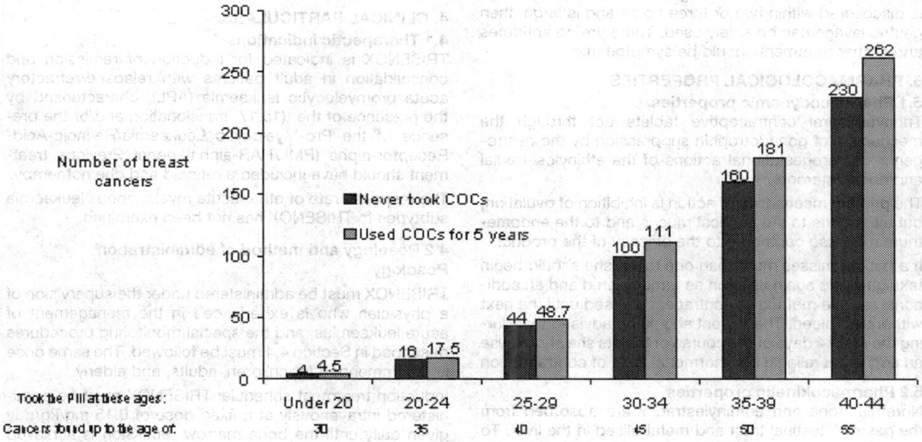

It can be definitely concluded, however, that if a risk of abnormality exists at all, it must be very small. Mothers who are breast feeding should be advised not to use the combined pill since this may reduce the amount of breast-milk, but may be advised instead to use a progestogen-only pill (POP).

4.7 Effects on ability to drive and use machines

Not applicable.

4.8 Undesirable effects

Various adverse reactions have been associated with oral contraceptive use. The first appearance of symptoms indicative of any one of these reactions necessitates immediate cessation of oral contraceptive use while appropriate diagnostic and therapeutic measures are undertaken.

Serious Adverse Reaction

There is a general opinion, based on statistical evidence that users of combined oral contraceptives experience more often than non-users various disorders of the circulation. How often these disorders occur in users of modern low-oestrogen oral contraceptives is unknown, but there are reasons for suggesting that they may occur less often than with the older types of pill which contain more oestrogen.

Various reports have associated oral contraceptive use with the occurrence of deep venous thrombosis, pulmonary embolism and other embolisms. Other investigations of these oral contraceptives have suggested an increased risk of oestrogen and/or progestogen dose-dependent coronary and cerebrovascular accidents, predominantly in heavy smokers. Thrombosis has very rarely been reported to occur in other veins or arteries, e.g. hepatic, mesenteric, renal or retinal.

It should be noted that there is no consensus about the often contradictory findings obtained in early studies. The physician should bear in mind, the possibility of vascular accidents occurring and that there may not be full recovery from such disorders and they may be fatal. The physician should take into account the presence of risk factors for arterial disease and deep venous thrombosis when prescribing oral contraceptives. Risk factors for arterial disease include smoking, the presence of hyperlipidaemia, hypertension, or diabetes.

Signs and symptoms of a thrombotic event may include: sudden severe pain in the chest, whether or not reaching to the left arm; sudden breathlessness; any unusual severe, prolonged headache, especially if it occurs for the first time or gets progressively worse, or is associated with any of the following symptoms: sudden partial or complete loss of vision or diplopia, aphasia, vertigo, a bad fainting attack or collapse with or without focal epilepsy, weakness or very marked numbness suddenly affecting one side or one part of the body, motor disturbances; severe pain in the calf of one leg; acute abdomen.

Cigarette smoking increases the risk of serious cardiovascular adverse reactions to oral contraceptive use. The risk increases with age and with heavy smoking and is more marked in women over 35 years of age. Women who use oral contraceptives should be strongly advised not to smoke.

The use of oestrogen-containing oral contraceptives may promote growth of existing sex steroid dependent tumours. For this reason, the use of these oral contraceptives in patients with such tumours is contraindicated. Numerous epidemiological studies have been reported on the risk of ovarian, endometrial, cervical and breast cancer in women using combined oral contraceptives.

The evidence is clear that combined oral contraceptives offer substantial protection against both ovarian and endometrial cancer. An increased risk of cervical cancer in long term users of combined oral contraceptives has been reported in some studies, but there continues to be controversy about the extent to which this is attributable to the confounding effects of sexual behaviour and other factors.

A meta-analysis from 54 epidemiological studies reported that there is a slightly increased relative risk (RR = 1.24) of having breast cancer diagnosed in women who are currently using combined oral contraceptives (COCs). The observed pattern of increased risk may be due to an earlier diagnosis of breast cancer in COC users, the biological effects of COCs or a combination of both. The additional breast cancers diagnosed in current users of COCs or in women who have used COCs in the last 10 years are more likely to be localised to the breast than those in women who never used COCs.

Breast cancer is rare among women under 40 years of age whether or not they take COCs. Whilst this background risk increases with age, the excess number of breast cancer diagnoses in current and recent COC users is small in relation to the overall risk of breast cancer (see bar chart).

The most important risk factor for breast cancer in COC users is the age women discontinue the COC; the older the age at stopping, the more breast cancers are diagnosed. Duration of use is less important and the excess risk gradually disappears during the course of the 10 years after stopping COC use such that by 10 years there appears to be no excess.

The possible increase in risk of breast cancer should be discussed with the user and weighed against the benefits of COCs taking into account the evidence that they offer substantial protection against the risk of developing certain other cancers (e.g. ovarian and endometrial cancer).

(see Figure 1 above)

Malignant hepatic tumours have been reported on rare occasions in long-term users of oral contraceptives. Benign hepatic tumours have also been associated with oral contraceptive usage. A hepatic tumour should be considered in the differential diagnosis when upper abdominal pain, enlarged liver or signs of intra abdominal haemorrhage occur.

The use of oral contraceptives may sometimes lead to the development of cholestatic jaundice or cholelithiasis.

On rare occasions the use of oral contraceptives may trigger or reactivate Systemic lupus erythematosus.

A further rare complication of oral contraceptive use is the occurrence of chorea which can be reversed by discontinuing the pill. The majority of cases of oral contraceptive-induced chorea show a pre-existing predisposition which often relates to acute rheumatism

Other Adverse Reactions

Cardiovascular system: Rise of blood pressure. If hypertension develops, treatment should be discontinued.

Genital tract: Intermenstrual bleeding, post-medication amenorrhoea, changes in cervical secretion, increase in size of uterine fibromyomata, aggravation of endometriosis, certain vaginal infections, e.g. candidiasis.

Breast: Tenderness, pain, enlargement, secretion.

Gastro- intestinal tract: Nausea, vomiting, cholelithiasis, cholestatic jaundice.

Skin: Erythema nodosum, rash, chloasma, erythema multiforme, hirsutism, loss of scalp hair.

Eyes: Discomfort of the cornea if contact lenses are used.

CNS: Headache, migraine, mood changes, depression.

Metabolic: Fluid retention, change in body weight, reduced glucose tolerance.

Other: Changes in libido, leg cramp, pre-menstrual-like syndrome.

4.9 Overdose

There have been no reports of serious ill-health from overdosage even when a considerable number of tablets have been taken by a small child. In general, it is therefore unnecessary to treat overdosage. However, if overdosage is discovered within two or three hours and is large, then gastric lavage can be safely used. There are no antidotes and further treatment should be symptomatic.

5. PHARMACOLOGICAL PROPERTIES

5.1 Pharmacodynamic properties

Trinovum oral contraceptive tablets act through the mechanism of gonadotrophin suppression by the oestrogenic and progestational actions of the ethinylosetradial and norethisterone.

The primary mechanism of action is inhibition of ovulation, but alterations to the cervical mucus and to the endometrium may also contribute to the efficacy of the product.

If a patient misses more than one tablet she should begin taking tablets again as soon as remembered and an additional reliable method of contraception used until the next withdrawal bleed. The patient should be advised that during the first 14 days of the course of tablets she should use an additional reliable non-hormonal form of contraception

5.2 Pharmacokinetic properties

Norethisterone and enthinylestradiol are absorbed from the gastro-intestinal tract and metabolised in the liver. To obtain maximal contraceptive effectiveness the tablet should be taken as directed and at approximately the same time each day. If the patient has vomiting or diarrhoea, absorption of the hormones will be impaired, making it advisable use an additional reliable method of contraception until her next menstrual Period.

Because the active ingredients are metabolised in the liver, reduced contraceptive efficacy has been associated with concomitant use of oral contraceptives and rifampicin.

A similar association has been suggested with oral contraceptives and barbiturates, phenytoin sodium, phenylbutazone griseofulvin and ampicillin.

5.3 Preclinical safety data

No relevant information additional to that contained elsewhere in the summary of characteristics

6. PHARMACEUTICAL PARTICULARS

6.1 List of excipients

White tablets:

Lactose, Pregelatinised starch, Magnesium stearate, Methanol* Purified water,

Light Peach tablet

Lactose, Pregelatinised starch, FD&C Yellow number6(-E110)Magnesium stearate. Methanol* Purified water

Peach Tablets:

Lactose, Pregelatinised starch, FD&C Yellow number6(-E110)Magnesium stearate. Methanol* Purified water(* not detected in final product)

6.2 Incompatibilities

None stated

6.3 Shelf life

2 years

6.4 Special precautions for storage

Do not store above 30°C. Protect from light.

6.5 Nature and contents of container

Clear uncoloured PVC/foil Blister strips of 21 tablets. Strips are packaged with a patient information leaflet with or without a plastic or card wallet in a cardboard carton. Park sizes:1x21*,3x21,6x21*,50x21* and 100x21*(* Not marketed)

6.6 Special precautions for disposal and other handling

None stated

7. MARKETING AUTHORISATION HOLDER

Janssen-Cilag Limited

50-100 Holmers Farm Way

High Wycombe

Buckinghamshire

HP12 4EG

UK

8. MARKETING AUTHORISATION NUMBER(S)

PL 00242/0279

9. DATE OF FIRST AUTHORISATION/RENEWAL OF THE AUTHORISATION

01 September 1995

10. DATE OF REVISION OF THE TEXT

17/07/2008

Trisenox 1 mg/ml concentrate for solution for infusion

(Cephalon (UK) Limited)

1. NAME OF THE MEDICINAL PRODUCT

TRISENOX 1 mg/ml, concentrate for solution for infusion

2. QUALITATIVE AND QUANTITATIVE COMPOSITION

One ml of TRISENOX contains 1 mg of Arsenic trioxide

For a full list of excipients, see section 6.1

3. PHARMACEUTICAL FORM

Concentrate for solution for infusion

Sterile, clear, colourless, aqueous solution.

4. CLINICAL PARTICULARS

4.1 Therapeutic indications

TRISENOX is indicated for induction of remission and consolidation in adult patients with relapsed/refractory acute promyelocytic leukaemia (APL), characterised by the presence of the t(15;17) translocation and/or the presence of the Pro-Myelocytic Leukaemia/Retinoic-Acid-Receptor-alpha (PML/RAR-alpha) gene. Previous treatment should have included a retinoid and chemotherapy.

The response rate of other acute myelogenous leukaemia subtypes to TRISENOX has not been examined.

4.2 Posology and method of administration

Posology

TRISENOX must be administered under the supervision of a physician who is experienced in the management of acute leukaemias, and the special monitoring procedures described in Section 4.4 must be followed. The same dose is recommended for children, adults, and elderly.

Induction treatment schedule: TRISENOX must be administered intravenously at a fixed dose of 0.15 mg/kg/day given daily until the bone marrow remission is achieved (less than 5% blasts present in cellular bone marrow with no evidence of leukaemic cells). If bone marrow remission has not occurred by day 50, dosing must be discontinued.

Consolidation schedule: Consolidation treatment must begin 3 to 4 weeks after completion of induction therapy. TRISENOX is to be administered intravenously at a dose of 0.15 mg/kg/day for 25 doses given 5 days per week, followed by 2 days interruption, repeated for 5 weeks.

Paediatric use: The experience in children is limited. Of 7 patients under 18 years of age (range 5 to 16 years) treated with TRISENOX at the recommended dose of 0.15 mg/kg/day, 5 patients achieved a complete response. Safety and effectiveness in paediatric patients under 5 years of age have not been studied.

Patients with hepatic and/or renal impairment:

Since limited data are available across all hepatic impairment groups and across all renal impairment groups, caution is advised in the use of TRISENOX in patients with hepatic and/or renal impairment.

Method of administration

TRISENOX must be administered intravenously over 1-2 hours. The infusion duration may be extended up to 4 hours if vasomotor reactions are observed. A central venous catheter is not required. Patients must be hospitalised at the beginning of treatment due to symptoms of disease and to ensure adequate monitoring.

4.3 Contraindications

Hypersensitivity to the active substance or any of the excipients.

4.4 Special warnings and precautions for use

Clinically unstable APL patients are especially at risk and will require more frequent monitoring of electrolyte and glycaemia levels as well as more frequent haematologic, hepatic, renal and coagulation parameter tests.

Leukocyte Activation Syndrome (APL Differentiation Syndrome): Twenty-five percent of patients with APL treated with TRISENOX have experienced symptoms similar to a syndrome called the retinoic-acid-acute promyelocytic leukaemia (RA-APL) or APL differentiation syndrome, characterised by fever, dyspnoea, weight gain, pulmonary infiltrates and pleural or pericardial effusions, with or without leukocytosis. This syndrome can be fatal. The management of the syndrome has not been fully studied, but high-dose steroids have been used at the first suspicion of the APL differentiation syndrome and appear to mitigate signs and symptoms. At the first signs that could suggest the syndrome (unexplained fever, dyspnoea and/or weight gain, abnormal chest auscultatory findings or radiographic abnormalities), high-dose steroids (dexamethasone 10 mg intravenously twice a day) must be immediately initiated, irrespective of the leukocyte count and continued for at least 3 days or longer until signs and symptoms have abated. The majority of patients do not require termination of TRISENOX therapy during treatment of the APL differentiation syndrome. It is recommended that chemotherapy not be added to treatment with steroids since there is no experience with administration of both steroids and chemotherapy during treatment of the leukocyte activation syndrome due to TRISENOX. Post-marketing experience suggests that a similar syndrome may occur in patients with other types of malignancy. Monitoring and management for these patients should be as described above.

Electrocardiogram (ECG) Abnormalities: Arsenic trioxide can cause QT interval prolongation and complete atrioventricular block. QT prolongation can lead to a torsade de pointes-type ventricular arrhythmia, which can be fatal. Previous treatment with anthracyclines may increase the risk of QT prolongation. The risk of torsade de pointes is related to the extent of QT prolongation, concomitant administration of QT prolonging medicinal products (such as class Ia and III antiarrythmics (e.g. quinidine, amiodarone, sotalol, dofetilide), antipsychotics (e.g. thioridazine), antidepressants (e.g. amitriptyline), some macrolides (e.g. erythromycin), some antihistamines (e.g. terfenadine and astemizole), some quinolone antibiotics (e.g. sparfloxacin), and other individual drugs known to increase QT interval (e.g. cisapride)), a history of torsade de pointes, pre-existing QT interval prolongation, congestive heart failure, administration of potassium-wasting diuretics, amphotericin B or other conditions that result in hypokalemia or hypomagnesaemia. In clinical trials, 40% of patients treated with TRISENOX experienced at least one QT corrected (QTc) interval prolongation greater than 500 msec. Prolongation of the QTc was observed between 1 and 5 weeks after TRISENOX infusion, and then returned to baseline by the end of 8 weeks after TRISENOX infusion. One patient (receiving multiple, concomitant medicinal products, including amphotericin B) had asymptomatic torsade de pointes during induction therapy for relapsed APL with arsenic trioxide.

ECG and Electrolyte Monitoring Recommendations: Prior to initiating therapy with TRISENOX, a 12-lead ECG must be performed and serum electrolytes (potassium, calcium, and magnesium) and creatinine must be assessed; preexisting electrolyte abnormalities must be corrected and, if possible, medicinal products that are known to prolong the QT interval must be discontinued. Patients with risk factors of QTc prolongation or risk factors of torsade de pointes should be monitored with continuous cardiac monitoring (ECG). For QTc greater than 500 msec, corrective measures must be completed and the QTc reassessed with serial ECGs prior to considering using TRISENOX. During therapy with TRISENOX, potassium concentrations must be kept above 4 mEq/l and magnesium concentrations must be kept above 1.8 mg/dl. Patients who reach an absolute QT interval value $>$ 500 msec must be reassessed and immediate action must be taken to correct concomitant risk factors, if any, while the risk/benefit of continuing versus suspending TRISENOX therapy must be considered. If syncope, rapid or irregular heartbeat develops, the patient must be hospitalised and monitored continuously, serum electrolytes must be assessed, TRISENOX therapy must be temporarily discontinued until the QTc interval regresses to below 460 msec, electrolyte abnormalities are corrected, and the syncope and irregular heartbeat cease. There are no data on the effect of TRISENOX on the QTc interval during the infusion. Electrocardiograms must be obtained twice weekly, and more frequently for clinically unstable patients, during induction and consolidation.

Dose Modification: Treatment with TRISENOX must be interrupted, adjusted, or discontinued before the scheduled end of therapy at any time that a toxicity grade 3 or greater on the National Cancer Institute Common Toxicity Criteria, Version 2 is observed and judged to be possibly related to TRISENOX treatment. Patients who experience such reactions that are considered TRISENOX related must resume treatment only after resolution of the toxic event or after recovery to baseline status of the abnormality that prompted the interruption. In such cases, treatment must resume at 50% of the preceding daily dose. If the toxic event does not recur within 3 days of restarting treatment at the reduced dose, the daily dose can be escalated back to 100% of the original dose. Patients who experience a recurrence of toxicity must be removed from treatment.

Laboratory tests: The patient's electrolyte and glycaemia levels, as well as haematologic, hepatic, renal and coagulation parameter tests must be monitored at least twice weekly, and more frequently for clinically unstable patients during the induction phase and at least weekly during the consolidation phase.

Patients with renal impairment:

Since limited data are available across all renal impairment groups, caution is advised in the use of TRISENOX in patients with renal impairment. The experience in patients with severe renal impairment is insufficient to determine if dose adjustment is required.

The use of TRISENOX in patients on dialysis has not been studied.

Patients with hepatic impairment:

Since limited data are available across all hepatic impairment groups, caution is advised in the use of TRISENOX in patients with hepatic impairment. The experience in patients with severe hepatic impairment is insufficient to determine if dose adjustment is required.

Elderly patients: There is limited clinical data on the use of TRISENOX in the elderly population. Caution is needed in these patients.

Hyperleukocytosis: Treatment with TRISENOX has been associated with the development of hyperleukocytosis ($\geqslant 10 \times 10^3/\mu l$) in some patients. There did not appear to be a relationship between baseline white blood cell (WBC) counts and development of hyperleukocytosis nor did there appear to be a correlation between baseline WBC count and peak WBC counts. Hyperleukocytosis was never treated with additional chemotherapy and resolved on continuation of TRISENOX. WBC counts during consolidation were not as high as during induction treatment and were $< 10 \times 10^3/\mu l$, except in one patient who had a WBC count of $22 \times 10^3/\mu l$ during consolidation. Twenty patients (50%) experienced leukocytosis; however, in all these patients, the WBC count was declining or had normalized by the time of bone marrow remission and cytotoxic chemotherapy or leukopheresis was not required.

4.5 Interaction with other medicinal products and other forms of interaction

No formal assessments of pharmacokinetic interactions between TRISENOX and other therapeutic medicinal products have been conducted. QT/QTc prolongation is expected during treatment with TRISENOX, and torsade de pointes and complete heart block have been reported. Patients who are receiving, or who have received, medicinal products known to cause hypokalemia or hypomagnesaemia, such as diuretics or amphotericin B, may be at higher risk for torsade de pointes. Caution is advised when TRISENOX is coadministered with other medicinal products known to cause QT/QTc interval prolongation such as macrolide antibiotics, the antipsychotic thioridazine, or medicinal products known to cause hypokalemia or hypomagnesaemia. Additional information about QT prolonging medicinal agents, is provided in Section 4.4. The influence of TRISENOX on the efficacy of other antileukaemic medicinal products is unknown.

4.6 Pregnancy and lactation

Arsenic trioxide has been shown to be embryotoxic and teratogenic in animal studies (see 5.3). There are no studies in pregnant women using TRISENOX. If this medicinal product is used during pregnancy or if the patient becomes pregnant while taking this product, the patient must be informed of the potential harm to the foetus. Men, and women of childbearing potential must use effective contraception during treatment with TRISENOX.

Arsenic is excreted in human milk. Because of the potential for serious adverse reactions in nursing infants from TRISENOX, breastfeeding must be discontinued prior to and throughout administration.

4.7 Effects on ability to drive and use machines

No studies on the effects on the ability to drive and use machines have been performed.

4.8 Undesirable effects

Related adverse reactions of CTC grade 3 and 4 occurred in 37% of patients in clinical trials. The most commonly reported reactions were hyperglycaemia, hypokalaemia, neutropenia, and increased alanine amino transferase (ALT). Leukocytosis occurred in 50% of patients with APL, as determined by haematology assessments, rather than adverse event reports.

Serious adverse reactions were common (1-10%) and not unexpected in this population. Those serious adverse reactions attributed to TRISENOX included APL differentiation syndrome (3), leukocytosis (3), prolonged QT interval (4, 1 with torsade de pointes), atrial fibrillation/atrial flutter (1), hyperglycaemia (2) and a variety of serious adverse reactions related to haemorrhage, infections, pain, diarrhoea, nausea.

In general, treatment-emergent adverse events tended to decrease over time, perhaps accounted for by amelioration of the underlying disease process. Patients tended to tolerate consolidation and maintenance treatment with less toxicity than in induction. This is probably due to the confounding of adverse events by the uncontrolled disease process early on in the treatment course and the myriad concomitant medicinal products required to control symptoms and morbidity.

The table below lists the related grade 3 and 4 adverse drug reactions for the 107 patients treated with TRISENOX in clinical trials (frequencies defined as: common $\geqslant 1/100$ to $< 1/10$, uncommon $\geqslant 1/1{,}000$ to $< 1/100$).

Within each frequency grouping, undesirable effects are presented in order of decreasing seriousness.

(see Table 1 below)

During TRISENOX treatment, 13 of the 52 patients in the APL studies had one or more symptoms of APL differentiation syndrome, characterised by fever, dyspnoea, weight gain, pulmonary infiltrates and pleural or pericardial effusions, with or without leukocytosis (see Section 4.4). Twenty-seven patients had leukocytosis (WBC $\geqslant 10 \times 10^3/\mu l$) during induction, 4 of whom had values above 100,000/µl. Baseline white blood cell (WBC) counts did not correlate with development of leukocytosis on study, and WBC counts during consolidation therapy were not as high as during induction. In these studies, leukocytosis was not treated with chemotherapeutic medicinal products. Medicinal products that are used to lower the white blood cell count often exacerbate the toxicities associated with leukocytosis, and no standard approach has proven effective. One patient treated under a compassionate use program died from cerebral infarct due to leukocytosis, following treatment with chemotherapeutic medicinal products to lower WBC count. Observation is the recommended approach with intervention only in selected cases.

Mortality in the pivotal studies from disseminated intravascular coagulation (DIC) associated haemorrhage was very common (> 10%), which is consistent with the early mortality reported in the literature.

Arsenic trioxide can cause QT interval prolongation (see Section 4.4). QT prolongation can lead to a torsade de pointes-type ventricular arrhythmia, which can be fatal. The risk of torsade de pointes is related to the extent of QT prolongation, concomitant administration of QT prolonging medicinal products, a history of torsade de pointes, preexisting QT interval prolongation, congestive heart failure, administration of potassium-wasting diuretics, or other conditions that result in hypokalaemia or hypomagnesaemia. One patient (receiving multiple, concomitant medicinal products, including amphotericin B) had asymptomatic torsade de pointes during induction therapy for relapsed APL with arsenic trioxide. She went onto consolidation without further evidence of QT prolongation.

Peripheral neuropathy, characterised by paresthesia/dysesthesia, is a common and well known effect of environmental arsenic. Only 2 patients discontinued treatment early due to this adverse event and one went on to receive additional TRISENOX on a subsequent protocol. Forty-four percent of patients experienced symptoms that could be associated with neuropathy; most were mild to moderate and were reversible upon cessation of treatment with TRISENOX.

Table 1

System Organ Class	Common	Uncommon
Blood and lymphatic system disorders	Neutropenia Thrombocytopenia	Febrile neutropenia Leucocytosis Leucopenia
Metabolism and nutrition disorders	Hyperglycaemia Hypokalaemia	Hypermagnesaemia Hypernatraemia Ketoacidosis
Nervous system disorders	Paraesthesia	
Cardiac disorders		Pericardial effusion Tachycardia
Vascular disorders		Vasculitis
Respiratory, thoracic and mediastinal disorders	Pleuritic pain Dyspnoea	Pulmonary alveolar haemorrhage Pleural effusion Hypoxia
Gastrointestinal disorders		Diarrhoea
Skin and subcutaneous tissue disorders		Pruritus Erythema
Musculoskeletal and connective tissue disorders	Bone pain Arthralgia	Myalgia
General disorders and administration site conditions	Pyrexia Fatigue	Chest pain Pain
Investigations	ECG QT prolonged ALT increased Aspartate amino transferase increased	Hyperbilirubinaemia Hypomagnesaemia

The following adverse events have been identified during the post-approval use of TRISENOX and have been included following consideration of the observed frequency, seriousness and possible causal relationship to TRISENOX. They are listed below by system organ class and frequency (frequencies are defined as: uncommon ($\geqslant 1/1{,}000$ to $< 1/100$), not known (cannot be estimated from the available data).

(see Table 2 on next page)

In post marketing experience, a differentiation syndrome, like retinoic acid syndrome, has also been reported for the treatment of malignancies other than APL with TRISENOX.

4.9 Overdose

If symptoms suggestive of serious acute arsenic toxicity (*e.g.* convulsions, muscle weakness and confusion) appear, TRISENOX must be immediately discontinued and chelating therapy with penicilamine at a daily dose $\leqslant$ 1 gm per day may be considered. The duration of treatment with penicillamine must be evaluated taking into account the urinary arsenic laboratory values. For patients who cannot take oral medication, dimercaprol administered at a dose of 3 mg/kg intramuscularly every 4 hours until any immediately life-threatening toxicity has subsided may be considered. Thereafter, penicillamine at a daily dose $\leqslant$ 1 gm per day may be given. In the presence of coagulopathy, the oral administration of the chelating agent Dimercaptosuccinic Acid Succimer (DCI) 10 mg/kg or 350 mg/m^2 every 8 hours during 5 days and then every 12 hours during 2 weeks is recommended. For patients with severe, acute arsenic overdose, dialysis should be considered

5. PHARMACOLOGICAL PROPERTIES

5.1 Pharmacodynamic properties

Pharmacotherapeutic group: Other antineoplastic agents, ATC code: L01XX27

TRISENOX has been authorised under "Exceptional Circumstances". This means that due to the rarity of the disease, it has not been possible to obtain complete information on this medicinal product. The European Medicines Agency (EMEA) will review any new information which may become available every year and this SPC will be updated as necessary.

Mechanism of action: The mechanism of action of TRISENOX is not completely understood. Arsenic trioxide causes morphological changes and deoxyribonucleic acid (DNA) fragmentation characteristic of apoptosis in NB4 human promyelocytic leukaemia cells *in vitro*. Arsenic trioxide also causes damage or degradation of the fusion protein Pro-Myelocytic Leukaemia/Retinoic Acid Receptor-alpha (PML/RAR alpha).

Clinical trials: TRISENOX has been investigated in 52 APL patients, previously treated with an anthracycline and a retinoid regimen, in two open-label, single-arm, non-comparative studies. One was a single investigator clinical study (n=12) and the other was a multicentre, 9-institution study (n=40). Patients in the first study received a median dose of 0.16 mg/kg/day of TRISENOX (range 0.06 to 0.20 mg/kg/day) and patients in the multicentre study received a fixed dose of 0.15 mg/kg/day. TRISENOX was administered intravenously over 1 to 2 hours until the bone marrow was free of leukaemic cells, up to a maximum of 60 days. Patients with complete remission received consolidation therapy with TRISENOX for 25 additional doses over a 5 week period. Consolidation therapy began 6 weeks (range, 3-8) after induction in the single institution study and 4 weeks (range, 3-6) in the multicentre study. Complete remission (CR) was defined as the absence of visible leukaemic cells in the bone marrow and peripheral recovery of platelets and white blood cells.

Patients in the single centre study had relapsed following 1-6 prior therapy regimens and 2 patients had relapsed following stem cell transplantation. Patients in the multicentre study had relapsed following 1-4 prior therapy regimens and 5 patients had relapsed following stem cell transplantation. The median age in the single centre study was 33 years (age range 9 to 75). The median age in the multicentre study was 40 years (age range 5 to 73).

The results are summarised in the table below.

	Single Centre Trial N=12	Multicentre Trial N=40
TRISENOX Dose, mg/kg/day (Median, Range)	0.16 (0.06 – 0.20)	0.15
Complete Remission	11 (92%)	34 (85%)
Time to Bone Marrow Remission (Median)	32 days	35 days
Time to CR (Median)	54 days	59 days
18-Month Survival	67%	66%

The single institution study included 2 paediatric patients (< 18 years old), both of whom achieved CR. The multicentre trial included 5 paediatric patients (< 18 years old), 3 of whom achieved CR. No children of less than 5 years of age were treated.

Table 2

System Organ Class	Uncommon	Not known
Infection and Infestations	Sepsis Pneumonia Herpes zoster	
Blood and Lymphatics System Disorders	Anaemia	Pancytopenia
Metabolism and Nutrition Disorders	Dehydration Fluid retention	
Psychiatric Disorders	Confusional state	
Nervous System Disorders	Convulsions Dizziness	
Eye Disorders	Vision blurred	
Cardiac Disorders	Cardiac failure Ventricular tachycardia Ventricular extrasystoles	
Vascular Disorders	Hypotension	
Respiratory, Thoracic and Mediastinal Disorders	Pneumonitis	Differentiation syndrome
Gastrointestinal Disorders	Vomiting Abdominal pain	
Skin and Subcutaneous Disorders	Face oedema Rash	
Renal and Urinary Disorders	Renal failure	
General Disorders and Administration Site Conditions	Oedema Chills	
Investigations	Blood creatinine increased Weight increased	

In a follow-up treatment after consolidation, 7 patients in the single institution study and 18 patients in the multicentre study received further maintenance therapy with TRISENOX. Three patients from the single institution study and 15 patients from the multicentre study had stem cell transplants after completing TRISENOX. The Kaplan-Meier median CR duration for the single institution study is 14 months and has not been reached for the multicentre study. At last follow-up, 6 of 12 patients in the single institution study were alive with a median follow-up time of 28 months (range 25 to 29). In the multicentre study 27 of 40 patients were alive with a median follow-up time of 16 months (range 9 to 25). Kaplan-Meier estimates of 18-month survival for each study are shown below.

(see Figure 1 opposite)

Cytogenetic confirmation of conversion to a normal genotype and Reverse Transcriptase - Polymerase Chain Reaction (RT-PCR) detection of PML/RARα conversion to normal are shown in the table below.

Cytogenetics after TRISENOX therapy

	Single Centre Pilot Trial N with CR = 11	Multicentre Trial N with CR = 34
Conventional Cytogenetics [t(15;17)]		
Absent	8 (73%)	31 (91%
Present	1 (9%)	0%
Not evaluable	2 (18%)	3 (9%)
RT-PCR for PML/ RARα		
Negative	8 (73%)	27 (79%)
Positive	3 (27%)	4 (12%)
Not evaluable	0	3 (9%)

Responses were seen across all age groups tested, ranging from 6 to 75 years. The response rate was similar for both genders. There is no experience on the effect of TRISENOX on the variant APL containing the t(11;17) and t(5;17) chromosomal translocations.

5.2 Pharmacokinetic properties

The inorganic, lyophilized form of arsenic trioxide, when placed into solution, immediately forms the hydrolysis product arsenious acid (As^{III}). As^{III} is the pharmacologically active species of arsenic trioxide.

In the total single dose range of 7 to 32 mg (administered as 0.15 mg/kg), systemic exposure (AUC) appears to be linear. The decline from peak plasma concentration of As^{III} occurs in a biphasic manner and is characterized by an initial rapid distribution phase followed by a slower terminal elimination phase. After administration at 0.15 mg/kg on a daily (n=6) or twice-weekly (n=3) regimen, an approximate 2-fold accumulation of As^{III} was observed as compared to a single infusion. This accumulation was slightly more than expected based on single-dose results.

Distribution:

The volume of distribution (V_d) for As^{III} is large (>400 L) indicating significant distribution into the tissues with negligible protein binding. V_d is also weight dependent, increasing with increasing body weight. Total arsenic accumulates mainly in the liver, kidney, and heart and, to a lesser extent, in the lung, hair, and nails.

Metabolism:

The metabolism of arsenic trioxide involves oxidation of arsenious acid (As^{III}), the active species of arsenic trioxide, to arsenic acid (As^{V}), as well as oxidative methylation to monomethylarsonic acid (MMA^{V}) and dimethylarsinic acid (DMA^{V}) by methyltransferases, primarily in the liver. The pentavalent metabolites, MMA^{V} and DMA^{V}, are slow to appear in plasma (approximately 10-24 hours after first administration of arsenic trioxide), but due to their longer half-life, accumulate more upon multiple dosing than does As^{III}. The extent of accumulation of these metabolites is dependent on the dosing regimen. Approximate accumulation ranged from 1.4- to 8-fold following multiple as compared to single dose administration. As^{V} is present in plasma only at relatively low levels.

In vitro enzymatic studies with human liver microsomes revealed that arsenic trioxide has no inhibitory activity on substrates of the major cytochrome P450 enzymes such as 1A2, 2A6, 2B6, 2C8, 2C9, 2C19, 2D6, 2E1, 3A4/5, 4A9/11. Drugs that are substrates for these P450 enzymes are not expected to interact with TRISENOX.

Elimination:

Approximately 15% of the administered TRISENOX dose is excreted in the urine as unchanged As^{III}. The methylated metabolites of As^{III} (MMA^{V}, DMA^{V}) are primarily excreted in the urine. The plasma concentration of As^{III} declines from peak plasma concentration in a biphasic manner with a mean terminal elimination half-life of 10 to 14 hours. The total clearance of As^{III} over the single-dose range of 7-32 mg (administered as 0.15 mg/kg) is 49 L/h and the renal clearance is 9 L/h. Clearance is not dependent on the weight of the subject or the dose administered over the dose range studied. The mean estimated terminal elimination half-lives of the metabolites MMA^{V} and DMA^{V} are 32 hours and 70 hours, respectively.

Renal Impairment:

Plasma clearance of As^{III} was not altered in patients with mild renal impairment (creatinine clearance of 50-80 mL/min) or moderate renal impairment (creatinine clearance of 30-49 mL/min). The plasma clearance of As^{III} in patients with severe renal impairment (creatinine clearance less than 30 mL/min) was 40% lower when compared with patients with normal renal function (see section 4.4).

Systemic exposure to MMA^{V} and DMA^{V} tended to be larger in patients with renal impairment; the clinical consequence of this is unknown but no increased toxicity was noted.

Hepatic Impairment:

Pharmacokinetic data from patients with hepatocellular carcinoma having mild to moderate hepatic impairment indicate that As^{III} or As^{V} do not accumulate following twice-weekly infusions. No clear trend toward an increase in systemic exposure to As^{III}, As^{V}, MMA^{V} or DMA^{V} was observed with decreasing level of hepatic function as assessed by dose-normalized (per mg dose) AUC.

5.3 Preclinical safety data

Limited reproductive toxicity studies of arsenic trioxide in animals indicate embryotoxicity and teratogenicity (neural tube defects, anophthalmia and microphthalmia) at administration of 1-10 times the recommended clinical dose (mg/m2). Fertility studies have not been conducted with TRISENOX. Arsenic compounds induce chromosomal aberrations and morphological transformations of mammalian cells *in vitro* and *in vivo*. No formal carcinogenicity studies of arsenic trioxide have been performed. However, arsenic trioxide and other inorganic arsenic compounds are recognised as human carcinogens.

6. PHARMACEUTICAL PARTICULARS

6.1 List of excipients

sodium hydroxide

hydrochloric acid as pH adjuster

water for injections

6.2 Incompatibilities

In the absence of incompatibility studies, this medicinal product must not be mixed with other medicinal products except those mentioned in 6.6.

Figure 1

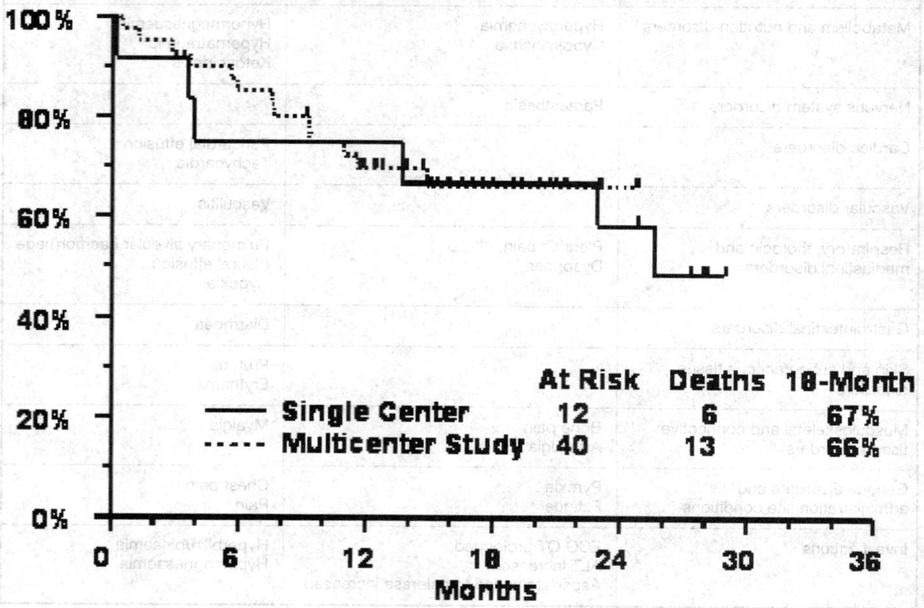

6.3 Shelf life

3 years.

After dilution in intravenous solutions, TRISENOX is chemically and physically stable for 24 hours at 15-30°C and 48 hours at refrigerated (2-8°C) temperatures. From a microbiological point of view, the product must be used immediately. If not used immediately, in-use storage times and conditions prior to use are the responsibility of the user and would normally not be longer than 24 hours at 2-8°C, unless dilution has taken place in controlled and validated aseptic conditions.

6.4 Special precautions for storage

Do not freeze.

6.5 Nature and contents of container

Type I borosilicate glass ampoule of 10 ml. Each pack contains 10 ampoules.

6.6 Special precautions for disposal and other handling

Preparation of TRISENOX

ASEPTIC TECHNIQUE MUST BE STRICTLY OBSERVED THROUGHOUT HANDLING OF TRISENOX SINCE NO PRESERVATIVE IS PRESENT.

TRISENOX must be diluted with 100 to 250 ml of glucose 50 mg/ml (5%) injection or sodium chloride 9 mg/ml (0.9%) injection immediately after withdrawal from the ampoule. For single use only. Unused portions of each ampoule must be discarded properly. Do not save any unused portions for later administration.

TRISENOX must not be mixed with or concomitantly administered in the same intravenous line with other medicinal products.

TRISENOX must be administered intravenously over 1-2 hours. The infusion duration may be extended up to 4 hours if vasomotor reactions are observed. A central venous catheter is not required.

The diluted solution must be clear and colourless. All parenteral solutions must be inspected visually for particulate matter and discoloration prior to administration. Do not use the preparation if foreign particulate matter is present.

Procedure for proper disposal

Any unused product, any items that come into contact with the product, and waste material must be disposed of in accordance with local requirements.

7. MARKETING AUTHORISATION HOLDER

Cephalon Europe
5 Rue Charles Martigny
94700 Maisons Alfort
FRANCE

8. MARKETING AUTHORISATION NUMBER(S)

EU/1/02/204/001

9. DATE OF FIRST AUTHORISATION/RENEWAL OF THE AUTHORISATION

Date of first authorisation: 05 March 2002

Date of last renewal: 05 March 2007

10. DATE OF REVISION OF THE TEXT

April 2009

Trisequens

(Novo Nordisk Limited)

1. NAME OF THE MEDICINAL PRODUCT

Trisequens®

2. QUALITATIVE AND QUANTITATIVE COMPOSITION

28 sequential tablets: 12 blue, 10 white, 6 red.

Active ingredients:

Blue tablets - Estradiol hemihydrate EP corresponding to estradiol 2mg

White tablets - Estradiol hemihydrate EP corresponding to estradiol 2mg

Norethisterone acetate EP 1mg

Red tablets - Estradiol hemihydrate EP corresponding to estradiol 1mg

Excipients: Lactose monohydrate. For a full list of excipients, see section 6.1.

3. PHARMACEUTICAL FORM

Film-coated tablets for oral administration.

4. CLINICAL PARTICULARS

4.1 Therapeutic indications

a) Hormone Replacement Therapy (HRT) for oestrogen deficiency symptoms.

b) Prevention of osteoporosis in postmenopausal women at high risk of future fractures who are intolerant of, or contraindicated for, other medicinal products approved for the prevention of osteoporosis.

See also section 4.4

The experience of treating women older than 65 years is limited.

4.2 Posology and method of administration

Trisequens is a continuous sequential preparation for hormone replacement therapy. The oestrogen is dosed continuously. The progestogen is added for 10 days in each 28 day cycle, in a sequential manner.

Trisequens is administered orally, without chewing, one tablet daily without interruption, starting with the blue tablets. After taking the last red tablet, treatment is continued with the first blue tablet of a new pack on the next day. A regular shedding of the endometrium is usually induced during the red tablet phase or at the end of the white tablet phase.

In menstruating women or women transferring from another sequential HRT, the first tablet should be taken on the fifth day of menstrual bleeding. If menstruation has stopped altogether or is infrequent and sporadic (2-4 monthly intervals) or in women transferring from a continuous-combined HRT product, the first tablet can be taken at any time.

For initiation and continuation of treatment of post menopausal symptoms, the lowest effective dose for the shortest duration (see also section 4.4) should be used.

A switch to a higher dose combination product could be indicated if the response after three months is insufficient for satisfactory symptom relief.

Unless there is a previous diagnosis of endometriosis, it is not recommended to add a progestogen in hysterectomised women.

If a patient forgets to take a tablet, the forgotten tablet should be taken within the next twelve hours. Otherwise the tablet should be discarded. Forgetting a tablet may increase the likelihood of breakthrough bleeding and spotting.

4.3 Contraindications

- Known, past or suspected breast cancer.
- Known or suspected oestrogen-dependent malignant tumours (e.g. endometrial cancer
- Undiagnosed genital bleeding.
- Untreated endometrial hyperplasia.
- Previous idiopathic or current venous thromboembolism (deep venous thrombosis, pulmonary embolism.
- Active or recent arterial thromboembolic disease (e.g. angina, myocardial infarction).
- Acute liver disease, or a history of liver disease as long as liver function tests have failed to return to normal.
- Known hypersensitivity to the active substances or any of the excipients.
- Porphyria.

4.4 Special warnings and precautions for use

For the treatment of postmenopausal symptoms, HRT should only be initiated for symptoms that adversely affect quality of life. In all cases, a careful appraisal of the risks and benefits should be undertaken at least annually and HRT should only be continued as long as the benefit outweighs the risk.

<u>Medical examination/follow-up</u>

Before initiating or reinstituting HRT, a complete personal and family medical history should be taken. Physical (including pelvic and breast) examination should be guided by this and by the contra-indications and warnings for use. During treatment, periodic check-ups are recommended of a frequency and nature adapted to the individual woman. Women should be advised what changes in their breasts should be reported to their doctor or nurse (see 'Breast cancer' below). Investigations, including mammography, should be carried out in accordance with currently accepted screening practices, modified to the clinical needs of the individual.

<u>Conditions which need supervision</u>

If any of the following conditions are present, have occurred previously, and/or have been aggravated during pregnancy or previous hormone treatment, the patient should be closely supervised. It should be taken into account that these conditions may recur or be aggravated during treatment with Trisequens, in particular:

- Leiomyoma (uterine fibroids) or endometriosis
- A history of, or risk factors for, thromboembolic disorders (see below)
- Risk factors for oestrogen dependent tumours, e.g. 1st degree heredity for breast cancer
- Hypertension
- Liver disorders (e.g. liver adenoma)
- Diabetes mellitus with or without vascular involvement
- Cholelithiasis
- Migraine or (severe) headache
- Systemic lupus erythematosus
- A history of endometrial hyperplasia (see below)
- Epilepsy
- Asthma
- Otosclerosis

<u>Reasons for immediate withdrawal of therapy</u>

Therapy should be discontinued in case a contra-indication is discovered and in the following situations:

- Jaundice or deterioration in liver function
- Significant increase in blood pressure
- New onset of migraine-type headache
- Pregnancy

<u>Endometrial hyperplasia</u>

- The risk of endometrial hyperplasia and carcinoma is increased when oestrogens are administered alone for prolonged periods (see section 4.8). The addition of a progestogen for 10 days per cycle in non-hysterectomised women reduces, but does not eliminate, this risk.
- Breakthrough bleeding and spotting may occur during the first months of treatment in women with intact uterus. If breakthrough bleeding or spotting appears after some time on therapy, or continues after treatment has been discontinued, the reason should be investigated, which may include endometrial biopsy to exclude endometrial malignancy.

<u>Breast Cancer</u>

A randomised placebo-controlled trial, the Women's Health Initiative study (WHI), and epidemiological studies, including the Million Women Study (MWS), have reported an increased risk of breast cancer in women taking oestrogens, oestrogen-progestogen combinations or tibolone for HRT for several years (see Section 4.8). For all HRT, an excess risk becomes apparent within a few years of use and increases with duration of intake but returns to baseline within a few (at most five) years after stopping treatment.

In the MWS, the relative risk of breast cancer with conjugated equine oestrogens (CEE) or estradiol (E2) was greater when a progestogen was added, either sequentially or continuously, and regardless of type of progestogen. There was no evidence of a difference in the risk between the different routes of administration.

In the WHI study, the continuous combined conjugated equine oestrogen and medroxyprogesterone acetate (CEE + MPA) product used was associated with breast cancers that were slightly larger in size and more frequently had local lymph node metastases compared to placebo.

HRT, especially oestrogen-progestogen combined treatment, increases the density of mammographic images which may adversely affect the radiological detection of breast cancer.

<u>Venous thromboembolism</u>

HRT is associated with a higher relative risk of developing venous thromboembolism (VTE), i.e. deep vein thrombosis or pulmonary embolism. One randomised controlled trial and epidemiological studies found a two- to three fold higher risk for users compared with non-users. For non-users it is estimated that the number of cases of VTE that will occur over a 5 year period is about 3 per 1000 women aged 50-59 years and 8 per 1000 women aged between 60-69 years. It is estimated that in healthy women who use HRT for 5 years, the number of additional cases of VTE over a 5 year period will be between 2 and 6 (best estimate = 4) per 1000 women aged 50-59 years and between 5 and 15 (best estimate = 9) per 1000 women aged 60-69 years. The occurrence of such an event is more likely in the first year of HRT than later.

Generally recognised risk factors for VTE include a personal history or family history, severe obesity ($BM > 30\ kg/m^2$) and systemic lupus erythematosus (SLE). There is no consensus about the possible role of varicose veins in VTE.

Patients with a history of VTE or known thrombophilic states have an increased risk of VTE. HRT may add to this risk. Personal or strong family history of thromboembolism, or recurrent spontaneous abortion, should be investigated in order to exclude a thrombophilic predisposition. Until a thorough evaluation of thrombophilic factors has been made or anticoagulant treatment initiated, use of HRT in such patients should be viewed as contraindicated. Those women already on anticoagulant treatment require careful consideration of the benefit-risk of use of HRT.

The risk of HRT may be temporarily increased with prolonged immobilisation, major trauma or major surgery. As in all postoperative patients, scrupulous attention should be given to prophylactic measures to prevent VTE following surgery. Where prolonged immobilisation is liable to follow elective surgery, particularly abdominal or orthopaedic surgery to the lower limbs, consideration should be given to temporarily stopping HRT 4 to 6 weeks earlier, if possible. Treatment should not be restarted until the woman is completely mobilised.

If VTE develops after initiating therapy, the drug should be discontinued. Patients should be told to contact their doctors immediately when they are aware of a potential thromboembolic symptom (e.g. painful swelling of a leg, sudden pain in the chest, dyspnoea).

<u>Coronary artery disease (CAD)</u>

There is no evidence from randomised controlled trials of cardiovascular benefit with continuous combined conjugated oestrogens and medroxyprogesterone acetate (MPA). Two large clinical trials (WHI and HERS i.e. Heart and Estrogen/progestin Replacement Study) showed a possible increased risk of cardiovascular morbidity in the first year of use and no overall benefit. For other HRT products there are only limited data from randomised controlled trials examining effects in cardiovascular morbidity or mortality. Therefore, it is uncertain whether these findings also extend to other HRT products.

Stroke

One large randomised clinical trial (WHI-trial) found, as a secondary outcome, an increased risk of ischaemic stroke in healthy women during treatment with continuous combined conjugated oestrogens and MPA. For women who do not use HRT, it is estimated that the number of cases of stroke that will occur over a 5 year period is about 3 per 1000 women aged 50-59 years and 11 per 1000 women aged 60-69 years. It is estimated that for women who use conjugated oestrogens and MPA for 5 years, the number of additional cases will be between 0 and 3 (best estimate = 1) per 1000 users aged 50-59 years and between 1 and 9 (best estimate = 4) per 1000 users aged 60-69 years. It is unknown whether the increased risk also extends to other HRT products.

Ovarian cancer

Long-term (at least 5 -10 years) use of combined HRTs and oestrogen-only HRT products has been associated with a slightly increased risk of ovarian cancer (see Section 4.8).

Other conditions

- Oestrogens may cause fluid retention, and therefore patients with cardiac or renal dysfunction should be carefully observed. Patients with terminal renal insufficiency should be closely observed since it is expected that the level of circulating active ingredients in Trisequens will be increased.

- Women with pre-existing hypertriglyceridemia should be followed closely during oestrogen replacement or hormone replacement therapy, since rare cases of large increases of plasma triglycerides leading to pancreatitis have been reported with oestrogen therapy in this condition.

- Oestrogens increase thyroid binding globulin (TGB), leading to increased circulating total thyroid hormone, as measured by protein-bound iodine (PBI), T4 levels (by column or by radio-immunoassay) or T3 levels (by radio-immunoassay). T3 resin uptake is decreased, reflecting the elevated TBG. Free T4 and free T3 concentrations are unaltered. Other binding proteins may be elevated in serum, i.e. corticoid binding globulin (CBG), sex-hormone-binding globulin (SHBG) leading to increased circulating corticosteroids and sex steroids, respectively. Free or biologically active hormone concentrations are unchanged. Other plasma proteins may be increased (angiotensinogen/renin substrate, alpha-1-antitrypsin, ceruloplasmin).

- There is no conclusive evidence for improvement of cognitive function. There is some evidence from the WHI trial of increased risk of probable dementia in women who start using continuous combined CEE and MPA after the age of 65. It is unknown whether the findings apply to younger post-menopausal women or other HRT products.

- Trisequens has no contraceptive effect. Patients using hormonal contraception should be advised to transfer to a non-hormonal method when taking Trisequens.

- Patients with rare hereditary problems of galactose intolerance, the Lapp lactase deficiency or glucose-galactose malabsorption should not take this medicine.

4.5 Interaction with other medicinal products and other forms of interaction

The metabolism of oestrogens and progestogens may be increased by concomitant use of substances known to induce drug-metabolising enzymes, specifically cytochrome P450 enzymes such as anticonvulsants (e.g. phenobarbital, phenytoin, carbamazepin) and anti-infectives (e.g. rifampicin, rifabutin, nevirapine, efavirenz).

Ritonavir and nelfinavir, although known as strong inhibitors, by contrast exhibit inducing properties when used concomitantly with steroid hormones. Herbal preparations containing St John's wort (Hypericum perforatum) may induce the metabolism of oestrogens and progestogens.

Clinically, an increased metabolism of oestrogens and progestogens may lead to decreased effect and changes in the uterine bleeding profile.

Drugs that inhibit the activity of hepatic microsomal drug metabolising enzymes, e.g. ketoconazole, may increase circulating levels of the active substances in Trisequens.

4.6 Pregnancy and lactation

Trisequens is not indicated during pregnancy. If pregnancy occurs during medication with Trisequens, treatment should be withdrawn immediately.

Data on a limited number of exposed pregnancies indicate adverse effects of norethisterone on the foetus. At dose levels higher than normally used in OC and HRT formulations masculinisation of female foetuses was observed. The results of most epidemiological studies to-date have not indicated a teratogenic or foetotoxic effect when combinations of oestrogens with progestogens at dose levels relevant for Trisequens were taken inadvertently during pregnancy.

Trisequens is not indicated during lactation.

4.7 Effects on ability to drive and use machines

No effects known.

4.8 Undesirable effects

Clinical experience:

The most frequently reported adverse events in the clinical trials with Trisequens were vaginal bleeding and breast pain/tenderness reported in approximately 10% to 20% of patients. Vaginal bleeding usually occurred in the first months of treatment. Breast pain usually disappears after a few months of therapy. All adverse events observed with a higher frequency in patients treated with Trisequens or similar HRT products as compared to placebo and which on an overall judgement were considered as possibly related to treatment are presented below.

(see Table 1 below)

Post-marketing experience:

In addition to the above-mentioned adverse drug reactions, those presented below have been spontaneously reported, and by an overall judgement considered possible related to Trisequens treatment. The reporting rate of these spontaneous adverse drug reactions is very rare (<1/10,000 patient years):

Neoplasms benign and malignant (incl. cysts and polyps): Endometrial cancer

Psychiatric disorders: Insomnia, anxiety, libido decreased, libido increased

Nervous system disorders: Dizziness, stroke

Eye disorders: Visual disturbances

Vascular disorders: Hypertension aggravated

Cardiac disorders: Myocardial infarction

Gastrointestinal disorders: Dyspepsia, vomiting

Hepatobiliary disorders: Gallbladder disease, cholelithiasis, cholelithiasis aggravated, cholelithiasis re-occurrence

Skin and subcutaneous tissue disorder: Seborrhoea, rash, angioneurotic oedema

Reproductive system and breast disorders: Vulvovaginal pruritus

Investigations: Weight decreased, blood pressure increased

The following adverse reactions have been reported in association with other oestrogen/progestogen treatment:

- Skin and subcutaneous disorders: chloasma, erythema multiforme, erythema nodosum, vascular purpura
- Probable dementia (see section 4.4).

Breast cancer

According to evidence from a large number of epidemiological studies and one randomised placebo-controlled trial, the Women's Health Initiative (WHI), the overall risk of breast cancer increases with increasing duration of HRT use in current or recent HRT users.

For *oestrogen-only* HRT, estimates of relative risk (RR) from a reanalysis of original data from 51 epidemiological studies (in which >80% of HRT use was oestrogen-only HRT) and from the epidemiological Million Women Study (MWS) are similar at 1.35 (95% CI: 1.21-1.49) and 1.30 (95% CI: 1.21-1.40), respectively.

For *oestrogen plus progestogen* combined HRT, several epidemiological studies have reported an overall higher risk for breast cancer than with oestrogens alone.

The MWS reported that, compared to never users, the use of various types of oestrogen-progestogen combined HRT was associated with a higher risk of breast cancer (RR = 2.00, 95% CI: 1.88-2.12) than use of oestrogens alone (RR = 1.30, 95% CI: 1.21-1.40) or use of tibolone (RR = 1.45, 95% CI: 1.25-1.68).

The WHI trial reported a risk estimate of 1.24 (95% CI: 1.01-1.54) after 5.6 years of use of oestrogen-progestogen combined HRT (CEE + MPA) in all users compared with placebo.

The absolute risks calculated from the MWS and the WHI trial are presented below:

The MWS has estimated, from the known average incidence of breast cancer in developed countries, that:

- For women not using HRT, about 32 in every 1000 are expected to have breast cancer diagnosed between the ages of 50 and 64 years.
- For 1000 current or recent users of HRT, the number of *additional* cases during the corresponding period will be
- For users of *oestrogen-only* replacement therapy,

- between 0 and 3 (best estimate = 1.5) for 5 years' use
- between 3 and 7 (best estimate = 5) for 10 years' use.

- For users of *oestrogen plus progestogen* combined HRT,

- between 5 and 7 (best estimate = 6) for 5 years' use
- between 18 and 20 (best estimate = 19) for 10 years use.

The WHI trial estimated that after 5.6 years of follow-up of women between the ages of 50 and 79 years, an *additional* 8 cases of invasive breast cancer would be due to *oestrogen-progestogen combined* HRT (CEE + MPA) per 10,000

Table 1

System organ class	Very common >1/10	Common >1/100; <1/10	Uncommon >1/1,000; <1/100	Rare >1/10,000; <1/1,000
Infections and infestations		Genital candidiasis or vaginitis, see also 'Reproductive system and breast disorders'		
Immune system disorders			Hypersensitivity, see also 'Skin and subcutaneous tissue disorders'	
Metabolism and nutrition disorders		Fluid retention, see also 'General disorders and administration site conditions'		
Psychiatric disorders		Depression or depression aggravated	Nervousness	
Nervous system disorders		Headache, migraine or migraine aggravated		
Vascular disorders			Thrombophlebitis superficial	Pulmonary embolism Deep vein thrombosis See also sections 4.3 and 4.4
Gastrointestinal disorders		Nausea Abdominal pain, abdominal distension or abdominal discomfort	Flatulence or bloating	
Skin and subcutaneous tissue disorders			Alopecia, hirsutism or acne Pruritus or urticaria	
Musuloskeletal, connective tissue and bone disorders		Back pain Leg cramps		
Reproductive system and breast disorders	Breast pain or breast tenderness Menstruation irregular or menorrhagia	Breast oedema or breast enlargement Uterine fibroids aggravated or uterine fibroids reoccurrence or uterine fibroids	Hyperplasia endometrial Dysmenorrhoea, see also back pain and abdominal pain	
General disorders and administration site conditions		Oedema peripheral	Drug ineffective	
Investigations		Weight increased		

women years. According to calculations from the trial data, it is estimated that:

- For 1000 women in the placebo group,

- about 16 cases of invasive breast cancer would be diagnosed in 5 years.

- For 1000 women who used oestrogen + progestogen combined HRT (CEE + MPA), the number of additional cases would be

- between 0 and 9 (best estimate = 4) for 5 years' use.

The number of additional cases of breast cancer in women who use HRT is broadly similar for women who start HRT irrespective of age at start of use (between the ages of 45-65) (see section 4.4).

Endometrial cancer

In women with an intact uterus, the risk of endometrial hyperplasia and endometrial cancer increases with increasing duration of use of unopposed oestrogens. According to data from epidemiological studies, the best estimate of the risk is that for women not using HRT, about 5 in every 1000 are expected to have endometrial cancer diagnosed between the ages of 50 and 65. Depending on the duration of treatment and oestrogen dose, the reported increase in endometrial cancer risk among unopposed oestrogen users varies from 2- to 12-fold greater compared with non-users. Adding a progestogen to oestrogen-only therapy greatly reduces this increased risk.

Ovarian cancer

Long-term use of oestrogen-only and combined oestrogen-progestogen HRT has been associated with a slightly increased risk of ovarian cancer. In the Million Women Study 5 years of HRT resulted in 1 extra case per 2500 users.

4.9 Overdose

Overdosage may be manifested by nausea and vomiting. Treatment should be symptomatic

5. PHARMACOLOGICAL PROPERTIES

5.1 Pharmacodynamic properties

ATC code GO3F BO5

Oestrogen and progestogen for continuous sequential hormone replacement therapy.

Estradiol: The active ingredient, synthetic 17 beta-estradiol, is chemically and biologically identical to endogenous human estradiol. It substitutes for the loss of oestrogen production in menopausal women, and alleviates menopausal symptoms.

Oestrogens prevent bone loss following menopause or ovariectomy.

Norethisterone acetate: As oestrogens promote the growth of the endometrium, unopposed oestrogens increase the risk of endometrial hyperplasia and cancer. The addition of a progestogen greatly reduces the oestrogen-induced risk of endometrial hyperplasia in non-hysterectomised women.

Relief of menopausal symptoms is achieved during the first few weeks of treatment.

Regular withdrawal bleeding occurred in 93% of women with a mean duration of 3-4 days.

Oestrogen deficiency at menopause is associated with an increasing bone turnover and decline in bone mass. The effect of oestrogens on the bone mineral density is dose-dependent. Protection appears to be effective for as long as treatment is continued. After discontinuation of HRT, bone mass is lost at a rate similar to that in untreated women.

Evidence from the WHI trial and meta-analysed trials shows that current use of HRT, alone or in combination with a progestogen – given to predominantly healthy women – reduces the risk of hip, vertebral, and other osteoporotic fractures. HRT may also prevent fractures in women with low bone density and/or established osteoporosis, but the evidence for that is limited.

Studies based on measurement of bone mineral content have shown that Trisequens is effective in the prevention of osteoporosis in postmenopausal women. After 2 years of treatment, bone mineral density in the spine had increased by 5.14% and in the hip by 3.21%.

5.2 Pharmacokinetic properties

Following oral administration of 17β-estradiol in micronised form, rapid absorption from the gastrointestinal tract occurs. It undergoes extensive first-pass metabolism in the liver and other enteric organs, and reaches a peak plasma concentration of approximately 44 pg/ml (range 30-35 pg/ml) within 5-8 hours after intake of 2mg. The half-life of 17β-estradiol is about 12-14 hours. It circulates bound to SHBG (37%) and to albumin (61%), while only approximately 1-2% is unbound. Metabolism of 17β-estradiol occurs mainly in the liver and the gut but also in target organs, and involves the formation of less active or inactive metabolites, including oestrone, catecholoestrogens and several oestrogen sulphates and glucuronides. Oestrogens are excreted with the bile, where they are hydrolysed and reabsorbed (enterohepatic circulation), and mainly in urine in biologically inactive form.

After oral administration norethisterone acetate is rapidly absorbed and transformed to norethisterone (NET). It undergoes first-pass metabolism in the liver and other enteric organs, and reaches a peak plasma concentration of approximately 9ng/ml (range 6-11 ng/ml) within 0.5 - 1.5 hours after intake of 1mg. The terminal half-life of NET is about 8-11 hours. NET binds to SHBG (36%) and to albumin (61%). The most important metabolites are isomers of 5α-dihydro-NET and of tetrahydro-NET, which are excreted mainly in the urine as sulphate or glucuronide conjugates.

The pharmacokinetics in the elderly have not been studied.

5.3 Preclinical safety data

Acute toxicity of oestrogens is low. Because of marked differences between animal species and between animal species and humans, preclinical results possess a limited predictive value for the use of oestrogens in humans.

In experimental animals estradiol and estradiol valerate displayed an embryolethal effect at relatively low doses; malformations of the urogenital tract and feminisation of male foetuses was observed.

Norethisterone, like other progestogens, caused virilisation of female foetuses in rats and monkeys. After high doses of norethisterone embryolethal effects were observed.

Preclinical data based on conventional studies of repeated dose toxicity, genotoxicity and carcinogenic potential revealed no particular human risks beyond those discussed in other sections of the SPC.

6. PHARMACEUTICAL PARTICULARS

6.1 List of excipients

Lactose monohydrate

Maize starch

Gelatin

Talc

Magnesium stearate

Hypromellose

Purified water

Blue tablets:	Indigo carmine (E132)
	Titanium dioxide (E171)
	Macrogol 400
White tablets:	Triacetin
Red tablets:	Iron oxide (E172)
	Titanium dioxide (E171)
	Propylene glycol

6.2 Incompatibilities

None known.

6.3 Shelf life

48 months.

6.4 Special precautions for storage

Store in a dry place, protected from light. Store below 25°C. Do not refrigerate.

6.5 Nature and contents of container

Polypropylene/polystyrene calendar dial pack containing 28 tablets. Calendar dial packs (3 × 28 tablets) are contained within outer carton.

6.6 Special precautions for disposal and other handling

Each carton contains a patient information leaflet with instructions for use of the calendar dial pack.

7. MARKETING AUTHORISATION HOLDER

Novo Nordisk Limited

Broadfield Park, Brighton Road

Crawley, West Sussex, RH11 9RT

8. MARKETING AUTHORISATION NUMBER(S)

PL 3132/0122.

9. DATE OF FIRST AUTHORISATION/RENEWAL OF THE AUTHORISATION

29 January 1998.

10. DATE OF REVISION OF THE TEXT

07/2009

LEGAL CATEGORY

Prescription-only medicine (POM).

Tritace Tablet Titration Pack

(sanofi-aventis)

1. NAME OF THE MEDICINAL PRODUCT

Tritace®Tablet Titration Pack

2. QUALITATIVE AND QUANTITATIVE COMPOSITION

Tritace®Tablet Titration Pack containing tablets of 2.5 mg, 5.0 mg and 10 mg ramipril.

For excipients see section 6.1

3. PHARMACEUTICAL FORM

2.5 mg:

Yellowish to yellow oblong tablets with score-line.

Upper stamp: 2.5 & logo

Lower stamp: HMR & 2.5

5.0 mg:

Pale red oblong tablets with score-line.

Upper stamp: 5 & logo

Lower stamp: HMP & 5

10 mg:

White to almost white oblong tablets with score-line.

Upper stamp: HMO/HMO

Lower stamp: Anonymous

4. CLINICAL PARTICULARS

4.1 Therapeutic indications

For reducing the risk of myocardial infarction, stroke, cardiovascular death or need for revascularisation procedures in patients of 55 years or more who have clinical evidence of cardiovascular disease (previous MI, unstable angina or multivessel CABG or multivessel PTCA), stroke or peripheral vascular disease.

Also for reducing the risk of myocardial infarction, stroke, cardiovascular death or need for revascularisation procedures in diabetic patients of 55 years or more who have one or more of the following clinical findings: hypertension (systolic blood pressure > 160mmHg or diastolic blood pressure > 90mmHg); high total cholesterol (>5.2 mmol/L); low HDL (<0.9 mmol/L); current smoker; known microalbuminuria; clinical evidence of previous vascular disease.

4.2 Posology and method of administration

Oral administration.

Dosage and Administration:

Tritace Tablets Titration Pack is a multi-strength pack containing a total of 35 tablets. The dose regimen is based on the fixed titration process to titrate the patient up to a maintenance dose of 10mg Tritace once a day, as shown below.

- Tritace 2.5mg once a day for 7 days
- Tritace 5mg once a day for 21 days
- Tritace 10mg once a day for 7 days

The patient opens the pack from the top to access the first week's treatment of Tritace 2.5mg. When this is finished the patient tears away the dividing cardboard layer to reach the next 3 weeks treatment of Tritace 5mg. The patient repeats this process to get to the final weeks worth of treatment of Tritace 10mg.

Tritace Tablets Titration Pack should only be used in patients for whom this titration schedule is thought to be suitable.

Caution is required in patients with concomitant use of diuretics, congestive heart failure, renal or hepatic insufficiency, incompletely corrected fluid or salt depletion, severe hypertension, or in patients in whom a hypotensive reaction would constitute a particular risk, (e.g., with relevant stenoses of the coronary or cerebral vessels). In these cases the fixed titration regimen may not be suitable and an individual titration schedule should be considered.

Elderly: Caution in all elderly patients.

Children: Tritace has not been studied in children, and therefore use in this age group is not recommended.

Tritace tablets should be swallowed, without chewing, with a glass of water. The absorption of ramipril is not affected by food and Tritace can therefore be taken before, during or after a meal.

4.3 Contraindications

Hypersensitivity to ramipril, any of the excipients of Tritace, or to any other ACE inhibitor.

History of angioedema.

Haemodynamically relevant bilateral renal artery stenosis or unilateral in the single kidney.

Hypotensive or haemodynamically unstable patients.

Pregnancy.

Breast-feeding women.

Concomitant use of ACE inhibitors and extracorporeal treatments leading to contact of blood with negatively charged surfaces must be avoided, since such use may lead to severe anaphylactoid reactions. Such extracorporeal treatments include dialysis or haemofiltration with certain high-flux (e.g. polyacrylonitril) membranes and low-density lipoprotein apheresis with dextran sulfate. This combination should therefore be avoided, either by use of alternative antihypertensive drugs or alternative membranes for dialysis.

4.4 Special warnings and precautions for use

Warnings:

Tritace Tablets Titration Pack should only be used in patients for whom this fixed dosage regimen is suitable. Those patients needing a lower starting dose or longer periods of time on the lower strengths of tablets should not be prescribed Tritace Tablet Titration Pack.

Angioneurotic oedema occurring during treatment with an ACE inhibitor necessitates immediate discontinuation of the drug. Angioneurotic oedema of the face, extremities, tongue, glottis or larynx has been reported in patients treated with ACE inhibitors and hospitalisation of the patient is advisable.

Intestinal angioedema has been reported in patients treated with ACE inhibitors.

These patients presented with abdominal pain (with or without nausea or vomiting); in some cases facial angioedema also occurred. The intestinal angioedema symptoms resolved after stopping the ACE inhibitor.

Tritace should not be used in patients with aortic or mitral valve stenosis or outflow obstruction (see Precautions section below).

Precautions:

Assessment of renal function: Evaluation of the patient should include assessment of renal function prior to initiation of therapy and during treatment.

Impaired renal function: Patients with renal insufficiency may require reduced or less frequent doses of Tritace; their renal function should be closely monitored. In the majority, renal function will not alter. There is a risk of impairment of renal function, particularly in patients with congestive heart failure or after a renal transplant, renal insufficiency, bilateral renal artery stenosis and unilateral renal artery stenosis in the single kidney. In the latter patient group, even a small increase in serum creatinine may be indicative of unilateral loss of renal function. If recognised early, such impairment of renal function is reversible upon discontinuation of therapy.

Patients haemodialysed using high flux polyacrylonitrile ('AN69') membranes are highly likely to experience anaphylactoid reactions if they are treated with ACE inhibitors. This combination should therefore be avoided, either by use of alternative antihypertensive drugs or alternative membranes for dialysis.

Similar reactions have been observed during low-density lipoprotein apheresis with dextran sulphate. This method should, therefore, not be used in patients treated with ACE inhibitors.

Some hypertensive patients with no apparent pre-existing renal disease may develop minor and usually transient increases in blood urea nitrogen and serum creatinine when Tritace is given, in particular concomitantly with a diuretic. Dosage reduction of Tritace and/or discontinuation of the diuretic may be required.

Impaired liver function: As ramipril is a prodrug metabolised to its active moiety in the liver, particular caution and close monitoring should be applied to patients with impaired liver function. The metabolism of the parent compound, and therefore the formation of the bioactive metabolite ramiprilat, may be diminished resulting in markedly elevated plasma levels of the parent compound (due to the reduced activity of esterases in the liver).

In patients in whom severe liver cirrhosis with oedema and/or ascites is present, the renin angiotensin system may be significantly activated; therefore, particular caution must be exercised in treating these patients (see also above and under "4.2 Posology and Method of Administration").

Agranulocytosis and bone marrow depression: In patients on angiotensin converting enzyme inhibitors agranulocytosis and bone marrow depression have been seen rarely, as well as a reduction in red cell count, haemoglobin content and platelet count. These are more frequent in patients with renal impairment, especially if they have a collagen vascular disease. Regular monitoring of white blood cell counts (to permit detection of a possible leucopenia) and protein levels in urine should be considered in patients with collagen vascular disease (e.g. lupus erythematosus and scleroderma), especially associated with impaired renal function and concomitant therapy particularly with corticosteroids and anti metabolites. Patients on allopurinol, immunosuppressants and other substances that may change the blood picture also have increased likelihood of other blood picture changes.

Hyperkalaemia: Elevated serum potassium has been observed very rarely in hypertensive patients. Risk factors for the development of hyperkalaemia include renal insufficiency, potassium sparing diuretics and the concomitant use of agents to treat hypokalaemia. It is recommended that serum potassium be monitored regularly. More frequent monitoring of serum potassium is necessary in patients with impaired renal function.

Patients with hyper-stimulated renin angiotensin system: In the treatment of patients with a hyper-stimulated renin angiotensin system, particular caution must be exercised (see also under "4.2 Posology and Method of Administration"). Such patients are at risk of an acute pronounced fall in blood pressure and deterioration of renal function due to ACE inhibition, especially when an ACE inhibitor or a concomitant diuretic is given for the first time or for the first time at an increased dose. Initial doses or initial dose increases must be accompanied by close blood pressure monitoring until such time as no further acute reduction in blood pressure is to be anticipated.

Significant activation of the renin angiotensin system is to be anticipated, for example:

– in patients with severe and/or with malignant hypertension.

– in patients with heart failure, particularly if severe or if treated with other substances having antihypertensive potential.

– in patients with haemodynamically relevant left-ventricular inflow or outflow obstruction (e.g., aortic or mitral valve stenosis).

– in patients pre-treated with diuretics.

– in patients with fluid or salt depletion, or in those in whom it may develop (as a result of insufficient fluid or salt intake, or as a result of, e.g., dialysis, diarrhoea, vomiting or excessive sweating in cases where salt and fluid replacement is inadequate).

Generally, it is recommended that dehydration, hypovolaemia or salt depletion be corrected before initiating treatment (in patients with heart failure, however, such corrective action must be carefully weighed against other risks of volume overload). When these conditions have become clinically relevant, treatment with Tritace must only be started or continued if appropriate steps are taken concurrently to prevent an excessive fall in blood pressure and deterioration of renal function.

For all of the above, the initial phase of treatment requires close medical supervision.

Patients at particular risk from a pronounced reduction in blood pressure: If symptomatic hypotension occurs, the patient should be placed in a supine position and, if necessary, receive an intravenous infusion of physiological saline. Intravenous atropine may be necessary if there is associated bradycardia. Treatment with Tritace may usually be continued following restoration of effective blood volume and blood pressure.

Surgery/anaesthesia: In patients undergoing surgery or during anaesthesia with agents producing hypotension, Tritace may block angiotensin II formation secondary to compensatory renin release. If hypotension occurs and is considered to be due to this mechanism, it can be corrected by appropriate treatment.

4.5 Interaction with other medicinal products and other forms of interaction

Vasopressor sympathomimetics: These may reduce the antihypertensive effect of Tritace. Particularly close blood pressure monitoring is recommended.

Allopurinol, immunosuppressants, corticosteroids, procainamide, cytostatics and other substances that may change the blood picture: Increased likelihood of haematological reactions (see also under "4.4 Special Warnings and Special Precautions for use").

Lithium Salts: Excretion of lithium may be reduced by ACE inhibitors. Such reduction may lead to increased serum lithium levels and increased lithium toxicity. Lithium levels must, therefore, be monitored.

Diuretics and other antihypertensive agents: Combination with diuretics or other antihypertensive agents may potentiate the antihypertensive response to Tritace. Potassium sparing diuretics (spironolactone, amiloride, triamterene) or potassium supplements may increase the risk of hyperkalaemia. Tritace may attenuate the potassium loss caused by thiazide-type diuretics. Regular monitoring of serum sodium and potassium is recommended in patients undergoing concurrent diuretic therapy. Adrenergic-blocking drugs should only be combined with ramipril under careful supervision.

Combination with antidiabetics: When antidiabetic agents (insulin and sulphonylurea derivatives) are used concurrently, the possibility of increased blood-sugar reduction must be considered. Particularly close blood glucose monitoring is therefore recommended in the initial phase of co-administration.

Combination with NSAIDs: When ACE inhibitors are administered simultaneously with non-steroidal anti-inflammatory drugs (e.g. acetylsalicylic acid and indomethacin), attenuation of the antihypertensive effect may occur. Furthermore, concomitant use of ACE inhibitors and NSAIDs may lead to an increased risk of worsening of renal function and an increase in serum potassium.

Heparin: Rise in serum potassium concentration possible.

Desensitisation therapy: The likelihood and severity of anaphylactic and anaphylactoid reactions to insect venoma is increased under ACE inhibition. It is assumed that this effect may also occur in connection with other allergens.

The protein binding of ramipril is about 73% and of ramiprilat about 56%.

4.6 Pregnancy and lactation

Tritace must not be taken during pregnancy. Therefore, pregnancy must be excluded before starting treatment. If the patient intends to become or becomes pregnant, treatment with ACE inhibitors must be discontinued, i.e. replaced by another form of treatment. Pregnancy must be avoided in cases where treatment with ACE inhibitors is indispensable.

It is not known if exposure limited to the first trimester only can harm the fetus. Exposure of the mother to ACE inhibitors in mid or late pregnancy has been associated with oligohydramnios and neonatal hypotension with anuria or renal failure.

From animal experiments it is known that use of ramipril may cause a decreased utero-placental perfusion. There is also a potential risk of fetal or post-natal effect as ACE inhibitors also influence the local renin-angiotensin system. In peri-post natal studies increased renal pelvic dilatation was observed in the first generation offspring. However, ramipril was not fetotoxic in our studies although ACE inhibitors have shown fetotoxicity in some species.

If treatment with Tritace is necessary during lactation, the patient must not breast feed in order to prevent the infant from ingesting small quantities of ramipril with breast milk.

4.7 Effects on ability to drive and use machines

In individual cases, as a result of a reduction in blood pressure, treatment with Tritace may affect the ability to drive and operate machinery. This occurs especially at the start of treatment, when changing over from other preparations and during concomitant use of alcohol. After the first dose or subsequent increases in dose it is not advisable to drive or operate machinery for several hours.

4.8 Undesirable effects

Generally, adverse reactions have been mild and transient, and do not require discontinuation of therapy. The most frequently reported adverse reactions are nausea, dizziness and headache. Uncommonly drowsiness, light-headedness or impaired reactions may occur.

Reactions such as peripheral oedema, tinnitus, fatigue, visual disturbances, sweating, disturbed hearing, disturbed orthostatic regulation are rare.

Cardiovascular: Symptomatic hypotension accompanied by dizziness, weakness and nausea may occur after the initial dose of Tritace and after an increase in the dose of Tritace. It has been rarely observed, but may occur in severely salt/volume-depleted patients such as those treated with diuretics, patients on dialysis and in patients with severe congestive heart failure. Syncope has also been observed rarely.

Myocardial infarction or cerebrovascular accident possibly secondary to severe hypotension in high risk patients, chest pain, palpitations, rhythm disturbances, angina pectoris may occur.

Renal: Treatment with Tritace may impair renal function and in isolated cases progression to acute renal failure may occur.

Gastrointestinal: Treatment with Tritace may be associated with symptoms in the digestive tract, e.g. rarely dryness of the mouth, glossitis, irritation or inflammation of the oral mucosa, digestive disturbances, constipation, diarrhoea, nausea, and vomiting, (gastritis-like) stomach pain, abdominal discomfort (sometimes with increased levels of pancreatic enzymes). Uncommonly, increases in hepatic enzymes and/or serum bilirubin, jaundice due to impaired excretion of bile pigment (cholestatic jaundice), acute hepatitis, potentially leading to liver failure.

Pancreatitis has been reported rarely in patients treated with ACE inhibitors; in some cases this has proved fatal.

Allergic: Hypersensitivity reactions accompanied by pruritus, rash, shortness of breath and sometimes fever may occur, but usually resolve spontaneously after withdrawal of Tritace.

In addition, the following cutaneous and mucosal reactions may occur: reddening of skin areas with accompanying heat sensation, conjunctivitis, itching, urticaria, other skin or mucosal eruptions (maculo-papular and lichenoid exanthema and enanthema, erythema multiforme), sometimes pronounced hair loss, exacerbation of disturbances due to vascular stenoses and precipitation or intensification of Raynaud's phenomenon. In isolated cases, pemphigus, exacerbation of psoriasis, psoriasiform and pemphigoid exanthema and enanthema, Stevens-Johnson syndrome, toxic epidermal necrolysis, hypersensitivity of the skin to light and onycholysis have been observed.

See Section 4.5 (Interactions) for advice on reactions to insect venoma.

Haematological reactions: Rarely, a mild - in isolated cases severe – reduction in the red blood cell count and haemoglobin content, white blood cell or blood platelet count may develop. In isolated cases, agranulocytosis, pancytopenia and bone marrow depression may occur.

In isolated cases haemolytic anaemia may develop.

Vasculitis, muscle and joint pains, fever, or eosinophilia may occur. Raised titres of antinuclear antibodies have been seen with other ACE inhibitors.

Angioedema: See Section 4.4 (Special Warnings and Special Precautions for Use). Uncommonly, pharmacologically mediated mild angioneurotic oedema may occur (the incidence of ACE inhibitor angioedema seems to be increased in black, i.e. Afro-Caribbean, patients as compared with non-black patients). Serious reactions of this type and other, non-pharmacologically mediated anaphylactic or anaphylactoid reactions to ramipril or any of the other ingredients are rare.

Respiratory tract: A dry tickling cough may occur. This is possibly due to the desired ACE inhibition as are the following adverse effects: rhinitis, sinusitis, bronchitis and, especially in patients with tickling cough, bronchospasm.

Other adverse reactions: Disturbances of balance, headache, nervousness, restlessness, tremor, sleep disorders, confusion, loss of appetite, depressed mood, feeling of anxiety, paraesthesiae, uncommonly disturbances of smell and taste or partial, sometimes complete, loss of taste, muscle cramps, erectile impotence and reduced sexual desire may occur.

Laboratory test findings: Increases in blood urea nitrogen and serum creatinine may occur, in particular with renal insufficiency or in patients pretreated with a diuretic. Pre-existing proteinuria may deteriorate (though ACE inhibitors usually reduce proteinuria), or there may be an increase in urinary output.

Sodium/Potassium serum levels– See Section 4.5 (Special warnings and special precautions for use).

4.9 Overdose

Symptoms

Overdosage may cause excessive peripheral vasodilatation (with marked hypotension, shock), bradycardia, electrolyte disturbances, and renal failure.

Management

General measures to ensure adequate ventilation and circulation should be taken.

Despite the benefits of gastric decontamination being uncertain, it is recommended to consider activated charcoal (50g for adults, 1g/kg for children) if the patient presents within 1 hour of ingestion of a potentially toxic amount (0.5mg/kg).

If severe hypotension occurs, the patient should be placed in the shock position and salt and volume supplementations should be given rapidly. In the event of prolonged hypotension, administration of inotropes (e.g. norepinephrine, dopamine) and angiotensin II (angiotensinamide) must be considered in addition to volume and salt substitution.

5. PHARMACOLOGICAL PROPERTIES

5.1 Pharmacodynamic properties

Pharmacotherapeutic group: ACE Inhibitor, plain. ATC Code: C09AA05

Ramipril is a prodrug which, after absorption from the gastrointestinal tract, is hydrolysed in the liver to form the active angiotensin converting enzyme (ACE) inhibitor, ramiprilat which is a potent and long acting ACE inhibitor. Administration of ramipril causes an increase in plasma renin activity and a decrease in plasma concentrations of angiotensin II and aldosterone. The beneficial haemodynamic effects resulting from ACE inhibition are a consequence of the reduction in angiotensin II causing dilation of peripheral vessels and reduction in vascular resistance. There is evidence suggesting that tissue ACE particularly in the vasculature, rather than circulating ACE, is the primary factor determining the haemodynamic effects.

Angiotensin converting enzyme is identical with kininase II, one of the enzymes responsible for the degradation of bradykinin. There is evidence that ACE inhibition by ramiprilat appears to have some effects on the kallikrein-kinin-prostaglandin systems. It is assumed that effects on these systems contribute to the hypotensive and metabolic activity of ramipril.

In a large endpoint study – HOPE - ramipril significantly reduced the incidence of stroke, myocardial infarction and/or cardiovascular death when compared with placebo. These benefits occurred largely in normotensive patients and were shown, using standard regression analysis techniques, to be only partially due to the relatively modest reductions in blood pressure demonstrated in the study. The 10mg dose, currently the highest safe dose level approved, was selected by the HOPE investigators from previous dose-ranging studies (SECURE, HEART) and was considered to be the most likely dose to effect full blockade of the renin-angiotensin-aldosterone system. This and other studies suggest that ACE inhibitors like ramipril are likely to have other direct effects on the cardiovascular system. These may include the antagonism of angiotensin II mediated vasoconstriction, the inhibition of proliferating vascular smooth muscle and plaque rupture, the enhancement of endothelial function, the reduction of LV hypertrophy and positive effects on fibrinolysis. Additional effects in diabetic patients may also contribute e.g. effects on insulin clearance and pancreatic blood flow.

5.2 Pharmacokinetic properties

Following oral administration ramipril is rapidly absorbed from the gastrointestinal tract; peak plasma concentrations of ramipril are reached within one hour. Peak plasma concentrations of the active metabolite, ramiprilat, are reached within 2 – 4 hours.

Plasma concentrations of ramiprilat decline in a polyphasic manner. The effective half-life of ramiprilat after multiple once daily administration of ramipril is 13 – 17 hours for 5 – 10 mg ramipril and markedly longer for lower doses, 1.25 – 2.5 mg ramipril. This difference is related to the long terminal phase of the ramiprilat concentration time curve observed at very low plasma concentrations. This terminal phase is independent of the dose, indicating a saturable capacity of the enzyme to bind ramiprilat. Steady-state plasma concentrations of ramiprilat after once daily dosing with the usual doses of ramipril are reached by about the fourth day of treatment.

Ramipril is almost completely metabolised and the metabolites are excreted mainly via the kidneys. In addition to the bioactive metabolite, ramiprilat, other, inactive metabolites have been identified, including diketopiperazine ester, diketopiperazine acid and conjugates.

5.3 Preclinical safety data

Reproduction toxicology studies in the rat, rabbit and monkey did not disclose any teratogenic properties. Fertility was not impaired either in male or in female rats. The administration of ramipril to female rats during the fetal period and lactation produced irreversible renal damage (dilation of the renal pelvis) in the offspring at daily doses of 50 mg/kg body weight and higher.

6. PHARMACEUTICAL PARTICULARS

6.1 List of excipients

Methylhydroxypropylcellulose, pregelatinised starch, microcrystalline cellulose, sodium stearyl fumarate; yellow ferric oxide E172 (2.5mg); red ferric oxide E172 (5mg).

6.2 Incompatibilities

None known.

6.3 Shelf life

48 months

6.4 Special precautions for storage

Store below 25°C

6.5 Nature and contents of container

PVC/Aluminium Blister packs of 35 tablets. 7 × 2.5mg, 21 × 5mg and 7 × 10mg tablets

6.6 Special precautions for disposal and other handling

None.

7. MARKETING AUTHORISATION HOLDER

Sanofi-aventis

One Onslow Street

Guildford

Surrey GU1 4YS

UK

8. MARKETING AUTHORISATION NUMBER(S)

PL 04425/0600

9. DATE OF FIRST AUTHORISATION/RENEWAL OF THE AUTHORISATION

March 2008

10. DATE OF REVISION OF THE TEXT

March 2008

Legal category; POM

Tritace Tablets

(sanofi-aventis)

1. NAME OF THE MEDICINAL PRODUCT

Tritace 1.25 mg Tablets

Tritace 2.5 mg Tablets

Tritace 5 mg Tablets

Tritace 10 mg Tablets

2. QUALITATIVE AND QUANTITATIVE COMPOSITION

1.25 mg ramipril.

2.5 mg ramipril.

5 mg ramipril

10 mg ramipril.

For excipients, see 6.1.

3. PHARMACEUTICAL FORM

Tablet

1.25mg: White to almost white oblong tablets with score-line.

Upper stamp: 1.25 & logo ( )

Lower stamp: HMN & 1.25

2.5mg: Yellowish to yellow oblong tablets with score-line.

Upper stamp: 2.5 & logo ( )

Lower stamp: HMR & 2.5

5mg: Pale red oblong tablets with score-line.

Upper stamp: 5 & logo ( )

Lower stamp: HMP & 5.

10mg: White to almost white, oblong tablets with a score-line

Upper stamp: HMO/HMO

4. CLINICAL PARTICULARS

4.1 Therapeutic indications

For reducing the risk of myocardial infarction, stroke, cardiovascular death or need for revascularisation procedures in patients of 55 years or more who have clinical evidence of cardiovascular disease (previous MI, unstable angina or multivessel CABG or multivessel PTCA), stroke or peripheral vascular disease.

Also for reducing the risk of myocardial infarction, stroke, cardiovascular death or need for revascularisation procedures in diabetic patients of 55 years or more who have one or more of the following clinical findings: hypertension (systolic blood pressure > 160mmHg or diastolic blood pressure > 90mmHg); high total cholesterol (>5.2 mmol/L); low HDL (<0.9 mmol/L); current smoker; known microalbuminuria; clinical evidence of previous vascular disease.

Tritace is indicated for the treatment of mild to moderate hypertension.

Congestive heart failure as adjunctive therapy to diuretics with or without cardiac glycosides.

Tritace has been shown to reduce mortality when given to patients surviving acute myocardial infarction with clinical evidence of heart failure.

4.2 Posology and method of administration

Oral administration.

Dosage and Administration:

Reducing the risk of myocardial infarction, stroke or cardiovascular death and/or the need for revascularisation procedures: The recommended initial dose is 2.5mg Tritace once a day. Depending on the tolerability, the dose should be gradually increased. It is therefore recommended that this dose is doubled after about one week of treatment then, after a further 3 weeks, it should be finally increased to 10mg. The usual maintenance dose is 10mg Tritace once a day. Patients already stabilised on lower doses of Tritace for other indications where possible should be titrated to 10mg Tritace once daily.

Hypertension: The recommended initial dosage in patients not on diuretics and without congestive heart failure is 1.25 mg Tritace once a day. Dosage should be increased incrementally at intervals of 1 - 2 weeks, based on patient response, up to a maximum of 10 mg once a day.

A 1.25 mg dose will only achieve a therapeutic response in a minority of patients. The usual maintenance dose is 2.5 - 5 mg as a single daily dose. If the patient response is still unsatisfactory at a dose of 10 mg Tritace, combination treatment is recommended.

In hypertensive patients who also have congestive heart failure, with or without associated renal insufficiency, symptomatic hypotension has been observed after treatment with ACE inhibitors. In these patients therapy should be started at a dose of 1.25 mg under close medical supervision in hospital.

Congestive heart failure: Recommended initial dose: In patients stabilised on diuretic therapy the initial dose is 1.25 mg once daily. Depending on the patient's response, the dose may be increased. It is recommended that the dose, if increased, be doubled at intervals of 1 to 2 weeks. If a daily dose of 2.5 mg or more is required, this may be taken as a single dose or as two divided doses. Maximum permitted daily dose: 10 mg.

Post myocardial infarction: Initiation of therapy: Treatment must be started in hospital between day 3 and day 10 following AMI. The starting dose is 2.5 mg twice a day with one taken in the morning and one in the evening. The dose can then be increased to 5 mg twice a day after 2 days. If the initial 2.5 mg dose is not tolerated a dose of 1.25 mg twice a day should be given for two days before increasing to 2.5 mg and 5.0 mg twice a day at intervals of 1 to 3 days.

If the dose cannot be increased to 2.5 mg twice a day treatment should be withdrawn.

Sufficient experience is still lacking in the treatment of patients with severe (NYHA IV) heart failure immediately after myocardial infarction. Should the decision be taken to treat these patients, it is recommended that therapy be started at 1.25mg once daily and that particular caution be exercised in any dose increase.

Maintenance dose: 2.5 to 5.0 mg twice a day.

Maximum daily dose: 10mg.

Patients on diuretics/Patients with salt depletion: In diuretic treated patients, the diuretic should be discontinued for 2-3 days (or longer depending on the duration of action of the diuretic), or at least the dose reduced, to reduce the likelihood of symptomatic hypotension. It may be resumed later if required. The initial daily dose in patients previously treated with a diuretic is generally 1.25mg Tritace.

In patients with incompletely corrected fluid or salt depletion, in patients with severe hypertension, as well as in patients in whom a hypotensive reaction would constitute a particular risk, (e.g., with relevant stenoses of the coronary or cerebral vessels), a reduced initial dose of 1.25mg Tritace should be considered.

Dosage adjustment in renal impairment: The usual dose of Tritace is recommended for patients with a creatinine clearance > 30 ml/min (serum creatinine < 165 µmol/l). For patients with a creatinine clearance < 30 ml/min (serum creatinine >165 µmol/l) the initial dose is 1.25 mg Tritace once daily and the maximum dose 5 mg Tritace once daily.

In patients with severe renal impairment (creatinine clearance < 10 ml/min and serum creatinine of 400-650 µmol/l), the recommended initial dose is also 1.25 mg Tritace once a day, but the maintenance dose should not exceed 2.5 mg Tritace once a day.

Dosage in hepatic impairment: In patients with impaired liver function the metabolism of the parent compound ramipril, and therefore the formation of the bioactive metabolite ramiprilat, is delayed due to a diminished activity of esterases in the liver, resulting in elevated plasma ramipril levels. Treatment with ramipril should therefore be initiated at a dose of 1.25 mg under close medical supervision in patients with impaired liver function.

Higher doses should be used with caution.

Elderly: Caution in all elderly patients especially those with concomitant use of diuretics, congestive heart failure or renal or hepatic insufficiency. A reduced initial dose of 1.25mg Tritace should be considered. The dose should then be titrated accordingly

Children: Tritace has not been studied in children, and therefore use in this age group is not recommended.

Tritace should be swallowed whole with a glass of water. The tablets must not be chewed or crushed. The absorption of ramipril is not affected by food and Tritace may therefore be taken before, during or after a meal.

4.3 Contraindications

Hypersensitivity to ramipril, any of the excipients of Tritace, or to any other ACE inhibitor.

History of angioedema.

Haemodynamically relevant bilateral renal artery stenosis or unilateral in the single kidney.

Hypotensive or haemodynamically unstable patients.

Pregnancy.

Breast-feeding women.

Concomitant use of ACE inhibitors and extracorporeal treatments leading to contact of blood with negatively charged surfaces must be avoided, since such use may lead to severe anaphylactoid reactions. Such extracorporeal treatments include dialysis or haemofiltration with certain high-flux (e.g. polyacrylonitril) membranes and low-density lipoprotein apheresis with dextran sulfate. This combination should therefore be avoided, either by use of alternative antihypertensive drugs or alternative membranes for dialysis.

4.4 Special warnings and precautions for use

Warnings:

Angioedema - Head, Neck or Extremities

Angioedema occurring during treatment with an ACE inhibitor necessitates immediate discontinuation of the drug. Angioedema of the face, extremities, lips, tongue, glottis or larynx has been reported in patients treated with ACE inhibitors and hospitalisation of the patient is advisable.

Angioedema – Intestinal

Intestinal angioedema has been reported in patients treated with ACE inhibitors.

These patients presented with abdominal pain (with or without nausea or vomiting); in some cases facial angioedema also occurred. The intestinal angioedema symptoms resolved after stopping the ACE inhibitor.

Tritace should not be used in patients with aortic or mitral valve stenosis or outflow obstruction (see Precautions section below).

Precautions:

Assessment of renal function: Evaluation of the patient should include assessment of renal function prior to initiation of therapy and during treatment.

Impaired renal function: Patients with renal insufficiency may require reduced or less frequent doses of Tritace; their renal function should be closely monitored. In the majority, renal function will not alter. There is a risk of impairment of renal function, particularly in patients with congestive heart failure or after a renal transplant, renal insufficiency and bilateral renal artery stenosis and unilateral renal artery stenosis in the single kidney. In the latter patient group, even a small increase in serum creatinine may be indicative of unilateral loss of renal function. If recognised early, such impairment of renal function is reversible upon discontinuation of therapy.

Patients haemodialysed using high flux polyacrylonitrile ('AN69') membranes are highly likely to experience anaphylactoid reactions if they are treated with ACE inhibitors. This combination should therefore be avoided, either by use of alternative antihypertensive drugs or alternative membranes for dialysis.

Similar reactions have been observed during low-density lipoprotein apheresis with dextran sulphate. This method should, therefore, not be used in patients treated with ACE inhibitors.

Some hypertensive patients with no apparent pre-existing renal disease may develop minor and usually transient increases in blood urea nitrogen and serum creatinine when Tritace is given, in particular concomitantly with a diuretic. Dosage reduction of Tritace and/or discontinuation of the diuretic may be required.

Impaired liver function: As ramipril is a prodrug metabolised to its active moiety in the liver, particular caution and close monitoring should be applied to patients with impaired liver function. The metabolism of the parent compound, and therefore the formation of the bioactive metabolite ramiprilat, may be diminished resulting in markedly elevated plasma levels of the parent compound (due to the reduced activity of esterases in the liver).

In patients in whom severe liver cirrhosis with oedema and/or ascites is present, the renin angiotensin system may be significantly activated; therefore, particular caution must be exercised in treating these patients (see also above and under "4.2 Posology and Method of Administration").

Symptomatic hypotension: In patients with uncomplicated hypertension, symptomatic hypotension has been observed rarely after the initial dose of Tritace as well as after increasing the dose of Tritace. It is more likely to occur in patients who have been volume- and salt-depleted by prolonged diuretic therapy, dietary salt restriction, dialysis, diarrhoea, vomiting or patients with severe heart failure. Therefore, in these patients, diuretic therapy should be discontinued and volume and/or salt depletion should be corrected before initiating therapy with Tritace.

Agranulocytosis and bone marrow depression: In patients on angiotensin converting enzyme inhibitors agranulocytosis and bone marrow depression have been seen rarely, as well as a reduction in red cell count, haemoglobin content and platelet count. These are more frequent in patients with renal impairment, especially if they have a collagen vascular disease. Regular monitoring of white blood cell counts (to permit detection of a possible leucopenia) and protein levels in urine should be considered in patients with collagen vascular disease (e.g. lupus erythematosus and scleroderma), especially associated with impaired renal function and concomitant therapy particularly with corticosteroids and anti metabolites. Patients on allopurinol, immunosuppressants and other substances that may change the blood picture also have increased likelihood of other blood picture changes.

Hyperkalaemia: Elevated serum potassium has been observed very rarely in hypertensive patients. Risk factors for the development of hyperkalaemia include renal insufficiency, potassium sparing diuretics and the concomitant use of agents to treat hypokalaemia. It is recommended that serum potassium be monitored regularly. More frequent monitoring of serum potassium is necessary in patients with impaired renal function.

Patients with hyper-stimulated renin angiotensin system: In the treatment of patients with a hyper-stimulated renin angiotensin system, particular caution must be exercised (see also under "4.2 Posology and Method of Administration"). Such patients are at risk of an acute pronounced fall in blood pressure and deterioration of renal function due to ACE inhibition, especially when an ACE inhibitor or a concomitant diuretic is given for the first time or for the first time at an increased dose. Initial doses or initial dose increases must be accompanied by close blood pressure monitoring until such time as no further acute reduction in blood pressure is to be anticipated.

Significant activation of the renin angiotensin system is to be anticipated, for example:

- in patients with severe and/or malignant hypertension.
- in patients with heart failure, particularly if severe or if treated with other substances having antihypertensive potential.
- in patients with haemodynamically relevant left-ventricular inflow or outflow obstruction (e.g., aortic or mitral valve stenosis).
- in patients pre-treated with diuretics.
- in patients with fluid or salt depletion, or in those whom it may develop (as a result of insufficient fluid or salt intake, or as a result of, e.g., dialysis, diarrhoea, vomiting or excessive sweating in cases where salt and fluid replacement is inadequate).

Generally, it is recommended that dehydration, hypovolaemia or salt depletion be corrected before initiating treatment (in patients with heart failure, however, such corrective action must be carefully weighed against other risks of volume overload). When these conditions have become clinically relevant, treatment with Tritace must only be started or continued if appropriate steps are taken concurrently to prevent an excessive fall in blood pressure and deterioration of renal function.

For all of the above, the initial phase of treatment requires close medical supervision.

Patients at particular risk from a pronounced reduction in blood pressure: If symptomatic hypotension occurs, the patient should be placed in a supine position and, if necessary, receive an intravenous infusion of physiological saline. Intravenous atropine may be necessary if there is associated bradycardia. Treatment with Tritace may usually be continued following restoration of effective blood volume and blood pressure.

Surgery/anaesthesia: In patients undergoing surgery or during anaesthesia with agents producing hypotension, Tritace may block angiotensin II formation secondary to compensatory renin release. If hypotension occurs and is considered to be due to this mechanism, it can be corrected by appropriate treatment.

4.5 Interaction with other medicinal products and other forms of interaction

Vasopressor sympathomimetics: These may reduce the antihypertensive effect of Tritace. Particularly close blood pressure monitoring is recommended.

Allopurinol, immunosuppressants, corticosteroids, procainamide, cytostatics and other substances that may change the blood picture: Increased likelihood of haematological reactions (see also under "4.4 Special Warnings and Special Precautions for use").

Lithium Salts: Excretion of lithium may be reduced by ACE inhibitors. Such reduction may lead to increased serum lithium levels and increased lithium toxicity. Lithium levels must, therefore, be monitored.

Diuretics and other antihypertensive agents: Combination with diuretics or other antihypertensive agents may potentiate the antihypertensive response to Tritace. Potassium sparing diuretics (spironolactone, amiloride, triamterene) or potassium supplements may increase the risk of hyperkalaemia. Tritace may attenuate the potassium loss caused by thiazide-type diuretics. Regular monitoring of serum sodium and potassium is recommended in patients undergoing concurrent diuretic therapy. Adrenergic-blocking drugs should only be combined with ramipril under careful supervision.

Combination with antidiabetics: When antidiabetic agents (insulin and sulphonylurea derivatives) are used concurrently, the possibility of increased blood-sugar reduction must be considered. Particularly close blood glucose monitoring is therefore recommended in the initial phase of co-administration.

Combination with NSAIDS: When ACE inhibitors are administered simultaneously with non-steroidal anti-inflammatory drugs (e.g. acetylsalicylic acid and indomethacin), attenuation of the antihypertensive effect may occur. Furthermore, concomitant use of ACE inhibitors and NSAIDs may lead to an increased risk of worsening of renal function and an increase in serum potassium.

Heparin: Rise in serum potassium concentration possible.

Desensitisation therapy: The likelihood and severity of anaphylactic and anaphylactoid reactions to insect venoma is increased under ACE inhibition. It is assumed that this effect may also occur in connection with other allergens.

The protein binding of ramipril is about 73% and of ramiprilat about 56%.

4.6 Pregnancy and lactation

Tritace must not be taken during pregnancy. Therefore, pregnancy must be excluded before starting treatment. If the patient intends to become or becomes pregnant, treatment with ACE inhibitors must be discontinued, i.e. replaced by another form of treatment. Pregnancy must be avoided in cases where treatment with ACE inhibitors is indispensable.

It is not known if exposure limited to the first trimester only can harm the fetus. Exposure of the mother to ACE inhibitors in mid or late pregnancy has been associated with oligohydramnios and neonatal hypotension with anuria or renal failure.

From animal experiments it is known that use of ramipril may cause a decreased utero-placental perfusion. There is also a potential risk of fetal or post-natal effect as ACE inhibitors also influence the local renin-angiotensin system. In peri-post natal studies increased renal pelvic dilation was observed in the first generation offspring. However, ramipril was not fetotoxic in our studies although ACE inhibitors have shown fetotoxicity in some species.

If treatment with Tritace is necessary during lactation, the patient must not breast feed in order to prevent the infant from ingesting small quantities of ramipril with breast milk.

4.7 Effects on ability to drive and use machines

In individual cases, as a result of a reduction in blood pressure, treatment with Tritace may affect the ability to drive and operate machinery. This occurs especially at the start of treatment, when changing over from other preparations and during concomitant use of alcohol. After the first dose or subsequent increases in dose it is not advisable to drive or operate machinery for several hours.

4.8 Undesirable effects

Generally, adverse reactions have been mild and transient, and do not require discontinuation of therapy. The most frequently reported adverse reactions are nausea, dizziness and headache. Uncommonly drowsiness, light-headedness or impaired reactions may occur.

Reactions such as peripheral oedema, tinnitus, fatigue, visual disturbances, sweating, disturbed hearing, disturbed orthostatic regulation are rare.

Cardiovascular: Symptomatic hypotension accompanied by dizziness, weakness and nausea may occur after the initial dose of Tritace and after an increase in the dose of Tritace. It has been rarely observed, but may occur in severely salt/volume-depleted patients such as those treated with diuretics, patients on dialysis and in patients with severe congestive heart failure. Syncope has also been observed rarely.

Myocardial infarction or cerebrovascular accident possibly secondary to severe hypotension in high risk patients, chest pain, palpitations, rhythm disturbances, angina pectoris may occur.

Renal: Treatment with Tritace may impair renal function and in isolated cases progression to acute renal failure may occur.

Gastrointestinal: Treatment with Tritace may be associated with symptoms in the digestive tract, e.g. rarely dryness of the mouth, glossitis, irritation or inflammation of the oral mucosa, digestive disturbances, constipation, diarrhoea, nausea, and vomiting, (gastritis-like) stomach pain, abdominal discomfort (sometimes with increased levels of pancreatic enzymes). Uncommonly increases in hepatic enzymes and/or serum bilirubin, jaundice due to impaired excretion of bile pigment (cholestatic jaundice), acute hepatitis, potentially leading to liver failure.

Pancreatitis has been reported rarely in patients treated with ACE inhibitors; in some cases this has proved fatal.

Allergic: Hypersensitivity reactions accompanied by pruritus, rash, shortness of breath and sometimes fever may occur, but usually resolve spontaneously after withdrawal of Tritace.

In addition, the following cutaneous and mucosal reactions may occur: reddening of skin areas with accompanying heat sensation, conjunctivitis, itching, urticaria, other skin or mucosal eruptions (maculo-papular and lichenoid exanthema and enanthema, erythema multiforme), sometimes pronounced hair loss, exacerbation of perfusion disturbances due to vascular stenoses and precipitation or intensification of Raynaud's phenomenon. In isolated cases, pemphigus, exacerbation of psoriasis, psoriasiform and pemphigoid exanthema and enanthema, Stevens-Johnson syndrome, toxic epidermal necrolysis, hypersensitivity of the skin to light, and onycholysis have been observed.

See Section 4.5 (Interactions) for advice on reactions to insect venoma.

Haematological reactions: Rarely, a mild - in isolated cases severe – reduction in the red blood cell count and haemoglobin content, white blood cell or blood platelet count may develop. In isolated cases, agranulocytosis, pancytopenia and bone marrow depression may occur.

In isolated cases haemolytic anaemia may develop.

Vasculitis, muscle and joint pains, fever, or eosinophilia may occur. Raised titres of antinuclear antibodies have been seen with other ACE inhibitors.

Angioedema: See Section 4.4 (Special Warnings and Special Precautions for use). Uncommonly, pharmacologically mediated mild angioedema may occur (the incidence of ACE inhibitor angioedema seems to be increased in black, i.e. Afro-Caribbean, patients as compared with non-black patients). Serious reactions of this type and other, non-pharmacologically mediated anaphylactic or anaphylactoid reactions to ramipril or any of the other ingredients are rare.

Respiratory tract: A dry tickling cough may occur. This is possibly due to the desired ACE inhibition as are the following adverse effects: rhinitis, sinusitis, bronchitis and, especially in patients with tickling cough, bronchospasm.

Other adverse reactions: Disturbances of balance, headache, nervousness, restlessness, tremor, sleep disorders, confusion, loss of appetite, depressed mood, feeling of anxiety, paraesthesiae, uncommonly, disturbances of smell and taste or partial, sometimes complete loss of taste, muscle cramps, erectile impotence and reduced sexual desire may occur.

Laboratory test findings: Increases in blood urea nitrogen and serum creatinine may occur, in particular with renal insufficiency or in patients pre-treated with a diuretic. Pre-existing proteinuria may deteriorate (though ACE inhibitors usually reduce proteinuria), or there may be an increase in urinary output.

Sodium/Potassium serum levels - See Section 4.5 (Special warnings and special precautions for use).

4.9 Overdose

Symptoms

Overdosage may cause excessive peripheral vasodilation (with marked hypotension, shock), bradycardia, electrolyte disturbances, and renal failure.

Management

General measures to ensure adequate ventilation and circulation should be taken.

Despite the benefits of gastric decontamination being uncertain, it is recommended to consider activated charcoal (50g for adults, 1g/kg for children) if the patient presents within 1 hour of ingestion of a potentially toxic amount (0.5mg/kg).

If severe hypotension occurs, the patient should be placed in the shock position and salt and volume supplementations should be given rapidly. In the event of prolonged hypotension that persists in spite of the above measures, administration of inotropes (e.g. dopamine, norepinephrine) or angiotensin II (angiotensinamide) must be considered in addition to volume and salt substitution.

5. PHARMACOLOGICAL PROPERTIES

5.1 Pharmacodynamic properties

Pharmacotherapeutic group: Converting Enzyme Blockers, ATC code CO2E A05.

Ramipril is a prodrug, which after absorption from the gastrointestinal tract, is hydrolysed in the liver to form the active angiotensin converting enzyme (ACE) inhibitor, ramiprilat, which is a potent and long acting ACE inhibitor. Administration of ramipril causes an increase in plasma renin activity and a decrease in plasma concentrations of angiotensin II and aldosterone. The beneficial haemodynamic effects resulting from ACE inhibition are a consequence of the reduction in angiotensin II causing dilation of peripheral vessels and reduction in vascular resistance. There is evidence suggesting that tissue ACE particularly in the vasculature, rather than circulating ACE, is the primary factor determining the haemodynamic effects.

Angiotensin converting enzyme is identical with kininase II, one of the enzymes responsible for the degradation of bradykinin. There is evidence that ACE inhibition by ramiprilat appears to have some effects on the kallikrein-kinin-prostaglandin systems. It is assumed that effects on these systems contribute to the hypotensive action of ramipril.

Administration of Tritace to hypertensive patients results in reduction of both supine and standing blood pressure. The antihypertensive effect is evident within one to two hours after the drug intake; peak effect occurs 3 - 6 hours after drug intake and has been shown to be maintained for at least 24 hours after usual therapeutic doses.

In a large endpoint study – HOPE - ramipril significantly reduced the incidence of stroke, myocardial infarction and/or cardiovascular death when compared with placebo. These benefits occurred largely in normotensive patients and were shown, using standard regression analysis techniques, to be only partially due to the relatively modest reductions in blood pressure demonstrated in the study. The 10mg dose, currently the highest safe dose level approved, was selected by the HOPE investigators from previous dose-ranging studies (SECURE, HEART) and was considered to be the most likely dose to effect full blockade of the renin-angiotensin-aldosterone system. This and other studies suggest that ACE inhibitors like ramipril are likely to have other direct effects on the cardiovascular system. These may include the antagonism of angiotensin II mediated vasoconstriction, the inhibition of proliferating vascular smooth muscle and plaque rupture, the enhancement of endothelial function, the reduction of LV hypertrophy and positive effects on fibrinolysis. Additional effects in diabetic patients may also contribute e.g. effects on insulin clearance and pancreatic blood flow.

5.2 Pharmacokinetic properties

Following oral administration ramipril is rapidly absorbed from the gastrointestinal tract; peak plasma concentrations of ramipril are reached within one hour. Peak plasma concentrations of the active metabolite, ramiprilat, are reached within 2 – 4 hours.

Plasma concentrations of ramiprilat decline in a polyphasic manner. The effective half-life of ramiprilat after multiple once daily administration of ramipril is 13 – 17 hours for 5 – 10 mg ramipril and markedly longer for lower doses, 1.25 – 2.5 mg ramipril. This difference is related to the long terminal phase of the ramiprilat concentration time curve observed at very low plasma concentrations. This terminal phase is independent of the dose, indicating a saturable capacity of the enzyme to bind ramiprilat. Steady-state plasma concentrations of ramiprilat after once daily dosing with the usual doses of ramipril are reached by about the fourth day of treatment.

Ramipril is almost completely metabolised and the metabolites are excreted mainly via the kidneys. In addition to the bioactive metabolite, ramiprilat, other, inactive metabolites have been identified, including diketopiperazine ester, diketopiperazine acid and conjugates.

5.3 Preclinical safety data

Reproduction toxicology studies in the rat, rabbit and monkey did not disclose any teratogenic properties. Fertility was not impaired either in male or in female rats. The administration of ramipril to female rats during the fetal period and lactation produced irreversible renal damage (dilation of the renal pelvis) in the offspring at daily doses of 50 mg/kg body weight and higher.

6. PHARMACEUTICAL PARTICULARS

6.1 List of excipients

1.25mg and 10mg: Methylhydroxypropylcellulose, pregelatinised starch, microcrystalline cellulose, sodium stearyl fumarate.

2.5mg: Methylhydroxypropylcellulose, pregelatinised starch, microcrystalline cellulose, sodium stearyl fumarate, yellow ferric oxide.

5mg: Methylhydroxypropylcellulose, pregelatinised starch, microcrystalline cellulose, sodium stearyl fumarate, red ferric oxide.

6.2 Incompatibilities

None known.

6.3 Shelf life

5 years (1.25mg, 2.5mg and 5mg tablets)

4 years (10mg tablets)

6.4 Special precautions for storage

Store below 25°C

6.5 Nature and contents of container

PVC aluminium blisters containing tablets. Available in packs of 28 tablets

6.6 Special precautions for disposal and other handling

None

7. MARKETING AUTHORISATION HOLDER

Sanofi-aventis

One Onslow Street

Guildford

Surrey GU1 4YS

UK

8. MARKETING AUTHORISATION NUMBER(S)

1.25mg: PL 04425/0356

2.5mg: PL 04425/0357

5mg: PL 04425/0358

10mg: PL 04425/0359

9. DATE OF FIRST AUTHORISATION/RENEWAL OF THE AUTHORISATION

30th September 2003

10. DATE OF REVISION OF THE TEXT

10 April 2007

Legal category: POM

Trizivir film-coated tablets

(GlaxoSmithKline UK)

1. NAME OF THE MEDICINAL PRODUCT

TRIZIVIR 300 mg/150 mg/300 mg film-coated tablets

2. QUALITATIVE AND QUANTITATIVE COMPOSITION

Each film-coated tablet contains 300 mg of abacavir (as sulfate), 150 mg lamivudine and 300 mg zidovudine.

For a full list of excipients see section 6.1.

3. PHARMACEUTICAL FORM

Film-coated tablet.

Blue-green capsule-shaped film-coated tablets engraved with "GX LL1" on one side.

4. CLINICAL PARTICULARS

4.1 Therapeutic indications

Trizivir is indicated for the treatment of Human Immunodeficiency Virus (HIV) infection in adults. This fixed combination replaces the three components (abacavir, lamivudine and zidovudine) used separately in similar dosages. It is recommended that treatment is started with abacavir, lamivudine, and zidovudine separately for the first 6-8 weeks (see section 4.4). The choice of this fixed combination should be based not only on potential adherence criteria, but mainly on expected efficacy and risk related to the three nucleoside analogues.

The demonstration of the benefit of Trizivir is mainly based on results of studies performed in treatment naive patients or moderately antiretroviral experienced patients with non-advanced disease. In patients with high viral load (> 100,000 copies/ml) choice of therapy needs special consideration (see section 5.1).

Before initiating treatment with abacavir, screening for carriage of the HLA-B*5701 allele should be performed in any HIV-infected patient, irrespective of racial origin. Abacavir should not be used in patients known to carry the HLA-B*5701 allele, unless no other therapeutic option is available in these patients, based on the treatment history and resistance testing (see section 4.4 and 4.8).

4.2 Posology and method of administration

Therapy should be prescribed by a physician experienced in the management of HIV infection.

The recommended dose of Trizivir in adults (18 years and over) is one tablet twice daily.

Trizivir can be taken with or without food.

Where discontinuation of therapy with one of the active substances of Trizivir is indicated, or where dose reduction is necessary separate preparations of abacavir, lamivudine and zidovudine are available.

Renal impairment: Whilst no dosage adjustment of abacavir is necessary in patients with renal dysfunction, lamivudine and zidovudine concentrations are increased in patients with renal impairment due to decreased clearance. Therefore, as dosage adjustments of these may be necessary, it is recommended that separate preparations of abacavir, lamivudine and zidovudine be administered to patients with reduced renal function (creatinine clearance ⩽ 50 ml/min). Physicians should refer to the individual summary of product characteristics of these medicinal products. Trizivir should not be administered to patients with end-stage renal disease (see sections 4.3 and 5.2).

Hepatic impairment: Trizivir is contra-indicated in patients with hepatic impairment (see sections 4.3 and 5.2).

Elderly: No pharmacokinetic data are currently available in patients over 65 years of age. Special care is advised in this age group due to age associated changes such as the decrease in renal function and alteration of haematological parameters.

Dosage adjustments in patients with haematological adverse reactions: Dosage adjustment of zidovudine may be necessary if the haemoglobin level falls below 9 g/dl or 5.59 mmol/l or the neutrophil count falls below 1.0×10^9/l (see sections 4.3 and 4.4). As dosage adjustment of Trizivir is not possible, separate preparations of abacavir, lamivudine and zidovudine should be used. Physicians should refer to the individual summary of product characteristics of these medicinal products.

4.3 Contraindications

Trizivir is contraindicated in patients with known hypersensitivity to abacavir, lamivudine or zidovudine, or to any of the excipients. See BOXED INFORMATION ON HYPERSENSITIVITY REACTIONS in section 4.4 and section 4.8.

Trizivir is contraindicated in patients with end-stage renal disease.

Trizivir is contraindicated in patients with hepatic impairment.

Due to the active substance zidovudine, Trizivir is contra-indicated in patients with abnormally low neutrophil counts (< 0.75×10^9/l), or abnormally low haemoglobin levels (< 7.5 g/dl or 4.65 mmol/l) (see section 4.4).

4.4 Special warnings and precautions for use

The special warnings and precautions relevant to abacavir, lamivudine and zidovudine are included in this section.

There are no additional precautions or warnings relevant to the combination Trizivir.

(see Table 1 opposite)

Mitochondrial dysfunction: nucleoside and nucleotide analogues have been demonstrated *in vitro* and *in vivo* to cause a variable degree of mitochondrial damage. There have been reports of mitochondrial dysfunction in HIV-negative infants exposed *in utero* and/or post-natally to nucleoside analogues. The main adverse events reported are haematological disorders (anaemia, neutropenia), metabolic disorders (hyperlactatemia, hyperlipasemia). These events are often transitory. Some late-onset neurological disorders have been reported (hypertonia, convulsion, abnormal behaviour). Whether the neurological disorders are transient or permanent is currently unknown. Any child exposed *in utero* to nucleoside and nucleotide analogues, even HIV-negative children, should have clinical and laboratory follow-up and should be fully investigated for possible mitochondrial dysfunction in case of relevant signs or symptoms. These findings do not affect current national recommendations to use antiretroviral therapy in pregnant women to prevent vertical transmission of HIV.

Lipodystrophy: combination antiretroviral therapy has been associated with the redistribution of body fat (lipodystrophy) in HIV patients. The long-term consequences of these events are currently unknown. Knowledge about the mechanism is incomplete. A connection between visceral lipomatosis and protease inhibitors (PIs) and lipoatrophy and nucleoside reverse transcriptase inhibitors (NRTIs) has been hypothesised. A higher risk of lipodystrophy has been associated with individual factors such as older age, and with drug related factors such as longer duration of antiretroviral treatment and associated metabolic disturbances. Clinical examination should include evaluation for physical signs of fat redistribution. Consideration should be given to the measurement of fasting serum lipids and blood glucose. Lipid disorders should be managed as clinically appropriate (see section 4.8).

Haematological adverse reactions: anaemia, neutropenia and leucopenia (usually secondary to neutropenia) can be expected to occur in patients receiving zidovudine. These occurred more frequently at higher zidovudine dosages (1200-1500 mg/day) and in patients with poor bone marrow reserve prior to treatment, particularly with advanced HIV disease. Haematological parameters should therefore be carefully monitored (see section 4.3) in patients receiving Trizivir. These haematological effects are not usually observed before four to six week's therapy. For patients with advanced symptomatic HIV disease, it is generally recommended that blood tests are performed at least every two weeks for the first three months of therapy and at least monthly thereafter.

In patients with early HIV disease haematological adverse reactions are infrequent. Depending on the overall condition of the patient, blood tests may be performed less often, for example every one to three months. Additionally dosage adjustment of zidovudine may be required if severe anaemia or myelosuppression occurs during treatment with Trizivir, or in patients with pre-existing bone marrow compromise e.g. haemoglobin < 9 g/dl (5.59 mmol/l) or neutrophil count < 1.0×10^9/l (see section 4.2). As dosage adjustment of Trizivir is not possible separate preparations of zidovudine, abacavir and lamivudine should be used. Physicians should refer to the individual prescribing information for these medicinal products.

Pancreatitis: cases of pancreatitis have occurred rarely in patients treated with abacavir, lamivudine and zidovudine. However it is not clear whether these cases were due to treatment with these medicinal products or to the underlying HIV disease. Treatment with Trizivir should be stopped immediately if clinical signs, symptoms or laboratory abnormalities suggestive of pancreatitis occur.

Liver disease: if lamivudine is being used concomitantly for the treatment of HIV and HBV, additional information relating to the use of lamivudine in the treatment of hepatitis B infection is available in the Zeffix SPC.

The safety and efficacy of Trizivir has not been established in patients with significant underlying liver disorders. Trizivir is contraindicated in patients with hepatic impairment (see section 4.3).

Patients with chronic hepatitis B or C and treated with combination antiretroviral therapy are at an increased risk of severe and potentially fatal hepatic adverse events. In case of concomitant antiviral therapy for hepatitis B or C, please refer also to the relevant product information for these medicinal products.

If Trizivir is discontinued in patients co-infected with hepatitis B virus, periodic monitoring of both liver function tests and markers of HBV replication is recommended, as withdrawal of lamivudine may result in an acute exacerbation of hepatitis (see Zeffix SPC).

Patients with pre-existing liver dysfunction including chronic active hepatitis have an increased frequency of liver function abnormalities during combination antiretroviral therapy and should be monitored according to standard practice. If there is evidence of worsening liver disease in such patients, interruption or discontinuation of treatment must be considered.

Table 1

Hypersensitivity Reaction (see also section 4.8):

In clinical studies approximately 5 % of subjects receiving abacavir (which is also the active substance of Ziagen) develop a hypersensitivity reaction. Some of these cases were life-threatening and resulted in a fatal outcome despite taking precautions.

Studies have shown that carriage of the HLA-B*5701 allele is associated with a significantly increased risk of a hypersensitivity reaction to abacavir. Based on the prospective study CNA106030 (PREDICT-1), use of pre-therapy screening for the HLA-B*5701 allele and subsequently avoiding abacavir in patients with this allele significantly reduced the incidence of abacavir hypersensitivity reactions. In populations similar to that enrolled in the PREDICT-1 study, it is estimated that 48% to 61% of patients with the HLA-B*5701 allele will develop a hypersensitivity reaction during the course of abacavir treatment compared with 0% to 4% of patients who do not have the HLA-B*5701 allele.

These results are consistent with those of prior retrospective studies.

As a consequence, before initiating treatment with abacavir, screening for carriage of the HLA-B*5701 allele should be performed in any HIV-infected patient, irrespective of racial origin. Abacavir should not be used in patients known to carry the HLA-B*5701 allele, unless no other therapeutic option is available based on the treatment history and resistance testing (see section 4.1).

In any patient treated with abacavir, the clinical diagnosis of suspected hypersensitivity reaction must remain the basis of clinical decision-making. It is noteworthy that among patients with a clinically suspected hypersensitivity reaction, a proportion did not carry HLA-B*5701. Therefore, even in the absence of HLA-B*5701 allele, it is important to permanently discontinue abacavir and not rechallenge with abacavir if a hypersensitivity reaction cannot be ruled out on clinical grounds, due to the potential for a severe or even fatal reaction.

Skin patch testing was used as a research tool for the PREDICT-1 study but has no utility in the clinical management of patients and therefore should not be used in the clinical setting.

• **Clinical Description**

Hypersensitivity reactions are characterised by the appearance of symptoms indicating multi-organ system involvement. Almost all hypersensitivity reactions will have fever and/or rash as part of the syndrome.

Other signs and symptoms may include respiratory signs and symptoms such as dyspnoea, sore throat, cough, and abnormal chest x-ray findings (predominantly infiltrates, which can be localised), gastrointestinal symptoms, such as nausea, vomiting, diarrhoea, or abdominal pain, **and may lead to misdiagnosis of hypersensitivity as respiratory disease (pneumonia, bronchitis, pharyngitis), or gastroenteritis.**

Other frequently observed signs or symptoms of the hypersensitivity reaction may include lethargy or malaise and musculoskeletal symptoms (myalgia, rarely myolysis, arthralgia).

The symptoms related to this hypersensitivity reaction worsen with continued therapy and can be life-threatening. These symptoms usually resolve upon discontinuation of abacavir.

• **Clinical Management**

Hypersensitivity reaction symptoms usually appear within the first six weeks of initiation of treatment with abacavir, although these reactions **may occur at any time during therapy**. Patients should be monitored closely, especially during the first two months of treatment with Trizivir, with consultation every two weeks.

Patients who are diagnosed with a hypersensitivity reaction whilst on therapy **MUST discontinue Trizivir immediately.**

Trizivir, or any other medicinal product containing abacavir (i.e. Kivexa, Ziagen), MUST NEVER be restarted in patients who have stopped therapy due to a hypersensitivity reaction.

Restarting abacavir following a hypersensitivity reaction results in a prompt return of symptoms within hours. This recurrence is usually more severe than on initial presentation, and may include life-threatening hypotension and death.

To avoid a delay in diagnosis and minimise the risk of a life-threatening hypersensitivity reaction, Trizivir must be permanently discontinued if hypersensitivity cannot be ruled out, even when other diagnoses are possible (respiratory diseases, flu-like illness, gastroenteritis or reactions to other medications).

Special care is needed for those patients simultaneously starting treatment with Trizivir and other medicinal products known to induce skin toxicity (such as non-nucleoside reverse transcriptase inhibitors - NNRTIs). This is because it is currently difficult to differentiate between rashes induced by these products and abacavir related hypersensitivity reactions.

• **Management after an interruption of Trizivir therapy**

If therapy with Trizivir has been discontinued for any reason and restarting therapy is under consideration, the reason for discontinuation must be established to assess whether the patient had any symptoms of a hypersensitivity reaction. **If a hypersensitivity reaction cannot be ruled out, Trizivir or any other medicinal product containing abacavir (i.e. Kivexa, Ziagen) must not be restarted.**

Hypersensitivity reactions with rapid onset, including life-threatening reactions have occurred after restarting abacavir in patients who had only one of the key symptoms of hypersensitivity (skin rash, fever, gastrointestinal, respiratory or constitutional symptoms such as lethargy and malaise) prior to stopping abacavir. The most common isolated symptom of a hypersensitivity reaction was a skin rash. Moreover, on very rare occasions hypersensitivity reactions have been reported in patients who have restarted therapy, and who had no preceding symptoms of a hypersensitivity reaction.

In both cases if a decision is made to restart Trizivir this must be done in a setting where medical assistance is readily available.

• **Essential patient information**

Prescribers must ensure that patients are fully informed regarding the following information on the hypersensitivity reaction:

- Patients must be made aware of the possibility of a hypersensitivity reaction to abacavir that may result in a life-threatening reaction or death.

- Patients developing signs or symptoms possibly linked with a hypersensitivity reaction **MUST CONTACT their doctor IMMEDIATELY.**

Patients who are hypersensitive to abacavir should be reminded that they must never

- take Trizivir or any other medicinal product containing abacavir (i.e. Kivexa, Ziagen) again.

- In order to avoid restarting Trizivir, patients who have experienced a hypersensitivity reaction should dispose of their remaining Trizivir tablets in their possession in accordance with the local requirements, and ask their doctor or pharmacist for advice.

- Patients who have stopped Trizivir for any reason, and particularly due to possible adverse

- reactions or illness, must be advised to contact their doctor before restarting.

- Patients should be advised of the importance of taking Trizivir regularly.

- Each patient should be reminded to read the Package Leaflet included in the Trizivir pack.

They should be reminded of the importance of removing the Alert Card included in the pack, and keeping it with them at all times.

Lactic acidosis:

lactic acidosis, usually associated with hepatomegaly and hepatic steatosis, has been reported with the use of nucleoside analogues. Early symptoms (symptomatic hyperlactatemia) include benign digestive symptoms (nausea, vomiting and abdominal pain), non-specific malaise, loss of appetite, weight loss, respiratory symptoms (rapid and/or deep breathing) or neurological symptoms (including motor weakness).

Lactic acidosis has a high mortality and may be associated with pancreatitis, liver failure, or renal failure.

Lactic acidosis generally occurred after a few or several months of treatment.

Treatment with nucleoside analogues should be discontinued in the setting of symptomatic hyperlactatemia and metabolic/lactic acidosis, progressive hepatomegaly, or rapidly elevating aminotransferase levels.

Caution should be exercised when administering nucleoside analogues to any patient (particularly obese women) with hepatomegaly, hepatitis or other known risk factors for liver disease and hepatic steatosis (including certain medicinal products and alcohol). Patients co-infected with hepatitis C and treated with alpha interferon and ribavirin may constitute a special risk.

Patients at increased risk should be followed closely.

Patients co-infected with hepatitis C virus:

The comcomitant use of ribavirin with zidovudine is not recommended due to an increased risk of anaemia (see section 4.5).

Children and adolescents: because insufficient data are available, the use of Trizivir in children or adolescents is not recommended. In this patient population, hypersensitivity reactions are particularly difficult to identify.

Immune Reactivation Syndrome: in HIV-infected patients with severe immune deficiency at the time of institution of combination antiretroviral therapy (CART), an inflammatory reaction to asymptomatic or residual opportunistic pathogens may arise and cause serious clinical conditions, or aggravation of symptoms. Typically, such reactions have been observed within the first few weeks or months of initiation of CART. Relevant examples are cytomegalovirus retinitis, generalised and/or focal mycobacterium infections, and Pneumocystis carinii pneumonia. Any inflammatory symptoms should be evaluated and treatment instituted when necessary.

Osteonecrosis: Although the etiology is considered to be multifactorial (including corticosteroid use, alcohol consumption, severe immunosuppression, higher body mass index), cases of osteonecrosis have been reported particularly in patients with advanced HIV-disease and/or long-term exposure to combination antiretroviral therapy (CART). Patients should be advised to seek medical advice if they experience joint aches and pain, joint stiffness or difficulty in movement.

Opportunistic infections: patients should be advised that Trizivir or any other antiretroviral therapy does not cure HIV infection and that they may still develop opportunistic infections and other complications of HIV infection. Therefore patients should remain under close clinical observation by physicians experienced in the treatment of these associated HIV diseases.

Myocardial Infarction: Observational studies have shown an association between myocardial infarction and the use of abacavir. Those studied were mainly antiretroviral experienced patients. Data from clinical trials showed limited numbers of myocardial infarction and could not exclude a small increase in risk. Overall the available data from observational cohorts and from randomised trials show some inconsistency so can neither confirm nor refute a causal relationship between abacavir treatment and the risk of myocardial infarction. To date, there is no established biological mechanism to explain a potential increase in risk. When prescribing Trizivir, action should be taken to try to minimize all modifiable risk factors (e.g. smoking, hypertension, and hyperlipidaemia).

Miscellaneous: patients should be advised that current antiretroviral therapy, including Trizivir, has not been proven to prevent the risk of transmission of HIV to others through sexual contact or blood contamination. Appropriate precautions should continue to be taken.

To date there are insufficient data on the efficacy and safety of Trizivir given concomitantly with NNRTIs or PIs (see section 5.1).

The concomitant use of stavudine with zidovudine should be avoided (see section 4.5).

4.5 Interaction with other medicinal products and other forms of interaction

As Trizivir contains abacavir, lamivudine and zidovudine, any interactions that have been identified with these agents individually may occur with Trizivir.

The likelihood of metabolic interactions with lamivudine is low due to limited metabolism and plasma protein binding, and almost complete renal clearance. Zidovudine is primarily eliminated by hepatic conjugation to an inactive glucuronidated metabolite. Medicinal products that are primarily eliminated by hepatic metabolism especially via glucuronidation may have the potential to inhibit metabolism of zidovudine. Based on the results of *in vitro* experiments and the known major metabolic pathways of abacavir, the potential for P450 mediated interactions with other medicinal products involving abacavir are low. Clinical studies have shown that there are no clinically significant interactions between abacavir, lamivudine and zidovudine.

The interactions listed below should not be considered exhaustive but are representative of the classes of medicinal products where caution should be exercised.

Interactions relevant to abacavir

Based on the results of *in vitro* experiments and the known major metabolic pathways of abacavir, the potential for P450 mediated interactions with other medicinal products involving abacavir is low. P450 does not play a major role in the metabolism of abacavir, and abacavir does not inhibit metabolism mediated by CYP 3A4. Abacavir has also been shown *in vitro* not to inhibit CYP 3A4, CYP 2C9 or CYP 2D6 enzymes at clinically relevant concentrations. Therefore, there is little potential for interactions with antiretroviral PIs and other medicinal products metabolised by major P450 enzymes.

Potent enzymatic inducers such as rifampicin, phenobarbital and phenytoin may via their action on UDP-glucuronyltransferases slightly decrease the plasma concentrations of abacavir.

The metabolism of abacavir is altered by concomitant ethanol resulting in an increase in AUC of abacavir of about 41 %. These findings are not considered clinically significant. Abacavir has no effect on the metabolism of ethanol.

Retinoid compounds are eliminated via alcohol dehydrogenase. Interaction with abacavir is possible but has not been studied.

In a pharmacokinetic study, coadministration of 600 mg abacavir twice daily with methadone showed a 35 % reduction in abacavir C_{max} and a 1 hour delay in t_{max}, but the AUC was unchanged. The changes in abacavir pharmacokinetics are not considered clinically relevant. In this study, abacavir increased the mean methadone systemic clearance by 22 %. The induction of drug metabolizing enzymes cannot therefore be excluded. Patients being treated with methadone and abacavir should be monitored for evidence of withdrawal symptoms indicating under dosing, as occasionally methadone re-titration may be required.

Interactions relevant to lamivudine

The possibility of interactions with other medicinal products administered concurrently with Trizivir should be considered, particularly when the main route of elimination is active renal secretion especially via the cationic transport system e.g. trimethoprim. Nucleoside analogues (e.g. zidovudine, didanosine and zalcitabine) and other medicinal products (e.g. ranitidine, cimetidine) are eliminated only in part by this mechanism and were shown not to interact with lamivudine.

Administration of trimethoprim/sulfamethoxazole 160 mg/800 mg results in a 40 % increase in lamivudine exposure, because of the trimethoprim component; the sulfamethoxazole component does not interact. However, unless the patient has renal impairment, no dosage adjustment of lamivudine is necessary (see section 4.2). Lamivudine has no effect on the pharmacokinetics of trimethoprim or sulfamethoxazole. When concomitant administration with co-trimoxazole is warranted, patients should be monitored clinically. Co-administration of Trizivir with high doses of co-trimoxazole for the treatment of *Pneumocystis carinii* pneumonia (PCP) and toxoplasmosis should be avoided.

Co-administration of lamivudine with intravenous ganciclovir or foscarnet is not recommended until further information is available.

Lamivudine may inhibit the intracellular phosphorylation of zalcitabine when the two medicinal products are used concurrently. Trizivir is therefore not recommended to be used in combination with zalcitabine.

Lamivudine metabolism does not involve CYP 3A, making interactions with medicinal products metabolised by this system (e.g. PIs and non-nucleosides) unlikely.

Interactions relevant to zidovudine

Limited data suggests that co-administration of zidovudine and rifampicin decreases the AUC of zidovudine by 48 % ± 34 %. However the clinical significance of this is unknown. Dose modifications of zidovudine in this situation have not been formally evaluated.

Limited data suggest that probenecid increases the mean half-life and area under the plasma concentration curve of zidovudine by decreasing glucuronidation. Renal excretion of the glucuronide (and possibly zidovudine itself) is reduced in the presence of probenecid. Patients receiving both drugs should be closely monitored for haematological toxicity.

Phenytoin blood levels have been reported to be low in some patients receiving zidovudine, while in one patient a high level was noted. These observations suggest that phenytoin concentrations should be carefully monitored in patients receiving Trizivir and phenytoin.

In a pharmacokinetic study co-administration of zidovudine and atovaquone tablets showed a decrease in zidovudine clearance after oral dosing leading to a 35 % ± 23 % increase in plasma zidovudine AUC. The mode of interaction is unknown and as higher concentrations of atovaquone can be achieved with atovaquone suspension it is possible that greater changes in the AUC values for zidovudine might be induced when atovaquone is administered as a suspension. Given the limited data available the clinical significance of this is unknown.

Valproic acid, fluconazole or methadone when co-administered with zidovudine have been shown to increase the AUC of zidovudine, with a corresponding decrease in its clearance. As only limited data are available the clinical significance of this is not known. If zidovudine is used concurrently with either valproic acid, fluconazole or methadone, patients should be monitored closely for potential toxicity of zidovudine.

Zidovudine and stavudine in combination are antagonistic *in vitro*, therefore, the concomitant use of stavudine with Trizivir should be avoided (see Section 4.4).

Exacerbation of anaemia due to ribavirin has been reported when zidovudine is part of the regimen used to treat HIV although the exact mechanism remains to be elucidated. The concomitant use of ribavirin with zidovudine is not recommended due to an increased risk of anaemia (see section 4.4). Consideration should be given to replacing zidovudine in a combination ART regimen if this is already established. This would be particularly important in patients with a known history of zidovudine induced anaemia.

Concomitant treatment, especially acute therapy, with potentially nephrotoxic or myelosuppressive medicinal products (e.g. systemic pentamidine, dapsone, pyrimethamine, co-trimoxazole, amphotericin, flucytosine, ganciclovir, interferon, vincristine, vinblastine and doxorubicin) may also increase the risk of adverse reactions to zidovudine. If concomitant therapy with Trizivir and any of these medicinal products is necessary then extra care should be taken in monitoring renal function and haematological parameters and, if required, the dosage of one or more agents should be reduced.

Limited data from clinical trials do not indicate a significantly increased risk of adverse reactions to zidovudine with co-trimoxazole (see interaction information above relating to lamivudine and cotrimoxazole) aerosolised pentamidine, pyrimethamine and acyclovir at doses used in prophylaxis.

Co-administration of Trizivir with high doses of co-trimoxazole for the treatment of *Pneumocystis carinii* pneumonia (PCP) and toxoplasmosis should be avoided.

Clarithromycin tablets reduce the absorption of zidovudine. This can be avoided by separating the administration of Trizivir and clarithromycin by at least two hours.

4.6 Pregnancy and lactation

Pregnancy

Trizivir is not recommended during pregnancy. There are no data on the use of Trizivir in pregnancy. Placental transfer of lamivudine and zidovudine occurs in humans, and for abacavir has been confirmed in animals. Studies with abacavir, lamivudine and zidovudine in animals have shown reproductive toxicity (see section 5.3). As the active substances of Trizivir may inhibit DNA replication any use, especially during the first trimester, presents a potential risk to the foetus.

Lactation

Both lamivudine and zidovudine are excreted in human milk at similar concentrations to those found in serum. It is expected that abacavir will also be secreted into human milk, although this has not been confirmed. It is therefore recommended that mothers do not breast-feed their babies while receiving treatment with Trizivir. Additionally, it is recommended that HIV infected women do not breast-feed their infants under any circumstances in order to avoid transmission of HIV.

4.7 Effects on ability to drive and use machines

No studies on the effects on the ability to drive and use machines have been performed. The clinical status of the patient and the adverse event profile of Trizivir should be borne in mind when considering the patient's ability to drive or operate machinery.

4.8 Undesirable effects

Overview

Adverse reactions have been reported with abacavir, lamivudine and zidovudine used separately or in combination for therapy of HIV disease. Because Trizivir contains abacavir, lamivudine and zidovudine, the adverse reactions associated with these compounds may be expected.

Hypersensitivity to abacavir (see also section 4.4):

In clinical studies, approximately 5 % of subjects receiving abacavir developed a hypersensitivity reaction; some of these were life-threatening and resulted in fatal outcome despite taking precautions. This reaction is characterised by the appearance of symptoms indicating multi-organ/body-system involvement.

Almost all patients developing hypersensitivity reactions will have fever and/or rash (usually maculopapular or urticarial) as part of the syndrome, however hypersensitivity reactions have occurred without rash or fever.

The signs and symptoms associated with hypersensitivity to abacavir are summarised in Table 1. These have been identified either from clinical studies or post marketing surveillance.

Some patients with hypersensitivity reactions were initially thought to have gastroenteritis, respiratory disease (pneumonia, bronchitis, pharyngitis) or a flu-like illness. This delay in diagnosis of hypersensitivity has resulted in abacavir being continued or re-introduced, leading to more severe hypersensitivity reactions or death. Therefore, the diagnosis of hypersensitivity reaction should be carefully considered for patients presenting with symptoms of these diseases.

Symptoms usually appeared within the first six weeks (median time to onset 11 days) of initiation of treatment with abacavir, although these reactions may occur at any time during therapy. Close medical supervision is necessary during the first two months, with consultations every two weeks.

It is likely that intermittent therapy may increase the risk of developing sensitisation and therefore occurrence of clinically significant hypersensitivity reactions. Consequently, patients should be advised of the importance of taking Trizivir regularly.

Restarting Trizivir, or any other medicinal product containing abacavir, following a hypersensitivity reaction would result in a prompt return of symptoms within hours. This recurrence of the hypersensitivity reaction was usually more severe than on initial presentation and may include life-threatening hypotension and death. **Patients who develop this hypersensitivity reaction must discontinue Trizivir and must never be rechallenged with Trizivir, or any other medicinal product containing abacavir (i.e. Kivexa, Ziagen).**

To avoid a delay in diagnosis and minimise the risk of a life-threatening hypersensitivity reaction, Trizivir must be permanently discontinued if hypersensitivity cannot be ruled out, even when other diagnoses are possible (respiratory disease, flu-like illness, gastroenteritis or reactions to other medications).

Hypersensitivity reactions with rapid onset, including life-threatening reactions have occurred after restarting abacavir in patients who had only one of the key symptoms of hypersensitivity (skin rash, fever, gastrointestinal, respiratory or constitutional symptoms such as lethargy and malaise) prior to stopping abacavir. The most common isolated symptom of a hypersensitivity reaction was a skin rash. Moreover, on very rare occasions hypersensitivity reactions have been reported in patients who have restarted therapy and who had no preceding symptoms of a hypersensitivity reaction. In both cases if a decision is made to restart Trizivir this must be done in a setting where medical assistance is readily available.

Each patient must be warned about this hypersensitivity reaction to abacavir.

Table 1: Summary of signs and symptoms associated with hypersensitivity to abacavir

(Signs and symptoms reported in at least 10 % of patients with a hypersensitivity reaction to abacavir are in **bold text**).

Body system	Adverse reactions
Gastrointestinal tract	**Nausea, vomiting, diarrhoea, abdominal pain,** mouth ulceration
Neurological/ psychiatry	**Headache**, paraesthesia
Haematological	Lymphopenia
Liver/pancreas	**Elevated liver function tests,** hepatitis, hepatic failure
Musculoskeletal	**Myalgia,** rarely myolysis, arthralgia, elevated creatine phosphokinase
Respiratory tract	**Dyspnoea,** sore throat, **cough,** adult respiratory distress syndrome, respiratory failure
Skin	**Rash** (usually maculopapular or urticarial)
Urology	Elevated creatinine, renal failure
Miscellaneous	**Fever, lethargy, malaise,** oedema, lymphadenopathy, hypotension, conjunctivitis, anaphylaxis

Undesirable effects reported with the individual substances

The adverse reactions reported with abacavir, lamivudine and zidovudine are presented in Table 2. They are listed by body system, organ class and absolute frequency. Frequencies are defined as very common (> 1/10), common (> 1/100, < 1/10), uncommon (> 1/1000, < 1/100), rare (> 1/10,000, < 1/1000), very rare (< 1/10,000). Care must be taken to eliminate the possibility of a hypersensitivity reaction if any of these symptoms occur.

Table 2: Adverse reactions reported with the individual components of Trizivir

(see Table 2 opposite)

Table 2 Adverse reactions reported with the individual components of Trizivir

Abacavir	Lamivudine	Zidovudine
IMPORTANT: for information on abacavir hypersensitivity, see the description above in the boxed information and Table 1		
Blood and lymphatic system disorders		
	Uncommon: neutropenia, anaemia (both occasionally severe), thrombocytopenia *Very rare:* pure red cell aplasia	*Common:* anaemia, neutropenia and leucopenia *Uncommon:* thrombocytopenia and pancytopenia with marrow hypoplasia *Rare:* pure red cell aplasia *Very rare:* aplastic anaemia
Immune system disorders		
Common: hypersensitivity		
Metabolism and nutrition disorders		
Common: anorexia		*Rare:* anorexia, lactic acidosis in the absence of hypoxaemia
Psychiatric disorders		
		Rare: anxiety, depression
Nervous system disorders		
Common: headache	*Common:* headache, insomnia *Very rare:* peripheral neuropathy (paraesthesiae)	*Very common:* headache *Common:* dizziness *Rare:* insomnia, paraesthesia, somnolence, loss of mental acuity, convulsions
Cardiac disorders		
		Rare: cardiomyopathy
Respiratory, thoracic and mediastinal disorders		
	Common: cough, nasal symptoms	*Uncommon:* dyspnoea *Rare:* cough
Gastrointestinal disorders		
Common: nausea, vomiting, diarrhoea *Rare:* pancreatitis	*Common:* nausea, vomiting, abdominal pain, diarrhoea *Rare:* rises in serum amylase, pancreatitis	*Very common:* Nausea *Common:* vomiting, abdominal pain, and diarrhoea *Uncommon:* flatulence *Rare:* oral mucosa pigmentation, taste disturbance dyspepsia, pancreatitis
Hepatobiliary disorders		
	Uncommon: transient rises in liver enzymes (AST, ALT) *Rare:* hepatitis	*Common:* raised blood levels of liver enzymes and bilirubin *Rare:* liver disorders such as severe hepatomegaly with steatosis,
Skin and subcutaneous tissue disorders		
Common: rash (without systemic symptoms) *Very rare:* erythema multiforme, Stevens-Johnson syndrome and toxic epidermal necrolysis	*Common:* rash, alopecia	*Uncommon:* rash and pruritus *Rare:* nail and skin pigmentation, urticaria and sweating
Musculoskeletal and connective tissue disorders		
	Common: arthralgia, muscle disorders *Rare:* rhabdomyolysis	*Common:* myalgia *Uncommon:* myopathy
Renal and urinary disorders		
		Rare: urinary frequency
Reproductive system and breast disorders		
		Rare: gynaecomastia
General disorders and administration site conditions		
Common: fever, lethargy, fatigue	*Common:* fatigue, malaise, fever	*Common:* malaise *Uncommon:* fever, generalised pain and asthenia *Rare:* chills, chest pain, and influenza-like syndrome

Adverse reactions associated with abacavir:

Many of the adverse reactions listed above occur commonly (nausea, vomiting, diarrhoea, fever, lethargy, rash) in patients with abacavir hypersensitivity. Therefore, patients with any of these symptoms should be carefully evaluated for the presence of this hypersensitivity reaction. If Trizivir has been discontinued in patients due to experiencing any one of these symptoms and a decision is made to restart a medicinal product containing abacavir, this must be done in a setting where medical assistance is readily available (see Section 4.4). Very rarely cases of erythema multiforme, Stevens Johnson syndrome or toxic epidermal necrolysis have been reported where abacavir hypersensitivity could not be ruled out. In such cases medicinal products containing abacavir should be permanently discontinued.

Haematological adverse reactions with zidovudine

Anaemia, neutropenia and leucopenia occurred more frequently at higher dosages (1200-1500 mg/day) and in patients with advanced HIV disease (especially when there is poor bone marrow reserve prior to treatment) and particularly in patients with CD4 cell counts less than 100/mm^3. Dosage reduction or cessation of therapy may become necessary (see section 4.4). The anaemia may necessitate transfusions.

The incidence of neutropenia was also increased in those patients whose neutrophil counts, haemoglobin levels and serum vitamin B_{12} levels were low at the start of zidovudine therapy.

Lactic acidosis

Treatment with nucleoside analogues has been associated with cases of lactic acidosis, sometimes fatal, usually associated with severe hepatomegaly and hepatic steatosis, (see section 4.4).

Lipodystrophy/metabolic abnormalities

Combination antiretroviral therapy has been associated with redistribution of body fat (lipodystrophy) in HIV patients including the loss of peripheral and facial subcutaneous fat, increased intra-abdominal and visceral fat, breast hypertrophy and dorsocervical fat accumulation (buffalo hump).

Combination antiretroviral therapy has been associated with metabolic abnormalities such as hypertriglyceridaemia, hypercholesterolaemia, insulin resistance, hyperglycaemia and hyperlactataemia (see section 4.4).

Immune Reactivation Syndrome

In HIV-infected patients with severe immune deficiency at the time of initiation of combination antiretroviral therapy (CART), an inflammatory reaction to asymptomatic or residual opportunistic infections may arise (see section 4.4).

Osteonecrosis

Cases of osteonecrosis have been reported, particularly in patients with generally acknowledged risk factors, advanced HIV disease or long-term exposure to combination antiretroviral therapy (CART). The frequency of this is unknown (see section 4.4).

4.9 Overdose

There is no experience of overdose with Trizivir. No specific symptoms or signs have been identified following acute overdose with zidovudine or lamivudine apart from those listed as undesirable effects. No fatalities occurred, and all patients recovered. Single doses up to 1200 mg and daily doses up to 1800 mg of abacavir have been administered to patients in clinical studies. No unexpected adverse reactions were reported. The effects of higher doses are not known.

If overdose occurs the patient should be monitored for evidence of toxicity (see section 4.8), and standard supportive treatment applied as necessary. Since lamivudine is dialysable, continuous haemodialysis could be used in the treatment of overdose, although this has not been studied. Haemodialysis and peritoneal dialysis appear to have a limited effect on elimination of zidovudine, but enhance the elimination of the glucuronide metabolite. It is not known whether abacavir can be removed by peritoneal dialysis or haemodialysis.

5. PHARMACOLOGICAL PROPERTIES

5.1 Pharmacodynamic properties

Pharmacotherapeutic group: Antivirals for treatment of HIV infections, combinations. ATC Code: J05AR04.

Mechanism of action: Abacavir, lamivudine and zidovudine are all NRTIs, and are potent selective inhibitors of HIV-1 and HIV-2. All three medicinal products are metabolised sequentially by intracellular kinases to the respective 5'-triphosphate (TP). Lamivudine-TP, carbovir-TP (the active triphosphate form of abacavir) and zidovudine-TP are substrates for and competitive inhibitors of HIV reverse transcriptase (RT). However, their main antiviral activity is through incorporation of the monophosphate form into the viral DNA chain, resulting in chain termination. Abacavir, lamivudine and zidovudine triphosphates show significantly less affinity for host cell DNA polymerases.

Lamivudine has been shown to be highly synergistic with zidovudine, inhibiting the replication of HIV in cell culture. Abacavir shows synergy *in vitro* in combination with nevirapine and zidovudine. It has been shown to be additive in combination with didanosine, stavudine and lamivudine.

In vitro resistance: HIV-1 resistance to lamivudine involves the development of a M184I or, more commonly, M184V amino acid change close to the active site of the viral RT.

Abacavir-resistant isolates of HIV-1 have been selected *in vitro* and are associated with specific genotypic changes in the RT codon region (codons M184V, K65R, L74V and Y115F). Viral resistance to abacavir develops relatively slowly *in vitro*, requiring multiple mutations for a clinically relevant increase in EC_{50} over wild-type virus.

In vivo resistance (Therapy naïve patients): The M184V or M184I variants arise in HIV-1 infected patients treated with lamivudine-containing antiretroviral therapy. Most patients experiencing virological failure with a regimen containing abacavir in a pivotal clinical trial with Combivir (fixed dose combination of lamivudine and zidovudine) showed either no NRTI-related changes from baseline (15%) or only M184V or M184I selection (78%). The overall selection frequency for M184V or M184I was high (85%), and selection of L74V, K65R and Y115F was not observed (see Table). Thymidine analogue mutations (TAMs) which are selected by zidovudine (ZDV) were also found (8%).

Therapy	Abacavir + Combivir
Number of Subjects	282
Number of Virological Failures	43
Number of On-Therapy Genotypes	40 (100%)
K65R	0
L74V	0
Y115F	0
M184V/I	34 (85%)
TAMs[1]	3 (8%)

1. Number of subjects with ⩾1 TAM.

TAMs might be selected when thymidine analogs are associated with abacavir. In a meta-analysis of six clinical trials, TAMs were not selected by regimens containing abacavir without zidovudine (0/127), but were selected by regimens containing abacavir and the thymidine analogue zidovudine (22/86, 26%). In addition, the selection of L74V and K65R was reduced when co-administered with ZDV (K65R: without ZDV: 13/127, 10%; with ZDV: 1/86, 1%; L74V: without ZDV: 51/127, 40%; with ZDV: 2/86, 2%).

In vivo resistance (Therapy experienced patients): The M184V or M184I variants arise in HIV-1 infected patients treated with lamivudine-containing antiretroviral therapy and confers high-level resistance to lamivudine. *In vitro* data tend to suggest that the continuation of lamivudine in anti-retroviral regimen despite the development of M184V might provide residual anti-retroviral activity (likely through impaired viral fitness). The clinical relevance of these findings is not established. Indeed, the available clinical data are very limited and preclude any reliable conclusion in the field. In any case, initiation of susceptible NRTIs should always be preferred to maintenance of lamivudine therapy. Therefore, maintaining lamivudine therapy despite emergence of M184V mutation should only be considered in cases where no other active NRTIs are available. Similarly, the presence of TAMs gives rise to resistance to ZDV.

Clinically significant reduction of susceptibility to abacavir has been demonstrated in clinical isolates of patients with uncontrolled viral replication, who have been pre-treated with and are resistant to other nucleoside inhibitors. In a meta-analysis of five clinical trials where abacavir was added to intensify therapy, of 166 subjects, 123 (74%) had M184V/I, 50 (30%) had T215Y/F, 45 (27%) had M41L, 30 (18%) had K70R and 25 (15%) had D67N. K65R was absent and L74V and Y115F were uncommon (⩽3%). Logistic regression modelling of the predictive value for genotype (adjusted for baseline plasma HIV-1 RNA [vRNA], CD4+ cell count, number and duration of prior antiretroviral therapies) showed that the presence of 3 or more NRTI resistance-associated mutations was associated with reduced response at Week 4 (p=0.015) or 4 or more mutations at median Week 24 (p⩽0.012). In addition, the 69 insertion complex or the Q151M mutation, usually found in combination with A62V, V75I, F77L and F116Y, cause a high level of resistance to abacavir.

(see Table 3 below)

Phenotypic resistance and cross-resistance: Phenotypic resistance to abacavir requires M184V with at least one other abacavir-selected mutation, or M184V with multiple TAMs. Phenotypic cross-resistance to other NRTIs with M184V or M184I mutation alone is limited. Zidovudine, didanosine, stavudine and tenofovir maintain their antiretroviral activities against such HIV-1 variants. The presence of M184V with K65R does give rise to cross-resistance between abacavir, tenofovir, didanosine and lamivudine, and M184V with L74V gives rise to cross-resistance between abacavir, didanosine and lamivudine. The presence of M184V with Y115F gives rise to cross-resistance between abacavir and lamivudine. Appropriate use of abacavir can be guided using currently recommended resistance algorithms.

Cross-resistance between abacavir, lamivudine or zidovudine and antiretrovirals from other classes e.g. PIs or NNRTIs is unlikely.

Clinical experience

One randomised, double blind, placebo controlled clinical study has compared the combination of abacavir, lamivudine and zidovudine to the combination of indinavir, lamivudine and zidovudine in treatment naive patients. Due to the high proportion of premature discontinuation (42 % of patients discontinued randomised treatment by week 48), no definitive conclusion can be drawn regarding the equivalence between the treatment regimens at week 48. Although a similar antiviral effect was observed between the abacavir and indinavir containing regimens in terms of proportion of patients with undetectable viral load (⩽ 400 copies/ml; intention to treat analysis (ITT), 47 % versus 49 %; as treated analysis (AT), 86 % versus 94 % for abacavir and indinavir combinations respectively), results favoured the indinavir combination, particularly in the subset of patients with high viral load (> 100,000 copies/ml at baseline; ITT, 46 % versus 55 %; AT, 84 % versus 93 % for abacavir and indinavir respectively).

ACTG5095 was a randomised (1:1:1), double-blind, placebo-controlled trial performed in 1147 antiretroviral naïve HIV-1 infected adults, comparing 3 regimens: zidovudine (ZDV), lamivudine (3TC), abacavir (ABC), efavirenz (EFV) vs ZDV/3TC/EFV vs ZDV/3TC/ABC. After a median follow-up of 32 weeks, the tritherapy with the three nucleosides ZDV/3TC/ABC was shown to be virologically inferior to the two other arms regardless of baseline viral load (< or > 100 000 copies/ml) with 26% of subjects on the ZDV/3TC/ABC arm, 16% on the ZDV/3TC/EFV arm and 13% on the 4 drug arm categorised as having virological failure (HIV RNA > 200 copies/ml). At week 48 the proportion of subjects with HIV RNA <50 copies/ml were 63%, 80% and 86% for the ZDV/3TC/ABC, ZDV/3TC/EFV and ZDV/3TC/ABC/EFV arms, respectively. The study Data Safety Monitoring Board stopped the ZDV/3TC/ABC arm at this time based on the higher proportion of patients with virologic failure. The remaining arms were continued in a blinded fashion. After a median follow-up of 144 weeks, 25% of subjects on the ZDV/3TC/ABC/EFV arm and 26% on the ZDV/3TC/EFV arm were categorised as having virological failure. There was no significant difference in the time to first virologic failure (p=0.73, log-rank test) between the 2 arms. In this study, addition of ABC to ZDV/3TC/EFV did not significantly improve efficacy.

(see Table 4 below)

In an ongoing clinical study over 16 weeks in treatment-naive patients, the combination of abacavir, lamivudine and zidovudine showed a similar antiviral effect to the combination with nelfinavir, lamivudine and zidovudine.

In antiretroviral-naïve patients the triple combination of abacavir, lamivudine and zidovudine was superior in terms of durability of viral load response over 48 weeks to lamivudine and zidovudine. In a similar patient population durability of antiviral response over 120 weeks was demonstrated in approximately 70 % of subjects.

In antiretroviral-naive patients treated with a combination of abacavir, lamivudine, zidovudine and efavirenz in a small, ongoing, open label pilot study, the proportion of patients with undetectable viral load (< 400 copies/ml) was approximately 90 % with 80 % having < 50 copies/ml after 24 weeks of treatment.

In patients with a low baseline viral load (< 5,000 copies/ml) and moderate exposure to antiretroviral therapy, addition of abacavir to previous treatment including lamivudine and zidovudine, produced a moderate impact on viral load at 48 weeks.

Currently there are no data on the use of Trizivir in heavily pre-treated patients, patients failing on other therapies or patients with advanced disease (CD4 cells < 50 cells/mm^3).

The degree of benefit of this nucleoside combination in heavily pre-treated patients will depend on the nature and duration of prior therapy that may have selected for HIV-1 variants with cross-resistance to abacavir, lamivudine or zidovudine.

To date there are insufficient data on the efficacy and safety of Trizivir given concomitantly with NNRTIs or PIs.

5.2 Pharmacokinetic properties

Absorption

Abacavir, lamivudine and zidovudine are rapidly and well absorbed from the gastro-intestinal tract following oral administration. The absolute bioavailability of oral abacavir, lamivudine and zidovudine in adults is about 83 %, 80 - 85 % and 60 - 70 % respectively.

In a pharmacokinetic study in HIV-1 infected patients, the steady state pharmacokinetic parameters of abacavir, lamivudine and zidovudine were similar when either Trizivir

Table 3

Baseline Reverse Transcriptase Mutation	Week 4 (n = 166)		
	n	Median Change vRNA (log_{10} c/mL)	Percent with <400 copies/mL vRNA
None	15	-0.96	40%
M184V alone	75	-0.74	64%
Any one NRTI mutation	82	-0.72	65%
Any two NRTI-associated mutations	22	-0.82	32%
Any three NRTI-associated mutations	19	-0.30	5%
Four or more NRTI-associated mutations	28	-0.07	11%

Table 4

		ZDV/3TC/ABC	ZDV/3TC/EFV	ZDV/3TC/ABC/EFV
Virologic failure (HIV RNA >200 copies/ml)	32 weeks	26%	16%	13%
	144 weeks	-	26%	25%
Virologic success (48 weeks HIV RNA < 50 copies/ml)		63%	80%	86%

alone or the combination tablet lamivudine/zidovudine and abacavir in combination were administered, and also similar to the values obtained in the bioequivalence study of Trizivir in healthy volunteers.

A bioequivalence study compared Trizivir with abacavir 300 mg, lamivudine 150 mg and zidovudine 300 mg taken together. The effect of food on the rate and extent of absorption was also studied. Trizivir was shown to be bioequivalent to abacavir 300 mg, lamivudine 150 mg and zidovudine 300 mg given as separate tablets for $AUC_{0-\infty}$ and C_{max}. Food decreased the rate of absorption of Trizivir (slight decrease C_{max} (mean 18 - 32 %) and increase t_{max} (approximately 1 hour), but not the extent of absorption ($AUC_{0-\infty}$). These changes are not considered clinically relevant and no food restrictions are recommended for administration of Trizivir.

At a therapeutic dosage (one Trizivir tablet twice daily) in patients, the mean (CV) steady-state C_{max} of abacavir, lamivudine and zidovudine in plasma are 3.49 μg/ml (45 %), 1.33 μg/ml (33 %) and 1.56 μg/ml (83 %), respectively. Corresponding values for C_{min} could not be established for abacavir and are 0.14 μg/ml (70 %) for lamivudine and 0.01 μg/ml (64 %) for zidovudine. The mean (CV) AUCs for abacavir, lamivudine and zidovudine over a dosing interval of 12 hours are 6.39 μg.h/ml (31 %), 5.73 μg.h/ml (31 %) and 1.50 μg.h/ml (47 %), respectively.

A modest increase in C_{max} (28 %) was observed for zidovudine when administered with lamivudine, however overall exposure (AUC) was not significantly altered. Zidovudine has no effect on the pharmacokinetics of lamivudine. An effect of abacavir is observed on zidovudine (C_{max} reduced with 20 %) and on lamivudine (C_{max} reduced with 35 %).

Distribution

Intravenous studies with abacavir, lamivudine and zidovudine showed that the mean apparent volume of distribution is 0.8, 1.3 and 1.6 l/kg respectively. Lamivudine exhibits linear pharmacokinetics over the therapeutic dose range and displays limited binding to the major plasma protein albumin (< 36 % serum albumin *in vitro*). Zidovudine plasma protein binding is 34 % to 38 %. Plasma protein binding studies *in vitro* indicate that abacavir binds only low to moderately (~ 49 %) to human plasma proteins at therapeutic concentrations. This indicates a low likelihood for interactions with other medicinal products through plasma protein binding displacement.

Interactions involving binding site displacement are not anticipated with Trizivir.

Data show that abacavir, lamivudine and zidovudine penetrate the central nervous system (CNS) and reach the cerebrospinal fluid (CSF). The mean ratios of CSF/serum lamivudine and zidovudine concentrations 2 - 4 hours after oral administration were approximately 0.12 and 0.5 respectively. The true extent of CNS penetration of lamivudine and its relationship with any clinical efficacy is unknown.

Studies with abacavir demonstrate a CSF to plasma AUC ratio of between 30 to 44 %. The observed values of the peak concentrations are 9 fold greater than the IC_{50} of abacavir of 0.08 μg/ml or 0.26 μM when abacavir is given at 600 mg twice daily.

Metabolism

Metabolism of lamivudine is a minor route of elimination. Lamivudine is predominately cleared by renal excretion of unchanged lamivudine. The likelihood of metabolic drug interactions with lamivudine is low due to the small extent of hepatic metabolism (5 - 10 %) and low plasma binding.

The 5'-glucuronide of zidovudine is the major metabolite in both plasma and urine, accounting for approximately 50 - 80 % of the administered dose eliminated by renal excretion. 3'-amino-3'-deoxythymidine (AMT) has been identified as a metabolite of zidovudine following intravenous dosing.

Abacavir is primarily metabolised by the liver with approximately 2 % of the administered dose being renally excreted, as unchanged compound. The primary pathways of metabolism in man are by alcohol dehydrogenase and by glucuronidation to produce the 5'-carboxylic acid and 5'-glucuronide which account for about 66 % of the dose excreted in the urine.

Elimination

The observed lamivudine half-life of elimination is 5 to 7 hours. The mean systemic clearance of lamivudine is approximately 0.32 l/h/kg, with predominantly renal clearance (> 70 %) via the organic cationic transport system. Studies in patients with renal impairment show lamivudine elimination is affected by renal dysfunction. Dose reduction is required for patients with creatinine clearance ⩽ 50 ml/min (see section 4.2).

From studies with intravenous zidovudine, the mean terminal plasma half-life was 1.1 hours and the mean systemic clearance was 1.6 l/h/kg. Renal clearance of zidovudine is estimated to be 0.34 l/h/kg, indicating glomerular filtration and active tubular secretion by the kidneys. Zidovudine concentrations are increased in patients with advanced renal failure.

The mean half-life of abacavir is about 1.5 hours. Following multiple oral doses of abacavir 300 mg twice a day there is no significant accumulation of abacavir. Elimination of abacavir is via hepatic metabolism with subsequent excretion of metabolites primarily in the urine. The metabolites and unchanged abacavir account for about 83 % of the administered abacavir dose in the urine the remainder is eliminated in the faeces.

Special populations

Hepatically impaired: There are no data available on the use of Trizivir in hepatically impaired patients. Limited data in patients with cirrhosis suggest that accumulation of zidovudine may occur in patients with hepatic impairment because of decreased glucuronidation. Data obtained in patients with moderate to severe hepatic impairment show that lamivudine pharmacokinetics are not significantly affected by hepatic dysfunction.

Abacavir is metabolised primarily by the liver. The pharmacokinetics of abacavir have been studied in patients with mild hepatic impairment (Child-Pugh score 5-6) receiving a single 600 mg dose. The results showed that there was a mean increase of 1.89 fold [1.32; 2.70] in the abacavir AUC, and 1.58 [1.22; 2.04] fold in the elimination half-life. No recommendation on dosage reduction is possible in patients with mild hepatic impairment due to substantial variability of abacavir exposure in this patient population. The pharmacokinetics of abacavir have not been studied in patients with moderate or severe hepatic impairment. Plasma concentrations of abacavir are expected to be variable and substantially increased in these patients (see section 4.3).

Renally impaired: The observed lamivudine half-life of elimination is 5 to 7 hours. The mean systemic clearance of lamivudine is approximately 0.32 l/h/kg, with predominantly renal clearance (> 70 %) via the organic cationic transport system. Studies in patients with renal impairment show lamivudine elimination is affected by renal dysfunction.

From studies with intravenous zidovudine, the mean terminal plasma half-life was 1.1 hours and the mean systemic clearance was 1.6 l/h/kg. Renal clearance of zidovudine is estimated to be 0.34 l/h/kg, indicating glomerular filtration and active tubular secretion by the kidneys. Zidovudine concentrations are increased in patients with advanced renal failure.

Abacavir is primarily metabolised by the liver with approximately 2 % of abacavir excreted unchanged in the urine. The pharmacokinetics of abacavir in patients with end-stage renal disease is similar to patients with normal renal function, and, therefore, no dose reduction is required in patients with renal impairment.

As dosage adjustments of lamivudine and zidovudine may be necessary it is recommended that separate preparations of abacavir, lamivudine and zidovudine be administered to patients with reduced renal function (creatinine clearance ⩽ 50 ml/min). Trizivir is contraindicated in patients with end-stage renal disease (see section 4.3).

Elderly: No pharmacokinetic data are available in patients over 65 years of age.

5.3 Preclinical safety data

There are no data available on treatment with the combination of abacavir, lamivudine and zidovudine in animals. The clinically relevant toxicological effects of these three medicinal products are anaemia, neutropenia and leucopenia.

Mutagenicity and carcinogenicity

Neither abacavir, lamivudine nor zidovudine is mutagenic in bacterial tests, but like many nucleoside analogues they show activity in the *in vitro* mammalian tests such as the mouse lymphoma assay. This is consistent with the known activity of other nucleoside analogues.

Lamivudine has not shown any genotoxic activity in the *in vivo* studies at doses that gave plasma concentrations up to 40 - 50 times higher than clinical plasma levels. Zidovudine showed clastogenic effects in oral repeated dose micronucleus tests in mice and rats. Peripheral blood lymphocytes from AIDS patients receiving zidovudine treatment have also been observed to contain higher numbers of chromosome breakages.

A pilot study has demonstrated that zidovudine is incorporated into leukocyte nuclear DNA of adults, including pregnant women, taking zidovudine as treatment for HIV-1 infection, or for the prevention of mother to child viral transmission. Zidovudine was also incorporated into DNA from cord blood leukocytes of infants from zidovudine-treated mothers. A transplacental genotoxicity study conducted in monkeys compared zidovudine alone with the combination of zidovudine and lamivudine at human-equivalent exposures. The study demonstrated that foetuses exposed *in utero* to the combination sustained a higher level of nucleoside analogue-DNA incorporation into multiple foetal organs, and showed evidence of more telomere shortening than in those exposed to zidovudine alone. The clinical significance of these findings is unknown.

Abacavir has a weak potential to cause chromosomal damage both *in vitro* and *in vivo* at high test concentrations and therefore any potential risk to man must be balanced against the expected benefits of treatment.

The carcinogenic potential of a combination of abacavir, lamivudine and zidovudine has not been tested. In long-term oral carcinogenicity studies in rats and mice, lamivudine did not show any carcinogenic potential. In oral carcinogenicity studies with zidovudine in mice and rats, late appearing vaginal epithelial tumours were observed. A subsequent intravaginal carcinogenicity study confirmed the hypothesis that the vaginal tumours were the result of long term local exposure of the rodent vaginal epithelium to high concentrations of unmetabolised zidovudine in urine. There were no other zidovudine-related tumours observed in either sex of either species.

In addition, two transplacental carcinogenicity studies have been conducted in mice. In one study, by the US National Cancer Institute, zidovudine was administered at maximum tolerated doses to pregnant mice from day 12 to 18 of gestation. One year postnatally, there was an increase in the incidence of tumours in the lung, liver and female reproductive tract of offspring exposed to the highest dose level (420 mg/kg term body weight).

In a second study, mice were administered zidovudine at doses up to 40 mg/kg for 24 months, with exposure beginning prenatally on gestation day 10. Treatment related findings were limited to late-occurring vaginal epithelial tumours, which were seen with a similar incidence and time of onset as in the standard oral carcinogenicity study. The second study thus provided no evidence that zidovudine acts as a transplacental carcinogen.

It is concluded that as the increase in incidence of tumours in the first transplacental carcinogenicity study represents a hypothetical risk, this should be balanced against the proven therapeutic benefit. Carcinogenicity studies with orally administered abacavir in mice and rats showed an increase in the incidence of malignant and non-malignant tumours. Malignant tumours occurred in the preputial gland of males and the clitoral gland of females of both species, and in rats in the thyroid gland of males and and in the liver, urinary bladder, lymph nodes and the subcutis of females.

The majority of these tumours occurred at the highest abacavir dose of 330 mg/kg/day in mice and 600 mg/kg/day in rats. The exception was the preputial gland tumour which occurred at a dose of 110 mg/kg in mice. The systemic exposure at the no effect level in mice and rats was equivalent to 3 and 7 times the human systemic exposure during therapy. While the carcinogenic potential in humans is unknown, these data suggest that a carcinogenic risk to humans is outweighed by the potential clinical benefit.

Repeat-dose toxicity:

In toxicology studies abacavir was shown to increase liver weights in rats and monkeys. The clinical relevance of this is unknown. There is no evidence from clinical studies that abacavir is hepatotoxic. Additionally, autoinduction of abacavir metabolism or induction of the metabolism of other medicinal products hepatically metabolised has not been observed in man.

Mild myocardial degeneration in the heart of mice and rats was observed following administration of abacavir for two years. The systemic exposures were equivalent to 7 to 24 times the expected systemic exposure in humans. The clinical relevance of this finding has not been determined.

Reproductive toxicology

Lamivudine was not teratogenic in animal studies but there were indications of an increase in early embryonic deaths in the rabbit at relatively low systemic exposures, comparable to those achieved in humans. A similar effect was not seen in rats even at very high systemic exposure.

Zidovudine had a similar effect in both species, but only at very high systemic exposures. At maternally toxic doses, zidovudine given to rats during organogenesis resulted in an increased incidence of malformations, but no evidence of foetal abnormalities was observed at lower doses.

Abacavir demonstrated toxicity to the developing embryo and foetus in rats, but not in rabbits. These findings included decreased foetal body weight, foetal oedema, and an increase in skeletal variations/malformations, early intra-uterine deaths and still births. No conclusion can be drawn with regard to the teratogenic potential of abacavir because of this embryo-foetal toxicity.

A fertility study in the rat has shown that abacavir had no effect on male or female fertility. Likewise, neither lamivudine nor zidovudine had any effect on fertility. Zidovudine has not been shown to affect the number of sperm, sperm morphology and motility in man.

6. PHARMACEUTICAL PARTICULARS

6.1 List of excipients

Core:

microcrystalline cellulose,

sodium starch glycollate (type A),

magnesium stearate.

Coating:

Opadry Green 03B11434 containing: hypromellose, titanium dioxide, polyethylene glycol, indigo carmine aluminium lake, iron oxide yellow.

6.2 Incompatibilities

Not applicable

6.3 Shelf life

2 years

6.4 Special precautions for storage

Do not store above 30°C

6.5 Nature and contents of container
Trizivir tablets are available in opaque PVC/Aclar blister packs containing 60 tablets or child-resistant HDPE bottles containing 60 tablets.

6.6 Special precautions for disposal and other handling
Any unused product should be disposed of in accordance with local requirements.

7. MARKETING AUTHORISATION HOLDER
Glaxo Group Ltd
Greenford
Middlesex UB6 0NN
United Kingdom

8. MARKETING AUTHORISATION NUMBER(S)
EU/1/00/156/002 - Blister pack (60 Tablets)
EU/1/00/156/003 -Bottle pack (60 Tablets)

9. DATE OF FIRST AUTHORISATION/RENEWAL OF THE AUTHORISATION
Date of first authorisation: 28 December 2000
Date of renewal: 28 December 2005

10. DATE OF REVISION OF THE TEXT
27 May 2009

Detailed information on this medicinal product is available on the website of the European Medicines Agency (EMEA) http://www.emea.europa.eu

Trosyl Nail Solution

(Pfizer Limited)

1. NAME OF THE MEDICINAL PRODUCT
TROSYL NAIL SOLUTION

2. QUALITATIVE AND QUANTITATIVE COMPOSITION
Tioconazole 283 mg/ml.
For excipients, see 6.1.

3. PHARMACEUTICAL FORM
Cutaneous solution. Clear pale yellow solution for topical application.

4. CLINICAL PARTICULARS

4.1 Therapeutic indications
Tioconazole is a broad spectrum imidazole antifungal agent. Trosyl Nail Solution is indicated for the topical treatment of nail infections due to susceptible fungi (dermatophytes and yeasts) and bacteria.

4.2 Posology and method of administration
Route of administration: Topical.

Adults The solution should be applied to the affected nails and immediately surrounding skin every twelve hours using the applicator brush supplied.

The duration of treatment is up to six months but may be extended to twelve months.

Use in the elderly No special precautions are required. Use the adult dose.

Use in children No special precautions are required. Use the adult dose.

4.3 Contraindications
Trosyl Nail Solution is contra-indicated in individuals who have been shown to be hypersensitive to imidazole antifungal agents, or to any of the components of the solution.

Use is contraindicated during pregnancy.

4.4 Special warnings and precautions for use
Trosyl Nail Solution is not for ophthalmic use.

4.5 Interaction with other medicinal products and other forms of interaction
None known.

4.6 Pregnancy and lactation
Use During Pregnancy: In animal studies tioconazole was not teratogenic. At high doses it increased the incidence of renal abnormalities in rat embryos, but this effect was minor and transient and was not evident in weaned animals.

There is insufficient evidence as to the drug's safety in human pregnancy although absorption after topical administration is negligible. Because of the extensive duration of treatment required for nail infections, the use of Trosyl Nail Solution is contra-indicated throughout pregnancy.

Use During Lactation: It is unknown whether this drug is excreted in human milk. Because many drugs are excreted in human milk, nursing should be temporarily discontinued while Trosyl is administered.

4.7 Effects on ability to drive and use machines
None known.

4.8 Undesirable effects
Trosyl Nail Solution is well tolerated upon local application. Symptoms of local irritation have been reported by some patients, but are usually seen during the first week of treatment and are transient and mild.

However, if a sensitivity reaction develops with the use of Trosyl Nail Solution, treatment should be discontinued and appropriate therapy instituted.

Skin and subcutaneous tissue disorders (at the application site): Bullous eruption, dermatitis, pruritis, pain, oedema, tingling/burning sensation, contact dermatitis, dry skin, nail disorder (including nail discoloration, periungual inflammation and nail pain), rash, skin exfoliation, skin irritation.

Immune system disorders: Allergic Reaction (including peripheral oedema, periorbital oedema and urticaria).

4.9 Overdose
No cases of overdosage with Trosyl Nail Solution have been reported. In the event of excessive oral ingestion, gastrointestinal symptoms may occur. Appropriate means of gastric lavage should be considered.

5. PHARMACOLOGICAL PROPERTIES

5.1 Pharmacodynamic properties
Pharmacotherapeutic group: Imidazole and triazole derivatives; ATC-code: D01AC07.

Tioconazole is an imidazole which is active against commonly occurring dermatophyte and yeast-like fungal species. It is fungicidal in murine models vs. Candida spp., *T. rubrum* and *T. mentacrophytes*. *In vitro* it is fungicidal to pathenogenic dermatophytes, yeasts and other fungi. All dermatophytes and Candida spp. were inhibited by 6.25 or 12.5 mg/l respectively. It is also inhibitory vs. Staph. spp. and Strep. spp. at 100 mg/l or less.

Oral doses (200 mg/kg) did not affect behaviour in rats but 25 mg/kg i.v. produced dose-related respiratory distress, gasping, tremors and prostration. Slight but dose-related impairment of performance of mice on the rotating rod occurred from 25 mg/kg. Slight anti-cholinergic and anti-histamine (H_1) activity was recorded *in vitro* but no effect on mice pupil size *in vivo*. Oral tioconazole prolonged alcohol and pentobarbital sleeping time at 150 and 37.5 mg/kg respectively.

In the anaesthetised cat i.v. tioconazole 2.5 - 10 mg/kg produced brief falls in blood pressure and increased heart rate, haematuria, tremors and twitches.

5.2 Pharmacokinetic properties
Absorption is rapid and extensive on oral administration to rats, monkeys and man, the major metabolite being a glucuronide conjugate of tioconazole. Tissue uptake in rat and monkey was highest in liver, kidney and intestinal tract with excretion in all species mainly in faeces.

Rat studies using oral, dermal and vaginal administration of C^{14} labelled tioconazole confirm significantly lower absorption via the topical route.

In man, oral formulations of tioconazole (500mg) gave plasma concentrations of 1300ng/ml. Topical administration of dermal cream 1% (20mg/day) for 28 days, or vaginal cream 2% (100mg/day) for 30 days gave negligible mean peak plasma levels, i.e. 10.1 and 11.5ng/ml respectively.

After single dose administration of tioconazole vaginal ointment 6.5% w/w (tioconazole 300mg) the mean peak plasma concentration was 18ng/ml in humans, achieved approximately 8 hours post dose.

5.3 Preclinical safety data
None relevant to the prescriber.

6. PHARMACEUTICAL PARTICULARS

6.1 List of excipients
Undecylenic acid, ethyl acetate.

6.2 Incompatibilities
Not applicable.

6.3 Shelf life
24 months.

6.4 Special precautions for storage
Do not store above 25°C. Avoid flame and heat. Do not refrigerate.

6.5 Nature and contents of container
Trosyl Nail Solution is contained in an amber glass bottle with a screw cap fitted with an applicator containing 12 ml.

6.6 Special precautions for disposal and other handling
No special instructions are required.

7. MARKETING AUTHORISATION HOLDER
Pfizer Limited
Ramsgate Road
Sandwich
Kent
CT13 9NJ
United Kingdom

8. MARKETING AUTHORISATION NUMBER(S)
PL 00057/0236

9. DATE OF FIRST AUTHORISATION/RENEWAL OF THE AUTHORISATION
21 July 1999

10. DATE OF REVISION OF THE TEXT
November 2007

LEGAL CATEGORY
POM

TY5_0

Trusopt 2% Eye drops, solution

(Merck Sharp & Dohme Limited)

1. NAME OF THE MEDICINAL PRODUCT
TRUSOPT ® 20 mg/ml Eye drops, solution

2. QUALITATIVE AND QUANTITATIVE COMPOSITION
Each ml contains 22.26 mg of dorzolamide hydrochloride corresponding to 20 mg of dorzolamide.

For a full list of excipients, see section 6.1.

3. PHARMACEUTICAL FORM
Eye drops, solution.
Clear, colourless to nearly colourless, slightly viscous, solution.

4. CLINICAL PARTICULARS

4.1 Therapeutic indications
TRUSOPT is indicated:

- as adjunctive therapy to beta-blockers,
- as monotherapy in patients unresponsive to beta-blockers or in whom beta-blockers are contraindicated, in the treatment of elevated intra-ocular pressure in:
- ocular hypertension,
- open-angle glaucoma,
- pseudo-exfoliative glaucoma.

4.2 Posology and method of administration
When used as monotherapy, the dose is one drop of dorzolamide in the conjunctival sac of the affected eye(s), three times daily.

When used as adjunctive therapy with an ophthalmic beta-blocker, the dose is one drop of dorzolamide in the conjunctival sac of the affected eye(s), two times daily.

When substituting dorzolamide for another ophthalmic anti-glaucoma agent, discontinue the other agent after proper dosing on one day, and start dorzolamide on the next day.

If more than one topical ophthalmic drug is being used, the drugs should be administered at least ten minutes apart.

Patients should be instructed to wash their hands before use and avoid allowing the tip of the container to come into contact with the eye or surrounding structures.

Patients should also be instructed that ocular solutions, if handled improperly, can become contaminated by common bacteria known to cause ocular infections. Serious damage to the eye and subsequent loss of vision may result from using contaminated solutions.

Patients should be informed of the correct handling of the OCUMETER PLUS bottles.

Usage instructions:

1. Before using the medication for the first time, be sure the Safety Strip on the front of the bottle is unbroken. A gap between the bottle and the cap is normal for an unopened bottle.
2. Tear off the Safety Strip to break the seal.
3. To open the bottle, unscrew the cap by turning as indicated by the arrows on the top of the cap. Do not pull the cap directly up and away from the bottle. Pulling the cap directly up will prevent your dispenser from operating properly.
4. Tilt your head back and pull your lower eyelid down slightly to form a pocket between your eyelid and eye.
5. Invert the bottle, and press lightly with the thumb or index finger over the "Finger Push Area" until a single drop is dispensed into the eye as directed by your doctor. DO NOT TOUCH YOUR EYE OR EYELID WITH THE DROPPER TIP.
6. If drop dispensing is difficult after opening for the first time, replace the cap on the bottle and tighten (do not overtighten) and then remove by turning the cap in the opposite directions as indicated by the arrows on the top of the cap.
7. Repeat steps 4 & 5 with the other eye if instructed to do so by your doctor.
8. Replace the cap by turning until it is firmly touching the bottle. The arrow on the left side of the cap must be aligned with the arrow on the left side of the bottle label for proper closure. Do not overtighten or you may damage the bottle and cap.
9. The dispenser tip is designed to provide a single drop; therefore, do NOT enlarge the hole of the dispenser tip.
10. After you have used all doses, there will be some TRUSOPT left in the bottle. You should not be concerned since an extra amount of TRUSOPT has been added and you will get the full amount of TRUSOPT that your doctor prescribed. Do not attempt to remove the excess medicine from the bottle.

Paediatric use:

Limited clinical data in paediatric patients with administration of dorzolamide three times a day are available. (For information regarding paediatric dosing see section 5.1).

4.3 Contraindications
Dorzolamide is contraindicated in patients who are hypersensitive to the active substance or to any of the excipients.

Dorzolamide has not been studied in patients with severe renal impairment (CrCl < 30 ml/min) or with hyperchloraemic acidosis. Because dorzolamide and its metabolites are excreted predominantly by the kidney, dorzolamide is therefore contra-indicated in such patients.

4.4 Special warnings and precautions for use

Dorzolamide has not been studied in patients with hepatic impairment and should therefore be used with caution in such patients.

The management of patients with acute angle-closure glaucoma requires therapeutic interventions in addition to ocular hypotensive agents. Dorzolamide has not been studied in patients with acute angle-closure glaucoma.

Dorzolamide contains a sulphonamido group, which also occurs in sulphonamides and although administered topically, is absorbed systemically. Therefore the same types of adverse reactions that are attributable to sulphonamides may occur with topical administration. If signs of serious reactions or hypersensitivity occur, discontinue the use of this preparation.

Therapy with oral carbonic anhydrase inhibitors has been associated with urolithiasis as a result of acid-base disturbances, especially in patients with a prior history of renal calculi. Although no acid-base disturbances have been observed with dorzolamide, urolithiasis has been reported infrequently. Because dorzolamide is a topical carbonic anhydrase inhibitor that is absorbed systemically, patients with a prior history of renal calculi may be at increased risk of urolithiasis while using dorzolamide.

If allergic reactions (e.g. conjunctivitis and eyelid reactions) are observed, discontinuation of treatment should be considered.

There is a potential for an additive effect on the known systemic effects of carbonic anhydrase inhibition in patients receiving an oral carbonic anhydrase inhibitor and dorzolamide. The concomitant administration of dorzolamide and oral carbonic anhydrase inhibitors is not recommended.

Corneal oedemas and irreversible corneal decompensations have been reported in patients with pre-existing chronic corneal defects and/or a history of intra-ocular surgery while using TRUSOPT. Topical dorzolamide should be used with caution in such patients.

Choroidal detachment concomitant with ocular hypotony have been reported after filtration procedures with administration of aqueous suppressant therapies.

TRUSOPT contains the preservative benzalkonium chloride, which may cause eye irritation. Contact lenses should be removed prior to application and wait at least 15 minutes before reinsertion. Benzalkonium chloride is known to discolour soft contact lenses.

Paediatric patients:

Dorzolamide has not been studied in patients less than 36 weeks gestational age and less than 1 week of age. Patients with significant renal tubular immaturity should only receive dorzolamide after careful consideration of the risk benefit balance because of the possible risk of metabolic acidosis.

4.5 Interaction with other medicinal products and other forms of interaction

Specific drug interaction studies have not been performed with dorzolamide.

In clinical studies, dorzolamide was used concomitantly with the following medications without evidence of adverse interactions: timolol ophthalmic solution, betaxolol ophthalmic solution and systemic medications, including ACE-inhibitors, calcium-channel blockers, diuretics, non-steroidal anti-inflammatory drugs including aspirin, and hormones (e.g. oestrogen, insulin, thyroxine).

Association between dorzolamide and miotics and adrenergic agonists has not been fully evaluated during glaucoma therapy.

4.6 Pregnancy and lactation

Use During Pregnancy

Dorzolamide should not be used during pregnancy. No adequate clinical data in exposed pregnancies are available. In rabbits, dorzolamide produced teratogenic effects at maternotoxic doses (See Section 5.3)

Use During Lactation

It is not know whether dorzolamide is excreted in human milk. In lactating rats, decreases in the body weight gain of offspring were observed. If treatment with dorzolamide is required, then lactation is not recommended.

4.7 Effects on ability to drive and use machines

No studies on the effects on the ability to drive and use machines have been performed. Possible side effects such as dizziness and visual disturbances may affect the ability to drive and use machines.

4.8 Undesirable effects

TRUSOPT was evaluated in more than 1400 individuals in controlled and uncontrolled clinical studies. In long-term studies of 1108 patients treated with TRUSOPT as monotherapy or as adjunctive therapy with an ophthalmic beta-blocker, the most frequent cause of discontinuation (approximately 3%) from treatment with TRUSOPT was drug-related ocular adverse reactions, primarily conjunctivitis and lid reactions.

The following adverse reactions have been reported either during clinical trials or during post-marketing experience:

[Very Common: (≥ 1/10), Common: (≥ 1/100 to < 1/10), Uncommon: (≥ 1/1,000 to < 1/100), Rare: (≥ 1/10,000 to < 1/1,000)]

Nervous system disorders:

Common: headache

Rare: dizziness, paraesthesia

Eye disorders:

Very Common: burning and stinging.

Common: superficial punctate keratitis, tearing, conjunctivitis, eyelid inflammation, eye itching, eyelid irritation, blurred vision

Uncommon: iridocyclitis

Rare: irritation including redness, pain, eyelid crusting, transient myopia (which resolved upon discontinuation of therapy), corneal oedema, ocular hypotony, choroidal detachment following filtration surgery

Respiratory, thoracic, and mediastinal disorders:

Rare: epistaxis

Gastrointestinal disorders:

Common: nausea, bitter taste

Rare: throat irritation, dry mouth

Skin and subcutaneous tissue disorders:

Rare: contact dermatitis

Renal and urinary disorders:

Rare: urolithiasis

General disorders and administration site conditions:

Common: asthenia/fatigue

Rare: Hypersensitivity: signs and symptoms of local reactions (palpebral reactions) and systemic allergic reactions including angioedema, urticaria and pruritus, rash, shortness of breath, rarely bronchospasm

Laboratory findings: dorzolamide was not associated with clinically meaningful electrolyte disturbances.

Paediatric patients:

See 5.1.

4.9 Overdose

Only limited information is available with regard to human overdose by accidental or deliberate ingestion of dorzolamide hydrochloride.

Symptoms

The following have been reported with oral ingestion: somnolence; topical application: nausea, dizziness, headache, fatigue, abnormal dreams, and dysphagia.

Treatment

Treatment should be symptomatic and supportive. Electrolyte imbalance, development of an acidotic state, and possible central nervous system effects may occur. Serum electrolyte levels (particularly potassium) and blood pH levels should be monitored.

5. PHARMACOLOGICAL PROPERTIES

5.1 Pharmacodynamic properties

Pharmacotherapuetic group: Antiglaucoma preparations and miotics, Carbonic Anhydrase Inhibitors, dorzolamide, ATC code: S01EC03

Mechanism of action

Carbonic anhydrase (CA) is an enzyme found in many tissues of the body including the eye. In humans, carbonic anhydrase exists as a number of isoenzymes, the most active being carbonic anhydrase II (CA-II) found primarily in red blood cells (RBCs) but also in other tissues. Inhibition of carbonic anhydrase in the ciliary processes of the eye decreases aqueous humor secretion. The result is a reduction in intra-ocular pressure (IOP).

TRUSOPT contains dorzolamide hydrochloride, a potent inhibitor of human carbonic anhydrase II. Following topical ocular administration, dorzolamide reduces elevated intra-ocular pressure, whether or not associated with glaucoma. Elevated intra-ocular pressure is a major risk factor in the pathogenesis of optic nerve damage and visual-field loss. Dorzolamide does not cause pupillary constriction and reduces intra-ocular pressure without side effects such as night blindness, accommodative spasm. Dorzolamide has minimal or no effect on pulse rate or blood pressure.

Topically applied beta-adrenergic blocking agents also reduce IOP by decreasing aqueous humor secretion but by a different mechanism of action. Studies have shown that when dorzolamide is added to a topical beta-blocker, additional reduction in IOP is observed; this finding is consistent with the reported additive effects of beta-blockers and oral carbonic anhydrase inhibitors.

Pharmacodynamic effects

Clinical effects:

Adult Patients

In patients with glaucoma or ocular hypertension, the efficacy of dorzolamide given t.i.d. as monotherapy (baseline IOP ≥23 mmHg) or given b.i.d. as adjunctive therapy while receiving ophthalmic beta-blockers (baseline IOP ≥22 mmHg) was demonstrated in large-scale clinical studies of up to one-year duration. The IOP-lowering effect of dorzolamide as monotherapy and as adjunctive therapy was demonstrated throughout the day and this effect was maintained during long-term administration. Efficacy during long-term monotherapy was similar to betaxolol and slightly less than timolol. When used as adjunctive therapy to ophthalmic beta-blockers, dorzolamide demonstrated additional IOP lowering similar to pilocarpine 2% q.i.d.

Paediatric Patients

A 3-month, double-masked, active-treatment controlled, multicentre study was undertaken in 184 (122 for dorzolamide) paediatric patients from 1 week of age to < 6 years of age with glaucoma or elevated intraocular pressure (baseline IOP ≥ 22 mmHg) to assess the safety of TRUSOPT when administered topically t.i.d. (three times a day). Approximately half the patients in both treatment groups were diagnosed with congenital glaucoma; other common aetiologies were Sturge Weber syndrome, iridocorneal mesenchymal dysgenesis, aphakic patients. The distribution by age and treatments in the monotherapy phase was as follows:

	Dorzolamide 2%	Timolol
Age cohort < 2 years	N=56 Age range: 1 to 23 months	Timolol GS 0.25% N=27 Age range: 0.25 to 22 months
Age cohort ≥ 2 - < 6 years	N=66 Age range: 2 to 6 years	Timolol 0.50% N=35 Age range: 2 to 6 years

Across both age cohorts approximately 70 patients received treatment for at least 61 days and approximately 50 patients received 81-100 days of treatment.

If IOP was inadequately controlled on dorzolamide or timolol gel-forming solution monotherapy, a change was made to open-label therapy according to the following: 30 patients < 2 years were switched to concomitant therapy with timolol gel-forming solution 0.25% daily and dorzolamide 2% t.i.d.; 30 patients ≥ 2 years were switched to 2% dorzolamide/0.5% timolol fixed combination b.i.d (twice a day).

Overall, this study did not reveal additional safety concerns in paediatric patients: approximately 26% (20% in dorzolamide monotherapy) of paediatric patients were observed to experience drug related adverse affects, the majority of which were local, non-serious ocular effects such as ocular burning and stinging, injection and eye pain. A small percentage < 4% was observed to have corneal oedema or haze. Local reactions appeared similar in frequency to comparator. In post marketing data, metabolic acidosis in the very young particularly with renal immaturity/impairment has been reported.

Efficacy results in paediatric patients suggest that the mean IOP decrease observed in the dorzolamide group was comparable to the mean IOP decrease observed in the timolol group even if a slight numeric advantage was observed for timolol.

Longer-term efficacy studies (> 12 weeks) are not available.

5.2 Pharmacokinetic properties

Unlike oral carbonic anhydrase inhibitors, topical administration of dorzolamide hydrochloride allows for the active substance to exert its effects directly in the eye at substantially lower doses and therefore with less systemic exposure. In clinical trials, this resulted in a reduction in IOP without the acid-base disturbances or alterations in electrolytes characteristic of oral carbonic anhydrase inhibitors.

When topically applied, dorzolamide reaches the systemic circulation. To assess the potential for systemic carbonic anhydrase inhibition following topical administration, active substance and metabolite concentrations in red blood cells (RBCs) and plasma and carbonic anhydrase inhibition in RBCs were measured. Dorzolamide accumulates in RBCs during chronic dosing as a result of selective binding to CA-II while extremely low concentrations of free active substance in plasma are maintained. The parent active substance forms a single N-desethyl metabolite that inhibits CA-II less potently than the parent active substance but also inhibits a less active isoenzyme (CA-I). The metabolite also accumulates in RBCs where it binds primarily to CA-I. Dorzolamide binds moderately to plasma proteins (approximately 33%). Dorzolamide is primarily excreted unchanged in the urine; the metabolite is also excreted in urine. After dosing ends, dorzolamide washes out of RBCs non linearly, resulting in a rapid decline of active substance concentration initially, followed by a slower elimination phase with a half-life of about four months.

When dorzolamide was given orally to simulate the maximum systemic exposure after long-term topical ocular administration, steady state was reached within 13 weeks. At steady state, there was virtually no free active substance or metabolite in plasma; CA inhibition in RBCs was less than that anticipated to be necessary for a pharmacological effect on renal function or respiration. Similar pharmacokinetic results were observed after chronic, topical administration of dorzolamide. However, some elderly patients with renal impairment (estimated CrCl 30-60 ml/min) had higher metabolite concentrations in RBCs, but no meaningful differences in carbonic anhydrase inhibition, and no clinically significant systemic side effects were directly attributable to this finding.

5.3 Preclinical safety data
The main findings in animal studies with dorzolamide hydrochloride administered orally were related to the pharmacological effects of systemic carbonic anhydrase inhibition. Some of these findings were species-specific and/or were a result of metabolic acidosis. In rabbits given maternotoxic doses of dorzolamide associated with metabolic acidosis, malformations of the vertebral bodies were observed.

In clinical studies, patients did not develop signs of metabolic acidosis or serum electrolyte changes that are indicative of systemic CA inhibition. Therefore, it is not expected that the effects noted in animal studies would be observed in patients receiving therapeutic doses of dorzolamide.

6. PHARMACEUTICAL PARTICULARS
6.1 List of excipients
Benzalkonium chloride

Hydroxyethyl cellulose

Mannitol (E421)

Sodium citrate (E331)

Sodium hydroxide (E524) for pH adjustment

Water for injections.

6.2 Incompatibilities
Not Applicable.

6.3 Shelf life
2 years.

TRUSOPT should be used no longer than 28 days after first opening the container.

6.4 Special precautions for storage
Store bottle in original carton, in order to protect from light.

6.5 Nature and contents of container
The OCUMETER Plus Ophthalmic Dispenser consists of a translucent, high-density polyethylene container with a sealed dropper tip, a flexible fluted side area which is depressed to dispense the drops, and a 2-piece cap assembly. The 2-piece cap mechanism punctures the sealed dropper tip upon initial use, then locks together to provide a single cap during the usage period. Tamper evidence is provided by a safety strip on the container label. The OCUMETER Plus Ophthalmic Dispenser contains 5 ml of solution.

TRUSOPT is available in the following packaging configurations:

1 × 5 ml (single 5-ml container)

3 × 5 ml (three 5-ml containers)

6 × 5 ml (six 5-ml containers)

Not all pack sizes may be marketed.

6.6 Special precautions for disposal and other handling
No special requirements.

7. MARKETING AUTHORISATION HOLDER
Merck Sharp & Dohme Limited, Hertford Road, Hoddesdon, Hertfordshire EN11 9BU, UK

8. MARKETING AUTHORISATION NUMBER(S)
PL 0025/0323.

9. DATE OF FIRST AUTHORISATION/RENEWAL OF THE AUTHORISATION
9 January 1995/ 10 November 2004.

10. DATE OF REVISION OF THE TEXT
June 2009

LEGAL CATEGORY
POM

MSD (logo)

Merck Sharp & Dohme Limited

Hertford Road, Hoddesdon, Hertfordshire EN11 9BU, UK

SPC.DZH.07.UK.2466 (II/37 + II/38)

Trusopt 2% Preservative-free eye drops solution

(Merck Sharp & Dohme Limited)

1. NAME OF THE MEDICINAL PRODUCT
TRUSOPT® Preservative-Free 20 mg/ml eye drops solution, single dose container

2. QUALITATIVE AND QUANTITATIVE COMPOSITION
Each ml contains 22.26 mg of dorzolamide hydrochloride corresponding to 20 mg of dorzolamide

For a full list of excipients, see section 6.1.

3. PHARMACEUTICAL FORM
Eye drops, solution, single dose container

Clear, colourless to nearly colourless, slightly viscous solution.

4. CLINICAL PARTICULARS
4.1 Therapeutic indications
TRUSOPT Preservative-Free is indicated:

- as adjunctive therapy to beta-blockers,
- as monotherapy in patients unresponsive to beta-blockers or in whom beta-blockers are contraindicated, in the treatment of elevated intra-ocular pressure in:
- ocular hypertension,
- open-angle glaucoma,
- pseudoexfoliative glaucoma.

4.2 Posology and method of administration
When used as monotherapy, the dose is one drop of dorzolamide in the conjunctival sac of the affected eye(s), three times daily.

When used as adjunctive therapy with an ophthalmic beta-blocker, the dose is one drop of dorzolamide in the conjunctival sac of the affected eye(s) two times daily.

When substituting dorzolamide for another ophthalmic anti-glaucoma agent, discontinue the other agent after proper dosing on one day, and start dorzolamide on the next day.

If more than one topical ophthalmic drug is being used, the drugs should be administered at least ten minutes apart.

Patients should be instructed to avoid allowing the tip of the container to come into contact with the eye or surrounding structures.

Patients should also be instructed that ocular solutions, if handled improperly, can become contaminated by common bacteria known to cause ocular infections. Serious damage to the eye and subsequent loss of vision may result from using contaminated solutions.

TRUSOPT Preservative-Free is a sterile solution that does not contain a preservative. The solution from one individual single-dose container is to be used immediately after opening for administration to the affected eye(s). Since sterility cannot be maintained after the individual single-dose container is opened, any remaining contents must be discarded immediately after administration. Each single dose container contains enough solution for both eyes.

Usage Instructions:

1. Open the sachet which contains 15 individual single-dose containers. There are three strips of 5 single-dose containers each in the sachet.
2. First wash your hands then break off one single-dose container from the strip and twist open the top.
3. Tilt your head back and pull your lower eyelid down slightly to form a pocket between your eyelid and eye.
4. Instill one drop in the affected eye(s) as directed by the physician.
5. After instillation, discard the used single-dose container even if there is solution remaining.
6. Store the remaining single-dose containers in the sachet; the remaining single-dose containers must be used within 15 days after opening of the sachet.

Paediatric use

Limited clinical data in paediatric patients with administration of dorzolamide (preserved formulation) three times a day are available. (For information regarding paediatric dosing see 5.1)

4.3 Contraindications
Dorzolamide is contraindicated in patients who are hypersensitive to the active substance or to any of the excipients.

Dorzolamide has not been studied in patients with severe renal impairment (CrCl < 30 ml/min) or with hyperchloraemic acidosis. Because dorzolamide and its metabolites are excreted predominantly by the kidney, dorzolamide is therefore contra-indicated in such patients.

4.4 Special warnings and precautions for use
Dorzolamide has not been studied in patients with hepatic impairment and should therefore be used with caution in such patients.

The management of patients with acute angle-closure glaucoma requires therapeutic interventions in addition to ocular hypotensive agents. Dorzolamide has not been studied in patients with acute angle-closure glaucoma.

Dorzolamide contains a sulphonamido group, which also occurs in sulphonamides and although administered topically, is absorbed systemically. Therefore the same types of adverse reactions that are attributable to sulphonamides may occur with topical administration. If signs of serious reactions or hypersensitivity occur, discontinue the use of this preparation.

Therapy with oral carbonic anhydrase inhibitors has been associated with urolithiasis as a result of acid-base disturbances, especially in patients with a prior history of renal calculi. Although no acid-base disturbances have been observed with dorzolamide, urolithiasis has been reported infrequently. Because dorzolamide is a topical carbonic anhydrase inhibitor that is absorbed systemically, patients with a prior history of renal calculi may be at increased risk of urolithiasis while using dorzolamide.

If allergic reactions (e.g. conjunctivitis and eyelid reactions) are observed, treatment discontinuation should be considered.

There is a potential for an additive effect on the known systemic effects of carbonic anhydrase inhibition in patients receiving an oral carbonic anhydrase inhibitor and dorzolamide. The concomitant administration of dorzolamide and oral carbonic anhydrase inhibitors is not recommended.

Corneal oedemas and irreversible corneal decompensations have been reported in patients with pre-existing chronic corneal defects and/or a history of intra-ocular surgery while using TRUSOPT multidose (preserved formulation). Topical dorzolamide should be used with caution in such patients.

Choroidal detachment concomitant with ocular hypotony have been reported after filtration procedures with administration of aqueous suppressant therapies.

TRUSOPT Preservative-Free has not been studied in patients wearing contact lenses.

Paediatric Patients

Dorzolamide has not been studied in patients less than 36 weeks gestational age and less than 1 week of age. Patients with significant renal tubular immaturity should only receive dorzolamide after careful consideration of the risk benefit balance because of the possible risk of metabolic acidosis.

4.5 Interaction with other medicinal products and other forms of interaction
Specific drug interaction studies have not been performed with dorzolamide.

In clinical studies, dorzolamide was used concomitantly with the following medications without evidence of adverse interactions: timolol ophthalmic solution, betaxolol ophthalmic solution and systemic medications including ACE-inhibitors, calcium channel blockers, diuretics, non-steroidal anti-inflammatory drugs including aspirin, and hormones (e.g. oestrogen, insulin, thyroxine).

Association between dorzolamide and miotics and adrenergic agonists has not been fully evaluated during glaucoma therapy.

4.6 Pregnancy and lactation
Use During Pregnancy

Dorzolamide should not be used during pregnancy. No adequate clinical data in exposed pregnancies are available. In rabbits, dorzolamide produced teratogenic effects at maternotoxic doses (see Section 5.3).

Use During Lactation

It is not known whether dorzolamide is excreted in human milk. In lactating rats, decreases in the body weight gain of offspring were observed. If treatment with dorzolamide is required, then lactation is not recommended.

4.7 Effects on ability to drive and use machines
No studies on the effects on the ability to drive and use machines have been performed. Possible side effects such as dizziness and visual disturbances may affect the ability to drive and use machines

4.8 Undesirable effects
In a multiple-dose, double-masked, active-treatment (TRUSOPT multidose) controlled, two period crossover multiclinic study, the safety profile of TRUSOPT Preservative-Free was similar to that of TRUSOPT multidose.

TRUSOPT multidose (preserved formulation) was evaluated in more than 1,400 individuals in controlled and uncontrolled clinical studies. In long term studies of 1,108 patients treated with TRUSOPT multidose as monotherapy or as adjunctive therapy with an ophthalmic beta-blocker, the most frequent cause of discontinuations from treatment were drug-related ocular adverse effects in approximately 3% of patients primarily conjunctivitis and eyelid reactions.

The following adverse effects have been reported either during clinical trials or during post-marketing experience with dorzolamide:

[Very Common: (≥ 1/10), Common: (≥ 1/100 to < 1/10), Uncommon: (≥ 1/1,000 to < 1/100), Rare: (≥ 1/10,000 to < 1/1,000)]

Nervous system disorders:

Common: headache

Rare: dizziness, paraesthesia

Eye disorders:

Very Common: burning and stinging,

Common: superficial punctate keratitis, tearing, conjunctivitis, eyelid inflammation, eye itching, eyelid irritation, blurred vision

Uncommon: iridocyclitis

Rare: irritation including redness, pain, eyelid crusting, transient myopia (which resolved upon discontinuation of therapy), corneal oedema, ocular hypotony, choroidal detachment following filtration surgery

Respiratory, thoracic, and mediastinal disorders:

Rare: epistaxis

Gastrointestinal disorders:

Common: nausea, bitter taste

Rare: throat irritation, dry mouth

Skin and subcutaneous tissue disorders:

Rare: contact dermatitis

Renal and urinary disorders:

Rare: urolithiasis

General disorders and administration site conditions:

Common: asthenia/fatigue

Rare: Hypersensitivity: signs and symptoms of local reactions (palpebral reactions) and systemic allergic reactions including angioedema, urticaria and pruritus, rash, shortness of breath, rarely bronchospasm

Laboratory Findings: dorzolamide was not associated with clinically meaningful electrolyte disturbances.

Paediatric patients:

See 5.1

4.9 Overdose

Only limited information is available with regard to human overdose by accidental or deliberate ingestion of dorzolamide hydrochloride.

Symptoms

The following have been reported with oral ingestion: somnolence; topical application: nausea, dizziness, headache, fatigue, abnormal dreams, and dysphagia.

Treatment

Treatment should be symptomatic and supportive. Electrolyte imbalance, development of an acidotic state, and possible central nervous system effects may occur. Serum electrolyte levels (particularly potassium) and blood pH levels should be monitored.

5. PHARMACOLOGICAL PROPERTIES

5.1 Pharmacodynamic properties

Pharmacotherapeutic group: Antiglaucoma preparations and miotics, Carbonic Anhydrase Inhibitors, dorzolamide, ATC code: S01EC03

Mechanism of action

Carbonic anhydrase (CA) is an enzyme found in many tissues of the body including the eye. In humans, carbonic anhydrase exists as a number of isoenzymes, the most active being carbonic anhydrase II (CA-II) found primarily in red blood cells (RBCs) but also in other tissues. Inhibition of carbonic anhydrase in the ciliary processes of the eye decreases aqueous humour secretion. The result is a reduction in intra-ocular pressure (IOP).

Single-dose TRUSOPT contains dorzolamide hydrochloride, a potent inhibitor of human carbonic anhydrase II. Following topical ocular administration, dorzolamide reduces elevated intra-ocular pressure, whether or not associated with glaucoma. Elevated intra-ocular pressure is a major risk factor in the pathogenesis of optic nerve damage and visual field loss. Dorzolamide does not cause pupillary constriction and reduces intra-ocular pressure without side effects such as night blindness or accommodative spasm. Dorzolamide has minimal or no effect on pulse rate or blood pressure.

Topically applied beta-adrenergic blocking agents also reduce IOP by decreasing aqueous humour secretion but by a different mechanism of action. Studies have shown that when dorzolamide is added to a topical beta-blocker, additional reduction in IOP is observed; this finding is consistent with the reported additive effects of beta-blockers and oral carbonic anhydrase inhibitors.

Pharmacodynamic effects

Clinical effects

Adult patients

In patients with glaucoma or ocular hypertension, the efficacy of dorzolamide given t.i.d. as monotherapy (baseline IOP ⩾23 mmHg) or given b.i.d. as adjunctive therapy while receiving ophthalmic beta-blockers (baseline IOP ⩾22 mmHg) was demonstrated in large-scale clinical studies of up to one-year duration. The IOP-lowering effect of dorzolamide as monotherapy and as adjunctive therapy was demonstrated throughout the day and this effect was maintained during long-term administration. Efficacy during long-term monotherapy was similar to betaxolol and slightly less than timolol. When used as adjunctive therapy to ophthalmic beta-blockers, dorzolamide demonstrated additional IOP lowering similar to pilocarpine 2% q.i.d.

In a multiple-dose, double-masked, active treatment (TRUSOPT multidose) controlled, two period crossover multiclinic study, in 152 patients with elevated baseline intraocular pressure (baseline IOP ⩾22 mmHg) in one or both eyes, TRUSOPT Preservative-Free had an IOP-lowering effect equivalent to that of TRUSOPT multidose. The safety profile of TRUSOPT Preservative-Free was similar to TRUSOPT multidose.

Paediatric Patients

A 3-month, double-masked, active-treatment controlled, multicentre study was undertaken in 184 (122 for dorzolamide) paediatric patients from 1week of age to <6 years of age with glaucoma or elevated intraocular pressure (baseline IOP ⩾22 mmHg) to assess the safety of TRUSOPT (preserved-formulation) when administered topically t.i.d. (three times a day). Approximately half the patients in both treatment groups were diagnosed with congenital glaucoma; other common etiologies were Sturge Weber syndrome, iridocorneal mesenchymal dysgenesis, aphakic patients. The distribution by age and treatments in the monotherapy phase was as follows:

	Dorzolamide 2%	Timolol
Age cohort <2 years	N=56 Age range: 1 to 23 months	Timolol GS 0.25% N=27 Age range: 0.25 to 22 months
Age cohort ⩾ 2 - <6 years	N=66 Age range: 2 to 6 years	Timolol 0.50% N=35 Age range: 2 to 6 years

Across both age cohorts approximately 70 patients received treatment for at least 61 days and approximately 50 patients received 81-100 days of treatment.

If IOP was inadequately controlled on dorzolamide or timolol gel-forming solution monotherapy, a change was made to open-label therapy according to the following: 30 patients <2 years were switched to concomitant therapy with timolol gel-forming solution 0.25% daily and dorzolamide 2% t.i.d.; 30 patients ⩾2 years were switched to 2% dorzolamide/0.5% timolol fixed combination b.i.d.(twice a day).

Overall, this study did not reveal additional safety concerns in paediatric patients: approximately 26% (20% in dorzolamide monotherapy) of paediatric patients were observed to experience drug related adverse effects, the majority of which were local, non serious ocular effects such as ocular burning and stinging, injection and eye pain. A small percentage <4%, was observed to have corneal oedema or haze. Local reactions appeared similar in frequency to comparator. In post marketing data, metabolic acidosis in the very young particularly with renal immaturity/impairment has been reported.

Efficacy results in paediatric patients suggest that the mean IOP decrease observed in the dorzolamide group was comparable to the mean IOP decrease observed in the timolol group even if a slight numeric advantage was observed for timolol.

Longer-term efficacy studies (>12 weeks) are not available.

5.2 Pharmacokinetic properties

Unlike oral carbonic anhydrase inhibitors, topical administration of dorzolamide hydrochloride allows for the active substance to exert its effects directly in the eye at substantially lower doses and therefore with less systemic exposure. In clinical trials with dorzolamide, this resulted in a reduction in IOP without the acid-base disturbances or alterations in electrolytes characteristic of oral carbonic anhydrase inhibitors.

When topically applied, dorzolamide reaches the systemic circulation. To assess the potential for systemic carbonic anhydrase inhibition following topical administration, active substance and metabolite concentrations in red blood cells (RBCs) and plasma and carbonic anhydrase inhibition in RBCs were measured. Dorzolamide accumulates in RBCs during chronic dosing as a result of selective binding to CA-II while extremely low concentrations of free active substance in plasma are maintained. The parent active substance forms a single N-desethyl metabolite that inhibits CA-II less potently than the parent active substance but also inhibits a less active isoenzyme (CA-I). The metabolite also accumulates in RBCs where it binds primarily to CA-I. Dorzolamide binds moderately to plasma proteins (approximately 33%). Dorzolamide is primarily excreted unchanged in the urine; the metabolite is also excreted in urine. After dosing ends, dorzolamide washes out of RBCs non-linearly, resulting in a rapid decline of active substance concentration initially, followed by a slower elimination phase with a half-life of about four months.

When dorzolamide was given orally to simulate the maximum systemic exposure after long-term topical ocular administration, steady state was reached within 13 weeks. At steady state, there was virtually no free active substance or metabolite in plasma; CA inhibition in RBCs was less than that anticipated to be necessary for a pharmacological effect on renal function or respiration. Similar pharmacokinetic results were observed after chronic, topical administration of dorzolamide.

However, some elderly patients with renal impairment (estimated CrCl 30-60 ml/min) had higher metabolite concentrations in RBCs, but no meaningful differences in carbonic anhydrase inhibition and no clinically significant systemic side effects were directly attributable to this finding.

5.3 Preclinical safety data

The main findings in animal studies with dorzolamide hydrochloride administered orally were related to the pharmacological effects of systemic carbonic anhydrase inhibition. Some of these findings were species-specific and/or were a result of metabolic acidosis. In rabbits given maternotoxic doses of dorzolamide associated with metabolic acidosis, malformation of the vertebral bodies were observed.

In clinical studies, patients did not develop signs of metabolic acidosis or serum electrolyte changes that are indicative of systemic CA inhibition. Therefore, it is not expected that the effects noted in animal studies would be observed in patients receiving a therapeutic dose of dorzolamide.

6. PHARMACEUTICAL PARTICULARS

6.1 List of excipients

Hydroxyethyl cellulose,

Mannitol (E421),

Sodium citrate (E331),

Sodium hydroxide (E524) for pH adjustment

Water for injections.

6.2 Incompatibilities

Not applicable.

6.3 Shelf life

2 years.

After first opening of the sachet: 15 days. Discard any unused single-dose containers after that time.

Discard the opened single dose container immediately after first use.

6.4 Special precautions for storage

Do not store above 30°C.

Do not freeze.

Store in the original package in order to protect from light.

6.5 Nature and contents of container

TRUSOPT Preservative-Free is available in 0.2 ml in low density polyethylene single- dose containers in an aluminum sachet containing 15 single-dose containers

Pack sizes:

30 × 0.2 ml (2 sachets with 15 single dose containers).

60 × 0.2 ml (4 sachets with 15 single dose containers)

120 × 0.2 ml (8 sachets with 15 single dose containers).

Not all pack sizes may be marketed.

6.6 Special precautions for disposal and other handling

No special requirements

7. MARKETING AUTHORISATION HOLDER

Merck Sharp & Dohme Limited

Hertford Road, Hoddesdon, Hertfordshire EN11 9BU, UK.

8. MARKETING AUTHORISATION NUMBER(S)

PL0025/0472

9. DATE OF FIRST AUTHORISATION/RENEWAL OF THE AUTHORISATION

19 December 2005

10. DATE OF REVISION OF THE TEXT

June 2009

LEGAL CATEGORY

POM

® denotes registered trademark of Merck & Co., Inc., Whitehouse Station, NJ, USA.

MSD (logo)

Merck Sharp & Dohme Limited

Hertford Road, Hoddesdon, Hertfordshire EN11 9BU, UK

SPC.TRUS-UD.07.UK.2467 (II/38 + II/39)

Truvada film-coated tablets

(Gilead Sciences Ltd)

1. NAME OF THE MEDICINAL PRODUCT

Truvada 200 mg/245 mg film-coated tablets.

2. QUALITATIVE AND QUANTITATIVE COMPOSITION

Each film-coated tablet contains 200 mg of emtricitabine and 245 mg of tenofovir disoproxil (equivalent to 300 mg of tenofovir disoproxil fumarate or 136 mg of tenofovir).

Excipient(s):

Each tablet contains 80 mg lactose monohydrate. For a full list of excipients, see section 6.1.

3. PHARMACEUTICAL FORM

Film-coated tablet.

Blue, capsule-shaped, film-coated tablet, debossed on one side with "GILEAD" and on the other side with "701".

4. CLINICAL PARTICULARS

4.1 Therapeutic indications

Truvada is a fixed dose combination of emtricitabine and tenofovir disoproxil fumarate. It is indicated in antiretroviral combination therapy for the treatment of HIV-1 infected adults.

The demonstration of the benefit of the combination emtricitabine and tenofovir disoproxil fumarate in antiretroviral therapy is based solely on studies performed in treatment-naïve patients (see section 5.1).

4.2 Posology and method of administration

Therapy should be initiated by a physician experienced in the management of HIV infection.

Posology

Adults: The recommended dose of Truvada is one tablet, taken orally, once daily. In order to optimise the absorption of tenofovir, it is recommended that Truvada should be taken with food. Even a light meal improves absorption of tenofovir from the combination tablet (see section 5.2).

Where discontinuation of therapy with one of the components of Truvada is indicated or where dose modification is necessary, separate preparations of emtricitabine and tenofovir disoproxil fumarate are available. Please refer to the Summary of Product Characteristics for these medicinal products.

Children and adolescents: Truvada is not recommended for use in children below the age of 18 years due to insufficient data on safety and efficacy (see section 5.2).

Elderly: No data are available on which to make a dose recommendation for patients over the age of 65 years. However, no adjustment in the recommended daily dose for adults should be required unless there is evidence of renal insufficiency.

Renal insufficiency: Emtricitabine and tenofovir are eliminated by renal excretion and the exposure to emtricitabine and tenofovir increases in patients with renal dysfunction. There are limited data on the safety and efficacy of Truvada in patients with moderate and severe renal impairment (creatinine clearance < 50 ml/min) and long term safety data has not been evaluated for mild renal impairment (creatinine clearance 50-80 ml/min). Therefore, in patients with renal impairment Truvada should only be used if the potential benefits of treatment are considered to outweigh the potential risks. Patients with renal impairment may require close monitoring of renal function (see section 4.4). Dose interval adjustments are recommended for patients with creatinine clearance between 30 and 49 ml/min. These dose adjustments have not been confirmed in clinical studies and the clinical response to treatment should be closely monitored in these patients (see sections 4.4 and 5.2).

Mild renal impairment (creatinine clearance 50-80 ml/min): Limited data from clinical studies support once daily dosing of Truvada in patients with mild renal impairment (see section 4.4).

Moderate renal impairment (creatinine clearance 30-49 ml/min): Administration of Truvada every 48 hours is recommended, based on modelling of single-dose pharmacokinetic data for emtricitabine and tenofovir disoproxil fumarate in non-HIV infected subjects with varying degrees of renal impairment (see section 4.4).*Severe renal impairment (creatinine clearance < 30 ml/min) and haemodialysis patients:* Truvada is not recommended for patients with severe renal impairment (creatinine clearance < 30 ml/min) and in patients who require haemodialysis because appropriate dose reductions cannot be achieved with the combination tablet.

Hepatic impairment: The pharmacokinetics of Truvada and emtricitabine have not been studied in patients with hepatic impairment. The pharmacokinetics of tenofovir have been studied in patients with hepatic impairment and no dose adjustment is required for tenofovir disoproxil fumarate in these patients. Based on minimal hepatic metabolism and the renal route of elimination for emtricitabine, it is unlikely that a dose adjustment would be required for Truvada in patients with hepatic impairment (see sections 4.4 and 5.2).

If Truvada is discontinued in patients co-infected with HIV and HBV, these patients should be closely monitored for evidence of exacerbation of hepatitis (see section 4.4).

Method of administration

If patients have difficulty in swallowing, Truvada can be disintegrated in approximately 100 ml of water, orange juice or grape juice and taken immediately.

4.3 Contraindications

Hypersensitivity to the active substances emtricitabine, tenofovir, tenofovir disoproxil fumarate or to any of the excipients.

4.4 Special warnings and precautions for use

Truvada should not be administered concomitantly with other medicinal products containing emtricitabine, tenofovir disoproxil (as fumarate) or other cytidine analogues, such as lamivudine and zalcitabine (see section 4.5).

Triple nucleoside therapy: There have been reports of a high rate of virological failure and of emergence of resistance at an early stage when tenofovir disoproxil fumarate was combined with lamivudine and abacavir as well as with lamivudine and didanosine as a once daily regimen. There is close structural similarity between lamivudine and emtricitabine and similarities in the pharmacokinetics and pharmacodynamics of these two agents. Therefore, the same problems may be seen if Truvada is administered with a third nucleoside analogue.

Patients receiving Truvada or any other antiretroviral therapy may continue to develop opportunistic infections and other complications of HIV infection, and therefore should remain under close clinical observation by physicians experienced in the treatment of patients with HIV associated diseases.

Patients must be advised that antiretroviral therapies, including Truvada, have not been proven to prevent the risk of transmission of HIV to others through sexual contact or contamination with blood. Appropriate precautions must continue to be used.

Renal impairment: Emtricitabine and tenofovir are primarily excreted by the kidneys by a combination of glomerular filtration and active tubular secretion. Renal failure, renal impairment, elevated creatinine, hypophosphataemia and proximal tubulopathy (including Fanconi syndrome) have been reported with the use of tenofovir disoproxil fumarate in clinical practice (see section 4.8).

It is recommended that creatinine clearance is calculated in all patients prior to initiating therapy with Truvada and renal function (creatinine clearance and serum phosphate) is also monitored every four weeks during the first year and then every three months. In patients at risk for renal impairment, including patients who have previously experienced renal events while receiving adefovir dipivoxil, consideration should be given to more frequent monitoring of renal function.

Patients with renal impairment (creatinine clearance < 80 ml/min), including haemodialysis patients: Renal safety with Truvada has only been studied to a very limited degree in patients with impaired renal function (creatinine clearance < 80 ml/min). Dose interval adjustments are recommended for patients with creatinine clearance 30-49 ml/min (see section 4.2). Limited clinical study data suggest that the prolonged dose interval is not optimal and could result in increased toxicity and possibly inadequate response. Furthermore, in a small clinical study, a subgroup of patients with creatinine clearance between 50 and 60 ml/min who received tenofovir disoproxil fumarate in combination with emtricitabine every 24 hours had a 2-4-fold higher exposure to tenofovir and worsening of renal function (see section 5.2). Therefore, a careful benefit-risk assessment is needed when Truvada is used in patients with creatinine clearance < 60 ml/min, and renal function should be closely monitored. In addition, the clinical response to treatment should be closely monitored in patients receiving Truvada at a prolonged dosing interval. The use of Truvada is not recommended in patients with severe renal impairment (creatinine clearance < 30 ml/min) and in patients who require haemodialysis since appropriate dose reductions cannot be achieved with the combination tablet (see sections 4.2 and 5.2).

If serum phosphate is < 1.5 mg/dl (0.48 mmol/l) or creatinine clearance is decreased to < 50 ml/min in any patient receiving Truvada, renal function should be re-evaluated within one week, including measurements of blood glucose, blood potassium and urine glucose concentrations (see section 4.8, proximal tubulopathy). Consideration should also be given to interrupting treatment with Truvada in patients with creatinine clearance decreased to < 50 ml/min or decreases in serum phosphate to < 1.0 mg/dl (0.32 mmol/l).

Use of Truvada should be avoided with concurrent or recent use of a nephrotoxic medicinal product (see section 4.5).

Truvada should be avoided in antiretroviral-experienced patients with HIV-1 harbouring the K65R mutation (see section 5.1).

Bone effects: In a 144-week controlled clinical study that compared tenofovir disoproxil fumarate with stavudine in combination with lamivudine and efavirenz in antiretroviral-naïve patients, small decreases in bone mineral density of the hip and spine were observed in both treatment groups. Decreases in bone mineral density of spine and changes in bone biomarkers from baseline were significantly greater in the tenofovir disoproxil fumarate treatment group at 144 weeks. Decreases in bone mineral density of hip were significantly greater in this group until 96 weeks. However, there was no increased risk of fractures or evidence for clinically relevant bone abnormalities over 144 weeks.

Bone abnormalities (infrequently contributing to fractures) may be associated with proximal renal tubulopathy (see section 4.8). If bone abnormalities are suspected then appropriate consultation should be obtained.

Patients with HIV and hepatitis B or C virus co-infection: Patients with chronic hepatitis B or C treated with antiretroviral therapy are at an increased risk for severe and potentially fatal hepatic adverse reactions.

Physicians should refer to current HIV treatment guidelines for the optimal management of HIV infection in patients co-infected with hepatitis B virus (HBV).

In case of concomitant antiviral therapy for hepatitis B or C, please refer also to the relevant Summary of Product Characteristics for these medicinal products.

The safety and efficacy of Truvada have not been established for the treatment of chronic HBV infection. Emtricitabine and tenofovir individually and in combination have shown activity against HBV in pharmacodynamic studies (see section 5.1). Limited clinical experience suggests that emtricitabine and tenofovir disoproxil fumarate have anti-HBV activity when used in antiretroviral combination therapy to control HIV infection.

Discontinuation of Truvada therapy in patients co-infected with HIV and HBV may be associated with severe acute exacerbations of hepatitis. Patients co-infected with HIV and HBV who discontinue Truvada should be closely monitored with both clinical and laboratory follow-up for at least several months after stopping treatment. If appropriate, resumption of hepatitis B therapy may be warranted. In patients with advanced liver disease or cirrhosis, treatment discontinuation is not recommended since post-treatment exacerbation of hepatitis may lead to hepatic decompensation.

Liver disease: The safety and efficacy of Truvada have not been established in patients with significant underlying liver disorders. The pharmacokinetics of Truvada and emtricitabine have not been studied in patients with hepatic impairment. The pharmacokinetics of tenofovir have been studied in patients with hepatic impairment and no dose adjustment is required in these patients. Based on minimal hepatic metabolism and the renal route of elimination for emtricitabine, it is unlikely that a dose adjustment would be required for Truvada in patients with hepatic impairment (see section 5.2).

Patients with pre-existing liver dysfunction, including chronic active hepatitis, have an increased frequency of liver function abnormalities during combination antiretroviral therapy and should be monitored according to standard practice. If there is evidence of worsening liver disease in such patients, interruption or discontinuation of treatment must be considered.

Lactic acidosis: Lactic acidosis, usually associated with hepatic steatosis, has been reported with the use of nucleoside analogues. Early symptoms (symptomatic hyperlactataemia) include benign digestive symptoms (nausea, vomiting and abdominal pain), non-specific malaise, loss of appetite, weight loss, respiratory symptoms (rapid and/or deep breathing) or neurological symptoms (including motor weakness). Lactic acidosis has a high mortality and may be associated with pancreatitis, liver failure or renal failure. Lactic acidosis generally occurred after a few or several months of treatment.

Treatment with nucleoside analogues should be discontinued in the setting of symptomatic hyperlactataemia and metabolic/lactic acidosis, progressive hepatomegaly, or rapidly elevating aminotransferase levels.

Caution should be exercised when administering nucleoside analogues to any patient (particularly obese women) with hepatomegaly, hepatitis or other known risk factors for liver disease and hepatic steatosis (including certain medicinal products and alcohol). Patients co-infected with hepatitis C and treated with alpha interferon and ribavirin may constitute a special risk.

Patients at increased risk should be followed closely.

Lipodystrophy: Combination antiretroviral therapy has been associated with the redistribution of body fat (lipodystrophy) in HIV patients. The long-term consequences of these events are currently unknown. Knowledge about the mechanism is incomplete. A connection between visceral lipomatosis and protease inhibitors and lipoatrophy and nucleoside reverse transcriptase inhibitors has been hypothesised. A higher risk of lipodystrophy has been associated with individual factors such as older age, and with drug related factors such as longer duration of antiretroviral treatment and associated metabolic disturbances. Clinical examination should include evaluation for physical signs of fat redistribution. Consideration should be given to the measurement of fasting serum lipids and blood glucose. Lipid disorders should be managed as clinically appropriate (see section 4.8).

Tenofovir is structurally related to nucleoside analogues hence the risk of lipodystrophy cannot be excluded. However, 144-week clinical data from antiretroviral-naïve patients indicate that the risk of lipodystrophy was lower with tenofovir disoproxil fumarate than with stavudine when administered with lamivudine and efavirenz.

Mitochondrial dysfunction: Nucleoside and nucleotide analogues have been demonstrated *in vitro* and *in vivo* to cause a variable degree of mitochondrial damage. There have been reports of mitochondrial dysfunction in HIV negative infants exposed *in utero* and/or postnatally to nucleoside analogues. The main adverse events reported are haematological disorders (anaemia, neutropenia), metabolic disorders (hyperlactataemia, hyperlipasaemia). These events are often transitory. Some late-onset neurological disorders have been reported (hypertonia, convulsion, abnormal behaviour). Whether the neurological disorders are transient or permanent is currently unknown. Any child exposed *in utero* to nucleoside and nucleotide analogues, even HIV negative children, should have clinical and laboratory follow-up and should be fully investigated for possible mitochondrial dysfunction in case of relevant signs or symptoms. These findings do not affect current national recommendations to use antiretroviral therapy in pregnant women to prevent vertical transmission of HIV.

Immune Reactivation Syndrome: In HIV infected patients with severe immune deficiency at the time of institution of combination antiretroviral therapy (CART), an inflammatory reaction to asymptomatic or residual opportunistic pathogens may arise and cause serious clinical conditions, or aggravation of symptoms. Typically, such reactions have been observed within the first few weeks or months of initiation of CART. Relevant examples are cytomegalovirus retinitis, generalised and/or focal mycobacterial infections, and *Pneumocystis jiroveci* pneumonia. Any inflammatory symptoms should be evaluated and treatment instituted when necessary.

Osteonecrosis: Although the etiology is considered to be multifactorial (including corticosteroid use, alcohol consumption, severe immunosuppression, higher body mass index), cases of osteonecrosis have been reported particularly in patients with advanced HIV-disease and/or long-term exposure to combination antiretroviral therapy (CART). Patients should be advised to seek medical advice if they experience joint aches and pain, joint stiffness or difficulty in movement.

Co-administration of tenofovir disoproxil fumarate and didanosine: is not recommended. Co-administration of tenofovir disoproxil fumarate and didanosine results in a 40-60% increase in systemic exposure to didanosine that may increase the risk of didanosine-related adverse events (see section 4.5). Rare cases of pancreatitis and lactic acidosis, sometimes fatal, have been reported. Co-administration of tenofovir disoproxil fumarate and didanosine at a dose of 400 mg daily has been associated with a significant decrease in CD4 cell count, possibly due to an intracellular interaction increasing phosphorylated (i.e. active) didanosine. A decreased dosage of 250 mg didanosine co-administered with tenofovir disoproxil fumarate therapy has been associated with reports of high rates of virological failure within several tested combinations.

Truvada contains lactose monohydrate. Consequently, patients with rare hereditary problems of galactose intolerance, the Lapp lactase deficiency, or glucose-galactose malabsorption should not take this medicine.

4.5 Interaction with other medicinal products and other forms of interaction

Interaction studies have only been performed in adults.

The steady-state pharmacokinetics of emtricitabine and tenofovir were unaffected when emtricitabine and tenofovir disoproxil fumarate were administered together *versus* each medicinal product dosed alone.

In vitro and clinical pharmacokinetic interaction studies have shown the potential for CYP450 mediated interactions involving emtricitabine and tenofovir disoproxil fumarate with other medicinal products is low.

Interactions relevant to emtricitabine:

In vitro, emtricitabine did not inhibit metabolism mediated by any of the following human CYP450 isoforms: 1A2, 2A6, 2B6, 2C9, 2C19, 2D6 and 3A4. Emtricitabine did not inhibit the enzyme responsible for glucuronidation.

There are no clinically significant interactions when emtricitabine is co-administered with indinavir, zidovudine, stavudine or famciclovir.

Emtricitabine is primarily excreted via glomerular filtration and active tubular secretion. With the exception of famciclovir and tenofovir disoproxil fumarate, the effect of co-administration of emtricitabine with medicinal products that are excreted by the renal route, or other medicinal products known to affect renal function, has not been evaluated. Co-administration of Truvada with medicinal products that are eliminated by active tubular secretion may lead to an increase in serum concentrations of either emtricitabine or a co-administered medicinal product due to competition for this elimination pathway.

There is no clinical experience with the co-administration of emtricitabine and cytidine analogues. Consequently, Truvada should not be administered in combination with lamivudine or zalcitabine for the treatment of HIV infection (see section 4.4).

Interactions relevant to tenofovir:

Co-administration of lamivudine, indinavir, efavirenz, nelfinavir or saquinavir (ritonavir boosted) with tenofovir disoproxil fumarate did not result in any clinically relevant interaction.

When tenofovir disoproxil fumarate was administered with lopinavir/ritonavir, no changes were observed in the pharmacokinetics of lopinavir and ritonavir. Tenofovir AUC was increased by approximately 30% when tenofovir disoproxil fumarate was administered with lopinavir/ritonavir. Higher tenofovir concentrations could potentiate tenofovir associated adverse events, including renal disorders.

When didanosine gastro-resistant capsules were administered 2 hours prior to or concurrently with tenofovir disoproxil fumarate, the AUC for didanosine was on average increased by 48% and 60% respectively. The mean increase in the AUC of didanosine was 44% when the buffered tablets were administered 1 hour prior to tenofovir. In both cases the pharmacokinetic parameters for tenofovir administered with a light meal were unchanged. The co-administration of tenofovir disoproxil fumarate and didanosine is not recommended (see section 4.4).

When tenofovir disoproxil fumarate was administered with atazanavir, a decrease in concentrations of atazanavir was observed (decrease of 25% and 40% of AUC and C_{min} respectively compared to atazanavir 400 mg). When ritonavir was added to atazanavir, the negative impact of tenofovir on atazanavir C_{min} was significantly reduced, whereas the decrease of AUC was of the same magnitude (decrease of 25% and 26% of AUC and C_{min} respectively compared to atazanavir/ritonavir 300/100 mg). The co-administration of atazanavir/ritonavir with tenofovir resulted in increased exposure to tenofovir. Higher tenofovir concentrations could potentiate tenofovir associated adverse events, including renal disorders.

Tenofovir is excreted renally, both by filtration and active secretion via the human organic anion transporter 1 (hOAT1). Co-administration of tenofovir disoproxil fumarate with other medicinal products that are also actively secreted via the anion transporter (e.g. cidofovir) may result in increased concentrations of tenofovir or of the co-administered medicinal product.

Tenofovir disoproxil fumarate has not been evaluated in patients receiving nephrotoxic medicinal products (e.g. aminoglycosides, amphotericin B, foscarnet, ganciclovir, pentamidine, vancomycin, cidofovir or interleukin-2). Use of tenofovir disoproxil fumarate should be avoided with concurrent or recent use of a nephrotoxic medicinal product. If concomitant use of Truvada and nephrotoxic agents is unavoidable, renal function should be monitored weekly (see section 4.4).

Co-administration of tenofovir disoproxil fumarate and methadone, ribavirin, rifampicin, adefovir dipivoxil or the hormonal contraceptive norgestimate/ethinyl oestradiol did not result in any pharmacokinetic interaction.

Interactions relevant to Truvada:

Co-administration of tacrolimus with the combination product emtricitabine/tenofovir disoproxil fumarate did not result in any clinically significant interactions.

4.6 Pregnancy and lactation

Pregnancy:

For emtricitabine and tenofovir disoproxil fumarate, insufficient data on exposed pregnancies are available.

Animal studies do not indicate direct or indirect harmful effects of emtricitabine or tenofovir disoproxil fumarate with respect to pregnancy, embryonal/foetal development, parturition or postnatal development (see section 5.3). However, Truvada should not be used during pregnancy unless no other alternative is available.

The use of Truvada must be accompanied by the use of effective contraception.

Lactation:

It is not known whether emtricitabine or tenofovir are excreted in human milk.

It is recommended that HIV infected women do not breast-feed their infants under any circumstances in order to avoid transmission of HIV to the infant.

4.7 Effects on ability to drive and use machines

No studies on the effects on the ability to drive and use machines have been performed. However, patients should be informed that dizziness has been reported during treatment with both emtricitabine and tenofovir disoproxil fumarate.

4.8 Undesirable effects

In an open-label randomised clinical study in antiretroviral-naïve patients (GS-01-934; see section 5.1), patients received emtricitabine, tenofovir disoproxil fumarate and efavirenz for 144 weeks (administered as the combination formulation Truvada, plus efavirenz from week 96). The safety profile of emtricitabine and tenofovir disoproxil fumarate was consistent with the previous experience with these agents when each was administered with other antiretroviral agents. The most frequently reported adverse reactions considered possibly or probably related to emtricitabine and/or tenofovir disoproxil fumarate were nausea (12%) and diarrhoea (7%).

The adverse reactions considered at least possibly related to treatment with the components of Truvada from clinical trial and post-marketing experience are listed below by body system organ class and absolute frequency. Within each frequency grouping, undesirable effects are presented in order of decreasing seriousness. Frequencies are defined as very common (≥ 1/10), common (≥ 1/100, < 1/10), uncommon (≥ 1/1,000, < 1/100), rare (≥ 1/10,000, < 1/1,000) or very rare (< 1/10,000) including isolated reports, or not known (identified through post-marketing safety surveillance and the frequency cannot be estimated from the available data).

Blood and lymphatic system disorders:

Common: neutropenia

Uncommon: anaemia

Immune system disorders:

Common: allergic reaction

Metabolism and nutrition disorders:

Very common: hypophosphataemia

Common: hyperglycaemia, hypertriglyceridaemia

Rare: lactic acidosis

Not known: hypokalaemia

Lactic acidosis, usually associated with hepatic steatosis, has been reported with the use of nucleoside analogues (see section 4.4).

Psychiatric disorders:

Common: insomnia, abnormal dreams

Nervous system disorders:

Very common: headache, dizziness

Respiratory, thoracic and mediastinal disorders:

Very rare: dyspnoea

Gastrointestinal disorders:

Very common: diarrhoea, vomiting, nausea

Common: elevated serum lipase, elevated amylase including elevated pancreatic amylase, abdominal pain, dyspepsia, flatulence

Rare: pancreatitis

Hepatobiliary disorders:

Common: increased transaminases, hyperbilirubinaemia

Very rare: hepatitis

Not known: hepatic steatosis

Skin and subcutaneous tissue disorders:

Common: urticaria, vesiculobullous rash, pustular rash, maculopapular rash, pruritus, rash and skin discolouration (increased pigmentation)

Musculoskeletal and connective tissue disorders:

Very common: elevated creatine kinase

Not known: rhabdomyolysis, osteomalacia (manifested as bone pain and infrequently contributing to fractures), muscular weakness, myopathy

Renal and urinary disorders:

Rare: renal failure (acute and chronic), proximal renal tubulopathy including Fanconi syndrome, increased creatinine, proteinuria

Very rare: acute tubular necrosis

Not known: nephritis (including acute interstitial nephritis), nephrogenic diabetes insipidus.

General disorders and administration site conditions:

Common: pain, asthenia

The following adverse reactions, listed under the body system headings above, may occur as a consequence of proximal renal tubulopathy: rhabdomyolysis, osteomalacia (manifested as bone pain and infrequently contributing to fractures), hypokalaemia, muscular weakness, myopathy and hypophosphataemia. These events are not considered to be causally associated with tenofovir disoproxil fumarate therapy in the absence of proximal renal tubulopathy.

In addition anaemia was common and skin discolouration (increased pigmentation) was very common when emtricitabine was administered to paediatric patients.

HIV/HBV or HCV co-infected patients: Only a limited number of patients were co-infected with HBV (n=13) or HCV (n=26) in study GS-01-934. The adverse reaction profile of emtricitabine and tenofovir disoproxil fumarate in patients co-infected with HIV/HBV or HIV/HCV was similar to that observed in patients infected with HIV without co-infection. However, as would be expected in this patient population, elevations in AST and ALT occurred more frequently than in the general HIV infected population.

Combination antiretroviral therapy has been associated with metabolic abnormalities such as hypertriglyceridaemia, hypercholesterolaemia, insulin resistance, hyperglycaemia and hyperlactataemia (see section 4.4).

Combination antiretroviral therapy has been associated with redistribution of body fat (lipodystrophy) in HIV patients including the loss of peripheral and facial subcutaneous fat, increased intra-abdominal and visceral fat, breast hypertrophy and dorsocervical fat accumulation (buffalo hump) (see section 4.4).

In HIV infected patients with severe immune deficiency at the time of initiation of combination antiretroviral therapy (CART), an inflammatory reaction to asymptomatic or residual opportunistic infections may arise (see section 4.4).

Cases of osteonecrosis have been reported, particularly in patients with generally acknowledged risk factors, advanced HIV disease or long-term exposure to combination antiretroviral therapy (CART). The frequency of this is unknown (see section 4.4).

4.9 Overdose

If overdose occurs the patient must be monitored for evidence of toxicity (see section 4.8), and standard supportive treatment applied as necessary.

Up to 30% of the emtricitabine dose and approximately 10% of the tenofovir dose can be removed by haemodialysis. It is not known whether emtricitabine or tenofovir can be removed by peritoneal dialysis.

5. PHARMACOLOGICAL PROPERTIES

5.1 Pharmacodynamic properties

Pharmacotherapeutic group: Nucleoside and nucleotide reverse transcriptase inhibitors, ATC code: J05AR03

Mechanism of action and pharmacodynamic effects: Emtricitabine is a nucleoside analogue of cytidine. Tenofovir disoproxil fumarate is converted *in vivo* to tenofovir, a nucleoside monophosphate (nucleotide) analogue of adenosine monophosphate. Both emtricitabine and tenofovir have activity that is specific to human immunodeficiency virus (HIV-1 and HIV-2) and hepatitis B virus.

Emtricitabine and tenofovir are phosphorylated by cellular enzymes to form emtricitabine triphosphate and tenofovir diphosphate, respectively. *In vitro* studies have shown that both emtricitabine and tenofovir can be fully phosphorylated when combined together in cells. Emtricitabine triphosphate and tenofovir diphosphate competitively inhibit HIV-1 reverse transcriptase, resulting in DNA chain termination.

Both emtricitabine triphosphate and tenofovir diphosphate are weak inhibitors of mammalian DNA polymerases and there was no evidence of toxicity to mitochondria *in vitro* and *in vivo*.

Antiviral activity in vitro: Synergistic antiviral activity was observed with the combination of emtricitabine and tenofovir *in vitro*. Additive to synergistic effects were observed in combination studies with protease inhibitors, and with nucleoside and non-nucleoside analogue inhibitors of HIV reverse transcriptase.

Resistance: Resistance has been seen *in vitro* and in some HIV-1 infected patients due to the development of the M184V/I mutation with emtricitabine or the K65R mutation with tenofovir. No other pathways of resistance to emtricitabine or tenofovir have been identified. Emtricitabine-resistant viruses with the M184V/I mutation were cross-resistant to lamivudine, but retained sensitivity to didanosine, stavudine, tenofovir, zalcitabine and zidovudine. The K65R mutation can also be selected by abacavir, didanosine or zalcitabine and results in reduced susceptibility to these agents plus lamivudine, emtricitabine and tenofovir. Tenofovir disoproxil fumarate should be avoided in patients with HIV-1 harbouring the K65R mutation.

Patients with HIV-1 expressing three or more thymidine analogue associated mutations (TAMs) that included either the M41L or L210W reverse transcriptase mutation showed reduced susceptibility to tenofovir disoproxil fumarate.

In vivo resistance (antiretroviral-naïve patients): In an open-label randomised clinical study (GS-01-934) in antiretroviral-naïve patients, genotyping was performed on plasma HIV-1 isolates from all patients with confirmed HIV RNA> 400 copies/ml at weeks 48, 96 or 144 or at the time of early study drug discontinuation. As of week 144:

- The M184V/I mutation developed in 2/19 (10.5%) isolates analysed from patients in the emtricitabine/tenofovir disoproxil fumarate/efavirenz group and in 10/29 (34.5%) isolates analysed from the lamivudine/zidovudine/efavirenz group (p-value < 0.05, Fisher's Exact test comparing the emtricitabine+tenofovir disoproxil fumarate group to the lamivudine/zidovudine group among all subjects).
- No virus analysed contained the K65R mutation.
- Genotypic resistance to efavirenz, predominantly the K103N mutation, developed in virus from 13/19 (68%) patients in the emtricitabine/tenofovir disoproxil fumarate/efavirenz group and in virus from 21/29 (72%) patients in the comparative group.

Clinical experience: In an open-label randomised clinical study (GS-01-934), antiretroviral-naïve HIV-1 infected patients received either a once daily regimen of emtricitabine, tenofovir disoproxil fumarate and efavirenz (n=255) or a fixed combination of lamivudine and zidovudine (Combivir) administered twice daily and efavirenz once daily (n=254). Patients in the emtricitabine and tenofovir disoproxil fumarate group were given Truvada and efavirenz from week 96 to week 144. At baseline the randomised groups had similar median plasma HIV-1 RNA (5.02 and 5.00 $\log_{10}$ copies/ml) and CD4 counts (233 and 241 cells/mm^3). The primary efficacy endpoint for this study was the achievement and maintenance of confirmed HIV-1 RNA concentrations < 400 copies/ml over 48 weeks. Secondary efficacy analyses over 144 weeks included the proportion of patients with HIV-1 RNA concentrations < 400 or < 50 copies/ml, and change from baseline in CD4 cell count.

The 48-week primary endpoint data showed that the combination of emtricitabine, tenofovir disoproxil fumarate and efavirenz provided superior antiviral efficacy as compared with the fixed combination of lamivudine and zidovudine (Combivir) with efavirenz as shown in Table 1. The 144 week secondary endpoint data are also presented in Table 1.

Table 1: 48- and 144-week efficacy data from study GS-01-934 in which emtricitabine, tenofovir disoproxil fumarate and efavirenz were administered to antiretroviral-naïve patients with HIV-1 infection

(see Table 1 below)

In a separate randomised clinical study (M02-418), one hundred and ninety antiretroviral-naïve adults were also treated once daily with emtricitabine and tenofovir disoproxil fumarate in combination with lopinavir/ritonavir given once or twice daily. At 48 weeks, 70% and 64% of patients demonstrated HIV-1 RNA < 50 copies/ml with the once and twice daily regimens of lopinavir/ritonavir, respectively. The mean changes in CD4 cell count from baseline were +185 cells/mm^3 and +196 cells/mm^3 with the once and twice daily regimens of lopinavir/ritonavir, respectively.

Limited clinical experience in patients co-infected with HIV and HBV suggests that treatment with emtricitabine or tenofovir disoproxil fumarate in antiretroviral combination therapy to control HIV infection also results in a reduction in HBV DNA (3 $\log_{10}$ reduction or 4 to 5 $\log_{10}$ reduction, respectively) (see section 4.4).

5.2 Pharmacokinetic properties

Absorption: The bioequivalence of one Truvada film-coated tablet with one emtricitabine 200 mg hard capsule and one tenofovir disoproxil fumarate 245 mg film-coated tablet was established following single dose administration to fasting healthy subjects. Following oral administration of Truvada to healthy subjects, emtricitabine and tenofovir disoproxil fumarate are rapidly absorbed and tenofovir disoproxil fumarate is converted to tenofovir. Maximum emtricitabine and tenofovir concentrations are observed in serum within 0.5 to 3.0 h of dosing in the fasted state. Administration of Truvada with food resulted in a delay of approximately three quarters of an hour in reaching maximum tenofovir concentrations and increases in tenofovir AUC and C_{max} of approximately 35% and 15%, respectively, when administered with a high fat or light meal, compared to administration in the fasted state. In order to optimise the absorption of tenofovir, it is recommended that Truvada should be taken with food.

Distribution: Following intravenous administration the volume of distribution of emtricitabine and tenofovir was approximately 1.4 l/kg and 800 ml/kg, respectively. After oral administration of emtricitabine or tenofovir disoproxil fumarate, emtricitabine and tenofovir are widely distributed throughout the body. *In vitro* binding of emtricitabine to human plasma proteins was < 4% and independent of concentration over the range of 0.02 to 200 μg/ml. *In vitro* protein binding of tenofovir to plasma or serum protein was less than 0.7 and 7.2%, respectively, over the tenofovir concentration range 0.01 to 25 μg/ml.

Biotransformation: There is limited metabolism of emtricitabine. The biotransformation of emtricitabine includes oxidation of the thiol moiety to form the 3'-sulphoxide diastereomers (approximately 9% of dose) and conjugation with glucuronic acid to form 2'-O-glucuronide (approximately 4% of dose). *In vitro* studies have determined that neither tenofovir disoproxil fumarate nor tenofovir are substrates for the CYP450 enzymes. Neither emtricitabine nor tenofovir inhibited *in vitro* drug metabolism mediated by any of the major human CYP450 isoforms involved in drug biotransformation. Also, emtricitabine did not inhibit uridine-5'-diphosphoglucuronyl transferase, the enzyme responsible for glucuronidation.

Elimination: Emtricitabine is primarily excreted by the kidneys with complete recovery of the dose achieved in urine (approximately 86%) and faeces (approximately 14%). Thirteen percent of the emtricitabine dose was recovered in urine as three metabolites. The systemic clearance of emtricitabine averaged 307 ml/min. Following oral administration, the elimination half-life of emtricitabine is approximately 10 hours.

Tenofovir is primarily excreted by the kidney by both filtration and an active tubular transport system with approximately 70-80% of the dose excreted unchanged in urine following intravenous administration. The apparent clearance of tenofovir averaged approximately 307 ml/min. Renal clearance has been estimated to be approximately 210 ml/min, which is in excess of the glomerular filtration rate. This indicates that active tubular secretion is an important part of the elimination of tenofovir. Following oral administration, the elimination half-life of tenofovir is approximately 12 to 18 hours.

Age, gender and ethnicity: Emtricitabine and tenofovir pharmacokinetics are similar in male and female patients. In general, the pharmacokinetics of emtricitabine in infants, children and adolescents (aged 4 months up to 18 years) are similar to those seen in adults. Pharmacokinetic studies have not been performed with tenofovir in children and adolescents (under 18 years). Pharmacokinetic studies have not been performed with emtricitabine or tenofovir in the elderly (over 65 years).

Renal impairment: Limited pharmacokinetic data are available for emtricitabine and tenofovir after co-administration of separate preparations or as Truvada in patients with renal impairment. Pharmacokinetic parameters were mainly determined following administration of single doses of emtricitabine 200 mg or tenofovir disoproxil 245 mg to non-HIV infected patients with varying degrees of renal impairment. The degree of renal impairment was defined according to baseline creatinine clearance (CrCl) (normal renal function when CrCl> 80 ml/min; mild impairment with CrCl = 50-79 ml/min; moderate impairment with CrCl = 30-49 ml/min and severe impairment with CrCl = 10-29 ml/min).

The mean (%CV) emtricitabine drug exposure increased from 12 (25%) μg•h/ml in subjects with normal renal function, to 20 (6%) μg•h/ml, 25 (23%) μg•h/ml and 34 (6%) μg•h/ml, in patients with mild, moderate and severe renal impairment, respectively.

The mean (%CV) tenofovir drug exposure increased from 2,185 (12%) ng•h/ml in patients with normal renal function, to 3,064 (30%) ng•h/ml, 6,009 (42%) ng•h/ml and 15,985 (45%) ng•h/ml, in patients with mild, moderate and severe renal impairment, respectively.

The increased dose interval for Truvada in patients with moderate renal impairment is expected to result in higher peak plasma concentrations and lower C_{min} levels as compared to patients with normal renal function. The clinical implications of this are unknown.

In patients with end-stage renal disease (ESRD) requiring haemodialysis, between dialysis drug exposures substantially increased over 72 hours to 53 (19%) μg•h/ml of emtricitabine, and over 48 hours to 42,857 (29%) ng•h/ml of tenofovir.

It is recommended that the dosing interval for Truvada is modified in patients with creatinine clearance between 30 and 49 ml/min. Truvada is not suitable for patients with CrCl < 30 ml/min or for those on haemodialysis (see section 4.2).

A small clinical study was conducted to evaluate the safety, antiviral activity and pharmacokinetics of tenofovir disoproxil fumarate in combination with emtricitabine in HIV infected patients with renal impairment. A subgroup of patients with baseline creatinine clearance between 50 and 60 ml/min, receiving once daily dosing, had a 2-4-fold increase in tenofovir exposure and worsening renal function.

Hepatic impairment: The pharmacokinetics of Truvada have not been studied in patients with hepatic impairment. However, it is unlikely that a dose adjustment would be required for Truvada in patients with hepatic impairment.

The pharmacokinetics of emtricitabine have not been studied in non-HBV infected subjects with varying degrees of hepatic insufficiency. In general, emtricitabine pharmacokinetics in HBV infected subjects were similar to those in healthy subjects and in HIV infected subjects.

A single 245 mg dose of tenofovir disoproxil was administered to non-HIV infected patients with varying degrees of hepatic impairment defined according to Child-Pugh-Turcotte (CPT) classification. Tenofovir pharmacokinetics were not substantially altered in subjects with hepatic impairment suggesting that no dose adjustment is required in these subjects. The mean (%CV) tenofovir C_{max} and $AUC_{0-\infty}$ values were 223 (34.8%) ng/ml and 2,050 (50.8%) ng•h/ml, respectively, in normal subjects compared with 289 (46.0%) ng/ml and 2,310 (43.5%) ng•h/ml in subjects with moderate hepatic impairment, and 305 (24.8%) ng/ml and 2,740 (44.0%) ng•h/ml in subjects with severe hepatic impairment.

5.3 Preclinical safety data

Non-clinical data on emtricitabine reveal no special hazard for humans based on conventional studies of safety pharmacology, repeated dose toxicity and genotoxicity.

Table 1 48- and 144-week efficacy data from study GS-01-934 in which emtricitabine, tenofovir disoproxil fumarate and efavirenz were administered to antiretroviral-naïve patients with HIV-1 infection

	GS-01-934 Treatment for 48 weeks		GS-01-934 Treatment for 144 weeks	
	Emtricitabine+ tenofovir disoproxil fumarate+efavirenz	Lamivudine+ zidovudine+ efavirenz	Emtricitabine+ tenofovir disoproxil fumarate+efavirenz*	Lamivudine+ zidovudine+ efavirenz
HIV-1 RNA < 400 copies/ml (TLOVR)	84% (206/244)	73% (177/243)	71% (161/227)	58% (133/229)
p-value	0.002**		0.004**	
% difference (95%CI)	11% (4% to 19%)		13% (4% to 22%)	
HIV-1 RNA < 50 copies/ml (TLOVR)	80% (194/244)	70% (171/243)	64% (146/227)	56% (130/231)
p-value	0.021**		0.082**	
% difference (95%CI)	9% (2% to 17%)		8% (-1% to 17%)	
Mean change from baseline in CD4 cell count (cells/mm^3)	+190	+158	+312	+271
p-value	0.002[a]		0.089[a]	
Difference (95%CI)	32 (9 to 55)		41 (4 to 79)	

* Patients receiving emtricitabine, tenofovir disoproxil fumarate and efavirenz were given Truvada plus efavirenz from week 96 to 144.

** The p-value based on the Cochran-Mantel-Haenszel Test stratified for baseline CD4 cell count

TLOVR=Time to Loss of Virologic Response

a: Van Elteren Test

Emtricitabine did not show any carcinogenic potential in long-term oral carcinogenicity studies in mice and rats.

Preclinical studies of tenofovir disoproxil fumarate conducted in rats, dogs and monkeys revealed target organ effects in gastrointestinal tract, kidney, bone and a decrease in serum phosphate concentration. Bone toxicity was diagnosed as osteomalacia (monkeys) and reduced bone mineral density (rats and dogs). Findings in the rat and monkey studies indicated that there was a substance-related decrease in intestinal absorption of phosphate with potential secondary reduction in bone mineral density. The mechanisms of these toxicities are not completely understood.

Conventional reproductive/developmental toxicity studies with emtricitabine and tenofovir disoproxil fumarate reveal no special hazard for humans.

Tenofovir disoproxil fumarate was positive in two out of three *in vitro* genotoxicity studies but negative in the *in vivo* micronucleus assay.

Tenofovir disoproxil fumarate did not show any carcinogenic potential in a long-term oral carcinogenicity study in rats. A long-term oral carcinogenicity study in mice showed a low incidence of duodenal tumours, considered likely related to high local concentrations in the gastrointestinal tract at a dose of 600 mg/kg/day. While the mechanism of tumour formation is uncertain, the findings are unlikely to be of relevance to humans.

The combination of emtricitabine and tenofovir disoproxil fumarate was positive in the *in vitro* mouse lymphoma assay, with comparable results to those obtained for tenofovir disoproxil fumarate alone. The combination of emtricitabine and tenofovir disoproxil fumarate was negative in the bacterial reverse mutation assay (Ames assay).

A one month dog study using the combination of emtricitabine and tenofovir disoproxil fumarate, found no exacerbation of toxicological effects compared to the separate components.

6. PHARMACEUTICAL PARTICULARS

6.1 List of excipients

Tablet core:

Croscarmellose sodium

Lactose monohydrate

Magnesium stearate (E572)

Microcrystalline cellulose (E460)

Pregelatinised starch (gluten free)

Film-coating:

Glycerol triacetate (E1518)

Hypromellose (E464)

Indigo carmine aluminium lake (E132)

Lactose monohydrate

Titanium dioxide (E171)

6.2 Incompatibilities

Not applicable.

6.3 Shelf life

4 years.

6.4 Special precautions for storage

Store in the original package in order to protect from moisture. Keep the bottle tightly closed.

6.5 Nature and contents of container

HDPE bottle with a child-resistant closure containing 30 film-coated tablets and a silica gel desiccant.

The following pack sizes are available: outer cartons containing 1 × 30 film-coated tablet and 3 × 30 film-coated tablet bottles. Not all pack sizes may be marketed.

6.6 Special precautions for disposal and other handling

Any unused product or waste material should be disposed of in accordance with local requirements.

7. MARKETING AUTHORISATION HOLDER

Gilead Sciences International Limited

Cambridge

CB21 6GT

United Kingdom

8. MARKETING AUTHORISATION NUMBER(S)

EU/1/04/305/001

EU/1/04/305/002

9. DATE OF FIRST AUTHORISATION/RENEWAL OF THE AUTHORISATION

21 February 2005

10. DATE OF REVISION OF THE TEXT

05/2009

Detailed information on this medicinal product is available on the website of the European Medicines Agency (EMEA) http://www.emea.europa.eu/.

Twinrix Adult Vaccine

(GlaxoSmithKline UK)

1. NAME OF THE MEDICINAL PRODUCT

Twinrix Adult, suspension for injection in prefilled syringe

Hepatitis A (inactivated) and hepatitis B(rDNA) (HAB) vaccine (adsorbed).

2. QUALITATIVE AND QUANTITATIVE COMPOSITION

1 dose (1 ml) contains:

Hepatitis A virus (inactivated)[1,2] 720 ELISA Units

Hepatitis B surface antigen[3,4] 20 micrograms

[1]Produced on human diploid (MRC-5) cells

[2]Adsorbed on aluminium hydroxide, hydrated 0.05 milligrams Al^{3+}

[3]Produced in yeast cells (*Saccharomyces cerevisiae*) by recombinant DNA technology

[4]Adsorbed on aluminium phosphate 0.4 milligrams Al^{3+}

For a full list of excipients, see section 6.1.

3. PHARMACEUTICAL FORM

Suspension for injection in prefilled syringe

Turbid white suspension

4. CLINICAL PARTICULARS

4.1 Therapeutic indications

Twinrix Adult is indicated for use in non immune adults and adolescents 16 years of age and above who are at risk of both hepatitis A and hepatitis B infection.

4.2 Posology and method of administration

Posology

- Dosage

A dose of 1.0 ml is recommended for adults and adolescents 16 years of age and above.

- Primary vaccination schedule

The standard primary course of vaccination with Twinrix Adult consists of three doses, the first administered at the elected date, the second one month later and the third six months after the first dose.

In exceptional circumstances in adults, when travel is anticipated within one month or more after initiating the vaccination course, but where insufficient time is available to allow the standard 0, 1, 6 month schedule to be completed, a schedule of three intramuscular injections given at 0, 7 and 21 days may be used. When this schedule is applied, a fourth dose is recommended 12 months after the first dose.

The recommended schedule should be adhered to. Once initiated, the primary course of vaccination should be completed with the same vaccine.

- Booster dose

Long-term antibody persistence data following vaccination with TWINRIX Adult are available up to 60 months after vaccination. The anti-HBs and anti-HAV antibody titres observed following a primary vaccination course with the combined vaccine are in the range of what is seen following vaccination with the monovalent vaccines. The kinetics of antibody decline are also similar. General guidelines for booster vaccination can therefore be drawn from experience with the monovalent vaccines.

Hepatitis B

The need for a booster dose of hepatitis B vaccine in healthy individuals who have received a full primary vaccination course has not been established; however some official vaccination programmes currently include a recommendation for a booster dose of hepatitis B vaccine and these should be respected.

For some categories of subjects or patients exposed to HBV (e.g; haemodialysis or immunocompromised patients) a precautionary attitude should be considered to ensure a protective antibody level ≥ 10IU/l.

Hepatitis A

It is not yet fully established whether immunocompetent individuals who have responded to hepatitis A vaccination will require booster doses as protection in the absence of detectable antibodies may be ensured by immunological memory. Guidelines for boosting are based on the assumption that antibodies are required for protection; anti-HAV antibodies have been predicted to persist for at least 10 years.

In situations where a booster dose of both hepatitis A and hepatitis B are desired, Twinrix Adult can be given. Alternatively, subjects primed with Twinrix Adult may be administered a booster dose of either of the monovalent vaccines.

Method of administration

Twinrix Adult is for intramuscular injection, preferably in the deltoid region.

Exceptionally the vaccine may be administered subcutaneously in patients with thrombocytopenia or bleeding disorders. However, this route of administration may result in suboptimal immune response to the vaccine. (see section 4.4).

4.3 Contraindications

Hypersensitivity to the active substances or to any of the excipients or neomycin.

Hypersensitivity after previous administration of hepatitis A and/or hepatitis B vaccines.

The administration of Twinrix Adult should be postponed in subjects suffering from acute severe febrile illness.

4.4 Special warnings and precautions for use

It is possible that subjects may be in the incubation period of a hepatitis A or hepatitis B infection at the time of vaccination. It is not known whether Twinrix Adult will prevent hepatitis A and hepatitis B in such cases.

The vaccine will not prevent infection caused by other agents such as hepatitis C and hepatitis E and other pathogens known to infect the liver.

Twinrix Adult is not recommended for postexposure prophylaxis (e.g. needle stick injury).

The vaccine has not been tested in patients with impaired immunity. In haemodialysis patients and persons with an impaired immune system, adequate anti-HAV and anti-HBs antibody titers may not be obtained after the primary immunisation course and such patients may therefore require administration of additional doses of vaccine.

Obesity (defined as BMI ≥ 30 kg/m^2) has been observed to reduce the immune response to hepatitis A vaccines. A number of factors have been observed to reduce the immune response to hepatitis B vaccines. These factors include older age, male gender, obesity, smoking, route of administration, and some chronic underlying diseases. Consideration should be given to serological testing of those subjects who may be at risk of not achieving seroprotection following a complete course of Twinrix Adult. Additional doses may need to be considered for persons who do not respond or have a sub-optimal response to a course of vaccinations.

As with all injectable vaccines, appropriate medical treatment and supervision should always be readily available in case of a rare anaphylactic event following the administration of the vaccine.

Since intradermal injection or intramuscular administration into the gluteal muscle could lead to a suboptimal response to the vaccine, these routes should be avoided. However, exceptionally Twinrix Adult can be administered subcutaneously to subjects with thrombocytopenia or bleeding disorders since bleeding may occur following an intramuscular administration to these subjects (see section 4.2.).

TWINRIX ADULT SHOULD UNDER NO CIRCUMSTANCES BE ADMINISTERED INTRAVASCULARLY.

As with any vaccine, a protective immune response may not be elicited in all vaccinees.

As with any injection procedure, vasovagal syncope can infrequently occur following administration of Twinrix Adult to adults and adolescents.

4.5 Interaction with other medicinal products and other forms of interaction

No data on concomitant administration of Twinrix Adult with specific hepatitis A immunoglobulin or hepatitis B immunoglobulin have been generated. However, when the monovalent hepatitis A and hepatitis B vaccines were administered concomitantly with specific immunoglobulins, no influence on seroconversion was observed although it may result in lower antibody titres.

Although the concomitant administration of Twinrix Adult and other vaccines has not specifically been studied, it is anticipated that, if different syringes and other injection sites are used, no interaction will be observed.

It may be expected that in patients receiving immunosuppressive treatment or patients with immunodeficiency, an adequate response may not be achieved.

4.6 Pregnancy and lactation

Pregnancy

The effect of Twinrix Adult on embryo-fetal, peri-natal and post-natal survival and development has been assessed in rats. This study did not indicate direct or indirect harmful effects with respect to fertility, pregnancy, embryonal/fetal development, parturition or post-natal development.

The effect of Twinrix Adult on embryo-fetal, peri-natal and post-natal survival and development has not been prospectively evaluated in clinical trials.

Data on outcomes of a limited number of pregnancies in vaccinated women do not indicate any adverse effects of Twinrix Adult on pregnancy or on the health of the fetus/newborn child. While it is not expected that recombinant hepatitis B virus surface antigen would have adverse effects on pregnancies or the fetus it is recommended that vaccination should be delayed until after delivery unless there is an urgent need to protect the mother against hepatitis B infection.

Lactation

It is unknown whether Twinrix Adult is excreted in human breast milk. The excretion of Twinrix Adult in milk has not been studied in animals. A decision on whether to continue/discontinue breast-feeding or to continue/discontinue therapy with Twinrix Adult should be made taking into account the benefit of breast-feeding to the child and the benefit of Twinrix Adult therapy to the woman.

4.7 Effects on ability to drive and use machines

Twinrix Adult has no or negligible influence on the ability to drive and use machines.

4.8 Undesirable effects

• Clinical trials

The current formulation of Twinrix does not contain thiomersal (an organomercuric compound) or any preservative. In a clinical study conducted with the current formulation, the incidence of pain, redness, swelling, fatigue, gastro-enteritis, headache and fever was comparable to the incidence observed with the former thiomersal and preservative containing vaccine formulation. The following undesirable effects have been reported following the widespread use of the former formulation.

The safety profile presented below is based on a pooled analysis of events per dose from more than 6,000 subjects who received either the standard 0, 1, 6 month schedule (n=5,683) or the accelerated 0, 7, 21 days schedule (n=320). In the two clinical trials in which Twinrix Adult was administered at 0, 7, 21 days, overall solicited general and local symptoms were reported with the same categories of frequency as defined below. After a fourth dose given at month 12, the incidence of systemic and local adverse reactions was comparable to that seen after vaccination at 0, 7, 21 days.

In comparative studies, it was noted that the frequency of solicited adverse events following the administration of Twinrix Adult is not different from the frequency of solicited adverse events following the administration of the monovalent vaccines.

Frequencies are reported as:

Very common: ≥ 1/10

Common: ≥ 1/100 to < 1/10

Uncommon: ≥ 1/1,000 to < 1/100

Rare: ≥ 1/10,000 to < 1/1,000

Very rare: < 1/10,000

* refers to adverse reactions observed in clinical trials performed with the paediatric formulation

Blood and lymphatic system disorders

Rare: lymphadenopathy

Nervous system disorders

Very common: headache

Uncommon: dizziness

Rare: hypoaesthesia, paraesthesia

Gastrointestinal disorders

Common: gastrointestinal symptoms, diarrhoea, nausea

Uncommon: vomiting, abdominal pain*

Skin and subcutaneous tissue disorders

Rare: rash, pruritus

Very rare: urticaria

Musculoskeletal and connective tissue disorders

Uncommon: myalgia

Rare: arthralgia

Metabolism and nutrition disorders

Rare: decreased appetite

Infections and infestations

Uncommon: upper respiratory tract infection

Vascular disorders

Rare: hypotension

General disorders and administration site conditions

Very common: pain and redness at the injection site, fatigue

Common: swelling at the injection site, injection site reactions (such as haematoma, pruritus and bruising), malaise

Uncommon: fever (≥ 37.5°C)

Rare: influenza like illness, chills

• Post-marketing surveillance

The following adverse reactions have been reported with either Twinrix or with GlaxoSmithKline monovalent hepatitis A or B vaccines:

Blood and lymphatic system disorders

Thrombocytopenia, thrombocytopenic purpura

Nervous system disorders

Encephalitis, encephalopathy, neuritis, neuropathy, paralysis, convulsions

Skin and subcutaneous tissue disorders

Angioneurotic oedema, lichen planus, erythema multiforme

Musculoskeletal and connective tissue disorders

Arthritis, muscular weakness

Infections and infestations

Meningitis

Vascular disorders

Vasculitis

Immune system disorders

Anaphylaxis, allergic reactions including anaphylactoid reactions and mimicking serum sickness

Following widespread use of the monovalent hepatitis A and/or hepatitis B vaccines, the following undesirable events have additionally been reported in temporal association with vaccination.

Investigations

Abnormal liver function tests

Nervous system disorders

Multiple sclerosis, myelitis, facial palsy, polyneuritis such as Guillain-Barré syndrome (with ascending paralysis), optic neuritis

4.9 Overdose

Cases of overdose have been reported during post-marketing surveillance. Adverse events reported following overdosage were similar to those reported with normal vaccine administration.

5. PHARMACOLOGICAL PROPERTIES

5.1 Pharmacodynamic properties

Pharmaco-therapeutic group: Hepatitis vaccines, ATC code J07BC20.

Twinrix Adult is a combined vaccine formulated by pooling bulk preparations of the purified, inactivated hepatitis A (HA) virus and purified hepatitis B surface antigen (HBsAg), separately adsorbed onto aluminium hydroxide and aluminium phosphate. The HA virus is propagated in MRC_5 human diploid cells. HBsAg is produced by culture, in a selective medium, of genetically engineered yeast cells.

Twinrix Adult confers immunity against HAV and HBV infection by inducing specific anti-HAV and anti-HBs antibodies.

Protection against hepatitis A and hepatitis B develops within 2-4 weeks. In the clinical studies, specific humoral antibodies against hepatitis A were observed in approximately 94% of the adults one month after the first dose and in 100% one month after the third dose (i.e. month 7). Specific humoral antibodies against hepatitis B were observed in 70% of the adults after the first dose and approximately 99% after the third dose.

The 0, 7 and 21 day primary schedule plus a fourth dose at month 12 is for use in exceptional circumstances in adults. In a clinical trial where Twinrix Adult was administered according to this schedule, 82% and 85% of vaccinees had seroprotective levels of anti-HBV antibodies at 1 and 5 weeks respectively following the third dose (i.e. at months 1 and 2 after the initial dose). The seroprotection rate against hepatitis B increased to 95.1% by three months after the first dose.

Seropositivity rates for anti-HAV antibodies were 100%, 99.5% and 100% at months 1, 2 and 3 after the initial dose. One month after the fourth dose, all vaccinees demonstrated seroprotective levels of anti-HBs antibodies and were seropositive for anti-HAV antibodies.

In a clinical study conducted in subjects over 40 years of age, the seropositivity rate for anti-HAV antibodies and seroprotection rate against hepatitis B of Twinrix Adult following a 0, 1, 6 months schedule were compared with the seropositivity and seroprotection rates of monovalent hepatitis A and B vaccines when administered in opposite arms.

The seroprotection rate against hepatitis B after the administration of Twinrix Adult was 92% and 87.5% at 7 and 12 months respectively, versus 80% and 74% after the GlaxoSmithKline Biologicals monovalent 20μg hepatitis B vaccine, and 71% and 56% after another licensed monovalent 10μg hepatitis B vaccine. However, anti-HBs antibody concentrations decreased as age and body mass index increased; they were also lower in male than in female subjects.

The seropositivity rate for anti-HAV antibodies after Twinrix Adult was 97% and 96% at 7 and 12 months respectively versus 99% and 98% after the GlaxoSmithKline Biologicals monovalent hepatitis A vaccine and 99% at both 7 and 12 months after another licensed monovalent hepatitis A vaccine.

In two long term clinical studies conducted in adults, persistence of anti-HAV and anti-HBs antibodies has been proven up to 60 months following the initiation of a primary vaccination course of Twinrix Adult in the majority of vaccinees. The kinetics of decline of anti-HAV and anti-HBs antibodies were shown to be similar to those of the monovalent vaccines.

These data were generated with the former Twinrix formulation containing thiomersal and a preservative. A clinical study conducted with the current formulation of Twinrix in adults showed that the current formulation elicited similar seroprotection and seroconversion rates as compared to the former formulation.

5.2 Pharmacokinetic properties

Evaluation of pharmacokinetic properties is not required for vaccines.

5.3 Preclinical safety data

Non-clinical data reveal no special hazard for humans based on general safety studies (see section 4.6).

6. PHARMACEUTICAL PARTICULARS

6.1 List of excipients

Sodium chloride

Water for injections

For adjuvants, see section 2.

6.2 Incompatibilities

In the absence of compatibility studies, this medicinal product must not be mixed with other medicinal products.

6.3 Shelf life

3 years.

6.4 Special precautions for storage

Store in a refrigerator (2°C - 8°C).

Do not freeze.

Store in the original package, in order to protect from light.

6.5 Nature and contents of container

1 ml of suspension in a prefilled syringe (type I glass) with a plunger stopper (rubber butyl).

Pack sizes of 1, 10 and 25 with or without needles.

Not all pack sizes may be marketed.

6.6 Special precautions for disposal and other handling

Upon storage, a fine white deposit with a clear colourless supernatant can be observed.

The vaccine should be well shaken to obtain a slightly opaque, white suspension and visually inspected for any foreign particulate matter and/or variation of physical aspect prior to administration. In the event of either being observed, discard the vaccine.

Any unused product of waste material should be disposed of in accordance with local requirements.

7. MARKETING AUTHORISATION HOLDER

GlaxoSmithKline Biologicals s.a.

rue de l'Institut 89

B-1330 Rixensart, Belgium

8. MARKETING AUTHORISATION NUMBER(S)

EU/1/96/020/001

EU/1/96/020/002

EU/1/96/020/003

EU/1/96/020/007

EU/1/96/020/008

EU/1/96/020/009

9. DATE OF FIRST AUTHORISATION/RENEWAL OF THE AUTHORISATION

Renewal of the Authorisation

Date of first authorisation: 20 September 1996

Date of latest renewal: 20 September 2006

10. DATE OF REVISION OF THE TEXT

19/06/2008

Twinrix Paediatric Vaccine

(GlaxoSmithKline UK)

1. NAME OF THE MEDICINAL PRODUCT

Twinrix Paediatric, suspension for injection in prefilled syringe

Hepatitis A (inactivated) and hepatitis B(rDNA) (HAB) vaccine ((adsorbed).

2. QUALITATIVE AND QUANTITATIVE COMPOSITION

1 dose (0.5 ml) contains:

Hepatitis A virus (inactivated)[1,2]	360 ELISA Units
Hepatitis B surface antigen[3,4]	10 micrograms

[1]Produced on human diploid (MRC-5) cells

[2]Adsorbed on aluminium hydroxide, hydrated — 0.025 milligrams Al^{3+}

[3]Produced in yeast cells (*Saccharomyces cerevisiae*) by recombinant DNA technology

[4]Adsorbed on aluminium phosphate — 0.2 milligrams Al^{3+}

For a full list of excipients, see section 6.1.

3. PHARMACEUTICAL FORM

Suspension for injection in prefilled syringe

Turbid white suspension.

4. CLINICAL PARTICULARS

4.1 Therapeutic indications

Twinrix Paediatric is indicated for use in non immune infants, children and adolescents from 1 year up to and including 15 years who are at risk of both hepatitis A and hepatitis B infection.

4.2 Posology and method of administration

Posology

- Dosage

The dose of 0.5 ml (360 ELISA Units HA/10 μg HBsAg) is recommended for infants, children and adolescents from 1 year up to and including 15 years of age.

- Primary vaccination schedule

The standard primary course of vaccination with Twinrix Paediatric consists of three doses, the first administered at the elected date, the second one month later and the third six months after the first dose. The recommended schedule should be adhered to. Once initiated, the primary course of vaccination should be completed with the same vaccine.

- Booster dose.

Long-term antibody persistence data following vaccination with Twinrix Paediatric are available up to 48 months after vaccination. The anti-HBs and anti-HAV antibody titres observed following a primary vaccination course with the combined vaccine are in the range of what is seen following vaccination with the monovalent vaccines. The kinetics of antibody decline are also similar. General guidelines for booster vaccination can therefore be drawn from experience with the monovalent vaccines.

Hepatitis B

The need for a booster dose of hepatitis B vaccine in healthy individuals who have received a full primary vaccination course has not been established; however some official vaccination programmes currently include a recommendation for a booster dose of hepatitis B vaccine and these should be respected.

For some categories of subjects or patients exposed to HBV (e.g. haemodialysis or immunocompromised patients) a precautionary attitude should be considered to ensure a protective antibody level ⩾ 10IU/l.

Hepatitis A

It is not yet fully established whether immunocompetent individuals who have responded to hepatitis A vaccination will require booster doses as protection in the absence of detectable antibodies may be insured by immunological memory. Guidelines for boosting are based on the assumption that antibodies are required for protection; anti-HAV antibodies have been predicted to persist for at least 10 years.

In situations where a booster dose of both hepatitis A and hepatitis B are desired, Twinrix Paediatric can be given. Alternatively, subjects primed with Twinrix Paediatric may be administered a booster dose of either of the monovalent vaccines.

Method of administration

Twinrix Paediatric is for intramuscular injection, preferably in the deltoid region in adolescents and children or in the anterolateral thigh in infants.

Exceptionally, the vaccine may be administered subcutaneously in patients with thrombocytopenia or bleeding disorders. However, this route of administration may result in suboptimal immune response to the vaccine. (see section 4.4)

4.3 Contraindications

Hypersensitivity to the active substances or to any of the excipients or neomycin.

Hypersensitivity after previous administration of hepatitis A and/or hepatitis B vaccines.

The administration of Twinrix Paediatric should be postponed in subjects suffering from acute severe febrile illness.

4.4 Special warnings and precautions for use

It is possible that subjects may be in the incubation period of a HA or HB infection at the time of vaccination. It is not known whether Twinrix Paediatric will prevent HA and HB in such cases.

The vaccine will not prevent infection caused by other agents such as hepatitis C and hepatitis E and other pathogens known to infect the liver.

Twinrix Paediatric is not recommended for postexposure prophylaxis (e.g. needle stick injury).

The vaccine has not been tested in patients with impaired immunity. In haemodialysis patients, patients receiving immunosuppressive treatment or patients with an impaired immune system, the anticipated immune response may not be achieved after the primary immunisation course. Such patients may require additional doses of vaccine; nevertheless immunocompromised patients may fail to demonstrate an adequate response.

As with all injectable vaccines, appropriate medical treatment and supervision should always be readily available in case of a rare anaphylactic event following the administration of the vaccine.

Since intradermal injection or intramuscular administration into the gluteal muscle could lead to a suboptimal response to the vaccine, these routes should be avoided. However, exceptionally Twinrix Paediatric can be administered subcutaneously to subjects with thrombocytopenia or bleeding disorders since bleeding may occur following an intramuscular administration to these subjects. (see section 4.2)

TWINRIX PAEDIATRIC SHOULD UNDER NO CIRCUMSTANCES BE ADMINISTERED INTRAVASCULARLY.

As with any injection procedure, vasovagal syncope can infrequently occur following administration of Twinrix Paediatric to adolescents.

4.5 Interaction with other medicinal products and other forms of interaction

No data on concomitant administration of Twinrix Paediatric with specific hepatitis A immunoglobulin or hepatitis B immunoglobulin have been generated. However, when the monovalent hepatitis A and hepatitis B vaccines were administered concomitantly with specific immunoglobulins, no influence on seroconversion was observed although it may result in lower antibody titers.

As the concomitant administration of Twinrix Paediatric and other vaccines has not specifically been studied it is advised that the vaccine should not be administered at the same time as other vaccines.

4.6 Pregnancy and lactation

Pregnancy

The effect of Twinrix Paediatrict on embryo-fetal, peri-natal and post-natal survival and development has been assessed in rats. This study did not indicate direct or indirect harmful effects with respect to fertility, pregnancy, embryonal/fetal development, parturition or post-natal development.

The effect of Twinrix Paediatric on embryo-fetal, peri-natal and post-natal survival and development has not been prospectively evaluated in clinical trials.

Data on outcomes of a limited number of pregnancies in vaccinated women do not indicate any adverse effects of Twinrix Paediatric on pregnancy or on the health of the fetus/newborn child. While it is not expected that recombinant hepatitis B virus surface antigen would have adverse effects on pregnancies or the fetus it is recommended that vaccination should be delayed until after delivery unless there is an urgent need to protect the mother against hepatitis B infection.

Lactation

It is unknown whether Twinrix Paediatric is excreted in human breast milk. The excretion of Twinrix Paediatric in milk has not been studied in animals. A decision on whether to continue/discontinue breast-feeding or to continue/discontinue therapy with Twinrix Paediatric should be made taking into account the benefit of breast-feeding to the child and the benefit of Twinrix Paediatric therapy to the woman.

4.7 Effects on ability to drive and use machines

Twinrix Paediatric has no or negligible influence on the ability to drive and use machines.

4.8 Undesirable effects

• Clinical trials

The current formulation of Twinrix does not contain thiomersal (an organomercuric compound) or any preservative. In a clinical study conducted with the current formulation, the incidence of pain, redness, swelling, fatigue, gastro-enteritis, headache and fever was comparable to the incidence observed with the former thiomersal and preservative containing vaccine formulation. The following undesirable events have been reported following the widespread use of the former formulation.

The safety profile presented below is based on data from approximately 800 subjects.

Frequencies are reported as:

Very common: ⩾ 1/10

Common: ⩾ 1/100 to < 1/10

Uncommon: ⩾ 1/1,000 to < 1/100

Rare: ⩾ 1/10,000 to < 1/1,000

Very rare: < 1/10,000

* refers to adverse reactions observed in clinical trials performed with the adult formulation

Blood and lymphatic system disorders

Rare: lymphadenopathy

Nervous system disorders

Common: drowsiness, headache

Rare: hypoaesthesia*, paraesthesia*, dizziness

Gastrointestinal disorders

Common: gastrointestinal symptoms, nausea

Uncommon: diarrhoea, vomiting, abdominal pain

Skin and subcutaneous tissue disorders

Uncommon: rash

Rare: urticaria, pruritus*

Musculoskeletal and connective tissue disorders

Uncommon: myalgia*

Rare: arthralgia*

Metabolism and nutrition disorders

Common: appetite lost

Infections and infestations

Uncommon: upper respiratory tract infection*

Vascular disorders

Rare: hypotension*

General disorders and administration site conditions

Very common: pain and redness at the injection site

Common: swelling at the injection site, injection site reaction (such as bruising), fatigue, malaise, fever (⩾ 37.5°C)

Rare: influenza like illness*, chills*

Psychiatric disorders

Common: irritability

• Post-marketing surveillance

The following adverse reactions have been reported with either Twinrix or with GlaxoSmithKline monovalent hepatitis A or B vaccines:

Blood and lymphatic system disorders

Thrombocytopenia, thrombocytopenic purpura

Nervous system disorders

Encephalitis, encephalopathy, neuritis, neuropathy, paralysis, convulsions

Skin and subcutaneous tissue disorders

Angioneurotic oedema, lichen planus, erythema multiforme

Musculoskeletal and connective tissue disorders

Arthritis, muscular weakness

Infections and infestations

Meningitis

Vascular disorders

Vasculitis

Immune system disorders

Anaphylaxis, allergic reactions including anaphylactoid reactions and mimicking serum sickness

Following widespread use of the monovalent hepatitis A and/or hepatitis B vaccines, the following undesirable events have additionally been reported in temporal association with vaccination.

Investigations

Abnormal liver function tests

Nervous system disorders

Multiple sclerosis, myelitis, facial palsy, polyneuritis such as Guillain-Barré syndrome (with ascending paralysis), optic neuritis

4.9 Overdose

Cases of overdose have been reported during post-marketing surveillance. Adverse events reported following overdosage were similar to those reported with normal vaccine administration.

5. PHARMACOLOGICAL PROPERTIES

5.1 Pharmacodynamic properties

Pharmaco-therapeutic group: Hepatitis vaccines, ATC code J07BC20.

Twinrix Paediatric is a combined vaccine formulated by pooling bulk preparations of the purified, inactivated hepatitis A (HA) virus and purified hepatitis B surface antigen (HBsAg), separately adsorbed onto aluminium hydroxide and aluminium phosphate.

The HA virus is propagated in MRC_5 human diploid cells. HBsAg is produced by culture, in a selective medium, of genetically engineered yeast cells.

Twinrix Paediatric confers immunity against HAV and HBV infection by inducing specific anti-HA and anti-HBs antibodies.

Protection against hepatitis A and hepatitis B develops within 2-4 weeks. In the clinical studies, specific humoral antibodies against hepatitis A were observed in approximately 89% of the subjects one month after the first dose and in 100% one month after the third dose (i.e. month 7). Specific humoral antibodies against hepatitis B were observed in approximately 67% of the subjects after the first dose and 100% after the third dose.

In a long term clinical trial, persistence of anti-HAV and anti-HBs antibodies has been demonstrated up to 48 months following the initiation of a primary vaccination course of Twinrix Paediatric in the majority of vaccinees (see section 4.2). The kinetics of decline of anti-HAV and anti-HBs antibodies were shown to be similar to those of the monovalent vaccines.

These data were generated with the former Twinrix formulation containing thiomersal and a preservative. A clinical study conducted with the current formulation of Twinrix in adults showed that the current formulation elicited similar seroprotection and seroconversion rates as compared to the former formulation.

5.2 Pharmacokinetic properties

Evaluation of pharmacokinetic properties is not required for vaccines.

5.3 Preclinical safety data

Non-clinical data reveal no special hazard for humans based on general safety studies (see section 4.6).

6. PHARMACEUTICAL PARTICULARS

6.1 List of excipients

Sodium chloride

Water for injections

For adjuvants, see section 2.

6.2 Incompatibilities

In the absence of compatibility studies, this medicinal product must not be mixed with other medicinal products.

6.3 Shelf life

3 years.

6.4 Special precautions for storage

Store in a refrigerator (2°C - 8°C).

Do not freeze.

Store in the original package, in order to protect from light.

6.5 Nature and contents of container

0.5 ml of suspension in a prefilled syringe (type I glass) with a plunger stopper (rubber butyl).

Pack sizes of 1, 10 and 50 with or without needles.

Not all pack sizes may be marketed.

6.6 Special precautions for disposal and other handling

Upon storage, a fine white deposit with a clear colourless supernatant can be observed.

The vaccine should be well shaken to obtain a slightly opaque, white suspension and visually inspected for any foreign particulate matter and/or variation of physical aspect prior to administration. In the event of either being observed, discard the vaccine.

Any unused product of waste material should be disposed of in accordance with local requirements.

7. MARKETING AUTHORISATION HOLDER

GlaxoSmithKline Biologicals s.a.

rue de l'Institut 89

B-1330 Rixensart, Belgium

8. MARKETING AUTHORISATION NUMBER(S)

EU/1/97/029/001

EU/1/97/029/002

EU/1/97/029/006

EU/1/97/029/007

EU/1/97/029/008

EU/1/97/029/009

EU/1/97/029/010

9. DATE OF FIRST AUTHORISATION/RENEWAL OF THE AUTHORISATION

Renewal of the Authorisation

Date of first authorisation: 10 February 1997

Date of latest renewal: 10 February 2007

10. DATE OF REVISION OF THE TEXT

19/06/2008

Tygacil 50mg powder for solution for infusion

(Wyeth Pharmaceuticals)

1. NAME OF THE MEDICINAL PRODUCT

Tygacil 50 mg ▼ powder for solution for infusion.

2. QUALITATIVE AND QUANTITATIVE COMPOSITION

Each 5 ml Tygacil vial contains 50 mg of tigecycline. After reconstitution, 1 ml contains 10 mg of tigecycline.

For a full list of excipients, see section 6.1.

3. PHARMACEUTICAL FORM

Powder for solution for infusion.

Lyophilised orange cake or powder.

4. CLINICAL PARTICULARS

4.1 Therapeutic indications

Tygacil is indicated for the treatment of the following infections (see sections 4.4 and 5.1):

- Complicated skin and soft tissue infections
- Complicated intra-abdominal infections

Consideration should be given to official guidance on the appropriate use of antibacterial agents.

4.2 Posology and method of administration

Posology

The recommended dose for adults is an initial dose of 100 mg followed by 50 mg every 12 hours for 5 to 14 days. The duration of therapy should be guided by the severity, site of the infection, and the patient's clinical response.

Hepatic insufficiency

No dosage adjustment is warranted in patients with mild to moderate hepatic impairment (Child Pugh A and Child Pugh B).

In patients with severe hepatic impairment (Child Pugh C), the dose of Tygacil should be reduced to 25 mg every 12 hours following the 100 mg loading dose. Patients with severe hepatic impairment (Child Pugh C) should be treated with caution and monitored for treatment response (see sections 4.4 and 5.2).

Renal insufficiency

No dosage adjustment is necessary in patients with renal impairment or in patients undergoing haemodialysis (see section 5.2).

Elderly patients

No dosage adjustment is necessary in elderly patients (see section 5.2).

Paediatric patients

Tygacil is not recommended for use in children and adolescents below 18 years due to the lack of data on safety and efficacy (see sections 5.2 and 4.4).

Method of administration:

Tygacil is administered only by intravenous infusion over 30 to 60 minutes (see section 6.6).

4.3 Contraindications

Hypersensitivity to the active substance or to any of the excipients. Patients hypersensitive to tetracycline class antibiotics may be hypersensitive to tigecycline.

4.4 Special warnings and precautions for use

Anaphylaxis/anaphylactoid reactions, potentially life-threatening, have been reported with tigecycline (see sections 4.3 and 4.8).

Cases of liver injury with a predominantly cholestatic pattern have been reported in patients receiving tigecycline treatment, including some cases of hepatic failure with a fatal outcome. Although hepatic failure may occur in patients treated with tigecycline due to the underlying conditions or concomitant medications, a possible contribution of tigecycline should be considered. (see section 4.8)

Glycylcycline class antibiotics are structurally similar to tetracycline class antibiotics. Tigecycline may have adverse reactions similar to tetracycline class antibiotics. Such reactions may include photosensitivity, pseudotumor cerebri, pancreatitis, and anti-anabolic action which has led to increased BUN, azotaemia, acidosis, and hyperphosphataemia (see section 4.8).

Acute pancreatitis, which can be serious, has occurred (frequency: uncommon) in association with tigecycline treatment (see section 4.8). The diagnosis of acute pancreatitis should be considered in patients taking tigecycline who develop clinical symptoms, signs, or laboratory abnormalities suggestive of acute pancreatitis. Most of the reported cases developed after at least one week of treatment. Cases have been reported in patients without known risk factors for pancreatitis. Patients usually improve after tigecycline discontinuation. Consideration should be given to the cessation of the treatment with tigecycline in cases suspected of having developed pancreatitis.

Experience in the use of tigecycline for treatment of infections in patients with severe underlying diseases is limited.

In clinical trials in complicated skin and soft tissue infections, the most common type of infection in tigecycline treated-patients was cellulitis (59 %), followed by major abscesses (27.5 %). Patients with severe underlying disease, such as those that were immunocompromised, patients with decubitus ulcer infections, or patients that had infections requiring longer than 14 days of treatment (for example, necrotizing fasciitis), were not enrolled. Few patients with diabetic foot infections (5%) were enrolled. A limited number of patients were enrolled with co-morbid factors such as diabetes (20 %), peripheral vascular disease (7 %), intravenous drug abuse (2 %), and HIV-positive infection (1 %). Limited experience is also available in treating patients with concurrent bacteraemia (3 %). Therefore, caution is advised when treating such patients.

In clinical trials in complicated intra-abdominal infections, the most common type of infection in tigecycline treated-patients was complicated appendicitis (51 %), followed by other diagnoses less commonly reported such as complicated cholecystitis (14 %), intra-abdominal abscess (10 %), perforation of intestine (10 %) and gastric or duodenal ulcer perforation less than 24 hours (5 %). Of these patients, 76 % had associated diffuse peritonitis (surgically-apparent peritonitis). There were a limited number of patients with severe underlying disease such as immunocompromised patients, patients with APACHE II scores > 15 (4 %), or with surgically apparent multiple intra-abdominal abscesses (10 %). Limited experience is also available in treating patients with concurrent bacteraemia (6 %). Therefore, caution is advised when treating such patients.

Consideration should be given to the use of combination antibacterial therapy whenever tigecycline is to be administered to severely ill patients with complicated intra-abdominal infections (cIAI) secondary to clinically apparent intestinal perforation or patients with incipient sepsis or septic shock (see section 4.8).

The effect of cholestasis in the pharmacokinetics of tigecycline has not been properly established. Biliary excretion accounts for approximately 50 % of the total tigecycline excretion. Therefore, patients presenting with cholestasis should be closely monitored.

Prothrombin time or other suitable anticoagulation test should be used to monitor patients if tigecycline is administered with anticoagulants (see section 4.5).

Pseudomembranous colitis has been reported with nearly all antibacterial agents and may range in severity from mild to life threatening. Therefore, it is important to consider this diagnosis in patients who present with diarrhoea during or subsequent to the administration of any antibacterial agent (see section 4.8).

The use of tigecycline may result in overgrowth of non-susceptible organisms, including fungi. Patients should be carefully monitored during therapy. If super infection occurs, appropriate measures should be taken (see section 4.8).

Results of studies in rats with tigecycline have shown bone discolouration. Tigecycline may be associated with permanent tooth discolouration in humans if used during tooth development (see section 4.8).

Tygacil should not be used in children under 8 years of age because of teeth discolouration, and is not recommended in adolescents below 18 years due to the lack of data on safety and efficacy (see sections 4.2 and 4.8).

4.5 Interaction with other medicinal products and other forms of interaction

Interaction studies have only been performed in adults.

Concomitant administration of tigecycline and warfarin (25 mg single-dose) to healthy subjects resulted in a decrease in clearance of R-warfarin and S-warfarin by 40 % and 23 %, and an increase in AUC by 68 % and 29 %, respectively. The mechanism of this interaction is still not elucidated. Available data does not suggest that this interaction may result in significant INR changes. However, since tigecycline may prolong both prothrombin time (PT) and activated partial thromboplastin time (aPTT), the relevant coagulation tests should be closely monitored when tigecycline is co-administered with anticoagulants (see section 4.4). Warfarin did not affect the pharmacokinetic profile of tigecycline.

Tigecycline is not extensively metabolised. Therefore, clearance of tigecycline is not expected to be affected by active substances that inhibit or induce the activity of the CYP450 isoforms. *In vitro*, tigecycline is neither a competitive inhibitor nor an irreversible inhibitor of CYP450 enzymes (see section 5.2).

Tigecycline in recommended dosage did not affect the rate or extent of absorption, or clearance of digoxin (0.5 mg followed by 0.25 mg daily) when administered in healthy adults. Digoxin did not affect the pharmacokinetic profile of tigecycline. Therefore, no dosage adjustment is necessary when tigecycline is administered with digoxin.

In *in vitro* studies, no antagonism has been observed between tigecycline and other commonly used antibiotic classes.

Concurrent use of antibiotics with oral contraceptives may render oral contraceptives less effective.

4.6 Pregnancy and lactation

There are no adequate data from the use of tigecycline in pregnant women. Results from animal studies have shown tigecycline may cause foetal harm when administered during pregnancy (see section 5.3). The potential risk for humans is unknown. As it is known for tetracycline class antibiotics, tigecycline may also induce permanent dental defects (discolouration and enamel defects) and a delay in ossification processes in foetuses, exposed *in utero* during the last half of gestation, and in children under eight years of age due to the enrichment in tissues with a high calcium turnover and formation of calcium chelate complexes (see section 4.4). Tigecycline should not be used during pregnancy unless clearly necessary.

It is not known whether this medicinal product is excreted in human milk. In animal studies tigecycline is excreted into milk of lactating rats. Because a potential risk to the breast-feeding infant cannot be ruled out, when treating with tigecycline, caution should be exercised and interruption of breast-feeding should be considered (see section 5.3).

4.7 Effects on ability to drive and use machines

No studies on the effects of tigecycline on the ability to drive and use machines have been performed. Dizziness may occur and this may have an effect on driving and use of machines (see section 4.8).

4.8 Undesirable effects

The total number of patients treated with tigecycline in Phase 3 clinical studies was 1415. Adverse reactions were reported in approximately 41 % of patients treated with tigecycline. Treatment was discontinued due to adverse reactions in 5 % of patients.

In clinical trials, the most common drug-related treatment emergent adverse reactions were reversible nausea (20 %) and vomiting (14 %), which usually occurred early (on treatment days 1-2) and were generally mild or moderate in severity.

Adverse reactions reported with Tygacil, including clinical trials and post-marketing experience, are listed below:

Frequency categories are expressed as: Very common (⩾1/10); Common (⩾1/100 to <1/10); Uncommon (⩾1/1,000 to <1/100); Rare (⩾1/10,000 to < 1/1,000); Very Rare (<1/10,000)

For adverse reactions identified from post-marketing experience with Tygacil derived from spontaneous reports for which the frequency cannot be estimated, the frequency grouping is categorized as not known.

Infections and infestations:

Common: Abscess, infections

Uncommon: Sepsis/septic shock

In Phase 3 clinical studies, infection-related serious adverse events were more frequently reported for subjects treated with tigecycline (6.7 %) vs comparators (4.6 %). Significant differences in sepsis/septic shock with tigecycline (1.5 %) vs comparators (0.5 %) were observed.

Blood and the lymphatic system disorders:

Common: Prolonged activated partial thromboplastin time (aPTT), Prolonged prothrombin time (PT)

Uncommon: Increased International Normalised Ratio (INR)

Not known: thrombocytopenia

Immune system disorders:

Not known: Anaphylaxis/anaphylactoid reactions (see sections 4.3 and 4.4)

Metabolism and nutrition disorders:

Uncommon: Hypoproteinaemia

Nervous system disorders:

Common: Dizziness

Vascular disorders:

Common: Phlebitis

Uncommon: Thrombophlebitis

Gastrointestinal disorders:

Very Common: Nausea, vomiting, diarrhoea

Common: Abdominal pain, dyspepsia, anorexia

Uncommon: Acute pancreatitis (see section 4.4)

Hepato-biliary disorders:

Common: Elevated aspartate aminotransferase (AST) in serum, and elevated alanine aminotransferase (ALT) in serum, hyperbilirubinaemia

AST and ALT abnormalities in Tygacil-treated patients were reported more frequently in the post therapy period than in those in comparator-treated patients, which occurred more often on therapy.

Uncommon: Jaundice, liver injury, mostly cholestatic

Not known: Hepatic failure(see section 4.4)

Skin and subcutaneous tissue disorders:

Common: Pruritus, rash

General disorders and administration site conditions:

Common: Headache

Uncommon: Injection site reaction, injection site inflammation, injection site pain, injection site oedema, injection site phlebitis

Investigations:

Common: Elevated amylase in serum, increased blood urea nitrogen (BUN)

In Phase 3 cSSSI and cIAI studies, death occurred in 2.3 % (32/1383) of patients receiving tigecycline and 1.6 % (22/1375) of patients receiving comparator drugs.

Antibiotic Class Effects:

Pseudomembranous colitis which may range in severity from mild to life threatening (see section 4.4)

Overgrowth of non-susceptible organisms, including fungi (see section 4.4)

Tetracycline Class Effects:

Glycylcycline class antibiotics are structurally similar to tetracycline class antibiotics. Tetracycline class adverse reactions may include photosensitivity, pseudotumour cerebri, pancreatitis, and anti-anabolic action which has led to increased BUN, azotaemia, acidosis, and hyperphosphataemia (see section 4.4).

Tigecycline may be associated with permanent tooth discolouration if used during tooth development (see section 4.4).

4.9 Overdose

No specific information is available on the treatment of overdosage. Intravenous administration of tigecycline at a single dose of 300 mg over 60 minutes in healthy volunteers resulted in an increased incidence of nausea and vomiting. Tigecycline is not removed in significant quantities by haemodialysis.

5. PHARMACOLOGICAL PROPERTIES

5.1 Pharmacodynamic properties

Pharmacotherapeutic group: Tetracyclines, ATC code: J01AA12.

Mode of action

Tigecycline, a glycylcycline antibiotic, inhibits protein translation in bacteria by binding to the 30S ribosomal subunit and blocking entry of amino-acyl tRNA molecules into the A site of the ribosome. This prevents incorporation of amino acid residues into elongating peptide chains.

In general, tigecycline is considered bacteriostatic. At 4 times the minimum inhibitory concentration (MIC), a 2-log reduction in colony counts was observed with tigecycline against *Enterococcus* spp., *Staphylococcus aureus*, and *Escherichia coli*.

Mechanism of resistance

Tigecycline is able to overcome the two major tetracycline resistance mechanisms, ribosomal protection and efflux. Cross-resistance between tigecycline and minocycline-resistant isolates among the *Enterobacteriacae* due to mulit-drug resistance (MDR) efflux pumps has been shown. There is no target-based cross-resistance between tigecycline and most classes of antibiotics.

Tigecycline is vulnerable to chromosomally-encoded multi-drug efflux pumps of *Proteeae* and *Psuedomonas aeruginosa*. Pathogens of the family *Proteeae* (*Proteus* spp., *Providencia* spp., and *Morganella* spp.) are generally less susceptible to tigecycline than other members of the *Enterobacteriaceae*. Decreased susceptibility in both groups has been attributed to the overexpression of the non-specific AcrAB multi-drug efflux pump. Decreased susceptibility in *Acinetobacter baumannii* has been attributed to the overexpression of the AdeABC efflux pump.

Breakpoints

Minimum inhibitory concentration (MIC) breakpoints established by the European Committee on Antimicrobial Susceptibility Testing (EUCAST) are as follows:

Staphylococcus spp. S ≤0.5 mg/L and R> 0.5 mg/L

Streptococcus spp. other than *S. pneumoniae* S ≤0.25 mg/L and R> 0.5 mg/L

Enterococcus spp. S ≤0.25 mg/L and R> 0.5 mg/L

Enterobacteriaceae S ≤1[^] mg/L and R> 2 mg/L

[^] Tigecycline has decreased *in vitro* activity against *Proteus, Providencia*, and *Morganella* spp.

For anaerobic bacteria there is clinical evidence of efficacy in polymicrobial intra-abdominal infections, but no correlation between MIC values, PK/PD data and clinical outcome. Therefore, no breakpoint for susceptibility is given. It should be noted that the MIC distributions for organisms of the genera *Bacteroides* and *Clostridium* are wide and may include values in excess of 2 mg/L tigecycline.

There is limited evidence of the clinical efficacy of tigecycline against enterococci. However, polymicrobial intra-abdominal infections have shown to respond to treatment with tigecycline in clinical trials.

Susceptibility

The prevalence of acquired resistance may vary geographically and with time for selected species, and local information on resistance is desirable, particularly when treating severe infections. As necessary, expert advice should be sought when the local prevalence of resistance is such that the utility of the agent in at least some types of infections is questionable.

Pathogen
Commonly Susceptible Species
Gram-positive Aerobes
Enterococcus spp.†
*Staphylococcus aureus**
Staphylococcus epidermidis
Staphylococcus haemolyticus
*Streptococcus agalactiae**
Streptococcus anginosus group*
(includes *S. anginosus, S. intermedius and S. constellatus*)
*Streptococcus pyogenes**
Viridans group streptococci
Gran-negative Aerobes
*Citrobacter freundii**
Citrobacter koseri
Escherichia coli*
*Klebsiella oxytoca**
Anaerobes
Clostridium perfringens†
Peptostreptococcus spp. †
Prevotella spp.
Species for which acquired resistance may be a problem
Gram-negative Aerobes
Acinetobacter baumannii
Burkholderia cepacia
Enterobacter aerogenes
*Enterobacter cloacae**
*Klebsiella pneumoniae**
Morganella morganii
Proteus spp.
Providencia spp.
Serratia marcescens
Stenotrophomonas maltophilia
Anaerobes
Bacteroides fragilis group†
Inherently resistant organisms
Gran-negative Aerobes
Pseudomonas aeruginosa

* denotes species against which it is considered that activity has been satisfactorily demonstrated in clinical studies.

† see section 5.1, *Breakpoints* above.

5.2 Pharmacokinetic properties

Absorption

Tigecycline is administered intravenously and therefore has 100 % bioavailability.

Distribution

The *in vitro* plasma protein binding of tigecycline ranges from approximately 71 % to 89 % at concentrations observed in clinical studies (0.1 to 1.0 μg/mL). Animal and human pharmacokinetic studies have demonstrated that tigecycline readily distributes to tissues.

In rats receiving single or multiple doses of ^{14}C-tigecycline, radioactivity was well distributed to most tissues, with the highest overall exposure observed in bone marrow, salivary glands, thyroid gland, spleen, and kidney. In humans, the steady-state volume of distribution of tigecycline averaged 500 to 700 L (7 to 9 L/kg), indicating that tigecycline is extensively distributed beyond the plasma volume and concentrates into tissues.

No data are available on whether tigecycline can cross the blood-brain barrier in humans.

In clinical pharmacology studies using the therapeutic dosage regimen of 100 mg followed by 50 mg q12h, serum tigecycline steady-state C_{max} was 866±233 ng/mL for 30-minute infusions and 634±97 ng/mL for 60-minute infusions. The steady-state $AUC_{0\text{-}12h}$ was 2349±850 ng•h/mL.

Metabolism

On average, it is estimated that less than 20 % of tigecycline is metabolised before excretion. In healthy male volunteers, following the administration of ^{14}C-tigecycline, unchanged tigecycline was the primary ^{14}C-labelled material recovered in urine and faeces, but a glucuronide, an N-acetyl metabolite and a tigecycline epimer were also present.

In vitro studies in human liver microsomes indicate that tigecycline does not inhibit metabolism mediated by any of the following 6 cytochrome P450 (CYP) isoforms: 1A2, 2C8, 2C9, 2C19, 2D6, and 3A4 by competitive inhibition. In addition, tigecycline did not show NADPH-dependency in the inhibition of CYP2C9, CYP2C19, CYP2D6 and CYP3A, suggesting the absence of mechanism-based inhibition of these CYP enzymes.

Elimination

The recovery of the total radioactivity in faeces and urine following administration of ^{14}C-tigecycline indicates that 59 % of the dose is eliminated by biliary/faecal excretion, and 33 % is excreted in urine. Overall, the primary route of elimination for tigecycline is biliary excretion of unchanged tigecycline. Glucuronidation and renal excretion of unchanged tigecycline are secondary routes.

The total clearance of tigecycline is 24 L/h after intravenous infusion. Renal clearance is approximately 13 % of total clearance. Tigecycline shows a polyexponential elimination from serum with a mean terminal elimination half-life after multiple doses of 42 hours although high interindividual variability exists.

Special populations

Hepatic Insufficiency

The single-dose pharmacokinetic disposition of tigecycline was not altered in patients with mild hepatic impairment. However, systemic clearance of tigecycline was reduced by 25 % and 55 % and the half-life of tigecycline was prolonged by 23 % and 43 % in patients with moderate or severe hepatic impairment (Child Pugh B and C), respectively (see section 4.2).

Renal Insufficiency

The single dose pharmacokinetic disposition of tigecycline was not altered in patients with renal insufficiency (creatinine clearance <30 mL/min, n=6). In severe renal impairment, AUC was 30 % higher than in subjects with normal renal function (see section 4.2).

Elderly Patients

No overall differences in pharmacokinetics were observed between healthy elderly subjects and younger subjects (see section 4.2).

Paediatric Patients

The pharmacokinetics of tigecycline in patients less than 18 years of age has not been established (see section 4.2).

Gender

There were no clinically relevant differences in the clearance of tigecycline between men and women. AUC was estimated to be 20 % higher in females than in males.

Race

There were no differences in the clearance of tigecycline based on race.

Weight

Clearance, weight-normalised clearance, and AUC were not appreciably different among patients with different body weights, including those weighing ≥125 kg. AUC was 24 % lower in patients weighing ≥125 kg. No data is available for patients weighing 140 kg and more.

5.3 Preclinical safety data

In repeated dose toxicity studies in rats and dogs, lymphoid depletion/atrophy of lymph nodes, spleen and thymus, decreased erythrocytes, reticulocytes, leukocytes, and platelets, in association with bone marrow hypocellularity, and adverse renal and gastrointestinal effects have been seen with tigecycline at exposures of 8 and 10 times the human daily dose based on AUC in rats and dogs, respectively. These alterations were shown to be reversible after two weeks of dosing.

Bone discolouring was observed in rats which was not reversible after two weeks of dosing.

Results of animal studies indicate that tigecycline crosses the placenta and is found in foetal tissues. In reproduction toxicity studies, decreased foetal weights in rats and rabbits (with associated delays in ossification) and foetal loss in rabbits have been observed with tigecycline. Tigecycline was not teratogenic in the rat or rabbit.

Results from animal studies using ^{14}C-labelled tigecycline indicate that tigecycline is excreted readily via the milk of lactating rats. Consistent with the limited oral bioavailability of tigecycline, there is little or no systemic exposure to tigecycline in the nursing pups as a result of exposure via maternal milk.

Lifetime studies in animals to evaluate the carcinogenic potential of tigecycline have not been performed, but short-term genotoxicity studies of tigecycline were negative.

Bolus intravenous administration of tigecycline has been associated with a histamine response in animal studies. These effects were observed at exposures of 14 and 3 times the human daily dose based on the AUC in rats and dogs respectively.

No evidence of photosensitivity was observed in rats following administration of tigecycline.

6. PHARMACEUTICAL PARTICULARS

6.1 List of excipients

Lactose monohydrate

Hydrochloric acid, sodium hydroxide (for pH adjustment)

6.2 Incompatibilities

The following active substances should not be administered simultaneously through the same Y-site as

Tygacil: Amphotericin B, amphotericin B lipid complex, diazepam, esomeprazole, omeprazole and intravenous solutions that could result in an increase of pH above 7.

Tygacil must not be mixed with other medicinal products for which compatibility data are not available (see section 6.6).

6.3 Shelf life
18 months.

Once reconstituted and diluted in the bag or other suitable infusion container (e.g. glass bottle), tigecycline should be used immediately.

6.4 Special precautions for storage
Store at or below 25°C.

For storage conditions of the reconstituted product see section 6.3.

6.5 Nature and contents of container
5 ml Type 1 clear glass vials fitted with grey butyl rubber stoppers and snap-off aluminium crimp seals. Tygacil is distributed in a ten vial tray pack.

6.6 Special precautions for disposal and other handling
The lyophilised powder should be reconstituted with 5.3 ml of sodium chloride 9 mg/ml (0.9 %) solution for injection or dextrose 50 mg/ml (5 %) solution for injection to achieve a concentration of 10 mg/ml of tigecycline. The vial should be gently swirled until the medicinal product is dissolved. Thereafter, 5 ml of the reconstituted solution should be immediately withdrawn from the vial and added to a 100 ml intravenous bag for infusion or other suitable infusion container (e.g., glass bottle).

For a 100 mg dose, reconstitute using two vials into a 100 ml intravenous bag or other suitable infusion container (e.g., glass bottle). Note: The vial contains a 6 % overage. Thus, 5 ml of reconstituted solution is equivalent to 50 mg of the active substance. The reconstituted solution should be yellow to orange in colour; if not, the solution should be discarded. Parenteral products should be inspected visually for particulate matter and discolouration (e.g., green or black) prior to administration.

Tygacil may be administered intravenously through a dedicated line or through a Y-site. If the same intravenous line is used for sequential infusion of several active substances, the line should be flushed before and after infusion of Tygacil with either sodium chloride 9 mg/ml (0.9 %) solution for injection or dextrose 50 mg/ml (5 %) solution for injection. Injection should be made with an infusion solution compatible with tigecycline and any other medicinal product(s) via this common line. (See section 6.2.)

This medicinal product is for single use only; any unused solution should be discarded.

Compatible intravenous solutions include: sodium chloride 9 mg/ml (0.9 %) solution for injection and dextrose 50 mg/ml (5 %) solution for injection.

When administered through a Y-site, compatibility of Tygacil diluted in sodium chloride 0.9 % for injection is demonstrated with the following medicinal products or diluents: amikacin, dobutamine, dopamine HCl, gentamicin, haloperidol, Lactacted Ringers's, lidocaine HCl, metoclopramide, morphine, norepinephrine, piperacillin/tazobactam (EDTA formulation), potassium chloride, propofol, ranitidine HCl, theophylline, and tobramycin.

7. MARKETING AUTHORISATION HOLDER
Wyeth Europa Ltd.
Huntercombe Lane South
Taplow, Maidenhead
Berkshire, SL6 0PH
United Kingdom

8. MARKETING AUTHORISATION NUMBER(S)
EU/1/06/336/001

9. DATE OF FIRST AUTHORISATION/RENEWAL OF THE AUTHORISATION
24 April 2006

10. DATE OF REVISION OF THE TEXT
07 July 2009

Detailed information on this medicinal product is available on the website of the European Medicines Agency (EMEA) http://www.emea.europa.eu/

Further information may be obtained from:
Wyeth Pharmaceuticals, Huntercombe Lane South,
Taplow, Maidenhead, Berkshire, SL6 0PH, UK
Telephone: 0845 367 0098

Tylex Capsules

(UCB Pharma Limited)

1. NAME OF THE MEDICINAL PRODUCT
Tylex Capsules or Medocodene 30/500 Capsules.

2. QUALITATIVE AND QUANTITATIVE COMPOSITION
Each capsule contains 500mg of paracetamol Ph.Eur and 30 mg of codeine phosphate hemihydrate Ph.Eur.

3. PHARMACEUTICAL FORM
Capsules.

4. CLINICAL PARTICULARS
4.1 Therapeutic indications
For the relief of severe pain.

4.2 Posology and method of administration
ADULTS

The capsules are given orally. The usual dose is one or two capsules every four hours as required. The total daily dose should not exceed 240 mg of codeine phosphate (i.e., not more than four doses per 24 hours should betaken)

ELDERLY

A reduced dose may be required.

CHILDREN

Use in children under 12 years of age is not recommended.

Dosage should be adjusted according to the severity of the pain and the response of the patient. However, it should be kept in mind that tolerance to codeine can develop with continued use and that the incidence of untoward effects is dose related. Doses of codeine higher than 60 mg fail to give commensurate relief of pain but merely prolong analgesia and are associated with an appreciably increased incidence of undesirable side effects.

4.3 Contraindications
These capsules should not be administered to patients who have previously exhibited hypersensitivity to either paracetamol or codeine, or to any of its excipients.

These capsules are not recommended for children under the age of 12 years.

4.4 Special warnings and precautions for use
The risk-benefit of continued use should be assessed regularly by the prescriber.

Because safety and effectiveness in the administration of paracetamol with codeine inchildren under 12 years of age have not been established, such use is not recommended.

These capsules contain sodium metabisulphite, a sulphite that may cause allergic reactions including anaphylactic symptoms and life threatening or less severe asthmatic episodes in certain susceptible people. The overall prevalence of sulphite sensitivity in the general population is unknown and probably low. Sulphite sensitivity is seen more frequently in asthmatic than non-asthmatic people.

These capsules should be used with caution in patients with head injuries, increased intracranial pressure, acute abdominal conditions, the elderly and debilitated, and those with severe impairment of hepatic or renal function, hypothyroidism, Addison's disease, prostatic hypertrophy or urethral stricture, myasthenia gravis, biliary tract disorders (including recent biliary tract surgery).

The hazard of overdose is greater in those with non-cirrhotic alcoholic liver disease.

Chronic heavy alcohol abusers may be at increased risk of liver toxicity from excessive paracetamol use, although reports of this event are rare. Reports almost invariably involve cases of severe chronic alcoholics and the dosages of paracetamol most often exceed recommended doses and often involve substantial overdose. Professionals should alert their patients who regularly consume large amounts of alcohol not to exceed recommended doses of paracetamol.

At high doses codeine has most of the disadvantages of morphine, including respiratory depression. Codeine can produce drug dependence of the morphine type, and therefore has the potential for being abused. Codeine may impair the mental and/or physical abilities required for the performance of potentially hazardous tasks.

Patients should be advised that immediate medical advice should be sought in the event of an overdose, because of the risk of delayed, serious liver damage. They should be advised not to exceed the recommended dose, not to take other paracetamol-containing products concurrently, to consult their doctor if symptoms persist and to keep the product out of the reach of children.

The leaflet will state in a prominent position in the 'before taking' section:

· Do not take for longer than directed by your prescriber

· Taking codeine regularly for a long time can lead to addiction, which might cause you to feel restless and irritable when you stop the tablets.

· Taking a painkiller for headaches too often or for too long can make them worse.

The label will state (To be displayed prominently on outer pack -not boxed):

· Do not take for longer than directed by your prescriber as taking codeine regularly for a long time can lead to addiction.

4.5 Interaction with other medicinal products and other forms of interaction
Patients receiving other central nervous system depressants (including otheropioid analgesics, tranquillisers, sedative hypnotics and alcohol) concomitantly with these capsules may exhibit an additive depressant effect. When such therapy is contemplated, the dose of one or both agents should be reduced.

Concurrent use of MAO inhibitors or tricyclic antidepressants with codeine may increase the effect of either the antidepressant or codeine. Concurrent use of anticholinergics and codeine may produce paralytic ileus.

The speed of absorption of paracetamol may be increased by metoclopramide or domperidone and absorption reduced by cholestyramine.

The anticoagulant effect of warfarin and other coumarins may be enhanced by prolonged regular daily use of paracetamol with increased risk of bleeding; occasional doses have no significant effect.

4.6 Pregnancy and lactation
These capsules are not recommended during pregnancy or lactation since safety in pregnant women or nursing mothers has not been established.

4.7 Effects on ability to drive and use machines
Patients should be advised not to drive or operate machinery if affected by dizziness or sedation.

4.8 Undesirable effects
Regular prolonged use of codeine is known to lead to addiction and tolerance. Symptoms of restlessness and irritability may result when treatment is stopped. Prolonged use of a painkiller for headaches can make them worse.

Reported adverse reactions seem more prominent in ambulatory than non-ambulatory patients and some of these effects may be alleviated if the patient lies down.

The most frequently observed reactions include light headedness, dizziness, sedation, shortness of breath, nausea and vomiting. These effects seem more prominent in ambulatory than non-ambulatory patients and some of these adverse reactions may be alleviated if the patient lies down. Other adverse reactions include allergic reactions, (including skin rash), euphoria, dysphoria, constipation, abdominal pain and pruritus.

In clinical use of paracetamol-containing products, there have been a few reports of blood dyscrasias including thrombocytopenia and agranulocytosis but these were not necessarily causally related to paracetamol.

4.9 Overdose
Paracetamol
Liver damage is possible in adults who have taken 10g or more of paracetamol. The following groups are at risk of liver damage from paracetamol doses of 5g or more:

- patients on long-term treatment with drugs which induce liver enzymes (e.g. barbiturates, St John's Wort);
- people who regularly drink excessive amounts of alcohol;
- patients with depleted glutathione levels (e.g. eating disorders, cystic fibrosis, HIV infection, starvation, cachexia).

Symptoms of paracetamol overdose include:

- pallor, nausea, vomiting, anorexia and abdominal pain within 24 hours of ingestion;
- liver damage may become apparent 12 to 48 hours after ingestion;
- abnormalities of glucose metabolism and metabolic acidosis may occur;
- in severe poisoning, hepatic failure may progress to encephalopathy, haemorrhage, hypoglycaemia, cerebral oedema and death;
- Acute renal failure with acute tubular necrosis (loin pain, haematuria and proteinuria), may develop regardless of severe liver damage;
- Cardiac arrhythmias and pancreatitis have been reported.

<u>Management</u>
Immediate treatment is essential. Despite a lack of significant early symptoms, patients should be referred to hospital urgently for immediate medical attention. Symptoms may be limited to nausea or vomiting and may not reflect the severity of overdose or the risk of organ damage. Management should be in accordance with established treatment guidelines (see BNF overdose section).

Treatment with activated charcoal should be considered within 1 hour of overdose. Plasma paracetamol concentration should be measured at 4 hours or more postingestion (to ensure the measurement is reliable). Treatment with N-acetylcysteine is most effective up to 8 hours after ingestion but may be used up to 24 hours after overdose. Antidote effectiveness declines sharply after 8 hours. If required, administer N-acetylcysteine intravenously, in line with the established dosage schedule. If vomiting is not a problem, oral methionine may be a suitable alternative for remote areas, outside hospital. Management of patients who present with serious hepatic dysfunction more than 24h after ingestion should be discussed with the NPIS or a liver unit.

Codeine
Simultaneous ingestion of alcohol and psychotropic drugs will potentiate the effects of overdosage.

Symptoms of codeine overdose may include:

- Central nervous system depression (including respiratory depression) but this is unlikely to be severe unless the overdose is large, or there is co-ingestion with other sedative agents or alcohol;

- pinpoint sized pupils;
- nausea and vomiting;
- hypotension and tachycardia are possible but unlikely.

Management

General symptomatic and supportive measures including a clear airway and monitoring of vital signs until stable. Consider activated charcoal if an adult presents within 1 hour after ingesting more than 350 mg or a child more than 5 mg/kg. Give naloxone if coma or respiratory depression is present. Naloxone is a competitive antagonist with a short half-life, so large and repeated doses may be required in a seriously poisoned patient. Observe patients for at least 4 hours after ingestion.

5. PHARMACOLOGICAL PROPERTIES

5.1 Pharmacodynamic properties

Paracetamol has analgesic and antipyretic actions similar to those of aspirin with weak anti-inflammatory effects. Paracetamol is only a weak inhibitor of prostaglandin biosynthesis, although there is some evidence to suggest that it may be more effective against enzymes in the CNS than those in the periphery. This fact may partly account for its well documented ability to reduce fever and to induce analgesia, effects that involve actions on neural tissues. Single or repeated therapeutic doses of paracetamol have no effect on the cardiovascular and respiratory systems. Acid-based changes do not occur and gastric irritation, erosion or bleeding is not produced as may occur after salicylates. There is only a weak effect upon platelets and no effect on bleeding time or the excretion of uric acid.

Codeine is an analgesic with uses similar to those of morphine but has only mild sedative effects. The major effect is on the CNS and the bowel. The effects are remarkably diverse and include analgesia, drowsiness, changes in mood, respiratory depression, decreased gastrointestinal motility, nausea, vomiting and alterations of the endocrine and autonomic nervous systems. The relief of pain is relatively selective, in that other sensory modalities, (touch, vibration, vision, hearing etc) are not obtunded.

5.2 Pharmacokinetic properties

Paracetamol is readily absorbed from the gastro-intestinal tract with peak plasma concentration occurring about 30 minutes to 2 hours after ingestion. It is metabolised in the liver and excreted in the urine mainly as the glucuronide and sulphate conjugates. Less than 5% is excreted as unchanged paracetamol. The elimination half-life varies from about 1 to 4 hours. Plasma-protein binding is negligible at usual therapeutic concentrations but increases with increasing concentrations.

A minor hydroxylated metabolite which is usually produced in very small amounts by mixed-function oxidases in the liver and which is usually detoxified by conjugation with liver glutathione may accumulate following paracetamol overdosage and cause liver damage.

Codeine and its salts are absorbed from the gastro intestinal tract. Ingestion of codeine phosphate produces peak plasma codeine concentrations in about one hour. Codeine is metabolised by O- & N-demethylation in the liver to morphine and norcodeine. Codeine and its metabolites are excreted almost entirely by the kidney, mainly as conjugates with glucuronic acid. The plasma half-life has been reported to be between 3 and 4 hours after administration by mouth or intravascular injection.

5.3 Preclinical safety data

None stated.

6. PHARMACEUTICAL PARTICULARS

6.1 List of excipients

Pregelatinized Starch

Calcium Stearate

Aerosol OT-B

Sodium metabisulphite

gelatin capsule

E171

E127

E132

Printing ink: Shellac, soya lecithin, 2-ethoxyethanol, dimethylpolysiloxane, E172

6.2 Incompatibilities

None pertinent

6.3 Shelf life

36 months- HDPE bottles and PVC/aluminium foil blisters.

36 months- PP securitainers

6.4 Special precautions for storage

Store at or below 25°C. Keep container in the outer carton.

6.5 Nature and contents of container

Tamper-evident high density polyethylene bottles fitted with low density polyethylene caps, containing 24, 100 or 500 capsules.

PVC/aluminium foil blister strips containing 1x7, 2x7, 4x7, 1x8, 3x8, 50x6, 100x6, 5x20, 10x10 capsules.

Polypropylene securitainers containing 8, 16, 24, 32, 56 or 64 capsules.

Not all pack sizes may be marketed.

6.6 Special precautions for disposal and other handling

None

7. MARKETING AUTHORISATION HOLDER

UCB Pharma Ltd

208 Bath Road

Slough

Berkshire SL1 3WE

United Kingdom

8. MARKETING AUTHORISATION NUMBER(S)

PL 00039/0749

9. DATE OF FIRST AUTHORISATION/RENEWAL OF THE AUTHORISATION

31/03/2008

10. DATE OF REVISION OF THE TEXT

14/06/2008

Tylex Effervescent

(UCB Pharma Limited)

1. NAME OF THE MEDICINAL PRODUCT

Tylex Effervescent.

2. QUALITATIVE AND QUANTITATIVE COMPOSITION

Each effervescent tablet contains 500mg of paracetamol Ph. Eur and 30 mg of codeine phosphate Ph.Eur.

3. PHARMACEUTICAL FORM

Effervescent tablets.

4. CLINICAL PARTICULARS

4.1 Therapeutic indications

For the relief of severe pain.

4.2 Posology and method of administration

ADULTS

The tablets are given orally and should be dissolved in at least half a tumblerful of water before taking. The usual dose is one or two tablets every four hours as required. The total daily dose should not exceed 240 mg of codeine phosphate (i.e., not more than eight tablets per 24 hours should be taken)

ELDERLY

A reduced dose may be required.

CHILDREN

Use in children under 12 years of age is not recommended.

Dosage should be adjusted according to the severity of the pain and the response of the patient. However, it should be kept in mind that tolerance to codeine can develop with continued use and that the incidence of untoward effects is dose related. Doses of codeine higher than 60 mg fail to give commensurate relief of pain but merely prolong analgesia and are associated with an appreciably increased incidence of undesirable side effects.

4.3 Contraindications

TYLEX EFFERVESCENT should not be administered to patients who have previously exhibited hypersensitivity to either paracetamol or codeine, or to any of its excipients.

TYLEX EFFERVESCENT is not recommended for children under the age of 12 years.

4.4 Special warnings and precautions for use

The risk-benefit of continued use should be assessed regularly by the prescriber.

Because safety and effectiveness in the administration of paracetamol with codeine in children under 12 years of age have not been established, such use is not recommended.

These tablets should be used with caution in patients with head injuries, increased intracranial pressure, acute abdominal conditions, the elderly and debilitated, and those with severe impairment of hepatic or renal function, hypothyroidism, Addison's disease, prostatic hypertrophy or urethral stricture, myasthenia gravis, biliary tract disorders (including recent biliary tract surgery).

The hazard of overdose is greater in those with non-cirrhotic alcoholic liver disease.

Chronic heavy alcohol abusers may be at increased risk of liver toxicity from excessive paracetamol use, although reports of this event are rare. Reports almost invariably involve cases of severe chronic alcoholics and the dosages of paracetamol most often exceed recommended doses and often involve substantial overdose. Professionals should alert their patients who regularly consume large amounts of alcohol not to exceed recommended doses of paracetamol.

These tablets contain 326.6 mg sodium/tablet and this should be taken into account when prescribing for patients for whom sodium restriction is indicated. The product also contains 25 mg aspartame/tablet and therefore care should be taken in phenylketonuria.

At high doses codeine has most of the disadvantages of morphine, including respiratory depression. Codeine can produce drug dependence of the morphine type, and therefore has the potential for being abused. Codeine may impair the mental/or physical abilities required for the performance of potentially hazardous tasks.

Patients should be advised that immediate medical advice should be sought in the event of an overdose, because of the risk of delayed, serious liver damage. They should be advised not to exceed the recommended dose, not to take other paracetamol-containing products concurrently, to consult their doctor if symptoms persist and to keep the product out of the reach of children.

The leaflet will state in a prominent position in the 'before taking' section:

· Do not take for longer than directed by your prescriber

· Taking codeine regularly for a long time can lead to addiction, which might cause you to feel restless and irritable when you stop the tablets.

· Taking a painkiller for headaches too often or for too long can make them worse.

The label will state (To be displayed prominently on outer pack -not boxed):

· Do not take for longer than directed by your prescriber as taking codeine regularly for a long time can lead to addiction

4.5 Interaction with other medicinal products and other forms of interaction

Patients receiving other central nervous system depressants (including other opioid analgesics, tranquillisers, sedative hypnotics and alcohol) concomitantly with TYLEX EFFERVESCENT may exhibit an additive depressant effect. When such therapy is contemplated, the dose of one or both agents should be reduced.

Concurrent use of MAO inhibitors or tricyclic antidepressants with codeine may increase the effect of either the antidepressant or codeine. Concurrent use of anticholinergics and codeine may produce paralytic ileus.

The speed of absorption of paracetamol may be increased by metoclopramide or domperidone and absorption reduced by cholestyramine.

The anticoagulant effect of warfarin and other coumarins may be enhanced by prolonged regular daily use of paracetamol with increased risk of bleeding; occasional doses have no significant effect.

4.6 Pregnancy and lactation

The use of TYLEX EFFERVESCENT is not recommended during pregnancy or lactation since safety in pregnant women or nursing mothers has not been established.

4.7 Effects on ability to drive and use machines

Patients should be advised not to drive or operate machinery if affected by dizziness or sedation.

4.8 Undesirable effects

Regular prolonged use of codeine is known to lead to addiction and tolerance. Symptoms of restlessness and irritability may result when treatment is stopped.

Prolonged use of a painkiller for headaches can make them worse.

Reported adverse reactions seem more prominent in ambulatory than non-ambulatory patients and some of these effects may be alleviated if the patient lies down.

The most frequently observed reactions include light headedness, dizziness, sedation, shortness of breath, nausea and vomiting. These effects seem more prominent in ambulatory than nonambulatory patients and some of these adverse reactions may be alleviated if the patient lies down. Other adverse reactions include allergic reactions, (including skin rash), euphoria, dysphoria, constipation, abdominal pain and pruritus.

In clinical use of paracetamol-containing products, there have been a few reports of blood dyscrasias including thrombocytopenia and agranulocytosis but these were not necessarily causally related to paracetamol.

4.9 Overdose

Paracetamol

Liver damage is possible in adults who have taken 10g or more of paracetamol. The following groups are at risk of liver damage from paracetamol doses of 5g or more:

- patients on long-term treatment with drugs which induce liver enzymes (e.g. barbiturates, St John's Wort);
- people who regularly drink excessive amounts of alcohol;
- patients with depleted glutathione levels (e.g. eating disorders, cystic fibrosis, HIV infection, starvation, cachexia).

Symptoms of paracetamol overdose include:

- pallor, nausea, vomiting, anorexia and abdominal pain within 24 hours of ingestion;
- liver damage may become apparent 12 to 48 hours after ingestion;
- abnormalities of glucose metabolism and metabolic acidosis may occur;
- in severe poisoning, hepatic failure may progress to encephalopathy, haemorrhage, hypoglycaemia, cerebral oedema and death;
- Acute renal failure with acute tubular necrosis (loin pain, haematuria and proteinuria), may develop regardless of severe liver damage;
- Cardiac arrhythmias and pancreatitis have been reported.

Management

Immediate treatment is essential. Despite a lack of significant early symptoms, patients should be referred to hospital urgently for immediate medical attention. Symptoms may be limited to nausea or vomiting and may not reflect the severity of overdose or the risk of organ damage. Management should be in accordance with established treatment guidelines (see BNF overdose section).

Treatment with activated charcoal should be considered within 1 hour of overdose. Plasma paracetamol concentration should be measured at 4 hours or more post-ingestion (to ensure the measurement is reliable). Treatment with N-acetylcysteine is most effective up to 8 hours after ingestion but may be used up to 24 hours after overdose. Antidote effectiveness declines sharply after 8 hours. If required, administer N-acetylcysteine intravenously, in line with the established dosage schedule. If vomiting is not a problem, oral methionine may be a suitable alternative for remote areas, outside hospital. Management of patients who present with serious hepatic dysfunction more than 24h after ingestion should be discussed with the NPIS or a liver unit.

Codeine

Simultaneous ingestion of alcohol and psychotropic drugs will potentiate the effects of overdosage.

Symptoms of codeine overdose may include:

- Central nervous system depression (including respiratory depression) but this is unlikely to be severe unless the overdose is large, or there is co-ingestion with other sedative agents or alcohol;
- pinpoint sized pupils;
- nausea and vomiting;
- hypotension and tachycardia are possible but unlikely.

Management

General symptomatic and supportive measures including a clear airway and monitoring of vital signs until stable. Consider activated charcoal if an adult presents within 1 hour after ingesting more than 350 mg or a child more than 5 mg/kg. Give naloxone if coma or respiratory depression is present. Naloxone is a competitive antagonist with a short half-life, so large and repeated doses may be required in a seriously poisoned patient. Observe patients for at least 4 hours after ingestion.

5. PHARMACOLOGICAL PROPERTIES

5.1 Pharmacodynamic properties

Paracetamol has analgesic and antipyretic actions similar to those of aspirin with weak anti-inflammatory effects. Paracetamol is only a weak inhibitor of prostaglandin biosynthesis, although there is some evidence to suggest that it may be more effective against enzymes in the CNS than those in the periphery. This fact may partly account for its well documented ability to reduce fever and to induce analgesia, effects that involve actions on neural tissues. Single or repeated therapeutic doses of paracetamol have no effect on the cardiovascular and respiratory systems. Acid-based changes do not occur and gastric irritation, erosion or bleeding is not produced as may occur after salicylates. There is only a weak effect upon platelets and no effect on bleeding time or the excretion of uric acid.

Codeine is an analgesic with uses similar to those of morphine but has only mild sedative effects. The major effect is on the CNS and the bowel. The effects are remarkably diverse and include analgesia, drowsiness, changes in mood, respiratory depression, decreased gastrointestinal motility, nausea, vomiting and alterations of the endocrine and autonomic nervous systems. The relief of pain is relatively selective, in that other sensory modalities, (touch, vibration, vision, hearing etc) are not obtunded.

5.2 Pharmacokinetic properties

Paracetamol is readily absorbed from the gastro-intestinal tract with peak plasma concentration occurring about 30 minutes to 2 hours after ingestion. It is metabolised in the liver and excreted in the urine mainly as the glucuronide and sulphate conjugates. Less than 5% is excreted as unchanged paracetamol. The elimination half-life varies from about 1 to 4 hours. Plasma-protein binding is negligible at usual therapeutic concentrations but increases with increasing concentrations.

A minor hydroylated metabolite which is usually produced in very small amounts by mixedfunction oxidases in the liver and which is usually detoxified by conjugation with liver glutathione may accumulate following paracetamol overdosage and cause liver damage.

Codeine and its salts are absorbed from the gastro intestinal tract. Ingestion of codeine phosphate produces peak plasma codeine concentrations in about one hour. Codeine is metabolised by O- & N-demethylation in the liver to morphine and norcodeine. Codeine and its metabolites are excreted almost entirely by the kidney, mainly as conjugates with glucuronic acid.

The plasma half-life has been reported to be between 3 and 4 hours after administration by mouth or intravascular injection.

5.3 Preclinical safety data

None stated

6. PHARMACEUTICAL PARTICULARS

6.1 List of excipients

Citric Acid Anhydrous

Sodium Bicarbonate

Sodium Carbonate Anhydrous

Aspartame

Polyethylene Glycol 6000

Magnesium Stearate

Ethanol 96 % (not detected in the finished product)

6.2 Incompatibilities

None pertinent

6.3 Shelf life

36 months

6.4 Special precautions for storage

Store at room temperature (at or below 25°C) in a dry place. Protect from light

6.5 Nature and contents of container

Paper/aluminium laminate blister strips packed in cardboard cartons.

Pack sizes: 1, 6, 8, 24, 30, 36, 42, 48, 90, 100 and 102 tablets.

Not all pack sizes may be marketed.

6.6 Special precautions for disposal and other handling

None

7. MARKETING AUTHORISATION HOLDER

SCHWARZ PHARMA Limited

5 Hercules Way

Leavesden Park

Watford

WD25 7GS

United Kingdom

8. MARKETING AUTHORISATION NUMBER(S)

PL 04438/0045

9. DATE OF FIRST AUTHORISATION/RENEWAL OF THE AUTHORISATION

27/02/2008

10. DATE OF REVISION OF THE TEXT

04/04/2008

Typherix

(GlaxoSmithKline UK)

1. NAME OF THE MEDICINAL PRODUCT

Typherix, solution for injection in a pre-filled syringe

Typhoid Polysaccharide vaccine.

2. QUALITATIVE AND QUANTITATIVE COMPOSITION

Each 0.5 ml dose of vaccine contains:

Vi polysaccharide of *Salmonella typhi (Ty2 strain)* 25 micrograms

For a full list of excipients, see section 6.1.

3. PHARMACEUTICAL FORM

Solution for injection in a pre-filled syringe.

Clear isotonic colourless solution.

4. CLINICAL PARTICULARS

4.1 Therapeutic indications

Typherix is indicated for active immunisation against typhoid fever for both adults and children two years of age and older.

4.2 Posology and method of administration

Posology

A single dose of 0.5 ml is recommended for both adults and children two years of age and older.

The vaccine should be administered at least two weeks prior to risk of exposure to typhoid fever.

Subjects who remain at risk of typhoid fever should be revaccinated using a single dose of vaccine with an interval of not more than 3 years.

Method of administration

Typherix is for **intramuscular** injection.

Typherix should under no circumstances be administered intravascularly.

4.3 Contraindications

Typherix should not be administered to subjects with known hypersensitivity to any component of the vaccine or to subjects having shown signs of hypersensitivity after previous administration.

As with other vaccines, the administration of Typherix should be postponed in subjects suffering from acute febrile illness. The presence of a minor infection, however, is not a contraindication for vaccination.

4.4 Special warnings and precautions for use

As with all injectable vaccines, appropriate medical treatment and supervision should always be readily available in case of a rare anaphylactic reaction following administration of the vaccine.

The vaccine protects against typhoid fever caused by *Salmonella typhi*. Protection is not conferred against disease caused by *Salmonella paratyphi* and other non-typhoidal Salmonellae.

Typherix has not been evaluated in children under 2 years of age. Polysaccharide vaccines in general have lower immunogenicity under this age.

Different injectable vaccines should always be administered at different injection sites.

Typherix should be administered with caution to subjects with thrombocytopenia or bleeding disorders since bleeding may occur following an intramuscular administration to these subjects: following injection, firm pressure should be applied to the site (without rubbing) for at least two minutes.

It may be expected that in patients receiving immunosuppressive treatment or patients with immunodeficiency, an adequate response may not be achieved.

4.5 Interaction with other medicinal products and other forms of interaction

In clinical studies in adults aged over 18 years, Typherix has been administered concomitantly in opposite arms with Havrix Monodose (1440), GlaxoSmithKline's inactivated hepatitis A vaccine.

There was no adverse impact on either the reactogenicity or immunogenicity of the vaccines when they were administered simultaneously in opposite arms.

No interaction studies with other vaccines have been performed.

4.6 Pregnancy and lactation

Pregnancy

The effect of Typherix on fetal development has not been assessed.

Typherix should only be used during pregnancy when there is a high risk of infection.

Lactation

The effect on breastfed infants of the administration of Typherix to their mothers has not been evaluated.

Typherix should therefore only be used in breastfeeding women when there is a high risk of infection.

4.7 Effects on ability to drive and use machines

Some of the effects mentioned under section 4.8 "Undesirable Effects" may affect the ability to drive or operate machinery.

4.8 Undesirable effects

During clinical studies, the most commonly reported adverse events after the first dose were reactions at the injection site, including soreness, redness and swelling.

Frequencies are reported as:

Common: (≥ 1/100 to < 1/10)

Very rare: (< 1/10,000)

Within each frequency grouping, undesirable effects are presented in order of decreasing seriousness.

General reactions that may occur in temporal association with Typherix vaccination include:

Clinical studies

Nervous system disorders:

Common: headache

Gastrointestinal disorders:

Common: nausea

Skin and subcutaneous tissue disorders:

Common: itching

General disorders and administration site conditions:

Common: fever, general aches, malaise

Following a second dose, there was an increased incidence of redness and soreness (>10%).

Local reactions were usually reported during the first 48 hours and systemic reactions were also transient.

Post-marketing

The following reactions have been reported in post-marketing experience:

Skin and subcutaneous tissue disorders:

Very rare: urticaria

Immune system disorders:

Very rare: anaphylaxis, allergic reactions, including anaphylactoid reactions

4.9 Overdose

Occasional reports of overdose have been received. The symptoms reported in these cases are not different from those reported following normal dosage.

5. PHARMACOLOGICAL PROPERTIES

5.1 Pharmacodynamic properties

Pharmacotherapeutic group: Bacterial vaccine, ATC code: J07AP03

In comparative clinical studies, the immune response to Typherix was shown to be equivalent to a licensed comparator Vi polysaccharide vaccine. Seroconversion was observed in >95% of Typherix recipients when measured at two weeks after administration. Two years after vaccination 61% were seropositive, and at three years 46%.

The protective efficacy of Typherix has not been investigated in clinical trials.

For individuals who remain at - or who may be reexposed to - risk of typhoid fever, it is recommended that they be revaccinated using a single dose of vaccine with an interval of not more than 3 years.

5.2 Pharmacokinetic properties
Evaluation of pharmacokinetic properties is not required for vaccines and formal pharmacokinetic studies have not been performed.

5.3 Preclinical safety data
No preclinical safety testing with the vaccine has been conducted.

6. PHARMACEUTICAL PARTICULARS

6.1 List of excipients
Sodium dihydrogen phosphate dihydrate

Disodium phosphate dihydrate

Sodium chloride

Phenol

Water for injection

6.2 Incompatibilities
In the absence of compatibility studies, this medicinal product must not be mixed with other medicinal products.

6.3 Shelf life
2 years.

6.4 Special precautions for storage
Store in a refrigerator (2°C-8°C)

Do not freeze.

Store in the original package, in order to protect from light.

6.5 Nature and contents of container
0.5 ml of solution in a pre-filled syringe (Type I glass) with an plunger stopper (elastomer rubber butyl) in pack sizes of 1, 10, 50 or 100.

Not all pack sizes may be marketed.

6.6 Special precautions for disposal and other handling
Vaccines should be inspected for any foreign particulate matter and/or variation of physical aspect. In the event of either being observed, discard the vaccine.

Shake before use.

Any unused product or waste material should be disposed of in accordance with local requirements.

7. MARKETING AUTHORISATION HOLDER
SmithKline Beecham plc

980 Great West Road

Brentford

Middlesex TW8 9BD

Trading as:

GlaxoSmithKline UK

Stockley Park West

Uxbridge

Middlesex, UB11 1BT

8. MARKETING AUTHORISATION NUMBER(S)
PL 10592/0126

9. DATE OF FIRST AUTHORISATION/RENEWAL OF THE AUTHORISATION
05/07/2008

10. DATE OF REVISION OF THE TEXT
05/07/2008
POM

TYSABRI 300 mg concentrate for solution for infusion

(Biogen Idec Ltd)

1. NAME OF THE MEDICINAL PRODUCT▼
TYSABRI ▼ 300 mg concentrate for solution for infusion.

2. QUALITATIVE AND QUANTITATIVE COMPOSITION
Concentrate: Each ml of concentrate contains 20 mg of natalizumab.

Natalizumab is a recombinant humanised anti-α4-integrin antibody produced in a murine cell line by recombinant DNA technology.

When diluted (see section 6.6), the solution for infusion contains approximately 2.6 mg/ml of natalizumab.

For a full list of excipients, see section 6.1.

3. PHARMACEUTICAL FORM
Concentrate for solution for infusion.

Colourless, clear to slightly opalescent solution.

4. CLINICAL PARTICULARS

4.1 Therapeutic indications
TYSABRI is indicated as single disease modifying therapy in highly active relapsing remitting multiple sclerosis for the following patient groups:

• Patients with high disease activity despite treatment with a beta-interferon (see section 5.1);

or

• Patients with rapidly evolving severe relapsing remitting multiple sclerosis (see section 5.1).

4.2 Posology and method of administration
TYSABRI therapy is to be initiated and supervised by specialised physicians experienced in the diagnosis and treatment of neurological conditions, in centres with timely access to MRI.

Patients treated with TYSABRI must be given the patient alert card.

Resources for the management of hypersensitivity reactions and access to MRI should be available.

After dilution (see section 6.6), the infusion is to be administered over approximately 1 hour and patients are to be observed during the infusion and for 1 hour after the completion of the infusion for signs and symptoms of hypersensitivity reactions.

TYSABRI must not be administered as a bolus injection.

Patients can switch directly from beta interferon or glatiramer acetate to natalizumab providing there are no signs of relevant treatment-related abnormalities e.g. neutropenia. If there are signs of treatment-related abnormalities these must return to normal before treatment with natalizumab is started.

Some patients may have been exposed to immunosuppressive medications (e.g. mitoxantrone, cyclophosphamide, azathioprine). These drugs have the potential to cause prolonged immunosuppression, even after dosing is discontinued. Therefore the physician must confirm that such patients are not immunocompromised before starting treatment with TYSABRI.

Continued therapy must be carefully reconsidered in patients who show no evidence of therapeutic benefit beyond 6 months.

Data on the safety and efficacy of natalizumab beyond 2 years are not available. Continued therapy beyond this time should be considered only following a reassessment of the potential for benefit and risk.

Adults
TYSABRI 300 mg is administered by intravenous infusion once every 4 weeks.

Elderly
TYSABRI is not recommended for use in patients aged over 65 due to a lack of data in this population.

Children and adolescents
TYSABRI is contraindicated in children and adolescents (see section 4.3).

Renal and hepatic impairment
Studies have not been conducted to examine the effects of renal or hepatic impairment.

The mechanism for elimination and results from population pharmacokinetics suggest that dose adjustment would not be necessary in patients with renal or hepatic impairment.

Readministration
The efficacy of re-administration has not been established, for safety see section 4.4.

4.3 Contraindications
Hypersensitivity to natalizumab or to any of the excipients.

Progressive multifocal leukoencephalopathy (PML).

Patients with increased risk for opportunistic infections, including immunocompromised patients (including those currently receiving immunosuppressive therapies or those immunocompromised by prior therapies, e.g. mitoxantrone or cyclophosphamide, see also sections 4.4 and 4.8).

Combination with beta-interferons or glatiramer acetate.

Known active malignancies, except for patients with cutaneous basal cell carcinoma.

Children and adolescents.

4.4 Special warnings and precautions for use
Progressive Multifocal Leukoencephalopathy (PML)
Use of TYSABRI has been associated with an increased risk of PML.

Before initiation of treatment with TYSABRI, a recent (usually within 3 months) Magnetic Resonance Image should be available. Patients must be monitored at regular intervals for any new or worsening neurological symptoms or signs that may be suggestive of PML.

If PML is suspected, further dosing must be suspended until PML has been excluded.

The clinician should evaluate the patient to determine if the symptoms are indicative of neurological dysfunction, and if so, whether these symptoms are typical of MS or possibly suggestive of PML. If any doubt exists, further evaluation, including MRI scan preferably with contrast (compared with pre-treatment MRI), CSF testing for JC Viral DNA and repeat neurological assessments, should be considered as described in the Physician Information and Management Guidelines (see educational guidance). Once the clinician has excluded PML (if necessary, by repeating clinical, imaging and/or laboratory investigations if clinical suspicion remains), dosing of natalizumab may resume.

The physician should be particularly alert to symptoms suggestive of PML that the patient may not notice (e.g. cognitive or psychiatric symptoms). Patients should also be advised to inform their partner or caregivers about their treatment, since they may notice symptoms that the patient is not aware of.

If a patient develops PML the dosing of TYSABRI must be permanently discontinued.

Following reconstitution of the immune system in immunocompromised patients with PML, stabilisation or improved outcome has been seen (see section 5.2). It remains unknown if early detection of PML and suspension of TYSABRI therapy may lead to similar stabilisation or improved outcome.

Other Opportunistic Infections
Other opportunistic infections have been reported with use of TYSABRI, primarily in patients with Crohn's disease who were immunocompromised or where significant co-morbidity existed, however increased risk of other opportunistic infections with use of TYSABRI in patients without these co-morbidities cannot currently be excluded. Opportunistic infections were also detected in MS patients treated with TYSABRI as a monotherapy (see section 4.8).

Prescribers should be aware of the possibility that other opportunistic infections may occur during TYSABRI therapy and should include them in the differential diagnosis of infections that occur in TYSABRI-treated patients. If an opportunistic infection is suspected, dosing with TYSABRI is to be suspended until such infections can be excluded through further evaluations.

If a patient receiving TYSABRI develops an opportunistic infection, dosing of TYSABRI must be permanently discontinued.

Educational guidance
All physicians who intend to prescribe TYSABRI must ensure they are familiar with the Physician Information and Management Guidelines.

Physicians must discuss the benefits and risks of TYSABRI therapy with the patient and provide them with a Patient Alert Card. Patients should be instructed that if they develop any infection then they should inform their physician that they are being treated with TYSABRI.

Physicians should counsel patients on the importance of uninterrupted dosing, particularly in the early months of treatment (see hypersensitivity).

Hypersensitivity
Hypersensitivity reactions have been associated with TYSABRI, including serious systemic reactions (see section 4.8). These reactions usually occurred during the infusion or up to 1 hour after completion of the infusion. The risk for hypersensitivity was greatest with early infusions and in patients re-exposed to TYSABRI following an initial short exposure (one or two infusions) and extended period (three months or more) without treatment. However, the risk of hypersensitivity reactions should be considered for every infusion administered.

Patients are to be observed during the infusion and for 1 hour after the completion of the infusion (see section 4.8). Resources for the management of hypersensitivity reactions should be available.

Discontinue administration of TYSABRI and initiate appropriate therapy at the first symptoms or signs of hypersensitivity.

Patients who have experienced a hypersensitivity reaction must be permanently discontinued from treatment with TYSABRI.

Concurrent or prior treatment with immunosuppressants
The safety and efficacy of TYSABRI in combination with other immunosuppressive and antineoplastic therapies have not been fully established. Concurrent use of these agents with TYSABRI may increase the risk of infections, including opportunistic infections, and is contraindicated (see section 4.3).

Patients with a treatment history of immunosuppressant medications, including cyclophosphamide and mitoxantrone, may experience prolonged immunosuppression and therefore may be at increased risk for PML. Care should be taken with patients who have previously received immunosuppressants to allow sufficient time for immune function recovery to occur. Physicians must evaluate each individual case to determine whether there is evidence of an immunocompromised state prior to commencing treatment with TYSABRI (see section 4.3).

In Phase 3 MS clinical trials, concomitant treatment of relapses with a short course of corticosteroids was not associated with an increased rate of infection. Short courses of corticosteroids can be used in combination with TYSABRI.

Immunogenicity
Disease exacerbations or infusion related events may indicate the development of antibodies against natalizumab. In these cases the presence of antibodies should be evaluated and if these remain positive in a confirmatory test after 6 weeks, treatment should be discontinued, as persistent antibodies are associated with a substantial decrease in efficacy of TYSABRI and an increased incidence of hypersensitivity reactions (see section 4.8).

Since patients who have received an initial short exposure to TYSABRI and then had an extended period without treatment are more at risk for hypersensitivity upon redosing, the presence of antibodies should be evaluated and if these remain positive in a confirmatory test after 6 weeks treatment should not be resumed.

Hepatic Events

Spontaneous serious adverse reactions of liver injury have been reported during the post marketing phase. These liver injuries may occur at any time during treatment, even after the first dose. In some instances, the reaction reoccurred when TYSABRI was reintroduced. Some patients with a past medical history of an abnormal liver test have experienced an exacerbation of abnormal liver test while on TYSABRI. Patients should be monitored as appropriate for impaired liver function, and be instructed to contact their physician in case signs and symptoms suggestive of liver injury occur, such as jaundice and vomiting. In cases of significant liver injury TYSABRI should be discontinued.

Stopping TYSABRI therapy

If a decision is made to stop treatment with natalizumab, the physician needs to be aware that natalizumab remains in the blood, and has pharmacodynamic effects (e.g increased lymphocyte counts) for approximately 12 weeks following the last dose. Starting other therapies during this interval will result in a concomitant exposure to natalizumab. For drugs such as interferon and glatiramer acetate, concomitant exposure of this duration was not associated with safety risks in clinical trials. No data are available in MS patients regarding concomitant exposure with immunosuppressant medication. Use of these medicines soon after the discontinuation of natalizumab may lead to an additive immunosuppressive effect. This should be carefully considered on a case-by-case basis, and a wash-out period of natalizumab might be appropriate. Short courses of steroids used to treat relapses were not associated with increased infections in clinical trials.

4.5 Interaction with other medicinal products and other forms of interaction

See section 4.3.

4.6 Pregnancy and lactation

There are no adequate data from the use of natalizumab in pregnant women. Studies in animals have shown reproductive toxicity (see section 5.3). The potential risk for humans is unknown. Natalizumab should not be used during pregnancy unless clearly necessary. If a woman becomes pregnant while taking TYSABRI, discontinuation of TYSABRI should be considered.

It is not known whether TYSABRI is excreted in human milk, but it has been observed in animal studies (see section 5.3). Patients receiving TYSABRI should not breastfeed their infants.

4.7 Effects on ability to drive and use machines

No studies on the effects on the ability to drive and use machines have been performed. Based on the pharmacological mechanism of action of natalizumab, the use of TYSABRI is not expected to affect patient's ability to drive and use machines.

4.8 Undesirable effects

In placebo-controlled trials in 1,617 MS patients treated with natalizumab for up to 2 years (placebo: 1,135), adverse events leading to discontinuation of therapy occurred in 5.8% of patients treated with natalizumab (placebo: 4.8%). Over the 2-year duration of the studies, 43.5% of patients treated with natalizumab reported adverse drug reactions (placebo: 39.6%)[1]. Adverse drug reactions reported with natalizumab with an incidence of 0.5% greater than reported with placebo are shown below. The reactions are reported as MedDRA preferred terms under the MedDRA primary system organ class. Frequencies were defined as follows:

Common (⩾ 1/100 to < 1/10), uncommon (⩾ 1/1,000 to < 1/100).

Within each frequency grouping, undesirable effects are presented in order of decreasing seriousness.

[1] An adverse event judged related to therapy by the investigating physician.

Nervous system disorders	
Common	Headache Dizziness
Gastrointestinal disorders	
Common	Vomiting Nausea
Musculoskeletal and connective tissue disorders	
Common	Arthralgia
Infections and infestations	
Common	Urinary tract infection Nasopharyngitis
General disorders and administration site conditions	
Common	Rigors Pyrexia Fatigue
Immune system disorders	
Common	Urticaria
Uncommon	Hypersensitivity

Infusion reactions

In 2-year controlled clinical trials in MS patients, an infusion-related event was defined as an adverse event occurring during the infusion or within 1 hour of the completion of the infusion. These occurred in 23.1% of MS patients treated with natalizumab (placebo: 18.7%). Events reported more commonly with natalizumab than with placebo included dizziness, nausea, urticaria and rigors.

Hypersensitivity reactions

In 2-year controlled clinical trials in MS patients, hypersensitivity reactions occurred in up to 4% of patients. Anaphylactic/anaphylactoid reactions occurred in less than 1% of patients receiving TYSABRI. Hypersensitivity reactions usually occurred during the infusion or within the 1-hour period after the completion of the infusion (See section 4.4). In post-marketing experience, there have been reports of hypersensitivity reactions which have occurred with one or more of the following associated symptoms: hypotension, hypertension, chest pain, chest discomfort, dyspnoea, angioedema, in addition to more usual symptoms such as rash and urticaria.

Immunogenicity

In 10% of patients antibodies against natalizumab were detected in 2-year controlled clinical trials in MS patients. Persistent anti-natalizumab antibodies (one positive test reproducible on retesting at least 6 weeks later) developed in approximately 6% of patients. Antibodies were detected on only one occasion in an additional 4% of patients. Persistent antibodies were associated with a substantial decrease in the effectiveness of TYSABRI and an increased incidence of hypersensitivity reactions. Additional infusion-related reactions associated with persistent antibodies included rigors, nausea, vomiting and flushing (see section 4.4).

If, after approximately 6 months of therapy, persistent antibodies are suspected, either due to reduced efficacy or due to occurrence of infusion-related events, they may be detected and confirmed with a subsequent test 6 weeks after the first positive test. Given that efficacy may be reduced or the incidence of hypersensitivity or infusion-related reactions may be increased in a patient with persistent antibodies, treatment should be discontinued in patients who develop persistent antibodies.

Infections, including PML and opportunistic infections

In 2-year controlled clinical trials in MS patients, the rate of infection was approximately 1.5 per patient-year in both natalizumab- and placebo-treated patients. The nature of the infections was generally similar in natalizumab- and placebo-treated patients. A case of *cryptosporidium* diarrhoea was reported in MS clinical trials. In other clinical trials, cases of additional opportunistic infections have been reported, some of which were fatal. In clinical trials, herpes infections (Varicella-Zoster virus, Herpes-simplex virus) occurred slightly more frequently in natalizumab-treated patients than in placebo-treated patients. In post marketing experience, there have been reports of serious cases, including one fatal case of herpes encephalitis. See section 4.4.

The majority of patients did not interrupt natalizumab therapy during infections and recovery occurred with appropriate treatment.

In clinical trials, cases of PML have been reported. PML usually leads to severe disability or death (see section 4.4). In pivotal clinical trials, two cases, including one fatality, occurred in MS patients who were being treated with concomitant interferon beta-1a therapy for more than 2 years. In another trial, one patient with Crohn's disease, who had a long history of treatment with immunosuppressants and associated lymphopenia also developed PML and died.

PML has been reported in post-marketing experience in patients treated with TYSABRI monotherapy.

Hepatic Events

Spontaneous cases of serious liver injuries, increased liver enzymes, hyperbilirubinaemia have been reported during the post marketing phase (see section 4.4).

Malignancies

No differences in incidence rates or the nature of malignancies between natalizumab- and placebo-treated patients were observed over 2 years of treatment. However, observation over longer treatment periods is required before any effect of natalizumab on malignancies can be excluded. See section 4.3.

Effects on laboratory tests

TYSABRI treatment was associated with increases in circulating lymphocytes, monocytes, eosinophils, basophils and nucleated red blood cells. Elevations in neutrophils were not seen. Increases from baseline for lymphocytes, monocytes, eosinophils and basophils ranged from 35% to 140% for individual cell types but mean cell counts remained within normal ranges. During treatment with TYSABRI, small reductions in haemoglobin (mean decrease 0.6 g/dl), haematocrit (mean decrease 2%) and red blood cell counts (mean decrease 0.1 × 10^6/l) were seen. All changes in haematological variables returned to pre-treatment values, usually within 16 weeks of last dose of TYSABRI and the changes were not associated with clinical symptoms.

4.9 Overdose

No case of overdose has been reported.

5. PHARMACOLOGICAL PROPERTIES

5.1 Pharmacodynamic properties

Pharmacotherapeutic group: Selective Immunosuppressive Agent, ATC code: L04AA23.

Pharmacodynamic properties

Natalizumab is a selective adhesion-molecule inhibitor and binds to the α4-subunit of human integrins, which is highly expressed on the surface of all leukocytes, with the exception of neutrophils. Specifically, natalizumab binds to the α4β1 integrin, blocking the interaction with its cognate receptor, vascular cell adhesion molecule-1 (VCAM-1), and ligands osteopontin, and an alternatively spliced domain of fibronectin, connecting segment-1 (CS-1). Natalizumab blocks the interaction of α4β7 integrin with the mucosal addressin cell adhesion molecule-1 (MadCAM-1). Disruption of these molecular interactions prevents transmigration of mononuclear leukocytes across the endothelium into inflamed parenchymal tissue. A further mechanism of action of natalizumab may be to suppress ongoing inflammatory reactions in diseased tissues by inhibiting the interaction of α4-expressing leukocytes with their ligands in the extracellular matrix and on parenchymal cells. As such, natalizumab may act to suppress inflammatory activity present at the disease site, and inhibit further recruitment of immune cells into inflamed tissues.

In MS, lesions are believed to occur when activated T-lymphocytes cross the blood-brain barrier (BBB). Leukocyte migration across the BBB involves interaction between adhesion molecules on inflammatory cells and endothelial cells of the vessel wall. The interaction between α4β1 and its targets is an important component of pathological inflammation in the brain and disruption of these interactions leads to reduced inflammation. Under normal conditions, VCAM-1 is not expressed in the brain parenchyma. However, in the presence of pro-inflammatory cytokines, VCAM-1 is upregulated on endothelial cells and possibly on glial cells near the sites of inflammation. In the setting of central nervous system (CNS) inflammation in MS, it is the interaction of α4β1 with VCAM-1, CS-1 and osteopontin that mediates the firm adhesion and transmigration of leukocytes into the brain parenchyma and may perpetuate the inflammatory cascade in CNS tissue. Blockade of the molecular interactions of α4β1 with its targets reduces inflammatory activity present in the brain in MS and inhibits further recruitment of immune cells into inflamed tissue, thus reducing the formation or enlargement of MS lesions.

Clinical efficacy

TYSABRI is indicated as a single disease modifying therapy in relapsing remitting multiple sclerosis to prevent relapses and delay progression of disability. Due to safety concerns (see sections 4.4 and 4.8) treatment is restricted to the following patient groups:

- Patients who have failed to respond to a full and adequate course of a beta-interferon. Patients should have had at least 1 relapse in the previous year while on therapy, and have at least 9 T2-hyperintense lesions in cranial MRI or at least 1 Gadolinium-enhancing lesion.

or

- Patients with rapidly evolving severe relapsing remitting multiple sclerosis, defined by 2 or more disabling relapses in one year, and with 1 or more Gadolinium enhancing lesions on brain MRI or a significant increase in T2 lesion load as compared to a previous recent MRI.

Efficacy as monotherapy has been evaluated in one randomised, double-blind, placebo-controlled study lasting 2 years (AFFIRM study) in relapsing-remitting MS patients who had experienced at least 1 clinical relapse during the year prior to entry and had a Kurtzke Expanded Disability Status Scale (EDSS) score between 0 and 5. Median age was 37 years, with a median disease duration of 5 years. The patients were randomised with a 2:1 ratio to receive TYSABRI 300 mg (n = 627) or placebo (n = 315) every 4 weeks for up to 30 infusions. Neurological evaluations were performed every 12 weeks and at times of suspected relapse. MRI evaluations for T1-weighted gadolinium (Gd)-enhancing lesions and T2-hyperintense lesions were performed annually.

Study features and results are presented in the table below.

AFFIRM study: Main features and results		
Design	Monotherapy; randomised double-blind placebo-controlled parallel-group trial for 120 weeks	
Subjects	RRMS (McDonald criteria)	
Treatment	Placebo / Natalizumab 300 mg i.v. every 4 weeks	
One year endpoint	Relapse rate	
Two year endpoint	Progression on EDSS	
Secondary endpoints	Relapse rate derived variables / MRI-derived variables	
Subjects	Placebo	Natalizumab
Randomised	315	627
Completing 1 years	296	609
Completing 2 years	285	589
Age yrs, median (range)	37 (19-50)	36 (18-50)

MS-history yrs, median (range)	6.0 (0-33)	5.0 (0-34)
Time since diagnosis, yrs median (range)	2.0 (0-23)	2.0 (0-24)
Relapses in previous 12 months, median (range)	1.0 (0-5)	1.0 (0-12)
EDSS-baseline, median (range)	2 (0-6.0)	2 (0-6.0)
RESULTS		
Annual relapse rate		
After one year (primary endpoint)	0.805	0.261
After two years	0.733	0.235
One year	Rate ratio 0.33 $CI_{95\%}$ 0.26; 0.41	
Two years	Rate ratio 0.32 $CI_{95\%}$ 0.26; 0.40	
Relapse free		
After one year	53%	76%
After two years	41%	67%
Disability		
Proportion progressed[1] (12-week confirmation; primary outcome)	29%	17%
	Hazard ratio 0.58, $CI_{95\%}$ 0.43; 0.73, $p<0.001$	
Proportion progressed[1] (24-week confirmation)	23%	11%
	Hazard ratio 0.46, $CI_{95\%}$ 0.33; 0.64, $p<0.001$	
MRI (0-2 years)		
Median % change in T2-hyperintense lesion volume	+8.8%	-9.4% ($p<0.001$)
Mean number of new or newly-enlarging T2-hyperintense lesions	11.0	1.9 ($p<0.001$)
Mean number of T1-hypointense lesions	4.6	1.1 ($p<0.001$)
Mean number of Gd-enhancing lesions	1.2	0.1 ($p<0.001$)

[1] Progression of disability was defined as at least a 1.0 point increase on the EDSS from a baseline EDSS >=1.0 sustained for 12 or 24 weeks or at least a 1.5 point increase on the EDSS from a baseline EDSS =0 sustained for 12 or 24 weeks.

In the sub-group of patients indicated for treatment of rapidly evolving relapsing remitting MS (patients with 2 or more relapses and 1 or more Gd+ lesion), the annualised relapse rate was 0.282 in the TYSABRI treated group (n = 148) and 1.455 in the placebo group (n = 61) (p <0.001). Hazard ratio for disability progression was 0.36 (95% CI: 0.17, 0.76) p = 0.008. These results were obtained from a *post hoc* analysis and should be interpreted cautiously. No information on the severity of the relapses before inclusion of patients in the study is available.

5.2 Pharmacokinetic properties

Following the repeat intravenous administration of a 300 mg dose of natalizumab to MS patients, the mean maximum observed serum concentration was 110 ± 52 μg/ml. Mean average steady-state trough natalizumab concentrations over the dosing period ranged from 23 μg/ml to 29 μg/ml. The predicted time to steady-state was approximately 36 weeks.

A population pharmacokinetics analysis was conducted on samples from over 1,100 MS patients receiving doses ranging from 3 to 6 mg/kg natalizumab. Of these, 581 patients received a fixed 300 mg dose as monotherapy. The mean ± SD steady-state clearance was 13.1 ± 5.0 ml/h, with a mean ± SD half-life of 16 ± 4 days. The analysis explored the effects of selected covariates including body weight, age, gender, hepatic and renal function, and presence of anti-natalizumab antibodies upon pharmacokinetics. Only body weight and the presence of anti-natalizumab antibodies were found to influence natalizumab disposition. Body weight was found to influence clearance in a less-than-proportional manner, such that a 43% change in body weight resulted in a 31% to 34% change in clearance. The change in clearance was not clinically significant. The presence of persistent anti-natalizumab antibodies increased natalizumab clearance approximately 3-fold, consistent with reduced serum natalizumab concentrations observed in persistently antibody-positive patients, (see section 4.8).

The pharmacokinetics of natalizumab in paediatric MS patients or in patients with renal or hepatic insufficiency has not been studied.

The effect of plasma exchange on natalizumab clearance and pharmacodynamics was evaluated in a study of 12 MS patients. Estimates of the total drug removal after 3 plasma exchanges (over a 5-8 day interval) was approximately 70-80%. This compares to approximately 40% seen in earlier studies in which measurements occurred after drug discontinuation over a similar period of observation. The impact of plasma exchange on the restitution of lymphocyte migration and ultimately its clinical usefulness is unknown.

5.3 Preclinical safety data

Non-clinical data reveal no special hazard for humans based on conventional studies of safety pharmacology, repeated dose toxicity and genotoxicity.

Consistent with the pharmacological activity of natalizumab, altered trafficking of lymphocytes was seen as white blood cell increases as well as increased spleen weights in most *in vivo* studies. These changes were reversible and did not appear to have any adverse toxicological consequences.

In studies conducted in mice, growth and metastasis of melanoma and lymphoblastic leukaemia tumour cells was not increased by the administration of natalizumab.

No clastogenic or mutagenic effects of natalizumab were observed in the Ames or human chromosomal aberration assays. Natalizumab showed no effects on *in vitro* assays of α4-integrin-positive tumour line proliferation or cytotoxicity.

Reductions in female guinea pig fertility were observed in one study at doses in excess of the human dose; natalizumab did not affect male fertility.

The effect of natalizumab on reproduction was evaluated in 5 studies, 3 in guinea pigs and 2 in *cynomolgus* monkeys. These studies showed no evidence of teratogenic effects or effects on growth of offspring. In one study in guinea pigs, a small reduction in pup survival was noted. In a study in monkeys, the number of abortions was doubled in the natalizumab 30 mg/kg treatment groups versus matching control groups. This was the result of a high incidence of abortions in treated groups in the first cohort that was not observed in the second cohort. No effects on abortion rates were noted in any other study. A study in pregnant *cynomolgus* monkeys demonstrated natalizumab-related changes in the foetus that included mild anaemia, reduced platelet counts, increased spleen weights and reduced liver and thymus weights. These changes were associated with increased splenic extramedullary haematopoiesis, thymic atrophy and decreased hepatic haematopoiesis. Platelet counts were also reduced in offspring born to mothers treated with natalizumab until parturition, however there was no evidence of anaemia in these offspring. All changes were observed at doses in excess of the human dose and were reversed upon clearance of natalizumab.

In *cynomolgus* monkeys treated with natalizumab until parturition, low levels of natalizumab were detected in the breast milk of some animals, indicating the possibility for transfer of natalizumab into breast milk in humans (see section 4.6).

6. PHARMACEUTICAL PARTICULARS

6.1 List of excipients

Sodium phosphate, monobasic, monohydrate

Sodium phosphate, dibasic, heptahydrate

Sodium chloride

Polysorbate 80 (E433)

Water for Injections.

6.2 Incompatibilities

TYSABRI must not be mixed with other medicinal products except those mentioned in section 6.6.

6.3 Shelf life

Concentrate

4 years

Diluted solution

After dilution, immediate use is recommended. If not used immediately, the diluted solution must be stored at 2°C - 8°C and infused within 8 hours of dilution. In-use storage times and conditions prior to use are the responsibility of the user.

6.4 Special precautions for storage

Concentrate

Store in a refrigerator (2°C - 8°C).

Do not freeze.

Keep the vial in the outer carton in order to protect from light.

For storage conditions of the diluted medicinal product see section 6.3.

6.5 Nature and contents of container

15 ml TYSABRI in a vial (type I glass) with a stopper (bromobutyl rubber) and a seal (aluminium) with a flip-off cap. Pack size of one vial per carton.

6.6 Special precautions for disposal and other handling

Instructions for use:

1. Inspect the TYSABRI vial for particles prior to dilution and administration. If particles are observed and/or the liquid in the vial is not colourless, clear to slightly opalescent, the vial must not be used.

2. Use aseptic technique when preparing TYSABRI solution for intravenous (IV) infusion. Remove flip-off cap from the vial. Insert the syringe needle into the vial through the centre of the rubber stopper and remove 15 ml concentrate for solution for infusion.

3. Add the 15 ml concentrate for solution for infusion to 100 ml sodium chloride 9 mg/ml (0.9%) solution for injection. Gently invert the TYSABRI solution to mix completely. Do not shake.

4. TYSABRI must not be mixed with other medicinal products or diluents.

5 Visually inspect the diluted product for particles or discolouration prior to administration. Do not use if it is discoloured or if foreign particles are seen.

6. The diluted product is to be used as soon as possible and within 8 hours of dilution. If the diluted product is stored at 2°C - 8°C (do not freeze), allow the solution to warm to room temperature prior to infusion.

7. The diluted solution is to be infused intravenously over 1 hour at a rate of approximately 2 ml/minute.

8. After the infusion is complete, flush the intravenous line with sodium chloride 9 mg/ml (0.9%) solution for injection.

9. Each vial is for single–use only.

10. Any unused product or waste material must be disposed of in accordance with local requirements.

7. MARKETING AUTHORISATION HOLDER

Elan Pharma International Ltd., Monksland, Athlone, County Westmeath, Ireland

8. MARKETING AUTHORISATION NUMBER(S)

EU/1/06/346/001

9. DATE OF FIRST AUTHORISATION/RENEWAL OF THE AUTHORISATION

27th June 2006

10. DATE OF REVISION OF THE TEXT

01/2009

Detailed information on this product is available on the website of the European Medicines Agency (EMEA) http://www.emea.europa.eu/.

Tyverb

(GlaxoSmithKline UK)

1. NAME OF THE MEDICINAL PRODUCT

Tyverb ▼ 250 mg film-coated tablets

2. QUALITATIVE AND QUANTITATIVE COMPOSITION

Each film-coated tablet contains lapatinib ditosylate monohydrate, equivalent to 250 mg lapatinib.

For a full list of excipients, see section 6.1.

3. PHARMACEUTICAL FORM

Film-coated tablet.

Oval, biconvex, yellow film-coated tablets, with "GS XJG" debossed on one side.

4. CLINICAL PARTICULARS

4.1 Therapeutic indications

Tyverb, in combination with capecitabine, is indicated for the treatment of patients with advanced or metastatic breast cancer whose tumours overexpress ErbB2 (HER2). Patients should have progressive disease following prior therapy which must include anthracyclines and taxanes and therapy with trastuzumab in the metastatic setting (see section 5.1).

4.2 Posology and method of administration

Lapatinib treatment should only be initiated by a physician experienced in the administration of anti-cancer agents.

ErbB2 overexpressing tumours are defined by IHC3+, or IHC2+ and gene amplification or gene amplification alone. Gene amplification should be performed using an accurate and validated assay.

Lapatinib is taken in combination with capecitabine.

The recommended dose of lapatinib is 1250 mg (i.e. five tablets) once daily continuously. The daily dose should not be divided. Lapatinib should be taken either at least one hour before, or at least one hour after food. To minimise variability in the individual patient, administration of lapatinib should be standardised in relation to food intake, for example always be taken before a meal (see sections 4.5 and 5.2 for information on absorption).

Missed doses should not be replaced and the dosing should resume with the next scheduled daily dose (see section 4.9).

The recommended dose of capecitabine is 2000 mg/m²/day taken in 2 doses 12 hours apart on days 1-14 in a 21 day cycle (see section 5.1). Capecitabine should be taken with food or within 30 minutes after food.

Dose delay and dose reduction

Cardiac events

Lapatinib should be discontinued in patients with symptoms associated with decreased left ventricular ejection fraction (LVEF) that are National Cancer Institute Common Terminology Criteria for Adverse Events (NCI CTCAE) grade 3 or greater or if their LVEF drops below the institutions lower limit of normal (see section 4.4). Lapatinib may be restarted at a reduced dose (1000 mg/day) after a minimum of 2 weeks and if the LVEF recovers to normal and the patient is asymptomatic.

Interstitial lung disease / pneumonitis

Lapatinib should be discontinued in patients who experience pulmonary symptoms which are NCI CTCAE grade 3 or greater (see section 4.4).

Other toxicities

Discontinuation or interruption of dosing with lapatinib may be considered when a patient develops toxicity greater than or equal to grade 2 on the National Cancer Institute Common Terminology Criteria for Adverse Events (NCI CTCAE). Dosing can be restarted at 1250 mg/day when the toxicity improves to grade 1 or less. If the toxicity recurs, then lapatinib should be restarted at a lower dose (1000 mg/day).

The prescribing information for capecitabine must be consulted for guidance on dose delay and dose reduction recommendations for capecitabine.

Renal impairment

No dose adjustment is necessary in patients with mild to moderate renal impairment. Caution is advised in patients with severe renal impairment as there is no experience of lapatinib in this population (see section 5.2).

Hepatic impairment

Lapatinib should be discontinued if changes in liver function are severe and patients should not be retreated (see section 4.4).

Administration of lapatinib to patients with moderate to severe hepatic impairment should be undertaken with caution due to increased exposure to the medicinal product. Insufficient data are available in patients with hepatic impairment to provide a dose adjustment recommendation (see section 5.2).

Paediatrics

Tyverb is not recommended for use in paediatrics due to insufficient data on safety and efficacy.

Elderly

There are limited data of the use of lapatinib in patients aged 65 years and older.

4.3 Contraindications

Hypersensitivity to the active substance or to any of the excipients.

Please refer to the capecitabine prescribing information for relevant contraindications and safety information when administering lapatinib in combination with capecitabine.

4.4 Special warnings and precautions for use

Lapatinib has been associated with reports of decreases in left ventricular ejection fraction (LVEF) (see section 4.8). Caution should be taken if lapatinib is to be administered to patients with conditions that could impair left ventricular function. LVEF should be evaluated in all patients prior to initiation of treatment with lapatinib to ensure that the patient has a baseline LVEF that is within the institutions normal limits. LVEF should continue to be evaluated during treatment with lapatinib to ensure that LVEF does not decline to an unacceptable level (see section 4.2).

Lapatinib has been associated with reports of pulmonary toxicity including interstitial lung disease and pneumonitis (see section 4.8). Patients should be monitored for symptoms of pulmonary toxicity (see section 4.2).

Hepatotoxicity has occurred with lapatinib use and may in rare cases be fatal. Liver function (transaminases, bilirubin and alkaline phosphatase) should be monitored before initiation of treatment and monthly thereafter, or as clinically indicated. Lapatinib dosing should be discontinued if changes in liver function are severe and patients should not be retreated.

Caution is warranted if lapatinib is prescribed to patients with moderate or severe hepatic impairment (see sections 4.2 and 5.2).

Caution is advised if lapatinib is prescribed to patients with severe renal impairment (see sections 4.2 and 5.2).

Diarrhoea, including severe diarrhoea, has been reported with lapatinib treatment (see section 4.8). Proactive management of diarrhoea with anti-diarrhoeal agents is important. Severe cases of diarrhoea may require administration of oral or intravenous electrolytes and fluids, and interruption or discontinuation of lapatinib therapy (see section 4.2 – dose delay and dose reduction – other toxicities).

Concomitant treatment with inducers of CYP3A4 should be avoided due to risk of decreased exposure to lapatinib (see section 4.5).

Concomitant treatment with strong inhibitors of CYP3A4 should be avoided due to risk of increased exposure to lapatinib (see section 4.5).

Grapefruit juice should be avoided during treatment with lapatinib (see section 4.5).

Coadministration of lapatinib with medicinal product with narrow therapeutic windows that are substrates of CYP3A4 or CYP2C8 should be avoided (see section 4.5).

Concomitant treatment with substances that increase gastric pH should be avoided, as lapatinib solubility and absorption may decrease (see section 4.5).

4.5 Interaction with other medicinal products and other forms of interaction

Effects of other medicinal products on lapatinib

Lapatinib is predominantly metabolised by CYP3A (see section 5.2).

In healthy volunteers receiving ketoconazole, a strong CYP3A4 inhibitor, at 200 mg twice daily for 7 days, systemic exposure to lapatinib (100 mg daily) was increased approximately 3.6–fold, and half-life increased 1.7–fold. Coadministration of lapatinib with strong inhibitors of CYP3A4 (e.g. ritonavir, saquinavir, telithromycin, ketoconazole, itraconazole, voriconazole, posaconazole, nefazodone) should be avoided. Coadministration of lapatinib with moderate inhibitors of CYP3A4 should proceed with caution and clinical adverse reactions should be carefully monitored.

In healthy volunteers receiving carbamazepine, a CYP3A4 inducer, at 100 mg twice daily for 3 days and 200 mg twice daily for 17 days, systemic exposure to lapatinib was decreased approximately 72%. Coadministration of lapatinib with known inducers of CYP3A4 (e.g. rifampicin, rifabutin, carbamazepine, phenytoin or Hypericum perforatum [St John's wort]) should be avoided.

Lapatinib is a substrate for the transport proteins Pgp and BCRP. Inhibitors (ketoconazole, itraconazole, quinidine, verapamil, cyclosporine, erythromycin) and inducers (rifampin, St John's Wort) of these proteins may alter the exposure and/or distribution of lapatinib (see section 5.2).

The solubility of lapatinib is pH-dependent. Concomitant treatment with substances that increase gastric pH should be avoided, as lapatinib solubility and absorption may decrease.

Effects of lapatinib on other medicinal products

Lapatinib inhibits CYP3A4 and CYP2C8 *in vitro* at clinically relevant concentrations. Coadministration of lapatinib with medicines with narrow therapeutic windows that are substrates of CYP3A4 (e.g. cisapride, pimozide and quinidine) or CYP2C8 (e.g. repaglinide) should be avoided (see sections 4.4 and 5.2).

If lapatinib is administered in combination with paclitaxel (175 mg/m^2 every three weeks), severe neutropenia may coincide with diarrhoea. This warrants monitoring and early treatment of diarrhoea.

Lapatinib inhibits the transport proteins Pgp, BCRP and OATP1B1 *in vitro*. The clinical relevance of this effect has not been evaluated. It cannot be excluded that lapatinib will affect the pharmacokinetics of substrates of Pgp (e.g. digoxin), BCRP (e.g. topotecan) and OATP1B1 (e.g. rosuvastatin) (see section 5.2).

Concomitant administration of lapatinib with capecitabine or trastuzumab did not meaningfully alter the pharmacokinetics of these agents (or the metabolites of capecitabine) or lapatinib.

Interactions with food and drink

The bioavailability of lapatinib is increased up to about 4 times by food, depending on e.g. the fat content in the meal (see sections 4.2 and 5.2).

Grapefruit juice may inhibit CYP3A4 in the gut wall and increase the bioavailability of lapatinib and should therefore be avoided during treatment with lapatinib.

4.6 Pregnancy and lactation

There are no adequate data from the use of lapatinib in pregnant women. Studies in animals have shown reproductive toxicity (see section 5.3). The potential risk for humans is not known.

Lapatinib should not be used during pregnancy unless clearly necessary. Women of childbearing potential should be advised to use adequate contraception and avoid becoming pregnant while receiving treatment with lapatinib.

The safe use of lapatinib during lactation has not been established. It is not known whether lapatinib is excreted in human milk. In rats, growth retardation was observed in pups which were exposed to lapatinib via breast milk. Breast feeding must be discontinued in women who are receiving therapy with lapatinib.

4.7 Effects on ability to drive and use machines

No studies on the effects on the ability to drive and use machines have been performed. A detrimental effect on such activities cannot be predicted from the pharmacology of lapatinib. The clinical status of the patient and the adverse event profile of lapatinib should be borne in mind when considering the patient's ability to perform tasks that require judgement, motor or cognitive skills.

4.8 Undesirable effects

Safety of lapatinib has been evaluated as monotherapy or in combination with other chemotherapies for various cancers including patients who received lapatinib in combination with capecitabine (see section 5.1).

The most common adverse reactions (>25%) during therapy with lapatinib plus capecitabine were gastrointestinal (diarrhoea, nausea, and vomiting) or dermatologic (palmar-plantar erythrodysesthesia [PPE] and rash). The incidence of PPE was similar in both lapatinib plus capecitabine and capecitabine alone treatment arms. Diarrhoea was the most common adverse reaction resulting in discontinuation of treatment and this had a similar incidence in both treatment groups (lapatinib plus capecitabine: 5%, capecitabine: 3%).

The following convention has been utilised for the classification of frequency: Very common ((≥1/10), Common (≥1/100 to <1/10), Uncommon (≥1/1,000 to <1/100), Rare (≥1/10,000 to <1/1,000) and Very rare (<1/10,000), not known (cannot be estimated from the available data).

Within each frequency grouping, undesirable effects are presented in order of decreasing seriousness.

The following adverse reactions have been reported to be associated with lapatinib:

Cardiac disorders	
Common	Decreased left ventricular ejection fraction (see section 4.2 - dose reduction – cardiac events and section 4.4)
Respiratory, thoracic and mediastinal disorders	
Uncommon	Interstitial lung disease/pneumonitis
Gastrointestinal disorders	
Very common	Diarrhoea, which may lead to dehydration (see section 4.2 - dose delay and dose reduction – other toxicities and section 4.4). Nausea Vomiting
Skin and subcutaneous tissue disorders	
Very common	Rash (including dermatitis acneiform) (see section 4.2 - dose delay and dose reduction – other toxicities)
Metabolism and nutrition disorders	
Very common	Anorexia
General disorders and administration site conditions	
Very common	Fatigue
Hepatobiliary disorders	
Common	Hyperbilirubinaemia, hepatotoxicity

The following additional adverse reactions have been reported to be associated with lapatinib in combination with capecitabine with a frequency difference of greater than 5% compared to capecitabine alone.

Gastrointestinal disorders	
Very common	Dyspepsia
Skin and subcutaneous tissue disorders	
Very common	Dry skin

In addition, the following adverse reactions were reported to be associated with lapatinib in combination with capecitabine but were seen at a similar frequency in the capecitabine alone arm.

Nervous system disorders	
Common	Headache
Gastrointestinal disorders	
Very common	Stomatitis, constipation, abdominal pain
Skin and subcutaneous tissue disorders	
Very common	Palmar-plantar erythrodysaesthesia
Musculoskeletal and connective tissue disorders	
Very common	Pain in extremity, back pain
General disorders and administrative site conditions	
Very common	Mucosal inflammation
Psychiatric disorders	
Very common	Insomnia

Decreased left ventricular ejection fraction

Left ventricular ejection fraction (LVEF) decreases have been reported in approximately 1% of patients receiving lapatinib and were asymptomatic in more than 90% of cases. LVEF decreases resolved or improved in more than 60% of cases on discontinuation of treatment with lapatinib. Symptomatic LVEF decreases were observed in approximately 0.1% of patients who received lapatinib monotherapy. Observed symptoms included dyspnoea, cardiac failure and palpitations. All events resolved promptly on discontinuation of lapatinib. LVEF decreases were reported in 2.5% of patients who received lapatinib in combination with capecitabine, as compared to 1.0% with capecitabine alone.

Diarrhoea

Diarrhoea occurred in approximately 65 % of patients who received lapatinib in combination with capecitabine. Most cases of diarrhoea were grade 1 or 2 and did not result in discontinuation of treatment with lapatinib. Diarrhoea responds well to proactive management (see section 4.4).

Rash

Rash occurred in approximately 28 % of patients who received lapatinib in combination with capecitabine. Rash was generally low grade and did not result in discontinuation of treatment with lapatinib.

4.9 Overdose

There is no specific antidote for the inhibition of EGFR (ErbB1) and/or ErbB2 (HER2) tyrosine phosphorylation. The maximum oral dose of lapatinib that has been administered in clinical trials is 1800 mg once daily.

There has been a report of one patient who took an overdose of 3000 mg of lapatinib for 10 days and suffered grade 3 diarrhoea and vomiting on day 10. The symptoms resolved following intravenous hydration and interruption of treatment with lapatinib and letrozole.

Lapatinib is not significantly renally excreted and is highly bound to plasma proteins, therefore haemodialysis would not be expected to be an effective method to enhance the elimination of lapatinib.

5. PHARMACOLOGICAL PROPERTIES

5.1 Pharmacodynamic properties

Pharmacotherapeutic group: Protein kinase inhibitor, ATC code: L01XE07

This medicinal product has been authorised under a so-called "conditional approval" scheme.

This means that furrther evidence on this medicinal product is awaited.

The European Medicines Agency (EMEA) will review new information on the product every year and this SPC will be updated as necessary.

Mechanism of action

Lapatinib a 4-anilinoquinazoline, is an inhibitor of the intracellular tyrosine kinase domains of both EGFR (ErbB1) and of ErbB2 (HER2) receptors (estimated Ki^{app} values of 3nM and 13nM, respectively) with a slow off-rate from these receptors (half-life greater than or equal to 300 minutes). Lapatinib inhibits ErbB-driven tumour cell growth *in vitro* and in various animal models.

The growth inhibitory effects of lapatinib were evaluated in trastuzumab-conditioned cell lines. Lapatinib retained significant activity against breast cancer cell lines selected for long-term growth in trastuzumab-containing medium *in vitro*.

Clinical studies

The efficacy and safety of lapatinib in combination with capecitabine in breast cancer patients with good performance status was evaluated in a randomized, phase III trial. Patients eligible for enrolment had ErbB2 (HER2)-over-expressing, locally advanced or metastatic breast cancer, progressing after prior treatment that included taxanes, anthracyclines and trastuzumab. LVEF was evaluated in all patients (using echocardiogram or MUGA) prior to initiation of treatment with lapatinib to ensure baseline LVEF was within the institutions normal limits. In clinical trials LVEF was monitored at approximately eight week intervals during treatment with lapatinib to ensure it did not decline to below the institutions lower limit of normal. The majority of LVEF decreases (greater than 60 %) were observed during the first nine weeks of treatment, however limited data was available for long term exposure.

Patients were randomized to receive either lapatinib 1250 mg once daily (continuously) plus capecitabine (2000 mg/m^2/day on days 1-14 every 21 days), or to receive capecitabine alone (2500 mg/m^2/day on days 1-14 every 21 days). The primary endpoint was time to progression (TTP). Assessments were undertaken by the study investigators and by an independent review panel, blinded to treatment. The study was halted based on the results of a pre-specified interim analysis that showed an improvement in TTP for patients receiving lapatinib plus capecitabine. An additional 75 patients were enrolled in the study between the time of the interim analysis and the end of the enrolment. Investigator analysis on data at the stop of enrolment is presented in the following table.

	Investigator assessment	
	Lapatinib (1,250 mg/day)+ capecitabine (2,000 mg/m^2/day)	**Capecitabine (2,500 mg/m^2/day)**
	(N = 198)	**(N = 201)**
Number of TTP events	121	126
Median TTP, weeks	23.9	18.3
Hazard Ratio	0.72	
(95% CI)	(0.56, 0.92)	
p value	0.008	

The independent assessment of the data also demonstrated that lapatinib when given in combination with capecitabine significantly increased time to progression (Hazard Ratio 0.57 [95 % CI 0.43, 0.77] p=0.0001) compared to capecitabine alone.

Results of an updated analysis of the overall survival data to 28 September 2007 are presented in the table below.

	Lapatinib (1,250 mg/day)+ capecitabine (2,000 mg/m^2/day)	**Capecitabine (2,500 mg/m^2/day)**
	(N = 207)	**(N = 201)**
Number of subjects who died	148	154
Median overall survival, weeks	74.0	65.9
Hazard Ratio	0.9	
(95% CI)	(0.71, 1.12)	
p value	0.3	

On the combination arm, there were 4 (2%) progressions in the central nervous system as compared with the 13 (6%) progressions on the capecitabine alone arm.

5.2 Pharmacokinetic properties

The absolute bioavailability following oral administration of lapatinib is unknown, but it is incomplete and variable (approximately 70% coefficient of variation in AUC). Serum concentrations appear after a median lag time of 0.25 hours (range 0 to 1.5 hours). Peak plasma concentrations (C_{max}) of lapatinib are achieved approximately 4 hours after administration. Daily dosing of 1250 mg produces steady state geometric mean (coefficient of variation) C_{max} values of 2.43 (76%) µg/ml and AUC values of 36.2 (79%) µg*hr/ml.

Systemic exposure to lapatinib is increased when administered with food. Lapatinib AUC values were approximately 3- and 4-fold higher (C_{max} approximately 2.5 and 3–fold higher) when administered with a low fat (5% fat [500 calories]) or with a high fat (50% fat [1,000 calories]) meal, respectively.

Lapatinib is highly bound (greater than 99%) to albumin and alpha-1 acid glycoprotein. *In vitro* studies indicate that lapatinib is a substrate for the transporters BCRP (ABCG1) and p-glycoprotein (ABCB1). Lapatinib has also been shown *in vitro* to inhibit these efflux transporters, as well as the hepatic uptake transporter OATP 1B1, at clinically relevant concentrations (IC_{50} values were equal to 2.3 µg/ml). The clinical significance of these effects on the pharmacokinetics of other medicinal products or the pharmacological activity of other anti-cancer agents is not known.

Lapatinib undergoes extensive metabolism, primarily by CYP3A4 and CYP3A5, with minor contributions from CYP2C19 and CYP2C8 to a variety of oxidated metabolites, none of which account for more than 14% of the dose recovered in the faeces or 10% of lapatinib concentration in plasma.

Lapatinib inhibits CYP3A (Ki 0.6 to 2.3 µg/ml) and CYP2C8 (0.3 µg/ml) *in vitro* at clinically relevant concentrations. Lapatinib did not significantly inhibit the following enzymes in human liver microsomes: CYP1A2, CYP2C9, CYP2C19, and CYP2D6 or UGT enzymes (*in vitro* IC_{50} values were greater than or equal to 6.9 µg/ml).

The half-life of lapatinib measured after single doses increases with increasing dose. However, daily dosing of lapatinib results in achievement of steady state within 6 to 7 days, indicating an effective half-life of 24 hours. Lapatinib is predominantly eliminated through metabolism by CYP3A4/5. Biliary excretion may also contribute to the elimination. The primary route of excretion for lapatinib and its metabolites is in faeces. Recovery of unchanged lapatinib in faeces accounts for a median 27% (range 3 to 67%) of an oral dose. Less than 2% of the administered oral dose (as lapatinib and metabolites) excreted in urine.

Lapatinib pharmacokinetics have not been specifically studied in patients with renal impairment or in patients undergoing haemodialysis. Available data suggest that no dose adjustment is necessary in patients with mild to moderate renal impairment.

The pharmacokinetics of lapatinib were examined in subjects with moderate (n = 8) or severe (n = 4) hepatic impairment (Child-Pugh scores of 7-9, or greater than 9, respectively) and in 8 healthy control subjects. Systemic exposure (AUC) to lapatinib after a single oral 100 mg dose increased approximately 56% and 85% in subjects with moderate and severe hepatic impairment, respectively. Administration of lapatinib in patients with hepatic impairment should be undertaken with caution (see sections 4.2 and 4.4).

5.3 Preclinical safety data

Lapatinib was studied in pregnant rats and rabbits given oral doses of 30, 60, and 120 mg/kg/day. There were no teratogenic effects; however, minor anomalies (left-sided umbilical artery, cervical rib and precocious ossification) occurred in rats at ⩾60 mg/kg/day (4 times the expected human clinical exposure). In rabbits, lapatinib was associated with maternal toxicity at 60 and 120 mg/kg/day (8% and 23% of the expected human clinical exposure, respectively) and abortions at 120 mg/kg/day. At ⩾60 mg/kg/day there were decreased foetal body weights, and minor skeletal variations. In the rat pre- and postnatal development study, a decrease in pup survival occurred between birth and postnatal day 21 at doses of 60 mg/kg/day or higher (5 times the expected human clinical exposure). The highest no-effect dose for this study was 20 mg/kg/day.

In oral carcinogenicity studies with lapatinib, severe skin lesions were seen at the highest doses tested which produced exposures based on AUC up to 2-fold in mice and male rats, and up to 15-fold in female rats, compared to humans given 1250 mg of lapatinib once daily. There was no evidence of carcinogenicity in mice. In rats, the incidence of benign haemangioma of the mesenteric lymph nodes was higher in some groups than in concurrent controls. There was also an increase in renal infarcts and papillary necrosis in female rats at exposures 7 and 10-fold compared to humans given 1250 mg of lapatinib once daily. The relevance of these findings for humans is uncertain.

There were no effects on male or female rat gonadal function, mating, or fertility at doses up to 120 mg/kg/day (females) and up to 180 mg/kg/day (males) (8 and 3 times the expected human clinical exposure, respectively). The effect on human fertility is unknown.

Lapatinib was not clastogenic or mutagenic in a battery of assays including the Chinese hamster chromosome aberration assay, the Ames assay, human lymphocyte chromosome aberration assay and an *in vivo* rat bone marrow chromosome aberration assay.

6. PHARMACEUTICAL PARTICULARS

6.1 List of excipients

Tablet core

Microcrystalline cellulose

Povidone (K30)

Sodium starch glycolate (Type A)

Magnesium stearate

Tablet coating

Hypromellose

Titanium dioxide (E171)

Macrogol 400

Polysorbate 80

Iron oxide yellow (E172)

Iron oxide red (E172)

6.2 Incompatibilities

Not applicable.

6.3 Shelf life

2 years

6.4 Special precautions for storage

Do not store above 30°C.

6.5 Nature and contents of container

Each pack of Tyverb contains 70 tablets in foil blisters (polyamide / aluminium / polyvinyl chloride / aluminium) of 10 tablets each. Each foil has a perforation down the middle to allow the blisters to be separated into a daily dose of 5 tablets.

6.6 Special precautions for disposal and other handling

Any unused product or waste material should be disposed of in accordance with local requirements.

7. MARKETING AUTHORISATION HOLDER

Glaxo Group Limited, Berkeley Avenue, Greenford, Middlesex UB6 0NN, United Kingdom.

8. MARKETING AUTHORISATION NUMBER(S)

EU/1/07/440/001

9. DATE OF FIRST AUTHORISATION/RENEWAL OF THE AUTHORISATION

Date of first authorisation: 10/06/2008

Date of last renewal: 12/06/2009

10. DATE OF REVISION OF THE TEXT

12/06/2009

Detailed information on this medicinal product is available on the website of the European Medicines Agency (EMEA) http://www.emea.europa.eu/.>

Ubretid

(sanofi-aventis)

1. NAME OF THE MEDICINAL PRODUCT
Ubretid™.

2. QUALITATIVE AND QUANTITATIVE COMPOSITION
Active ingredient Distigmine bromide 5mg.

3. PHARMACEUTICAL FORM
Tablets.

4. CLINICAL PARTICULARS

4.1 Therapeutic indications
Anticholinesterase. Post-operative urinary retention. Post operative ileus and intestinal atony. To assist emptying of the neurogenic bladder. As an adjunct in the treatment of myasthenia gravis.

4.2 Posology and method of administration
Adults

In prevention of urinary retention, ileus or intestinal atony following surgery:
One Ubretid tablet daily, half an hour before breakfast.

In neurogenic bladder:
One Ubretid tablet daily or on alternate days, half an hour before breakfast, on an empty stomach.

In myasthenia gravis:
Dosage to be individualised for each patient, dependent upon the severity of the condition, the degree and duration of response and the side effects encountered. The tablets should always be taken on an empty stomach half an hour before breakfast. Dosage should commence at 1 tablet daily and may be adjusted at intervals of three to four days to a total not exceeding 4 tablets daily.

Children
Up to 2 tablets daily according to age.

Elderly
No dosage adjustment is necessary for elderly patients.

Ubretid tablets are for oral administration.

4.3 Contraindications
Ubretid is contraindicated in cases of severe post operative shock, serious circulatory insufficiency, severe constipation, serious spastic and mechanical ileus, asthma and mechanical urinary obstruction.

4.4 Special warnings and precautions for use
Caution should be taken in conditions where the potentiation of the effects of acetylcholine is undesirable, eg cardiac dysfunction, bronchospasm, peptic ulcer, oesophagitis, epilepsy and Parkinsonism. The patient should be supervised in the early stages of dosage titration to guard against the possibility of myasthenic crisis or cholinergic crisis.

4.5 Interaction with other medicinal products and other forms of interaction
Use with caution in patients receiving concomitantly drugs acting on the cardiovascular system, e.g. beta blockers, drugs with local anaesthetic properties and muscle relaxants. In myasthenia gravis, where short acting cholinergic drugs are taken concurrently, their dosage should be reduced to the minimum required to control symptoms.

4.6 Pregnancy and lactation
Ubretid should be avoided during pregnancy. No information is available on lactation.

4.7 Effects on ability to drive and use machines
None stated.

4.8 Undesirable effects
The following side effects may occur infrequently: bradycardia, AV block, hypotension, bronchospasm, dyspnoea, increased bronchial secretions, sweating, salivation and lacrimation, muscle twitching, abdominal cramps, diarrhoea, urinary frequency and miosis. These effects of Ubretid may be controlled with atropine, giving 2mg intramuscularly; atropinisation should be maintained for at least 24 hours.

4.9 Overdose
Overdosage of Ubretid may also produce skeletal muscle fatigue, weakness and eventually paralysis. The muscarinic effects of overdosage may be controlled with atropine 2mg intramuscularly repeated at intervals indicated by the clinical response until signs of mild atropinisation (dry mouth, mydriasis) appear. The patient should be kept fully atropinised for at least 24 hours.

5. PHARMACOLOGICAL PROPERTIES

5.1 Pharmacodynamic properties
Distigmine is an inhibitor of cholinesterase by the formation of complexes with the enzyme. This process is reversible. Specific cholinesterase or acetylcholinesterase is inhibited more strongly than pseudo or plasma cholinesterase.

5.2 Pharmacokinetic properties
Maximum inhibition of plasma cholinesterase occurs 9 hours after a single intramuscular dose and persists for about 24 hours.
Tritium labelled Ubretid was used to determine the urinary and biliary excretion of the drug in the rat. Activity in the urine was demonstrated quickly, amounting to 43% after 8 hours. Biliary excretion was shown to be insignificant. In man, results suggested that about 50% of a 0.5mg 1ml dose was excreted in 24 hours.

5.3 Preclinical safety data
There are no preclinical data of relevance to the prescriber which are additional to that already included in other sections of the SPC.

6. PHARMACEUTICAL PARTICULARS

6.1 List of excipients
Lactose

Maize starch

Purified talc

Magnesium stearate

6.2 Incompatibilities
None stated.

6.3 Shelf life
36 months.

6.4 Special precautions for storage
Store in a dry place below 25°C.

6.5 Nature and contents of container
Blisters of 20μm aluminium foil and 250μm UPVC/PVdC opaque white film containing 30 tablets.

6.6 Special precautions for disposal and other handling
None.

7. MARKETING AUTHORISATION HOLDER
Sanofi-aventis

One Onslow Street

Guildford

Surrey

GU1 4YS, UK

8. MARKETING AUTHORISATION NUMBER(S)
PL 04425/0617

9. DATE OF FIRST AUTHORISATION/RENEWAL OF THE AUTHORISATION
7 February 2009

10. DATE OF REVISION OF THE TEXT
February 2009

11 LEGAL CLASSIFICATION
POM

Ucerax Syrup 10mg/5ml

(UCB Pharma Limited)

1. NAME OF THE MEDICINAL PRODUCT
Ucerax Syrup 10 mg/5ml.

2. QUALITATIVE AND QUANTITATIVE COMPOSITION
Hydroxyzine hydrochloride 2 mg/ml.

For excipients, see 6.1.

3. PHARMACEUTICAL FORM
Syrup.

4. CLINICAL PARTICULARS

4.1 Therapeutic indications
Ucerax is indicated to assist in the management of anxiety.

Ucerax is indicated to assist in the management of pruritus associated with acute and chronic urticaria, including cholinergic and physical types, and in atopic and contact dermatosis in adults and children.

4.2 Posology and method of administration
Adults:

Anxiety.

50 mg/day in 3 separate administrations of 12.5-12.5-25mg. In more severe cases, doses up to 300mg/day can be used.

Pruritus.

Starting dose of 25 mg at night, increasing as necessary to 25 mg three or four times daily.

The maximum single dose in adults should not exceed 200mg whereas the maximum daily doses should not exceed 300mg.

Children:

Children aged from 12 months to 6 years: 1mg/kg/day up to 2.5mg/kg/day in divided doses.

Children aged over 6 years: 1mg/kg/day up to 2mg/kg/day in divided doses.

The dosage should be adjusted according to the patient's response to therapy.

In the elderly, it is advised to start with half the recommended dose due to the prolonged action.

In patients with hepatic dysfunction, it is recommended to reduce the daily dose by 33%.

Dosage should be reduced in patients with moderate or severe renal impairment due to decreased excretion of its metabolite cetirizine.

4.3 Contraindications
Ucerax is contra-indicated in patients with a history of hypersensitivity to any of its constituents, to cetirizine, to other piperazine derivatives, to aminophylline, or to ethylenediamine.

Ucerax is contra-indicated during pregnancy and lactation.
Ucerax is contra-indicated in patients with porphyria.

4.4 Special warnings and precautions for use
Ucerax should be administered cautiously in patients with increased potential for convulsions.

Young children are more susceptible to develop adverse events related to the central nervous system (see section 4.8). In children, convulsions have been more frequently reported than in adults.

Because of its potential anticholinergic effects, Ucerax should be used cautiously in patients suffering from glaucoma, bladder outflow obstruction, decreased gastro-intestinal motility, myasthenia gravis, or dementia.

Dosage adjustments may be required if Ucerax is used simultaneously with other central nervous system depressant drugs or with drugs having anticholinergic properties (see section 4.5).

The concomitant use of alcohol and Ucerax should be avoided (see section 4.5).

Caution is needed in patients who have a known predisposing factor to cardiac arrhythmia, or who are concomitantly treated with a potentially arrhythmogenic drug.

In the elderly, it is advised to start with half the recommended dose due to a prolonged action.

Ucerax dosage should be reduced in patients with hepatic dysfunction and in patients with moderate or severe renal impairment (see section 4.2).

The treatment should be stopped at least 5 days before allergy testing or methacholine bronchial challenge, to avoid effects on the test results.

This product contains ethanol (alcohol), less than 100mg per dose.

This product also contains sucrose and as such care is required in patients with diabetes mellitus. It may be harmful to the teeth.

Due to the presence of sucrose, patients with rare hereditary problems of fructose intolerance, glucose-galactose malabsorption or sucrase-isomaltase insufficiency should not take this medicine.

4.5 Interaction with other medicinal products and other forms of interaction
Patients should be informed that Ucerax may potentiate the effects of barbiturates, other CNS depressants or drugs having anticholinergic properties.

Alcohol also potentiates the effects of Ucerax.

Ucerax antagonizes the effects of betahistine, and of anticholinesterase drugs.

The treatment should be stopped at least 5 days before allergy testing or methacholine bronchial challenge, to avoid effects on the test results.

Simultaneous administration of Ucerax with monoamine oxidase inhibitors should be avoided.

Ucerax counteracts the epinephrine pressor action.

In rats, hydroxyzine antagonised the anticonvulsant action of phenytoin.

Cimetidine 600 mg bid has been shown to increase the serum concentrations of hydroxyzine by 36% and to decrease peak concentrations of the metabolite cetirizine by 20%.

Ucerax is an inhibitor of cytochrome P450 2D6 (Ki: 3.9 μM; 1.7 μg/ml) and may cause at high doses drug-drug interactions with CYP2D6 substrates.

Ucerax has no inhibitory effect at 100 μM on UDP-glucuronyl transferase isoforms 1A1 and 1A6 in human liver microsomes. It inhibits cytochrome P_{450} 2C9/C10, 2C19 and 3A4 isoforms at concentrations (IC_{50} : 19 to 140 μM; 7 to 52 μg/ml) well above peak plasma concentrations. The metabolite cetirizine at 100 μM has no inhibitory effect on human liver cytochrome P_{450} (1A2, 2A6, 2C9/C10, 2C19, 2D6, 2E1 and 3A4) and UDP-glucuronyl transferase isoforms. Therefore, Ucerax is unlikely to impair the metabolism of drugs which are substrates for these enzymes.

As hydroxyzine is metabolized in the liver, an increase in hydroxyzine blood concentrations may be expected when hydroxyzine is co-administered with other drugs known to be potent inhibitors of liver enzymes.

4.6 Pregnancy and lactation

Animal studies have shown reproductive toxicity.

Hydroxyzine crosses the placental barrier leading to higher fetal than maternal concentrations.

To date, no relevant epidemiological data are available relating to exposure to Ucerax during pregnancy.

In neonates whose mothers received Ucerax during late pregnancy and/or labour, the following events were observed immediately or only a few hours after birth: hypotonia, movement disorders including extrapyramidal disorders, clonic movements, CNS depression, neonatal hypoxic conditions, or urinary retention.

Therefore, Ucerax should not be used during pregnancy.

Ucerax is contra-indicated during lactation. Breast-feeding should be stopped if Ucerax therapy is needed.

4.7 Effects on ability to drive and use machines

Alertness or reaction time may be impaired by Ucerax therefore patients' driving capacity or ability to use machines may be reduced. Concomitant use of Ucerax with alcohol or other sedative drugs should be avoided as it aggravates these effects.

4.8 Undesirable effects

Undesirable effects are mainly related to CNS depressant or paradoxical CNS stimulation effects, to anticholinergic activity, or to hypersensitivity reactions. The following adverse reactions, in MedDRA terms, have been spontaneously reported:

Cardiac disorders:

Tachycardia NOS

Eye disorders:

Accommodation disorder, vision blurred

Gastrointestinal disorders:

Constipation, dry mouth, nausea, vomiting NOS

General disorders and administration site conditions:

Fatigue, malaise, pyrexia

Immune system disorders:

Anaphylactic shock, hypersensitivity NOS

Investigations:

Liver function tests NOS abnormal

Nervous system disorders:

Convulsions NOS, dizziness, dyskinesia NEC, headache NOS, insomnia NEC, sedation, somnolence, tremor NEC

Psychiatric disorders:

Agitation, confusion, disorientation, hallucination NOS

Renal and urinary disorders:

Urinary retention

Respiratory, thoracic and mediastinal disorders:

Bronchospasm NOS

Skin and subcutaneous tissue disorders:

Angioneurotic oedema, dermatitis NOS, pruritus NOS, rash erythematous, rash maculo-papular, sweating increased, urticaria NOS

Vascular disorders:

Hypotension NOS.

4.9 Overdose

Symptoms observed after an important overdose are mainly associated with excessive anticholinergic load, CNS depression or CNS paradoxical stimulation. They include nausea, vomiting, tachycardia, pyrexia, somnolence, impaired pupillary reflex, tremor, confusion, or hallucination. This may be followed by depressed level of consciousness, respiratory depression, convulsions, hypotension, or cardiac arrhythmia. Deepening coma and cardiorespiratory collapse may ensue.

Airway, breathing and circulatory status must be closely monitored with continuous ECG recording and an adequate oxygen supply should be available. Cardiac and blood pressure monitoring should be maintained until the patient is free of symptoms for 24 hours. Patients with altered mental status should be checked for simultaneous intake of other drugs or alcohol and should be given oxygen, naloxone, glucose, and thiamine if deemed necessary.

Norepinephrine or metaraminol should be used if vasopressor is needed. Epinephrine should not be used.

Syrup of ipecac should not be administered in symptomatic patients or those who could rapidly become obtunded, comatose or convulsing, as this could lead to aspiration pneumonitis. Gastric lavage with prior endotracheal intubation may be performed if a clinically significant ingestion has occurred. Activated charcoal may be left in the stomach but there are scant data to support its efficacy.

It is doubtful that hemodialysis or hemoperfusion would be of any value.

There is no specific antidote.

Literature data indicate that, in the presence of severe, life-threatening, intractable anticholinergic effects unresponsive to other agents, a therapeutic trial dose of physostigmine may be useful. Physostigmine should not be used just to keep the patient awake. If cyclic antidepressants have been coingested, use of physostigmine may precipitate seizures and intractable cardiac arrest. Also avoid physostigmine in patients with cardiac conduction defects.

5. PHARMACOLOGICAL PROPERTIES

5.1 Pharmacodynamic properties

Hydroxyzine is an anxiolytic compound with a rapid onset of action and a wide margin of safety. It is unrelated chemically to the phenothiazines, reserpine, meprobamate or benzodiazepines.

Its action may be due to a suppression of activity in certain key regions of the subcortical area of the CNS.

Hydroxyzine also has potent antihistaminic properties.

5.2 Pharmacokinetic properties

In man a mean maximum hydroxyzine plasma concentration of about 30 to 80 ng/ml occurs about 2 to 5 hours after single oral doses of 25 to 100 mg. The drug and its metabolites are widely distributed in the tissues. Hydroxyzine crosses the blood - brain barrier and the placental barrier. Elimination is biphasic with a terminal half-life of about 20 hours.

5.3 Preclinical safety data

There is no pre-clincal data of relevance to the subscriber additional to that noted in other sections of this SPC.

6. PHARMACEUTICAL PARTICULARS

6.1 List of excipients

Sucrose.

Ethyl alcohol.

Sodium benzoate.

Menthol.

Imitation hazelnut flavour.

Purified water.

6.2 Incompatibilities

None.

6.3 Shelf life

3 years

6.4 Special precautions for storage

Do not store above 25 °C. Keep container in the outer carton.

6.5 Nature and contents of container

Amber glass bottle, with a polypropylene screw cap and polyethylene inner liner, containing 100 or 200 ml of syrup

6.6 Special precautions for disposal and other handling

Not applicable.

7. MARKETING AUTHORISATION HOLDER

UCB Pharma Limited

208 Bath Road

Slough

Berkshire

SL1 3WE

8. MARKETING AUTHORISATION NUMBER(S)

PL 00039/0537

9. DATE OF FIRST AUTHORISATION/RENEWAL OF THE AUTHORISATION

16.08.2001.

10. DATE OF REVISION OF THE TEXT

February 2006

Ucerax Tablets 25 mg

(UCB Pharma Limited)

1. NAME OF THE MEDICINAL PRODUCT

Ucerax Tablets 25 mg.

2. QUALITATIVE AND QUANTITATIVE COMPOSITION

Hydroxyzine hydrochloride 25 mg.

For excipients, see 6.1.

3. PHARMACEUTICAL FORM

Film-coated tablets.

4. CLINICAL PARTICULARS

4.1 Therapeutic indications

Ucerax is indicated to assist in the management of anxiety.

Ucerax is indicated to assist in the management of pruritus associated with acute and chronic urticaria, including cholinergic and physical types, and in atopic and contact dermatosis in adults and children.

4.2 Posology and method of administration

Adults:

Anxiety.

50 mg/day in 3 separate administrations of 12.5-12.5-25mg. In more severe cases, doses up to 300mg/day can be used.

Pruritus.

Starting dose of 25 mg at night, increasing as necessary to 25 mg three or four times daily.

The maximum single dose in adults should not exceed 200mg whereas the maximum daily doses should not exceed 300mg.

Children:

Children aged from 12 months to 6 years: 1mg/kg/day up to 2.5mg/kg/day in divided doses.

Children aged over 6 years:1mg/kg/day up to 2mg/kg/day in divided doses.

The dosage should be adjusted according to the patient's response to therapy.

In the elderly, it is advised to start with half the recommended dose due to the prolonged action.

In patients with hepatic dysfunction, it is recommended to reduce the daily dose by 33%.

Dosage should be reduced in patients with moderate or severe renal impairment due to decreased excretion of its metabolite cetirizine.

4.3 Contraindications

Ucerax is contra-indicated in patients with a history of hypersensitivity to any of its constituents, to cetirizine, to other piperazine derivatives, to aminophylline, or to ethylenediamine.

Ucerax is contra-indicated during pregnancy and lactation.

Ucerax is contra-indicated in patients with porphyria.

4.4 Special warnings and precautions for use

Ucerax should be administered cautiously in patients with increased potential for convulsions.

Young children are more susceptible to develop adverse events related to the central nervous system (see section 4.8). In children, convulsions have been more frequently reported than in adults.

Because of its potential anticholinergic effects, Ucerax should be used cautiously in patients suffering from glaucoma, bladder outflow obstruction, decreased gastro-intestinal motility, myasthenia gravis, or dementia.

Dosage adjustments may be required if Ucerax is used simultaneously with other central nervous system depressant drugs or with drugs having anticholinergic properties (see section 4.5).

The concomitant use of alcohol and Ucerax should be avoided (see section 4.5).

Caution is needed in patients who have a known predisposing factor to cardiac arrhythmia, or who are concomitantly treated with a potentially arrhythmogenic drug.

In the elderly, it is advised to start with half the recommended dose due to a prolonged action.

Ucerax dosage should be reduced in patients with hepatic dysfunction and in patients with moderate or severe renal impairment (see section 4.2).

The treatment should be stopped at least 5 days before allergy testing or methacholine bronchial challenge, to avoid effects on the test results.

Due to the presence of lactose, patients with rare hereditary problems of galactose intolerance, the Lapp lactase deficiency or glucose-galactose malabsorption should not take this medicine.

4.5 Interaction with other medicinal products and other forms of interaction

Patients should be informed that Ucerax may potentiate the effects of barbiturates, other CNS depressants or drugs having anticholinergic properties.

Alcohol also potentiates the effects of Ucerax.

Ucerax antagonizes the effects of betahistine, and of anticholinesterase drugs.

The treatment should be stopped at least 5 days before allergy testing or methacholine bronchial challenge, to avoid effects on the test results.

Simultaneous administration of Ucerax with monoamine oxidase inhibitors should be avoided.

Ucerax counteracts the epinephrine pressor action.

In rats, hydroxyzine antagonised the anticonvulsant action of phenytoin.

Cimetidine 600 mg bid has been shown to increase the serum concentrations of hydroxyzine by 36% and to decrease peak concentrations of the metabolite cetirizine by 20%.

Ucerax is an inhibitor of cytochrome P450 2D6 (Ki: 3.9 μM; 1.7 μg/ml) and may cause at high doses drug-drug interactions with CYP2D6 substrates.

Ucerax has no inhibitory effect at 100 μM on UDP-glucuronyl transferase isoforms 1A1 and 1A6 in human liver microsomes. It inhibits cytochrome P_{450} 2C9/C10, 2C19 and 3A4 isoforms at concentrations (IC_{50} : 19 to 140 μM; 7 to 52 μg/ml) well above peak plasma concentrations. The metabolite cetirizine at 100 μM has no inhibitory effect on human liver cytochrome P_{450} (1A2, 2A6, 2C9/C10, 2C19, 2D6, 2E1 and 3A4) and UDP-glucuronyl transferase isoforms. Therefore, Ucerax is unlikely to impair the metabolism of drugs which are substrates for these enzymes.

As hydroxyzine is metabolized in the liver, an increase in hydroxyzine blood concentrations may be expected when hydroxyzine is co-administered with other drugs known to be potent inhibitors of liver enzymes.

4.6 Pregnancy and lactation
Animal studies have shown reproductive toxicity.

Hydroxyzine crosses the placental barrier leading to higher fetal than maternal concentrations.

To date, no relevant epidemiological data are available relating to exposure to Ucerax during pregnancy.

In neonates whose mothers received Ucerax during late pregnancy and/or labour, the following events were observed immediately or only a few hours after birth: hypotonia, movement disorders including extrapyramidal disorders, clonic movements, CNS depression, neonatal hypoxic conditions, or urinary retention.

Therefore, Ucerax should not be used during pregnancy.

Ucerax is contra-indicated during lactation. Breast-feeding should be stopped if Ucerax therapy is needed.

4.7 Effects on ability to drive and use machines
Alertness or reaction time may be impaired by Ucerax therefore patients' driving capacity or ability to use machines may be reduced. Concomitant use of Ucerax with alcohol or other sedative drugs should be avoided as it aggravates these effects.

4.8 Undesirable effects
Undesirable effects are mainly related to CNS depressant or paradoxical CNS stimulation effects, to anticholinergic activity, or to hypersensitivity reactions. The following adverse reactions, in MedDRA terms, have been spontaneously reported:

Cardiac disorders:
Tachycardia NOS

Eye disorders:
Accommodation disorder, vision blurred

Gastrointestinal disorders:
Constipation, dry mouth, nausea, vomiting NOS

General disorders and administration site conditions:
Fatigue, malaise, pyrexia

Immune system disorders:
Anaphylactic shock, hypersensitivity NOS

Investigations:
Liver function tests NOS abnormal

Nervous system disorders:
Convulsions NOS, dizziness, dyskinesia NEC, headache NOS, insomnia NEC, sedation, somnolence, tremor NEC

Psychiatric disorders:
Agitation, confusion, disorientation, hallucination NOS

Renal and urinary disorders:
Urinary retention

Respiratory, thoracic and mediastinal disorders:
Bronchospasm NOS

Skin and subcutaneous tissue disorders:
Angioneurotic oedema, dermatitis NOS, pruritus NOS, rash erythematous, rash maculo-papular, sweating increased, urticaria NOS

Vascular disorders:
Hypotension NOS

4.9 Overdose
Symptoms observed after an important overdose are mainly associated with excessive anticholinergic load, CNS depression or CNS paradoxical stimulation. They include nausea, vomiting, tachycardia, pyrexia, somnolence, impaired pupillary reflex, tremor, confusion, or hallucination. This may be followed by depressed level of consciousness, respiratory depression, convulsions, hypotension, or cardiac arrhythmia. Deepening coma and cardiorespiratory collapse may ensue.

Airway, breathing and circulatory status must be closely monitored with continuous ECG recording and an adequate oxygen supply should be available. Cardiac and blood pressure monitoring should be maintained until the patient is free of symptoms for 24 hours. Patients with altered mental status should be checked for simultaneous intake of other drugs or alcohol and should be given oxygen, naloxone, glucose, and thiamine if deemed necessary.

Norepinephrine or metaraminol should be used if vasopressor is needed. Epinephrine should not be used.

Syrup of ipecac should not be administered in symptomatic patients or those who could rapidly become obtunded, comatose or convulsing, as this could lead to aspiration pneumonitis. Gastric lavage with prior endotracheal intubation may be performed if a clinically significant ingestion has occurred. Activated charcoal may be left in the stomach but there are scant data to support its efficacy.

It is doubtful that hemodialysis or hemoperfusion would be of any value.

There is no specific antidote.

Literature data indicate that, in the presence of severe, life-threatening, intractable anticholinergic effects unresponsive to other agents, a therapeutic trial dose of physostigmine may be useful. Physostigmine should not be used just to keep the patient awake. If cyclic antidepressants have been coingested, use of physostigmine may precipitate seizures and intractable cardiac arrest. Also avoid physostigmine in patients with cardiac conduction defects.

5. PHARMACOLOGICAL PROPERTIES

5.1 Pharmacodynamic properties
Hydroxyzine is an anxiolytic compound with a rapid onset of action and a wide margin of safety. It is unrelated chemically to the phenothiazines, reserpine, meprobamate or benzodiazepines.

Its action may be due to a suppression of activity in certain key regions of the subcortical area of the CNS.

Hydroxyzine also has potent antihistaminic properties.

5.2 Pharmacokinetic properties
In man a mean maximum hydroxyzine plasma concentration of about 30 to 80 ng/ml occurs about 2 to 5 hours after single oral doses of 25 to 100 mg. The drug and its metabolites are widely distributed in the tissues. Hydroxyzine crosses the blood - brain barrier and the placental barrier. Elimination is biphasic with a terminal half-life of about 20 hours.

5.3 Preclinical safety data
There is no pre-clinical data of relevance to the subscriber additional to that noted in other sections of this SPC.

6. PHARMACEUTICAL PARTICULARS

6.1 List of excipients
Lactose monohydrate.

Microcrystalline cellulose

Magnesium stearate

Anhydrous colloidal silica

Purified water

Opadry® Y-1-7000 containing:

Titanium dioxide

Hydroxypropylmethylcellulose 2910 5cP

Macrogol 400.

6.2 Incompatibilities
None.

6.3 Shelf life
5 years.

6.4 Special precautions for storage
Keep container in the outer pack.

6.5 Nature and contents of container
Aluminium foil / PVC blister packs containing 25, 30, 50 or 60 tablets.

6.6 Special precautions for disposal and other handling
Not applicable.

7. MARKETING AUTHORISATION HOLDER
UCB Pharma Limited

208 Bath Road

Slough

Berkshire

SL1 3WE

8. MARKETING AUTHORISATION NUMBER(S)
PL 00039/0538

9. DATE OF FIRST AUTHORISATION/RENEWAL OF THE AUTHORISATION
16 August 2001

10. DATE OF REVISION OF THE TEXT
February 2006

Uftoral Hard Capsules

(Merck Serono)

1. NAME OF THE MEDICINAL PRODUCT
Uftoral 100 mg/224 mg hard capsules

2. QUALITATIVE AND QUANTITATIVE COMPOSITION
Each Uftoral capsule contains tegafur (100 mg) and uracil (224 mg).

For excipients, see 6.1.

3. PHARMACEUTICAL FORM
Capsule, hard

The capsules are white, opaque and imprinted with the code TC434.

4. CLINICAL PARTICULARS

4.1 Therapeutic indications
Uftoral is indicated for first-line treatment of metastatic colorectal cancer in combination with calcium folinate (see 5.1).

4.2 Posology and method of administration
Adults: the dose of Uftoral is 300 mg/m^2/day tegafur and 672 mg/m^2/day uracil combined with 90 mg/day oral calcium folinate, given in three divided doses (preferably every 8 hours). Calcium folinate should be taken at the same time as Uftoral. Doses should be taken at least one hour before or one hour after meals for 28 consecutive days. Subsequent cycles should start after 7 days without Uftoral/calcium folinate (i.e. 35 days per treatment cycle). The daily dose per body surface area (BSA) is presented below:

(see Table 1 on next page)

Dose modification: to manage toxicity, the following dose reduction and stopping guidelines are provided:

	Worst Common Toxicity Criteria (CTC) Grade Toxicity	Uftoral Dose Modification †
Non-Haematologic Toxicity (including diarrhoea)	0 - 1	No change
	2	Therapy withheld until toxicity resolves to resolves to ⩽ grade 1. No change in subsequent dose
	3 - 4	Therapy withheld until toxicity resolves to resolves to ⩽ grade 1. Decrease subsequent dose by 1 capsule/day. Dose reduction maintained for ongoing cycle and remainder of therapy
Haematologic Toxicity (based on granulocyte or platelet count)	0 - 1	No change
	2 - 4	Therapy withheld until granulocytes ⩾ 1500/mm^3 and platelets ⩾ 100,000/mm^3
Haematologic Toxicity: Retreatment	0 - 2	No change
	3 - 4	Decrease subsequent dose by 1 capsule/day. Dose reduction maintained for ongoing cycle and remainder of therapy

† Calcium folinate dose remains unchanged, even if < 3 Uftoral capsules/day are required. If Uftoral therapy is interrupted, calcium folinate must also be stopped. When Uftoral therapy is interrupted, doses that are missed during 28 consecutive days of treatment should not be taken later.

Adolescents, children, and infants: the safety and efficacy of the Uftoral and calcium folinate combination has not been established and should not be used in these patient populations (see 4.3).

Elderly: the elderly population has been well studied as 45% of patients studied were at least 65 years old and 26% of these were at least 75 years old. However, elderly patients should be monitored for age-related impaired renal-, hepatic- or cardiac function or for concomitant medications or diseases (see 4.4 and 4.8).

Renal impairment: the effect of renal impairment on the excretion of Uftoral has not been assessed. Although the primary route of elimination for Uftoral is not renal, caution should be exercised in patients with impaired renal function. These patients should be monitored closely for any emergent toxicities (see 4.4).

Hepatic impairment: the effect of hepatic impairment on the elimination of Uftoral has not been assessed (see 4.3 and 4.4).

4.3 Contraindications
Uftoral is contraindicated in patients who:

- have a known hypersensitivity to 5-FU, tegafur, uracil, or any of the excipients;
- are pregnant or attempting to become pregnant;
- are breast feeding;
- are adolescents, children or infants;
- have severe hepatic impairment;
- present with evidence of bone marrow suppression from previous radiotherapy or antineoplastic agents;
- have a known deficiency of hepatic CYP2A6;

- have a known or suspected dihydropyrimidine dehydrogenase deficiency;

- are treated or have recently been treated with dihydropyrimidine dehydrogenase inhibitors such as brivudine (see 4.5).

4.4 Special warnings and precautions for use
Patient compliance with oral therapy: the physician should instruct the patient on the importance of full compliance with the posology and method of administration of this medicinal product. Specific guidance on the importance of following physician recommendations for dose reductions or treatment interruptions in cases of emerging toxicities should be provided (see 4.2 and 4.8). Individual patient characteristics that may negatively impact on this compliance should be considered in the selection of therapy for this disease.

Patients receiving the Uftoral/calcium folinate combination should be monitored by a physician experienced in the use

Table 1

BSA (m^2)	Uftoral (capsules/day)	Daily schedule (number of capsules)		
		Morning	Midday	Evening
< 1.17	3	1	1	1
1.17 - 1.49	4	2	1	1
1.50 - 1.83	5	2	2	1
> 1.83	6	2	2	2

of cytotoxic agents and who has the facilities for regular monitoring of clinical, biochemical and haematological effects during and after administration of chemotherapy. Any emergent toxicity should be handled as described in dose modifications (see 4.2).

The Uftoral/calcium folinate combination should be used with caution in patients with, renal or hepatic impairment, signs and symptoms of bowel obstruction and in elderly patients.

Patients treated with coumarin anticoagulants (such as warfarin) concomitantly with Uftoral should be monitored regularly for alterations in prothrombin time or International Normalised Ratio.

Patients taking phenytoin concomitantly with Uftoral should be regularly monitored for increased phenytoin plasma concentrations.

Hepatic disorders: since hepatic disorders, including fatal fulminant hepatitis, have been reported in patients receiving single agent Uftoral, appropriate testing should be performed on any patient receiving the Uftoral/calcium folinate combination who presents signs and symptoms of hepatitis, other liver disease or hepatic impairment. Liver function should be monitored during treatment in patients with mild to moderate hepatic dysfunction.

Renal insufficiency: there is no experience with the Uftoral/calcium folinate combination in patients with renal impairment. Physicians should exercise caution when Uftoral/calcium folinate is administered to such patients.

Diarrhoea: Uftoral/calcium folinate often induces diarrhoea, however, this is mild in the majority of cases. Patients with severe diarrhoea should be carefully monitored and given fluid and electrolyte replacement to avoid the potentially fatal complications of dehydration (see 4.2). Special attention should also be paid to the requirement to withhold therapy with Uftoral/calcium folinate upon occurrence of grade 2 or worse diarrhoea.

Significant cardiac disease: caution should also be exercised in patients with a history of significant cardiac disease as myocardial ischaemia and angina have been associated with fluoropyrimidine-based therapy and rare cardiac events of uncertain causality, including myocardial infarction, have been reported in patients receiving Uftoral.

4.5 Interaction with other medicinal products and other forms of interaction

Pharmacokinetic interactions of Uftoral with other concomitantly administered medications have not been formally investigated.

Co-administration of 5-fluorouracil or its pro-drugs with medicinal products that inhibit dihydropyrimidine dehydrogenase, an enzyme responsible for the catabolism of endogenous and fluorinated pyrimidines, may lead to increased fluoropyrimidine toxicity which is potentially fatal. Therefore, Uftoral must not be co-administered with dihydropyrimidine dehydrogenase inhibitors such as brivudine. In patients treated with brivudine, a time interval of 4 weeks must be respected before administration of Uftoral to allow for recovery of enzyme activity.

Marked elevations in prothrombin time (PT) or International Normalised Ratio (INR) have been reported in patients stabilised on warfarin therapy following initiation of Uftoral therapy.

Increased phenytoin plasma concentrations resulting in symptoms of phenytoin intoxication have been reported with the concomitant use of Uftoral and phenytoin (see 4.4).

In vitro, tegafur is partially metabolised by CYP2A6 (see 4.3). Uftoral should be administered with caution in combination with substrates or inhibitors of this enzyme. e.g. coumarin, methoxypsoralen, clotrimazole, ketoconazole, miconazole. Neither tegafur nor uracil significantly inhibits the *in vitro* activity of CYP3A4 or CYP2D6. Furthermore, *in vitro*, tegafur is not metabolised by CYP1A1, -1A2, -2B6, -2C8, -2C9, -2C19, -2D6, -2E1, or -3A4 suggesting it is unlikely that there will be interactions with medications metabolised by these enzymes.

The absorption of Uftoral is affected by food (see 5.2).

4.6 Pregnancy and lactation

Pregnancy: for Uftoral, no clinical data on exposed pregnancies are available. Uracil/tegafur is suspected to cause serious birth defects when administered during pregnancy. Uftoral is therefore contraindicated (see 4.3) in pregnancy. Contraceptive measures must be taken by both male and female patients during (and up to 3 months after) treatment. If pregnancy occurs during treatment with Uftoral, genetic counselling would be considered.

Lactation: it is not known whether tegafur, uracil, and 5-FU are excreted in human milk following Uftoral administration. Because of the potential for serious adverse reactions in nursing infants, the use of Uftoral in lactating women is contraindicated (see 4.3).

4.7 Effects on ability to drive and use machines

The Uftoral/calcium folinate combination has not been demonstrated to interfere with the ability to drive or use machines. However, as confusion has occasionally been reported (see 4.8), patients should be advised to exercise caution.

4.8 Undesirable effects

Unless otherwise indicated, the undesirable effect information relates to the 594 patients that have been treated with Uftoral/calcium folinate combination in two Phase III trials with a median of 3 to 3.5 courses (see 5.1).

As with all cytotoxic agents, adverse reactions can be expected in the majority of patients. Most undesirable effects observed, including diarrhoea, nausea and vomiting were reversible and rarely required permanent discontinuation of therapy, although doses were withheld or reduced in some patients (see 4.2). The most common severe and clinically relevant adverse events, regardless of attribution to Uftoral/calcium folinate were diarrhoea (20%), nausea/vomiting (12%), abdominal pain (12%) and asthenia (9%).

Approximately 45% of these patients were ≥ 65 years of age, and about 26% of these were ≥ 75 years. No clinically relevant differences in safety were observed, although older patients tended to have a higher incidence of anaemia, diarrhoea and stomatitis/mucositis.

The following information specifies undesirable effects of any severity, reported at a frequency of ≥ 1% and attributed to Uftoral/calcium folinate. Additionally, terms are (*) when severe and clinically relevant undesirable effects, regardless of treatment attribution to Uftoral/calcium folinate, were reported in a proportion of patients at a frequency of ≥ 0.1%.

[MedDRA convention: very common (≥ 10%), common (≥ 1% to < 10%) or uncommon (≥ 0.1% to < 1%)]:

Infections and infestations:

• common: moniliasis

• uncommon: infection *, sepsis *

Blood and lymphatic system disorders:

• very common: myelosuppression, anaemia, trombocytopenia, leukopenia, neutropenia

• uncommon: coagulation disorder *, febrile neutropenia

Metabolism and nutrition disorders:

• common: dehydration * cachexia *

Nervous system disorders:

• common: taste perversion *, taste loss, somnolence, dizziness, insomnia, depression, paresthesia, confusion *

Eye disorders:

• common: lacrimation, conjunctivitis

Cardiac disorders:

• common: peripheral oedema *

• uncommon: arrhythmia *, congestive heart failure *, myocardial infarction *, heart arrest *

Vascular disorders:

• common: deep thrombophlebitis *

• uncommon: shock *

Respiratory, thoracic and mediastinal disorders:

• common: dyspnoea *, increased coughing, pharyngitis

• uncommon: pulmonary embolism *

Gastrointestinal disorders:

• very common: diarrhoea *, nausea *, stomatitis *, anorexia, vomiting *, abdominal pain *

• common: constipation *, flatulence, dyspepsia, mucositis *, dry mouth, eructation, anorexia *, intestinal obstruction *

• uncommon: enteritis *, gastritis *, ileitis *, intestinal perforation *

Hepato-biliary disorders:

• uncommon: hepatitis *, jaundice *, liver failure *

Skin and subcutaneous tissue disorders:

• common: alopecia, rash, exfoliative dermatitis, skin discoloration, pruritus, photosensitivity, sweating, dry skin, nail disorder

Musculoskeletal, connective tissue and bone disorders:

• common: myalgia, back pain *, arthralgia *

Renal and urinary disorders:

• uncommon: abnormal kidney function *, urinary retention *, haematuria *

Reproductive system and breast disorders:

• uncommon: impotence *

General disorders and administration site conditions:

• very common: asthenia *

• common: fever *, headache, malaise, chills, pain *

• uncommon: chest pain *

Investigations:

• very common: increased alkaline phosphatase, increased ALT, increased AST, increased total bilirubin **

• common: weight loss *

(**)Hyperbilirubinaemia was reported approximately twice as often when compared with the bolus 5-FU/calcium folinate control arm. When reported, it was usually isolated, reversible and not associated with an adverse clinical outcome.

After marketing the following additional adverse reactions, have been reported for single-agent Uftoral. Only those adverse reactions that are not described in the Uftoral plus CF clinical trial experience are noted.

Infections and infestations:

• rare: leukoencephalopathy

Blood and lymphatic system disorders:

• very rare: haemolytic anaemia, myelodysplastic syndrome, acute myeloic leukaemia, acute promyelocytic leukaemia, agranulocytosis, pancytopenia, disseminated intravascular coagulation

Nervous system disorders:

• rare: anosmia, parosmia

• very rare: memory loss, movement disorders including extrapyramidal symptoms and paralysis in the extremities, speech disturbance, gait disturbance, disturbance of consciousness, hypoesthesia

Cardiac disorders:

• very rare: angina

Respiratory, thoracic and mediastinal disorders:

• rare: interstitial pneumonia

• very rare: pneumonia

Gastrointestinal disorders:

• very rare: acute pancreatitis, gastro/duodenal ulcer, enterocolitis, ileus paralytic, ascites, ischemic colitis

Hepato-biliary disorders:

• very rare: hepatic cirrhosis, fulminant hepatitis, hepatic fibrosis ***

Skin and subcutaneous tissue disorders:

• very rare: discoid lupus erythematosus-like eruption, skin dyscrasia (including blistering, and dermatitis), urticaria, Stevens Jonhson syndrome, palmar-plantar erythrodysaesthesia

Renal and urinary disorders:

• very rare: acute renal failure, nephrotic syndrome, urinary incontinence

General disorders and administration site conditions:

• rare: fatigue

• very rare: multi-organ failure

(***) Very rare cases of mild to moderate hepatic fibrosis without elevation of serum transaminase levels have been reported in patients with elevated serum 7S collagen and PIIINP levels receiving Uftoral alone.

4.9 Overdose

In case of overdosing, the frequency and severity of undesirable effects can increase, leading to possibly fatal conditions. Anticipated manifestations include nausea, vomiting, diarrhoea, gastrointestinal ulceration, bleeding, and bone marrow suppression (thrombocytopenia, leukopenia, and agranulocytosis). No specific antidote is available; supportive care should be provided.

5. PHARMACOLOGICAL PROPERTIES

5.1 Pharmacodynamic properties

Pharmacotherapeutic group/ATC code: antineoplastic agents, antimetabolites, pyrimidine analogues. L01B C.

Uftoral, an orally administered dihydropyrimidine dehydrogenase (DPD) inhibitory fluoropyrimidine, is a fixed molar ratio (1:4) of tegafur and uracil. Uracil is a competitive inhibitor of 5-FU degradation.

The combined individual activities of uracil and calcium folinate give rise to dual biomodulation:

• Tegafur is an oral prodrug of 5-FU and uracil reversibly inhibits DPD, the primary catabolic enzyme for 5-FU, and

• Calcium folinate enhances the cytotoxicity of 5-FU via one of its intracellular metabolites, 5,10-methylenetetrahydrofolate.

5-FU undergoes intracellular activation into its active metabolites, 5-fluoro-deoxyuridine-monophosphate (FdUMP) and 5-fluorouridine-triphosphate (FUTP). FdUMP inhibits DNA synthesis by forming inhibitory tertiary complexes with thymidylate synthetase (TS) and reduced intracellular folates. FUTP is integrated into cellular RNA, causing disruption of RNA function. Following competitive inhibition of DPD by uracil, tegafur-derived plasma concentrations of 5-FU are elevated.

The efficacy of the Uftoral/calcium folinate combination in metastatic colorectal carcinoma has been established in 2 randomised and comparative phase III trials vs. the Mayo regimen (IV 5-FU [425 mg/m^2/day] and calcium folinate [20 mg/m^2/day]) administered for 5 days every 4 weeks (study-011) or every 5 weeks (study-012).

In study -011 (n= 816), there was no statistically significant difference in the primary endpoint of survival between the two treatment arms. The median survival time was 12.4 months (95% CI: 11.2-13.6 months) and 13.4 months (95% CI: 11.6-15.4 months) in the Uftoral/calcium folinate and the 5FU/calcium folinate treatment groups, respectively. The hazard ratio for 5-FU/calcium folinate over Uftoral/calcium folinate was 0.96 (95% CI: 0.83-1.13). The assessment of the secondary endpoint of time to progression in this study was complicated by the difference in cycle duration between the two treatment arms. The median time to progression was 3.5 months (95% CI: 3.0-4.4 months) and 3.8 months (95% CI: 3.6-5.0 months) in the Uftoral/calcium folinate and 5-FU/calcium folinate treatment groups, respectively (p= 0.01).

In study -012 (n= 380), there was no statistically significant difference in the primary endpoint of time to progression nor in the secondary endpoint of survival between the two treatment arms. The median time to progression was 3.4 months (95% CI: 2.6-3.8 months) and 3.3 months (95% CI: 2.5-3.7 months) in the Uftoral/calcium folinate and 5-FU/calcium folinate treatment groups, respectively. The median survival time was 12.2 months (95% CI: 10.4-13.8 months) and 10.3 months (95% CI: 8.2-13.0 months) in the Uftoral/calcium folinate and 5-FU/calcium folinate treatment groups, respectively. The hazard ratio for 5-FU/calcium folinate over Uftoral/calcium folinate was 1.14 (95% CI: 0.92-1.42).

In the first-line treatment of metastatic colorectal carcinoma, combinations of novel agents with 5-FU have been authorised. However, the use of Uftoral in combination with novel agents is still under investigation.

5.2 Pharmacokinetic properties

The single dose and steady-state plasma pharmacokinetics of oral Uftoral have been evaluated in patients with colorectal cancer.

Absorption

Following Uftoral administration, tegafur and uracil are rapidly absorbed. C_{max} of tegafur, uracil, and 5-FU were achieved within 1 to 2 hours. Concurrent administration of oral calcium folinate with Uftoral did not significantly alter the plasma pharmacokinetics of tegafur, uracil, or 5-FU. Similarly, Uftoral did not affect the absorption of oral calcium folinate. Following a high-fat meal, plasma AUC for uracil and 5-FU were 66% and 37% lower, respectively, compared with Uftoral under fasting conditions. Plasma tegafur AUC was not significantly altered. C_{max} was reduced and delayed for tegafur, uracil, and 5-FU.

Distribution

Following oral administration of Uftoral, plasma concentrations over time for Uftoral and uracil generally display monoexponential absorption and elimination processes. The mean apparent oral volume of distribution for tegafur and uracil following Uftoral dosing at steady state are 59 and 474 L, respectively. Serum protein binding is 52% for tegafur but negligible for uracil.

Metabolism

Conversion of tegafur to 5-FU occurs via C-5' oxidation (microsomal enzymes) and C-2' hydrolysis (cytosolic enzymes). Microsomal oxidation of tegafur is partially mediated by CYP2A6. The cytosolic enzymes responsible for the metabolism of tegafur are not known. Other metabolic products of tegafur include 3'-hydroxy tegafur, 4'-hydroxy tegafur, and dihydro tegafur which are all significantly less cytotoxic than 5-FU. The metabolism of 5-FU formed from tegafur follows the intrinsic *de novo* pathways for the naturally occurring pyrimidine, uracil.

Neither tegafur, uracil or 5-FU inhibited the catalytic conversion of cDNA-derived cytochrome P450 CYP1A2, -2C9, -2C19, -2D6 and -3A4 at concentrations of at least 100 μM. This data suggests that Uftoral is unlikely to significantly alter the metabolic clearance of drugs metabolised by these routes.

Elimination

Less than 20% of tegafur is excreted intact into the urine. The terminal elimination half-lives of tegafur and uracil following Uftoral are approximately 11 hours and 20-40 minutes, respectively. The three hydroxy metabolites of tegafur are excreted in the urine. The plasma half-life for S-tegafur (10.3 hours) is 4.4 times longer relative to R-tegafur (2.4 hours).

Following Uftoral 300 mg/m^2/day, in three divided doses, tegafur plasma concentrations of > 1,000 ng/mL are maintained, whereas uracil concentrations decline rapidly following C_{max} 5-FU plasma concentrations peak in 30 to 60 minutes at approximately 200 ng/mL, and remain detectable (> 1 ng/mL) over each 8-hour dosing interval. No significant accumulation of tegafur, uracil or 5-FU occurred over a 28-day course of Uftoral therapy.

Linearity/Non-Linearity

Following single dose Uftoral (100 to 400 mg), increases in plasma exposures (C_{max} and AUC) of tegafur were generally in proportion to dose. Increases in uracil and 5-FU plasma exposures were greater than in proportion to dose.

Pharmacokinetics in Special Populations

A pooled statistical analysis of single dose Uftoral (200 mg) pharmacokinetic data (C_{max} and AUC) from three studies (46 patients, average age 60 years, 28 male, 18 female) did not identify clinically significant associations between patient age, gender and presence of metastatic liver involvement and the pharmacokinetics of tegafur, uracil or 5-FU following single dose Uftoral. In view of the predominant reliance of hepatic processes for the metabolism and elimination of both tegafur and uracil, renal abnormalities are unlikely to have significant effect on the pharmacokinetics of Uftoral.

5.3 Preclinical safety data

In rats and dogs, repeated dosing with Uftoral produces toxicity in the gastrointestinal tract, lymphoid organs, bone marrow, liver, kidney and testes. Round vacuoles, were observed histologically in the cerebrum of dogs that did not exhibit any clinical signs. With the exception of testicular changes and the vacuoles in the cerebrum of dogs, all of these findings were reversible.

Following Uftoral administration, tegafur, uracil and 5-FU are excreted in breast milk in rats. Also in rats, Uftoral showed maternal toxicity and a decrease in conception rate. Embryomortality, foetal toxicity and teratogenicity were observed in rats, mice and rabbits. Uftoral was not mutagenic in bacterial strains but did induce chromosomal aberrations in Chinese Hamster Ovary cells and was genotoxic in a rat micronucleus test. Long-term animal carcinogenicity studies have not been conducted. However, the positive mutagenicity data are indicative of a carcinogenic potential.

6. PHARMACEUTICAL PARTICULARS

6.1 List of excipients

Low-substituted hydroxypropylcellulose, sodium laurilsulfate.

Capsule shell: gelatin and titanium dioxide (E171).

Capsule shell imprints (edible ink): titanium dioxide (E171), synthetic iron oxide red (E172), carnauba wax, shellac and glyceryl monooleate.

6.2 Incompatibilities

Not applicable.

6.3 Shelf life

2 years

6.4 Special precautions for storage

Do not store above 25°C

6.5 Nature and contents of container

PVC/PVDC/Aluminium blisters.

Packs of 21, 28, 35, 36, 42, 56, 70, 84, 112, 120, 140 or 168 capsules.

Not all pack sizes may be marketed.

6.6 Special precautions for disposal and other handling

Procedures for the proper handling and disposal of cytotoxic drugs should be followed.

7. MARKETING AUTHORISATION HOLDER

Merck Ltd

t/a Merck Pharmaceuticals (A division of Merck Ltd)

Harrier House

High Street

West Drayton

Middlesex

UB7 7QG

8. MARKETING AUTHORISATION NUMBER(S)

PL 11648/0065

9. DATE OF FIRST AUTHORISATION/RENEWAL OF THE AUTHORISATION

31 October 2005

10. DATE OF REVISION OF THE TEXT

16 October 2008

Ultiva Injection

(GlaxoSmithKline UK)

1. NAME OF THE MEDICINAL PRODUCT

Ultiva (remifentanil hydrochloride) for Injection 1 mg

Ultiva (remifentanil hydrochloride) for Injection 2 mg

Ultiva (remifentanil hydrochloride) for Injection 5 mg

2. QUALITATIVE AND QUANTITATIVE COMPOSITION

Ultiva is a sterile, endotoxin-free, preservative-free, white to off white, lyophilized powder, to be reconstituted before use.

When reconstituted as directed, solutions of Ultiva are clear and colourless and contain 1mg/ml of remifentanil base as remifentanil hydrochloride.

Ultiva for injection is available in glass vials containing 1 mg, 2 mg or 5 mg of remifentanil base.

3. PHARMACEUTICAL FORM

Lyophilized powder for reconstitution for intravenous administration.

4. CLINICAL PARTICULARS

4.1 Therapeutic indications

Ultiva is indicated as an analgesic agent for use during induction and/or maintenance of general anaesthesia under close supervision.

Ultiva is indicated for provision of analgesia and sedation in mechanically ventilated intensive care patients 18 years of age and over.

4.2 Posology and method of administration

Ultiva should be administered only in a setting fully equipped for the monitoring and support of respiratory and cardiovascular function and by persons specifically trained in the use of anaesthetic drugs and the recognition and management of the expected adverse effects of potent opioids, including respiratory and cardiac resuscitation. Such training must include the establishment and maintenance of a patent airway and assisted ventilation.

Ultiva is for intravenous use only and must not be administered by epidural or intrathecal injection (see section 4.3 Contraindications).

There is a potential for the development of tolerance during administration of μ-opioid agonists.

Ultiva may be given by target controlled infusion (TCI) with an approved infusion device incorporating the Minto pharmacokinetic model with covariates for age and lean body mass (LBM) (Anesthesiology 1997;86;10-23)

Ultiva is stable for 24 hours at room temperature after reconstitution and further dilution with one of the following IV fluids listed below:

Sterilised Water for Injections

5% Dextrose Injection

5% Dextrose and 0.9% Sodium Chloride Injection

0.9% Sodium Chloride Injection0.45% Sodium Chloride Injection

For manually-controlled infusion Ultiva can be diluted to concentrations of 20 to 250 micrograms/ml (50 micrograms/ml is the recommended dilution for adults and 20 to 25 micrograms/ml for paediatric patients aged 1 year and over).

For TCI the recommended dilution of Ultiva is 20 to 50 micrograms/ml.

(See Section 6.6 Instructions for use/handling for additional information, including tables to help titrate Ultiva to the patient's anaesthetic needs).

General Anaesthesia - Adults

Administration by Manually-Controlled Infusion

The administration of Ultiva must be individualised based on the patient's response. Specific dosing guidelines for patients undergoing cardiac surgery are provided in the section headed 'Cardiac Surgery' below.

The following table summarises the starting infusion rates and dose range:

DOSING GUIDELINES FOR ADULTS

(see Table 1 on next page)

When given by bolus injection at induction Ultiva should be administered over not less than 30 seconds.

At the doses recommended above, remifentanil significantly reduces the amount of hypnotic agent required to maintain anaesthesia. Therefore, isoflurane and propofol should be administered as recommended above to avoid excessive depth of anaesthesia (see Concomitant medication below).

Induction of anaesthesia: Ultiva should be administered with an hypnotic agent, such as propofol, thiopentone, or isoflurane, for the induction of anaesthesia. Administering Ultiva after an hypnotic agent will reduce the incidence of muscle rigidity. Ultiva can be administered at an infusion rate of 0.5 to 1 microgram/kg/min, with or without an initial bolus injection of 1 microgram/kg given over not less than 30 seconds. If endotracheal intubation is to occur more than 8 to 10 minutes after the start of the infusion of Ultiva, then a bolus injection is not necessary.

Maintenance of anaesthesia in ventilated patients: After endotracheal intubation, the infusion rate of Ultiva should be decreased, according to anaesthetic technique, as indicated in the above table. Due to the fast onset and short duration of action of Ultiva, the rate of administration during anaesthesia can be titrated upward in 25% to 100% increments or downward in 25% to 50% decrements, every 2 to 5 minutes to attain the desired level of μ-opioid response. In response to light anaesthesia, supplemental bolus injections may be administered every 2 to 5 minutes.

Table 1 DOSING GUIDELINES FOR ADULTS

INDICATION	BOLUS INJECTION (microgram/kg)	CONTINUOUS INFUSION (microgram/kg/min)	
		Starting Rate	Range
Induction of anaesthesia	1(give over not less than 30 seconds)	0.5 to 1	
Maintenance of anaesthesia in ventilated patients			
• Nitrous oxide (66%)	0.5 to 1	0.4	0.1 to 2
• Isoflurane (starting dose 0.5MAC)	0.5 to 1	0.25	0.05 to 2
• Propofol (Starting dose 100 microgram/kg/min)	0.5 to 1	0.25	0.05 to 2

Anaesthesia in spontaneously breathing anaesthetised patients with a secured airway (e.g. laryngeal mask anaesthesia): In spontaneously breathing anaesthetised patients with a secured airway respiratory depression is likely to occur. Special care is needed to adjust the dose to the patient requirements and ventilatory support may be required. The recommended starting infusion rate for supplemental analgesia in spontaneously breathing anaesthetised patients is 0.04 microgram/kg/min with titration to effect. A range of infusion rates from 0.025 to 0.1 microgram/kg/min has been studied. Bolus injections are not recommended in spontaneously breathing anaesthetised patients.

Concomitant medication: Ultiva decreases the amounts or doses of inhaled anaesthetics, hypnotics and benzodiazepines required for anaesthesia (see Section 4.5 Interaction with other medicaments and other forms of interaction).

Doses of the following agents used in anaesthesia: isoflurane, thiopentone, propofol and temazepam have been reduced by up to 75% when used concurrently with remifentanil.

Guidelines for discontinuation: Due to the very rapid offset of action of Ultiva no residual opioid activity will be present within 5 to 10 minutes after discontinuation. For those patients undergoing surgical procedures where post-operative pain is anticipated, analgesics should be administered prior to discontinuation of Ultiva. Sufficient time must be allowed to reach the maximum effect of the longer acting analgesic. The choice of analgesic should be appropriate for the patient's surgical procedure and the level of post-operative care.

Care should be taken to avoid inadvertent administration of Ultiva remaining in IV lines and cannulae (see section 4.4 Special warnings and precautions for use).

Guidance on provision of analgesia and sedation in mechanically ventilated intensive care patients is provided below (see Intensive Care).

Administration by Target-Controlled Infusion

Induction and maintenance of anaesthesia in ventilated patients: Ultiva TCI should be used in association with an intravenous or inhalational hypnotic agent during the induction and maintenance of anaesthesia in ventilated adult patients (see the table in *Dosing Guidelines For Adults* under *4.2 Posology and method of administration – General Anaesthesia – Adults - Administration by Manually-Controlled Infusion*). In association with these agents, adequate analgesia for induction of anaesthesia and surgery can generally be achieved with target blood remifentanil concentrations ranging from 3 to 8 nanograms/ml. Ultiva should be titrated to individual patient response. For particularly stimulating surgical procedures target blood concentrations up to 15 nanograms/ml may be required.

At the doses recommended above, remifentanil significantly reduces the amount of hypnotic agent required to maintain anaesthesia. Therefore, isoflurane and propofol should be administered as recommended above to avoid excessive depth of anaesthesia (see *Dosing Guidelines for Adults* and *Concomitant Medication* under *4.2 Posology and method of administration – General Anaesthesia – Adults - Administration by Manually-Controlled Infusion).*

For information on blood remifentanil concentrations achieved with manually-controlled infusion see Table 5.

There are insufficient data to make recommendations on the use of TCI for spontaneous ventilation anaesthesia.

Guidelines for discontinuation/continuation into the immediate post-operative period: At the end of surgery when the TCI infusion is stopped or the target concentration reduced, spontaneous respiration is likely to return at calculated remifentanil concentrations in the region of 1 to 2 nanograms/ml. As with manually-controlled infusion, post-operative analgesia should be established before the end of surgery with longer acting analgesics (see *Guidelines for discontinuation* under *4.2 Posology and method of administration – General Anaesthesia – Adults - Administration by Manually-Controlled Infusion*)

As there are insufficient data, the administration of Ultiva by TCI for the management of post-operative analgesia is not recommended.

General Anaesthesia - Paediatric patients (1 to12 years of age)

Co-administration of Ultiva with induction agents has not been studied. Ultiva TCI has not been studied in paediatric patients.

When given by bolus injection Ultiva should be administered over not less than 30 seconds. Surgery should not commence until at least 5 minutes after the start of the Ultiva infusion, if a simultaneous bolus dose has not been given. Paediatric patients should be monitored and the dose titrated to the depth of analgesia appropriate for the surgical procedure.

Induction of anaesthesia: The use of remifentanil for induction of anaesthesia in patients aged 1 to12 years is not recommended as there are no data available in this patient population.

Maintenance of anaesthesia: The following doses of Ultiva are recommended for maintenance of anaesthesia:

DOSING GUIDELINES FOR PAEDIATRIC PATIENTS (1 to12 years of age)

(see Table 2 below)

Concomitant medication: At the doses recommended above, remifentanil significantly reduces the amount of hypnotic agent required to maintain anaesthesia. Therefore, isoflurane, halothane and sevoflurane should be administered as recommended above to avoid excessive depth of anaesthesia. No data are available for dosage recommendations for simultaneous use of other hypnotics with remifentanil (see section 4.2. Posology and method of administration, General Anaesthesia – Adults, Concomitant medication).

Guidelines for patient management in the immediate post-operative period/ Establishment of alternative analgesia prior to discontinuation of Ultiva: Due to the very rapid offset of action of Ultiva, no residual activity will be present within 5 to 10 minutes after discontinuation. For those patients undergoing surgical procedures where post-operative pain is anticipated, analgesics should be administered prior to discontinuation of Ultiva. Sufficient time must be allowed to reach the therapeutic effect of the longer acting analgesic. The choice of agent(s), the dose and the time of administration should be planned in advance and individually tailored to be appropriate for the patient's surgical procedure and the level of post-operative care anticipated (see section 4.4. Special warnings and precautions for use).

Neonates/infants (aged less than 1 year):

The pharmacokinetic profile of remifentanil in neonates/ infants (aged less than 1 year) is comparable to that seen in adults after correction for body weight differences. However, there are insufficient clinical data to make dosage recommendations for this age group.

Elderly (over 65 years of age):

General anaesthesia: Caution should be exercised in the administration of Ultiva in this population. The initial starting dose of Ultiva administered to patients over 65 should be half the recommended adult dose and then titrated to individual patient need as an increased sensitivity to the pharmacodynamic effects of remifentanil has been seen in this patient population.

Because of the increased sensitivity of elderly patients to Ultiva, when administering Ultiva by TCI in this population the initial target concentration should be 1.5 to 4 nanograms/ml with subsequent titration to response.

Cardiac anaesthesia: No initial dose reduction is required (See Cardiac Surgery below).

Intensive Care: No initial dose reduction is required (see Intensive Care).

Cardiac Surgery

Administration by Manually-Controlled Infusion

DOSING GUIDELINES FOR CARDIAC ANAESTHESIA

(see Table 3 below)

Ultiva is not recommended for use in patients with poor left ventricular function (left ventricular ejection fraction less than 0.35), since the safe use of the product in this patient group has not been established. There are no data available on use in patients under 18 years of age undergoing cardiac surgery.

Induction period of anaesthesia: After administration of hypnotic to achieve loss of consciousness, Ultiva should be administered at an initial infusion rate of 1 microgram/ kg/min. The use of bolus injections of Ultiva during induction in cardiac surgical patients is not recommended. Endotracheal intubation should not occur until at least 5 minutes after the start of the infusion.

Maintenance period of anaesthesia: After endotracheal intubation the infusion rate of Ultiva can be titrated upward in 25% to 100% increments, or downward in 25% to 50% decrements, every 2 to 5 minutes according to patient need. Supplemental bolus doses, administered over not less than 30 seconds, may also be given every 2 to 5 minutes as required. High risk cardiac patients, such as those undergoing valve surgery, should be administered a maximum bolus dose of 0.5 microgram/kg. These dosing recommendations also apply during hypothermic cardiopulmonary bypass (see section 5.2 Pharmacokinetic properties - Cardiac anaesthesia).

Concomitant medication: At the doses recommended above, remifentanil significantly reduces the amount of hypnotic agent required to maintain anaesthesia. Therefore, isoflurane and propofol should be administered as recommended above to avoid excessive depth of anaesthesia. No data are available for dosage recommendations for simultaneous use of other hypnotics with remifentanil (see above under General Anaesthesia - Adults - Concomitant medication).

Continuation of Ultiva post-operatively to provide analgesia prior to weaning for extubation: It is recommended that the infusion of Ultiva should be maintained at the final intra-operative rate during transfer of patients to

Table 2 DOSING GUIDELINES FOR PAEDIATRIC PATIENTS (1 to12 years of age)

* CONCOMITANT ANAESTHETIC AGENT	BOLUS INJECTION (microgram/kg)	CONTINUOUS INFUSION (microgram/kg/min)	
		Starting Rate	Range
Halothane (starting dose 0.3MAC)	1	0.25	0.05 to 1.3
Sevoflurane (starting dose 0.3MAC)	1	0.25	0.05 to 0.9
Isoflurane (starting dose 0.5MAC)	1	0.25	0.06 to 0.9

*co-administered with nitrous oxide/oxygen in a ratio of 2:1

Table 3 DOSING GUIDELINES FOR CARDIAC ANAESTHESIA

INDICATION	BOLUS INJECTION (microgram/kg)	CONTINUOUS INFUSION (microgram/kg/min)	
		Starting Rate	Range
Induction of anaesthesia	Not recommended	1	_
Maintenance of anaesthesia in ventilated patients:			
• Isoflurane (starting dose 0.4MAC)	0.5 to 1	1	0.003 to 4
• Propofol (Starting dose 50 microgram/kg/min)	0.5 to 1	1	0.01 to 4.3
Continuation of post-operative analgesia, prior to extubation	Not recommended	1	0 to 1

the post-operative care area. Upon arrival into this area, the patient's level of analgesia and sedation should be closely monitored and the Ultiva infusion rate adjusted to meet the individual patient's requirements (see Intensive care, below, for further information on management of intensive care patients.

Establishment of alternative analgesia prior to discontinuation of Ultiva: Due to the very rapid offset of action of Ultiva, no residual opioid activity will be present within 5 to 10 minutes after discontinuation. Prior to discontinuation of Ultiva, patients must be given alternative analgesic and sedative agents at a sufficient time in advance to allow the therapeutic effects of these agents to become established. It is therefore recommended that the choice of agent(s), the dose and the time of administration are planned, before weaning the patient from the ventilator. When other opioid agents are administered as part of the regimen for transition to alternative analgesia, the patient must be carefully monitored. The benefit of providing adequate post-operative analgesia must always be balanced against the potential risk of respiratory depression with these agents.

Guidelines for discontinuation of Ultiva: Due to the very rapid offset of action of Ultiva, hypertension, shivering and aches have been reported in cardiac patients immediately following discontinuation of Ultiva (see section 4.8 Undesirable effects). To minimise the risk of these occurring, adequate alternative analgesia must be established (as described above), before the Ultiva infusion is discontinued. The infusion rate should be reduced by 25% decrements in at least 10-minute intervals until the infusion is discontinued. During weaning from the ventilator the Ultiva infusion should not be increased and only down titration should occur, supplemented as required with alternative analgesics. Haemodynamic changes such as hypertension and tachycardia should be treated with alternative agents as appropriate.

Administration by Target-Controlled Infusion

Induction and maintenance of anaesthesia: Ultiva TCI should be used in association with an intravenous or inhalational hypnotic agent during the induction and maintenance of anaesthesia in ventilated adult patients (see the table in *Dosing Guidelines for Cardiac Anaesthesia* under *4.2 Posology and method of administration – Cardiac Surgery - Administration by Manually-Controlled Infusion*). In association with these agents, adequate analgesia for cardiac surgery is generally achieved at the higher end of the range of target blood remifentanil concentrations used for general surgical procedures. Following titration of remifentanil to individual patient response, blood concentrations as high as 20 nanograms/ml have been used in clinical studies. At the doses recommended above, remifentanil significantly reduces the amount of hypnotic agent required to maintain anaesthesia. Therefore, isoflurane and propofol should be administered as recommended above to avoid excessive depth of anaesthesia (see table in *Dosing Guidelines for Cardiac Anaesthesia* and *Concomitant medication* paragraph under *4.2 Posology and method of administration - Cardiac Surgery -Administration by Manually-Controlled Infusion*).

For information on blood remifentanil concentrations achieved with manually-controlled infusion see Table 5.

Guidelines for discontinuation/continuation into the immediate post-operative period: At the end of surgery when the TCI infusion is stopped or the target concentration reduced, spontaneous respiration is likely to return at calculated remifentanil concentrations in the region of 1 to 2 nanograms/ml. As with manually-controlled infusion, post-operative analgesia should be established before the end of surgery with longer acting analgesics (see *Guidelines for discontinuation* under *4.2 Posology and method of administration – Cardiac Surgery - Administration by Manually-Controlled Infusion*)

As there are insufficient data, the administration of Ultiva by TCI for the management of post-operative analgesia is not recommended.

Intensive Care - Adults

Ultiva can be initially used alone for the provision of analgesia and sedation in mechanically ventilated intensive care patients.

It is recommended that Ultiva is initiated at an infusion rate of 0.1 microgram/kg/min (6 microgram/kg/h) to 0.15 microgram/kg/min (9 microgram/kg/h). The infusion rate should be titrated in increments of 0.025 microgram/kg/min (1.5 microgram/kg/h) to achieve the desired level of sedation and analgesia. A period of at least 5 minutes should be allowed between dose adjustments. The level of sedation and analgesia should be carefully monitored, regularly reassessed and the Ultiva infusion rate adjusted accordingly. If an infusion rate of 0.2 microgram/kg/min (12 microgram/kg/h) is reached and the desired level of sedation is not achieved, it is recommended that dosing with an appropriate sedative agent is initiated (see below). The dose of sedative agent should be titrated to obtain the desired level of sedation. Further increases to the Ultiva infusion rate in increments of 0.025 microgram/kg/min (1.5 microgram/kg/h) may be made if additional analgesia is required.

Ultiva has been studied in intensive care patients in well controlled clinical trials for up to three days. As patients were not studied beyond three days, no evidence of safety and efficacy for longer treatment has been established.

The following table summarises the starting infusion rates and typical dose range for provision of analgesia and sedation in individual patients:

DOSING GUIDELINES FOR USE OF ULTIVA WITHIN THE INTENSIVE CARE SETTING

CONTINUOUS INFUSION microgram/kg/min (microgram/kg/h)	
Starting Rate	Range
0.1 (6) to 0.15 (9)	0.006 (0.36) to 0.74 (44.4)

Bolus doses of Ultiva are not recommended in the intensive care setting.

The use of Ultiva will reduce the dosage requirement of any concomitant sedative agents. Typical starting doses for sedative agents, if required, are given below:

RECOMMENDED STARTING DOSE OF SEDATIVE AGENTS, IF REQUIRED

Sedative Agent	Bolus (mg/kg)	Infusion (mg/kg/h)
Propofol	Up to 0.5	0.5
Midazolam	Up to 0.03	0.03

To allow separate titration of the respective agents sedative agents should not be administered as an admixture.

Additional analgesia for ventilated patients undergoing stimulating procedures: An increase in the existing Ultiva infusion rate may be required to provide additional analgesic cover for ventilated patients undergoing stimulating and/or painful procedures such as endotracheal suctioning, wound dressing and physiotherapy. It is recommended that an Ultiva infusion rate of at least 0.1 microgram/kg/min (6 microgram/kg/h) should be maintained for at least 5 minutes prior to the start of the stimulating procedure. Further dose adjustments may be made every 2 to 5 minutes in increments of 25%-50% in anticipation of, or in response to, additional requirement for analgesia. A mean infusion rate of 0.25 microgram/kg/min (15 microgram/kg/h), maximum 0.75 microgram/kg/min (45 microgram/kg/h), has been administered for provision of additional analgesia during stimulating procedures.

Establishment of alternative analgesia prior to discontinuation of Ultiva: Due to the very rapid offset of action of Ultiva, no residual opioid activity will be present within 5 to 10 minutes after discontinuation regardless of the duration of infusion. Prior to discontinuation of Ultiva, patients must be given alternative analgesic and sedative agents at a sufficient time in advance to allow the therapeutic effects of these agents to become established. It is therefore recommended that the choice of agent(s), the dose and the time of administration are planned prior to discontinuation of Ultiva.

Guidelines for extubation and discontinuation of Ultiva: In order to ensure a smooth emergence from an Ultiva-based regimen it is recommended that the infusion rate of Ultiva is titrated in stages to 0.1 microgram/kg/min (6 microgram/kg/h) over a period up to 1 hour prior to extubation.

Following extubation, the infusion rate should be reduced by 25% decrements in at least 10-minute intervals until the infusion is discontinued. During weaning from the ventilator the Ultiva infusion should not be increased and only down titration should occur, supplemented as required with alternative analgesics.

Upon discontinuation of Ultiva, the IV cannula should be cleared or removed to prevent subsequent inadvertent administration.

When other opioid agents are administered as part of the regimen for transition to alternative analgesia, the patient must be carefully monitored. The benefit of providing adequate analgesia must always be balanced against the potential risk of respiratory depression.

Ultiva TCI has not been studied in intensive care patients

Intensive Care - Paediatric patients

The use of remifentanil in intensive care patients under the age of 18 years is not recommended as there are no data available in this patient population.

Renally-impaired intensive care patients

No adjustments to the doses recommended above are necessary in renally-impaired patients, including those undergoing renal replacement therapy (see Section 5.2 Pharmacokinetic properties).

Neurosurgery

Limited clinical experience in patients undergoing neurosurgery has shown that no special dosage recommendations are required.

ASA III/IV patients

General anaesthesia: As the haemodynamic effects of potent opioids can be expected to be more pronounced in ASA III/IV patients, caution should be exercised in the administration of Ultiva in this population. Initial dosage reduction and subsequent titration to effect is therefore recommended.

For TCI, a lower initial target of 1.5 to 4 nanograms/ml should be used in ASA III or IV patients and subsequently titrated to response.

Cardiac anaesthesia: No initial dose reduction is required.

Obese patients

For manually-controlled infusion it is recommended that for obese patients the dosage of Ultiva should be reduced and based upon ideal body weight as the clearance and volume of distribution of remifentanil are better correlated with ideal body weight than actual body weight.

With the calculation of lean body mass (LBM) used in the Minto model, LBM is likely to be underestimated in female patients with a body mass index (BMI) greater than 35 kg/m^2 and in male patients with BMI greater than 40 kg/m^2. To avoid underdosing in these patients, remifentanil TCI should be titrated carefully to individual response.

Renal impairment

On the basis of investigations carried out to date, a dose adjustment in patients with impaired renal function, including intensive care patients, is not necessary.

Hepatic impairment

No adjustment of the initial dose, relative to that used in healthy adults, is necessary as the pharmacokinetic profile of remifentanil is unchanged in this patient population. However, patients with severe hepatic impairment may be slightly more sensitive to the respiratory depressant effects of remifentanil. These patients should be closely monitored and the dose of Ultiva titrated to individual patient need.

4.3 Contraindications

As glycine is present in the formulation Ultiva is contra-indicated for epidural and intrathecal use.

Ultiva is contra-indicated in patients with known hypersensitivity to any component of the preparation and other fentanyl analogues.

Ultiva is contra-indicated for use as the sole agent for induction of anaesthesia.

4.4 Special warnings and precautions for use

Ultiva should be administered only in a setting fully equipped for the monitoring and support of respiratory and cardiovascular function, and by persons specifically trained in the use of anaesthetic drugs and the recognition and management of the expected adverse effects of potent opioids, including respiratory and cardiac resuscitation. Such training must include the establishment and maintenance of a patent airway and assisted ventilation.

Rapid offset of action

Due to the very rapid offset of action of Ultiva, patients may emerge rapidly from anaesthesia and no residual opioid activity will be present within 5-10 minutes after the discontinuation of Ultiva. For those patients undergoing surgical procedures where post-operative pain is anticipated, analgesics should be administered prior to discontinuation of Ultiva. Sufficient time must be allowed to reach the maximum effect of the longer acting analgesic. The choice of analgesic should be appropriate for the patient's surgical procedure and the level of post-operative care. When other opioid agents are administered as part of the regimen for transition to alternative analgesia, the benefit of providing adequate post-operative analgesia must always be balanced against the potential risk of respiratory depression with these agents.

Discontinuation of Treatment

Common post-operative events associated with the emergence from general anaesthesia, such as shivering, agitation, tachycardia, hypertension, may occur earlier following discontinuation of Ultiva.

Symptoms including tachycardia, hypertension and agitation have been reported infrequently upon abrupt cessation, particularly after prolonged administration of Ultiva. Where reported, re-introduction and tapering of the infusion has been beneficial.

Inadvertent administration

A sufficient amount of Ultiva may be present in the dead space of the IV line and/or cannula to cause respiratory depression, apnoea and/or muscle rigidity if the line is flushed with IV fluids or other drugs. This may be avoided by administering Ultiva into a fast flowing IV line or via a dedicated IV line which is removed when Ultiva is discontinued.

Muscle rigidity - prevention and management

At the doses recommended muscle rigidity may occur. As with other opioids, the incidence of muscle rigidity is related to the dose and rate of administration. Therefore, bolus injections should be administered over not less than 30 seconds.

Muscle rigidity induced by remifentanil must be treated in the context of the patient's clinical condition with appropriate supporting measures including ventilatory support. Excessive muscle rigidity occurring during the induction of anaesthesia should be treated by the administration of a neuromuscular blocking agent and/or additional hypnotic agents. Muscle rigidity seen during the use of remifentanil as an analgesic may be treated by stopping or decreasing the rate of administration of remifentanil. Resolution of muscle rigidity after discontinuing the infusion of remifentanil occurs within minutes. Alternatively an opioid antagonist may be administered, however this may reverse or attenuate the analgesic effect of remifentanil.

Respiratory depression - management

As with all potent opioids, profound analgesia is accompanied by marked respiratory depression. Therefore, remifentanil should only be used in areas where facilities for monitoring and dealing with respiratory depression are available. The appearance of respiratory depression should be managed appropriately, including decreasing the rate of infusion by 50%, or by a temporary discontinuation of the infusion. Unlike other fentanyl analogues, remifentanil has not been shown to cause recurrent respiratory depression even after prolonged administration. However, as many factors may affect post-operative recovery it is important to ensure that full consciousness and adequate spontaneous ventilation are achieved before the patient is discharged from the recovery area.

Cardiovascular effects

Hypotension and bradycardia (see section 4.8 Undesirable Effects) may be managed by reducing the rate of infusion of Ultiva or the dose of concurrent anaesthetics or by using IV fluids, vasopressor or anticholinergic agents as appropriate.

Debilitated, hypovolaemic, and elderly patients may be more sensitive to the cardiovascular effects of remifentanil.

Drug abuse

As with other opioids remifentanil may produce dependency.

4.5 Interaction with other medicinal products and other forms of interaction

Remifentanil is not metabolised by plasmacholinesterase, therefore, interactions with drugs metabolised by this enzyme are not anticipated.

As with other opioids remifentanil, whether given by manually-controlled infusion or TCI, decreases the amounts or doses of inhaled and IV anaesthetics, and benzodiazepines required for anaesthesia (see section 4.2 Posology and method of administration, General Anaesthesia – Adults, Paediatric Patients, and Cardiac Surgery). If doses of concomitantly administered CNS depressant drugs are not reduced patients may experience an increased incidence of adverse effects associated with these agents.

The cardiovascular effects of Ultiva (hypotension and bradycardia), may be exacerbated in patients receiving concomitant cardiac depressant drugs, such as beta-blockers and calcium channel blocking agents.

4.6 Pregnancy and lactation

There are no adequate and well-controlled studies in pregnant women. Ultiva should be used during pregnancy only if the potential benefit justifies the potential risk to the foetus.

It is not known whether remifentanil is excreted in human milk. However, because fentanyl analogues are excreted in human milk and remifentanil-related material was found in rat milk after dosing with remifentanil, caution should be exercised when remifentanil is administered to a nursing mother.

For a summary of the reproductive toxicity study findings please refer to Section 5.3 Preclinical safety data.

Labour and delivery

The safety profile of remifentanil during labour or delivery has not been demonstrated. There are insufficient data to recommend remifentanil for use during labour and Caesarean section. Remifentanil crosses the placental barrier and fentanyl analogues can cause respiratory depression in the child.

4.7 Effects on ability to drive and use machines

If an early discharge is envisaged, following treatment using anaesthetic agents, patients should be advised not to drive or operate machinery.

4.8 Undesirable effects

The most common adverse events associated with remifentanil are direct extensions of μ-opioid agonist pharmacology. These are acute respiratory depression, bradycardia, hypotension and/or skeletal muscle rigidity. These adverse events resolve within minutes of discontinuing or decreasing the rate of remifentanil administration.

Post-operative shivering, apnoea, hypertension, hypoxia, pruritis, constipation, aches, sedation, nausea and vomiting have also been reported.

Very rarely, allergic reactions including anaphylaxis have been reported in patients receiving remifentanil in conjunction with one or more anaesthetic agents.

In common with other opioids, very rare cases of asystole, usually preceded by severe bradycardia, have been reported in patients receiving remifentanil in conjunction with other anaesthetic agents.

4.9 Overdose

As with all potent opioid analgesics, overdose would be manifested by an extension of the pharmacologically predictable actions of remifentanil. Due to the very short duration of action of Ultiva, the potential for deleterious effects due to overdose is limited to the immediate time period following drug administration. Response to discontinuation of the drug is rapid, with return to baseline within ten minutes.

Table 4 Ultiva for Injection Infusion Rates (ml/kg/h)

Drug Delivery Rate (microgram/kg/min)	Infusion Delivery Rate (ml/kg/h) for Solution Concentrations of 25 microgram/ml 1mg/40ml	50 microgram/ml 1mg/20ml	250 microgram/ml 10mg/40ml
0.0125	0.03	0.015	Not recommended
0.025	0.06	0.03	Not recommended
0.05	0.12	0.06	0.012
0.075	0.18	0.09	0.018
0.1	0.24	0.12	0.024
0.15	0.36	0.18	0.036
0.2	0.48	0.24	0.048
0.25	0.6	0.3	0.06
0.5	1.2	0.6	0.12
0.75	1.8	0.9	0.18
1.0	2.4	1.2	0.24
1.25	3.0	1.5	0.3
1.5	3.6	1.8	0.36
1.75	4.2	2.1	0.42
2.0	4.8	2.4	0.48

In the event of overdose, or suspected overdose, take the following actions: discontinue administration of Ultiva, maintain a patent airway, initiate assisted or controlled ventilation with oxygen, and maintain adequate cardiovascular function. If depressed respiration is associated with muscle rigidity, a neuromuscular blocking agent may be required to facilitate assisted or controlled respiration. Intravenous fluids and vasopressor agents for the treatment of hypotension and other supportive measures may be employed.

Intravenous administration of an opioid antagonist such as naloxone may be given as a specific antidote in addition to ventilatory support to manage severe respiratory depression. The duration of respiratory depression following overdose with Ultiva is unlikely to exceed the duration of action of the opioid antagonist.

5. PHARMACOLOGICAL PROPERTIES

5.1 Pharmacodynamic properties

Remifentanil is a selective μ-opioid agonist with a rapid onset and very short duration of action. The μ-opioid activity, of remifentanil, is antagonised by narcotic antagonists, such as naloxone.

Assays of histamine in patients and normal volunteers have shown no elevation in histamine levels after administration of remifentanil in bolus doses up to 30 microgram/kg.

5.2 Pharmacokinetic properties

Following administration of the recommended doses of remifentanil, the effective biological half-life is 3-10 minutes. The average clearance of remifentanil in young healthy adults is 40ml/min/kg, the central volume of distribution is 100ml/kg and the steady-state volume of distribution is 350ml/kg. In children aged 1 to 12 years, remifentanil clearance and volume of distribution decreases with increasing age; the values of these parameters in neonates are approximately twice those of healthy young adults.

Blood concentrations of remifentanil are proportional to the dose administered throughout the recommended dose range. For every 0.1 microgram/kg/min increase in infusion rate, the blood concentration of remifentanil will rise 2.5nanograms/ml. Remifentanil is approximately 70% bound to plasma proteins.

Metabolism

Remifentanil is an esterase metabolised opioid that is susceptible to metabolism by non-specific blood and tissue esterases. The metabolism of remifentanil results in the formation of an essentially inactive carboxylic acid metabolite (1/4600th as potent as remifentanil). The half life of the metabolite in healthy adults is 2 hours. Approximately 95% of remifentanil is recovered in the urine as the carboxylic acid metabolite. Remifentanil is not a substrate for plasma cholinesterase.

Cardiac anaesthesia

The clearance of remifentanil is reduced by approximately 20% during hypothermic (28°C) cardiopulmonary bypass. A decrease in body temperature lowers elimination clearance by 3% per degree centigrade.

Renal impairment

The rapid recovery from remifentanil-based sedation and analgesia is unaffected by renal status.

The pharmacokinetics of remifentanil are not significantly changed in patients with varying degrees of renal impairment even after administration for up to 3 days in the intensive care setting.

The clearance of the carboxylic acid metabolite is reduced in patients with renal impairment. In intensive care patients with moderate/severe renal impairment, the concentration of the carboxylic acid metabolite is expected to reach approximately 100-fold the level of remifentanil at steady-state. Clinical data demonstrate that the accumulation of the metabolite does not result in clinically relevant μ-opioid effects even after administration of remifentanil infusions for up to 3 days in these patients.

There is no evidence that remifentanil is extracted during renal replacement therapy.

The carboxylic acid metabolite is extracted during haemodialysis by 25 - 35 %.

Hepatic impairment

The pharmacokinetics of remifentanil are not changed in patients with severe hepatic impairment awaiting liver transplant, or during the anhepatic phase of liver transplant surgery. Patients with severe hepatic impairment may be slightly more sensitive to the respiratory depressant effects of remifentanil. These patients should be closely monitored and the dose of remifentanil should be titrated to the individual patient need.

Paediatric patients

The average clearance and steady state volume of distribution of remifentanil are increased in younger children and decline to young healthy adult values by age 17. The elimination half-life of remifentanil in neonates is not significantly different from that of young healthy adults. Changes in analgesic effect after changes in infusion rate of remifentanil should be rapid and similar to those seen in young healthy adults. The pharmacokinetics of the carboxylic acid metabolite in paediatric patients 2-17 years of age are similar to those seen in adults after correcting for differences in body weight.

Elderly

The clearance of remifentanil is slightly reduced (approximately 25%) in elderly patients >65 years) compared to young patients. The pharmacodynamic activity of remifentanil increases with increasing age. Elderly patients have a remifentanil EC50 for formation of delta waves on the electroencephalogram (EEG) that is 50% lower than young patients; therefore, the initial dose of remifentanil should be reduced by 50% in elderly patients and then carefully titrated to meet the individual patient need.

5.3 Preclinical safety data

Intrathecal administration of the glycine formulation without remifentanil to dogs caused agitation, pain and hind limb dysfunction and incoordination. These effects are believed to be secondary to the glycine excipient. Glycine is a commonly used excipient in intravenous products and this finding has no relevance for intravenous administration of Ultiva.

Reproductive toxicity studies

Remifentanil has been shown to reduce fertility in male rats when administered daily by intravenous injection for at least 70 days at a dose of 0.5mg/kg, or approximately

250 times the maximum recommended human bolus dose of 2 microgram/kg. The fertility of female rats was not affected at doses up to 1mg/kg when administered for at least 15 days prior to mating. No teratogenic effects have been observed with remifentanil at doses up to 5mg/kg in rats and 0.8mg/kg in rabbits. Administration of remifentanil to rats throughout late gestation and lactation at doses up to 5mg/kg IV had no significant effect on the survival, development, or reproductive performance of the F1 generation.

Genotoxicity

Remifentanil was devoid of genotoxic activity in bacteria and in rat liver or mouse bone marrow cells in vivo. However, a positive response was seen in vitro in different mammalian cell systems in the presence of a metabolic activation system. This activity was seen only at concentrations more than three orders of magnitude higher than therapeutic blood levels.

6. PHARMACEUTICAL PARTICULARS

6.1 List of excipients

Glycine Ph. Eur.

Hydrochloric acid Ph. Eur.

6.2 Incompatibilities

Ultiva should only be admixed with those infusion solutions recommended (see section 6.6 Instructions for use/handling).

It should not be admixed with Lactated Ringer's Injection or Lactated Ringer's and 5% Dextrose Injection.

Ultiva should not be mixed with propofol in the same intravenous admixture solution.

Administration of Ultiva into the same intravenous line with blood/serum/plasma is not recommended. Non-specific esterases in blood products may lead to the hydrolysis of remifentanil to its inactive metabolite.

Ultiva should not be mixed with other therapeutic agents prior to administration.

6.3 Shelf life

Ultiva for Injection 1mg: 18 months

Ultiva for Injection 2mg: 2 years

Ultiva for Injection 5mg: 3 years

6.4 Special precautions for storage

Store at or below 25°C.

The reconstituted solution of Ultiva is chemically and physically stable for 24 hours at room temperature. However, Ultiva does not contain an antimicrobial preservative and thus care must be taken to assure the sterility of prepared solutions, reconstituted product should be used promptly, and any unused material discarded.

6.5 Nature and contents of container

Ultiva for Injection 1mg for intravenous use is available as 1mg of Remifentanil lyophilised powder in 3ml vials, in cartons of 5.

Ultiva for Injection 2mg for intravenous use is available as 2mg of Remifentanil lyophilised powder in 5ml vials, in cartons of 5.

Ultiva for Injection 5mg for intravenous use is available as 5mg of Remifentanil lyophilised powder in 10ml vials, in cartons of 5.

6.6 Special precautions for disposal and other handling

Ultiva is stable for 24 hours at room temperature after reconstitution and further dilution with one of the following IV fluids listed below:

Sterilised Water for Injections

5% Dextrose Injection

5% Dextrose and 0.9% Sodium Chloride Injection

0.9% Sodium Chloride Injection

0.45% Sodium Chloride Injection

For manually-controlled infusion Ultiva can be diluted to concentrations of 20 to 250 micrograms/ml (50 micrograms/ml is the recommended dilution for adults and 20 to 25 micrograms/ml for paediatric patents aged 1 year and over).

For TCI the recommended dilution of Ultiva is 20 to 50 micrograms/ml.

Ultiva has been shown to be compatible with the following intravenous fluids when administered into a running IV catheter:

Lactated Ringer's Injection

Lactated Ringer's and 5% Dextrose Injection

Ultiva has been shown to be compatible with propofol when administered into a running IV catheter.

The following tables give guidelines for infusion rates of Ultiva for manually-controlled infusion:

Table 4 Ultiva for Injection Infusion Rates (ml/kg/h)

(see Table 4 on previous page)

Table 5 Ultiva for Injection Infusion Rates (ml/h) for a 25 microgram/ml Solution

(see Table 5 above)

Table 6. Ultiva for Injection Infusion Rates (ml/h) for a 50 microgram/ml Solution

(see Table 6 above)

Table 5 Ultiva for Injection Infusion Rates (ml/h) for a 25 microgram/ml Solution

Infusion Rate	Patient Weight (kg)									
(microgram /kg/min)	10	20	30	40	50	60	70	80	90	100
0.0125	0.3	0.6	0.9	1.2	1.5	1.8	2.1	2.4	2.7	3.0
0.025	0.6	1.2	1.8	2.4	3.0	3.6	4.2	4.8	5.4	6.0
0.05	1.2	2.4	3.6	4.8	6.0	7.2	8.4	9.6	10.8	12.0
0.075	1.8	3.6	5.4	7.2	9.0	10.8	12.6	14.4	16.2	18.0
0.1	2.4	4.8	7.2	9.6	12.0	14.4	16.8	19.2	21.6	24.0
0.15	3.6	7.2	10.8	14.4	18.0	21.6	25.2	28.8	32.4	36.0
0.2	4.8	9.6	14.4	19.2	24.0	28.8	33.6	38.4	43.2	48.0

Table 6 Ultiva for Injection Infusion Rates (ml/h) for a 50 microgram/ml Solution

Infusion Rate	Patient Weight (kg)							
(microgram/kg/min)	30	40	50	60	70	80	90	100
0.025	0.9	1.2	1.5	1.8	2.1	2.4	2.7	3.0
0.05	1.8	2.4	3.0	3.6	4.2	4.8	5.4	6.0
0.075	2.7	3.6	4.5	5.4	6.3	7.2	8.1	9.0
0.1	3.6	4.8	6.0	7.2	8.4	9.6	10.8	12.0
0.15	5.4	7.2	9.0	10.8	12.6	14.4	16.2	18.0
0.2	7.2	9.6	12.0	14.4	16.8	19.2	21.6	24.0
0.25	9.0	12.0	15.0	18.0	21.0	24.0	27.0	30.0
0.5	18.0	24.0	30.0	36.0	42.0	48.0	54.0	60.0
0.75	27.0	36.0	45.0	54.0	63.0	72.0	81.0	90.0
1.0	36.0	48.0	60.0	72.0	84.0	96.0	108.0	120.0
1.25	45.0	60.0	75.0	90.0	105.0	120.0	135.0	150.0
1.5	54.0	72.0	90.0	108.0	126.0	144.0	162.0	180.0
1.75	63.0	84.0	105.0	126.0	147.0	168.0	189.0	210.0
2.0	72.0	96.0	120.0	144.0	168.0	192.0	216.0	240.0

Table 7 Ultiva for Injection Infusion Rates (ml/h) for a 250 microgram/ml Solution

Infusion Rate	Patient Weight (kg)							
(microgram/kg/min)	30	40	50	60	70	80	90	100
0.1	0.72	0.96	1.20	1.44	1.68	1.92	2.16	2.40
0.15	1.08	1.44	1.80	2.16	2.52	2.88	3.24	3.60
0.2	1.44	1.92	2.40	2.88	3.36	3.84	4.32	4.80
0.25	1.80	2.40	3.00	3.60	4.20	4.80	5.40	6.00
0.5	3.60	4.80	6.00	7.20	8.40	9.60	10.80	12.00
0.75	5.40	7.20	9.00	10.80	12.60	14.40	16.20	18.00
1.0	7.20	9.60	12.00	14.40	16.80	19.20	21.60	24.00
1.25	9.00	12.00	15.00	18.00	21.00	24.00	27.00	30.00
1.5	10.80	14.40	18.00	21.60	25.20	28.80	32.40	36.00
1.75	12.60	16.80	21.00	25.20	29.40	33.60	37.80	42.00
2.0	14.40	19.20	24.00	28.80	33.60	38.40	43.20	48.00

Table 7. Ultiva for Injection Infusion Rates (ml/h) for a 250 microgram/ml Solution

(see Table 7 above)

The following table provides the equivalent blood remifentanil concentration using a TCI approach for various manually-controlled infusion rates at steady state:

Table 8. Remifentanil Blood Concentrations (nanograms/ml) estimated using the Minto (1997) Pharmacokinetic Model in a 70 kg, 170 cm, 40 Year Old Male Patient for Various Manually-Controlled Infusion rates (micrograms /kg/min) at Steady State.

Ultiva Infusion Rate (micrograms /kg/min)	Remifentanil Blood Concentration (nanograms/ml)
0.05	1.3
0.10	2.6
0.25	6.3
0.40	10.4
0.50	12.6
1.0	25.2
2.0	50.5

7. MARKETING AUTHORISATION HOLDER

GlaxoSmithKline UK Ltd

980 Great West Rd

Brentford

Middlesex

TW8 9GS

8. MARKETING AUTHORISATION NUMBER(S)

19494/0026 < Ultiva for Injection 1mg >

19494/0027 <Ultiva for Injection 2mg >

19494/0028 < Ultiva for Injection 5mg >

9. DATE OF FIRST AUTHORISATION/RENEWAL OF THE AUTHORISATION

01 May 2004

10. DATE OF REVISION OF THE TEXT

27/4/09

Uniphyllin Continus tablets

(Napp Pharmaceuticals Limited)

1. NAME OF THE MEDICINAL PRODUCT

UNIPHYLLIN®CONTINUS® 200, 300 and 400 mg prolonged release tablets

2. QUALITATIVE AND QUANTITATIVE COMPOSITION
Tablets containing 200, 300 or 400 mg of Theophylline PhEur.

For excipients, see 6.1

3. PHARMACEUTICAL FORM
Prolonged release tablets

200 mg	Capsule shaped, white tablet with a scoreline on one side and U200 on the other.
300 mg	Capsule shaped, white tablet with a scoreline on one side and U300 on the other.
400 mg	Capsule shaped, white tablet with UNIPHYLLIN on one side and the Napp logo and U400 on either side of a scoreline on the reverse.

4. CLINICAL PARTICULARS
4.1 Therapeutic indications
For the treatment and prophylaxis of bronchospasm associated with asthma, chronic obstructive pulmonary disease and chronic bronchitis. Also indicated for the treatment of left ventricular and congestive cardiac failure.

4.2 Posology and method of administration
Route of Administration

Oral

The tablets should be swallowed whole and not crushed or chewed. Crushing or chewing the tablets may lead to a rapid release of theophylline with the potential for toxicity. Patients vary in their response to xanthines and it may be necessary to titrate the dose on an individual basis.

The usual maintenance dose for adults and elderly patients is 200 mg 12 hourly. This may be titrated to either 300 mg or 400 mg dependent on the therapeutic response. Plasma theophylline concentrations should ideally be maintained between 5 and 15 mg/l. A plasma level of 5 mg/l probably represents the lower level of clinical effectiveness. Significant adverse reactions are usually seen at plasma theophylline levels greater than 20 mg/l. Patients may require monitoring of plasma theophylline levels when higher dosages are prescribed or when co-administered with medication that reduces theophylline clearance.

Children: The maintenance dose is 9 mg/kg twice daily. Some children with chronic asthma require and tolerate much higher doses (10-16 mg/kg twice daily). Lower dosages (based on usual adult dose) may be required for adolescents.

It may be appropriate to administer a larger evening or morning dose in some patients, in order to achieve optimum therapeutic effect when symptoms are most severe e.g. at the time of the 'morning dip' in lung function.

In patients whose night time or day time symptoms persist despite other therapy and who are not currently receiving theophylline, then the total daily requirement of UNIPHYLLIN CONTINUS tablets (as specified above) may be added to their treatment regimen as either a single evening or morning dose.

4.3 Contraindications
Porphyria; hypersensitivity to xanthines or any of the tablet constituents; concomitant administration with ephedrine in children.

4.4 Special warnings and precautions for use
The patient's response to therapy should be carefully monitored – worsening of asthma symptoms requires medical attention.

Use with caution in patients with cardiac arrhythmias, peptic ulcer, hyperthyroidism, severe hypertension, hepatic dysfunction, chronic alcoholism or acute febrile illness.

The half-life of theophylline may be prolonged in the elderly and in patients with heart failure, hepatic impairment or viral infections. Toxic accumulation may occur (see Section 4.9 Overdose). A reduction of dosage may be necessary in the elderly patient.

The hypokalaemia resulting from beta agonist therapy, steroids, diuretics and hypoxia may be potentiated by xanthines. Particular care is advised in patients suffering from severe asthma who require hospitalisation. It is recommended that serum potassium levels are monitored in such situations.

Severe side effects (hypertonia, convulsions, supraventricular tachycardia) may indicate serum concentrations of theophylline above therapeutic levels. Serum concentrations should be checked urgently and a decrease in the dose of theophylline may be required.

Alternative treatment is advised for patients with a history of seizure activity.

It is not possible to ensure bioequivalence between different prolonged release theophylline products. Therefore patients, once titrated to an effective dose, should not be changed from one prolonged release theophylline preparation to a different prolonged release preparation without re-titration and clinical assessment.

4.5 Interaction with other medicinal products and other forms of interaction
The following increase clearance and it may therefore be necessary to increase dosage to ensure a therapeutic effect: aminoglutethimide, carbamazepine, isoprenaline, moracizine, phenytoin, rifampicin, ritonavir, sulphinpyrazone, barbiturates and hypericum perforatum. Plasma concentrations of theophylline can be reduced by concomitant use of the herbal remedy St John's Wort (hypericum perforatum). Smoking and alcohol consumption can also increase clearance of theophylline.

The following reduce clearance and a reduced dosage may therefore be necessary to avoid side-effects: allopurinol, carbimazole, cimetidine, ciprofloxacin, clarithromycin, diltiazem, disulfiram, erythromycin, fluconazole, interferon, isoniazid, methotrexate, mexiletine, nizatidine, norfloxacin, oxpentifylline, propafenone, propranolol, ofloxacin, thiabendazole, verapamil, viloxazine hydrochloride and oral contraceptives (see Section 4.9 Overdose). The concomitant use of theophylline and fluvoxamine should usually be avoided. Where this is not possible, patients should have their theophylline dose halved and plasma theophylline should be monitored closely.

Factors such as viral infections, liver disease and heart failure also reduce theophylline clearance (see Section 4.9 Overdose). There are conflicting reports concerning the potentiation of theophylline by influenza vaccine and physicians should be aware that interaction may occur. A reduction in dosage may be necessary in elderly patients. Thyroid disease or associated treatment may alter theophylline plasma levels. There is also a pharmacological interaction with adenosine, benzodiazepines, halothane, lomustine and lithium and these drugs should be used with caution.

Theophylline may decrease steady state phenytoin levels.

Xanthines can potentiate hypokalaemia resulting from $beta_2$ agonist therapy, steroids, diuretics and hypoxia. Particular caution is advised in severe asthma. It is recommended that serum potassium levels are monitored in such situations.

Co-administration with β-blockers may cause antagonism of bronchodilation; with ketamine may cause reduced convulsive threshold; with doxapram may cause increased CNS stimulation.

4.6 Pregnancy and lactation
There are no adequate data from well controlled studies of the use of theophylline in pregnant women. Theophylline has been reported to give rise to teratogenic effects in mice, rats and rabbits (See section 5.3). The potential risk for humans is unknown. Theophylline should not be administered during pregnancy unless clearly necessary. Theophylline is secreted in breast milk, and may be associated with irritability in the infant, therefore it should only be given to breast feeding women when the anticipated benefits outweigh the risk to the child.

4.7 Effects on ability to drive and use machines
No known effects.

4.8 Undesirable effects
The risk of side-effects usually associated with theophylline and xanthine derivatives such as nausea, gastric irritation, headache, CNS stimulation, tachycardia, palpitations, hypertonia, arrhythmias and convulsions is significantly reduced when UNIPHYLLIN CONTINUS tablet preparations are given (see Section 4.9 Overdose).

4.9 Overdose
Over 3 g could be serious in an adult (40 mg/kg in a child). The fatal dose may be as little as 4.5 g in an adult (60 mg/kg in a child), but is generally higher.

Symptoms
Warning: Serious features may develop as long as 12 hours after overdosage with prolonged release formulations.

Alimentary features: Nausea, vomiting (which is often severe), epigastric pain and haematemesis. Consider pancreatitis if abdominal pain persists.

Neurological features: Restlessness, hypertonia, exaggerated limb reflexes and convulsions. Coma may develop in very severe cases.

Cardiovascular features: Sinus tachycardia is common. Ectopic beats and supraventricular and ventricular tachycardia may follow.

Metabolic features: Hypokalaemia due to shift of potassium from plasma into cells is common, can develop rapidly and may be severe. Hyperglycaemia, hypomagnesaemia and metabolic acidosis may also occur. Rhabdomyolysis may also occur.

Management
Activated charcoal or gastric lavage should be considered if a significant overdose has been ingested within 1-2 hours. Repeated doses of activated charcoal given by mouth can enhance theophylline elimination. Measure the plasma potassium concentration urgently, repeat frequently and correct hypokalaemia. BEWARE! If large amounts of potassium have been given, serious hyperkalaemia may develop during recovery. If plasma potassium is low, then the plasma magnesium concentration should be measured as soon as possible.

In the treatment of ventricular arrhythmias, proconvulsant antiarrhythmic agents such as lignocaine (lidocaine) should be avoided because of the risk of causing or exacerbating seizures.

Measure the plasma theophylline concentration regularly when severe poisoning is suspected, until concentrations are falling. Vomiting should be treated with an antiemetic such as metoclopramide or ondansetron.

Tachycardia with an adequate cardiac output is best left untreated. Beta-blockers may be given in extreme cases but not if the patient is asthmatic. Control isolated convulsions with intravenous diazepam. Exclude hypokalaemia as a cause.

5. PHARMACOLOGICAL PROPERTIES
5.1 Pharmacodynamic properties
Theophylline is a bronchodilator. In addition it affects the function of a number of cells involved in the inflammatory processes associated with asthma and chronic obstructive airways disease. Of most importance may be enhanced suppressor, T-lymphocyte activity and reduction of eosinophil and neutrophil function. These actions may contribute to an anti-inflammatory prophylactic activity in asthma and chronic obstructive airways disease. Theophylline stimulates the myocardium and produces a diminution of venous pressure in congestive heart failure leading to marked increase in cardiac output.

5.2 Pharmacokinetic properties
Theophylline is well absorbed from UNIPHYLLIN CONTINUS tablets and at least 60% may be bound to plasma proteins. The main urinary metabolites are 1,3-dimethyl uric acid and 3-methylxanthine. About 10% is excreted unchanged.

5.3 Preclinical safety data
In studies in which mice, rats and rabbits were dosed during the period of organogenesis, theophylline produced teratogenic effects.

6. PHARMACEUTICAL PARTICULARS
6.1 List of excipients
Hydroxyethylcellulose

Povidone (K25)

Cetostearyl Alcohol

Macrogol 6000

Talc

Magnesium Stearate

6.2 Incompatibilities
Not applicable.

6.3 Shelf life
Three years.

6.4 Special precautions for storage
Do not store above 25°C.

6.5 Nature and contents of container
Blister packs consisting of aluminium foil sealed to 250 µm PVC with a PVdC coating of at least 40 gsm thickness, containing 56 tablets.

6.6 Special precautions for disposal and other handling
None.

7. MARKETING AUTHORISATION HOLDER
Napp Pharmaceuticals Ltd

Cambridge Science Park

Milton Road

Cambridge CB4 0GW

8. MARKETING AUTHORISATION NUMBER(S)
PL 16950/0066-0068

9. DATE OF FIRST AUTHORISATION/RENEWAL OF THE AUTHORISATION
200 mg - 23 August 1979/15 May 2003

300 mg – 22 February 1988/15 May 2003

400 mg – 29 October 1982/15 May 2003

10. DATE OF REVISION OF THE TEXT
June 2009

11 LEGAL CATEGORY
P

® UNIPHYLLIN, CONTINUS and the Napp Device are Registered Trade Marks.

Univer Capsules 120, 180 and 240mg hard-capsules

(Cephalon Limited)

1. NAME OF THE MEDICINAL PRODUCT
Univer 120mg Prolonged-release Hard Capsules

Univer 180mg Prolonged-release Hard Capsules

Univer 240mg Prolonged-release Hard Capsules

2. QUALITATIVE AND QUANTITATIVE COMPOSITION
Verapamil hydrochloride 120 mg.

Verapamil hydrochloride 180 mg.

Verapamil hydrochloride 240 mg.

For excipients, see 6.1.

3. PHARMACEUTICAL FORM
Prolonged-release capsule, hard.

Capsules are blue and yellow and printed with V120.

Capsules are yellow and printed with V180.

Capsules are blue and yellow and printed with V240.

4. CLINICAL PARTICULARS

4.1 Therapeutic indications

Mild to moderate hypertension. Angina pectoris.

4.2 Posology and method of administration

For oral administration only. The capsules should be swallowed whole and not chewed.

The bioequivalence of Univer to other prolonged release verapamil formulations may not have been evaluated. As such, this product should not be directly substituted for other non-identical formulations of verapamil and vice-versa.

Adults:

Mild to moderate hypertension: Initial dose in adult patients new to verapamil therapy should be 120 mg once daily. This can be increased to 240 mg once daily which is the normal maintenance dosage. The dose may be further increased to a maximum of 480 mg once daily if required.

Angina: The usual adult dose is 360 mg once daily. Dosage may be increased to a maximum of 480 mg daily if required.

Elderly: Elderly patients show enhanced bioavailability of verapamil and therapeutic control may be achieved with lower doses in this patient population.

Children: Not recommended in children and adolescents under the age of 18 years.

Hepatic impairment: Verapamil is extensively metabolised in the liver and for those patients with impaired liver function, the dose should be reduced and carefully titrated.

Renal impairment: About 70% of an administered dose of verapamil is excreted as metabolites in the urine. Verapamil should be prescribed cautiously when renal function is impaired. Careful patient monitoring is recommended.

4.3 Contraindications

- Acute myocardial infarction with complications such as bradycardia, hypotension, left ventricular decompensation or congestive heart failure.
- Second or third degree atrioventricular block without pacemaker.
- Sick sinus syndrome, sino-atrial block, or severe sinus bradycardia (except in patients with functioning artificial ventricular pacemaker).
- Uncompensated cardiac failure.
- Atrial flutter or atrial fibrillation associated with an accessory pathway (e.g. Wolff-Parkinson-White, Lown-Ganong-Levine syndrome).
- Porphyria.
- Hypotension (systolic pressure <90 mm Hg) or cardiogenic shock.
- Intravenous dantrolene (see section 4.5).
- Known hypersensitivity to any of the ingredients.
- Concomitant ingestion of grapefruit juice.

4.4 Special warnings and precautions for use

Special care should be taken in hypotension (see section 4.3), especially in acute myocardial infarction as this is a condition where atrioventricular conduction defects may develop and contractility may be impaired.

Use with caution in patients with first degree atrioventricular block.

Left ventricular contractility may be affected and although the effect is small, cardiac failure may be precipitated or aggravated. Hence incipient cardiac failure should be controlled using appropriate therapy before verapamil is given.

Verapamil is extensively metabolised in the liver and special care should be taken in cases where liver damage exists, as plasma levels of verapamil may be increased (see section 4.2).

4.5 Interaction with other medicinal products and other forms of interaction

Concomitant use contra-indicated

Dantrolene: the association of this muscle relaxant given intravenously and verapamil is potentially dangerous (can cause fatal ventricular fibrillation in animals) and is contra-indicated.

Intravenous beta-blockers should not be given to patients under treatment with verapamil.

Concomitant use not recommended

The combination of verapamil and beta-blockers, antiarrhythmic agents or inhaled anaesthetics may lead to additive cardiovascular effects (e.g. AV block, bradycardia, hypotension, heart failure). A period between stopping beta-blocking therapy and starting therapy with this product may be advisable. Concomitant use of verapamil and beta-blockers or antiarrhythmics, if necessary, should only be administered to patients in a closely monitored clinical setting.

Other pharmacodynamic interactions

The effects of verapamil may be additive to other hypotensive agents.

Lithium toxicity may be enhanced. Lithium can enhance neuromuscular block during anaesthesia and hence verapamil with lithium may potentiate the neuromuscular blocking effect.

Interactions involving CYP3A4

Verapamil is metabolised by CYP3A4. Inhibitors of CYP3A4 such as ketoconazole, erythromycin and ritonavir may increase plasma levels of verapamil.

Conversely, inducers of CYP3A4 such as rifampicin, phenytoin and phenobarbital may reduce plasma levels of verapamil.

Verapamil is also a moderate inhibitor of CYP3A4. Caution is required when verapamil is given with theophylline, midazolam, ciclosporin, carbamazepine and simvastatin as plasma levels of these drugs may rise, which may result in an increased frequency or seriousness of adverse effects associated with these drugs.

Interactions involving P-glycoprotein

Verapamil is an inhibitor of P-glycoprotein and this can contribute to clinically significant drug interactions. In particular, verapamil may increase digoxin levels.

Other relevant interactions

Alcohol: an increase in blood alcohol and slowed elimination has been reported.

Grapefruit juice – an increase in verapamil serum level has been reported.

4.6 Pregnancy and lactation

Animal studies have shown no teratogenic effects and data on a limited number of exposed pregnancies showed no adverse effects on the health of the foetus or newborn child.

Caution should be exercised, however, when prescribing to pregnant women and verapamil should be avoided in the first trimester unless the benefits clearly outweigh the risks.

Verapamil is excreted in breast milk and rare hypersensitivity reactions have been reported. Verapamil should only be used during lactation if, in the clinicians judgement, it is essential for the welfare of the patient.

4.7 Effects on ability to drive and use machines

It is possible that a patient's ability to drive a vehicle or operate machinery may be impaired, particularly when starting treatment.

Verapamil has been shown to increase the blood levels of alcohol and slow its elimination. Therefore, the effects of alcohol may be exaggerated.

4.8 Undesirable effects

Occasionally, particularly in high doses or with prior myocardial damage, cardiovascular effects may be larger than desired giving rise to bradycardic arrhythmias, such as sinus bradycardia, second and third degree atrioventricular block, bradyarrhythmia in atrial fibrillation, transient asystole, hypotension, heart failure.

Constipation may occur. Headaches, dizziness, fatigue and ankle oedema are uncommon. Very infrequently nausea, vomiting, flushing and allergic reactions have been observed. Reversible impairment of liver function has been rarely reported and is most likely a hypersensitivity reaction.

There have been rare reports of gynaecomastia, gingival hyperplasia, erythromelalgia, paraesthesia and elevated prolactin levels.

4.9 Overdose

Normal resuscitation procedures should be initiated in the event of cardiovascular collapse, i.e. if atrioventricular conduction defects such as second or third degree block develop these should be treated in the usual way using atropine, isoprenaline or the temporary insertion of a pacemaker, as required. Hypotension may be observed and, if persistent, and in the absence of a conduction defect, treatment with systemic dopaminergic agents, e.g. dopamine, dobutamine or noradrenaline should be started. Specific antidote may be given, e.g. slow intravenous injection, or an infusion, of 10-20 ml calcium gluconate 10% solution. Overdose with modified-release preparations may result in prolonged toxicity of delayed onset.

5. PHARMACOLOGICAL PROPERTIES

5.1 Pharmacodynamic properties

Verapamil is a phenylalkylamine calcium antagonist with effects upon arterial smooth muscle, myocardial cells and cells of the cardiac conduction system. It lowers heart rate, increases myocardial perfusion and reduces coronary spasm. It decreases vascular peripheral resistance and lowers blood pressure by vasodilation without reflex tachycardia. The effects are more pronounced on high blood pressure than on normal pressure because of its use-dependent action on the voltage-operated calcium channel.

5.2 Pharmacokinetic properties

Approximately 90% of verapamil is absorbed following oral administration and is subject to extensive first pass metabolism in the liver. There is considerable interindividual variation in plasma concentrations. About 70% of the oral dose is excreted by the kidneys and 16% with the faeces. Where liver damage exists plasma levels of verapamil may be increased. Renal failure does not significantly alter the kinetics of the drug. Elderly subjects show enhanced bioavailability of verapamil.

Univer provides prolonged release of verapamil in the gastrointestinal tract and a pharmacokinetic profile consistent with a prolonged release formulation. A study in healthy volunteers compared the pharmacokinetics of Univer 240 mg administered once daily and immediate-release verapamil 80 mg administered three times daily. The comparative steady state kinetic data are shown below:

Steady State	Univer, dose 240 mg	Verapamil immediate release, dose 80 mg
C_{max} (ng/ml)	117.60	172.23
T_{max} (hr)	7.68	1.16
AUC_{0-8hr} (ng × hr/ml)	—	694.15
AUC_{0-24hr} (ng × hr/ml)	1572.98	—
Half-life (hr)	9.01	6.38
Elimination Rate (hr^{-1})	0.08	0.12

5.3 Preclinical safety data

There is no evidence of teratogenicity or carcinogenicity with verapamil. There are no additional preclinical safety data of relevance to the prescriber.

6. PHARMACEUTICAL PARTICULARS

6.1 List of excipients

Capsule contents:

Fumaric acid

Sugar spheres (containing sucrose and maize starch)

Talc

Povidone

Shellac

Capsule shell:

Gelatin

Titanium dioxide (E171)

Erythrosine (E127)

Indigotine (E132)

Yellow iron oxide (E172)

Printing ink:

Titanium dioxide (E171)

Black iron oxide (E172)

Shellac

Propylene glycol (E1520)

6.2 Incompatibilities

None stated.

6.3 Shelf life

2 years.

6.4 Special precautions for storage

Do not store above 25°C. Store in the original package.

6.5 Nature and contents of container

PVC/aluminium blister packs of 4, 8, 28 or 56 capsules.

Containers of 100 or 500.

6.6 Special precautions for disposal and other handling

None

7. MARKETING AUTHORISATION HOLDER

Cephalon Limited

1 Albany Place

Hyde Way

Welwyn Garden City

Hertfordshire

AL7 3BT

8. MARKETING AUTHORISATION NUMBER(S)

Univer 120 mg – PL 21799/0011

Univer 180 mg – PL 21799/0012

Univer 240 mg – PL 21799/0013

9. DATE OF FIRST AUTHORISATION/RENEWAL OF THE AUTHORISATION

30 December 2005

10. DATE OF REVISION OF THE TEXT

17.09.2008

11. LEGAL CATEGORY

POM

Ursofalk Capsules

(Dr. Falk Pharma UK Ltd)

1. NAME OF THE MEDICINAL PRODUCT

Ursofalk

2. QUALITATIVE AND QUANTITATIVE COMPOSITION

Each capsule of Ursofalk contains the following active ingredient:

Ursodeoxycholic Acid 250mg

3. PHARMACEUTICAL FORM

White, opaque, hard gelatine capsule

4. CLINICAL PARTICULARS

4.1 Therapeutic indications

Ursofalk is indicated in the treatment of primary biliary cirrhosis (PBC) and for the dissolution of radiolucent gallstones in patients with a functioning gall bladder.

4.2 Posology and method of administration

Method of administration: Oral

Primary Biliary Cirrhosis

Adults and the Elderly: 10-15mg ursodeoxycholic acid (UDCA) per kg per day in two to four divided doses. The following dosage regimen is recommended:

Body Weight (kg)	Capsules Daily (in 2-4 divided doses)	1 Mg (UDCA)/kg/day
50 - 62	2 - 4	10.0 - 16.1
63 - 85	3 - 5	11.9 - 14.7
86 - 120	4 - 7	11.6 - 14.6

Children: Dosage should be related to bodyweight.

Dissolution of gallstones

Adults: 8-12mg ursodeoxycholic acid (UDCA) per kg per day in two divided doses. The following dosage regimen is recommended:

Body Weight (kg)	Capsules Daily (in 2 divided doses)	1 Mg (UDCA)/kg/day
50 - 62	2	8.1 - 10
63 - 85	3	8.8 - 11.9
86 - 120	4	8.3 - 11.6

If doses are unequal the larger dose should be taken in late evening to counteract the rise in biliary cholesterol saturation which occurs in the early morning. The late evening dose may usefully be taken with food to help maintain bile flow overnight.

The time required for dissolution of gallstones is likely to range from 6 to 24 months depending on stone size and composition. Follow-up cholecystograms or ultrasound investigation may be useful at 6 month intervals until the gallstones have disappeared.

Treatment should be continued until 2 successive cholecystograms and/or ultrasound investigations 4-12 weeks apart have failed to demonstrate gallstones. This is because these techniques do not permit reliable visualisation of stones less than 2mm in diameter.

The likelihood of recurrence of gallstones after dissolution by bile acid treatment has been estimated as up to 50% at 5 years.

The efficiency of Ursofalk in treating radio-opaque or partially radio opaque gallstones has not been tested but these are generally thought to be less soluble than radiolucent stones.

Non-cholesterol stones account for 10-15% radiolucent stones and may not be dissolved by bile acids.

Elderly: There is no evidence to suggest that any alteration in the adult dose is needed but the relevant precautions should be taken into account.

Children: Cholesterol rich gallstones are rare in children but when they occur, dosage should be related to bodyweight.

4.3 Contraindications

Ursofalk is not suitable for the dissolution of radio-opaque gallstones and should not be used in patients with a non-functioning gall bladder.

4.4 Special warnings and precautions for use

A product of this class has been found to be carcinogenic in animals. The relevance of these findings to the clinical use of Ursofalk has not been established.

4.5 Interaction with other medicinal products and other forms of interaction

Some drugs, such as cholestyramine, charcoal, colestipol and certain antacids (e.g. aluminium hydroxide) bind bile acids *in vitro*. They could therefore have a similar effect *in vivo* and may interfere with the absorption of Ursofalk.

Drugs which increase cholesterol elimination in bile, such as oestrogenic hormones, oestrogen-rich contraceptive agents and certain blood cholesterol lowering agents, such as Clofibrate, should not be taken with Ursofalk.

UDCA may increase the absorption of cyclosporin in transplantation patients.

4.6 Pregnancy and lactation

Ursofalk should not be used in pregnancy. When treating women of childbearing potential, non-hormonal or low oestrogen oral contraceptive measures are recommended.

4.7 Effects on ability to drive and use machines

Ursofalk is not expected to affect ability to drive and use machines.

4.8 Undesirable effects

Diarrhoea may occur rarely.

4.9 Overdose

Serious adverse effects are unlikely to occur in overdosage. However, liver function should be monitored. If necessary, ion-exchange resins may be used to bind bile acids in the intestines.

5. PHARMACOLOGICAL PROPERTIES

5.1 Pharmacodynamic properties

UDCA is a bile acid which effects a reduction in cholesterol in biliary fluid primarily by dispersing the cholesterol and forming a liquid-crystal phase.

5.2 Pharmacokinetic properties

Ursodeoxycholic acid occurs naturally in the body. When given orally it is rapidly and completely absorbed. It is 96-98% bound to plasma proteins and efficiently extracted by the liver and excreted in the bile as glycine and taurine conjugates. In the intestine some of the conjugates are deconjugated and reabsorbed. The conjugates may also be dehydroxylated to lithocholic acid, part of which is absorbed, sulphated by the liver and excreted via the biliary tract.

5.3 Preclinical safety data

Not applicable.

6. PHARMACEUTICAL PARTICULARS

6.1 List of excipients

Ursofalk contains the following excipients:

Maize starch, colloidal anhydrous silica, magnesium stearate, gelatin, titanium dioxide.

6.2 Incompatibilities

None known.

6.3 Shelf life

36 months.

6.4 Special precautions for storage

None.

6.5 Nature and contents of container

Clear PVC blister strips with aluminium foil backing packed in cardboard cartons. Available in cartons containing 60 capsules packaged in six blister strips of 10 capsules or 100 capsules packaged in 4 blister strips of 25 capsules.

6.6 Special precautions for disposal and other handling

None.

7. MARKETING AUTHORISATION HOLDER

Dr Falk Pharma UK Ltd

Unit K

Bourne End Business Park

Cores End Road

Bourne End

Bucks

SL8 5AS

United Kingdom

8. MARKETING AUTHORISATION NUMBER(S)

PL 10341/0006

9. DATE OF FIRST AUTHORISATION/RENEWAL OF THE AUTHORISATION

31st December 2004

10. DATE OF REVISION OF THE TEXT

Ursofalk Suspension

(Dr. Falk Pharma UK Ltd)

1. NAME OF THE MEDICINAL PRODUCT

Ursofalk Suspension.

2. QUALITATIVE AND QUANTITATIVE COMPOSITION

5ml (=1 measuring spoon) of Ursofalk Suspension contains the following active ingredient: ursodeoxycholic acid 250mg.

3. PHARMACEUTICAL FORM

Suspension for oral administration.

4. CLINICAL PARTICULARS

4.1 Therapeutic indications

Ursofalk Suspension is indicated in the treatment of primary biliary cirrhosis (PBC) and for the dissolution of radiolucent gallstones in patients with a functioning gall bladder.

4.2 Posology and method of administration

Method of administration: Oral.

Primary Biliary Cirrhosis

Adults and the elderly: 10-15mg ursodeoxycholic acid (UDCA) per kg per day in two to four divided doses. The following dosage regimen is recommended:

Body Weight (kg)	Spoonfuls (5ml) (in 2 - 4 divided doses)	mg (UDCA) / kg/day
50 - 62	2 - 4	10.0 - 16.1
63 - 85	3 - 5	11.9 - 14.7
86 - 120	4 - 7	11.6 - 14.6

Children: Dosage should be related to bodyweight.

Dissolution of Gallstones

Adults: 8 - 12mg ursodeoxycholic acid (UDCA) per kg per day in two divided doses. The following dosage regimen is recommended:

Body Weight (kg)	Spoonfuls (5ml) (in 2 divided doses)	mg (UDCA) / kg/day
50 - 62	2	8.1 - 10.0
63 - 85	3	8.8 - 11.9
86 - 120	4	8.3 - 11.6

If doses are unequal the larger dose should be taken in late evening to counteract the rise in biliary cholesterol saturation which occurs in the early morning. The late evening dose may usefully be taken with food to help maintain bile flow overnight.

The time required for dissolution of gallstones is likely to range from 6 to 24 months depending on stone size and composition.

Follow-up cholecystograms or ultrasound investigation may be useful at 6 month intervals until the gallstones have disappeared.

Treatment should be continued until 2 successive cholecystograms and/or ultrasound investigations

4 - 12 weeks apart have failed to demonstrate gallstones. This is because these techniques do not permit reliable visualisation of stones less than 2mm in diameter.

The likelihood of recurrence of gallstones after dissolution by bile acid treatment has been estimated as up to 50% at 5 years.

The efficiency of Ursofalk Suspension in treating radio-opaque or partially radio-opaque gallstones has not been tested but these are generally thought to be less soluble than radiolucent stones.

Non-cholesterol stones account for 10-15% of radiolucent stones and may not be dissolved by bile acids.

Elderly: There is no evidence to suggest that any alteration in the adult dose is needed but the relevant precautions should be taken into account.

Children: Cholesterol rich gallstones are rare in children but when they occur, dosage should be related to bodyweight.

4.3 Contraindications

Ursofalk Suspension is not suitable for the dissolution of radio-opaque gallstones and should not be used in patients with a non-functioning gall bladder.

4.4 Special warnings and precautions for use

A product of this class has been found to be carcinogenic in animals.

The relevance of these findings to the clinical use of Ursofalk Suspension has not been established.

4.5 Interaction with other medicinal products and other forms of interaction

Some drugs, such as cholestyramine, charcoal, colestipol and certain antacids (e.g. aluminium hydroxide) bind bile acids in vitro. They could therefore have a similar effect in vivo and may interfere with the absorption of Ursofalk Suspension.

Drugs which increase cholesterol elimination in bile, such as oestrogenic hormones, oestrogen-rich contraceptive agents and certain blood cholesterol lowering agents, such as clofibrate, should not be taken with Ursofalk Suspension.

UDCA may increase the absorption of cyclosporin in transplantation patients.

4.6 Pregnancy and lactation

Ursofalk Suspension should not be used in pregnancy. When treating women of childbearing potential, non-hormonal or low oestrogen oral contraceptive measures are recommended.

4.7 Effects on ability to drive and use machines

Ursofalk Suspension is not expected to affect ability to drive and use machines.

4.8 Undesirable effects

Diarrhoea may occur rarely.

4.9 Overdose
Serious adverse effects are unlikely to occur in overdosage. However, liver function should be monitored. If necessary, ion-exchange resins may be used to bind bile acids in the intestines.

5. PHARMACOLOGICAL PROPERTIES

5.1 Pharmacodynamic properties
UDCA is a bile acid which effects a reduction in cholesterol in biliary fluid primarily by dispersing the cholesterol and forming a liquid-crystal phase. UDCA affects the enterohepatic circulation of bile salts by reducing the ileal reabsorption of endogenous more hydrophobic and potentially toxic salts such as cholic and chenodeoxycholic acids.

In-vitro studies show that UDCA has a direct hepatoprotective effect and reduces the hepatotoxicity of hydrophobic bile salts. Immunological effects have also been demonstrated with a reduction in abnormal expression of HLS Class I antigens on hepatocytes as well as suppression of cytokine and interleukin production.

5.2 Pharmacokinetic properties
Ursodeoxycholic acid occurs naturally in the body. When given orally it is rapidly and completely absorbed. It is 96 - 98% bound to plasma proteins and efficiently extracted by the liver and excreted in the bile as glycine and taurine conjugates. In the intestine some of the conjugates are deconjugated and reabsorbed. The conjugates may also be dehydroxylated to lithocholic acid, part of which is absorbed, sulphated by the liver and excreted via the biliary tract.

5.3 Preclinical safety data
None Stated.

6. PHARMACEUTICAL PARTICULARS

6.1 List of excipients
Ursofalk Suspension contains the following excipients:

Benzoic acid (E210), microcrystalline cellulose and carboxymethyl-cellulose sodium, sodium chloride, sodium citrate, citric acid anhydrous, glycerol, propylene glycol, xylitol, sodium cyclamate, lemon flavouring (Givaudan 87017) and purified water.

6.2 Incompatibilities
None known other than the interactions identified in Section 4.5.

6.3 Shelf life
48 months.

6.4 Special precautions for storage
Do not refrigerate or freeze.

6.5 Nature and contents of container
Amber glass bottle closed with a plastic screw cap, containing 250ml of suspension.

6.6 Special precautions for disposal and other handling
Shake well before use. After opening the bottle, do not use after 4 months.

7. MARKETING AUTHORISATION HOLDER
Dr Falk Pharma UK Ltd
Unit K
Bourne End Business Park
Cores End Road
Bourne End
Bucks
SL8 5AS
United Kingdom

8. MARKETING AUTHORISATION NUMBER(S)
PL 10341/0007

9. DATE OF FIRST AUTHORISATION/RENEWAL OF THE AUTHORISATION
31st December 2004

10. DATE OF REVISION OF THE TEXT
November 2006

Utinor Tablets 400mg
(Merck Sharp & Dohme Limited)

1. NAME OF THE MEDICINAL PRODUCT
UTINOR® 400 mg Tablets

2. QUALITATIVE AND QUANTITATIVE COMPOSITION
'Utinor' contains 400 mg of the active ingredient, norfloxacin.

For excipients, see 6.1

3. PHARMACEUTICAL FORM
'Utinor' is supplied as off-white oval tablets marked 'MSD 705'.

4. CLINICAL PARTICULARS

4.1 Therapeutic indications
Norfloxacin is a broad-spectrum, quinolone bactericidal agent indicated for the treatment of:

Upper and lower, complicated and uncomplicated, acute and chronic urinary tract infections. These infections include cystitis, pyelitis, pyelonephritis, chronic prostatitis and those urinary infections associated with urological surgery, neurogenic bladder or nephrolithiasis caused by bacteria susceptible to 'Utinor'.

Consideration should be given to official local guidance (e.g. national recommendations) on the appropriate use of bacterial agents.

Susceptibility of the causative organism to the treatment should be tested (if possible), although therapy may be initiated before the results are available.

4.2 Posology and method of administration
'Utinor' should be taken with a glass of water at least one hour before or two hours after a meal or milk ingestion. Multivitamins, products containing iron or zinc, antacids containing magnesium and aluminium, sucralfate or products containing didanosine should not be taken within 2 hours of administration of norfloxacin.

Susceptibility of the causative organism to 'Utinor' should be tested. However, therapy may be initiated before obtaining the results of these tests.

Diagnosis	Dosage	Therapy duration
Uncomplicated lower urinary tract infections (e.g. cystitis)*	400 mg twice daily	3 days
Urinary tract infections	400 mg twice daily	7-10 days
Chronic relapsing urinary tract infection**	400 mg twice daily	Up to 12 weeks

* Trials in over 600 patients have demonstrated the efficacy and tolerability of 'Utinor' in the three-day treatment of uncomplicated urinary tract infections.

** If adequate suppression is obtained within the first four weeks of therapy, the dose of 'Utinor' may be reduced to 400 mg daily.

Patients with renal impairment
'Utinor' is suitable for the treatment of patients with renal impairment. In studies involving patients whose creatinine clearance was less than 30 ml/min/1.73m^2, but who did not require haemodialysis, the plasma half-life of norfloxacin was approximately eight hours. Clinical studies showed there was no difference in the mean half-life of norfloxacin in patients with a creatinine clearance of less than 10 ml/min/1.73m^2, compared to patients with creatinine clearance of 10-30 ml/min/1.73m^2. Hence, for these patients, the recommended dose is one 400 mg tablet once daily. At this dosage, concentrations in appropriate body tissues or fluids exceed the MICs for most pathogens sensitive to norfloxacin.

Use in the elderly
Pharmacokinetic studies have shown no appreciable changes when compared to younger patients, apart from a slight prolongation of half-life. In the absence of renal impairment, no adjustment of dosage is necessary. Limited clinical studies have shown 'Utinor' to be well tolerated.

4.3 Contraindications
Hypersensitivity to any component of this product or any chemically related quinolone antibacterials.

'Utinor' is contra-indicated in prepubertal children and growing adolescents.

4.4 Special warnings and precautions for use
As with other drugs in this class, 'Utinor' should not be used in patients with a history of convulsions or known factors that predispose to seizures unless there is an overwhelming clinical need. Convulsions have been reported rarely with norfloxacin.

Tendinitis and/or tendon rupture, particularly affecting the Achilles tendon, may occur with quinolone antibiotics. Such reactions have been observed, particularly in older patients and in those treated concurrently with corticosteroids. At the first sign of pain or inflammation, patients should discontinue 'Utinor' and rest the affected limbs.

Photosensitivity reactions have been observed in patients who are exposed to excessive sunlight while receiving some members of this drug class. Excessive sunlight should be avoided. Therapy should be discontinued if photosensitivity occurs.

Quinolones, including norfloxacin, may exacerbate the signs of myasthenia gravis and lead to life threatening weakness of the respiratory muscles. Caution should be exercised when using quinolones, including 'Utinor', in patients with myasthenia gravis (see section 4.8 'Undesirable effects').

Rarely, haemolytic reactions have been reported in patients with latent or actual defects in glucose-6-phosphate dehydrogenase activity who take quinolone antibacterial agents, including norfloxacin (see 4.8 'Undesirable effects').

Very rarely, some quinolones have been associated with prolongation of the QTc interval on the electrocardiogram and infrequent cases of arrhythmia (including extremely rare cases of torsade de pointes) have been observed. As with other agents associated with prolongation of the QTc interval, caution should be exercised when using 'Utinor' in patients with hypokalaemia, significant bradycardia or undergoing concurrent treatment with class Ia or class III anti-arrhythmics.

Some quinolones including 'Utinor' should be used with caution in patients using cisapride, erythromycin, antipsychotics, tricyclic antidepressants or who have any personal or family history of QTc prolongation.

Pseudomembranous colitis has been reported with nearly all antibacterial agents, including 'Utinor', and may range in severity from mild to life-threatening. Therefore it is important to consider this diagnosis in patients who present with diarrhoea subsequent to the administration of antibacterial agents. Studies indicte that a toxin produced by *Clostridium difficile* is a primary cause of "antibiotic-associated colitis".

If CDAD is suspected or confirmed, ongoing antibiotic use not directed against *C.difficile* may need to be discontinued. Appropriate fluid and electrolyte management, protein supplementation, antibiotic treatment of *C.difficile*, and surgical evaluation should be instituted as clinically indicated.

Use in children
As with other quinolones, 'Utinor' has been shown to cause arthropathy in immature animals. The safety of 'Utinor' in children has not been adequately explored and therefore the use of 'Utinor' in prepubertal children or growing adolescents is contra-indicated.

4.5 Interaction with other medicinal products and other forms of interaction
Co-administration of probenecid does not affect serum concentrations of norfloxacin, but urinary excretion of the drug diminishes.

As with other organic acid antibacterials, antagonism has been demonstrated *in vitro* between 'Utinor' and nitrofurantoin.

Quinolones, including norfloxacin, have been shown *in vitro* to inhibit CYP1A2. Concomitant use with drugs metabolised by CYP1A2 (e.g. caffeine clozapine, ropinirole, theophylline, tizadine) may result in increased levels of these drugs, with the potential risk of increased toxicity. Patients taking any concomitant drugs metabolised by CYP1A2 should be carefully monitored.

Specifically in relation to this interaction:

Monitoring of theophylline plasma levels should be considered and dosage of theophylline adjusted as required.

The dose of clozapine or ropinirole may need to be adjusted in patients already taking these medications if norfloxacin is introduced or withdrawn.

Co-administration of tizanidine and norfloxacin is not recommended.

Elevated serum levels of ciclosporin have been reported with concomitant use of norfloxacin. Ciclosporin serum levels should be monitored and appropriate ciclosporin dosage adjustments made when these drugs are used concomitantly.

Quinolones, including norfloxacin, may enhance the effects of the anticoagulant warfarin, or its derivatives, by displacing significant amounts from serum albumin-binding sites. When concomitant administration of these products cannot be avoided, measurements of prothrombin time or other suitable coagulation tests should be carried out.

The concomitant administration of quinolones including norfloxacin with glibenclamide (a sulphonylurea agent) has, on occasions, resulted in severe hypoglycaemia. Therefore monitoring of blood glucose is recommended when these agents are co-administered.

Multivitamins, products containing iron or zinc, antacids or sucralfate should not be administered concomitantly with, or within two hours of, the administration of norfloxacin because they may interfere with absorption, resulting in lower serum and urine levels of norfloxacin.

Products containing didanosine should not be administered concomitantly with, or within 2 hours of the administration of norfloxacin, because the products may interfere with absorption resulting in lower serum and urine levels of norfloxacin.

The concomitant administration of a non-steroidal anti-inflammatory drug (NSAID) with a quinolone including norfloxacin, may increase the risk of CNS stimulation and convulsive seizures. Therefore 'Utinor' should be used with caution in individuals receiving NSAIDS concomitantly.

Animal data have shown that quinolones in combination with fenbufen can lead to convulsions. Therefore, concomitant administration of quinolones and fenbufen should be avoided.

4.6 Pregnancy and lactation
There is no evidence from animal studies that norfloxacin has any teratogenic or mutagenic effects. Embryotoxicity secondary to maternotoxicity was observed after large doses in rabbits. Embryonic losses were observed in cynomolgus monkeys without any teratogenic effects. The relevance of these findings for humans is uncertain.

The safe use of 'Utinor' in pregnant women has not been established; however, as with other quinolones, norfloxacin has been shown to cause arthropathy in immature animals and therefore its use during pregnancy is not recommended.

It is not known whether 'Utinor' is excreted in human milk; administration to breast-feeding mothers is thus not recommended.

4.7 Effects on ability to drive and use machines
Norfloxacin may cause dizziness and lightheadedness and, therefore, patients should know how they react to norfloxacin before they drive or operate machinery or engage in activities requiring mental alertness and coordination.

4.8 Undesirable effects
The overall incidence of drug-related side effects reported during clinical trials was approximately 3%.

The most common side effects have been gastro-intestinal, neuropsychiatric and skin reactions, and include nausea, headache, dizziness, rash, heartburn, abdominal pain/cramps, and diarrhoea.

Less commonly, other side effects such as anorexia, sleep disturbances, depression, anxiety/nervousness, irritability, euphoria, disorientation, hallucination, tinnitus, and epiphora have been reported.

Abnormal laboratory side effects observed during clinical trials included:

leucopenia, elevation of ALAT (SGPT), ASAT (SGOT), eosinophilia, neutropenia, thrombocytopenia.

With more widespread use the following additional side effects have been reported:

Hypersensitivity reactions

Hypersensitivity reactions including anaphylaxis, angioedema, dyspnoea, vasculitis, urticaria, arthritis, myalgia, arthralgia and interstitial nephritis.

Skin

Photosensitivity, Stevens-Johnson syndrome, toxic epidermal necrolysis, exfoliative dermatitis, erythema multiforme, pruritus.

Gastro-intestinal

Pseudomembranous colitis, pancreatitis (rare), hepatitis, jaundice including cholestatic jaundice and elevated liver-function tests.

Musculoskeletal

Tendinitis, tendon rupture, exacerbation of myasthenia gravis, elevated creatinine kinase (CK).

Nervous system/psychiatric

Polyneuropathy including Guillaine-Barré syndrome, confusion, paraesthesia, hypoaesthesia, psychic disturbances including psychotic reactions, convulsions, tremors, myoclonus.

Haematological

Agranulocytosis, haemolytic anaemia, sometimes associated with glucose-6-phosphate dehydrogenase deficiency.

Genito-urinary

Vaginal candidiasis.

Renal function

Renal failure.

Special senses

Dysgeusia, visual disturbances, hearing loss.

Cardiovascular

Very rarely: prolonged QTc interval and ventricular arrhythmia (including torsade de pointes) may occur with some quinolones including norfloxacin.

4.9 Overdose
No information is available at present.

In the event of recent acute overdosage, the stomach should be emptied by induced vomiting or by gastric lavage and the patient carefully observed and given symptomatic and supportive treatment. Adequate hydration must be maintained.

5. PHARMACOLOGICAL PROPERTIES

5.1 Pharmacodynamic properties
Pharmacotherapeutic group: Fluoroquinolone

ATC code

JO1MA06

Mode of Action

Norfloxacin inhibits bacterial deoxyribonucleic acid synthesis and is bactericidal. At the molecular level, three specific events were attributed to norfloxacin in *Escherichia coli* cells:

(1) Inhibition of the ATP-dependent DNA supercoiling reaction catalysed by DNA gyrase

(2) Inhibition of the relaxation of supercoiled DNA

(3) Promotion of double-stranded DNA breakage.

'Utinor' has a broad spectrum of antibacterial activity against Gram-positive and Gram-negative aerobic pathogens. The fluorine atom at the 6 position provides increased potency against Gram-negative organisms and the piperazine moiety at the 7 position is responsible for the anti-pseudomonal activity.

PK/PD relationship

Efficacy is mainly dependent upon the C_{max} (maximum serum concentration): MIC (minimum inhibitory concentration) ratio of the pathogen and the AUC (area under the curve): MIK ratio of the pathogen, respectively.

Mechanism/s of Resistance

The major mechanism of resistance to the quinolones, including norfloxacin, is through mutations in the genes that encode for DNA gyrase and topoisomerase IV, the targets of quinolone action. Additional mechanisms of resistance include mutations in the cell membrane proteins, which alter membrane permeability and the development of efflux pumps.

There is no cross-resistance between norfloxacin and structurally unrelated antibacterial agents such as penicillins, cephalosporins, tetracyclines, macrolides, aminocyclitols and sulphonamides, 2, 4 diaminopyrimidines, or combinations thereof (e.g. co-trimoxazole).

Break points

EUCAST clinical MIC breakpoints to separate susceptible (S) pathogens from resistant (R) pathogens are:

Entero-bacteriaceae S < 0.5mcg/ml, R > 1mcg/ml

For *Neisseria gonorrhoeae* and other species MIC breakpoint not defined.

Susceptibility

The prevalence of resistance may vary geographically and with time for selected species and local information on resistance is desirable, particularly when treating severe infections. The information below gives only approximate guidance on the probability as to whether the micro-organism will be susceptible to norfloxacin or not.

Commonly susceptible species:
Gram-negative aerobes:
Aeromonas hydrophilia
Proteus vulgaris
Providencia rettgeri
Salmonella spp.
Shigella spp.
Species for which acquired resistance may be a problem:
Gram-positive aerobes:
Enterococcus faecalis
Staphylococcus aureus (including penicillinase-producing strains)
Staphylococcus epidermidis
Staphylococcus saprophyticus
Streptococcus agalactiae
Gram-negative aerobes:
Citrobacter freundii
Enterobacter aerogenes
Enterobacter cloacae
Escherichia coli
Klebsiella oxytoca
Klebsiella pneumoniae
Morganella morganii
Proteus mirabilis
Providencia stuartii
Pseudomonas aeruginosa
Serratia marcescens

5.2 Pharmacokinetic properties
Norfloxacin is rapidly absorbed following oral administration. In healthy volunteers, at least 30-40% of an oral dose of norfloxacin is absorbed. This results in a serum concentration of 1.5 mcg/ml being attained approximately 1 hour after administration of a 400 mg dose. Mean serum half-life is 3 to 4 hours, and is independent of dose.

The following are mean concentrations of norfloxacin in various fluids and tissues measured 1 to 4 hours post-dose after the two 400 mg doses, unless otherwise indicated:

Renal parenchyma	7.3 mcg/g
Prostate	2.5 mcg/g
Seminal fluid	2.7 mcg/ml
Testicle	1.6 mcg/g
Uterus/cervix	3.0 mcg/g
Vagina	4.3 mcg/g
Fallopian tube	1.9 mcg/g
Bile	6.9 mcg/ml (after 2 × 200 mg doses).

Norfloxacin is eliminated through metabolism, biliary excretion and renal excretion. After a single 400 mg dose of norfloxacin, mean antimicrobial activities equivalent to 278, 773 and 82 mcg of norfloxacin/g of faeces were obtained at 12, 24 and 48 hours, respectively.

Renal excretion occurs by both glomerular filtration and net tubular secretion, as evidenced by the high rate of renal clearance (approximately 275 ml/min). After a single 400 mg dose, urinary concentrations reach a value of 200 or more mcg/ml in healthy volunteers and remain above 30 mcg/ml for at least 12 hours. In the first 24 hours, 33-48% of the drug is recovered in the urine.

Norfloxacin exists in the urine as norfloxacin and six active metabolites of lesser antimicrobial potency. The parent compound accounts for over 70% of total excretion. The bactericidal potency of norfloxacin is not affected by the pH of urine.

Protein binding is less than 15%.

5.3 Preclinical safety data
Norfloxacin, when administered to 3- to 5-month-old dogs at doses four or more times the usual human dose, produced blister formation and eventual erosion of the articular cartilage of the weight-bearing joints. Similar changes have been produced by other structurally related drugs. Dogs six months or older were not susceptible to these changes.

Teratology studies in mice and rats and fertility studies in mice at oral doses of 30 to 50 times the usual dose for humans did not reveal teratogenic or foetal toxic effects. Embryotoxicity was observed in rabbits at doses of 100 mg/kg/day. This was secondary to maternal toxicity and it is a non-specific antimicrobial effect in the rabbit due to an unusual sensitivity to antibiotic-induced changes in the gut microflora.

Although the drug was not teratogenic in cynomolgus monkeys at several times the therapeutic human dosage, an increased percentage of embryonic losses was observed.

6. PHARMACEUTICAL PARTICULARS

6.1 List of excipients
'Utinor' contains the following inactive ingredients:

Croscarmellose sodium USNF
Magnesium stearate Ph Eur
Microcrystalline cellulose Ph Eur
Hydroxypropylcellulose Ph Eur
Hypromellose Ph Eur
Titanium dioxide Ph Eur
Carnauba wax Ph Eur

6.2 Incompatibilities
None

6.3 Shelf life
36 months shelf-life for blister packs.

6.4 Special precautions for storage
Store below 25°C, in a dry place protected from light.

6.5 Nature and contents of container
'Utinor' is available as blister packs of 6, 7 and 14 tablets.

6.6 Special precautions for disposal and other handling
None.

7. MARKETING AUTHORISATION HOLDER
Merck Sharp & Dohme Limited
Hertford Road, Hoddesdon, Hertfordshire EN11 9BU, UK

8. MARKETING AUTHORISATION NUMBER(S)
PL 0025/0254

9. DATE OF FIRST AUTHORISATION/RENEWAL OF THE AUTHORISATION
Authorisation first granted 3 August 1990. Licence last renewed 4 December 2001.

10. DATE OF REVISION OF THE TEXT
March 2009

® denotes registered trademark of Merck & Co., Inc., Whitehouse Station, NJ, USA.

SPC.NRX.08.UK.2827

Utovlan Tablets

(Pharmacia Limited)

1. NAME OF THE MEDICINAL PRODUCT
Utovlan.

2. QUALITATIVE AND QUANTITATIVE COMPOSITION
Each tablet contains 5mg norethisterone Ph Eur.

For excipients see Section 6.1.

3. PHARMACEUTICAL FORM

White, flat, circular, bevel-edged tablet inscribed 'SEARLE' on one side and 'U' on the other.

4. CLINICAL PARTICULARS

4.1 Therapeutic indications

At low dose: Dysfunctional uterine bleeding, endometriosis, polymenorrhoea, menorrhagia, metropathia, haemorrhagia, postponement of menstruation and premenstrual syndrome.

At high dose: Disseminated carcinoma of the breast.

4.2 Posology and method of administration

Oral Administration

Low dose

Dysfunctional uterine bleeding, polymenorrhoea, menorrhagia, dysmenorrhoea and metropathia haemorrhagia: 1 tablet three times daily for 10 days; bleeding usually stops within 48 hours. Withdrawal bleeding resembling true menstruation occurs a few days after the end of treatment. One tablet twice daily, from days 19 to 26 of the two subsequent cycles, should be given to prevent recurrence of the condition.

Endometriosis: 1 tablet three times daily for a minimum treatment period of six months. The dosage should be increased to 4 or 5 tablets a day if spotting occurs. The initial dosage should be resumed when bleeding or spotting stops.

Postponement of menstruation: 1 tablet three times daily, starting three days before the expected onset of menstruation. Menstruation usually follows within three days of finishing the treatment.

Pre-menstrual syndrome: 1 tablet daily from days 16 to 25 of the menstrual cycle.

High dose

For disseminated breast carcinoma the starting dose is 8 tablets (40mg) per day increasing to 12 tablets (60mg) if no regression is noted.

4.3 Contraindications

Pregnancy

Previous idiopathic or current venous thromboembolism (deep vein thrombosis, pulmonary embolism)

Active or recent arterial thromboembolic disease (e.g. angina, myocardial infarction)

Disturbance of liver function

History during pregnancy of idiopathic jaundice

Severe pruritus or pemphigoid gestationis

Undiagnosed irregular vaginal bleeding

Porphyria

Known hypersensitivity to norethisterone or any of the excipients

4.4 Special warnings and precautions for use

If menstrual bleeding should fail to follow a course of Utovlan, the possibility of pregnancy must be excluded before a further course is given.

Therapy should be discontinued if the following occur:

- Jaundice or deterioration in liver function
- Significant increase in blood pressure
- New onset of migraine-type headache

Progestogens may cause fluid retention. Special care should be taken when prescribing norethisterone in patients with conditions which might be aggravated by this factor:

- Epilepsy
- Migraine
- Asthma
- Cardiac dysfunction
- Renal dysfunction

Risk of venous thromboembolism (VTE)

Long term use of low dose progestogens as part of combined oral contraception or combined hormone replacement therapy has been associated with an increased risk of venous thromboembolism, although the role of progestogens in this aetiology is uncertain. A patient who develops symptoms suggestive of thromboembolic complications should have her status and need for treatment carefully assessed before continuing therapy.

Any patient who develops an acute impairment of vision, proptosis, diplopia or migraine headache should be carefully evaluated ophthalmologically to exclude papilloedema or retinal vascular lesions before continuing medication.

Generally recognised risk factors for VTE include a personal history or family history, severe obesity (BMI >30 kg/m^2) and systemic lupus erythematosus (SLE). There is no consensus about the possible role of varicose veins in VTE.

Treatment with steroid hormones may add to these risk factors. Personal or strong family history of thromboembolism or recurrent spontaneous abortion should be investigated in order to exclude a thrombophillic predisposition. Until a thorough evaluation of thrombophillic factors has been made or anticoagulant treatment initiated, use of progestogens in these patients should be viewed as contraindicated. Where a patient is already taking anticoagulants, the risks and benefits of progestogen therapy should be carefully considered.

The risk of VTE may be temporarily increased with prolonged immobilisation, major trauma or major surgery. As in all post-operative patients, scrupulous attention should be given to prophylactic measures to prevent VTE. Where prolonged immobilisation is likely to follow elective surgery, particularly abdominal or orthopaedic surgery to the lower limbs, consideration should be given to stopping progestogen therapy 4-6 weeks pre-operatively. Treatment should not be restarted until the patient is fully remobilised.

If VTE develops after initiating therapy the drug should be withdrawn. Patients should be advised to contact their doctor immediately if they become aware of a potential thromboembolic symptom (e.g., painful swelling in the leg, sudden pain in the chest, dyspnoea).

4.5 Interaction with other medicinal products and other forms of interaction

Interaction with other medicines

The metabolism of progestogens may be increased by concommitant administration of compounds known to induce drug-metabolising enzymes, specifically cytochrome P450 enzymes. These compopunds include anticonvulsants (e.g., phenobarbital, phenytoin, carbamezapin) and anti-infectives (e.g., rifampicin, rifabutin, nevirapine, efavirenz, tetracyclines, ampicillin, oxacillin and cotrimoxazole)

Ritonavir and nelfinavir, although known as strong inhibitors, by contrast exhibit inducing properties when used concomitantly with steroid hormones. Herbal preparations containing St John's Wort (Hypericum Perforatum) may induce the metabolism of progestogens. Progestogen levels may therefore be reduced.

Aminoglutethimide has been reported to decrease plasma levels of some progestogens.

Concurrent administration of cyclosporin and norethisterone has been reported to lead to increased plasma cyclosporin levels and/or decreased plamsa norethisterone levels.

When used in combination with cytotoxic drugs, it is possible that progestogens may reduce the haematological toxicity of chemotherapy.

Special care should be taken when progestogens are administered with other drugs which also cause fluid retention, such as NSAIDs and vasodilators.

Other forms of interaction

Progestogens can influence certain laboratory tests (e.g., tests for hepatic function, thyroid function and coagulation).

4.6 Pregnancy and lactation

Contra-indicated in pregnancy.

4.7 Effects on ability to drive and use machines

None.

4.8 Undesirable effects

Progestogens given alone at low doses have been associated with the following undesirable effects:

Genitourinary	breakthrough bleeding, spotting, amenorrhoea, abnormal uterine bleeding, (irregular, increase, decrease), alterations of cervical secretions, cervical erosions, prolonged anovulation
Breast	Galactorrhoea, mastodynia, tenderness
Central Nervous System	depression, headache, dizziness, fatigue, insomnia, nervousness, somnolence, confusion, euphoria, loss of concentration, vision disorders
Gastrointestinal/ Hepatobiliary	nausea, vomiting, cholestatic icterus/jaundice, constipation, diarrhoea, dry mouth, disturbed liver function
Metabolic & Nutritional	altered serum lipid and lipoprotein profiles, increased fasting glucose levels, increased fasting insulin levels, decreased glucose tolerance, adrenergic-like effects (e.g., fine hand tremors, sweating, cramps in calves at night), corticoid-like effects (e.g., Cushingoid syndrome), diabetic cataract, exacerbation of diabetes mellitus, glycosuria
Cardiovascular	thrombo-embolic disorders, cerebral and myocardial infarction, congestive heart failure, increased blood pressure, palpitations, pulmonary embolism, retinal thrombosis, tachycardia, thrombophlebitis
Skin & Mucous Membranes	acne, hirsutism, alopecia, pruritis, rash, urticaria
Allergy	hypersensitivity reactions (e.g., anaphylaxis & anaphylactoid reactions, angioedema)
Miscellaneous	oedema/fluid retention, bloating, weight gain, pyrexia, change in appetite, change in libido, hypercalcaemia, malaise

4.9 Overdose

Overdosage may be manifested by nausea, vomiting, breast enlargement and later vaginal bleeding. There is no specific antidote and treatment should be symptomatic.

Gastric lavage may be employed if the overdosage is large and the patient is seen sufficiently early (within four hours).

5. PHARMACOLOGICAL PROPERTIES

Pharmotherapeutic group (ATC code) L02A B.

5.1 Pharmacodynamic properties

Norethisterone given at intermediate doses (5-10mg) suppresses ovulation via its effect on the pituitary. The endogenous production of oestrogens and progesterones are also suppressed, and the ectopic endometrium is converted to a decidua resembling that of pregnancy. In carcinoma norethisterone may act by pituitary inhibition or by direct action on tumour deposits.

5.2 Pharmacokinetic properties

Norethisterone is rapidly and completely absorbed after oral administration, peak plasma concentration occurring in the majority of subjects between 1 and 3 hours. Due to first-pass metabolism, blood levels after oral administration are 60% of those after i.v. administration. The half life of elimination varies from 5 to 12 hours, with a mean of 7.6 hours. Norethisterone is metabolised mainly in the liver. Approximately 60% of the administered dose is excreted as metabolites in urine and faeces.

5.3 Preclinical safety data

The toxicity of norethisterone is very low. Reports of teratogenic effects in animals are uncommon. No carcinogenic effects have been found even in long-term studies.

6. PHARMACEUTICAL PARTICULARS

6.1 List of excipients

maize starch

polyvidone

magnesium stearate

lactose

6.2 Incompatibilities

None stated.

6.3 Shelf life

The shelf life of Utovlan tablets is 3 years.

6.4 Special precautions for storage

Store in a dry place, below 25°C, away from direct sunlight.

6.5 Nature and contents of container

Utovlan tablets are supplied in pvc/foil blister packs of 30 and 90 tablets.

6.6 Special precautions for disposal and other handling

None.

Administrative Data

7. MARKETING AUTHORISATION HOLDER

Pharmacia Limited

Ransgate Road

Sandwich

Kent CT13 9NJ, UK

8. MARKETING AUTHORISATION NUMBER(S)

PL 00032/0423

9. DATE OF FIRST AUTHORISATION/RENEWAL OF THE AUTHORISATION

15th July 2002/15th February 2003

10. DATE OF REVISION OF THE TEXT

May 2007

Company Ref: UT 2_0

Utrogestan 100mg Capsules

(Ferring Pharmaceuticals Ltd)

1. NAME OF THE MEDICINAL PRODUCT

UTROGESTAN 100MG CAPSULES

2. QUALITATIVE AND QUANTITATIVE COMPOSITION

Each capsule contains 100 mg micronised progesterone (INN). For excipients, see 6.1.

3. PHARMACEUTICAL FORM

Capsules, soft

White

4. CLINICAL PARTICULARS

4.1 Therapeutic indications

Adjunctive use with estrogen in post-menopausal women with an intact uterus. (HRT)

4.2 Posology and method of administration

Posology

In women receiving estrogen replacement therapy there is an increased risk of endometrial cancer which can be countered by progesterone administration. The recommended dose is 200 mg daily at bedtime, for twelve days in the last half of each therapeutic cycle (beginning on day 15 of the cycle and ending on day 26). Withdrawal bleeding may occur in the following week. Alternatively 100 mg can be given at bedtime from day 1 to day 25 of each therapeutic cycle, withdrawal bleeding being less with this treatment schedule.

Children: Not applicable.

Elderly: As for adults

Method of Administration: Oral. Utrogestan 100mg Capsules should not be taken with food

4.3 Contraindications

Known allergy or hypersensitivity to progesterone or to any of the excipients. The capsules contain arachis oil (peanut oil) and should never be used by patients allergic to peanuts. Severe hepatic dysfunction. Undiagnosed vaginal bleeding. Mammary or genital tract carcinoma. Thrombophlebitis. Thromboembolic disorders. Cerebral haemorrhage. Porphyria.

4.4 Special warnings and precautions for use

Warnings:

Utrogestan 100mg Capsules are not a treatment for premature labour.

Prescription of progesterone beyond the first trimester of pregnancy may reveal gravidic cholestasis.

Utrogestan 100mg Capsules are not suitable for use as a contraceptive.

If unexplained, sudden or gradual, partial or complete loss of vision, proptosis or diplopia, papilloedema, retinal vascular lesions or migraine occur during therapy, the drug should be discontinued and appropriate diagnostic and therapeutic measures instituted.

Utrogestan 100mg Capsules are intended to be co-prescribed with an estrogen product as HRT. Epidemiological evidence suggests that the use of HRT is associated with an increased risk of developing deep vein thrombosis (DVT) or pulmonary embolism. The prescribing information for the co-prescribed estrogen product should be referred to for information about the risks of venous thromboembolism.

There is suggestive evidence of a small increased risk of breast cancer with estrogen replacement therapy. It is not known whether concurrent progesterone influences the risk of cancer in post-menopausal women taking hormone replacement therapy. The prescribing information for the co-prescribed estrogen product should be referred to for information about the risks of breast cancer.

Precautions

Prior to taking hormone replacement therapy (and at regular intervals thereafter) each woman should be assessed. A personal and family medical history should be taken and physical examination should be guided by this and by the contraindications and warnings for this product.

Utrogestan 100mg Capsules should not be taken with food and should be taken at bedtime. Concomitant food ingestion increases the bioavailability of Utrogestan 100mg Capsules.

Utrogestan 100mg Capsules should be used cautiously in patients with conditions that might be aggravated by fluid retention (e.g. hypertension, cardiac disease, renal disease, epilepsy, migraine, asthma); in patients with a history of depression, diabetes, mild to moderate hepatic dysfunction, migraine or photosensitivity and in breast-feeding mothers.

Clinical examination of the breasts and pelvic examination should be performed where clinically indicated rather than as a routine procedure. Women should be encouraged to participate in the national breast cancer screening programme (mammography) and the national cervical cancer screening programme (cervical cytology) as appropriate for their age. Breast awareness should also be encouraged and women advised to report any changes in their breasts to their doctor or nurse.

4.5 Interaction with other medicinal products and other forms of interaction

Utrogestan 100mg Capsules may interfere with the effects of bromocriptine and may raise the plasma concentration of ciclosporin. Utrogestan 100mg Capsules may affect the results of laboratory tests of hepatic and/or endocrine functions.

Metabolism of Utrogestan 100mg Capsules is accelerated by rifamycin an antibacterial agent.

The metabolism of progesterone by human liver microsomes was inhibited by ketoconazole (IC_{50} <0.1 μM Ketoconazole is a known inhibitor of cytochrome P450 3A4. These data therefore suggest that ketoconazole may increase the bioavailability of progesterone. The clinical relevance of the in vitro findings is unknown.

4.6 Pregnancy and lactation

Pregnancy

Utrogestan 100mg Capsules are not indicated during pregnancy. If pregnancy occurs during medication, Utrogestan 100mg Capsules should be withdrawn immediately.

Lactation

Detectable amounts of progesterone enter the breast milk. There is no indication for prescribing HRT during lactation.

4.7 Effects on ability to drive and use machines

Utrogestan 100mg Capsules may cause drowsiness and/or dizziness in a minority of patients; therefore caution is advised in drivers and users of machines. Taking the capsules at bedtime should reduce these effects during the day.

4.8 Undesirable effects

Somnolence or transient dizziness may occur 1 to 3 hours after intake of the drug. Bedtime dosing and reduction of the dose may reduce these effects.

Shortening of the cycle or breakthrough bleeding may occur. If this occurs, the dose of Utrogestan 100mg Capsules can be reduced and taken at bedtime from day 1 to day 26 of each therapeutic cycle.

Acne, urticaria, rashes, fluid retention, weight changes, gastro-intestinal disturbances, changes in libido, breast discomfort, premenstrual symptoms, menstrual disturbances; also chloasma, depression, pyrexia, insomnia, alopecia, hirsutism; rarely jaundice.

Venous thromboembolism, i.e. deep leg or pelvic venous thrombosis and pulmonary embolism, is more frequent among hormone replacement therapy users than among non-users.

4.9 Overdose

Symptoms of overdosage may include somnolence, dizziness, euphoria or dysmenorrhoea. Treatment is observation and, if necessary, symptomatic and supportive measures should be provided.

5. PHARMACOLOGICAL PROPERTIES

5.1 Pharmacodynamic properties

Pharmacotherapeutic group (ATC code: G03D)

Progesterone is a natural progestogen, the main hormone of the corpus luteum and the placenta. It acts on the endometrium by converting the proliferating phase to the secretory phase. Utrogestan 100mg Capsules have all the properties of endogenous progesterone with induction of a full secretory endometrium and in particular gestagenic, antiestrogenic, slightly anti-androgenic and antialdosterone effects.

5.2 Pharmacokinetic properties

Absorption

Micronised progesterone is absorbed by the digestive tract. Pharmacokinetic studies conducted in healthy volunteers have shown that after oral administration of 2 capsules (200mg), plasma progesterone levels increased to reach the Cmax of 13.8ng/ml +/- 2.9ng/ml in 2.2 +/- 1.4 hours. The elimination half-life observed was 16.8+/- 2.3 hours.

Although there were inter-individual variations, the individual pharmacokinetic characteristics were maintained over several months, indicating predictable responses to the drug.

Distribution

Progesterone is approximately 96%-99% bound to serum proteins, primarily to serum albumin (50%-54%) and transcortin (43%-48%).

Elimination

Urinary elimination is observed for 95% in the form of glycuroconjugated metabolites, mainly 3 α, 5 β-pregnanediol (pregnandiol).

Metabolism

Progesterone is metabolised primarily by the liver. The main plasma metabolites are 20 α hydroxy- Δ 4 α- prenolone and 5 α-dihydroprogesterone. Some progesterone metabolites are excreted in the bile and these may be deconjugated and further metabolised in the gut via reduction, dehydroxylation and epimerisation. The main plasma and urinary metabolites are similar to those found during the physiological secretion of the corpus luteum.

5.3 Preclinical safety data

Preclinical data revealed no special hazard for humans based on conventional studies of safety pharmacology and toxicity.

6. PHARMACEUTICAL PARTICULARS

6.1 List of excipients

Arachis oil

Soya lecithin

Gelatin

Glycerol

Titanium dioxide

6.2 Incompatibilities

None.

6.3 Shelf life

3 years.

6.4 Special precautions for storage

No special precautions for storage.

6.5 Nature and contents of container

The product is supplied in PVC/Aluminium blisters contained in cartons.

Pack size: 30 capsules

6.6 Special precautions for disposal and other handling

Not applicable.

7. MARKETING AUTHORISATION HOLDER

Laboratoires BESINS INTERNATIONAL

3, rue du Bourg l'Abbé

75003

Paris

France

8. MARKETING AUTHORISATION NUMBER(S)

PL 16468/0001

9. DATE OF FIRST AUTHORISATION/RENEWAL OF THE AUTHORISATION

10 January 2003

10. DATE OF REVISION OF THE TEXT

Feburary 2006

Utrogestan 200mg Capsules

(Ferring Pharmaceuticals Ltd)

1. NAME OF THE MEDICINAL PRODUCT

Utrogestan 200mg capsules

2. QUALITATIVE AND QUANTITATIVE COMPOSITION

Each capsule contains 200 mg micronised progesterone (INN). For excipients, see 6.1.

3. PHARMACEUTICAL FORM

Capsules, soft

White

4. CLINICAL PARTICULARS

4.1 Therapeutic indications

Adjunctive use with estrogen in post-menopausal women with an intact uterus. (HRT)

4.2 Posology and method of administration

Posology

In women receiving estrogen replacement therapy there is an increased risk of endometrial cancer which can be countered by progesterone administration. The recommended dose is 200 mg daily at bedtime, for twelve days in the last half of each therapeutic cycle (beginning on day 15 of the cycle and ending on day 26). Withdrawal bleeding may occur in the following week. Alternatively 100 mg can be given at bedtime from day 1 to day 25 of each therapeutic cycle, withdrawal bleeding being less with this treatment schedule.

Children: Not applicable.

Elderly: As for adults

Method of Administration: Oral. Utrogestan 200mg Capsules should not be taken with food

4.3 Contraindications

Known allergy or hypersensitivity to progesterone or to any of the excipients. The capsules contain arachis oil (peanut oil) and should never be used by patients allergic to peanuts. Severe hepatic dysfunction. Undiagnosed vaginal bleeding. Mammary or genital tract carcinoma. Thrombophlebitis. Thromboembolic disorders. Cerebral haemorrhage. Porphyria.

4.4 Special warnings and precautions for use

Warnings:

Utrogestan 200mg Capsules are not a treatment for premature labour.

Prescription of progesterone beyond the first trimester of pregnancy may reveal gravidic cholestasis.

Utrogestan 200mg Capsules are not suitable for use as a contraceptive.

If unexplained, sudden or gradual, partial or complete loss of vision, proptosis or diplopia, papilloedema, retinal vascular lesions or migraine occur during therapy, the drug should be discontinued and appropriate diagnostic and therapeutic measures instituted.

Utrogestan 200mg Capsules are intended to be co-prescribed with an estrogen product as HRT. Epidemiological evidence suggests that the use of HRT is associated with an increased risk of developing deep vein thrombosis (DVT) or pulmonary embolism. The prescribing information for the co-prescribed estrogen product should be referred to for information about the risks of venous thromboembolism.

There is suggestive evidence of a small increased risk of breast cancer with estrogen replacement therapy. It is not known whether concurrent progesterone influences the risk of cancer in post-menopausal women taking hormone replacement therapy. The prescribing information for the co-prescribed estrogen product should be referred to for information about the risks of breast cancer.

Precautions

Prior to taking hormone replacement therapy (and at regular intervals thereafter) each woman should be assessed. A personal and family medical history should be taken and physical examination should be guided by this and by the contraindications and warnings for this product.

Utrogestan 200mg Capsules should not be taken with food and should be taken at bedtime. Concomitant food ingestion increases the bioavailability of Utrogestan 100mg Capsules.

Utrogestan 200mg Capsules should be used cautiously in patients with conditions that might be aggravated by fluid retention (e.g. hypertension, cardiac disease, renal disease, epilepsy, migraine, asthma); in patients with a history of depression, diabetes, mild to moderate hepatic dysfunction, migraine or photosensitivity and in breast-feeding mothers.

Clinical examination of the breasts and pelvic examination should be performed where clinically indicated rather than as a routine procedure. Women should be encouraged to participate in the national breast cancer screening programme (mammography) and the national cervical cancer screening programme (cervical cytology) as appropriate for their age. Breast awareness should also be encouraged and women advised to report any changes in their breasts to their doctor or nurse.

4.5 Interaction with other medicinal products and other forms of interaction

Utrogestan 200mg Capsules may interfere with the effects of bromocriptine and may raise the plasma concentration of cyclosporine. Utrogestan 200mg Capsules may affect the results of laboratory tests of hepatic and/or endocrine functions.

Metabolism of Utrogestan 200mg Capsules is accelerated by rifamycin an antibacterial agent.

The metabolism of progesterone by human liver microsomes was inhibited by ketoconazole ($IC_{50} < 0.1$ μM Ketoconazole is a known inhibitor of cytochrome P450 3A4. These data therefore suggest that ketoconazole may increase the bioavailability of progesterone. The clinical relevance of the in vitro findings is unknown.

4.6 Pregnancy and lactation

Pregnancy

Utrogestan 200mg Capsules are not indicated during pregnancy. If pregnancy occurs during medication, Utrogestan 200mg Capsules should be withdrawn immediately.

Lactation

Detectable amounts of progesterone enter the breast milk. There is no indication for prescribing HRT during lactation.

4.7 Effects on ability to drive and use machines

Utrogestan 200mg Capsules may cause drowsiness and/or dizziness in a minority of patients; therefore caution is advised in drivers and users of machines. Taking the capsules at bedtime should reduce these effects during the day.

4.8 Undesirable effects

Somnolence or transient dizziness may occur 1 to 3 hours after intake of the drug. Bedtime dosing and reduction of the dose may reduce these effects.

Shortening of the cycle or breakthrough bleeding may occur. If this occurs, the dose of Utrogestan 200mg Capsules can be reduced and taken at bedtime from day 1 to day 26 of each therapeutic cycle.

Acne, urticaria, rashes, fluid retention, weight changes, gastro-intestinal disturbances, changes in libido, breast discomfort, premenstrual symptoms, menstrual disturbances; also chloasma, depression, pyrexia, insomnia, alopecia, hirsutism; rarely jaundice.

Venous thromboembolism, i.e. deep leg or pelvic venous thrombosis and pulmonary embolism, is more frequent among hormone replacement therapy users than among non-users.

4.9 Overdose

Symptoms of overdosage may include somnolence, dizziness, euphoria or dysmenorrhoea. Treatment is observation and, if necessary, symptomatic and supportive measures should be provided.

5. PHARMACOLOGICAL PROPERTIES

5.1 Pharmacodynamic properties

Pharmacotherapeutic group (ATC code: G03D)

Progesterone is a natural progestogen, the main hormone of the corpus luteum and the placenta. It acts on the endometrium by converting the proliferating phase to the secretory phase. Utrogestan 200mg Capsules have all the properties of endogenous progesterone with induction of a full secretory endometrium and in particular gestagenic, antiestrogenic, slightly anti-androgenic and antialdosterone effects.

5.2 Pharmacokinetic properties

Absorption

Micronised progesterone is absorbed by the digestive tract. Pharmacokinetic studies conducted in healthy volunteers have shown that after oral administration of 2 capsules (200mg), plasma progesterone levels increased to reach the Cmax of 13.8ng/ml +/- 2.9ng/ml in 2.2 +/- 1.4 hours. The elimination half-life observed was 16.8+/- 2.3 hours.

Although there were inter-individual variations, the individual pharmacokinetic characteristics were maintained over several months, indicating predictable responses to the drug.

Distribution

Progesterone is approximately 96%-99% bound to serum proteins, primarily to serum albumin (50%-54%) and transcortin (43%-48%).

Elimination

Urinary elimination is observed for 95% in the form of glycuroconjugated metabolites, mainly 3 α, 5 β–pregnanediol (pregnandiol).

Metabolism

Progesterone is metabolised primarily by the liver. The main plasma metabolites are 20 α hydroxy- Δ 4 α- prenolone and 5 α-dihydroprogesterone. Some progesterone metabolites are excreted in the bile and these may be deconjugated and further metabolised in the gut via reduction, dehydroxylation and epimerisation. The main plasma and urinary metabolites are similar to those found during the physiological secretion of the corpus luteum.

5.3 Preclinical safety data

Preclinical data revealed no special hazard for humans based on conventional studies of safety pharmacology and toxicity.

6. PHARMACEUTICAL PARTICULARS

6.1 List of excipients

Arachis oil

Soya lecithin

Gelatin

Glycerol

Titanium dioxide

6.2 Incompatibilities

None.

6.3 Shelf life

3 years.

6.4 Special precautions for storage

No special precautions for storage.

6.5 Nature and contents of container

The product is supplied in PVC/Aluminium blisters contained in cartons.

Pack size: 15 capsules per carton

6.6 Special precautions for disposal and other handling

Not applicable.

7. MARKETING AUTHORISATION HOLDER

Laboratoires BESINS INTERNATIONAL

3, rue du Bourg l'Abbé

75003

Paris

France

8. MARKETING AUTHORISATION NUMBER(S)

PL 16468/0007

9. DATE OF FIRST AUTHORISATION/RENEWAL OF THE AUTHORISATION

6th January 2005

10. DATE OF REVISION OF THE TEXT

February 2006

Vagifem 25 μg film-coated tablets

(Novo Nordisk Limited)

1. NAME OF THE MEDICINAL PRODUCT

Vagifem® 25 micrograms film-coated vaginal tablets

2. QUALITATIVE AND QUANTITATIVE COMPOSITION

One vaginal tablet contains:

Estradiol hemihydrate equivalent to estradiol 25 micrograms.

Excipients:

For a full list of excipients, see section 6.1

3. PHARMACEUTICAL FORM

Film-coated vaginal tablet inset in disposable applicator.

4. CLINICAL PARTICULARS

4.1 Therapeutic indications

Hormone replacement therapy for the treatment of vaginal atrophy due to oestrogen deficiency.

The experience of treating women older than 65 years is limited.

4.2 Posology and method of administration

4.2.1 Dosage

Vagifem® is administered intravaginally using the applicator. An initial dose of one tablet daily for two weeks will usually improve vaginal atrophy and associated symptoms; a maintenance dose of two tablets per week should then be instituted.

Treatment may be started on any convenient day.

If a dose is forgotten, it should be administered as soon as the patient remembers. A double dose should be avoided.

For initiation and continuation of treatment of postmenopausal symptoms, the lowest effective dose for the shortest duration (see also section 4.4) should be used.

Vagifem® may be used in women with or without an intact uterus.

The addition of a progestogen is not recommended during treatment with Vagifem® (but see section 4.4)

Not intended for children or males.

Use in the elderly: there are no special dosage requirements.

4.2.2 Administration

The applicator is inserted into the vagina up to the end of the smooth part of the applicator (approximately 9 cms). The tablet is released by pressing the plunger. The applicator is then withdrawn and disposed of.

4.3 Contraindications

Known, past or suspected breast cancer.

Known, past or suspected oestrogen-dependent malignant tumours (eg endometrial cancer).

Undiagnosed genital bleeding.

Untreated endometrial hyperplasia.

Previous idiopathic or current venous thromboembolism (deep venous thrombosis, pulmonary embolism).

Active or recent arterial thromboembolic disease (e.g. angina, myocardial infarction.

Acute liver disease or history of liver disease as long as liver function tests have failed to return to normal.

Known hypersensitivity to the active substance or to any of the excipients.

Porphyria.

4.4 Special warnings and precautions for use

For the treatment of postmenopausal symptoms, HRT should only be initiated for symptoms that adversely affect quality of life. In all cases, a careful appraisal of the risks and benefits should be undertaken annually and HRT should only be continued as long as the benefit outweighs the risk.

Medical examination/follow-up

Before initiating or reinstituting HRT, a complete personal and family medical history should be taken. Physical (including pelvic and breast) examination should be guided by this and by the contra-indications and warnings for use. During treatment, periodic check-ups are recommended of a frequency and nature adapted to the individual woman. Women should be advised what changes in their breasts should be reported to their doctor or nurse. Investigations, including mammography, should be carried out in accordance with currently accepted screening practices, modified to the clinical needs of the individual.

Vaginal infections should be treated before initiation of Vagifem® therapy.

Due to the intermittent administration of low dose estradiol in Vagifem®, low systemic exposure of estradiol is expected (see section 5.2), however being an HRT product the following need to be considered especially for long-term or repeated use of this product.

Conditions which need supervision

If any of the following conditions are present, have occurred previously, and/or have been aggravated during pregnancy or previous hormone treatment, the patient should be closely supervised. It should be taken into account that these conditions may recur or be aggravated during systemic oestrogen treatment, in particular:

- Leiomyoma (uterine fibroids) or endometriosis
- A history of, or risk factors for, thromboembolic disorders (see below)
- Risk factors for oestrogen dependent tumours, e.g. 1st degree heredity for breast cancer
- Hypertension
- Liver disorders (e.g. liver adenoma)
- Diabetes mellitus with or without vascular involvement
- Cholelithiasis
- Migraine or (severe) headache
- Systemic lupus erythematosus
- A history of endometrial hyperplasia (see below)
- Epilepsy
- Asthma
- Otosclerosis

Reasons for immediate withdrawal of therapy

Therapy should be discontinued in case a contra-indication is discovered and in the following situations:

- Jaundice or deterioration in liver function
- Significant increase in blood pressure
- New onset of migraine-type headache
- Pregnancy

Endometrial hyperplasia

The risk of endometrial hyperplasia and carcinoma is increased when systemic oestrogens are administered for prolonged periods of time. The endometrial safety of long-term or repeated use of topical vaginal oestrogens is uncertain. Therefore, if repeated, treatment should be reviewed at least annually, with special consideration given to any symptoms of endometrial hyperplasia or carcinoma.

If bleeding or spotting appears at any time on therapy, the reason should be investigated, which may include endometrial biopsy to exclude endometrial malignancy.

Unopposed oestrogen stimulation may lead to premalignant or malignant transformation in the residual foci of endometriosis. Therefore caution is advised when using this product in women who have undergone hysterectomy because of endometriosis, especially if they are known to have residual endometriosis.

Vagifem® is a local low dose preparation and therefore the occurrence of the below mentioned conditions is less likely than that with systemic oestrogen treatment.

Breast cancer

A randomised placebo-controlled trial, the Women's Health Initiative study (WHI), and epidemiological studies, including the Million Women Study (MWS), have reported an increased risk of breast cancer in women taking estrogens, estrogen-progestagen combinations or tibolone for HRT for several years (see section 4.8). For all HRT, an excess risk becomes apparent within a few years of use and increases with duration of intake but returns to baseline within a few (at most five) years after stopping treatment.

In the MWS, the relative risk of breast cancer with conjugated equine estrogens (CEE) or estradiol (E2) was greater when a progestagen was added, either sequentially or continuously, and regardless of type of progestagen. There was no evidence of a difference in risk between the different routes of administration.

In the WHI study, the continuous combined conjugated equine estrogen and medroxyprogesterone acetate (CEE + MPA) product used was associated with breast cancers that were slightly larger in size and more frequently had local lymph node metastases compared to placebo. HRT, especially estrogen-progestagen combined treatment, increases the density of mammographic images which may adversely affect the radiological detection of breast cancer.

Venous thromboembolism

Systemic HRT is associated with a higher relative risk of developing venous thromboembolism (VTE), i.e. deep vein thrombosis or pulmonary embolism. One randomised controlled trial and epidemiological studies found a two- to threefold higher risk for users compared with non-users. For non-users it is estimated that the number of cases of VTE that will occur over a 5 year period is about 3 per 1000 women aged 50-59 years and 8 per 1000 women aged between 60-69 years. It is estimated that in healthy women who use HRT for 5 years, the number of additional cases of VTE over a 5 year period will be between 2 and 6 (best estimate = 4) per 1000 women aged 50-59 years and between 5 and 15 (best estimate = 9) per 1000 women aged 60-69 years. The occurrence of such an event is more likely in the first year of HRT than later.

Generally recognised risk factors for VTE include a personal history or family history, severe obesity (BMI > 30 kg/m^2) and systemic lupus erythematosus (SLE). There is no consensus about the possible role of varicose veins in VTE.

Patients with a history of VTE or known thrombophilic states have an increased risk of VTE. HRT may add to this risk. Personal or strong family history of thromboembolism, or recurrent spontaneous abortion, should be investigated in order to exclude a thrombophilic predisposition. Until a thorough evaluation of thrombophilic factors has been made or anticoagulant treatment initiated, use of HRT in such patients should be viewed as contraindicated. Those women already on anticoagulant treatment require careful consideration of the benefit-risk of use of HRT.

The risk of VTE may be temporarily increased with prolonged immobilisation, major trauma or major surgery. As in all postoperative patients, scrupulous attention should be given to prophylactic measures to prevent VTE following surgery. Where prolonged immobilisation is liable to follow elective surgery, particularly abdominal or orthopaedic surgery to the lower limbs, consideration should be given to temporarily stopping HRT 4 to 6 weeks earlier, if possible. Treatment should not be restarted until the woman is completely mobilised.

If VTE develops after initiating therapy, the drug should be discontinued. Patients should be told to contact their doctors immediately when they are aware of a potential thromboembolic symptom (e.g. painful swelling of a leg, sudden pain in the chest, dyspnoea).

Coronary artery disease (CAD)

There is no evidence from randomised controlled trials of cardiovascular benefit with continuous combined conjugated estrogens and medroxyprogesterone acetate (MPA). Two large clinical trials (WHI and HERS i.e. Heart and Estrogen/progestin Replacement Study) showed a possible increased risk of cardiovascular morbidity in the first year of use and no overall benefit. For other HRT products there are only limited data from randomised controlled trials examining effects in cardiovascular morbidity or mortality. Therefore, it is uncertain whether these findings also extend to other HRT products.

Stroke

One large randomised clinical trial (WHI-trial) found, as a secondary outcome, an increased risk of ischaemic stroke in healthy women during treatment with continuous combined conjugated oestrogens and medroxyprogesterone acetate (MPA). For women who do not use HRT, it is estimated that the number of cases of stroke that will occur over a 5 year period is about 3 per 1000 women aged 50-59 years and 11 per 1000 women aged 60-69 years. It is estimated that for women who use conjugated oestrogens and MPA for 5 years, the number of additional cases will be between 0 and 3 (best estimate = 1) per 1000 users aged 50-59 years and between 1 and 9 (best estimate = 4) per 1000 users aged 60-69 years. It is unknown whether the increased risk also extends to other HRT products.

Ovarian cancer

Long-term (at least 5 -10 years) use of oestrogen-only HRT products in hysterectomised women has been associated with an increased risk of ovarian cancer in some epidemiological studies. It is uncertain whether long-term use of combined HRT confers a different risk than oestrogen-only products.

Other conditions

Oestrogens may cause fluid retention, and therefore patients with cardiac or renal dysfunction should be carefully observed. Patients with terminal renal insufficiency should be closely observed, since the level of circulating active ingredient in Vagifem® may be increased.

Systemic oestrogens have been reported to increase thyroid binding globulin (TBG), leading to increased circulating total thyroid hormone as measured by protein-bound iodine (PBI), T4 levels (by column or by radio-immunoassay) or T3 levels (by radio-immunoassay). T3 resin uptake is decreased, reflecting the elevated TBG. Free T4 and free T3 concentrations are unaltered. Other binding proteins may be elevated in serum, i.e. corticoid binding globulin (CBG), sex-hormone-binding globulin (SHBG), leading to increased circulating corticosteroids and sex steroids respectively. Free or biologically active hormone concentrations are unchanged. Other plasma proteins may be increased (angiotensinogen/renin substrate, alpha-1-antitrypsin, ceruloplasmin). The systemic exposure of estradiol with intermittent administration of low dose estradiol in Vagifem® (see section 5.2) may result in less pronounced effects on plasma binding proteins than with oral hormones

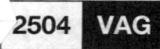

Women with pre-existing hypertriglyceridaemia should be followed closely during oestrogen replacement or hormone replacement therapy, since rare cases of large increases in plasma triglycerides leading to pancreatitis have been reported with oestrogen therapy in this condition.

There is no conclusive evidence for improvement of cognitive function. There is some evidence from the WHI trial of increased risk of probable dementia in women who start using continuous combined CEE and MPA after the age of 65. It is unknown whether the findings apply to younger post-menopausal women or other HRT products.

4.5 Interaction with other medicinal products and other forms of interaction

None reported.

4.6 Pregnancy and lactation

Vagifem® is not indicated during pregnancy. If pregnancy occurs during medication with Vagifem®, treatment should be withdrawn immediately. The results of most epidemiological studies to-date relevant to inadvertent foetal exposure to oestrogens indicate no teratogenic or foetotoxic effects.

Vagifem® is not indicated during lactation.

4.7 Effects on ability to drive and use machines

No effects known.

4.8 Undesirable effects

More than 640 patients have been treated with Vagifem® in clinical trials, including over 200 patients treated for between 28 and 64 weeks. Well known oestrogen-related adverse effects which occurred with a higher frequency in the treated group as compared with the placebo group are presented as "Common (>1/100, <1/10)"

The spontaneous reporting rate on Vagifem® corresponds to approximately 1 case per 10,000 patient years. Adverse events for which an increased frequency has not been observed in clinical trials, but which have been spontaneously reported and which on an overall judgement are considered possibly related to Vagifem® treatment are therefore presented as "Very rare (<1/10,000)"

Post marketing experience is subject to under-reporting especially with regard to trivial and well-known adverse drug reactions. The presented frequencies should be interpreted in that light.

The most commonly reported adverse drug reactions are: vaginal discharge and vaginal discomfort. Oestrogen-related adverse events such as breast pain, peripheral oedema and postmenopausal bleedings are most likely to present at the beginning of Vagifem® treatment.

(see Table 1 below)

Table 1

System organ class	Common >1/100; <1/10	Uncommon >1/1000; <1/100	Rare >1/10,000; <1/1000	Very rare <1/10,000 incl. isolated reports
Neoplasms benign and malignant (incl. cysts and polyps)				Breast cancer Endometrial cancer
Immune system disorders				Hypersensitivity, NOS
Psychiatric disorders				Insomnia Depression
Nervous system disorders	Headache			Migraine aggravated
Vascular disorders				Deep venous thrombosis
Gastrointestinal disorders	Nausea Abdominal pain, abdominal distension or abdominal discomfort Dyspepsia Vomiting Flatulence			Diarrhoea
Skin and subcutaneous tissue disorders				Urticaria Rash erythematous Rash NOS Rash pruritic General pruritus
Reproductive system and breast disorders	Genital candidiasis or vaginitis Vaginal haemorrhage, vaginal discharge or vaginal discomfort Breast oedema, breast enlargement, breast pain or breast tenderness			Hyperplasia endometrial Vaginal irritation, vaginal pain, vaginismus, vaginal ulceration
General disorders and administration site conditions	Oedema peripheral			Fluid retention Drug ineffective
Investigations				Weight increased Blood oestrogen increased

Breast cancer

According to evidence from a large number of epidemiological studies and one randomised placebo-controlled trial, the Women's Health Initiative (WHI), the overall risk of breast cancer increases with increasing duration of HRT use in current or recent HRT users.

For oestrogen-only HRT, estimates of relative risk (RR) from a reanalysis of original data from 51 epidemiological studies (in which >80% of HRT use was oestrogen-only HRT) and from the epidemiological Million Women Study (MWS) are similar at 1.35 (95%CI 1.21 – 1.49) and 1.30 (95%CI 1.21 – 1.40), respectively.

For oestrogen plus progestagen combined HRT, several epidemiological studies have reported an overall higher risk for breast cancer than with oestrogens alone.

The MWS reported that, compared to never users, the use of various types of oestrogen-progestagen combined HRT was associated with a higher risk of breast cancer (RR = 2.00, 95%CI: 1.88 – 2.12) than use of oestrogens alone (RR = 1.30, 95%CI: 1.21 – 1.40) or use of tibolone (RR=1.45; 95%CI 1.25-1.68).

The WHI trial reported a risk estimate of 1.24 (95%CI 1.01 – 1.54) after 5.6 years of use of oestrogen-progestagen combined HRT (CEE + MPA) in all users compared with placebo.

The absolute risks calculated from the MWS and the WHI trial are presented below:

The MWS has estimated, from the known average incidence of breast cancer in developed countries, that:

• For women not using HRT, about 32 in every 1000 are expected to have breast cancer diagnosed between the ages of 50 and 64 years.

• For 1000 current or recent users of HRT, the number of additional cases during the corresponding period will be

o For users of oestrogen-only replacement therapy

• between 0 and 3 (best estimate = 1.5) for 5 years' use
• between 3 and 7 (best estimate = 5) for 10 years' use.

o For users of oestrogen plus progestagen combined HRT,

• between 5 and 7 (best estimate = 6) for 5 years' use
• between 18 and 20 (best estimate = 19) for 10 years' use.

The WHI trial estimated that after 5.6 years of follow-up of women between the ages of 50 and 79 years, an additional 8 cases of invasive breast cancer would be due to oestrogen-progestagen combined HRT (CEE + MPA) per 10,000 women years.

According to calculations from the trial data, it is estimated that:

• For 1000 women in the placebo group,

o about 16 cases of invasive breast cancer would be diagnosed in 5 years.

• For 1000 women who used oestrogen + progestagen combined HRT (CEE + MPA), the number of additional cases would be

o between 0 and 9 (best estimate = 4) for 5 years' use.

The number of additional cases of breast cancer in women who use HRT is broadly similar for women who start HRT irrespective of age at start of use (between the ages of 45-65) (see section 4.4).

The following adverse reactions have been reported in association with other oestrogen treatment:

- Myocardial infarction, stroke
- Gallbladder disease
- Skin and subcutaneous disorders: chloasma, erythema multiforme, erythema nodosum, vascular purpura, pruritus
- Risk of development of endometrial cancer (see section 4.4), endometrial hyperplasia or increase in size of uterine fibroids*
- Probable dementia (see section 4.4).

* In non-hysterectomised women.

4.9 Overdose

Symptoms that may occur in the case of an acute overdose of oestrogen are nausea and vomiting. If necessary a symptomatic treatment should be instituted.

5. PHARMACOLOGICAL PROPERTIES

5.1 Pharmacodynamic properties

Pharmacotherapeutic group: ATC code G03C A03

Natural and semisynthetic oestrogens, plain (for vaginal use).

The active ingredient in Vagifem® is synthetic 17β-estradiol which is chemically and biologically identical to endogenous human estradiol.

17β-estradiol is the principal and most active of the naturally occurring human oestrogens. It has pharmacological actions in common with all oestrogenic compounds. The action on the vagina is to increase maturation of vaginal epithelial cells and increase cervical secretory activity.

5.2 Pharmacokinetic properties

Estrogen drug products are well absorbed through the skin, mucous membranes, and the gastrointestinal tract. After treatment with Vagifem®, marginal elevations of plasma estradiol and conjugated oestrogens as well as suppression of pituitary gonadotrophins have been observed. The vaginal delivery of estrogens circumvents first-pass metabolism.

A single-centre randomised, double-blind two period cross-over study was performed to evaluate the pharmacokinetics of Vagifem®. Peak levels were approximately 175 pmol/L (48pg/ml) following a single dose of Vagifem®. After 14 days of treatment, only marginal absorption of estradiol could be detected, with mean levels in the post-menopausal range.

Another study in younger patients, mean age 52 years, showed that vaginal administration of Vagifem® over a 12 week course demonstrated a mean C_{max} of estradiol of 50 pg/ml and that there was no significant accumulation of estradiol as measured by the AUC_{0-24} (see table 2 below). The average estradiol concentrations at each time point were within the normal postmenopausal range.

Table 2: Mean (± standard deviation) pharmacokinetic parameters for estradiol

(see Table 2 on next page)

The levels of oestrone seen during 12 weeks of Vagifem® administration do not show any accumulation of oestrone, and the observed values are within the postmenopausal range.

Oestrogen metabolites are primarily excreted in the urine as glucuronides and sulphates.

5.3 Preclinical safety data

As 17β-estradiol is a well known substance in humans, described in the pharmacotoxicological literature, no further studies have been performed.

6. PHARMACEUTICAL PARTICULARS

6.1 List of excipients

Tablet core:

Hypromellose

Lactose monohydrate

Maize starch

Magnesium stearate

Film-coating:

Hypromellose

Macrogol 6000

6.2 Incompatibilities

None known

Table 2: Mean (± standard deviation) pharmacokinetic parameters for estradiol

	Week 0	Week 2	Week 12
AUC (pg.hr/ml)	538 (±265)	567 (±246)	563 (±341)
C_{max} (pg/ml)	51 (±34)	47 (±21)	49 (±27)

6.3 Shelf life
36 months

6.4 Special precautions for storage
Store in a dry place, protect from light. Store below 25°C. Do not refrigerate.

6.5 Nature and contents of container
Laminated bubble strips containing 5 applicators with inset tablet. Packed in cartons containing 3 strips (15 tablets and applicators).

6.6 Special precautions for disposal and other handling
No special requirements

7. MARKETING AUTHORISATION HOLDER
Novo Nordisk A/S
Novo Alle
DK-2880 Bagsvaerd
Denmark
The registered office in the UK is:-
Novo Nordisk Limited
Broadfield Park
Crawley
West Sussex
RH11 9RT
Tel: (01293) 613555

8. MARKETING AUTHORISATION NUMBER(S)
PL 4668/0026

9. DATE OF FIRST AUTHORISATION/RENEWAL OF THE AUTHORISATION
First authorised August 1990
Authorisation renewed 10/03/2009

10. DATE OF REVISION OF THE TEXT
24/03/2009

Valcyte 450mg film-coated tablets

(Roche Products Limited)

1. NAME OF THE MEDICINAL PRODUCT
Valcyte 450 mg film-coated tablets

2. QUALITATIVE AND QUANTITATIVE COMPOSITION
Each tablet contains 496.3 mg of valganciclovir hydrochloride equivalent to 450 mg of valganciclovir (as free base).

For a full list of excipients, see section 6.1.

3. PHARMACEUTICAL FORM
Film-coated tablets

Pink, convex oval film-coated tablets, with "VGC" embossed on one side and "450" on the other side.

4. CLINICAL PARTICULARS

4.1 Therapeutic indications
Valcyte is indicated for the induction and maintenance treatment of cytomegalovirus (CMV) retinitis in patients with acquired immunodeficiency syndrome (AIDS).

Valcyte is indicated for the prevention of CMV disease in CMV-negative patients who have received a solid organ transplant from a CMV-positive donor.

4.2 Posology and method of administration
Caution – Strict adherence to dosage recommendations is essential to avoid overdose; see sections 4.4 and 4.9.

Valganciclovir is rapidly and extensively metabolised to ganciclovir after oral dosing. Oral valganciclovir 900 mg b.i.d. is therapeutically equivalent to intravenous ganciclovir 5 mg/kg b.i.d.

Standard dosage in adults

Induction treatment of CMV retinitis:

For patients with active CMV retinitis, the recommended dose is 900 mg valganciclovir (two Valcyte 450 mg tablets) twice a day for 21 days and, whenever possible, taken with food. Prolonged induction treatment may increase the risk of bone marrow toxicity (see section 4.4).

Maintenance treatment of CMV retinitis:

Following induction treatment, or in patients with inactive CMV retinitis, the recommended dose is 900mg valganciclovir (two Valcyte 450 mg tablets) once daily and, whenever possible, taken with food. Patients whose retinitis worsens may repeat induction treatment; however, consideration should be given to the possibility of viral drug resistance.

Prevention of CMV disease in solid organ transplantation:

For patients who have received a transplant, the recommended dose is 900 mg (two Valcyte 450 mg tablets) once daily, starting within 10 days of transplantation and continuing until 100 days post-transplantation. Whenever possible, the tablets should be taken with food.

Special dosage instructions

Patients with renal impairment:

Serum creatinine levels or creatinine clearance should be monitored carefully. Dosage adjustment is required according to creatinine clearance, as shown in the table below (see sections 4.4 and 5.2).

An estimated creatinine clearance (mL/min) can be related to serum creatinine by the following formulae:

$$\text{For males} = \frac{(140 - \text{age [years]}) \times (\text{body weight [kg]})}{(72) \times (0.011 \times \text{serum creatinine [micromol/L]})}$$

For females = 0.85 × male value

CrCl (mL/min)	Induction dose of valganciclovir	Maintenance/ Prevention dose of valganciclovir
⩾ 60	900 mg (2 tablets) twice daily	900 mg (2 tablets) once daily
40 – 59	450 mg (1 tablet) twice daily	450 mg (1 tablet) once daily
25 – 39	450 mg (1 tablet) once daily	450 mg (1 tablet) every 2 days
10 – 24	450 mg (1 tablet) every 2 days	450 mg (1 tablet) twice weekly

Patients undergoing haemodialysis:

For patients on haemodialysis (CrCl < 10 mL/min) a dose recommendation cannot be given. Thus Valcyte should not be used in these patients (see sections 4.4 and 5.2).

Patients with hepatic impairment:

Safety and efficacy of Valcyte tablets have not been studied in patients with hepatic impairment (see section 5.2).

Paediatric patients:

Valcyte is not recommended for use in the paediatric population due to insufficient data on safety and efficacy (see sections 4.4 and 5.3)

Elderly patients:

Safety and efficacy have not been established in this patient population.

Patients with severe leucopenia, neutropenia, anaemia, thrombocytopenia and pancytopenia;

See section 4.4 before initiation of therapy.

If there is a significant deterioration of blood cell counts during therapy with Valcyte, treatment with haematopoietic growth factors and/or dose interruption should be considered (see sections 4.4 and 4.8).

Method of administration

Valcyte is administered orally, and whenever possible, should be taken with food (see section 5.2).

The tablets should not be broken or crushed. Since Valcyte is considered a potential teratogen and carcinogen in humans, caution should be observed in handling broken tablets (see section 4.4). Avoid direct contact of broken or crushed tablets with skin or mucous membranes. If such contact occurs, wash thoroughly with soap and water, rinse eyes thoroughly with sterile water, or plain water if sterile water is unavailable.

4.3 Contraindications
Valcyte is contra-indicated in patients with hypersensitivity to valganciclovir, ganciclovir or to any of the excipients.

Due to the similarity of the chemical structure of Valcyte and that of aciclovir and valaciclovir, a cross-hypersensitivity reaction between these drugs is possible. Therefore, Valcyte is contra-indicated in patients with hypersensitivity to aciclovir and valaciclovir.

Valcyte is contra-indicated during lactation, refer to section 4.6.

4.4 Special warnings and precautions for use
Prior to the initiation of valganciclovir treatment, patients should be advised of the potential risks to the foetus. In animal studies, ganciclovir was found to be mutagenic, teratogenic, aspermatogenic and carcinogenic, and a suppressor of female fertility. Valcyte should, therefore, be considered a potential teratogen and carcinogen in humans with the potential to cause birth defects and cancers (see section 5.3). It is also considered likely that Valcyte causes temporary or permanent inhibition of spermatogenesis. Women of child bearing potential must be advised to use effective contraception during treatment. Men must be advised to practise barrier contraception during treatment, and for at least 90 days thereafter, unless it is certain that the female partner is not at risk of pregnancy (see sections 4.6, 4.8 and 5.3).

The use of Valcyte in children and adolescents is not recommended because the pharmacokinetic characteristics of Valcyte have not been established in these patient populations (see section 4.2). Furthermore, valganciclovir has the potential to cause carcinogenicity and reproductive toxicity in the long term.

Severe leucopenia, neutropenia, anaemia, thrombocytopenia, pancytopenia, bone marrow depression and aplastic anaemia have been observed in patients treated with Valcyte (and ganciclovir). Therapy should not be initiated if the absolute neutrophil count is less than 500 cells/µL, or the platelet count is less than 25000/µL, or the haemoglobin level is less than 8 g/dL (see sections 4.2 and 4.8).

Valcyte should be used with caution in patients with pre-existing haematological cytopenia or a history of drug-related haematological cytopenia and in patients receiving radiotherapy.

It is recommended that complete blood counts and platelet counts be monitored during therapy. Increased haematological monitoring may be warranted in patients with renal impairment. In patients developing severe leucopenia, neutropenia, anaemia and/or thrombocytopenia, it is recommended that treatment with haematopoietic growth factors and/or dose interruption be considered (see sections 4.2 and 4.8).

The bioavailability of ganciclovir after a single dose of 900 mg valganciclovir is approximately 60 %, compared with approximately 6 % after administration of 1000 mg oral ganciclovir (as capsules). Excessive exposure to ganciclovir may be associated with life-threatening adverse reactions. Therefore, careful adherence to the dose recommendations is advised when instituting therapy, when switching from induction to maintenance therapy, and in patients who may switch from oral ganciclovir to valganciclovir as Valcyte cannot be substituted for ganciclovir capsules on a one-to-one basis. Patients switching from ganciclovir capsules should be advised of the risk of overdosage if they take more than the prescribed number of Valcyte tablets (see sections 4.2 and 4.9).

In patients with impaired renal function, dosage adjustments based on creatinine clearance are required (see sections 4.2and 5.2).

Valcyte should not be used in patients on haemodialysis (see sections 4.2 and 5.2).

Convulsions have been reported in patients taking imipenem-cilastatin and ganciclovir. Valcyte should not be used concomitantly with imipenem-cilastatin unless the potential benefits outweigh the potential risks (see section 4.5).

Patients treated with Valcyte and (a) didanosine, (b) drugs that are known to be myelosuppressive (e.g. zidovudine), or (c) substances affecting renal function, should be closely monitored for signs of added toxicity (see section 4.5).

The controlled clinical study using valganciclovir for the prophylactic treatment of CMV disease in transplantation, as detailed in section 5.1 did not include lung and intestinal transplant patients. Therefore, experience in these transplant patients is limited.

4.5 Interaction with other medicinal products and other forms of interaction

Drug interactions with valganciclovir

In-vivo drug interaction studies with Valcyte have not been performed. Since valganciclovir is extensively and rapidly metabolised to ganciclovir; drug interactions associated with ganciclovir will be expected for valganciclovir.

Effects of other medicinal products on ganciclovir

Imipenem-cilastatin

Convulsions have been reported in patients taking ganciclovir and imipenem-cilastatin concomitantly. These drugs should not be used concomitantly unless the potential benefits outweigh the potential risks (see section 4.4).

Probenecid

Probenecid given with oral ganciclovir resulted in statistically significantly decreased renal clearance of ganciclovir (20 %) leading to statistically significantly increased exposure (40 %). These changes were consistent with a mechanism of interaction involving competition for renal tubular secretion. Therefore, patients taking probenecid and Valcyte should be closely monitored for ganciclovir toxicity.

Effects of ganciclovir on other medicinal products

Zidovudine

When zidovudine was given in the presence of oral ganciclovir there was a small (17 %), but statistically significant increase in the AUC of zidovudine. There was also a trend towards lower ganciclovir concentrations when administered with zidovudine, although this was not statistically significant. However, since both zidovudine and ganciclovir have the potential to cause neutropenia and anaemia, some patients may not tolerate concomitant therapy at full dosage (see section 4.4).

Didanosine

Didanosine plasma concentrations were found to be consistently raised when given with ganciclovir (both intravenous and oral). At ganciclovir oral doses of 3 and 6 g/day, an increase in the AUC of didanosine ranging from 84 to 124 % has been observed, and likewise at intravenous doses of 5 and 10 mg/kg/day, an increase in the AUC of didanosine ranging from 38 to 67 % has been observed. There was no clinically significant effect on ganciclovir concentrations. Patients should be closely monitored for didanosine toxicity (see section 4.4).

Mycophenolate Mofetil

Based on the results of a single dose administration study of recommended doses of oral mycophenolate mofetil (MMF) and intravenous ganciclovir and the known effects of renal impairment on the pharmacokinetics of MMF and ganciclovir, it is anticipated that co-administration of these agents (which have the potential to compete for renal tubular secretion) will result in increases in phenolic glucuronide of mycophenolic acid (MPAG) and ganciclovir concentration. No substantial alteration of mycophenolic acid (MPA) pharmacokinetics is anticipated and MMF dose adjustment is not required. In patients with renal impairment to whom MMF and ganciclovir are co-administered, the dose recommendation of ganciclovir should be observed and the patients monitored carefully. Since both MMF and ganciclovir have the potential to cause neutropenia and leucopenia, patients should be monitored for additive toxicity.

Zalcitabine

No clinically significant pharmacokinetic changes were observed after concomitant administration of ganciclovir and zalcitabine. Both valganciclovir and zalcitabine have the potential to cause peripheral neuropathy and patients should be monitored for such events.

Stavudine

No clinically significant interactions were observed when stavudine and oral ganciclovir were given in combination.

Trimethoprim

No clinically significant pharmacokinetic interaction was observed when trimethoprim and oral ganciclovir were given in combination. However, there is a potential for toxicity to be enhanced since both drugs are known to be myelosuppressive and therefore both drugs should be used concomitantly only if the potential benefits outweigh the risks.

Other antiretrovirals

At clinically relevant concentrations, there is unlikely to be either a synergistic or antagonistic effect on the inhibition of either HIV in the presence of ganciclovir or CMV in the presence of a variety of antiretroviral drugs. Metabolic interactions with, for example, protease inhibitors and non-nucleoside reverse transcriptase inhibitors (NNRTIs) are unlikely due to the lack of P450 involvement in the metabolism of either valganciclovir or ganciclovir.

Other potential drug interactions

Toxicity may be enhanced when valganciclovir is co-administered with, or is given immediately before or after, other drugs that inhibit replication of rapidly dividing cell populations such as occur in the bone marrow, testes and germinal layers of the skin and gastrointestinal mucosa. Examples of these types of drugs are dapsone, pentamidine, flucytosine, vincristine, vinblastine, adriamycin, amphotericin B, trimethoprim/sulpha combinations, nucleoside analogues and hydroxyurea.

Since ganciclovir is excreted through the kidney (section 5.2), toxicity may also be enhanced during co-administration of valganciclovir with drugs that might reduce the renal clearance of ganciclovir and hence increase its exposure. The renal clearance of ganciclovir might be inhibited by two mechanisms: (a) nephrotoxicity, caused by drugs such as cidofovir and foscarnet, and (b) competitive inhibition of active tubular secretion in the kidney by, for example, other nucleoside analogues.

Therefore, all of these drugs should be considered for concomitant use with valganciclovir only if the potential benefits outweigh the potential risks (see section 4.4).

4.6 Pregnancy and lactation

There are no data from the use of Valcyte in pregnant women. Its active metabolite, ganciclovir, readily diffuses across the human placenta. Based on its pharmacological mechanism of action and reproductive toxicity observed in animal studies with ganciclovir (see section 5.3) there is a theoretical risk of teratogenicity in humans.

Valcyte should not be used in pregnancy unless the therapeutic benefit for the mother outweighs the potential risk of teratogenic damage to the child.

Women of child-bearing potential must be advised to use effective contraception during treatment. Male patients must be advised to practise barrier contraception during, and for at least 90 days following treatment with Valcyte unless it is certain that the female partner is not at risk of pregnancy (see section 5.3).

It is unknown if ganciclovir is excreted in breast milk, but the possibility of ganciclovir being excreted in the breast milk and causing serious adverse reactions in the nursing infant cannot be discounted. Therefore, breast-feeding must be discontinued.

Table 1

Body System	Very Common (≥1/10)	Common (≥1/100 <1/10)	Uncommon (≥1/1000 < 1/100)
Infections and infestations		Oral candidiasis, sepsis (bacteraemia, viraemia), cellulitis, urinary tract infection	
Blood and lymphatic system disorders	(severe) neutropenia, anaemia	Severe anaemia, (severe) thrombocytopenia, (severe) leucopenia, (severe) pancytopenia	Bone marrow depression
Immune system disorders			Anaphylactic reaction
Metabolic and nutrition disorders		Appetite decreased, anorexia	
Psychiatric disorders		Depression, anxiety, confusion, abnormal thinking	Agitation, psychotic disorder
Nervous system disorders		Headache, insomnia, dysgeusia, (taste disturbance), hypoaesthesia, paraesthesia, peripheral neuropathy, dizziness (excluding vertigo), convulsions	tremor
Eye disorders		Macular oedema, retinal detachment, vitreous floaters, eye pain	Vision abnormal, conjunctivitis
Ear and labyrinth disorders		Ear pain	Deafness
Cardiac disorders			Arrhythmias
Vascular disorders			Hypotension
Respiratory, thoracic and mediastinal disorders	Dyspnoea	Cough	
Gastrointestinal disorders	Diarrhoea	Nausea, vomiting, abdominal pain, abdominal pain upper, dyspepsia, constipation, flatulence, dysphagia	Abdominal distension, mouth ulcerations, pancreatitis
Hepato-biliary disorders		(severe) hepatic function abnormal, blood alkaline phosphatase increased, aspartate aminotransferase increased	Alanine aminotransferase increased
Skin and subcutaneous disorders		Dermatitis, night sweats, pruritis	Alopecia, urticaria, dry skin
Musculoskeletal, connective tissue and bone disorders		Back pain, myalgia, arthralgia, muscle cramps	
Renal and urinary disorder		Creatinine clearance renal decreased, renal impairment	Haematuria, renal failure
Reproductive system and breast disorders			Male infertility
General disorders and administration site conditions		Fatigue, pyrexia, rigors, pain, chest pain, malaise, asthenia	
Investigations		Weight decreased, blood creatinine increased	

4.7 Effects on ability to drive and use machines

No studies on the effects on ability to drive and use machines have been performed.

Convulsions, sedation, dizziness, ataxia, and/or confusion have been reported with the use of Valcyte and/or ganciclovir. If they occur, such effects may affect tasks requiring alertness, including the patient's ability to drive and operate machinery.

4.8 Undesirable effects

Valganciclovir is a prodrug of ganciclovir, which is rapidly and extensively metabolised to ganciclovir after oral administration. The undesirable effects known to be associated with ganciclovir usage can be expected to occur with valganciclovir. All of the undesirable effects observed in valganciclovir clinical studies have been previously observed with ganciclovir. The most commonly reported adverse drug reactions following administration of valganciclovir are neutropenia, anaemia and diarrhoea.

The oral formulations, valganciclovir and ganciclovir, are associated with a higher risk of diarrhoea compared to intravenous ganciclovir. In addition, valganciclovir is associated with a higher risk of neutropenia and leucopenia compared to oral ganciclovir.

Severe neutropenia (< 500 ANC/μL) is seen more frequently in CMV retinitis patients undergoing treatment with valganciclovir than in solid organ transplant patients receiving valganciclovir or oral ganciclovir.

The frequency of adverse reactions reported in clinical trials with either valganciclovir, oral ganciclovir, or intravenous ganciclovir is presented in the table below. Frequencies are defined as very common (≥1/10), common (≥1/100 <1/10), uncommon (≥1/1000 < 1/100), rare (≥1/10,000 <1/1000) and very rare (<1/10,000). The adverse reactions listed were reported in clinical trials in patients with AIDS for the induction or maintenance treatment of CMV retinitis, or in liver, kidney or heart transplant patients for the prophylaxis of CMV disease. No reactions with rare or very rare frequencies have been identified from clinical experience. The term (severe) in parenthesis in the table indicates that the adverse reaction has been reported in patients at both mild/moderate intensity and severe/life-threatening intensity at that specific frequency.

(see Table 1 above)

4.9 Overdose

Overdose experience with Valganciclovir

One adult developed fatal bone marrow depression (medullary aplasia) after several days of dosing that was at least 10-fold greater than recommended for the patient's degree of renal impairment (decreased creatinine clearance).

It is expected that an overdose of valganciclovir could also possibly result in increased renal toxicity (see sections 4.2 and 4.4).

Haemodialysis and hydration may be of benefit in reducing blood plasma levels in patients who receive an overdose of valganciclovir (see section 5.2).

Overdose experience with intravenous ganciclovir

Reports of overdoses with intravenous ganciclovir have been received from clinical trials and during post-marketing experience. In some of these cases no adverse events were reported. The majority of patients experienced one or more of the following adverse events:

- *Haematological toxicity:* pancytopenia, bone marrow depression, medullary aplasia, leucopenia, neutropenia, granulocytopenia.

- *Hepatotoxicity*: hepatitis, liver function disorder.

- *Renal toxicity*: worsening of haematuria in a patient with pre-existing renal impairment, acute renal failure, elevated creatinine.

Table 2

Parameter	Ganciclovir (5 mg/kg, i.v.) n = 18	Valganciclovir (900 mg, p.o.) n = 25	
		Ganciclovir	Valganciclovir
AUC(0 - 12 h) (μg.h/ml)	28.6 ± 9.0	32.8 ± 10.1	0.37 ± 0.22
C_{max} (μg/ml)	10.4 ± 4.9	6.7 ± 2.1	0.18 ± 0.06

- *Gastrointestinal toxicity*: abdominal pain, diarrhoea, vomiting.
- *Neurotoxicity*: generalised tremor, convulsion.

5. PHARMACOLOGICAL PROPERTIES

5.1 Pharmacodynamic properties

Pharmacotherapeutic group: ATC code: J05A B14 (anti-infectives for systemic use, antivirals for systemic use, direct acting antivirals).

Mechanism of action:

Valganciclovir is an L-valyl ester (prodrug) of ganciclovir. After oral administration, valganciclovir is rapidly and extensively metabolised to ganciclovir by intestinal and hepatic esterases. Ganciclovir is a synthetic analogue of 2'-deoxyguanosine and inhibits replication of herpes viruses *in vitro* and *in vivo*. Sensitive human viruses include human cytomegalovirus (HCMV), herpes simplex virus-1 and -2 (HSV-1 and HSV-2), human herpes virus -6, -7 and -8 (HHV-6, HHV-7, HHV8), Epstein-Barr virus (EBV), varicella-zoster virus (VZV) and hepatitis B virus (HBV).

In CMV-infected cells, ganciclovir is initially phosphorylated to ganciclovir monophosphate by the viral protein kinase, pUL97. Further phosphorylation occurs by cellular kinases to produce ganciclovir triphosphate, which is then slowly metabolised intracellularly. Triphosphate metabolism has been shown to occur in HSV- and HCMV- infected cells with half-lives of 18 and between 6 and 24 hours respectively, after the removal of extracellular ganciclovir. As the phosphorylation is largely dependent on the viral kinase, phosphorylation of ganciclovir occurs preferentially in virus-infected cells.

The virustatic activity of ganciclovir is due to inhibition of viral DNA synthesis by: (a) competitive inhibition of incorporation of deoxyguanosine-triphosphate into DNA by viral DNA polymerase, and (b) incorporation of ganciclovir triphosphate into viral DNA causing termination of, or very limited, further viral DNA elongation.

Antiviral Activity

The in-vitro anti-viral activity, measured as IC_{50} of ganciclovir against CMV, is in the range of 0.08 μM (0.02 μg/mL) to 14 μM (3.5 μg/mL).

The clinical antiviral effect of Valcyte has been demonstrated in the treatment of AIDS patients with newly diagnosed CMV retinitis (Clinical trial WV15376). CMV shedding was decreased in urine from 46 % (32/69) of patients at study entry to 7 % (4/55) of patients following four weeks of Valcyte treatment.

Clinical efficacy

Treatment of CMV retinitis:

Patients with newly diagnosed CMV retinitis were randomised in one study to induction therapy with either Valcyte 900mg b.i.d or intravenous ganciclovir 5 mg/kg b.i.d. The proportion of patients with photographic progression of CMV retinitis at week 4 was comparable in both treatment groups, 7/70 and 7/71 patients progressing in the intravenous ganciclovir and valganciclovir arms respectively.

Following induction treatment dosing, all patients in this study received maintenance treatment with Valcyte given at the dose of 900mg daily. The mean (median) time from randomisation to progression of CMV retinitis in the group receiving induction and maintenance treatment with Valcyte was 226 (160) days and in the group receiving induction treatment with intravenous ganciclovir and maintenance treatment with Valcyte was 219 (125) days.

Prevention of CMV disease in transplantation:

A double-blind, double-dummy clinical active comparator study has been conducted in heart, liver and kidney transplant patients (lung and gastro-intestinal transplant patients were not included in the study) at high-risk of CMV disease (D+/R-) who received either Valcyte (900 mg od) or oral ganciclovir (1000 mg tid) starting within 10 days of transplantation until Day 100 post-transplant. The incidence of CMV disease (CMV syndrome + tissue invasive disease) during the first 6 months post-transplant was 12.1 % in the Valcyte arm (n=239) compared with 15.2 % in the oral ganciclovir arm (n=125). The large majority of cases occurred following cessation of prophylaxis (post-Day 100) with cases in the valganciclovir arm occurring on average later than those in the oral ganciclovir arm. The incidence of acute rejection in the first 6 months was 29.7 % in patients randomised to valganciclovir compared with 36.0 % in the oral ganciclovir arm, with the incidence of graft loss being equivalent, occurring in 0.8 % of patients, in each arm.

Viral Resistance

Virus resistant to ganciclovir can arise after chronic dosing with valganciclovir by selection of mutations in the viral kinase gene (UL97) responsible for ganciclovir monophosphorylation and/or the viral polymerase gene (UL54). Viruses containing mutations in the UL97 gene are resistant to ganciclovir alone, whereas viruses with mutations in the UL54 gene are resistant to ganciclovir but may show cross-resistance to other antivirals that also target the viral polymerase.

Treatment of CMV retinitis:

Genotypic analysis of CMV in polymorphonuclear leucocytes (PMNL) isolates from 148 patients with CMV retinitis enrolled in one clinical study has shown that 2.2 %, 6.5 %, 12.8 %, and 15.3 % contain UL97 mutations after 3, 6, 12 and 18 months, respectively, of valganciclovir treatment.

Prevention of CMV disease in transplantation:

Resistance was studied by genotypic analysis of CMV in PMNL samples collected i) on Day 100 (end of study drug prophylaxis) and ii) in cases of suspected CMV disease up to 6 months after transplantation. From the 245 patients randomised to receive valganciclovir, 198 Day 100 samples were available for testing and no ganciclovir resistance mutations were observed. This compares with 2 ganciclovir resistance mutations detected in the 103 samples tested (1.9 %) for patients in the oral ganciclovir comparator arm.

Of the 245 patients randomised to receive valganciclovir, samples from 50 patients with suspected CMV disease were tested and no resistance mutations were observed. Of the 127 patients randomised on the ganciclovir comparator arm, samples from 29 patients with suspected CMV disease were tested, from which two resistance mutations were observed, giving an incidence of resistance of 6.9 %.

5.2 Pharmacokinetic properties

The pharmacokinetic properties of valganciclovir have been evaluated in HIV- and CMV-seropositive patients, patients with AIDS and CMV retinitis and in solid organ transplant patients.

Absorption

Valganciclovir is a prodrug of ganciclovir. It is well absorbed from the gastrointestinal tract and rapidly and extensively metabolised in the intestinal wall and liver to ganciclovir. Systemic exposure to valganciclovir is transient and low. The absolute bioavailability of ganciclovir from valganciclovir is approximately 60 % across all the patient populations studied and the resultant exposure to ganciclovir is similar to that after its intravenous administration (please see below). For comparison, the bioavailability of ganciclovir after administration of 1000mg oral ganciclovir (as capsules) is 6 - 8 %.

Valganciclovir in HIV+, CMV+ patients:

Systemic exposure of HIV+, CMV+ patients after twice daily administration of ganciclovir and valganciclovir for one week is:

(see Table 2 above)

The efficacy of ganciclovir in increasing the time-to-progression of CMV retinitis has been shown to correlate with systemic exposure (AUC).

Valganciclovir in solid organ transplant patients:

Steady state systemic exposure of solid organ transplant patients to ganciclovir after daily oral administration of ganciclovir and valganciclovir is:

Parameter	Ganciclovir (1000 mg tid.) n = 82	Valganciclovir (9 00mg, od) n = 161
		Ganciclovir
AUC(0 - 24 h) (μg.h/ml)	28.0 ± 10.9	46.3 ± 15.2
C_{max} (μg/ml)	1.4 ± 0.5	5.3 ± 1.5

The systemic exposure of ganciclovir to heart, kidney and liver transplant recipients was similar after oral administration of valganciclovir according to the renal function dosing algorithm.

Food effect:

Dose proportionality with respect to ganciclovir AUC following administration of valganciclovir in the dose range 450 to 2625mg was demonstrated only under fed conditions. When valganciclovir was given with food at the recommended dose of 900 mg, higher values were seen in both mean ganciclovir AUC (approximately 30 %) and mean ganciclovir C_{max} values (approximately 14 %) than in the fasting state. Also, the inter-individual variation in exposure of ganciclovir decreases when taking Valcyte with food. Valcyte has only been administered with food in clinical studies. Therefore, it is recommended that Valcyte be administered with food (see section 4.2).

Distribution:

Because of rapid conversion of valganciclovir to ganciclovir, protein binding of valganciclovir was not determined. Plasma protein binding of ganciclovir was 1 – 2 % over concentrations of 0.5 and 51 μg/mL. The steady state volume of distribution of ganciclovir after intravenous administration was 0.680 ± 0.161 L/kg (n=114).

Metabolism

Valganciclovir is rapidly and extensively metabolised to ganciclovir; no other metabolites have been detected. No metabolite of orally administered radiolabelled ganciclovir (1000 mg single dose) accounted for more than 1 – 2 % of the radioactivity recovered in the faeces or urine.

Elimination

Following dosing with Valcyte, renal excretion, as ganciclovir, by glomerular filtration and active tubular secretion is the major route of elimination of valganciclovir. Renal clearance accounts for 81.5 % ± 22 % (n=70) of the systemic clearance of ganciclovir. The half-life of ganciclovir from valganciclovir is 4.1 ± 0.9 hours in HIV- and CMV-seropositive patients.

Pharmacokinetics in special clinical situations

Patients with renal impairment

Decreasing renal function resulted in decreased clearance of ganciclovir from valganciclovir with a corresponding increase in terminal half-life. Therefore, dosage adjustment is required for renally impaired patients (see sections 4.2 and 4.4).

Patients undergoing haemodialysis

For patients receiving haemodialysis dose recommendations for Valcyte 450 mg film-coated tablets cannot be given. This is because an individual dose of Valcyte required for these patients is less than the 450 mg tablet strength. Thus, Valcyte should not be used in these patients (see sections 4.2 and 4.4).

Patients with hepatic impairment

The safety and efficacy of Valcyte tablets have not been studied in patients with hepatic impairment. Hepatic impairment should not affect the pharmacokinetics of ganciclovir since it is excreted renally and, therefore, no specific dose recommendation is made.

5.3 Preclinical safety data

Valganciclovir is a pro-drug of ganciclovir and therefore effects observed with ganciclovir apply equally to valganciclovir. Toxicity of valganciclovir in pre-clinical safety studies was the same as that seen with ganciclovir and was induced at ganciclovir exposure levels comparable to, or lower than, those in humans given the induction dose.

These findings were gonadotoxicity (testicular cell loss) and nephrotoxicity (uraemia, cell degeneration), which were irreversible; myelotoxicity (anaemia, neutropenia, lymphocytopenia) and gastrointestinal toxicity (mucosal cell necrosis), which were reversible.

Further studies have shown ganciclovir to be mutagenic, carcinogenic, teratogenic, embryotoxic, aspermatogenic (i.e. impairs male fertility) and to suppress female fertility.

6. PHARMACEUTICAL PARTICULARS

6.1 List of excipients

Tablet core	Tablet film-coat
Povidone K30	Opadry Pink 15B24005 containing:
Crospovidone	Hypromellose
Microcrystalline cellulose	Titanium dioxide (E171
Stearic acid	Macrogol 400)
	Red iron oxide (E172)
	Polysorbate 80

6.2 Incompatibilities

Not applicable.

6.3 Shelf life

3 years

6.4 Special precautions for storage

This medicinal product does not require any special storage conditions.

6.5 Nature and contents of container

High density polyethylene (HDPE) bottle, with child-resistant polypropylene closure, and cotton pad enclosed.

60 tablets.

6.6 Special precautions for disposal and other handling

Any unused product or waste material should be disposed of in accordance with local requirements.

7. MARKETING AUTHORISATION HOLDER

Roche Products Limited, 6 Falcon Way, Shire Park, Welwyn Garden City, AL7 1TW, United Kingdom.

8. MARKETING AUTHORISATION NUMBER(S)

UK: PL 00031/0599

Ireland: PA 50/150/1

9. DATE OF FIRST AUTHORISATION/RENEWAL OF THE AUTHORISATION

UK: April 2002 / 20th Sep 2006

Ireland: September 2002 / 20th Sep 2006

10. DATE OF REVISION OF THE TEXT

September 2007

LEGAL STATUS

POM

Valcyte Powder for Oral Solution

(Roche Products Limited)

1. NAME OF THE MEDICINAL PRODUCT

VALCYTE 50 mg/ml powder for oral solution.

2. QUALITATIVE AND QUANTITATIVE COMPOSITION

Each bottle contains 5.5 g valganciclovir hydrochloride per 12 g powder for oral solution.

Each ml of the reconstituted solution contains 50 mg valganciclovir (as hydrochloride).

For a full list of excipients, see section 6.1.

3. PHARMACEUTICAL FORM

Powder for oral solution.

The powder is a granulate with a white to slightly yellow colour.

When the powder is dissolved, it forms a clear, colourless to brown solution.

4. CLINICAL PARTICULARS

4.1 Therapeutic indications

VALCYTE is indicated for the induction and maintenance treatment of cytomegalovirus (CMV) retinitis in patients with acquired immunodeficiency syndrome (AIDS).

VALCYTE is indicated for the prevention of CMV disease in CMV-negative patients who have received a solid organ transplant from a CMV-positive donor.

4.2 Posology and method of administration

Caution – Strict adherence to dosage recommendations is essential to avoid overdose (see sections 4.4 and 4.9).

Valganciclovir is rapidly and extensively metabolised to ganciclovir after oral dosing. Oral valganciclovir 900 mg taken twice daily is therapeutically equivalent to intravenous ganciclovir 5 mg/kg taken twice daily. The ganciclovir systemic exposure following administration of 900 mg valganciclovir oral solution is equivalent to valganciclovir 900 mg tablets.

Standard dosage in adults

Induction treatment of CMV retinitis:

For patients with active CMV retinitis, the recommended dose is 900 mg valganciclovir twice a day for 21 days. Prolonged induction treatment may increase the risk of bone marrow toxicity (see section 4.4).

Maintenance treatment of CMV retinitis:

Following induction treatment, or in patients with inactive CMV retinitis, the recommended dose is 900 mg valganciclovir once daily. Patients whose retinitis worsens may repeat induction treatment; however, consideration should be given to the possibility of viral drug resistance.

Prevention of CMV disease in solid organ transplantation:

For patients who have received a transplant, the recommended dose is 900 mg once daily, starting within 10 days of transplantation and continuing until 100 days post transplantation.

Special dosage instructions

Patients with renal impairment

Serum creatinine levels or creatinine clearance should be monitored carefully. Dosage adjustment is required according to creatinine clearance, as shown in the Table below (see sections 4.4 and 5.2).

An estimated creatinine clearance (ml/min) can be related to serum creatinine by the following formulae:

$$\text{For males} = \frac{(140 - \text{age [years]}) \times (\text{body weight [kg]})}{(72) \times (0.011 \times \text{serum creatinine [micromol/1]})}$$

$$\text{For females} = 0.85 \times \text{male value}$$

CrCl (ml/min)	Induction dose of valganciclovir	Maintenance/ Prevention dose of valganciclovir
≥ 60	900 mg twice daily	900 mg once daily
40 – 59	450 mg twice daily	450 mg once daily
25 – 39	450 mg once daily	225 mg once daily
10 – 24	225 mg once daily	125 mg once daily
<10	200 mg three times a week after dialysis	100 mg three times a week after dialysis

Patients undergoing haemodialysis:

Dosage adjustment is necessary for patients on haemodialysis (CrCl <10ml/min) (see sections 4.4 5.2) and a dosing recommendation is given in the Table above.

Patients with hepatic impairment

Safety and efficacy of VALCYTE have not been studied in patients with hepatic impairment (see sections 4.4 and 5.2).

Children and adolescents (less than 18 years of age):

Valcyte is not recommended for use in children below 18 years of age due to lack of data on safety and efficacy in this patient population (see section 4.4).

Elderly patients:

Safety and efficacy of VALCYTE have not been established in this patient population.

Patients with severe leucopenia, neutropenia, anaemia, thrombocytopenia and pancytopenia:

see section 4.4 before initiation of therapy.

If there is a significant deterioration of blood cell counts during therapy with VALCYTE, treatment with haematopoietic growth factors and/or dose interruption should be considered (see section 4.4).

Method of administration

VALCYTE is administered orally, and whenever possible, should be taken with food (see section 5.2).

VALCYTE powder for oral solution requires reconstitution prior to oral administration (see section 6.6). Two oral dosing dispensers with graduations in 25 mg up to 500 mg are provided. It is recommended that patients use the dispenser.

4.3 Contraindications

VALCYTE is contraindicated in patients with hypersensitivity to valganciclovir, ganciclovir or to any of the excipients.

Due to the similarity of the chemical structure of VALCYTE and that of aciclovir and valaciclovir, a cross-hypersensitivity reaction between these drugs is possible. Therefore, VALCYTE is contraindicated in patients with hypersensitivity to aciclovir and valaciclovir.

VALCYTE is contraindicated during lactation (see section 4.6).

4.4 Special warnings and precautions for use

Owing to the teratogenic character, the VALCYTE powder and reconstituted solution should be handled with caution. Inhalation should be avoided. If the powder or solution make direct contact with skin, the area should be washed thoroughly with soap and water. If the solution gets into the eye, the eye should be thouroghly washed with water immediately.

Prior to the initiation of valganciclovir treatment, patients should be advised of the potential risks to the foetus. In animal studies, ganciclovir was found to be mutagenic, teratogenic, aspermatogenic and carcinogenic, and a suppressor of female fertility. VALCYTE should, therefore, be considered a potential teratogen and carcinogen in humans with the potential to cause birth defects and cancers (see section 5.3). It is also considered likely that VALCYTE causes temporary or permanent inhibition of spermatogenesis. Women of child bearing potential must be advised to use effective contraception during treatment. Men must be advised to practise barrier contraception during treatment, and for at least 90 days thereafter, unless it is certain that the female partner is not at risk of pregnancy (see sections 4.6, 4.8 and 5.3).

Severe leucopenia, neutropenia, anaemia, thrombocytopenia, pancytopenia, bone marrow depression and aplastic anaemia have been observed in patients treated with VALCYTE (and ganciclovir). Therapy should not be initiated if the absolute neutrophil count is less than 500 cells/µl, or the platelet count is less than 25000/µl, or the haemoglobin level is less than 8g/dl (see sections 4.2 and 4.8).

VALCYTE should be used with caution in patients with pre-existing haematological cytopenia or a history of drug-related haematological cytopenia and in patients receiving radiotherapy.

It is recommended that complete blood counts and platelet counts be monitored during therapy. Increased haematological monitoring may be warranted in patients with renal impairment. In patients developing severe leucopenia, neutropenia, anaemia and/or thrombocytopenia, it is recommended that treatment with haematopoietic growth factors and/or dose interruption be considered (see sections 4.2 and 4.8).

In patients with impaired renal function, dosage adjustments based on creatinine clearance are required (see sections 4.2 and 5.2).

Convulsions have been reported in patients taking imipenem-cilastatin and ganciclovir. VALCYTE should not be used concomitantly with imipenem-cilastatin unless the potential benefits outweigh the potential risks (see section 4.5).

Patients treated with VALCYTE and (a) didanosine, (b) drugs that are known to be myelosuppressive (e.g. zidovudine), or (c) substances affecting renal function, should be closely monitored for signs of added toxicity (see section 4.5).

The controlled clinical study using valganciclovir for the prophylactic treatment of CMV disease in transplantation, as detailed in section 5.1, did not include lung and intestinal transplant patients. Therefore, experience in these transplant patients is limited.

For patients on a sodium-controlled diet, this medicinal product contains a total of 0.188 mg/ml sodium.

4.5 Interaction with other medicinal products and other forms of interaction

Drug interactions with valganciclovir

In-vivo drug interaction studies with VALCYTE have not been performed. Since valganciclovir is extensively and rapidly metabolised to ganciclovir; drug interactions associated with ganciclovir will be expected for valganciclovir.

Drug interactions with ganciclovir

Imipenem-cilastatin

Convulsions have been reported in patients taking ganciclovir and imipenem-cilastatin concomitantly. These drugs should not be used concomitantly unless the potential benefits outweigh the potential risks (see section 4.4).

Probenecid

Probenecid given with oral ganciclovir resulted in statistically significantly decreased renal clearance of ganciclovir (20%) leading to statistically significantly increased exposure (40%). These changes were consistent with a mechanism of interaction involving competition for renal tubular secretion. Therefore, patients taking probenecid and VALCYTE should be closely monitored for ganciclovir toxicity.

Zidovudine

When zidovudine was given in the presence of oral ganciclovir there was a small (17%), but statistically significant increase in the AUC of zidovudine. There was also a trend towards lower ganciclovir concentrations when administered with zidovudine, although this was not statistically significant. However, since both zidovudine and ganciclovir have the potential to cause neutropenia and anaemia, some patients may not tolerate concomitant therapy at full dosage (see section 4.4).

Didanosine

Didanosine plasma concentrations were found to be consistently raised when given with ganciclovir (both intravenous and oral). At ganciclovir oral doses of 3 and 6g/day, an increase in the AUC of didanosine ranging from 84 to 124% has been observed, and likewise at intravenous doses of 5 and 10 mg/kg/day, an increase in the AUC of didanosine ranging from 38 to 67% has been observed. There was no clinically significant effect on ganciclovir concentrations. Patients should be closely monitored for didanosine toxicity (see section 4.4).

Mycophenolate Mofetil

Based on the results of a single dose administration study of recommended doses of oral mycophenolate mofetil (MMF) and intravenous ganciclovir and the known effects of renal impairment on the pharmacokinetics of MMF and ganciclovir, it is anticipated that co-administration of these agents (which have the potential to compete for renal tubular secretion) will result in increases in phenolic glucuronide of mycophenolic acid (MPAG) and ganciclovir concentration. No substantial alteration of mycophenolic acid (MPA) pharmacokinetics is anticipated and MMF dose adjustment is not required. In patients with renal impairment to whom MMF and ganciclovir are co-administered, the dose recommendation of ganciclovir should be observed and the patients monitored carefully. Since both MMF and ganciclovir have the potential to cause neutropenia and leucopenia, patients should be monitored for additive toxicity.

Zalcitabine

No clinically significant pharmacokinetic changes were observed after concomitant administration of ganciclovir and zalcitabine. Both valganciclovir and zalcitabine have the potential to cause peripheral neuropathy and patients should be monitored for such events.

Stavudine

No clinically significant interactions were observed when stavudine and oral ganciclovir were given in combination.

Trimethoprim

No clinically significant pharmacokinetic interaction was observed when trimethoprim and oral ganciclovir were given in combination. However, there is a potential for toxicity to be enhanced since both drugs are known to be myelosuppressive and therefore both drugs should be used concomitantly only if the potential benefits outweigh the risks.

Other antiretrovirals

At clinically relevant concentrations, there is unlikely to be either a synergistic or antagonistic effect on the inhibition of either human immunodeficiency virus (HIV) in the presence of ganciclovir or CMV in the presence of a variety of antiretroviral drugs. Metabolic interactions with, for example, protease inhibitors and non-nucleoside reverse transcriptase inhibitors (NNRTIs) are unlikely due to the lack of P450 involvement in the metabolism of either valganciclovir or ganciclovir.

Other potential drug interactions

Toxicity may be enhanced when valganciclovir is co-administered with, or is given immediately before or after, other drugs that inhibit replication of rapidly dividing cell populations such as occur in the bone marrow, testes and germinal layers of the skin and gastrointestinal mucosa. Examples of these types of drugs are dapsone, pentamidine, flucytosine, vincristine, vinblastine, adriamycin, amphotericin B, trimethoprim/sulpha combinations, nucleoside analogues and hydroxyurea.

Since ganciclovir is excreted through the kidney (section 5.2), toxicity may also be enhanced during co-administration of valganciclovir with drugs that might reduce the renal clearance of ganciclovir and hence increase its exposure. The renal clearance of ganciclovir might be inhibited by two mechanisms: (a) nephrotoxicity, caused by drugs such as cidofovir and foscarnet, and (b) competitive inhibition of active tubular secretion in the kidney by, for example, other nucleoside analogues.

Therefore, all of these drugs should be considered for concomitant use with valganciclovir only if the potential benefits outweigh the potential risks (see section 4.4).

4.6 Pregnancy and lactation

There are no adequate data from the use of VALCYTE in pregnant women. Its active metabolite, ganciclovir, readily diffuses across the human placenta. Based on its pharmacological mechanism of action and reproductive toxicity observed in animal studies with ganciclovir (see section 5.3) there is a theoretical risk of teratogenicity in humans.

VALCYTE should not be used in pregnancy unless the therapeutic benefit for the mother outweighs the potential risk of teratogenic damage to the child.

Women of child-bearing potential must be advised to use effective contraception during treatment. Male patients must be advised to practise barrier contraception during, and for at least 90 days following treatment with VALCYTE unless it is certain that the female partner is not at risk of pregnancy (see section 5.3).

It is unknown if ganciclovir is excreted in breast milk, but the possibility of ganciclovir being excreted in the breast milk and causing serious adverse reactions in the nursing infant cannot be discounted. Therefore, breast-feeding must be discontinued (see section 4.3).

4.7 Effects on ability to drive and use machines

No studies on the effects on the ability to drive and use machines have been performed.

Convulsions, sedation, dizziness, ataxia, and/or confusion have been reported with the use of VALCYTE and/or ganciclovir. If they occur, such effects may affect the patient's ability to drive and operate machinery.

4.8 Undesirable effects

Valganciclovir is a prodrug of ganciclovir, which is rapidly and extensively metabolised to ganciclovir after oral administration. The undesirable effects known to be associated with ganciclovir use can be expected to occur with valganciclovir. All of the undesirable effects observed with valganciclovir clinical studies have been previously observed with ganciclovir. The most commonly reported adverse drug reactions following administration of valganciclovir in adults are neutropenia, anaemia and diarrhoea.

Valganciclovir is associated with a higher risk of diarrhoea compared to intravenous ganciclovir. In addition, valganciclovir is associated with a higher risk of neutropenia and leucopenia compared to oral ganciclovir.

Severe neutropenia (< 500 ANC/µl) is seen more frequently in CMV retinitis patients undergoing treatment with valganciclovir than in solid organ transplant patients receiving valganciclovir.

The frequency of adverse reactions reported in clinical trials with either valganciclovir, oral ganciclovir, or intravenous ganciclovir is presented in the Table below. The adverse reactions listed were reported in clinical trials in patients with AIDS for the induction or maintenance treatment of CMV retinitis, or in liver, kidney or heart transplant patients for the prophylaxis of CMV disease. The term (severe) in parenthesis in the Table indicates that the adverse reaction has been reported in patients at both mild/moderate intensity and severe/life-threatening intensity at that specific frequency.

Within each frequency grouping, undesirable effects are presented in order of decreasing seriousness.

(see Table 1 below)

Severe thrombocytopenia may be associated with potentially life-threatening bleeding.

4.9 Overdose

Overdose experience with valganciclovir

One adult developed fatal bone marrow depression (medullary aplasia) after several days of dosing that was at least 10-fold greater than recommended for the patient's degree of renal impairment (decreased creatinine clearance).

It is expected that an overdose of valganciclovir could also possibly result in increased renal toxicity (see section 4.2 and section 4.4).

Haemodialysis and hydration may be of benefit in reducing blood plasma levels in patients who receive an overdose of valganciclovir (see section 5.2)

Overdose experience with intravenous ganciclovir

Reports of overdoses with intravenous ganciclovir have been received from clinical trials and during post-marketing experience. In some of these cases no adverse events were reported. The majority of patients experienced one or more of the following adverse events:

Haematological toxicity: pancytopenia, bone marrow depression, medullary aplasia, leucopenia, neutropenia, granulocytopenia

– *Hepatotoxicity*: hepatitis, liver function disorder

Renal toxicity: worsening of haematuria in a patient with pre-existing renal impairment, acute renal failure, elevated creatinine

– *Gastrointestinal toxicity*: abdominal pain, diarrhoea, vomiting

– *Neurotoxicity:* generalised tremor, convulsion

5. PHARMACOLOGICAL PROPERTIES

5.1 Pharmacodynamic properties

Pharmacotherapeutic group: nucleosides and nucleotides excl. reverse transcriptase inhibitors, ATC code: J05A B14

Mechanism of action

Valganciclovir is an L-valyl ester (prodrug) of ganciclovir. After oral administration, valganciclovir is rapidly and extensively metabolised to ganciclovir by intestinal and hepatic esterases. Ganciclovir is a synthetic analogue of

Table 1

Body System	Very Common (≥ 1/10)	Common (≥ 1/100, < 1/10)	Uncommon (≥ 1/1000, < 1/100)	Rare (≥ 1/10,000, < 1/1000)
Investigations		blood creatinine increased, weight decreased		
Cardiac disorders			arrhythmia	
Blood and lymphatic system disorders	(severe) neutropenia, anaemia	(severe) pancytopenia, (severe) leucopenia, (severe) anaemia, (severe) thrombocytopenia	bone marrow failure	aplastic anaemia
Nervous system disorders		convulsion, neuropathy peripheral, insomnia, hypoaesthesia, paraesthesia, dizziness, dysgeusia (taste disturbance), headache	tremor	
Eye disorders		retinal detachment, macular oedema, eye pain, vitreous floaters	visual disturbance, conjunctivitis	
Ear and labyrinth disorders		ear pain	deafness	
Respiratory, thoracic and mediastinal disorders	Dyspnoea	Cough		
Gastrointestinal disorders	diarrhea	nausea, vomiting, abdominal pain, abdominal pain upper, constipation, dysphagia, dyspepsia, flatulence	pancreatitis, abdominal distension, mouth ulceration	
Renal and urinary disorders		renal impairment, creatinine renal clearance decreased	renal failure, haematuria	
Skin and subcutaneous tissue disorders		dermatitis, night sweats, pruritus	alopecia, urticaria, dry skin	
Musculoskeletal and connective tissue disorders		back pain, myalgia, arthralgia, muscle spasms		
Metabolism and nutrition disorders		anorexia, decreased appetite		
Infections and infestations		sepsis (bacteraemia, viraemia), cellulitis, urinary tract infection, oral candidiasis		
Vascular disorders			hypotension	
General disorders and administration site conditions		fatigue, pyrexia, chills, pain, chest pain, malaise, asthenia		
Immune system disorders			anaphylactic reaction	
Hepatobiliary disorders		(severe) hepatic function abnormal, blood alkaline phosphatase increased, aspartate aminotransferase increased	alanine aminotransferase increased	
Reproductive system and breast disorders			infertility male	
Psychiatric disorders		depression, anxiety, confusional state, thinking abnormal	psychotic disorder, hallucination, agitation	

Table 2

Parameter	Ganciclovir (5 mg/kg, IV) n = 18	Valganciclovir (900 mg, p.o.) n = 25	
		Ganciclovir	Valganciclovir
AUC(0 - 12 h) (μg.h/ml)	28.6 ± 9.0	32.8 ± 10.1	0.37 ± 0.22
C_{max} (μg/ml)	10.4 ± 4.9	6.7 ± 2.1	0.18 ± 0.06

2'-deoxyguanosine and inhibits replication of herpes viruses *in vitro* and *in vivo*. Sensitive human viruses include human cytomegalovirus (HCMV), herpes simplex virus-1 and -2 (HSV-1 and HSV-2), human herpes virus -6, -7 and -8 (HHV-6, HHV-7, HHV-8), Epstein-Barr virus (EBV), varicella-zoster virus (VZV) and hepatitis B virus (HBV).

In CMV-infected cells, ganciclovir is initially phosphorylated to ganciclovir monophosphate by the viral protein kinase, pUL97. Further phosphorylation occurs by cellular kinases to produce ganciclovir triphosphate, which is then slowly metabolised intracellularly. Triphosphate metabolism has been shown to occur in HSV- and HCMV- infected cells with half-lives of 18 and between 6 and 24 hours respectively, after the removal of extracellular ganciclovir. As the phosphorylation is largely dependent on the viral kinase, phosphorylation of ganciclovir occurs preferentially in virus-infected cells.

The virustatic activity of ganciclovir is due to inhibition of viral DNA synthesis by: (a) competitive inhibition of incorporation of deoxyguanosine-triphosphate into DNA by viral DNA polymerase, and (b) incorporation of ganciclovir triphosphate into viral DNA causing termination of, or very limited, further viral DNA elongation.

Antiviral Activity

The *in-vitro* anti-viral activity, measured as IC_{50} of ganciclovir against CMV, is in the range of 0.08μM (0.02μg/ml) to 14μM (3.5μg/ml).

The clinical antiviral effect of VALCYTE has been demonstrated in the treatment of AIDS patients with newly diagnosed CMV retinitis. CMV shedding was decreased in urine from 46% (32/69) of patients at study entry to 7% (4/55) of patients following four weeks of VALCYTE treatment.

Clinical efficacy

Treatment of CMV retinitis:

Patients with newly diagnosed CMV retinitis were randomised in one study to induction therapy with either VALCYTE 900 mg (twice daily) or intravenous ganciclovir 5 mg/kg (twice daily). The proportion of patients with photographic progression of CMV retinitis at week 4 was comparable in both treatment groups, 7/70 and 7/71 patients progressing in the intravenous ganciclovir and valganciclovir arms respectively.

Following induction treatment dosing, all patients in this study received maintenance treatment with VALCYTE given at the dose of 900 mg once daily. The mean (median) time from randomisation to progression of CMV retinitis in the group receiving induction and maintenance treatment with VALCYTE was 226 (160) days and in the group receiving induction treatment with intravenous ganciclovir and maintenance treatment with VALCYTE was 219 (125) days.

Prevention of CMV disease in transplantation

A double-blind, double-dummy clinical active comparator study has been conducted in heart, liver and kidney transplant patients (lung and gastro-intestinal transplant patients were not included in the study) at high-risk of CMV disease (D+/R-) who received either VALCYTE (900 mg once daily) or oral ganciclovir (1000 mg three times daily) starting within 10 days of transplantation until Day 100 post-transplant. The incidence of CMV disease (CMV syndrome + tissue invasive disease) during the first 6 months post-transplant was 12.1% in the VALCYTE arm (n=239) compared with 15.2% in the oral ganciclovir arm (n=125). The large majority of cases occurred following cessation of prophylaxis (post-Day 100) with cases in the valganciclovir arm occurring on average later than those in the oral ganciclovir arm. The incidence of acute rejection in the first 6 months was 29.7% in patients randomised to valganciclovir compared with 36.0% in the oral ganciclovir arm, with the incidence of graft loss being equivalent, occurring in 0.8% of patients, in each arm.

Viral Resistance

Virus resistant to ganciclovir can arise after chronic dosing with valganciclovir by selection of mutations in the viral kinase gene (UL97) responsible for ganciclovir monophosphorylation and/or the viral polymerase gene (UL54). Viruses containing mutations in the UL97 gene are resistant to ganciclovir alone, whereas viruses with mutations in the UL54 gene are resistant to ganciclovir but may show cross-resistance to other antivirals that also target the viral polymerase.

Treatment of CMV retinitis:

Genotypic analysis of CMV in polymorphonuclear leucocytes (PMNL) isolates from 148 patients with CMV retinitis enrolled in one clinical study has shown that 2.2%, 6.5%, 12.8%, and 15.3% contain UL97 mutations after 3, 6, 12 and 18 months, respectively, of valganciclovir treatment.

Prevention of CMV disease in transplantation:

Resistance was studied by genotypic analysis of CMV in PMNL samples collected i) on Day 100 (end of study drug prophylaxis) and ii) in cases of suspected CMV disease up to 6 months after transplantation. From the 245 patients randomised to receive valganciclovir, 198 Day 100 samples were available for testing and no ganciclovir resistance mutations were observed. This compares with 2 ganciclovir resistance mutations detected in the 103 samples tested (1.9%) for patients in the oral ganciclovir comparator arm.

Of the 245 patients randomised to receive valganciclovir, samples from 50 patients with suspected CMV disease were tested and no resistance mutations were observed. Of the 127 patients randomised on the ganciclovir comparator arm, samples from 29 patients with suspected CMV disease were tested, from which two resistance mutations were observed, giving an incidence of resistance of 6.9%.

5.2 Pharmacokinetic properties

The pharmacokinetic properties of valganciclovir have been evaluated in HIV- and CMV-seropositive patients, patients with AIDS and CMV retinitis and in solid organ transplant patients.

Absorption

Valganciclovir is a prodrug of ganciclovir. It is well absorbed from the gastrointestinal tract and rapidly and extensively metabolised in the intestinal wall and liver to ganciclovir. Systemic exposure to valganciclovir is transient and low. The absolute bioavailability of ganciclovir from valganciclovir is approximately 60% across all the patient populations studied and the resultant exposure to ganciclovir is similar to that after its intravenous administration (please see below).

Valganciclovir in HIV positive, CMV positive patients:

Systemic exposure of HIV positive, CMV positive patients after twice daily administration of ganciclovir and valganciclovir for one week is:

(see Table 2 above)

The efficacy of ganciclovir in increasing the time-to-progression of CMV retinitis has been shown to correlate with systemic exposure (AUC).

Valganciclovir in solid organ transplant patients:

Steady state systemic exposure of solid organ transplant patients to ganciclovir after daily oral administration of ganciclovir and valganciclovir is:

Parameter	Ganciclovir (1000 mg three times daily) n = 82	Valganciclovir (900 mg, once daily) n = 161
		Ganciclovir
AUC(0 - 24 h) (μg.h/ml)	28.0 ± 10.9	46.3 ± 15.2
C_{max} (μg/ml)	1.4 ± 0.5	5.3 ± 1.5

The systemic exposure of ganciclovir to heart, kidney and liver transplant recipients was similar after oral administration of valganciclovir according to the renal function dosing algorithm.

Following the administration of valganciclovir as an oral solution, equivalent systemic ganciclovir exposures were obtained compared to the tablet formulation.

Food effect:

Dose proportionality with respect to ganciclovir AUC following administration of valganciclovir in the dose range 450 to 2625 mg was demonstrated only under fed conditions. When valganciclovir was given with food at the recommended dose of 900 mg, higher values were seen in both mean ganciclovir AUC (approximately 30%) and mean ganciclovir C_{max} values (approximately 14%) than in the fasting state. Also, the inter-individual variation in exposure of ganciclovir decreases when taking VALCYTE with food. VALCYTE has only been administered with food in clinical studies. Therefore, it is recommended that VALCYTE be administered with food (see section 4.2).

Distribution:

Because of rapid conversion of valganciclovir to ganciclovir, protein binding of valganciclovir was not determined. Plasma protein binding of ganciclovir was 1 - 2% over concentrations of 0.5 and 51μg/ml. The steady state volume of distribution (V_d) of ganciclovir after intravenous administration was 0.680 ± 0.161 L/kg (n=114).

Metabolism

Valganciclovir is rapidly and extensively metabolised to ganciclovir; no other metabolites have been detected. No metabolite of orally administered radiolabelled ganciclovir (1000 mg single dose) accounted for more than 1 - 2% of the radioactivity recovered in the faeces or urine.

Elimination

Following dosing with VALCYTE, renal excretion, as ganciclovir, by glomerular filtration and active tubular secretion is the major route of elimination of valganciclovir. Renal clearance accounts for 81.5% ± 22% (n=70) of the systemic clearance of ganciclovir. Post-hoc Bayesian estimates for population mean apparent clearance of ganciclovir in patients with CrCl> 60 ml/min is 14.05 ± 4.13 L/h. In patients with renal impairment, the mean apparent clearance of ganciclovir is 8.46 ± 1.67 L/h (CrCl between 40 and 60 mL/min) and 7.00 ± 1.08 L/h (CrCl between 25 and 40 ml/min).

The half-life of ganciclovir from valganciclovir is 4.1 ± 0.9 hours in HIV- and CMV-seropositive patients.

Pharmacokinetics in special clinical situations

Patients with renal impairment

Decreasing renal function resulted in decreased clearance of ganciclovir from valganciclovir with a corresponding increase in terminal half-life. Therefore, dosage adjustment is required for renally impaired patients (see section 4.2 and 4.4).

Patients undergoing haemodialysis

For patients receiving haemodialysis VALCYTE powder for oral solution is recommended to provide an individualised dose (see sections 4.2 and 4.4).

Patients with hepatic impairment

The safety and efficacy of VALCYTE have not been studied in patients with hepatic impairment. Hepatic impairment should not significantly affect the pharmacokinetics of ganciclovir since it is excreted renally and, therefore, no specific dose recommendation is made.

5.3 Preclinical safety data

Valganciclovir is a pro-drug of ganciclovir and therefore effects observed with ganciclovir apply equally to valganciclovir. Toxicity of valganciclovir in pre-clinical safety studies was the same as that seen with ganciclovir and was induced at ganciclovir exposure levels comparable to, or lower than, those in humans given the induction dose.

These findings were gonadotoxicity (testicular cell loss) and nephrotoxicity (uraemia, cell degeneration), which were irreversible; myelotoxicity (anaemia, neutropenia, lymphocytopenia) and gastrointestinal toxicity (mucosal cell necrosis), which were reversible.

Further studies have shown ganciclovir to be mutagenic, carcinogenic, teratogenic, embryotoxic, aspermatogenic (i.e. impairs male fertility) and to suppress female fertility.

6. PHARMACEUTICAL PARTICULARS

6.1 List of excipients

povidone

fumaric acid

sodium benzoate (E211)

sodium saccharin

mannitol

Tutti-frutti flavour:

maltodextrins (maize)

propylene glycol

arabic gum E414 and natural flavouring substances mainly consisting of banana, pineapple and peach flavour

6.2 Incompatibilities

Not applicable.

6.3 Shelf life

Powder for oral solution: 2 years.

Reconstituted solution: 49 days. Store in a refrigerator (2°C - 8°C)

6.4 Special precautions for storage

This medicinal product does not require any special storage condition.

For storage conditions of the reconstituted medicinal product, see section 6.3.

6.5 Nature and contents of container

Carton containing a 100 ml amber glass bottle with a child-resistant plastic screw cap, a plastic bottle adapter and a plastic bag containing 2 plastic oral dispensers graduated to 500 mg with graduations of 25 mg.

Each bottle contains 12 g of powder for oral solution. When reconstituted, the volume of the solution is 100 ml, providing a minimal usable volume of 88 ml.

6.6 Special precautions for disposal and other handling

Since VALCYTE is considered a potential teratogen and carcinogen in humans, caution should be observed in handling the powder and the reconstituted solution (see section 4.4). Avoid inhalation and direct contact of the powder and solution with skin and mucous membranes. If such contact occurs, wash thoroughly with soap and water. If the powder or solution gets into the eyes, rinse eyes thoroughly with water.

It is recommended that VALCYTE powder for oral solution be reconstituted by the pharmacist prior to dispensing to the patient.

Preparation of oral solution

1. Measure 91 ml of water in a graduated cylinder.

2. Remove the child resistant cap, add the water to the bottle, then close the bottle with the child resistant cap. Shake the closed bottle until the powder is dissolved forming a clear, colourless to brown solution.

3. Remove the child resistant cap and push the bottle adapter into the neck of the bottle.

4. Close the bottle with the child resistant cap tightly. This will assure the proper seating of the bottle adapter in the bottle and child resistant status of the cap.

5. Write the date of expiration of the reconstituted solution on the bottle label (see section 6.3).

Any unused product or waste material should be disposed of in accordance with local requirements.

7. MARKETING AUTHORISATION HOLDER

Roche Products Limited, 6 Falcon Way, Shire Park,

Welwyn Garden City. AL7 1TW

United Kingdom

8. MARKETING AUTHORISATION NUMBER(S)

UK: PL 00031/0829

IRL: PA 50/150/2

9. DATE OF FIRST AUTHORISATION/RENEWAL OF THE AUTHORISATION

UK: 09/09/08

IRL: 15/08/08

10. DATE OF REVISION OF THE TEXT

POM

Valdoxan

(Servier Laboratories Limited)

1. NAME OF THE MEDICINAL PRODUCT

▼ Valdoxan 25 mg film-coated tablets

2. QUALITATIVE AND QUANTITATIVE COMPOSITION

Each film-coated tablet contains 25 mg of agomelatine.

Excipient: lactose monohydrate 61.84 mg

For a full list of excipients, see section 6.1.

3. PHARMACEUTICAL FORM

Film-coated tablet [tablet].

Orange-yellow, oblong, film-coated tablet with blue imprint of company logo on one side.

4. CLINICAL PARTICULARS

4.1 Therapeutic indications

Treatment of major depressive episodes in adults

4.2 Posology and method of administration

The recommended dose is 25 mg once daily taken orally at bedtime.

After two weeks of treatment, if there is no improvement of symptoms, the dose may be increased to 50 mg once daily, i.e. two 25 mg tablets, taken together at bedtime.

Liver function tests should be performed in all patients: at initiation of treatment, and then periodically after around six weeks (end of acute phase), twelve weeks and twenty four weeks (end of maintenance phase) and thereafter when clinically indicated (see also section 4.4).

Patients with depression should be treated for a sufficient period of at least 6 months to ensure that they are free of symptoms.

Valdoxan tablets may be taken with or without food.

Children and adolescents:

Valdoxan is not recommended for use in children and adolescents below 18 years of age due to a lack of data on safety and efficacy (see section 4.4).

Elderly patients:

Efficacy has not been clearly demonstrated in the elderly (⩾ 65 years). Only limited clinical data is available on the use of Valdoxan in elderly patients ⩾ 65 years old with major depressive episodes. Therefore, caution should be exercised when prescribing Valdoxan to these patients (see section 4.4).

Patients with renal impairment:

No relevant modification in agomelatine pharmacokinetic parameters in patients with severe renal impairment has been observed. However, only limited clinical data on the use of Valdoxan in depressed patients with severe or moderate renal impairment with major depressive episodes is available. Therefore, caution should be exercised when prescribing Valdoxan to these patients.

Patients with hepatic impairment:

Valdoxan is contra-indicated in patients with hepatic impairment (see sections 4.3, 4.4 and 5.2).

Treatment discontinuation:

No dosage tapering is needed on treatment discontinuation.

4.3 Contraindications

Hypersensitivity to the active substance or to any of the excipients.

Hepatic impairment (i.e. cirrhosis or active liver disease) (see sections 4.2 and 4.4).

Concomitant use of potent CYP1A2 inhibitors (e.g. fluvoxamine, ciprofloxacin) (see section 4.5).

4.4 Special warnings and precautions for use

Use in children and adolescents:

Valdoxan is not recommended in the treatment of depression in patients under 18 years of age since safety and efficacy of Valdoxan have not been established in this age group. In clinical trials among children and adolescents treated with other antidepressants, suicide-related behaviour (suicide attempt and suicidal thoughts), and hostility (predominantly aggression, oppositional behaviour and anger) were more frequently observed compared to those treated with placebo.

Use in elderly patients with dementia:

Valdoxan should not be used for the treatment of major depressive episodes in elderly patients with dementia since the safety and efficacy of Valdoxan have not been established in these patients.

Mania / Hypomania:

Valdoxan should be used with caution in patients with a history of mania or hypomania and should be discontinued if a patient develops manic symptoms.

Suicide/suicidal thoughts:

Depression is associated with an increased risk of suicidal thoughts, self-harm and suicide (suicide-related events). This risk persists until significant remission occurs. As improvement may not occur during the first few weeks or more of treatment, patients should be closely monitored until such improvement occurs. It is general clinical experience that the risk of suicide may increase in the early stages of recovery.

Patients with a history of suicide-related events or those exhibiting a significant degree of suicidal ideation prior to commencement of treatment are known to be at greater risk of suicidal thoughts or suicide attempts, and should receive careful monitoring during treatment. A meta-analysis of placebo-controlled clinical trials of antidepressants in adult patients with psychiatric disorders showed an increased risk of suicidal behaviour with antidepressants compared to placebo, in patients less than 25 years old.

Close supervision of patients and in particular those at high risk should accompany treatment especially in early treatment and following dose changes. Patients (and caregivers of patients) should be alerted to the need to monitor for any clinical worsening, suicidal behaviour or thoughts and unusual changes in behaviour and to seek medical advice immediately if these symptoms present.

Combination with CYP1A2 inhibitors (see sections 4.3 and 4.5)

Combination with potent CYP1A2 inhibitors is contra-indicated. Caution should be exercised when prescribing Valdoxan with moderate CYP1A2 inhibitors (*e.g.* propranolol, grepafloxacin, enoxacin) which may result in increased exposure of agomelatine.

Increased serum transaminases:

In clinical studies, elevations of serum transaminases (>3 times the upper limit of the normal range) have been observed in patients treated with Valdoxan particularly on a 50 mg dose (see section 4.8). When Valdoxan was discontinued in these patients, the serum transaminases usually returned to normal levels. Liver function tests should be performed in all patients: at initiation of treatment and then periodically after around six weeks (end of acute phase), after around twelve and twenty four weeks (end of maintenance phase) and thereafter when clinically indicated. Any patient who develops increased serum transaminases should have his/her liver function tests repeated within 48 hours. Therapy should be discontinued if the increase in serum transaminases exceeds 3X upper limit of normal and liver function tests should be performed regularly until serum transaminases return to normal.

If any patient develops symptoms suggesting hepatic dysfunction liver function tests should be performed. The decision whether to continue the patient on therapy with Valdoxan should be guided by clinical judgement pending laboratory evaluations. If jaundice is observed therapy should be discontinued.

Caution should be exercised when Valdoxan is administered to patients who consume substantial quantities of alcohol or who are treated with medicinal products associated with risk of hepatic injury.

Lactose intolerance:

Valdoxan contains lactose. Patients with rare hereditary problems of galactose intolerance, the Lapp lactase deficiency or glucose-galactose malabsorption should not take this medicine.

4.5 Interaction with other medicinal products and other forms of interaction

Potential interactions affecting agomelatine:

Agomelatine is metabolised mainly by cytochrome P450 1A2 (CYP1A2) (90%) and by CYP2C9/19 (10%). Medicinal products that interact with these isoenzymes may decrease or increase the bioavailability of agomelatine.

Fluvoxamine, a potent CYP1A2 and moderate CYP2C9 inhibitor markedly inhibits the metabolism of agomelatine resulting in a 60-fold (range 12-412) increase of agomelatine exposure.

Consequently, co-administration of Valdoxan with potent CYP1A2 inhibitors (e.g. fluvoxamine, ciprofloxacin) is contra-indicated.

Combination of agomelatine with oestrogens (moderate CYP1A2 inhibitors) results in a several fold increased exposure of agomelatine. While there was no specific safety signal in the 800 patients treated in combination with oestrogens, caution should be exercised when prescribing agomelatine with other moderate CYP1A2 inhibitors (e.g. propranolol, grepafloxacin, enoxacin) until more experience has been gained (see section 4.4)

Potential for agomelatine to affect other medicinal products:

In vivo, agomelatine does not induce CYP450 isoenzymes. Agomelatine inhibits neither CYP1A2 *in vivo* nor the other CYP450 *in vitro*. Therefore, agomelatine will not modify exposure to medicinal products metabolised by CYP 450.

Medicinal products highly bound to plasma protein:

Agomelatine does not modify free concentrations of medicinal products highly bound to plasma proteins or *vice versa*.

Other medicinal products:

No evidence of pharmacokinetic or pharmacodynamic interaction with medicinal products which could be prescribed concomitantly with Valdoxan in the target population was found in phase I clinical trials: benzodiazepines, lithium, paroxetine, fluconazole and theophylline.

Alcohol:

The combination of Valdoxan and alcohol is not advisable.

Electroconvulsive therapy (ECT):

There is no experience of concurrent use of agomelatine with ECT. Animal studies have not shown proconvulsant properties (see section 5.3). Therefore, clinical consequences of ECT concomitant treatment with Valdoxan are considered to be unlikely.

4.6 Pregnancy and lactation

For agomelatine, no clinical data on exposed pregnancies are available. Animal studies do not indicate direct or indirect harmful effects with respect to pregnancy, embryonal/foetal development, parturition or postnatal development (see section 5.3). Caution should be exercised when prescribing to pregnant women.

It is not known whether agomelatine is excreted into human milk. Agomelatine or its metabolites are excreted in the milk of lactating rats. Potential effects of agomelatine on the breast-feeding infant have not been established. If treatment with Valdoxan is considered necessary, breast-feeding should be discontinued.

4.7 Effects on ability to drive and use machines

No studies on the effects on the ability to drive and use machines have been performed.

However, considering that dizziness and somnolence are common adverse reactions patients should be cautioned about their ability to drive a car or operate machinery.

4.8 Undesirable effects

In clinical trials, over 3,900 depressed patients have received Valdoxan.

Adverse reactions were usually mild or moderate and occurred within the first two weeks of treatment. The most common adverse reactions were nausea and dizziness.

These adverse reactions were usually transient and did not generally lead to cessation of therapy.

Depressed patients display a number of symptoms that are associated with the illness itself. It is therefore sometimes difficult to ascertain which symptoms are a result of the illness itself and which are a result of treatment with Valdoxan.

Adverse reactions are listed below using the following convention: very common (⩾1/10); common (⩾1/100 to <1/10); uncommon (⩾1/1,000 to <1/100); rare (⩾1/10,000 to <1/1,000); very rare (<1/10,000), not known (cannot be estimated from the available data). The frequencies have not been corrected for placebo.

Nervous system disorders:

Common: headache, dizziness, somnolence, insomnia, migraine,

Uncommon: paraesthesia

Eye disorders:

Uncommon: blurred vision

Gastrointestinal disorders:

Common: nausea, diarrhoea, constipation, upper abdominal pain

Skin and subcutaneous tissue disorders

Common: hyperhidrosis

Uncommon: eczema

Rare: erythematous rash

Musculoskeletal and connective tissue disorders

Common: back pain

General disorders and administration site conditions:

Common: fatigue

Hepato-biliary disorders:

Common increases (>3 times the upper limit of the normal range) in ALAT and/or ASAT (i.e. 1.1% on agomelatine 25/50 mg vs 0.7% on placebo).

Rare: hepatitis

Psychiatric disorders:

Common: anxiety

Frequency not known: Suicidal thoughts or behaviour (see section 4.4)

4.9 Overdose

There is limited experience with agomelatine overdose. During the clinical development, there were a few reports of agomelatine overdose, taken alone (up to 450 mg) or in combination (up to 525 mg) with other psychotropic medicinal products. Signs and symptoms of overdose were limited and included drowsiness and epigastralgia.

No specific antidotes for agomelatine are known. Management of overdose should consist of treatment of clinical symptoms and routine monitoring. Medical follow-up in a specialised environment is recommended.

5. PHARMACOLOGICAL PROPERTIES

5.1 Pharmacodynamic properties

Pharmacotherapeutic group: Other antidepressants, ATC-code: NO6AX22

Agomelatine is a melatonergic agonist (MT_1 and MT_2 receptors) and $5\text{-}HT_{2C}$ antagonist. Binding studies indicate that agomelatine has no effect on monoamine uptake and no affinity for α, β adrenergic, histaminergic, cholinergic, dopaminergic and benzodiazepine receptors.

Agomelatine resynchronises circadian rhythms in animal models of circadian rhythm disruption. Agomelatine increases noradrenaline and dopamine release specifically in the frontal cortex and has no influence on the extracellular levels of serotonin.

Agomelatine has shown an antidepressant-like effect in animal models of depression (learned helplessness test, despair test, chronic mild stress) as well as in models with circadian rhythm desynchronisation and in models related to stress and anxiety.

In humans, Valdoxan has positive phase shifting properties; it induces a phase advance of sleep, body temperature decline and melatonin onset.

The efficacy and safety of Valdoxan in major depressive episodes have been studied in a clinical programme including 5,800 patients of whom 3,900 were treated with Valdoxan.

Six placebo controlled trials have been performed to investigate the short term efficacy of Valdoxan in major depressive disorder: two flexible dose studies and four fixed dose studies. At the end of treatment (over 6 or 8 weeks), significant efficacy of agomelatine 25-50 mg was demonstrated in 3 of the six short-term double-blind placebo-controlled studies. Agomelatine failed to differentiate from placebo in one study where the active control fluoxetine showed assay sensitivity. In two other studies, it was not possible to draw any conclusions because the active controls, paroxetine and fluoxetine, failed to differentiate from placebo.

Efficacy was also observed in more severely depressed patients (baseline HAM-D ⩾ 25) in all positive placebo-controlled studies.

Response rates were statistically significantly higher with Valdoxan compared with placebo.

The maintenance of antidepressant efficacy was demonstrated in a relapse prevention study. Patients responding to 8/10-weeks of acute treatment with open-label Valdoxan 25-50 mg once daily were randomised to either Valdoxan 25-50 mg once daily or placebo for further 6-months. Valdoxan 25-50 mg once daily demonstrated a statistically significant superiority compared to placebo (p=0.0001) on the primary outcome measure, the prevention of depressive relapse, as measured by time to relapse. The incidence of relapse during the 6-months double-blind follow up period was 22% and 47% for Valdoxan and placebo, respectively.

Valdoxan does not alter daytime vigilance and memory in healthy volunteers. In depressed patients, treatment with Valdoxan 25 mg increased slow wave sleep without modification of REM (Rapid Eye Movement) sleep amount or REM latency. Valdoxan 25 mg also induced an advance of the time of sleep onset and of minimum heart rate. From the first week of treatment, onset of sleep and the quality of sleep were significantly improved without daytime clumsiness as assessed by patients.

In a specific sexual dysfunction comparative study with remitted depressed patients, there was a numerical trend (not statistically significant) towards less sexual emergent dysfunction than venlafaxine for Sex Effects Scale (SEXFX) drive arousal or orgasm scores on Valdoxan. The pooled analysis of studies using the Arizona Sexual Experience Scale (ASEX) showed that Valdoxan was not associated with sexual dysfunction. In healthy volunteers Valdoxan preserved sexual function in comparison with paroxetine.

Valdoxan had neutral effect on body weight, heart rate and blood pressure in clinical studies.

In a study designed to assess discontinuation symptoms by the Discontinuation Emergent Signs and Symptoms (DESS) check-list in patients with remitted depression, Valdoxan did not induce discontinuation syndrome after abrupt treatment cessation.

Valdoxan has no abuse potential as measured in healthy volunteer studies on a specific visual analogue scale or the Addiction Research Centre Inventory (ARCI) 49 check-list.

5.2 Pharmacokinetic properties

Absorption and bioavailability:

Agomelatine is rapidly and well (⩾ 80%) absorbed after oral administration. Absolute bioavailability is low (< 5% at the therapeutic oral dose) and the interindividual variability is substantial. The bioavailability is increased in women compared to men. The bioavailability is increased by intake of oral contraceptives and reduced by smoking. The peak plasma concentration is reached within 1 to 2 hours.

In the therapeutic dose-range, agomelatine systemic exposure increases proportionally with dose. At higher doses, a saturation of the first-pass effect occurs.

Food intake (standard meal or high fat meal) does not modify the bioavailability or the absorption rate. The variability is increased with high fat food.

Distribution:

Steady state volume of distribution is about 35 l and plasma protein binding is 95% irrespective of the concentration and is not modified with age and in patients with renal impairment but the free fraction is doubled in patients with hepatic impairment.

Biotransformation:

Following oral administration, agomelatine is rapidly metabolised mainly via hepatic CYP1A2; CYP2C9 and CYP2C19 isoenzymes are also involved but with a low contribution.

The major metabolites, hydroxylated and demethylated agomelatine, are not active and are rapidly conjugated and eliminated in the urine.

Elimination:

Elimination is rapid, the mean plasma half-life is between 1 and 2 hours and the clearance is high (about 1,100 ml/min) and essentially metabolic.

Excretion is mainly (80%) urinary and in the form of metabolites, whereas unchanged compound recovery in urine is negligible.

Kinetics are not modified after repeated administration.

Renal impairment:

No relevant modification of pharmacokinetic parameters in patients with severe renal impairment has been observed (n=8, single dose of 25 mg) but caution should be exercised in patients with severe or moderate renal impairment as only limited clinical data are available in these patients (see section 4.2).

Hepatic impairment:

In a specific study involving cirrhotic patients with chronic mild (Child-Pugh type A) or moderate (Child-Pugh type B) liver impairment, exposure to agomelatine 25 mg was substantially increased (70-times and 140-times, respectively), compared to matched volunteers (age, weight and smoking habit) with no liver failure (see section 4.2, 4.3 and 4.4).

Ethnic groups:

There is no data on the influence of race on agomelatine pharmacokinetics.

5.3 Preclinical safety data

In mice, rats and monkeys sedative effects were observed after single and repeated administration at high doses.

In rodents, a marked induction of CYP2B and a moderate induction of CYP1A and CYP3A were seen from 125 mg/kg/day whereas in monkeys the induction was slight for CYP2B and CYP3A at 375 mg/kg/day. No hepatotoxicity was observed in rodents and monkeys in the repeat dose toxicity studies.

Agomelatine passes into the placenta and foetuses of pregnant rats.

Reproduction studies in the rat and the rabbit showed no effect of agomelatine on fertility, embryofoetal development and pre- and post natal development.

A battery of *in vitro* and *in vivo* standard genotoxicity assays concludes to no mutagenic or clastogenic potential of agomelatine.

In carcinogenicity studies agomelatine induced an increase in the incidence of liver tumours in the rat and the mouse, at a dose at least 110-fold higher than the therapeutic dose. Liver tumours are most likely related to enzyme induction specific to rodents. The frequency of benign mammary fibroadenomas observed in the rat was increased with high exposures (60-fold the exposure at the therapeutic dose) but remains in the range of that of controls.

Safety pharmacology studies showed no effect of agomelatine on hERG (human Ether à-go-go Related Gene) current or on dog Purkinje cells action potential. Agomelatine did not show proconvulsive properties at ip doses up to 128 mg/kg in mice and rats.

6. PHARMACEUTICAL PARTICULARS

6.1 List of excipients

Tablet core:

- Lactose monohydrate
- Maize starch
- Povidone
- Sodium starch glycolate type A
- Stearic acid
- Magnesium stearate
- Silica, colloidal anhydrous

Film-coating:

- Hypromellose
- Yellow iron oxide (E172)
- Glycerol
- Macrogol
- Magnesium stearate
- Titanium dioxide (E171)

Printing ink containing shellac, propylene glycol and indigotine (E132) aluminium lake.

6.2 Incompatibilities

Not applicable.

6.3 Shelf life

3 years.

6.4 Special precautions for storage

This medicinal product does not require any special storage conditions.

6.5 Nature and contents of container

Aluminium/PVC blister packed in cardboard boxes (calendar).

Packs containing 7, 14, 28, 42, 56, 84 and 98 film-coated tablets.

Packs of 100 film-coated tablets for hospital use.

Not all pack sizes may be marketed.

6.6 Special precautions for disposal and other handling

No special requirements.

7. MARKETING AUTHORISATION HOLDER

Les Laboratoires Servier

22, rue Garnier

F-92200 Neuilly-sur-Seine

France

8. MARKETING AUTHORISATION NUMBER(S)

EU/01/08/499/001 (Pack of 7 tablets)

EU/01/08/499/002 (Pack of 14 tablets)

EU/01/08/499/003 (Pack of 28 tablets)

EU/01/08/499/004 (Pack of 42 tablets)

EU/01/08/499/005 (Pack of 56 tablets)

EU/01/08/499/006 (Pack of 84 tablets)

EU/01/08/499/007 (Pack of 98 tablets)

EU/01/08/499/008 (Pack of 100 tablets)

9. DATE OF FIRST AUTHORISATION/RENEWAL OF THE AUTHORISATION

19 February 2009

10. DATE OF REVISION OF THE TEXT

February 2009

Detailed information on this medicinal product is available on the website of the European Medicines Agency (EMEA) http://www.emea.europa.eu

Valtrex Tablets 250mg

(GlaxoSmithKline UK)

1. NAME OF THE MEDICINAL PRODUCT

Valtrex™ Tablets 250mg.

2. QUALITATIVE AND QUANTITATIVE COMPOSITION

250mg of valaciclovir

3. PHARMACEUTICAL FORM

Film coated tablets

4. CLINICAL PARTICULARS

4.1 Therapeutic indications

Valtrex is indicated for the treatment of herpes zoster (shingles).

Valtrex is indicated for the treatment of herpes simplex infections of the skin and mucous membranes, including initial and recurrent genital herpes.

Valtrex is indicated for the suppression (prevention) of recurrent herpes simplex infections of the skin and mucous membranes, including genital herpes.

Valtrex can reduce transmission of genital herpes when taken as suppressive therapy and combined with safer sex practices (particularly the use of condoms).

Valtrex is indicated for the prophylaxis of cytomegalovirus (CMV) infection and disease, following renal transplantation.

4.2 Posology and method of administration

Route of administration: oral

DOSAGE IN ADULTS:

• **Treatment of herpes zoster:**

1000 mg of Valtrex to be taken 3 times daily for 7 days.

• **Treatment of herpes simplex:**

Valtrex can prevent lesion development when taken at the first signs and symptoms of an HSV recurrence.

500 mg of Valtrex to be taken twice daily. For recurrent episodes, treatment should be for 5 days. For initial episodes, which can be more severe, treatment may have to be extended to 10 days. Dosing should begin as early as possible. For recurrent episodes of herpes simplex, this should ideally be during the prodromal period or immediately the first signs or symptoms appear.

• **Suppression (prevention) of herpes simplex infection:**

In immunocompetent patients, 500mg of Valtrex is to be taken once daily.

Some patients with very frequent recurrences (e.g. more than 10 per year) may benefit from taking 500mg as a divided dose (250mg twice daily).

For immunocompromised patients the dose is 500mg twice daily.

• **Reduction of transmission of genital herpes:**

In immunocompetent heterosexual adult patients with 9 or fewer recurrences per year, 500 mg of Valtrex to be taken once daily by the infected partner in order to reduce transmission to a sexual partner negative for HSV-2 antibodies. Safer sex practices (particularly condom use) should be maintained, and sexual contact avoided if lesions are present.

There are no data on the reduction of transmission beyond 8 months in other patient populations.

• **Prophylaxis of cytomegalovirus infection (CMV) and disease**

Dosage in adults and adolescents (from 12 years of age):

The dosage of Valtrex is 2g four times a day, to be initiated within 72 hours post-transplant, or as soon as oral medication can be tolerated. This dose should be reduced according to creatinine clearance (see Dosage in renal impairment below).

The duration of treatment will usually be 90 days.

DOSAGE IN CHILDREN:

There are no data available on the use of Valtrex in children.

DOSAGE IN THE ELDERLY:

The possibility of renal impairment in the elderly must be considered and the dosage should be adjusted accordingly (see Renal impairment below). Adequate hydration should be maintained.

DOSAGE IN RENAL IMPAIRMENT:

• **Herpes zoster treatment and herpes simplex treatment, suppression and reduction of transmission:**

Caution is advised when administering Valtrex to patients with impaired renal function. Adequate hydration should be maintained.

The dosage of Valtrex should be reduced in patients with significantly impaired renal function as shown in Table 1 below:

Table 1

Therapeutic indication	Creatinine clearance ml/min	Valtrex dosage
Herpes zoster	15-30 less than 15	1 g twice a day 1 g once a day
Herpes simplex (treatment)	less than 15	500 mg once a day
Herpes simplex prevention (suppression):		
- immunocompetent patients	less than 15	250 mg once a day
- immunocompromised patients	less than 15	500 mg once a day
Reduction of transmission of genital herpes:	less than 15	250 mg once a day

In patients on haemodialysis, the Valtrex dosage recommended for patients with a creatinine clearance of less than 15 ml/min should be used, but this should be administered after the haemodialysis has been performed.

• ***CMV prophylaxis:***

Caution is advised when administering Valtrex to patients with impaired renal function. Adequate hydration should be maintained.

The dosage of Valtrex should be reduced in patients with impaired renal function as shown in Table 2 below:

Table 2

Creatinine clearance ml/min	Valtrex dosage
75 or greater	*2 g four times a day*
50 to less than 75	*1.5 g four times a day*
25 to less than 50	*1.5 g three times a day*
10 to less than 25	*1.5 g twice a day*
less than 10 or dialysis	*1.5 g once a day*

In patients on haemodialysis, the Valtrex dosage should be administered after the haemodialysis has been performed.

The creatinine clearance should be monitored frequently, and the Valtrex dosage adjusted accordingly. It is recommended that creatinine clearance is monitored daily for optimum dose adjustments, especially during the first 10 days post-transplant, and at least twice weekly during hospitalisation, and as considered necessary thereafter.

DOSAGE IN HEPATIC IMPAIRMENT:

Studies with 1g unit dose of Valtrex show that dose modification is not required in patients with mild or moderate cirrhosis (hepatic synthetic function maintained). Pharmacokinetic data in patients with advanced cirrhosis, (impaired hepatic synthetic function and evidence of portal-systemic shunting) do not indicate the need for dosage adjustment; however, clinical experience is limited.

There are no data available on the use of higher doses of Valtrex (for CMV prophylaxis) in patients with liver disease. However, following a 1g unit dose of Valtrex, aciclovir AUCs were elevated in patients with moderate or severe cirrhosis. Therefore, caution should be exercised when administering higher doses of Valtrex to patients with hepatic impairment.

4.3 Contraindications

Valtrex is contra-indicated in patients known to be hypersensitive to valaciclovir, aciclovir or any components of formulations of Valtrex.

4.4 Special warnings and precautions for use

Hydration status:

Care should be taken to ensure adequate fluid intake in patients who are at risk of dehydration, particularly the elderly.

Use in patients with renal impairment and in elderly patients:

Aciclovir is eliminated by renal clearance, therefore the dose of Valtrex must be reduced in patients with renal impairment (see 4.2 Dosage and Administration). Elderly patients are likely to have reduced renal function and therefore the need for dose reduction must be considered in this group of patients. Both elderly patients and patients with renal impairment are at increased risk of developing neurological side effects and should be closely monitored for evidence of these effects. In the reported cases, these reactions were generally reversible on discontinuation of treatment (see 4.8 Adverse Reactions).

Use of high dose Valtrex in hepatic impairment:

There are no data available on the use of higher doses of Valtrex (for CMV prophylaxis) in patients with liver disease. However, following a 1g unit dose of Valtrex, aciclovir AUCs were elevated in patients with moderate or severe cirrhosis. Therefore, caution should be exercised when administering higher doses of Valtrex to patients with hepatic impairment.

Use in genital herpes: Suppressive therapy with Valtrex reduces the risk of transmitting genital herpes. It does not cure genital herpes or completely eliminate the risk of transmission. In addition to therapy with Valtrex, it is recommended that patients use safer sex practices (particularly the use of condoms).

4.5 Interaction with other medicinal products and other forms of interaction

No clinically significant interactions have been identified.

Cimetidine and probenecid increase the AUC of aciclovir by reducing its renal clearance: however no dosage adjustment is necessary because of the wide therapeutic index of aciclovir. Other drugs which affect renal physiology could affect plasma levels of aciclovir.

In patients receiving high dose Valtrex (4g/day) for CMV prophylaxis, caution is required during concurrent administration with drugs which compete with aciclovir elimination, because of the potential for increased plasma levels of one or both drugs or their metabolites. Following 1g Valtrex, cimetidine and probenecid increase the AUC of aciclovir by this mechanism, and reduce aciclovir renal clearance. However, no dosage adjustment is necessary at this dose of 1g because of the wide therapeutic index of aciclovir. Alternative agents, which do not interact with other agents excreted primarily via the kidney, may be considered for the management of excess gastric acid production and urate-lowering therapy when administering high dose valaciclovir.

Increases in plasma AUCs of aciclovir and of the inactive metabolite of mycophenolate mofetil, an immunosuppressant agent used in transplant patients, have been shown when the drugs are coadministered; there is limited clinical experience with the use of this combination.

Care is also required, with monitoring for changes in renal function (see 4.2, Posology and Method of Administration), if administering high-doses of Valtrex (4g or more/day) with drugs which affect other aspects of renal physiology (e.g.ciclosporin, tacrolimus).

4.6 Pregnancy and lactation

Teratogenicity:

Valaciclovir was not teratogenic in rats or rabbits. Valaciclovir is almost completely metabolised to aciclovir. Subcutaneous administration of aciclovir in internationally accepted tests did not produce teratogenic effects in rats or rabbits. In additional studies in rats, foetal abnormalities were observed at subcutaneous doses that produced plasma levels of 100 µg/ml and maternal toxicity.

Fertility:

Valaciclovir did not affect fertility in male or female rats dosed by the oral route.

Pregnancy:

There are limited data on the use of Valtrex in pregnancy. Valtrex should only be used in pregnancy if the potential benefits of treatment outweigh the potential risk.

A post-marketing acyclovir pregnancy registry has documented pregnancy outcomes in women exposed to Valtrex or any formulation of Zovirax (aciclovir, the inactive metabolite of valaciclovir). The birth defects described amongst aciclovir exposed subjects have not shown any uniqueness or consistent pattern to suggest a common cause.

Given the small number of women enrolled into the valaciclovir pregnancy registry, reliable and definitive conclusions could not be reached regarding the safety of valaciclovir in pregnancy (see also 5.2 Pharmacokinetic Properties).

The daily aciclovir AUC (area under plasma concentration-time curve) following Valtrex 1000 mg and 8000 mg daily would be approximately 2 and 9 times greater than that expected with oral aciclovir 1000 mg daily, respectively.

Lactation:

Aciclovir, the principle metabolite of valaciclovir, is excreted in breast milk. Following oral administration of a 500 mg dose of valaciclovir, peak aciclovir concentrations (Cmax) in breast milk ranged from 0.5 to 2.3 (median 1.4) times the corresponding maternal aciclovir serum concentrations. The aciclovir breast milk to maternal serum AUC ratios ranged from 1.4 to 2.6 (median 2.2). The median aciclovir concentration in breast milk was 2.24 µg/ml (9.95 µM). With a maternal valaciclovir dosage of 500 mg twice daily, this level would expose a nursing infant to a daily oral aciclovir dosage of about 0.61 mg/kg/day. The elimination half-life of aciclovir from breast milk was similar to that for serum.

Unchanged valaciclovir was not detected in maternal serum, breast milk, or infant urine.

Caution is advised if Valtrex is to be administered to a nursing woman. However, aciclovir is used to treat neonatal herpes simplex at intravenous doses of 30 mg/kg /day.

4.7 Effects on ability to drive and use machines

No special precautions necessary.

4.8 Undesirable effects

Adverse reactions are listed below by MedDRA body system organ class and by frequency.

The frequency categories used are:

Very common ⩾ 1 in 10,

Common ⩾ 1 in 100 and < 1 in 10,

Uncommon ⩾ 1 in 1,000 and < 1 in 100,

Rare ⩾ 1 in 10,000 and < 1 in 1,000,

Very rare < 1 in 10,000.

Blood and lymphatic system disorders

Very rare: Leukopenia / Neutropenia, thrombocytopenia.

Leukopenia / Neutropenia is mainly reported in immunocompromised patients.

Immune system disorders

Very rare: Anaphylaxis.

Psychiatric and nervous system disorders

Common: *Headache

Rare: Dizziness, confusion, hallucinations, decreased consciousness.

Very rare: Agitation, tremor, ataxia, dysarthria, psychotic symptoms, convulsions, encephalopathy, coma.

The above events are generally reversible and usually seen in patients with renal impairment or with other predisposing factors (see 4.4 Special Warnings & Precautions for Use). In renal transplant patients receiving high doses (8 g daily) of Valtrex for CMV prophylaxis, psychiatric reactions (confusion, hallucinations and thinking disorders) occurred more frequently compared with lower doses for other indications. They were mainly mild to moderate in nature, reversible upon dose adjustment, and occurred mainly in the immediate post-transplant period. Therefore, it is important to monitor creatinine clearance frequently in these patients, and to adjust the dose accordingly (see 4.2 Posology and Method of Administration). The cause of these events appears to be multi-factorial, including the over-exposure to aciclovir, renal impairment, dialysis, administration of psychotropic agents, and other underlying medical conditions.

Respiratory, thoracic and mediastinal disorders

Uncommon: Dyspnoea.

Gastrointestinal disorders

Common: *Nausea

Rare: Abdominal discomfort, vomiting, diarrhoea.

Hepato-biliary disorders

Very rare: Reversible increases in liver function tests.

These are occasionally described as hepatitis.

Skin and subcutaneous tissue disorders

Uncommon: Rashes including photosensitivity.

Rare: Pruritus.

Very rare: Urticaria, angioedema.

Renal and urinary disorders

Rare: Renal impairment.

Very rare: Acute renal failure, renal pain.

Renal pain may be associated with renal failure.

Other: There have been reports of renal insufficiency, microangiopathic haemolytic anaemia and thrombocytopenia (sometimes in combination) in severely immunocompromised patients, particularly those with advanced HIV disease, receiving high doses (8 g daily) of valaciclovir for prolonged periods in clinical trials. These findings have been observed in patients not treated with valaciclovir who have the same underlying or concurrent conditions.

* Clinical trial data have been used to assign frequency categories to these adverse reactions. For all other adverse events, spontaneous post-marketing data has been used as a basis for allocating frequency.

4.9 Overdose

Symptoms and signs:

Acute renal failure and neurological symptoms, including confusion, hallucinations, agitation, decreased consciousness and coma, have been reported in patients receiving overdoses of Valtrex. Nausea and vomiting may also occur. Caution is required to prevent inadvertent overdosing. Many of the reported cases involved renally impaired and elderly patients receiving repeated overdoses, due to lack of appropriate dosage reduction.

Management:

Patients should be observed closely for signs of toxicity. Haemodialysis significantly enhances the removal of aciclovir from the blood and may, therefore, be considered a management option in the event of symptomatic overdose.

5. PHARMACOLOGICAL PROPERTIES

5.1 Pharmacodynamic properties

Pharmacotherapeutic group:

Valaciclovir, an antiviral, is the L-valine ester of aciclovir. Aciclovir is a purine (guanine) nucleoside analogue.

Mode of action:

Valaciclovir is rapidly and almost completely converted in man to aciclovir and valine, probably by the enzyme referred to as valaciclovir hydrolase.

Aciclovir is a specific inhibitor of the herpes viruses with in vitro activity against herpes simplex viruses (HSV) type 1 and type 2, varicella zoster virus (VZV), cytomegalovirus (CMV), Epstein-Barr Virus (EBV), and human herpes virus 6 (HHV-6). Aciclovir inhibits herpes virus DNA synthesis once it has been phosphorylated to the active triphosphate form.

The first stage of phosphorylation requires the activity of a virus-specific enzyme. In the case of HSV, VZV and EBV this enzyme is the viral thymidine kinase (TK), which is only present in virus infected cells. Selectivity is maintained in CMV with phosphorylation, at least in part, being mediated through the phosphotransferase gene product of UL97. This requirement for activation of aciclovir by a virus specific enzyme largely explains its selectivity.

The phosphorylation process is completed (conversion from mono to triphosphate) by cellular kinases. Aciclovir triphosphate competitively inhibits the virus DNA polymerase and incorporation of this nucleoside analogue results in obligate chain termination, halting virus DNA synthesis and thus blocking virus replication.

CMV prophylaxis with Valtrex significantly reduces HSV disease in renal transplant patients.

Extensive monitoring of clinical isolates from patients receiving aciclovir therapy or prophylaxis has revealed that virus with reduced sensitivity to aciclovir is extremely rare in the immunocompetent and is only found infrequently in severely immunocompromised individuals e.g. solid organ or bone marrow transplant recipients, patients receiving chemotherapy for malignant disease and people infected with the human immunodeficiency virus (HIV).

Resistance is normally due to a thymidine kinase deficient phenotype which results in a virus which is profoundly disadvantaged in the natural host. Infrequently, reduced sensitivity to aciclovir has been described as a result of subtle alterations in either the virus thymidine kinase or DNA polymerase. The virulence of these variants resembles that of the wild-type virus.

5.2 Pharmacokinetic properties

General characteristics:

After oral administration valaciclovir is well absorbed and rapidly and almost completely converted to aciclovir and valine. This conversion is probably mediated by an enzyme isolated from human liver referred to as valaciclovir hydrolase.

The bioavailability of aciclovir from 1000 mg valaciclovir is 54%, and is not reduced by food. Mean peak aciclovir concentrations are 10-25 μM (2.2-5.7μg/ml) following single doses of 250 -1000 mg valaciclovir, and occur at a median time of 1.50 hours post dose.

Peak plasma concentrations of valaciclovir are only 4% of aciclovir levels, occur at a median time of 30 to 60 minutes post dose, and are below measurable concentrations 3 hours after dosing. The valaciclovir and aciclovir pharmacokinetic profiles are similar after single and repeat dosing. Binding of valaciclovir to plasma proteins is very low (15%).

The elimination plasma half-life of aciclovir after both single and multiple dosing with valaciclovir is approximately 3 hours. Less than 1% of the administered dose of valaciclovir is recovered in the urine. Valaciclovir is eliminated principally as aciclovir and the known aciclovir metabolite, 9-carboxymethoxymethylguanine (CMMG), in the urine.

Characteristics in patients:

Herpes zoster and herpes simplex do not significantly alter the pharmacokinetics of valaciclovir and aciclovir after oral administration of Valtrex.

In renal transplant recipients receiving valaciclovir 2g 4 times daily, aciclovir peak concentrations are similar to or greater than those in healthy volunteers with comparable doses and renal function. However, the estimated daily AUCs are appreciably greater.

In patients with HIV infection, the disposition and pharmacokinetic characteristics of aciclovir after oral administration of single or multiple doses of 1000 mg or 2000 mg Valtrex are unaltered compared with healthy subjects.

5.3 Preclinical safety data

Mutagenicity:

The results of mutagenicity tests in vitro and in vivo indicate that valaciclovir is unlikely to pose a genetic risk to humans.

Carcinogenicity:

Valaciclovir was not carcinogenic in bio-assays performed in mice and rats.

6. PHARMACEUTICAL PARTICULARS

6.1 List of excipients

Tablet core:

Microcrystalline cellulose

Crospovidone

Povidone K90

Magnesium stearate

Colloidal silicon dioxide

Film coat:

White Colour Concentrate OY-S-28861 containing;

Hydroxypropylmethylcellulose

Titanium dioxide

Polyethylene glycol 400

Purified water

Printing ink:

Brilliant Blue Printing Ink FT203 containing Brilliant Blue, E133

Polish:

Carnauba wax

6.2 Incompatibilities

No data.

6.3 Shelf life

Two years

6.4 Special precautions for storage

Store below 30°C

6.5 Nature and contents of container

Tablets are packed in blister packs prepared from unplasticised polyvinyl chloride and aluminium foil.

Pack size: 60 × 250mg

6.6 Special precautions for disposal and other handling

No special instructions for use.

Administrative Data

7. MARKETING AUTHORISATION HOLDER

The Wellcome Foundation Ltd

Glaxo Wellcome House

Berkeley Avenue

Greenford

Middlesex UB6 0NN

Trading as GlaxoSmithKline UK, StockleyPark West, Uxbridge, Middlesex UB11 1BT

8. MARKETING AUTHORISATION NUMBER(S)

PL 00003/0371

9. DATE OF FIRST AUTHORISATION/RENEWAL OF THE AUTHORISATION

5 June 1998

10. DATE OF REVISION OF THE TEXT

11 August 2008

11. Legal Status

POM

Valtrex Tablets 500mg

(GlaxoSmithKline UK)

1. NAME OF THE MEDICINAL PRODUCT

Valtrex™ Tablets 500mg

2. QUALITATIVE AND QUANTITATIVE COMPOSITION

500mg of valaciclovir

3. PHARMACEUTICAL FORM

Film coated tablets

4. CLINICAL PARTICULARS

4.1 Therapeutic indications

Valtrex is indicated for the treatment of herpes zoster (shingles).

Valtrex is indicated for the treatment of herpes simplex infections of the skin and mucous membranes, including initial and recurrent genital herpes.

Valtrex is indicated for the suppression (prevention) of recurrent herpes simplex infections of the skin and mucous membranes, including genital herpes.

Valtrex can reduce transmission of genital herpes when taken as suppressive therapy and combined with safer sex practices (particularly the use of condoms).

Valtrex is indicated for the prophylaxis of cytomegalovirus (CMV) infection and disease, following renal transplantation.

4.2 Posology and method of administration

Route of administration: oral

DOSAGE IN ADULTS:

- **Treatment of herpes zoster:**

1000 mg of Valtrex to be taken 3 times daily for 7 days.

- **Treatment of herpes simplex:**

Valtrex can prevent lesion development when taken at the first signs and symptoms of an HSV recurrence.

500 mg of Valtrex to be taken twice daily. For recurrent episodes, treatment should be for 5 days. For initial episodes, which can be more severe, treatment may have to be extended to 10 days. Dosing should begin as early as possible. For recurrent episodes of herpes simplex, this should ideally be during the prodromal period or immediately the first signs or symptoms appear.

- **Suppression (prevention) of herpes simplex infection:**

In immunocompetent patients, 500mg of Valtrex is to be taken once daily.

Some patients with very frequent recurrences (e.g. more than 10 per year) may benefit from taking 500mg as a divided dose (250mg twice daily).

For immunocompromised patients the dose is 500mg twice daily.

- **Reduction of transmission of genital herpes:**

In immunocompetent heterosexual adult patients with 9 or fewer recurrences per year, 500 mg of Valtrex to be taken once daily by the infected partner in order to reduce transmission to a sexual partner negative for HSV-2 antibodies. Safer sex practices (particularly condom use) should be maintained, and sexual contact avoided if lesions are present.

There are no data on the reduction of transmission beyond 8 months in other patient populations.

- **Prophylaxis of cytomegalovirus infection (CMV) and disease**

Dosage in adults and adolescents (from 12 years of age):

The dosage of Valtrex is 2g four times a day, to be initiated within 72 hours post-transplant, or as soon as oral medication can be tolerated. This dose should be reduced according to creatinine clearance (see Dosage in renal impairment below).

The duration of treatment will usually be 90 days.

DOSAGE IN CHILDREN:

There are no data available on the use of Valtrex in children.

DOSAGE IN THE ELDERLY:

The possibility of renal impairment in the elderly must be considered and the dosage should be adjusted accordingly (see Renal impairment below).

Adequate hydration should be maintained.

DOSAGE IN RENAL IMPAIRMENT:

- **Herpes zoster treatment and herpes simplex treatment, suppression and reduction of transmission:**

Caution is advised when administering Valtrex to patients with impaired renal function. Adequate hydration should be maintained.

The dosage of Valtrex should be reduced in patients with significantly impaired renal function as shown in Table 1 below:

Table 1

Therapeutic indication	**Creatinine clearance ml/min**	**Valtrex dosage**
Herpes zoster	15-30	1 g twice a day
	less than 15	1 g once a day
Herpes simplex (treatment)	less than 15	500 mg once a day
Herpes simplex prevention (suppression):		
- immunocompetent patients	less than 15	250 mg once a day
- immunocompromised patients	less than 15	500 mg once a day
Reduction of transmission of genital herpes:	less than 15	250 mg once a day

In patients on haemodialysis, the Valtrex dosage recommended for patients with a creatinine clearance of less than 15 ml/min should be used, but this should be administered after the haemodialysis has been performed.

• **CMV prophylaxis:**

Caution is advised when administering Valtrex to patients with impaired renal function. Adequate hydration should be maintained.

The dosage of Valtrex should be reduced in patients with impaired renal function as shown in Table 2 below:

Table 2

Creatinine clearance ml/min	**Valtrex dosage**
75 or greater	*2 g four times a day*
50 to less than 75	*1.5 g four times a day*
25 to less than 50	*1.5 g three times a day*
10 to less than 25	*1.5 g twice a day*
less than 10 or dialysis	*1.5 g once a day*

In patients on haemodialysis, the Valtrex dosage should be administered after the haemodialysis has been performed.

The creatinine clearance should be monitored frequently, and the Valtrex dosage adjusted accordingly. It is recommended that creatinine clearance is monitored daily for optimum dose adjustments, especially during the first 10 days post-transplant, and at least twice weekly during hospitalisation, and as considered necessary thereafter.

DOSAGE IN HEPATIC IMPAIRMENT:

Studies with a 1g unit dose of Valtrex show that dose modification is not required in patients with mild or moderate cirrhosis (hepatic synthetic function maintained). Pharmacokinetic data in patients with advanced cirrhosis (impaired hepatic synthetic function and evidence of portal-systemic shunting) do not indicate the need for dosage adjustment. However, clinical experience is limited.

There are no data available on the use of higher doses of Valtrex (for CMV prophylaxis) in patients with liver disease. However, following a 1g unit dose of Valtrex, aciclovir AUCs were elevated in patients with moderate or severe cirrhosis. Therefore, caution should be exercised when administering higher doses of Valtrex to patients with hepatic impairment.

4.3 Contraindications

Valtrex is contra-indicated in patients known to be hypersensitive to valaciclovir, aciclovir or any components of formulations of Valtrex.

4.4 Special warnings and precautions for use

Hydration status:

Care should be taken to ensure adequate fluid intake in patients who are at risk of dehydration, particularly the elderly.

Use in patients with renal impairment and elderly patients:

Aciclovir is eliminated by renal clearance, therefore the dose of Valtrex must be reduced in patients with renal impairment (see 4.2 Dosage and Administration). Elderly patients are likely to have reduced renal function and therefore the need for dose reduction must be considered in this group of patients. Both elderly patients and patients with renal impairment are at increased risk of developing neurological side effects and should be closely monitored for evidence of these effects. In the reported cases, these reactions were generally reversible on discontinuation of treatment (see 4.8 Adverse Reactions).

Use of high dose Valtrex in hepatic impairment:

There are no data available on the use of higher doses of Valtrex (for CMV prophylaxis) in patients with liver disease. However, following a 1g unit dose of Valtrex, aciclovir AUCs were elevated in patients with moderate or severe cirrhosis. Therefore, caution should be exercised when administering higher doses of Valtrex to patients with hepatic impairment.

Use in genital herpes: Suppressive therapy with Valtrex reduces the risk of transmitting genital herpes. It does not cure genital herpes or completely eliminate the risk of transmission. In addition to therapy with Valtrex, it is recommended that patients use safer sex practices (particularly the use of condoms).

4.5 Interaction with other medicinal products and other forms of interaction

No clinically significant interactions have been identified.

Aciclovir is eliminated primarily unchanged in the urine via active tubular secretion. Any drugs administered concurrently that compete with this mechanism for elimination may increase aciclovir plasma concentrations following Valtrex administration.

In patients receiving high dose Valtrex (4g/day) for CMV prophylaxis, caution is required during concurrent administration with drugs which compete with aciclovir elimination, because of the potential for increased plasma levels of one or both drugs or their metabolites. Following 1g Valtrex, cimetidine and probenecid increase the AUC of aciclovir by this mechanism, and reduce aciclovir renal clearance. However, no dosage adjustment is necessary at this dose of 1g because of the wide therapeutic index of aciclovir. Alternative agents, which do not interact with other agents excreted primarily via the kidney, may be considered for the management of excess gastric acid production and urate-lowering therapy when administering high dose valaciclovir.

Increases in plasma AUCs of aciclovir and of the inactive metabolite of mycophenolate mofetil, an immunosuppressant agent used in transplant patients, have been shown when the drugs are coadministered; there is limited clinical experience with the use of this combination.

Care is also required, with monitoring for changes in renal function (see 4.2, Posology and Method of Administration), if administering high-doses of Valtrex (4g or more/day) with drugs which affect other aspects of renal physiology (e.g.ciclosporin, tacrolimus).

4.6 Pregnancy and lactation

Teratogenicity:

Valaciclovir was not teratogenic in rats or rabbits. Valaciclovir is almost completely metabolised to aciclovir. Subcutaneous administration of aciclovir in internationally accepted tests did not produce teratogenic effects in rats or rabbits. In additional studies in rats, foetal abnormalities were observed at subcutaneous doses that produced plasma levels of 100 μg/ml and maternal toxicity.

Fertility:

Valaciclovir did not affect fertility in male or female rats dosed by the oral route.

Pregnancy:

There are limited data on the use of Valtrex in pregnancy. Valtrex should only be used in pregnancy if the potential benefits of treatment outweigh the potential risk.

A post-marketing acyclovir pregnancy registry has documented pregnancy outcomes in women exposed to Valtrex or any formulation of Zovirax (aciclovir, the inactive metabolite of valaciclovir). The birth defects described amongst aciclovir exposed subjects have not shown any uniqueness or consistent pattern to suggest a common cause.

Given the small number of women enrolled into the valaciclovir pregnancy registry, reliable and definitive conclusions could not be reached regarding the safety of valaciclovir in pregnancy (see also 5.2 Pharmacokinetic Properties).

The daily aciclovir AUC (area under plasma concentration-time curve) following Valtrex 1000 mg and 8000 mg daily would be approximately 2 and 9 times greater than that expected with oral aciclovir 1000 mg daily, respectively.

Lactation:

Aciclovir, the principle metabolite of valaciclovir, is excreted in breast milk. Following oral administration of a 500 mg dose of valaciclovir, peak aciclovir concentrations (Cmax) in breast milk ranged from 0.5 to 2.3 (median 1.4) times the corresponding maternal aciclovir serum concentrations. The aciclovir breast milk to maternal serum AUC ratios ranged from 1.4 to 2.6 (median 2.2). The median aciclovir concentration in breast milk was 2.24 μg/ml (9.95 μM). With a maternal valaciclovir dosage of 500 mg twice daily, this level would expose a nursing infant to a daily oral aciclovir dosage of about 0.61 mg/kg/day. The elimination half-life of aciclovir from breast milk was similar to that for serum.

Unchanged valaciclovir was not detected in maternal serum, breast milk, or infant urine.

Caution is advised if Valtrex is to be administered to a nursing woman. However, aciclovir is used to treat neonatal herpes simplex at intravenous doses of 30 mg/kg /day.

4.7 Effects on ability to drive and use machines

No special precautions necessary.

4.8 Undesirable effects

Adverse reactions are listed below by MedDRA body system organ class and by frequency.

The frequency categories used are:

Very common ⩾ 1 in 10,

Common ⩾ 1 in 100 and < 1 in 10,

Uncommon ⩾ 1 in 1,000 and < 1 in 100,

Rare ⩾ 1 in 10,000 and < 1 in 1,000,

Very rare < 1 in 10,000.

Blood and lymphatic system disorders

Very rare: Leukopenia / Neutropenia, thrombocytopenia.

Leukopenia / Neutropenia is mainly reported in immunocompromised patients.

Immune system disorders

Very rare: Anaphylaxis.

Psychiatric and nervous system disorders

Common: *Headache

Rare: Dizziness, confusion, hallucinations, decreased consciousness.

Very rare: Agitation, tremor, ataxia, dysarthria, psychotic symptoms convulsions, encephalopathy, coma.

The above events are generally reversible and usually seen in patients with renal impairment or with other predisposing factors (see 4.4 Special Warnings & Precautions for Use). In renal transplant patients receiving high doses (8 g daily) of Valtrex for CMV prophylaxis, psychiatric reactions (confusion, hallucinations and thinking disorders) occurred more frequently compared with lower doses for other indications. They were mainly mild to moderate in nature, reversible upon dose adjustment, and occurred mainly in the immediate post-transplant period. Therefore, it is important to monitor creatinine clearance frequently in these patients, and to adjust the dose accordingly (see 4.2 Posology and Method of Administration). The cause of these events appears to be multi-factorial, including over-exposure to aciclovir, renal impairment, dialysis, administration of psychotropic agents, and other underlying medical conditions.

Respiratory, thoracic and mediastinal disorders

Uncommon: Dyspnoea.

Gastrointestinal disorders

Common: *Nausea

Rare: Abdominal discomfort, vomiting, diarrhoea.

Hepato-biliary disorders

Very rare: Reversible increases in liver function tests.

These are occasionally described as hepatitis.

Skin and subcutaneous tissue disorders

Uncommon: Rashes including photosensitivity.

Rare: Pruritus.

Very rare: Urticaria, angioedema.

Renal and urinary disorders

Rare: Renal impairment.

Very rare: Acute renal failure, renal pain.

Renal pain may be associated with renal failure.

Other: There have been reports of renal insufficiency, microangiopathic haemolytic anaemia and thrombocytopenia (sometimes in combination) in severely immunocompromised patients, particularly those with advanced HIV disease, receiving high doses (8 g daily) of valaciclovir for prolonged periods in clinical trials. These findings have been observed in patients not treated with valaciclovir who have the same underlying or concurrent conditions.

* Clinical trial data have been used to assign frequency categories to these adverse reactions. For all other adverse events, spontaneous post-marketing data has been used as a basis for allocating frequency.

4.9 Overdose

Symptoms and signs:

Acute renal failure and neurological symptoms, including confusion, hallucinations, agitation, decreased consciousness and coma, have been reported in patients receiving overdoses of Valtrex. Nausea and vomiting may also occur. Caution is required to prevent inadvertent overdosing. Many of the reported cases involved renally impaired and elderly patients receiving repeated overdoses, due to lack of appropriate dosage reduction.

Management:

Patients should be observed closely for signs of toxicity. Haemodialysis significantly enhances the removal of aciclovir from the blood and may, therefore, be considered a management option in the event of symptomatic overdose.

5. PHARMACOLOGICAL PROPERTIES

5.1 Pharmacodynamic properties

Pharmacotherapeutic group:

Valaciclovir, an antiviral, is the L-valine ester of aciclovir. Aciclovir is a purine (guanine) nucleoside analogue.

Mode of action:

Valaciclovir is rapidly and almost completely converted in man to aciclovir and valine, probably by the enzyme referred to as valaciclovir hydrolase.

Aciclovir is a specific inhibitor of the herpes viruses with in vitro activity against herpes simplex viruses (HSV) type 1 and type 2, varicella zoster virus (VZV), cytomegalovirus

(CMV), Epstein-Barr Virus (EBV), and human herpes virus 6 (HHV-6). Aciclovir inhibits herpes virus DNA synthesis once it has been phosphorylated to the active triphosphate form.

The first stage of phosphorylation requires the activity of a virus-specific enzyme. In the case of HSV, VZV and EBV this enzyme is the viral thymidine kinase (TK), which is only present in virus infected cells. Selectivity is maintained in CMV with phosphorylation, at least in part, being mediated through the phosphotransferase gene product of UL97. This requirement for activation of aciclovir by a virus specific enzyme largely explains its selectivity.

The phosphorylation process is completed (conversion from mono- to triphosphate) by cellular kinases. Aciclovir triphosphate competitively inhibits the virus DNA polymerase and incorporation of this nucleoside analogue results in obligate chain termination, halting virus DNA synthesis and thus blocking virus replication.

CMV prophylaxis with Valtrex significantly reduces HSV disease in renal transplant patients.

Extensive monitoring of clinical HSV and VZV isolates from patients receiving aciclovir therapy or prophylaxis has revealed that virus with reduced sensitivity to aciclovir is extremely rare in the immunocompetent and is only found infrequently in severely immunocompromised individuals e.g. solid organ or bone marrow transplant recipients, patients receiving chemotherapy for malignant disease and people infected with the human immunodeficiency virus (HIV).

Resistance is normally due to a thymidine kinase deficient phenotype, which results in a virus that is profoundly disadvantaged in the natural host. Infrequently, reduced sensitivity to aciclovir has been described as a result of subtle alterations in either the virus thymidine kinase or DNA polymerase. The virulence of these variants resembles that of the wild-type virus.

5.2 Pharmacokinetic properties

General characteristics:

After oral administration valaciclovir is well absorbed and rapidly and almost completely converted to aciclovir and valine. This conversion is probably mediated by an enzyme isolated from human liver referred to as valaciclovir hydrolase.

The bioavailability of aciclovir from 1000 mg valaciclovir is 54%, and is not reduced by food. Mean peak aciclovir concentrations are 10-37 µM (2.2-8.3µg/ml) following single doses of 250-2000 mg valaciclovir to healthy subjects with normal renal function, and occur at a median time of 1.00 –2.00 hours post dose.

Peak plasma concentrations of valaciclovir are only 4% of aciclovir levels, occur at a median time of 30 to 100 minutes post dose, and are at or below the limit of quantification 3 hours after dosing. The valaciclovir and aciclovir pharmacokinetic profiles are similar after single and repeat dosing. Binding of valaciclovir to plasma proteins is very low (15%).

In patients with normal renal function, the elimination plasma half-life of aciclovir after both single and multiple dosing with valaciclovir is approximately 3 hours. In patients with end-stage renal disease, the average elimination half-life of aciclovir after valaciclovir administration is approximately 14 hours. Less than 1% of the administered dose of valaciclovir is recovered in the urine as unchanged drug. Valaciclovir is eliminated principally as aciclovir (greater than 80% of the recovered dose) and the known aciclovir metabolite, 9-carboxymethoxymethylguanine (CMMG), in the urine.

Characteristics in patients:

Herpes zoster and herpes simplex do not significantly alter the pharmacokinetics of valaciclovir and aciclovir after oral administration of Valtrex.

In patients with HIV infection, the disposition and pharmacokinetic characteristics of aciclovir after oral administration of single or multiple doses of 1000 mg or 2000 mg Valtrex are unaltered compared with healthy subjects.

In renal transplant recipients receiving valaciclovir 2g 4 times daily, aciclovir peak concentrations are similar to or greater than those in healthy volunteers with comparable doses and renal function. However, the estimated daily AUCs are appreciably greater.

5.3 Preclinical safety data

Mutagenicity:

The results of mutagenicity tests in vitro and in vivo indicate that valaciclovir is unlikely to pose a genetic risk to humans.

Carcinogenicity:

Valaciclovir was not carcinogenic in bio-assays performed in mice and rats.

6. PHARMACEUTICAL PARTICULARS

6.1 List of excipients

Tablet core:

Microcrystalline cellulose

Crospovidone

Povidone K90

Magnesium stearate

Colloidal silicon dioxide

Purified water

Film coat:

White Colour Concentrate YS-1-18043 containing;

Hydroxypropylmethylcellulose

Titanium dioxide

Polyethylene glycol 400

Polysorbate 80

Purified water

Printing ink:

Brilliant Blue Printing Ink FT203 containing Brilliant Blue, E133

Polish:

Carnauba wax

6.2 Incompatibilities

No data.

6.3 Shelf life

Three years

6.4 Special precautions for storage

Store below 30°C

6.5 Nature and contents of container

Tablets are packed into blister packs prepared from unplasticised polyvinyl chloride and aluminium foil.

Pack sizes 4 × 500mg

10 × 500mg

42 × 500mg

Tablets are packed into polypropylene containers with polyethylene snap-fitting caps Pack size: 500 × 500mg

6.6 Special precautions for disposal and other handling

No special instructions for use.

Administrative Data

7. MARKETING AUTHORISATION HOLDER

The Wellcome Foundation Ltd

Glaxo Wellcome House

Berkeley Avenue

Greenford

Middlesex

UB6 0NN

8. MARKETING AUTHORISATION NUMBER(S)

PL 00003/0352

9. DATE OF FIRST AUTHORISATION/RENEWAL OF THE AUTHORISATION

20 January 1995

10. DATE OF REVISION OF THE TEXT

11 August 2008

11. Legal Status

POM

Vantas 50 mg Implant

(Orion Pharma (UK) Limited)

1. NAME OF THE MEDICINAL PRODUCT

Vantas▼50 mg implant

2. QUALITATIVE AND QUANTITATIVE COMPOSITION

Each implant contains 50 mg histrelin acetate.

For a full list of excipients, see section 6.1.

3. PHARMACEUTICAL FORM

Implant.

The implant is in the form of a small, thin flexible tube. The histrelin acetate core is placed in a non-biodegradable 34.5 mm × 3.15 mm cylindrically shaped hydrogel reservoir.

4. CLINICAL PARTICULARS

4.1 Therapeutic indications

Palliative treatment of advanced prostate cancer.

4.2 Posology and method of administration

The recommended dose of Vantas™ is one implant for 12 months. An average of 50 µg histrelin acetate is delivered daily. The implant is inserted subcutaneously in the inner aspect of the upper arm.

The implant must be removed after 12 months of treatment. At the time the implant is removed a new implant may be inserted in order to continue the treatment. Please see insertion and removal procedures below.

The safety and efficacy of Vantas™ in paediatric patients and in women have not been established.

Hepatic impairment and Renal impairment

Vantas™ has not been studied adequately in patients with impaired liver function.

In patients with mild to moderate renal impairment (CLcr: 15-60 ml/min), no adjustments in drug dosing are warranted. Vantas™ has not been studied in prostate cancer patients with severe renal impairment.

4.3 Contraindications

Vantas™ is contraindicated in patients with hypersensitivity to histrelin or to any of the excipients in the implant, GnRH, GnRH-agonists/- analogues, or stearic acid. Anaphylactic reactions to synthetic LH-RH or LH-RH-agonists/-analogues, have also been reported.

Vantas™ is contraindicated in women.

Vantas™ is contraindicated in children due to a lack of data on safety and efficacy

4.4 Special warnings and precautions for use

Histrelin, causes a transient increase in serum concentrations of testosterone during the first week of treatment. Patients may experience a worsening of symptoms or onset of new symptoms, including joint pain, bone pain, neuropathy, haematuria, or ureteral or bladder outlet obstruction. Cases of ureteral obstruction and spinal cord compression, which may lead to paralysis with or without fatal complications, have been reported in connection with LH-RH-agonists. Patients with metastatic vertebral lesions and/or urinary tract obstruction should be closely observed during the first few weeks of therapy. These patients should be considered for prohylactic treatment with anti-androgens. If spinal cord compression or renal impairment occurs, the standard treatment for these complications should be initiated.

Insertion of an implant is a surgical procedure. Only Vantas implantation device can be used for insertion of the implant. Careful adherence to the recommended procedures for insertion and removal is recommended in order to reduce the risk of complications and implant expulsion (see section 6.6).

In cases where the implant is difficult to locate by palpation, ultrasound or CT scan may be used. Reactions to the treatment with Vantas™ should be monitored by regular measurement of serum concentrations of testosterone and prostate-specific antigen, especially if the anticipated clinical or biochemical response to treatment has not been achieved.

The results of the testosterone determinations are dependent on the method of analysis. It is advisable to be aware of the type and precision of the assay methodology to ensure the correct clinical and therapeutic decisions.

The container of this medicinal product contains latex rubber. May cause severe allergic reactions.

4.5 Interaction with other medicinal products and other forms of interaction

No pharmacokinetic-based drug-drug interaction studies have been performed with Vantas™.

Treatment with histrelin results in suppression of the pituitary-gonadal system. Results of diagnostic tests of pituitary/gonadotropic and gonadal functions conducted during or after histrelin treatment may be affected.

4.6 Pregnancy and lactation

Due to its indication, Vantas™ has not been studied in pregnant or breast-feeding women and is not for use in women.

4.7 Effects on ability to drive and use machines

No studies on the effects on the ability to drive and use machines have been performed.

4.8 Undesirable effects

The safety of Vantas™ was evaluated in 171 patients with prostate cancer treated for up to 36 months in two clinical trials. Vantas™, like other LH-RH-analogues, caused a transient increase in serum testosterone concentrations during the first week of treatment. Therefore, potential exacerbations of the signs and symptoms of the disease during the first few weeks of treatment are a factor in patients with vertebral metastases and/or urinary obstruction or hematuria. If these conditions are aggravated, it may lead to neurological problem such as weakness and/or paraesthesia of the lower limbs or worsening of urinary tract symptoms (see section 4.4).

In the first 12 months after insertion of the implant(s), an implant extruded through the incision site in eight out of 171 patients in the clinical trial. In a pivotal study, a detailed evaluation of implant site reactions was also conducted. Insertion site reactions were very common and were experienced by 13.8 % of the patients in the study. All these local site reactions were reported as mild in severity. The majority of these reactions were associated with initial insertion or removal/insertion of a new implant and began and resolved within the first two weeks following implant insertion. Reactions persisted in 2.8 % of the patients, and an additional 2.8 % developed insertion-site reactions after the first two weeks following implantation.

Of 138 patients in a pivotal study, 2 patients developed a local skin infection and inflammation. The one instance resolved after treatment with oral antibiotics, and the other without treatment. Local reactions following insertion of a subsequent implant were comparable to those seen after initial insertion.

The following possibly or probably related systemic adverse events occurred during clinical trials after up to 24 months treatment with Vantas™. The reported undesirable effect during Vantas treatment in clinical trials are stated in Table 1 below according to the organ system and frequence.

Very common (≥1/10)

Common (≥1/100 to <1/10)

Uncommon (≥1/1,000 to <1/100)

Table 1 The incidence of possible or probably related undesirable effects reported by patients treated with Vantas up to 24 months

Organ group	Very common	Common	Uncommon	Rare
Infections and infestations				Skin infection
Blood and lymphatic system disorders			Anaemia	
Metabolism and nutrition disorders			Fluid retention, hypercalcemia, hypercholesterolaemia, food cravings, increased appetite	
Psychiatric disorders		Depression, decreased libido, insomnia		
Nervous system disorders		Dizziness, headache	Tremor, lethargy	
Cardiac disorders			Palpitations, ventricular extrasystoles	
Vascular disorders	Hot flushes*	Blushing	Haematoma	
Respiratory, thoracic and mediastinal disorders		Exercise induced dyspnoea		
Gastrointestinal disorders		Constipation	Abdominal discomfort, nausea	
Hepatobiliary disorders		Hepatic disorder		
Skin and subcutaneous tissue disorders		Hypertrichosis	Night sweats, pruritus, hyperhidrosis	
Musculoskelatal and connective tissue disorders		Arthralgia, pain in the extremities	Back pain, muscle spasm, muscle infiltration, neck pain	
Renal and urinary disorders		Pollakisuria, impaired renal function**, urinary retention	Renal failure, nephrolithiasis, dysuria, haematuria	
Reproductive system and breast disorders		Erectile dysfunction*, testicular atrophy*, gynecomastia*	Sexual dysfunction, breast pain, breast tenderness, genital pruritus (males)	
General disorders and administration site conditions		Injury at the application site, erythema at the application site, asthenia, fatigue, reaction at the application site, pain, tenderness,	Peripheral edema, pain (exacerbated), swelling, pain (non specific), malaise, feelings of cold, irritability	Inflammation
Injury, poisoning and procedural complications			Stent occlusion, bruising	
Investigations		Weight gain, elevated blood glucose	Elevated aspartate-aminotransferase, elevated blood lactate dehydrogenase, elevated blood testosterone, lowered creatinine clearance, elevated acid phosphatase in the prostate, weight loss	

*Anticipated pharmacological reaction to inhibition of testosterone

** 5 of 8 patients experienced a single instance of mildly impaired renal function (defined as creatinine clearance ⩾ 30 ml/min and < 60 ml/min), which resolved to the normal range by the next medical consultation.

Rare (⩾1/10,000 to <1/1,000)

Very rare (<1/10,000), not known (cannot be estimated from the available data)

Within each frequency grouping, undesirable effects are presented in order of decreasing seriousness.

Table 1: The incidence of possible or probably related undesirable effects reported by patients treated with Vantas up to 24 months.

(see Table 1 above)

Decreased bone density has been reported in the medical literature in men who have had orchiectomy or who have been treated with an LH-RH agonist analogue. It can be anticipated that long periods of medical castration in men will have effects on bone density.

4.9 Overdose

Not relevant.

5. PHARMACOLOGICAL PROPERTIES

5.1 Pharmacodynamic properties

Pharmacotherapeutic group: Gonadotropin-releasing hormones. ATC code: H01CA03.

Histrelin is a synthetic analogue of a naturally occurring LHRH. After implantation of Vantas™, histrelin is diffused into the tissue, resulting in inhibition of pituitary LH secretion leading to a fall in serum testosterone concentrations in males. The effect is reversible on discontinuation of therapy. Initially, Vantas™ like other LHRH agonists may transiently increase serum testosterone concentration.

By one month after the implantation, testosterone concentrations have fallen to within castrate range and remain suppressed while Vantas™ is present. This inhibition leads to prostate tumour regression and symptomatic improvement in the majority of patients.

The implant is inserted subcutaneously and remains in place for 12 months whilst the drug is released through the hydrogel reservoir at approximately 50 µg histrelin daily.

The implant's hydrogel reservoir determines the diffusion rate in the water-based environment. Hydrogel is not dissolved, but is similar to living tissue in composition, which contributes to its biocompatibility as it lessens the mechanical irritation of surrounding cells and tissue. It also displays low surface tension in vivo, which lessens the tendency for proteins to be absorbed and gather on the surface. This is important for the prevention of thrombosis and other biological rejection processes.

5.2 Pharmacokinetic properties

Absorption:

Following subcutaneous insertion of one Vantas™ 50 mg implant in patients with advanced prostate cancer (n = 17), peak serum concentrations of 1.10 ± 0.375 ng/ml (mean value ± SD) occurred at a median of 12 hours. Continuous subcutaneous release was evident as serum levels were sustained throughout the entire 52-week dosing period. The mean serum histrelin concentration at the end of the 52-week treatment period was 0.13 ± 0.065 ng/ml. When histrelin serum concentrations were measured following a second implant inserted after 52 weeks, the observed serum concentrations over 8 weeks following insertion of the second implant were comparable to the level in the same period following the first implant. The average rate of subcutaneous drug release from 41 implants, assayed for residual drug content, was 56.7 ± 7.71 µg/day over the 52-week dosing period. The relative bioavailability for the Vantas™ implant in prostate cancer patients with normal renal- and hepatic function compared to a subcutaneous bolus dose in healthy male volunteers was 92 %. Serum histrelin concentrations were proportional to dose after one, two or four 50 mg Vantas™ implants (50, 100 or 200 mg as histrelin acetate) in 42 prostate cancer patients.

Distribution:

The apparent volume of distribution of histrelin following a subcutaneous bolus dose (500 µg) in healthy adult volunteers was 58.4 ± 7.86 L. The fraction of drug unbound in plasma measured in vitro was 29.5 % ± 8.9 % (mean value ± SD).

Biotransformation:

An in vitro drug metabolism study using human hepatocytes identified a single histrelin metabolite resulting from C-terminal dealkylation. Peptide fragments resulting from hydrolysis are also likely metabolites. Following a subcutaneous bolus dose in healthy volunteers, the apparent clearance of histrelin was 179 ± 37.8 ml/min (mean value ± SD), and the terminal half-life was 3.92 ± 1.01 hr (mean value ± SD). The apparent clearance following insertion of a 50 mg (as histrelin acetate) Vantas™ implant in 17 prostate cancer patients was 174 ± 56.5 ml/min (mean value ± SD).

Elimination:

No drug excretion study has been conducted with Vantas™ 50 mg implants.

Luteinizing hormone (LH) returned to normal level 1 to 6 weeks after extraction of the implant. The testosterone level also returned to normal level within 2 weeks of the increase in LH-level, which indicated that the inhibition is reversible.

Special populations:

Geriatrics

The majority (89.9 %) of the 138 patients studied in the primary clinical trial were 65 years or older.

Paediatrics

Safety and efficacy for Vantas™ in paediatric patients have not been established (see section 4.3).

Race

When serum histrelin concentrations were compared for 7 Latin-American, 30 Black and 77 Caucasian patients, average histrelin concentrations were similar.

Renal impairment:

When average serum histrelin concentrations were compared between 42 prostate cancer patients with mild to moderate renal impairment (CLcr: 15-60 ml/min) and 92 patients with no renal or hepatic impairment, the levels were approximately 50 % higher in those patients with renal impairment (0.392 ng/ml versus 0.264 ng/ml). Greater concentrations were noted in patients with a greater degree of renal impairment. There is no data in patients with severe renal impairment. These changes as a result of renal impairment are not considered to be clinically relevant. Therefore, no adjustments in drug dosing are warranted for these patient subpopulations.

Hepatic insufficiency

The influence of hepatic insufficiency on the pharmacokinetics of histrelin has not been adequately studied.

5.3 Preclinical safety data

Non-clinical data reveal no special hazard for humans based on conventional studies of safety pharmacology, repeated dose toxicity, genotoxicity, carcinogenic potential and toxicity to reproduction. Local studies show that Vantas™ is a mild irritant and becomes encapsulated over time. Mineralization occurred in rats, rabbits and dogs, but not in apes.

6. PHARMACEUTICAL PARTICULARS

6.1 List of excipients

The drug core contains stearic acid.

The acrylic copolymer shell consists of:

2-hydroxyethyl methacrylate

2-hydroxyropyl methacrylate

trimethylolpropan trimethacrylate.

6.2 Incompatibilities

Not applicable

6.3 Shelf life

2 years

6.4 Special precautions for storage

Implant

Store in a refrigerator (2 °C-8 °C). Do not freeze.

Store in the original package in order to protect from light.

Implantation device

The implantation device supplied is sterile in its pouch.

Store at room temperature (20 °C – 25 °C), and keep out of direct sunlight.

6.5 Nature and contents of container

The implant is contained in a type 1 glass vial and supplied with a Teflon-coated bung and an aluminium seal. The implant is stored in 2 ml of 1.8 % sterile NaCl.

Vantas™ is supplied in a carton with an amber plastic bag, which contains the glass vial with the implant.

The sterile implantation device is supplied in a self-sealing Tyvek-bag for sterilization, which is placed in a carton.

6.6 Special precautions for disposal and other handling

Packaging and any unused product or waste material should be disposed of in accordance with local requirements.

Insertion procedure

It is important that aseptic technique be used in order to minimize the risk of infection. Sterile gloves are required for insertion and removal of the implant.

Identification of the insertion site

The patient should lie on his back with the arm that is least used (i.e. the left arm in a right-handed person) flexed so the physician has ready access to the inner aspect of the upper arm. Prop the arm with pillows so the patient can easily hold that position. The optimum site for insertion is approximately half way between the shoulder and the elbow in the crease between the biceps and triceps muscle.

Preparation of the implantation device

Prepare the implantation device before preparation of the insertion site and prior to insertion. Remove the implantation device from its sterile bag. The device is supplied with the cannula fully extended. Verify this by inspecting the position of the green retraction button. The button should be all the way forwards, toward the cannula, and away from the handle.

Remove the metal band from the glass vial, remove the rubber stopper and use a mosquito clamp to grasp either tip of the implant. Avoid grasping or clamping the middle of the implant to prevent distortion of the implant.

Insert the implant into the implantation device. The implant will lie in the cannula in such a way that just the tip is visible at the bottom of the bevel.

Inserting the implant

Swab the insertion site with povidone-iodine and place a fenestrated drape over the site.

Anesthetic

Ensure that the patient is not allergic to lidocaine/adrenaline. Inject a few ml of the anesthetic, starting at the planned incision site and then infiltrating up to the length of the implant, 32 mm, in a fan-like fashion.

Incision

Using a scalpel make a 2-3 mm shallow skin incision on in the inner aspect of the upper arm perpendicular to length of the biceps.

Insertion

Grasp the implantation device by its handle.

Insert the tip of the device into the incision with the bevel upward, and advance the device subcutaneously along the path of the anaesthetic up to the inscribed line on the cannula. To ensure subcutaneous placement, the implantation device should visibly raise the skin at all times during insertion. Make sure that the implantation device does not enter muscle tissue.

Hold the device in place at the same time as you move your thumb toward the green retraction button. Press the button down to release the locking mechanism, then draw the button back to the back-stop whilst holding the device in place. The cannula is withdrawn from the incision leaving the implant in the dermis. Withdraw the implantation device from the incision. The freed implant can be checked by palpation.

Note: Do not attempt to push the device deeper once the retraction process has started to avoid severing the implant. If you wish to re-start the procedure, withdraw the device, grasp the implant by the tip to extract it, reset the retraction button to the most forward position, reload the implant and start the procedure again.

Closing the incision

Close the incision using one or two sutures (optional) with the knots facing inside the incision. Apply a thin layer of antibiotic ointment directly onto the incision. Close the incision with two surgical steri-strips. Apply a gauze dressing over the incision and secure it with a bandage.

Removal procedure and insertion of new implant

The Vantas™ implant must be removed after 12 months of treatment.

Locating the implant

The implant can be located by palpating the area near the incision of the previous year. The implant is normally readily palpated. Press on the distal end of the implant to determine the proximal tip location relative to the old incision.

If the implant is difficult to locate, ultrasound may be used. If the implant cannot be located by ultrasound, other imaging techniques such as CT or MRI may be used to locate it.

Preparation of the insertion site

Patient position and preparation of the implantation site are the same as for the initial implantation. Swab the area above and around the implant with povidone-iodine. Drape the area with a fenestrated drape.

Anesthetic

First determine that the patient is not allergic to lidocaine/adrenaline then press down on the tip of the implant furthest from the original incision. Inject a small amount of lidocaine/adrenaline at the tip near the incision, then advance the cannula along the length, but beneath the implant, steadily injecting a small amount of anesthetic into the skin. The anesthetic will raise up the implant within the dermis. If a new implant is to be inserted, you have the option of placing the implant in the same "pocket" as the removed one, or of using the same incision and inserting the implant in the opposite direction. If you place the implant in the opposite direction, inject the anesthetic along the length of the new implant prior to explantation.

Incision/explantation

Use a scalpel to make a 2-3 mm incision near the tip and approximately 1-2 mm deep. Generally, the tip of the implant will be visible through a thin pseudo-capsule of tissue. If the implant is not visible, press down on the distal tip of the implant and massage it forward towards the incision. Carefully "nick" the pseudo-capsule to reveal the polymer tip.

Grasp the tip with a mosquito clamp and extract the implant.

If inserting a new implant, proceed as per the initial instructions. The new implant may be placed through the same incision site. Alternatively, the opposite arm may be used.

Patient instructions – aftercare

Give the patient the information leaflet. Instruct the patient to avoid wetting the arm containing the implant for 24 hours. The pressure bandage can be removed after 24 hours. The patient must not remove the surgical steri-strips. These strips should be allowed to fall off by themselves after several days. Patients should avoid lifting heavy objects and participating in strenuous physical activity involving the treated arm for 7 days to allow the incision to fully close.

7. MARKETING AUTHORISATION HOLDER

Orion Corporation

Orionintie 1

FI-02200 Espoo

Finland

8. MARKETING AUTHORISATION NUMBER(S)

PL 27925/0047

9. DATE OF FIRST AUTHORISATION/RENEWAL OF THE AUTHORISATION

01/09/2008

10. DATE OF REVISION OF THE TEXT

April 2009

Varilrix

(GlaxoSmithKline UK)

1. NAME OF THE MEDICINAL PRODUCT

Varilrix®▼, 10 $^{3.3}$ PFU/0.5ml, powder and solvent for solution for injection.

2. QUALITATIVE AND QUANTITATIVE COMPOSITION

One dose (0.5 ml) contains:

Live attenuated varicella-zoster (Oka strain) virus* $10^{3.3}$ plaque forming units (PFU)

*propagated in MRC5 human diploid cells

For excipients, see 6.1.

3. PHARMACEUTICAL FORM

Powder and solvent for solution for injection.

Clear peach to pink coloured solution.

4. CLINICAL PARTICULARS

4.1 Therapeutic indications

Varilrix is indicated for active immunisation against varicella in healthy adults and adolescents (≥ 13 years) who have been found to be seronegative with respect to the varicella-zoster virus and are, therefore, at risk of developing chickenpox.

Varilrix is not indicated for routine use in children. However, it may be administered to seronegative healthy children of 1-12 years of age who are close contacts (e.g. household) of persons considered to be at high risk of severe varicella infections.

4.2 Posology and method of administration

Posology

Children 1-12 years, adolescents (≥ 13 years) and adults

Two doses (each of 0.5 ml of reconstituted vaccine) should be given, with an interval between doses of at least 6 weeks but in no circumstances less than 4 weeks.

One dose of Varilrix may be administered after a first dose of another varicella containing vaccine (see section 5.1).

There are insufficient data to determine the long-term protective efficacy of the vaccine. However, there is currently no evidence that further doses are routinely required following completion of a two-dose regimen in healthy adolescents and adults (see section 5.1).

If Varilrix is to be administered to seronegative subjects before a period of planned or possible future immunosuppression (such as those awaiting organ transplantation and those in remission from malignant disease), the timing of the vaccinations should take into account the delay after the second dose before maximal protection might be expected (see also sections 4.3, 4.4 and 5.1).

Varilrix should not be administered to children aged less than one year.

Elderly

There are no data on immune responses to Varilrix in the elderly.

Method of administration

Varilrix is for subcutaneous administration only. The upper arm (deltoid region) is the preferred site of injection.

Varilrix should not be administered intradermally.

Varilrix must under no circumstances be administered intravascularly.

Varilrix must not be mixed with any other medicinal product in the same syringe (see also sections 4.5 and 6.2).

4.3 Contraindications

Varilrix is contra-indicated in subjects who have a history of hypersensitivity to neomycin, or to any of the excipients in the vaccine, or to any other varicella vaccine.

A second dose of Varilrix is contra-indicated in subjects who have had a hypersensitivity reaction following the first dose.

Varilrix is contra-indicated during pregnancy and breast-feeding (see also sections 4.4 and 4.6).

Varilrix must not be administered to subjects with primary or acquired immunodeficiency states with a total lymphocyte count less than 1,200 per mm^3 or presenting other evidence of lack of cellular immune competence, such as subjects with leukaemias, lymphomas, blood dyscrasias, clinically manifest HIV infection, or patients receiving immunosuppressive therapy (including high dose corticosteroids).

Administration of Varilrix must be postponed in subjects suffering from acute, severe febrile illness. In healthy subjects the presence of a minor infection, however, is not a contraindication.

4.4 Special warnings and precautions for use

As with all injectable vaccines, appropriate medical treatment and supervision should always be readily available in case of a rare anaphylactic reaction following the administration of the vaccine.

Varilrix contains a live attenuated varicella-zoster virus and administration is contra-indicated during pregnancy (see sections 4.3 and 4.6). Due to an unknown degree of risk to the mother and to the fetus, female candidates for vaccination must be advised to take adequate precautions to prevent pregnancy occurring between the two doses and for three months after the second dose.

Serological studies of efficacy and post-marketing experience indicate that the vaccine does not completely protect all individuals from naturally-acquired varicella and cannot be expected to provide maximal protection against infection with varicella-zoster virus until about six weeks after the second dose (see section 5.1).

Administration of Varilrix to subjects who are in the incubation period of the infection cannot be expected to protect against clinically manifest varicella or to modify the course of the disease.

The rash produced during naturally-acquired primary infection with varicella-zoster may be more severe in those with existing severe skin damage, including severe eczematous conditions. It is not known if there is an increased risk of vaccine-associated skin lesions in such persons, but this possibility should be taken into consideration before vaccination.

Transmission of the vaccine viral strain

Transmission of vaccine viral strain has been shown to occur from healthy vaccinees to healthy contacts, to pregnant contacts and to immunosuppressed contacts. However, transmission to any of these groups occurs rarely or very rarely and has not been confirmed to occur in the absence of vaccine-associated cutaneous lesions in the vaccinee (see section 4.8).

In healthy contacts of vaccinees, seroconversion has sometimes occurred in the absence of any clinical manifestations of infection. Clinically apparent infections due to transmission of the vaccine viral strain have been associated with few skin lesions and minimal systemic upset.

However, contact with the following groups must be avoided if the vaccinee develops a cutaneous rash thought likely to be vaccine-related (especially vesicular or papulovesicular) within four to six weeks of the first or second dose and until this rash has completely disappeared (see also sections 4.6 and 5.1).

- varicella-susceptible pregnant women and

- individuals at high risk of severe varicella, such as those with primary and acquired immunodeficiency states. These include individuals with leukaemias, lymphomas, blood dyscrasias, clinically manifest HIV infections, and patients who are receiving immunosuppressive therapy, including high dose corticosteroids.

In the absence of a rash in the vaccinee, the risk of transmission of the vaccine viral strain to contacts in the above groups appears to be extremely small. Nevertheless, vaccinees (*e.g.* healthcare workers) who are very likely to come into contact with persons in the above groups should preferably avoid any such contact during the period between vaccinations and for 4-6 weeks after the second dose. If this is not feasible, then vaccinees should be vigilant regarding the reporting of any skin rash during this period, and should take steps as above if a rash is discovered.

Healthy seronegative children may be vaccinated if they are close contacts of persons who are at high risk of severe varicella infection (see sections 4.1 and 4.2). In these circumstances, continued contact between the vaccinee and the person at risk may be unavoidable. Therefore, the risk of transmission of the attenuated vaccine viral strain from the vaccinee should be weighed against the potential for acquisition of wild-type varicella-zoster by the at-risk person.

The Oka vaccine viral strain has recently been shown to be sensitive to acyclovir.

4.5 Interaction with other medicinal products and other forms of interaction

In subjects who have received immune globulins or a blood transfusion, vaccination should be delayed for at least three months because of the likelihood of vaccine failure due to passively acquired antibody to the varicella-zoster virus.

Aspirin and systemic salicylates should not be given to children under the age of 16, except under medical supervision, because of the risk of Reye's syndrome. Reye's syndrome has been reported in children treated with aspirin during natural varicella infection. However, there is no evidence to suggest that vaccination with Varilrix should be contrainidicated for older age-groups who need to take aspirin.

In a study in which Varilrix was administered to toddlers at the same time as, but at a different site to, a combined measles, mumps and rubella vaccine, there was no evidence of significant immune interference between the live viral antigens.

If a measles containing vaccine is not given at the same time as Varilrix, it is recommended that an interval of at least one month between vaccinations is respected, since it is recognised that measles vaccination may cause short-term suppression of the cell-mediated response.

If it is considered necessary to administer another live vaccine at the same time as Varilrix, the vaccines must be given as separate injections and at different body sites.

4.6 Pregnancy and lactation

Pregnancy

Varicella-zoster virus may cause severe clinical disease in pregnant individuals and may adversely affect the fetus and/or result in perinatal varicella, depending on the gestational stage when the infection occurs. Because the possible effects of infection with the vaccine viral strain on the mother and on the fetus are unknown, Varilrix must not be administered to pregnant women.

Furthermore, female candidates for vaccination must be advised to take adequate precautions to avoid pregnancy occurring between the two vaccine doses and for three months following the second dose.

Lactation

The infants of seronegative women would not have acquired transplacental antibody to varicella-zoster virus. Therefore, due to the theoretical risk of transmission of the vaccine viral strain from mother to infant, women should not be vaccinated while breastfeeding.

4.7 Effects on ability to drive and use machines

It would not be expected that vaccination would affect the ability to drive or operate machinery.

4.8 Undesirable effects

Clinical trials in healthy subjects

More than 7,900 individuals have participated in clinical trials evaluating the reactogenicity profile of the vaccine administered alone or concomitantly with other vaccines.

The safety profile presented below is based on a total of 5369 doses of Varilrix administered alone to children, adolescents and adults.

The most common adverse reactions observed after vaccine administration were injection site pain (23.8%), redness (19.9%) and swelling (12.1%).

Frequencies are reported as:

Very common: ≥10%

Common: ≥1% and <10%

Uncommon: ≥0.1% and <1%

Rare: ≥0.01% and <0.1%

Very rare: <0.01%

Blood and lymphatic system disorders

Uncommon: lymphadenopathy

Nervous system disorders

Uncommon: headache, somnolence

Very rare: dizziness

Eye disorders

Rare: conjunctivitis

Respiratory, thoracic and mediastinal disorders

Uncommon: cough, rhinitis

Gastrointestinal disorders

Uncommon: nausea, vomiting

Rare: abdominal pain, diarrhoea

Skin and subcutaneous tissue disorders

Common: rash

Uncommon: varicella-like rash, pruritus

Rare: urticaria

Musculoskeletal and connective tissue disorders

Uncommon: arthralgia, myalgia

Infections and infestations

Uncommon: upper respiratory tract infection, pharyngitis

General disorders and administration site conditions

Very common: pain, redness and swelling at the injection site*, fever (oral/axillary temperature ≥ 37.5°C or rectal temperature ≥ 38.0°C)*

Uncommon: fever (oral/axillary temperature > 39.0°C or rectal temperature > 39.5°C), fatigue, malaise

Very rare: face oedema

Psychiatric disorders

Uncommon: irritability

* Swelling at the injection site and fever were commonly reported in studies conducted in children ≤ 12 years.

In general, the reactogenicity profile after the second dose was comparable to that after the first dose. However, the rates of injection site reactions (primarily redness and swelling) were higher after the second dose in children aged ≤12 years.

No differences were seen in the reactogenicity profile between initially seropositive and initially seronegative subjects.

Post-marketing surveillance

Nervous system disorders

Febrile and non-febrile convulsions, cerebellar ataxia**

Infections and infestations

Herpes zoster**

Immune system disorders

Hypersensitivity, anaphylactic reactions

** This reaction reported after vaccination is also a consequence of wild-type varicella infection. There is no indication of an increased risk of its occurrence following vaccination compared with wild-type disease.

Transmission of the vaccine virus from healthy vaccinees to healthy contacts has been shown to occur very rarely.

4.9 Overdose

Cases of accidental administration of more than the recommended dose of Varilrix have been reported. Amongst these cases, the following adverse events were reported: lethargy and convulsions. In other cases, no associated adverse events were reported.

5. PHARMACOLOGICAL PROPERTIES

5.1 Pharmacodynamic properties

ATC code J07B K01

The Oka strain virus contained in Varilrix was initially obtained from a child with natural varicella; the virus was then attenuated through sequential passage in tissue culture.

Natural infection induces a cellular and humoral immune response to the varicella-zoster virus, which can be rapidly detected following infection. IgG, IgM and IgA directed against viral proteins usually appear at the same time that a cellular immune response can be demonstrated, making the relative contribution of humoral and cellular immunity to disease progression difficult to ascertain. Vaccination has been shown to induce both humoral and cell-mediated types of immunity.

In clinical trials, the immune response to vaccination was routinely measured using an immunofluorescence assay. Antibody titres of ≥ 1:4 (the detection level of the test) were considered as positive.

In clinical trials that enrolled 211 adolescents and 213 adults, all vaccinees had detectable levels of antibodies in blood samples taken six weeks after the second vaccine dose. Virtually all (98.7%) of the 1637 children tested had detectable antibodies six weeks after immunisation with one dose of vaccine.

Virtually all (≥98.7%) children aged 9 months to 12 years tested had antibody levels ≥ 4 (dil-1) six weeks after immunisation with one dose of Varilrix.

All of 659 children aged 9 months to 6 years, who received a second dose of Varilrix or received Varilrix after a first dose of another varicella vaccine, had antibody levels ≥ 4 (dil-1) at 6-18 weeks following vaccination. There was a large increase in GMT (up to 13-fold) between post-dose 1 and post-dose 2.

However, the safety and immunogenicity of a second dose of Varilrix in adolescents (≥13 years) and adults primed with another varicella-containing vaccine has not been specifically studied in clinical trials.

In a follow-up study over 2 years in 159 vaccinated adult health care workers, 2 out of 72 (3%) vaccinees reporting contacts with wild-type chickenpox experienced mild breakthrough disease. Approximately one-third of the vaccinees showed an increase in antibody titre over the follow-up period, indicative of contact with the virus, without clinical evidence of varicella infection.

The percentage of vaccinees who will later experience herpes-zoster due to reactivation of the Oka strain virus is currently unknown. However, the risk of zoster after vaccination is currently thought to be much lower than would be expected after wild-type virus infection, due to attenuation of the vaccine strain.

5.2 Pharmacokinetic properties

Evaluation of pharmacokinetic properties is not required for vaccines.

5.3 Preclinical safety data

There is no other relevant information that has not already been stated above.

6. PHARMACEUTICAL PARTICULARS

6.1 List of excipients

Amino acids

Human albumin

Lactose

Neomycin sulphate

Mannitol

Sorbitol

6.2 Incompatibilities

Varilrix should not be mixed with other vaccines in the same syringe.

6.3 Shelf life

2 years.

The vaccine should be used immediately after reconstitution. If not used immediately, in-use storage times and conditions prior to use are the responsibility of the user and should normally not be longer than 1 hour at +2°C to +8°C (in a refrigerator). Do not freeze.

6.4 Special precautions for storage

Store at +2°C to +8°C (in a refrigerator).

The lyophilised vaccine is not affected by freezing.

6.5 Nature and contents of container

Powder for reconstitution

Cream to yellowish or pinkish coloured cake or powder in 3 ml vials (Type I glass) with stopper (bromobutyl rubber) and flip-off cap (aluminium).

Solvent for reconstitution

Water for Injections in 1 ml ampoule (Type I glass).

Packs of one.

6.6 Special precautions for disposal and other handling

Due to minor variations of its pH, the colour of the reconstituted vaccine may vary from peach to pink. The diluent and the reconstituted vaccine should be inspected visually for any foreign particulate matter and/or variation of physical appearance prior to administration. In the event of either being observed, discard the diluent or the reconstituted vaccine.

Varilrix must be reconstituted by adding the contents of the supplied container of water for injections diluent to the vial containing the pellet. After the addition of the diluent to the pellet, the mixture should be well shaken until the pellet is completely dissolved in the diluent.

Biochemical and physical in-use stability has been demonstrated on the reconstituted vaccine for 90 minutes at room temperature or for 8 hours at 2°C-8°C.

From a microbiological point of view, the product should be used immediately. If not used immediately, in-use storage times and conditions prior to use are the responsibility of the user and would not normally be longer than 8 hours at 2°C-8°C, unless reconstitution has taken place in controlled and validated aseptic conditions.

Alcohol and other disinfecting agents must be allowed to evaporate from the skin before injection of the vaccine since they may inactivate the virus.

Any unused product or waste material should be disposed of in accordance with local requirements.

7. MARKETING AUTHORISATION HOLDER

SmithKline Beecham plc

980, Great West Road

Brentford

Middlesex TW8 9GS

United Kingdom

Trading as:

GlaxoSmithKline UK
Stockley Park West
Uxbridge
Middlesex UB11 1BT
United Kingdom

8. MARKETING AUTHORISATION NUMBER(S)

Vaccine: PL 10592/0121

Diluent: PL 10592/0021

9. DATE OF FIRST AUTHORISATION/RENEWAL OF THE AUTHORISATION

25 June 2002

10. DATE OF REVISION OF THE TEXT

27 February 2009

Vascace

(Roche Products Limited)

1. NAME OF THE MEDICINAL PRODUCT

Vascace

2. QUALITATIVE AND QUANTITATIVE COMPOSITION

One film coated tablet 0.5mg contains:

Cilazapril, anhydrous 0.5mg, in the form of the monohydrate (cilazapril 0.522mg).

Excipients include lactose monohydrate 82.028 mg.

One film coated tablet 1.0mg contains:

Cilazapril, anhydrous 1.0mg, in the form of the monohydrate (cilazapril 1.044mg).

Excipients include lactose monohydrate 81.506 mg.

One film coated tablet 2.5mg contains:

Cilazapril, anhydrous 2.5mg, in the form of the monohydrate (cilazapril 2.61mg).

Excipients include lactose monohydrate 124.39 mg.

One film coated tablet 5.0mg contains:

Cilazapril, anhydrous 5.0mg, in the form of the monohydrate (cilazapril 5.22mg).

Excipients include lactose monohydrate 121.78 mg.

For warnings related to lactose monohydrate, see section *4.4 Special warnings and precautions for use*.

For full list of excipients, see section *6.1*.

3. PHARMACEUTICAL FORM

Tablets.

4. CLINICAL PARTICULARS

4.1 Therapeutic indications

Vascace is indicated in treatment of all grades of essential hypertension. Vascace is also indicated in the treatment of chronic heart failure, usually as an adjunctive therapy with digitalis and/or diuretics.

4.2 Posology and method of administration

Vascace should be administered once-daily. As food intake has no clinically significant influence on absorption, Vascace can be administered before or after a meal. The dose should always be taken at about the same time of day.

Special Dosage Instructions:

Essential hypertension

The recommended initial dosage is 1mg once a day. Dosage should be adjusted individually in accordance with the blood pressure response until control is achieved. Most patients can be maintained on between 2.5 and 5.0mg/day. If the blood pressure is not adequately controlled with 5mg Vascace once daily, a low dose of a non-potassium-sparing diuretic may be administered concomitantly to enhance the anti-hypertensive effect.

Hypertensive patients receiving diuretics

The diuretic should be discontinued two to three days before beginning therapy with Vascace to reduce the likelihood of symptomatic hypotension. It may be resumed later if required. The recommended starting dose in these patients is 0.5mg once daily.

Chronic heart failure

Vascace can be used as adjunctive therapy with digitalis and/or diuretics in patients with chronic heart failure. Therapy with Vascace should be initiated with a recommended starting dose of 0.5mg once daily under close medical supervision. The dose should be increased to the lowest maintenance dose of 1mg daily according to tolerability and clinical status. Further titration within the usual maintenance dose of 1mg to 2.5mg daily should be carried out based on patients response, clinical status and tolerability. The usual maximum dose is 5mg once daily.

Results from clinical trials showed that clearance of cilazaprilat in patients with chronic heart failure is correlated with creatinine clearance. Thus in patients with chronic heart failure and impaired renal function special dosage recommendation as given under "Impaired Renal Function" should be followed.

Impaired renal function

Reduced dosages may be required for patients with renal impairment, depending on their creatinine clearance (see section *4.4 Special warnings and precautions for use*).

The following dose schedules are recommended:

Creatinine clearance	Initial dose of Vascace	Maximal dose of Vascace
> 40ml/min	1mg once daily	5mg once daily
10 - 40ml/min	0.5mg once daily	2.5mg once daily
< 10ml/min	Not recommended	

In patients requiring haemodialysis, Vascace should be administered on days when dialysis is not performed and the dosage should be adjusted according to blood pressure response.

Impaired hepatic function

In the unlikely event that a patient with liver cirrhosis should require treatment with cilazapril, it should be initiated with caution, at a dose of 0.5 mg or less once daily, because significant hypotension may occur (see section *4.4 Special warnings and precautions for use*).

Vascace is contraindicated in patients with ascites (see section *4.3 Contraindications*).

Elderly

In the treatment of hypertension, Vascace should be initiated with between 0.5mg and 1mg once daily. Thereafter, the maintenance dose must be adapted to individual response.

In the treatment of chronic heart failure, Vascace should be initiated with a dose of 0.5mg daily. The maintenance dose of 1mg to 2.5mg must be adapted to individual tolerability, response and clinical status.

In elderly patients with chronic heart failure on high diuretic dosage the recommended starting dose of Vascace 0.5mg must be strictly followed.

Children

Safety and efficacy in children have not been established therefore there is no recommendation for administration of cilazapril to children.

4.3 Contraindications

Vascace is contraindicated in patients who are hypersensitive to cilazapril, other ACE-inhibitors or any of the product excipients, in patients with ascites and in the second and third trimesters of pregnancy (see section *4.4 Special warnings and precautions for use* and section *4.6 Pregnancy and lactation*).

Vascace is also contraindicated in patients with a history of angioedema after treatment with other ACE-inhibitors.

4.4 Special warnings and precautions for use

(See also *Special Dosage Instructions* under section *4.2 Posology and method of administration*)

Vascace should be used with caution in patients with aortic stenosis, hypertrophic cardiomyopathy or outflow obstruction.

In elderly patients with chronic heart failure on high diuretic dosage the recommended starting dose of Vascace 0.5mg must be strictly followed.

Hypersensitivity/angioneurotic oedema

Angioneurotic oedema has been reported in patients being treated with ACE-inhibitors (see section *4.8 Undesirable effects*).

Haemodyalysis/anaphylaxis

Although the mechanism involved has not been definitely established, there is clinical evidence that haemodialysis with polyacrylonitrile methallyl sulphate high-flux membranes (e.g. AN69), haemofiltration or LDL-apheresis, if performed in patients being treated with ACE-inhibitors, including cilazapril, can lead to the provocation of anaphylaxis/anaphylactoid reactions including life-threatening shock. The above-mentioned procedures must therefore be avoided in such patients.

Symptomatic hypotension

Occasionally, symptomatic hypotension has been reported with ACE-inhibitor therapy, particularly in patients with sodium or volume depletion in connection with conditions such as vomiting, diarrhoea, pre-treatment with diuretics, low sodium diet or after dialysis. In patients with angina pectoris or cerebrovascular disease, treatment with ACE-inhibitors should be started under close medical supervision, as excessive hypotension could result in myocardial infarction or cerebrovascular accident.

Patients with chronic heart failure, especially those taking high doses of loop diuretics, may experience a pronounced blood pressure decrease in response to ACE-inhibitors. This should be treated by having the patient rest in the supine position and may require infusion of normal saline or volume expanders. After volume repletion, Vascace therapy may be continued. However, if symptoms persist, the dosage should be reduced or the drug discontinued.

Renal impairment

Reduced dosages may be required for patients with renal impairment, depending on their creatinine clearance (see section *4.2 Special dosage instruc-tions*). Treatment with ACE-inhibitors may produce increases in blood urea nitrogen and/or serum creatinine. Although these alterations are usually reversible upon discontinuation of Vascace and/or diuretic therapy, cases of severe renal dysfunction and, rarely, acute renal failure have been reported.

In this patient population, renal function should be monitored during the first weeks of therapy.

For haemodialysis using high-flux polyacrylonitrile (AN69) membranes please see above statement under the heading of *Special warnings and special precautions for use*.

Hepatic impairment

In patients with severe liver function impairment, hypotension may occur.

Hepatic failure

Rarely, ACE-inhibitors have been associated with hepatotoxicity including cholestatic and hepatocellular hepatitis. More severe reactions such as fulminant hepatic necrosis have also been reported. Patients receiving ACE-inhibitors who develop jaundice or elevations of hepatic enzymes should discontinue the ACE-inhibitor and receive appropriate medical follow-up.

Serum potassium

Concomitant administration of potassium-sparing diuretics, potassium supplements or potassium containing salt substitutes may lead to increases in serum potassium, particularly in patients with renal impairment (see section *4.5 Interaction with other medicinal products and other forms of interaction* and section *5.1 Pharmacodynamic properties*). Therefore, if concomitant use for such agents is indicated, their dosage should be reduced when Vascace is initiated and serum potassium and renal function should be monitored carefully.

Surgery anaesthesia

The use of ACE-inhibitors in combination with anaesthetic drugs in surgery that also have blood-pressure-lowering effects, can produce arterial hypotension. If this occurs, volume expansion by means of intravenous infusion or - if resistant to these measures - angiotensin II infusion is indicated.

Neutropenia

Neutropenia and agranulocytosis have been rarely reported with ACE-inhibitors. Periodic monitoring of white blood cell counts should be considered in patients with collagen vascular disease and renal disease such as systemic lupus erythematosus and scleroderma, or in patients receiving immunosuppressive therapy, especially when they also have impaired renal function.

Pregnancy

ACE-inhibitors should not be initiated during pregnancy. Unless continued ACE-inhibitor therapy is considered essential, patients planning pregnancy should be changed to alternative antihypertensive treatments which have an established safety profile for use in pregnancy. When pregnancy is diagnosed, treatment with ACE-inhibitors should be stopped immediately, and, if appropriate, alternative therapy should be started (see section *4.3 Contraindications* and section *4.6 Pregnancy and lactation*).

Owing to the presence of lactose monohydrate, patients with rare hereditary problems of galactose intolerance, the Lapp lactase deficiency or glucose-galactose malabsorption should not take this medicine.

4.5 Interaction with other medicinal products and other forms of interaction

There was no increase in plasma digoxin concentrations when Vascace was administered concomitantly with digoxin. No clinically significant drug interactions were observed when Vascace was administered concomitantly with nitrates, oral antidiabetics, H2-receptor blockers and coumarin anticoagulants. No significant pharmacokinetic drug interactions between Vascace and furosemide or thiazides were noted. An additive effect may be observed when Vascace is administered in combination with other blood-pressure-lowering agents.

Potassium-sparing diuretics, potassium supplements or potassium containing salt substitutes administered together with Vascace can lead to increases in serum potassium, particularly in patients with renal impairment (see section *4.4 Special warnings and precautions for use* and section *5.1 Pharmacodynamic properties*).

As with other ACE-inhibitors, use of Vascace concomitantly with a non-steroidal anti-inflammatory drug (NSAID) may diminish the anti-hypertensive effect of Vascace.

Anaphylactic reactions can occur in patients undergoing desensitisation therapy with wasp or bee venom while receiving an ACE-inhibitor. Cilazapril must therefore be interrupted before the start of desensitisation therapy. Additionally, in this situation, cilazapril must not be replaced by a beta blocker.

Concomitant administration of ACE-inhibitors and antidiabetic medicines (insulin, oral hypoglycaemic agents) may cause an increased blood glucose lowering effect with the risk of hypoglycaemia. This phenomenon may be more likely to occur during the first weeks of combined treatment and in patients with renal impairment.

Lithium should generally not be given with ACE-inhibitors. ACE-inhibitors reduce the renal clearance of lithium and add a risk of lithium toxicity.

Concomitant administration of allopurinol, cytostatic or immunosuppressive agents, systemic corticosteroids or procainamide with ACE-inhibitors may lead to an increased risk of leucopenia.

Alcohol can enhance the hypotensive effect of ACE-inhibitors.

4.6 Pregnancy and lactation

The use of ACE-inhibitors is not recommended during the first trimester of pregnancy (see section *4.4 Special warnings and precautions for use*). The use of ACE-inhibitors is contraindicated during the second and third trimester of pregnancy (see section *4.3 Contraindications* and section *4.4 Special warnings and precautions for use*).

Epidemiological evidence regarding the risk of teratogenicity following exposure to ACE-inhibitors during the first trimester of pregnancy has not been conclusive; however a small increase in risk cannot be excluded. Unless continued ACE-inhibitor therapy is considered essential, patients planning pregnancy should be changed to alternative antihypertensive treatments which have an established safety profile for use in pregnancy. When pregnancy is diagnosed, treatment with ACE-inhibitors should be stopped immediately, and, if appropriate, alternative therapy should be started.

Exposure to ACE-inhibitor therapy during the second and third trimesters is known to induce human foetotoxicity (decreased renal function, oligohydramnios, skull ossification retardation) and neonatal toxicity (renal failure, hypotension, hyperkalaemia). Should exposure to an ACE-inhibitor have occurred from the second trimester of pregnancy, ultrasound check of renal function and skull is recommended. Infants whose mothers have taken ACE-inhibitors should be closely observed for hypotension (see section *4.3 Contraindications* and section *4.4 Special warnings and precautions for use*).

Lactation

Because no information is available regarding the use of Vascace during breast-feeding, Vascace is not recommended, and alternative treatments with better established safety profiles during breast-feeding are preferable, especially while nursing a newborn or preterm infant.

4.7 Effects on ability to drive and use machines

There are no studies on the effect of Vascace on the ability to drive. When driving vehicles or operating machinery it should be taken into account that occasionally dizziness or fatigue may occur (see section *4.8 Undesirable effects*). These effects may be enhanced by the concomitant use of alcohol (see section *4.5 Interaction with other medicinal products and other forms of interaction*).

4.8 Undesirable effects

In most cases undesirable effects are transient, mild or moderate in degree, and do not require discontinuation of therapy. The most common adverse effects include dry cough, rash, hypotension, dizziness, fatigue, headache and nausea, dyspepsia and other gastrointestinal disturbances.

Blood and lymphatic system disorders

Blood disorders have been reported with ACE-inhibitors and include neutropenia and agranulocytosis (especially in patients with renal failure and those with collagen vascular disorders such as systemic lupus erythematosus and scleroderma), thrombocytopenia and anaemia.

Cardiac disorders

Pronounced hypotension may occur at the start of therapy with ACE-inhibitors, particularly in patients with heart failure and in sodium- or volume-depleted patients. Myocardial infarction and stroke have been reported and may relate to severe falls in blood pressure in patients with ischaemic heart disease or cerbrovascular disease. Other cardiovascular effects that have occurred include tachycardia, palpitations and chest pain.

Hepatobiliary disorders

Single cases of liver function disorders, such as increased liver function tests (transaminases, bilirubin, alkaline phosphatase, gamma GT) and cholestatic hepatitis with or without necrosis, have been reported.

Immune system disorders

ACE-inhibitors have been documented to induce cough in a substantial number of patients. Rarely dyspnoea, sinusitis, rhinitis, glossitis, bronchitis and bronchospasm have been reported.

As with other ACE-inhibitors, angioneurotic oedema has been reported, although rarely, in patients receiving Vascace. Angioedema involving the tongue, glottis or larynx may be **fatal**. If involvement of the face, lips, tongue, glottis and/or larynx occurs Vascace should be discontinued, replaced by an agent belonging to another class of drugs and appropriate therapy instituted without delay. Emergency therapy should be given including, but not necessarily limited to, immediate intramuscular adrenaline (epinephrine) solution 1:1000 (0.3 to 0.5ml) or slow intravenous adrenaline 1mg/ml (observing dilution instructions) with control of ECG and blood pressure. The patient should be hospitalised and observed for at least 12 to 24 hours and should not be discharged until complete resolution of symptoms has occurred.

Gastrointestinal disorders

Pancreatitis has been reported rarely in patients treated with ACE-inhibitors (including Vascace); in some cases this has proved fatal.

Skin and subcutaneous tissue disorders

Skin rashes (including erythema multiforme and toxic epidermal necrolysis) may occur; photosensitivity, alopecia and other hypersensitivity reactions have also been reported.

Laboratory test findings

Clinically relevant changes in laboratory test values possibly or probably related to Vascace treatment have been observed only rarely.

Minor, mostly reversible increases in serum creatinine/urea have been observed in patients treated with Vascace. Such changes are likely to occur in patients with renal artery stenosis or with renal impairment (see section *4.4 Special warnings and precautions for use*), but they have also occasionally been observed in patients with normal renal function, particularly in those receiving concomitant diuretics.

Renal and urinary disorders

Isolated cases of acute renal failure have been reported in patients with severe heart failure, renal artery stenosis or renal disorders (see section *4.4 Special warnings and precautions for use*).

4.9 Overdose

While single doses of up to 160mg Vascace have been administered to normal healthy volunteers without untoward effects on blood pressure, only a few data on overdose are available in patients.

The most likely symptoms of overdosage are hypotension, which may be severe, shock, stupor, bradycardia, hyperkalaemia, hyponatraemia and renal impairment with metabolic acidosis.

Treatment should be mainly symptomatic and supportive.

After ingestion of an overdose, the patient should be kept under close supervision, preferably in an intensive care unit. Serum electrolytes and creatinine should be monitored frequently. Therapeutic measures depend on the nature and severity of the symptoms. Measurements to prevent absorption such as gastric lavage, administration of adsorbents and sodium sulphate within 30 minutes after intake, and to hasten elimination should be applied if ingestion is recent. If hypotension occurs, the patient should be placed in the shock position and salt and volume supplementation should be given, rapidly. Treatment with angiotensin II may be considered if conventional therapy is ineffective. Bradycardia or extensive vagal reactions should be treated by administering atropine. The use of a pacemaker may be considered. ACE-inhibitors may be removed from the circulation by haemodialysis. The use of high-flux polyacrylonitrile membranes should be avoided.

5. PHARMACOLOGICAL PROPERTIES

5.1 Pharmacodynamic properties

Pharmacotherapeutic group: ACE inhibitors, plain, ATC code: C09AA08.

Vascace (cilazapril) is a specific, long-acting angiotensin-converting enzyme (ACE) inhibitor which suppresses the renin-angiotensin-aldosterone system and thereby the conversion of the inactive angiotensin I to angiotensin II which is a potent vasoconstrictor. At recommended doses, the effect of Vascace in hypertensive patients and in patients with chronic heart failure is maintained for up to 24 hours.

In patients with normal renal function, serum potassium usually remains within the normal range during Vascace treatment. In patients concomitantly taking potassium-sparing diuretics, potassium levels may rise (see section *4.4 Special warnings and precautions for use* and section *4.5 Interaction with other medicinal products and other forms of interaction*).

Hypertension

Vascace induces a reduction of both supine and standing systolic and diastolic blood pressure, usually with no orthostatic component. It is effective in all degrees of essential hypertension as well as in renal hypertension. The antihypertensive effect of Vascace is usually apparent within the first hour after administration, with maximum effect observed between three and seven hours after dosing. In general the heart rate remains unchanged. Reflex tachycardia is not induced, although small, clinically insignificant alterations of heart rate may occur. In some patients blood pressure reduction may diminish toward the end of the dosage interval.

The initial dosage seldom achieves the desired therapeutic response. Blood pressure should be assessed and dosage adjusted as required. Should the effect of Vascace at the top of the recommended dose be insufficient it can be combined with non-potassium-sparing diuretics.

The anti-hypertensive effect of Vascace is maintained during long-term therapy. No rapid increase in blood pressure has been observed after abrupt withdrawal of Vascace.

In hypertensive patients with moderate to severe renal impairment, the glomerular filtration rate and renal blood flow remained in general unchanged with Vascace despite a clinically significant blood pressure reduction.

As with other ACE-inhibitors, the blood pressure-lowering effect of Vascace in black patients may be less pronounced than in non-blacks. However, racial differences in response are no longer evident when Vascace is administered in combination with hydrochlorothiazide.

Chronic heart failure

In patients with chronic heart failure the renin-angiotensin-aldosterone and the sympathetic nervous systems are generally activated leading to enhanced systemic vasoconstriction and to the promotion of sodium and water retention. By suppressing the renin-angiotensin-aldosterone system, Vascace improves loading conditions in the failing heart by reducing systemic vascular resistance (afterload) and pulmonary capillary wedge pressure (preload) in patients on diuretics and/or digitalis. Furthermore, the exercise tolerance of these patients increases significantly showing an improvement in quality of life. The haemodynamic and clinical effects occur promptly and persist.

5.2 Pharmacokinetic properties

Cilazapril is efficiently absorbed and rapidly converted to the active form, cilazaprilat. Ingestion of food immediately prior to Vascace administration, delays and reduces the absorption to a minor extent which, however, is therapeutically irrelevant. The bioavailability of cilazaprilat from oral cilazapril approximates 60% based on urinary recovery data. Maximum plasma concentrations are reached within two hours after administration and are directly related to dosage.

Cilazaprilat is eliminated unchanged by the kidneys, with an effective half-life of nine hours after once-daily dosing with Vascace.

Renal impairment

In patients with renal impairment, higher plasma concentrations of cilazaprilat are observed than in patients with normal renal function, since drug clearance is reduced when creatinine clearance is lower. There is no elimination in patients with complete renal failure, but haemodialysis reduces concentrations of both cilazapril and cilazaprilat to a limited extent.

Elderly patients

In elderly patients whose renal function is normal for age, plasma concentrations of cilazaprilat may be up to 40% higher, and the clearance 20% lower than in younger patients.

Hepatic impairment

In patients with liver cirrhosis, increased plasma concentrations and reduced plasma and renal clearance were observed, with a greater effect on cilazapril than on its active metabolite cilazaprilat.

Chronic heart failure

In patients with chronic heart failure the clearance of cilazaprilat is correlated with the creatinine clearance. Thus, dosage adjustments beyond those recommended for patients with impaired renal function (see section *4.2 Special Dosage Instructions*) should not be necessary.

5.3 Preclinical safety data

Teratogenicity

Foetotoxicity has been observed for ACE-inhibitors in animals.

6. PHARMACEUTICAL PARTICULARS

6.1 List of excipients

In the tablet core:

Lactose monohydrate

Maize starch

Hypromellose 3cp

Talc

Sodium stearyl fumarate

In the film coat:

Hypromellose 6cp

Talc

Titanium dioxide E171

Iron oxide red E172 (2.5mg and 5.0mg only)

Iron oxide yellow E172 (1.0mg and 2.5mg only)

6.2 Incompatibilities

Not applicable.

6.3 Shelf life

3 years.

6.4 Special precautions for storage

Do not store above 25°C.

6.5 Nature and contents of container

Glass Bottles and Aluminium Blisters

0.5mg: 2, 28, 30 or 100 tablets

1.0mg: 2, 28, 30 or 100 tablets

2.5mg: 4, 28, 30, 98 or 100 tablets

5.0mg: 28, 30, 98 or 100 tablets

Not all pack sizes may be marketed.

6.6 Special precautions for disposal and other handling

None stated.

7. MARKETING AUTHORISATION HOLDER

Roche Products Limited, 6 Falcon Way, Shire Park, Welwyn Garden City, AL7 1TW, United Kingdom.

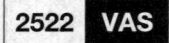

8. MARKETING AUTHORISATION NUMBER(S)

PL 0031/0244	0.5mg Tablets
PL 0031/0245	1.0mg Tablets
PL 0031/0246	2.5mg Tablets
PL 0031/0247	5.0mg Tablets

9. DATE OF FIRST AUTHORISATION/RENEWAL OF THE AUTHORISATION

26 October 1990/7 December 2001

10. DATE OF REVISION OF THE TEXT

March 2009

LEGAL STATUS

POM

Vascace is a registered trade mark

Vascalpha 10mg Prolonged Release Tablet

(Actavis UK Ltd)

1. NAME OF THE MEDICINAL PRODUCT

VASCALPHA 10 mg PROLONGED RELEASE TABLETS (FELODIPINE)

2. QUALITATIVE AND QUANTITATIVE COMPOSITION

One prolonged release tablet contains 10mg of felodipine.

Lactose monohydrate 21.45mg

For excipients, see 6.1.

3. PHARMACEUTICAL FORM

Prolonged release tablet.

Reddish brown, round, biconvex, film coated prolonged release tablets with imprint 10.

4. CLINICAL PARTICULARS

4.1 Therapeutic indications

Essential hypertension

4.2 Posology and method of administration

Vascalpha (felodipine) prolonged release tablets should usually be administered as follows:

The recommended starting dose is 5 mg felodipine once daily.

If necessary, the dose may be increased to 10 mg felodipine once daily or another antihypertensive agent added. Dose increases should occur at intervals of at least 2 weeks. The usual maintenance dose is 5-10mg once daily.

The maximum daily dose is 10 mg felodipine.

The dose should be adjusted to the individual requirements of the patient.

Elderly

The recommended starting dose should be 2.5mg.

Subsequent dose increases should be undertaken with particular caution.

Impaired hepatic function

In patients with mild to moderate hepatic impairment, the recommended starting dose should be lowered to the minimal therapeutic effective dose of felodipine.

The dose should only be increased after carefully balancing the benefits against the risks (see 5.2 Pharmacokinetic properties). It is contraindicated in patients with severe hepatic impairment.

Impaired renal function

The pharmacokinetics are not significantly affected in patients with mild to moderate impaired renal function. Caution should be taken in patients with severe renal impairment (see section 4.4 Special warnings and precautions for use and section 5.2. Pharmacokinetic properties).

Children

Felodipine is not recommended for use in children due to lack of data on safety and efficacy.

Administration

The prolonged release tablets should be taken in the morning with a sufficient amount of fluid (e.g. a glass of water, but it should NOT be taken with grapefruit juice!) (see 4.5 Interaction with other medicinal products and other forms of interaction).

The prolonged release tablets should be swallowed whole and not chewed or crushed. The tablets may be taken on an empty stomach or with a light meal, however a high fat meal should be avoided (see 5.2 Pharmacokinetic properties).

4.3 Contraindications

Felodipine is contra-indicated in patients with:

- hypersensitivity to felodipine (or other dihydropyridines) or to any of the excipients
- cardiogenic shock
- severe aortic and mitral stenosis
- obstructive hyperthrophic cardiomyopathy
- unstable angina pectoris
- acute myocardial infarction (within 4-8 weeks of a myocardial infarction)
- decompensated heart failure
- severe hepatic impairment
- pregnancy (see section 4.6)

4.4 Special warnings and precautions for use

Felodipine should be used with caution in patients with:

- conduction disorders, compensated heart failure, tachycardia and aortic or mitral valve stenosis.
- mild to moderate hepatic impairment, as the anti-hypertensive effect may be enhanced. Adjustment of the dosage should be considered.
- severe renal impairment (GFR <30ml/min)
- AV block of the second or third degree

If treatment with felodipine is discontinued abruptly, a hypertensive crisis may occur in individual cases.

Felodipine could cause significant hypotension (vasodilation effect) with consecutive tachycardia, leading to myocardial ischaemia in sensitive patients, therefore predisposed patients may suffer from myocardial infarction (see section 5.1 Pharmacodynamic properties).

Dihydropyridines may cause acute hypotension. In some cases there is a risk of hypoperfusion accompanied by reflex tachycardia (paradoxical angor) (see section 5.1 Pharmacodynamic properties).

Patients with rare hereditary problems of galactose intolerance, the lapp lactase deficiency or glucose-galactose malabsorption should not take this medicinal product.

4.5 Interaction with other medicinal products and other forms of interaction

Felodipine is a CYP3A4 substrate. Drugs that induce or inhibit CYP3A4 will have large influence on felodipine concentrations.

The anti-hypertensive effect of felodipine may be enhanced by other anti-hypertensives and tricyclic antidepressants.

The concomitant intake of felodipine and drugs which inhibit the cytochrome P450 isoenzyme 3A4 of the liver (such as cimetidine, azole antifungals [itraconazole or ketoconazole], macrolide antibiotics [erythromycin, clarithromycin, telithromycin] or HIV protease inhibitors leads to increased felodipine plasma levels (see section 4.4 Special warnings and precautions for use). Grapefruit juice results in increased peak plasma levels and bioavailability possibly due to interaction with flavanoids in the fruit juice. Therefore grapefruit juice should not be taken together with felodipine.

Cocomitant treatment with drugs such as carbamazepine, phenytoin and barbiturates (e.g. phenobarbital) and rifampicin reduces the plasma levels of felodipine via enzyme induction in the liver (cytochrome P450 System). A similar effect is expected with St John's Wort. Therefore a dose increase of felodipine may be necessary.

Hydrochlorothiazide may enhance the antihypertensive effect of felodipine.

Felodipine can induce an increase of Cmax of ciclosporin. Additionally, ciclosporin may inhibit felodipine metabolism, which may create a potential risk of felodipine toxicity.

Blood levels of digoxin increase during concomitant administration of felodipine. Therefore, decreasing of digoxin dosage should be taken into account when the two drugs are administered concurrently.

4.6 Pregnancy and lactation

Pregnancy

Felodipine is contra-indicated during the entire duration of pregnancy, as animal experiments have demonstrated foetal damage (see 5.3 Preclinical safety data). Pregnancy must be excluded before starting treatment with felodipine.

Lactation

Felodipine is excreted in breast milk. If the breast-feeding mother is taking therapeutic doses of felodipine, a fully breast-fed infant absorbs only a very low dose of the active substance with the breast milk. There is no experience of the risk this may pose to the newborn, therefore as a precaution breast-feeding should be discontinued during treatment.

4.7 Effects on ability to drive and use machines

Felodipine can cause dizziness or tiredness. These adverse effects are more likely to occur after initiation of the treatment, after dose increases, or after concomitant ingestion of alcohol. Should they occur, one should refrain from driving and other activities requiring alertness.

4.8 Undesirable effects

Adverse drug reactions are listed below by system organ class and frequency. Frequencies are defined as: very common (≥ 1/10), common (≥ 1/100, < 1/10), uncommon (≥ 1/1,000, < 1/100), rare (≥ 1/10,000, < 1/1,000), very rare (< 1/10,000), not known (cannot be estimated from the available data).

Nervous system disorders

Very common: Headache (particularly at the beginning of treatment, when the dose is increased or when high doses are administered). Generally, those effects subside on continued treatment.

Uncommon: Paraesthesia, dizziness, fatigue, syncope, restlessness

Ear and labyrinth disorders

Very common: Tinnitus (particularly at the beginning of treatment, when the dose is increased or when high doses are administered). Generally, those effects subside on continued treatment.

Cardiac disorders

Common: Particularly at the beginning of treatment, angina pectoris attacks may occur, or in patients with pre-existing angina pectoris there may be an increase in the frequency, duration and severity of the attacks.

Uncommon: Palpitations, tachycardia, hypotension.

Very rare: Myocardial infarction

Vascular disorders

Rare: Leucocytoclastic vasculitis

Respiratory, thoracic and mediastinal disorders

Uncommon: Dyspnoea

Gastrointestinal disorders

Uncommon: Nausea, vomiting, diarrhoea, constipation.

Hepatobiliary disorders

Very rare: Hepatic function disorders (elevated transaminase levels).

Skin and subcutaneous tissue disorders

Very common: Flushing (particularly at the beginning of treatment, when the dose is increased or when high doses are administered). Generally, those effects subside on continued treatment.

Uncommon: Skin and hypersensitivity reactions such as pruritus, urticaria, exanthema, photosensitisation. Gingival hyperplasia and gingivitis

Very rare: Exfoliative dermatitis

Musculoskeletal and connective tissue disorders

Uncommon: Myalgia, arthralgia, tremors

Renal and urinary disorders

Uncommon: Pollakisuria

Reproductive system and breast disorders

Very rare: Erection disorders, gynaecomastia, menorrhagia.

General disorders and administration site conditions

Common: Peripheral oedema (The degree of ankle swelling is dose related).

Uncommon: Weight gain, sweating

Very rare: Angioedema, fever

4.9 Overdose

Symptoms of intoxication

Overdose may lead to excessive peripheral vasodilatation with marked hypotension and in rare cases bradycardia.

Management of intoxication

The therapeutic measures should focus on elimination of the active ingredient (e.g. administration of charcoal, bowel irrigation) and monitoring of the vital signs. If severe hypotension occurs, symptomatic treatment should be provided, the patient should be placed supine with the legs elevated. In case of accompanying bradycardia, atropine (0.5 – 1.0 mg) should be given intravenously. Additional intravenous fluids should be cautiously administered under haemodynamic supervision to prevent cardiac overloading. Sympathomimetic drugs with predominant effect on the α_1-adrenoreceptor (such as dobutamine, dopamine, noradrenaline (norepinephrine) or adrenaline (epinephrine)) may also be given. Dosage depends on the efficacy obtained.

Felodipine is only dialysable to a minimal extent (approx. 9%).

5. PHARMACOLOGICAL PROPERTIES

5.1 Pharmacodynamic properties

Pharmacotherapeutic group: 1,4-didydropyridine derivative/calcium antagonist

ATC code: C08C A02

Felodipine is a calcium antagonist of the dihydropyridine class of calcium channel blockers. Calcium antagonists interfere with the voltage-dependent L-type (slow) calcium channels in the plasma membranes of smooth muscle cells and reduce the inflow of calcium ions. This results in vasodilatation.

Felodipine has a greater selectivity for vascular smooth muscle than myocardial muscle. Felodipine selectively dilates arterioles with no effects on venous vessels. Felodipine leads to a dose-related lowering of blood pressure via vasodilatation and consequently a reduction of peripheral vascular resistance. It reduces both systolic and diastolic blood pressure. The haemodynamic effect of felodipine is accompanied by reflex (baroreceptor-mediated) tachycardia. In therapeutic doses, felodipine has no direct effect on either cardiac contractility or cardiac conduction. Felodipine reduces renal vascular resistance. The glomerular filtration rate remains unchanged.

Felodipine has a weak natriuretic/diuretic effect and does not provoke fluid retention.

Felodipine can be used as a monotherapy but also concomitantly with beta-blockers, diuretics and ACE inhibitors.

5.2 Pharmacokinetic properties

Absorption

Felodipine is completely absorbed following oral administration. Peak plasma levels are reached with the prolonged release formulation after 3 – 5 hours and result in even felodipine plasma concentrations within the therapeutic range for 24 hours. Steady state is reached approx. 3 days after starting treatment. Due to an extensive first-pass effect, only approx. 15 % of the administered dose is systemically available.

Distribution

The plasma protein binding of felodipine is > 99 %. The volume of distribution is approximately 10 l/kg at steady state, so that felodipine is indicating large tissue distribution. There is no significant accumulation during long-term treatment.

Metabolism

Felodipine is extensively metabolised in the liver by CYP3A4. All identified metabolites are inactive.

Elimination

No unchanged parent substance is detectable in the urine. The average half-life of felodipine in the terminal phase is 25 hours. The inactive hydrophilic metabolites formed by hepatic biotransformation are mainly eliminated renally (to approx. 70 %), and the remainder is excreted in the faeces. The mean plasma clearance is 1100 ml/l and depends on the hepatic blood flow.

Elderly

Increased plasma concentrations have been measured in elderly patients.

Impaired hepatic function

Increased plasma concentrations of up to 100% have been measured in patients with impaired hepatic function.

Impaired renal function

Renal impairment does not affect the pharmacokinetics of felodipine, although accumulation of inactive metabolites occurs in renal failure.

Effect of food

The rate, but not the extent of absorption is affected by the simultaneous ingestion of fatty food. Cmax was 2 to 2.5 times higher following intake of a high-fat meal compared to a fasting state.

5.3 Preclinical safety data

Preclinical data reveal no special hazard for humans based on conventional studies of safety pharmacology, repeated dose toxicity, genotoxicity and carcinogenic potential. In animal studies with respect to the reproduction, adverse effects were found. Effects in rats (prolonged duration of pregnancy and difficult labour) and rabbits (impaired development of distal phalanges, presumably due to decreased uteroplacental perfusion) revealed no evidence of a direct teratogenic effect, but indicate secondary consequences of the pharmacodynamic effect. In monkeys, an abnormal position of the distal phalanges was found. The significance of these observations for humans is unknown.

6. PHARMACEUTICAL PARTICULARS

6.1 List of excipients

Tablet core:

Lactose monohydrate, microcrystalline cellulose, hypromellose, povidone K25, propyl gallate (PhEur), colloidal anhydrous silica, magnesium stearate (PhEur)

Tablet coat:

Hypromellose, talcum, propylene glycol, titanium dioxide (E171), iron oxide red (E172), iron oxide yellow (E172).

6.2 Incompatibilities

Not applicable.

6.3 Shelf life

48 months

6.4 Special precautions for storage

Do not store above 25°C.

6.5 Nature and contents of container

PVC/PE/PVDC aluminium blister.

Pack sizes: 10, 14, 20, 28, 30, 50, 56, 60, 90, 98, 100, 250, 500 and 1000 prolonged release tablets.

Not all pack sizes may be marketed.

6.6 Special precautions for disposal and other handling

No special requirements

7. MARKETING AUTHORISATION HOLDER

Actavis UK Limited (Trading style: Actavis)

Whiddon Valley

BARNSTAPLE

N Devon EX32 8NS

8. MARKETING AUTHORISATION NUMBER(S)

PL 00142/0542

9. DATE OF FIRST AUTHORISATION/RENEWAL OF THE AUTHORISATION

21 July 2003

10. DATE OF REVISION OF THE TEXT

June 2007

Vascalpha 5mg Prolonged Release Tablet

(Actavis UK Ltd)

1. NAME OF THE MEDICINAL PRODUCT

VASCALPHA 5 mg PROLONGED RELEASE TABLETS (FELODIPINE)

2. QUALITATIVE AND QUANTITATIVE COMPOSITION

One prolonged release tablet contains 5mg of felodipine.

Lactose monohydrate 23.95mg

For excipients, see 6.1

3. PHARMACEUTICAL FORM

Prolonged release tablet.

Light pink, round, biconvex, film-coated prolonged release tablets with imprint 5.

4. CLINICAL PARTICULARS

4.1 Therapeutic indications

Essential hypertension

4.2 Posology and method of administration

Vascalpha (felodipine) prolonged release tablets should usually be administered as follows:

The recommended starting dose is 5 mg felodipine once daily.

If necessary, the dose may be increased to 10 mg felodipine once daily or another antihypertensive agent added. Dose increases should occur at intervals of at least 2 weeks. The usual maintenance dose is 5-10mg once daily.

The maximum daily dose is 10 mg felodipine.

The dose should be adjusted to the individual requirements of the patient.

Elderly

The recommended starting dose should be 2.5mg.

Subsequent dose increases should be undertaken with particular caution.

Impaired hepatic function

In patients with mild to moderate hepatic impairment, the recommended starting dose should be lowered to the minimal therapeutic effective dose of felodipine.

The dose should only be increased after carefully balancing the benefits against the risks (see 5.2 Pharmacokinetic properties). It is contraindicated in patients with severe hepatic impairment.

Impaired renal function

The pharmacokinetics are not significantly affected in patients with mild to moderate impaired renal function. Caution should be taken in patients with severe renal impairment (see section 4.4 Special warnings and precautions for use and section 5.2. Pharmacokinetic properties).

Children

Felodipine is not recommended for use in children due to lack of data on safety and efficacy.

Administration

The prolonged release tablets should be taken in the morning with a sufficient amount of fluid (e.g. a glass of water, but it should NOT be taken with grapefruit juice!) (see 4.5 Interaction with other medicinal products and other forms of interaction).

The prolonged release tablets should be swallowed whole and not chewed or crushed. The tablets may be taken on an empty stomach or with a light meal, however a high fat meal should be avoided (see 5.2 Pharmacokinetic properties).

4.3 Contraindications

Felodipine is contra-indicated in patients with:

- hypersensitivity to felodipine (or other dihydropyridines) or to any of the excipients
- cardiogenic shock
- severe aortic and mitral stenosis
- obstructive hypertrophic cardiomyopathy
- unstable angina pectoris
- acute myocardial infarction (within 4-8 weeks of a myocardial infarction)
- decompensated heart failure
- severe hepatic impairment
- pregnancy (see section 4.6)

4.4 Special warnings and precautions for use

Felodipine should be used with caution in patients with:

- conduction disorders, compensated heart failure, tachycardia and aortic or mitral valve stenosis.
- mild to moderate hepatic impairment, as the anti-hypertensive effect may be enhanced. Adjustment of the dosage should be considered.
- severe renal impairment (GFR <30ml/min)
- AV block of the second or third degree

If treatment with felodipine is discontinued abruptly, a hypertensive crisis may occur in individual cases.

Felodipine could cause significant hypotension (vasodilation effect) with consecutive tachycardia, leading to myocardial ischaemia in sensitive patients, therefore predisposed patients may suffer from myocardial infarction (see section 5.1 Pharmacodynamic properties).

Dihydropyridines may cause acute hypotension. In some cases there is a risk of hypoperfusion accompanied by reflex tachycardia (paradoxical angor) (see section 5.1 Pharmacodynamic properties).

Patients with rare hereditary problems of galactose intolerance, the lapp lactase deficiency or glucose-galactose malabsorption should not take this medicinal product.

4.5 Interaction with other medicinal products and other forms of interaction

Felodipine is a CYP3A4 substrate. Drugs that induce or inhibit CYP3A4 will have large influence on felodipine concentrations.

The anti-hypertensive effect of felodipine may be enhanced by other anti-hypertensives and tricyclic antidepressants.

The concomitant intake of felodipine and drugs which inhibit the cytochrome P450 isoenzyme 3A4 of the liver (such as cimetidine, azole antifungals [itraconazole or ketoconazole], macrolide antibiotics [erythromycin clarithromycin, telithromycin] or HIV protease inhibitors leads to increased felodipine plasma levels (see section 4.4 Special warnings and precautions for use). Grapefruit juice results in increased peak plasma levels and bioavailability possibly due to interaction with flavanoids in the fruit juice. Therefore grapefruit juice should not be taken together with felodipine.

Cocomitant treatment with drugs such as carbamazepine, phenytoin and barbiturates (e.g. phenobarbital) and rifampicin reduces the plasma levels of felodipine via enzyme induction in the liver (cytochrome P450 System). A similar effect is expected with St John's Wort. Therefore a dose increase of felodipine may be necessary.

Hydrochlorothiazide may enhance the antihypertensive effect of felodipine.

Felodipine can induce an increase of Cmax of ciclosporin. Additionally, ciclosporin may inhibit felodipine metabolism, which may create a potential risk of felodipine toxicity.

Blood levels of digoxin increase during concomitant administration of felodipine. Therefore, decreasing of digoxin dosage should be taken into account when the two drugs are administered concurrently.

4.6 Pregnancy and lactation

Pregnancy

Felodipine is contra-indicated during the entire duration of pregnancy, as animal experiments have demonstrated foetal damage (see 5.3 Preclinical safety data). Pregnancy must be excluded before starting treatment with felodipine.

Lactation

Felodipine is excreted in breast milk. If the breast-feeding mother is taking therapeutic doses of felodipine, a fully breast-fed infant absorbs only a very low dose of the active substance with the breast milk. There is no experience of the risk this may pose to the newborn, therefore as a precaution breast-feeding should be discontinued during treatment.

4.7 Effects on ability to drive and use machines

Felodipine can cause dizziness or tiredness. These adverse effects are more likely to occur after initiation of the treatment, after dose increases, or after concomitant ingestion of alcohol. Should they occur, one should refrain from driving and other activities requiring alertness.

4.8 Undesirable effects

Adverse drug reactions are listed below by system organ class and frequency. Frequencies are defined as: very common (≥ 1/10), common (≥ 1/100, < 1/10), uncommon (≥ 1/1,000, < 1/100), rare (≥ 1/10,000, < 1/1,000), very rare (< 1/10,000), not known (cannot be estimated from the available data).

Nervous system disorders

Very common: Headache (particularly at the beginning of treatment, when the dose is increased or when high doses are administered). Generally, those effects subside on continued treatment.

Uncommon: Paraesthesia, dizziness, fatigue, syncope, restlessness

Ear and labyrinth disorders

Very common: Tinnitus (particularly at the beginning of treatment, when the dose is increased or when high doses are administered). Generally, those effects subside on continued treatment.

Cardiac disorders

Common: Particularly at the beginning of treatment, angina pectoris attacks may occur, or in patients with pre-existing angina pectoris there may be an increase in the frequency, duration and severity of the attacks.

Uncommon: Palpitations, tachycardia, hypotension.

Very rare: Myocardial infarction

Vascular disorders

Rare: Leucocytoclastic vasculitis

Respiratory, thoracic and mediastinal disorders

Uncommon: Dyspnoea

Gastrointestinal disorders

Uncommon: Nausea, vomiting, diarrhoea, constipation.

Hepatobiliary disorders

Very rare: Hepatic function disorders (elevated transaminase levels).

Skin and subcutaneous tissue disorders

Very common: Flushing (particularly at the beginning of treatment, when the dose is increased or when high doses are administered). Generally, those effects subside on continued treatment.

Uncommon: Skin and hypersensitivity reactions such as pruritus, urticaria, exanthema, photosensitisation. Gingival hyperplasia and gingivitis

Very rare: Exfoliative dermatitis

Musculoskeletal and connective tissue disorders

Uncommon: Myalgia, arthralgia, tremors

Renal and urinary disorders

Uncommon: Pollakisuria

Reproductive system and breast disorders

Very rare: Erection disorders, gynaecomastia, menorrhagia.

General disorders and administration site conditions

Common: Peripheral oedema (The degree of ankle swelling is dose related).

Uncommon: Weight gain, sweating

Very rare: Angioedema, fever

4.9 Overdose

Symptoms of intoxication

Overdose may lead to excessive peripheral vasodilatation with marked hypotension and in rare cases bradycardia.

Management of intoxication

The therapeutic measures should focus on elimination of the active ingredient (e.g. administration of charcoal, bowel irrigation) and monitoring of the vital signs. If severe hypotension occurs, symptomatic treatment should be provided, the patient should be placed supine with the legs elevated. In case of accompanying bradycardia, atropine (0.5 – 1.0 mg) should be given intravenously. Additional intravenous fluids should be cautiously administered under haemodynamic supervision to prevent cardiac overloading. Sympathomimetic drugs with predominant effect on the α_1-adrenoreceptor (such as dobutamine, dopamine, noradrenaline (norepinephrine) or adrenaline (epinephrine)) may also be given. Dosage depends on the efficacy obtained.

Felodipine is only dialysable to a minimal extent (approx. 9%).

5. PHARMACOLOGICAL PROPERTIES

5.1 Pharmacodynamic properties

Pharmacotheraputic group: 1,4-didydropyridine derivative/calcium antagonist

ATC code: C08C A02

Felodipine is a calcium antagonist of the dihydropyridine class of calcium channel blockers. Calcium antagonists interfere with the voltage-dependent L-type (slow) calcium channels in the plasma membranes of smooth muscle cells and reduce the inflow of calcium ions. This results in vasodilatation.

Felodipine has a greater selectivity for vascular smooth muscle than myocardial muscle. Felodipine selectively dilates arterioles with no effects on venous vessels. Felodipine leads to a dose-related lowering of blood pressure via vasodilatation and consequently a reduction of peripheral vascular resistance. It reduces both systolic and diastolic blood pressure. The haemodynamic effect of felodipine is accompanied by reflex (baroreceptor-mediated) tachycardia. In therapeutic doses, felodipine has no direct effect on either cardiac contractility or cardiac conduction. Felodipine reduces renal vascular resistance. The glomerular filtration rate remains unchanged.

Felodipine has a weak natriuretic/diuretic effect and does not provoke fluid retention.

Felodipine can be used as a monotherapy but also concomitantly with beta-blockers, diuretics and ACE inhibitors.

5.2 Pharmacokinetic properties

Absorption

Felodipine is completely absorbed following oral administration. Peak plasma levels are reached with the prolonged release formulation after 3 – 5 hours and result in even felodipine plasma concentrations within the therapeutic range for 24 hours. Steady state is reached approx. 3 days after starting treatment. Due to an extensive first-pass effect, only approx. 15 % of the administered dose is systemically available.

Distribution

The plasma protein binding of felodipine is > 99 %. The volume of distribution is approximately 10 l/kg at steady state, so that felodipine is indicating large tissue distribution. There is no significant accumulation during long-term treatment.

Metabolism

Felodipine is extensively metabolised in the liver by CYP3A4. All identified metabolites are inactive.

Elimination

No unchanged parent substance is detectable in the urine. The average half-life of felodipine in the terminal phase is 25 hours. The inactive hydrophilic metabolites formed by hepatic biotransformation are mainly eliminated renally (to approx. 70 %), and the remainder is excreted in the faeces. The mean plasma clearance is 1100 ml/l and depends on the hepatic blood flow.

Elderly

Increased plasma concentrations have been measured in elderly patients.

Impaired hepatic function

Increased plasma concentrations of up to 100% have been measured in patients with impaired hepatic function.

Impaired renal function

Renal impairment does not affect the pharmacokinetics of felodipine, although accumulation of inactive metabolites occurs in renal failure.

Effect of food

The rate, but not the extent of absorption is affected by the simultaneous ingestion of fatty food. Cmax was 2 to 2.5 times higher following intake of a high-fat meal compared to a fasting state.

5.3 Preclinical safety data

Preclinical data reveal no special hazard for humans based on conventional studies of safety pharmacology, repeated dose toxicity, genotoxicity and carcinogenic potential. In animal studies with respect to the reproduction, adverse effects were found. Effects in rats (prolonged duration of pregnancy and difficult labour) and rabbits (impaired development of distal phalanges, presumably due to decreased uteroplacental perfusion) revealed no evidence of a direct teratogenic effect, but indicate secondary consequences of the pharmacodynamic effect. In monkeys, an abnormal position of the distal phalanges was found. The significance of these observations for humans is unknown.

6. PHARMACEUTICAL PARTICULARS

6.1 List of excipients

Tablet core:

Lactose monohydrate, microcrystalline cellulose, hypromellose, povidone K25, propyl gallate (PhEur), colloidal anhydrous silica, magnesium stearate (PhEur)

Tablet coat:

Hypromellose, talcum, propylene glycol, titanium dioxide (E171), iron oxide red (E172), iron oxide yellow (E172).

6.2 Incompatibilities

Not applicable.

6.3 Shelf life

48 months

6.4 Special precautions for storage

Do not store above 25°C.

6.5 Nature and contents of container

PVC/PE/PVDC aluminium blister.

Pack sizes: 10, 14, 20, 28, 30, 50, 56, 60, 90, 98, 100, 250, 500 and 1000 prolonged release tablets.

Not all pack sizes may be marketed.

6.6 Special precautions for disposal and other handling

No special requirements

7. MARKETING AUTHORISATION HOLDER

Actavis UK Limited (Trading style: Actavis)

Whiddon Valley

BARNSTAPLE

N Devon EX32 8NS

8. MARKETING AUTHORISATION NUMBER(S)

PL 00142/0541

9. DATE OF FIRST AUTHORISATION/RENEWAL OF THE AUTHORISATION

21 July 2003

10. DATE OF REVISION OF THE TEXT

June 2007

Vasogen Cream

(Forest Laboratories UK Limited)

1. NAME OF THE MEDICINAL PRODUCT

VASOGEN CREAM

2. QUALITATIVE AND QUANTITATIVE COMPOSITION

Dimethicone (as silicone fluid 200) BP 20.0% w/w

Zinc oxide Ph.Eur. 7.5% w/w

Calamine BP 1.5% w/w

3. PHARMACEUTICAL FORM

Cream

4. CLINICAL PARTICULARS

4.1 Therapeutic indications

The prevention and treatment of nappy rash and bedsores. Local protection of skin around the stoma after ileostomy and colostomy.

4.2 Posology and method of administration

Vasogen is applied topically to the skin and may be either rubbed in gently or applied thinly and left to dry. Further application can be made as required.

4.3 Contraindications

Use in patients with known hypersensitivity to the product or any of its ingredients, e.g. lanolin or phenonip. Vasogen should not be applied when it is considered that free drainage is necessary, e.g. weeping dermatitis.

4.4 Special warnings and precautions for use

None

4.5 Interaction with other medicinal products and other forms of interaction

None known

4.6 Pregnancy and lactation

No restrictions

4.7 Effects on ability to drive and use machines

Not applicable

4.8 Undesirable effects

Side-effects such as local sensitivity reactions are extremely rare.

4.9 Overdose

Not applicable

5. PHARMACOLOGICAL PROPERTIES

5.1 Pharmacodynamic properties

Dimethicone is an inert polymer which has a low surface tension and is a water repellent. It is widely used in barrier creams. Zinc oxide is a mild astringent and antiseptic. Calamine has a mild astringent activity and is widely used in various dermatological conditions.

5.2 Pharmacokinetic properties

Not applicable

5.3 Preclinical safety data

There are no preclinical data of relevance to the prescriber which are additional to that already included in other sections of the SPC.

6. PHARMACEUTICAL PARTICULARS

6.1 List of excipients

Aluminium Hydroxide (wet gel)

Lanolin (anhydrous)

Methylcellulose

Phenonip

Purified Water

6.2 Incompatibilities

None known.

6.3 Shelf life

3 years

6.4 Special precautions for storage

Do not store above 25°C.

6.5 Nature and contents of container

White low-density polyethylene tube with white polypropylene cap.

Pack sizes 14, 50 and 100g.

6.6 Special precautions for disposal and other handling

None

7. MARKETING AUTHORISATION HOLDER

Forest Laboratories UK Limited

Bourne Road

Bexley

Kent DA5 1NX

8. MARKETING AUTHORISATION NUMBER(S)

PL 0108/5033R

9. DATE OF FIRST AUTHORISATION/RENEWAL OF THE AUTHORISATION

29 August 1989/26 March 1996

10. DATE OF REVISION OF THE TEXT

January 2001

11. Legal Category

GSL

Vectavir Cold Sore Cream

(Novartis Consumer Health)

1. NAME OF THE MEDICINAL PRODUCT

Vectavir Cold Sore Cream

2. QUALITATIVE AND QUANTITATIVE COMPOSITION

Each gram of the cream contains:

Active substance: 10 mg penciclovir

Excipients: cetostearyl alcohol, propylene glycol.

For a full list of excipients, see section 6.1.

3. PHARMACEUTICAL FORM

Cream

Smooth white cream of homogeneous appearance.

4. CLINICAL PARTICULARS

4.1 Therapeutic indications

Vectavir Cold Sore Cream is indicated for the treatment of cold sores (herpes labialis).

4.2 Posology and method of administration

Adults (including the elderly) and children over 12 years of age:

Vectavir Cold Sore Cream should be applied at approximately two hourly intervals during waking hours. Vectavir Cold Sore Cream may be applied with a clean finger or with a single-use applicator (for packages which contain applicators), in the amount required for the size of the affected area of skin. Treatment should be continued for 4 days.

Treatment should be started as early as possible after the first sign of an infection.

Children (under 12 years):

No work has been carried out in children below 12 years of age.

4.3 Contraindications

Known hypersensitivity to penciclovir, famciclovir or the other constituents of the formulation, eg. propylene glycol.

4.4 Special warnings and precautions for use

The cream should only be used on cold sores on the lips and around the mouth. It is not recommended for application to mucous membranes. Particular care should be taken to avoid application in or near the eyes.

Severely immunocompromised patients (eg AIDs patients or bone marrow transplant recipients) should be encouraged to consult a physician in case oral therapy is indicated.

The cream contains cetostearyl alcohol, which may cause local skin reactions (e.g. contact dermatitis). It also contains propylene glycol, which may cause skin irritation.

4.5 Interaction with other medicinal products and other forms of interaction

Clinical trial experience has not identified any interactions resulting from concomitant administration of topical or systemic drugs with Vectavir Cold Sore Cream.

4.6 Pregnancy and lactation

There is unlikely to be any cause for concern regarding adverse effects when the cream is used in pregnant and/or lactating women as systemic absorption of penciclovir following topical administration of Vectavir Cold Sore Cream has been shown to be minimal (see Section 5.2).

Animal studies have not shown any embryotoxic or teratogenic effects with penciclovir given intravenously (at doses greater than 1200 times those recommended for clinical use via topical application), nor were there any effects on male and female fertility and general reproductive performance (at doses greater than 1600 times those recommended for clinical use via topical application). Studies in rats show that penciclovir is excreted in the breast milk of lactating females given oral famciclovir (famciclovir; the oral form of penciclovir, is converted in vivo to penciclovir). There is no information on excretion of penciclovir in human milk.

Since the safety of penciclovir in human pregnancy has not been established, Vectavir Cold Sore Cream should only be used during pregnancy or in nursing mothers on the advice of a doctor, if the potential benefits are considered to outweigh the potential risks associated with treatment.

4.7 Effects on ability to drive and use machines

Adverse effects on the ability to drive or operate machinery have not been observed.

4.8 Undesirable effects

Vectavir Cold Sore Cream has been well-tolerated in human studies. Clinical trial experience has shown that there was no difference between Vectavir Cold Sore Cream and placebo in the rate or type of adverse reactions reported. In particular, application site reactions (eg transient burning, stinging, numbness) occurred in less than 3% of patients in each group in the pivotal clinical trials.

Post-marketing surveillance has revealed isolated cases of hypersensitivity-type reactions, such as allergic dermatitis, rash, urticaria, pruritus and oedema (all reactions were either localised or generalised).

No cases of photosensitivity were reported in the pivotal clinical trials.

4.9 Overdose

No untoward effects would be expected even if the entire contents of a container of Vectavir Cold Sore Cream were ingested orally; penciclovir is poorly absorbed following oral administration. However, some irritation in the mouth could occur. No specific treatment is necessary if accidental oral ingestion occurs.

5. PHARMACOLOGICAL PROPERTIES

5.1 Pharmacodynamic properties

Penciclovir has demonstrable in vivo and in vitro activity against herpes simplex viruses (types 1 and 2) and varicella zoster virus. In virus-infected cells penciclovir is rapidly and efficiently converted into a triphosphate (mediated via virus-induced thymidine kinase). Penciclovir triphosphate persists in infected cells for more than 12 hours where it inhibits replication of viral DNA and has a half-life of 9, 10 and 20 hours in cells infected with varicella zoster virus, herpes simplex virus type 1 and herpes simplex virus type 2 respectively. In uninfected cells treated with penciclovir, concentrations of penciclovir triphosphate are only barely detectable. Accordingly, uninfected cells are unlikely to be affected by therapeutic concentrations of penciclovir.

In clinical studies, Vectavir Cold Sore Cream treated patients healed 30% faster than placebo (up to one day earlier), pain resolution was 25-30% faster (median improvement of up to one day) and infectivity resolved up to 40% faster (one day earlier) than placebo.

5.2 Pharmacokinetic properties

Following application of Vectavir Cold Sore Cream in a human volunteer study at a daily dose of 180mg penciclovir (approximately 67 times the proposed daily clinical dose), to occluded and abraded skin for 4 days, penciclovir was not quantifiable in plasma and urine.

5.3 Preclinical safety data

General toxicology

Topical application of 5% Vectavir Cold Sore Cream for 4 weeks to rats and rabbits was well tolerated. There was no evidence of contact sensitisation in guinea pigs.

A full programme of studies has been completed using intravenous penciclovir. These studies did not raise any safety concerns regarding topical use of Vectavir Cold Sore Cream. There is a minimal systemic absorption of penciclovir following topical administration.

The results of a wide range of mutagenicity studies in vitro and in vivo indicates that penciclovir does not pose a genotoxic risk to man.

6. PHARMACEUTICAL PARTICULARS

6.1 List of excipients

White soft paraffin

Liquid paraffin

Cetostearyl alcohol (see section 4.4 'Special warnings and precautions for use')

Propylene glycol (see section 4.4 'Special warnings and precautions for use')

Cetomacrogol 1000

Purified water

6.2 Incompatibilities

Not applicable.

6.3 Shelf life

2g and 5g aluminium tubes - 3 years.

2g plastic airless pump dispenser - 2 years.

6.4 Special precautions for storage

Store at temperatures not exceeding 30°C.

Do not freeze.

6.5 Nature and contents of container

2g and 5g aluminium tube. May be supplied with 20 single-use Low Density Polyethylene (LDPE) applicators.

2g plastic airless pump dispenser.

Not all pack sizes may be marketed.

6.6 Special precautions for disposal and other handling

No special requirements.

7. MARKETING AUTHORISATION HOLDER

Novartis Consumer Health (UK) Limited

Wimblehurst Road

Horsham

West Sussex RH12 5AB

UK

Trading as: Novartis Consumer Health

8. MARKETING AUTHORISATION NUMBER(S)

PL 00030/0210

9. DATE OF FIRST AUTHORISATION/RENEWAL OF THE AUTHORISATION

Date of first authorisation: 2 June 2003

Date of last renewal: 16 April 2006

10. DATE OF REVISION OF THE TEXT

9 September 2008

Legal category

POM

Velcade

(Janssen-Cilag Ltd)

1. NAME OF THE MEDICINAL PRODUCT

VELCADE ▼ 3.5 mg powder for solution for injection

2. QUALITATIVE AND QUANTITATIVE COMPOSITION

Each vial contains 3.5 mg bortezomib (as a mannitol boronic ester).

After reconstitution, 1 ml of solution for injection contains 1 mg bortezomib.

For a full list of excipients, see section 6.1.

3. PHARMACEUTICAL FORM

Powder for solution for injection.

White to off-white cake or powder.

4. CLINICAL PARTICULARS

4.1 Therapeutic indications

VELCADE in combination with melphalan and prednisone is indicated for the treatment of patients with previously untreated multiple myeloma who are not eligible for high-dose chemotherapy with bone marrow transplant.

VELCADE is indicated as monotherapy for the treatment of progressive multiple myeloma in patients who have received at least 1 prior therapy and who have already undergone or are unsuitable for bone marrow transplantation.

4.2 Posology and method of administration

Treatment must be initiated and administered under the supervision of a physician qualified and experienced in the use of chemotherapeutic agents.

Posology for monotherapy

The recommended starting dose of bortezomib is 1.3 mg/m^2 body surface area twice weekly for two weeks (days 1, 4, 8, and 11) followed by a 10-day rest period (days 12-21). This 3-week period is considered a treatment cycle. At least 72 hours should elapse between consecutive doses of VELCADE.

It is recommended that patients with a confirmed complete response receive 2 additional cycles of VELCADE beyond a confirmation. It is also recommended that responding patients who do not achieve a complete remission receive a total of 8 cycles of VELCADE therapy.

Currently there are limited data concerning re-treatment with VELCADE.

Dose adjustments during treatment and re-initiation of treatment for monotherapy

VELCADE treatment must be withheld at the onset of any Grade 3 non-haematological or any Grade 4 haematological toxicities, excluding neuropathy as discussed below (see also section 4.4). Once the symptoms of the toxicity have resolved, VELCADE treatment may be re-initiated at a 25% reduced dose (1.3 mg/m^2 reduced to 1.0 mg/m^2; 1.0 mg/m^2 reduced to 0.7 mg/m^2). If the toxicity is not resolved or if it recurs at the lowest dose, discontinuation of VELCADE must be considered unless the benefit of treatment clearly outweighs the risk.

Patients who experience bortezomib-related neuropathic pain and/or peripheral neuropathy are to be managed as presented in Table 1 (see section 4.4). Patients with pre-existing severe neuropathy may be treated with VELCADE only after careful risk/benefit assessment.

Table 1: Recommended posology modifications for bortezomib-related neuropathy.*

Severity of neuropathy	Posology modification
Grade 1 (paraesthesia, weakness and/or loss of reflexes) with no pain or loss of function	No action
Grade 1 with pain or Grade 2 (interfering with function but not with activities of daily living)	Reduce to 1.0 mg/m^2
Grade 2 with pain or Grade 3 (interfering with activities of daily living)	Withhold VELCADE treatment until symptoms of toxicity have resolved. When toxicity resolves re-initiate VELCADE treatment and reduce dose to 0.7 mg/m^2 and change treatment schedule to once per week.
Grade 4 (sensory neuropathy which is disabling or motor neuropathy that is life threatening or leads to paralysis) and/or severe autonomic neuropathy	Discontinue VELCADE

* Based on posology modifications in Phase II and III multiple myeloma studies and post-marketing experience.

Paediatric patients

VELCADE is not intended for use in children below age 18 due to a lack of data on safety and efficacy (see sections 5.1 and 5.2).

Elderly patients

There is no evidence to suggest that dose adjustments are necessary in patients over 65 years of age (see section 4.8).

Renal impairment

The pharmacokinetics of bortezomib are not influenced in patients with mild to moderate renal impairment (Creatinine Clearance (CrCL)> 20 ml/min/1.73 m^2); therefore, dose adjustments are not necessary for these patients. It is unknown if the pharmacokinetics of bortezomib are influenced in patients with severe renal impairment not undergoing dialysis (CrCL < 20 ml/min/1.73 m^2). Since dialysis may reduce bortezomib concentrations, VELCADE should

Table 2: Recommended Posology for VELCADE in combination with melphalan and prednisone for patients with previously untreated multiple myeloma

Twice weekly VELCADE (cycles 1-4)												
Week	**1**				**2**		**3**	**4**		**5**		**6**
Vc (1.3 mg/m^2)	Day 1	–	–	Day 4	Day 8	Day 11	rest period	Day 22	Day 25	Day 29	Day 32	rest period
M (9 mg/m^2) P (60 mg/m^2)	Day 1	Day 2	Day 3	Day 4	–		rest period	–	–	–	–	rest period
Once weekly VELCADE (cycles 5-9)												
Week	**1**				**2**		**3**	**4**		**5**		**6**
Vc (1.3 mg/m^2)	Day 1	–	–	–	Day 8		rest period	Day 22		Day 29		rest period
M (9 mg/m^2) P (60 mg/m^2)	Day 1	Day 2	Day 3	Day 4	–		rest period	–				rest period

Vc = VELCADE; M = melphalan, P=prednisone

be administered after the dialysis procedure (see section 5.2).

Hepatic impairment

VELCADE has not been studied in patients with impaired hepatic function. Significant hepatic impairment may have an impact on the elimination of bortezomib and may increase the likelihood of interactions with other active substances. Patients with impaired liver function should be treated with extreme caution and a dose reduction should be considered (see sections 4.3 and 4.4).

Posology for combination therapy

VELCADE (bortezomib) is administered in combination with oral melphalan and oral prednisone for nine 6-week treatment cycles as shown in Table 2. In Cycles 1-4, VELCADE is administered twice weekly (days 1, 4, 8, 11, 22, 25, 29 and 32). In Cycles 5-9, VELCADE is administered once weekly (days 1, 8, 22 and 29). Melphalan and prednisone should both be given orally on days 1, 2, 3 and 4 of the first week of each cycle.

Table 2: Recommended Posology for VELCADE in combination with melphalan and prednisone for patients with previously untreated multiple myeloma

(see Table 2 above)

Dose adjustments for combination therapy

Dose modification and re-initiation of therapy when VELCADE is administered in combination with melphalan and prednisone

Prior to initiating a new cycle of therapy:

- Platelet counts should be ⩾70 × 10^9/l and the absolute neutrophils count should be ⩾ 1.0 × 10^9/l
- Non-haematological toxicities should have resolved to Grade 1 or baseline

Table3: Posology modifications during subsequent cycles

Toxicity	**Posology modification or delay**
Haematological toxicity during a cycle • If prolonged Grade 4 neutropenia or thrombocytopenia, or thrombocytopenia with bleeding is observed in the previous cycle	Consider reduction of the melphalan dose by 25% in the next cycle.
• If platelet counts ⩽30 × 10^9/l or ANC ⩽0.75 × 10^9/l on a VELCADE dosing day (other than Day 1)	VELCADE therapy should be withheld
• If several VELCADE doses in a cycle are withheld (⩾ 3 doses during twice weekly administration or ⩾ 2 doses during weekly administration)	VELCADE dose should be reduced by 1 dose level (from 1.3 mg/m^2 to 1 mg/m^2, or from 1 mg/m^2 to 0.7 mg/m^2)
Grade ⩾ 3 non-haematological toxicities	VELCADE therapy should be withheld until symptoms of the toxicity have resolved to Grade 1 or baseline. Then, VELCADE may be reinitiated with one dose level reduction (from 1.3 mg/m^2 to 1 mg/m^2, or from 1 mg/m^2 to 0.7 mg/m^2). For VELCADE-related neuropathic pain and/or peripheral neuropathy, hold and/or modify VELCADE as outlined in Table 1.

For additional information concerning melphalan and prednisone, see the corresponding Summary of Product Characteristics.

Method of administration

The reconstituted solution is administered as a 3-5 second bolus intravenous injection through a peripheral or central intravenous catheter followed by a flush with sodium chloride 9 mg/ml (0.9%) solution for injection.

4.3 Contraindications

Hypersensitivity to bortezomib, boron or to any of the excipients.

Severe hepatic impairment (see section 4.4).

Acute diffuse infiltrative pulmonary and pericardial disease.

4.4 Special warnings and precautions for use

Gastrointestinal toxicity

Gastrointestinal toxicity, including nausea, diarrhoea, vomiting and constipation are very common with VELCADE treatment. Cases of ileus have been uncommonly reported (see section 4.8), therefore patients who experience constipation should be closely monitored.

Haematological toxicity

VELCADE treatment is very commonly associated with haematological toxicities (thrombocytopenia, neutropenia and anaemia). The most common haematologic toxicity is transient thrombocytopenia. Platelets were lowest at Day 11 of each cycle of VELCADE treatment. There was no evidence of cumulative thrombocytopenia, including in the Phase II extension study. The mean platelet count nadir measured was approximately 40% of baseline. In patients with advanced myeloma the severity of thrombocytopenia was related to pre-treatment platelet count: for baseline platelet counts <75,000/μl, 90% of 21 patients had a count ⩽25,000/μl during the study, including 14% <10,000/μl; in contrast, with a baseline platelet count >75,000/μl, only 14% of 309 patients had a count ⩽25 × 10^9/l during the study. Platelet counts should be monitored prior to each dose of VELCADE. Therapy should be held when the platelet count is <25,000/μl and re-initiated at a reduced dose after resolution (see section 4.2). Potential benefit of the treatment should be carefully weighed against the risks, particularly in case of moderate to severe thrombocytopenia and risk factors for bleeding.

Therefore, complete blood counts (CBC) including platelet counts should be frequently monitored throughout treatment with VELCADE.

Peripheral neuropathy

Treatment with VELCADE is very commonly associated with peripheral neuropathy, which is predominantly sensory. However, cases of severe motor neuropathy with or without sensory peripheral neuropathy have been reported. The incidence of peripheral neuropathy increases early in the treatment and has been observed to peak during cycle 5.

It is recommended that patients be carefully monitored for symptoms of neuropathy such as a burning sensation, hyperesthesia, hypoesthesia, paraesthesia, discomfort, neuropathic pain or weakness. Patients experiencing new or worsening peripheral neuropathy should undergo neurological evaluation and may require the dose and schedule of VELCADE to be modified (see section 4.2). Neuropathy has been managed with supportive care and other therapies. Improvement in, or resolution of, peripheral neuropathy was reported in 51% of patients with ⩾ Grade 2 peripheral neuropathy in the single-agent Phase III multiple myeloma study and 71% of patients with grade 3 or 4 peripheral neuropathy or peripheral neuropathy leading to discontinuation of treatment in Phase II studies, respectively.

In addition to peripheral neuropathy, there may be a contribution of autonomic neuropathy to some adverse reactions such as postural hypotension and severe constipation with ileus. Information on autonomic neuropathy and its contribution to these undesirable effects is limited.

Seizures

Seizures have been uncommonly reported in patients without previous history of seizures or epilepsy. Special care is required when treating patients with any risk factors for seizures.

Hypotension

VELCADE treatment is commonly associated with orthostatic/postural hypotension. Most undesirable effects are mild to moderate in nature and are observed throughout treatment. Patients developing orthostatic hypotension on VELCADE did not have evidence of orthostatic hypotension prior to treatment with VELCADE. Most patients required treatment for their orthostatic hypotension. A minority of patients with orthostatic hypotension experienced syncopal events. Orthostatic/postural hypotension was not acutely related to bolus infusion of VELCADE. The mechanism of this event is unknown although a component may be due to autonomic neuropathy. Autonomic neuropathy may be related to bortezomib or bortezomib may aggravate an underlying condition such as diabetic or amyloidotic neuropathy. Caution is advised when treating patients with a history of syncope receiving medicinal products known to be associated with hypotension; or who are dehydrated due to recurrent diarrhoea or vomiting. Management of orthostatic/postural hypotension may include adjustment of antihypertensive medicinal products, rehydration or administration of mineralocorticosteroids and/or sympathomimetics. Patients should be instructed to seek medical advice if they experience symptoms of dizziness, light-headedness or fainting spells.

Heart failure

Acute development or exacerbation of congestive heart failure, and/or new onset of decreased left ventricular ejection fraction has been reported during bortezomib treatment. In a single-agent Phase III randomised, comparative study the incidence of heart failure in the VELCADE group was similar to that in the dexamethasone group. Fluid retention may be a predisposing factor for signs and symptoms of heart failure. Patients with risk factors for or existing heart disease should be closely monitored.

ECG investigations

There have been isolated cases of QT-interval prolongation in clinical studies, causality has not been established.

Pulmonary disorders

There have been rare reports of acute diffuse infiltrative pulmonary disease of unknown aetiology such as pneumonitis, interstitial pneumonia, lung infiltration, and acute respiratory distress syndrome (ARDS) in patients receiving VELCADE (see section 4.8). Some of these events have been fatal. A pre-treatment chest radiograph is recommended to determine if any additional diagnostic measures are necessary and to serve as a baseline for potential post-treatment pulmonary changes.

In the event of new or worsening pulmonary symptoms (e.g. cough, dyspnoea), a prompt diagnostic evaluation should be performed and patients treated appropriately. The benefit/risk ratio should be considered prior to continuing VELCADE therapy.

In a clinical trial, two patients (out of 2) given high-dose cytarabine (2 g/m^2 per day) by continuous infusion over 24 hours with daunorubicin and VELCADE for relapsed acute myelogenous leukaemia died of ARDS early in the course of therapy, and the study was terminated. Therefore, this specific regimen with concomitant administration with high-dose cytarabine (2g/m^2 per day) by continuous infusion over 24 hours is not recommended.

Renal impairment

Renal complications are frequent in patients with multiple myeloma. Such patients should be monitored closely (see sections 4.2 and 5.2).

Hepatic impairment

Patients with hepatic impairment should be treated with extreme caution and a dose reduction should be considered (see sections 4.2, 4.3 and 5.2).

Hepatic reactions

Rare cases of acute liver failure have been reported in patients receiving multiple concomitant medications and with serious underlying medical conditions. Other reported hepatic reactions include increases in liver enzymes, hyperbilirubinaemia, and hepatitis. Such changes may be reversible upon discontinuation of bortezomib (see section 4.8).

Tumour lysis syndrome

Because bortezomib is a cytotoxic agent and can rapidly kill malignant plasma cells, the complications of tumour lysis syndrome may occur. The patients at risk of tumour lysis syndrome are those with high tumour burden prior to treatment. These patients should be monitored closely and appropriate precautions taken.

Amyloidosis

The impact of proteasome inhibition by bortezomib on disorders associated with protein accumulation such as amyloidosis is unknown. Caution is advised in these patients.

Concomitant medicinal products

Patients should be closely monitored when given bortezomib in combination with potent CYP3A4-inhibitors. Caution should be exercised when bortezomib is combined with CYP3A4- or CYP2C19 substrates (see section 4.5).

Normal liver function should be confirmed and caution should be exercised in patients receiving oral hypoglycemics (see section 4.5).

Potentially immunocomplex-mediated reactions

Potentially immunocomplex-mediated reactions, such as serum-sickness-type reaction, polyarthritis with rash and proliferative glomerulonephritis have been reported uncommonly. Bortezomib should be discontinued if serious reactions occur.

4.5 Interaction with other medicinal products and other forms of interaction

In vitro studies indicate that bortezomib is a weak inhibitor of the cytochrome P450 (CYP) isozymes 1A2, 2C9, 2C19, 2D6 and 3A4. Based on the limited contribution (7%) of CYP2D6 to the metabolism of bortezomib, the CYP2D6 poor metabolizer phenotype is not expected to affect the overall disposition of bortezomib.

An interaction study based on data from 12 patients, assessing the effect of ketoconazole, a potent CYP3A4 inhibitor, showed a bortezomib AUC mean increase of 35% ($CI_{90\%}$ [1.032 to 1.772]). Therefore patients should be closely monitored when given bortezomib in combination with potent CYP3A4 inhibitors (e.g. ketoconazole, ritonavir).

In an interaction study based on data from 17 patients, assessing the effect of omeprazole, a potent CYP2C19 inhibitor, there was no significant effect on the pharmacokinetics of bortezomib.

Patients should be closely monitored when given bortezomib in combination with CYP2C19-inhibitors (e.g. fluoxetine).

In the absence of interaction studies investigating the effect of CYP3A4 inducers on the pharmacokinetics of bortezomib, patients should be closely monitored when given bortezomib in combination with potent CYP3A4 inducers (e.g. rifampicin).

An interaction study assessing the effect of melphalan-prednisone on bortezomib showed a 17% increase in mean bortezomib AUC based on data from 21 patients. This is not considered clinically relevant.

During clinical trials, hypoglycemia and hyperglycemia were uncommonly and commonly reported in diabetic patients receiving oral hypoglycemics. Patients on oral antidiabetic agents receiving VELCADE treatment may require close monitoring of their blood glucose levels and adjustment of the dose of their antidiabetics.

4.6 Pregnancy and lactation

The teratogenic potential of bortezomib has not been fully investigated.

In non-clinical studies, bortezomib had no effects on embryonal/foetal development in rats and rabbits at the highest maternally tolerated doses. Animal studies to determine the effects of bortezomib parturition and postnatal development were not conducted (see section 5.3). VELCADE should not be used during pregnancy unless clearly necessary.

For VELCADE no clinical data with regard to exposure during pregnancy are available. Male and female patients of childbearing potential must use effective contraceptive measures during and for 3 months following treatment. If VELCADE is used during pregnancy, or if the patient becomes pregnant while receiving this medicinal product, the patient should be informed of potential for hazard to the foetus.

It is not known whether bortezomib is excreted in human milk. Because of the potential for serious undesirable effects in breast-fed infants, lactation should be discontinued during treatment with VELCADE.

4.7 Effects on ability to drive and use machines

VELCADE may have a moderate influence on the ability to drive and use machines. VELCADE may be associated with fatigue very commonly, dizziness commonly, syncope uncommonly, orthostatic/postural hypotension or blurred vision commonly. Therefore, patients must be cautious when operating machinery, or when driving (see section 4.8).

4.8 Undesirable effects

The following undesirable effects were considered by the investigators to have at least a possible or probable causal relationship to VELCADE during the conduct of 5 non-comparative Phase II studies and 1 comparative Phase III trial VELCADE vs dexamethasone in 663 patients with relapsed or refractory multiple myeloma, of whom 331 received VELCADE as single agent. The safety database comprises data from patients with multiple myeloma or

Table 4: Adverse reactions in patients with relapsed/refractory multiple myeloma

Infections and infestations *Very common*: herpes zoster (including disseminated). *Common*: pneumonia, bronchitis, sinusitis, nasopharyngitis, herpes simplex. *Uncommon*: sepsis, bacteraemia, pneumonia pneumococcal, bronchopneumonia, upper and lower respiratory tract infection, catheter related infection, pleural infection, haemophilus infection, cytomegalovirus infection, influenza, infectious mononucleosis, varicella, urinary tract infection, gastroenteritis, candidal infection, fungal infection, post herpetic neuralgia, oral candidiasis, blepharitis, infection.
Neoplasms benign and malignant (including cysts and polyps) *Uncommon*: tumour lysis syndrome (see section 4.4).
Blood and lymphatic system disorders (see section 4.4) *Very common*: thrombocytopenia, neutropenia, anaemia. *Common*: leukopenia, lymphopenia. *Uncommon*: pancytopenia, febrile neutropenia, haemolytic anaemia, thrombocytopenic purpura, lymphadenopathy.
Immune system disorders *Uncommon*: hypersensitivity, immunocomplex mediated hypersensitivity, potentially immunocomplex-mediated reactions, such as serum-sickness-type reaction, polyarthritis with rash and proliferative glomerulonephritis (see section 4.4).
Endocrine disorders *Uncommon*: inappropriate antidiuretic hormone (ADH) secretion.
Metabolism and nutrition disorders *Very common*: appetite decreased. *Common*: dehydration, hypokalaemia, hyperglycaemia. Uncommon: hyperkalaemia, cachexia, hypercalcaemia, hypocalcaemia, hypernatraemia, hyponatraemia, hypoglycaemia, hyperuricaemia, vitamin B12 deficiency, appetite increased, hypomagnesaemia, hypophosphataemia.
Psychiatric disorders *Common*: confusion, depression, insomnia, anxiety. *Uncommon*: agitation, delirium, hallucinations, restlessness, mood swings, mental status changes, sleep disorder, irritability, abnormal dreams.
Nervous system disorders(see sections 4.4 and 4.7) *Very common:* peripheral neuropathy, peripheral sensory neuropathy (see section 4.4), paraesthesia, headache. *Common*: polyneuropathy, peripheral neuropathy aggravated, dizziness (excluding vertigo), dysgeusia, dysaesthesia, hypoaesthesia, tremor. *Uncommon*: paraplegia, intracranial haemorrhage, subarachnoid haemorrhage convulsions (see section 4.4), peripheral motor neuropathy, syncope, paresis, disturbance in attention, increased activity, ageusia, somnolence, migraine, cognitive disorder, jerky movements, dizziness postural, sciatica, mononeuropathy, speech disorder, restless leg syndrome.
Eye disorders *Common*: vision blurred (see section 4.7), eye pain. *Uncommon*: eye haemorrhage, vision abnormal, dry eye, conjunctivitis, eye discharge, photophobia, eye irritation, lacrimation increased, conjunctival hyperaemia, eye swelling.
Ear and labyrinth disorders *Common*: vertigo. *Uncommon*: deafness, tinnitus, hypoacusis, hearing impaired.
Cardiac disorders *Uncommon*: cardiac arrest, cardiogenic shock, myocardial infarction, angina pectoris, angina unstable, development or exacerbation of congestive heart failure (see section 4.4), cardiac failure, ventricular hypokinesia, pulmonary oedema and acute pulmonary oedema, sinus arrest, atrioventricular block complete, tachycardia, sinus tachycardia, supraventricular tachycardia, arrhythmia, atrial fibrillation, palpitations. *Rare*: new onset of decreased left ventricular ejection fraction.
Vascular disorders *Common*: hypotension, orthostatic and postural hypotension (see sections 4.4 and 4.7), phlebitis, haematoma, hypertension. *Uncommon*: cerebral hemorrhage, vasculitis, cerebrovascular accident, pulmonary hypertension, petechiae, ecchymosis, purpura, vein discolouration, vein distended, wound hemorrhage, flushing, hot flushes.
Respiratory, thoracic and mediastinal disorders *Very Common*: dyspnoea. *Common*: dyspnoea exertional, epistaxis, cough, rhinorrhoea. *Uncommon*: respiratory arrest, hypoxia, pulmonary congestion, pleural effusion, asthma, respiratory alkalosis, tachypnoea, wheezing, nasal congestion, hoarseness, rhinitis, hyperventilation, orthopnoea, chest wall pain, sinus pain, throat tightness, productive cough.
Gastrointestinal disorders (see section 4.4) *Very common:* vomiting, diarrhoea, nausea, constipation. *Common*: abdominal pain, stomatitis, dyspepsia, loose stools, abdominal pain upper, flatulence, abdominal distension, hiccups, mouth ulceration, pharyngolaryngeal pain, dry mouth. *Uncommon*: acute pancreatitis, ileus paralytic, antibiotic associated colitis, colitis, haematemesis, diarrhoea haemorrhagic, gastrointestinal haemorrhage, rectal haemorrhage, enteritis, dysphagia, abdominal discomfort, eructation, gastrointestinal motility disorder, oral pain, retching, change in bowel habit, spleen pain, oesophagitis, gastritis, gastro-oesophageal reflux disease, gastrointestinal pain, gingival bleeding, gingival pain, hiatus hernia, irritable bowel syndrome, oral mucosal petechiae, salivary hypersecretion, tongue coated, tongue discolouration, faecal impaction.
Hepato-biliary disorders (see section 4.4) *Uncommon:* hepatitis, hepatic haemorrhage, hypoproteinaemia, hyperbilirubinaemia.
Skin and subcutaneous tissue disorders *Very common:* rash. *Common*: periorbital oedema, urticaria, rash pruritic, pruritus, erythema, sweating increased, dry skin, eczema. *Uncommon*: vasculitic rash, rash erythematous, photosensitivity reaction, contusion, pruritus generalised, rash macular, rash papular, psoriasis, rash generalized, eyelid oedema, face oedema, dermatitis, alopecia, nail disorder, skin discolouration, dermatitis atopic, hair texture abnormal, heat rash, night sweats, pressure sore, ichthyosis, skin nodule.
Musculoskeletal, connective tissue and bone disorders *Very Common*: myalgia. *Common*: muscle weakness, musculoskeletal pain, pain in limb, muscle cramps, arthralgia, bone pain, back pain, peripheral swelling. *Uncommon*: muscle spasms, muscle twitching or sensation of heaviness, muscle stiffness, joint swelling, joint stiffness, buttock pain, swelling, pain in jaw.
Renal and urinary disorders *Common*: renal impairment, dysuria. *Uncommon*: renal failure acute, renal failure, oliguria, renal colic, haematuria, proteinuria, urinary retention, urinary frequency, difficulty in micturition, loin pain, urinary incontinence, micturition urgency.
Reproductive system and breast disorders *Uncommon*: testicular pain, erectile dysfunction.
General disorders and administration site conditions *Very Common*: fatigue (see section 4.7), pyrexia. *Common*: asthenia, weakness, lethargy, rigors, malaise, influenza like illness, oedema peripheral, chest pain, pain, oedema. *Uncommon*: fall, mucosal haemorrhage, mucosal inflammation, neuralgia, injection site phlebitis, extravasation inflammation tenderness, injection site erythema, feeling cold, chest pressure sensation, chest discomfort, groin pain, chest tightness.
Investigations *Common*: weight decreased, blood lactate dehydrogenase increased. *Uncommon*: alanine aminotransferase increased, aspartate aminotransferase increased, blood bilirubin increased, blood alkaline phosphatase increased, blood creatinine increased, blood urea increased, gamma-glutamyltransferase increased, blood amylase increased, liver function tests abnormal, red blood cell count decreased, white blood cell count decreased, blood bicarbonate decreased, heart rate irregular, C-reactive protein increased, blood phosphate decreased, weight increased.
Injury and poisoning *Uncommon*: catheter related complications, post procedural pain, post procedural haemorrhage, burns.

Table 5: Treatment emergent drug-related adverse reactions reported in ≥ 10% of patients treated with VELCADE in combination with melphalan and prednisone

	Vc+M+P			M+P		
	(n=340)			(n=337)		
MedDRA System Organ Class	Total	Toxicity Grade, n (%)		Total	Toxicity Grade, n (%)	
Preferred Term	n (%)	3	≥4	n (%)	3	≥4
Infections and Infestations						
Herpes Zoster	39 (11)	11 (3)	0	9 (3)	4 (1)	0
Blood and lymphatic system disorders						
Thrombocytopenia	164 (48)	60 (18)	57 (17)	140 (42)	48 (14)	39 (12)
Neutropenia	160 (47)	101 (30)	33 (10)	143 (42)	77 (23)	42 (12)
Anaemia	109 (32)	41 (12)	4 (1)	156 (46)	61 (18)	18 (5)
Leukopenia	108 (32)	64 (19)	8 (2)	93 (28)	53 (16)	11 (3)
Lymphopenia	78 (23)	46 (14)	17 (5)	51 (15)	26 (8)	7 (2)
Metabolism and nutrition disorders						
Anorexia	64 (19)	6 (2)	0	19 (6)	0	0
Psychiatric disorders						
Insomnia	35 (10)	1 (<1)	0	21 (6)	0	0
Nervous system disorders						
Peripheral Neuropathy	156 (46)	42 (12)	2 (1)	4 (1)	0	0
Neuralgia	117 (34)	27 (8)	2 (1)	1 (<1)	0	0
Paraesthesia	42 (12)	6 (2)	0	4 (1)	0	0
Gastrointestinal disorders						
Nausea	134 (39)	10 (3)	0	70 (21)	1 (<1)	0
Diarrhoea	119 (35)	19 (6)	2 (1)	20 (6)	1 (<1)	0
Vomiting	87 (26)	13 (4)	0	41 (12)	2 (1)	0
Constipation	77 (23)	2 (1)	0	14 (4)	0	0
Abdominal Pain Upper	34 (10)	1 (<1)	0	20 (6)	0	0
Skin and subcutaneous tissue disorders						
Rash	38 (11)	2 (1)	0	7 (2)	0	0
General disorders and administration site conditions						
Fatigue	85 (25)	19 (6)	2 (1)	48 (14)	4 (1)	0
Asthenia	54 (16)	18 (5)	0	23 (7)	3 (1)	0
Pyrexia	53 (16)	4 (1)	0	19 (6)	1 (<1)	1 (<1)

B-cell lymphocytic leukemia (CLL). Patients were treated with VELCADE as a single agent, or in combination with dexamethasone.

Adverse reactions are listed below by system organ class and frequency grouping. Frequencies are defined as: Very common (≥1/10); common (≥1/100 to <1/10); uncommon (≥1/1,000 to <1/100); rare (≥1/10,000 to <1/1,000); very rare (<1/10,000), not known (cannot be estimated from the available data). Within each frequency grouping, undesirable effects are presented in order of decreasing seriousness.

Table 4: Adverse reactions in patients with relapsed/refractory multiple myeloma

(see Table 4 on previous page)

Summary of safety data in patients with previously untreated multiple myeloma:

The following table 5 describes safety data from 340 patients with previously untreated multiple myeloma who received VELCADE (1.3 mg/m^2) in combination with melphalan (9 mg/m^2) and prednisone (60 mg/m^2) in a prospective Phase III study.

Overall, the safety profile of patients treated with VELCADE in monotherapy was similar to that observed in patients treated with VELCADE in combination with melphalan and prednisone.

Table 5: Treatment emergent drug-related adverse reactions reported in ≥ 10% of patients treated with VELCADE in combination with melphalan and prednisone

(see Table 5 above)

Herpes zoster virus reactivation

Antiviral prophylaxis should be considered in patients being treated with VELCADE. In the Phase III study in patients with previously untreated multiple myeloma, the overall incidence of herpes zoster reactivation was more common in patients treated with Vc+M+P compared with M+P (14% vs 4% respectively). Antiviral prophylaxis was administered to 26% of the patients in the VcMP arm. The incidence of herpes zoster among patients in the VcMP treatment group was 17% for patients not administered antiviral prophylaxis compared to 3% for patients administered antiviral prophylaxis.

Post Marketing Experience

Clinically significant adverse reactions are listed in Table 6, if they have been reported during post approval use of VELCADE and may or may not have been reported in clinical trials. Their frequency is not known.

Table 6: Adverse reactions from post-marketing reports

Infections and infestations	
Not known:	Herpes meningoencephalitis, septic shock
Immune system disorders	
Not known:	Angioedema
Nervous system disorders	
Not known:	Encephalopathy, autonomic neuropathy
Eye disorders	
Not known:	Ophthalmic herpes
Cardiac disorders	
Not known:	Cardiac tamponade, pericarditis, cardiac and cardiopulmonary arrest, ventricular arrhythmias, atrio-ventricular block complete, atrial fibrillation, tachycardia, sinus and ventricular tachycardia
Respiratory, thoracic and mediastinal disorders (see section 4.4)	
Not known:	Pneumonitis, pneumonia, interstitial pneumonia, Acute Respiratory Distress Syndrome (ARDS), acute diffuse infiltrative pulmonary disease, pulmonary hypertension, respiratory failure, pulmonary alveolar haemorrhage, acute pulmonary oedema, pulmonary oedema, pulmonary embolism, peripheral embolism
Gastrointestinal disorders	
Not known:	Ischemic colitis
Hepatobiliary disorders	
Not known:	Liver failure
Skin and subcutaneous tissue disorders	
Not known:	Stevens-Johnson Syndrome, toxic epidermal necrolysis

4.9 Overdose

In patients, overdose more than twice the recommended dose has been associated with the acute onset of symptomatic hypotension and thrombocytopenia with fatal outcomes. For preclinical cardiovascular safety pharmacology studies, see section 5.3.

There is no known specific antidote for bortezomib overdose. In the event of an overdose, the patient's vital signs should be monitored and appropriate supportive care given to maintain blood pressure (such as fluids, pressors, and/or inotropic agents) and body temperature (see sections 4.2 and 4.4).

5. PHARMACOLOGICAL PROPERTIES

5.1 Pharmacodynamic properties

Pharmacotherapeutic group: Other antineoplastic agent, ATC code: L01XX32

This medicinal product has been authorised under "Exceptional Circumstances". This means that for scientific reasons it has not been possible to obtain complete information on this medicinal product.

The European Medicines Agency (EMEA) will review any new information which may become available every year and this SPC will be updated as necessary.

Mechanism of action

Bortezomib is a proteasome inhibitor. It is specifically designed to inhibit the chymotrypsin-like activity of the 26S proteasome in mammalian cells. The 26S proteasome is a large protein complex that degrades ubiquitinated proteins. The ubiquitin-proteasome pathway plays an essential role in regulating the turnover of specific proteins, thereby maintaining homeostasis within cells. Inhibition of the 26S proteasome prevents this targeted proteolysis and affects multiple signalling cascades within the cell, ultimately resulting in cancer cell death.

Bortezomib is highly selective for the proteasome. At 10 μM concentrations, bortezomib does not inhibit any of a wide variety of receptors and proteases screened and is more than 1500-fold more selective for the proteasome than for its next preferable enzyme. The kinetics of proteasome inhibition were evaluated *in vitro*, and bortezomib was shown to dissociate from the proteasome with a $t_{1/2}$ of 20 minutes, thus demonstrating that proteasome inhibition by bortezomib is reversible.

Bortezomib mediated proteasome inhibition affects cancer cells in a number of ways, including, but not limited to, altering regulatory proteins, which control cell cycle progression and nuclear factor kappa B (NF-kB) activation. Inhibition of the proteasome results in cell cycle arrest and apoptosis. NF-kB is a transcription factor whose activation is required for many aspects of tumourigenesis, including cell growth and survival, angiogenesis, cell-cell interactions, and metastasis. In myeloma, bortezomib affects the ability of myeloma cells to interact with the bone marrow microenvironment.

Experiments have demonstrated that bortezomib is cytotoxic to a variety of cancer cell types and that cancer cells are more sensitive to the proapoptotic effects of proteasome inhibition than normal cells. Bortezomib causes reduction of tumour growth *in vivo* in many preclinical tumour models, including multiple myeloma.

Clinical efficacy in previously untreated multiple myeloma

A prospective Phase III, international, randomized (1:1), open-label clinical study (VISTA) of 682 patients was conducted to determine whether VELCADE (1.3 mg/m^2) in combination with melphalan (9 mg/m^2) and prednisone (60 mg/m^2) resulted in improvement in time to progression (TTP) when compared to melphalan (9 mg/m^2) and prednisone (60 mg/m^2) in patients with previously untreated multiple myeloma. Treatment was administered for a maximum of 9 cycles (approximately 54 weeks) and was discontinued early for disease progression or unacceptable toxicity. Baseline demographics and patient characteristics are summarized in Table 7.

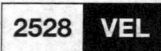

Table 7: Summary of baseline patient and disease characteristics in the VISTA study

Patient Characteristics	Vc+M+P n=344	M+P n=338
Median age in years (range)	71.0 (57, 90)	71.0 (48, 91)
Gender: male/female	51% / 49%	49% / 51%
Race: Caucasian/asian/ black/other	88% / 10% / 1% / 1%	87% / 11% / 2% / 0%
Karnofsky performance status score ⩽70	35%	33%
Hemoglobin <100 g/l	37%	36%
Platelet count <75 × 10^9/l	<1%	1%
Disease Characteristics		
Type of myeloma (%): IgG/IgA/Light chain	64% / 24% / 8%	62% / 26% / 8%
Median β2-microglobulin (mg/l)	4.2	4.3
Median albumin (g/l)	33.0	33.0
Creatinine clearance ⩽30 ml/min [n (%)]	20 (6%)	16 (5%)

At the time of a pre-specified interim analysis, the primary endpoint, time to progression, was met and patients in the M+P arm were offered Vc+M+P treatment. Survival continued to be followed after the interim analysis. Median follow-up was 16.3 months. Efficacy results are presented in Table 8:

Table 8: Summary of Efficacy Analyses in the VISTA study

Efficacy endpoint	Vc+M+P n=344	M+P n=338
Time to progression Events n (%)	101 (29)	152 (45)
Median[a] (95% CI)	20.7 mo (17.6, 24,7)	15.0 mo (14.1, 17.9)
Hazard ratio[b] (95% CI)	0.54 (0.42, 0.70)	
p-value [c]	0.000002	
Progression-free survival Events n (%)	135 (39)	190 (56)
Median[a] (95% CI)	18.3 mo (16.6, 21.7)	14.0 mo (11.1, 15.0)
Hazard ratio[b] (95% CI)	0.61 (0.49, 0.76)	
p-value [c]	0.00001	
Overall survival Events (deaths) n (%)	45 (13)	76 (23)
Hazard ratio[b] (95% CI)	0.61 (0.42, 0.88)	
p-value [c]	0.00782	
Response rate population[e] n = 668	n=337	n=331
CR[f] n (%)	102 (30)	12 (4)
PR[f] n (%)	136 (40)	103 (31)
nCR n (%)	5 (1)	0
CR + PR[f] n (%)	238 (71)	115 (35)
p-value[d]	$<10^{-10}$	
Reduction in serum M-protein population[g] n=667	n=336	n=331
>=90% n (%)	151 (45)	34 (10)
Time to first response in CR + PR		
Median	1.4 mo	4.2 mo
Median[a] response duration		
CR[f]	24.0 mo	12.8 mo
CR + PR[f]	19.9 mo	13.1 mo
Time to next therapy Events n (%)	73 (21)	127 (38)
Median[a] (95% CI)	NE (26.1, NE)	20.8 mo (18.3, 28.5)
Hazard ratio[b] (95% CI)	0.52 (0.39, 0.70)	
p-value [c]	0.000009	

[a] Kaplan-Meier estimate.

[b] Hazard ratio estimate is based on a Cox proportional-hazard model adjusted for stratification factors: β_2-microglobulin, albumin, and region. A hazard ratio less than 1 indicates an advantage for VMP

[c] p-value based on the stratified log-rank test adjusted for stratification factors: β_2-microglobulin, albumin, and region

[d] p-value for Response Rate (CR + PR) from the Cochran-Mantel-Haenszel chi-square test adjusted for the stratification factors

[e] Response population includes patients who had measurable disease at baseline

[f] EBMT criteria

[g] All randomized patients with secretory disease

NE: Not estimable

Clinical efficacy in relapsed or refractory multiple myeloma

The safety and efficacy of VELCADE were evaluated in 2 studies at the recommended dose of 1.3 mg/m^2: a Phase III randomized, comparative study, versus dexamethasone (Dex), of 669 patients with relapsed or refractory multiple myeloma who had received 1-3 prior lines of therapy, and a Phase II single-arm study of 202 patients with relapsed and refractory multiple myeloma, who had received at least 2 prior lines of treatment and who were progressing on their most recent treatment. (see Tables 9, 10 and 11).

Table 9: Dosing regimens in Phase II and Phase III studies

(see Table 9 below)

Table 10: Patient characteristics in Phase II and Phase III studies

(see Table 10 below)

Table 11: Patient exposure to treatment with VELCADE during Phase II and III studies

(see Table 11 on next page)

In the Phase III study, treatment with VELCADE led to a significantly longer time to progression, a significantly prolonged survival and a significantly higher response rate, compared to treatment with dexamethasone (see Table 12), in all patients as well as in patients who have received 1 prior line of therapy. As a result of a preplanned interim analysis, the dexamethasone arm was halted at the recommendation of the data monitoring committee and all patients randomised to dexamethasone were then offered VELCADE, regardless of disease status. Due to this early crossover, the median duration of follow-up for surviving patients is 8.3 months. Both in patients who were refractory to their last prior therapy and those who were not refractory, overall survival was significantly longer and response rate was significantly higher on the VELCADE arm.

Of the 669 patients enrolled, 245 (37%) were 65 years of age or older. Response parameters as well as TTP remained significantly better for VELCADE independently of age. Regardless of β_2- microglobulin levels at baseline, all efficacy parameters (time to progression and overall survival, as well as response rate) were significantly improved on the VELCADE arm.

In the refractory population of the Phase II study, responses were determined by an independent review committee and the response criteria were those of the European Bone Marrow Transplant Group. The median survival of all patients enrolled was 17 months (range

Table 9 : Dosing regimens in Phase II and Phase III studies

Phase/arm	Treatment schedule	Dose	Regimen
II	Vc: Day 1,4,8,11, (rest Day 12-21)	1.3 mg/m^2 (intravenous bolus)	Q3 weeks × 8 cycles (extension**)
III	Vc* a) Days 1,4,8,11, (Rest Day 12-21) b) Days 1,8,15,22	1.3 mg/m^2 (intravenous bolus)	a) Q3weeks × 8, then b) Q5 weeks × 3
III	Dex a) Days 1–4, 9–12, 17–20 b) Days 1–4	40 mg (oral)	a) Q5 week × 4 b) Q4 week × 5
II	Add Dex***	20 mg (oral) (Days 1,2,4,5,8,9, 11,12)	Q3 weeks

*a) is the initial treatment, a) and b) represent a full course of treatment

**An extension study authorised patients benefiting from treatment to continue receiving VELCADE

***If after 2 or 4 cycles of VELCADE, the patients had progressive disease or stable disease, respectively, they could receive dexamethasone

Table 10: Patient characteristics in Phase II and Phase III studies

	Phase II Vc	Phase III Vc	Phase III Dex
Patient number, ITT analysis	202	333	336
Male %	60	56	60
Median age, yrs (range)	59 (34-84)	61 (33-84)	61 (27-86)
Caucasian	81 %	90 %	88 %
Karnofsky PS>80%	80 %	87 %	84 %
Platelets < 75,000/μl	21 %	6 %	4 %
Hemoglobin < 100g/l	44 %	32 %	28 %
Median Creatinine Clearance, ml/min (range)	74 (14-221)	73.3 (15.6-170.7)	73.3 (15.3-261.1)
Myeloma IgG	60 %	60 %	59 %
Myeloma IgA	24 %	23 %	24 %
Myeloma light chain	14 %	12 %	13 %
Median duration since diagnosis (yrs)	4.0	3.5	3.1
Chromosome 13 abnormalities	15 %	25.7 %	25.0 %
Median β_2 microglobulin (mg/l)	3.5	3.7	3.6
Median number prior treatment lines* (range)	6 (2-15)	2 (1-7)	2 (1-8)
1 prior line > 1 prior line	0	n =132 (40 %) n = 186 (60 %)	n = 119 (35 %) n = 194 (65 %)

*Including steroids, alkylating agents, anthracyclines, thalidomide and stem cell transplants

Table 11: Patient exposure to treatment with VELCADE during Phase II and III studies

	Phase II Vc	Phase III Vc	Phase III Dex
Received at least 1 dose	n = 202	n =331	n = 332
Completed 4 cycles a) all initial cycles (number) b) full course (number) c) extension *	62 % 27 % (8 cycles) NA n = 63 pts (median 7 cycles) or total median 14 cycles (range 7-32)	69 % 29 % (8 cycles) 9 % (11 cycles) NA	 36 % (4 cycles) 5 % (9 cycles) NA

*Patients could continue on treatment after completing 8 cycles, in case of benefit

NA = not applicable

Table 12: Summary of Disease Outcomes from the Phase III and Phase II studies

	Phase III All patients		Phase III 1 Prior line of therapy		Phase III >1 Prior line of therapy		Phase II ≥ 2 prior lines
Time related events	**Vc n =333[a]**	**Dex n =336[a]**	**Vc n =132[a]**	**Dex n =119[a]**	**Vc n =200[a]**	**Dex n =217[a]**	**Vc n =202[a]**
TTP, days [95% CI]	189[b] [148, 211]	106[b] [86, 128]	212[d] [188, 267]	169[d] [105, 191]	148[b] [129, 192]	87[b] [84, 107]	210 [154, 281]
1 year survival, % [95% CI]	80[d] [74,85]	66[d] [59,72]	89[d] [82,95]	72[d] [62,83]	73 [64,82]	62 [53,71]	60
Best response (%)	**Vc n =315[c]**	**Dex n =312[c]**	**Vc n =128**	**Dex n =110**	**Vc n =187**	**Dex n =202**	**Vc n=193**
CR	20 (6) [b]	2 (<1) [b]	8 (6)	2 (2)	12 (6)	0 (0)	(4)**
CR + nCR	41 (13) [b]	5 (2) [b]	16 (13)	4 (4)	25 (13)	1 (<1)	(10)**
CR+ nCR + PR	121 (38) [b]	56 (18) [b]	57 (45) [d]	29 (26) [d]	64 (34) [b]	27 (13) [b]	(27)**
CR + nCR+ PR+MR	146 (46)	108 (35)	66 (52)	45 (41)	80 (43)	63 (31)	(35)**
Median duration Days (months)	242 (8.0)	169 (5.6)	246 (8.1)	189 (6.2)	238 (7.8)	126 (4.1)	385*
Time to response CR + PR (days)	43	43	44	46	41	27	38*

[a] Intent to Treat (ITT) population

[b] p-value from the stratified log-rank test; analysis by line of therapy excludes stratification for therapeutic history; $p<0.0001$

[c] Response population includes patients who had measurable disease at baseline and received at least 1 dose of study drug.

[d] p-value from the Cochran-Mantel-Haenszel chi-square test adjusted for the stratification factors; analysis by line of therapy excludes stratification for therapeutic history

*CR+PR+MR **CR=CR, (IF-); nCR=CR (IF+)

NA = not applicable, NE = not estimated

<1 to 36+ months). This survival was greater than the six-to-nine month median survival anticipated by consultant clinical investigators for a similar patient population. By multivariate analysis, the response rate was independent of myeloma type, performance status, chromosome 13 deletion status, or the number or type of previous therapies. Patients who had received 2 to 3 prior therapeutic regimens had a response rate of 32% (10/32) and patients who received greater than 7 prior therapeutic regimens had a response rate of 31% (21/67).

Table 12: Summary of Disease Outcomes from the Phase III and Phase II studies

(see Table 12 above)

In the Phase II study, patients who did not obtain an optimal response to therapy with VELCADE alone were able to receive high-dose dexamethasone in conjunction with VELCADE (see Table 9). The protocol allowed patients to receive dexamethasone if they had had a less than optimal response to VELCADE alone. A total of 74 evaluable patients were administered dexamethasone in combination with VELCADE. Eighteen percent of patients achieved, or had an improved response (MR (11%) or PR (7%)) with combination treatment.

5.2 Pharmacokinetic properties

Following intravenous bolus administration of a 1.0 mg/m^2 and 1.3 mg/m^2 dose to 11 patients with multiple myeloma and creatinine clearance values greater than 50 ml/min, the mean first-dose maximum plasma concentrations of bortezomib were 57 and 112 ng/ml, respectively. In subsequent doses, mean maximum observed plasma concentrations ranged from 67 to 106 ng/ml for the 1.0 mg/m^2 dose and 89 to 120 ng/ml for the 1.3 mg/m^2 dose.

Distribution

The mean distribution volume (V_d) of bortezomib ranged from 1659 l to 3294 l following single- or repeated-dose administration of 1.0 mg/m^2 or 1.3 mg/m^2 to patients with multiple myeloma. This suggests that bortezomib distributes widely to peripheral tissues. Over a bortezomib concentration range of 0.01 to 1.0 µg/ml, the *in vitro* protein binding averaged 82.9% in human plasma. The fraction of bortezomib bound to plasma proteins was not concentration-dependent.

Metabolism

In vitro studies with human liver microsomes and human cDNA-expressed cytochrome P450 isozymes indicate that bortezomib is primarily oxidatively metabolized via cytochrome P450 enzymes, 3A4, 2C19, and 1A2. The major metabolic pathway is deboronation to form two deboronated metabolites that subsequently undergo hydroxylation to several metabolites. Deboronated-bortezomib metabolites are inactive as 26S proteasome inhibitors.

Elimination

The mean elimination half-life of bortezomib upon multiple dosing ranged from 40-193 hours. Bortezomib is eliminated more rapidly following the first dose compared to subsequent doses. Mean total body clearances were 102 and 112 l/h following the first dose for doses of 1.0 mg/m^2 and 1.3 mg/m^2, respectively, and ranged from 15 to 32 l/h and 18 to 32 l/h following subsequent doses for doses of 1.0 mg/m^2 and 1.3 mg/m^2, respectively.

Special populations

Hepatic impairment

Formal studies in patients with severely impaired hepatic function have not been conducted to date (see section 4.4). In the absence of data VELCADE is contraindicated in patients with severe liver impairment (see section 4.3).

Renal impairment

A pharmacokinetic study was conducted in patients with various degrees of renal impairment who were classified according to their creatinine clearance values (CrCL) into the following groups: Normal (CrCL ≥ 60 ml/min/1.73 m^2, n=12), Mild (CrCL = 40-59 ml/min/1.73 m^2, n = 10), Moderate (CrCL = 20-39 ml/min/1.73 m^2, n = 9), and Severe (CrCL < 20 ml/min/1.73 m^2, n = 3). A group of dialysis patients who were dosed after dialysis was also included in the study (n = 8). Patients were administered intravenous doses of 0.7 to 1.3 mg/m^2 of VELCADE twice weekly. Exposure of VELCADE (dose-normalized AUC and Cmax) was comparable among all the groups (see section 4.2).

5.3 Preclinical safety data

Bortezomib was positive for clastogenic activity (structural chromosomal aberrations) in the *in vitro* chromosomal aberration assay using Chinese hamster ovary cells (CHO) at concentrations as low as 3.125 µg/ml, which was the lowest concentration evaluated. Bortezomib was not genotoxic when tested in the *in vitro* mutagenicity assay (Ames assay) and *in vivo* micronucleus assay in mice.

Developmental toxicity studies in the rat and rabbit have shown embryo-fetal lethality at maternally toxic dosages, but no direct embryo-foetal toxicity below maternally toxic dosages. Fertility studies were not performed but evaluation of reproductive tissues has been performed in the general toxicity studies. In the 6-month rat study, degenerative effects in both the testes and the ovary have been observed. It is, therefore, likely that bortezomib could have a potential effect on either male or female fertility. Peri- and postnatal development studies were not conducted.

In multi-cycle general toxicity studies conducted in the rat and monkey, the principal target organs included the gastrointestinal tract, resulting in vomiting and/or diarrhoea, haematopoietic and lymphatic tissues resulting in peripheral blood cytopenias, lymphoid tissue atrophy and hematopoietic bone marrow hypocellularity: peripheral neuropathy (observed in monkeys, mice and dogs) involving sensory nerve axons; and mild changes in the kidneys. All these target organs have shown partial to full recovery following discontinuation of treatment.

Based on animal studies, the penetration of bortezomib through the blood-brain barrier appears to be limited, if any and the relevance to humans is unknown.

Cardiovascular safety pharmacology studies in monkeys and dogs show that intravenous doses approximately two to three times the recommended clinical dose on a mg/m^2 basis are associated with increases in heart rate, decreases in contractility, hypotension and death. In dogs, the decreased cardiac contractility and hypotension responded to acute intervention with positive inotropic or pressor agents. Moreover, in dog studies, a slight increase in the corrected QT interval was observed.

6. PHARMACEUTICAL PARTICULARS

6.1 List of excipients

Mannitol (E 421)

Nitrogen.

6.2 Incompatibilities

This medicinal product must not be mixed with other medicinal products except those mentioned in section 6.6.

6.3 Shelf life

3 years

Reconstituted solution:

The reconstituted solution should be used immediately after preparation. If the reconstituted solution is not used immediately, in-use storage times and conditions prior to use are the responsibility of the user. However, the chemical and physical in-use stability of the reconstituted solution has been demonstrated for 8 hours at 25 °C stored in the original vial and/or a syringe prior to administration, with a maximum of 8 hours in the syringe.

6.4 Special precautions for storage

Do not store above 30°C. Keep the vial in the outer carton in order to protect from light.

For storage conditions of the reconstituted medicinal product, see section 6.3.

6.5 Nature and contents of container

Type 1 glass 10 ml-vial with a grey bromobutyl stopper and an aluminium seal, with a royal blue cap.

The vial is contained in a transparent blister pack consisting of a tray with a lid.

Pack containing 1 single-use vial.

6.6 Special precautions for disposal and other handling

General precautions

Bortezomib is a cytotoxic agent. Therefore, caution should be used during handling and preparation of VELCADE. Use of gloves and other protective clothing to prevent skin contact is recommended.

Aseptic technique must be strictly observed throughout handling of VELCADE, since it contains no preservative.

Instructions for reconstitution

Each 10 ml vial must be reconstituted with 3.5 ml of sodium chloride 9 mg/ml (0.9%) for injection. Dissolution of the lyophilised powder is completed in less than 2 minutes.

After reconstitution, each ml solution contains 1 mg bortezomib. The reconstituted solution is clear and colourless, with a final pH of 4 to 7.

The reconstituted solution must be inspected visually for particulate matter and discolouration prior to administration. If any discolouration or particulate matter is observed, the reconstituted solution must be discarded.

Disposal

For single use only.

Any unused product or waste material should be disposed of in accordance with local requirements.

7. MARKETING AUTHORISATION HOLDER
JANSSEN-CILAG INTERNATIONAL NV
Turnhoutseweg, 30
B-2340 Beerse
Belgium

8. MARKETING AUTHORISATION NUMBER(S)
EU/1/04/274/001

9. DATE OF FIRST AUTHORISATION/RENEWAL OF THE AUTHORISATION
Date of first authorization: 26/04/2004
Date of latest renewal: 26/04/2009

10. DATE OF REVISION OF THE TEXT
29th May 2009

Venofer 20 mg/ml Solution for Injection

(Syner-Med (Pharmaceutical Products) Ltd)

1. NAME OF THE MEDICINAL PRODUCT
Venofer 20 mg iron per ml, solution for injection or concentrate for solution for infusion.

2. QUALITATIVE AND QUANTITATIVE COMPOSITION
Each 5 ml ampoule of Venofer contains 100 mg iron as iron sucrose (iron(III)-hydroxide sucrose complex; 20 mg iron per ml)

For excipients, see 6.1.

3. PHARMACEUTICAL FORM
Solution for injection or concentrate for solution for infusion.

Venofer is a dark brown, non transparent, aqueous solution.

4. CLINICAL PARTICULARS
4.1 Therapeutic indications
Venofer is indicated for the treatment of iron deficiency in the following indications:

- where there is a clinical need to deliver iron rapidly to iron stores,
- in patients who cannot tolerate oral iron therapy or who are non-compliant,
- in active inflammatory bowel disease where oral iron preparations are ineffective.

The diagnosis of iron deficiency must be based on appropriate laboratory tests (e.g. Hb, serum ferritin, serum iron, etc.).

4.2 Posology and method of administration
Adults and the elderly: The total cumulative dose of Venofer, equivalent to the total iron deficit (mg), is determined by the haemoglobin level and body weight. The dose for Venofer must be individually determined for each patient according to the total iron deficit calculated with the following formula:

Total iron deficit [mg]= body weight [kg] × (target Hb - actual Hb) [g/l] × 0.24* + depot iron [mg]

- Below 35 kg body weight: target Hb = 130 g/l and depot iron = 15 mg/kg body weight
- 35 kg body weight and above: target Hb = 150 g/l and depot iron = 500 mg

*Factor 0.24 = 0.0034 × 0.07 × 1000 (Iron content of haemoglobin 0.34%; Blood volume 7% of body weight; Factor 1000 = conversion from g to mg)

The total amount of Venofer required is determined from either the above calculation or the following dosage table:

(see Table 1 below)

Dosage: The total single dose must not exceed 200 mg of iron given not more than three times per week. If the total necessary dose exceeds the maximum allowed single dose, then the administration has to be split.

Children: The use of Venofer has not been adequately studied in children and, therefore, Venofer is not recommended for use in children.

Administration: Venofer must only be administered by the intravenous route. This may be by a slow intravenous injection or by an intravenous drip infusion. Before administering the first dose to a new patient, a test dose of Venofer should be given.

Venofer must not be used for intramuscular injection.

Intravenous drip infusion: Venofer must be diluted only in sterile 0.9% m/V sodium chloride solution:

- 5 ml Venofer (100 mg iron)

in max. 100 ml sterile 0.9% m/V sodium chloride solution

- 10 ml Venofer (200 mg iron)

in max. 200 ml sterile 0.9% m/V sodium chloride solution

For stability reasons, dilutions to lower Venofer concentrations are not permissible.

Dilution must take place immediately prior to infusion and the solution should be administered as follows:

- 100 mg iron (5 ml Venofer) in at least 15 minutes
- 200 mg iron (10 ml Venofer) in at least 30 minutes

The first 25 mg of iron (i.e. 25 ml of solution) should be infused as a test dose over a period of 15 minutes. If no adverse reactions occur during this time then the remaining portion of the infusion should be given at an infusion rate of not more than 50 ml in 15 minutes.

Intravenous injection: Venofer may be administered by slow intravenous injection at a rate of 1 ml undiluted solution per minute (i.e. 5 minutes per ampoule) and not exceeding 2 ampoules Venofer (200 mg iron) per injection.

Before administering a slow intravenous injection, a test dose of 1 ml (20 mg of iron) should be injected slowly over a period of 1 to 2 minutes. If no adverse events occur within 15 minutes of completing the test dose, then the remaining portion of the injection may be given.

Injection into dialyser: Venofer may be administered during a haemodialysis session directly into the venous limb of the dialyser under the same procedures as those outlined for intravenous injection.

4.3 Contraindications
The use of Venofer is contra-indicated in cases of:

- known hypersensitivity to Venofer or any of its excipients
- anaemias not attributable to iron deficiency
- iron overload or disturbances in utilisation of iron
- patients with a history of asthma, eczema or other atopic allergy, because they are more susceptible to experience allergic reactions
- pregnancy first trimester.

4.4 Special warnings and precautions for use
Parenterally administered iron preparations can cause allergic or anaphylactoid reactions, which may be potentially fatal. Therefore, treatment for serious allergic reactions and facilities with the established cardio-pulmonary resuscitation procedures should be available.

In patients with liver dysfunction, parenteral iron should only be administered after careful risk/benefit assessment. Parenteral iron administration should be avoided in patients with hepatic dysfunction where iron overload is a precipitating factor, in particular Porphyria Cutanea Tarda (PCT). Careful monitoring of iron status is recommended to avoid iron overload.

Parenteral iron must be used with caution in case of acute or chronic infection. It is recommended that the administration of iron sucrose is stopped in patients with ongoing bacteraemia. In patients with chronic infection a risk/benefit evaluation has to be performed, taking into account the suppression of erythropoiesis.

Hypotensive episodes may occur if the injection is administered too rapidly. Allergic reactions, sometimes involving arthralgia, have been more commonly observed when the recommended dose is exceeded.

Paravenous leakage must be avoided because leakage of Venofer at the injection site may lead to pain, inflammation, tissue necrosis and brown discoloration of the skin.

4.5 Interaction with other medicinal products and other forms of interaction
As with all parenteral iron preparations, Venofer should not be administered concomitantly with oral iron preparations since the absorption of oral iron is reduced. Therefore, oral iron therapy should be started at least 5 days after the last injection of Venofer.

4.6 Pregnancy and lactation
Data on a limited number of exposed pregnancies indicated no adverse effects of Venofer on pregnancy or on the health of the foetus/newborn child. No well-controlled studies in pregnant women are available to date. Animal studies do not indicate direct or indirect harmful effects with respect to pregnancy, embryonal/foetal development, parturition or postnatal development.

Nevertheless, risk/benefit evaluation is required.

Venofer should only be used in pregnant women in whom oral iron is ineffective or cannot be tolerated and the level of anaemia is judged sufficient to put the mother or foetus at risk.

Pregnancy first trimester see contra-indications.

Non metabolised Venofer is unlikely to pass into the mother's milk. No well-controlled clinical studies are available to date. Animal studies do not indicate direct or indirect harmful effects to the nursing child.

4.7 Effects on ability to drive and use machines
In the case of symptoms of dizziness, confusion or light headedness following the administration of Venofer, patients should not drive or use machinery until the symptoms have ceased.

4.8 Undesirable effects
The most frequently reported adverse drug reactions (ADRs) of Venofer in clinical trials were transient taste perversion, hypotension, fever and shivering, injection site reactions and nausea, occurring in 0.5 to 1.5% of the patients. Non-serious anaphylactoid reactions occurred rarely.

In general anaphylactoid reactions are potentially the most serious adverse reactions (see "Special warnings and Precautions for Use" section 4.4).

In clinical trials, the following adverse drug reactions have been reported in temporal relationship with the administration of Venofer, with at least a possible causal relationship:

Nervous system disorders
Common (> 1/100, < 1/10): transient taste perversions (in particular metallic taste).

Uncommon (> 1/1000, < 1/100): headache; dizziness.

Rare (> 1/10000, < 1/1000): paraesthesia.

Cardio-vascular disorders
Uncommon (> 1/1000, < 1/100): hypotension and collapse; tachycardia and palpitations.

Respiratory, thoracic and mediastinal disorders
Uncommon (> 1/1000, < 1/100): bronchospasm, dyspnoea.

Gastrointestinal disorders
Uncommon (> 1/1000, < 1/100): nausea; vomiting; abdominal pain; diarrhoea.

Skin and subcutaneous tissue disorders
Uncommon(> 1/1000, < 1/100): pruritus; urticaria; rash, exanthema, erythema.

Musculoskeletal, connective tissue and bone disorders
Uncommon(> 1/1000, < 1/100): muscle cramps, myalgia.

General disorders and administration site disorders
Uncommon (> 1/1000, < 1/100): fever, shivering, flushing; chest pain and tightness. Injection site disorders such as superficial phlebitis, burning, swelling.

Rare (> 1/10000, < 1/1000): anaphylactoid reactions (rarely involving arthralgia); peripheral oedema; fatigue, asthenia; malaise.

Moreover, in spontaneous reports the following adverse reactions have been reported:

Isolated cases: reduced level of consciousness, light-headed feeling, confusion; angio-oedema; swelling of joints, hyperhidrosis, back pain.

4.9 Overdose
Overdosage can cause acute iron overloading which may manifest itself as haemosiderosis. Overdosage should be treated, if required, with an iron chelating agent.

5. PHARMACOLOGICAL PROPERTIES
5.1 Pharmacodynamic properties
The ferrokinetics of Venofer labelled with ^{59}Fe and ^{52}Fe were assessed in 5 patients with anaemia and chronic renal failure. Plasma clearance of ^{52}Fe was in the range of 60 to 100 minutes. ^{52}Fe was distributed to the liver, spleen and bone marrow. At two weeks after administration, the

Table 1

Body Weight [kg]	Total number of ampoules Venofer to be administered: (1 ampoule of Venofer corresponds to 5 ml)			
	Hb 60 g/l	Hb 75 g/l	Hb 90 g/l	Hb 105 g/l
30	9.5	8.5	7.5	6.5
35	12.5	11.5	10	9
40	13.5	12	11	9.5
45	15	13	11.5	10
50	16	14	12	10.5
55	17	15	13	11
60	18	16	13.5	11.5
65	19	16.5	14.5	12
70	20	17.5	15	12.5
75	21	18.5	16	13
80	22.5	19.5	16.5	13.5
85	23.5	20.5	17	14
90	24.5	21.5	18	14.5

To convert Hb (mM) to Hb (g/l), multiply the former by 16.1145.

maximum red blood cell utilisation of ^{59}Fe ranged from 62% to 97%.

5.2 Pharmacokinetic properties

Following intravenous injection of a single dose of Venofer containing 100 mg iron in healthy volunteers, maximum iron levels, averaging 538 μmol/l, were obtained 10 minutes after injection. The volume of distribution of the central compartment corresponded well to the volume of plasma (approximately 3 litres).

The iron injected was rapidly cleared from the plasma, the terminal half-life being approx. 6 h. The volume of distribution at steady state was about 8 litres, indicating a low iron distribution in the body fluid. Due to the lower stability of iron sucrose in comparison to transferrin, a competitive exchange of iron to transferrin was observed. This resulted in iron transport of approx. 31 mg iron/24 h.

Renal elimination of iron, occurring in the first 4 h after injection, corresponds to less than 5% of the total body clearance. After 24 h the plasma levels of iron were reduced to the pre-dose iron level and about 75% of the dosage of sucrose was excreted.

5.3 Preclinical safety data

There are no preclinical data of relevance to the prescriber that are additional to information already in other sections of the SPC.

6. PHARMACEUTICAL PARTICULARS

6.1 List of excipients

Water for injections

Sodium hydroxide

6.2 Incompatibilities

Venofer must only be mixed with sterile 0.9% m/V sodium chloride solution. No other solutions and therapeutic agents should be used as there is the potential for precipitation and/or interaction. The compatibility with containers other than glass, polyethylene and PVC is not known.

6.3 Shelf life

Shelf life of the product as packaged for sale:

3 years.

Shelf life after first opening of the container:

From a microbiological point of view, the product should be used immediately.

Shelf life after dilution with sterile 0.9% m/V sodium chloride solution:

From a microbiological point of view, the product should be used immediately after dilution with sterile 0.9% m/V sodium chloride solution.

6.4 Special precautions for storage

Store in original carton. Do not store above 25°C. Do not freeze.

6.5 Nature and contents of container

5 ml solution in one ampoule (type I glass) in pack sizes of 5.

6.6 Special precautions for disposal and other handling

Ampoules should be visually inspected for sediment and damage before use. Only those with sediment free and homogenous solution must be used.

The diluted solution must appear as brown and clear.

See also 6.3 shelf-life.

Any unused product or waste material should be disposed of in accordance with local requirements.

7. MARKETING AUTHORISATION HOLDER

Vifor France SA

123, rue Jules Guesde

92300 Levallois-Perret

France

8. MARKETING AUTHORISATION NUMBER(S)

UK: PL 15240/0001

Ireland: PA 949/1/1

9. DATE OF FIRST AUTHORISATION/RENEWAL OF THE AUTHORISATION

UK: 08.06.1998 / 08.06.2003

Ireland: 20.03.2000 / 08.06.2003

10. DATE OF REVISION OF THE TEXT

August 2006

Ventolin Accuhaler

(Allen & Hanburys)

1. NAME OF THE MEDICINAL PRODUCT

Ventolin™ Accuhaler™

2. QUALITATIVE AND QUANTITATIVE COMPOSITION

Ventolin Accuhaler is a plastic inhaler device containing a foil strip with 60 regularly spaced blisters each containing a mixture of 200 micrograms of microfine salbutamol (as sulphate) and larger particle lactose.

3. PHARMACEUTICAL FORM

Multi-dose dry powder inhalation device.

4. CLINICAL PARTICULARS

4.1 Therapeutic indications

Ventolin Accuhaler can be used in the management of asthma, bronchospasm and/or reversible airways obstruction.

Ventolin Accuhaler is particularly suitable for the relief of asthma symptoms. It should be used to relieve symptoms when they occur, and to prevent them in those circumstances recognised by the patient to precipitate an asthma attack (e.g. before exercise or unavoidable allergen exposure).

Ventolin Accuhaler is particularly valuable as relief medication in mild, moderate or severe asthma, provided that reliance on it does not delay the introduction and use of regular inhaled corticosteroid therapy.

4.2 Posology and method of administration

Ventolin Accuhaler is for inhalation use only. Ventolin Accuhaler is suitable for many patients including those who cannot use a metered-dose inhaler successfully.

Adults (including the elderly): For the relief of acute bronchospasm, 200 micrograms as a single dose. The maximum daily dose is 200 micrograms four times a day.

To prevent allergen- or exercise-induced symptoms, 200 micrograms should be taken 10-15 minutes before challenge.

Children: The recommended dose for relief of acute bronchospasm or before allergen exposure or exercise is 200 micrograms. The maximum daily dose is 200 micrograms four times a day.

On-demand use of Ventolin Accuhaler should not exceed four times daily. Reliance on such frequent supplementary use, or a sudden increase in dose, indicates poorly controlled or deteriorating asthma (see section 4.4).

4.3 Contraindications

Although intravenous salbutamol, and occasionally salbutamol tablets, are used in the management of premature labour uncomplicated by conditions such as placenta praevia, ante-partum haemorrhage, or toxaemia of pregnancy, inhaled salbutamol preparations are not appropriate for managing premature labour. Salbutamol preparations should not be used for threatened abortion.

Ventolin Accuhaler is contra-indicated in patients with a history of hypersensitivity to any of the components. (see section 6.1).

4.4 Special warnings and precautions for use

Bronchodilators should not be the only or main treatment in patients with severe or unstable asthma. Severe asthma requires regular medical assessment, including lung-function testing, as patients are at risk of severe attacks and even death. Physicians should consider using the maximum recommended dose of inhaled corticosteroid and/or oral corticosteroid therapy in these patients.

The dosage or frequency of administration should only be increased on medical advice.

Increasing use of bronchodilators, in particular short-acting inhaled β_2-agonists to relieve symptoms, indicates deterioration of asthma control. The patient should be instructed to seek medical advice if short-acting relief bronchodilator treatment becomes less effective, or more inhalations than usual are required. In this situation the patient should be assessed and consideration given to the need for increased anti-inflammatory therapy (e.g. higher doses of inhaled corticosteroid or a course of oral corticosteroid).

Severe exacerbations of asthma must be treated in the normal way.

Cardiovascular effects may be seen with sympathomimetic drugs, including salbutamol. There is some evidence from post-marketing data and published literature of rare occurrences of myocardial ischaemia associated with salbutamol. Patients with underlying severe heart disease (e.g. ischaemic heart disease, arrhythmia or severe heart failure) who are receiving salbutamol should be warned to seek medical advice if they experience chest pain or other symptoms of worsening heart disease. Attention should be paid to assessment of symptoms such as dyspnoea and chest pain, as they may be of either respiratory or cardiac origin.

Salbutamol should be administered cautiously to patients suffering from thyrotoxicosis.

Potentially serious hypokalaemia may result from β_2-agonist therapy, mainly from parenteral and nebulised administration. Particular caution is advised in acute severe asthma as this effect may be potentiated by hypoxia and by concomitant treatment with xanthine derivatives, steroids and diuretics. Serum potassium levels should be monitored in such situations.

4.5 Interaction with other medicinal products and other forms of interaction

Salbutamol and non-selective β-blocking drugs such as propranolol, should not usually be prescribed together.

4.6 Pregnancy and lactation

Pregnancy: Administration of drugs during pregnancy should only be considered if the expected benefit to the mother is greater than any possible risk to the fetus. As with the majority of drugs, there is little published evidence of the safety of salbutamol in the early stages of human pregnancy, but in animal studies there was evidence of some harmful effects on the fetus at very high dose levels.

Lactation: As salbutamol is probably secreted in breast milk, its use in nursing mothers requires careful consideration. It is not known whether salbutamol has a harmful effect on the neonate, and so its use should be restricted to situations where it is felt that the expected benefit to the mother is likely to outweigh any potential risk to the neonate.

4.7 Effects on ability to drive and use machines

None reported.

4.8 Undesirable effects

Adverse events are listed below by system organ class and frequency. Frequencies are defined as: very common (≥1/10), common (≥1/100 and <1/10), uncommon (≥1/1000 and <1/100), rare (≥1/10,000 and <1/1000) and very rare (<1/10,000) including isolated reports. Very common and common events were generally determined from clinical trial data. Rare, very rare and unknown events were generally determined from spontaneous data.

Immune system disorders

Very rare: Hypersensitivity reactions including angioedema, urticaria, bronchospasm, hypotension and collapse

Metabolism and nutrition disorders

Rare: Hypokalaemia.

Potentially serious hypokalaemia may result from $beta_2$ agonist therapy.

Nervous system disorders

Common: Tremor, headache.

Very rare: Hyperactivity.

Cardiac disorders

Common: Tachycardia.

Uncommon: Palpitations.

Very rare: Cardiac arrhythmias including atrial fibrillation, supraventricular tachycardia and extrasystoles

Unknown: Myocardial ischaemia* (see section 4.4)

Vascular disorders

Rare: Peripheral vasodilatation.

Respiratory, thoracic and mediastinal disorders

Very rare: Paradoxical bronchospasm.

As with other inhalation therapy, paradoxical bronchospasm may occur with an immediate increase in wheezing after dosing. This should be treated immediately with an alternative presentation or a different fast-acting inhaled bronchodilator. Ventolin Accuhaler should be discontinued immediately, the patient assessed, and, if necessary, alternative therapy instituted.

Gastrointestinal disorders

Uncommon: Mouth and throat irritation.

Musculoskeletal and connective tissue disorders

Uncommon: Muscle cramps.

* reported spontaneously in post-marketing data therefore frequency regarded as unknown

4.9 Overdose

The most common signs and symptoms of overdose with salbutamol are transient beta agonist pharmacologically mediated events, including tachycardia, tremor, hyperactivity and metabolic effects including hypokalaemia (see sections 4.4 and 4.8).

Hypokalaemia may occur following overdose with salbutamol. Serum potassium levels should be monitored.

Consideration should be given to discontinuation of treatment and appropriate symptomatic therapy such as cardio-selective beta-blocking agents in patients presenting with cardiac symptoms (e.g. tachycardia, palpitations). Beta-blocking drugs should be used with caution in patients with a history of bronchospasm.

5. PHARMACOLOGICAL PROPERTIES

5.1 Pharmacodynamic properties

Salbutamol is a selective β_2-adrenoceptor agonist. At therapeutic doses it acts on the β_2-adrenoceptors of bronchial muscle, with little or no action on the β_1-adrenoceptors of cardiac muscle.

Salbutamol provides short-acting (4-6 hour) bronchodilatation with a fast onset (within 5 minutes) in reversible airways obstruction.

5.2 Pharmacokinetic properties

Salbutamol administered intravenously has a half-life of 4 to 6 hours and is cleared partly renally, and partly by metabolism to the inactive 4'-O-sulphate (phenolic sulphate) which is also excreted primarily in the urine. The faeces are a minor route of excretion. After administration by the inhaled route between 10 and 20% of the dose reaches the lower airways. The remainder is retained in the delivery system or is deposited in the oropharynx from where it is swallowed. The fraction deposited in the airways is absorbed into the pulmonary tissues and circulation, but is not metabolised by the lung. On reaching the systemic circulation it becomes accessible to hepatic metabolism and is excreted, primarily in the urine, as unchanged drug and as the phenolic sulphate. The swallowed portion of an inhaled dose is absorbed from the gastrointestinal tract and undergoes considerable first-pass metabolism to the phenolic sulphate. Both unchanged drug and conjugate are excreted primarily in the urine. Almost all of a dose of salbutamol given intravenously, orally or by inhalation is excreted within 72 hours. Salbutamol is bound to plasma proteins to the extent of 10%.

5.3 Preclinical safety data
In common with other potent selective β_2-receptor agonists, salbutamol has been shown to be teratogenic in mice when given subcutaneously. In a reproductive study, 9.3% of fetuses were found to have cleft palate at 2.5mg/kg, 4 times the maximum human oral dose. In rats, treatment at the levels of 0.5, 2.32, 10.75 and 50mg/kg/day orally throughout pregnancy resulted in no significant fetal abnormalities. The only toxic effect was an increase in neonatal mortality at the highest dose level as the result of lack of maternal care. A reproductive study in rabbits revealed cranial malformations in 37% of fetuses at 50mg/kg/day, 78 times the maximum human oral dose.

6. PHARMACEUTICAL PARTICULARS
6.1 List of excipients
Lactose (which contains milk protein)

6.2 Incompatibilities
None reported.

6.3 Shelf life
24 months.

6.4 Special precautions for storage
Do not store above 30°C. Keep in the original container

6.5 Nature and contents of container
The powder mix of salbutamol (as sulphate) and lactose is filled into a blister strip consisting of a formed base foil with a peelable foil laminate lid. The foil strip is contained within the Accuhaler device.

6.6 Special precautions for disposal and other handling
The powdered medicine is inhaled through the mouth into the lungs.

The Accuhaler device contains the medicine in individual blisters which areopened as the device is manipulated.

For detailed instructions for use refer to the Patient Information Leaflet in every pack.

Adminstrative Details
7. MARKETING AUTHORISATION HOLDER
Glaxo Wellcome UK Ltd,
trading as Allen & Hanburys,
Stockley Park West,
Uxbridge, Middlesex,
UB11 1BT.

8. MARKETING AUTHORISATION NUMBER(S)
10949/0252

9. DATE OF FIRST AUTHORISATION/RENEWAL OF THE AUTHORISATION
December 1995

10. DATE OF REVISION OF THE TEXT
02 July 2009

Ventolin Evohaler

(Allen & Hanburys)

1. NAME OF THE MEDICINAL PRODUCT
Ventolin$_{TM}$ Evohaler$_{TM}$.

2. QUALITATIVE AND QUANTITATIVE COMPOSITION
Ventolin Evohaler is a pressurised metered-dose inhaler delivering 100 micrograms of salbutamol (as Salbutamol Sulphate BP) per actuation. Ventolin Evohaler contains a new propellant (HFA 134a) and does not contain any chlorofluorocarbons.

3. PHARMACEUTICAL FORM
Aerosol.

4. CLINICAL PARTICULARS
4.1 Therapeutic indications
Ventolin Evohaler provides short-acting (4 to 6 hour) bronchodilatation with fast onset (within 5 minutes) in reversible airways obstruction.

It is particularly suitable for the relief and prevention of asthma symptoms. It should be used to relieve symptoms when they occur, and to prevent them in those circumstances recognised by the patient to precipitate an asthma attack (e.g. before exercise or unavoidable allergen exposure).

Ventolin Evohaler is particularly valuable as relief medication in mild, moderate or severe asthma, provided that reliance on it does not delay the introduction and use of regular inhaled corticosteroid therapy.

4.2 Posology and method of administration
Ventolin Evohaler is for oral inhalation use only. Ventolin Evohaler may be used with a Volumatic™ spacer device by patients who find it difficult to synchronise aerosol actuation with inspiration of breath.

Adults (including the elderly): For the relief of acute asthma symptoms including bronchospasm, one inhalation (100 micrograms) may be administered as a single minimum starting dose. This may be increased to two inhalations if necessary. To prevent allergen- or exercise-induced symptoms, two inhalations should be taken 10-15 minutes before challenge.

For chronic therapy, two inhalations up to four times a day.

Children: For the relief of acute asthma symptoms including bronchospasm, or before allergen exposure or exercise, one inhalation, or two if necessary.

For chronic therapy, two inhalations up to four times a day.

The Babyhaler$_{TM}$ spacer device may be used to facilitate administration to children under 5 years of age.

On-demand use of Ventolin Evohaler should not exceed 8 inhalations in any 24 hours. Reliance on such frequent supplementary use, or a sudden increase in dose, indicates poorly controlled or deteriorating asthma (see section 4.4).

4.3 Contraindications
Although intravenous salbutamol, and occasionally salbutamol tablets, are used in the management of premature labour uncomplicated by conditions such as placenta praevia, ante-partum haemorrhage or toxaemia of pregnancy, inhaled salbutamol preparations are not appropriate for managing premature labour. Salbutamol preparations should not be used for threatened abortion.

Ventolin Evohaler is contra-indicated in patients with a history of hypersensitivity to any of the components.

4.4 Special warnings and precautions for use
Patients inhaler technique should be checked to make sure that aerosol actuation is synchronised with inspiration of breath for optimum delivery of drug to the lungs. Patients should be warned that they may experience a different taste upon inhalation compared to their previous inhaler.

Bronchodilators should not be the only or main treatment in patients with severe or unstable asthma. Severe asthma requires regular medical assessment, including lung-function testing, as patients are at risk of severe attacks and even death. Physicians should consider using the maximum recommended dose of inhaled corticosteroid and/or oral corticosteroid therapy in these patients.

The dosage or frequency of administration should only be increased on medical advice. If a previously effective dose of inhaled salbutamol fails to give relief lasting at least three hours, the patient should be advised to seek medical advice.

Increasing use of bronchodilators, in particular short-acting inhaled β_2-agonists, to relieve symptoms, indicates deterioration of asthma control. The patient should be instructed to seek medical advice if short-acting relief bronchodilator treatment becomes less effective, or more inhalations than usual are required. In this situation the patient should be assessed and consideration given to the need for increased anti-inflammatory therapy (e.g. higher doses of inhaled corticosteroid or a course of oral corticosteroid).

Severe exacerbations of asthma must be treated in the normal way.

Cardiovascular effects may be seen with sympathomimetic drugs, including salbutamol. There is some evidence from post-marketing data and published literature of rare occurrences of myocardial ischaemia associated with salbutamol. Patients with underlying severe heart disease (e.g. ischaemic heart disease, arrhythmia or severe heart failure) who are receiving salbutamol should be warned to seek medical advice if they experience chest pain or other symptoms of worsening heart disease. Attention should be paid to assessment of symptoms such as dyspnoea and chest pain, as they may be of either respiratory or cardiac origin.

Salbutamol should be administered cautiously to patients with thyrotoxicosis.

Potentially serious hypokalaemia may result from β_2-agonist therapy, mainly from parenteral and nebulised administration. Particular caution is advised in acute severe asthma as this effect may be potentiated by hypoxia and by concomitant treatment with xanthine derivatives, steroids and diuretics. Serum potassium levels should be monitored in such situations.

4.5 Interaction with other medicinal products and other forms of interaction
Salbutamol and non-selective β-blocking drugs such as propranolol, should not usually be prescribed together.

4.6 Pregnancy and lactation
Studies in animals have shown reproductive toxicity (see section 5.3). Safety in pregnant women has not been established. No controlled clinical trials with salbutamol have been conducted in pregnant women. Rare reports of various congenital anomalies following intrauterine exposure to salbutamol (including cleft palate, limb defects and cardiac disorders) have been received. Some of the mothers were taking multiple medications during their pregnancies. Ventolin Evohaler should not be used during pregnancy unless clearly necessary.

As salbutamol is probably secreted in breast milk, its use in nursing mothers requires careful consideration. It is not known whether salbutamol has a harmful effect on the neonate, and so its use should be restricted to situations where it is felt that the expected benefit to the mother is likely to outweigh any potential risk to the neonate.

4.7 Effects on ability to drive and use machines
None reported.

4.8 Undesirable effects
Adverse events are listed below by system organ class and frequency. Frequencies are defined as: very common (≥1/10), common (≥1/100 and <1/10), uncommon (≥1/1000 and <1/100), rare (≥1/10,000 and <1/1000) and very rare (<1/10,000) including isolated reports. Very common and common events were generally determined from clinical trial data. Rare, very rare and unknown events were generally determined from spontaneous data.

Immune system disorders
Very rare: Hypersensitivity reactions including angioedema, urticaria, bronchospasm, hypotension and collapse.

Metabolism and nutrition disorders
Rare: Hypokalaemia.
Potentially serious hypokalaemia may result from *beta*$_2$ agonist therapy.

Nervous system disorders
Common: Tremor, headache.
Very rare: Hyperactivity.

Cardiac disorders
Common: Tachycardia.
Uncommon: Palpitations.
Very rare: Cardiac arrhythmias (including atrial fibrillation, supraventricular tachycardia and extrasystoles).
Unknown: Myocardial ischaemia* (see section 4.4)

Vascular disorders
Rare: Peripheral vasodilatation.

Respiratory, thoracic and mediastinal disorders
Very rare: Paradoxical bronchospasm.

As with other inhalation therapy, paradoxical bronchospasm may occur with an immediate increase in wheezing after dosing. This should be treated immediately with an alternative presentation or a different fast-acting inhaled bronchodilator. EVOHALER should be discontinued immediately, the patient assessed, and, if necessary, alternative therapy instituted.

Gastrointestinal disorders
Uncommon: Mouth and throat irritation.

Musculoskeletal and connective tissue disorders
Uncommon: Muscle cramps.

* reported spontaneously in post-marketing data therefore frequency regarded as unknown

4.9 Overdose
The most common signs and symptoms of overdose with salbutamol are transient beta agonist pharmacologically mediated events, including tachycardia, tremor, hyperactivity and metabolic effects including hypokalaemia (see sections 4.4 and 4.8).

Hypokalaemia may occur following overdose with salbutamol. Serum potassium levels should be monitored.

Consideration should be given to discontinuation of treatment and appropriate symptomatic therapy such as cardio-selective beta-blocking agents in patients presenting with cardiac symptoms (e.g. tachycardia, palpitations). Beta-blocking drugs should be used with caution in patients with a history of bronchospasm.

5. PHARMACOLOGICAL PROPERTIES
5.1 Pharmacodynamic properties
Salbutamol is a selective β_2-adrenoceptor agonist. At therapeutic doses it acts on the β_2-adrenoceptors of bronchial muscle providing short acting (4-6 hour) bronchodilatation with a fast onset (within 5 minutes) in reversible airways obstruction.

5.2 Pharmacokinetic properties
Salbutamol administered intravenously has a half life of 4 to 6 hours and is cleared partly renally and partly by metabolism to the inactive 4'-O-sulphate (phenolic sulphate) which is also excreted primarily in the urine. The faeces are a minor route of excretion.

After administration by the inhaled route between 10 and 20% of the dose reaches the lower airways. The remainder is retained in the delivery system or is deposited in the oropharynx from where it is swallowed. The fraction deposited in the airways is absorbed into the pulmonary tissues and circulation, but is not metabolised by the lung. On reaching the systemic circulation it becomes accessible to hepatic metabolism and is excreted, primarily in the urine, as unchanged drug and as the phenolic sulphate.

The swallowed portion of an inhaled dose is absorbed from the gastrointestinal tract and undergoes considerable first-pass metabolism to the phenolic sulphate. Both unchanged drug and conjugate are excreted primarily in the urine. Most of a dose of salbutamol given intravenously, orally or by inhalation is excreted within 72 hours. Salbutamol is bound to plasma proteins to the extent of 10%.

5.3 Preclinical safety data
In common with other potent selective β_2-agonists, salbutamol has been shown to be teratogenic in mice when given subcutaneously. In a reproductive study, 9.3% of fetuses were found to have cleft palate at 2.5mg/kg dose. In rats, treatment at the levels of 0.5, 2.32, 10.75 and 50mg/kg/day orally throughout pregnancy resulted in no

significant fetal abnormalities. The only toxic effect was an increase in neonatal mortality at the highest dose level as the result of lack of maternal care. Reproductive studies in the rabbit at doses of 50mg/kg/day orally (i.e. much higher than the normal human dose) have shown fetuses with treatment related changes; these included open eyelids (ablepharia), secondary palate clefts (palatoschisis), changes in ossification of the frontal bones of the cranium (cranioschisis) and limb flexure. Reformulation of the Ventolin Evohaler has not altered the known toxicological profile of salbutamol.

The non-CFC propellant, HFA 134a, has been shown to have no toxic effect at very high vapour concentrations, far in excess of those likely to be experienced by patients, in a wide range of animal species exposed daily for periods of two years.

6. PHARMACEUTICAL PARTICULARS

6.1 List of excipients
HFA 134a.

6.2 Incompatibilities
None reported.

6.3 Shelf life
24 months when stored below 30°C.

6.4 Special precautions for storage
Store below 30°C (86°F).

Protect from frost and direct sunlight.

As with most inhaled medications in aerosol canisters, the therapeutic effect of this medication may decrease when the canister is cold.

The canister should not be broken, punctured or burnt, even when apparently empty.

Replace the mouthpiece cover firmly and snap it into position.

6.5 Nature and contents of container
An inhaler comprising an aluminium alloy can sealed with a metering valve, actuator and dust cap. Each canister contains 200 metered actuations providing 100 micrograms of salbutamol (as Salbutamol Sulphate BP).

6.6 Special precautions for disposal and other handling
The aerosol spray is inhaled through the mouth into the lungs. After shaking the inhaler, the mouthpiece is placed in the mouth and the lips closed around it. The actuator is depressed to release a spray, which must coincide with inspiration of breath.

For detailed instructions for use refer to the Patient Information Leaflet in every pack.

7. MARKETING AUTHORISATION HOLDER
Glaxo Wellcome UK Ltd trading as Allen & Hanburys

Stockley Park West

Uxbridge

Middlesex, UB11 1BT

8. MARKETING AUTHORISATION NUMBER(S)
PL 10949/0274.

9. DATE OF FIRST AUTHORISATION/RENEWAL OF THE AUTHORISATION
28 June 2003

10. DATE OF REVISION OF THE TEXT
02 July 2009

Ventolin Injection 500mcg

(Allen & Hanburys)

1. NAME OF THE MEDICINAL PRODUCT
Ventolin Injection 500 micrograms (0.5mg) in 1ml

2. QUALITATIVE AND QUANTITATIVE COMPOSITION
Ventolin Injection 500 micrograms (0.5mg) in 1ml (500 micrograms/ml) is presented as ampoules of 1ml, each containing 500 micrograms salbutamol as salbutamol sulphate BP in a sterile isotonic solution.

3. PHARMACEUTICAL FORM
A colourless or faintly straw coloured solution for injection.

4. CLINICAL PARTICULARS

4.1 Therapeutic indications
Ventolin Injection provides short-acting (4-6 hour) bronchodilatation with a fast onset (within 5 minutes) in reversible airways obstruction. It is indicated for the relief of severe bronchospasm.

4.2 Posology and method of administration
Ventolin Injection may be administered by the subcutaneous, intramuscular or intravenous route, under the direction of a physician.

Adults:

Subcutaneous route: 500 micrograms (8 micrograms/kg body weight) and repeated every four hours as required.

Intramuscular route: 500 micrograms (8 micrograms/kg body weight) and repeated every four hours as required.

Slow intravenous injection:

250 micrograms (4 micrograms/kg bodyweight) injected slowly. If necessary the dose may be repeated.

The use of Ventolin Injection 500 micrograms in 1ml (500 micrograms/ml, for intravenous administration may be facilitated by dilution to 10ml with Water for Injection BP (final concentration of 50 micrograms/ml) and 5mls of the diluted preparation (250 micrograms/5ml) administered by slow intravenous injection.

Children:

At present there are insufficient data to recommend a dosage regimen for routine use.

Instructions to open the ampoule

Ampoules are equipped with the OPC (One Point Cut) opening system and must be opened using the following instructions:

hold with one hand the bottom part of the ampoule as indicated in Picture 1

put the other hand on the top of the ampoule positioning the thumb above the coloured point and press as indicated in Picture 2

Picture 1

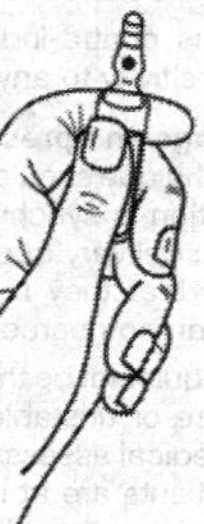

Picture 2

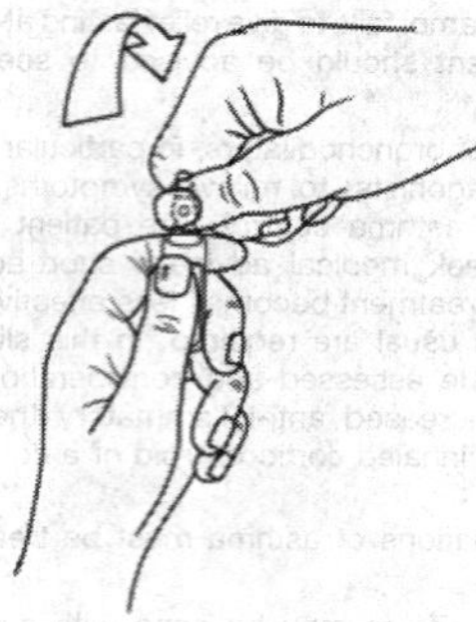

4.3 Contraindications
Although intravenous salbutamol, and occasionally salbutamol tablets, are used in the management of premature labour uncomplicated by conditions such as placenta praevia, ante-partum haemorrhage or toxaemia of pregnancy, salbutamol preparations should not be used for threatened abortion.

Ventolin Injection is contra-indicated in patients with a history of hypersensitivity to any of the components.

4.4 Special warnings and precautions for use
Bronchodilators should not be the only or main treatment in patients with severe or unstable asthma. Severe asthma requires regular medical assessment, including lung-function testing, as patients are at risk of severe attacks and even death. Physicians should consider using the maximum recommended dose of inhaled corticosteroid and/or oral corticosteroid therapy in these patients.

The dosage or frequency of administration should only be increased on medical advice.

Patients being treated with Ventolin Injection may also be receiving short-acting inhaled bronchodilators to relieve symptoms. Increasing use of bronchodilators, in particular short-acting inhaled β_2-agonists to relieve symptoms, indicates deterioration of asthma control.

The patient should be instructed to seek medical advice if short-acting relief bronchodilator treatment becomes less effective, or more inhalations than usual are required. In this situation the patient should be assessed and consideration given to the need for increased anti-inflammatory therapy (e.g. higher doses of inhaled corticosteroid or a course of oral corticosteroid).

Cardiovascular effects may be seen with sympathomimetic drugs, including salbutamol. There is some evidence from post-marketing data and published literature of rare occurrences of myocardial ischaemia associated with salbutamol. Patients with underlying severe heart disease (e.g. ischaemic heart disease, arrhythmia or severe heart failure) who are receiving salbutamol should be warned to seek medical advice if they experience chest pain or other symptoms of worsening heart disease. Attention should be paid to assessment of symptoms such as dyspnoea and chest pain, as they may be of either respiratory or cardiac origin.

Salbutamol should be administered cautiously to patients suffering from thyrotoxicosis.

Potentially serious hypokalaemia may result from β_2-agonist therapy, mainly from parenteral and nebulised administration. Particular caution is advised in acute severe asthma as this effect may be potentiated by hypoxia and by concomitant treatment with xanthine derivatives, steroids and diuretics. Serum potassium levels should be monitored in such situations.

Severe exacerbations of asthma must be treated in the normal way.

The use of Ventolin Injection in the treatment of severe bronchospasm does not obviate the requirement for corticosteroid therapy as appropriate. When practicable, administration of oxygen concurrently with Ventolin Injection is recommended. In common with other β-adrenoceptor agonists, salbutamol can induce reversible metabolic changes such as hypokalaemia and increased blood glucose levels. Diabetic patients may be unable to compensate for the increase in blood glucose and the development of ketoacidosis has been reported. Concurrent administration of corticosteroids can exaggerate this effect.

Lactic acidosis has been reported in association with high therapeutic doses of intravenous and nebulised short-acting beta-agonist therapy, mainly in patients being treated for an acute asthma exacerbation (see Section 4.8). Increase in lactate levels may lead to dyspnoea and compensatory hyperventilation, which could be misinterpreted as a sign of asthma treatment failure and lead to inappropriate intensification of short-acting beta-agonist treatment. It is therefore recommended that patients are monitored for the development of elevated serum lactate and consequent metabolic acidosis in this setting.

As maternal pulmonary oedema has been reported during or following management of premature labour with β_2-agonists, careful attention should be given to fluid balance and cardio-respiratory function should be monitored. If signs of pulmonary oedema develop, discontinuation of treatment should be considered (see section 4.8).

4.5 Interaction with other medicinal products and other forms of interaction
Salbutamol and non-selective beta-blocking drugs such as propranolol, should not usually be prescribed together.

4.6 Pregnancy and lactation
Administration of drugs during pregnancy should only be considered if the expected benefit to the mother is greater than any possible risk to the foetus.

As with the majority of drugs, there is little published evidence of the safety of salbutamol in the early stages of human pregnancy, but in animal studies there was evidence of some harmful effects on the foetus at very high dose levels.

As salbutamol is probably secreted in breast milk its use in nursing mothers is not recommended unless the expected benefits outweigh any potential risk. In such situations the use of the inhaled route may be preferable although it is not known whether salbutamol has a harmful effect on the neonate.

4.7 Effects on ability to drive and use machines
Not applicable.

4.8 Undesirable effects
Adverse events are listed below by system organ class and frequency. Frequencies are defined as: very common (≥1/10), common (≥1/100 and <1/10), uncommon (≥1/1000 and <1/100), rare (≥1/10,000 and <1/1000) and very rare (<1/10,000). Very common and common events were generally determined from clinical trial data. Rare, very rare and unknown events were generally determined from spontaneous data.

Immune system disorders

Very rare: Hypersensitivity reactions including angioedema, urticaria, bronchospasm, hypotension and collapse.

Metabolism and nutrition disorders

Rare: Hypokalaemia.

Potentially serious hypokalaemia may result from beta-agonist therapy.

Unknown: Lactic acidosis (see section 4.4)

Nervous system disorders

Very common: Tremor.

Common: Headache.

Very rare: Hyperactivity.

Cardiac disorders

Very common: Tachycardia.

Common: Palpitations.

Rare: Cardiac arrhythmias including atrial fibrillation, supraventricular tachycardia and extrasystoles.

Unknown: Myocardial ischaemia* (see section 4.4)

Vascular disorders

Rare: Peripheral vasodilatation.

Respiratory, thoracic and mediastinal disorders

Uncommon: Pulmonary oedema.

In the management of pre-term labour, Ventolin Injection has uncommonly been associated with pulmonary oedema. Patients with predisposing factors including multiple pregnancies, fluid overload, maternal infection and pre-eclampsia may have an increased risk of developing pulmonary oedema.

Gastrointestinal disorders

Unknown: Nausea, vomiting *.

Musculoskeletal and connective tissue disorders

Common: Muscle cramps.

Injury, poisoning and procedural complications

Unknown: Slight pain or stinging on i.m. use of undiluted injection*.

* reported spontaneously in post-marketing data therefore frequency regarded as unknown.

4.9 Overdose

The most common signs and symptoms of overdose with salbutamol are transient beta agonist pharmacologically mediated events, including tachycardia, tremor, hyperactivity and metabolic effects including hypokalaemia and lactic acidosis (see sections 4.4 and 4.8).

Hypokalaemia may occur following overdose with salbutamol. Serum potassium levels should be monitored.

Nausea, vomiting and hyperglycaemia have been reported, predominantly in children and when salbutamol overdose has been taken via the oral route.

Consideration should be given to discontinuation of treatment and appropriate symptomatic therapy such as cardio-selective beta-blocking agents in patients presenting with cardiac symptoms (e.g. tachycardia, palpitations). Beta-blocking drugs should be used with caution in patients with a history of bronchospasm.

5. PHARMACOLOGICAL PROPERTIES

5.1 Pharmacodynamic properties

Salbutamol is a selective β_2-adrenoceptor agonist. At therapeutic doses it acts on β_2-adrenoceptors of bronchial muscle providing short-acting (4-6 hour) bronchodilation with a fast onset (within 5 minutes) in reversible airways obstruction.

5.2 Pharmacokinetic properties

Salbutamol administered intravenously has a half-life of 4 to 6 hours and is cleared partly renally and partly by metabolism to the inactive 4'-O-sulphate (phenolic sulphate) which is also excreted primarily in the urine. The faeces are a minor route of excretion. The majority of a dose of salbutamol given intravenously, orally or by inhalation is excreted within 72 hours. Salbutamol is bound to plasma proteins to the extent of 10%.

5.3 Preclinical safety data

There are no additional preclinical safety data other than are provided in the other sections of the Summary of Product Characteristics.

6. PHARMACEUTICAL PARTICULARS

6.1 List of excipients

Sodium chloride

Sodium hydroxide pellets

Dilute sulphuric acid

Water for injections

Nitrogen (oxygen free)

6.2 Incompatibilities

None stated

6.3 Shelf life

36 months

24 hours – shelf life of admixtures with infusion fluids.

6.4 Special precautions for storage

Store below 30°C and keep the ampoule in the outer container.

6.5 Nature and contents of container

Clear, neutral glass ampoules, packed in plastic trays with a cardboard sleeve over the trays.

Pack size: 1ml ampoules in plastic trays of 5.

6.6 Special precautions for disposal and other handling

The only recommended diluents for Ventolin Injection are water for injections BP, sodium chloride injection BP, sodium chloride and dextrose injection BP or dextrose injection BP.

All unused admixtures of Ventolin Injection should be discarded 24 hours after preparation.

Ventolin Injection should not be administered in the same syringe as any other medication.

Administrative Data

7. MARKETING AUTHORISATION HOLDER

Glaxo Wellcome UK Ltd

trading as Allen & Hanburys

Stockley Park West

Uxbridge

Middlesex

UB11 1BT

8. MARKETING AUTHORISATION NUMBER(S)

PL 10949/0084

9. DATE OF FIRST AUTHORISATION/RENEWAL OF THE AUTHORISATION

6 September 2000

10. DATE OF REVISION OF THE TEXT

31 July 2009

Ventolin Nebules 2.5mg, 5mg

(Allen & Hanburys)

1. NAME OF THE MEDICINAL PRODUCT

Ventolin Nebules 2.5mg.

Ventolin Nebules 5 mg.

2. QUALITATIVE AND QUANTITATIVE COMPOSITION

Plastic ampoule containing 2.5ml of a sterile 0.1% or 0.2% w/v solution of salbutamol (as Salbutamol Sulphate BP) in normal saline.

3. PHARMACEUTICAL FORM

Solution for inhalation via a nebuliser.

4. CLINICAL PARTICULARS

4.1 Therapeutic indications

Salbutamol is a selective β2-agonist providing short-acting (4-6 hour) bronchodilatation with a fast onset (within 5 minutes) in reversible airways obstruction.

Ventolin Nebules are indicated for use in the routine management of chronic bronchospasm unresponsive to conventional therapy, and in the treatment of acute severe asthma.

4.2 Posology and method of administration

Ventolin Nebules are for inhalation use only, to be breathed in through the mouth, under the direction of a physician, using a suitable nebuliser.

The solution should not be injected or swallowed.

Adults (including the elderly): 2.5mg to 5mg salbutamol up to four times a day. Up to 40mg per day can be given under strict medical supervision in hospital.

Children 4 years and above: 2.5mg to 5mg up to four times a day.

Children 18 months to 4 years: 2.5mg up to four times a day. The dose may be increased to 5mg if necessary, but medical assessment should be considered since alternative therapy may be indicated.

Infants under 18 months old: 1.25mg (0.25mg/kg) to 2.5mg up to four times a day. As transient hypoxia may occur supplemental oxygen therapy should be considered.

Ventolin Nebules are intended to be used undiluted. However, if prolonged delivery time (more than 10 minutes) is required, the solution may be diluted with sterile normal saline.

4.3 Contraindications

Although intravenous salbutamol, and occasionally salbutamol tablets, are used in the management of premature labour uncomplicated by conditions such as placenta praevia, ante-partum haemorrhage or toxaemia of pregnancy, inhaled salbutamol preparations are not appropriate for managing premature labour. Salbutamol preparations should not be used for threatened abortion.

Ventolin Nebules are contra-indicated in patients with a history of hypersensitivity to any of the components.

4.4 Special warnings and precautions for use

Ventolin Nebules must only be used by inhalation, to be breathed in through the mouth, and must not be injected or swallowed.

Bronchodilators should not be the only or main treatment in patients with severe or unstable asthma. Severe asthma requires regular medical assessment, including lung-function testing, as patients are at risk of severe attacks and even death. Physicians should consider using the maximum recommended dose of inhaled corticosteroid and/or oral corticosteroid therapy in these patients.

Patients receiving treatment at home should seek medical advice if treatment with Ventolin Nebules becomes less effective. The dosage or frequency of administration should only be increased on medical advice.

Patients being treated with Ventolin Nebules may also be receiving other dosage forms of short-acting inhaled bronchodilators to relieve symptoms. Increasing use of bronchodilators, in particular short-acting inhaled β2-agonists to relieve symptoms, indicates deterioration of asthma control. The patient should be instructed to seek medical advice if short-acting relief bronchodilator treatment becomes less effective or more inhalations than usual are required. In this situation patients should be assessed and consideration given to the need for increased anti-inflammatory therapy (e.g. higher doses of inhaled corticosteroid or a course of oral corticosteroid).

Severe exacerbations of asthma must be treated in the normal way.

Salbutamol should be administered cautiously to patients suffering from thyrotoxicosis.

Cardiovascular effects may be seen with sympathomimetic drugs, including salbutamol. There is some evidence from post-marketing data and published literature of rare occurrences of myocardial ischaemia associated with salbutamol. Patients with underlying severe heart disease (e.g. ischaemic heart disease, arrhythmia or severe heart failure) who are receiving salbutamol should be warned to seek medical advice if they experience chest pain or other symptoms of worsening heart disease. Attention should be paid to assessment of symptoms such as dyspnoea and chest pain, as they may be of either respiratory or cardiac origin.

Ventolin Nebules should be used with care in patients known to have received large doses of other sympathomimetic drugs.

Potentially serious hypokalaemia may result from β2-agonist therapy, mainly from parenteral and nebulised administration. Particular caution is advised in acute severe asthma as this effect may be potentiated by hypoxia and by concomitant treatment with xanthine derivatives, steroids and diuretics. Serum potassium levels should be monitored in such situations.

In common with other β-adrenoceptor agonists, salbutamol can induce reversible metabolic changes such as increased blood glucose levels. Diabetic patients may be unable to compensate for the increase in blood glucose and the development of ketoacidosis has been reported. Concurrent administration of corticosteroids can exaggerate this effect.

Lactic acidosis has been reported in association with high therapeutic doses of intravenous and nebulised short-acting beta-agonist therapy, mainly in patients being treated for an acute asthma exacerbation (see Section 4.8). Increase in lactate levels may lead to dyspnoea and compensatory hyperventilation, which could be misinterpreted as a sign of asthma treatment failure and lead to inappropriate intensification of short-acting beta-agonist treatment. It is therefore recommended that patients are monitored for the development of elevated serum lactate and consequent metabolic acidosis in this setting.

A small number of cases of acute angle-closure glaucoma have been reported in patients treated with a combination of nebulised salbutamol and ipratropium bromide. A combination of nebulised salbutamol with nebulised anticholinergics should therefore be used cautiously. Patients should receive adequate instruction in correct administration and be warned not to let the solution or mist enter the eye.

4.5 Interaction with other medicinal products and other forms of interaction

Salbutamol and non-selective β-blocking drugs such as propranolol, should not usually be prescribed together.

4.6 Pregnancy and lactation

Administration of drugs during pregnancy should only be considered if the expected benefit to the mother is greater than any possible risk to the fetus. As with the majority of drugs, there is little published evidence of the safety of salbutamol in the early stages of human pregnancy, but in animal studies there was evidence of some harmful effects on the fetus at very high dose levels.

As salbutamol is probably secreted in breast milk, its use in nursing mothers requires careful consideration. It is not known whether salbutamol has a harmful effect on the neonate, and so its use should be restricted to situations where it is felt that the expected benefit to the mother is likely to outweigh any potential risk to the neonate.

4.7 Effects on ability to drive and use machines

None reported.

4.8 Undesirable effects

Adverse events are listed below by system organ class and frequency. Frequencies are defined as: very common ($\geq$1/10), common ($\geq$1/100 and $<$1/10), uncommon ($\geq$1/1000 and $<$1/100), rare ($\geq$1/10,000 and $<$1/1000) and very rare ($<$1/10,000). Very common and common events were generally determined from clinical trial data. Rare, very rare and unknown events were generally determined from spontaneous data.

Immune system disorders

Very rare: Hypersensitivity reactions including angioedema, urticaria, bronchospasm, hypotension and collapse

Metabolism and nutrition disorders

Rare: Hypokalaemia.

Potentially serious hypokalaemia may result from beta$_2$ agonist therapy.

Unknown: Lactic acidosis (see section 4.4)

Nervous system disorders

Common: Tremor, headache.

Very rare: Hyperactivity.

Cardiac disorders

Common: Tachycardia.

Uncommon: Palpitations

Very rare: Cardiac arrhythmias including atrial fibrillation, supraventricular tachycardia and extrasystoles

Unknown: Myocardial ischaemia* (see section 4.4)

Vascular disorders

Rare: Peripheral vasodilatation.

Respiratory, thoracic and mediastinal disorders

Very rare: Paradoxical bronchospasm.

As with other inhalation therapy, paradoxical bronchospasm may occur with an immediate increase in wheezing after dosing. This should be treated immediately with an alternative presentation or a different fast-acting inhaled bronchodilator. Ventolin Nebules should be discontinued immediately, the patient assessed, and, if necessary, alternative therapy instituted.

Gastrointestinal disorders

Uncommon: Mouth and throat irritation.

Musculoskeletal and connective tissue disorders

Uncommon: Muscle cramps.

* reported spontaneously in post-marketing data therefore frequency regarded as unknown

4.9 Overdose

The most common signs and symptoms of overdose with salbutamol are transient beta agonist pharmacologically mediated events, including tachycardia, tremor, hyperactivity and metabolic effects including hypokalaemia and lactic acidosis (see sections 4.4 and 4.8).

Hypokalaemia may occur following overdose with salbutamol. Serum potassium levels should be monitored.

Consideration should be given to discontinuation of treatment and appropriate symptomatic therapy such as cardio-selective beta-blocking agents in patients presenting with cardiac symptoms (e.g. tachycardia, palpitations). Beta-blocking drugs should be used with caution in patients with a history of bronchospasm.

5. PHARMACOLOGICAL PROPERTIES

5.1 Pharmacodynamic properties

Salbutamol is a selective β2-agonist providing short-acting (4-6 hour) bronchodilatation with a fast onset (within 5 minutes) in reversible airways obstruction. At therapeutic doses it acts on the β2-adrenoceptors of bronchial muscle. With its fast onset of action, it is particularly suitable for the management and prevention of attack in asthma.

5.2 Pharmacokinetic properties

Salbutamol administered intravenously has a half-life of 4 to 6 hours and is cleared partly renally, and partly by metabolism to the inactive 4'-O-sulphate (phenolic sulphate) which is also excreted primarily in the urine. The faeces are a minor route of excretion. Most of a dose of salbutamol given intravenously, orally or by inhalation is excreted within 72 hours. Salbutamol is bound to plasma proteins to the extent of 10%.

After administration by the inhaled route between 10 and 20% of the dose reaches the lower airways. The remainder is retained in the delivery system or is deposited in the oropharynx from where it is swallowed. The fraction deposited in the airways is absorbed into the pulmonary tissues and circulation, but is not metabolised by the lung. On reaching the systemic circulation it becomes accessible to hepatic metabolism and is excreted, primarily in the urine, as unchanged drug and as the phenolic sulphate.

The swallowed portion of an inhaled dose is absorbed from the gastrointestinal tract and undergoes considerable first-pass metabolism to the phenolic sulphate. Both unchanged drug and conjugate are excreted primarily in the urine.

5.3 Preclinical safety data

No additional preclinical safety data are included here.

6. PHARMACEUTICAL PARTICULARS

6.1 List of excipients

Sodium chloride

Sulphuric acid if required to adjust pH

Purified water

6.2 Incompatibilities

None known.

6.3 Shelf life

3 years if unopened.

3 months after removal from the foil overwrap, (see below).

6.4 Special precautions for storage

Ventolin Nebules should be stored below 30°C. The Nebules should be protected from light after removal from the foil tray.

6.5 Nature and contents of container

Low density polyethylene ampoules available in boxes of 20 or 40 in strips of 5 or 10. Sample pack of 5.

6.6 Special precautions for disposal and other handling

The nebulised solution may be inhaled through a face mask, T-piece or via an endotracheal tube. Intermittent positive pressure ventilation (IPPV) may be used but is rarely necessary. When there is a risk of anoxia through hypoventilation, oxygen should be added to the inspired air.

As many nebulisers operate on a continuous flow basis, it is likely that some nebulised drug will be released into the local environment. Ventolin Nebules should therefore be administered in a well-ventilated room, particularly in hospitals when several patients may be using nebulisers at the same time.

Dilution: Ventolin Nebules may be diluted with sterile normal saline. Solutions in nebulisers should be replaced daily.

Administrative Data

7. MARKETING AUTHORISATION HOLDER

Allen & Hanburys

Stockley Park West

Uxbridge

Middlesex UB11 1BT

8. MARKETING AUTHORISATION NUMBER(S)

Ventolin Nebules 2.5mgPL10949/0085

Ventolin Nebules 5 mg. PL10949/0086

9. DATE OF FIRST AUTHORISATION/RENEWAL OF THE AUTHORISATION

10th July 2002

10. DATE OF REVISION OF THE TEXT

02 July 2009

Ventolin Respirator Solution

(Allen & Hanburys)

1. NAME OF THE MEDICINAL PRODUCT

Ventolin™ Respirator Solution.

2. QUALITATIVE AND QUANTITATIVE COMPOSITION

Aqueous, colourless to light yellow solution, pH 3.5, providing 5mg/ml of salbutamol (as Salbutamol Sulphate BP).

3. PHARMACEUTICAL FORM

Solution for nebulisation.

4. CLINICAL PARTICULARS

4.1 Therapeutic indications

Ventolin Respirator Solution is indicated for use in the routine management of chronic bronchospasm unresponsive to conventional therapy, and in the treatment of acute severe asthma.

4.2 Posology and method of administration

Ventolin Respirator Solution is for inhalation use only, to be breathed in through the mouth, under the direction of a physician, using a suitable nebuliser. The solution should not be injected or swallowed. Ventolin Respirator Solution may be administered intermittently or continuously. Salbutamol has a duration of action of 4 to 6 hours in most patients.

Intermittent administration

Adults: Ventolin Respirator solution 0.5ml (2.5mg of salbutamol) should be diluted to a final volume of 2ml with sterile normal saline. This may be increased to 1ml (5mg of salbutamol) diluted to a final volume of 2.5ml. The resulting solution is inhaled from a suitably driven nebuliser until aerosol generation ceases. Using a correctly matched nebuliser and driving source this should take about ten minutes.

Ventolin Respirator Solution may be used undiluted for intermittent administration. For this, 2ml of Ventolin Respirator Solution (10mg of salbutamol) is placed in the nebuliser and the patient allowed to inhale the nebulised solution until bronchodilatation is achieved. This usually takes 3 - 5 minutes. Some adult patients may require higher doses of salbutamol up to 10mg, in which case nebulisation of the undiluted solution may continue until aerosol generation ceases.

Children: The same mode of administration for intermittent administration is also applicable to children. The minimum starting dosage for children under the age of twelve years is 0.5ml (2.5mg of salbutamol) diluted to 2 to 2.5ml with sterile normal saline. Some children may, however, require higher doses of salbutamol up to 5mg. Intermittent treatment may be repeated up to four times daily.

Continuous administration

Ventolin Respirator Solution is diluted with sterile normal saline to contain 50-100 micrograms of salbutamol per ml, (1-2ml solution made up to 100ml with diluent). The diluted solution is administered as an aerosol by a suitably driven nebuliser. The usual rate of administration is 1-2mg per hour.

In infants under 18 months the clinical efficacy of nebulised salbutamol is uncertain. As transient hypoxaemia may occur supplemental oxygen therapy should be considered.

4.3 Contraindications

Hypersensitivity.

Threatened abortion.

4.4 Special warnings and precautions for use

Ventolin Respirator Solution must only be used by inhalation, to be breathed in through the mouth, and must not be injected or swallowed.

Bronchodilators should not be the only or main treatment in patients with severe or unstable asthma. Severe asthma requires regular medical assessment, including lung-function testing, as patients are at risk of severe attacks and even death. Physicians should consider using the maximum recommended dose of inhaled corticosteroid and/or oral corticosteroid therapy in these patients.

Patients receiving treatment at home should be warned to seek medical advice if treatment with Ventolin Respirator Solution becomes less effective. As there may be adverse effects associated with excessive dosing the dosage or frequency of administration should only be increased on medical advice.

Patients being treated with Ventolin Respirator Solution may also be receiving other dosage forms of short-acting inhaled bronchodilators to relieve symptoms.

Increasing use of bronchodilators, in particular short-acting inhaled β2-agonists, to relieve symptoms, indicates deterioration of asthma control. The patient should be instructed to seek medical advice if short-acting relief bronchodilator treatment becomes less effective, or more inhalations than usual are required. In this situation the patient should be assessed and consideration given to the need for increased anti-inflammatory therapy (e.g. higher doses of inhaled corticosteroid or a course of oral corticosteroid).

Severe exacerbations of asthma must be treated in the normal way.

Cardiovascular effects may be seen with sympathomimetic drugs, including salbutamol. There is some evidence from post-marketing data and published literature of rare occurrences of myocardial ischaemia associated with salbutamol. Patients with underlying severe heart disease (e.g. ischaemic heart disease, arrhythmia or severe heart failure) who are receiving salbutamol should be warned to seek medical advice if they experience chest pain or other symptoms of worsening heart disease. Attention should be paid to assessment of symptoms such as dyspnoea and chest pain, as they may be of either respiratory or cardiac origin.

Ventolin Respirator Solution should be used with care in patients known to have received large doses of other sympathomimetic drugs.

Potentially serious hypokalaemia may result from β_2-agonist therapy, mainly from parenteral and nebulised administration. Particular caution is advised in acute severe asthma as this effect may be potentiated by hypoxia and by concomitant treatment with xanthine derivatives, steroids and diuretics. Serum potassium levels should be monitored in such situations.

In common with other β-adrenoceptor agonists, salbutamol can induce reversible metabolic changes such as increased blood glucose levels. Diabetic patients may be unable to compensate for the increase in blood glucose and the development of ketoacidosis has been reported. Concurrent administration of corticosteroids can exaggerate this effect.

Lactic acidosis has been reported in association with high therapeutic doses of intravenous and nebulised short-acting beta-agonist therapy, mainly in patients being treated for an acute asthma exacerbation (see Section 4.8). Increase in lactate levels may lead to dyspnoea and compensatory hyperventilation, which could be misinterpreted as a sign of asthma treatment failure and lead to inappropriate intensification of short-acting beta-agonist treatment. It is therefore recommended that patients are monitored for the development of elevated serum lactate and consequent metabolic acidosis in this setting.

A small number of cases of acute angle-closure glaucoma have been reported in patients treated with a combination of nebulised salbutamol and ipratropium bromide. A combination of nebulised salbutamol with nebulised anticholinergics should therefore be used cautiously. Patients should receive adequate instruction in correct administration and be warned not to let the solution or mist enter the eye.

Salbutamol should be administered cautiously to patients suffering from thyrotoxicosis.

4.5 Interaction with other medicinal products and other forms of interaction

Should not normally be prescribed with non-selective β-blocking drugs such as propranolol.

4.6 Pregnancy and lactation

Administration of drugs during pregnancy should only be considered if the expected benefit to the mother is greater than any possible risk to the foetus. As with the majority of drugs, there is little published evidence of the safety of salbutamol in the early stages of human pregnancy, but in animal studies there was evidence of some harmful effects on the foetus at very high dose levels.

As salbutamol is probably secreted in breast milk, its use in nursing mothers requires careful consideration. It is not known whether salbutamol has a harmful effect on the neonate, and so its use should be restricted to situations where it is felt that the expected benefit to the mother is likely to outweigh any potential risk to the neonate.

4.7 Effects on ability to drive and use machines

None reported.

4.8 Undesirable effects

Adverse events are listed below by system organ class and frequency. Frequencies are defined as: very common (≥1/10), common (≥1/100 and <1/10), uncommon (≥1/1000 and <1/100), rare (≥1/10,000 and <1/1000) and very rare (<1/10,000). Very common and common events were generally determined from clinical trial data. Rare, very rare and unknown events were generally determined from spontaneous data.

Immune system disorders

Very rare: Hypersensitivity reactions including angioedema, urticaria, bronchospasm, hypotension and collapse

Metabolism and nutrition disorders

Rare: Hypokalaemia.

Potentially serious hypokalaemia may result from beta$_2$ agonist therapy.

Unknown: Lactic acidosis (see section 4.4)

Nervous system disorders

Common: Tremor, headache.

Very rare: Hyperactivity.

Cardiac disorders

Common: Tachycardia.

Uncommon: Palpitations

Very rare: Cardiac arrhythmias including atrial fibrillation, supraventricular tachycardia and extrasystoles

Unknown: Myocardial ischaemia* (see section 4.4)

Vascular disorders

Rare: Peripheral vasodilatation.

Respiratory, thoracic and mediastinal disorders

Very rare: Paradoxical bronchospasm.

As with other inhalation therapy, paradoxical bronchospasm may occur with an immediate increase in wheezing after dosing. This should be treated immediately with an alternative presentation or a different fast-acting inhaled bronchodilator. Ventolin Respirator Solution should be discontinued immediately, the patient assessed, and, if necessary, alternative therapy instituted.

Gastrointestinal disorders

Uncommon: Mouth and throat irritation.

Musculoskeletal and connective tissue disorders

Uncommon: Muscle cramps.

* reported spontaneously in post-marketing data therefore frequency regarded as unknown

4.9 Overdose

The most common signs and symptoms of overdose with salbutamol are transient beta agonist pharmacologically mediated events, including tachycardia, tremor, hyperactivity and metabolic effects including hypokalaemia and lactic acidosis (see sections 4.4 and 4.8).

Hypokalaemia may occur following overdose with salbutamol. Serum potassium levels should be monitored.

Consideration should be given to discontinuation of treatment and appropriate symptomatic therapy such as cardioselective beta-blocking agents in patients presenting with cardiac symptoms (e.g. tachycardia, palpitations). Beta-blocking drugs should be used with caution in patients with a history of bronchospasm.

5. PHARMACOLOGICAL PROPERTIES

5.1 Pharmacodynamic properties

Salbutamol is a selective β2-agonist providing short-acting (4-6 hour) bronchodilatation with a fast onset (within 5 minutes) in reversible airways obstruction. At therapeutic doses it acts on the β$_2$-adrenoceptors of bronchial muscle. With its fast onset of action, it is particularly suitable for the management and prevention of attack in asthma.

5.2 Pharmacokinetic properties

Salbutamol administered intravenously has a half-life of 4 to 6 hours and is cleared partly renally and partly by metabolism to the inactive 4'-0-sulphate (phenolic sulphate) which is also excreted primarily in the urine. The faeces are a minor route of excretion. Most of a dose of salbutamol given intravenously, orally or by inhalation is excreted within 72 hours. Salbutamol is bound to plasma proteins to the extent of 10%.

After administration by the inhaled route between 10 and 20% of the dose reaches the lower airways. The remainder is retained in the delivery system or is deposited in the oropharynx from where it is swallowed. The fraction deposited in the airways is absorbed into the pulmonary tissues and circulation, but is not metabolised by the lung. On reaching the systemic circulation it becomes accessible to hepatic metabolism and is excreted, primarily in the urine, as unchanged drug and as the phenolic sulphate.

The swallowed portion of an inhaled dose is absorbed from the gastrointestinal tract and undergoes considerable first-pass metabolism to the phenolic sulphate. Both unchanged drug and conjugate are excreted primarily in the urine.

5.3 Preclinical safety data

No additional preclinical safety data are included here.

6. PHARMACEUTICAL PARTICULARS

6.1 List of excipients

Preservative: Benzalkonium chloride. Sulphuric acid if required to adjust to pH 3.5.

Purified water.

6.2 Incompatibilities

None known.

6.3 Shelf life

Unopened: 3 years. Following opening for the first time: 28 days.

6.4 Special precautions for storage

Store below 25°C. Protect from light. Discard any contents remaining one month after opening the bottle.

6.5 Nature and contents of container

Screw-capped 10ml amber glass bottle.

Screw-capped 20ml amber glass bottle.

6.6 Special precautions for disposal and other handling

Inhalation use only, using a suitable nebuliser.

The nebulised solution may be inhaled through a face mask, "T" piece or via an endotracheal tube. Intermittent positive pressure ventilation (IPPV) may be used, but is rarely necessary. When there is a risk of anoxia through hypoventilation, oxygen should be added to the inspired air.

As many nebulisers operate on a continuous flow basis, it is likely that nebulised drug will be released into the local environment. Ventolin Respirator Solution should therefore be administered in a well ventilated room, particularly in hospitals when several patients may be using nebulisers at the same time.

Administrative Data

7. MARKETING AUTHORISATION HOLDER

Glaxo Wellcome UK Ltd

trading as Allen & Hanburys

Stockley Park West

Uxbridge

Middlesex UB11 1BT.

8. MARKETING AUTHORISATION NUMBER(S)

PL 10949/0244

9. DATE OF FIRST AUTHORISATION/RENEWAL OF THE AUTHORISATION

06 July 2000

10. DATE OF REVISION OF THE TEXT

02 July 2009

Ventolin Solution for IV Infusion

(Allen & Hanburys)

1. NAME OF THE MEDICINAL PRODUCT

Ventolin™ Solution for Intravenous Infusion 5mg in 5ml (1mg/ml).

2. QUALITATIVE AND QUANTITATIVE COMPOSITION

Ventolin Solution for Intravenous Infusion 5mg in 5ml (1mg/ml) is presented as ampoules of 5ml, each containing 5mg salbutamol as Salbutamol Sulphate BP in a sterile isotonic solution.

3. PHARMACEUTICAL FORM

Clear, colourless or pale straw-coloured solution for intravenous infusion.

4. CLINICAL PARTICULARS

4.1 Therapeutic indications

Ventolin Solution for Intravenous Infusion should be administered under the direction of a physician. It is indicated for two distinct clinical situations:

a) For the relief of severe bronchospasm.

b) In the management of premature labour; to arrest uncomplicated labour between 24 and 33 weeks of gestation in patients with no medical or obstetric contra-indication to tocolytic therapy. Data suggest that the main effect of tocolytic therapy is a delay in delivery of up to 48 hours. This delay may be used to administer glucocorticoids or to implement other measures known to improve perinatal health.

4.2 Posology and method of administration

Ventolin Solution for Intravenous Infusion is used to prepare an infusion solution. It should not be injected undiluted. Ventolin Solution for Intravenous Infusion should not be administered in the same syringe or infusion as any other medication.

1) In severe bronchospasm.

Adults: A suitable solution for infusion providing 10 micrograms salbutamol/ml is prepared by diluting 5ml Ventolin Solution for Intravenous Infusion to 500ml with an infusion solution such as Sodium Chloride and Dextrose Injection BP. Other suitable diluents are Water for Injections BP, Sodium Chloride Injection BP or Dextrose Injection BP.

Infusion rates providing 3 to 20 micrograms salbutamol/minute (0.3 to 2ml/minute of the above infusion solution) are usually adequate. Higher doses have been used with success in patients with respiratory failure. Children: There are insufficient data to recommend a dosage regime for routine use.

2. In the management of premature labour.

The infusion, prepared as described below, should be administered as early as possible after the diagnosis of premature labour, and after evaluation of the patient to eliminate any contra-indications to the use of salbutamol (see section 4.3).

During infusion the maternal pulse rate should be monitored and the infusion rate adjusted to avoid excessive maternal heart rate (above 140 beats/minute).

It is essential that the volume of infusion fluid is kept to a minimum to control the level of hydration and so avoid the risk of maternal pulmonary oedema. Treatment discontinuation should be considered should signs of pulmonary oedema or myocardial ischaemia develop (see section 4.8)

A controlled infusion device, preferably a syringe pump, should be used.

Infusion rates providing 10 to 45 micrograms salbutamol/minute are generally adequate to control uterine contractions. A starting rate of 10 micrograms/minute is recommended, increasing the rate at 10-minute intervals until there is evidence of patient response shown by diminution in strength, frequency or duration of contractions. Thereafter, the infusion rate may be increased slowly until contractions cease. Careful attention should be given to cardio-respiratory function and fluid balance monitored. Once uterine contractions have ceased the infusion rate should be maintained at the same level for one hour and then reduced by 50% decrements at six hourly intervals. If labour progresses despite treatment the infusion should be stopped. If contractions have been successfully inhibited by the infusion, treatment may be continued orally with Ventolin Tablets 4mg given three or four times daily.

Dilution: The recommended diluent is 5% Dextrose (see section 4.3 for precautions with diabetic patients).

For use in a syringe pump: Prepare a solution providing 200 micrograms salbutamol/ml by diluting 10ml Ventolin Solution for Intravenous Infusion with 40ml diluent. An infusion rate of 10 to 45 micrograms/minute is equivalent to 0.05 to 0.225ml/minute of this solution.

Other infusion methods: Prepare a solution providing 20 micrograms salbutamol/ml by diluting 10ml Ventolin Solution for Intravenous Infusion with 490ml diluent. An infusion rate of 10 to 45 micrograms/minute is equivalent to 0.5 to 2.25ml/minute of this solution.

Instructions to open the ampoule

Ampoules are equipped with the OPC (One Point Cut) opening system and must be opened using the following instructions:

- hold with one hand the bottom part of the ampoule as indicated in Picture 1
- put the other hand on the top of the ampoule positioning the thumb above the coloured point and press as indicated in Picture 2

Picture 1

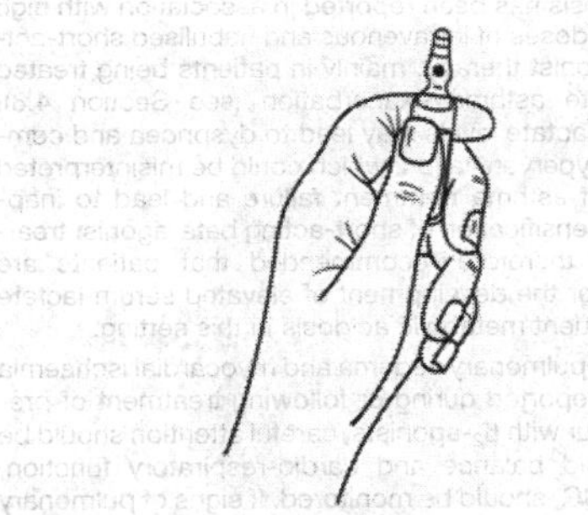

Picture 2

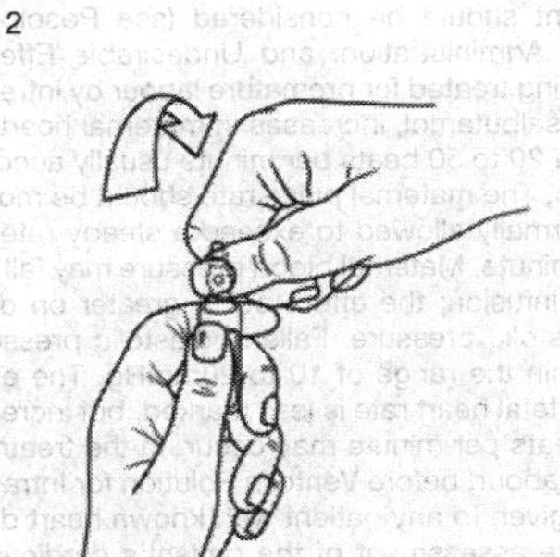

4.3 Contraindications

Although Ventolin Solution for Intravenous Infusion and occasionally salbutamol tablets, are used in the management of premature labour uncomplicated by conditions such as placenta praevia, ante-partum haemorrhage or toxaemia of pregnancy, salbutamol preparations should not be used for threatened abortion.

Ventolin Solution for Intravenous Infusion is contra-indicated in patients with a history of hypersensitivity to any of the components.

4.4 Special warnings and precautions for use

Bronchodilators should not be the only or main treatment in patients with severe or unstable asthma. Severe asthma requires regular medical assessment, including lung-function testing, as patients are at risk of severe attacks and even death. Physicians should consider using the maximum recommended dose of inhaled corticosteroid and/or oral corticosteroid therapy in these patients.

The dosage or frequency of administration should only be increased on medical advice.

Patients being treated with Ventolin Solution for Intravenous Infusion may also be receiving short-acting inhaled bronchodilators to relieve symptoms. Increasing use of bronchodilators, in particular short-acting inhaled β_2-agonists to relieve symptoms, indicates deterioration of asthma control.

The patient should be instructed to seek medical advice if short-acting relief bronchodilator treatment becomes less effective, or more inhalations than usual are required. In this situation the patient should be assessed and consideration given to the need for increased anti-inflammatory therapy (e.g. higher doses of inhaled corticosteroid or a course of oral corticosteroid). Severe exacerbations of asthma must be treated in the normal way. The use of Ventolin Solution for Intravenous Infusion in the treatment of severe bronchospasm does not obviate the requirement for corticosteroid therapy as appropriate. When practicable, administration of oxygen concurrently with parenteral Ventolin is recommended, particularly when it is given by intravenous infusion to hypoxic patients. In common with other β-adrenoceptor agonists, salbutamol can induce reversible metabolic changes such as hypokalaemia and increased blood glucose levels. Diabetic patients may be unable to compensate for the increase in blood glucose and the development of ketoacidosis has been reported. Concurrent administration of corticosteroids can exaggerate this effect.

Therefore, diabetic patients and those concurrently receiving corticosteroids should be monitored frequently during intravenous infusion of Ventolin so that remedial steps (e.g. an increase in insulin dosage) can be taken to counter any metabolic change occurring. For these patients it may be preferable to dilute Ventolin Solution for Intravenous Infusion in Sodium Chloride Injection BP rather than in diluents containing dextrose.

Salbutamol should be administered cautiously to patients suffering from thyrotoxicosis.

Potentially serious hypokalaemia may result from β_2-agonist therapy, mainly from parenteral and nebulised administration. Particular caution is advised in acute severe asthma as this effect may be potentiated by hypoxia and by concomitant treatment with xanthine derivatives, steroids and diuretics. Serum potassium levels should be monitored in such situations.

Lactic acidosis has been reported in association with high therapeutic doses of intravenous and nebulised short-acting beta-agonist therapy, mainly in patients being treated for an acute asthma exacerbation (see Section 4.8). Increase in lactate levels may lead to dyspnoea and compensatory hyperventilation, which could be misinterpreted as a sign of asthma treatment failure and lead to inappropriate intensification of short-acting beta-agonist treatment. It is therefore recommended that patients are monitored for the development of elevated serum lactate and consequent metabolic acidosis in this setting.

As maternal pulmonary oedema and myocardial ischaemia have been reported during or following treatment of premature labour with β_2-agonists, careful attention should be given to fluid balance and cardio-respiratory function, including ECG, should be monitored. If signs of pulmonary oedema or myocardial ischaemia develop, discontinuation of treatment should be considered (see Posology and Method of Administration, and Undesirable Effects). In patients being treated for premature labour by intravenous infusion of salbutamol, increases in maternal heart rate of the order of 20 to 50 beats per minute usually accompany the infusion. The maternal pulse rate should be monitored and not normally allowed to exceed a steady rate of 140 beats per minute. Maternal blood pressure may fall slightly during the infusion; the effect being greater on diastolic than on systolic pressure. Falls in diastolic pressure are usually within the range of 10 to 20mmHg. The effect of infusion on fetal heart rate is less marked, but increases of up to 20 beats per minute may occur. In the treatment of premature labour, before Ventolin Solution for Intravenous Infusion is given to any patient with known heart disease, an adequate assessment of the patient's cardiovascular status should be made by a physician experienced in cardiology. In order to minimise the risk of hypotension associated with tocolytic therapy, special care should be taken to avoid caval compression by keeping the patient in the left or right lateral positions throughout the infusion.

4.5 Interaction with other medicinal products and other forms of interaction

Ventolin Solution for Intravenous Infusion should not be administered in the same syringe or infusion as any other medication.

Salbutamol and non-selective β-blocking drugs such as propranolol, should not usually be prescribed together.

4.6 Pregnancy and lactation

Administration of drugs during pregnancy should only be considered if the expected benefit to the mother is greater than any possible risk to the fetus. As with the majority of drugs, there is little published evidence of the safety of salbutamol in the early stages of human pregnancy, but in animal studies there was evidence of some harmful effects on the fetus at very high dose levels. As salbutamol is probably secreted in breast milk, its use in nursing mothers requires careful consideration. It is not known whether salbutamol has a harmful effect on the neonate, and so its use should be restricted to situations where it is felt that the expected benefit to the mother is likely to outweigh any potential risk to the neonate.

4.7 Effects on ability to drive and use machines

None reported.

4.8 Undesirable effects

Adverse events are listed below by system organ class and frequency. Frequencies are defined as: very common (≥ 1/10), common (≥ 1/100 and < 1/10), uncommon (≥ 1/1000 and < 1/100), rare (≥ 1/10,000 and < 1/1000) and very rare (< 1/10,000). Very common and common events were generally determined from clinical trial data. Rare, very rare and unknown events were generally determined from spontaneous data.

Immune system disorders

Very rare: Hypersensitivity reactions including angioedema, urticaria, bronchospasm, hypotension and collapse.

Metabolism and nutrition disorders

Rare: Hypokalaemia.

Potentially serious hypokalaemia may result from β_2-agonist therapy.

Unknown: Lactic acidosis(see section 4.4)

Nervous system disorders

Very common: Tremor.

Common: Headache.

Very rare: Hyperactivity.

Cardiac disorders

Very common: Tachycardia.

Common: Palpitations.

Unknown: Myocardial ischaemia* (see section 4.4)

Rare: Cardiac arrhythmias including atrial fibrillation, supraventricular tachycardia and extrasystoles.

* In the management of pre-term labour with salbutamol solution for infusion.

Vascular disorders

Rare: Peripheral vasodilatation.

Respiratory, thoracic and mediastinal disorders

Uncommon: Pulmonary oedema.

In the management of pre-term labour, Ventolin Solution for Intravenous Infusion has uncommonly been associated with pulmonary oedema. Patients with predisposing factors including multiple pregnancies, fluid overload, maternal infection and pre-eclampsia may have an increased risk of developing pulmonary oedema.

Gastrointestinal disorders

Unknown: Nausea, vomiting.

In the management of premature labour, intravenous infusion of Ventolin has very rarely been associated with nausea and vomiting.

Musculoskeletal and connective tissue disorders

Common: Muscle cramps.

4.9 Overdose

The most common signs and symptoms of overdose with salbutamol are transient beta agonist pharmacologically mediated events, including tachycardia, tremor, hyperactivity and metabolic effects including hypokalaemia and lactic acidosis (see sections 4.4 and 4.8).

Hypokalaemia may occur following overdose with salbutamol. Serum potassium levels should be monitored.

Nausea, vomiting and hyperglycaemia have been reported, predominantly in children and when salbutamol overdose has been taken via the oral route.

Consideration should be given to discontinuation of treatment and appropriate symptomatic therapy such as cardio-selective beta-blocking agents in patients presenting with cardiac symptoms (e.g. tachycardia, palpitations). Beta-blocking drugs should be used with caution in patients with a history of bronchospasm.

5. PHARMACOLOGICAL PROPERTIES

5.1 Pharmacodynamic properties

Salbutamol is a selective β_2-agonist which acts on the β_2-adrenoceptors of the bronchi and uterus.

5.2 Pharmacokinetic properties

Salbutamol administered intravenously has a half-life of 4 to 6 hours and is cleared partly renally and partly by metabolism to the inactive 4'-0-sulphate (phenolic sulphate) which is also excreted primarily in the urine. The faeces are a minor route of excretion. Most of a dose of salbutamol given intravenously, orally or by inhalation is excreted within 72 hours. Salbutamol is bound to plasma proteins to the extent of 10%.

5.3 Preclinical safety data

No additional preclinical safety data are included here.

6. PHARMACEUTICAL PARTICULARS

6.1 List of excipients

Sodium chloride, sodium hydroxide, sulphuric acid and Water for Injections.

6.2 Incompatibilities

None stated.

6.3 Shelf life

36 months.

24 hours after mixing with infusion fluids.

6.4 Special precautions for storage

Store below 30°C and keep container in the outer carton.

6.5 Nature and contents of container

Clear, neutral glass ampoules, available in boxes of 10 ampoules or 5 ampoules.

6.6 Special precautions for disposal and other handling

Ventolin Solution for Intravenous Infusion must be diluted before use. The recommended diluents are Water for Injections BP, Sodium Chloride Injection BP, Sodium Chloride and Dextrose Injection BP and Dextrose Injection BP (see section 4.2).

All unused admixtures of Ventolin Solution for Intravenous Infusion with infusion fluids should be discarded twenty-four hours after preparation.

Administrative Data

7. MARKETING AUTHORISATION HOLDER

Glaxo Wellcome UK Ltd,

trading as Allen & Hanburys,

Stockley Park West,

Uxbridge,

Middlesex,

UB11 1BT.

8. MARKETING AUTHORISATION NUMBER(S)

PL 10949/0087

9. DATE OF FIRST AUTHORISATION/RENEWAL OF THE AUTHORISATION

11 September 2000

10. DATE OF REVISION OF THE TEXT

31 July 2009

Ventolin(TM) is a trade mark of the Glaxo Wellcome Group of Companies

Ventolin Syrup

(Allen & Hanburys)

1. NAME OF THE MEDICINAL PRODUCT

Ventolin Syrup

2. QUALITATIVE AND QUANTITATIVE COMPOSITION

Each 5 ml contains 2 mg Salbutamol (as Salbutamol Sulphate BP).

3. PHARMACEUTICAL FORM

Syrup

4. CLINICAL PARTICULARS

4.1 Therapeutic indications

Salbutamol is a selective beta-2 adrenoceptor agonist providing short-acting (4-6 hour) bronchodilatation in reversible airways obstruction. Ventolin syrup can be used in the management of asthma, bronchospasm and/or reversible airways obstruction.

Relief of bronchospasm in bronchial asthma of all types.

Ventolin syrup is suitable oral therapy for children and adults who are unable to use an inhaler device.

4.2 Posology and method of administration

Route of administration: oral

Adults

The minimum starting dose is 2mg three times a day given as 5ml syrup. The usual effective dose is 4mg (10ml syrup) three or four times a day, which may be increased to a maximum of 8mg (20ml syrup) three or four times a day if adequate bronchodilatation is not obtained.

Elderly

In elderly patients or in those known to be unusually sensitive to beta-adrenergic stimulant drugs, it is advisable to initiate treatment with the minimum starting dose.

Children

2 - 6 years: the minimum starting dose is 1mg as 2.5ml of syrup three times daily. This may be increased to 2mg as 5ml of syrup three or four times daily.

6-12 years: the minimum starting dose is 2mg as 5ml syrup three times daily. This may be increased to four times daily.

Over 12 years: the minimum starting dose is 2mg three times daily given as 5ml syrup. This may be increased to 4mg as 10ml syrup three or four times daily.

Ventolin is well tolerated by children so that, if necessary, these doses may be cautiously increased to the maximum dose.

For lower doses the syrup may be diluted with freshly prepared purified water BP.

4.3 Contraindications

Although intravenous salbutamol and occasionally salbutamol tablets are used in the management of premature labour, uncomplicated by conditions such as placenta praevia, ante-partum haemorrhage, or toxaemia of pregnancy, salbutamol presentations should not be used for threatened abortion.

Ventolin oral preparations are contra-indicated in patients with a history of hypersensitivity to any of their components.

4.4 Special warnings and precautions for use
Bronchodilators should not be the only or main treatment in patients with severe or unstable asthma. Severe asthma requires regular medical assessment including lung function testing as patients are at risk of severe attacks and even death. Physicians should consider using oral corticosteroid therapy and/or the maximum recommended dose of inhaled corticosteroid in those patients.

Patients should seek medical advice if treatment with Ventolin syrup becomes less effective.

The dosage or frequency of administration should only be increased on medical advice.

Patients taking Ventolin syrup may also be receiving short-acting inhaled bronchodilators to relieve symptoms.

Increasing use of bronchodilators in particular short-acting inhaled beta$_2$-agonists to relieve symptoms indicates deterioration of asthma control. The patient should be instructed to seek medical advice if short-acting relief bronchodilator treatment becomes less effective or they need more inhalations than usual.

In this situation patients should be reassessed and consideration given to the need for increased anti-inflammatory therapy (eg. Higher doses of inhaled corticosteroids or a course of oral corticosteroid). Severe exacerbations of asthma must be treated in the normal way.

Patients should be warned that if either the usual relief with Ventolin oral preparations is diminished or the usual duration of action reduced, they should not increase the dose or its frequency of administration, but should seek medical advice.

Ventolin syrup and non-selective beta-blocking drugs, such as propranolol, should not usually be prescribed together.

Cardiovascular effects may be seen with sympathomimetic drugs, including salbutamol. There is some evidence from post-marketing data and published literature of rare occurrences of myocardial ischaemia associated with salbutamol. Patients with underlying severe heart disease (e.g. ischaemic heart disease, arrhythmia or severe heart failure) who are receiving salbutamol should be warned to seek medical advice if they experience chest pain or other symptoms of worsening heart disease. Attention should be paid to assessment of symptoms such as dyspnoea and chest pain, as they may be of either respiratory or cardiac origin.

Salbutamol should be administered cautiously to patients suffering from thyrotoxicosis.

Potentially serious hypokalaemia may result from beta-2 agonist therapy mainly from parenteral and nebulised administration. Particular caution is advised in acute severe asthma as this effect may be potentiated by hypoxia and by concomitant treatment with xanthine derivatives, steroids. It is recommended that serum potassium levels are monitored is such situations.

In common with other β-adrenoceptor agonists, salbutamol can induce reversible metabolic changes such as increased blood glucose levels. Diabetic patients may be unable to compensate for the increase in blood glucose and the development of ketoacidosis has been reported. Concurrent administration of corticosteroids can exaggerate this effect.

4.5 Interaction with other medicinal products and other forms of interaction
None known.

4.6 Pregnancy and lactation
Administration of drugs during pregnancy should only be considered if the expected benefit to the mother is greater than any possible risk to the foetus.

As with the majority of drugs, there is little published evidence of its safety in the early stages of human pregnancy, but in animal studies there was evidence of some harmful effects on the foetus at very high dose levels.

As salbutamol is probably secreted in breast milk its use in nursing mothers requires careful consideration. It is not known whether salbutamol has a harmful effect on the neonate, and so its use should be restricted to situations where it is felt that the expected benefit to the mother is likely to outweigh any potential risk to the neonate.

4.7 Effects on ability to drive and use machines
None known.

4.8 Undesirable effects
Adverse events are listed below by system organ class and frequency. Frequencies are defined as: very common (≥1/10), common (≥1/100 and <1/10), uncommon (≥1/1000 and <1/100), rare (≥1/10,000 and <1/1000) and very rare (<1/10,000) including isolated reports. Very common and common events were generally determined from clinical trial data. Rare, very rare and unknown events were generally determined from spontaneous data.

Immune system disorders

Very rare: Hypersensitivity reactions including angioedema, urticaria, bronchospasm, hypotension and collapse.

Metabolism and nutrition disorders

Rare: Hypokalaemia.

Potentially serious hypokalaemia may result from beta agonist therapy.

Nervous system disorders

Very common: Tremor.

Common: Headache.

Very rare: Hyperactivity.

Cardiac disorders

Common: Tachycardia, palpitations.

Rare: Cardiac arrhythmias including atrial fibrillation, supraventricular tachycardia and extrasystoles

Unknown: Myocardial ischaemia* (see section 4.4)

Vascular disorders

Rare: Peripheral vasodilatation.

Musculoskeletal and connective tissue disorders

Common: Muscle cramps.

Very rare: Feeling of muscle tension.

* reported spontaneously in post-marketing data therefore frequency regarded as unknown

4.9 Overdose
The most common signs and symptoms of overdose with salbutamol are transient beta agonist pharmacologically mediated events, including tachycardia, tremor, hyperactivity and metabolic effects including hypokalaemia and lactic acidosis (see sections 4.4 and 4.8).

Hypokalaemia may occur following overdose with salbutamol. Serum potassium levels should be monitored.

Nausea, vomiting and hyperglycaemia have been reported, predominantly in children and when salbutamol overdose has been taken via the oral route.

Consideration should be given to discontinuation of treatment and appropriate symptomatic therapy such as cardio-selective beta-blocking agents in patients presenting with cardiac symptoms (e.g. tachycardia, palpitations). Beta-blocking drugs should be used with caution in patients with a history of bronchospasm.

5. PHARMACOLOGICAL PROPERTIES

5.1 Pharmacodynamic properties
Salbutamol is a selective beta-2 adrenoceptor agonist. At therapeutic doses it acts on the beta-2 adrenoceptors of bronchial muscle.

5.2 Pharmacokinetic properties
Salbutamol administered intravenously has a half life of 4 to 6 hours and is cleared partly renally and partly by metabolism to the inactive 4' -O-sulphate (phenolic sulphate) which is also excreted primarily in the urine. The faeces are a minor route of excretion. The majority of a dose of salbutamol given intravenously, orally or by inhalation is excreted within 72 hours. Salbutamol is bound to plasma proteins to the extent of 10%.

After oral administration, salbutamol is absorbed from the gastrointestinal tract and undergoes considerable first-pass metabolism to the phenolic sulphate. Both unchanged drug and conjugate are excreted primarily in the urine. The bioavailability of orally administered salbutamol is about 50%.

5.3 Preclinical safety data
There are no preclinical data of relevance to the prescriber which are additional to that in other sections of the SmPC.

6. PHARMACEUTICAL PARTICULARS

6.1 List of excipients
Sodium citrate

Citric acid monohydrate

Hydroxypropyl methylcellulose

Sodium benzoate

Saccharin sodium

Sodium chloride

Orange flavour IFF 17.42.8187

Purified water

6.2 Incompatibilities
None known.

Ventolin syrup is sugar free. If dilution is required freshly prepared Purified Water BP should be used. The diluted mixture must be protected from light and stored below 25°C.

6.3 Shelf life
36 months.

6.4 Special precautions for storage
Store at a temperature not exceeding 30°C.

Protect from light.

Ventolin syrup may be diluted with freshly Purified Water BP. The diluted mixture must be protected from light and stored below 25°C. Discard after 28 days.

6.5 Nature and contents of container
Amber glass bottle.

Closure (150ml): plastic tamper evident, child resistant or plastic child resistant or ROPP aluminium (lacquered internally and externally) with either PVdC faced EPE or LDPE faced PVdC/EPE OR LLDPE/PVdC-PVC/LLDPE/EPE (single or double faced) wad.

Closure (2000ml): polypropylene cap with wadding as for 150ml.

Pack size: 150ml, 2000ml.

6.6 Special precautions for disposal and other handling
Ventolin syrup may be diluted with Purified Water BP (50%v/v). The resulting mixture should be protected from light and used within 28 days.

A 50% v/v dilution of Ventolin syrup has been shown to be adequately preserved against microbial contamination.

Admixture of Ventolin syrup with other liquid preparation is not recommended.

Administrative Data

7. MARKETING AUTHORISATION HOLDER
Glaxo Wellcome UK Ltd
trading as Allen & Hanburys
Stockley Park West
Uxbridge
Middlesex, UB11 1BT

8. MARKETING AUTHORISATION NUMBER(S)
PL 10949/0088

9. DATE OF FIRST AUTHORISATION/RENEWAL OF THE AUTHORISATION
14 October 2005

10. DATE OF REVISION OF THE TEXT
31 July 2009

Vermox Suspension

(Janssen-Cilag Ltd)

1. NAME OF THE MEDICINAL PRODUCT
Vermox® Suspension

2. QUALITATIVE AND QUANTITATIVE COMPOSITION
Each 5 ml of suspension contains mebendazole PhEur 100 mg.

3. PHARMACEUTICAL FORM
White homogeneous oral suspension.

4. CLINICAL PARTICULARS

4.1 Therapeutic indications
Broad spectrum gastrointestinal anthelmintic indicated for the treatment of:

Enterobius vermicularis (threadworm/pinworm)

Oxyuris vermicularis

Trichuris trichuria (whipworm)

Ascaris lumbricoides (large roundworm)

Ancylostoma duodenale (common hookworm)

Necator americanus (American hookworm)

There is no evidence that Vermox Suspension is effective in the treatment of cysticercosis.

4.2 Posology and method of administration
Method of administration.

Oral Use

Adults and children over 2 years:

Enterobiasis:

1 × 5 ml (1 dosing cup).

It is highly recommended that a second dose is taken after two weeks, if reinfection is suspected.

Ascariasis, trichuriasis, ancylostomiasis, necatoriasis and mixed infections:

1 × 5 ml (1 dosing cup) bd for three days.

4.3 Contraindications
Vermox is contra-indicated in pregnancy and in patients who have shown hypersensitivity to the product or any components.

4.4 Special warnings and precautions for use
Not recommended in the treatment of children under 2 years.

A case-control study of a single outbreak of Stevens-Johnson syndrome /toxic epidermal necrolysis (SJS/TEN) suggested a possible association with the concomitant use of metronidazole with mebendazole. Although there are no additional data on this potential interaction, concomitant use of mebendazole and metronidazole should be avoided.

4.5 Interaction with other medicinal products and other forms of interaction
Concomitant treatment with cimetidine may inhibit the metabolism of mebendazole in the liver, resulting in increased plasma concentrations of the drug.

Concomitant use of mebendazole and metronidazole should be avoided (see section 4.4).

4.6 Pregnancy and lactation
Since Vermox is contra-indicated in pregnancy, patients who think they are or may be pregnant should not take this preparation.

As it is not known whether mebendazole is excreted in human milk, it is not advisable to breast feed following administration of Vermox.

4.7 Effects on ability to drive and use machines
None known.

4.8 Undesirable effects
At the recommended dose, Vermox is generally well tolerated. However, patients with high parasitic burdens when treated with Vermox have manifested diarrhoea and abdominal pain.

Post-marketing experience

Within each system organ class, the adverse drug reactions are ranked under the headings of reporting frequency, using the following convention:

Very common (> 1/10) Common (> 1/100, < 1/10) Uncommon (> 1/1000, < 1/100) Rare (> 1/10000, < 1/1000) Very rare (< 1/10000) including isolated reports.

Immune system disorders

Very rare: hypersensitivity reactions such as anaphylactic and anaphylactoid reactions.

Nervous system disorders

Very rare: convulsions in infants.

Gastrointestinal disorders

Very rare: abdominal pain, diarrhoea (these symptoms can also be the result of the worm infestation itself).

Skin and subcutaneous tissue disorders

Very rare: toxic epidermal necrolysis, Stevens-Johnson syndrome (see also section 4.4), exanthema, angioedema, urticaria, rash.

Adverse drug reactions reported with prolonged use at dosages substantially above those recommended

Liver function disturbances, hepatitis, glomerulonephritis and neutropenia.

4.9 Overdose
Symptoms

In the event of accidental overdosage, abdominal cramps, nausea, vomiting and diarrhoea may occur.

See also section 4.8. subheading 'Adverse drug reactions reported with prolonged use at dosages substantially above those recommended'.

Treatment

There is no specific antidote. Within the first hour after ingestion, gastric lavage may be performed. Activated charcoal may be given if considered appropriate.

5. PHARMACOLOGICAL PROPERTIES

5.1 Pharmacodynamic properties
In vitro and *in vivo* work suggests that mebendazole blocks the uptake of glucose by adult and larval forms of helminths, in a selective and irreversible manner. Inhibition of glucose uptake appears to lead to endogenous depletion of glycogen stores within the helminth. Lack of glycogen leads to decreased formation of ATP and ultrastructural changes in the cells.

There is no evidence that Vermox is effective in the treatment of cysticercosis.

5.2 Pharmacokinetic properties
Using a tracer dose of ^{3}H-mebendazole, the pharmacokinetics and bioavailability of a solution and IV drug have been examined. After oral administration, the half life was 0.93 hours. Absorption of this tracer dose was almost complete but low availability indicated a high first pass effect. At normal therapeutic doses, it is very hard to measure levels in the plasma.

5.3 Preclinical safety data
No relevant information additional to that contained elsewhere in the Summary of Product Characteristics.

6. PHARMACEUTICAL PARTICULARS

6.1 List of excipients
Sucrose

Microcrystalline cellulose and sodium carboxymethyl cellulose

Methylcellulose 15 mPa.s

Methylparaben

Propylparaben

Sodium lauryl sulphate

Banana 1

Citric acid, monohydrate

Purified water

6.2 Incompatibilities
None known.

6.3 Shelf life
5 years.

6.4 Special precautions for storage
Shake well before use.

Keep out of reach and sight of children.

6.5 Nature and contents of container
Amber glass flask containing 30 ml suspension, with either:

• Pilfer-proof screw cap. Cork insert in cap is coated on both sides with polyvinylchloride

or

• Child-resistant polypropylene screw cap, lined inside with a LDPE insert.

A 5 ml natural polypropylene (food-grade) dosing cup is also provided, graduated for 2.5 ml and 5 ml.

6.6 Special precautions for disposal and other handling
Not applicable.

7. MARKETING AUTHORISATION HOLDER
Janssen-Cilag Ltd
50-100 Holmers Farm Way
High Wycombe
Buckinghamshire
HP12 4EG
UK

8. MARKETING AUTHORISATION NUMBER(S)
PL 0242/0050

9. DATE OF FIRST AUTHORISATION/RENEWAL OF THE AUTHORISATION
Date of First Authorisation: 17 November 1977
Date of Renewal of Authorisation: 15 December 2002

10. DATE OF REVISION OF THE TEXT
September 2008

Vermox Tablets

(Janssen-Cilag Ltd)

1. NAME OF THE MEDICINAL PRODUCT
Vermox tablets

2. QUALITATIVE AND QUANTITATIVE COMPOSITION
Each tablet contains mebendazole 100 mg.

3. PHARMACEUTICAL FORM
Tablet.

4. CLINICAL PARTICULARS

4.1 Therapeutic indications
For the treatment of *Trichuris trichuria* (whipworm), *Enterobius vermicularis* (pinworm or threadworm), *Ascaris lumbricoides* (roundworm), *Ancylostoma duodenale* (common hookworm), *Necator americanus* (American hookworm) in single or mixed gastrointestinal infestations.

There is no evidence that Vermox Tablets are effective in the treatment of cysticercosis.

4.2 Posology and method of administration
Adults and children over 2 years:

For the control of trichuriasis, ascariasis and hookworm infections, one tablet twice a day for three consecutive days.

For the control of enterobiasis a single tablet is administered. It is highly recommended that a second tablet is taken after two weeks, if re-infection is suspected.

Tablets may be chewed or swallowed whole. Crush the tablet before giving it to a young child. Always supervise a child while they are taking this medicine.

Method of Administration

Oral use.

4.3 Contraindications
Vermox is contraindicated in pregnancy and in patients who have shown hypersensitivity to the product or any components.

4.4 Special warnings and precautions for use
Not recommended in the treatment of children under 2 years.

A case-control study of a single outbreak of Stevens-Johnson syndrome /toxic epidermal necrolysis (SJS/TEN) suggested a possible association with the concomitant use of metronidazole with mebendazole. Although there are no additional data on this potential interaction, concomitant use of mebendazole and metronidazole should be avoided.

4.5 Interaction with other medicinal products and other forms of interaction
Concomitant treatment with cimetidine may inhibit the metabolism of mebendazole in the liver, resulting in increased plasma concentrations of the drug.

Concomitant use of mebendazole and metronidazole should be avoided (see section 4.4).

4.6 Pregnancy and lactation
Since Vermox is contra-indicated in pregnancy, patients who think they are, or may be, pregnant should not take this preparation.

Lactation

As it is not known whether mebendazole is excreted in human milk, it is not advisable to breast feed following administration of Vermox.

4.7 Effects on ability to drive and use machines
None stated.

4.8 Undesirable effects
At the recommended dose, Vermox is generally well tolerated. However, patients with high parasitic burdens when treated with Vermox have manifested diarrhoea and abdominal pain.

Post-marketing experience

Within each system organ class, the adverse drug reactions are ranked under the headings of reporting frequency, using the following convention:

Very common (≥ 1/10) Common (≥ 1/100, < 1/10) Uncommon (≥ 1/1000, < 1/100) Rare (≥ 1/10000, < 1/1,000) Very rare (< 1/10,000) including isolated reports.

Immune system disorders

Very rare: hypersensitivity reactions such as anaphylactic and anaphylactoid reactions.

Nervous system disorders

Very rare: convulsions in infants.

Gastrointestinal disorders

Very rare: abdominal pain, diarrhoea (these symptoms can also be the result of the worm infestation itself).

Skin and subcutaneous tissue disorders

Very rare: toxic epidermal necrolysis, Stevens-Johnson syndrome (see also section 4.4), exanthema, angioedema, urticaria, rash.

Adverse drug reactions reported with prolonged use at dosages substantially above those recommended

Liver function disturbances, hepatitis, glomerulonephritis and neutropenia.

4.9 Overdose
Symptoms

In the event of accidental overdosage, abdominal cramps, nausea, vomiting and diarrhoea may occur.

See also section 4.8. subheading 'Adverse drug reactions reported with prolonged use at dosages substantially above those recommended'.

Treatment

There is no specific antidote. Within the first hour after ingestion, gastric lavage may be performed. Activated charcoal may be given if considered appropriate.

5. PHARMACOLOGICAL PROPERTIES

5.1 Pharmacodynamic properties
In vitro and *in vivo* work suggests that mebendazole blocks the uptake of glucose by adult and larval forms of helminths, in a selective and irreversible manner. Inhibition of glucose uptake appears to lead to endogenous depletion of glycogen stores within the helminth. Lack of glycogen leads to decreased formation of ATP and ultrastructural changes in the cells.

There is no evidence that Vermox is effective in the treatment of cysticercosis.

5.2 Pharmacokinetic properties
Using a tracer dose of ^{3}H-mebendazole, the pharmacokinetics and bioavailability of a solution and IV drug have been examined. After oral administration, the half life was 0.93 hours. Absorption of this tracer dose was almost complete but low availability indicated a high first pass effect. At normal therapeutic doses, it is very hard to measure levels in the plasma.

5.3 Preclinical safety data
No relevant information additional to that contained elsewhere in the Summary of Product Characteristics.

6. PHARMACEUTICAL PARTICULARS

6.1 List of excipients
Microcrystalline cellulose

Sodium starch glycolate

Talc

Maize starch

Sodium saccharin

Magnesium stearate

Hydrogenated vegetable oil

Orange flavour

Colloidal anhydrous silica

Sodium lauryl sulphate

Orange yellow S

Purified water*

2-propanol*

* Not present in the final product.

6.2 Incompatibilities
Not applicable.

6.3 Shelf life
36 months.

6.4 Special precautions for storage
None.

6.5 Nature and contents of container
Blister strips of PVC genotherm glass clear aluminium foil coated on the inside with a heat seal lacquer.

Pack sizes: 1 and 6 tablet packs.

6.6 Special precautions for disposal and other handling
Not applicable

7. MARKETING AUTHORISATION HOLDER
Janssen-Cilag Ltd
50-100 Holmers Farm Way
High Wycombe
Buckinghamshire
HP12 4EG
UK

8. MARKETING AUTHORISATION NUMBER(S)
PL 0242/0011

9. DATE OF FIRST AUTHORISATION/RENEWAL OF THE AUTHORISATION
Date of First Authorisation: 9 April 1975
Date of Renewal of Authorisation: 30 September 2003

10. DATE OF REVISION OF THE TEXT
01 May 2009

LEGAL CATEGORY POM

Versatis 5% Medicated Plaster

(Grunenthal Ltd)

1. NAME OF THE MEDICINAL PRODUCT
Versatis 5% medicated plaster

2. QUALITATIVE AND QUANTITATIVE COMPOSITION
Each 10 cm × 14 cm plaster contains 700 mg (5% w/w) lidocaine
(50 mg lidocaine per gram adhesive base)
Excipients:
Methyl parahydroxybenzoate 14 mg
Propyl parahydroxybenzoate 7 mg
Propylene glycol 700 mg
For a full list of excipients, see section 6.1.

3. PHARMACEUTICAL FORM
Medicated plaster
White hydrogel plaster containing adhesive material, which is applied to a non-woven polyethylene terephthalate backing embossed with "Lidocaine 5%" and covered with a polyethylene terephthalate film release liner.

4. CLINICAL PARTICULARS
4.1 Therapeutic indications
Versatis is indicated for the symptomatic relief of neuropathic pain associated with previous herpes zoster infection (post-herpetic neuralgia, PHN).

4.2 Posology and method of administration
Adults and elderly patients
The painful area should be covered with the plaster once daily for up to 12 hours within a 24 hours period. Only the number of plasters that are needed for an effective treatment should be used. When needed, the plasters may be cut into smaller sizes with scissors prior to removal of the release liner. In total, not more than three plasters should be used at the same time.

The plaster must be applied to intact, dry, non-irritated skin (after healing of the shingles).

Each plaster must be worn no longer than 12 hours. The subsequent plaster-free interval must be at least 12 hours.

The plaster must be applied to the skin immediately after removal from the sachet and following removal of the release liner from the gel surface. Hairs in the affected area must be cut off with a pair of scissors (not shaved).

Treatment outcome should be re-evaluated after 2-4 weeks. If there has been no response to Versatis after this period or if any relieving effect can solely be related to the skin protective properties of the plaster, treatment must be discontinued as potential risks may outweigh benefits in this context (see sections 4.4 and 5.1). Treatment should be reassessed at regular intervals to decide whether the amount of plasters needed to cover the painful area can be reduced, or if the plaster-free period can be extended.

Use for patients under the age of 18 is not recommended because of the lack of data in this group.

4.3 Contraindications
Hypersensitivity to the active substance or to any of the excipients. The plaster is also contraindicated in patients with known hypersensitivity to other local anaesthetics of the amide type e.g. bupivacaine, etidocaine, mepivacaine and prilocaine.

The plaster must not be applied to inflamed or injured skin, such as active herpes zoster lesions, atopic dermatitis or wounds.

4.4 Special warnings and precautions for use
The plaster should not be applied to mucous membranes. Eye contact with the plaster should be avoided.

The plaster contains propylene glycol which may cause skin irritation. It also contains methyl parahydroxybenzoate and propyl parahydroxybenzoate which may cause allergic reactions (possibly delayed).

The plaster should be used with caution in patients with severe cardiac impairment, severe renal impairment or severe hepatic impairment.

One of the lidocaine metabolites, 2,6 xylidine, has been shown to be genotoxic and carcinogenic in rats (see section 5.3). Secondary metabolites have been shown to be mutagenic. The clinical significance of this finding is unknown. Consequently long term treatment with Versatis is only justified if there is a therapeutic benefit for the patient (see section 4.2).

4.5 Interaction with other medicinal products and other forms of interaction
No interaction studies have been performed. No clinically relevant interactions have been observed in clinical studies with the plaster.

Since the maximum lidocaine plasma concentrations observed in clinical trials with the plaster were low (see section 5.2), a clinically relevant pharmacokinetic interaction is unlikely.

Although normally the absorption of lidocaine from the skin is low, the plaster must be used with caution in patients receiving Class I antiarrhythmic medicinal products (e.g. tocainide, mexiletine) and other local anaesthetics since the risk of additive systemic effects cannot be excluded.

4.6 Pregnancy and lactation
Pregnancy
Lidocaine crosses the placenta. However, there are no adequate data from the use of lidocaine in pregnant women.

Animal studies are incomplete with respect to effects on pregnancy, embryo-foetal development, parturition or postnatal development (see section 5.3).

The potential risk for humans is unknown. Therefore, Versatis should not be used during pregnancy unless clearly necessary.

Lactation
Lidocaine is excreted in breast milk. However, there are no studies of the plaster in breast-feeding women. Since the metabolism of lidocaine occurs relatively fast and almost completely in the liver, only very low levels of lidocaine are expected to be excreted into human milk.

4.7 Effects on ability to drive and use machines
No studies on the effects on the ability to drive and use machines have been performed. An effect on the ability to drive and use machines is unlikely because systemic absorption is minimal (see section 5.2)

4.8 Undesirable effects
Within each frequency grouping, undesirable effects are presented in order of decreasing seriousness.

Approximately 16% of patients can be expected to experience adverse reactions. These are localised reactions due to the nature of the medicinal product.

The most commonly reported adverse reactions were administration site reactions including erythema, rash, application site pruritus, application site burning, application site dermatitis, application site erythema, application site vesicles, dermatitis, skin irritation, and pruritus.

The table below lists adverse reactions that have been reported in studies of post herpetic neuralgia patients receiving the plaster. They are listed by system organ class and frequency. Frequencies are defined as very common (≥1/10); common (≥1/100 to <1/10); uncommon (≥1/1,000 to <1/100); rare (≥1/10,000 to <1/1,000); very rare (<1/10,000), not known (cannot be estimated from the available data).

Body system	Adverse drug reaction
Skin and subcutaneous tissues disorders	
uncommon	Skin lesion
Injury, poisoning and procedural complications	
uncommon	Skin injury
General disorders and administration site conditions	
Very common	Administration site reactions

The following reactions have been observed in patients receiving the plaster under post-marketing conditions:

Body system	Adverse drug reaction
Injury, poisoning and procedural complications	
Very rare	Open wound
Immune system disorders	
Very rare	Anaphylactic reaction, hypersensitivity

All adverse reactions were predominantly of mild and moderate intensity. Of those less than 5% lead to treatment discontinuation.

Systemic adverse reactions following the appropriate use of the plaster are unlikely since the systemic concentration of lidocaine is very low (see section 5.2). Systemic adverse reactions to lidocaine are similar in nature to those observed with other amide local anaesthetic agents (see section 4.9).

4.9 Overdose
Overdose with the plaster is unlikely but it cannot be excluded that inappropriate use, such as use of a higher number of plasters at the same time, with prolonged application period, or using the plaster on broken skin might result in higher than normal plasma concentrations. Possible signs of systemic toxicity will be similar in nature to those observed after administration of lidocaine as a local anaesthetic agent, and may include the following signs and symptoms:
dizziness, vomiting drowsiness, seizures, mydriasis, bradycardia, arrhythmia, and shock.

In addition, known drug interactions related to systemic lidocaine concentrations with beta-blockers, CYP3A4 inhibitors (e.g. imidazole derivatives, macrolides) and antiarrhythmic agents might become relevant with overdose.

In case of suspected overdose the plaster should be removed and supportive measures taken as clinically needed. There is no antidote to lidocaine.

5. PHARMACOLOGICAL PROPERTIES
5.1 Pharmacodynamic properties
Pharmacotherapeutic group: local anaesthetics, amides
ATC code: N01 BB02
Mechanism of action
Lidocaine when applied topically in the form of the plaster, has been shown in studies to produce a local analgesic effect. The mechanism by which this occurs is due to stabilisation of neuronal membranes, which is thought to cause down regulation of sodium channels resulting in pain reduction.
Clinical efficacy
Pain management in PHN is difficult. There is evidence of efficacy with Versatis in the symptomatic relief from the allodynic component of PHN in some cases (see section 4.2).

Efficacy of Versatis has been shown in post-herpetic neuralgia studies. Other models of neuropathic pain have not been studied.

There were two main controlled studies carried out to assess the efficacy of the lidocaine 5% medicated plaster.

In the first study, patients were recruited from a population who were already considered to respond to the product. It was a cross over design of 14 days treatment with lidocaine 5% medicated plaster followed by placebo, or vice versa. The primary endpoint was the time to exit, where patients withdrew because their pain relief was two points lower than their normal response on a six point scale (ranging from worse to complete relief). There were 32 patients, of whom 30 completed. The median time to exit for placebo was 4 days and for active was 14 days (p value < 0.001); none of those on active discontinued during the two week treatment period.

In the second study 265 patients with post-herpetic neuralgia were recruited and allocated eight weeks of open label active treatment with lidocaine 5% medicated plaster. In this uncontrolled setting approximately 50% of patients responded to treatment as measured by two points lower than their normal response on a six point scale (ranging from worse to complete relief). A total of 71 patients were randomised to receive either placebo or lidocaine 5% medicated plaster given for 2-14 days. The primary endoint was defined as lack of efficacy on two consecutive days leading to withdrawal of treatment. There were 9/36 patients on active and 16/35 patients on placebo who withdrew because of lack of treatment benefit.

Post hoc analyses of the second study showed that the initial response was independent of the duration of pre-existing PHN. However, the notion that patients with longer duration of PHN (> 12 months) do benefit more from active treatment is supported by the finding that this group of patients was more likely to drop out due to lack of efficacy when switched to placebo during the double-blind withdrawal part of this study.

5.2 Pharmacokinetic properties
Absorption
When lidocaine 5% medicated plaster is used according to the maximum recommended dose (3 plasters applied simultaneously for 12 h) about 3 ± 2% of the total applied lidocaine dose is systemically available and similar for single and multiple administrations.

A population kinetics analysis of the clinical efficacy studies in patients suffering from PHN revealed a mean maximum concentration for lidocaine of 45 ng/ml after application of 3 plasters simultaneously 12 h per day after repeated application for up to one year. This concentration is in accordance with the observation in pharmacokinetic studies in PHN patients (52 ng/ml) and in healthy volunteers (85 ng/ml and 125 ng/ml).

For lidocaine and its metabolites MEGX, GX, and 2,6-xylidine no tendency for accumulation was found, steady state concentrations were reached within the first four days.

The population kinetic analysis indicated that when increasing the number from 1 to 3 plasters worn simultaneously, the systemic exposure increased less than proportionally to the number of used plasters.

Distribution

After intravenous administration of lidocaine to healthy volunteers, the volume of distribution was found to be 1.3 ± 0.4 l/kg (mean ± S.D., n = 15). The lidocaine distribution volume showed no age-dependency, it is decreased in patients with congestive heart failure and increased in patients with liver disease. At plasma concentrations produced by application of the plaster approximately 70 % of lidocaine is bound to plasma proteins. Lidocaine crosses the placental and blood brain barriers presumably by passive diffusion.

Biotransformation

Lidocaine is metabolised rapidly in the liver to a number of metabolites. The primary metabolic route for lidocaine is N-dealkylation to monoethylglycinexylidide (MEGX) and glycinexylidide (GX), both of which are less active than lidocaine and available in low concentrations. These are hydrolyzed to 2,6-xylidine, which is converted to conjugated 4-hydroxy-2,6-xylidine.

The metabolite, 2,6-xylidine, has unknown pharmacological activity but shows carcinogenic potential in rats (see section 5.3). A population kinetics analysis revealed a mean maximum concentration for 2,6-xylidine of 9 ng/ml after repeated daily applications for up to one year This finding is confirmed by a phase I pharmacokinetic study. Data on lidocaine metabolism in the skin are not available.

Elimination

Lidocaine and its metabolites are excreted by the kidneys. More than 85 % of the dose is found in the urine in the form of metabolites or active substance. Less than 10 % of the lidocaine dose is excreted unchanged. The main metabolite in urine is a conjugate of 4-hydroxy-2,6-xylidine, accounting for about 70 to 80% of the dose excreted in the urine. 2,6-xylidine is excreted in the urine in man at a concentration of less than 1% of the dose. The elimination half-life of lidocaine after plaster application in healthy volunteers is 7.6 hours. The excretion of lidocaine and its metabolites may be delayed in cardiac, renal or hepatic insufficiency.

5.3 Preclinical safety data

Effects in non-clinical studies were observed only at exposures considered sufficiently in excess of the maximum human exposure indicating little relevance to clinical use.

In toxicological studies described in the literature using systemic administration of lidocaine, cardiovascular effects (tachycardia or bradycardia, decreases in cardiac output and blood pressure, cardiac arrest) and central nervous system effects (convulsion, coma, respiratory arrest) were observed at exposures considered sufficiently in excess of the maximum human exposure following treatment with Versatis. This indicates that these effects have little relevance to clinical use.

Lidocaine HCl has shown no genotoxicity when investigated *in vitro* or *in vivo*. Its hydrolysis product and metabolite, 2,6-xylidine, showed mixed genotoxic activity in several assays particularly after metabolic activation.

Carcinogenicity studies have not been performed with lidocaine. Studies performed with the metabolite 2,6-xylidine mixed in the diet of male and female rats resulted in treatment-related cytotoxicity and hyperplasia of the nasal olfactory epithelium and carcinomas and adenomas in the nasal cavity were observed. Tumorigenic changes were also found in the liver and subcutis. Because the risk to humans is unclear, long-term treatment with high doses of lidocaine should be avoided.

Lidocaine had no effect on general reproductive performance or female fertility in rats at plasma concentrations up to 130-fold those observed in patients. No adverse effects were seen in an embryo-foetal/teratogenicity study in rats at plasma concentrations more than 200-fold that observed in humans.

Animal studies are incomplete with respect to effects on pregnancy, embryofoetal development, parturition or post-natal development.

6. PHARMACEUTICAL PARTICULARS

6.1 List of excipients

Self-adhesive layer:

glycerol,

liquid sorbitol, crystallising,

carmellose sodium,

propylene glycol (E1520),

urea,

heavy kaolin,

tartaric acid,

gelatin,

polyvinyl alcohol,

aluminium glycinate,

disodium edetate,

methyl parahydroxybenzoate (E218),

propyl parahydroxybenzoate (E216),

polyacrylic acid,

sodium polyacrylate,

purified water.

Backing fabric:

Polyethylene terephthalate (PET)

Release liner:

Polyethylene terephthalate

6.2 Incompatibilities

Not applicable.

6.3 Shelf life

3 years.

After first opening the sachet, the plasters must be used within 14 days.

6.4 Special precautions for storage

Do not refrigerate or freeze.

After first opening: Keep the sachet tightly closed.

6.5 Nature and contents of container

Re-sealable sachet composed of paper/polyethylene/aluminium/ethylene meta-acrylic acid co-polymer containing 5 plasters.

Each carton contains 5, 10, 20, 25 or 30 plasters. Not all pack sizes may be marketed.

6.6 Special precautions for disposal and other handling

After use the plaster still contains active substance. After removal, the used plasters should be folded in half, adhesive side inwards so that the self-adhesive layer is not exposed, and the plaster should be discarded.

Any unused product or waste material should be disposed of in accordance with local requirements.

7. MARKETING AUTHORISATION HOLDER

Grünenthal Ltd

Regus Lakeside House

1 Furzeground Way

Stockley Park East

Uxbridge

Middlesex UB11 1BD

United Kingdom

8. MARKETING AUTHORISATION NUMBER(S)

PL 21727/0016

9. DATE OF FIRST AUTHORISATION/RENEWAL OF THE AUTHORISATION

05 January 2007

10. DATE OF REVISION OF THE TEXT

04 September 2009

Vesanoid 10mg soft capsules

(Roche Products Limited)

1. NAME OF THE MEDICINAL PRODUCT

VESANOID®10 mg soft capsules

2. QUALITATIVE AND QUANTITATIVE COMPOSITION

Active substance:

1 capsule contains 10 mg of tretinoin

Excipients:

1 capsule contains 107.92 mg of soya-bean oil.

The capsule-shell contains between 0.96 – 1.46 mg of sorbitol (E420).

For the full list of excipients, see section 6.1

3. PHARMACEUTICAL FORM

Capsule, soft

Bi-coloured orange-yellow / reddish-brown capsules.

4. CLINICAL PARTICULARS

4.1 Therapeutic indications

VESANOID (tretinoin) is indicated for induction of remission in acute promyelocytic leukaemia (APL; FAB classification AML-M3).

This treatment is intended for previously untreated patients as well as patients who relapse after a standard chemotherapy (anthracycline and cytosine arabinoside or equivalent therapies) or patients who are refractory to chemotherapy.

The association of tretinoin with chemotherapy increases the duration of survival and reduces the risk of relapse compared to chemotherapy alone.

4.2 Posology and method of administration

A total daily dose of 45 mg/m^2 body surface divided in two equal doses is recommended for oral administration. This is approximately 8 capsules per adult dose.

Capsules should be swallowed together with water. Capsules should not be chewed. It is recommended to take the capsules with a meal or shortly thereafter.

There is limited safety and efficacy information on the use of tretinoin in children.

Pediatric patients can be treated with 45 mg/m^2 unless severe toxicity becomes apparent. Dose reduction should be particularly considered for children with intractable headache.

Treatment should be continued until complete remission has been achieved or up to a maximum of 90 days.

Due to limited information on patients with hepatic and/or renal insufficiency, the dose will be decreased to 25 mg/m^2 as a precautionary measure.

Full-dose anthracycline-based chemotherapy should be added to the tretinoin regimen as follows (see section 4.4):

- When the leukocyte count at start of therapy is greater than 5 × 10^9/L, chemotherapy should be started together with tretinoin on day one.
- When the leukocyte count at start of therapy is less than 5 × 10^9/L but rapidly increases during tretinoin therapy, chemotherapy should be **immediately** added to the tretinoin regimen if the leukocyte count reaches greater than 6 × 10^9/L by day five, or greater than 10 × 10^9/L by day ten, or greater than 15 × 10^9/L by day 28.
- All other patients should receive chemotherapy immediately after complete remission is attained.

If chemotherapy is added to tretinoin because of hyperleukocytosis, it is not necessary to modify the dose of tretinoin.

After completion of tretinoin therapy and the first chemotherapy course, consolidation anthracycline-based chemotherapy should be given, for example, a further two courses at 4 to 6 week intervals.

In some patients the plasma levels of tretinoin may fall significantly in spite of continued administration.

4.3 Contraindications

Known allergy to tretinoin, retinoids or to any of the excipients.

Pregnancy (see section 4.6).

Lactation (see section 4.6).

Tetracyclines (see section 4.5).

Vitamin A (see section 4.5).

Vesanoid contains soya-bean oil, therefore Vesanoid is contraindicated in patients allergic to soya or peanut.

4.4 Special warnings and precautions for use

Tretinoin should be administered to patients with acute promyelocytic leukaemia only under the strict supervision of a physician who is experienced in the treatment of hematological / oncological diseases.

Supportive care appropriate for patients with acute promyelocytic leukaemia, for example prophylaxis for bleeding and prompt therapy for infection, should be maintained during therapy with tretinoin. The patient's hematologic profile, coagulation profile, liver function test results, and triglyceride and cholesterol levels should be monitored frequently.

During clinical trials hyperleukocytosis has been frequently observed (in 75% of the cases), sometimes associated with the "Retinoic Acid Syndrome". Retinoic acid syndrome has been reported in many acute promyelocytic leukaemia patients (up to 25% in some centers) treated with tretinoin.

Retinoic acid syndrome is characterized by fever, dyspnoea, acute respiratory distress, pulmonary infiltrates, pleural and pericardial effusions, hypotension, oedema, weight gain, hepatic, renal and multi-organ failure.

Retinoic acid syndrome is frequently associated with hyperleukocytosis and may be fatal.

The incidence of the retinoic acid syndrome is diminished when full dose chemotherapy is added to the tretinoin regimen based on the white blood cell count. The current therapeutic treatment recommendations and method of administration are detailed in section 4.2.

Immediate treatment with dexamethasone (10 mg every 12 hours for up to maximum 3 days or until resolution of the symptoms) should be given, if the patient presents any symptom(s) or sign(s) of this syndrome.

In cases of moderate and severe retinoic acid syndrome, temporary interruption of Vesanoid therapy should be considered.

Vesanoid may cause pseudotumour cerebri. This condition should be treated according to standard medical practice. Temporary discontinuation of Vesanoid should be considered in patients not responding to treatment.

Sweet's syndrome or acute febrile neutrophilic dermatitis responded dramatically to corticosteroid treatment.

There is a risk of thrombosis (both venous and arterial) which may involve any organ system, during the first month of treatment (see section 4.8). Therefore, caution should be exercised when treating patients with the combination of Vesanoid and anti-fibrinolytic agents, such as tranexamic acid, aminocaproic acid or aprotinin (see section 4.5).

Because hypercalcaemia may occur during therapy, serum calcium levels should be monitored.

Micro-dosed progesterone preparations ("minipill") are an inadequate method of contraception during treatment with tretinoin (see section 4.6).

Vesanoid contains sorbitol, therefore patients with rare hereditary problems of fructose intolerance should not take Vesanoid.

4.5 Interaction with other medicinal products and other forms of interaction

Tetracyclines: systemic treatment with retinoids may cause elevation of the intracranial pressure. As tetracyclines may also cause elevation of the intracranial pressure, patients must not be treated with tretinoin and tetracyclines at the same time (see section 4.3).

Vitamin A: As with other retinoids, tretinoin must not be administered in combination with vitamin A because symptoms of hypervitaminosis A could be aggravated (see section 4.3).

The effect of food on the bioavailability of tretinoin has not been characterised. Since the bioavailability of retinoids, as a class, is known to increase in the presence of food, it is recommended that tretinoin be administered with a meal or shortly thereafter.

As tretinoin is metabolised by the hepatic P450 system, there is the potential for alteration of pharmacokinetics parameters in patients administered concomitant medications that are also inducers or inhibitors of this system. Medications that generally induce hepatic P450 enzymes include rifampicin, glucocorticoids, phenobarbital and pentobarbital. Medications that generally inhibit hepatic P450 enzymes include ketoconazole, cimetidine, erythromycin, verapamil, diltiazem and ciclosporin. There are no data to suggest that co-use with these medications increases or decreases either efficacy or toxicity of tretinoin.

Cases of fatal thrombotic complications have been reported rarely in patients concomitantly treated with all-trans retinoic acid and anti-fibrinolytic agents such as tranexamic acid, aminocaproic acid and aprotinin (see section 4.4). Therefore, caution should be exercised when administering all-trans retinoic acid concomitantly with these agents.

There are no data on a possible pharmacokinetic interaction between tretinoin and daunorubicin or AraC.

4.6 Pregnancy and lactation

All the measures listed below should be considered in relationship to the severity of the disease and the urgency of the treatment.

Pregnancy: Vesanoid contains a retinoid similar to vitamin A. Therefore Vesanoid should not be used by women who are pregnant or likely to become pregnant. Tretinoin causes serious birth defects when administered during pregnancy. Its use is contraindicated in pregnant women and women who might become pregnant during the treatment with tretinoin and within one month after cessation of treatment, unless the benefit of tretinoin treatment outweighs the risk of foetal abnormalities due to the severity of the patient's condition and the urgency of treatment.

There is a very high risk for any exposed foetus that a deformed infant will result if pregnancy occurs while taking tretinoin, irrespective of the dose or duration of the treatment.

Therapy with tretinoin should only be started in female patients of child-bearing age if each of the following conditions is met:

- She is informed by her physician of the hazards of becoming pregnant during and one month after treatment with tretinoin.
- She is willing to comply with the mandatory effective contraception measures: to use a reliable contraception method without interruption during therapy and for one month after discontinuation of treatment with tretinoin (see section 4.4).
- Pregnancy tests must be performed at monthly intervals during therapy.

In spite of these precautions, should pregnancy occur during treatment with tretinoin or up to one month after its discontinuation, there is a high risk of severe malformation of the foetus, particularly when tretinoin is given during the first trimester of pregnancy.

Lactation: Nursing must be discontinued if therapy with tretinoin is initiated.

4.7 Effects on ability to drive and use machines

Vesanoid has minor or moderate influence on the ability to drive and use machines, particularly if patients are experiencing dizziness or severe headache.

4.8 Undesirable effects

In patients treated with the recommended daily doses of tretinoin the most frequent undesirable effects are consistent with the signs and symptoms of the hypervitaminosis A syndrome (as for other retinoids).

Retinoic acid syndrome has been reported in many acute promyelocytic leukaemia patients (up to 25% in some centers) treated with tretinoin. Retinoic acid syndrome is characterised by fever, dyspnoea, acute respiratory distress, pulmonary infiltrates, pleural and pericardial effusions, hypotension, oedema, weight gain, hepatic, renal and multi-organ failure. Retinoic acid syndrome is frequently associated with hyperleukocytosis and may be fatal. For prevention and treatment of retinoic acid syndrome see section 4.4.

In addition, the following adverse reactions have been reported in clinical studies and during the post-marketing period.

("Frequency not known" corresponds to post marketing experience)

Infections and infestations:

Frequency not known: Necrotizing fasciitis.

Blood and lymphatic system disorders:

Frequency not known: Thrombocythaemia, basophilia.

Metabolism and nutrition disorders:

Very common (≥ 1/10): Decreased appetite.

Frequency not known: Hypercalcaemia.

Psychiatric disorders:

Very common (≥ 1/10): Confusional state, anxiety, depression, insomnia.

Nervous system disorders:

Very common (≥ 1/10): Headache, intracranial pressure increased, benign intracranial hypertension, dizziness, paraesthesia.

Frequency not known: Cerebrovascular accident.

Eye disorders:

Very common (≥ 1/10): Visual disturbances, conjunctival disorders.

Ear and labyrinth disorders:

Very common (≥ 1/10): Hearing impaired.

Cardiac disorders:

Very common (≥ 1/10): Arrhythmia.

Frequency not known: Myocardial infarction.

Vascular disorders:

Very common (≥ 1/10): Flushing.

Frequency not known: Thrombosis, vasculitis.

Respiratory, thoracic and mediastinal disorders:

Very common (≥ 1/10): Respiratory failure, nasal dryness, asthma.

Gastrointestinal disorders:

Very common (≥ 1/10): Dry mouth, nausea, vomiting, abdominal pain, diarrhoea, constipation, pancreatitis, cheilitis.

Skin and subcutaneous tissue disorders:

Very common (≥ 1/10): Erythema, rash, pruritus, alopecia, hyperhidrosis.

Frequency not known: Erythema nodosum, acute febrile neutrophilic dermatosis.

Musculoskeletal and connective tissue disorders:

Very common (≥ 1/10): Bone pain.

Frequency not known: Myositis.

Renal and urinary disorders:

Frequency not known: Renal infarct.

Reproductive system and breast disorders:

Frequency not known: Genital ulceration.

General disorders and administration site conditions:

Very common (≥ 1/10): Chest pain, chills, malaise.

Investigations:

Very common (≥ 1/10): Blood triglyceride increased, blood creatinine increased, blood cholesterol increased, transaminases increased.

Frequency not known: Histamine level increased.

The decision to interrupt or continue therapy should be based on an evaluation of the benefit of the treatment versus the severity of the side-effects.

Teratogenicity: See section 4.6.

There is limited safety information on the use of tretinoin in children. There have been some reports of increased toxicity in children treated with tretinoin, particularly increased pseudotumour cerebri.

4.9 Overdose

In case of overdose with all-trans retinoic, reversible signs of hyper-vitaminosis A (headache, nausea, vomiting, mucocutaneous symptoms) can appear.

The recommended dose in acute promyelocytic leukaemia is one-quarter of the maximum tolerated dose in solid tumor patients and below the maximum tolerated dose in children.

There is no specific treatment in the case of an overdose, however it is important that the patient be treated in a special haematological unit.

5. PHARMACOLOGICAL PROPERTIES

5.1 Pharmacodynamic properties

Pharmacotherapeutic group: Cytostatic-differentiating agent, ATC code: L01XX14.

Tretinoin is a natural metabolite of retinol and belongs to the class of retinoids, comprising natural and synthetic analogs.

In vitro studies with tretinoin have demonstrated induction of differentiation and inhibition of cell proliferation in transformed haemopoietic cell lines, including human myeloid leukaemia cell lines.

The mechanism of action in acute promyelocytic leukaemia is not known but it may be due to a modification in binding of tretinoin to a nuclear retinoic acid receptor (RAR) given that the α-receptor of retinoic acid is altered by fusion with a protein called PML.

5.2 Pharmacokinetic properties

Tretinoin is an endogenous metabolite of vitamin A which is normally present in plasma.

After oral administration, tretinoin is absorbed by the digestive tract and maximum plasma concentrations in healthy volunteers are attained after 3 hours.

There is a large inter-patient and intra-patient variation in plasma levels of tretinoin.

Tretinoin is extensively bound to plasma proteins. Following peak levels, plasma concentrations decline with a mean elimination half life of 0.7 hours. Plasma concentrations return to endogenous levels after 7 to 12 hours following a single 40 mg dose. No accumulation is seen after multiple doses and tretinoin is not retained in body tissues.

After an oral dose of radiolabelled tretinoin, about 60% of the radioactivity was excreted in urine and about 30% in faeces. The metabolites found in urine were formed by oxidation and glucuronidation.

During continuous administration a marked decrease in plasma concentration can occur, possibly due to cytochrome P-450 enzyme induction which increases clearance and decreases bioavailability after oral doses.

At present there are no data on a possible interaction between tretinoin and daunorubicin.

The requirement for dosage adjustment in patients with renal or hepatic insufficiency has not been investigated. As a precautionary measure, the dose will be decreased (see section 4.2).

5.3 Preclinical safety data

Oral administration of tretinoin to animals indicated that the compound had very low acute toxicity in all species investigated.

In animal experimental tests it was shown that in all investigated species the acute toxicity of tretinoin administered orally is low. After a longer period of administration rats exhibit a dose- and time-dependent bone matrix dissolution, a decrease in erythrocyte count and toxic alterations in kidney and testes.

Dogs mainly exhibited disorders concerning spermatogenesis and hyperplasia of the bone marrow.

The major metabolites of tretinoin (4-oxo-tretinoin, isotretinoin and 4-oxo-isotretinoin) are less effective than tretinoin in inducing differentiation of human leukaemic cells (HL-60)

Subchronic and chronic toxicity studies in rats indicated that the no effect oral dose was at or below 1 mg/kg/day; in dogs, 30 mg/kg/day was associated with toxic effects including weight loss, dermatological and testicular changes.

Reproduction studies in animals have demonstrated the teratogenic activity of tretinoin.

No evidence of mutagenicity has been found.

6. PHARMACEUTICAL PARTICULARS

6.1 List of excipients

Capsule contents:

Yellow beeswax

Hydrogenated soya-bean oil

Partially hydrogenated soya-bean oil

Soya-bean oil

Capsule shell:

Gelatin

Glycerol (E 422)

Karion 83: Sorbitol (E 420), Mannitol (E 421), Starch (maize)

Titanium dioxide (E 171)

Iron oxide yellow (E 172)

Iron oxide red (E 172)

6.2 Incompatibilities

Not applicable.

6.3 Shelf life

3 years

6.4 Special precautions for storage

Bottles:

Do not store above 30°C.

Keep the bottle tightly closed in order to protect from moisture.

Keep the bottle in the outer carton in order to protect from light.

Blister packs:

Do not store above 30°C.

Keep the blisters in the outer carton in order to protect from light.

6.5 Nature and contents of container

Amber glass bottles of 100 capsules.

PVC/PE/PVDC/Aluminium blister packs of 100 capsules.

Not all pack sizes may be marketed.

6.6 Special precautions for disposal and other handling

Use and handling: No special requirements.

Disposal: Any unused product or waste material should be disposed of in accordance with local requirements.

7. MARKETING AUTHORISATION HOLDER

Roche Products Limited
6 Falcon Way
Shire Park
Welwyn Garden City
AL7 1TW
United Kingdom

8. MARKETING AUTHORISATION NUMBER(S)
00031/0618

9. DATE OF FIRST AUTHORISATION/RENEWAL OF THE AUTHORISATION
17/08/2006

10. DATE OF REVISION OF THE TEXT
24/10/08

Vesicare 5mg & 10mg film-coated tablets

(Astellas Pharma Ltd)

1. NAME OF THE MEDICINAL PRODUCT
Vesicare® 5 mg, film-coated tablet
Vesicare® 10 mg, film-coated tablet

2. QUALITATIVE AND QUANTITATIVE COMPOSITION
Vesicare 5 mg film-coated tablet: Each tablet contains 5 mg solifenacin succinate, corresponding to 3.8 mg solifenacin.

Vesicare 10 mg film-coated tablet: Each tablet contains 10 mg solifenacin succinate, corresponding to 7.5 mg solifenacin.

Excipients: lactose monohydrate 107.5mg (5mg), 102.5mg (10mg)

For a full list of excipients, see Section 6.1.

3. PHARMACEUTICAL FORM
Film-coated tablets

Vesicare 5 mg film-coated tablet: Each 5 mg tablet is a round, light-yellow tablet marked with the company logo and "150" on the same side.

Vesicare 10 mg film-coated tablet: Each 10 mg tablet is a round, light-pink tablet marked with the company logo and "151" on the same side.

4. CLINICAL PARTICULARS

4.1 Therapeutic indications
Symptomatic treatment of urge incontinence and/or increased urinary frequency and urgency as may occur in patients with overactive bladder syndrome.

4.2 Posology and method of administration
Posology
Adults, including the elderly
The recommended dose is 5 mg solifenacin succinate once daily. If needed, the dose may be increased to 10 mg solifenacin succinate once daily.

Children and adolescents
Safety and effectiveness in children have not yet been established. Therefore, Vesicare should not be used in children.

Special Populations
Patients with renal impairment
No dose adjustment is necessary for patients with mild to moderate renal impairment (creatinine clearance > 30 ml/min). Patients with severe renal impairment (creatinine clearance ≤ 30 ml/min) should be treated with caution and receive no more than 5 mg once daily (see Section 5.2).

Patients with hepatic impairment
No dose adjustment is necessary for patients with mild hepatic impairment. Patients with moderate hepatic impairment (Child-Pugh score of 7 to 9) should be treated with caution and receive no more than 5 mg once daily (see Section 5.2).

Potent inhibitors of cytochrome P450 3A4
The maximum dose of Vesicare should be limited to 5 mg when treated simultaneously with ketoconazole or therapeutic doses of other potent CYP3A4 inhibitors e.g. ritonavir, nelfinavir, itraconazole (see Section 4.5).

Method of administration
Vesicare should be taken orally and should be swallowed whole with liquids. It can be taken with or without food.

4.3 Contraindications
- Solifenacin is contraindicated in patients with urinary retention, severe gastrointestinal condition (including toxic megacolon), myasthenia gravis or narrow-angle glaucoma and in patients at risk for these conditions.
- Patients hypersensitive to the active substance or to any of the excipients.
- Patients undergoing haemodialysis (see Section 5.2).
- Patients with severe hepatic impairment (see Section 5.2).
- Patients with severe renal impairment or moderate hepatic impairment and who are on treatment with a potent CYP3A4 inhibitor, e.g. ketoconazole (see Section 4.5).

4.4 Special warnings and precautions for use
Other causes of frequent urination (heart failure or renal disease) should be assessed before treatment with Vesicare. If urinary tract infection is present, an appropriate antibacterial therapy should be started.

Vesicare should be used with caution in patients with:
- clinically significant bladder outflow obstruction at risk of urinary retention.
- gastrointestinal obstructive disorders.
- risk of decreased gastrointestinal motility.
- severe renal impairment (creatinine clearance ≤ 30 ml/min; see Section 4.2 and 5.2) and doses should not exceed 5 mg for these patients.
- moderate hepatic impairment (Child-Pugh score of 7 to 9; see Section 4.2 and 5.2) and doses should not exceed 5 mg for these patients.
- concomitant use of a potent CYP3A4 inhibitor, e.g. ketoconazole (see 4.2 and 4.5).
- hiatus hernia/gastroesophageal reflux and/or who are concurrently taking medicinal products (such as bisphosphonates) that can cause or exacerbate oesophagitis.
- autonomic neuropathy.

Safety and efficacy have not yet been established in patients with a neurogenic cause for detrusor overactivity.

Patients with rare hereditary problems of galactose intolerance, the Lapp lactase deficiency or glucose-galactose malabsorption should not take this medicinal product.

The maximum effect of Vesicare can be determined after 4 weeks at the earliest.

4.5 Interaction with other medicinal products and other forms of interaction
Pharmacological interactions
Concomitant medication with other medicinal products with anticholinergic properties may result in more pronounced therapeutic effects and undesirable effects. An interval of approximately one week should be allowed after stopping treatment with Vesicare before commencing other anticholinergic therapy. The therapeutic effect of solifenacin may be reduced by concomitant administration of cholinergic receptor agonists.

Solifenacin can reduce the effect of medicinal products that stimulate the motility of the gastrointestinal tract, such as metoclopramide and cisapride.

Pharmacokinetic interactions
In vitro studies have demonstrated that at therapeutic concentrations, solifenacin does not inhibit CYP1A1/2, 2C9, 2C19, 2D6, or 3A4 derived from human liver microsomes. Therefore, solifenacin is unlikely to alter the clearance of drugs metabolised by these CYP enzymes.

Effect of other medicinal products on the pharmacokinetics of solifenacin
Solifenacin is metabolised by CYP3A4. Simultaneous administration of ketoconazole (200 mg/day), a potent CYP3A4 inhibitor, resulted in a two-fold increase of the AUC of solifenacin, while ketoconazole at a dose of 400 mg/day resulted in a three-fold increase of the AUC of solifenacin. Therefore, the maximum dose of Vesicare should be restricted to 5 mg when used simultaneously with ketoconazole or therapeutic doses of other potent CYP3A4 inhibitors (e.g. ritonavir, nelfinavir, itraconazole) (see Section 4.2). Simultaneous treatment of solifenacin and a potent CYP3A4 inhibitor is contraindicated in patients with severe renal impairment or moderate hepatic impairment.

The effects of enzyme induction on the pharmacokinetics of solifenacin and its metabolites have not been studied as well as the effect of higher affinity CYP3A4 substrates on solifenacin exposure. Since solifenacin is metabolised by CYP3A4, pharmacokinetic interactions are possible with other CYP3A4 substrates with higher affinity (e.g. verapamil, diltiazem) and CYP3A4 inducers (e.g. rifampicin, phenytoin, carbamazepine).

Effect of solifenacin on the pharmacokinetics of other medicinal products
Oral Contraceptives
Intake of Vesicare showed no pharmacokinetic interaction of solifenacin on combined oral contraceptives (ethinylestradiol/levonorgestrel).

Warfarin
Intake of Vesicare did not alter the pharmacokinetics of *R*-warfarin or *S*-warfarin or their effect on prothrombin time.

Digoxin
Intake of Vesicare showed no effect on the pharmacokinetics of digoxin.

4.6 Pregnancy and lactation
Pregnancy
No clinical data are available from women who became pregnant while taking solifenacin. Animal studies do not indicate direct harmful effects on fertility, embryonal / foetal development or parturition (see Section 5.3). The potential risk for humans is unknown. Caution should be exercised when prescribing to pregnant women.

Lactation
No data on the excretion of solifenacin in human milk are available. In mice, solifenacin and/or its metabolites was excreted in milk, and caused a dose dependent failure to thrive in neonatal mice (see Section 5.3). The use of Vesicare should therefore be avoided during breast-feeding.

4.7 Effects on ability to drive and use machines
Since solifenacin, like other anticholinergics may cause blurred vision, and, uncommonly, somnolence and fatigue (see section 4.8. Undesirable effects), the ability to drive and use machines may be negatively affected.

4.8 Undesirable effects
Due to the pharmacological effect of solifenacin, Vesicare may cause anticholinergic undesirable effects of (in general) mild or moderate severity. The frequency of anticholinergic undesirable effects is dose related. The most commonly reported adverse reaction with Vesicare was dry mouth. It occurred in 11% of patients treated with 5 mg once daily, in 22% of patients treated with 10 mg once daily and in 4% of placebo-treated patients. The severity of dry mouth was generally mild and only occasionally led to discontinuation of treatment. In general, medicinal product compliance was very high (approximately 99%) and approximately 90% of the patients treated with Vesicare completed the full study period of 12 weeks treatment.

(see Table 1 below)

4.9 Overdose
Overdosage with solifenacin succinate can potentially result in severe anticholinergic effects. The highest dose of solifenacin succinate accidentally given to a single patient was 280 mg in a 5 hour period, resulting in mental status changes not requiring hospitalisation.

In the event of overdose with solifenacin succinate, the patient should be treated with activated charcoal. Gastric lavage is useful if performed within 1 hour, but vomiting should not be induced.

Table 1

MedDRA system organ class	Very common > 1/10	Common > 1/100, < 1/10	Uncommon > 1/1000, < 1/100	Rare > 1/10000, < 1/1000	Very rare < 1/10,000, not known (cannot be estimated from the available data)
Gastrointestinal disorders	Dry mouth	Constipation Nausea Dyspepsia Abdominal pain	Gastroesophageal reflux diseases Dry throat	Colonic obstruction Faecal impaction	Vomiting
Infections and infestations			Urinary tract infection Cystitis		
Nervous system disorders			Somnolence Dysgeusia		Dizziness, headache
Psychiatric disorders					Hallucinations
Eye disorders		Blurred vision	Dry eyes		
General disorders and administration site conditions			Fatigue Peripheral oedema		
Respiratory, thoracic and mediastinal disorders			Nasal dryness		
Skin and subcutaneous tissue disorders			Dry skin		Pruritus, rash, urticaria
Renal and urinary disorders			Difficulty in micturition	Urinary retention	

Table 2 Results (pooled data) of four controlled Phase 3 studies with a treatment duration of 12 weeks

	Placebo	Vesicare 5 mg o.d.	Vesicare 10 mg o.d.	Tolterodine 2 mg b.i.d.
No. of micturitions/24 h				
Mean baseline	11.9	12.1	11.9	12.1
Mean reduction from baseline	1.4	2.3	2.7	1.9
% change from baseline	(12%)	(19%)	(23%)	(16%)
n	1138	552	1158	250
p-value*		<0.001	<0.001	0.004
No. of urgency episodes/24 h				
Mean baseline	6.3	5.9	6.2	5.4
Mean reduction from baseline	2.0	2.9	3.4	2.1
% change from baseline	(32%)	(49%)	(55%)	(39%)
n	1124	548	1151	250
p-value*		<0.001	<0.001	0.031
No. of incontinence episodes/24 h				
Mean baseline	2.9	2.6	2.9	2.3
Mean reduction from baseline	1.1	1.5	1.8	1.1
% change from baseline	(38%)	(58%)	(62%)	(48%)
n	781	314	778	157
p-value*		<0.001	<0.001	0.009
No. of nocturia episodes/24 h				
Mean baseline	1.8	2.0	1.8	1.9
Mean reduction from baseline	0.4	0.6	0.6	0.5
% change from baseline	(22%)	(30%)	(33%)	(26%)
n	1005	494	1035	232
p-value*		0.025	<0.001	0.199
Volume voided/micturition				
Mean baseline	166 ml	146 ml	163 ml	147 ml
Mean increase from baseline	9 ml	32 ml	43 ml	24 ml
% change from baseline	(5%)	(21%)	(26%)	(16%)
n	1135	552	1156	250
p-value*		<0.001	<0.001	<0.001
No. of pads/24 h				
Mean baseline	3.0	2.8	2.7	2.7
Mean reduction from baseline	0.8	1.3	1.3	1.0
% change from baseline	(27%)	(46%)	(48%)	(37%)
n	238	236	242	250
p-value*		<0.001	<0.001	0.010

Note: In 4 of the pivotal studies, Vesicare 10 mg and placebo were used. In 2 out of the 4 studies also Vesicare 5 mg was used and one of the studies included tolterodine 2 mg bid.
Not all parameters and treatment groups were evaluated in each individual study. Therefore, the numbers of patients listed may deviate per parameter and treatment group.
* P-value for the pair-wise comparison to placebo

As for other anticholinergics, symptoms can be treated as follows:

- Severe central anticholinergic effects such as hallucinations or pronounced excitation: treat with physostigmine or carbachol.
- Convulsions or pronounced excitation: treat with benzodiazepines.
- Respiratory insufficiency: treat with artificial respiration.
- Tachycardia: treat with beta-blockers.
- Urinary retention: treat with catheterisation.
- Mydriasis: treat with pilocarpine eye drops and/or place patient in a dark room.

As with other antimuscarinics, in case of overdosing, specific attention should be paid to patients with known risk for QT-prolongation (i.e. hypokalaemia, bradycardia and concurrent administration of medicinal products known to prolong QT-interval) and relevant pre-existing cardiac diseases (i.e. myocardial ischaemia, arrhythmia, congestive heart failure).

5. PHARMACOLOGICAL PROPERTIES

5.1 Pharmacodynamic properties

Pharmacotherapeutic group: Urinary antispasmodics, ATC code: G04B D08.

Mechanism of action:

Solifenacin is a competitive, specific cholinergic-receptor antagonist.

The urinary bladder is innervated by parasympathetic cholinergic nerves. Acetylcholine contracts the detrusor smooth muscle through muscarinic receptors of which the M_3 subtype is predominantly involved. *In vitro* and *in vivo* pharmacological studies indicate that solifenacin is a competitive inhibitor of the muscarinic M_3 subtype receptor. In addition, solifenacin showed to be a specific antagonist for muscarinic receptors by displaying low or no affinity for various other receptors and ion channels tested.

Pharmacodynamic effects:

Treatment with Vesicare in doses of 5 mg and 10 mg daily was studied in several double-blind, randomised, controlled clinical trials in men and women with overactive bladder.

As shown in the table below, both the 5 mg and 10 mg doses of Vesicare produced statistically significant improvements in the primary and secondary endpoints compared with placebo. Efficacy was observed within one week of starting treatment and stabilised over a period of 12 weeks. A long-term open- label study demonstrated that efficacy was maintained for at least 12 months. After 12 weeks of treatment, approximately 50% of patients suffering from incontinence before treatment were free of incontinence episodes, and in addition 35% of patients achieved a micturition frequency of less than 8 micturitions per day. Treatment of the symptoms of overactive bladder also results in a benefit on a number of Quality of Life measures, such as general health perception, incontinence impact, role limitations, physical limitations, social limitations, emotions, symptom severity, severity measures and sleep/energy.

Results (pooled data) of four controlled Phase 3 studies with a treatment duration of 12 weeks

(see Table 2 above)

5.2 Pharmacokinetic properties

General characteristics

Absorption

After intake of Vesicare tablets, maximum solifenacin plasma concentrations (C_{max}) are reached after 3 to 8 hours. The t_{max} is independent of the dose. The C_{max} and area under the curve (AUC) increase in proportion to the dose between 5 to 40 mg. Absolute bioavailability is approximately 90%. Food intake does not affect the C_{max} and AUC of solifenacin.

Distribution

The apparent volume of distribution of solifenacin following intravenous administration is about 600 L. Solifenacin is to a great extent (approximately 98%) bound to plasma proteins, primarily α_1-acid glycoprotein.

Metabolism

Solifenacin is extensively metabolised by the liver, primarily by cytochrome P450 3A4 (CYP3A4). However, alternative metabolic pathways exist, that can contribute to the metabolism of solifenacin. The systemic clearance of solifenacin is about 9.5 L/h and the terminal half life of solifenacin is 45 - 68 hours. After oral dosing, one pharmacologically active (4*R*-hydroxy solifenacin) and three inactive metabolites (*N*-glucuronide, *N*-oxide and 4*R*- hydroxy-*N*-oxide of solifenacin) have been identified in plasma in addition to solifenacin.

Excretion

After a single administration of 10 mg [^{14}C-labelled]-solifenacin, about 70% of the radioactivity was detected in urine and 23% in faeces over 26 days. In urine, approximately 11% of the radioactivity is recovered as unchanged active substance; about 18% as the *N*-oxide metabolite, 9% as the 4*R*-hydroxy- *N*-oxide metabolite and 8% as the 4*R*-hydroxy metabolite (active metabolite).

Dose Proportionality

Pharmacokinetics are linear in the therapeutic dose range.

Characteristics in patients

Age

No dosage adjustment based on patient age is required. Studies in the elderly have shown that the exposure to solifenacin, expressed as the AUC, after administration of solifenacin succinate (5 mg and 10 mg once daily) was similar in healthy elderly subjects (aged 65 - 80 years) and healthy young subjects (aged less than 55 years). The mean rate of absorption expressed as t_{max} was slightly slower in the elderly and the terminal half-life was approximately 20% longer in elderly subjects. These modest differences were considered not clinically significant.

The pharmacokinetics of solifenacin have not been established in children and adolescents.

Gender

The pharmacokinetics of solifenacin are not influenced by gender.

Race

The pharmacokinetics of solifenacin are not influenced by race.

Renal impairment

The AUC and C_{max} of solifenacin in mild and moderate renally impaired patients was not significantly different from that found in healthy volunteers. In patients with severe renal impairment (creatinine clearance $\leqslant$ 30 ml/min), exposure to solifenacin was significantly greater than in the controls, with increases in C_{max} of about 30%, AUC of more than 100% and $t_{1/2}$ of more than 60%. A statistically significant relationship was observed between creatinine clearance and solifenacin clearance.

Pharmacokinetics in patients undergoing haemodialysis have not been studied.

Hepatic impairment

In patients with moderate hepatic impairment (Child-Pugh score of 7 to 9) the C_{max} is not affected, AUC increased by 60% and $t_{1/2}$ doubled. Pharmacokinetics of solifenacin in patients with severe hepatic impairment have not been studied.

5.3 Preclinical safety data

Preclinical data reveal no special hazard for humans based on conventional studies of safety pharmacology, repeated dose toxicity, fertility, embryofetal development, genotoxicity, and carcinogenic potential. In the pre- and postnatal development study in mice, solifenacin treatment of the mother during lactation caused dose-dependent lower postpartum survival rate, decreased pup weight and slower physical development at clinically relevant levels.

6. PHARMACEUTICAL PARTICULARS

6.1 List of excipients

Core tablet:

Maize starch

Lactose monohydrate

Hypromellose

Magnesium stearate

Film Coating:

Macrogol 8000

Talc

Hypromellose

Titanium dioxide (E171)

Yellow ferric oxide (E172) - Vesicare 5 mg

Red ferric oxide (E172) - Vesicare 10 mg

6.2 Incompatibilities

Not applicable.

6.3 Shelf life

3 years.

6.4 Special precautions for storage

This medicinal product does not require any special storage conditions.

6.5 Nature and contents of container

Container:

The tablets are packed in PVC/Aluminium blisters.

Pack sizes:

3, 5, 10, 20, 30, 50, 60, 90 or 100 tablets (not all pack sizes may be marketed).

6.6 Special precautions for disposal and other handling

No special requirements.

7. MARKETING AUTHORISATION HOLDER

Astellas Pharma Limited
Lovett House
Lovett Road
Staines
TW18 3AZ
United Kingdom

8. MARKETING AUTHORISATION NUMBER(S)

PL 00166/0197 Vesicare 5 mg
PL 00166/0198 Vesicare 10 mg

9. DATE OF FIRST AUTHORISATION/RENEWAL OF THE AUTHORISATION

16 August 2004

10. DATE OF REVISION OF THE TEXT

10 September 2008

11. LEGAL CATEGORY

POM

VFEND 50 mg and 200 mg film-coated tablets, VFEND 200 mg powder for solution for infusion, VFEND 40 mg/ml powder for oral suspension

(Pfizer Limited)

1. NAME OF THE MEDICINAL PRODUCT

VFEND 50 mg and 200 mg film-coated tablets.

VFEND 200 mg powder for solution for infusion.

VFEND 40 mg/ml powder for oral suspension.

2. QUALITATIVE AND QUANTITATIVE COMPOSITION

Film-coated tablets:

Each tablet contains 50 mg or 200 mg voriconazole.

Excipient: lactose monohydrate 63.42 mg or 253.675 mg

For a full list of excipients, see section 6.1.

Powder for solution for infusion:

Each ml contains 10 mg of voriconazole after reconstitution (see section 6.6) - once reconstituted further dilution is required before administration. Each vial contains 200 mg of voriconazole.

Excipient: each vial contains 217.6 mg sodium

For a full list of excipients, see section 6.1.

Powder for oral suspension:

Each ml of oral suspension contains 40 mg of voriconazole when reconstituted with water (see section 6.6). Each bottle contains 3 g of voriconazole.

Excipient: Each ml of suspension contains 0.54 g of sucrose

For a full list of excipients, see section 6.1.

3. PHARMACEUTICAL FORM

Film-coated tablets:

White, round tablets, debossed "Pfizer" on one side and "VOR50" on the reverse.

White, capsule-shaped tablets, debossed "Pfizer" on one side and "VOR200" on the reverse.

Powder for solution for infusion:

White lyophilised powder

Powder for oral suspension:

White to off-white powder

4. CLINICAL PARTICULARS

4.1 Therapeutic indications

Voriconazole, is a broad spectrum, triazole antifungal agent and is indicated as follows:

- Treatment of invasive aspergillosis.
- Treatment of candidaemia in non-neutropenic patients
- Treatment of fluconazole-resistant serious invasive *Candida* infections (including *C. krusei*).
- Treatment of serious fungal infections caused by *Scedosporium* spp. and *Fusarium* spp.

VFEND should be administered primarily to patients with progressive, possibly life-threatening infections.

4.2 Posology and method of administration

Film-coated tablets (50mg and 200mg):

VFEND film-coated tablets are to be taken at least one hour before, or one hour following, a meal.

Powder for oral suspension:

VFEND oral suspension (40mg/mL) is to be taken at least one hour before, or two hours following, a meal.

Powder for solution for infusion:

VFEND requires reconstitution and dilution (see section 6.6) prior to administration as an intravenous infusion. Not for bolus injection.

It is recommended that VFEND is administered at a maximum rate of 3 mg/kg per hour over 1 to 2 hours.

Electrolyte disturbances such as hypokalaemia, hypomagnesaemia and hypocalcaemia should be monitored and corrected, if necessary, prior to initiation and during voriconazole therapy (see section 4.4).

VFEND must not be infused into the same line or cannula concomitantly with other intravenous products. VFEND must not be administered simultaneously with any blood product or any short-term infusion of concentrated solutions of electrolytes, even if the two infusions are running in separate lines. Total parenteral nutrition (TPN) need *not* be discontinued when prescribed with VFEND, but does need to be infused through a separate line (see section 6.2).

Use in adults and adolescents (12 to 16 years of age)

Therapy must be initiated with the specified loading dose regimen of either intravenous or oral VFEND to achieve plasma concentrations on Day 1 that are close to steady state. On the basis of the high oral bioavailability (96 %; see section 5.2), switching between intravenous and oral administration is appropriate when clinically indicated.

Detailed information on dosage recommendations is provided in the following table:

(see Table 1 below)

Dosage adjustment

Film-coated tablets & Powder for oral suspension:

If patient response is inadequate, the maintenance dose may be increased to 300 mg twice daily for oral administration. For patients less than 40 kg the oral dose may be increased to 150 mg twice daily.

If patients are unable to tolerate treatment at these higher doses reduce the oral dose by 50 mg steps to the 200 mg twice daily (or 100 mg twice daily for patients less than 40 kg) maintenance dose.

Phenytoin may be co-administered with voriconazole if the maintenance dose of voriconazole is increased from 200 mg to 400 mg orally, twice daily (100 mg to 200 mg orally, twice daily in patients less than 40 kg), see sections 4.4 and 4.5.

Rifabutin may be co-administered with voriconazole if the maintenance dose of voriconazole is increased from 200 mg to 350 mg orally, twice daily (100 mg to 200 mg orally, twice daily in patients less than 40 kg), see sections 4.4 and 4.5.

Efavirenz may be co-administered with voriconazole if the maintenance dose of voriconazole is increased to 400 mg every 12 hours and the efavirenz dose is reduced by 50%, i.e. to 300 mg once daily. When treatment with voriconazole is stopped, the initial dosage of efavirenz should be restored (see sections 4.4 and 4.5).

Treatment duration depends upon patients' clinical and mycological response.

Powder for solution for infusion:

If patients are unable to tolerate treatment at 4 mg/kg twice daily, reduce the intravenous dose to 3 mg/kg twice daily.

Rifabutin or phenytoin may be co-administered with voriconazole if the maintenance dose of voriconazole is increased to 5 mg/kg intravenously twice daily, see sections 4.4 and 4.5.

Efavirenz may be co-administered with voriconazole if the maintenance dose of voriconazole is increased to 400 mg every 12 hours and the efavirenz dose is reduced by 50%, i.e. to 300 mg once daily. When treatment with voriconazole is stopped, the initial dosage of efavirenz should be restored (see sections 4.4 and 4.5).

Treatment duration depends upon patients' clinical and mycological response. The duration of treatment with the intravenous formulation should be no longer than 6 months (see section 5.3).

Use in the elderly

No dose adjustment is necessary for elderly patients (see section 5.2).

Use in patients with renal impairment

Film-coated tablets & Powder for oral suspension:

The pharmacokinetics of orally administered voriconazole are not affected by renal impairment. Therefore, no adjustment is necessary for oral dosing for patients with mild to severe renal impairment (see section 5.2).

Voriconazole is haemodialysed with a clearance of 121 ml/min. A four hour haemodialysis session does not remove a sufficient amount of voriconazole to warrant dose adjustment.

Powder for solution for infusion:

In patients with moderate to severe renal dysfunction (creatinine clearance < 50 ml/min), accumulation of the intravenous vehicle, SBECD, occurs. Oral voriconazole should be administered to these patients, unless an assessment of the risk benefit to the patient justifies the use of intravenous voriconazole. Serum creatinine levels should be closely monitored in these patients and, if increases occur, consideration should be given to changing to oral voriconazole therapy (see section 5.2).

Voriconazole is haemodialysed with a clearance of 121 ml/min. A 4 hour haemodialysis session does not remove a sufficient amount of voriconazole to warrant dose adjustment.

The intravenous vehicle, SBECD, is haemodialysed with a clearance of 55 ml/min.

Use in patients with hepatic impairment

No dose adjustment is necessary in patients with acute hepatic injury, manifested by elevated liver function tests (ALAT, ASAT) (but continued monitoring of liver function tests for further elevations is recommended).

It is recommended that the standard loading dose regimens be used but that the maintenance dose be halved in patients with mild to moderate hepatic cirrhosis (Child-Pugh A and B) receiving VFEND (see section 5.2).

VFEND has not been studied in patients with severe chronic hepatic cirrhosis (Child-Pugh C).

VFEND has been associated with elevations in liver function tests and clinical signs of liver damage, such as jaundice, and must only be used in patients with severe hepatic impairment if the benefit outweighs the potential risk. Patients with hepatic impairment must be carefully monitored for drug toxicity (see also section 4.8).

Use in children

VFEND is not recommended for use in children below 2 years due to insufficient data on safety and efficacy (see also sections 4.8 and 5.1).

Film-coated tablets, Powder for oral suspension & Powder for solution for infusion:

The recommended maintenance dosing regimen in paediatric patients aged 2 to <12 years is as follows:

	Intravenous*	Oral (Tablets and suspension) **
Loading Dose Regimen	No oral or intravenous loading dose is recommended	
Maintenance Dose	7 mg/kg twice daily	200 mg (5 ml) twice daily

*Based on a population pharmacokinetic analysis in 82 immunocompromised patients aged 2 to <12 years

**Based on a population pharmacokinetic analysis in 47 immunocompromised patients aged 2 to <12 years

Use in paediatric patients aged 2 to <12 years with hepatic or renal insufficiency has not been studied (see section 4.8 and section 5.2).

Adolescents (12 to 16 years of age): should be dosed as adults.

Film-coated tablets and Powder for oral suspension:

These paediatric dose recommendations are based on studies in which VFEND was administered as the powder for oral suspension. Bioequivalence between the powder for oral suspension and tablets has not been investigated in a paediatric population. Considering the assumed limited gastro-enteric transit time in paediatrics, the absorption of the tablets may be different in paediatric compared to adult patients. It is therefore recommended to use the oral suspension formulation in children aged 2 to <12 years.

Powder for solution for infusion:

If paediatric patients are unable to tolerate an intravenous dose of 7mg/kg twice daily, a dose reduction from 7mg/kg to 4mg/kg twice daily may be considered based on the population pharmacokinetic analysis and previous clinical experience. This provides equivalent exposure to 3mg/kg twice daily in adults (see section 4.2 use in adults).

4.3 Contraindications

Hypersensitivity to the active substance or to any of the excipients.

Co-administration of the CYP3A4 substrates, terfenadine, astemizole, cisapride, pimozide or quinidine with VFEND is contraindicated since increased plasma concentrations of these medicinal products can lead to QTc prolongation and rare occurrences of *torsades de pointes* (see section 4.5).

Table 1

	Intravenous	Oral (Tablets and Suspension)	
		Patients 40 kg and above	Patients less than 40 kg
Loading Dose Regimen (first 24 hours)	6 mg/kg every 12 hours (for the first 24 hours)	400 mg (10 ml) every 12 hours (for the first 24 hours)	200 mg (5 ml) every 12 hours (for the first 24 hours)
Maintenance Dose (after first 24 hours)	4 mg/kg twice daily	200 mg (5 ml) twice daily	100 mg (2.5 ml) twice daily

Co-administration of VFEND with rifampicin, carbamazepine and phenobarbital is contraindicated since these medicinal products are likely to decrease plasma voriconazole concentrations significantly (see section 4.5).

Co-administration of VFEND with high dose ritonavir (400 mg and above twice daily) is contraindicated because ritonavir significantly decreases plasma voriconazole concentrations in healthy subjects at this dose. (see section 4.5, for lower doses see section 4.4).

Co-administration of ergot alkaloids (ergotamine, dihydroergotamine), which are CYP3A4 substrates, is contraindicated since increased plasma concentrations of these medicinal products can lead to ergotism (see section 4.5).

Co-administration of voriconazole and sirolimus is contraindicated, since voriconazole is likely to increase plasma concentrations of sirolimus significantly (see section 4.5).

The concomitant use of voriconazole with St John's Wort is contraindicated (see section 4.5).

4.4 Special warnings and precautions for use

Hypersensitivity: Caution should be used in prescribing VFEND to patients with hypersensitivity to other azoles (see also section 4.8).

Cardiovascular:

Some azoles, including voriconazole have been associated with QT interval prolongation. There have been rare cases of torsades de pointes in patients taking voriconazole who had risk factors, such as history of cardiotoxic chemotherapy, cardiomyopathy, hypokalaemia and concomitant medications that may have been contributory. Voriconazole should be administered with caution to patients with potentially proarrhythmic conditions, such as

- Congenital or acquired QT-prolongation
- Cardiomyopathy, in particular when heart failure is present
- Sinus bradycardia
- Existing symptomatic arrhythmias
- Concomitant medication that is known to prolong QT interval.

Electrolyte disturbances such as hypokalaemia, hypomagnesaemia and hypocalcaemia should be monitored and corrected, if necessary, prior to initiation and during voriconazole therapy (see section 4.2). A study has been conducted in healthy volunteers which examined the effect on QT interval of single doses of voriconazole up to 4 times the usual daily dose. No subject experienced an interval exceeding the potentially clinically relevant threshold of 500 msec (see section 5.1).

Infusion-related reactions: Infusion-related reactions, predominantly flushing and nausea, have been observed during administration of the intravenous formulation of voriconazole. Depending on the severity of symptoms, consideration should be given to stopping treatment (see section 4.8).

Hepatic toxicity: In clinical trials, there have been uncommon cases of serious hepatic reactions during treatment with VFEND (including clinical hepatitis, cholestasis and fulminant hepatic failure, including fatalities). Instances of hepatic reactions were noted to occur primarily in patients with serious underlying medical conditions (predominantly haematological malignancy). Transient hepatic reactions, including hepatitis and jaundice, have occurred among patients with no other identifiable risk factors. Liver dysfunction has usually been reversible on discontinuation of therapy (see section 4.8).

Monitoring of hepatic function: Monitoring of hepatic function should be carried out in both children and adults. Patients at the beginning of therapy with voriconazole and patients who develop abnormal liver function tests during VFEND therapy must be routinely monitored for the development of more severe hepatic injury. Patient management should include laboratory evaluation of hepatic function (particularly liver function tests and bilirubin). Discontinuation of VFEND should be considered if clinical signs and symptoms are consistent with liver disease development. Monitoring of hepatic function should be carried out in both children and adults.

Visual adverse events: There have been rare reports of prolonged visual adverse events, including blurred vision, optic neuritis and papilloedema (see section 4.8).

Renal adverse events: Acute renal failure has been observed in severely ill patients undergoing treatment with VFEND. Patients being treated with voriconazole are likely to be treated concomitantly with nephrotoxic medications and have concurrent conditions that may result in decreased renal function (see section 4.8).

Monitoring of renal function: Patients should be monitored for the development of abnormal renal function. This should include laboratory evaluation, particularly serum creatinine.

Monitoring of pancreatic function: Patients, especially children, with risk factors for acute pancreatitis (e.g. recent chemotherapy, hematopoietic stem cell transplantation (HSCT)), should be monitored closely during Vfend treatment. Monitoring of serum amylase or lipase may be considered in this clinical situation.

Dermatological reactions: Patients have rarely developed exfoliative cutaneous reactions, such as Stevens-Johnson syndrome, during treatment with VFEND. If patients develop a rash they should be monitored closely and VFEND discontinued if lesions progress.

In addition VFEND has been associated with photosensitivity skin reaction especially during long term therapy. It is recommended that patients should be informed to avoid sunlight during the treatment.

Paediatric use: Safety and effectiveness in paediatric subjects below the age of two years has not been established (see also sections 4.8 and 5.1). Voriconazole is indicated for paediatric patients aged two years or older. Hepatic function should be monitored in both children and adults. Oral bioavailability may be limited in paediatric patients aged 2 to <12 years with malabsorption and very low body weight for age. In that case, intravenous voriconazole administration is recommended.

Phenytoin (CYP2C9 substrate and potent CYP450 inducer): Careful monitoring of phenytoin levels is recommended when phenytoin is co-administered with voriconazole. Concomitant use of voriconazole and phenytoin should be avoided unless the benefit outweighs the risk (see section 4.5).

Rifabutin (CYP450 inducer): Careful monitoring of full blood counts and adverse reactions to rifabutin (e.g. uveitis) is recommended when rifabutin is co-administered with voriconazole. Concomitant use of voriconazole and rifabutin should be avoided unless the benefit outweighs the risk (see section 4.5).

Methadone (CYP3A4 substrate). Frequent monitoring for adverse events and toxicity related to methadone, including QTc prolongation, is recommended when co-administered with voriconazole since methadone levels increased following co-administration of voriconazole. Dose reduction of methadone may be needed (see section 4.5).

Short Acting Opiates (CYP3A4 substrate): Reduction in the dose of alfentanil and other short acting opiates similar in structure to alfentanil and metabolised by CYP3A4 (e.g. fentanyl and sufentanil) should be considered when co-administered with voriconazole (see section 4.5). As the half-life of alfentanil is prolonged in a four-fold manner when alfentanil is co-administered with voriconazole, a longer respiratory monitoring period may be necessary.

Ritonavir (potent CYP450 inducer; CYP3A4 inhibitor and substrate): Co-administration of voriconazole and low dose ritonavir (100mg twice daily) should be avoided unless an assessment of the benefit/risk justifies the use of voriconazole. (see section 4.5, for higher doses see section 4.3).

Efavirenz (CYP450 inducer; CYP3A4 inhibitor and substrate): When voriconazole is co-administered with efavirenz the dose of voriconazole should be increased to 400 mg every 12 hours and that of efavirenz should be decreased to 300 mg every 24 hours (see sections 4.2 and 4.5).

VFEND tablets contain lactose and should not be given to patients with rare hereditary problems of galactose intolerance, Lapp lactase deficiency or glucose-galactose malabsorption.

VFEND oral suspension contains sucrose and should not be given to patients with rare hereditary problems of fructose intolerance, sucrase-isomaltase deficiency or glucose-galactose malabsorption.

Sodium content: Each vial of VFEND powder for infusion contains 217.6 mg of sodium. This should be taken into consideration for patients on a controlled sodium diet.

4.5 Interaction with other medicinal products and other forms of interaction

Unless otherwise specified, drug interaction studies have been performed in healthy adult male subjects using multiple dosing to steady state with oral voriconazole at 200 mg twice daily. These results are relevant to other populations and routes of administration.

This section addresses the effects of other medicinal products on voriconazole, the effects of voriconazole on other medicinal products and two-way interactions. The interactions for the first two sections are presented in the following order: contraindications, those requiring dosage adjustment and careful clinical and/or biological monitoring and finally those that have no significant pharmacokinetic interaction but may be of clinical interest in this therapeutic field.

Effects of other medicinal products on voriconazole

Voriconazole is metabolised by cytochrome P450 isoenzymes, CYP2C19, CYP2C9 and CYP3A4. Inhibitors or inducers of these isoenzymes may increase or decrease voriconazole plasma concentrations respectively.

Rifampicin (CYP450 inducer): Rifampicin (600 mg once daily) decreased the C_{max} (maximum plasma concentration) and AUC_{τ} (area under the plasma concentration time curve within a dose interval) of voriconazole by 93 % and 96 %, respectively. Co-administration of voriconazole and rifampicin is contraindicated (see section 4.3).

Ritonavir (potent CYP450 inducer; CYP3A4 inhibitor and substrate): The effect of the co-administration of oral voriconazole (200 mg twice daily) and high dose (400 mg) and low dose (100 mg) oral ritonavir was investigated in two separate studies in healthy volunteers. High doses of ritonavir (400 mg twice daily) decreased the steady state C_{max} and AUC_{τ} of oral voriconazole by an average of 66 % and 82 %, whereas low doses of ritonavir (100mg twice daily) decreased the C_{max} and AUC_{τ} of voriconazole by an average of 24 % and 39 % respectively. Administration of voriconazole did not have a significant effect on mean C_{max} and AUC_{τ} of ritonavir in the high dose study, although a minor decrease in steady state C_{max} and AUC_{τ} of ritonavir with an average of 25 % and 13 % respectively was observed in the low dose ritonavir interaction study. One outlier subject with raised voriconazole levels was identified in each of the ritonavir interaction studies. Co-administration of voriconazole and high doses of ritonavir (400 mg and above twice daily) is contraindicated. Co-administration of voriconazole and low dose ritonavir (100 mg twice daily) should be avoided, unless an assessment of the benefit/risk to the patient justifies the use of voriconazole (see section 4.3 and 4.4).

Carbamazepine and phenobarbital (potent CYP450 inducers): Although not studied, carbamazepine or phenobarbital are likely to significantly decrease plasma voriconazole concentrations. Co-administration of voriconazole with carbamazepine and phenobarbital is contraindicated (see section 4.3).

Cimetidine (non-specific CYP450 inhibitor and increases gastric pH): Cimetidine (400 mg twice daily) increased voriconazole C_{max} and AUC_{τ} by 18 % and 23 %, respectively. No dosage adjustment of voriconazole is recommended.

Ranitidine (increases gastric pH): Ranitidine (150 mg twice daily) had no significant effect on voriconazole C_{max} and AUC_{τ}.

Macrolide antibiotics: Erythromycin (CYP3A4 inhibitor; 1 g twice daily) and azithromycin (500 mg once daily) had no significant effect on voriconazole C_{max} and AUC_{τ}.

St John's Wort (CYP450 inducer; P-gp inducer): In a clinical study in healthy volunteers, St John's Wort exhibited a short initial inhibitory effect followed by induction of voriconazole metabolism. After 15 days of treatment with St John's Wort (300 mg three times daily), plasma exposure following a single 400 mg dose of voriconazole decreased by 40-60%. Therefore, concomitant use of voriconazole with St John's Wort is contraindicated (see section 4.3).

Effects of voriconazole on other medicinal products

Voriconazole inhibits the activity of cytochrome P450 isoenzymes, CYP2C19, CYP2C9 and CYP3A4. Therefore there is potential for voriconazole to increase the plasma levels of substances metabolised by these CYP450 isoenzymes.

Voriconazole should be administered with caution in patients with concomitant medication that is known to prolong QT interval. When there is also a potential for voriconazole to increase the plasma levels of substances metabolised by CYP3A4 isoenzymes (certain antihistamines, quinidine, cisapride, pimozide) co-administration is contraindicated (see below and section 4.3)

Terfenadine, astemizole, cisapride, pimozide and quinidine (CYP3A4 substrates): Although not studied, co-administration of voriconazole with terfenadine, astemizole, cisapride, pimozide, or quinidine is contraindicated, since increased plasma concentrations of these medicinal products can lead to QTc prolongation and rare occurrences of *torsades de pointes* (see section 4.3).

Sirolimus (CYP3A4 substrate): Voriconazole increased sirolimus (2 mg single dose) C_{max} and AUC_{τ} by 556 % and 1014 %, respectively. Co-administration of voriconazole and sirolimus is contraindicated (see section 4.3).

Ergot alkaloids (CYP3A4 substrates): Although not studied, voriconazole may increase the plasma concentrations of ergot alkaloids (ergotamine and dihydroergotamine) and lead to ergotism. Co-administration of voriconazole with ergot alkaloids is contraindicated (see section 4.3).

Cyclosporin (CYP3A4 substrate): In stable, renal transplant recipients, voriconazole increased cyclosporin C_{max} and AUC_{τ} by at least 13 % and 70 %, respectively. When initiating voriconazole in patients already receiving cyclosporin it is recommended that the cyclosporin dose be halved and cyclosporin level carefully monitored. Increased cyclosporin levels have been associated with nephrotoxicity. When voriconazole is discontinued, cyclosporin levels must be carefully monitored and the dose increased as necessary.

Methadone (CYP3A4 substrate): In subjects receiving a methadone maintenance dose (32-100 mg once daily) co-administration of oral voriconazole (400 mg twice daily for 1 day, then 200 mg twice daily for four days) increased the C_{max} and AUC_{τ} of pharmacologically active R-methadone by 31 % and 47 %, respectively, whereas the C_{max} and AUC_{τ} of the S-enantiomer increased by approximately 65 % and 103 %, respectively. Voriconazole plasma concentrations during co-administration of methadone were comparable to voriconazole levels (historical data) in healthy subjects without any comedication. Frequent monitoring for adverse events and toxicity related to increased plasma concentrations of methadone, including QT prolongation, is recommended during co-administration. Dose reduction of methadone may be needed.

Short Acting Opiates (CYP3A4 substrate): Steady-state administration of oral voriconazole increased the AUCτ of a single dose of alfentanil by 6-fold. Reduction in the dose of alfentanil and other short acting opiates similar in structure to alfentanil and metabolised by CYP3A4 (e.g. fentanyl and sufentanil), should be considered when co-administered with voriconazole (see section 4.4).

Tacrolimus (CYP3A4 substrate): Voriconazole increased tacrolimus (0.1 mg/kg single dose) C_{max} and AUC_t (area under the plasma concentration time curve to the last quantifiable measurement) by 117 % and 221 %, respectively. When initiating voriconazole in patients already receiving tacrolimus, it is recommended that the tacrolimus dose be reduced to a third of the original dose and tacrolimus level carefully monitored. Increased tacrolimus levels have been associated with nephrotoxicity. When voriconazole is discontinued, tacrolimus levels must be carefully monitored and the dose increased as necessary.

Oral anticoagulants:

Warfarin (CYP2C9 substrate): Co-administration of voriconazole (300 mg twice daily) with warfarin (30 mg single dose) increased maximum prothrombin time by 93 %. Close monitoring of prothrombin time is recommended if warfarin and voriconazole are co-administered.

Other oral anticoagulants e.g. phenprocoumon, acenocoumarol (CYP2C9, CYP3A4 substrates): Although not studied, voriconazole may increase the plasma concentrations of coumarins and therefore may cause an increase in prothrombin time. If patients receiving coumarin preparations are treated simultaneously with voriconazole, the prothrombin time should be monitored at close intervals and the dosage of anticoagulants adjusted accordingly.

Sulphonylureas (CYP2C9 substrates): Although not studied, voriconazole may increase the plasma levels of sulphonylureas, (e.g. tolbutamide, glipizide, and glyburide) and therefore cause hypoglycaemia. Careful monitoring of blood glucose is recommended during co-administration.

Statins (CYP3A4 substrates): Although not studied clinically, voriconazole has been shown to inhibit lovastatin metabolism *in vitro* (human liver microsomes). Therefore, voriconazole is likely to increase plasma levels of statins that are metabolised by CYP3A4. It is recommended that dose adjustment of the statin be considered during co-administration. Increased statin levels have been associated with rhabdomyolysis.

Benzodiazepines (CYP3A4 substrates): Although not studied clinically, voriconazole has been shown to inhibit midazolam metabolism *in vitro* (human liver microsomes). Therefore, voriconazole is likely to increase the plasma levels of benzodiazepines that are metabolised by CYP3A4 (e.g. midazolam and triazolam) and lead to a prolonged sedative effect. It is recommended that dose adjustment of the benzodiazepine be considered during co-administration.

Vinca Alkaloids (CYP3A4 substrates): Although not studied, voriconazole may increase the plasma levels of the vinca alkaloids (e.g. vincristine and vinblastine) and lead to neurotoxicity.

Prednisolone (CYP3A4 substrate): Voriconazole increased C_{max} and AUC_τ of prednisolone (60 mg single dose) by 11 % and 34 %, respectively. No dosage adjustment is recommended.

Digoxin (P-glycoprotein mediated transport): Voriconazole had no significant effect on C_{max} and AUC_τ of digoxin (0.25 mg once daily).

Mycophenolic acid (UDP-glucuronyl transferase substrate): Voriconazole had no effect on the C_{max} and AUC_t of mycophenolic acid (1 g single dose).

Non-Steroidal Anti-Inflammatory Drugs (CYP2C9 substrates): Voriconazole increased Cmax and AUC of ibuprofen (400 mg single dose) by 20% and 100%, respectively. Voriconazole increased Cmax and AUC of diclofenac (50 mg single dose) by 114% and 78%, respectively. Frequent monitoring for adverse events and toxicity related to NSAIDs is recommended. Adjustment of dosage of NSAIDs may be needed.

Two-way interactions

Phenytoin (CYP2C9 substrate and potent CYP450 inducer): Concomitant use of voriconazole and phenytoin should be avoided unless the benefit outweighs the risk.

Phenytoin (300 mg once daily) decreased the C_{max} and AUC_τ of voriconazole by 49 % and 69 %, respectively. Voriconazole (400 mg twice daily, see section 4.2) increased C_{max} and AUC_τ of phenytoin (300 mg once daily) by 67 % and 81 %, respectively. Careful monitoring of phenytoin plasma levels is recommended when phenytoin is co-administered with voriconazole.

Phenytoin may be co-administered with voriconazole if the maintenance dose of voriconazole is increased to 5 mg /kg intravenously twice daily or from 200 mg to 400 mg orally, twice daily (100 mg to 200 mg orally, twice daily in patients less than 40 kg), see section 4.2.

Rifabutin (CYP450 inducer): Concomitant use of voriconazole and rifabutin should be avoided unless the benefit outweighs the risk.

Rifabutin (300 mg once daily) decreased the C_{max} and AUC_τ of voriconazole at 200 mg twice daily by 69 % and 78 %, respectively. During co-administration with rifabutin, the C_{max} and AUC_τ of voriconazole at 350 mg twice daily were 96 % and 68 % of the levels when administered alone at 200 mg twice daily. At a voriconazole dose of 400 mg twice daily C_{max} and AUC_τ were 104 % and 87 % higher, respectively, compared with voriconazole alone at 200 mg twice daily. Voriconazole at 400 mg twice daily increased C_{max} and AUC_τ of rifabutin by 195 % and 331 %, respectively.

If rifabutin co-administration with voriconazole is justified then the maintenance dose of voriconazole may be increased to 5 mg/kg intravenously twice daily or from 200 mg to 350 mg orally, twice daily (100 mg to 200 mg orally, twice daily in patients less than 40 kg) (see section 4.2). Careful monitoring of full blood counts and adverse reactions to rifabutin (e.g. uveitis) is recommended when rifabutin is co-administered with voriconazole.

Omeprazole (CYP2C19 inhibitor; CYP2C19 and CYP3A4 substrate): Omeprazole (40 mg once daily) increased voriconazole C_{max} and AUC_τ by 15 % and 41 %, respectively. No dosage adjustment of voriconazole is recommended. Voriconazole increased omeprazole C_{max} and AUC_τ by 116 % and 280 %, respectively. When initiating voriconazole in patients already receiving omeprazole, it is recommended that the omeprazole dose be halved. The metabolism of other proton pump inhibitors which are CYP2C19 substrates may also be inhibited by voriconazole.

Oral Contraceptives Co-administration of voriconazole and an oral contraceptive (1 mg norethisterone and 0.035mg ethinylestradiol; once daily) in healthy female subjects resulted in increases in the Cmax and AUC_τ of ethinylestradiol (36 % and 61 % respectively) and norethisterone (15 % and 53 % respectively). Voriconazole Cmax and AUC_τ increased by 14 % and 46 % respectively. It is expected that the voriconazole levels will return to standard levels during the pill-free week. As the ratio between norethisterone and ethinylestradiol remained similar during interaction with voriconazole, their contraceptive activity would probably not be affected. Although no increase in the incidence of hormonal-related adverse events was observed in the clinical interaction study, higher estrogen and progestagen levels may cause notably nausea and menstrual disorders. Oral contraceptives containing doses other than 1mg norethisterone and 0.035 mg ethinylestradiol have not been studied.

Antiretroviral agents:

Indinavir (CYP3A4 inhibitor and substrate): Indinavir (800 mg three times daily) had no significant effect on voriconazole C_{max}, C_{min} and AUC_τ. Voriconazole did not have a significant effect on C_{max} and AUC_τ of indinavir (800 mg three times daily).

Other HIV protease inhibitors (CYP3A4 inhibitors): *In vitro* studies suggest that voriconazole may inhibit the metabolism of HIV protease inhibitors (e.g. saquinavir, amprenavir and nelfinavir). *In vitro* studies also show that the metabolism of voriconazole may be inhibited by HIV protease inhibitors. However results of the combination of voriconazole with other HIV protease inhibitors cannot be predicted in humans only from *in vitro* studies. Patients should be carefully monitored for any occurrence of drug toxicity and/or loss of efficacy during the co- administration of voriconazole and HIV protease inhibitors.

Efavirenz (a non-nucleoside reverse transcriptase inhibitor) (CYP450 inducer; CYP3A4 inhibitor and substrate)): Standard doses of voriconazole and standard doses of efavirenz must not be co-administered. Steady-state efavirenz (400 mg orally once daily) decreased the steady state C_{max} and AUC_τ of voriconazole by an average of 61 % and 77 %, respectively, in healthy subjects. In the same study voriconazole at steady state increased the steady state C_{max} and AUC_τ of efavirenz by an average of 38 % and 44 % respectively, in healthy subjects.

In a separate study in healthy subjects, voriconazole dose of 300mg BID in combination with low dose efavirenz (300 mg once daily) did not lead to sufficient voriconazole exposure.

Following co-administration of voriconazole 400 mg twice daily with efavirenz 300 mg orally once daily, in healthy subjects, the AUC_τ of voriconazole was decreased by 7 % and Cmax was increased by 23 %, compared to voriconazole 200 mg twice daily alone. (The AUC_τ of efavirenz was increased by 17 % and Cmax was equivalent compared to efavirenz 600 mg once daily alone). These differences were not considered to be clinically significant.

When voriconazole is co-administered with efavirenz, voriconazole maintenance dose should be increased to 400 mg twice daily and the efavirenz dose should be reduced by 50 %, i.e. to 300 mg once daily (see section 4.2). When treatment with voriconazole is stopped, the initial dosage of efavirenz should be restored.

Non-nucleoside reverse transcriptase inhibitors (NNRTI)(CYP3A4 substrates, inhibitors or CYP450 inducers): *In vitro* studies show that the metabolism of voriconazole may be inhibited by delavirdine. Although not studied, the metabolism of voriconazole may be induced by nevirapine. An in-vivo study showed that voriconazole inhibited the metabolism of efavirenz. Voriconazole may also inhibit the metabolism of NNRTIs besides efavirenz. Patients should be carefully monitored for any occurrence of drug toxicity and/or lack of efficacy during the co-administration of voriconazole and NNRTIs. Dose adjustments are required when voriconazole is co-administered with efavirenz (see sections 4.2 and 4.4).

4.6 Pregnancy and lactation

Pregnancy

No adequate information on the use of VFEND in pregnant women is available.

Studies in animals have shown reproductive toxicity (see section 5.3). The potential risk forhumans is unknown.

VFEND must not be used during pregnancy unless the benefit to the mother clearly outweighs the potential risk to the foetus.

Women of child-bearing potential

Women of child-bearing potential must always use effective contraception during treatment.

Lactation

The excretion of voriconazole into breast milk has not been investigated. Breast-feeding must be stopped on initiation of treatment with VFEND.

4.7 Effects on ability to drive and use machines

VFEND may have a moderate influence on the ability to drive and use machines. It may cause transient and reversible changes to vision, including blurring, altered/enhanced visual perception and/or photophobia. Patients must avoid potentially hazardous tasks, such as driving or operating machinery while experiencing these symptoms.

4.8 Undesirable effects

The safety profile of voriconazole is based on an integrated safety database of more than 2000 subjects (1655 patients in therapeutic trials). This represents a heterogeneous population, containing patients with haematological malignancy, HIV infected patients with oesophageal candidiasis and refractory fungal infections, non-neutropenic patients with candidaemia or aspergillosis and healthy volunteers. Five hundred and sixty one patients had a duration of voriconazole therapy of greater than 12 weeks, with 136 patients receiving voriconazole for over 6 months.

In the table below, since the majority of the studies were of an open nature all causality adverse events, by system organ class and frequency (very common $\geqslant 1/10$, common $\geqslant 1/100$ and $< 1/10$, uncommon $\geqslant 1/1000$ and $< 1/100$, rare, $\geqslant 1/10\,000$ and $< 1/1000$ and very rare, $< 1/10\,000$) if possibly causally related are listed. Within each frequency grouping, undesirable effects are presented in order of decreasing seriousness. The most commonly reported adverse events were visual disturbances, pyrexia, rash, vomiting, nausea, diarrhoea, headache, peripheral oedema and abdominal pain. The severity of the adverse events was generally mild to moderate. No clinically significant differences were seen when the safety data were analysed by age, race, or gender.

Undesirable effects reported in subjects receiving voriconazole

System Organ Class	Adverse drug reactions
Investigations	
Common	Elevated liver function tests (including ASAT, ALAT, alkaline phosphatase, GGT, LDH, bilirubin), blood creatinine increased
Uncommon	Electrocardiogram QT corrected interval prolonged, blood urea increased, blood cholesterol increased
Cardiac disorders	
Very common	Oedema peripheral
Uncommon	Ventricular fibrillation, ventricular arrhythmia, syncope, supraventricular arrhythmia, supraventricular tachycardia, tachycardia, bradycardia
Rare	Torsades de pointes, ventricular tachycardia, atrioventricular complete block, bundle branch block, nodal rhythm
Blood and Lymphatic system disorders	
Common	Pancytopenia, bone marrow depression, leukopenia, thrombocytopenia, purpura, anaemia
Uncommon	Disseminated intravascular coagulation, agranulocytosis, lymphadenopathy, eosinophilia
Nervous system disorders	
Very common	Headache
Common	Dizziness, confusional state, tremor, agitation, paraesthesia
Uncommon	Brain oedema, ataxia, diplopia, vertigo, hypoaesthesia
Rare	Convulsion, encephalopathy, Guillain-Barre syndrome, extrapyramidal symptoms, somnolence during infusion

Eye disorders	
Very common	Visual disturbances [including blurred vision (see section 4.4), chromatopsia and photophobia]
Uncommon	Papilloedema (see section 4.4), optic nerve disorder (including optic neuritis, see section 4.4), nystagmus, scleritis, blepharitis
Rare	Retinal haemorrhage, optic atrophy, oculogyration, corneal opacity
Ear and labyrinth disorders	
Rare	Hypoacusis, tinnitus
Respiratory, thoracic and mediastinal disorders	
Common	Acute respiratory distress syndrome, pulmonary oedema, respiratory distress, chest pain
Gastrointestinal disorders	
Very common	Abdominal pain, nausea, vomiting, diarrhoea
Uncommon	Pancreatitis, peritonitis, duodenitis, gingivitis, glossitis, swollen tongue, dyspepsia, constipation
Rare	Dysgeusia
Renal and urinary disorders	
Common	Renal failure acute, haematuria
Uncommon	Nephritis, proteinuria
Rare	Renal tubular necrosis
Skin and subcutaneous tissue disorders	
Very common	Rash
Common	Exfoliative dermatitis, face oedema, photosensitivity reaction, maculo-papular rash, macular rash, papular rash, cheilitis, pruritus, alopecia, erythema
Uncommon	Stevens-Johnson syndrome, angioneurotic oedema, allergic dermatitis, urticaria, drug hypersensitivity, psoriasis
Rare	Toxic epidermal necrolysis, erythema multiforme, discoid lupus erythematosis
Musculoskeletal and connective tissue disorders	
Common	Back pain
Uncommon	Arthritis
Rare	Hypertonia
Endocrine disorders	
Uncommon	Adrenal insufficiency
Rare	Hyperthyroidism, hypothyroidism
Metabolism and nutrition system disorders	
Common	Hypoglycaemia, hypokalaemia
Infections and infestation	
Common	Gastroenteritis, influenza-like illness
Rare	Pseudomembranous colitis
Vascular disorders	
Common	Hypotension, thrombophlebitis, phlebitis
Rare	Lymphangitis
General disorders and administrative site conditions	
Very common	Pyrexia
Common	Injection site reaction / inflammation, chills, asthenia,
Immune system disorders	
Common	Sinusitis
Uncommon	Anaphylactoid reaction, hypersensitivity
Hepato-biliary disorders	
Common	Jaundice, cholestatic jaundice
Uncommon	Hepatic failure, hepatitis, hepatomegaly, cholecystitis, cholelithiasis
Rare	Hepatic coma
Psychiatric disorders	
Common	Depression, anxiety, hallucination
Rare	Insomnia

Altered taste perception

In the combined data from three bioequivalence studies using the powder for oral suspension formulation, treatment related taste perversion was recorded in 12 (14 %) of subjects.

Visual disturbances

In clinical trials, voriconazole treatment-related visual disturbances were very common. In these studies, short-term as well as long-term treatment, approximately 30 % of subjects experienced altered/enhanced visual perception, blurred vision, colour vision change or photophobia. These visual disturbances were transient and fully reversible, with the majority spontaneously resolving within 60 minutes and no clinically significant long-term visual effects were observed. There was evidence of attenuation with repeated doses of voriconazole. The visual disturbances were generally mild, rarely resulted in discontinuation and were not been associated with long-term sequelae. Visual disturbances may be associated with higher plasma concentrations and/or doses.

The mechanism of action is unknown, although the site of action is most likely to be within the retina. In a study in healthy volunteers investigating the impact of voriconazole on retinal function, voriconazole caused a decrease in the electroretinogram (ERG) waveform amplitude. The ERG measures electrical currents in the retina. The ERG changes did not progress over 29 days of treatment and were fully reversible on withdrawal of voriconazole.

Dermatological reactions

Dermatological reactions were common in patients treated with voriconazole in clinical trials, but these patients had serious underlying diseases and were receiving multiple concomitant medications. The majority of rashes were of mild to moderate severity. Patients have rarely developed serious cutaneous reactions, including Stevens-Johnson syndrome, toxic epidermal necrolysis and erythema multiforme during treatment with VFEND.

If patients develop a rash they should be monitored closely and VFEND discontinued if lesions progress.

Photosensitivity reactions have been reported, especially during long-term therapy (see also section 4.4).

Liver function tests

The overall incidence of clinically significant transaminase abnormalities in the voriconazole clinical programme was 13.4 % (200/1493) of subjects treated with voriconazole. Liver function test abnormalities may be associated with higher plasma concentrations and/or doses. The majority of abnormal liver function tests either resolved during treatment without dose adjustment or following dose adjustment, including discontinuation of therapy.

Voriconazole has been infrequently associated with cases of serious hepatic toxicity in patients with other serious underlying conditions. This includes cases of jaundice, and rare cases of hepatitis and hepatic failure leading to death (see section 4.4).

Infusion-related reactions

During infusion of the intravenous formulation of voriconazole in healthy subjects, anaphylactoid-type reactions, including flushing, fever, sweating, tachycardia, chest tightness, dyspnoea, faintness, nausea, pruritus and rash have occurred. Symptoms appeared immediately upon initiating the infusion (see also section 4.4).

Paediatric Use

The safety of voriconazole was investigated in 245 paediatric patients aged 2 to <12 years who were treated with voriconazole in pharmacokinetic studies (87 paediatric patients) and in compassionate use programs (158 paediatric patients). The adverse event profile of these 245 paediatric patients was similar to that in adults, although post-marketing data suggest there might be a higher occurrence of skin reactions (esp. erythema) in the paediatric population compared to adults. In the 22 patients less than 2 years old who received voriconazole in a compassionate use programme, the following adverse events (for which a relationship to voriconazole could not be excluded) were reported: photosensitivity reaction (1), arrhythmia (1), pancreatitis (1), blood bilirubin increased (1), hepatic enzymes increased (1), rash (1) and papilloedema (1).

There have been post-marketing reports of pancreatitis in paediatric patients.

4.9 Overdose

In clinical trials there were 3 cases of accidental overdose. All occurred in paediatric patients, who received up to five times the recommended intravenous dose of voriconazole. A single adverse reaction of photophobia of 10 minutes duration was reported.

There is no known antidote to voriconazole.

Voriconazole is haemodialysed with a clearance of 121 ml/min. The intravenous vehicle, SBECD, is haemodialysed with a clearance of 55 ml/min. In an overdose, haemodialysis may assist in the removal of voriconazole and SBECD from the body.

5. PHARMACOLOGICAL PROPERTIES

5.1 Pharmacodynamic properties

Pharmacotherapeutic group: ATC code: J02A C03

Antimycotics for Systemic Use – Triazole derivatives

Mechanism of action

In vitro, voriconazole displays broad-spectrum antifungal activity with antifungal potency against *Candida* species (including fluconazole resistant *C. krusei* and resistant strains of *C. glabrata* and *C. albicans*) and fungicidal activity against all *Aspergillus* species tested. In addition voriconazole shows *in vitro* fungicidal activity against emerging fungal pathogens, including those such as *Scedosporium* or *Fusarium* which have limited susceptibility to existing antifungal agents. Its mode of action is inhibition of fungal cytochrome P450-mediated 14α-sterol demethylation, an essential step in ergosterol biosynthesis.

In animal studies there is a correlation between minimum inhibitory concentration values and efficacy against experimental mycoses. By contrast, in clinical studies, there appears to be no correlation between minimum inhibitory concentration values and clinical outcome. Furthermore, there does not appear to be a correlation between plasma levels and clinical outcome. This is typical of azole antimycotics.

Microbiology

Clinical efficacy (with partial or complete response, see below under Clinical Experience) has been demonstrated for *Aspergillus* spp. including *A. flavus, A. fumigatus, A. terreus, A. niger, A. nidulans, Candida* spp., including *C. albicans, C. glabrata, C. krusei, C. parapsilosis* and *C. tropicalis* and limited numbers of *C. dubliniensis, C. inconspicua* and *C. guilliermondii, Scedosporium* spp., including *S. apiospermum, S. prolificans* and *Fusarium* spp.

Other treated fungal infections (with often partial or complete response, see below under Clinical Experience) included isolated cases of *Alternaria* spp., *Blastomyces dermatitidis, Blastoschizomyces capitatus, Cladosporium* spp., *Coccidioides immitis, Conidiobolus coronatus, Cryptococcus neoformans, Exserohilum rostratum, Exophiala spinifera, Fonsecaea pedrosoi, Madurella mycetomatis, Paecilomyces lilacinus, Penicillium* spp. including *P. marneffei, Phialophora richardsiae, Scopulariopsis brevicaulis* and *Trichosporon* spp. including *T. beigelii* infections.

In vitro activity against clinical isolates has been observed for *Acremonium* spp., *Alternaria* spp., *Bipolaris* spp., *Cladophialophora* spp., *Histoplasma capsulatum*, with most strains being inhibited by concentrations of voriconazole in the range 0.05 to 2 μg/ml.

In vitro activity against the following pathogens has been shown, but the clinical significance is unknown: *Curvularia* spp. and *Sporothrix* spp.

Specimens for fungal culture and other relevant laboratory studies (serology, histopathology) should be obtained prior to therapy to isolate and identify causative organisms. Therapy may be instituted before the results of the cultures and other laboratory studies are known; however, once these results become available, anti-infective therapy should be adjusted accordingly.

Clinical isolates with decreased susceptibility to voriconazole have been identified. However, elevated minimum inhibitory concentrations did not always correlate with clinical failure and clinical success has been observed in patients infected with organisms resistant to other azoles. Correlation of *in vitro* activity with clinical outcome is difficult owing to the complexity of the patients studied in clinical trials; breakpoints for voriconazole remain to be established.

Clinical Experience

Successful outcome in this section is defined as complete or partial response.

***Aspergillus* infections – efficacy in aspergillosis patients with poor prognosis**

Voriconazole has *in vitro* fungicidal activity against *Aspergillus* spp. The efficacy and survival benefit of voriconazole versus conventional amphotericin B in the primary treatment of acute invasive aspergillosis was demonstrated in an open, randomised, multicentre study in 277 immunocompromised patients treated for 12 weeks. A satisfactory global response (complete or partial resolution of all attributable symptoms signs, radiographic/bronchoscopic abnormalities present at baseline) was seen in 53 % of voriconazole-treated patients compared to 31 % of patients treated with comparator. The 84-day survival rate for voriconazole was statistically significantly higher than that for the comparator and a clinically and statistically significant benefit was shown in favour of voriconazole for both time to death and time to discontinuation due to toxicity.

This study confirmed findings from an earlier, prospectively designed study where there was a positive outcome in subjects with risk factors for a poor prognosis, including graft versus host disease, and, in particular, cerebral infections (normally associated with almost 100 % mortality).

The studies included cerebral, sinus, pulmonary and disseminated aspergillosis in patients with bone marrow and solid organ transplants, haematological malignancies, cancer and AIDS.

Candidaemia in non-neutropenic patients

The efficacy of voriconazole compared to the regimen of amphotericin B followed by fluconazole in the primary treatment of candidaemia was demonstrated in an open, comparative study. Three hundred and seventy non-neutropenic patients (above 12 years of age) with documented candidaemia were included in the study, of whom 248 were treated with voriconazole. Nine subjects in the voriconazole group and five in the amphotericin B followed by fluconazole group also had mycologically proven infection in deep tissue. Patients with renal failure were excluded from this study. The median treatment duration was 15 days in both treatment arms. In the primary analysis, successful response as assessed by a Data Review Committee (DRC) blinded to study medication was defined as resolution/improvement in all clinical signs and symptoms of infection with eradication of *Candida* from blood and infected deep tissue sites at 12 weeks after the end of therapy (EOT). Patients who did not have an assessment 12 weeks after EOT were counted as failures. In this analysis a successful response was seen in 41 % of patients in both treatment arms.

In a secondary analysis, which utilised *DRC* assessments at the latest evaluable time point (EOT, or 2, 6, or 12 weeks after EOT) voriconazole and the regimen of amphotericin B followed by fluconazole had successful response rates of 65 % and 71 %, respectively. The Investigator's assessment of successful outcome at each of these time points is shown in the following table.

Timepoint	*Voriconazole (N=248)*	*Amphotericin B → fluconazole (N=122)*
EOT	*178 (72 %)*	*88 (72 %)*
2 weeks after EOT	*125 (50 %)*	*62 (51 %)*
6 weeks after EOT	*104 (42 %)*	*55 (45 %)*
12 weeks after EOT	*104 (42 %)*	*51 (42 %)*

Serious refractory *Candida* infections

The study comprised 55 patients with serious refractory systemic *Candida* infections (including candidaemia, disseminated and other invasive candidiasis) where prior antifungal treatment, particularly with fluconazole, had been ineffective. Successful response was seen in 24 patients (15 complete, 9 partial responses). In fluconazole-resistant non *albicans* species, a successful outcome was seen in 3/3 *C. krusei* (complete responses) and 6/8 *C. glabrata* (5 complete, 1 partial response) infections. The clinical efficacy data were supported by limited susceptibility data.

***Scedosporium* and *Fusarium* infections**

Voriconazole was shown to be effective against the following rare fungal pathogens:

Scedosporium spp.: Successful response to voriconazole therapy was seen in 16 (6 complete, 10 partial responses) of 28 patients with *S. apiospermum* and in 2 (both partial responses) of 7 patients with *S. prolificans* infection. In addition, a successful response was seen in 1 of 3 patients with infections caused by more than one organism including *Scedosporium* spp.

Fusarium spp.: Seven (3 complete, 4 partial responses) of 17 patients were successfully treated with voriconazole. Of these 7 patients, 3 had eye, 1 had sinus, and 3 had disseminated infection. Four additional patients with fusariosis had an infection caused by several organisms; two of them had a successful outcome.

The majority of patients receiving voriconazole treatment of the above mentioned rare infections were intolerant of, or refractory to, prior antifungal therapy.

Duration of treatment

In clinical trials, 561 patients received voriconazole therapy for greater than 12 weeks, with 136 patients receiving voriconazole for over 6 months.

Experience in paediatric patients

Sixty one paediatric patients aged 9 months up to 15 years who had definite or probable invasive fungal infections, were treated with voriconazole. This population included 34 patients 2 to < 12 years old and 20 patients 12 to 15 years of age.

The majority (57/61) had failed previous antifungal therapies. Therapeutic studies included 5 patients aged 12 to15 years, the remaining patients received voriconazole in the compassionate use programmes. Underlying diseases in these patients included haematological malignancies and aplastic anaemia (27 patients) and chronic granulomatous disease (14 patients). The most commonly treated fungal infection was aspergillosis (43/61; 70 %).

Clinical Studies Examining QT Interval

A placebo-controlled, randomized, single-dose, crossover study to evaluate the effect on the QT interval of healthy volunteers was conducted with three oral doses of voriconazole and ketoconazole. The placebo-adjusted mean maximum increases in QTc from baseline after 800, 1200 and 1600 mg of voriconazole were 5.1, 4.8, and 8.2 msec, respectively and 7.0 msec for ketoconazole 800 mg. No subject in any group had an increase in QTc of ⩾60 msec from baseline. No subject experienced an interval exceeding the potentially clinically relevant threshold of 500 msec.

5.2 Pharmacokinetic properties

General pharmacokinetic characteristics

The pharmacokinetics of voriconazole have been characterised in healthy subjects, special populations and patients. During oral administration of 200 mg or 300 mg twice daily for 14 days in patients at risk of aspergillosis (mainly patients with malignant neoplasms of lymphatic or haematopoietic tissue), the observed pharmacokinetic characteristics of rapid and consistent absorption, accumulation and non-linear pharmacokinetics were in agreement with those observed in healthy subjects.

The pharmacokinetics of voriconazole are non-linear due to saturation of its metabolism. Greater than proportional increase in exposure is observed with increasing dose. It is estimated that, on average, increasing the oral dose from 200 mg twice daily to 300 mg twice daily leads to a 2.5-fold increase in exposure (AUC_τ). When the recommended intravenous or oral loading dose regimens are administered, plasma concentrations close to steady state are achieved within the first 24 hours of dosing. Without the loading dose, accumulation occurs during twice daily multiple dosing with steady-state plasma voriconazole concentrations being achieved by day 6 in the majority of subjects.

Absorption

Voriconazole is rapidly and almost completely absorbed following oral administration, with maximum plasma concentrations (C_{max}) achieved 1-2 hours after dosing. The absolute bioavailability of voriconazole after oral administration is estimated to be 96 %.

Bioequivalence was established between the 200 mg tablets and the 40mg/ml oral suspension when administered as a 200 mg dose. When multiple doses of voriconazole are administered with high fat meals, C_{max} and AUC_τ are reduced by 34 % and 24 %, respectively. The absorption of voriconazole is not affected by changes in gastric pH.

Distribution

The volume of distribution at steady state for voriconazole is estimated to be 4.6 l/kg, suggesting extensive distribution into tissues. Plasma protein binding is estimated to be 58 %. Cerebrospinal fluid samples from eight patients in a compassionate programme showed detectable voriconazole concentrations in all patients.

Metabolism

In vitro studies showed that voriconazole is metabolised by the hepatic cytochrome P450 isoenzymes, CYP2C19, CYP2C9 and CYP3A4.

The inter-individual variability of voriconazole pharmacokinetics is high.

In vivo studies indicated that CYP2C19 is significantly involved in the metabolism of voriconazole. This enzyme exhibits genetic polymorphism. For example, 15-20 % of Asian populations may be expected to be poor metabolisers. For Caucasians and Blacks the prevalence of poor metabolisers is 3-5 %. Studies conducted in Caucasian and Japanese healthy subjects have shown that poor metabolisers have, on average, 4-fold higher voriconazole exposure (AUC_τ) than their homozygous extensive metaboliser counterparts. Subjects who are heterozygous extensive metabolisers have on average 2-fold higher voriconazole exposure than their homozygous extensive metaboliser counterparts.

The major metabolite of voriconazole is the N-oxide, which accounts for 72 % of the circulating radiolabelled metabolites in plasma. This metabolite has minimal antifungal activity and does not contribute to the overall efficacy of voriconazole.

Excretion

Voriconazole is eliminated via hepatic metabolism with less than 2 % of the dose excreted unchanged in the urine.

After administration of a radiolabelled dose of voriconazole, approximately 80 % of the radioactivity is recovered in the urine after multiple intravenous dosing and 83 % in the urine after multiple oral dosing. The majority (> 94 %) of the total radioactivity is excreted in the first 96 hours after both oral and intravenous dosing.

The terminal half-life of voriconazole depends on dose and is approximately 6 hours at 200 mg (orally). Because of non-linear pharmacokinetics, the terminal half-life is not useful in the prediction of the accumulation or elimination of voriconazole.

Pharmacokinetic-Pharmacodynamic relationships

In 10 therapeutic studies, the median for the average and maximum plasma concentrations in individual subjects across the studies was 2425 ng/ml (inter-quartile range 1193 to 4380 ng/ml) and 3742 ng/ml (inter-quartile range 2027 to 6302 ng/ml), respectively. A positive association between mean, maximum or minimum plasma voriconazole concentration and efficacy in therapeutic studies was not found.

Pharmacokinetic-Pharmacodynamic analyses of clinical trial data identified positive associations between plasma voriconazole concentrations and both liver function test abnormalities and visual disturbances.

Pharmacokinetics in special patient groups

Gender

In an oral multiple dose study, C_{max} and AUC_τ for healthy young females were 83 % and 113 % higher, respectively, than in healthy young males (18-45 years). In the same study, no significant differences in C_{max} and AUC_τ were observed between healthy elderly males and healthy elderly females (⩾ 65 years).

In the clinical programme, no dosage adjustment was made on the basis of gender. The safety profile and plasma concentrations observed in male and female patients were similar. Therefore, no dosage adjustment based on gender is necessary.

Elderly

In an oral multiple dose study C_{max} and AUC_τ in healthy elderly males (⩾ 65 years) were 61 % and 86 % higher, respectively, than in healthy young males (18-45 years). No significant differences in C_{max} and AUC_τ were observed between healthy elderly females (⩾ 65 years) and healthy young females (18- 45 years).

In the therapeutic studies no dosage adjustment was made on the basis of age. A relationship between plasma concentrations and age was observed. The safety profile of voriconazole in young and elderly patients was similar and, therefore, no dosage adjustment is necessary for the elderly (see section 4.2).

Paediatrics

Film-coated tablets & Powder for oral suspension:

The recommended oral dose in paediatrics is based on a population pharmacokinetic analysis of data obtained from 47 immunocompromised paediatric patients aged 2 to <12 years old who were evaluated in a pharmacokinetic study examining multiple oral suspension doses of 4 and 6 mg/kg twice daily. A comparison of the paediatric and adult population pharmacokinetic data indicated that in order to obtain comparable exposures to those obtained in adults following a maintenance dose of 200 mg twice daily, 200 mg of oral suspension twice daily is required in paediatric patients, independent of body weight. In paediatric patients there is a general trend towards low bioavailability at lower body weights and high bioavailability at higher body weights (approaching the extent demonstrated in adults). Based on the population pharmacokinetic analysis, no dosage adjustment according to age or weight is warranted in patients aged 2 to <12 years old at the 200 mg b.i.d. oral solution dosing regimen. A loading dose is not indicated in paediatric patients. Oral bioavailability may, however, be limited in paediatric patients with malabsorption and very low body weight for their age. In that case, intravenous voriconazole administration is recommended.

Powder for Solution for Infusion:

The recommended intravenous dose in paediatric patients is based on a population pharmacokinetic analysis of data pooled from 82 immunocompromised paediatric patients aged 2 to <12 years old who were evaluated in three pharmacokinetic studies (examining single intravenous doses of 3 and 4 mg/kg twice daily, multiple intravenous doses of 3, 4, 6 and 8mg/kg twice daily and multiple oral suspension doses of 4 and 6 mg/kg twice daily). The majority of patients received more than one dose level with a maximum duration of dosing of 30 days.

A comparison of the paediatric and adult population pharmacokinetic data indicated that in order to obtain comparable exposures to those obtained in adults following intravenous maintenance doses of 4 mg/kg twice daily, intravenous maintenance doses of 7 mg/kg twice daily are required in paediatric patients. The higher intravenous maintenance dose in paediatric patients relative to adults reflects the higher elimination capacity in paediatric patients due to a greater liver mass to body mass ratio. In order to obtain comparable exposures to those obtained in adults following intravenous maintenance doses of 3mg/kg twice daily, intravenous maintenance doses of 4 mg/kg twice daily are required in paediatric patients.

Based on the population pharmacokinetic analysis, no loading dose or dosage adjustment according to age is warranted in patients aged 2 to <12 years old.

Renal impairment

Film-coated tablets:

In an oral single dose (200 mg) study in subjects with normal renal function and mild (creatinine clearance 41-60 ml/min) to severe (creatinine clearance < 20 ml/min) renal impairment, the pharmacokinetics of voriconazole were not significantly affected by renal impairment. The plasma protein binding of voriconazole was similar in subjects with different degrees of renal impairment. See dosing and monitoring recommendations under sections 4.2 and 4.4.

Powder for solution for infusion:

In patients with moderate to severe renal dysfunction (serum creatinine levels >2.5 mg /dl), accumulation of the intravenous vehicle, SBECD, occurs. See dosing and monitoring recommendations under sections 4.2 and 4.4.

Hepatic impairment

After an oral single dose (200 mg), AUC was 233 % higher in subjects with mild to moderate hepatic cirrhosis (Child-Pugh A and B) compared with subjects with normal hepatic function. Protein binding of voriconazole was not affected by impaired hepatic function.

In an oral multiple dose study, AUC_τ was similar in subjects with moderate hepatic cirrhosis (Child-Pugh B) given a maintenance dose of 100 mg twice daily and subjects with normal hepatic function given 200 mg twice daily. No pharmacokinetic data are available for patients with severe hepatic cirrhosis (Child-Pugh C). See dosing and monitoring recommendations under sections 4.2 and 4.4.

5.3 Preclinical safety data

Repeated-dose toxicity studies with voriconazole indicated the liver to be the target organ. Hepatotoxicity occurred at plasma exposures similar to those obtained at therapeutic doses in humans, in common with other antifungal agents. In rats, mice and dogs, voriconazole also induced minimal adrenal changes. Conventional studies of safety pharmacology, genotoxicity or carcinogenic potential did not reveal a special hazard for humans.

In reproduction studies, voriconazole was shown to be teratogenic in rats and embryotoxic in rabbits at systemic exposures equal to those obtained in humans with therapeutic doses. In the pre and postnatal development study in rats at exposures lower than those obtained in humans with therapeutic doses, voriconazole prolonged the duration of gestation and labour and produced dystocia with consequent maternal mortality and reduced perinatal survival of pups. The effects on parturition are probably mediated by species-specific mechanisms, involving reduction of oestradiol levels, and are consistent with those observed with other azole antifungal agents.

Preclinical data on the intravenous vehicle, SBECD indicated that the main effects were vacuolation of urinary tract epithelium and activation of macrophages in the liver and lungs in the repeated-dose toxicity studies. As GPMT (guinea pig maximisation test) result was positive, prescribers should be aware of the hypersensitivity potential of the intravenous formulation. Standard genotoxicity and reproduction studies with the excipient SBECD reveal no special hazard for humans. Carcinogenicity studies were not performed with SBECD. An impurity, present in SBECD, has been shown to be an alkylating mutagenic agent with evidence for carcinogenicity in rodents. This impurity should be considered a substance with carcinogenic potential in humans. In the light of these data the duration of treatment of the intravenous formulation should be no longer than 6 months.

6. PHARMACEUTICAL PARTICULARS

6.1 List of excipients

Film-coated tablets:

Tablet core:

Lactose Monohydrate

Pregelatinised Starch

Croscarmellose Sodium

Povidone

Magnesium Stearate

Film-coat:

Hypromellose

Titanium Dioxide (E171)

Lactose Monohydrate

Glycerol Triacetate

Powder for solution for infusion:

Sulphobutylether beta cyclodextrin sodium (SBECD)

Powder for oral suspension:

Sucrose Silica, Colloidal

Titanium Dioxide (E171)

Xanthan Gum

Sodium Citrate

Sodium Benzoate (E211)

Citric Acid

Natural Orange Flavour (containing orange oil, maltodextrin and tocopherol)

6.2 Incompatibilities

Film-coated tablets:

Not applicable

Powder for solution for infusion:

VFEND must not be infused into the same line or cannula concomitantly with other intravenous products. When the VFEND infusion is complete, the line may be used for administration of other intravenous products.

Blood products and short-term infusion of concentrated solutions of electrolytes:

Electrolyte disturbances such as hypokalemia, hypomagnesemia and hypocalcemia should be corrected prior to initiation of voriconazole therapy (see section 4.2 and section 4.4). VFEND must not be administered simultaneously with any blood product or any short-term infusion of concentrated solutions of electrolytes, even if the two infusions are running in separate lines.

Total parenteral nutrition:

Total parenteral nutrition (TPN) need *not* be discontinued when prescribed with VFEND, but does need to be infused through a separate line. If infused through a multiple-lumen catheter, TPN needs to be administered using a different port from the one used for VFEND.

VFEND must not be diluted with 4.2 % Sodium Bicarbonate Infusion.

Compatibility with other concentrations is unknown.

This medicinal product must not be mixed with other medicinal products except those mentioned in section 6.6.

Powder for oral suspension:

This medicinal product must not be mixed with other medicinal products except those mentioned in 6.6. It is not intended that the suspension be further diluted with water or other vehicles.

6.3 Shelf life

VFEND film-coated tablets: 3 years.

VFEND powder for solution for infusion: 3 years.

VFEND is a single dose unpreserved sterile lyophile. Therefore, from a microbiological point of view, once reconstituted, the product must be used immediately. If not used immediately, in-use storage times and conditions prior to use are the responsibility of the user and would normally not be longer than 24 hours at 2°C to 8°C, unless reconstitution has taken place in controlled and validated aseptic conditions.

Chemical and physical in-use stability has been demonstrated for 24 hours at 2°C to 8°C.

Powder for oral suspension:

The shelf-life of the powder for oral suspension is 2 years.

The shelf-life of the constituted suspension is 14 days.

Constituted suspension: Do not store above 30°C, do not refrigerate or freeze.

6.4 Special precautions for storage

Film-coated tablets:

No special precautions for storage.

Powder for solution for infusion:

Reconstituted concentrate: Store at 2°C-8°C for up to 24 hours (in a refrigerator).

For storage conditions of the reconstituted medicinal product, see section 6.3.

Powder for oral suspension:

Powder for oral suspension: Store at 2°C - 8°C (in a refrigerator) before constitution.

For storage conditions of the constituted suspension see section 6.3.

Constituted suspension: Do not store above 30°C, do not refrigerate or freeze.

Keep the container tightly closed.

6.5 Nature and contents of container

Film-coated tablets:

HDPE tablet containers of 2, 30 and 100. Not all bottle sizes may be marketed.

PVC / Aluminium blister in cartons of 2, 10, 14, 20, 28, 30, 50, 56 and 100.

Not all pack sizes may be marketed.

Powder for solution for infusion:

Packs of 1 single use 30 ml clear Type I glass vials with rubber stoppers and aluminium caps with plastic seals.

Powder for oral suspension:

One 100 ml high-density polyethylene (HDPE) bottle (with a polypropylene child resistant closure) contains 45 g of powder for oral suspension. Following constitution, the volume of the suspension is 75 ml, providing a usable volume of 70 ml.

A measuring cup (graduated to indicate 23 ml), 5 ml oral syringe and a press-in bottle adaptor are also provided.

Pack size: 1 bottle.

6.6 Special precautions for disposal and other handling

Film-coated tablets:

No special requirements.

Powder for solution for infusion:

Any unused product or waste material should be disposed of in accordance with local requirements.

The powder is reconstituted with 19 ml of Water for Injections to obtain an extractable volume of 20 ml of clear concentrate containing 10 mg/ml of voriconazole. Discard the VFEND vial if vacuum does not pull the diluent into the vial. It is recommended that a standard 20 ml (non-automated) syringe be used to ensure that the exact amount (19.0 ml) of Water for Injections is dispensed. This medicinal product is for single use only and any unused solution should be discarded and only clear solutions without particles should be used.

For administration, the required volume of the reconstituted concentrate is added to a recommended compatible infusion solution (detailed below) to obtain a final voriconazole solution containing 0.5-5 mg/ml.

Required Volumes of 10 mg/ml VFEND Concentrate (see Table 2 below)

Voriconazole is a single dose unpreserved sterile lyophile. Therefore, from a microbiological point of view, the reconstituted solution must be used immediately. If not used immediately, in-use storage times and conditions prior to use are the responsibility of the user and would normally not be longer than 24 hours at 2 to 8°C, unless reconstitution has taken place in controlled and validated aseptic conditions.

The reconstituted solution can be diluted with:

9 mg/ml (0.9 %) Sodium Chloride for Infusion

Lactated Ringer's Intravenous Infusion

5 % Glucose and Lactated Ringer's Intravenous Infusion

5 % Glucose and 0.45 % Sodium Chloride Intravenous Infusion

5 % Glucose Intravenous Infusion

Table 2 Required Volumes of 10 mg/ml VFEND Concentrate

Body Weight (kg)	Volume of VFEND Concentrate (10mg/ml) required for:			
	3mg/kg dose (number of vials)	4mg/kg dose (number of vials)	6mg/kg dose (number of vials)	7mg/kg dose (number of vials)
10	-	4.0ml (1)	-	7.0ml (1)
15	-	6.0ml (1)	-	10.5ml (1)
20	-	8.0ml (1)	-	14.0ml (1)
25	-	10.0ml (1)	-	17.5ml (1)
30	9.0ml (1)	12.0ml (1)	18.0ml (1)	21.0ml (2)
35	10.5ml (1)	14.0ml (1)	21.0ml (2)	24.5ml (2)
40	12.0ml (1)	16.0ml (1)	24.0ml (2)	28.0ml (2)
45	13.5ml (1)	18.0ml (1)	27.0ml (2)	31.5ml (2)
50	15.0ml (1)	20.0ml (1)	30.0ml (2)	35.0ml (2)
55	16.5ml (1)	22.0ml (2)	33.0ml (2)	-
60	18.0ml (1)	24.0ml (2)	36.0ml (2)	-
65	19.5ml (1)	26.0ml (2)	39.0ml (2)	-
70	21.0ml (2)	28.0ml (2)	42.0ml (3)	-
75	22.5ml (2)	30.0ml (2)	45.0ml (3)	-
80	24.0ml (2)	32.0ml (2)	48.0ml (3)	-
85	25.5ml (2)	34.0ml (2)	51.0ml (3)	-
90	27.0 ml (2)	36.0 ml (2)	54.0 ml (3)	-
95	28.5 ml (2)	38.0 ml (2)	57.0 ml (3)	-
100	30.0 ml (2)	40.0 ml (2)	60.0 ml (3)	-

5 % Glucose in 20 mEq Potassium Chloride Intravenous Infusion

0.45 % Sodium Chloride Intravenous Infusion

5% Glucose and 0.9 % Sodium Chloride Intravenous Infusion

The compatibility of voriconazole with diluents other than described above or in section 6.2 is unknown.

Powder for oral suspension:

Any unused product or waste material should be disposed of in accordance with local requirements.

Any remaining suspension should be discarded 14 days after constitution.

Constitution instructions:

1. Tap the bottle to release the powder.
2. Measure 23 ml of water by filling the measuring cup to the top of the marked line. Add the water to the bottle. Using the cup measure another 23 ml of water and add this to the bottle.
3. Shake the closed bottle vigorously for about 1 minute.
4. Remove child-resistant cap. Press bottle adaptor into the neck of the bottle.
5. Replace the cap.
6. Write the date of expiration of the constituted suspension on the bottle label (the shelf-life of the constituted suspension is 14 days).

Instructions for use:

Shake the closed bottle of constituted suspension for approximately 10 seconds before each use.

Once constituted, VFEND oral suspension should only be administered using the oral syringe supplied with each pack. Refer to the patient leaflet for more detailed instructions for use.

7. MARKETING AUTHORISATION HOLDER

Pfizer Limited, Ramsgate Road, Sandwich, Kent CT13 9NJ, United Kingdom

8. MARKETING AUTHORISATION NUMBER(S)

EU/1/02/212/001 VFEND 50 mg Film-coated tablets; Pack size 2 tablets; Blister

EU/1/02/212/002 VFEND 50 mg Film-coated tablets; Pack size 10 tablets; Blister

EU/1/02/212/003 VFEND 50 mg Film-coated tablets; Pack size 14 tablets; Blister

EU/1/02/212/004 VFEND 50 mg Film-coated tablets; Pack size 20 tablets; Blister

EU/1/02/212/005 VFEND 50 mg Film-coated tablets; Pack size 28 tablets; Blister

EU/1/02/212/006 VFEND 50 mg Film-coated tablets; Pack size 30 tablets; Blister

EU/1/02/212/007 VFEND 50 mg Film-coated tablets; Pack size 50 tablets; Blister

EU/1/02/212/008 VFEND 50 mg Film-coated tablets; Pack size 56 tablets; Blister

EU/1/02/212/009 VFEND 50 mg Film-coated tablets; Pack size 100 tablets; Blister

EU/1/02/212/010 VFEND 50 mg Film-coated tablets; Pack size 2 tablets; Bottle

EU/1/02/212/011 VFEND 50 mg Film-coated tablets; Pack size 30 tablets; Bottle

EU/1/02/212/012 VFEND 50 mg Film-coated tablets; Pack size 100 tablets; Bottle

EU/1/02/212/013 VFEND 200 mg Film-coated tablets; Pack size 2 tablets; Blister

EU/1/02/212/014 VFEND 200 mg Film-coated tablets; Pack size 10 tablets; Blister

EU/1/02/212/015 VFEND 200 mg Film-coated tablets; Pack size 14 tablets; Blister

EU/1/02/212/016 VFEND 200 mg Film-coated tablets; Pack size 20 tablets; Blister

EU/1/02/212/017 VFEND 200 mg Film-coated tablets; Pack size 28 tablets; Blister

EU/1/02/212/018 VFEND 200 mg Film-coated tablets; Pack size 30 tablets; Blister

EU/1/02/212/019 VFEND 200 mg Film-coated tablets; Pack size 50 tablets; Blister

EU/1/02/212/020 VFEND 200 mg Film-coated tablets; Pack size 56 tablets; Blister

EU/1/02/212/021 VFEND 200 mg Film-coated tablets; Pack size 100 tablets; Blister

EU/1/02/212/022 VFEND 200 mg Film-coated tablets; Pack size 2 tablets; Bottle

EU/1/02/212/023 VFEND 200 mg Film-coated tablets; Pack size 30 tablets; Bottle

EU/1/02/212/024 VFEND 200 mg Film-coated tablets; Pack size 100 tablets; Bottle

EU/1/02/212/025 VFEND 200 mg Powder for solution for infusion; Vial

EU/1/02/212/026 VFEND 40 mg/ml Powder for oral suspension; Bottle

9. DATE OF FIRST AUTHORISATION/RENEWAL OF THE AUTHORISATION

Date of first authorisation: 21 March 2002

Date of last renewal: 21 March 2007

10. DATE OF REVISION OF THE TEXT

1 September 2009

LEGAL CATEGORY

POM

Ref: VF 20_0

Detailed information on this medicinal product is available on the website of the European Medicines Agency (EMEA) http://www.emea.europa.eu

Viagra 25mg, 50mg, 100mg

(Pfizer Limited)

1. NAME OF THE MEDICINAL PRODUCT

VIAGRA ® 25 mg film-coated tablets.

VIAGRA ® 50 mg film-coated tablets.

VIAGRA ® 100 mg film-coated tablets.

2. QUALITATIVE AND QUANTITATIVE COMPOSITION

Each tablet contains 25mg, 50mg or 100mg of sildenafil (as citrate).

Excipient: Lactose.

For a full list of excipients, see Section 6.1.

3. PHARMACEUTICAL FORM

Film-coated tablet.

25 mg: Blue rounded diamond-shaped tablets, marked "PFIZER" on one side and "VGR 25" on the other.

50 mg: Blue rounded diamond-shaped tablets, marked "PFIZER" on one side and "VGR 50" on the other.

100 mg: Blue rounded diamond-shaped tablets, marked "PFIZER" on one side and "VGR 100" on the other.

4. CLINICAL PARTICULARS

4.1 Therapeutic indications

Treatment of men with erectile dysfunction, which is the inability to achieve or maintain a penile erection sufficient for satisfactory sexual performance.

In order for VIAGRA to be effective, sexual stimulation is required.

4.2 Posology and method of administration

For oral use.

Use in adults

The recommended dose is 50mg taken as needed approximately one hour before sexual activity. Based on efficacy and toleration, the dose may be increased to 100mg or decreased to 25mg. The maximum recommended dose is 100 mg. The maximum recommended dosing frequency is once per day. If VIAGRA is taken with food, the onset of activity may be delayed compared to the fasted state (see Section 5.2).

Use in the elderly

Dosage adjustments are not required in elderly patients.

Use in patients with impaired renal function

The dosing recommendations described in "Use in adults" apply to patients with mild to moderate renal impairment (creatinine clearance = 30-80 ml/min).

Since sildenafil clearance is reduced in patients with severe renal impairment (creatinine clearance < 30 ml/min) a 25mg dose should be considered. Based on efficacy and toleration, the dose may be increased to 50mg and 100mg.

Use in patients with impaired hepatic function

Since sildenafil clearance is reduced in patients with hepatic impairment (e.g. cirrhosis) a 25mg dose should be considered. Based on efficacy and toleration, the dose may be increased to 50mg and 100mg.

Use in children and adolescents

VIAGRA is not indicated for individuals below 18 years of age.

Use in patients using other medicines

With the exception of ritonavir for which co-administration with sildenafil is not advised (see Section 4.4) a starting dose of 25mg should be considered in patients receiving concomitant treatment with CYP3A4 inhibitors (see Section 4.5).

In order to minimise the potential for developing postural hypotension, patients should be stable on alpha-blocker therapy prior to initiating sildenafil treatment. In addition, initiation of sildenafil at a dose of 25 mg should be considered (see Sections 4.4 and 4.5).

4.3 Contraindications

Hypersensitivity to the active substance or to any of the excipients.

Consistent with its known effects on the nitric oxide/cyclic guanosine monophosphate (cGMP) pathway (see Section 5.1), sildenafil was shown to potentiate the hypotensive effects of nitrates, and its co-administration with nitric oxide donors (such as amyl nitrite) or nitrates in any form is therefore contraindicated.

Agents for the treatment of erectile dysfunction, including sildenafil, should not be used in men for whom sexual activity is inadvisable (e.g. patients with severe cardiovascular disorders such as unstable angina or severe cardiac failure).

VIAGRA is contraindicated in patients who have loss of vision in one eye because of non-arteritic anterior ischaemic optic neuropathy (NAION), regardless of whether this episode was in connection or not with previous PDE5 inhibitor exposure (see section 4.4).

The safety of sildenafil has not been studied in the following sub-groups of patients and its use is therefore contraindicated: severe hepatic impairment, hypotension (blood pressure < 90/50 mmHg), recent history of stroke or myocardial infarction and known hereditary degenerative retinal disorders such as retinitis pigmentosa (a minority of these patients have genetic disorders of retinal phosphodiesterases).

4.4 Special warnings and precautions for use

A medical history and physical examination should be undertaken to diagnose erectile dysfunction and determine potential underlying causes, before pharmacological treatment is considered.

Prior to initiating any treatment for erectile dysfunction, physicians should consider the cardiovascular status of their patients, since there is a degree of cardiac risk associated with sexual activity. Sildenafil has vasodilator properties, resulting in mild and transient decreases in blood pressure (see Section 5.1). Prior to prescribing sildenafil, physicians should carefully consider whether their patients with certain underlying conditions could be adversely affected by such vasodilatory effects, especially in combination with sexual activity. Patients with increased susceptibility to vasodilators include those with left ventricular outflow obstruction (e.g., aortic stenosis, hypertrophic obstructive cardiomyopathy), or those with the rare syndrome of multiple system atrophy manifesting as severely impaired autonomic control of blood pressure.

VIAGRA potentiates the hypotensive effect of nitrates (see Section 4.3).

Serious cardiovascular events, including myocardial infarction, unstable angina, sudden cardiac death, ventricular arrhythmia, cerebrovascular haemorrhage, transient ischaemic attack, hypertension and hypotension have been reported post-marketing in temporal association with the use of VIAGRA. Most, but not all, of these patients had pre-existing cardiovascular risk factors. Many events were reported to occur during or shortly after sexual intercourse and a few were reported to occur shortly after the use of VIAGRA without sexual activity. It is not possible to determine whether these events are related directly to these factors or to other factors.

Agents for the treatment of erectile dysfunction, including sildenafil, should be used with caution in patients with anatomical deformation of the penis (such as angulation, cavernosal fibrosis or Peyronie's disease), or in patients who have conditions which may predispose them to priapism (such as sickle cell anaemia, multiple myeloma or leukaemia).

The safety and efficacy of combinations of sildenafil with other treatments for erectile dysfunction have not been studied. Therefore the use of such combinations is not recommended.

Visual defects and cases of non-arteritic anterior ischaemic optic neuropathy have been reported in connection with the intake of sildenafil and other PDE5 inhibitors. The patient should be advised that in case of sudden visual defect, he should stop taking VIAGRA and consult a physician immediately (see section 4.3).

Co-administration of sildenafil with ritonavir is not advised (see Section 4.5).

Caution is advised when sildenafil is administered to patients taking an alpha-blocker, as the coadministration may lead to symptomatic hypotension in a few susceptible individuals (see Section 4.5). This is most likely to occur within 4 hours post sildenafil dosing. In order to minimise the potential for developing postural hypotension, patients should be hemodynamically stable on alpha-blocker therapy prior to initiating sildenafil treatment. Initiation of sildenafil at a dose of 25 mg should be considered (see Section 4.2). In addition, physicians should advise patients what to do in the event of postural hypotensive symptoms.

Studies with human platelets indicate that sildenafil potentiates the antiaggregatory effect of sodium nitroprusside *in vitro*. There is no safety information on the administration of sildenafil to patients with bleeding disorders or active peptic ulceration. Therefore sildenafil should be administered to these patients only after careful benefit-risk assessment.

The film coating of the VIAGRA tablet contains lactose. VIAGRA should not be administered to men with rare hereditary problems of galactose intolerance, Lapp lactase deficiency or glucose-galactose malabsorption.

VIAGRA is not indicated for use by women.

4.5 Interaction with other medicinal products and other forms of interaction

Effects of other medicinal products on sildenafil

***In vitro* studies:**

Sildenafil metabolism is principally mediated by the cytochrome P450 (CYP) isoforms 3A4 (major route) and 2C9 (minor route). Therefore, inhibitors of these isoenzymes may reduce sildenafil clearance.

***In vivo* studies:**

Population pharmacokinetic analysis of clinical trial data indicated a reduction in sildenafil clearance when co-administered with CYP3A4 inhibitors (such as ketoconazole, erythromycin, cimetidine). Although no increased incidence of adverse events was observed in these patients, when sildenafil is administered concomitantly with CYP3A4 inhibitors, a starting dose of 25mg should be considered.

Co-administration of the HIV protease inhibitor ritonavir, which is a highly potent P450 inhibitor, at steady state (500mg twice daily) with sildenafil (100mg single dose) resulted in a 300% (4-fold) increase in sildenafil C_{max} and a 1,000% (11-fold) increase in sildenafil plasma AUC. At 24 hours, the plasma levels of sildenafil were still approximately 200ng/ml, compared to approximately 5ng/ml when sildenafil was administeredalone. This is consistent with ritonavir's marked effects on a broad range of P450 substrates. Sildenafil had no effect on ritonavir pharmacokinetics. Based on these pharmacokinetic results co-administration of sildenafil with ritonavir is not advised (see Section 4.4) and in any event the maximum dose of sildenafil should under no circumstances exceed 25mg within 48 hours.

Co-administration of the HIV protease inhibitor saquinavir, a CYP3A4 inhibitor, at steady state (1200mg three times a day) with sildenafil (100mg single dose) resulted in a 140% increase in sildenafil C_{max} and a 210% increase in sildenafil AUC. Sildenafil had no effect on saquinavir pharmacokinetics (see Section 4.2). Stronger CYP3A4 inhibitors such as ketoconazole and itraconazole would be expected to have greater effects.

When a single 100mg dose of sildenafil was administered with erythromycin, a specific CYP3A4 inhibitor, at steady state (500mg twice daily for 5 days), there was a 182% increase in sildenafil systemic exposure (AUC). In normal healthy male volunteers, there was no evidence of an effect of azithromycin (500mg daily for 3 days) on the AUC, C_{max}, T_{max}, elimination rate constant, or subsequent half-life of sildenafil or its principal circulating metabolite. Cimetidine (800mg), a cytochrome P450 inhibitor and non-specific CYP3A4 inhibitor, caused a 56% increase in plasma sildenafil concentrations when co-administered with sildenafil (50mg) to healthy volunteers.

Grapefruit juice is a weak inhibitor of CYP3A4 gut wall metabolism and may give rise to modest increases in plasma levels of sildenafil.

Single doses of antacid (magnesium hydroxide/aluminium hydroxide) did not affect the bioavailability of sildenafil.

Although specific interaction studies were not conducted for all medicinal products, population pharmacokinetic analysis showed no effect of concomitant medication on sildenafil pharmacokinetics when grouped as CYP2C9 inhibitors (such as tolbutamide, warfarin, phenytoin), CYP2D6 inhibitors (such as selective serotonin reuptake inhibitors, tricyclic antidepressants), thiazide and related diuretics, loop and potassium sparing diuretics, angiotensin converting enzyme inhibitors, calcium channel blockers, beta-adrenoreceptor antagonists or inducers of CYP450 metabolism (such as rifampicin, barbiturates).

Nicorandil is a hybrid of potassium channel activator and nitrate. Due to the nitrate component it has the potential to have serious interaction with sildenafil.

Effects of sildenafil on other medicinal products

***In vitro* studies:**

Sildenafil is a weak inhibitor of the cytochrome P450 isoforms 1A2, 2C9, 2C19, 2D6, 2E1 and 3A4 ($IC_{50} > 150\ \mu M$). Given sildenafil peak plasma concentrations of approximately 1 μM after recommended doses, it is unlikely that VIAGRA will alter the clearance of substrates of these isoenzymes.

There are no data on the interaction of sildenafil and non-specific phosphodiesterase inhibitors such as theophylline or dipyridamole.

***In vivo* studies:**

Consistent with its known effects on the nitric oxide/cGMP pathway (see Section 5.1), sildenafil was shown to potentiate the hypotensive effects of nitrates, and its co-administration with nitric oxide donors or nitrates in any form is therefore contraindicated (see Section 4.3).

Concomitant administration of sildenafil to patients taking alpha-blocker therapy may lead to symptomatic hypotension in a few susceptible individuals. This is most likely to occur within 4 hours post sildenafil dosing (see Sections 4.2 and 4.4). In three specific drug-drug interaction studies, the alpha-blocker doxazosin (4 mg and 8 mg) and sildenafil (25 mg, 50 mg, or 100 mg) were administered simultaneously to patients with benign prostatic hyperplasia (BPH) stabilized on doxazosin therapy. In these study populations, mean additional reductions of supine blood pressure of 7/7 mmHg, 9/5 mmHg, and 8/4 mmHg, and mean additional reductions of standing blood pressure of 6/6 mmHg, 11/4 mmHg, and 4/5 mmHg, respectively, were observed. When sildenafil and doxazosin were administered simultaneously to patients stabilized on doxazosin therapy, there were infrequent reports of patients who experienced symptomatic postural hypotension. These reports included dizziness and light-headedness, but not syncope.

No significant interactions were shown when sildenafil (50mg) was co-administered with tolbutamide (250mg) or warfarin (40mg), both of which are metabolised by CYP2C9.

Sildenafil (50mg) did not potentiate the increase in bleeding time caused by acetyl salicylic acid (150mg).

Sildenafil (50mg) did not potentiate the hypotensive effects of alcohol in healthy volunteers with mean maximum blood alcohol levels of 80 mg/dl.

Pooling of the following classes of antihypertensive medication; diuretics, beta-blockers, ACE inhibitors, angiotensin II antagonists, antihypertensive medicinal products (vasodilator and centrally-acting), adrenergic neurone blockers, calcium channel blockers and alpha-adrenoceptor blockers, showed no difference in the side effect profile in patients taking sildenafil compared to placebo treatment. In a specific interaction study, where sildenafil (100mg) was co-administered with amlodipine in hypertensive patients, there was an additional reduction on supine systolic blood pressure of 8 mmHg. The corresponding additional reduction in supine diastolic blood pressure was 7 mmHg. These additional blood pressure reductions were of a similar magnitude to those seen when sildenafil was administered alone to healthy volunteers (see Section 5.1).

Sildenafil (100mg) did not affect the steady state pharmacokinetics of the HIV protease inhibitors, saquinavir and ritonavir, both of which are CYP3A4 substrates.

4.6 Pregnancy and lactation

VIAGRA is not indicated for use by women.

No relevant adverse effects were found in reproduction studies in rats and rabbits following oral administration of sildenafil.

4.7 Effects on ability to drive and use machines

No studies on the effects on the ability to drive and use machines have been performed.

As dizziness and altered vision were reported in clinical trials with sildenafil, patients should be aware of how they react to VIAGRA, before driving or operating machinery.

4.8 Undesirable effects

The safety profile of VIAGRA is based on 8691 patients who received the recommended dosing regimen in 67 placebo-controlled clinical studies. The most commonly reported adverse reactions in clinical studies among sildenafil treated patients were headache, flushing, dyspepsia, visual disorders, nasal congestion, dizziness and visual colour distortion.

Adverse reactions from post-marketing surveillance has been gathered covering an estimated period >9 years. Because not all adverse reactions are reported to the Marketing Authorisation Holder and included in the safety database, the frequencies of these reactions cannot be reliably determined.

In the table below all medically important adverse reactions, which occurred in clinical trials at an incidence greater than placebo are listed by system organ class and frequency (very common (≥1/10), common (≥1/100 to <1/10), uncommon (≥1/1,000 to <1/100), rare (≥1/10,000 to, 1/1,000).

In addition, the frequency of medically important adverse reactions reported from post-marketing experience is included as not known.

Within each frequency grouping, undesirable effects are presented in order of decreasing seriousness.

Table 1: Medically important adverse reactions reported at an incidence greater than placebo in controlled clinical studies and medically important adverse reactions reported through post-marketing surveillance

MedDRA System Organ Class	Adverse Reaction
Immune system disorders	
Rare	Hypersensitivity reactions
Nervous system disorders	
Very common	Headache
Common	Dizziness
Uncommon	Somnolence, Hypoaesthesia
Rare	Cerebrovascular accident, Syncope
Not known	Transient ischaemic attack, Seizure, Seizure recurrence
Eye disorders	
Common	Visual disorders, Visual colour distortion
Uncommon	Conjunctival disorders, Eye disorders, Lacrimation disorders, Other eye disorders
Not known	Non-arteritic anterior ischaemic optic neuropathy (NAION), Retinal vascular occlusion, Visual field defect.
Ear and labyrinth disorders	
Uncommon	Vertigo, Tinnitus
Rare	Deafness*
Vascular disorders	
Common	Flushing
Rare	Hypertension, Hypotension
Cardiac disorders	
Uncommon	Palpitations, Tachycardia
Rare	Myocardial infarction, Atrial fibrillation
Unknown	Ventricular arrhythmia, Unstable angina, Sudden cardiac death
Respiratory, thoracic and mediastinal disorders	
Common	Nasal congestion
Rare	Epistaxis
Gastrointestinal disorders	
Common	Dyspepsia
Uncommon	Vomiting, Nausea, Dry mouth
Skin, subcutaneous and soft tissue disorders	
Uncommon	Skin rash
Musculoskeletal and connective tissue disorders	
System Organ Class	**Adverse Reactions**
Uncommon	Myalgia
Reproductive system and breast disorders	
Not known	Priapism, Prolonged erection
General disorders and administration site conditions	
Uncommon	Chest pain, Fatigue
Investigations	
Uncommon	Heart rate increased

* Ear disorders: Sudden deafness. Sudden decrease or loss of hearing has been reported in a small number of post-marketing and clinical trial cases with the use of all PDE5 inhibitors, including sildenafil.

4.9 Overdose

In single dose volunteer studies of doses up to 800mg, adverse reactions were similar to those seen at lower doses, but the incidence rates and severities were increased. Doses of 200mg did not result in increased efficacy but the incidence of adverse reactions (headache, flushing, dizziness, dyspepsia, nasal congestion, altered vision) was increased.

In cases of overdose, standard supportive measures should be adopted as required. Renal dialysis is not expected to accelerate clearance as sildenafil is highly bound to plasma proteins and not eliminated in the urine.

5. PHARMACOLOGICAL PROPERTIES

5.1 Pharmacodynamic properties

Pharmacotherapeutic group: Drugs used in erectile dysfunction. ATC Code: G04B E03.

Sildenafil is an oral therapy for erectile dysfunction. In the natural setting, i.e. with sexual stimulation, it restores impaired erectile function by increasing blood flow to the penis.

The physiological mechanism responsible for erection of the penis involves the release of nitric oxide (NO) in the corpus cavernosum during sexual stimulation. Nitric oxide then activates the enzyme guanylate cyclase, which results in increased levels of cyclic guanosine monophosphate (cGMP), producing smooth muscle relaxation in the corpus cavernosum and allowing inflow of blood.

Sildenafil is a potent and selective inhibitor of cGMP specific phosphodiesterase type 5 (PDE5) in the corpus cavernosum, where PDE5 is responsible for degradation of cGMP. Sildenafil has a peripheral site of action on erections. Sildenafil has no direct relaxant effect on isolated human corpus cavernosum but potently enhances the relaxant effect of NO on this tissue. When the NO/cGMP pathway is activated, as occurs with sexual stimulation, inhibition of PDE5 by sildenafil results in increased corpus cavernosum levels of cGMP. Therefore sexual stimulation is required in order for sildenafil to produce its intended beneficial pharmacological effects.

Studies *in vitro* have shown that sildenafil is selective for PDE5, which is involved in the erection process. Its effect is more potent on PDE5 than on other known phosphodiesterases. There is a 10-fold selectivity over PDE6 which is involved in the phototransduction pathway in the retina. At maximum recommended doses, there is an 80-fold selectivity over PDE1, and over 700-fold over PDE 2, 3, 4, 7, 8, 9, 10 and 11. In particular, sildenafil has greater than

4,000-fold selectivity for PDE5 over PDE3, the cAMP-specific phosphodiesterase isoform involved in the control of cardiac contractility.

Two clinical studies were specifically designed to assess the time window after dosing during which sildenafil could produce an erection in response to sexual stimulation. In a penile plethysmography (RigiScan) study of fasted patients, the median time to onset for those who obtained erections of 60% rigidity (sufficient for sexual intercourse) was 25 minutes (range 12-37 minutes) on sildenafil. In a separate RigiScan study, sildenafil was still able to produce an erection in response to sexual stimulation 4-5 hours post-dose.

Sildenafil causes mild and transient decreases in blood pressure which, in the majority of cases, do not translate into clinical effects. The mean maximum decreases in supine systolic blood pressure following 100mg oral dosing of sildenafil was 8.4 mmHg. The corresponding change in supine diastolic blood pressure was 5.5 mmHg. These decreases in blood pressure are consistent with the vasodilatory effects of sildenafil, probably due to increased cGMP levels in vascular smooth muscle. Single oral doses of sildenafil up to 100mg in healthy volunteers produced no clinically relevant effects on ECG.

In a study of the hemodynamic effects of a single oral 100mg dose of sildenafil in 14 patients with severe coronary artery disease (CAD) (>70% stenosis of at least one coronary artery), the mean resting systolic and diastolic blood pressures decreased by 7% and 6% respectively compared to baseline. Mean pulmonary systolic blood pressure decreased by 9%. Sildenafil showed no effect on cardiac output, and did not impair blood flow through the stenosed coronary arteries.

No clinical relevant differences were demonstrated in time to limiting angina for sildenafil when compared with placebo in a double blind, placebo controlled exercise stress trial in 144 patients with erectile dysfunction and chronic stable angina, who were taking on a regular basis anti-anginal medications (except nitrates).

Mild and transient differences in colour discrimination (blue/green) were detected in some subjects using the Farnsworth-Munsell 100 hue test at 1 hour following a 100mg dose, with no effects evident after 2 hours post-dose. The postulated mechanism for this change in colour discrimination is related to inhibition of PDE6, which is involved in the phototransduction cascade of the retina. Sildenafil has no effect on visual acuity or contrast sensitivity. In a small size placebo-controlled study of patients with documented early age-related macular degeneration (n=9), sildenafil (single dose, 100mg) demonstrated no significant changes in visual tests conducted (visual acuity, Amsler grid, colour discrimination simulated traffic light, Humphrey perimeter and photostress).

There was no effect on sperm motility or morphology after single 100mg oral doses of sildenafil in healthy volunteers.

Further information on clinical trials

In clinical trials sildenafil was administered to more than 8000 patients aged 19-87. The following patient groups were represented: elderly (19.9%), patients with hypertension (30.9%), diabetes mellitus (20.3%), ischaemic heart disease (5.8%), hyperlipidaemia (19.8%), spinal cord injury (0.6%), depression (5.2%), transurethral resection of the prostate (3.7%), radical prostatectomy (3.3%). The following groups were not well represented or excluded from clinical trials: patients with pelvic surgery, patients post-radiotherapy, patients with severe renal or hepatic impairment and patients with certain cardiovascular conditions (see Section 4.3).

In fixed dose studies, the proportions of patients reporting that treatment improved their erections were 62% (25mg), 74% (50mg) and 82% (100mg) compared to 25% on placebo. In controlled clinical trials, the discontinuation rate due to sildenafil was low and similar to placebo.

Across all trials, the proportion of patients reporting improvement on sildenafil were as follows: psychogenic erectile dysfunction (84%), mixed erectile dysfunction (77%), organic erectile dysfunction (68%), elderly (67%), diabetes mellitus (59%), ischaemic heart disease (69%), hypertension (68%), TURP (61%), radical prostatectomy (43%), spinal cord injury (83%), depression (75%). The safety and efficacy of sildenafil was maintained in long term studies.

5.2 Pharmacokinetic properties

Absorption

Sildenafil is rapidly absorbed. Maximum observed plasma concentrations are reached within 30 to 120 minutes (median 60 minutes) of oral dosing in the fasted state. The mean absolute oral bioavailability is 41% (range 25-63%). After oral dosing of sildenafil AUC and C_{max} increase in proportion with dose over the recommended dose range (25-100mg).

When sildenafil is taken with food, the rate of absorption is reduced with a mean delay in T_{max} of 60 minutes and a mean reduction in C_{max} of 29%.

Distribution

The mean steady state volume of distribution (V_d) for sildenafil is 105 l, indicating distribution into the tissues. After a single oral dose of 100 mg, the mean maximum total plasma concentration of sildenafil is approximately 440 ng/ml (CV 40%). Since sildenafil (and its major circulating N-desmethyl metabolite) is 96% bound to plasma proteins, this results in the mean maximum free plasma concentration for sildenafil of 18 ng/ml (38 nM). Protein binding is independent of total drug concentrations.

In healthy volunteers receiving sildenafil (100mg single dose), less than 0.0002% (average 188ng) of the administered dose was present in ejaculate 90 minutes after dosing.

Metabolism

Sildenafil is cleared predominantly by the CYP3A4 (major route) and CYP2C9 (minor route) hepatic microsomal isoenzymes. The major circulating metabolite results from N-demethylation of sildenafil. This metabolite has a phosphodiesterase selectivity profile similar to sildenafil and an *in vitro* potency for PDE5 approximately 50% that of the parent drug. Plasma concentrations of this metabolite are approximately 40% of those seen for sildenafil. The N-desmethyl metabolite is further metabolised, with a terminal half life of approximately 4 h.

Elimination

The total body clearance of sildenafil is 41 l/h with a resultant terminal phase half life of 3-5 h. After either oral or intravenous administration, sildenafil is excreted as metabolites predominantly in the faeces (approximately 80% of administered oral dose) and to a lesser extent in the urine (approximately 13% of administered oral dose).

Pharmacokinetics in special patient groups

Elderly

Healthy elderly volunteers (65 years or over) had a reduced clearance of sildenafil, resulting in approximately 90% higher plasma concentrations of sildenafil and the active N-desmethyl metabolite compared to those seen in healthy younger volunteers (18-45 years). Due to age-differences in plasma protein binding, the corresponding increase in free sildenafil plasma concentration was approximately 40%.

Renal insufficiency

In volunteers with mild to moderate renal impairment (creatinine clearance = 30-80 ml/min), the pharmacokinetics of sildenafil were not altered after receiving a 50mg single oral dose. The mean AUC and C_{max} of the N-desmethyl metabolite increased 126% and 73% respectively, compared to age-matched volunteers with no renal impairment. However, due to high inter-subject variability, these differences were not statistically significant. In volunteers with severe renal impairment (creatinine clearance < 30 ml/min), sildenafil clearance was reduced, resulting in mean increases in AUC and C_{max} of 100% and 88% respectively compared to age-matched volunteers with no renal impairment. In addition, N-desmethyl metabolite AUC and C_{max} values were significantly increased 79% and 200% respectively.

Hepatic insufficiency

In volunteers with mild to moderate hepatic cirrhosis (Child-Pugh A and B) sildenafil clearance was reduced, resulting in increases in AUC (84%) and C_{max} (47%) compared to age-matched volunteers with no hepatic impairment. The pharmacokinetics of sildenafil in patients with severely impaired hepatic function have not been studied.

5.3 Preclinical safety data

Non-clinical data revealed no special hazard for humans based on conventional studies of safety pharmacology, repeated dose toxicity, genotoxicity, carcinogenic potential, and toxicity to reproduction.

6. PHARMACEUTICAL PARTICULARS

6.1 List of excipients

Tablet core: microcrystalline cellulose, calcium hydrogen phosphate (anhydrous), croscarmellose sodium, magnesium stearate.

Film coat: hypromellose, titanium dioxide (E171), lactose, triacetin, indigo carmine aluminium lake (E132).

6.2 Incompatibilities

Not applicable.

6.3 Shelf life

5 years.

6.4 Special precautions for storage

Do not store above 30°C.

Store in the original package, in order to protect from moisture.

6.5 Nature and contents of container

PVC/Aluminium foil blisters in cartons of 2, 4, 8 or 12 tablets. Not all pack sizes may be marketed.

6.6 Special precautions for disposal and other handling

No special requirements.

7. MARKETING AUTHORISATION HOLDER

Pfizer Limited, Sandwich, Kent, CT13 9NJ, United Kingdom.

8. MARKETING AUTHORISATION NUMBER(S)

EU/1/98/077/013 - Viagra tablets 25 mg; pack size 2 tablets

EU/1/98/077/002 - Viagra tablets 25 mg; pack size 4 tablets

EU/1/98/077/003 - Viagra tablets 25 mg; pack size 8 tablets

EU/1/98/077/004 - Viagra tablets 25 mg; pack size 12 tablets

EU/1/98/077/014- Viagra tablets 50 mg; pack size 2 tablets

EU/1/98/077/006 - Viagra tablets 50 mg; pack size 4 tablets

EU/1/98/077/007 - Viagra tablets 50 mg; pack size 8 tablets

EU/1/98/077/008 - Viagra tablets 50 mg; pack size 12 tablets

EU/1/98/077/015 - Viagra tablets 100 mg; pack size 2 tablets

EU/1/98/077/010 - Viagra tablets 100 mg; pack size 4 tablets

EU/1/98/077/011 - Viagra tablets 100 mg; pack size 8 tablets

EU/1/98/077/012 - Viagra tablets 100 mg; pack size 12 tablets

9. DATE OF FIRST AUTHORISATION/RENEWAL OF THE AUTHORISATION

Date of first authorisation: 14 September 1998

Date of last renewal: 26 August 2008

10. DATE OF REVISION OF THE TEXT

29 January 2009

11. LEGAL CATEGORY

POM

Detailed information on this medicinal product is available on the website of the European Medicines Agency (EMEA) http://www.emea.eu.int/

Ref: VI 18_0

Viazem XL 120mg

(Genus Pharmaceuticals)

1. NAME OF THE MEDICINAL PRODUCT

VIAZEM XL

2. QUALITATIVE AND QUANTITATIVE COMPOSITION

Diltiazem hydrochloride: 120 mg capsule.

For excipients, see section 6.1

3. PHARMACEUTICAL FORM

Prolonged release capsule, hard.

Lavender opaque capsule. Each capsule is printed on the caps and body, in white ink Viazem XL 120

4. CLINICAL PARTICULARS

4.1 Therapeutic indications

VIAZEM XL is indicated for the management of stable angina pectoris and the treatment of mild to moderate hypertension.

4.2 Posology and method of administration

Dosage requirements may differ between patients with angina and patients with hypertension. In addition individual patients response may vary, necessitating careful titration. The range of strengths facilitates titration to the optimal dose.

One capsule of VIAZEM XL is to be taken before or during a meal. The dose should be taken at approximately the same time each day.

The capsule should not be chewed but swallowed whole, with a glass of water.

Due to the variability of release profile in individual patients, when changing from one type of sustained release diltiazem preparation to another, it may be necessary to adjust the dose.

Adults:

Hypertension: The usual starting dose is 180 mg once daily. The dose may be increased after 2-4 weeks according to the patient's response and the usual maintenance dose is 240mg-360mg once daily. The maximum daily dose is 360 mg. However, the single daily doses of 300 mg and 360 mg should only be administered to patients when no satisfactory therapeutic effect has been effected with lower doses and after the benefit risk-ratio has been carefully assessed by the doctor.

Angina: Care should be taken when titrating patients with stable angina in order to establish the optimal dose. The usual starting dose is 180 mg once daily. The dose may be increased after 2-4 weeks according to the patient's response. The maximum daily dose is 360 mg. However, the single daily doses of 300 mg and 360 mg should only be administered to patients when no satisfactory therapeutic effect has been effected with lower doses and after the benefit risk-ratio has been carefully assessed by the doctor.

Elderly and patients with impaired hepatic or renal function:

Plasma levels of diltiazem can be increased in the elderly, and in patients with impaired hepatic renal or hepatic function. In these cases, the starting dose should be one 120mg VIAZEM XL capsule once daily. Heart rate should be monitored and if it falls below 50 beats per minute, the dose should not be increased. Dose adjustment may be required to obtain a satisfactory clinical response.

Children:

Safety and efficacy in children have not been established.

4.3 Contraindications

Diltiazem depresses atrioventricular node conduction and is therefore contraindicated in patients with severe bradycardia (less than 50 bpm), sick sinus syndrome, congestive heart failure, and left ventricular failure with second or third degree AV or sino-atrial block, except in the presence of a functioning pacemaker. Diltiazem is also contraindicated in left ventricular failure with pulmonary stasis as diltiazem may have mild negative effects on contractility.

Diltiazem is contraindicated in acute complicated myocardial infarction (e.g. bradycardia hypotension, congestive heart failure/reduced LV function), pulmonary congestion, hypotension (<90 mmHg systolic) cerebrovascular accident, cardiac shock and unstable angina pectoris.

Diltiazem is contraindicated in pre-excitation syndrome (e.g. WPW) accompanied with atrial flutter, fibrillation and in digitalis intoxication, as diltiazem may precipitate ventricular tachycardia.

Diltiazem should not be used in patients with known hypersensitivity to diltiazem.

Diltiazem should not be used during pregnancy, by women of child-bearing potential, or by women who are breastfeeding.

4.4 Special warnings and precautions for use

Patients treated with beta-adrenoreceptor blocking drugs and patients with conduction disturbances (bradycardia, bundle branch block, first degree AV block, prolonged PR interval) should only be treated with VIAZEM XL after special consideration due to the risk of serious bradyarrhythmias.

This product should be used with caution in patients with hepatic dysfunction. Abnormalities of liver function may appear during therapy. The higher single daily doses of VIAZEM XL capsules 300mg and 360mg should not be administered to patients with impaired renal and/or hepatic function and to elderly patients (prolonged half life of elimination) because there is no experience on the use of such high dosages in these patient categories.

In patients undergoing long-term therapy with cyclosporin, plasma levels of cyclosporin should be monitored when concurrent administration of diltiazem is initiated, or discontinued or if the dose of diltiazem is changed.

Abnormally short transit time through the gastrointestinal tract could lead to incomplete release of contents of the capsule e.g. in chronic conditions with associated diarrhoea such as Crohns disease or ulcerative colitis.

4.5 Interaction with other medicinal products and other forms of interaction

Combinations contraindicated as a safety measure:

In animals, fatal ventricular fibrillations are constantly seen during administration of verapamil and dantrolene via the i.v. route. The combination of a calcium antagonist and dantrolene is therefore potentially dangerous. The concurrent iv administration of beta-adrenergic blocking agents with diltiazem should be avoided because an additive effect on SA and AV conduction and ventricular function will occur. The use of such a combination requires ECG monitoring especially at the beginning of treatment.

Combinations requiring safety precautions:

In common with other calcium antagonists, when diltiazem is used with drugs which may induce bradycardia or with antiarrhythmic drugs (e.g. amiodarone) or other antihypertensive drugs, the possibility of an additive effect should be borne in mind. Inhalation anaesthetics should be used with caution during diltiazem therapy. Tri/tetracyclic antidepressants and neuroleptics may increase the antihypertensive effects of diltiazem whilst the concomitant use of lithium with diltiazem may lead to neurotoxicity (extrapyramidal effects). Rifampin and other hepatic enzyme inducers may reduce the bioavailability of diltiazem and high doses of Vitamin D and/or high intake of calcium salts leading to elevated serum calcium levels may reduce the response to diltiazem.

Diltiazem is metabolised by CYP3A4 and could, by competitive inhibition of CYP3A4, affect the pharmacokinetics of other drugs metabolised by this enzyme. In addition inhibitors and inducers of CYP3A4 may affect the pharmacokinetics of diltiazem.

Diltiazem prolongs the sedative effect of medazolam and triazolam via metabolic interaction and decreases nifedipine clearance by 50%. Diltiazem may cause increases in the levels of digitoxin. Diltiazem has been shown to increase the bioavailability of imipramine by 30% probably due to inhibition of its first pass metabolism.

Diltiazem has been used safely in combination with diuretics, ACE-inhibitors and other anti-hypertensive agents. It is recommended that patients receiving these combinations should be regularly monitored. Concomitant use of diltiazem with alpha-blockers such as prazosin should be strictly monitored because of the possible synergistic hypotensive effect of the combination.

Case reports have suggested that blood levels of carbamazepine, cyclosporin, theophylline and phenytoin may be increased when given concurrently with diltiazem. Care should be exercised in patients taking these drugs. In common with other calcium antagonists diltiazem may cause small increases in plasma levels of digoxin. In patients taking H_2-antagonists concurrently with diltiazem there may be increased levels of diltiazem.

Magnification of the hypotensive and lipothymic effects (summation of vasodilator properties) of nitrate derivatives can occur. In patients on calcium inhibitors, prescriptions of nitrate derivatives should be made at progressively increasing doses. Diltiazem treatment has been continued without problem during anaesthesia, but diltiazem may potentiate the activity of curare-like and depolarising neuromuscular blocking agents, therefore the anaesthetist should be informed that the patient is receiving a calcium antagonist.

4.6 Pregnancy and lactation

Pregnancy:

Diltiazem should not be taken during pregnancy. Women of child bearing-potential should exclude the possibility of pregnancy before commencing treatment by taking suitable contraceptive measures if necessary. In animal tests, Diltiazem was found to have a tetratogenic effects in some species of animal.

Diltiazem may suppress the contractility of the uterus. Definite evidence that this will prolong partus in full-term pregnancy is lacking. A risk of hypoxia in the foetus may arise in the event of hypotension in the mother and reduced perfusion of the uterus due to redistribution of blood flow due to peripheral vasodilatation. In animal experiments diltiazem has exhibited teratogenic effects in some animal species. In the absence of adequate evidence of safety in human pregnancy, VIAZEM XL should not be used in pregnancy or in women of childbearing potential.

Lactation:

Diltiazem is excreted in breast milk in concentrations similar to those in serum. If the use of diltiazem is considered essential, an alternative method of infant feeding should be instituted.

4.7 Effects on ability to drive and use machines

There are no studies on the effect of diltiazem when driving vehicles or operating machines. It should be taken into account that occasionally asthenia/fatigue and dizziness may occur. Treatment of hypertension with this medicinal product requires regular monitoring. Individual different reactions may affect the ability to drive. This risk should be considered especially at the beginning of treatment, when changing the drug, or in combination with alcohol.

4.8 Undesirable effects

Certain undesirable effects may lead to suspension of treatment: sinus bradycardia, sino-atrial heart block, 2nd and 3rd degree atrioventricular heart block, skin rash, oedema of the lower limbs.

In hypertensive patients, adverse effects are generally mild and transient and are most commonly vasodilatory related events.

The following have been described in decreasing order of frequency: lower limb oedema, headache, hot flushes/flushing, asthenia/fatigue, palpitations, malaise, minor gastro-intestinal disorders (dyspepsia, abdominal pain, dry mouth, nausea, vomiting, diarrhoea, constipation) and skin rash. Erythema multiform and Stevens Johnson syndrome have been reported infrequently in patients receiving diltiazem hydrochloride. Vasodilatory related events (in particular, oedema) are dose-dependent and appear to be more frequent in elderly subjects.

Rare cases of symptomatic bradycardia and exceptionally sino-atrial block and atrioventricular block, hypotension, syncope, reduced left ventricular function have also been recorded. Isolated cases of hallucinations, depression, insomnia, hyperglycaemia and impotence have been reported.

Experience with use in other indications and with other formulations has shown that skin rashes are usually localised and are limited to cases of erythemia, urticaria or occasionally desquamative erthema, with or without fever, which regress when treatment is discontinued.

Isolated cases of moderate and transient elevations of liver transaminases have been observed at the start of treatment. Isolated cases of clinical hepatitis have been reported which resolved with cessation of therapy.

Dizziness, pruritis, nervousness, paraesthesia, articular/muscular pain, photo sensitisation, hypotension, gingival hyperplasia, and gynaecomastia, have also been observed.

4.9 Overdose

The clinical consequences of overdose can be severe hypotension leading to collapse, and sinus bradycardia which may be accompanied by isorhythmic dissociation and atrioventricular conduction disturbances. Observation in a coronary care unit is advisable. Vasopressors such as adrenaline may be indicated in patients exhibiting profound hypotension. Calcium gluconate may help reverse the effects of calcium entry blockade. Atropine administration and temporary cardiac pacing may be required to manage bradycardia and/or conduction disturbances.

Glucagon can be used in cases of established hypoglycaemia.

Diltiazem and its metabolites are very poorly dialysable.

5. PHARMACOLOGICAL PROPERTIES

5.1 Pharmacodynamic properties

Diltiazem is classified as a calcium channel blocker, benziothiazepine derivative, C08DB01, under the ATC classification. It selectively reduces calcium entry through voltage-dependent calcium-n channels into vascular smooth muscle cells and myocardial cells. This lowers the concentration of intracellular calcium which is available to activate contractile proteins. This action of diltiazem results in dilation of coronary arteries causing an increase in myocardial oxygen supply. It reduces cardiac work by moderating the heart rate and by reducing systemic vascular resistance thus reducing oxygen demand. Diltiazem also prolongs AV conduction and has mild effects on contractility. Clinical data on morbidity and mortality are not available.

5.2 Pharmacokinetic properties

Multiple dose pharmacokinetic studies have shown that the kinetics of VIAZEM XL are non-linear within the 120mg-360mg dosage range. Diltiazem is well absorbed, but has a highly saturable first pass effect leading to a variable absolute bioavailability, which is on average 35%. The saturable first pass effect results in higher than expected systemic exposure with increasing doses.

The protein binding is 80 to 85% and the volume of distribution is 5.0 l/kg.

Diltiazem is metabolised by CYP3A4 in the liver and 70% of the dose is excreted in urine, mainly as metabolites. The plasma levels of the two main metabolites, N-monodesmethyldiltiazem and desacetyldiltiazem, represent 35% and 15% of diltiazem levels respectively. The metabolites contribute around 50% of the clinical effect. Plasma clearance of diltiazem is approximately 0.5 l/h/kg. Plasma half-life of diltiazem is approximately 5-7 hours.

VIAZEM XL capsules allow a prolonged absorption of diltiazem and maximum levels are reached within 6 to 12 hours. Concomitant food intake with VIAZEM XL does not influence the pharmacokinetics of diltiazem. For most patients, chronic administration of VIAZEM XL 300mg once daily, results in therapeutic diltiazem levels (50-200ng/ml) over 24 hours. However, the inter-individual variability is high and individual dose adjustment based on therapeutic response is therefore necessary.

5.3 Preclinical safety data

Tests on reproductive functions in animals show that diltiazem decreases fertility in rats and that it is teratogenic in mice, rats and rabbits. Exposure during late pregnancy induces dystocia and a decrease in the number of live newborns in rats.

Detailed mutagenicity and carcinogenicity tests performed negative.

6. PHARMACEUTICAL PARTICULARS

6.1 List of excipients

- Sucrose Stearate
- Microcrystalline cellulose
- Povidone
- Magnesium Stearate
- Talc
- Titanium dioxide
- Hypromellose
- Polysorbate 80
- Polyacrylate dispersion 30% (dry)
- Simethicone emulsion
- Gelatine capsule

Gelatin capsule colours

	Capsule body	Capsule cap
120 mg	Lavender opaque[1]	Lavender opaque[1]

1 = Colour is composed of Azorubine E122, Indigotine E132, Titanium Dioxide E171

Gelatin capsule markings:

	Capsule body	Capsule cap
120 mg (Capsule Size 3)	Viazem XL 120 (white ink EEC approved)	Viazem XL 120 (white ink EEC approved)

White printing ink contains:

Shellac, Ethyl Alcohol, Isopropyl Alcohol, n-Butyl, Propylene Glycol, Sodium Hydroxide, Polyvinylpyrrolidone, Titanium Dioxide

6.2 Incompatibilities

Not applicable.

6.3 Shelf life

3 years

6.4 Special precautions for storage

Do not store above 25°C. Store in original package in a dry place away from any heat source, e.g. direct sunlight, heaters, steam, etc.

6.5 Nature and contents of container

The capsules are packed in PVC/aluminium blisters. Pack sizes are 28 capsules per blister.

6.6 Special precautions for disposal and other handling

Swallow capsules whole, with a glass of water do not chew.

7. MARKETING AUTHORISATION HOLDER
Stada Arzneimittel AG
Stadastrasse 2-18
61118 Bad Vilbel, Germany

8. MARKETING AUTHORISATION NUMBER(S)
PL 11204/0090

9. DATE OF FIRST AUTHORISATION/RENEWAL OF THE AUTHORISATION
2nd April 1997

10. DATE OF REVISION OF THE TEXT
7 August 2008

Viazem XL 180mg

(Genus Pharmaceuticals)

1. NAME OF THE MEDICINAL PRODUCT
VIAZEM XL

2. QUALITATIVE AND QUANTITATIVE COMPOSITION
Diltiazem hydrochloride: 180 mg capsule.

For excipients, see section 6.1

3. PHARMACEUTICAL FORM
Prolonged release capsule, hard.

White and blue-green opaque capsules. Each capsule is printed on the cap and body, in black ink, with Viazem XL 180.

4. CLINICAL PARTICULARS

4.1 Therapeutic indications
VIAZEM XL is indicated for the management of stable angina pectoris and the treatment of mild to moderate hypertension.

4.2 Posology and method of administration
Dosage requirements may differ between patients with angina and patients with hypertension. In addition individual patients response may vary, necessitating careful titration. The range of strengths facilitates titration to the optimal dose.

One capsule of VIAZEM XL is to be taken before or during a meal. The dose should be taken at approximately the same time each day.

The capsule should not be chewed but swallowed whole, with a glass of water.

Due to the variability of release profile in individual patients, when changing from one type of sustained release diltiazem preparation to another, it may be necessary to adjust the dose.

Adults:

Hypertension: The usual starting dose is 180 mg once daily. The dose may be increased after 2-4 weeks according to the patient's response and the usual maintenance dose is 240mg-360mg once daily. The maximum daily dose is 360 mg. However, the single daily doses of 300 mg and 360 mg should only be administered to patients when no satisfactory therapeutic effect has been effected with lower doses and after the benefit risk-ratio has been carefully assessed by the doctor.

Angina: Care should be taken when titrating patients with stable angina in order to establish the optimal dose. The usual starting dose is 180 mg once daily. The dose may be increased after 2-4 weeks according to the patient's response. The maximum daily dose is 360 mg. However, the single daily doses of 300 mg and 360 mg should only be administered to patients when no satisfactory therapeutic effect has been effected with lower doses and after the benefit risk-ratio has been carefully assessed by the doctor.

Elderly and patients with impaired hepatic or renal function:
Plasma levels of diltiazem can be increased in the elderly, and in patients with impaired hepatic renal or hepatic function. In these cases, the starting dose should be one 120mg VIAZEM XL capsule once daily. Heart rate should be monitored and if it falls below 50 beats per minute, the dose should not be increased. Dose adjustment may be required to obtain a satisfactory clinical response.

Children:
Safety and efficacy in children have not been established.

4.3 Contraindications
Diltiazem depresses atrioventricular node conduction and is therefore contraindicated in patients with severe bradycardia (less than 50 bpm), sick sinus syndrome, congestive heart failure, and left ventricular failure with second or third degree AV or sino-atrial block, except in the presence of a functioning pacemaker. Diltiazem is also contraindicated in left ventricular failure with pulmonary stasis as diltiazem may have mild negative effects on contractility.

Diltiazem is contraindicated in acute complicated myocardial infarction (e.g. bradycardia hypotension, congestive heart failure/reduced LV function), pulmonary congestion, hypotension (<90 mmHg systolic) cerebrovascular accident, cardiac shock and unstable angina pectoris.

Diltiazem is contraindicated in pre-excitation syndrome (e.g. WPW) accompanied with atrial flutter, fibrillation and in digitalis intoxication, as diltiazem may precipitate ventricular tachycardia.

Diltiazem should not be used in patients with known hypersensitivity to diltiazem.

Diltiazem should not be used during pregnancy, by women of child-bearing potential, or by women who are breast-feeding.

4.4 Special warnings and precautions for use
Patients treated with beta-adrenoreceptor blocking drugs and patients with conduction disturbances (bradycardia, bundle branch block, first degree AV block, prolonged PR interval) should only be treated with VIAZEM XL after special consideration due to the risk of serious bradyarrhythmias.

This product should be used with caution in patients with hepatic dysfunction. Abnormalities of liver function may appear during therapy. The higher single daily doses of VIAZEM XL capsules 300mg and 360mg should not be administered to patients with impaired renal and/or hepatic function and to elderly patients (prolonged half life of elimination) because there is no experience on the use of such high dosages in these patient categories.

In patients undergoing long-term therapy with cyclosporin, plasma levels of cyclosporin should be monitored when concurrent administration of diltiazem is initiated, or discontinued or if the dose of diltiazem is changed.

Abnormally short transit time through the gastrointestinal tract could lead to incomplete release of contents of the capsule e.g. in chronic conditions with associated diarrhoea such as Crohns disease or ulcerative colitis.

4.5 Interaction with other medicinal products and other forms of interaction
Combinations contraindicated as a safety measure:

In animals, fatal ventricular fibrillations are constantly seen during administration of verapamil and dantrolene via the i.v. route. The combination of a calcium antagonist and dantrolene is therefore potentially dangerous. The concurrent iv administration of beta-adrenergic blocking agents with diltiazem should be avoided because an additive effect on SA and AV conduction and ventricular function will occur. The use of such a combination requires ECG monitoring especially at the beginning of treatment.

Combinations requiring safety precautions:

In common with other calcium antagonists, when diltiazem is used with drugs which may induce bradycardia or with antiarrhythmic drugs (e.g. amiodarone) or other antihypertensive drugs, the possibility of an additive effect should be borne in mind. Inhalation anaesthetics should be used with caution during diltiazem therapy. Tri/tetracyclic antidepressants and neuroleptics may increase the antihypertensive effects of diltiazem whilst the concomitant use of lithium with diltiazem may lead to neurotoxicity (extrapyramidal effects). Rifampin and other hepatic enzyme inducers may reduce the bioavailability of diltiazem and high doses of Vitamin D and/or high intake of calcium salts leading to elevated serum calcium levels may reduce the response to diltiazem.

Diltiazem is metabolised by CYP3A4 and could, by competitive inhibition of CYP3A4, affect the pharmacokinetics of other drugs metabolised by this enzyme. In addition inhibitors and inducers of CYP3A4 may affect the pharmacokinetics of diltiazem.

Diltiazem prolongs the sedative effect of medazolam and triazolam via metabolic interaction and decreases nifedipine clearance by 50%. Diltiazem may cause increases in the levels of digitoxin. Diltiazem has been shown to increase the bioavailability of imipramine by 30% probably due to inhibition of its first pass metabolism.

Diltiazem has been used safely in combination with diuretics, ACE-inhibitors and other anti-hypertensive agents. It is recommended that patients receiving these combinations should be regularly monitored. Concomitant use of diltiazem with alpha-blockers such as prazosin should be strictly monitored because of the possible synergistic hypotensive effect of the combination.

Case reports have suggested that blood levels of carbamazepine, cyclosporin, theophylline and phenytoin may be increased when given concurrently with diltiazem. Care should be exercised in patients taking these drugs. In common with other calcium antagonists diltiazem may cause small increases in plasma levels of digoxin. In patients taking H_2-antagonists concurrently with diltiazem there may be increased levels of diltiazem.

Magnification of the hypotensive and lipothymic effects (summation of vasodilator properties) of nitrate derivatives can occur. In patients on calcium inhibitors, prescriptions of nitrate derivatives should be made at progressively increasing doses. Diltiazem treatment has been continued without problem during anaesthesia, but diltiazem may potentiate the activity of curare-like and depolarising neuromuscular blocking agents, therefore the anaesthetist should be informed that the patient is receiving a calcium antagonist.

4.6 Pregnancy and lactation
Pregnancy:

Diltiazem should not be taken during pregnancy. Women of child bearing-potential should exclude the possibility of pregnancy before commencing treatment by taking suitable contraceptive measures if necessary. In animal tests, Diltiazem was found to have a tetratogenic effects in some species of animal.

Diltiazem may suppress the contractility of the uterus. Definite evidence that this will prolong partus in full-term pregnancy is lacking. A risk of hypoxia in the foetus may arise in the event of hypotension in the mother and reduced perfusion of the uterus due to redistribution of blood flow due to peripheral vasodilatation. In animal experiments diltiazem has exhibited teratogenic effects in some animal species. In the absence of adequate evidence of safety in human pregnancy, VIAZEM XL should not be used in pregnancy or in women of childbearing potential.

Lactation:

Diltiazem is excreted in breast milk in concentrations similar to those in serum. If the use of diltiazem is considered essential, an alternative method of infant feeding should be instituted.

4.7 Effects on ability to drive and use machines
There are no studies on the effect of diltiazem when driving vehicles or operating machines. It should be taken into account that occasionally asthenia/fatigue and dizziness may occur. Treatment of hypertension with this medicinal product requires regular monitoring. Individual different reactions may affect the ability to drive. This risk should be considered especially at the beginning of treatment, when changing the drug, or in combination with alcohol.

4.8 Undesirable effects
Certain undesirable effects may lead to suspension of treatment: sinus bradycardia, sino-atrial heart block, 2nd and 3rd degree atrioventricular heart block, skin rash, oedema of the lower limbs.

In hypertensive patients, adverse effects are generally mild and transient and are most commonly vasodilatory related events.

The following have been described in decreasing order of frequency: lower limb oedema, headache, hot flushes/flushing, asthenia/fatigue, palpitations, malaise, minor gastro-intestinal disorders (dyspepsia, abdominal pain, dry mouth, nausea, vomiting, diarrhoea, constipation) and skin rash. Erythema multiform and Stevens Johnson syndrome have been reported infrequently in patients receiving diltiazem hydrochloride. Vasodilatory related events (in particular, oedema) are dose-dependent and appear to be more frequent in elderly subjects.

Rare cases of symptomatic bradycardia and exceptionally sino-atrial block and atrioventricular block, hypotension, syncope, reduced left ventricular function have also been recorded. Isolated cases of hallucinations, depression, insomnia, hyperglycaemia and impotence have been reported.

Experience with use in other indications and with other formulations has shown that skin rashes are usually localised and are limited to cases of erythemia, urticaria or occasionally desquamative erthema, with or without fever, which regress when treatment is discontinued.

Isolated cases of moderate and transient elevations of liver transaminases have been observed at the start of treatment. Isolated cases of clinical hepatitis have been reported which resolved with cessation of therapy.

Dizziness, pruritis, nervousness, paraesthesia, articular/muscular pain, photo sensitisation, hypotension, gingival hyperplasia, and gynaecomastia, have also been observed.

4.9 Overdose
The clinical consequences of overdose can be severe hypotension leading to collapse, and sinus bradycardia which may be accompanied by isorhythmic dissociation and atrioventricular conduction disturbances. Observation in a coronary care unit is advisable. Vasopressors such as adrenaline may be indicated in patients exhibiting profound hypotension. Calcium gluconate may help reverse the effects of calcium entry blockade. Atropine administration and temporary cardiac pacing may be required to manage bradycardia and/or conduction disturbances.

Glucagon can be used in cases of established hypoglycaemia.

Diltiazem and its metabolites are very poorly dialysable.

5. PHARMACOLOGICAL PROPERTIES

5.1 Pharmacodynamic properties
Diltiazem is classified as a calcium channel blocker, benziothiazepine derivative, C08DB01, under the ATC classification. It selectively reduces calcium entry through voltage-dependent calcium-n channels into vascular smooth muscle cells and myocardial cells. This lowers the concentration of intracellular calcium which is available to activate contractile proteins. This action of diltiazem results in dilation of coronary arteries causing an increase in myocardial oxygen supply. It reduces cardiac work by moderating the heart rate and by reducing systemic vascularly resistance thus reducing oxygen demand. Diltiazem also prolongs AV conduction and has mild effects on contractility. Clinical data on morbidity and mortality are not available.

5.2 Pharmacokinetic properties
Multiple dose pharmacokinetic studies have shown that the kinetics of VIAZEM XL are non-linear within the 120mg-360mg dosage range. Diltiazem is well absorbed, but has a

highly saturable first pass effect leading to a variable absolute bioavailability, which is on average 35%. The saturable first pass effect results in higher than expected systemic exposure with increasing doses.

The protein binding is 80 to 85% and the volume of distribution is 5.0 l/kg.

Diltiazem is metabolised by CYP3A4 in the liver and 70% of the dose is excreted in urine, mainly as metabolites. The plasma levels of the two main metabolites, N-monodesmethyldiltiazem and desacetyldiltiazem, represent 35% and 15% of diltiazem levels respectively. The metabolites contribute around 50% of the clinical effect. Plasma clearance of diltiazem is approximately 0.5 l/h/kg. Plasma half-life of diltiazem is approximately 5-7 hours.

VIAZEM XL capsules allow a prolonged absorption of diltiazem and maximum levels are reached within 6 to 12 hours. Concomitant food intake with VIAZEM XL does not influence the pharmacokinetics of diltiazem. For most patients, chronic administration of VIAZEM XL 300mg once daily, results in therapeutic diltiazem levels (50-200ng/ml) over 24 hours. However, the inter-individual variability is high and individual dose adjustment based on therapeutic response is therefore necessary.

5.3 Preclinical safety data

Tests on reproductive functions in animals show that diltiazem decreases fertility in rats and that it is teratogenic in mice, rats and rabbits. Exposure during late pregnancy induces dystocia and a decrease in the number of live newborns in rats.

Detailed mutagenicity and carcinogenicity tests proved negative.

6. PHARMACEUTICAL PARTICULARS

6.1 List of excipients

- Sucrose Stearate
- Microcrystalline cellulose
- Povidone
- Magnesium Stearate
- Talc
- Titanium dioxide
- Hypromellose
- Polysorbate 80
- Polyacrylate dispersion 30% (dry)
- Simethicone emulsion
- Gelatine capsule

Gelatin capsule colours

	Capsule body	Capsule cap
180 mg	White opaque[1]	Blue Green opaque[2]

1 = Colour is composed of Titanium Dioxide E171

2 = Colour is composed of Quinoline Yellow E104, Indigotine E132, Titanium Dioxide E171

Gelatin capsule markings:

	Capsule body	Capsule cap
180 mg (Capsule Size 2)	Viazem XL 180 (black ink EEC approved)	Viazem XL 180 (black ink EEC approved)

Black printing ink contains:

Shellac, Ethyl Alcohol, Isopropyl Alcohol, n-Butyl, Propylene Glycol, Water (Purified) Ammonium Hydroxide, Potassium Hydroxide, Black Iron Oxide

6.2 Incompatibilities

Not applicable.

6.3 Shelf life

3 years

6.4 Special precautions for storage

Do not store above 25°C. Store in original package in a dry place away from any heat source, e.g. direct sunlight, heaters, steam, etc.

6.5 Nature and contents of container

The capsules are packed in PVC/aluminium blisters. Pack sizes are 28 capsules per blister.

6.6 Special precautions for disposal and other handling

Swallow capsules whole, with a glass of water do not chew.

7. MARKETING AUTHORISATION HOLDER

Stada Arzneimittel AG

Stadastrasse 2-18

61118 Bad Vilbel, Germany

8. MARKETING AUTHORISATION NUMBER(S)

PL 11201/0091

9. DATE OF FIRST AUTHORISATION/RENEWAL OF THE AUTHORISATION

2nd April 1997

10. DATE OF REVISION OF THE TEXT

7 September 2008

Viazem XL 240mg

(Genus Pharmaceuticals)

1. NAME OF THE MEDICINAL PRODUCT

VIAZEM XL

2. QUALITATIVE AND QUANTITATIVE COMPOSITION

Diltiazem hydrochloride: 240 mg capsule.

For excipients, see section 6.1

3. PHARMACEUTICAL FORM

Prolonged release capsule, hard.

Blue-green and lavender opaque colourless. Each capsule is printed on the cap and body, in white ink, with Viazem XL 240.

4. CLINICAL PARTICULARS

4.1 Therapeutic indications

VIAZEM XL is indicated for the management of stable angina pectoris and the treatment of mild to moderate hypertension.

4.2 Posology and method of administration

Dosage requirements may differ between patients with angina and patients with hypertension. In addition individual patients response may vary, necessitating careful titration. The range of strengths facilitates titration to the optimal dose.

One capsule of VIAZEM XL is to be taken before or during a meal. The dose should be taken at approximately the same time each day.

The capsule should not be chewed but swallowed whole, with a glass of water.

Due to the variability of release profile in individual patients, when changing from one type of sustained release diltiazem preparation to another, it may be necessary to adjust the dose.

Adults:

Hypertension: The usual starting dose is 180 mg once daily. The dose may be increased after 2-4 weeks according to the patient's response and the usual maintenance dose is 240mg-360mg once daily. The maximum daily dose is 360 mg. However, the single daily doses of 300 mg and 360 mg should only be administered to patients when no satisfactory therapeutic effect has been effected with lower doses and after the benefit risk-ratio has been carefully assessed by the doctor.

Angina: Care should be taken when titrating patients with stable angina in order to establish the optimal dose. The usual starting dose is 180 mg once daily. The dose may be increased after 2-4 weeks according to the patient's response. The maximum daily dose is 360 mg. However, the single daily doses of 300 mg and 360 mg should only be administered to patients when no satisfactory therapeutic effect has been effected with lower doses and after the benefit risk-ratio has been carefully assessed by the doctor.

Elderly and patients with impaired hepatic or renal function:

Plasma levels of diltiazem can be increased in the elderly, and in patients with impaired hepatic renal or hepatic function. In these cases, the starting dose should be one 120mg VIAZEM XL capsule once daily. Heart rate should be monitored and if it falls below 50 beats per minute, the dose should not be increased. Dose adjustment may be required to obtain a satisfactory clinical response.

Children:

Safety and efficacy in children have not been established.

4.3 Contraindications

Diltiazem depresses atrioventricular node conduction and is therefore contraindicated in patients with severe bradycardia (less than 50 bpm), sick sinus syndrome, congestive heart failure, and left ventricular failure with second or third degree AV or sino-atrial block, except in the presence of a functioning pacemaker. Diltiazem is also contraindicated in left ventricular failure with pulmonary stasis as diltiazem may have mild negative effects on contractility.

Diltiazem is contraindicated in acute complicated myocardial infarction (e.g. bradycardia hypotension, congestive heart failure/reduced LV function), pulmonary congestion, hypotension (<90 mmHg systolic) cerebrovascular accident, cardiac shock and unstable angina pectoris.

Diltiazem is contraindicated in pre-excitation syndrome (e.g. WPW) accompanied with atrial flutter, fibrillation and in digitalis intoxication, as diltiazem may precipitate ventricular tachycardia.

Diltiazem should not be used in patients with known hypersensitivity to diltiazem.

Diltiazem should not be used during pregnancy, by women of child-bearing potential, or by women who are breast-feeding.

4.4 Special warnings and precautions for use

Patients treated with beta-adrenoreceptor blocking drugs and patients with conduction disturbances (bradycardia, bundle branch block, first degree AV block, prolonged PR interval) should only be treated with VIAZEM XL after special consideration due to the risk of serious bradyarrhythmias.

This product should be used with caution in patients with hepatic dysfunction. Abnormalities of liver function may appear during therapy. The higher single daily doses of VIAZEM XL capsules 300mg and 360mg should not be administered to patients with impaired renal and/or hepatic function and to elderly patients (prolonged half life of elimination) because there is no experience on the use of such high dosages in these patient categories.

In patients undergoing long-term therapy with cyclosporin, plasma levels of cyclosporin should be monitored when concurrent administration of diltiazem is initiated, or discontinued or if the dose of diltiazem is changed.

Abnormally short transit time through the gastrointestinal tract could lead to incomplete release of contents of the capsule e.g. in chronic conditions with associated diarrhoea such as Crohns disease or ulcerative colitis.

4.5 Interaction with other medicinal products and other forms of interaction

Combinations contraindicated as a safety measure:

In animals, fatal ventricular fibrillations are constantly seen during administration of verapamil and dantrolene via the i.v. route. The combination of a calcium antagonist and dantrolene is therefore potentially dangerous. The concurrent iv administration of beta-adrenergic blocking agents with diltiazem should be avoided because an additive effect on SA and AV conduction and ventricular function will occur. The use of such a combination requires ECG monitoring especially at the beginning of treatment.

Combinations requiring safety precautions:

In common with other calcium antagonists, when diltiazem is used with drugs which may induce bradycardia or with antiarrhythmic drugs (e.g. amiodarone) or other antihypertensive drugs, the possibility of an additive effect should be borne in mind. Inhalation anaesthetics should be used with caution during diltiazem therapy. Tri/tetracyclic antidepressants and neuroleptics may increase the antihypertensive effects of diltiazem whilst the concomitant use of lithium with diltiazem may lead to neurotoxicity (extrapyramidal effects). Rifampin and other hepatic enzyme inducers may reduce the bioavailability of diltiazem and high doses of Vitamin D and/or high intake of calcium salts leading to elevated serum calcium levels may reduce the response to diltiazem.

Diltiazem is metabolised by CYP3A4 and could, by competitive inhibition of CYP3A4, affect the pharmacokinetics of other drugs metabolised by this enzyme. In addition inhibitors and inducers of CYP3A4 may affect the pharmacokinetics of diltiazem.

Diltiazem prolongs the sedative effect of medazolam and triazolam via metabolic interaction and decreases nifedipine clearance by 50%. Diltiazem may cause increases in the levels of digitoxin. Diltiazem has been shown to increase the bioavailability of imipramine by 30% probably due to inhibition of its first pass metabolism.

Diltiazem has been used safely in combination with diuretics, ACE-inhibitors and other anti-hypertensive agents. It is recommended that patients receiving these combinations should be regularly monitored. Concomitant use of diltiazem with alpha-blockers such as prazosin should be strictly monitored because of the possible synergistic hypotensive effect of the combination.

Case reports have suggested that blood levels of carbamazepine, cyclosporin, theophylline and phenytoin may be increased when given concurrently with diltiazem. Care should be exercised in patients taking these drugs. In common with other calcium antagonists diltiazem may cause small increases in plasma levels of digoxin. In patients taking H_2-antagonists concurrently with diltiazem there may be increased levels of diltiazem.

Magnification of the hypotensive and lipothymic effects (summation of vasodilator properties) of nitrate derivatives can occur. In patients on calcium inhibitors, prescriptions of nitrate derivatives should be made at progressively increasing doses. Diltiazem treatment has been continued without problem during anaesthesia, but diltiazem may potentiate the activity of curare-like and depolarising neuromuscular blocking agents, therefore the anaesthetist should be informed that the patient is receiving a calcium antagonist.

4.6 Pregnancy and lactation

Pregnancy:

Diltiazem should not be taken during pregnancy. Women of child bearing-potential should exclude the possibility of pregnancy before commencing treatment by taking suitable contraceptive measures if necessary. In animal tests, Diltiazem was found to have a tetratogenic effects in some species of animal.

Diltiazem may suppress the contractility of the uterus. Definite evidence that this will prolong partus in full-term pregnancy is lacking. A risk of hypoxia in the foetus may arise in the event of hypotension in the mother and reduced perfusion of the uterus due to redistribution of blood flow due to peripheral vasodilatation. In animal experiments diltiazem has exhibited teratogenic effects in some animal species. In the absence of adequate evidence of safety in human pregnancy, VIAZEM XL should not be used in pregnancy or in women of childbearing potential.

Lactation:

Diltiazem is excreted in breast milk in concentrations similar to those in serum. If the use of diltiazem is considered essential, an alternative method of infant feeding should be instituted.

4.7 Effects on ability to drive and use machines

There are no studies on the effect of diltiazem when driving vehicles or operating machines. It should be taken into account that occasionally asthenia/fatigue and dizziness may occur. Treatment of hypertension with this medicinal product requires regular monitoring. Individual different reactions may affect the ability to drive. This risk should be considered especially at the beginning of treatment, when changing the drug, or in combination with alcohol.

4.8 Undesirable effects

Certain undesirable effects may lead to suspension of treatment: sinus bradycardia, sino-atrial heart block, 2nd and 3rd degree atrioventricular heart block, skin rash, oedema of the lower limbs.

In hypertensive patients, adverse effects are generally mild and transient and are most commonly vasodilatory related events.

The following have been described in decreasing order of frequency: lower limb oedema, headache, hot flushes/flushing, asthenia/fatigue, palpitations, malaise, minor gastro-intestinal disorders (dyspepsia, abdominal pain, dry mouth, nausea, vomiting, diarrhoea, constipation) and skin rash. Erythema multiform and Stevens Johnson syndrome have been reported infrequently in patients receiving diltiazem hydrochloride. Vasodilatory related events (in particular, oedema) are dose-dependent and appear to be more frequent in elderly subjects.

Rare cases of symptomatic bradycardia and exceptionally sino-atrial block and atrioventricular block, hypotension, syncope, reduced left ventricular function have also been recorded. Isolated cases of hallucinations, depression, insomnia, hyperglycaemia and impotence have been reported.

Experience with use in other indications and with other formulations has shown that skin rashes are usually localised and are limited to cases of erythemia, urticaria or occasionally desquamative erthema, with or without fever, which regress when treatment is discontinued.

Isolated cases of moderate and transient elevations of liver transaminases have been observed at the start of treatment. Isolated cases of clinical hepatitis have been reported which resolved with cessation of therapy.

Dizziness, pruritis, nervousness, paraesthesia, articular/muscular pain, photo sensitisation, hypotension, gingival hyperplasia, and gynaecomastia, have also been observed.

4.9 Overdose

The clinical consequences of overdose can be severe hypotension leading to collapse, and sinus bradycardia which may be accompanied by isorhythmic dissociation and atrioventricular conduction disturbances. Observation in a coronary care unit is advisable. Vasopressors such as adrenaline may be indicated in patients exhibiting profound hypotension. Calcium gluconate may help reverse the effects of calcium entry blockade. Atropine administration and temporary cardiac pacing may be required to manage bradycardia and/or conduction disturbances.

Glucagon can be used in cases of established hypoglycaemia.

Diltiazem and its metabolites are very poorly dialysable.

5. PHARMACOLOGICAL PROPERTIES

5.1 Pharmacodynamic properties

Diltiazem is classified as a calcium channel blocker, benziothiazepine derivative, C08DB01, under the ATC classification. It selectively reduces calcium entry through voltage-dependent calcium-n channels into vascular smooth muscle cells and myocardial cells. This lowers the concentration of intracellular calcium which is available to activate contractile proteins. This action of diltiazem results in dilation of coronary arteries causing an increase in myocardial oxygen supply. It reduces cardiac work by moderating the heart rate and by reducing systemic vascular resistance thus reducing oxygen demand. Diltiazem also prolongs AV conduction and has mild effects on contractility. Clinical data on morbidity and mortality are not available.

5.2 Pharmacokinetic properties

Multiple dose pharmacokinetic studies have shown that the kinetics of VIAZEM XL are non-linear within the 120mg-360mg dosage range. Diltiazem is well absorbed, but has a highly saturable first pass effect leading to a variable absolute bioavailability, which is on average 35%. The saturable first pass effect results in higher than expected systemic exposure with increasing doses.

The protein binding is 80 to 85% and the volume of distribution is 5.0 l/kg.

Diltiazem is metabolised by CYP3A4 in the liver and 70% of the dose is excreted in urine, mainly as metabolites. The plasma levels of the two main metabolites, N-monodesmethyldiltiazem and desacetyldiltiazem, represent 35% and 15% of diltiazem levels respectively. The metabolites contribute around 50% of the clinical effect. Plasma clearance of diltiazem is approximately 0.5 l/h/kg. Plasma half-life of diltiazem is approximately 5-7 hours.

VIAZEM XL capsules allow a prolonged absorption of diltiazem and maximum levels are reached within 6 to 12 hours. Concomitant food intake with VIAZEM XL does not influence the pharmacokinetics of diltiazem. For most patients, chronic administration of VIAZEM XL 300mg once daily, results in therapeutic diltiazem levels (50-200ng/ml) over 24 hours. However, the inter-individual variability is high and individual dose adjustment based on therapeutic response is therefore necessary.

5.3 Preclinical safety data

Tests on reproductive functions in animals show that diltiazem decreases fertility in rats and that it is teratogenic in mice, rats and rabbits. Exposure during late pregnancy induces dystocia and a decrease in the number of live newborns in rats.

Detailed mutagenicity and carcinogenicity tests proved negative.

6. PHARMACEUTICAL PARTICULARS

6.1 List of excipients

- Sucrose Stearate
- Microcrystalline cellulose
- Povidone
- Magnesium Stearate
- Talc
- Titanium dioxide
- Hypromellose
- Polysorbate 80
- Polyacrylate dispersion 30% (dry)
- Simethicone emulsion
- Gelatine capsule

Gelatin capsule colours

	Capsule body	Capsule cap
240 mg	Blue Green opaque[1]	Lavender opaque[2]

1 = Colour is composed of Quinoline Yellow E104, Indigotine E132, Titanium Dioxide E171

2 = Colour is composed of Azorubine E122, Indigotine E132, Titanium Dioxide E171

Gelatin capsule markings:

	Capsule body	Capsule cap
240 mg	Viazem XL 240	Viazem XL 240
(Capsule Size 1)	(White ink EEC approved)	(White ink EEC approved)

White printing ink contains:

Shellac, Ethyl Alcohol, Isopropyl Alcohol, n-Butyl, Propylene Glycol, Sodium Hydroxide, Polyvinylpyrrolidone, Titanium Dioxide

6.2 Incompatibilities

Not applicable.

6.3 Shelf life

3 years

6.4 Special precautions for storage

Do not store above 25°C. Store in original package in a dry place away from any heat source, e.g. direct sunlight, heaters, steam, etc.

6.5 Nature and contents of container

The capsules are packed in PVC/aluminium blisters. Pack sizes are 28 capsules per blister.

6.6 Special precautions for disposal and other handling

Swallow capsules whole, with a glass of water do not chew.

7. MARKETING AUTHORISATION HOLDER

Stada Arzneimittel AG

Stadastrasse 2-18

61118 Bad Vilbel, Germany

8. MARKETING AUTHORISATION NUMBER(S)

PL 11204/0092

9. DATE OF FIRST AUTHORISATION/RENEWAL OF THE AUTHORISATION

2nd April 1997

10. DATE OF REVISION OF THE TEXT

07 September 2008

Viazem XL 300mg

(Genus Pharmaceuticals)

1. NAME OF THE MEDICINAL PRODUCT

VIAZEM XL

2. QUALITATIVE AND QUANTITATIVE COMPOSITION

Diltiazem hydrochloride: 300 mg capsule.

For excipients, see section 6.1

3. PHARMACEUTICAL FORM

Prolonged release capsule, hard.

White and lavender opaque capsules. Each capsule is printed on the cap and body, in black ink, with Viazem XL 300.

4. CLINICAL PARTICULARS

4.1 Therapeutic indications

VIAZEM XL is indicated for the management of stable angina pectoris and the treatment of mild to moderate hypertension.

4.2 Posology and method of administration

Dosage requirements may differ between patients with angina and patients with hypertension. In addition individual patients response may vary, necessitating careful titration. The range of strengths facilitates titration to the optimal dose.

One capsule of VIAZEM XL is to be taken before or during a meal. The dose should be taken at approximately the same time each day.

The capsule should not be chewed but swallowed whole, with a glass of water.

Due to the variability of release profile in individual patients, when changing from one type of sustained release diltiazem preparation to another, it may be necessary to adjust the dose.

Adults:

Hypertension: The usual starting dose is 180 mg once daily. The dose may be increased after 2-4 weeks according to the patient's response and the usual maintenance dose is 240mg-360mg once daily. The maximum daily dose is 360 mg. However, the single daily doses of 300 mg and 360 mg should only be administered to patients when no satisfactory therapeutic effect has been effected with lower doses and after the benefit risk-ratio has been carefully assessed by the doctor.

Angina: Care should be taken when titrating patients with stable angina in order to establish the optimal dose. The usual starting dose is 180 mg once daily. The dose may be increased after 2-4 weeks according to the patient's response. The maximum daily dose is 360 mg. However, the single daily doses of 300 mg and 360 mg should only be administered to patients when no satisfactory therapeutic effect has been effected with lower doses and after the benefit risk-ratio has been carefully assessed by the doctor.

Elderly and patients with impaired hepatic or renal function:

Plasma levels of diltiazem can be increased in the elderly, and in patients with impaired hepatic renal or hepatic function. In these cases, the starting dose should be one 120mg VIAZEM XL capsule once daily. Heart rate should be monitored and if it falls below 50 beats per minute, the dose should not be increased. Dose adjustment may be required to obtain a satisfactory clinical response.

Children:

Safety and efficacy in children have not been established.

4.3 Contraindications

Diltiazem depresses atrioventricular node conduction and is therefore contraindicated in patients with severe bradycardia (less than 50 bpm), sick sinus syndrome, congestive heart failure, and left ventricular failure with second or third degree AV or sino-atrial block, except in the presence of a functioning pacemaker. Diltiazem is also contraindicated in left ventricular failure with pulmonary stasis as diltiazem may have mild negative effects on contractility.

Diltiazem is contraindicated in acute complicated myocardial infarction (e.g. bradycardia hypotension, congestive heart failure/reduced LV function), pulmonary congestion, hypotension (<90 mmHg systolic) cerebrovascular accident, cardiac shock and unstable angina pectoris.

Diltiazem is contraindicated in pre-excitation syndrome (e.g. WPW) accompanied with atrial flutter, fibrillation and in digitalis intoxication, as diltiazem may precipitate ventricular tachycardia.

Diltiazem should not be used in patients with known hypersensitivity to diltiazem.

Diltiazem should not be used during pregnancy, by women of child-bearing potential, or by women who are breast-feeding.

4.4 Special warnings and precautions for use

Patients treated with beta-adrenoreceptor blocking drugs and patients with conduction disturbances (bradycardia, bundle branch block, first degree AV block, prolonged PR interval) should only be treated with VIAZEM XL after special consideration due to the risk of serious bradyarrhythmias.

This product should be used with caution in patients with hepatic dysfunction. Abnormalities of liver function may appear during therapy. The higher single daily doses of VIAZEM XL capsules 300mg and 360mg should not be administered to patients with impaired renal and/or hepatic function and to elderly patients (prolonged half life of elimination) because there is no experience on the use of such high dosages in these patient categories.

In patients undergoing long-term therapy with cyclosporin, plasma levels of cyclosporin should be monitored when concurrent administration of diltiazem is initiated, or discontinued or if the dose of diltiazem is changed.

Abnormally short transit time through the gastrointestinal tract could lead to incomplete release of contents of the capsule e.g. in chronic conditions with associated diarrhoea such as Crohns disease or ulcerative colitis.

4.5 Interaction with other medicinal products and other forms of interaction

Combinations contraindicated as a safety measure:

In animals, fatal ventricular fibrillations are constantly seen during administration of verapamil and dantrolene via the i.v. route. The combination of a calcium antagonist and dantrolene is therefore potentially dangerous. The concurrent iv administration of beta-adrenergic blocking agents with diltiazem should be avoided because an additive effect on SA and AV conduction and ventricular function will occur. The use of such a combination requires ECG monitoring especially at the beginning of treatment.

Combinations requiring safety precautions:

In common with other calcium antagonists, when diltiazem is used with drugs which may induce bradycardia or with antiarrhythmic drugs (e.g. amiodarone) or other antihypertensive drugs, the possibility of an additive effect should be borne in mind. Inhalation anaesthetics should be used with caution during diltiazem therapy. Tri/tetracyclic antidepressants and neuroleptics may increase the antihypertensive effects of diltiazem whilst the concomitant use of lithium with diltiazem may lead to neurotoxicity (extrapyramidal effects). Rifampin and other hepatic enzyme inducers may reduce the bioavailability of diltiazem and high doses of Vitamin D and/or high intake of calcium salts leading to elevated serum calcium levels may reduce the response to diltiazem.

Diltiazem is metabolised by CYP3A4 and could, by competitive inhibition of CYP3A4, affect the pharmacokinetics of other drugs metabolised by this enzyme. In addition inhibitors and inducers of CYP3A4 may affect the pharmacokinetics of diltiazem.

Diltiazem prolongs the sedative effect of midazolam and triazolam via metabolic interaction and decreases nifedipine clearance by 50%. Diltiazem may cause increases in the levels of digitoxin. Diltiazem has been shown to increase the bioavailability of imipramine by 30% probably due to inhibition of its first pass metabolism.

Diltiazem has been used safely in combination with diuretics, ACE-inhibitors and other anti-hypertensive agents. It is recommended that patients receiving these combinations should be regularly monitored. Concomitant use of diltiazem with alpha-blockers such as prazosin should be strictly monitored because of the possible synergistic hypotensive effect of the combination.

Case reports have suggested that blood levels of carbamazepine, cyclosporin, theophylline and phenytoin may be increased when given concurrently with diltiazem. Care should be exercised in patients taking these drugs. In common with other calcium antagonists diltiazem may cause small increases in plasma levels of digoxin. In patients taking H_2-antagonists concurrently with diltiazem there may be increased levels of diltiazem.

Magnification of the hypotensive and lipothymic effects (summation of vasodilator properties) of nitrate derivatives can occur. In patients on calcium inhibitors, prescriptions of nitrate derivatives should be made at progressively increasing doses. Diltiazem treatment has been continued without problem during anaesthesia, but diltiazem may potentiate the activity of curare-like and depolarising neuromuscular blocking agents, therefore the anaesthetist should be informed that the patient is receiving a calcium antagonist.

4.6 Pregnancy and lactation

Pregnancy:

Diltiazem should not be taken during pregnancy. Women of child bearing-potential should exclude the possibility of pregnancy before commencing treatment by taking suitable contraceptive measures if necessary. In animal tests, Diltiazem was found to have a tetratogenic effects in some species of animal.

Diltiazem may suppress the contractility of the uterus. Definite evidence that this will prolong partus in full-term pregnancy is lacking. A risk of hypoxia in the foetus may arise in the event of hypotension in the mother and reduced perfusion of the uterus due to redistribution of blood flow due to peripheral vasodilatation. In animal experiments diltiazem has exhibited teratogenic effects in some animal species. In the absence of adequate evidence of safety in human pregnancy, VIAZEM XL should not be used in pregnancy or in women of childbearing potential.

Lactation:

Diltiazem is excreted in breast milk in concentrations similar to those in serum. If the use of diltiazem is considered essential, an alternative method of infant feeding should be instituted.

4.7 Effects on ability to drive and use machines

There are no studies on the effect of diltiazem when driving vehicles or operating machines. It should be taken into account that occasionally asthenia/fatigue and dizziness may occur. Treatment of hypertension with this medicinal product requires regular monitoring. Individual different reactions may affect the ability to drive. This risk should be considered especially at the beginning of treatment, when changing the drug, or in combination with alcohol.

4.8 Undesirable effects

Certain undesirable effects may lead to suspension of treatment: sinus bradycardia, sino-atrial heart block, 2nd and 3rd degree atrioventricular heart block, skin rash, oedema of the lower limbs.

In hypertensive patients, adverse effects are generally mild and transient and are most commonly vasodilatory related events.

The following have been described in decreasing order of frequency: lower limb oedema, headache, hot flushes/flushing, asthenia/fatigue, palpitations, malaise, minor gastro-intestinal disorders (dyspepsia, abdominal pain, dry mouth, nausea, vomiting, diarrhoea, constipation) and skin rash. Erythema multiform and Stevens Johnson syndrome have been reported infrequently in patients receiving diltiazem hydrochloride. Vasodilatory related events (in particular, oedema) are dose-dependent and appear to be more frequent in elderly subjects.

Rare cases of symptomatic bradycardia and exceptionally sino-atrial block and atrioventricular block, hypotension, syncope, reduced left ventricular function have also been recorded. Isolated cases of hallucinations, depression, insomnia, hyperglycaemia and impotence have been reported.

Experience with use in other indications and with other formulations has shown that skin rashes are usually localised and are limited to cases of erythemia, urticaria or occasionally desquamative erthema, with or without fever, which regress when treatment is discontinued.

Isolated cases of moderate and transient elevations of liver transaminases have been observed at the start of treatment. Isolated cases of clinical hepatitis have been reported which resolved with cessation of therapy.

Dizziness, pruritis, nervousness, paraesthesia, articular/muscular pain, photo sensitisation, hypotension, gingival hyperplasia, and gynaecomastia, have also been observed.

4.9 Overdose

The clinical consequences of overdose can be severe hypotension leading to collapse, and sinus bradycardia which may be accompanied by isorhythmic dissociation and atrioventricular conduction disturbances. Observation in a coronary care unit is advisable. Vasopressors such as adrenaline may be indicated in patients exhibiting profound hypotension. Calcium gluconate may help reverse the effects of calcium entry blockade. Atropine administration and temporary cardiac pacing may be required to manage bradycardia and/or conduction disturbances.

Glucagon can be used in cases of established hypoglycaemia.

Diltiazem and its metabolites are very poorly dialysable.

5. PHARMACOLOGICAL PROPERTIES

5.1 Pharmacodynamic properties

Diltiazem is classified as a calcium channel blocker, benziothiazepine derivative, C08DB01, under the ATC classification. It selectively reduces calcium entry through voltage-dependent calcium-n channels into vascular smooth muscle cells and myocardial cells. This lowers the concentration of intracellular calcium which is available to activate contractile proteins. This action of diltiazem results in dilation of coronary arteries causing an increase in myocardial oxygen supply. It reduces cardiac work by moderating the heart rate and by reducing systemic vascular resistance thus reducing oxygen demand. Diltiazem also prolongs AV conduction and has mild effects on contractility. Clinical data on morbidity and mortality are not available.

5.2 Pharmacokinetic properties

Multiple dose pharmacokinetic studies have shown that the kinetics of VIAZEM XL are non-linear within the 120mg-360mg dosage range. Diltiazem is well absorbed, but has a highly saturable first pass effect leading to a variable absolute bioavailability, which is on average 35%. The saturable first pass effect results in higher than expected systemic exposure with increasing doses.

The protein binding is 80 to 85% and the volume of distribution is 5.0 l/kg.

Diltiazem is metabolised by CYP3A4 in the liver and 70% of the dose is excreted in urine, mainly as metabolites. The plasma levels of the two main metabolites, N-monodesmethyldiltiazem and desacetyldiltiazem, represent 35% and 15% of diltiazem levels respectively. The metabolites contribute around 50% of the clinical effect. Plasma clearance of diltiazem is approximately 0.5 l/h/kg. Plasma half-life of diltiazem is approximately 5-7 hours.

VIAZEM XL capsules allow a prolonged absorption of diltiazem and maximum levels are reached within 6 to 12 hours. Concomitant food intake with VIAZEM XL does not influence the pharmacokinetics of diltiazem. For most patients, chronic administration of VIAZEM XL 300mg once daily, results in therapeutic diltiazem levels (50-200ng/ml) over 24 hours. However, the inter-individual variability is high and individual dose adjustment based on therapeutic response is therefore necessary.

5.3 Preclinical safety data

Tests on reproductive functions in animals show that diltiazem decreases fertility in rats and that it is teratogenic in mice, rats and rabbits. Exposure during late pregnancy induces dystocia and a decrease in the number of live newborns in rats.

Detailed mutagenicity and carcinogenicity tests proved negative.

6. PHARMACEUTICAL PARTICULARS

6.1 List of excipients

- Sucrose Stearate
- Microcrystalline cellulose
- Povidone
- Magnesium Stearate
- Talc
- Titanium dioxide
- Hypromellose
- Polysorbate 80
- Polyacrylate dispersion 30% (dry)
- Simethicone emulsion
- Gelatine capsule

Gelatin capsule colours

	Capsule body	Capsule cap
300 mg	White opaque[1]	Lavender opaque[2]

1 =	Colour is composed of	Titanium Dioxide E171
2 =	Colour is composed of	Azorubine E122 Indigotine E132 Titanium Dioxide E171

Gelatin capsule markings:

	Capsule body	Capsule cap
300 mg	Viazem XL 300	Viazem XL 300
(Capsule Size 0)	(Black ink EEC approved)	(Black ink EEC approved)

Black printing ink contains:

Shellac, Ethyl Alcohol, Isopropyl Alcohol, n-Butyl, Propylene Glycol, Water (Purified) Ammonium Hydroxide, Potassium Hydroxide, Black Iron Oxide

6.2 Incompatibilities

Not applicable.

6.3 Shelf life

3 years

6.4 Special precautions for storage

Do not store above 25°C. Store in original package in a dry place away from any heat source, e.g. direct sunlight, heaters, steam, etc.

6.5 Nature and contents of container

The capsules are packed in PVC/aluminium blisters. Pack sizes are 28 capsules per blister.

6.6 Special precautions for disposal and other handling

Swallow capsules whole, with a glass of water do not chew.

7. MARKETING AUTHORISATION HOLDER

Stada Arzneimittel AG

Stadastrasse 2-18

61118 Bad Vilbel, Germany

8. MARKETING AUTHORISATION NUMBER(S)

VIAZEM XL 300 mg PL 11204/0093

9. DATE OF FIRST AUTHORISATION/RENEWAL OF THE AUTHORISATION

2nd April 1997

10. DATE OF REVISION OF THE TEXT

7 September 2008

Viazem XL 360mg

(Genus Pharmaceuticals)

1. NAME OF THE MEDICINAL PRODUCT

VIAZEM XL

2. QUALITATIVE AND QUANTITATIVE COMPOSITION

Diltiazem hydrochloride: 360 mg capsule.

For excipients see section 6.1

3. PHARMACEUTICAL FORM

Prolonged release capsule, hard.

Blue-green opaque capsules. Each capsule is printed on the cap and body, in white ink, with Viazem XL 360.

4. CLINICAL PARTICULARS

4.1 Therapeutic indications

VIAZEM XL is indicated for the management of stable angina pectoris and the treatment of mild to moderate hypertension.

4.2 Posology and method of administration

Dosage requirements may differ between patients with angina and patients with hypertension. In addition individual patients response may vary, necessitating careful titration. The range of strengths facilitates titration to the optimal dose.

One capsule of VIAZEM XL is to be taken before or during a meal. The dose should be taken at approximately the same time each day.

The capsule should not be chewed but swallowed whole, with a glass of water.

Due to the variability of release profile in individual patients, when changing from one type of sustained release diltiazem preparation to another, it may be necessary to adjust the dose.

Adults:

Hypertension: The usual starting dose is 180 mg once daily. The dose may be increased after 2-4 weeks according to the patient's response and the usual maintenance dose is 240mg-360mg once daily. The maximum daily dose is 360 mg. However, the single daily doses of 300 mg and 360 mg should only be administered to patients when no satisfactory therapeutic effect has been effected with lower doses and after the benefit risk-ratio has been carefully assessed by the doctor.

Angina: Care should be taken when titrating patients with stable angina in order to establish the optimal dose. The usual starting dose is 180 mg once daily. The dose may be increased after 2-4 weeks according to the patient's response. The maximum daily dose is 360 mg. However, the single daily doses of 300 mg and 360 mg should only be administered to patients when no satisfactory therapeutic effect has been effected with lower doses and after the benefit risk-ratio has been carefully assessed by the doctor.

Elderly and patients with impaired hepatic or renal function:

Plasma levels of diltiazem can be increased in the elderly, and in patients with impaired hepatic renal or hepatic function. In these cases, the starting dose should be one 120mg VIAZEM XL capsule once daily. Heart rate should be monitored and if it falls below 50 beats per minute, the dose should not be increased. Dose adjustment may be required to obtain a satisfactory clinical response.

Children:

Safety and efficacy in children have not been established.

4.3 Contraindications

Diltiazem depresses atrioventricular node conduction and is therefore contraindicated in patients with severe bradycardia (less than 50 bpm), sick sinus syndrome, congestive heart failure, and left ventricular failure with second or third degree AV or sino-atrial block, except in the presence of a functioning pacemaker. Diltiazem is also contraindicated in left ventricular failure with pulmonary stasis as diltiazem may have mild negative effects on contractility.

Diltiazem is contraindicated in acute complicated myocardial infarction (e.g. bradycardia hypotension, congestive heart failure/reduced LV function), pulmonary congestion, hypotension (<90 mmHg systolic) cerebrovascular accident, cardiac shock and unstable angina pectoris.

Diltiazem is contraindicated in pre-excitation syndrome (e.g. WPW) accompanied with atrial flutter, fibrillation and in digitalis intoxication, as diltiazem may precipitate ventricular tachycardia.

Diltiazem should not be used in patients with known hypersensitivity to diltiazem.

Diltiazem should not be used during pregnancy, by women of child-bearing potential, or by women who are breast-feeding.

4.4 Special warnings and precautions for use

Patients treated with beta-adrenoreceptor blocking drugs and patients with conduction disturbances (bradycardia, bundle branch block, first degree AV block, prolonged PR interval) should only be treated with VIAZEM XL after special consideration due to the risk of serious bradyarrhythmias.

This product should be used with caution in patients with hepatic dysfunction. Abnormalities of liver function may appear during therapy. The higher single daily doses of VIAZEM XL capsules 300mg and 360mg should not be administered to patients with impaired renal and/or hepatic function and to elderly patients (prolonged half life of elimination) because there is no experience on the use of such high dosages in these patient categories.

In patients undergoing long-term therapy with cyclosporin, plasma levels of cyclosporin should be monitored when concurrent administration of diltiazem is initiated, or discontinued or if the dose of diltiazem is changed.

Abnormally short transit time through the gastrointestinal tract could lead to incomplete release of contents of the capsule e.g. in chronic conditions with associated diarrhoea such as Crohns disease or ulcerative colitis.

4.5 Interaction with other medicinal products and other forms of interaction

Combinations contraindicated as a safety measure:

In animals, fatal ventricular fibrillations are constantly seen during administration of verapamil and dantrolene via the i.v. route. The combination of a calcium antagonist and dantrolene is therefore potentially dangerous. The concurrent iv administration of beta-adrenergic blocking agents with diltiazem should be avoided because an additive effect on SA and AV conduction and ventricular function will occur. The use of such a combination requires ECG monitoring especially at the beginning of treatment.

Combinations requiring safety precautions:

In common with other calcium antagonists, when diltiazem is used with other drugs which may induce bradycardia or with antiarrhythmic drugs (e.g. amiodarone) or other antihypertensive drugs, the possibility of an additive effect should be borne in mind. Inhalation anaesthetics should be used with caution during diltiazem therapy. Tri/tetracyclic antidepressants and neuroleptics may increase the antihypertensive effects of diltiazem whilst the concomitant use of lithium with diltiazem may lead to neurotoxicity (extrapyramidal effects). Rifampin and other hepatic enzyme inducers may reduce the bioavailability of diltiazem and high doses of Vitamin D and/or high intake of calcium salts leading to elevated serum calcium levels may reduce the response to diltiazem.

Diltiazem is metabolised by CYP3A4 and could, by competitive inhibition of CYP3A4, affect the pharmacokinetics of other drugs metabolised by this enzyme. In addition inhibitors and inducers of CYP3A4 may affect the pharmacokinetics of diltiazem.

Diltiazem prolongs the sedative effect of medazolam and triazolam via metabolic interaction and decreases nifedipine clearance by 50%. Diltiazem may cause increases in the levels of digitoxin. Diltiazem has been shown to increase the bioavailability of imipramine by 30% probably due to inhibition of its first pass metabolism.

Diltiazem has been used safely in combination with diuretics, ACE-inhibitors and other anti-hypertensive agents. It is recommended that patients receiving these combinations should be regularly monitored. Concomitant use of diltiazem with alpha-blockers such as prazosin should be strictly monitored because of the possible synergistic hypotensive effect of the combination.

Case reports have suggested that blood levels of carbamazepine, cyclosporin, theophylline and phenytoin may be increased when given concurrently with diltiazem. Care should be exercised in patients taking these drugs. In common with other calcium antagonists diltiazem may cause small increases in plasma levels of digoxin. In patients taking H_2-antagonists concurrently with diltiazem there may be increased levels of diltiazem.

Magnification of the hypotensive and lipothymic effects (summation of vasodilator properties) of nitrate derivatives can occur. In patients on calcium inhibitors, prescriptions of nitrate derivatives should be made at progressively increasing doses. Diltiazem treatment has been continued without problem during anaesthesia, but diltiazem may potentiate the activity of curare-like and depolarising neuromuscular blocking agents, therefore the anaesthetist should be informed that the patient is receiving a calcium antagonist.

4.6 Pregnancy and lactation

Pregnancy:

Diltiazem should not be taken during pregnancy. Women of child bearing-potential should exclude the possibility of pregnancy before commencing treatment by taking suitable contraceptive measures if necessary. In animal tests, Diltiazem was found to have a tetratogenic effects in some species of animal.

Diltiazem may suppress the contractility of the uterus. Definite evidence that this will prolong partus in full-term pregnancy is lacking. A risk of hypoxia in the foetus may arise in the event of hypotension in the mother and reduced perfusion of the uterus due to redistribution of blood flow due to peripheral vasodilatation. In animal experiments diltiazem has exhibited teratogenic effects in some animal species. In the absence of adequate evidence of safety in human pregnancy, VIAZEM XL should not be used in pregnancy or in women of childbearing potential.

Lactation:

Diltiazem is excreted in breast milk in concentrations similar to those in serum. If the use of diltiazem is considered essential, an alternative method of infant feeding should be instituted.

4.7 Effects on ability to drive and use machines

There are no studies on the effect of diltiazem when driving vehicles or operating machines. It should be taken into account that occasionally asthenia/fatigue and dizziness may occur. Treatment of hypertension with this medicinal product requires regular monitoring. Individual different reactions may affect the ability to drive. This risk should be considered especially at the beginning of treatment, when changing the drug, or in combination with alcohol.

4.8 Undesirable effects

Certain undesirable effects may lead to suspension of treatment: sinus bradycardia, sino-atrial heart block, 2nd and 3rd degree atrioventricular heart block, skin rash, oedema of the lower limbs.

In hypertensive patients, adverse effects are generally mild and transient and are most commonly vasodilatory related events.

The following have been described in decreasing order of frequency: lower limb oedema, headache, hot flushes/flushing, asthenia/fatigue, palpitations, malaise, minor gastro-intestinal disorders (dyspepsia, abdominal pain, dry mouth, nausea, vomiting, diarrhoea, constipation) and skin rash. Erythema multiform and Stevens Johnson syndrome have been reported infrequently in patients receiving diltiazem hydrochloride. Vasodilatory related events (in particular, oedema) are dose-dependent and appear to be more frequent in elderly subjects.

Rare cases of symptomatic bradycardia and exceptionally sino-atrial block and atrioventricular block, hypotension, syncope, reduced left ventricular function have also been recorded. Isolated cases of hallucinations, depression, insomnia, hyperglycaemia and impotence have been reported.

Experience with use in other indications and with other formulations has shown that skin rashes are usually localised and are limited to cases of erythemia, urticaria or occasionally desquamative erthema, with or without fever, which regress when treatment is discontinued.

Isolated cases of moderate and transient elevations of liver transaminases have been observed at the start of treatment. Isolated cases of clinical hepatitis have been reported which resolved with cessation of therapy.

Dizziness, pruritis, nervousness, paraesthesia, articular/muscular pain, photo sensitisation, hypotension, gingival hyperplasia, and gynaecomastia, have also been observed.

4.9 Overdose

The clinical consequences of overdose can be severe hypotension leading to collapse, and sinus bradycardia which may be accompanied by isorhythmic dissociation and atrioventricular conduction disturbances. Observation in a coronary care unit is advisable. Vasopressors such as adrenaline may be indicated in patients exhibiting profound hypotension. Calcium gluconate may help reverse the effects of calcium entry blockade. Atropine administration and temporary cardiac pacing may be required to manage bradycardia and/or conduction disturbances.

Glucagon can be used in cases of established hypoglycaemia.

Diltiazem and its metabolites are very poorly dialysable.

5. PHARMACOLOGICAL PROPERTIES

5.1 Pharmacodynamic properties

Diltiazem is classified as a calcium channel blocker, benziothiazepine derivative, C08DB01, under the ATC classification. It selectively reduces calcium entry through voltage-dependent calcium-n channels into vascular smooth muscle cells and myocardial cells. This lowers the concentration of intracellular calcium which is available to activate contractile proteins. This action of diltiazem results in dilation of coronary arteries causing an increase in myocardial oxygen supply. It reduces cardiac work by moderating the heart rate and by reducing systemic vascular resistance thus reducing oxygen demand. Diltiazem also prolongs AV conduction and has mild effects on contractility. Clinical data on morbidity and mortality are not available.

5.2 Pharmacokinetic properties

Multiple dose pharmacokinetic studies have shown that the kinetics of VIAZEM XL are non-linear within the 120mg-360mg dosage range. Diltiazem is well absorbed, but has a highly saturable first pass effect leading to a variable absolute bioavailability, which is on average 35%. The saturable first pass effect results in higher than expected systemic exposure with increasing doses.

The protein binding is 80 to 85% and the volume of distribution is 5.0 l/kg.

Diltiazem is metabolised by CYP3A4 in the liver and 70% of the dose is excreted in urine, mainly as metabolites. The plasma levels of the two main metabolites, N-monodesmethyldiltiazem and desacetyldiltiazem, represent 35% and 15% of diltiazem levels respectively. The metabolites contribute around 50% of the clinical effect. Plasma clearance of diltiazem is approximately 0.5 l/h/kg. Plasma half-life of diltiazem is approximately 5-7 hours.

VIAZEM XL capsules allow a prolonged absorption of diltiazem and maximum levels are reached within 6 to 12 hours. Concomitant food intake with VIAZEM XL does not influence the pharmacokinetics of diltiazem. For most patients, chronic administration of VIAZEM XL 300mg once daily, results in therapeutic diltiazem levels (50-200ng/ml) over 24 hours. However, the inter-individual variability is high and individual dose adjustment based on therapeutic response is therefore necessary.

5.3 Preclinical safety data

Tests on reproductive functions in animals show that diltiazem decreases fertility in rats and that it is teratogenic in mice, rats and rabbits. Exposure during late pregnancy induces dystocia and a decrease in the number of live newborns in rats.

Detailed mutagenicity and carcinogenicity tests proved negative.

6. PHARMACEUTICAL PARTICULARS

6.1 List of excipients

- Sucrose Stearate
- Microcrystalline cellulose
- Povidone
- Magnesium Stearate
- Talc
- Titanium dioxide
- Hypromellose
- Polysorbate 80
- Polyacrylate dispersion 30% (dry)
- Simethicone emulsion
- Gelatine capsule

Gelatin capsule colours

	Capsule body	Capsule cap
360 mg	Blue Green opaque[1]	Blue Green opaque[1]

1 = Colour is composed of Quinoline Yellow E104, Indigotine E132, Titanium Dioxide E171

Gelatin capsule markings (printed radially):

	Capsule body	Capsule cap
360 mg	Viazem XL 360	Viazem XL 360
(Capsule Size 0)	(White ink EEC approved)	(White ink EEC approved)

White printing ink contains:

Shellac, Ethyl Alcohol, Isopropyl Alcohol, n-Butyl, Propylene Glycol, Sodium Hydroxide, Polyvinylpyrrolidone, Titanium Dioxide

6.2 Incompatibilities
Not applicable.

6.3 Shelf life
3 years

6.4 Special precautions for storage
Do not store above 25°C. Store in original package in a dry place away from any heat source, e.g. direct sunlight, heaters, steam, etc.

6.5 Nature and contents of container
The capsules are packed in PVC/aluminium blisters. Pack sizes are 28 capsules per blister.

6.6 Special precautions for disposal and other handling
Swallow capsules whole, with a glass of water do not chew.

7. MARKETING AUTHORISATION HOLDER
Stada Arzneimittel AG
Stadastrasse 2-18
61118 Bad Vilbel, Germany

8. MARKETING AUTHORISATION NUMBER(S)
PL 11204/0094

9. DATE OF FIRST AUTHORISATION/RENEWAL OF THE AUTHORISATION
2nd April 1997

10. DATE OF REVISION OF THE TEXT
7 September 2008

Vibramycin 50 CAPSULES

(Pfizer Limited)

1. NAME OF THE MEDICINAL PRODUCT
VIBRAMYCIN 50

2. QUALITATIVE AND QUANTITATIVE COMPOSITION
Active Ingredient: doxycycline.

Vibramycin 50 Capsules contain 50mg doxycycline as doxycycline hyclate Ph. Eur.

3. PHARMACEUTICAL FORM
Vibramycin 50 capsules are green and ivory, coded 'Pfizer' and 'VBM 50'.

4. CLINICAL PARTICULARS
4.1 Therapeutic indications
Vibramycin has been found clinically effective in the treatment of a variety of infections caused by susceptible strains of Gram-positive and Gram-negative bacteria and certain other micro-organisms.

Respiratory tract infections Pneumonia and other lower respiratory tract infections due to susceptible strains of *Streptococcus pneumoniae*, *Haemophilus influenzae*, *Klebsiella pneumoniae* and other organisms. *Mycoplasma pneumoniae* pneumonia. Treatment of chronic bronchitis, sinusitis.

Urinary tract infections caused by susceptible strains of Klebsiella species, Enterobacter species, *Escherichia coli*, *Streptococcus faecalis* and other organisms.

Sexually transmitted diseases Infections due to *Chlamydia trachomatis* including uncomplicated urethral, endocervical or rectal infections. Non-gonococcal urethritis caused by *Ureaplasma urealyticum* (T-mycoplasma). Vibramycin is also indicated in chancroid, granuloma inguinale and lymphogranuloma venereum. Vibramycin is an alternative drug in the treatment of gonorrhoea and syphilis.

Skin infections Acne vulgaris, when antibiotic therapy is considered necessary.

Since Vibramycin is a member of the tetracycline series of antibiotics, it may be expected to be useful in the treatment of infections which respond to other tetracyclines, such as:

Ophthalmic infections Due to susceptible strains of gonococci, staphylococci and *Haemophilus influenzae*. Trachoma, although the infectious agent, as judged by immunofluorescence, is not always eliminated. Inclusion conjunctivitis may be treated with oral Vibramycin alone or in combination with topical agents.

Rickettsial infections Rocky Mountain spotted fever, typhus group, Q fever, Coxiella endocarditis and tick fevers.

Other infections Psittacosis, brucellosis (in combination with streptomycin), cholera, bubonic plague, louse and tick-borne relapsing fever, tularaemia glanders, melioidosis, chloroquine-resistant falciparum malaria and acute intestinal amoebiasis (as an adjunct to amoebicides).

Vibramycin is an alternative drug in the treatment of leptospirosis, gas gangrene and tetanus.

Vibramycin is indicated for prophylaxis in the following conditions: Scrub typhus, travellers' diarrhoea (enterotoxigenic *Escherichia coli)*, leptospirosis and malaria. Prophylaxis of malaria should be used in accordance to current guidelines, as resistance is an ever changing problem.

4.2 Posology and method of administration
Adults
The usual dosage of Vibramycin for the treatment of acute infections in adults is 200mg on the first day (as a single dose or in divided doses) followed by a maintenance dose of 100mg/day. In the management of more severe infections, 200mg daily should be given throughout treatment. Capsules are for oral administration only.

Vibramycin capsules should be administered with adequate amounts of fluid. This should be done in the sitting or standing position and well before retiring at night to reduce the risk of oesophageal irritation and ulceration. If gastric irritation occurs, it is recommended that Vibramycin be given with food or milk. Studies indicate that the absorption of Vibramycin is not notably influenced by simultaneous ingestion of food or milk.

Exceeding the recommended dosage may result in an increased incidence of side effects. Therapy should be continued for at least 24 to 48 hours after symptoms and fever have subsided.

When used in streptococcal infections, therapy should be continued for 10 days to prevent the development of rheumatic fever or glomerulonephritis.

Dosage recommendations in specific infections:

Acne vulgaris 50mg daily with food or fluid for 6 to 12 weeks.

Sexually transmitted diseases 100mg twice daily for 7 days is recommended in the following infections: uncomplicated gonococcal infections (except anorectal infections in men); uncomplicated urethral, endocervical or rectal infection caused by *Chlamydia trachomatis*; non-gonococcal urethritis caused by *Ureaplasma urealyticum*. Acute epididymo-orchitis caused by *Chlamydia trachomatis* or *Neisseria gonorrhoea* 100mg twice daily for 10 days. Primary and secondary syphilis: Non-pregnant penicillin-allergic patients who have primary or secondary syphilis can be treated with the following regimen: doxycycline 200mg orally twice daily for two weeks, as an alternative to penicillin therapy.

Louse and tick-borne relapsing fevers A single dose of 100 or 200mg according to severity.

Treatment of chloroquine-resistant falciparum malaria 200mg daily for at least 7 days. Due to the potential severity of the infection, a rapid-acting schizonticide such as quinine should always be given in conjunction with Vibramycin; quinine dosage recommendations vary in different areas.

Prophylaxis of malaria 100mg daily in adults and children over the age of 12 years. Prophylaxis can begin 1-2 days before travel to malarial areas. It should be continued daily during travel in the malarial areas and for 4 weeks after the traveller leaves the malarial area. For current advice on geographical resistance patterns and appropriate chemoprophylaxis, current guidelines or the Malaria Reference Laboratory should be consulted, details of which can be found in the British National Formulary (BNF).

For the prevention of scrub typhus 200mg as a single dose.

For the prevention of travellers' diarrhoea in adults 200mg on the first day of travel (administered as a single dose or as 100mg every 12 hours) followed by 100mg daily throughout the stay in the area. Data on the use of the drug prophylactically are not available beyond 21 days.

For the prevention of leptospirosis 200mg once each week throughout the stay in the area and 200mg at the completion of the trip. Data on the use of the drug prophylactically are not available beyond 21 days.

Use for children See under "Contra-indications".

Use in the elderly Vibramycin may be prescribed in the elderly in the usual dosages with no special precautions. No dosage adjustment is necessary in the presence of renal impairment.

Use in patients with impaired hepatic function See under "Special warnings and precautions for use".

Use in patients with renal impairment Studies to date have indicated that administration of Vibramycin at the usual recommended doses does not lead to accumulation of the antibiotic in patients with renal impairment see under " Special warnings and precautions for use".

4.3 Contraindications
Persons who have shown hypersensitivity to doxycycline, any of its inert ingredients or to any of the tetracyclines.

The use of drugs of the tetracycline class during tooth development (pregnancy, infancy and childhood to the age of 12 years) may cause permanent discolouration of the teeth (yellow-grey-brown). This adverse reaction is more common during long-term use of the drugs but has been observed following repeated short-term courses. Enamel hypoplasia has also been reported. Vibramycin is therefore contra-indicated in these groups of patients.

Pregnancy Vibramycin is contra-indicated in pregnancy. It appears that the risks associated with the use of tetracyclines during pregnancy are predominantly due to effects on teeth and skeletal development. (See above about use during tooth development).

Nursing mothers Tetracyclines are excreted into milk and are therefore contra-indicated in nursing mothers. (See above about use during tooth development).

Children Vibramycin is contra-indicated in children under the age of 12 years. As with other tetracyclines, Vibramycin forms a stable calcium complex in any bone-forming tissue. A decrease in the fibula growth rate has been observed in prematures given oral tetracyclines in doses of 25mg/kg every 6 hours. This reaction was shown to be reversible when the drug was discontinued. (See above about use during tooth development).

4.4 Special warnings and precautions for use
Use in patients with impaired hepatic function Vibramycin should be administered with caution to patients with hepatic impairment or those receiving potentially hepatotoxic drugs.

Abnormal hepatic function has been reported rarely and has been caused by both the oral and parenteral administration of tetracyclines, including doxycycline.

Use in patients with renal impairment Excretion of doxycycline by the kidney is about 40%/72 hours in individuals with normal renal function. This percentage excretion may fall to a range as low as 1-5%/72 hours in individuals with severe renal insufficiency (creatinine clearance below 10ml/min). Studies have shown no significant difference in the serum half-life of doxycycline in individuals with normal and severely impaired renal function. Haemodialysis does not alter the serum half-life of doxycycline. The anti-anabolic action of the tetracyclines may cause an increase in blood urea. Studies to date indicate that this anti-anabolic effect does not occur with the use of Vibramycin in patients with impaired renal function.

Photosensitivity Photosensitivity manifested by an exaggerated sunburn reaction has been observed in some individuals taking tetracyclines, including doxycycline. Patients likely to be exposed to direct sunlight or ultraviolet light should be advised that this reaction can occur with tetracycline drugs and treatment should be discontinued at the first evidence of skin erythema.

Microbiological overgrowth The use of antibiotics may occasionally result in the overgrowth of non-susceptible organisms including Candida. If a resistant organism appears, the antibiotic should be discontinued and appropriate therapy instituted.

Pseudomembranous colitis has been reported with nearly all antibacterial agents, including doxycycline, and has ranged in severity from mild to life-threatening. It is important to consider this diagnosis in patients who present with diarrhoea subsequent to the administration of antibacterial agents.

Oesophagitis Instances of oesophagitis and oesophageal ulcerations have been reported in patients receiving capsule and tablet forms of drugs in the tetracycline class, including doxycycline. Most of these patients took medications immediately before going to bed or with inadequate amounts of fluid.

Bulging fontanelles in infants and benign intracranial hypertension in juveniles and adults have been reported in individuals receiving full therapeutic dosages. These conditions disappeared rapidly when the drug was discontinued.

Porphyria There have been rare reports of porphyria in patients receiving tetracyclines.

Venereal disease When treating venereal disease, where co-existent syphilis is suspected, proper diagnostic procedures including dark-field examinations should be utilised. In all such cases monthly serological tests should be made for at least four months.

Beta-haemolytic streptococci infections Infections due to group A beta-haemolytic streptococci should be treated for at least 10 days.

Myasthenia gravis Due to a potential for weak neuromuscular blockade, care should be taken in administering tetracyclines to patients with myasthenia gravis.

Systemic lupus erythematosus Tetracyclines can cause exacerbation of SLE.

Methoxyflurane Caution is advised in administering tetracyclines with methoxyflurane. See section 4.5.

4.5 Interaction with other medicinal products and other forms of interaction
The absorption of doxycycline may be impaired by concurrently administered antacids containing aluminium, calcium, magnesium or other drugs containing these cations; oral zinc, iron salts or bismuth preparations. Dosages should be maximally separated.

Since bacteriostatic drugs may interfere with the bactericidal action of penicillin, it is advisable to avoid giving Vibramycin in conjunction with penicillin.

There have been reports of prolonged prothrombin time in patients taking warfarin and doxycycline. Tetracyclines depress plasma prothrombin activity and reduced doses of concomitant anticoagulants may be necessary.

The serum half-life of doxycycline may be shortened when patients are concurrently receiving barbiturates, carbamazepine or phenytoin. An increase in the daily dosage of Vibramycin should be considered.

Alcohol may decrease the half-life of doxycycline.

A few cases of pregnancy or breakthrough bleeding have been attributed to the concurrent use of tetracycline antibiotics with oral contraceptives.

Doxycycline may increase the plasma concentration of cyclosporin. Co-administration should only be undertaken with appropriate monitoring.

The concurrent use of tetracyclines and methoxyflurane has been reported to result in fatal renal toxicity. See section 4.4

Laboratory test interactions

False elevations of urinary catecholamine levels may occur due to interference with the fluorescence test.

4.6 Pregnancy and lactation

See "Contra-indications".

4.7 Effects on ability to drive and use machines

The effect of doxycycline on the ability to drive or operate heavy machinery has not been studied. There is no evidence to suggest that doxycycline may affect these abilities.

4.8 Undesirable effects

The following adverse reactions have been observed in patients receiving tetracyclines, including doxycycline.

Autonomic nervous system Flushing.

Body as a whole Hypersensitivity reactions, including anaphylactic shock, anaphylaxis, anaphylactoid reaction, anaphylactoid purpura, hypotension, pericarditis, angioneurotic oedema, exacerbation of systemic lupus erythematosus, dyspnoea, serum sickness, peripheral oedema, tachycardia and urticaria.

Central and Peripheral nervous system Headache. Bulging fontanelles in infants and benign intracranial hypertension in juveniles and adults have been reported in individuals receiving full therapeutic dosages of tetracyclines. In relation to benign intracranial hypertension, symptoms included blurring of vision, scotomata and diplopia. Permanent visual loss has been reported.

Gastro-intestinal Gastro-intestinal symptoms are usually mild and seldom necessitate discontinuation of treatment. Abdominal pain, anorexia, nausea, vomiting, diarrhoea, dyspepsia and rarely dysphagia. Oesophagitis and oesophageal ulceration have been reported in patients receiving Vibramycin. A significant proportion of these occurred with the hyclate salt in the capsule form. (See 'Special warnings and precautions for use' section).

Hearing/Vestibular Tinnitus.

Haemopoietic Haemolytic anaemia, thrombocytopenia, neutropenia, porphyria, and eosinophilia have been reported with tetracyclines.

Liver/Biliary Transient increases in liver function tests, hepatitis, jaundice, hepatic failure and pancreatitis have been reported rarely.

Musculo-Skeletal Arthralgia and myalgia.

Skin Rashes including maculopapular and erythematous rashes, exfoliative dermatitis, erythema multiforme, Steven-Johnson syndrome and toxic epidermal necrolysis. Photosensitivity skin reactions (see 'Special warnings and precautions for use' section).

Superinfection As with all antibiotics, overgrowth of non-susceptible organisms may cause candidiasis, glossitis, staphylococcal enterocolitis, pseudomembranous colitis (with *Clostridium difficile* overgrowth) and inflammatory lesions (with candidal overgrowth) in the anogenital region. Similarly there have been reports for products in the tetracycline class of stomatitis and vaginitis.

Urinary system Increased blood urea. (See 'Special warnings and precautions for use' section.)

Other When given over prolonged periods, tetracyclines have been reported to produce brown-black microscopic discolouration of thyroid tissue. No abnormalities of thyroid function are known to occur.

Tetracyclines may cause discoloration of teeth and enamel hypoplasia, but usually only after long-term use.

4.9 Overdose

Acute overdosage with antibiotics is rare. In the event of overdosage discontinue medication. Gastric lavage plus appropriate supportive treatment is indicated.

Dialysis does not alter serum half-life and thus would not be of benefit in treating cases of overdosage.

5. PHARMACOLOGICAL PROPERTIES

5.1 Pharmacodynamic properties

Vibramycin is primarily bacteriostatic and is believed to exert its antimicrobial effect by the inhibition of protein synthesis. Vibramycin is active against a wide range of Gram-positive and Gram-negative bacteria and certain other micro-organisms.

5.2 Pharmacokinetic properties

Tetracyclines are readily absorbed and are bound to plasma proteins in varying degrees. They are concentrated by the liver in the bile and excreted in the urine and faeces at high concentrations and in a biologically active form. Doxycycline is virtually completely absorbed after oral administration. Studies reported to date indicate that the absorption of doxycycline, unlike certain other tetracyclines, is not notably influenced by the ingestion of food or milk. Following a 200mg dose, normal adult volunteers averaged peak serum levels of 2.6 micrograms/ml of doxycycline at 2 hours decreasing to 1.45 micrograms/ml at 24 hours. Doxycycline has a high degree of lipid solubility and a low affinity for calcium. It is highly stable in normal human serum. Doxycycline will not degrade into an epianhydro form.

6. PHARMACEUTICAL PARTICULARS

6.1 List of excipients

Vibramycin 50mg capsules: Maize Starch Ph.Eur., Lactose Ph.Eur., alginic acid, Magnesium Stearate NF, Sodium Lauryl Sulphate Ph Eur. In addition the capsule shell cap contains: Gelatin BP, titanium dioxide (E171), patent blue V (E131) and quinoline yellow (E104) and the body contains yellow iron oxide (E172), indigotine (E132) and titanium dioxide (E171).

6.2 Incompatibilities

None stated.

6.3 Shelf life

Vibramycin 50mg capsules 48 months.

6.4 Special precautions for storage

Store below 25°C.

6.5 Nature and contents of container

Vibramycin 50 Capsules 50mg are available as:

Calendar Packs of 28 Capsules. Aluminium/PVC blister strips, 14 capsules per strip, 2 strips in a carton box.

6.6 Special precautions for disposal and other handling

No special requirements.

7. MARKETING AUTHORISATION HOLDER

Pfizer Limited

Ramsgate Road

Sandwich

Kent CT13 9NJ

United Kingdom

8. MARKETING AUTHORISATION NUMBER(S)

Vibramycin Capsules 50mg

0057/0238

9. DATE OF FIRST AUTHORISATION/RENEWAL OF THE AUTHORISATION

Vibramycin Capsules 50mg

29/10/00

10. DATE OF REVISION OF THE TEXT

May 2008

Legal Category

POM

Ref: VM 9_0

Vibramycin-D Dispersible Tablets 100 mg

(Pfizer Limited)

1. NAME OF THE MEDICINAL PRODUCT

VIBRAMYCIN™-D DISPERSIBLE TABLETS

2. QUALITATIVE AND QUANTITATIVE COMPOSITION

100 mg doxycycline as doxycycline monohydrate.

3. PHARMACEUTICAL FORM

Vibramycin-D Dispersible Tablets are light yellow, round tablets scored on one face and coded 'VN' on the other.

4. CLINICAL PARTICULARS

4.1 Therapeutic indications

Vibramycin has been found clinically effective in the treatment of a variety of infections caused by susceptible strains of Gram-positive and Gram-negative bacteria and certain other micro-organisms.

Respiratory tract infections Pneumonia and other lower respiratory tract infections due to susceptible strains of *Streptococcus pneumoniae, Haemophilus influenzae, Klebsiella pneumoniae* and other organisms. *Mycoplasma pneumoniae* pneumonia. Treatment of chronic bronchitis, sinusitis.

Urinary tract infections caused by susceptible strains of Klebsiella species, Enterobacter species, *Escherichia coli, Streptococcus faecalis* and other organisms.

Sexually transmitted diseases Infections due to *Chlamydia trachomatis* including uncomplicated urethral, endocervical or rectal infections. Non-gonococcal urethritis caused by *Ureaplasma urealyticum* (T-mycoplasma). Vibramycin is also indicated in chancroid, granuloma inguinale and lymphogranuloma venereum. Vibramycin is an alternative drug in the treatment of gonorrhoea and syphilis.

Skin infections Acne vulgaris, when antibiotic therapy is considered necessary.

Since Vibramycin is a member of the tetracycline series of antibiotics, it may be expected to be useful in the treatment of infections which respond to other tetracyclines, such as:

Ophthalmic infections Due to susceptible strains of gonococci, staphylococci and Haemophilus influenzae. Trachoma, although the infectious agent, as judged by immunofluorescence, is not always eliminated. Inclusion conjunctivitis may be treated with oral Vibramycin alone or in combination with topical agents.

Rickettsial infections Rocky Mountain spotted fever, typhus group, Q fever, Coxiella endocarditis and tick fevers.

Other infections Psittacosis, brucellosis (in combination with streptomycin), cholera, bubonic plague, louse and tick-borne relapsing fever, tularaemia glanders, melioidosis, chloroquine-resistant falciparum malaria and acute intestinal amoebiasis (as an adjunct to amoebicides).

Vibramycin is an alternative drug in the treatment of leptospirosis, gas gangrene and tetanus.

Vibramycin is indicated for prophylaxis in the following conditions: Scrub typhus, travellers' diarrhoea (enterotoxigenic *Escherichia coli*), leptospirosis and malaria. Prophylaxis of malaria should be used in accordance to current guidelines, as resistance is an ever changing problem.

4.2 Posology and method of administration

Adults

The usual dosage of Vibramycin for the treatment of acute infections in adults is 200 mg on the first day (as a single dose or in divided doses) followed by a maintenance dose of 100 mg/day. In the management of more severe infections, 200 mg daily should be given throughout treatment.

Dispersible Tablets are for oral administration only.

Vibramycin-D tablets are administered by drinking a suspension of the tablets in a small amount of water. This should be done in the sitting or standing position and well before retiring at night to reduce the risk of oesophageal irritation and ulceration. If gastric irritation occurs, it is recommended that Vibramycin be given with food or milk. Studies indicate that the absorption of Vibramycin is not notably influenced by simultaneous ingestion of food or milk.

Exceeding the recommended dosage may result in an increased incidence of side effects. Therapy should be continued for at least 24 to 48 hours after symptoms and fever have subsided.

When used in streptococcal infections, therapy should be continued for 10 days to prevent the development of rheumatic fever or glomerulonephritis.

Dosage recommendations in specific infections:

Acne vulgaris 50 mg daily with food or fluid for 6 to 12 weeks.

Sexually transmitted diseases 100 mg twice daily for 7 days is recommended in the following infections: uncomplicated gonococcal infections (except anorectal infections in men); uncomplicated urethral, endocervical or rectal infection caused by Chlamydia trachomatis; non-gonococcal urethritis caused by Ureaplasma urealyticum. Acute epididymo-orchitis caused by Chlamydia trachomatis or Neisseria gonorrhoea 100 mg twice daily for 10 days. Primary and secondary syphilis: Non-pregnant penicillin-allergic patients who have primary or secondary syphilis can be treated with the following regimen: doxycycline 200 mg orally twice daily for two weeks, as an alternative to penicillin therapy.

Louse and tick-borne relapsing fevers A single dose of 100 or 200 mg according to severity.

Treatment of chloroquine-resistant falciparum malaria 200 mg daily for at least 7 days. Due to the potential severity of the infection, a rapid-acting schizonticide such as quinine should always be given in conjunction with Vibramycin; quinine dosage recommendations vary in different areas.

Prophylaxis of malaria 100 mg daily in adults and children over the age of 12 years. Prophylaxis can begin 1-2 days before travel to malarial areas. It should be continued daily during travel in the malarial areas and for 4 weeks after the traveller leaves the malarial area. For current advice on geographical resistance patterns and appropriate chemoprophylaxis, current guidelines or the Malaria Reference Laboratory should be consulted, details of which can be found in the British National Formulary (BNF).

For the prevention of scrub typhus 200 mg as a single dose.

For the prevention of travellers' diarrhoea in adults 200 mg on the first day of travel (administered as a single dose or as 100 mg every 12 hours) followed by 100 mg daily throughout the stay in the area. Data on the use of the drug prophylactically are not available beyond 21 days.

For the prevention of leptospirosis 200 mg once each week throughout the stay in the area and 200 mg at the completion of the trip. Data on the use of the drug prophylactically are not available beyond 21 days.

Use for children See under "Contra-indications".

Use in the elderly Vibramycin may be prescribed in the elderly in the usual dosages with no special precautions. No dosage adjustment is necessary in the presence of renal impairment. The Vibramycin-D dispersible tablet may be preferred for the elderly since it is less likely to be associated with oesophageal irritation and ulceration.

Use in patients with impaired hepatic function See under " Special warnings and precautions for use".

Use in patients with renal impairmentStudies to date have indicated that administration of Vibramycin at the usual recommended doses does not lead to accumulation of the antibiotic in patients with renal impairment see under "Special warnings and precautions for use".

4.3 Contraindications

Persons who have shown hypersensitivity to doxycycline, any of its inert ingredients or to any of the tetracyclines.

The use of drugs of the tetracycline class during tooth development (pregnancy, infancy and childhood to the age of 12 years) may cause permanent discolouration of the teeth (yellow-grey-brown). This adverse reaction is more common during long-term use of the drugs but has been observed following repeated short-term courses. Enamel hypoplasia has also been reported. Vibramycin is therefore contra-indicated in these groups of patients.

Pregnancy Vibramycin is contra-indicated in pregnancy. It appears that the risks associated with the use of tetracyclines during pregnancy are predominantly due to effects on teeth and skeletal development. (See above about use during tooth development).

Nursing mothers Tetracyclines are excreted into milk and are therefore contra-indicated in nursing mothers. (See above about use during tooth development).

Children Vibramycin is contra-indicated in children under the age of 12 years. As with other tetracyclines, Vibramycin forms a stable calcium complex in any bone-forming tissue. A decrease in the fibula growth rate has been observed in prematures given oral tetracyclines in doses of 25 mg/kg every 6 hours. This reaction was shown to be reversible when the drug was discontinued. (See above about use during tooth development).

4.4 Special warnings and precautions for use

Use in patients with impaired hepatic function Vibramycin should be administered with caution to patients with hepatic impairment or those receiving potentially hepatotoxic drugs.

Abnormal hepatic function has been reported rarely and has been caused by both the oral and parenteral administration of tetracyclines, including doxycycline.

Use in patients with renal impairment Excretion of doxycycline by the kidney is about 40%/72 hours in individuals with normal renal function. This percentage excretion may fall to a range as low as 1-5%/72 hours in individuals with severe renal insufficiency (creatinine clearance below 10ml/min). Studies have shown no significant difference in the serum half-life of doxycycline in individuals with normal and severely impaired renal function. Haemodialysis does not alter the serum half-life of doxycycline. The anti-anabolic action of the tetracyclines may cause an increase in blood urea. Studies to date indicate that this anti-anabolic effect does not occur with the use of Vibramycin in patients with impaired renal function.

Photosensitivity Photosensitivity manifested by an exaggerated sunburn reaction has been observed in some individuals taking tetracyclines, including doxycycline. Patients likely to be exposed to direct sunlight or ultraviolet light should be advised that this reaction can occur with tetracycline drugs and treatment should be discontinued at the first evidence of skin erythema.

Microbiological overgrowth The use of antibiotics may occasionally result in the overgrowth of non-susceptible organisms including Candida. If a resistant organism appears, the antibiotic should be discontinued and appropriate therapy instituted.

Pseudomembranous colitis has been reported with nearly all antibacterial agents, including doxycycline, and has ranged in severity from mild to life-threatening. It is important to consider this diagnosis in patients who present with diarrhoea subsequent to the administration of antibacterial agents.

Clostridium difficile associated diarrhoea (CDAD) has been reported with use of nearly all antibacterial agents, including doxycycline, and may range in severity from mild diarrhoea to fatal colitis. Treatment with antibacterial agents alters the normal flora of the colon leading to overgrowth of *C. difficile*.

C. difficile produces toxins A and B which contribute to the development of CDAD.

Hypertoxin producing strains of *C. difficile* cause increased morbidity and mortality, as these infections can be refractory to antimicrobial therapy and may require colectomy. CDAD must be considered in all patients who present with diarrhoea following antibiotic use. Careful medical history is necessary since CDAD has been reported to occur over two months after the administration of antibacterial agents.

Oesophagitis Instances of oesophagitis and oesophageal ulcerations have been reported in patients receiving capsule and tablet forms of drugs in the tetracycline class, including doxycycline. Most of these patients took medications immediately before going to bed or with inadequate amounts of fluid.

Bulging fontanelles in infants and benign intracranial hypertension in juveniles and adults have been reported in individuals receiving full therapeutic dosages. These conditions disappeared rapidly when the drug was discontinued.

Porphyria There have been rare reports of porphyria in patients receiving tetracyclines.

Venereal disease When treating venereal disease, where co-existent syphilis is suspected, proper diagnostic procedures including dark-field examinations should be utilised. In all such cases monthly serological tests should be made for at least four months.

Beta-haemolytic streptococci infections Infections due to group A beta-haemolytic streptococci should be treated for at least 10 days.

Myasthenia gravis Due to a potential for weak neuromuscular blockade, care should be taken in administering tetracyclines to patients with myasthenia gravis.

Systemic lupus erythematosus Tetracyclines can cause exacerbation of SLE.

Methoxyflurane Caution is advised in administering tetracyclines with methoxyflurane. See section 4.5.

4.5 Interaction with other medicinal products and other forms of interaction

The absorption of doxycycline may be impaired by concurrently administered antacids containing aluminium, calcium, magnesium or other drugs containing these cations; oral zinc, iron salts or bismuth preparations. Dosages should be maximally separated.

Since bacteriostatic drugs may interfere with the bactericidal action of penicillin, it is advisable to avoid giving Vibramycin in conjunction with penicillin.

There have been reports of prolonged prothrombin time in patients taking warfarin and doxycycline. Tetracyclines depress plasma prothrombin activity and reduced doses of concomitant anticoagulants may be necessary.

The serum half-life of doxycycline may be shortened when patients are concurrently receiving barbiturates, carbamazepine or phenytoin. An increase in the daily dosage of Vibramycin should be considered.

Alcohol may decrease the half-life of doxycycline.

A few cases of pregnancy or breakthrough bleeding have been attributed to the concurrent use of tetracycline antibiotics with oral contraceptives.

Doxycycline may increase the plasma concentration of cyclosporin. Co-administration should only be undertaken with appropriate monitoring.

The concurrent use of tetracyclines and methoxyflurane has been reported to result in fatal renal toxicity. See section 4.4.

Laboratory test interactions

False elevations of urinary catecholamine levels may occur due to interference with the fluorescence test.

4.6 Pregnancy and lactation

See "Contra-indications".

4.7 Effects on ability to drive and use machines

The effect of doxycycline on the ability to drive or operate heavy machinery has not been studied. There is no evidence to suggest that doxycycline may affect these abilities.

4.8 Undesirable effects

The following adverse reactions have been observed in patients receiving tetracyclines, including doxycycline.

Autonomic nervous system Flushing.

Body as a whole Hypersensitivity reactions, including anaphylactic shock, anaphylaxis, anaphylactoid reaction, anaphylactoid purpura, hypotension, pericarditis, angioneurotic oedema, exacerbation of systemic lupus erythematosus, dyspnoea, serum sickness, peripheral oedema, tachycardia and urticaria.

Central and Peripheral nervous system Headache. Bulging fontanelles in infants and benign intracranial hypertension in juveniles and adults have been reported in individuals receiving full therapeutic dosages of tetracyclines. In relation to benign intracranial hypertension, symptoms included blurring of vision, scotomata and diplopia. Permanent visual loss has been reported.

Gastro-intestinalGastro-intestinal symptoms are usually mild and seldom necessitate discontinuation of treatment. Abdominal pain, anorexia, nausea, vomiting, diarrhoea, dyspepsia and rarely dysphagia. Oesophagitis and oesophageal ulceration have been reported in patients receiving Vibramycin. A significant proportion of these occurred with the hyclate salt in the capsule form. (See 'Special warnings and precautions for use' section).

Hearing/Vestibular Tinnitus.

Haemopoietic Haemolytic anaemia, thrombocytopenia, neutropenia, porphyria, and eosinophilia have been reported with tetracyclines.

Hepatobiliary Disorders There have been rare reports of hepatotoxicity with transient increases in liver function tests, hepatitis, jaundice hepatic failure and pancreatitis.

Musculo-Skeletal Arthralgia and myalgia.

Skin and Subcutaneous Tissue Disorders Rashes including maculopapular and erythematous rashes, exfoliative dermatitis, erythema multiforme, Steven-Johnson syndrome, toxic epidermal necrolysis, photosensitivity skin reactions (see 'Special warnings and precautions for use' section) and photo-onycholysis.

Superinfection As with all antibiotics, overgrowth of non-susceptible organisms may cause candidiasis, glossitis, staphylococcal enterocolitis, pseudomembranous colitis (with *Clostridium difficile* overgrowth) and inflammatory lesions (with candidal overgrowth) in the anogenital region. Similarly there have been reports for products in the tetracycline class of stomatitis and vaginitis.

Urinary system Increased blood urea. (See 'Special warnings and precautions for use' section.)

Other When given over prolonged periods, tetracyclines have been reported to produce brown-black microscopic discolouration of thyroid tissue. No abnormalities of thyroid function are known to occur.

Tetracyclines may cause discoloration of teeth and enamel hypoplasia, but usually only after long-term use.

4.9 Overdose

Acute overdosage with antibiotics is rare. In the event of overdosage discontinue medication. Gastric lavage plus appropriate supportive treatment is indicated.

Dialysis does not alter serum half-life and thus would not be of benefit in treating cases of overdosage.

5. PHARMACOLOGICAL PROPERTIES

5.1 Pharmacodynamic properties

Vibramycin is primarily bacteriostatic and is believed to exert its antimicrobial effect by the inhibition of protein synthesis. Vibramycin is active against a wide range of Gram-positive and Gram-negative bacteria and certain other micro-organisms.

5.2 Pharmacokinetic properties

Tetracyclines are readily absorbed and are bound to plasma proteins in varying degrees. They are concentrated by the liver in the bile and excreted in the urine and faeces at high concentrations and in a biologically active form. Doxycycline is virtually completely absorbed after oral administration. Studies reported to date indicate that the absorption of doxycycline, unlike certain other tetracyclines, is not notably influenced by the ingestion of food or milk. Following a 200 mg dose, normal adult volunteers averaged peak serum levels of 2.6 micrograms/ml of doxycycline at 2 hours decreasing to 1.45 micrograms/ml at 24 hours. Doxycycline has a high degree of lipid solubility and a low affinity for calcium. It is highly stable in normal human serum. Doxycycline will not degrade into an epianhydro form.

6. PHARMACEUTICAL PARTICULARS

6.1 List of excipients

Vibramycin-D Dispersible tablets: Anhydrous colloidal silica Ph.Eur., microcrystalline cellulose Ph.Eur. and Magnesium Stearate Ph.Eur.

6.2 Incompatibilities

None stated.

6.3 Shelf life

Vibramycin-D Dispersible tablets: 48 months

6.4 Special precautions for storage

Store below 25°C.

6.5 Nature and contents of container

Packs of 8 Tablets. Aluminium/PVC blister strips, a single strip of 8 tablets in a carton box.

6.6 Special precautions for disposal and other handling

No special requirements.

7. MARKETING AUTHORISATION HOLDER

Pfizer Limited

Ramsgate Road

Sandwich

Kent CT13 9NJ

United Kingdom

8. MARKETING AUTHORISATION NUMBER(S)

00057/0188

9. DATE OF FIRST AUTHORISATION/RENEWAL OF THE AUTHORISATION

29/10/00, 29/10/2005, 15/12/2008

10. DATE OF REVISION OF THE TEXT

December 2008

VM9_0

Victanyl 100 micrograms/hour Transdermal Patch (Actavis UK Ltd)

(Actavis UK Ltd)

1. NAME OF THE MEDICINAL PRODUCT

Victanyl 100 micrograms/hour Transdermal Patch

fentanyl

2. QUALITATIVE AND QUANTITATIVE COMPOSITION

Each patch releases 100 micrograms fentanyl per hour. Each patch of 30 cm2 contains 16.5 mg fentanyl.

For a full list of excipients, see section 6.1.

3. PHARMACEUTICAL FORM

Transdermal patch

Transparent and colourless patch with blue imprint on the backing foil: "fentanyl 100 µg/h".

4. CLINICAL PARTICULARS

4.1 Therapeutic indications

The product is indicated in severe chronic pain which can be adequately managed only with opioid analgesics.

4.2 Posology and method of administration

The dosing is individual and based on the patient's opioid history and takes into account:

• the possible development of tolerance,

• the current general condition, the medical status of the patient, and

• the degree of severity of the disorder.

The required fentanyl dosage is adjusted individually and should be assessed regularly after each administration.

Patients receiving opioid treatment for the first time

Patches with a release rate of 12.5 micrograms/hour are available and should be used for initial dosing. In very elderly or weak patients, it is not recommended to initiate an opioid treatment with *Victanyl*, due to their known susceptibility to opioid treatments. In these cases, it would be preferable to initiate a treatment with low doses of immediate release morphine and to prescribe *Victanyl* after determination of the optimal dosage.

Switching from other opioids

When changing over from oral or parenteral opioids to fentanyl treatment, the initial dosage should be calculated as follows:

1. The quantity of analgesics required over the last 24 hours should be determined.

2. The obtained sum should be converted to correspond the oral morphine dosage using Table 1.

3. The corresponding fentanyl dosage should be determined as follows:

a) using Table 2 for patients who have a need for opioid rotation (conversion ratio of oral morphine to transdermal fentanyl equal to150:1)

b) using Table 3 for patients on stable and well tolerated opioid therapy (conversion ratio of oral morphine to transdermal fentanyl equal to 100:1)

Table 1: Equianalgesic potency conversion

All dosages given in the table are equivalent in analgesic effect to 10 mg parenteral morphine.

	Equianalgesic doses (mg)	
Active substance	**Parenteral (im)**	**Oral**
Morphine	10	30-40
Hydromorphone	1.5	7.5
Oxycodone	10-15	20-30
Methadone	10	20
Levorphanol	2	4
Oxymorphine	1	10 (rectal)
Diamorphine	5	60
Pethidine	75	-
Codeine	-	200
Buprenorphine	0.4	0.8 (sublingual)
Ketobemidone	10	20-30

Table 2: Recommended __initial dose__ of transdermal fentanyl based on daily oral morphine dose (for patients who have a need for opioid rotation)

Oral morphine dose (mg/24 h)	Transdermal fentanyl release (micrograms/h)
< 44	12.5
45-134	25
135-224	50
225-314	75
315-404	100
405-494	125
495-584	150
585-674	175
675-764	200
765-854	225
855-944	250
945-1034	275
1035-1124	300

Table 3: Recommended __initial dose__ of transdermal fentanyl based on daily oral morphine dose (for patients on stable and well tolerated opioid therapy)

Oral morphine dose (mg/24 h)	Transdermal fentanyl release (micrograms/h)
< 60	12.5
60-89	25
90-149	50
150-209	75
210-269	100
270-329	125
330-389	150
390-449	175
450-509	200
510-569	225
570-629	250
630-689	275
690-749	300

By combining several transdermal patches, a fentanyl release rate of over 100 micrograms/h can be achieved.

The initial evaluation of the maximum analgesic effect of *Fentanyl transdermal patch* should not be made before the patch has been worn for 24 hours. This is due to the gradual increase in serum fentanyl concentrations during the first 24 hours after application of the patch.

In the first 12 hours after changing to *Fentanyl transdermal patch* the patient continues to receive the previous analgesic at the previous dose; over the next 12 hours this analgesic is administered according to need.

Dose titration and maintenance therapy

The patch should be replaced every 72 hours. The dose should be titrated individually until analgesic efficacy is attained. In patients who experience a marked decrease in the period 48-72 hours after application, replacement of fentanyl after 48 hours may be necessary.

Patches with a release rate of 12.5 microgram/hour are available and are appropriate for dose titration in the lower dosage area. If analgesia is insufficient at the end of the initial application period, the dose may be increased after 3 days until the desired effect is obtained for each patient. Additional dose adjustment should normally be performed in 25 micrograms/hour increments, although the supplementary analgesic requirements and pain status of the patient should be taken into account. Patients may require periodic supplemental doses of a short-acting analgesic for breakthrough pain. Additional or alternative methods of analgesia or alternative administration of opioids should be considered when the *Fentanyl transdermal patch* dose exceeds 300 micrograms/hour.

Withdrawal symptoms have been reported when changing from long-term treatment with Morphine to transdermal fentanyl despite adequate analgesic efficacy. In case of withdrawal symptoms it is recommended to treat those with short-acting Morphine in low doses.

Changing or ending therapy

If discontinuation of the patch is necessary, any replacement with other opioids should be gradual, starting at a low dose and increasing slowly. This is because fentanyl levels fall gradually after the patch is removed; it takes at least 17 hours for the fentanyl serum concentration to decrease by 50%. As a general rule, the discontinuation of opioid analgesia should be gradual, in order to prevent withdrawal symptoms (nausea, vomiting, diarrhoea, anxiety and muscular tremor). Tables 2 and 3 should not be used to switch from transdermal fentanyl to a morphine treatment.

Method of administration

Directly after removal from the pack and the release liner, *Fentanyl transdermal patch* is applied to a non-hairy area of skin on the upper body (chest, back, upper arm). To remove hair, scissors should be used instead of razors.

Prior to application, the skin should be carefully washed with clean water (no cleaning agents) and thoroughly dried. The transdermal patch is then applied using slight pressure with the palm of the hand for approximately 10-30 seconds. The skin area to which the patch is applied should be free of microlesions (e.g. due to irradiation or shaving) and skin irritation.

As the transdermal patch is protected by an outer waterproof backing film, it can also be worn while showering.

Occasionally, additional adhesion of the patch may be required.

If progressive dose increases are made, the active surface area required may reach a point where no further increase is possible.

Duration of administration

The patch should be changed after 72 hours. If an earlier change becomes necessary in individual cases, no change should be made before 48 hours have elapsed, otherwise a rise in mean fentanyl concentrations may occur. A new skin area must be selected for each application. A period of 7 days should be allowed to elapse before applying a new patch to the same area of skin. The analgesic effect may persist for some time after removal of the transdermal patch.

If traces of the transdermal patch remain on the skin after its removal, these can be cleaned off using copious amounts of soap and water. No alcohol or other solvents may be used for cleaning, as these may penetrate the skin due to the effect of the patch.

Paediatric population

The experience in children under 12 years of age is limited. *Victanyl* should not be used in this population.

Use in elderly patients

Elderly should be observed carefully and the dose reduced if necessary (see sections 4.4 and 5.2).

Hepatic and renal impairment

Patients with hepatic or renal impairment should be observed carefully and the dose reduced if necessary (see section 4.4).

4.3 Contraindications

- Hypersensitivity to the active substance or to any of the excipients.

- Acute or postoperative pain, since dosage titration is not possible during short-term use.

- Severe impairment of the central nervous system.

4.4 Special warnings and precautions for use

The product should be used only as part of an integrated treatment of pain in cases where the patient is adequately assessed medically, socially and psychologically.

Treatment with *Fentanyl transdermal patch* should only be initiated by an experienced physician familiar with the pharmacokinetics of Fentanyl transdermal patches and the risk for severe hypoventilation.

After exhibiting a serious adverse reaction a patient should be monitored for 24 hours following removal of a transdermal patch due to the half life of fentanyl (see section 5.2).

In chronic non-cancer pain, it might be preferable to initiate the treatment with immediate-release strong opoids (e.g. morphine) and to prescribe fentanyl transdermal patch after determination of the efficacy and the optimal dosage of the strong opioid.

The transdermal patch should not be cut, since no information is available on the quality, efficacy and safety of such divided patches.

If higher dosages than 500 mg morphine-equivalent are needed, a reassessment of opioid-therapy is recommended.

The most common adverse reactions following administration at usual doses are drowsiness, confusion, nausea, vomiting and constipation. The first of these are transient and their cause should be investigated if symptoms persist. Constipation, on the other hand, does not stop if treatment continues. All of these effects can be expected and should, therefore, be anticipated in order to optimise treatment, especially constipation. Corrective treatment may often be required (see section 4.8).

The concomitant use of buprenorphine, nalbuphine or pentazocine is not recommended (see also section 4.5).

Breakthrough pain

Studies have shown that almost all patients, despite treatment with a fentanyl patch, require supplemental medication with potent rapid-release drugs to arrest breakthrough pain.

Respiratory depression

As with all potent opioids some patients may experience respiratory depression with the *Fentanyl transdermal patch*, and patients must be observed for this effect. Respiratory depression may persist beyond the removal of the patch. The incidence of respiratory depression increases as the fentanyl dose is increased. CNS active active substances may worsen the respiratory depression (see sections 4.5).

In patients with existing respiratory depression, fentanyl should only be used with caution and at a lower dose.

Chronic pulmonary disease

In patients with chronic obstructive or other pulmonary diseases fentanyl may have more severe adverse reactions, in such patients opioids may decrease respiratory drive and increase airway resistance.

Drug dependence

Tolerance and physical and psychological dependence may develop upon repeated administration of opioids, but is rare in treatment of cancer related pain.

Increased intracranial pressure

Fentanyl transdermal patch should be used with caution in patients who may be particularly susceptible to the intracranial effects of CO_2 retention such as those with evidence of increased intracranial pressure, impaired consciousness or coma.

Cardiac disease

Opioids may cause hypotonia, especially in patients with hypovolemia. Caution should therefore be taken in treatment of patients with hypotonia and/or patients with hypovolemia. Fentanyl may produce bradycardia. *Fentanyl transdermal patch* should therefore not be administered to patients with bradyarrhythmias.

Impaired liver function

Fentanyl is metabolised to inactive metabolites in the liver, so patients with hepatic disease might have a delayed elimination. Patients with hepatic impairment should be observed carefully and the dose reduced if necessary.

Renal impairment

Less than 10 % of fentanyl is excreted unchanged by the kidneys, and unlike morphine, there are no known active metabolites eliminated by the kidneys. Data obtained with intravenous fentanyl in patients with renal failure suggest that the volume of distribution of fentanyl may be changed by dialysis. This may affect serum concentrations. If patients with renal impairment receive transdermal fentanyl they should be observed carefully for signs of fentanyl toxicity and the dose reduced if necessary.

Patients with fever/external heat

Patients who develop fever should be monitored for opioid adverse reactions since significant increases in body temperature can potentially increase fentanyl absorption rate. The patch application site should not be exposed to heat from external heat sources, e.g. sauna.

Elderly patients

Data from intravenous studies with fentanyl suggest that the elderly patients may have reduced clearance, a prolonged half-life. Moreover elderly patients may be more sensitive to the active substance than younger patients. However, studies of Fentanyl transdermal patch in elderly patients demonstrated fentanyl pharmacokinetics which did not differ significantly from young patients although serum concentrations tended to be higher. Elderly or cachectic patients should be observed carefully and the dose reduced if necessary.

Paediatric patients

Due to limited experience in children under 12 years of age, *Victanyl* should be used in this age group only after careful consideration has been given to the benefit versus risk ratio.

Lactation

As fentanyl is excreted into breast milk, lactation should be discontinued under treatment with *Victanyl* (see also section 4.6).

Patients with myasthenia gravis

Non-epileptic (myo)clonic reactions can occur. Caution should be exercised when treating patients with myasthenia gravis.

Interactions

Combination with barbituric acid derivatives, buprenorphine, nalbuphine and pentazocine should in general be avoided (see section 4.5).

4.5 Interaction with other medicinal products and other forms of interaction

The concomitant use of barbituric acid derivatives should be avoided, since the respiratory depressing effect of fentanyl may be increased.

The concomitant use of buprenorphine, nalbuphine or pentazocine is not recommended. They have high affinity to opioid receptors with relatively low intrinsic activity and therefore partially antagonise the analgesic effect of fentanyl and may induce withdrawal symptoms in opioid dependant patients (see also section 4.4).

The concomitant use of other CNS depressants, may produce additive depressant effects and hypoventilation, hypotension as well as profound sedation or coma may occur. The CNS depressants mentioned above include:

- opioids
- anxiolytics and tranquilizers
- hypnotics
- general anaesthetics
- phenothiazines
- skeletal muscle relaxants
- sedating antihistamines
- alcoholic beverages

Therefore, the use of any of the above mentioned concomitant medicinal products and active substances require observation of the patient.

MAO-inhibitors have been reported to increase the effect of narcotic analgesics, especially in patients with cardiac failure. Therefore, fentanyl should not be used within 14 days after discontinuation of treatment with MAO-inhibitors.

Fentanyl, a high clearance active substance, is rapidly and extensively metabolised mainly by CYP3A4.

Itraconazole (a potent CYP3A4 inhibitor) at 200 mg/day given orally for four days had no significant effect on the pharmacokinetics of intravenous fentanyl. Increased plasma concentrations were, however, observed in individual subjects. Oral administration of ritonavir (one of the most potent CYP3A4 inhibitors) reduced the clearance of intravenous fentanyl by two thirds and doubled the half-life. Concomitant use of potent CYP3A4-inhibitors (e.g. ritonavir) with transdermally administered fentanyl may result in increased plasma concentrations of fentanyl. This may increase or prolong both the therapeutic effects and the adverse reactions, which may cause severe respiratory depression. In such cases increased care and observation of the patient should be undertaken. Combined use of ritonavir or other potent CYP3A4-inhibitors with transdermal fentanyl is not recommended, unless the patient is carefully observed.

4.6 Pregnancy and lactation

The safety of fentanyl in pregnancy has not been established. Studies in animals have shown reproductive toxicity (see section 5.3). The potential risk for humans is unknown. Fentanyl should only be used during pregnancy when clearly necessary.

Long-term treatment during pregnancy may cause withdrawal symptoms in the infant.

It is advised not to use fentanyl during labour and delivery (including caesarean section) since fentanyl passes the placenta and may cause respiratory depression in the foetus or in the infant.

Fentanyl is excreted into breast milk and may cause sedation and respiratory depression in the breast-fed infant. Lactation should therefore be discontinued for at least 72 hours after the removal of *Victanyl* (see also section 4.4).

4.7 Effects on ability to drive and use machines

Victanyl has major influence on the ability to drive and use machines. This has to be expected especially at the beginning of treatment, at any change of dosage as well as in connection with alcohol or tranquilizers. Patients stabilized on a specific dosage will not necessarily be restricted. Therefore, patients should consult their physician as to whether driving or use of machines is permitted.

4.8 Undesirable effects

The following frequencies are used for the description of the occurrence of adverse reactions:

Very common ($\geq$1/10), Common ($\geq$1/100, $<$1/10), Uncommon ($\geq$1/1000, $<$1/100), Rare ($\geq$1/10,000, $<$1/1000), Very rare ($<$1/10,000)

The most serious undesirable effect of fentanyl is respiratory depression.

Cardiac disorders

Uncommon: tachycardia, bradycardia.

Rare: arrhythmia.

Nervous system disorders

Very common: headache, dizziness.

Uncommon: tremor, paraesthesia, speech disorder.

Very rare: ataxia, seizures (including clonic and grand mal seizures).

Eye disorders

Very rare: amblyopia.

Respiratory, thoracic and mediastinal disorders

Uncommon: dyspnoea, hypoventilation.

Very rare: respiratory depression, apnoea.

Gastrointestinal disorders

Very common: nausea, vomiting, constipation.

Common: xerostomia, dyspepsia.

Uncommon: diarrhoea.

Rare: hiccup.

Very rare: painful flatulence, ileus.

Renal and urinary disorders

Uncommon: urinary retention.

Very rare: cystalgia, oliguria.

Skin and subcutaneous tissue disorders

Very common: sweating, pruritus.

Common: skin reactions on the application site.

Uncommon: exanthema, erythema.

Rash, erythema and pruritus will usually disappear within one day after the patch has been removed.

Vascular disorders

Uncommon: hypertension, hypotension.

Rare: vasodilatation.

General disorders

Rare: oedema, cold feeling.

Immune system disorders

Very rare: anaphylaxis.

Psychiatric disorders

Very common: somnolence.

Common: sedation, nervousness, loss of appetite.

Uncommon: euphoria, amnesia, insomnia, hallucinations, agitation.

Very rare: delusional ideas, states of excitement, asthenia, depression, anxiety, confusion, sexual dysfunction, withdrawal symptoms.

Other undesirable effects

Not known (cannot be estimated from the available data): Long-term use of fentanyl can lead to development of tolerance and physical and psychological dependence. After switching from previously prescribed opioid analgesics to *Victanyl* or after abrupt discontinuation of therapy patients may show opioid withdrawal symptoms (for instance: nausea, vomiting, diarrhoea, anxiety and shivering).

4.9 Overdose

Symptoms

The symptoms of fentanyl overdose are an extension of its pharmacological actions, e.g. lethargy, coma, respiratory depression with Cheyne-Stokes respiration and/or cyanosis. Other symptoms may be hypothermia, decreased muscle tonus, bradycardia, hypotonia. Signs of toxicity are deep sedation, ataxia, miosis, convulsions and respiratory depression, which is the main symptom.

Treatment

For management of respiratory depression immediate countermeasures should be started, including removing the patch and physically or verbally stimulating the patient. These actions can be followed by administration of a specific opioid antagonist such as naloxone.

A starting dose of 0.4-2 mg naloxone hydrochloride i.v. is recommended for adults. If needed, a similar dose can be given every 2 or 3 minutes, or be administered as continued infusion as 2 mg in 500 ml sodium chloride 9 mg/ml (0.9 %) solution for injection or glucose 50 mg/ml (5 %) solution. The infusion rate should be adjusted according to previous bolus injections and the individual response of the patient. If intravenous administration is impossible, naloxone hydrochloride can also be given intramuscularly or subcutaneously. Following intramuscular or subcutaneous administration the onset of action will be slower compared with intravenous administration. Intramuscular administration will give a more prolonged effect than intravenous administration. Respiratory depression due to overdose can persist longer than the effect of the opioid antagonist. Reversing the narcotic effect can give rise to acute pain and release of catecholamines. Intensive care unit treatment is important, if required by the patient's clinical condition. If severe or persistent hypotension occurs, hypovolemia should be considered, and the condition should be managed with appropriate parenteral fluid therapy.

5. PHARMACOLOGICAL PROPERTIES

5.1 Pharmacodynamic properties

Pharmacotherapeutic group: opioids; Phenylpiperidine derivatives

ATC code: N02AB03

Fentanyl is an opioid analgesic which interacts predominantly with the μ-receptor. Its principal therapeutic effects are analgesia and sedation. The serum concentrations of fentanyl that cause a minimal analgesic effect in opioid-naive patients fluctuate between 0.3–1.5 ng/ml; an increased incidence of adverse effects is observed if serum levels exceed 2 ng/ml.

Both the lowest effective fentanyl concentration and the concentration causing adverse reactions will increase with the development of increasing tolerance. The tendency to develop tolerance varies considerably between individuals.

5.2 Pharmacokinetic properties

Following administration of *Fentanyl transdermal patch*, fentanyl is continuously absorbed through the skin over a period of 72 hours. Due to the polymer matrix and the diffusion of fentanyl through the skin layers, the release rate remains relatively constant.

Absorption

After the first application of *Fentanyl transdermal patch*, serum fentanyl concentrations increase gradually, generally levelling off between 12 and 24 hours, and remaining relatively constant for the remainder of the 72-hour application period. The serum fentanyl concentrations attained are dependant on the Fentanyl transdermal patch size. For all practical purposes by the second 72-hour application, a steady state serum concentration is reached and is maintained during subsequent applications of a patch of the same size.

Distribution

The plasma protein binding for fentanyl is 84 %.

Biotransformation

Fentanyl is metabolized primarily in the liver via CYP3A4. The major metabolite, norfentanyl, is inactive.

Elimination

When treatment with Fentanyl transdermal patches is withdrawn, serum fentanyl concentrations decline gradually, falling approximately 50 % in 13-22 hours in adults or 22-25 hours in children, respectively. Continued absorption of fentanyl from the skin accounts for a slower reduction in serum concentration than is seen after an intravenous infusion.

Around 75 % of fentanyl is excreted into the urine, mostly as metabolites, with less than 10 % as unchanged drug. About 9 % of the dose is recovered in the faeces, primarily as metabolites.

Pharmacokinetics in special groups

Elderly and debilitated patients may have reduced clearance of fentanyl leading to prolonged terminal half life. In patients with renal or hepatic impairment, clearance of fentanyl may be altered because of changes of plasma proteins and metabolic clearance resulting in increased serum concentrations.

5.3 Preclinical safety data

Non-clinical data reveal no special hazard for humans based on conventional studies of safety pharmacology, repeated dose toxicity and genotoxicity.

Animal studies have shown reduced fertility and increased mortality in rat foetuses. Teratogenic effects have, however, not been demonstrated.

Long-term carcinogenicity studies have not been performed.

6. PHARMACEUTICAL PARTICULARS

6.1 List of excipients

Adhesive layer

Polyacrylate adhesive layer

Backing film

Polypropylene foil

Blue printing ink

Release liner

Polyethylene terephthalate foil (siliconised)

6.2 Incompatibilities

Not applicable.

6.3 Shelf life

18 months

6.4 Special precautions for storage

Do not store above 25°C.

6.5 Nature and contents of container

Each transdermal patch is packed in a separate sachet. The Composite foil containing the following layers from outside to inside: coated Kraft paper, low density polyethylene foil, aluminium foil, Surlyn

Pack containing 3 transdermal patches

Pack containing 4 transdermal patches

Pack containing 5 transdermal patches

Pack containing 8 transdermal patches

Pack containing 10 transdermal patches

Pack containing 16 transdermal patches

Pack containing 20 transdermal patches

Not all pack sizes may be marketed.

6.6 Special precautions for disposal and other handling

High quantities of fentanyl remain in the transdermal patches even after use. Used transdermal patches should be folded with the adhesive surfaces inwards and discarded or whenever possible returned to the pharmacy. Any unused medicinal product should be discarded or returned to the pharmacy.

7. MARKETING AUTHORISATION HOLDER

Actavis Group PTC ehf

Reykjavikurvegur 76-78

220 IS Hafnarfjordur

Iceland

8. MARKETING AUTHORISATION NUMBER(S)

PL 30306/0134

9. DATE OF FIRST AUTHORISATION/RENEWAL OF THE AUTHORISATION

27/06/08

10. DATE OF REVISION OF THE TEXT

09/07/08

11. DOSIMETRY

Not applicable.

12 INSTRUCTIONS FOR PREPARATION OF RADIOPHARMACEUTICALS (IF APPLICABLE)

Not applicable.

Victanyl 25 micrograms/hour Transdermal Patch (Actavis UK Ltd)

(Actavis UK Ltd)

1. NAME OF THE MEDICINAL PRODUCT

Victanyl 25 micrograms/hour Transdermal Patch

fentanyl

2. QUALITATIVE AND QUANTITATIVE COMPOSITION

Each patch releases 25 micrograms fentanyl per hour. Each patch of 7.5 cm^2 contains 4.125 mg fentanyl.

For a full list of excipients, see section 6.1.

3. PHARMACEUTICAL FORM

Transdermal patch

Transparent and colourless patch with blue imprint on the backing foil: "fentanyl 25 μg/h".

4. CLINICAL PARTICULARS

4.1 Therapeutic indications

The product is indicated in severe chronic pain which can be adequately managed only with opioid analgesics.

4.2 Posology and method of administration

The dosing is individual and based on the patient's opioid history and takes into account:

- the possible development of tolerance,
- the current general condition, the medical status of the patient, and
- the degree of severity of the disorder.

The required fentanyl dosage is adjusted individually and should be assessed regularly after each administration.

Patients receiving opioid treatment for the first time

Patches with a release rate of 12.5 micrograms/hour are available and should be used for initial dosing. In very elderly or weak patients, it is not recommended to initiate an opioid treatment with *Victanyl*, due to their known susceptibility to opioid treatments. In these cases, it would be preferable to initiate a treatment with low doses of immediate release morphine and to prescribe *Victanyl* after determination of the optimal dosage.

Switching from other opioids

When changing over from oral or parenteral opioids to fentanyl treatment, the initial dosage should be calculated as follows:

1. The quantity of analgesics required over the last 24 hours should be determined.

2. The obtained sum should be converted to correspond the oral morphine dosage using Table 1.

3. The corresponding fentanyl dosage should be determined as follows:

a) using Table 2 for patients who have a need for opioid rotation (conversion ratio of oral morphine to transdermal fentanyl equal to150:1)

b) using Table 3 for patients on stable and well tolerated opioid therapy (conversion ratio of oral morphine to transdermal fentanyl equal to 100:1)

Table 1: Equianalgesic potency conversion

All dosages given in the table are equivalent in analgesic effect to 10 mg parenteral morphine.

	Equianalgesic doses (mg)	
Active substance	**Parenteral (im)**	**Oral**
Morphine	10	30-40
Hydromorphone	1.5	7.5
Oxycodone	10-15	20-30
Methadone	10	20
Levorphanol	2	4
Oxymorphine	1	10 (rectal)
Diamorphine	5	60
Pethidine	75	
Codeine	-	200
Buprenorphine	0.4	0.8 (sublingual)
Ketobemidone	10	20-30

Table 2: Recommended initial dose of transdermal fentanyl based on daily oral morphine dose (for patients who have a need for opioid rotation)

Oral morphine dose (mg/24h)	Transdermal fentanyl release (micrograms/h)
< 44	12.5
45-134	25
135-224	50
225-314	75
315-404	100
405-494	125
495-584	150
585-674	175
675-764	200
765-854	225
855-944	250
945-1034	275
1035-1124	300

Table 3: Recommended initial dose of transdermal fentanyl based on daily oral morphine dose (for patients on stable and well tolerated opioid therapy)

Oral morphine dose (mg/24 h)	Transdermal fentanyl release (micrograms/h)
< 60	12.5
60-89	25
90-149	50
150-209	75
210-269	100
270-329	125
330-389	150
390-449	175
450-509	200
510-569	225
570-629	250
630-689	275
690-749	300

By combining several transdermal patches, a fentanyl release rate of over 100 micrograms/h can be achieved.

The initial evaluation of the maximum analgesic effect of *Fentanyl transdermal patch* should not be made before the patch has been worn for 24 hours. This is due to the gradual increase in serum fentanyl concentrations during the first 24 hours after application of the patch.

In the first 12 hours after changing to *Fentanyl transdermal patch* the patient continues to receive the previous analgesic at the previous dose; over the next 12 hours this analgesic is administered according to need.

Dose titration and maintenance therapy

The patch should be replaced every 72 hours. The dose should be titrated individually until analgesic efficacy is attained. In patients who experience a marked decrease in the period 48-72 hours after application, replacement of fentanyl after 48 hours may be necessary.

Patches with a release rate of 12.5 micrograms/hour are available and are appropriate for dose titration in the lower dosage area. If analgesia is insufficient at the end of the initial application period, the dose may be increased after 3 days until the desired effect is obtained for each patient. Additional dose adjustment should normally be performed in 25 micrograms/hour increments, although the supplementary analgesic requirements and pain status of the patient should be taken into account. Patients may require periodic supplemental doses of a short-acting analgesic for breakthrough pain. Additional or alternative methods of analgesia or alternative administration of opioids should be considered when the *Fentanyl transdermal patch* dose exceeds 300 micrograms/hour.

Withdrawal symptoms have been reported when changing from long-term treatment with Morphine to transdermal fentanyl despite adequate analgesic efficacy. In case of withdrawal symptoms it is recommended to treat those with short-acting Morphine in low doses.

Changing or ending therapy

If discontinuation of the patch is necessary, any replacement with other opioids should be gradual, starting at a low dose and increasing slowly. This is because fentanyl levels fall gradually after the patch is removed; it takes at least 17 hours for the fentanyl serum concentration to decrease by 50%. As a general rule, the discontinuation of opioid analgesia should be gradual, in order to prevent withdrawal symptoms (nausea, vomiting, diarrhoea, anxiety and muscular tremor). Tables 2 and 3 should not be used to switch from transdermal fentanyl to a morphine treatment.

Method of administration

Directly after removal from the pack and the release liner, *Fentanyl transdermal patch* is applied to a non-hairy area of skin on the upper body (chest, back, upper arm). To remove hair, scissors should be used instead of razors.

Prior to application, the skin should be carefully washed with clean water (no cleaning agents) and thoroughly dried. The transdermal patch is then applied using slight pressure with the palm of the hand for approximately 10-30 seconds. The skin area to which the patch is applied should be free of microlesions (e.g. due to irradiation or shaving) and skin irritation.

As the transdermal patch is protected by an outer waterproof backing film, it can also be worn while showering.

Occasionally, additional adhesion of the patch may be required.

If progressive dose increases are made, the active surface area required may reach a point where no further increase is possible.

Duration of administration

The patch should be changed after 72 hours. If an earlier change becomes necessary in individual cases, no change should be made before 48 hours have elapsed, otherwise a rise in mean fentanyl concentrations may occur. A new skin area must be selected for each application. A period of 7 days should be allowed to elapse before applying a new patch to the same area of skin. The analgesic effect may persist for some time after removal of the transdermal patch.

If traces of the transdermal patch remain on the skin after its removal, these can be cleaned off using copious amounts of soap and water. No alcohol or other solvents may be used for cleaning, as these may penetrate the skin due to the effect of the patch.

Paediatric population

The experience in children under 12 years of age is limited. *Victanyl* should not be used in this population.

Use in elderly patients

Elderly should be observed carefully and the dose reduced if necessary (see sections 4.4 and 5.2).

Hepatic and renal impairment

Patients with hepatic or renal impairment should be observed carefully and the dose reduced if necessary (see section 4.4).

4.3 Contraindications

- Hypersensitivity to the active substance or to any of the excipients.

- Acute or postoperative pain, since dosage titration is not possible during short-term use.

- Severe impairment of the central nervous system.

4.4 Special warnings and precautions for use

The product should be used only as part of an integrated treatment of pain in cases where the patient is adequately assessed medically, socially and psychologically.

Treatment with *Fentanyl transdermal patch* should only be initiated by an experienced physician familiar with the pharmacokinetics of Fentanyl transdermal patches and the risk for severe hypoventilation.

After exhibiting a serious adverse reaction a patient should be monitored for 24 hours following removal of a transdermal patch due to the half life of fentanyl (see section 5.2).

In chronic non-cancer pain, it might be preferable to initiate the treatment with immediate-release strong opoids (e.g. morphine) and to prescribe fentanyl transdermal patch after determination of the efficacy and the optimal dosage of the strong opioid.

The transdermal patch should not be cut, since no information is available on the quality, efficacy and safety of such divided patches.

If higher dosages than 500 mg morphine-equivalent are needed, a reassessment of opioid-therapy is recommended.

The most common adverse reactions following administration at usual doses are drowsiness, confusion, nausea, vomiting and constipation. The first of these are transient and their cause should be investigated if symptoms persist. Constipation, on the other hand, does not stop if treatment continues. All of these effects can be expected and should, therefore, be anticipated in order to optimise treatment, especially constipation. Corrective treatment may often be required (see section 4.8).

The concomitant use of buprenorphine, nalbuphine or pentazocine is not recommended (see also section 4.5).

Breakthrough pain

Studies have shown that almost all patients, despite treatment with a fentanyl patch, require supplemental medication with potent rapid-release drugs to arrest breakthrough pain.

Respiratory depression

As with all potent opioids some patients may experience respiratory depression with the *Fentanyl transdermal patch*, and patients must be observed for this effect. Respiratory depression may persist beyond the removal of the patch. The incidence of respiratory depression increases as the fentanyl dose is increased. CNS active substances may worsen the respiratory depression (see sections 4.5).

In patients with existing respiratory depression, fentanyl should only be used with caution and at a lower dose.

Chronic pulmonary disease

In patients with chronic obstructive or other pulmonary diseases fentanyl may have more severe adverse reactions, in such patients opioids may decrease respiratory drive and increase airway resistance.

Drug dependence

Tolerance and physical and psychological dependence may develop upon repeated administration of opioids, but is rare in treatment of cancer related pain.

Increased intracranial pressure

Fentanyl transdermal patch should be used with caution in patients who may be particularly susceptible to the intracranial effects of CO_2 retention such as those with evidence of increased intracranial pressure, impaired consciousness or coma.

Cardiac disease

Opioids may cause hypotonia, especially in patients with hypovolemia. Caution should therefore be taken in treatment of patients with hypotonia and/or patients with hypovolemia. Fentanyl may produce bradycardia. *Fentanyl transdermal patch* should therefore not be administered to patients with bradyarrhythmias.

Impaired liver function

Fentanyl is metabolised to inactive metabolites in the liver, so patients with hepatic disease might have a delayed elimination. Patients with hepatic impairment should be observed carefully and the dose reduced if necessary.

Renal impairment

Less than 10 % of fentanyl is excreted unchanged by the kidneys, and unlike morphine, there are no known active metabolites eliminated by the kidneys. Data obtained with intravenous fentanyl in patients with renal failure suggest that the volume of distribution of fentanyl may be changed by dialysis. This may affect serum concentrations. If patients with renal impairment receive transdermal fentanyl they should be observed carefully for signs of fentanyl toxicity and the dose reduced if necessary.

Patients with fever/external heat

Patients who develop fever should be monitored for opioid adverse reactions since significant increases in body temperature can potentially increase fentanyl absorption rate. The patch application site should not be exposed to heat from external heat sources, e.g. sauna.

Elderly patients

Data from intravenous studies with fentanyl suggest that the elderly patients may have reduced clearance, a prolonged half-life. Moreover elderly patients may be more sensitive to the active substance than younger patients. However, studies of Fentanyl transdermal patch in elderly patients demonstrated fentanyl pharmacokinetics which did not differ significantly from young patients although serum concentrations tended to be higher. Elderly or cachectic patients should be observed carefully and the dose reduced if necessary.

Paediatric patients

Due to limited experience in children under 12 years of age, *Victanyl* should be used in this age group only after careful consideration has been given to the benefit versus risk ratio.

Lactation

As fentanyl is excreted into breast milk, lactation should be discontinued under treatment with *Victanyl* (see also section 4.6).

Patients with myasthenia gravis

Non-epileptic (myo)clonic reactions can occur. Caution should be exercised when treating patients with myasthenia gravis.

Interactions

Combination with barbituric acid derivatives, buprenorphine, nalbuphine and pentazocine should in general be avoided (see section 4.5).

4.5 Interaction with other medicinal products and other forms of interaction

The concomitant use of barbituric acid derivatives should be avoided, since the respiratory depressing effect of fentanyl may be increased.

The concomitant use of buprenorphine, nalbuphine or pentazocine is not recommended. They have high affinity to opioid receptors with relatively low intrinsic activity and therefore partially antagonise the analgesic effect of fentanyl and may induce withdrawal symptoms in opioid dependant patients (see also section 4.4).

The concomitant use of other CNS depressants, may produce additive depressant effects and hypoventilation, hypotension as well as profound sedation or coma may occur. The CNS depressants mentioned above include:

- opioids
- anxiolytics and tranquilizers
- hypnotics
- general anaesthetics
- phenothiazines
- skeletal muscle relaxants
- sedating antihistamines
- alcoholic beverages

Therefore, the use of any of the above mentioned concomitant medicinal products and active substances require observation of the patient.

MAO-inhibitors have been reported to increase the effect of narcotic analgesics, especially in patients with cardiac failure. Therefore, fentanyl should not be used within 14 days after discontinuation of treatment with MAO-inhibitors.

Fentanyl, a high clearance active substance, is rapidly and extensively metabolised mainly by CYP3A4.

Itraconazole (a potent CYP3A4 inhibitor) at 200 mg/day given orally for four days had no significant effect on the pharmacokinetics of intravenous fentanyl. Increased plasma concentrations were, however, observed in individual subjects. Oral administration of ritonavir (one of the most potent CYP3A4 inhibitors) reduced the clearance of intravenous fentanyl by two thirds and doubled the half-life. Concomitant use of potent CYP3A4-inhibitors (e.g. ritonavir) with transdermally administered fentanyl may result in increased plasma concentrations of fentanyl. This may increase or prolong both the therapeutic effects and the adverse reactions, which may cause severe respiratory depression. In such cases increased care and observation of the patient should be undertaken. Combined use of ritonavir or other potent CYP3A4-inhibitors with transdermal fentanyl is not recommended, unless the patient is carefully observed.

4.6 Pregnancy and lactation

The safety of fentanyl in pregnancy has not been established. Studies in animals have shown reproductive toxicity (see section 5.3). The potential risk for humans is unknown. Fentanyl should only be used during pregnancy when clearly necessary.

Long-term treatment during pregnancy may cause withdrawal symptoms in the infant.

It is advised not to use fentanyl during labour and delivery (including caesarean section) since fentanyl passes the placenta and may cause respiratory depression in the foetus or in the infant.

Fentanyl is excreted into breast milk and may cause sedation and respiratory depression in the breast-fed infant. Lactation should therefore be discontinued for at least 72 hours after the removal of *Victanyl* (see also section 4.4).

4.7 Effects on ability to drive and use machines

Victanyl has major influence on the ability to drive and use machines. This has to be expected especially at the beginning of treatment, at any change of dosage as well as in connection with alcohol or tranquilizers. Patients stabilized on a specific dosage will not necessarily be restricted. Therefore, patients should consult their physician as to whether driving or use of machines is permitted.

4.8 Undesirable effects

The following frequencies are used for the description of the occurrence of adverse reactions:

Very common ($\geqslant$1/10), Common ($\geqslant$1/100, $<$1/10), Uncommon ($\geqslant$1/1000, $<$1/100), Rare ($\geqslant$1/10,000, $<$1/1000), Very rare ($<$1/10,000)

The most serious undesirable effect of fentanyl is respiratory depression.

Cardiac disorders

Uncommon: tachycardia, bradycardia.

Rare: arrhythmia.

Nervous system disorders

Very common: headache, dizziness.

Uncommon: tremor, paraesthesia, speech disorder.

Very rare: ataxia, seizures (including clonic and grand mal seizures).

Eye disorders

Very rare: amblyopia.

Respiratory, thoracic and mediastinal disorders

Uncommon: dyspnoea, hypoventilation.

Very rare: respiratory depression, apnoea.

Gastrointestinal disorders

Very common: nausea, vomiting, constipation.

Common: xerostomia, dyspepsia.

Uncommon: diarrhoea.

Rare: hiccup.

Very rare: painful flatulence, ileus.

Renal and urinary disorders

Uncommon: urinary retention.

Very rare: cystalgia, oliguria.

Skin and subcutaneous tissue disorders

Very common: sweating, pruritus.

Common: skin reactions on the application site.

Uncommon: exanthema, erythema.

Rash, erythema and pruritus will usually disappear within one day after the patch has been removed.

Vascular disorders

Uncommon: hypertension, hypotension.

Rare: vasodilatation.

General disorders

Rare: oedema, cold feeling.

Immune system disorders

Very rare: anaphylaxis.

Psychiatric disorders

Very common: somnolence.

Common: sedation, nervousness, loss of appetite.

Uncommon: euphoria, amnesia, insomnia, hallucinations, agitation.

Very rare: delusional ideas, states of excitement, asthenia, depression, anxiety, confusion, sexual dysfunction, withdrawal symptoms.

Other undesirable effects

Not known (cannot be estimated from the available data): Long-term use of fentanyl can lead to development of tolerance and physical and psychological dependence. After switching from previously prescribed opioid analgesics to *Victanyl* or after abrupt discontinuation of therapy patients may show opioid withdrawal symptoms (for instance: nausea, vomiting, diarrhoea, anxiety and shivering).

4.9 Overdose

Symptoms

The symptoms of fentanyl overdose are an extension of its pharmacological actions, e.g. lethargy, coma, respiratory depression with Cheyne-Stokes respiration and/or cyanosis. Other symptoms may be hypothermia, decreased muscle tonus, bradycardia, hypotonia. Signs of toxicity are deep sedation, ataxia, miosis, convulsions and respiratory depression, which is the main symptom.

Treatment

For management of respiratory depression immediate countermeasures should be started, including removing the patch and physically or verbally stimulating the patient. These actions can be followed by administration of a specific opioid antagonist such as naloxone.

A starting dose of 0.4-2 mg naloxone hydrochloride i.v. is recommended for adults. If needed, a similar dose can be given every 2 or 3 minutes, or be administered as continued infusion as 2 mg in 500 ml sodium chloride 9 mg/ml (0.9 %) solution for injection or glucose 50 mg/ml (5 %) solution. The infusion rate should be adjusted according to previous bolus injections and the individual response of the patient. If intravenous administration is impossible, naloxone hydrochloride can also be given intramuscularly or subcutaneously. Following intramuscular or subcutaneous administration the onset of action will be slower compared with intravenous administration. Intramuscular administration will give a more prolonged effect than intravenous administration. Respiratory depression due to overdose can persist longer than the effect of the opioid antagonist. Reversing the narcotic effect can give rise to acute pain and release of catecholamines. Intensive care unit treatment is important, if required by the patient's clinical condition. If severe or persistent hypotension occurs, hypovolemia should be considered, and the condition should be managed with appropriate parenteral fluid therapy.

5. PHARMACOLOGICAL PROPERTIES

5.1 Pharmacodynamic properties

Pharmacotherapeutic group: opioids; Phenylpiperidine derivatives

ATC code: N02AB03

Fentanyl is an opioid analgesic which interacts predominantly with the μ-receptor. Its principal therapeutic effects are analgesia and sedation. The serum concentrations of fentanyl that cause a minimal analgesic effect in opioid-naive patients fluctuate between 0.3–1.5 ng/ml; an increased incidence of adverse effects is observed if serum levels exceed 2 ng/ml.

Both the lowest effective fentanyl concentration and the concentration causing adverse reactions will increase with the development of increasing tolerance. The tendency to develop tolerance varies considerably between individuals.

5.2 Pharmacokinetic properties

Following administration of *Fentanyl transdermal patch*, fentanyl is continuously absorbed through the skin over a period of 72 hours. Due to the polymer matrix and the diffusion of fentanyl through the skin layers, the release rate remains relatively constant.

Absorption

After the first application of *Fentanyl transdermal patch*, serum fentanyl concentrations increase gradually, generally levelling off between 12 and 24 hours, and remaining relatively constant for the remainder of the 72-hour application period. The serum fentanyl concentrations attained are dependant on the Fentanyl transdermal patch size. For all practical purposes by the second 72-hour application, a steady state serum concentration is reached and is maintained during subsequent applications of a patch of the same size.

Distribution

The plasma protein binding for fentanyl is 84 %.

Biotransformation

Fentanyl is metabolized primarily in the liver via CYP3A4. The major metabolite, norfentanyl, is inactive.

Elimination

When treatment with Fentanyl transdermal patches is withdrawn, serum fentanyl concentrations decline gradually, falling approximately 50 % in 13-22 hours in adults or 22-25 hours in children, respectively. Continued absorption of fentanyl from the skin accounts for a slower reduction in serum concentration than is seen after an intravenous infusion.

Around 75 % of fentanyl is excreted into the urine, mostly as metabolites, with less than 10 % as unchanged drug. About 9 % of the dose is recovered in the faeces, primarily as metabolites.

Pharmacokinetics in special groups

Elderly and debilitated patients may have reduced clearance of fentanyl leading to prolonged terminal half life. In patients with renal or hepatic impairment, clearance of fentanyl may be altered because of changes of plasma proteins and metabolic clearance resulting in increased serum concentrations.

5.3 Preclinical safety data

Non-clinical data reveal no special hazard for humans based on conventional studies of safety pharmacology, repeated dose toxicity and genotoxicity.

Animal studies have shown reduced fertility and increased mortality in rat foetuses. Teratogenic effects have, however, not been demonstrated.

Long-term carcinogenicity studies have not been performed.

6. PHARMACEUTICAL PARTICULARS

6.1 List of excipients

Adhesive layer

Polyacrylate adhesive layer

Backing film

Polypropylene foil

Blue printing ink

Release liner

Polyethylene terephthalate foil (siliconised)

6.2 Incompatibilities

Not applicable.

6.3 Shelf life

18 months

6.4 Special precautions for storage

Do not store above 25°C.

6.5 Nature and contents of container

Each transdermal patch is packed in a separate sachet. The Composite foil containing the following layers from outside to inside: coated Kraft paper, low density polyethylene foil, aluminium foil, Surlyn

Pack containing 3 transdermal patches

Pack containing 4 transdermal patches

Pack containing 5 transdermal patches

Pack containing 8 transdermal patches

Pack containing 10 transdermal patches

Pack containing 16 transdermal patches

Pack containing 20 transdermal patches

Not all pack sizes may be marketed.

6.6 Special precautions for disposal and other handling

High quantities of fentanyl remain in the transdermal patches even after use. Used transdermal patches should be folded with the adhesive surfaces inwards and discarded or whenever possible returned to the pharmacy. Any unused medicinal product should be discarded or returned to the pharmacy.

7. MARKETING AUTHORISATION HOLDER

Actavis Group PTC ehf

Reykjavikurvegur 76-78

220 IS Hafnarfjordur

Iceland

8. MARKETING AUTHORISATION NUMBER(S)

PL 30306/0131

9. DATE OF FIRST AUTHORISATION/RENEWAL OF THE AUTHORISATION

27/06/08

10. DATE OF REVISION OF THE TEXT

09/07/08

11. DOSIMETRY

Not applicable.

12 INSTRUCTIONS FOR PREPARATION OF RADIOPHARMACEUTICALS (IF APPLICABLE)

Not applicable.

Victanyl 50 micrograms/hour Transdermal Patch (Actavis UK Ltd)

(Actavis UK Ltd)

1. NAME OF THE MEDICINAL PRODUCT

Victanyl 50 micrograms/hour Transdermal Patch

fentanyl

2. QUALITATIVE AND QUANTITATIVE COMPOSITION

Each patch releases 50 micrograms fentanyl per hour. Each patch of 15 cm2 contains 8.25 mg fentanyl.

For a full list of excipients, see section 6.1.

3. PHARMACEUTICAL FORM

Transdermal patch

Transparent and colourless patch with blue imprint on the backing foil: "fentanyl 50 μg/h".

4. CLINICAL PARTICULARS

4.1 Therapeutic indications

The product is indicated in severe chronic pain which can be adequately managed only with opioid analgesics.

4.2 Posology and method of administration

The dosing is individual and based on the patient's opioid history and takes into account:

- the possible development of tolerance,
- the current general condition, the medical status of the patient, and
- the degree of severity of the disorder.

The required fentanyl dosage is adjusted individually and should be assessed regularly after each administration.

Patients receiving opioid treatment for the first time

Patches with a release rate of 12.5 micrograms/hour are available and should be used for initial dosing. In very elderly or weak patients, it is not recommended to initiate an opioid treatment with *Victanyl*, due to their known susceptibility to opioid treatments. In these cases, it would be preferable to initiate a treatment with low doses of immediate release morphine and to prescribe *Victanyl* after determination of the optimal dosage.

Switching from other opioids

When changing over from oral or parenteral opioids to fentanyl treatment, the initial dosage should be calculated as follows:

1. The quantity of analgesics required over the last 24 hours should be determined.

2. The obtained sum should be converted to correspond the oral morphine dosage using Table 1.

3. The corresponding fentanyl dosage should be determined as follows:

a) using Table 2 for patients who have a need for opioid rotation (conversion ratio of oral morphine to transdermal fentanyl equal to150:1)

b) using Table 3 for patients on stable and well tolerated opioid therapy (conversion ratio of oral morphine to transdermal fentanyl equal to 100:1)

Table 1: Equianalgesic potency conversion

All dosages given in the table are equivalent in analgesic effect to 10 mg parenteral morphine.

	Equianalgesic doses (mg)	
Active substance	**Parenteral (im)**	**Oral**
Morphine	10	30-40
Hydromorphone	1.5	7.5
Oxycodone	10-15	20-30
Methadone	10	20
Levorphanol	2	4
Oxymorphine	1	10 (rectal)
Diamorphine	5	60
Pethidine	75	-
Codeine		200
Buprenorphine	0.4	0.8 (sublingual)
Ketobemidone	10	20-30

Table 2: Recommended <u>initial dose</u> of transdermal fentanyl based on daily oral morphine dose (for patients who have a need for opioid rotation)

Oral morphine dose (mg/24 h)	Transdermal fentanyl release (micrograms/h)
< 44	12.5
45-134	25
135-224	50
225-314	75
315-404	100
405-494	125

495-584	150
585-674	175
675-764	200
765-854	225
855-944	250
945-1034	275
1035-1124	300

Table 3: Recommended initial dose of transdermal fentanyl based on daily oral morphine dose (for patients on stable and well tolerated opioid therapy)

Oral morphine dose (mg/24 h)	Transdermal fentanyl release (micrograms/h)
< 60	12.5
60-89	25
90-149	50
150-209	75
210-269	100
270-329	125
330-389	150
390-449	175
450-509	200
510-569	225
570-629	250
630-689	275
690-749	300

By combining several transdermal patches, a fentanyl release rate of over 100 micrograms/h can be achieved.

The initial evaluation of the maximum analgesic effect of *Fentanyl transdermal patch* should not be made before the patch has been worn for 24 hours. This is due to the gradual increase in serum fentanyl concentrations during the first 24 hours after application of the patch.

In the first 12 hours after changing to *Fentanyl transdermal patch* the patient continues to receive the previous analgesic at the previous dose; over the next 12 hours this analgesic is administered according to need.

Dose titration and maintenance therapy

The patch should be replaced every 72 hours. The dose should be titrated individually until analgesic efficacy is attained. In patients who experience a marked decrease in the period 48-72 hours after application, replacement of fentanyl after 48 hours may be necessary.

Patches with a release rate of 12.5 micrograms/hour are available and are appropriate for dose titration in the lower dosage area. If analgesia is insufficient at the end of the initial application period, the dose may be increased after 3 days until the desired effect is obtained for each patient. Additional dose adjustment should normally be performed in 25 micrograms/hour increments, although the supplementary analgesic requirements and pain status of the patient should be taken into account. Patients may require periodic supplemental doses of a short-acting analgesic for breakthrough pain. Additional or alternative methods of analgesia or alternative administration of opioids should be considered when the *Fentanyl transdermal patch* dose exceeds 300 micrograms/hour.

Withdrawal symptoms have been reported when changing from long-term treatment with Morphine to transdermal fentanyl despite adequate analgesic efficacy. In case of withdrawal symptoms it is recommended to treat those with short-acting Morphine in low doses.

Changing or ending therapy

If discontinuation of the patch is necessary, any replacement with other opioids should be gradual, starting at a low dose and increasing slowly. This is because fentanyl levels fall gradually after the patch is removed; it takes at least 17 hours for the fentanyl serum concentration to decrease by 50%. As a general rule, the discontinuation of opioid analgesia should be gradual, in order to prevent withdrawal symptoms (nausea, vomiting, diarrhoea, anxiety and muscular tremor). Tables 2 and 3 should not be used to switch from transdermal fentanyl to a morphine treatment.

Method of administration

Directly after removal from the pack and the release liner, *Fentanyl transdermal patch* is applied to a non-hairy area of skin on the upper body (chest, back, upper arm). To remove hair, scissors should be used instead of razors.

Prior to application, the skin should be carefully washed with clean water (no cleaning agents) and thoroughly dried. The transdermal patch is then applied using slight pressure with the palm of the hand for approximately 10-30 seconds. The skin area to which the patch is applied should be free of microlesions (e.g. due to irradiation or shaving) and skin irritation.

As the transdermal patch is protected by an outer waterproof backing film, it can also be worn while showering.

Occasionally, additional adhesion of the patch may be required.

If progressive dose increases are made, the active surface area required may reach a point where no further increase is possible.

Duration of administration

The patch should be changed after 72 hours. If an earlier change becomes necessary in individual cases, no change should be made before 48 hours have elapsed, otherwise a rise in mean fentanyl concentrations may occur. A new skin area must be selected for each application. A period of 7 days should be allowed to elapse before applying a new patch to the same area of skin. The analgesic effect may persist for some time after removal of the transdermal patch.

If traces of the transdermal patch remain on the skin after its removal, these can be cleaned off using copious amounts of soap and water. No alcohol or other solvents may be used for cleaning, as these may penetrate the skin due to the effect of the patch.

Paediatric population

The experience in children under 12 years of age is limited. *Victanyl* should not be used in this population.

Use in elderly patients

Elderly should be observed carefully and the dose reduced if necessary (see sections 4.4 and 5.2).

Hepatic and renal impairment

Patients with hepatic or renal impairment should be observed carefully and the dose reduced if necessary (see section 4.4).

4.3 Contraindications

- Hypersensitivity to the active substance or to any of the excipients.
- Acute or postoperative pain, since dosage titration is not possible during short-term use.
- Severe impairment of the central nervous system.

4.4 Special warnings and precautions for use

The product should be used only as part of an integrated treatment of pain in cases where the patient is adequately assessed medically, socially and psychologically.

Treatment with *Fentanyl transdermal patch* should only be initiated by an experienced physician familiar with the pharmacokinetics of Fentanyl transdermal patches and the risk for severe hypoventilation.

After exhibiting a serious adverse reaction a patient should be monitored for 24 hours following removal of a transdermal patch due to the half life of fentanyl (see section 5.2).

In chronic non-cancer pain, it might be preferable to initiate the treatment with immediate-release strong opoids (e.g. morphine) and to prescribe fentanyl transdermal patch after determination of the efficacy and the optimal dosage of the strong opioid.

The transdermal patch should not be cut, since no information is available on the quality, efficacy and safety of such divided patches.

If higher dosages than 500 mg morphine-equivalent are needed, a reassessment of opioid-therapy is recommended.

The most common adverse reactions following administration at usual doses are drowsiness, confusion, nausea, vomiting and constipation. The first of these are transient and their cause should be investigated if symptoms persist. Constipation, on the other hand, does not stop if treatment continues. All of these effects can be expected and should, therefore, be anticipated in order to optimise treatment, especially constipation. Corrective treatment may often be required (see section 4.8).

The concomitant use of buprenorphine, nalbuphine or pentazocine is not recommended (see also section 4.5).

Breakthrough pain

Studies have shown that almost all patients, despite treatment with a fentanyl patch, require supplemental medication with potent rapid-release drugs to arrest breakthrough pain.

Respiratory depression

As with all potent opioids some patients may experience respiratory depression with the *Fentanyl transdermal patch*, and patients must be observed for this effect. Respiratory depression may persist beyond the removal of the patch. The incidence of respiratory depression increases as the fentanyl dose is increased. CNS active active substances may worsen the respiratory depression (see sections 4.5).

In patients with existing respiratory depression, fentanyl should only be used with caution and at a lower dose.

Chronic pulmonary disease

In patients with chronic obstructive or other pulmonary diseases fentanyl may have more severe adverse reactions, in such patients opioids may decrease respiratory drive and increase airway resistance.

Drug dependence

Tolerance and physical and psychological dependence may develop upon repeated administration of opioids, but is rare in treatment of cancer related pain.

Increased intracranial pressure

Fentanyl transdermal patch should be used with caution in patients who may be particularly susceptible to the intracranial effects of CO_2 retention such as those with evidence of increased intracranial pressure, impaired consciousness or coma.

Cardiac disease

Opioids may cause hypotonia, especially in patients with hypovolemia. Caution should therefore be taken in treatment of patients with hypotension and/or patients with hypovolemia. Fentanyl may produce bradycardia. *Fentanyl transdermal patch* should therefore not be administered to patients with bradyarrhythmias.

Impaired liver function

Fentanyl is metabolised to inactive metabolites in the liver, so patients with hepatic disease might have a delayed elimination. Patients with hepatic impairment should be observed carefully and the dose reduced if necessary.

Renal impairment

Less than 10 % of fentanyl is excreted unchanged by the kidneys, and unlike morphine, there are no known active metabolites eliminated by the kidneys. Data obtained with intravenous fentanyl in patients with renal failure suggest that the volume of distribution of fentanyl may be changed by dialysis. This may affect serum concentrations. If patients with renal impairment receive transdermal fentanyl they should be observed carefully for signs of fentanyl toxicity and the dose reduced if necessary.

Patients with fever/external heat

Patients who develop fever should be monitored for opioid adverse reactions since significant increases in body temperature can potentially increase fentanyl absorption rate. The patch application site should not be exposed to heat from external heat sources, e.g. sauna.

Elderly patients

Data from intravenous studies with fentanyl suggest that the elderly patients may have reduced clearance, a prolonged half-life. Moreover elderly patients may be more sensitive to the active substance than younger patients. However, studies of Fentanyl transdermal patch in elderly patients demonstrated fentanyl pharmacokinetics which did not differ significantly from young patients although serum concentrations tended to be higher. Elderly or cachectic patients should be observed carefully and the dose reduced if necessary.

Paediatric patients

Due to limited experience in children under 12 years of age, *Victanyl* should be used in this age group only after careful consideration has been given to the benefit versus risk ratio.

Lactation

As fentanyl is excreted into breast milk, lactation should be discontinued under treatment with *Victanyl* (see also section 4.6).

Patients with myasthenia gravis

Non-epileptic (myo)clonic reactions can occur. Caution should be exercised when treating patients with myasthenia gravis.

Interactions

Combination with barbituric acid derivatives, buprenorphine, nalbuphine and pentazocine should in general be avoided (see section 4.5).

4.5 Interaction with other medicinal products and other forms of interaction

The concomitant use of barbituric acid derivatives should be avoided, since the respiratory depressing effect of fentanyl may be increased.

The concomitant use of buprenorphine, nalbuphine or pentazocine is not recommended. They have high affinity to opioid receptors with relatively low intrinsic activity and therefore partially antagonise the analgesic effect of fentanyl and may induce withdrawal symptoms in opioid dependant patients (see also section 4.4).

The concomitant use of other CNS depressants, may produce additive depressant effects and hypoventilation, hypotension as well as profound sedation or coma may occur. The CNS depressants mentioned above include:

- opioids
- anxiolytics and tranquilizers
- hypnotics
- general anaesthetics
- phenothiazines
- skeletal muscle relaxants
- sedating antihistamines
- alcoholic beverages

Therefore, the use of any of the above mentioned concomitant medicinal products and active substances require observation of the patient.

MAO-inhibitors have been reported to increase the effect of narcotic analgesics, especially in patients with cardiac failure. Therefore, fentanyl should not be used within 14 days after discontinuation of treatment with MAO-inhibitors.

Fentanyl, a high clearance active substance, is rapidly and extensively metabolised mainly by CYP3A4.

Itraconazole (a potent CYP3A4 inhibitor) at 200 mg/day given orally for four days had no significant effect on the pharmacokinetics of intravenous fentanyl. Increased plasma concentrations were, however, observed in individual subjects. Oral administration of ritonavir (one of the most potent CYP3A4 inhibitors) reduced the clearance of intravenous fentanyl by two thirds and doubled the half-life. Concomitant use of potent CYP3A4-inhibitors (e.g. ritonavir) with transdermally administered fentanyl may result in increased plasma concentrations of fentanyl. This may increase or prolong both the therapeutic effects and the adverse reactions, which may cause severe respiratory depression. In such cases increased care and observation of the patient should be undertaken. Combined use of ritonavir or other potent CYP3A4-inhibitors with transdermal fentanyl is not recommended, unless the patient is carefully observed.

4.6 Pregnancy and lactation

The safety of fentanyl in pregnancy has not been established. Studies in animals have shown reproductive toxicity (see section 5.3). The potential risk for humans is unknown. Fentanyl should only be used during pregnancy when clearly necessary.

Long-term treatment during pregnancy may cause withdrawal symptoms in the infant.

It is advised not to use fentanyl during labour and delivery (including caesarean section) since fentanyl passes the placenta and may cause respiratory depression in the foetus or in the infant.

Fentanyl is excreted into breast milk and may cause sedation and respiratory depression in the breast-fed infant. Lactation should therefore be discontinued for at least 72 hours after the removal of *Victanyl* (see also section 4.4).

4.7 Effects on ability to drive and use machines

Victanyl has major influence on the ability to drive and use machines. This has to be expected especially at the beginning of treatment, at any change of dosage as well as in connection with alcohol or tranquilizers. Patients stabilized on a specific dosage will not necessarily be restricted. Therefore, patients should consult their physician as to whether driving or use of machines is permitted.

4.8 Undesirable effects

The following frequencies are used for the description of the occurrence of adverse reactions:

Very common (≥1/10), Common (≥1/100, <1/10), Uncommon (≥1/1000, <1/100), Rare (≥1/10,000, <1/1000), Very rare (<1/10,000)

The most serious undesirable effect of fentanyl is respiratory depression.

Cardiac disorders

Uncommon: tachycardia, bradycardia.

Rare: arrhythmia.

Nervous system disorders

Very common: headache, dizziness.

Uncommon: tremor, paraesthesia, speech disorder.

Very rare: ataxia, seizures (including clonic and grand mal seizures).

Eye disorders

Very rare: amblyopia.

Respiratory, thoracic and mediastinal disorders

Uncommon: dyspnoea, hypoventilation.

Very rare: respiratory depression, apnoea.

Gastrointestinal disorders

Very common: nausea, vomiting, constipation.

Common: xerostomia, dyspepsia.

Uncommon: diarrhoea.

Rare: hiccup.

Very rare: painful flatulence, ileus.

Renal and urinary disorders

Uncommon: urinary retention.

Very rare: cystalgia, oliguria.

Skin and subcutaneous tissue disorders

Very common: sweating, pruritus.

Common: skin reactions on the application site.

Uncommon: exanthema, erythema.

Rash, erythema and pruritus will usually disappear within one day after the patch has been removed.

Vascular disorders

Uncommon: hypertension, hypotension.

Rare: vasodilatation.

General disorders

Rare: oedema, cold feeling.

Immune system disorders

Very rare: anaphylaxis.

Psychiatric disorders

Very common: somnolence.

Common: sedation, nervousness, loss of appetite.

Uncommon: euphoria, amnesia, insomnia, hallucinations, agitation.

Very rare: delusional ideas, states of excitement, asthenia, depression, anxiety, confusion, sexual dysfunction, withdrawal symptoms.

Other undesirable effects

Not known (cannot be estimated from the available data): Long-term use of fentanyl can lead to development of tolerance and physical and psychological dependence. After switching from previously prescribed opioid analgesics to *Victanyl* or after abrupt discontinuation of therapy patients may show opioid withdrawal symptoms (for instance: nausea, vomiting, diarrhoea, anxiety and shivering).

4.9 Overdose

Symptoms

The symptoms of fentanyl overdose are an extension of its pharmacological actions, e.g. lethargy, coma, respiratory depression with Cheyne-Stokes respiration and/or cyanosis. Other symptoms may be hypothermia, decreased muscle tonus, bradycardia, hypotonia. Signs of toxicity are deep sedation, ataxia, miosis, convulsions and respiratory depression, which is the main symptom.

Treatment

For management of respiratory depression immediate countermeasures should be started, including removing the patch and physically or verbally stimulating the patient. These actions can be followed by administration of a specific opioid antagonist such as naloxone.

A starting dose of 0.4-2 mg naloxone hydrochloride i.v. is recommended for adults. If needed, a similar dose can be given every 2 or 3 minutes, or be administered as continued infusion as 2 mg in 500 ml sodium chloride 9 mg/ml (0.9 %) solution for injection or glucose 50 mg/ml (5 %) solution. The infusion rate should be adjusted according to previous bolus injections and the individual response of the patient. If intravenous administration is impossible, naloxone hydrochloride can also be given intramuscularly or subcutaneously. Following intramuscular or subcutaneous administration the onset of action will be slower compared with intravenous administration. Intramuscular administration will give a more prolonged effect than intravenous administration. Respiratory depression due to overdose can persist longer than the effect of the opioid antagonist. Reversing the narcotic effect can give rise to acute pain and release of catecholamines. Intensive care unit treatment is important, if required by the patient's clinical condition. If severe or persistent hypotension occurs, hypovolemia should be considered, and the condition should be managed with appropriate parenteral fluid therapy.

5. PHARMACOLOGICAL PROPERTIES

5.1 Pharmacodynamic properties

Pharmacotherapeutic group: opioids; Phenylpiperidine derivatives

ATC code: N02AB03

Fentanyl is an opioid analgesic which interacts predominantly with the μ-receptor. Its principal therapeutic effects are analgesia and sedation. The serum concentrations of fentanyl that cause a minimal analgesic effect in opioid-naive patients fluctuate between 0.3–1.5 ng/ml; an increased incidence of adverse effects is observed if serum levels exceed 2 ng/ml.

Both the lowest effective fentanyl concentration and the concentration causing adverse reactions will increase with the development of increasing tolerance. The tendency to develop tolerance varies considerably between individuals.

5.2 Pharmacokinetic properties

Following administration of *Fentanyl transdermal patch*, fentanyl is continuously absorbed through the skin over a period of 72 hours. Due to the polymer matrix and the diffusion of fentanyl through the skin layers, the release rate remains relatively constant.

Absorption

After the first application of *Fentanyl transdermal patch*, serum fentanyl concentrations increase gradually, generally levelling off between 12 and 24 hours, and remaining relatively constant for the remainder of the 72-hour application period. The serum fentanyl concentrations attained are dependant on the Fentanyl transdermal patch size. For all practical purposes by the second 72-hour application, a steady state serum concentration is reached and is maintained during subsequent applications of a patch of the same size.

Distribution

The plasma protein binding for fentanyl is 84 %.

Biotransformation

Fentanyl is metabolized primarily in the liver via CYP3A4. The major metabolite, norfentanyl, is inactive.

Elimination

When treatment with Fentanyl transdermal patches is withdrawn, serum fentanyl concentrations decline gradually, falling approximately 50 % in 13-22 hours in adults or 22-25 hours in children, respectively. Continued absorption of fentanyl from the skin accounts for a slower reduction in serum concentration than is seen after an intravenous infusion.

Around 75 % of fentanyl is excreted into the urine, mostly as metabolites, with less than 10 % as unchanged drug. About 9 % of the dose is recovered in the faeces, primarily as metabolites.

Pharmacokinetics in special groups

Elderly and debilitated patients may have reduced clearance of fentanyl leading to prolonged terminal half life. In patients with renal or hepatic impairment, clearance of fentanyl may be altered because of changes of plasma proteins and metabolic clearance resulting in increased serum concentrations.

5.3 Preclinical safety data

Non-clinical data reveal no special hazard for humans based on conventional studies of safety pharmacology, repeated dose toxicity and genotoxicity.

Animal studies have shown reduced fertility and increased mortality in rat foetuses. Teratogenic effects have, however, not been demonstrated.

Long-term carcinogenicity studies have not been performed.

6. PHARMACEUTICAL PARTICULARS

6.1 List of excipients

Adhesive layer

Polyacrylate adhesive layer

Backing film

Polypropylene foil

Blue printing ink

Release liner

Polyethylene terephthalate foil (siliconised)

6.2 Incompatibilities

Not applicable.

6.3 Shelf life

18 months

6.4 Special precautions for storage

Do not store above 25°C.

6.5 Nature and contents of container

Each transdermal patch is packed in a separate sachet. The Composite foil containing the following layers from outside to inside: coated Kraft paper, low density polyethylene foil, aluminium foil, Surlyn

Pack containing 3 transdermal patches

Pack containing 4 transdermal patches

Pack containing 5 transdermal patches

Pack containing 8 transdermal patches

Pack containing 10 transdermal patches

Pack containing 16 transdermal patches

Pack containing 20 transdermal patches

Not all pack sizes may be marketed.

6.6 Special precautions for disposal and other handling

High quantities of fentanyl remain in the transdermal patches even after use. Used transdermal patches should be folded with the adhesive surfaces inwards and discarded or whenever possible returned to the pharmacy. Any unused medicinal product should be discarded or returned to the pharmacy.

7. MARKETING AUTHORISATION HOLDER

Actavis Group PTC ehf

Reykjavikurvegur 76-78

220 IS Hafnarfjordur

Iceland

8. MARKETING AUTHORISATION NUMBER(S)

PL 30306/0132

9. DATE OF FIRST AUTHORISATION/RENEWAL OF THE AUTHORISATION

27/06/08

10. DATE OF REVISION OF THE TEXT

09/07/08

11. DOSIMETRY

Not applicable.

12 INSTRUCTIONS FOR PREPARATION OF RADIOPHARMACEUTICALS (IF APPLICABLE)

Not applicable.

Victanyl 75 micrograms/hour Transdermal Patch (Actavis UK Ltd)

(Actavis UK Ltd)

1. NAME OF THE MEDICINAL PRODUCT

Victanyl 75 micrograms/hour Transdermal Patch

fentanyl

2. QUALITATIVE AND QUANTITATIVE COMPOSITION
Each patch releases 75 micrograms fentanyl per hour. Each patch of 22.5 cm2 contains 12.375 mg fentanyl.

For a full list of excipients, see section 6.1.

3. PHARMACEUTICAL FORM
Transdermal patch

Transparent and colourless patch with blue imprint on the backing foil: "fentanyl 75 μg/h".

4. CLINICAL PARTICULARS

4.1 Therapeutic indications
The product is indicated in severe chronic pain which can be adequately managed only with opioid analgesics.

4.2 Posology and method of administration
The dosing is individual and based on the patient's opioid history and takes into account:

- the possible development of tolerance,
- the current general condition, the medical status of the patient, and
- the degree of severity of the disorder.

The required fentanyl dosage is adjusted individually and should be assessed regularly after each administration.

Patients receiving opioid treatment for the first time

Patches with a release rate of 12.5 micrograms/hour are available and should be used for initial dosing. In very elderly or weak patients, it is not recommended to initiate an opioid treatment with *Victanyl*, due to their known susceptibility to opioid treatments. In these cases, it would be preferable to initiate a treatment with low doses of immediate release morphine and to prescribe *Victanyl* after determination of the optimal dosage.

Switching from other opioids

When changing over from oral or parenteral opioids to fentanyl treatment, the initial dosage should be calculated as follows:

1. The quantity of analgesics required over the last 24 hours should be determined.

2. The obtained sum should be converted to correspond the oral morphine dosage using Table 1.

3. The corresponding fentanyl dosage should be determined as follows:

a) using Table 2 for patients who have a need for opioid rotation (conversion ratio of oral morphine to transdermal fentanyl equal to150:1)

b) using Table 3 for patients on stable and well tolerated opioid therapy (conversion ratio of oral morphine to transdermal fentanyl equal to 100:1)

Table 1: Equianalgesic potency conversion

All dosages given in the table are equivalent in analgesic effect to 10 mg parenteral morphine.

	Equianalgesic doses (mg)	
Active substance	**Parenteral (im)**	**Oral**
Morphine	10	30-40
Hydromorphone	1.5	7.5
Oxycodone	10-15	20-30
Methadone	10	20
Levorphanol	2	4
Oxymorphine	1	10 (rectal)
Diamorphine	5	60
Pethidine	75	-
Codeine	-	200
Buprenorphine	0.4	0.8 (sublingual)
Ketobemidone	10	20-30

Table 2: Recommended <u>initial dose</u> of transdermal fentanyl based on daily oral morphine dose (for patients who have a need for opioid rotation)

Oral morphine dose (mg/24 h)	Transdermal fentanyl release (micrograms/h)
< 44	12.5
45-134	25
135-224	50
225-314	75
315-404	100
405-494	125
495-584	150
585-674	175
675-764	200
765-854	225
855-944	250
945-1034	275
1035-1124	300

Table 3: Recommended <u>initial dose</u> of transdermal fentanyl based on daily oral morphine dose (for patients on stable and well tolerated opioid therapy)

Oral morphine dose (mg/24 h)	Transdermal fentanyl release (micrograms/h)
< 60	12.5
60-89	25
90-149	50
150-209	75
210-269	100
270-329	125
330-389	150
390-449	175
450-509	200
510-569	225
570-629	250
630-689	275
690-749	300

By combining several transdermal patches, a fentanyl release rate of over 100 micrograms/h can be achieved.

The initial evaluation of the maximum analgesic effect of *Fentanyl transdermal patch* should not be made before the patch has been worn for 24 hours. This is due to the gradual increase in serum fentanyl concentrations during the first 24 hours after application of the patch.

In the first 12 hours after changing to *Fentanyl transdermal patch* the patient continues to receive the previous analgesic at the previous dose; over the next 12 hours this analgesic is administered according to need.

Dose titration and maintenance therapy

The patch should be replaced every 72 hours. The dose should be titrated individually until analgesic efficacy is attained. In patients who experience a marked decrease in the period 48-72 hours after application, replacement of fentanyl after 48 hours may be necessary.

Patches with a release rate of 12.5 micrograms/hour are available and are appropriate for dose titration in the lower dosage area. If analgesia is insufficient at the end of the initial application period, the dose may be increased after 3 days until the desired effect is obtained for each patient. Additional dose adjustment should normally be performed in 25 micrograms/hour increments, although the supplementary analgesic requirements and pain status of the patient should be taken into account. Patients may require periodic supplemental doses of a short-acting analgesic for breakthrough pain. Additional or alternative methods of analgesia or alternative administration of opioids should be considered when the *Fentanyl transdermal patch* dose exceeds 300 micrograms/hour.

Withdrawal symptoms have been reported when changing from long-term treatment with Morphine to transdermal fentanyl despite adequate analgesic efficacy. In case of withdrawal symptoms it is recommended to treat those with short-acting Morphine in low doses.

Changing or ending therapy

If discontinuation of the patch is necessary, any replacement with other opioids should be gradual, starting at a low dose and increasing slowly. This is because fentanyl levels fall gradually after the patch is removed; it takes at least 17 hours for the fentanyl serum concentration to decrease by 50%. As a general rule, the discontinuation of opioid analgesia should be gradual, in order to prevent withdrawal symptoms (nausea, vomiting, diarrhoea, anxiety and muscular tremor). Tables 2 and 3 should not be used to switch from transdermal fentanyl to a morphine treatment.

Method of administration

Directly after removal from the pack and the release liner, *Fentanyl transdermal patch* is applied to a non-hairy area of skin on the upper body (chest, back, upper arm). To remove hair, scissors should be used instead of razors.

Prior to application, the skin should be carefully washed with clean water (no cleaning agents) and thoroughly dried. The transdermal patch is then applied using slight pressure with the palm of the hand for approximately 10-30 seconds. The skin area to which the patch is applied should be free of microlesions (e.g. due to irradiation or shaving) and skin irritation.

As the transdermal patch is protected by an outer waterproof backing film, it can also be worn while showering.

Occasionally, additional adhesion of the patch may be required.

If progressive dose increases are made, the active surface area required may reach a point where no further increase is possible.

Duration of administration

The patch should be changed after 72 hours. If an earlier change becomes necessary in individual cases, no change should be made before 48 hours have elapsed, otherwise a rise in mean fentanyl concentrations may occur. A new skin area must be selected for each application. A period of 7 days should be allowed to elapse before applying a new patch to the same area of skin. The analgesic effect may persist for some time after removal of the transdermal patch.

If traces of the transdermal patch remain on the skin after its removal, these can be cleaned off using copious amounts of soap and water. No alcohol or other solvents may be used for cleaning, as these may penetrate the skin due to the effect of the patch.

Paediatric population

The experience in children under 12 years of age is limited. *Victanyl* should not be used in this population.

Use in elderly patients

Elderly should be observed carefully and the dose reduced if necessary (see sections 4.4 and 5.2).

Hepatic and renal impairment

Patients with hepatic or renal impairment should be observed carefully and the dose reduced if necessary (see section 4.4).

4.3 Contraindications

- Hypersensitivity to the active substance or to any of the excipients.

- Acute or postoperative pain, since dosage titration is not possible during short-term use.

- Severe impairment of the central nervous system.

4.4 Special warnings and precautions for use

The product should be used only as part of an integrated treatment of pain in cases where the patient is adequately assessed medically, socially and psychologically.

Treatment with *Fentanyl transdermal patch* should only be initiated by an experienced physician familiar with the pharmacokinetics of Fentanyl transdermal patches and the risk for severe hypoventilation.

After exhibiting a serious adverse reaction a patient should be monitored for 24 hours following removal of a transdermal patch due to the half life of fentanyl (see section 5.2).

In chronic non-cancer pain, it might be preferable to initiate the treatment with immediate-release strong opoids (e.g. morphine) and to prescribe fentanyl transdermal patch after determination of the efficacy and the optimal dosage of the strong opioid.

The transdermal patch should not be cut, since no information is available on the quality, efficacy and safety of such divided patches.

If higher dosages than 500 mg morphine-equivalent are needed, a reassessment of opioid-therapy is recommended.

The most common adverse reactions following administration at usual doses are drowsiness, confusion, nausea, vomiting and constipation. The first of these are transient and their cause should be investigated if symptoms persist. Constipation, on the other hand, does not stop if treatment continues. All of these effects can be expected and should, therefore, be anticipated in order to optimise treatment, especially constipation. Corrective treatment may often be required (see section 4.8).

The concomitant use of buprenorphine, nalbuphine or pentazocine is not recommended (see also section 4.5).

Breakthrough pain

Studies have shown that almost all patients, despite treatment with a fentanyl patch, require supplemental medication with potent rapid-release drugs to arrest breakthrough pain.

Respiratory depression

As with all potent opioids some patients may experience respiratory depression with the *Fentanyl transdermal patch*, and patients must be observed for this effect. Respiratory depression may persist beyond the removal of the patch. The incidence of respiratory depression increases as the fentanyl dose is increased. CNS active active substances may worsen the respiratory depression (see sections 4.5).

In patients with existing respiratory depression, fentanyl should only be used with caution and at a lower dose.

Chronic pulmonary disease

In patients with chronic obstructive or other pulmonary diseases fentanyl may have more severe adverse reactions, in such patients opioids may decrease respiratory drive and increase airway resistance.

Drug dependence

Tolerance and physical and psychological dependence may develop upon repeated administration of opioids, but is rare in treatment of cancer related pain.

Increased intracranial pressure

Fentanyl transdermal patch should be used with caution in patients who may be particularly susceptible to the intracranial effects of CO_2 retention such as those with evidence of increased intracranial pressure, impaired consciousness or coma.

Cardiac disease

Opioids may cause hypotonia, especially in patients with hypovolemia. Caution should therefore be taken in treatment of patients with hypotonia and/or patients with hypovolemia. Fentanyl may produce bradycardia. *Fentanyl transdermal patch* should therefore not be administered to patients with bradyarrhythmias.

Impaired liver function

Fentanyl is metabolised to inactive metabolites in the liver, so patients with hepatic disease might have a delayed elimination. Patients with hepatic impairment should be observed carefully and the dose reduced if necessary.

Renal impairment

Less than 10 % of fentanyl is excreted unchanged by the kidneys, and unlike morphine, there are no known active metabolites eliminated by the kidneys. Data obtained with intravenous fentanyl in patients with renal failure suggest that the volume of distribution of fentanyl may be changed by dialysis. This may affect serum concentrations. If patients with renal impairment receive transdermal fentanyl they should be observed carefully for signs of fentanyl toxicity and the dose reduced if necessary.

Patients with fever/external heat

Patients who develop fever should be monitored for opioid adverse reactions since significant increases in body temperature can potentially increase fentanyl absorption rate. The patch application site should not be exposed to heat from external heat sources, e.g. sauna.

Elderly patients

Data from intravenous studies with fentanyl suggest that the elderly patients may have reduced clearance, a prolonged half-life. Moreover elderly patients may be more sensitive to the active substance than younger patients. However, studies of Fentanyl transdermal patch in elderly patients demonstrated fentanyl pharmacokinetics which did not differ significantly from young patients although serum concentrations tended to be higher. Elderly or cachectic patients should be observed carefully and the dose reduced if necessary.

Paediatric patients

Due to limited experience in children under 12 years of age, *Victanyl* should be used in this age group only after careful consideration has been given to the benefit versus risk ratio.

Lactation

As fentanyl is excreted into breast milk, lactation should be discontinued under treatment with *Victanyl* (see also section 4.6).

Patients with myasthenia gravis

Non-epileptic (myo)clonic reactions can occur. Caution should be exercised when treating patients with myasthenia gravis.

Interactions

Combination with barbituric acid derivatives, buprenorphine, nalbuphine and pentazocine should in general be avoided (see section 4.5).

4.5 Interaction with other medicinal products and other forms of interaction

The concomitant use of barbituric acid derivatives should be avoided, since the respiratory depressing effect of fentanyl may be increased.

The concomitant use of buprenorphine, nalbuphine or pentazocine is not recommended. They have high affinity to opioid receptors with relatively low intrinsic activity and therefore partially antagonise the analgesic effect of fentanyl and may induce withdrawal symptoms in opioid dependant patients (see also section 4.4).

The concomitant use of other CNS depressants, may produce additive depressant effects and hypoventilation, hypotension as well as profound sedation or coma may occur. The CNS depressants mentioned above include:

- opioids
- anxiolytics and tranquilizers
- hypnotics
- general anaesthetics
- phenothiazines
- skeletal muscle relaxants
- sedating antihistamines
- alcoholic beverages

Therefore, the use of any of the above mentioned concomitant medicinal products and active substances require observation of the patient.

MAO-inhibitors have been reported to increase the effect of narcotic analgesics, especially in patients with cardiac failure. Therefore, fentanyl should not be used within 14 days after discontinuation of treatment with MAO-inhibitors.

Fentanyl, a high clearance active substance, is rapidly and extensively metabolised mainly by CYP3A4.

Itraconazole (a potent CYP3A4 inhibitor) at 200 mg/day given orally for four days had no significant effect on the pharmacokinetics of intravenous fentanyl. Increased plasma concentrations were, however, observed in individual subjects. Oral administration of ritonavir (one of the most potent CYP3A4 inhibitors) reduced the clearance of intravenous fentanyl by two thirds and doubled the half-life. Concomitant use of potent CYP3A4-inhibitors (e.g. ritonavir) with transdermally administered fentanyl may result in increased plasma concentrations of fentanyl. This may increase or prolong both the therapeutic effects and the adverse reactions, which may cause severe respiratory depression. In such cases increased care and observation of the patient should be undertaken. Combined use of ritonavir or other potent CYP3A4-inhibitors with transdermal fentanyl is not recommended, unless the patient is carefully observed.

4.6 Pregnancy and lactation

The safety of fentanyl in pregnancy has not been established. Studies in animals have shown reproductive toxicity (see section 5.3). The potential risk for humans is unknown. Fentanyl should only be used during pregnancy when clearly necessary.

Long-term treatment during pregnancy may cause withdrawal symptoms in the infant.

It is advised not to use fentanyl during labour and delivery (including caesarean section) since fentanyl passes the placenta and may cause respiratory depression in the foetus or in the infant.

Fentanyl is excreted into breast milk and may cause sedation and respiratory depression in the breast-fed infant. Lactation should therefore be discontinued for at least 72 hours after the removal of *Victanyl* (see also section 4.4).

4.7 Effects on ability to drive and use machines

Victanyl has major influence on the ability to drive and use machines. This has to be expected especially at the beginning of treatment, at any change of dosage as well as in connection with alcohol or tranquilizers. Patients stabilized on a specific dosage will not necessarily be restricted. Therefore, patients should consult their physician as to whether driving or use of machines is permitted.

4.8 Undesirable effects

The following frequencies are used for the description of the occurrence of adverse reactions:

Very common ($\geqslant$1/10), Common ($\geqslant$1/100, <1/10), Uncommon ($\geqslant$1/1000, <1/100), Rare ($\geqslant$1/10,000, <1/1000), Very rare (<1/10,000)

The most serious undesirable effect of fentanyl is respiratory depression.

Cardiac disorders

Uncommon: tachycardia, bradycardia.

Rare: arrhythmia.

Nervous system disorders

Very common: headache, dizziness.

Uncommon: tremor, paraesthesia, speech disorder.

Very rare: ataxia, seizures (including clonic and grand mal seizures).

Eye disorders

Very rare: amblyopia.

Respiratory, thoracic and mediastinal disorders

Uncommon: dyspnoea, hypoventilation.

Very rare: respiratory depression, apnoea.

Gastrointestinal disorders

Very common: nausea, vomiting, constipation.

Common: xerostomia, dyspepsia.

Uncommon: diarrhoea.

Rare: hiccup.

Very rare: painful flatulence, ileus.

Renal and urinary disorders

Uncommon: urinary retention.

Very rare: cystalgia, oliguria.

Skin and subcutaneous tissue disorders

Very common: sweating, pruritus.

Common: skin reactions on the application site.

Uncommon: exanthema, erythema.

Rash, erythema and pruritus will usually disappear within one day after the patch has been removed.

Vascular disorders

Uncommon: hypertension, hypotension.

Rare: vasodilatation.

General disorders

Rare: oedema, cold feeling.

Immune system disorders

Very rare: anaphylaxis.

Psychiatric disorders

Very common: somnolence.

Common: sedation, nervousness, loss of appetite.

Uncommon: euphoria, amnesia, insomnia, hallucinations, agitation.

Very rare: delusional ideas, states of excitement, asthenia, depression, anxiety, confusion, sexual dysfunction, withdrawal symptoms.

Other undesirable effects

Not known (cannot be estimated from the available data): Long-term use of fentanyl can lead to development of tolerance and physical and psychological dependence. After switching from previously prescribed opioid analgesics to *Victanyl* or after abrupt discontinuation of therapy patients may show opioid withdrawal symptoms (for instance: nausea, vomiting, diarrhoea, anxiety and shivering).

4.9 Overdose

Symptoms

The symptoms of fentanyl overdose are an extension of its pharmacological actions, e.g. lethargy, coma, respiratory depression with Cheyne-Stokes respiration and/or cyanosis. Other symptoms may be hypothermia, decreased muscle tonus, bradycardia, hypotonia. Signs of toxicity are deep sedation, ataxia, miosis, convulsions and respiratory depression, which is the main symptom.

Treatment

For management of respiratory depression immediate countermeasures should be started, including removing the patch and physically or verbally stimulating the patient. These actions can be followed by administration of a specific opioid antagonist such as naloxone.

A starting dose of 0.4-2 mg naloxone hydrochloride i.v. is recommended for adults. If needed, a similar dose can be given every 2 or 3 minutes, or be administered as continued infusion as 2 mg in 500 ml sodium chloride 9 mg/ml (0.9 %) solution for injection or glucose 50 mg/ml (5 %) solution. The infusion rate should be adjusted according to previous bolus injections and the individual response of the patient. If intravenous administration is impossible, naloxone hydrochloride can also be given intramuscularly or subcutaneously. Following intramuscular or subcutaneous administration the onset of action will be slower compared with intravenous administration. Intramuscular administration will give a more prolonged effect than intravenous administration. Respiratory depression due to overdose can persist longer than the effect of the opioid antagonist. Reversing the narcotic effect can give rise to acute pain and release of catecholamines. Intensive care unit treatment is important, if required by the patient's clinical condition. If severe or persistent hypotension occurs, hypovolemia should be considered, and the condition should be managed with appropriate parenteral fluid therapy.

5. PHARMACOLOGICAL PROPERTIES

5.1 Pharmacodynamic properties

Pharmacotherapeutic group: opioids; Phenylpiperidine derivatives

ATC code: N02AB03

Fentanyl is an opioid analgesic which interacts predominantly with the μ-receptor. Its principal therapeutic effects are analgesia and sedation. The serum concentrations of fentanyl that cause a minimal analgesic effect in opioid-naive patients fluctuate between 0.3–1.5 ng/ml; an increased incidence of adverse effects is observed if serum levels exceed 2 ng/ml.

Both the lowest effective fentanyl concentration and the concentration causing adverse reactions will increase with the development of increasing tolerance. The tendency to develop tolerance varies considerably between individuals.

5.2 Pharmacokinetic properties

Following administration of *Fentanyl transdermal patch*, fentanyl is continuously absorbed through the skin over a period of 72 hours. Due to the polymer matrix and the diffusion of fentanyl through the skin layers, the release rate remains relatively constant.

Absorption

After the first application of *Fentanyl transdermal patch*, serum fentanyl concentrations increase gradually, generally levelling off between 12 and 24 hours, and remaining relatively constant for the remainder of the 72-hour application period. The serum fentanyl concentrations attained are dependant on the Fentanyl transdermal patch size. For all practical purposes by the second 72-hour application, a steady state serum concentration is reached and is maintained during subsequent applications of a patch of the same size.

Distribution

The plasma protein binding for fentanyl is 84 %.

Biotransformation

Fentanyl is metabolized primarily in the liver via CYP3A4. The major metabolite, norfentanyl, is inactive.

Elimination

When treatment with Fentanyl transdermal patches is withdrawn, serum fentanyl concentrations decline gradually, falling approximately 50 % in 13-22 hours in adults or 22-25 hours in children, respectively. Continued absorption of fentanyl from the skin accounts for a slower reduction in serum concentration than is seen after an intravenous infusion.

Around 75 % of fentanyl is excreted into the urine, mostly as metabolites, with less than 10 % as unchanged drug. About 9 % of the dose is recovered in the faeces, primarily as metabolites.

Pharmacokinetics in special groups

Elderly and debilitated patients may have reduced clearance of fentanyl leading to prolonged terminal half life. In patients with renal or hepatic impairment, clearance of fentanyl may be altered because of changes of plasma proteins and metabolic clearance resulting in increased serum concentrations.

5.3 Preclinical safety data

Non-clinical data reveal no special hazard for humans based on conventional studies of safety pharmacology, repeated dose toxicity and genotoxicity.

Animal studies have shown reduced fertility and increased mortality in rat foetuses. Teratogenic effects have, however, not been demonstrated.

Long-term carcinogenicity studies have not been performed.

6. PHARMACEUTICAL PARTICULARS

6.1 List of excipients

Adhesive layer

Polyacrylate adhesive layer

Backing film

Polypropylene foil

Blue printing ink

Release liner

Polyethylene terephthalate foil (siliconised)

6.2 Incompatibilities

Not applicable.

6.3 Shelf life

18 months

6.4 Special precautions for storage

Do not store above 25°C.

6.5 Nature and contents of container

Each transdermal patch is packed in a separate sachet. The Composite foil containing the following layers from outside to inside: coated Kraft paper, low density polyethylene foil, aluminium foil, Surlyn

Pack containing 3 transdermal patches

Pack containing 4 transdermal patches

Pack containing 5 transdermal patches

Pack containing 8 transdermal patches

Pack containing 10 transdermal patches

Pack containing 16 transdermal patches

Pack containing 20 transdermal patches

Not all pack sizes may be marketed.

6.6 Special precautions for disposal and other handling

High quantities of fentanyl remain in the transdermal patches even after use. Used transdermal patches should be folded with the adhesive surfaces inwards and discarded or whenever possible returned to the pharmacy. Any unused medicinal product should be discarded or returned to the pharmacy.

7. MARKETING AUTHORISATION HOLDER

Actavis Group PTC ehf

Reykjavikurvegur 76-78

220 IS Hafnarfjordur

Iceland

8. MARKETING AUTHORISATION NUMBER(S)

PL 30306/0133

9. DATE OF FIRST AUTHORISATION/RENEWAL OF THE AUTHORISATION

27/06/08

10. DATE OF REVISION OF THE TEXT

09/07/08

11. DOSIMETRY

Not applicable.

12 INSTRUCTIONS FOR PREPARATION OF RADIOPHARMACEUTICALS (IF APPLICABLE)

Not applicable.

Victoza 6 mg/ml solution for injection in pre-filled pen

(Novo Nordisk Limited)

1. NAME OF THE MEDICINAL PRODUCT

Victoza ▼ 6 mg/ml solution for injection in pre-filled pen

2. QUALITATIVE AND QUANTITATIVE COMPOSITION

One ml of solution contains 6 mg of liraglutide*. One pre-filled pen contains 18 mg liraglutide in 3 ml.

* human glucagon-like peptide-1 (GLP-1) analogue produced by recombinant DNA technology in *Saccharomyces cerevisiae*.

For a full list of excipients, see section 6.1.

3. PHARMACEUTICAL FORM

Solution for injection in pre-filled pen (injection).

Clear, colourless, isotonic solution; pH=8.15.

4. CLINICAL PARTICULARS

4.1 Therapeutic indications

Victoza is indicated for treatment of adults with type 2 diabetes mellitus to achieve glycaemic control:

In combination with:

– Metformin or a sulphonylurea, in patients with insufficient glycaemic control despite maximal tolerated dose of monotherapy with metformin or sulphonylurea.

In combination with:

– Metformin and a sulphonylurea or metformin and a thiazolidinedione in patients with insufficient glycaemic control despite dual therapy.

4.2 Posology and method of administration

Posology

To improve gastro-intestinal tolerability, the starting dose is 0.6 mg liraglutide daily. After at least one week, the dose should be increased to 1.2 mg. Some patients are expected to benefit from an increase in dose from 1.2 mg to 1.8 mg and based on clinical response, after at least one week the dose can be increased to 1.8 mg to further improve glycaemic control. Daily doses higher than 1.8 mg are not recommended.

Victoza can be added to existing metformin or to a combination of metformin and thiazolidinedione therapy. The current dose of metformin and thiazolidinedione can be continued unchanged.

Victoza can be added to existing sulphonylurea or to a combination of metformin and sulphonylurea therapy. When Victoza is added to sulphonylurea therapy, a reduction in the dose of sulphonylurea should be considered to reduce the risk of hypoglycaemia (see section 4.4).

Self-monitoring of blood glucose is not needed in order to adjust the dose of Victoza. However, when initiating treatment with Victoza in combination with a sulphonylurea, blood glucose self-monitoring may become necessary to adjust the dose of the sulphonylurea.

Special populations

Elderly (>65 years old): No dose adjustment is required based on age. Therapeutic experience in patients ⩾75 years of age is limited (see section 5.2).

Renal impairment: No dose adjustment is required for patients with mild renal impairment (creatinine clearance ⩽60-90 ml/min). There is very limited therapeutic experience in patients with moderate renal impairment (creatinine clearance of 30-59 ml/min) and no therapeutic experience in patients with severe renal impairment (creatinine clearance below 30 ml/min). Victoza can currently not be recommended for use in patients with moderate and severe renal impairment including patients with end-stage renal disease (see section 5.2).

Hepatic impairment: The therapeutic experience in patients with all degrees of hepatic impairment is currently too limited to recommend the use in patients with mild, moderate or severe hepatic impairment (see section 5.2).

Paediatric population: Victoza is not recommended for use in children below 18 years of age due to lack of data on its safety and efficacy.

Method of administration

Victoza should **not** be administered intravenously or intramuscularly.

Victoza is administered once daily at any time, independent of meals, and can be injected subcutaneously in the abdomen, in the thigh or in the upper arm. The injection site and timing can be changed without dose adjustment. However, it is preferable that Victoza is injected around the same time of the day, when the most convenient time of the day has been chosen. For further instructions on administration, see section 6.6.

4.3 Contraindications

Hypersensitivity to the active substance or to any of the excipients.

4.4 Special warnings and precautions for use

Victoza should not be used in patients with type 1 diabetes mellitus or for the treatment of diabetic ketoacidosis.

There is limited experience in patients with congestive heart failure New York Heart Association (NYHA) class I-II. There is no experience in patients with congestive heart failure NYHA class III-IV.

There is limited experience in patients with inflammatory bowel disease and diabetic gastroparesis and Victoza is therefore not recommended in these patients. The use of Victoza is associated with transient gastrointestinal adverse reactions, including nausea, vomiting and diarrhoea.

Use of other GLP-1 analogues has been associated with the risk of pancreatitis. There have been few reported events of acute pancreatitis. Patients should be informed of the characteristic symptom of acute pancreatitis: persistent, severe abdominal pain. If pancreatitis is suspected, Victoza and other potentially suspect medicinal products should be discontinued.

Thyroid adverse events, including increased blood calcitonin, goitre and thyroid neoplasm have been reported in clinical trials in particular in patients with pre-existing thyroid disease (see section 4.8).

Patients receiving Victoza in combination with a sulphonylurea may have an increased risk of hypoglycaemia (see section 4.8). The risk of hypoglycaemia can be lowered by a reduction in the dose of sulphonylurea.

4.5 Interaction with other medicinal products and other forms of interaction

In vitro, liraglutide has shown very low potential to be involved in pharmacokinetic interactions with other active substances related to cytochrome P450 and plasma protein binding.

The small delay of gastric emptying with liraglutide may influence absorption of concomitantly administered oral medicinal products. Interaction studies did not show any clinically relevant delay of absorption. Few patients treated with liraglutide reported at least one episode of severe diarrhoea. Diarrhoea may affect the absorption of concomitant oral medicinal products.

Paracetamol

Liraglutide did not change the overall exposure of paracetamol following a single dose of 1000 mg. Paracetamol C_{max} was decreased by 31% and median t_{max} was delayed up to 15 min. No dose adjustment for concomitant use of paracetamol is required.

Atorvastatin

Liraglutide did not change the overall exposure of atorvastatin to a clinical relevant degree following single dose administration of atorvastatin 40 mg. Therefore, no dose adjustment of atorvastatin is required when given with liraglutide. Atorvastatin C_{max} was decreased by 38% and median t_{max} was delayed from 1 h to 3 h with liraglutide.

Griseofulvin

Liraglutide did not change the overall exposure of griseofulvin following administration of a single dose of griseofulvin 500 mg. Griseofulvin C_{max} increased by 37% while median t_{max} did not change. Dose adjustments of griseofulvin and other compounds with low solubility and high permeability are not required.

Lisinopril and digoxin

Single dose administration of lisinopril 20 mg or digoxin 1 mg with liraglutide showed a reduction of lisinopril and digoxin AUC by 15% and 16%, respectively; C_{max} decreased by 27% and 31%, respectively. Lisinopril median t_{max} was delayed from 6 h to 8 h with liraglutide; whereas digoxin median t_{max} was delayed from 1 h to 1.5 h. No adjustment of lisinopril or digoxin dose is required based on these results.

Oral contraceptives

Liraglutide lowered ethinyloestradiol and levonorgestrel C_{max} by 12 and 13%, respectively, following administration of a single dose of an oral contraceptive product. T_{max} was delayed by 1.5 h with liraglutide for both compounds. There was no clinically relevant effect on the overall exposure of either ethinyloestradiol or levonorgestrel. The contraceptive effect is therefore anticipated to be unaffected when co-administered with liraglutide.

Warfarin

No interaction study has been performed. A clinically relevant interaction with active substances with poor solubility or with narrow therapeutic index such as warfarin cannot be excluded. Upon initiation of liraglutide treatment in patients on warfarin more frequent monitoring of INR (International Normalised Ratio) is recommended.

Insulin

Combination of liraglutide with insulin has not been evaluated and is therefore not recommended.

4.6 Pregnancy and lactation

Pregnancy

There are no adequate data from the use of Victoza in pregnant women. Studies in animals have shown reproductive toxicity (see section 5.3). The potential risk for humans is unknown.

Victoza should not be used during pregnancy, and the use of insulin is recommended instead. If a patient wishes to become pregnant, or pregnancy occurs, treatment with Victoza should be discontinued.

Lactation

It is not known whether liraglutide is excreted in human milk. Animal studies have shown that the transfer of liraglutide and metabolites of close structural relationship into milk is low. Non-clinical studies have shown a treatment-related reduction of neonatal growth in suckling rat pups (see section 5.3). Because of lack of experience, Victoza should not be used during breast-feeding.

4.7 Effects on ability to drive and use machines

No studies on the effects on the ability to drive and use machines have been performed. Patients should be advised to take precautions to avoid hypoglycaemia while driving and using machines, in particular when Victoza is used in combination with a sulphonylurea.

4.8 Undesirable effects

In five large long-term clinical trials over 2500 patients have received treatment with Victoza alone or in combination with metformin, a sulphonylurea (with or without metformin) or metformin plus rosiglitazone.

Frequencies are defined as: Very common (⩾1/10); common (⩾1/100 to <1/10); uncommon (⩾1/1,000 to <1/100); rare (⩾1/10,000 to <1/1,000); very rare (<1/10,000); not known (cannot be estimated from the available data). Within each frequency grouping, undesirable effects are presented in order of decreasing seriousness.

The most frequently reported adverse reactions during clinical trials were gastrointestinal disorders: nausea and diarrhoea were very common, whereas vomiting, constipation, abdominal pain, and dyspepsia were common. At the beginning of Victoza therapy, these gastrointestinal adverse reactions may occur more frequently. These reactions usually diminish within a few days or weeks on continued treatment. Headache and nasopharyngitis were also common. Furthermore, hypoglycaemia was common, and very common when Victoza is used in combination with a sulphonylurea. Major hypoglycaemia has primarily been observed when combined with a sulphonylurea.

Table 1 lists related adverse reactions identified from Phase III combination-studies with Victoza. The table presents adverse reactions that occurred with a frequency >5% if the frequency was higher among Victoza-treated patients than patients treated with comparator. The table also includes adverse reactions with a frequency ⩾2% if the frequency was >2 times the frequency for comparator-treated subjects.

Table 1 Adverse reactions identified from long-term controlled phase III studies

(see Table 1 below)

In a clinical trial with Victoza as monotherapy rates of hypoglycaemia reported with Victoza were lower than rates reported for patients treated with active comparator (glimepiride). The most frequently reported adverse events were gastrointestinal and infections and infestations.

Hypoglycaemia

Most episodes of confirmed hypoglycaemia in clinical studies were minor. No episodes of major hypoglycaemia were observed in the study with Victoza used as monotherapy. Major hypoglycaemia may occur uncommonly and has primarily been observed when Victoza is combined with a sulphonylurea (0.02 events/subject year). Very few episodes (0.001 events/subject year) were observed with administration of Victoza in combination with oral antidiabetics other than sulphonylureas.

Gastrointestinal adverse reactions

When combining Victoza with metformin, 20.7% of patients reported at least one episode of nausea, and 12.6% of patients reported at least one episode of diarrhoea. When combining Victoza with a sulphonylurea, 9.1% of patients reported at least one episode of nausea and 7.9% of patients reported at least one episode of diarrhoea. Most episodes were mild to moderate and occurred in a dose-dependent fashion. With continued therapy, the frequency and severity decreased in most patients who initially experienced nausea.

Patients >70 years may experience more gastrointestinal effects when treated with liraglutide.

Patients with mild renal impairment (creatinine clearance ⩽60-90 ml/min) may experience more gastrointestinal effects when treated with liraglutide.

Withdrawal

The incidence of withdrawal due to adverse reactions was 7.8% for Victoza-treated patients and 3.4% for comparator-treated patients in the long-term controlled trials (26 weeks or longer). The most frequent adverse reactions leading to withdrawal for Victoza-treated patients were nausea (2.8% of patients) and vomiting (1.5%).

Immunogenicity

Consistent with the potentially immunogenic properties of medicinal products containing proteins or peptides, patients may develop anti-liraglutide antibodies following treatment with Victoza. On average, 8.6% of patients developed antibodies. Antibody formation has not been associated with reduced efficacy of Victoza.

Few cases (0.05%) of angioedema have been reported during all long-term clinical trials with Victoza.

Injection site reactions

Injection site reaction has been reported in approximately 2% of subjects receiving Victoza in long-term (26 weeks or longer) controlled trials. These reactions have usually been mild and did not lead to discontinuation of Victoza.

Pancreatitis

Few cases (<0.2%) of acute pancreatitis have been reported during long-term clinical trials with Victoza. A causal relationship between Victoza and pancreatitis can neither be established nor excluded.

Thyroid events

The overall rates of thyroid adverse events in all intermediate and long-term trials are 33.5, 30.0 and 21.7 events per 1000 subject years of exposure for total liraglutide, placebo and total comparators; 5.4, 2.1 and 0.8 events, respectively concern serious thyroid adverse events.

In liraglutide-treated patients, thyroid neoplasms, increased blood calcitonin and goiters are the most frequently thyroid adverse events and were reported in 0.5%, 1% and 0.8% of patients respectively.

4.9 Overdose

In a clinical study of Victoza, one patient with type 2 diabetes experienced a single overdose of 17.4 mg subcutaneous (10 times the maximal recommended maintenance dose of 1.8 mg). Effects of the overdose included severe nausea and vomiting, but not hypoglycaemia. The patient recovered without complications.

In the event of overdose, appropriate supportive treatment should be initiated according to the patient's clinical signs and symptoms.

5. PHARMACOLOGICAL PROPERTIES

5.1 Pharmacodynamic properties

Pharmacotherapeutic group: Other blood glucose lowering drugs, excl. insulins. ATC code: A10BX07

Mechanism of action

Liraglutide is a GLP-1 analogue with 97% sequence homology to human GLP-1 that binds to and activates the GLP-1 receptor. The GLP-1 receptor is the target for native GLP-1, an endogenous incretin hormone that potentiates glucose-dependent insulin secretion from the pancreatic beta cells. Unlike native GLP-1, liraglutide has a pharmacokinetic and pharmacodynamic profile in humans suitable for once daily administration. Following subcutaneous administration, the protracted action profile is based on three mechanisms: self-association, which results in slow absorption; binding to albumin; and higher enzymatic stability towards the dipeptidyl peptidase IV (DPP-IV) and neutral endopeptidase (NEP) enzymes, resulting in a long plasma half-life.

Liraglutide action is mediated via a specific interaction with GLP-1 receptors, leading to an increase in cyclic adenosine monophosphate (cAMP). Liraglutide stimulates insulin secretion in a glucose-dependent manner. Simultaneously, liraglutide lowers inappropriately high glucagon secretion, also in a glucose-dependent manner. Thus, when blood glucose is high, insulin secretion is stimulated and glucagon secretion is inhibited. Conversely, during hypoglycaemia liraglutide diminishes insulin secretion and does not impair glucagon secretion. The mechanism of blood glucose lowering also involves a minor delay in gastric emptying. Liraglutide reduces body weight and body fat mass through mechanisms involving reduced hunger and lowered energy intake.

Pharmacodynamic effects

Liraglutide has 24-hour duration of action and improves glycaemic control by lowering fasting and postprandial blood glucose in patients with type 2 diabetes mellitus.

Clinical efficacy

Five double-blind, randomised, controlled clinical trials were conducted to evaluate the effects of Victoza on glycaemic control. Treatment with Victoza produced clinically and statistically significant improvements in glycosylated haemoglobin A_{1c} (HbA_{1c}), fasting plasma glucose and post-prandial glucose compared with placebo.

These studies included 3,978 exposed patients with type 2 diabetes (2,501 subjects treated with Victoza), 53.7% men and 46.3% women, 797 subjects (508 treated with Victoza) were ⩾65 years of age and 113 subjects (66 treated with Victoza) were ⩾75 years of age.

There was an additional open-label randomised controlled study comparing liraglutide with exenatide.

Glycaemic control

Victoza in combination therapy, for 26 weeks, with metformin, glimepiride or metformin and rosiglitazone resulted

Table 1 Adverse reactions identified from long-term controlled phase III studies

Adverse reaction	Frequency of adverse reaction by treatment group			
	Liraglutide with metformin	**Liraglutide with glimepiride**	**Liraglutide with metformin and glimepiride**	**Liraglutide with metformin and rosiglitazone**
Infections and infestations				
Nasopharyngitis		Common		Common
Bronchitis			Common	
Metabolism and nutrition disorders				
Hypoglycaemia		Common	Very common	Common
Anorexia	Common	Common	Common	Common
Appetite decreased	Common			Common
Nervous system disorders				
Headache	Very common		Common	Common
Dizziness	Common			
Gastrointestinal disorders				
Nausea	Very common	Common	Very common	Very common
Diarrhoea	Very common	Common	Very common	Very common
Vomiting	Common	Common	Common	Very common
Dyspepsia	Common	Common	Common	Common
Abdominal pain upper			Common	
Constipation		Common	Common	Common
Gastritis	Common			
Flatulence				Common
Abdominal distension				Common
Gastroesophageal reflux disease				Common
Abdominal discomfort		Common		
Toothache			Common	
Gastroenteritis viral				Common
General disorders and administration site conditions				
Fatigue				Common
Pyrexia				Common

Table 2 Results of two 26 week trials. Victoza in combination with metformin and Victoza in combination with glimepiride

Metformin add-on therapy	1.8 mg liraglutide + metformin[3]	1.2 mg liraglutide + metformin[3]	Placebo + metformin[3]	Glimepiride[2] + metformin[3]
N	242	240	121	242
Mean HbA_{1c} (%)				
Baseline	8.4	8.3	8.4	8.4
Change from baseline	-1.00	-0.97	0.09	-0.98
Patients (%) achieving HbA_{1c} <7%				
All patients	42.4	35.3	10.8	36.3
Previous OAD monotherapy	66.3	52.8	22.5	56.0
Mean body weight (kg)				
Baseline	88.0	88.5	91.0	89.0
Change from baseline	-2.79	-2.58	-1.51	0.95
Glimepiride add-on therapy	**1.8 mg liraglutide + glimepiride[2]**	**1.2 mg liraglutide + glimepiride[2]**	**Placebo + glimepiride[2]**	**rosiglitazone[1] + glimepiride[2]**
N	234	228	114	231
Mean HbA_{1c} (%)				
Baseline	8.5	8.5	8.4	8.4
Change from baseline	-1.13	-1.08	0.23	-0.44
Patients (%) achieving HbA_{1c} <7%				
All patients	41.6	34.5	7.5	21.9
Previous OAD monotherapy	55.9	57.4	11.8	36.1
Mean body weight (kg)				
Baseline	83.0	80.0	81.9	80.6
Change from baseline	-0.23	0.32	-0.10	2.11

[1] Rosiglitazone 4 mg/day; [2] glimepiride 4 mg/day; [3] metformin 2000 mg/day

in statistically significant ($p < 0.0001$) and sustained reductions in HbA_{1c} compared with patients receiving placebo (Tables 2 and 3).

Table 2 Results of two 26 week trials. Victoza in combination with metformin and Victoza in combination with glimepiride.

(see Table 2 above)

Table 3 Results of two 26 week trials. Victoza in combination with metformin + rosiglitazone and Victoza in combination with glimepiride + metformin.

(see Table 3 opposite)

Guideline for titration of insulin glargine

Self-measured FPG	Increase in insulin glargine dose (IU)
≤5.5 mmol/l (≤100 mg/dl) Target	No adjustment
>5.5 and <6.7 mmol/l (>100 and <120 mg/dl)	0 – 2 IU[a]
≥6.7 mmol/l (≥120 mg/dl)	2 IU

[a] According to the individualised recommendation by the investigator at the previous visit for example depending on whether subject has experienced hypoglycaemia.

[2] Metformin 2000 mg/day; [3] rosiglitazone 4 mg twice daily; [4] glimepiride 4 mg/day.

Proportion of patients achieving reductions in HbA_{1c}

Victoza in combination with metformin, glimepiride, or metformin and rosiglitazone resulted in a statistically significant ($p \leqslant 0.0001$) greater proportion of patients achieving an $HbA_{1c} \leqslant 6.5\%$ at 26 weeks compared with patients receiving these agents alone.

Fasting plasma glucose

Treatment with Victoza alone or in combination with one or two oral antidiabetic drugs resulted in a reduction in fasting plasma glucose of 13-43.5 mg/dl (0.72-2.42 mmol/l). This reduction was observed within the first two weeks of treatment.

Post-prandial glucose

Victoza reduces post-prandial glucose across all three daily meals by 31-49 mg/dl (1.68-2.71 mmol/l).

Beta-cell function

Clinical studies with Victoza indicate improved beta-cell function based on measures such as the homeostasis model assessment for beta-cell function (HOMA-B) and the proinsulin to insulin ratio. Improved first and second phase insulin secretion after 52 weeks treatment with Victoza was demonstrated in a subset of patients with type 2 diabetes (N=29).

Body weight

Victoza in combination with metformin, metformin and glimepiride or metformin and rosiglitazone was associated with sustained weight reduction over the duration of studies in a range from 1.0 kg to 2.8 kg.

Larger weight reduction was observed with increasing body mass index (BMI) at baseline.

Blood pressure

Over the duration of the studies Victoza decreased the systolic blood pressure on average of 2.3 to 6.7 mmHg from baseline and compared to active comparator the decrease was 1.9 to 4.5 mmHg

5.2 Pharmacokinetic properties

Absorption

The absorption of liraglutide following subcutaneous administration is slow, reaching maximum concentration 8-12 hours post dosing. Estimated maximum liraglutide concentration was 9.4 nmol/l for a subcutaneous single dose of liraglutide 0.6 mg. At 1.8 mg liraglutide, the average steady state concentration of liraglutide ($AUC_{\tau/24}$) reached approximately 34 nmol/l. Liraglutide exposure increased proportionally with dose. The intra-subject coefficient of variation for liraglutide AUC was 11% following single dose administration.

Absolute bioavailability of liraglutide following subcutaneous administration is approximately 55%.

Distribution

The apparent volume of distribution after subcutaneous administration is 11-17 l. The mean volume of distribution after intravenous administration of liraglutide is 0.07 l/kg. Liraglutide is extensively bound to plasma proteins (>98%).

Metabolism

During 24 hours following administration of a single radiolabelled [^{3}H]-liraglutide dose to healthy subjects, the major component in plasma was intact liraglutide. Two minor plasma metabolites were detected (≤9% and ≤5% of total plasma radioactivity exposure). Liraglutide is metabolised in a similar manner to large proteins without a specific organ having been identified as major route of elimination.

Elimination

Following a [^{3}H]-liraglutide dose, intact liraglutide was not detected in urine or faeces. Only a minor part of the administered radioactivity was excreted as liraglutide-related metabolites in urine or faeces (6% and 5%, respectively). The urine and faeces radioactivity was mainly excreted during the first 6-8 days, and corresponded to three minor metabolites, respectively.

The mean clearance following subcutaneous administration of a single dose liraglutide is approximately 1.2 l/h with an elimination half-life of approximately 13 hours.

Special populations

Elderly: Age had no clinically relevant effect on the pharmacokinetics of liraglutide based on the results from a pharmacokinetic study in healthy subjects and population pharmacokinetic data analysis of patients (18 to 80 years).

Table 3 Results of two 26 week trials. Victoza in combination with metformin + rosiglitazone and Victoza in combination with glimepiride + metformin

Metformin + rosiglitazone add-on therapy	1.8 mg liraglutide + metformin[2] + rosiglitazone[3]	1.2mg liraglutide + metformin[2] + rosiglitazone[3]	placebo + metformin[2] + rosiglitazone[3]	N/A
N	178	177	175	
Mean HbA_{1c} (%)				
Baseline	8.56	8.48	8.42	
Change from baseline	-1.48	-1.48	-0.54	
Patients (%) achieving HbA_{1c} <7%				
All patients	53.7	57.5	28.1	
Mean body weight (kg)				
Baseline	94.9	95.3	98.5	
Change from baseline	-2.02	-1.02	0.60	
Metformin + glimepiride add-on therapy	**1.8 mg liraglutide + metformin[2] + glimepiride[4]**	**N/A**	**Placebo + metformin[2] + glimepiride[4]**	**insulin glargine[1] + metformin[2] + glimepiride[4]**
N	230		114	232
Mean HbA_{1c} (%)				
Baseline	8.3		8.3	8.1
Change from baseline	-1.33		-0.24	-1.09
Patients (%) achieving HbA_{1c} <7%				
All patients	53.1		15.3	45.8
Mean body weight (kg)				
Baseline	85.8		85.4	85.2
Change from baseline	-1.81		-0.42	1.62

[1] The dosing of insulin glargine was open-labelled and was applied according to the following titration guideline. Titration of the insulin glargine dose was managed by the patient after instruction by the investigator.

Gender: Gender had no clinically meaningful effect on the pharmacokinetics of liraglutide based on the results of population pharmacokinetic data analysis of male and female patients and a pharmacokinetic study in healthy subjects.

Ethnic origin: Ethnic origin had no clinically relevant effect on the pharmacokinetics of liraglutide based on the results of population pharmacokinetic analysis which included subjects of White, Black, Asian and Hispanic groups.

Obesity: Population pharmacokinetic analysis suggests that body mass index (BMI) has no significant effect on the pharmacokinetics of liraglutide.

Hepatic impairment: The pharmacokinetics of liraglutide was evaluated in subjects with varying degree of hepatic impairment in a single-dose trial. Liraglutide exposure was decreased by 13-23% in subjects with mild to moderate hepatic impairment compared to healthy subjects.

Exposure was significantly lower (44%) in subjects with severe hepatic impairment (Child Pugh score >9).

Renal impairment: Liraglutide exposure was reduced in subjects with renal impairment compared to individuals with normal renal function. Liraglutide exposure was lowered by 33%, 14%, 27% and 28%, respectively, in subjects with mild (creatinine clearance, CrCL 50-80 ml/min), moderate (CrCL 30-50 ml/min), and severe (CrCL <30 ml/min) renal impairment and in end-stage renal disease requiring dialysis.

5.3 Preclinical safety data

Non-clinical data reveal no special hazards for humans based on conventional studies of safety pharmacology, repeat-dose toxicity, or genotoxicity.

Non-lethal thyroid C-cell tumours were seen in 2-year carcinogenicity studies in rats and mice. In rats, a no observed adverse effect level (NOAEL) was not observed. These tumours were not seen in monkeys treated for 20 months. These findings in rodents are caused by a non-genotoxic, specific GLP-1 receptor-mediated mechanism to which rodents are particularly sensitive. The relevance for humans is likely to be low but cannot be completely excluded. No other treatment-related tumours have been found.

Animal studies did not indicate direct harmful effects with respect to fertility but slightly increased early embryonic deaths at the highest dose. Dosing with Victoza during mid-gestation caused a reduction in maternal weight and foetal growth with equivocal effects on ribs in rats and skeletal variation in the rabbit. Neonatal growth was reduced in rats while exposed to Victoza, and persisted in the post-weaning period in the high dose group. It is unknown whether the reduced pup growth is caused by reduced pup milk intake due to a direct GLP-1 effect or reduced maternal milk production due to decreased caloric intake.

6. PHARMACEUTICAL PARTICULARS

6.1 List of excipients

Disodium phosphate dihydrate

Propylene glycol

Phenol

Water for injections

6.2 Incompatibilities

Substances added to Victoza may cause degradation of liraglutide. In the absence of compatibility studies, this medicinal product must not be mixed with other medicinal products.

6.3 Shelf life

30 months.

After first use: 1 month

6.4 Special precautions for storage

Store in a refrigerator (2°C - 8°C).

Do not freeze.

Store away from the freezer compartment.

After first use: Store below 30°C or store in a refrigerator (2°C - 8°C). Do not freeze.

Keep the cap on the pen in order to protect from light.

6.5 Nature and contents of container

Cartridge (type 1 glass) with a plunger (bromobutyl) and a stopper (bromobutyl/polyisoprene) contained in a pre-filled multidose disposable pen made of polyolefin and polyacetal.

Each pen contains 3 ml solution, delivering 30 doses of 0.6 mg, 15 doses of 1.2 mg or 10 doses of 1.8 mg.

Pack sizes of 1, 2, 3, 5 or 10 pre-filled pens.

Not all pack sizes may be marketed.

6.6 Special precautions for disposal and other handling

Victoza should not be used if it does not appear clear and colourless.

Victoza should not be used if it has been frozen.

Victoza can be administered with needles up to a length of 8 mm and as thin as 32G. The pen is designed to be used with NovoFine or NovoTwist disposable needles.

Injection needles are not included.

The patient should be advised to discard the injection needle in accordance with local requirements after each injection and store the Victoza pen without an injection needle attached. This prevents contamination, infection, and leakage. It also ensures that the dosing is accurate.

7. MARKETING AUTHORISATION HOLDER

Novo Nordisk A/S

Novo Allé

DK-2880 Bagsværd

Denmark

8. MARKETING AUTHORISATION NUMBER(S)

EU/1/09/529/001

EU/1/09/529/002

EU/1/09/529/003

EU/1/09/529/004

EU/1/09/529/005

9. DATE OF FIRST AUTHORISATION/RENEWAL OF THE AUTHORISATION

Date of first authorisation: 30 June 2009

10. DATE OF REVISION OF THE TEXT

06/2009

Detailed information on this medicinal product is available on the website of the European Medicines Agency (EMEA) http://www.emea.europa.eu/.

Vimpat 50 mg, 100 mg, 150 mg & 200 mg film-coated tablets, 15 mg/ml syrup and 10 mg/ml solution for infusion

(UCB Pharma Limited)

1. NAME OF THE MEDICINAL PRODUCT

Vimpat 50 mg film-coated tablets ▼

Vimpat 100 mg film-coated tablets

Vimpat 150 mg film-coated tablets

Vimpat 200 mg film-coated tablets

Vimpat 15 mg/ml syrup

Vimpat 10 mg/ml solution for infusion

2. QUALITATIVE AND QUANTITATIVE COMPOSITION

Tablets:

Each film-coated tablet contains 50 mg lacosamide, 100 mg lacosamide, 150 mg lacosamide or 200 mg lacosamide and 0.17 mg, 0.34 mg, 0.50 mg or 0.67 mg, respectively, of the excipient soya-lecithin.

Syrup:

Each ml of syrup contains 15 mg lacosamide.

1 bottle of 200 ml contains 3000 mg lacosamide.

Excipients: each ml of Vimpat syrup contains 280 mg sorbitol (E420), 0.2 mg sodium propylparahydroxybenzoate (E217), 2.0 mg sodium methylparahydroxybenzoate (E219), 0.05 mg aspartame (E951) and 1.89 mg sodium.

Solution for infusion:

Each ml of solution for infusion contains 10 mg lacosamide.

1 vial of 20 ml solution for infusion contains 200 mg lacosamide.

Excipient: each ml of solution for infusion contains 2.99 mg sodium.

For a full list of excipients, see section 6.1.

3. PHARMACEUTICAL FORM

Tablets:

Film-coated tablet

50 mg: Pinkish, oval film-coated tablet debossed with 'SP' on one side and '50' on the other side.

100 mg: Dark yellow, oval film-coated tablet debossed with 'SP' on one side and '100' on the other side.

150 mg: Salmon, oval film-coated tablet debossed with 'SP' on one side and '150' on the other side.

200 mg: Blue, oval film-coated tablet debossed with 'SP' on one side and '200' on the other side.

Syrup:

Clear solution, slightly yellow to yellow-brown in colour.

Solution for infusion:

Clear, colourless solution.

4. CLINICAL PARTICULARS

4.1 Therapeutic indications

Vimpat is indicated as adjunctive therapy in the treatment of partial-onset seizures with or without secondary generalisation in patients with epilepsy aged 16 years and older.

Solution for infusion:

Vimpat solution for infusion is an alternative for patients when oral administration is temporarily not feasible.

4.2 Posology and method of administration

Vimpat must be taken twice a day. The recommended starting dose is 50 mg twice a day which should be increased to an initial therapeutic dose of 100 mg twice a day after one week.

Depending on response and tolerability, the maintenance dose can be further increased by 50 mg twice a day every week, to a maximum recommended daily dose of 400 mg (200 mg twice a day). Vimpat may be taken with or without food.

Vimpat therapy can be initiated with either oral or i.v. administration.

In accordance with current clinical practice, if Vimpat has to be discontinued, it is recommended this be done gradually (e.g. taper the daily dose by 200 mg/week).

Syrup:

Vimpat syrup is provided with a measuring cup with graduation marks and instructions for use in the package leaflet.

Solution for infusion:

The solution for infusion is infused over a period of 15 to 60 minutes twice daily. Vimpat solution for infusion can be administered i.v. without further dilution. Conversion to or from oral and i.v. administration can be done directly without titration. The total daily dose and twice daily administration should be maintained.

There is experience with twice daily infusions of Vimpat up to 5 days.

<u>Use in patients with renal impairment</u>

No dose adjustment is necessary in mildly and moderately renally impaired patients (CL_{CR}>30 ml/min). A maximum dose of 250 mg/day is recommended for patients with severe renal impairment ($CL_{CR} \leq 30$ ml/min) and in patients with endstage renal disease. For patients requiring haemodialysis a supplement of up to 50% of the divided daily dose directly after the end of haemodialysis is recommended. Treatment of patients with end-stage renal disease should be made with caution as there is little clinical experience and accumulation of a metabolite (with no known pharmacological activity). In all patients with renal impairment, the dose titration should be performed with caution (see section 5.2).

<u>Use in patients with hepatic impairment</u>

No dose adjustment is needed for patients with mild to moderate hepatic impairment.

The dose titration in these patients should be performed with caution considering co-existing renal impairment. The pharmacokinetics of lacosamide has not been evaluated in severely hepatic impaired patients (see section 5.2).

<u>Use in elderly (over 65 years of age)</u>

No dose reduction is necessary in elderly patients. The experience with lacosamide in elderly patients with epilepsy is limited. Age associated decreased renal clearance with an increase in AUC levels should be considered in elderly patients (see 'Use in patients with renal impairment' above and section 5.2).

<u>Paediatric patients</u>

Vimpat is not recommended for use in children and adolescents below the age of 16 as there is no data on safety and efficacy in these age groups.

4.3 Contraindications

Tablets:

Hypersensitivity to the active substance or to peanuts or soya or to any of the excipients.

Known second- or third-degree atrioventricular (AV) block.

Syrup and Solution for infusion:

Hypersensitivity to the active substance or to any of the excipients.

Known second- or third-degree atrioventricular (AV) block.

4.4 Special warnings and precautions for use

Treatment with lacosamide has been associated with dizziness which could increase the occurrence of accidental injury or falls. Therefore, patients should be advised to exercise caution until they are familiar with the potential effects of the medicine (see section 4.8).

Prolongations in PR interval with lacosamide have been observed in clinical studies. Lacosamide should be used with caution in patients with known conduction problems or severe cardiac disease such as a history of myocardial infarction or heart failure. Caution should especially be exerted when treating elderly patients as they may be at an increased risk of cardiac disorders or when lacosamide is used in combination with products known to be associated with PR prolongation.

Suicidal ideation and behaviour have been reported in patients treated with anti-epileptic agents in several indications. A meta-analysis of randomised placebo controlled trials of anti-epileptic drugs has also shown a small increased risk of suicidal ideation and behaviour. The mechanism of this risk is not known and the available data do not exclude the possibility of an increased risk for lacosamide.

Therefore patients should be monitored for signs of suicidal ideation and behaviours and appropriate treatment should be considered. Patients (and caregivers of patients) should be advised to seek medical advice should signs of suicidal ideation or behaviour emerge.

Syrup:

Vimpat syrup contains sodium propylhydroxybenzoate (E217) and sodium methylhydroxybenzoate (E219), which may cause allergic reactions (possibly delayed). It contains 3.7 g sorbitol (E420) per dose (200 mg lacosamide), corresponding to a calorific value of 9.7 kcal. Patients with rare hereditary problems of fructose intolerance should not take this medicine. The syrup contains aspartame (E951), a source of phenylalanine, which may be harmful for people with phenylketonuria. It contains 1.06 mmol (or 25.2 mg) sodium per dose (200 mg lacosamide). To be taken into consideration for patients on a controlled sodium diet.

Solution for infusion:

This medicinal product contains 2.6 mmol (or 59.8 mg) sodium per vial. To be taken into consideration for patients on a controlled sodium diet.

4.5 Interaction with other medicinal products and other forms of interaction

Lacosamide should be used with caution in patients treated with medicinal products known to be associated with PR prolongation (e.g. carbamazepine, lamotrigine, pregabalin) and in patients treated with class I antiarrhythmic drugs. However, subgroup analysis did not identify an increased magnitude of PR prolongation in patients with concomitant administration of carbamazepine or lamotrigine in clinical trials.

Data generally suggest that lacosamide has a low interaction potential. *In vitro* studies indicate that the enzymes CYP1A2, 2B6, and 2C9 are not induced and that CYP1A1, 1A2, 2A6, 2B6, 2C8, 2C9, 2D6, and 2E1 are not inhibited by lacosamide at plasma concentrations observed in clinical trials. An *in vitro* study indicated that lacosamide is not transported by P-glycoprotein in the intestine. Lacosamide does not inhibit or induce the enzyme CYP2C19 in vivo.

In vitro studies indicate that lacosamide may be a weak inhibitor and inducer of CYP3A4. The clinical relevance of this is presently unknown. An interaction study with carbamazepine does not indicate a marked inhibitory effect of lacosamide on CYP3A4 catalysed metabolism at therapeutic doses.

Strong enzyme inducers such as rifampicin or St John's wort (Hypericum perforatum) may moderately reduce the systemic exposure of lacosamide. Therefore, starting or ending treatment with these enzyme inducers should be done with caution.

Antiepileptic drugs

In interaction trials lacosamide did not significantly affect the plasma concentrations of carbamazepine and valproic acid. Lacosamide plasma concentrations were not affected by carbamazepine and by valproic acid. A population PK analysis estimated that concomitant treatment with other anti-epileptic drugs known to be enzyme inducers (carbamazepine, phenytoin, phenobarbital, in various doses) decreased the overall systemic exposure of lacosamide by 25%.

Oral contraceptives

In an interaction trial there was no clinically relevant interaction between lacosamide and the oral contraceptives ethinylestradiol and levonorgestrel. Progesterone concentrations were not affected when the medicinal products were co-administered.

Others

Interaction trials showed that lacosamide had no effect on the pharmacokinetics of digoxin. There was no clinically relevant interaction between lacosamide and metformin.

Omeprazole 40 mg q.d. increased the AUC of lacosamide by 19%. The effect probably lacks clinical relevance. Lacosamide did not affect the single-dose pharmacokinetics of omeprazole.

No data on the interaction of lacosamide with alcohol are available.

Lacosamide has a low protein binding of less than 15%. Therefore, clinically relevant interactions with other drugs through competition for protein binding sites are considered unlikely.

4.6 Pregnancy and lactation

Pregnancy

Risk related to epilepsy and antiepileptic medicinal products in general

For all anti-epileptic drugs, it has been shown that in the offspring of women treated with epilepsy, the prevalence of malformations is two to three times greater than the rate of approximately 3% in the general population. In the treated population, an increase in malformations has been noted with polytherapy, however, the extent to which the treatment and/or the illness is responsible has not been elucidated.

Moreover, effective anti-epileptic therapy must not be interrupted, since the aggravation of the illness is detrimental to both the mother and the foetus.

Risk related to lacosamide

There are no adequate data from the use of lacosamide in pregnant women. Studies in animals did not indicate any teratogenic effects in rats or rabbits, but embryotoxicity was observed in rats and rabbits at maternal toxic doses (see section 5.3). The potential risk for humans is unknown.

Lacosamide should not be used during pregnancy unless clearly necessary (if the benefit to the mother clearly outweighs the potential risk to the foetus). If women decide to become pregnant, the use of this product should be carefully re-evaluated.

Lactation

It is unknown whether lacosamide is excreted in human breast milk. Animal studies have shown excretion of lacosamide in breast milk. For precautionary measures, breastfeeding should be discontinued during treatment with lacosamide.

4.7 Effects on ability to drive and use machines

Vimpat may have minor to moderate influence on the ability to drive and use machines. Vimpat treatment has been associated with dizziness or blurred vision.

Accordingly, patients should be advised not to drive a car or to operate other potentially hazardous machinery until they are familiar with the effects of Vimpat on their ability to perform such activities.

4.8 Undesirable effects

Based on the analysis of pooled placebo-controlled clinical trials in 1,308 patients with partial-onset seizures, a total of 61.9% of patients randomized to lacosamide and 35.2% of patients randomized to placebo reported at least 1 adverse reaction. The most frequently reported adverse reactions with lacosamide treatment were dizziness, headache, nausea and diplopia. They were usually mild to moderate in intensity. Some were dose-related and could be alleviated by reducing the dose. Incidence and severity of CNS and gastrointestinal (GI) adverse reactions usually decreased over time.

Over all controlled studies, the discontinuation rate due to adverse reactions was 12.2% for patients randomized to lacosamide and 1.6% for patients randomized to placebo. The most common adverse reaction resulting in discontinuation of lacosamide therapy was dizziness.

The table below shows the frequencies of adverse reactions which have been reported in pooled placebo-controlled clinical trials. The frequencies are defined as follows: very common (≥1/10), common (≥1/100 to <1/10), uncommon (≥1/1,000 to <1/100). Within each frequency grouping, undesirable effects are presented in order of decreasing seriousness.

System organ class	Very common	Common
Psychiatric disorders		Depression
Nervous system disorders	Dizziness Headache	Balance disorder Coordination abnormal Memory impairment Cognitive disorder Somnolence Tremor Nystagmus
Eye disorders	Diplopia	Vision blurred
Ear and labyrinth disorders		Vertigo
Gastrointestinal disorders	Nausea	Vomiting Constipation Flatulence
Skin and subcutaneous tissue disorders		Pruritus
General disorders and administration site conditions		Gait disturbance Asthenia Fatigue
Injury, poisoning and procedural complications		Fall Skin laceration

The use of lacosamide is associated with dose-related increase in the PR interval. Adverse reactions associated with PR interval prolongation (e.g. atrioventricular block, syncope, bradycardia) may occur.

In epilepsy patients the incidence rate of reported first degree AV Block is uncommon, 0.7%, 0%, 0.5% and 0% for lacosamide 200 mg, 400 mg, 600 mg or placebo, respectively. No second or higher degree AV Block was seen in lacosamide treated patients.

The incidence rate for syncope is uncommon and did not differ between lacosamide treated epilepsy patients (0.1%) and placebo treated epilepsy patients (0.3%).

4.9 Overdose

There is limited clinical experience with lacosamide overdose in humans. Clinical symptoms (dizziness and nausea) following doses of 1200 mg/day were mainly related to the central nervous system and the gastrointestinal system and resolved with dose adjustments.

The highest reported overdose in the clinical development program for lacosamide was 12 g taken in conjunction with toxic doses of multiple other antiepileptic drugs. The subject was initially comatose and then fully recovered without permanent sequelae.

There is no specific antidote for overdose with lacosamide. Treatment of lacosamide overdose should include general supportive measures and may include haemodialysis if necessary (see section 5.2).

5. PHARMACOLOGICAL PROPERTIES

5.1 Pharmacodynamic properties

Pharmacotherapeutic group: other antiepileptics, ATC code: N03AX18

The active substance, lacosamide (R-2-acetamido-N-benzyl-3-methoxypropionamide) is a functionalised amino acid.

Mechanism of action

The precise mechanism by which lacosamide exerts its antiepileptic effect in humans remains to be fully elucidated. Two observations that may be of relevance for the observed therapeutic effects are:

In vitro electrophysiological studies have shown that lacosamide selectively enhances slow inactivation of voltage-gated sodium channels, resulting in stabilization of hyperexcitable neuronal membranes. Further, lacosamide binds to collapsin response mediator protein-2 (CRMP-2), a phosphoprotein which is mainly expressed in the nervous system and is involved in neuronal differentiation and control of axonal outgrowth.

Pharmacodynamic effects

Lacosamide protected against seizures in a broad range of animal models of partial and primary generalized seizures and delayed kindling development.

In non-clinical experiments lacosamide in combination with levetiracetam, carbamazepine, phenytoin, valproate, lamotrigine, topiramate or gabapentin showed synergistic or additive anticonvulsant effects.

Clinical experience

The efficacy of Vimpat as adjunctive therapy at recommended doses (200 mg/day, 400 mg/day) was established in 3 multicenter, randomized, placebo-controlled clinical trials with a 12-week maintenance period. Vimpat 600 mg/day was also shown to be effective in controlled adjunctive therapy trials, although the efficacy was similar to 400 mg/day and patients were less likely to tolerate this dose because of CNS- and gastrointestinal-related adverse reactions. Thus, the 600 mg/day dose is not recommended. The maximum recommended dose is 400 mg/day. These trials, involving 1308 patients with a history of an average of 23 years of partial-onset seizures, were designed to evaluate the efficacy and safety of lacosamide when administered concomitantly with 1-3 antiepileptic drugs in patients with uncontrolled partial-onset seizures with or without secondary generalisation. Overall the proportion of subjects with a 50% reduction in seizure frequency was 23%, 34%, and 40% for placebo, lacosamide 200 mg/day and lacosamide 400 mg/day.

There are insufficient data regarding the withdrawal of concomitant antiepileptic medicinal products to achieve monotherapy with lacosamide.

5.2 Pharmacokinetic properties

Absorption

Tablets and Syrup:

Lacosamide is rapidly and completely absorbed after oral administration. The oral bioavailability of lacosamide tablets is approximately 100%. Following oral administration, the plasma concentration of unchanged lacosamide increases rapidly and reaches C_{max} about 0.5 to 4 hours post-dose. Vimpat tablets and oral syrup are bioequivalent. Food does not affect the rate and extent of absorption.

Solution for infusion:

After i.v. administration, C_{max} is reached at the end of infusion. The plasma concentration increases proportionally with dose after oral (100-800 mg) and i.v. (50-300 mg) administration.

Distribution

The volume of distribution is approximately 0.6 L/kg. Lacosamide is less than 15% bound to plasma proteins.

Metabolism

95% of the dose is excreted in the urine as drug and metabolites. The metabolism of lacosamide has not been completely characterised.

The major compounds excreted in urine are unchanged lacosamide (approximately 40% of the dose) and its O-desmethyl metabolite less than 30%.

A polar fraction proposed to be serine derivatives accounted for approximately 20% in urine, but was detected only in small amounts (0-2%) in human plasma of some subjects. Small amounts (0.5-2%) of additional metabolites were found in the urine.

CYP2C19 is mainly responsible for the formation of the O-desmethyl metabolite. However, no clinically relevant difference in lacosamide exposure was observed comparing its pharmacokinetics in extensive metabolisers (EMs, with a functional CYP2C19) and poor metabolisers (PMs, lacking a functional CYP2C19). Furthermore an interaction trial with omeprazole (CYP2C19-inhibitor) demonstrated no clinically relevant changes in lacosamide plasma concentrations indicating that the importance of this pathway is minor. No other enzymes have been identified to be involved in the metabolism of lacosamide.

The plasma concentration of O-desmethyl-lacosamide is approximately 15% of the concentration of lacosamide in plasma. This major metabolite has no known pharmacological activity.

Elimination

Lacosamide is primarily eliminated from the systemic circulation by renal excretion and biotransformation. After oral and intravenous administration of radiolabeled lacosamide, approximately 95% of radioactivity administered was recovered in the urine and less than 0.5% in the faeces. The elimination half-life of the unchanged drug is approximately 13 hours. The pharmacokinetics is dose-proportional and constant over time, with low intra- and inter-subject variability. Following twice daily dosing, steady state plasma concentrations are achieved after a 3 day period. The plasma concentration increases with an accumulation factor of approximately 2.

Pharmacokinetics in special patient groups

Gender

Clinical trials indicate that gender does not have a clinically significant influence on the plasma concentrations of lacosamide.

Renal impairment

The AUC of lacosamide was increased by approximately 30% in mildly and moderately and 60% in severely renal impaired patients and patients with endstage renal disease requiring hemodialysis compared to healthy subjects, whereas c_{max} was unaffected.

Lacosamide is effectively removed from plasma by haemodialysis. Following a 4-hour haemodialysis treatment, AUC of lacosamide is reduced by approximately 50%. Therefore dosage supplementation following haemodialysis is recommended (see section 4.2). The exposure of the O-desmethyl metabolite was several-fold increased in patients with moderate and severe renal impairment. In absence of haemodialysis in patients with endstage renal disease, the levels were increased and continuously rising during the 24-hour sampling. It is unknown whether the increased metabolite exposure in endstage renal disease subjects could give rise to adverse effects but no pharmacological activity of the metabolite has been identified.

Hepatic impairment

Subjects with moderate hepatic impairment (Child-Pugh B) showed higher plasma concentrations of lacosamide (approximately 50% higher AUC_{norm}). The higher exposure was partly due to a reduced renal function in the studied subjects. The decrease in non-renal clearance in the patients of the study was estimated to give a 20% increase in the AUC of lacosamide. The pharmacokinetics of lacosamide has not been evaluated in severe hepatic impairment (see section 4.2).

Elderly (over 65 years of age)

In a study in elderly men and women including 4 patients >75 years of age, AUC was about 30 and 50% increased compared to young men, respectively. This is partly related to lower body weight. The body weight normalized difference is 26 and 23%, respectively. An increased variability in exposure was also observed. The renal clearance of lacosamide was only slightly reduced in elderly subjects in this study.

A general dose reduction is not considered to be necessary unless indicated due to reduced renal function (see section 4.2).

5.3 Preclinical safety data

In the toxicity studies, the plasma concentrations of lacosamide obtained were similar or only marginally higher than those observed in patients, which leaves low or non-existing margins to human exposure.

A safety pharmacology study with intravenous administration of lacosamide in anesthetized dogs showed transient increases in PR interval and QRS complex duration and decreases in blood pressure most likely due to a cardiodepressant action. These transient changes started in the same concentration range as after maximum recommended clinical dosing. In anesthetized dogs and Cynomolgus monkeys, at intravenous doses of 15-60 mg/kg, slowing of atrial and ventricular conductivity, atrioventricular block and atrioventricular dissociation were seen.

In the repeated dose toxicity studies, mild reversible liver changes were observed in rats starting at about 3 times the clinical exposure. These changes included an increased organ weight, hypertrophy of hepatocytes, increases in serum concentrations of liver enzymes and increases in total cholesterol and triglycerides. Apart from the hypertrophy of hepatocytes, no other histopathologic changes were observed.

In reproductive and developmental toxicity studies in rodents and rabbits, no teratogenic effects but an increase in numbers of stillborn pups and pup deaths in the peripartum period, and slightly reduced live litter sizes and pup body weights were observed at maternal toxic doses in rats corresponding to systemic exposure levels similar to the expected clinical exposure. Since higher exposure levels could not be tested in animals due to maternal toxicity, data are insufficient to fully characterise the embryofetotoxic and teratogenic potential of lacosamide.

Studies in rats revealed that lacosamide and/or its metabolites readily crossed the placental barrier.

6. PHARMACEUTICAL PARTICULARS

6.1 List of excipients

Tablets:

Tablet core:

microcrystalline cellulose

hydroxypropylcellulose

hydroxypropylcellulose (low substituted)

silica, colloidal, anhydrous

crospovidone

magnesium stearate

Tablet coat:

polyvinyl alcohol

polyethylene glycol 400, 3350 and 8000

talc

soya-lecithin

hypromellose

titanium dioxide (E171)

50 mg tablet: red iron oxide (E172), black iron oxide (E172), indigo carmine aluminium lake (E132)

100 mg tablet: yellow iron oxide (E172)

150 mg tablet: yellow iron oxide (E172), red iron oxide (E172), black iron oxide (E172)

200 mg tablet: indigo carmine aluminium lake (E132)

Syrup:

glycerol (E422)

carmellose sodium

sorbitol liquid (crystallizing) (E420)

polyethylene glycol 4000

sodium chloride

citric acid, anhydrous

acesulfame potassium (E950)

sodium propylparahydroxybenzoate (E217)

sodium methylparahydroxybenzoate (E219)

strawberry flavour (contains propylene glycol, maltol)

masking flavour (contains propylene glycol, aspartame (E951), acesulfame potassium (E950), maltol, deionised water)

purified water

Solution for infusion:

water for injection

sodium chloride

hydrochloric acid (for pH adjustment)

6.2 Incompatibilities

Tablets and Syrup:

Not applicable.

Solution for infusion:

This medicinal product must not be mixed with other medicinal products except those mentioned in section 6.6.

6.3 Shelf life

Tablets:

3 years.

Syrup:

2 years

After first opening: 4 weeks.

Solution for infusion:

3 years.

Chemical and physical in-use stability has been demonstrated for 24 hours at temperatures up to 25° C for product mixed with the diluents mentioned in 6.6.

From a microbiological point of view, the product should be used immediately. If not used immediately, in-use storage times and conditions prior to use are the responsibility of the user and would not be longer than 24 hours at 2 to 8°C, unless dilution has taken place in controlled and validated aseptic conditions.

6.4 Special precautions for storage

Tablets:

This medicinal product does not require any special storage conditions.

Syrup:

Do not store above 30°C.

Solution for infusion:

Do not store above 25°C.

6.5 Nature and contents of container

Tablets:

PVC/PVDC blister sealed with an aluminium foil.

50 mg & 100 mg: Packs of 14, 56 and 168 film-coated tablets.

150 mg & 200 mg: Packs of 14, 56 and 168 film-coated tablets (multipacks containing 3 packs of 56 tablets).

The treatment initiation pack contains 4 cartons, each carton with 14 tablets of 50 mg, 100 mg, 150 mg and 200 mg

Not all pack sizes may be marketed.

Syrup:

200 ml and 465 ml amber type III glass or polyethylene terephthalate (PET) bottles with a polypropylene screw cap and a measuring cup.

Not all pack sizes may be marketed.

Solution for infusion:

1x20 ml colourless type I glass vial with a chlorobutyl rubber closure coated with a fluoropolymer.

6.6 Special precautions for disposal and other handling

Tablets and Syrup:

No special requirements.

Solution for infusion:

This medicinal product is for single use only, any unused solution should be discarded.

Product with particulate matter or discolouration should not be used. Vimpat solution for infusion was found to be physically compatible and chemically stable when mixed with the following diluents for at least 24 hours and stored in glass or PVC bags at temperatures up to 25°C.

Diluents:

sodium chloride 9 mg/ml (0.9%) solution for injection

glucose 50 mg/ml (5%) solution for injection

lactated Ringer's solution for injection.

7. MARKETING AUTHORISATION HOLDER

UCB Pharma SA

Allée de la Recherche 60

B-1070 Bruxelles

Belgium

8. MARKETING AUTHORISATION NUMBER(S)

50 mg × 14 tabs: EU/1/08/470/001

100 mg × 14 tabs: EU/1/08/470/004

100 mg × 56 tabs: EU/1/08/470/005

150 mg × 14 tabs: EU/1/08/470/007

150 mg × 56 tabs: EU/1/08/470/008

200 mg × 56 tabs: EU/1/08/470/011

Syrup (15 mg/ml) × 200 ml: EU/1/08/470/014

Solution for Infusion (10 mg/ml) × 20 ml: EU/1/08/470/016

9. DATE OF FIRST AUTHORISATION/RENEWAL OF THE AUTHORISATION

Date of first authorisation: 29 August 2008

10. DATE OF REVISION OF THE TEXT

02/2009

Detailed information on this medicine is available on the European Medicines Agency (EMEA) web site: http://www.emea.europa.eu/.

Vinorelbine 10 mg/ml Concentrate for solution for infusion

(medac GmbH)

1. NAME OF THE MEDICINAL PRODUCT

Vinorelbine 10 mg/ml Concentrate for solution for infusion

2. QUALITATIVE AND QUANTITATIVE COMPOSITION

Vinorelbine (as tartrate) 10 mg/ml

Each 1 ml vial contains a total content of vinorelbine (as tartrate) of 10 mg

Each 5 ml vial contains a total content of vinorelbine (as tartrate) of 50 mg

For excipients, see section 6.1.

3. PHARMACEUTICAL FORM

Concentrate for solution for infusion

Clear, colourless to pale yellow solution.

4. CLINICAL PARTICULARS

4.1 Therapeutic indications

- As a single agent or in combination for the first line treatment of stage 3 or 4 non small cell lung cancer.
- Treatment of advanced breast cancer stage 3 and 4 relapsing after or refractory to an anthracycline containing regimen.

4.2 Posology and method of administration

Vinorelbine must be administered under the supervision of a doctor experienced in the use of chemotherapy.

Strictly by intravenous injection through an infusion line.

The use of intrathecal route is contra-indicated.

In adults:

- Vinorelbine is usually given at 25-30 mg/m^2 weekly.

Vinorelbine may be administered by slow bolus (5-10 minutes) after dilution in 20 – 50 ml of normal saline or glucose 50 mg/ml (5%) solution or by a short infusion (20-30 minutes) after dilution in 125 ml of normal saline or glucose 50 mg/ml (5%) solution. Administration should always be followed by a normal saline infusion to flush the vein.

Dose modifications:

Vinorelbine metabolism and clearance are mostly hepatic: only 18.5% is excreted unchanged in the urine. No prospective study relating altered metabolism of the active substance to its pharmacodynamic effects is available in order to establish guidelines for vinorelbine dose reduction in patients with impaired liver or kidney function.

Hepatic Impairment

In breast cancer-patients, vinorelbine clearance is not altered in the presence of moderate liver metastases (i.e. 75% of liver volume replaced by the tumour). In these patients, there is no pharmacokinetic rationale for reducing vinorelbine doses.

In patients with massive liver metastases (i.e. >75% of liver volume replaced by the tumour), the real impact of impaired drug elimination capacity of the liver has not been characterised. In these patients, it is empirically suggested that the dose be reduced by 1/3 and the haematological toxicity closely followed-up.

Renal impairment

There is no pharmacokinetic rationale for reducing vinorelbine dose in patients with impaired kidney function.

The dose limiting toxicity of vinorelbine is mainly neutropenia. This usually occurs between day 8 and day 12 after administration of the medicinal product, is short-lived, and is not cumulative. If the neutrophil count is $<2000/mm^3$ and/or platelet number is $<75000/mm^3$, then the treatment should be delayed until recovery. Administration of the medicinal product is expected to be delayed by 1 week in about 35% of treatment courses.

The maximum tolerated dose per administration: 35.4 mg/m^2 body surface area

The maximum total dose per administration: 60 mg

The safety and efficacy in children and adolescents have not been demonstrated.

4.3 Contraindications

- Hypersensitivity to vinorelbine or other vinca alkaloids
- Neutrophil count $<2000/mm^3$ or severe current or recent infection (within the last 2 weeks)
- Platelet count less than 75.000/mm^3
- Severe hepatic impairment not related to the tumoural process
- In combination with yellow fever vaccine
- Pregnancy (see section 4.6)
- Lactation (see section 4.6)

4.4 Special warnings and precautions for use

- Vinorelbine must only be administered by the intravenous route. The use of intrathecal route is contra-indicated. Administration should always be followed by a normal saline infusion to flush the vein.
- Vinorelbine must be administered intravenously with great precision: It is very important to make sure that the cannula has been accurately placed into the vein before starting to infuse vinorelbine. If vinorelbine extravasates during intravenous administration, this can cause considerable local irritation. In this case, the infusion must be stopped immediately, the vein flushed through with physiological saline solution and the rest of the dose should be administered in another vein. In the event of extravasation glucosteroids can be given intravenously in order to reduce the risk of phlebitis.
- Treatment should be undertaken with close haematological monitoring (determination of haemoglobin level and number of leukocytes, granulocytes and platelets before each new injection). If the neutrophil count is $<2000/mm^3$ and/or thrombocyte count is below $75000/mm^3$, treatment should be delayed until recovery and the patient should be observed (see section 4.2).
- If the patients present signs or symptoms suggestive of infection, a prompt investigation should be carried out.
- If there is significant hepatic impairment the dose should be reduced: caution is recommended and careful monitoring of haematological parameters required (see section 4.2).
- In case of renal impairment, because of the low level of renal excretion, no dose modification is necessary (see section 4.2 and 5.2).
- Vinorelbine should not be given concomitantly with radiotherapy if the treatment field includes the liver.
- This product is generally not recommended in combination with live attenuated vaccines.
- All contact with the eyes should be strictly avoided: risk of severe irritation and even corneal ulceration if the medicinal product is sprayed under pressure. Immediate liberal washing of the eye with normal saline solution should be undertaken if any contact occurs.
- Vinorelbine can have genotoxic effects. Therefore, men being treated with vinorelbine are advised not to father a child during and up to six months after treatment. Women of childbearing potential must use an effective method of contraception during treatment and three months thereafter.

4.5 Interaction with other medicinal products and other forms of interaction

The combination of vinorelbine and cisplatin (a very common combination) does not affect the pharmacokinetic parameters. However, there is an increased incidence of granulocytopenia in the combination of vinorelbine and cisplatin than in vinorelbine as monotherapy.

As the metabolism of vinorelbine mainly involves CYP3A4, combinations with inductors (e.g. phenytoin, rifampicin) or inhibitors of this enzyme (e.g. itraconazole, ketoconazole) can modify the pharmacokinetics of vinorelbine.

Concomitant use of vinca alkaloids and mitomycin C increases the risk of bronchospasm and dyspnoea. In rare cases, particularly in combination with mitomycin, an interstitial pneumonitis has been observed.

Vinorelbine is a P-glycoprotein substrate and concomitant use with inhibitors or inducers of this transport protein can affect the concentration of vinorelbine.

4.6 Pregnancy and lactation

- Pregnancy

There are insufficient data from the use of vinorelbine in pregnant women. In animal reproductive studies vinorelbine was embryo- and feto-lethal and teratogenic. Women should not become pregnant during treatment with vinorelbine. This product should not be used during pregnancy. If pregnancy should occur during the treatment, the possibility of genetic counselling should be considered.

Women of childbearing potential must be advised to use effective contraception during treatment and three months thereafter and should inform their doctor if they become pregnant.

- Lactation

There are no data on the excretion of vinorelbine into breast milk. Breast-feeding must therefore be discontinued before treatment with this medicinal product.

4.7 Effects on ability to drive and use machines

No studies of the effects on the ability to drive and use machines have been performed.

4.8 Undesirable effects

Bone marrow toxicity and gastrointestinal symptoms are the most frequent and relevant undesirable effects of vinorelbine in monotherapy and combined therapy.

In combined chemotherapy of vinorelbine with other antineoplastic medicinal products it has to be considered, that the listed undesirable effect can occur more frequently and more severe than those undesirable effects observed during and after monotherapy. Moreover, the additional specific undesirable effects of the other medicinal products have to be considered.

Frequencies

Very common (>1/10)

Common (>1/100, <1/10)

Uncommon (>1/1,000, <1/100)

Rare (>1/10,000, <1/1,000)

Very rare (<1/10,000), including isolated reports

Infections and infestations	Common Infection
Blood and lymphatic system disorders	Very common Neutropenia, anaemia Common Thrombocytopenia, febrile neutropenia, neutropenic sepsis with potential fatal outcome
Immune system disorders	Common Allergic reactions (skin reactions, respiratory reactions)
Metabolism and nutrition disorders	Rare Severe hyponatraemia Very rare SIADH-syndrome
Nervous system disorders	Very common Constipation (see also „Gastrointestinal disorders"), loss of deep tendon reflexes Common Paraesthesia, neurosensory and neuromotor disorders, Guillain-Barré syndrome Rare Weakness of lower extremities, paralytic ileus (see also „Gastrointestinal disorders")
Cardiac disorders	Rare Ischaemic heart disease like angina pectoris, transitory electrocardiogram modifications, myocardial infarction
Respiratory, thoracic and mediastinal disorders	Common Dyspnoea, bronchospasm Rare Interstitial lung disease
Gastrointestinal disorders	Very common Constipation (see also "Nervous system disorders"), nausea, vomiting, diarrhoea, stomatitis, oesophagitis, anorexia Rare Pancreatitis, paralytic ileus (see also "Nervous system disorders")
Hepatobiliary disorders	Very common Abnormal liver function values (total bilirubin increased, alkaline phosphatase increased, aspartate aminotransferase increased, alanine aminotransferase increased)
Skin and subcutaneous tissue disorders	Very common Alopecia Common Skin reactions Rare Generalised skin reactions
Musculoskeletal and connective tissue disorders	Common Myalgia, Arthralgia Rare Jaw pain
Renal and urinary disorders	Common Creatinine increased
General disorders and administration site conditions	Very common Fatigue, fever, pain in different locations, asthenia, injection site erythema, injection site pain, injection site discolouration, injection site phlebitis Rare Injection site necrosis

Grades (G) of toxicity according to WHO classification

Infections and infestations

- Infections can develop commonly, mainly due to bone marrow suppression.

Blood and lymphatic system disorders

- The limiting toxicity is bone marrow depression which is manifested, in particular, as neutropenia (G1: 9.7%; G2: 15.2%; G3: 24.3%, G4: 27.8%), which is reversible within 5-7 days and non-cumulative; the neutrophil count is usually at its lowest 7-14 days after administration.
- Febrile neutropenia and neutropenic sepsis which in some cases (1.2%) had a fatal outcome can occur.
- Anaemia (G1-2: 61.2%; G3-4: 7.4% in monotherapy) and thrombocytopenia (G1-2: 5.1%; G3-4: 2.5% in monotherapy) can occur but are rarely severe.

Immune system disorders

- Allergic reactions (skin reactions, respiratory reactions) are common.

Metabolism and nutrition disorders

- Rare cases of severe hyponatraemia and in very rare cases SIADH-syndrome (syndrome of inappropriate antidiuretic hormone secretion) have been reported.

Nervous system disorders

Peripheral nervous system

Neurological conditions will normally be restricted to loss of deep tendon reflexes.

Development of severe paraesthesias, neurosensory and neuromotor disorders can occur (G1: 17.2%, G2: 3.6%, G3: 2.6%, G4: 0.1%). Very rarely Guillain-Barré syndrome.

Weakness of the lower extremities has been reported after long-term treatment. These symptoms are generally reversible.

Autonomic nervous system

The main symptom is constipation due to intestinal paresis (G1: 16.9%; G2: 4.9%; G3: 2%; G4: 0.7%), but it rarely progresses to paralytic ileus (see also "Gastrointestinal disorders"). The incidence of such reactions can increase when vinorelbine is combined with other chemotherapy.

Cardiac disorders

- Ischaemic heart disease (angina pectoris and/or transitory electrocardiogram modifications, myocardial infarction) has been reported in rare cases.

Respiratory system, thoracic and mediastinal disorders

- As with other vinca alkaloids, vinorelbine can cause dyspnoea and bronchospasm. Rare cases of interstitial lung disease have been reported, especially in patients treated with vinorelbine in combination with mitomycin.

Gastrointestinal disorders

- Very commonly nausea and vomiting is observed (G1: 19.9%; G2: 8.3%). Severe nausea and vomiting can occur commonly (G3: 1.9%; G4: 0.3%). The incidence of nausea and vomiting can increase when vinorelbine is combined with other chemotherapy. Antiemetic treatment can reduce the frequency.
- Constipation and paralytic ileus (see also "Autonomous nervous system"). The treatment can be resumed after recovery of normal intestinal function.
- Stomatitis as well as diarrhoea (G1: 7.6%; G2: 3.6%; G3: 0.7%; G4: 0.1%) and oesophagitis can occur. Severe diarrhoea is uncommon.
- Anorexia is observed very commonly (G1-2: 14%; G3: 1%).
- Rare cases of pancreatitis have been reported.

Hepatobiliary disorders

Temporary elevation of liver parameters without clinical symptoms has been reported: total bilirubin, alkaline phosphatase, aspartate aminotransferase, alanine aminotransferase.

Skin and subcutaneous tissue disorders

Mild alopecia may commonly occur which progresses if the treatment is continued (G1-2: 21%; G3-4: 4.1% in monotherapy). Commonly vinorelbine can cause skin reactions and in rare cases generalised skin reactions.

Musculoskeletal and connective tissue disorders

Arthralgia including jaw pain and myalgia have been reported in patients being treated with vinorelbine.

Renal and urinary disorders

Increased blood creatinine was observed commonly.

General disorders and administration site conditions

Patients being treated with vinorelbine can have fatigue, asthenia, fever and pain in different locations such as chest pain and pain in the tumor.

Reactions at the injection site can include erythema, smarting pains, discoloration of the vein and local phlebitis (G1: 12.3%; G2: 8.2%, G3: 3.6%; G4: 0.1% in monotherapy). As other vinca alkaloids vinorelbine has vesicant power. In rare cases local necrosis due to extravasation has been observed. This undesirable effect can be limited by correct positioning of the intravenous cannula or catheter and bolus injection, followed by liberal flushing of the vein.

4.9 Overdose

Cases of accidental acute overdose have been reported in humans: Such cases can result in bone marrow hypoplasia and are sometimes associated with infection, fever and paralytic ileus. Supporting treatment such as blood transfusion or broad-spectrum antibiotic treatment is normally initiated at the doctor's discretion. There is no known antidote.

As there is no specific antidote for the overdosage of vinorelbine given intravenously, symptomatic measures are necessary in case of an overdosage, e.g.:

- Continuous control of vital signs and careful monitoring of the patient.
- Daily control of blood count to observe the need of blood transfusions, of growth factors and to detect the need of intensive care and to minimize the risk of infections.
- Measures for prevention or for therapy of paralytic ileus
- Control of circulation system and of liver function
- Broad spectrum antibiotic therapy may be necessary in case of complications due to infections. In case of a paralytic ileus, decompression by a probe may be necessary.

5. PHARMACOLOGICAL PROPERTIES

5.1 Pharmacodynamic properties

Pharmacotherapeutic group: Antineoplastic and immunmodulating agents, vinca alkaloids

ATC code: L 01 CA 04

Vinorelbine is an antineoplastic active substance of the vinca alkaloid family, but in contrast to all other vinca alkaloids the catharanthine portion of vinorelbine has undergone a structural modification. On the molecular level it affects the dynamic equilibrium of tubulin in the microtubular system of the cell.

Vinorelbine inhibits tubulin polymerisation and binds preferentially to mitotic microtubules, only affecting axonal microtubules at high concentrations. Spiralisation of the tubulin is induced to a lesser degree than with vincristine. Vinorelbine blocks mitosis in phase G2-M, causing cell death in interphase or at the following mitosis.

5.2 Pharmacokinetic properties

After intravenous bolus injection or infusion in patients, the plasma concentration of vinorelbine is characterised by a three exponential elimination curve. The terminal elimination phase reflects a long half-life greater than 40 hours. Total clearance of vinorelbine is high (0.97-1.26 l/h/kg).

The active ingredient is widely distributed in the body with a volume of distribution ranging from 25.4-40.1 l/kg. Penetration of vinorelbine into pulmonary tissue is significant with tissue/plasma concentration ratios of greater than 300 in a study involving surgical biopsy. There is moderate binding to plasma proteins (13.5 %) but strong binding to platelets (78%). Linear pharmacokinetics have been shown for intravenously administered vinorelbine up to a dose of 45 mg/m^2.

Vinorelbine is primarily metabolised by CYP3A4 of cytochrome P450. All metabolites have been identified and none are active with the exception of 4-O-deacetylvinorelbine, which is the principal metabolite in the blood.

Renal elimination is low (<20% of the dose). Small concentrations of deacetyl vinorelbine have been recovered in humans, but vinorelbine is principally detected as the unchanged compound in urine. Elimination of the active substance is mainly via the bile duct and consists of the metabolites and mainly of unchanged vinorelbine.

The effect of kidney dysfunction on the disposition of vinorelbine has not been studied, but dose reduction is not indicated because of the low degree of renal excretion. In patients with liver metastases changes only occurred in the mean clearance of vinorelbine when over 75% of the liver was affected. In 6 cancer patients with moderate liver dysfunction (bilirubin $\leq 2 \times$ ULN and aminotransferases $\leq 5 \times$ ULN) treated with up to 25 mg/m^2 and 8 cancer patients with severe liver dysfunction (bilirubin $> 2 \times$ ULN and/or aminotransferases $> 5 \times$ ULN) treated with up to 20 mg/m^2, mean total clearance in the two groups were similar to that in patients with normal liver function. These data may however not be representative for patients with reduced drug elimination capacity of the liver and therefore caution is recommended in patients with severe hepatic impairment and careful monitoring of haematological parameters required (see section 4.2 and 4.4).

5.3 Preclinical safety data

The limiting toxicity in animals is bone marrow depression. In animal studies, vinorelbine induced aneuploidy and polyploidy.

It can be assumed that vinorelbine can also cause genotoxic effects in humans (induction of aneuploidy and polyploidy).

The results of studies for carcinogenic potential in mice and rats were negative but only low doses have been tested.

In animal reproductive studies, effects were observed at subtherapeutic dosages. Embryo- and fetotoxicity were seen, such as intra-uterine growth retardation and delayed ossification. Teratogenicity (fusion of the vertebrae, missing ribs) was observed at maternally toxic doses. In addition, spermatogenesis and secretion of prostate and seminal vesicles were reduced, but fertility in rats was not diminished.

6. PHARMACEUTICAL PARTICULARS

6.1 List of excipients

Water for injections.

6.2 Incompatibilities

- Vinorelbine 10 mg/ml concentrate for solution for infusion should not be diluted with alkaline solutions (risk for precipitation).
- This medicinal product must not be mixed with other medicinal products except those mentioned in section 6.6.

6.3 Shelf life

In unopened packaging: 36 months.

After dilution:

Chemical and physical in use stability has been demonstrated for 24 hours at 2-8°C and at 25°C.

From a microbiological point of view, the product should be used immediately. If not used immediately, in-use storage times and conditions prior to use are the responsibility of the user and would not normally be longer than 24 hours at 2-8°C, unless opening and dilution has taken place in controlled and validated aseptic conditions.

6.4 Special precautions for storage

Store in a refrigerator (2°C - 8°C).

Store in the original package in order to protect from light.

Do not freeze.

6.5 Nature and contents of container

Glass vial type I with fluoropolymer-coated bromobutyl rubber stoppers and aluminium cap.

Pack sizes: 1 ml or 5 ml concentrate in packs of 1 or 10 vials. Not all pack sizes may be marketed.

6.6 Special precautions for disposal and other handling

The preparation and administration of vinorelbine should be carried out only by trained personnel. Suitable protective goggles, disposable gloves and disposable clothing must be worn. Spills and leakages must be wiped up.

Any contact with the eyes must be strictly avoided. If the solution does come into contact with the eyes they must be rinsed immediately with plenty of physiological saline.

After preparation, any exposed surface must be thoroughly cleaned and hands and face washed.

There is no incompatibility between the contents and container for Vinorelbine 10 mg/ml Concentrate for solution for infusion and a neutral glass bottle, PVC bag, vinylacetate bag or infusion set with PVC tubes.

It is recommended to administer vinorelbine as an infusion over the course of 5-10 minutes after dilution in 20-50 ml physiological saline or glucose 50 mg/ml (5%) solution or by a short infusion (20-30 minutes) after dilution in 125 ml of normal saline or glucose 50 mg/ml (5%) solution. After administration the vein must be flushed through thoroughly with at least 250 ml isotonic solution.

Unused medicinal product and waste must be disposed of in accordance with local requirements.

7. MARKETING AUTHORISATION HOLDER

medac
Gesellschaft für klinische
Spezialpräparate mbH
Fehlandtstraβe 3
D-20354 Hamburg
Germany
Telefon: +49 4103 8006 0
Fax: +49 4103 8006 100

8. MARKETING AUTHORISATION NUMBER(S)

11587/0036

9. DATE OF FIRST AUTHORISATION/RENEWAL OF THE AUTHORISATION

20/07/2006

10. DATE OF REVISION OF THE TEXT

01/08/2006

Viracept Film-coated Tablets

(Roche Products Limited)

1. NAME OF THE MEDICINAL PRODUCT

VIRACEPT 250 mg film-coated tablets.

2. QUALITATIVE AND QUANTITATIVE COMPOSITION

Each film-coated tablet contains nelfinavir mesilate corresponding to 250 mg of nelfinavir.

Excipients:

For a full list of excipients, see section 6.1.

3. PHARMACEUTICAL FORM

Blue, oblong biconvex film-coated tablets.

4. CLINICAL PARTICULARS

4.1 Therapeutic indications

VIRACEPT is indicated in antiretroviral combination treatment of human immunodeficiency virus (HIV-1) infected adults, adolescents and children of 3 years of age and older.

In protease inhibitor (PI) experienced patients the choice of nelfinavir should be based on individual viral resistance testing and treatment history.

See section 5.1.

4.2 Posology and method of administration

Therapy with VIRACEPT should be initiated by a physician experienced in the management of HIV infection.

VIRACEPT is administered orally and should always be ingested with food (see section 5.2).

Patients older than 13 years: the recommended dosage of VIRACEPT film-coated tablets is 1250 mg (five 250 mg tablets) twice a day (BID) or 750 mg (three 250 mg tablets) three times a day (TID) by mouth.

The efficacy of the BID (twice daily) regimen has been evaluated versus the TID (three times daily) regimen primarily in patients naïve to PIs (see section 5.1).

Patients aged 3 to 13 years: for children, the recommended starting dose is 50-55 mg/kg BID or, if using a TID regimen, 25 – 30 mg/kg body weight per dose. For children unable to take tablets, VIRACEPT oral powder may be administered (see Summary of Product Characteristics for VIRACEPT oral powder).

The recommended dose of VIRACEPT film-coated tablets to be administered **BID to children aged 3 to 13 years** is as follows:

Body Weight kg	Number of VIRACEPT 250 mg film-coated tablets per dose*
18 to < 22	4
≥ 22	5

The recommended dose of VIRACEPT film-coated tablets to be administered **TID to children aged 3 to 13 years** is as follows:

Body Weight kg	Number of VIRACEPT 250 mg film-coated tablets per dose*
18 to < 23	2
≥ 23	3

*see Summary of Product Characteristics for VIRACEPT oral powder for patients with less than 18 kg body weight.

Renal and hepatic impairment: there are no data specific for patients with renal impairment and therefore specific dosage recommendations cannot be made. Nelfinavir is principally metabolised and eliminated by the liver. There are not sufficient data from patients with liver impairment and therefore specific dose recommendations cannot be made (see section 5.2). Caution should be used when administering VIRACEPT to patients with impaired renal or hepatic function.

4.3 Contraindications

Hypersensitivity to the active substance or to any of the excipients.

Co-administration with medicinal products with narrow therapeutic windows and which are substrates of CYP3A4 [e.g., terfenadine, astemizole, cisapride, amiodarone, quinidine, pimozide, triazolam, orally administered midazolam (for caution on parenterally administered midazolam, see section 4.5), ergot derivatives; see section 4.5].

Potent inducers of CYP3A (e.g., rifampicin, phenobarbital and carbamazepine) reduce nelfinavir plasma concentrations.

Co-administration with rifampicin is contra-indicated due to a reduction in exposure to nelfinavir. Physicians should not use potent CYP3A4 in combination with Viracept and should consider using alternatives when a patient is taking VIRACEPT (see section 4.5).

Herbal preparations containing St. John's wort *(Hypericum perforatum)* must not be used while taking nelfinavir due to the risk of decreased plasma concentrations and reduced clinical effects of nelfinavir (see section 4.5).

VIRACEPT should not be co-administered with omeprazole due to a reduction in exposure to nelfinavir and its active metabolite M8 (Tert-butyl hydroxyl nelfinavir). This may lead to a loss of virologic response and possible resistance to VIRACEPT (see section 4.5).

4.4 Special warnings and precautions for use

Patients should be instructed that VIRACEPT is not a cure for HIV infection, that they may continue to develop infections or other illnesses associated with HIV disease, and that VIRACEPT has not been shown to reduce the risk of

Table 1 Interactions and dose recommendations with other medical products

Medicinal product by therapeutic areas (dose of nelfinavir used in study)	Effects on drug levels % Change	Recommendations concerning coadministration
Antiretrovirals		
NRTIs		
		Clinically significant interactions have not been observed between nelfinavir and nucleoside analogues. At present, there is no evidence of inadequate efficacy of zidovudine in the CNS that could be associated with the modest reduction in plasma levels of zidovudine when co-administered with nelfinavir. Since it is recommended that didanosine be administered on an empty stomach, VIRACEPT should be administered (with food) one hour after or more than 2 hours before didanosine.
Protease Inhibitors		
Ritonavir 500 mg single dose (nelfinavir 750 mg tid 6 days)	Ritonavir AUC ↔ Ritonavir Cmax ↔ Nelfinavir concentrations not measured	No dosage adjustment for needed for either product
Ritonavir 500 mg BID, 3 doses (nelfinavir 750 single dose)	Ritonavir concentrations not measured Nelfinavir AUC ↑ 152 %	No dosage adjustment for needed for either product
Ritonavir 100 mg or 200 mg BID (nelfinavir 1250 mg BID morning administration)	Ritonavir concentrations not measured Nelfinavir AUC ↑ 20% M8 metabolite AUC ↑ 74%	There were no significant differences between low doses of ritonavir (either 100 or 200 mg BID) for effects on AUCs of nelfinavir and M8. The clinical relevance of these findings has not been established.
Ritonavir 100 mg or 200 mg BID (nelfinavir 1250 mg BID evening administration)	Ritonavir concentrations not measured Nelfinavir AUC ↑ 39 % M8 metabolite AUC ↑ 86%	
Indinavir 800 mg single dose (nelfinavir 750 mg TID X 7 days)	Indinavir AUC ↑ 51% Indinavir Cmax ↔ Nelfinavir concentrations not measured	The safety of the combination indinavir + nelfinavir has not been established
Indinavir 800 mg Q8H X 7 days (nelfinavir 750 mg single dose)	Indinavir concentrations not measured Nelfinavir AUC ↑ 83%	
Saquinavir 1200 mg single dose (nelfinavir 750 mg TID X 4 days)	Saquinavir AUC ↑ 392% Nelfinavir concentrations not measured	
Saquinavir 1200 mg TID (nelfinavir 750 mg single dose)	Saquinavir concentrations not measured Nelfinavir AUC ↑ 30%	
Amprenavir 800 mg TID (nelfinavir 750 mg TID)	Amprenavir AUC ↔ Amprenavir Cmin ↑ 189 % Nelfinavir AUC ↔	No dosage adjustment for needed for either product
Non-nucleoside Analogue Reverse Transcriptase Inhibitors (NNRTIs)		
Efavirenz 600 mg QD (Nelfinavir 750 mg TID)	Efavirenz AUC ↔ Nelfinavir AUC ↓ 20 %	No dosage adjustment for needed for either product
Delavirdine 400 mg TID (Nelfinavir 750 mg TID)	Delavirdine AUC ↓ 31 % Nelfinavir AUC ↑ 107 %	Safety of combination not established; combination not recommended
Nevirapine		Dose adjustment is not needed when nevirapine is administered with nelfinavir.
Anti infective Agents		
Rifabutin 300 mg QD (Nelfinavir 750 mg TID)	Rifabutin AUC ↑ 207 % Nelfinavir AUC ↓ 32 %	Dosage reduction of rifabutin to 150 mg QD is necessary when nelfinavir 750 mt TID or 1250 mg BID and rifabutin are co-administered.
Rifabutin 150 mg QD (Nelfinavir 750 mg TID)	Rifabutin AUC ↑ 83 % Nelfinavir AUC ↓ 23 %	Dosage reduction of rifabutin to 150 mg QD is necessary when nelfinavir 750 mg TID or 1250 mg BID and rifabutin are co-administered
Rifampin 600 mg qd × 7 days (Nelfinavir 750 mg q8h × 5-6 days)	Rifampin concentrations not measured Nelfinavir AUC ↓82%	Concomitant use of rifampin is contraindicated with nelfinavir
Ketoconazole	Ketoconazole concentrations not measured Nelfinavir AUC ↑35%	Coadministration of nelfinavir and a strong inhibitor of CYP3A, ketoconazole, resulted in a 35 % increase in nelfinavir plasma AUC. The changes in nelfinavir concentrations are not considered clinically significant and no dose adjustment is needed when ketoconazole and nelfinavir are co-administered.
Oral Contraceptives		
17 α-Ethinyl estradiol 35 µg qd × 15 days (Nelfinavir 750 mg q8h × 7 days)	Ethinyl estradiol AUC ↓47% Nelfinavir concentrations not measured	Contraceptives with ethinyl estradiol should not be coadministered with nelfinavir. Alternative contraceptive measures should be considered.
Norethindrone 0.4 mg qd × 15 days (Nelfinavir 750 mg q8h × 7 days)	Norethindrone AUC ↓18% Nelfinavir concentrations not measured	Contraceptives with norethindrone should not be coadministered with nelfinavir. Alternative contraceptive measures should be considered.
HMG-CoA reductase inhibitors		
		Since increased concentrations of HMG-CoA reductase inhibitors may cause myopathy, including rhabdomyolysis, the combination of these medicinal products with nelfinavir is not recommended.
Simvastatin 20 mg qd (Nelfinavir 1250 mg bid)	Simvastatin AUC ↑ 506 % Nelfinavir concentrations not measured	Combination of simvastatin and nelfinavir is not recommended.
Atorvastatin 10 mg qd (Nelfinavir 1250 mg bid)	Atorvastatin AUC ↑ 74 % Nelfinavir concentrations not measured	Atorvastatin is less dependent on CYP3A4 for metabolism. When used with nelfinavir, the lowest possible dose of atorvastatin should be administered.
Pravastatin, fluvastatin		The metabolism of pravastatin and fluvastatin is not dependent on CYP3A4, and interactions are not expected with PIs. If treatment with HMG-CoA reductase inhibitors is indicated in combination with nelfinavir, pravastatin or fluvastatin is recommended.

Medicinal product by therapeutic areas (dose of nelfinavir used in study)	Effects on drug levels % Change	Recommendations concerning coadministration
Anticonvulsants		
Phenytoin 300 mg qd × 7 days (Nelfinavir 1250 mg bid × 14 days)	Phenytoin AUC ↓29% Free Phenytoin ↓28%	No dose adjustment for nelfinavir is recommended. Nelfinavir may lead to decreased AUC of phenytoin; therefore phenytoin concentrations should be monitored during concomitant use with nelfinavir.
Proton Pump Inhibitors		
Omeprazole 20 mg bid × 4 days administered 30 minutes before nelfinavir (Nelfinavir 1250 mg bid × 4 days)	Omeprazole concentrations not measured Nelfinavir AUC ↓36% Nelfinavir Cmax ↓37% Nelfinavir Cmin ↓39% M8 metabolite AUC ↓92% M8 metabolite Cmax ↓89% M8 metabolite Cmin ↓75%	Omeprazole should not be co-administered with nelfinavir. The absorption of nelfinavir may be reduced in situations where the gastric pH is increased irrespective of cause. Co-administration of nelfinavir with omeprazole may lead to a loss of virologic response and therefore concomitant use is contra-indicated. Caution is recommended when nelfinavir is co-administered with other proton pump inhibitors
Sedatives/ Anxiolytics		
Midazolam	No drug interaction study has been performed for the co-administration of nelfinavir with benzodiazepines.	Midazolam is extensively metabolised by CYP3A4. Co-administration of midazolam with nelfinavir may cause a large increase in the concentration of this benzodiazepine. Based on data for other CYP3A4 inhibitors, plasma concentrations of midazolam are expected to be significantly higher when midazolam is given orally. Therefore nelfinavir should not be co-administered with orally administered midazolam. If nelfinavir is co-administered with parenteral midazolam, it should be done in an intensive care unit (ICU) or similar setting which ensures close clinical monitoring and appropriate medical management in case of respiratory depression and/or prolonged sedation. Dosage adjustment for midazolam should be considered, especially if more than a single dose of midazolam is administered
H1 Receptor Antagonists, 5-HT Agonists		
Terfenadine, astemizole, cisapride	Nelfinavir increases terfenadine plasma concentrations. Similar interactions are likely with astemizole and cisapride.	Nelfinavir must not be administered concurrently with terfenadine, astemizole or cisapride because of the potential for serious and/or life-threatening cardiac arrhythmias.
Analgesics		
Methadone 80 mg ± 21 mg qd > 1 month (Nelfinavir 1250mg bid × 8 days	Methadone AUC ↓47%	None of the subjects experienced withdrawal symptoms in this study; however, due to the pharmacokinetic changes, it should be expected that some patients who received this combination may experience withdrawal symptoms and require an upward adjustment of the methadone dose. Methadone AUC may be decreased when co-administered with nelfinavir; therefore upward adjustment of methadone dose may be required during concomitant use with nelfinavir.
Herbal Products		
St. John's wort	Plasma levels of nelfinavir can be reduced by concomitant use of the herbal preparation St. John's wort *(Hypericum perforatum)*. This is due to induction of drug metabolising enzymes and/or transport proteins by St. John's wort.	Herbal preparations containing St. John's wort must not be used concomitantly with nelfinavir. If a patient is already taking St. John's wort, stop St. John's wort, check viral levels and if possible nelfinavir levels. Nelfinavir levels may increase on stopping St. John's wort, and the dose of nelfinavir may need adjusting. The inducing effect of St. John's wort may persist for at least 2 weeks after cessation of treatment.

↑ Indicates increase, ↓ indicates decrease, ↔ indicates minimal change (< 10 %)

transmission of HIV disease through sexual contact or blood contamination.

Immune Reactivation Syndrome: In HIV-infected patients with severe immune deficiency at the time of institution of combination antiretroviral therapy (CART), an inflammatory reaction to asymptomatic or residual opportunistic pathogens may arise and cause serious clinical conditions, or aggravation of symptoms. Typically, such reactions have been observed within the first few weeks or months of initiation of CART. Relevant examples are cytomegalovirus retinitis, generalised and/or focal mycobacterium infections, and *Pneumocystis carinii* pneumonia. Any inflammatory symptoms should be evaluated and treatment instituted when necessary.

Liver Disease: The safety and efficacy of nelfinavir has not been established in patients with significant underlying liver disorders. Patients with chronic hepatitis B or C and treated with combination antiretroviral therapy are at an increased risk for severe and potentially fatal hepatic adverse events. In case of concomitant antiviral therapy for hepatitis B or C, please refer also to the relevant product information for these medicinal products.

Patients with pre-existing liver dysfunction including chronic active hepatitis have an increased frequency of liver function abnormalities during combination antiretroviral therapy and should be monitored according to standard practice. If there is evidence of worsening liver disease in such patients, interruption or discontinuation of treatment must be considered. The use of nelfinavir in patients with moderate hepatic impairment has not been studied. In the absence of such studies, caution should be exercised, as increases in nelfinavir levels and/or increases in liver enzymes may occur.

Osteonecrosis: Although the aetiology is considered to be multifactorial (including corticosteroid use, alcohol consumption, severe immunosuppression, higher body mass index), cases of osteonecrosis have been reported particularly in patients with advanced HIV-disease and/or long-term exposure to combination antiretroviral therapy (CART). Patients should be advised to seek medical advice if they experience joint aches and pain, joint stiffness or difficulty in movement.

Renal Impairment: Since nelfinavir is highly bound to plasma proteins, it is unlikely that it will be significantly removed by haemodialysis or peritoneal dialysis. Therefore, no special precautions or dose adjustments are required in these patients.

Diabetes mellitus and hyperglycaemia: New onset diabetes mellitus, hyperglycaemia or exacerbation of existing diabetes mellitus has been reported in patients receiving PIs. In some of these the hyperglycaemia was severe and in some cases also associated with ketoacidosis. Many patients had confounding medical conditions, some of which required therapy with agents that have been associated with the development of diabetes or hyperglycaemia.

Patients with haemophilia: There have been reports of increased bleeding, including spontaneous skin haematomas and haemarthroses, in haemophiliac patients type A and B treated with PIs. In some patients additional factor VIII was given. In more than half of the reported cases, treatment with PIs was continued or reintroduced if treatment had been discontinued. A causal relationship has been evoked, although the mechanism of action has not been elucidated. Haemophiliac patients should therefore be made aware of the possibility of increased bleeding.

Lipodystrophy: Combination antiretroviral therapy has been associated with the redistribution of body fat (acquired lipodystrophy) in HIV patients. The long-term consequences of these events are currently unknown. Knowledge about the mechanism is incomplete. A connection between visceral lipomatosis and PIs and lipoatrophy and nucleoside analogue reverse transcriptase inhibitors (NRTIs) has been hypothesised. A higher risk of lipodystrophy has been associated with individual factors such as older age, and with drug related factors such as longer duration of antiretroviral treatment and associated metabolic disturbances. Clinical examination should include evaluation for physical signs of fat redistribution. Consideration should be given to the measurement of fasting serum lipids and blood glucose. Lipid disorders should be managed as clinically appropriate (see section 4.8).

4.5 Interaction with other medicinal products and other forms of interaction

Combination with other medicinal products: Caution is advised whenever VIRACEPT is co-administered with medicinal products which are inducers or inhibitors and/or substrates of CYP3A4; such combinations may require dose adjustment (see also sections 4.3 and 4.8).

Co-administration of a PI with sildenafil is expected to substantially increase sildenafil concentration and may result in an increase in sildenafil associated adverse events, including hypotension, visual changes, and priapism.

Potent inducers of CYP3A (e.g., phenobarbital and carbamazepine) may reduce nelfinavir plasma concentrations. Physicians should consider using alternatives when a patient is taking VIRACEPT (see section 4.3.)

Interactions of nelfinavir with selected compounds that describe the impact of nelfinavir on the pharmacokinetics of the co-administered compound and the impact of other drugs on pharmacokinetics of nelfinavir are listed in Table 1.

Nelfinavir is primarily metabolised via the cytochrome P450 isoenzymes CYP3A and CYP2C19 (see section 5.2). Co-administration with the following medicinal products that are substrates for CYP3A4 and which have narrow therapeutic windows is contraindicated (see section 4.3 and below): terfenadine, astemizole, cisapride, amiodarone, quinidine, ergot derivatives, pimozide, oral midazolam and triazolam.

Metabolic enzyme inducers: Caution should be used when co-administering medicinal products that induce CYP3A or potentially toxic medicinal products which are themselves metabolised by CYP3A (see section 4.3). Based on *in vitro* data, nelfinavir is unlikely to inhibit other cytochrome P450 isoforms at concentrations in the therapeutic range.

Metabolic enzyme inhibitors: Co-administration of nelfinavir with inhibitors of CYP2C19 (e.g., fluconazole, fluoxetine, paroxetine, lansoprazole, imipramine, amitriptyline and diazepam) may be expected to reduce the conversion of nelfinavir to its major active metabolite M8 (*tert-butyl* hydroxy nelfinavir) with a concomitant increase in plasma nelfinavir levels (see section 5.2). Limited clinical trial data from patients receiving one or more of these medicinal products with nelfinavir indicated that a clinically significant effect on safety and efficacy is not expected. However, such an effect cannot be ruled out.

Table 1: Interactions and dose recommendations with other medical products

(see Table 1 on page 2581)

4.6 Pregnancy and lactation

No treatment-related adverse reactions were seen in animal reproductive toxicity studies in rats at doses providing systemic exposure comparable to that observed with the clinical dose. Clinical experience in pregnant women is limited. VIRACEPT should be given during pregnancy only if the expected benefit justifies the possible risk to the foetus.

It is recommended that HIV-infected women must not breast-feed their infants under any circumstances in order to avoid transmission of HIV. Studies in lactating rats showed that nelfinavir is excreted in breast milk. There is no data available on nelfinavir excretion into human breast milk. Mothers must be instructed to discontinue breast-feeding if they are receiving VIRACEPT.

4.7 Effects on ability to drive and use machines

VIRACEPT has no or negligible influence on the ability to drive and use machines.

4.8 Undesirable effects

The safety of the VIRACEPT 250 mg tablet was studied in controlled clinical trials with over 1300 patients. The majority of patients in these studies received either 750 mg TID either alone or in combination with nucleoside analogues or 1250 mg BID in combination with nucleoside analogues. The following adverse events with an at least possible relationship to nelfinavir (i.e. adverse reactions) were reported most frequently: diarrhoea, nausea, and rash. Within each frequency grouping, undesirable effects are presented in order of decreasing seriousness.

Adverse reactions from clinical trials with nelfinavir

Adverse reactions in clinical studies are summarised in Table 2. The list also includes marked laboratory abnormalities that have been observed with nelfinavir (at 48 weeks).

Table2: Incidences of Adverse Reactions and marked laboratory abnormalities from the phase II and phase III studies. (Very common (⩾ 10 %); common (⩾ 1 % and < 10 %))

Body System Frequency of Reaction	Adverse Reactions	
	Grades 3&4	All Grades
Gastrointestinal disorders		
Very common		Diarrhoea
Common		Nausea, flatulence,
Skin and subcutaneous tissue disorders		
Common		Rash
Investigations		
Common		Increased alanine aminotransferase, increased aspartate aminotransferase, neutropenia, blood creatinine phosphokinase increased, neutrophil count decreased

Children and neonates:

A total of approximately 400 patients received nelfinavir in paediatric treatment trials (Studies 524, 556, PACTG 377/725, and PENTA-7) for up to 96 weeks. The adverse reaction profile seen during paediatric clinical trials was similar to that for adults. Diarrhoea was the most commonly reported adverse event in children. Neutropenia/leucopenia was the most frequently observed laboratory abnormality. During these trials less than 13% of patients in total discontinued treatment due to adverse events.

Post-marketing experience with nelfinavir

Serious and non-serious adverse reactions from post-marketing spontaneous reports (where nelfinavir was taken as the sole protease inhibitor or in combination with other antiretroviral therapy), not mentioned previously in section 4.8, for which a causal relationship to nelfinavir cannot be excluded, are summarised below. As these data come from the spontaneous reporting system, the frequency of the adverse reactions is not confirmed.

Immune system disorders:

Uncommon (⩾ 0.1 % - ⩽ 1 %): hypersensitivity including bronchospasm, pyrexia, pruritus, facial oedema and rash maculo-papular or dermatitis bullous.

Metabolism and nutrition disorders:

Uncommon - rare (⩾ 0.01 % - ⩽ 1 %): Combination antiretroviral therapy has been associated with redistribution of body fat (Lipodystrophy acquired) in HIV patients including the loss of peripheral and facial subcutaneous fat, increased intra-abdominal and visceral fat, breast hypertrophy and dorsocervical fat accumulation (lypohypertrophy buffalo hump).

Rare (⩾ 0.01 % - ⩽ 0.1 %): new onset diabetes mellitus, or exacerbation of existing diabetes mellitus.

Gastrointestinal disorders:

Uncommon (⩾ 0.1 % - ⩽ 1 %): vomiting, pancreatitis/blood amylase increased.

Rare (⩾ 0.01 % - ⩽ 0.1 %): abdominal distension,

Hepatobiliary disorders:

Rare (⩾ 0.01 % - ⩽ 0.1 %): hepatitis, hepatic enzymes increased and jaundice when nelfinavir is used in combination with other antiretroviral agents.

Musculoskeletal and connective tissue disorders:

Rare (⩾ 0.01 % - ⩽ 0.1 %): Blood creatine phosphokinase increased, myalgia, myositis and rhabdomyolysis have been reported with PIs, particularly in combination with nucleoside analogues.

Vascular disorders:

Rare (⩾ 0.01 % - ⩽ 0.1 %): increased spontaneous haemorrhage bleeding in patients with haemophilia.

Skin and subcutaneous tissue disorders:

Very rare (⩽ 0.01 %), including isolated reports: Erythema multiforme.

Paediatric population:

Additional adverse reactions have been reported in the post-marketing experience and are listed below. As these data come from the spontaneous reporting system, the frequency of the adverse reactions is unknown: hypertriglyceridaemia, anaemia, blood lactic acid increased, and pneumonia.

Cases of osteonecrosis have been reported, particularly in patients with generally acknowledged risk factors, advanced HIV disease or long-term exposure to combination antiretroviral therapy (CART). The frequency of this is unknown (see section 4.4).

Combination antiretroviral therapy has been associated with metabolic abnormalities such as blood triglycerides increased, blood cholesterol increased, insulin resistance, hyperglycaemia and hyperlactaemia. The frequency of this is unknown (see section 4.4).

In HIV-infected patients with severe immune deficiency at the time of initiation of combination antiretroviral therapy (CART), an inflammatory reaction to asymptomatic or residual opportunistic infections may arise. The frequency of this is unknown (see section 4.4).

4.9 Overdose

Human experience of acute overdose with VIRACEPT is limited. There is no specific antidote for overdose with nelfinavir. If indicated, elimination of unabsorbed nelfinavir should be achieved by emesis or gastric lavage. Administration of activated charcoal may also be used to aid removal of unabsorbed nelfinavir. Since nelfinavir is highly protein bound, dialysis is unlikely to significantly remove it from blood.

Overdoses of nelfinavir could theoretically be associated with prolongation of the QT-interval of the ECG (see also section 5.3). Monitoring of overdosed patients is warranted.

5. PHARMACOLOGICAL PROPERTIES

5.1 Pharmacodynamic properties

Pharmacotherapeutic group: direct acting antivirals, ATC code: J05AE04

Mechanism of action: HIV protease is an enzyme required for the proteolytic cleavage of the viral polyprotein precursors to the individual proteins found in infectious HIV. The cleavage of these viral polyproteins is essential for the maturation of infectious virus. Nelfinavir reversibly binds to the active site of HIV protease and prevents cleavage of the polyproteins resulting in the formation of immature non-infectious viral particles.

Antiviral activity in vitro: the antiviral activity of nelfinavir *in vitro* has been demonstrated in both HIV acute and chronic infections in lymphoblastoid cell lines, peripheral blood lymphocytes and monocytes/macrophages. Nelfinavir was found to be active against a broad range of laboratory strains and clinical isolates of HIV-1 and the HIV-2 strain ROD. The EC_{95} (95 % effective concentration) of nelfinavir ranged from 7 to 111 nM (mean of 58 nM). Nelfinavir demonstrated additive to synergistic effects against HIV in combination with reverse transcriptase inhibitors zidovudine (ZDV), lamivudine (3TC), didanosine (ddI), zalcitabine (ddC) and stavudine (d4T) without enhanced cytotoxicity.

Resistance: Viral escape from nelfinavir can occur via viral protease mutations at amino acid positions 30, 88 and 90.

In vitro: HIV isolates with reduced susceptibility to nelfinavir have been selected *in vitro*. HIV isolates from selected patients treated with nelfinavir alone or in combination with reverse transcriptase inhibitors were monitored for phenotypic (n=19) and genotypic (n=195, 157 of which were assessable) changes in clinical trials over a period of 2 to 82 weeks. One or more viral protease mutations at amino acid positions 30, 35, 36, 46, 71, 77 and 88 were detected in > 10 % of patients with assessable isolates. Of 19 patients for whom both phenotypic and genotypic analyses were performed on clinical isolates, 9 patients isolates showed reduced susceptibility (5- to 93-fold) to nelfinavir *in vitro*. Isolates from all 9 patients possessed one or more mutations in the viral protease gene. Amino acid position 30 appeared to be the most frequent mutation site.

Cross resistance in vitro: HIV isolates obtained from 5 patients during nelfinavir therapy showed a 5- to 93-fold decrease in nelfinavir susceptibility *in vitro* when compared to matched baseline isolates but did not demonstrate a concordant decrease in susceptibility to indinavir, ritonavir, saquinavir or amprenavir *in vitro*. Conversely, following ritonavir therapy, 6 of 7 clinical isolates with decreased ritonavir susceptibility (8- to 113-fold) *in vitro* compared to baseline also exhibited decreased susceptibility to nelfinavir *in vitro* (5- to 40 fold). An HIV isolate obtained from a patient receiving saquinavir therapy showed decreased susceptibility to saquinavir (7- fold) but did not demonstrate a concordant decrease in susceptibility to nelfinavir. Cross-resistance between nelfinavir and reverse transcriptase inhibitors is unlikely because different enzyme targets are involved. Clinical isolates (n=5) with decreased susceptibility to zidovudine, lamivudine, or nevirapine remain fully susceptible to nelfinavir *in vitro*.

In vivo: The overall incidence of the D30N mutation in the viral protease of assessable isolates (n=157) from patients receiving nelfinavir monotherapy or nelfinavir in combination with zidovudine and lamivudine or stavudine was 54.8 %. The overall incidence of other mutations associated with primary PI resistance was 9.6 % for the L90M substitution where as substitutions at 48, 82 and 84 were not observed.

Clinical pharmacodynamic data: treatment with nelfinavir alone or in combination with other antiretroviral agents has been documented to reduce viral load and increase CD4 cell counts in HIV-1 seropositive patients. Decreases in HIV RNA observed with nelfinavir monotherapy were less pronounced and of shorter duration. The effects of nelfinavir (alone or combined with other antiretroviral agents) on biological markers of disease activity, CD4 cell count and viral RNA, were evaluated in several studies involving HIV-1 infected patients.

The efficacy of the BID regimen has been evaluated versus the TID regimen with VIRACEPT 250 mg tablets primarily in patients naïve to PIs. A randomised open-label study compared the HIV RNA suppression of nelfinavir 1250 mg BID versus nelfinavir 750 mg TID in PI naïve patients also receiving stavudine (30-40 mg BID) and lamivudine (150 mg BID).

(see Table 3 on next page)

The BID regimen produced statistically significantly higher peak nelfinavir plasma levels versus the TID regimen. Small, non-statistically significant differences were observed in other pharmacokinetic parameters with no trend favouring one regimen over the other. Although study 542 showed no statistically significant differences between the two regimens in efficacy in a predominantly antiretroviral naïve patient population, the significance of these findings for antiretroviral experienced patients is unknown.

In a study of 297 HIV-1 seropositive patients receiving zidovudine and lamivudine plus nelfinavir (2 different doses) or zidovudine and lamivudine alone, the mean baseline CD4 cell count was 288 cells/mm^3 and the mean baseline plasma HIV RNA was 5.21 log^{10} copies/ml (160,394 copies/ml). The mean decrease in plasma HIV RNA using a PCR assay (< 400 copies/ml) at 24 weeks was 2.33 log^{10} in patients receiving combination therapy with nelfinavir 750 mg TID, compared to 1.34 log^{10} in patients receiving zidovudine and lamivudine alone. At 24 weeks, the percentage of patients whose plasma HIV RNA levels had decreased to below the limit of detection of the assay (< 400 copies/ml) were 81 % and 8 % for the

Table 3

Proportion of patients with HIV RNA below LOQ (sensitive and ultrasensitive assays) at Week 48

Assay	Analysis	Viracept BID (%)	Viracept TID (%)	95 % CI
Sensitive	Observed data	135/164 (82 %)	146/169 (86 %)	(-12, +4)
	LOCF	145/200 (73 %)	161/206 (78 %)	(-14, +3)
	ITT (NC = F)	135/200 (68 %)	146/206 (71 %)	(-12, +6)
Ultrasensitive	Observed data	114/164 (70 %)	125/169 (74 %)	(-14, +5)
	LOCF	121/200 (61 %)	136/206 (66 %)	(-15, +4)
	ITT (NC = F)	114/200 (57 %)	125/206 (61 %)	(-13, +6)

LOCF= Last observation carried forward
ITT = Intention to Treat
NC = F: non-completers = failures

groups treated with nelfinavir 750 mg TID plus zidovudine and lamivudine or zidovudine and lamivudine, respectively. Mean CD4 cell counts at 24 weeks were increased by 150 and 95 cells/mm^3 for the groups treated with nelfinavir 750 mg TID plus zidovudine and lamivudine or zidovudine and lamivudine, respectively. At 48 weeks, approximately 75 % of the patients treated with nelfinavir 750 mg TID plus zidovudine and lamivudine remained below the level of detection of the assay (< 400 copies/ml); mean increase in CD4 cell counts was 198 cells/mm^3 at 48 weeks in this group.

No important differences in safety or tolerability were observed between the BID and TID dosing groups, with the same proportion of patients in each arm experiencing adverse events of any intensity, irrespective of relationship to trial medication.

Plasma levels of certain HIV-1 protease inhibitors, which are metabolised predominantly by CYP3A4, can be increased by the co-administration of low-dose ritonavir, which is an inhibitor of this metabolism. Treatment paradigms for several protease inhibitors, which are subject to this interaction, require the co-administration of low-dose ritonavir ('boosting') in order to enhance plasma levels and optimise antiviral efficacy. Plasma levels of nelfinavir, which is metabolised predominantly by CYP2C19 and only partially by CYP3A4, are not greatly increased by co-administration with ritonavir, and therefore nelfinavir does not require co-administration with low-dose ritonavir. Two studies have compared the safety and efficacy of nelfinavir (unboosted) with ritonavir- boosted protease inhibitors, each in combination with other antiretroviral agents.

Study M98-863 is a randomised, double blind trial of 653 antiretroviral-naïve patients investigating lopinavir/ritonavir (400/100 mg BID n=326) compared to nelfinavir (750 mg TID n=327), each in combination with lamivudine (150 mg twice daily) and stavudine (40 mg twice daily). Median baseline HIV-1 RNA was 4.98 log^{10} copies/ml and 5.01 log^{10} copies/ml in the nelfinavir and lopinavir/ritonavir treatment groups respectively. Median baseline CD4+ cell count was 232 cells/mm^3 in both groups. At week 48, 63 % nelfinavir and 75 % lopinavir/ritonavir patients had HIV-1 RNA < 400 copies/ml, whereas 52 % nelfinavir and 67 % lopinavir/ritonavir patients had HIV-1 RNA <50 copies/ml (intent-to-treat, missing = failure). The mean increase from baseline in CD4+ cell count at week 48 was 195 cells/mm^3 and 207 cells/mm^3 in the nelfinavir and lopinavir/ritonavir groups respectively. Through 48 weeks of therapy, a statistically significantly higher proportion of patients in the lopinavir/ritonavir arm had HIV-1 RNA < 50 copies/ml compared to the nelfinavir arm.

Study APV30002 is a randomised, open-label trial of 649 antiretroviral treatment naïve patients with advanced HIV-disease, investigating fosamprenavir/ritonavir (1400 mg/ 200 mg QD n=322) compared to nelfinavir (1250 mg BID n=327), each in combination with lamivudine (150 mg twice daily) and abacavir (300 mg twice daily). Median baseline HIV-1 RNA was 4.8 log^{10} copies/ml in both treatment groups. Median baseline CD4+ cell counts were 177 and 166 x10^6 cells/l for the nelfinavir and fosamprenavir/ritonavir groups respectively. At week 48, non-inferiority was shown with 68 % of patients in the group treated with nelfinavir and 69 % patients treated with fosamprenavir/ritonavir having plasma HIV-1 RNA <400 copies/ml whereas 53 % in the nelfinavir and 55 % in the fosamprenavir/ritonavir patients had HIV-1 RNA <50 copies/ml (intent-to-treat, rebound/discontinuation = failure). The median increase from baseline in CD4+ cell count over 48 weeks was 207 cells/mm^3 and 203 cells/mm^3 in the nelfinavir and fosamprenavir/ritonavir groups respectively. The virological failure was greater in the nelfinavir group (17 %) than in the fosamprenavir/ritonavir group (7 %). Treatment emergent NRTI resistance was significantly less frequent with fosamprenavir/ritonavir compared to nelfinavir (13 % versus 57 %; $p<0.001$).

5.2 Pharmacokinetic properties

The pharmacokinetic properties of nelfinavir have been evaluated in healthy volunteers and HIV-infected patients. No substantial differences have been observed between healthy volunteers and HIV-infected patients.

__Absorption:__ after single or multiple oral doses of 500 to 750 mg (two to three 250 mg tablets) with food, peak nelfinavir plasma concentrations were typically achieved in 2 to 4 hours.

After multiple dosing with 750 mg every 8 hours for 28 days (steady-state), peak plasma concentrations (C_{max}) averaged 3-4 µg/ml and plasma concentrations prior to the next dose (trough) were 1-3 µg/ml. A greater than dose-proportional increase in nelfinavir plasma concentrations was observed after single doses; however, this was not observed after multiple dosing.

A pharmacokinetic study in HIV-positive patients compared multiple doses of 1250 mg twice daily (BID) with multiple doses of 750 mg three times daily (TID) for 28 days. Patients receiving VIRACEPT BID (n=10) achieved nelfinavir C_{max} of 4.0 ± 0.8 µg/ml and morning and evening trough concentrations of 2.2 ± 1.3 µg/ml and 0.7 ± 0.4 µg/ml, respectively. Patients receiving VIRACEPT TID (n=11) achieved nelfinavir peak plasma concentrations (C_{max}) of 3.0 ± 1.6 µg/ml and morning and evening trough concentrations of 1.4 ± 0.6 µg/ml and 1.0 ± 0.5 µg/ml, respectively. The difference between morning and afternoon or evening trough concentrations for the TID and BID regimens was also observed in healthy volunteers who were dosed at precise 8- or 12-hour intervals.

The pharmacokinetics of nelfinavir are similar during BID and TID administration. In patients, the nelfinavir AUC_{0-24} with 1250 mg BID administration was 52.8 ± 15.7 µg•h/ml (n=10) and with 750 mg TID administration was 43.6 ± 17.8 µg•h/ml (n=11). Trough drug exposures remain at least twenty fold greater than the mean IC_{95} throughout the dosing interval for both regimens. The clinical relevance of relating *in vitro* measures to drug potency and clinical outcome has not been established. A greater than dose-proportional increase in nelfinavir plasma concentrations was observed after single doses; however, this was not observed after multiple dosing.

The absolute bioavailability of VIRACEPT has not been determined.

__Effect of food on gastrointestinal absorption:__ maximum plasma concentrations and area under the plasma concentration-time curve were consistently 2 to 3-fold higher under fed conditions compared to fasting. The increased plasma concentrations with food were independent of fat content of the meals. The effect of meal content on nelfinavir exposure was investigated in a study using the 250 mg film-coated tablets formulation. Steady state nelfinavir AUC and C_{max} were respectively 15 % and 20 % higher when doses followed a 800 kcal/50 % fat meal compared to those following a light meal (350 kcal/33 % fat), suggesting that meal content has less effect on nelfinavir exposures during multiple dosing than would be anticipated based on data from single dose studies.

__Distribution:__ Nelfinavir in serum is extensively protein-bound (≥ 98 %). The estimated volumes of distribution in both animals and humans is 2-7 l/kg which exceeded total body water and suggests extensive penetration of nelfinavir into tissues.

__Metabolism:__ *In vitro* studies demonstrated that multiple cytochrome P-450 isoforms including CYP3A, CYP2C19/C9 and CYP2D6 are responsible for the metabolism of nelfinavir. One major and several minor oxidative metabolites were found in plasma. The major oxidative metabolite, M8 (*tert-butyl* hydroxy nelfinavir), has *in vitro* antiviral activity equal to the parent drug and its formation is catalysed by the polymorphic cytochrome CYP2C19. The further degradation of M8 appears to be catalysed by CYP3A4. In subjects with normal CYP2C19 activity, plasma levels of this metabolite are approximately 25 % of the total plasma nelfinavir-related concentration. It is expected that in CYP2C19 poor metabolisers or in patients receiving concomitantly strong CYP2C19 inhibitors (see section 4.5), nelfinavir plasma levels would be elevated whereas levels of *tert-butyl* hydroxy nelfinavir would be negligible or non-measurable.

__Elimination:__ oral clearance estimates after single doses (24-33 l/h) and multiple doses (26-61 l/h) indicate that nelfinavir exhibits medium to high hepatic bioavailability. The terminal half-life in plasma was typically 3.5 to 5 hours. The majority (87 %) of an oral 750 mg dose containing ^{14}C-nelfinavir was recovered in the faeces; total faecal radioactivity consisted of nelfinavir (22 %) and numerous oxidative metabolites (78 %). Only 1-2 % of the dose was recovered in urine, of which unchanged nelfinavir was the major component.

__Pharmacokinetics in special clinical situations:__

__Children:__

In children between the ages of 2 and 13 years, the clearance of orally administered nelfinavir is approximately 2 to 3 times higher than in adults, with large intersubject variability. Administration of VIRACEPT oral powder or film-coated tablets with food at a dose of approximately 25-30 mg/kg TID achieves steady-state plasma concentrations similar to adult patients receiving 750 mg TID.

In an open prospective study, the pharmacokinetics of BID and TID VIRACEPT regimens in 18 HIV infected children aged 2-14 years were investigated. Children weighing less than 25 kg received 30-37 mg/kg nelfinavir TID or 45-55 mg/kg nelfinavir BID. Children over 25 kg received 750 mg TID or 1250 mg BID.

The C_{min}, C_{max} and AUC_{0-24} were all significantly higher with the BID regimen compared with the TID regimen. In addition, in twice daily application, 14 out of 18 (78 %) and 11 out of 18 (61 %) reached C_{min} values of 1-3 µg/ml and C_{max} values of 3-4 µg/ml, whereas in TID application only 4 out of 18 (22 %) and 7 out of 18 (39 %) reached these values.

__Elderly:__

There are no data available in the elderly.

__Hepatic impairment:__

Pharmacokinetics of nelfinavir after a single dose of 750 mg was studied in patients with liver impairment and healthy volunteers. A 49 %-69 % increase was observed in AUC of nelfinavir in the hepatically impaired groups with impairment (Child-Turcotte Classes A to C) compared to the healthy group. Specific dose recommendations for nelfinavir cannot be made based on the results of this study.

5.3 Preclinical safety data

During *in vitro* studies, cloned human cardiac potassium channels (hERG) were inhibited by high concentrations of nelfinavir and its active metabolite M8. hERG potassium channels were inhibited by 20 % at nelfinavir and M8 concentrations that are about four- to five-fold and seventy-fold, respectively, above the average free therapeutic levels in humans. By contrast, no effects suggesting prolongation of the QT-interval of the ECG were observed at similar doses in dogs or in isolated cardiac tissue. The clinical relevance of these *in vitro* data is unknown. However, based on data from products known to prolong the QT-interval, a block of hERG potassium channels of > 20 % may be clinically relevant. Therefore the potential for QT prolongation should be considered in cases of overdose (see section 4.9).

__Acute and chronic toxicity:__ oral acute and chronic toxicity studies were conducted in the mouse (500 mg/kg/day), rat (up to 1,000 mg/kg/day) and monkey (up to 800 mg/kg/day). There were increased liver weights and dose-related thyroid follicular cell hypertrophy in rats. Weight loss and general physical decline was observed in monkeys together with general evidence of gastrointestinal toxicity.

__Mutagenicity:__ *in vitro* and *in vivo* studies with and without metabolic activation have shown that nelfinavir has no mutagenic or genotoxic activity.

__Carcinogenicity:__ Two year oral carcinogenicity studies with nelfinavir mesilate were conducted in mice and rats. In mice, administration of up to 1000 mg/kg/day did not result in any evidence for an oncogenic effect. In rats administration of 1000 mg/kg/day resulted in increased incidences of thyroid follicular cell adenoma and carcinoma, relative to those for controls. Systemic exposures were 3 to 4 times those for humans given therapeutic doses. Administration of 300 mg/kg/day resulted in an increased incidence of thyroid follicular cell adenoma. Chronic nelfinavir treatment of rats has been demonstrated to produce effects consistent with enzyme induction, which predisposed rats, but not humans, to thyroid neoplasms. The weight of evidence indicates that nelfinavir is unlikely to be a carcinogen in humans.

6. PHARMACEUTICAL PARTICULARS

6.1 List of excipients

Each tablet contains the following excipients:

Tablet core:

Calcium silicate,

Crospovidone,

Magnesium stearate,

Indigo carmine (E132) as powder.

Tablet coat:

Hypromellose,

Glycerol triacetate.

6.2 Incompatibilities

Not applicable.

6.3 Shelf life

3 years.

6.4 Special precautions for storage
Store in the original container. Do not store above 30°C.

6.5 Nature and contents of container
VIRACEPT film-coated tablets are provided in HDPE plastic bottles containing either 270 or 300 tablets, fitted with HDPE child resistant closures with polyethylene liners. Not all pack sizes may be marketed.

6.6 Special precautions for disposal and other handling
No special requirements.

7. MARKETING AUTHORISATION HOLDER
Roche Registration Limited
6 Falcon Way
Shire Park
Welwyn Garden City
AL7 1TW
United Kingdom

8. MARKETING AUTHORISATION NUMBER(S)
EU/1/97/054/004 - EU/1/97/054/005

9. DATE OF FIRST AUTHORISATION/RENEWAL OF THE AUTHORISATION
Date of first authorisation: 22 January 1998
Date of latest renewal: 23 January 2008

10. DATE OF REVISION OF THE TEXT
28 July 2008

Viramune 200mg Tablets

(Boehringer Ingelheim Limited)

1. NAME OF THE MEDICINAL PRODUCT
VIRAMUNE 200 mg tablets

2. QUALITATIVE AND QUANTITATIVE COMPOSITION
Each tablet contains 200 mg of nevirapine (as anhydrate).

Excipient: each tablet contains 318 mg of lactose monohydrate.

For a full list of excipients, see section 6.1.

3. PHARMACEUTICAL FORM
Tablet
White, oval, biconvex tablets. One side is embossed with the code "54 193", with a single bisect separating the "54" and "193". The opposite side is marked with the company symbol. The tablet should not be divided.

4. CLINICAL PARTICULARS

4.1 Therapeutic indications
VIRAMUNE is indicated in combination with other antiretroviral medicinal products for the treatment of HIV-1 infected adults, adolescents, and children of any age (see section 4.4.).

Most of the experience with VIRAMUNE is in combination with nucleoside reverse transcriptase inhibitors (NRTIs). The choice of a subsequent therapy after VIRAMUNE should be based on clinical experience and resistance testing (see section 5.1).

4.2 Posology and method of administration
VIRAMUNE should be administered by physicians who are experienced in the treatment of HIV infection.

Patients 16 years and older

The recommended dose of VIRAMUNE is one 200 mg tablet daily for the first 14 days (this lead-in period should be used because it has been found to lessen the frequency of rash), followed by one 200 mg tablet twice daily, in combination with at least two additional antiretroviral agents.

Paediatric (adolescent) patients

VIRAMUNE 200 mg tablets, following the dosing schedule described above, are suitable for larger children, particularly adolescents, below the age of 16 who weigh more than 50 kg or whose body surface area is above 1.25 m^2 according to the Mosteller formula. An oral suspension dosage form, which can be dosed according to body weight or body surface area, is available for children in this age group weighing less than 50 kg or whose body surface area is below 1.25 m^2 (please refer to the Summary of Product Characteristics of VIRAMUNE oral suspension).

VIRAMUNE may be taken with or without food.

Renal impairment

For patients with renal dysfunction requiring dialysis an additional 200 mg dose of VIRAMUNE following each dialysis treatment is recommended. Patients with CLcr ≥ 20 ml/min do not require a dose adjustment, see section 5.2.

Hepatic impairment

VIRAMUNE should not be used in patients with severe hepatic impairment (Child-Pugh C, see section 4.3). No dose adjustment is necessary in patients with mild to moderate hepatic impairment (see sections 4.4 and 5.2).

Elderly:

VIRAMUNE has not been specifically investigated in patients over the age of 65.

Dose management considerations

Patients experiencing rash during the 14-day lead-in period of 200 mg/day should not have their VIRAMUNE dose increased until the rash has resolved. The isolated rash should be closely monitored (please refer to section 4.4). The 200 mg once daily dosing regimen should not be continued beyond 28 days at which point in time an alternative treatment should be sought due to the possible risk of underexposure and resistance.

Patients who interrupt VIRAMUNE dosing for more than 7 days should restart the recommended dosing regimen using the two week lead-in period.

For toxicities that require interruption of VIRAMUNE therapy, see section 4.4.

4.3 Contraindications
Hypersensitivity to the active substance or to any of the excipients.

VIRAMUNE must not be readministered to patients who have required permanent discontinuation for severe rash, rash accompanied by constitutional symptoms, hypersensitivity reactions, or clinical hepatitis due to nevirapine.

VIRAMUNE must not be used in patients with severe hepatic impairment (Child-Pugh C) or pre-treatment ASAT or ALAT > 5 ULN until baseline ASAT/ALAT are stabilised < 5 ULN.

VIRAMUNE must not be readministered in patients who previously had ASAT or ALAT > 5 ULN during VIRAMUNE therapy and had recurrence of liver function abnormalities upon readministration of VIRAMUNE (see section 4.4).

Herbal preparations containing St John's wort (*Hypericum perforatum*) must not be used while taking VIRAMUNE due to the risk of decreased plasma concentrations and reduced clinical effects of nevirapine (see section 4.5).

4.4 Special warnings and precautions for use
VIRAMUNE should only be used with at least two other antiretroviral agents (see section 5.1).

VIRAMUNE should not be used as the sole active antiretroviral, as monotherapy with any antiretroviral has shown to result in viral resistance.

The first 18 weeks of therapy with VIRAMUNE are a critical period which requires close monitoring of patients to disclose the potential appearance of severe and life-threatening skin reactions (including cases of Stevens-Johnson syndrome (SJS) and toxic epidermal necrolysis (TEN)) or serious hepatitis/ hepatic failure. The greatest risk of hepatic events and skin reactions occurs in the first 6 weeks of therapy. However, the risk of any hepatic event continues past this period and monitoring should continue at frequent intervals. Female gender and higher CD4 counts at the initiation of therapy place patients at greater risk of hepatic adverse events. Unless the benefit outweighs the risk VIRAMUNE should not be initiated in adult females with CD4 cell counts greater than 250 cells/mm^3 or in adult males with CD4 cell counts greater than 400 cells/mm^3. This is based on the occurrence of serious and life threatening hepatotoxicity in controlled and uncontrolled studies.

In some cases, hepatic injury has progressed despite discontinuation of treatment. Patients developing signs or symptoms of hepatitis, severe skin reaction or hypersensitivity reactions must discontinue VIRAMUNE and seek medical evaluation immediately. Viramune must not be restarted following severe hepatic, skin or hypersensitivity reactions (see section 4.3).

The dosage must be strictly adhered to, especially the 14-days lead-in period (see section 4.2).

Cutaneous reactions

Severe and life-threatening skin reactions, including fatal cases, have occurred in patients treated with VIRAMUNE mainly during the first 6 weeks of therapy. These have included cases of Stevens-Johnson syndrome, toxic epidermal necrolysis and hypersensitivity reactions characterised by rash, constitutional findings and visceral involvement. Patients should be intensively monitored during the first 18 weeks of treatment. Patients should be closely monitored if an isolated rash occurs. VIRAMUNE must be permanently discontinued in any patient experiencing severe rash or a rash accompanied by constitutional symptoms (such as fever, blistering, oral lesions, conjunctivitis, facial oedema, muscle or joint aches, or general malaise), including Stevens-Johnson syndrome, or toxic epidermal necrolysis. VIRAMUNE must be permanently discontinued in any patient experiencing hypersensitivity reaction (characterised by rash with constitutional symptoms, plus visceral involvement, such as hepatitis, eosinophilia, granulocytopenia, and renal dysfunction), see section 4.4.

VIRAMUNE administration above the recommended dose might increase the frequency and seriousness of skin reactions, such as Stevens-Johnson syndrome and toxic epidermal necrolysis.

Rhabdomyolysis has been observed in patients experiencing skin and/or liver reactions associated with VIRAMUNE use.

Concomitant prednisone use (40 mg/day for the first 14 days of VIRAMUNE administration) has been shown not to decrease the incidence of VIRAMUNE-associated rash, and may be associated with an increase in incidence and severity of rash during the first 6 weeks of VIRAMUNE therapy.

Some risk factors for developing serious cutaneous reactions have been identified, they include failure to follow the initial dosing of 200 mg daily during the lead-in period and a long delay between the initial symptoms and medical consultation. Women appear to be at higher risk than men of developing rash, whether receiving VIRAMUNE or non-VIRAMUNE containing therapy.

Patients should be instructed that a major toxicity of VIRAMUNE is rash. They should be advised to promptly notify their physician of any rash and avoid delay between the initial symptoms and medical consultation. The majority of rashes associated with VIRAMUNE occur within the first 6 weeks of initiation of therapy. Therefore, patients should be monitored carefully for the appearance of rash during this period. Patients should be instructed that dose escalation is not to occur if any rash occurs during the two-week lead-in dosing period, until the rash resolves. The 200 mg once daily dosing regimen should not be continued beyond 28 days at which point in time an alternative treatment should be sought due to the possible risk of underexposure and resistance.

Any patient experiencing severe rash or a rash accompanied by constitutional symptoms such as fever, blistering, oral lesions, conjunctivitis, facial oedema, muscle or joint aches, or general malaise should discontinue the medicinal product and immediately seek medical evaluation. In these patients VIRAMUNE must not be restarted.

If patients present with a suspected VIRAMUNE-associated rash, liver function tests should be performed. Patients with moderate to severe elevations (ASAT or ALAT > 5 ULN) should be permanently discontinued from VIRAMUNE.

If a hypersensitivity reaction occurs, characterised by rash with constitutional symptoms such as fever, arthralgia, myalgia and lymphadenopathy, plus visceral involvement, such as hepatitis, eosinophilia, granulocytopenia, and renal dysfunction, VIRAMUNE must be permanently stopped and not be re-introduced (see section 4.3).

Hepatic reactions

Severe and life-threatening hepatoxicity, including fatal fulminant hepatitis, has occurred in patients treated with VIRAMUNE. The first 18 weeks of treatment is a critical period which requires close monitoring. The risk of hepatic events is greatest in the first 6 weeks of therapy. However the risk continues past this period and monitoring should continue at frequent intervals throughout treatment.

Rhabdomyolysis has been observed in patients experiencing skin and/or liver reactions associated with VIRAMUNE use.

Increased ASAT or ALAT levels ≥ 2.5 ULN and/or co-infection with hepatitis B and/or C at the start of antiretroviral therapy is associated with greater risk of hepatic adverse reactions during antiretroviral therapy in general, including VIRAMUNE containing regimens.

Female gender and patients with higher CD4 counts are at increased risk of hepatic adverse events. Women have a three fold higher risk than men for symptomatic, often rash-associated, hepatic events (5.8% versus 2.2%), and patients with higher CD4 counts at initiation of VIRAMUNE therapy are at higher risk for symptomatic hepatic events with VIRAMUNE. In a retrospective review, women with CD4 counts > 250 cells/mm^3 had a 12 fold higher risk of symptomatic hepatic adverse events compared to women with CD4 counts < 250 cells/mm^3 (11.0% versus 0.9%). An increased risk was observed in men with CD4 counts > 400 cells/mm^3 (6.3% versus 1.2% for men with CD4 counts < 400 cells/mm^3).

Patients should be informed that hepatic reactions are a major toxicity of VIRAMUNE requiring close monitoring during the first 18 weeks. They should be informed that occurrence of symptoms suggestive of hepatitis should lead them to discontinue VIRAMUNE and immediately seek medical evaluation, which should include liver function tests.

Liver monitoring

Clinical chemistry tests, which include liver function tests, should be performed prior to initiating VIRAMUNE therapy and at appropriate intervals during therapy.

Abnormal liver function tests have been reported with VIRAMUNE, some in the first few weeks of therapy.

Asymptomatic elevations of liver enzymes are frequently described and are not necessarily a contraindication to use VIRAMUNE. Asymptomatic GGT elevations are not a contraindication to continue therapy.

Monitoring of hepatic tests should be done every two weeks during the first 2 months of treatment, at the 3rd month and then regularly thereafter. Liver test monitoring should be performed if the patient experiences signs or symptoms suggestive of hepatitis and/or hypersensitivity.

If ASAT or ALAT ≥ 2.5 ULN before or during treatment, then liver tests should be monitored more frequently during regular clinic visits. VIRAMUNE must not be administered to patients with pre-treatment ASAT or ALAT > 5 ULN until baseline ASAT/ALAT are stabilised < 5 ULN (see section 4.3).

Physicians and patients should be vigilant for prodromal signs or findings of hepatitis, such as anorexia, nausea, jaundice, bilirubinuria, acholic stools, hepatomegaly or liver tenderness. Patients should be instructed to seek medical attention promptly if these occur.

If ASAT or ALAT increase to > 5 ULN during treatment, VIRAMUNE should be immediately stopped. If ASAT and ALAT return to baseline values and if the patient had no clinical signs or symptoms of hepatitis, rash, constitutional symptoms or other findings suggestive of organ dysfunction, it may be possible to reintroduce VIRAMUNE, on a case by case basis, at the starting dosage regimen of 200 mg/day for 14 days followed by 400 mg/day. In these cases, more frequent liver monitoring is required. If liver function abnormalities recur, VIRAMUNE should be permanently discontinued.

If clinical hepatitis occurs, characterised by anorexia, nausea, vomiting, icterus AND laboratory findings (such as moderate or severe liver function test abnormalities (excluding GGT), VIRAMUNE must be permanently stopped. VIRAMUNE must not be readministered to patients who have required permanent discontinuation for clinical hepatitis due to nevirapine.

Liver Disease

The safety and efficacy of VIRAMUNE has not been established in patients with significant underlying liver disorders. VIRAMUNE is contraindicated in patients with severe hepatic impairment (Child-Pugh C, see section 4.3). Pharmacokinetic results suggest caution should be exercised when VIRAMUNE is administered to patients with moderate hepatic dysfunction (Child-Pugh B). Patients with chronic hepatitis B or C and treated with combination antiretroviral therapy are at an increased risk for severe and potentially fatal hepatic adverse events. In the case of concomitant antiviral therapy for hepatitis B or C, please refer also to the relevant product information for these medicinal products.

Patients with pre-existing liver dysfunction including chronic active hepatitis have an increased frequency of liver function abnormalities during combination antiretroviral therapy and should be monitored according to standard practice. If there is evidence of worsening liver disease in such patients, interruption or discontinuation of treatment must be considered.

Other warnings

Post-Exposure-Prophylaxis: Serious hepatotoxicity, including liver failure requiring transplantation, has been reported in HIV-uninfected individuals receiving multiple doses of VIRAMUNE in the setting of post-exposure-prophylaxis (PEP), an unapproved use. The use of VIRAMUNE has not been evaluated within a specific study on PEP, especially in term of treatment duration and therefore, is strongly discouraged.

Combination therapy with VIRAMUNE is not a curative treatment of patients infected with HIV-1; patients may continue to experience illnesses associated with advanced HIV-1 infection, including opportunistic infections.

Combination therapy with VIRAMUNE has not been shown to reduce the risk of transmission of HIV-1 to others through sexual contact or contaminated blood.

Hormonal methods of birth control other than DMPA should not be used as the sole method of contraception in women taking VIRAMUNE, since nevirapine might lower the plasma concentrations of these medications. For this reason, and to reduce the risk of HIV transmission, barrier contraception (e.g., condoms) is recommended. Additionally, when postmenopausal hormone therapy is used during administration of VIRAMUNE, its therapeutic effect should be monitored.

Combination antiretroviral therapy has been associated with the redistribution of body fat (lipodystrophy) in HIV infected patients. The long-term consequences of these events are currently unknown. Knowledge about the mechanism is incomplete. A connection between visceral lipomatosis and PIs and lipoatrophy and NRTIs has been hypothesised. A higher risk of lipodystrophy has been associated with individual factors such as older age, and with drug related factors such as longer duration of antiretroviral treatment and associated metabolic disturbances. Clinical examination should include evaluation for physical signs of fat redistribution. Consideration should be given to the measurement of fasting serum lipids and blood glucose. Lipid disorders should be managed as clinically appropriate (see section 4.8).

In clinical studies, VIRAMUNE has been associated with an increase in HDL- cholesterol and an overall improvement in the total to HDL-cholesterol ratio. However, in the absence of specific studies with VIRAMUNE on modifying the cardiovascular risk in HIV infected patients, the clinical impact of these findings is not known. The selection of antiretroviral drugs must be guided primarily by their antiviral efficacy.

Osteonecrosis: Although the etiology is considered to be multifactorial (including corticosteroid use, alcohol consumption, severe immunosuppression, higher body mass index), cases of osteonecrosis have been reported particularly in patients with advanced HIV-disease and/or long-term exposure to combination antiretroviral therapy (CART). Patients should be advised to seek medical advice if they experience joint aches and pain, joint stiffness or difficulty in movement.

Immune Reactivation Syndrome: In HIV-infected patients with severe immune deficiency at the time of institution of combination antiretroviral therapy (CART), an inflammatory reaction to asymptomatic or residual opportunistic pathogens may arise and cause serious clinical conditions, or aggravation of symptoms. Typically, such reactions have been observed within the first few weeks or months of initiation of CART. Relevant examples are cytomegalovirus retinitis, generalised and/or focal mycobacterial infections, and Pneumocystis jiroveci pneumonia. Any inflammatory symptoms should be evaluated and treatment instituted when necessary.

The available pharmacokinetic data suggest that the concomitant use of rifampicin and VIRAMUNE is not recommended (please also refer to section 4.5).

Lactose: VIRAMUNE tablets contain 636 mg of lactose per maximum recommended daily dose.

Patients with rare hereditary problems of galactose intolerance e.g. galactosaemia, the Lapp lactase deficiency or glucose-galactose malabsorption should not take this medicine.

4.5 Interaction with other medicinal products and other forms of interaction

Nevirapine is an inducer of CYP3A and potentially CYP2B6, with maximal induction occurring within 2-4 weeks of initiating multiple-dose therapy.

Compounds using this metabolic pathway may have decreased plasma concentrations when co-administered with VIRAMUNE. Careful monitoring of the therapeutic effectiveness of P450 metabolised medicinal products is recommended when taken in combination with VIRAMUNE.

The absorption of nevirapine is not affected by food, antacids or medicinal products which are formulated with an alkaline buffering agent.

The interaction data is presented as geometric mean value with 90% confidence interval (90% CI) whenever these data were available. ND = Not Determined, ↑ = Increased, ↓ = Decreased, ↔ = No Effect

(see Table 1 on next page)

Other information:

Nevirapine metabolites: Studies using human liver microsomes indicated that the formation of nevirapine hydroxylated metabolites was not affected by the presence of dapsone, rifabutin, rifampicin, and trimethoprim/sulfamethoxazole. Ketoconazole and erythromycin significantly inhibited the formation of nevirapine hydroxylated metabolites.

4.6 Pregnancy and lactation

Current available data on pregnant women indicate no malformative or foeto/neonatal toxicity. To date no other relevant epidemiological data are available. No observable teratogenicity was detected in reproductive studies performed in pregnant rats and rabbits (see section 5.3). There are no adequate and well-controlled studies in pregnant women. Caution should be exercised when prescribing VIRAMUNE to pregnant women (see section 4.4). As hepatotoxicity is more frequent in women with CD4 cell counts above 250 cells/mm^3, these conditions should be taken into consideration on therapeutic decision (see section 4.4).

Women of childbearing potential should not use oral contraceptives as the sole method for birth control, since nevirapine might lower the plasma concentrations of these medications (see sections 4.4 & 4.5).

Nevirapine readily crosses the placenta and is found in breast milk.

It is recommended that HIV-infected mothers do not breast-feed their infants to avoid risking postnatal transmission of HIV and that mothers should discontinue breast-feeding if they are receiving VIRAMUNE.

4.7 Effects on ability to drive and use machines

No studies on the effects on the ability to drive and use machines have been performed.

4.8 Undesirable effects

The most frequently reported adverse reactions related to VIRAMUNE therapy, across all clinical trials, were rash, allergic reactions, hepatitis, abnormal liver function tests, nausea, vomiting, diarrhoea, abdominal pain, fatigue, fever, headache and myalgia.

The postmarketing experience has shown that the most serious adverse reactions are Stevens-Johnson syndrome and toxic epidermal necrolysis and serious hepatitis/hepatic failure and hypersensitivity reactions, characterised by rash with constitutional symptoms such as fever, arthralgia, myalgia and lymphadenopathy, plus visceral involvement, such as hepatitis, eosinophilia, granulocytopenia, and renal dysfunction. The first 18 weeks of treatment is a critical period which requires close monitoring (see section 4.4).

The following adverse reactions which may be causally related to the administration of VIRAMUNE have been reported. The frequencies estimated are based on pooled clinical trial data for events considered related to VIRAMUNE treatment.

Frequency is defined using the following convention: very common (≥1/10); common (≥1/100 to <1/10); uncommon (≥1/1,000 to <1/100); rare (≥1/10,000 to <1/1,000); very rare (<1/10,000), not known (cannot be estimated from the available data).

Investigations

Common liver function tests abnormal

Blood and lymphatic system disorders

Common granulocytopenia*

Uncommon anaemia

* In study 1100.1090, from which the majority of related adverse events (n=28) were received, patients on placebo had a higher incidence of events of granulocytopenia (3.3%) than patients on nevirapine (2.5%).

Nervous system disorders

Common headache

Gastrointestinal disorders

Common vomiting, diarrhoea, abdominal pain, nausea

Skin and subcutaneous tissue disorders

Very common rash (13.6%)

Uncommon Stevens Johnson Syndrome/toxic epidermal necrolysis (0.1%), angioneurotic oedema, urticaria

Musculoskeletal and connective tissue disorders

Common myalgia

Uncommon arthralgia

General disorders and administration site conditions

Common fever, fatigue

Immune system disorders

Common hypersensitivity

Not known drug rash with eosinophilia and systemic symptoms, anaphylaxis

Hepatobiliary disorders

Common hepatitis (1.4%)

Uncommon jaundice

Rare hepatitis fulminant

Combination antiretroviral therapy has been associated with redistribution of body fat (lipodystrophy) in HIV infected patients including the loss of peripheral and facial subcutaneous fat, increased intra-abdominal and visceral fat, breast hypertrophy and dorsocervical fat accumulation (buffalo hump).

Combination antiretroviral therapy has been associated with metabolic abnormalities such as hypertriglyceridaemia, hypercholesterolaemia, insulin resistance, hyperglycaemia and hyperlactataemia (see section 4.4).

The following events have also been reported when VIRAMUNE has been used in combination with other antiretroviral agents: pancreatitis, peripheral neuropathy and thrombocytopaenia. These events are commonly associated with other antiretroviral agents and may be expected to occur when VIRAMUNE is used in combination with other agents; however it is unlikely that these events are due to VIRAMUNE treatment. Hepatic-renal failure syndromes have been reported rarely.

In HIV-infected patients with severe immune deficiency at the time of initiation of combination antiretroviral therapy (CART), an inflammatory reaction to asymptomatic or residual opportunistic infections may arise (see section 4.4).

Cases of osteonecrosis have been reported, particularly in patients with generally acknowledged risk factors, advanced HIV disease or long-term exposure to combination antiretroviral therapy (CART). The frequency of this is unknown (see section 4.4).

Skin and subcutaneous tissues

The most common clinical toxicity of VIRAMUNE is rash, with VIRAMUNE attributable rash occurring in 13.6% of patients in combination regimens in controlled studies.

Rashes are usually mild to moderate, maculopapular erythematous cutaneous eruptions, with or without pruritus, located on the trunk, face and extremities. Allergic reactions (anaphylaxis, angioedema and urticaria) have been reported. Rashes occur alone or in the context of hypersensitivity reactions, characterised by rash with constitutional symptoms such as fever, arthralgia, myalgia and lympadenopathy, plus visceral involvement, such as hepatitis, eosinophilia, granulocytopenia, and renal dysfunction.

Severe and life-threatening skin reactions have occurred in patients treated with VIRAMUNE, including Stevens-Johnson syndrome (SJS) and toxic epidermal necrolysis (TEN). Fatal cases of SJS, TEN and hypersensitivity reactions have been reported. The majority of severe rashes occurred within the first 6 weeks of treatment and some required hospitalisation, with one patient requiring surgical intervention (see section 4.4).

Hepato-biliary

The most frequently observed laboratory test abnormalities are elevations in liver function tests (LFTs), including ALAT, ASAT, GGT, total bilirubin and alkaline phosphatase. Asymptomatic elevations of GGT levels are the most

Table 1

Medicinal products by therapeutic areas	Interaction	Recommendations concerning co-administration
ANTI-INFECTIVES		
ANTIRETROVIRALS		
NRTIs		
Didanosine 100-150 mg BID	Didanosine AUC ↔ 1.08 (0.92-1.27) Didanosine C_{min} ND Didanosine C_{max}↔ 0.98 (0.79-1.21)	Didanosine and VIRAMUNE can be co-administered without dose adjustments.
Lamivudine 150 mg BID	No changes to lamivudine apparent clearance and volume of distribution, suggesting no induction effect of nevirapine on lamivudine clearance.	Lamivudine and VIRAMUNE can be co-administered without dose adjustments.
Stavudine: 30/40 mg BID	Stavudine AUC ↔ 0.96 (0.89-1.03) Stavudine C_{min} ND Stavudine C_{max} ↔ 0.94 (0.86-1.03) Nevirapine: compared to historical controls, levels appeared to be unchanged.	Stavudine and VIRAMUNE can be co-administered without dose adjustments.
Tenofovir 300 mg QD	Tenofovir plasma levels remain unchanged when co-administered with Nevirapine. Nevirapine plasma levels were not altered by co-administration of tenofovir.	Tenofovir and VIRAMUNE can be co-administered without dose adjustments.
Zidovudine 100-200 mg TID	Zidovudine AUC ↓ 0.72 (0.60-0.96) Zidovudine C_{min} ND Zidovudine C_{max}↓ 0.70 (0.49-1.04) Nevirapine: Zidovudine had no effect its pharmacokinetics.	Zidovudine and VIRAMUNE can be co-administered without dose adjustments
NNRTIs		
Efavirenz 600 mg QD	Efavirenz AUC ↓ 0.72 (0.66-0.86) Efavirenz C_{min}↓ 0.68 (0.65-0.81) Efavirenz C_{max}↓ 0.88 (0.77-1.01)	It is not recommended to co-administer efavirenz and VIRAMUNE, because of additive toxicity and no benefit in terms of efficacy over either NNRTI alone.
PIs		
Atazanavir/ritonavir 300/100 mg QD 400/100 mg QD	Atazanavir/r 300/100mg: Atazanavir/r AUC ↓ 0.58 (0.48-0.71) Atazanavir/r C_{min} ↓ 0.28 (0.20-0.40) Atazanavir/r C_{max}↓ 0.72 (0.60-0.86) Atazanavir/r 400/100mg: Atazanavir/r AUC ↓ 0.81 (0.65-1.02) Atazanavir/r C_{min}↓ 0.41 (0.27-0.60) Atazanavir/r C_{max} ↔ 1.02 (0.85–1.24) (compared to 300/100mg without nevirapine) Nevirapine AUC ↑ 1.25 (1.17-1.34) Nevirapine C_{min} ↑ 1.32 (1.22–1.43) Nevirapine C_{max} ↑ 1.17 (1.09-1.25)	It is not recommended to co-administer atazanavir/ritonavir and VIRAMUNE.
Darunavir/ritonavir 400/100 mg BID	Darunavir AUC ↑ 1.24 (0.97-1.57) Darunavir C_{min} ↔ 1.02 (0.79-1.32) Darunavir C_{max} ↑ 1.40 (1.14-1.73) Nevirapine AUC ↑ 1.27 (1.12-1.44) Nevirapine C_{min} ↑ 1.47 (1.20-1.82) Nevirapine C_{max} ↑ 1.18 (1.02-1.37)	Darunavir and VIRAMUNE can be co-administered without dose adjustments.
Fosamprenavir 1400 mg BID,	Amprenavir AUC ↓ 0.67 (0.55-0.80) Amprenavir C_{min}↓ 0.65 (0.49-0.85) Amprenavir C_{max}↓ 0.75 (0.63-0.89) Nevirapine AUC ↑ 1.29 (1.19-1.40) Nevirapine C_{min} ↑ 1.34 (1.21-1.49) Nevirapine C_{max} ↑ 1.25 (1.14-1.37)	It is not recommended to co-administer fosamprenavir and VIRAMUNE if fosamprenavir is not co-administered with ritonavir.
Fosamprenavir/ritonavir 700/100 mg BID	Amprenavir AUC ↔ 0.89 (0.77-1.03) Amprenavir C_{min}↓ 0.81 (0.69-0.96) Amprenavir C_{max}↔ 0.97 (0.85-1.10) Nevirapine AUC ↑ 1.14 (1.05-1.24) Nevirapine C_{min} ↑ 1.22 (1.10-1.35) Nevirapine C_{max} ↑ 1.13 (1.03-1.24)	Fosamprenavir/ritonavir and VIRAMUNE can be co-administered without dose adjustments
Lopinavir/ritonavir (capsules) 400/100 mg BID	patients: Lopinavir AUC ↓ 0.73 (0.53-0.98) Lopinavir C_{min}↓ 0.54 (0.28-0.74) Lopinavir C_{max}↓ 0.81 (0.62-0.95)	An increase in the dose of lopinavir/ritonavir to 533/133 mg (4 capsules) or 500/125 mg (5 tablets with 100/25 mg each) twice daily with food is recommended in combination with VIRAMUNE. Dose adjustment of VIRAMUNE is not required when co-administered with lopinavir.
Lopinavir/ritonavir (oral solution) 300/75 mg/m² BID	Paediatric patients: Lopinavir AUC ↓ 0.78 (0.56-1.09) Lopinavir C_{min}↓ 0.45 (0.25-0.82) Lopinavir C_{max}↓ 0.86 (0.64-1.16)	For children, increase of the dose of lopinavir/ritonavir to 300/75 mg/m² twice daily with food should be considered when used in combination with VIRAMUNE, particularly for patients in whom reduced susceptibility to lopinavir/ritonavir is suspected.
Nelfinavir 750 mg TID	Nelfinavir AUC ↔ 1.06 (0.78-1.14) C_{min}↔ 0.68 (0.50-1.5) C_{max} ↔ 1.06 (0.92-1.22) Nelfinavir metabolite M8: AUC ↓ 0.38 (0.30–0.47) C_{min}↓ 0.34 (0.26–0.45) C_{max} ↓ 0.41 (0.32–0.52) Nevirapine: compared to historical controls, levels appeared to be unchanged.	Nelfinavir and VIRAMUNE can be co-administered without dose adjustments.

Medicinal products by therapeutic areas	Interaction	Recommendations concerning co-administration
Ritonavir 600 mg BID	Ritonavir AUC↔ 0.92 (0.79-1.07) Ritonavir C_{min}↔ 0.93 (0.76-1.14) Ritonavir C_{max} ↔ 0.93 (0.78-1.07) Nevirapine: Co-administration of ritonavir does not lead to any clinically relevant change in nevirapine plasma levels.	Ritonavir and VIRAMUNE can be co-administered without dose adjustments.
Saquinavir/ritonavir	The limited data available with saquinavir soft gel capsule boosted with ritonavir do not suggest any clinically relevant interaction between saquinavir boosted with ritonavir and Nevirapine	Saquinavir/ritonavir and VIRAMUNE can be co-administered without dose adjustments.
Tipranavir/ritonavir 500/200 mg BID	No specific drug-drug interaction study has been performed. The limited data available from a phase IIa study in HIV-infected patients have shown a clinically non significant 20% decrease of TPV C_{min}.	Tipranavir and VIRAMUNE can be co-administered without dose adjustments.
ENTRY INHIBITORS		
Enfuvirtide	Due to the metabolic pathway no clinically significant pharmacokinetic interactions are expected between enfuvirtide and nevirapine.	Enfuvirtide and VIRAMUNE can be co-administered without dose adjustments.
Maraviroc 300 mg QD	Maraviroc AUC ↔ 1.01 (0.6 -1.55) Maraviroc C_{min} ND Maraviroc C_{max}↔ 1.54 (0.94-2.52) compared to historical controls Nevirapine concentrations not measured, no effect is expected.	Maraviroc and VIRAMUNE can be co-administered without dose adjustments.
INTEGRASE INHIBITORS		
Raltegravir 400 mg BID	No clinical data available. Due to the metabolic pathway of raltegravir no interaction is expected.	Raltegravir and VIRAMUNE can be co-administered without dose adjustments.
ANTIBIOTICS		
Clarithromycin 500 mg BID	Clarithromycin AUC ↓ 0.69 (0.62-0.76) Clarithromycin C_{min}↓ 0.44 (0.30-0.64) Clarithromycin C_{max}↓ 0.77 (0.69-0.86) Metabolite 14-OH clarithromycin AUC ↑ 1.42 (1.16-1.73) Metabolite 14-OH clarithromycin C_{min} ↔ 0 (0.68-1.49) Metabolite 14-OH clarithromycin C_{max} ↑ 1.47 (1.21-1.80) Nevirapine AUC ↑ 1.26 Nevirapine C_{min} ↑ 1.28 Nevirapine C_{max} ↑ 1.24 compared to historical controls.	Clarithromycin exposure was significantly decreased, 14-OH metabolite exposure increased. Because the clarithromycin active metabolite has reduced activity against *Mycobacterium avium-intracellulare complex* overall activity against the pathogen may be altered. Alternatives to clarithromycin, such as azithromycin should be considered. Close monitoring for hepatic abnormalities is recommended
Rifabutin 150 or 300 mg QD	Rifabutin AUC ↑ 1.17 (0.98-1.40) Rifabutin C_{min}↔ 1.07 (0.84-1.37) Rifabutin C_{max} ↑ 1.28 (1.09-1.51) Metabolite 25-O-desacetylrifabutin AUC ↑ 1.24 (0.84-1.84) Metabolite 25-O-desacetylrifabutin C_{min} ↑ 1.22 (0.86-1.74) Metabolite 25-O-desacetylrifabutin C_{max} ↑ 1.29 (0.98-1.68) A clinically not relevant increase in the apparent clearance of nevirapine (by 9%) compared to historical data was reported.	No significant effect on rifabutin and VIRAMUNE mean PK parameters is seen. Rifabutin and VIRAMUNE can be co-administered without dose adjustments. However, due to the high intersubject variability some patients may experience large increases in rifabutin exposure and may be at higher risk for rifabutin toxicity. Therefore, caution should be used in concomitant administration.
Rifampicin 600 mg QD	Rifampicin AUC ↔ 1.11 (0.96-1.28) Rifampicin C_{min} ND Rifampicin C_{max}↔ 1.06 (0.91-1.22) Nevirapine AUC ↓ 0.42 Nevirapine C_{min}↓ 0.32 Nevirapine C_{max}↓ 0.50 compared to historical controls.	It is not recommended to co-administer rifampicin and VIRAMUNE (see section 4.4). Physicians needing to treat patients co-infected with tuberculosis and using a VIRAMUNE containing regimen may consider co-administration of rifabutin instead.
ANTIFUNGALS		
Fluconazole 200 mg QD	Fluconazole AUC ↔ 0.94 (0.88-1.01) Fluconazole C_{min}↔ 0.93 (0.86-1.01) Fluconazole C_{max}↔ 0.92 (0.85-0.99) Nevirapine: exposure: ↑100% compared with historical data where nevirapine was administered alone.	Because of the risk of increased exposure to VIRAMUNE, caution should be exercised if the medicinal products are given concomitantly and patients should be monitored closely.
Itraconazole 200 mg QD	Itraconazole AUC ↓ 0.39 Itraconazole C_{min}↓ 0.13 Itraconazole C_{max}↓ 0.62 Nevirapine: there was no significant difference in Nevirapine pharmacokinetic parameters.	A dose increase for itraconazole should be considered when these two agents are administered concomitantly.
Ketoconazole 400 mg QD	Ketoconazole AUC ↓ 0.28 (0.20-0.40) Ketoconazole C_{min} ND Ketoconazole C_{max}↓ 0.56 (0.42-0.73) Nevirapine: plasma levels: ↑ 1.15-1.28 compared to historical controls.	It is not recommended to co-administer ketoconazole and VIRAMUNE.
ANTACIDS		
Cimetidine	Cimetidine: no significant effect on cimetidine PK parameters is seen. Nevirapine C_{min} ↑ 1.07	Cimetidine and VIRAMUNE can be co-administered without dose adjustments.
ANTITHROMBOTICS		
Warfarin	The interaction between Nevirapine and the antithrombotic agent warfarin is complex, with the potential for both increases and decreases in coagulation time when used concomitantly.	Close monitoring of anticoagulation levels is warranted.

Medicinal products by therapeutic areas	Interaction	Recommendations concerning co-administration
CONTRACEPTIVES		
Depo-medroxyprogesterone acetate (DMPA) 150 mg every 3 months	DMPA AUC ↔ DMPA C_{min}↔ DMPA C_{max}↔ Nevirapine AUC ↑ 1.20 Nevirapine C_{max} ↑ 1.20	Viramune co-administration did not alter the ovulation suppression effects of DMPA. DMPA and VIRAMUNE can be co-administered without dose adjustments.
Ethinyl estradiol (EE) 0.035 mg	EE AUC ↓ 0.80 (0.67 - 0.97) EE C_{min} ND EE C_{max}↔ 0.94 (0.79 - 1.12)	Oral hormonal contraceptives should not be used as the sole method of contraception in women taking VIRAMUNE (see section 4.4). Appropriate doses for hormonal contraceptives (oral or other forms of application) other than DMPA in combination with VIRAMUNE have not been established with respect to safety and efficacy.
Norethindrone (NET) 1.0 mg QD	NET AUC ↓ 0.81 (0.70 - 0.93) NET C_{min} ND NET C_{max}↓ 0.84 (0.73 - 0.97)	
DRUG ABUSE		
Methadone Individual Patient Dosing	Methadone AUC ↓ 0.40 (0.31 - 0.51) Methadone C_{min} ND Methadone C_{max}↓ 0.58 (0.50 - 0.67)	Methadone-maintained patients beginning VIRAMUNE therapy should be monitored for evidence of withdrawal and methadone dose should be adjusted accordingly.
HERBAL PRODUCTS		
St. John's Wort	Serum levels of Nevirapine can be reduced by concomitant use of the herbal preparation St. John's Wort (*Hypericum perforatum*). This is due to induction of drug metabolism enzymes and/or transport proteins by St. John's Wort.	Herbal preparations containing St. John's Wort and VIRAMUNE must not be co-administered (see section 4.3). If a patient is already taking St. John's Wort check nevirapine and if possible viral levels and stop St John's Wort. Nevirapine levels may increase on stopping St John's Wort. The dose of VIRAMUNE may need adjusting. The inducing effect may persist for at least 2 weeks after cessation of treatment with St. John's Wort.

frequent. Cases of jaundice have been reported. Cases of hepatitis (severe and life-threatening hepatotoxicity, including fatal fulminant hepatitis) have been reported in patients treated with VIRAMUNE. The best predictor of a serious hepatic event was elevated baseline liver function tests. The first 18 weeks of treatment is a critical period which requires close monitoring (see section 4.4).

Paediatric population

Based on clinical trial experience of 361 paediatric patients the majority of which received combination treatment with ZDV or/and ddI, the most frequently reported adverse events related to VIRAMUNE were similar to those observed in adults. Granulocytopenia was more frequently observed in children. In an open-label clinical trial (ACTG 180) granulocytopenia assessed as drug-related occurred in 5/37 (13.5%) of patients. In ACTG 245, a double-blind placebo controlled study, the frequency of serious drug-related granulocytopenia was 5/305 (1.6%). Isolated cases of Stevens-Johnson syndrome or Stevens-Johnson/toxic epidermal necrolysis transition syndrome have been reported in this population.

4.9 Overdose

There is no known antidote for VIRAMUNE overdosage. Cases of VIRAMUNE overdose at doses ranging from 800 to 6000 mg per day for up to 15 days have been reported. Patients have experienced oedema, erythema nodosum, fatigue, fever, headache, insomnia, nausea, pulmonary infiltrates, rash, vertigo, vomiting, increase in transaminases and weight decrease. All of these effects subsided following discontinuation of VIRAMUNE.

5. PHARMACOLOGICAL PROPERTIES

5.1 Pharmacodynamic properties

Pharmacotherapeutic group: NNRTI (non-nucleoside reverse transcriptase inhibitors), ATC code J05AG01.

Mechanism of Action

Nevirapine is a NNRTI of HIV-1. Nevirapine is a non-competitive inhibitor of the HIV-1 reverse transcriptase, but it does not have a biologically significant inhibitory effect on the HIV-2 reverse transcriptase or on eukaryotic DNA polymerases α, β, γ, or δ.

Antiviral activity *in vitro*

Nevirapine had a median EC_{50} value (50% inhibitory concentration) of 63 nM against a panel of group M HIV-1 isolates from clades A, B, C, D, F, G, and H, and circulating recombinant forms (CRF), CRF01_AE, CRF02_AG and CRF12_BF replicating in human embryonic kidney 293 cells. In a panel of 2,923 predominantly subtype B HIV-1 clinical isolates, the mean EC_{50} value was 90nM. Similar EC_{50} values are obtained when the antiviral activity of nevirapine is measured in peripheral blood mononuclear cells, monocyte derived macrophages or lymphoblastoid cell line. Nevirapine had no antiviral activity in cell culture against group O HIV-1 isolates or HIV-2 isolates.

Nevirapine in combination with efavirenz exhibited a strong antagonistic anti-HIV-1 activity *in vitro* (see section 4.5) and was additive to antagonistic with the protease inhibitor ritonavir or the fusion inhibitor enfuvirtide. Nevirapine exhibited additive to synergistic anti-HIV-1 activity in combination with the protease inhibitors amprenavir, atazanavir, indinavir, lopinavir, nelfinavir, saquinavir and tipranavir, and the NRTIs abacavir, didanosine, emtricitabine, lamivudine, stavudine, tenofovir and zidovudine. The anti-HIV-1 activity of nevirapine was antagonized by the anti-HBV drug adefovir and by the anti-HCV drug ribavirin *in vitro*.

Resistance

HIV-1 isolates with reduced susceptibility (100-250-fold) to nevirapine emerge in cell culture. Genotypic analysis showed mutations in the HIV-1 RT gene Y181C and/or V106A depending upon the virus strain and cell line employed. Time to emergence of nevirapine resistance in cell culture was not altered when selection included nevirapine in combination with several other NNRTIs.

Phenotypic and genotypic changes in HIV-1 isolates from treatment-naïve patients receiving either nevirapine (n=24) or nevirapine and ZDV (n=14) were monitored in Phase I/II trials over 1 to ⩾ 12 weeks. After 1 week of nevirapine monotherapy, isolates from 3/3 patients had decreased susceptibility to nevirapine in cell culture. One or more of the RT mutations resulting in amino acid substitutions K103N, V106A, V108I, Y181C, Y188C and G190A were detected in HIV-1 isolates from some patients as early as 2 weeks after therapy initiation. By week eight of nevirapine monotherapy, 100% of the patients tested (n=24) had HIV-1 isolates with a >100-fold decrease in susceptibility to nevirapine in cell culture compared to baseline, and had one or more of the nevirapine-associated RT resistance mutations. Nineteen of these patients (80%) had isolates with Y181C substitutions regardless of dose.

Genotypic analysis of isolates from antiretroviral naïve patients experiencing virologic failure

(n=71) receiving nevirapine once daily (n=25) or twice daily (n=46) in combination with lamivudine and stavudine for 48 weeks showed that isolates from 8/25 and 23/46 patients, respectively, contained one or more of the following NNRTI resistance-associated substitutions:

Y181C, K101E, G190A/S, K103N, V106A/M, V108I, Y188C/L, A98G, F227L and M230L.

Cross-resistance

Rapid emergence of HIV-strains which are cross-resistant to NNRTIs has been observed in vitro. Cross resistance to delavirdine and efavirenz is expected after virologic failure with nevirapine. Depending on resistance testing results, an etravirine-containing regimen may be used subsequently. Cross-resistance between nevirapine and either HIV protease inhibitors, HIV integrase inhibitors or HIV entry inhibitors is unlikely because the enzyme targets involved are different. Similarly the potential for cross-resistance between nevirapine and NRTIs is low because the molecules have different binding sites on the reverse transcriptase.

Clinical results

VIRAMUNE has been evaluated in both treatment naïve and treatment experienced patients.

Studies in treatment naïve patients

2NN study

The double non-nucleoside study 2 NN was a randomised, open-label, multicentre prospective study comparing the NNRTIs VIRAMUNE, efavirenz and both drugs given together.

1216 antiretroviral-therapy naïve patients with plasma HIV-1 RNA> 5000 copies/ml at baseline were assigned to VIRAMUNE 400 mg once daily, VIRAMUNE 200 mg twice daily, efavirenz 600 mg once daily, or VIRAMUNE (400 mg) and efavirenz (800 mg) once daily, plus stavudine and lamivudine for 48 weeks.

The primary endpoint, treatment failure, was defined as less than 1 log_{10} decline in plasma HIV-1 RNA in the first 12 weeks, or two consecutive measurements of more than 50 copies/ ml from week 24 onwards, or disease progression (new Centers for Disease Control and Prevention grade C event or death), or change of allocated treatment.

Median age was 34 years and about 64% were male patients, median CD4 cell count was 170 and 190 cells per mm^3 in the VIRAMUNE twice daily and efavirenz groups, respectively. There were no significant differences in demographic and baseline characteristics between the treatment groups.

Table 2: Number of patients with treatment failure, components of treatment failure, and number of patients with plasma HIV-RNA concentration < 50 c/ml, at week 48 (Intention-To-Treat (ITT) Analysis)

	VIRAMUNE 200 mg twice daily (n = 387)	Efavirenz 600 mg once daily (n = 400)
Treatment failure on or before week 48, % (95% IC)	43.7% (38.7-48.8)	37.8% (33.0-42.7)
Components of failure (%)		
Virological	18.9%	15.3%
Progression	2.8%	2.5%
Change of treatment	22.0%	20.0%
Permanent change of NNRTI (n)	61	51
Temporary discontinuation of NNRTI (n)	13	8
Additional antiretroviral drugs (n)	1	1
Non-allowable change of NNRTI (n)	1	1
Never started ART* (n)	9	19
Plasma HIV-1 RNA concentration <50 c/mL at 48 weeks, %(95% IC)	65.4% (60.4-70.1)	70.0% (65.2-74.5)

* ART = antiretroviral therapy

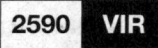

The predetermined primary efficacy comparison was between the VIRAMUNE twice daily and the efavirenz treatment groups. Details of the primary efficacy comparison are given in table 2.

Table 2: Number of patients with treatment failure, components of treatment failure, and number of patients with plasma HIV-RNA concentration < 50 c/ml, at week 48 (Intention-To-Treat (ITT) Analysis).

(see Table 2 on previous page)

Although, overall, treatment failure was numerically lower in the efavirenz group than in the nevirapine-only groups, the findings of this study show no evidence that efavirenz is superior to nevirapine twice daily in terms of treatment failure. However, equivalence within the 10% limits of these treatment groups was not shown even though the study was adequately powered for such an analysis. The nevirapine twice daily regimen and the efavirenz regimen were not significantly different (p= 0.091) in terms of efficacy as measured by incidence of treatment failure. There was also no significant difference between VIRAMUNE twice daily and efavirenz regarding any components of treatment failure including virological failure.

The simultaneous use of nevirapine (400 mg) plus efavirenz (800 mg) was associated with the highest frequency of clinical adverse events and with the highest rate of treatment failure (53.1%). As the regimen of nevirapine plus efavirenz did not have additional efficacy and caused more adverse events than each drug separately, this regimen is not recommended.

Twenty per cent of patients assigned to nevirapine twice daily and 18% of patients assigned to efavirenz had at least one grade 3 or 4 clinical adverse event. Clinical hepatitis reported as clinical adverse event occurred in 10 (2.6%) and 2 (0.5%) patients in the nevirapine twice daily and efavirenz groups respectively. The proportion of patients with at least one grade 3 or 4 liver-associated laboratory toxicity was 8.3% for nevirapine twice daily and 4.5% for efavirenz. Of the patients with grade 3 or 4 liver-associated laboratory toxicity, the proportions coinfected with hepatitis B or hepatitis C virus were 6.7% and 20.0% in the nevirapine twice daily group, 5.6% and 11.1% in the efavirenz group.

2NN Three-year follow-up-study

This is a retrospective multicentre study comparing the 3-year antiviral efficacy of VIRAMUNE and efavirenz in combination with stavudine and lamivudine in 2NN patients from week 49 to week 144.

Patients who participated in the 2NN study and were still under active follow-up at week 48 when the study closed and were still being treated at the study clinic, were asked to participate in this study. Primary study endpoints (percentage of patients with treatment failures) and secondary study endpoints as well as backbone therapy were similar to the original 2NN study.

Table 3 shows the main efficacy results of this study.

Table 3: Number of patients with treatment failure, components of treatment failure, and number of patients with plasma HIV-RNA concentration < 400 copies/ml, between week 49 to 144 (ITT analysis).

	VIRAMUNE 200 mg twice daily (n=224)	Efavirenz 600 mg once daily (n=223)
Treatment failure (%)	35.7	35.0
Virologic failure >400 c/ml) (%)	5.8	4.9
pVL <400 c/ml at week 144 (%)	87.2	87.4
CD4 increase (cells/mm3)	+135	+130
Disease progression / death (%)	5.8	6.3

A durable response to VIRAMUNE for at least three years was documented in this study. Equivalence within a 10% range was demonstrated between VIRAMUNE 200 mg twice daily and efavirenz with respect to treatment failure. Both, the primary (p = 0.92) and secondary endpoints showed no statistically significant differences between efavirenz and VIRAMUNE 200 mg twice daily.

Studies in treatment experienced patients

NEFA study

The NEFA trial is a controlled prospective randomised study which evaluated treatment options for patients who switch from protease inhibitor (PI) based regimen with undetectable load to either VIRAMUNE, efavirenz or abacavir.

The study randomly assigned 460 adults who were taking two nucleoside reverse-transcriptase inhibitors and at least one PI and whose plasma HIV-1 RNA levels had been less than 200 c/ml for at least the previous six months to switch from the PI to VIRAMUNE (155 patients), efavirenz (156), or abacavir (149).

Table 4: Outcome of Therapy 12 months after switch from PI based therapy

	VIRAMUNE (n=155)	Efavirenz (n=156)	Abacavir (n=149)
	Number of patients		
Death	1	2	1
Progression to AIDS	0	0	2
Virologic failure While taking study medication After switching study medication	14 8 6	7 5 2	16 16 0
Lost to follow-up	3	6	8
Switched study medication without virologic failure	20	29	9
Response; still taking study medication at 12 months	117	112	113

The primary study endpoint was death, progression to the acquired immunodeficiency syndrome, or an increase in HIV-1 RNA levels to 200 copies or more per millilitre. The main results regarding the primary endpoint are given in table 4.

Table 4: Outcome of Therapy 12 months after switch from PI based therapy

(see Table 4 above)

At 12 months, the Kaplan–Meier estimates of the likelihood of reaching the endpoint were 10 % in the VIRAMUNE group, 6 % in the efavirenz group, and 13 percent in the abacavir group (P=0.10 according to an intention-to-treat analysis).

The overall incidence of adverse events was significantly lower (61 patients, or 41%) in the abacavir group than in the nevirapine group (83 patients, or 54%) or the efavirenz group (89 patients, or 57%). Significantly fewer patients in the abacavir group (9 patients, or 6%) than in the nevirapine group (26 patients, or 17%) or the efavirenz group (27 patients, or 17%) discontinued the study medication because of adverse events (see table below).

(see Table 5 on next page)

Perinatal Transmission

The HIVNET 012 study conducted in Kampala (Uganda) evaluated the efficacy of VIRAMUNE to prevent vertical transmission of HIV-1 infection. Mothers received only study antiretroviral therapy during these trials. Mother-infant pairs were randomised to receive oral VIRAMUNE (mother: 200 mg at the onset of labour; infant: 2 mg/kg within 72 hours of birth), or an ultra-short oral zidovudine regimen (mother: 600 mg at the onset of labour and 300 mg every 3 hours until delivery; infant: 4 mg/kg twice daily for 7 days). The cumulative HIV-1 infant infection rate at 14-16 weeks was 13.1% (n = 310) in the VIRAMUNE group, versus 25.1% (n = 308 in the ultra-short zidovudine group (p = 0.00063).

From a study in which infants of HIV infected mothers received either placebo or single dose nevirapine, 30 HIV infected infants, 15 who have received placebo and 15 who have received nevirapine, were subsequently treated with nevirapine combined with other anti-retroviral drugs. Virologic failure after 6 months of treatment with nevirapine combined with other anti-retroviral drugs occurred in significantly more infants who had previously received a single dose of nevirapine (10 of 15) than in infants who had received placebo previously (1 of 15). This indicates that in infants previously treated with single-dose nevirapine alone for prevention of mother to child transmission of HIV-1, the efficacy of VIRAMUNE as part of a combination therapy which they receive for their own health may be reduced.

In a study in which women who had received single dose nevirapine for prevention of mother-to-child transmission were treated with VIRAMUNE combined with other antiretroviral drugs for their own health, 29 of 123, or 24% experienced virologic failure, and five (38%) of 13 women with HIV-1 detected baseline resistance to VIRAMUNE experienced virologic failure. This indicates that in women previously treated with single-dose nevirapine alone for prevention of mother to child transmission of HIV-1, the efficacy of VIRAMUNE as part of a combination therapy which the women receive for their own health may be reduced.

A blinded randomized clinical trial in women already taking antiretroviral therapy throughout pregnancy (PACTG 316) demonstrated no further reduction of vertical HIV-1 transmission when the mother and the child received a single VIRAMUNE dose during labour and after birth respectively. HIV-1 transmission rates were similarly low in both treatment groups (1.3% in the VIRAMUNE group, 1.4% in the placebo group). The vertical transmission decreased neither in women with HIV-1 RNA below the limit of quantification nor in women with HIV-1 RNA above the limit of quantification prior to partus. Of the 95 women who received intrapartum VIRAMUNE, 15% developed nevirapine resistance mutations at 6 weeks post partus.

The clinical relevance of these data in European populations has not been established. Furthermore, in the case VIRAMUNE is used as single dose to prevent vertical transmission of HIV-1 infection, the risk of hepatotoxicity in mother and child cannot be excluded.

5.2 Pharmacokinetic properties

VIRAMUNE tablets and oral suspension have been shown to be comparably bioavailable and interchangeable at doses up to 200 mg.

Absorption: Nevirapine is readily absorbed (> 90%) after oral administration in healthy volunteers and in adults with HIV-1 infection. Absolute bioavailability in 12 healthy adults following single-dose administration was 93 ± 9% (mean SD) for a 50 mg tablet and 91 ± 8% for an oral solution. Peak plasma nevirapine concentrations of 2 ± 0.4 µg/ml (7.5 µM) were attained by 4 hours following a single 200 mg dose. Following multiple doses, nevirapine peak concentrations appear to increase linearly in the dose range of 200 to 400 mg/day. Data reported in the literature from 20 HIV infected patients suggest a steady state C_{max} of 5.74 µg/ml (5.00-7.44) and C_{min} of 3.73 µg/ml (3.20-5.08) with an AUC of 109.0 h·µg/ml (96.0-143.5) in patients taking 200 mg of nevirapine bid. Other published data support these conclusions. Long-term efficacy appears to be most likely in patients whose nevirapine trough levels exceed 3.5 µg/ml.

Distribution: Nevirapine is lipophilic and is essentially non-ionized at physiologic pH. Following intravenous administration to healthy adults, the volume of distribution (Vdss) of nevirapine was 1.21 ± 0.09 l/kg, suggesting that nevirapine is widely distributed in humans. Nevirapine readily crosses the placenta and is found in breast milk. Nevirapine is about 60% bound to plasma proteins in the plasma concentration range of 1-10 µg/ml. Nevirapine concentrations in human cerebrospinal fluid (n = 6) were 45% (± 5%) of the concentrations in plasma; this ratio is approximately equal to the fraction not bound to plasma protein.

Biotransformation and elimination: *In vivo* studies in humans and *in vitro* studies with human liver microsomes have shown that nevirapine is extensively biotransformed via cytochrome P450 (oxidative) metabolism to several hydroxylated metabolites. *In vitro* studies with human liver microsomes suggest that oxidative metabolism of nevirapine is mediated primarily by cytochrome P450 isozymes from the CYP3A family, although other isozymes may have a secondary role. In a mass balance/excretion study in eight healthy male volunteers dosed to steady state with nevirapine 200 mg given twice daily followed by a single 50 mg dose of 14C-nevirapine, approximately 91.4 ± 10.5% of the radiolabelled dose was recovered, with urine (81.3 ± 11.1%) representing the primary route of excretion compared to faeces (10.1 ± 1.5%). Greater than 80% of the radioactivity in urine was made up of glucuronide conjugates of hydroxylated metabolites. Thus cytochrome P450 metabolism, glucuronide conjugation, and urinary excretion of glucuronidated metabolites represent the primary route of nevirapine biotransformation and elimination in humans. Only a small fraction (< 5%) of the radioactivity in urine (representing < 3% of the total dose) was made up of parent compound; therefore, renal excretion plays a minor role in elimination of the parent compound.

Nevirapine has been shown to be an inducer of hepatic cytochrome P450 metabolic enzymes. The pharmacokinetics of autoinduction are characterised by an approximately 1.5 to 2 fold increase in the apparent oral clearance of nevirapine as treatment continues from a single dose to two-to-four weeks of dosing with 200-400 mg/day. Autoinduction also results in a corresponding decrease in the terminal phase half-life of nevirapine in plasma from approximately 45 hours (single dose) to approximately 25-30 hours following multiple dosing with 200-400 mg/day.

Special populations:

Renal dysfunction: The single-dose pharmacokinetics of nevirapine have been compared in 23 subjects with either mild (50 ⩽ CLcr < 80 ml/min), moderate (30 ⩽ CLcr < 50 ml/min) or severe renal dysfunction (CLcr < 30 ml/min), renal impairment or end-stage renal disease (ESRD) requiring dialysis, and 8 subjects with normal renal function (CLcr > 80 ml/min). Renal impairment (mild, moderate and severe) resulted in no significant change in the pharmacokinetics of nevirapine. However, subjects with ESRD

Table 5 Number of patients who had one or more adverse events*

Adverse Event	Nevirapine (N=155)			Efavirenz (N=156)			Abacavir (N=149)		
	Any adverse event	Grade 3 or 4 adverse event	Adverse event leading to discontinuation	Any adverse event	Grade 3 or 4 adverse event	Adverse event leading to discontinuation	Any adverse event	Grade 3 or 4 adverse event	Adverse event leading to discontinuation
	Number of patients (percent)								
Clinical									
- Neuropsychiatric	11	6	6	48	22	19	14	1	0
- Cutaneous	20	13	12	11	3	3	7	0	0
- Gastrointestinal	6	2	0	8	4	4	12	2	1
- Systemic**	7	1	1	5	2	0	10	8	8
- Other	25	8	1	11	5	1	12	3	0
Laboratory									
- Increased aminotransferase levels	12	6	4	4	1	0	5	1	0
- Hyperglycemia	2	2	2	2	2	0	1	1	0
Total	83 (54) ***	38	26 (17) ****	89 (57) ***	39	27 (17) ****	61 (41) ***	16	9 (6)****

* A grade 3 event was defined as severe, and a grade 4 event as life-threatening

** Systemic adverse events included hypersensitivity reactions

*** P=0.02 by the chi-square test

**** P=0.01 by the chi-square test

requiring dialysis exhibited a 43.5% reduction in nevirapine AUC over a one-week exposure period. There was also accumulation of nevirapine hydroxy-metabolites in plasma. The results suggest that supplementing VIRAMUNE therapy with an additional 200 mg dose of VIRAMUNE following each dialysis treatment would help offset the effects of dialysis on nevirapine clearance. Otherwise patients with CLcr ⩾ 20 ml/min do not require an adjustment in VIRAMUNE dosing.

Hepatic dysfunction: A steady state study comparing 46 patients with

mild (n=17: Ishak Score 1-2),

moderate (n=20; Ishak Score 3-4),

or severe (n=9; Ishak Score 5-6, Child-Pugh A in 8 pts., for 1 Child-Pugh score not applicable)

liver fibrosis as a measure of hepatic impairment was conducted.

The patients studied were receiving antiretroviral therapy containing Viramune 200 mg twice daily for at least 6 weeks prior to pharmacokinetic sampling, with a median duration of therapy of 3.4 years. In this study, the multiple dose pharmacokinetic disposition of nevirapine and the five oxidative metabolites were not altered.

However, approximately 15% of these patients with hepatic fibrosis had nevirapine trough concentrations above 9,000 ng/ml (2 fold the usual mean trough). Patients with hepatic impairment should be monitored carefully for evidence of drug induced toxicity.

In a 200 mg nevirapine single dose pharmacokinetic study of HIV-negative patients with mild and moderate hepatic impairment (Child-Pugh A, n=6; Child-Pugh B, n=4), a significant increase in the AUC of nevirapine was observed in one Child-Pugh B patient with ascites suggesting that patients with worsening hepatic function and ascites may be at risk of accumulating nevirapine in the systemic circulation. Because nevirapine induces its own metabolism with multiple dosing, this single dose study may not reflect the impact of hepatic impairment on multiple dose pharmacokinetics (see section 4.4).

In the multinational 2NN study, a population pharmacokinetic substudy of 1077 patients was performed that included 391 females. Female patients showed a 13.8% lower clearance of nevirapine than did male patients. This difference is not considered clinically relevant. Since neither body weight nor Body Mass Index (BMI) had influence on the clearance of nevirapine, the effect of gender cannot be explained by body size. Nevirapine pharmacokinetics in HIV-1 infected adults do not appear to change with age (range 19-68 years) or race (Black, Hispanic, or Caucasian). VIRAMUNE has not been specifically investigated in patients over the age of 65.

Paediatric patients: Data concerning the pharmacokinetics of nevirapine has been derived from two major sources: a 48 week paediatric trial in South Africa (BI 1100.1368) involving 123 HIV-1 positive, antiretroviral naïve patients aged 3 months to 16 years; and a consolidated analysis of five Paediatric AIDS Clinical Trials Group (PACTG) protocols comprising 495 patients aged 14 days to 19 years.

The results of the 48 week analysis of the South African study BI 1100.1368 confirmed that the 4/7 mg/kg and 150 mg/m^2 nevirapine dose groups were well tolerated and effective in treating antiretroviral naïve paediatric patients. A marked improvement in the CD4+ cell percent was observed through week 48 for both dose groups. Also, both dosing regimens were effective in reducing the viral load. In this 48 week study no unexpected safety findings were observed in either dosing group.

Pharmacokinetic data on 33 patients (age range 0.77 – 13.7 years) in the intensive sampling group demonstrated that clearance of nevirapine increased with increasing age in a manner consistent with increasing body surface area. Dosing of nevirapine at 150 mg/m^{2}BID (after a two-week lead in at 150 mg/m^2 QD) produced geometric mean or mean trough nevirapine concentrations between 4-6 μg/ml (as targeted from adult data). In addition, the observed trough nevirapine concentrations were comparable between the two methods.

The consolidated analysis of Paediatric AIDS Clinical Trials Group (PACTG) protocols 245, 356, 366, 377, and 403 allowed for the evaluation of paediatric patients less than 3 months of age (n=17) enrolled in these PACTG studies. The plasma nevirapine concentrations observed were within the range observed in adults and the remainder of the paediatric population, but were more variable between patients, particularly in the second month of age.

5.3 Preclinical safety data

Non-clinical data reveal no special hazard for humans other than those observed in clinical studies based on conventional studies of safety, pharmacology, repeated dose toxicity, and genotoxicity. In reproductive toxicology studies, evidence of impaired fertility was seen in rats. In carcinogenicity studies, nevirapine induces hepatic tumours in rats and mice. These findings are most likely related to nevirapine being a strong inducer of liver enzymes, and not due to a genotoxic mode of action.

6. PHARMACEUTICAL PARTICULARS

6.1 List of excipients

Microcrystalline cellulose

Lactose monohydrate

Povidone K25

Sodium starch glycolate

Colloidal silicon dioxide

Magnesium stearate

6.2 Incompatibilities

Not applicable.

6.3 Shelf life

3 years

6.4 Special precautions for storage

This medicinal product does not require any special storage conditions.

6.5 Nature and contents of container

Treatment initiation pack:

Polyvinyl chloride (PVC)/aluminium foil push-through blister units (blister card of 7 tablets). Cartons containing 2 blister cards (14 tablets).

Maintenance packs:

Polyvinyl chloride (PVC)/aluminium foil push-through blister units (blister card of 10 tablets). Cartons containing 6 or 12 blister cards (60 or 120 tablets).

Not all pack sizes may be marketed.

6.6 Special precautions for disposal and other handling

Any unused product or waste material should be disposed of in accordance with local requirements.

7. MARKETING AUTHORISATION HOLDER

Boehringer Ingelheim International GmbH

Binger Strasse 173

55216 Ingelheim am Rhein, Germany

8. MARKETING AUTHORISATION NUMBER(S)

EU/1/97/055/001 (60 tablets)

EU/1/97/055/003 (120 tablets)

EU/1/97/055/004 (14 tablets)

9. DATE OF FIRST AUTHORISATION/RENEWAL OF THE AUTHORISATION

Date of first authorisation: 5 February 1998

Date of latest renewal: 10 January 2008

10. DATE OF REVISION OF THE TEXT

29 May 2009

Detailed information on this product is available on the website of the European Medicines Agency (EMEA) http://www.emea.europa.eu

Viread 245 mg film-coated tablets

(Gilead Sciences Ltd)

1. NAME OF THE MEDICINAL PRODUCT

Viread ▼ 245 mg film-coated tablets

2. QUALITATIVE AND QUANTITATIVE COMPOSITION

Each film-coated tablet contains 245 mg of tenofovir disoproxil (as fumarate), equivalent to 300 mg of tenofovir disoproxil fumarate, or 136 mg of tenofovir.

Excipient(s):

Each tablet contains 153.33 mg lactose monohydrate. For a full list of excipients, see section 6.1.

3. PHARMACEUTICAL FORM

Film-coated tablet.

Light blue, almond-shaped, film-coated tablets, debossed on one side with the markings "GILEAD" and "4331" and on the other side with the marking "300".

4. CLINICAL PARTICULARS

4.1 Therapeutic indications

HIV-1 infection: Viread is indicated in combination with other antiretroviral medicinal products for the treatment of HIV-1 infected adults over 18 years of age.

The demonstration of benefit of Viread in HIV-1 infection is based on results of one study in treatment-naïve patients, including patients with a high viral load (> 100,000 copies/

ml) and studies in which Viread was added to stable background therapy (mainly tritherapy) in antiretroviral pre-treated patients experiencing early virological failure (< 10,000 copies/ml, with the majority of patients having < 5,000 copies/ml).

The choice of Viread to treat antiretroviral experienced patients with HIV-1 infection should be based on individual viral resistance testing and/or treatment history of patients.

Hepatitis B infection: Viread is indicated for the treatment of chronic hepatitis B in adults with compensated liver disease, with evidence of active viral replication, persistently elevated serum alanine aminotransferase (ALT) levels and histological evidence of active inflammation and/or fibrosis.

This indication is based on histological, virological, biochemical and serological responses mainly in adult nucleoside-naïve patients with HBeAg positive and HBeAg negative chronic hepatitis B with compensated liver function.

4.2 Posology and method of administration

Therapy should be initiated by a physician experienced in the management of HIV infection and/or treatment of chronic hepatitis B.

In exceptional circumstances in patients having particular difficulty in swallowing, Viread can be administered following disintegration of the tablet in at least 100 ml of water, orange juice or grape juice.

Adults: The recommended dose for the treatment of HIV or for the treatment of chronic hepatitis B is 245 mg (one tablet) once daily taken orally with food.

Chronic hepatitis B: The optimal duration of treatment is unknown. Treatment discontinuation may be considered as follows:

- In HBeAg positive patients without cirrhosis, treatment should be administered for at least 6-12 months after HBe seroconversion (HBeAg loss and HBV DNA loss with anti-HBe detection) is confirmed or until HBs seroconversion or there is loss of efficacy (see section 4.4). Serum ALT and HBV DNA levels should be followed regularly after treatment discontinuation to detect any late virological relapse.

- In HBeAg negative patients without cirrhosis, treatment should be administered at least until HBs seroconversion or there is evidence of loss of efficacy. With prolonged treatment for more than 2 years, regular reassessment is recommended to confirm that continuing the selected therapy remains appropriate for the patient.

Paediatric patients: Viread is not recommended for use in children below the age of 18 years due to insufficient data on safety and efficacy (see section 5.2).

Elderly: No data are available on which to make a dose recommendation for patients over the age of 65 years (see section 4.4).

Renal insufficiency: Tenofovir is eliminated by renal excretion and the exposure to tenofovir increases in patients with renal dysfunction. There are limited data on the safety and efficacy of tenofovir disoproxil fumarate in patients with moderate and severe renal impairment (creatinine clearance < 50 ml/min) and long term safety data has not been evaluated for mild renal impairment (creatinine clearance 50-80 ml/min). Therefore, in patients with renal impairment tenofovir disoproxil fumarate should only be used if the potential benefits of treatment are considered to outweigh the potential risks. Dose interval adjustments are recommended for patients with creatinine clearance < 50 ml/min.

Mild renal impairment (creatinine clearance 50-80 ml/min): Limited data from clinical studies support once daily dosing of tenofovir disoproxil fumarate in patients with mild renal impairment.

Moderate renal impairment (creatinine clearance 30-49 ml/min): Administration of 245 mg tenofovir disoproxil (as fumarate) every 48 hours is recommended based on modelling of single-dose pharmacokinetic data in non-HIV and non-HBV infected subjects with varying degrees of renal impairment, including end-stage renal disease requiring haemodialysis, but has not been confirmed in clinical studies. Therefore, clinical response to treatment and renal function should be closely monitored in these patients (see sections 4.4 and 5.2).

Severe renal impairment (creatinine clearance < 30 ml/min) and haemodialysis patients: Adequate dose adjustments cannot be applied due to lack of alternative tablet strengths, therefore use in this group of patients is not recommended. If no alternative treatment is available, prolonged dose intervals may be used as follows:

Severe renal impairment: 245 mg tenofovir disoproxil (as fumarate) may be administered every 72-96 hours (dosing twice a week).

Haemodialysis patients: 245 mg tenofovir disoproxil (as fumarate) may be administered every 7 days following completion of a haemodialysis session*.

These dose adjustments have not been confirmed in clinical studies. Simulations suggest that the prolonged dose interval is not optimal and could result in increased toxicity and possibly inadequate response. Therefore clinical response to treatment and renal function should be closely monitored (see sections 4.4 and 5.2).

* Generally, once weekly dosing assuming three haemodialysis sessions per week, each of approximately 4 hours duration or after 12 hours cumulative haemodialysis.

No dosing recommendations can be given for non-haemodialysis patients with creatinine clearance < 10 ml/min.

Hepatic impairment: No dose adjustment is required in patients with hepatic impairment (see sections 4.4 and 5.2).

If Viread is discontinued in patients with chronic hepatitis B with or without HIV co-infection, these patients should be closely monitored for evidence of exacerbation of hepatitis (see section 4.4).

4.3 Contraindications

Hypersensitivity to the active substance or to any of the excipients.

4.4 Special warnings and precautions for use

General: Tenofovir disoproxil fumarate has not been studied in patients under the age of 18 or in patients over the age of 65. Elderly patients are more likely to have decreased renal function, therefore caution should be exercised when treating elderly patients with tenofovir disoproxil fumarate (see below).

HIV antibody testing should be offered to all HBV infected patients before initiating tenofovir disoproxil fumarate therapy (see below *Co-infection with HIV-1 and hepatitis B*).

Patients must be advised that tenofovir disoproxil fumarate has not been proven to prevent the risk of transmission of HIV or HBV to others through sexual contact or contamination with blood. Appropriate precautions must continue to be used.

Viread contains lactose monohydrate. Consequently, patients with rare hereditary problems of galactose intolerance, the Lapp lactase deficiency, or glucose-galactose malabsorption should not take this medicinal product.

Co-administration of other medicinal products:

- Viread should not be administered with any other medicinal products containing tenofovir disoproxil fumarate (Truvada or Atripla).

- Viread should also not be administered concurrently with adefovir dipivoxil.

- Co-administration of tenofovir disoproxil fumarate and didanosine is not recommended. Co-administration of tenofovir disoproxil fumarate and didanosine results in a 40-60% increase in systemic exposure to didanosine that may increase the risk of didanosine-related adverse events (see section 4.5). Rare cases of pancreatitis and lactic acidosis, sometimes fatal, have been reported. Co-administration of tenofovir disoproxil fumarate and didanosine at a dose of 400 mg daily has been associated with a significant decrease in CD4 cell count, possibly due to an intracellular interaction increasing phosphorylated (i.e. active) didanosine. A decreased dosage of 250 mg didanosine co-administered with tenofovir disoproxil fumarate therapy has been associated with reports of high rates of virological failure within several tested combinations for the treatment of HIV-1 infection.

Triple therapy with nucleosides/nucleotides: There have been reports of a high rate of virological failure and of emergence of resistance at early stage in HIV patients when tenofovir disoproxil fumarate was combined with lamivudine and abacavir as well as with lamivudine and didanosine as a once daily regimen.

Renal function: Tenofovir is principally eliminated via the kidney. Renal failure, renal impairment, elevated creatinine, hypophosphataemia and proximal tubulopathy (including Fanconi syndrome) have been reported with the use of tenofovir disoproxil fumarate in clinical practice (see section 4.8).

Renal safety with tenofovir has only been studied to a very limited degree in patients with impaired renal function (CrCl < 80 ml/min).

It is recommended that creatinine clearance is calculated in all patients prior to initiating therapy with tenofovir disoproxil fumarate and renal function (creatinine clearance and serum phosphate) is also monitored every four weeks during the first year, and then every three months. In patients at risk for renal impairment, including patients who have previously experienced renal events while receiving adefovir dipivoxil, consideration should be given to more frequent monitoring of renal function.

Patients with creatinine clearance < 50 ml/min, including haemodialysis patients: There are limited data on the safety and efficacy of tenofovir disoproxil fumarate in patients with impaired renal function. Therefore, tenofovir disoproxil fumarate should only be used if the potential benefits of treatment are considered to outweigh the potential risks. In patients with severe renal impairment (creatinine clearance < 30 ml/min) use of tenofovir is not recommended. If no alternative treatment is available, the dosing interval must be adjusted and renal function should be closely monitored (see sections 4.2 and 5.2).

If serum phosphate is < 1.5 mg/dl (0.48 mmol/l) or creatinine clearance is decreased to < 50 ml/min in any patient receiving tenofovir disoproxil fumarate, renal function should be re-evaluated within one week, including measurements of blood glucose, blood potassium and urine glucose concentrations (see section 4.8, proximal tubulopathy). Consideration should also be given to interrupting treatment with tenofovir disoproxil fumarate in patients with creatinine clearance decreased to < 50 ml/min or decreases in serum phosphate to < 1.0 mg/dl (0.32 mmol/l).

Use of tenofovir disoproxil fumarate should be avoided with concurrent or recent use of a nephrotoxic medicinal product (e.g. aminoglycosides, amphotericin B, foscarnet, ganciclovir, pentamidine, vancomycin, cidofovir or interleukin-2). If concomitant use of tenofovir disoproxil fumarate and nephrotoxic agents is unavoidable, renal function should be monitored weekly.

Tenofovir disoproxil fumarate has not been clinically evaluated in patients receiving medicinal products which are secreted by the same renal pathway, including the transport proteins human organic anion transporter (hOAT) 1 and 3 or MRP 4 (e.g. cidofovir, a known nephrotoxic medicinal product). These renal transport proteins may be responsible for tubular secretion and in part, renal elimination of tenofovir and cidofovir. Consequently, the pharmacokinetics of these medicinal products which are secreted by the same renal pathway including transport proteins hOAT 1 and 3 or MRP 4 might be modified if they are co-administered. Unless clearly necessary, concomitant use of these medicinal products which are secreted by the same renal pathway is not recommended, but if such use is unavoidable, renal function should be monitored weekly (see section 4.5).

Bone effects: In HIV infected patients, in a 144-week controlled clinical study that compared tenofovir disoproxil fumarate with stavudine in combination with lamivudine and efavirenz in antiretroviral-naïve patients, small decreases in bone mineral density of the hip and spine were observed in both treatment groups. Decreases in bone mineral density of spine and changes in bone biomarkers from baseline were significantly greater in the tenofovir disoproxil fumarate treatment group at 144 weeks. Decreases in bone mineral density of hip were significantly greater in this group until 96 weeks. However, there was no increased risk of fractures or evidence for clinically relevant bone abnormalities over 144 weeks.

Bone abnormalities (infrequently contributing to fractures) may be associated with proximal renal tubulopathy (see section 4.8). If bone abnormalities are suspected then appropriate consultation should be obtained.

Liver disease: The safety of tenofovir in patients with decompensated liver disease is being studied. At present the safety in this patient population has not been thoroughly evaluated.

No safety and efficacy data are available in liver transplant patients.

Exacerbations of hepatitis:

Flares on treatment: Spontaneous exacerbations in chronic hepatitis B are relatively common and are characterised by transient increases in serum ALT. After initiating antiviral therapy, serum ALT may increase in some patients as serum HBV DNA levels decline (see section 4.8). Among tenofovir-treated patients on-treatment exacerbations typically occurred after 4-8 weeks of therapy. In patients with compensated liver disease, these increases in serum ALT are generally not accompanied by an increase in serum bilirubin concentrations or hepatic decompensation. Patients with cirrhosis may be at a higher risk for hepatic decompensation following hepatitis exacerbation, and therefore should be monitored closely during therapy.

Flares after treatment discontinuation: Acute exacerbation of hepatitis has also been reported in patients who have discontinued hepatitis B therapy. Post-treatment exacerbations are usually associated with rising HBV DNA, and the majority appears to be self-limited. However, severe exacerbations, including fatalities, have been reported. Hepatic function should be monitored at repeated intervals with both clinical and laboratory follow-up for at least 6 months after discontinuation of hepatitis B therapy. If appropriate, resumption of hepatitis B therapy may be warranted. In patients with advanced liver disease or cirrhosis, treatment discontinuation is not recommended since post-treatment exacerbation of hepatitis may lead to hepatic decompensation.

Liver flares are especially serious, and sometimes fatal in patients with decompensated liver disease.

Co-infection with hepatitis C or D: There are no data on the efficacy of tenofovir in patients co-infected with hepatitis C or D virus.

Co-infection with HIV-1 and hepatitis B: Due to the risk of development of HIV resistance, tenofovir disoproxil fumarate should only be used as part of an appropriate antiretroviral combination regimen in HIV/HBV co-infected patients. Patients with pre-existing liver dysfunction including chronic active hepatitis have an increased frequency of liver function abnormalities during combination antiretroviral therapy and should be monitored according to standard practice. If there is evidence of worsening liver disease in such patients, interruption or discontinuation of treatment must be considered. However, it should be noted that increases of ALT can be part of HBV clearance during therapy with tenofovir, see above *Exacerbations of hepatitis*.

Lactic acidosis: Lactic acidosis, usually associated with hepatic steatosis, has been reported with the use of nucleoside analogues. The preclinical and clinical data suggest that the risk of occurrence of lactic acidosis, a class effect of nucleoside analogues, is low for tenofovir disoproxil fumarate. However, as tenofovir is structurally related to nucleoside analogues, this risk cannot be excluded. Early symptoms (symptomatic hyperlactatemia) include benign digestive symptoms (nausea, vomiting and abdominal pain), non-specific malaise, loss of appetite, weight loss, respiratory symptoms (rapid and/or deep breathing) or neurological symptoms (including motor weakness). Lactic acidosis has a high mortality and may be associated with pancreatitis, liver failure or renal failure. Lactic acidosis generally occurred after a few or several months of treatment.

Treatment with nucleoside analogues should be discontinued in the setting of symptomatic hyperlactatemia and metabolic/lactic acidosis, progressive hepatomegaly, or rapidly elevating aminotransferase levels.

Caution should be exercised when administering nucleoside analogues to any patient (particularly obese women) with hepatomegaly, hepatitis or other known risk factors for liver disease and hepatic steatosis (including certain medicinal products and alcohol). Patients co-infected with hepatitis C and treated with alpha interferon and ribavirin may constitute a special risk.

Patients at increased risk should be followed closely.

Lipodystrophy (lipoatrophy/lipomatosis): In HIV infected patients, combination antiretroviral therapy has been associated with the redistribution of body fat (lipodystrophy). The long-term consequences of these events are currently unknown. Knowledge about the mechanism is incomplete. A connection between visceral lipomatosis and protease inhibitors and lipoatrophy and nucleoside reverse transcriptase inhibitors has been hypothesised. A higher risk of lipodystrophy has been associated with individual factors such as older age, and with drug related factors such as longer duration of antiretroviral treatment and associated metabolic disturbances. Clinical examination should include evaluation for physical signs of fat redistribution. Consideration should be given to the measurement of fasting serum lipids and blood glucose. Lipid disorders should be managed as clinically appropriate (see section 4.8).

Tenofovir is structurally related to nucleoside analogues hence the risk of lipodystrophy cannot be excluded. However, 144-week clinical data from antiretroviral-naïve HIV infected patients indicate that the risk of lipodystrophy was lower with tenofovir disoproxil fumarate than with stavudine when administered with lamivudine and efavirenz.

Mitochondrial dysfunction: Nucleoside and nucleotide analogues have been demonstrated *in vitro* and *in vivo* to cause a variable degree of mitochondrial damage. There have been reports of mitochondrial dysfunction in HIV negative infants exposed *in utero* and/or postnatally to nucleoside analogues. The main adverse events reported are haematological disorders (anaemia, neutropenia), metabolic disorders (hyperlactataemia, hyperlipasaemia). These events are often transitory. Some late-onset neurological disorders have been reported (hypertonia, convulsion, abnormal behaviour). Whether the neurological disorders are transient or permanent is currently unknown. Any child exposed *in utero* to nucleoside and nucleotide analogues, even HIV negative children, should have clinical and laboratory follow-up and should be fully investigated for possible mitochondrial dysfunction in case of relevant signs or symptoms. These findings do not affect current national recommendations to use antiretroviral therapy in pregnant women to prevent vertical transmission of HIV.

Immune Reactivation Syndrome: In HIV infected patients with severe immune deficiency at the time of institution of combination antiretroviral therapy (CART), an inflammatory reaction to asymptomatic or residual opportunistic pathogens may arise and cause serious clinical conditions, or aggravation of symptoms. Typically, such reactions have been observed within the first few weeks or months of initiation of CART. Relevant examples are cytomegalovirus retinitis, generalised and/or focal mycobacterium infections, and *Pneumocystis jiroveci* pneumonia. Any inflammatory symptoms should be evaluated and treatment instituted when necessary.

Osteonecrosis: Although the etiology is considered to be multifactorial (including corticosteroid use, alcohol consumption, severe immunosuppression, higher body mass index), cases of osteonecrosis have been reported particularly in patients with advanced HIV-disease and/or long-term exposure to combination antiretroviral therapy (CART). Patients should be advised to seek medical advice if they experience joint aches and pain, joint stiffness or difficulty in movement.

4.5 Interaction with other medicinal products and other forms of interaction

Interaction studies have only been performed in adults.

Based on the results of *in vitro* experiments and the known elimination pathway of tenofovir, the potential for CYP450 mediated interactions involving tenofovir with other medicinal products is low.

Concomitant use not recommended:

Viread should not be administered with any other medicinal products containing tenofovir disoproxil fumarate (Truvada or Atripla).

Viread should also not be administered concurrently with adefovir dipivoxil.

Didanosine: Co-administration of tenofovir disoproxil fumarate and didanosine is not recommended (see section 4.4 and Table 1).

Renally eliminated medicinal products: Since tenofovir is primarily eliminated by the kidneys, co-administration of tenofovir disoproxil fumarate with medicinal products that reduce renal function or compete for active tubular secretion via transport proteins hOAT 1, hOAT 3 or MRP 4 (e.g. cidofovir) may increase serum concentrations of tenofovir and/or the co-administered medicinal products.

Use of tenofovir disoproxil fumarate should be avoided with concurrent or recent use of a nephrotoxic medicinal product. Some examples include, but are not limited to, aminoglycosides, amphotericin B, foscarnet, ganciclovir, pentamidine, vancomycin, cidofovir or interleukin-2 (see section 4.4).

Given that tacrolimus can affect renal function, close monitoring is recommended when it is co-administered with tenofovir disoproxil fumarate.

Other interactions:

Interactions between tenofovir disoproxil fumarate and protease inhibitors and antiretroviral agents other than protease inhibitors are listed in Table 1 below (increase is indicated as "↑", decrease as "↓", no change as "↔", twice daily as "b.i.d.", and once daily as "q.d.").

Table 1: Interactions between tenofovir disoproxil fumarate and other medicinal products

(see Table 1 below)

Studies conducted with other medicinal products: There were no clinically significant pharmacokinetic interactions when tenofovir disoproxil fumarate was co-administered with emtricitabine, lamivudine, indinavir, efavirenz, nelfinavir, saquinavir (ritonavir boosted), methadone, ribavirin, rifampicin, tacrolimus, or the hormonal contraceptive norgestimate/ethinyl oestradiol.

Tenofovir disoproxil fumarate must be taken with food, as food enhances the bioavailability of tenofovir (see section 5.2).

4.6 Pregnancy and lactation

Pregnancy

For tenofovir disoproxil fumarate limited clinical data on exposed pregnancies are available.

Animal studies do not indicate direct or indirect harmful effects of tenofovir disoproxil fumarate with respect to pregnancy, foetal development, parturition or postnatal development (see section 5.3).

Tenofovir disoproxil fumarate should be used during pregnancy only if the potential benefit justifies the potential risk to the foetus.

Given that the potential risks to developing human foetuses are unknown, the use of tenofovir disoproxil fumarate in women of childbearing potential must be accompanied by the use of effective contraception.

Lactation

In animal studies it has been shown that tenofovir is excreted into milk. It is not known whether tenofovir is excreted in human milk. Therefore, it is recommended that mothers being treated with tenofovir disoproxil fumarate do not breast-feed their infants.

As a general rule, it is recommended that HIV and HBV infected women do not breast-feed their infants in order to avoid transmission of HIV and HBV to the infant.

Table 1: Interactions between tenofovir disoproxil fumarate and other medicinal products

Medicinal product by therapeutic areas (dose in mg)	Effects on drug levels Mean percent change in AUC, C_{max}, C_{min}	Recommendation concerning co-administration with tenofovir disoproxil fumarate 300 mg
ANTI-INFECTIVES		
Antiretrovirals		
Protease inhibitors		
Atazanavir/Ritonavir (300 q.d./100 q.d./300 q.d.)	Atazanavir: AUC: ↓ 25% C_{max}: ↓ 28% C_{min}: ↓ 26% Tenofovir: AUC: ↑ 37% C_{max}: ↑ 34% C_{min}: ↑ 29%	No dose adjustment is recommended. The increased exposure of tenofovir could potentiate tenofovir associated adverse events, including renal disorders. Renal function should be closely monitored (see section 4.4).
Lopinavir/Ritonavir (400 b.i.d./100 b.i.d./300 q.d.)	Lopinavir/ritonavir: No significant effect on lopinavir/ritonavir PK parameters. Tenofovir: AUC: ↑ 32% C_{max}: ↔ C_{min}: ↑ 51%	No dose adjustment is recommended. The increased exposure of tenofovir could potentiate tenofovir associated adverse events, including renal disorders. Renal function should be closely monitored (see section 4.4).
Darunavir/Ritonavir (300/100 b.i.d./300 q.d.)	Darunavir: No significant effect on darunavir/ritonavir PK parameters. Tenofovir: AUC: ↑ 22% C_{min}: ↑ 37%	No dose adjustment is recommended. The increased exposure of tenofovir could potentiate tenofovir associated adverse events, including renal disorders. Renal function should be closely monitored (see section 4.4).
NRTIs		
Didanosine	Co-administration of tenofovir disoproxil fumarate and didanosine results in a 40-60% increase in systemic exposure to didanosine that may increase the risk for didanosine-related adverse events. Rare cases of pancreatitis and lactic acidosis, sometimes fatal, have been reported. Co-administration of tenofovir disoproxil fumarate and didanosine at a dose of 400 mg daily has been associated with a significant decrease in CD4 cell count, possibly due to an intracellular interaction increasing phosphorylated (i.e. active) didanosine. A decreased dosage of 250 mg didanosine co-administered with tenofovir disoproxil fumarate therapy has been associated with reports of high rates of virological failure within several tested combinations for the treatment of HIV-1 infection.	Co-administration of tenofovir disoproxil fumarate and didanosine is not recommended (see section 4.4).
Adefovir dipivoxil	AUC: ↔ C_{max}: ↔	Tenofovir disoproxil fumarate should not be administered concurrently with adefovir dipivoxil (see section 4.4).
Entecavir	AUC: ↔ C_{max}: ↔	No clinically significant pharmacokinetic interactions when tenofovir disoproxil fumarate was co-administered with entecavir.

4.7 Effects on ability to drive and use machines

No studies on the effects on the ability to drive and use machines have been performed. However, patients should be informed that dizziness has been reported during treatment with tenofovir disoproxil fumarate.

4.8 Undesirable effects

HIV-1: Assessment of adverse reactions from clinical study data is based on experience in two studies in 653 treatment-experienced patients receiving treatment with tenofovir disoproxil fumarate (n = 443) or placebo (n = 210) in combination with other antiretroviral medicinal products for 24 weeks and also in a double-blind comparative controlled study in which 600 treatment-naïve patients received treatment with tenofovir disoproxil 245 mg (as fumarate) (n = 299) or stavudine (n = 301) in combination with lamivudine and efavirenz for 144 weeks.

Approximately one third of patients can be expected to experience adverse reactions following treatment with tenofovir disoproxil fumarate in combination with other antiretroviral agents. These reactions are usually mild to moderate gastrointestinal events.

The adverse reactions with suspected (at least possible) relationship to treatment are listed below by body system organ class and absolute frequency. Within each frequency grouping, undesirable effects are presented in order of decreasing seriousness. Frequencies are defined as very common ($\geq$ 1/10) or common ($\geq$ 1/100, < 1/10). See also *Post-marketing experience* below.

Metabolism and nutrition disorders:

Very common: hypophosphataemia

Nervous system disorders:

Very common: dizziness

Gastrointestinal disorders:

Very common: diarrhoea, vomiting, nausea

Common: flatulence

Approximately 1% of tenofovir disoproxil fumarate-treated patients discontinued treatment due to the gastrointestinal events.

Combination antiretroviral therapy has been associated with metabolic abnormalities such as hypertriglyceridaemia, hypercholesterolaemia, insulin resistance, hyperglycaemia and hyperlactataemia (see section 4.4).

Combination antiretroviral therapy has been associated with redistribution of body fat (lipodystrophy) in HIV patients including the loss of peripheral and facial subcutaneous fat, increased intra-abdominal and visceral fat, breast hypertrophy and dorsocervical fat accumulation (buffalo hump).

In a 144-week controlled clinical study in antiretroviral-naïve patients that compared tenofovir disoproxil fumarate with stavudine in combination with lamivudine and efavirenz, patients who received tenofovir disoproxil had a significantly lower incidence of lipodystrophy compared with patients who received stavudine. The tenofovir disoproxil fumarate arm also had significantly smaller mean increases in fasting triglycerides and total cholesterol than the comparator arm.

In HIV infected patients with severe immune deficiency at the time of initiation of combination antiretroviral therapy (CART), an inflammatory reaction to asymptomatic or residual opportunistic infections may arise (see section 4.4).

Cases of osteonecrosis have been reported, particularly in patients with generally acknowledged risk factors, advanced HIV disease or long-term exposure to combination antiretroviral therapy (CART). The frequency of this is unknown (see section 4.4).

Hepatitis B: Assessment of adverse reactions from clinical study data is primarily based on experience in two double-blind comparative controlled studies (GS-US-174-0102 and GS-US-174-0103) in which 641 patients with chronic hepatitis B and compensated liver disease received treatment with tenofovir disoproxil 245 mg (as fumarate) daily (n = 426) or adefovir dipivoxil 10 mg daily (n = 215) for 48 weeks.

The adverse reactions with suspected (at least possible) relationship to treatment are listed below by body system organ class and frequency. Frequencies are defined as common ($\geq$ 1/100, < 1/10). See also *Post-marketing experience* below.

Nervous system disorders:

Common: headache

Gastrointestinal disorders:

Common: diarrhoea, vomiting, abdominal pain, nausea, abdominal distension, flatulence

Hepatobiliary disorders:

Common: ALT increase

General disorders and administration site conditions:

Common: fatigue

Treatment beyond 48 weeks: Continued treatment with tenofovir disoproxil fumarate for 96 weeks, in studies GS-US-174-0102 and GS-US-174-0103, did not reveal any new adverse reactions and no change in the tolerability profile (nature or severity of adverse events).

Exacerbations during treatment: In studies with nucleoside-naïve patients, on-treatment ALT elevations > 10 times ULN (upper limit of normal) and > 2 times baseline occurred in 2.6% of tenofovir disoproxil fumarate-treated patients *versus* 1.9% of adefovir dipivoxil-treated patients. Among tenofovir disoproxil fumarate-treated patients, on-treatment ALT elevations had a median time to onset of 8 weeks, resolved with continued treatment, and, in a majority of cases, were associated with a $\geq 2 \log_{10}$ copies/ml reduction in viral load that preceded or coincided with the ALT elevation. Periodic monitoring of hepatic function is recommended during treatment.

Post-marketing experience: In addition to adverse reaction reports from clinical studies the following possible adverse reactions have also been identified during post-marketing safety surveillance of tenofovir disoproxil fumarate. Frequencies are defined as rare ($\geq$ 1/10,000, < 1/1,000) or very rare (< 1/10,000) including isolated reports. Because these events have been reported voluntarily from a population of unknown size, estimates of frequency cannot always be made.

Metabolism and nutrition disorders:

Rare: lactic acidosis

Not known: hypokalaemia

Respiratory, thoracic and mediastinal disorders:

Very rare: dyspnoea

Gastrointestinal disorders:

Rare: pancreatitis

Hepatobiliary disorders:

Rare: increased transaminases

Very rare: hepatitis

Not known: hepatic steatosis

Skin and subcutaneous tissue disorders:

Rare: rash

Musculoskeletal and connective tissue disorders:

Not known: rhabdomyolysis, osteomalacia (manifested as bone pain and infrequently contributing to fractures), muscular weakness, myopathy

Renal and urinary disorders:

Rare: acute renal failure, renal failure, proximal renal tubulopathy (including Fanconi syndrome), increased creatinine

Very rare: acute tubular necrosis

Not known: nephritis (including acute interstitial nephritis), nephrogenic diabetes insipidus

General disorders and administration site conditions:

Very rare: asthenia

The following adverse reactions, listed under the body system headings above, may occur as a consequence of proximal renal tubulopathy: rhabdomyolysis, osteomalacia (manifested as bone pain and infrequently contributing to fractures), hypokalaemia, muscular weakness, myopathy and hypophosphataemia. These events are not considered to be causally associated with tenofovir disoproxil fumarate therapy in the absence of proximal renal tubulopathy.

In HBV infected patients, clinical and laboratory evidence of exacerbations of hepatitis have occurred after discontinuation of HBV therapy (see section 4.4).

4.9 Overdose

If overdose occurs the patient must be monitored for evidence of toxicity (see sections 4.8 and 5.3), and standard supportive treatment applied as necessary.

Tenofovir can be removed by haemodialysis; the median haemodialysis clearance of tenofovir is 134 ml/min. The elimination of tenofovir by peritoneal dialysis has not been studied.

5. PHARMACOLOGICAL PROPERTIES

5.1 Pharmacodynamic properties

Pharmacotherapeutic group: Nucleoside and nucleotide reverse transcriptase inhibitors, ATC code: J05AF07

Mechanism of action: Tenofovir disoproxil fumarate is the fumarate salt of the prodrug tenofovir disoproxil. Tenofovir disoproxil is absorbed and converted to the active substance tenofovir, which is a nucleoside monophosphate (nucleotide) analogue. Tenofovir is then converted to the active metabolite, tenofovir diphosphate, an obligate chain terminator, by constitutively expressed cellular enzymes. Tenofovir diphosphate has an intracellular half-life of 10 hours in activated and 50 hours in resting peripheral blood mononuclear cells (PBMCs). Tenofovir diphosphate inhibits HIV-1 reverse transcriptase and the HBV polymerase by direct binding competition with the natural deoxyribonucleotide substrate and, after incorporation into DNA, by DNA chain termination. Tenofovir diphosphate is a weak inhibitor of cellular polymerases α, β, and γ. At concentrations of up to 300 μmol/l, tenofovir has also shown no effect on the synthesis of mitochondrial DNA or the production of lactic acid in *in vitro* assays.

Data pertaining to HIV:

HIV antiviral activity in vitro: The concentration of tenofovir required for 50% inhibition (EC_{50}) of the wild-type laboratory strain HIV-1_{IIIB} is 1-6 μmol/l in lymphoid cell lines and 1.1 μmol/l against primary HIV-1 subtype B isolates in PBMCs. Tenofovir is also active against HIV-1 subtypes A, C, D, E, F, G, and O and against HIV_{BaL} in primary monocyte/macrophage cells. Tenofovir shows activity *in vitro* against HIV-2, with an EC_{50} of 4.9 μmol/l in MT-4 cells.

Resistance: Strains of HIV-1 with reduced susceptibility to tenofovir and a K65R mutation in reverse transcriptase have been selected *in vitro* and in some patients (see *Clinical results*). Tenofovir disoproxil fumarate should be avoided in antiretroviral experienced patients with strains harbouring the K65R mutation (see section 4.4).

Clinical studies in treatment-experienced patients have assessed the anti-HIV activity of tenofovir disoproxil 245 mg (as fumarate) against strains of HIV-1 with resistance to nucleoside inhibitors. The results indicate that patients whose HIV expressed 3 or more thymidine-analogue associated mutations (TAMs) that included either the M41L or L210W reverse transcriptase mutation showed reduced response to tenofovir disoproxil 245 mg (as fumarate) therapy.

Clinical results: The effects of tenofovir disoproxil fumarate in treatment-experienced and treatment-naïve HIV-1 infected adults have been demonstrated in trials of 48 weeks duration in treatment-experienced HIV-1 infected adults.

In study GS-99-907, 550 treatment-experienced patients were treated with placebo or tenofovir disoproxil 245 mg (as fumarate) for 24 weeks. The mean baseline CD4 cell count was 427 cells/mm^3, the mean baseline plasma HIV-1 RNA was 3.4 $\log_{10}$ copies/ml (78% of patients had a viral load of < 5,000 copies/ml) and the mean duration of prior HIV treatment was 5.4 years. Baseline genotypic analysis of HIV isolates from 253 patients revealed that 94% of patients had HIV-1 resistance mutations associated with nucleoside reverse transcriptase inhibitors, 58% had mutations associated with protease inhibitors and 48% had mutations associated with non-nucleoside reverse transcriptase inhibitors.

At week 24 the time-weighted average change from baseline in $\log_{10}$ plasma HIV-1 RNA levels ($DAVG_{24}$) was -0.03 $\log_{10}$ copies/ml and -0.61 $\log_{10}$ copies/ml for the placebo and tenofovir disoproxil 245 mg (as fumarate) recipients ($p < 0.0001$). A statistically significant difference in favour of tenofovir disoproxil 245 mg (as fumarate) was seen in the time-weighted average change from baseline at week 24 ($DAVG_{24}$) for CD4 count (+13 cells/mm^3 for tenofovir disoproxil 245 mg (as fumarate) *versus*-11 cells/mm^3 for placebo, p-value = 0.0008). The antiviral response to tenofovir disoproxil fumarate was durable through 48 weeks ($DAVG_{48}$ was -0.57 $\log_{10}$ copies/ml, proportion of patients with HIV-1 RNA below 400 or 50 copies/ml was 41% and 18% respectively). Eight (2%) tenofovir disoproxil 245 mg (as fumarate) treated patients developed the K65R mutation within the first 48 weeks.

The 144-week, double-blind, active controlled phase of study GS-99-903 evaluated the efficacy and safety of tenofovir disoproxil 245 mg (as fumarate) *versus* stavudine when used in combination with lamivudine and efavirenz in HIV-1 infected patients naïve to antiretroviral therapy. The mean baseline CD4 cell count was 279 cells/mm^3, the mean baseline plasma HIV-1 RNA was 4.91 $\log_{10}$ copies/ml, 19% of patients had symptomatic HIV-1 infection and 18% had AIDS. Patients were stratified by baseline HIV-1 RNA and CD4 count. Forty-three percent of patients had baseline viral loads > 100,000 copies/ml and 39% had CD4 cell counts < 200 cells/ml.

By intent to treat analysis (Missing data and switch in antiretroviral therapy (ART) considered as failure), the proportion of patients with HIV-1 RNA below 400 copies/ml and 50 copies/ml at 48 weeks of treatment was 80% and 76% respectively in the tenofovir disoproxil 245 mg (as fumarate) arm, compared to 84% and 80% in the stavudine arm. At 144 weeks, the proportion of patients with HIV-1 RNA below 400 copies/ml and 50 copies/ml was 71% and 68% respectively in the tenofovir disoproxil 245 mg (as fumarate) arm, compared to 64% and 63% in the stavudine arm.

The average change from baseline for HIV-1 RNA and CD4 count at 48 weeks of treatment was similar in both treatment groups (-3.09 and -3.09 $\log_{10}$ copies/ml; +169 and 167 cells/mm^3 in the tenofovir disoproxil 245 mg (as fumarate) and stavudine groups, respectively). At 144 weeks of treatment, the average change from baseline remained similar in both treatment groups (-3.07 and -3.03 $\log_{10}$ copies/ml; +263 and +283 cells/mm^3 in the tenofovir disoproxil 245 mg (as fumarate) and stavudine groups, respectively). A consistent response to treatment with tenofovir disoproxil 245 mg (as fumarate) was seen regardless of baseline HIV-1 RNA and CD4 count.

The K65R mutation occurred in a slightly higher percentage of patients in the tenofovir disoproxil fumarate group than the active control group (2.7% *versus* 0.7%). Efavirenz or lamivudine resistance either preceded or was coincident with the development of K65R in all cases. Eight patients had HIV that expressed K65R in the tenofovir disoproxil 245 mg (as fumarate) arm, 7 of these occurred during the first 48 weeks of treatment and the last one at week 96. No further K65R development was observed up to week 144. From both the genotypic and phenotypic analyses there was no evidence for other pathways of resistance to tenofovir.

Data pertaining to HBV:

HBV antiviral activity in vitro: The *in vitro* antiviral activity of tenofovir against HBV was assessed in the HepG2 2.2.15 cell line. The EC_{50} values for tenofovir were in the range of 0.14 to 1.5 μmol/l, with CC_{50} (50% cytotoxicity concentration) values > 100 μmol/l.

Resistance: No HBV mutations associated with tenofovir disoproxil fumarate resistance have been identified (see *Clinical results*). In cell based assays, HBV strains expressing the rtV173L, rtL180M, and rtM204I/V mutations associated with resistance to lamivudine and telbivudine showed a susceptibility to tenofovir ranging from 0.7- to 3.4-fold that of wild-type virus. HBV strains expressing the rtL180M, rtT184G, rtS202G/I, rtM204V and rtM250V mutations associated with resistance to entecavir showed a susceptibility to tenofovir ranging from 0.6- to 6.9-fold that of wild-type virus. HBV strains expressing the adefovir-associated resistance mutations rtA181V and rtN236T showed a susceptibility to tenofovir ranging from 2.9- to 10-fold that of wild-type virus. Viruses containing the rtA181T mutation remained susceptible to tenofovir with EC_{50} values 1.5-fold that of wild-type virus.

Clinical results: The demonstration of benefit of tenofovir disoproxil fumarate is based on histological, virological, biochemical and serological responses mainly in treatment-naïve adults with HBeAg positive and HBeAg negative chronic hepatitis B with compensated liver disease.

Experience in patients with compensated liver disease at 48 weeks (studies GS-US-174-0102 and GS-US-174-0103): Results through 48 weeks from two randomised, phase 3 double-blind studies comparing tenofovir disoproxil fumarate to adefovir dipivoxil in patients with compensated liver disease are presented in Table 2 below. Study GS-US-174-0103 was conducted in 266 (randomised and treated) HBeAg positive patients while study GS-US-174-0102 was conducted in 375 (randomised and treated) patients negative for HBeAg and positive for HBeAb.

In both of these studies tenofovir disoproxil fumarate was significantly superior to adefovir dipivoxil for the primary efficacy endpoint of complete response (defined as HBV DNA levels < 400 copies/ml and Knodell necroinflammatory score improvement of at least 2 points without worsening in Knodell fibrosis). Treatment with tenofovir disoproxil 245 mg (as fumarate) was also associated with significantly greater proportions of patients with HBV DNA < 400 copies/ml, when compared to adefovir dipivoxil 10 mg treatment. Both treatments produced similar results with regard to histological response (defined as Knodell necroinflammatory score improvement of at least 2 points without worsening in Knodell fibrosis) at week 48 (see Table 2 below).

In study GS-US-174-0103 a significantly greater proportion of patients in the tenofovir disoproxil fumarate group than in the adefovir dipivoxil group had normalised ALT and achieved HBsAg loss at week 48 (see Table 2 below).

Table 2: Efficacy parameters in compensated HBeAg positive and HBeAg negative patients at week 48

(see Table 2 below)

Tenofovir disoproxil fumarate was associated with significantly greater proportions of patients with undetectable HBV DNA (< 169 copies/ml [< 29 IU/ml]; the limit of quantification of the Roche Cobas Taqman HBV assay), when compared to adefovir dipivoxil (study GS-US-174-0102; 91%, 56% and study GS-US-174-0103; 69%, 9%), respectively.

Response to treatment with tenofovir disoproxil fumarate was comparable in nucleoside-experienced (n = 51) and nucleoside-naïve (n = 375) patients and in patients with normal ALT (n = 21) and abnormal ALT (n = 405) at baseline when studies GS-US-174-0102 and GS-US-174-0103 were combined. Forty-nine of the 51 nucleoside-experienced patients were previously treated with lamivudine.

Table 3: Efficacy parameters in compensated HBeAg positive and HBeAg negative patients at week 96 open-label treatment

	Study 174-0102 (HBeAg negative)		Study 174-0103 (HBeAg positive)	
Parameter[a]	Tenofovir disoproxil 245 mg (as fumarate) 96 weeks[b] n = 250	Adefovir dipivoxil 10 mg roll over to tenofovir disoproxil 245 mg (as fumarate)[c] n = 125	Tenofovir disoproxil 245 mg (as fumarate) 96 weeks[b] n = 176	Adefovir dipivoxil 10 mg roll over to tenofovir disoproxil 245 mg (as fumarate)[c] n = 90
HBV DNA (%) < 400 copies/ml (< 69 IU/ml)	90	89	76	74
ALT (%) Normalised ALT[d]	72	68	60	65
Serology (%) HBeAg loss/ seroconversion	N/A	N/A	26/23	24/20
HBsAg loss/ seroconversion	0/0	0/0	5/4	6/5

[a] Based upon Long Term Evaluation algorithm (LTE Analysis) - Patients who discontinued the study at any time prior to week 96 due to a protocol defined endpoint, as well as those completing week 96, are included in the denominator, [b] 48 weeks double-blind tenofovir disoproxil fumarate followed by 48 weeks open-label, [c] 48 weeks double-blind adefovir dipivoxil followed by 48 weeks open-label tenofovir disoproxil fumarate, [d] The population used for analysis of ALT normalisation included only patients with ALT above ULN at baseline, N/A= not applicable.

Seventy-three percent of nucleoside-experienced and 69% of nucleoside-naïve patients achieved complete response to treatment; 90% of nucleoside-experienced and 88% of nucleoside-naïve patients achieved HBV DNA suppression < 400 copies/ml. All patients with normal ALT at baseline and 88% of patients with abnormal ALT at baseline achieved HBV DNA suppression < 400 copies/ml.

Experience beyond 48 weeks in studies GS-US-174-0102 and GS-US-174-0103: In studies GS-US-174-0102 and GS-US-174-0103, after receiving double-blind treatment for 48 weeks (either tenofovir disoproxil 245 mg (as fumarate) or adefovir dipivoxil 10 mg), patients rolled over with no interruption in treatment to open-label tenofovir disoproxil fumarate through week 96. In study GS-US-174-0102, 90% and 88% of patients and in study GS-US-174-0103, 82% and 92% of patients who were randomised to tenofovir disoproxil fumarate or adefovir dipivoxil, respectively, completed 96 weeks of treatment. At week 96, viral suppression, biochemical and serological responses were maintained with continued tenofovir disoproxil fumarate treatment (see Table 3 above).

Table 3: Efficacy parameters in compensated HBeAg positive and HBeAg negative patients at week 96 open-label treatment

(see Table 3 above)

In a randomised, 48-week double-blind, controlled study of tenofovir disoproxil 245 mg (as fumarate) in patients co-infected with HIV-1 and chronic hepatitis B with prior lamivudine experience (study ACTG 5127), the mean serum HBV DNA levels at baseline in patients randomised to the tenofovir arm were 9.45 $\log_{10}$ copies/ml (n = 27). Treatment with tenofovir disoproxil 245 mg (as fumarate) was associated with a mean change in serum HBV DNA from baseline, in the patients for whom there was 48-week data, of -5.74 $\log_{10}$ copies/ml (n = 18). In addition, 61% of patients had normal ALT at week 48.

Experience in patients with persistent viral replication: The efficacy and safety of tenofovir disoproxil 245 mg (as fumarate) or tenofovir disoproxil 245 mg (as fumarate) plus 200 mg emtricitabine has been evaluated in a randomised, double-blind study (study GS-US-174-0106), in HBeAg positive and HBeAg negative patients who had persistent viraemia (HBV DNA ⩾ 1,000 copies/ml) while receiving adefovir dipivoxil 10 mg for more than 24 weeks. At baseline, 57% of patients randomised to tenofovir disoproxil fumarate *versus* 60% of patients randomised to emtricitabine plus tenofovir disoproxil fumarate treatment group had previously been treated with lamivudine. Overall at week 24, treatment with tenofovir disoproxil fumarate resulted in 66% (35/53) of patients with HBV DNA < 400 copies/ml (< 69 IU/ml) *versus* 69% (36/52) of patients treated with emtricitabine plus tenofovir disoproxil fumarate ($p = 0.672$). In addition 55% (29/53) of patients treated with tenofovir disoproxil fumarate had undetectable HBV DNA (< 169 copies/ml [< 29 IU/ml]; the limit of quantification of the Roche Cobas TaqMan HBV assay) *versus* 60% (31/52) of patients treated with emtricitabine plus tenofovir disoproxil fumarate ($p = 0.504$). Comparisons between treatment groups beyond week 24 are difficult to interpret since investigators had the option to intensify treatment to open-label emtricitabine plus tenofovir disoproxil. Long-term studies to evaluate the benefit/risk of bitherapy with emtricitabine plus tenofovir disoproxil fumarate in HBV monoinfected patients are ongoing.

Clinical resistance: Four hundred and twenty-six HBeAg negative (GS-US-174-0102, n = 250) and HBeAg positive (GS-US-174-0103, n = 176) patients were evaluated for genotypic changes in HBV polymerase from baseline. Genotypic evaluations were performed on all patients with HBV DNA > 400 copies/ml at week 48 (n = 39) and week 96 (n = 24). No mutations associated with tenofovir disoproxil fumarate resistance have been identified.

Table 2: Efficacy parameters in compensated HBeAg positive and HBeAg negative patients at week 48

	Study 174-0102 (HBeAg negative)		Study 174-0103 (HBeAg positive)	
Parameter	Tenofovir disoproxil 245 mg (as fumarate) n = 250	Adefovir dipivoxil 10 mg n = 125	Tenofovir disoproxil 245 mg (as fumarate) n = 176	Adefovir dipivoxil 10 mg n = 90
Complete response (%)[a]	71*	49	67*	12
Histology				
Histological response (%)[b]	72	69	74	68
MedianHBV DNA reduction from baseline[c] ($\log_{10}$ copies/ml)	-4.7*	-4.0	-6.4*	-3.7
HBV DNA (%) < 400 copies/ml (< 69 IU/ml)	93*	63	76*	13
ALT (%) Normalised ALT[d]	76	77	68*	54
Serology (%) HBeAg loss/seroconversion	N/A	N/A	22/21	18/18
HBsAg loss/seroconversion	0/0	0/0	3*/1	0/0

* p-value *versus* adefovir dipivoxil < 0.05, [a] Complete response defined as HBV DNA levels < 400 copies/ml and Knodell necroinflammatory score improvement of at least 2 points without worsening in Knodell fibrosis, [b] Knodell necroinflammatory score improvement of at least 2 points without worsening in Knodell fibrosis, [c] Median change from baseline HBV DNA merely reflects the difference between baseline HBV DNA and the limit of detection (LOD) of the assay, [d] The population used for analysis of ALT normalisation included only patients with ALT above ULN at baseline. N/A= not applicable.

5.2 Pharmacokinetic properties

Tenofovir disoproxil fumarate is a water soluble ester prodrug which is rapidly converted *in vivo* to tenofovir and formaldehyde.

Tenofovir is converted intracellularly to tenofovir monophosphate and to the active component, tenofovir diphosphate.

Absorption

Following oral administration of tenofovir disoproxil fumarate to HIV infected patients, tenofovir disoproxil fumarate is rapidly absorbed and converted to tenofovir. Administration of multiple doses of tenofovir disoproxil fumarate with a meal to HIV infected patients resulted in mean (%CV) tenofovir C_{max}, $AUC_{0-\infty}$, and C_{min} values of 326 (36.6%) ng/ml, 3,324 (41.2%) ng·h/ml and 64.4 (39.4%) ng/ml, respectively. Maximum tenofovir concentrations are observed in serum within one hour of dosing in the fasted state and within two hours when taken with food. The oral bioavailability of tenofovir from tenofovir disoproxil fumarate in fasted patients was approximately 25%. Administration of tenofovir disoproxil fumarate with a high fat meal enhanced the oral bioavailability, with an increase in tenofovir AUC by approximately 40% and C_{max} by approximately 14%. Following the first dose of tenofovir disoproxil fumarate in fed patients, the median C_{max} in serum ranged from 213 to 375 ng/ml. However, administration of tenofovir disoproxil fumarate with a light meal did not have a significant effect on the pharmacokinetics of tenofovir.

Distribution

Following intravenous administration the steady-state volume of distribution of tenofovir was estimated to be approximately 800 ml/kg. After oral administration of tenofovir disoproxil fumarate, tenofovir is distributed to most tissues with the highest concentrations occurring in the kidney, liver and the intestinal contents (preclinical studies). *In vitro* protein binding of tenofovir to plasma or serum protein was less than 0.7 and 7.2%, respectively, over the tenofovir concentration range 0.01 to 25 μg/ml.

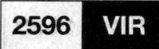

Biotransformation

In vitro studies have determined that neither tenofovir disoproxil fumarate nor tenofovir are substrates for the CYP450 enzymes. Moreover, at concentrations substantially higher (approximately 300-fold) than those observed *in vivo*, tenofovir did not inhibit *in vitro* drug metabolism mediated by any of the major human CYP450 isoforms involved in drug biotransformation (CYP3A4, CYP2D6, CYP2C9, CYP2E1, or CYP1A1/2). Tenofovir disoproxil fumarate at a concentration of 100 μmol/l had no effect on any of the CYP450 isoforms, except CYP1A1/2, where a small (6%) but statistically significant reduction in metabolism of CYP1A1/2 substrate was observed. Based on these data, it is unlikely that clinically significant interactions involving tenofovir disoproxil fumarate and medicinal products metabolised by CYP450 would occur.

Elimination

Tenofovir is primarily excreted by the kidney by both filtration and an active tubular transport system with approximately 70-80% of the dose excreted unchanged in urine following intravenous administration. Total clearance has been estimated to be approximately 230 ml/h/kg (approximately 300 ml/min). Renal clearance has been estimated to be approximately 160 ml/h/kg (approximately 210 ml/min), which is in excess of the glomerular filtration rate. This indicates that active tubular secretion is an important part of the elimination of tenofovir. Following oral administration the terminal half-life of tenofovir is approximately 12 to 18 hours.

Studies have established the pathway of active tubular secretion of tenofovir to be influx into proximal tubule cell by the human organic anion transporters (hOAT) 1 and 3 and efflux into the urine by the multidrug resistant protein 4 (MRP 4).

Linearity/non-linearity

The pharmacokinetics of tenofovir were independent of tenofovir disoproxil fumarate dose over the dose range 75 to 600 mg and were not affected by repeated dosing at any dose level.

Age and gender

Limited data on the pharmacokinetics of tenofovir in women indicate no major gender effect.

Pharmacokinetic studies have not been performed in children and adolescents (under 18) or in the elderly (over 65).

Pharmacokinetics have not been specifically studied in different ethnic groups.

Renal impairment

Pharmacokinetic parameters of tenofovir were determined following administration of a single dose of tenofovir disoproxil 245 mg to 40 non-HIV, non-HBV infected patients with varying degrees of renal impairment defined according to baseline creatinine clearance (CrCl) (normal renal function when CrCl > 80 ml/min; mild with CrCl = 50-79 ml/min; moderate with CrCl = 30-49 ml/min and severe with CrCl = 10-29 ml/min). Compared with patients with normal renal function, the mean (%CV) tenofovir exposure increased from 2,185 (12%) ng·h/ml in subjects with CrCl > 80 ml/min to respectively 3,064 (30%) ng·h/ml, 6,009 (42%) ng·h/ml and 15,985 (45%) ng·h/ml in patients with mild, moderate and severe renal impairment. The dosing recommendations in patients with renal impairment, with increased dosing interval, are expected to result in higher peak plasma concentrations and lower C_{min} levels in patients with renal impairment compared with patients with normal renal function. The clinical implications of this are unknown.

In patients with end-stage renal disease (ESRD) (CrCl < 10 ml/min) requiring haemodialysis, between dialysis tenofovir concentrations substantially increased over 48 hours achieving a mean C_{max} of 1,032 ng/ml and a mean AUC_{0-48h} of 42,857 ng·h/ml.

It is recommended that the dosing interval for tenofovir disoproxil 245 mg (as fumarate) is modified in patients with creatinine clearance < 50 ml/min or in patients who already have ESRD and require dialysis (see section 4.2).

The pharmacokinetics of tenofovir in non-haemodialysis patients with creatinine clearance < 10 ml/min and in patients with ESRD managed by peritoneal or other forms of dialysis have not been studied.

Hepatic impairment

A single 245 mg dose of tenofovir disoproxil was administered to non-HIV, non-HBV infected patients with varying degrees of hepatic impairment defined according to Child-Pugh-Turcotte (CPT) classification. Tenofovir pharmacokinetics were not substantially altered in subjects with hepatic impairment suggesting that no dose adjustment is required in these subjects. The mean (%CV) tenofovir C_{max} and $AUC_{0-\infty}$ values were 223 (34.8%) ng/ml and 2,050 (50.8%) ng·h/ml, respectively, in normal subjects compared with 289 (46.0%) ng/ml and 2,310 (43.5%) ng·h/ml in subjects with moderate hepatic impairment, and 305 (24.8%) ng/ml and 2,740 (44.0%) ng·h/ml in subjects with severe hepatic impairment.

Intracellular pharmacokinetics

In non-proliferating human peripheral blood mononuclear cells (PBMCs) the half-life of tenofovir diphosphate was found to be approximately 50 hours, whereas the half-life in phytohaemagglutinin-stimulated PBMCs was found to be approximately 10 hours.

5.3 Preclinical safety data

Preclinical studies conducted in rats, dogs and monkeys revealed target organ effects in gastrointestinal tract, kidney, bone and a decrease in serum phosphate concentration. Bone toxicity was diagnosed as osteomalacia (monkeys) and reduced bone mineral density (rats and dogs). Findings in the rat and monkey studies indicated that there was a substance-related decrease in intestinal absorption of phosphate with potential secondary reduction in bone mineral density. However, no conclusion could be drawn on the mechanism(s) underlying these toxicities.

Reproductive studies were conducted in rats and rabbits. There were no effects on mating or fertility parameters or on any pregnancy or foetal parameter. There were no gross foetal alterations of soft or skeletal tissues. Tenofovir disoproxil fumarate reduced the viability index and weight of pups in peri-post natal toxicity studies.

Genotoxicity studies have shown that tenofovir disoproxil fumarate was negative in the *in vivo* mouse bone marrow micronucleus assay but was positive for inducing forward mutations in the *in vitro* L5178Y mouse lymphoma cell assay in the presence or absence of S9 metabolic activation. Tenofovir disoproxil fumarate was positive in the Ames test (strain TA 1535) in two out of three studies, once in the presence of S9 mix (6.2- to 6.8-fold increase) and once without S9 mix. Tenofovir disoproxil fumarate was also weakly positive in an *in vivo / in vitro* unscheduled DNA synthesis test in primary rat hepatocytes.

Tenofovir disoproxil fumarate did not show any carcinogenic potential in a long-term oral carcinogenicity study in rats. A long-term oral carcinogenicity study in mice showed a low incidence of duodenal tumours, considered likely related to high local concentrations of tenofovir disoproxil fumarate in the gastrointestinal tract at a dose of 600 mg/kg/day. While the mechanism of tumour formation is uncertain, the findings are unlikely to be of relevance to humans.

6. PHARMACEUTICAL PARTICULARS

6.1 List of excipients

Core:

Microcrystalline cellulose (E460)

Pregelatinised starch (gluten free)

Croscarmellose sodium

Lactose monohydrate

Magnesium stearate (E572)

Coating:

Lactose monohydrate

Hypromellose (E464)

Titanium dioxide (E171)

Glycerol triacetate (E1518)

Indigo carmine aluminium lake (E132)

6.2 Incompatibilities

Not applicable.

6.3 Shelf life

4 years

6.4 Special precautions for storage

This medicinal product does not require any special storage conditions.

6.5 Nature and contents of container

Viread is supplied in high density polyethylene (HDPE) bottles with a child-resistant closure containing 30 film-coated tablets with a silica gel desiccant.

The following pack sizes are available: outer cartons containing 1 × 30 film-coated tablet and 3 × 30 film-coated tablet bottles. Not all pack sizes may be marketed.

6.6 Special precautions for disposal and other handling

Any unused product or waste material should be disposed of in accordance with local requirements.

7. MARKETING AUTHORISATION HOLDER

Gilead Sciences International Limited

Cambridge

CB21 6GT

United Kingdom

8. MARKETING AUTHORISATION NUMBER(S)

EU/1/01/200/001

EU/1/01/200/002

9. DATE OF FIRST AUTHORISATION/RENEWAL OF THE AUTHORISATION

Date of first authorisation: 5 February 2002

Date of last renewal: 7 February 2007

10. DATE OF REVISION OF THE TEXT

07/2009

Detailed information on this medicinal product is available on the website of the European Medicines Agency (EMEA) http://www.emea.europa.eu/.

Viridal 10 Duo

(UCB Pharma Limited)

1. NAME OF THE MEDICINAL PRODUCT

VIRIDAL 10 DUO

2. QUALITATIVE AND QUANTITATIVE COMPOSITION

1 double-chamber glass cartridge containing dry substance (47.8 mg) composed of alprostadil 10 micrograms (used as 1:1 clathrate complex with alfadex) and diluent (1 ml).

Diluent:

1 ml sterile sodium chloride solution 0.9% (w/v) PhEur.

3. PHARMACEUTICAL FORM

Double chamber glass cartridge containing lyophilised powder and diluent for reconstitution.

Administration devices

1 reusable injector (starter kit)

1 double-chamber cartridge with dry substance and 1 ml 0.9% sterile sodium chloride solution

1 injection needle 29 G × ½ (0.33 mm × 12.7 mm)

1 alcohol swab to be obtained for each injection.

Route of administration

For injection into the penile cavernous body.

4. CLINICAL PARTICULARS

4.1 Therapeutic indications

As an adjunct to the diagnostic evaluation of erectile dysfunction in adult males.

Treatment of erectile dysfunction in adult males.

4.2 Posology and method of administration

The drug solution should be prepared shortly before the injection.

Prior to injection the needle should be screwed onto the tip of the injector. After disinfecting the tip of the cartridge with one of the alcohol swabs, the cartridge should then be inserted into the injector. By screwing the thread part clockwise, the cartridge is fixed in the injector. Then, the dry substance, which is inside the front chamber of the cartridge, is reconstituted with 1 ml sterile sodium chloride solution 0.9% in the bottom chamber. While holding the device in a vertical position with the needle upwards, the thread part should be screwed slowly until it will not go any further. The solvent will by-pass the upper stopper into the front chamber and dissolve the dry substance within a few seconds. As soon as the dry substance is reconstituted, the larger external and the smaller inner protective cap have to be removed from the needle. The air should then be expelled out of the cartridge and the prescribed dose adjusted precisely.

Unused solution must be discarded immediately.

Viridal Duo is injected into either the right or the left cavernous body of the penile shaft. Once the needle is in the cavernous body, the injection should be done within 5 to 10 seconds and is very easy without much resistance if the needle is in the correct position.

The development of an erection will start approximately 5 – 15 minutes after the injection.

Dosage for injection in the clinic

Injections for diagnostic evaluation and dose titration must be performed by the attending physician. He will determine an individual dose suitable to produce an erectile response for diagnostic purposes.

The recommended starting dose is 2.5 mcg Viridal Duo in patients with primary psychogenic or neurogenic origin of erectile dysfunction. In all other patients with erectile dysfunction 5 mcg Viridal Duo should be used as a starting dose. Dose adjustments may be performed in increments of about 2.5 mcg to 5 mcg Viridal Duo. Most of the patients require between 10 and 20 mcg per injection. Some patients may need to be titrated to higher doses. Doses exceeding 20 mcg should be prescribed with particular care in patients with cardiovascular risk factors. The dose per injection should never exceed 40 mcg.

Dosage for self-injection therapy at home

Before starting treatment at home, each patient or the patient's partner has to be taught by a physician how to prepare the drug and perform the injection. In no cases should the injection therapy be started without precise instructions by the physician. The patient should only use his optimum individual dosage, which has been pre-determined by his physician using the above-mentioned procedure. This dose should allow the patient to have an erection at home, which should not last longer than one hour. If he experiences prolonged erections beyond 2 hours but less than 4 hours, the patient is recommended to contact his physician to re-establish the dose of the drug. Maximum injection frequency recommended is 2 or 3 times a week with an interval of at least 24 hours between the injections.

Follow-up

After the first injections and at regular intervals, e.g. every three months, the physician should re-evaluate the patient. Any local adverse reaction, e.g. haematoma, fibrosis or nodules should be noted and controlled. Following discussion with the patient, an adjustment of dosage may be necessary.

4.3 Contraindications
Hypersensitivity to alprostadil and/or alfadex (ingredients of Viridal Duo).

Patients with diseases causing priapism e.g. sickle-cell disease, leukaemia and multiple myeloma or patients with anatomical deformation of the penis as cavernosal fibrosis or Peyronie's disease. Patients with penis implants should not use Viridal Duo.

Viridal Duo should not be used in men for whom sexual activity is contraindicated.

4.4 Special warnings and precautions for use
The physician should carefully select patients suitable for self-injection therapy.

Sexual stimulation and intercourse can lead to cardiac and/or pulmonary events in patients with coronary heart disease, congestive heart failure or pulmonary disease. Viridal Duo should be used with care in these patient groups and patients should be examined and cleared for stress resistance by a cardiologist before treatment.

Viridal Duo should be used with care in patients who have experienced transient ischaemic attacks.

Patients who experience a prolonged erection lasting longer than four hours should contact their physician immediately. Therefore it is recommended that the patient has an emergency telephone number of his attending physician or of a clinic experienced in therapy of erectile dysfunction. Prolonged erection may damage penile erectile tissue and lead to irreversible erectile dysfunction.

A benefit-risk evaluation is neccesary before using Viridal Duo in patients with pre-existing scarring, e.g. nodules of the cavernous body or pre-existing penile deviation or Peyronie's disease or clinically relevant phimosis, e.g. phimosis with risk of paraphimosis these patients should be treated with particular care, e.g. more frequent re-evaluation of the patient's condition.

Patients who have to be treated with alpha-adrenergic drugs due to prolonged erections (see: overdose) may in the case of concomitant therapy with monoamino-oxidase-inhibitors, develop a hypertensive crisis.

Other intracavernous drugs e.g. smooth muscle relaxing agents or alpha-adrenergic blocking agents may lead to prolonged erection and must not be used concomitantly. The effects of a combination therapy of alprostadil with oral, intraurethral or topical medicinal products for erectile dysfunction are currently unknown.

Patients with blood clotting disorders or patients on therapy influencing blood clotting parameters should be treated with special care, e.g. monitoring of the clotting parameters and advice to the patient to exercise sufficient manual pressure on the injection site. This is because of the increased risk of bleeding.

To prevent abuse, self-injection therapy with Viridal Duo should not be used by patients with drug addiction and/or disturbances of psychological or intellectual development.

In cases of excessive use, e.g. higher frequencies than recommended, an increased risk of penile scarring cannot be excluded.

Use of intracavernous alprostadil offers no protection from the transmission of sexually transmitted diseases. Individuals who use alprostadil should be counselled about the protective measures that are necessary to guard against the spread of sexually transmitted diseases, including the human immunodeficiency virus (HIV). In some patients, injection of Viridal Duo can induce a small amount of bleeding at the injection site. In patients infected with blood borne diseases, this could increase the transmission of such diseases to the partner. For this reason we recommend that a condom is used for intercourse after injecting Viridal Duo.

Viridal Duo is for intracavernous injection. Subcutaneous injection or injections at areas of the penis other than the cavernous body should be avoided.

The injection should be performed under hygienic conditions to avoid infections. In any condition that precludes safe self-injection like poor manual dexterity, poor visual acuity or morbid obesity, the partner should be trained in the injection technique and should perform the injection.

Up to now, there is no clinical experience in patients under 18 and over 75 years of age.

Viridal Duo does not interfere with ejaculation and fertility.

4.5 Interaction with other medicinal products and other forms of interaction
Concomitant use of smooth muscle relaxing drugs like papaverine or other drugs inducing erection like alpha-adrenergic blocking agents may lead to prolonged erection and should not be used in parallel with Viridal Duo.

Risks exist when using alpha-adrenergic drugs to terminate prolonged erections in patients with cardiovascular disorders or receiving MAO inhibitors.

The effects of blood pressure lowering and vasodilating drugs may be increased.

4.6 Pregnancy and lactation
Not applicable.

Alprostadil did not cause any adverse effects on fertility or general reproductive performance in male and female rats treated with 40-200 mcg/kg/day. The high dose of 200 mcg/kg/day is about 300 times the maximum recommended human dose on a body weight basis (MHRD < 1 mcg/kg).

Alprostadil was not fetotoxic or teratogenic at doses up to 5000 mcg/kg/day (7500 times the MHRD) in rats, 200 mcg/kg/day (300 times the MHRD) in rabbits and doses up to 20 mcg/kg/day (30 times the MHRD) in guinea pigs or monkeys.

4.7 Effects on ability to drive and use machines
Viridal Duo may rarely induce hypotension with subsequent impairment of reactivity.

4.8 Undesirable effects
A burning sensation during injection is common (< 10 %) and generally subsides shortly afterwards. A sensation of tension in the penis and pain at the site of injection are common (< 10 %) and mostly of mild intensity. Spotlike haemorrhage/ spotlike bruises at the site of puncture occur uncommonly (< 1 %). Haemosiderin deposits, reddening and swellings at the site of injection are also uncommon (< 1 %). Other uncommon (< 1 %) reactions are swellings of the preputium or the glans, and headache.

Prolonged erections of more than 4 hours duration are uncommon (< 1 %) and are mainly seen during dose titration.

During long-term treatment, fibrotic alterations (e.g. fibrotic nodules, plaques at the site of injection or in the corpus cavernosum) may occur commonly (< 10 %) in follow up periods of up to 4 years. This may be associated with slight penile axis deviations in uncommon (< 1 %) cases. In rare cases (< 0.1%), fibrotic changes of the cavernous body may occur during treatment lasting up to 4 years.

Rare cases (< 0.1%) of circulatory effects such as short periods of hypotension and/or vertigo or dizziness have been observed after the intracavernous injection of Viridal Duo.

In rare cases (< 0.1%) allergic reactions ranging from cutaneous hypersensitivity such as rash, erythema, urticaria to anaphylactic/anaphylactoid reactions may occur.

4.9 Overdose
Symptoms

Full rigid erections lasting more than four hours.

If the patient experiences a prolonged erection, he is advised to contact his attending physician or a urologic clinic nearby immediately.

Treatment strategy
Treatment of prolonged erection should be done by a physician experienced in the field of erectile dysfunction. If prolonged erection occurs, the following is recommended:

If the erection has lasted less than six hours:

– observation of the erection because spontaneous flaccidity frequently occurs.

If the erection has lasted longer than six hours:

– cavernous body injection of alpha-adrenergic substances (e.g. phenylephrine or epinephrine (adrenaline)). Risks exist when using drugs in patients with cardiovascular disorders or receiving MAO inhibitors. All patients should be monitored for cardiovascular effects when these drugs are used to terminate prolonged erections.

or

– aspiration of blood from the cavernous body.

Accidental systemic injection of high doses
Single dose rising tolerance studies in healthy volunteers indicated that single intravenous doses of alprostadil from 1 to 120 mcg were well tolerated. Starting with a 40 mcg bolus intravenous dose, the frequency of drug-related adverse events increased in a dose-dependent manner, characterised mainly by facial flushing.

5. PHARMACOLOGICAL PROPERTIES

5.1 Pharmacodynamic properties
ATC Code: Other urologicals G04BX 05

Alprostadil [Prostaglandin E_1 (PGE_1)], the active ingredient of Viridal Duo, is an endogenous compound derived from the essential fatty acid dihomogammalinolenic acid. Alprostadil is a potent smooth muscle relaxant that produces vasodilation and occurs in high concentrations in the human seminal fluid. Pre-contracted isolated preparations of the human corpus cavernosum, corpus spongiosum and cavernous artery were relaxed by alprostadil, while other prostanoids were less effective. Alprostadil has been shown to bind to specific receptors in the cavernous tissue of human and non-human primates.

The binding of alprostadil to its receptors is accompanied by an increase in intracellular cAMP levels. Human cavernosal smooth muscle cells respond to alprostadil by releasing intracellular calcium. Since relaxation of smooth muscle is associated with a reduction of the cytoplasmic free calcium concentration, this effect may contribute to the relaxing activity of this prostanoid.

Intracavernous injection of alprostadil in healthy monkeys resulted in penile elongation and tumescence without rigidity. The cavernous arterial blood flow was increased for a mean duration of 20 min. In contrast, intracavernous application of alprostadil to rabbits and dogs caused no erectile response.

Systemic intravascular administration of alprostadil leads to a vasodilation and reduction of systemic peripheral vascular resistance. A decrease in blood pressure can be observed after administration of high doses. Alprostadil has also been shown in animal and *in vitro* tests to reduce platelet reactivity and neutrophil activation. Additional alprostadil activity has been reported: increase in fibrinolytic activity of fibroblasts, improvement of erythrocyte deformability and inhibition of erythrocyte aggregation; inhibition of the proliferative and mitotic activity of non-striated myocytes; inhibition of cholesterol synthesis and LDL-receptor activity; and an increase in the supply of oxygen and glucose to ischaemic tissue along with improved tissue utilisation of these substrates.

5.2 Pharmacokinetic properties
After reconstitution, alprostadil (PGE_1) dissociates from the α-cyclodextrin clathrate, and the two components have independent fates.

In symptomatic volunteers, systemic mean endogenous PGE_1 venous plasma concentrations measured before intracavernous injection are approximately 1pg/ml. After injection of 20 mcg of alprostadil, the PGE_1 venous plasma concentrations increase rapidly to concentrations of about 10-20 pg/ml. The PGE_1 plasma concentrations return to concentrations close to the baseline within a few minutes. Approximately 90% of PGE_1 found in plasma is protein-bound.

Metabolism
Enzymatic oxidation of the C15-hydroxy group and reduction of the C13,14 double bond produce the primary metabolites, 15-keto-PGE_1, PGE_o (13,14-dihydro-PGE_1) and 15-keto-PGE_o. Only PGE_o and 15-keto-PGE_o have been detected in human plasma. Unlike the 15-keto metabolites, which are less pharmacologically active than the parent compound, PGE_o has a potency similar to that of PGE_1 in most respects.

In symptomatic volunteers, the mean endogenous PGE_o venous plasma concentrations measured before an intracavernous injection are approximately 1 pg/ml. After the injection of 20 mcg of alprostadil, the PGE_o plasma concentrations increase to concentrations of about 5 pg/ml.

Excretion
After further degradation of the primary metabolites by beta and omega oxidation, the resulting, more polar metabolites are excreted primarily with the urine (88%) and the faeces (12%) and there is no evidence of tissue retention of PGE_1 or its metabolites.

5.3 Preclinical safety data
Studies on local tolerance following single and repeated intracavernous injections of alprostadil or alprostadil alfadex in rabbits and/or monkeys, in monkeys up to 6 months with daily injection revealed in general good local tolerance. Possible adverse effects like haematomas and inflammations are more likely related to the injection procedure.

Within the 6 months study in male monkeys, there were no adverse effects of alprostadil alfadex on male reproductive organs.

Mutagenicity studies with alprostadil alfadex revealed no risk of mutagenicity.

6. PHARMACEUTICAL PARTICULARS

6.1 List of excipients
Powder for injection:

Lactose monohydrates

Alfadex

Diluent:

Sodium chloride

Water for injection.

6.2 Incompatibilities
No incompatibilities have so far been demonstrated.

6.3 Shelf life
Shelf life for the product as packaged for sale: 4 years.

Shelf life after reconstitution: for immediate use only.

6.4 Special precautions for storage
Do not store above 25°C. Store in the original packaging.

6.5 Nature and contents of container
1. Cartons containing one colourless glass double-chamber cartridge, one injection needle 29 G × ½ (0.33 mm × 12.7 mm) and one reusable injector (starter kit).

2. Cartons containing two colourless glass double-chamber cartridges, two injection needles 29 G × ½ (0.33 mm × 12.7 mm) and one reusable injector (starter kit).

3. Cartons containing one, two or six colourless glass double-chamber cartridges and corresponding number of injection needles 29 G × ½ (0.33 mm × 12.7 mm) without reusable injector.

6.6 Special precautions for disposal and other handling
Fix the injection needle onto the front part of the injector.

Disinfect the tip of the cartridge with one of the alcohol swabs. Insert the cartridge into the re-usable injector and fix it by screwing the thread part. Dissolve the drug substance in the front chamber of the cartridge by completely screwing the thread-part into the injector thus moving both rubber stoppers to the top of the cartridge and allowing the solvent in to the bottom chamber to reach the dry substance via the bypass of the cartridge. Shake slightly until a clear solution is produced.

Expel the air and adjust the prescribed dosage precisely prior to intracavernous injection.

After preparation of the solution, the injection must be performed using aseptic procedures into either the left or right cavernous body of the penile shaft. Care should be taken not to inject into penile vessels or nerves on the upper side of the penis and into the urethra on the under side. The injection should be completed within 5 to 10 seconds and manual pressure should be applied to the injection site for 2 to 3 minutes.

Unused solution must be discarded immediately.

Advice

The content of the front chamber of the cartridge consists of a white, dry powder, which forms a compact layer, approximately 8 mm in height. The layer may show cracks and crumble slightly.

In case of damage to the cartridge, the usually dry content of the front chamber becomes moist and sticky and extensively loses volume. Viridal Duo must not be used in this case.

The bottom chamber contains the clear, colourless sodium chloride solvent solution.

The dry substance dissolves immediately after addition of the sodium chloride solution. Initially after reconstitution the solution may appear slightly opaque due to the presence of bubbles. This is of no relevance and disappears within a short time to give a clear solution.

7. MARKETING AUTHORISATION HOLDER

SCHWARZ PHARMA Limited

5 Hercules Way

Leavesden Park

Watford

WD25 7GS

United Kingdom

8. MARKETING AUTHORISATION NUMBER(S)

PL 04438/0049

9. DATE OF FIRST AUTHORISATION/RENEWAL OF THE AUTHORISATION

23 May 1997

10. DATE OF REVISION OF THE TEXT

July 2006

Viridal 20 Duo

(UCB Pharma Limited)

1. NAME OF THE MEDICINAL PRODUCT

VIRIDAL 20 DUO

2. QUALITATIVE AND QUANTITATIVE COMPOSITION

1 double-chamber glass cartridge containing dry substance (48.2 mg) composed of alprostadil 20 micrograms (used as 1:1 clathrate complex with alfadex) and diluent (1 ml).

Diluent:

1 ml sterile sodium chloride solution 0.9% (w/v) Ph Eur.

3. PHARMACEUTICAL FORM

Double chamber glass cartridge containing lyophilised powder and diluent for reconstitution.

Administration devices

1 reusable injector (starter kit)

1 double-chamber cartridge with dry substance and 1 ml 0.9% sterile sodium chloride solution

1 injection needle 29 G × ½ (0.33 mm × 12.7 mm)

1 alcohol swab to be obtained for each injection

Route of administration

For injection into the penile cavernous body.

4. CLINICAL PARTICULARS

4.1 Therapeutic indications

As an adjunct to the diagnostic evaluation of erectile dysfunction in adult males.

Treatment of erectile dysfunction in adult males.

4.2 Posology and method of administration

The drug solution should be prepared shortly before the injection.

Prior to injection the needle should be screwed onto the tip of the injector. After disinfecting the tip of the cartridge with one of the alcohol swabs, the cartridge should then be inserted into the injector. By screwing the thread part clockwise, the cartridge is fixed in the injector. Then, the dry substance, which is inside the front chamber of the cartridge, is reconstituted with 1 ml sterile sodium chloride solution 0.9% in the bottom chamber. While holding the device in a vertical position with the needle upwards, the thread part should be screwed slowly until it will not go any further. The solvent will by-pass the upper stopper into the front chamber and dissolve the dry substance within a few seconds. As soon as the dry substance is reconstituted, the larger external and the smaller inner protective cap have to be removed from the needle. The air should then be expelled out of the cartridge and the prescribed dose adjusted precisely.

Unused solution must be discarded immediately.

Viridal Duo is injected into either the right or the left cavernous body of the penile shaft. Once the needle is in the cavernous body, the injection should be done within 5 to 10 seconds and is very easy without much resistance if the needle is in the correct position.

The development of an erection will start approximately 5 – 15 minutes after the injection.

Dosage for injection in the clinic

Injections for diagnostic evaluation and dose titration must be performed by the attending physician. He will determine an individual dose suitable to produce an erectile response for diagnostic purposes.

The recommended starting dose is 2.5 mcg Viridal Duo in patients with primary psychogenic or neurogenic origin of erectile dysfunction. In all other patients with erectile dysfunction 5 mcg Viridal Duo should be used as a starting dose. Dose adjustments may be performed in increments of about 2.5 mcg to 5 mcg Viridal Duo. Most of the patients require between 10 and 20 mcg per injection. Some patients may need to be titrated to higher doses. Doses exceeding 20 mcg should be prescribed with particular care in patients with cardiovascular risk factors. The dose per injection should never exceed 40 mcg.

Dosage for self-injection therapy at home

Before starting treatment at home, each patient or the patient's partner has to be taught by a physician how to prepare the drug and perform the injection. In no cases should the injection therapy be started without precise instructions by the physician. The patient should only use his optimum individual dosage which has been pre-determined by his physician using the above-mentioned procedure. This dose should allow the patient to have an erection at home which should not last longer than one hour. If he experiences prolonged erections beyond 2 hours but less than 4 hours, the patient is recommended to contact his physician to re-establish the dose of the drug. Maximum injection frequency recommended is 2 or 3 times a week with an interval of at least 24 hours between the injections.

Follow-up

After the first injections and at regular intervals, e.g. every three months, the physician should re-evaluate the patient. Any local adverse reaction, e.g. haematoma, fibrosis or nodules should be noted and controlled. Following discussion with the patient, an adjustment of dosage may be necessary.

4.3 Contraindications

Hypersensitivity to alprostadil and/or alfadex (ingredients of Viridal Duo).

Patients with diseases causing priapism e.g. sickle-cell disease, leukaemia and multiple myeloma or patients with anatomical deformation of the penis as cavernosal fibrosis or Peyronie's disease. Patients with penis implants should not use Viridal Duo.

Viridal Duo should not be used in men for whom sexual activity is contraindicated.

4.4 Special warnings and precautions for use

The physician should carefully select patients suitable for self-injection therapy.

Sexual stimulation and intercourse can lead to cardiac and/or pulmonary events in patients with coronary heart disease, congestive heart failure or pulmonary disease. Viridal Duo should be used with care in these patient groups and patients should be examined and cleared for stress resistance by a cardiologist before treatment.

Viridal Duo should be used with care in patients who have experienced transient ischaemic attacks.

Patients who experience a prolonged erection lasting longer than four hours should contact their physician immediately. Therefore it is recommended that the patient has an emergency telephone number of his attending physician or of a clinic experienced in therapy of erectile dysfunction. Prolonged erection may damage penile erectile tissue and lead to irreversible erectile dysfunction.

A benefit-risk evaulation is neccesary before using Viridal Duo in patients with pre-existing scarring, e.g. nodules of the cavernous body or pre-existing penile deviation or Peyronie's disease or clinically relevant phimosis, e.g. phimosis with risk of paraphimosis these patients should be treated with particular care, e.g. more frequent re-evaluation of the patient's condition.

Patients who have to be treated with alpha-adrenergic drugs due to prolonged erections (see: overdose) may in the case of concomitant therapy with monoamino-oxidase-inhibitors, develop a hypertensive crisis.

Other intracavernous drugs e.g. smooth muscle relaxing agents or alpha-adrenergic blocking agents may lead to prolonged erection and must not be used concomitantly.

The effects of a combination therapy of alprostadil with oral, intraurethral or topical medicinal products for erectile dysfunction are currently unknown.

Patients with blood clotting disorders or patients on therapy influencing blood clotting parameters should be treated with special care, e.g. monitoring of the clotting parameters and advice to the patient to exercise sufficient manual pressure on the injection site. This is because of the increased risk of bleeding.

To prevent abuse, self-injection therapy with Viridal Duo should not be used by patients with drug addiction and/or disturbances of psychological or intellectual development.

In cases of excessive use, e.g. higher frequencies than recommended, an increased risk of penile scarring cannot be excluded.

Use of intracavernous alprostadil offers no protection from the transmission of sexually transmitted diseases. Individuals who use alprostadil should be counselled about the protective measures that are necessary to guard against the spread of sexually transmitted diseases, including the human immunodeficiency virus (HIV). In some patients, injection of Viridal Duo can induce a small amount of bleeding at the injection site. In patients infected with blood borne diseases, this could increase the transmission of such diseases to the partner. For this reason we recommend that a condom is used for intercourse after injecting Viridal Duo.

Viridal Duo is for intracavernous injection. Subcutaneous injection or injections at areas of the penis other than the cavernous body should be avoided.

The injection should be performed under hygienic conditions to avoid infections. In any condition that precludes safe self-injection like poor manual dexterity, poor visual acuity or morbid obesity, the partner should be trained in the injection technique and should perform the injection.

Up to now, there is no clinical experience in patients under 18 and over 75 years of age.

Viridal Duo does not interfere with ejaculation and fertility.

4.5 Interaction with other medicinal products and other forms of interaction

Concomitant use of smooth muscle relaxing drugs like papaverine or other drugs inducing erection like alpha-adrenergic blocking agents may lead to prolonged erection and should not be used in parallel with Viridal Duo.

Risks exist when using alpha-adrenergic drugs to terminate prolonged erections in patients with cardiovascular disorders or receiving MAO inhibitors.

The effects of blood pressure lowering and vasodilating drugs may be increased.

4.6 Pregnancy and lactation

Not applicable.

Alprostadil did not cause any adverse effects on fertility or general reproductive performance in male and female rats treated with 40-200 mcg/kg/day. The high dose of 200 mcg/kg/day is about 300 times the maximum recommended human dose on a body weight basis (MHRD < 1 mcg/kg).

Alprostadil was not fetotoxic or teratogenic at doses up to 5000 mcg/kg/day (7500 times the MHRD) in rats, 200 mcg/kg/day (300 times the MHRD) in rabbits and doses up to 20 mcg/kg/day (30 times the MHRD) in guinea pigs or monkeys.

4.7 Effects on ability to drive and use machines

Viridal Duo may rarely induce hypotension with subsequent impairment of reactivity.

4.8 Undesirable effects

A burning sensation during injection is common (< 10 %) and generally subsides shortly afterwards. A sensation of tension in the penis and pain at the site of injection are common (< 10 %) and mostly of mild intensity. Spotlike haemorrhage/ spotlike bruises at the site of puncture occur uncommonly (< 1 %). Haemosiderin deposits, reddening and swellings at the site of injection are also uncommon (< 1 %). Other uncommon (< 1 %) reactions are swellings of the preputium or the glans, and headache.

Prolonged erections of more than 4 hours duration are uncommon (< 1 %) and are mainly seen during dose titration.

During long-term treatment, fibrotic alterations (e.g. fibrotic nodules, plaques at the site of injection or in the corpus cavernosum) may occur commonly (< 10 %) in follow up periods of up to 4 years. This may be associated with slight penile axis deviations in uncommon (< 1 %) cases. In rare cases (< 0.1%), fibrotic changes of the cavernous body may occur during treatment lasting up to 4 years.

Rare cases (< 0.1%) of circulatory effects such as short periods of hypotension and/or vertigo or dizziness have been observed after the intracavernous injection of Viridal Duo.

In rare cases (< 0.1%) allergic reactions ranging from cutaneous hypersensitivity such as rash, erythema, urticaria to anaphylactic/anaphylactoid reactions may occur.

4.9 Overdose

Symptoms

Full rigid erections lasting more than four hours.

If the patient experiences a prolonged erection, he is advised to contact his attending physician or a urologic clinic nearby immediately.

Treatment strategy

Treatment of prolonged erection should be done by a physician experienced in the field of erectile dysfunction.

If prolonged erection occurs, the following is recommended:

If the erection has lasted less than six hours:

– observation of the erection because spontaneous flaccidity frequently occurs.

If the erection has lasted longer than six hours:

– cavernous body injection of alpha-adrenergic substances (e.g. phenylephrine or epinephrine (adrenaline)). Risks exist when using drugs in patients with cardiovascular disorders or receiving MAO inhibitors. All patients should be monitored for cardiovascular effects when these drugs are used to terminate prolonged erections.

or

– aspiration of blood from the cavernous body.

Accidental systemic injection of high doses

Single dose rising tolerance studies in healthy volunteers indicated that single intravenous doses of alprostadil from 1 to 120 mcg were well tolerated. Starting with a 40 mcg bolus intravenous dose, the frequency of drug-related adverse events increased in a dose-dependent manner, characterised mainly by facial flushing.

5. PHARMACOLOGICAL PROPERTIES

5.1 Pharmacodynamic properties

ATC Code: Other urologicals G04BX 05

Alprostadil [Prostaglandin E_1 (PGE_1)], the active ingredient of Viridal Duo, is an endogenous compound derived from the essential fatty acid dihomogammalinolenic acid. Alprostadil is a potent smooth muscle relaxant that produces vasodilation and occurs in high concentrations in the human seminal fluid. Pre-contracted isolated preparations of the human corpus cavernosum, corpus spongiosum and cavernous artery were relaxed by alprostadil, while other prostanoids were less effective.

Alprostadil has been shown to bind to specific receptors in the cavernous tissue of human and non-human primates.

The binding of alprostadil to its receptors is accompanied by an increase in intracellular cAMP levels. Human cavernosal smooth muscle cells respond to alprostadil by releasing intracellular calcium. Since relaxation of smooth muscle is associated with a reduction of the cytoplasmic free calcium concentration, this effect may contribute to the relaxing activity of this prostanoid.

Intracavernous injection of alprostadil in healthy monkeys resulted in penile elongation and tumescence without rigidity. The cavernous arterial blood flow was increased for a mean duration of 20 min. In contrast, intracavernous application of alprostadil to rabbits and dogs caused no erectile response.

Systemic intravascular administration of alprostadil leads to a vasodilation and reduction of systemic peripheral vascular resistance. A decrease in blood pressure can be observed after administration of high doses. Alprostadil has also been shown in animal and *in vitro* tests to reduce platelet reactivity and neutrophil activation. Additional alprostadil activity has been reported: increase in fibrinolytic activity of fibroblasts, improvement of erythrocyte deformability and inhibition of erythrocyte aggregation; inhibition of the proliferative and mitotic activity of non-striated myocytes; inhibition of cholesterol synthesis and LDL-receptor activity; and an increase in the supply of oxygen and glucose to ischaemic tissue along with improved tissue utilisation of these substrates.

5.2 Pharmacokinetic properties

After reconstitution, alprostadil (PGE_1) dissociates from the α-cyclodextrin clathrate, and the two components have independent fates.

In symptomatic volunteers, systemic mean endogenous PGE_1 venous plasma concentrations measured before intracavernous injection are approximately 1pg/ml. After injection of 20 mcg of alprostadil, the PGE_1 venous plasma concentrations increase rapidly to concentrations of about 10-20 pg/ml. The PGE_1 plasma concentrations return to concentrations close to the baseline within a few minutes. Approximately 90% of PGE_1 found in plasma is protein-bound.

Metabolism

Enzymatic oxidation of the C15-hydroxy group and reduction of the C13,14 double bond produce the primary metabolites, 15-keto- PGE_1, PGE (13,14-dihydro-PGE_1) and 15-keto-PGE_0. Only PGE_0 and 15-keto-PGE_0 have been detected in human plasma. Unlike the 15-keto metabolites, which are less pharmacologically active than the parent compound, PGE_0 has a potency similar to that of PGE_1 in most respects.

In symptomatic volunteers, the mean endogenous PGE_0 venous plasma concentrations measured before an intracavernous injection are approximately 1 pg/ml. After the injection of 20 mcg of alprostadil, the PGE_0 plasma concentrations increase to concentrations of about 5 pg/ml.

Excretion

After further degradation of the primary metabolites by beta and omega oxidation, the resulting, more polar metabolites are excreted primarily with the urine (88%) and the faeces (12%) and there is no evidence of tissue retention of PGE_1 or its metabolites.

5.3 Preclinical safety data

Studies on local tolerance following single and repeated intracavernous injections of alprostadil or alprostadil alfadex in rabbits and/or monkeys, in monkeys up to 6 months with daily injection revealed in general good local tolerance. Possible adverse effects like haematomas and inflammations are more likely related to the injection procedure.

Within the 6 months study in male monkeys, there were no adverse effects of alprostadil alfadex on male reproductive organs.

Mutagenicity studies with alprostadil alfadex revealed no risk of mutagenicity.

6. PHARMACEUTICAL PARTICULARS

6.1 List of excipients

Powder for injection:

Lactose monohydrate

Alfadex

Diluent:

Sodium chloride

Water for injection.

6.2 Incompatibilities

No incompatibilities have so far been demonstrated.

6.3 Shelf life

Shelf life for the product as packaged for sale: 4 years.

Shelf life after reconstitution: for immediate use only.

6.4 Special precautions for storage

Do not store above 25°C. Store in the original packaging.

6.5 Nature and contents of container

1. Cartons containing one colourless glass double-chamber cartridge, one injection needle 29 G × ½ (0.33 mm × 12.7 mm) and one reusable injector (starter kit).

2. Cartons containing two colourless glass double-chamber cartridges, two injection needles 29 G × ½ (0.33 mm × 12.7 mm) and one reusable injector (starter kit).

3. Cartons containing one, two or six colourless glass double-chamber cartridges and corresponding number of injection needles 29 G × ½ (0.33 mm × 12.7 mm) without reusable injector.

6.6 Special precautions for disposal and other handling

Fix the injection needle onto the front part of the injector.

Disinfect the tip of the cartridge with one of the alcohol swabs. Insert the cartridge into the reusable injector and fix it by screwing the thread part. Dissolve the drug substance in the front chamber of the cartridge by completely screwing the thread-part into the injector thus moving both rubber stoppers to the top of the cartridge and allowing the solvent in to the bottom chamber to reach the dry substance via the bypass of the cartridge. Shake slightly until a clear solution is produced.

Expel the air and adjust the prescribed dosage precisely prior to intracavernous injection.

After preparation of the solution, the injection must be performed using aseptic procedures into either the left or right cavernous body of the penile shaft. Care should be taken not to inject into penile vessels or nerves on the upper side of the penis and into the urethra on the under side. The injection should be completed within 5 to 10 seconds and manual pressure should be applied to the injection site for 2 to 3 minutes.

Unused solution must be discarded immediately.

Advice

The content of the front chamber of the cartridge consists of a white, dry powder, which forms a compact layer, approximately 8 mm in height. The layer may show cracks and crumble slightly.

In case of damage to the cartridge, the usually dry content of the front chamber becomes moist and sticky and extensively loses volume. Viridal Duo must not be used in this case.

The bottom chamber contains the clear, colourless sodium chloride solvent solution.

The dry substance dissolves immediately after addition of the sodium chloride solution. Initially after reconstitution the solution may appear slightly opaque due to the presence of bubbles. This is of no relevance and disappears within a short time to give a clear solution.

7. MARKETING AUTHORISATION HOLDER

SCHWARZ PHARMA Limited

5 Hercules Way

Leavesden Park

Watford

WD25 7GS

United Kingdom

8. MARKETING AUTHORISATION NUMBER(S)

PL 04438/0050

9. DATE OF FIRST AUTHORISATION/RENEWAL OF THE AUTHORISATION

23 May 1997

10. DATE OF REVISION OF THE TEXT

July 2006

Viridal 40 Duo

(UCB Pharma Limited)

1. NAME OF THE MEDICINAL PRODUCT

VIRIDAL 40 DUO

2. QUALITATIVE AND QUANTITATIVE COMPOSITION

1 double-chamber glass cartridge containing dry substance (48.8 mg) composed of alprostadil 40 micrograms (used as 1:1 clathrate complex with alfadex) and diluent (1 ml).

Diluent:

1 ml sterile sodium chloride solution 0.9% (w/v) Ph Eur

3. PHARMACEUTICAL FORM

Double chamber glass cartridge containing lyophilised powder and diluent for reconstitution.

Administration devices

1 reusable injector (starter kit)

1 double-chamber cartridge with dry substance and 1 ml 0.9% sterile sodium chloride solution

1 injection needle 29 G × ½ (0.33 mm × 12.7 mm)

1 alcohol swab to be obtained for each injection

Route of administration

For injection into the penile cavernous body.

4. CLINICAL PARTICULARS

4.1 Therapeutic indications

As an adjunct to the diagnostic evaluation of erectile dysfunction in adult males.

Treatment of erectile dysfunction in adult males.

4.2 Posology and method of administration

The drug solution should be prepared shortly before the injection.

Prior to injection the needle should be screwed onto the tip of the injector. After disinfecting the tip of the cartridge with one of the alcohol swabs, the cartridge should then be inserted into the injector. By screwing the thread part clockwise, the cartridge is fixed in the injector. Then, the dry substance, which is inside the front chamber of the cartridge, is reconstituted with 1 ml sterile sodium chloride solution 0.9% in the bottom chamber. While holding the device in a vertical position with the needle upwards, the thread part should be screwed slowly until it will not go any further. The solvent will by-pass the upper stopper into the front chamber and dissolve the dry substance within a few seconds. As soon as the dry substance is reconstituted, the larger external and the smaller inner protective cap have to be removed from the needle. The air should then be expelled out of the cartridge and the prescribed dose adjusted precisely.

Unused solution must be discarded immediately.

Viridal Duo is injected into either the right or the left cavernous body of the penile shaft. Once the needle is in the cavernous body, the injection should be done within 5 to 10 seconds and is very easy without much resistance if the needle is in the correct position.

The development of an erection will start approximately 5 – 15 minutes after the injection.

Dosage for injection in the clinic

Injections for diagnostic evaluation and dose titration must be performed by the attending physician. He will determine an individual dose suitable to produce an erectile response for diagnostic purposes.

The recommended starting dose is 2.5 mcg Viridal Duo in patients with primary psychogenic or neurogenic origin of erectile dysfunction. In all other patients with erectile dysfunction 5 mcg Viridal Duo should be used as a starting dose. Dose adjustments may be performed in increments of about 2.5 mcg to 5 mcg Viridal Duo. Most of the patients require between 10 and 20 mcg per injection. Some patients may need to be titrated to higher doses. Doses exceeding 20 mcg should be prescribed with particular care in patients with cardiovascular risk factors. The dose per injection should never exceed 40 mcg.

Dosage for self-injection therapy at home

Before starting treatment at home, each patient or the patient's partner has to be taught by a physician how to prepare the drug and perform the injection. In no cases should the injection therapy be started without precise instructions by the physician. The patient should only use his optimum individual dosage which has been pre-determined by his physician using the above-mentioned procedure. This dose should allow the patient to have an erection at home which should not last longer than one hour. If he experiences prolonged erections beyond 2 hours but less than 4 hours, the patient is recommended to contact his physician to re-establish the dose of the drug. Maximum injection frequency recommended is 2 or 3 times a week with an interval of at least 24 hours between the injections.

Follow-up

After the first injections and at regular intervals, e.g. every three months, the physician should re-evaluate the patient. Any local adverse reaction, e.g. haematoma, fibrosis or nodules should be noted and controlled. Following discussion with the patient, an adjustment of dosage may be necessary.

4.3 Contraindications

Hypersensitivity to alprostadil and/or alfadex (ingredients of Viridal Duo).

Patients with diseases causing priapism e.g. sickle-cell disease, leukaemia and multiple myeloma or patients with anatomical deformation of the penis as cavernosal fibrosis or Peyronie's disease. Patients with penis implants should not use Viridal Duo.

Viridal Duo should not be used in men for whom sexual activity is contraindicated.

4.4 Special warnings and precautions for use

The physician should carefully select patients suitable for self-injection therapy.

Sexual stimulation and intercourse can lead to cardiac and/or pulmonary events in patients with coronary heart disease, congestive heart failure or pulmonary disease.

Viridal Duo should be used with care in these patient groups and patients should be examined and cleared for stress resistance by a cardiologist before treatment.

Viridal Duo should be used with care in patients who have experienced transient ischaemic attacks.

Patients who experience a prolonged erection lasting longer than four hours should contact their physician immediately. Therefore it is recommended that the patient has an emergency telephone number of his attending physician or of a clinic experienced in therapy of erectile dysfunction. Prolonged erection may damage penile erectile tissue and lead to irreversible erectile dysfunction.

A benefit-risk evaulation is neccesary before using Viridal Duo in patients with pre-existing scarring, e.g. nodules of the cavernous body or pre-existing penile deviation or Peyronie's disease or clinically relevant phimosis, e.g. phimosis with risk of paraphimosis these patients should be treated with particular care, e.g. more frequent re-evaluation of the patient's condition.

Patients who have to be treated with alpha-adrenergic drugs due to prolonged erections (see: overdose) may in the case of concomitant therapy with monoamino-oxidase-inhibitors, develop a hypertensive crisis.

Other intracavernous drugs e.g. smooth muscle relaxing agents or alpha-adrenergic blocking agents may lead to prolonged erection and must not be used concomitantly.

The effects of a combination therapy of alprostadil with oral, intraurethral or topical medicinal products for erectile dysfunction are currently unknown.

Patients with blood clotting disorders or patients on therapy influencing blood clotting parameters should be treated with special care, e.g. monitoring of the clotting parameters and advice to the patient to exercise sufficient manual pressure on the injection site. This is because of the increased risk of bleeding.

To prevent abuse, self-injection therapy with Viridal Duo should not be used by patients with drug addiction and/or disturbances of psychological or intellectual development.

In cases of excessive use, e.g. higher frequencies than recommended, an increased risk of penile scarring cannot be excluded.

Use of intracavernous alprostadil offers no protection from the transmission of sexually transmitted diseases. Individuals who use alprostadil should be counselled about the protective measures that are necessary to guard against the spread of sexually transmitted diseases, including the human immunodeficiency virus (HIV). In some patients, injection of Viridal Duo can induce a small amount of bleeding at the injection site. In patients infected with blood borne diseases, this could increase the transmission of such diseases to the partner. For this reason we recommend that a condom is used for intercourse after injecting Viridal Duo.

Viridal Duo is for intracavernous injection. Subcutaneous injection or injections at areas of the penis other than the cavernous body should be avoided.

The injection should be performed under hygienic conditions to avoid infections. In any condition that precludes safe self-injection like poor manual dexterity, poor visual acuity or morbid obesity, the partner should be trained in the injection technique and should perform the injection.

Up to now, there is no clinical experience in patients under 18 and over 75 years of age.

Viridal Duo does not interfere with ejaculation and fertility.

4.5 Interaction with other medicinal products and other forms of interaction

Concomitant use of smooth muscle relaxing drugs like papaverine or other drugs inducing erection like alpha-adrenergic blocking agents may lead to prolonged erection and should not be used in parallel with Viridal Duo.

Risks exist when using alpha-adrenergic drugs to terminate prolonged erections in patients with cardiovascular disorders or receiving MAO inhibitors.

The effects of blood pressure lowering and vasodilating drugs may be increased.

4.6 Pregnancy and lactation

Not applicable.

Alprostadil did not cause any adverse effects on fertility or general reproductive performance in male and female rats treated with 40-200 mcg/kg/day. The high dose of 200 mcg/kg/day is about 300 times the maximum recommended human dose on a body weight basis (MHRD < 1 mcg/kg).

Alprostadil was not fetotoxic or teratogenic at doses up to 5000 mcg/kg/day (7500 times the MHRD) in rats, 200 mcg/kg/day (300 times the MHRD) in rabbits and doses up to 20 mcg/kg/day (30 times the MHRD) in guinea pigs or monkeys.

4.7 Effects on ability to drive and use machines

Viridal Duo may rarely induce hypotension with subsequent impairment of reactivity.

4.8 Undesirable effects

A burning sensation during injection is common (< 10 %) and generally subsides shortly afterwards. A sensation of tension in the penis and pain at the site of injection are common (< 10 %) and mostly of mild intensity. Spotlike haemorrhage/ spotlike bruises at the site of puncture occur uncommonly (< 1 %). Haemosiderin deposits, reddening and swellings at the site of injection are also uncommon (< 1 %). Other uncommon (< 1 %) reactions are swellings of the preputium or the glans, and headache.

Prolonged erections of more than 4 hours duration are uncommon (< 1 %) and are mainly seen during dose titration.

During long-term treatment, fibrotic alterations (e.g. fibrotic nodules, plaques at the site of injection or in the corpus cavernosum) may occur commonly (< 10 %) in follow up periods of up to 4 years. This may be associated with slight penile axis deviations in uncommon (< 1 %) cases. In rare cases (< 0.1%), fibrotic changes of the cavernous body may occur during treatment lasting up to 4 years.

Rare cases (< 0.1%) of circulatory effects such as short periods of hypotension and/or vertigo or dizziness have been observed after the intracavernous injection of Viridal Duo.

In rare cases (< 0.1%) allergic reactions ranging from cutaneous hypersensitivity such as rash, erythema, urticaria to anaphylactic/anaphylactoid reactions may occur.

4.9 Overdose

Symptoms

Full rigid erections lasting more than four hours.

If the patient experiences a prolonged erection, he is advised to contact his attending physician or a urologic clinic nearby immediately.

Treatment strategy

Treatment of prolonged erection should be done by a physician experienced in the field of erectile dysfunction. If prolonged erection occurs, the following is recommended:

If the erection has lasted less than six hours:

– observation of the erection because spontaneous flaccidity frequently occurs.

If the erection has lasted longer than six hours:

– cavernous body injection of alpha-adrenergic substances (e.g. phenylephrine or epinephrine (adrenaline)). Risks exist when using drugs in patients with cardiovascular disorders or receiving MAO inhibitors. All patients should be monitored for cardiovascular effects when these drugs are used to terminate prolonged erections.

or

– aspiration of blood from the cavernous body.

Accidental systemic injection of high doses

Single dose rising tolerance studies in healthy volunteers indicated that single intravenous doses of alprostadil from 1 to 120 mcg were well tolerated. Starting with a 40 mcg bolus intravenous dose, the frequency of drug-related adverse events increased in a dose-dependent manner, characterised mainly by facial flushing.

5. PHARMACOLOGICAL PROPERTIES

5.1 Pharmacodynamic properties

ATC Code: Other urologicals G04BX 05

Alprostadil [Prostaglandin E_1 (PGE_1)], the active ingredient of Viridal Duo, is an endogenous compound derived from the essential fatty acid dihomogammalinolenic acid. Alprostadil is a potent smooth muscle relaxant that produces vasodilation and occurs in high concentrations in the human seminal fluid. Pre-contracted isolated preparations of the human corpus cavernosum, corpus spongiosum and cavernous artery were relaxed by alprostadil, while other prostanoids were less effective. Alprostadil has been shown to bind to specific receptors in the cavernous tissue of human and non-human primates.

The binding of alprostadil to its receptors is accompanied by an increase in intracellular cAMP levels. Human cavernosal smooth muscle cells respond to alprostadil by releasing intracellular calcium. Since relaxation of smooth muscle is associated with a reduction of the cytoplasmic free calcium concentration, this effect may contribute to the relaxing activity of this prostanoid.

Intracavernous injection of alprostadil in healthy monkeys resulted in penile elongation and tumescence without rigidity. The cavernous arterial blood flow was increased for a mean duration of 20 min. In contrast, intracavernous application of alprostadil to rabbits and dogs caused no erectile response.

Systemic intravascular administration of alprostadil leads to a vasodilation and reduction of systemic peripheral vascular resistance. A decrease in blood pressure can be observed after administration of high doses. Alprostadil has also been shown in animal and *in vitro* tests to reduce platelet reactivity and neutrophil activation. Additional alprostadil activity has been reported: increase in fibrinolytic activity of fibroblasts, improvement of erythrocyte deformability and inhibition of erythrocyte aggregation; inhibition of the proliferative and mitotic activity of non-striated myocytes; inhibition of cholesterol synthesis and LDL-receptor activity; and an increase in the supply of oxygen and glucose to ischaemic tissue along with improved tissue utilisation of these substrates.

5.2 Pharmacokinetic properties

After reconstitution, alprostadil (PGE_1) dissociates from the α-cyclodextrin clathrate, and the two components have independent fates.

In symptomatic volunteers, systemic mean endogenous PGE_1 venous plasma concentrations measured before intracavernous injection are approximately 1 pg/ml. After injection of 20 mcg of alprostadil, the PGE_1 venous plasma concentrations increase rapidly to concentrations of about 10-20 pg/ml. The PGE_1 plasma concentrations return to concentrations close to the baseline within a few minutes. Approximately 90% of PGE_1 found in plasma is protein-bound.

Metabolism

Enzymatic oxidation of the C15-hydroxy group and reduction of the C13,14 double bond produce the primary metabolites, 15-keto-PGE_1, PGE (13,14-dihydro-PGE_1) and 15-keto-PGE_o. Only PGE_o and 15-keto-PGE_o have been detected in human plasma. Unlike the 15-keto metabolites, which are less pharmacologically active than the parent compound, PGE_o has a potency similar to that of PGE_1 in most respects.

In symptomatic volunteers, the mean endogenous PGE_o venous plasma concentrations measured before an intracavernous injection are approximately 1 pg/ml. After the injection of 20 mcg of alprostadil, the PGE_o plasma concentrations increase to concentrations of about 5 pg/ml.

Excretion

After further degradation of the primary metabolites by beta and omega oxidation, the resulting, more polar metabolites are excreted primarily with the urine (88%) and the faeces (12%) and there is no evidence of tissue retention of PGE_1 or its metabolites.

5.3 Preclinical safety data

Studies on local tolerance following single and repeated intracavernous injections of alprostadil or alprostadil alfadex in rabbits and/or monkeys, in monkeys up to 6 months with daily injection revealed in general good local tolerance. Possible adverse effects like haematomas and inflammations are more likely related to the injection procedure.

Within the 6 months study in male monkeys, there were no adverse effects of alprostadil alfadex on male reproductive organs.

Mutagenicity studies with alprostadil alfadex revealed no risk of mutagenicity.

6. PHARMACEUTICAL PARTICULARS

6.1 List of excipients

Powder for injection:

Lactose monohydrate

Alfadex

Diluent:

Sodium chloride

Water for injection.

6.2 Incompatibilities

No incompatibilities have so far been demonstrated.

6.3 Shelf life

Shelf life for the product as packaged for sale: 4 years.

Shelf life after reconstitution: for immediate use only.

6.4 Special precautions for storage

Do not store above 25°C. Store in the original packaging.

6.5 Nature and contents of container

1. Cartons containing one colourless glass double-chamber cartridge, one injection needle 29 G × ½ (0.33 mm × 12.7 mm) and one reusable injector (starter kit).

2. Cartons containing two colourless glass double-chamber cartridges, two injection needles 29 G × ½ (0.33 mm × 12.7 mm) and one reusable injector (starter kit).

3. Cartons containing one, two or six colourless glass double-chamber cartridges and corresponding number of injection needles 29 G × ½ (0.33 mm × 12.7 mm) without reusable injector.

6.6 Special precautions for disposal and other handling

Fix the injection needle onto the front part of the injector.

Disinfect the tip of the cartridge with one of the alcohol swabs. Insert the cartridge into the reusable injector and fix it by screwing the thread part. Dissolve the drug substance in the front chamber of the cartridge by completely screwing the thread-part into the injector thus moving both rubber stoppers to the top of the cartridge and allowing the solvent in to the bottom chamber to reach the dry substance via the bypass of the cartridge. Shake slightly until a clear solution is produced.

Expel the air and adjust the prescribed dosage precisely prior to intracavernous injection.

After preparation of the solution, the injection must be performed using aseptic procedures into either the left or right cavernous body of the penile shaft. Care should be taken not to inject into penile vessels or nerves on the upper side of the penis and into the urethra on the under side. The injection should be completed within 5 to 10 seconds and manual pressure should be applied to the injection site for 2 to 3 minutes.

Unused solution must be discarded immediately.

Advice

The content of the front chamber of the cartridge consists of a white, dry powder, which forms a compact layer, approximately 8 mm in height. The layer may show cracks and crumble slightly.

In case of damage to the cartridge, the usually dry content of the front chamber becomes moist and sticky and extensively loses volume. Viridal Duo must not be used in this case.

The bottom chamber contains the clear, colourless sodium chloride solvent solution.

The dry substance dissolves immediately after addition of the sodium chloride solution. Initially after reconstitution the solution may appear slightly opaque due to the presence of bubbles. This is of no relevance and disappears within a short time to give a clear solution.

7. MARKETING AUTHORISATION HOLDER

SCHWARZ PHARMA Limited

5 Hercules Way

Leavesden Park

Watford

WD25 7GS

United Kingdom

8. MARKETING AUTHORISATION NUMBER(S)

PL 04438/0051

9. DATE OF FIRST AUTHORISATION/RENEWAL OF THE AUTHORISATION

7 October 1998

10. DATE OF REVISION OF THE TEXT

July 2006

Vistabel

(Allergan Ltd)

1. NAME OF THE MEDICINAL PRODUCT

VISTABEL, 4 Allergan Units/0.1ml, powder for solution for injection

2. QUALITATIVE AND QUANTITATIVE COMPOSITION

Botulinum toxin type A[1] 4 Allergan units per 0.1ml of reconstituted solution.

[1]of *Clostridium botulinum*

Allergan units are not interchangeable with other preparations of botulinum toxin.

Vial of 50 units.

For a full list of excipients, see section 6.1.

3. PHARMACEUTICAL FORM

Powder for solution for injection.

White Powder

4. CLINICAL PARTICULARS

4.1 Therapeutic indications

VISTABEL is indicated for the temporary improvement in the appearance of moderate to severe vertical lines between the eyebrows seen at frown, in adults <65 years old, when the severity of these lines has an important psychological impact for the patient.

4.2 Posology and method of administration

<u>Considering that botulinum toxin units are different depending on the medicinal products, doses of botulinum toxin are not interchangeable from one product to another.</u>

There is limited phase 3 clinical data with VISTABEL in patients older than 65 years (see section 5.1). Until more studies have been performed in this age group, VISTABEL is not recommended in patients older than 65 years.

The safety and effectiveness of VISTABEL in the treatment of vertical lines between the eyebrows (known as glabellar lines) in individuals under 18 years of age have not been demonstrated. The use of VISTABEL is not recommended in individuals under 18 years (see section 4.4).

<u>VISTABEL should only be administered by physicians with appropriate qualifications and expertise in this treatment and having the required equipment.</u>

<u>VISTABEL, after reconstitution, must be used only for one session of injection(s) per patient.</u>

The recommended injection volume per muscle site is 0.1 ml. See also dilution table in section 6.6.

For instructions for use, handling and disposal of the vials, see section 6.6.

Care should be taken to ensure that VISTABEL is not injected into a blood vessel when it is injected in the vertical lines between the eyebrows also called Glabellar Lines.

Reconstituted VISTABEL (50 U/1.25 mL) is injected using a sterile 30 gauge needle. 0.1 mL (4 U) is administered in each of the 5 injection sites: 2 injections in each corrugator muscle and 1 injection in the procerus muscle for a total dose of 20 U.

Before injection, the thumb or index finger are to be placed firmly below the orbital rim in order to prevent extravasation below the orbital rim. The needle should be oriented superiorly and medially during the injection. In order to reduce the risk of ptosis, injections near the levator palpebrae superioris muscle must be avoided, particularly in patients with larger brow-depressor complexes (depressor supercilii). Injections in the corrugator muscle must be done in the central part of that muscle, at least 1 cm above the arch of the eyebrows.

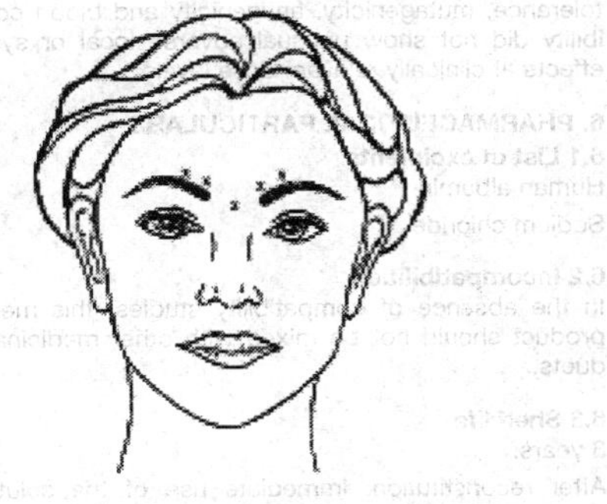

Improvement of severity of vertical lines between the eyebrows (glabellar lines) generally occurs within one week after treatment. The effect was demonstrated for up to 4 months after injection.

Treatment intervals should not be more frequent than every three months. In the event of treatment failure or diminished effect following repeat injections, alternative treatment methods should be employed.

<u>**General information**</u>

In case of treatment failure after the first treatment session, i.e. in the absence, at one month after injection, of significant improvement from baseline, the following approaches may be considered:

- Analysis of the causes of failure, e.g. incorrect muscles injected, injection technique, formation of toxin-neutralising antibodies, insufficient dose;
- Re-evaluation of the relevance of treatment with botulinum toxin type A;

In case of insufficient dose and in the absence of any undesirable effects secondary to the first treatment session, initiate a second treatment session as follows:

i) Consider adjusting the total dose up to 40 or 50 units, taking into account the analysis of the previous treatment failure;

ii) At least a three-month interval between the two treatment sessions should be maintained.

4.3 Contraindications

VISTABEL is contraindicated,

- In individuals with a known hypersensitivity to botulinum toxin type A or to any of the excipients of the formulation;

- In the presence of myasthenia gravis or Eaton Lambert Syndrome;

- In the presence of infection at the proposed injection sites.

4.4 Special warnings and precautions for use

It is mandatory that VISTABEL is used for one single patient treatment only during a single session. The excess of unused product must be disposed of as detailed in section 6.6. Particular precautions should be taken for product preparation and administration as well as for the inactivation and disposal of the remaining unused solution (see section 6.6).

This medicinal product contains less than 1 mmol sodium (23 mg) per dose, i.e. essentially "sodium free".

The relevant anatomy, and any alterations to the anatomy due to prior surgical procedures, must be understood prior to administering VISTABEL. The recommended dosage and frequency of administration of VISTABEL should not be exceeded.

An anaphylactic reaction may occur very rarely after injection of botulinum toxin. Epinephrine (adrenaline) or any other anti-anaphylactic measures should therefore be available.

Adverse reactions possibly related to the spread of toxin distant from the site of administration have been reported very rarely with botulinum toxin (see section 4.8). Patients treated with therapeutic doses may experience exaggerated muscle weakness. Injection of VISTABEL is not recommended in patients with a history of dysphagia and aspiration.

Patients or caregivers should be advised to seek immediate medical care if swallowing, speech or respiratory disorders arise.

Too frequent or excessive dosing may enhance the risk of antibody formation. Antibody formation may lead to treatment failure of botulinum toxin type A even for other indications.

Caution should be taken when VISTABEL is used in the presence of inflammation at the proposed injection site(s) or when the targeted muscle shows excessive weakness or atrophy. Caution should also be exercised when VISTABEL is used for treatment of patients with amyotrophic lateral sclerosis or with peripheral neuromuscular disorders.

The effect of administering different botulinum neurotoxin serotypes at the same time or within several months of each other is unknown. Excessive neuromuscular weakness may be exacerbated by administration of another botulinum toxin prior to the resolution of the effects of a previously administered botulinum toxin.

The use of VISTABEL is not recommended in individuals under 18 years and in patients older than 65 years.

4.5 Interaction with other medicinal products and other forms of interaction

Theoretically, the effect of botulinum toxin may be potentiated by aminoglycoside antibiotics, spectinomycin, or other medicinal products that interfere with neuromuscular transmission (e.g. tubocurarine-type muscle relaxants).

No specific tests have been carried out to establish the possibility of clinical interaction with other medicinal products. No other interactions of clinical significance have been reported in this indication.

4.6 Pregnancy and lactation

<u>**Pregnancy**</u>

There are no adequate data from the use of botulinum toxin type A in pregnant women. Studies in animals have shown reproductive toxicity (see section 5.3). The potential risk for humans is unknown. VISTABEL should not be used during pregnancy unless clearly necessary.

<u>**Lactation**</u>

There is no information on whether VISTABEL is excreted in human milk. The use of VISTABEL during lactation cannot be recommended.

4.7 Effects on ability to drive and use machines

Attention is drawn in vehicle drivers and users of machines to the potential risks of asthenia, muscle weakness, dizziness and visual disturbance linked with the use of this medicinal product, which could make driving or using machines dangerous.

4.8 Undesirable effects

a) <u>General</u>

Based on controlled clinical trial data, the proportion of patients that would be expected to experience an adverse reaction after treatment with VISTABEL is 23,5% (placebo: 19,2%). These adverse reactions may be related to treatment, injection technique or both.

In general, adverse reactions occur within the first few days following injection and are transient. Most adverse events reported were of mild to moderate severity.

The expected pharmacological action of botulinum toxin is a local muscle weakness. Blepharoptosis, which may be technique-related, is consistent with the pharmacological action of VISTABEL. As is expected for any injection procedure, pain/burning/stinging, oedema and/or bruising may be observed in association with the injection.

b) <u>Adverse reactions - frequency</u>

The frequency is defined as follows: Very Common (≥ 1/10); Common (≥ 1/100, <1/10); Uncommon (≥ 1/1,000, <1/100); Rare (≥ 1/10,000, <1/1,000); Very Rare (<1/10,000).

Infections and infestations

Uncommon: Infection

Psychiatric disorders

Uncommon: Anxiety

Nervous system disorders

Common: Headache

Uncommon: Paresthesia, dizziness

Eye disorders

Common: Eyelid ptosis

Uncommon: Blepharitis, eye pain, visual disturbance

Gastrointestinal disorders

Uncommon: Nausea, oral dryness

Skin and subcutaneous tissue disorders

Common: Erythema

Uncommon: Skin tightness, oedema (face, eyelid, periorbital), photosensitivity reaction, pruritus, dry skin

Musculoskeletal and connective tissue disorders

Common: Localised muscle weakness

Uncommon: Muscle twitching

General disorders and administration site conditions

Common: Face pain

Uncommon: Flu syndrome, asthenia, fever

c) Post-Marketing data (frequency not known)

The following adverse reactions have been reported rarely since the drug has been marketed for the treatment of Glabellar Lines and other clinical indications: rash, urticaria, pruritus, erythema multiforme, psoriasiform eruption, anaphylactic reaction (angiodema, bronchospasm), alopecia, madarosis, tinnitus and hypoacousia.

Adverse reactions possibly related to the spread of toxin distant from the site of administration have been reported very rarely with botulinum toxin (e.g. muscle weakness, dysphagia, or aspiration pneumonia which can be fatal) (see section 4.4).

4.9 Overdose

No cases of systemic toxicity resulting from accidental injection of botulinum toxin type A have been observed. No cases of ingestion of botulinum toxin type A have been reported. Signs of overdose are not apparent immediately post-injection. Should accidental injection or ingestion occur, the patient should be medically supervised for several days for signs and symptoms of general weakness or muscle paralysis.

Admission to hospital should be considered in patients presenting symptoms of botulinum toxin type A poisoning (generalised weakness, ptosis, diplopia, swallowing and speech disorders, or paresis of the respiratory muscles).

5. PHARMACOLOGICAL PROPERTIES

5.1 Pharmacodynamic properties

Pharmacotherapeutic group: Muscle relaxants, peripherally acting agents,

ATC code: M03A X01.

Botulinum toxin type A *(Clostridium botulinum* neurotoxin) blocks peripheral acetylcholine release at presynaptic cholinergic nerve terminals by cleaving SNAP-25, a protein integral to the successful docking and release of acetylcholine from vesicles situated within the nerve endings leading to denervation of the muscle and therefore to a paralysis.

After injection, there is an initial rapid high-affinity binding of toxin to specific cell surface receptors. This is followed by transfer of the toxin across the plasma membrane by receptor-mediated endocytosis. Finally, the toxin is released into the cytosol. This latter process is accompanied by progressive inhibition of acetylcholine release, clinical signs are manifest within 2-3 days, with peak effect seen within 5-6 weeks of injection.

Recovery after intramuscular injection takes place normally within 12 weeks of injection as nerve terminals sprout and reconnect with the endplates.

Clinical data:

537 patients with moderate to severe vertical lines between the eyebrows (glabellar lines) at maximum frown have been included in clinical studies.

VISTABEL injections significantly reduced the severity of glabellar lines for up to 4 months, as measured by the investigator assessment of glabellar line severity at maximum frown and by subject's global assessment of change in appearance of his/her vertical lines between the eyebrows (glabellar lines). None of the clinical endpoints included an objective evaluation of the psychological impact. Thirty days after injection 80% (325/405) of VISTABEL-treated patients were considered by investigators as treatment responders (none or mild severity at maximum frown), compared to 3% (4/132) of placebo-treated patients. At this same timepoint, 89% (362/405) of VISTABEL-treated patients felt they had a moderate or better improvement, compared to 7% (9/132) of placebo-treated patients.

VISTABEL injections also significantly reduced the severity of glabellar lines at rest. Of the 537 patients enrolled, 39% (210/537) had moderate to severe glabellar lines at rest (15% had no lines at rest). Of these, 74% (119/161) of VISTABEL-treated patients were considered treatment responders (none or mild severity) thirty days after injection, compared with 20% (10/49) of placebo-treated patients.

There is limited phase 3 clinical data with VISTABEL in patients older than 65 years. Only 6.0% (32/537) of subjects were >65 years old and efficacy results obtained were lower in this population.

5.2 Pharmacokinetic properties

a) General characteristics of the active substance:

Distribution studies in rats indicate slow muscular diffusion of ^{125}I-botulinum neurotoxin A complex in the gastrocnemius muscle after injection, followed by rapid systemic metabolism and urinary excretion. The amount of radiolabeled material in the muscle declined with a half-life of approximately 10 hours. At the injection site, the radioactivity was bound to large protein molecules, whereas in the plasma it was bound to small molecules, suggesting rapid systemic metabolism of the substrate. Within 24 hours of dosing, 60% of the radioactivity was excreted in the urine. Toxin is probably metabolised by proteases and the molecular components recycled through normal metabolic pathways.

Classical absorption, distribution, biotransformation and elimination (ADME) studies on the active substance have not been performed due to the nature of this product.

b) Characteristics in patients:

It is believed that at therapeutic doses, low systemic distribution of VISTABEL occurs. Clinical studies using single fibre electromyographic techniques have shown increased electrophysiologic neuromuscular activity in muscles distant to the injection site, with no associated clinical signs or symptoms.

5.3 Preclinical safety data

In reproductive studies in mice, rats, and rabbits, embryo toxicity was observed with high doses (delayed ossification and reduced foetal bodyweight). No teratogenic effects were observed in these species. In rats adverse effects on male fertility and female estrous cycling and fertility occurred only at high doses.

Studies on acute toxicity, repeated dose toxicity, local tolerance, mutagenicity, antigenicity and blood compatibility did not show unusual adverse local or systemic effects at clinically relevant dose levels.

6. PHARMACEUTICAL PARTICULARS

6.1 List of excipients

Human albumin

Sodium chloride

6.2 Incompatibilities

In the absence of compatibility studies, this medicinal product should not be mixed with other medicinal products.

6.3 Shelf life

3 years.

After reconstitution, immediate use of the solution is recommended; however, stability has been demonstrated for 4 hours at 2°C - 8°C.

6.4 Special precautions for storage

Store in a refrigerator (2°C - 8°C).

For storage conditions of the reconstituted medicinal product, see section 6.3.

6.5 Nature and contents of container

Powder in a vial (Type I glass) fitted with a stopper (chlorobutyl rubber) and a seal (aluminium);

Vial of 50 Allergan Units of Botulinum toxin type A – pack of one or pack of two

NOT ALL PACK SIZES MAY BE MARKETED

6.6 Special precautions for disposal and other handling

Reconstitution should be performed in accordance with good practices rules, particularly for the respect of asepsis. VISTABEL has to be reconstituted with a 0.9% preservative free sodium chloride solution for injection. As per the dilution table below, the requested amount of sodium chloride 9mg/ml (0.9%) solution for injection has to be drawn up into a syringe in order to obtain a reconstituted solution at a concentration of 4U/0.1 ml;

Amount of solvent added (0.9% sodium chloride solution) to a 50 U vial	Resulting dose (Units per 0.1 ml)
1.25 ml	4.0 U

The central part of the rubber cap has to be cleaned with alcohol.

To avoid VISTABEL denaturation, the solution is prepared by injecting the solvent slowly into the vial and by gently rotating the vial avoiding bubble formation. The vial has to be discarded if the vacuum does not pull the solvent into the vial. Once reconstituted, the solution should be visually inspected prior to use. Only clear, colourless to slightly yellow solution without particles should be used.

<u>It is mandatory that VISTABEL is used for one single patient treatment only during a single session.</u>

<u>Procedure to follow for a safe disposal of vials, syringes and materials used:</u>

Immediately after use, and prior to disposal, unused reconstituted VISTABEL solution in the vial and/or the syringe must be inactivated, with 2 ml of dilute sodium hypochlorite solution at 0.5% or 1 % and should be disposed of in accordance with local requirements.

Used vials, syringes and materials should not be emptied and must be discarded into appropriate containers and disposed of as a Medical Biohazardous Waste in accordance with local requirements.

<u>Recommendations in the event of an accident when handling botulinum toxin.</u>

In the event of an accident when handling the product, whether in the vacuum-dried state or reconstituted, the appropriate measures described below must be initiated immediately.

- The toxin is very sensitive to heat and certain chemical agents
- Any spillage must be wiped up: either with an absorbent material soaked in a solution of sodium hypochlorite (Javel solution) in the case of the vacuum-dried product, or with a dry absorbent material in the case of the reconstituted product.
- Contaminated surfaces must be cleaned with an absorbent material soaked in a solution of sodium hypochlorite (Javel solution) and then dried.
- If a vial is broken, carefully collect up the pieces of glass and wipe up the product as stated above, avoiding cutting the skin.
- If splashed, wash with a solution of sodium hypochlorite and then rinse thoroughly with plenty of water.
- If splashed into the eyes, rinse one's eyes thoroughly with plenty of water or with an eye wash solution.
- If the operator injures himself (cuts, pricks himself), proceed as above and take the appropriate medical steps according to the dose injected.

<u>This instruction for use and handling, and disposal should be strictly followed.</u>

7. MARKETING AUTHORISATION HOLDER

Allergan Pharmaceuticals Ireland

Castlebar Road

Westport

County Mayo

Ireland

8. MARKETING AUTHORISATION NUMBER(S)

PL 05179/0010

9. DATE OF FIRST AUTHORISATION/RENEWAL OF THE AUTHORISATION

Date of first authorisation: 12 January 2006

Date of last renewal: 16 May 2008

10. DATE OF REVISION OF THE TEXT

16 May 2008

Vistide

(Gilead Sciences Ltd)

1. NAME OF THE MEDICINAL PRODUCT

VISTIDE 75 mg/ml concentrate for solution for infusion.

2. QUALITATIVE AND QUANTITATIVE COMPOSITION

Each ml contains 75 mg cidofovir anhydrous. Each vial contains 375 mg/5ml cidofovir anhydrous as the active substance.

Each vial contains approximately 2.5 mmol (or 57 mg) sodium per vial (5 ml) as a constituent of the excipients.

The formulation is adjusted to pH 7.4.

For a full list of excipients, see 6.1.

3. PHARMACEUTICAL FORM

Concentrate for solution for infusion.

4. CLINICAL PARTICULARS

4.1 Therapeutic indications

VISTIDE is indicated for the treatment of CMV retinitis in patients with acquired immunodeficiency syndrome (AIDS) and without renal dysfunction. VISTIDE should be used only when other agents are considered unsuitable.

4.2 Posology and method of administration

The therapy should be prescribed by a physician experienced in the management of HIV infection.

Before each administration of VISTIDE, serum creatinine and urine protein levels should be investigated. VISTIDE must be administered with oral probenecid and intravenous saline as described below (see section 4.4 for appropriate recommendations, and under section 6.6 for information on obtaining probenecid).

The recommended dosage, frequency, or infusion rate must not be exceeded. VISTIDE must be diluted in 100 millilitres 0.9% (normal) saline prior to administration. To minimise potential nephrotoxicity, oral probenecid and intravenous saline prehydration must be administered with each VISTIDE infusion.

<u>Dosage in adults</u>

<u>Induction treatment.</u> The recommended dose of cidofovir is 5 mg/kg body weight (given as an intravenous infusion at a constant rate over 1 hour) administered once weekly for two consecutive weeks.

<u>Maintenance treatment.</u> Beginning two weeks after the completion of induction treatment, the recommended maintenance dose of cidofovir is 5 mg/kg body weight (given as an intravenous infusion at a constant rate over 1 hour) administered once every two weeks.

Suspension of maintenance treatment with cidofovir should be considered in accordance with local recommendations for the management of HIV-infected patients.

Dosage in elderly

The safety and efficacy of VISTIDE have not been established for the treatment of CMV disease in patients over 60 years of age. Since elderly individuals frequently have reduced glomerular function, particular attention should be paid to assessing renal function before and during administration of VISTIDE.

Dosage in children and neonates

VISTIDE is not recommended for use in children below 18 years of age due to a lack of data on safety and efficacy.

Dosage in renal insufficiency

Renal insufficiency [creatinine clearance ≤ 55 ml/min or ≥ 2+ proteinuria (≥ 100 mg/dl)] is a contraindication for the use of VISTIDE (see section 4.3 and 4.4).

Dosage in hepatic insufficiency

The safety and efficacy of VISTIDE have not been established in patients with hepatic disease and therefore it should be used with caution in this patient population.

4.3 Contraindications

Hypersensitivity to the active substance (cidofovir) or to any excipients.

Cidofovir administration is contraindicated in patients unable to receive probenecid or other sulfa-containing medication (see section 4.4 Prevention of nephrotoxicity).

VISTIDE is contraindicated in patients with renal insufficiency (see section 4.2).

Concomitant administration of VISTIDE and other potentially nephrotoxic agents is contraindicated (see section 4.4).

Direct intraocular injection of VISTIDE is contraindicated; direct injection may be associated with significant decreases in intraocular pressure and impairment of vision.

4.4 Special warnings and precautions for use

VISTIDE is formulated for intravenous infusion only and must not be administered by intraocular injection. VISTIDE should be infused only into veins with adequate blood flow to permit rapid dilution and distribution.

Renal insufficiency/Haemodialysis

Treatment with VISTIDE must not be initiated in patients with creatinine clearance ≤ 55 ml/min, or ≥ 2+ Proteinuria (≥ 100 mg/dl), as the optimum induction and maintenance doses for patients with moderate to severe renal impairment are not known. The efficacy and safety of cidofovir in such conditions has not been established.

High flux haemodialysis has been shown to reduce the serum levels of cidofovir by approximately 75%. The fraction of the dose extracted during haemodialysis is 51.9 ± 11.0%.

Nephrotoxicity

Dose-dependent nephrotoxicity is the major dose-limiting toxicity related to administration of cidofovir. The safety of cidofovir has not been evaluated in patients receiving other known potentially nephrotoxic agents (e.g. tenofovir, aminoglycosides, amphotericin B, foscarnet, intravenous pentamidine, adefovir and vancomycin). It is recommended to discontinue potentially nephrotoxic agents at least 7 days before starting cidofovir. (See section 4.8).

Patients treated at 3.0 mg/kg, 5.0 mg/kg or 10 mg/kg without concomitant probenecid developed evidence of proximal tubular cell injury, including glycosuria, and decreases in serum phosphate, uric acid and bicarbonate, and elevations in serum creatinine. The signs of nephrotoxicity were partially reversible in some patients. Concomitant use of probenecid is essential for reducing the pronounced nephrotoxicity of cidofovir to an extent that results in an acceptable benefit/risk balance of cidofovir therapy.

Prevention of nephrotoxicity

Therapy must be accompanied by administration of oral probenecid and adequate intravenous saline prehydration (see 6.6 for information on obtaining probenecid) with each cidofovir dose. All clinical trials relevant to clinical efficacy evaluation were performed using probenecid concomitantly with cidofovir. Two grams of probenecid should be administered 3 hours prior to the cidofovir dose and one gram administered at 2 and again at 8 hours after completion of the 1 hour cidofovir infusion (for a total of 4 grams). In order to reduce the potential for nausea and/or vomiting associated with administration of probenecid, patients should be encouraged to eat food prior to each dose of probenecid. The use of an anti-emetic may be necessary.

In patients who develop allergic or hypersensitivity symptoms to probenecid (e.g., rash, fever, chills and anaphylaxis), prophylactic or therapeutic use of an appropriate antihistamine and/or paracetamol should be considered.

Cidofovir administration is contraindicated in patients unable to receive probenecid because of a clinically significant hypersensitivity to the active substance or medicinal product or to other sulfa-containing medicines. Use of cidofovir without concomitant probenecid has not been clinically investigated. A probenecid desensitisation program is not recommended for use.

In addition to probenecid, patients must receive a total of one litre of 0.9% (normal) saline solution intravenously immediately prior to each infusion of cidofovir. Patients who can tolerate the additional fluid load may receive up to a total of 2 litres of 0.9% saline intravenously with each dose of cidofovir. The first litre of saline solution should be infused over a 1 hour period immediately before the cidofovir infusion, and the second litre, if given, infused over a 1-3 hour period beginning simultaneously with the cidofovir infusion or starting immediately after the infusion of cidofovir.

Cidofovir therapy should be discontinued and intravenous hydration is advised if serum creatinine increases by ≥ 44 μmol/l (≥ 0.5 mg/dl), or if persistent proteinuria ≥ 2+ develops. In patients exhibiting ≥ 2+ proteinuria, intravenous hydration should be performed and the test repeated. If following hydration, a ≥ 2+ proteinuria is still observed, cidofovir therapy should be discontinued. Continued administration of cidofovir to patients with persistent ≥ 2+ proteinuria following intravenous hydration may result in further evidence of proximal tubular injury, including glycosuria, decreases in serum phosphate, uric acid and bicarbonate, and elevations in serum creatinine.

Interruption, and possibly discontinuation, is required for changes in renal function. For those patients who fully recover from cidofovir associated renal toxicity, the benefits-risk balance of reintroducing cidofovir has not yet been evaluated.

Patient Monitoring

Proteinuria appears to be an early and sensitive indicator of cidofovir-induced nephrotoxicity. Patients receiving cidofovir must have their serum creatinine and urine protein levels determined on specimens obtained within 24 hours prior to the administration of each dose of cidofovir. Differential white blood cell counts should also be performed prior to each dose of cidofovir (see section 4.8).

Ocular Events

Patients receiving cidofovir should be advised to have regular follow-up ophthalmologic examinations for possible occurrence of Uveitis/ Iritis and Ocular Hypotony. In case of Uveitis/Iritis cidofovir should be discontinued if there is no response to treatment with a topical corticosteroid or the condition worsens, or if iritis/uveitis reoccurs after successful treatment.

Other

Cidofovir should be considered a potential carcinogen in humans (see section 5.3 Preclinical safety data).

Caution should be applied when considering cidofovir treatment of patients with diabetes mellitus due to the potential increased risk of developing ocular hypotony.

Male patients should be advised that cidofovir caused reduced testes weight and hypospermia in animals. Although not observed in clinical studies of cidofovir, such changes may occur in humans and cause infertility.

Appropriate precautions should continue to be employed to prevent transmission of HIV.

4.5 Interaction with other medicinal products and other forms of interaction

Probenecid increases the AUC of zidovudine. Patients receiving both drugs should be closely monitored for zidovudine induced haematological toxicity.

For other NRTI drugs administered concomitantly with probenecid, reference should be made to their respective prescribing information for any appropriate recommendations.

Interactions of cidofovir/probenecid and anti-HIV drugs or drugs used to treat common chronic viral infections in this population, such as HCV and HBV-related hepatitis, have not been investigated in clinical trials.

Probenecid is known to increase the exposure of many substances (e.g., paracetamol, acyclovir, angiotensin-converting enzyme inhibitors, aminosalicyclic acid, barbiturates, benzodiazepines, bumetanide, clofibrate, methotrexate, famotidine, furosemide, nonsteroidal anti-inflammatory agents, theophylline, and zidovudine).

Therefore, when co-prescribing cidofovir/probenecid with other agents, it is important for prescribers to consult the current probenecid SPC (or an appropriate drug reference source) and the respective prescribing information of the other co-administered products for full information regarding drug interactions and other features of that product.

4.6 Pregnancy and lactation

Cidofovir is embryotoxic in rats and rabbits at subtherapeutic dose levels. A significantly increased foetal incidence of external, soft tissue and skeletal anomalies occurred in rabbits at 1.0 mg/kg/day, which was also maternally toxic.

Pregnancy

There are no studies of cidofovir in pregnant women. VISTIDE should not be used during pregnancy.

Women of childbearing potential should be advised to use effective contraception during and after treatment with cidofovir.

Lactation

It is not known whether cidofovir is excreted in human milk. Because many substances are excreted in human milk, nursing mothers should be instructed to discontinue cidofovir or discontinue nursing if they continue to receive cidofovir. Passage of the placenta barrier of cidofovir-related compound was observed in pregnant rats. Excretion of cidofovir-related material into milk of lactating animals was not examined.

Refer to section 4.4 for further information

4.7 Effects on ability to drive and use machines

Adverse reactions such as asthenia may occur during cidofovir therapy. The physician is advised to discuss this issue with the patient, and based upon the condition of the disease and the tolerance of medication, give his recommendation in the individual case.

4.8 Undesirable effects

The table below lists the adverse reactions identified through clinical trials or post-marketing surveillance by system organ class (SOC) and frequency. Within each frequency grouping, adverse reactions are presented in order of decreasing seriousness. Frequencies are defined as: very common (≥ 1/10), common (≥ 1/100 to < 1/10), uncommon (≥ 1/1000 to < 1/100) or not known (cannot be estimated from the available data). Adverse reactions identified from post-marketing experience are included in italics.

Adverse reactions possibly or probably related to cidofovir based on clinical trial experience and post-marketing surveillance

System Organ Class	Adverse reactions
Blood and lymphatic system disorders	
Very common	Neutropenia
Nervous system disorders	
Very common	Headache
Eye disorders	
Common	Iritis, uveitis, hypotony of the eye (see Section 4.4)
Ear and labyrinth disorders	
Not known	*Hearing impaired*
Respiratory, thoracic and mediastinal disorders	
Common	Dyspnea
Gastrointestinal disorders	
Very common Not known	Nausea, Vomiting *Pancreatitis*
Skin and subcutaneous tissue disorders	
Very common	Alopecia, rash
Renal and urinary disorders	
Very common Common Uncommon	Proteinuria, blood creatinine increased (see Section 4.4) *Renal failure* *Fanconi syndrome acquired*
General disorders and administration site conditions	
Very common Common	Asthenia, fever Chills

Reports of renal failure (plus events possibly caused by renal failure, e.g. blood creatinine increased, proteinuria, glycosuria) received during post-marketing surveillance include some which were fatal. Cases of acute renal failure have been reported after only one or two doses of cidofovir.

The finding of any glycosuria, proteinuria/aminoaciduria, hypouricemia, hypophosphatemia and/or hypokalemia, should prompt for the consideration of cidofovir-related Fanconi syndrome.

The following table lists adverse reactions possibly or probably related to probenecid based on clinical trial experience:

System Organ Class	Adverse reactions
Nervous system disorders	
Common	Headache
Gastrointestinal disorders	
Very common	Nausea, vomiting
Skin and subcutaneous tissue disorders	
Very common	Rash
General disorders and administration site conditions	
Very common Common	Fever Asthenia, chills

In addition probenecid may also cause other adverse reactions including anorexia, gingival pain, flushing, alopecia, dizziness, anaemia, and pollakiuria. Hypersensitivity reactions, with dermatitis, pruritus, urticaria and, rarely, anaphylaxis, and Stevens-Johnson syndrome have occurred. There have been reports of leukopenia, hepatic necrosis, nephrotic syndrome, and aplastic anaemia. Haemolytic anaemia has also occurred, and may be associated with G6DP deficiency. Therefore, when co-prescribing probenecid with cidofovir, it is important for prescribers to consult the current probenecid SmPC (or an appropriate drug reference source) for full information on the safety profile and other features of that product.

4.9 Overdose

Two cases of cidofovir overdose have been reported. In both cases, the overdose occurred during the first induction dose and no additional cidofovir therapy was administered. One patient received a single dose of 16.4 mg/kg and the other patient received a single dose of 17.3 mg/kg. Both patients were hospitalised and received prophylactic oral probenecid and vigorous hydration for 3 to 7 days. One of these patients experienced a minor transient change in renal function, while the other patient had no change in renal function (see section 4.4).

5. PHARMACOLOGICAL PROPERTIES

5.1 Pharmacodynamic properties

Pharmacotherapeutic group: Antiviral for systemic use, ATC Code: J05AB12

General

Cidofovir is a cytidine analogue with *in vitro* and *in vivo* activity against human cytomegalovirus (HCMV). HCMV strains resistant to ganciclovir may still be susceptible to cidofovir.

Mechanism of action

Cidofovir suppresses HCMV replication by selective inhibition of viral DNA synthesis. Biochemical data support selective inhibition of HSV-1, HSV-2 and HCMV DNA polymerases by cidofovir diphosphate, the active intracellular metabolite of cidofovir.

Cidofovir diphosphate inhibits these viral polymerases at concentrations that are 8- to 600-fold lower than those needed to inhibit human cellular DNA polymerases alpha, beta, and gamma. Incorporation of cidofovir into viral DNA results in reductions in the rate of viral DNA synthesis.

Cidofovir enters cells by fluid-phase endocytosis and is phosphorylated to cidofovir monophosphate and subsequently to cidofovir diphosphate. Prolonged antiviral effects of cidofovir are related to the half-lives of its metabolites; cidofovir diphosphate persists inside cells with a half-life of 17-65 hours and a cidofovir phosphate-choline adduct has a half-life of 87 hours.

Antiviral activity

Cidofovir is active *in vitro* against HCMV, a member of the herpesviridae family. Antiviral activity is seen at concentrations significantly below those which cause cell death.

The *in vitro* sensitivity to cidofovir is shown in the following table:

Cidofovir Inhibition of Virus Multiplication in Cell Culture	
Virus	IC_{50} (μM)
wild-type CMV isolates	0.7 (± 0.6)
ganciclovir-resistant CMV isolates	7.5 (± 4.3)
foscarnet-resistant CMV isolates	0.59 (± 0.07)

In vivo activity against HCMV was confirmed with controlled clinical studies of cidofovir for the treatment of CMV retinitis in patients with AIDS, which demonstrated statistically significant delays in time to CMV retinitis progression for patients on cidofovir when compared to control patients. The median times to retinitis progression in the two efficacy studies (GS-93-106 and GS-93-105), were 120 days and not reached for the treatment arms vs. 22 days and 21 days for the untreated (deferred treatment) arms, respectively.

In study GS-93-107 conducted in patients who had relapsed after treatment with other agents, the median time to retinitis progression was 115 days.

Viral resistance

Following *in vitro* selection of ganciclovir-resistant HCMV isolates, cross-resistance between ganciclovir and cidofovir was seen with ganciclovir-selected mutations in the HCMV DNA polymerase gene but not with mutations in the UL97 gene. No cross-resistance between foscarnet and cidofovir was seen with foscarnet-selected mutants. Cidofovir-selected mutants had a mutation in the DNA polymerase gene and were cross-resistant to ganciclovir, but susceptible to foscarnet.

5.2 Pharmacokinetic properties

The major route of elimination of cidofovir was by renal excretion of unchanged drug by a combination of glomerular filtration and tubular secretion. In patients with normal renal function, 80 to 100% of the intravenous dose was recovered in the urine over 24 hours as unchanged cidofovir. No metabolites of cidofovir have been detected in serum or urine of patients.

At the end of a one-hour infusion of cidofovir 5 mg/kg administered with concomitant oral probenecid, the mean (± SD) serum concentration of cidofovir was 19.6 (± 7.18) mcg/ml. The mean values of total serum clearance, volume of distribution at steady-state and terminal elimination half-life were 138 (± 36) ml/hr/kg, 388 (± 125) ml/kg and 2.2 (±0.5) hour, respectively.

Dose-independent kinetics were demonstrated with single doses of cidofovir given over the dose range 3 to 7.5 mg/kg.

In vitro protein binding

In vitro protein binding of cidofovir to plasma or serum protein was 10% or less over the cidofovir concentration range 0.25 to 25 mcg/ml.

5.3 Preclinical safety data

Preclinical animal studies demonstrated that nephrotoxicity was the major dose-limiting toxicity of cidofovir. Evidence for a nephroprotective effect for probenecid was shown in a 52-week study conducted in cynomolgus monkeys administered cidofovir 2.5 mg/kg once weekly intravenously with 1 g of probenecid given orally.

Carcinogenesis

In a 26-week intravenous toxicity study, a significant increase in incidence of mammary adenocarcinomas was seen in female rats and of Zymbal's gland carcinomas in male and female rats at subtherapeutic plasma levels of cidofovir. In a separate study, once weekly subcutaneous injections of cidofovir for 19 consecutive weeks resulted in mammary adenocarcinomas in female rats at doses as low as 0.6 mg/kg/week. In both studies, tumours were observed within 3 months of dosing. No tumours were observed in cynomolgus monkeys administered cidofovir intravenously once weekly for 52 weeks at doses up to 2.5 mg/kg/week.

Mutagenicity and reproductive toxicology

Studies have shown that cidofovir is clastogenic *in vitro* at 100 μg/ml and is embryotoxic in rats and rabbits.

No mutagenic response was elicited by cidofovir at dose levels up to 5 mg/plate, in the presence and absence of metabolic activation by rat liver S-9 fraction, in microbial assays involving *Salmonella typhimurium* for base pair substitutions or frameshift mutations (Ames) and *Escherichia coli* for reverse mutations.

An increase in formation of micronucleated polychromatic erythrocytes was observed *in vivo* in mice receiving a high, toxic intraperitoneal dose of cidofovir (≥ 2000 mg/kg).

Cidofovir induced chromosomal aberrations in human peripheral blood lymphocytes *in vitro* without metabolic activation (S-9 fraction). At the 4 cidofovir levels (12.5 to 100 μg/ml) tested, the percentage of damaged metaphases and number of aberrations per cell increased in a concentration-dependent manner.

No adverse effects on fertility or general reproduction were seen following once weekly intravenous injections of cidofovir in male rats for 13 consecutive weeks at doses up to 15 mg/kg/week. Female rats dosed intravenously once weekly at 1.2 mg/kg/week or higher for up to 6 weeks prior to mating and for 2 weeks post mating had decreased litter sizes and live births per litter and increased early resorptions per litter. Peri- and post-natal development studies in which female rats received subcutaneous injections of cidofovir once daily at doses up to 1.0 mg/kg/day from day 7 of gestation through day 21 postpartum (approximately 5 weeks) resulted in no adverse effects on viability, growth, behaviour, sexual maturation or reproductive capacity in the offspring. Daily intravenous administration of cidofovir during the period of organogenesis led to reduced fetal body weights when administered to pregnant rats at 1.5 mg/kg/day and to pregnant rabbits at 1.0 mg/kg/day. The no-observable-effect dosages for embryotoxicity was 0.5 mg/kg/day in rats and 0.25 mg/kg/day in rabbits.

6. PHARMACEUTICAL PARTICULARS

6.1 List of excipients

Sodium Hydroxide

Hydrochloric Acid

Water for Injection

6.2 Incompatibilities

This medicinal product must not be mixed with other medicinal products or diluents except those mentioned in section 6.6.

6.3 Shelf life

3 years

From a microbiological point of view, the product must be used immediately.

Chemical and physical in-use stability has been demonstrated for up to 24 hours at 2 – 8°C when dilution is performed under controlled and validated aseptic conditions. Storage beyond 24 hours or freezing is not recommended. Refrigerated solutions should be allowed to warm to room temperature prior to use.

6.4 Special precautions for storage

Do not store above 30°C. Do not refrigerate or freeze.

For storage conditions of the diluted medicinal product see section 6.3

6.5 Nature and contents of container

5 ml clear glass vials with a 5 ml nominal fill volume. The container/closure components include: Type I clear borosilicate glass vials, Teflon faced grey butyl plug stoppers, and aluminium crimp seals with a flip off plastic tab. Each pack contains one 5 ml vial.

VISTIDE is supplied in single-use vials. Partially used vials should be discarded.

6.6 Special precautions for disposal and other handling

Method of preparation and administration

VISTIDE vials should be visually inspected for particulate matter and discolouration prior to administration.

With a syringe, transfer under aseptic conditions the appropriate dose of VISTIDE from the vial to an infusion bag containing 100 ml 0.9% (normal) saline solution, and mix thoroughly. The entire volume should be infused intravenously into the patient at a constant rate over a period of 1 hour by use of a standard infusion pump. VISTIDE should be administered by health care professionals adequately experienced in the care of AIDS patients.

The chemical and physical stability of VISTIDE admixed with saline has been demonstrated in glass bottles, in infusion bags composed of either polyvinyl chloride (PVC) or ethylene/propylene copolymer, and in PVC based vented I.V. administration sets. Other types of I.V. set tubing and infusion bags have not been studied.

Compatibility with Ringer's Solution, Lactated Ringer's Solution or bacteriostatic infusion fluids has not been evaluated.

Handling and disposal

Adequate precautions including the use of appropriate safety equipment are recommended for the preparation, administration and disposal of VISTIDE. The preparation of VISTIDE reconstituted solution should be done in a laminar flow biological safety cabinet. Personnel preparing the reconstituted solution should wear surgical gloves, safety glasses and a closed front surgical-type gown with knit cuffs. If VISTIDE contacts the skin, wash membranes and flush thoroughly with water. Excess VISTIDE and all other materials used in the admixture preparation and administration should be placed in a leak-proof, puncture-proof container for disposal. Any unused product or waste material should be disposed of in accordance with local requirements.

Obtaining probenecid

Probenecid is not supplied with VISTIDE and should be obtained via the Marketing Authorisation Holder of probenecid. However, in case of difficulty in obtaining probenecid the local representative of the Marketing Authorisation Holder of VISTIDE should be contacted for information (See also sections 4.2 and 4.4).

7. MARKETING AUTHORISATION HOLDER

Gilead Sciences International Limited

Cambridge

CB21 6GT

United Kingdom

8. MARKETING AUTHORISATION NUMBER(S)

EU/1/97/037/001

9. DATE OF FIRST AUTHORISATION/RENEWAL OF THE AUTHORISATION

Date of first authorisation: 23 April 1997

Date of last renewal.: 08 June 2007

10. DATE OF REVISION OF THE TEXT

01/2009

Detailed information on this product is available on the website of the European Medicines Agency (EMEA) http://www.emea.europa.eu/.

Vitamin E Suspension 100mg/ml

(Cambridge Laboratories)

1. NAME OF THE MEDICINAL PRODUCT

Vitamin E Suspension 100mg/ml

2. QUALITATIVE AND QUANTITATIVE COMPOSITION

Each 5ml of suspension contains 500mg of DL-alpha-tocopheryl acetate.

3. PHARMACEUTICAL FORM

Oral Suspension

4. CLINICAL PARTICULARS

4.1 Therapeutic indications

For the correction of Vitamin E deficiency occurring in malabsorption disorders ie. cystic fibrosis, chronic cholestasis and abetalipoproteinaemia.

4.2 Posology and method of administration

Route of administration: For oral use.

Adults (including the elderly)

For the treatment of malabsorption disorders the following doses should be administered:

Cystic fibrosis 100-200mg/day

Abetalipoproteinaemia 50-100mg/kg/day

Children

For the treatment of cystic fibrosis a dose of 50mg/day should be given to children less than 1 year and 100mg/day to children 1 year and over.

The adult dosage should be used for the treatment of abetalipoproteinaemia (50-100mg/kg/day).

Infants with vitamin E deficiency which is secondary to chronic cholestasis may be treated with doses of 150-200mg/kg/day.

4.3 Contraindications
Use in patients with a known hypersensitivity to Vitamin E.

4.4 Special warnings and precautions for use
Vitamin E has been reported to increase the risk of thrombosis in patients predisposed to this condition, including patients taking oestrogens. This finding has not been confirmed but should be borne in mind when selecting patients for treatment, in particular women taking oral contraceptives containing oestrogens.

A higher incidence of necrotising enterocolitis has been noted in lower weight premature infants (less than 1.5kg) treated with vitamin E.

4.5 Interaction with other medicinal products and other forms of interaction
Vitamin E may increase the risk of thrombosis in patients taking oestrogens (see 4.4 above).

4.6 Pregnancy and lactation
There is no evidence of the safety of high doses of vitamin E in pregnancy nor is there evidence from animal work that it is free from hazard, therefore do not use in pregnancy especially in the first trimester. No information is available on excretion in breast milk, therefore it is advisable not to use during lactation.

4.7 Effects on ability to drive and use machines
None known.

4.8 Undesirable effects
Diarrhoea and abdominal pain may occur with doses greater than 1g daily.

4.9 Overdose
Transient gastro-intestinal disturbances have been reported with doses greater than 1g daily and where necessary, general supportive measures should be employed.

5. PHARMACOLOGICAL PROPERTIES

5.1 Pharmacodynamic properties
The exact role of vitamin E in the animal organism has not yet been established. Vitamin E is known to exert an important physiological function as an antioxidant for fats, with a sparing action on vitamin A, carotenoids and on unsaturated fatty acids. Other work has demonstrated that vitamin E is connected with the maintenance of certain factors essential for the normal metabolic cycle.

5.2 Pharmacokinetic properties
Vitamin E is absorbed from the gastrointestinal tract. Most of the vitamin appears in the lymph and is then widely distributed to all tissues. Most of the dose is slowly excreted in the bile and the remainder is eliminated in the urine as glucuronides of tocopheronic acid or other metabolites.

5.3 Preclinical safety data
There are no pre-clinical data of relevance to the prescriber which are additional to that already included in other sections of the SPC.

6. PHARMACEUTICAL PARTICULARS

6.1 List of excipients
Castor oil polyethylene glycol ether

Benzoic acid

Sorbic acid

Glycerol

Syrup

Flavour raspberry

Purified Water

6.2 Incompatibilities
None.

6.3 Shelf life
Unopened: Two years.

After first opening: One month (The product will be stable after opening for the normal duration of treatment providing the cap is replaced after use and the recommended storage conditions on the label are observed).

6.4 Special precautions for storage
Store below 25°C.

6.5 Nature and contents of container
Amber glass bottles with aluminium screw caps or Vistop tamper-evident caps.

6.6 Special precautions for disposal and other handling
Vitamin E Suspension may be diluted with Syrup BP but should be used immediately and not stored.

7. MARKETING AUTHORISATION HOLDER
Cambridge Laboratories Limited

Deltic House

Kingfisher Way

Silverlink Business Park

Wallsend

Tyne & Wear

NE28 9NX

8. MARKETING AUTHORISATION NUMBER(S)
PL 12070/0010

9. DATE OF FIRST AUTHORISATION/RENEWAL OF THE AUTHORISATION
8 March 1993

10. DATE OF REVISION OF THE TEXT
March 2000

Vivaglobin 160mg/ml solution for injection (subcutaneous use)

(CSL Behring UK Limited)

1. NAME OF THE MEDICINAL PRODUCT
Vivaglobin®, 160mg/ml solution for injection (subcutaneous use)

2. QUALITATIVE AND QUANTITATIVE COMPOSITION
1ml contains:

Human normal immunoglobulin (subcutaneous) 160mg

Corresponding to the total protein content of which at least 95% is IgG.

Distribution of IgG subclasses:

IgG_1	ca. 61 %
IgG_2	ca. 28 %
IgG_3	ca. 5 %
IgG_4	ca. 6 %
IgA	max. 1.7 mg/ml

Excipients:

Sodium (as chloride and hydroxide): 0.8 to 1.6 mg/ml

For a full list of excipients, see section 6.1.

3. PHARMACEUTICAL FORM
Solution for injection (subcutaneous use).

Vivaglobin is a clear solution. The colour can vary from colourless to pale yellow up to light brown during shelf life.

4. CLINICAL PARTICULARS

4.1 Therapeutic indications
Replacement therapy in adults and children in primary immunodeficiency (PID) syndromes such as:

– Congenital agammaglobulinaemia and hypogammaglobulinaemia

– Common variable immunodeficiency

– Severe combined immunodeficiency

– IgG subclass deficiencies with recurrent infections

Replacement therapy in myeloma or chronic lymphatic leukaemia with severe secondary hypogammaglobulinaemia and recurrent infections.

4.2 Posology and method of administration

Posology
The dosage may need to be individualized for each patient dependent on the pharmacokinetic and clinical response. The following dosage regimens are given as a guideline. The dosage regimen using the subcutaneous route should achieve a sustained plasma level of IgG.

A loading dose of at least 0.2 to 0.5 g/kg (1.3 to 3.1 ml/kg) bodyweight – divided over several days with a maximal daily dose of 0.1 to 0.15 g/kg bodyweight and as indicated by the treating physician - may be required. After steady state IgG levels have been attained, maintenance doses are administered at repeated intervals, ideally weekly, to reach a cumulative monthly dose of about 0.4 to 0.8 g/kg (2.5 to 5 ml/kg) bodyweight.

Trough levels of IgG should be measured in order to adjust the dose and dosage interval of Vivaglobin.

Method of administration
Vivaglobin should be administered via the subcutaneous route (see section 3. 'Pharmaceutical form' and 6.6 'Special precautions for disposal and other handling').

Subcutaneous infusion for home treatment should be initiated and monitored by a physician experienced in the treatment of immunodeficiency and in the guidance of patients for home treatment. The patient will be instructed in the use of a syringe driver, infusion techniques, the keeping of a treatment diary and measures to be taken in case of severe adverse events. The recommended infusion rate is 22 ml/hour. In a clinical study with 53 patients evaluated, during the training phase under supervision of a physician, the infusion rate was increased from initially 10 ml to 22 ml/hour.

Vivaglobin should preferentially be administered in the abdominal wall, thigh and/or buttocks. No more than 15ml should be injected into a single site. Doses over 15 ml should be divided and injected into 2 or more sites.

4.3 Contraindications
Hypersensitivity to any of the components of the product.

Vivaglobin must not be given intravascularly.

It must also not be administered intramuscularly in case of severe thrombocytopenia and in other disorders of haemostasis.

4.4 Special warnings and precautions for use
Do not inject intravascularly! If Vivaglobin is accidentally administered into a blood vessel, patients could develop an anaphylactic shock.

The recommended infusion rate of Vivaglobin stated under '4.2 *Method of administration*' should be adhered to. Patients should be closely monitored and carefully observed for any adverse event throughout the infusion period.

Certain adverse reactions may occur more frequently in patients who receive human normal immunoglobulin for the first time or, in rare cases, when the product is switched or when treatment has been interrupted for more than eight weeks.

True hypersensitivity reactions are rare. They can occur in the very rare cases of IgA deficiency with anti-IgA antibodies and these patients should be treated with caution. Rarely, Vivaglobin can induce a fall in blood pressure with anaphylactic reaction, even in patients who had tolerated previous treatment with normal human immunoglobulin.

Potential complications can often be avoided by ensuring:

- that patients are not sensitive to human normal immunoglobulin, by first infusing the product slowly (see '4.2 *Method of administration*');

- that patients are carefully monitored for any symptoms throughout the infusion period. In particular, patients should be monitored during the first infusion and for the first hour thereafter, in order to detect potential adverse reactions in the following situations:

  - patients naïve to human normal immunoglobulin,
  - patients switched from an alternative product, or,
  - when there has been a long interval since the previous infusion.

All other patients should be observed for at least 20 minutes after administration.

On suspicion of an allergic or anaphylactic reaction the administration has to be discontinued immediately. In case of shock, the current medical standards for shock treatment have to be applied.

Important information about some of the ingredients of Vivaglobin
This medicine contains up to 110 mg sodium per dose (bodyweight 75 kg) if the maximal daily dose (11.25 g = 70.3 ml) is applied. To be taken into consideration in patients on a controlled sodium diet.

Virus safety
Standard measures to prevent infections resulting from the use of medicinal products prepared from human blood or plasma include selection of donors, screening of individual donations and plasma pools for specific markers of infection, and the inclusion of effective manufacturing steps for the inactivation/removal of viruses. Despite this, when medicinal products prepared from human blood or plasma are administered, the possibility of transmitting infective agents cannot be totally excluded. This also applies to unknown or emerging viruses and other pathogens.

The measures are considered effective for enveloped viruses such as HIV, HBV and HCV, and for the non-enveloped viruses, HAV and parvovirus B19.

There is reassuring clinical experience regarding the lack of hepatitis A or parvovirus B19 transmission with immunoglobulins and it is also assumed that the antibody content makes an important contribution to the virus safety.

It is strongly recommended that every time that Vivaglobin is administered to a patient, the name and batch number of the product are recorded in order to maintain a link between the patient and the batch of the product.

4.5 Interaction with other medicinal products and other forms of interaction

Live attenuated virus vaccines
Immunoglobulin administration may impair, for a period of at least 6 weeks and up to 3 months, the efficacy of live attenuated virus vaccines such as measles, rubella, mumps, and varicella vaccines. After administration of Vivaglobin, an interval of at least 3 months should elapse before vaccination with live attenuated virus vaccines.

In the case of measles, this impairment may persist for up to 1 year. Therefore, patients receiving measles vaccine should have their antibody status checked.

Interference with serological testing
It has to be considered that when serological test results are interpreted, the transitory rise of passively transferred antibodies after immunoglobulin injection may result in misleading positive test results.

Passive transmission of antibodies to erythrocyte antigens, e.g., A, B and D, may interfere with some serological tests for red cell allo-antibodies (e.g. Coombs test), reticulocyte count and haptoglobin.

4.6 Pregnancy and lactation
The safety of this medicinal product for use in human pregnancy has not been established in controlled clinical trials and therefore should only be given with caution to pregnant women or breast-feeding mothers. Clinical experience with immunoglobulins suggests that no harmful effects on the course of pregnancy, or on the foetus and the neonate are to be expected.

4.7 Effects on ability to drive and use machines
There are no indications that Vivaglobin may impair the ability to drive or use machines.

4.8 Undesirable effects
In a clinical study with s.c. administration in 60 subjects the following undesirable effects have been reported. The following standard categories of frequency are used:

Very common	≥ 1/10
Common	≥ 1/100 and < 1/10
Uncommon	≥ 1/1,000 and < 1/100
Rare	≥ 1/10,000 and < 1/1,000
Very rare	< 1/10,000 (including reported single cases)

•***Local reactions at the injection/infusion site***
Very common: swelling, soreness, redness, induration, local heat, itching, bruising or rash.

The frequency declined very rapidly within the first ten infusions, when patients became used to the subcutaneous form of treatment. (In study patients who were treated with subcutaneous immunoglobulin for years before the trial, injection site reactions were not reported.)

•***Immune system disorders***
In single cases: Allergic reactions including fall in blood pressure

•***General disorders***
In single cases: Generalized reactions such as chills, fever, headache, malaise, moderate back pain, syncope, dizziness, rash, bronchospasm.

Adverse reactions reported from post-marketing surveillance are similar to the reactions which have also been observed during the clinical trials as listed above. In addition, the following have also been reported during post-marketing surveillance:

•***Immune system disorders***
Allergic/anaphylactic reactions including dyspnoea, cutaneous reactions, in isolated cases reaching as far as anaphylactic shock, even when the patient has shown no hypersensitivity to previous administration

•***General disorders***
Generalized reactions such as nausea, vomiting, arthralgia

•***Cardiovascular disorders***
Cardiovascular reactions particularly if the product is inadvertently injected intravascularly

For information on infectious disease risk, see 4.4 subsection '*Virus safety*'.

4.9 Overdose
Consequences of an overdose are not known.

5. PHARMACOLOGICAL PROPERTIES

5.1 Pharmacodynamic properties
Pharmacotherapeutic group: immune sera and immunoglobulins: immunoglobulins, normal human for extravascular administration, ATC code: J06B A01.

Human normal immunoglobulin contains mainly immunoglobulin G (IgG) having a broad spectrum of antibodies against various infectious agents.

Vivaglobin contains the immunoglobulin G antibodies present in the normal population. It is usually prepared from pooled plasma of at least 1,000 donors. It has a distribution of immunoglobulin G subclasses closely proportional to that in native human plasma.

Adequate doses of this medicinal product may restore abnormally low immunoglobulin G levels to the normal range.

5.2 Pharmacokinetic properties
With subcutaneous administration of human normal immunoglobulin, peak levels are achieved in the recipient's circulation after a delay of approximately 2 days. Data from a clinical study (n=60) show that trough levels of approximately 8 to 9 g/l (n=53) in the plasma can be maintained by weekly doses between 0.05 and 0.15 g (0.3 to 0.9 ml/kg) Vivaglobin per kg bodyweight. This is commensurate to a monthly cumulative dosage of 0.2 to 0.6 g per kg bodyweight.

IgG and IgG-complexes are broken down in cells of the reticuloendothelial system.

5.3 Preclinical safety data
There are no preclinical data considered relevant to clinical safety beyond data included in other sections of the SPC.

6. PHARMACEUTICAL PARTICULARS

6.1 List of excipients
Glycine, sodium chloride, hydrochloric acid or sodium hydroxide (in small amounts for pH adjustment), water for injections.

6.2 Incompatibilities
In the absence of compatibility studies this medicinal product must not be mixed with other medicinal products.

6.3 Shelf life
3 years

Once an ampoule or injection vial has been opened its contents are to be used immediately.

6.4 Special precautions for storage
Store in a refrigerator (+2 °C to + 8 °C) in the outer carton in order to protect from light. Do not freeze!

The product may be stored at room temperature (up to 25 °C) for a limited period of three months or until the expiry date (whichever date comes first) without being refrigerated again during this period. The new expiry date at room temperature should be noted on the carton. At the end of this period the product has to be used or discarded.

6.5 Nature and contents of container
3 ml of solution in a vial (Type I glass) with a stopper (chlorobutyl) – pack of 1 or 10 vials

5ml of solution in an ampoule (Type I glass) – pack size of 1 ampoule

10 ml of solution in a vial (Type I glass) with a stopper (chlorobutyl) – pack of 1, 10 or 20 vials

20 ml of solution in a vial (Type I glass) with a stopper (chlorobutyl) – pack of 1 vial

Not all pack sizes may be marketed.

6.6 Special precautions for disposal and other handling
Vivaglobin is a ready-for-use solution and should be administered at body temperature. Do not use solutions that are cloudy or have deposits.

The product must be inspected visually prior to administration and should not be used if there is any variation of physical appearance (see also section 3 'Pharmaceutical form').

Any unused product or waste material should be disposed of in accordance with local requirements.

7. MARKETING AUTHORISATION HOLDER
CSL Behring GmbH
Emil-von-Behring-Strasse 76
35041 Marburg
Germany

8. MARKETING AUTHORISATION NUMBER(S)
PL 15036/0016

9. DATE OF FIRST AUTHORISATION/RENEWAL OF THE AUTHORISATION
21 February 2005

10. DATE OF REVISION OF THE TEXT
31 March 2008

Volibris

(GlaxoSmithKline UK)

1. NAME OF THE MEDICINAL PRODUCT
5 mg film-coated tablets
Volibris ▼ 5 mg film-coated tablets
10 mg film-coated tablets
Volibris ▼ 10 mg film-coated tablets

2. QUALITATIVE AND QUANTITATIVE COMPOSITION
5 mg film-coated tablets
Each tablet contains 5 mg of ambrisentan.
10 mg film-coated tablets
Each tablet contains 10 mg of ambrisentan.

Excipients *5 mg film-coated tablets*
Each tablet contains lactose monohydrate (approximately 95 mg), Lecithin (Soya) (E322) (approximately 0.25 mg) and Allura red AC Aluminium Lake (E129) (approximately 0.11 mg).

10 mg film-coated tablets
Each tablet contains lactose monohydrate (approximately 90 mg), Lecithin (Soya) (E322) (approximately 0.25 mg) and Allura red AC Aluminium Lake (E129) (approximately 0.45 mg).

For a full list of excipients, see section 6.1.

3. PHARMACEUTICAL FORM
Film-coated tablet.
5 mg film-coated tablets
Pale-pink, square, convex, film-coated tablet with "GS" debossed on one side and "K2C" on the other side.
10 mg film-coated tablets
Deep-pink, oval, convex, film-coated tablet with "GS" debossed on one side and "KE3" on the other side.

4. CLINICAL PARTICULARS

4.1 Therapeutic indications
Volibris is indicated for the treatment of patients with pulmonary arterial hypertension (PAH) classified as WHO functional class II and III, to improve exercise capacity (see section 5.1). Efficacy has been shown in idiopathic PAH (IPAH) and in PAH associated with connective tissue disease.

4.2 Posology and method of administration
Treatment must be initiated by a physician experienced in the treatment of PAH.

Volibris is to be taken orally at a dose of 5 mg once daily. It is recommended that the tablet is swallowed whole and it can be taken with or without food.

Some additional efficacy has been observed with 10 mg Volibris in patients with class III symptoms, however an increase in peripheral oedema has also been observed. Patients with PAH associated with connective tissue disease may require 10 mg Volibris for optimal efficacy. Confirm that the 5 mg dose is well tolerated before considering an increase in dose to 10 mg Volibris in these patients (see sections 4.4 and 4.8).

Limited data suggest that the abrupt discontinuation of Volibris is not associated with rebound worsening of PAH.

Children and adolescents

Volibris is not recommended for use in patients below 18 years of age due to a lack of data on safety and efficacy.

Elderly

No dose adjustment is required in patients over the age of 65 (see section 5.2).

Patients with renal impairment

No dose adjustment is required in patients with renal impairment (see section 5.2). There is limited experience with Volibris in individuals with severe renal impairment (creatinine clearance <30 ml/min); initiate therapy cautiously in this subgroup and take particular care if the dose is increased to 10 mg Volibris.

Patients with hepatic impairment

Volibris has not been studied in individuals with severe hepatic impairment (with or without cirrhosis). Since the main routes of metabolism of ambrisentan are glucuronidation and oxidation with subsequent elimination in the bile, hepatic impairment would be expected to increase exposure (C_{max} and AUC) to ambrisentan. Therefore Volibris should not be initiated in patients with severe hepatic impairment, or clinically significant elevated hepatic aminotransferases (greater than 3 times the Upper Limit of Normal (>3xULN); see sections 4.3 and 4.4).

4.3 Contraindications
• Hypersensitivity to the active substance, to soya, or to any of the excipients (see sections 4.4 and 6.1).
• Pregnancy (see section 4.6).
• Women of child-bearing potential who are not using reliable contraception (see sections 4.4 and 4.6).
• Lactation (see section 4.6).
• Severe hepatic impairment (with or without cirrhosis) (see section 4.2).
• Baseline values of hepatic aminotransferases (aspartate aminotransferases (AST) and/or alanine aminotransferases (ALT)) >3xULN (see sections 4.2 and 4.4).

4.4 Special warnings and precautions for use
Volibris has not been studied in a sufficient number of patients to establish the benefit/risk balance in WHO functional class I PAH.

The efficacy of Volibris as monotherapy has not been established in patients with WHO functional class IV PAH. Therapy that is recommended at the severe stage of the disease (e.g. epoprostenol) should be considered if the clinical condition deteriorates.

Liver function

Liver function abnormalities have been associated with PAH. Hepatic enzyme elevations potentially related to therapy have been observed with endothelin receptor antagonists (ERAs) (see section 5.1). Therefore hepatic aminotransferases (ALT and AST) should be evaluated prior to initiation of Volibris. Volibris treatment should not be initiated in patients with baseline values of ALT and/or AST >3xULN (see section 4.3).

Monthly monitoring of ALT and AST is recommended. If patients develop sustained, unexplained, clinically significant ALT and/or AST elevation, or if ALT and/or AST elevation is accompanied by signs or symptoms of hepatic injury (e.g. jaundice), Volibris therapy should be discontinued.

In patients without clinical symptoms of hepatic injury or of jaundice, re-initiation of Volibris may be considered following resolution of hepatic enzyme abnormalities. The advice of a hepatologist is recommended.

Haemoglobin concentration

Reductions in haemoglobin concentrations and haematocrit have been associated with ERAs including Volibris (see section 4.8). Most of these decreases were detected during the first 4 weeks of treatment and haemoglobin generally stabilised thereafter.

Initiation of Volibris is not recommended for patients with clinically significant anaemia. It is recommended that haemoglobin and/or haematocrit levels are measured during treatment with Volibris, for example at 1 month, 3 months and periodically thereafter in line with clinical practice. If a clinically significant decrease in haemoglobin or haematocrit is observed, and other causes have been excluded, dose reduction or discontinuation of treatment should be considered.

Fluid retention

Peripheral oedema has been observed with ERAs including ambrisentan. Most cases of peripheral oedema in clinical studies with ambrisentan were mild to moderate in severity, although it appeared to occur with greater frequency and severity in patients ⩾65 years. Peripheral oedema was reported more frequently with 10 mg ambrisentan (see section 4.8).

Post-marketing reports of fluid retention occurring within weeks after starting ambrisentan have been received and, in some cases, have required intervention with a diuretic or hospitalisation for fluid management or decompensated heart failure. If patients have pre-existing fluid overload, this should be managed as clinically appropriate prior to starting ambrisentan.

If clinically significant fluid retention develops during therapy with ambrisentan, with or without associated weight gain, further evaluation should be undertaken to determine the cause, such as ambrisentan or underlying heart failure, and the possible need for specific treatment or discontinuation of ambrisentan therapy.

Women of child-bearing potential

Volibris treatment must not be initiated in women of child-bearing potential unless the result of a pre-treatment pregnancy test is negative and reliable contraception is practiced. If there is any doubt on what contraceptive advice should be given to the individual patient, consultation with a gynaecologist should be considered. Monthly pregnancy tests during treatment with Volibris are recommended (see sections 4.3 and 4.6).

Excipients

Volibris tablets contain lactose monohydrate. Patients with rare hereditary problems of galactose intolerance, the Lapp lactase deficiency or glucose-galactose malabsorption should not take this medicine.

Volibris tablets contain the azo colouring agent Allura red AC Aluminium Lake (E129), which can cause allergic reactions.

4.5 Interaction with other medicinal products and other forms of interaction

Ambrisentan does not inhibit or induce phase I or II drug metabolizing enzymes at clinically relevant concentrations in *in vitro* and *in vivo* non-clinical studies, suggesting a low potential for ambrisentan to alter the profile of medicinal products metabolized by these pathways.

The potential for ambrisentan to induce CYP3A4 activity was explored in healthy volunteers with results suggesting a lack of inductive effect of ambrisentan on the CYP3A4 isoenzyme.

Co-administration of ambrisentan with a phosphodiesterase inhibitor, either sildenafil or tadalafil (both substrates of CYP3A4) in healthy volunteers did not significantly affect the pharmacokinetics of the phosphodiesterase inhibitor or ambrisentan (see section 5.2).

Steady state administration of ketoconazole (a strong inhibitor of CYP3A4) did not result in a clinically significant increase in exposure to ambrisentan (see section 5.2).

The impact of the co-administration of Volibris with inducers of CYP3A4 and 2C19 is unknown.

Ambrisentan had no effects on the steady state pharmacokinetics and anti-coagulant activity of warfarin in a healthy volunteer study (see section 5.2). Warfarin also had no clinically significant effects on the pharmacokinetics of ambrisentan. In addition, in patients, ambrisentan had no overall effect on the weekly warfarin-type anticoagulant dose, prothrombin time (PT) and international normalized ratio (INR).

Cyclosporine A is an inhibitor of multiple metabolic enzymes and transporters. Use caution when Volibris is co-administered with cyclosporine A.

In a clinical study in healthy volunteers, steady-state dosing with ambrisentan 10 mg once daily did not significantly affect the single-dose pharmacokinetics of the ethinyl estradiol and norethindrone components of a combined oral contraceptive (see section 5.2). Based on this pharmacokinetic study, ambrisentan would not be expected to significantly affect exposure to oestrogen- or progestogen-based contraceptives.

The efficacy and safety of Volibris when co-administered with other treatments for PAH (e.g. prostanoids and phosphodiesterase type V inhibitors) has not been specifically studied in controlled clinical trials (see section 5.1). Therefore, caution is recommended in the case of co-administration.

Effect of ambrisentan on xenobiotic transporters

In vitro, ambrisentan has no inhibitory effect on the P-glycoprotein (Pgp)-mediated efflux of digoxin and is a weak substrate for Pgp-mediated efflux. Additional *in vitro* studies in rat and human hepatocytes showed that ambrisentan did not inhibit sodium-taurocholate co-transporter (NTCP), organic anion export pump (OATP), bile salt export pump (BSEP) and multi-drug resistance protein isoform-2 (MRP2). *In vitro* studies in rat hepatocytes also showed that ambrisentan has no inductive effects on Pgp, BSEP or MRP2.

Steady-state administration of ambrisentan in healthy volunteers had no clinically relevant effects on the single-dose pharmacokinetics of digoxin, a substrate for Pgp (see section 5.2).

4.6 Pregnancy and lactation

Pregnancy

Volibris is contraindicated in pregnancy (see section 4.3). Animal studies have shown that ambrisentan is teratogenic. There is no experience in humans.

Volibris treatment must not be initiated in women of child-bearing potential unless the result of a pre-treatment pregnancy test is negative and reliable contraception is practiced. Monthly pregnancy tests during treatment with Volibris are recommended.

Women receiving Volibris must be advised of the risk of foetal harm and alternative therapy initiated if pregnancy occurs (see sections 4.3, 4.4 and 5.3).

Lactation

It is not known whether ambrisentan is excreted in human breast milk. The excretion of ambrisentan in milk has not been studied in animals. Therefore lactation is contraindicated in patients taking Volibris (see section 4.3).

Male fertility

The development of testicular tubular atrophy in male animals has been linked to the chronic administration of ERAs, including ambrisentan (see section 5.3). The effect on male human fertility is not known. Chronic administration of ambrisentan was not associated with a change in plasma testosterone in clinical studies.

4.7 Effects on ability to drive and use machines

No studies on the effects on the ability to drive and use machines have been performed.

4.8 Undesirable effects

Experience from clinical studies

Safety of Volibris has been evaluated in clinical trials of more than 483 patients with PAH (see section 5.1). Adverse drug reactions (ADR) identified from 12 week placebo controlled clinical trial data are listed below by system organ class and frequency. With longer observation in uncontrolled studies (mean observation of 79 weeks), the safety profile was similar to that observed in the short term studies. Frequencies are defined as: very common (⩾ 1/10); common (⩾ 1/100 to < 1/10); uncommon (⩾1/1,000 to < 1/100); rare (⩾1/10,000 to < 1/1,000); very rare (< 1/10,000). For dose-related adverse reactions the frequency category reflects the higher dose of Volibris. Frequency categories do not account for other factors including varying study duration, pre-existing conditions and baseline patient characteristics. Adverse reaction frequency categories assigned based on clinical trial experience may not reflect the frequency of adverse events occurring during normal clinical practice. Within each frequency grouping, undesirable effects are presented in order of decreasing seriousness.

Cardiac disorders	
Palpitation	Common
Blood and lymphatic system disorders	
Anaemia (decreased haemoglobin, decreased haematocrit)	Common
Nervous system disorders	
Headache (including sinus headache, migraine)[1]	Very common
Respiratory, thoracic and mediastinal disorders	
Upper respiratory (e.g. nasal[2], sinus) congestion, sinusitis, nasopharyngitis, rhinitis	Common
Gastrointestinal disorders	
Abdominal pain	Common
Constipation	Common
Vascular disorders	
Flushing	Common
General disorders and administration site conditions	
Peripheral oedema, fluid retention[3]	Very common
Chest pain/discomfort	Common
Immune system disorders	
Hypersensitivity reactions (e.g. angioedema, rash, pruritus)	Uncommon

[1] The frequency of headache appeared higher with 10 mg Volibris.

[2] The incidence of nasal congestion was dose related during Volibris therapy.

[3] Peripheral oedema was reported more frequently with 10 mg Volibris. In clinical studies peripheral oedema was reported more commonly and tended to be more severe in patients ⩾65 years (see section 4.4).

Laboratory abnormalities

Decreased haemoglobin (see section 4.4).

The frequency of decreased haemoglobin (anaemia) was higher with 10 mg Volibris. Across the 12 week placebo controlled Phase III clinical studies, mean haemoglobin concentrations decreased for patients in the Volibris groups and were detected as early as week 4 (decrease by 0.83 g/dl); mean changes from baseline appeared to stabilise over the subsequent 8 weeks. A total of 17 patients (6.5%) in the Volibris treatment groups had decreases in haemoglobin of ⩾15% from baseline and which fell below the lower limit of normal.

Post-marketing data

In addition to adverse reactions identified from clinical studies, the following adverse reactions were identified during post-approval use of Volibris. Frequencies are defined as: 'not known' (cannot be estimated from the available data).

Nervous system disorders	
Dizziness	Not known
Cardiac disorders	
Cardiac failure[4]	Not known
Respiratory, thoracic and mediastinal disorders	
Dyspnoea[5]	Not known

[4]Most of the reported cases of cardiac failure were associated with fluid retention.

[5]Cases of worsening dyspnoea of unclear aetiology have been reported shortly after starting Volibris therapy.

4.9 Overdose

There is no experience in PAH patients of Volibris at daily doses greater than 10 mg. In healthy volunteers, single doses of 50 and 100 mg (5 to 10 times the maximum recommended dose) were associated with headache, flushing, dizziness, nausea and nasal congestion.

Due to the mechanism of action, an overdose of Volibris could potentially result in hypotension (see section 5.3). In the case of pronounced hypotension, active cardiovascular support may be required. No specific antidote is available.

5. PHARMACOLOGICAL PROPERTIES

5.1 Pharmacodynamic properties

Pharmacotherapeutic group: other anti-hypertensives, ATC code: C02KX02.

Mechanism of action

Ambrisentan is an orally active, propanoic acid-class, ERA selective for the endothelin A (ET_A) receptor. Endothelin plays a significant role in the pathophysiology of PAH.

– Ambrisentan blocks the ET_A receptor subtype, localized predominantly on vascular smooth muscle cells and cardiac myocytes. This prevents endothelin-mediated activation of second messenger systems that result in vasoconstriction and smooth muscle cell proliferation.

– The selectivity of ambrisentan for the ET_A over the ET_B receptor is expected to retain ET_B receptor mediated production of the vasodilators nitric oxide and prostacyclin.

Efficacy

Two randomised, double-blind, multi-centre, placebo controlled, Phase 3 pivotal studies were conducted (ARIES-1 and 2). ARIES-1 included 201 patients and compared Volibris 5 mg and 10 mg with placebo. ARIES-2 included 192 patients and compared Volibris 2.5 mg and 5 mg with placebo. In both studies, Volibris was added to patients' supportive/background medication, which could have included a combination of digoxin, anticoagulants, diuretics, oxygen and vasodilators (calcium channel blockers, ACE inhibitors). Patients enrolled had IPAH or PAH associated with connective tissue disease. The majority of patients had WHO functional Class II (38.4%) or Class III (55.0%) symptoms. Patients with pre-existent hepatic disease (cirrhosis or clinically significantly elevated aminotransferases) and patients using other targeted therapy for PAH (e.g. prostanoids) were excluded. Haemodynamic parameters were not assessed in these studies.

The primary endpoint defined for the Phase 3 studies was improvement in exercise capacity assessed by change from baseline in 6 minute walk distance (6MWD) at 12 weeks. In both studies, treatment with Volibris resulted in a significant improvement in 6MWD for each dose of Volibris.

The placebo-adjusted improvement in mean 6MWD at week 12 compared to baseline was 30.6 m (95% CI: 2.9 to 58.3; p=0.008) and 59.4 m (95% CI: 29.6 to 89.3; p<0.001) for the 5 mg group, in ARIES 1 and 2 respectively. The placebo-adjusted improvement in mean 6MWD at week 12 in patients in the 10 mg group in ARIES-1 was 51.4 m (95% CI: 26.6 to 76.2; p <0.001).

A pre-specified combined analysis of the Phase 3 studies (ARIES-C) was conducted. The placebo-adjusted mean improvement in 6MWD was 44.6 m (95% CI: 24.3 to 64.9; p<0.001) for the 5 mg dose, and 52.5 m (95% CI: 28.8 to 76.2; p<0.001) for the 10 mg dose.

In ARIES-2, Volibris (combined dose group) significantly delayed the time to clinical worsening of PAH compared to placebo ($p < 0.001$), the hazard ratio demonstrated a 80% reduction (95% CI: 47% to 92%). The measure included: death, lung transplantation, hospitalisation for PAH, atrial septostomy, addition of other PAH therapeutic agents and early escape criteria. A statistically significant increase (3.41 ± 6.96) was observed for the combined dose group in the physical functioning scale of the SF-36 Health Survey compared with placebo (-0.20 ± 8.14, p=0.005). Treatment with Volibris led to a statistically significant improvement in Borg Dyspnea Index (BDI) at week 12 (placebo-adjusted BDI of -1.1 (95% CI: -1.8 to -0.4; p=0.019; combined dose group)).

Long term data

Patients enrolled into ARIES 1 and 2 were eligible to enter a long term open label extension study ARIES E (n=383).

The effect of Volibris on the outcome of the disease is unknown. The observed probability of survival at 1 year for subjects receiving Volibris (combined Volibris dose group) was 95% and at 2 years was 84%.

In an open label study (AMB222), Volibris was studied in 36 patients to evaluate the incidence of increased serum aminotransferase concentrations in patients who had previously discontinued other ERA therapy due to aminotransferase abnormalities. During a mean of 53 weeks of treatment with Volibris, none of the patients enrolled had a confirmed serum ALT > 3xULN that required permanent discontinuation of treatment. Fifty percent of patients had increased from 5 mg to 10 mg Volibris during this time.

The cumulative incidence of serum aminotransferase abnormalities > 3xULN in all Phase 2 and 3 studies (including respective open label extensions) was 17 of 483 subjects over a mean exposure duration of 79.5 weeks. This is an event rate of 2.3 events per 100 patient years of exposure for Volibris.

Other clinical information

An improvement in haemodynamic parameters was observed in patients with PAH after 12 weeks (n=29) in a Phase 2 study (AMB220). Treatment with Volibris resulted in an increase in mean cardiac index, a decrease in mean pulmonary artery pressure, and a decrease in mean pulmonary vascular resistance.

No clinically meaningful effects on the pharmacokinetics of ambrisentan or sildenafil were seen during a drug-drug interaction study in healthy volunteers, and the combination was well tolerated. The number of patients who received concomitant Volibris and sildenafil in ARIES-E and AMB222 was 22 patients (5.7%) and 17 patients (47%), respectively. No additional safety concerns were identified in these patients.

5.2 Pharmacokinetic properties

Absorption

Ambrisentan is absorbed rapidly in humans. After oral administration, maximum plasma concentrations (C_{max}) of ambrisentan typically occur around 1.5 hours post-dose under both fasted and fed conditions. C_{max} and area under the plasma concentration-time curve (AUC) increase dose proportionally over the therapeutic dose range. Steady-state is generally achieved following 4 days of repeat dosing.

A food-effect study involving administration of ambrisentan to healthy volunteers under fasting conditions and with a high-fat meal indicated that the C_{max} was decreased 12% while the AUC remained unchanged. This decrease in peak concentration is not clinically significant, and therefore ambrisentan can be taken with or without food.

Distribution

Ambrisentan is highly plasma protein bound. The *in vitro* plasma protein binding of ambrisentan was, on average, 98.8% and independent of concentration over the range of 0.2 – 20 microgram/ml. Ambrisentan is primarily bound to albumin (96.5%) and to a lesser extent to alpha$_1$-acid glycoprotein.

The distribution of ambrisentan into red blood cells is low, with a mean blood: plasma ratio of 0.57 and 0.61 in males and females, respectively.

Metabolism

Ambrisentan is a non-sulphonamide (propanoic acid) ERA. Ambrisentan is glucuronidated via several UGT isoenzymes (UGT1A9S, UGT2B7S and UGT1A3S) to form ambrisentan glucuronide (13%). Ambrisentan also undergoes oxidative metabolism mainly by CYP3A4 and to a lesser extent by CYP3A5 and CYP2C19 to form 4-hydroxymethyl ambrisentan (21%) which is further glucuronidated to 4-hydroxymethyl ambrisentan glucuronide (5%). The binding affinity of 4-hydroxymethyl ambrisentan for the human endothelin receptor is 65-fold less than ambrisentan. Therefore at concentrations observed in the plasma (approximately 4% relative to parent ambrisentan), 4-hydroxymethyl ambrisentan is not expected to contribute to pharmacological activity of ambrisentan.

In vitro data have shown that at therapeutic concentrations, ambrisentan does not inhibit UGT1A1, UGT1A6, UGT1A9, UGT2B7 or cytochrome P450 enzymes 1A2, 2A6, 2B6, 2C8, 2C9, 2C19, 2D6, 2E1 and 3A4. Additional *in vitro* studies showed that ambrisentan does not inhibit NTCP, OATP or BSEP. Furthermore, ambrisentan does not induce MRP2, Pgp or BSEP.

The effects of steady-state ambrisentan (10 mg once daily) on the pharmacokinetics and pharmacodynamics of a single dose of warfarin (25 mg), as measured by PT and INR, were investigated in 20 healthy volunteers. Ambrisentan did not have any clinically relevant effects on the pharmacokinetics or pharmacodynamics of warfarin. Similarly, co-administration with warfarin did not affect the pharmacokinetics of ambrisentan (see section 4.5).

The effect of 7-day dosing of sildenafil (20 mg three times daily) on the pharmacokinetics of a single dose of ambrisentan, and the effects of 7-day dosing of ambrisentan (10 mg once daily) on the pharmacokinetics of a single dose of sildenafil were investigated in 19 healthy volunteers. With the exception of a 13% increase in sildenafil C_{max} following co-administration with ambrisentan, there were no other changes in the pharmacokinetic parameters of sildenafil, N-desmethyl-sildenafil and ambrisentan. This slight increase in sildenafil C_{max} is not considered clinically relevant (see section 4.5).

The effects of steady-state ambrisentan (10 mg once daily) on the pharmacokinetics of a single dose of tadalafil, and the effects of steady-state tadalafil (40 mg once daily) on the pharmacokinetics of a single dose of ambrisentan were studied in 23 healthy volunteers. Ambrisentan did not have any clinically relevant effects on the pharmacokinetics of tadalafil. Similarly, co-administration with tadalafil did not affect the pharmacokinetics of ambrisentan (see section 4.5).

The effects of repeat dosing of ketoconazole (400 mg once daily) on the pharmacokinetics of a single dose of 10 mg ambrisentan were investigated in 16 healthy volunteers. Exposures of ambrisentan as measured by $AUC_{(0-inf)}$ and C_{max} were increased by 35% and 20%, respectively. This change in exposure is unlikely to be of any clinical relevance and therefore Volibris may be co-administered with ketoconazole.

The effects of repeat dosing of ambrisentan (10 mg) on the pharmacokinetics of single dose digoxin were studied in 15 healthy volunteers. Multiple doses of ambrisentan resulted in slight increases in digoxin AUC_{0-last} and trough concentrations, and a 29% increase in digoxin C_{max}. The increase in digoxin exposure observed in the presence of multiple doses of ambrisentan was not considered clinically relevant, and no dose adjustment of digoxin is warranted (see section 4.5).

The effects of 12 days dosing with ambrisentan (10 mg once daily) on the pharmacokinetics of a single dose of oral contraceptive containing ethinyl estradiol (35 μg) and norethindrone (1 mg) were studied in healthy female volunteers. The Cmax and AUC(0–∞) were slightly decreased for ethinyl estradiol (8% and 4%, respectively), and slightly increased for norethindrone (13% and 14 %, respectively). These changes in exposure to ethinyl estradiol or norethindrone were small and are unlikely to be clinically significant (see section 4.5).

Elimination

Ambrisentan and its metabolites are eliminated primarily in the bile following hepatic and/or extra-hepatic metabolism. Approximately 22% of the administered dose is recovered in the urine following oral administration with 3.3% being unchanged ambrisentan. Plasma elimination half-life in humans ranges from 13.6 to 16.5 hours.

Special populations

Based on the results of a population pharmacokinetic analysis in healthy volunteers and patients with PAH, the pharmacokinetics of ambrisentan were not significantly influenced by gender or age (see section 4.2).

Renal impairment

Ambrisentan does not undergo significant renal metabolism or renal clearance (excretion). In a population pharmacokinetic analysis, creatinine clearance was found to be a statistically significant covariate affecting the oral clearance of ambrisentan. The magnitude of the decrease in oral clearance is modest (20-40%) in patients with moderate renal impairment and therefore is unlikely to be of any clinical relevance. However, caution should be used in patients with severe renal impairment (see section 4.2).

Hepatic impairment

The main routes of metabolism of ambrisentan are glucuronidation and oxidation with subsequent elimination in the bile and therefore hepatic impairment would be expected to increase exposure (C_{max} and AUC) of ambrisentan. In a population pharmacokinetic analysis, the oral clearance was shown to be decreased as a function of increasing bilirubin levels. However, the magnitude of effect of bilirubin is modest (compared to the typical patient with a bilirubin of 0.6 mg/dl, a patient with an elevated bilirubin of 4.5 mg/dl would have approximately 30% lower oral clearance of ambrisentan). The pharmacokinetics of ambrisentan in patients with severe hepatic impairment (with or without cirrhosis) has not been studied. Therefore Volibris should not be initiated in patients with severe hepatic impairment or clinically significant elevated hepatic aminotransferases (> 3xULN) (see sections 4.3 and 4.4).

5.3 Preclinical safety data

Due to the class primary pharmacologic effect, a large single dose of ambrisentan (i.e. an overdose) could lower arterial pressure and have the potential for causing hypotension and symptoms related to vasodilation.

Ambrisentan was not shown to be an inhibitor of bile acid transport or to produce overt hepatotoxicity.

Inflammation and changes in the nasal cavity epithelium have been seen in rodents after chronic administration at exposures below the therapeutic levels in humans. In dogs, slight inflammatory responses were observed following chronic high dose administration of ambrisentan at exposures greater than 20-fold that observed in patients.

Nasal bone hyperplasia of the ethmoid turbinates has been observed in the nasal cavity of rats treated with ambrisentan, at exposure levels 3-fold the clinical AUC. Nasal bone hyperplasia has not been observed with ambrisentan in mice or dogs. In the rat, hyperplasia of nasal turbinate bone is a recognised response to nasal inflammation, based on experience with other compounds.

Ambrisentan was clastogenic when tested at high concentrations in mammalian cells *in vitro*. No evidence for mutagenic or genotoxic effects of ambrisentan were seen in bacteria or in two *in vivo* rodent studies.

There were no treatment-related increases in the incidence of tumours in 2 year oral studies in rats and mice.

Testicular tubular atrophy, which was occasionally associated with aspermia, was observed in oral repeat dose toxicity and fertility studies with male rats and mice without safety margin. The testicular changes were not fully recoverable during the off-dose periods evaluated. However no testicular changes were observed in dog studies of up to 39 weeks duration at an exposure 35-fold that seen in humans based on AUC. The effect of ambrisentan on male human fertility is not known.

Ambrisentan has been shown to be teratogenic in rats and rabbits. Abnormalities of the lower jaw, tongue, and/or palate were seen at all doses tested. In addition, interventricular septal defects, trunk vessel defects, thyroid and thymus abnormalities, ossification of the basisphenoid bone and increased incidence of left umbilical artery were seen in the rat study. Teratogenicity is a suspected class effect of ERAs.

Administration of ambrisentan to female rats from late-pregnancy through lactation caused adverse events on maternal behaviour, reduced pup survival and impairment of the reproductive capability of the offspring (with observation of small testes at necropsy), at exposure 3-fold the AUC at the maximum recommended human dose.

6. PHARMACEUTICAL PARTICULARS

6.1 List of excipients

5 mg film-coated tablets

Tablet core

Lactose monohydrate

Microcrystalline cellulose

Croscarmellose sodium

Magnesium stearate

5 mg film-coated tablets

Film coat

Polyvinyl alcohol (Partially Hydrolyzed)

Talc (E553b)

Titanium dioxide (E171)

Macrogol / PEG 3350

Lecithin (Soya) (E322)

Allura red AC Aluminium Lake (E129)

10 mg film-coated tablets

Tablet core

Lactose monohydrate

Microcrystalline cellulose

Croscarmellose sodium

Magnesium stearate

10 mg film-coated tablets

Film coat

Polyvinyl alcohol (Partially Hydrolyzed)

Talc (E553b)

Titanium dioxide (E171)

Macrogol / PEG 3350

Allura red AC Aluminium Lake (E129)

Lecithin (Soya) (E322)

6.2 Incompatibilities

Not applicable.

6.3 Shelf life

2 years.

6.4 Special precautions for storage

This medicinal product does not require any special storage conditions.

6.5 Nature and contents of container

PVC/PVDC/aluminium foil blisters. Pack sizes of 10 or 30 film-coated tablets. Not all pack sizes may be marketed.

6.6 Special precautions for disposal and other handling

No special requirements.

7. MARKETING AUTHORISATION HOLDER

Glaxo Group Ltd

Greenford

Middlesex

UB6 0NN

United Kingdom

8. MARKETING AUTHORISATION NUMBER(S)

5 mg film-coated tablets

EU/1/08/451/001

EU/1/08/451/002

10 mg film-coated tablets

EU/1/08/451/003

EU/1/08/451/004

9. DATE OF FIRST AUTHORISATION/RENEWAL OF THE AUTHORISATION

21/04/2008

10. DATE OF REVISION OF THE TEXT

28 August 2009

Detailed information on this medicinal product is available on the website of the European Medicines Agency (EMEA) http://www.emea.europa.eu/.

Volmax Tablets 4mg, 8mg

(Allen & Hanburys)

1. NAME OF THE MEDICINAL PRODUCT

VOLMAX Tablets 4mg.

VOLMAX Tablets 8mg.

2. QUALITATIVE AND QUANTITATIVE COMPOSITION

Salbutamol Sulphate BP 4.82mg equivalent to Salbutamol 4mg per tablet.

Salbutamol Sulphate BP 9.64mg equivalent to Salbutamol 8mg per tablet.

3. PHARMACEUTICAL FORM

Controlled Release Tablets.

4. CLINICAL PARTICULARS

4.1 Therapeutic indications

Salbutamol is a selective Beta-2 adrenoceptor agonist.

Volmax Tablets are indicated for the treatment of asthma, bronchospasm and/or reversible airways obstruction.

Volmax Tablets are suitable oral therapy for children and adults who are unable to use an inhaler device. In these patients, the controlled-release formulation makes Volmax Tablets helpful in the management of nocturnal asthma.

4.2 Posology and method of administration

Volmax Tablets must be swallowed whole with a glass of water and not chewed or crushed.

Volmax Tablets sustain bronchodilation over a 12 hour period.

Adults

The recommended dose is one 8mg tablet twice daily. There is not need to adjust the dose in the elderly.

Children

In children aged 3 - 12 years, the recommended dose is one 4mg tablet twice daily.

For oral administration.

4.3 Contraindications

Although intravenous salbutamol and occasionally salbutamol tablets are used in the management of premature labour, uncomplicated by conditions such as placenta praevia, antepartum haemorrhage or toxaemia of pregnancy, salbutamol presentations should not be used for threatened abortion.

Volmax Tablets are contra-indicated in patients with a history of hypersensitivity to any of their components.

4.4 Special warnings and precautions for use

Bronchodilators should not be the only or main treatment in patients with severe or unstable asthma. Severe asthma requires regular medical assessment including lung function testing as patients are at risk of severe attacks and even death. Physicians should consider using oral corticosteroid therapy and/or the maximum recommended dose of inhaled corticosteroid in these patients.

Patients taking Volmax Tablets may also be receiving short-acting inhaled bronchodilators to relieve symptoms. Increasing use of bronchodilators, in particular short-acting inhaled Beta2-agonists to relieve symptoms, indicates deterioration of asthma control. If patients find that short acting relief bronchodilator treatment becomes less effective or they need more inhalations than usual, medical attention must be sought. Similarly, if patients find that treatment with Volmax becomes less effective, medical attention must be sought.

In these situations, patients should be reassessed and consideration given to the need for increased anti-inflammatory therapy (e.g. higher doses of inhaled corticosteroids or a course of oral corticosteroids). Severe exacerbations of asthma must be treated in the normal way.

Salbutamol and non-selective beta-blocking drugs, such as propranolol, should not usually be prescribed together.

Cardiovascular effects may be seen with sympathomimetic drugs, including salbutamol. There is some evidence from post-marketing data and published literature of rare occurrences of myocardial ischaemia associated with salbutamol. Patients with underlying severe heart disease (e.g. ischaemic heart disease, arrhythmia or severe heart failure) who are receiving salbutamol should be warned to seek medical advice if they experience chest pain or other symptoms of worsening heart disease. Attention should be paid to assessment of symptoms such as dyspnoea and chest pain, as they may be of either respiratory or cardiac origin.

Salbutamol should be administered cautiously to patients with thyrotoxicosis.

Potentially serious hypokalaemia may result from Beta-2 agonist therapy mainly from parenteral and nebulised administration. Particular caution is advised in acute severe asthma as this effect may be potentiated by concomitant treatment with xanthine derivatives, steroids, diuretics and hypoxia. It is recommended that serum potassium levels are monitored in such situations.

In common with other β-adrenoceptor agonists, salbutamol can induce reversible metabolic changes such as increased blood glucose levels. Diabetic patients may be unable to compensate for the increase in blood glucose and the development of ketoacidoses has been reported. Concurrent administration of corticosteroids can exaggerate this effect.

4.5 Interaction with other medicinal products and other forms of interaction

None known.

4.6 Pregnancy and lactation

Administration of drugs during pregnancy should only be considered if the expected benefit to the mother is greater than any possible risk to the foetus.

As with the majority of drugs, there is little published evidence of the safety of salbutamol in the early stages of human pregnancy but in animal studies, there was evidence of some harmful effects on the foetus at very high dose levels.

As salbutamol is probably secreted in breast milk, its use in nursing mothers requires careful consideration. It is not known whether salbutamol has a harmful effect on the neonate and so its use should be restricted to situations where it is felt that the expected benefit to the mother is likely to outweigh any potential risk to the neonate.

4.7 Effects on ability to drive and use machines

None known.

4.8 Undesirable effects

Adverse events are listed below by system organ class and frequency. Frequencies are defined as: very common (≥1/10), common (≥1/100 and <1/10), uncommon (≥1/1000 and <1/100), rare (≥1/10,000 and <1/1000) and very rare (<1/10,000) including isolated reports. Very common and common events were generally determined from clinical trial data. Rare, very rare and unknown events were generally determined from spontaneous data.

Immune System Disorders

Very rare: Hypersensitivity reactions including angioedema, urticaria, bronchospasm, hypotension and collapse.

Metabolism and Nutrition Disorders

Rare: Hypokalaemia.

Potentially serious hypokalaemia may result from *beta$_2$* agonist therapy.

Nervous System Disorders

Very common: Tremor

Common: Headache

Very rare: Hyperactivity.

Cardiac Disorders

Common: Tachycardia, palpitations

Rare: Cardiac arrhythmias including atrial fibrillation, supraventricular tachycardia and extrasystoles.

Unknown: Myocardial ischaemia* (see section 4.4)

Vascular Disorders

Rare: Peripheral vasodilatation

Musculoskeletal and Connective Tissue Disorders

Common: Muscle cramps.

Very rare: Feeling of muscle tension

* reported spontaneously in post-marketing data therefore frequency regarded as unknown

4.9 Overdose

The preferred antidote for overdosage with salbutamol is a cardio-selective beta-blocking agent but beta-blocking drugs should be used with caution in patients with a history of bronchospasm.

Hypokalaemia may occur following overdose with salbutamol. Serum potassium levels should be monitored.

5. PHARMACOLOGICAL PROPERTIES

5.1 Pharmacodynamic properties

Salbutamol is a selective Beta-2 adrenoceptor agonist. At therapeutic doses, it acts on the Beta-2 adrenoceptors of bronchial muscle.

Volmax Tablets are a controlled release formulation of salbutamol.

5.2 Pharmacokinetic properties

Salbutamol administered intravenously has a half-life of 4 to 6 hours and is cleared partly renally and partly by metabolism to the inactive 4' - 0 - sulphate (phenolic sulphate) which is also excreted primarily in the urine. The faeces are a minor route of excretion, salbutamol is bound to plasma proteins to the extent of 10%.

After oral administration, salbutamol is absorbed from the gastrointestinal tract and undergoes considerable first-pass metabolism to the phenolic sulphate. Both unchanged drug and conjugate are excreted primarily in the urine. The bioavailability of orally administered salbutamol is about 50%.

Volmax Tablets are designed to deliver 90% of their salbutamol content in vitro over 9 hours. This corresponds to a release rate of 0.8mg/h for the 8mg tablet and 0.4mg/h for the 4mg tablet.

5.3 Preclinical safety data

There are no pre-clinical data of relevance to the prescriber which are additional to that already included in other sections of the SmPC.

6. PHARMACEUTICAL PARTICULARS

6.1 List of excipients

Tablet Core:

Sodium Chloride PhEur.

Povidone BP

Croscarmellose Sodium Type A USNF

Silica Gel USNF

Magnesium Stearate PhEur.

Industrial Methylated Spirit 99% HSE

or

Ethanol IP

Purified Water PhEur.

Membrane:

Cellulose Acetate 398-10 USNF

Cellulose Acetate 320S USNF

Methylhydroxypropylcellulose PhEur.

Methylene Chloride USNF

Methyl Alcohol USNF

Colour:

Methylhydroxypropylcellulose PhEur.

Opaspray K-1-7000 HSE

Methylene Chloride USNF

Methyl Alcohol USNF

Printing Ink:

Opacode S-1-4362 HSE

6.2 Incompatibilities

None known.

6.3 Shelf life

36 months.

6.4 Special precautions for storage

Store at temperatures not exceeding 30° C.

6.5 Nature and contents of container

Double foil blister pack with a push through lid.

Pack size: 14 or 56 tablets.

6.6 Special precautions for disposal and other handling

No special instructions.

Administrative Data

7. MARKETING AUTHORISATION HOLDER

Glaxo Wellcome UK Ltd

trading as Allen & Hanburys

Stockley Park West

Uxbridge

Middlesex UB11 1BT

8. MARKETING AUTHORISATION NUMBER(S)

VOLMAX Tablets 4mg PL10949/0089

VOLMAX Tablets 8mg PL10949/0090

9. DATE OF FIRST AUTHORISATION/RENEWAL OF THE AUTHORISATION

1 August 1994.

10. DATE OF REVISION OF THE TEXT

5 June 2007

Voltarol Emulgel

(Novartis Consumer Health)

1. NAME OF THE MEDICINAL PRODUCT

Voltarol® 1.16% Emulgel®, gel

2. QUALITATIVE AND QUANTITATIVE COMPOSITION

Diethylammonium-{-o-[2,6-dichlorophenyl)-amino]-phenyl}-acetate.

1g of Voltarol Emulgel contains 11.6mg of the active substance diclofenac diethylammonium, which corresponds to 10mg diclofenac sodium.

For full list of excipients, see section 6.1

3. PHARMACEUTICAL FORM

Gel for topical administration

Oil emulsion in an aqueous gel. White to off white, soft, homogeneous, cream like

4. CLINICAL PARTICULARS

4.1 Therapeutic indications

For the local symptomatic relief of pain and inflammation in:

- trauma of the tendons, ligaments, muscles and joints, e.g. due to sprains, strains and bruises

- localised forms of soft tissue rheumatism

It is recommended that treatment be reviewed after 14 days in these indications.

For the treatment of osteoarthritis of superficial joints such as the knee.

In the treatment of osteoarthritis, therapy should be reviewed after 4 weeks.

4.2 Posology and method of administration

Adults: Voltarol Emulgel should be rubbed gently into the skin. Depending on the size of the affected site to be treated 2-4g (a circular shaped mass approximately 2.0-2.5cm in diameter) should be applied 3 - 4 times a daily. After application, the hands should be washed unless they are the site being treated.

Use in the elderly: The usual adult dosage may be used.

Children: Voltarol Emulgel is not recommended for use in children as dosage recommendations and indications for use in this group of patients have not been established.

Voltarol Emulgel is suitable for the transmission of ultrasound and may be used as a couplant in combination with ultrasound therapy. If large areas of the body are covered with gel, systemic absorption will be greater and the risk of side-effects increased, especially if the therapy is used frequently.

4.3 Contraindications

• Patients with or without chronic asthma in whom attacks of asthma, urticaria or acute rhinitis are precipitated by aspirin or other non-steroidal anti-inflammatory agents (NSAIDs).

• Hypersensitivity to the active substance or any of the excipients,

• Hypersensitivity to propylene glycol, isopropanol or other components of the gel base.

4.4 Special warnings and precautions for use

Warnings

The likelihood of systemic side effects with topical diclofenac is small compared to the frequency of side effects in patients using oral diclofenac. However when Voltarol Emulgel is applied to relatively large areas of skin over a prolonged period of time, as described in the product information on systemic forms the possibility of systemic side effects cannot be excluded.

Voltarol Emulgel contains propylene glycol, which may cause mild, localised skin irritation in some people.

Precautions

Concomitant use of oral NSAID's should be cautioned as the incidence of untoward effects, particularly systemic side effects, may increase. (See also 'Interactions')

Voltarol Emulgel should not be co-administered with other products containing diclofenac.

Voltarol Emulgel should be applied only to intact, non-diseased skin and not to skin wounds or open injuries. It should be not be used with occlusion. It should not be allowed to come into contact with the eyes or mucous membranes, and should never be taken by mouth.

Some possibility of gastro-intestinal bleeding in those with a significant history of this condition has been reported in isolated cases.

4.5 Interaction with other medicinal products and other forms of interaction

Systemic absorption of Voltarol Emulgel is low and hence the risk of an interaction is small. There are no known interactions with Voltarol Emulgel but for a list of interactions known with oral diclofenac the data sheet for oral dosage forms should be consulted.

4.6 Pregnancy and lactation

Pregnancy

Since no experience has been acquired with Voltarol Emulgel in pregnancy or lactation, it is not recommended for use in these circumstances.

During the last trimester of pregnancy the use of prostaglandin synthetase inhibitors may result in premature closure of the ductus arteriosus, or in uterine inertia.

Animal data has shown an increased incidence of dystonia and delayed parturition when drug administration is continued into late pregnancy (see section 5.3 Preclinical safety data).

Lactation

It is not known whether topical diclofenac is excreted in human milk, and Voltarol Emulgel is therefore not recommended during breast-feeding, if there are compelling reasons for using Voltarol Emugel during breast feeding it should not be applied to the breast or to large areas of skin, nor should it be used for a prolonged period.

4.7 Effects on ability to drive and use machines

None known.

4.8 Undesirable effects

Adverse reactions (Table 1) are ranked under heading of frequency, the most frequent first, using the following convention: common (≥ 1/100, < 1/10); uncommon (≥ 1/1,000, < 1/100); rare (≥ 1/10,000, < 1/1,000); very rare (< 1/10,000), including isolated reports.

Table 1

Infections and infestations:	
Very rare:	Rash pustular.
Immune system disorders:-	
Very rare cases:	Hypersensitivity, angioneurotic oedema.
Respiratory, thoracic and mediastinal disorders	
Very rare:	Asthma.
Skin and subcutaneous tissue disorders	
Common:	Rash, eczema, erythema, dermatitis (including dermatitis contact)
Rare:	Dermatitis bullous
Very rare cases:	Photosensitivity reactions (patients should be warned against excessive exposure to sunlight in order to reduce the incidence of photosensitivity)

4.9 Overdose

Signs and symptoms

The low systemic absorption of Voltarol Emulgel renders overdosage extremely unlikely. However, undesirable effects, similar to those observed following an overdose of Voltarol tablets, can be expected if Voltarol Emulgel is inadvertently ingested (1 tube of 100g contains the equivalent of 1000mg of diclofenac sodium). In the event of accidental ingestion, resulting in significant systemic side-effects, general therapeutic measures normally adopted to treat poisoning with non-steroidal anti-inflammatory drugs should be used.

Treatment

Management of overdosage with NSAIDs essentially consists of supportive and symptomatic measures. There is no typical clinical picture resulting from Voltarol overdosage. Supportive and symptomatic treatment should be given for complications such as hypotension, renal failure, convulsions, gastro-intestinal irritation, and respiratory depression; specific therapies such as forced diuresis, dialysis or haemoperfusion are probably of no help in eliminating NSAIDs due to their high rate of protein binding and extensive metabolism.

5. PHARMACOLOGICAL PROPERTIES

5.1 Pharmacodynamic properties

Pharmacotherapeutic group: Topical products for joint and muscular pain, anti inflammatory preparations, non-steroids for topical use (ATC code M02A A15)

Voltarol Emulgel is a non-steroidal anti-inflammatory (NSAID) and analgesic preparation designed for external application. Due to an aqueous-alcoholic base the gel exerts a soothing and cooling effect.

5.2 Pharmacokinetic properties

When Voltarol Emulgel is applied locally, the active substance is absorbed through the skin. In healthy volunteers approximately 6% of the dose applied is absorbed, as determined by urinary excretion of diclofenac and its hydroxylated metabolites. Findings in patients confirm that diclofenac penetrates inflamed areas following local application of Voltarol Emulgel.

After topical administration of Voltarol Emulgel to hand and knee joints diclofenac can be measured in plasma, synovial tissue and synovial fluid. Maximum plasma concentrations of diclofenac are about 100 times lower than after oral administration of Voltarol.

5.3 Preclinical safety data

None known

6. PHARMACEUTICAL PARTICULARS

6.1 List of excipients

Diethylamine, carbomer, macrogol cetostearyl ether, cocyl caprylocaprate, isopropyl alcohol, liquid paraffin heavy, perfume creme 45, propylene glycol dist., and water.

6.2 Incompatibilities

None known.

6.3 Shelf life

Three years.

6.4 Special precautions for storage

Protect from heat (store below 30°C).

Voltarol Emulgel should be kept out of reach and sight of children.

6.5 Nature and contents of container

Aluminium tubes with protective inner coating, available in packs of 20g and 100g

6.6 Special precautions for disposal and other handling

None

7. MARKETING AUTHORISATION HOLDER

Novartis Consumer Health UK Ltd.

Trading as:

Novartis Consumer Health

Wimblehurst Road

Horsham

West Sussex

RH12 5AB

8. MARKETING AUTHORISATION NUMBER(S)

PL 00030/0420

9. DATE OF FIRST AUTHORISATION/RENEWAL OF THE AUTHORISATION

11 July 1997

10. DATE OF REVISION OF THE TEXT

24 January 2007

Legal Category

POM

Voltarol Gel Patch

(Novartis Consumer Health)

1. NAME OF THE MEDICINAL PRODUCT

Voltarol® Gel Patch 1 %, medicated plaster

2. QUALITATIVE AND QUANTITATIVE COMPOSITION

Each 10 cm × 14 cm medicated plaster contains diclofenac epolamine corresponding to 140 mg of diclofenac sodium (1% w/w).

For excipients, see 6.1.

3. PHARMACEUTICAL FORM

Medicated plaster.

White to pale yellow paste spread as a uniform layer onto unwoven support.

4. CLINICAL PARTICULARS

4.1 Therapeutic indications

Local symptomatic treatment of pain in epicondylitis and ankle sprain.

4.2 Posology and method of administration

Cutaneous use only

Article I. Posology

Adults

- Treatment of ankle sprains: 1 application a day

- Treatment of epicondylitis: 1 application morning and evening

Article II. Duration of administration

Voltarol Gel Patch is to be used for as short as possible depending on the indication:

- Treatment of ankle sprains: 3 days

- Treatment of epicondylitis: max. 14 days.

If there is no improvement, during the recommended duration of treatment, a doctor should be consulted.

Elderly

This medication should be used with caution in elderly patients who are more prone to adverse events. See also Section 4.4.

Children

Since no specific study has been performed, the use of Voltarol Gel Patch in children under 15 years old is not recommended.

Patients with hepatic or renal insufficiency

For the use of Voltarol Gel Patch in patients with hepatic or renal insufficiency see section 4.4.

Article III. Method of administration

Cut the envelope containing the medicated plaster as indicated. Remove one medicated plaster, remove the plastic film used to protect the adhesive surface and apply it to painful joint or region. If necessary it can be held in place with an elastic net. Carefully reseal the envelope with the sliding closure.

The plaster should be used whole.

4.3 Contraindications

This medicinal product is contraindicated in the following cases:

- Hypersensitivity to diclofenac, acetylsalicylic acid or other non-steroidal anti-inflammatory drugs (NSAIDs) or any excipients of the finished medicinal product.

- damaged skin, whatever the lesion involved: exudative dermatitis, eczema, infected lesion, burn or wound.

- from the beginning of the 6th month of pregnancy (see 4.6 Pregnancy and lactation).

- Patients with active peptic ulceration.

4.4 Special warnings and precautions for use

- The medicated plaster should not come into contact with or be applied to the mucosae or the eyes.

- Not for use with occlusive dressing.

- Discontinue the treatment immediately if a skin rash develops after applying the medicated plaster.

- Do not administer concurrently, by either the topical or the systemic route, any medicinal product containing diclofenac or other NSAIDs.

- Although systemic effects should be low, the plaster should be used with caution in patients with renal, cardiac or hepatic impairment, history of peptic ulceration or inflammatory bowel disease or bleeding diathesis. Non-steroidal anti-inflammatory drugs should be used with particular caution in elderly patients who are more prone to adverse events.

- This medicinal product contains methylparahydroxybenzoate and propylparahydroxybenzoate. It may cause allergic reactions (possibly delayed). It also contains propylene glycol, which may cause skin irritation.

- Patients should be warned against exposure to direct and solarium sunlight in order to reduce the risk of photosensitivity.

- Bronchospasm may be precipitated in patients suffering from or with a previous history of bronchial asthma or allergenic disease or allergy to acetylsalicylic acid or other NSAID. The medicated plaster should be used with caution in patients with or without chronic asthma in whom attacks of asthma, urticaria or acute rhinitis are precipitated by aspirin or other nonsteroidal anti-inflammatory agents (see 4.3 Contraindications).

4.5 Interaction with other medicinal products and other forms of interaction

In view of the low rate of systemic transfer during normal use of the medicated plasters, the drug interactions reported for oral diclofenac are unlikely to be observed.

4.6 Pregnancy and lactation

By analogy with the other routes of administration

Pregnancy

There is insufficient experience for the use during pregnancy. Animal studies have shown reproductive toxicity (see section 5.3). The potential risk for humans is unknown. Therefore Voltarol Gel Patch should be avoided during the first 5 months of pregnancy and is contra-indicated from the beginning of the 6th month of pregnancy.

During the last trimester of pregnancy, the use of prostaglandine synthetase inhibitors may result in:

- Inhibition of uterine contractions, prolongation of pregnancy and delivery
- Pulmonary and cardiac toxicity in the foetus (pulmonary hypertension with preterm closing of the ductus arteriosus)
- Renal insufficiency in the foetus with oligohydramnios
- Increased possibility of bleeding in the mother and child and increased oedema formation in the mother.

Lactation

Experimental data regarding excretion of diclofenac epolamine in human or animal milk are not available therefore, Voltarol Gel Patch is not recommended in nursing mothers.

4.7 Effects on ability to drive and use machines

Patients who experienced dizziness or other central nervous disturbances while taking NSAID's should refrain from driving or operating machinery, but this would be very unlikely using topical preparations such as Voltarol Gel Patch.

4.8 Undesirable effects

Skin disorders are commonly reported.

Skin: pruritus, redness, erythema (including in very rare cases erythema bullosum), rashes, application site reactions, allergic dermatitis.

1252 patients were treated with Voltarol Gel Patch and 734 with Placebo in clinical trials. The following adverse drug reactions were reported:

(see Table 1 below)

Undesirable effects may be reduced by using the minimum effective dose for the shortest possible duration.

In patients using topical NSAID preparations, in isolated cases, generalised skin rash, hypersensitivity reactions such as angioedema and reactions of anaphylactic type and photosensitivity reactions have been reported.

Systemic absorption of diclofenac is very low compared with plasma levels obtained following administration of oral forms of diclofenac and the likelihood of systemic side-effects reactions (like gastric and renal disorders) occurring with topical diclofenac is very small compared with the frequency of side-effects associated with oral diclofenac. However, where Voltarol Gel Patch is applied to a relatively large area of skin and over a prolonged period, the possibility of systemic side-effects cannot be excluded.

4.9 Overdose

Not applicable

5. PHARMACOLOGICAL PROPERTIES

5.1 Pharmacodynamic properties

Pharmacotherapeutic group: Antiinflammatory preparations, non-steroids for topical use.

ATC Code: M02AA15

Diclofenac hydroxyethylpyrrolidine or diclofenac epolamine is a water soluble salt of diclofenac.

Diclofenac is a nonsteroidal anti-inflammatory drug derived from phenylacetic acid which belongs to the aryl carboxylic acid group of compounds.

In the form of a medicated plaster, it has topical anti-inflammatory and analgesic activity.

5.2 Pharmacokinetic properties

Following cutaneous application of the medicated plaster, diclofenac epolamine is absorbed through the skin.

The absorption kinetics at steady state show a prolonged release of the active ingredient with a maximum diclofenac plasma level (Cmax) of 17.4 ±13.5 ng/ml, which is reached after about 5 hours (Tmax 5.4±3.7 hours).

Diclofenac is extensively bound to plasma protein (about 99 %).

Systemic transfer in healthy volunteers when using the medicated plaster, compared with oral forms of diclofenac, is of the order of 2%, as estimated from the urinary excretion of the drug and its metabolites and from a between study comparison.

5.3 Preclinical safety data

In the rat and rabbit, diclofenac epolamine, epolamine monosubstance and N-oxide epolamine (main metabolite of epolamine in humans) have caused embryotoxicity and increased embryolethality after oral use.

Other preclinical data reveal no special hazard for humans, beyond the information included in other sections of the SPC.

6. PHARMACEUTICAL PARTICULARS

6.1 List of excipients

Supporting layer:

Unwoven polyester support.

Adhesive layer (active Gel):

Gelatin, povidone (K90), liquid sorbitol (non crystallising), heavy kaolin, titanium dioxide (E171), propylene glycol, methyl parahydroxybenzoate (E218), propyl parahydroxybenzoate (E216), disodium edetate (E385), tartaric acid, aluminium glycinate, carmellose sodium, sodium polyacrylate, 1,3-butylene glycol, polysorbate 80, Dalin PH perfume (propylene glycol, benzyl salicylate, phenylethyl alcohol, alpha amylcinnamic aldehyde, hydroxycitronellal, phenyethyl phenylacetate, cinnamyl acetate, benzyl acetate, terpineol, cinnamic alcohol, cyclamenaldehyde), purified water.

6.2 Incompatibilities

Not applicable.

6.3 Shelf life

3 years.

After first opening the sealed envelope: 3 months.

6.4 Special precautions for storage

Do not store above 25°C.

6.5 Nature and contents of container

Sealed envelopes made of paper/PE/aluminium/ethylene and methacrylic acid copolymer contain 2 or 5 medicated plasters.

Pack size: 2, 5, 10 and 14 medicated plasters per box.

Not all pack sizes may be marketed.

6.6 Special precautions for disposal and other handling

Remaining active ingredient of the plaster may pose a risk to the aquatic environment. Do not flush used plasters down the toilet. The plasters should be disposed of according to local requirements.

7. MARKETING AUTHORISATION HOLDER

Novartis Consumer Health
Wimblehurst Road
Horsham, West Sussex
RH12 5AB

8. MARKETING AUTHORISATION NUMBER(S)

PL 00030/ 0206

9. DATE OF FIRST AUTHORISATION/RENEWAL OF THE AUTHORISATION

10 March 2004

10. DATE OF REVISION OF THE TEXT

14 November 2005

Legal category

POM

Table 1

System Organ Class	Very Common (>1/10)	Common (>1/100, <1/10)	Uncommon (>1/1000, <1/100)	Rare (>1/10'000, <1/1000)
Skin and subcutaneous tissue disorders		2.95%		
- Pruritus		2.3%		
- Redness			0.3%	
- Erythema				0.05%
- Dermatitis allergic			0.15%	
- Petechiae			0.1%	
- Dry skin				0.05%
General disorders and administration site conditions		1.05%		
- Application site rash			0.5%	
- Application site reaction			0.4%	
- Feeling hot			0.1%	
- Application site edema				0.05%

Voltarol Pain-eze® Tablets

(Novartis Consumer Health)

1. NAME OF THE MEDICINAL PRODUCT

Voltarol Pain-eze® Tablets

2. QUALITATIVE AND QUANTITATIVE COMPOSITION

Each tablet contains 12.5 mg of diclofenac potassium.

For a full list of excipients, see section 6.1.

3. PHARMACEUTICAL FORM

White capsule-shaped film-coated tablet

4. CLINICAL PARTICULARS

4.1 Therapeutic indications

Short term relief of headache, dental pain, period pain, rheumatic pain, muscular pain and backache and the symptoms of colds and flu, including fever.

4.2 Posology and method of administration

Adults and children aged 14 years and over:

Initially two tablets, followed by one or two tablets every 4 to 6 hours as needed. No more than 6 tablets (75 mg) should be taken in any 24 hour period.

Voltarol Pain-eze Tablets should not be used for longer than 3 days. If symptoms persist or worsen consult your doctor.

The tablets should be swallowed whole with a drink of water.

Children and Adolescents:

Voltarol Pain-eze Tablets are not to be used in children and adolescents under 14 years of age.

4.3 Contraindications

- Known hypersensitivity to diclofenac or to any of the excipients. Patients in whom attacks of asthma, urticaria, angioedema, or acute rhinitis are precipitated by aspirin or other non-steroidal anti-inflammatory drugs such as ibuprofen.
- Gastric or intestinal ulcer, bleeding or perforation.
- Pregnancy or breastfeeding (see section 4.6 Pregnancy and lactation).
- Severe hepatic, renal or cardiac failure (see section 4.4 Special warnings and special precautions for use).
- Concomitant use of anticoagulants and antiplatelets (see section 4.5 Interactions)
- Use with concomitant NSAIDs including cyclo-oxygenase-2 specific inhibitors (see section 4.5 Interactions)

4.4 Special warnings and precautions for use

Warnings

Gastrointestinal bleeding, ulceration or perforation, which can be fatal, have been reported with all NSAIDs and may occur at any time during treatment, with or without warning symptoms or a previous history of serious gastrointestinal events. They generally have more serious consequences in the elderly. If gastrointestinal bleeding or ulceration occur in patients receiving diclofenac, the medicinal product should be withdrawn.

Serious skin reactions, some of them fatal, including exfoliative dermatitis, Stevens-Johnson syndrome and toxic epidermal necrolysis, have been reported very rarely in association with the use of NSAIDs, including diclofenac (see section 4.8 Undesirable effects). Patients appear to be at highest risk of these reactions early in the course of therapy, the onset of the reaction occurring in the majority of cases within the first month of treatment. Diclofenac should be discontinued at the first appearance of skin rash, mucosal lesions or any other sign of hypersensitivity.

As with other NSAIDs, allergic reactions, including anaphylactic/anaphylactoid reactions, can occur in rare cases without earlier exposure to diclofenac.

In common with other NSAIDs, diclofenac may mask the signs and symptoms of infection due to its pharmacodynamic properties.

Precautions

General

Undesirable effects may be minimised by using the lowest effective dose for the shortest duration necessary to control symptoms (see *GI* and *Cardiovascular* risks below).

The concomitant use of diclofenac with systemic NSAIDs, including cyclooxygenase-2 selective inhibitors, should be avoided due to the absence of any evidence demonstrating synergistic benefits and the potential for additive undesirable effects.

Caution is indicated in the elderly. In particular, it is recommended that the lowest effective dose be used in frail elderly patients or those with a low body weight.

Voltarol Pain-eze Tablets contain lactose and therefore are not recommended for patients with rare hereditary problems of galactose intolerance, of severe lactase deficiency or of glucose-galactose malabsorption.

Caution (discussion with doctor or pharmacist) is required prior to starting treatment in patients with a history of hypertension and/or heart failure as fluid retention, hypertension and oedema have been reported in association with NSAIDs therapy (see *Renal effects* below).

Pre-existing asthma

In patients with asthma, seasonal allergic rhinitis, swelling of nasal mucosa (i.e. nasal polypus), chronic obstructive pulmonary disease or chronic infection of the respiratory tract (especially if linked to allergic rhinitis-like symptoms), reactions to NSAIDs such as asthma exacerbations (so-called intolerance to analgesics / analgesics-asthma), angioedema or urticaria are more frequent than in other patients.

Gastrointestinal effects

As with all NSAIDs, close medical surveillance is imperative and caution should be exercised when prescribing diclofenac in patients with symptoms indicative of gastrointestinal (GI) disorders or with a history suggestive of gastric or intestinal ulceration, bleeding or perforation (see section 4.8 Undesirable effects). The risk of GI bleeding is higher with increasing NSAID doses and in patients with a history of ulcer, particularly if complicated with haemorrhage or perforation and in the elderly.

Patients with a history of GI toxicity, particularly the elderly, should report any unusual abdominal symptoms (especially GI bleeding). Caution is recommended in patients receiving concomitant medications which could increase the risk of ulceration or bleeding, such as systemic corticosteroids, anticoagulants, anti-platelet agents or selective serotonin-reuptake inhibitors (see section 4.5 Interaction with other medicinal products and other forms of interaction).

Close medical surveillance should also be exercised in patients with ulcerative colitis or Crohn's disease, as their condition may be exacerbated (see section 4.8 Undesirable effects).

Cardiovascular and cerebrovascular effects

Clinical trial and epidemiological data suggest that use of diclofenac, particularly at high doses (150 mg daily) and in long-term treatment may be associated with a small increased risk of arterial thrombotic events (for example myocardial infarction or stroke). Available data do not suggest an increased risk with use of low dose diclofenac (up to 75 mg/day) up to 3 days for relief of pain or fever.

Hepatic effects

Close medical surveillance is required when prescribing diclofenac to patients with impaired hepatic function, as their condition may be exacerbated.

As with other NSAIDs, values of one or more liver enzymes may increase. In the case of diclofenac being prescribed for a prolonged period, regular monitoring of hepatic function is indicated as a precautionary measure. If abnormal liver function tests persist or worsen, if clinical signs or symptoms consistent with liver disease develop, or if other manifestations occur (e.g. eosinophilia, rash), diclofenac should be discontinued. Hepatitis may occur without prodromal symptoms.

Caution is called for when using diclofenac in patients with hepatic porphyria, since it may trigger an attack.

Renal effects

Caution is called for in patiens with impaired renal function, particularly the elderly and patients receiving concomitant treatment with diuretics or medicinal products that can significantly impact renal function and in those patients with substantial extracellular volume depletion.

As fluid retention and oedema have been reported in association with NSAID therapy, particular caution is called for in elderly patients receiving concomitant treatment with diuretics or medicinal products that can significantly impact renal function, and in those patients with substantial extracellular volume depletion from any cause, e.g. before or after major surgery (see section 4.3 Contraindications). Monitoring of renal function is recommended as a precautionary measure when using diclofenac in such cases. Discontinuation of therapy is usually followed by recovery to the pre-treatment state.

Haematological effects

Like other NSAIDs, diclofenac may temporarily inhibit platelet aggregation. Patients with defects of haemostasis should be carefully monitored.

Dermatological effects

Serious skin reactions, some of them fatal, including exfoliative dermatitis, Stevens Johnson syndrome, and toxic epidermal necrolysis, have been reported very rarely in association with the use of NSAIDs (see section 4.8). Patients appear to be at highest risk for these reactions early in the course of therapy: the onset of the reaction occurring in the majority of cases within the first month of treatment. Voltarol Pain-eze Tablets should be discontinued at the first appearance of skin rash, mucosal lesions, or any other sign of hypersensitivity.

The label will state:

Read the enclosed leaflet before taking this medicine.

Do not take if you:

- have or have ever had a stomach ulcer, perforation or bleeding
- are allergic to diclofenac or any other ingredient of the product, acetylsalicylic acid, ibuprofen or other related painkillers
- are taking other NSAID painkillers, or aspirin
- are pregnant or breastfeeding

Speak to a pharmacist or your doctor before taking this product if you:

- have or have had asthma, diabetes, high cholesterol, high blood pressure, a stroke, liver, heart, kidney or bowel problems
- are intolerant to some sugars
- are on a controlled potassium diet
- are a smoker

If symptoms persist or worsen, consult your doctor.

4.5 Interaction with other medicinal products and other forms of interaction

Lithium and digoxin: Diclofenac may increase plasma concentrations of lithium and digoxin.

Diuretics and antihypertensive agents: Like other NSAIDs, concomitant use of diclofenac with diuretics or antihypertensive agents (e.g. beta-blockers, angiotensin converting enzyme (ACE) inhibitors) may cause a decrease in their antihypertensive effect. Therefore, the combination should be administered with caution and patients, especially the elderly, should have their blood pressure periodically monitored. Patients should be adequately hydrated and consideration should be given to monitoring of renal function after initiation of concomitant therapy and periodically thereafter, particularly for diuretics and ACE inhibitors due to the increased risk of nephrotoxicity. Concomitant treatment with potassium-sparing diuretics may be associated with increased serum potassium levels, which should therefore be monitored frequently (see section 4.4 Special warnings and special precautions for use).

Other NSAIDs** including* cyclooxygenase-2 selective inhibitors ***and corticosteroids:

Co-administration of diclofenac with aspirin or corticosteroids may increase the risk of gastrointestinal bleeding or ulceration. Avoid concomitant use of two or more NSAIDs (see section 4.4 Special warnings and special precautions for use).

Selective serotonin reuptake inhibitors (SSRIs) and anti-platelet agents: Increased risk of gastrointestinal bleeding (see section 4.4 Special warnings and special precautions for use).

Antidiabetics: Clinical studies have shown that diclofenac can be given together with oral antidiabetic agents without influencing their clinical effect. However, there have been isolated reports of both hypoglycaemic and hyperglycaemic effects necessitating changes in the dosage of the antidiabetic agents during treatment with diclofenac. Monitoring of the blood glucose level is recommended as a precautionary measure during concomitant therapy.

Methotrexate: Caution is recommended when NSAIDs are administered less than 24 hours before or after treatment with methotrexate, since blood concentrations of methotrexate may rise and the toxicity of this substance be increased.

Ciclosporin and tacrolimus: Diclofenac, like other NSAIDs, may increase the nephrotoxicity of ciclosporin due to the effect on renal prostaglandins. Therefore, it should be given at doses lower than those that would be used in patients not receiving ciclosporin or tacrolimus.

Quinolone antibacterials: There have been isolated reports of convulsions which may have been due to concomitant use of quinolones and NSAIDs.

4.6 Pregnancy and lactation

Pregnancy

The use of diclofenac in pregnant women has not been studied. Therefore, Voltarol Pain-eze Tablets should not be used during pregnancy except on the advice of a doctor.

Lactation

Like other NSAIDs, diclofenac passes into the breast milk in small amounts. Therefore, Voltarol Pain-eze Tablets should not be administered during breast feeding in order to avoid undesirable effects in the infant.

Fertility

As with other NSAIDs, the use of diclofenac may impair female fertility and is not recommended in women attempting to conceive. In women who have difficulties conceiving or who are undergoing investigation of infertility, withdrawal of diclofenac should be considered.

4.7 Effects on ability to drive and use machines

Usually there is no effect at the recommended low-dose and short duration of treatment. However patients experiencing visual disturbances, dizziness, vertigo, somnolence or other central nervous system disturbances while taking diclofenac should refrain from driving or using machines.

4.8 Undesirable effects

Adverse reactions (Table 1) are ranked under heading of frequency, the most frequent first, using the following convention: common (≥ 1/100, < 1/10); uncommon (≥ 1/1,000, < 1/100); rare (≥ 1/10,000, < 1/1,000); very rare (< 1/10,000), including isolated reports.

Available data do not suggest an increased risk with use of low dose diclofenac (up to 75 mg/day) for up to 3 days treatment for the relief of pain or fever

Table 1

Blood and lymphatic system disorders	
Very rare:	Thrombocytopenia, leukopenia, anaemia (including haemolytic anaemia and aplastic anaemia), agranulocytosis.
Immune system disorders	
Rare:	Hypersensitivity, anaphylactic and anaphylactoid reaction (including hypotension and shock).
Very rare:	Angioneurotic oedema (including face oedema).
Psychiatric disorders	
Very rare:	Disorientation, depression, insomnia, nightmare, irritability, psychotic disorder.
Nervous system disorders	
Common:	Headache, dizziness.
Rare:	Somnolence.
Very rare:	Paraesthesia, memory impairment, convulsion, anxiety, tremor, aseptic meningitis, taste disturbances, cerebrovascular accident.
Eye disorders	
Very rare:	Visual disturbance, vision blurred, diplopia.
Ear and labyrinth disorders	
Common:	Vertigo.
Very rare:	Tinnitus, hearing impaired.
Cardiac disorders	
Very rare:	Palpitations, chest pain, cardiac failure, myocardial infarction.
Vascular disorders	
Very rare:	Hypertension, vasculitis.
Respiratory, thoracic and mediastinal disorders	
Rare:	Asthma (including dyspnoea).
Very rare:	Pneumonitis.
Gastrointestinal disorders	
Common:	Nausea, vomiting, diarrhoea, dyspepsia, abdominal pain, flatulence, anorexia.

Rare:	Gastritis, gastrointestinal haemorrhage, Haematemesis, diarrhoea, hemorrhagic melaena, gastrointestinal ulcer (with or without bleeding or perforation).
Very rare:	Colitis, (including haemorrhagic colitis and exacerbation of ulcerative colitis or Crohn's disease), constipation, stomatitis, glossitis, oesophageal disorder, diaphragm-like intestinal strictures, pancreatitis.
Hepatobiliary disorders	
Common:	Transaminases increased.
Rare:	Hepatitis, jaundice, liver disorder.
Very rare:	Fulminant hepatitis
Skin and subcutaneous tissue disorders	
Common:	Rash.
Rare:	Urticaria.
Very rare:	Bullous eruptions, eczema, erythema, erythema multiforme, Stevens-Johnson syndrome, toxic epidermal necrolysis (Lyell's syndrome), dermatitis exfoliative, loss of hair, photosensitivity reaction, purpura, allergic purpura, pruritus.
Renal and urinary disorders	
Very rare:	Acute renal failure, haematuria, proteinuria, nephrotic syndrome, interstitial nephritis, renal papillary necrosis.
General disorders and administration site conditions	
Rare:	Oedema.

Clinical trial and epidemiological data suggest that use of diclofenac (particularly at high doses 150 mg daily and in long-term treatment) may be associated with a small increased risk of arterial thrombotic events (for example myocardial infarction or stroke) (see section 4.4).

4.9 Overdose

Symptoms

There is no typical clinical picture resulting from diclofenac overdosage. Overdose can cause symptoms such as vomiting, gastrointestinal haemorrhage, diarrhoea, dizziness, tinnitus or convulsions. In the event of significant poisoning, acute renal failure and liver damage are possible.

Therapeutic measures

Management of acute poisoning with NSAIDs essentially consists of supportive measures and symptomatic treatment. These should be given for complications such as hypotension, renal failure, convulsions, gastrointestinal disorder, and respiratory depression.

Special measures such as forced diuresis, dialysis or haemoperfusion are probably of no help in eliminating NSAIDs due to the high protein binding and extensive metabolism.

Activated charcoal may be considered in case of a potentially toxic overdose, and gastric decontamination (e.g. vomiting, gastric lavage) in case of a potentially life-threatening overdose.

5. PHARMACOLOGICAL PROPERTIES

5.1 Pharmacodynamic properties

Pharmacotherapeutic group: Anti-inflammatory and anti-rheumatic products, non-steroids, acetic acid derivatives and related substances (ATC code M01A B05).

Voltarol Pain-eze Tablets contain diclofenac potassium, a non-steroidal anti-inflammatory drug (NSAID) with pronounced analgesic, anti-inflammatory and antipyretic properties. Inhibition of prostaglandin biosynthesis is considered fundamental to its mechanism of action. Prostaglandins play a major role in causing inflammation, pain and fever.

Diclofenac potassium in vitro does not suppress proteoglycan biosynthesis in cartilage at concentrations equivalent to those reached in humans.

5.2 Pharmacokinetic properties

Absorption

Diclofenac is rapidly and completely absorbed. Following ingestion of two 12.5 mg coated tablets, mean peak plasma concentrations of 2.15 μmol/L are attained after approximately 30 minutes (median Tmax).

The amount absorbed is in linear proportion to the size of the dose.

Since about half of diclofenac is metabolised during its first passage through the liver ("first pass" effect), the area under the concentration curve is about half as large following oral administration as it is following a parenteral dose of equal size.

Pharmacokinetic behaviour does not change after repeated administration. No accumulation occurs provided the recommended dosage intervals are observed.

Distribution

99.7% of diclofenac binds to serum proteins, mainly to albumin (99.4%). The apparent volume of distribution is 0.12 to 0.17 L/kg.

Diclofenac enters the synovial fluid, where maximum concentrations are measured 2 to 4 hours after peak plasma values have been reached. The apparent half-life for elimination from the synovial fluid is 3 to 6 hours. Two hours after reaching peak plasma levels, concentrations of the active substance are already higher in the synovial fluid than in the plasma, and they remain higher for up to 12 hours.

Biotransformation

Biotransformation of diclofenac takes place partly by glucuronidation of the intact molecule, but mainly by single and multiple hydroxylation and methoxylation, resulting in several phenolic metabolites, most of which are converted to glucuronide conjugates. Two of these phenolic metabolites are biologically active, but to a much lesser extent than diclofenac.

Elimination

Total systemic clearance of diclofenac from plasma is 263 ± 56 mL/min. The terminal half-life in plasma is 1 to 2 hours. Four of the metabolites, including the two active ones, also have short plasma half-lives of 1 to 3 hours. A fifth metabolite, 3'-hydroxy-4'-methoxy-diclofenac, has a much longer plasma half-life. This metabolite is virtually inactive.

About 60% of the administered dose is excreted in the urine as the glucuronide conjugate of the intact molecule and as metabolites, most of which are also converted to glucuronide conjugates. Less than 1% is excreted as unchanged substance. The rest of the dose is eliminated as metabolites through the bile in the faeces.

Characteristics in patients

No relevant age-dependent differences in the drug's absorption, metabolism, or excretion have been observed.

In patients suffering from renal impairment, no accumulation of the unchanged active substance can be inferred from the single dose kinetics when applying the usual dosage schedule. At a creatinine clearance of less than 10 mL/min, the calculated steady-state plasma levels of the hydroxy metabolites are about 4 times higher than in normal subjects. However, the metabolites are ultimately cleared through the bile.

In patients with chronic hepatitis or non-decompensated cirrhosis, the kinetics and metabolism of diclofenac are the same as in patients without liver disease.

5.3 Preclinical safety data

Preclinical data from acute and repeated dose toxicity studies, as well as from genotoxicity, mutagenicity, and carcinogenicity studies with diclofenac revealed no specific hazard for humans at the intended therapeutic doses. There was no evidence that diclofenac had a teratogenic potential in mice, rats or rabbits.

6. PHARMACEUTICAL PARTICULARS

6.1 List of excipients

Core: silica, lactose, maize starch, sodium starch glycolate, polyvidone, microcrystalline cellulose, magnesium stearate.

Coating: methylhydroxypropylcellulose, titanium dioxide, Macrogol, polysorbate, maltodextrin.

6.2 Incompatibilities

Not applicable

6.3 Shelf life

3 years

6.4 Special precautions for storage

Do not store above 25°C.

6.5 Nature and contents of container

PVC/PE/PVDC/Aluminium blisters.

Pack size: 18 tablets

6.6 Special precautions for disposal and other handling

No special requirements

7. MARKETING AUTHORISATION HOLDER

Novartis Consumer Health

Wimblehurst Road

Horsham

West Sussex, RH12 5AB

8. MARKETING AUTHORISATION NUMBER(S)

PL 00030/0073

9. DATE OF FIRST AUTHORISATION/RENEWAL OF THE AUTHORISATION

17 June 2008

10. DATE OF REVISION OF THE TEXT

17 June 2008

Legal category: P

Warticon Cream

(Stiefel Laboratories (UK) Limited)

1. NAME OF THE MEDICINAL PRODUCT
Warticon 0.15% w/w Cream

2. QUALITATIVE AND QUANTITATIVE COMPOSITION
Podophyllotoxin 1.5 mg/g (0.15% w/w).

For excipients, see 6.1

3. PHARMACEUTICAL FORM
Topical cream

A homogenous white cream.

4. CLINICAL PARTICULARS
4.1 Therapeutic indications
Route of administration: Topical

For the topical treatment of condylomata acuminata affecting the penis and the external female genitalia.

4.2 Posology and method of administration
The affected area should be thoroughly washed with soap and water, and dried prior to application.

Using a fingertip, the cream is applied twice daily for 3 days using only enough cream to just cover each wart.

Residual warts should be treated with further courses of twice daily applications for three days at weekly intervals, if necessary for a total of 4 weeks of treatment.

Where lesions are greater than 4 cm^2, it is recommended that treatment takes place under the direct supervision of medical staff.

4.3 Contraindications
Known hypersensitivity to any of the ingredients

Open wounds eg. Following surgical procedures.

Use in children.

Hypersensitivity to podophyllotoxin.

Concomitant use with other podophyllotoxin containing preparations.

Pregnancy and lactation.

4.4 Special warnings and precautions for use
Avoid contact with eyes. Should the cream accidentally come into the eye, the eye should be thoroughly rinsed with water.

The hands should be thoroughly washed after each application. Prolonged contact with healthy skin must be avoided since cream contains an active pharmaceutical substance which could be harmful on healthy skin.

4.5 Interaction with other medicinal products and other forms of interaction
None presently known.

4.6 Pregnancy and lactation
The product is not for use in pregnancy or lactation.

Reproduction toxicity studies in animals have not given evidence of an increased incidence of foetal damage or other deleterious effects on the reproductive process. However, since podophyllotoxin is a mitosis inhibitor, Warticon Cream should not be used during pregnancy or lactation.

It is not known if the substance is excreted into breast milk.

Observations in man indicate that podophyllin, a crude mixture of lignans, can be harmful to pregnancy. Such observations have not been reported in patients treated with podophyllotoxin.

4.7 Effects on ability to drive and use machines
None presently known.

4.8 Undesirable effects
Local irritation may occur on the second or third day of application associated with the start of wart necrosis. In most cases the reactions are mild. Tenderness, itching, smarting, erythema, superficial epithelial ulceration and balanoposthitis have been reported. Local irritation decreases after treatment.

4.9 Overdose
There have been no reported overdosages with Warticon cream. However, excessive use of podophyllotoxin 0.5% solution has been reported as causing two cases of severe local reactions. In cases of excessive use of Warticon cream resulting in severe local reaction, the treatment should be stopped, the area washed and symptomatic treatment introduced.

No specific antidote is known. In the event of accidental ingestion, give emetic or stomach washout. Treatment should be symptomatic and in severe oral overdose ensure the airway is clear and give fluids. Check and correct electrolyte balance, monitor blood gases and liver function. Blood count should be monitored for at least 5 days.

5. PHARMACOLOGICAL PROPERTIES
5.1 Pharmacodynamic properties
Pharmaco-therapeutic group, D06BB antivirals

Podophyllotoxin is a metaphase inhibitor in dividing cells binding to at least one binding site on tubulin. Binding prevents tubulin polymerisation required for microtubule assembly. At higher concentrations, podophyllotoxin also inhibits nucleoside transport through the cell membrane.

The chemotherapeutic action of podophyllotoxin is assumed to be due to inhibition of growth and the ability to invade the tissue of the viral infected cells.

5.2 Pharmacokinetic properties
Systemic absorption of podophyllotoxin after topical application with a higher strength, 0.3% is low. Thus no study was performed on the present strength, 0.15%. The C_{max} (1.0 – 4.7 ng/ml) and T_{max} (0.5 – 36 hrs) are comparable for the 0.3% cream and 0.5% solution in both males and females.

5.3 Preclinical safety data
No relevant findings

6. PHARMACEUTICAL PARTICULARS
6.1 List of excipients
Purified Water

Methyl parahydroxybenzoate E218

Propyl parahydroxybenzoate E216

Sorbic acid

Phosphoric acid

Stearyl alcohol

Cetyl alcohol

Isopropyl myristate

Paraffin, liquid

Fractionated coconut oil

Butylhydroxyanisole (BHA) E320

Macrogol -7 stearyl ether

Macrogol – 10 stearyl ether

6.2 Incompatibilities
None known

6.3 Shelf life
3 years

6.4 Special precautions for storage
This medicinal product does not require any special storage precautions.

6.5 Nature and contents of container
A collapsible aluminium tube with imperforate nozzle membrane and internally coated with a protective lacquer. Tube cap of polyethylene with a spike on the upper end aimed to perforate the membrane when opening the tube for the first time. Size 5g.

6.6 Special precautions for disposal and other handling
No special requirements.

7. MARKETING AUTHORISATION HOLDER
Stiefel Laboratories (UK) Ltd.

Holtspur Lane,

Wooburn Green,

High Wycombe,

Bucks.

HP10 0AU

8. MARKETING AUTHORISATION NUMBER(S)
PL 00174/0210

9. DATE OF FIRST AUTHORISATION/RENEWAL OF THE AUTHORISATION
26 April 1999/18 January 2005

10. DATE OF REVISION OF THE TEXT
February 2005

Warticon Solution

(Stiefel Laboratories (UK) Limited)

1. NAME OF THE MEDICINAL PRODUCT
Warticon

2. QUALITATIVE AND QUANTITATIVE COMPOSITION
Podophyllotoxin 5 mg/ml (0.5% w/v). The quality of podophyllotoxin fulfills in-house specification.

3. PHARMACEUTICAL FORM
Topical solution

4. CLINICAL PARTICULARS
4.1 Therapeutic indications
For the topical treatment of condylomata acuminata affecting the penis and the external female genitalia.

4.2 Posology and method of administration
The affected area should be thoroughly washed with soap and water, and dried prior to application.

Warticon is applied twice daily for 3 days. If residual warts persist, this 3-day treatment may be repeated weekly, if necessary, for a total of 4 weeks of treatment.

Where lesions are greater than 4 cm^2, it is recommended that treatment takes place under the direct supervision of medical staff.

4.3 Contraindications
Open wounds following surgical procedures should not be treated with podophyllotoxin.

Hypersensitivity to podophyllotoxin is a contra-indication.

Use in children.

Concomitant use with other podophyllotoxin containing preparations.

Pregnancy and lactation.

4.4 Special warnings and precautions for use
Avoid contact with eyes. Should the solution accidentally come into contact with the eye, the eye should be thoroughly rinsed with water.

The hands should be thoroughly washed after each application. Prolonged contact with healthy skin must be avoided since the solution contains an active pharmaceutical substance which could be harmful on healthy skin.

4.5 Interaction with other medicinal products and other forms of interaction
None presently known.

4.6 Pregnancy and lactation
The product is not for use in pregnancy or lactation.

Reproduction toxicity studies in animals have not given evidence of an increased incidence of foetal damage or other deleterious effects on the reproductive process. However, since podophyllotoxin is a mitosis inhibitor, Warticon Solution should not be used during pregnancy or lactation.

It is not known if the substance is excreted into breast milk.

Observations in man indicate that podophyllin, a crude mixture of lignans, can be harmful to pregnancy. Such observations have not been reported in patients treated with podophyllotoxin.

4.7 Effects on ability to drive and use machines
None presently known.

4.8 Undesirable effects
Local irritation may occur on the second or third day of application associated with the start of wart necrosis. In most cases the reactions are mild. Tenderness, itching, smarting, erythema, superficial epithelial ulceration and balanoposthitis have been reported. Local irritation decreases after treatment.

4.9 Overdose
There have been no reported overdosages with Warticon Solution. However, excessive use of podophyllotoxin 0.5% solution has been reported as causing two cases of severe local reactions. In cases of excessive use of Warticon Solution resulting in severe local reaction, the treatment should be stopped, the area washed and symptomatic treatment introduced. No specific antidote is known. In the event of accidental ingestion, give emetic or stomach washout. Treatment should be symptomatic and in severe oral overdose ensure the airway is clear and give fluids. Check and correct electrolyte balance, monitor blood gases and liver function. Blood count should be monitored for at least 5 days.

5. PHARMACOLOGICAL PROPERTIES
5.1 Pharmacodynamic properties
Pharmaco-therapeutic group: D06B B Antivirals

Podophyllotoxin is a metaphase inhibitor in dividing cells binding to at least one binding site on tubulin. Binding prevents tubulin polymerisation required for microtubule assembly. At higher concentrations podophyllotoxin also inhibits nucleoside transport through the cell membrane.

The chemotherapeutic action of podophyllotoxin is assumed to be due to inhibition of growth and the ability to invade the tissue of the viral infected cells.

5.2 Pharmacokinetic properties
Topical Administration of a 0.5% solution of ethanolic podophyllotoxin in the majority of cases only requires volumes in the range of 0.1 ml to 0.2 ml. Studies monitoring serum drug level reveal that topical application of a twice daily dose of 100MCL to the penile preputial cavity in 10 patients resulted in a maximum serum concentration of 0.25 ng/ml.

5.3 Preclinical safety data
No relevant findings

6. PHARMACEUTICAL PARTICULARS

6.1 List of excipients

Phosphoric acid Ph Eur

Ethanol BP

Purified Water Ph Eur

Patent Blue V (E131)

6.2 Incompatibilities

None known.

6.3 Shelf life

36 months

6.4 Special precautions for storage

Should be stored below 25°C.

6.5 Nature and contents of container

An amber glass bottle with plastic child-proof cap. Each bottle contains 3 ml of Warticon Solution. The outer carton also includes a tube containing plastic applicators. Each loop will carry approximately 5µl Warticon Solution.

6.6 Special precautions for disposal and other handling

The solution is applied by the plastic applicators provided.

7. MARKETING AUTHORISATION HOLDER

Stiefel Laboratories (UK) Ltd

Eurasia Headquarters

Concorde Road

Maidenhead

SL6 4BY

UK

8. MARKETING AUTHORISATION NUMBER(S)

PL0174/0211

9. DATE OF FIRST AUTHORISATION/RENEWAL OF THE AUTHORISATION

21st June 1999 / 8th October 2003

10. DATE OF REVISION OF THE TEXT

August 2009

Waxsol Ear Drops

(Norgine Limited)

1. NAME OF THE MEDICINAL PRODUCT

WAXSOL Ear Drops, Ducosate sodium BP 0.5% w/v

2. QUALITATIVE AND QUANTITATIVE COMPOSITION

WAXSOL Ear Drops contain the following active ingredient:

Docusate Sodium BP 0.5% w/v.

3. PHARMACEUTICAL FORM

Ear drops.

4. CLINICAL PARTICULARS

4.1 Therapeutic indications

WAXSOL Ear Drops are indicated as an aid in the removal of ear wax.

4.2 Posology and method of administration

Recommended dose and dosage schedules:

Adults (including the elderly): The application of ear drops sufficient to fill the affected ear on not more than two consecutive nights, prior to attending for syringing if this is necessary.

Children: As for adult dose.

4.3 Contraindications

Perforation of the ear drum or inflammation of the ear.

4.4 Special warnings and precautions for use

If pain or inflammation is experienced, treatment should be discontinued.

4.5 Interaction with other medicinal products and other forms of interaction

None known.

4.6 Pregnancy and lactation

There is no evidence to suggest that WAXSOL Ear Drops should not be used during pregnancy and lactation.

4.7 Effects on ability to drive and use machines

None known.

4.8 Undesirable effects

Rarely transient stinging or irritation may occur.

4.9 Overdose

None known.

5. PHARMACOLOGICAL PROPERTIES

5.1 Pharmacodynamic properties

The so-called "wax" which often obstructs the external auditory meatus of the ear contains less than 50% of fatty matter derived from secretions of the sebaceous ceruminous glands. The majority of the wax consists of desquamated epithelium, foreign matter and shed hairs. This non-fatty material forms a matrix holding together the granules of fatty matter to form the ceruminous mass.

The addition of oils or solvents binds the mass more firmly together, but aqueous solutions, if they are able to penetrate the matrix, cause a disintegration of the ceruminous mass.

WAXSOL Ear Drops, because of their low surface tension and miscibility, rapidly penetrate the dry matrix of the ceruminous mass, reducing the solid material to a semi-solid debris. This can be syringed away readily, or in less severe or chronic cases, is ejected by normal physiological processes.

5.2 Pharmacokinetic properties

Not applicable.

5.3 Preclinical safety data

None.

6. PHARMACEUTICAL PARTICULARS

6.1 List of excipients

Glycerin

Phenonip (solution of esters of 4-hydroxybenzoic acid in phenoxetol)

Water

6.2 Incompatibilities

None known.

6.3 Shelf life

The shelf life is 3 years.

6.4 Special precautions for storage

Store below 25°C.

6.5 Nature and contents of container

Amber glass bottle with a dropper applicator, containing 10 or 11 ml of WAXSOL solution.

6.6 Special precautions for disposal and other handling

The dropper applicator must be filled before dripping WAXSOL Ear Drops into the affected ear.

7. MARKETING AUTHORISATION HOLDER

Norgine Limited

Chaplin House

Widewater Place

Moorhall Road

Harefield

UXBRIDGE

Middlesex, UB9 6NS

United Kingdom

8. MARKETING AUTHORISATION NUMBER(S)

PL 00322/5016R

9. DATE OF FIRST AUTHORISATION/RENEWAL OF THE AUTHORISATION

27/09/2006

10. DATE OF REVISION OF THE TEXT

27/09/2006

Legal Category: **P**

Wellvone 750mg/5ml oral suspension

(GlaxoSmithKline UK)

1. NAME OF THE MEDICINAL PRODUCT

Wellvone 750 mg/5 ml oral suspension

2. QUALITATIVE AND QUANTITATIVE COMPOSITION

Each ml of suspension contains 150 mg atovaquone

A unit dose of 5 ml contains 750 mg atovaquone.

For a full list of excipients, see section 6.1.

3. PHARMACEUTICAL FORM

Oral suspension.

Wellvone oral suspension is a bright yellow liquid

4. CLINICAL PARTICULARS

4.1 Therapeutic indications

Wellvone Suspension is indicated for:

Acute treatment of mild to moderate Pneumocystis pneumonia (PCP, caused by *Pneumocystis jiroveci*, formerly classified as *P. carinii*) (alveolar - arterial oxygen tension difference [(A-a) DO_2] $\leq$ 45 mmHg (6 kPa) and oxygen tension in arterial blood (PaO_2) $\geqslant$ 60 mmHg (8 kPa) breathing room air) in patients who are intolerant of co-trimoxazole therapy (see section 4.4).

4.2 Posology and method of administration

The importance of taking the full prescribed dose of Wellvone with food should be stressed to patients. The presence of food, particularly high fat food, increases bioavailability two to three fold.

Dosage in adults

Pneumocystis pneumonia:

The recommended oral dose is 750 mg twice a day (1 × 5 ml morning and evening) administered with food each day for 21 days.

Higher doses may be more effective in some patients (see section 5.2).

Dosage in Children

Clinical efficacy has not been studied.

Dosage in the Elderly

There have been no studies of Wellvone in the elderly (see section 4.4).

Renal or hepatic impairment

Wellvone has not been specifically studied in patients with significant hepatic or renal impairment (see section 5.2 for pharmacokinetics in adults). If it is necessary to treat such patients with Wellvone, caution is advised and administration should be closely monitored.

4.3 Contraindications

Wellvone Suspension is contra-indicated in individuals with known hypersensitivity to atovaquone or to any components of the formulation.

4.4 Special warnings and precautions for use

Diarrhoea at the start of treatment has been shown to be associated with significantly lower atovaquone plasma levels. These in turn correlated with a higher incidence of therapy failures and a lower survival rate. Therefore, alternative therapies should be considered for such patients and for patients who have difficulty taking Wellvone with food.

The concomitant administration of atovaquone and rifampicin or rifabutin is not recommended (see section 4.5).

The efficacy of Wellvone has not been systematically evaluated i) in patients failing other PCP therapy, including co-trimoxazole, ii) for treatment of severe episodes of PCP [(A-a) DO_2 > 45 mmHg (6kPa)], iii) as a prophylactic agent for PCP, or iv) versus intravenous pentamidine for treatment of PCP.

No data are available in non-HIV immuno-compromised patients suffering with PCP.

No clinical experience of atovaquone treatment has been gained in elderly patients. Therefore use in the elderly should be closely monitored.

Patients with pulmonary disease should be carefully evaluated for causes of disease other than PCP and treated with additional agents as appropriate. Wellvone is not expected to be effective therapy for other fungal, bacterial, mycobacterial or viral diseases.

4.5 Interaction with other medicinal products and other forms of interaction

As experience is limited, care should be taken when combining other drugs with Wellvone.

Concomitant administration of rifampicin or rifabutin is known to reduce atovaquone levels by approximately 50% and 34%, respectively, and could result in sub therapeutic plasma concentrations in some patients (see section 4.4).

Concomitant treatment with tetracycline or metoclopramide has been associated with significant decreases in plasma concentrations of atovaquone. Caution should be exercised in prescribing these drugs with Wellvone until the potential interaction has been further studied.

In clinical trials of Wellvone small decreases in plasma concentrations of atovaquone (mean < 3 µg/ml) were associated with concomitant administration of paracetamol, benzodiazepines, acyclovir, opiates, cephalosporins, anti-diarrhoeals and laxatives. The causal relationship between the change in plasma concentrations of atovaquone and the administration of the drugs mentioned above is unknown.

Clinical trials have evaluated the interaction of Wellvone Tablets with:

Zidovudine -Zidovudine does not appear to affect the pharmacokinetics of atovaquone. However, pharmacokinetic data have shown that atovaquone appears to decrease the rate of metabolism of zidovudine to its glucuronide metabolite (steady state AUC of zidovudine was increased by 33% and peak plasma concentration of the glucuronide was decreased by 19%). At zidovudine dosages of 500 or 600 mg/day it would seem unlikely that a three week, concomitant course of Wellvone for the treatment of acute PCP would result in an increased incidence of adverse reactions attributable to higher plasma concentrations of zidovudine.

Didanosine (ddI) - ddI does not affect the pharmacokinetics of atovaquone as determined in a prospective multi-dose drug interaction study of atovaquone and ddI. However, there was a 24% decrease in the AUC for ddI when co-administered with atovaquone which is unlikely to be of clinical significance.

Nevertheless, the modes of interaction being unknown, the effects of atovaquone administration on zidovudine and ddI may be greater with atovaquone suspension. The higher concentrations of atovaquone possible with the suspension might induce greater changes in the AUC values for zidovudine or ddI than those observed. Patients receiving atovaquone and zidovudine should be regularly monitored for zidovudine associated adverse effects.

Concomitant administration of Wellvone and indinavir results in a significant decrease in the C_{min} of indinavir (23% decrease; 90% CI 8-35%) and the AUC (9% decrease; 90% CI 1-18%). Caution should be exercised on the potential risk of failure of indinavir treatment if co-administered with atovaquone. No data are available regarding potential interactions of Wellvone and other protease inhibitor drugs.

In clinical trials of Wellvone the following medications were not associated with a change in steady state plasma concentrations of atovaquone: fluconazole, clotrimazole, ketoconazole, antacids, systemic corticosteroids, non-steroidal anti-inflammatory drugs, anti-emetics (excluding metoclopramide) and H_2-antagonists.

Atovaquone is highly bound to plasma proteins and caution should be used when administering Wellvone concurrently with other highly plasma protein bound drugs with narrow therapeutic indices. Atovaquone does not affect the pharmacokinetics, metabolism or extent of protein binding of phenytoin *in vivo*. *In vitro* there is no plasma protein binding interaction between atovaquone and quinine, phenytoin, warfarin, sulfamethoxazole, indometacin or diazepam.

4.6 Pregnancy and lactation

There is no information on the effects of atovaquone administration during human pregnancy. Atovaquone should not be used during pregnancy unless the benefit of treatment to the mother outweighs any possible risk to the developing foetus.

Insufficient data are available from animal experiments to assess the possible risk to reproductive potential or performance.

It is not known whether atovaquone is excreted in human milk, and therefore breast feeding is not recommended.

4.7 Effects on ability to drive and use machines

There have been no studies to investigate the effect of Wellvone on driving performance or the ability to operate machinery but a detrimental effect on such activities is not predicted from the pharmacology of the drug.

4.8 Undesirable effects

Patients participating in clinical trials with Wellvone have often had complications of advanced Human Immunodeficiency Virus (HIV) disease and therefore the causal relationship between the adverse experiences and atovaquone is difficult to evaluate.

The following convention is used for frequencies: very common ($\geqslant$ 1/10); common ($\geqslant$ 1/100 to $<$ 1/10); uncommon ($\geqslant$ 1/1 000 to $<$ 1/100); rare ($\geqslant$ 1/10 000 to $<$ 1/1 000); very rare ($<$ 1/10 000); not known (cannot be estimated from the available data).

Blood and the lymphatic system disorders

Common: anaemia, neutropenia

Metabolism and nutrition disorders

Common: hyponatraemia

Psychiatric disorders

Common: insomnia

Nervous system disorders

Common: headache

Gastrointestinal disorders

Very common: nausea

Common: diarrhoea, vomiting

Hepatobiliary disorders

Common: elevated liver enzymes levels

Immune System Disorders

Common: hypersensitivity reactions including angioedema, bronchospasm and throat tightness

Skin and subcutaneous tissue disorders

Very common: rash, pruritus

Common: urticaria

Not known: erythema multiforme, Stevens-Johnson Syndrome

General disorders and administration site conditions

Common: fever

Investigations

Uncommon: elevated amylase levels

4.9 Overdose

There is insufficient experience to predict the consequences or suggest specific management of atovaquone overdose. However, in the reported cases of overdosage, the observed effects were consistent with known undesirable effects of the drug. If overdosage occurs, the patient should be monitored and standard supportive treatment applied.

5. PHARMACOLOGICAL PROPERTIES

5.1 Pharmacodynamic properties

Pharmacotherapeutic group: Antiprotozoals,

ATC Code: P01A X06.

Mode of Action

Atovaquone is a selective and potent inhibitor of the eukaryotic mitochondrial electron transport chain in a number of parasitic protozoa and the parasitic fungus *P. jiroveci*. The site of action appears to be the cytochrome bc1 complex (complex III). The ultimate metabolic effect of such blockade is likely to be inhibition of nucleic acid and ATP synthesis.

Microbiology

Atovaquone has potent activity against *Pneumocystic* sp, both *in vitro* and in animal models, (IC_{50} 0.5-8µg/mL).

5.2 Pharmacokinetic properties

Atovaquone is a highly lipophilic compound with a low aqueous solubility. It is 99.9% bound to plasma proteins. The bioavailability of the drug demonstrates a relative decrease with single doses above 750 mg, and shows considerable inter-individual variability. Average absolute bioavailablility of a 750 mg single dose of atovaquone suspension administered with food to adult HIV positive males is 47% (compared to 23% for Wellvone tablets). Following the intravenous administration, the volume of distribution and clearance were calculated to be 0.62±0.19 l/kg and 0.15±0.09 ml/min/kg, respectively.

The bioavailability of atovaquone is greater when administered with food than in the fasting state. In healthy volunteers, a standardized breakfast (23 g fat; 610 kCal) increased bioavailability two to three-fold following a single 750 mg dose. The mean area under the atovaquone plasma concentration-time curve (AUC) was increased 2.5 fold and the mean C_{max} was increased 3.4 fold. The mean (±SD) AUC values for suspension were 324.3 (±115.0) µg/ml.h fasted and 800.6 (±319.8) µg/ml.h with food.

In a safety and pharmacokinetic study in patients with PCP, the following results were obtained:

Dose regimen	750 mg twice daily	1000 mg twice daily
Number of Patients	18	9
C avg, ss (range)	22 µg/ml (6-41)	25.7 µg/ml (15-36)
% of patients with C avg, ss $>$15 µg/ml	67%	100%

In a small safety and pharmacokinetic study of two higher dosing regimens [750 mg three times daily (n=8) and 1500 mg twice daily (n=8)] in HIV infected volunteers with severity criteria comparable to patients with PCP, similar Cavg were reached with the two doses [respectively for the 750 mg tid and 1500 mg bid doses: 24.8 (7-40) and 23.4 µg/ml (7-35). Moreover, for both doses a Cavg, ss $>$15 µg/ml was reached in 87.5% of patients.

Average steady state concentrations above 15 µg/ml are predictive of a high ($>$90%) success rate.

In healthy volunteers and patients with AIDS, atovaquone has a half-life of 2 to 3 days.

In healthy volunteers there is no evidence that the drug is metabolised and there is negligible excretion of atovaquone in the urine, with parent drug being predominantly ($>$90%) excreted unchanged in faeces.

5.3 Preclinical safety data

Carcinogenicity

Oncogenicity studies in mice showed an increased incidence of hepatocellular adenomas and carcinomas without determination of the no observed adverse effect level. No such findings were observed in rats and mutagenicity tests were negative. These findings appear to be due to the inherent susceptibility of mice to atovaquone and are not predictive of a risk in the clinical situation.

Reproductive toxicity

In the dosage range of 600 to 1200 mg/kg studies in rabbits gave indications of maternal and embryotoxic effects.

6. PHARMACEUTICAL PARTICULARS

6.1 List of excipients

Benzyl alcohol

Xanthan Gum

Poloxamer 188

Saccharin Sodium

Purified water

Tutti Frutti Flavour (Firmenich 51.880/A) containing sweet orange oil, concentrated orange oil, propylene glycol, benzyl alcohol, vanillin, acetic aldehyde, amyl acetate and ethyl butyrate.

6.2 Incompatibilities

Not applicable

6.3 Shelf life

2 years

After first opening, the suspension may be stored for up to 21 days.

6.4 Special precautions for storage

Do not store above 25°C.

Do not freeze.

6.5 Nature and contents of container

A 240 ml high density polyethylene bottle with child resistant polypropylene closure, containing 226 ml of atovaquone suspension.

A 5 ml measuring spoon (polypropylene) is included.

6.6 Special precautions for disposal and other handling

Do not dilute

7. MARKETING AUTHORISATION HOLDER

Glaxo Wellcome UK Ltd

trading as

GlaxoSmithKline UK

Stockley Park West

Uxbridge, Middlesex

UB11 1BT

8. MARKETING AUTHORISATION NUMBER(S)

PL 10949/0271

9. DATE OF FIRST AUTHORISATION/RENEWAL OF THE AUTHORISATION

Date of first authorisation: 25 March 1997

Date of last renewal: 21 May 2006

10. DATE OF REVISION OF THE TEXT

19 March 2008

Woodward's Gripe Water

(SSL International plc)

1. NAME OF THE MEDICINAL PRODUCT

Woodward's Gripe Water- Alcohol Free & Sugar Free.

2. QUALITATIVE AND QUANTITATIVE COMPOSITION

Terpeneless Dill Seed Oil 2.3mg/5ml; Sodium Hydrogen Carbonate BP 52.5mg/5ml.

3. PHARMACEUTICAL FORM

Oral solution.

4. CLINICAL PARTICULARS

4.1 Therapeutic indications

For the symptomatic relief of distress associated with wind in infants up to one year old.

4.2 Posology and method of administration

For oral use. Adults including the elderly: not applicable. Children 1-6 months: one 5ml spoonful.

Children 6-12 months: two 5ml spoonsful. Children under 1 month: not to be used. These doses may be given during or after each feed or up to six times in 24 hours.

4.3 Contraindications

Should not be used where impaired kidney function or hypersensitivity to hydroxybenzoates exists.

4.4 Special warnings and precautions for use

If symptoms persist, medical advice should be sought. Keep all medicines out of the reach of children.

4.5 Interaction with other medicinal products and other forms of interaction

None known.

4.6 Pregnancy and lactation

Not applicable.

4.7 Effects on ability to drive and use machines

Not applicable.

4.8 Undesirable effects

None known.

4.9 Overdose

Symptoms following overdose are rare and are generally due to the effects of sodium hydrogen carbonate. These may include diarrhoea, metabolic alkalosis and hypernatraemia. In the event of severe overdosing, medical advice should be sought immediately. Symptoms of hypernatraemia may include drowsiness and irritability, pyrexia and tachypnoea. In more severe instances of acute sodium overload, signs of dehydration and convulsions may occur. The treatment of hypernatraemia includes repair of any dehydration present and gradual reduction of the plasma sodium. The alkalosis, if present, will respond usually to the treatment of hypernatraemia. At all times intensive monitoring of the electrolytes, and patients circulatory and central nervous system are necessary.

5. PHARMACOLOGICAL PROPERTIES

5.1 Pharmacodynamic properties

Sodium hydrogen carbonate has a well established antacid action. Dill seed oil is a widely used aromatic carminative especially for use in the treatment of flatulence in children.

5.2 Pharmacokinetic properties

Not applicable.

5.3 Preclinical safety data

Not applicable.

6. PHARMACEUTICAL PARTICULARS

6.1 List of excipients

Glycerol; Maltitol Liquid; Propylene Glycol; Nipasept Sodium; Disodium Edetate; Purified Water.

6.2 Incompatibilities

None known.

6.3 Shelf life

18 months unopened; 14 days after opening.

6.4 Special precautions for storage

Do not store above 25°C.

6.5 Nature and contents of container

Clear, white, flint glass bottle with an expanded polyethylene wadded cap containing 150ml of product.

6.6 Special precautions for disposal and other handling

None.

7. MARKETING AUTHORISATION HOLDER

Seton Products Limited, Tubiton House, Oldham, Lancashire, OL1 3HS.

8. MARKETING AUTHORISATION NUMBER(S)

PL 11314/0139.

9. DATE OF FIRST AUTHORISATION/RENEWAL OF THE AUTHORISATION

2nd December 1999. / 15/04/2005

10. DATE OF REVISION OF THE TEXT

April 2005

Xagrid 0.5mg hard capsule

(Shire Pharmaceuticals Limited)

1. NAME OF THE MEDICINAL PRODUCT

Xagrid ▼ 0.5mg hard capsule

2. QUALITATIVE AND QUANTITATIVE COMPOSITION

Each capsule contains 0.5 mg anagrelide (as 0.61 mg anagrelide hydrochloride)

For a full list of excipients, see section 6.1

3. PHARMACEUTICAL FORM

Capsule, hard

An opaque white hard capsule imprinted with S 063

4. CLINICAL PARTICULARS

4.1 Therapeutic indications

Xagrid is indicated for the reduction of elevated platelet counts in at risk essential thrombocythaemia (ET) patients who are intolerant to their current therapy or whose elevated platelet counts are not reduced to an acceptable level by their current therapy.

An at risk patient

An at risk essential thrombocythaemia patient is defined by one or more of the following features:

>60 years of age or

A platelet count $>1000 \times 10^9$/l or

A history of thrombo-haemorrhagic events.

4.2 Posology and method of administration

Treatment with Xagrid capsules should be initiated by a clinician with experience in the management of essential thrombocythaemia.

The recommended starting dosage of anagrelide is 1mg/day, which should be administered orally in two divided doses (0.5mg/dose).

The starting dose should be maintained for at least one week. After one week the dosage may be titrated, on an individual basis, to achieve the lowest effective dosage required to reduce and/or maintain a platelet count below 600×10^9/l and ideally at levels between 150×10^9/l and 400×10^9/l. The dosage increment must not exceed more than 0.5mg/day in any one-week and the recommended maximum single dose should not exceed 2.5mg (see section 4.9). During clinical development dosages of 10mg/day have been used.

The effects of treatment with anagrelide must be monitored on a regular basis (see section 4.4). If the starting dose is >1mg/day platelet counts should be performed every two days during the first week of treatment and at least weekly thereafter until a stable maintenance dose is reached. Typically, a fall in the platelet count will be observed within 14 to 21 days of starting treatment and in most patients an adequate therapeutic response will be observed and maintained at a dosage of 1 to 3mg/day (for further information on the clinical effects refer to section 5.1).

Elderly

The observed pharmacokinetic differences between elderly and young patients with ET (see section 5.2) do not warrant using a different starting regimen or different dose titration step to achieve an individual patient-optimised anagrelide regimen.

During clinical development approximately 50% of the patients treated with anagrelide were over 60 years of age and no age specific alterations in dosage were required in these patients. However, as expected, patients in this age group had twice the incidence of serious adverse events (mainly cardiac).

Renal impairment

Currently, there are no specific pharmacokinetic data for this patient population and the potential risks and benefits of anagrelide therapy in a patient with impairment of renal function should be assessed before treatment is commenced.

Hepatic impairment

Currently, there are no specific pharmacokinetic data for this patient population. However, hepatic metabolism represents the major route of drug clearance and liver function may therefore be expected to influence this process. Therefore it is recommended that patients with moderate or severe hepatic impairment are not treated with anagrelide. The potential risks and benefits of anagrelide therapy in a patient with mild impairment of hepatic function should be assessed before treatment is commenced (see sections 4.3 and 4.4).

Children and adolescents:

The experience in children is limited.

4.3 Contraindications

Hypersensitivity to anagrelide or to any of the excipients of the medicinal product.

Patients with moderate or severe hepatic impairment. Patients with moderate or severe renal impairment (creatinine clearance <50ml/min).

4.4 Special warnings and precautions for use

Hepatic impairment: (see sections 4.2 and 4.3) the potential risks and benefits of anagrelide therapy in a patient with mild impairment of hepatic function should be assessed before treatment is commenced. It is not recommended in patients with elevated transaminases (>5 times the upper limit of normal).

Renal impairment: (see sections 4.2 and 4.3) the potential risks and benefits of anagrelide therapy in a patient with impairment of renal function should be assessed before treatment is commenced.

General: therapy requires close clinical supervision of the patient which will include a full blood count (haemoglobin and white blood cell and platelet counts), and assessment of liver function (ALT and AST) and renal function (serum creatinine and urea) tests.

Platelets: the platelet count will increase within 4 days of stopping treatment with Xagrid capsules and will return to pre-treatment levels within 10 to 14 days.

Cardiovascular: Cases of cardiomegaly and congestive heart failure have been reported (see section 4.8). Anagrelide should be used with caution in patients of any age with known or suspected heart disease, and only if the potential benefits of therapy outweigh the potential risks. Anagrelide is an inhibitor of cyclic AMP phosphodiesterase III and because of its positive inotropic effects, a pre-treatment cardiovascular examination (including further investigation such as echocardiography, electrocardiogram) is recommended. Patients should be monitored during treatment for evidence of cardiovascular effects that may require further cardiovascular examination and investigation.

Paediatric patients: (see section 5.1) limited data are available on the use of anagrelide in the paediatric population and anagrelide should be used in this patient group with caution.

Clinically relevant interactions: anagrelide is an inhibitor of cyclic AMP phosphodiesterase III (PDE III). Concomitant use of anagrelide with other PDE III inhibitors such as milrinone, amrinone, enoximone, olprinone and cilostazol is not recommended.

Excipients: This product contains lactose. Patients with rare hereditary problems of galactose intolerance, the Lapp lactase deficiency or glucose-galactose malabsorption should not take this medicine.

4.5 Interaction with other medicinal products and other forms of interaction

Limited pharmacokinetic and/or pharmacodynamic studies investigating possible interactions between anagrelide and other medicinal products have been conducted.

Drug interactions: effects of other substances on anagrelide

- Anagrelide is primarily metabolised by CYP1A2. It is known that CYP1A2 is inhibited by several medicinal products, including fluvoxamine and omeprazole, and such medicinal products could theoretically adversely influence the clearance of anagrelide.
- *In vivo* interaction studies in humans have demonstrated that digoxin and warfarin do not affect the pharmacokinetic properties of anagrelide.

Drug interactions: effects of anagrelide on other substances

- Anagrelide demonstrates some limited inhibitory activity towards CYP1A2 which may present a theoretical potential for interaction with other co-administered medicinal products sharing that clearance mechanism e.g. theophylline.
- Anagrelide is an inhibitor of PDE III. The effects of medicinal products with similar properties such as the inotropes milrinone, enoximone, amrinone, olprinone and cilostazol may be exacerbated by anagrelide.
- *In vivo* interaction studies in humans have demonstrated that anagrelide does not affect the pharmacokinetic properties of digoxin or warfarin.
- At the doses recommended for use in the treatment of essential thrombocythaemia, anagrelide may theoretically potentiate the effects of other medicinal products that inhibit or modify platelet function e.g. acetylsalicylic acid.
- A clinical interaction study performed in healthy subjects showed that co-administration of repeat-dose anagrelide 1mg once daily and acetylsalicylic acid 75mg once daily may enhance the anti-platelet aggregation effects of each drug compared with administration of acetylsalicylic acid alone. Therefore, due to the lack of data in ET patients, the potential risks of the concomitant use of anagrelide with acetylsalicylic acid should be assessed, particularly in patients with a high risk profile for haemorrhage before treatment is initiated.
- Anagrelide may cause intestinal disturbance in some patients and compromise the absorption of hormonal oral contraceptives.

Food interactions:

- Food delays the absorption of anagrelide but does not significantly alter systemic exposure.
- The effects of food on bioavailability are not considered clinically relevant to the use of anagrelide.

4.6 Pregnancy and lactation

Pregnancy:

There are no adequate data from the use of anagrelide in pregnant women.

Studies in animals have shown reproductive toxicity (see section 5.3). The potential risk for humans is unknown.

Use of Xagrid during pregnancy is not recommended. If Xagrid is used during pregnancy, or if the patient becomes pregnant while using the drug, she should be advised of the potential risk to the foetus.

Women of child-bearing potential should use adequate birth-control measures during treatment with anagrelide.

Lactation: It is not known whether anagrelide hydrochloride is excreted in milk. Since many medicinal products are excreted in human milk and because of the potential for adverse reactions in breast-feeding infants, mothers should discontinue breast-feeding when taking Xagrid.

4.7 Effects on ability to drive and use machines

No studies on the effects on the ability to drive and use machines have been performed. In clinical development, dizziness was commonly reported.

Patients are advised not to drive or operate machinery while taking Xagrid if dizziness is experienced.

4.8 Undesirable effects

The safety of anagrelide has been examined in 4 open label clinical studies. In 3 of the studies 942 patients who received anagrelide at a mean dose of approximately 2mg/day were assessed for safety. In these studies 22 patients received anagrelide for up to 4 years.

In the later study 3660 patients who received anagrelide at a mean dose of approximately 2mg/day were assessed for safety. In this study 34 patients received anagrelide for up to 5 years.

The most commonly reported drug related adverse reactions were headache occurring at approximately 14%, palpitations occurring at approximately 9%, fluid retention and nausea both occurring at approximately 6%, and diarrhoea occurring at 5%. These adverse drug reactions are expected based on the pharmacology of anagrelide (inhibition of PDE III). Gradual dose titration may help diminish these effects (see section 4.2).

The following convention was used for frequency of adverse drug reactions: very common ($>1/10$); common ($>1/100$, $<1/10$); uncommon ($>1/1{,}000$, $<1/100$); rare ($>1/10{,}000$, $<1/1{,}000$); not known (cannot be estimated from the available data).

Blood and lymphatic system disorders

Common: Anaemia

Uncommon: Thrombocytopenia, pancytopenia, ecchymosis, haemorrhage

Metabolism and nutrition disorders

Common: Fluid retention

Uncommon: Oedema, weight loss

Rare: Weight gain

Nervous system disorders

Very common: Headache

Common: Dizziness

Uncommon: Paraesthesia, insomnia, depression, confusion, hypoaesthesia, nervousness, dry mouth, amnesia

Rare: Somnolence, abnormal coordination, dysarthria, migraine

Special senses

Rare: Vision abnormal, tinnitus, diplopia

Cardiac disorders

Common: Palpitations, tachycardia

Uncommon: Congestive heart failure, hypertension, arrhythmia, atrial fibrillation, supraventricular tachycardia, ventricular tachycardia, syncope

Rare: Angina pectoris, myocardial infarction, cardiomegaly, cardiomyopathy, pericardial effusion, vasodilatation, postural hypotension

Respiratory and thoracic disorders

Uncommon: Dyspnoea, epistaxis, pleural effusion, pneumonia

Rare: Pulmonary hypertension, pulmonary infiltrates

Not known: Allergic alveolitis

Gastrointestinal disorders

Common: Nausea, diarrhoea, abdominal pain, flatulence, vomiting

Uncommon: Dyspepsia, anorexia, pancreatitis, constipation, gastrointestinal haemorrhage, gastrointestinal disorder

Rare: Colitis, gastritis, gingival bleeding

Hepatobiliary disorders

Uncommon: Hepatic enzymes increased

Skin and subcutaneous tissue

Common: Rash

Uncommon: Alopecia, skin discoloration, pruritus

Rare: Dry skin

Musculoskeletal and connective tissue disorders

Uncommon: Myalgia, arthralgia, back pain

Urogenital

Uncommon: Impotence

Rare: Nocturia, renal failure

Investigations

Rare: Blood creatinine increased

General disorders and administration site conditions

Common: Fatigue

Uncommon: Chest pain, weakness, chills, malaise, fevery

Rare: Asthenia, pain, flu-like syndrome

4.9 Overdose

There have been a small number of post-marketing case reports of intentional overdose with anagrelide. Reported symptoms include sinus tachycardia and vomiting. Symptoms resolved with conservative management.

A specific antidote for anagrelide has not been identified. In case of overdose, close clinical supervision of the patient is required; this includes monitoring of the platelet count for thrombocytopenia. Dosage should be decreased or stopped, as appropriate, until the platelet count returns to within the normal range.

Xagrid, at higher than recommended doses, has been shown to produce reductions in blood pressure with occasional instances of hypotension. A single 5mg dose of anagrelide can lead to a fall in blood pressure usually accompanied by dizziness.

5. PHARMACOLOGICAL PROPERTIES

5.1 Pharmacodynamic properties

Pharmacotherapeutic group:

ATC Code: L01XX35 (Other Antineoplastic Agents)

The specific mechanism of action by which anagrelide reduces platelet count is not yet fully understood although it has been confirmed that anagrelide is platelet selective from *in vitro* and *in vivo* study information.

In vitro studies of human megakaryocytopoiesis established that anagrelide's inhibitory actions on platelet formation in man are mediated via retardation of maturation of megakaryocytes, and reducing their size and ploidy. Evidence of similar *in vivo* actions was observed in bone marrow biopsy samples from treated patients.

Anagrelide is an inhibitor of cyclic AMP phosphodiesterase III.

The safety and efficacy of anagrelide as a platelet lowering agent have been evaluated in four open-label, non-controlled clinical trials (study numbers 700-012, 700-014, 700-999 and 13970-301) including more than 4000 patients with myeloproliferative disorders (MPDs). In patients with essential thrombocythaemia complete response was defined as a decrease in platelet count to $\leqslant 600 \times 10^9$/l or a $\geqslant 50\%$ reduction from baseline and maintenance of the reduction for at least 4 weeks. In studies 700-012, 700-014, 700-999 and study 13970-301 the time to complete response ranged from 4 to 12 weeks. Clinical benefit in terms of thrombohaemorrhagic events has not been convincingly demonstrated.

Children and adolescents:

An open label clinical study with a 3 month treatment period did not raise any safety concerns for anagrelide in 17 children/adolescent patients with ET (age range 7-14 years) compared to 18 adult patients. Earlier during clinical development a limited number (12) of children (age range 5 - 17 years) with essential thrombocythaemia were treated with anagrelide.

5.2 Pharmacokinetic properties

Following oral administration of anagrelide in man, at least 70% is absorbed from the gastrointestinal tract. In fasted subjects, peak plasma levels occur about 1 hour after a 0.5mg dose; the plasma half-life is short, approximately 1.3 hours. Dose proportionality has been found in the dose range 0.5mg to 2mg.

Anagrelide is primarily metabolised by CYP1A2; less than 1% is recovered in the urine as anagrelide. Two major urinary metabolites, 2-amino-5, 6-dichloro-3, 4-dihydroquinazoline and N-(5,6-dichloro-3,4-dihydroquinazalin-2-yl)-2-oxoacetamide have been identified. The mean recovery of 2-amino-5, 6-dichloro-3, 4-dihydroquinazoline in urine is approximately 18-35% of the administered dose.

Pharmacokinetic data from healthy subjects established that food decreases the C_{max} of anagrelide by 14%, but increases the AUC by 20%. Food had a more significant effect on the active metabolite and decreased the C_{max} by 29%, although it had no effect on the AUC.

As expected from its half-life, there is no evidence for anagrelide accumulation in the plasma. Additionally these results show no evidence of auto-induction of the anagrelide clearance.

Special populations

Children and adolescents

Pharmacokinetic data from fasting children and adolescents (age range 7 - 14 years) with essential thrombocythaemia indicate that dose and body weight normalised exposure, Cmax and AUC, of anagrelide were lower in children/adolescents compared to adults. There was also a trend to lower exposure to the active metabolite. These observations may be a reflection of more efficient metabolic clearance in younger subjects.

Elderly

Pharmacokinetic data from fasting elderly patients with ET (age range 65-75 years) compared to fasting adult patients (age range 22-50 years) indicate that the C_{max} and AUC of anagrelide were 36% and 61% higher respectively in elderly patients, but that the C_{max} and AUC of the active metabolite, 2-amino-5, 6-dichloro-3, 4-dihydroquinazoline, were 42% and 37% lower respectively in the elderly patients. These differences were likely to be caused by lower presystemic metabolism of anagrelide to 2-amino-5, 6-dichloro-3, 4-dihydroquinazoline in the elderly patients.

5.3 Preclinical safety data

Repeated dose toxicity.

Following repeated administration of anagrelide, at doses of 1mg/kg/day or higher, subendocardial haemorrhage and focal myocardial necrosis occurred in dogs.

Reproductive toxicology.

Maternally toxic doses of anagrelide (60 mg/kg/day and above) in rats and rabbits were associated with increased embryo resorption and foetal mortality.

Mutagenic and carcinogenic potential.

Studies on the genotoxic potential of anagrelide did not identify any mutagenic or clastogenic effects.

In a two-year rat carcinogenicity study, non-neoplastic and neoplastic findings were observed and related or attributed to an exaggerated pharmacological effect. Among them, the incidence of adrenal phaeochromocytomas was increased relative to control in males at all dose levels ($\geqslant$ 3 mg/kg/day) and in females receiving 10 mg/kg/day and above. The lowest dose in males (3 mg/kg/day) corresponds to 37 times the human AUC exposure after a 1 mg twice daily dose. Uterine adenocarcinomas, of epigenetic origin, could be related to an enzyme induction of CYP1 family. They were observed in females receiving 30 mg/kg/day, corresponding to 572 times the human AUC exposure after a 1 mg twice daily dose.

Currently, there is no clinical evidence that these findings are of relevance to human use.

6. PHARMACEUTICAL PARTICULARS

6.1 List of excipients

Capsule contents

Povidone (E1201)

Anhydrous lactose

Lactose monohydrate

Microcrystalline cellulose (E460)

Crospovidone

Magnesium stearate

Capsule shell

Gelatin

Titanium dioxide (E171)

Printing ink

Shellac

Strong ammonium solution

Potassium hydroxide (E525)

Black iron oxide (E172)

6.2 Incompatibilities

Not applicable

6.3 Shelf life

3 years

6.4 Special precautions for storage

No special precautions for storage

6.5 Nature and contents of container

High-density polyethylene (HDPE) bottles containing desiccant with child-resistant closures containing 100 capsules

6.6 Special precautions for disposal and other handling

No special requirements

7. MARKETING AUTHORISATION HOLDER

Shire Pharmaceutical Contracts Ltd

Hampshire International Business Park

Chineham

Basingstoke

Hampshire RG24 8EP

United Kingdom

8. MARKETING AUTHORISATION NUMBER(S)

EU/1/04/295/001

9. DATE OF FIRST AUTHORISATION/RENEWAL OF THE AUTHORISATION

16/11/2004

10. DATE OF REVISION OF THE TEXT

02/2009

Xalacom eye drops, solution

(Pharmacia Limited)

1. NAME OF THE MEDICINAL PRODUCT

Xalacom eye drops, solution.

2. QUALITATIVE AND QUANTITATIVE COMPOSITION

1ml solution contains latanoprost 50 micrograms and timolol maleate 6.8 mg equivalent to 5 mg timolol.

For a full list of excipients, see section 6.1.

3. PHARMACEUTICAL FORM

Eye drops, solution

The solution is a clear colourless liquid.

4. CLINICAL PARTICULARS

4.1 Therapeutic indications

Reduction of intraocular pressure (IOP) in patients with open angle glaucoma and ocular hypertension who are insufficiently responsive to topical beta-blockers or prostaglandin analogues.

4.2 Posology and method of administration

Recommended dosage for adults (including the elderly):

Recommended therapy is one eye drop in the affected eye(s) once daily.

If one dose is missed, treatment should continue with the next dose as planned. The dose should not exceed one drop in the affected eye(s) daily.

Administration:

Contact lenses should be removed before instillation of the eye drops and may be reinserted after 15 minutes (see section 4.4).

If more than one topical ophthalmic drug is being used, the drugs should be administered at least five minutes apart.

Use in children and adolescents:

Safety and effectiveness in children and adolescents has not been established.

4.3 Contraindications

Xalacom is contraindicated in patients with:

- Reactive airway disease including bronchial asthma or a history of bronchial asthma, severe chronic obstructive pulmonary disease.

- Sinus bradycardia, second or third degree atrioventricular block, overt cardiac failure, cardiogenic shock.

- Hypersensitivity to the active substances or to any of the excipients.

4.4 Special warnings and precautions for use

Systemic effects

Like other topically applied ophthalmic agents, Xalacom may be absorbed systemically. Due to the beta-adrenergic component timolol, the same types of cardiovascular and pulmonary adverse reactions as seen with systemic beta-blockers may occur. Cardiac failure should be adequately controlled before beginning therapy with timolol. Patients with a history of severe cardiac disease should be watched for signs of cardiac failure and have their pulse rates checked. Respiratory reactions and cardiac reactions, including death due to bronchospasm in patients with asthma and, rarely, death in association with cardiac failures, have been reported following administration of timolol maleate. Beta-blockers should be administered with caution in patients subject to spontaneous hypoglycaemia or to patients with labile insulin-dependant diabetes, as beta-blockers may mask the signs and symptoms of acute hypoglycaemia. Beta-blockers may also mask the signs of hyperthyroidism and cause worsening of Prinzmetal angina, severe peripheral and central circulatory disorders and hypotension.

Anaphylactic reactions

While taking beta-blockers, patients with a history of atopy or a history of severe anaphylactic reaction to a variety of allergens may be unresponsive to the usual doses of adrenaline used to treat anaphylactic reactions.

Concomitant therapy

Timolol may interact with other drugs, see 4.5 Interaction with other medicinal products and other forms of interaction.

The effect on intraocular pressure or the known effects of systemic beta-blockade may be potentiated when Xalacom is given to patients already receiving an oral beta-blocking agent. The use of two local beta-blockers or two local prostaglandins is not recommended.

Ocular effects

Latanoprost may gradually change the eye colour by increasing the amount of brown pigment in the iris. Similar to experience with latanoprost eye drops, increased iris pigmentation was seen in 16-20% of all patients treated with Xalacom for up to one year (based on photographs). This effect has predominantly been seen in patients with mixed coloured irides, i.e. green-brown, yellow-brown or blue/grey-brown, and is due to increased melanin content in the stromal melanocytes of the iris. Typically the brown pigmentation around the pupil spreads concentrically towards the periphery in affected eyes, but the entire iris or parts of it may become more brownish. In patients with homogeneously blue, grey, green or brown eyes, the change has only rarely been seen during two years of treatment in clinical trials with latanoprost.

The change in iris colour occurs slowly and may not be noticeable for several months to years and it has not been associated with any symptom or pathological changes.

No further increase in brown iris pigment has been observed after discontinuation of treatment, but the resultant colour change may be permanent.

Neither naevi nor freckles of the iris have been affected by treatment.

Accumulation of pigment in the trabecular meshwork or elsewhere in the anterior chamber has not been observed but patients should be examined regularly and, depending on the clinical situation, treatment may be stopped if increased iris pigmentation ensues.

Before treatment is instituted patients should be informed of the possibility of a change in eye colour. Unilateral treatment can result in permanent heterochromia.

There is no documented experience with latanoprost in inflammatory, neovascular, chronic angle closure or congenital glaucoma, in open angle glaucoma of pseudophakic patients and in pigmentary glaucoma.

Latanoprost has no or little effect on the pupil but there is no documented experience in acute attacks of closed angle glaucoma. It is recommended, therefore, that Xalacom should be used with caution in these conditions until more experience is obtained.

Macular oedema, including cystoid macular oedema, has been reported during treatment with latanoprost. These reports have mainly occurred in aphakic patients, in pseudophakic patients with a torn posterior lens capsule, or in patients with known risk factors for macular oedema. Xalacom should be used with caution in these patients.

Choroidal detachment has been reported with administration of aqueous suppressant therapy (e.g. timolol, acetazolamide) after filtration procedures.

Use of contact lenses

Xalcom contains benzalkonium chloride, which is commonly used as a preservative in ophthalmic products. Benzalkonium chloride has been reported to cause punctate keratopathy and/or toxic ulcerative keratopathy, may cause eye irritation and is known to discolour soft contact lenses. Close monitoring is required with frequent or prolonged use of Xalcom in dry eye patients, or in conditions where the cornea is compromised. Contact lenses may absorb benzalkonium chloride and these should be removed before applying Xalcom but may be reinserted after 15 minutes (see section 4.2 Posology and Method of Administration).

4.5 Interaction with other medicinal products and other forms of interaction

Specific medicinal product interaction studies have not been performed with Xalacom.

There have been reports of paradoxical elevations in intraocular pressure following the concomitant ophthalmic administration of two prostaglandin analogues. Therefore, the use of two or more prostaglandins, prostaglandin analogues, or prostaglandin derivatives is not recommended.

The effect on intraocular pressure or the known effects of systemic beta-blockade may be potentiated when Xalacom is given to patients already receiving an oral beta-adrenergic blocking agent, and the use of two or more topical beta-adrenergic blocking agents is not recommended.

Mydriasis has occasionally been reported when timolol was given with epinephrine.

There is a potential for additive effects resulting in hypotension and/or marked bradycardia when eye drops with timolol are administered concomitantly with oral calcium channel blockers, guanethidine or beta-blocking agents, antiarrhythmics, digitalis glycosides or parasympathomimetics.

The hypertensive reaction to sudden withdrawal of clonidine can be potentiated when taking beta-blockers.

Beta-blockers may increase the hypoglycaemic effect of antidiabetic agents. Beta-blockers can mask the signs and symptoms of hypoglycaemia (see 4.4, Special warnings and special precautions for use).

4.6 Pregnancy and lactation

PREGNANCY

Latanoprost:

There are no adequate data from the use of lantanoprost in pregnant women. Studies in animals have shown reproductive toxicity (see 5.3). The potential risk for humans is unknown.

Timolol:

Well controlled epidemiological studies with systemic use of beta-blockers did not indicate malformative effects, but some pharmacological effects such as bradycardia have already been observed in foetuses or neonates.

Consequently Xalacom should not be used during pregnancy (see 5.3).

LACTATION

Timolol is excreted into breast milk. Latanoprost and its metabolites may pass into breast milk. Xalacom should therefore not be used in women who are breast-feeding.

4.7 Effects on ability to drive and use machines

Instillation of eye drops may cause transient blurring of vision. Until this is resolved, patients should not drive or use machines.

4.8 Undesirable effects

For latanoprost, the majority of adverse events relate to the ocular system. In data from the extension phase of the Xalacom pivotal trials, 16 - 20% of patients developed increased iris pigmentation, which may be permanent. In an open 5 year latanoprost safety study, 33% of patients developed iris pigmentation (see 4.4). Other ocular adverse events are generally transient and occur on dose administration. For timolol, the most serious adverse events are systemic in nature, including bradycardia, arrhythmia, congestive heart failure, bronchospasm and allergic reactions.

Treatment related adverse events seen in clinical trials with Xalacom are listed below.

Adverse events are categorized by frequency as follows: very common (≥1/10), common (≥1/100, <1/10), uncommon (≥1/1000, <1/100), rare (≥1/10,0000, <1/1000) and very rare (<1/10,000).

Nervous System Disorders:

Uncommon: Headache.

Eye Disorders:

Very common: Increased iris pigmentation.

Common: Eye irritation (including stinging, burning and itching), Eye pain.

Uncommon: Eye hyperaemia, Conjunctivitis, Vision blurred, Lacrimation increased, Blepharitis, Corneal disorders.

Skin and Subcutaneous Tissue Disorders:

Uncommon: Skin rash, Pruritus.

Additional adverse events have been reported specific to the use of the individual components of Xalacom in either in clinical studies, spontaneous reports or in the available literature.

For latanoprost, these are:

Nervous System Disorders:

Dizziness.

Eye Disorders:

Eyelash and vellus hair changes (increased length, thickness, pigmentation, and number), Punctate epithelial erosions, periorbital oedema, iritis/uveitis, macular oedema (in aphakic, pseudophakic patients with torn posterior lens capsules or in patients with known risk factors for macular oedema), Dry eye, Keratitis, Corneal oedema and erosions, Misdirected eyelashes sometimes resulting in eye irritation.

Cardiac Disorders:

Aggravation of angina in patients with pre-existing disease, Palpitations.

Respiratory, Thoracic and Mediastinal Disorders

Asthma, Asthma aggravation, Dysponea.

Skin and Subcutaneous Tissue Disorders:

Darkening of palpebral skin.

Musculoskeletal, Connective Tissue and Bone Disorders:

Joint pain, Muscle pain.

General disorders and Administration Site Conditions:

Chest pain

For timolol, these are:

Immune System Disorders:

Signs and symptoms of systemic allergic reactions including angioedema, urticaria, and localized and generalized rash.

Psychiatric Disorders:

Depression, Memory loss, Decreased libido, Insomnia, Nightmares.

Nervous System Disorders:

Dizziness, Paraesthesia, Cerebral ischemia, Cerebrovascular accident, Increase in signs and symptoms of myasthenia gravis, Syncope.

Eye Disorders:

Signs and symptoms of ocular irritation including keratitis, decreased corneal sensitivity and dry eyes, Visual disturbances including refractive changes (due to withdrawal of miotic therapy in some cases), Diplopia, Ptosis, Choroidal detachment (following filtration surgery).

Ear and Labyrinth Disorders:

Tinnitus

Cardiac Disorders:

Palpitation, Arrhythmia, Bradycardia, Cardiac arrest, Heart block, Congestive heart failure.

Vascular Disorders:

Hypotension, Raynaud's phenomenon, Cold hands and feet.

Respiratory, Thoracic and Mediastinal Disorders:

bronchospasm (predominantly in patients with pre-existing bronchospastic disease), Dyspnoea, Cough.

Gastrointestinal Disorders:

Nausea, Diarrhoea, Dyspepsia, Dry mouth.

Skin and Subcutaneous Tissue Disorders:

Alopecia, Psoriasiform rash or exacerbation of psoriasis.

General Disorders and Administration Site Conditions:

Asthenia/fatigue, Chest pain, Oedema.

4.9 Overdose

No data are available in humans with regard to overdose with Xalacom.

Symptoms of systemic timolol overdose are: bradycardia, hypotension, bronchospasm and cardiac arrest. If such symptoms occur the treatment should be symptomatic and supportive. Studies have shown that timolol does not dialyse readily.

Apart from ocular irritation and conjunctival hyperaemia no other ocular or systemic side effects are known if latanoprost is overdosed.

If latanoprost is accidentally ingested orally the following information may be useful: Treatment: Gastric lavage if needed. Symptomatic treatment. Latanoprost is extensively metabolised during the first pass through the liver. Intravenous infusion of 3 micrograms/kg in healthy volunteers induced no symptoms but a dose of 5.5-10 micrograms/kg caused nausea, abdominal pain, dizziness, fatigue, hot flushes and sweating. These events were mild to moderate in severity and resolved without treatment, within 4 hours after terminating the infusion.

5. PHARMACOLOGICAL PROPERTIES

5.1 Pharmacodynamic properties

Pharmacotherapeutic group:

Ophthalmological-betablocking agents - timolol, combinations

ATC code: S01ED51

Mechanism of action

Xalacom consists of two components: latanoprost and timolol maleate. These two components decrease elevated intraocular pressure (IOP) by different mechanisms of action and the combined effect results in additional IOP reduction compared to either compound administered alone.

Latanoprost, a prostaglandin F_{2alpha} analogue, is a selective prostanoid FP receptor agonist that reduces the IOP by increasing the outflow of aqueous humour. The main mechanism of action is increased uveoscleral outflow. Additionally, some increase in outflow facility (decrease in trabecular outflow resistance) has been reported in man. Latanoprost has no significant effect on the production of aqueous humour, the blood-aqueous barrier or the intraocular blood circulation. Chronic treatment with latanoprost in monkey eyes, which had undergone extracapsular lens extraction, did not affect the retinal blood vessels as determined by fluorescein angiography. Latanoprost has not induced fluorescein leakage in the posterior segment of pseudophakic human eyes during short-term treatment.

Timolol is a beta-1 and beta-2 (non-selective) adrenergic receptor blocking agent that has no significant intrinsic sympathomimetic, direct myocardial depressant or membrane-stabilising activity. Timolol lowers IOP by decreasing the formation of aqueous in the ciliary epithelium. The precise mechanism of action is not clearly established, but inhibition of the increased cyclic AMP synthesis caused by endogenous beta-adrenergic stimulation is probable. Timolol has not been found to significantly affect the permeability of the blood-aqueous barrier to plasma proteins. In rabbits, timolol was without effect on the regional ocular blood flow after chronic treatment.

Pharmacodynamic effects

Clinical effects

In dose finding studies, Xalacom produced significantly greater decreases in mean diurnal IOP compared to latanoprost and timolol administered once daily as monotherapy. In two well controlled, double masked six-month clinical studies the IOP reducing effect of Xalacom was compared with latanoprost and timolol monotherapy in patients with an IOP of at least 25 mm Hg or greater. Following a 2-4 week run-in with timolol (mean decrease in IOP from enrollment of 5 mm Hg), additional decreases in mean diurnal IOP of 3.1, 2.0 and 0.6 mm Hg were observed after 6 months of treatment for Xalacom, latanoprost and timolol (twice daily), respectively. The IOP lowering effect of Xalacom was maintained in 6 month open label extensions of these studies.

Existing data suggest that evening dosing may be more effective in IOP lowering than morning dosing. However, when considering a recommendation of either morning or evening dosing, sufficient consideration should be given to the lifestyle of the patient and their likely compliance.

It should be kept in mind that in case of insufficient efficacy of the fixed combination, results from studies indicate that the use of unfixed administration of Timolol bid and latanoprost once a day might be still efficient.

Onset of action of Xalacom is within one hour and maximal effect occurs within six to eight hours. Adequate IOP reducing effect has been shown to be present up to 24 hours post dosage after multiple treatments.

5.2 Pharmacokinetic properties

Latanoprost

Latanoprost is an isopropyl ester prodrug, which *per se* is inactive, but after hydrolysis by esterases in the cornea to the acid of latanoprost, becomes biologically active. The prodrug is well absorbed through the cornea and all drug that enters the aqueous humor is hydrolysed during the passage through the cornea. Studies in man indicate that the maximum concentration in the aqueous humour, approximately 15-30 ng/ml, is reached about 2 hours after topical administration of latanoprost alone. After topical application in monkeys latanoprost is distributed primarily in the anterior segment, the conjunctiva and the eyelids.

The acid of latanoprost has a plasma clearance of 0.40 l/h/kg and a small volume of distribution, 0.16 l/kg, resulting in a rapid half life in plasma, 17 minutes. After topical ocular administration the systemic bioavailability of the acid of latanoprost is 45%. The acid of latanoprost has a plasma protein binding of 87%.

There is practically no metabolism of the acid of latanoprost in the eye. The main metabolism occurs in the liver. The main metabolites, the 1,2-dinor and 1,2,3,4- tetranor metabolites, exert no or only weak biological activity in animal studies and are excreted primarily in the urine.

Timolol

The maximum concentration of timolol in the aqueous humor is reached about 1 hour after topical administration of eye drops. Part of the dose is absorbed systemically and a maximum plasma concentration of 1 ng/ml is reached 10-20 minutes after topical administration of one eye drop to each eye once daily (300 micrograms/day). The half life of timolol in plasma is about 6 hours. Timolol is extensively metabolised in the liver. The metabolites are excreted in the urine together with some unchanged timolol.

Xalacom

No pharmacokinetic interactions between latanoprost and timolol were observed although there was an approximate 2-fold increased concentration of the acid of latanoprost in aqueous humour 1-4 hours after administration of Xalacom compared to monotherapy.

5.3 Preclinical safety data

The ocular and systemic safety profile of the individual components is well established. No adverse ocular or systemic effects were seen in rabbits treated topically with the fixed combination or with concomitantly administered latanoprost and timolol ophthalmic solutions. Safety pharmacology, genotoxicity and carcinogenicity studies with each of the components revealed no special hazards for humans. Latanoprost did not affect corneal wound healing in the rabbit eye, whereas timolol inhibited the process in the rabbit and the monkey eye when administered more frequently than once a day.

For latanoprost, no effects on male and female fertility in rats and no teratogenic potential in rats and rabbits have been established. No embryotoxicity was observed in rats after intravenous doses of up to 250 micrograms/kg/day. Latanoprost, however, caused embryofetal toxicity, characterised by increased incidence of late resorption and abortion and by reduced foetal weight, in rabbits at intravenous doses of 5 micrograms/kg/day (approximately 100 times the clinical dose) and above. Timolol showed no effects on male and female fertility in rats or teratogenic potential in mice, rats and rabbits.

6. PHARMACEUTICAL PARTICULARS

6.1 List of excipients

Sodium chloride

Benzalkonium chloride

Sodium dihydrogen phosphate monohydrate

Disodium phosphate anhydrous

Hydrochloric acid solution (for adjustment to pH 6.0)

Sodium hydroxide solution (for adjustment to pH 6.0)

Water for injections

6.2 Incompatibilities

In vitro studies have shown that precipitation occurs when eye drops containing thiomersal are mixed with Xalatan. If such drugs are used concomitantly with Xalacom, the eye drops should be administered with an interval of at least five minutes.

6.3 Shelf life

2 years

After opening of container: 4 weeks

6.4 Special precautions for storage

Store in a refrigerator (2°C - 8°C).

Opened bottle: Do not store above 25 °C.

Keep the bottle in the outer carton.

6.5 Nature and contents of container

LDPE bottle (5 ml) and dropper applicator (dropper tip), HDPE screw cap, tamper evident LDPE overcap.

Each bottle contains 2.5 ml eye drop solution.

Pack sizes:	1 × 2.5 ml
	3 × 2.5 ml
	6 × 2.5 ml

Not all pack sizes may be marketed.

6.6 Special precautions for disposal and other handling

The tamper evident overcap should be removed before use.

Administrative Data

7. MARKETING AUTHORISATION HOLDER

Pharmacia Limited

Ramsgate Road, Sandwich

Kent

CT 13 9NJ

United Kingdom

8. MARKETING AUTHORISATION NUMBER(S)

PL 00032/0288

9. DATE OF FIRST AUTHORISATION/RENEWAL OF THE AUTHORISATION

16th February 2007

10. DATE OF REVISION OF THE TEXT

November 2007

XM9_1

Xalatan 0.005% eye drops solution

(Pharmacia Limited)

1. NAME OF THE MEDICINAL PRODUCT

Xalatan® 0.005% w/v eye drops solution.

2. QUALITATIVE AND QUANTITATIVE COMPOSITION

100 ml eye drops solution contains 0.005 g latanoprost.

One drop contains approximately 1.5 micrograms latanoprost.

Excipient: Benzalkonium chloride 0.02% w/v is included as a preservative.

For a full list of excipients, see section 6.1.

3. PHARMACEUTICAL FORM

Eye drops, solution.

The solution is a clear colourless liquid.

4. CLINICAL PARTICULARS

4.1 Therapeutic indications

Reduction of elevated intraocular pressure in patients with open angle glaucoma and ocular hypertension.

4.2 Posology and method of administration

Recommended dosage for adults (including the elderly):

Recommended therapy is one eye drop in the affected eye(s) once daily. Optimal effect is obtained if Xalatan is administered in the evening.

The dosage of Xalatan should not exceed once daily since it has been shown that more frequent administration decreases the intraocular pressure lowering effect.

If one dose is missed, treatment should continue with the next dose as normal.

As with any eye drops, to reduce possible systemic absorption, it is recommended that the lachrymal sac be compressed at the medial canthus (punctal occlusion) for one minute. This should be performed immediately following the instillation of each drop.

Contact lenses should be removed before instillation of the eye drops and may be reinserted after 15 minutes.

If more than one topical ophthalmic drug is being used, the drugs should be administered at least five minutes apart.

Children:

Safety and effectiveness in children has not been established. Therefore, Xalatan is not recommended for use in children.

4.3 Contraindications

Known hypersensitivity to any component in Xalatan.

4.4 Special warnings and precautions for use

Xalatan may gradually change eye colour by increasing the amount of brown pigment in the iris. Before treatment is instituted, patients should be informed of the possibility of a permanent change in eye colour. Unilateral treatment can result in permanent heterochromia.

This change in eye colour has predominantly been seen in patients with mixed coloured irides, i.e. blue-brown, grey-brown, yellow-brown and green-brown. In studies with latanoprost, the onset of the change is usually within the first 8 months of treatment, rarely during the second or third year, and has not been seen after the fourth year of treatment. The rate of progression of iris pigmentation decreases with time and is stable for five years. The effect of increased pigmentation beyond five years has not been evaluated. In an open 5-year latanoprost safety study, 33% of patients developed iris pigmentation (see 4.8). The iris colour change is slight in the majority of cases and often not observed clinically. The incidence in patients with mixed colour irides ranged from 7 to 85%, with yellow-brown irides having the highest incidence. In patients with homogeneously blue eyes, no change has been observed and in patients with homogeneously grey, green or brown eyes, the change has only rarely been seen.

The colour change is due to increased melanin content in the stromal melanocytes of the iris and not to an increase in number of melanocytes. Typically, the brown pigmentation around the pupil spreads concentrically towards the periphery in affected eyes, but the entire iris or parts of it may become more brownish. No further increase in brown iris pigment has been observed after discontinuation of treatment. It has not been associated with any symptom or pathological changes in clinical trials to date.

Neither naevi nor freckles of the iris have been affected by treatment. Accumulation of pigment in the trabecular meshwork or elsewhere in the anterior chamber has not been observed in clinical trials. Based on 5 years clinical experience, increased iris pigmentation has not been shown to have any negative clinical sequelae and Xalatan can be continued if iris pigmentation ensues. However, patients should be monitored regularly and if the clinical situation warrants, Xalatan treatment may be discontinued.

There is limited experience of Xalatan in chronic angle closure glaucoma, open angle glaucoma of pseudophakic patients and in pigmentary glaucoma. There is no experience of Xalatan in inflammatory and neovascular glaucoma, inflammatory ocular conditions, or congenital glaucoma. Xalatan has no or little effect on the pupil, but there is no experience in acute attacks of closed angle glaucoma. Therefore, it is recommended that Xalatan should be used with caution in these conditions until more experience is obtained.

There are limited study data on the use of Xalatan during the peri-operative period of cataract surgery. Xalatan should be used with caution in these patients.

Reports of macular oedema have occurred (see 4.8) mainly in aphakic patients, in pseudophakic patients with torn posterior lens capsule or anterior chamber lenses, or in patients with known risk factors for cystoid macular oedema (such as diabetic retinopathy and retinal vein occlusion). Xalatan should be used with caution in aphakic patients, in pseudophakic patients with torn posterior lens capsule or anterior chamber lenses, or in patients with known risk factors for cystoid macular oedema.

In patients with known predisposing risk factors for iritis/uveitis, Xalatan can be used with caution.

There is limited experience from patients with asthma, but some cases of exacerbation of asthma and/or dyspnoea were reported in post marketing experience. Asthmatic patients should therefore be treated with caution until there is sufficient experience, see also 4.8.

Periorbital skin discolouration has been observed, the majority of reports being in Japanese patients. Experience to date shows that periorbital skin discolouration is not permanent and in some cases has reversed while continuing treatment with Xalatan.

Latanoprost may gradually change eyelashes and vellus hair in the treated eye and surrounding areas; these changes include increased length, thickness, pigmentation, number of lashes or hairs and misdirected growth of eyelashes. Eyelash changes are reversible upon discontinuation of treatment.

Xalatan contains benzalkonium chloride, which is commonly used as a preservative in ophthalmic products. Benzalkonium chloride has been reported to cause punctate keratopathy and/or toxic ulcerative keratopathy, may cause eye irritation and is known to discolour soft contact lenses. Close monitoring is required with frequent or prolonged use of Xalatan in dry eye patients, or in conditions where the cornea is compromised. Contact lenses may absorb benzalkonium chloride and these should be removed before applying Xalatan but may be reinserted after 15 minutes (see section 4.2 Posology and Method of Administration).

4.5 Interaction with other medicinal products and other forms of interaction

Definitive drug interaction data are not available.

There have been reports of paradoxical elevations in intraocular pressure following the concomitant ophthalmic administration of two prostaglandin analogues. Therefore, the use of two or more prostaglandins, prostaglandin analogues or prostaglandin derivatives is not recommended.

4.6 Pregnancy and lactation

Pregnancy

The safety of this medicinal product for use in human pregnancy has not been established. It has potential hazardous pharmacological effects with respect to the course of pregnancy, to the unborn or the neonate. Therefore, Xalatan should not be used during pregnancy.

Lactation

Latanoprost and its metabolites may pass into breast milk and Xalatan should therefore not be used in nursing women or breast feeding should be stopped.

4.7 Effects on ability to drive and use machines

In common with other eye preparations, instillation of eye drops may cause transient blurring of vision.

4.8 Undesirable effects

The majority of adverse events relate to the ocular system. In an open 5-year latanoprost safety study, 33% of patients developed iris pigmentation (see 4.4). Other ocular adverse events are generally transient and occur on dose administration.

Adverse events are categorized by frequency as follows: very common (≥ 1/10), common (≥ 1/100, < 1/10), uncommon (≥ 1/1000, < 1/100), rare (≥ 1/10,0000, < 1/1000) and very rare (< 1/10,000). Frequencies for events reported post-marketing are not known.

Eye Disorders:

Very common: Increased iris pigmentation; mild to moderate conjunctival hyperaemia eye irritation (burning grittiness, itching, stinging and foreign body sensation); eyelash and vellus hair changes (increased length, thickness, pigmentation and number) (vast majority of reports in Japanese population).

Common: transient punctate epithelial erosions, mostly without symptoms; blepharitis; eye pain.

Uncommon: Eyelid oedema: dry eye; keratitus; vision blurred; conjunctivitis.

Rare: Iritis/uveitis (the majority of reports in patients with concomitant predisposing factors); macular oedema; symptomatic corneal oedema and erosions; periorbital oedema; misdirected eyelashes sometimes resulting in eye irritation; extra row of cilia at the aperture of the meibomian glands (distichiasis).

Cardiac Disorders:

Very rare: Aggravation of angina in patients with pre-existing disease.

Respiratory, Thoracic and Mediastinal Disorders:

Rare: Asthma, asthma exacerbation and dyspnoea.

Skin and Subcutaneous Tissue Disorders:

Uncommon: Skin rash.

Rare: Localised skin reaction on the eyelids; darkening of the palpebral skin of the eyelids.

General Disorders and Administration Site Conditions:

Very rare: Chest pain.

There have been additional post-marketing spontaneous reports of the following:

Nervous System Disorders:

Headache, Dizziness.

Cardiac Disorders:

Palpitations.

Musculoskeletal and Connective Tissue Disorders:

Myalgia; Arthralgia.

4.9 Overdose

Apart from ocular irritation and conjunctival hyperaemia, no other ocular side effects are known if Xalatan is overdosed.

If Xalatan is accidentally ingested the following information may be useful: One bottle contains 125 micrograms latanoprost. More than 90% is metabolised during the first pass through the liver. Intravenous infusion of 3 micrograms/kg in healthy volunteers induced no symptoms, but a dose of 5.5-10 micrograms/kg caused nausea, abdominal pain, dizziness, fatigue, hot flushes and sweating. In monkeys, latanoprost has been infused intravenously in doses of up to 500 micrograms/kg without major effects on the cardiovascular system.

Intravenous administration of latanoprost in monkeys has been associated with transient bronchoconstriction. However, in patients with moderate bronchial asthma, bronchoconstriction was not induced by latanoprost when applied topically on the eyes in a dose of seven times the clinical dose of Xalatan.

If overdosage with Xalatan occurs, treatment should be symptomatic.

5. PHARMACOLOGICAL PROPERTIES

5.1 Pharmacodynamic properties

Pharmacotherapeutic group (ATC code): S 01 E E 01

The active substance latanoprost, a prostaglandin $F_{2\alpha}$ analogue, is a selective prostanoid FP receptor agonist which reduces the intraocular pressure by increasing the outflow of aqueous humour. Reduction of the intraocular pressure in man starts about three to four hours after administration and maximum effect is reached after eight to twelve hours. Pressure reduction is maintained for at least 24 hours.

Studies in animals and man indicate that the main mechanism of action is increased uveoscleral outflow, although some increase in outflow facility (decrease in outflow resistance) has been reported in man.

Pivotal studies have demonstrated that Xalatan is effective as monotherapy. In addition, clinical trials investigating combination use have been performed. These include studies that show that latanoprost is effective in combination with beta-adrenergic antagonists (timolol). Short-term (1 or 2 weeks) studies suggest that the effect of latanoprost is additive in combination with adrenergic agonists (dipivalyl epinephrine), oral carbonic anhydrase inhibitors (acetazolamide) and at least partly additive with cholinergic agonists (pilocarpine).

Clinical trials have shown that latanoprost has no significant effect on the production of aqueous humour. Latanoprost has not been found to have any effect on the blood-aqueous barrier.

Latanoprost has no or negligible effects on the intraocular blood circulation when used at the clinical dose and studied in monkeys. However, mild to moderate conjunctival or episcleral hyperaemia may occur during topical treatment.

Chronic treatment with latanoprost in monkey eyes, which had undergone extracapsular lens extraction, did not affect the retinal blood vessels as determined by fluorescein angiography.

Latanoprost has not induced fluorescein leakage in the posterior segment of pseudophakic human eyes during short-term treatment.

Latanoprost in clinical doses has not been found to have any significant pharmacological effects on the cardiovascular or respiratory system.

5.2 Pharmacokinetic properties

Latanoprost (mw 432.58) is an isopropyl ester prodrug which per se is inactive, but after hydrolysis to the acid of latanoprost becomes biologically active.

The prodrug is well absorbed through the cornea and all drug that enters the aqueous humour is hydrolysed during the passage through the cornea.

Studies in man indicate that the peak concentration in the aqueous humour is reached about two hours after topical administration. After topical application in monkeys, latanoprost is distributed primarily in the anterior segment, the conjunctivae and the eyelids. Only minute quantities of the drug reach the posterior segment.

There is practically no metabolism of the acid of latanoprost in the eye. The main metabolism occurs in the liver. The half life in plasma is 17 minutes in man. The main metabolites, the 1,2-dinor and 1,2,3,4-tetranor metabolites, exert no or only weak biological activity in animal studies and are excreted primarily in the urine.

5.3 Preclinical safety data

The ocular as well as systemic toxicity of latanoprost has been investigated in several animal species. Generally, latanoprost is well tolerated with a safety margin between clinical ocular dose and systemic toxicity of at least 1000 times. High doses of latanoprost, approximately 100 times the clinical dose/kg body weight, administered intravenously to unanaesthetised monkeys have been shown to increase the respiration rate probably reflecting bronchoconstriction of short duration. In animal studies, latanoprost has not been found to have sensitising properties.

In the eye, no toxic effects have been detected with doses of up to 100 micrograms/eye/day in rabbits or monkeys (clinical dose is approximately 1.5 micrograms/eye/day). In monkeys, however, latanoprost has been shown to induce increased pigmentation of the iris.

The mechanism of increased pigmentation seems to be stimulation of melanin production in melanocytes of the iris with no proliferative changes observed. The change in iris colour may be permanent.

In chronic ocular toxicity studies, administration of latanoprost 6 micrograms/eye/day has also been shown to induce increased palpebral fissure. This effect is reversible and occurs at doses above the clinical dose level. The effect has not been seen in humans.

Latanoprost was found negative in reverse mutation tests in bacteria, gene mutation in mouse lymphoma and mouse micronucleus test. Chromosome aberrations were observed in vitro with human lymphocytes. Similar effects were observed with prostaglandin $F_{2\alpha}$, a naturally occurring prostaglandin, and indicates that this is a class effect.

Additional mutagenicity studies on in vitro/in vivo unscheduled DNA synthesis in rats were negative and indicate that latanoprost does not have mutagenic potency. Carcinogenicity studies in mice and rats were negative.

Latanoprost has not been found to have any effect on male or female fertility in animal studies. In the embryotoxicity study in rats, no embryotoxicity was observed at intravenous doses (5, 50 and 250 micrograms/kg/day) of latanoprost. However, latanoprost induced embryolethal effects in rabbits at doses of 5 micrograms/kg/day and above.

The dose of 5 micrograms/kg/day (approximately 100 times the clinical dose) caused significant embryofoetal toxicity characterised by increased incidence of late resorption and abortion and by reduced foetal weight.

No teratogenic potential has been detected.

6. PHARMACEUTICAL PARTICULARS

6.1 List of excipients

Sodium chloride

Benzalkonium chloride

Sodium dihydrogen phosphate monohydrate

Anhydrous disodium phosphate

Water for injections

6.2 Incompatibilities

In vitro studies have shown that precipitation occurs when eye drops containing thiomersal are mixed with Xalatan. If such drugs are used, the eye drops should be administered with an interval of at least five minutes.

6.3 Shelf life

Before first opening: 3 years for the dropper container with clear tamper-evident overcap and white inner screw cap

2 years for the dropper container with white screw cap and tamper evident ring

After first opening of container: 4 weeks (for both dropper containers)

6.4 Special precautions for storage

Store in a refrigerator (2°C – 8°C).

Keep the bottle in the outer carton in order to protect from light.

After first opening the bottle: do not store above 25°C and use within four weeks.

6.5 Nature and contents of container

Dropper container (5 ml) of polyethylene with either a screw cap and tamper evident overcap of polyethylene or with a screw cap and tamper-evident ring

Each dropper container contains 2.5 ml eye drops solution corresponding to approximately 80 drops of solution.

Pack sizes: 1 × 2.5 ml, 3 × 2.5 ml, 6 × 2.5 ml.

Not all pack sizes may be marketed.

6.6 Special precautions for disposal and other handling

No special requirements.

7. MARKETING AUTHORISATION HOLDER

Pharmacia Limited

Ramsgate Road

Sandwich

Kent

CT13 9NJ

United Kingdom

8. MARKETING AUTHORISATION NUMBER(S)

PL 00032/0220

9. DATE OF FIRST AUTHORISATION/RENEWAL OF THE AUTHORISATION

16 December 1996/16 December 2006

10. DATE OF REVISION OF THE TEXT

July 2009

XN 11_0

Xamiol gel

(Leo Laboratories Limited)

1. NAME OF THE MEDICINAL PRODUCT

Xamiol 50 microgram/g + 0.5 mg/g gel

2. QUALITATIVE AND QUANTITATIVE COMPOSITION

One gram of gel contains 50 microgram of calcipotriol (as monohydrate) and 0.5 mg of betamethasone (as dipropionate).

Excipient: 160 microgram butylated hydroxytoluene/g gel.

For a full list of excipients, see section 6.1.

3. PHARMACEUTICAL FORM

Gel.

An almost clear, colourless to slightly off-white gel.

4. CLINICAL PARTICULARS

4.1 Therapeutic indications

Topical treatment of scalp psoriasis.

4.2 Posology and method of administration

Xamiol gel should be applied to affected areas of the scalp once daily. The recommended treatment period is 4 weeks. After this period repeated treatment with Xamiol gel can be initiated under medical supervision.

All the affected scalp areas may be treated with Xamiol gel. Usually an amount between 1 g and 4 g per day is sufficient for treatment of the scalp (4g corresponds to one teaspoon).

When using calcipotriol containing products, the maximum daily dose should not exceed 15 g, and the maximum weekly dose should not exceed 100 g. The body surface area treated with calcipotriol containing products **should not exceed** 30% (see section 4.4).

Shake the bottle before use. In order to achieve optimal effect, it is recommended that the hair is not washed immediately after application of Xamiol gel. Xamiol gel should remain on the scalp during the night or during the day.

Paediatric patients:

Xamiol gel is not recommended for use in children below 18 years due to lack of data on safety and efficacy.

4.3 Contraindications

Hypersensitivity to the active substances or to any of the excipients.

Due to the content of calcipotriol, Xamiol gel is contraindicated in patients with known disorders of calcium metabolism.

Due to the content of corticosteroid, Xamiol gel is contraindicated in the following conditions: Viral (e.g. herpes or varicella) lesions of the skin, fungal or bacterial skin infections, parasitic infections, skin manifestations in relation to tuberculosis or syphilis, perioral dermatitis, atrophic skin, striae atrophicae, fragility of skin veins, ichthyosis, acne vulgaris, acne rosacea, rosacea, ulcers and wounds.

Xamiol gel is contraindicated in guttate, erythrodermic, exfoliative and pustular psoriasis.

Xamiol gel is contraindicated in patients with severe renal insufficiency or severe hepatic disorders.

4.4 Special warnings and precautions for use

Xamiol gel contains a potent group III steroid and concurrent treatment with other steroids on the scalp must be avoided. Adverse effects found in connection with systemic corticosteroid treatment, such as adrenocortical suppression or impact on the metabolic control of diabetes mellitus, may occur also during topical corticosteroid treatment due to systemic absorption. Application under occlusive dressings should be avoided since it increases the systemic absorption of corticosteroids.

In a study in patients with both extensive scalp and extensive body psoriasis using a combination of high doses of Xamiol gel (scalp application) and high doses of Dovobet ointment (body application), 5 of 32 patients showed a borderline decrease in cortisol response to adrenocorticotropic hormone (ACTH) challenge after 4 weeks of treatment (see section 5.1).

Due to the content of calcipotriol, hypercalcaemia may occur if the maximum weekly dose (100 g) is exceeded. Serum calcium is, however, quickly normalised when treatment is discontinued. The risk of hypercalcaemia is minimal when the recommendations relevant to calcipotriol are followed.

Efficacy and safety of use of this product on areas other than the scalp have not been established. Treatment of more than 30% of the body surface should be avoided (see section 4.2). Application on large areas of damaged skin or on mucous membranes or in skin folds should be avoided since it increases the systemic absorption of corticosteroids (see section 4.8). Skin of the face and genitals are very sensitive to corticosteroids. These areas should only be treated with weaker corticosteroids. Uncommon local adverse reactions (such as eye irritation or irritation of facial skin) were observed, when the drug was accidentally administered in the area of face, or accidentally to the eyes or conjunctives (see sections 4.8 and 5.1). The patient must be instructed in correct use of the product to avoid application and accidental transfer to the face, mouth and eyes. Hands must be washed after each application to avoid accidental transfer to these areas.

When lesions become secondarily infected, they should be treated with antimicrobiological therapy. However, if infection worsens, treatment with corticosteroids should be stopped.

When treating psoriasis with topical corticosteroids, there may be a risk of generalised pustular psoriasis or of rebound effects when discontinuing treatment. Medical supervision should therefore continue in the post-treatment period.

With long-term use there is an increased risk of local and systemic corticosteroid undesirable effects. The treatment should be discontinued in case of undesirable effects related to long-term use of corticosteroid (see section 4.8).

There is no experience with concurrent use of other anti-psoriatic products administered systemically or with phototherapy.

During Xamiol gel treatment, physicians are recommended to advise patients to limit or avoid excessive exposure to either natural or artificial sunlight. Topical calcipotriol should be used with UVR only if the physician and patient consider that the potential benefits outweigh the potential risks (see section 5.3).

Xamiol gel contains butylated hydroxytoluene (E321), which may cause local skin reactions (e.g. contact dermatitis), or irritation to the eyes and mucous membranes.

4.5 Interaction with other medicinal products and other forms of interaction

No interaction studies have been performed.

4.6 Pregnancy and lactation

Pregnancy

There are no adequate data from the use of Xamiol gel in pregnant women. Studies in animals with glucocorticoids have shown reproductive toxicity (see section 5.3), but a number of epidemiological studies have not revealed congenital anomalies among infants born to women treated with corticosteroids during pregnancy. The potential risk for humans is uncertain. Therefore, during pregnancy, Xamiol gel should only be used when the potential benefit justifies the potential risk.

Lactation

Betamethasone passes into breast milk, but risk of an adverse effect on the infant seems unlikely with therapeutic doses. There are no data on the excretion of calcipotriol in breast milk. Caution should be exercised when prescribing Xamiol gel to women who breast-feed.

4.7 Effects on ability to drive and use machines

Xamiol gel has no influence on the ability to drive and use machines.

4.8 Undesirable effects

The following terminologies have been used in order to classify the frequencies of adverse drug reactions:

Very common	≥1/10
Common	≥1/100 and <1/10
Uncommon	≥1/1,000 and <1/100
Rare	≥1/10,000 and <1/1,000
Very rare	<1/10,000

Not known (cannot be estimated from the available data)

The clinical trial programme for Xamiol gel has so far included more than 4,400 patients of whom more than 1,900 were treated with Xamiol gel. Approximately 8% of patients treated with Xamiol gel experienced a non-serious adverse drug reaction.

Based on data from clinical trials the only known common adverse drug reaction is pruritus. Uncommon adverse drug reactions are burning sensation of skin, skin pain or irritation, folliculitis, dermatitis, erythema, acne, dry skin, exacerbation of psoriasis, rash, pustular rash, and eye irritation. These adverse drug reactions were all non-serious local reactions.

The adverse drug reactions are listed by MedDRA SOC, and the individual adverse drug reactions are listed starting with the most frequently reported.

• **Eye disorders**

Uncommon:	Eye irritation

• **Skin and subcutaneous tissue disorders**

Common:	Pruritus
Uncommon:	Burning sensation of skin
Uncommon:	Skin pain or irritation
Uncommon:	Folliculitis
Uncommon:	Dermatitis
Uncommon:	Erythema
Uncommon:	Acne
Uncommon:	Dry skin
Uncommon:	Exacerbation of psoriasis
Uncommon:	Rash
Uncommon:	Pustular rash

Adverse drug reactions observed for calcipotriol and betamethasone, respectively:

Calcipotriol

Adverse drug reactions include application site reactions, pruritus, skin irritation, burning and stinging sensation, dry skin, erythema, rash, dermatitis, eczema, psoriasis aggravated, photosensitivity and hypersensitivity reactions including very rare cases of angioedema and facial oedema. Systemic effects after topical use may appear very rarely causing hypercalcaemia or hypercalciuria (see section 4.4).

Betamethasone (as dipropionate)

Local reactions can occur after topical use, especially during prolonged application, including skin atrophy, telangiectasia, striae, folliculitis, hypertrichosis, perioral dermatitis, allergic contact dermatitis, depigmentation and colloid milia. When treating psoriasis, there may be a risk of generalised pustular psoriasis.

Systemic effects due to topical use of corticosteroids are rare in adults, however, they can be severe. Adrenocortical suppression, cataract, infections and increase of intraocular pressure can occur, especially after long-term treatment. Systemic effects occur more frequently when applied under occlusion (plastic, skin folds), when applied on large areas and during long-term treatment (see section 4.4).

4.9 Overdose

Use above the recommended dose may cause elevated serum calcium which should rapidly subside when treatment is discontinued.

Excessive prolonged use of topical corticosteroids may suppress the pituitary-adrenal functions, resulting in secondary adrenal insufficiency which is usually reversible. In such cases, symptomatic treatment is indicated.

In case of chronic toxicity, the corticosteroid treatment must be discontinued gradually.

It has been reported that due to misuse one patient with extensive erythrodermic psoriasis treated with 240 g of Dovobet ointment weekly (maximum dose 100 g weekly) for 5 months developed Cushing's syndrome and pustular psoriasis after abruptly stopping treatment.

5. PHARMACOLOGICAL PROPERTIES

5.1 Pharmacodynamic properties

Pharmacotherapeutic group: Other antipsoriatics for topical use, Calcipotriol, combinations

ATC Code: D05AX52

Calcipotriol is a vitamin D analogue. In vitro data suggest that calcipotriol induces differentiation and suppresses proliferation of keratinocytes. This is the proposed basis for its effect in psoriasis.

Like other topical corticosteroids, betamethasone dipropionate has anti-inflammatory, antipruritic, vasoconstrictive and immunosuppresive properties, however, without curing the underlying condition. Through occlusion the effect can be enhanced due to increased penetration of the stratum corneum. The incidence of adverse events will increase because of this. In general, the mechanism of the anti-inflammatory activity of the topical steroids is unclear.

Adrenal response to ACTH was determined by measuring serum cortisol levels in patients with both extensive scalp and body psoriasis, using up to 106 g per week combined Xamiol gel and Dovobet ointment. A borderline decrease in cortisol response at 30 minutes post ACTH challenge was seen in 5 of 32 patients (15.6%) after 4 weeks of treatment and in 2 of 11 patients (18.2%) who continued treatment until 8 weeks. In all cases, the serum cortisol levels were normal at 60 minutes post ACTH challenge. There was no evidence of change of calcium metabolism observed in these patients.

The efficacy of once daily use of Xamiol gel was investigated in two randomised, double-blind, 8-week clinical studies including a total of more than 2,900 patients with scalp psoriasis of at least mild severity according to the Investigator's Global Assessment of disease severity (IGA). Comparators were betamethasone dipropionate in the gel vehicle, calcipotriol in the gel vehicle and (in one of the studies) the gel vehicle alone, all used once daily. Results for the primary response criterion (absent or very mild disease according to the IGA at week 8) showed that Xamiol gel was statistically significantly more effective than the comparators. Results for speed of onset based on similar data at week 2 also showed Xamiol gel to be statistically significantly more effective than the comparators.

(see Table 1 below)

Another randomised, investigator-blinded clinical study including 312 patients with scalp psoriasis of at least moderate severity according to the IGA investigated use of Xamiol gel once daily compared with Dovonex Scalp solution twice daily for up to 8 weeks. Results for the primary response criterion (absent or very mild disease according to the IGA at week 8) showed that Xamiol gel was statistically significantly more effective than Dovonex Scalp solution.

% of patients with absent or very mild disease	Xamiol gel (n=207)	Dovonex Scalp solution (n=105)
week 8	68.6%	31.4%[1]

[1] Statistically significantly less effective than Xamiol gel ($P<0.001$)

A randomised, double-blind long-term clinical study including 873 patients with scalp psoriasis of at least moderate severity (according to the IGA) investigated the use of Xamiol gel compared with calcipotriol in the gel vehicle. Both treatments were applied once daily, intermittently as required, for up to 52 weeks. Adverse events possibly related to long-term use of corticosteroids on the scalp, were identified by an independent, blinded panel of dermatologists. There was no difference in the percentages of patients experiencing such adverse events between the treatment groups (2.6% in the Xamiol gel group and 3.0% in the calcipotriol group; P=0.73). No cases of skin atrophy were reported.

5.2 Pharmacokinetic properties

The systemic exposure to calcipotriol and betamethasone dipropionate from topically applied Xamiol gel is comparable to Dovobet ointment in rats and minipigs. Clinical studies with radiolabelled ointment indicate that the systemic absorption of calcipotriol and betamethasone from Dovobet ointment formulation is less than 1% of the dose (2.5 g) when applied to normal skin (625 cm^2) for 12 hours. Application to psoriasis plaques and under occlusive dressings may increase the absorption of topical corticosteroids.

Following systemic exposure, both active ingredients – calcipotriol and betamethasone dipropionate – are rapidly and extensively metabolised. The main route of excretion of calcipotriol is via faeces (rats and minipigs) and for

Table 1

% of patients with absent or very mild disease	Xamiol gel (n=1,108)	Beta-methasone dipropionate (n=1,118)	Calcipotriol (n=558)	Gel vehicle (n=136)
week 2	53.2%	42.8%[1]	17.2%[1]	11.8%[1]
week 8	69.8%	62.5%[1]	40.1%[1]	22.8%[1]

[1] Statistically significantly less effective than Xamiol gel ($P<0.001$)

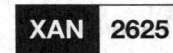

betamethasone dipropionate it is via urine (rats and mice). In rats, tissue distribution studies with radiolabelled calcipotriol and betamethasone dipropionate, respectively, showed that the kidney and liver had the highest level of radioactivity.

Calcipotriol and betamethasone dipropionate were below the lower limit of quantification in all blood samples of 34 patients treated for 4 or 8 weeks with both Xamiol gel and Dovobet ointment for extensive psoriasis involving the body and scalp. One metabolite of calcipotriol and one metabolite of betamethasone dipropionate were quantifiable in some of the patients.

5.3 Preclinical safety data

Studies of corticosteroids in animals have shown reproductive toxicity (cleft palate, skeletal malformations). In reproduction toxicity studies with long-term oral administration of corticosteroids to rats, prolonged gestation and prolonged and difficult labour were detected. Moreover, reduction in offspring survival, body weight and body weight gain was observed. There was no impairment of fertility. The relevance for humans is unknown.

A dermal carcinogenicity study with calcipotriol in mice revealed no special hazard to humans.

In a photo(co)carcinogenicity study, albino hairless mice were repeatedly exposed to both UVR and dermally administered calcipotriol solution for 40 weeks at dose levels corresponding to 9, 30 and 90 μg/m^2/day (equivalent to 0.25, 0.84, 2.5 times the maximum recommended daily dose for a 60 kg adult, respectively). A reduction in the time required for UVR to induce the formation of skin tumours was observed (statistically significant in males only), suggesting that calcipotriol may enhance the effect of UVR to induce skin tumours. In a supplementary study, mice of the same strain were treated repeatedly with either calcipotriol solution or calcipotriol/ betamethasone gel, followed by irradiation with UVR and measurement of recognised cellular indicators of skin photocarcinogenicity. This study showed a similar enhancing effect of calcipotriol alone on the photobiological response of the skin but indicated no effect of the calcipotriol/betamethasone combination. The clinical relevance of these findings is unknown.

No carcinogenicity or photocarcinogenicity studies have been performed with betamethasone dipropionate.

In local tolerability studies in rabbits, Xamiol gel caused mild to moderate skin irritation and a slight transient irritation of the eye.

6. PHARMACEUTICAL PARTICULARS

6.1 List of excipients

Paraffin, liquid

Polyoxypropylene-15 stearyl ether

Castor oil, hydrogenated

Butylhydroxytoluene (E321)

All-rac-α-tocopherol

6.2 Incompatibilities

In the absence of compatibility studies, this medicinal product must not be mixed with other medicinal products.

6.3 Shelf life

2 years.

After first opening: 3 months.

6.4 Special precautions for storage

Do not refrigerate. Keep the bottle in the outer carton in order to protect from light.

6.5 Nature and contents of container

High-density polyethylene bottles with low-density polyethylene nozzle and a high-density polyethylene screw cap. The bottles are placed in cartons.

Pack sizes: 15, 30, 60 and 2 × 60 g.

Not all pack sizes may be marketed.

6.6 Special precautions for disposal and other handling

Any unused product or waste material should be disposed of in accordance with local requirements.

7. MARKETING AUTHORISATION HOLDER

LEO Pharmaceutical Products Ltd. A/S

Industriparken 55

DK-2750 Ballerup

Denmark

8. MARKETING AUTHORISATION NUMBER(S)

PL 05293/0006

9. DATE OF FIRST AUTHORISATION/RENEWAL OF THE AUTHORISATION

25/09/2008

10. DATE OF REVISION OF THE TEXT

25/09/2008

Xanax Tablets 250 micrograms & 500 micrograms

(Pharmacia Limited)

1. NAME OF THE MEDICINAL PRODUCT

Xanax® Tablets 250 and 500 micrograms

2. QUALITATIVE AND QUANTITATIVE COMPOSITION

Alprazolam 250 and 500 micrograms

3. PHARMACEUTICAL FORM

White, oval, biconvex tablets containing 250 microgram (0.25 mg) alprazolam, scored on one side and marked "Upjohn 29" on the other.

Pink, oval, biconvex tablets containing 500 microgram (0.5 mg) alprazolam, scored on one side and marked "Upjohn 55" on the other.

4. CLINICAL PARTICULARS

4.1 Therapeutic indications

Xanax is indicated for the short-term treatment of moderate or severe anxiety states and anxiety associated with depression. It is only indicated when the disorder is severe, disabling or subjecting the individual to extreme distress.

Xanax should not be used to treat short-term mild anxiety, such as anxiety or tension associated with the stress of everyday life. As the efficacy of Xanax in depression and in phobic or obsessional states has yet to be established, specific treatment may have to be considered.

4.2 Posology and method of administration

Treatment should be as short as possible. It is recommended that the patient be reassessed at the end of no longer than 4 weeks' treatment and the need for continued treatment established, especially in case the patient is symptom free. The overall duration of treatment should not be more than 8-12 weeks, including a tapering off process.

In certain cases extension beyond the maximum treatment period may be necessary; if so, it should not take place without re-evaluation of the patient's status with special expertise. As with all benzodiazepines, physicians should be aware that long-term use might lead to dependence in certain patients.

The optimum dosage of Xanax should be based upon the severity of the symptoms and individual patient response. The lowest dose which can control symptoms should be used. Dosage should be reassessed at intervals of no more than 4 weeks. The usual dosage is stated below; in the few patients who require higher doses, the dosage should be increased cautiously to avoid adverse effects. When higher dosage is required, the evening dose should be increased before the daytime doses. In general, patients who have not previously received psychotropic medications will require lower doses than those so treated, or those with a history of chronic alcoholism.

Treatment should always be tapered off gradually. During discontinuation of alprazolam treatment, the dosage should be reduced slowly in keeping with good medical practice. It is suggested that the daily dosage of alprazolam be decreased by no more than 0.5 mg every three days. Some patients may require an even slower dosage reduction

There is a reduced clearance of the drug and, as with other benzodiazepines, an increased sensitivity to the drug in elderly patients.

Anxiety: 250 micrograms (0.25 mg) to 500 micrograms (0.5 mg) three times daily increasing if required to a total of 3 mg daily.

Geriatric patients or in the presence of debilitating disease: 250 micrograms (0.25 mg) two to three times daily to be gradually increased if needed and tolerated.

Children: Not recommended.

If side-effects occur, the dose should be lowered. It is advisable to review treatment regularly and to discontinue use as soon as possible. Should longer term treatment be necessary, then intermittent treatment may be considered to minimize the risk of dependence.

4.3 Contraindications

Myasthenia gravis Hypersensitivity to benzodiazepines or any of the other constituents of the tablet Severe respiratory insufficiency Sleep apnoea syndrome Severe hepatic insufficiency

4.4 Special warnings and precautions for use

Tolerance

Some loss of efficacy to the hypnotic effects of benzodiazepines may develop after repeated use for a few weeks.

Dependence

Use of benzodiazepines may lead to the development of physical and psychic dependence upon these products. The risk of dependence increases with dose and duration of treatment; it is also greater in patients with a history of alcohol and drug abuse.

Once physical dependence has developed, abrupt termination of treatment will be accompanied by withdrawal symptoms. These may consist of headaches, muscle pain, extreme anxiety, tension, restlessness, confusion and irritability. In severe cases the following symptoms may occur: derealization, depersonalisation, hyperacusis, numbness and tingling of the extremities, hypersensitivity to light, noise and physical contact, hallucinations or epileptic seizures.

Rebound insomnia and anxiety: a transient syndrome whereby the symptoms that led to treatment with a benzodiazepine recur in an enhanced form may occur on withdrawal of treatment. It may be accompanied by other reactions including mood changes, anxiety or sleep disturbances and restlessness. Since the risk of withdrawal phenomena/rebound phenomena is greater after abrupt discontinuation of treatment, it is recommended that the dosage be decreased gradually by no more than 0.5 mg every three days. Some patients may require an even slower dose reduction.

Duration of treatment

The duration of treatment should bed as short as possible (see posology) depending on the indication, but should not exceed eight to twelve weeks including tapering off process. Extension beyond these periods should not take place without re-evaluation of the situation.

It may be useful to inform the patient when treatment is started that it will be of limited duration and to explain precisely how the dosage will be progressively decreased. Moreover it is important that the patient should be aware of the possibility of rebound phenomena, thereby minimising anxiety over such symptoms should they occur while the medicinal product is being discontinued.

There are indications, that in the case of benzodiazepines with a short duration of action, withdrawal phenomena can become manifest within the dosage interval, especially when the dosage is high. When benzodiazepines with a long duration of action are being used it is important to warn against changing to a benzodiazepine with a short duration of action, as withdrawal symptoms may develop.

Amnesia

Benzodiazepines may induce anterograde amnesia. The condition occurs most often several hours after ingesting the product and therefore to reduce the risk patients should ensure that they will be able to have uninterrupted sleep of 7-8 ours (see also undesirable effects).

Psychiatric and 'paradoxical' reactions

Reactions like restlessness, agitation, irritability, aggressiveness, delusion, rages, nightmares, hallucinations, psychoses, inappropriate behaviour and other adverse behavioural effects are known to occur when using benzodiazepines. Should this occur, use of the drug should be discontinued.

They are more likely to occur in children and the elderly.

Specific patient groups

Benzodiazepines should not be given to children without careful assessment of the need to do so; the duration of treatment must be kept to a minimum. The elderly should be given a reduced dose (see posology). A lower dose is also recommended for patients with chronic respiratory insufficiency due to risk of respiratory depression.

Benzodiazepines are not indicated to treat patients with severe hepatic insufficiency as they may precipitate encephalopathy. Caution is recommended when treating patients with impaired renal or hepatic function.

Benzodiazepines are not recommended for the primary treatment of psychotic illness.

Benzodiazepines should not be used alone to treat depression of anxiety associated with depression (suicide may be precipitated in such patients). Administration to severely depressed or suicidal patients should be done with appropriate precautions and appropriate size of the prescription.

Benzodiazepines should be used with extreme caution in patients with a history of alcohol or drug abuse.

4.5 Interaction with other medicinal products and other forms of interaction

Not recommended: Concomitant intake with alcohol

The sedative effects may be enhanced when the product is used in combination with alcohol. This affects the ability to drive or use machines.

Take into account: Combination with CNS depressants

Enhancement of the central depressive effect may occur in cases of concomitant use with antipsychotics (neuroleptics), hypnotics, anxiolytics/sedatives, antidepressant agents, narcotic analgesics, anti-epileptic drugs, anaesthetics and sedative antihistamines.

Pharmacokinetic interactions can occur when alprazolam is administered along with drugs that interfere with its metabolism. Compounds that inhibit certain hepatic enzymes (particularly cytochrome P450 3A4) may increase the concentration of alprazolam and enhance it's activity. Data from clinical studies with alprazolam, in-vitro studies with alprazolam and clinical studies with drugs metabolised similarly to alprazolam provide evidence for varying degrees of interaction and possible interaction with alprazolam for a number of drugs. Based on the degree of interaction and the type of data available, the following recommendations are made:

The co-administration of alprazolam with ketoconazole, itraconazole, or other azole-type antifungals is not recommended.

Caution and consideration of dose reduction is recommended when alprazolam is co-administered with nefazodone, fluvoxamine and cimetidine.

Caution is recommended when alprazolam is co-administered with fluoxetine, propoxyphene, oral contraceptives, sertraline, diltiazem, or macrolide antibiotics such as erythromycin and troleandomycin.

Interactions involving HIV protease inhibitors (e.g. ritonavir) and alprazolam are complex and time dependent. Low doses of ritonavir resulted in a large impairment of alprazolam clearance, prolonged its elimination half-life and enhanced clinical effects, however, upon extended exposure to ritonavir, CYP3A induction offset this inhibition. This interaction will require a dose-adjustment or discontinuation of alprazolam.

4.6 Pregnancy and lactation
If the product is prescribed to a woman of childbearing potential, she should be warned to contact her physician regarding discontinuance of the product if she intends to become or suspects that she is pregnant. The data concerning teratogenicity and effects on postnatal development and behaviour following benzodiazepine treatment are inconsistent. There is evidence from some early studies with other members of the benzodiazepine class that in utero exposure may be associated with malformations. Later studies with the benzodiazepine class of drugs have provided no clear evidence of any type of defect.

If, for compelling medical reasons, the product is administered during the late phase of pregnancy or during labour, effects on the neonate such as hypothermia, hypotonia and moderate respiratory depression, can be expected, due to the pharmacological action of the compound.

Infants born to mothers who took benzodiazepines chronically during the latter stages of pregnancy may have developed physical dependence and may be at some risk of developing withdrawal symptoms in the postnatal period.

Since benzodiazepines are found in the breast milk, benzodiazepines should not be given to breast feeding mothers.

4.7 Effects on ability to drive and use machines
Sedation, amnesia, impaired concentration and impaired muscle function may adversely affect the ability to drive or use machines. If insufficient sleep occurs, the likelihood of impaired alertness may be increased (see also interactions).

These effects are potentiated by alcohol (see also interactions).

Patients should be cautioned about operating motor vehicles or engaging in other dangerous activities while taking Xanax.

4.8 Undesirable effects
Sedation/drowsiness, light-headedness, numbed emotions, reduced alertness, confusion, fatigue, headache, dizziness, muscle weakness, ataxia, double or blurred vision, insomnia, nervousness/anxiety, tremor, change in weight. These phenomena occur predominantly at the start of therapy and usually disappear with repeated administration. Other side effects like gastrointestinal disturbances, changes in libido or skin reactions have been reported occasionally.

In addition, the following adverse events have been reported in association with the use of alprazolam: dystonia, anorexia, slurred speech, jaundice, musculoskeletal weakness, sexual dysfunction/changes in libido, menstrual irregularities, incontinence, urinary retention, abnormal liver function and hyperprolactinaemia. Increased intraocular pressure has been rarely reported.

Withdrawal symptoms have occurred following rapid decrease or abrupt discontinuance of benzodiazepines including alprazolam. These can range from mild dysphoria and insomnia to a major syndrome, which may include abdominal and muscle cramps, vomiting, sweating, tremor and convulsions. In addition, withdrawal seizures have occurred upon rapid decrease or abrupt discontinuation of therapy with alprazolam.

Amnesia
Anterograde amnesia may occur at therapeutic dosages, the risk increasing at higher dosages. Amnesic effects may be associated with inappropriate behaviour (see warnings and precautions).

Depression
Pre-existing depression may be unmasked during benzodiazepam use.

Psychiatric and 'paradoxical' reactions
Reactions like restlessness, agitation, irritability, aggressiveness, delusion, rages, nightmares, hallucinations, psychoses, inappropriate behaviour and other adverse behavioural effects are known to occur when using benzodiazepines or benzodiazepine-like agents. They may be quite severe with this product. They are more likely to occur in children and the elderly.

In many of the spontaneous case reports of adverse behavioural effects, patients were receiving other CNS drugs concomitantly and/or were described as having underlying psychiatric conditions. Patients who have borderline personality disorder, a prior history of violent or aggressive behaviour, or alcohol or substance abuse may be at risk of such events. Instances of irritability, hostility and intrusive thoughts have been reported during discontinuance of alprazolam in patients with post-traumatic stress disorder.

Dependence
Use (even at therapeutic doses) may lead to the development of physical dependence: discontinuation of the therapy may result in withdrawal or rebound phenomena (see warnings and precautions). Psychic dependence may occur. Abuse of benzodiazepines have been reported.

4.9 Overdose
As with other benzodiazepines, overdose should not present a threat to life unless combined with other CNS depressants (including alcohol). In the management of overdose with any medicinal product, it should be borne in mind that multiple agents have been taken.

Following overdose with any medicinal product, vomiting may be induced (within 1 hour) if the patient is conscious or gastric lavage undertaken with the airway protected if the patient is unconscious. If there is no advantage in emptying the stomach, activated charcoal should be given to reduce absorption.

Special attention should be paid to respiratory and cardiovascular functions in intensive care.

Symptoms of overdose are extensions of its pharmacological activity and usually manifested by slurring of speech, motor incoordination and degrees of central nervous system depression ranging from drowsiness to coma. In mild cases, symptoms include drowsiness, mental confusion and lethargy, in more serious cases, symptoms may include ataxia, hypotonia, hypotension, respiratory depression, rarely coma and very rarely death.

Flumazenil may be useful as an antidote.

5. PHARMACOLOGICAL PROPERTIES

5.1 Pharmacodynamic properties
Alprazolam, like other benzodiazepines, has a high affinity for the benzodiazepine binding site in the brain. It facilitates the inhibitory neurotransmitter action of gamma-aminobutyric acid, which mediates both pre- and post synaptic inhibition in the central nervous system (CNS).

5.2 Pharmacokinetic properties
Alprazolam is readily absorbed. Following oral administration peak concentration in the plasma occurs after 1 - 2 hours.

The mean half-life is 12 - 15 hours. Repeated dosage may lead to accumulation and this should be borne in mind in elderly patients and those with impaired renal or hepatic function. Alprazolam and its metabolites are excreted primarily in the urine.

In vitro alprazolam is bound (80%) to human serum protein.

5.3 Preclinical safety data
None given

6. PHARMACEUTICAL PARTICULARS

6.1 List of excipients
Lactose monohydrate, microcrystalline cellulose, colloidal anhydrous silica, maize starch, magnesium stearate and docusate sodium with sodium benzoate.

6.2 Incompatibilities
None known.

6.3 Shelf life
5 years.

6.4 Special precautions for storage
Do not store above 25°C.

Blister pack: Keep container in the outer carton.

Bottle pack only: Store in the original container.

6.5 Nature and contents of container
Clear PVC/aluminium foil blister strips of 10 tablets, packed 6 strips to a box. Glass bottle with metal screw cap or HDPE bottle with LDPE tamper evident cap containing 100 or 1000 tablets.

6.6 Special precautions for disposal and other handling
Not applicable.

Administrative Data

7. MARKETING AUTHORISATION HOLDER
Pharmacia Limited
Ramsgate Road
Sandwich
Kent
CT13 9NJ
United Kingdom

8. MARKETING AUTHORISATION NUMBER(S)
PL 00032/0092 and 0093

9. DATE OF FIRST AUTHORISATION/RENEWAL OF THE AUTHORISATION
27 August 1982/23 January 2003

10. DATE OF REVISION OF THE TEXT
June 2006

Legal category: POM

Ref: XX 2_0

Xatral

(sanofi-aventis)

1. NAME OF THE MEDICINAL PRODUCT
Xatral 2.5 mg film coated tablet

2. QUALITATIVE AND QUANTITATIVE COMPOSITION
Each tablet contains 2.5mg alfuzosin hydrochloride.

Excipient: Lactose

For a full list of excipients, see section 6.1

3. PHARMACEUTICAL FORM
Film coated tablet.

White round tablet marked Xatral 2.5 on one side.

4. CLINICAL PARTICULARS

4.1 Therapeutic indications
Treatment of the functional symptoms of benign prostatic hypertrophy.

4.2 Posology and method of administration
Xatral tablets should be swallowed whole. The first dose should be given just before bedtime.

Adults

The usual dose is one tablet three times daily. The dose may be increased to a maximum of 4 tablets (10mg) per day depending on the clinical response.

Elderly and treated hypertensive patients

As a routine precaution when prescribing alfuzosin to elderly patients (aged over 65 years) and the treated hypertensive patient, the initial dose should be 1 tablet in the morning and 1 tablet in the evening.

Renal insufficiency

In patients with renal insufficiency, as a precaution, it is recommended that the dosing be started at Xatral 2.5mg twice daily adjusted according to clinical response.

Hepatic insufficiency

In patients with mild to moderate hepatic insufficiency, it is recommended that therapy should commence with a single dose of Xatral 2.5mg/day to be increased to Xatral 2.5mg twice daily according to clinical response.

4.3 Contraindications
Hypersensitivity to the active substance or any of the excipients. History of orthostatic hypotension. Combination with other α-blockers. Severe hepatic insufficiency.

4.4 Special warnings and precautions for use
As with all alpha-1-blockers, in some subjects, in particular patients receiving antihypertensive medications, postural hypotension with or without symptoms (dizziness, fatigue, sweating) may develop within a few hours following administration. In such cases, the patient should lie down until the symptoms have completely disappeared.

These effects are transient and do not usually prevent the continuation of treatment after adjustment of the dose. The patient should be warned of the possible occurrence of such events.

Treatment should be initiated gradually in patients with hypersensitivity to alpha-1-blockers. Xatral should be administered carefully to patients being treated with antihypertensives. Blood pressure should be monitored regularly, especially at the beginning of treatment.

In patients with coronary insufficiency specific anti-anginal therapy should be continued, but if the angina reappears or worsens Xatral should be discontinued.

Patients with rare hereditary problems of galactose intolerance, the Lapp lactase deficiency or glucose-galactose malabsorption should not take this medicine.

The 'Intraoperative Floppy Iris Syndrome' (IFIS, a variant of small pupil syndrome) has been observed during cataract surgery in some patients on or previously treated with tamsulosin. Isolated reports have also been received with other alpha-1 blockers and the possibility of a class effect cannot be excluded. As IFIS may lead to increased procedural complications during the cataract operation current or past use of alpha-1 blockers should be made known to the ophthalmic surgeon in advance of surgery.

4.5 Interaction with other medicinal products and other forms of interaction
Combinations contraindicated:

- Alpha-1-receptor blockers (see section 4.3)

Combinations to be taken into account:

- Antihypertensive drugs (see section 4.4.2)
- Nitrates
- potent CYP3A4 inhibitors such as ketoconazole, itraconazole and ritonavir.

Repeated 200 mg daily dosing of ketoconazole, for seven days resulted in a 2.1-fold increase in Cmax and a 2.5-fold increase in exposure of alfuzosin 10 mg when administered as a single dose under fed conditions (high fat meal). Other parameters such as tmax and $t_{1/2}$ were not modified. Cmax and AUC of alfuzosin 10 mg, when administered as a single dose under fed conditions, increased 2.3- fold and 3.0-fold, respectively following 8-day repeated 400 mg ketoconazole daily dosing (see section 5.2)

The administration of general anaesthetics to patients receiving Xatral could cause profound hypotension. It is recommended that Xatral be withdrawn 24 hours before surgery.

Other forms of interaction
No pharmacodynamic or pharmacokinetic interaction has been observed in healthy volunteers between alfuzosin and the following drugs: warfarin, digoxin, hydrochlorothiazide and atenolol.

4.6 Pregnancy and lactation

Due to the type of indication this section is not applicable.

4.7 Effects on ability to drive and use machines

There are no data available on the effect on driving vehicles. Adverse reactions such as vertigo, dizziness and asthenia may occur. This has to be taken into account when driving vehicles and operating machinery.

4.8 Undesirable effects

Classification of expected frequencies:

Very common ($\geq$1/10), common ($\geq$1/100 to $<$1/10), uncommon ($\geq$1/1,000 to $<$1/100), rare ($\geq$1/10,000 to $<$1/1,000), very rare ($<$1/10,000)), not known (cannot be estimated from the available data).

Within each frequency grouping, undesirable effects are presented in order of decreasing seriousness.

- Nervous system disorders

Common: faintness/dizziness, vertigo, malaise, headache

Uncommon: drowsiness

- Eye disorders

Uncommon: vision abnormal

Unknown: intraoperative floppy iris syndrome

- Cardiac disorders

Common: hypotension (postural)

Uncommon: tachycardia, palpitations, syncope

Very rare: New onset, aggravation or recurrence of angina pectoris in patients with pre-existing coronary artery disease (see section 4.4.)

- Respiratory, thoracic and mediastinal disorders

Uncommon: rhinitis

- Gastro-intestinal disorders

Common: nausea, abdominal pain, diarrhoea, dry mouth

- Hepatobiliary disorders

Not known: hepatocellular injury, cholestatic liver disease

- Skin and subcutaneous tissue disorders

Uncommon: rash, pruritus

Very rare: urticaria, angioedema

- General disorders and administration site conditions

Common: asthenia

Uncommon: flushes, oedema, chest pain

Although only reported in isolated cases with alfuzosin, occurrence of priapism can not be excluded as it is generally accepted as being attributable to all other alpha adrenoreceptor blockers.

4.9 Overdose

In case of overdosage, the patient should be hospitalised, kept in the supine position, and conventional treatment of hypotension should take place.

Alfuzosin is not easily dialysable because of its high degree of protein binding.

5. PHARMACOLOGICAL PROPERTIES

5.1 Pharmacodynamic properties

Alfuzosin is an orally active quinazoline derivative. It is a selective, peripherally acting antagonist of post synaptic α_1-adrenoceptors.

Pharmacotherapeutic group: alpha-adrenoreceptor antagonists

ATC code: G04CA01

<u>In vitro</u> pharmacological studies have documented the selectivity of alfuzosin for the alpha$_1$-adrenoreceptors located in the prostate, bladder base and prostatic urethra.

Clinical manifestations of Benign Prostatic Hypertrophy are associated with infra vesical obstruction which is triggered by both anatomical (static) and functional (dynamic) factors. The functional component of obstruction arises from the tension of prostatic smooth muscle which is mediated by α-adrenoceptors. Activation of α_1-adrenoceptors stimulates smooth muscle contraction, thereby increasing the tone of the prostate, prostatic capsule, prostatic urethra and bladder base, and, consequently, increasing the resistance to bladder outflow. This in turn leads to outflow obstruction and possible secondary bladder instability.

Alpha-blockade decreases infra vesical obstruction via a direct action on prostatic smooth muscle.

<u>In vivo</u>, animal studies have shown that alfuzosin decreases urethral pressure and therefore, resistance to urine flow during micturition. Moreover, alfuzosin inhibits the hypertonic response of the urethra more readily than that of vascular muscle and shows functional uroselectivity in conscious normotensive rats by decreasing urethral pressure at doses that do not affect blood pressure.

In man, alfuzosin improves voiding parameters by reducing urethral tone and bladder outlet resistance, and facilitates bladder emptying.

In placebo controlled studies in BPH patients, alfuzosin:

significantly increases peak flow rate (Qmax) in patients with Qmax $\leq$ 15ml/s by a mean of 30%. This improvement is observed from the first dose, significantly reduces the detrusor pressure and increases the volume producing a strong desire to void, significantly reduces the residual urine volume.

These favourable urodynamic effects lead to an improvement of lower urinary tract symptoms ie. Filling (irritative) as well as voiding (obstructive) symptoms.

Alfuzosin may cause moderate antihypertensive effects.

5.2 Pharmacokinetic properties

Xatral is well absorbed with a mean bioavailability of 64%, peak plasma levels are generally reached in 0.5-3 hours. Kinetics within the therapeutic range are linear. The kinetic profile is characterised by large interindividual fluctuations in plasma concentrations. The terminal half-life is 3-5 hours. Alfuzosin is 90% protein bound in plasma, 68.2% to human serum albumin and 52.5% to human serum alpha-glycoprotein. It is partially metabolised and excreted mainly in the bile and faeces.

None of the metabolites found in man has any pharmacodynamic activity. The pharmacokinetic profile is not affected by taking Xatral with food.

In subjects over 75 years, absorption is more rapid and peak plasma levels are higher. Bioavailability may be increased and in some patients the volume of distribution is reduced. The elimination half-life does not change.

The volume of distribution and clearance of alfuzosin are increased in renal insufficiency, with or without dialysis, owing to an increase in the free fraction. Chronic renal insufficiency even when severe (creatinine clearance between 15 and 40 mls/min) is not adversely affected by alfuzosin.

In patients with severe hepatic insufficiency, the elimination half-life is prolonged. A two-fold increase in Cmax values and a three-fold increase in the AUC is observed. Bioavailability is increased compared with healthy volunteers.

The pharmacokinetic profile of alfuzosin is not affected by chronic cardiac insufficiency.

Metabolic interactions: CYP3A4 is the principal hepatic enzyme isoform involved in the metabolism of alfuzosin (see section 4.5)

5.3 Preclinical safety data

No data of therapeutic relevance.

6. PHARMACEUTICAL PARTICULARS

6.1 List of excipients

Tablet core:

Microcrystalline Cellulose

Lactose

Povidone

Sodium Starch Glycollate

Magnesium Stearate

Coating:

Methylhydroxypropylcellulose

Macrogol 400

Titanium Dioxide (E171)

6.2 Incompatibilities

Not known.

6.3 Shelf life

3 years.

6.4 Special precautions for storage

Store in a dry place at or below 30°C.

6.5 Nature and contents of container

Boxes with 60 tablets in pvc/foil blister strips.

6.6 Special precautions for disposal and other handling

No special requirements

7. MARKETING AUTHORISATION HOLDER

Sanofi-aventis

One Onslow Street

Guildford

Surrey,

GU1 4YS

8. MARKETING AUTHORISATION NUMBER(S)

PL 04425/0655

9. DATE OF FIRST AUTHORISATION/RENEWAL OF THE AUTHORISATION

09th February 2009

10. DATE OF REVISION OF THE TEXT

February 2009

Legal Status

POM

Xatral XL 10mg

(sanofi-aventis)

1. NAME OF THE MEDICINAL PRODUCT

Xatral XL 10 mg prolonged release tablets

2. QUALITATIVE AND QUANTITATIVE COMPOSITION

Each tablet contains 10mg alfuzosin hydrochloride.

Excipient: Hydrogenated castor oil

For a full list of excipients, see section 6.1

3. PHARMACEUTICAL FORM

Prolonged release tablet.

Round biconvex, three layer tablet: one white layer between two yellow layers.

4. CLINICAL PARTICULARS

4.1 Therapeutic indications

Treatment of the functional symptoms of benign prostatic hypertrophy (BPH).

For information on use in acute urinary retention (AUR) related to BPH see sections 4.2 and 5.1.

4.2 Posology and method of administration

Xatral XL should be swallowed whole (see section 4.4).

BPH: The recommended dose is one 10mg tablet to be taken once daily after a meal.

AUR: In patients 65 years and older, one 10 mg tablet daily after a meal to be taken from the first day of catheterisation. The treatment should be administered for 3-4 days, 2-3 days during catheterisation and 1 day after its removal. In this indication no benefit has been established in patients under 65 years of age or if treatment is extended beyond 4 days.

4.3 Contraindications

Hypersensitivity to the active substance or to any of the excipients. History of orthostatic hypotension. Combination with other alpha-blockers. Hepatic insufficiency.

4.4 Special warnings and precautions for use

As with all alpha-1-blockers in some subjects, in particular patients receiving antihypertensive medications, postural hypotension with or without symptoms (dizziness, fatigue, sweating) may develop within a few hours following administration. In such cases, the patient should lie down until the symptoms have completely disappeared.

These effects are transient and do not usually prevent the continuation of treatment after adjustment of the dose. The patient should be warned of the possible occurrence of such events.

Treatment should be initiated gradually in patients with hypersensitivity to alpha-1-blockers. Xatral XL should be administered carefully to patients being treated with antihypertensives. Blood pressure should be monitored regularly, especially at the beginning of treatment.

In patients with coronary insufficiency specific anti-anginal therapy should be continued, but if the angina reappears or worsens Xatral XL should be discontinued.

Experience in patients with severe renal impairment is limited and cautious use in these patients is recommended.

Patients should be warned that the tablet should be swallowed whole. Any other mode of administration, such as crunching, crushing, chewing, grinding or pounding to powder should be prohibited. These actions may lead to inappropriate release and absorption of the drug and therefore possible early adverse reactions.

The excipient hydrogenated castor oil may cause stomach upset and diarrhoea.

The 'Intraoperative Floppy Iris Syndrome' (IFIS, a variant of small pupil syndrome) has been observed during cataract surgery in some patients on or previously treated with tamsulosin. Isolated reports have also been received with other alpha-1 blockers and the possibility of a class effect cannot be excluded. As IFIS may lead to increased procedural complications during the cataract operation current or past use of alpha-1 blockers should be made known to the ophthalmic surgeon in advance of surgery.

4.5 Interaction with other medicinal products and other forms of interaction

<u>Combinations contra-indicated:</u>

- Alpha-1-receptor blockers (see section 4.3).

<u>Combinations to be taken into account:</u>

- Antihypertensive drugs (see section 4.4).
- Nitrates
- potent CYP3A4 inhibitors such as ketoconazole, itraconazole and ritonavir.

Repeated 200 mg daily dosing of ketoconazole, for seven days resulted in a 2.1-fold increase in Cmax and a 2.5-fold increase in exposure of alfuzosin 10 mg when administered as a single dose under fed conditions (high fat meal). Other parameters such as tmax and $t_{1/2}$ were not modified.

Cmax and AUC of alfuzosin 10 mg, when administered as a single dose under fed conditions, increased 2.3- fold and 3.0- fold, respectively following 8-day repeated 400 mg ketoconazole daily dosing i (see section 5.2).

The administration of general anaesthetics to patients receiving Xatral XL could cause profound hypotension. It is recommended that the tablets be withdrawn 24 hours before surgery.

Other forms of interaction

No pharmacodynamic or pharmacokinetic interaction has been observed in healthy volunteers between alfuzosin and the following drugs: warfarin, digoxin, hydrochlorothiazide and atenolol.

4.6 Pregnancy and lactation

Due to the type of indication this section is not applicable

Table 1

Age	Placebo N (%)	Alfuzosin N (%)	Relative difference vs placebo 95%CI	p value
65 years and above	30 (35.7%)	88 (56.1%)	1.57 (1.14-2.16)	0.003
Below 65 years	28 (75.7%)	58 (73.4%)	0.97 (0.77-1.22)	0.80
All patients (50 years and above)	58 (47.8%)	146 (61.9%)	1.29 (1.04-1.60)	0.012

4.7 Effects on ability to drive and use machines

There are no data available on the effect on driving vehicles. Adverse reactions such as vertigo, dizziness and asthenia may occur. This has to be taken into account when driving vehicles and operating machinery.

4.8 Undesirable effects

Classification of expected frequencies:

Very common (≥1/10), common (≥1/100 to <1/10), uncommon (≥1/1,000 to <1/100), rare (≥1/10,000 to <1/1,000), very rare (<1/10,000), not known (cannot be estimated from the available data).

Within each frequency grouping, undesirable effects are presented in order of decreasing seriousness.

• **Nervous system disorders**

Common: faintness/dizziness, headache

Uncommon: vertigo, malaise, drowsiness

• **Eye disorders**

Uncommon: vision abnormal

Not known: intraoperative floppy iris syndrome (see section 4.4)

• **Cardiac disorders**

Uncommon: tachycardia, palpitations, hypotension (postural), syncope

Very rare: New onset, aggravation or recurrence of angina pectoris in patients with pre-existing coronary artery disease. (see section 4.4.)

• **Respiratory, thoracic and mediastinal disorders**

Uncommon: rhinitis

• **Gastro-intestinal disorders**

Common: nausea, abdominal pain

Uncommon: diarrhoea, dry mouth, vomiting

• **Hepatobiliary disorders**

Not known: hepatocellular injury, cholestatic liver disease.

• **Skin and subcutaneous tissue disorders**

Uncommon: rash, pruritus

Very rare: urticaria, angioedema

• **General disorders and administration site conditions**

Common: asthenia

Uncommon: flushes, oedema, chest pain

Although only reported in isolated cases with alfuzosin, occurrence of priapism can not be excluded as it is generally accepted as being attributable to all other alpha adrenoreceptor blockers.

4.9 Overdose

In case of overdosage, the patient should be hospitalized, kept in the supine position, and conventional treatment of hypotension should take place.

Alfuzosin is not dialysable because of its high degree of protein binding.

5. PHARMACOLOGICAL PROPERTIES

5.1 Pharmacodynamic properties

Pharmacotherapeutic group: alpha-adrenoreceptor antagonists

ATC code: G04CA01

Alfuzosin is an orally active quinazoline derivative. It is a selective, peripherally acting antagonist of postsynaptic alpha-1-adrenoceptors.

In vitro pharmacological studies have documented the selectivity of alfuzosin for the alpha-1-adrenoreceptors located in the prostate, bladder base and prostatic urethra.

Clinical manifestations of Benign Prostatic Hypertrophy are associated with infra vesical obstruction which is triggered by both anatomical (static) and functional (dynamic) factors. The functional component of obstruction arises from the tension of prostatic smooth muscle which is mediated by alpha-adrenoceptors. Activation of alpha-1-adrenoceptors stimulates smooth muscle contraction, thereby increasing the tone of the prostate, prostatic capsule, prostatic urethra and bladder base, and, consequently, increasing the resistance to bladder outflow. This in turn leads to outflow obstruction and possible secondary bladder instability.

Alpha-blockade decreases infra vesical obstruction via a direct action on prostatic smooth muscle.

In vivo, animal studies have shown that alfuzosin decreases urethral pressure and therefore, resistance to urine flow during micturition. Moreover, alfuzosin inhibits the hypertonic response of the urethra more readily than that of vascular muscle and shows functional uroselectivity in conscious normotensive rats by decreasing urethral pressure at doses that do not affect blood pressure.

In man, alfuzosin improves voiding parameters by reducing urethral tone and bladder outlet resistance, and facilitates bladder emptying.

In placebo controlled studies in BPH patients, alfuzosin:

• significantly increases peak flow rate (Qmax) in patients with Qmax ≤ 15ml/s by a mean of 30%. This improvement is observed from the first dose,

• significantly reduces the detrusor pressure and increases the volume producing a strong desire to void,

• significantly reduces the residual urine volume.

These favourable urodynamic effects lead to an improvement of lower urinary tract symptoms ie. filling (irritative) as well as voiding (obstructive) symptoms.

Alfuzosin may cause moderate antihypertensive effects.

A lower frequency of acute urinary retention is observed in the alfuzosin treated patient than in the untreated patient.

AUR (related to BPH):

In the ALFAUR study, the effect of alfuzosin on the return of normal voiding was evaluated in 357 men over 50 years, presenting with a first episode of acute urinary retention (AUR), related to BPH. In this multicentre, randomised double blind parallel group study comparing alfuzosin 10mg/day and placebo, the evaluation of voiding was performed 24 hours after catheter removal, the morning after 2-3 days of treatment.

In men aged 65 years and over alfuzosin significantly increased the success rate of spontaneous voiding after catheter removal – see table. No benefit has been established in patients under 65 years of age or if treatment is extended beyond 4 days.

ALFAUR study: Percentage of patients (ITT population) successfully voiding post-catheter removal

(see Table 1 above)

5.2 Pharmacokinetic properties

Prolonged-release formulation:

The mean value of the relative bioavailability is 104.4 % versus the immediate release formulation (2.5 mg tid) in middle-aged healthy volunteers and the maximum plasma concentration is being achieved 9 hours after administration compared to 1 hour for the immediate release formulation.

The apparent elimination half-life is 9.1 hours.

Studies have shown that consistent pharmacokinetic profiles are obtained when the product is administered after a meal.

Under fed conditions, mean Cmax and Ctrough values are 13.6 (SD=5.6) and 3.2 (SD=1.6) ng/ml respectively. Mean AUC_{0-24} is 194 (SD=75) ng.h/ml. A plateau of concentration is observed from 3 to 14 hours with concentrations above 8.1 ng/ml (Cav) for 11 hours.

Compared to healthy middle aged volunteers, the pharmacokinetic parameters (Cmax and AUC) are not increased in elderly patients.

Compared to subjects with normal renal function, mean Cmax and AUC values are moderately increased in patients with renal impairment, without modification of the apparent elimination half-life. This change in the pharmacokinetic profile is not considered clinically relevant. Therefore, this does not necessitate a dosing adjustment.

The binding of alfuzosin to plasma proteins is about 90%. Alfuzosin undergoes extensive metabolism by the liver, with only 11 % of the parent compound being excreted unchanged in the urine. The majority of the metabolites (which are inactive) are excreted in the faeces (75 to 91 %).

The pharmacokinetic profile of alfuzosin is not affected by chronic cardiac insufficiency.

Metabolic interactions: CYP3A4 is the main hepatic enzyme isoform involved in the metabolism of alfuzosin (see section 4.5)

5.3 Preclinical safety data

No data of therapeutic relevance.

6. PHARMACEUTICAL PARTICULARS

6.1 List of excipients

Ethylcellulose

Hydrogenated Castor Oil

Hypromellose

Yellow Ferric Oxide (E172)

Magnesium Stearate

Microcrystalline Cellulose

Povidone

Silica Colloidal Hydrated

Mannitol.

6.2 Incompatibilities

None known.

6.3 Shelf life

3 years.

6.4 Special precautions for storage

No special precautions for storage.

Store in the original container.

6.5 Nature and contents of container

Boxes with 10 and 30 tablets in pvc/foil blister strips.

6.6 Special precautions for disposal and other handling

No special requirements

7. MARKETING AUTHORISATION HOLDER

Sanofi-aventis

One Onslow Street

Guildford

Surrey, GU1 4YS, UK

8. MARKETING AUTHORISATION NUMBER(S)

PL 04425/0657

9. DATE OF FIRST AUTHORISATION/RENEWAL OF THE AUTHORISATION

02 April 2009

10. DATE OF REVISION OF THE TEXT

April 2009

Legal Status

POM

Xeloda

(Roche Products Limited)

1. NAME OF THE MEDICINAL PRODUCT

Xeloda 150 mg and 500 mg film-coated tablets.

2. QUALITATIVE AND QUANTITATIVE COMPOSITION

150 mg or 500 mg capecitabine.

Excipient: 15.6 mg anhydrous lactose (150 mg tablet).

Excipient: 52 mg anhydrous lactose (500 mg tablet).

For a full list of excipients, see section 6.1.

3. PHARMACEUTICAL FORM

Film-coated tablet

Light peach film-coated tablet of biconvex, oblong shape with the marking '150' on the one side and 'Xeloda' on the other side.

Peach film-coated tablet of biconvex, oblong shape with the marking '500' on the one side and 'Xeloda' on the other side.

4. CLINICAL PARTICULARS

4.1 Therapeutic indications

Xeloda is indicated for the adjuvant treatment of patients following surgery of stage III (Dukes' stage C) colon cancer (see section 5.1).

Xeloda is indicated for the treatment of metastatic colorectal cancer (see section 5.1).

Xeloda is indicated for first-line treatment of advanced gastric cancer in combination with a platinum-based regimen (see section 5.1).

Xeloda in combination with docetaxel (see section 5.1) is indicated for the treatment of patients with locally advanced or metastatic breast cancer after failure of cytotoxic chemotherapy. Previous therapy should have included an anthracycline. Xeloda is also indicated as monotherapy for the treatment of patients with locally advanced or metastatic breast cancer after failure of taxanes and an anthracycline-containing chemotherapy regimen or for whom further anthracycline therapy is not indicated.

4.2 Posology and method of administration

Xeloda should only be prescribed by a qualified physician experienced in the utilisation of anti-neoplastic agents. Xeloda tablets should be swallowed with water within 30 minutes after a meal. Treatment should be discontinued if progressive disease or intolerable toxicity is observed. Standard and reduced dose calculations according to body surface area for starting doses of Xeloda of 1250 mg/m^2 and 1000 mg/m^2 are provided in tables 1 and 2, respectively.

Recommended posology (see section 5.1):

Monotherapy

Colon, colorectal and breast cancer

Given as single agent, the recommended starting dose for Xeloda in the adjuvant treatment of colon cancer, in the treatment of metastatic colorectal cancer or of locally advanced or metastatic breast cancer is 1250 mg/m^2 administered twice daily (morning and evening; equivalent to 2500 mg/m^2 total daily dose) for 14 days followed by a 7-day rest period. Adjuvant treatment in patients with stage III colon cancer is recommended for a total of 6 months.

Combination therapy

Colorectal and gastric cancer

In combination treatment, the recommended starting dose of Xeloda should be reduced to 800 – 1000 mg/m^2 when administered twice daily for 14 days followed by a 7-day rest period, or to 625 mg/m^2 twice daily when administered continuously (see section 5.1). The inclusion of biological agents in a combination regimen has no effect on the starting dose of Xeloda. Premedication to maintain adequate hydration and anti-emesis according to the cisplatin summary of product characteristics should be started prior to cisplatin administration for patients receiving the Xeloda plus cisplatin combination.

Breast cancer

In combination with docetaxel, the recommended starting dose of Xeloda in the treatment of metastatic breast cancer is 1250 mg/m^2 twice daily for 14 days followed by a 7-day rest period, combined with docetaxel at 75 mg/m^2 as a 1 hour intravenous infusion every 3 weeks. Pre-medication with an oral corticosteroid such as dexamethasone according to the docetaxel summary of product characteristics should be started prior to docetaxel administration for patients receiving the Xeloda plus docetaxel combination.

Xeloda Dose Calculations

Table 1 Standard and reduced dose calculations according to body surface area for a starting dose of Xeloda of 1250 mg/m^2

(see Table 1 opposite)

Table 2 Standard and reduced dose calculations according to body surface area for a starting dose of Xeloda of 1000 mg/m^2

(see Table 2 opposite)

Posology adjustments during treatment:

General

Toxicity due to Xeloda administration may be managed by symptomatic treatment and/or modification of the dose (treatment interruption or dose reduction). Once the dose has been reduced, it should not be increased at a later time. For those toxicities considered by the treating physician to be unlikely to become serious or life-threatening, e.g. alopecia, altered taste, nail changes, treatment can be continued at the same dose without reduction or interruption. Patients taking Xeloda should be informed of the need to interrupt treatment immediately if moderate or severe toxicity occurs. Doses of Xeloda omitted for toxicity are not replaced. The following are the recommended dose modifications for toxicity:

Table 3 Xeloda Dose Reduction Schedule (3-weekly Cycle or Continuous Treatment)

Toxicity grades*	Dose changes within a treatment cycle	Dose adjustment for next cycle/dose (% of starting dose)
• *Grade 1*	Maintain dose level	Maintain dose level
• *Grade 2*		
-1st appearance	Interrupt until resolved to grade 0-1	100%
-2nd appearance		75%
-3rd appearance		50%
-4th appearance	Discontinue treatment permanently	Not applicable
• *Grade 3*		
-1st appearance	Interrupt until resolved to grade 0-1	75%
-2nd appearance		50%
-3rd appearance	Discontinue treatment permanently	Not applicable
• *Grade 4*		
-1st appearance	Discontinue permanently *or* If physician deems it to be in the patient's best interest to continue, interrupt until resolved to grade 0-1	50%
-2nd appearance	Discontinue permanently	Not applicable

*According to the National Cancer Institute of Canada Clinical Trial Group (NCIC CTG) Common Toxicity Criteria (version 1) or the Common Terminology Criteria for Adverse Events (CTCAE) of the Cancer Therapy Evaluation Program, US National Cancer Institute, version 3.0. For hand-foot syndrome and hyperbilirubinaemia, see section 4.4.

Haematology: Patients with baseline neutrophil counts of $<1.5 \times 10^9$/L and/or thrombocyte counts of $<100 \times 10^9$/L should not be treated with Xeloda. If unscheduled laboratory assessments during a treatment cycle show that the neutrophil count drops below 1.0×10^9/L or that the platelet count drops below 75×10^9/L, treatment with Xeloda should be interrupted.

Dose modifications for toxicity when Xeloda is used as a 3 weekly cycle in combination with other agents:

Dose modifications for toxicity when Xeloda is used as a 3 weekly cycle in combination with other agents should be made according to Table 3 above for Xeloda and according to the appropriate summary of product characteristics for the other agent(s).

At the beginning of a treatment cycle, if a treatment delay is indicated for either Xeloda or the other agent(s), then administration of all agents should be delayed until the requirements for restarting all drugs are met.

During a treatment cycle for those toxicities considered by the treating physician not to be related to Xeloda, Xeloda should be continued and the dose of the other agent should be adjusted according to the appropriate Prescribing Information.

If the other agent(s) have to be discontinued permanently, Xeloda treatment can be resumed when the requirements for restarting Xeloda are met.

This advice is applicable to all indications and to all special populations.

Dose modifications for toxicity when Xeloda is used continuously in combination with other agents:

Dose modifications for toxicity when Xeloda is used continuously in combination with other agents should be made according to Table 3 above for Xeloda and according to the appropriate summary of product characteristics for the other agent(s).

Posology adjustments for special populations:

Hepatic impairment: insufficient safety and efficacy data are available in patients with hepatic impairment to provide a dose adjustment recommendation. No information is available on hepatic impairment due to cirrhosis or hepatitis.

Table 1 Standard and reduced dose calculations according to body surface area for a starting dose of Xeloda of 1250 mg/m^2

	Dose level 1250 mg/m^2 (twice daily)				
	Full dose 1250 mg/m^2	Number of 150 mg tablets and/or 500 mg tablets per administration (each administration to be given morning and evening)		Reduced dose (75%) 950 mg/m^2	Reduced dose (50%) 625 mg/m^2
Body Surface Area (m^2)	Dose per administration (mg)	150 mg	500 mg	Dose per administration (mg)	Dose per administration (mg)
≤1.26	1500	-	3	1150	800
1.27 - 1.38	1650	1	3	1300	800
1.39 - 1.52	1800	2	3	1450	950
1.53 - 1.66	2000	-	4	1500	1000
1.67 - 1.78	2150	1	4	1650	1000
1.79 - 1.92	2300	2	4	1800	1150
1.93 - 2.06	2500	-	5	1950	1300
2.07 - 2.18	2650	1	5	2000	1300
≥2.19	2800	2	5	2150	1450

Table 2 Standard and reduced dose calculations according to body surface area for a starting dose of Xeloda of 1000 mg/m^2

	Dose level 1000 mg/m^2 (twice daily)				
	Full dose 1000 mg/m^2	Number of 150 mg tablets and/or 500 mg tablets per administration (each administration to be given morning and evening)		Reduced dose (75%) 750 mg/m^2	Reduced dose (50%) 500 mg/m^2
Body Surface Area (m^2)	Dose per administration (mg)	150 mg	500 mg	Dose per administration (mg)	Dose per administration (mg)
≤1.26	1150	1	2	800	600
1.27 - 1.38	1300	2	2	1000	600
1.39 - 1.52	1450	3	2	1100	750
1.53 - 1.66	1600	4	2	1200	800
1.67 - 1.78	1750	5	2	1300	800
1.79 - 1.92	1800	2	3	1400	900
1.93 - 2.06	2000	-	4	1500	1000
2.07 - 2.18	2150	1	4	1600	1050
≥2.19	2300	2	4	1750	1100

Renal impairment: Xeloda is contraindicated in patients with severe renal impairment (creatinine clearance below 30 ml/min [Cockcroft and Gault] at baseline). The incidence of grade 3 or 4 adverse reactions in patients with moderate renal impairment (creatinine clearance 30-50 ml/min at baseline) is increased compared to the overall population. In patients with moderate renal impairment at baseline, a dose reduction to 75% for a starting dose of 1250 mg/m^2 is recommended. In patients with moderate renal impairment at baseline, no dose reduction is required for a starting dose of 1000 mg/m^2. In patients with mild renal impairment (creatinine clearance 51-80 ml/min at baseline) no adjustment of the starting dose is recommended. Careful monitoring and prompt treatment interruption is recommended if the patient develops a grade 2, 3 or 4 adverse event during treatment and subsequent dose adjustment as outlined in Table 3 above. If the calculated creatinine clearance decreases during treatment to a value below 30 ml/min, Xeloda should be discontinued. These dose adjustment recommendations for renal impairment apply both to monotherapy and combination use (see also section "Elderly" below).

There is no experience in children (under 18 years).

Elderly:

During Xeloda monotherapy, no adjustment of the starting dose is needed. However, grade 3 or 4 treatment-related adverse reactions were more frequent in patients ≥60 years of age compared to younger patients.

When Xeloda was used in combination with other agents, elderly patients (≥65 years) experienced more grade 3 and grade 4 adverse drug reactions, including those leading to discontinuation, compared to younger patients. Careful monitoring of patients ≥60 years of age is advisable.

- *In combination with docetaxel*: an increased incidence of grade 3 or 4 treatment-related adverse reactions and treatment-related serious adverse reactions were observed in patients 60 years of age or more (see section 5.1). For patients 60 years of age or more, a starting dose reduction of Xeloda to 75% (950 mg/m^2 twice daily) is recommended.

If no toxicity is observed in patients ⩾60 years of age treated with a reduced Xeloda starting dose in combination with docetaxel, the dose of Xeloda may be cautiously escalated to 1250 mg/m^2 twice daily.

- *In combination with irinotecan*: for patients 65 years of age or more, a starting dose reduction of Xeloda to 800 mg/m^2 twice daily is recommended.

4.3 Contraindications

• History of severe and unexpected reactions to fluoropyrimidine therapy,

• Hypersensitivity to capecitabine or to any of the excipients or fluorouracil,

• In patients with known dihydropyrimidine dehydrogenase (DPD) deficiency,

• During pregnancy and lactation,

• In patients with severe leucopenia, neutropenia, or thrombocytopenia,

• In patients with severe hepatic impairment,

• In patients with severe renal impairment (creatinine clearance below 30 ml/min),

• Treatment with sorivudine or its chemically related analogues, such as brivudine (see section 4.5),

• If contraindications exist to any of the agents in the combination regimen, that agent should not be used.

4.4 Special warnings and precautions for use

Dose limiting toxicities include diarrhoea, abdominal pain, nausea, stomatitis and hand-foot syndrome (hand-foot skin reaction, palmar-plantar erythrodysaesthesia). Most adverse reactions are reversible and do not require permanent discontinuation of therapy, although doses may need to be withheld or reduced.

Diarrhoea. Patients with severe diarrhoea should be carefully monitored and given fluid and electrolyte replacement if they become dehydrated. Standard antidiarrhoeal treatments (e.g. loperamide) may be used. NCIC CTC grade 2 diarrhoea is defined as an increase of 4 to 6 stools/day or nocturnal stools, grade 3 diarrhoea as an increase of 7 to 9 stools/day or incontinence and malabsorption. Grade 4 diarrhoea is an increase of ⩾10 stools/day or grossly bloody diarrhoea or the need for parenteral support. Dose reduction should be applied as necessary (see section 4.2).

Dehydration. Dehydration should be prevented or corrected at the onset. Patients with anorexia, asthenia, nausea, vomiting or diarrhoea may rapidly become dehydrated. If Grade 2 (or higher) dehydration occurs, Xeloda treatment should be immediately interrupted and the dehydration corrected. Treatment should not be restarted until the patient is rehydrated and any precipitating causes have been corrected or controlled. Dose modifications applied should be applied for the precipitating adverse event as necessary (see section 4.2).

Hand-foot syndrome (also known as hand-foot skin reaction or palmar-plantar erythrodysaesthesia or chemotherapy induced acral erythema). Grade 1 hand- foot syndrome is defined as numbness, dysaesthesia/paraesthesia, tingling, painless swelling or erythema of the hands and/or feet and/or discomfort which does not disrupt the patient's normal activities.

Grade 2 hand- foot syndrome is painful erythema and swelling of the hands and/or feet and/or discomfort affecting the patient's activities of daily living.

Grade 3 hand- foot syndrome is moist desquamation, ulceration, blistering and severe pain of the hands and/or feet and/or severe discomfort that causes the patient to be unable to work or perform activities of daily living. If grade 2 or 3 hand- foot syndrome occurs, administration of Xeloda should be interrupted until the event resolves or decreases in intensity to grade 1. Following grade 3 hand- foot syndrome, subsequent doses of Xeloda should be decreased. When Xeloda and cisplatin are used in combination, the use of vitamin B6 (pyridoxine) is not advised for symptomatic or secondary prophylactic treatment of hand-foot syndrome, because of published reports that it may decrease the efficacy of cisplatin.

Cardiotoxicity. Cardiotoxicity has been associated with fluoropyrimidine therapy, including myocardial infarction, angina, dysrhythmias, cardiogenic shock, sudden death and electrocardiographic changes. These adverse reactions may be more common in patients with a prior history of coronary artery disease. Cardiac arrhythmias, angina pectoris, myocardial infarction, heart failure and cardiomyopathy have been reported in patients receiving Xeloda. Caution must be exercised in patients with history of significant cardiac disease, arrhythmias and angina pectoris (See section 4.8).

Hypo- or hypercalcaemia. Hypo- or hypercalcaemia has been reported during Xeloda treatment. Caution must be exercised in patients with pre-existing hypo- or hypercalcaemia (see section 4.8).

Central or peripheral nervous system disease. Caution must be exercised in patients with central or peripheral nervous system disease, e.g. brain metastasis or neuropathy (see section 4.8).

Diabetes mellitus or electrolyte disturbances. Caution must be exercised in patients with diabetes mellitus or electrolyte disturbances, as these may be aggravated during Xeloda treatment.

Coumarin-derivative anticoagulation. In a drug interaction study with single-dose warfarin administration, there was a significant increase in the mean AUC (+57%) of S-warfarin. These results suggest an interaction, probably due to an inhibition of the cytochrome P450 2C9 isoenzyme system by capecitabine. Patients receiving concomitant Xeloda and oral coumarin-derivative anticoagulant therapy should have their anticoagulant response (INR or prothrombin time) monitored closely and the anticoagulant dose adjusted accordingly (see section 4.5).

Hepatic impairment. In the absence of safety and efficacy data in patients with hepatic impairment, Xeloda use should be carefully monitored in patients with mild to moderate liver dysfunction, regardless of the presence or absence of liver metastasis. Administration of Xeloda should be interrupted if treatment-related elevations in bilirubin of >3.0 × ULN or treatment-related elevations in hepatic aminotransferases (ALT, AST) of >2.5 × ULN occur. Treatment with Xeloda monotherapy may be resumed when bilirubin decreases to ⩽3.0 × ULN or hepatic aminotransferases decrease to ⩽ 2.5 × ULN.

Renal impairment. The incidence of grade 3 or 4 adverse reactions in patients with moderate renal impairment (creatinine clearance 30-50 ml/min) is increased compared to the overall population (see section 4.2 and 4.3).

As this medicinal product contains anhydrous lactose as an excipient, patients with rare hereditary problems of galactose intolerance, the Lapp lactase deficiency or glucose-galactose malabsorption should not take this medicine.

4.5 Interaction with other medicinal products and other forms of interaction

Interaction studies have only been performed in adults.

Interaction with other medicinal products:

Coumarin-derivative anticoagulants: altered coagulation parameters and/or bleeding have been reported in patients taking Xeloda concomitantly with coumarin-derivative anticoagulants such as warfarin and phenprocoumon. These reactions occurred within several days and up to several months after initiating Xeloda therapy and, in a few cases, within one month after stopping Xeloda. In a clinical pharmacokinetic interaction study, after a single 20 mg dose of warfarin, Xeloda treatment increased the AUC of S-warfarin by 57% with a 91% increase in INR value. Since metabolism of R-warfarin was not affected, these results indicate that capecitabine down-regulates isozyme 2C9, but has no effect on isozymes 1A2 and 3A4. Patients taking coumarin-derivative anticoagulants concomitantly with Xeloda should be monitored regularly for alterations in their coagulation parameters (PT or INR) and the anti-coagulant dose adjusted accordingly.

Phenytoin: increased phenytoin plasma concentrations resulting in symptoms of phenytoin intoxication in single cases have been reported during concomitant use of Xeloda with phenytoin. Patients taking phenytoin concomitantly with Xeloda should be regularly monitored for increased phenytoin plasma concentrations.

Folinic acid: a combination study with Xeloda and folinic acid indicated that folinic acid has no major effect on the pharmacokinetics of Xeloda and its metabolites. However, folinic acid has an effect on the pharmacodynamics of Xeloda and its toxicity may be enhanced by folinic acid: the maximum tolerated dose (MTD) of Xeloda alone using the intermittent regimen is 3000 mg/m^2 per day whereas it is only 2000 mg/m^2 per day when Xeloda was combined with folinic acid (30 mg orally bid).

Sorivudine and analogues: a clinically significant drug-drug interaction between sorivudine and 5-FU, resulting from the inhibition of dihydropyrimidine dehydrogenase by sorivudine, has been described. This interaction, which leads to increased fluoropyrimidine toxicity, is potentially fatal. Therefore, Xeloda must not be administered concomitantly with sorivudine or its chemically related analogues, such as brivudine (see section 4.3). There must be at least a 4-week waiting period between end of treatment with sorivudine or its chemically related analogues such as brivudine and start of Xeloda therapy.

Antacid: the effect of an aluminum hydroxide and magnesium hydroxide-containing antacid on the pharmacokinetics of capecitabine was investigated. There was a small increase in plasma concentrations of capecitabine and one metabolite (5'-DFCR); there was no effect on the 3 major metabolites (5'-DFUR, 5-FU and FBAL).

Allopurinol: interactions with allopurinol have been observed for 5-FU; with possible decreased efficacy of 5-FU. Concomitant use of allopurinol with Xeloda should be avoided.

Interaction with cytochrome P-450: For potential interactions with isozymes 1A2, 2C9 and 3A4, see interactions with coumarin-derivative anticoagulation.

Interferon alpha: the MTD of Xeloda was 2000 mg/m^2 per day when combined with interferon alpha-2a (3 MIU/m^2 per day) compared to 3000 mg/m^2 per day when Xeloda was used alone.

Radiotherapy: the MTD of Xeloda alone using the intermittent regimen is 3000 mg/m^2 per day, whereas, when combined with radiotherapy for rectal cancer, the MTD of Xeloda is 2000 mg/m^2 per day using either a continuous schedule or given daily Monday through Friday during a 6-week course of radiotherapy.

Oxaliplatin: no clinically significant differences in exposure to capecitabine or its metabolites, free platinum or total platinum occurred when capecitabine was administered in combination with oxaliplatin or in combination with oxaliplatin and bevacizumab.

Bevacizumab: there was no clinically significant effect of bevacizumab on the pharmacokinetic parameters of capecitabine or its metabolites in the presence of oxaliplatin.

Food interaction: In all clinical trials, patients were instructed to administer Xeloda within 30 minutes after a meal. Since current safety and efficacy data are based upon administration with food, it is recommended that Xeloda be administered with food. Administration with food decreases the rate of capecitabine absorption (see section 5.2).

4.6 Pregnancy and lactation

There are no studies in pregnant women using Xeloda; however, it should be assumed that Xeloda may cause foetal harm if administered to pregnant women. In reproductive toxicity studies in animals, Xeloda administration caused embryolethality and teratogenicity. These findings are expected effects of fluoropyrimidine derivatives. Xeloda is contraindicated during pregnancy. Women of childbearing potential should be advised to avoid becoming pregnant while receiving treatment with Xeloda. If the patient becomes pregnant while receiving Xeloda, the potential hazard to the foetus must be explained.

It is not known whether Xeloda is excreted in human breast milk. In lactating mice, considerable amounts of capecitabine and its metabolites were found in milk. Breast-feeding should be discontinued while receiving treatment with Xeloda.

4.7 Effects on ability to drive and use machines

Xeloda has minor or moderate influence on the ability to drive and use machines. Xeloda may cause dizziness, fatigue and nausea.

4.8 Undesirable effects

a. Summary of the safety profile

The overall safety profile of Xeloda is based on data from over 3000 patients treated with Xeloda as monotherapy or Xeloda in combination with different chemotherapy regimens in multiple indications. The safety profiles of Xeloda monotherapy for the metastatic breast cancer, metastatic colorectal cancer and adjuvant colon cancer populations are comparable. See section 5.1 for details of major studies, including study designs and major efficacy results.

The most commonly reported and/or clinically relevant treatment-related adverse drug reactions (ADRs) were gastrointestinal disorders (especially diarrhoea, nausea, vomiting, abdominal pain, stomatitis), hand-foot syndrome (palmar-plantar erythrodysaesthesia), fatigue, asthenia, anorexia, cardiotoxicity, increased renal dysfunction in those with preexisting compromised renal function, and thrombosis/embolism.

b. Tabulated summary of adverse reactions

ADRs considered by the investigator to be possibly, probably, or remotely related to the administration of Xeloda are listed in Table 4 for Xeloda given as a single agent and in Table 5 for Xeloda given in combination with different chemotherapy regimens in multiple indications. The following headings are used to rank the ADRs by frequency: very common (⩾ 1/10), common (⩾ 1/100, < 1/10) and uncommon (⩾ 1/1,000, < 1/100). Within each frequency grouping, ADRs are presented in order of decreasing seriousness.

Xeloda Monotherapy:

Table 4 lists ADRs associated with the use of Xeloda monotherapy based on a pooled analysis of safety data from three major studies including over 1900 patients (studies M66001, SO14695, and SO14796). ADRs are added to the appropriate frequency grouping according to the overall incidence from the pooled analysis.

Table 4 Summary of related ADRs reported in patients treated with Xeloda monotherapy

(see Table 4 on next page)

Xeloda in combination therapy:

Table 5 lists ADRs associated with the use of Xeloda in combination with different chemotherapy regimens in multiple indications based on safety data from over 1400 patients. ADRs are added to the appropriate frequency grouping (Very common or Common) according to the highest incidence seen in any of the major clinical trials and are only added when they were seen **in addition to** those seen with Xeloda monotherapy or seen at **a higher frequency grouping** compared to Xeloda monotherapy (see Table 4). Uncommon ADRs reported for Xeloda in combination therapy are consistent with the ADRs reported for Xeloda monotherapy or reported for monotherapy with the combination agent (in literature and/or respective summary of product characteristics).

Some of the ADRs are reactions commonly seen with the combination agent (e.g. peripheral sensory neuropathy with docetaxel or oxaliplatin, hypertension seen with bevacizumab); however an exacerbation by Xeloda therapy can not be excluded.

Table 5 Summary of related ADRs reported in patients treated with Xeloda in combination treatment **in addition**

Table 4 Summary of related ADRs reported in patients treated with Xeloda monotherapy

Body System	Very Common	Common	Uncommon
	All grades	*All grades*	*Severe and/or Life-threatening (grade 3-4) or considered medically relevant*
Infections and infestations	-	Herpes viral infection, Nasopharyngitis, Lower respiratory tract infection	Sepsis, Urinary tract infection, Cellulitis, Tonsillitis, Pharyngitis, Oral candidiasis, Influenza, Gastroenteritis, Fungal infection, Infection, Tooth abscess
Neoplasm benign, malignant and unspecified			Lipoma
Blood and lymphatic system disorders	-	Neutropenia, Anaemia	Febrile neutropenia, Pancytopenia, Granulocytopenia, Thrombocytopenia, Leucopenia, Haemolytic anaemia, International normalised Ratio (INR) increased/Prothrombin time prolonged
Immune system disorders	-	-	Hypersensitivity
Metabolism and nutrition disorders	Anorexia	Dehydration, Decreased appetite, Weight decreased	Diabetes, Hypokalaemia, Appetite disorder, Malnutrition, Hypertriglyceridaemia,
Psychiatric disorders		Insomnia, Depression	Confusional state, Panic attack, Depressed mood, Libido decreased
Nervous system disorders	-	Headache, Lethargy Dizziness, Paraesthesia Dysgeusia	Aphasia, Memory impairment, Ataxia, Syncope, Balance disorder, Sensory disorder, Neuropathy peripheral
Eye disorders	-	Lacrimation increased, Conjunctivitis, Eye irritation	Visual acuity reduced, Diplopia
Ear and labyrinth disorders	-	-	Vertigo, Ear pain
Cardiac disorders	-		Angina unstable, Angina pectoris, Myocardial ischaemia, Atrial fibrillation, Arrhythmia, Tachycardia, Sinus tachycardia, Palpitations
Vascular disorders	-	Thrombophlebitis	Deep vein thrombosis, Hypertension, Petechiae, Hypotension, Hot flush, Peripheral coldness
Respiratory, thoracic and mediastinal disorders	-	Dyspnoea, Epistaxis, Cough, Rhinorrhoea	Pulmonary embolism, Pneumothorax, Haemoptysis, Asthma, Dyspnoea exertional
Gastrointestinal disorders	Diarrhoea, Vomiting, Nausea, Stomatitis, Abdominal pain	Gastrointestinal haemorrhage, Constipation, Upper abdominal pain, Dyspepsia, Flatulence, Dry mouth	Intestinal obstruction, Ascites, Enteritis, Gastritis, Dysphagia, Abdominal pain lower, Oesophagitis, Abdominal discomfort, Gastroesophageal reflux disease, Colitis, Blood in stool
Hepatobiliary Disorders	-	Hyperbilirubinaemia, Liver function test abnormalities	Jaundice
Skin and subcutaneous tissue disorders	Palmar-plantar erythrodysaesthesia syndrome	Rash, Alopecia, Erythema, Dry skin, Pruritus, Skin hyper-pigmentation, Rash macular, Skin desquamation, Dermatitis, Pigmentation disorder, Nail disorder	Skin ulcer, Rash, Urticaria, Photosensitivity reaction, Palmar erythema, Swelling face, Purpura
Muskuloskeletal and connective tissue disorders	-	Pain in extremity, Back pain, Arthralgia	Joint swelling, Bone pain, Facial pain, Musculoskeletal stiffness, Muscular weakness
Renal and urinary disorders	-	-	Hydronephrosis, Urinary incontinence, Haematuria, Nocturia, Blood creatinine increased
Reproductive system and breast disorders	-	-	Vaginal haemorrhage
General disorders and administration site conditions	Fatigue, Asthenia	Pyrexia, Lethargy, Oedema peripheral, Malaise, Chest pain	Oedema, Chills, Influenza like illness, Rigors, Body temperature increased
Injury, poisoning and procedural complications	-	-	Blister, Overdose

to those seen with Xeloda monotherapy or seen at **a higher frequency grouping** compared to Xeloda monotherapy

(see Table 5 on next page)

Post-Marketing Experience:

The following additional serious adverse reactions have been identified during post-marketing exposure:

- Very rare: lacrimal duct stenosis
- Very rare: hepatic failure and cholestatic hepatitis have been reported during clinical trials and post-marketing exposure

c. Description of selected adverse reactions

Hand-foot syndrome (see section 4.4):

For the capecitabine dose of 1250 mg/m^2 twice daily on days 1 to 14 every 3 weeks, a frequency of 53% to 60% of all-grades HFS was observed in capecitabine monotherapy trials (comprising studies in adjuvant therapy in colon cancer, treatment of metastatic colorectal cancer, and treatment of breast cancer) and a frequency of 63% was observed in the capecitabine/docetaxel arm for the treatment of metastatic breast cancer. For the capecitabine dose of 1000 mg/m^2 twice daily on days 1 to 14 every 3 weeks, a frequency of 22% to 30% of all-grade HFS was observed in capecitabine combination therapy

A meta-analysis of 13 clinical trials with data from over 3800 patients treated with capecitabine monotherapy or capecitabine in combination with different chemotherapy regimens in multiple indications (colon, colorectal, gastric and breast cancer) showed that HFS (all grades) occurred in 1788 (47%) patients after a median time of 155 [95% CI 135, 187] days after starting treatment with capecitabine. In all studies combined, the following covariates were statistically significantly associated with an increased risk of developing HFS: increasing capecitabine starting dose (gram), decreasing cumulative capecitabine dose (0.1*kg), increasing relative dose intensity in the first six weeks, increasing duration of study treatment (weeks), increasing age (by 10 year increments), female gender, and good ECOG performance status at baseline (0 versus ≥1).

Diarrhoea (see section 4.4):

Xeloda can induce the occurrence of diarrhoea, which has been observed in up to 50% of patients.

The results of a meta-analysis of 13 clinical trials with data from over 3800 patients treated with capecitabine showed that in all studies combined, the following covariates were statistically significantly associated with an increased risk of developing diarrhoea: increasing capecitabine starting dose (gram), increasing duration of study treatment (weeks), increasing age (by 10 year increments), and female gender. The following covariates were statistically significantly associated with a decreased risk of developing diarrhoea: increasing cumulative capecitabine dose (0.1*kg) and increasing relative dose intensity in the first six weeks.

Cardiotoxicity (see section 4.4):

In addition to the ADRs described in Tables 4 and 5, the following ADRs with an incidence of less than 0.1% were associated with the use of Xeloda monotherapy based on a pooled analysis from clinical safety data from 7 clinical trials including 949 patients (2 phase III and 5 phase II clinical trials in metastatic colorectal cancer and metastatic breast cancer): cardiomyopathy, cardiac failure, sudden death, and ventricular extrasystoles.

Encephalopathy:

In addition to the ADRs described in Tables 4 and 5, and based on the above pooled analysis from clinical safety data from 7 clinical trials, encephalopathy was also associated with the use of Xeloda monotherapy with an incidence of less than 0.1%.

d. Special populations

Elderly patients (see section 4.2):

An analysis of safety data in patients ≥60 years of age treated with Xeloda monotherapy and an analysis of patients treated with Xeloda plus docetaxel combination therapy showed an increase in the incidence of treatment-related grade 3 and 4 adverse reactions and treatment-related serious adverse reactions compared to patients <60 years of age. Patients ≥60 years of age treated with Xeloda plus docetaxel also had more early withdrawals from treatment due to adverse reactions compared to patients <60 years of age.

The results of a meta-analysis of 13 clinical trials with data from over 3800 patients treated with capecitabine showed that in all studies combined, increasing age (by 10 year increments) was statistically significantly associated with an increased risk of developing HFS and diarrhoea and with a decreased risk of developing neutropenia.

Gender

The results of a meta-analysis of 13 clinical trials with data from over 3800 patients treated with capecitabine showed that in all studies combined, female gender was statistically significantly associated with an increased risk of developing HFS and diarrhoea and with a decreased risk of developing neutropenia.

Patients with renal impairment (see section 4.2, 4.4, and 5.2):

An analysis of safety data in patients treated with Xeloda monotherapy (colorectal cancer) with baseline renal

Table 5 Summary of related ADRs reported in patients treated with Xeloda in combination treatment in addition to those seen with Xeloda monotherapy or seen at **a higher frequency grouping** compared to Xeloda monotherapy

Body System	**Very common** ***All grades***	**Common** ***All grades***
Infections and infestations	-	Herpes zoster, Urinary tract infection, Oral candidiasis, Upper respiratory tract infection, Rhinitis, Influenza, +Infection
Blood and lymphatic system disorders	+Neutropenia, +Leucopenia, +Anaemia, +Neutropenic fever, Thrombocytopenia	Bone marrow depression, +Febrile Neutropenia
Immune system disorders	-	Hypersensitivity
Metabolism and nutrition disorders	Appetite decreased	Hypokalaemia, Hyponatraemia, Hypomagnesaemia, Hypocalcaemia, Hyperglycaemia
Psychiatric disorders	-	Sleep disorder, Anxiety
Nervous system disorders	Taste disturbance, Paraesthesia and dysaesthesia, Peripheral neuropathy, Dysgeusia, Headache	Neurotoxicity, Tremor, Neuralgia, Hypersensitivity reaction
Eye disorders	Lacrimation increased	Visual disorders, Dry eye
Ear and labyrinth disorders	-	Tinnitus, Hypoacusis
Cardiac disorders	-	Atrial fibrillation, Cardiac ischaemia/ infarction
Vascular disorders	Lower limb oedema, Hypertension, +Embolism and thrombosis	Flushing, Hypotension, Hypertensive crisis
Respiratory, thoracic and mediastinal system disorders	Sore throat, Dysaesthesia pharynx	Hiccups, Pharyngolaryngeal pain, Dysphonia
Gastrointestinal disorders	Constipation, Dyspepsia	Upper gastrointestinal haemorrhage, Mouth ulceration, Gastritis, Abdominal distension, Gastroesophageal reflux disease, Oral pain, Dysphagia, Rectal haemorrhage, Abdominal pain lower
Hepatobiliary disorders	-	Hepatic function abnormal
Skin and subcutaneous tissue disorders	Alopecia, Nail disorder	Hyperhidrosis, Rash erythematous, Urticaria, Night sweats
Musculoskeletal and connective tissue disorders	Myalgia, Arthralgia, Pain in extremity	Pain in jaw, Muscle spasms, Trismus, Muscular weakness
Renal and urinary disorder	-	Haematuria, Proteinuria, Creatinine renal clearance decreased
General disorders and administration site conditions	Pyrexia, Weakness, +Lethargy	Mucosal inflammation, Pain in limb, Pain, Temperature intolerance, Chills, Chest pain, Influenza-like illness, +Fever
Injury, poisoning and procedural complications	-	Contusion

+ For each term, the frequency count was based on ADRs of all grades. For terms marked with a "+", the frequency count was based on grade 3-4 ADRs. ADRs are added according to the highest incidence seen in any of the major combination trials.

impairment showed an increase in the incidence of treatment-related grade 3 and 4 adverse reactions compared to patients with normal renal function (36% in patients without renal impairment n=268, vs. 41% in mild n=257 and 54% in moderate n=59, respectively) (see section 5.2). Patients with moderately impaired renal function show an increased rate of dose reduction (44%) vs. 33% and 32% in patients with no or mild renal impairment and an increase in early withdrawals from treatment (21% withdrawals during the first two cycles) vs. 5% and 8% in patients with no or mild renal impairment.

4.9 Overdose

The manifestations of acute overdose include nausea, vomiting, diarrhoea, mucositis, gastrointestinal irritation and bleeding, and bone marrow depression. Medical management of overdose should include customary therapeutic and supportive medical interventions aimed at correcting the presenting clinical manifestations and preventing their possible complications.

5. PHARMACOLOGICAL PROPERTIES

5.1 Pharmacodynamic properties

Pharmacotherapeutic group: cytostatic (antimetabolite), ATC code: L01BC06

Capecitabine is a non-cytotoxic fluoropyrimidine carbamate, which functions as an orally administered precursor of the cytotoxic moiety 5-fluorouracil (5-FU). Capecitabine is activated via several enzymatic steps (see section 5.2). The enzyme involved in the final conversion to 5-FU, thymidine phosphorylase (ThyPase), is found in tumour tissues, but also in normal tissues, albeit usually at lower levels. In human cancer xenograft models capecitabine demonstrated a synergistic effect in combination with docetaxel, which may be related to the upregulation of thymidine phosphorylase by docetaxel.

There is evidence that the metabolism of 5-FU in the anabolic pathway blocks the methylation reaction of deoxyuridylic acid to thymidylic acid, thereby interfering with the synthesis of deoxyribonucleic acid (DNA). The incorporation of 5-FU also leads to inhibition of RNA and protein synthesis. Since DNA and RNA are essential for cell division and growth, the effect of 5-FU may be to create a thymidine deficiency that provokes unbalanced growth and death of a cell. The effects of DNA and RNA deprivation are most marked on those cells which proliferate more rapidly and which metabolise 5-FU at a more rapid rate.

Colon and colorectal cancer:

Adjuvant Therapy with Xeloda in colon cancer

Data from one multicentre, randomised, controlled phase III clinical trial in patients with stage III (Dukes' C) colon cancer supports the use of Xeloda for the adjuvant treatment of patients with colon cancer (XACT Study; M66001). In this trial, 1987 patients were randomised to treatment with Xeloda (1250 mg/m^2 twice daily for 2 weeks followed by a 1-week rest period and given as 3-week cycles for 24 weeks) or 5-FU and leucovorin (Mayo Clinic regimen: 20 mg/m^2 leucovorin IV followed by 425 mg/m^2 IV bolus 5-FU, on days 1 to 5, every 28 days for 24 weeks). Xeloda was at least equivalent to IV 5-FU/LV in disease-free survival in per protocol population (hazard ratio 0.92; 95% CI 0.80-1.06). In the all-randomised population, tests for difference of Xeloda vs 5-FU/LV in disease-free and overall survival showed hazard ratios of 0.88 (95% CI 0.77 – 1.01; p = 0.068) and 0.86 (95% CI 0.74 – 1.01; p = 0.060), respectively. The median follow up at the time of the analysis was 6.9 years. In a preplanned multivariate Cox analysis, superiority of Xeloda compared with bolus 5-FU/LV was demonstrated. The following factors were pre-specified in the statistical analysis plan for inclusion in the model: age, time from surgery to randomisation, gender, CEA levels at baseline, lymph nodes at baseline, and country. In the all-randomised population, Xeloda was shown to be superior to 5FU/LV for disease-free survival (hazard ratio 0.849; 95% CI 0.739 - 0.976; p = 0.0212), as well as for overall survival (hazard ratio 0.828; 95% CI 0.705 - 0.971; p = 0.0203). Currently, data on the use of Xeloda in combination with other chemotherapeutic agents in adjuvant therapy of colon cancer is not available.

Monotherapy with Xeloda in metastatic colorectal cancer

Data from two identically-designed, multicentre, randomised, controlled phase III clinical trials (SO14695; SO14796) support the use of Xeloda for first line treatment of metastatic colorectal cancer. In these trials, 603 patients were randomised to treatment with Xeloda (1250 mg/m^2 twice daily for 2 weeks followed by a 1-week rest period and given as 3-week cycles). 604 patients were randomised to treatment with 5-FU and leucovorin (Mayo regimen: 20 mg/m^2 leucovorin IV followed by 425 mg/m^2 IV bolus 5-FU, on days 1 to 5, every 28 days). The overall objective response rates in the all-randomised population (investigator assessment) were 25.7% (Xeloda) vs. 16.7% (Mayo regimen); p <0.0002. The median time to progression was 140 days (Xeloda) vs. 144 days (Mayo regimen). Median survival was 392 days (Xeloda) vs. 391 days (Mayo regimen). Currently, no comparative data are available on Xeloda monotherapy in colorectal cancer in comparison with first line combination regimens.

Combination therapy in first-line treatment of metastatic colorectal cancer

Data from a multicentre, randomised, controlled phase III clinical study (NO16966) support the use of Xeloda in combination with oxaliplatin or in combination with oxaliplatin and bevacizumab for the first-line treatment of metastatic colorectal cancer. The study contained two parts: an initial 2-arm part in which 634 patients were randomised to two different treatment groups, including XELOX or FOLFOX-4, and a subsequent 2x2 factorial part in which 1401 patients were randomised to four different treatment groups, including XELOX plus placebo, FOLFOX-4 plus placebo, XELOX plus bevacizumab, and FOLFOX-4 plus bevacizumab. See Table 6 for treatment regimens.

Table 6 Treatment Regimens in Study NO16966 (mCRC)

(see Table 6 on next page)

Non-inferiority of the XELOX-containing arms compared with the FOLFOX-4-containing arms in the overall comparison was demonstrated in terms of progression-free survival in the eligible patient population and the intent-to-treat population (see Table 7). The results indicate that XELOX is equivalent to FOLFOX-4 in terms of overall survival (see Table 7). A comparison of XELOX plus bevacizumab versus FOLFOX-4 plus bevacizumab was a pre-specified exploratory analysis. In this treatment subgroup comparison, XELOX plus bevacizumab was similar compared to FOLFOX-4 plus bevacizumab in terms of progression-free survival (hazard ratio 1.01; 97.5% CI 0.84 - 1.22). The median follow up at the time of the primary analyses in the intent-to-treat population was 1.5 years; data from analyses following an additional 1 year of follow up are also included in Table 7. However, the on-treatment PFS analysis did not confirm the results of the general PFS and OS analysis: the hazard ratio of XELOX versus FOLFOX-4 was 1.24 with 97.5% CI 1.07 - 1.44. Although sensitivity analyses show that differences in regimen schedules and timing of tumour assessments impact the on-treatment PFS analysis, a full explanation for this result has not been found.

Table 7 Key efficacy results for the non-inferiority analysis of Study NO16966

(see Table 7 on next page)

Data from a randomised, controlled phase III study (CAIRO) support the use of Xeloda at a starting dose of 1000 mg/m^2 for 2 weeks every 3 weeks in combination with irinotecan for the first-line treatment of patients with metastatic colorectal cancer. 820 Patients were randomized to receive either sequential treatment (n=410) or combination treatment (n=410). Sequential treatment consisted of first-line treatment with Xeloda (1250 mg/m2 twice daily for 14 days), second-line irinotecan (350 mg/m2 on day 1), and third-line combination of capecitabine (1000 mg/m2 twice daily for 14 days) with oxaliplatin (130 mg/m2 on day 1). Combination treatment consisted of first-line treatment of Xeloda (1000 mg/m2 twice daily for 14 days) combined with irinotecan (250 mg /m2 on day 1) (XELIRI) and second-line capecitabine (1000 mg/m2 twice daily for 14 days) plus oxaliplatin (130 mg/m2 on day 1). All treatment cycles were administered at intervals of 3 weeks. In first-line treatment the median progression-free survival in the intent-to-treat population was 5.8 months (95%CI 5.1 - 6.2 months) for Xeloda monotherapy and 7.8 months (95%CI 7.0 - 8.3 months; p=0.0002) for XELIRI.

Data from an interim analysis of a multicentre, randomised, controlled phase II study (AIO KRK 0604) support the use of

Table 6 Treatment Regimens in Study NO16966 (mCRC)

	Treatment	Starting Dose	Schedule
FOLFOX-4 or FOLFOX-4 + Bevacizumab	Oxaliplatin	85 mg/m^2 IV 2 hr	Oxaliplatin on Day 1, every 2 weeks
	Leucovorin	200 mg/m^2 IV 2 hr	Leucovorin on Days 1 and 2, every 2 weeks
	5-Fluorouracil	400 mg/m^2 IV bolus, followed by 600 mg/ m^2 IV 22 hr	5-fluorouracil IV bolus/infusion, each on Days 1 and 2, every 2 weeks
	Placebo or Bevacizumab	5 mg/kg IV 30-90 mins	Day 1, prior to FOLFOX-4, every 2 weeks
XELOX or XELOX+ Bevacizumab	Oxaliplatin	130 mg/m^2 IV 2 hr	Oxaliplatin on Day 1, every 3 weeks
	Capecitabine	1000 mg/m^2 oral twice daily	Capecitabine oral twice daily for 2 weeks (followed by 1 week off- treatment)
	Placebo or Bevacizumab	7.5 mg/kg IV 30-90 mins	Day 1, prior to XELOX, every 3 weeks
5-Fluorouracil: IV bolus injection immediately after leucovorin			

Table 7 Key efficacy results for the non-inferiority analysis of Study NO16966

PRIMARY ANALYSIS			
	XELOX/XELOX+P / XELOX+BV (EPP*: N=967; ITT**: N=1017)	FOLFOX-4/FOLFOX-4+P / FOLFOX-4+BV (EPP*: N = 937; ITT**: N= 1017)	
Population	Median Time to Event (Days)		HR (97.5% CI)
Parameter: Progression-free Survival			
EPP ITT	241 244	259 259	1.05 (0.94; 1.18) 1.04 (0.93; 1.16)
Parameter: Overall Survival			
EPP ITT	577 581	549 553	0.97 (0.84; 1.14) 0.96 (0.83; 1.12)
ADDITIONAL 1 YEAR OF FOLLOW UP			
Population	Median Time to Event (Days)		HR (97.5% CI)
Parameter: Progression-free Survival			
EPP ITT	242 244	259 259	1.02 (0.92; 1.14) 1.01 (0.91; 1.12)
Parameter: Overall Survival			
EPP ITT	600 602	594 596	1.00 (0.88; 1.13) 0.99 (0.88; 1.12)

*EPP=eligible patient population; **ITT=intent-to-treat population

Xeloda at a starting dose of 800 mg/m^2 for 2 weeks every 3 weeks in combination with irinotecan and bevacizumab for the first-line treatment of patients with metastatic colorectal cancer. 115 Patients were randomised to treatment with Xeloda combined with irinotecan (XELIRI) and bevacizumab: Xeloda (800 mg/m2 twice daily for two weeks followed by a 7-day rest period), irinotecan (200 mg/m2 as a 30 minute infusion on day 1 every 3 weeks), and bevacizumab (7.5 mg/kg as a 30 to 90 minute infusion on day 1 every 3 weeks); a total of 118 patients were randomised to treatment with Xeloda combined with oxaliplatin plus bevacizumab: Xeloda (1000 mg/m2 twice daily for two weeks followed by a 7-day rest period), oxaliplatin (130 mg/m2 as a 2 hour infusion on day 1 every 3 weeks), and bevacizumab (7.5 mg/kg as a 30 to 90 minute infusion on day 1 every 3 weeks). Progression-free survival at 6 months in the intent-to-treat population was 80% (XELIRI plus bevacizumab) versus 74% (XELOX plus bevacizumab). Overall response rate (complete response plus partial response) was 45% (XELOX plus bevacizumab) versus 47% (XELIRI plus bevacizumab).

Combination therapy in second-line treatment of metastatic colorectal cancer

Data from a multicentre, randomised, controlled phase III clinical study (NO16967) support the use of Xeloda in combination with oxaliplatin for the second-line treatment of metastatic colorectal cancer. In this trial, 627 patients with metastatic colorectal carcinoma who have received prior treatment with irinotecan in combination with a fluoropyrimidine regimen as first line therapy were randomised to treatment with XELOX or FOLFOX-4. For the dosing schedule of XELOX and FOLFOX-4 (without addition of placebo or bevacizumab), refer to Table 6. XELOX was demonstrated to be non-inferior to FOLFOX-4 in terms of progression-free survival in the per-protocol population and intent-to-treat population (see Table 8). The results indicate that XELOX is equivalent to FOLFOX-4 in terms of overall survival (see Table 8). The median follow up at the time of the primary analyses in the intent-to-treat population was 2.1 years; data from analyses following an additional 6 months of follow up are also included in Table 8.

Table 8 Key efficacy results for the non-inferiority analysis of Study NO16967

(see Table 8 below)

Advanced gastric cancer:

Data from a multicentre, randomised, controlled phase III clinical trial in patients with advanced gastric cancer supports the use of Xeloda for the first-line treatment of advanced gastric cancer (ML17032). In this trial, 160 patients were randomised to treatment with Xeloda (1000 mg/m^2 twice daily for 2 weeks followed by a 7-day rest period) and cisplatin (80 mg/m^2 as a 2-hour infusion every 3 weeks). A total of 156 patients were randomised to treatment with 5-FU (800 mg/m^2 per day, continuous infusion on days 1 to 5 every 3 weeks) and cisplatin (80 mg/m^2 as a 2-hour infusion on day 1, every 3 weeks). Xeloda in combination with cisplatin was non-inferior to 5-FU in combination with cisplatin in terms of progression-free survival in the per protocol analysis (hazard ratio 0.81; 95% CI 0.63 - 1.04). The median progression-free survival was 5.6 months (Xeloda + cisplatin) versus 5.0 months (5-FU + cisplatin). The hazard ratio for duration of survival (overall survival) was similar to the hazard ratio for progression-free survival (hazard ratio 0.85; 95% CI 0.64 - 1.13). The median duration of survival was 10.5 months (Xeloda + cisplatin) versus 9.3 months (5-FU + cisplatin).

Data from a randomised multicentre, phase III study comparing capecitabine to 5-FU and oxaliplatin to cisplatin in patients with advanced gastric cancer supports the use of Xeloda for the first-line treatment of advanced gastric cancer (REAL-2). In this trial, 1002 patients were randomised in a 2x2 factorial design to one of the following 4 arms:

- ECF: epirubicin (50 mg/ m^2 as a bolus on day 1 every 3 weeks), cisplatin (60 mg/m^2 as a two hour infusion on day 1 every 3 weeks) and 5-FU (200 mg/m^2 daily given by continuous infusion via a central line).
- ECX: epirubicin (50 mg/m^2 as a bolus on day 1 every 3 weeks), cisplatin (60 mg/m^2 as a two hour infusion on day 1 every 3 weeks), and Xeloda (625 mg/m^2 twice daily continuously).
- EOF: epirubicin (50 mg/m^2 as a bolus on day 1 every 3 weeks), oxaliplatin (130 mg/m^2 given as a 2 hour infusion on day 1 every three weeks), and 5-FU (200 mg/m^2 daily given by continuous infusion via a central line).
- EOX: epirubicin (50 mg/m^2 as a bolus on day 1 every 3 weeks), oxaliplatin (130 mg/m^2 given as a 2 hour infusion on day 1 every three weeks), and Xeloda (625 mg/m^2 twice daily continuously).

The primary efficacy analyses in the per protocol population demonstrated non-inferiority in overall survival for capecitabine- vs 5-FU-based regimens (hazard ratio 0.86; 95% CI 0.8 - 0.99) and for oxaliplatin- vs cisplatin-based regimens (hazard ratio 0.92; 95% CI 0.80 - 1.1). The median overall survival was 10.9 months in capecitabine-based regimens and 9.6 months in 5-FU based regimens. The median overall survival was 10.0 months in cisplatin-based regimens and 10.4 months in oxaliplatin-based regimens.

Table 8 Key efficacy results for the non-inferiority analysis of Study NO16967

PRIMARY ANALYSIS			
	XELOX (PPP*: N=251; ITT**: N=313)	FOLFOX-4 (PPP*: N = 252; ITT**: N= 314)	
Population	Median Time to Event (Days)		HR (95% CI)
Parameter: Progression-free Survival			
PPP ITT	154 144	168 146	1.03 (0.87; 1.24) 0.97 (0.83; 1.14)
Parameter: Overall Survival			
PPP ITT	388 363	401 382	1.07 (0.88; 1.31) 1.03 (0.87; 1.23)
ADDITIONAL 6 MONTHS OF FOLLOW UP			
Population	Median Time to Event (Days)		HR (95% CI)
Parameter: Progression-free Survival			
PPP ITT	154 143	166 146	1.04 (0.87; 1.24) 0.97 (0.83; 1.14)
Parameter: Overall Survival			
PPP ITT	393 363	402 382	1.05 (0.88; 1.27) 1.02 (0.86; 1.21)

*PPP=per-protocol population; **ITT=intent-to-treat population

Xeloda has also been used in combination with oxaliplatin for the treatment of advanced gastric cancer. Studies with Xeloda monotherapy indicate that Xeloda has activity in advanced gastric cancer.

Colon, colorectal and advanced gastric cancer: meta-analysis

A meta-analysis of six clinical trials (studies SO14695, SO14796, M66001, NO16966, NO16967, M17032) supports Xeloda replacing 5-FU in mono- and combination treatment in gastrointestinal cancer. The pooled analysis includes 3097 patients treated with Xeloda-containing regimens and 3074 patients treated with 5-FU-containing regimens. Median overall survival time was 703 days (95% CI: 671; 743) in patients treated with Xeloda-containing regimens and 683 days (95% CI: 648; 715) in patients treated with 5-FU-containing regimens. The hazard ratio for overall survival was 0.96 (95% CI: 0.90; 1.02) indicating that Xeloda-containing regimens are equivalent to 5-FU-containing regimens.

Breast cancer:

Combination therapy with Xeloda and docetaxel in locally advanced or metastatic breast cancer

Data from one multicentre, randomised, controlled phase III clinical trial support the use of Xeloda in combination with docetaxel for treatment of patients with locally advanced or metastatic breast cancer after failure of cytotoxic chemotherapy, including an anthracycline. In this trial, 255 patients were randomised to treatment with Xeloda (1250 mg/m^2 twice daily for 2 weeks followed by 1-week rest period and docetaxel 75 mg/m^2 as a 1 hour intravenous infusion every 3 weeks). 256 patients were randomised to treatment with docetaxel alone (100 mg/m^2 as a 1 hour intravenous infusion every 3 weeks). Survival was superior in the Xeloda + docetaxel combination arm (p=0.0126). Median survival was 442 days (Xeloda + docetaxel) vs. 352 days (docetaxel alone). The overall objective response rates in the all-randomised population (investigator assessment) were 41.6% (Xeloda + docetaxel) vs. 29.7% (docetaxel alone); p = 0.0058. Time to progressive disease was superior in the Xeloda + docetaxel combination arm (p < 0.0001). The median time to progression was 186 days (Xeloda + docetaxel) vs. 128 days (docetaxel alone).

Monotherapy with Xeloda after failure of taxanes, anthracycline containing chemotherapy, and for whom anthracycline therapy is not indicated

Data from two multicentre phase II clinical trials support the use of Xeloda monotherapy for treatment of patients after failure of taxanes and an anthracycline-containing chemotherapy regimen or for whom further anthracycline therapy is not indicated. In these trials, a total of 236 patients were treated with Xeloda (1250 mg/m^2 twice daily for 2 weeks followed by 1-week rest period). The overall objective response rates (investigator assessment) were 20% (first trial) and 25% (second trial). The median time to progression was 93 and 98 days. Median survival was 384 and 373 days.

All indications:

A meta-analysis of 13 clinical trials with data from over 3800 patients treated with Xeloda monotherapy or Xeloda in combination with different chemotherapy regimens in multiple indications (colon, colorectal, gastric and breast cancer) showed that patients on Xeloda who developed hand-foot syndrome (HFS) had a longer overall survival compared to patients who did not develop HFS: median overall survival 29.0 months (95% CI 26.0; 31.6) vs 15.9 months (95% CI 15.0; 17.0) with a hazard ratio of 0.59 (95% CI 0.54; 0.64).

5.2 Pharmacokinetic properties

The pharmacokinetics of capecitabine have been evaluated over a dose range of 502-3514 mg/m^2/day. The parameters of capecitabine, 5'-deoxy-5-fluorocytidine (5'-DFCR) and 5'-deoxy-5-fluorouridine (5'-DFUR) measured on days 1 and 14 were similar. The AUC of 5-FU was 30%-35% higher on day 14. Capecitabine dose reduction decreases systemic exposure to 5-FU more than dose-proportionally, due to non-linear pharmacokinetics for the active metabolite.

Absorption: after oral administration, capecitabine is rapidly and extensively absorbed, followed by extensive conversion to the metabolites, 5'-DFCR and 5'-DFUR. Administration with food decreases the rate of capecitabine absorption, but only results in a minor effect on the AUC of 5'-DFUR, and on the AUC of the subsequent metabolite 5-FU. At the dose of 1250 mg/m^2 on day 14 with administration after food intake, the peak plasma concentrations (C_{max} in μg/ml) for capecitabine, 5'-DFCR, 5'-DFUR, 5-FU and FBAL were 4.67, 3.05, 12.1, 0.95 and 5.46 respectively. The time to peak plasma concentrations (T_{max} in hours) were 1.50, 2.00, 2.00, 2.00 and 3.34. The $AUC_{0-\infty}$ values in μg•h/ml were 7.75, 7.24, 24.6, 2.03 and 36.3.

Protein binding: in vitro human plasma studies have determined that capecitabine, 5'-DFCR, 5'-DFUR and 5-FU are 54%, 10%, 62% and 10% protein bound, mainly to albumin.

Metabolism: capecitabine is first metabolised by hepatic carboxylesterase to 5'-DFCR, which is then converted to 5'-DFUR by cytidine deaminase, principally located in the liver and tumour tissues. Further catalytic activation of 5'-DFUR then occurs by thymidine phosphorylase (ThyPase). The enzymes involved in the catalytic activation are found in tumour tissues but also in normal tissues, albeit usually at lower levels. The sequential enzymatic biotransformation of capecitabine to 5-FU leads to higher concentrations within tumour tissues. In the case of colorectal tumours, 5-FU generation appears to be in large part localised in tumour stromal cells. Following oral administration of capecitabine to patients with colorectal cancer, the ratio of 5-FU concentration in colorectal tumours to adjacent tissues was 3.2 (ranged from 0.9 to 8.0). The ratio of 5-FU concentration in tumour to plasma was 21.4 (ranged from 3.9 to 59.9, n=8) whereas the ratio in healthy tissues to plasma was 8.9 (ranged from 3.0 to 25.8, n=8). Thymidine phosphorylase activity was measured and found to be 4 times greater in primary colorectal tumour than in adjacent normal tissue. According to immunohistochemical studies, thymidine phosphorylase appears to be in large part localised in tumour stromal cells.

5-FU is further catabolised by the enzyme dihydropyrimidine dehydrogenase (DPD) to the much less toxic dihydro-5-fluorouracil (FUH_2). Dihydropyrimidinase cleaves the pyrimidine ring to yield 5-fluoro-ureidopropionic acid (FUPA). Finally, β-ureido-propionase cleaves FUPA to α-fluoro-β-alanine (FBAL) which is cleared in the urine. Dihydropyrimidine dehydrogenase (DPD) activity is the rate limiting step. Deficiency of DPD may lead to increased toxicity of capecitabine (see section 4.3 and 4.4).

Elimination: the elimination half-life ($t_{1/2}$ in hours) of capecitabine, 5'-DFCR, 5'-DFUR, 5-FU and FBAL were 0.85, 1.11, 0.66, 0.76 and 3.23 respectively. Capecitabine and its metabolites are predominantly excreted in urine; 95.5% of administered capecitabine dose is recovered in urine. Faecal excretion is minimal (2.6%). The major metabolite excreted in urine is FBAL, which represents 57% of the administered dose. About 3% of the administered dose is excreted in urine as unchanged drug.

Combination therapy: Phase I studies evaluating the effect of Xeloda on the pharmacokinetics of either docetaxel or paclitaxel and vice versa showed no effect by Xeloda on the pharmacokinetics of docetaxel or paclitaxel (C_{max} and AUC) and no effect by docetaxel or paclitaxel on the pharmacokinetics of 5'-DFUR.

Pharmacokinetics in special populations: A population pharmacokinetic analysis was carried out after Xeloda treatment of 505 patients with colorectal cancer dosed at 1250 mg/m^2 twice daily. Gender, presence or absence of liver metastasis at baseline, Karnofsky Performance Status, total bilirubin, serum albumin, ASAT and ALAT had no statistically significant effect on the pharmacokinetics of 5'-DFUR, 5-FU and FBAL.

Patients with hepatic impairment due to liver metastases: According to a pharmacokinetic study in cancer patients with mild to moderate liver impairment due to liver metastases, the bioavailability of capecitabine and exposure to 5-FU may increase compared to patients with no liver impairment. There are no pharmacokinetic data on patients with severe hepatic impairment.

Patients with renal impairment: Based on a pharmacokinetic study in cancer patients with mild to severe renal impairment, there is no evidence for an effect of creatinine clearance on the pharmacokinetics of intact drug and 5-FU. Creatinine clearance was found to influence the systemic exposure to 5'-DFUR (35% increase in AUC when creatinine clearance decreases by 50%) and to FBAL (114% increase in AUC when creatinine clearance decreases by 50%). FBAL is a metabolite without antiproliferative activity.

Elderly: Based on the population pharmacokinetic analysis, which included patients with a wide range of ages (27 to 86 years) and included 234 (46%) patients greater or equal to 65, age has no influence on the pharmacokinetics of 5'-DFUR and 5-FU. The AUC of FBAL increased with age (20% increase in age results in a 15% increase in the AUC of FBAL). This increase is likely due to a change in renal function.

Ethnic factors: Following oral administration of 825 mg/m^2 capecitabine twice daily for 14 days, Japanese patients (n=18) had about 36% lower C_{max} and 24% lower AUC for capecitabine than Caucasian patients (n=22). Japanese patients had also about 25% lower C_{max} and 34% lower AUC for FBAL than Caucasian patients. The clinical relevance of these differences is unknown. No significant differences occurred in the exposure to other metabolites (5'-DFCR, 5'-DFUR, and 5-FU).

5.3 Preclinical safety data

In repeat-dose toxicity studies, daily oral administration of capecitabine to cynomolgus monkeys and mice produced toxic effects on the gastrointestinal, lymphoid and haemopoietic systems, typical for fluoropyrimidines. These toxicities were reversible. Skin toxicity, characterised by degenerative/regressive changes, was observed with capecitabine. Capecitabine was devoid of hepatic and CNS toxicities. Cardiovascular toxicity (e.g. PR- and QT-interval prolongation) was detectable in cynomolgus monkeys after intravenous administration (100 mg/kg) but not after repeated oral dosing (1379 mg/m^2/day).

A two-year mouse carcinogenicity study produced no evidence of carcinogenicity by capecitabine.

During standard fertility studies, impairment of fertility was observed in female mice receiving capecitabine; however, this effect was reversible after a drug-free period. In addition, during a 13-week study, atrophic and degenerative changes occurred in reproductive organs of male mice; however these effects were reversible after a drug-free period.

In embryotoxicity and teratogenicity studies in mice, dose-related increases in foetal resorption and teratogenicity were observed. In monkeys, abortion and embryolethality were observed at high doses, but there was no evidence of teratogenicity.

Capecitabine was not mutagenic *in vitro* to bacteria (Ames test) or mammalian cells (Chinese hamster V79/HPRT gene mutation assay). However, similar to other nucleoside analogues (ie, 5-FU), capecitabine was clastogenic in human lymphocytes (*in vitro*) and a positive trend occurred in mouse bone marrow micronucleus tests (*in vivo*).

6. PHARMACEUTICAL PARTICULARS

6.1 List of excipients

Tablet core:

anhydrous lactose,

croscarmellose sodium,

hypromellose,

microcrystalline cellulose,

magnesium stearate.

Tablet coating:

hypromellose,

titanium dioxide (E171),

yellow and red iron oxide (E172),

talc.

6.2 Incompatibilities

Not applicable.

6.3 Shelf life

3 years.

6.4 Special precautions for storage

Do not store above 30°C.

6.5 Nature and contents of container

Nature: PVC/PVDC blisters

Content: 150 mg: 60 film-coated tablets (6 blisters of 10 tablets)

500 mg: 120 film-coated tablets (12 blisters of 10 tablets)

6.6 Special precautions for disposal and other handling

No special requirements.

7. MARKETING AUTHORISATION HOLDER

Roche Registration Limited

6 Falcon Way

Shire Park

Welwyn Garden City

AL7 1TW

United Kingdom

8. MARKETING AUTHORISATION NUMBER(S)

EU/1/00/163/001 – 150 mg film-coated tablets

EU/1/00/163/002 – 500 mg film-coated tablets

9. DATE OF FIRST AUTHORISATION/RENEWAL OF THE AUTHORISATION

Date of first authorisation: 02 February 2001

Date of first renewal: 02 February 2006

10. DATE OF REVISION OF THE TEXT

31 October 2008

Detailed information on this medicinal product is available on the website of the European Medicines Agency (EMEA) http://www.emea.europa.eu/.

Xenazine 25

(Cambridge Laboratories)

1. NAME OF THE MEDICINAL PRODUCT

Xenazine™ 25

2. QUALITATIVE AND QUANTITATIVE COMPOSITION

Each tablet contains 25mg Tetrabenazine.

3. PHARMACEUTICAL FORM

Tablets.

4. CLINICAL PARTICULARS

4.1 Therapeutic indications

Movement disorders associated with organic central nervous system conditions, e.g. Huntington's chorea, hemiballismus and senile chorea.

Xenazine™ 25 is also indicated for the treatment of moderate to severe tardive dyskinesia, which is disabling and/or socially embarrassing. The condition should be persistent despite withdrawal of antipsychotic therapy, or in cases where withdrawal of antipsychotic medication is not a realistic option; also where the condition persists despite reduction in dosage of antipsychotic medication or switching to atypical antipsychotic medication.

4.2 Posology and method of administration

The tablets are for oral administration.

Organic Central Nervous System Movement Disorders

Adults

Dosage and administration are variable and only a guide is given. An initial starting dose of 25mg three times a day is recommended. This can be increased by 25mg a day every three or four days until 200mg a day is being given or the limit of tolerance, as dictated by unwanted effects, is reached, whichever is the lower dose.

If there is no improvement at the maximum dose in seven days, it is unlikely that the compound will be of benefit to the patient, either by increasing the dose or by extending the duration of treatment.

Tardive Dyskinesia

Recommended starting dose of 12.5mg a day, subsequently titrated according to response. Medication should be discontinued if there is no clear benefit or if the side-effects cannot be tolerated

The elderly

No specific studies have been performed in the elderly, but Xenazine™ 25 has been administered to elderly patients in standard dosage without apparent ill effect.

Children

No specific dosage recommendations are made for the administration of Xenazine™ 25 to children, although it has been used without ill effect.

4.3 Contraindications

Xenazine™ 25 blocks the action of reserpine.

4.4 Special warnings and precautions for use

Tardive Dyskinesia

The condition should be persistent despite withdrawal of antipsychotic therapy, or in cases where withdrawal of antipsychotic medication is not a realistic option; also where the condition persists despite reduction in dosage of antipsychotic medication or switching to atypical antipsychotic medication.

4.5 Interaction with other medicinal products and other forms of interaction

Levodopa should be administered with caution in the presence of Xenazine™ 25.

4.6 Pregnancy and lactation

There is inadequate evidence of safety of the drug in human pregnancy and no evidence from animal work, but it has been in wide use for many years without apparent ill consequence. Tetrabenazine should be avoided in breast-feeding mothers.

4.7 Effects on ability to drive and use machines

Patients should be advised that Xenazine™ 25 may cause drowsiness and therefore may modify their performance at skilled tasks (driving ability, operation of machinery, etc.) to a varying degree, depending on dose and individual susceptibility.

4.8 Undesirable effects

Side-effects are usually mild with little hypotensive action and few digestive disorders. The main unwanted effect reported to date has been drowsiness, which occurs with higher doses. If depression occurs, it can be controlled by reducing the dose or by giving antidepressant drugs such as the monoamine oxidase inhibitors. However, Xenazine™ 25 should not be given immediately after a course of any of the monoamine oxidase inhibitors as such treatment may lead to a state of restlessness, disorientation and confusion. In man, a Parkinsonian-like syndrome has been reported on rare occasions, usually in doses above 200mg per day, but this disappears on reducing the dose.

Neuroleptic malignant syndrome (NMS) associated with the use of Tetrabenazine has been reported rarely. This may occur soon after initiation of therapy, following an increase in dosage or after prolonged treatment. The clinical features usually include hyperthermia, severe extrapyramidal symptoms including muscular rigidity, autonomic dysfunction and altered levels of consciousness. Skeletal muscle damage may occur. If NMS is suspected Xenazine™ 25 should be withdrawn and appropriate supportive therapy instituted; treatment with Dantrolene and Bromocriptine may be effective.

4.9 Overdose

Signs and symptoms of overdosage may include drowsiness, sweating, hypotension and hypothermia. Treatment is symptomatic.

5. PHARMACOLOGICAL PROPERTIES

Pharmacotherapeutic group: Other nervous system drugs, ATC Code: N07XX

5.1 Pharmacodynamic properties

The central effects of Xenazine™ 25 closely resemble those of Reserpine, but it differs from the latter in having less peripheral activity and being much shorter acting.

5.2 Pharmacokinetic properties

Tetrabenazine has a low and erratic bioavailability. It appears to be extensively metabolised by first-pass metabolism. The major metabolite, hydroxytetrabenazine, is formed by reduction. Little unchanged Tetrabenazine can be detected in the urine. Since hydroxytetrabenazine is reported to be as active as Tetrabenazine in depleting brain amines, it is likely that this is the major therapeutic agent.

5.3 Preclinical safety data

It is known from animal experiments that Tetrabenazine intervenes in the metabolism of biogenic amines, such as serotonin and noradrenaline, and that this activity is mainly limited to the brain. It is thought that the effect of Tetrabenazine on brain amines explains its clinical effects in man.

6. PHARMACEUTICAL PARTICULARS

6.1 List of excipients

Starch BP

Lactose BP

Talc BP

Magnesium stearate BP

Iron oxide yellow E172

6.2 Incompatibilities

None known.

6.3 Shelf life

5 years.

6.4 Special precautions for storage

The recommended maximum storage temperature is 30°C.

6.5 Nature and contents of container

White HDPE bottle, pack size 112 tablets.

6.6 Special precautions for disposal and other handling

None.

7. MARKETING AUTHORISATION HOLDER

Lifehealth Limited

23 Winkfield Road

Windsor

BERKS

SL4 4BA

8. MARKETING AUTHORISATION NUMBER(S)

PL 14576/0005

9. DATE OF FIRST AUTHORISATION/RENEWAL OF THE AUTHORISATION

23 October 1995

10. DATE OF REVISION OF THE TEXT

February 2008

Xenical 120mg hard capsules

(Roche Products Limited)

1. NAME OF THE MEDICINAL PRODUCT

Xenical 120 mg hard capsules

2. QUALITATIVE AND QUANTITATIVE COMPOSITION

Each hard capsule contains 120 mg orlistat.

For a full list of excipients, see 6.1.

3. PHARMACEUTICAL FORM

Hard capsule.

The capsule has a turquoise cap and turquoise body bearing the imprint of "ROCHE XENICAL 120".

4. CLINICAL PARTICULARS

4.1 Therapeutic indications

Xenical is indicated in conjunction with a mildly hypocaloric diet for the treatment of obese patients with a body mass index (BMI) greater or equal to 30 kg/m^2, or overweight patients (BMI $\geq$ 28 kg/m^2) with associated risk factors.

Treatment with orlistat should be discontinued after 12 weeks if patients have been unable to lose at least 5 % of the body weight as measured at the start of therapy.

4.2 Posology and method of administration

Adults

The recommended dose of orlistat is one 120 mg capsule taken with water immediately before, during or up to one hour after each main meal. If a meal is missed or contains no fat, the dose of orlistat should be omitted.

The patient should be on a nutritionally balanced, mildly hypocaloric diet that contains approximately 30 % of calories from fat. It is recommended that the diet should be rich in fruit and vegetables. The daily intake of fat, carbohydrate and protein should be distributed over three main meals.

Doses of orlistat above 120 mg three times daily have not been shown to provide additional benefit.

The effect of orlistat results in an increase in faecal fat as early as 24 to 48 hours after dosing. Upon discontinuation of therapy, faecal fat content usually returns to pre-treatment levels, within 48 to 72 hours.

Special populations

The effect of orlistat in patients with hepatic and/or renal impairment, children and elderly patients has not been studied.

There is no relevant indication for use of Xenical in children.

4.3 Contraindications

- Hypersensitivity to the active substance or to any of the excipients.
- Chronic malabsorption syndrome.
- Cholestasis.
- Breast-feeding.

4.4 Special warnings and precautions for use

In clinical trials, the decrease in bodyweight with orlistat treatment was less in type II diabetic patients than in non-diabetic patients. Antidiabetic medicinal product treatment may have to be closely monitored when taking orlistat.

Co-administration of orlistat with ciclosporin is not recommended (see section 4.5).

Patients should be advised to adhere to the dietary recommendations they are given (see section 4.2).

The possibility of experiencing gastrointestinal adverse reactions (see section 4.8) may increase when orlistat is taken with a diet high in fat (e.g. in a 2000 kcal/day diet, > 30 % of calories from fat equates to > 67 g of fat). The daily intake of fat should be distributed over three main meals. If orlistat is taken with a meal very high in fat, the possibility of gastrointestinal adverse reactions may increase.

Cases of rectal bleeding have been reported with Xenical. Prescribers should investigate further in case of severe and/or persistent symptoms.

The use of an additional contraceptive method is recommended to prevent possible failure of oral contraception that could occur in case of severe diarrhoea (see section 4.5).

Coagulation parameters should be monitored in patients treated with concomitant oral anticoagulants (see section 4.5 and 4.8).

The use of orlistat may be associated with hyperoxaluria and oxalate nephropathy in patients with underlying chronic kidney disease and/or volume depletion (see section 4.8).

Rare occurrence of hypothyroidism and/or reduced control of hypothyroidism may occur. The mechanism, although not proven, may involve a decreased absorption of iodine salts and/or levothyroxine (see section 4.5).

Antiepileptics patient: Orlistat may unbalance anticonvulsivant treatment by decreasing the absorption of antiepileptic drugs, leading to convulsions (see section 4.5).

4.5 Interaction with other medicinal products and other forms of interaction

Ciclosporin

A decrease in ciclosporin plasma levels has been observed in a drug-drug-interaction study and also reported in several cases, when orlistat was administered concomitantly. This can lead to a decrease of immunosuppressive efficacy. Therefore the combination is not recommended (see section 4.4). However, if such concomitant use is unavoidable, more frequent monitoring of ciclosporin blood levels should be performed both after addition of orlistat and upon discontinuation of orlistat in ciclosporin treated patients. Ciclosporin blood levels should be monitored until stabilised.

Acarbose

In the absence of pharmacokinetic interaction studies, the concomitant administration of orlistat with acarbose should be avoided.

Oral anticoagulants

When warfarin or other anticoagulants are given in combination with orlistat, international normalised ratio (INR) values should be monitored (see section 4.4).

Fat soluble vitamins

Treatment with orlistat may potentially impair the absorption of fat-soluble vitamins (A, D, E and K).

The vast majority of patients receiving up to four full years of treatment with orlistat in clinical studies had vitamin A, D, E and K and beta-carotene levels that stayed within normal range. In order to ensure adequate nutrition, patients on a weight control diet should be advised to have a diet rich in fruit and vegetables and use of a multivitamin supplement could be considered. If a multivitamin supplement is recommended, it should be taken at least two hours after the administration of orlistat or at bedtime.

Amiodarone

A slight decrease in plasma levels of amiodarone, when given as a single dose, has been observed in a limited number of healthy volunteers who received orlistat concomitantly. In patients receiving amiodarone treatment, the clinical relevance of this effect remains unknown but may become clinically relevant in some cases. In patients receiving concomitant amiodarone treatment, reinforcement of clinical and ECG monitoring is warranted.

Convulsions have been reported in patients treated concomitantly with orlistat and antiepileptic drugs e.g. valproate, lamotrigine, for which a causal relationship to an interaction cannot be excluded. Therefore, these patients should be monitored for possible changes in the frequency and/or severity of convulsions.

Rare occurrence of hypothyroidism and/or reduced control of hypothyroidism may occur. The mechanism, although not proven, may involve a decreased absorption of iodine salts and/or levothyroxine (see section 4.4).

Lack of interactions

No interactions with amitriptyline, atorvastatin, biguanides, digoxin, fibrates, fluoxetine, losartan, phenytoin, phentermine, pravastatin, nifedipine Gastrointestinal Therapeutic System (GITS), nifedipine slow release, sibutramine or alcohol have been observed. The absence of these interactions has been demonstrated in specific drug-drug-interaction studies.

The absence of an interaction between oral contraceptives and orlistat has been demonstrated in specific drug-drug interaction studies. However, orlistat may indirectly reduce the availability of oral contraceptives and lead to unexpected pregnancies in some individual cases. An additional contraceptive method is recommended in case of severe diarrhoea (see section 4.4).

4.6 Pregnancy and lactation

For orlistat no clinical data on exposed pregnancies are available.

Animal studies do not indicate direct or indirect harmful effects with respect to pregnancy, embryonal/foetal development, parturition or postnatal development (see section 5.3).

Caution should be exercised when prescribing to pregnant women.

As it is not known whether orlistat is secreted into human milk, orlistat is contra-indicated during breast-feeding.

4.7 Effects on ability to drive and use machines

Xenical has no influence on the ability to drive and use machines.

4.8 Undesirable effects

Adverse reactions to orlistat are largely gastrointestinal in nature. The incidence of adverse events decreased with prolonged use of orlistat.

Adverse events are listed below by system organ class and frequency. Frequencies are defined as: very common (≥1/10), common (≥1/100 to <1/10), uncommon (≥1/1,000 to <1/100), rare (≥1/10,000 to <1/1,000) and very rare (<1/10,000) including isolated reports.

Within each frequency grouping, undesirable effects are presented in order of decreasing seriousness.

The following table of undesirable effects (first year of treatment) is based on adverse events that occurred at a frequency of > 2 % and with an incidence ≥ 1 % above placebo in clinical trials of 1 and 2 years duration:

System organ class	Adverse reaction/event
Nervous system disorders	
Very common:	Headache
Respiratory, thoracic and mediastinal disorders	
Very common:	Upper respiratory infection
Common:	Lower respiratory infection
Gastrointestinal disorders	
Very common:	Abdominal pain/discomfort Oily spotting from the rectum Flatus with discharge Faecal urgency Fatty/oily stool Flatulence Liquid stools Oily evacuation Increased defecation
Common:	Rectal pain/discomfort Soft stools Faecal incontinence Abdominal distension* Tooth disorder Gingival disorder
Renal and urinary disorders	
Common:	Urinary tract infection
Metabolism and nutrition disorders	
Very common:	Hypoglycaemia*
Infections and infestations	
Very common:	Influenza
General disorders and administration site conditions	
Common:	Fatigue
Reproductive system and breast disorders	
Common:	Menstrual irregularity
Psychiatric disorders	
Common:	Anxiety

* only unique treatment adverse events that occurred at a frequency of > 2 % and with an incidence ≥ 1 % above placebo in obese type 2 diabetic patients.

In a 4 year clinical trial, the general pattern of adverse event distribution was similar to that reported for the 1 and 2 year studies with the total incidence of gastrointestinal related adverse events occurring in year 1 decreasing year on year over the four year period.

The following table of undesirable effects is based on post-marketing spontaneous reports, and therefore the frequency remains unknown:

System organ class	Adverse reaction
Investigations	Increase in liver transaminases and in alkaline phosphatase. Decreased prothrombin, increased INR and unbalanced anticoagulant treatment resulting in variations of haemostatic parameters have been reported in patients treated with anticoagulants in association with orlistat (see section 4.4 and 4.5)
Gastrointestinal disorders	Rectal bleeding Diverticulitis Pancreatitis
Skin and subcutaneous tissue disorders	Bullous eruptions
Immune system disorders	Hypersensitivity (e.g. pruritus, rash, urticaria, angioedema, bronchospasm and anaphylaxis)
Hepatobiliary disorders	Cholelithiasis Hepatitis that may be serious
Renal and urinary disorders	Oxalate nephropathy

4.9 Overdose

Single doses of 800 mg orlistat and multiple doses of up to 400 mg three times daily for 15 days have been studied in normal weight and obese subjects without significant adverse findings. In addition, doses of 240 mg tid have been administered to obese patients for 6 months. The majority of orlistat overdose cases received during post-marketing reported either no adverse events or adverse events that are similar to those reported with recommended dose.

Should a significant overdose of orlistat occur, it is recommended that the patient be observed for 24 hours. Based on human and animal studies, any systemic effects attributable to the lipase-inhibiting properties of orlistat should be rapidly reversible.

5. PHARMACOLOGICAL PROPERTIES

5.1 Pharmacodynamic properties

Pharmaco-therapeutic group: Peripherally acting antiobesity agent, ATC code A08AB01.

Orlistat is a potent, specific and long-acting inhibitor of gastrointestinal lipases. It exerts its therapeutic activity in the lumen of the stomach and small intestine by forming a covalent bond with the active serine site of the gastric and pancreatic lipases. The inactivated enzyme is thus unavailable to hydrolyse dietary fat, in the form of triglycerides, into absorbable free fatty acids and monoglycerides.

In the 2-year studies and the 4-year study, a hypocaloric diet was used in association with treatment in both the orlistat and the placebo treated groups.

Pooled data from five 2 year studies with orlistat and a hypocaloric diet showed that 37 % of orlistat patients and 19 % of placebo patients demonstrated a loss of at least 5 % of their baseline body weight after 12 weeks of treatment. Of these, 49 % of orlistat treated patients and 40 % of placebo treated patients went on to lose ≥ 10 % of their baseline body weight at one year. Conversely, of patients failing to demonstrate a loss of 5 % of their baseline body weight after 12 weeks of treatment, only 5 % of orlistat treated patients and 2 % of placebo treated patients went on to lose ≥ 10 % of their baseline body weight at one year. Overall, after one year of treatment, the percentage of patients taking 120 mg orlistat who lost 10 % or more of their body weight was 20 % with orlistat 120 mg compared to 8 % of patients taking placebo. The mean difference in weight loss with the drug compared to placebo was 3.2 kg.

Data from the 4-year XENDOS clinical trial showed that 60 % of orlistat patients and 35 % of placebo patients demonstrated a loss of at least 5 % of their baseline body weight after 12 weeks of treatment. Of these, 62 % of orlistat treated patients and 52 % of placebo treated patients went on to lose ≥ 10 % of their baseline body weight at one year. Conversely, of patients failing to demonstrate a loss of 5 % of their baseline body weight after 12 weeks of treatment, only 5 % of orlistat treated patients and 4 % of placebo treated patients went on to lose ≥ 10 % of their baseline body weight at one year. After 1 year of treatment, 41 % of the orlistat treated patients versus 21 % of placebo treated patients lost ≥ 10 % of body weight with a mean difference of 4.4 kg between the two groups. After 4 years of treatment 21 % of the orlistat treated patients compared to 10 % of the placebo treated patients had lost ≥ 10 % of body weight, with a mean difference of 2.7 kg.

More patients on orlistat or placebo lost baseline body weight of at least 5 % at 12 weeks or 10 % at one year in the XENDOS study than in the five 2-year studies. The reason for this difference is that the five 2-year studies included a 4-week diet and placebo lead-in period during which patients lost on average 2.6 kg prior to commencing treatment.

Data from the 4-year clinical trial also suggested that weight loss achieved with orlistat delayed the development of type 2 diabetes during the study (cumulative diabetes cases incidences: 3.4 % in the orlistat group compared to 5.4 % in the placebo-treated group). The great majority of diabetes cases came from the subgroup of patients with impaired glucose tolerance at baseline, which represented 21 % of the randomised patients. It is not known whether these findings translate into long-term clinical benefits.

In obese type 2 diabetic patients insufficiently controlled by antidiabetic agents, data from four one-year clinical trials showed that the percentage of responders (≥ 10 % of body weight loss) was 11.3 % with orlistat as compared to 4.5 % with placebo. In orlistat-treated patients, the mean difference from placebo in weight loss was 1.83 kg to 3.06 kg and the mean difference from placebo in HbA1c reduction was 0.18 % to 0.55 %. It has not been demonstrated that the effect on HbA1c is independent from weight reduction.

In a multi-centre (US, Canada), parallel-group, double-blind, placebo-controlled study, 539 obese adolescent patients were randomised to receive either 120 mg orlistat (n=357) or placebo (n=182) three times daily as an adjunct to a hypocaloric diet and exercise for 52 weeks. Both populations received multivitamin supplements. The primary endpoint was the change in body mass index (BMI) from baseline to the end of the study.

The results were significantly superior in the orlistat group (difference in BMI of 0.86 kg/m^2 in favour of orlistat). 9.5 % of the orlistat treated patients versus 3.3 % of the placebo treated patients lost ≥ 10 % of body weight after 1 year with a mean difference of 2.6 kg between the two groups. The difference was driven by the outcome in the group of patients with ≥ 5 % weight loss after 12 weeks of treatment with orlistat representing 19 % of the initial population. The side effects were generally similar to those observed in adults. However, there was an unexplained increase in the incidence of bone fractures (6 % versus 2.8 % in the orlistat and placebo groups, respectively).

5.2 Pharmacokinetic properties

Absorption

Studies in normal weight and obese volunteers have shown that the extent of absorption of orlistat was minimal. Plasma concentrations of intact orlistat were non-measurable (< 5 ng/ml) eight hours following oral administration of orlistat.

In general, at therapeutic doses, detection of intact orlistat in plasma was sporadic and concentrations were extremely low (< 10 ng/ml or 0.02 μmol), with no evidence of accumulation, which is consistent with minimal absorption.

Distribution

The volume of distribution cannot be determined because the drug is minimally absorbed and has no defined systemic pharmacokinetics. *In vitro* orlistat is > 99 % bound to plasma proteins (lipoproteins and albumin were the major binding proteins). Orlistat minimally partitions into erythrocytes.

Metabolism

Based on animal data, it is likely that the metabolism of orlistat occurs mainly within the gastrointestinal wall. Based on a study in obese patients, of the minimal fraction of the dose that was absorbed systemically, two major metabolites, M1 (4-member lactone ring hydrolysed) and M3 (M1 with N-formyl leucine moiety cleaved), accounted for approximately 42 % of the total plasma concentration.

M1 and M3 have an open beta-lactone ring and extremely weak lipase inhibitory activity (1000 and 2500 fold less than orlistat respectively). In view of this low inhibitory activity and the low plasma levels at therapeutic doses (average of 26 ng/ml and 108 ng/ml respectively), these metabolites are considered to be pharmacologically inconsequential.

Elimination

Studies in normal weight and obese subjects have shown that faecal excretion of the unabsorbed drug was the major route of elimination. Approximately 97 % of the administered dose was excreted in faeces and 83 % of that as unchanged orlistat.

The cumulative renal excretion of total orlistat-related materials was < 2 % of the given dose. The time to reach complete excretion (faecal plus urinary) was 3 to 5 days. The disposition of orlistat appeared to be similar between normal weight and obese volunteers. Orlistat, M1 and M3 are all subject to biliary excretion.

5.3 Preclinical safety data

Non-clinical data reveal no special hazard for humans based on conventional studies of safety pharmacology, repeated dose toxicity, genotoxicity, carcinogenic potential, and toxicity to reproduction.

In animal reproductive studies, no teratogenic effect was observed. In the absence of a teratogenic effect in animals, no malformative effect is expected in man. To date, active substances responsible for malformations in man have been found teratogenic in animals when well-conducted studies were performed in two species.

6. PHARMACEUTICAL PARTICULARS

6.1 List of excipients

Capsule filling:

microcrystalline cellulose (E460)

sodium starch glycollate

povidone (E1201)

sodium lauryl sulphate

talc

Capsule shell:

gelatine

indigo carmine (E132)

titanium dioxide (E171)

edible printing ink (black iron oxide, ammonium hydroxide, potassium hydroxide, shellac)

6.2 Incompatibilities

Not applicable.

6.3 Shelf life

3 years.

6.4 Special precautions for storage

Blisters: Do not store above 25 °C. Store in original package in order to protect from moisture.

Bottles: Do not store above 30 °C. Keep the container tightly closed in order to protect from moisture.

6.5 Nature and contents of container

PVC/PE/PVDC blisters containing 21, 42 and 84 hard capsules.

Glass bottles with desiccant containing 21, 42 and 84 hard capsules.

Not all pack sizes may be marketed.

6.6 Special precautions for disposal and other handling

No special requirements.

7. MARKETING AUTHORISATION HOLDER

Roche Registration Limited
6 Falcon Way
Shire Park
Welwyn Garden City
AL7 1TW
United Kingdom

8. MARKETING AUTHORISATION NUMBER(S)

EU/1/98/071/001-006

9. DATE OF FIRST AUTHORISATION/RENEWAL OF THE AUTHORISATION

Date of first authorisation: 29 July 1998

Date of latest renewal: 29 July 2008

10. DATE OF REVISION OF THE TEXT

25 March 2009

LEGAL STATUS

POM

Xeomin

(Merz Pharma UK Ltd)

1. NAME OF THE MEDICINAL PRODUCT

Xeomin 100 LD_{50} units powder for solution for injection ▼

2. QUALITATIVE AND QUANTITATIVE COMPOSITION

1 vial contains 100 LD_{50} units* of Clostridium Botulinum neurotoxin type A (150 kD), free of complexing proteins.

* One unit corresponds to the median lethal dose (LD_{50}) when the reconstituted product is injected intraperitoneally into mice under defined conditions.

Due to differences in the LD_{50} assay, these units are specific to Xeomin and are not interchangeable with other Botulinum toxin preparations.

Excipient(s):

For a full list of excipients, see section 6.1.

3. PHARMACEUTICAL FORM

Powder for solution for injection

White powder

4. CLINICAL PARTICULARS

4.1 Therapeutic indications

Xeomin is indicated for the symptomatic management of blepharospasm and cervical dystonia of a predominantly rotational form (spasmodic torticollis) in adults.

4.2 Posology and method of administration

Unit doses recommended for Xeomin are not interchangeable with those for other preparations of Botulinum toxin.

Xeomin may only be used by physicians with suitable qualifications and proven experience in the application of Botulinum toxin and in the use of the necessary equipment, e.g. EMG (electromyography).

Reconstituted Xeomin is intended for intramuscular injection.

The optimum dosage and number of injection sites in the treated muscle should be determined by the physician individually for each patient. A titration of the dose should be performed.

For instructions on reconstitution / dilution of the vials, see section 6.6. After reconstitution, Xeomin should be used for only one injection session and for only one patient.

A decrease or increase in the Xeomin dose is possible by administering a smaller or larger injection volume. The smaller the injection volume the less pressure sensation and the less spread of Botulinum neurotoxin type A in the injected muscle occurs. This is of benefit in reducing effects on nearby muscles when small muscle groups are being injected.

Blepharospasm

After reconstitution, the Xeomin solution is injected using a suitable sterile needle (e.g. 27-30 gauge/0.30-0.40 mm). Electromyographic guidance is not necessary. An injection volume of approximately 0.05 to 0.1 ml is recommended.

Xeomin is injected into the medial and lateral orbicularis oculi of the upper lid and the lateral orbicularis oculi of the lower lid. Additional sites in the brow area, the lateral orbicularis and in the upper facial area may also be injected if spasms here interfere with vision.

The initial recommended dose is 1.25-2.5 U (0.05-0.1 ml volume) at each site. The initial dose should not exceed 25 U per eye. In the management of blepharospasm, total dosing should not exceed 100 U every 12 weeks.

Injections near the levator palpebrae superioris should be avoided to reduce the occurrence of ptosis. Diplopia may develop as a result of Botulinum neurotoxin type A diffusion into the inferior oblique. Avoiding medial injections into the lower lid may reduce this adverse reaction.

The median first onset of effect is observed within four days after injection. The effect of each treatment generally lasts approximately 3-4 months, however, it may last significantly longer or shorter. The treatment can be repeated if required.

At repeat treatment sessions, the dose may be increased up to two-fold if the response to the initial treatment is considered insufficient – usually defined as an effect that does not last longer than two months. However, there appears to be no additional benefit obtainable from injecting more than 5.0 U per site. Normally, no additional benefit is conferred by treating more frequently than every three months.

Spasmodic torticollis

In the management of spasmodic torticollis, Xeomin dosing must be tailored to the individual patient, based on the patient's head and neck position, location of possible pain, muscle hypertrophy, patient's body weight, and response to the injection. A suitable sterile needle (e.g. 25-30 gauge/ 0.30-0.50 mm) is used for injections into superficial muscles, and an e.g. 22 gauge/0.70 mm needle may be used for injections into deeper musculature. An injection volume of approximately 0.1 to 0.5 ml is recommended.

In the management of spasmodic torticollis, Xeomin is usually injected into the sternocleidomastoid, levator scapulae, scalenus, splenius capitis, and/or the trapezius muscle(s). This list is not exhaustive as any of the muscles responsible for controlling head position may be involved and therefore require treatment. If difficulties arise isolating single muscles, injections should be performed using electromyographic guidance. The muscle mass and the degree of hypertrophy or atrophy are factors to be taken into consideration when selecting the appropriate dose.

In practice, the maximum total dose is usually not more than 200 U. Doses of up to 300 U may be given. No more than 50 U should be given at any one injection site.

Multiple injection sites permit Xeomin more uniform coverage of the innervated areas of the dystonic muscle and are especially useful in larger muscles. The optimum number of injection sites is dependent upon the size of the muscle to be chemically denervated.

The sternocleidomastoid should not be injected bilaterally as there is an increased risk of adverse reactions (in particular dysphagia) when bilateral injections or doses in excess of 100 U are administered into this muscle.

The median first onset of effect is observed within seven days after injection. The effect of each treatment generally lasts approximately 3-4 months, however, it may last significantly longer or shorter. The period between each treatment session should be at least 10 weeks.

All indications

If no treatment effect occurs within a month after the initial injection, the following measures should be taken:

- clinical verification of the neurotoxin effect on the injected muscle: e.g. an electromyographic investigation in a specialised facility
- analysis of the reason for non-response, e.g. poor isolation of the muscles intended to be injected, too low dose, poor injection technique, fixed contracture, too weak antagonist, possible development of antibodies
- review of Botulinum neurotoxin type A treatment as an adequate therapy
- if no adverse reactions have occurred during the initial treatment, an additional course of treatment can be performed under the following conditions: 1) dose adjustment with regard to analysis of the most recent failure to respond, 2) EMG-guidance, 3) the recommended minimum interval between the initial and repeat treatment is not exceeded

The patient should be regarded as a primary non-responder in cases of first injection failure. It has not been investigated whether secondary non-response due to the development of antibodies is less frequent under Xeomin therapy than under treatment with conventional preparations containing the Botulinum toxin type A complex. In cases of non-response, alternative therapies should be considered.

Xeomin has not been studied in the paediatric population and is therefore not recommended in the paediatric age group until further data become available.

4.3 Contraindications

Hypersensitivity to the active substance Botulinum neurotoxin type A or to any of the excipients.

Generalised disorders of muscle activity (e.g. myasthenia gravis, Lambert-Eaton syndrome).

Presence of infection at the proposed injection site.

4.4 Special warnings and precautions for use

Side effects related to spread of Botulinum toxin distant from the site of administration have been reported (see section 4.8), sometimes resulting in death, which in some cases was associated with dysphagia, pneumonia and/or significant debility.

Patients treated with therapeutic doses may experience exaggerated muscle weakness. Patients with underlying neurological disorders including swallowing difficulties are at increased risk of these side effects. The Botulinum toxin product should be used under specialist supervision in these patients and should only be used if the benefit of treatment is considered to outweigh the risk. Patients with a history of dysphagia and aspiration should be treated with extreme caution.

Patients or caregivers should be advised to seek immediate medical care if swallowing, speech or respiratory disorders arise.

An anaphylactic reaction may occur rarely after injection of Botulinum neurotoxin type A (see section 4.8). Adrenaline and other medical aids for treating anaphylaxis should be available.

Prior to administering Xeomin the physician must make himself familiar with the patient's anatomy and any alterations to the anatomy due to prior surgical procedures. Extra caution is required when injecting at sites close to sensitive structures such as the carotid artery and lung apices.

There is limited experience in treatment-naïve patients and long-term treatment.

Xeomin should be used with caution:

- if bleeding disorders of any type occur
- in patients receiving anticoagulant therapy
- in patients suffering from amyotrophic lateral sclerosis or other diseases which result in peripheral neuromuscular dysfunction
- in targeted muscles which display pronounced weakness or atrophy.

The recommended single doses of Xeomin should not be exceeded and the intervals between injections should not be shortened.

The clinical effects of Botulinum neurotoxin type A can increase or decrease by repeated injections. The possible reasons are different techniques of reconstitution, the chosen injection intervals, the injected muscles and marginally varying toxin activity resulting from the biological testing procedure employed or secondary non-response.

Too frequent dosing of Botulinum toxin may result in antibody formation which may lead to resistance to treatment (see section 4.2).

Previously akinetic or sedentary patients should be reminded to gradually resume activities following the injection of Xeomin.

Xeomin contains albumin, a derivative of human blood. Standard measures to prevent infections resulting from the use of medicinal products prepared from human blood or plasma include careful selection of donors, screening of individual donations and plasma pools for specific markers of infection and the inclusion of effective manufacturing steps for the inactivation/removal of viruses. Despite this, when medicinal products prepared from human blood or plasma are administered, the possibility of transmitting infective agents cannot be totally excluded. This also applies to unknown or emerging viruses and other pathogens. There are no reports of viral transmissions with albumin manufactured to European Pharmacopoeia specifications by established processes.

Blepharospasm

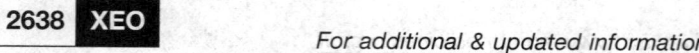

Because of the anticholinergic effect of Botulinum neurotoxin type A, Xeomin should be used with caution in patients at risk of developing an angle closure glaucoma.

In order to prevent ectropion, injections into the lower lid area should be avoided, and vigorous treatment of any epithelial defect is necessary. This may require protective drops, ointments, soft bandage contact lenses, or closure of the eye by patching or similar means.

Reduced blinking following Xeomin injection into the orbicularis muscle can lead to corneal exposure, persistent epithelial defects and corneal ulceration, especially in patients with cranial nerve disorders (facial nerve). Careful testing of corneal sensation should be performed in patients with previous eye operations.

Ecchymosis easily occurs in the soft tissues of the eyelid. Immediate gentle pressure at the injection site can limit that risk.

Spasmodic torticollis

Patients should be informed that injections of Xeomin for the management of spasmodic torticollis may cause mild to severe dysphagia with the risk of aspiration and dyspnoea. Medical intervention may be necessary (e.g. in the form of a gastric feeding tube) (see also section 4.8). Dysphagia can last for up to two to three weeks after injection, but a duration of up to five months has been reported in one case. Limiting the dose injected into the sternocleidomastoid muscle to less than 100 U may decrease the occurrence of dysphagia. Patients with smaller neck muscle mass, or patients who require bilateral injections into the sternocleidomastoid muscles are at greater risk. The occurrence of dysphagia is attributable to the spread of the pharmacological effect of Xeomin as the result of the neurotoxin spread into the oesophageal musculature.

4.5 Interaction with other medicinal products and other forms of interaction

Theoretically, the effect of Botulinum neurotoxin may be potentiated by aminoglycoside antibiotics or other medicinal products that interfere with neuromuscular transmission e.g. tubocurarine-type muscle relaxants.

Therefore the concomitant use of Xeomin with aminoglycosides or spectinomycin requires special care. Peripheral muscle relaxants should be used with caution, if necessary reducing the starting dose of relaxant, or using an intermediate-acting substance such as vecuronium or atracurium rather than substances with longer lasting effects.

4-Aminochinolines may reduce the effect of Xeomin.

4.6 Pregnancy and lactation

There are no adequate data from the use of Botulinum neurotoxin type A in pregnant women. Studies in animals have shown reproductive toxicity (see section 5.3). The potential risk for humans is unknown.

Therefore, Xeomin should not be used during pregnancy unless clearly necessary and unless the potential benefit justifies the risk.

It is not known whether Botulinum neurotoxin type A is excreted into the breast milk. Therefore, the use of Xeomin during lactation cannot be recommended.

4.7 Effects on ability to drive and use machines

Xeomin has minor or moderate influence on the ability to drive and use machines.

Due to the nature of the diseases being treated, the ability to drive and to operate machines can be reduced. Due to the latency of onset, some of the therapeutic and/or adverse effects of Xeomin may also interfere with the ability to drive and operate machinery. Consequently affected persons should avoid these tasks until their faculties are fully recovered.

4.8 Undesirable effects

Undesirable effects may occur from misplaced injections of Botulinum neurotoxin type A temporarily paralysing nearby muscle groups. Large doses may cause paralysis in muscles distant to the injection site. Usually, undesirable effects are observed within the first week after treatment and are temporary in nature. They may be restricted to the area around the injection site (e.g. local pain, tenderness at the injection site, and injection site haemorrhage).

Frequency by different indications

Based on clinical experience information on the frequency of adverse reactions for the individual indications is given below. The frequency categories are defined as follows: very common (≥1/10); common (≥1/100, <1/10); uncommon (≥1/1,000, <1/100), rare (≥1/10,000, <1/1,000); very rare (<1/10,000).

Blepharospasm

The following adverse reactions were reported with Xeomin:

Nervous system disorders

Uncommon: paraesthesia, headache

Eye disorders

Common: ptosis, dry eyes

Uncommon: conjunctivitis

Gastrointestinal disorders

Uncommon: dry mouth

Skin and subcutaneous tissue disorders

Uncommon: skin rash

Musculoskeletal and connective tissue disorders

Uncommon: muscle weakness

Injury, poisoning and procedural complications

Uncommon: inflicted injury

Additionally, the following undesirable effects and accordingly their frequencies are known for the comparative compound containing conventional Botulinum toxin type A complex used in clinical trials with Xeomin. It is possible that these undesirable effects may also occur with Xeomin.

Nervous system disorders

Uncommon: dizziness, facial paralysis

Eye disorders

Common: superficial punctate keratitis, lagophthalmos, eye irritation, photophobia, lacrimation

Uncommon: keratitis, ectropion, diplopia, entropion, visual disturbance, blurred vision

Rare: swelling of eyelid

Very rare: angle closure glaucoma, corneal ulceration

Skin and subcutaneous tissue disorders

Uncommon: dermatitis

Musculoskeletal and connective tissue disorders

Uncommon: facial muscle weakness

General disorders and administration site conditions

Uncommon: tiredness

Spasmodic torticollis

The following adverse reactions were reported with Xeomin:

Nervous system disorders

Uncommon: headache, tremor

Eye disorders

Uncommon: eye pain

Respiratory, thoracic and mediastinal disorders

Uncommon: dysphonia

Gastrointestinal disorders

Common: dysphagia

Uncommon: diarrhoea, dry mouth, vomiting, colitis

Skin and subcutaneous tissue disorders

Uncommon: skin rash, erythema, pruritus, sweating increased

Musculoskeletal and connective tissue disorders

Common: muscle weakness, back pain

Uncommon: skeletal pain, myalgia

General disorders and administration site conditions

Uncommon: asthenia, injection site inflammation, injection site tenderness

Additionally, the following undesirable effects and accordingly their frequencies are known for the comparative compound containing conventional Botulinum toxin type A complex used in clinical trials with Xeomin. It is possible that these undesirable effects may also occur with Xeomin.

Nervous system disorders

Common: dizziness, numbness, drowsiness

Eye disorders

Uncommon: diplopia, ptosis

Respiratory, thoracic and mediastinal disorders

Common: rhinitis, upper respiratory tract infection

Uncommon: dyspnoea, voice alteration

Gastrointestinal disorders

Common: nausea, oral dryness

Skin and subcutaneous tissue disorders

Common: skin sores

Musculoskeletal and connective tissue disorders

Common: stiffness, hypertonia

General disorders and administration site conditions

Very common: pain, local weakness

Common: generalised weakness, flu like symptoms, malaise

Uncommon: fever

The management of spasmodic torticollis may cause dysphagia with varying degrees of severity with the potential for aspiration which may require medical intervention. Dysphagia may persist for two to three weeks after injection, but has been reported in one case to last five months. Dysphagia appears to be dose-dependent. In clinical trials with Botulinum toxin type A complex it was reported that dysphagia occurs less frequently with total doses below 200 U per treatment session.

General

The following additional information is based on publications on conventional preparations containing the Botulinum toxin type A complex.

Side effects related to spread of toxin distant from the site of administration have been reported very rarely (exaggerated muscle weakness, dysphagia, aspiration pneumonitis with fatal outcome in some cases) (see section 4.4).

Dysphagia has been reported following injection to sites other than the cervical musculature.

There have been rare reports of undesirable effects related to cardiovascular system, such as arrhythmia and myocardial infarction, some with fatal outcomes. It remains unclear whether these deaths were induced by conventional preparations containing the Botulinum toxin type A complex or caused by pre-existing cardiovascular disease.

A case of peripheral neuropathy has been reported in a male after receiving four sets of injections of a conventional preparation containing the Botulinum toxin type A complex (for neck and back spasm, and severe pain) over an 11 week period.

A female patient developed brachial plexopathy two days after injection of a conventional preparation containing the Botulinum toxin type A complex for the treatment of cervical dystonia, with recovery after five months.

Erythema multiforme, urticaria, psoriasis-like rash, pruritus, and allergic reactions have been described with the use of conventional preparations containing the Botulinum toxin type A complex, but their causal relationship remains unclear.

Following injection of conventional Botulinum toxin type A complex, EMG showed increased jitter in some distant muscles which was not associated with muscle weakness or other types of electrophysiological abnormalities.

4.9 Overdose

Symptoms of overdose:

Increased doses of Botulinum neurotoxin type A may result in pronounced neuromuscular paralysis distant from the injection site. Symptoms of overdose are not immediately apparent post-injection and may include general weakness, ptosis, diplopia, swallowing and speech difficulties or paralysis of the respiratory muscles resulting in an aspiration pneumonia.

Measures in cases of overdose:

In case of an overdose the patient must be monitored medically for several days. If signs of intoxication appear, hospitalisation with general supportive measures is necessary. Intubation and assisted ventilation will become necessary until improvement if paralysis of the respiratory muscles occurs.

5. PHARMACOLOGICAL PROPERTIES

5.1 Pharmacodynamic properties

Pharmacotherapeutic group: Muscle relaxant, peripherally acting agent, ATC code: M03AX01

Botulinum neurotoxin type A blocks cholinergic transmission at the neuromuscular junction by inhibiting the release of acetylcholine. The nerve terminals of the neuromuscular junction no longer respond to nerve impulses, and secretion of the neurotransmitter is prevented (chemical denervation). Recovery of impulse transmission is re-established by the formation of new nerve terminals and motor endplates.

The mechanism of action by which Botulinum neurotoxin type A exerts its effects on cholinergic nerve terminals can be described by a three-step sequential process which includes the following steps:

a) binding to the cholinergic nerve terminals

b) entry or internalisation into the nerve terminal and

c) inhibition of acetylcholine release by intracellular poisoning within the nerve terminal.

The heavy chain of the Botulinum neurotoxin type A binds with an exceptionally high selectivity and affinity to receptors only found on cholinergic terminals. After internalisation of the neurotoxin the light chain cleaves very specifically a target protein (SNAP 25) that is essential for the release of acetylcholine.

Recovery after injection normally takes place within 3-4 months as nerve terminals sprout and reconnect with the endplate.

5.2 Pharmacokinetic properties

a) General characteristics of the active substance:

Classic kinetic and distribution studies cannot be conducted with Botulinum neurotoxin type A because the active substance is applied in such small quantities (picograms per injection), and because it binds so rapidly and irreversibly to cholinergic nerve terminals.

Native Botulinum toxin is a high molecular weight complex, which, in addition to the neurotoxin (150 kD) contains other non-toxic proteins, like haemagglutinins and non-haemagglutinins. In contrast to conventional preparations containing the Botulinum toxin type A complex, Xeomin contains pure (150 kD) neurotoxin since it is free of complexing proteins.

Like many other proteins of its size, Botulinum neurotoxin type A has been shown to undergo retrograde axonal transport after intramuscular injection. Retrograde transsynaptic passage of active Botulinum neurotoxin type A into the central nervous system however has not been found.

Receptor-bound Botulinum neurotoxin type A is endocytosed into the nerve terminal prior to reaching its target (SNAP 25) and will eventually be degraded intracellularly. Free circulating Botulinum neurotoxin type A molecules which have not bound to presynaptic cholinergic nerve terminal receptors will be phagocytosed or pinocytosed and degraded like any other free circulating protein.

b) Distribution of the active substance in patients:

Human pharmacokinetic studies with Xeomin have not been performed for the reasons detailed above.

5.3 Preclinical safety data

Non-clinical data reveal no special hazard for humans based on conventional studies of cardiovascular safety pharmacology.

The findings made in repeat-dose toxicity studies conducted with Xeomin were mainly related to its pharmacodynamic action.

No evidence of local intolerability was noted. Reproductive toxicity studies with Xeomin, performed in rabbits, did not show adverse effects on male or female fertility nor direct effects on embryo-foetal development. However, the administration of Xeomin at dose levels exhibiting clear maternal toxicity at weekly to biweekly intervals increased the number of abortions in a prenatal toxicity study in rabbits. A continuous systemic exposure of the dams during the (unknown) sensitive phase of the organogenesis as a pre-requisite for the induction of teratogenic effects cannot necessarily be assumed.

No genotoxicity, carcinogenicity and pre- and postnatal development studies have been conducted with Xeomin.

6. PHARMACEUTICAL PARTICULARS

6.1 List of excipients

Human albumin

Sucrose

6.2 Incompatibilities

This medicinal product must not be mixed with other medicinal products except those mentioned in section 6.6.

6.3 Shelf life

Unopened vial: 4 years

Reconstituted solution: Chemical and physical in-use stability has been demonstrated for 24 hours at 2 to 8°C. From a microbiological point of view, the product should be used immediately.

6.4 Special precautions for storage

Unopened vial: Do not store above 25°C

For storage conditions of the reconstituted medicinal product, see section 6.3.

6.5 Nature and contents of container

Vial (type 1 glass) with rubber stopper (bromobutyl rubber) and tamper-proof seal (aluminium) in pack sizes of 1 (single unit pack), 2, 3 or 6 vials (multi-packs). A clinical pack is also available with 6 vials.

Not all pack sizes may be marketed.

6.6 Special precautions for disposal and other handling

Xeomin is reconstituted prior to use with sterile unpreserved sodium chloride 9 mg/ml (0.9%) solution for injection. Reconstitution and dilution should be performed with good practice, particularly with respect to asepsis.

It is good practice to perform vial reconstitution and syringe preparation over plastic-lined paper towels to catch any spillage. An appropriate amount of solvent (see dilution table) is drawn up into a syringe. The exposed portion of the rubber stopper of the vial is cleaned with alcohol (70%) prior to insertion of the needle. The solvent must be injected gently into the vial. The vial must be discarded, if the vacuum does not pull the solvent into the vial. Reconstituted Xeomin is a clear colourless solution free of particulate matter.

Xeomin should not be used if the reconstituted solution (prepared as above) has a cloudy appearance or contains floccular or particulate matter.

The recommended dilutions are indicated in the following table:

Solvent added (sodium chloride 9 mg/ml (0.9%) solution for injection)	Resulting dose in units per 0.1 ml	
0.5 ml	20.0	U
1.0 ml	10.0	U
2.0 ml	5.0	U
4.0 ml	2.5	U
8.0 ml	1.25	U

Any solution for injection that has been stored for more than 24 hours as well as any unused solution for injection should be discarded.

For safe disposal, unused vials should be reconstituted with a small amount of water and then autoclaved. Any used vials, syringes, and spillage etc. should be autoclaved and any residual Xeomin inactivated using diluted sodium hydroxide solution (0.1 N NaOH).

7. MARKETING AUTHORISATION HOLDER

Merz Pharmaceuticals GmbH

Eckenheimer Landstraβe 100

60318 Frankfurt/Main

Germany

P.O. Box 11 13 53

60048 Frankfurt/Main

Germany

Phone: +49-69/15 03-1

Fax: +49-69/15 03-200

8. MARKETING AUTHORISATION NUMBER(S)

PL 29978/0001

9. DATE OF FIRST AUTHORISATION/RENEWAL OF THE AUTHORISATION

20/12/2007

10. DATE OF REVISION OF THE TEXT

04/09/2008

Xigris 20mg powder for solution for infusion, 5mg powder for solution for infusion

(Eli Lilly and Company Limited)

1. NAME OF THE MEDICINAL PRODUCT

XIGRIS* 5mg powder for solution for infusion.

XIGRIS 20mg powder for solution for infusion.

2. QUALITATIVE AND QUANTITATIVE COMPOSITION

XIGRIS 5mg: Each vial contains 5mg of drotrecogin alfa (activated).

After reconstitution with 2.5ml of Water for Injection each ml contains 2mg of Drotrecogin alfa (activated).

Excipient: Each vial contains approximately 17mg sodium.

XIGRIS 20mg: Each vial contains 20mg of drotrecogin alfa (activated).

After reconstitution with 10ml of Water for Injection, each ml contains 2mg of Drotrecogin alfa (activated).

Excipient: Each vial contains approximately 68mg sodium.

Drotrecogin alfa (activated) is a recombinant version of the endogenous activated Protein C and is produced by genetic engineering from an established human cell line.

For a full list of excipients, see section 6.1.

3. PHARMACEUTICAL FORM

Powder for solution for infusion. XIGRIS is supplied as a lyophilised, white to off-white powder.

4. CLINICAL PARTICULARS

4.1 Therapeutic indications

XIGRIS is indicated for the treatment of adult patients with severe sepsis with multiple organ failure when added to best standard care. The use of XIGRIS should be considered mainly in situations when therapy can be started within 24 hours after the onset of organ failure (for further information see section 5.1).

4.2 Posology and method of administration

XIGRIS should be used by experienced doctors in institutions skilled in the care of patients with severe sepsis.

Treatment should be started within 48 hours, and preferably within 24 hours, of onset of the first documented sepsis-induced organ dysfunction (see section 5.1).

The recommended dose of XIGRIS is 24µg/kg/hr (based on actual body weight) given as a continuous intravenous infusion for a total duration of 96 hours. It is recommended that XIGRIS be infused with an infusion pump to accurately control the infusion rate. If the infusion is interrupted for any reason, XIGRIS should be restarted at the 24µg/kg/hr infusion rate and continued to complete the full recommended 96 hours of dosing administration. Dose escalation or bolus doses of XIGRIS are not necessary to account for the interruption in the infusion.

No dose adjustments are required in adult patients with severe sepsis with regard to age, gender, hepatic function (as measured by transaminase levels), renal function, obesity or co-administration of prophylactic heparin. The pharmacokinetics of drotrecogin alfa (activated) have not been studied in patients with severe sepsis and pre-existing end-stage renal disease and chronic hepatic disease.

Paediatrics: Data from a placebo-controlled clinical trial, which was stopped for futility after 477 patients 0 to 17 years old had received the study treatment, did not establish efficacy of XIGRIS in paediatric patients and showed a higher rate of central nervous system bleeding in the XIGRIS versus placebo group. Therefore, no dosage recommendation can be made and the use of XIGRIS is not recommended in children below the age of 18 (see section 4.4).

4.3 Contraindications

Hypersensitivity to the active substance, to any of the excipients, or to bovine thrombin (a trace residue from the manufacturing process).

Because drotrecogin alfa (activated) may increase the risk of bleeding, XIGRIS is contra-indicated in the following situations:

- Active internal bleeding.
- Patients with intracranial pathology; neoplasm or evidence of cerebral herniation.
- Concurrent heparin therapy ⩾15 international units/kg/hr.
- Known bleeding diathesis except for acute coagulopathy related to sepsis.
- Chronic severe hepatic disease.
- Platelet count $<30,000 \times 10^6$/l, even if the platelet count is increased after transfusions.
- Patients at increased risk for bleeding (for example):

a) Any major surgery, defined as surgery that requires general or spinal anaesthesia, performed within the 12-hour period immediately preceding drug infusion, or any postoperative patient who demonstrates evidence of active bleeding, or any patient with planned or anticipated surgery during the drug infusion period.

b) History of severe head trauma that required hospitalisation, intracranial or intraspinal surgery, or haemorrhagic stroke within the previous 3 months, or any history of intracerebral arteriovenous malformation, cerebral aneurysm, or central nervous system mass lesion; patients with an epidural catheter or who are anticipated to receive an epidural catheter during drug infusion.

c) History of congenital bleeding diatheses.

d) Gastro-intestinal bleeding within the last 6 weeks that has required medical intervention unless definitive surgery has been performed.

e) Trauma patients at increased risk of bleeding.

4.4 Special warnings and precautions for use

Patients With Single Organ Dysfunction and Recent Surgery

XIGRIS is not approved for the treatment of patients with single organ dysfunction and should not be used in this particular subgroup of patients, especially if they had recent surgery (within 30 days). In each of two randomised, placebo-controlled trials, PROWESS and ADDRESS (see section 5.1), 28-day and in-hospital mortality were higher in patients treated with drotrecogin alfa (activated) compared to placebo for the sub-population of patients with single organ dysfunction and recent surgery (n = 98 in PROWESS and n = 636 in ADDRESS).

Bleeding

Drotrecogin alfa (activated) increases the risk of bleeding. In the following conditions, the risks of the administration of XIGRIS should be weighed against the anticipated benefits:

- Recent administration (within 3 days) of thrombolytic therapy.
- Recent administration (within 7 days) of oral anticoagulants.
- Recent administration (within 7 days) of aspirin or other platelet inhibitors.
- Recent (within 3 months) ischaemic stroke.
- Any other condition in which the physician considers significant bleeding is likely.

For procedures with an inherent bleeding risk, discontinue XIGRIS for 2 hours prior to the start of the procedure. XIGRIS may be restarted 12 hours after major invasive procedures or surgery if adequate haemostasis has been achieved. The incidence of serious bleeding events with XIGRIS was higher in patients with recent (within 30 days) surgery than in "medical" patients without surgery (see section 4.8). Bleeding risk should be taken into account when considering the risk benefit for individual patients. XIGRIS may be restarted immediately after uncomplicated less invasive procedures if adequate haemostasis has been achieved.

As a component of routine care, measures of haemostasis (e.g., activated partial thromboplastin time [APTT], prothrombin time [PT], and platelet count) should be obtained during the infusion of XIGRIS. If sequential tests of haemostasis indicate an uncontrolled or worsening coagulopathy that significantly increases the risk of bleeding, the benefits of continuing the infusion must be weighed against the potential increased risk of bleeding for that patient.

Laboratory Tests

Drotrecogin alfa (activated) has minimal effect on the PT. Prolongation of the APTT in patients with severe sepsis receiving XIGRIS may be due to the underlying coagulopathy, the pharmacodynamic effect of drotrecogin alfa (activated), and/or the effect of other concurrent medicinal products. The pharmacodynamic effect of drotrecogin alfa (activated) on the APTT assay is dependent on the reagent and instrument used to perform the assay and the time that elapses between sample acquisition and assay performance. Drotrecogin alfa (activated) that is present in a blood or plasma sample drawn from a patient who is being infused with the drug will be gradually neutralised by endogenous plasma protease inhibitors present in the sample. Virtually no measurable activity of drotrecogin alfa (activated) is present 2 hours after obtaining the blood sample. Due to these biological and analytical variables, the APTT should not be used to assess the pharmacodynamic effect of drotrecogin alfa (activated). In addition, approximately 2 hours after terminating the infusion of the drug, there is virtually no measurable activity of drotrecogin alfa (activated) remaining in the circulation of the patient; blood samples drawn for APTT determination after this point are no longer affected by the drug. The interpretation of sequential determinations of the PT and/or APTT should take these variables into consideration.

Because drotrecogin alfa (activated) may affect the APTT assays, drotrecogin alfa (activated) present in plasma samples may interfere with one-stage coagulation assays based on the APTT (such as Factor VIII, IX, and XI assays). Drotrecogin alfa (activated) present in plasma samples does not interfere with one-stage factor assays based on the PT (such as Factor II, V, VII and X assays).

If sequential measures of coagulopathy (including platelet count) indicate severe or worsening coagulopathy, the risk of continuing the infusion should be weighed against the expected benefit.

Immunogenicity

In adult patients in severe sepsis clinical studies, the frequency of anti-human Activated Protein C IgA/IgG/IgM antibodies or neutralising antibodies is low and is similar between drotrecogin alfa (activated) and placebo-treated patients tested. In patients developing antibodies adverse events were not more frequent in drotrecogin alfa (activated) than in placebo patients. There was no evidence that the antibodies detected represented a specific immune response to drotrecogin alfa (activated) therapy.

There have been no clinical trials in severe sepsis specifically studying drotrecogin alfa (activated) re-administration. However, a small number of patients in severe sepsis controlled clinical trials received a prior course of drotrecogin alfa (activated). No hypersensitivity reactions were reported in these patients. Samples available were subsequently tested and all were negative for anti-human Activated Protein C antibody.

No anti-activated Protein C antibody formation was detected in healthy subjects, even after repeat administration.

However, the possibility of allergic reactions to constituents of the preparation cannot be completely excluded in certain predisposed patients. If allergic or anaphylactic reactions occur, treatment should be discontinued immediately and appropriate therapy initiated. If XIGRIS is readministered to patients, caution should be employed.

Paediatric Patients

XIGRIS is not recommended in children below the age of 18 and therefore it should not be used in children.

Data from a placebo-controlled clinical trial did not establish efficacy of XIGRIS in paediatric patients suffering from severe sepsis, acute infection, systemic inflammation and respiratory and cardiovascular organ dysfunction. This trial was stopped for futility after 477 patients had received the study drug (out of 600 patients intended).

A planned interim analysis (with 400 patients enrolled) showed a low likelihood of demonstrating a significant difference in the primary endpoint of "Composite Time to Complete Organ Failure Resolution" (CTCOFR score of 9.8 versus 9.7 mean days over 14 days). There was also no difference in 28-day mortality (17.1% versus 17.3% in the XIGRIS and placebo groups, respectively).

Investigators attributed 2 deaths in the XIGRIS group and 5 deaths in the placebo group to bleeding events. There was a higher rate of central nervous system (CNS) bleeding in the drotrecogin alfa (activated) versus the placebo group. Over the infusion period (study days 0-6) the number of patients experiencing CNS bleeding was 5 versus 1 (2.1% versus 0.4%) for the overall population (drotrecogin alfa [activated] versus placebo), with 4 of the 5 events in the drotrecogin alfa (activated) group occurring in patients ≤60 days old or ≤3.5 kg bodyweight. Fatal CNS bleeding events, serious bleeding events (over the infusion period and over the 28-day study period), serious adverse events, and major amputations were similar in the drotrecogin alfa (activated) and placebo groups.

XIGRIS 5mg: This medicinal product contains approximately 17mg sodium per vial. To be taken into consideration by patients on a controlled sodium diet.

XIGRIS 20mg: This medicinal product contains approximately 68mg sodium per vial. To be taken into consideration by patients on a controlled sodium diet.

4.5 Interaction with other medicinal products and other forms of interaction

Caution should be employed when XIGRIS is used with other drugs that affect haemostasis (see sections 4.3 and 4.4), including Protein C, thrombolytics (e.g., streptokinase, tPA, rPA and urokinase), oral anticoagulants (e.g., warfarin), hirudins, antithrombin, aspirin and other antiplatelets agents, e.g., non-steroidal anti-inflammatory drugs, ticlopidine and clopidogrel, glycoprotein IIb/IIIa antagonists (such as abciximab, eptifibatide, tirofiban) and prostacyclins, such as iloprost.

Co-administration of Low-dose Heparin for Prophylaxis of Venous Thrombotic Events (VTE)

Low-dose heparin for VTE prophylaxis may be co-administered with drotrecogin alfa (activated). In a randomised study of heparin versus placebo (XPRESS) in 1,935 adult severe sepsis patients, all treated with drotrecogin alfa (activated), prophylactic heparin did not adversely affect mortality (heparin 28.3% versus placebo 31.9% in the overall ITT population, and heparin 30.3% versus placebo 26.9% in patients with multiple organ dysfunction treated within 24 hours of their first sepsis-induced organ dysfunction (n=890)). In the subgroup of 885 patients who were already receiving prophylactic heparin at study entry, mortality was 26.9% in the group randomised to continue heparin versus 35.6% in the group whose randomisation (to placebo) led to the discontinuation of heparin. However, the reasons for this difference are unknown and could be related to other factors. Additionally, there was no increased risk of serious bleeding, including central nervous system (CNS) bleeding. Prophylactic heparin increased the risk of non-serious bleeding (see section 4.8). There was no statistical difference in the rates of VTE between study arms.

4.6 Pregnancy and lactation

Animal studies with respect to effects on pregnancy, embryonal/foetal development, parturition, and post-natal development have not been conducted with XIGRIS. Therefore, the potential risk for humans is unknown. XIGRIS should not be used during pregnancy unless clearly necessary.

It is not known whether XIGRIS is excreted in human milk or if there is a potential effect on the breast-fed infant. Therefore, the patient should not breast-feed whilst treated with XIGRIS.

4.7 Effects on ability to drive and use machines

Not relevant.

4.8 Undesirable effects

XIGRIS increases the risk of bleeding.

The Phase 3 international, multi-centre, randomised, double-blind, placebo-controlled clinical trial (PROWESS) involved 850 drotrecogin alfa (activated)-treated and 840 placebo-treated patients. The percentage of patients experiencing at least one bleeding event in the two treatment groups was 24.9% and 17.7%, respectively. In both treatment groups, the majority of bleeding events were ecchymosis or gastro-intestinal tract bleeding. The difference in the incidence of serious bleeding events between the two treatment groups occurred primarily during study drug administration.

A total of 2,378 adult patients with severe sepsis received drotrecogin alfa (activated) in a Phase 3b, international, single-arm, open-label clinical trial (ENHANCE).

The incidence of serious bleeding events in the PROWESS and ENHANCE studies is provided below. In these studies, serious bleeding events included any intracranial haemorrhage, any life-threatening or fatal bleed, any bleeding event requiring the administration of ≥3 units of packed red blood cells per day for 2 consecutive days, or any bleeding event assessed as serious by the investigator.

A Phase 3b, international, multi-centre, randomised, double-blind, placebo-controlled clinical trial (ADDRESS) of adult severe sepsis patients at low risk of death involved 1,317 drotrecogin alfa (activated)-treated and 1,293 placebo-treated patients. The percentage of patients experiencing at least one bleeding event in the two treatment groups was 10.9% and 6.4%, respectively ($P < 0.001$). Bleeding events included serious bleeding events, bleeding events assessed as possibly study drug related by the investigator, bleeding events associated with the need for a red blood cell transfusion, and bleeding events that led to permanent discontinuation of the study drug. In the ADDRESS trial, serious bleeding events included any fatal bleed, any life-threatening bleed, any CNS bleed, or any bleeding event assessed as serious by the investigator.

Serious Bleeding Events During the Infusion Period

The following table lists the percentage of patients in PROWESS and ENHANCE experiencing serious bleeding events by site of haemorrhage during the study drug infusion period (defined as the duration of infusion plus the next full calendar day following the end of the infusion).

(see Table 1 below)

During the infusion period in PROWESS and ENHANCE, the incidence of serious bleeding events with XIGRIS was numerically higher in patients with recent (within 30 days) surgery than in patients without surgery (PROWESS: 3.3% versus 2.0%; ENHANCE: 5.0% versus 3.1% respectively. Placebo rates in PROWESS 0.4% versus 1.2% respectively).

In ADDRESS, the percentage of treated patients experiencing a serious bleeding event by site of haemorrhage was similar to that observed in PROWESS. The incidence of serious bleeding events during infusion (defined as study day 0 through study day 6) was 31 (2.4%) and 15 (1.2%) in drotrecogin alfa (activated)-treated and placebo-treated patients, respectively ($P = 0.02$). The incidence of CNS bleeds during infusion was 4 (0.3%) and 3 (0.2%) for drotrecogin alfa (activated)-treated and placebo-treated patients, respectively. Recent surgery (within 30 days prior to study entry) was associated with a numerically higher risk of serious bleeding during infusion in both the XIGRIS-treated and the placebo-treated patients (XIGRIS: 3.6% in patients with recent surgery versus 1.6% in patients without recent surgery; placebo: 1.6% versus 0.9%, respectively).

In XPRESS, a randomised study of prophylactic heparin versus placebo in adult severe sepsis patients, all treated with drotrecogin alfa (activated), serious bleeding rates were consistent with those observed in previous studies over the treatment period of 0-6 days, and prophylactic heparin did not increase the risk of serious bleeding compared to placebo (2.3% versus 2.5%, respectively), including CNS bleeding (0.3% on both arms). However, prophylactic heparin increased the risk of non-serious bleeding compared with placebo (8.7% versus 5.7%, respectively; $P = 0.0116$).

Serious Bleeding Events During the 28-Day Study Period

In PROWESS, the incidence of serious bleeding events during the 28-day study period was 3.5% and 2.0% in drotrecogin alfa (activated)-treated and placebo-treated patients, respectively. The incidence of CNS bleeds during the 28-day study period was 0.2% and 0.1% for drotrecogin alfa (activated)-treated and placebo-treated patients, respectively. The risk of CNS bleeding may increase with severe coagulopathy and severe thrombocytopenia (see sections 4.3 and 4.4).

In the open-label ENHANCE study, the incidence of serious bleeding events during the 28-day study period was 6.5%, and the incidence of CNS bleeds during the 28-day study period was 1.5%.

In the placebo-controlled ADDRESS study, the incidence of serious bleeding events during the 28-day study period was 51 (3.9%) and 28 (2.2%) in drotrecogin alfa (activated)-treated and placebo-treated patients, respectively ($P = 0.01$). The incidence of CNS bleeds during the 28-day study period was 6 (0.5%) and 5 (0.4%) for drotrecogin alfa (activated)-treated and placebo-treated patients, respectively.

In XPRESS, serious bleeding rates were consistent with those observed in previous studies during the 28-day study period (days 0-28). Prophylactic heparin did not increase the risk of serious bleeding compared to placebo (3.9% versus 5.2%, respectively), including CNS bleeding (1.0% versus 0.7%, respectively).

In the Phase 1 studies, adverse events with a frequency of ≥5% included headache (30.9%), ecchymosis (23.0%), and pain (5.8%).

Table 1

Site of Haemorrhage	Drotrecogin Alfa (Activated) [PROWESS] n = 850	Placebo [PROWESS] n = 840	Drotrecogin Alfa (Activated) [ENHANCE] n = 2,378
Gastro-intestinal	5 (0.6%)	4 (0.5%)	19 (0.8%)
Intra-abdominal	2 (0.2%)	3 (0.4%)	18 (0.8%)
Intra-thoracic	4 (0.5%)	0	11 (0.5%)
Retroperitoneal	3 (0.4%)	0	4 (0.2%)
Central nervous system (CNS)[1]	2 (0.2%)	0	15 (0.6%)
Genito-urinary	2 (0.2%)	0	0
Skin/soft tissue	1 (0.1%)	0	16 (0.7%)
Nasopharyngeal	0	0	4 (0.2%)
Joint/bone	0	0	1 (0.04%)
Site unknown[2]	1 (0.1%)	1 (0.1%)	6 (0.3%)
Total	20 (2.4%)	8 (1.0%)	85[3] (3.6%)

[1]CNS bleeding is defined as any bleed in the central nervous system, including the following types of haemorrhage: petechial, parenchymal, subarachnoid, subdural, and stroke with haemorrhagic transformation.

[2]Patients requiring the administration of ≥3 units of packed red blood cells per day for 2 consecutive days without an identified site of bleeding.

[3]In ENHANCE, six patients experienced multiple serious bleeding events during the study drug infusion period (94 events observed in 85 patients).

4.9 Overdose

In clinical trials and in post-marketing experience there have been reports of accidental overdosing. In the majority of cases, no reactions have been observed. For the other reports, the observed events were consistent with known undesirable effects of the drug (see section 4.8), effects of the drug on laboratory tests (see section 4.4), or consequences of the underlying condition of sepsis.

There is no known antidote for drotrecogin alfa (activated). In case of overdose, immediately stop the infusion (see section 5.2).

5. PHARMACOLOGICAL PROPERTIES

5.1 Pharmacodynamic properties

Pharmacotherapeutic group: Antithrombotic agents, enzymes. *ATC code:* B01AD10.

This medicinal product has been authorised under "Exceptional Circumstances". This means that for scientific reasons it has not been possible to obtain complete information on this medicinal product. The European Medicines Agency (EMEA) will review any new information which may become available every year, and this SPC will be updated as necessary.

Mechanism of Action

XIGRIS is a recombinant version of the natural plasma-derived Activated Protein C, from which it differs only by unique oligosaccharides in the carbohydrate portion of the molecule. Activated Protein C is a crucial coagulation regulator. It limits thrombin formation by inactivating Factors Va and VIIIa, thereby providing negative feedback regulation of coagulation. Excessive coagulation activation in the microcirculatory bed plays a significant part in the pathophysiology of severe sepsis. Furthermore, Activated Protein C is an important modulator of the systemic response to infection and has antithrombotic and profibrinolytic properties. XIGRIS has similar properties to those of endogenous human Activated Protein C.

Pharmacodynamic Effects

In placebo-controlled clinical trials in patients with severe sepsis, XIGRIS exerted an antithrombotic effect by limiting thrombin generation and improved sepsis-associated coagulopathy, as shown by a more rapid improvement in markers of coagulation and fibrinolysis. XIGRIS caused a more rapid decline in thrombotic markers, such as D-dimer, prothrombin F1.2, and thrombin-antithrombin levels, and a more rapid increase in Protein C and antithrombin levels. XIGRIS also restored endogenous fibrinolytic potential, as evidenced by a more rapid trend toward normalisation in plasminogen levels and a more rapid decline in plasminogen activator inhibitor-1 levels. Additionally, patients with severe sepsis treated with XIGRIS had a more rapid decline in interleukin-6 levels, a global marker of inflammation, consistent with a reduction in the inflammatory response.

Clinical Efficacy

XIGRIS was studied in one Phase 3, international, multi-centre, randomised, double-blind, placebo-controlled trial (PROWESS) in 1,690 patients with severe sepsis. Severe sepsis is defined as sepsis associated with acute organ dysfunction. Patients meeting the clinical diagnosis of severe sepsis had: a) known or suspected infection; b) clinical evidence of systemic response to infection, including fever or hypothermia, leucopenia or leucocytosis, tachycardia and tachypnoea; and c) acute organ dysfunction. Organ dysfunction was defined as shock, hypotension or the need for vasopressor support despite adequate fluid resuscitation, relative hypoxemia (ratio of partial pressure of oxygen in arterial blood in mmHg to the percentage of oxygen in the inspired air expressed as a decimal [PaO_2/FiO_2 ratio] <250), oliguria despite adequate fluid resuscitation, marked reduction in blood platelet counts, and/or elevated lactic acid concentrations.

Exclusion criteria encompassed patients at high risk of bleeding (see sections 4.3 and 4.4), patients who were not expected to survive for 28 days due to a pre-existing, non-sepsis related medical condition, HIV positive patients whose most recent CD_4 count was ⩽50/mm^3, patients on chronic dialysis, and patients who had undergone bone marrow, lung, liver, pancreas, or small bowel transplantation, and patients with acute clinical pancreatitis without a proven source of infection.

In the PROWESS trial, treatment was initiated within 48 hours of onset of the first sepsis-induced organ dysfunction. The median duration of organ dysfunction prior to treatment was 18 hours. Patients were given a 96-hour constant rate infusion of XIGRIS at 24µg/kg/hr (n = 850) or placebo (n = 840). XIGRIS was added to best standard care. Best standard care includes adequate antibiotics, source control and supportive treatment (fluids, inotropes, vasopressors and support of failing organs, as required).

Patients treated with XIGRIS experienced improved 28-day survival compared to those treated with placebo. At 28 days, the overall mortality rates were 24.7% for the XIGRIS-treated group and 30.8% for the placebo-treated group (*P* = 0.005).

Significant absolute death reduction was limited to the subgroup of patients with greater disease severity, i.e., baseline APACHE II score ⩾25 or at least 2 acute organ dysfunctions at baseline. (The APACHE II score is designed to assess the risk of mortality based on acute physiology and chronic health evaluation.) In the subgroup of patients with an APACHE II score ⩾25 at baseline, the mortality was 31% in the XIGRIS group (128 out of 414) and 44% in the placebo group (176 out of 403). No death reduction was observed in the subgroup of patients with lower disease severity. In the subgroup of patients with at least 2 acute organ dysfunctions at baseline, the mortality was 26.5% in the XIGRIS group (168 out of 634) and 33.9% in the placebo group (216 out of 637). No significant death reduction was observed in the subgroup of patients with less than 2 acute organ dysfunctions at baseline.

A consistent treatment effect on mortality with XIGRIS administration was observed across patient subgroups defined by age, gender, and infection type.

PROWESS Follow-Up Study

Survival status was assessed in a follow-up study of PROWESS survivors. In-hospital and 3-month survival status was reported for 98% and 94% of the 1,690 PROWESS subjects, respectively. In the overall population, the in-hospital mortality was significantly lower in patients on XIGRIS than in patients on placebo (29.4% versus 34.6%; *P* = 0.023). Survival through 3 months was also better in the XIGRIS group compared to placebo (log rank *P* = 0.048). These data confirmed that the benefit of XIGRIS is limited to the more severely affected sepsis patients, such as patients with multiple organ failure and shock.

Further Clinical Experience

In a Phase 3b, international, single-arm, open-label clinical trial (ENHANCE), 2,378 adult patients with severe sepsis received drotrecogin alfa (activated). The entry criteria were similar to those employed in PROWESS. Patients received drotrecogin alfa (activated) within 48 hours of onset of the first sepsis-induced organ dysfunction. The median duration of organ dysfunction prior to treatment was 25 hours. At 28 days, the mortality rate in the Phase 3b study was 25.3%. The mortality rate was lower for patients treated within 24 hours of organ dysfunction compared to those treated after 24 hours, even after adjustment for differences in disease severity.

A total of 2,640 adult patients with severe sepsis who were at low risk of death (e.g., patients with APACHE II <25 or with only one sepsis-induced organ failure) were enrolled in a randomised, double-blind, placebo-controlled trial (ADDRESS). The trial was stopped after an interim analysis due to a low likelihood of demonstrating a significant difference in 28-day mortality by the end of the trial.

The ADDRESS trial did enrol 872 patients with multiple organ dysfunction. Compared to multiple organ dysfunction patients in PROWESS, those in ADDRESS had organ dysfunction for longer prior to receiving study drug (median 25 versus 18 hours), had lower APACHE II scores (median 20 versus 25), and were more likely to have two organ dysfunctions (76% versus 43%). At 28 days, the mortality rates for multiple organ dysfunction patients in ADDRESS were 20.7% versus 21.9% for drotrecogin alfa (activated)-treated and placebo-treated patients, respectively. In-hospital mortality rates were 23.1% and 25.3%, respectively. In the subgroup with two organ dysfunctions, the results were similar to those seen in the PROWESS trial.

In placebo-controlled clinical trials, the treatment effect was most evident at sites enrolling larger numbers of patients.

5.2 Pharmacokinetic properties

Drotrecogin alfa (activated) and endogenous human Activated Protein C are inactivated in plasma by endogenous protease inhibitors, but the mechanism by which they are cleared from plasma is unknown. Plasma concentrations of endogenous Activated Protein C in healthy subjects and patients with severe sepsis are usually below detection limits (<5ng/ml) and do not significantly influence the pharmacokinetic properties of drotrecogin alfa (activated).

In healthy subjects, greater than 90% of the steady-state condition is attained within 2 hours following the start of a constant-rate intravenous infusion of XIGRIS. Following the completion of an infusion, the decline in plasma drotrecogin alfa (activated) concentrations is biphasic and is comprised of a rapid initial phase ($t_{½α}$ = 13 minutes) and a slower second phase ($t_{½β}$ = 1.6 hours). The short half-life of 13 minutes accounts for approximately 80% of the area under the plasma concentration curve and governs the initial rapid accrual of plasma drotrecogin alfa (activated) concentrations towards the steady-state. Plasma drotrecogin alfa (activated) steady-state concentrations are proportional to the infusion rate over a range of infusion rates from 12µg/kg/hr to 48µg/kg/hr. The mean steady-state plasma concentration of drotrecogin alfa (activated) in healthy subjects receiving 24µg/kg/hr is 72ng/ml.

In patients with severe sepsis, infusion of drotrecogin alfa (activated) from 12µg/kg/hr to 30µg/kg/hr rapidly produced steady-state plasma concentrations that were proportional to infusion rates. In the Phase 3 trial, the pharmacokinetics of drotrecogin alfa (activated) were evaluated in 342 patients with severe sepsis administered a 96-hour continuous infusion at 24µg/kg/hr. The pharmacokinetics of drotrecogin alfa (activated) were characterised by attainment of steady-state plasma concentration within 2 hours following the start of the infusion. In the majority of patients, measurements of Activated Protein C beyond 2 hours after termination of the infusion were below the quantifiable limit, suggesting rapid elimination of drotrecogin alfa (activated) from the systemic circulation. The plasma clearance of drotrecogin alfa (activated) is approximately 41.8 l/hr in sepsis patients as compared with 28.1 l/hr in healthy subjects.

In patients with severe sepsis, the plasma clearance of drotrecogin alfa (activated) was significantly decreased by renal impairment and hepatic dysfunction, but the magnitude of the differences in clearance (<30%) does not warrant any dosage adjustment.

5.3 Preclinical safety data

Changes observed in monkeys at, or in small excess of, the maximum human exposure during repeated dose studies were all related to the pharmacological effect of XIGRIS and include, beside the expected prolongation of APTT, decreases in haemoglobin, erythrocytes and haematocrit and increases in reticulocyte count and PT.

Drotrecogin alfa (activated) was not mutagenic in an *in vivo* micronucleus study in mice or in an *in vitro* chromosomal aberration study in human peripheral blood lymphocytes with or without rat liver metabolic activation.

Carcinogenicity studies and animal reproduction studies have not been conducted with XIGRIS. However, with respect to the latter, the potential risk for humans being unknown, XIGRIS should not be used during pregnancy unless clearly necessary (see section 4.6).

6. PHARMACEUTICAL PARTICULARS

6.1 List of excipients

Sucrose

Sodium chloride

Sodium citrate

Citric acid

Hydrochloric acid

Sodium hydroxide

6.2 Incompatibilities

This medicinal product must not be mixed with other medicinal products except those mentioned in section 6.6.

6.3 Shelf life

3 years.

After reconstitution, immediate use is recommended. However, the reconstituted solution in the vial may be held for up to 3 hours at room temperature (15 °C- 30°C). After preparation, the intravenous infusion solution can be used at room temperature (15 °C- 30°C) for a period up to 14 hours.

6.4 Special precautions for storage

Store in a refrigerator (2°C-8°C). Keep the vial in the outer carton in order to protect it from light.

6.5 Nature and contents of container

Powder in Type I glass vial. Pack of 1 vial.

6.6 Special precautions for disposal and other handling

1. Use appropriate aseptic technique during the preparation of XIGRIS for intravenous administration.

2. Calculate the dose and the number of XIGRIS vials needed.

XIGRIS 5mg: Each XIGRIS vial contains 5mg of drotrecogin alfa (activated).

XIGRIS 20mg: Each XIGRIS vial contains 20mg of drotrecogin alfa (activated).

The vial contains an excess of drotrecogin alfa (activated) to facilitate delivery of the label amount.

3. *XIGRIS 5mg:* Prior to administration, 5mg vials of XIGRIS must be reconstituted with 2.5ml of sterile water for injection, resulting in a solution with a concentration of approximately 2mg/ml drotrecogin alfa (activated).

XIGRIS 20mg: Prior to administration, 20mg vials of XIGRIS must be reconstituted with 10ml of sterile water for injection, resulting in a solution with a concentration of approximately 2mg/ml drotrecogin alfa (activated).

Slowly add the sterile water for injection to the vial and avoid inverting or shaking the vial. Gently swirl each vial until the powder is completely dissolved.

4. The solution of reconstituted XIGRIS must be further diluted with sterile 0.9% sodium chloride injection to a final concentration of between 100µg/ml and 200µg/ml. Slowly withdraw the appropriate amount of reconstituted drotrecogin alfa (activated) solution from the vial. Add the reconstituted drotrecogin alfa (activated) into a prepared infusion bag of sterile 0.9% sodium chloride injection. When adding the reconstituted drotrecogin alfa (activated) into the infusion bag, direct the stream to the side of the bag to minimise the agitation of the solution. Gently invert the infusion bag to obtain a homogeneous solution. Do not transport the infusion bag between locations using mechanical delivery systems.

5. After reconstitution, immediate use is recommended. However, the reconstituted solution in the vial may be held for up to 3 hours at room temperature (15 to 30°C).

After preparation, the intravenous infusion solution can be used at room temperature (15 to 30°C) for a period up to 14 hours.

6. Parenteral drug products should be inspected visually for particulate matter and discolouration prior to administration.

7. **It is recommended that XIGRIS be infused with an infusion pump to accurately control the infusion rate.**

The solution of reconstituted XIGRIS should be diluted into an infusion bag containing sterile 0.9% sodium chloride injection to a final concentration of between 100μg/ml and 200μg/ml.

8. When administering drotrecogin alfa (activated) at low flow rates (less than approximately 5ml/hr), the infusion set must be primed for approximately 15 minutes at a flow rate of approximately 5ml/hr.

9. XIGRIS should be administered via a dedicated intravenous line or a dedicated lumen of a multi-lumen central venous catheter. The ONLY other solutions that can be administered through the same line are 0.9% sodium chloride injection, lactated Ringer's injection, dextrose, or dextrose and saline mixtures.

10. Avoid exposing drotrecogin alfa (activated) solutions to heat and/or direct sunlight. No incompatibilities have been observed between drotrecogin alfa (activated) and glass infusion bottles or infusion bags made of polyvinylchloride, polyethylene, polypropylene, or polyolefin. The use of other types of infusion sets could have a negative impact on the amount and potency of drotrecogin alfa (activated) administered.

11. Care should be taken to administer XIGRIS at the appropriate rate, calculated based on kg of bodyweight and infused for the correct duration. It is recommended that the bag be labelled accordingly.

7. MARKETING AUTHORISATION HOLDER
Eli Lilly Nederland BV, Grootslag 1-5, 3991 RA Houten, The Netherlands.

8. MARKETING AUTHORISATION NUMBER(S)
5mg vial: EU/1/02/225/001
20mg vial: EU/1/02/225/002

9. DATE OF FIRST AUTHORISATION/RENEWAL OF THE AUTHORISATION
Date of first authorisation: 22 August 2002
Date of latest renewal: 22 August 2007

10. DATE OF REVISION OF THE TEXT
04 December 2008

LEGAL CATEGORY
POM

Detailed information on this product is available on the website of the European Medicines Agency (EMEA): http://www.emea.europa.eu/

*XIGRIS (drotrecogin alfa [activated]) is a trademark of Eli Lilly and Company.

XIG11M

Xismox 60 XL Prolonged Release Tablets
(Genus Pharmaceuticals)

1. NAME OF THE MEDICINAL PRODUCT
ISIB 60 XL Prolonged Release Tablets
and
CIBRAL 60 XL Prolonged Release Tablets and
XISMOX 60 XL Prolonged Release Tablets

2. QUALITATIVE AND QUANTITATIVE COMPOSITION
Isosorbide mononitrate 60.0 mg
For excipients, see section 6.1.

3. PHARMACEUTICAL FORM
Prolonged Release Tablets
Light yellow, biconvex, oval-shaped, prolonged release tablets, scored on both sides and marked "DX 31" on one side.

4. CLINICAL PARTICULARS
4.1 Therapeutic indications
Prophylaxis of angina pectoris

4.2 Posology and method of administration
Adults: The recommended dose is one 60 mg tablet once daily to be taken in the morning. The dose may be increased to 120 mg (two tablets) daily, both to be taken once daily in the morning. The dose can be titrated, by initiating treatment with 30 mg (half tablet) for the first 2-4 days to minimize the possibility of headache.

Children: The safety and efficacy in children has not been established.

Elderly: No evidence of a need for routine dosage adjustment in the elderly has been found, but special care may be needed in those with increased susceptibility to hypotension or marked hepatic or renal insufficiency.

There is a risk of tolerance developing when nitrate therapy is given. For this reason it is important that the tablets are taken once a day to achieve an interval with low nitrate concentration, thereby reducing the risk of tolerance development.

When necessary the product may be used in combination with beta-adrenoreceptor blockers and calcium antagonists. Dose adjustments of either class of agent may be necessary.

The tablets must not be chewed or crushed. They should be swallowed with half a glass of water.

4.3 Contraindications
Hypersensitivity to isosorbide mononitrate, or to any of the excipients.

Sildenafil has been shown to potentiate the hypotensive effects of nitrates, and its co-administration with nitrates or nitric oxide donors is therefore contra-indicated.

Isosorbide mononitrate is contraindicated in constrictive pericarditis and pericardial tamponade.

4.4 Special warnings and precautions for use
Use with extreme caution in hypotension with or without other signs of shock and in cases of cerebrovascular insufficiency.

Other special warnings and precautions with Isosorbide mononitrate:

Significant aortic or mitral valve stenosis.

Hypertrophic obstructive cardiomyopathy.

Anaemia. Hypoxaemia, Hypothyroidism.

The tablets are not indicated for relief of acute angina attacks.

Patients with rare hereditary problems of fructose or galactose intolerance, the Lapp lactase deficiency, sucrase-isomaltase insufficiency or glucose-galactose malabsorption should not take this medicine.

4.5 Interaction with other medicinal products and other forms of interaction
Isosorbide mononitrate may act as a physiological antagonist to noradrenaline, acetylcholine, histamine and many other agents. The effect of anti-hypertensive drugs may be enhanced. Alcohol may enhance the hypotensive effects of isosorbide mononitrate.

The hypotensive effects of nitrates are potentiated by concurrent administration of sildenafil.

4.6 Pregnancy and lactation
The tablets should not be used during pregnancy and lactation.

4.7 Effects on ability to drive and use machines
Patients experiencing headache or dizziness following initial treatment with the tablets should become stabilised on treatment before driving or using machines.

4.8 Undesirable effects
Most of the adverse reactions are pharmacodynamically mediated and dose dependent. Headache may occur when treatment is initiated but usually disappears after continued treatment. Hypotension with symptoms such as dizziness and nausea has occasionally been reported. These symptoms generally disappear during long-term treatment. Less common are vomiting and diarrhoea. Uncommon is fainting.

Skin rashes (dry rash, exfoliative dermatitis) and pruritus have been reported rarely with isosorbide mononitrate. Myalgia has been reported very rarely.

4.9 Overdose
Symptoms: Pulsing headache. More serious symptoms are excitation, flushing, cold perspiration, nausea, vomiting, vertigo, syncope, tachycardia and a fall in blood pressure. Very large doses may give rise to methaemoglobinaemia (Very rare).

Treatment: Induction of emesis, activated charcoal. In case of pronounced hypotension the patient should first be placed in the supine position with legs raised. If necessary, fluid should be administered intravenously. (In cases of cyanosis as a result of methaemoglobinaemia, methyl thionine (methylene blue) 1 -2mg/Kg, slow intravenous delivery). Expert advice should be sought.

5. PHARMACOLOGICAL PROPERTIES
5.1 Pharmacodynamic properties
Pharmacotherapeutic group: Organic nitrates, ATC code: C01D A14.

Isosorbide mononitrate is an organic nitrate, the major active metabolite of isosorbide dinitrate and an active vasodilator in its own right. The mechanism of action of Isosorbide mononitrate, like other organic nitrates, is believed to involve peripheral vasodilation, both venous and arterial. Maximal venous dilatation is usually achieved with lower doses of the nitrate, while higher doses cause progressive dilatation of the arterial vasculature. Nitrates thus lead to pooling of blood in the veins and reduced left ventricular and diastolic pressure. As arterial vascular resistance is also decreased, arterial blood pressure is reduced. Isosorbide mononitrate is an effective antianginal agent because it improves exertional angina by reducing myocardial oxygen demand, secondary to reduced preload and afterload. Organic nitrates release nitric oxide (NO), which induces protein phosphorylations, finally resulting in vascular smooth muscle relaxation.

In comparison to an immediate release product taken on a multiple dose basis, this prolonged release product has the advantage of both lowering the incidence of tolerance and increasing patient compliance.

5.2 Pharmacokinetic properties
Isosorbide mononitrate is completely absorbed after oral administration. The absorption is not affected by simultaneous food intake. Contrary to many other nitrates, Isosorbide mononitrate is not subject to first pass metabolism and its oral bioavailability is therefore close to 100%. This feature probably contributes to the relatively small inter-subject variability in plasma levels that are achieved following ingestion of the drug. Peak plasma concentrations of Isosorbide mononitrate after oral ingestion of a prolonged release tablet usually occur within 3.1-4.5 hours. Isosorbide mononitrate's volume of distribution is about 0.6 litres/kg, and its plasma protein binding is negligible (about 4%). Isosorbide mononitrate is metabolised to form several inactive compounds. Elimination is primarily by denitration and conjugation in the liver. The metabolites are excreted mainly via the kidneys. About 2% of the dose is excreted intact via the kidneys. The half-life of Isosorbide mononitrate in the plasma of healthy volunteers as well as in most patients is about 6.5 hours after administration of prolonged release tablets. Neither renal nor hepatic disease influence the pharmacokinetic of isosorbide mononitrate. The tablets are a prolonged release formulation. The active substance is released independently of pH.

5.3 Preclinical safety data
Isosorbide mononitrate is a well-established drug for which there is adequate published safety data.

6. PHARMACEUTICAL PARTICULARS
6.1 List of excipients
Hypromellose 2208

Lactose monohydrate

Compressible Sugar (composed of Sucrose and Maltodextrin)

Magnesium stearate

Colloidal anhydrous silica

Iron oxide yellow.

6.2 Incompatibilities
Not applicable.

6.3 Shelf life
3 years

6.4 Special precautions for storage
Do not store above 25°C.

6.5 Nature and contents of container
Blister pack PVDC- or ACLAR-coated-PVC/Aluminium 28, 30 or 98 tablets.

Not all pack sizes may be marketed.

6.6 Special precautions for disposal and other handling
No special requirements.

7. MARKETING AUTHORISATION HOLDER
Dexcel-Pharma Ltd.

1 Cottesbrooke Park

Heartlands Business Park, Daventry

Northamptonshire NN1 1 8YL, England

8. MARKETING AUTHORISATION NUMBER(S)
PL 14017/0096

9. DATE OF FIRST AUTHORISATION/RENEWAL OF THE AUTHORISATION
27th October 2004.

10. DATE OF REVISION OF THE TEXT
9 June 2005.

Xomolix® 2.5mg/ml solution for injection
(ProStrakan)

1. NAME OF THE MEDICINAL PRODUCT
Xomolix® 2.5 mg/ml solution for injection

2. QUALITATIVE AND QUANTITATIVE COMPOSITION
Each millilitre of the solution contains 2.5 mg droperidol.

Excipient: sodium < 23 mg per ml.

For a full list of excipients, see section 6.1.

3. PHARMACEUTICAL FORM
Solution for injection.

Clear colourless solution, free from visible particles.

The pH of droperidol solution for injection is 3.0 – 3.8 and has an osmolarity of approximately 300 millimosmol /kg water.

4. CLINICAL PARTICULARS
4.1 Therapeutic indications
• Prevention and treatment of post-operative nausea and vomiting in adults and, as second line, in children and adolescents.

• Prevention of nausea and vomiting induced by morphine derivates during post-operative patient controlled analgesia (PCA) in adults.

Certain precautions are required when administering droperidol: see sections 4.2, 4.3, and 4.4.

4.2 Posology and method of administration
For intravenous use.

Prevention and treatment of post-operative nausea and vomiting (PONV).

Adults: 0.625 mg to 1.25 mg (0.25 to 0.5 ml).

Elderly: 0.625 mg (0.25 ml)

Renal/hepatic impairment: 0.625 mg (0.25 ml)

Children (over the age of 2 years) and adolescents: 20 to 50 microgram/kg (up to a maximum of 1.25 mg).

Children (below the age of 2 years): not recommended.

Administration of droperidol is recommended 30 minutes before the anticipated end of surgery. Repeat doses may be given every 6 hours as required.

The dosage should be adapted to each individual case. The factors to be considered here include age, body weight, use of other medicinal products, type of anaesthesia and surgical procedure.

Prevention of nausea and vomiting induced by morphine derivatives during post-operative patient controlled analgesia (PCA).

Adults: 15 to 50 micrograms droperidol per mg of morphine, up to a maximum daily dose of 5 mg droperidol.

Elderly, renal and hepatic impairment: no data in PCA available.

Children (over the age of 2 years) and adolescents: not indicated in PCA.

Continuous pulse oximetry should be performed in patients with identified or suspected risk of ventricular arrhythmia and should continue for 30 minutes following single i.v. administration.

For instructions on dilution of the product before administration, see section 6.6.

See also sections 4.3, 4.4 and 5.1.

4.3 Contraindications

Droperidol is contraindicated in patients with:

- Hypersensitivity to droperidol or to any of the excipients;
- Hypersensitivity to butyrophenones;
- Known or suspected prolonged QT interval (QTc of > 450 msec in females and > 440 msec in males). This includes patients with congenitally long QT interval, patients who have a family history of congenital QT prolongation and those treated with medicinal products known to prolong the QT interval (see section 4.5);
- Hypokalaemia or hypomagnesaemia;
- Bradycardia (< 55 heartbeats per minute);
- Known concomitant treatment leading to bradycardia;
- Phaeochromocytoma;
- Comatose states;
- Parkinson's Disease;
- Severe depression.

4.4 Special warnings and precautions for use

Central Nervous System

Droperidol may enhance CNS depression produced by other CNS-depressant drugs. Any patient subjected to anaesthesia and receiving potent CNS depressant medicinal products or showing symptoms of CNS depression should be monitored closely.

Concomitant use of metoclopramide and other neuroleptics may lead to an increase in extrapyramidal symptoms and should be avoided (see section 4.5).

Use with caution in patients with epilepsy (or a history of epilepsy) and conditions predisposing to epilepsy or convulsions.

Cardiovascular

Mild to moderate hypotension and occasionally (reflex) tachycardia have been observed following the administration of droperidol. This reaction usually subsides spontaneously. However, should hypotension persist, the possibility of hypovolaemia should be considered and appropriate fluid replacement administered.

Patients with, or suspected of having, the following risk factors for cardiac arrhythmia should be carefully evaluated prior to administration of droperidol:

- a history of significant cardiac disease including serious ventricular arrhythmia, second or third degree atrio-ventricular block, sinus node dysfunction, congestive heart failure, ischemic heart disease and left ventricular hypertrophy;
- family history of sudden death;
- renal failure (particularly when on chronic dialysis);
- significant chronic obstructive pulmonary disease and respiratory failure;
- risk factors for electrolyte disturbances, as seen in patients taking laxatives, glucocorticoids, potassium-wasting diuretics, in association with the administration of insulin in acute settings, or in patients with prolonged vomiting and/or diarrhoea.

Patients at risk for cardiac arrhythmia should have serum electrolytes and creatinine levels assessed and the presence of QT prolongation excluded prior to administration of droperidol.

Continuous pulse oximetry should be performed in patients with identified or suspected risk of ventricular arrhythmia and should continue for 30 minutes following single i.v. administration.

General

To prevent QT prolongation, caution is necessary when patients are taking medicinal products likely to induce electrolyte imbalance (hypokalaemia and/or hypomagnesaemia) e.g. potassium-wasting diuretics, laxatives and glucocorticoids.

Substances inhibiting the activity of cytochrome P450 isoenzymes (CYP) CYP1A2, CYP3A4 or both could decrease the rate at which droperidol is metabolised and prolong its pharmacological action. Hence, caution is advised if droperidol is given concomitantly with strong CYP1A2 and CYP3A4 inhibitors (see section 4.5).

Patients who have, or are suspected of having, a history of alcohol abuse or recent high intakes, should be thoroughly assessed before droperidol is administered.

In case of unexplained hyperthermia, it is essential to discontinue treatment, since this sign may be one of the elements of malignant syndrome reported with neuroleptics.

The dose should be reduced in the elderly and those with impaired renal and hepatic function (see section 4.2).

This medicinal product contains less than 1 mmol sodium (23 mg) per 1 ml, i.e. essentially 'sodium-free'.

4.5 Interaction with other medicinal products and other forms of interaction

Contraindicated for concomitant use

Medicinal products known to prolong the QTc interval should not be concomitantly administered with droperidol. Examples include certain antiarrhythmics, such as those of Class IA (e.g. quinidine, disopyramide, procainamide) and Class III (e.g. amiodarone, sotalol); macrolide antibiotics (e.g. azithromycin, erythromycin, clarithromycin), fluoroquinolone antibiotics (e.g. sparfloxacin); certain antihistamines (e.g. astemizole, terfenadine); tricyclic antidepressants (e.g. amitriptyline); certain tetracyclic antidepressants (e.g. maprotiline); certain antipsychotic medications (e.g. amisulpride, chlorpromazine, haloperidol, melperone, phenothiazines, pimozide, sulpiride, sertindole, tiapride); SSRIs (e.g. fluoxetine, sertraline, fluvoxamine); anti-malaria agents (e.g. quinine, chloroquine, halofantrine); cisapride, pentamidine, tacrolimus, tamoxifen, and vincamine.

Concomitant use of medicinal products that induce extrapyramidal symptoms, e.g. metoclopramide and other neuroleptics, may lead to an increased incidence of these symptoms and should therefore be avoided.

Consumption of alcoholic beverages and medicines should be avoided.

Caution is advised for concomitant use

To prevent QT prolongation, caution is necessary when patients are taking medicinal products likely to induce electrolyte imbalance (hypokalaemia and/or hypomagnesaemia) e.g. potassium-wasting diuretics, laxatives and glucocorticoids.

Droperidol may potentiate the action of sedatives (barbiturates, benzodiazepines, morphine derivatives). The same applies to antihypertensive agents, so that orthostatic hypotension may ensue.

Like other sedatives, droperidol may potentiate respiratory depression caused by opioids.

Since droperidol blocks dopamine receptors, it may inhibit the action of dopamine agonists, such as bromocriptine, lisuride, and of L-dopa.

Substances inhibiting the activity of cytochrome P450 isoenzymes (CYP) CYP1A2, CYP3A4 or both could decrease the rate at which droperidol is metabolised and prolong its pharmacological action. Hence, caution is advised if droperidol is given concomitantly with CYP1A2 (e.g. ciprofloxacin, ticlopidine), CYP3A4 inhibitors (e.g. diltiazem, erythromycin, fluconazole, indinavir, itraconazole, ketoconazole, nefazodone, nelfinavir, ritonavir, saquinavir, verapamil) or both (e.g. cimetidine, mibefradil).

4.6 Pregnancy and lactation

Pregnancy

In a prospective study, 80 patients suffering from hyperemesis gravidarum received high doses of droperidol (average 1 mg/h over 50 hours) to control nausea and vomiting. Gestational age at delivery, mean birth weight, incidence of pre-term birth and incidence of 'small for gestational age' were comparable to a historic control group. Another study, in which 28 patients received droperidol 1 mg/hour over 40 hours on average, showed no statistically significant differences between treatment and historic control groups for spontaneous abortions, elective abortions, Apgar scores, gestational age at delivery and birth weight.

Droperidol has not been shown to be teratogenic in rats. Animal studies are insufficient with respect to the effects on pregnancy and embryonal/foetal, parturition and postnatal development.

In newborn babies from mothers under long-term treatment and high doses of neuroleptics, temporary neurological disturbances of extrapyramidal nature have been described.

In practice, as a precautionary measure, it is preferable not to administer droperidol during pregnancy. In late pregnancy, if its administration is necessary, monitoring of the newborn's neurological functions is recommended.

Lactation

Neuroleptics of the butyrophenone type are known to be excreted in breast milk; treatment with droperidol should be limited to a single administration. Repeat administration is not recommended.

4.7 Effects on ability to drive and use machines

Droperidol has major influence on the ability to drive and use machines.

Patients should not drive or operate a machine for 24 hours after droperidol administration.

4.8 Undesirable effects

The most frequently reported events during clinical experience are incidents of drowsiness and sedation. In addition, less frequent reports of hypotension, cardiac arrhythmias, neuroleptic malignant syndrome (NMS) and symptoms associated with NMS, plus movement disorders, such as dyskinesias, plus incidents of anxiety or agitation have occurred.

(see Table 1 on next page)

Symptoms potentially associated with NMS have occasionally been reported i.e. changes in body temperature, stiffness and fever. An alteration in mental status with confusion or agitation and altered consciousness, have been seen. Autonomic instability may manifest as tachycardia, fluctuating blood pressure, excessive sweating/salivation and tremor. In extreme cases NMS may lead to coma, or renal and/or hepato-biliary problems.

Isolated cases of amenorrhoea, galactorrhoea, gynaecomastia, hyperprolactinaemia, and oligomenorrhoea have been associated with prolonged exposure in psychiatric indications.

4.9 Overdose

Symptoms

The manifestations of droperidol overdose are an extension of its pharmacologic actions.

Symptoms of accidental overdose are psychic indifference with a transition to sleep, sometimes in association with lowered blood pressure.

At higher doses or in sensitive patients, extrapyramidal disorders may occur (salivation, abnormal movements, sometimes muscle rigidity). Convulsions may occur at toxic doses.

Cases of QT-interval prolongation, ventricular arrhythmias and sudden death have been reported rarely.

Treatment

No specific antidote is known. However, when extrapyramidal reactions occur, an anticholinergic should be administered.

Patients with droperidol overdose should be closely monitored for signs of QT interval prolongation.

Factors which predispose to torsades de pointes, e.g. electrolyte disturbances (especially hypokalaemia or hypomagnesaemia) and bradycardia should be taken into consideration.

Pronounced hypotension should be treated by boosting circulation volume and taking other appropriate measures. Clear airways and adequate oxygenation should be maintained; an oropharyngeal airway or endotracheal tube might be indicated.

If required, the patient should be observed carefully for 24 hours or longer; body warmth and adequate fluid intake should be maintained.

5. PHARMACOLOGICAL PROPERTIES

5.1 Pharmacodynamic properties

Pharmacotherapeutic group: Butyrophenone derivatives. ATC code: N05AD08.

Droperidol is a butyrophenone neuroleptic. Its pharmacologic profile is characterised mainly by dopamine-blocking and weak α_1-adrenolytic effects. Droperidol is devoid of anticholinergic and antihistaminic activity.

Droperidol's inhibitory action on dopaminergic receptors in the chemotrigger zone in the area postrema, gives it a potent antiemetic effect, especially useful for the prevention and treatment of postoperative nausea and vomiting and/or induced by opioid analgesics.

At a dose of 0.15 mg/kg, droperidol induces a fall in mean blood pressure (MBP), due to a decrease in cardiac output in a first phase, and then subsequently due to a decrease in pre-load. These changes occur independently of any alteration in myocardial contractility or vascular resistance. Droperidol does not affect myocardial contractility or heart rate, therefore has no negative inotropic effect. Its weak α_1-adrenergic blockade can cause a modest hypotension and decreased peripheral vascular resistance and may decrease pulmonary arterial pressure (particularly if it is abnormally high). It may also reduce the incidence of epinephrine-induced arrhythmia, but it does not prevent other forms of cardiac arrhythmia.

Droperidol has a specific antiarrhythmic effect at a dose of 0.2 mg/kg by an effect on myocardial contractility (prolongation of the refractory period) and a decrease in blood pressure.

Two studies (one placebo-controlled and one comparative active treatment-controlled) performed in the general anaesthesia setting and designed to better identify the QTc changes associated with postoperative nausea and vomiting treatment by small dose of droperidol (0.625 and 1.25 mg intravenous, and 0.75 mg intravenous, respectively) identified a QT interval prolongation at 3-6 min after

Table 1

System Organ Class	Common ≥1/100 to < 1/10	Uncommon ≥1/1,000 to < 1/100	Rare ≥1/10,000 to < 1/1,000	Very Rare < 1/10,000	Not known (cannot be estimated from the available data)
Blood and lymphatic systems disorders				Blood dyscrasias	
Immune system disorders			Anaphylactic reaction; Angioneurotic oedema; Hypersensitivity		
Metabolism and nutrition disorders					Inappropriate anti-diuretic hormone secretion
Psychiatric disorders		Anxiety; Restlessness/ Akathisia;	Confusional states; Agitation	Dysphoria	Hallucinations
Nervous system disorders	Drowsiness	Dystonia; Oculogyration		Extra-pyramidal disorder; Convulsions; Tremor	Epileptic fits; Parkinson's disease; Psychomotor hyperactivity; Coma
Cardiac disorders		Tachycardia; Dizziness	Cardiac arrhythmias, including ventricular arrhythmias	Cardiac arrest	*Torsade de pointes*; Electrogram QT prolonged
Vascular disorders	Hypotension				Syncope
Respiratory, thoracic and mediastinal disorders					Broncho-spasm; Laryngospasm
Skin and subcutaneous system disorders			Rash		
General disorders and administration site conditions			Neuroleptic malignant syndrome (NMS)	Sudden death	

administration of 0.625 and 1.25 mg droperidol (respectively 15 ± 40 and 22 ± 41 ms), but these changes did not differ significantly from that seen with saline (12 ± 35 ms). There were no statistically significant differences amongst the droperidol and saline groups in the number of patients with greater than 10% prolongation in QTc versus baseline. There was no evidence of droperidol-induced QTc prolongation after surgery.

No ectopic heartbeats were reported from the electrocardiographic records or 12-lead recordings during the perioperative period. The comparative active-treatment study with 0.75 mg intravenous droperidol identified a significant QTc interval prolongation (maximal of 17 ± 9 ms at the second minute after droperidol injection when compared with pre-treatment QTc measurement), with the QTc interval significantly lower after the 90th minute.

5.2 Pharmacokinetic properties

The action of a single intravenous dose commences 2-3 minutes following administration. The tranquillising and sedative effects tend to persist for 2 to 4 hours, although alertness may be affected for up to 12 hours.

Distribution

Following intravenous administration, plasma concentrations fall rapidly during the first 15 minutes. Plasma protein binding amounts to 85 – 90 %. The distribution volume is approximately 1.5 l/kg.

Metabolism

Droperidol is extensively metabolised in the liver, and undergoes oxidation, dealkylation, demethylation and hydroxylation by cytochrome P450 isoenzymes 1A2 and 3A4, and to a lesser extent by 2C19. The metabolites are devoid of neuroleptic activity.

Elimination

Elimination occurs mainly through metabolism; 75% are excreted via the kidneys. Only 1% of the active substance is excreted unchanged with urine, and 11% with faeces. Plasma clearance is 0.8 (0.4 - 1.8) l/min. The elimination half-life ($t_{1/2\beta}$) is 134 ± 13 min.

5.3 Preclinical safety data

Non-clinical data reveal no special hazard for humans based on conventional studies of repeated dose toxicity, carcinogenic potential, and reproductive toxicity.

Droperidol was not mutagenic *in vitro* in an Ames test using 5 bacterial strains and was negative *in vivo* for induction of micronuclei in a rat bone marrow test following intravenous injection. In an *in vitro* test using L5178Y mouse lymphoma cells, there was no significant mutagenic activity in either of the two independent assays without metabolic activation (-S9), but a biologically significant positive result in the second assay with S9. Within this class of compounds conflicting results are found in reported studies (haloperidol) and it is not possible to conclude whether the positive gene mutation result in the recent *in vitro* mouse lymphoma assay with droperidol could represent a class effect.

Electrophysiological *in vitro* and *in vivo* studies indicate an overall risk of droperidol to prolong the QT interval in humans.

In humans, the free peak plasma concentration estimated above is approximately 4-fold higher to 25-fold lower than the droperidol concentrations affecting the endpoints examined in the different *in vitro* and *in vivo* test systems used to assess the impact of this drug on cardiac repolarisation. Plasma levels fall by about one order of magnitude over the first twenty minutes after administration.

6. PHARMACEUTICAL PARTICULARS

6.1 List of excipients

Mannitol

Tartaric acid

Sodium hydroxide (for pH adjustment)

Water for injections

6.2 Incompatibilities

Incompatible with barbiturates. This medicinal product must not be mixed with other medicinal products except those mentioned in section 6.6.

6.3 Shelf life

Unopened: 3 years.

After first opening: For immediate use.

Following dilution: Compatibility of droperidol with morphine sulphate in 0.9% sodium chloride (14 days at room temperature) has been demonstrated in plastic syringes. From a microbiological point of view, the diluted product should be used immediately. If not used immediately, in-use storage times and conditions prior to use are the responsibility of the user and would normally not be longer than 24 hours at 2 to 8 °C, unless dilution has taken place in controlled and validated aseptic conditions.

6.4 Special precautions for storage

Store in the original package.

6.5 Nature and contents of container

Type I amber glass ampoules containing 1 ml solution for injection, in packs of 5 and 10 ampoules.

Not all pack sizes may be marketed.

6.6 Special precautions for disposal and other handling

For single use only. Any unused solution should be discarded.

The solution should be inspected visually prior to use. Only clear and colourless solutions free from visible particles should be used.

For use in PCA: Draw droperidol and morphine into a syringe and make up the volume with 0.9% sodium chloride for injection.

Any unused product or waste material should be disposed of in accordance with local requirements.

7. MARKETING AUTHORISATION HOLDER

ProStrakan Ltd

Galabank Business Park

Galashiels

TD1 1QH

United Kingdom

Tel. +44 (0)1896 664000

8. MARKETING AUTHORISATION NUMBER(S)

PL 16508/0036

9. DATE OF FIRST AUTHORISATION/RENEWAL OF THE AUTHORISATION

28.01.2008

10. DATE OF REVISION OF THE TEXT

28.01.2008

11. LEGAL CLASSIFICATION

POM

Xylocaine 1% and 2% with Adrenaline

(AstraZeneca UK Limited)

1. NAME OF THE MEDICINAL PRODUCT

Xylocaine 1% with Adrenaline (Epinephrine) 1:200,000.

Xylocaine 2% with Adrenaline (Epinephrine) 1:200,000.

2. QUALITATIVE AND QUANTITATIVE COMPOSITION

Xylocaine 1% with Adrenaline (Epinephrine) 1:200,000:

Each ml of solution for injection contains lidocaine hydrochloride monohydrate Ph. Eur., equivalent to 10 mg of lidocaine hydrochloride anhydrous (200 mg per 20 ml vial), 5 micrograms of adrenaline (epinephrine) as the acid tartrate (100 micrograms per 20 ml vial).

Xylocaine 2% with Adrenaline (Epinephrine) 1:200,000:

Each ml of solution for injection contains lidocaine hydrochloride monohydrate Ph. Eur., equivalent to 20 mg of lidocaine hydrochloride anhydrous (400 mg per 20 ml vial), 5 micrograms of adrenaline (epinephrine) as the acid tartrate (100 micrograms per 20 ml vial).

For excipients see 6.1

3. PHARMACEUTICAL FORM

Solution for injection

4. CLINICAL PARTICULARS

4.1 Therapeutic indications

Xylocaine with Adrenaline is indicated for the production of local anaesthesia by the following techniques:

- Local infiltration

- Minor and major nerve blocks

4.2 Posology and method of administration

Adults and children above 12 years of age

The dosage is adjusted according to the response of the patient and the site of administration. The lowest concentration and smallest dose producing the required effect should be given (see section 4.4). The maximum single dose of Xylocaine when given with adrenaline is 500 mg.

The following table is a guide for the more commonly used techniques in the average adult. The figures reflect the expected average dose range needed. Standard textbooks should be consulted for factors affecting specific block techniques and for individual patient requirements.

The clinician's experience and knowledge of the patient's physical status are of importance in calculating the required dose. Elderly or debilitated patients require smaller doses, commensurate with age and physical status.

(see Table 1 on next page)

Please note: Preservative containing solutions i.e. those supplied in multidose vials should not be used for intrathecal and epidural anaesthesia or in doses more than 15 ml for other types of blockades.

In general, surgical anaesthesia requires the use of higher concentrations and doses. When a less intense block is required, the use of a lower concentration is indicated. The volume of drug used will affect the extent and spread of anaesthesia.

Table 1

Type of block	% Conc.	Each dose ml	Each dose mg	Indication
Field Block (e.g. minor nerve blocks and infiltration)				
Infiltration	1	up to 15	up to 150	Surgical operations
Intercostals (per nerve)	1	2-5 Max. 15 ml	20-50 Max. 150 mg	Surgical operations Postoperative pain and fractured ribs
Pudendal	1	10	100	Instrumental delivery
Major Nerve Block				
Paracervical (each side)	1	10	100	Surgical operations and dilatation of cervix Obstetric pain relief
Sciatic	2	15	300	Surgical operations

Care should be taken to prevent acute toxic reactions by avoiding intravascular injection. Careful aspiration before and during the injection is recommended. An accidental intravascular injection may be recognised by a temporary increase in heart rate. The main dose, should be injected slowly, at a rate of 100-200 mg/min, or in incremental doses, while keeping in constant verbal contact with the patient. If toxic symptoms occur, the injection should be stopped immediately.

4.3 Contraindications

Hypersensitivity to local anaesthetics of the amide type, or to any of the excipients.

Hypersensitivity to methyl and/or propyl parahydroxybenzoate (methyl-/propyl paraben), or to their metabolite para amino benzoic acid (PABA). Formulations of lidocaine containing parabens should be avoided in patients allergic to ester local anaesthetics or their metabolite PABA.

The use of a vasoconstrictor is contra-indicated for anaesthesia of fingers, toes, tip of nose, ears and penis.

4.4 Special warnings and precautions for use

Regional anaesthetic procedures should always be performed in a properly equipped and staffed area. Equipment and drugs necessary for monitoring and emergency resuscitation should be immediately available. When performing major blocks, or using large doses, an IV cannula should be inserted before the local anaesthetic is injected. Clinicians should have received adequate and appropriate training in the procedure to be performed and should be familiar with the diagnosis and treatment of side effects, systemic toxicity or other complications (see sections 4.8 and 4.9).

Xylocaine with Adrenaline should not be given intravenously.

The effect of local anaesthetics may be reduced if an injection is made into an inflamed or infected area.

Attempts should be made to optimise the patient's condition before major blocks.

Although regional anaesthesia is frequently the optimal anaesthetic technique, some patients require special attention in order to reduce the risk of dangerous side effects:

- Patients with epilepsy.
- Patients with impaired respiratory function.
- The elderly and patients in poor general condition.
- Patients with partial or complete heart conduction block - due to the fact that local anaesthetics may depress myocardial conduction.
- Patients with advanced liver disease or severe renal dysfunction.
- Patients treated with anti-arrhythmic drugs class III (e.g. amiodarone) should be under close surveillance and ECG monitoring considered, since cardiac effects may be additive (see section 4.5).
- Patients with acute porphyria. Xylocaine solution for injection is probably porphyrinogenic and should only be prescribed to patients with acute porphyria on strong or urgent indications. Appropriate precautions should be taken for all porphyric patients.

Certain local anaesthetic procedures may be associated with serious adverse reactions, regardless of the local anaesthetic drug used, e.g.:

- Injections in the head and neck regions may be made inadvertently into an artery, causing cerebral symptoms even at low doses.
- Paracervical block can sometimes cause foetal bradycardia/tachycardia, and careful monitoring of the foetal heart rate is necessary.

Solutions containing adrenaline should be used with caution in patients with hypertension, cardiac disease, cerebrovascular insufficiency hyperthyroidism, advanced diabetes and any other pathological condition that may be aggravated by the effects of adrenaline.

Xylocaine with adrenaline contains sodium metabisulphite, which may cause allergic reactions including anaphylactic symptoms and life-threatening or less severe asthmatic episodes in certain susceptible people. The overall prevalence of sulphite sensitivity in the general population is unknown and probably low. Sulphite sensitivity is seen more frequently in asthmatic than non-asthmatic people.

Preservative containing solutions, i.e. those supplied in multidose vials should not be used for intrathecal and epidural anaesthesia or in doses more than 15 ml for other types of blockades.

4.5 Interaction with other medicinal products and other forms of interaction

Lidocaine should be used with caution in patients receiving other local anaesthetics or agents structurally related to amide-type local anaesthetics e.g. certain anti-arrhythmics, such as mexilitine, since the systemic toxic effects are additive. Specific interaction studies with lidocaine and anti-arrhythmic drugs class III (e.g. amiodarone) have not been performed, but caution is advised (see also section 4.4).

Drugs that reduce the clearance of lidocaine (e.g. cimetidine or betablockers) may cause potentially toxic plasma concentrations when lidocaine is given in repeated high doses over a long time period. Such interactions should be of no clinical importance following short term treatment with lidocaine at recommended doses.

Solutions containing adrenaline should be used cautiously in patients taking tricyclic antidepressants, monoamine oxidase inhibitors or receiving potent general anaesthetic agents since severe, prolonged hypertension may be the result. In addition, the concurrent use of adrenaline-containing solutions and oxytocic drugs of the ergot type may cause severe, persistent hypertension and possibly cerebrovascular and cardiac accidents. Phenothiazines and butyrophenones may oppose the vasoconstrictor effects of adrenaline giving rise to hypotensive responses and tachycardia.

Solutions containing adrenaline should be used with caution in patients undergoing general anaesthesia with inhalation agents, such as halothane and enflurane, due to the risk of serious cardiac arrhythmias.

Non-cardioselective betablockers such as propranolol enhance the pressor effects of adrenaline, which may lead to severe hypertension and bradycardia.

4.6 Pregnancy and lactation

Although there is no evidence from animal studies of harm to the foetus, as with all drugs, Xylocaine should not be given during early pregnancy unless the benefits are considered to outweigh the risks.

The addition of adrenaline may potentially decrease uterine blood flow and contractility, especially after inadvertent injection into maternal blood vessels.

Foetal adverse effects due to local anaesthetics, such as foetal bradycardia, seem to be most apparent in paracervical block anaesthesia. Such effects may be due to high concentrations of anaesthetic reaching the foetus.

Lidocaine may enter the mother's milk, but in such small amounts that there is generally no risk of this affecting the neonate. It is not known whether adrenaline enters breast milk or not, but it is unlikely to affect the breast-fed child.

4.7 Effects on ability to drive and use machines

Besides the direct anaesthetic affect, local anaesthetics may have a very mild effect on mental function and co-ordination, even in the absence of overt CNS toxicity, and may temporarily impair locomotion and alertness.

4.8 Undesirable effects

In common with other local anaesthetics, adverse reactions to Xylocaine with Adrenaline are rare and are usually the result of excessively high blood concentrations due to inadvertent intravascular injection, excessive dosage, rapid absorption or occasionally to hypersensitivity, idiosyncrasy or diminished tolerance on the part of the patient. In such circumstances systemic effects occur involving the central nervous system and/or the cardiovascular system.

The following table gives a list of the frequencies of undesirable effects:

Common (>1/100 <1/10)	Vascular disorders: Hypotension, hypertension Gastrointestinal disorders: Nausea, vomiting Nervous system disorders: paraesthesia, dizziness Cardiac disorders: bradycardia
Uncommon (>1/1000 <1/100)	Nervous system disorders: Signs and symptoms of CNS toxicity (Convulsions, Numbness of tongue and Paraesthesia circumoral, Tinnitus, Tremor, Dysarthria, Hyperacusis, Visual disturbances, CNS depression)
Rare (<1/1000)	Cardiac disorders: Cardiac arrest, Cardiac arrhythmias Immune system disorders: Allergic reactions, Anaphylactic reaction Respiratory disorders: Respiratory depression Nervous system disorders: Neuropathy, peripheral nerve injury, Arachnoiditis Eye disorders: Diplopia

4.8.1 Acute systemic toxicity

Systemic toxic reactions primarily involve the central nervous system (CNS) and the cardiovascular system (CVS). Such reactions are caused by high blood concentrations of a local anaesthetic, which may appear due to (accidental) intravascular injection, overdose or exceptionally rapid absorption from highly vascularised areas (see section 4.9). CNS reactions are similar for all amide local anaesthetics, while cardiac reactions are more dependent on the drug, both quantitatively and qualitatively. Signs of toxicity in the central nervous system generally precede cardiovascular toxic effects, unless the patient is receiving a general anaesthetic or is heavily sedated with drugs such as benzodiazepine or barbiturate.

Central nervous system toxicity is a graded response with symptoms and signs of escalating severity. The first symptoms are usually, circumoral paraesthesia, numbness of the tongue, light-headedness, hyperacusis, tinnitus and visual disturbances. Dysarthria, muscular twitching or tremors are more serious and precede the onset of generalised convulsions. These signs must not be mistaken for a neurotic behaviour. Unconsciousness and grand mal convulsions may follow which may last from a few seconds to several minutes. Hypoxia and hypercarbia occur rapidly following convulsions due to the increased muscular activity, together with the interference with respiration and possible loss of functional airways. In severe cases apnoea may occur. Acidosis hyperkalaemia, hypocalcaemia and hypoxia increase and extend the toxic effects of local anaesthetics.

Recovery is due to redistribution of the local anaesthetic drug from the central nervous system and subsequent metabolism and excretion. Recovery may be rapid unless large amounts of the drug have been injected.

Cardiovascular system toxicity may be seen in severe cases and is generally preceded by signs of toxicity in the central nervous system. In patients under heavy sedation or receiving a general anaesthetic, prodromal CNS symptoms may be absent. Hypotension, bradycardia, arrhythmia and even cardiac arrest may occur as a result of high systemic concentrations of local anaesthetics, but in rare cases cardiac arrest has occurred without prodromal CNS effects.

In children, early signs of local anaesthetic toxicity may be difficult to detect in cases where the block is given during general anaesthesia.

4.8.2 Treatment of acute toxicity

If signs of acute systemic toxicity appear, injection of the local anaesthetic should be stopped immediately and CNS symptoms (convulsion, CNS depression) must promptly be treated with appropriate airway/respiratory support and the administration of anticonvulsant drugs.

If circulatory arrest should occur, immediate cardiopulmonary resuscitation should be instituted. Optimal oxygenation and ventilation and circulatory support as well as treatment of acidosis are of vital importance.

If cardiovascular depression occurs (hypotension, bradycardia), appropriate treatment with intravenous fluids, vasopressor, chronotropic and or inotropic agents should be considered. Children should be given doses commensurate with age and weight.

4.9 Overdose

Accidental intravascular injections of local anaesthetics may cause immediate (within seconds to a few minutes) systemic toxic reactions. In the event of overdose, systemic toxicity appears later (15–60 minutes after injection) due to the slower increase in local anaesthetic blood concentration (see section 4.8.1 and 4.8.2).

5. PHARMACOLOGICAL PROPERTIES

5.1 Pharmacodynamic properties

ATC code: N01B B52

Lidocaine is a local anaesthetic of the amide type. At high doses lidocaine has a quinidine like action on the myocardium i.e. cardiac depressant. All local anaesthetics stimulate the CNS and may produce anxiety, restlessness and tremors.

5.2 Pharmacokinetic properties

Lidocaine is readily absorbed from the gastro-intestinal tract, from mucous membranes and through damaged skin. It is rapidly absorbed from injection sites including muscle.

Elimination half-life is 2 hours.

Lidocaine undergoes first pass metabolism in the liver.

Less than 10% of a dose is excreted unchanged via the kidneys.

The speed of onset and duration of action of lidocaine are increased by the addition of a vasoconstrictor and absorption into the site of injection is reduced.

5.3 Preclinical safety data

Lidocaine and adrenaline are well-established active ingredients.

In animal studies, the signs and symptoms of toxicity noted after high doses of lidocaine are the results of effects on the central nervous and cardiovascular systems. No drug related adverse effects were seen in the reproduction toxicity studies, neither did lidocaine show any mutagenic potential in either in vitro or in vivo mutagenicity tests. Cancer studies have not been performed with lidocaine, due to the area and duration of therapeutic use for this drug.

6. PHARMACEUTICAL PARTICULARS

6.1 List of excipients

Sodium chloride, sodium metabisulphite, methylparahydroxybenzoate, sodium hydroxide, hydrochloric acid and water for injections.

6.2 Incompatibilities

None

6.3 Shelf life

Two years.

Use within 3 days of first opening.

6.4 Special precautions for storage

Store between 2°C and 8°C.

6.5 Nature and contents of container

Multiple dose vials - 20 ml and 50 ml.

6.6 Special precautions for disposal and other handling

None

7. MARKETING AUTHORISATION HOLDER

AstraZeneca UK Ltd,

600 Capability Green,

Luton, LU1 3LU, UK.

8. MARKETING AUTHORISATION NUMBER(S)

Xylocaine 1% with Adrenaline (Epinephrine) 1:200,000: PL 17901/0174

Xylocaine 2% with Adrenaline (Epinephrine) 1:200,000: PL 17901/0175

9. DATE OF FIRST AUTHORISATION/RENEWAL OF THE AUTHORISATION

21st May 2002

10. DATE OF REVISION OF THE TEXT

7th July 2009

Xylocaine Spray

(AstraZeneca UK Limited)

1. NAME OF THE MEDICINAL PRODUCT

Xylocaine Spray

2. QUALITATIVE AND QUANTITATIVE COMPOSITION

Lidocaine Ph. Eur. 10 mg/dose.

For excipients see 6.1.

3. PHARMACEUTICAL FORM

Topical anaesthetic pump spray.

4. CLINICAL PARTICULARS

4.1 Therapeutic indications

For the prevention of pain associated with the following procedures:

Otorhinolaryngology

– Puncture of the maxillary sinus and minor surgical procedures in the nasal cavity, pharynx and epipharynx.

– Paracentesis.

Obstetrics

During the final stages of delivery and before episiotomy and perineal suturing as supplementary pain control.

Introduction of instruments and catheters into the respiratory and digestive tract

Provides surface anaesthesia for the oropharyngeal and tracheal areas to reduce reflex activity, attenuate haemodynamic response and to facilitate insertion of the tube or the passage of instruments during endotracheal intubation, laryngoscopy, bronchoscopy and oesophagoscopy.

Dental practice

Before injections, dental impressions, X-ray photography, removal of calculus.

4.2 Posology and method of administration

As with any local anaesthetic, reactions and complications are best averted by employing the minimal effective dosage. Debilitated or elderly patients and children should be given doses commensurate with their age and physical condition.

Xylocaine Spray should not be used on cuffs of endotracheal tubes (ETT) made of plastic (see also section 4.4).

Each activation of the metered dose valve delivers 10 mg lidocaine base. It is unnecessary to dry the site prior to application. No more than 20 spray applications should be used in any adult to produce the desired anaesthetic effect.

The number of sprays depend on the extent of the area to be anaesthetised.

– Dental practice

1–5 applications to the mucous membranes.

– Otorhinolaryngology

3 applications for puncture of the maxillary sinus.

– During delivery

Up to 20 applications (200 mg lidocaine base).

– Introduction of instruments and catheters into the respiratory and digestive tract

Up to 20 applications (200 mg lidocaine base) for procedures in pharynx, larynx, and trachea.

4.3 Contraindications

Known history of hypersensitivity to local anaesthetics of the amide-type or to other components of the spray solution.

4.4 Special warnings and precautions for use

Absorption from wound surfaces and mucous membranes is relatively high, especially in the bronchial tree. Xylocaine Spray should be used with caution in patients with traumatised mucosa and/or sepsis in the region of the proposed application.

If the dose or site of administration is likely to result in high blood levels, lidocaine, in common with other local anaesthetics, should be used with caution in patients with epilepsy, cardiovascular disease and heart failure, impaired cardiac conduction, bradycardia, severe renal dysfunction, impaired hepatic function and in severe shock. Lidocaine should also be used with caution in the elderly and patients in poor general health.

In paralysed patients under general anaesthesia, higher blood concentrations may occur than in spontaneously breathing patients. Unparalysed patients are more likely to swallow a large proportion of the dose, which then undergoes considerable first-pass hepatic metabolism following absorption from the gut.

The oropharyngeal use of topical anaesthetic agents may interfere with swallowing and thus enhance the danger of aspiration. This is particularly important in children because of their frequency of eating. Numbness of the tongue or buccal mucosa may increase the danger of biting trauma.

Avoid contact with the eyes.

Patients treated with antiarrhythmic drugs class III (e.g. amiodarone) should be under close surveillance and ECG monitoring considered, since cardiac effects may be additive.

Xylocaine Spray should not be used on cuffs of endotracheal tubes (ETT) made of plastic. Lidocaine base in contact with both PVC and non-PVC cuffs of endotracheal tubes may cause damage of the cuff. This damage is described as pinholes, which may cause leakage that could lead to pressure loss in the cuff.

Xylocaine Spray is probably porphyrinogenic and should only be prescribed to patients with acute porphyria on strong or urgent indications. Appropriate precautions should be taken for all porphyric patients.

4.5 Interaction with other medicinal products and other forms of interaction

Lidocaine should be used with caution in patients receiving other local anaesthetics or agents structurally related to amide-type local anaesthetics e.g. antiarrhythmic drugs such as mexiletine, since the toxic effects are additive.

Specific interaction studies with lidocaine and antiarrhythmic drugs class III (e.g. amiodarone) have not been performed, but caution is advised (see also section 4.4).

Drugs that reduce the clearance of lidocaine (e.g. cimetidine or beta-blockers) may cause potentially toxic plasma concentrations when lidocaine is given in repeated high doses over a long time period. Such interactions should therefore be of no clinical importance following short-term treatment with lidocaine (e.g. Xylocaine Spray) at recommended doses.

4.6 Pregnancy and lactation

There is no, or inadequate evidence of safety of the drug in human pregnancy but it has been in wide use for many years without apparent ill consequence, and animal studies have shown no hazard. If drug therapy is needed in pregnancy, this drug can be used if there is no safer alternative.

Lidocaine enters the mother's milk, but in such small quantities that there is generally no risk of the child being affected at therapeutic dose levels.

4.7 Effects on ability to drive and use machines

Depending on the dose, local anaesthetics may have a very mild effect on mental function and may temporarily impair locomotion and co-ordination.

4.8 Undesirable effects

In extremely rare cases amide-type local anaesthetic preparations have been associated with allergic reactions (in the most severe instances anaphylactic shock).

Local irritation at the application site has been described. Following application to laryngeal mucosa before endotracheal intubation, reversible symptoms such as "sore throat", "hoarseness" and "loss of voice" have been reported. The use of Xylocaine pump spray provides surface anaesthesia during an endotracheal procedure but does not prevent post-intubation soreness.

Systemic adverse reactions are rare and may result from high plasma levels due to excessive dosage or rapid absorption (e.g. following application to areas below the vocal chords) or from hypersensitivity, idiosyncrasy or reduced tolerance on the part of the patient. Such reactions involve the central nervous system and/or the cardiovascular system.

CNS reactions are excitatory and/or depressant and may be characterised by nervousness, dizziness, convulsions, unconsciousness and possibly respiratory arrest. The excitatory reactions may be very brief or may not occur at all, in which case the first manifestations of toxicity may be drowsiness, merging into unconsciousness and respiratory arrest.

Cardiovascular reactions are depressant and may be characterised by hypotension, myocardial depression, bradycardia and possibly cardiac arrest.

4.9 Overdose

Acute systemic toxicity

Toxic reactions originate mainly in the central nervous and the cardiovascular systems.

Central nervous system toxicity is a graded response with symptoms and signs of escalating severity. The first symptoms are circumoral paraesthesia, numbness of the tongue, light-headedness, hyperacusis and tinnitus. Visual disturbance and muscular tremors are more serious and precede the onset of generalized convulsions. Unconsciousness and grand mal convulsions may follow, which may last from a few seconds to several minutes. Hypoxia and hypercarbia occur rapidly following convulsions due to the increased muscular activity, together with the interference with normal respiration. In severe cases, apnoea may occur. Acidosis increases the toxic effects of local anaesthetics.

Cardiovascular effects are only seen in cases with high systemic concentrations. Severe hypotension, bradycardia, arrhythmia and cardiovascular collapse may be the result in such cases.

Cardiovascular toxic effects are generally preceded by signs of toxicity in the central nervous system, unless the patient is receiving a general anaesthetic or is heavily sedated with drugs such as a benzodiazepine or barbiturate.

Recovery is due to redistribution and metabolism of the local anaesthetic drug from the central nervous system. Recovery may be rapid unless large amounts of the drug have been administered.

Treatment of acute toxicity

The treatment of a patient with toxic manifestations consists of ensuring adequate ventilation and arresting convulsions. Ventilation should be maintained with oxygen by assisted or controlled respiration as required.

An anticonvulsant should be given i.v. if the convulsions do not stop spontaneously in 15–30 sec. Thiopentone sodium 1–3 mg/kg i.v. will abort the convulsions rapidly. Alternatively, diazepam 0.1 mg/kg body-weight i.v. may be used, although its action will be slow. Prolonged convulsions may jeopardise the patient's ventilation and oxygenation. If so, injection of a muscle relaxant (e.g. succinylcholine 1 mg/kg body-weight) will facilitate ventilation, and oxygenation can be controlled. Early endotracheal intubation must be considered in such situations.

If cardiovascular depression is evident (hypotension, bradycardia), ephedrine 5–10 mg i.v. should be given and repeated, if necessary, after 2–3 minutes.

Should circulatory arrest occur, immediate cardiopulmonary resuscitation should be instituted. Optimal oxygenation and ventilation and circulatory support as well as treatment of acidosis are of vital importance, since hypoxia and acidosis will increase the systemic toxicity of local anaesthetics.

Children should be given doses commensurate with their age and weight.

5. PHARMACOLOGICAL PROPERTIES

5.1 Pharmacodynamic properties

ATC code: N01B B02

Lidocaine, like other local anaesthetics, causes a reversible blockade of impulse propagation along nerve fibres by preventing the inward movement of sodium ions through the nerve membrane. Local anaesthetics of the amide-type are thought to act within the sodium channels of the nerve membrane.

Local anaesthetic drugs may also have similar effects on excitable membranes in the brain and myocardium. If excessive amounts of drug reach the systemic circulation rapidly, symptoms and signs of toxicity will appear, emanating from the central nervous and cardiovascular systems.

Central nervous system toxicity usually precedes the cardiovascular effects since it occurs at lower plasma concentrations. Direct effects of local anaesthetics on the heart include slow conduction, negative inotropism and eventually cardiac arrest.

5.2 Pharmacokinetic properties

Lidocaine is absorbed following topical administration to mucous membranes; its rate and extent of absorption being dependent upon the concentration and total dose administered, the specific site of application, and duration of exposure. In general, the rate of absorption of local anaesthetic agents following topical application is most rapid after intratracheal and bronchial administration. Lidocaine is also well absorbed from the gastrointestinal tract, although little of the intact drug appears in the circulation because of biotransformation in the liver.

The plasma protein binding of lidocaine is dependent on the drug concentration, and the fraction bound decreases with increasing concentration. At concentrations of 1 to 4 microgram of free base per ml, 60 to 80 percent of lidocaine is protein-bound. Binding is also dependent on the plasma concentration of the alpha-1-acid glycoprotein.

Lidocaine crosses the blood-brain and placental barriers, presumably by passive diffusion.

Lidocaine is metabolised rapidly by the liver, and metabolites and unchanged drug are excreted by the kidneys. Biotransformation includes oxidative N-dealkylation, ring hydroxylation, cleavage of the amide linkage and conjugation. N-dealkylation, a major pathway of biotransformation, yields the metabolites monoethylglycinexylidide and glycinexylidide. The pharmacological/toxicological actions of these metabolites are similar to, but less potent than, those of lidocaine. Approximately 90% of lidocaine administered is excreted in the form of various metabolites, and less than 10% is excreted unchanged. The primary metabolite in urine is a conjugate of 4-hydroxy-2,6-dimethylaniline.

The elimination half-life of lidocaine following an intravenous bolus injection is typically 1.5 to 2.0 hours. Because of the rapid rate at which lidocaine is metabolised, any condition that affects liver function may alter lidocaine kinetics. The half-life may be prolonged two-fold or more in patients with liver dysfunction. Renal dysfunction does not affect lidocaine kinetics but may increase the accumulation of metabolites.

Factors such as acidosis and the use of CNS stimulants and depressants affect the CNS levels of lidocaine required to produce overt systemic effects. Objective adverse manifestations become increasingly apparent with increasing venous plasma levels above 6.0 microgram free base per ml.

5.3 Preclinical safety data

Lidocaine is a well-established active ingredient.

6. PHARMACEUTICAL PARTICULARS

6.1 List of excipients

Ethanol, Macrogol 400, Essence of Banana, Menthol natural, Saccharin and Water purified.

6.2 Incompatibilities

None known.

6.3 Shelf life

3 years.

6.4 Special precautions for storage

Do not store above 25°C. During storage at temperatures below +8°C precipitation may occur. The precipitate dissolves on warming up to room temperature.

6.5 Nature and contents of container

50 ml spray bottles (approx. 500 spray doses) with a metering valve with applicator.

Each depression of the metered valve delivers 10 mg lidocaine base. The contents of the spray bottles are sufficient to provide approximately 500 sprays.

6.6 Special precautions for disposal and other handling

The spray nozzle is bent to ensure correct spray function. Do not try to alter the shape as this could affect its performance.

The nozzle must not be shortened, as it will affect the spray function.

To clean the nozzle, submerge in boiling water for 5 minutes.

7. MARKETING AUTHORISATION HOLDER

AstraZeneca UK Ltd.,

600 Capability Green,

Luton, LU1 3LU, UK.

8. MARKETING AUTHORISATION NUMBER(S)

PL 17901/0177

9. DATE OF FIRST AUTHORISATION/RENEWAL OF THE AUTHORISATION

7th May 2002

10. DATE OF REVISION OF THE TEXT

27th March 2008

Xyloproct Ointment

(AstraZeneca UK Limited)

1. NAME OF THE MEDICINAL PRODUCT

Xyloproct Ointment

2. QUALITATIVE AND QUANTITATIVE COMPOSITION

Composition for: 100 g:

Lidocaine 5 g

Hydrocortisone Acetate micro Ph. Eur. 0.275 g

For excipients, see 6.1

3. PHARMACEUTICAL FORM

Ointment.

4. CLINICAL PARTICULARS

4.1 Therapeutic indications

For the relief of symptoms such as anal and peri-anal pruritus, pain and inflammation associated with haemorrhoids, anal fissure, fistulas and proctitis. Pruritus vulva.

4.2 Posology and method of administration

Route of administration: Topical.

To be applied several times daily according to the severity of the condition. For intrarectal use, apply the ointment with the special applicator. Cleanse the applicator thoroughly after use.

A daily dose of 6 g ointment is well within safety limits. The duration of treatment may vary between ten days and three weeks. If the treatment is prolonged, a free interval can be recommended, especially if it is suspected that irritation due to lidocaine or hydrocortisone has occurred. If the local irritation disappears after the cessation of treatment, the possibility of sensitivity to lidocaine or hydrocortisone can be investigated, e.g. by a patch test.

Debilitated or elderly patients and children should be given doses commensurate with their age, weight and physical condition.

4.3 Contraindications

Known hypersensitivity to local anaesthetics of the amide type or any of the other ingredients. Use on atrophic skin. Xyloproct Ointment should not be used in patients with untreated infections of bacterial, viral, pathogenic fungal or parasitic origin. Xyloproct should not be used by patients being treated with a class III anti-arrhythmic drug outside of hospital (see sections 4.4 and 4.5).

4.4 Special warnings and precautions for use

Xyloproct is intended for use for limited periods. Excessive dosage of lidocaine or short intervals between doses, may result in high plasma levels of lidocaine and serious adverse effects. Patients should be instructed to strictly adhere to recommended dosage.

Hospitalised patients treated with anti-arrhythmic drugs class III (e.g. amiodarone or sotalol) should be kept under close surveillance and ECG monitoring considered, since cardiac effects may be additive (see sections 4.3 and 4.5).

Appropriate antibacterial, antiviral or antifungal therapy should be given with Xyloproct if infection is present at the site of application.

The possibility of malignancy should be excluded before use.

If irritation or rectal bleeding develops treatment should be discontinued.

When using the special applicator, care should be taken to avoid instillation of excessive amounts of Xyloproct Ointment into the rectum. This is of particular importance in infants and children.

Systemic absorption of lidocaine may occur from the rectum, and large doses may result in CNS side-effects. On rare occasions convulsions have occurred in children.

Prolonged and excessive use of hydrocortisone use may produce systemic corticosteroid effects or local effects such as skin atrophy. With the recommended dosage systemic effects of hydrocortisone are unlikely.

Xyloproct ointment is possibly porphyrinogenic and should only be prescribed to patients with acute porphyria when no safer alternative is available. Appropriate precautions should be taken for vulnerable patients.

4.5 Interaction with other medicinal products and other forms of interaction

Lidocaine should be used with caution in patients receiving anti-arrhythmic drugs, local anaesthetics or agents structurally related to local anaesthetics, since the toxic effects of these compounds are additive (see sections 4.3 and 4.4).

4.6 Pregnancy and lactation

Do not use in pregnancy unless considered essential by the physician.

Lidocaine and hydrocortisone acetate are excreted into breast milk but in such small quantities that adverse effects on the child are unlikely at therapeutic doses.

4.7 Effects on ability to drive and use machines

Depending on the dose local anaesthetics may have a very mild effect on mental function and coordination even in the absence of overt CNS toxicity and may temporarily impair locomotion and alertness. With the recommended doses of Xyloproct adverse effects on the CNS are unlikely.

4.8 Undesirable effects

Contact sensitivity to lidocaine has been reported after perianal use. Contact sensitivity may also occur after the use of topical hydrocortisone.

In extremely rare cases amide-type local anaesthetic preparations have been associated with allergic reactions (in the most severe instances anaphylactic shock).

4.9 Overdose

When using the special applicator care should be taken to avoid instillation of excessive amounts of Xyloproct Ointment into the rectum. This is of particular importance in infants and children.

Systemic absorption of lidocaine may occur from the rectum, and large doses may result in CNS side effects. On rare occasions convulsions have occurred in children.

5. PHARMACOLOGICAL PROPERTIES

5.1 Pharmacodynamic properties

ATC code: C05A A01

Lidocaine exerts a local anaesthetic effect by stabilising the neural membrane and preventing the initiation and conduction of nerve impulses.

Hydrocortisone acetate belongs to the mild group of corticosteroids and is effective because of its anti-inflammatory and anti-pruritic action.

5.2 Pharmacokinetic properties

The onset of action of lidocaine is 3–5 minutes on mucous membranes. Lidocaine can be absorbed following application to mucous membranes with metabolism taking place in the liver. Metabolites and unchanged drug are excreted in the urine.

Absorption of hydrocortisone may occur from normal intact skin and mucous membranes. Corticosteroids are metabolised mainly in the liver but also in the kidney, and are excreted in the urine.

5.3 Preclinical safety data

Lidocaine and hydrocortisone acetate are well established active ingredients.

In animal studies the toxicity noted after high doses of lidocaine consisted of effects on the central nervous and cardiovascular systems. No drug-related adverse effects were seen in reproduction toxicity studies, neither did lidocaine show a mutagenic potential in either in vitro or in vivo mutagenicity tests. Cancer studies have not been performed with lidocaine, due to the area and duration of therapeutic use for this drug.

6. PHARMACEUTICAL PARTICULARS

6.1 List of excipients

Zinc oxide

Aluminium acetate

Stearyl alcohol

Cetyl alcohol

Water purified

Macrogol (3350 and 400)

6.2 Incompatibilities

None known

6.3 Shelf life

The shelf-life of this product is 2 years when stored between 2°C and 8°C and 2 months when stored up to 25°C.

6.4 Special precautions for storage

Store at 2°C–8°C (in a refrigerator). The patient may store the product at temperatures up to 25°C for 2 months whilst in use. The remaining ointment should then be discarded.

6.5 Nature and contents of container

Aluminium tube 20 g.

6.6 Special precautions for disposal and other handling

None

7. MARKETING AUTHORISATION HOLDER

AstraZeneca UK Ltd.,

600 Capability Green,

Luton,

LU1 3LU,

UK.

8. MARKETING AUTHORISATION NUMBER(S)

PL 17901/0179

9. DATE OF FIRST AUTHORISATION/RENEWAL OF THE AUTHORISATION

18th March 2002

10. DATE OF REVISION OF THE TEXT

05th June 2008

Xyrem 500 mg/ml oral solution

(UCB Pharma Limited)

1. NAME OF THE MEDICINAL PRODUCT

Xyrem 500 mg/ml oral solution.▼

2. QUALITATIVE AND QUANTITATIVE COMPOSITION

One ml Xyrem contains 500 mg of sodium oxybate.

For a full list of excipients, see section 6.1.

3. PHARMACEUTICAL FORM

Oral solution.

The oral solution is clear to slightly opalescent.

4. CLINICAL PARTICULARS

4.1 Therapeutic indications

Treatment of narcolepsy with cataplexy in adult patients.

4.2 Posology and method of administration

Treatment should be initiated by and remain under the guidance of a physician experienced in the treatment of sleep disorders. Due to the well known potential of abuse of sodium oxybate, physicians should evaluate patients for a history of drug abuse (see section 4.4).

The recommended starting dose is 4.5 g/day sodium oxybate divided into two equal doses of 2.25 g/dose. The dose should be titrated to effect based on efficacy and tolerability (see Section 4.4) up to a maximum of 9 g/day divided into two equal doses of 4.5g/dose by adjusting up or down in dose increments of 1.5 g/day (i.e. 0.75 g/dose). A minimum of one to two weeks is recommended between dosage increments. The dose of 9g/day should not be exceeded due to the possible occurrence of severe symptoms at doses of 18 g/day or above (see section 4.4).

A 10ml measuring syringe and two 90 ml dosing cups are provided with Xyrem. Each dose of Xyrem must be diluted with 60 ml of water in the dosing cup prior to ingestion.

Single doses of 4.5g should not be given unless the patient has been titrated previously to that dose level.

Because food significantly reduces the bioavailability of sodium oxybate, patients should eat at least several (2-3) hours before taking the first dose of Xyrem at bedtime. Patients should always observe the same timing of dosing in relation to meals.

Using Xyrem

Xyrem should be taken orally upon getting into bed and again between 2.5 to 4 hours later. It is recommended that both doses of Xyrem should be made up at the same time upon retiring to bed.

Xyrem is provided for use with a graduated measuring syringe and dosing cup with child resistant cap. Each measured dose of Xyrem must be dispensed into the dosing cup and diluted with 60 ml of water prior to ingestion.

Discontinuation of Xyrem

The discontinuation effects of sodium oxybate have not been systematically evaluated in controlled clinical trials (see Section 4.4).

If the patient stops medication for more than 14 consecutive days, titration should be restarted from the lowest dose

Patients with hepatic impairment

The starting dose should be halved in patients with hepatic impairment, and response to dose increments monitored closely (see section 4.4).

Patients with renal impairment

Patients with impaired renal function should consider a dietary recommendation to reduce sodium intake (see section 4.4).

Elderly patients

Elderly patients should be monitored closely for impaired motor and/or cognitive function when taking Sodium oxybate (see section 4.4).

Paediatric patients

Safety and effectiveness in children and adolescents has not been established, therefore use in patients under 18 years of age is not recommended.

4.3 Contraindications

Hypersensitivity to sodium oxybate or to any of the excipients.

Sodium oxybate is contraindicated in patients with succinic semialdehyde dehydrogenase deficiency.

Sodium oxybate is contraindicated in patients being treated with opoids or barbiturates.

4.4 Special warnings and precautions for use

Xyrem has the potential to induce respiratory depression

Abuse potential and dependance

The active substance in Xyrem is sodium oxybate, which is as the sodium salt of gamma hydroxybutyrate (GHB), a CNS depressant active substance with well known abuse potential. Physicians should evaluate patients for a history of drug abuse and follow such patients closely.

There have been case reports of dependence after illicit use of GHB at frequent repeated doses (18 to 250 g/day) in excess of the therapeutic dose range. Whilst there is no clear evidence of emergence of dependence in patients taking sodium oxybate at therapeutic doses, this possibility cannot be excluded.

CNS depression

The combined use of alcohol or any CNS depressant drug with sodium oxybate may result in potentiation of the CNS-depressant effects of sodium oxybate. Therefore, patients should be warned against the use of alcohol in conjunction with sodium oxybate.

Patients with porphyria

Sodium oxybate is considered to be unsafe in patients with porphyria because it has been shown to be porphyrogenic in animals or in-vitro systems.

Respiratory depression

Sodium oxybate also has the potential to induce respiratory depression. Apnoea and respiratory depression have been observed in a fasting healthy subject after a single intake of 4.5g (twice the recommended starting dose). Patients should be questioned regarding signs of CNS or respiratory depression. Special caution should be observed in patients with an underlying respiratory disorder.

Approximately 80% of patients who received sodium oxybate during clinical trials maintained CNS stimulant use. Whether this affected respiration during the night is unknown. Before increasing the sodium oxybate dose (see section 4.2), prescribers should be aware that sleep apnoea occurs in up to 50% of patients with narcolepsy.

Benzodiazepines

Given the possibility of increasing the risk of respiratory depression, the concomitant use of benzodiazepines and Xyrem should be avoided.

Neuropsychiatric events

Patients may become confused while being treated with sodium oxybate. If this occurs, they should be evaluated fully, and appropriate intervention considered on an individual basis. Other neuropsychiatric events include psychosis, paranoia, hallucinations, and agitation. The emergence of thought disorders and/or behavioural abnormalities when patients are treated with sodium oxybate requires careful and immediate evaluation.

The emergence of depression when patients are treated with sodium oxybate requires careful and immediate evaluation. Patients with a previous history of a depressive illness and/or suicide attempt should be monitored especially carefully for the emergence of depressive symptoms while taking sodium oxybate.

If a patient experiences urinary or faecal incontinence during sodium oxybate therapy, the prescriber should consider pursuing investigations to rule out underlying aetiologies.

Sleepwalking has been reported in patients treated in clinical trials with sodium oxybate. It is unclear if some or all of these episodes correspond to true somnambulism (a parasomnia occurring during non-REM sleep) or to any other specific medical disorder. The risk of injury or self-harm should be borne in mind in any patient with sleepwalking. Therefore, episodes of sleepwalking should be fully evaluated and appropriate interventions considered.

Sodium intake

Patients taking sodium oxybate will have an additional daily intake of sodium that ranges from 0.82g (for a 4.5g/day Xyrem dose) to 1.6g (for a 9g/day Xyrem dose). A dietary recommendation to reduce sodium intake should be carefully considered in the management of patients with heart failure, hypertension or compromised renal function. (see section 4.2).

Patients with compromised liver function

Patients with compromised liver function will have an increased elimination half-life and systemic exposure to sodium oxybate (see Section 5.2). The starting dose should therefore be halved in such patients, and response to dose increments monitored closely (see section 4.2).

Elderly

There is very limited experience with sodium oxybate in the elderly. Therefore, elderly patients should be monitored closely for impaired motor and/or cognitive function when taking sodium oxybate.

Childhood and adolescence

Safety and effectiveness in children and adolescents has not been established, therefore use in patients under 18 years of age is not recommended.

Epileptic patients

Seizures have been observed in patients treated with sodium oxybate. In patients with epilepsy, the safety and efficacy of sodium oxybate has not been established, therefore use is not recommended.

Rebound effects and withdrawal syndrome

The discontinuation effects of sodium oxybate have not been systematically evaluated in controlled clinical trials. In some patients, cataplexy may return at a higher frequency on cessation of sodium oxybate therapy, however this may be due to the normal variability of the disease. Although the clinical trial experience with sodium oxybate in narcolepsy/cataplexy patients at therapeutic doses does not show clear evidence of a withdrawal syndrome, in rare cases, events such as insomnia, headache, anxiety, dizziness, sleep disorder, somnolence, hallucination, and psychotic disorders were observed after GHB discontinuation.

4.5 Interaction with other medicinal products and other forms of interaction

The combined use of alcohol with sodium oxybate may result in potentiation of the central nervous system-depressant effects of sodium oxybate. Patients should be warned against the use of any alcoholic beverages in conjunction with sodium oxybate.

Sodium oxybate should not be used in combination with sedative hypnotics or other CNS depressants.

Drug interaction studies in healthy adults demonstrated no pharmacokinetic interactions between sodium oxybate and protriptyline hydrochloride (an antidepressant), zolpidem tartrate (a hypnotic), and modafinil (a stimulant). However, pharmacodynamic interactions with these drugs have not been assessed.

The co-administration of omeprazole (a drug that alters gastric pH) has no clinically significant effect on the pharmacokinetics of sodium oxybate. The dosage of sodium oxybate therefore does not require adjustment when given concomitantly with proton pump inhibitors.

Studies *in vitro* with pooled human liver microsomes indicate that sodium oxybate does not significantly inhibit the activities of the human isoenzymes (see section 5.2).

Since sodium oxybate is metabolised by GHB dehydrogenase there is a potential risk of an interaction with drugs that stimulate or inhibit this enzyme (e.g. valproate, phenytoin or ethosuximide). No interaction studies have been conducted in human subjects

Sodium oxybate has been administered concomitantly with CNS stimulant agents in approximately 80 % of patients in clinical studies. Whether this affected respiration during the night is unknown.

Antidepressants have been used in the treatment of cataplexy. A possible additive effect of antidepressants and sodium oxybate cannot be excluded. The rate of adverse events have increased when sodium oxybate is co-administered with tricyclic antidepressants.

4.6 Pregnancy and lactation

Pregnancy

Animal studies have shown no evidence of teratogenicity but embryolethality was seen in both rat and rabbit studies (see section 5.3).

There are no adequate data on the use of sodium oxybate during the first trimester of pregnancy. Limited data from pregnant patients during second and third trimester indicate no malformative nor foeto/neonatal toxicity of sodium oxybate.

Sodium oxybate is not recommended during pregnancy.

Lactation

It is not known whether sodium oxybate is excreted into breast milk. Breastfeeding is not recommended when treating with Xyrem.

4.7 Effects on ability to drive and use machines

Sodium oxybate has a major influence on the ability to drive and use machines.

For at least 6 hours after taking sodium oxybate, patients must not undertake activities requiring complete mental alertness or motor co-ordination, such as operating machinery or driving.

When patients first start taking sodium oxybate, until they know whether this medicinal product will still have some carryover effect on them the next day, they should use extreme care while driving a car, operating heavy machines, or performing any other task that could be dangerous or require full mental alertness.

4.8 Undesirable effects

The most commonly reported adverse drug reactions are dizziness, nausea, and headache, all occurring in 10 % to 20 % of patients.

Frequency estimate: very common ($\geqslant$ 1/10); common ($\geqslant$ 1/100 to < 1/10); uncommon ($\geqslant$ 1/1000 to < 1/100); rare ($\geqslant$ 1/10,000 to < 1/1000); very rare (< 1/10,000); not known (cannot be estimated from the available data).

Immune system disorders:

Not known: hypersensitivity

Metabolism and nutrition disorders:

Common: anorexia

Psychiatric disorders:

Common: abnormal dreams, confusion, disorientation, nightmares, sleepwalking, depression, sleep disorder, cataplexy, anxiety, insomnia, middle insomnia, nervousness

Uncommon: psychosis, paranoia, abnormal thinking, hallucination, agitation, suicide attempt, initial insomnia

Not known: suicidal ideation

Nervous system disorders:

Very common: dizziness, headache

Common: sleep paralysis, somnolence, tremor, balance disorder, disturbance in attention, hypoaesthesia, paraesthesia, sedation

Uncommon: myoclonus, amnesia, restless legs syndrome

Not known: convulsion

Eye disorders:

Common: blurred vision

Vascular disorders:

Common: hypertension

Respiratory, thoracic and mediastinal disorders:

Common: dyspnoea, snoring

Not known: respiratory depression

Gastrointestinal disorders:

Very common: nausea (the frequency of nausea is higher in women than men)

Common: vomiting, upper abdominal pain, diarrhoea

Uncommon: faecal incontinence

Skin and subcutaneous tissue disorders:

Common: sweating

Uncommon: rash

Not known: urticaria

Musculoskeletal, connective tissue and bone disorders:

Common: muscle cramps, arthralgia

Renal and urinary disorders:

Common: enuresis nocturna, urinary incontinence

General disorders and administration site conditions:

Common: asthenia, fatigue, feeling drunk, oedema peripheral

Investigations:

Uncommon: weight decreased, blood pressure increased

Injury, poisoning and procedural complications

Common: fall

In some patients, cataplexy may return at a higher frequency on cessation of sodium oxybate therapy, however this may be due to the normal variability of the disease. Although the clinical trial experience with sodium oxybate in narcolepsy/cataplexy patients at therapeutic doses does not show clear evidence of a withdrawal syndrome, in rare cases, adverse events such as insomnia, headache, anxiety, dizziness, sleep disorder, somnolence, hallucination, and psychotic disorders were observed after GHB discontinuation.

4.9 Overdose

Information about signs and symptoms associated with overdosage with sodium oxybate is limited. Most data derives from the illicit use of GHB. Sodium oxybate is the sodium salt of GHB. Events associated with withdrawal syndrome have been observed outside the therapeutic range.

Patients have exhibited varying degrees of depressed consciousness that may fluctuate rapidly between a confusional, agitated combative state with ataxia and coma. Emesis (even with impaired consciousness), diaphoresis, headache, and impaired psychomotor skills may be observed. Blurred vision has been reported. An increasing depth of coma has been observed at higher doses. Myoclonus and tonic-clonic seizures have been reported. There are reports of compromise in the rate and depth of respiration and of life-threatening respiratory depression, necessitating intubation and ventilation. Cheyne-Stokes respiration and apnoea have been observed. Bradycardia and hypothermia may accompany unconsciousness, as well as muscular hypotonia, but tendon reflexes remain intact. Bradycardia has been responsive to atropine intravenous administration.

Gastric lavage may be considered if co-ingestants are suspected. Because emesis may occur in the presence of impaired consciousness, appropriate posture (left lateral recumbent position) and protection of the airway by intubation may be warranted. Although gag reflex may be absent in deeply comatose patients, even unconscious patients may become combative to intubation, and rapid sequence induction (without the use of sedative) should be considered.

No reversal of the central depressant effects of sodium oxybate can be expected from flumazenil administration. There is insufficient evidence to recommend the use of naloxone in the treatment of overdose with GHB. The use of haemodialysis and other forms of extracorporeal drug removal have not been studied in sodium oxybate overdose. However, due to the rapid metabolism of sodium oxybate, these measures are not warranted.

5. PHARMACOLOGICAL PROPERTIES

5.1 Pharmacodynamic properties

Pharmacotherapeutic group: Other Nervous System Drugs, ATC code: N07XX04 hydroxybutyric acid

Sodium oxybate is a central nervous system depressant which reduces excessive daytime sleepiness and cataplexy in patients with narcolepsy and modifies sleep architecture reducing fragmented nighttime sleep. The precise mechanism by which sodium oxybate produces an effect is unknown, however sodium oxybate is thought to act by promoting slow (delta) wave sleep and consolidating nighttime sleep. Sodium oxybate administered before nocturnal sleep increases Stages 3 and 4 sleep and increases sleep latency, whilst reducing the frequency of sleep onset REM periods (SOREMPs). Other mechanisms, which have yet to be elucidated, may also be involved.

In the clinical trial database, greater than 80 % of patients maintained concomitant stimulant use.

The effectiveness of sodium oxybate for the treatment of narcolepsy symptoms was established in four multicentre, randomised, double-blind, placebo-controlled, parallel-group trials (Trial 1, 2, 3 and 4) in patients with narcolepsy with cataplexy except for trial 2 where cataplexy was not required for enrolment Concomitant stimulant use was permitted in all trials (except for the active-treatment phase of Trial 2); antidepressants were withdrawn prior to active treatment in all trials with the exception of Trial 2. In each trial, the daily dose was divided into two equal doses. The first dose each night was taken at bedtime and the second dose was taken 2.5 to 4 hours later.

Table 1 Summary of Clinical Trials Performed Using Sodium Oxybate for the Treatment of Narcolepsy

Trial	Primary Efficacy	*N=*	Secondary Efficacy	Duration	Active treatment and Dose (g/d)
Trial 1	EDS (ESS); CGIc	246	MWT/Sleep Architecture/ Cataplexy/ Naps/FOSQ	8 weeks	Xyrem 4.5 - 9
Trial 2	EDS (MWT)	231	Sleep Architecture/ ESS/CGIc/Naps	8 weeks	Xyrem 6 – 9 Modafinil 200-600 mg
Trial 3	Cataplexy	136	EDS (ESS)/CGIc/Naps	4 weeks	Xyrem 3 - 9
Trial 4	Cataplexy	55	None	4 weeks	Xyrem 3 - 9

EDS – Excessive daytime sleepiness; ESS – Epworth Sleepiness Scale; MWT – Maintenance of Wakefulness Test; Naps – Number of inadvertent daytime naps; CGIc – Clinical Global Impression of Change; FOSQ – Functional Outcomes of Sleep Questionnaire

Trial 1 enrolled 246 patients with narcolepsy and incorporated a 1 week up-titration period. The primary measures of efficacy were changes in excessive daytime sleepiness as measured by the Epworth Sleepiness Scale (ESS), and the change in the overall severity of the patient's narcolepsy symptoms as assessed by the investigator using the Clinical Global Impressions of Change (CGI-c) measure.

Table 2 Summary of ESS in Trial 1

Epworth Sleepiness Scale (ESS; range 0-24)				
Dose Group [g/d (n)]	Baseline	Endpoint	Median Change from Baseline	Change from Baseline Compared to Placebo **(p-value)**
Placebo (60)	17.3	16.7	-0.5	-
4.5 (68)	17.5	15.7	-1.0	0.119
6 (63)	17.9	15.3	-2.0	**0.001**
9 (55)	17.9	13.1	-2.0	< **0.001**

Table 3 Summary of CGI-c in Trial 1

Clinical Global Impressions of Change (CGI-c)		
Dose Group [g/d (n)]	Responders* N (%)	Change from Baseline Compared to Placebo **(p-value)**
Placebo (60)	13 (21.7)	-
4.5 (68)	32 (47.1)	**0.002**
6 (63)	30 (47.6)	< **0.001**
9 (55)	30 (54.4)	< **0.001**

* The CGI-c data were analysed by defining responders as those patients who were very much improved or much improved.

Trial 2 compared the effects of orally administered sodium oxybate, modafinil and sodium oxybate + modafinil, with placebo in the treatment of daytime sleepiness in narcolepsy. During the 8 week double-blind period, patients took modafinil at their established dose or placebo equivalent. The sodium oxybate or placebo equivalent dose was 6g/day for the first 4 weeks and was increased to 9g/day for the remaining 4 weeks. The primary measure of efficacy was excessive daytime sleepiness as measured by objective response in MWT.

Table 4 Summary of MWT in Trial 2

(see Table 4 on next page)

Trial 3 enrolled 136 narcoleptic patients with moderate to severe cataplexy (median of 21 cataplexy attacks per week) at baseline. The primary efficacy measure in this trial was the frequency of cataplexy attacks.

Table 5 Summary of Outcomes in Trial 3

(see Table 5 on next page)

Trial 4 enrolled 55 narcoleptic patients who had been taking open-label sodium oxybate for 7 to 44 months. Patients were randomised to continued treatment with sodium oxybate at their stable dose or to placebo. Trial 4 was designed specifically to evaluate the continued efficacy of sodium oxybate after long-term use. The primary efficacy measure in this trial was the frequency of cataplexy attacks.

Table 6 Summary of outcome in Trial 4

(see Table 6 on next page)

In Trial 4, the response was numerically similar for patients treated with doses of 6 to 9 g/day, but there was no effect seen in patients treated with doses less than 6 g/day.

5.2 Pharmacokinetic properties

Sodium oxybate is rapidly but incompletely absorbed after oral administration; absorption is delayed and decreased by a high fat meal. It is eliminated mainly by metabolism with a half-life of 0.5 to 1 hour. Pharmacokinetics are nonlinear with the area under the plasma concentration curve (AUC) versus time curve increasing 3.8-fold as dose is doubled from 4.5g to 9g. The pharmacokinetics are not altered with repeat dosing.

Absorption: Sodium oxybate is absorbed rapidly following oral administration with an absolute bioavailability of about 25 %. The average peak plasma concentrations (1st and 2nd peak) following administration of a 9 g daily dose divided into two equivalent doses given four hours apart were 78 and 142 μg/ml, respectively. The average time to peak plasma concentration (T_{max}) ranged from 0.5 to 2 hours in eight pharmacokinetic studies. Following oral administration, the plasma levels of sodium oxybate increase more than proportionally with increasing dose. Single doses greater than 4.5 g have not been studied. Administration of sodium oxybate immediately after a high fat meal resulted in delayed absorption (average T_{max} increased from 0.75 hr to 2.0 hr) and a reduction in peak plasma level (C_{max}) by a mean of 58% and of systemic exposure (AUC) by 37%.

Distribution: Sodium oxybate is a hydrophilic compound with an apparent volume of distribution averaging 190-384 ml/kg. At sodium oxybate concentrations ranging from 3 to 300 μg/ml, less than 1 % is bound to plasma proteins.

Metabolism: Animal studies indicate that metabolism is the major elimination pathway for sodium oxybate, producing carbon dioxide and water via the tricarboxylic acid (Krebs) cycle and secondarily by β-oxidation. The primary pathway involves a cytosolic $NADP^+$-linked enzyme, GHB dehydrogenase, that catalyses the conversion of sodium oxybate to succinic semialdehyde, which is then biotransformed to succinic acid by the enzyme succinic semialdehyde dehydrogenase. Succinic acid enters the Krebs cycle where it is metabolised to carbon dioxide and water. A second mitochondrial oxidoreductase enzyme, a transhydrogenase, also catalyses the conversion to succinic semialdehyde in the presence of α-ketoglutarate. An alternate pathway of biotransformation involves β-oxidation via 3,4-dihydroxybutyrate to Acetyl CoA, which also enters the citric acid

Table 4 Summary of MWT in Trial 2

TRIAL 2				
Dose Group	Baseline	Endpoint	Mean Change from Baseline	Endpoint Compared to Placebo
Placebo (56)	9.9	6.9	-2.7	-
Sodium Oxybate (55)	11.5	11.3	0.16	$<$0.001
Modafinil (63)	10.5	9.8	-0.6	**0.004**
Sodium Oxybate + Modafinil (57)	10.4	12.7	2.3	$<$0.001

Table 5 Summary of Outcomes in Trial 3

Dosage	Number of Subjects	Cataplexy Attacks		
Trial 3		Baseline	Median Change from Baseline	Change from Baseline Compared to Placebo (p-value)
		Median attacks/week		
Placebo	33	20.5	-4	-
3.0 g/day	33	20.0	-7	0.5235
6.0 g/day	31	23.0	-10	**0.0529**
9.0 g/day	33	23.5	-16	**0.0008**

Table 6 Summary of outcome in Trial 4

	Number of Subjects	Baseline	Median Change from Baseline	Change from Baseline Compared to Placebo (p-value)
Trial 4		Median attacks/two weeks		
Placebo	29	4.0	21.0	-
Sodium oxybate	26	1.9	0	**p $<$0.001**

cycle to result in the formation of carbon dioxide and water. No active metabolites have been identified.

Studies *in vitro* with pooled human liver microsomes indicate that sodium oxybate does not significantly inhibit the activities of the human isoenzymes: CYP1A2, CYP2C9, CYP2C19, CYP2D6, CYP2E1, or CYP3A up to the concentration of 3 mM (378 μg/ml). These levels are considerably higher than levels achieved with therapeutic doses.

Elimination: The clearance of sodium oxybate is almost entirely by biotransformation to carbon dioxide, which is then eliminated by expiration. On average, less than 5% of unchanged drug appears in human urine within 6 to 8 hours after dosing. Faecal excretion is negligible.

Special Populations:

Elderly patients: The pharmacokinetics of sodium oxybate in patients greater than the age of 65 years have not been studied.

Paediatric patients: The pharmacokinetics of sodium oxybate in paediatric patients under the age of 18 years have not been studied.

Renal Impairment: Because the kidney does not have a significant role in the excretion of sodium oxybate, no pharmacokinetic study in patients with renal dysfunction has been conducted; no effect of renal function on sodium oxybate pharmacokinetics would be expected.

Hepatic Disease: Sodium oxybate undergoes significant presystemic (hepatic first-pass) metabolism. After a single oral dose of 25 mg/kg, AUC values were double in cirrhotic patients, with apparent oral clearance reduced from 9.1 in healthy adults to 4.5 and 4.1 ml/min/kg in Class A (without ascites) and Class C (with ascites) patients, respectively. Elimination half-life was significantly longer in Class C and Class A patients than in control subjects (mean $t_{1/2}$ of 59 and 32 versus 22 minutes). It is prudent to reduce the starting dose of sodium oxybate by one-half in patients with liver dysfunction (see Section 4.2).

Race

The effect of race on metabolism of sodium oxybate has not been evaluated.

5.3 Preclinical safety data

Repeat administration of sodium oxybate to rats (90 days and 26 weeks) and dogs (52 weeks) did not result in any significant findings in clinical chemistry and micro- and macro pathology. Treatment-related clinical signs were mainly related to sedation, reduced food consumption and secondary changes in body weight, body weight gain and organ weights. The rat and dog exposures at the NOEL were lower (~50%) than that in humans. Sodium oxybate was non-mutagenic and non-clastogenic in in vitro and in vivo assays.

Gamma Butyrolactone (GBL), a pro-drug of GHB tested at exposures similar to the expected in man (1.21-1.64 times) has been classified by NTP as non-carcinogenic in rats and equivocal carcinogen in mice, due to slight increase of pheochromocytomas which was difficult to interpret due to high mortality in the high dose group. In a rat carcinogenicity study with oxybate no compound-related tumours were identified.

GHB had no effect on mating, general fertility or sperm parameters and did not produce embryo-foetal toxicity in rats exposed to up 1000 mg/kg/day GHB (1.64 times the human exposure calculated in nonpregnant animals). Perinatal mortality was increased and mean pup weight was decreased during the lactation period in high-dose F_1 animals. The association of these developmental effects with maternal toxicity could not be established. In rabbits, slight foetotoxicity was observed.

Drug discrimination studies show that GHB produces a unique discriminative stimulus that in some respects is similar to that of alcohol, morphine and certain GABA-mimetic drugs. Self-administration studies in rats, mice and monkeys have produced conflicting results, whereas tolerance to GHB as well as cross-tolerance to alcohol have been clearly demonstrated in rodents.

6. PHARMACEUTICAL PARTICULARS

6.1 List of excipients

Purified water

Malic acid for pH adjustment

Sodium Hydroxide for pH adjustment

6.2 Incompatibilities

This medicinal product must not be mixed with other medicinal products.

6.3 Shelf life

5 years

After First opening: 40 days

After dilution in the dosing cups (see Section 4.2), the preparation should be used within 24 hours.

6.4 Special precautions for storage

This medicinal product does not require any special storage conditions.

6.5 Nature and contents of container

Amber oval PET bottle with a child resistant closure composed of HDPE/polypropylene with a LDPE liner fitted with a PVC tamper evident seal.

Each carton contains one bottle of 180ml Xyrem, a press-in bottle adaptor consisting of an LDPE bottle-well housing, a Silastic Biomedical ETR Elastomer valve, an acrylonitrile butadiene styrene terpolymer valve retainer and LDPE tubing, a graduated 10ml measuring device (polypropylene syringe), two polypropylene dosing cups and two HDPE child resistant screw closures.

6.6 Special precautions for disposal and other handling

No special requirements

7. MARKETING AUTHORISATION HOLDER

UCB Pharma Ltd

208 Bath Road

Slough

Berkshire

SL1 3WE

UK

8. MARKETING AUTHORISATION NUMBER(S)

EU/1/05/312/001

9. DATE OF FIRST AUTHORISATION/RENEWAL OF THE AUTHORISATION

13/10/2005

10. DATE OF REVISION OF THE TEXT

22/07/2008

Detailed information on this product is available on the website of the European Medicines Agency (EMEA) http://www.emea.europa.eu/

Xyzal 5 mg film-coated tablets, Xyzal 0.5 mg/ml oral solution

(UCB Pharma Limited)

1. NAME OF THE MEDICINAL PRODUCT

Xyzal 5 mg film coated Tablets and Xyzal 0.5 mg/ml oral solution

2. QUALITATIVE AND QUANTITATIVE COMPOSITION

Tablets:

Each film-coated tablet contains 5 mg levocetirizine dihydrochloride.

Excipients: 63.50 mg lactose monohydrate / tablet

Solution:

1 ml of oral solution contains 0.5 mg levocetirizine dihydrochloride.

Excipients: 0.675 mg methyl parahydroxybenzoate/ml
0.075 mg propyl parahydroxybenzoate/ml
0.4 g maltitol/ml

For a full list of excipients, see section 6.1.

3. PHARMACEUTICAL FORM

Film-coated tablet.

White to off-white, oval, film-coated tablet with a Y logo on one side.

Oral solution

Clear and colorless liquid

4. CLINICAL PARTICULARS

4.1 Therapeutic indications

Symptomatic treatment of allergic rhinitis (including persistent allergic rhinitis) and chronic idiopathic urticaria.

4.2 Posology and method of administration

Tablets:

The film-coated tablet must be taken orally, swallowed whole with liquid and may be taken with or without food. It is recommended to take the daily dose in one single intake.

Adults and adolescents 12 years and above:

The daily recommended dose is 5 mg (1 film-coated tablet).

Elderly:

Adjustment of the dose is recommended in elderly patients with moderate to severe renal impairment (see Patients with renal impairment below).

Children aged 6 to 12 years:

The daily recommended dose is 5 mg (1 film-coated tablet).

For children aged 2 to 6 years no adjusted dosage is possible with the film-coated tablet formulation. It is recommended to use a paediatric formulation of levocetirine.

Solution:

Instruction for use

A dosing oral syringe is included in the package. The appropriate volume of oral solution should be measured with the oral syringe, and poured in a spoon or in a glass of water. The oral solution must be taken orally immediately after dilution, and may be taken with or without food.

Adults and adolescents 12 years and above:

The daily recommended dose is 5 mg (10 ml of solution).

Elderly:

Adjustment of the dose is recommended in elderly patients with moderate to severe renal impairment (see Patients with renal impairment below).

Children aged 6 to 12 years:

The daily recommended dose is 5 mg (10 ml of solution).

Children aged 2 to 6 years:

The daily recommended dose is 2.5 mg to be administered in 2 intakes of 1.25 mg (2.5 ml of solution twice daily).

Due to the lack of data in this population, the administration of the product to infants and toddlers aged less than 2 years is not recommended (see also section 4.4).

Tablets & Solution:

Adult patients with renal impairment:

The dosing intervals must be individualised according to renal function. Refer to the following table and adjust the dose as indicated. To use this dosing table, an estimate of the patient's creatinine clearance (CLcr) in ml/min is needed. The CLcr (ml/min) may be estimated from serum creatinine (mg/dl) determination using the following formula:

$$CL_{cr} = \frac{[140 - age(years)] \, x \, weight \, (kg)}{72 \, x \, serum \, creatinine \, (mg/dl)} \, (x \, 0.85 \, for \, women)$$

Dosing Adjustments for Patients with Impaired Renal Function:

Group	Creatinine clearance (ml/min)	Dosage and frequency
Normal	≥80	5 mg once daily
Mild	50 – 79	5 mg once daily
Moderate	30 – 49	5 mg once every 2 days
Severe	< 30	5 mg once every 3 days
End-stage renal disease - Patients undergoing dialysis	< 10-	Contra-indicated

In paediatric patients suffering from renal impairment, the dose will have to be adjusted on an individual basis taking into account the renal clearance of the patient and his body weight. There are no specific data for children with renal impairment.

Patients with hepatic impairment:

No dose adjustment is needed in patients with solely hepatic impairment. In patients with hepatic impairment and renal impairment, adjustment of the dose is recommended (see Patients with renal impairment above).

Duration of use:

Intermittent allergic rhinitis (symptoms <4days/week or during less than 4 weeks) has to be treated according to the disease and its history; it can be stopped once the symptoms have disappeared and can be restarted again when symptoms reappear. In case of persistent allergic rhinitis (symptoms >4days/week and during more than 4 weeks), continuous therapy can be proposed to the patient during the period of exposure to allergens. Clinical experience with 5 mg levocetirizine as a film-coated tablet formulation is currently available for a 6-month treatment period. For chronic urticaria and chronic allergic rhinitis, up to one year's clinical experience is available for the racemate.

4.3 Contraindications

Tablets:

Hypersensitivity to levocetirizine, to other piperazine derivatives, or to any of the excipients.

Patients with rare hereditary problems of galactose intolerance, the Lapp lactase deficiency or glucose-galactose malabsorption should not take this medicine.

Solution:

Hypersensitivity to levocetirizine, to any piperazine derivative, methyl parahydroxybenzoate, propyl parahydroxybenzoate, or any of the other excipients.

Xyzal 0.5 mg/ml oral solution contains maltitol: Patients with rare hereditary problems of fructose intolerance should not take this medicine.

Tablets & Solution:

Severe renal impairment at less than 10 ml/min creatinine clearance.

4.4 Special warnings and precautions for use

The use of the film-coated tablet formulation is not recommended in children aged less than 6 years since this formulation does not allow for appropriate dose adaptation. It is recommended to use a paediatric formulation of levocetirine.

The administration of levocetirizine to infants and toddlers aged less than 2 years is not recommended.

Precaution is recommended with intake of alcohol (see Interactions).

Solution:

The presence of methyl parahydroxybenzoate and propyl parahydroxybenzoate may cause allergic reactions (possibly delayed).

Due to the lack of data in this population, the administration of the product to infants and toddlers aged less than 2 years is not recommended.

4.5 Interaction with other medicinal products and other forms of interaction

No interaction studies have been performed with levocetirizine (including no studies with CYP3A4 inducers); studies with the racemate compound cetirizine demonstrated that there were no clinically relevant adverse interactions (with pseudoephedrine, cimetidine, ketoconazole, erythromycin, azithromycin, glipizide and diazepam). A small decrease in the clearance of cetirizine (16%) was observed in a multiple dose study with theophylline (400 mg once a day); while the disposition of theophylline was not altered by concomitant cetirizine administration.

The extent of absorption of levocetirizine is not reduced with food, although the rate of absorption is decreased.

In sensitive patients the simultaneous administration of cetirizine or levocetirizine and alcohol or other CNS depressants may have effects on the central nervous system, although it has been shown that the racemate cetirizine does not potentiate the effect of alcohol.

4.6 Pregnancy and lactation

For levocetirizine no clinical data on exposed pregnancies are available. Animal studies do not indicate direct or indirect harmful effects with respect to pregnancy, embryonal/fetal development, parturition or postnatal development. Caution should be exercised when prescribing to pregnant or lactating women.

4.7 Effects on ability to drive and use machines

Comparative clinical trials have revealed no evidence that levocetirizine at the recommended dose impairs mental alertness, reactivity or the ability to drive.

Nevertheless, some patients could experience somnolence, fatigue and asthenia under therapy with Levocetirizine. Therefore, patients intending to drive, engage in potentially hazardous activities or operate machinery should take their response to the medicinal product into account.

4.8 Undesirable effects

In therapeutic studies in women and men aged 12 to 71 years, 15.1% of the patients in the levocetirizine 5 mg group had at least one adverse drug reaction compared to 11.3% in the placebo group. 91.6 % of these adverse drug reactions were mild to moderate.

In therapeutic trials, the drop out rate due to adverse events was 1.0% (9/935) with levocetirizine 5 mg and 1.8% (14/771) with placebo.

Clinical therapeutic trials with levocetirizine included 935 subjects exposed to the drug at the recommended dose of 5 mg daily. From this pooling, following incidence of adverse drug reactions were reported at rates of 1 % or greater (common: >1/100, <1/10) under levocetirizine 5 mg or placebo:

Preferred Term (WHOART)	Placebo (n =771)	Levocetirizine 5 mg (n = 935)
Headache	25 (3.2 %)	24 (2.6 %)
Somnolence	11 (1.4 %)	49 (5.2 %)
Mouth dry	12 (1.6%)	24 (2.6%)
Fatigue	9 (1.2 %)	23 (2.5 %)

Further uncommon incidences of adverse reactions (uncommon >1/1000, <1/100) like asthenia or abdominal pain were observed.

The incidence of sedating adverse drug reactions such as somnolence, fatigue, and asthenia was altogether more common (8.1 %) under levocetirizine 5 mg than under placebo (3.1%).

In addition to the adverse reactions reported during clinical studies and listed above, very rare cases of the following adverse drug reactions have been reported in post-marketing experience.

- Immune system disorders: hypersensitivity including anaphylaxis
- Psychiatric disorders: aggression, agitation
- Nervous system disorders: convulsion
- Eyes disorders: visual disturbances
- Cardiac disorders: palpitations
- Respiratory, thoracic, and mediastinal disorders: dyspnoea
- Gastrointestinal disorders: nausea
- Hepatobiliary disorders: hepatitis
- Skin and subcutaneous tissue disorders: angioneurotic oedema, fixed drug eruption, pruritus, rash, urticaria
- Musculoskeletal, connective tissues, and bone disorders: myalgia
- Investigations: weight increased, abnormal liver function tests

4.9 Overdose

a) Symptoms

Symptoms of overdose may include drowsiness in adults and initially agitation and restlessness, followed by drowsiness in children.

b) Management of overdoses

There is no known specific antidote to levocetirizine.

Should overdose occur, symptomatic or supportive treatment is recommended. Gastric lavage should be considered following short-term ingestion. Levocetirizine is not effectively removed by haemodialysis.

5. PHARMACOLOGICAL PROPERTIES

5.1 Pharmacodynamic properties

Pharmacotherapeutic group: antihistamine for systemic use, piperazine derivative, ATC code: R06A E09.

Levocetirizine, the (R) enantiomer of cetirizine, is a potent and selective antagonist of peripheral H1-receptors.

Binding studies revealed that levocetirizine has high affinity for human H1-receptors (Ki = 3.2 nmol/l). Levocetirizine has an affinity 2-fold higher than that of cetirizine (Ki = 6.3 nmol/l). Levocetirizine dissociates from H1-receptors with a half-life of 115 ± 38 min. After single administration, levocetirizine shows a receptor occupancy of 90% at 4 hours and 57% at 24 hours.

Pharmacodynamic studies in healthy volunteers demonstrate that, at half the dose, levocetirizine has comparable activity to cetirizine, both in the skin and in the nose.

The pharmacodynamic activity of levocetirizine has been studied in randomised, controlled trials:

In a study comparing the effects of levocetirizine 5mg, desloratadine 5mg, and placebo on histamine-induced wheal and flare, levocetirizine treatment resulted in significantly decreased wheal and flare formation which was highest in the first 12 hours and lasted for 24 hours, ($p<0.001$) compared with placebo and desloratadine.

The onset of action of levocetirizine 5 mg in controlling pollen-induced symptoms has been observed at 1 hour post drug intake in placebo controlled trials in the model of the allergen challenge chamber.

In vitro studies (Boyden chambers and cell layers techniques) show that levocetirizine inhibits eotaxin-induced eosinophil transendothelial migration through both dermal and lung cells. A pharmacodynamic experimental study *in vivo* (skin chamber technique) showed three main inhibitory effects of levocetirizine 5 mg in the first 6 hours of pollen-induced reaction, compared with placebo in 14 adult patients: inhibition of VCAM-1 release, modulation of vascular permeability and a decrease in eosinophil recruitment.

The efficacy and safety of levocetirizine has been demonstrated in several double-blind, placebo controlled, clinical trials performed in adult patients suffering from seasonal allergic rhinitis, perennial allergic rhinitis, or persistent allergic rhinitis. Levocetirizine has been shown to significantly improve symptoms of allergic rhinitis, including nasal obstruction in some studies.

A 6-month clinical study in 551 adult patients (including 276 levocetirizine-treated patients) suffering from persistent allergic rhinitis (symptoms present 4 days a week for at least 4 consecutive weeks) and sensitized to house dust mites and grass pollen demonstrated that levocetirizine 5 mg was clinically and statistically significantly more potent than placebo on the relief from the total symptom score of allergic rhinitis throughout the whole duration of the study, without any tachyphylaxis. During the whole duration of the study, levocetirizine significantly improved the quality of life of the patients.

The paediatric safety and efficacy of levocetirizine tablets has been studied in two placebo controlled clinical trials including patients aged 6 to 12 years and suffering from seasonal and perennial allergic rhinitis, respectively. In both trials, levocetirizine significantly improved symptoms and increased health-related quality of life.

In a placebo-controlled clinical trial including 166 patients suffering from chronic idiopathic urticaria, 85 patients were treated with placebo and 81 patients with levocetirizine 5mg once daily over six weeks. Treatment with levocetirizine resulted in significant decrease in pruritus severity over the first week and over the total treatment period as compared to placebo. Levocetirizine also resulted in a larger improvement of health-related quality of life as assessed by the Dermatology Life Quality Index as compared to placebo.

Pharmacokinetic / pharmacodynamic relationship:

The action on histamine-induced skin reactions is out of phase with the plasma concentrations.

ECGs did not show relevant effects of levocetirizine on QT interval.

5.2 Pharmacokinetic properties

The pharmacokinetics of levocetirizine are linear with dose- and time-independent with low inter-subject variability. The pharmacokinetic profile is the same when given as the single enantiomer or when given as cetirizine. No chiral inversion occurs during the process of absorption and elimination.

Absorption:

Levocetirizine is rapidly and extensively absorbed following oral administration. Peak plasma concentrations are achieved 0.9 h after dosing. Steady state is achieved after two days. Peak concentrations are typically 270 ng/ml and 308 ng/ml following a single and a repeated 5 mg o.d. dose, respectively. The extent of absorption is dose-independent and is not altered by food, but the peak concentration is reduced and delayed.

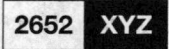

Distribution:

No tissue distribution data are available in humans, neither concerning the passage of levocetirizine through the blood-brain-barrier. In rats and dogs, the highest tissue levels are found in liver and kidneys, the lowest in the CNS compartment.

Levocetirizine is 90% bound to plasma proteins. The distribution of levocetirizine is restrictive, as the volume of distribution is 0.4 l/kg.

Biotransformation:

The extent of metabolism of levocetirizine in humans is less than 14% of the dose and therefore differences resulting from genetic polymorphism or concomitant intake of enzyme inhibitors are expected to be negligible. Metabolic pathways include aromatic oxidation, N- and O- dealkylation and taurine conjugation. Dealkylation pathways are primarily mediated by CYP 3A4 while aromatic oxidation involved multiple and/or unidentified CYP isoforms. Levocetirizine had no effect on the activities of CYP isoenzymes 1A2, 2C9, 2C19, 2D6, 2E1 and 3A4 at concentrations well above peak concentrations achieved following a 5 mg oral dose.

Due to its low metabolism and absence of metabolic inhibition potential, the interaction of levocetirizine with other substances, or vice-versa, is unlikely.

Elimination:

The plasma half-life in adults is 7.9 ± 1.9 hours. The mean apparent total body clearance is 0.63 ml/min/kg. The major route of excretion of levocetirizine and metabolites is via urine, accounting for a mean of 85.4% of the dose. Excretion via feces accounts for only 12.9% of the dose. Levocetirizine is excreted both by glomerular filtration and active tubular secretion.

Renal impairment:

The apparent body clearance of levocetirizine is correlated to the creatinine clearance. It is therefore recommended to adjust the dosing intervals of levocetirizine, based on creatinine clearance in patients with moderate and severe renal impairment. In anuric end stage renal disease subjects, the total body clearance is decreased by approximately 80% when compared to normal subjects. The amount of levocetirizine removed during a standard 4-hour hemodialysis procedure was < 10%.

5.3 Preclinical safety data

Non-clinical data reveal no special hazard for humans based on conventional studies of safety pharmacology, repeated dose toxicity, toxicity to reproduction, genotoxicity or carcinogenicity.

6. PHARMACEUTICAL PARTICULARS

6.1 List of excipients

Tablets:

Core
Microcrystalline cellulose
Lactose monohydrate
Colloidal anhydrous silica
Magnesium stearate
Coating
Opadry® Y-1-7000 consisting of:
Hypromellose (E464)
Titanium dioxide (E 171)
Macrogol 400
Solution:
Sodium acetate trihydrate (for pH adjustment)
Glacial acetic acid (for pH adjustment)
Methyl parahydroxybenzoate (E218)
Propyl parahydroxybenzoate (E216)
Glycerol 85%
Maltitol (E965)
Saccharin sodium
Tutti frutti flavor
Triacetin (E1518)
benzaldehyde
orange oil
vanilin
ethyl butyrate
orange oil concentrated
isoamyl acetate
allyl hexanoate
gamma-undecalactone
citral
geraniol
citronellol
alpha tocopherol (E307)
Purified water

6.2 Incompatibilities

Not applicable.

6.3 Shelf life

Tablets:

3 years

Solution:

2 years.

3 months after first opening.

6.4 Special precautions for storage

This medicinal product does not require any special storage conditions.

6.5 Nature and contents of container

Tablets:

Aluminium – OPA/aluminium/PVCblister

Pack sizes of 1, 2, 4, 5, 7, 10, 2 × 10, 10 × 10, 14, 15, 20, 21, 28, 30 40, 50, 60, 70, 90, 100.

Solution:

Type III 200 ml amber glass bottle closed with a white polypropylene child-resistant closure in a cardboard box also containing a graduated 10 ml oral syringe (polyethylene, polystyrene) and a patient information leaflet.

6.6 Special precautions for disposal and other handling

No special requirements.

7. MARKETING AUTHORISATION HOLDER

UCB Pharma Ltd
208 Bath Rd
Slough
SL1 3WE

8. MARKETING AUTHORISATION NUMBER(S)

Tablets: PL 00039/0539

Solution: PL 00039/0731

9. DATE OF FIRST AUTHORISATION/RENEWAL OF THE AUTHORISATION

Tablets: 02/2001, 02/2006

Solution: 05/2006

10. DATE OF REVISION OF THE TEXT

08/2007

Yentreve 20mg and 40mg hard gastro-resistant capsules

(Eli Lilly and Company Limited)

1. NAME OF THE MEDICINAL PRODUCT

YENTREVE*▼ 20mg and 40mg hard gastro-resistant capsules.

2. QUALITATIVE AND QUANTITATIVE COMPOSITION

Each 20mg capsule contains 20mg of duloxetine (as hydrochloride).

Excipients 20mg: Each capsule contains 5.7mg sucrose.

Each 40mg capsule contains 40mg of duloxetine (as hydrochloride).

Excipients 40mg: Each capsule contains 11.5mg sucrose.

For a full list of excipients, see section 6.1.

3. PHARMACEUTICAL FORM

Hard gastro-resistant capsule.

The 20mg capsule has an opaque blue body, imprinted with '20mg', and an opaque blue cap, imprinted with '9544'.

The 40mg capsule has an opaque orange body, imprinted with '40mg', and an opaque blue cap, imprinted with '9545'.

4. CLINICAL PARTICULARS

4.1 Therapeutic indications

YENTREVE is indicated for women for the treatment of moderate to severe stress urinary incontinence (SUI) (see section 5.1).

4.2 Posology and method of administration

The recommended dose of YENTREVE is 40mg twice daily, without regard to meals. After 2-4 weeks of treatment, patients should be re-assessed in order to evaluate the benefit and tolerability of the therapy. Some patients may benefit from starting treatment at a dose of 20mg twice daily for two weeks before increasing to the recommended dose of 40mg twice daily. Dose escalation may decrease, though not eliminate, the risk of nausea and dizziness. However, limited data are available to support the efficacy of YENTREVE 20mg twice daily. A 20 mg capsule is also available.

The efficacy of YENTREVE has not been evaluated for longer than 3 months in placebo-controlled studies. The benefit of treatment should be re-assessed at regular intervals.

Combining YENTREVE with a pelvic floor muscle training (PFMT) programme may be more effective than either treatment alone. It is recommended that consideration be given to concomitant PFMT.

Hepatic impairment

YENTREVE must not be used in women with liver disease resulting in hepatic impairment (see section 4.3).

Renal impairment

No dosage adjustment is necessary for patients with mild or moderate renal dysfunction (creatinine clearance 30 to 80ml/min). YENTREVE must not be used in patients with severe renal impairment (creatinine clearance <30 ml/min; see section 4.3).

Method of administration

For oral use.

Elderly

Caution should be exercised when treating the elderly.

Children and Adolescents

Duloxetine is not recommended for use in children and adolescents due to insufficient data on safety and efficacy (see section 4.4).

Discontinuation of Treatment

Abrupt discontinuation should be avoided. When stopping treatment with YENTREVE the dose should be gradually reduced over a period of at least one to two weeks in order to reduce the risk of withdrawal reactions (see sections 4.4 and 4.8). If intolerable symptoms occur following a decrease in the dose or upon discontinuation of treatment, then resuming the previously prescribed dose may be considered. Subsequently, the physician may continue decreasing the dose, but at a more gradual rate.

4.3 Contraindications

Hypersensitivity to the active substance or to any of the excipients.

Liver disease resulting in hepatic impairment (see section 5.2).

YENTREVE should not be used in combination with non-selective, irreversible monoamine oxidase inhibitors (MAOIs) (see section 4.5).

YENTREVE should not be used in combination with CYP1A2 inhibitors, like fluvoxamine, ciprofloxacin, or enoxacine, since the combination results in elevated plasma concentrations of duloxetine (see section 4.5).

Severe renal impairment (creatinine clearance <30ml/min) (see section 4.4).

The initiation of treatment with YENTREVE is contra-indicated in patients with uncontrolled hypertension that could expose patients to a potential risk of hypertensive crisis (see sections 4.4 and 4.8).

4.4 Special warnings and precautions for use

Mania and Seizures

YENTREVE should be used with caution in patients with a history of mania or a diagnosis of bipolar disorder, and/or seizures.

Use with Antidepressants

The use of YENTREVE in combination with antidepressants (especially with SSRI, SNRI, and reversible MAOIs) is not recommended (see below, '*Depression, suicidal ideation and behaviour*', and section 4.5).

St John's Wort

Adverse reactions may be more common during concomitant use of YENTREVE and herbal preparations containing St John's Wort (*Hypericum perforatum*).

Mydriasis

Mydriasis has been reported in association with duloxetine; therefore, caution should be used when prescribing duloxetine in patients with increased intra-ocular pressure, or those at risk of acute narrow-angle glaucoma.

Blood Pressure and Heart Rate

Duloxetine has been associated with an increase in blood pressure and clinically significant hypertension in some patients. This may be due to the noradrenergic effect of duloxetine. Cases of hypertensive crisis have been reported with duloxetine, especially in patients with pre-existing hypertension. Therefore, in patients with known hypertension and/or other cardiac disease, blood pressure monitoring is recommended, especially during the first month of treatment. Duloxetine should be used with caution in patients whose conditions could be compromised by an increased heart rate or by an increase in blood pressure. Caution should also be exercised when duloxetine is used with medicinal products that may impair its metabolism (see section 4.5). For patients who experience a sustained increase in blood pressure while receiving duloxetine, either dose reduction or gradual discontinuation should be considered (see section 4.8). In patients with uncontrolled hypertension, duloxetine should not be initiated (see section 4.3).

Renal Impairment

Increased plasma concentrations of duloxetine occur in patients with severe renal impairment on haemodialysis (creatinine clearance <30ml/min). For patients with severe renal impairment, see section 4.3. See section 4.2 for information on patients with mild or moderate renal dysfunction.

Haemorrhage

There have been reports of bleeding abnormalities, such as ecchymoses, purpura, and gastro-intestinal haemorrhage, with selective serotonin reuptake inhibitors (SSRIs) and serotonin/noradrenaline reuptake inhibitors (SNRIs). Caution is advised in patients taking anticoagulants and/or medicinal products known to affect platelet function, and in patients with known bleeding tendencies.

Discontinuation of Treatment

Withdrawal symptoms when treatment is discontinued are common, particularly if discontinuation is abrupt (see section 4.8). In a clinical trial, adverse events seen on abrupt treatment discontinuation occurred in approximately 44% of patients treated with YENTREVE and 24% of patients taking placebo.

The risk of withdrawal symptoms seen with SSRIs and SNRIs may be dependent on several factors, including the duration and dose of therapy and the rate of dose reduction. The most commonly reported reactions are listed in section 4.8. Generally, the symptoms are mild to moderate; however, in some patients they may be severe in intensity. They usually occur within the first few days of discontinuing treatment, but there have been very rare reports of such symptoms in patients who have inadvertently missed a dose. Generally, these symptoms are self-limiting and usually resolve within 2 weeks, though in some individuals they may be prolonged (2-3 months or more). It is therefore advised that duloxetine should be gradually tapered when discontinuing treatment over a period of no less than 2 weeks, according to the patient's needs (see section 4.2).

Hyponatraemia

Hyponatraemia has been reported rarely, predominantly in the elderly, when administering YENTREVE. Caution is required in patients at increased risk for hyponatraemia, such as elderly, cirrhotic, or dehydrated patients, or patients treated with diuretics. Hyponatraemia may be due to a syndrome of inappropriate anti-diuretic hormone secretion (SIADH).

Depression, Suicidal Ideation and Behaviour

Although YENTREVE is not indicated for the treatment of depression, its active ingredient (duloxetine) also exists as an antidepressant medicinal product. Depression is associated with an increased risk of suicidal thoughts, self-harm and suicide (suicide-related events). This risk persists until significant remission occurs. As improvement may not occur during the first few weeks or more of treatment, patients should be closely monitored until such improvement occurs. It is general clinical experience that the risk of suicide may increase in the early stages of recovery. Patients with a history of suicide-related events or those exhibiting a significant degree of suicidal thoughts prior to commencement of treatment are known to be at a greater risk of suicidal thoughts or suicidal behaviour, and should receive careful monitoring during treatment. A meta-analysis of placebo-controlled clinical trials of antidepressant medicinal products in psychiatric disorders showed an increased risk of suicidal behaviour with antidepressants compared to placebo in patients less than 25 years old. Cases of suicidal thoughts and suicidal behaviours have been reported during duloxetine therapy or early after treatment discontinuation (see section 4.8). Physicians should encourage patients to report any distressing thoughts or feelings or depressive symptoms at any time. If, while on YENTREVE therapy, the patient develops agitation or depressive symptoms, specialised medical advice should be sought, as depression is a serious medical condition. If a decision to initiate antidepressant pharmacological therapy is taken, the gradual discontinuation of YENTREVE is recommended (see section 4.2).

Use in Children and Adolescents Under 18 Years of Age

No clinical trials have been conducted with duloxetine in paediatric populations. YENTREVE should not be used in the treatment of children and adolescents under the age of 18 years. Suicide-related behaviours (suicide attempts and suicidal thoughts) and hostility (predominantly aggression, oppositional behaviour, and anger) were more frequently observed in clinical trials among children and adolescents treated with antidepressants compared to those treated with placebo. Long-term safety data in children and adolescents concerning growth, maturation, and cognitive and behavioural development are lacking.

Medicinal Products Containing Duloxetine

Duloxetine is used under different trademarks in several indications (treatment of diabetic neuropathic pain, major depressive episodes, generalised anxiety disorder as well as stress urinary incontinence). The use of more than one of these products concomitantly should be avoided.

Hepatitis/Increased Liver Enzymes

Cases of liver injury, including severe elevations of liver enzymes (>10-times upper limit of normal), hepatitis, and jaundice, have been reported with duloxetine (see section 4.8). Most of them occurred during the first months of treatment. The pattern of liver damage was predominantly hepatocellular. Duloxetine should be used with caution in patients treated with other medicinal products associated with hepatic injury.

Akathisia/Psychomotor Restlessness

The use of duloxetine has been associated with the development of akathisia, characterised by a subjectively unpleasant or distressing restlessness and need to move, often accompanied by an inability to sit or stand still. This is most likely to occur within the first few weeks of treatment. In patients who develop these symptoms, increasing the dose may be detrimental.

Sucrose

YENTREVE hard gastro-resistant capsules contain sucrose. Patients with rare hereditary problems of fructose intolerance, glucose-galactose malabsorption or sucrose-isomaltase insufficiency should not take this medicine.

4.5 Interaction with other medicinal products and other forms of interaction

Monoamine oxidase inhibitors (MAOIs): Due to the risk of serotonin syndrome, duloxetine should not be used in combination with non-selective, irreversible monoamine oxidase inhibitors (MAOIs), or within at least 14 days of discontinuing treatment with an MAOI. Based on the half-life of duloxetine, at least 5 days should be allowed after stopping YENTREVE before starting an MAOI (see section 4.3).

Serotonin syndrome: In rare cases, serotonin syndrome has been reported in patients using SSRIs concomitantly with serotonergic medicinal products. The use of YENTREVE in combination with serotonergic antidepressants like SSRIs, tricyclics like clomipramine or amitriptyline, venlafaxine, or triptans, tramadol and tryptophan is not recommended.

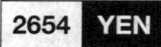

CNS medicinal products: Caution is advised when YENTREVE is taken in combination with other centrally acting medicinal products or substances, including alcohol and sedative medicinal products (benzodiazepines, morphinomimetics, antipsychotics, phenobarbital, sedative antihistamines).

Effect of Duloxetine on Other Medicinal Products

Medicinal products metabolised by CYP1A2: The pharmacokinetics of theophylline, a CYP1A2 substrate, were not significantly affected by co-administration with duloxetine (60mg twice daily).

Medicinal products metabolised by CYP2D6: Duloxetine is a moderate inhibitor of CYP2D6. When duloxetine was administered at a dose of 60mg twice daily with a single dose of desipramine, a CYP2D6 substrate, the AUC of desipramine increased 3-fold. The co-administration of duloxetine (40mg twice daily) increases steady-state AUC of tolterodine (2mg twice daily) by 71%, but does not affect the pharmacokinetics of its active 5-hydroxyl metabolite and no dosage adjustment is recommended. Caution is advised if YENTREVE is co-administered with medicinal products that are predominantly metabolised by CYP2D6 (risperidone, tricyclic antidepressants [TCAs], such as nortriptyline, amitriptyline, and imipramine), particularly if they have a narrow therapeutic index (such as flecainide, propafenone, and metoprolol).

Oral contraceptives and other steroidal agents: Results of *in vitro* studies demonstrate that duloxetine does not induce the catalytic activity of CYP3A. Specific *in vivo* drug interaction studies have not been performed.

Anticoagulants and antiplatelet agents: Caution should be exercised when duloxetine is combined with oral anticoagulants or antiplatelet agents due to a potential increased risk of bleeding attributable to a pharmacodynamic interaction. Furthermore, increases in INR values have been reported when duloxetine was co-administered to patients treated with warfarin. However, concomitant administration of duloxetine with warfarin under steady state conditions, in healthy volunteers, as part of a clinical pharmacology study, did not result in a clinically significant change in INR from baseline or in the pharmacokinetics of R- or S-warfarin.

Effects of Other Medicinal Products on Duloxetine

Antacids and H_2-antagonists: Co-administration of YENTREVE with aluminium- and magnesium-containing antacids or with famotidine had no significant effect on the rate or extent of duloxetine absorption after administration of a 40mg oral dose.

Inhibitors of CYP1A2: Because CYP1A2 is involved in duloxetine metabolism, concomitant use of YENTREVE with potent inhibitors of CYP1A2 is likely to result in higher concentrations of duloxetine. Fluvoxamine (100mg once daily), a potent inhibitor of CYP1A2, decreased the apparent plasma clearance of duloxetine by about 77% and increased AUC_{0-t} 6-fold. Therefore, YENTREVE should not be administered in combination with potent inhibitors of CYP1A2 like fluvoxamine (see section 4.3).

Inducers of CYP1A2: Population pharmacokinetic studies analyses have shown that smokers have almost 50% lower plasma concentrations of duloxetine compared with non-smokers.

4.6 Pregnancy and lactation

Pregnancy: There are no adequate data on the use of duloxetine in pregnant women. Studies in animals have shown reproductive toxicity at systemic exposure levels (AUC) of duloxetine lower than the maximum clinical exposure (see section 5.3). The potential risk for humans is unknown. As with other serotoninergic medicinal products, discontinuation symptoms may occur in the neonate after maternal duloxetine use near term. YENTREVE should be used in pregnancy only if the potential benefit justifies the potential risk to the foetus. Women should be advised to notify their physician if they become pregnant, or intend to become pregnant, during therapy.

Breast-feeding: Duloxetine is very weakly excreted into human milk based on a study of 6 lactating patients who did not breast feed their children. The estimated daily infant dose on a mg/kg basis is approximately 0.14% of the maternal dose (see section 5.2). As the safety of duloxetine in infants is not known, the use of YENTREVE while breast-feeding is not recommended.

4.7 Effects on ability to drive and use machines

No studies on the effects on the ability to drive and use machines have been performed. YENTREVE may be associated with sedation and dizziness. Patients should be instructed that if they experience sedation or dizziness they should avoid potentially hazardous tasks such as driving or operating machinery.

4.8 Undesirable effects

Table 1 gives the adverse reactions observed from spontaneous reporting and in placebo-controlled clinical trials (comprising a total of 8241 patients, 4504 on duloxetine and 3737 on placebo) in SUI and other lower urinary tract disorders.

The most commonly reported adverse events in patients treated with YENTREVE in clinical trials in SUI and other lower urinary tract disorders were nausea, dry mouth, fatigue and constipation. The data analysis of four 12-week, placebo-controlled clinical trials in patients with

Table 1 Adverse reactions

Very common	Common	Uncommon	Rare	Very Rare	Frequency not known
Infections and infestations					
		Laryngitis			
Immune system disorders					
		Hyper-sensitivity disorder	Anaphylactic reaction		
Endocrine disorders					
		Hypo-thyroidism			
Metabolism and Nutrition Disorders					
	Appetite decreased	Dehydration	Hyperglycaemia (reported especially in diabetic patients) Hyponatraemia		SIADH
Psychiatric Disorders					
	Insomnia Anxiety Sleep disorder Agitation Libido decreased	Disorientation Abnormal dreams Apathy Bruxism Orgasm abnormal	Hallucinations		Suicidal behaviour Suicidal ideation[4] Mania Aggression and anger[5]
Nervous System Disorders					
	Headache Dizziness Tremor Lethargy Somnolence Paraesthesia	Poor quality sleep Disturbance in attention Nervousness Dysgeusia	Dyskinesia Myoclonus Restless legs syndrome		Serotonin syndrome Psychomotor restlessness Convulsions[1] Akathisia Extrapyramidal symptoms
Eye Disorders					
	Blurred vision	Visual disturbance Mydriasis	Glaucoma		
Ear and Labyrinth Disorders					
	Vertigo	Tinnitus[1] Ear pain			
Cardiac Disorders					
		Palpitations Tachycardia			Supra-ventricular arrhythmia, mainly atrial fibrillation
Vascular Disorders					
	Flushing	Syncope[2] Blood pressure increase	Hypertensive crisis Orthostatic hypotension[2] Peripheral coldness		Hypertension
Respiratory, Thoracic and Mediastinal Disorders					
		Yawning	Epistaxis Throat tightness		
Gastrointestinal Disorders					
Nausea (22.8%) Dry mouth (12.1%) Constipation (10.3%)	Diarrhoea Vomiting Dyspepsia	Gastroenteritis Stomatitis Gastritis Flatulence Eructation Breath odour	Haematochezia		Gastrointestinal haemorrhage
Hepato-biliary Disorders					
		Hepatitis[3] Elevated liver enzymes (ALT, AST, alkaline phosphatase) Acute liver injury			Hepatic failure Jaundice
Skin and Subcutaneous Tissue Disorders					
	Sweating increased	Rash Increased tendency to bruise Night sweats Cold sweat Dermatitis contact Urticaria	Photo-sensitivity reactions		Stevens-Johnson Syndrome Angioneurotic oedema
Musculoskeletal and Connective Tissue Disorders					
		Muscle spasm Muscle tightness Musculo-skeletal pain Trismus	Muscle twitching		

Very common	Common	Uncommon	Rare	Very Rare	Frequency not known
Renal and Urinary Disorders					
		Urinary hesitation Dysuria Nocturia Urine odour abnormal	Urine flow decreased Polyuria		Urinary retention
Reproductive System and Breast Disorders					
		Menopausal symptoms Gynaecological haemorrhage			
General Disorders and Administration Site Conditions					
Fatigue (10.9%)	Abdominal pain Asthenia Chills	Malaise Feeling abnormal Feeling cold Feeling hot Thirst	Gait disturbance		Chest pain
Investigations					
		Weight decrease Weight increase Blood cholesterol increased Creatine phosphokinase increased			

[1] Cases of convulsion and cases of tinnitus have also been reported after treatment discontinuation.

[2] Cases of orthostatic hypotension and syncope have been reported especially at the initiation of treatment.

[3] See section 4.4.

[4] Cases of suicidal ideation and suicidal behaviours have been reported during duloxetine therapy or early after treatment discontinuation (see section 4.4).

[5] Cases of aggression and anger have been reported particularly early in treatment or after treatment discontinuation.

SUI, including 958 duloxetine-treated and 955 placebo-treated patients, showed that the onset of the reported adverse events typically occurred in the first week of therapy. However, the majority of the most frequent adverse events were mild to moderate and resolved within 30 days of occurrence (e.g., nausea).

Table 1: Adverse reactions

Frequencies are defined as: Very common (≥1/10), common (≥1/100 to <1/10), uncommon (≥1/1,000 to <1/100), rare (≥1/10,000 and <1/1,000), very rare (<1/10,000), not known (cannot be estimated from the available data).

Within each frequency grouping, undesirable effects are presented in order of decreasing seriousness.

(see Table 1 on previous page)

Discontinuation of duloxetine (particularly when abrupt) commonly leads to withdrawal symptoms. Dizziness, sensory disturbances (including paraesthesia), sleep disturbances (including insomnia and intense dreams), agitation or anxiety, nausea and/or vomiting, tremor, headache, irritability, diarrhoea, hyperhydrosis and vertigo are the most commonly reported reactions.

Generally, for SSRIs and SNRIs, these events are mild to moderate and self-limiting; however, in some patients they may be severe and/or prolonged. It is therefore advised that when duloxetine treatment is no longer required, gradual discontinuation by dose tapering should be carried out (see sections 4.2 and 4.4).

The heart rate-corrected QT interval in duloxetine-treated patients did not differ from that seen in placebo-treated patients. No clinically significant differences were observed for QT, PR, QRS, or QTcB measurements between duloxetine-treated and placebo-treated patients.

In the 12-week acute phase of three clinical trials of duloxetine in patients with diabetic neuropathic pain, small but statistically significant increases in fasting blood glucose were observed in duloxetine-treated patients. HbA_{1c} was stable in both duloxetine-treated and placebo-treated patients. In the extension phase of these studies, which lasted up to 52 weeks, there was an increase in HbA_{1c} in both the duloxetine and routine care groups, but the mean increase was 0.3% greater in the duloxetine-treated group. There was also a small increase in fasting blood glucose and in total cholesterol in duloxetine-treated patients, while those laboratory tests showed a slight decrease in the routine care group.

4.9 Overdose

Cases of overdoses, alone or in combination with other medicinal products, with duloxetine doses of 5400mg were reported. Some fatalities have occurred, primarily with mixed overdoses, but also with duloxetine alone at a dose of approximately 1000 mg. Signs and symptoms of overdose (duloxetine alone or in combination with other medicinal products) included somnolence, coma, serotonin syndrome, seizures, vomiting and tachycardia.

No specific antidote for duloxetine is known but if serotonin syndrome ensues, specific treatment (such as with cyproheptadine and/or temperature control) may be considered. A free airway should be established. Monitoring of cardiac and vital signs is recommended, along with appropriate symptomatic and supportive measures. Gastric lavage may be indicated if performed soon after ingestion or in symptomatic patients. Activated charcoal may be useful in limiting absorption. Duloxetine has a large volume of distribution and forced diuresis, haemoperfusion, and exchange perfusion are unlikely to be beneficial.

5. PHARMACOLOGICAL PROPERTIES

5.1 Pharmacodynamic properties

Pharmacotherapeutic group: Other antidepressants. *ATC code:* N06AX21.

Duloxetine is a combined serotonin (5-HT) and noradrenaline (NA) reuptake inhibitor. It weakly inhibits dopamine reuptake, with no significant affinity for histaminergic, dopaminergic, cholinergic, and adrenergic receptors.

In animal studies, increased levels of 5-HT and NE in the sacral spinal cord lead to increased urethral tone via enhanced pudendal nerve stimulation to the urethral striated sphincter muscle only during the storage phase of the micturition cycle. A similar mechanism in women is believed to result in stronger urethral closure during urine storage with physical stress that could explain the efficacy of duloxetine in the treatment of women with SUI.

The efficacy of duloxetine 40mg given twice daily in the treatment of SUI was established in four double-blind, placebo-controlled studies that randomised 1,913 women (22 to 83 years) with SUI; of these, 958 patients were randomised to duloxetine and 955 to placebo. The primary efficacy measures were incontinence episode frequency (IEF) from diaries and an incontinence specific Quality of Life Questionnaire score (I-QoL).

Incontinence episode frequency: In all four studies the duloxetine-treated group had a 50% or greater median decrease in IEF compared with 33% in the placebo-treated group. Differences were observed at each visit after 4 weeks (duloxetine 54% and placebo 22%), 8 weeks (52% and 29%), and 12 weeks (52% and 33%) of medication.

In an additional study limited to patients with severe SUI, all responses with duloxetine were achieved within 2 weeks.

The efficacy of YENTREVE has not been evaluated for longer than 3 months in placebo-controlled studies. The clinical benefit of YENTREVE compared with placebo has not been demonstrated in women with mild SUI, defined in randomised trials as those with IEF <14 per week. In these women, YENTREVE may provide no benefit beyond that afforded by more conservative behavioural interventions.

Quality of Life: Incontinence Quality of Life (I-QoL) Questionnaire scores were significantly improved in the duloxetine-treated patient group compared with the placebo-treated group (9.2 versus 5.9 score improvement; $P < 0.001$). Using a global improvement scale (PGI), significantly more women using duloxetine considered their symptoms of stress incontinence to be improved with treatment compared with women using placebo (64.6% versus 50.1%; $P < 0.001$).

YENTREVE and prior continence surgery: There are limited data that suggest that the benefits of YENTREVE are not diminished in women with stress urinary incontinence who have previously undergone continence surgery.

YENTREVE and pelvic floor muscle training (PFMT): During a 12-week blinded, randomised, controlled study, YENTREVE demonstrated greater reductions in IEF compared with either placebo treatment or with PFMT alone. Combined therapy (duloxetine + PFMT) showed greater improvement in both pad use and condition-specific quality of life measures than YENTREVE alone or PFMT alone.

5.2 Pharmacokinetic properties

Duloxetine is administered as a single enantiomer. Duloxetine is extensively metabolised by oxidative enzymes (CYP1A2 and the polymorphic CYP2D6), followed by conjugation. The pharmacokinetics of duloxetine demonstrate large intersubject variability (generally 50-60%), partly due to gender, age, smoking status, and CYP2D6 metaboliser status.

Absorption: Duloxetine is well absorbed after oral administration, with a C_{max} occurring 6 hours post-dose. The absolute oral bioavailability of duloxetine ranged from 32% to 80% (mean of 50%). Food delays the time to reach the peak concentration from 6 to 10 hours and it marginally decreases the extent of absorption (approximately 11 %). These changes do not have any clinical significance.

Distribution: Duloxetine is approximately 96% bound to human plasma proteins. Duloxetine binds to both albumin and $alpha_1$ acid glycoprotein. Protein binding is not affected by renal or hepatic impairment.

Biotransformation: Duloxetine is extensively metabolised and the metabolites are excreted principally in urine. Both cytochromes P450-2D6 and 1A2 catalyse the formation of the two major metabolites, glucuronide conjugate of 4-hydroxy duloxetine and sulphate conjugate of 5-hydroxy 6-methoxy duloxetine. Based upon *in vitro* studies, the circulating metabolites of duloxetine are considered pharmacologically inactive. The pharmacokinetics of duloxetine in patients who are poor metabolisers with respect to CYP2D6 has not been specifically investigated. Limited data suggest that the plasma levels of duloxetine are higher in these patients.

Elimination: The elimination half-life of duloxetine ranges from 8 to 17 hours (mean of 12 hours). After an intravenous dose, the plasma clearance of duloxetine ranges from 22 l/hr to 46 l/hr (mean of 36 l/hr). After an oral dose, the apparent plasma clearance of duloxetine ranges from 33 to 261 l/hr (mean 101 l/hr).

Special Populations

Gender: pharmacokinetic differences have been identified between males and females (apparent plasma clearance is approximately 50% lower in females). Based upon the overlap in the range of clearance, gender-based pharmacokinetic differences do not justify the recommendation for using a lower dose for female patients.

Age: Pharmacokinetic differences have been identified between younger and elderly females (≥65 years) (AUC increases by about 25% and half-life is about 25% longer in the elderly), although the magnitude of these changes is not sufficient to justify adjustments to the dose. As a general recommendation, caution should be exercised when treating the elderly (see sections 4.2 and 4.4).

Renal impairment: End stage renal disease (ESRD) patients receiving dialysis had a 2-fold higher duloxetine C_{max} and AUC values compared to healthy subjects. Pharmacokinetic data on duloxetine is limited in patients with mild or moderate renal impairment.

Hepatic impairment: Moderate liver disease (Child-Pugh Class B) affected the pharmacokinetics of duloxetine. Compared with healthy subjects, the apparent plasma clearance of duloxetine was 79% lower, the apparent terminal half-life was 2.3-times longer, and the AUC was 3.7-times higher in patients with moderate liver disease. The pharmacokinetics of duloxetine and its metabolites have not been studied in patients with mild or severe hepatic insufficiency.

Breast-feeding mothers: The disposition of duloxetine was studied in 6 lactating women who were at least 12- weeks postpartum. Duloxetine is detected in breast milk, and steady-state concentrations in breast milk are about one-fourth those in plasma. The amount of duloxetine in breast milk is approximately 7μg/day while on 40mg twice daily dosing. Lactation did not influence duloxetine pharmacokinetics.

5.3 Preclinical safety data

Duloxetine was not genotoxic in a standard battery of tests and was not carcinogenic in rats. Multinucleated cells were seen in the liver in the absence of other histopathological changes in the rat carcinogenicity study. The underlying mechanism and the clinical relevance are unknown.

Female mice receiving duloxetine for 2 years had an increased incidence of hepatocellular adenomas and carcinomas at the high dose only (144mg/kg/day), but these were considered to be secondary to hepatic microsomal enzyme induction. The relevance of this mouse data to humans is unknown. Female rats receiving duloxetine before and during mating and early pregnancy had a decrease in maternal food consumption and body weight, oestrous cycle disruption, decreased live birth indices and progeny survival, and progeny growth retardation at systemic exposure levels estimated to be at the most at maximum clinical exposure (AUC). In an embryotoxicity study in the rabbit, a higher incidence of cardiovascular and skeletal malformations was observed at systemic exposure levels below the maximum clinical exposure (AUC). No malformations were observed in another study testing a higher dose of a different salt of duloxetine. In a prenatal/postnatal toxicity study in the rat, duloxetine induced adverse behavioural effects in the offspring at systemic exposure levels below maximum clinical exposure (AUC).

6. PHARMACEUTICAL PARTICULARS

6.1 List of excipients

Capsule content:

Hypromellose

Hypromellose acetate succinate

Sucrose

Sugar spheres

Talc

Titanium dioxide (E171)

Triethyl citrate

Capsule shell (20mg):

Gelatin, sodium lauryl sulphate, titanium dioxide (E171), indigo carmine (E132), edible black ink.

Capsule shell (40mg):

Gelatin, sodium lauryl sulphate, titanium dioxide (E171), indigo carmine (E132), red iron oxide (E172), yellow iron oxide (E172), edible black ink.

Edible ink: Black iron oxide - synthetic (E172), propylene glycol, shellac.

6.2 Incompatibilities

Not applicable.

6.3 Shelf life

3 years.

6.4 Special precautions for storage

Store in the original package in order to protect from moisture. Do not store above 30°C.

6.5 Nature and contents of container

Polyvinylchloride (PVC), polyethylene (PE), and polychlorotrifluoroethylene (PCTFE) blister sealed with an aluminium foil.

20 mg capsules:

Packs of 28, 56 and 98 capsules.

40 mg capsules:

Packs of 28, 56, 98, 140 and 196 (2 × 98) capsules.

Not all pack sizes may be marketed.

6.6 Special precautions for disposal and other handling

No special requirements.

7. MARKETING AUTHORISATION HOLDER

Eli Lilly Nederland BV, Grootslag 1-5, NL-3991 RA Houten, The Netherlands.

8. MARKETING AUTHORISATION NUMBER(S)

20mg, 28 capsules: EU/1/04/280/007

20mg, 56 capsules: EU/1/04/280/001

20mg, 98 capsules: EU/1/04/280/008

40mg, 28 capsules: EU/1/04/280/002

40mg, 56 capsules: EU/1/04/280/003

40mg, 98 capsules: EU/1/04/280/004

40mg, 140 capsules: EU/1/04/280/005

40mg, 98 × 2 capsules: EU/1/04/280/006

9. DATE OF FIRST AUTHORISATION/RENEWAL OF THE AUTHORISATION

Date of first authorisation: 11 August 2004

Date of latest renewal: 24 June 2009

10. DATE OF REVISION OF THE TEXT

07 July 2009

Detailed information on this medicine is available on the European Medicines Agency (EMEA) web site: http://www.emea.europa.eu

LEGAL CATEGORY

POM

*YENTREVE (duloxetine) is a trademark of Eli Lilly and Company. YEN10M

Yondelis 0.25 mg powder for concentrate for solution for infusion/Yondelis 1 mg powder for concentrate for solution for infusion

(Pharma Mar, S.A.)

1. NAME OF THE MEDICINAL PRODUCT

0.25 mg vial

▼Yondelis 0.25 mg powder for concentrate for solution for infusion.

1 mg vial

▼Yondelis 1 mg powder for concentrate for solution for infusion.

2. QUALITATIVE AND QUANTITATIVE COMPOSITION

0.25 mg vial

Each vial contains 0.25 mg of trabectedin.

1 mg vial

Each vial contains 1 mg of trabectedin.

0.25 mg and 1 mg vials

1 ml of reconstituted solution contains 0.05 mg of trabectedin.

Excipients:

0.25 mg vial

Each vial contains 2 mg of potassium and 0.1 g of sucrose.

1 mg vial

Each vial contains 8 mg of potassium and 0.4 g of sucrose.

0.25 mg and 1 mg vials

For a full list of excipients, see section 6.1.

3. PHARMACEUTICAL FORM

Powder for concentrate for solution for infusion.

White to off-white powder.

4. CLINICAL PARTICULARS

4.1 Therapeutic indications

Yondelis is indicated for the treatment of patients with advanced soft tissue sarcoma, after failure of anthracyclines and ifosfamide, or who are unsuited to receive these agents. Efficacy data are based mainly on liposarcoma and leiomyosarcoma patients.

4.2 Posology and method of administration

Yondelis must be administered under the supervision of a physician experienced in the use of chemotherapy. Its use should be confined to qualified oncologists or other health professionals specialised in the administration of cytotoxic agents.

The recommended dose is 1.5 mg/m^2 body surface area, administered as an intravenous infusion over 24 hours with a three-week interval between cycles. Administration through a central venous line is strongly recommended (see section 6.6).

All patients must receive 20 mg of dexamethasone intravenously 30 minutes prior to Yondelis; not only as antiemetic prophylaxis, but also because it appears to provide hepatoprotective effects. Additional anti-emetics may be administered as needed.

The following criteria are required to allow treatment with Yondelis:

- Absolute neutrophil count (ANC) ≥ 1,500/mm^3
- Platelet count ≥ 100,000/mm^3
- Bilirubin ≤ upper limit of normal (ULN)
- Alkaline phosphatase ≤ 2.5 ULN (consider hepatic isoenzymes 5-nucleotidase or GGT, if the elevation could be osseous in origin).
- Albumin ≥ 25 g/l.
- Alanine aminotransferase (ALT) and Aspartate aminotransferase (AST) ≤ 2.5 × ULN
- Creatinine clearance ≥ 30 ml/min
- Creatine phosphokinase (CPK) ≤ 2.5 ULN
- Haemoglobin ≥ 9 g/dl

The same criteria as above must be met prior to re-treatment. Otherwise treatment must be delayed for up to 3 weeks until the criteria are met.

Additional monitoring of haematological parameters bilirubin, alkaline phosphatase, aminotransferases and CPK should occur weekly during the first two cycles of therapy, and at least once between treatments in subsequent cycles.

The same dose should be given for all cycles provided that no grade 3-4 toxicities are seen and that the patient fulfils the re-treatment criteria.

Dose adjustments during treatment

Prior to re-treatment, patients must fulfil the baseline criteria defined above. If any of the following events occur at any time between cycles, the dose must be reduced to 1.2 mg/m^2 for subsequent cycles:

- Neutropenia < 500/mm^3 lasting for more than 5 days or associated with fever or infection
- Thrombocytopenia < 25,000/mm^3
- Increase of bilirubin > ULN and/or alkaline phosphatase > 2.5 × ULN
- Increase of aminotransferases (AST or ALT) > 2.5 × ULN which has not recovered by day 21
- Any other grade 3 or 4 adverse reactions (such as nausea, vomiting, fatigue)

Once a dose has been reduced because of toxicity, dose escalation in the subsequent cycles is not recommended. If any of these toxicities reappear in subsequent cycles in a patient exhibiting clinical benefit, the dose may be further reduced to 1 mg/m^2. In the event that further dose reductions are necessary, treatment discontinuation should be considered.

Duration of treatment

In clinical trials, there were no pre-defined limits to the number of cycles administered. Treatment continued whilst clinical benefit was noted. Trabectedin has been administered for 6 or more cycles in 168 out of 569 (29.5%) patients treated with the proposed dose and schedule. This regime has been used for up to 38 cycles. No cumulative toxicities have been observed in patients treated with multiple cycles.

Special patient populations

Paediatric patients

The safety and efficacy of trabectedin in paediatric patients have not yet been established. Therefore, this medicinal product must not be used in children and adolescents until further data become available.

Elderly patients

No specific studies in elderly patients have been performed. Overall 20% of the 1164 patients in the integrated safety analysis were over 65 years. No relevant differences in the safety profile were seen in this patient population. It seems that plasma clearance and distribution volume of trabectedin are not influenced by age. Therefore, dose adjustments based uniquely on age criteria are not routinely recommended.

Patients with impaired hepatic function

No studies with the proposed regime have been conducted in patients with liver dysfunction. Thus, data are not available to recommend a lower starting dose in patients with hepatic impairment. However, special caution is advised and dose adjustments may be necessary in these patients since systemic exposure is probably increased and the risk of hepatotoxicity might be increased. Patients with elevated bilirubin must not be treated with Yondelis (see section 4.4).

Patients with impaired renal function

Studies including patients with severe renal insufficiency (creatinine clearance < 30 ml/min) have not been conducted and therefore Yondelis must not be used in this patient population (see section 4.4). Considering the pharmacokinetic characteristics of trabectedin (see section 5.2), no dose adjustments are warranted in patients with mild or moderate renal impairment.

For instructions on reconstitution and dilution of the medicinal product before administration, see section 6.6.

4.3 Contraindications

- Hypersensitivity to trabectedin or to any of the excipients
- Concurrent serious or uncontrolled infection
- Breast-feeding (see section 4.6)
- Combination with yellow fever vaccine (see section 4.4)

4.4 Special warnings and precautions for use

Hepatic impairment

Patients must meet specific criteria on hepatic function parameters to start treatment with Yondelis. Since systemic exposure to trabectedin is probably increased due to hepatic impairment and therefore the risk of hepatotoxicity might be increased, patients with clinically relevant liver diseases, such as active chronic hepatitis, must be closely monitored and the dose adjusted if needed. Patients with elevated bilirubin must not be treated with trabectedin (see section 4.2).

Renal impairment

Creatinine clearance must be monitored prior to and during treatment. Trabectedin must not be used in patients with creatinine clearance < 30 ml/min (see section 4.2).

Neutropenia and thrombocytopenia

Grades 3 or 4 neutropenia and thrombocytopenia associated with trabectedin therapy have been very commonly reported. A full blood cell count including differential and platelet count must be performed at baseline, weekly for the first two cycles and then once between cycles (see section 4.2). Patients who develop fever should promptly seek medical attention. If this occurs, active supportive therapy should be started immediately.

Nausea and vomiting

Anti-emetic prophylaxis with dexamethasone must be administered to all patients (see section 4.2).

Rhabdomyolysis and severe CPK elevations (> 10 × ULN)

Trabectedin must not be used in patients with CPK> 2.5 ULN (see section 4.2). Rhabdomyolysis has been uncommonly reported, usually in association with myelotoxicity, severe liver function test abnormalities and/or renal failure. Therefore, CPK should be closely monitored whenever a patient may be experiencing any of these toxicities. If rhabdomyolysis occurs, supportive measures such as parenteral hydration, urine alkalinisation and dialysis should be promptly established, as indicated. Treatment with Yondelis should be discontinued until the patient fully recovers.

Caution should be taken if medicinal products associated with rhabdomyolysis (e.g. statins), are administered concomitantly with trabectedin, since the risk of rhabdomyolysis may be increased

Liver Function Test (LFT) abnormalities

Reversible acute increases in aspartate aminotransferase (AST) and alanine aminotransferase (ALT) have been reported in most patients. Yondelis must not be used in patients with elevated bilirubin. Patients with increases in AST, ALT and alkaline phosphatase between cycles may necessitate dose reduction (see section 4.2).

Injection site reactions

The use of central venous access is strongly recommended (see section 4.2). Patients may develop a potentially severe injection site reaction when trabectedin is administered through a peripheral venous line.

Trabectedin extravasation may cause tissue necrosis requiring debridement. There is no specific antidote for extravasation of trabectedin. Extravasation should be managed by local standard practice.

Others

Co-administration of Yondelis with potent inhibitors of the enzyme CYP3A4 should be avoided (see section 4.5). If this is not possible, close monitoring of toxicities are required and dose reductions of trabectedin should be considered.

Caution should be taken if medicinal products associated with hepatotoxicity are administered concomitantly with trabectedin, since the risk of hepatotoxicity may be increased.

Concomitant use of trabectedin with phenytoin may reduce phenytoin absorption leading to an exacerbation of convulsions. Combination of trabectedin with phenytoin or live attenuated vaccines is not recommended and with yellow fever vaccine is specifically contraindicated (see section 4.3).

The concomitant use of trabectedin with alcohol must be avoided (see section 4.5).

Men in fertile age and women of childbearing potential must use effective contraception during treatment and 3 months thereafter for women and immediately inform the treating physician if a pregnancy occurs, and 5 months after treatment for men (see section 4.6).

This medicine contains potassium, less than 1 mmol (39 mg) per vial, i.e. essentially "potassium-free".

4.5 Interaction with other medicinal products and other forms of interaction

Effects of other substances on trabectedin

In vivo interaction studies have not been performed. Since trabectedin is metabolised mainly by CYP3A4, co-administration of substances that inhibit this isoenzyme e.g. ketoconazole, fluconazole ritonavir, clarithromycin or aprepitant could decrease metabolism and increase trabectedin concentrations. If such combinations are needed, close monitoring of toxicities is required (see section 4.4). Likewise co-administration with potent inducers of this enzyme (e.g. rifampicin, phenorbarbital, Saint John's Wort) may decrease the systemic exposure to trabectedin.

Alcohol consumption must be avoided during treatment with trabectedin due to the hepatotoxicity of the medicinal product (see section 4.4).

Preclinical data have demonstrated that trabectedin is a substrate to P-gp. Concomitant administration of inhibitors of P-gp, e.g. cyclosporine and verapamil, may alter trabectedin distribution and/or elimination. The relevance of this interaction e.g. CNS toxicity has not been established. Caution should be taken in such situations.

4.6 Pregnancy and lactation

Pregnancy

No sufficient clinical data on exposed pregnancies are available. However, based on its known mechanism of action, trabectedin may cause serious birth defects when administered during pregnancy. Trabectedin should not be used during pregnancy unless clearly necessary. If it is used during pregnancy, the patient must be informed of the potential risk to the foetus (see section 5.3) and be monitored carefully. If trabectedin is used at the end of pregnancy, potential adverse reactions should be monitored carefully in the newborns.

Fertility

Men in fertile age and women of childbearing potential must use effective contraception during treatment and 3 months thereafter for women and immediately inform the treating physician if a pregnancy occurs (see section 5.3) and 5 months after treatment for men (see section 4.4).

Trabectedin can have genotoxic effects. Advice on conservation of sperm should be sought prior to treatment because of the possibility of irreversible infertility due to therapy with Yondelis.

If pregnancy occurs during treatment the possibility of genetic counselling should be considered. Genetic counselling is also recommended for patients wishing to have children after therapy.

Lactation

It is not known whether trabectedin is excreted in human milk. The excretion of trabectedin in milk has not been studied in animals. Breast-feeding is contraindicated during treatment and 3 months thereafter (see section 4.3).

4.7 Effects on ability to drive and use machines

No studies on the effects of the ability to drive and to use machines have been performed. However, fatigue and/or asthenia have been reported in patients receiving trabectedin. Patients who experience any of these events during therapy must not drive or operate machines.

4.8 Undesirable effects

Unless otherwise specified, the following safety profile of Yondelis is based on the evaluation in clinical trials of 569 patients treated up to April 2007 with the recommended treatment regime in several cancer types including soft tissue sarcoma, breast cancer, osteosarcoma, ovarian cancer, GIST, melanoma and renal carcinoma.

Approximately 91% of patients can be expected to have adverse reactions of any grade. Around 40% of patients are expected to have adverse reactions of grade 3 or 4 severity. The most common adverse reactions of any severity grade were nausea, fatigue, vomiting, anorexia, neutropenia, and increases in AST/ALT.

Fatal adverse reactions have occurred in 1.9% of patients. They were often the result of a combination of events including pancytopenia, febrile neutropenia, some of them with sepsis, hepatic involvement, renal failure and rhabdomyolysis.

Adverse reactions

The frequencies of the adverse reactions reported below are classified as very common (≥ 1/10), common (≥ 1/100 to < 1/10) and uncommon (≥ 1/1000 to < 1/100).

The table below displays the adverse reactions reported in ≥ 1% of patients according to the standard MedDRA system organ class. Both adverse events and laboratory values have been used to provide frequencies. Within each frequency grouping, undesirable effects are presented in order of decreasing seriousness.

System Organ Class	Adverse reactions reported in ≥ 1% of patients in clinical trials at the recommended regime [1.5mg/m^2, 24 hour infusion every 3 weeks (24-h q3wk)]
Investigations	**Very Common** Blood creatine phosphokinase increased, Blood creatinine increased, Blood albumin decreased **Common** Weight decreased
Blood and Lymphatic System Disorders	**Very Common** Neutropenia, Thrombocytopenia, Anaemia, Leukopenia **Common** Febrile neutropenia
Nervous System Disorders	**Very Common** Headache **Common** Peripheral sensory neuropathy, Dysgeusia, Dizziness, Paraesthesia
Respiratory, Thoracic and Mediastinal Disorders	**Common** Dyspnoea, Cough
Gastrointestinal disorders	**Very Common** Vomiting, Nausea, Constipation **Common** Diarrhoea, Stomatitis, Abdominal pain, Dyspepsia, Upper abdominal pain
Skin and Subcutaneous Tissue Disorders	**Common** Alopecia
Musculoskeletal and Connective Tissue Disorders	**Common** Myalgia, Arthralgia, Back pain
Metabolism and Nutrition Disorders	**Very Common** Anorexia **Common** Dehydration, Decreased appetite, Hypokalaemia
Infections and Infestations	**Common** Infection
Vascular Disorders	**Common** Hypotension, Flushing
General Disorders and Administration Site Conditions	**Very Common** Fatigue, Asthenia **Common** Pyrexia, Oedema, Oedema peripheral, Injection site reaction
Hepatobiliary Disorders	**Very Common** Hyperbilirubinemia, Alanine aminotransferase increased, Aspartate aminotransferase increased, Blood alkaline phosphatase increased, Gamma-glutamyltransferase increased
Psychiatric Disorders	**Common** Insomnia

Most frequent adverse reactions

Blood and Lymphatic system disorders

Neutropenia: Neutropenia occurred in 77% of patients. Grade 3 and 4 neutropenia occurred in 26% and 24% of patients respectively. The analysis per cycle showed that neutropenia of grade 3 and 4 occurred in approximately 19% and 8% of cycles respectively Febrile neutropenia occurred in 2% of patients and in < 1% of cycles.

Neutropenia followed a predictable pattern of rapid onset and reversibility, and was rarely associated with fever or infection.

Thrombocytopenia: Grade 3 and 4 thrombocytopenia occurred in 11% and 2% of patients respectively. The analysis per cycle showed that thrombocytopenia of grade 3 and 4 occurred in approximately 3% and < 1% of cycles respectively. Bleeding events associated to thrombocytopenia occurred in < 1% of patients.

Anaemia: Anaemia occurred in 93% of patients although 46% of patients were anaemic at baseline. Grade 3 and 4 anaemia occurred in 10% and 3% of patients respectively. The analysis per cycle showed that anaemia of grade 3 and 4 occurred in approximately 3% and 1% of cycles respectively.

Hepatobiliary disorders

AST/ALT increases: Transient grade 3 increases of aspartate aminotransferase (AST) and alanine aminotransferase (ALT) were observed in 38% and 44% of the patients and grade 4 elevations in 3% and 7% of the patients, respectively. The median time to reach the peak values was 5 days for both AST and ALT. Most of the values had decreased to grade 1 or resolved by day 14-15 (see section 4.4). Grade 3 elevations of AST and ALT occurred in 12% and 20% of cycles respectively. Grade 4 elevations of AST and ALT occurred in 1% and 2% of cycles respectively. Most transaminase elevations improved to grade 1 or to pre-retreatment levels within 15 days, and less than 2% of cycles had recovering times longer than 25 days. ALT and AST increases did not follow a cumulative pattern but showed a tendency towards less severe elevations over time.

Hyperbilirubinemia: Grades 1 to 2 bilirubin increases were observed in 23% of the patients. Grade 3 hyperbilirubinemia occurred in 1% of patients. Bilirubin peaks approximately a week after onset and resolves approximately two weeks after onset.

Clinical manifestations of severe hepatic injury were uncommon with a lower than 1% incidence of individual signs and symptoms including jaundice, hepatomegaly or liver pain. Mortality in the presence of hepatic injury occurred in less than 1% of patients.

Other adverse reactions

Nausea, vomiting, diarrhoea and constipation: Nausea and vomiting were reported in 63 and 38.5% of patients respectively. Grade 3-4 *nausea and vomiting were* reported in 6% and 6.5% of patients, respectively. Grade 3-4 *diarrhoea* and *constipation were reported* in less than 1% of patients.

Stomatitis: Grade 3-4 mucositis was reported in less than 1% of the patients.

Fatigue/Asthenia: Grade 3-4 fatigue/asthenia occurred in 9 and 1% of patients respectively.

Anorexia: Grade 3-4 anorexia occurred in less than 1% of the patients.

CPK elevations and rhabdomyolysis: CPK elevations of any grade were observed in 26% of patients. Grade 3 or 4 increases of CPK were observed in 4% of patients. CPK increases in association with rhabdomyolysis were reported in less than 1% of patients.

Dyspnoea: Grade 3-4 dyspnoea reported as trabectedin related occurred in 2% of the patients.

Alopecia: Alopecia was reported in approximately 3% of all patients, of which the majority was grade 1 alopecia.

Post-marketing experience

During post-marketing surveillance few cases of trabectedin extravasation with subsequent *tissue necrosis* requiring debridement have been reported (see section 4.4).

4.9 Overdose

There is limited data on the effects of trabectedin overdose. The major anticipated toxicities are gastrointestinal, bone marrow suppression and hepatic toxicity. There is no specific antidote for trabectedin currently available. In the event of an overdose, patients should be closely monitored and symptomatic supportive care measures instituted as required.

5. PHARMACOLOGICAL PROPERTIES

5.1 Pharmacodynamic properties

Pharmacotherapeutic group: Antineoplastic agent, ATC code: L01CX01.

Mechanism of action

Trabectedin binds to the minor groove of DNA, bending the helix to the major groove. This binding to DNA triggers a cascade of events affecting several transcription factors, DNA binding proteins, and DNA repair pathways, resulting in perturbation of the cell cycle. Trabectedin has been shown to exert antiproliferative *in vitro* and *in vivo* activity against a range of human tumour cell lines and experimental tumours, including malignancies such as sarcoma, breast, non-small cell lung, ovarian and melanoma.

Clinical efficacy

The efficacy and safety of trabectedin is based in a randomised trial in patients with locally advanced or metastatic liposarcoma or leiomyosarcoma, whose disease had progressed or relapsed after treatment with at least anthracyclines and ifosfamide. In this trial trabectedin was administered either at 1.5 mg/m^2 as a 24-hour intravenous infusion every 3 weeks or at 0.58 mg/m^2 weekly as a 3-hour intravenous infusion for 3-weeks of a 4-week cycle. The protocol specified final time to progression (TTP) analysis showed a 26.6% reduction in the relative risk of progression for patients treated in the 24-h q3wk group (Hazard Ratio = 0.734 CI 0.554-0.974). Median TTP values were 3.7 months (CI: 2.1-5.4 m) in the 24-h q3wk group and 2.3 months (CI: 2.0-3.5 m) in the 3-h qwk group (p=0.0302). No significant differences were detected in overall survival (OS). Median OS with the 24-h q3wk regime was 13.9 months (CI: 12.5-18.6) and 60.2% of patients were alive at 1 year (CI: 52.0-68.5%).

Additional efficacy data are available from 3 single-arm Phase II trials with similar populations treated with the same regime. These trials evaluated a total of 100 patients with lipo and leiomyosarcoma and 83 patients with other types of sarcoma.

This medicinal product has been authorised under "Exceptional Circumstances". This means that due to the rarity of the disease it has not been possible to obtain complete information on this medicinal product.

The European Medicines Agency (EMEA) will review any new information which may become available every year and this SPC will be updated as necessary.

5.2 Pharmacokinetic properties

Systemic exposure after administration as a 24 hour constant rate intravenous infusion is dose proportional at doses up to and including 1.8 mg/m^2. Trabectedin pharmacokinetic profile is consistent with a multiple-compartment disposition model.

Following intravenous administration, trabectedin demonstrates a high apparent volume of distribution, consistent with extensive tissue and plasma protein binding (94 to 98% of trabectedin in plasma is protein bound). The distribution volume at steady state of trabectedin in human subjects exceeds 5000 l.

Cytochrome P450 3A4 is the major cytochrome P450 isozyme responsible for the oxidative metabolism of trabectedin at clinically relevant concentrations. Other P450 enzymes may contribute to metabolism. Trabectedin does not induce or inhibit major cytochrome P450 enzymes.

Renal elimination of unchanged trabectedin in humans is low (less than 1%). The terminal half-life is long (population value of the terminal elimination phase: 180-hr). After a dose of radiolabelled trabectedin administered to cancer patients, faecal mean (SD) recovery of total radioactivity is 58% (17%), and urinary mean (SD) recovery is 5.8% (1.73%). Based on the population estimate for plasma clearance of trabectedin (31.5 l/h) and blood/plasma ratio (0.89), the clearance of trabectedin in whole blood is approximately 35 l/h. This value is approximately one-half the rate of human hepatic blood flow. Thus the trabectedin extraction ratio can be considered moderate. The inter-patient variability of the population estimate for plasma clearance of trabectedin was 51% and intra-patient variability was 28%.

Special populations

A population pharmacokinetic analysis indicated that the plasma clearance of trabectedin is not influenced by age (range 19-83 years), or gender. The effects of race and ethnicity on trabectedin pharmacokinetics have not been studied.

Impaired renal function

There is no relevant influence of renal function measured by creatinine clearance on trabectedin pharmacokinetics within the range of values (≥ 34.4 ml/min) present in the patients included in the clinical studies. No data are available in patients with a creatinine clearance of less than 34.4 ml/min. The low recovery (< 9% in all studied patients) of total radioactivity in the urine after a single dose of ^{14}C-labelled trabectedin indicates that renal impairment has little influence on the elimination of trabectedin or its metabolites.

Impaired hepatic function

Although the population analysis showed no relationship between the serum liver enzymes concentrations and the plasma clearance of trabectedin, systemic exposure to trabectedin may be increased in patients with hepatic impairment; therefore close monitoring of toxicity is warranted.

5.3 Preclinical safety data

Preclinical data indicate that trabectedin has limited effect on the cardiovascular, respiratory and central nervous system at exposures below the therapeutic clinical range, in terms of AUC.

The effects of trabectedin on cardiovascular and respiratory function have been investigated *in vivo* (anesthetised Cynomolgus monkeys). A 1 hour infusion schedule was selected to attain maximum plasma levels (C_{max} values) in the range of those observed in the clinic. The plasma trabectedin levels attained were 10.6 ± 5.4 (C_{max}), higher than those reached in patients after infusion of 1500 μg/m^2 for 24 (C_{max} of 1.8 ± 1.1 ng/ml) and similar to those reached after administration of the same dose by 3 hour infusion (C_{max} of 10.8 ± 3.7 ng/ml).

Myelosupression and hepatoxicity were identified as the primary toxicity for trabectedin. Findings observed included haematopoietic toxicity (severe leukopenia, anaemia, and lymphoid and bone marrow depletion) as well as increases in liver function tests, hepatocellular degeneration, intestinal epithelial necrosis, and severe local reactions at the injection site. Renal toxicological findings were detected in multi-cycle toxicity studies conducted in monkeys. These findings were secondary to severe local reaction at the administration site, and therefore uncertainly attributable to trabectedin; however, caution must be guaranteed in the interpretation of these renal findings, and treatment-related toxicity cannot be excluded.

Trabectedin is genotoxic both *in vitro* and *in vivo*. Long-term carcinogenicity studies have not been performed.

Fertility studies with trabectedin were not performed but limited histopathological changes were observed in the gonads in the repeat dose toxicity studies. Considering the nature of the compound (cytotoxic and mutagenic), it is likely to affect the reproductive capacity.

6. PHARMACEUTICAL PARTICULARS

6.1 List of excipients

Sucrose.

Potassium dihydrogen phosphate.

Phosphoric acid (for pH-adjustment).

Potassium hydroxide (for pH-adjustment).

6.2 Incompatibilities

Yondelis must not be mixed or diluted with other medicinal products except those mentioned in section 6.6.

6.3 Shelf life

Unopened vials: 36 months.

After reconstitution, chemical and physical stability has been demonstrated for 30 hours up to 25°C.

From a microbiological point of view, the reconstituted solution should be diluted and used immediately. If not diluted and used immediately, in-use storage times and conditions prior to use of the reconstituted product are the responsibility of the user and would normally not be longer than 24 hours at 2°C to 8°C, unless reconstitution has taken place in controlled and validated aseptic conditions.

After dilution, chemical and physical stability has been demonstrated for 30 hours up to 25°C.

6.4 Special precautions for storage

Store in a refrigerator (2°C - 8°C).

For storage conditions of the reconstituted and diluted medicinal product, see section 6.3.

6.5 Nature and contents of container

Yondelis is supplied in a Type I colourless glass vial with a bromobutyl rubber stopper covered with an aluminium flip-off seal.

0.25 mg vial

Each vial contains 0.25 mg of trabectedin.

1 mg vial

Each vial contains 1 mg of trabectedin.

0.25 mg and 1 mg vials

Each outer carton contains one vial.

6.6 Special precautions for disposal and other handling

Preparation for intravenous infusion

0.25 mg vial

Appropriate aseptic techniques must be used. Yondelis must be reconstituted and further diluted prior to infusion. Each vial containing 0.25 mg of trabectedin is reconstituted with 5 ml of sterile water for injections. The solution obtained has a concentration of 0.05 mg/ml and is for single-use only.

Instructions for reconstitution

A syringe is used to inject 5 ml of sterile water for injections into the vial. Shake the vial until complete dissolution. The reconstituted solution results in a clear, colourless or slightly yellowish solution, essentially free of visible particles.

1 mg vial

Appropriate aseptic techniques must be used. Yondelis must be reconstituted and further diluted prior to infusion. Each vial containing 1 mg of trabectedin is reconstituted with 20 ml of sterile water for injections. The solution obtained has a concentration of 0.05 mg/ml and is for single-use only.

Instructions for reconstitution

A syringe is used to inject 20 ml of sterile water for injections into the vial. Shake the vial until complete dissolution. The reconstituted solution results in a clear, colourless or slightly yellowish solution, essentially free of visible particles.

0.25 mg and 1 mg vials

This reconstituted solution contains 0.05 mg/ml of trabectedin. It requires further dilution and is for single-use only

Instructions for dilution

The reconstituted solution should be diluted with sodium chloride 9 mg/ml (0.9%) solution for infusion or glucose 50 mg/ml (5%) solution for infusion. The required volume should be calculated as follows:

$$\text{Volume (ml)} = \frac{\text{BSA (m}^2\text{)} \times \text{individual dose (mg/m}^2\text{)}}{0.05 \text{ mg/ml}}$$

BSA = Body Surface Area

If administration is to be made through a central venous line, the appropriate amount of reconstituted solution should be withdrawn from the vial and added to an infusion bag containing ≥ 50 ml of diluent (sodium chloride 9 mg/ml (0.9%) solution for infusion or glucose 50 mg/ml (5%) solution for infusion), the concentration of trabectedin in the infusion solution being ≤ 0.030 mg/ml.

If central venous access is not feasible and a peripheral venous line has to be used, the reconstituted solution should be added to an infusion bag containing ≥ 1,000 ml of diluent (sodium chloride 9 mg/ml (0.9%) solution for infusion or glucose 50 mg/ml (5%) solution for infusion).

Parenteral solutions should be inspected visually for particles prior to administration. Once the infusion is prepared, it should be administered immediately.

Instructions for handling and disposal

Yondelis is a cytotoxic anticancer medicinal product and, as with other potentially toxic compounds, caution should be exercised during handling. Procedures for proper handling and disposal of cytotoxic medicinal products must be followed. Personnel should be trained in the correct techniques to reconstitute and dilute the medicinal product and should wear protective clothing including mask, goggles and gloves during the reconstitution and dilution. Pregnant staff must be excluded from working with this medicinal product.

Accidental contact with the skin, eyes or mucous membranes must be treated immediately with copious amounts of water.

Any unused product or waste material should be disposed of in accordance with local requirements for cytotoxic medicinal products.

No incompatibilities have been observed between Yondelis and type I glass bottles, polyvinylchloride (PVC) and polyethylene (PE) bags and tubing, polyisoprene reservoirs and titanium implantable vascular access systems.

7. MARKETING AUTHORISATION HOLDER

Pharma Mar, S.A.

Avda. de los Reyes 1, Polígono Industrial La Mina

28770 Colmenar Viejo (Madrid)

Spain

8. MARKETING AUTHORISATION NUMBER(S)

Yondelis 0.25 mg vial

EU/1/07/417/001

Yondelis 1 mg vial

EU/1/07/417/002

9. DATE OF FIRST AUTHORISATION/RENEWAL OF THE AUTHORISATION

17 September 2007

10. DATE OF REVISION OF THE TEXT

22 June 2009

Zacin Cream 0.025%

(Cephalon Limited)

1. NAME OF THE MEDICINAL PRODUCT
Zacin 0.025% w/w Cream

2. QUALITATIVE AND QUANTITATIVE COMPOSITION
Capsaicin 0.025% w/w

3. PHARMACEUTICAL FORM
Cream for topical application

4. CLINICAL PARTICULARS

4.1 Therapeutic indications
For the symptomatic relief of pain associated with osteoarthritis.

4.2 Posology and method of administration
Adults and the elderly:

For topical administration to unbroken skin. Apply only a small amount of cream (pea size) to affected area 4 times daily. These applications should be evenly spaced throughout the waking hours and not more often than every 4 hours. The cream should be gently rubbed in, there should be no residue left on the surface. Hands should be washed immediately after application of Zacin unless hands and fingers are being treated. Zacin should not be applied near the eyes. Pain relief usually begins within the first week of treatment and increases with continuing regular application for the next two to eight weeks.

Not suitable for use in children.

4.3 Contraindications
Zacin cream is contra-indicated on broken or irritated skin.

Zacin Cream is contra-indicated in patients with known hypersensitivity to capsaicin or any of the excipients used in this product.

4.4 Special warnings and precautions for use
The hands should be washed immediately after application of the cream, unless the hands are the treated areas, in which case, they should be washed 30 minutes after application

Patients should avoid taking a hot bath or shower just before or after applying Zacin, as it can enhance the burning sensation.

Keep Zacin away from the eyes.

Medical advice should be sought if the condition worsens, or clears up then recurs.

Tight bandages should not be applied on top of Zacin cream.

4.5 Interaction with other medicinal products and other forms of interaction
Not applicable.

4.6 Pregnancy and lactation
The safety of Zacin during pregnancy and lactation has not been established, in either humans or animals. However, in the small amounts absorbed transdermally from Zacin Cream, it is considered unlikely that capsaicin will cause any adverse effects in humans.

4.7 Effects on ability to drive and use machines
Not applicable.

4.8 Undesirable effects
Zacin may cause transient burning on application. This burning is observed more frequently when application schedules of less than 4 times daily are utilised. The burning can be enhanced if too much cream is used and if it is applied just before or after a bath or shower.

Irritation of the mucous membranes of the eyes and respiratory tract (such as coughing, sneezing, and runny eyes) on application of Zacin cream has been reported rarely. These events are usually mild and self-limiting. There have been a few reports of dyspnoea, wheezing and exacerbation of asthma.

4.9 Overdose
Not applicable.

5. PHARMACOLOGICAL PROPERTIES

5.1 Pharmacodynamic properties
Although the precise mechanism of action of capsaicin is not fully understood, current evidence suggests that capsaicin exerts an analgesic effect by depleting and preventing reaccumulation of Substance P in peripheral sensory neurons. Substance P is thought to be the principal chemomediator of pain impulses from the periphery to the central nervous system.

5.2 Pharmacokinetic properties
Absorption after topical application is unknown. Average consumption of dietary spice from capsicum fruit has been estimated at 2.5g/person/day in India and 5.0g/person/day in Thailand. Capsaicin content in capsicum fruit is approximately 1% therefore dietary intake of capsaicin may range from 0.5-1mg/kg/day for a 50kg person. Application of two tubes of Zacin Cream 0.025% (90g) each week results in 3.21mg/day topical exposure. Assuming 100% absorption in a 50kg person, daily exposure would be 0.064mg/kg which is approximately one seventh to one eighth of the above mentioned dietary intake.

5.3 Preclinical safety data
The available animal toxicity data relating to capsicum, capsicum extracts and capsaicin do not suggest that, in usual doses, they pose any significant toxicity hazard to man. Thus, in both single and repeat dosing studies which have been reported, capsicum extracts and capsicum are generally well-tolerated at many times even the highest estimated human intakes. The safety of Zacin for use in human pregnancy has not been established since no formal reproduction studies have been performed in either animals or man. However, there is no reason to suspect from human or animal studies currently available that any adverse effects in humans are likely.

Studies reported in the published literature which relate to potential genotoxic and carcinogenic action of capsaicin have produced inconclusive and conflicting data. However, it is unlikely that capsaicin, in the quantities absorbed transdermally from Zacin cream, will pose any significant hazard to humans.

6. PHARMACEUTICAL PARTICULARS

6.1 List of excipients
Purified Water
Sorbitol Solution
Isopropyl Myristate
Cetyl Alcohol
White Soft Paraffin
Glyceryl Stearate and Peg-100
Stearate (Arlacel 165)
Benzyl Alcohol

6.2 Incompatibilities
Not applicable.

6.3 Shelf life
3 years

6.4 Special precautions for storage
Store below 25°C.

Return any unused cream to your doctor or pharmacist.

6.5 Nature and contents of container
Aluminium tubes with epoxyphenolic lining and polypropylene spiked cap containing 45g of Zacin Cream 0.025%.

6.6 Special precautions for disposal and other handling
Not applicable.

7. MARKETING AUTHORISATION HOLDER
Cephalon Limited
1 Albany Place
Hyde Way
Welwyn Garden City
Hertfordshire
AL7 3BT

8. MARKETING AUTHORISATION NUMBER(S)
PL 21799/0014

9. DATE OF FIRST AUTHORISATION/RENEWAL OF THE AUTHORISATION
31st December 2006

10. DATE OF REVISION OF THE TEXT
5th August 2009

11. Legal Category
POM

Zanaflex 2 and 4mg tablets

(Cephalon Limited)

1. NAME OF THE MEDICINAL PRODUCT
Zanaflex®

2. QUALITATIVE AND QUANTITATIVE COMPOSITION
Zanaflex tablets containing 2 mg of tizanidine as the hydrochloride.

Zanaflex tablets containing 4 mg of tizanidine as the hydrochloride.

For excipients, see 6.1

3. PHARMACEUTICAL FORM
Tablet

White to off-white, circular flat bevelled edge tablet. Scored on one side, 'A' and 592 on the other side.

White to off-white, circular flat bevelled edge tablet. Cross scored on one side, 'A' and 594 on the other side.

4. CLINICAL PARTICULARS

4.1 Therapeutic indications
Treatment of spasticity associated with multiple sclerosis or with spinal cord injury or disease.

4.2 Posology and method of administration
For oral administration

The effect of Zanaflex on spasticity is maximal within 2-3 hours of dosing and it has a relatively short duration of action. The timing and frequency of dosing should therefore be tailored to the individual, and Zanaflex should be given in divided doses, up to 3-4 times daily, depending on the patient's needs. There is considerable variation in response between patients so careful titration is necessary. Care should be taken not to exceed the dose producing the desired therapeutic effect. It is usual to start with a single dose of 2 mg increasing by 2 mg increments at no less than half-weekly intervals.

The total daily dose should not exceed 36 mg, although it is usually not necessary to exceed 24 mg daily. Secondary pharmacological effects (see section 4.8 Undesirable Effects) may occur at therapeutic doses but these can be minimised by slow titration so that in the large majority of patients they are not a limiting factor.

Elderly

Experience in the elderly is limited and use of Zanaflex is not recommended unless the benefit of treatment clearly outweighs the risk. Pharmacokinetic data suggest that renal clearance in the elderly may be decreased by up to three fold.

Children

Experience with Zanaflex in patients under the age of 18 years is limited. Zanaflex is not recommended for use in children.

Patients with Renal impairment

In patients with renal insufficiency (creatinine clearance < 25mL/min) treatment should be started with 2 mg once daily with slow titration to achieve the effective dose. Dosage increases should be in increments of no more than 2 mg according to tolerability and effectiveness. It is advisable to slowly increase the once-daily dose before increasing the frequency of administration. Renal function should be monitored as appropriate in these patients.

Patients with Hepatic Impairment

Zanaflex is contraindicated in patients with significantly impaired hepatic function.

4.3 Contraindications
Hypersensitivity to tizanidine or any other component of the product (see section 6.1 List of excipients).

The use of Zanaflex in patients with significantly impaired hepatic function is contraindicated, because tizanidine is extensively metabolised by the liver (see section 5.2 Pharmacodynamic properties).

Concomitant use of tizanidine with fluvoxamine or ciprofloxacin is contra-indicated (see section 4.5 Interaction with other medicinal products and other forms of interaction and section 4.4 Special warnings and special precautions for use).

4.4 Special warnings and precautions for use
Concomitant use of tizanidine with CYP1A2 inhibitors is not recommended (see section 4.3 Contraindications and section 4.5 Interaction with other medicaments and other forms of interaction).

Hypotension may occur during treatment with tizanidine (see section 4.8 Undesirable effects) and also as a result of drug interactions with CYP1A2 inhibitors and/or antihypertensive drugs (see section 4.5 Interaction with other medicinal products and other forms of interaction). Severe manifestations of hypotension such as loss of consciousness and circulatory collapse have also been observed.

Rebound hypertension and tachycardia have been observed after sudden withdrawal of tizanidine, when it had been used chronically, and/or in high daily dosages, and/or concomitantly with antihypertensive drugs (see also section 4.5 Interaction with other medicinal products and other forms of interaction). In extreme cases, rebound hypertension might lead to cerebrovascular accident. Tizanidine should not be stopped abruptly, but rather gradually, and blood pressure should be monitored regularly on withdrawal.

Use in Renal Impairment

Patients with renal impairment may require lower doses and therefore caution should be exercised when using Zanaflex in these patients (see section 4.2 Posology and Method of Administration).

Liver Function

Hepatic dysfunction has been reported in association with Zanaflex. It is recommended that liver function tests should be monitored monthly for the first four months in all patients and in those who develop symptoms suggestive of liver dysfunction such as unexplained nausea, anorexia or tiredness. Treatment with Zanaflex should be discontinued if serum levels of SGPT and/or SGOT are persistently above three times the upper limit of normal range.

Zanaflex tablets contain lactose. This medicine is not recommended in patients with the rare hereditary problem of galactose intolerance, of severe lactase deficiency or of glucose-galactose malabsorption.

Zanaflex should be kept out of the reach and sight of children.

4.5 Interaction with other medicinal products and other forms of interaction

As Zanaflex may induce hypotension (see 4.4 Special warnings and precautions for use) it may potentiate the effect of antihypertensive drugs, including diuretics, and caution should therefore be exercised in patients receiving blood pressure lowering drugs.

Caution should also be exercised when Zanaflex is used concurrently with β-adrenoceptor blocking drugs or digoxin as the combination may potentiate hypotension or bradycardia.

Caution should be exercised when Zanaflex is prescribed with drugs known to increase the QT interval.

Concomitant use of tizanidine with fluvoxamine or ciprofloxacin, both CYP450 1A2 inhibitors in man, is contraindicated. Concomitant use of tizanidine with fluvoxamine or ciprofloxacin resulted in a 33-fold and 10-fold increase in tizanidine AUC, respectively. Clinically significant and prolonged hypotension may result along with somnolence, dizziness and decreased psychomotor performance (see section 4.3 Contraindications and section 4.4 Special warnings and precautions for use). Co-administration of tizanidine with other inhibitors of CYP1A2 such as some antiarrhythmics (amiodarone, mexiletine, propafenone), cimetidine, some fluoroquinolones (enoxacin, norfloxacin) and ticlopidine is not recommended (see section 4.4 Special warnings and special precautions for use).

The increased plasma levels of tizanidine may result in overdose symptoms such as QT(c) prolongation (see also section 4.9 Overdose).

Pharmacokinetic data following single and multiple doses of Zanaflex suggested that clearance of Zanaflex was reduced by approximately 50% in women who were concurrently taking oral contraceptives. Although no specific pharmacokinetic study has been conducted to investigate a potential interaction between oral contraceptives and Zanaflex, the possibility of a clinical response and/or adverse effects occurring at lower doses of Zanaflex should be borne in mind when prescribing Zanaflex to a patient taking the contraceptive pill. Clinically significant drug-drug interactions have not been reported in clinical trials.

Alcohol or sedatives may enhance the sedative action of Zanaflex.

4.6 Pregnancy and lactation

Reproductive studies in rats and rabbits indicate that Zanaflex does not have embryotoxic or teratogenic potential but at maternally toxic doses of 10-100 mg/kg per day Zanaflex can retard foetal development due to its pharmacodynamic effects. Zanaflex and/or its metabolites have been found in the milk of rodents (see section 5.3 preclinical safety data). The safety of Zanaflex in pregnancy has not been established and its safety in breast-fed infants of mothers receiving Zanaflex is not known. Therefore Zanaflex should not be used in pregnant or nursing mothers unless the likely benefit clearly outweighs the risk.

4.7 Effects on ability to drive and use machines

Patients experiencing drowsiness, dizziness or any signs or symptoms of hypotension should be advised against activities requiring a high degree of alertness, e.g. driving a vehicle or operating machinery.

4.8 Undesirable effects

The most frequently reported adverse events occurring in association with Zanaflex include drowsiness, fatigue, dizziness, dry mouth, nausea, gastrointestinal disturbances, and a reduction in blood pressure. With slow upward titration of the dose of Zanaflex these effects are usually not severe enough to require discontinuation of treatment. Insomnia, bradycardia and hallucinations have also been reported. The hallucinations are self-limiting, without evidence of psychosis, and have invariably occurred in patients concurrently taking potentially hallucinogenic drugs, e.g. anti-depressants. Increases in hepatic serum transaminases, which are reversible on stopping treatment, have occurred. Infrequent cases of acute hepatitis and hepatic failure have been reported. Muscle weakness has been reported infrequently, although in controlled clinical trials it was clearly demonstrated that Zanaflex does not adversely affect muscle strength. Allergic reactions (e.g. pruritus and rash) have rarely been reported.

Rebound hypertension on withdrawal may lead in severe cases to a cerebrovascular event.

4.9 Overdose

Clinical experience is limited. In one adult case, who ingested 400mg Zanaflex, recovery was uneventful. This patient received mannitol and frusemide.

Symptoms: Nausea, vomiting, hypotension, QT(c) prolongation, dizziness, miosis, respiratory distress, coma, restlessness, somnolence.

Treatment: General supportive measures are indicated and an attempt should be made to remove uningested drug from the gastro-intestinal tract using gastric lavage or activated charcoal. The patient should be well hydrated.

5. PHARMACOLOGICAL PROPERTIES

5.1 Pharmacodynamic properties

Tizanidine is an α_2-adrenergic receptor agonist within the central nervous system at supra-spinal and spinal levels. This effect results in inhibition of spinal polysynaptic reflex activity. Tizanidine has no direct effect on skeletal muscle, the neuromuscular junction or on monosynaptic spinal reflexes.

In humans, tizanidine reduces pathologically increased muscle tone, including resistance to passive movements and alleviates painful spasms and clonus.

5.2 Pharmacokinetic properties

Tizanidine is rapidly absorbed, reaching peak plasma concentration in approximately 1 hour. Tizanidine is only about 30% bound to plasma proteins and, in animal studies, was found to readily cross the blood-brain barrier. Although tizanidine is well absorbed, first pass metabolism limits plasma availability to 34% of that of an intravenous dose. Tizanidine undergoes rapid and extensive metabolism in the liver and the pattern of biotransformation in animals and humans is qualitatively similar. The metabolites are primarily excreted via the renal route (approximately 70% of the administered dose) and appear to be inactive. Renal excretion of the parent compound is approximately 53% after a single 5 mg dose and 66% after dosing with 4 mg three times daily. The elimination half-life of tizanidine from plasma is 2-4 hours in patients.

Concomitant food intake has no influence on the pharmacokinetic profile of tizanidine tablets.

5.3 Preclinical safety data

Acute toxicity

Tizanidine possesses a low order of acute toxicity. Signs of overdosage were seen after single doses >40 mg/kg in animals and are related to the pharmacological action of the drug.

Repeat dose toxicity

The toxic effects of tizanidine are mainly related to its pharmacological action. At doses of 24 and 40 mg/kg per day in subchronic and chronic rodent studies, the α_2-agonist effects resulted in CNS stimulation, e.g. motor excitation, aggressiveness, tremor and convulsions.

Signs related to centrally mediated muscle relaxation, e.g. sedation and ataxia, were frequently observed at lower dose levels in subchronic and chronic oral studies with dogs. Such signs, related to the myotonolytic activity of the drug, were noted at 1 to 4 mg/kg per day in a 13 week dog study, and at 1.5 mg/kg per day in a 52-week dog study.

Prolongation of the QT interval and bradycardia were noted in chronic toxicity studies in dogs at doses of 1.0 mg/kg per day and above.

Slight increases in hepatic serum transaminases were observed in a number of toxicity studies at higher dose levels. They were not consistently associated with histopathological changes in the liver.

Mutagenicity

Various in vitro assays as well as in vivo assays produced no evidence of mutagenic potential of tizanidine.

Carcinogenicity

No evidence for carcinogenicity was demonstrated in two long-term dietary studies in mice (78 weeks) and rats (104 weeks), at dose levels up to 9 mg/kg per day in rats and up to 16 mg/kg per day in mice. At these dose levels, corresponding to the maximum tolerated dose, based on reductions in growth rate, no neoplastic or pre-neoplastic pathology, attributable to treatment, was observed.

Reproductive toxicity

No embryotoxicity or teratogenicity occurred in pregnant rats and rabbits at dose levels up to 30 mg/kg per day of tizanidine. However, doses of 10-100 mg/kg per day in rats were maternally toxic and resulted in developmental retardation of foetuses as seen by lower foetal body weights and retarded skeletal ossification.

In female rats, treated prior to mating through lactation or during late pregnancy until weaning of the young, a dose-dependent (10 and 30 mg/kg per day) prolongation of gestation time and dystocia occurred, resulting in an increased foetal mortality and delayed development. These effects were attributed to the pharmacological effect of tizanidine. No developmental effects occurred at 3mg/kg per day although sedation was induced in the treated dams.

Passage of tizanidine and/or its metabolites into milk of rodents is known to occur.

6. PHARMACEUTICAL PARTICULARS

6.1 List of excipients

silica, colloidal anhydrous

stearic acid

cellulose, microcrystalline

lactose, anhydrous.

6.2 Incompatibilities

None known.

6.3 Shelf life

5 years in both temperate and hot climates, and 5 years in tropical climate.

6.4 Special precautions for storage

No special precautions for storage

6.5 Nature and contents of container

PVC/PVDC/Al foil blisters. Carton containing 4 blister strips of 30 tablets to give pack size of 120.

6.6 Special precautions for disposal and other handling

Not applicable.

7. MARKETING AUTHORISATION HOLDER

Cephalon Limited

1 Albany Place

Hyde Way

Welwyn Garden City

Hertfordshire

AL7 3BT

8. MARKETING AUTHORISATION NUMBER(S)

Zanaflex 2 mg – PL 21799/0015

Zanaflex 4 mg – PL 21799/0016

9. DATE OF FIRST AUTHORISATION/RENEWAL OF THE AUTHORISATION

Zanaflex 2 mg – 15 September 2005

Zanaflex 4 mg – 30 January 2006

10. DATE OF REVISION OF THE TEXT

August 2009

Legal Category

POM

Zantac Effervescent Tablets 150mg

(GlaxoSmithKline UK)

1. NAME OF THE MEDICINAL PRODUCT

Zantac Effervescent Tablets 150 mg

2. QUALITATIVE AND QUANTITATIVE COMPOSITION

Each tablet contains ranitidine 150 mg (as the hydrochloride) and 14.3 mEq (328 mg) of sodium.

3. PHARMACEUTICAL FORM

Effervescent Tablet.

4. CLINICAL PARTICULARS

4.1 Therapeutic indications

Adults

Duodenal ulcer and benign gastric ulcer, including that associated with non-steroidal anti-inflammatory agents.

Prevention of non-steroidal anti-inflammatory drug (including aspirin) associated duodenal ulcers, especially in patients with a history of peptic ulcer disease.

Treatment of duodenal ulcers associated with *Helicobacter pylori* infection.

Post-operative ulcer.

Oesophageal reflux disease.

Symptom relief in gastro-oesophageal reflux disease.

Zollinger-Ellison Syndrome.

Chronic episodic dyspepsia, characterised by pain (epigastric or retrosternal) which is related to meals or disturbs sleep but not associated with the above conditions.

Prophylaxis of stress ulceration in seriously ill patients.

Prophylaxis of recurrent haemorrhage from peptic ulcer.

Prophylaxis of Mendelson's syndrome.

Children (3 to 18 years)

Short term treatment of peptic ulcer

Treatment of gastro-oesophageal reflux, including reflux oesophagitis and symptomatic relief of gastro-oesophageal reflux disease.

4.2 Posology and method of administration

Adults (including the elderly) / Adolescents (12 years and over)

Duodenal ulcer and benign gastric ulcer:

Acute treatment:

The standard dosage regimen for duodenal or benign gastric ulcer is 150 mg twice daily or 300 mg nocte. In most cases of duodenal ulcer or benign gastric ulcer healing occurs within 4 weeks. Healing usually occurs after a further 4 weeks in those not fully healed after the initial 4 weeks.

Long-term management:

For the long-term management of duodenal or benign gastric ulcer the usual dosage regimen is 150 mg nocte.

In duodenal ulcer 300 mg twice daily for 4 weeks results in healing rates which are higher than those at 4 weeks with ranitidine 150 mg twice daily or 300 mg nocte. The increased dose has not been associated with an increased incidence of unwanted effects.

NSAID associated peptic ulceration:

Acute treatment:

In ulcers following non-steroidal anti-inflammatory drug therapy, or associated with continued non-steroidal anti-inflammatory drugs, 8-12 weeks treatment may be necessary with 150 mg twice daily or 300 mg nocte.

Prophylaxis:

For the prevention of non-steroidal anti-inflammatory drug associated duodenal ulcers ranitidine 150 mg twice daily may be given concomitantly with non-steroidal anti-inflammatory drug therapy.

For duodenal ulcers associated with *Helicobacter pylori* infection, ranitidine 300 mg at bedtime or 150 mg twice daily may be given with oral amoxicillin 750 mg three times daily and metronidazole 500 mg three times daily for two weeks. Therapy with ranitidine should continue for a further two weeks. This dose regimen significantly reduces the frequency of duodenal ulcer recurrence.

Postoperative ulcer:

The standard dosage regimen for postoperative ulcer is 150mg twice daily. Most cases heal within 4 weeks. Those not fully healed after the initial 4 weeks usually do so after a further 4 weeks.

Gastro-oesophageal reflux disease:

Symptom relief in gastro-oesophageal reflux disease.

In patients with gastro-oesophageal reflux disease, a dose regimen of 150 mg twice daily for 2 weeks is recommended and this can be repeated in patients in whom the initial symptomatic response is inadequate.

In the management of oesophageal reflux disease, the recommended course of treatment is either 150 mg twice daily or 300 mg at bedtime for up to 8 weeks or 12 weeks if necessary.

In patients with moderate to severe oesophagitis, the dosage of ranitidine may be increased to 150 mg 4 times daily for up to 12 weeks. The increased dose has not been associated with an increased incidence of unwanted effects.

Zollinger-Ellison syndrome:

The initial dosage regimen for Zollinger-Ellison syndrome is 150 mg three times daily, but this may be increased as necessary. Doses up to 6 grams per day have been well tolerated.

Chronic episodic dyspepsia:

The standard dosage regimen for patients with chronic episodic dyspepsia is 150 mg twice daily for up to 6 weeks. Anyone not responding or relapsing shortly afterwards should be investigated.

Prophylaxis of haemorrhage from stress ulceration in seriously ill patients or prophylaxis of recurrent haemorrhage in patients bleeding from peptic ulceration:

150 mg twice daily may be substituted for the injection once oral feeding commences.

Prophylaxis of Mendelson's syndrome:

150 mg 2 hours before anaesthesia, and preferably 150 mg the previous evening. Alternatively, the injection is also available. In obstetric patients in labour 150 mg every 6 hours, but if general anaesthesia is required it is recommended that a non-particulate antacid (e.g. sodium citrate) be given in addition.

Children from 3 to 11 years and over 30 kg of weight

See section 5.2 Pharmacokinetic Properties (Special Patient Populations)

Peptic Ulcer Acute Treatment

The recommended oral dose for the treatment of peptic ulcer in children is 4 mg/kg/day to 8 mg/kg/day administered as two divided doses to a maximum of 300 mg ranitidine per day for a duration of 4 weeks. For those patients with incomplete healing, another 4 weeks of therapy is indicated, as healing usually occurs after eight weeks of treatment.

Gastro-Oesophageal Reflux

The recommended oral dose for the treatment of gastro-oesophageal reflux in children is 5 mg/kg/day to 10 mg/kg/day administered as two divided doses in a maximum dose of 600 mg (the maximum dose is likely to apply to heavier children or adolescents with severe symptoms).

Safety and efficacy in new-born patients has not been established.

Renal Impairment:

Accumulation of ranitidine with resulting elevated plasma concentrations will occur in patients with severe renal impairment (creatinine clearance less than 50 ml/min). It is recommended that the daily dose of ranitidine in such patients should be 150 mg.

For oral administration.

4.3 Contraindications

Ranitidine is contra-indicated in patients known to have hypersensitivity to any component of the preparation.

4.4 Special warnings and precautions for use

Malignancy:

The possibility of malignancy should be excluded before commencement of therapy in patients with gastric ulcer (and if indications include dyspepsia; patients of middle age and over with new or recently changed dyspeptic symptoms) as treatment with ranitidine may mask symptoms of gastric carcinoma.

Renal Disease:

Ranitidine is excreted via the kidney and so plasma levels of the drug are increased in patients with severe renal impairment.

The dosage should be adjusted as detailed above under Dosage in Renal Impairment.

Regular supervision of patients who are taking non-steroidal anti-inflammatory drugs concomitantly with ranitidine is recommended, especially in the elderly and in those with a history of peptic ulcer.

Rare clinical reports suggest that ranitidine may precipitate acute porphyric attacks. Ranitidine should therefore be avoided in patients with a history of acute porphyria.

In patients such as the elderly, persons with chronic lung disease, diabetes or the immunocompromised, there may be an increased risk of developing community acquired pneumonia. A large epidemiological study showed an increased risk of developing community acquired pneumonia in current users of H_2 receptor antagonists versus those who had stopped treatment, with an observed adjusted relative risk increase of 1.63 (95% CI, 1.07–2.48).

Zantac Effervescent Tablets contain sodium. Care should therefore be taken in treating patients in whom sodium restriction is indicated.

Zantac Effervescent Tablets contain aspartame. They should be used with caution in patients with phenylketonuria.

4.5 Interaction with other medicinal products and other forms of interaction

Ranitidine has the potential to affect the absorption, metabolism or renal excretion of other drugs. The altered pharmacokinetics may necessitate dosage adjustment of the affected drug or discontinuation of treatment

Interactions occur by several mechanisms including:

1) Inhibition of cytochrome P450-linked mixed function oxygenase system: Ranitidine at usual therapeutic doses does not potentiate the actions of drugs which are inactivated by this enzyme system such as diazepam, lidocaine, phenytoin, propanolol and theophylline.

There have been reports of altered prothrombin time with coumarin anticoagulants (e.g. warfarin). Due to the narrow therapeutic index, close monitoring of increased or decreased prothrombin time is recommended during concurrent treatment with ranitidine.

2) Competition for renal tubular secretion:

Since ranitidine is partially eliminated by the cationic system, it may affect the clearance of other drugs eliminated by this route. High doses of ranitidine (e.g. such as those used in the treatment of Zollinger-Ellison syndrome) may reduce the excretion of procainamide and N-acetylprocainamide resulting in increased plasma level of these drugs.

3) Alteration of gastric pH:

The bioavailability of certain drugs may be affected. This can result in either an increase in absorption (e.g. triazolam, midazolam, glipizide) or a decrease in absorption (e.g. ketoconazole, atazanavir, delaviridine, gefitnib).

There is no evidence of an interaction between ranitidine and amoxicillin or metronidazole.

4.6 Pregnancy and lactation

Ranitidine crosses the placenta and is excreted in human breast milk.

Like other drugs it should only be used during pregnancy and nursing if considered essential.

4.7 Effects on ability to drive and use machines

None reported.

4.8 Undesirable effects

The following convention has been utilised for the classification of undesirable effects: very common (≥1/10), common (≥1/100, <1/10), uncommon (≥1/1000, ≤1/100), rare (≥1/10,000, ≤1/1000), very rare (≤1/10,000), unknown (cannot be estimated from the available data).

Blood & Lymphatic System Disorders

Unknown:

Blood count changes (leucopenia, thrombocytopenia). These are usually reversible. Agranulocytosis or pancytopenia, sometimes with marrow hypoplasia or marrow aplasia.

Immune System Disorders

Uncommon:

Hypersensitivity reactions (urticaria, angioneurotic oedema, fever, bronchospasm, hypotension and chest pain).

Unknown:

Anaphylactic shock.

These events have been reported after a single dose.

Psychiatric Disorders

Very Rare:

Depression.

Unknown:

Reversible mental confusion and hallucinations.

These have been reported predominantly in severely ill and elderly patients.

Nervous System Disorders

Common:

Headache (sometimes severe) anddizziness.

Unknown:

Reversible involuntary movement disorders.

Eye Disorders

Uncommon:

Reversible blurred vision.

There have been reports of blurred vision, which is suggestive of a change in accommodation.

Cardiac Disorders

Unknown:

As with other H_2 receptor antagonists bradycardia and A-V Block.

Vascular Disorders

Unknown:

Vasculitis.

Gastrointestinal Disorders

Common:

Diarrhoea.

Unknown:

Acute pancreatitis.

Hepatobiliary Disorders

Very Rare:

Transient and reversible changes in liver function tests.

Unknown:

Hepatitis (hepatocellular, hepatocanalicular or mixed) with or without jaundice, these were usually reversible.

Skin and Subcutaneous Tissue Disorders

Uncommon:

Skin Rash.

Unknown:

Erythema multiforme, alopecia.

Musculoskeletal and Connective Tissue Disorders

Unknown:

Musculoskeletal symptoms such as arthralgia and myalgia.

Renal and Urinary Disorders

Unknown:

Acute interstitial nephritis.

Reproductive System and Breast Disorders

Unknown:

Reversible impotence, breast symptoms and breast conditions (such as gynaecomastia and galactorrhoea).

The safety of ranitidine has been assessed in children aged 0 to 16 years with acid-related disease and was generally well tolerated with an adverse event profile resembling that in adults. There are limited long term safety data available, in particular regarding growth and development.

4.9 Overdose

Ranitidine is very specific in action and accordingly no particular problems are expected following overdosage with the drug, clinicians should be aware of the sodium content (see Section 4.4 Special Warnings and Precautions for Use). Symptomatic and supportive therapy should be given as appropriate

5. PHARMACOLOGICAL PROPERTIES

5.1 Pharmacodynamic properties

Ranitidine is a specific rapidly acting histamine H_2-antagonist. It inhibits basal and stimulated secretion of gastric acid, reducing both the volume and the acid and pepsin content of the secretion. Ranitidine has a relatively long duration of action and so a single 150 mg dose effectively suppresses gastric acid secretion for twelve hours.

5.2 Pharmacokinetic properties

The bioavailability of ranitidine is consistently about 50%. Absorption of ranitidine after oral administration is rapid and peak plasma concentrations are usually achieved 2-3 hours after administration. Absorption is not significantly impaired by food or antacids. Ranitidine is not extensively metabolised. Elimination of the drug is primarily by tubular secretion. The elimination half-life of ranitidine is 2-3 hours. In balance studies with 150 mg ^{3}H-ranitidine 60-70% of an oral dose was excreted in urine and 26% in faeces. Analysis of urine excreted in the first 24 hours after dosing showed that 35% of the oral dose was eliminated unchanged. About 6% of the dose is excreted as the N-Oxide, 2% as the S-Oxide, 2% as desmethyl ranitidine and 1-2% as the furoic acid analogue.

Special Patient Populations

Children (3 years and above)

Limited pharmacokinetic data have shown that there is no significant differences in half-life (range for children 3 years and above: 1.7 - 2.2 h) and plasma clearance (range for children 3 years and above: 9 - 22 ml/min/kg) between children and healthy adults receiving oral ranitidine when correction is made for body weight.

5.3 Preclinical safety data
No additional data of relevance.

6. PHARMACEUTICAL PARTICULARS
6.1 List of excipients
Monosodium Citrate Anhydrous
Sodium Bicarbonate
Aspartame
Povidone
Sodium Benzoate
Orange Flavour (IFF No. 6)
Grapefruit Flavour (IFF 18C 222)
Pharmaceutical Industrial Alcohol or Ethanol

6.2 Incompatibilities
None.

6.3 Shelf life
2 years.

6.4 Special precautions for storage
Store below 30°C in a dry place.

6.5 Nature and contents of container
Polypropylene tubes with polyethylene tamper evident cap, each tube contains 15 tablets packed in cartons of 15 or 60 tablets.

Aluminium foil strips of six tablets packed in cartons of 6 or 30 tablets.

6.6 Special precautions for disposal and other handling
Place the tablets in half a glass of water (minimum 75 ml) and allow to dissolve completely before swallowing.

Administrative Data
7. MARKETING AUTHORISATION HOLDER
Glaxo Wellcome UK Limited
trading as GlaxoSmithKline UK
Stockley Park West
Uxbridge
Middlesex
UB11 1BT

8. MARKETING AUTHORISATION NUMBER(S)
PL 10949/0137.

9. DATE OF FIRST AUTHORISATION/RENEWAL OF THE AUTHORISATION
28 April 2002

10. DATE OF REVISION OF THE TEXT
10 March 2009

11. Legal Status
POM

Zantac Effervescent Tablets 300mg

(GlaxoSmithKline UK)

1. NAME OF THE MEDICINAL PRODUCT
Zantac Effervescent Tablets 300 mg

2. QUALITATIVE AND QUANTITATIVE COMPOSITION
Each tablet contains ranitidine 300 mg (as the hydrochloride) and 20.8 mEq (479 mg) of sodium.

3. PHARMACEUTICAL FORM
Effervescent Tablet.

4. CLINICAL PARTICULARS
4.1 Therapeutic indications
Adults
- Duodenal ulcer and benign gastric ulcer, including that associated with non-steroidal anti-inflammatory agents.
- Treatment of duodenal ulcers associated with *Helicobacter pylori* infection.
- Post-operative ulcer.
- Oesophageal reflux disease.
- Zollinger-Ellison Syndrome.
- Chronic episodic dyspepsia, characterised by pain (epigastric or retrosternal) which is related to meals or disturbs sleep but not associated with the above conditions.
- Prophylaxis of stress ulceration in seriously ill patients.
- Prophylaxis of recurrent haemorrhage from peptic ulcer.
- Prophylaxis of Mendelson's syndrome.

Children (3 to 18 years)
Short term treatment of peptic ulcer
Treatment of gastro-oesophageal reflux, including reflux oesophagitis and symptomatic relief of gastro-oesophageal reflux disease.

4.2 Posology and method of administration
Adults (including the elderly) / Adolescents (12 years and over)
Duodenal ulcer and benign gastric ulcer:
- Acute treatment:
The standard dosage regimen for duodenal or benign gastric ulcer is 150 mg twice daily or 300 mg nocte. In most cases of duodenal ulcer or benign gastric ulcer healing occurs within 4 weeks. Healing usually occurs after a further 4 weeks in those not fully healed after the initial 4 weeks.
- Long-term management:
For the long-term management of duodenal or benign gastric ulcer the usual dosage regimen is 150 mg nocte.
In duodenal ulcer 300 mg twice daily for 4 weeks results in healing rates which are higher than those at 4 weeks with ranitidine 150 mg twice daily or 300 mg nocte. The increased dose has not been associated with an increased incidence of unwanted effects.
NSAID associated peptic ulceration:
- Acute treatment:
In ulcers following non-steroidal anti-inflammatory drug therapy, or associated with continued non-steroidal anti-inflammatory drugs, 8-12 weeks treatment may be necessary with 150 mg twice daily or 300 mg nocte.
For duodenal ulcers associated with *Helicobacter pylori* infection, ranitidine 300 mg at bedtime or 150 mg twice daily may be given with oral amoxycillin 750mg three times daily and metronidazole 500 mg three times daily for two weeks. Therapy with ranitidine should continue for a further two weeks. This dose regimen significantly reduces the frequency of duodenal ulcer recurrence.
Postoperative ulcer:
The standard dosage regimen for postoperative ulcer is 150 mg twice daily. Most cases heal within 4 weeks. Those not fully healed after the initial 4 weeks usually do so after a further 4 weeks.
In the management of oesophageal reflux disease, the recommended course of treatment is either 150 mg twice daily or 300 mg at bedtime for up to 8 weeks or 12 weeks if necessary.
Zollinger-Ellison syndrome:
The initial dosage regimen for Zollinger-Ellison syndrome is 150 mg three times daily, but this may be increased as necessary. Doses up to 6 grams per day have been well tolerated.
Chronic episodic dyspepsia:
The standard dosage regimen for patients with chronic episodic dyspepsia is 150 mg twice daily for up to 6 weeks. Anyone not responding or relapsing shortly afterwards should be investigated.
Prophylaxis of haemorrhage from stress ulceration in seriously ill patients or prophylaxis of recurrent haemorrhage in patients bleeding from peptic ulceration:
150 mg twice daily may be substituted for the injection once oral feeding commences.
Prophylaxis of Mendelson's syndrome:
150 mg 2 hours before anaesthesia, and preferably 150 mg the previous evening. Alternatively, the injection is also available. In obstetric patients in labour 150 mg every 6 hours, but if general anaesthesia is required it is recommended that a non-particulate antacid (e.g. sodium citrate) be given in addition.
Children from 3 to 11 years and over 30 kg of weight
See section 5.2 Pharmacokinetic Properties (Special Patient Populations)
Peptic Ulcer Acute Treatment
The recommended oral dose for the treatment of peptic ulcer in children is 4 mg/kg/day to 8 mg/kg/day administered as two divided doses to a maximum of 300 mg ranitidine per day for a duration of 4 weeks. For those patients with incomplete healing, another 4 weeks of therapy is indicated, as healing usually occurs after eight weeks of treatment.
Gastro-Oesophageal Reflux
The recommended oral dose for the treatment of gastro-oesophageal reflux in children is 5 mg/kg/day to 10 mg/kg/day administered as two divided doses in a maximum of 600 mg (the maximum dose is likely to apply to heavier children or adolescents with severe symptoms).
Safety and efficacy in new-born patients has not been established.
Renal Impairment:
Accumulation of ranitidine with resulting elevated plasma concentrations will occur in patients with severe renal impairment (creatinine clearance less than 50 ml/min). It is recommended that the daily dose of ranitidine in such patients should be 150 mg.

4.3 Contraindications
Ranitidine is contra-indicated in patients known to have hypersensitivity to any component of the preparation.

4.4 Special warnings and precautions for use
Malignancy:
The possibility of malignancy should be excluded before commencement of therapy in patients with gastric ulcer (and if indications include dyspepsia; patients of middle age and over with new or recently changed dyspeptic symptoms) as treatment with ranitidine may mask symptoms of gastric carcinoma.
Renal Disease:
Ranitidine is excreted via the kidney and so plasma levels of the drug are increased in patients with severe renal impairment.
The dosage should be adjusted as detailed above under Dosage in Renal Impairment.
Regular supervision of patients who are taking non-steroidal anti-inflammatory drugs concomitantly with ranitidine is recommended, especially in the elderly and in those with a history of peptic ulcer.
Rare clinical reports suggest that ranitidine may precipitate acute porphyric attacks. Ranitidine should therefore be avoided in patients with a history of acute porphyria.
In patients such as the elderly, persons with chronic lung disease, diabetes or the immunocompromised, there may be an increased risk of developing community acquired pneumonia. A large epidemiological study showed an increased risk of developing community acquired pneumonia in current users of H_2 receptor antagonists versus those who had stopped treatment, with an observed adjusted relative risk increase of 1.63 (95% CI, 1.07–2.48).
Zantac Effervescent Tablets contain sodium. Care should therefore be taken in treating patients in whom sodium restriction is indicated.
Zantac Effervescent Tablets contain aspartame. They should be used with caution in patients with phenylketonuria.

4.5 Interaction with other medicinal products and other forms of interaction
Ranitidine has the potential to affect the absorption, metabolism or renal excretion of other drugs. The altered pharmacokinetics may necessitate dosage adjustment of the affected drug or discontinuation of treatment
Interactions occur by several mechanisms including:
1) Inhibition of cytochrome P450-linked mixed function oxygenase system: Ranitidine at usual therapeutic doses does not potentiate the actions of drugs which are inactivated by this enzyme system such as diazepam, lidocaine, phenytoin, propanolol and theophylline.
There have been reports of altered prothrombin time with coumarin anticoagulants (e.g. warfarin). Due to the narrow therapeutic index, close monitoring of increased or decreased prothrombin time is recommended during concurrent treatment with ranitidine.
2) Competition for renal tubular secretion:
Since ranitidine is partially eliminated by the cationic system, it may affect the clearance of other drugs eliminated by this route. High doses of ranitidine (e.g. such as those used in the treatment of Zollinger-Ellison syndrome) may reduce the excretion of procainamide and N-acetylprocainamide resulting in increased plasma level of these drugs.
3) Alteration of gastric pH:
The bioavailability of certain drugs may be affected. This can result in either an increase in absorption (e.g. triazolam, midazolam, glipizide) or a decrease in absorption (e.g. ketoconazole, atazanavir, delaviridine, gefitnib).
There is no evidence of an interaction between ranitidine and amoxycillin or metronidazole.

4.6 Pregnancy and lactation
Ranitidine crosses the placenta and is excreted in human breast milk.
Like other drugs it should only be used during pregnancy and nursing if considered essential.

4.7 Effects on ability to drive and use machines
None reported.

4.8 Undesirable effects
The following convention has been utilised for the classification of undesirable effects: very common ($\geq$1/10), common ($\geq$1/100, $<$1/10), uncommon ($\geq$1/1000, $\leq$1/100), rare ($>$1/10,000, $<$1/1000), very rare ($\leq$1/10,000), unknown (cannot be estimated from the available data.
Blood & Lymphatic System Disorders
Unknown: Blood count changes (leucopenia, thrombocytopenia). These are usually reversible. Agranulocytosis or pancytopenia, sometimes with marrow hypoplasia or marrow aplasia.
Immune System Disorders
Uncommon: Hypersensitivity reactions (urticaria, angioneurotic oedema, fever, bronchospasm, hypotension and chest pain).
Unknown: Anaphylactic shock
These events have been reported after a single dose.
Psychiatric Disorders
Very Rare: Depression.
Unknown: Reversible mental confusion and hallucinations.
These have been reported predominantly in severely ill and elderly patients.
Nervous System Disorders
Common: Headache (sometimes severe) and dizziness.
Unknown: Reversible involuntary movement disorders.
Eye Disorders
Uncommon: Reversible blurred vision.
There have been reports of blurred vision, which is suggestive of a change in accommodation.
Cardiac Disorders
Unknown: As with other H_2 receptor antagonists bradycardia and A-V Block.

Vascular Disorders
Unknown: Vasculitis.

Gastrointestinal Disorders
Common: Diarrhoea.
Unknown: Acute pancreatitis.

Hepatobiliary Disorders
Very Rare: Transient and reversible changes in liver function tests.
Unknown: Hepatitis (hepatocellular, hepatocanalicular or mixed) with or without jaundice, these were usually reversible.

Skin and Subcutaneous Tissue Disorders
Uncommon: Skin Rash.
Unknown: Erythema multiforme, alopecia.

Musculoskeletal and Connective Tissue Disorders
Unknown: Musculoskeletal symptoms such as arthralgia and myalgia.

Renal and Urinary Disorders
Unknown: Acute interstitial nephritis.

Reproductive System and Breast Disorders
Unknown: Reversible impotence, breast symptoms and breast conditions (such as gynaecomastia and galactorrhoea).

The safety of ranitidine has been assessed in children aged 0 to 16 years with acid-related disease and was generally well tolerated with an adverse event profile resembling that in adults. There are limited long term safety data available, in particular regarding growth and development.

4.9 Overdose
Ranitidine is very specific in action and accordingly no particular problems are expected following overdosage with the drug, clinicians should be aware of the sodium content (see Precautions section). Symptomatic and supportive therapy should be given as appropriate.

5. PHARMACOLOGICAL PROPERTIES

5.1 Pharmacodynamic properties
Ranitidine is a specific rapidly acting histamine H_2-antagonist. It inhibits basal and stimulated secretion of gastric acid, reducing both the volume and the acid and pepsin content of the secretion. Ranitidine has a relatively long duration of action and so a single 150 mg dose effectively suppresses gastric acid secretion for twelve hours.

5.2 Pharmacokinetic properties
The bioavailability of ranitidine is consistently about 50%. Absorption of ranitidine after oral administration is rapid and peak plasma concentrations are usually achieved 2-3 hours after administration. Absorption is not significantly impaired by food or antacids. Ranitidine is not extensively metabolised. Elimination of the drug is primarily by tubular secretion. The elimination half-life of ranitidine is 2-3 hours. In balance studies with 150mg 3H-ranitidine 60-70% of an oral dose was excreted in urine and 26% in faeces. Analysis of urine excreted in the first 24 hours after dosing showed that 35% of the oral dose was eliminated unchanged. About 6% of the dose is excreted as the N-Oxide, 2% as the S-Oxide, 2% as desmethyl ranitidine and 1-2% as the furoic acid analogue.

Special Patient Populations

Children (3 years and above)

Limited pharmacokinetic data have shown that there are no significant differences in half-life (range for children 3 years and above: 1.7 - 2.2 h) and plasma clearance (range for children 3 years and above: 9 - 22 ml/min/kg) between children and healthy adults receiving oral ranitidine when correction is made for body weight.

5.3 Preclinical safety data
No additional data of relevance.

6. PHARMACEUTICAL PARTICULARS

6.1 List of excipients
Monosodium Citrate Anhydrous
Sodium Bicarbonate
Aspartame
Povidone
Sodium Benzoate
Orange Flavour (IFF No. 6)
Grapefruit Flavour (IFF 18C 222)
Pharmaceutical Industrial Alcohol or Ethanol

6.2 Incompatibilities
None.

6.3 Shelf life
2 years.

6.4 Special precautions for storage
Store below 30°C in a dry place.

6.5 Nature and contents of container
Polypropylene tubes with polyethylene tamper evident cap, each tube contains 15 tablets packed in cartons of 30 tablets.

Aluminium foil strips of six tablets packed in cartons of 30 tablets.

6.6 Special precautions for disposal and other handling
Place the tablets in half a glass of water (minimum 75 ml) and allow to dissolve completely before swallowing.

Administrative Data

7. MARKETING AUTHORISATION HOLDER
Glaxo Wellcome UK Limited
Stockley Park West
Uxbridge
Middlesex UB11 1BT
Trading as: GlaxoSmithKline UK

8. MARKETING AUTHORISATION NUMBER(S)
PL 10949/0138.

9. DATE OF FIRST AUTHORISATION/RENEWAL OF THE AUTHORISATION
26 January 2000

10. DATE OF REVISION OF THE TEXT
10 March 2009

11. Legal Status
POM

Zantac Injection 50mg/2ml

(GlaxoSmithKline UK)

1. NAME OF THE MEDICINAL PRODUCT
Zantac Injection 50 mg/2ml

2. QUALITATIVE AND QUANTITATIVE COMPOSITION
Ranitidine Hydrochloride HSE 56.0 mg/2ml equivalent to Ranitidine 50.0 mg/2ml.

3. PHARMACEUTICAL FORM
Injection (Aqueous solution)

A clear colourless to pale yellow liquid, practically free from particles.

4. CLINICAL PARTICULARS

4.1 Therapeutic indications

Adults:

Zantac Injection is indicated for the treatment of duodenal ulcer, benign gastric ulcer, post - operative ulcer, reflux oesophagitis, Zollinger - Ellison Syndrome and the following conditions where reduction of gastric secretion and acid output is desirable:

The prophylaxis of gastrointestinal haemorrhage from stress ulceration in seriously ill patients, the prophylaxis of recurrent haemorrhage in patients with bleeding peptic ulcers and before general anaesthesia in patients considered to be at risk of acid aspiration (Mendelson's Syndrome), particularly obstetric patients during labour. For appropriate cases, Zantac tablets are also available.

Children (6 months to 18 years):

Zantac Injection is indicated for the short term treatment of peptic ulcer and the treatment of gastro-oesophageal reflux, including reflux oesophagitis and symptomatic relief of gastro-oesophageal reflux disease.

4.2 Posology and method of administration
(See Section 5.2 Pharmacokinetic Properties – Special patient Populations)

Adults (including elderly) / Adolescents (12 years and over)

Zantac Injection may be given either as a slow (over 2 minutes) intravenous injection up to a maximum of 50 mg, after dilution to a volume of 20 ml per 50 mg dose, which may be repeated every 6 to 8 hours; or as an intermittent intravenous infusion at a rate of 25 mg per hour for two hours; the infusion may be repeated at 6 to 8 hour intervals, or as an intramuscular injection of 50 mg (2 ml) every 6 to 8 hours.

Prophylaxis of haemorrhage from stress ulceration or recurrent haemorrhage:

In the prophylaxis of haemorrhage from stress ulceration in seriously ill patients or the prophylaxis of recurrent haemorrhage in patients bleeding from peptic ulceration, parenteral administration may be continued until oral feeding commences. Patients considered to be still at risk may then be treated with Zantac tablets 150 mg twice daily.

In the prophylaxis of upper gastro-intestinal haemorrhage from stress ulceration in seriously ill patients a priming dose of 50 mg as a slow intravenous injection followed by a continuous intravenous infusion of 0.125 - 0.250 mg/kg/hr may be preferred.

Prophylaxis of Mendleson's syndrome:

In patients considered to be at risk of developing acid aspiration syndrome, Zantac Injection 50 mg may be given intramuscularly or by slow intravenous injection 45 to 60 minutes before induction of general anaesthesia.

Children / Infants (6 months to 11 years)

(See Section 5.2 Pharmacokinetic Properties) – Special Patient Populations

Zantac injection may be given as a slow (over 2 minutes) i.v. injection up to a maximum of 50 mg every 6 to 8 hours.

Peptic Ulcer Acute Treatment and Gastro-Oesophageal Reflux

Intravenous therapy in children with peptic ulcer disease is indicated only when oral therapy is not possible.

For acute treatment of peptic ulcer disease and gastro-oesophageal reflux in paediatric patients, Zantac injection may be administered at doses that have been shown to be effective for these diseases in adults and effective for acid suppression in critically ill children. The initial dose (2.0 mg/kg or 2.5 mg/kg, maximum 50 mg) may be administered as a slow intravenous infusion over 10 minutes, either with a syringe pump followed by a 3 mL flush with normal saline over 5 min, or following dilution with normal saline to 20 mL. Maintenance of pH > 4.0 can be achieved by intermittent infusion of 1.5 mg/kg every 6 h to 8 h. Alternatively treatment can be continuous, administering a loading dose of 0.45 mg/kg followed by a continuous infusion of 0.15 mg/kg/hr.

Prophylaxis of stress ulceration in seriously ill patients

The recommended dose for prophylaxis of stress ulceration is 1mg/kg (maximum 50 mg) every 6h to 8h.

Alternatively treatment can be continuous, administering 125 - 250 micrograms/kg/hr as continuous infusion.

Neonates (under 1 month)

(See Section 5.2 – Pharmacokinetic Properties – Special Patient Populations)

Renal Impairment:

Accumulation of ranitidine with resulting elevated plasma concentrations will occur in patients with severe renal impairment (creatinine clearance less than 50 ml/min). Accordingly, it is recommended in such patients that ranitidine be administered in doses of 25 mg.

Route of Administration

Intravenous or intramuscular injection

4.3 Contraindications
Ranitidine is contraindicated for patients known to have hypersensitivity to any component of the preparation.

4.4 Special warnings and precautions for use
Treatment with a histamine H_2-antagonist may mask the symptoms associated with carcinoma of the stomach and may therefore delay diagnosis of the condition. Accordingly, where gastric ulcer is suspected, the possibility of malignancy should be excluded before therapy with Zantac is instituted.

Ranitidine is excreted via the kidney and so plasma levels of the drug are increased in patients with renal impairment. The dosage should be adjusted as detailed under Dosage in Renal Impairment.

Bradycardia in association with rapid administration of Zantac Injection has been reported rarely, usually in patients with factors predisposing to cardiac rhythm disturbances. Recommended rates of administration should not be exceeded.

It has been reported that the use of higher than recommended doses of intravenous H_2-antagonists has been associated with rises in liver enzymes when treatment has been extended beyond five days.

Although clinical reports of acute intermittent porphyria associated with ranitidine administration have been rare and inconclusive, ranitidine should be avoided in patients with a history of this condition.

In patients such as the elderly, persons with chronic lung disease, diabetes or the immunocompromised, there may be an increased risk of developing community acquired pneumonia. A large epidemiological study showed an increased risk of developing community acquired pneumonia in current users of H_2 receptor antagonists versus those who had stopped treatment, with an observed adjusted relative risk increase of 1.63 (95% CI, 1.07–2.48).

4.5 Interaction with other medicinal products and other forms of interaction
Ranitidine has the potential to affect the absorption, metabolism or renal excretion of other drugs. The altered pharmacokinetics may necessitate dosage adjustment of the affected drug or discontinuation of treatment

Interactions occur by several mechanisms including:

1) Inhibition of cytochrome P450-linked mixed function oxygenase system: Ranitidine at usual therapeutic doses does not potentiate the actions of drugs which are inactivated by this enzyme system such as diazepam, lidocaine, phenytoin, propanolol and theophylline.

There have been reports of altered prothrombin time with coumarin anticoagulants (e.g. warfarin). Due to the narrow therapeutic index, close monitoring of increased or decreased prothrombin time is recommended during concurrent treatment with ranitidine.

2) Competition for renal tubular secretion:

Since ranitidine is partially eliminated by the cationic system, it may affect the clearance of other drugs eliminated by this route. High doses of ranitidine (e.g. such as those used in the treatment of Zollinger-Ellison syndrome) may reduce the excretion of procainamide and N-acetylprocainamide resulting in increased plasma level of these drugs.

3) Alteration of gastric pH:

The bioavailability of certain drugs may be affected. This can result in either an increase in absorption (e.g. triazolam, midazolam, glipizide) or a decrease in absorption (e.g. ketoconazole, atazanavir, delaviridine, gefitnib).

4.6 Pregnancy and lactation

Zantac crosses the placenta but therapeutic doses administered to obstetric patients in labour or undergoing caesarean section have been without any adverse effect on labour, delivery or subsequent neonatal progress. Zantac is also excreted in human breast milk. Like other drugs, Zantac should only be used during pregnancy and nursing if considered essential.

4.7 Effects on ability to drive and use machines

None known.

4.8 Undesirable effects

The following convention has been utilised for the classification of undesirable effects: very common ($\geqslant$1/10), common ($\geqslant$1/100, <1/10), uncommon ($\geqslant$1/1000, $\leqslant$1/100), rare ($\geqslant$1/10,000, $\leqslant$1/1000), very rare ($\leqslant$1/10,000), unknown (cannot be estimated from the available data).

Blood & Lymphatic System Disorders

Unknown: Blood count changes (leucopenia, thrombocytopenia). These are usually reversible. Agranulocytosis or pancytopenia, sometimes with marrow hypoplasia or marrow aplasia.

Immune System Disorders

Uncommon: Hypersensitivity reactions (urticaria, angioneurotic oedema, fever, bronchospasm, hypotension and chest pain).

Unknown: Anaphylactic shock.

These events have been reported after a single dose.

Psychiatric Disorders

Very Rare: Depression.

Unknown: Reversible mental confusion and hallucinations.

These have been reported predominantly in severely ill and elderly patients.

Nervous System Disorders

Common: Headache (sometimes severe) and dizziness.

Unknown: Reversible involuntary movement disorders.

Eye Disorders

Uncomon: Reversible blurred vision.

There have been reports of blurred vision, which is suggestive of a change in accommodation.

Cardiac Disorders

Unknown: As with other H_2 receptor antagonists bradycardia and A-V Block.

Vascular Disorders

Unknown: Vasculitis.

Gastrointestinal Disorders

Common: Diarrhoea.

Uknown: Acute pancreatitis.

Hepatobiliary Disorders

Very Rare: Transient and reversible changes in liver function tests.

Unknown: Hepatitis (hepatocellular, hepatocanalicular or mixed) with or without jaundice, these were usually reversible.

Skin and Subcutaneous Tissue Disorders

Uncommon: Skin Rash.

Unknown: Erythema multiforme, alopecia.

Musculoskeletal and Connective Tissue Disorders

Unknown: Musculoskeletal symptoms such as arthralgia and myalgia.

Renal and Urinary Disorders

Unknown: Acute interstitial nephritis.

Reproductive System and Breast Disorders

Unknown: Reversible impotence, breast symptoms and breast conditions (such as gynaecomastia and galactorrhoea).

The safety of ranitidine has been assessed in children aged 0 to 16 years with acid-related disease and was generally well tolerated with an adverse event profile resembling that in adults. There are limited long term safety data available, in particular regarding growth and development.

4.9 Overdose

Zantac is very specific in action and accordingly, no particular problems are expected following overdosage with the drug. Symptomatic and supportive therapy should be given as appropriate.

5. PHARMACOLOGICAL PROPERTIES

5.1 Pharmacodynamic properties

Ranitidine is a specific, rapidly acting histamine H_2-antagonist. It inhibits basal and stimulated secretion of gastric acid, reducing both the volume and the acid and pepsin content of the secretion.

The clinical data available mentions the use of ranitidine in children to prevent stress ulcers. No direct evidence for prevention of stress ulcers is available. Treatment for these patients is based on the observation that pH is above 4 after administration of ranitidine. The value of this surrogate parameter in children with stress ulcers remains to be established.

5.2 Pharmacokinetic properties

Absorption of ranitidine after intramuscular injection is rapid and peak plasma concentrations are usually achieved within 15 minutes of administration. Ranitidine is not extensively metabolised. The elimination of the drug is primarily by tubular secretion. The elimination half-life of ranitidine is 2-3 hours. In balance, studies with 150mg 3H-ranitidine, 93% of an intravenous dose was excreted in urine and 5% in faeces. Analysis of urine excreted in the first 24 hours after dosing showed that 70% of the intravenous dose was eliminated unchanged. About 6% of the dose is excreted in the urine as the N-oxide, 2% as desmethyl ranitidine and 1-2% as the furoic acid analogue.

Special Patient Populations

Children/infants (6 months and above)

Limited pharmacokinetic data show that there were no significant differences in half-life (range for children 3 years and above: 1.7 - 2.2 h) and plasma clearance (range for children 3 years and above: 9 - 22 ml/min/kg) between children and healthy adults receiving intravenous ranitidine when correction is made for body weight. Pharmacokinetic data in infants is extremely limited but appears to be in line with that for older children.

Neonates (under 1 month)

Limited pharmacokinetic data from term babies undergoing treatment with Extracorporeal Membrane Oxygenation (EMCO) suggests that plasma clearance following iv administration may be reduced (1.5-8.2 ml/min/kg) and the half-life increased in the new-born. Clearance of ranitidine appeared to be related to the estimated glomerular filtration rate in the neonates.

5.3 Preclinical safety data

There are no pre-clinical data of relevance to the prescriber which are additional to that already included in other sections of the SmPC.

6. PHARMACEUTICAL PARTICULARS

6.1 List of excipients

Sodium chloride	BP
Potassium Dihydrogen Orthophosphate	HSE
Disodium Hydrogen Orthophosphate	HSE
Water for Injection	BP

6.2 Incompatibilities

See 6.6 Instructions for Use/Handling.

6.3 Shelf life

36 months unopened.

6.4 Special precautions for storage

Store below 25°C, protect from light.

Zantac Injection should not be autoclaved.

6.5 Nature and contents of container

2 ml colourless Type I glass ampoules, Pack size: 5 ampoules.

6.6 Special precautions for disposal and other handling

Zantac Injection has been shown to be compatible with the following intravenous infusion fluids:-

0.9% Sodium Chloride BP

5% Dextrose BP

0.18% Sodium Chloride and 4% Dextrose BP

4.2% Sodium Bicarbonate BP

Hartmann's Solution.

All unused admixtures of Zantac Injection with infusion fluids should be discarded 24 hours after preparation.

Although compatibility studies have only been undertaken in polyvinyl chloride infusion bags (in glass for Sodium Bicarbonate BP) and a polyvinyl chloride administration set it is considered that adequate stability would be conferred by the use of a polyethylene infusion bag.

Administrative Data

7. MARKETING AUTHORISATION HOLDER

Glaxo Wellcome UK Ltd

T/A GlaxoSmithKline UK

Stockley Park West

Uxbridge

Middlesex, UB11 1BT

8. MARKETING AUTHORISATION NUMBER(S)

PL 10949/0109

9. DATE OF FIRST AUTHORISATION/RENEWAL OF THE AUTHORISATION

25 March 1998

10. DATE OF REVISION OF THE TEXT

10 March 2009

11. Legal Status

POM.

Zantac Syrup

(GlaxoSmithKline UK)

1. NAME OF THE MEDICINAL PRODUCT

Zantac Syrup

2. QUALITATIVE AND QUANTITATIVE COMPOSITION

Ranitidine Hydrochloride 168.0 mg (Equivalent to Ranitidine 150.0 mg)

3. PHARMACEUTICAL FORM

Syrup

4. CLINICAL PARTICULARS

4.1 Therapeutic indications

Adults

Zantac syrup is indicated for the treatment of duodenal ulcer and benign gastric ulcer, including that associated with non-steroidal anti-inflammatory agents. In addition, Zantac syrup is indicated for the prevention of NSAID associated duodenal ulcers. Zantac syrup is also indicated for the treatment of post-operative ulcer, Zollinger-Ellison Syndrome and oesophageal reflux disease including long term management of healed oesophagitis. Other patients with chronic episodic dyspepsia, characterised by pain (epigastric or retrosternal) which is related to meals or disturbs sleep but is not associated with the preceding conditions may benefit from ranitidine treatment. Zantac syrup is indicated for the following conditions where reduction of gastric secretion and acid output is desirable; the prophylaxis of gastro-intestinal haemorrhage from stress ulceration in seriously ill patients, the prophylaxis of recurrent haemorrhage in patients with bleeding peptic ulcers and before general anaesthesia in patients considered to be at risk of acid aspiration (Mendelson's Syndrome), particularly obstetric patients during labour. For appropriate cases Zantac injection is also available (see separate SPC).

Children (3 to 18 years):

Short term treatment of peptic ulcer. Treatment of gastro-oesophageal reflux, including reflux oesophagitis and symptomatic relief of gastro-oesophageal reflux disease.

See section 4.4 Special warnings and precautions for use.

4.2 Posology and method of administration

Route of administration: Oral

Adults (including the elderly) / Adolescents (12 years and over)

The usual dosage is 150 mg twice daily, taken in the morning and evening. Alternatively, patients with duodenal ulceration, gastric ulceration or oesophageal reflux disease may be treated with a single bedtime dose of 300 mg. It is not necessary to time the dose in relation to meals.

Duodenal ulcer, benign gastric ulcer and post-operative ulcer:

In most cases of duodenal ulcer, benign gastric ulcer and post operative ulcer, healing occurs in four weeks. Healing usually occurs after a further 4 weeks of treatment in those patients whose ulcers have not fully healed after the initial course of therapy.

NSAID associated peptic ulceration, including prophylaxis of duodenal ulcers:

In ulcers following non-steroidal anti-inflammatory drug therapy or associated with continued non-steroidal anti-inflammatory drugs, 8 weeks treatment may be necessary.

For the prevention of non-steroidal anti-inflammatory drug associated duodenal ulcers ranitidine 150 mg twice daily may be given concomitantly with non-steroidal anti-inflammatory drug therapy.

In duodenal ulcer 300 mg twice daily for 4 weeks results in healing rates which are higher than those at 4 weeks with ranitidine 150 mg twice daily or 300 mg nocte. The increased dose has not been associated with an increased incidence of unwanted effects.

Maintenance treatment at a reduced dosage of 150 mg at bedtime is recommended for patients who have responded to short term therapy, particularly those with a history of recurrent ulcer.

Gastro-oesophageal reflux disease:

In the management of oesophageal reflux disease, the recommended course of treatment is either 150 mg twice daily or 300 mg at bedtime for up to 8 weeks or if necessary 12 weeks.

In patients with moderate to severe oesophagitis, the dosage of ranitidine may be increased to 150 mg four times daily for up to twelve weeks. The increased dose has not been associated with an incidence of unwanted effects.

For the long-term management of oesophagitis the recommended adult oral dose is 150 mg twice daily. Long-term treatment is not indicated in the management of patients with unhealed oesophagitis with or without barrett's epithelium.

Zollinger-Ellison syndrome:

In patients with Zollinger-Ellison Syndrome, the starting dose is 150 mg three times daily and this may be increased as necessary. Patients with this syndrome have been given increasing doses up to 6 g per day and these doses have been well tolerated.

Chronic episodic dyspepsia:

For patients with chronic episodic dyspepsia the recommended course of treatment is 150 mg twice daily for up to six weeks. Anyone not responding or relapsing shortly afterwards should be investigated.

Prophylaxis of haemorrhage from stress ulceration or recurrent haemorrhage:

In the prophylaxis of haemorrhage from stress ulceration in seriously ill patients or in the prophylaxis of recurrent haemorrhage in patients bleeding from peptic ulceration, treatment with Zantac tablets 150 mgs twice daily may be substituted for Zantac injection once oral feeding commences in patients considered to be still at risk from these conditions.

Prophylaxis of Mendelson's syndrome:

In patients thought to be at risk of acid aspiration syndrome an oral dose of 150 mg can be given 2 hours before induction of general anaesthesia, and preferably also 150 mg the previous evening.

In obstetric patients at commencement of labour, an oral dose of 150 mg may be given followed by 150 mg at six hourly intervals. It is recommended that since gastric emptying and drug absorption are delayed during labour, any patient requiring emergency general anaesthesia should be given, in addition, a non-particulate antacid (eg sodium citrate) prior to induction of anaesthesia. The usual precautions to avoid acid aspiration should also be taken.

Children (3 to 11 years):

See Section 5.2 Pharmacokinetic Properties (Special Patient Population)

Zantac syrup contains approximately 7.5%w/v ethanol. Therefore an alternative formulation of ranitidine may be considered necessary for at-risk groups, including children (see section 4.4 Special warnings and precautions for use).

Peptic Ulcer Acute Treatment

The recommended oral dose for the treatment of peptic ulcer in children is 4 mg/kg/day to 8 mg/kg/day administered as two divided doses to a maximum of 300 mg ranitidine per day for a duration of 4 weeks. For those patients with incomplete healing, another 4 weeks of therapy is indicated, as healing usually occurs after eight weeks of treatment.

Gastro-Oesophageal Reflux

The recommended oral dose for the treatment of gastro-oesophageal reflux in children is 5 mg/kg/day to 10 mg/kg/day administered as two divided doses to a maximum of 600 mg (the maximum dose is likely to apply to heavier children or adolescents with severe symptoms).

Safety and efficacy in new-born patients has not been established.

Renal Impairment:

Accumulation of ranitidine with resulting elevated plasma concentrations will occur in patients with severe renal impairment (creatinine clearance less than 50 ml/min). Accordingly, it is recommended that the daily dose of ranitidine in such patients be 150 mg at night for 4 to 8 weeks. The same dose should be used for maintenance treatment if necessary. If an ulcer has not healed after treatment, the standard dosage regimen of 150 mg twice daily should be instituted, followed, if need be, by maintenance treatment at 150 mg at night.

4.3 Contraindications

Ranitidine is contraindicated for patients known to have hypersensitivity to any component of the preparation.

4.4 Special warnings and precautions for use

Treatment with a histamine H_2-antagonist may mask symptoms associated with carcinoma of the stomach and may therefore delay diagnosis of the condition. Accordingly, where gastric ulcer has been diagnosed or in patients of middle age and over with new or recently changed dyspeptic symptoms the possibility of malignancy should be excluded before therapy with Zantac is instituted.

Ranitidine is excreted via the kidney and so plasma levels of the drug are increased in patients with severe renal impairment. The dosage should be adjusted as detailed under Dosage in Renal Impairment.

Regular supervision of patients who are taking non-steroidal anti-inflammatory drugs concomitantly with ranitidine is recommended, especially in the elderly. Current evidence shows that ranitidine protects against NSAID associated ulceration in the duodenum and not in the stomach.

Although clinical reports of acute intermittent porphyria associated with ranitidine administration have been rare and inconclusive, ranitidine should be avoided in patients with a history of this condition.

Rates of healing of ulcers in clinical trial patients aged 65 and over have not been found to differ from those in younger patients. Additionally, there was no difference in the incidence of adverse effects.

Zantac syrup contains approximately 7.5% w/v ethanol (alcohol), i.e. up to 405 mg per 5 ml spoonful which is equivalent to about 11 ml of beer or 5 ml of wine. It is harmful for those suffering from alcoholism. It should be taken into account in pregnant or lactating women, high-risk groups (those suffering from alcoholism, liver disease, epilepsy, brain injury or disease) and children (see section 4.2). It may modify or increase the effects of other medicines.

Alternative formulation of Zantac may be considered preferential in these populations.

In patients such as the elderly, persons with chronic lung disease, diabetes or the immunocompromised, there may be an increased risk of developing community acquired pneumonia. A large epidemiological study showed an increased risk of developing community acquired pneumonia in current users of H_2 receptor antagonists versus those who had stopped treatment, with an observed adjusted relative risk increase of 1.63 (95% CI, 1.07-2.48).

4.5 Interaction with other medicinal products and other forms of interaction

Ranitidine has the potential to affect the absorption, metabolism or renal excretion of other drugs. The altered pharmacokinetics may necessitate dosage adjustment of the affected drug or discontinuation of treatment

Interactions occur by several mechanisms including:

1) Inhibition of cytochrome P450-linked mixed function oxygenase system: Ranitidine at usual therapeutic doses does not potentiate the actions of drugs which are inactivated by this enzyme system such as diazepam, lidocaine, phenytoin, propanolol and theophylline.

There have been reports of altered prothrombin time with coumarin anticoagulants (e.g. warfarin). Due to the narrow therapeutic index, close monitoring of increased or decreased prothrombin time is recommended during concurrent treatment with ranitidine.

2) Competition for renal tubular secretion:

Since ranitidine is partially eliminated by the cationic system, it may affect the clearance of other drugs eliminated by this route. High doses of ranitidine (e.g. such as those used in the treatment of Zollinger-Ellison syndrome) may reduce the excretion of procainamide and N-acetylprocainamide resulting in increased plasma level of these drugs.

3) Alteration of gastric pH:

The bioavailability of certain drugs may be affected. This can result in either an increase in absorption (e.g. triazolam, midazolam, glipizide) or a decrease in absorption (e.g. ketoconazole, atazanavir, delaviridine, gefitnib).

4.6 Pregnancy and lactation

Zantac crosses the placenta but therapeutic doses administered to obstetric patients in labour or undergoing caesarean section have been without any adverse effect on labour, delivery or subsequent neonatal progress. Zantac is also excreted in human breast milk. Like other drugs, Zantac should only be used during pregnancy and nursing if considered essential.

4.7 Effects on ability to drive and use machines

Not applicable

4.8 Undesirable effects

The following convention has been utilised for the classification of undesirable effects: very common ($\geqslant$1/10), common ($\geqslant$1/100, $<$1/10), uncommon ($\geqslant$1/1000, $\leqslant$1/100), rare ($\geqslant$1/10,000, $\leqslant$1/1000), very rare ($\leqslant$1/10,000), unknown (cannot be estimated from the available data).

Blood & Lymphatic System Disorders

Unknown: Blood count changes (leucopenia, thrombocytopenia). These are usually reversible. Agranulocytosis or pancytopenia, sometimes with marrow hypoplasia or marrow aplasia.

Immune System Disorders

Uncommon: Hypersensitivity reactions (urticaria, angioneurotic oedema, fever, bronchospasm, hypotension and chest pain).

Unknown: Anaphylactic shock

These events have been reported after a single dose.

Psychiatric Disorders

Very Rare: Depression.

Unknown: Reversible mental confusion and hallucinations.

These have been reported predominantly in severely ill and elderly patients.

Nervous System Disorders

Common: Headache (sometimes severe) and dizziness.

Unknown: Reversible involuntary movement disorders.

Eye Disorders

Uncommon: Reversible blurred vision.

There have been reports of blurred vision, which is suggestive of a change in accommodation.

Cardiac Disorders

Unknown: As with other H_2 receptor antagonists bradycardia and A-V Block.

Vascular Disorders

Unknown: Vasculitis.

Gastrointestinal Disorders

Common: Diarrhoea.

Unknown: Acute pancreatitis.

Hepatobiliary Disorders

Very Rare: Transient and reversible changes in liver function tests.

Unknown: Hepatitis (hepatocellular, hepatocanalicular or mixed) with or without jaundice, these were usually reversible.

Skin and Subcutaneous Tissue Disorders

Uncommon: Skin Rash.

Unknown: Erythema multiforme, alopecia.

Musculoskeletal and Connective Tissue Disorders

Unknown: Musculoskeletal symptoms such as arthralgia and myalgia.

Renal and Urinary Disorders

Unknown: Acute interstitial nephritis.

Reproductive System and Breast Disorders

Unknown: Reversible impotence, breast symptoms and breast conditions (such as gynaecomastia and galactorrhoea).

The safety of ranitidine has been assessed in children aged 0 to 16 years with acid-related disease and was generally well tolerated with an adverse event profile resembling that in adults. There are limited long term safety available, in particular regarding growth and development.

4.9 Overdose

Zantac is very specific in action and accordingly no particular problems are expected following overdosage with the drug. Symptomatic and supportive therapy should be given as appropriate.

5. PHARMACOLOGICAL PROPERTIES

5.1 Pharmacodynamic properties

Zantac is a specific, rapidly acting H_2-antagonist. It inhibits basal and stimulated secretion of gastric acid, reducing both the volume of the acid and pepsin content of the secretion. Zantac has a relatively long duration of action and a single 150 mg dose effectively suppresses gastric acid secretion for twelve hours.

5.2 Pharmacokinetic properties

The bioavailability of Ranitidine is consistently about 50 %. Absorption of ranitidine after oral administration is rapid and peak plasma concentrations are usually achieved 2-3 hours after administration. absorption is not significantly impaired by foods or antacids. Ranitidine is not extensively metabolised. Elimination of the drug is primarily by tubular secretion. The elimination half-life of ranitidine is 2-3 hours. In balance studies with 150 mg 3H-ranitidine 60-70% of an oral dose was excreted in urine and 26% in faeces. Analysis of urine excreted in the first 24 hours after dosing showed that 35% of the oral dose was eliminated unchanged. About 6% of the dose is excreted as the N-oxide, 2% as the S-oxide, 2% as desmethyl ranitidine and 1-2% as the furoic acid analogue.

Special Patient Populations

Children (3 years and above)

Limited pharmacokinetic data show that there are no significant differences in half-life (range for children 3 years and above: 1.7 - 2.2 h) and plasma clearance (range for children 3 years and above: 9 - 22 ml/min/kg) between children and healthy adults receiving oral ranitidine when correction is made for body weight.

5.3 Preclinical safety data

No clinically relevant findings were observed in preclinical studies.

6. PHARMACEUTICAL PARTICULARS

6.1 List of excipients

Hydroxypropyl methylcellulose USP

2906 or 2910

Ethanol (96%) BP

Propyl hydroxybenzoate BP

Butyl hydroxybenzoate BP

Potassium dihydrogen

OrthophosphateAR

Disodium hydrogen orthophosphat

Anhydrous AR

Sodium chloride BP

Saccharin sodium BP

Sorbitol solution 1973 BPC

Mint flavour IFF 17: 42: 3632

Purified water BP

6.2 Incompatibilities

Not applicable.

6.3 Shelf life

24 months.

6.4 Special precautions for storage

Zantac syrup should be stored at a temperature not exceeding 25°C.

6.5 Nature and contents of container

Amber glass bottles with polypropylene child resistant caps, or plastic child resistant closures, or plastic child resistant tamper evident closures with either pet faced/al foil/epe wads, or pet faced/al foil/folding box board

Pack sizes: 300 ml, 2 × 150 ml.

6.6 Special precautions for disposal and other handling

None.

Administrative Data

7. MARKETING AUTHORISATION HOLDER

Glaxo Wellcome UK Ltd., trading as GlaxoSmithKline UK

Stockley Park West,

Uxbridge,

Middlesex, UB11 1BT

8. MARKETING AUTHORISATION NUMBER(S)

PL 10949/0108

9. DATE OF FIRST AUTHORISATION/RENEWAL OF THE AUTHORISATION
17 April 2003

10. DATE OF REVISION OF THE TEXT
10 March 2009

11. Legal Status
POM

Zantac Tablets 150mg

(GlaxoSmithKline UK)

1. NAME OF THE MEDICINAL PRODUCT
Zantac Tablets 150 mg

2. QUALITATIVE AND QUANTITATIVE COMPOSITION
Each tablet contains ranitidine 150 mg (as the hydrochloride).

3. PHARMACEUTICAL FORM
Tablet.

4. CLINICAL PARTICULARS

4.1 Therapeutic indications

Adults

Duodenal ulcer and benign gastric ulcer, including that associated with non-steroidal anti-inflammatory agents.

Prevention of non-steroidal anti-inflammatory drug associated duodenal ulcers.

Treatment of duodenal ulcers associated with *Helicobacter pylori* infection.

Post-operative ulcer.

Oesophageal reflux disease including long term management of healed oesophagitis.

Symptomatic relief in gastro-oesophageal reflux disease.

Zollinger-Ellison Syndrome.

Chronic episodic dyspepsia, characterised by pain (epigastric or retrosternal) which is related to meals or disturbs sleep but not associated with the above conditions.

Prophylaxis of gastrointestinal haemorrhage from stress ulceration in seriously ill patients

Prophylaxis of recurrent haemorrhage with bleeding peptic ulcers.

Before general anaesthesia in patients at risk of acid aspiration (Mendelson's syndrome), particularly obstetric patients during labour.

For appropriate cases, Zantac injection is also available (see separate SPC).

Children (3 to 18 years)

Short term treatment of peptic ulcer

Treatment of gastro-oesophageal reflux, including reflux oesophagitis and symptomatic relief of gastro-oesophageal reflux disease.

4.2 Posology and method of administration

Adults (including the elderly) / Adolescents (12 years and over)

Usual dosage is 150 mg twice daily, taken in the morning and evening.

Duodenal ulcer, gastric ulcer:

The standard dosage regimen is 150 mg twice daily or 300 mg at night. It is not necessary to time the dose in relation to meals.

In most cases of duodenal ulcer, benign gastric ulcer and post-operative ulcer, healing occurs within 4 weeks. Healing usually occurs after a further 4 weeks of treatment in those not fully healed after the initial course of therapy.

Ulcers following NSAID therapy or associated with continued NSAIDs:

8 weeks treatment may be necessary

Prevention of NSAID associated duodenal ulcers:

150 mg twice daily may be given concomitantly with NSAID therapy.

In duodenal ulcer, 300 mg twice daily for 4 weeks results in healing rates which are higher than those at 4 weeks with ranitidine 150 mg twice daily or 300 mg at night. The increased dose has not been associated with an increased incidence of unwanted effects.

Duodenal ulcers associated with *Helicobacter pylori* infection:

For duodenal ulcers associated with *Helicobacter pylori* infection, ranitidine 300 mg at bedtime or 150 mg twice daily may be given with oral amoxicillin 750 mg three times daily and metronidazole 500 mg three times daily for two weeks. Therapy with ranitidine should continue for a further two weeks. This dose regimen significantly reduces the frequency of duodenal ulcer recurrence.

Maintenance treatment at a reduced dosage of 150 mg at bedtime is recommended for patients who have responded to short term therapy, particularly those with a history of recurrent ulcer.

Gastro-oesophageal reflux disease:

Symptom relief in gastro-oesophageal reflux disease. In patients with gastro-oesophageal reflux disease, a dose regimen of 150 mg twice daily for 2 weeks is recommended and this can be repeated in patients in whom the initial symptomatic response is inadequate

Oesophageal reflux disease:

In the management of oesophageal reflux disease, the recommended course of treatment is either 150 mg twice daily or 300 mg at bedtime for up to 8 weeks or 12 weeks if necessary.

In patients with moderate to severe oesophagitis, the dosage of ranitidine may be increased to 150 mg 4 times daily for up to 12 weeks. The increased dose has not been associated with an increased incidence of unwanted effects.

Healed oesophagitis:

For long term treatment, recommended adult dose is 150 mg twice daily. Long term treatment is not indicated in management of patients with unhealed oesophagitis with or without Barrett's epithelium.

Zollinger-Ellison syndrome:

The starting dose for Zollinger-Ellison syndrome is 150 mg three times daily, and this may be increased as necessary. Doses up to 6 grams per day have been well tolerated.

Chronic episodic dyspepsia:

The standard dosage regimen for patients with chronic episodic dyspepsia is 150 mg twice daily for up to 6 weeks. Anyone not responding or relapsing shortly afterwards should be investigated.

Prophylaxis of haemorrhage from stress ulceration in seriously ill patients or prophylaxis of recurrent haemorrhage in patients bleeding from peptic ulceration:

150 mg twice daily may be substituted for the injection once oral feeding commences.

Prophylaxis of acid aspiration (Mendelson's) syndrome:

150 mg oral dose can be given 2 hours before anaesthesia, and preferably also 150 mg the previous evening. Alternatively, the injection is also available. In obstetric patients in labour 150 mg every 6 hours, but if general anaesthesia is required it is recommended that a non-particulate antacid (e.g. sodium citrate) be given in addition. The usual precautions to avoid acid aspiration should also be taken.

Children from 3 to 11 years and over 30 kg of weight

See Section 5.2 Pharmacokinetic Properties (Special Patient Population)

Peptic Ulcer Acute Treatment

The recommended oral dose for the treatment of peptic ulcer in children is 4 mg/kg/day to 8 mg/kg/day administered as two divided doses to a maximum of 300 mg ranitidine per day for a duration of 4 weeks. For those patients with complete healing, another 4 weeks of therapy is indicated, as healing usually occurs after eight weeks of treatment.

Gastro-Oesophageal Reflux

The recommended oral dose for the treatment of gastro-oesophageal reflux in children is 5 mg/kg/day to 10 mg/kg/day administered as two divided doses to a maximum of 600 mg (the maximum dose is likely to apply to heavier children or adolescents with severe symptoms).

Safety and efficacy in new-born patients has not been established.

Renal Impairment:

Accumulation of ranitidine with resulting elevated plasma concentrations will occur in patients with severe renal impairment (creatinine clearance less than 50 ml/min). Accordingly, it is recommended that the daily dose of ranitidine in such patients should be 150 mg at night for 4-8 weeks. The same dose should be used for maintenance treatment, if necessary. If an ulcer has not healed after treatment, 150 mg twice daily dosage should be instituted followed, if need be, by maintenance treatment of 150 mg at night.

4.3 Contraindications

Ranitidine is contra-indicated in patients known to have hypersensitivity to any component of the preparation.

4.4 Special warnings and precautions for use

Malignancy:

The possibility of malignancy should be excluded before commencement of therapy in patients with gastric ulcer (and if indications include dyspepsia, patients of middle age and over with new or recently changed dyspeptic symptoms) as treatment with ranitidine may mask symptoms of gastric carcinoma.

Renal Disease:

Ranitidine is excreted via the kidney and so plasma levels of the drug are increased in patients with severe renal impairment. The dosage should be adjusted as detailed under Dosage in Renal Impairment.

Regular supervision of patients who are taking non-steroidal anti-inflammatory drugs concomitantly with ranitidine is recommended, especially in the elderly and in those with a history of peptic ulcer.

Rare clinical reports suggest that ranitidine may precipitate acute porphyric attacks. Ranitidine should therefore be avoided in patients with a history of acute porphyria.

Use in elderly patients:

Rates of healing of ulcers in clinical trial patients aged 65 and over have not been found to differ from those in younger patients. Additionally there was no difference in the incidence of adverse effects.

In patients such as the elderly, persons with chronic lung disease, diabetes or the immunocompromised, there may be an increased risk of developing community acquired pneumonia. A large epidemiological study showed an increased risk of developing community acquired pneumonia in current users of H_2 receptor antagonists versus those who had stopped treatment, with an observed adjusted relative risk increase of 1.63 (95% CI, 1.07–2.48).

4.5 Interaction with other medicinal products and other forms of interaction

Ranitidine has the potential to affect the absorption, metabolism or renal excretion of other drugs. The altered pharmacokinetics may necessitate dosage adjustment of the affected drug or discontinuation of treatment

Interactions occur by several mechanisms including:

1) Inhibition of cytochrome P450-linked mixed function oxygenase system: Ranitidine at usual therapeutic doses does not potentiate the actions of drugs which are inactivated by this enzyme system such as diazepam, lidocaine, phenytoin, propanolol and theophylline.

There have been reports of altered prothrombin time with coumarin anticoagulants (e.g. warfarin). Due to the narrow therapeutic index, close monitoring of increased or decreased prothrombin time is recommended during concurrent treatment with ranitidine.

2) Competition for renal tubular secrection:

Since ranitidine is partially eliminated by the cationic system, it may affect the clearance of other drugs eliminated by this route. High doses of ranitidine (e.g. such as those used in the treatment of Zollinger-Ellison syndrome) may reduce the excretion of procainamide and N-acetylprocainamide resulting in increased plasma level of these drugs.

3) Alteration of gastric pH:

The bioavailability of certain drugs may be affected. This can result in either an increase in absorption (e.g. triazolam, midazolam, glipizide) or a decrease in absorption (e.g. ketoconazole, atazanavir, delaviridine, gefitnib).

There is no evidence of an interaction between ranitidine and -amoxicillin or metronidazole

4.6 Pregnancy and lactation

Ranitidine crosses the placenta but therapeutic doses administered to obstetric patients in labour or undergoing caesarean section have been without any adverse effect on labour, delivery or subsequent neonatal progress. It is excreted in human breast milk.

Like other drugs it should only be used during pregnancy and nursing if considered essential.

4.7 Effects on ability to drive and use machines

Not applicable.

4.8 Undesirable effects

The following convention has been utilised for the classification of undesirable effects: very common ($\geqslant$1/10), common ($\geqslant$1/100, $<$1/10), uncommon ($\geqslant$1/1000, $\leqslant$1/100), rare ($\geqslant$1/10,000, $\leqslant$1/1000), very rare ($\leqslant$1/10,000), unknown (cannot be estimated from the available data).

Blood & Lymphatic System Disorders

Unknown:

Blood count changes (leucopenia, thrombocytopenia). These are usually reversible. Agranulocytosis or pancytopenia, sometimes with marrow hypoplasia or marrow aplasia.

Immune System Disorders

Uncommon:

Hypersensitivity reactions (urticaria, angioneurotic oedema, fever, bronchospasm, hypotension and chest pain).

Unknown:

Anaphylactic shock.

These events have been reported after a single dose.

Psychiatric Disorders

Very Rare:

Depression.

Unknown:

Reversible mental confusion and hallucinations.

These have been reported predominantly in severely ill and elderly patients.

Nervous System Disorders

Common:

Headache (sometimes severe) and dizziness.

Unknown:

Reversible involuntary movement disorders.

Eye Disorders

Uncommon:

Reversible blurred vision.

There have been reports of blurred vision, which is suggestive of a change in accommodation.

Cardiac Disorders

Unknown:

As with other H_2 receptor antagonists bradycardia and A-V Block.

Vascular Disorders

Unknown:

Vasculitis.

Gastrointestinal Disorders

Common:

Diarrhoea.

Unknown:

Acute pancreatitis.

Hepatobiliary Disorders

Very Rare:

Transient and reversible changes in liver function tests.

Unknown:

Hepatitis (hepatocellular, hepatocanalicular or mixed) with or without jaundice, these were usually reversible.

Skin and Subcutaneous Tissue Disorders

Uncommon:

Skin Rash.

Unknown:

Erythema multiforme, alopecia.

Musculoskeletal and Connective Tissue Disorders

Unknown:

Musculoskeletal symptoms such as arthralgia and myalgia.

Renal and Urinary Disorders

Unknown:

Acute interstitial nephritis.

Reproductive System and Breast Disorders

Unknown:

Reversible impotence, breast symptoms and breast conditions (such as gynaecomastia and galactorrhoea).

The safety of ranitidine has been assessed in children aged 0 to 16 years with acid-related disease and was generally well tolerated with an adverse event profile resembling that in adults. There are limited long term safety data available, in particular regarding growth and development.

4.9 Overdose

Ranitidine is very specific in action and accordingly no particular problems are expected following overdosage. Symptomatic and supportive therapy should be given as appropriate.

5. PHARMACOLOGICAL PROPERTIES

5.1 Pharmacodynamic properties

Ranitidine is a specific rapidly acting histamine H_2-antagonist. It inhibits basal and stimulated secretion of gastric acid, reducing both the volume and the acid and pepsin content of the secretion. Ranitidine has a relatively long duration of action and so a single 150 mg dose effectively suppresses gastric acid secretion for twelve hours.

5.2 Pharmacokinetic properties

Absorption of ranitidine after oral administration is rapid and peak plasma concentrations are usually achieved within two hours of administration. Absorption is not significantly impaired by food or antacids. The elimination half-life of ranitidine is approximately 2 hours. Ranitidine is excreted via the kidneys mainly as the free drug and in minor amounts as metabolites Its major metabolite is an N-oxide and there are smaller quantities of S-oxide and desmethyl ranitidine. The 24 hour urinary recovery of free ranitidine and its metabolites is about 40% with orally administered drug.

Special Patient Populations

Children (3 years and above)

Limited pharmacokinetic data show that there are no significant differences in half-life (range for children 3 years and above: 1.7 - 2.2 h) and plasma clearance (range for children 3 years and above: 9 - 22 ml/min/kg) between children and healthy adults receiving oral ranitidine when correction is made for body weight.

5.3 Preclinical safety data

No additional data of relevance.

6. PHARMACEUTICAL PARTICULARS

6.1 List of excipients

Tablet core:

Microcrystalline cellulose NF

Magnesium stearate EP

Methylhydroxypropyl cellulose (E464) EP

Film coat:

Titanium Dioxide E171 EP

Triacetin NF

6.2 Incompatibilities

None.

6.3 Shelf life

60 months.

6.4 Special precautions for storage

None necessary.

6.5 Nature and contents of container

Cartons of 30, 60 or 90 tablets, in aluminium foil strips or push through double foil blister packs.

6.6 Special precautions for disposal and other handling

No special instructions.

Administrative Data

7. MARKETING AUTHORISATION HOLDER

Glaxo Wellcome UK Limited

Trading as GlaxoSmithKline UK

Stockley Park West

Uxbridge

Middlesex

UB11 1BT

8. MARKETING AUTHORISATION NUMBER(S)

PL 10949/0042

9. DATE OF FIRST AUTHORISATION/RENEWAL OF THE AUTHORISATION

27 March 2002

10. DATE OF REVISION OF THE TEXT

10 March 2009

11. Legal Status

POM

Zantac Tablets 300mg

(GlaxoSmithKline UK)

1. NAME OF THE MEDICINAL PRODUCT

Zantac Tablets 300 mg

2. QUALITATIVE AND QUANTITATIVE COMPOSITION

Each tablet contains ranitidine 300 mg (as the hydrochloride).

3. PHARMACEUTICAL FORM

Tablet.

4. CLINICAL PARTICULARS

4.1 Therapeutic indications

Adults

Zantac Tablets are indicated for:

- treatment of duodenal ulcer and benign gastric ulcer, including that associated with non-steroidal anti-inflammatory agents.
- treatment of duodenal ulcers associated with *Helicobacter pylori* infection.
- treatment of post-operative ulcer
- Zollinger-Ellison syndrome
- oesophageal reflux disease
- chronic episodic dyspepsia, characterised by pain (epigastric or retrosternal) which is related to meals or disturbs sleep but is not associated with the preceding conditions may benefit from ranitidine treatment.

Zantac Tablets are indicated for the following conditions where reduction of gastric secretion and acid output is desirable:

- prophylaxis of gastrointestinal haemorrhage from stress ulceration in seriously ill patients
- prophylaxis of recurrent haemorrhage in patients with bleeding peptic ulcers
- before general anaesthesia in patients considered to be at risk of acid aspiration (Mendelson's syndrome), particularly obstetric patients during labour.

For appropriate cases Zantac Injection is also available (see separate SPC).

Children (3 to 18 years)

Short term treatment of peptic ulcer

Treatment of gastro-oesophageal reflux, including reflux oesophagitis and symptomatic relief of gastro-oesophageal reflux disease.

4.2 Posology and method of administration

Adults (including the elderly) / Adolescents (12 years and over)

The usual dosage is 150 mg twice daily, taken in the morning and evening.

Patients with duodenal ulceration, gastric ulceration or oesophageal reflux disease may be treated with a single bedtime dose of 300 mg. It is not necessary to time the dose in relation to meals.

Duodenal ulcer, benign gastric ulcer and post operative ulcer:

In most cases of duodenal ulcer, benign gastric ulcer and post operative ulcer, healing occurs in four weeks. Healing usually occurs after a further four weeks of treatment in those patients whose ulcers have not fully healed after the initial course of therapy.

NSAID associated peptic ulceration, including prophylaxis of duodenal ulcers:

In ulcers following non-steroidal anti-inflammatory drug therapy or associated with continued non-steroidal anti-inflammatory drugs, eight weeks treatment may be necessary.

In duodenal ulcer 300 mg twice daily for 4 weeks results in healing rates which are higher than those at 4 weeks with ranitidine 150 mg twice daily or 300 mg nocte. The increased dose has not been associated with an increased incidence of unwanted effects.

Duodenal ulcers associated with *Helicobacter pylori* infection:

For duodenal ulcers associated with *Helicobacter pylori* infection ranitidine 300 mg at bedtime or 150 mg twice daily may be given with oral amoxicillin 750 mg three times daily and metronidazole 500 mg three times daily for two weeks. Therapy with ranitidine should continue for a further 2 weeks. This dose regimen significantly reduces the frequency of duodenal ulcer recurrence.

Maintenance treatment at a reduced dosage of 150 mg at bedtime is recommended for patients who have responded to short-term therapy, particularly those with a history of recurrent ulcer.

Oesophageal reflux disease

In the management of oesophageal reflux disease, the recommended course of treatment is either 150 mg twice daily or 300 mg at bedtime for up to 8 weeks or if necessary 12 weeks.

Zollinger-Ellison syndrome:

In patients with Zollinger-Ellison syndrome, the starting dose is 150 mg three times daily and this may be increased as necessary. Patients with this syndrome have been given increasing doses up to 6 g per day and these doses have been well tolerated.

Chronic episodic dyspepsia:

For patients with chronic episodic dyspepsia the recommended course of treatment is 150 mg twice daily for up to six weeks. Anyone not responding or relapsing shortly afterwards should be investigated.

In the prophylaxis of haemorrhage from stress ulceration in seriously ill patients or the prophylaxis of recurrent haemorrhage in patients bleeding from peptic ulceration, treatment with Zantac Tablets 150 mg twice daily may be substituted for Zantac Injection (see separate SPC) once oral feeding commences in patients considered to be still at risk from these conditions.

Prophylaxis of acid aspiration (Mendleson's syndrome):

In patients thought to be at risk of acid aspiration syndrome an oral dose of 150 mg can be given 2 hours before induction of general anaesthesia, and preferably also 150 mg the previous evening.

In obstetric patients at commencement of labour, an oral dose of 150 mg may be given followed by 150 mg at six hourly intervals. It is recommended that since gastric emptying and drug absorption are delayed during labour, any patient requiring emergency general anaesthesia should be given, in addition, a non-particulate antacid (e.g. sodium citrate) prior to induction of anaesthesia. The usual precautions to avoid acid aspiration should also be taken.

Children from 3 to 11 years and over 30kg of weight

See Section 5.2 Pharmacokinetic Properties (Special Patient Populations)

Peptic Ulcer Acute Treatment

The recommended oral dose for treatment of peptic ulcer in children is 4 mg/kg/day to 8 mg/kg/day administered as two divided doses to a maximum of 300 mg ranitidine per day for a duration of 4 weeks. For those patients with incomplete healing, another 4 weeks of therapy is indicated, as healing usually occurs after eight weeks of treatment.

Gastro-Oesophageal Reflux

The recommended oral dose for the treatment of gastro-oesophageal reflux in children is 5 mg/kg/day to 10 mg/kg/day administered as two divided doses to a maximum of 600 mg (the maximum dose is likely to apply to heavier children or adolescents with severe symptoms).

Safety and efficacy in new-born patients has not been established.

Renal Impairment

Accumulation of ranitidine with resulting elevated plasma concentrations will occur in patients with severe renal impairment (creatinine clearance less than 50 ml/min). Accordingly, it is recommended that the daily dose of ranitidine in such patients should be 150 mg at night for 4-8 weeks. The same dose should be used for maintenance treatment, if necessary. If an ulcer has not healed after treatment, 150 mg twice daily dosage should be instituted followed, if need be, by maintenance treatment of 150 mg at night.

4.3 Contraindications

Ranitidine is contra-indicated in patients known to have hypersensitivity to any component of the preparation.

4.4 Special warnings and precautions for use

Treatment with a histamine H_2-antagonist may mask symptoms associated with carcinoma of the stomach and may therefore delay diagnosis of the condition. Accordingly, where gastric ulcer has been diagnosed or in patients of middle age and over with new or recently changed dyspeptic symptoms the possibility of malignancy should be excluded before therapy with Zantac Tablets is instituted.

Ranitidine is excreted via the kidney and so plasma levels of the drug are increased in patients with severe renal impairment. The dose should be adjusted as detailed under Dosage in Renal Impairment.

Regular supervision of patients who are taking non-steroidal anti-inflammatory drugs concomitantly with ranitidine is recommended, especially in the elderly. Current evidence shows that ranitidine protects against NSAID associated ulceration in the duodenum and not in the stomach.

Although clinical reports of acute intermittent porphyria associated with ranitidine administration have been rare and inconclusive, ranitidine should be avoided in patients with a history of this condition.

Use in elderly patients:

Rates of healing of ulcers in clinical trial patients aged 65 and over have not been found to differ from those in younger patients. Additionally, there was no difference in the incidence of adverse effects.

In patients such as the elderly, persons with chronic lung disease, diabetes or the immunocompromised, there may be an increased risk of developing community acquired pneumonia. A large epidemiological study showed an increased risk of developing community acquired pneumonia in current users of H_2 receptor antagonists versus those who had stopped treatment, with an observed adjusted relative risk increase of 1.63 (95% CI, 1.07–2.48).

4.5 Interaction with other medicinal products and other forms of interaction

Ranitidine has the potential to affect the absorption, metabolism or renal excretion of other drugs. The altered pharmacokinetics may necessitate dosage adjustment of the affected drug or discontinuation of treatment

Interactions occur by several mechanisms including:

1) Inhibition of cytochrome P450-linked mixed function oxygenase system: Ranitidine at usual therapeutic doses does not potentiate the actions of drugs which are inactivated by this enzyme system such as diazepam, lidocaine, phenytoin, propanolol and theophylline.

There have been reports of altered prothrombin time with coumarin anticoagulants (e.g. warfarin). Due to the narrow therapeutic index, close monitoring of increased or decreased prothrombin time is recommended during concurrent treatment with ranitidine.

2) Competition for renal tubular secretion:

Since ranitidine is partially eliminated by the cationic system, it may affect the clearance of other drugs eliminated by this route. High doses of ranitidine (e.g. such as those used in the treatment of Zollinger-Ellison syndrome) may reduce the excretion of procainamide and N-acetylprocainamide resulting in increased plasma level of these drugs.

3) Alteration of gastric pH:

The bioavailability of certain drugs may be affected. This can result in either an increase in absorption (e.g. triazolam, midazolam, glipizide) or a decrease in absorption (e.g. ketoconazole, atazanavir, delaviridine, gefitnib).

There is no evidence of an interaction between ranitidine and amoxicillin or metronidazole.

4.6 Pregnancy and lactation

Zantac crosses the placenta but therapeutic doses administered to obstetric patients in labour or undergoing caesarean section have been without any adverse effect on labour, delivery or subsequent neonatal progress. Zantac is also excreted in human breast milk.

Like other drugs, Zantac should only be used during pregnancy and nursing if considered essential.

4.7 Effects on ability to drive and use machines

Not applicable.

4.8 Undesirable effects

The following convention has been utilised for the classification of undesirable effects: very common ($\geqslant$1/10), common ($\geqslant$1/100, $<$1/10), uncommon ($\geqslant$1/1000, $\leqslant$1/100), rare ($\geqslant$1/10,000, $\leqslant$1/1000), very rare ($\leqslant$1/10,000).

Blood & Lymphatic System Disorders

Unknown: Blood count changes (leucopenia, thrombocytopenia). These are usually reversible. Agranulocytosis or pancytopenia, sometimes with marrow hypoplasia or marrow aplasia.

Immune System Disorders

Uncommon: Hypersensitivity reactions (urticaria, angioneurotic oedema, fever, bronchospasm, hypotension and chest pain).

Unknown: Anaphylactic shock.

These events have been reported after a single dose.

Psychiatric Disorders

Very Rare: Depression.

Unknown: Reversible mental confusion and hallucinations.

These have been reported predominantly in severely ill and elderly patients.

Nervous System Disorders

Common: Headache (sometimes severe) and dizziness.

Unknown: Reversible involuntary movement disorders.

Eye Disorders

Uncommon: Reversible blurred vision.

There have been reports of blurred vision, which is suggestive of a change in accommodation.

Cardiac Disorders

Unknown: As with other H_2 receptor antagonists bradycardia and A-V Block.

Vascular Disorders

Unknown: Vasculitis.

Gastrointestinal Disorders

Common: Diarrhoea.

Unknown: Acute pancreatitis.

Hepatobiliary Disorders

Very Rare: Transient and reversible changes in liver function tests.

Unknown: Hepatitis (hepatocellular, hepatocanalicular or mixed) with or without jaundice, these were usually reversible.

Skin and Subcutaneous Tissue Disorders

Uncommon: Skin Rash.

Unknown: Erythema multiforme, alopecia.

Musculoskeletal and Connective Tissue Disorders

Unknown: Musculoskeletal symptoms such as arthralgia and myalgia.

Renal and Urinary Disorders

Unknown: Acute interstitial nephritis.

Reproductive System and Breast Disorders

Unknown: Reversible impotence, breast symptoms and breast conditions (such as gynaecomastia and galactorrhoea).

The safety of ranitidine has been assessed in children ages 0 to 16 years with acid-related disease and was generally well tolerated with an adverse event profile resembling that in adults. There are limited long term data available, in particular regarding growth and development.

4.9 Overdose

Zantac is very specific in action and accordingly no particular problems are expected following overdosage. Symptomatic and supportive therapy should be given as appropriate.

5. PHARMACOLOGICAL PROPERTIES

5.1 Pharmacodynamic properties

Ranitidine is a specific rapidly acting histamine H_2-antagonist. It inhibits basal and stimulated secretion of gastric acid, reducing both the volume and the acid and pepsin content of the secretion. Ranitidine has a relatively long duration of action and so a single 150 mg dose effectively suppresses gastric acid secretion for twelve hours.

5.2 Pharmacokinetic properties

The bioavailability of ranitidine is consistently about 50%. Absorption of ranitidine after oral administration is rapid and peak plasma concentrations are usually achieved within 2-3 hours of administration. Absorption is not significantly impaired by food or antacids. Ranitidine is not extensively metabolised. Elimination of the drug is primarily by tubular secretion. The elimination half-life of ranitidine is 2-3 hours. In balanced studies with 150 mg 3H-Ranitidine 60-70% of an oral dose was excreted in urine and 25% in faeces. Analysis of urine excretion in the first 24 hours after dosing showed that 35% of the oral dose was eliminated unchanged. About 6% of the dose is excreted as the N-oxide, 2% as the S-oxide, 2% as desmethyl ranitidine and 1-2% as the furoic acid analogue.

Special Patient Populations

Children (3 years and above)

Limited pharmacokinetic data have shown that there are no significant differences in half-life (range for children 3 years and above: 1.7 - 2.2 h) and plasma clearance (range for children 3 years and above: 9 - 22 ml/min/kg) between children and healthy adults receiving oral ranitidine when correction is made for body weight.

5.3 Preclinical safety data

No additional data of relevance.

6. PHARMACEUTICAL PARTICULARS

6.1 List of excipients

Tablet core:

Microcrystalline cellulose

Croscarmellose sodium

Magnesium stearate

Film coat:

Methylhydroxypropyl cellulose (E464)

Titanium Dioxide (E171)

Triacetin

6.2 Incompatibilities

None.

6.3 Shelf life

3 years

6.4 Special precautions for storage

None necessary.

6.5 Nature and contents of container

Cartons of 30 tablets in aluminium foil strips or push through double foil blister packs.

6.6 Special precautions for disposal and other handling

No special instructions.

Administrative Data

7. MARKETING AUTHORISATION HOLDER

Glaxo Wellcome UK Limited

Trading as GlaxoSmithKline UK

Stockley Park West

Uxbridge

Middlesex

UB11 1BT

8. MARKETING AUTHORISATION NUMBER(S)

PL 10949/0043

9. DATE OF FIRST AUTHORISATION/RENEWAL OF THE AUTHORISATION

03 October 2000

10. DATE OF REVISION OF THE TEXT

10 March 2009

11. Legal Status

POM

Zarontin Syrup 250mg/5ml

(Pfizer Limited)

1. NAME OF THE MEDICINAL PRODUCT

Zarontin Syrup 250mg/ 5ml

2. QUALITATIVE AND QUANTITATIVE COMPOSITION

Each 5 ml syrup contains: Ethosuximide 250 mg.

3. PHARMACEUTICAL FORM

Syrup

4. CLINICAL PARTICULARS

4.1 Therapeutic indications

Primarily useful in absence seizures. When generalised tonic clonic seizures (grand mal) and other forms of epilepsy co-exist with absence seizures, Zarontin may be administered in combination with other antiepileptic drugs.

4.2 Posology and method of administration

For oral use.

Adults (including the elderly) and children over six years

Initially two 5 ml spoonfuls daily and adjusted thereafter to the patient's needs; daily dosage should be increased by small increments, for example, by 5 ml every 4 to 7 days until control is achieved with minimal side effects. Although 20-30 ml daily in divided doses often produces control of seizures, higher doses up to 40 ml daily may occasionally be required.

Infants and children under six years

The initial dose is 5 ml daily which is adjusted by small increments until control is achieved with minimal side effects. The optimal dose for most children is 20mg/kg/day. This dose has given average plasma levels within the accepted therapeutic range of 40 to 100mg/l.

4.3 Contraindications

Hypersensitivity to succinimides, ethosuximide or any of the components of this medication.

Zarontin Syrup contains sucrose. Patients with rare hereditary problems of fructose intolerance, glucose-galactose malabsorption or sucrase-isomaltase insufficiency should not take this medicine.

4.4 Special warnings and precautions for use

General

Suicidal ideation and behaviour have been reported in patients treated with anti-epileptic agents in several indications. A meta-analysis of randomised placebo controlled trials of anti-epileptic drugs has also shown a small increased risk of suicidal ideation and behaviour. The mechanism of this risk is not known and the available data do not exclude the possibility of an increased risk for ethosuximide.

Therefore patients should be monitored for signs of suicidal ideation and behaviours and appropriate treatment should be considered. Patients (and caregivers of patients) should be advised to seek medical advice should signs of suicidal ideation or behaviour emerge.

Ethosuximide when used alone in mixed types of epilepsy, may increase the frequency of generalised tonic-clonic (grand mal) seizures in some patients.

As with other anticonvulsants, it is important to proceed slowly when increasing or decreasing dosage, as well as when adding or eliminating other medication. Abrupt withdrawal of anticonvulsant medication may precipitate absence (petit mal) seizures.

Haemopoietic Effect

Blood dyscrasias including some with fatal outcome have been reported to be associated with the use of ethosuximide; therefore, periodic blood count determinations should be performed. Should symptoms and/or signs of infection (e.g. sore throat, fever) develop, blood count determinations should be performed at that point.

Hepatic/Renal Impairment

Zarontin should be used with extreme caution in patients with impaired hepatic or renal function. Periodic urinalysis and liver function studies are advised for all patients receiving the drug. Ethosuximide is capable of producing morphological and functional changes in the animal liver. In humans, abnormal liver and renal function studies have been reported.

Autoimmune Disorders

Cases of systemic lupus erythematosus have been reported with the use of ethosuximide. The physician should be alert to this possibility. Additionally, lupus-like reactions have been reported in children given ethosuximide. They vary in severity from systemic immunological disorders, which include the nephrotic syndrome, to the asymptomatic presence of antinuclear antibodies. The nephrotic syndrome is rare and a complete recovery has usually been reported on drug withdrawal

Information for Patients

Patients taking taking ethosuximide should be advised of the importance of adhering strictly to the prescribed dosage regimen.

Patients should be instructed to promptly contact their physician if they develop signs and/or symptoms (eg., sore throat, fever) suggesting an infection (See Haemopoietic Effect above)

4.5 Interaction with other medicinal products and other forms of interaction

Since ethosuximide may interact with concurrently administered antiepileptic drugs, periodic serum level determinations of these drugs may be necessary (e.g. ethosuximide may elevate phenytoin serum levels and valproic acid has been reported to both increase and decrease ethosuximide levels).

4.6 Pregnancy and lactation

Pregnancy

Ethosuximide crosses the placenta. Reports suggest an association between the use of other anticonvulsant drugs by women with epilepsy and an elevated incidence of birth defects in children born to those women. Cases of birth defects have been reported with ethosuximide. The prescribing physician should weigh the benefit versus risk of ethosuximide in treating or counselling epileptic women of childbearing potential.

Lactation

Ethosuximide is excreted in breast milk. Because the effects of ethosuximide on the nursing infant are unknown, caution should be exercised when ethosuximide is administered to a nursing mother. Ethosuximide should be used in nursing mothers only if the benefits clearly outweigh the risks. Breast feeding is best avoided.

4.7 Effects on ability to drive and use machines

Ethosuximide may impair the mental and/or physical abilities required for the performance of potentially hazardous tasks such as driving or other such activities requiring alertness. Therefore, the patient should be cautioned accordingly.

4.8 Undesirable effects

Blood and lymphatic system disorders: Agranulocytosis, aplastic anaemia, eosinophilia, leucopenia and pancytopenia, with or without bone marrow suppression. In most cases of leucopenia, the blood picture has been restored to normal on reduction of the dosage or discontinuation of the drug. Where leucopenia has occurred with other drugs, the polymorph count has in some cases increased steadily after starting treatment with ethosuximide and discontinuing the previous medication (See also section 4.4 Special Warnings and Precautions for Use –Hemopoietic Effect.). Monocytosis, leucocytosis and transitory mild eosinophilia have also been noted.

Immune system disorders: Allergic reaction, systemic lupus erythematosus (See also section 4.4 Special Warnings and Precautions for Use – Autoimmune Disorders.)

Metabolism and nutrition disorders: Weight loss.

Psychiatric disorders: Psychiatric or psychological aberrations associated with ethosuximide administration have included aggressiveness, disturbances of sleep, inability to concentrate and night terrors. These effects may be noted particularly in patients who have previously exhibited psychological abnormalities. There have been rare reports of increased libido.

Nervous system disorders: Fatigue, headache. Neurologic and sensory reactions reported during therapy with ethosuximide have included ataxia, dizziness, drowsiness, euphoria, extrapyramidal side effects, hyperactivity, irritability and lethargy.

Eye disorders: Myopia.

Respiratory, thoracic and mediastinal disorders: Hiccups.

Gastrointestinal disorders: Abdominal pain, gastrointestinal symptoms occur frequently and include anorexia, cramps, diarrhoea, epigastric pain, nausea, vague gastric upset and vomiting. There have been reports of gum hypertrophy and swelling of the tongue. (See also section 4.4 Special Warnings and Precautions for Use – Hepatic/ Renal Impairment).

Skin and subcutaneous tissue disorders: Pruritic erythematous rashes, Stevens-Johnson syndrome, urticaria.and alopecia

Renal and urnary disorders: Haematuria. (See also section 4.4 Special Warnings and Precautions for Use – Hepatic/ Renal Impairment.)

Reproductive system and breast disorders: Vaginal bleeding.

4.9 Overdose

Acute overdoses may produce nausea, vomiting and CNS depression including coma with respiratory depression. A relationship between ethosuximide toxicity and its plasma levels has not been established.

If less than 2g have been taken, fluids should be given by mouth. If a larger dose has been taken the stomach should be emptied, respiration maintained and any other symptoms treated accordingly. Activated charcoal and purgatives are known to be used in the treatment of overdosage. Haemodialysis may be useful. Forced diuresis and exchange transfusions are ineffective.

5. PHARMACOLOGICAL PROPERTIES

5.1 Pharmacodynamic properties

Ethosuximide is an anticonvulsant.

Ethosuximide suppresses the paroxysmal spike and wave pattern common to absence (petit mal) seizures. The frequency of epileptiform attacks is reduced, apparently by depression of the motor cortex and elevation of the threshold of the central nervous system to convulsive stimuli. Compared with other succinimide anticonvulsants, ethosuximide is more specific for pure absence seizures.

5.2 Pharmacokinetic properties

Ethosuximide is given by mouth. It is completely and rapidly absorbed from the gastrointestinal tract. Peak serum levels occur 1 to 7 hours after a single oral dose. Ethosuximide is not significantly bound to plasma proteins and therefore the drug is present in saliva and CSF in concentrations that approximate to that of the plasma. Therapeutic concentrations are in the range of 40 to 100 micrograms/ml. Ethosuximide is extensively metabolised to at least 3 plasma metabolites. Only between 12% and 20% of the drug is excreted unchanged in the urine. The elimination half life of ethosuximide is long, 40 to 60 hours in adults and 30 hours in children.

5.3 Preclinical safety data

The results of the preclinical tests do not add anything of further significance to the prescriber.

6. PHARMACEUTICAL PARTICULARS

6.1 List of excipients

Zarontin Syrup contains the following excipients:

Sodium citrate, sodium benzoate (E211), saccharin sodium, sucrose, glycerol, raspberry flavour, citric acid monohydrate and purified water.

6.2 Incompatibilities

None known.

6.3 Shelf life

3 years.

6.4 Special precautions for storage

Store below 25°C

6.5 Nature and contents of container

Amber round bottle stoppered with aluminium screw cap equipped with expanded PE disk surfaced on each face with PE films or stoppered with high density polyethylene plastic cap equipped with polyethylene/ aluminium/polyethylene terephtalate liner containing 200 ml.

6.6 Special precautions for disposal and other handling

No special instructions needed.

7. MARKETING AUTHORISATION HOLDER

Pfizer Limited

Ramsgate Road

Sandwich

Kent

CT13 9NJ

United Kingdom

8. MARKETING AUTHORISATION NUMBER(S)

Zarontin Syrup: PL 00057/0545

9. DATE OF FIRST AUTHORISATION/RENEWAL OF THE AUTHORISATION

1 March 2003

10. DATE OF REVISION OF THE TEXT

October 2008

Ref: Syrup: ZA6_0 UK

Zarzio Solution for Injection

(Sandoz Limited)

1. NAME OF THE MEDICINAL PRODUCT

Zarzio ▼ 30 MU/0.5 ml solution for injection or infusion in pre-filled syringe

Zarzio ▼ 48 MU/0.5 ml solution for injection or infusion in pre-filled syringe

2. QUALITATIVE AND QUANTITATIVE COMPOSITION

Zarzio 30 MU/0.5 ml solution for injection or infusion in pre-filled syringe:

Each ml of solution contains 60 million units (MU) [equivalent to 600 micrograms (μg)] filgrastim*.

Each pre-filled syringe contains 30 MU (equivalent to 300 μg) filgrastim in 0.5 ml.

Zarzio 48 MU/0.5 ml solution for injection or infusion in pre-filled syringe:

Each ml of solution contains 96 million units (MU) [equivalent to 960 micrograms (μg)] filgrastim*.

Each pre-filled syringe contains 48 MU (equivalent to 480 μg) filgrastim in 0.5 ml.

* recombinant methionylated human granulocyte-colony stimulating factor (G-CSF) produced in *E. coli* by recombinant DNA technology.

Excipient: Each ml of solution contains 50 mg sorbitol (E420).

For a full list of excipients, see section 6.1.

3. PHARMACEUTICAL FORM

Solution for injection or infusion in pre-filled syringe

Clear, colourless to slightly yellowish solution.

4. CLINICAL PARTICULARS

4.1 Therapeutic indications

- Reduction in the duration of neutropenia and the incidence of febrile neutropenia in patients treated with established cytotoxic chemotherapy for malignancy (with the exception of chronic myeloid leukaemia and myelodysplastic syndromes) and reduction in the duration of neutropenia in patients undergoing myeloablative therapy followed by bone marrow transplantation considered to be at increased risk of prolonged severe neutropenia.

The safety and efficacy of filgrastim are similar in adults and children receiving cytotoxic chemotherapy.

- Mobilisation of peripheral blood progenitor cells (PBPC).

- In children and adults with severe congenital, cyclic, or idiopathic neutropenia with an absolute neutrophil count (ANC) of $\leqslant 0.5 \times 10^9$/l, and a history of severe or recurrent infections, long term administration of filgrastim is indicated to increase neutrophil counts and to reduce the incidence and duration of infection-related events.

- Treatment of persistent neutropenia (ANC $\leqslant 1.0 \times 10^9$/l) in patients with advanced HIV infection, in order to reduce the risk of bacterial infections when other therapeutic options are inappropriate.

4.2 Posology and method of administration

Filgrastim therapy should only be given in collaboration with an oncology centre which has experience in granulocyte-colony stimulating factor (G-CSF) treatment and haematology and has the necessary diagnostic facilities.

The mobilisation and apheresis procedures should be performed in collaboration with an oncology-haematology centre with acceptable experience in this field and where the monitoring of haematopoietic progenitor cells can be correctly performed.

Zarzio is available in strengths of 30 MU/0.5 ml and 48 MU/ 0.5 ml.

Established cytotoxic chemotherapy

The recommended dose of filgrastim is 0.5 MU/kg/day (5 μg/kg/day). The first dose of filgrastim should not be administered less than 24 hours following cytotoxic chemotherapy.

Daily dosing with filgrastim should continue until the expected neutrophil nadir is passed and the neutrophil count has recovered to the normal range. Following established chemotherapy for solid tumours, lymphomas, and lymphoid leukaemias, it is expected that the duration of treatment required to fulfil these criteria will be up to 14 days. Following induction and consolidation treatment for acute myeloid leukaemia the duration of treatment may be substantially longer (up to 38 days) depending on the type, dose and schedule of cytotoxic chemotherapy used.

In patients receiving cytotoxic chemotherapy, a transient increase in neutrophil counts is typically seen 1 - 2 days after initiation of filgrastim therapy. However, for a sustained therapeutic response, filgrastim therapy should not be discontinued before the expected nadir has passed and the neutrophil count has recovered to the normal range. Premature discontinuation of filgrastim therapy, prior to the time of the expected neutrophil nadir, is not recommended.

Patients treated with myeloablative therapy followed by bone marrow transplantation

The recommended starting dose of filgrastim is 1.0 MU/kg/ day (10 μg/kg/day). The first dose of filgrastim should not be administered less than 24 hours following cytotoxic chemotherapy and within 24 hours of bone marrow infusion.

Dose adjustments: Once the neutrophil nadir has been passed, the daily dose of filgrastim should be titrated against the neutrophil response as follows:

Absolute neutrophil count	Filgrastim dose adjustment
ANC> 1.0 × 10^9/l for 3 consecutive days	Reduce to 0.5 MU/kg/day (5 µg/kg/day)
Then, if ANC remains > 1.0 × 10^9/l for 3 more consecutive days	Discontinue filgrastim
If the ANC decreases to < 1.0 × 10^9/l during the treatment period, the dose of filgrastim should be re-escalated according to the above steps	

Mobilisation of PBPC

Patients undergoing myelosuppressive or myeloablative therapy followed by autologous PBPC transplantation

The recommended dose of filgrastim for PBPC mobilisation when used alone is 1.0 MU/kg/day (10 µg/kg/day) for 5 - 7 consecutive days. Timing of leukapheresis: 1 or 2 leukaphereses on days 5 and 6 are often sufficient. In other circumstances, additional leukaphereses may be necessary. Filgrastim dosing should be maintained until the last leukapheresis.

The recommended dose of filgrastim for PBPC mobilisation after myelosuppressive chemotherapy is 0.5 MU/kg/day (5 µg/kg/day) given daily from the first day after completion of chemotherapy until the expected neutrophil nadir is passed and the neutrophil count has recovered to the normal range. Leukapheresis should be performed during the period when the ANC rises from < 0.5 × 10^9/l to > 5.0 × 10^9/l. For patients who have not had extensive chemotherapy, one leukapheresis is often sufficient. In other circumstances, additional leukaphereses are recommended.

There are no prospectively randomised comparisons of the two recommended mobilisation methods (filgrastim alone or in combination with myelosuppressive chemotherapy) within the same patient population. The degree of variation between individual patients and between laboratory assays of $CD34^+$ cells means that direct comparison between different studies is difficult. It is therefore difficult to recommend an optimum method. The choice of mobilisation method should be considered in relation to the overall objectives of treatment for an individual patient.

Normal donors prior to allogeneic PBPC transplantation

For PBPC mobilisation in normal donors prior to allogeneic PBPC transplantation, filgrastim should be administered at 1.0 MU/kg/day (10 µg/kg/day) for 4 - 5 consecutive days. Leukapheresis should be started at day 5 and continued until day 6 if needed in order to collect 4 × 10^6 CD34+ cells/kg recipient bodyweight (BW).

Severe chronic neutropenia (SCN)

Congenital neutropenia

The recommended starting dose is 1.2 MU/kg/day (12 µg/kg/day) as a single dose or in divided doses.

Idiopathic or cyclic neutropenia

The recommended starting dose is 0.5 MU/kg/day (5 µg/kg/day) as a single dose or in divided doses.

Dose adjustments

Filgrastim should be administered daily until the neutrophil count has reached and can be maintained at more than 1.5 × 10^9/l. When the response has been obtained, the minimal effective dose to maintain this level should be established. Long-term daily administration is required to maintain an adequate neutrophil count.

After 1 - 2 weeks of therapy, the initial dose may be doubled or halved depending upon the patient's response. Subsequently the dose may be individually adjusted every 1 - 2 weeks to maintain the average neutrophil count between 1.5 × 10^9/l and 10 × 10^9/l. A faster schedule of dose escalation may be considered in patients presenting with severe infections. In clinical studies, 97% of patients who responded had a complete response at doses of ≤ 2.4 MU/kg/day (24 µg/kg/day). The long-term safety of filgrastim administration above 2.4 MU/kg/day (24 µg/kg/day) in patients with SCN has not been established.

HIV infection

Reversal of neutropenia

The recommended starting dose of filgrastim is 0.1 MU/kg/day (1 µg/kg/day) given daily with titration up to a maximum of 0.4 MU/kg/day (4 µg/kg/day) until a normal neutrophil count is reached and can be maintained (ANC> 2.0 × 10^9/l). In clinical studies, > 90% of patients responded at these doses, achieving reversal of neutropenia in a median of 2 days.

In a small number of patients (< 10%), doses up to 1.0 MU/kg/day (10 µg/kg/day) were required to achieve reversal of neutropenia.

Maintenance of normal neutrophil counts

When reversal of neutropenia has been achieved, the minimal effective dose to maintain a normal neutrophil count should be established. Initial dose adjustment to alternate day dosing with 30 MU/day (300 µg/day) is recommended. Further dose adjustment may be necessary, as determined by the patient's ANC, to maintain the neutrophil count at > 2.0 × 10^9/l. In clinical studies, dosing with 30 MU/day (300 µg/day) on 1 - 7 days per week was required to maintain the ANC> 2.0 × 10^9/l, with the median dose frequency being 3 days per week. Long-term administration may be required to maintain the ANC> 2.0 × 10^9/l.

Special populations

Patients with renal/hepatic impairment

Studies of filgrastim in patients with severe impairment of renal or hepatic function demonstrate that it exhibits a similar pharmacokinetic and pharmacodynamic profile to that seen in normal individuals. Dose adjustment is not required in these circumstances.

Paediatric patients in the SCN and cancer settings

In clinical studies 65% of patients treated for SCN were younger than 18 years. For this age-group, which mostly includes patients with congenital neutropenia, efficacy was proven. There were no differences in the safety profiles for paediatric patients treated for SCN in comparison to adults.

Data from clinical studies in paediatric patients indicate that the safety and efficacy of filgrastim are similar in both adults and children receiving cytotoxic chemotherapy.

The dosage recommendations in paediatric patients are the same as those in adults receiving myelosuppressive cytotoxic chemotherapy.

Elderly patients

In clinical investigations with filgrastim a small number of elderly patients was included. No specific studies have been performed for this patient population. Therefore, specific posology recommendations for these patients cannot be made.

Method of administration

Established cytotoxic chemotherapy

Filgrastim may be administered as a daily subcutaneous injection or alternatively as a daily intravenous infusion over 30 minutes. For further instructions on dilution with glucose 50 mg/ml (5%) solution prior to infusion see section 6.6. The subcutaneous route is preferred in most cases. There is some evidence from a study of single dose administration that intravenous dosing may shorten the duration of effect. The clinical relevance of this finding to multiple dose administration is not clear. The choice of route should depend on the individual clinical circumstance. In randomised clinical studies, a subcutaneous dose of 23 MU/m^2/day (230 µg/m^2/day) or rather 0.4 - 0.84 MU/kg/day (4 - 8.4 µg/kg/day) was used.

Patients treated with myeloablative therapy followed by bone marrow transplantation

Filgrastim is administered as an intravenous short-term infusion over 30 minutes or as a subcutaneous or intravenous continuous infusion over 24 hours, in each case after dilution in 20 ml of glucose 50 mg/ml (5%) solution. For further instructions on dilution with glucose 50 mg/ml (5%) solution prior to infusion see section 6.6.

Mobilisation of PBPC

Subcutaneous injection.

For the mobilisation of PBPC in patients undergoing myelosuppressive or myeloablative therapy followed by autologous PBPC transplantation the recommended dose of filgrastim may also be administered as a 24 hour subcutaneous continuous infusion. For infusions filgrastim should be diluted in 20 ml of glucose 50 mg/ml (5%) solution. For further instructions on dilution with glucose 50 mg/ml (5%) solution prior to infusion see section 6.6.

SCN/HIV infection

Subcutaneous injection.

4.3 Contraindications

Hypersensitivity to the active substance or to any of the excipients.

4.4 Special warnings and precautions for use

Special warnings

Filgrastim should not be used to increase the dose of cytotoxic chemotherapy beyond established posology regimens (see below).

Filgrastim should not be administered to patients with severe congenital neutropenia (Kostmann's syndrome) with abnormal cytogenetics (see below).

Established cytotoxic chemotherapy

Malignant cell growth

Since investigations showed that G-CSF can promote growth of myeloid cells *in vitro* the following warnings should be considered.

The safety and efficacy of filgrastim administration in patients with myelodysplastic syndrome, or chronic myelogenous leukaemia have not been established. Therefore filgrastim is not indicated for use in these conditions. Particular care should be taken to distinguish the diagnosis of blast transformation of chronic myeloid leukaemia from acute myeloid leukaemia.

In view of limited safety and efficacy data in patients with secondary AML, filgrastim should be administered with caution.

The safety and efficacy of filgrastim administration in *de novo* AML patients aged < 55 years with good cytogenetics [t(8;21), t(15;17), and inv(16)] have not been established.

Leucocytosis

White blood cell counts of 100 × 10^9/l or greater have been observed in less than 5% of patients receiving filgrastim at doses above 0.3 MU/kg/day (3 µg/kg/day). No undesirable effects directly attributable to this degree of leucocytosis have been reported. However, in view of the potential risks associated with severe leucocytosis, a white blood cell count should be performed at regular intervals during filgrastim therapy. If leukocyte counts exceed 50 × 10^9/l after the expected nadir, filgrastim should be discontinued immediately. However, during the period of administration of filgrastim for PBPC mobilisation, it should be discontinued or its dose should be reduced if the leukocyte counts rise to > 70 × 10^9/l.

Risks associated with increased doses of chemotherapy

Special caution should be used when treating patients with high-dose chemotherapy because improved tumour outcome has not been demonstrated and intensified doses of chemotherapeutic agents may lead to increased toxicities including cardiac, pulmonary, neurologic, and dermatologic effects (please refer to the Summary of Product Characteristics of the specific chemotherapy agents used).

Treatment with filgrastim alone does not preclude thrombocytopenia and anaemia due to myelosuppressive chemotherapy. Because of the potential of receiving higher doses of chemotherapy (e.g. full doses on the prescribed schedule) the patient may be at greater risk of thrombocytopenia and anaemia. Regular monitoring of platelet count and haematocrit is recommended. Special care should be taken when administering single or combination chemotherapeutic agents which are known to cause severe thrombocytopenia.

The use of filgrastim-mobilised PBPCs has been shown to reduce the depth and duration of thrombocytopenia following myelosuppressive or myeloablative chemotherapy.

Other special precautions

The effects of filgrastim in patients with substantially reduced myeloid progenitors have not been studied. Filgrastim acts primarily on neutrophil precursors to exert its effect in elevating neutrophil counts. Therefore, in patients with reduced precursors, neutrophil response may be diminished (such as those treated with extensive radiotherapy or chemotherapy, or those with bone marrow infiltration by tumour).

There have been reports of Graft versus Host Disease (GvHD) and fatalities in patients receiving G-CSF after allogeneic bone marrow transplantation (see section 5.1).

Mobilisation of PBPC

Prior exposure to cytotoxic agents

Patients who have undergone very extensive prior myelosuppressive therapy, followed by administration of filgrastim for mobilisation of PBPCs, may not show sufficient mobilisation of these blood cells to achieve the recommended minimum yield (≥ 2.0 × 10^6 CD34+ cells/kg) or acceleration of platelet recovery to the same degree.

Some cytotoxic agents exhibit particular toxicities to the haematopoietic progenitor pool and may adversely affect progenitor mobilisation. Agents such as melphalan, carmustine (BCNU) and carboplatin, when administered over prolonged periods prior to attempts at progenitor mobilisation may reduce progenitor yield. However, the administration of melphalan, carboplatin or BCNU together with filgrastim has been shown to be effective for progenitor mobilisation. When a PBPC transplantation is envisaged it is advisable to plan the stem cell mobilisation procedure early in the treatment course of the patient. Particular attention should be paid to the number of progenitors mobilised in such patients before the administration of high-dose chemotherapy. If yields are inadequate, as measured by the criteria above, alternative forms of treatment not requiring progenitor support should be considered.

Assessment of progenitor cell yields

In assessing the number of progenitor cells harvested in patients treated with filgrastim, particular attention should be paid to the method of quantitation. The results of flow cytometric analysis of CD34+ cell numbers vary depending on the precise methodology used and therefore, recommendations of numbers based on studies in other laboratories need to be interpreted with caution.

Statistical analysis of the relationship between the number of CD34+ cells re-infused and the rate of platelet recovery after high-dose chemotherapy indicates a complex but continuous relationship. The recommendation of a minimum yield of ≥ 2.0 × 10^6 CD34+ cells/kg is based on published experience resulting in adequate haematologic reconstitution. Yields in excess of this minimum yield appear to correlate with more rapid recovery, those below with slower recovery.

Normal donors prior to allogeneic PBPC transplantation

Mobilisation of PBPC does not provide a direct clinical benefit to normal donors and should only be considered for the purposes of allogeneic stem cell transplantation.

PBPC mobilisation should be considered only in donors who meet normal clinical and laboratory eligibility criteria for stem cell donation with special attention to haematological values and infectious disease.

The safety and efficacy of filgrastim have not been assessed in normal donors < 16 years or > 60 years.

Transient thrombocytopenia (platelets < 100 × 10^9/l) following filgrastim administration and leukapheresis was observed in 35% of subjects studied. Among these, two cases of platelets < 50 × 10^9/l were reported and attributed to the leukapheresis procedure. If more than one leukapheresis is required, particular attention should be paid to donors with platelets < 100 × 10^9/l prior to leukapheresis; in general apheresis should not be performed if platelets < 75 × 10^9/l.

Leukapheresis should not be performed in donors who are anticoagulated or who have known defects in haemostasis.

Filgrastim administration should be discontinued or its posology should be reduced if the leukocyte counts rise to > 70 × 10^9/l.

Donors who receive G-CSFs for PBPC mobilisation should be monitored until haematological indices return to normal. Long-term safety follow-up of donors is ongoing. For up to 4 years, there have been no reports of abnormal haematopoiesis in normal donors. Nevertheless, a risk of promotion of a malignant myeloid clone can not be excluded. It is recommended that the apheresis centre perform a systematic record and tracking of the stem cell donors to ensure monitoring of long-term safety.

Transient cytogenic modifications have been observed in normal donors following G-CSF use. The significance of these changes in terms of the development of haematological malignancy is unknown. Common but generally asymptomatic cases of splenomegaly and very rare cases of splenic rupture have been reported in healthy donors and patients following administration of G-CSFs. Some cases of splenic rupture were fatal. Therefore, spleen size should be carefully monitored (e.g. clinical examination, ultrasound). A diagnosis of splenic rupture should be considered in donors and/or patients reporting left upper abdominal pain or shoulder tip pain.

In normal donors, pulmonary adverse events (haemoptysis, pulmonary haemorrhage, pulmonary infiltrates, dyspnoea and hypoxia) have been reported very rarely in post marketing experience. In case of suspected or confirmed pulmonary adverse events, discontinuation of treatment with filgrastim should be considered and appropriate medical care given.

Recipients of allogeneic PBPCs mobilised with filgrastim

Current data indicate that immunological interactions between the allogeneic PBPC graft and the recipient may be associated with an increased risk of acute and chronic GvHD when compared with bone marrow transplantation.

SCN

Blood cell counts

Platelet counts should be monitored closely, especially during the first few weeks of filgrastim therapy. Consideration should be given to intermittent cessation or decreasing the dose of filgrastim in patients who develop thrombocytopenia, i.e. platelets consistently < 100,000/mm^3.

Other blood cell changes occur, including anaemia and transient increases in myeloid progenitors, which require close monitoring of cell counts.

Transformation to leukaemia or myelodysplastic syndrome

Special care should be taken in the diagnosis of SCNs to distinguish them from other haematopoietic disorders such as aplastic anaemia, myelodysplasia, and myeloid leukaemia. Complete blood cell counts with differential and platelet counts, and an evaluation of bone marrow morphology and karyotype should be performed prior to treatment.

There was a low frequency (approximately 3%) of myelodysplastic syndromes (MDS) or leukaemia in clinical study patients with SCN treated with filgrastim. This observation has only been made in patients with congenital neutropenia. MDS and leukaemias are natural complications of the disease and are of uncertain relation to filgrastim therapy. A subset of approximately 12% of patients who had normal cytogenetic evaluations at baseline were subsequently found to have abnormalities, including monosomy 7, on routine repeat evaluation. If patients with SCN develop abnormal cytogenetics, the risks and benefits of continuing filgrastim should be carefully weighed; Filgrastim should be discontinued if MDS or leukaemia occurs. It is currently unclear whether long-term treatment of patients with SCN will predispose patients to cytogenetic abnormalities, MDS or leukaemic transformation. It is recommended to perform morphologic and cytogenetic bone marrow examinations in patients at regular intervals (approximately every 12 months).

Other special precautions

Causes of transient neutropenia, such as viral infections should be excluded.

Splenic enlargement is a direct effect of treatment with filgrastim. 31% of patients in studies were documented as having palpable splenomegaly. Increases in volume, measured radiographically, occurred early during Filgrastim therapy and tended to plateau. Dose reductions were noted to slow or stop the progression of splenic enlargement, and in 3% of patients a splenectomy was required. Spleen size should be evaluated regularly. Abdominal palpation should be sufficient to detect abnormal increases in splenic volume.

Haematuria/proteinuria occurred in a small number of patients. Regular urine analyses should be performed to monitor this event.

The safety and efficacy in neonates and patients with autoimmune neutropenia have not been established.

HIV infection

Blood cell counts

ANC should be monitored closely, especially during the first few weeks of filgrastim therapy. Some patients may respond very rapidly and with a considerable increase in neutrophil count to the initial dose of filgrastim. It is recommended that the ANC is measured daily for the first 2 - 3 days of filgrastim administration. Thereafter, it is recommended that the ANC is measured at least twice per week for the first 2 weeks and subsequently once per week or once every other week during maintenance therapy. During intermittent dosing with 30 MU/day (300 μg/day) of filgrastim, there can be wide fluctuations in the patient's ANC over time. In order to determine a patient's trough or nadir ANC, it is recommended that blood samples are taken for ANC measurement immediately prior to any scheduled dosing with filgrastim.

Risk associated with increased doses of myelosuppressive medicinal products

Treatment with filgrastim alone does not preclude thrombocytopenia and anaemia due to myelosuppressive treatments. As a result of the potential to receive higher doses or a greater number of these medicinal products with filgrastim therapy, the patient may be at higher risk of developing thrombocytopenia and anaemia. Regular monitoring of blood counts is recommended (see above).

Infections and malignancies causing myelosuppression

Neutropenia may be due to bone marrow-infiltrating opportunistic infections such as Mycobacterium avium complex or malignancies such as lymphoma. In patients with known bone marrow-infiltrating infections or malignancy, consider appropriate therapy for treatment of the underlying condition in addition to administration of filgrastim for treatment of neutropenia. The effects of filgrastim on neutropenia due to bone marrow-infiltrating infection or malignancy have not been well established.

Other special precautions

Rare pulmonary adverse reactions, in particular interstitial pneumonia, have been reported after G-CSF administration (see section 4.8). Patients with a recent history of pulmonary infiltrates or pneumonia may be at higher risk. The onset of pulmonary signs, such as cough, fever and dyspnoea in association with radiological signs of pulmonary infiltrates and deterioration in pulmonary function may be preliminary signs of Adult Respiratory Distress Syndrome (ARDS). Filgrastim should be discontinued and appropriate treatment given in these cases.

Monitoring of bone density may be indicated in patients with underlying osteoporotic bone diseases who undergo continuous therapy with filgrastim for more than 6 months.

Sickle cells crises, in some cases fatal, have been reported with the use of filgrastim in subjects with sickle cell disease. Physicians should exercise caution when considering the use of filgrastim in patients with sickle cell disease, and only after careful evaluation of the potential risks and benefits.

Increased haematopoietic activity of the bone marrow in response to growth factor therapy has been associated with transient positive bone-imaging findings. This should be considered when interpreting bone imaging results.

Excipients

Zarzio contains sorbitol. Patients with rare hereditary problems of fructose intolerance should not use this medicinal product.

4.5 Interaction with other medicinal products and other forms of interaction

The safety and efficacy of filgrastim given on the same day as myelosuppressive cytotoxic chemotherapy have not been definitively established. In view of the sensitivity of rapidly dividing myeloid cells to myelosuppressive cytotoxic chemotherapy, the use of filgrastim is not recommended in the period from 24 hours before to 24 hours after chemotherapy. Preliminary evidence from a small number of patients treated concomitantly with filgrastim and 5-fluorouracil indicates that the severity of neutropenia may be exacerbated.

Possible interactions with other haematopoietic growth factors and cytokines have not yet been investigated in clinical studies.

Since lithium promotes the release of neutrophils, lithium is likely to potentiate the effect of filgrastim. Although this interaction has not been formally investigated, there is no evidence that such an interaction is harmful.

4.6 Pregnancy and lactation

There are no adequate data from the use of filgrastim in pregnant women. There are reports in the literature where the transplacental passage of filgrastim in pregnant women has been demonstrated. There is no evidence from studies in rats and rabbits that filgrastim is teratogenic. An increased incidence of embryo-loss has been observed in rabbits, but no malformation has been seen.

In pregnancy, the possible risk of filgrastim use to the foetus must be weighed against the expected therapeutic benefit.

It is not known whether filgrastim is excreted in human milk, therefore it is not recommended for use in breast-feeding women.

4.7 Effects on ability to drive and use machines

Filgrastim has no influence on the ability to drive and use machines.

4.8 Undesirable effects

The most commonly reported adverse reactions to filgrastim are mild to moderate musculoskeletal pain occurring in more than 10% of patients. Musculoskeletal pain is usually controlled with standard analgesics.

Adverse reactions listed below are classified according to frequency and system organ class. Frequency groupings are defined according to the following convention: Very common (⩾ 1/10), common (⩾ 1/100 to < 1/10), uncommon (⩾ 1/1,000 to < 1/100), rare (⩾ 1/10,000 to < 1/1,000), very rare (< 1/10,000), not known (cannot be estimated from the available data).

Table 1. Adverse reactions in clinical trials in cancer patients

Immune system disorders	
Very rare:	Allergic-type reactions*, including anaphylaxis, skin rash, urticaria, angioedema, dyspnoea and hypotension
Vascular disorders	
Uncommon:	Hypotension (transient)
Rare:	Vascular disorders* including venoocclusive disease and fluid volume disturbances
Respiratory, thoracic and mediastinal disorders	
Very rare:	Pulmonary oedema*, interstitial pneumonia*, pulmonary infiltrates*
Skin and subcutaneous tissue disorders	
Very rare:	Sweet's Syndrome*, cutaneous vasculitis
Musculoskeletal, connective tissue and bone disorders	
Very common:	Musculoskeletal pain (mild or moderate)
Common:	Musculoskeletal pain (severe)
Very rare:	Rheumatoid arthritis exacerbation
Renal and urinary disorders	
Very rare:	Micturition disorders (predominantly dysuria)
Investigations	
Very common:	Blood alkaline phosphatase, blood lactate dehydrogenase (LDH), gamma-glutamyltransferase (GGT) and blood uric acid increased (reversible, dose-dependent, mild or moderate)

* see below

Table 2. Adverse reactions in clinical trials in normal donors undergoing PBPC mobilisation

Immune system disorders	
Uncommon:	Severe allergic reaction: anaphylaxis, angioedema, urticaria, rash
Blood and the lymphatic system disorders	
Very common:	Leucocytosis (WBC > 50 × 10^9/l), thrombocytopenia (platelets < 100 × 10^9/l; transient)
Common:	Splenomegaly (generally asymptomatic, also in patients)
Uncommon:	Spleen disorder
Very rare:	Splenic rupture (also in patients)
Nervous system disorders	
Very common:	Headache
Respiratory, thoracic and mediastinal disorders	
Very rare:	Haemoptysis*, pulmonary haemorrhage*, pulmonary infiltrates*, dyspnoea*, hypoxia*

Musculoskeletal, connective tissue and bone disorders	
Very common:	Musculoskeletal pain (mild to moderate, transient)
Uncommon:	Rheumatoid arthritis and arthritic symptoms exacerbation
Investigations	
Common:	Blood alkaline phosphatase and LDH increased (transient, minor)
Uncommon:	Aspartate aminotransferase (AST) and blood uric acid increased (transient, minor)

* see below

Table 3. Adverse reactions in clinical trials in SCN patients

Blood and the lymphatic system disorders	
Very common:	Anaemia, splenomegaly (may be progressive in a minority of cases)
Common:	Thrombocytopenia
Uncommon:	Spleen disorder
Nervous system disorders	
Common:	Headache
Respiratory, thoracic and mediastinal disorders	
Very common:	Epistaxis
Gastrointestinal disorders	
Common:	Diarrhoea
Hepato-biliary disorders	
Common:	Hepatomegaly
Skin and subcutaneous tissue disorders	
Common:	Cutaneous vasculitis (during long term use), alopecia, rash
Musculoskeletal, connective tissue and bone disorders	
Very common:	General musculoskeletal pain, bone pain
Common:	Osteoporosis, arthralgia
Renal and urinary disorders	
Uncommon:	Haematuria, proteinuria
General disorders and administration site conditions	
Common:	Injection site pain
Investigations	
Very common:	Blood alkaline phosphatase, LDH and blood uric acid increased (transient), blood glucose decreased (transient, moderate)

Table 4. Adverse reactions in clinical trials in HIV Patients

Blood and lymphatic system disorders	
Common:	Spleen disorder, splenomegaly*
Musculoskeletal, connective tissue and bone disorders	
Very common:	Musculoskeletal pain (mild to moderate)

* see below

In randomised, placebo-controlled clinical studies, filgrastim did not increase the incidence of undesirable effects associated with cytotoxic chemotherapy. Undesirable effects reported with equal frequency in patients treated with filgrastim/chemotherapy and placebo/chemotherapy included nausea and vomiting, alopecia, diarrhoea, fatigue, anorexia, mucositis, headache, cough, skin rash, chest pain, generalised weakness, sore throat, constipation and unspecified pain.

Allergic reactions occurred on initial or subsequent treatment in patients receiving filgrastim. Overall, reports were more common after intravenous administration. In some cases, symptoms have recurred with rechallenge, suggesting a causal relationship. Filgrastim should be permanently discontinued in patients who experience a serious allergic reaction.

Vascular disorders have been reported in patients undergoing high dose chemotherapy followed by autologous bone marrow transplantation. The causal association with filgrastim has not been established.

Pulmonary adverse reactions have in some cases been reported with an outcome of respiratory failure or adult respiratory distress syndrome (ARDS), which may be fatal. In normal donors, pulmonary adverse events (haemoptysis, pulmonary haemorrhage, pulmonary infiltrates, dyspnoea and hypoxia) have been reported very rarely in post marketing experience (see section 4.4).

The occurrence of Sweet's syndrome (acute febrile neutrophilic dermatosis) has been reported occasionally in cancer patients. However, since a significant percentage of these patients were suffering from leukaemia, a condition known to be associated with Sweet's syndrome, a causal relationship with filgrastim has not been established.

Isolated cases of sickle cells crises have been reported in patients with sickle cell disease (see section 4.4). The frequency is not known.

In all cases of splenic enlargement in HIV patients this was mild or moderate on physical examination and the clinical course was benign; no patients had a diagnosis of hypersplenism and no patients underwent splenectomy. As splenic enlargement is a common finding in patients with HIV infection and is present to varying degrees in most patients with AIDS, the relationship to filgrastim treatment is unclear.

Immunogenicity

In four clinical studies none of the healthy volunteers or cancer patients developed anti-rhG-CSF antibodies (neither binding nor neutralising) upon treatment with Zarzio.

4.9 Overdose

The effects of filgrastim overdose have not been established.

5. PHARMACOLOGICAL PROPERTIES

5.1 Pharmacodynamic properties

Pharmacotherapeutic group: Colony stimulating factors, ATC Code: L03AA02

Human G-CSF is a glycoprotein which regulates the production and release of functional neutrophils from the bone marrow. Zarzio containing r-metHuG-CSF (filgrastim) causes marked increases in peripheral blood neutrophil counts within 24 hours, with minor increases in monocytes. In some SCN patients filgrastim can also induce a minor increase in the number of circulating eosinophils and basophils relative to baseline; some of these patients may present with eosinophilia or basophilia already prior to treatment. Elevations of neutrophil counts are dose-dependent at recommended doses. Neutrophils produced in response to filgrastim show normal or enhanced function as demonstrated by tests of chemotactic and phagocytic function. Following termination of filgrastim therapy, circulating neutrophil counts decrease by 50% within 1 - 2 days, and to normal levels within 1 - 7 days. As with other haematopoietic growth factors, G-CSF has shown *in vitro* stimulating properties on human endothelial cells, which have specific receptors for G-CSF. Accordingly, G-CSF has been shown to induce endothelial cell functions related to angiogenesis. Additionally, G-CSF has been shown to increase neutrophil migration across the vascular endothelium.

Use of filgrastim in patients undergoing cytotoxic chemotherapy leads to significant reductions in the incidence, severity and duration of neutropenia and febrile neutropenia. Treatment with filgrastim significantly reduces the duration of febrile neutropenia, antibiotic use and hospitalisation after induction chemotherapy for acute myelogenous leukaemia or myeloablative therapy followed by bone marrow transplantation. The incidence of fever and documented infections were not reduced in either setting. The duration of fever was not reduced in patients undergoing myeloablative therapy followed by bone marrow transplantation.

Use of filgrastim, either alone, or after chemotherapy, mobilises haematopoietic progenitor cells into peripheral blood. These autologous PBPCs may be harvested and infused after high-dose cytotoxic therapy, either in place of, or in addition to bone marrow transplantation. Infusion of PBPCs accelerates haematopoietic recovery reducing the duration of risk for haemorrhagic complications and the need for platelet transfusions.

One retrospective European study evaluating the use of G-CSF after allogeneic bone marrow transplantation in patients with acute leukaemias suggested an increase in the risk of GvHD, treatment related mortality (TRM) and mortality when G-CSF was administered. In a separate retrospective international study in patients with acute and chronic myelogenous leukaemias, no effect on the risk of GvHD, TRM and mortality was seen. A meta-analysis of allogeneic transplant studies, including the results of nine prospective randomized trials, 8 retrospective studies and 1 case-controlled study, did not detect an effect on the risks of acute GvHD, chronic GvHD or early treatment-related mortality.

(see Table 5 below)

Use of filgrastim for the mobilisation of PBPCs in normal donors prior to allogeneic PBPC transplantation

In normal donors, a 1 MU/kg/day (10 μg/kg/day) dose administered subcutaneously for 4 - 5 consecutive days allows a collection of $\geqslant 4 \times 10^6$ CD34+ cells/kg recipient BW in the majority of the donors after two leukaphereses.

Recipients of allogeneic PBPCs mobilised with filgrastim experienced significantly more rapid haematological recovery, leading to a significant decrease in time to unsupported platelet recovery when compared with allogeneic bone marrow transplantation.

Use of filgrastim in children or adults with SCN (severe congenital, cyclic, and idiopathic neutropenia) induces a sustained increase in ACNs in peripheral blood and a reduction of infection and related events.

Use of filgrastim in patients with HIV infection maintains normal neutrophil counts to allow scheduled dosing of antiviral and/or other myelosuppressive treatments. There is no evidence that patients with HIV infection treated with filgrastim show an increase in HIV replication.

5.2 Pharmacokinetic properties

Randomised, double-blind, single and multiple dose, crossover studies in 146 healthy volunteers showed that the pharmacokinetic profile of Zarzio was comparable to that of the reference product after subcutaneous and intravenous administration.

Absorption

A single subcutaneous dose of 0.5 MU/kg (5 μg/kg) resulted in maximum serum concentrations after a t_{max} of 4.5 ± 0.9 hours (mean ± SD).

Distribution

The volume of distribution in blood is approximately 150 ml/kg. Following subcutaneous administration of recommended doses, serum concentrations were maintained above 10 ng/ml for 8 - 16 hours. There is a positive linear correlation between the dose and the serum concentration of filgrastim, whether administered intravenously or subcutaneously.

Elimination

The elimination of filgrastim is non-linear with respect to dose, the serum clearance decreases with increasing dose. Filgrastim appears to be mainly eliminated by neutrophil mediated clearance, which becomes saturated at higher doses. However, the serum clearance increases with repeated dosing while the neutrophil count increases. The median serum elimination half-life ($t_{1/2}$) of filgrastim after single subcutaneous doses ranged from 2.7 hours (1.0 MU/kg, 10 μg/kg) to 5.7 hours (0.25 MU/kg, 2.5 μg/kg) and was prolonged after 7 days of dosing to 8.5 - 14 hours, respectively.

Continuous infusion with filgrastim over a period of up to 28 days, in patients recovering from autologous bone-marrow transplantation, resulted in no evidence of drug accumulation and comparable elimination half-lives.

5.3 Preclinical safety data

There are no preclinical data of relevance to the prescriber which are additional to that already included in other sections of the Summary of Product Characteristics.

6. PHARMACEUTICAL PARTICULARS

6.1 List of excipients

Glutamic acid

Sorbitol (E420)

Polysorbate 80

Water for injections

Table 5

Relative Risk (95% CI) of GvHD and TRM Following treatment with G-CSF after bone marrow transplantation

Publication	Period of Study	N	Acute Grade II - IV GvHD	Chronic GvHD	TRM
Meta-Analysis (2003)	1986 - 2001[a]	1198	1.08 (0.87, 1.33)	1.02 (0.82, 1.26)	0.70 (0.38, 1.31)
European Retrospective Study (2004)	1992 - 2002[b]	1789	1.33 (1.08, 1.64)	1.29 (1.02, 1.61)	1.73 (1.30, 2.32)
International Retrospective Study (2006)	1995 - 2000[b]	2110	1.11 (0.86, 1.42)	1.10 (0.86, 1.39)	1.26 (0.95, 1.67)

[a]Analysis includes studies involving BM transplant during this period; some studies used GM-CSF

[b]Analysis includes patients receiving BM transplant during this period

6.2 Incompatibilities

Zarzio must not be diluted with sodium chloride solutions.

This medicinal product must not be mixed with other medicinal products except those mentioned in section 6.6.

Diluted filgrastim may be adsorbed to glass and plastic materials, unless it is diluted in glucose 50 mg/ml (5%) solution (see section 6.6).

6.3 Shelf life

30 months.

After dilution: Chemical and physical in-use stability of the diluted solution for infusion has been demonstrated for 24 hours at 2°C to 8°C. From a microbiological point of view, the product should be used immediately. If not used immediately, in-use storage times and conditions prior to use are the responsibility of the user and would normally not be longer than 24 hours at 2°C to 8°C, unless dilution has taken place in controlled and validated aseptic conditions.

6.4 Special precautions for storage

Store in a refrigerator (2°C - 8°C).

Keep the pre-filled syringe in the outer carton in order to protect from light.

For storage conditions of the diluted medicinal product, see section 6.3.

6.5 Nature and contents of container

Pre-filled syringe (type I glass) with injection needle (stainless steel), with or without a needle safety guard, containing 0.5 ml solution.

Pack sizes of 1, 3, 5 or 10 pre-filled syringes.

Not all pack sizes may be marketed.

6.6 Special precautions for disposal and other handling

The solution should be visually inspected prior to use. Only clear solutions without particles should be used. Accidental exposure to freezing temperatures does not adversely affect the stability of Zarzio.

Zarzio contains no preservative: In view of the possible risk of microbial contamination, Zarzio syringes are for single use only.

Dilution prior to administration (optional)

If required, Zarzio may be diluted in glucose 50 mg/ml (5%) solution.

Dilution to a final concentration < 0.2 MU/ml (2 µg/ml) is not recommended at any time.

For patients treated with filgrastim diluted to concentrations < 1.5 MU/ml (15 µg/ml), human serum albumin (HSA) should be added to a final concentration of 2 mg/ml.

Example: In a final volume of 20 ml, total doses of filgrastim less than 30 MU (300 µg) should be given with 0.2 ml of human serum albumin 200 mg/ml (20%) solution Ph. Eur. added.

When diluted in glucose 50 mg/ml (5%) solution, filgrastim is compatible with glass and a variety of plastics including polyvinylchloride, polyolefin (a copolymer of polypropylene and polyethylene) and polypropylene.

Using the pre-filled syringe with a needle safety guard

The needle safety guard covers the needle after injection to prevent needle stick injury. This does not affect normal operation of the syringe. Depress the plunger slowly and evenly until the entire dose has been given and the plunger cannot be depressed any further. While maintaining pressure on the plunger, remove the syringe from the patient. The needle safety guard will cover the needle when releasing the plunger.

Using the pre-filled syringe without a needle safety guard

Administer the dose as per standard protocol.

Disposal

Any unused product or waste material should be disposed of in accordance with local requirements.

7. MARKETING AUTHORISATION HOLDER

Sandoz GmbH

Biochemiestrasse 10

A-6250 Kundl

Austria

8. MARKETING AUTHORISATION NUMBER(S)

Zarzio 30 MU/0.5 ml solution for injection or infusion in pre-filled syringe

EU/1/08/495/001 – pack of 1 syringe

EU/1/08/495/002 – pack of 3 syringes

EU/1/08/495/003 – pack of 5 syringes

EU/1/08/495/004 – pack of 10 syringes

Zarzio 48 MU/0.5 ml solution for injection or infusion in pre-filled syringe

EU/1/08/495/005 – pack of 1 syringe

EU/1/08/495/006 – pack of 3 syringes

EU/1/08/495/007 – pack of 5 syringes

EU/1/08/495/008 – pack of 10 syringes

9. DATE OF FIRST AUTHORISATION/RENEWAL OF THE AUTHORISATION

6 February 2009

10. DATE OF REVISION OF THE TEXT

6 February 2009

Detailed information on this medicinal product is available on the website of the European Medicines Agency (EMEA) http://www.emea.europa.eu/.

Zavedos Capsules 5mg, 10mg and 25mg

(Pharmacia Limited)

1. NAME OF THE MEDICINAL PRODUCT

Zavedos Capsules 5 mg

Zavedos Capsules 10 mg

Zavedos Capsules 25mg

2. QUALITATIVE AND QUANTITATIVE COMPOSITION

Idarubicin Hydrochloride 5.0 mg HSE

Idarubicin Hydrochloride 10.0 mg HSE

Idarubicin Hydrochloride 25.0 mg HSE

3. PHARMACEUTICAL FORM

Zavedos capsules 5 mg -Opaque red cap and body, self-locking, hard gelatin capsule, size no. 4, containing an orange powder.

Zavedos capsules 10mg -Opaque red cap and white body, self-locking, hard gelatin capsule, size no. 4, containing an orange powder.

Zavedos capsules 25 mg - Opaque white cap and body, self-locking, hard gelatin capsule, size no. 2, containing an orange powder.

4. CLINICAL PARTICULARS

4.1 Therapeutic indications

Acute non-lymphocytic leukaemia (ANLL).

Whenever intravenous idarubicin cannot be employed e.g. for medical, psychological or social reasons, oral idarubicin can be used for remission induction in patients with previously untreated, relapsed or refractory acute non-lymphocytic leukaemia.

Zavedos may be used in combination chemotherapy regimens involving other cytotoxic agents.

As a single agent in the treatment of advanced breast cancer after failure of front line chemotherapy not including anthracyclines.

4.2 Posology and method of administration

Route of Administration: Oral

Dosage is usually calculated on the basis of body surface area.

In adult ANLL the recommended dose schedule suggested is 30 mg/m^2 orally given daily for 3 days as a single agent, or between 15 and 30 mg/m^2 orally daily for 3 days in combination with other anti-leukaemic agents.

In advanced breast cancer the recommended dose schedule as single agent is 45 mg/m^2 orally given either on a single day or divided over 3 consecutive days, to be repeated every 3 or 4 weeks based on the haematological recovery.

A maximum cumulative dose of 400 mg/m^2 is recommended.

These dosage schedules should, however, take into account the haematological status of the patient and the dosages of other cytotoxic drugs when used in combination.

In patients with hepatic impairment a dose reduction of Zavedos should be considered. (See special warnings).

The capsules should be swallowed whole with some water and should not be sucked, bitten or chewed. Zavedos Capsules may also be taken with a light meal.

4.3 Contraindications

- hypersensitivity to idarubicin or any other component of the product, other anthracyclines or anthracenediones
- severe hepatic impairment
- severe renal impairment
- uncontrolled infections
- severe myocardial insufficiency
- recent myocardial infarction
- severe arrhythmias
- persistent myelosuppression
- previous treatment with maximum cumulative doses of idarubicin and/or other anthracyclines and anthracenediones (See section **4.4**)
- Breast-feeding should be stopped during drug therapy (See section **4.6**)

4.4 Special warnings and precautions for use

General

Idarubicin should be administered only under the supervision of physicians experienced in the use of cytotoxic chemotherapy.

This ensures that immediate and effective treatment of severe complications of the disease and/or its treatment (e.g. haemorrhage, overwhelming infections) may be carried out.

Patients should recover from acute toxicities of prior cytotoxic treatment (such as stomatitis, neutropenia, thrombocytopenia, and generalized infections) before beginning treatment with idarubicin.

Cardiac Function

Cardiotoxicity is a risk of anthracycline treatment that may be manifested by early (i.e., acute) or late (i.e., delayed) events.

Early (i.e. Acute) Events

Early cardiotoxicity of idarubicin consists mainly of sinus tachycardia and/or electrocardiogram (ECG) abnormalities, such as non-specific ST-T wave changes. Tachyarrhythmias, including premature ventricular contractions and ventricular tachycardia, bradycardia, as well as atrioventricular and bundle-branch block have also been reported. These effects do not usually predict subsequent development of delayed cardiotoxicity, are rarely of clinical importance, and are generally not a reason for the discontinuation of idarubicin treatment.

Late (i.e. Delayed) Events

Delayed cardiotoxicity usually develops late in the course of therapy or within 2 to 3 months after treatment termination, but later events, several months to years after completion of treatment have also been reported. Delayed cardiomyopathy is manifested by reduced left ventricular ejection fraction (LVEF) and/or signs and symptoms of congestive heart failure (CHF) such as dyspnoea, pulmonary oedema, dependent oedema, cardiomegaly, hepatomegaly, oliguria, ascites, pleural effusion, and gallop rhythm. Subacute effects such as pericarditis/myocarditis have also been reported. Life-threatening CHF is the most severe form of anthracycline-induced cardiomyopathy and represents the cumulative dose-limiting toxicity of the drug.

Cumulative dose limits for IV or oral idarubicin have not been defined. However, idarubicin-related cardiomyopathy was reported in 5% of patients who received cumulative IV doses of 150 to 290 mg/m2. Available data on patients treated with oral idarubicin total cumulative doses up to 400 mg/m2 suggest a low probability of cardiotoxicity.

Cardiac function should be assessed before patients undergo treatment with idarubicin and must be monitored throughout therapy to minimize the risk of incurring severe cardiac impairment. The risk may be decreased through regular monitoring of LVEF during the course of treatment with prompt discontinuation of idarubicin at the first sign of impaired function. The appropriate quantitative method for repeated assessment of cardiac function (evaluation of LVEF) includes Multiple Gated Acquisition (MUGA) scan or echocardiography (ECHO). A baseline cardiac evaluation with an ECG and either a MUGA scan or an ECHO is recommended, especially in patients with risk factors for increased cardiotoxicity. Repeated MUGA or ECHO determinations of LVEF should be performed, particularly with higher, cumulative anthracycline doses. The technique used for assessment should be consistent throughout follow-up.

Risk factors for cardiac toxicity include active or dormant cardiovascular disease, prior or concomitant radiotherapy to the mediastinal/pericardial area, previous therapy with other anthracyclines or anthracenediones, and concomitant use of drugs with the ability to suppress cardiac contractility or cardiotoxic drugs (e.g., trastuzumab). Anthracyclines including idarubicin should not be administered in combination with other cardiotoxic agents unless the patient's cardiac function is closely monitored. Patients receiving anthracyclines after stopping treatment with other cardiotoxic agents, especially those with long half-lives such as trastuzumab, may also be at an increased risk of developing cardiotoxicity. The half-life of trastuzumab is approximately 28.5 days and may persist in the circulation for up to 24 weeks. Therefore, physicians should avoid anthracycline-based therapy for up to 24 weeks after stopping trastuzumab when possible. If anthracyclines are used before this time, careful monitoring of cardiac function is recommended.

Cardiac function monitoring must be particularly strict in patients receiving high cumulative doses and in those with risk factors. However, cardiotoxicity with idarubicin may occur at lower cumulative doses whether or not cardiac risk factors are present.

In infants and children there appears to be a greater susceptibility to anthracycline induced cardiac toxicity, and a long-term periodic evaluation of cardiac function has to be performed. It is probable that the toxicity of idarubicin and other anthracyclines or anthracenediones is additive.

Hematologic Toxicity

Idarubicin is a potent bone marrow suppressant. Severe myelosuppression will occur in all patients given a therapeutic dose of this agent. Hematologic profiles should be assessed before and during each cycle of therapy with idarubicin, including differential white blood cell (WBC) counts. A dose-dependent, reversible leukopenia and/or granulocytopenia (neutropenia) is the predominant manifestation of idarubicin hematologic toxicity and is the most common acute dose-limiting toxicity of this drug. Leukopenia and neutropenia are usually severe; thrombocytopenia and anaemia may also occur. Neutrophil and platelet counts usually reach their nadir 10 to 14 days after drug administration; however, cell counts generally return to normal levels during the third week. Clinical consequences of severe myelosuppression include fever, infections, sepsis/septicaemia, septic shock, haemorrhage, tissue hypoxia, or death.

Secondary Leukaemia

Secondary leukaemia, with or without a preleukemic phase, has been reported in patients treated with anthracyclines, including idarubicin. Secondary leukaemia is more common when such drugs are given in combination with DNA damaging antineoplastic agents, when patients have been heavily pre-treated with cytotoxic drugs, or when doses of the anthracyclines have been escalated. These leukemias can have a 1- to 3-year latency period.

Gastrointestinal

Idarubicin is emetigenic. Mucositis (mainly stomatitis, less often esophagitis) generally appears early after drug administration and, if severe, may progress over a few days to mucosal ulcerations. Most patients recover from this adverse event by the third week of therapy.

Occasionally, episodes of serious gastrointestinal events (such as perforation or bleeding) have been observed in patients receiving oral idarubicin who had acute leukaemia or a history of other pathologies or had received medications known to lead to gastrointestinal complications. In patients with active gastrointestinal disease with increased risk of bleeding and/or perforation, the physician must balance the benefit of oral idarubicin therapy against the risk.

Hepatic and/or Renal Function

Since hepatic and/or renal function impairment can affect the disposition of idarubicin, liver and kidney function should be evaluated with conventional clinical laboratory tests (using serum bilirubin and serum creatinine as indicators) prior to, and during, treatment. In a number of Phase III clinical trials, treatment was contraindicated if bilirubin and/or creatinine serum levels exceeded 2.0-mg %. With other anthracyclines a 50% dose reduction is generally used if bilirubin levels are in the range 1.2 to 2.0-mg %

Tumor Lysis Syndrome

Idarubicin may induce hyperuricemia as a consequence of the extensive purine catabolism that accompanies rapid drug-induced lysis of neoplastic cells ('tumor lysis syndrome'). Blood uric acid levels, potassium, calcium phosphate, and creatinine should be evaluated after initial treatment. Hydration, urine alkalinization, and prophylaxis with allopurinol to prevent hyperuricemia may minimize potential complications of tumor lysis syndrome.

Immunosuppressant Effects/Increased Susceptibility to Infections

Administration of live or live-attenuated vaccines in patients immunocompromised by chemotherapeutic agents, including idarubicin, may result in serious or fatal infections. Vaccination with a live vaccine should be avoided in patients receiving idarubicin. Killed or inactivated vaccines may be administered; however, the response to such vaccines may be diminished.

Reproductive system

Men treated with idarubicin hydrochloride are advised to adopt contraceptive measures during therapy and, if appropriate and available, to seek advice on sperm preservation due to the possibility of irreversible infertility caused by the therapy.

Other

As with other cytotoxic agents, thrombophlebitis and thromboembolic phenomena, including pulmonary embolism have been coincidentally reported with the use of idarubicin.

Patients with rare hereditary problems of galactose intolerance, the Lapp lactose deficiency or glucose-galactose malabsorption should not take this medicine

4.5 Interaction with other medicinal products and other forms of interaction

Idarubicin is a potent myelosuppressant and combination chemotherapy regimens including other agents with similar action may be expected to induce additive myelosuppressant effects (See Section 4.4). The use of idarubicin in combination chemotherapy with other potentially cardiotoxic drugs, as well as the concomitant use of other cardioactive compounds (e.g., calcium channel blockers), requires monitoring of cardiac function throughout treatment.

Changes in hepatic or renal function induced by concomitant therapies may affect idarubicin metabolism, pharmacokinetics, and therapeutic efficacy and/or toxicity (See section **4.4**).

An additive myelosuppressant effect may occur when radiotherapy is given concomitantly or within 2-3 weeks prior to treatment with idarubicin.

4.6 Pregnancy and lactation

Impairment of Fertility

Idarubicin can induce chromosomal damage in human spermatozoa. For this reason, males undergoing treatment with idarubicin should use effective contraceptive methods (See section **4.4**).

Pregnancy

The embryotoxic potential of idarubicin has been demonstrated in both in vitro and in vivo studies. However, there are no adequate and well-controlled studies in pregnant women. Women of childbearing potential should be advised not to become pregnant during treatment and adopt adequate contraceptive measures during therapy as suggested by a physician. Idarubicin should be used during pregnancy only if the potential benefit justifies the potential risk to the fetus. The patient should be informed of the potential hazard to the fetus. Patients desiring to have children after completion of therapy should be advised to obtain genetic counselling first if appropriate and available.

Lactation

It is not known whether idarubicin or its metabolites are excreted in human milk. Mothers should not breast-feed during treatment with idarubicin hydrochloride.

4.7 Effects on ability to drive and use machines

The effect of idarubicin on the ability to drive or use machinery has not been systematically evaluated

4.8 Undesirable effects

The frequencies of undesirable effects are based on the following categories:

Very common (≥1/10)

Common (≥1/100 to <1/10)

Uncommon (≥1/1,000 to <1/100)

Rare (≥1/10,000 to <1/1,000)

Very rare (<1/10,000)

Not known (cannot be estimated from the available data)

Infections and infestations	
Very common	Infections
Uncommon	Sepsis, septicaemia
Neoplasms benign, malignant and unspecified (including cysts and polyps)	
Uncommon	Secondary leukaemia (acute myeloid leukaemia and myelodysplastic syndrome)
Blood and lymphatic system disorders	
Very common	Anaemia, severe leukopenia and neutropenia, thrombocytopenia
Immune system disorders	
Very rare	Anaphylaxis
Endocrine disorders	
Very common	Anorexia
Uncommon	Hyperuricemia
Nervous system disorders	
Rare	Cerebral haemorrhages
Cardiac disorders	
Common	Bradycardia, sinus tachycardia, tachyarrhythmia, asymptomatic reduction of left ventricular ejection fraction, congestive heart failure
Uncommon	ECG abnormalities (e.g. non-specific ST segment changes), myocardial infarction
Very rare	Pericarditis, myocarditis, atrioventricular and bundle branch block
Vascular disorders	
Common	Local phlebitis, thrombophlebitis
Uncommon	Shock
Very rare	Thromboembolism, flush
Gastrointestinal disorders	
Very common	Nausea, vomiting, mucositis/stomatitis, diarrhea, abdominal pain or burning sensation
Common	Gastrointestinal tract bleeding, bellyache
Uncommon	Esophagitis, colitis (including severe enterocolitis / neutropenic enterocolitis with perforation)
Very rare	Gastric erosions or ulcerations
Hepatobiliary disorders	
Common	Elevation of the liver enzymes and bilirubin
Skin and subcutaneous tissue disorders	
Very common	Alopecia
Common	Rash, Itch, hypersensitivity of irradiated skin ('radiation recall reaction')
Uncommon	Skin and nail hyperpigmentation, urticaria
Very rare	Acral erythema
Renal and urinary disorders	
Very common	Red coloration of the urine for 1 – 2 days after the treatment.
General disorders and administration site conditions	
Very common	Fever
Common	Hemorrhages
Uncommon	Dehydration

Hematopoietic system

Pronounced myelosuppression is the most severe adverse effect of idarubicin treatment. However, this is necessary for the eradication of leukaemic cells (See section **4.4**)

Leukocyte and thrombocyte counts usually reach their nadir 10 - 14 days after the administration of idarubicin hydrochloride. Cell counts generally return to normal levels during the third week. During the phase of severe myelosuppression, deaths due to infections and/or haemorrhages have been reported.

Clinical consequences of myelosuppression may be fever, infections, sepsis, septic shock, haemorrhages, and tissue hypoxia, which can lead to death. If febrile neutropenia occurs, treatment with an IV antibiotic is recommended.

Cardiotoxicity

Life-threatening CHF is the most severe form of anthracycline-induced cardiomyopathy and represents the cumulative dose-limiting toxicity of the drug (See section **4.4**).

4.9 Overdose

Very high doses of idarubicin may be expected to cause acute myocardial toxicity within 24 hours and severe myelosuppression within one to two weeks.

Delayed cardiac failure has been seen with anthracyclines for up to several months after the overdose.

Patients treated with oral idarubicin should be observed for possible gastrointestinal haemorrhage and severe mucosal damage.

5. PHARMACOLOGICAL PROPERTIES

5.1 Pharmacodynamic properties

Idarubicin is an antimitotic and cytotoxic agent which intercalates with DNA and interacts with topoisomerase II and has an inhibitory effect on nucleic acid synthesis.

The compound has a high lipophilicity which results in an increased rate of cellular uptake compared with doxorubicin and daunorubicin. Idarubicin has been shown to have a higher potency with respect to daunorubicin and to be an effective agent against murine leukaemia and lymphomas both by i.v. and oral routes. Studies *in-vitro* on human and murine anthracycline-resistant cells have shown a lower degree of cross-resistance for idarubicin compared with doxorubicin and daunorubicin. Cardiotoxicity studies in animals have indicated that idarubicin has a better therapeutic index than daunorubicin and doxorubicin. The main metabolite, idarubicinol, has shown *in-vitro* and *in-vivo* antitumoral activity in experimental models. In the rat, idarubicinol, administered at the same doses as the parent drug, is clearly less cardiotoxic than idarubicin.

5.2 Pharmacokinetic properties

After oral administration to patients with normal renal and hepatic function, idarubicin is rapidly absorbed, with a peak time of 2-4 H., is eliminated from systemic circulation with a terminal plasma T½ ranging between 10-35 H and is extensively metabolized to an active metabolite, idarubicinol, which is more slowly eliminated with a plasma T½ ranging between 33 and 60 H. The drug is mostly eliminated by biliary excretion, mainly in the form of idarubicinol, urinary excretion accounting for 1-2% of the dose as unchanged drug and for up to 4.6% as idarubicinol.

Average values of absolute bioavailability have been shown to range between 18 and 39% (individual values observed in the studies ranging between 3 and 77%), whereas the average values calculated on the data from the active metabolite, idarubicinol, are somewhat higher (29 - 58%; extremes 12 - 153%).

Studies of cellular (nucleated blood and bone marrow cells) drug concentrations in leukaemic patients have shown that uptake is rapid and almost parallels the appearance of the drug in plasma. Idarubicin and idarubicinol concentrations in nucleated blood and bone marrow cells are more than two hundred times the plasma concentrations. Idarubicin and idarubicinol disappearance rates in plasma and cells were almost comparable.

5.3 Preclinical safety data

No further preclinical safety data are available.

6. PHARMACEUTICAL PARTICULARS

6.1 List of excipients

Microcrystalline cellulose Ph. Eur.

Glyceryl palmito-stearate HSE

Capsule shell:

Red iron oxide (E172) FP

Titanium dioxide (E171) Ph. Eur.

Gelatin Ph. Eur.

Sodium dodecyl sulphate Ph. Eur.

6.2 Incompatibilities

Not known.

6.3 Shelf life

36 months.

6.4 Special precautions for storage

Store in a dry place

6.5 Nature and contents of container

Type III amber glass bottles closed with an aluminium screw cap with a polyethylene gasket and a polyethylene cover cap. Aluminium/aluminium strips. Pack size: 1.

6.6 Special precautions for disposal and other handling

None stated.

Administrative Data

7. MARKETING AUTHORISATION HOLDER

Pharmacia Limited

Ramsgate Road

Sandwich

Kent CT13 9NJ

UK

8. MARKETING AUTHORISATION NUMBER(S)

PL 0032/0439 - 10mg

PL 00032/0440 - 25mg

PL 00032/0441 - 5mg

9. DATE OF FIRST AUTHORISATION/RENEWAL OF THE AUTHORISATION

10th May 2002

25 March 2002

10. DATE OF REVISION OF THE TEXT

February 2009

ZD4_0

Zavedos Injection 5mg/10mg

(Pharmacia Limited)

1. NAME OF THE MEDICINAL PRODUCT

Zavedos 5 mg Powder for Solution for Injection

Zavedos 10 mg Powder for Solution for Injection

2. QUALITATIVE AND QUANTITATIVE COMPOSITION

Each vial contains 5mg idarubicin hydrochloride

Each vial contains10mg idarubicin hydrochloride

The reconstituted solution contains 1mg/ml.

For a full list of excipients, see section 6.1:

3. PHARMACEUTICAL FORM

Powder for Solution for Injection

Sterile, pyrogen-free, orange-red, freeze-dried powder in vial containing 5 mg of idarubicin hydrochloride, with 50 mg of lactose monohydrate

Sterile, pyrogen-free, orange-red, freeze-dried powder in vial containing 10 mg of idarubicin hydrochloride, with 100 mg of lactose monohydrate.

4. CLINICAL PARTICULARS

4.1 Therapeutic indications

For the treatment of acute non-lymphoblastic leukaemia (ANLL) in adults, for remission induction in untreated patients or for remission induction in relapsed or refractory patients.

In the treatment of relapsed acute lymphoblastic leukaemia (ALL) as second line treatment in adults and children.

Zavedos may be used in combination chemotherapy regimens involving other cytotoxic agents.

4.2 Posology and method of administration

For intravenous use only.

Not for intrathecal use.

Dosage is calculated on the basis of body surface area.

Acute non-lymphoblastic leukaemia (ANLL)

Adults

- 12 mg/m^2/day i.v. daily for 3 days in combination with cytarabine.

or

- 8 mg/m^2/day i.v. daily for 5 days with/without combination.

Acute lymphoblastic leukaemia (ALL)

Adults

As single agent in *ALL* the suggested dose in adults is 12 mg/m^2 i.v. daily for 3 days.

Children

10 mg/m^2 i.v. daily for 3 days, as a single agent.

All of these dosage schedules should, however, take into account the haematological status of the patient and the dosages of other cytotoxic drugs when used in combination.

Administration of the second course should be delayed in patients who develop severe mucositis until recovery from this toxicity has occurred and a dose reduction of 25% is recommended.

For instruction on dilution of the product before administration, see section 6.6.

4.3 Contraindications

- Hypersensitivity to idarubicin or to any other component of the product, other anthracyclines or anthracenediones
- Severe hepatic impairment
- Severe renal impairment
- Uncontrolled infections
- Severe myocardial insufficiency
- Recent myocardial infarction
- Severe arrhythmias
- Persistent myelosuppression
- Previous treatment with maximum cumulative doses of idarubicin and/ or other anthracyclines and anthracenediones (See section **4.4**)
- Breast-feeding should be stopped during drug therapy (See section **4.6**)

4.4 Special warnings and precautions for use

General: Idarubicin should be administered only under the supervision of physicians experienced in the use of cytotoxic chemotherapy.

This ensures that immediate and effective treatment of severe complications of the disease and/or its treatment (e.g. haemorrhage, overwhelming infections) may be carried out.

Patients should recover from acute toxicities of prior cytotoxic treatment (such as stomatitis, neutropenia, thrombocytopenia, and generalized infections) before beginning treatment with idarubicin.

Haematological Toxicity: Idarubicin is a potent bone marrow suppressant. Severe myelosuppression will occur in all patients given a therapeutic dose of this agent.

Haematological profiles should be assessed before and during each cycle of therapy with idarubicin, including differential white blood cell (WBC) counts.

A dose-dependant reversible luekopenia and/or granulocytopenia (neutropenia) is the predominant manifestation of idarubicin hematologic toxicity and is the most common acute dose-limiting toxicity of this drug. Leukopenia and neutropenia are usually severe; thrombocytopenia and anaemia may also occur. Neutrophil and platelet counts usually reach their nadir 10 to 14 days after drug administration; however, cell counts generally return to normal levels during the third week. Clinical consequences of severe myelosuppression include fever, infections, sepsis/septicaemia, septic shock, haemorrhage, tissue hypoxia or death.

Secondary Leukaemia: Secondary leukaemia, with or without a preleukaemic phase, has been reported in patients treated with anthracyclines, including idarubicin. Secondary leukaemia is more common when such drugs are given in combination with DNA-damaging antineoplastic agents, when patients have been heavily pretreated with cytotoxic drugs, or when doses of the anthracyclines have been escalated. These leukaemias can have a 1 to 3 year latency period.

Cardiac Function: Cardiotoxicity is a risk of anthracycline treatment that may be manifested by early (i.e., acute) or late (i.e., delayed) events.

Early (i.e. Acute) Events: Early cardiotoxicity of idarubicin consists mainly of sinus tachycardia and/ or electrocardiogram (ECG) abnormalities, such as non-specific ST-T wave changes. Tachyarrhythmias, including premature ventricular contractions and ventricular tachycardia, bradycardia, as well as atrioventricular and bundle-branch block have also been reported. These effects do not usually predict subsequent development of delayed cardiotoxicity, are rarely of clinical importance, and are generally not a reason for the discontinuation of idarubicin treatment.

Late (i.e. Delayed) Events: Delayed cardiotoxicity usually develops late in the course of therapy or within 2 to 3 months after treatment termination, but later events, several months to years after completion of treatment have also been reported. Delayed cardiomyopathy is manifested by reduced left ventricular ejection fraction (LVEF) and/ or signs and symptoms of congestive heart failure (CHF) such as dyspnoea, pulmonary oedema, dependent oedema, cardiomegaly, hepatomegaly, oliguira, ascitres, pleural effusion, and gallop rhythm. Subacute effects such as pericarditis/myocarditis have also been reported. Life-threatening CHF is the most severe form of anthracycline-induced cardiomyopathy and represents the cumulative dose-limiting toxicity of the drug.

Cumulative dose limits for IV or oral idarubicin have not been defined. However, idarubicin-related cardiomyopathy was reported in 5% of patients who received cumulative IV doses of 150 to 290mg/m^2. Available data on patients treated with oral idarubicin total cumulative doses up to 400 mg/m^2 suggest a low probability of cardiotoxicity.

Cardiac function should be assessed before patients undergo treatment with idarubicin and must be monitored throughout therapy to minimize the risk of incurring severe cardiac impairment. The risk may be decreased through regular monitoring of LVEF during the course of treatment with prompt discontinuation of idarubicin at the first sign of impaired function. The appropriate quantitative method for repeated assessment of cardiac function (evaluation of LVEF) includes multi-gated radionuclide angiography (MUGA) scan or echocardiography (ECHO). A baseline cardiac evaluation with an ECG and either a MUGA scan or an ECHO is recommended, especially in patients with risk factors for increased cardiotoxicity. Repeated MUGA or ECHO determinations of LVEF should be performed, particularly with higher, cumulative anthracycline doses. The technique used for assessment should be consistent throughout follow-up. Risk factors for cardiac toxicity include active or dormant cardiovascular disease, prior or concomitant radiotherapy to the mediastinal/pericardial area, previous therapy with other anthracyclines or anthracenediones, and concomitant use of drugs with the ability to suppress cardiac contractility or cardiotoxic drugs (e.g., trastuzumab). Anthracyclines including idarubicin should not be administered in combination with other cardiotoxic agents unless the patient's cardiac function is closely monitored. Patients receiving anthracyclines after stopping treatment with other cardiotoxic agents, especially those with long half-lives such as trastuzumab, may also be at an increased risk of developing cardiotoxicity. The half-life of trastuzumab is approximately 28.5 days and may persist in the circulation for up to 24 weeks. Therefore, physicians should avoid anthracycline-based therapy for up to 24 weeks after stopping trastuzumab when possible. If anthracyclines are used before this time, careful monitoring of cardiac function is recommended.

Cardiac function monitoring must be particularly strict in patients receiving high cumulative doses and in those with risk factors. However, cardiotoxicity with idarubicin may occur at lower cumulative doses whether or not cardiac risk factors are present.

In infants and children there appears to be a greater susceptibility to anthracycline induced cardiac toxicity, and a long-term periodic evaluation of cardiac function has to be performed. It is probable that the toxicity of idarubicin and other anthracyclines or anthracenediones is additive.

Hepatic and renal function: Since hepatic and/or renal function impairment can affect the disposition of idarubicin, liver and kidney function should be evaluated with conventional clinical laboratory tests (using serum bilirubin and serum creatinine as indicators) prior to, and during, treatment. In a number of Phase III clinical trials, treatment was contraindicated if bilirubin and/or creatinine serum levels exceeded 2.0-mg%. With other anthracyclines a 50% dose reduction is generally used if bilirubin levels are in the range 1.2 - 2.0 mg%.

Gastrointestinal: Idarubicin is emetigenic. Mucositis (mainly stomatitis, less often esophagitis) generally appears early after drug administration and, if severe, may progress over a few days to mucosal ulcerations. Most patients recover from this adverse event by the third week of therapy. Occasionally, episodes of serious gastrointestinal events (such as perforation or bleeding) have been observed in patients receiving oral idarubicin who had acute leukaemia or a history of other pathologies or had received medications known to lead to gastrointestinal complications. In patients with active gastrointestinal disease with increased risk of bleeding and/or perforation, the physician must balance the benefit of oral idarubicin therapy against the risk.

Effects at site of injection: Phlebosclerosis may result from an injection into a small vessel or from previous injections into the same vein. Following the recommended administration procedures may minimize the risk of phlebitis/thrombophlebitis at the injection site.

Extravasation: Extravasation of idarubicin during intravenous injection may cause local pain, severe tissue lesions (vesication, severe cellulitis), and necrosis. Should signs or symptoms of extravasation occur during intravenous administration of idarubicin, the drug infusion should be immediately stopped.

Tumour Lysis Syndrome: Idarubicin may induce hyperuricaemia as a consequence of the extensive purine catabolism that accompanies rapid drug-induced lysis of neoplastic cells ('tumour lysis syndrome'). Blood uric acid levels, potassium, calcium, phosphate and creatinine should be evaluated after initial treatment. Hydration, urine alkalinization, and prophylaxis with allopurinol to prevent hyperuricaemia may minimize potential complications of tumour lysis syndrome.

Immunosuppressant Effects/Increased Susceptibility to Infections: Administration of live or live-attenuated vaccines in patients immunocompromised by chemotherapeutic agents including idarubicin may result in serious or fatal infections. Vaccination with a live vaccine should be avoided in patients receiving idarubicin. Killed or inactivated vaccines may be administered; however, the response to such vaccines may be diminished.

Reproductive system: Men treated with idarubicin hydrochloride are advised to adopt contraceptive measures during therapy and, if appropriate and available, to seek advice on sperm preservation due to the possibility of irreversible infertility caused by the therapy.

Other: As with other cytotoxic agents, thrombophlebitis and thromboembolic phenomena, including pulmonary embolism have been coincidentally reported with the use of idarubicin.

Patients with rare hereditary problems of galactose intolerance, the Lapp lactose deficiency or glucose-galactose malabsorption should not take this medicine.

4.5 Interaction with other medicinal products and other forms of interaction

Idarubicin is a potent myelosuppressant and combination chemotherapy regimens including other agents with similar action may be expected to induce to additive myelosuppressive effects (See section 4.4).

Changes in hepatic or renal function induced by concomitant therapies may affect idarubicin metabolism, pharmacokinetics, and therapeutic efficacy and/or toxicity (See section **4.4**).

The use of idarubicin in combination chemotherapy with other potentially cardiotoxic drugs, as well as the concomitant use of other cardioactive compounds (e.g., calcium channel blockers), requires monitoring of cardiac function throughout treatment.

An additive myelosuppressant effect may occur when radiotherapy is given concomitantly or within 2-3 weeks prior to treatment with idarubicin.

4.6 Pregnancy and lactation

Impairment of Fertility: Idarubicin can induce chromosomal damage in human spermatozoa. For this reason, males undergoing treatment with idarubicin should use effective contraceptive methods (See section **4.4**).

Pregnancy: The embryotoxic potential of idarubicin has been demonstrated in both in vitro and in vivo studies. However, there are no adequate and well-controlled studies in pregnant women. Women of child bearing potential should be advised not to become pregnant during treatment and adopt adequate contraceptive measures during therapy as suggested by a physician. Idarubicin should be used during pregnancy only if the potential benefit justifies the potential risk to the foetus. The patient should be informed of the potential hazard to the foetus. Patients desiring to have children after completion of therapy should be advised to obtain genetic counselling first if appropriate and available.

Lactation: It is not known whether idarubicin or its metabolites are excreted in human milk. Mothers should not breast-feed during treatment with idarubicin hydrochloride

4.7 Effects on ability to drive and use machines

The effect of idarubicin on the ability to drive or use machinery has not been systematically evaluated.

4.8 Undesirable effects

The frequencies of undesirable effects are based on the following categories:

Very common ($\geq$1/10)

Common ($\geq$1/100 to $<$1/10)

Uncommon ($\geq$1/1,000 to $<$1/100)

Rare ($\geq$1/10,000 to $<$1/1,000)

Very rare ($<$1/10,000)

Not known (cannot be estimated from the available data)

Infections and infestations

Very common	Infections
Uncommon	Sepsis, septicaemia

Neoplasms benign, malignant and unspecified (including cysts and polyps)

Uncommon	Secondary leukaemia (acute myeloid leukaemia and myelodysplastic syndrome)

Blood and lymphatic system disorders

Very common	Anaemia, severe leukopenia and neutropenia, thrombocytopenia

Immune system disorders

Very rare	Anaphylaxis

Endocrine disorders

Very common	Anorexia
Uncommon	Hyperuricemia

Nervous system disorders

Rare	Cerebral haemorrhages

Cardiac disorders

Common	Bradycardia, sinus tachycardia, tachyarrhythmia, asymptomatic reduction of left ventricular ejection fraction, congestive heart failure
Uncommon	ECG abnormalities (e.g. non-specific ST segment changes), myocardial infarction
Very rare	Pericarditis, myocarditis, atrioventricular and bundle branch block

Vascular disorders

Common	Local phlebitis, thrombophlebitis
Uncommon	Shock
Very rare	Thromboembolism, flush

Gastrointestinal disorders

Very common	Nausea, vomiting, mucositis/stomatitis, diarrhoea, abdominal pain or burning sensation
Common	Gastrointestinal tract bleeding, bellyache
Uncommon	Esophagitis, colitis (including severe enterocolitis / neutropenic enterocolitis with perforation)
Very rare	Gastric erosions or ulcerations

Hepatobiliary disorders

Common	Elevation of the liver enzymes and bilirubin

Skin and subcutaneous tissue disorders

Very common	Alopecia
Common	Rash, Itch, hypersensitivity of irradiated skin ('radiation recall reaction')
Uncommon	Skin and nail hyperpigmentation, urticaria
Very rare	Acral erythema

Renal and urinary disorders

Very common	Red coloration of the urine for 1 – 2 days after the treatment

General disorders and administration site conditions

Very common	Fever
Common	Haemorrhages
Uncommon	Dehydration

Hematopoietic system

Pronounced myelosuppression is the most severe adverse effect of idarubicin treatment. However, this is necessary for the eradication of leukaemic cells (See section **4.4**)

Leukocyte and thrombocyte counts usually reach their nadir 10 - 14 days after the administration of idarubicin hydrochloride. Cell counts generally return to normal levels during the third week. During the phase of severe myelosuppression, deaths due to infections and/or haemorrhages have been reported.

Clinical consequences of myelosuppression may be fever, infections, sepsis, septic shock, haemorrhages, and tissue hypoxia, which can lead to death. If febrile neutropenia occurs, treatment with an IV antibiotic is recommended.

Cardiotoxicity

Life-threatening CHF is the most severe form of anthracycline-induced cardiomyopathy and represents the cumulative dose-limiting toxicity of the drug (See section **4.4**).

4.9 Overdose

Very high doses of idarubicin may be expected to cause acute myocardial toxicity within 24 hours and severe myelosuppression within one to two weeks. Delayed cardiac failure has been seen with the anthracyclines for up to several months after the overdose. Patients treated with oral idarubicin should be observed for possible gastrointestinal haemorrhage and severe mucosal damage.

5. PHARMACOLOGICAL PROPERTIES

5.1 Pharmacodynamic properties

Pharmacotherapeutic group: Anthracyclines and related substances

ATC Code: L01DB06

Idarubicin is a DNA intercalating anthracycline which interacts with the enzyme topoisomerase II and has an inhibitory effect on nucleic acid synthesis.

The modification of position 4 of the anthracycline structure gives the compound a high lipophilicity which results in an increased rate of cellular uptake compared with doxorubicin and daunorubicin.

Idarubicin has been shown to have a higher potency with respect to daunorubicin and to be an effective agent against murine leukaemia and lymphomas both by i.v. and oral routes. Studies *in-vitro* on human and murine anthracycline-resistant cells have shown a lower degree of cross-resistance for idarubicin compared with doxorubicin and daunorubicin. Cardiotoxicity studies in animals have indicated that idarubicin has a better therapeutic index than daunorubicin and doxorubicin. The main metabolite, idarubicinol, has shown *in-vitro* and *in-vivo*, antitumoural activity in experimental models. In the rat, idarubicinol administered at the same doses as the parent drug, is clearly less cardiotoxic than idarubicin.

In vitro studies have shown plasma protein binding of at least 95% for this product. This fact should be borne in mind when considering its use in combination with other drugs.

5.2 Pharmacokinetic properties

After i.v administration to patients with normal renal and hepatic function, idarubicin is eliminated from systemic circulation (terminal plasma $T_{½}$ ranging between 11 - 25 hours) and is extensively metabolised to an active metabolite, idarubicinol, which is slowly eliminated with a plasma $T_{½}$ ranging between 41 - 69 hours). The drug is eliminated by biliary and renal excretion, mostly in the form or idarubicinol.

Studies of cellular (nucleated blood and bone marrow cells) in leukaemic patients have shown that peak cellular idarubicin concentrations are reached a few minutes after injection. Idarubicin and idarubicinol concentrations in nucleated blood and bone marrow cells are more than a hundred times the plasma concentrations. Idarubicin disappearance rates in plasma and cells were comparable, with a terminal half-life of about 15 hours. The terminal half-life of idarubicinol in cells was about 72 hours.

5.3 Preclinical safety data

Idarubicin has mutagenic properties and it is carcinogenic in rats.

Reproduction studies in animals have shown that idarubicin is embryotoxic and teratogenic in rats but not rabbits.

6. PHARMACEUTICAL PARTICULARS

6.1 List of excipients

Lactose monohydrate

6.2 Incompatibilities

Prolonged contact with any solution of an alkaline pH should be avoided as it will result in degradation of the drug. Zavedos should not be mixed with heparin as a precipitate may form and it is not recommended that it be mixed with other drugs.

6.3 Shelf life

The shelf-life expiry date for this product shall not exceed three years from the date of its manufacture.

6.4 Special precautions for storage

Unreconstituted solution: No special storage conditions

Reconstituted solution: The reconstituted solution is chemically stable when stored for at least 48 hours at 2-8°C and 24 hours at room temperature (20°C - 25°C); however, it is recommended that, in line with good pharmaceutical practice, the solution should not normally be stored for longer than 24 hours at 2-8°C.

The product does not contain any antibacterial preservative. Therefore of aseptic preparation cannot be ensured, the product must be prepared immediately before use and any unused portion discarded.

6.5 Nature and contents of container

Colourless glass vial, type I, with chlorobutyl rubber bung and aluminium seal with insert yellow polypropylene disk.

Zavedos 10mg Powder for Solution for Injection vials are available as single vials.

6.6 Special precautions for disposal and other handling

The following protective recommendations are given due to the toxic nature of this substance:

• This product should be handled only by personnel who have been trained in the safe handling of such preparations.

• Pregnant staff should be excluded from working with this drug

• Personnel handling idarubicin should wear protective clothing: goggles, gowns and disposable gloves and masks

• All items used for administration or cleaning, including gloves, should be placed in high risk, waste disposal bags for high temperature incineration.

• The reconstituted solution is hypotonic and the recommended administration procedure described below must be followed.

Reconstitute with 10ml of Water for Injections to produce a 1mg/ml solution for injection (i.v). The reconstituted solution is clear red-orange solution, essentially free from visible foreign matter, see section 6.4 also.

Intravenous administration: Zavedos, as the reconstituted solution, must be administered only by the intravenous route. A slow administration over 5 to 10 minutes via the tubing of a freely running intravenous infusion of 0.9% sodium chloride must be followed. A direct push injection is not recommended due to the risk of extravasation, which may occur even in the presence of adequate blood return upon needle aspiration, see section 4.4.

Spillage or leakage should be treated with dilute sodium hypochlorite (1% available chlorine) solution, preferably by soaking, and then with water.

All cleaning materials should be disposed of as indicated previously. Accidental contact with the skin and eyes should be treated immediately by copious lavage with water, or sodium bicarbonate solution, medical attention should be sought.

Discard any unused solution

7. MARKETING AUTHORISATION HOLDER

Pharmacia Limited

Ramsgate Road

Sandwich

Kent CT13 9NJ, UK

8. MARKETING AUTHORISATION NUMBER(S)

PL 00032/0349

PL 00032/0438

9. DATE OF FIRST AUTHORISATION/RENEWAL OF THE AUTHORISATION

10th May 2002

10. DATE OF REVISION OF THE TEXT

February 2009

ZD4_0

Zeffix 100mg film-coated tablets

(GlaxoSmithKline UK)

1. NAME OF THE MEDICINAL PRODUCT

Zeffix 100 mg film-coated tablets

2. QUALITATIVE AND QUANTITATIVE COMPOSITION

Zeffix film-coated tablets contain 100 mg lamivudine

For a full list of excipients see section 6.1.

3. PHARMACEUTICAL FORM

Film-coated tablet

Butterscotch coloured, film-coated, capsule shaped, biconvex and engraved "GX CG5" on one face.

4. CLINICAL PARTICULARS

4.1 Therapeutic indications

Zeffix is indicated for the treatment of chronic hepatitis B in adults with:

• compensated liver disease with evidence of active viral replication, persistently elevated serum alanine aminotransferase (ALT) levels and histological evidence of active liver inflammation and/or fibrosis.

• decompensated liver disease.

4.2 Posology and method of administration

Therapy with Zeffix should be initiated by a physician experienced in the management of chronic hepatitis B.

Adults: the recommended dosage of Zeffix is 100 mg once daily. Zeffix can be taken with or without food.

Duration of treatment: The optimal duration of treatment is unknown.

• In patients with HBeAg positive chronic hepatitis B (CHB) without cirrhosis, treatment should be administered for at least 6-12 months after HBeAg seroconversion (HBeAg and HBV DNA loss with HBeAb detection) is confirmed, to limit the risk of virological relapse, or until HBsAg seroconversion or there is loss of efficacy (see section 4.4). Serum ALT and HBV DNA levels should be followed regularly after treatment discontinuation to detect any late virological relapse.

• In patients with HBeAg negative CHB (pre-core mutant) without cirrhosis, treatment should be administered at least until HBs seroconversion or there is evidence of loss of efficacy. With prolonged treatment, regular reassessment is recommended to confirm that continuation of the selected therapy remains appropriate for the patient.

• In patients with either HBeAg positive or HBeAg negative CHB, the development of YMDD (tyrosine-methionine-aspartate-aspartate) variant HBV may result in a diminished therapeutic response to lamivudine, indicated by a rise in HBV DNA and ALT from previous on-treatment levels. In patients with YMDD variant HBV, a switch to or addition of an alternative agent should be considered (see section 5.1).

• In patients with decompensated liver disease or cirrhosis and in liver transplant recipients, treatment cessation is not recommended. If there is a loss of efficacy attributable to the emergence of YMDD variant HBV in these patients, additional or alternative therapies should be considered (see section 5.1).

If Zeffix is discontinued, patients should be periodically monitored for evidence of recurrent hepatitis (see section 4.4).

Children and adolescents: Zeffix is not recommended for use in children and adolescents below 18 years of age due to lack of data on safety and efficacy (see section 5.2).

Renal impairment: lamivudine serum concentrations (AUC) are increased in patients with moderate to severe renal impairment due to decreased renal clearance. The dosage should therefore be reduced for patients with a creatinine clearance of < 50 ml/minute. When doses below 100 mg are required Zeffix oral solution should be used (see Table 1 below).

Table 1: Dosage of Zeffix in patients with decreased renal clearance.

Creatinine clearance ml/min	First Dose of Zeffix oral solution *	Maintenance Dose Once daily
30 to < 50	20 ml (100 mg)	10 ml (50 mg)
15 to < 30	20 ml (100 mg)	5 ml (25 mg)
5 to < 15	7 ml (35 mg)	3 ml (15 mg)
< 5	7 ml (35 mg)	2 ml (10 mg)

* Zeffix oral solution containing 5 mg/ml lamivudine.

Data available in patients undergoing intermittent haemodialysis (for less than or equal to 4 hrs dialysis 2-3 times weekly), indicate that following the initial dosage reduction of lamivudine to correct for the patient's creatinine clearance, no further dosage adjustments are required while undergoing dialysis.

Hepatic impairment: data obtained in patients with hepatic impairment, including those with end-stage liver disease awaiting transplant, show that lamivudine pharmacokinetics are not significantly affected by hepatic dysfunction. Based on these data, no dose adjustment is necessary in patients with hepatic impairment unless accompanied by renal impairment.

4.3 Contraindications

Hypersensitivity to the active substance or to any of the excipients.

4.4 Special warnings and precautions for use

Lamivudine has been administered to children (2 years and above) and adolescents with compensated chronic hepatitis B. However, due to limitations of the data, the administration of lamivudine to this patient population is not currently recommended (see section 5.1).

The efficacy of lamivudine in patients co-infected with Delta hepatitis or hepatitis C has not been established and caution is advised.

Data are limited on the use of lamivudine in HBeAg negative (pre-core mutant) patients and in those receiving concurrent immunosuppressive regimes, including cancer chemotherapy. Lamivudine should be used with caution in these patients.

During treatment with Zeffix patients should be monitored regularly. Serum ALT levels should be monitored at 3 month intervals and HBV DNA and HBeAg should be assessed every 6 months.

Exacerbations of hepatitis

HBV viral subpopulations with reduced susceptibility to lamivudine (YMDD variant HBV) have been identified with extended therapy. In some patients the development of YMDD variant HBV can lead to exacerbation of hepatitis, primarily detected by serum ALT elevations and re-emergence of HBV DNA. In patients who have YMDD variant HBV and worsening liver disease (increasing ALT with or without decompensated cirrhosis) or recurrent hepatitis B after liver transplantation, a switch to or addition of an alternative agent should be considered.

If Zeffix is discontinued or there is a loss of efficacy due to the development of YMDD variant HBV (see section 4.2), some patients may experience clinical or laboratory evidence of recurrent hepatitis. If Zeffix is discontinued, patients should be periodically monitored both clinically and by assessment of serum liver function tests (ALT and bilirubin levels), for at least four months, and then as clinically indicated. Exacerbation of hepatitis has primarily been detected by serum ALT elevations, in addition to the re-emergence of HBV DNA. See Table 3 in section 5.1 for more information regarding frequency of post treatment ALT elevations. Most events have been self-limited, however some fatalities have been observed.

For patients who develop evidence of recurrent hepatitis post-treatment, there are insufficient data on the benefits of re-initiation of lamivudine treatment.

Transplantation recipients and patients with advanced liver disease are at greater risk from active viral replication. Due to the marginal liver function in these patients, hepatitis reactivation at discontinuation of lamivudine or loss of efficacy during treatment may induce severe and even fatal decompensation. These patients should be monitored for clinical, virological and serological parameters associated with hepatitis B, liver and renal function, and antiviral response during treatment (at least every month), and, if treatment is discontinued for any reason, for at least 6 months after treatment. Laboratory parameters to be monitored should include (as a minimum) serum ALT, bilirubin, albumin, blood urea nitrogen, creatinine, and virological status: HBV antigen/antibody, and serum HBV DNA concentrations when possible. Patients experiencing signs of hepatic insufficiency during or post-treatment should be monitored more frequently as appropriate.

HIV co-infection

For the treatment of patients who are co-infected with HIV and are currently receiving or plan to receive treatment with lamivudine or the combination lamivudine-zidovudine, the dose of lamivudine prescribed for HIV infection (usually 150 mg/twice daily in combination with other antiretrovirals) should be maintained. For HIV co-infected patients not requiring anti-retroviral therapy, there is a risk of HIV mutation when using lamivudine alone for treating chronic hepatitis B.

Transmission of hepatitis B

There is no information available on maternal-foetal transmission of hepatitis B virus in pregnant women receiving treatment with lamivudine. The standard recommended procedures for hepatitis B virus immunisation in infants should be followed.

Patients should be advised that therapy with lamivudine has not been proven to reduce the risk of transmission of hepatitis B virus to others and therefore, appropriate precautions should still be taken.

Lactic acidosis and severe hepatomegaly with steatosis

Occurrences of lactic acidosis (in the absence of hypoxaemia), sometimes fatal, usually associated with severe hepatomegaly and hepatic steatosis, have been reported with the use of nucleoside analogues. As Zeffix is a nucleoside analogue, this risk cannot be excluded. Treatment with nucleoside analogues should be discontinued when rapidly elevating aminotransferase levels, progressive hepatomegaly or metabolic/lactic acidosis of unknown aetiology occur. Benign digestive symptoms, such as nausea, vomiting and abdominal pain, might be indicative of lactic acidosis development. Severe cases, sometimes with fatal outcome, were associated with pancreatitis, liver failure/hepatic steatosis, renal failure and higher levels of serum lactate. Caution should be exercised when prescribing nucleoside analogues to any patient (particularly obese women) with hepatomegaly, hepatitis or other known risk factors for liver disease and hepatic steatosis (including certain medicinal products and alcohol). Patients co-infected with hepatitis C and treated with alpha interferon and ribivirin may constitute a special risk. These patients should be followed closely.

Mitochondrial dysfunction

Nucleoside and nucleotide analogues have been demonstrated *in vitro* and *in vivo* to cause a variable degree of mitochondrial damage. There have been reports of mitochondrial dysfunction in infants exposed in utero and/or post-natally to nucleoside analogues. The main adverse events reported are haematological disorders (anaemia, neutropenia), metabolic disorders (hyperlactatemia, hyperlipasemia). Some late-onset neurological disorders have been reported (hypertonia, convulsion, abnormal behaviour). The neurological disorders might be transient or permanent. Any child exposed *in utero* to nucleoside and nucleotide analogues, should have clinical and laboratory follow-up and should be fully investigated for possible mitochondrial dysfunction in cases which have relevant signs or symptoms.

Zeffix should not be taken with any other medicinal products containing lamivudine or medicinal products containing emtricitabine.

4.5 Interaction with other medicinal products and other forms of interaction

Interaction studies have only been performed in adults.

The likelihood of metabolic interactions is low due to limited metabolism and plasma protein binding and almost complete renal elimination of unchanged substance.

Lamivudine is predominantly eliminated by active organic cationic secretion. The possibility of interactions with other medicinal products administered concurrently should be considered, particularly when their main route of elimination is active renal secretion via the organic cationic transport system e.g. trimethoprim. Other medicinal products (e.g. ranitidine, cimetidine) are eliminated only in part by this mechanism and were shown not to interact with lamivudine.

Substances shown to be predominately excreted either via the active organic anionic pathway, or by glomerular filtration are unlikely to yield clinically significant interactions with lamivudine.

Administration of trimethoprim/sulphamethoxazole 160 mg/800 mg increased lamivudine exposure by about 40 %. Lamivudine had no effect on the pharmacokinetics of trimethoprim or sulphamethoxazole. However, unless the patient has renal impairment, no dosage adjustment of lamivudine is necessary.

A modest increase in C_{max} (28 %) was observed for zidovudine when administered with lamivudine, however overall exposure (AUC) was not significantly altered. Zidovudine had no effect on the pharmacokinetics of lamivudine (see section 5.2).

Lamivudine has no pharmacokinetic interaction with alpha-interferon when the two medicinal products are concurrently administered. There were no observed clinically significant adverse interactions in patients taking lamivudine concurrently with commonly used immunosuppressant medicinal products (e.g. cyclosporin A). However, formal interaction studies have not been performed.

Lamivudine may inhibit the intracellular phosphorylation of zalcitabine when the two medicinal products are used concurrently. Zeffix is therefore not recommended to be used in combination with zalcitabine.

4.6 Pregnancy and lactation

A large amount of data on pregnant women (more than 1000 exposed outcomes) indicate no malformative toxicity. Zeffix can be used during pregnancy if clinically needed.

For patients who are being treated with lamivudine and subsequently become pregnant consideration should be given to the possibility of a recurrence of hepatitis on discontinuation of lamivudine.

Following oral administration, lamivudine was excreted in breast milk at similar concentrations to those found in serum. It is therefore recommended that mothers taking lamivudine do not breast feed their infants.

Mitochondrial dysfunction:

Nucleoside and nucleotide analogues have been demonstrated in vitro and in vivo to cause a variable degree of mitochondrial damage. There have been reports of mitochondrial dysfunction in infants exposed in utero and/or post-natally to nucleoside analogues (see section 4.4).

4.7 Effects on ability to drive and use machines

No studies on the effects on the ability to drive and use machines have been performed.

4.8 Undesirable effects

The incidence of adverse reactions and laboratory abnormalities (with the exception of elevations of ALT and CPK, see below) were similar between placebo and lamivudine treated patients). The most common adverse reactions reported were malaise and fatigue, respiratory tract infections, throat and tonsil discomfort, headache, abdominal discomfort and pain, nausea, vomiting and diarrhoea.

Adverse reactions are listed below by system organ class and frequency. Frequency categories are only assigned to those adverse reactions considered to be at least possibly causally related to lamivudine. Frequencies are defined as: very common (⩾ 1/10), common (⩾ 1/100 to < 1/10), uncommon (⩾ 1/1000 to < 1/100), rare (⩾ 1/10,000 to < 1/1000) and very rare (< 1/10,000).

The frequency categories assigned to the adverse reactions below are estimates: for most reactions, suitable data for calculating incidence are not available. Very common and common adverse drug reaction frequency categories were determined from clinical trial data and the background incidence in placebo groups was not taken into account.

Blood and lymphatic system disorders	
Not known	Thrombocytopenia
Immune system disorders:	
Not known	Angioedema
Hepatobiliary disorders	
Very common	ALT elevations (see section 4.4)
Exacerbations of hepatitis, primarily detected by serum ALT elevations, have been reported 'on-treatment' and following lamivudine withdrawal. Most events have been self-limited, however fatalities have been observed very rarely (see section 4.4).	
Skin and subcutaneous tissue disorders	
Common	Rash, pruritus
Musculoskeletal and connective tissue disorders	
Common	Elevations of CPK
Not known	Muscle disorders, including myalgia, cramps and rhabdomyolysis

In patients with HIV infection, cases of pancreatitis and peripheral neuropathy (or paresthesia) have been reported. In patients with chronic hepatitis B there was no observed difference in incidence of these events between placebo and lamivudine treated patients.

Cases of lactic acidosis, sometimes fatal, usually associated with severe hepatomegaly and hepatic steatosis, have been reported with the use of combination nucleoside analogue therapy in patients with HIV. There have been rare reports of lactic acidosis in patients receiving lamivudine for hepatitis B.

4.9 Overdose

Administration of lamivudine at very high dose levels in acute animal studies did not result in any organ toxicity. Limited data are available on the consequences of ingestion of acute overdoses in humans. No fatalities occurred, and the patients recovered. No specific signs or symptoms have been identified following such overdose.

If overdose occurs the patient should be monitored and standard supportive treatment applied as required. Since lamivudine is dialysable, continuous haemodialysis could be used in the treatment of overdose, although this has not been studied.

5. PHARMACOLOGICAL PROPERTIES

5.1 Pharmacodynamic properties

Pharmacotherapeutic group - nucleoside and nucleotide reverse transcriptase inhibitors, ATC Code: J05AF05.

Lamivudine is an antiviral agent which is active against hepatitis B virus in all cell lines tested and in experimentally infected animals.

Lamivudine is metabolised by both infected and uninfected cells to the triphosphate (TP) derivative which is the active form of the parent compound. The intracellular half life of the triphosphate in hepatocytes is 17-19 hours *in vitro*. Lamivudine-TP acts as a substrate for the HBV viral polymerase.

The formation of further viral DNA is blocked by incorporation of lamivudine-TP into the chain and subsequent chain termination.

Lamivudine-TP does not interfere with normal cellular deoxynucleotide metabolism. It is also only a weak inhibitor of mammalian DNA polymerases alpha and beta. Furthermore, lamivudine-TP has little effect on mammalian cell DNA content.

Table 2: Efficacy results 5 years by YMDD status (Asian Study) NUCB3018

	Subjects, % (no.)			
YMDD variant HBV status	YMDD[1]		Non-YMDD[1]	
HBeAg seroconversion				
- All patients	38	(15/40)	72	(13/18)
- Baseline ALT ⩽ 1 × ULN[2]	9	(1/11)	33	(2/6)
- Baseline ALT > 2 × ULN	60	(9/15)	100	(11/11)
Undetectable HBV DNA				
- Baseline [3]	5	(2/40)	6	(1/18)
- Week 260 [4] negative	8	(2/25)	0	
positive < baseline	92	(23/25)	100	(4/4)
positive > baseline	0		0	
ALT normalisation				
- Baseline				
normal	28	(11/40)	33	(6/18)
above normal	73	(29/40)	67	(12/18)
- Week 260				
normal	46	(13/28)	50	(2/4)
above normal < baseline	21	(6/28)	0	
above normal > baseline	32	(9/28)	50	(2/4)

1 Patients designated as YMDD variant were those with ⩾5% YMDD variant HBV at any annual time-point during the 5-year period. Patients categorised as non-YMDD variant were those with > 95% wild-type HBV at all annual time-points during the 5-year study period

2 Upper limit of normal

3 Abbott Genostics solution hybridisation assay (LLOD < 1.6 pg/ml

4 Chiron Quantiplex assay (LLOD 0.7 Meq/ml)

In assays relating to potential substance effects on mitochondrial structure and DNA content and function, lamivudine lacked appreciable toxic effects. It has a very low potential to decrease mitochondrial DNA content, is not permanently incorporated into mitochondrial DNA, and does not act as an inhibitor of mitochondrial DNA polymerase gamma.

Clinical experience

Experience in patients with HBeAg positive CHB and compensated liver disease: in controlled studies, 1 year of lamivudine therapy significantly suppressed HBV DNA replication [34-57 % of patients were below the assay detection limits (Abbott Genostics solution hybridization assay, LLOD < 1.6pg/ml)}, normalised ALT level (40-72 % of patients), induced HBeAg seroconversion (HBeAg loss and HBeAb detection with HBV DNA loss [by conventional assay], 16-18 % of patients), improved histology (38-52 % of patients had a ⩾ 2 point decrease in the Knodell Histologic Activity Index [HAI]) and reduced progression of fibrosis (in 3-17 % of patients) and progression to cirrhosis.

Continued lamivudine treatment for an additional 2 years in patients who had failed to achieve HBeAg seroconversion in the initial 1 year controlled studies resulted in further improvement in bridging fibrosis. In patients with YMDD variant HBV, 41/82 (50 %) patients had improvement in liver inflammation and 40/56 (71 %) patients without YMDD variant HBV had improvement. Improvement in bridging fibrosis occurred in 19/30 (63 %) patients without YMDD variant and 22/44 (50 %) patients with the variant. Five percent (3/56) of patients without the YMDD variant and 13 % (11/82) of patients with YMDD variant showed worsening in liver inflammation compared to pre-treatment. Progression to cirrhosis occurred in 4/68 (6 %) patients with the YMDD variant, whereas no patients without the variant progressed to cirrhosis.

In an extended treatment study in Asian patients (NUCB3018) the HBeAg seroconversion rate and ALT normalisation rate at the end of the 5 year treatment period was 48 % (28/58) and 47 % (15/32), respectively. HBeAg seroconversion was increased in patients with elevated ALT levels; 77 % (20/26) of patients with pre-treatment ALT> 2 × ULN seroconverted. At the end of 5 years, all patients had HBV DNA levels that were undetectable or lower than pre-treatment levels.

Further results from the trial by YMDD variant status are summarised in Table 2.

Table 2: Efficacy results 5 years by YMDD status (Asian Study) NUCB3018

(see Table 2 above)

Comparative data according to YMDD status were also available for histological assessment but only up to three years. In patients with YMDD variant HBV, 18/39 (46 %) had improvements in necroinflammatory activity and 9/39 (23 %) had worsening. In patients without the variant, 20/27 (74 %) had improvements in necroinflammatory activity and 2/27 (7 %) had worsening.

Following HBeAg seroconversion, serologic response and clinical remission are generally durable after stopping lamivudine. However, relapse following seroconversion can occur. In a long-term follow-up study of patients who had previously seroconverted and discontinued lamivudine, late virological relapse occurred in 39 % of the subjects. Therefore, following HBeAg seroconversion, patients should be periodically monitored to determine that serologic and clinical responses are being maintained. In patients who do not maintain a sustained serological response, consideration should be given to retreatment with either lamivudine or an alternative antiviral agent for resumption of clinical control of HBV.

In patients followed for up to 16 weeks after discontinuation of treatment at one year, post-treatment ALT elevations were observed more frequently in patients who had received lamivudine than in patients who had received placebo. A comparison of post-treatment ALT elevations between weeks 52 and 68 in patients who discontinued lamivudine at week 52 and patients in the same studies who received placebo throughout the treatment course is shown in Table 3. The proportion of patients who had post-treatment ALT elevations in association with an increase in bilirubin levels was low and similar in patients receiving either lamivudine or placebo.

Table 3: Post-treatment ALT Elevations in 2 Placebo-Controlled Studies in Adults

	Patients with ALT Elevation/ Patients with Observations*	
Abnormal Value	Lamivudine	Placebo
ALT ⩾ 2 × baseline value	37/137 (27 %)	22/116 (19 %)
ALT ⩾ 3 × baseline value†	29/137 (21 %)	9/116 (8 %)
ALT ⩾ 2 × baseline value and absolute ALT> 500 IU/l	21/137 (15 %)	8/116 (7 %)
ALT ⩾2 × baseline value; and bilirubin >2 × ULN and ⩾2 × baseline value	1/137 (0.7 %)	1/116 (0.9 %)

*Each patient may be represented in one or more category.

†Comparable to a Grade 3 toxicity in accordance with modified WHO criteria.

ULN = Upper limit of normal.

Experience in patients with HBeAg negative CHB: initial data indicate the efficacy of lamivudine in patients with HBeAg negative CHB is similar to patients with HBeAg positive CHB, with 71 % of patients having HBV DNA suppressed below the detection limit of the assay, 67 % ALT normalisation and 38 % with improvement in HAI after one year of treatment. When lamivudine was discontinued, the majority of patients (70 %) had a return of viral replication. Data is available from an extended treatment study in HBeAg negative patients (NUCAB3017) treated with lamivudine. After two years of treatment in this study, ALT normalisation and undetectable HBV DNA occurred in 30/69 (43 %) and 32/68 (47 %) patients respectively and improvement in necroinflammatory score in 18/49 (37 %) patients. In patients without YMDD variant HBV, 14/22 (64 %) showed improvement in necroinflammatory score and 1/22 (5 %) patients worsened compared to pre-treatment. In patients with the variant, 4/26 (15 %) patients showed improvement in necroinflammatory score and 8/26 (31 %) patients worsened compared to pre-treatment. No patients in either group progressed to cirrhosis.

Frequency of emergence of YMDD variant HBV and impact on the treatment response: lamivudine monotherapy results in the selection of YMDD variant HBV in approximately 24 % of patients following one year of therapy, increasing to 67 % following 4 years of therapy. Development of YMDD variant HBV is associated with reduced treatment response in some patients, as evidenced by increased HBV DNA levels and ALT elevations from previous on-therapy levels, progression of signs and symptoms of hepatitis disease and/or worsening of hepatic necroinflammatory findings. The optimal therapeutic management of patients with YMDD variant HBV has not yet been established (see section 4.4).

In a double-blind study in CHB patients with YMDD variant HBV and compensated liver disease (NUC20904), with a reduced virological and biochemical response to lamivudine (n=95), the addition of adefovir dipivoxil 10 mg once daily to ongoing lamivudine 100mg for 52 weeks resulted in a median decrease in HBV DNA of 4.6 log_{10} copies/ml compared to a median increase of 0.3 log_{10} copies/ml in those patients receiving lamivudine monotherapy. Normalisation of ALT levels occurred in 31 % (14/45) of patients receiving combined therapy versus 6 % (3/47) receiving lamivudine alone.

Forty patients (HBeAg negative or HBeAg positive) with either decompensated liver disease or recurrent HBV following liver transplantation and YMDD variant were also enrolled into an open label arm of the study. Addition of 10 mg adefovir dipivoxil once daily to ongoing lamivudine 100mg for 52 weeks resulted in a median decrease in HBV DNA of 4.6 log_{10} copies/ml. Improvement in liver function was also seen after one year of therapy

Experience in patients with decompensated liver disease: placebo controlled studies have been regarded as inappropriate in patients with decompensated liver disease, and have not been undertaken. In non-controlled studies, where lamivudine was administered prior to and during transplantation, effective HBV DNA suppression and ALT normalisation was demonstrated. When lamivudine therapy was continued post transplantation there was reduced graft re-infection by HBV, increased HBsAg loss and on one-year survival rate of 76 – 100 %.

As anticipated due to the concomitant immunosuppression, the rate of emergence of YMDD variant HBV after 52 weeks treatment was higher (36 % - 64 %) in the liver transplant population than in the immunocompetent CHB patients (14 % - 32 %).

Experience in CHB patients with advanced fibrosis or cirrhosis: in a placebo-controlled study in 651 patients with clinically compensated chronic hepatitis B and histologically confirmed fibrosis or cirrhosis, lamivudine treatment (median duration 32 months) significantly reduced the rate of overall disease progression (34/436, 7.8 % for lamivudine versus 38/215, 17.7 % for placebo, p=0.001), demonstrated by a significant reduction in the proportion of patients having increased Child-Pugh scores (15/436, 3.4 % versus 19/215, 8.8 %, p=0.023) or developing hepatocellular carcinoma (17/436, 3.9 % versus 16/215, 7.4 %, p=0.047). The rate of overall disease progression in the lamivudine group was higher for subjects with detectable YMDD variant HBV DNA (23/209, 11 %) compared to those without detectable YMDD variant HBV (11/221, 5 %). However, disease progression in YMDD subjects in the lamivudine group was lower than the disease progression in the placebo group (23/209, 11 % versus 38/214, 18 % respectively). Confirmed HBeAg seroconversion occurred in 47 % (118/252) of subjects treated with lamivudine and 93 % (320/345) of subjects receiving lamivudine became HBV DNA negative (VERSANT [version 1], bDNA assay, LLOD < 0.7 MEq/ml) during the study.

Experience in children and adolescents: lamivudine has been administered to children and adolescents with compensated CHB in a placebo controlled study of 286 patients aged 2 to 17 years. This population primarily consisted of children with minimal hepatitis B. A dose of 3 mg/kg once daily (up to a maximum of 100 mg daily) was used in children aged 2 to 11 years and a dose of 100 mg once daily in adolescents aged 12 years and above. This dose needs to be further substantiated. The difference in the HBeAg seroconversion rates (HBeAg and HBV DNA loss with HBeAb detection) between placebo and lamivudine was not statistically significant in this population (rates after one year were 13 % (12/95) for placebo versus 22 % (42/191) for lamivudine; p=0.057). The incidence of YMDD variant HBV was similar to that observed in adults, ranging from 19 % at week 52 up to 45 % in patients treated continuously for 24 months.

5.2 Pharmacokinetic properties

Absorption: Lamivudine is well absorbed from the gastrointestinal tract, and the bioavailability of oral lamivudine in adults is normally between 80 and 85 %. Following oral administration, the mean time (t_{max}) to maximal serum concentrations (C_{max}) is about an hour. At therapeutic dose levels i.e. 100 mg once daily, C_{max} is in the order of 1.1-1.5 μg/ml and trough levels were 0.015-0.020 μg/ml.

Co-administration of lamivudine with food resulted in a delay of t_{max} and a lower C_{max} (decreased by up to 47 %). However, the extent (based on the AUC) of lamivudine absorbed was not influenced, therefore lamivudine can be administered with or without food.

Distribution: From intravenous studies the mean volume of distribution is 1.3 l/kg. Lamivudine exhibits linear pharmacokinetics over the therapeutic dose range and displays low plasma protein binding to albumin.

Limited data shows lamivudine penetrates the central nervous system and reaches the cerebro-spinal fluid (CSF). The mean lamivudine CSF/serum concentration ratio 2-4 hours after oral administration was approximately 0.12.

Metabolism: Lamivudine is predominately cleared by renal excretion of unchanged substance. The likelihood of metabolic substance interactions with lamivudine is low due to the small (5-10 %) extent of hepatic metabolism and the low plasma protein binding.

Elimination: The mean systemic clearance of lamivudine is approximately 0.3 l/h/kg. The observed half-life of elimination is 5 to 7 hours. The majority of lamivudine is excreted unchanged in the urine via glomerular filtration and active secretion (organic cationic transport system). Renal clearance accounts for about 70 % of lamivudine elimination.

Special populations:

Studies in patients with renal impairment show lamivudine elimination is affected by renal dysfunction. Dose reduction in patients with a creatinine clearance of < 50 ml/min is necessary (see section 4.2).

The pharmacokinetics of lamivudine are unaffected by hepatic impairment. Limited data in patients undergoing liver transplantation, show that impairment of hepatic function does not impact significantly on the pharmacokinetics of lamivudine unless accompanied by renal dysfunction.

In elderly patients the pharmacokinetic profile of lamivudine suggests that normal ageing with accompanying renal decline has no clinically significant effect on lamivudine exposure, except in patients with creatinine clearance of < 50 ml/min (see section 4.2).

5.3 Preclinical safety data

Administration of lamivudine in animal toxicity studies at high doses was not associated with any major organ toxicity. At the highest dosage levels, minor effects on indicators of liver and kidney function were seen together with occasional reduction in liver weights. Reduction of erythrocytes and neutrophil counts were identified as the effects most likely to be of clinical relevance. These events were seen infrequently in clinical studies.

Lamivudine was not mutagenic in bacterial tests but, like many nucleoside analogues showed activity in an *in vitro* cytogenetic assay and the mouse lymphoma assay. Lamivudine was not genotoxic *in vivo* at doses that gave plasma concentrations around 60-70 times higher than the anticipated clinical plasma levels. As the *in vitro* mutagenic activity of lamivudine could not be confirmed by *in vivo* tests, it is concluded that lamivudine should not represent a genotoxic hazard to patients undergoing treatment.

Reproductive studies in animals have not shown evidence of teratogenicity and showed no effect on male or female fertility. Lamivudine induces early embryolethality when administered to pregnant rabbits at exposure levels comparable to those achieved in man, but not in the rat even at very high systemic exposures.

The results of long term carcinogenicity studies with lamivudine in rats and mice did not shown any carcinogenic potential.

6. PHARMACEUTICAL PARTICULARS

6.1 List of excipients

Tablet core:

Microcrystalline cellulose

Sodium starch glycolate

Magnesium stearate

Tablet film coat:

Hypromellose

Titanium dioxide

Macrogol 400

Polysorbate 80

Synthetic yellow and red iron oxides

6.2 Incompatibilities

Not applicable

6.3 Shelf life

3 years

6.4 Special precautions for storage

Do not store above 30°C.

6.5 Nature and contents of container

Boxes containing 28 or 84 film-coated tablets in double foil blisters, laminated with polyvinyl chloride.

Not all pack-sizes may be marketed.

6.6 Special precautions for disposal and other handling

Any unused product should be disposed of in accordance with local requirements.

7. MARKETING AUTHORISATION HOLDER

Glaxo Group Ltd

Greenford Road

Greenford

Middlesex UB6 0NN

United Kingdom

8. MARKETING AUTHORISATION NUMBER(S)

EU/1/99/114/001

EU/1/99/114/002

9. DATE OF FIRST AUTHORISATION/RENEWAL OF THE AUTHORISATION

Date of first authorisation: 29 July 1999

Date of latest renewal: 29 July 2004

10. DATE OF REVISION OF THE TEXT

27 August 2009

Detailed information on this medicinal product is available on the website of the European Medicines Agency (EMEA) http://www.emea.europa.eu

Zeffix 5mg/ml oral solution

(GlaxoSmithKline UK)

1. NAME OF THE MEDICINAL PRODUCT

Zeffix 5 mg/ml oral solution

2. QUALITATIVE AND QUANTITATIVE COMPOSITION

Each ml of the oral solution contains 5 mg lamivudine

Excipients:

Sucrose 20 % (4 g/20 ml)

Methyl parahydroxybenzoate (E218) 1.5 mg/ml

Propyl parahydroxybenzoate (E216) 0.18 mg/ml

For a full list of excipients see section 6.1.

3. PHARMACEUTICAL FORM

Oral solution

Clear, colourless to pale yellow in colour.

4. CLINICAL PARTICULARS

4.1 Therapeutic indications

Zeffix is indicated for the treatment of chronic hepatitis B in adults with:

- compensated liver disease with evidence of active viral replication, persistently elevated serum alanine aminotransferase (ALT) levels and histological evidence of active liver inflammation and/or fibrosis.
- decompensated liver disease.

4.2 Posology and method of administration

Therapy with Zeffix should be initiated by a physician experienced in the management of chronic hepatitis B.

Adults: the recommended dosage of Zeffix is 100 mg once daily. Zeffix can be taken with or without food.

Duration of treatment: The optimal duration of treatment is unknown.

- In patients with HBeAg positive chronic hepatitis B (CHB) without cirrhosis, treatment should be administered for at least 6-12 months after HBeAg seroconversion (HBeAg and HBV DNA loss with HBeAb detection) is confirmed, to limit the risk of virological relapse, or until HBsAg seroconversion or there is loss of efficacy (see section 4.4). Serum ALT and HBV DNA levels should be followed regularly after treatment discontinuation to detect any late virological relapse.
- In patients with HBeAg negative CHB (pre-core mutant), without cirrhosis, treatment should be administered at least until HBs seroconversion or there is evidence of loss of efficacy. With prolonged treatment, regular reassessment is recommended to confirm that continuation of the selected therapy remains appropriate for the patient.
- In patients with either HBeAg positive or HBeAg negative CHB the development of YMDD (tyrosine-methionine-aspartate-aspartate) variant HBV may result in a diminished therapeutic response to lamivudine, indicated by a rise in HBV DNA and ALT from previous on-treatment levels. In patients with YMDD variant HBV, a switch to or addition of an alternative agent should be considered (see section 5.1).
- In patients with decompensated liver disease or cirrhosis and in liver transplant recipients, treatment cessation is not recommended. If there is a loss of efficacy attributable to the emergence of YMDD variant HBV in these patients, additional or alternative therapies should be considered (see section 5.1).

If Zeffix is discontinued, patients should be periodically monitored for evidence of recurrent hepatitis (see section 4.4).

Children and adolescents: Zeffix is not recommended for use in children and adolescents below 18 years of age due to lack of data on safety and efficacy (see section 5.2).

Renal impairment: lamivudine serum concentrations (AUC) are increased in patients with moderate to severe renal impairment due to decreased renal clearance. The dosage should therefore be reduced for patients with a creatinine clearance of < 50 ml/minute. When doses below 100 mg are required Zeffix oral solution should be used (see Table 1 below).

Table 1: Dosage of Zeffix in patients with decreased renal clearance.

Creatinine clearanceml/min	First Dose of Zeffixoral solution	Maintenance DoseOnce daily
30 to < 50	20 ml (100 mg)	10 ml (50 mg)

15 to < 30	20 ml (100 mg)	5 ml (25 mg)
5 to < 15	7 ml (35 mg)	3 ml (15 mg)
< 5	7 ml (35 mg)	2 ml (10 mg)

Data available in patients undergoing intermittent haemodialysis (for less than or equal to 4 hrs dialysis 2-3 times weekly), indicate that following the initial dosage reduction of lamivudine to correct for the patient's creatinine clearance, no further dosage adjustments are required while undergoing dialysis.

Hepatic impairment: data obtained in patients with hepatic impairment, including those with end-stage liver disease awaiting transplant, show that lamivudine pharmacokinetics are not significantly affected by hepatic dysfunction. Based on these data, no dose adjustment is necessary in patients with hepatic impairment unless accompanied by renal impairment.

4.3 Contraindications
Hypersensitivity to the active substance or to any of the excipients.

4.4 Special warnings and precautions for use
Lamivudine has been administered to children (2 years and above) and adolescents with compensated chronic hepatitis B. However, due to limitations of the data, the administration of lamivudine to this patient population is not currently recommended (see section 5.1).

The efficacy of lamivudine in patients co-infected with Delta hepatitis or hepatitis C has not been established and caution is advised.

Data are limited on the use of lamivudine in HBeAg negative (pre-core mutant) patients and in those receiving concurrent immunosuppressive regimes, including cancer chemotherapy. Lamivudine should be used with caution in these patients.

During treatment with Zeffix patients should be monitored regularly. Serum ALT levels should be monitored at 3 month intervals and HBV DNA and HBeAg should be assessed every 6 months.

Exacerbations of hepatitis
HBV viral subpopulations with reduced susceptibility to lamivudine (YMDD variant HBV) have been identified with extended therapy. In some patients the development of YMDD variant HBV can lead to exacerbation of hepatitis, primarily detected by serum ALT elevations and re-emergence of HBV DNA. In patients who have YMDD variant HBV and worsening liver disease (increasing ALT with or without decompensated cirrhosis) or recurrent hepatitis B after liver transplantation, a switch to or addition of an alternative agent should be considered.

If Zeffix is discontinued or there is a loss of efficacy due to the development of YMDD variant HBV (see section 4.2), some patients may experience clinical or laboratory evidence of recurrent hepatitis. If Zeffix is discontinued, patients should be periodically monitored both clinically and by assessment of serum liver function tests (ALT and bilirubin levels), for at least four months, and then as clinically indicated. Exacerbation of hepatitis has primarily been detected by serum ALT elevations, in addition to the re-emergence of HBV DNA. See Table 3 in section 5.1 for more information regarding frequency of post treatment ALT elevations. Most events have been self-limited, however some fatalities have been observed.

For patients who develop evidence of recurrent hepatitis post-treatment, there are insufficient data on the benefits of re-initiation of lamivudine treatment.

Transplantation recipients and patients with advanced liver disease are at greater risk from active viral replication. Due to the marginal liver function in these patients, hepatitis reactivation at discontinuation of lamivudine or loss of efficacy during treatment may induce severe and even fatal decompensation. These patients should be monitored for clinical, virological and serological parameters associated with hepatitis B, liver and renal function, and antiviral response during treatment (at least every month), and, if treatment is discontinued for any reason, for at least 6 months after treatment. Laboratory parameters to be monitored should include (as a minimum) serum ALT, bilirubin, albumin, blood urea nitrogen, creatinine, and virological status: HBV antigen/antibody, and serum HBV DNA concentrations when possible. Patients experiencing signs of hepatic insufficiency during or post-treatment should be monitored more frequently as appropriate.

HIV co-infection
For the treatment of patients who are co-infected with HIV and are currently receiving or plan to receive treatment with lamivudine or the combination lamivudine-zidovudine, the dose of lamivudine prescribed for HIV infection (usually 150 mg/twice daily in combination with other antiretrovirals) should be maintained. For HIV co-infected patients not requiring anti-retroviral therapy, there is a risk of HIV mutation when using lamivudine alone for treating chronic hepatitis B.

Transmission of hepatitis B
There is no information available on maternal-foetal transmission of hepatitis B virus in pregnant women receiving treatment with lamivudine. The standard recommended procedures for hepatitis B virus immunisation in infants should be followed.

Patients should be advised that therapy with lamivudine has not been proven to reduce the risk of transmission of hepatitis B virus to others and therefore, appropriate precautions should still be taken.

Patients with rare hereditary problems of fructose intolerance, glucose-galactose malabsorption or sucrase-isomaltase insufficiency should not take this medicine.

Diabetic patients should be advised that each dose of oral solution (100 mg = 20 ml) contains 4 g of sucrose.

The oral solution contains propyl and methyl parahydroxybenzoate. These products may cause an allergic reaction in some individuals. This reaction may be delayed.

Lactic acidosis and severe hepatomegaly with steatosis
Occurrences of lactic acidosis (in the absence of hypoxaemia), sometimes fatal, usually associated with severe hepatomegaly and hepatic steatosis, have been reported with the use of nucleoside analogue. As Zeffix is a nucleoside analogue, this risk cannot be excluded. Treatment with nucleoside analogues should be discontinued when rapidly elevating aminotransferase levels, progressive hepatomegaly or metabolic/lactic acidosis of unknown aetiology occur. Benign digestive symptoms, such as nausea, vomiting and abdominal pain, might be indicative of lactic acidosis development. Severe cases, sometimes with fatal outcome, were associated with pancreatitis, liver failure/hepatic steatosis, renal failure and higher levels of serum lactate. Caution should be exercised when prescribing nucleoside analogues to any patient (particularly obese women) with hepatomegaly, hepatitis or other known risk factors for liver disease and hepatic steatosis (including certain medicinal products and alcohol). Patients co-infected with hepatitis C and treated with alpha interferon and ribivirin may constitute a special risk. These patients should be followed closely.

Mitochondrial dysfunction
Nucleoside and nucleotide analogues have been demonstrated *in vitro* and *in vivo* to cause a variable degree of mitochondrial damage. There have been reports of mitochondrial dysfunction in infants exposed in utero and/or post-natally to nucleoside analogues. The main adverse events reported are haematological disorders (anaemia, neutropenia), metabolic disorders (hyperlactatemia, hyperlipasemia). Some late-onset neurological disorders have been reported (hypertonia, convulsion, abnormal behaviour). The neurological disorders might be transient or permanent. Any child exposed *in utero* to nucleoside and nucleotide analogues, should have clinical and laboratory follow-up and should be fully investigated for possible mitochondrial dysfunction in cases which have relevant signs or symptoms.

Zeffix should not be taken with any other medicinal products containing lamivudine or medicinal products containing emtricitabine.

4.5 Interaction with other medicinal products and other forms of interaction
Interaction studies have only been performed in adults.

The likelihood of metabolic interactions is low due to limited metabolism and plasma protein binding and almost complete renal elimination of unchanged substance.

Lamivudine is predominantly eliminated by active organic cationic secretion. The possibility of interactions with other medicinal products administered concurrently should be considered, particularly when their main route of elimination is active renal secretion via the organic cationic transport system e.g. trimethoprim. Other medicinal products (e.g. ranitidine, cimetidine) are eliminated only in part by this mechanism and were shown not to interact with lamivudine.

Substances shown to be predominately excreted either via the active organic anionic pathway, or by glomerular filtration are unlikely to yield clinically significant interactions with lamivudine.

Administration of trimethoprim/sulphamethoxazole 160 mg/800 mg increased lamivudine exposure by about 40 %. Lamivudine had no effect on the pharmacokinetics of trimethoprim or sulphamethoxazole. However, unless the patient has renal impairment, no dosage adjustment of lamivudine is necessary.

A modest increase in C_{max} (28 %) was observed for zidovudine when administered with lamivudine, however overall exposure (AUC) was not significantly altered. Zidovudine had no effect on the pharmacokinetics of lamivudine (see section 5.2).

Lamivudine has no pharmacokinetic interaction with alpha-interferon when the two medicinal products are concurrently administered. There were no observed clinically significant adverse interactions in patients taking lamivudine concurrently with commonly used immunosuppressant medicinal products (e.g. cyclosporin A). However, formal interaction studies have not been performed.

Lamivudine may inhibit the intracellular phosphorylation of zalcitabine when the two medicinal products are used concurrently. Zeffix is therefore not recommended to be used in combination with zalcitabine.

4.6 Pregnancy and lactation
A large amount of data on pregnant women (more than 1000 exposed outcomes) indicate no malformative toxicity. Zeffix can be used in pregnancy if clinically needed.

For patients who are being treated with lamivudine and subsequently become pregnant consideration should be given to the possibility of a recurrence of hepatitis on discontinuation of lamivudine.

Following oral administration, lamivudine was excreted in breast milk at similar concentrations to those found in serum. It is therefore recommended that mothers taking lamivudine do not breast feed their infants.

Mitochondrial dysfunction:

Nucleoside and nucleotide analogues have been demonstrated in vitro and in vivo to cause a variable degree of mitochondrial damage. There have been reports of mitochondrial dysfunction in infants exposed in utero and/or post-natally to nucleoside analogues (see section 4.4).

4.7 Effects on ability to drive and use machines
No studies on the effects on the ability to drive and use machines have been performed.

4.8 Undesirable effects
The incidence of adverse reactions and laboratory abnormalities (with the exception of elevations of ALT and CPK, see below) were similar between placebo and lamivudine treated patients). The most common adverse reactions reported were malaise and fatigue, respiratory tract infections, throat and tonsil discomfort, headache, abdominal discomfort and pain, nausea, vomiting and diarrhoea.

Adverse reactions are listed below by system organ class and frequency. Frequency categories are only assigned to those adverse reactions considered to be at least possibly causally related to lamivudine. Frequencies are defined as: very common (≥ 1/10), common (≥ 1/100 to < 1/10), uncommon (≥ 1/1000 to < 1/100), rare (≥ 1/10,000 to < 1/1000) and very rare (< 1/10,000).

The frequency categories assigned to the adverse reactions below are estimates: for most reactions, suitable data for calculating incidence are not available. Very common and common adverse drug reaction frequency categories were determined from clinical trial data and the background incidence in placebo groups was not taken into account.

Blood and lymphatic system disorders	
Not known	Thrombocytopenia
Immune system disorders:	
Not known	Angioedema
Hepatobiliary disorders	
Very common	ALT elevations (see section 4.4)
Exacerbations of hepatitis, primarily detected by serum ALT elevations, have been reported 'on-treatment' and following lamivudine withdrawal. Most events have been self-limited, however fatalities have been observed very rarely (see section 4.4).	
Skin and subcutaneous tissue disorders	
Common	Rash, pruritus
Musculoskeletal and connective tissue disorders	
Common	Elevations of CPK
Not known	Muscle disorders, including myalgia, cramps and rhabdomyolysis

In patients with HIV infection, cases of pancreatitis and peripheral neuropathy (or paresthesia) have been reported. In patients with chronic hepatitis B there was no observed difference in incidence of these events between placebo and lamivudine treated patients.

Cases of lactic acidosis, sometimes fatal, usually associated with severe hepatomegaly and hepatic steatosis, have been reported with the use of combination nucleoside analogue therapy in patients with HIV. There have been rare reports of lactic acidosis in patients receiving lamivudine for hepatitis B.

4.9 Overdose
Administration of lamivudine at very high dose levels in acute animal studies did not result in any organ toxicity. Limited data are available on the consequences of ingestion of acute overdoses in humans. No fatalities occurred, and the patients recovered. No specific signs or symptoms have been identified following such overdose.

If overdose occurs the patient should be monitored, and standard supportive treatment applied as required. Since lamivudine is dialysable, continuous haemodialysis could be used in the treatment of overdose, although this has not been studied.

5. PHARMACOLOGICAL PROPERTIES

5.1 Pharmacodynamic properties
Pharmacotherapeutic group - nucleoside and nucleotide reverse transcriptase inhibitors, ATC Code: J05AF05.

Lamivudine is an antiviral agent which is active against hepatitis B virus in all cell lines tested and in experimentally infected animals.

Table 2: Efficacy results 5 years by YMDD status (Asian Study) NUCB3018

	Subjects, % (no.)			
YMDD variant HBV status	YMDD[1]		Non-YMDD[1]	
HBeAg seroconversion				
- All patients	38	(15/40)	72	(13/18)
- Baseline ALT ⩽ 1 × ULN[2]	9	(1/11)	33	(2/6)
- Baseline ALT > 2 × ULN	60	(9/15)	100	(11/11)
Undetectable HBV DNA				
- Baseline [3]	5	(2/40)	6	(1/18)
- Week 260 [4]				
negative	8	(2/25)	0	
positive < baseline	92	(23/25)	100	(4/4)
positive > baseline	0		0	
ALT normalisation				
- Baseline				
normal	28	(11/40)	33	(6/18)
above normal	73	(29/40)	67	(12/18)
- Week 260				
normal	46	(13/28)	50	(2/4)
above normal < baseline	21	(6/28)	0	
above normal > baseline	32	(9/28)	50	(2/4)

1 Patients designated as YMDD variant were those with ⩾5% YMDD variant HBV at any annual time-point during the 5-year period. Patients categorised as non-YMDD variant were those with > 95% wild-type HBV at all annual time-points during the 5-year study period

2 Upper limit of normal

3 Abbott Genostics solution hybridisation assay (LLOD < 1.6 pg/ml

4 Chiron Quantiplex assay (LLOD 0.7 Meq/ml)

Lamivudine is metabolised by both infected and uninfected cells to the triphosphate (TP) derivative which is the active form of the parent compound. The intracellular half life of the triphosphate in hepatocytes is 17-19 hours *in vitro*. Lamivudine-TP acts as a substrate for the HBV viral polymerase.

The formation of further viral DNA is blocked by incorporation of lamivudine-TP into the chain and subsequent chain termination.

Lamivudine-TP does not interfere with normal cellular deoxynucleotide metabolism. It is also only a weak inhibitor of mammalian DNA polymerases alpha and beta. Furthermore, lamivudine-TP has little effect on mammalian cell DNA content.

In assays relating to potential substance effects on mitochondrial structure and DNA content and function, lamivudine lacked appreciable toxic effects. It has a very low potential to decrease mitochondrial DNA content, is not permanently incorporated into mitochondrial DNA, and does not act as an inhibitor of mitochondrial DNA polymerase gamma.

Clinical experience

Experience in patients with HBeAg positive CHB and compensated liver disease: in controlled studies, 1 year of lamivudine therapy significantly suppressed HBV DNA replication (34-57 % of patients were below the assay detection limits (Abbott Genostics solution hybridization assay, LLOD < 1.6pg/ml)], normalised ALT level (40-72 % of patients), induced HBeAg seroconversion (HBeAg loss and HBeAb detection with HBV DNA loss [by conventional assay], 16-18 % of patients), improved histology (38-52 % of patients had a ⩾ 2 point decrease in the Knodell Histologic Activity Index [HAI]) and reduced progression of fibrosis (in 3-17 % of patients) and progression to cirrhosis.

Continued lamivudine treatment for an additional 2 years in patients who had failed to achieve HBeAg seroconversion in the initial 1 year controlled studies resulted in further improvement in bridging fibrosis. In patients with YMDD variant HBV, 41/82 (50 %) patients had improvement in liver inflammation and 40/56 (71 %) patients without YMDD variant HBV had improvement. Improvement in bridging fibrosis occurred in 19/30 (63 %) patients without YMDD variant and 22/44 (50 %) patients with the variant. Five percent (3/56) of patients without the YMDD variant and 13 % (11/82) of patients with YMDD variant showed worsening in liver inflammation compared to pre-treatment. Progression to cirrhosis occurred in 4/68 (6 %) patients with the YMDD variant, whereas no patients without the variant progressed to cirrhosis.

In an extended treatment study in Asian patients (NUCB3018) the HBeAg seroconversion rate and ALT normalisation rate at the end of the 5 year treatment period was 48 % (28/58) and 47 % (15/32), respectively. HBeAg seroconversion was increased in patients with elevated ALT levels; 77 % (20/26) of patients with pre-treatment ALT> 2 × ULN seroconverted. At the end of 5 years, all patients had HBV DNA levels that were undetectable or lower than pre-treatment levels.

Further results from the trial by YMDD variant status are summarised in Table 2.

Table 2: Efficacy results 5 years by YMDD status (Asian Study) NUCB3018

(see Table 2 above)

Comparative data according to YMDD status were also available for histological assessment but only up to three years. In patients with YMDD variant HBV, 18/39 (46 %) had improvements in necroinflammatory activity and 9/39 (23 %) had worsening. In patients without the variant, 20/27 (74 %) had improvements in necroinflammatory activity and 2/27 (7 %) had worsening.

Following HBeAg seroconversion, serologic response and clinical remission are generally durable after stopping lamivudine. However, relapse following seroconversion can occur. In a long-term follow-up study of patients who had previously seroconverted and discontinued lamivudine, late virological relapse occurred in 39 % of the subjects. Therefore, following HBeAg seroconversion, patients should be periodically monitored to determine that serologic and clinical responses are being maintained. In patients who do not maintain a sustained serological response, consideration should be given to retreatment with either lamivudine or an alternative antiviral agent for resumption of clinical control of HBV.

In patients followed for up to 16 weeks after discontinuation of treatment at one year, post-treatment ALT elevations were observed more frequently in patients who had received lamivudine than in patients who had received placebo. A comparison of post-treatment ALT elevations between weeks 52 and 68 in patients who discontinued lamivudine at week 52 and patients in the same studies who received placebo throughout the treatment course is shown in Table 3. The proportion of patients who had post-treatment ALT elevations in association with an increase in bilirubin levels was low and similar in patients receiving either lamivudine or placebo.

Table 3: Post-treatment ALT Elevations in 2 Placebo-Controlled Studies in Adults

	Patients with ALT Elevation/ Patients with Observations*	
Abnormal Value	Lamivudine	Placebo
ALT ⩾ 2 × baseline value	37/137 (27 %)	22/116 (19 %)
ALT ⩾ 3 × baseline value[†]	29/137 (21 %)	9/116 (8 %)
ALT ⩾ 2 × baseline value and absolute ALT> 500 IU/l	21/137 (15 %)	8/116 (7 %)
ALT ⩾ 2 × baseline value; and bilirubin > 2 × ULN and ⩾ 2 × baseline value	1/137 (0.7 %)	1/116 (0.9 %)

*Each patient may be represented in one or more category.

[†]Comparable to a Grade 3 toxicity in accordance with modified WHO criteria.

ULN = Upper limit of normal.

Experience in patients with HBeAg negative CHB: initial data indicate the efficacy of lamivudine in patients with HBeAg negative CHB is similar to patients with HBeAg positive CHB, with 71 % of patients having HBV DNA suppressed below the detection limit of the assay, 67 % ALT normalisation and 38 % with improvement in HAI after one year of treatment. When lamivudine was discontinued, the majority of patients (70 %) had a return of viral replication. Data is available from an extended treatment study in HBeAg negative patients (NUCAB3017) treated with lamivudine. After two years of treatment in this study, ALT normalisation and undetectable HBV DNA occurred in 30/69 (43 %) and 32/68 (47 %) patients respectively and improvement in necroinflammatory score in 18/49 (37 %) patients. In patients without YMDD variant HBV, 14/22 (64 %) showed improvement in necroinflammatory score and 1/22 (5 %) patients worsened compared to pre-treatment. In patients with the variant, 4/26 (15%) patients showed improvement in necroinflammatory score and 8/26 (31 %) patients worsened compared to pre-treatment. No patients in either group progressed to cirrhosis.

Frequency of emergence of YMDD variant HBV and impact on the treatment response: lamivudine monotherapy results in the selection of YMDD variant HBV in approximately 24 % of patients following one year of therapy, increasing to 67 % following 4 years of therapy. Development of YMDD variant HBV is associated with reduced treatment response in some patients, as evidenced by increased HBV DNA levels and ALT elevations from previous on-therapy levels, progression of signs and symptoms of hepatitis disease and/or worsening of hepatic necroinflammatory findings. The optimal therapeutic management of patients with YMDD variant HBV has not yet been established (see section 4.4).

In a double-blind study in CHB patients with YMDD variant HBV and compensated liver disease (NUC20904), with a reduced virological and biochemical response to lamivudine (n=95), the addition of adefovir dipivoxil 10 mg once daily to ongoing lamivudine 100mg for 52 weeks resulted in a median decrease in HBV DNA of 4.6 $\log_{10}$ copies/ml compared to a median increase of 0.3 $\log_{10}$ copies/ml in those patients receiving lamivudine monotherapy. Normalisation of ALT levels occurred in 31 % (14/45) of patients receiving combined therapy versus 6 % (3/47) receiving lamivudine alone.

Forty patients (HBeAg negative or HBeAg positive) with either decompensated liver disease or recurrent HBV following liver transplantation and YMDD variant were also enrolled into an open label arm of the study. Addition of 10 mg adefovir dipivoxil once daily to ongoing lamivudine 100mg for 52 weeks resulted in a median decrease in HBV DNA of 4.6 $\log_{10}$ copies/ml. Improvement in liver function was also seen after one year of therapy.

Experience in patients with decompensated liver disease: placebo controlled studies have been regarded as inappropriate in patients with decompensated liver disease, and have not been undertaken. In non-controlled studies, where lamivudine was administered prior to and during transplantation, effective HBV DNA suppression and ALT normalisation was demonstrated. When lamivudine therapy was continued post transplantation there was reduced graft re-infection by HBV, increased HBsAg loss and on one-year survival rate of 76 – 100 %.

As anticipated due to the concomitant immunosuppression, the rate of emergence of YMDD variant HBV after 52 weeks treatment was higher (36 % - 64 %) in the liver transplant population than in the immunocompetent CHB patients (14 % - 32 %).

Experience in CHB patients with advanced fibrosis or cirrhosis: in a placebo-controlled study in 651 patients with clinically compensated chronic hepatitis B and histologically confirmed fibrosis or cirrhosis, lamivudine treatment (median duration 32 months) significantly reduced the rate of overall disease progression (34/436, 7.8 % for lamivudine versus 38/215, 17.7 % for placebo, p=0.001), demonstrated by a significant reduction in the proportion of patients having increased Child-Pugh scores (15/436, 3.4 % versus 19/215, 8.8 %, p=0.023) or developing hepatocellular carcinoma (17/436, 3.9 % versus 16/215, 7.4 %, p=0.047). The rate of overall disease progression in the lamivudine group was higher for subjects with detectable YMDD variant HBV DNA (23/209, 11 %) compared to those without detectable YMDD variant HBV (11/221, 5 %). However, disease progression in YMDD subjects in the lamivudine group was lower than the disease progression in the placebo group (23/209, 11 % versus 38/214, 18 % respectively). Confirmed HBeAg seroconversion occurred in 47 % (118/252) of subjects treated with lamivudine and 93 %

(320/345) of subjects receiving lamivudine became HBV DNA negative (VERSANT [version 1], bDNA assay, LLOD < 0.7 MEq/ml) during the study.

Experience in children and adolescents: lamivudine has been administered to children and adolescents with compensated CHB in a placebo controlled study of 286 patients aged 2 to 17 years. This population primarily consisted of children with minimal hepatitis B. A dose of 3 mg/kg once daily (up to a maximum of 100 mg daily) was used in children aged 2 to 11 years and a dose of 100 mg once daily in adolescents aged 12 years and above. This dose needs to be further substantiated. The difference in the HBeAg seroconversion rates (HBeAg and HBV DNA loss with HBeAb detection) between placebo and lamivudine was not statistically significant in this population (rates after one year were 13 % (12/95) for placebo versus 22 % (42/191) for lamivudine; p=0.057). The incidence of YMDD variant HBV was similar to that observed in adults, ranging from 19 % at week 52 up to 45 % in patients treated continuously for 24 months.

5.2 Pharmacokinetic properties

Absorption: Lamivudine is well absorbed from the gastrointestinal tract, and the bioavailability of oral lamivudine in adults is normally between 80 and 85 %. Following oral administration, the mean time (t_{max}) to maximal serum concentrations (C_{max}) is about an hour. At therapeutic dose levels i.e. 100 mg once daily, C_{max} is in the order of 1.1-1.5 µg/ml and trough levels were 0.015-0.020 µg/ml.

Co-administration of lamivudine with food resulted in a delay of t_{max} and a lower C_{max} (decreased by up to 47 %). However, the extent (based on the AUC) of lamivudine absorbed was not influenced, therefore lamivudine can be administered with or without food.

Distribution: From intravenous studies the mean volume of distribution is 1.3 l/kg. Lamivudine exhibits linear pharmacokinetics over the therapeutic dose range and displays low plasma protein binding to albumin.

Limited data shows lamivudine penetrates the central nervous system and reaches the cerebro-spinal fluid (CSF). The mean lamivudine CSF/serum concentration ratio 2-4 hours after oral administration was approximately 0.12.

Metabolism: Lamivudine is predominately cleared by renal excretion of unchanged substance. The likelihood of metabolic substance interactions with lamivudine is low due to the small (5-10 %) extent of hepatic metabolism and the low plasma protein binding.

Elimination: The mean systemic clearance of lamivudine is approximately 0.3 l/h/kg. The observed half-life of elimination is 5 to 7 hours. The majority of lamivudine is excreted unchanged in the urine via glomerular filtration and active secretion (organic cationic transport system). Renal clearance accounts for about 70 % of lamivudine elimination.

Special populations:

Studies in patients with renal impairment show lamivudine elimination is affected by renal dysfunction. Dose reduction in patients with a creatinine clearance of < 50 ml/min is necessary (see section 4.2).

The pharmacokinetics of lamivudine are unaffected by hepatic impairment. Limited data in patients undergoing liver transplantation, show that impairment of hepatic function does not impact significantly on the pharmacokinetics of lamivudine unless accompanied by renal dysfunction.

In elderly patients the pharmacokinetic profile of lamivudine suggests that normal ageing with accompanying renal decline has no clinically significant effect on lamivudine exposure, except in patients with creatinine clearance of < 50 ml/min (see section 4.2).

5.3 Preclinical safety data

Administration of lamivudine in animal toxicity studies at high doses was not associated with any major organ toxicity. At the highest dosage levels, minor effects on indicators of liver and kidney function were seen together with occasional reduction in liver weights. Reduction of erythrocytes and neutrophil counts were identified as the effects most likely to be of clinical relevance. These events were seen infrequently in clinical studies.

Lamivudine was not mutagenic in bacterial tests but, like many nucleoside analogues showed activity in an *in vitro* cytogenetic assay and the mouse lymphoma assay. Lamivudine was not genotoxic *in vivo* at doses that gave plasma concentrations around 60-70 times higher than the anticipated clinical plasma levels. As the *in vitro* mutagenic activity of lamivudine could not be confirmed by *in vivo* tests, it is concluded that lamivudine should not represent a genotoxic hazard to patients undergoing treatment.

Reproductive studies in animals have not shown evidence of teratogenicity and showed no effect on male or female fertility. Lamivudine induces early embryolethality when administered to pregnant rabbits at exposure levels comparable to those achieved in man, but not in the rat even at very high systemic exposures.

The results of long term carcinogenicity studies with lamivudine in rats and mice did not shown any carcinogenic potential.

6. PHARMACEUTICAL PARTICULARS

6.1 List of excipients

Sucrose (20 % w/v)

Methyl Parahydroxybenzoate (E218)

Propyl Parahydroxybenzoate (E216)

Citric Acid (anhydrous)

Propylene Glycol

Sodium Citrate

Artificial strawberry flavour

Artificial banana flavour

Purified water

6.2 Incompatibilities

Not applicable

6.3 Shelf life

2 years

After first opening: 1 month

6.4 Special precautions for storage

Do not store above 25°C.

6.5 Nature and contents of container

Cartons containing 240 ml lamivudine oral solution in an opaque, white, high-density polyethylene (HDPE) bottle with a polypropylene child resistant closure. The pack includes a clear polypropylene oral dosing syringe and a polyethylene syringe-adapter.

The oral dosing syringe is provided for accurate measurement of the prescribed dose of oral solution. Instructions for use are included in the pack.

6.6 Special precautions for disposal and other handling

Any unused product should be disposed of in accordance with local requirements.

7. MARKETING AUTHORISATION HOLDER

Glaxo Group Ltd

Greenford Road

Greenford

Middlesex UB6 0NN

United Kingdom

8. MARKETING AUTHORISATION NUMBER(S)

EU/1/99/114/003

9. DATE OF FIRST AUTHORISATION/RENEWAL OF THE AUTHORISATION

Date of first authorisation: 29 July 1999

Date of latest renewal: 29 July 2004

10. DATE OF REVISION OF THE TEXT

27 August 2009

Detailed information on this medicinal product is available on the website of the European Medicines Agency (EMEA) http://www.emea.europa.eu

Zelapar

(Cephalon Limited)

1. NAME OF THE MEDICINAL PRODUCT

Zelapar 1.25 mg Oral Lyophilisate.

2. QUALITATIVE AND QUANTITATIVE COMPOSITION

Each Zelapar Oral Lyophilisate contains 1.25 mg of selegiline hydrochloride, equivalent to 1.05 mg selegiline free base. For excipients, see section 6.1.

Each tablet contains 1.25mg of aspartame (source of Phenylalanine)

3. PHARMACEUTICAL FORM

Oral lyophilisate.

A pale yellow round tablet with the letter A on one side.

4. CLINICAL PARTICULARS

4.1 Therapeutic indications

Adjunctive therapy in combination with levodopa (with a peripheral decarboxylase inhibitor) in the treatment of Parkinson's disease. Zelapar in combination with maximal levodopa therapy is indicated particularly in patients who experience fluctuations in their condition such as 'end-dose' type fluctuations, 'on-off' symptoms or other dyskinesias.

Zelapar may be used alone in early Parkinson's disease for symptomatic relief and/or to delay the need for levodopa.

4.2 Posology and method of administration

When prescribed as monotherapy for the first time in the early stage of Parkinson's disease or as an adjuvant to levodopa, the dose of Zelapar is one 1.25 mg unit placed on the tongue in the morning, at least five minutes before breakfast and allowed to dissolve. The unit will dissolve rapidly (in less than 10 seconds) in the mouth. The patient should not eat, drink, rinse or wash-out out their mouth for five minutes after taking their medicine to enable selegiline to be absorbed pre-gastrically.

When Zelapar adjunctive therapy is prescribed a reduction (10 to 30%) in the dose of levodopa is usually required. Reduction of the levodopa dose should be gradual in steps of 10% every 3 to 4 days.

No dosage adjustment is required for patients with renal or hepatic impairment.

Do not push the Zelapar tablet through the foil blister. Peel back the foil and carefully remove the unit.

Unused tablets must be disposed of after three months of a sachet opening.

4.3 Contraindications

Zelapar is contra-indicated in patients with known hypersensitivity (including severe dizziness or hypotension) to conventional selegiline tablets or liquid or any of the excipients used in this product.

Zelapar is contra-indicated in patients receiving treatment with serotonin-agonists (e.g. sumatriptan, naratriptan, zolmitriptan and rizatriptan).

Zelapar is contra-indicated in patients with phenylketonuria due to the content of aspartame, a source of phenylalanine.

Selegiline is also contra-indicated for concomitant use with pethidine and other opioids.

Selegiline should not be used in patients with other extrapyramidal disorders not related to dopamine deficiency.

Selegiline should not be used in patients with active duodenal or gastric ulcer.

Selegiline should not be used in patients who are being treated with antidepressant drugs, including MAO inhibitors and selective serotonin reuptake inhibitors (e.g citalopram, escitalopram, fluoxetine, fluvoxamine, paroxetine, sertraline and venlafaxine. See section 4.5 interactions).

Selegiline should also not be used with other drugs which are also monoamine oxidase inhibitors, e.g. linezolid.

Selegiline in combination with levodopa is contra-indicated in severe cardiovascular disease, arterial hypertension, hyperthyroidism, phaeochromocytoma, narrow-angle glaucoma, prostatic adenoma with appearance of residual urine, tachycardia, arrhythmias, severe angina pectoris, psychoses, advanced dementia and thyrotoxicosis.

4.4 Special warnings and precautions for use

One unit of Zelapar contains 1.25 mg selegiline. It is recommended that patients be warned that the correct dose of Zelapar is one oral lyophilisate.

Special care should be taken when administering selegiline to patients who have labile hypertension, cardiac arrhythmias, severe angina pectoris, psychosis or a history of peptic ulceration.

Although serious hepatic toxicity has not been observed, caution is recommended in patients with a history of hepatic dysfunction. Transient or continuing abnormalities with a tendency for elevated plasma concentrations of liver enzymes have been described during long-term therapy with conventional tablets of selegiline.

The selectivity for MAO-B following administration of conventional selegiline tablets may be diminished with doses above 10 mg/day. A non-selective dose of Zelapar above 10 mg/day has not been determined. The precise dose at which selegiline becomes a non-selective inhibitor of all MAO has not been determined, but with doses higher than 10 mg/day there is a theoretical risk of hypertension after ingestion of tyramine-rich food.

Concomitant treatment with medicines which inhibit MAO-A, (or non-selective MAO inhibitors) can cause hypotensive reactions. Hypotension, sometimes sudden in onset, has been reported with conventional selegiline.

Since selegiline potentiates the effects of levodopa, the adverse effects of levodopa may be increased. When selegiline is added to the maximum tolerated dose of levodopa, involuntary movements and agitation may occur. Levodopa should be reduced by about 10 to 30% when selegiline is added to the treatment (see section 4.2 Posology and Method of Administration). When an optimum dose of levodopa is reached, adverse effects from the combination are less than those observed with levodopa on its own.

Although conventional tablets of selegiline, at doses of 5 to 10 mg/day, have been in widespread use for many years, the full spectrum of possible responses to Zelapar may not have been observed to date. Therefore patients should be observed closely for atypical responses.

Mouth ulcers may occur during treatment with Zelapar 1.25 mg oral lyophilisate.

4.5 Interaction with other medicinal products and other forms of interaction

Selegiline should not be administered with any type of antidepressant.

When selegiline is used at its recommended dose, it selectively inhibits MAO-B. The combined use of the SSRI, fluoxetine and Zelapar, should only be used under clinical supervision. Use of Zelapar beyond the recommended dose could lead to non-selectivity and serious adverse effects.

Serious reactions with signs and symptoms that may include diaphoresis, flushing, ataxia, tremor, hyperthermia, hyper/hypotension, seizures, palpitation, dizziness and mental changes that include agitation, confusion and hallucinations progressing to delirium and coma have been reported in some patients receiving a combination of selegiline and fluoxetine. Similar experience has been reported in patients receiving selegiline and two other serotonin reuptake inhibitors, sertraline and paroxetine. There is a potential risk of interaction with fluvoxamine and venlafaxine.

Death has been reported to occur following the initiation of therapy with non-selective MAO inhibitors shortly after discontinuation of fluoxetine. Fluoxetine and its active metabolite have long half-lives; therefore MAO inhibitor therapy should not be started until at least 5 weeks after discontinuation of fluoxetine. Selegiline should not be started until 2 weeks after stopping sertraline. For all other serotonin reuptake inhibitors, a time interval of 1 week is recommended between discontinuation of the serotonin reuptake inhibitor and initiation of selegiline. In general, selegiline should not be introduced after a drug that is known to interact with selegiline, until after 5 half lives of that drug have elapsed.

At least 14 days should lapse between the discontinuation of selegiline and initiation of treatment with any drug known to interact with selegiline.

A time interval of 24 hours is recommended between the discontinuation of selegiline and initiation of serotonin agonists.

Patients being treated with selegiline currently or within the past 2 weeks should receive dopamine only after careful risk-benefit assessment, as this combination enhances the risk of hypertensive reactions.

Selegiline should not be given in conjunction with non-specific MAO inhibitors, e.g. linezolid.

Severe CNS toxicity has been reported in patients with the combination of tricyclic antidepressants and selegiline. In one patient receiving amitriptyline and selegiline this included hyperpyrexia and death, and another patient receiving protriptyline and selegiline experienced tremor, agitation, and restlessness followed by unresponsiveness and death two weeks after selegiline was added.

Other adverse reactions occasionally reported in patients receiving a combination of selegiline with various tricyclic antidepressants include hyper/hypotension, dizziness, diaphoresis, tremor, seizures and changes in behavioural and mental status.

Concomitant use of sympathomimetics, nasal decongestants, hypertensive agents, anti-hypertensives, psychostimulants, central suppressant drugs (sedatives, hypnotics) and alcohol should be avoided.

The combination of selegiline and oral contraceptives or drugs for hormone replacement therapy, should be avoided, as this combination may multiply the bioavailability of selegiline.

Foodstuffs containing tyramine have not been found to cause hypertensive reactions during therapy with conventional selegiline tablets at dosages recommended for the treatment of Parkinson's disease. As the selectivity of action of Zelapar for MAO-B is identical to that of conventional tablets of selegiline given in the same dosage (10 mg), no adverse interactions with foodstuffs containing tyramine are anticipated with Zelapar.

Concomitant administration of amantadine and anticholinergic drugs can lead to an increased occurrence of side-effects.

In view of the high degree of binding to plasma proteins by selegiline particular attention must be given to patients who are being treated with medicines with a narrow therapeutic margin such as digitalis and/or anticoagulants.

Four patients receiving altretamine and a monamine oxidase inhibitor experienced symptomatic hypotension after four to seven days of concomitant therapy.

Interactions between non-selective MAO-inhibitors and pethidine as well as selegiline and pethidine have been described. The mechanism of this interaction is not fully understood and therefore, use of pethidine concomitantly with selegiline should be avoided (see contra-indications).

4.6 Pregnancy and lactation
Selegiline is indicated for the treatment of Parkinson's disease which, in most cases, is a disease occurring after childbearing age. As no work has been done to assess the effects of selegiline on pregnancy and lactation, it should not be used in such cases.

Selegiline should not be used by mothers when breast-feeding as information is lacking concerning whether selegiline passes into breast milk.

4.7 Effects on ability to drive and use machines
Even when used correctly, this medicine can affect reaction capacity to the extent that driving or operating machinery is affected and therefore patients should avoid these activities.

4.8 Undesirable effects
The following undesirable effects have been reported with Zelapar during clinical trials and/or post-marketing use. They are listed below as MedDRA preferred term by system organ class and frequency. Frequencies are defined as: undesirable effects very common (>1/10), common (⩾1/100 and <1/10), uncommon (⩾1/1000 and <1/100).

System Organ Class	Frequency	Undesirable effects
Psychiatric disorders	common	Confusion, depression, hallucinations, insomnia,
	uncommon	abnormal dreams, agitation, anxiety, psychoses
Nervous system disorders	common	Dizziness, dyskinesia (including akinesia, bradykinesia), headache, impaired balance, tremor,
Ear and labyrinth disorders	common	vertigo
Cardiac disorders	uncommon	angina pectoris
Vascular disorders	common	Hypertension, hypotension
Respiratory, thoracic and mediastinal disorders	common	nasal congestion, sore throat
	uncommon	dyspnoea
Gastrointestinal disorders	very common	stomatitis
	common	constipation, diarrhoea, dry mouth, mouth ulceration, nausea
Skin and subcutaneous tissue disorders	common	sweating increased
Muskuloskeletal and lymphatic system disorders	common	arthralgia, back pain, muscle cramps
General disorders and administration site conditions	common	fatigue
	uncommon	chest pain, irritability
Injury, poisoning and procedural complications	common	fall

The following undesirable effects have been reported with selegiline, with an uncommon frequency (⩾1/1000 and <1/100). Undesirable effects are listed below as MedDRA preferred term by system organ class.

System Organ Class	Undesirable effects
Infections and infestations	pharyngitis
Blood and lymphatic system disorders	Leucocytopenia, thrombocytopenia
Metabolism and nutrition disorders	loss of appetite
Eye disorders	blurred vision
Cardiac disorders	Arrhythmias, palpitations
Vascular disorders	orthostatic hypotension
Skin and subcutaneous tissue disorders	hair loss, skin eruptions
Muskuloskeletal and lymphatic system disorders	myopathy
Renal and urinary disorders	micturition disorders
General disorders and administration site conditions	ankle oedema
Investigations	transient transaminase increase (ALAT), transient increase in liver enzyme values

In the first 5 years of marketing experience with Zelapar, the following adverse reactions were reported: nausea, confusional state, dizziness, hallucinations and vertigo.

As selegiline potentiates the effect of levodopa, the side-effects of levodopa may be emphasised unless the dosage of levodopa is reduced. The most common undesirable effect reported for conventional tablets is dyskinesia (4% of patients). Once the optimum levodopa dose level has been established, the side-effects produced by the combination will usually be less than those caused by the levodopa therapy on its own.

4.9 Overdose
Zelapar is rapidly metabolised and the metabolites rapidly excreted. In cases of suspected overdosage the patient should be kept under observation for 24 to 48 hours.

No specific information is available about clinically significant overdoses with Zelapar. However, experience gained in use of conventional tablets of selegiline reveals that some individuals exposed to doses of 60 mg/day suffered severe hypotension and psychomotor agitation.

Since the selective inhibition of MAO-B by selegiline hydrochloride is achieved only at doses in the range recommended for the treatment of Parkinson's disease, overdoses are likely to cause significant inhibition of both MAO-A and MAO-B. Consequently, the signs and symptoms of overdose may resemble those observed with non-selective MAOIs (e.g. tranylcypromine, isocarboxazide and phenelzine) and are dizziness, ataxia, irritability, pyrexia, tremor, convulsions, hypomania, psychosis, convulsions, euphoria, respiratory depression, hypotension, hypertension (sometimes with sub-arachnoid haemorrhage), coma and extra-pyramidal symptoms.

5. PHARMACOLOGICAL PROPERTIES
5.1 Pharmacodynamic properties
ATC Code: N04B D01

Zelapar selectively inhibits MAO-B. It prevents dopamine and β-phenylethylamine breakdown in the brain. Selegiline can be used as monotherapy and permits the initiation of treatment with levodopa to be significantly postponed. It potentiates and prolongs the effect of concomitantly administered levodopa. Since it does not interfere with the breakdown of 5-hydroxytryptamine (serotonin) or noradrenaline, it does not cause any hypertensive crises or changes in the plasma or urinary metabolites of these monoamines. Although dietary restrictions are not necessary during Zelapar treatment, the inhibition of MAO-B in blood platelets can lead to a slight potentiation of the circulatory effects of any tyramine not broken down by gastrointestinal MAO-A during absorption. This effect is no greater with Zelapar than with conventional selegiline in equal doses.

The magnitude of increase in the urinary excretion of β-phenylethylamine over 24 hours is simply related to the area under the selegiline plasma concentration-time curve after any selegiline product. Urinary β-phenylethylamine increase reflects the degree of inhibition of MAO-B. Zelapar gives rise to a similar increase in β-phenylethylamine as 10 mg conventional selegiline tablets.

Combined with levodopa therapy selegiline reduces, in particular, fluctuation in the condition of patients who suffer from parkinsonism, e.g. on-off symptoms or end-of-dose akinesia.

In a clinical trial where patients were switched from 10 mg conventional selegiline tablets to 1.25 mg Zelapar oral lyophilisate, control of motor symptoms was maintained.

Zelapar may be useful in those patients with Parkinson's disease who experience difficulties in swallowing.

5.2 Pharmacokinetic properties
Zelapar dissolves completely within 10 seconds of placing on the tongue and, in contrast to conventional tablets, selegiline is absorbed primarily pregastrically.

The plasma concentrations of selegiline following single doses of Zelapar 1.25 mg are of the same order as those obtained with conventional 10 mg tablets of selegiline, but are much less variable. The range of AUCs for plasma selegiline is 0.22 to 2.82 ng.h/ml for Zelapar 1.25 mg and 0.05 to 23.64 ng.h/ml for conventional 10 mg tablets. The Cmax ranges are 0.32 to 4.58 ng/ml and 0.07 to 16.0 ng/ml respectively.

After Zelapar 1.25 mg, plasma concentrations of selegiline metabolites, *N*-desmethylselegiline, *l*-methamphetamine and *l*-amphetamine, were reduced by between 88% and 92% in comparison with the concentrations reached after conventional selegiline tablets 10 mg.

Ninety-four per cent of plasma selegiline is reversibly bound to plasma protein. Selegiline is mainly eliminated by metabolism. It is excreted mainly in the urine as metabolites (mainly *l*-methamphetamine) and the remainder in the faeces.

5.3 Preclinical safety data
Selegiline has not been sufficiently tested for reproductive toxicity. Studies with selegiline revealed no evidence of mutagenic or carcinogenic effects. The only safety concerns for human use derived from animal studies were effects associated with an exaggerated pharmacological action.

6. PHARMACEUTICAL PARTICULARS
6.1 List of excipients
Gelatin

Mannitol

Glycine

Aspartame

Citric Acid anhydrous

Grapefruit flavour

Yellow Colouring (yellow iron oxide [E172], hypromellose [E464]).

6.2 Incompatibilities
Not applicable.

6.3 Shelf life
Sealed sachets - 3 years.

Opened sachets - 3 months.

6.4 Special precautions for storage
Do not store above 25°C.

6.5 Nature and contents of container
PVC/PE/PVdC blister packs sealed with aluminium foil enclosed in a paper/PE/aluminium foil/PE sachet. Each pack contains 10, 30, 60 or 100 oral lyophilisates. Not all pack sizes may be marketed.

6.6 Special precautions for disposal and other handling
No special requirements.

7. MARKETING AUTHORISATION HOLDER
Cephalon Limited
1 Albany Place
Hyde Way
Welwyn Garden City
Hertfordshire
AL7 3BT
United Kingdom

8. MARKETING AUTHORISATION NUMBER(S)
PL 21799/0017

9. DATE OF FIRST AUTHORISATION/RENEWAL OF THE AUTHORISATION
18/09/2008

10. DATE OF REVISION OF THE TEXT
18/09/2008

Zemplar 5 microgram/ml Solution for Injection

(Abbott Laboratories Limited)

1. NAME OF THE MEDICINAL PRODUCT
Zemplar▼ 5 microgram/ml Solution for Injection

2. QUALITATIVE AND QUANTITATIVE COMPOSITION
Each ml of solution for injection contains 5 micrograms of paricalcitol.

Each 2 ml of solution for injection contains 10 micrograms of paricalcitol.

For excipients, see section 6.1.

3. PHARMACEUTICAL FORM
Solution for Injection
A clear and colourless aqueous solution

4. CLINICAL PARTICULARS

4.1 Therapeutic indications
Paricalcitol is indicated for the prevention and treatment of secondary hyperparathyroidism in patients with chronic renal failure undergoing haemodialysis.

4.2 Posology and method of administration
Zemplar solution for injection is administered via haemodialysis access.

Adults
1) Initial Dose should be calculated based on baseline parathyroid hormone (PTH) levels:

The initial dose of paricalcitol is based on the following formula:

(see Formula 1 below)

and administered as an intravenous (IV) bolus dose no more frequently then every other day at any time during dialysis.

The maximum dose safely administered in clinical studies was as high as 40 µg.

2) Titration Dose:

The currently accepted target range for PTH levels in end-stage renal failure subjects undergoing dialysis is no more than 1.5 to 3 times the non-uremic upper limit of normal, 15.9 to 31.8 pmol/l (150-300 pg/ml), for intact PTH. Close monitoring and individual dose titration are necessary to reach appropriate physiological endpoints. If hypercalcaemia or a persistently elevated corrected Ca × P product greater than 5.2 mmol^2/l^2 (65 mg^2/dl^2) is noted, the dosage should be reduced or interrupted until these parameters are normalised. Then, paricalcitol administration should be reinitiated at a lower dose. Doses may need to be decreased as the PTH levels decrease in response to therapy.

The following table is a suggested approach for dose titration:

Suggested Dosing Guidelines (Dose adjustments at 2 to 4 week intervals)

IPTH Level Relative to Baseline	Paricalcitol Dose Adjustment
Same or increased	Increase by 2 to 4 micrograms
Decreased by < 30%	
Decreased by ⩾30%, ⩽60%	Maintain
Decreased > 60%	Decrease by 2 to 4 micrograms
IPTH < 15.9 pmol/l (150 pg/mL)	

Once dosage has been established, serum calcium and phosphate should be measured at least monthly. Serum intact PTH measurements are recommended every three months. During dose adjustment with paricalcitol, laboratory tests may be required more frequently.

Hepatic insufficiency

Unbound concentrations of paricalcitol in patients with mild to moderate hepatic impairment are similar to healthy subjects and dose adjustment is not necessary in this patient population. There is no experience in patients with severe hepatic impairment.

Pediatric Use

Data in pediatric patients are limited and no data for children under the age of 5 are available. See Section 5.1 for study results.

Geriatric Use

There is a limited amount of experience with patients 65 years of age or over receiving paricalcitol in the phase III studies. In these studies, no overall differences in efficacy or safety were observed between patients 65 years or older and younger patients.

4.3 Contraindications
Hypersensitivity to paricalcitol or any of the excipients
Vitamin D toxicity
Hypercalcemia

4.4 Special warnings and precautions for use
Over suppression of parathyroid hormone may result in elevations of serum calcium levels and may lead to metabolic bone disease. Patient monitoring and individualized dose titration is required to reach appropriate physiological endpoints.

Digitalis toxicity is potentiated by hypercalcemia of any cause, so caution should be applied when digitalis is prescribed concomitantly with paricalcitol.

If clinically significant hypercalcemia develops, and the patient is receiving a calcium-based phosphate binder, the dose of the calcium-based phosphate binder should be reduced or interrupted.

This medicinal product contains 20% v/v of ethanol (alcohol). Each dose may contain up to 1.3g ethanol. Harmful for those suffering from alcoholism.

To be taken into account in pregnant or breast-feeding women, children and high risk groups such as patients with liver disease or epilepsy.

Caution should be exercised if co-administering paricalcitol with ketoconazole.

4.5 Interaction with other medicinal products and other forms of interaction
Specific interaction studies were not performed. Digitalis toxicity is potentiated by hypercalcaemia of any cause, so caution should be applied when digitalis is prescribed concomitantly with paricalcitol.

Phosphate or vitamin D-related medicinal products should not be taken concomitantly with paricalcitol, due to an increased risk of hypercalcaemia and Ca × P product elevation.

Aluminium-containing preparations (e.g., antacids, phosphate-binders) should not be administered chronically with Vitamin D medicinal products, as increased blood levels of aluminium and aluminium bone toxicity may occur.

High doses of calcium-containing preparations or thiazide diuretics may increase the risk of hypercalcaemia.

Magnesium-containing preparations (e.g. antacids) should not be taken concomitantly with vitamin D preparations, because hypermagnesemia may occur.

Ketoconazole: The effect of multiple doses of ketaconazole administered as 200 mg, twice daily (BID) for 5 days on the pharmacokinetics of paricalcitol capsule has been studied in healthy subjects. The Cmax of paricalcitol was minimally affected, but AUC0-∞ approximately doubled in the presence of ketoconazole. The mean half-life of paricalcitol was 17.0 hours in the presence of ketoconazole as compared to 9.8 hours, when paricalcitol was administered alone (See PRECAUTIONS Section 4.4)

4.6 Pregnancy and lactation
There is no adequate data on the use of paricalcitol in pregnant women. Animal studies have shown reproductive toxicity (see section 5.3). Potential risk in human use is not known, therefore paricalcitol should be not be used unless clearly necessary.

Lactation: It is not known whether paricalcitol is excreted in human milk. Because many active substances are excreted in human milk, caution should be exercised when paricalcitol is administered to a nursing woman.

4.7 Effects on ability to drive and use machines
No studies on the effects on the ability to drive a car and use machines have been performed.

4.8 Undesirable effects
Approximately 600 patients were treated with Zemplar in Phase II/III/IV clinical trials. Overall, 6% of the Zemplar treated patients reported adverse reactions.

The most common adverse reaction associated with Zemplar therapy was hypercalcaemia, occurring in 4.7% of patients. Hypercalcaemia is dependent on the level of PTH oversuppression and can be minimised by proper dose titration.

Adverse reactions from clinical trials that were possibly, probably or definitely related to paricalcitol are presented in the following table by body system and frequency. The following frequency categories are used: Very common (>1/10); common (>1/100, <1/10); uncommon (>1/1000, <1/100); rare (>1/10,000, <1/1000); very rare (<1/10000, including isolated reports).

Body System	Frequency	Adverse Reaction
Endocrine system	Common	parathyroid disorder
Haematological and lymphatic system	Uncommon	Anaemia, leucopoenia, lymphadenopathy, increased bleeding time
Immune system disorder	Common	pruritus
	Uncommon	allergic reaction, rash
Metabolic and nutrition disorders	Common	Hypercalcemia, hyperphosphatemia,
	Uncommon	oedema, peripheral oedema, increased AST, and weight loss
Nervous system	Uncommon	confusion, delirium, dizziness, abnormal gait, agitation, depersonalisation, hypesthesia, insomnia, myoclonus, nervousness, paraesthesia and stupor
Special senses	Common	taste perversion,
	Uncommon	conjunctivitis, ear disorder, and glaucoma
Cardiovascular system	Uncommon	Hypotension, arrhythmia, atrial flutter, cerebral ischaemia, cerebrovascular accident, cardiac arrest, hypertension, and syncope
Respiratory System	Uncommon	asthma, increased cough, dyspnoea, epistaxis, pulmonary oedema, pharyngitis, and pneumonia
Digestive system	Uncommon	anorexia, colitis, constipation, diarrhoea, dry mouth, dysphagia, gastrointestinal disorder, gastritis, rectal haemorrhage, thirst, nausea, vomiting, dyspepsia

Formula 1

$$\text{Initial dose (micrograms)} = \frac{\text{baseline intact PTH level in pmol/l}}{8}$$

OR

$$= \frac{\text{baseline intact PTH level in pg/mL}}{80}$$

Skin and Appendages	Uncommon	alopecia, hirsutism, rash, sweating, and vesiculobullous,
Musculoskeletal System	Uncommon	arthralgia, myalgia, joint disorder, and twitching
Urogenitial system	Uncommon	Impotence, breast carcinoma, breast pain, and vaginitis
Body as a whole	Common	Headache
	Uncommon	injection site pain, pain, asthenia, back pain, chest pain, fever, flu syndrome, infection, malaise, and sepsis

Post -Marketing Adverse Reactions

Immune system disorders, hypersensitivity.

Angioedema, laryngeal oedema and urticaria have been reported rarely.

4.9 Overdose

Overdosage of paricalcitol may lead to hypercalcemia.

Treatment of patients with clinically significant hypercalcaemia consists of immediate dose reduction or interruption of paricalcitol therapy and includes a low calcium diet, withdrawal of calcium supplements, patient mobilisation, attention to fluid and electrolyte imbalances, assessment of electrocardiographic abnormalities (critical in patients receiving digitalis), and haemodialysis or peritoneal dialysis against a calcium-free dialysate, as warranted.

Serum calcium levels should be monitored frequently until normocalcaemia ensues

Paricalcitol is not significantly removed by dialysis.

Zemplar solution for injection contains 30% v/v of propyleneglycol as an excipient. Isolated cases of Central Nervous System depression, haemolysis and lactic acidosis have been reported as toxic effect associated with propyleneglycol administration at high doses. Although they are not expected to be found with Zemplar administration as propyleneglycol is eliminated during the dialysis process, the risk of toxic effect in overdosing situations has to be taken into account.

5. PHARMACOLOGICAL PROPERTIES

5.1 Pharmacodynamic properties

Pharmaco-therapeutic group: Vitamin D and analogues - ATC code: A11CC

Mechanism of action:

Paricalcitol is a synthetic, biologically active vitamin D analog of calcitriol with modifications to the side chain (D_2) and the A (19-nor) ring allowing for selective vitamin D receptor (VDR) activation. Paricalcitol selectively upregulates the VDR in the parathyroid glands without increasing VDR in the intestine and is less active on bone resorption. Paricalcitol also upregulates the calcium sensing receptor (CaSR) in the parathyroid glands. As a result, paricalcitol reduces parathyroid hormone (PTH) levels by inhibiting parathyroid proliferation and decreasing PTH synthesis and secretion, with minimal impact on calcium and phosphorus levels, and can act directly on bone cells to maintain bone volume and improve mineralization surfaces. Correcting abnormal PTH levels, with normalization of calcium and phosphorus homeostasis, may prevent or treat the metabolic bone disease associated with chronic kidney disease.

Paediatric clinical data: The safety and effectiveness of Zemplar were examined in a 12-week randomised, double-blind, placebo-controlled study of 29 pediatric patients, aged 5-19 years, with end-stage renal disease on hemodialysis. The six youngest Zemplar-treated patients in the study were 5 - 12 years old. The initial dose of Zemplar was 0.04 mcg/kg 3 times per week, based on baseline iPTH level of less than 500 pg/mL, or 0.08 mcg/kg 3 times a week based on baseline iPTH level of ⩾ 500 pg/mL, respectively. The dose of Zemplar was adjusted in 0.04 mcg/kg increments based on the levels of serum iPTH, calcium, and Ca × P. 67% of the Zemplar-treated patients and 14% placebo-treated patients completed the trial. 60% of the subjects in the Zemplar group had 2 consecutive 30% decreases from baseline iPTH compared with 21% patients in the placebo group. 71% of the placebo patients were discontinued due to excessive elevations in iPTH levels. No subjects in either the Zemplar group or placebo group developed hypercalcemia. No data are available for patients under the age of 5.

5.2 Pharmacokinetic properties

Distribution

The pharmacokinetics of paricalcitol have been studied in patients with chronic renal failure (CRF) requiring haemodialysis. Paricalcitol is administered as an intravenous bolus injection. Within two hours after administering doses ranging from 0.04 to 0.24 microgram/kg, concentrations of paricalcitol decreased rapidly; thereafter, concentrations of paricalcitol declined log-linearly with a mean half-life of about 15 hours. No accumulation of paricalcitol was observed with multiple dosing.

Elimination

In healthy subjects, a study was conducted with a single 0.16 microgram/kg intravenous bolus dose of ^{3}H-paricalcitol (n=4), plasma radioactivity was attributed to parent substance. Paricalcitol was eliminated primarily by hepatobiliary excretion, as 74% of the radioactive dose was recovered in faeces and only 16% was found in urine.

Metabolism

Several unknown metabolites were detected in both the urine and faeces, with no detectable paricalcitol in the urine. These metabolites have not been characterised and have not been identified. Together, these metabolites contributed 51% of the urinary radioactivity and 59% of the faecal radioactivity. *In vitro* plasma protein binding of paricalcitol was extensive (>99.9%) and nonsaturable over the concentration range of 1 to 100 ng/mL.

Paricalcitol Pharmacokinetic Characteristics in CRF Patients (0.24 μ g/kg dose)		
Parameter	**N**	**Values (Mean ± SD)**
C_{max} (5 minutes after bolus)	6	1850± 664 (pg/mL)
$AUC_{0-\infty}$	5	27382 ± 8230 (pg•hr/mL)
CL	5	0.72 ± 0.24 (L/hr)
V_{ss}	5	6 ± 2 (L)

Special Populations

Gender, Race and Age: No age or gender related pharmacokinetic differences have been observed in adult patients studied. Pharmacokinetic differences due to race have not been identified.

Hepatic insufficiency: Unbound concentrations of paricalcitol in patients with mild to moderate hepatic impairment is similar to healthy subjects and dose adjustment is not necessary in this patient population. There is no experience in patients with severe hepatic impairment.

5.3 Preclinical safety data

Salient findings in the repeat dose toxicology studies in rodents and dogs were generally attributed to paricalcitol's calcaemic activity. Effects not clearly related to hypercalcaemia included decreased white blood cell counts and thymic atrophy in dogs, and altered APTT values (increased in dogs, decreased in rats). WBC changes were not observed in clinical trials of paricalcitol.

Paricalcitol did not affect fertility in rats and there was no evidence of teratogenic activity in rats or rabbits. High doses of other vitamin D preparations applied during pregnancy in animals lead to teratogenesis. Paricalcitol was shown to affect foetal viability, as well as to promote a significant increase of peri-natal and post-natal mortality of newborn rats, when administered at maternally toxic doses.

Paricalcitol did not exhibit genotoxic potential in a set of *in-vitro* and *in-vivo* genotoxicity assays

Carcinogenicity studies in rodents did not indicate any special risks for human use.

Doses administered and/or systemic exposures to paricalcitol were slightly higher than therapeutic doses/systemic exposures.

6. PHARMACEUTICAL PARTICULARS

6.1 List of excipients

Ethanol (20 % v/v)

Propylene glycol

Water for Injections

6.2 Incompatibilities

Propylene glycol interacts with heparin and neutralises its effect. Zemplar solution for injection contains propylene glycol as an excipient and should be administered through a different injection port than heparin.

This medicinal product must not be mixed with other medicinal products.

6.3 Shelf life

2 years.

After opening, use immediately

6.4 Special precautions for storage

This medicinal product does not require any special storage conditions.

6.5 Nature and contents of container

Zemplar solution for injection 1 ml or 2 ml in Type I glass ampoule; box of 5.

6.6 Special precautions for disposal and other handling

Parenteral medicinal products should be inspected visually for particulate matter and discoloration prior to administration. The solution is clear and colourless.

For single use only. Any unused solution should be discarded.

7. MARKETING AUTHORISATION HOLDER

Abbott Laboratories Limited

Queenborough

Kent

ME11 5EL

8. MARKETING AUTHORISATION NUMBER(S)

PL 00037/0403

9. DATE OF FIRST AUTHORISATION/RENEWAL OF THE AUTHORISATION

Date of first authorisation: 9 August 2002

Date of Last renewal: 9 August 2007

10. DATE OF REVISION OF THE TEXT

4 October 2007

Zemplar Soft Capsules 1, 2 and 4 mcg

(Abbott Laboratories Limited)

1. NAME OF THE MEDICINAL PRODUCT

Zemplar▼ 1 microgram capsules, soft

Zemplar ▼2 micrograms capsules, soft

Zemplar ▼ 4 micrograms capsules, soft

2. QUALITATIVE AND QUANTITATIVE COMPOSITION

Each capsule, soft contains

	Paricalcitol	Excipients (Ethanol)
Zemplar 1 microgram	1 microgram	0.71 mg
Zemplar 2 micrograms	2 micrograms	1.42 mg
Zemplar 4 micrograms	4 micrograms	1.42 mg

For a full list of excipients, see section 6.1.

3. PHARMACEUTICAL FORM

Capsule, soft

1 microgram capsule: oval, gray soft capsule imprinted with and ZA

2 micrograms capsule: oval, orange-brown soft capsule imprinted with and ZF

4 micrograms capsule: oval, gold soft capsule imprinted with and ZK

4. CLINICAL PARTICULARS

4.1 Therapeutic indications

Zemplar is indicated for the prevention and treatment of secondary hyperparathyroidism associated with chronic renal insufficiency (chronic kidney disease Stages 3 and 4) patients and chronic renal failure (chronic kidney disease Stage 5) patients on haemodialysis or peritoneal dialysis.

4.2 Posology and method of administration

Zemplar can be taken with or without food.

Chronic Kidney Disease (CKD) Stages 3 and 4

Zemplar should be administered once a day, either daily or three times a week taken every other day.

Initial Dose

The initial dose is based on baseline intact parathyroid hormone (iPTH) levels.

Table 1. Initial Dose		
Baseline iPTH Level	**Daily Dose**	**Three Times a Week Dose***
⩽ 500 pg/mL (56 pmol/L)	1 microgram	2 micrograms
> 500 pg/mL (56 pmol/L)	2 micrograms	4 micrograms

* To be administered no more frequently than every other day

Dose Titration

Dosing must be individualised based on serum or plasma iPTH levels, with monitoring of serum calcium and serum phosphorus. Table 2 presents a suggested approach for dose titration.

Table 2. Dose Titration		
iPTH Level Relative to Baseline	**Dose Adjustment at 2 to 4 Week Intervals**	
	Daily Dose	**Three Times a Week Dose**[1]
The same or increased	Increase 1 microgram	Increase 2 micrograms
Decreased by < 30%		
Decreased by ⩾30%, ⩽60%	Maintain	Maintain

Decreased $> 60\%$	Decrease[2] 1 microgram	Decrease[2] 2 micrograms
iPTH < 60 pg/mL (7 pmol/L)		

[1] To be administered no more frequently than every other day.
[2] If a patient is taking the lowest dose on the daily or three times a week regimen, and a dose reduction is needed, dosing frequency can be decreased.

Serum calcium levels should be closely monitored after initiation of the treatment and during dose titration periods. If hypercalcemia or a persistently elevated calcium-phosphorus product greater than 55 mg^2/dL^2 (4.4 $mmol^2/L^2$) is observed, the dose of calcium based phosphate binders should be reduced or withheld. Alternatively, the dose of Zemplar may be reduced or temporarily interrupted. If interrupted, the drug should be restarted at a lower dose, when serum calcium and calcium-phosphorus product are in the target range.

__Chronic Kidney Disease (CKD), Stage 5__

Zemplar should be administered three times a week every other day.

Initial Dose

The initial dose of Zemplar in micrograms is based on a baseline iPTH level (pg/mL)/60 [(pmol/L)/7], up to an initial maximum dose of 32 micrograms.

Dose Titration

Subsequent dosing should be individualised and based on iPTH, serum calcium and phosphorus levels. A suggested dose titration of paricalcitol capsules is based on the following formula:

(see Formula 1 below)

Serum calcium and phosphorus levels should be closely monitored after initiation, during dose titration periods, and with co-administration of strong P450 3A inhibitors. If an elevated serum calcium or elevated Ca × P is observed and the patient is on a calcium-based phosphate binder, the binder dose may be decreased or withheld, or the patient may be switched to a non-calcium-based phosphate binder.

If serum calcium > 11.0 mg/dL (2.8 mmol/L) or Ca × P > 70 mg^2/dL^2 (5.6 $mmol^2/L^2$) or iPTH ≤ 150 pg/mL, the dose should be decreased by 2 to 4 micrograms with respect to that calculated by the most recent iPTH/60 (pg/mL) [iPTH/7 (pmol/L)]. If further adjustment is required, the dose of paricalcitol capsules should be reduced or interrupted until these parameters are normalised.

As iPTH approaches the target range (150-300 pg/mL), small, individualised dose adjustments may be necessary in order to achieve a stable iPTH. In situations where monitoring of iPTH, Ca or P occurs less frequently than once per week, a more modest initial and dose titration ratio may be warranted.

Special Populations

Hepatic Impairment:

No dose adjustment is required in patients with mild to moderate hepatic impairment.

There is no experience in patients with severe hepatic impairment (see Section 5.2).

Paediatric population:

Safety and efficacy of Zemplar Capsules in paediatric patients have not been established (see Section 5.1).

Elderly:

No overall differences in safety and effectiveness were observed between elderly patients (65 – 75 years) with regard to younger patients, but greater sensitivity of some older individuals cannot be ruled out.

4.3 Contraindications

Paricalcitol should not be given to patients with evidence of vitamin D toxicity, hypercalcaemia, or hypersensitivity to paricalcitol or any of the excipients in this medicinal product.

4.4 Special warnings and precautions for use

Over suppression of parathyroid hormone may result in elevations of serum calcium levels and may lead to low-turnover bone disease. Patient monitoring and individualised dose titration is required to reach appropriate physiological endpoints.

If clinically significant hypercalcaemia develops and the patient is receiving a calcium-based phosphate binder, the dose of the calcium-based phosphate binder should be reduced or interrupted.

Digitalis toxicity is potentiated by hypercalcemia of any cause, so caution should be applied when digitalis is prescribed concomitantly with paricalcitol (see Section 4.5).

Caution should be exercised if co-administering paricalcitol with ketoconazole (see Section 4.5).

Warning for excipients:

This medicinal product contains small amounts of ethanol (alcohol), less than 100 mg per 1 mcg, 2 mcg and 4 mcg capsule which may be harmful to those suffering from alcoholism (refer to sections 2 and 4.2). To be taken into account in pregnant or breast-feeding women, children and high risk groups such as patients with liver disease or epilepsy.

4.5 Interaction with other medicinal products and other forms of interaction

Ketoconazole: Ketoconazole is known to be a nonspecific inhibitor of several cytochrome P450 enzymes. The available *in vivo* and *in vitro* data suggest that ketoconazole may interact with enzymes that are responsible for the metabolism of paricalcitol and other vitamin D analogs. Caution should be taken while dosing paricalcitol with ketoconazole. The effect of multiple doses of ketaconazole administered as 200 mg, twice daily (BID) for 5 days on the pharmacokinetics of paricalcitol capsule has been studied in healthy subjects. The Cmax of paricalcitol was minimally affected, but AUC0-∞ approximately doubled in the presence of ketoconazole. The mean half-life of paricalcitol was 17.0 hours in the presence of ketoconazole as compared to 9.8 hours, when paricalcitol was administered alone (see PRECAUTIONS Section 4.4). The results of this study indicate that following either oral or intravenous administration of paricalcitol the maximum amplification of the paricalcitol AUCINF from a drug interaction with ketoconazole is not likely to be greater than about two-fold.

Specific interaction studies were not performed. Digitalis toxicity is potentiated by hypercalcaemia of any cause, so caution should be applied when digitalis is prescribed concomitantly with paricalcitol.

Prescription-based phosphate or vitamin D-related medicinal products should not be taken concomitantly with paricalcitol due to an increased risk of hypercalcaemia and Ca × P product elevation.

High doses of calcium-containing preparation or thiazide diuretics may increase the risk of hypercalcaemia.

Magnesium-containing preparations (e.g. antacids) should not be taken concomitantly with vitamin D preparations, because hypermagnesemia may occur.

Aluminium-containing preparations (e.g. antacids, phosphate-binders) should not be administered chronically with Vitamin D medicinal products, as increased blood levels of aluminium and aluminium bone toxicity may occur.

4.6 Pregnancy and lactation

There is no adequate data on the use of paricalcitol in pregnant women. Animal studies have shown reproductive toxicity (see section 5.3). Potential risk in human use is not known, therefore paricalcitol should be not be used unless clearly necessary.

Lactation: It is not known whether paricalcitol is excreted in human milk. Animal studies have shown excretion of paricalcitol or its metabolites in breast milk, in small amounts. A decision on whether to continue/discontinue breastfeeding or to continue/discontinue therapy with Zemplar should be made taking into account the benefit of breastfeeding to the child and the benefit of Zemplar therapy to the woman.

4.7 Effects on ability to drive and use machines

No studies on the effects on the ability to drive or use machines have been performed, however, paricalcitol is expected to have negligible effect on the ability to drive or use machines.

4.8 Undesirable effects

__Chronic Kidney Disease, Stages 3 and 4__

The safety of paricalcitol capsules has been evaluated in three 24-week, double-blind, placebo-controlled, multicentre clinical trials involving 220 CKD Stage 3 and 4 patients. There were no statistically significant differences between the paricalcitol-treated patients and placebo-treated patients in the incidence of hypercalcaemia Zemplar (2/106, 2 %) vs placebo (0/111, 0 %) or elevated calcium phosphorus product Zemplar (13/106, 12%) vs placebo (7/111, 6%).

The most commonly reported adverse reaction for paricalcitol treated patients was rash, occurring in 2% of patients.

All adverse events at least possibly related to paricalcitol, both clinical and laboratory, are displayed in Table 3 by MedDRA System Organ Class, Preferred Term and frequency. The following frequency groupings are used: very common (≥1/10); common (≥1/100 to <1/10); uncommon (≥1/1,000 to <1/100); rare (≥1/10,000 to <1/1,000); very rare (<1/10,000), not known (cannot be estimated from the available data).

Table 3. Adverse Reactions Reported in Stages 3 and 4 CKD Clinical Studies

System Organ Class	Preferred Term	Frequency
Investigations	Hepatic Enzyme Abnormal	Uncommon
Nervous system disorders	Dizziness Dysgeusia	Uncommon Uncommon
Gastrointestinal disorders	Stomach discomfort Constipation Dry mouth	Common Uncommon Uncommon
Skin and subcutaneous tissue disorders	Rash Pruritus Urticaria	Common Uncommon Uncommon
Musculoskeletal and connective tissue disorders	Muscle spasms	Uncommon
Immune system disorders	Hypersensitivity	Uncommon

__Chronic Kidney Disease, Stage 5__

The safety of paricalcitol capsules has been evaluated in one 12-week, double-blind, placebo-controlled, multi-centre clinical trial involving 88 CKD Stage 5 patients. There were no statistically significant differences between the paricalcitol-treated patients and placebo-treated patients in the incidence of hypercalcaemia Zemplar (1/61, 2%) vs placebo (0/26, 0.0%), or elevated calcium phosphorus product Zemplar (6/61, 10%) vs placebo (1/26, 4%).

All adverse events at least possibly related to paricalcitol, both clinical and laboratory, are displayed in Table 4 by MedDRA System Organ Class, Preferred Term and frequency. The following frequency groupings are used: very common (≥1/10); common (≥1/100 to <1/10); uncommon (≥1/1,000 to <1/100); rare (≥1/10,000 to <1/1,000); very rare (<1/10,000), not known (cannot be estimated from the available data).

Table 4. Adverse Reactions Reported in Stage 5 CKD pivotal phase III Study

System Organ Class	Preferred Term	Frequency
Nervous system disorders	Dizziness	Common
Gastrointestinal disorders	Diarrhoea Gastroesophageal reflux disease	Common Common
Skin and subcutaneous tissue disorders	Acne	Common
Metabolism and nutrition disorders	Hypercalcaemia Hypocalcaemia Decreased appetite	Common Common Common
Reproductive system and breast disorders	Breast tenderness	Common

The following additional adverse reactions have been seen in clinical trials with Zemplar injection.

Common

Nervous system disorders: headache, dysgeusia

Skin and subcutaneous tissue disorders: pruritis

Endocrine disorders: hypoparathyroidism

Metabolism and nutrition disorders: hyperphosphataemia, hypercalcaemia

Uncommon

Investigations: heart rate irregular, bleeding time prolonged, aspartate aminotransferase increased, weight decreased

Cardiac disorders: cardiac arrest, atrial flutter, arrhythmia

Blood and lymphatic system disorders: neutropenia, leukopenia, anaemia, lymphadenopathy

Nervous system disorders: cerebrovascular accident, transient ischemic attack, coma, syncope, dizziness, myoclonus, paraesthesia, hypoesthesia

Eye disorders: glaucoma, conjunctivitis, ocular hyperaemia

Formula 1

$$\text{Titration dose (micrograms)} = \frac{\text{most recent iPTH level (pg/mL)}}{60}$$

OR

$$\text{Titration dose (micrograms)} = \frac{\text{most recent iPTH level (pmol/L)}}{7}$$

Ear and labyrinth disorders: ear discomfort

Respiratory, thoracic and mediastinal disorders: pulmonary oedema, epistaxis, dyspnoea, orthopnoea, wheezing, cough

Gastrointestinal disorders: intestinal ischaemia, rectal haemmorrhage, gastritis, dysphagia, irritable bowel syndrome, diarrhoea, constipation, dyspepsia, vomiting, nausea, dry mouth, stomach discomfort

Skin and subcutaneous tissue disorders: rash pruritic, rash, blister, alopecia, hirsutism, night sweats, injection site pain, skin burning sensation,

Musculoskeletal and connective tissue disorders: arthralgia, myalgia, back pain, joint stiffness, muscle twitching

Endocrine disorders: hyperparathyroidism

Metabolism and nutrition disorders: anorexia, decreased appetite

Infections and infestations: sepsis, pneumonia, influenza, upper respiratory tract infection, nasopharyngitis, vaginal infection

Neoplasms benign, malignant, unspecified (including cysts and polyps): breast cancer

Vascular disorders: hypotension, hypertension

General disorders and administration site conditions: chest pain, gait disturbance, oedema, peripheral, oedema, swelling, chest discomfort, pyrexia, asthenia, pain, fatigue, malaise, thirst, feeling abnormal, Immune system disorders: hypersensitivity

Reproductive system and breast disorders: breast pain, erectile dysfunction

Psychiatric disorders: delirium, confusional state, agitation, sleep disorder, insomnia, nervousness, restlessness.

Post-marketing adverse reactions reported with Zemplar injection:

Immune system disorders: hypersensitivity

Skin and subcutaneous tissue disorders: angioedema, laryngeal oedema, urticaria.

4.9 Overdose

Excessive administration of Zemplar capsules can cause hypercalcaemia, hypercalciuria, hyperphosphataemia, and over suppression of parathyroid hormone. High intake of calcium and phosphate concomitant with Zemplar capsules may lead to similar abnormalities.

Treatment of patients with clinically significant hypercalcaemia consists of immediate dose reduction or interruption of paricalcitol therapy and includes a low calcium diet, withdrawal of calcium supplements, patient mobilisation, attention to fluid and electrolyte imbalances, assessment of electrocardiographic abnormalities (critical in patients receiving digitalis), and haemodialysis or peritoneal dialysis against a calcium-free dialysate, as warranted.

Signs and symptoms of vitamin D intoxication associated with hypercalcaemia include:

Early: Weakness, headache, somnolence, nausea, vomiting, dry mouth, constipation, muscle pain, bone pain and metallic taste.

Late: Anorexia, weight loss, conjunctivitis (calcific), pancreatitis, photophobia, rhinorrhoea, pruritis, hyperthermia, decreased libido, elevated BUN, hypercholesterolaemia, elevated AST and ALT, ectopic calcification, hypertension, cardiad arrhythmias, somnolence, death and rarely, overt psychosis.

Serum calcium levels should be monitored frequently until normocalcaemia ensues.

Paricalcitol is not significantly removed by dialysis.

5. PHARMACOLOGICAL PROPERTIES

5.1 Pharmacodynamic properties

Pharmacotherapeutic group: vitamin D analog, ATC code: A11CC07

Mechanism of Action

Paricalcitol is a synthetic, biologically active vitamin D analog of calcitriol with modifications to the side chain (D_2) and the A (19-nor) ring allowing for selective vitamin D receptor (VDR) activation. Paricalcitol selectively upregulates the VDR in the parathyroid glands without increasing VDR in the intestine and is less active on bone resorption. Paricalcitol also upregulates the calcium sensing receptor in the parathyroid glands. As a result, paricalcitol reduces parathyroid hormone (PTH) levels by inhibiting parathyroid proliferation and decreasing PTH synthesis and secretion, with minimal impact on calcium and phosphorus levels, and can act directly on bone cells to maintain bone volume and improve mineralization surfaces. Correcting abnormal PTH levels, with normalisation of calcium and phosphorus homeostasis, may prevent or treat the metabolic bone disease associated with chronic kidney disease.

Clinical Efficacy

Chronic Kidney Disease, Stages 3-4

The primary efficacy endpoint of at least two consecutive $\geqslant$ 30 % reductions from baseline iPTH was achieved by 91% of paricalcitol capsules-treated patients and 13% of the placebo patients ($p < 0.001$). Serum bone specific alkaline phosphatase like serum osteocalcin were significantly reduced ($p < 0.001$) in patients treated with paricalcitol capsules compared to placebo, which is associated with a correction of the high bone turnover due to secondary hyperparathyroidism. No deterioration in the kidney function parameters of estimated glomerular filtration rate (via MDRD formula) and serum creatinine was detected in paricalcitol capsules treated patients in comparison to placebo treated patients. Significantly more of paricalcitol capsules treated patients experienced a reduction in urinary protein, as measured by semiquantitative dipstick, compared to placebo treated patients.

Chronic kidney disease, Stage 5

The primary efficacy endpoint of at least two consecutive $\geqslant$ 30 % reductions from baseline iPTH was achieved by 88% of paricalcitol capsules treated patients and 13% of the placebo patients ($p < 0.001$).

Paediatric clinical data with Zemplar Injection (IV)

The safety and effectiveness of Zemplar IV were examined in a 12-week randomised, double-blind, placebo-controlled study of 29 pediatric patients, aged 5-19 years, with end-stage renal disease on hemodialysis. The six youngest Zemplar IV-treated patients in the study were 5 - 12 years old. The initial dose of Zemplar IV was 0.04 mcg/kg 3 times per week, based on baseline iPTH level of less than 500 pg/mL, or 0.08 mcg/kg 3 times a week based on baseline iPTH level of $\geqslant$ 500 pg/mL, respectively. The dose of Zemplar IV was adjusted in 0.04 mcg/kg increments based on the levels of serum iPTH, calcium, and Ca $\times$ P. 67% of the Zemplar IV-treated patients and 14% placebo-treated patients completed the trial. 60% of the subjects in the Zemplar IV group had 2 consecutive 30% decreases from baseline iPTH compared with 21% patients in the placebo group. 71% of the placebo patients were discontinued due to excessive elevations in iPTH levels. No subjects in either the Zemplar IV group or placebo group developed hypercalcemia. No data are available for patients under the age of 5.

5.2 Pharmacokinetic properties

Absorption

Paricalcitol is well absorbed. In healthy subjects, following oral administration of paricalcitol at 0.24 micrograms/kg, the mean absolute bioavailability was approximately 72%; the maximum plasma concentration (C_{max}) was 0.630 ng/mL (1.512 pmol/mL) at 3 hours and area under the concentration time curve ($AUC_{0-\infty}$) was 5.25 ng•h/mL (12.60 pmol•h/mL). The mean absolute bioavailability of paricalcitol in hemodialysis (HD) and peritoneal dialysis (PD) patients is 79% and 86%, respectively, with the upper bound of 95% confidence interval of 93% and 112%, respectively. A food interaction study in healthy subjects indicated that the C_{max} and $AUC_{0-\infty}$ were unchanged when paricalcitol was administered with a high fat meal compared to fasting. Therefore, Zemplar Capsules may be taken without regard to food.

The C_{max} and $AUC_{0-\infty}$ of paricalcitol increased proportionally over the dose range of 0.06 to 0.48 micrograms/kg in healthy subjects. Following multiple dosing, either as daily or three times a week in healthy subjects, steady-state exposure was reached within seven days.

Distribution

Paricalcitol is extensively bound to plasma proteins (> 99%). The ratio of blood paricalcitol to plasma paricalcitol concentration averaged 0.54 over the concentration range of 0.01 to 10 ng/mL (0.024 to 24 pmol/mL) indicating that very little drug associated with blood cells. The mean apparent volume of distribution following a 0.24 micrograms/kg dose of paricalcitol in healthy subjects was 34 litres.

Metabolism and Excretion

After oral administration of a 0.48 micrograms/kg dose of ^{3}H-paricalcitol, parent drug was extensively metabolised, with only about 2% of the dose eliminated unchanged in the faeces, and no parent drug found in the urine. Approximately 70% of the radioactivity was eliminated in the faeces and 18% was recovered in the urine. Most of the systemic exposure was from the parent drug. Two minor metabolites, relative to paricalcitol, were detected in human plasma. One metabolite was identified as 24(R)-hydroxy paricalcitol, while the other metabolite was unidentified. The 24(R)-hydroxy paricalcitol is less active than paricalcitol in an *in vivo* rat model of PTH suppression.

In vitro data suggest that paricalcitol is metabolised by multiple hepatic and non-hepatic enzymes, including mitochondrial CYP24, as well as CYP3A4 and UGT1A4. The identified metabolites include the product of 24(R)-hydroxylation, as well as 24,26- and 24,28-dihydroxylation and direct glucuronidation.

Elimination

In healthy subjects, the mean elimination half-life of paricalcitol is five to seven hours over the studied dose range of 0.06 to 0.48 micrograms/kg. The degree of accumulation was consistent with the half-life and dosing frequency. Haemodialysis procedure has essentially no effect on paricalcitol elimination.

Special Populations

Elderly

The pharmacokinetics of paricalcitol have not been investigated in patients greater than 65 years.

Paediatric

The pharmacokinetics of paricalcitol have not been investigated in patients less than 18 years of age.

Gender

The pharmacokinetics of paricalcitol following single doses over 0.06 to 0.48 micrograms/kg dose range were gender independent.

Hepatic Impairment

In a study performed with Zemplar intravenous, the disposition of paricalcitol (0.24 micrograms/kg) was compared in patients with mild (n = 5) and moderate (n = 5) hepatic impairment (in accordance with the Child-Pugh method) and subjects with normal hepatic function (n = 10). The pharmacokinetics of unbound paricalcitol was similar across the range of hepatic function evaluated in this study. No dosing adjustment is required in patients with mild to moderate hepatic impairment. The influence of severe hepatic impairment on the pharmacokinetics of paricalcitol has not been evaluated.

Renal Impairment

Paricalcitol pharmacokinetics following single dose administration were characterised in patients with CKD Stage 3 or moderate renal impairment (n = 15, GFR = 36.9 to 59.1 mL/min/1.73 m^2), CKD Stage 4 or severe renal impairment (n = 14, GFR = 13.1 to 29.4 mL/min/1.73 m^2), and CKD 5 or end-stage renal disease [n = 14 in haemodialysis (HD) and n = 8 in peritoneal dialysis (PD)]. Similar to endogenous 1,25$(OH)_2$ D_3, the pharmacokinetics of paricalcitol following oral administration were affected significantly by renal impairment, as shown in Table 5. Compared to healthy subjects results obtained, Chronic Kidney Disease, Stage 3, 4, and 5 patients showed decreased CL/F and increased half-life.

Table 5. Comparison of Mean ± SD Pharmacokinetic Parameters in Different Stages of Renal Impairment *versus* Healthy Subjects

(see Table 5 on next page)

Following oral administration of paricalcitol capsules, the pharmacokinetic profile of paricalcitol for Chronic kidney disease, Stages 3 to 5 was comparable. Therefore, no special dosing adjustments are required other than those recommended (see section 4.2).

5.3 Preclinical safety data

Salient findings in the repeat-dose toxicology studies in rodents and dogs were generally attributed to paricalcitol's calcaemic activity. Effects not clearly related to hypercalcaemia included decreased white blood cell counts and thymic atrophy in dogs, and altered APTT values (increased in dogs, decreased in rats). WBC changes were not observed in clinical trials of paricalcitol.

Paricalcitol did not affect fertility in rats and there was no evidence of teratogenic activity in rats or rabbits. High doses of other vitamin D preparations applied during pregnancy in animals lead to teratogenesis. Paricalcitol was shown to affect fetal viability, as well as to promote a significant increase of peri-natal and post-natal mortality of newborn rats, when administered at maternally toxic doses.

Paricalcitol did not exhibit genotoxic potential in a set of *in-vitro* and *in-vivo* genotoxicity assays.

Carcinogenicity studies in rodents did not indicate any special risks for human use.

Doses administered and/or systemic exposures to paricalcitol were slightly higher than therapeutic doses/systemic exposures.

6. PHARMACEUTICAL PARTICULARS

6.1 List of excipients

Capsule contents:

Medium chain triglycerides

Ethanol

Butylhydroxytoluene

Capsule shell:

1 microgram	2 microgram	4 microgram
Gelatin	Gelatin	Gelatin
Glycerol	Glycerol	Glycerol
Water	Water	Water
Titanium dioxide (E171)	Titanium dioxide (E171)	Titanium dioxide (E171)
Iron oxide black (E172)	Iron oxide red (E172) Iron oxide yellow (E172)	Iron oxide yellow (E172)

Black Ink:

Propylene glycol

Black iron oxide (E172)

Polyvinyl acetate phthalate

Polyethylene glycol 400

Ammonium hydroxide

6.2 Incompatibilities

Not applicable.

6.3 Shelf life

2 years

6.4 Special precautions for storage

This medicinal product does not require any special storage conditions.

Table 5. Comparison of Mean ± SD Pharmacokinetic Parameters in Different Stages of Renal Impairment *versus* Healthy Subjects

Pharmacokinetic Parameter	Healthy Subjects	CKD Stage 3	CKD Stage 4	CKD Stage 5	
				HD	PD
N	25	15	14	14	8
Dose (micrograms/kg)	0.240	0.047	0.036	0.240	0.240
CL/F (L/h)	3.6 ± 1.0	1.8 ± 0.5	1.5 ± 0.4	1.8 ± 0.8	1.8 ± 0.8
$t_{1/2}$(h)	5.9 ± 2.8	16.8 ± 2.6	19.7 ± 7.2	13.9 ± 5.1	17.7 ± 9.6
f_u* (%)	0.06 ± 0.01	0.06 ± 0.01	0.07 ± 0.02	0.09 ± 0.04	0.13 ± 0.08

* Measured at 15 nM paricalcitol concentration.

6.5 Nature and contents of container
High-density polyethylene (HDPE) bottles closed with polypropylene caps. Each bottle contains 30 capsules.

PVC/fluoropolymer/aluminium blister packs containing 7 or 28 capsules. Each carton contains 1 or 4 blisters. Each blister foil card contains 7 capsules.

Not all pack sizes may be marketed.

6.6 Special precautions for disposal and other handling
No special requirements.

7. MARKETING AUTHORISATION HOLDER
Abbott Laboratories Limited,
Queenborough,
Kent ME11 5EL,
United Kingdom

8. MARKETING AUTHORISATION NUMBER(S)
Zemplar 1 microgram capsules, soft: PL 00037/0626

Zemplar 2 micrograms capsules, soft: PL 00037/0627

Zemplar 4 micrograms capsules, soft: PL 00037/0628

9. DATE OF FIRST AUTHORISATION/RENEWAL OF THE AUTHORISATION
6 December 2007

10. DATE OF REVISION OF THE TEXT

Zeridame SR Prolonged Release Tablets 100mg

(Actavis UK Ltd)

1. NAME OF THE MEDICINAL PRODUCT
Zeridame SR 100mg Prolonged Release Tablets

2. QUALITATIVE AND QUANTITATIVE COMPOSITION
One prolonged-release tablet contains 100mg tramadol hydrochloride.

For a full list of excipients, see section 6.1.

3. PHARMACEUTICAL FORM
Prolonged-release tablet.

Zeridame SR 100mg Prolonged Release Tablets are off white, round biconvex tablets, 9.1 mm diameter.

4. CLINICAL PARTICULARS
4.1 Therapeutic indications
Treatment of moderate to severe pain.

4.2 Posology and method of administration
Route of Administration

Oral use

Posology

The dose should be adjusted to the severity of the pain and the individual clinical response of the patient.

For doses not realisable / practicable with this medicinal product, other strengths of this medicinal product are available.

Unless otherwise prescribed, Zeridame SR Prolonged Release Tablets should be given as follows:

Adults and adolescents older than 12 years:

The usual initial dose is 100mg, twice daily, in the morning and evening.

Dependent upon the needs of the patient, subsequent doses may be administered earlier than 12 hours, but must not be administered earlier than 8 hours after the previous dose. **Under no circumstances should more than two doses be taken in any one 24 hour period.**

If the painkilling is insufficient, the dose may be increased to:

150mg, twice daily or

200mg, twice daily.

Zeridame SR Prolonged Release Tablets should be swallowed completely, without breaking or chewing, independent of meals, with sufficient liquid.

The smallest effective analgesic dose should always be used. Daily doses of 400 mg of active substance must not be exceeded, unless exceptional medical reasons require so.

Under no circumstances should Zeridame SR be used for longer than absolutely necessary.

If long-term pain treatment with tramadol is necessary in view of the nature and severity of the illness, then careful and regular monitoring should be carried out (if necessary with breaks in treatment) to establish whether, and to what extent, further treatment is necessary.

Children

Zeridame SR is not suitable for children under the age of 12 years.

Elderly

As a rule adjustment of the dose, in elderly patients (up to 75 years) without any clinical manifestations of hepatic or renal impairment, is not necessary.

In elderly patients (over 75 years) elimination may be prolonged. Therefore, if necessary the dosage interval is to be extended according to the patient's requirements.

Renal impairment, dialysis and hepatic impairment

In patients with serious renal or hepatic impairment the use of Zeridame SR is not recommended. In moderate cases, an adjustment of the dosage interval may be considered.

4.3 Contraindications
Zeridame SR Prolonged Release Tablets must not be used in:

- hypersensitivity to tramadol hydrochloride, or to any of the excipients in the medicinal product (see section 6.1),

- in acute intoxication with alcohol, hypnotics, analgesics, opioids or psychotropic drugs.

- in patients receiving MAO – inhibitors, or within 2 weeks of their withdrawal.

- in patients with epilepsy not adequately controlled by treatment

Zeridame SR Prolonged Release Tablets should not be used for opioid withdrawal treatment.

4.4 Special warnings and precautions for use
Zeridame SR should only be used following a strict benefit – risk evaluation and appropriate precautionary measures in the following cases: in patients dependent on opioids, patients suffering head injuries, shock, decreased level of consciousness of unknown origin, disturbances of the respiratory centre or function, or increased intracranial pressure, patients with moderate to severe impaired liver or kidney function.

Zeridame SR should not be used in combination with alcohol.

In patients sensitive for opioids the medicine should be used cautiously.

Convulsions have been reported at therapeutic doses and the risk may be increased at doses exceeding the usual upper daily dose limit (400 mg).

The risk on convulsions may increase in patients taking tramadol and concomitant medication that can lower the seizure threshold. (see section 4.5). Patients with a history of epilepsy or those susceptible to seizures should only be treated with tramadol if there are compelling reasons.

Tramadol has a low dependence potential. On long-term use tolerance, psychic and physical dependence may develop. In patients with a tendency to drug abuse or dependence, treatment should be for short periods under strict medical supervision.

Tramadol is not a suitable substitute in opioid dependent patients. The product does not suppress morphine withdrawal symptoms although it is an opioid agonist.

4.5 Interaction with other medicinal products and other forms of interaction
Tramadol / MAO – inhibitors

Zeridame SR should not be combined with MAO-inhibitors (see section 4.3). Life threatening interactions affecting the central nervous system as well as respiratory and cardiovascular function have been observed in patients who have been treated with MAO inhibitors within 14 days prior to the administration of the opioid pethidine. The same interactions with Zeridame SR as with MAO inhibitors cannot be ruled out.

Tramadol / Other centrally acting active substances

In concomitant use of Zeridame SR and other centrally acting drugs, including alcohol, a potentiation of CNS effects should be taken into consideration (See section 4.8).

Tramadol / Enzyme inhibitor / inducer

The results of pharmacokinetic research, so far, showed that no interactions need to be expected in concomitant or prior use of cimetidine (enzyme inhibitor).

The concomitant or prior use of carbamazepine (enzyme inducer) may reduce the analgesic effectiveness and shorten the duration of the action.

Tramadol / Mixed opioid agonists / antagonists

The combination of mixed agonists/antagonists (e.g. buprenorphine, nalbuphine, pentazocine) and tramadol is not recommended because it is theoretically possible that the analgesic effect of a pure agonist is attenuated under these circumstances.

Tramadol / Seizure threshold lowering drugs

Tramadol may induce convulsions and may increase the potential for selective serotonin re-uptake inhibitors, tricyclic antidepressants, anti-psychotics and other seizure threshold lowering drugs to cause convulsions.

Tramadol / Serotonergic agents

Isolated cases of serotonergic syndrome have been reported with the therapeutic use of tramadol in combination with other serotonergic agents such as selective serotonin re-uptake inhibitors (SSRIs). Serotonergic syndrome can be manifested by symptoms such as confusion, restlessness, fever, sweating, ataxia, hyperreflexia, myoclonia and diarrhoea. Withdrawal of the serotonergic agent produces a rapid improvement. It depends on the nature and severity of symptoms whether medicinal treatment is to be considered.

Tramadol / Coumarin derivatives

Caution should be exercised during concomitant treatment with tramadol and coumarin derivatives (e.g. warfarin) due to reports of increased INR and ecchymoses in some patients.

Tramadol / CYP3A4 Inhibitors

Other medicinal products with a known inhibiting effect on CYP3A4, such as ketoconazole and erythromycin, could inhibit the metabolism of tramadol (N-demethylation) and probably also the metabolism of the active O-demethyl-metabolite. The clinical relevancy of this interaction has not been investigated. (See section 4.8).

Tramadol / Ondansetron

In a limited number of studies the pre – or postoperative application of the antiemetic 5 – HT_3 antagonist ondansetron increased the requirement of tramadol in patients with postoperative pain.

4.6 Pregnancy and lactation
Animal tests with very large concentrations of tramadol showed effects on the development of the organs, bone formation and mortality of the neonate.

Teratogenic effects have not been found. Tramadol crosses the placenta, insufficient experience is available on the chronic use of tramadol during pregnancy. The repeated administration of tramadol during pregnancy can lead to increased tolerance of tramadol in the foetus and consequently to withdrawal symptoms in the new borne infant after birth, as a consequence of habituation. Therefore Zeridame SR should not be used during pregnancy.

Tramadol – administered before or during birth – does not affect uterine contractility. In neonates it may induce changes in the respiratory rate which are usually not clinically relevant.

When breastfeeding about 0.1 % of the tramadol dose administered is excreted in milk. Administration of Zeridame SR is not advised while breastfeeding.

In case of a once only administration of tramadol it is usually not required to discontinue breastfeeding.

4.7 Effects on ability to drive and use machines
Zeridame SR has minor or moderate influence on the ability to drive and use machines. It may cause drowsiness and blurred vision. This is especially applicable in combination with other psychotropic drugs, and alcohol. Ambulant patients should be warned not to drive or operate machinery if affected.

4.8 Undesirable effects
The most commonly reported adverse drug reactions are nausea and dizziness, both occurring in ≥ 1 / 10 of patients, very common.

Cardiovascular disorders:

Uncommon (≥ 1 / 1000 to 1 / 100): effects on cardiovascular regulation (palpitation, tachycardia, postural hypotension or cardiovascular collapse). These adverse effects may occur especially on intravenous administration and in patients who are physically stressed.

Rare (≥ 1 / 10000 to < 1 / 1000): bradycardia, increase in blood pressure.

Nervous system disorders:

Very common (≥ 1 / 10): dizziness

Common (≥ 1 / 100 to < 1 / 10): headache, drowsiness

Rare (≥1 / 10000 to < 1 / 1000): changes in appetite, paraesthesia, tremor, respiratory depression, epileptiform convulsions, involuntary muscle contractions, and syncope.

If the recommended doses are considerably exceeded and other centrally depressant substances are administered concomitantly (see section 4.5) respiratory depression may occur.

Epileptiform convulsions occurred mainly after administration of high doses of tramadol or after concomitant treatment with drugs, which can lower the seizure threshold or themselves induce cerebral convulsions (see section 4.4 and section 4.5)

Psychiatric disorders:

Rare (≥ 1 / 10000 to < 1 / 1000): hallucinations, confusion, anxiety, sleep distubances and nightmares. Psychic side-effects may vary individually in intensity and nature (depending on personality and duration of medication). These include changes in mood (usually elation, occasionally dysphoria), changes in activity (usually suppression, occasionally increase) and changes in cognitive and sensorial capacity (e.g. decision behaviour, perception disorders).

Dependence, abuse and addiction may occur.

Eye disorders:

Rare (≥ 1 / 10000 to < 1 / 1000): blurred vision

Respiratory disorders:

Worsening of asthma has also been reported, though a causal relationship has not been established.

Gastrointestinal disorders:

Very common (≥ 1 / 10): nausea

Common (≥ 1 / 100 to < 1 / 10): vomiting, constipation, dry mouth.

Uncommon (≥ 1 / 1000 to < 1 / 100): Retching, gastro-intestinal irritation (a feeling of pressure in the stomach, bloating).

Skin and subcutaneous tissue disorders:

Common (≥ 1 / 100 to < 1 / 10): sweating

Uncommon (≥ 1 / 1000 to < 1 / 100): dermal reactions (e.g. pruritus, rash, urticaria)

Musculoskeletal disorders:

Rare (≥ 1 / 10000 to < 1 / 1000): motorial weakness

Hepato-biliary disorders:

Very rare (< 1 / 10000) an increase in liver enzyme values has been reported after use of tramadol.

Renal and urinary system disorders:

Rare (≥ 1 / 10000 to < 1 / 1000): micturition disorders (difficulty in passing urine and urinary retention).

Immune system disorders:

Rare (≥ 1 / 10000 to < 1 / 1000): Allergic reactions (e.g. dyspnoea, bronchospasm, wheezing, angioneurotic oedema) and anaphylaxis;

General disorders:

Common (≥ 1 / 100 to < 1 / 10): fatigue.

Physical Dependence

Dependence, abuse, addiction, and withdrawal reactions may occur. Symptoms which occur on withdrawal, identical to withdrawal symptoms in opioids, may be: agitation, anxiety, nervousness, insomnia, hyperkinesia, tremor and gastro intestinal symptoms. Very rare (< 1/10000) atypical withdrawal symptoms have been reported: panic attack, severe anxiety, hallucinations, paraesthesia, tinnitus, and other unusual central nervous system symptoms.

4.9 Overdose

Symptoms

In tramadol intoxication, in principle, the same symptoms occur as for all other central acting analgesics (opioids). In particular, these include miosis, vomiting, cardiovascular collapse, narrowing of consciousness leading to coma, convulsions, respiratory depression leading to respiratory failure.

Treatment

General emergency measures are applicable.

Maintenance of the airway (aspiration), maintenance of respiration and cardiovascular circulation depending on the symptoms.

Emptying of the stomach by means of vomiting (patient to be conscious) or by means of pumping the stomach. Consideration should also be given to the administration of activated charcoal, if necessary via the stomach pump tube. Depending how long has elapsed from ingestion, administration of a suitable laxative to speed up elimination should be considered. In the event that the patient's conciousness is reduced, intubation prior to performing these procedures is essential.

The antidote for respiratory depression is naloxone.

In animal tests naloxone proved to be ineffective against convulsions.

In that case diazepam should be administered intravenously.

Tramadol is only minimally removed from plasma using haemodialysis, haemofiltration or haemoperfusion.

Therefore treatment of acute overdose of tramadol using haemodialysis or haemofiltration alone is not a suitable way of detoxification. Administration of a suitable laxative may help to speed up elimination of unabsorbed tramadol, if administered early after overdose.

5. PHARMACOLOGICAL PROPERTIES

5.1 Pharmacodynamic properties

ATC code N 02 AX 02: Pharmacotherapeutic group: Analgesics, other opioids

Tramadol is a centrally acting opioid analgesic.

It is a non-selective, partial agonist of μ-, δ- and κ-opioid receptors with a higher affinity for μ-receptors. Other mechanisms contributing to the analgesic effect are the inhibition of the neural noradrenaline reuptake, and an enhanced release of serotonin.

Tramadol has an antitussive action.

Contrary to morphine tramadol does not suppress respiration in analgetic doses over a large range.

The action on the cardiovascular system is minimal.

The potency of tramadol is reported to be 1 / 10 to 1 / 6 of morphine.

5.2 Pharmacokinetic properties

More than 90% of tramadol is absorbed after oral administration.

The mean absolute bioavailability is approximately 70 %, irrespective of concomitant intake of food.

The difference between absorbed and non – metabolised available tramadol is probably due to low first – pass effect. The first pass – effect after oral administration is a maximum of 30 %.

Tramadol has a high tissue affinity ($V_{d,\beta}$ = 203 ± 40 l). Protein binding is about 20 %.

After administration of Minular 100 mg SR Tablets the maximum peak plasma concentration C_{max} 141 ± 40 ng / ml is reached after 4.9 hours. After administration of Minular 200 mg SR Tablets a C_{max} 260 ± 62 ng / ml is reached after 4.8 hours.

Tramadol passes the blood – brain and placenta barrier. Very small amounts of the substance and its O – demethyl derivative are found in the breast – milk (0.1 % and 0.02 % respectively of the applied dose).

Elimination of half-life $t_{½\beta}$ is approximately 6 h, irrespective of the mode of administration. In patients above 75 years of age it may be prolonged by a factor of 1.4.

In humans tramadol is mainly metabolised by means of N – and O – demethylation and conjugation of the O – demethylation products with glucuronic acid. Only O – desmethyltramadol is pharmacologically active. There are considerable interindividual quantitative differences between the other metabolites. So far, eleven metabolites have been found in the urine. Animal experiments have shown that O – desmethyltramadol is more potent than the parent substance by the factor 2 – 4. Its half life $t_{½\beta}$ (6 healthy volunteers) is 7.9 h (range 5.4 – 9.6 h) and is approximately that of tramadol.

The inhibition of one or both cytochrome p450 isoenzymes, cyp3a4 and cyp2d6 involved in the metabolism of tramadol, may affect the plasma concentration of tramadol or its active metabolite. The clinical consequences of any such interactions are not known.

Tramadol and its metabolites are almost completely excreted via the kidneys. Cumulative urinary excretion is 90 % of the total radioactivity of the administered dose. In cases of impaired hepatic and renal function the half – life may be slightly prolonged. In patients with cirrhosis of the liver, elimination half – lives of 13.3 ± 4.9 h (tramadol) and 18.5 ± 9.4 h (O – desmethyltramadol), in an extreme case 22.3 h and 36 h respectively have been determined. In patients with renal insufficiency (creatinine clearance < 5 ml / min) the values were 11 ± 3.2 h and 16.9 ± 3 h, in an extreme case 19.5 h and 43.2 h, respectively.

Tramadol has a linear pharmacokinetic profile within the therapeutic dosage range.

The relationship between serum concentrations and the analgesic effect is dose – dependent, but varies considerably in isolated cases. A serum concentration of 100 – 300 ng / ml is usually effective.

5.3 Preclinical safety data

In repeated oral and parenteral administration of tramadol during 6 to 26 weeks to rats and dogs, as also during 12 months to dogs, there are no indications for changes caused by the substance in haematological, clinical – chemical and histological experiments.

Only after high doses, far above the therapeutic doses, central symptoms occurred: restlessness, salivation, convulsion, reduced increase in weight.

Rats and dogs tolerate the oral dose of 20 mg / kg resp 10 mg / kg bodyweight, dogs also tolerate 20 mg / kg bodyweight, rectally administered.

Tramadol doses as from 50 mg / kg / day cause intoxication of the mother, in rats, and result in an increased mortality in newborn rats.

In young rats development disorders occurred as ossification disturbances, delayed opening of the vagina and eyes.

The fertility of male rats was not influenced.

However the percentage of females with young reduced after high dosages (as of 50 mg / kg / day).

In rabbits, toxic effects occurred as of 125 mg / kg in the mother and skeletal anomalies in the offspring.

In some *in – vitro* test systems there is report on mutagenic effects.

In *in – vivo* experiments there was no indication for mutagenic effects.

On the basis of the knowledge available up till now it is unclear whether tramadol possesses mutagenic potential.

Experiments have been performed on rats and mice with regard to the tumuorigenic potential of tramadol.

From tests in rats it could not be shown that the substance increases the chance of tumours.

In tests in mice an increased incidence of liver – cell adenomas in males (depending on the dose, with an insignificant increase as of 15 mg / kg) and an increased chance of lung tumours in females in all dose selections (significant, but not dose dependent) was found.

6. PHARMACEUTICAL PARTICULARS

6.1 List of excipients

Calcium hydrogen phosphate dihydrate (E341),
Hydroxypropylcellulose (E463),
Colloidal anhydrous silica (E551),
Magnesium stearate (E470b).

6.2 Incompatibilities

Not applicable.

6.3 Shelf life

3 years

PP / PE tablet container: 6 months after opening

6.4 Special precautions for storage

Store in the original package in order to protect from moisture.

6.5 Nature and contents of container

Al / clear PVC blisters in carton boxes in packs of 10, 20, 30, 50, 60, 90, 100, 120, 180, and 500 tablets.

Al / opaque PVC child resistant blisters in carton boxes in packs of 10, 20, 30, 50, 60, 90, 100, 120, 180, and 500 tablets.

Polypropylene tablet container with polyethylene tamper evident closure containing 10, 20, 30, 50, 60, 90, 100, 120, 180, and 500 tablets.

Not all pack sizes may be marketed.

6.6 Special precautions for disposal and other handling

Any unused product or waste material should be disposed of in accordance with local requirements.

7. MARKETING AUTHORISATION HOLDER

Actavis Group hf
Reykjavíkurvegur 76-78
220 Hafnarfjordur
Iceland

8. MARKETING AUTHORISATION NUMBER(S)

PL 21231/0013

9. DATE OF FIRST AUTHORISATION/RENEWAL OF THE AUTHORISATION

10/08/2007

10. DATE OF REVISION OF THE TEXT

10/08/2007

Zeridame SR Prolonged Release Tablets 150mg

(Actavis UK Ltd)

1. NAME OF THE MEDICINAL PRODUCT

Zeridame SR 150mg Prolonged Release Tablets

2. QUALITATIVE AND QUANTITATIVE COMPOSITION

One prolonged-release tablet contains 150mg tramadol hydrochloride.

For a full list of excipients, see section 6.1.

3. PHARMACEUTICAL FORM

Prolonged-release tablet.

Zeridame SR 150mg Prolonged Release Tablets are off white, capsule shaped tablets, 14.3 mm long.

4. CLINICAL PARTICULARS

4.1 Therapeutic indications

Treatment of moderate to severe pain.

4.2 Posology and method of administration

Route of Administration

Oral use

Posology

The dose should be adjusted to the severity of the pain and the individual clinical response of the patient.

For doses not realisable / practicable with this medicinal product, other strengths of this medicinal product are available.

Unless otherwise prescribed, Zeridame SR Prolonged Release Tablets should be given as follows:

Adults and adolescents older than 12 years:

The usual initial dose is 100mg, twice daily, in the morning and evening.

Dependent upon the needs of the patient, subsequent doses may be administered earlier than 12 hours, but must not be administered earlier than 8 hours after the previous dose. **Under no circumstances should more than two doses be taken in any one 24 hour period.**

If the painkilling is insufficient, the dose may be increased to:

150mg, twice daily or 200mg, twice daily.

Zeridame SR Prolonged Release Tablets should be swallowed completely, without breaking or chewing, independent of meals, with sufficient liquid.

The smallest effective analgesic dose should always be used. Daily doses of 400 mg of active substance must not be exceeded, unless exceptional medical reasons require so.

Under no circumstances should Zeridame SR be used for longer than absolutely necessary.

If long-term pain treatment with tramadol is necessary in view of the nature and severity of the illness, then careful and regular monitoring should be carried out (if necessary with breaks in treatment) to establish whether, and to what extent, further treatment is necessary.

Children

Zeridame SR is not suitable for children under the age of 12 years.

Elderly

As a rule adjustment of the dose, in elderly patients (up to 75 years) without any clinical manifestations of hepatic or renal impairment, is not necessary.

In elderly patients (over 75 years) elimination may be prolonged. Therefore, if necessary the dosage interval is to be extended according to the patient's requirements.

Renal impairment, dialysis and hepatic impairment

In patients with serious renal or hepatic impairment the use of Zeridame SR is not recommended. In moderate cases, an adjustment of the dosage interval may be considered.

4.3 Contraindications

Zeridame SR Prolonged Release Tablets must not be used in:

- hypersensitivity to tramadol hydrochloride, or to any of the excipients in the medicinal product (see section 6.1),
- in acute intoxication with alcohol, hypnotics, analgesics, opioids or psychotropic drugs.
- in patients receiving MAO – inhibitors, or within 2 weeks of their withdrawal.
- in patients with epilepsy not adequately controlled by treatment

Zeridame SR Prolonged Release Tablets should not be used for opioid withdrawal treatment.

4.4 Special warnings and precautions for use

Zeridame SR should only be used following a strict benefit – risk evaluation and appropriate precautionary measures in the following cases: in patients dependent on opioids, patients suffering head injuries, shock, decreased level of consciousness of unknown origin, disturbances of the respiratory centre or function, or increased intracranial pressure, patients with moderate to severe impaired liver or kidney function.

Zeridame SR should not be used in combination with alcohol.

In patients sensitive for opioids the medicine should be used cautiously.

Convulsions have been reported at therapeutic doses and the risk may be increased at doses exceeding the usual upper daily dose limit (400 mg).

The risk on convulsions may increase in patients taking tramadol and concomitant medication that can lower the seizure threshold. (see section 4.5). Patients with a history of epilepsy or those susceptible to seizures should only be treated with tramadol if there are compelling reasons.

Tramadol has a low dependence potential. On long-term use tolerance, psychic and physical dependence may develop. In patients with a tendency to drug abuse or dependence, treatment should be for short periods under strict medical supervision.

Tramadol is not a suitable substitute in opioid dependent patients. The product does not suppress morphine withdrawal symptoms although it is an opioid agonist.

4.5 Interaction with other medicinal products and other forms of interaction

Tramadol / MAO – inhibitors

Zeridame SR should not be combined with MAO-inhibitors (see section 4.3). Life threatening interactions affecting the central nervous system as well as respiratory and cardiovascular function have been observed in patients who have been treated with MAO inhibitors within 14 days prior to the administration of the opioid pethidine. The same interactions with Zeridame SR as with MAO inhibitors cannot be ruled out.

Tramadol / Other centrally acting active substances

In concomitant use of Zeridame SR and other centrally acting drugs, including alcohol, a potentiation of CNS effects should be taken into consideration (See section 4.8).

Tramadol / Enzyme inhibitor / inducer

The results of pharmacokinetic research, so far, showed that no interactions need to be expected in concomitant or prior use of cimetidine (enzyme inhibitor).

The concomitant or prior use of carbamazepine (enzyme inducer) may reduce the analgesic effectiveness and shorten the duration of the action.

Tramadol / Mixed opioid agonists / antagonists

The combination of mixed agonists/antagonists (e.g. buprenorphine, nalbuphine, pentazocine) and tramadol is not recommended because it is theoretically possible that the analgesic effect of a pure agonist is attenuated under these circumstances.

Tramadol / Seizure threshold lowering drugs

Tramadol may induce convulsions and may increase the potential for selective serotonin re-uptake inhibitors, tricyclic antidepressants, anti-psychotics and other seizure threshold lowering drugs to cause convulsions.

Tramadol / Serotonergic agents

Isolated cases of serotonergic syndrome have been reported with the therapeutic use of tramadol in combination with other serotonergic agents such as selective serotonin re-uptake inhibitors (SSRIs). Serotonergic syndrome can be manifested by symptoms such as confusion, restlessness, fever, sweating, ataxia, hyperreflexia, myoclonia and diarrhoea. Withdrawal of the serotonergic agent produces a rapid improvement. It depends on the nature and severity of symptoms whether medicinal treatment is to be considered.

Tramadol / Coumarin derivatives

Caution should be exercised during concomitant treatment with tramadol and coumarin derivatives (e.g. warfarin) due to reports of increased INR and ecchymoses in some patients.

Tramadol / CYP3A4 Inhibitors

Other medicinal products with a known inhibiting effect on CYP3A4, such as ketoconazole and erythromycin, could inhibit the metabolism of tramadol (N-demethylation) and probably also the metabolism of the active O-demethylmetabolite. The clinical relevancy of this interaction has not been investigated. (See section 4.8).

Tramadol / Ondansetron

In a limited number of studies the pre – or postoperative application of the antiemetic 5 – HT_3 antagonist ondansetron increased the requirement of tramadol in patients with postoperative pain.

4.6 Pregnancy and lactation

Animal tests with very large concentrations of tramadol showed effects on the development of the organs, bone formation and mortality of the neonate.

Teratogenic effects have not been found. Tramadol crosses the placenta, insufficient experience is available on the chronic use of tramadol during pregnancy. The repeated administration of tramadol during pregnancy can lead to increased tolerance of tramadol in the foetus and consequently to withdrawal symptoms in the new borne infant after birth, as a consequence of habituation.

Therefore Zeridame SR should not be used during pregnancy.

Tramadol – administered before or during birth – does not affect uterine contractility. In neonates it may induce changes in the respiratory rate which are usually not clinically relevant.

When breastfeeding about 0.1 % of the tramadol dose administered is excreted in milk. Administration of Zeridame SR is not advised while breastfeeding.

In case of a once only administration of tramadol it is usually not required to discontinue breastfeeding.

4.7 Effects on ability to drive and use machines

Zeridame SR has minor or moderate influence on the ability to drive and use machines. It may cause drowsiness and blurred vision. This is especially applicable in combination with other psychotropic drugs, and alcohol. Ambulant patients should be warned not to drive or operate machinery if affected.

4.8 Undesirable effects

The most commonly reported adverse drug reactions are nausea and dizziness, both occurring in ≥ 1 / 10 of patients, very common.

Cardiovascular disorders:

Uncommon (≥ 1 / 1000 to 1 / 100): effects on cardiovascular regulation (palpitation, tachycardia, postural hypotension or cardiovascular collapse). These adverse effects may occur especially on intravenous administration and in patients who are physically stressed.

Rare (≥ 1 / 10000 to < 1 / 1000): bradycardia, increase in blood pressure.

Nervous system disorders:

Very common (≥ 1 / 10): dizziness

Common (≥ 1 / 100 to < 1 / 10): headache, drowsiness

Rare (≥1 / 10000 to < 1 / 1000): changes in appetite, paraesthesia, tremor, respiratory depression, epileptiform convulsions, involuntary muscle contractions, and syncope.

If the recommended doses are considerably exceeded and other centrally depressant substances are administered concomitantly (see section 4.5) respiratory depression may occur.

Epileptiform convulsions occurred mainly after administration of high doses of tramadol or after concomitant treatment with drugs, which can lower the seizure threshold or themselves induce cerebral convulsions (see section 4.4 and section 4.5)

Psychiatric disorders:

Rare (≥ 1 / 10000 to < 1 / 1000): hallucinations, confusion, anxiety, sleep distubances and nightmares. Psychic side-effects may vary individually in intensity and nature (depending on personality and duration of medication). These include changes in mood (usually elation, occasionally dysphoria), changes in activity (usually suppression, occasionally increase) and changes in cognitive and sensorial capacity (e.g. decision behaviour, perception disorders).

Dependence, abuse and addiction may occur.

Eye disorders:

Rare (≥ 1 / 10000 to < 1 / 1000): blurred vision

Respiratory disorders:

Worsening of asthma has also been reported, though a causal relationship has not been established.

Gastrointestinal disorders:

Very common (≥ 1 / 10): nausea

Common (≥ 1 / 100 to < 1 / 10): vomiting, constipation, dry mouth.

Uncommon (≥ 1 / 1000 to < 1 / 100): Retching, gastrointestinal irritation (a feeling of pressure in the stomach, bloating).

Skin and subcutaneous tissue disorders:

Common (≥ 1 / 100 to < 1 / 10): sweating

Uncommon (≥ 1 / 1000 to < 1 / 100): dermal reactions (e.g. pruritus, rash, urticaria)

Musculoskeletal disorders:

Rare (≥ 1 / 10000 to < 1 / 1000): motorial weakness

Hepato-biliary disorders:

Very rare (< 1 / 10000) an increase in liver enzyme values has been reported after use of tramadol.

Renal and urinary system disorders:

Rare (≥ 1 / 10000 to < 1 / 1000): micturition disorders (difficulty in passing urine and urinary retention).

Immune system disorders:

Rare (≥ 1 / 10000 to < 1 / 1000): Allergic reactions (e.g. dyspnoea, bronchospasm, wheezing, angioneurotic oedema) and anaphylaxis;

General disorders:

Common (≥ 1 / 100 to < 1 / 10): fatigue.

Physical Dependence

Dependence, abuse, addiction, and withdrawal reactions may occur. Symptoms which occur on withdrawal, identical to withdrawal symptoms in opioids, may be: agitation, anxiety, nervousness, insomnia, hyperkinesia, tremor and gastro intestinal symptoms. Very rare (< 1 / 10000) atypical withdrawal symptoms have been reported: panic attack, severe anxiety, hallucinations, paraesthesia, tinnitus, and other unusual central nervous system symptoms.

4.9 Overdose

Symptoms

In tramadol intoxication, in principle, the same symptoms occur as for all other central acting analgesics (opioids). In particular, these include miosis, vomiting, cardiovascular collapse, narrowing of consciousness leading to coma, convulsions, respiratory depression leading to respiratory failure.

Treatment

General emergency measures are applicable.

Maintenance of the airway (aspiration), maintenance of respiration and cardiovascular circulation depending on the symptoms.

Emptying of the stomach by means of vomiting (patient to be conscious) or by means of pumping the stomach. Consideration should also be given to the administration of activated charcoal, if necessary via the stomach pump tube. Depending how long has elapsed from ingestion, administration of a suitable laxative to speed up elimination should be considered. In the event that the patient's conciousness is reduced, intubation prior to performing these procedures is essential.

The antidote for respiratory depression is naloxone.

In animal tests naloxone proved to be ineffective against convulsions.

In that case diazepam should be administered intravenously.

Tramadol is only minimally removed from plasma using haemodialysis, haemofiltration or haemoperfusion.

Therefore treatment of acute overdose of tramadol using haemodialysis or haemofiltration alone is not a suitable way of detoxification. Administration of a suitable laxative may help to speed up elimination of unabsorbed tramadol, if administered early after overdose.

5. PHARMACOLOGICAL PROPERTIES

5.1 Pharmacodynamic properties

ATC code N 02 AX 02: Pharmacotherapeutic group: Analgesics, other opioids

Tramadol is a centrally acting opioid analgesic.

It is a non-selective, partial agonist of μ-, δ- and κ-opioid receptors with a higher affinity for μ-receptors. Other mechanisms contributing to the analgesic effect are the inhibition of the neural noradrenaline reuptake, and an enhanced release of serotonin.

Tramadol has an antitussive action.

Contrary to morphine tramadol does not suppress respiration in analgetic doses over a large range.

The action on the cardiovascular system is minimal.

The potency of tramadol is reported to be 1 / 10 to 1 / 6 of morphine.

5.2 Pharmacokinetic properties

More than 90% of tramadol is absorbed after oral administration.

The mean absolute bioavailability is approximately 70 %, irrespective of concomitant intake of food.

The difference between absorbed and non – metabolised available tramadol is probably due to low first – pass effect. The first pass – effect after oral administration is a maximum of 30 %.

Tramadol has a high tissue affinity ($V_{d,\beta}$ = 203 ± 40 l). Protein binding is about 20 %.

After administration of Minular 100 mg SR Tablets the maximum peak plasma concentration C_{max} 141 ± 40 ng / ml is reached after 4.9 hours. After administration of Minular 200 mg SR Tablets a C_{max} 260 ± 62 ng / ml is reached after 4.8 hours.

Tramadol passes the blood – brain and placenta barrier. Very small amounts of the substance and its O – demethyl derivative are found in the breast – milk (0.1 % and 0.02 % respectively of the applied dose).

Elimination of half-life $t_{½\beta}$ is approximately 6 h, irrespective of the mode of administration. In patients above 75 years of age it may be prolonged by a factor of 1.4.

In humans tramadol is mainly metabolised by means of N – and O – demethylation and conjugation of the O – demethylation products with glucuronic acid. Only O – desmethyltramadol is pharmacologically active. There are considerable interindividual quantitative differences between the other metabolites. So far, eleven metabolites have been found in the urine. Animal experiments have shown that O – desmethyltramadol is more potent than the parent substance by the factor 2 – 4. Its half life $t_{½\beta}$ (6 healthy volunteers) is 7.9 h (range 5.4 – 9.6 h) and is approximately that of tramadol.

The inhibition of one or both cytochrome p450 isoenzymes, cyp3a4 and cyp2d6 involved in the metabolism of tramadol, may affect the plasma concentration of tramadol or its active metabolite. The clinical consequences of any such interactions are not known.

Tramadol and its metabolites are almost completely excreted via the kidneys. Cumulative urinary excretion is 90 % of the total radioactivity of the administered dose. In cases of impaired hepatic and renal function the half – life may be slightly prolonged. In patients with cirrhosis of the liver, elimination half – lives of 13.3 ± 4.9 h (tramadol) and 18.5 ± 9.4 h (O – desmethyltramadol), in an extreme case 22.3 h and 36 h respectively have been determined. In patients with renal insufficiency (creatinine clearance < 5 ml / min) the values were 11 ± 3.2 h and 16.9 ± 3 h, in an extreme case 19.5 h and 43.2 h, respectively.

Tramadol has a linear pharmacokinetic profile within the therapeutic dosage range.

The relationship between serum concentrations and the analgesic effect is dose – dependent, but varies considerably in isolated cases. A serum concentration of 100 – 300 ng / ml is usually effective.

5.3 Preclinical safety data

In repeated oral and parenteral administration of tramadol during 6 to 26 weeks to rats and dogs, as also during 12 months to dogs, there are no indications for changes caused by the substance in haematological, clinical – chemical and histological experiments.

Only after high doses, far above the therapeutic doses, central symptoms occurred: restlessness, salivation, convulsion, reduced increase in weight.

Rats and dogs tolerate the oral dose of 20 mg / kg resp 10 mg / kg bodyweight, dogs also tolerate 20 mg / kg bodyweight, rectally administered.

Tramadol doses as from 50 mg / kg / day cause intoxication of the mother, in rats, and result in an increased mortality in newborn rats.

In young rats development disorders occurred as ossification disturbances, delayed opening of the vagina and eyes.

The fertility of male rats was not influenced.

However the percentage of females with young reduced after high dosages (as of 50 mg / kg / day).

In rabbits, toxic effects occurred as of 125 mg / kg in the mother and skeletal anomalies in the offspring.

In some *in – vitro* test systems there is report on mutagenic effects.

In *in – vivo* experiments there was no indication for mutagenic effects.

On the basis of the knowledge available up till now it is unclear whether tramadol possesses mutagenic potential.

Experiments have been performed on rats and mice with regard to the tumuorigenic potential of tramadol.

From tests in rats it could not be shown that the substance increases the chance of tumours.

In tests in mice an increased incidence of liver – cell adenomas in males (depending on the dose, with an insignificant increase as of 15 mg / kg) and an increased chance of lung tumours in females in all dose selections (significant, but not dose dependent) was found.

6. PHARMACEUTICAL PARTICULARS

6.1 List of excipients

Calcium hydrogen phosphate dihydrate (E341),

Hydroxypropylcellulose (E463),

Colloidal anhydrous silica (E551),

Magnesium stearate (E470b).

6.2 Incompatibilities

Not applicable.

6.3 Shelf life

3 years

PP / PE tablet container: 6 months after opening

6.4 Special precautions for storage

Store in the original package in order to protect from moisture.

6.5 Nature and contents of container

Al / clear PVC blisters in carton boxes in packs of 10, 20, 30, 50, 60, 90, 100, 120, 180, and 500 tablets.

Al / opaque PVC child resistant blisters in carton boxes in packs of 10, 20, 30, 50, 60, 90, 100, 120, 180, and 500 tablets.

Polypropylene tablet container with polyethylene tamper evident closure containing 10, 20, 30, 50, 60, 90, 100, 120, 180, and 500 tablets.

Not all pack sizes may be marketed.

6.6 Special precautions for disposal and other handling

Any unused product or waste material should be disposed of in accordance with local requirements.

7. MARKETING AUTHORISATION HOLDER

Actavis Group hf

Reykjavíkurvegur 76-78

220 Hafnarfjordur

Iceland

8. MARKETING AUTHORISATION NUMBER(S)

PL 21231/0014

9. DATE OF FIRST AUTHORISATION/RENEWAL OF THE AUTHORISATION

10/08/2007

10. DATE OF REVISION OF THE TEXT

10/08/2007

Zeridame SR Prolonged Release Tablets 200mg

(Actavis UK Ltd)

1. NAME OF THE MEDICINAL PRODUCT

Zeridame SR 200mg Prolonged Release Tablets

2. QUALITATIVE AND QUANTITATIVE COMPOSITION

One prolonged-release tablet contains 200mg tramadol hydrochloride.

For a full list of excipients, see section 6.1.

3. PHARMACEUTICAL FORM

Prolonged-release tablet.

Zeridame SR 200mg Prolonged Release Tablets are off white, capsule shaped tablets 17.1 mm long.

4. CLINICAL PARTICULARS

4.1 Therapeutic indications

Treatment of moderate to severe pain.

4.2 Posology and method of administration

Route of Administration

Oral use

Posology

The dose should be adjusted to the severity of the pain and the individual clinical response of the patient.

For doses not realisable / practicable with this medicinal product, other strengths of this medicinal product are available.

Unless otherwise prescribed, Zeridame SR Prolonged Release Tablets should be given as follows:

Adults and adolescents older than 12 years:

The usual initial dose is 100mg, twice daily, in the morning and evening.

Dependent upon the needs of the patient, subsequent doses may be administered earlier than 12 hours, but must not be administered earlier than 8 hours after the previous dose. **Under no circumstances should more than two doses be taken in any one 24 hour period.**

If the painkilling is insufficient, the dose may be increased to:

150mg, twice daily or

200mg, twice daily.

Zeridame SR Prolonged Release Tablets should be swallowed completely, without breaking or chewing, independent of meals, with sufficient liquid.

The smallest effective analgesic dose should always be used. Daily doses of 400 mg of active substance must not be exceeded, unless exceptional medical reasons require so.

Under no circumstances should Zeridame SR be used for longer than absolutely necessary.

If long-term pain treatment with tramadol is necessary in view of the nature and severity of the illness, then careful and regular monitoring should be carried out (if necessary with breaks in treatment) to establish whether, and to what extent, further treatment is necessary.

Children

Zeridame SR is not suitable for children under the age of 12 years.

Elderly

As a rule adjustment of the dose, in elderly patients (up to 75 years) without any clinical manifestations of hepatic or renal impairment, is not necessary.

In elderly patients (over 75 years) elimination may be prolonged. Therefore, if necessary the dosage interval is to be extended according to the patient's requirements.

Renal impairment, dialysis and hepatic impairment

In patients with serious renal or hepatic impairment the use of Zeridame SR is not recommended. In moderate cases, an adjustment of the dosage interval may be considered.

4.3 Contraindications

Zeridame SR Prolonged Release Tablets must not be used in:

- hypersensitivity to tramadol hydrochloride, or to any of the excipients in the medicinal product (see section 6.1),
- in acute intoxication with alcohol, hypnotics, analgesics, opioids or psychotropic drugs.
- in patients receiving MAO – inhibitors, or within 2 weeks of their withdrawal.
- in patients with epilepsy not adequately controlled by treatment

Zeridame SR Prolonged Release Tablets should not be used for opioid withdrawal treatment.

4.4 Special warnings and precautions for use

Zeridame SR should only be used following a strict benefit – risk evaluation and appropriate precautionary measures in the following cases: in patients dependent on opioids, patients suffering head injuries, shock, decreased level of consciousness of unknown origin, disturbances of the respiratory centre or function, or increased intracranial pressure, patients with moderate to severe impaired liver or kidney function.

Zeridame SR should not be used in combination with alcohol.

In patients sensitive for opioids the medicine should be used cautiously.

Convulsions have been reported at therapeutic doses and the risk may be increased at doses exceeding the usual upper daily dose limit (400 mg).

The risk on convulsions may increase in patients taking tramadol and concomitant medication that can lower the seizure threshold. (see section 4.5). Patients with a history of epilepsy or those susceptible to seizures should only be treated with tramadol if there are compelling reasons.

Tramadol has a low dependence potential. On long-term use tolerance, psychic and physical dependence may develop. In patients with a tendency to drug abuse or dependence, treatment should be for short periods under strict medical supervision.

Tramadol is not a suitable substitute in opioid dependent patients. The product does not suppress morphine withdrawal symptoms although it is an opioid agonist.

4.5 Interaction with other medicinal products and other forms of interaction

Tramadol / MAO – inhibitors

Zeridame SR should not be combined with MAO-inhibitors (see section 4.3). Life threatening interactions affecting the central nervous system as well as respiratory and cardiovascular function have been observed in patients who have been treated with MAO inhibitors within 14 days prior to the administration of the opioid pethidine. The same interactions with Zeridame SR as with MAO inhibitors cannot be ruled out.

Tramadol / Other centrally acting active substances

In concomitant use of Zeridame SR and other centrally acting drugs, including alcohol, a potentiation of CNS effects should be taken into consideration (See section 4.8).

Tramadol / Enzyme inhibitor / inducer

The results of pharmacokinetic research, so far, showed that no interactions need to be expected in concomitant or prior use of cimetidine (enzyme inhibitor).

The concomitant or prior use of carbamazepine (enzyme inducer) may reduce the analgesic effectiveness and shorten the duration of the action.

Tramadol / Mixed opioid agonists / antagonists

The combination of mixed agonists/antagonists (e.g. buprenorphine, nalbuphine, pentazocine) and tramadol is not recommended because it is theoretically possible that the analgesic effect of a pure agonist is attenuated under these circumstances.

Tramadol / Seizure threshold lowering drugs

Tramadol may induce convulsions and may increase the potential for selective serotonin re-uptake inhibitors, tricyclic antidepressants, anti-psychotics and other seizure threshold lowering drugs to cause convulsions.

Tramadol / Serotonergic agents

Isolated cases of serotonergic syndrome have been reported with the therapeutic use of tramadol in combination with other serotonergic agents such as selective serotonin re-uptake inhibitors (SSRIs). Serotonergic syndrome can be manifested by symptoms such as confusion, restlessness, fever, sweating, ataxia, hyperreflexia, myoclonia and diarrhoea. Withdrawal of the serotonergic agent produces a rapid improvement. It depends on the nature and severity of symptoms whether medicinal treatment is to be considered.

Tramadol / Coumarin derivatives

Caution should be exercised during concomitant treatment with tramadol and coumarin derivatives (e.g. warfarin) due to reports of increased INR and ecchymoses in some patients.

Tramadol / CYP3A4 Inhibitors

Other medicinal products with a known inhibiting effect on CYP3A4, such as ketoconazole and erythromycin, could inhibit the metabolism of tramadol (N-demethylation) and probably also the metabolism of the active O-demethyl-metabolite. The clinical relevancy of this interaction has not been investigated. (See section 4.8).

Tramadol / Ondansetron

In a limited number of studies the pre – or postoperative application of the antiemetic 5 – HT_3 antagonist ondansetron increased the requirement of tramadol in patients with postoperative pain.

4.6 Pregnancy and lactation

Animal tests with very large concentrations of tramadol showed effects on the development of the organs, bone formation and mortality of the neonate.

Teratogenic effects have not been found. Tramadol crosses the placenta, insufficient experience is available on the chronic use of tramadol during pregnancy. The repeated administration of tramadol during pregnancy can lead to increased tolerance of tramadol in the foetus and consequently to withdrawal symptoms in the new borne infant after birth, as a consequence of habituation. Therefore Zeridame SR should not be used during pregnancy.

Tramadol – administered before or during birth – does not affect uterine contractility. In neonates it may induce changes in the respiratory rate which are usually not clinically relevant.

When breastfeeding about 0.1 % of the tramadol dose administered is excreted in milk. Administration of Zeridame SR is not advised while breastfeeding.

In case of a once only administration of tramadol it is usually not required to discontinue breastfeeding.

4.7 Effects on ability to drive and use machines

Zeridame SR has minor or moderate influence on the ability to drive and use machines. It may cause drowsiness and blurred vision. This is especially applicable in combination with other psychotropic drugs, and alcohol. Ambulant patients should be warned not to drive or operate machinery if affected.

4.8 Undesirable effects

The most commonly reported adverse drug reactions are nausea and dizziness, both occurring in ≥ 1 / 10 of patients, very common.

Cardiovascular disorders:

Uncommon (≥ 1 / 1000 to 1 / 100): effects on cardiovascular regulation (palpitation, tachycardia, postural hypotension or cardiovascular collapse). These adverse effects may occur especially on intravenous administration and in patients who are physically stressed.

Rare (≥ 1 / 10000 to < 1 / 1000): bradycardia, increase in blood pressure.

Nervous system disorders:

Very common (≥ 1 / 10): dizziness

Common (≥ 1 / 100 to < 1 / 10): headache, drowsiness

Rare (≥1 / 10000 to < 1 / 1000): changes in appetite, paraesthesia, tremor, respiratory depression, epileptiform convulsions, involuntary muscle contractions, and syncope.

If the recommended doses are considerably exceeded and other centrally depressant substances are administered concomitantly (see section 4.5) respiratory depression may occur.

Epileptiform convulsions occurred mainly after administration of high doses of tramadol or after concomitant treatment with drugs, which can lower the seizure threshold or themselves induce cerebral convulsions (see section 4.4 and section 4.5)

Psychiatric disorders:

Rare (≥ 1 / 10000 to < 1 / 1000): hallucinations, confusion, anxiety, sleep distubances and nightmares. Psychic side-effects may vary individually in intensity and nature (depending on personality and duration of medication). These include changes in mood (usually elation, occasionally dysphoria), changes in activity (usually suppression, occasionally increase) and changes in cognitive and sensorial capacity (e.g. decision behaviour, perception disorders).

Dependence, abuse and addiction may occur.

Eye disorders:

Rare (≥ 1 / 10000 to < 1 / 1000): blurred vision

Respiratory disorders:

Worsening of asthma has also been reported, though a causal relationship has not been established.

Gastrointestinal disorders:

Very common (≥ 1 / 10): nausea

Common (≥ 1 / 100 to < 1 / 10): vomiting, constipation, dry mouth.

Uncommon (≥ 1 / 1000 to < 1 / 100): Retching, gastrointestinal irritation (a feeling of pressure in the stomach, bloating).

Skin and subcutaneous tissue disorders:

Common (≥ 1 / 100 to < 1 / 10): sweating

Uncommon (≥ 1 / 1000 to < 1 / 100): dermal reactions (e.g. pruritus, rash, urticaria)

Musculoskeletal disorders:

Rare (≥ 1 / 10000 to < 1 / 1000): motorial weakness

Hepato-biliary disorders:

Very rare (< 1 / 10000) an increase in liver enzyme values has been reported after use of tramadol.

Renal and urinary system disorders:

Rare (≥ 1 / 10000 to < 1 / 1000): micturition disorders (difficulty in passing urine and urinary retention).

Immune system disorders:

Rare (≥ 1 / 10000 to < 1 / 1000): Allergic reactions (e.g. dyspnoea, bronchospasm, wheezing, angioneurotic oedema) and anaphylaxis;

General disorders:

Common (≥ 1 / 100 to < 1 / 10): fatigue.

Physical Dependence

Dependence, abuse, addiction, and withdrawal reactions may occur. Symptoms which occur on withdrawal, identical to withdrawal symptoms in opioids, may be: agitation, anxiety, nervousness, insomnia, hyperkinesia, tremor and gastro intestinal symptoms. Very rare (< 1 / 10000) atypical withdrawal symptoms have been reported: panic attack, severe anxiety, hallucinations, paraesthesia, tinnitus, and other unusual central nervous system symptoms.

4.9 Overdose

Symptoms

In tramadol intoxication, in principle, the same symptoms occur as for all other central acting analgesics (opioids). In particular, these include miosis, vomiting, cardiovascular collapse, narrowing of consciousness leading to coma, convulsions, respiratory depression leading to respiratory failure.

Treatment

General emergency measures are applicable.

Maintenance of the airway (aspiration), maintenance of respiration and cardiovascular circulation depending on the symptoms.

Emptying of the stomach by means of vomiting (patient to be conscious) or by means of pumping the stomach. Consideration should also be given to the administration of activated charcoal, if necessary via the stomach pump tube. Depending how long has elapsed from ingestion, administration of a suitable laxative to speed up elimination should be considered. In the event that the patient's consciousness is reduced, intubation prior to performing these procedures is essential.

The antidote for respiratory depression is naloxone.

In animal tests naloxone proved to be ineffective against convulsions.

In that case diazepam should be administered intravenously.

Tramadol is only minimally removed from plasma using haemodialysis, haemofiltration or haemoperfusion.

Therefore treatment of acute overdose of tramadol using haemodialysis or haemofiltration alone is not a suitable way of detoxification. Administration of a suitable laxative may help to speed up elimination of unabsorbed tramadol, if administered early after overdose.

5. PHARMACOLOGICAL PROPERTIES

5.1 Pharmacodynamic properties

ATC code N 02 AX 02: Pharmacotherapeutic group: Analgesics, other opioids

Tramadol is a centrally acting opioid analgesic.

It is a non-selective, partial agonist of μ-, δ- and κ-opioid receptors with a higher affinity for μ-receptors. Other mechanisms contributing to the analgesic effect are the inhibition of the neural noradrenaline reuptake, and an enhanced release of serotonin.

Tramadol has an antitussive action.

Contrary to morphine tramadol does not suppress respiration in analgetic doses over a large range.

The action on the cardiovascular system is minimal.

The potency of tramadol is reported to be 1 / 10 to 1 / 6 of morphine.

5.2 Pharmacokinetic properties

More than 90% of tramadol is absorbed after oral administration.

The mean absolute bioavailability is approximately 70 %, irrespective of concomitant intake of food.

The difference between absorbed and non – metabolised available tramadol is probably due to low first – pass effect. The first pass – effect after oral administration is a maximum of 30 %.

Tramadol has a high tissue affinity ($V_{d,\beta}$ = 203 ± 40 l). Protein binding is about 20 %.

After administration of Minular 100 mg SR Tablets the maximum peak plasma concentration C_{max} 141 ± 40 ng / ml is reached after 4.9 hours. After administration of Minular 200 mg SR Tablets a C_{max} 260 ± 62 ng / ml is reached after 4.8 hours.

Tramadol passes the blood – brain and placenta barrier. Very small amounts of the substance and its O – demethyl derivative are found in the breast – milk (0.1 % and 0.02 % respectively of the applied dose).

Elimination of half-life $t_{½\beta}$ is approximately 6 h, irrespective of the mode of administration. In patients above 75 years of age it may be prolonged by a factor of 1.4.

In humans tramadol is mainly metabolised by means of N – and O – demethylation and conjugation of the O – demethylation products with glucuronic acid. Only O – desmethyltramadol is pharmacologically active. There are considerable interindividual quantitative differences between the other metabolites. So far, eleven metabolites have been found in the urine. Animal experiments have shown that O – desmethyltramadol is more potent than the parent substance by the factor 2 – 4. Its half life $t_{½\beta}$ (6 healthy volunteers) is 7.9 h (range 5.4 – 9.6 h) and is approximately that of tramadol.

The inhibition of one or both cytochrome p450 isoenzymes, cyp3a4 and cyp2d6 involved in the metabolism of tramadol, may affect the plasma concentration of tramadol or its active metabolite. The clinical consequences of any such interactions are not known.

Tramadol and its metabolites are almost completely excreted via the kidneys. Cumulative urinary excretion is 90 % of the total radioactivity of the administered dose. In cases of impaired hepatic and renal function the half – life may be slightly prolonged. In patients with cirrhosis of the liver, elimination half – lives of 13.3 ± 4.9 h (tramadol) and 18.5 ± 9.4 h (O – desmethyltramadol), in an extreme case 22.3 h and 36 h respectively have been determined. In patients with renal insufficiency (creatinine clearance < 5 ml / min) the values were 11 ± 3.2 h and 16.9 ± 3 h, in an extreme case 19.5 h and 43.2 h, respectively.

Tramadol has a linear pharmacokinetic profile within the therapeutic dosage range.

The relationship between serum concentrations and the analgesic effect is dose – dependent, but varies considerably in isolated cases. A serum concentration of 100 – 300 ng / ml is usually effective.

5.3 Preclinical safety data

In repeated oral and parenteral administration of tramadol during 6 to 26 weeks to rats and dogs, as also during 12 months to dogs, there are no indications for changes caused by the substance in haematological, clinical – chemical and histological experiments.

Only after high doses, far above the therapeutic doses, central symptoms occurred: restlessness, salivation, convulsion, reduced increase in weight.

Rats and dogs tolerate the oral dose of 20 mg / kg resp 10 mg / kg bodyweight, dogs also tolerate 20 mg / kg bodyweight, rectally administered.

Tramadol doses as from 50 mg / kg / day cause intoxication of the mother, in rats, and result in an increased mortality in newborn rats.

In young rats development disorders occurred as ossification disturbances, delayed opening of the vagina and eyes.

The fertility of male rats was not influenced.

However the percentage of females with young reduced after high dosages (as of 50 mg / kg / day).

In rabbits, toxic effects occurred as of 125 mg / kg in the mother and skeletal anomalies in the offspring.

In some *in – vitro* test systems there is report on mutagenic effects.

In *in – vivo* experiments there was no indication for mutagenic effects.

On the basis of the knowledge available up till now it is unclear whether tramadol possesses mutagenic potential.

Experiments have been performed on rats and mice with regard to the tumuorigenic potential of tramadol.

From tests in rats it could not be shown that the substance increases the chance of tumours.

In tests in mice an increased incidence of liver – cell adenomas in males (depending on the dose, with an insignificant increase as of 15 mg / kg) and an increased chance of lung tumours in females in all dose selections (significant, but not dose dependent) was found.

6. PHARMACEUTICAL PARTICULARS

6.1 List of excipients

Calcium hydrogen phosphate dihydrate (E341),

Hydroxypropylcellulose (E463),

Colloidal anhydrous silica (E551),

Magnesium stearate (E470b).

6.2 Incompatibilities

Not applicable.

6.3 Shelf life

3 years

PP / PE tablet container: 6 months after opening

6.4 Special precautions for storage

Store in the original package in order to protect from moisture.

6.5 Nature and contents of container

Al / clear PVC blisters in carton boxes in packs of 10, 20, 30, 50, 60, 90, 100, 120, 180, and 500 tablets.

Al / opaque PVC child resistant blisters in carton boxes in packs of 10, 20, 30, 50, 60, 90, 100, 120, 180, and 500 tablets.

Polypropylene tablet container with polyethylene tamper evident closure containing 10, 20, 30, 50, 60, 90, 100, 120, 180, and 500 tablets.

Not all pack sizes may be marketed.

6.6 Special precautions for disposal and other handling

Any unused product or waste material should be disposed of in accordance with local requirements.

7. MARKETING AUTHORISATION HOLDER

Actavis Group hf

Reykjavíkurvegur 76-78

220 Hafnarfjordur

Iceland

8. MARKETING AUTHORISATION NUMBER(S)

PL 21231/0015

9. DATE OF FIRST AUTHORISATION/RENEWAL OF THE AUTHORISATION

10/08/2007

10. DATE OF REVISION OF THE TEXT

10/08/2007

Zestoretic 10

(AstraZeneca UK Limited)

1. NAME OF THE MEDICINAL PRODUCT

'Zestoretic' 10.

2. QUALITATIVE AND QUANTITATIVE COMPOSITION

Each tablet contains lisinopril dihydrate (equivalent to 10 mg anhydrous lisinopril) and hydrochlorothiazide Ph. Eur. 12.5 mg.

3. PHARMACEUTICAL FORM

Tablet.

4. CLINICAL PARTICULARS

4.1 Therapeutic indications

'Zestoretic' 10 is indicated in the management of mild to moderate hypertension in patients who have been stabilised on the individual components given in the same proportions.

4.2 Posology and method of administration

The usual dosage is one tablet, administered once daily. As with all other medication taken once daily, 'Zestoretic' 10 should be taken at approximately the same time each day.

In general, if the desired therapeutic effect cannot be achieved in a period of 2 to 4 weeks at this dose level, the dose can be increased to two tablets administered once daily.

No adjustment of dosage is required in the elderly.

Safety and effectiveness in children have not been established.

Dosage in Renal Insufficiency

Thiazides may not be appropriate diuretics for use in patients with renal impairment and are ineffective at creatinine clearance values of 30 ml/min or below (i.e. moderate or severe renal insufficiency).

'Zestoretic' 10 is not to be used as initial therapy in any patient with renal insufficiency.

In patients with creatinine clearance of >30 and <80 ml/min, 'Zestoretic' 10 may be used, but only after titration of the individual components.

Prior Diuretic Therapy

Symptomatic hypotension may occur following the initial dose of 'Zestoretic' 10; this is more likely in patients who are volume and/or salt depleted as a result of prior diuretic therapy. The diuretic therapy should be discontinued for 2-3 days prior to initiation of therapy with 'Zestoretic' 10. If this is not possible, treatment should be started with lisinopril alone, in a 2.5 mg dose.

4.3 Contraindications

'Zestoretic' 10 is contraindicated in pregnancy and treatment should be stopped if pregnancy is suspected (see also Section 4.6).

'Zestoretic' 10 is contraindicated in patients with anuria.

'Zestoretic' 10 is contraindicated in patients who are hypersensitive to any component of this product and in patients with a history of angioneurotic oedema relating to previous treatment with an angiotensin-converting enzyme inhibitor and in patients with hereditary or idiopathic angioedema.

'Zestoretic' 10 is contraindicated in patients who are hypersensitive to other sulphonamide-derived drugs.

4.4 Special warnings and precautions for use

Hypotension and Electrolyte/Fluid Imbalance

As with all antihypertensive therapy, symptomatic hypotension may occur in some patients. This was rarely seen in uncomplicated hypertensive patients but is more likely in the presence of fluid or electrolyte imbalance, eg. volume depletion, hyponatraemia, hypochloraemic alkalosis, hypomagnesaemia or hypokalaemia which may occur from prior diuretic therapy, dietary salt restriction, dialysis, or during intercurrent diarrhoea or vomiting. Periodic determination of serum electrolytes should be performed at appropriate intervals in such patients.

In patients at increased risk of symptomatic hypotension, initiation of therapy and dose adjustment should be monitored under close medical supervision.

Particular consideration should be given when therapy is administered to patients with ischaemic heart or cerebrovascular disease because an excessive fall in blood pressure could result in a myocardial infarction or cerebrovascular accident.

If hypotension occurs, the patient should be placed in the supine position and, if necessary, should receive an intravenous infusion of normal saline. A transient hypotensive response is not a contraindication to further doses. Following restoration of effective blood volume and pressure, reinstitution of therapy at reduced dosage may be possible; or either of the components may be used appropriately alone.

As with other vasodilators, 'Zestoretic' 10 should be given with caution to patients with aortic stenosis or hypertrophic cardiomyopathy.

Renal Function Impairment

Thiazides may not be appropriate diuretics for use in patients with renal impairment and are ineffective at creatinine clearance values of 30ml/min or below (i.e. moderate or severe renal insufficiency).

'Zestoretic' 10 should not be administered to patients with renal insufficiency (creatinine clearance ≤80 ml/min) until titration of the individual components has shown the need for the doses present in the combination tablet.

In some patients with bilateral renal artery stenosis or stenosis of the artery to a solitary kidney, who have been treated with angiotensin converting enzyme inhibitors, increases in blood urea and serum creatinine, usually reversible upon discontinuation of therapy have been seen. This is especially likely in patients with renal insufficiency. If renovascular hypertension is also present there is an increased risk of severe hypotension and renal insufficiency. In these patients, treatment should be started under close medical supervision with low doses and careful dose titration. Since treatment with diuretics may be a contributory factor to the above, renal function should be monitored during the first few weeks of 'Zestoretic' 10 therapy.

Some hypertensive patients with no apparent pre-existing renal disease have developed usually minor and transient increases in blood urea and serum creatinine when lisinopril has been given concomitantly with a diuretic. If this occurs during therapy with 'Zestoretic' 10, the combination should be discontinued. Reinstitution of therapy at reduced dosage may be possible; or either of the components may be used appropriately alone.

Hepatic Disease

Thiazides should be used with caution in patients with impaired hepatic function or progressive liver disease, since minor alterations of fluid and electrolyte balance may precipitate hepatic coma.

Surgery/Anaesthesia

In patients undergoing major surgery or during anaesthesia with agents that produce hypotension, lisinopril may block angiotensin II formation secondary to compensatory renin release. If hypotension occurs and is considered to be due to this mechanism, it can be corrected by volume expansion.

Metabolic and Endocrine Effects

Thiazide therapy may impair glucose tolerance. Dosage adjustment of antidiabetic agents, including insulin, may be required.

Thiazides may decrease urinary calcium excretion and may cause intermittent and slight elevation of serum calcium. Marked hypercalcaemia may be evidence of hidden hyperparathyroidism. Thiazides should be discontinued before carrying out tests for parathyroid function.

Increases in cholesterol and triglyceride levels may be associated with thiazide diuretic therapy.

Thiazide therapy may precipitate hyperuricaemia and/or gout in certain patients. However, lisinopril may increase urinary uric acid and thus may attenuate the hyperuricaemic effect of hydrochlorothiazide.

Hypersensitivity/Angioneurotic Oedema

Angioneurotic oedema of the face, extremities, lips, tongue, glottis and/or larynx has been reported rarely in patients treated with angiotensin converting enzyme inhibitors, including lisinopril. In such cases, 'Zestoretic' 10 should be discontinued promptly and appropriate monitoring should be instituted to ensure complete resolution of symptoms prior to dismissing the patient. In those instances where swelling has been confined to the face and lips, the condition generally resolved without treatment, although antihistamines have been useful in relieving symptoms.

Angioneurotic oedema associated with laryngeal oedema may be fatal. Where there is involvement of the tongue, glottis or larynx, likely to cause airway obstruction, appropriate emergency therapy should be administered promptly. This may include administration of adrenaline and/or the maintenance of a patent airway. The patient should be under close medical supervision until complete and sustained resolution of symptoms has occurred. Angioedema may also affect the intestines and present with acute abdominal pain, nausea, vomiting and diarrhoea.

Angiotensin converting enzyme inhibitors cause a higher rate of angioedema in black patients than in non-black patients.

Patients with a history of angioedema unrelated to ACE inhibitor therapy may be at increased risk of angioedema while receiving an ACE inhibitor. (See also Section 4.3).

In patients receiving thiazides, sensitivity reactions may occur with or without a history of allergy or bronchial asthma. Exacerbation or activation of systemic lupus erythematosus has been reported with the use of thiazides.

Race

Angiotensin converting enzyme inhibitors cause a higher rate of angioedema in black patients than in non-black patients.

Desensitisation

Patients receiving ACE inhibitors during desensitisation treatment (eg. hymenoptera venom) have sustained anaphylactoid reactions. In the same patients, these reactions have been avoided when ACE inhibitors were temporarily withheld but they reappeared upon inadvertent rechallenge.

Haemodialysis Membranes

See Section 4.5

Cough

Cough has been reported with the use of ACE inhibitors. Characteristically, the cough is non-productive, persistent and resolves after discontinuation of therapy. ACE inhibitor-induced cough should be considered as part of the differential diagnosis of cough.

Paediatric Use

Safety and effectiveness in children have not been established.

Use in the Elderly

In clinical studies the efficacy and tolerability of lisinopril and hydrochlorothiazide, administered concomitantly, were similar in both elderly and younger hypertensive patients.

4.5 Interaction with other medicinal products and other forms of interaction

Prior Diuretic Therapy

Symptomatic hypotension may occur following the initial dose of 'Zestoretic' 10; this is more likely in patients who are volume and/or salt depleted as a result of prior diuretic therapy. The diuretic therapy should be discontinued for 2-3 days prior to initiation of therapy with 'Zestoretic' 10. If this is not possible, treatment should be started with lisinopril alone, in a 2.5 mg dose.

Haemodialysis Membranes

The use of 'Zestoretic' 10 is not indicated in patients requiring dialysis for renal failure. A high incidence of anaphylactoid reactions have been reported in patients dialysed with high-flux membranes (eg. AN 69) and treated concomitantly with an ACE inhibitor. This combination should therefore be avoided.

Serum Potassium

The potassium losing effect of thiazide diuretics is usually attenuated by the potassium conserving effect of lisinopril. The use of potassium supplements, potassium-sparing agents or potassium-containing salt substitutes, particularly in patients with impaired renal function, may lead to a significant increase in serum potassium. If concomitant use of 'Zestoretic' 10 and any of these agents is deemed appropriate, they should be used with caution and with frequent monitoring of serum potassium.

Lithium

Lithium generally should not be given with diuretics or ACE inhibitors. Diuretic agents and ACE inhibitors reduce the renal clearance of lithium and add a high risk of lithium toxicity. Refer to the prescribing information for lithium preparations before use of such preparations.

Other Agents

Indomethacin may diminish the antihypertensive effect of concomitantly-administered 'Zestoretic' 10. In some patients with compromised renal function who are being treated with non-steroidal anti-inflammatory drugs (NSAIDs), the co-administration of lisinopril may result in a further deterioration of renal function.

The antihypertensive effect of 'Zestoretic' 10 may be potentiated when given concomitantly with other agents likely to cause postural hypotension.

Thiazides may increase the responsiveness to tubocurarine.

4.6 Pregnancy and lactation

'Zestoretic' 10 is contraindicated in pregnancy and treatment should be stopped if pregnancy is suspected.

ACE inhibitors can cause foetal and neonatal morbidity and mortality when administered to pregnant women during the second and third trimesters. Use of ACE inhibitors during this period has been associated with foetal and neonatal injury including hypotension, renal failure, hyperkalaemia and/or skull hypoplasia in the newborn. Maternal oligohydramnios, presumably representing decreased foetal renal function, has occurred and may result in limb contractures, craniofacial deformations and hypoplastic lung development.

These adverse effects to the embryo and foetus do not appear to have resulted from intrauterine ACE inhibitor exposure limited to the first trimester.

Infants whose mothers have taken lisinopril should be closely observed for hypotension, oliguria and hyperkalaemia. Lisinopril, which crosses the placenta, has been removed from the neonatal circulation by peritoneal dialysis with some clinical benefit, and theoretically may be removed by exchange transfusion. There is no experience with the removal of hydrochlorothiazide, which also crosses the placenta, from the neonatal circulation.

Nursing Mothers

It is not known whether lisinopril is secreted in human milk; however, thiazides do appear in human milk. Because of the potential for serious reactions in breast-fed infants, a decision should be made whether to discontinue breast feeding or to discontinue 'Zestoretic' 10, taking into account the importance of the drug to the mother.

4.7 Effects on ability to drive and use machines

None known.

4.8 Undesirable effects

Side Effects with the Combination

'Zestoretic' 10 is usually well tolerated. In clinical studies, side effects have usually been mild and transient, and in most instances have not required interruption of therapy. The side effects that have been observed have been limited to those reported previously with lisinopril or hydrochlorothiazide.

One of the most common clinical side effects was dizziness, which generally responded to dosage reduction and seldom required discontinuation of therapy.

Other side effects were headache, dry cough, fatigue and hypotension including orthostatic hypotension.

Less common were diarrhoea, nausea, vomiting, dry mouth, rash, gout, palpitations, chest discomfort, muscle cramps and weakness, paraesthesia, asthenia and impotence.

Pancreatitis has been reported rarely with lisinopril and with hydrochlorothiazide and, therefore, is a potential side effect of 'Zestoretic' 10.

Hypersensitivity/Angioneurotic Oedema

Angioneurotic oedema of the face, extremities, lips, tongue, glottis and/or larynx has been reported rarely (see Section 4.4). In very rare cases, intestinal angioedema has been reported.

A symptom complex has been reported which may include one or more of the following: fever, vasculitis, myalgia, arthralgia/arthritis, a positive ANA, elevated ESR, eosinophilia and leucocytosis, rash, photosensitivity, or other dermatological manifestations.

Laboratory Test Findings

Laboratory side effects have rarely been of clinical importance. Occasional hyperglycaemia, hyperuricaemia and hyper- or hypokalaemia have been noted. Usually minor and transient increases in blood urea nitrogen and serum creatinine have been seen in patients without evidence of pre-existing renal impairment. If such increases persist, they are usually reversible upon discontinuation of 'Zestoretic' 10. Bone marrow depression, manifest as anaemia and/or thrombocytopenia and/or leucopenia has been reported. Agranulocytosis has been rarely reported. Small decreases in haemoglobin and haematocrit have been reported frequently in hypertensive patients treated with 'Zestoretic' 10 but were rarely of clinical importance unless another cause of anaemia co-existed. Rarely, elevations of liver enzymes and/or serum bilirubin have occurred, but a causal relationship to 'Zestoretic' 10 has not been established.

Other Side Effects Reported with the Individual Components Alone

These may be potential side effects with 'Zestoretic' 10 and include:

Hydrochlorothiazide: anorexia, gastric irritation, constipation, jaundice (intrahepatic cholestatic jaundice), pancreatitis, sialoadenitis, vertigo, xanthopsia, leucopenia, agranulocytosis, thrombocytopenia, aplastic anaemia, haemolytic anaemia, purpura, photosensitivity, urticaria, necrotizing angiitis (vasculitis) (cutaneous vasculitis), fever, respiratory distress including pneumonitis and pulmonary oedema, anaphylactic reactions, hyperglycaemia, glycosuria, hyperuricaemia, electrolyte imbalance including hyponatraemia, muscle spasm, restlessness, transient blurred vision, renal failure, renal dysfunction and interstitial nephritis.

Lisinopril: myocardial infarction or cerebrovascular accident possibly secondary to excessive hypotension in high risk patients, tachycardia, abdominal pain and indigestion, mood alterations, mental confusion, vertigo have occurred; as with other angiotensin converting enzyme inhibitors, taste disturbance and sleep disturbance have been reported; bronchospasm, rhinitis, sinusitis, alopecia, urticaria, diaphoresis, pruritus, psoriasis and severe skin disorders, (including pemphigus, toxic epidermal necrolysis, Stevens-Johnson Syndrome and erythema multiforme), have been reported; hyponatraemia, uraemia, oliguria/anuria, renal dysfunction, acute renal failure, hepatitis (hepatocellular or cholestatic), jaundice and haemolytic anaemia.

4.9 Overdose

No specific information is available on the treatment of overdosage with 'Zestoretic' 10. Treatment is symptomatic and supportive. Therapy with 'Zestoretic' 10 should be discontinued and the patient should be kept under very close supervision. Therapeutic measures depend on the nature and severity of the symptoms. Measures to prevent absorption and methods to speed elimination should be employed.

Lisinopril: The most likely features of overdosage would be hypotension, electrolyte disturbance and renal failure. If severe hypotension occurs, the patient should be placed in the shock position and an intravenous infusion of normal saline should be given rapidly. Treatment with angiotensin II (if available) may be considered. Angiotensin converting enzyme inhibitors may be removed from the general circulation by haemodialysis. The use of high-flux polyacrylonitrile dialysis membranes should be avoided. Serum electrolytes and creatinine should be monitored frequently.

Hydrochlorothiazide: The most common signs and symptoms observed are those caused by electrolyte depletion (hypokalaemia, hypochloraemia, hyponatraemia) and dehydration resulting from excessive diuresis. If digitalis has also been administered hypokalaemia may accentuate cardiac arrhythmias.

5. PHARMACOLOGICAL PROPERTIES

5.1 Pharmacodynamic properties

'Zestoretic' 10 is a fixed dose combination product containing lisinopril, an inhibitor of angiotensin converting enzyme (ACE) and hydrochlorothiazide, a thiazide diuretic. Both components have complementary modes of action and exert an additive antihypertensive effect.

Lisinopril is a peptidyl dipeptidase inhibitor. It inhibits the angiotensin converting enzyme (ACE) that catalyses the conversion of angiotensin I to the vasoconstrictor peptide, angiotensin II. Angiotensin II also stimulates aldosterone secretion by the adrenal cortex. Inhibition of ACE results in decreased concentrations of angiotensin II which results in decreased vasopressor activity and reduced aldosterone secretion. The latter decrease may result in an increase in serum potassium concentration. While the mechanism through which lisinopril lowers blood pressure is believed to be primarily suppression of the renin-angiotensin-aldosterone system, lisinopril is antihypertensive even in patients with low-renin hypertension. ACE is identical to kininase II, an enzyme that degrades bradykinin. Whether increased levels of bradykinin, a potent vasodilatory peptide, play a role in the therapeutic effects of lisinopril remains to be elucidated.

Hydrochlorothiazide is a diuretic and an antihypertensive agent. It affects the distal renal tubular mechanism of electrolyte reabsorption and increases excretion of sodium and chloride in approximately equivalent amounts. Natriuresis may be accompanied by some loss of potassium and bicarbonate. The mechanism of the antihypertensive effect of the thiazides is unknown. Thiazides do not usually affect normal blood pressure.

When combined with other antihypertensive agents, additive falls in blood pressure may occur.

5.2 Pharmacokinetic properties

Concomitant administration of lisinopril and hydrochlorothiazide has little or no effect on the bioavailability of either drug. The combination tablet is bioequivalent to concomitant administration of the separate entities.

Lisinopril

Following oral administration of lisinopril, peak serum concentrations occur within about 7 hours. On multiple dosing lisinopril has an effective half life of accumulation of 12.6 hours. Declining serum concentrations exhibit a prolonged terminal phase which does not contribute to drug accumulation. This terminal phase probably represents saturable binding to ACE and is not proportional to dose. Lisinopril does not appear to bind to other serum proteins.

Impaired renal function decreases elimination of lisinopril, which is excreted via the kidneys, but this decrease becomes clinically important only when the glomerular filtration rate is below 30 ml/min. Older patients have higher blood levels and higher values for the area under the plasma concentration time curve than younger patients. Lisinopril can be removed by dialysis.

Based on urinary recovery, the mean extent of absorption of lisinopril is approximately 25%, with interpatient variability (6-60%) at all doses tested (5-80 mg).

Lisinopril does not undergo metabolism and absorbed drug is excreted unchanged entirely in the urine. Lisinopril absorption is not affected by the presence of food in the gastrointestinal tract.

Studies in rats indicate that lisinopril crosses the blood-brain barrier poorly.

Hydrochlorothiazide

When plasma levels have been followed for at least 24 hours, the plasma half-life has been observed to vary between 5.6 and 14.8 hours. At least 61% of the dose is eliminated unchanged within 24 hours. After oral hydrochlorothiazide, diuresis begins within 2 hours, peaks in about 4 hours and lasts 6 to 12 hours. Hydrochlorothiazide crosses the placental but not the blood-brain barrier.

5.3 Preclinical safety data

Lisinopril and hydrochlorthiazide are both drugs on which extensive clinical experience has been obtained, both separately and in combination. All relevant information for the prescriber is provided elsewhere in the Summary of Product Characteristics.

6. PHARMACEUTICAL PARTICULARS

6.1 List of excipients

Calcium Hydrogen Phosphate Dihydrate Ph. Eur.

Iron Oxide E172.

Magnesium Stearate Ph. Eur.

Maize Starch Ph. Eur.

Mannitol Ph. Eur.

Pregelatinised Starch Ph. Eur.

6.2 Incompatibilities

None known, but see Section 4.5.

6.3 Shelf life

2.5 years stored in the sales package.

6.4 Special precautions for storage

Store below 30°C and protect from light. If blister packs are removed from the carton, they should be protected from light.

6.5 Nature and contents of container

Blister packs of 28 tablets

6.6 Special precautions for disposal and other handling

Not applicable.

7. MARKETING AUTHORISATION HOLDER

AstraZeneca UK Limited,

600 Capability Green,

Luton, LU1 3LU, UK.

8. MARKETING AUTHORISATION NUMBER(S)

PL 17901/0058

9. DATE OF FIRST AUTHORISATION/RENEWAL OF THE AUTHORISATION

8 June 2000

10. DATE OF REVISION OF THE TEXT

4th March 2004

Zestoretic 20

(AstraZeneca UK Limited)

1. NAME OF THE MEDICINAL PRODUCT

'Zestoretic' 20.

2. QUALITATIVE AND QUANTITATIVE COMPOSITION

Each tablet contains lisinopril dihydrate (equivalent to 20 mg anhydrous lisinopril) and hydrochlorothiazide Ph. Eur. 12.5 mg.

3. PHARMACEUTICAL FORM

Tablet.

4. CLINICAL PARTICULARS

4.1 Therapeutic indications

'Zestoretic' 20 is indicated in the management of mild to moderate hypertension in patients who have been stabilised on the individual components given in the same proportions.

4.2 Posology and method of administration

The usual dosage is one tablet, administered once daily. As with all other medication taken once daily, 'Zestoretic' 20 should be taken at approximately the same time each day.

In general, if the desired therapeutic effect cannot be achieved in a period of 2 to 4 weeks at this dose level, the dose can be increased to two tablets administered once daily.

Use in the elderly

In clinical studies the efficacy and tolerability of lisinopril and hydrochlorothiazide, administered concomitantly, were similar in both elderly and younger hypertensive patients.

Lisinopril was equally effective in elderly (65 years or older) and non-elderly hypertensive patients. In elderly hypertensive patients, monotherapy with lisinopril was as effective in reducing diastolic blood pressure as monotherapy with either hydrochlorothiazide or atenolol in clinical studies, age did not affect the tolerability of lisinopril.

Safety and effectiveness in children have not been established.

Dosage in Renal Insufficiency

Thiazides may not be appropriate diuretics for use in patients with renal impairment and are ineffective at creatinine clearance values of 30 ml/min or below (i.e. moderate or severe renal insufficiency).

'Zestoretic' 20 is not to be used as initial therapy in any patient with renal insufficiency.

In patients with creatinine clearance of >30 and <80 ml/min, 'Zestoretic' 20 may be used, but only after titration of the individual components.

Prior Diuretic Therapy

Symptomatic hypotension may occur following the initial dose of 'Zestoretic' 20; this is more likely in patients who are volume and/or salt depleted as a result of prior diuretic therapy. The diuretic therapy should be discontinued for 2-3 days prior to initiation of therapy with 'Zestoretic' 20. If this is not possible, treatment should be started with lisinopril alone, in a 2.5 mg dose.

4.3 Contraindications

'Zestoretic' 20 is contraindicated in pregnancy and treatment should be stopped if pregnancy is suspected (see also Section 4.6).

'Zestoretic' 20 is contraindicated in patients with anuria.

'Zestoretic' 20 is contraindicated in patients who are hypersensitive to any component of this product and in patients with a history of angioneurotic oedema relating to previous treatment with an angiotensin-converting enzyme inhibitor and in patients with hereditary or idiopathic angioedema.

'Zestoretic' 20 is contraindicated in patients who are hypersensitive to other sulphonamide-derived drugs.

4.4 Special warnings and precautions for use

Hypotension and Electrolyte/Fluid Imbalance

As with all antihypertensive therapy, symptomatic hypotension may occur in some patients. This was rarely seen in uncomplicated hypertensive patients but is more likely in the presence of fluid or electrolyte imbalance, eg. volume depletion, hyponatraemia, hypochloraemic alkalosis, hypomagnesaemia or hypokalaemia which may occur from prior diuretic therapy, dietary salt restriction, dialysis, or during intercurrent diarrhoea or vomiting. Periodic determination of serum electrolytes should be performed at appropriate intervals in such patients.

In patients at increased risk of symptomatic hypotension, initiation of therapy and dose adjustment should be monitored under close medical supervision.

Particular consideration should be given when therapy is administered to patients with ischaemic heart or cerebrovascular disease because an excessive fall in blood pressure could result in a myocardial infarction or cerebrovascular accident.

If hypotension occurs, the patient should be placed in the supine position and, if necessary, should receive an intravenous infusion of normal saline. A transient hypotensive response is not a contraindication to further doses. Following restoration of effective blood volume and pressure, reinstitution of therapy at reduced dosage may be possible; or either of the components may be used appropriately alone.

As with other vasodilators, 'Zestoretic' 20 should be given with caution to patients with aortic stenosis or hypertrophic cardiomyopathy.

Renal Function Impairment

Thiazides may not be appropriate diuretics for use in patients with renal impairment and are ineffective at creatinine clearance values of 30ml/min or below (i.e. moderate or severe renal insufficiency).

'Zestoretic' 20 should not be administered to patients with renal insufficiency (creatinine clearance ≤80 ml/min) until titration of the individual components has shown the need for the doses present in the combination tablet.

In some patients with bilateral renal artery stenosis or stenosis of the artery to a solitary kidney, who have been treated with angiotensin enzyme inhibitors, increases in blood urea and serum creatinine, usually reversible upon discontinuation of therapy, have been seen. This is especially likely in patients with renal insufficiency. If renovascular hypertension is also present there is an increased risk of severe hypotension and renal insufficiency. In these patients, treatment should be started under close medical supervision with low doses and careful dose titration. Since treatment with diuretics may be a contributory factor to the above, renal function should be monitored during the first few weeks of 'Zestoretic' 20 therapy.

Some hypertensive patients with no apparent pre-existing renal disease have developed usually minor and transient increases in blood urea and serum creatinine when lisinopril has been given concomitantly with a diuretic. If this occurs during therapy with 'Zestoretic' 20, the combination should be discontinued. Reinstitution of therapy at reduced dosage may be possible; or either of the components may be used appropriately alone.

Hepatic Disease

Thiazides should be used with caution in patients with impaired hepatic function or progressive liver disease, since minor alterations of fluid and electrolyte balance may precipitate hepatic coma.

Surgery/Anaesthesia

In patients undergoing major surgery or during anaesthesia with agents that produce hypotension, lisinopril may block angiotensin II formation secondary to compensatory renin release. If hypotension occurs and is considered to be due to this mechanism, it can be corrected by volume expansion.

Metabolic and Endocrine Effects

Thiazide therapy may impair glucose tolerance. Dosage adjustment of antidiabetic agents, including insulin, may be required.

Thiazides may decrease urinary calcium excretion and may cause intermittent and slight elevation of serum calcium. Marked hypercalcaemia may be evidence of hidden hyperparathyroidism. Thiazides should be discontinued before carrying out tests for parathyroid function.

Increases in cholesterol and triglyceride levels may be associated with thiazide diuretic therapy.

Thiazide therapy may precipitate hyperuricaemia and/or gout in certain patients. However, lisinopril may increase urinary uric acid and thus may attenuate the hyperuricaemic effect of hydrochlorothiazide.

Hypersensitivity/Angioneurotic Oedema

Angioneurotic oedema of the face, extremities, lips, tongue, glottis and/or larynx has been reported rarely in patients treated with angiotensin converting enzyme inhibitors, including lisinopril. In such cases, 'Zestoretic' 20 should be discontinued promptly and appropriate monitoring should be instituted to ensure complete resolution of symptoms prior to dismissing the patient. In those instances where swelling has been confined to the face and lips, the condition generally resolved without treatment, although antihistamines have been useful in relieving symptoms.

Angioneurotic oedema associated with laryngeal oedema may be fatal. Where there is involvement of the tongue, glottis or larynx, likely to cause airway obstruction, appropriate emergency therapy should be administered promptly. This may include administration of adrenaline and/or the maintenance of a patent airway. The patient should be under close medical supervision until complete and sustained resolution of symptoms has occurred. Angioedema may also affect the intestines and present with acute abdominal pain, nausea, vomiting and diarrhoea.

Angiotensin converting enzyme inhibitors cause a higher rate of angioedema in black patients than in non-black patients.

Patients with a history of angioedema unrelated to ACE inhibitor therapy may be at increased risk of angioedema while receiving an ACE inhibitor. (See also Section 4.3).

In patients receiving thiazides, sensitivity reactions may occur with or without a history of allergy or bronchial asthma. Exacerbation or activation of systemic lupus erythematosus has been reported with the use of thiazides.

Race

Angiotensin converting enzyme inhibitors cause a higher rate of angioedema in black patients than in non-black patients.

Desensitisation

Patients receiving ACE inhibitors during desensitisation treatment (e.g. hymenoptera venom) have sustained anaphylactoid reactions. In the same patients, these reactions have been avoided when ACE inhibitors were temporarily withheld but they reappeared upon inadvertent rechallenge.

Haemodialysis Membranes

(See Section 4.5).

Cough

Cough has been reported with the use of ACE inhibitors. Characteristically, the cough is non-productive, persistent and resolves after discontinuation of therapy. ACE inhibitor-induced cough should be considered as part of the differential diagnosis of cough.

Paediatric Use

Safety and effectiveness in children have not been established.

Use in the Elderly

In clinical studies the efficacy and tolerability of lisinopril and hydrochlorothiazide, administered concomitantly, were similar in both elderly and younger hypertensive patients.

4.5 Interaction with other medicinal products and other forms of interaction

Prior Diuretic Therapy

Symptomatic hypotension may occur following the initial dose of 'Zestoretic' 20; this is more likely in patients who are volume and/or salt depleted as a result of prior diuretic therapy. The diuretic therapy should be discontinued for 2-3 days prior to initiation of therapy with 'Zestoretic' 20. If this is not possible, treatment should be started with lisinopril alone, in a 2.5 mg dose.

Haemodialysis Membranes

The use of 'Zestoretic' 20 is not indicated in patients requiring dialysis for renal failure. A high incidence of anaphylactoid reactions have been reported in patients dialysed with high-flux membranes (e.g. AN 69) and treated concomitantly with an ACE inhibitor. This combination should therefore be avoided.

Serum Potassium

The potassium losing effect of thiazide diuretics is usually attenuated by the potassium conserving effect of lisinopril. The use of potassium supplements, potassium-sparing agents or potassium-containing salt substitutes, particularly in patients with impaired renal function, may lead to a significant increase in serum potassium. If concomitant use of 'Zestoretic' 20 and any of these agents is deemed appropriate, they should be used with caution and with frequent monitoring of serum potassium.

Lithium

Lithium generally should not be given with diuretics or ACE inhibitors. Diuretic agents and ACE inhibitors reduce the renal clearance of lithium and add a high risk of lithium toxicity. Refer to the prescribing information for lithium preparations before use of such preparations.

Other Agents

Indomethacin may diminish the antihypertensive effect of concomitantly administered 'Zestoretic' 20. In some patients with compromised renal function who are being treated with non-steroidal anti-inflammatory drugs (NSAIDs), the co-administration of lisinopril may result in a further deterioration of renal function.

The antihypertensive effect of 'Zestoretic' 20 may be potentiated when given concomitantly with other agents likely to cause postural hypotension.

Thiazides may increase the responsiveness to tubocurarine.

4.6 Pregnancy and lactation

'Zestoretic' 20 is contraindicated in pregnancy and treatment should be stopped if pregnancy is suspected.

ACE inhibitors can cause foetal and neonatal morbidity and mortality when administered to pregnant women during the second and third trimesters. Use of ACE inhibitors during this period has been associated with foetal and neonatal injury including hypotension, renal failure, hyperkalaemia and/or skull hypoplasia in the newborn. Maternal oligohydramnios, presumably representing decreased foetal renal function, has occurred and may result in limb contractures, craniofacial deformations and hypoplastic lung development.

These adverse effects to the embryo and foetus do not appear to have resulted from intrauterine ACE inhibitor exposure limited to the first trimester.

Infants whose mothers have taken lisinopril should be closely observed for hypotension, oliguria and hyperkalaemia. Lisinopril, which crosses the placenta, has been removed from the neonatal circulation by peritoneal dialysis with some clinical benefit, and theoretically may be removed by exchange transfusion. There is no experience with the removal of hydrochlorothiazide, which also crosses the placenta, from the neonatal circulation.

Nursing Mothers

It is not known whether lisinopril is secreted in human milk; however, thiazides do appear in human milk. Because of the potential for serious reactions in breast-fed infants, a decision should be made whether to discontinue breast feeding or to discontinue 'Zestoretic' 20, taking into account the importance of the drug to the mother.

4.7 Effects on ability to drive and use machines

None known.

4.8 Undesirable effects

Side Effects with the Combination

'Zestoretic' 20 is usually well tolerated. In clinical studies, side effects have usually been mild and transient, and in most instances have not required interruption of therapy. The side effects that have been observed have been limited to those reported previously with lisinopril or hydrochlorothiazide.

One of the most common clinical side effects was dizziness, which generally responded to dosage reduction and seldom required discontinuation of therapy.

Other side effects were headache, dry cough, fatigue and hypotension including orthostatic hypotension.

Less common were diarrhoea, nausea, vomiting, dry mouth, rash, gout, palpitations, chest discomfort, muscle cramps and weakness, paraesthesia, asthenia and impotence.

Pancreatitis has been reported rarely with lisinopril and with hydrochlorothiazide and, therefore, is a potential side effect of 'Zestoretic' 20.

Hypersensitivity/Angioneurotic Oedema

Angioneurotic oedema of the face, extremities, lips, tongue, glottis and/or larynx has been reported rarely (see Section 4.4). In very rare cases, intestinal angioedema has been reported.

A symptom complex has been reported which may include one or more of the following: fever, vasculitis, myalgia, arthralgia/arthritis, a positive ANA, elevated ESR, eosinophilia and leucocytosis, rash, photosensitivity, or other dermatological manifestations.

Laboratory Test Findings

Laboratory side effects have rarely been of clinical importance. Occasional hyperglycaemia, hyperuricaemia and hyper- or hypokalaemia have been noted. Usually minor and transient increases in blood urea nitrogen and serum creatinine have been seen in patients without evidence of pre-existing renal impairment. If such increases persist, they are usually reversible upon discontinuation of 'Zestoretic' 20. Bone marrow depression, manifest as anaemia and/or thrombocytopenia and/or leucopenia has been reported. Agranulocytosis has been rarely reported. Small decreases in haemoglobin and haematocrit have been reported frequently in hypertensive patients treated with 'Zestoretic' 20 but were rarely of clinical importance unless another cause of anaemia co-existed. Rarely, elevations of liver enzymes and/or serum bilirubin have occurred, but a causal relationship to 'Zestoretic' 20 has not been established.

Other Side Effects Reported with the Individual Components Alone

These may be potential side effects with 'Zestoretic' 20 and include:

Hydrochlorothiazide: anorexia, gastric irritation, constipation, jaundice (intrahepatic cholestatic jaundice), pancreatitis, sialoadenitis, vertigo, xanthopsia, leucopenia, agranulocytosis, thrombocytopenia, aplastic anaemia, haemolytic anaemia, purpura, photosensitivity, urticaria, necrotizing angiitis (vasculitis) (cutaneous vasculitis), fever, respiratory distress including pneumonitis and pulmonary oedema, anaphylactic reactions, hyperglycaemia, glycosuria, hyperuricaemia, electrolyte imbalance including hyponatraemia, muscle spasm, restlessness, transient blurred vision, renal failure, renal dysfunction and interstitial nephritis.

Lisinopril: myocardial infarction or cerebrovascular accident possibly secondary to excessive hypotension in high risk patients, tachycardia, abdominal pain and indigestion, mood alterations, mental confusion, vertigo have occurred; as with other angiotensin converting enzyme inhibitors, taste disturbance and sleep disturbance have been reported; bronchospasm, rhinitis, sinusitis, alopecia, urticaria, diaphoresis, pruritus, psoriasis and severe skin disorders, (including pemphigus, toxic epidermal necrolysis, Stevens-Johnson Syndrome and erythema multiforme), have been reported; hyponatraemia, uraemia, oliguria/anuria, renal dysfunction, acute renal failure, hepatitis (hepatocellular or cholestatic), jaundice and haemolytic anaemia.

4.9 Overdose

No specific information is available on the treatment of overdosage with 'Zestoretic' 20. Treatment is symptomatic and supportive. Therapy with 'Zestoretic' 20 should be discontinued and the patient should be kept under very close supervision. Therapeutic measures depend on the nature and severity of the symptoms. Measures to prevent absorption and methods to speed elimination should be employed.

Lisinopril: The most likely features of overdosage would be hypotension, electrolyte disturbance and renal failure. If severe hypotension occurs, the patient should be placed in the shock position and an intravenous infusion of normal saline should be given rapidly. Treatment with angiotensin II (if available) may be considered. Angiotensin converting enzyme inhibitors may be removed from the general circulation by haemodialysis. The use of high-flux polyacrylonitrile dialysis membranes should be avoided. Serum electrolytes and creatinine should be monitored frequently.

Hydrochlorothiazide: The most common signs and symptoms observed are those caused by electrolyte depletion (hypokalaemia, hypochloraemia, hyponatraemia) and dehydration resulting from excessive diuresis. If digitalis has also been administered hypokalaemia may accentuate cardiac arrhythmias.

5. PHARMACOLOGICAL PROPERTIES

5.1 Pharmacodynamic properties

'Zestoretic' 20 is a fixed dose combination product containing lisinopril, an inhibitor of angiotensin converting enzyme (ACE) and hydrochlorothiazide, a thiazide diuretic. Both components have complementary modes of action and exert an additive antihypertensive effect.

Lisinopril is a peptidyl dipeptidase inhibitor. It inhibits the angiotensin converting enzyme (ACE) that catalyses the conversion of angiotensin I to the vasoconstrictor peptide, angiotensin II. Angiotensin II also stimulates aldosterone secretion by the adrenal cortex. Inhibition of ACE results in decreased concentrations of angiotensin II which results in decreased vasopressor activity and reduced aldosterone secretion. The latter decrease may result in an increase in serum potassium concentration.

While the mechanism through which lisinopril lowers blood pressure is believed to be primarily suppression of the renin-angiotensin-aldosterone system, lisinopril is antihypertensive even in patients with low-renin hypertension. ACE is identical to kininase II, an enzyme that degrades bradykinin. Whether increased levels of bradykinin, a potent vasodilatory peptide, play a role in the therapeutic effects of lisinopril remains to be elucidated.

Hydrochlorothiazide is a diuretic and an antihypertensive agent. It affects the distal renal tubular mechanism of electrolyte reabsorption and increases excretion of sodium and chloride in approximately equivalent amounts. Natriuresis may be accompanied by some loss of potassium and bicarbonate. The mechanism of the antihypertensive effect of the thiazides is unknown. Thiazides do not usually affect normal blood pressure.

When combined with other antihypertensive agents, additive falls in blood pressure may occur.

5.2 Pharmacokinetic properties

Concomitant administration of lisinopril and hydrochlorothiazide has little or no effect on the bioavailability of either drug. The combination tablet is bioequivalent to concomitant administration of the separate entities.

Lisinopril:

Following oral administration of lisinopril, peak serum concentrations occur within about 7 hours. On multiple dosing lisinopril has an effective half life of accumulation of 12.6 hours. Declining serum concentrations exhibit a prolonged terminal phase which does not contribute to drug accumulation. This terminal phase probably represents saturable binding to ACE and is not proportional to dose. Lisinopril does not appear to bind to other serum proteins.

Impaired renal function decreases elimination of lisinopril, which is excreted via the kidneys, but this decrease becomes clinically important only when the glomerular filtration rate is below 30 ml/min. Older patients have higher blood levels and higher values for the area under the plasma concentration time curve than younger patients. Lisinopril can be removed by dialysis.

Based on urinary recovery, the mean extent of absorption of lisinopril is approximately 25%, with interpatient variability (6-60%) at all doses tested (5-80 mg).

Lisinopril does not undergo metabolism and absorbed drug is excreted unchanged entirely in the urine. Lisinopril absorption is not affected by the presence of food in the gastrointestinal tract.

Studies in rats indicate that lisinopril crosses the blood-brain barrier poorly.

Hydrochlorothiazide:

When plasma levels have been followed for at least 24 hours, the plasma half-life has been observed to vary between 5.6 and 14.8 hours. At least 61% of the dose is eliminated unchanged within 24 hours. After oral hydrochlorothiazide, diuresis begins within 2 hours, peaks in about 4 hours and lasts 6 to 12 hours. Hydrochlorothiazide crosses the placental but not the blood-brain barrier.

5.3 Preclinical safety data

Lisinopril and hydrochlorthiazide are both drugs on which extensive clinical experience has been obtained, both separately and in combination. All relevant information for the prescriber is provided elsewhere in the Summary of Product Characteristics.

6. PHARMACEUTICAL PARTICULARS

6.1 List of excipients

Calcium Hydrogen Phosphate Dihydrate Ph. Eur.

Magnesium Stearate Ph. Eur

Maize Starch Ph. Eur.

Mannitol Ph. Eur.

Pregelatinised Maize Starch Ph. Eur.

6.2 Incompatibilities

None known, but see Section 4.5.

6.3 Shelf life

2.5 years stored in the sales package.

6.4 Special precautions for storage

Store below 30°C and protect from light.

6.5 Nature and contents of container

Blister packs of 28 tablets

6.6 Special precautions for disposal and other handling

Not applicable.

7. MARKETING AUTHORISATION HOLDER

AstraZeneca UK Limited,

600 Capability Green,

Luton, LU1 3LU, UK.

8. MARKETING AUTHORISATION NUMBER(S)

PL 17901/0059

9. DATE OF FIRST AUTHORISATION/RENEWAL OF THE AUTHORISATION

8 June 2000

10. DATE OF REVISION OF THE TEXT

4th March 2004

Zestril 2.5mg, 5mg, 10mg, and 20mg tablets.

(AstraZeneca UK Limited)

1. NAME OF THE MEDICINAL PRODUCT

Zestril 2.5 mg, 5 mg, 10 mg, and 20 mg tablets.

2. QUALITATIVE AND QUANTITATIVE COMPOSITION

Each tablet contains lisinopril dihydrate equivalent to 2.5 mg, 5 mg, 10 mg, or 20 mg anhydrous lisinopril.

For excipients, see 6.1 List of excipients.

3. PHARMACEUTICAL FORM

2.5 mg tablets are white, round and biconvex. They have a diameter of 6 mm.

5 mg tablets are pink, round and biconvex. They have a diameter of 6 mm.

10 mg tablets are pink, round and biconvex. They have a diameter of 8 mm.

20 mg tablets are pink, round and biconvex. They have a diameter of 8 mm.

All tablets are marked on one side with a number denoting the tablet strength.

4. CLINICAL PARTICULARS

4.1 Therapeutic indications

Hypertension

Treatment of hypertension.

Heart failure

Treatment of symptomatic heart failure.

Acute myocardial infarction

Short-term (6 weeks) treatment of haemodynamically stable patients within 24 hours of an acute myocardial infarction.

Renal complications of diabetes mellitus

Treatment of renal disease in hypertensive patients with Type 2 diabetes mellitus and incipient nephropathy (see section 5.1).

4.2 Posology and method of administration

Zestril should be administered orally in a single daily dose. As with all other medication taken once daily, Zestril should be taken at approximately the same time each day. The absorption of Zestril tablets is not affected by food.

The dose should be individualised according to patient profile and blood pressure response (see section 4.4).

Hypertension

Zestril may be used as monotherapy or in combination with other classes of antihypertensive therapy.

Starting dose

In patients with hypertension the usual recommended starting dose is 10 mg. Patients with a strongly activated renin-angiotensin-aldosterone system (in particular, renovascular hypertension, salt and /or volume depletion, cardiac decompensation, or severe hypertension) may experience an excessive blood pressure fall following the initial dose. A starting dose of 2.5-5 mg is recommended in such patients and the initiation of treatment should take place under medical supervision. A lower starting dose is required in the presence of renal impairment (see Table 1 below).

Maintenance dose

The usual effective maintenance dosage is 20 mg administered in a single daily dose. In general, if the desired therapeutic effect cannot be achieved in a period of 2 to 4 weeks on a certain dose level, the dose can be further increased. The maximum dose used in long-term, controlled clinical trials was 80 mg/day.

Diuretic-treated patients

Symptomatic hypotension may occur following initiation of therapy with Zestril. This is more likely in patients who are being treated currently with diuretics. Caution is recommended therefore, since these patients may be volume and/or salt depleted. If possible, the diuretic should be discontinued 2 to 3 days before beginning therapy with Zestril. In hypertensive patients in whom the diuretic cannot be discontinued, therapy with Zestril should be initiated with a 5 mg dose. Renal function and serum potassium should be monitored. The subsequent dosage of Zestril should be adjusted according to blood pressure response. If required, diuretic therapy may be resumed (see section 4.4 and section 4.5).

Dosage adjustment in renal impairment

Dosage in patients with renal impairment should be based on creatinine clearance as outlined in Table 1 below.

Table 1 Dosage adjustment in renal impairment

Creatinine Clearance (ml/min)	Starting Dose (mg/day)
Less than 10 ml/min (including patients on dialysis)	2.5 mg*
10-30 ml/min	2.5-5 mg
31-80 ml/min	5-10 mg

* Dosage and/or frequency of administration should be adjusted depending on the blood pressure response.

The dosage may be titrated upward until blood pressure is controlled or to a maximum of 40 mg daily.

Heart failure

In patients with symptomatic heart failure, Zestril should be used as adjunctive therapy to diuretics and, where appropriate, digitalis or beta-blockers. Zestril may be initiated at a starting dose of 2.5 mg once a day, which should be administered under medical supervision to determine the initial effect on the blood pressure. The dose of Zestril should be increased:

- By increments of no greater than 10 mg
- At intervals of no less than 2 weeks
- To the highest dose tolerated by the patient up to a maximum of 35 mg once daily.

Dose adjustment should be based on the clinical response of individual patients.

Patients at high risk of symptomatic hypotension, e.g. patients with salt depletion with or without hyponatraemia, patients with hypovolaemia or patients who have been receiving vigorous diuretic therapy should have these conditions corrected, if possible, prior to therapy with Zestril. Renal function and serum potassium should be monitored (see section 4.4).

Acute myocardial infarction

Patients should receive, as appropriate, the standard recommended treatments such as thrombolytics, aspirin, and beta-blockers. Intravenous or transdermal glyceryl trinitrate may be used together with Zestril.

Starting dose (first 3 days after infarction)

Treatment with Zestril may be started within 24 hours of the onset of symptoms. Treatment should not be started if systolic blood pressure is lower than 100 mm Hg. The first dose of Zestril is 5 mg given orally, followed by 5 mg after 24 hours, 10 mg after 48 hours and then 10 mg once daily. Patients with a low systolic blood pressure (120 mm Hg or less) when treatment is started or during the first 3 days after the infarction should be given a lower dose - 2.5 mg orally (see section 4.4).

In cases of renal impairment (creatinine clearance <80 ml/min), the initial Zestril dosage should be adjusted according to the patient's creatinine clearance (see Table 1).

Maintenance dose

The maintenance dose is 10 mg once daily. If hypotension occurs (systolic blood pressure less than or equal to 100 mm Hg) a daily maintenance dose of 5 mg may be given with temporary reductions to 2.5 mg if needed. If prolonged hypotension occurs (systolic blood pressure less than 90 mm Hg for more than 1 hour) Zestril should be withdrawn.

Treatment should continue for 6 weeks and then the patient should be re-evaluated. Patients who develop symptoms of heart failure should continue with Zestril (see section 4.2).

Renal complications of diabetes mellitus

In hypertensive patients with type 2 diabetes mellitus and incipient nephropathy, the dose is 10 mg Zestril once daily which can be increased to 20 mg once daily, if necessary, to achieve a sitting diastolic blood pressure below 90 mm Hg.

In cases of renal impairment (creatinine clearance <80 ml/min), the initial Zestril dosage should be adjusted according to the patient's creatinine clearance (see Table 1).

Paediatric use

Efficacy and safety of use in children has not been fully established. Therefore, use in children is not recommended.

Use in the elderly

In clinical studies, there was no age-related change in the efficacy or safety profile of the drug. When advanced age is associated with decrease in renal function, however, the guidelines set out in Table 1 should be used to determine the starting dose of Zestril. Thereafter, the dosage should be adjusted according to the blood pressure response.

Use in kidney transplant patients

There is no experience regarding the administration of Zestril in patients with recent kidney transplantation. Treatment with Zestril is therefore not recommended.

4.3 Contraindications

- Hypersensitivity to Zestril, to any of the excipients or any other angiotensin converting enzyme (ACE) inhibitor
- History of angioedema associated with previous ACE inhibitor therapy
- Hereditary or idiopathic angioedema
- Second and third trimesters of pregnancy (see sections 4.4 and 4.6).

4.4 Special warnings and precautions for use

Symptomatic hypotension

Symptomatic hypotension is seen rarely in uncomplicated hypertensive patients. In hypertensive patients receiving Zestril, hypotension is more likely to occur if the patient has been volume-depleted, e.g. by diuretic therapy, dietary salt restriction, dialysis, diarrhoea or vomiting, or has severe renin-dependent hypertension (see section 4.5 and section 4.8). In patients with heart failure, with or without associated renal insufficiency, symptomatic hypotension has been observed. This is most likely to occur in those patients with more severe degrees of heart failure, as reflected by the use of high doses of loop diuretics, hyponatraemia or functional renal impairment. In patients at increased risk of symptomatic hypotension, initiation of therapy and dose adjustment should be closely monitored. Similar considerations apply to patients with ischaemic heart or cerebrovascular disease in whom an excessive fall in blood pressure could result in a myocardial infarction or cerebrovascular accident.

If hypotension occurs, the patient should be placed in the supine position and, if necessary, should receive an intravenous infusion of normal saline. A transient hypotensive response is not a contraindication to further doses, which can be given usually without difficulty once the blood pressure has increased after volume expansion.

In some patients with heart failure who have normal or low blood pressure, additional lowering of systemic blood pressure may occur with Zestril. This effect is anticipated and is not usually a reason to discontinue treatment. If hypotension becomes symptomatic, a reduction of dose or discontinuation of Zestril may be necessary.

Hypotension in acute myocardial infarction

Treatment with Zestril must not be initiated in acute myocardial infarction patients who are at risk of further serious haemodynamic deterioration after treatment with a vasodilator. These are patients with systolic blood pressure of 100 mm Hg or lower, or those in cardiogenic shock. During the first 3 days following the infarction, the dose should be reduced if the systolic blood pressure is 120 mm Hg or lower. Maintenance doses should be reduced to 5 mg or temporarily to 2.5 mg if systolic blood pressure is 100 mm Hg or lower. If hypotension persists (systolic blood pressure less than 90 mm Hg for more than 1 hour) then Zestril should be withdrawn.

Aortic and mitral valve stenosis / hypertrophic cardiomyopathy

As with other ACE inhibitors, Zestril should be given with caution to patients with mitral valve stenosis and obstruction in the outflow of the left ventricle such as aortic stenosis or hypertrophic cardiomyopathy.

Renal function impairment

In cases of renal impairment (creatinine clearance <80 ml/min), the initial Zestril dosage should be adjusted according to the patient's creatinine clearance (see Table 1 in section 4.2), and then as a function of the patient's response to treatment. Routine monitoring of potassium and creatinine is part of normal medical practice for these patients.

In patients with heart failure, hypotension following the initiation of therapy with ACE inhibitors may lead to some further impairment in renal function. Acute renal failure, usually reversible, has been reported in this situation.

In some patients with bilateral renal artery stenosis or with a stenosis of the artery to a solitary kidney, who have been treated with angiotensin-converting enzyme inhibitors, increases in blood urea and serum creatinine, usually reversible upon discontinuation of therapy, have been seen. This is especially likely in patients with renal insufficiency. If renovascular hypertension is also present there is an increased risk of severe hypotension and renal insufficiency. In these patients, treatment should be started under close medical supervision with low doses and careful dose titration. Since treatment with diuretics may be a contributory factor to the above, they should be discontinued and renal function should be monitored during the first weeks of Zestril therapy.

Some hypertensive patients with no apparent pre-existing renal vascular disease have developed increases in blood urea and serum creatinine, usually minor and transient, especially when Zestril has been given concomitantly with a diuretic. This is more likely to occur in patients with pre-existing renal impairment. Dosage reduction and/or discontinuation of the diuretic and/or Zestril may be required.

In acute myocardial infarction, treatment with Zestril should not be initiated in patients with evidence of renal dysfunction, defined as serum creatinine concentration exceeding 177 micromol/l and/or proteinuria exceeding 500 mg/24 h. If renal dysfunction develops during treatment with Zestril (serum creatinine concentration exceeding 265 micromol/l or a doubling from the pre-treatment value) then the physician should consider withdrawal of Zestril.

Hypersensitivity/Angioedema

Angioedema of the face, extremities, lips, tongue, glottis and/or larynx has been reported uncommonly in patients treated with angiotensin-converting enzyme inhibitors, including Zestril. This may occur at any time during therapy. In such cases, Zestril should be discontinued promptly and appropriate treatment and monitoring should be instituted to ensure complete resolution of symptoms prior to dismissing the patients. Even in those instances where swelling of only the tongue is involved, without respiratory distress, patients may require prolonged observation since treatment with antihistamines and corticosteroids may not be sufficient.

Very rarely, fatalities have been reported due to angioedema associated with laryngeal oedema or tongue oedema. Patients with involvement of the tongue, glottis or larynx, are likely to experience airway obstruction, especially those with a history of airway surgery. In such cases emergency therapy should be administered promptly. This may include the administration of adrenaline and/or the maintenance of a patent airway. The patient should be under close medical supervision until complete and sustained resolution of symptoms has occurred.

Angiotensin-converting enzyme inhibitors cause a higher rate of angioedema in black patients than in non-black patients.

Patients with a history of angioedema unrelated to ACE inhibitor therapy may be at increased risk of angioedema while receiving an ACE inhibitor (see section 4.3).

Anaphylactoid reactions in haemodialysis patients

Anaphylactoid reactions have been reported in patients dialysed with high flux membranes (e.g. AN 69) and treated concomitantly with an ACE inhibitor. In these patients, consideration should be given to using a different type of dialysis membrane or different class of antihypertensive agent.

Anaphylactoid reactions during low-density lipoproteins (LDL) apheresis

Rarely, patients receiving ACE inhibitors during low-density lipoproteins (LDL) apheresis with dextran sulphate have experienced life-threatening anaphylactoid reactions. These reactions were avoided by temporarily withholding ACE inhibitor therapy prior to each apheresis.

Desensitisation

Patients receiving ACE inhibitors during desensitisation treatment (e.g. hymenoptera venom) have sustained anaphylactoid reactions. In the same patients, these reactions have been avoided when ACE inhibitors were temporarily withheld but they have reappeared upon inadvertent re-administration of the medicinal product.

Hepatic failure

Very rarely, ACE inhibitors have been associated with a syndrome that starts with cholestatic jaundice and progresses to fulminant necrosis and (sometimes) death. The mechanism of this syndrome is not understood. Patients receiving Zestril who develop jaundice or marked elevations of hepatic enzymes should discontinue Zestril and receive appropriate medical follow-up.

Neutropenia/Agranulocytosis

Neutropenia/agranulocytosis, thrombocytopenia and anaemia have been reported in patients receiving ACE inhibitors. In patients with normal renal function and no other complicating factors, neutropenia occurs rarely. Neutropenia and agranulocytosis are reversible after discontinuation of the ACE inhibitor. Zestril should be used with extreme caution in patients with collagen vascular disease, immunosuppressant therapy, treatment with allopurinol or procainamide, or a combination of these complicating factors, especially if there is pre-existing impaired renal function. Some of these patients developed serious infections, which in a few instances did not respond to intensive antibiotic therapy. If Zestril is used in such patients, periodic monitoring of white blood cell counts is advised and patients should be instructed to report any sign of infection.

Race

Angiotensin-converting enzyme inhibitors cause a higher rate of angioedema in black patients than in non-black patients.

As with other ACE inhibitors, Zestril may be less effective in lowering blood pressure in black patients than in non-blacks, possibly because of a higher prevalence of low-renin states in the black hypertensive population.

Cough

Cough has been reported with the use of ACE inhibitors. Characteristically, the cough is non-productive, persistent and resolves after discontinuation of therapy. ACE inhibitor-induced cough should be considered as part of the differential diagnosis of cough.

Surgery/Anaesthesia

In patients undergoing major surgery or during anaesthesia with agents that produce hypotension, Zestril may block angiotensin II formation secondary to compensatory renin release. If hypotension occurs and is considered to be due to this mechanism, it can be corrected by volume expansion.

Hyperkalaemia

Elevations in serum potassium have been observed in some patients treated with ACE inhibitors, including Zestril. Patients at risk for the development of hyperkalaemia include those with renal insufficiency, diabetes mellitus, or those using concomitant potassium-sparing diuretics, potassium supplements or potassium-containing salt substitutes, or those patients taking other drugs associated with increases in serum potassium (e.g. heparin). If concomitant use of the above-mentioned agents is deemed appropriate, regular monitoring of serum potassium is recommended (see section 4.5).

Diabetic patients

In diabetic patients treated with oral antidiabetic agents or insulin, glycaemic control should be closely monitored during the first month of treatment with an ACE inhibitor (see 4.5 Interaction with other medicinal products and other forms of interaction).

Lithium

The combination of lithium and Zestril is generally not recommended (see section 4.5).

Pregnancy and lactation

ACE inhibitors should not be initiated during pregnancy. Unless continued ACE inhibitor therapy is considered essential, patients planning pregnancy should be changed to alternative antihypertensive treatments which have an established safety profile for use in pregnancy. When pregnancy is diagnosed, treatment with ACE inhibitors should be stopped immediately, and, if appropriate, alternative therapy should be started (see sections 4.3 and 4.6).

Use of lisinopril is not recommended during breast-feeding.

4.5 Interaction with other medicinal products and other forms of interaction

Diuretics

When a diuretic is added to the therapy of a patient receiving Zestril the antihypertensive effect is usually additive.

Patients already on diuretics and especially those in whom diuretic therapy was recently instituted, may occasionally experience an excessive reduction of blood pressure when Zestril is added. The possibility of symptomatic hypotension with Zestril can be minimised by discontinuing the diuretic prior to initiation of treatment with Zestril (see section 4.4 and section 4.2).

Potassium supplements, potassium-sparing diuretics or potassium-containing salt substitutes

Although in clinical trials, serum potassium usually remained within normal limits, hyperkalaemia did occur in some patients. Risk factors for the development of hyperkalaemia include renal insufficiency, diabetes mellitus, and concomitant use of potassium-sparing diuretics (e.g. spironolactone, triamterene or amiloride), potassium supplements or potassium-containing salt substitutes. The use of potassium supplements, potassium-sparing diuretics or potassium-containing salt substitutes, particularly in patients with impaired renal function, may lead to a significant increase in serum potassium. If Zestril is given with a potassium-losing diuretic, diuretic-induced hypokalaemia may be ameliorated.

Lithium

Reversible increases in serum lithium concentrations and toxicity have been reported during concomitant administration of lithium with ACE inhibitors. Concomitant use of thiazide diuretics may increase the risk of lithium toxicity and enhance the already increased lithium toxicity with ACE inhibitors. Use of Zestril with lithium is not recommended, but if the combination proves necessary, careful monitoring of serum lithium levels should be performed (see section 4.4).

Non-steroidal anti-inflammatory drugs (NSAIDs) including acetylsalicylic acid $\geqslant$ 3 g/day

Chronic administration of NSAIDs may reduce the antihypertensive effect of an ACE inhibitor. NSAIDs and ACE inhibitors exert an additive effect on the increase in serum potassium and may result in a deterioration of renal function. These effects are usually reversible. Rarely, acute renal failure may occur, especially in patients with compromised renal function such as the elderly or dehydrated.

Gold

Nitritoid reactions (symptoms of vasodilatation including flushing, nausea, dizziness and hypotension, which can be very severe) following injectable gold (for example, sodium aurothiomalate) have been reported more frequently in patients receiving ACE inhibitor therapy.

Other antihypertensive agents

Concomitant use of these agents may increase the hypotensive effects of Zestril. Concomitant use with glyceryl trinitrate and other nitrates, or other vasodilators, may further reduce blood pressure.

Tricyclic antidepressants / Antipsychotics / Anaesthetics

Concomitant use of certain anaesthetic medicinal products, tricyclic antidepressants and antipsychotics with ACE inhibitors may result in further reduction of blood pressure (see section 4.4).

Sympathomimetics

Sympathomimetics may reduce the antihypertensive effects of ACE inhibitors.

Antidiabetics

Epidemiological studies have suggested that concomitant administration of ACE inhibitors and antidiabetic medicines (insulins, oral hypoglycaemic agents) may cause an increased blood glucose-lowering effect with risk of hypoglycaemia. This phenomenon appeared to be more likely to occur during the first weeks of combined treatment and in patients with renal impairment.

Acetylsalicylic acid, thrombolytics, beta-blockers, nitrates

Zestril may be used concomitantly with acetylsalicylic acid (at cardiologic doses), thrombolytics, beta-blockers and/or nitrates.

4.6 Pregnancy and lactation

Pregnancy

The use of ACE inhibitors is not recommended during the first trimester of pregnancy (see section 4.4). The use of ACE inhibitors is contra-indicated during the second and third trimester of pregnancy (see sections 4.3 and 4.4).

Epidemiological evidence regarding the risk of teratogenicity following exposure to ACE inhibitors during the first trimester of pregnancy has not been conclusive; however a small increase in risk cannot be excluded. Unless continued ACE inhibitors therapy is considered essential, patients planning pregnancy should be changed to alternative anti-hypertensive treatments which have an established safety profile for use in pregnancy. When pregnancy is diagnosed, treatment with ACE inhibitors should be stopped immediately, and, if appropriate, alternative therapy should be started.

Exposure to ACE inhibitor therapy during the second and third trimesters is known to induce human foetotoxicity (decreased renal function, oligohydramnios, skull ossification retardation) and neonatal toxicity (renal failure, hypotension, hyperkalaemia). (See section 5.3).

Should exposure to ACE inhibitors have occurred from the second trimester of pregnancy, ultrasound check of renal function and skull is recommended.

Infants whose mothers have taken ACE inhibitors should be closely observed for hypotension (see sections 4.3 and 4.4).

Lactation

It is not known whether Zestril is excreted into human breast milk. Lisinopril is excreted into the milk of lactating rats. The use of Zestril is not recommended in women who are breast-feeding.

4.7 Effects on ability to drive and use machines

When driving vehicles or operating machines it should be taken into account that occasionally dizziness or tiredness may occur.

4.8 Undesirable effects

The following undesirable effects have been observed and reported during treatment with Zestril and other ACE inhibitors with the following frequencies: Very common ($\geqslant$1/10), common ($\geqslant$1/100 to <1/10), uncommon ($\geqslant$1/1,000 to <1/100), rare ($\geqslant$1/10,000 to <1/1,000), very rare (<1/10,000), not known (cannot be estimated from the available data).

Blood and the lymphatic system disorders

rare: decreases in haemoglobin, decreases in haematocrit

very rare: bone marrow depression, anaemia, thrombocytopenia, leucopenia, neutropenia, agranulocytosis (see section 4.4), haemolytic anaemia, lymphadenopathy, autoimmune disease.

Metabolism and nutrition disorders

very rare: hypoglycaemia.

Nervous system and psychiatric disorders

common: dizziness, headache

uncommon: mood alterations, paraesthesia, vertigo, taste disturbance, sleep disturbances

rare: mental confusion

frequency not known: depressive symptoms, syncope.

Cardiac and vascular disorders

common: orthostatic effects (including hypotension)

uncommon: myocardial infarction or cerebrovascular accident, possibly secondary to excessive hypotension in high risk patients (see section 4.4), palpitations, tachycardia, Raynaud's phenomenon.

Respiratory, thoracic and mediastinal disorders

common: cough

uncommon: rhinitis

very rare: bronchospasm, sinusitis, allergic alveolitis/eosinophilic pneumonia.

Gastrointestinal disorders

common: diarrhoea, vomiting

uncommon: nausea, abdominal pain and indigestion

rare: dry mouth

very rare: pancreatitis, intestinal angioedema, hepatitis - either hepatocellular or cholestatic, jaundice and hepatic failure (see section 4.4).

Skin and subcutaneous tissue disorders

uncommon: rash, pruritus, hypersensitivity/angioneurotic oedema: angioneurotic oedema of the face, extremities, lips, tongue, glottis, and/or larynx (see section 4.4)

rare: urticaria, alopecia, psoriasis

very rare: diaphoresis, pemphigus, toxic epidermal necrolysis, Stevens-Johnson Syndrome, erythema multiforme, cutaneous pseudolymphoma.

A symptom complex has been reported which may include one or more of the following: fever, vasculitis, myalgia, arthralgia/arthritis, positive antinuclear antibodies (ANA), elevated red blood cell sedimentation rate (ESR), eosinophilia and leucocytosis, rash, photosensitivity or other dermatological manifestations may occur.

Renal and urinary disorders

common: renal dysfunction

rare: uraemia, acute renal failure

very rare: oliguria/anuria.

Reproductive system and breast disorders

uncommon: impotence

rare: gynaecomastia.

General disorders and administration site conditions

uncommon: fatigue, asthenia.

Investigations

uncommon: increases in blood urea, increases in serum creatinine, increases in liver enzymes, hyperkalaemia

rare: increases in serum bilirubin, hyponatraemia.

4.9 Overdose

Limited data are available for overdose in humans. Symptoms associated with overdosage of ACE inhibitors may include hypotension, circulatory shock, electrolyte disturbances, renal failure, hyperventilation, tachycardia, palpitations, bradycardia, dizziness, anxiety and cough.

The recommended treatment of overdose is intravenous infusion of normal saline solution. If hypotension occurs, the patient should be placed in the shock position. If available, treatment with angiotensin II infusion and/or intravenous catecholamines may also be considered. If ingestion is recent, take measures aimed at eliminating Zestril (e.g. emesis, gastric lavage, administration of absorbents and sodium sulphate). Zestril may be removed from the general circulation by haemodialysis (see 4.4 Special warnings and Precautions for use). Pacemaker therapy is indicated for therapy-resistant bradycardia. Vital signs, serum electrolytes and creatinine concentrations should be monitored frequently.

5. PHARMACOLOGICAL PROPERTIES

5.1 Pharmacodynamic properties

Pharmacotherapeutic group: Angiotensin-converting enzyme inhibitors, ATC code: C09A A03.

Zestril is a peptidyl dipeptidase inhibitor. It inhibits the angiotensin-converting enzyme (ACE) that catalyses the conversion of angiotensin I to the vasoconstrictor peptide, angiotensin II. Angiotensin II also stimulates aldosterone secretion by the adrenal cortex. Inhibition of ACE results in decreased concentrations of angiotensin II which results in decreased vasopressor activity and reduced aldosterone secretion. The latter decrease may result in an increase in serum potassium concentration.

Whilst the mechanism through which lisinopril lowers blood pressure is believed to be primarily suppression of the renin-angiotensin-aldosterone system, lisinopril is antihypertensive even in patients with low renin hypertension. ACE is identical to kininase II, an enzyme that degrades bradykinin. Whether increased levels of bradykinin, a potent vasodilatory peptide, play a role in the therapeutic effects of lisinopril remains to be elucidated.

The effect of Zestril on mortality and morbidity in heart failure has been studied by comparing a high dose (32.5 mg or 35 mg once daily) with a low dose (2.5 mg or 5 mg once daily). In a study of 3164 patients, with a median follow-up period of 46 months for surviving patients, high dose Zestril produced a 12% risk reduction in the combined endpoint of all-cause mortality and all-cause hospitalisation (p = 0.002) and an 8% risk reduction in all-cause mortality and cardiovascular hospitalisation (p = 0.036) compared with low dose. Risk reductions for all-cause mortality (8%; p = 0.128) and cardiovascular mortality (10%; p = 0.073) were observed. In a post-hoc analysis, the number of hospitalisations for heart failure was reduced by 24% (p=0.002) in patients treated with high-dose Zestril compared with low dose. Symptomatic benefits were similar in patients treated with high and low doses of Zestril.

The results of the study showed that the overall adverse event profiles for patients treated with high or low dose Zestril were similar in both nature and number. Predictable events resulting from ACE inhibition, such as hypotension or altered renal function, were manageable and rarely led to treatment withdrawal. Cough was less frequent in patients treated with high dose Zestril compared with low dose.

In the GISSI-3 trial, which used a 2x2 factorial design to compare the effects of Zestril and glyceryl trinitrate given alone or in combination for 6 weeks versus control in 19,394 patients who were administered the treatment within 24 hours of an acute myocardial infarction, Zestril produced a statistically significant risk reduction in mortality of 11% versus control (2p=0.03). The risk reduction with glyceryl trinitrate was not significant but the combination of Zestril and glyceryl trinitrate produced a significant risk reduction in mortality of 17% versus control (2p=0.02). In the sub-groups of elderly (age > 70 years) and females, pre-defined as patients at high risk of mortality, significant benefit was observed for a combined endpoint of mortality and cardiac function. The combined endpoint for all patients, as well as the high-risk subgroups at 6 months, also showed significant benefit for those treated with Zestril or Zestril plus glyceryl trinitrate for 6 weeks, indicating a prevention effect for Zestril. As would be expected from any vasodilator treatment, increased incidences of hypotension and renal dysfunction were associated with Zestril treatment but these were not associated with a proportional increase in mortality.

In a double-blind, randomised, multicentre trial which compared Zestril with a calcium channel blocker in 335 hypertensive Type 2 diabetes mellitus subjects with incipient nephropathy characterised by microalbuminuria, Zestril 10 mg to 20 mg administered once daily for 12 months, reduced systolic/diastolic blood pressure by 13/10 mmHg and urinary albumin excretion rate by 40%. When compared with the calcium channel blocker, which produced a similar reduction in blood pressure, those treated with Zestril showed a significantly greater reduction in urinary albumin excretion rate, providing evidence that the ACE inhibitory action of Zestril reduced microalbuminuria by a direct mechanism on renal tissues in addition to its blood pressure-lowering effect.

Lisinopril treatment does not affect glycaemic control as shown by a lack of significant effect on levels of glycated haemoglobin (HbA_{1c}).

5.2 Pharmacokinetic properties

Lisinopril is an orally active non-sulphydryl-containing ACE inhibitor.

Absorption

Following oral administration of lisinopril, peak serum concentrations occur within about 7 hours, although there was a trend to a small delay in time taken to reach peak serum concentrations in acute myocardial infarction patients. Based on urinary recovery, the mean extent of absorption of lisinopril is approximately 25% with interpatient variability of 6-60% over the dose range studied (5-80 mg). The absolute bioavailability is reduced approximately 16% in patients with heart failure. Lisinopril absorption is not affected by the presence of food.

Distribution

Lisinopril does not appear to be bound to serum proteins other than to circulating angiotensin-converting enzyme (ACE). Studies in rats indicate that lisinopril crosses the blood-brain barrier poorly.

Elimination

Lisinopril does not undergo metabolism and is excreted entirely unchanged into the urine. On multiple dosing, lisinopril has an effective half-life of accumulation of 12.6 hours. The clearance of lisinopril in healthy subjects is approximately 50 ml/min. Declining serum concentrations exhibit a prolonged terminal phase, which does not contribute to drug accumulation. This terminal phase probably represents saturable binding to ACE and is not proportional to dose.

Hepatic Impairment

Impairment of hepatic function in cirrhotic patients resulted in a decrease in lisinopril absorption (about 30% as determined by urinary recovery), but an increase in exposure (approximately 50%) compared to healthy subjects due to decreased clearance.

Renal impairment

Impaired renal function decreases elimination of lisinopril, which is excreted via the kidneys, but this decrease becomes clinically important only when the glomerular filtration rate is below 30 ml/min. In mild to moderate renal impairment (creatinine clearance 30-80 ml/min), mean AUC was increased by 13% only, while a 4.5- fold increase in mean AUC was observed in severe renal impairment (creatinine clearance 5-30 ml/min).

Lisinopril can be removed by dialysis. During 4 hours of haemodialysis, plasma lisinopril concentrations decreased on average by 60%, with a dialysis clearance between 40 and 55 ml/min.

Heart failure

Patients with heart failure have a greater exposure of lisinopril when compared to healthy subjects (an increase in AUC on average of 125%), but based on the urinary recovery of lisinopril, there is reduced absorption of approximately 16% compared to healthy subjects.

Elderly

Older patients have higher blood levels and higher values for the area under the plasma concentration-time curve (increased approximately 60%) compared with younger subjects.

5.3 Preclinical safety data

Preclinical data reveal no special hazard for humans based on conventional studies of general pharmacology, repeated dose toxicity, genotoxicity, and carcinogenic potential. Angiotensin-converting enzyme inhibitors, as a class, have been shown to induce adverse effects on the late foetal development, resulting in foetal death and congenital effects, in particular affecting the skull. Foetotoxicity, intrauterine growth retardation and patent ductus arteriosus have also been reported. These developmental anomalies are thought to be partly due to a direct action of ACE inhibitors on the foetal renin-angiotensin system and partly due to ischaemia resulting from maternal hypotension and decreases in foetal-placental blood flow and oxygen/nutrients delivery to the foetus.

6. PHARMACEUTICAL PARTICULARS

6.1 List of excipients

Mannitol

Calcium Hydrogen Phosphate dihydrate

Red Iron Oxide, in all except the 2.5 mg (E172)

Maize Starch

Pregelatinised Starch

Magnesium Stearate

6.2 Incompatibilities

Not applicable.

6.3 Shelf life

4 years.

6.4 Special precautions for storage

2.5 mg tablets: Do not store above 25°C.

5, 10, 20 and 30 mg tablets: Do not store above 30°C.

6.5 Nature and contents of container

2.5 mg Tablets: Aluminium/PVC-PVDC or Aluminium/PVC foil blister packs of 14, 20, 28, 30, 50, 84, 100 and 400 tablets.

HDPE bottle packs of 20, 30, 50, 100 and 400 tablets.

5 mg Tablets: Aluminium/PVC-PVDC, Aluminium/PVC or Aluminium/Aluminium foil blister packs of 14, 20, 28, 28x1, 30, 42, 50, 56, 60, 84, 98, 100, 400 and 500 tablets.

HDPE bottle packs of 20, 30, 50, 100 and 400 tablets.

10 mg Tablets: Aluminium/PVC-PVDC or Aluminium/PVC foil blister packs of 14, 20, 28, 30, 50, 56, 84, 98, 100 and 400 tablets.

HDPE bottle packs of 20, 30, 50, 100 and 400 tablets.

20 mg Tablets: Aluminium/PVC-PVDC, Aluminium/PVC or Aluminium/Aluminium foil blister packs of 14, 20, 28, 30, 42, 50, 56, 56x1 60, 84, 98, 100, 400 and 500 tablets.

HDPE bottle packs of 20, 30, 50, 100 and 400 tablets.

Not all pack sizes may be marketed.

6.6 Special precautions for disposal and other handling

No special requirements.

7. MARKETING AUTHORISATION HOLDER

AstraZeneca UK Limited,

600 Capability Green,

Luton, LU1 3LU, UK.

8. MARKETING AUTHORISATION NUMBER(S)

2.5 mg: PL 17901/0060

5 mg: PL 17901/0061

10 mg: PL 17901/0062

20 mg: PL 17901/0063

9. DATE OF FIRST AUTHORISATION/RENEWAL OF THE AUTHORISATION

Date of first authorisation:8 June 2000

Date of first renewal: 01 August 2005

10. DATE OF REVISION OF THE TEXT

20th November 2008

Ziagen 20 mg/ml Oral Solution

(GlaxoSmithKline UK)

1. NAME OF THE MEDICINAL PRODUCT

Ziagen 20 mg/ml oral solution

2. QUALITATIVE AND QUANTITATIVE COMPOSITION

Each ml of oral solution contains 20 mg of abacavir (as sulfate).

Excipients:

Sorbitol (E420) 340 mg/ml

Methyl parahydroxybenzoate (E218) 1.5 mg/ml

Propyl parahydroxybenzoate (E216) 0.18 mg/ml

For a full list of excipients see section 6.1.

3. PHARMACEUTICAL FORM

Oral solution

The oral solution is clear to slightly opalescent yellowish, aqueous solution.

4. CLINICAL PARTICULARS

4.1 Therapeutic indications

Ziagen is indicated in antiretroviral combination therapy for the treatment of Human Immunodeficiency Virus (HIV) infection.

The demonstration of the benefit of Ziagen is mainly based on results of studies performed in treatment-naïve adult patients on combination therapy with a twice daily regimen (see section 5.1).

Before initiating treatment with abacavir, screening for carriage of the HLA-B*5701 allele should be performed in any HIV-infected patient, irrespective of racial origin. Abacavir should not be used in patients known to carry the HLA-B*5701 allele, unless no other therapeutic option is available in these patients, based on the treatment history and resistance testing (see section 4.4 and 4.8).

4.2 Posology and method of administration

Ziagen should be prescribed by physicians experienced in the management of HIV infection.

Adults and adolescents: the recommended dose of Ziagen is 600 mg daily (30 ml). This may be administered as either 300 mg (15 ml) twice daily or 600 mg (30 ml) once daily (see sections 4.4 and 5.1).

Patients changing to the once daily regimen should take 300 mg (15 ml) twice a day and switch to 600 mg (30 ml) once a day the following morning. Where an evening once daily regimen is preferred, 300 mg (15 ml) of Ziagen should be taken on the first morning only, followed by 600 mg (30 ml) in the evening. When changing back to a twice daily regimen, patients should complete the day's treatment and start 300 mg (15 ml) twice a day the following morning.

Children from three months to 12 years: the recommended dose is 8 mg/kg twice daily up to a maximum of 600 mg (30 ml) daily.

Children less than three months: the experience in children aged less than three months is limited (see section 5.2).

Ziagen can be taken with or without food.

Ziagen is also available as a tablet formulation.

Renal impairment: no dosage adjustment of Ziagen is necessary in patients with renal dysfunction. However, Ziagen is not recommended for patients with end-stage renal disease (see section 5.2).

Hepatic impairment: abacavir is primarily metabolised by the liver. No dose recommendation can be made in patients with mild hepatic impairment. In patients with moderate hepatic impairment, no data are available, therefore the use of abacavir is not recommended unless judged necessary. If abacavir is used in patients with mild or moderate hepatic impairment, then close monitoring is required, and if feasible, monitoring of abacavir plasma levels is recommended (see section 5.2). Abacavir is contraindicated in patients with severe hepatic impairment (see section 4.3 and 4.4).

Elderly: no pharmacokinetic data is currently available in patients over 65 years of age.

4.3 Contraindications

Hypersensitivity to the active substance or to any of the excipients. See BOXED INFORMATION ON HYPERSENSITIVITY REACTIONS in sections 4.4. and 4.8.

Severe hepatic impairment.

4.4 Special warnings and precautions for use

(see Table 1 on next page)

Lactic acidosis: lactic acidosis, usually associated with hepatomegaly and hepatic steatosis, has been reported with the use of nucleoside analogues. Early symptoms (symptomatic hyperlactatemia) include benign digestive symptoms (nausea, vomiting and abdominal pain), non-specific malaise, loss of appetite, weight loss, respiratory symptoms (rapid and/or deep breathing) or neurological symptoms (including motor weakness).

Lactic acidosis has a high mortality and may be associated with pancreatitis, liver failure, or renal failure.

Lactic acidosis generally occurred after a few or several months of treatment.

Treatment with nucleoside analogues should be discontinued in the setting of symptomatic hyperlactatemia and metabolic/lactic acidosis, progressive hepatomegaly, or rapidly elevating aminotransferase levels.

Caution should be exercised when administering nucleoside analogues to any patient (particularly obese women) with hepatomegaly, hepatitis or other known risk factors for liver disease and hepatic steatosis (including certain medicinal products and alcohol). Patients co-infected with hepatitis C and treated with alpha interferon and ribavirin may constitute a special risk.

Patients at increased risk should be followed closely.

Mitochondrial dysfunction: nucleoside and nucleotide analogues have been demonstrated *in vitro* and *in vivo* to cause a variable degree of mitochondrial damage. There have been reports of mitochondrial dysfunction in HIV-negative infants exposed *in utero* and/or post-natally to nucleoside analogues. The main adverse reactions reported are haematological disorders (anaemia, neutropenia), metabolic disorders (hyperlactatemia, hyperlipasemia). These events are often transitory. Some late-onset neurological disorders have been reported (hypertonia, convulsion, abnormal behaviour). Whether the neurological disorders are transient or permanent is currently unknown. Any child exposed *in utero* to nucleoside and nucleotide analogues, even HIV-negative children, should have

Table 1

Hypersensitivity reaction (see also section 4.8):

In clinical studies approximately 5% of subjects receiving abacavir develop a hypersensitivity reaction; some of these cases were life-threatening and resulted in a fatal outcome despite taking precautions.

Studies have shown that carriage of the HLA-B*5701 allele is associated with a significantly increased risk of a hypersensitivity reaction to abacavir. Based on the prospective study CNA106030 (PREDICT-1), use of pre-therapy screening for the HLA-B*5701 allele and subsequently avoiding abacavir in patients with this allele significantly reduced the incidence of abacavir hypersensitivity reactions. In populations similar to that enrolled in the PREDICT-1 study, it is estimated that 48% to 61% of patients with the HLA-B*5701 allele will develop a hypersensitivity reaction during the course of abacavir treatment compared with 0% to 4% of patients who do not have the HLA-B*5701 allele.

These results are consistent with those of prior retrospective studies.

As a consequence, before initiating treatment with abacavir, screening for carriage of the HLA-B*5701 allele should be performed in any HIV-infected patient, irrespective of racial origin. Abacavir should not be used in patients known to carry the HLA-B*5701 allele, unless no other therapeutic option is available based on the treatment history and resistance testing (see section 4.1).

In any patient treated with abacavir, the clinical diagnosis of suspected hypersensitivity reaction must remain the basis of clinical decision-making. It is noteworthy that among patients with a clinically suspected hypersensitivity reaction, a proportion did not carry HLA-B*5701. Therefore, even in the absence of HLA-B*5701 allele, it is important to permanently discontinue abacavir and not rechallenge with abacavir if a hypersensitivity reaction cannot be ruled out on clinical grounds, due to the potential for a severe or even fatal reaction.

Skin patch testing was used as a research tool for the PREDICT-1 study but has no utility in the clinical management of patients and therefore should not be used in the clinical setting.

• **Clinical description**

Hypersensitivity reactions are characterised by the appearance of symptoms indicating multi-organ system involvement. Almost all hypersensitivity reactions will have fever and/or rash as part of the syndrome.

Other signs and symptoms may include respiratory signs and symptoms such as dyspnoea, sore throat, cough and abnormal chest x-ray findings (predominantly infiltrates, which can be localised), gastrointestinal symptoms, such as nausea, vomiting, diarrhoea, or abdominal pain, **and may lead to misdiagnosis of hypersensitivity as respiratory disease (pneumonia, bronchitis, pharyngitis), or gastroenteritis.**
Other frequently observed signs or symptoms of the hypersensitivity reaction may include lethargy or malaise and musculoskeletal symptoms (myalgia, rarely myolysis, arthralgia).

The symptoms related to this hypersensitivity reaction worsen with continued therapy and can be life-threatening. These symptoms usually resolve upon discontinuation of Ziagen.

• **Clinical management**

Hypersensitivity reaction symptoms usually appear within the first six weeks of initiation of treatment with abacavir, although these reactions **may occur at any time during therapy.**
Patients should be monitored closely, especially during the first two months of treatment with Ziagen, with consultation every two weeks.

Patients who are diagnosed with a hypersensitivity reaction whilst on therapy **MUST discontinue Ziagen immediately.**

Ziagen, or any other medicinal product containing abacavir (e.g. Kivexa, Trizivir), MUST NEVER be restarted in patients who have stopped therapy due to a hypersensitivity reaction.
Restarting abacavir following a hypersensitivity reaction results in a prompt return of symptoms within hours. This recurrence is usually more severe than on initial presentation, and may include life-threatening hypotension and death.

To avoid a delay in diagnosis and minimise the risk of a life-threatening hypersensitivity reaction, Ziagen must be permanently discontinued if hypersensitivity cannot be ruled out, even when other diagnoses are possible (respiratory diseases, flu-like illness, gastroenteritis or reactions to other medications).

Special care is needed for those patients simultaneously starting treatment with Ziagen and other medicinal products known to induce skin toxicity (such as non-nucleoside reverse transcriptase inhibitors - NNRTIs). This is because it is currently difficult to differentiate between rashes induced by these products and abacavir related hypersensitivity reactions.

• **Management after an interruption of Ziagen therapy**

If therapy with Ziagen has been discontinued for any reason and restarting therapy is under consideration, the reason for discontinuation must be established to assess whether the patient had any symptoms of a hypersensitivity reaction. **If a hypersensitivity reaction cannot be ruled out, Ziagen or any other medicinal product containing abacavir (e.g. Kivexa, Trizivir) must not be restarted.**

Hypersensitivity reactions with rapid onset, including life-threatening reactions have occurred after restarting Ziagen in patients who had only one of the key symptoms of hypersensitivity (skin rash, fever, gastrointestinal, respiratory or constitutional symptoms such as lethargy and malaise) prior to stopping Ziagen. The most common isolated symptom of a hypersensitivity reaction was a skin rash. Moreover, on very rare occasions hypersensitivity reactions have been reported in patients who have restarted therapy, and who had no preceding symptoms of a hypersensitivity reaction.
In both cases, if a decision is made to restart Ziagen this must be done in a setting where medical assistance is readily available.

• **Essential patient information**

Prescribers must ensure that patients are fully informed regarding the following information on the hypersensitivity reaction:

- patients must be made aware of the possibility of a hypersensitivity reaction to abacavir that may result in a life-threatening reaction or death.

- patients developing signs or symptoms possibly linked with a hypersensitivity reaction **MUST CONTACT their doctor IMMEDIATELY.**

- patients who are hypersensitive to abacavir should be reminded that they must never take Ziagen or any other medicinal product containing abacavir (e.g. Kivexa, Trizivir)

- in order to avoid restarting Ziagen, patients who have experienced a hypersensitivity reaction should be asked to return the remaining Ziagen tablets or oral solution to the pharmacy.

- patients who have stopped Ziagen for any reason, and particularly due to possible adverse reactions or illness, must be advised to contact their doctor before restarting.

- each patient should be reminded to read the Package Leaflet included in the Ziagen pack. They should be reminded of the importance of removing the Alert Card included in the pack, and keeping it with them at all times.

clinical and laboratory follow-up and should be fully investigated for possible mitochondrial dysfunction in case of relevant signs or symptoms. These findings do not affect current national recommendations to use antiretroviral therapy in pregnant women to prevent vertical transmission of HIV.

Lipodystrophy: combination antiretroviral therapy has been associated with the redistribution of body fat (lipodystrophy) in HIV patients. The long-term consequences of these events are currently unknown. Knowledge about the mechanism is incomplete. A connection between visceral lipomatosis and protease inhibitors (PIs) and lipoatrophy and nucleoside reverse transcriptase inhibitors (NRTIs) has been hypothesised. A higher risk of lipodystrophy has been associated with individual factors such as older age, and with drug related factors such as longer duration of antiretroviral treatment and associated metabolic disturbances. Clinical examination should include evaluation for physical signs of fat redistribution. Consideration should be given to the measurement of fasting serum lipids and blood glucose. Lipid disorders should be managed as clinically appropriate (see section 4.8).

Pancreatitis: pancreatitis has been reported, but a causal relationship to abacavir treatment is uncertain.

Triple nucleoside therapy: in patients with high viral load (>100,000 copies/ml) the choice of a triple combination with abacavir, lamivudine and zidovudine needs special consideration (see section 5.1).

There have been reports of a high rate of virological failure and of emergence of resistance at an early stage when abacavir was combined with tenofovir disoproxil fumarate and lamivudine as a once daily regimen.

Liver disease: the safety and efficacy of Ziagen has not been established in patients with significant underlying liver disorders. Ziagen is contraindicated in patients with severe hepatic impairment (see section 4.3). Patients with chronic hepatitis B or C and treated with combination antiretroviral therapy are at an increased risk of severe and potentially fatal hepatic adverse reactions. In case of concomitant antiviral therapy for hepatitis B or C, please refer also to the relevant product information for these medicinal products.

Patients with pre-existing liver dysfunction, including chronic active hepatitis, have an increased frequency of liver function abnormalities during combination antiretroviral therapy, and should be monitored according to standard practice. If there is evidence of worsening liver disease in such patients, interruption or discontinuation of treatment must be considered.

A pharmacokinetic study has been performed in patients with mild hepatic impairment. However, a definitive recommendation on dose reduction is not possible due to substantial variability of drug exposure in this patient population (see section 5.2). The clinical safety data available with abacavir in hepatically impaired patients is very limited. Due to the potential increases in exposure (AUC) in some patients, close monitoring is required. No data are available in patients with moderate or severe hepatic impairment. Plasma concentrations of abacavir are expected to substantially increase in these patients. Therefore, the use of abacavir in patients with moderate hepatic impairment is not recommended unless judged necessary and requires close monitoring of these patients.

Renal disease: Ziagen should not be administered to patients with end-stage renal disease (see section 5.2).

Excipients: Ziagen oral solution contains 340 mg/ml of sorbitol. When taken according to the dosage recommendations each 15 ml dose contains approximately 5 g of sorbitol. Patients with rare hereditary problems of fructose intolerance should not take this medicine. Sorbitol can have a mild laxative effect. The calorific value of sorbitol is 2.6 kcal/g.

Ziagen oral solution also contains methyl parahydroxybenzoate and propyl parahydroxybenzoate which may cause allergic reactions (possibly delayed).

Immune Reactivation Syndrome: In HIV-infected patients with severe immune deficiency at the time of institution of combination antiretroviral therapy (CART), an inflammatory reaction to asymptomatic or residual opportunistic pathogens may arise and cause serious clinical conditions, or aggravation of symptoms. Typically, such reactions have been observed within the first few weeks or months of initiation of CART. Relevant examples are cytomegalovirus retinitis, generalised and/or focal mycobacterium infections, and Pneumocystis carinii pneumonia. Any inflammatory symptoms should be evaluated and treatment instituted when necessary.

Osteonecrosis: Although the aetiology is considered to be multifactorial (including corticosteroid use, alcohol consumption, severe immunosuppression, higher body mass index), cases of osteonecrosis have been reported particularly in patients with advanced HIV-disease and/or long-term exposure to combination antiretroviral therapy (CART). Patients should be advised to seek medical advice if they experience joint aches and pain, joint stiffness or difficulty in movement.

Opportunistic infections: patients receiving Ziagen or any other antiretroviral therapy may still develop opportunistic infections and other complications of HIV infection. Therefore patients should remain under close clinical

Table 2

Hypersensitivity (see also section 4.4): In clinical studies, approximately 5% of subjects receiving abacavir developed a hypersensitivity reaction. In clinical studies with abacavir 600 mg once daily the reported rate of hypersensitivity remained within the range recorded for abacavir 300 mg twice daily. Some of these hypersensitivity reactions were life-threatening and resulted in fatal outcome despite taking precautions. This reaction is characterised by the appearance of symptoms indicating multi-organ/body-system involvement. Almost all patients developing hypersensitivity reactions will have fever and/or rash (usually maculopapular or urticarial) as part of the syndrome, however reactions have occurred without rash or fever. The signs and symptoms of this hypersensitivity reaction are listed below. These have been identified either from clinical studies or post marketing surveillance. Those reported **in at least 10% of patients** with a hypersensitivity reaction are in bold text.	
Skin	**Rash** (usually maculopapular or urticarial)
Gastrointestinal tract	**Nausea, vomiting, diarrhoea, abdominal pain**, mouth ulceration
Respiratory tract	**Dyspnoea, cough**, sore throat, adult respiratory distress syndrome, respiratory failure
Miscellaneous	**Fever, lethargy, malaise**, oedema, lymphadenopathy, hypotension, conjunctivitis, anaphylaxis
Neurological/Psychiatry	**Headache**, paraesthesia
Haematological	Lymphopenia
Liver/pancreas	**Elevated liver function tests**, hepatitis, hepatic failure
Musculoskeletal	**Myalgia**, rarely myolysis, arthralgia, elevated creatine phosphokinase
Urology	Elevated creatinine, renal failure
Rash (81% vs 67% respectively) and gastrointestinal manifestations (70% vs 54% respectively) were more frequently reported in children compared to adults. Some patients with hypersensitivity reactions were initially thought to have gastroenteritis, respiratory disease (pneumonia, bronchitis, pharyngitis) or a flu-like illness. This delay in diagnosis of hypersensitivity has resulted in Ziagen being continued or re-introduced, leading to more severe hypersensitivity reactions or death. Therefore, the diagnosis of hypersensitivity reaction should be carefully considered for patients presenting with symptoms of these diseases. Symptoms usually appeared within the first six weeks (median time to onset 11 days) of initiation of treatment with abacavir, although these reactions may occur at any time during therapy. Close medical supervision is necessary during the first two months, with consultations every two weeks. It is likely that intermittent therapy may increase the risk of developing sensitisation and therefore occurrence of clinically significant hypersensitivity reactions. Consequently, patients should be advised of the importance of taking Ziagen regularly. Restarting Ziagen following a hypersensitivity reaction results in a prompt return of symptoms within hours. This recurrence of the hypersensitivity reaction was usually more severe than on initial presentation, and may include life-threatening hypotension and death. **Patients who develop this hypersensitivity reaction must discontinue Ziagen and must never be rechallenged with Ziagen, or any other medicinal product containing abacavir (e.g. Kivexa, Trizivir).** To avoid a delay in diagnosis and minimise the risk of a life-threatening hypersensitivity reaction, Ziagen must be permanently discontinued if hypersensitivity cannot be ruled out, even when other diagnoses are possible (respiratory diseases, flu-like illness, gastroenteritis or reactions to other medications). **Hypersensitivity reactions with rapid onset, including life-threatening reactions have occurred after restarting Ziagen in patients who had only one of the key symptoms of hypersensitivity (skin rash, fever, gastrointestinal, respiratory or constitutional symptoms such as lethargy and malaise) prior to stopping Ziagen. The most common isolated symptom of a hypersensitivity reaction was a skin rash. Moreover,on very rare occasions hypersensitivity reactions have been reported in patients who have restarted therapy and who had <u>no preceding symptoms</u> of a hypersensitivity reaction.** In both cases, if a decision is made to restart Ziagen this must be done in a setting where medical assistance is readily available. Each patient must be warned about this hypersensitivity reaction to abacavir.	

observation by physicians experienced in the treatment of these associated HIV diseases.

Transmission: patients should be advised that current antiretroviral therapy, including Ziagen, have not been proven to prevent the risk of transmission of HIV to others through sexual contact or blood contamination. Appropriate precautions should continue to be taken.

Mycoardial Infarction: Observational studies have shown an association between myocardial infarction and the use of abacavir. Those studied were mainly antiretroviral experienced patients. Data from clinical trials showed l imited numbers of myocardial infarction and could not exclude a small increase in risk. Overall the available data from observational cohorts and from randomised trials show some inconsistency so can neither confirm nor refute a causal relationship between abacavir treatment and the risk of myocardial infarction. To date, there is no established biological mechanism to explain a potential increase in risk. When prescribing Ziagen, action should be taken to try to minimize all modifiable risk factors (e.g. smoking, hypertension, and hyperlipidaemia).

4.5 Interaction with other medicinal products and other forms of interaction

Based on the results of *in vitro* experiments and the known major metabolic pathways of abacavir, the potential for P450 mediated interactions with other medicinal products involving abacavir is low. P450 does not play a major role in the metabolism of abacavir, and abacavir does not inhibit metabolism mediated by CYP 3A4. Abacavir has also been shown *in vitro* not to inhibit CYP 3A4, CYP2C9 or CYP2D6 enzymes at clinically relevant concentrations. Induction of hepatic metabolism has not been observed in clinical studies. Therefore, there is little potential for interactions with antiretroviral PIs and other medicinal products metabolised by major P450 enzymes. Clinical studies have shown that there are no clinically significant interactions between abacavir, zidovudine, and lamivudine.

Potent enzymatic inducers such as rifampicin, phenobarbital and phenytoin may via their action on UDP-glucuronyltransferases slightly decrease the plasma concentrations of abacavir.

Ethanol: the metabolism of abacavir is altered by concomitant ethanol resulting in an increase in AUC of abacavir of about 41%. These findings are not considered clinically significant. Abacavir has no effect on the metabolism of ethanol.

Methadone: in a pharmacokinetic study, co-administration of 600 mg abacavir twice daily with methadone showed a 35% reduction in abacavir C_{max} and a one hour delay in t_{max} but the AUC was unchanged. The changes in abacavir pharmacokinetics are not considered clinically relevant. In this study abacavir increased the mean methadone systemic clearance by 22%. The induction of drug metabolising enzymes cannot therefore be excluded. Patients being treated with methadone and abacavir should be monitored for evidence of withdrawal symptoms indicating under dosing, as occasionally methadone re-titration may be required.

Retinoids: retinoid compounds are eliminated via alcohol dehydrogenase. Interaction with abacavir is possible but has not been studied.

4.6 Pregnancy and lactation

Ziagen is not recommended during pregnancy. The safe use of abacavir in human pregnancy has not been established. Placental transfer of abacavir and/or its related metabolites has been shown to occur in animals. Toxicity to the developing embryo and foetus occurred in rats, but not in rabbits (see section 5.3). The teratogenic potential of abacavir could not be established from studies in animals.

Abacavir and its metabolites are secreted into the milk of lactating rats. It is expected that these will also be secreted into human milk, although this has not been confirmed. There are no data available on the safety of abacavir when administered to babies less than three months old. It is therefore recommended that mothers do not breast-feed their babies while receiving treatment with abacavir. Additionally, it is recommended that HIV infected women do not breast-feed their infants under any circumstances in order to avoid transmission of HIV.

4.7 Effects on ability to drive and use machines

No studies on the effects on ability to drive and use machines have been performed.

4.8 Undesirable effects

(see Table 2)

For many of the other adverse reactions reported, it is unclear whether they are related to Ziagen, to the wide range of medicinal products used in the management of HIV infection or as a result of the disease process.

Many of those listed below occur commonly (nausea, vomiting, diarrhoea, fever, lethargy, rash) in patients with abacavir hypersensitivity. Therefore, patients with any of these symptoms should be carefully evaluated for the presence of this hypersensitivity reaction. If Ziagen has been discontinued in patients due to experiencing any one of these symptoms and a decision is made to restart a medicinal product containing abacavir, this must be done in a setting where medical assistance is readily available (see section 4.4.). Very rarely cases of erythema multiforme, Stevens Johnson syndrome or toxic epidermal necrolysis have been reported where abacavir hypersensitivity could not be ruled out. In such cases medicinal products containing abacavir should be permanently discontinued.

Many of the adverse reactions have not been treatment limiting. The following convention has been used for their classification: very common (>1/10), common (>1/100 to <1/10), uncommon (>1/1,000 to <1/100), rare (>1/10,000 to <1/1,000) very rare (<1/10,000).

<u>Metabolism and nutrition disorders</u>

Common: anorexia

<u>Nervous system disorders</u>

Common: headache

<u>Gastrointestinal disorders</u>

Common: nausea, vomiting, diarrhoea

Rare: pancreatitis

<u>Skin and subcutaneous tissue disorders</u>

Common: rash (without systemic symptoms)

Very rare: erythema multiforme, Stevens-Johnson syndrome and toxic epidermal necrolysis

<u>General disorders and administration site conditions</u>

Common: fever, lethargy, fatigue

Cases of lactic acidosis, sometimes fatal, usually associated with severe hepatomegaly and hepatic steatosis, have been reported with the use of nucleoside analogues(-see section 4.4).

Combination antiretroviral therapy has been associated with redistribution of body fat (lipodystrophy) in HIV patients including the loss of peripheral and facial subcutaneous fat, increased intra-abdominal and visceral fat, breast hypertrophy and dorsocervical fat accumulation (buffalo hump).

Combination antiretroviral therapy has been associated with metabolic abnormalities such as hypertriglyceridaemia, hypercholesterolaemia, insulin resistance, hyperglycaemia and hyperlactataemia (see section 4.4).

In HIV-infected patients with severe immune deficiency at the time of initiation of combination antiretroviral therapy (CART) an inflammatory reaction to asymptomatic or residual opportunistic infections may arise (see section 4.4).

Cases of osteonecrosis have been reported, particularly in patients with generally acknowledged risk factors, advanced HIV disease or long-term exposure to combination antiretroviral therapy (CART). The frequency of this is unknown (see section 4.4).

<u>*Laboratory abnormalities*</u>

In controlled clinical studies laboratory abnormalities related to Ziagen treatment were uncommon, with no differences in incidence observed between Ziagen treated patients and the control arms.

4.9 Overdose

Single doses up to 1200 mg and daily doses up to 1800 mg of Ziagen have been administered to patients in clinical studies. No additional adverse reactions to those reported for normal doses were reported. The effects of higher doses are not known. If overdose occurs the patient should be monitored for evidence of toxicity (see section 4.8), and standard supportive treatment applied as necessary. It is not known whether abacavir can be removed by peritoneal dialysis or haemodialysis.

5. PHARMACOLOGICAL PROPERTIES

5.1 Pharmacodynamic properties

Pharmacotherapeutic group: nucleoside reverse transcriptase inhibitors, ATC Code: J05AF06

Table 3

Therapy	Abacavir + Combivir[1]	Abacavir + lamivudine + NNRTI	Abacavir + lamivudine + PI (or PI/ritonavir)	Total
Number of Subjects	282	1094	909	2285
Number of Virological Failures	43	90	158	306
Number of On-Therapy Genotypes	40 (100%)	51 (100%)[2]	141 (100%)	232 (100%)
K65R	0	1 (2%)	2 (1%)	3 (1%)
L74V	0	9 (18%)	3 (2%)	12 (5%)
Y115F	0	2 (4%)	0	2 (1%)
M184V/I	34 (85%)	22 (43%)	70 (50%)	126 (54%)
TAMs[3]	3 (8%)	2 (4%)	4 (3%)	9 (4%)

1. Combivir is a fixed dose combination of lamivudine and zidovudine
2. Includes three non-virological failures and four unconfirmed virological failures.
3. Number of subjects with ⩾1 Thymidine Analogue Mutations (TAMs).

Mechanism of action: Abacavir is a NRTI. It is a potent selective inhibitor of HIV-1 and HIV-2. Abacavir is metabolised intracellularly to the active moiety, carbovir 5'-triphosphate (TP). *In vitro* studies have demonstrated that its mechanism of action in relation to HIV is inhibition of the HIV reverse transcriptase enzyme, an event which results in chain termination and interruption of the viral replication cycle. Abacavir shows synergy *in vitro* in combination with nevirapine and zidovudine. It has been shown to be additive in combination with didanosine, lamivudine and stavudine.

In vitro resistance: Abacavir-resistant isolates of HIV-1 have been selected *in vitro* and are associated with specific genotypic changes in the reverse transcriptase (RT) codon region (codons M184V, K65R, L74V and Y115F). Viral resistance to abacavir develops relatively slowly *in vitro*, requiring multiple mutations for a clinically relevant increase in EC_{50} over wild-type virus.

In vivo resistance (Therapy naïve patients) Isolates from most patients experiencing virological failure with a regimen containing abacavir in pivotal clinical trials showed either no NRTI-related changes from baseline (45%) or only M184V or M184I selection (45%). The overall selection frequency for M184V or M184I was high (54%), and less common was the selection of L74V (5%), K65R (1%) and Y115F (1%). The inclusion of zidovudine in the regimen has been found to reduce the frequency of L74V and K65R selection in the presence of abacavir (with zidovudine: 0/40, without zidovudine: 15/192, 8%).

(see Table 3 above)

TAMs might be selected when thymidine analogs are associated with abacavir. In a meta-analysis of six clinical trials, TAMs were not selected by regimens containing abacavir without zidovudine (0/127), but were selected by regimens containing abacavir and the thymidine analogue zidovudine (22/86, 26%).

In vivo resistance (Therapy experienced patients): Clinically significant reduction of susceptibility to abacavir has been demonstrated in clinical isolates of patients with uncontrolled viral replication, who have been pre-treated with and are resistant to other nucleoside inhibitors. In a meta-analysis of five clinical trials where abacavir was added to intensify therapy, of 166 subjects, 123 (74%) had M184V/I, 50 (30%) had T215Y/F, 45 (27%) had M41L, 30 (18%) had K70R and 25 (15%) had D67N. K65R was absent and L74V and Y115F were uncommon (⩽3%). Logistic regression modelling of the predictive value for genotype (adjusted for baseline plasma HIV-1 RNA [vRNA], CD4+ cell count, number and duration of prior antiretroviral therapies), showed that the presence of 3 or more NRTI resistance-associated mutations was associated with reduced response at Week 4 (p=0.015) or 4 or more mutations at median Week 24 (p⩽0.012). In addition, the 69 insertion complex or the Q151M mutation, usually found in combination with A62V, V75I, F77L and F116Y, cause a high level of resistance to abacavir.

(see Table 4 opposite)

Phenotypic resistance and cross-resistance: Phenotypic resistance to abacavir requires M184V with at least one other abacavir-selected mutation, or M184V with multiple TAMs. Phenotypic cross-resistance to other NRTIs with M184V or M184I mutation alone is limited. Zidovudine, didanosine, stavudine and tenofovir maintain their antiretroviral activities against such HIV-1 variants. The presence of M184V with K65R does give rise to cross-resistance between abacavir, tenofovir, didanosine and lamivudine, and M184V with L74V gives rise to cross-resistance between abacavir, didanosine and lamivudine. The presence of M184V with Y115F gives rise to cross-resistance between abacavir and lamivudine. Appropriate use of abacavir can be guided using currently recommended resistance algorithms.

Cross-resistance between abacavir and antiretrovirals from other classes (e.g. PIs or NNRTIs) is unlikely.

Clinical Experience

The demonstration of the benefit of Ziagen is mainly based on results of studies performed in adult treatment-naïve patients using a regimen of Ziagen 300 mg twice daily in combination with zidovudine and lamivudine.

Twice daily (300 mg) administration:

• *Therapy naïve adults*

In adults treated with abacavir in combination with lamivudine and zidovudine the proportion of patients with undetectable viral load (<400 copies/ml) was approximately 70% (intention to treat analysis at 48 weeks) with corresponding rise in CD4 cells.

One randomised, double blind, placebo controlled clinical study in adults has compared the combination of abacavir, lamivudine and zidovudine to the combination of indinavir, lamivudine and zidovudine. Due to the high proportion of premature discontinuation (42% of patients discontinued randomised treatment by week 48), no definitive conclusion can be drawn regarding the equivalence between the treatment regimens at week 48. Although a similar antiviral effect was observed between the abacavir and indinavir containing regimens in terms of proportion of patients with undetectable viral load (⩽400 copies/ml; intention to treat analysis (ITT), 47% versus 49%; as treated analysis (AT), 86% versus 94% for abacavir and indinavir combinations respectively), results favoured the indinavir combination, particularly in the subset of patients with high viral load (>100,000 copies/ml at baseline; ITT, 46% versus 55%; AT, 84% versus 93% for abacavir and indinavir respectively).

In a multicentre, double-blind, controlled study (CNA30024), 654 HIV-infected, antiretroviral therapy-naïve patients were randomised to receive either abacavir 300 mg twice daily or zidovudine 300 mg twice daily, both in combination with lamivudine 150 mg twice daily and efavirenz 600 mg once daily. The duration of double-blind treatment was at least 48 weeks. In the intent-to-treat (ITT) population, 70% of patients in the abacavir group, compared to 69% of patients in the zidovudine group, achieved a virologic response of plasma HIV-1 RNA ⩽50 copies/ml by Week 48 (point estimate for treatment difference: 0.8, 95% CI -6.3, 7.9). In the as treated (AT) analysis the difference between both treatment arms was more noticeable (88% of patients in the abacavir group, compared to 95% of patients in the zidovudine group (point estimate for treatment difference: -6.8, 95% CI -11.8; -1.7). However, both analyses were compatible with a conclusion of non-inferiority between both treatment arms.

ACTG5095 was a randomised (1:1:1), double-blind, placebo-controlled trial performed in 1147 antiretroviral naïve HIV-1 infected adults, comparing 3 regimens: zidovudine (ZDV), lamivudine (3TC), abacavir (ABC), efavirenz (EFV) vs ZDV/3TC/EFV vs ZDV/3TC/ABC. After a median follow-up of 32 weeks, the tritherapy with the three nucleosides ZDV/3TC/ABC was shown to be virologically inferior to the two other arms regardless of baseline viral load (< or > 100 000 copies/ml) with 26% of subjects on the ZDV/3TC/ABC arm, 16% on the ZDV/3TC/EFV arm and 13% on the 4 drug arm categorised as having virological failure (HIV RNA>200 copies/ml). At week 48 the proportion of subjects with HIV RNA <50 copies/ml were 63%, 80% and 86% for the ZDV/3TC/ABC, ZDV/3TC/EFV and ZDV/3TC/ABC/EFV arms, respectively. The study Data Safety Monitoring Board stopped the ZDV/3TC/ABC arm at this time based on the higher proportion of patients with virologic failure. The remaining arms were continued in a blinded fashion. After a median follow-up of 144 weeks, 25% of subjects on the ZDV/3TC/ABC/EFV arm and 26% on the ZDV/3TC/EFV arm were categorised as having virological failure. There was no significant difference in the time to first virologic failure (p=0.73, log-rank test) between the 2 arms. In this study, addition of ABC to ZDV/3TC/EFV did not significantly improve efficacy.

(see Table 5 below)

• *Therapy naïve children*

In a study comparing the unblinded NRTI combinations (with or without blinded nelfinavir) in children, a greater proportion treated with abacavir and lamivudine (71%) or abacavir and zidovudine (60%) had HIV-1 RNA ⩽400 copies/ml at 48 weeks, compared with those treated with lamivudine and zidovudine (47%)[p=0.09, intention to treat analysis]. Similarly, greater proportions of children treated with the abacavir containing combinations had HIV-1 RNA ⩽50 copies/ml at 48 weeks (53%, 42% and 28% respectively, p=0.07).

• *Therapy experienced patients*

In adults moderately exposed to antiretroviral therapy the addition of abacavir to combination antiretroviral therapy provided modest benefits in reducing viral load (median change 0.44 log_{10} copies/ml at 16 weeks).

In heavily NRTI pretreated patients the efficacy of abacavir is very low. The degree of benefit as part of a new combination regimen will depend on the nature and duration of prior therapy which may have selected for HIV-1 variants with cross-resistance to abacavir.

Once daily (600 mg) administration:

• *Therapy naïve adults*

The once daily regimen of abacavir is supported by a 48 weeks multi-centre, double-blind, controlled study (CNA30021) of 770 HIV-infected, therapy-naïve adults. These were primarily asymptomatic HIV infected patients (CDC stage A). They were randomised to receive either abacavir 600 mg once daily or 300 mg twice daily, in combination with efavirenz and lamivudine given once daily. Similar clinical success (point estimate for treatment difference -1.7, 95% CI -8.4, 4.9) was observed for both regimens. From these results, it can be concluded with 95% confidence that the true difference is no greater than 8.4% in favour of the twice daily regimen. This potential difference is sufficiently small to draw an overall conclusion

Table 4

Baseline Reverse Transcriptase Mutation	Week 4 (n = 166) n	Median Change vRNA (log_{10} c/mL)	Percent with <400 copies/mL vRNA
None	15	-0.96	40%
M184V alone	75	-0.74	64%
Any one NRTI mutation	82	-0.72	65%
Any two NRTI-associated mutations	22	-0.82	32%
Any three NRTI-associated mutations	19	-0.30	5%
Four or more NRTI-associated mutations	28	-0.07	11%

Table 5

		ZDV/3TC/ABC	ZDV/3TC/EFV	ZDV/3TC/ABC/EFV
Virologic failure (HIV RNA>200 copies/ml)	32 weeks	26%	16%	13%
	144 weeks	-	26%	25%
Virologic success (48 weeks HIV RNA < 50 copies/ml)		63%	80%	86%

of non-inferiority of abacavir once daily over abacavir twice daily.

There was a low, similar overall incidence of virologic failure (viral load >50 copies/ml) in both the once and twice daily treatment groups (10% and 8% respectively). In the small sample size for genotypic analysis, there was a trend toward a higher rate of NRTI-associated mutations in the once daily versus the twice daily abacavir regimens. No firm conclusion could be drawn due to the limited data derived from this study. Long term data with abacavir used as a once daily regimen (beyond 48 weeks) are currently limited.

•*Therapy experienced patients*

In study CAL30001, 182 treatment-experienced patients with virologic failure were randomised and received treatment with either the fixed-dose combination of abacavir/lamivudine (FDC) once daily or abacavir 300 mg twice daily plus lamivudine 300 mg once daily, both in combination with tenofovir and a PI or an NNRTI for 48 weeks. Results indicate that the FDC group was non-inferior to the abacavir twice daily group, based on similar reductions in HIV-1 RNA as measured by average area under the curve minus baseline (AAUCMB, -1.65 log_{10} copies/ml versus -1.83 log_{10} copies/ml respectively, 95% CI -0.13, 0.38). Proportions with HIV-1 RNA < 50 copies/ml (50% versus 47%) and < 400 copies/ml (54% versus 57%) were also similar in each group (ITT population). However, as there were only moderately experienced patients included in this study with an imbalance in baseline viral load between the arms, these results should be interpreted with caution.

In study ESS30008, 260 patients with virologic suppression on a first line therapy regimen containing abacavir 300 mg plus lamivudine 150 mg, both given twice daily and a PI or NNRTI, were randomised to continue this regimen or switch to abacavir/lamivudine FDC plus a PI or NNRTI for 48 weeks. Results indicate that the FDC group was associated with a similar virologic outcome (non-inferior) compared to the abacavir plus lamivudine group, based on proportions of subjects with HIV-1 RNA < 50 copies/ml (90% and 85% respectively, 95% CI -2.7, 13.5).

Additional information:

The safety and efficacy of Ziagen in a number of different multidrug combination regimens is still not completely assessed (particularly in combination with NNRTIs).

Abacavir penetrates the cerebrospinal fluid (CSF) (see section 5.2), and has been shown to reduce HIV-1 RNA levels in the CSF. However, no effects on neuropsychological performance were seen when it was administered to patients with AIDS dementia complex.

5.2 Pharmacokinetic properties

Absorption: abacavir is rapidly and well absorbed following oral administration. The absolute bioavailability of oral abacavir in adults is about 83%. Following oral administration, the mean time (t_{max}) to maximal serum concentrations of abacavir is about 1.5 hours for the tablet formulation and about 1.0 hour for the solution formulation.

There are no differences observed between the AUC for the tablet or solution. At therapeutic dosages a dosage of 300 mg twice daily, the mean (CV) steady state C_{max} and C_{min} of abacavir are approximately 3.00 μg/ml (30%) and 0.01 μg/ml (99%), respectively. The mean (CV) AUC over a dosing interval of 12 hours was 6.02 μg.h/ml (29%), equivalent to a daily AUC of approximately 12.0 μg.h/ml. The C_{max} value for the oral solution is slightly higher than the tablet. After a 600 mg abacavir tablet dose, the mean (CV) abacavir C_{max} was approximately 4.26 μg/ml (28%) and the mean (CV) AUC_{∞} was 11.95 μg.h/ml (21%).

Food delayed absorption and decreased C_{max} but did not affect overall plasma concentrations (AUC). Therefore Ziagen can be taken with or without food.

Distribution: following intravenous administration, the apparent volume of distribution was about 0.8 l/kg, indicating that abacavir penetrates freely into body tissues.

Studies in HIV infected patients have shown good penetration of abacavir into the cerebrospinal fluid (CSF), with a CSF to plasma AUC ratio of between 30 to 44%. The observed values of the peak concentrations are 9 fold greater than the IC_{50} of abacavir of 0.08 μg/ml or 0.26 μM when abacavir is given at 600 mg twice daily.

Plasma protein binding studies *in vitro* indicate that abacavir binds only low to moderately (~49%) to human plasma proteins at therapeutic concentrations. This indicates a low likelihood for interactions with other medicinal products through plasma protein binding displacement.

Metabolism: abacavir is primarily metabolised by the liver with approximately 2% of the administered dose being renally excreted, as unchanged compound. The primary pathways of metabolism in man are by alcohol dehydrogenase and by glucuronidation to produce the 5'-carboxylic acid and 5'-glucuronide which account for about 66% of the administered dose. The metabolites are excreted in the urine.

Elimination: the mean half-life of abacavir is about 1.5 hours. Following multiple oral doses of abacavir 300 mg twice a day there is no significant accumulation of abacavir. Elimination of abacavir is via hepatic metabolism with subsequent excretion of metabolites primarily in the urine. The metabolites and unchanged abacavir account for about 83% of the administered abacavir dose in the urine. The remainder is eliminated in the faeces.

Intracellular pharmacokinetics

In a study of 20 HIV-infected patients receiving abacavir 300 mg twice daily, with only one 300 mg dose taken prior to the 24 hour sampling period, the geometric mean terminal carbovir-TP intracellular half-life at steady-state was 20.6 hours, compared to the geometric mean abacavir plasma half-life in this study of 2.6 hours. In a crossover study in 27 HIV-infected patients, intracellular carbovir-TP exposures were higher for the abacavir 600 mg once daily regimen ($AUC_{24,ss}$ + 32 %, $C_{max24,ss}$ + 99 % and C_{trough} + 18 %) compared to the 300 mg twice daily regimen. Overall, these data support the use of abacavir 600 mg once daily for the treatment of HIV infected patients. Additionally, the efficacy and safety of abacavir given once daily has been demonstrated in a pivotal clinical study (CNA30021- See section 5.1 Clinical experience).

Special populations

Hepatically impaired: abacavir is metabolised primarily by the liver. The pharmacokinetics of abacavir have been studied in patients with mild hepatic impairment (Child-Pugh score 5-6) receiving a single 600 mg dose. The results showed that there was a mean increase of 1.89 fold [1.32; 2.70] in the abacavir AUC, and 1.58 [1.22; 2.04] fold in the elimination half-life. No recommendation on dosage reduction is possible in patients with mild hepatic impairment due to the substantial variability of abacavir exposure.

Renally impaired: abacavir is primarily metabolised by the liver with approximately 2% of abacavir excreted unchanged in the urine. The pharmacokinetics of abacavir in patients with end-stage renal disease is similar to patients with normal renal function. Therefore no dosage reduction is required in patients with renal impairment. Based on limited experience Ziagen should be avoided in patients with end-stage renal disease.

Children: according to clinical trials performed in children abacavir is rapidly and well absorbed from an oral solution administered to children. The overall pharmacokinetic parameters in children are comparable to adults, with greater variability in plasma concentrations. The recommended dose for children from three months to 12 years is 8 mg/kg twice daily. This will provide slightly higher mean plasma concentrations in children, ensuring that the majority will achieve therapeutic concentrations equivalent to 300 mg twice daily in adults.

There are insufficient safety data to recommend the use of Ziagen in infants less than three months old. The limited data available indicate that a dose of 2 mg/kg in neonates less than 30 days old provides similar or greater AUCs, compared to the 8 mg/kg dose administered to older children.

Elderly: the pharmacokinetics of abacavir have not been studied in patients over 65 years of age.

5.3 Preclinical safety data

Abacavir was not mutagenic in bacterial tests but showed activity *in vitro* in the human lymphocyte chromosome aberration assay, the mouse lymphoma assay, and the *in vivo* micronucleus test. This is consistent with the known activity of other nucleoside analogues. These results indicate that abacavir has a weak potential to cause chromosomal damage both *in vitro* and *in vivo* at high test concentrations.

Carcinogenicity studies with orally administered abacavir in mice and rats showed an increase in the incidence of malignant and non-malignant tumours. Malignant tumours occurred in the preputial gland of males and the clitoral gland of females of both species, and in rats in the thyroid gland of males and the liver, urinary bladder, lymph nodes and the subcutis of females.

The majority of these tumours occurred at the highest abacavir dose of 330 mg/kg/day in mice and 600 mg/kg/day in rats. The exception was the preputial gland tumour which occurred at a dose of 110 mg/kg in mice. The systemic exposure at the no effect level in mice and rats was equivalent to 3 and 7 times the human systemic exposure during therapy. While the carcinogenic potential in humans is unknown, these data suggest that a carcinogenic risk to humans is outweighed by the potential clinical benefit.

In pre-clinical toxicology studies, abacavir treatment was shown to increase liver weights in rats and monkeys. The clinical relevance of this is unknown. There is no evidence from clinical studies that abacavir is hepatotoxic. Additionally, autoinduction of abacavir metabolism or induction of the metabolism of other medicinal products hepatically metabolised has not been observed in man.

Mild myocardial degeneration in the heart of mice and rats was observed following administration of abacavir for two years. The systemic exposures were equivalent to 7 to 24 times the expected systemic exposure in humans. The clinical relevance of this finding has not been determined.

In reproductive toxicity studies, embryo and foetal toxicity have been observed in rats but not in rabbits. These findings included decreased foetal body weight, foetal oedema, and an increase in skeletal variations/malformations, early intra-uterine deaths and still births. No conclusion can be drawn with regard to the teratogenic potential of abacavir because of this embryo-foetal toxicity.

A fertility study in the rat has shown that abacavir had no effect on male or female fertility.

6. PHARMACEUTICAL PARTICULARS

6.1 List of excipients

Sorbitol 70% (E420)

Saccharin sodium

Sodium citrate

Citric acid anhydrous

Methyl parahydroxybenzoate (E218)

Propyl parahydroxybenzoate (E216)

Propylene glycol (E1520)

Maltodextrin

Lactic acid

Glyceryl triacetate

Natural and artificial strawberry and banana flavours

Purified water

Sodium hydroxide and/or hydrochloric acid for pH adjustment.

6.2 Incompatibilities

Not applicable

6.3 Shelf life

2 years

After first opening the container: 2 months

6.4 Special precautions for storage

Do not store above 30°C

6.5 Nature and contents of container

Ziagen oral solution is supplied in high density polyethylene bottles with child-resistant closures, containing 240 ml of oral solution.

A 10 ml polypropylene oral dosing syringe and a polyethylene adapter are also included in the pack.

6.6 Special precautions for disposal and other handling

A plastic adapter and oral dosing syringe are provided for accurate measurement of the prescribed dose of oral solution. The adapter is placed in the neck of the bottle and the syringe attached to this. The bottle is inverted and the correct volume withdrawn.

Any unused product or waste material should be disposed of in accordance with local requirements.

7. MARKETING AUTHORISATION HOLDER

Glaxo Group Ltd

Greenford

Middlesex UB6 0NN

United Kingdom

8. MARKETING AUTHORISATION NUMBER(S)

EU/1/99/112/002

9. DATE OF FIRST AUTHORISATION/RENEWAL OF THE AUTHORISATION

Date of first authorisation: 8 July 1999

Date of latest renewal: 8 July 2004

10. DATE OF REVISION OF THE TEXT

08 June 2009

Detailed information on this medicinal product is available on the website of the European Medicines Agency (EMEA) http://www.emea.europa.eu

Ziagen 300 mg Film Coated Tablets

(GlaxoSmithKline UK)

1. NAME OF THE MEDICINAL PRODUCT

Ziagen 300 mg film-coated tablets

2. QUALITATIVE AND QUANTITATIVE COMPOSITION

Each film-coated tablet contains 300 mg of abacavir (as sulfate).

For a full list of excipients see section 6.1.

3. PHARMACEUTICAL FORM

Film-coated tablet (tablets)

The scored tablets are yellow, biconvex, capsule shaped and are engraved with 'GX 623' on both sides.

The tablet can be divided into equal halves.

4. CLINICAL PARTICULARS

4.1 Therapeutic indications

Ziagen is indicated in antiretroviral combination therapy for the treatment of Human Immunodeficiency Virus (HIV) infection.

The demonstration of the benefit of Ziagen is mainly based on results of studies performed with a twice daily regimen, in treatment-naïve adult patients on combination therapy (see section 5.1).

Before initiating treatment with abacavir, screening for carriage of the HLA-B*5701 allele should be performed in any HIV-infected patient, irrespective of racial origin. Abacavir should not be used in patients known to carry the HLA-B*5701 allele, unless no other therapeutic option is available in these patients, based on the treatment history and resistance testing (see section 4.4 and 4.8).

4.2 Posology and method of administration

Ziagen should be prescribed by physicians experienced in the management of HIV infection.

Ziagen can be taken with or without food.

To ensure administration of the entire dose, the tablet(s) should ideally be swallowed without crushing.

Ziagen is also available as an oral solution for use in children over three months of age and weighing less than 14 kg and for those patients for whom the tablets are inappropriate.

Alternatively, for patients who are unable to swallow tablets, the tablet(s) may be crushed and added to a small amount of semi-solid food or liquid, all of which should be consumed immediately (see section 5.2).

Adults and adolescents (over 12 years of age): the recommended dose of Ziagen is 600 mg daily. This may be administered as either 300 mg (one tablet) twice daily or 600 mg (two tablets) once daily (see sections 4.4 and 5.1).

Patients changing to the once daily regimen should take 300 mg twice a day and switch to 600 mg once a day the following morning. Where an evening once daily regimen is preferred, 300 mg of Ziagen should be taken on the first morning only, followed by 600 mg in the evening. When changing back to a twice daily regimen, patients should complete the day's treatment and start 300 mg twice a day the following morning.

Children (under 12 years of age):

A dosing according to weight bands is recommended for Ziagen tablets. This dosing regimen for paediatric patients weighing 14-30 kg is based primarily on pharmacokinetic modelling. A pharmacokinetic overexposure of abacavir can occur since accurate dosing can not be achieved with this formulation. Therefore a close safety monitoring is warranted in these patients.

Children weighing at least 30 kg: the adult dosage of 300 mg twice daily should be taken.

Children weighing > 21 kg to < 30 kg: one half of a Ziagen tablet taken in the morning and one whole tablet taken in the evening.

Children weighing 14 to 21 kg: one half of a Ziagen tablet twice daily.

Children less than three months: the experience in children aged less than three months is limited (see section 5.2).

Renal impairment: no dosage adjustment of Ziagen is necessary in patients with renal dysfunction. However, Ziagen is not recommended for patients with end-stage renal disease (see section 5.2).

Hepatic impairment: abacavir is primarily metabolised by the liver. No dose recommendation can be made in patients with mild hepatic impairment. In patients with moderate hepatic impairment, no data are available, therefore the use of abacavir is not recommended unless judged necessary. If abacavir is used in patients with mild or moderate hepatic impairment, then close monitoring is required, and if feasible, monitoring of abacavir plasma levels is recommended (see section 5.2). Abacavir is contraindicated in patients with severe hepatic impairment (see section 4.3 and 4.4).

Elderly: no pharmacokinetic data is currently available in patients over 65 years of age.

4.3 Contraindications

Hypersensitivity to the active substance or to any of the excipients. See BOXED INFORMATION ON HYPERSENSITIVITY REACTIONS in sections 4.4. and 4.8.

Severe hepatic impairment.

4.4 Special warnings and precautions for use
(see Table 1 opposite)

Lactic acidosis: lactic acidosis, usually associated with hepatomegaly and hepatic steatosis, has been reported with the use of nucleoside analogues. Early symptoms (symptomatic hyperlactatemia) include benign digestive symptoms (nausea, vomiting and abdominal pain), non-specific malaise, loss of appetite, weight loss, respiratory symptoms (rapid and/or deep breathing) or neurological symptoms (including motor weakness).

Lactic acidosis has a high mortality and may be associated with pancreatitis, liver failure, or renal failure.

Lactic acidosis generally occurred after a few or several months of treatment.

Treatment with nucleoside analogues should be discontinued in the setting of symptomatic hyperlactatemia and metabolic/lactic acidosis, progressive hepatomegaly, or rapidly elevating aminotransferase levels.

Caution should be exercised when administering nucleoside analogues to any patient (particularly obese women) with hepatomegaly, hepatitis or other known risk factors for liver disease and hepatic steatosis (including certain medicinal products and alcohol).

Patients co-infected with hepatitis C and treated with alpha interferon and ribavirin may constitute a special risk.

Patients at increased risk should be followed closely.

Table 1

Hypersensitivity reaction (see also section 4.8):

In clinical studies approximately 5% of subjects receiving abacavir develop a hypersensitivity reaction; some of these cases were life-threatening and resulted in a fatal outcome despite taking precautions.

Studies have shown that carriage of the HLA-B*5701 allele is associated with a significantly increased risk of a hypersensitivity reaction to abacavir. Based on the prospective study CNA106030 (PREDICT-1), use of pre-therapy screening for the HLA-B*5701 allele and subsequently avoiding abacavir in patients with this allele significantly reduced the incidence of abacavir hypersensitivity reactions. In populations similar to that enrolled in the PREDICT-1 study, it is estimated that 48% to 61% of patients with the HLA-B*5701 allele will develop a hypersensitivity reaction during the course of abacavir treatment compared with 0% to 4% of patients who do not have the HLA-B*5701 allele.

These results are consistent with those of prior retrospective studies.

As a consequence, before initiating treatment with abacavir, screening for carriage of the HLA-B*5701 allele should be performed in any HIV-infected patient, irrespective of racial origin. Abacavir should not be used in patients known to carry the HLA-B*5701 allele, unless no other therapeutic option is available based on the treatment history and resistance testing (see section 4.1).

In any patient treated with abacavir, the clinical diagnosis of suspected hypersensitivity reaction must remain the basis of clinical decision-making. It is noteworthy that among patients with a clinically suspected hypersensitivity reaction, a proportion did not carry HLA-B*5701. Therefore, even in the absence of HLA-B*5701 allele, it is important to permanently discontinue abacavir and not rechallenge with abacavir if a hypersensitivity reaction cannot be ruled out on clinical grounds, due to the potential for a severe or even fatal reaction.

Skin patch testing was used as a research tool for the PREDICT-1 study but has no utility in the clinical management of patients and therefore should not be used in the clinical setting.

- **Clinical description**

Hypersensitivity reactions are characterised by the appearance of symptoms indicating multi-organ system involvement. Almost all hypersensitivity reactions will have fever and/or rash as part of the syndrome.

Other signs and symptoms may include respiratory signs and symptoms such as dyspnoea, sore throat, cough and abnormal chest x-ray findings (predominantly infiltrates, which can be localised), gastrointestinal symptoms, such as nausea, vomiting, diarrhoea, or abdominal pain, **and may lead to misdiagnosis of hypersensitivity as respiratory disease (pneumonia, bronchitis, pharyngitis), or gastroenteritis.**

Other frequently observed signs or symptoms of the hypersensitivity reaction may include lethargy or malaise and musculoskeletal symptoms (myalgia, rarely myolysis, arthralgia).

The symptoms related to this hypersensitivity reaction worsen with continued therapy and can be life-threatening. These symptoms usually resolve upon discontinuation of Ziagen.

- **Clinical management**

Hypersensitivity reaction symptoms usually appear within the first six weeks of initiation of treatment with abacavir, although these reactions **may occur at any time during therapy.**

Patients should be monitored closely, especially during the first two months of treatment with Ziagen, with consultation every two weeks.

Patients who are diagnosed with a hypersensitivity reaction whilst on therapy **MUST discontinue Ziagen immediately. Ziagen, or any other medicinal product containing abacavir (e.g. Kivexa, Trizivir), MUST NEVER be restarted in patients who have stopped therapy due to a hypersensitivity reaction.**

Restarting abacavir following a hypersensitivity reaction results in a prompt return of symptoms within hours. This recurrence is usually more severe than on initial presentation, and may include life-threatening hypotension and death.

To avoid a delay in diagnosis and minimise the risk of a life-threatening hypersensitivity reaction, Ziagen must be permanently discontinued if hypersensitivity cannot be ruled out, even when other diagnoses are possible (respiratory diseases, flu-like illness, gastroenteritis or reactions to other medications).

Special care is needed for those patients simultaneously starting treatment with Ziagen and other medicinal products known to induce skin toxicity (such as non-nucleoside reverse transcriptase inhibitors - NNRTIs). This is because it is currently difficult to differentiate between rashes induced by these products and abacavir related hypersensitivity reactions.

- **Management after an interruption of Ziagen therapy**

If therapy with Ziagen has been discontinued for any reason and restarting therapy is under consideration, the reason for discontinuation must be established to assess whether the patient had any symptoms of a hypersensitivity reaction. **If a hypersensitivity reaction cannot be ruled out, Ziagen or any other medicinal product containing abacavir (e.g. Kivexa, Trizivir) must not be restarted.**

Hypersensitivity reactions with rapid onset, including life-threatening reactions have occurred after restarting Ziagen in patients who had only one of the key symptoms of hypersensitivity (skin rash, fever, gastrointestinal, respiratory or constitutional symptoms such as lethargy and malaise) prior to stopping Ziagen. The most common isolated symptom of a hypersensitivity reaction was a skin rash. Moreover, on very rare occasions hypersensitivity reactions have been reported in patients who have restarted therapy, and who had no preceding symptoms of a hypersensitivity reaction.

In both cases, if a decision is made to restart Ziagen this must be done in a setting where medical assistance is readily available.

- **Essential patient information**

Prescribers must ensure that patients are fully informed regarding the following information on the hypersensitivity reaction:

- patients must be made aware of the possibility of a hypersensitivity reaction to abacavir that may result in a life-threatening reaction or death.

- patients developing signs or symptoms possibly linked with a hypersensitivity reaction **MUST CONTACT their doctor IMMEDIATELY.**

- patients who are hypersensitive to abacavir should be reminded that they must never take Ziagen or any other medicinal product containing abacavir (e.g. Kivexa, Trizivir)

- in order to avoid restarting Ziagen, patients who have experienced a hypersensitivity reaction should be asked to return the remaining Ziagen tablets or oral solution to the pharmacy.

- patients who have stopped Ziagen for any reason, and particularly due to possible adverse reactions or illness, must be advised to contact their doctor before restarting.

- each patient should be reminded to read the Package Leaflet included in the Ziagen pack. They should be reminded of the importance of removing the Alert Card included in the pack, and keeping it with them at all times.

Mitochondrial dysfunction: nucleoside and nucleotide analogues have been demonstrated *in vitro* and *in vivo* to cause a variable degree of mitochondrial damage. There have been reports of mitochondrial dysfunction in HIV-negative infants exposed *in utero* and/or post-natally to nucleoside analogues. The main adverse reactions reported are haematological disorders (anaemia, neutropenia), metabolic disorders (hyperlactatemia, hyperlipasemia). These events are often transitory. Some late-onset neurological disorders have been reported (hypertonia, convulsion, abnormal behaviour). Whether the neurological disorders are transient or permanent is currently unknown. Any child exposed *in utero* to nucleoside and nucleotide analogues, even HIV-negative children, should have clinical and laboratory follow-up and should be fully investigated for possible mitochondrial dysfunction in case of relevant signs or symptoms. These findings do not affect current national recommendations to use antiretroviral therapy in pregnant women to prevent vertical transmission of HIV.

Lipodystrophy: combination antiretroviral therapy has been associated with the redistribution of body fat (lipodystrophy) in HIV patients. The long-term consequences of these events are currently unknown. Knowledge about the mechanism is incomplete. A connection between visceral lipomatosis and protease inhibitors (PIs) and lipoatrophy and nucleoside reverse transcriptase inhibitors (NRTIs) has been hypothesised. A higher risk of lipodystrophy has been associated with individual factors such as older age, and with drug related factors such as longer duration of antiretroviral treatment and associated metabolic disturbances. Clinical examination should include evaluation for physical signs of fat redistribution. Consideration should be given to the measurement of fasting serum lipids and blood glucose. Lipid disorders should be managed as clinically appropriate (see section 4.8).

Pancreatitis: pancreatitis has been reported, but a causal relationship to abacavir treatment is uncertain.

Triple nucleoside therapy: in patients with high viral load (>100,000 copies/ml) the choice of a triple combination with abacavir, lamivudine and zidovudine needs special consideration (see section 5.1).

There have been reports of a high rate of virological failure and of emergence of resistance at an early stage when abacavir was combined with tenofovir disoproxil fumarate and lamivudine as a once daily regimen.

Liver disease: the safety and efficacy of Ziagen has not been established in patients with significant underlying liver disorders. Ziagen is contraindicated in patients with severe hepatic impairment (see section 4.3). Patients with chronic hepatitis B or C and treated with combination antiretroviral therapy are at an increased risk of severe and potentially fatal hepatic adverse reactions. In case of concomitant antiviral therapy for hepatitis B or C, please refer also to the relevant product information for these medicinal products.

Patients with pre-existing liver dysfunction, including chronic active hepatitis, have an increased frequency of liver function abnormalities during combination antiretroviral therapy, and should be monitored according to standard practice. If there is evidence of worsening liver disease in such patients, interruption or discontinuation of treatment must be considered.

A pharmacokinetic study has been performed in patients with mild hepatic impairment. However, a definitive recommendation on dose reduction is not possible due to substantial variability of drug exposure in this patient population (see section 5.2). The clinical safety data available with abacavir in hepatically impaired patients is very limited. Due to the potential increases in exposure (AUC) in some patients, close monitoring is required. No data are available in patients with moderate or severe hepatic impairment. Plasma concentrations of abacavir are expected to substantially increase in these patients. Therefore, the use of abacavir in patients with moderate hepatic impairment is not recommended unless judged necessary and requires close monitoring of these patients.

Renal disease: Ziagen should not be administered to patients with end-stage renal disease (see section 5.2).

Immune Reactivation Syndrome: In HIV-infected patients with severe immune deficiency at the time of institution of combination antiretroviral therapy (CART), an inflammatory reaction to asymptomatic or residual opportunistic pathogens may arise and cause serious clinical conditions, or aggravation of symptoms. Typically, such reactions have been observed within the first few weeks or months of initiation of CART. Relevant examples are cytomegalovirus retinitis, generalised and/or focal mycobacterium infections, and Pneumocystis carinii pneumonia. Any inflammatory symptoms should be evaluated and treatment instituted when necessary.

Osteonecrosis: Although the aetiology is considered to be multifactorial (including corticosteroid use, alcohol consumption, severe immunosuppression, higher body mass index), cases of osteonecrosis have been reported particularly in patients with advanced HIV-disease and/or long-term exposure to combination antiretroviral therapy (CART). Patients should be advised to seek medical advice if they experience joint aches and pain, joint stiffness or difficulty in movement.

Opportunistic infections: patients receiving Ziagen or any other antiretroviral therapy may still develop opportunistic infections and other complications of HIV infection. Therefore patients should remain under close clinical observation by physicians experienced in the treatment of these associated HIV diseases.

Transmission: patients should be advised that current antiretroviral therapy, including Ziagen, have not been proven to prevent the risk of transmission of HIV to others through sexual contact or blood contamination. Appropriate precautions should continue to be taken.

Myocardial Infarction: Observational studies have shown an association between myocardial infarction and the use of abacavir. Those studied were mainly antiretroviral experienced patients. Data from clinical trials showed limited numbers of myocardial infarction and could not exclude a small increase in risk. Overall the available data from observational cohorts and from randomised trials show some inconsistency so can neither confirm nor refute a causal relationship between abacavir treatment and the risk of myocardial infarction. To date, there is no established biological mechanism to explain a potential increase in risk. When prescribing Ziagen, action should be taken to try to minimize all modifiable risk factors (e.g. smoking, hypertension, and hyperlipidaemia).

4.5 Interaction with other medicinal products and other forms of interaction

Based on the results of *in vitro* experiments and the known major metabolic pathways of abacavir, the potential for P450 mediated interactions with other medicinal products involving abacavir is low. P450 does not play a major role in the metabolism of abacavir, and abacavir does not inhibit metabolism mediated by CYP 3A4. Abacavir has also been shown *in vitro* not to inhibit CYP 3A4, CYP2C9 or CYP2D6 enzymes at clinically relevant concentrations. Induction of hepatic metabolism has not been observed in clinical studies. Therefore, there is little potential for interactions with antiretroviral PIs and other medicinal products metabolised by major P450 enzymes. Clinical studies have shown that there are no clinically significant interactions between abacavir, zidovudine, and lamivudine.

Potent enzymatic inducers such as rifampicin, phenobarbital and phenytoin may via their action on UDP-glucuronyltransferases slightly decrease the plasma concentrations of abacavir.

Ethanol: the metabolism of abacavir is altered by concomitant ethanol resulting in an increase in AUC of abacavir of about 41%. These findings are not considered clinically significant. Abacavir has no effect on the metabolism of ethanol.

Methadone: in a pharmacokinetic study, co-administration of 600 mg abacavir twice daily with methadone showed a 35% reduction in abacavir C_{max} and a one hour delay in t_{max} but the AUC was unchanged. The changes in abacavir pharmacokinetics are not considered clinically relevant. In this study abacavir increased the mean methadone systemic clearance by 22%. The induction of drug metabolising enzymes cannot therefore be excluded. Patients being treated with methadone and abacavir should be monitored for evidence of withdrawal symptoms indicating under dosing, as occasionally methadone re-titration may be required.

Retinoids: retinoid compounds are eliminated via alcohol dehydrogenase. Interaction with abacavir is possible but has not been studied.

4.6 Pregnancy and lactation

Ziagen is not recommended during pregnancy. The safe use of abacavir in human pregnancy has not been established. Placental transfer of abacavir and/or its related metabolites has been shown to occur in animals. Toxicity to the developing embryo and foetus occurred in rats, but not in rabbits (see section 5.3). The teratogenic potential of abacavir could not be established from studies in animals.

Abacavir and its metabolites are secreted into the milk of lactating rats. It is expected that these will also be secreted into human milk, although this has not been confirmed. There are no data available on the safety of abacavir when administered to babies less than three months old. It is therefore recommended that mothers do not breast-feed their babies while receiving treatment with abacavir. Additionally, it is recommended that HIV infected women do not breast-feed their infants under any circumstances in order to avoid transmission of HIV.

4.7 Effects on ability to drive and use machines

No studies on the effects on ability to drive and use machines have been performed.

4.8 Undesirable effects

(see Table 2 on next page)

For many of the other adverse reactions reported, it is unclear whether they are related to Ziagen, to the wide range of medicinal products used in the management of HIV infection or as a result of the disease process.

Many of those listed below occur commonly (nausea, vomiting, diarrhoea, fever, lethargy, rash) in patients with abacavir hypersensitivity. Therefore, patients with any of these symptoms should be carefully evaluated for the presence of this hypersensitivity reaction. If Ziagen has been discontinued in patients due to experiencing any one of these symptoms and a decision is made to restart a medicinal product containing abacavir, this must be done in a setting where medical assistance is readily available (see section 4.4.). Very rarely cases of erythema multiforme, Stevens Johnson syndrome or toxic epidermal necrolysis have been reported where abacavir hypersensitivity could not be ruled out. In such cases medicinal products containing abacavir should be permanently discontinued.

Many of the adverse reactions have not been treatment limiting. The following convention has been used for their classification: very common (> 1/10), common (> 1/100 to < 1/10), uncommon (> 1/1,000 to < 1/100), rare (> 1/10,000 to < 1/1,000) very rare (< 1/10,000).

<u>Metabolism and nutrition disorders</u>

Common: anorexia

<u>Nervous system disorders</u>

Common: headache

<u>Gastrointestinal disorders</u>

Common: nausea, vomiting, diarrhoea

Rare: pancreatitis

<u>Skin and subcutaneous tissue disorders</u>

Common: rash (without systemic symptoms)

Very rare: erythema multiforme, Stevens-Johnson syndrome and toxic epidermal necrolysis

<u>General disorders and administration site conditions</u>

Common: fever, lethargy, fatigue

Cases of lactic acidosis, sometimes fatal, usually associated with severe hepatomegaly and hepatic steatosis, have been reported with the use of nucleoside analogues (see section 4.4).

Combination antiretroviral therapy has been associated with redistribution of body fat (lipodystrophy) in HIV patients including the loss of peripheral and facial subcutaneous fat, increased intra-abdominal and visceral fat, breast hypertrophy and dorsocervical fat accumulation (buffalo hump).

Combination antiretroviral therapy has been associated with metabolic abnormalities such as hypertriglyceridaemia, hypercholesterolaemia, insulin resistance, hyperglycaemia and hyperlactataemia (see section 4.4).

In HIV-infected patients with severe immune deficiency at the time of initiation of combination antiretroviral therapy (CART) an inflammatory reaction to asymptomatic or residual opportunistic infections may arise (see section 4.4).

Cases of osteonecrosis have been reported, particularly in patients with generally acknowledged risk factors, advanced HIV disease or long-term exposure to combination antiretroviral therapy (CART). The frequency of this is unknown (see section 4.4).

<u>*Laboratory abnormalities*</u>

In controlled clinical studies laboratory abnormalities related to Ziagen treatment were uncommon, with no differences in incidence observed between Ziagen treated patients and the control arms.

4.9 Overdose

Single doses up to 1200 mg and daily doses up to 1800 mg of Ziagen have been administered to patients in clinical studies. No additional adverse reactions to those reported for normal doses were reported. The effects of higher doses are not known. If overdose occurs the patient should be monitored for evidence of toxicity (see section 4.8), and standard supportive treatment applied as necessary. It is not known whether abacavir can be removed by peritoneal dialysis or haemodialysis.

5. PHARMACOLOGICAL PROPERTIES

5.1 Pharmacodynamic properties

Pharmacotherapeutic group: nucleoside reverse transcriptase inhibitors, ATC Code: J05AF06

Mechanism of action: Abacavir is a NRTI. It is a potent selective inhibitor of HIV-1 and HIV-2. Abacavir is metabolised intracellularly to the active moiety, carbovir 5'-triphosphate (TP). *In vitro* studies have demonstrated that its mechanism of action in relation to HIV is inhibition of the HIV reverse transcriptase enzyme, an event which results in chain termination and interruption of the viral replication cycle. Abacavir shows synergy *in vitro* in combination with nevirapine and zidovudine. It has been shown to be additive in combination with didanosine, lamivudine and stavudine.

In vitro resistance: Abacavir-resistant isolates of HIV-1 have been selected *in vitro* and are associated with specific genotypic changes in the reverse transcriptase (RT) codon region (codons M184V, K65R, L74V and Y115F). Viral resistance to abacavir develops relatively slowly *in vitro*, requiring multiple mutations for a clinically relevant increase in EC_{50} over wild-type virus.

In vivo resistance (Therapy naïve patients) Isolates from most patients experiencing virological failure with a regimen containing abacavir in pivotal clinical trials showed either no NRTI-related changes from baseline (45%) or only M184V or M184I selection (45%). The overall selection frequency for M184V or M184I was high (54%), and less common was the selection of L74V (5%), K65R (1%) and Y115F (1%). The inclusion of zidovudine in the regimen has been found to reduce the frequency of L74V and K65R

Table 2

Hypersensitivity (see also section 4.4):

In clinical studies, approximately 5% of subjects receiving abacavir developed a hypersensitivity reaction. In clinical studies with abacavir 600 mg once daily the reported rate of hypersensitivity remained within the range recorded for abacavir 300 mg twice daily.

Some of these hypersensitivity reactions were life-threatening and resulted in fatal outcome despite taking precautions. This reaction is characterised by the appearance of symptoms indicating multi-organ/body-system involvement.

Almost all patients developing hypersensitivity reactions will have fever and/or rash (usually maculopapular or urticarial) as part of the syndrome, however reactions have occurred without rash or fever.

The signs and symptoms of this hypersensitivity reaction are listed below. These have been identified either from clinical studies or post marketing surveillance. Those reported **in at least 10% of patients** with a hypersensitivity reaction are in bold text.

Skin	**Rash** (usually maculopapular or urticarial)
Gastrointestinal tract	**Nausea, vomiting, diarrhoea, abdominal pain**, mouth ulceration
Respiratory tract	**Dyspnoea, cough**, sore throat, adult respiratory distress syndrome, respiratory failure
Miscellaneous	**Fever, lethargy, malaise**, oedema, lymphadenopathy, hypotension, conjunctivitis, anaphylaxis
Neurological/Psychiatry	**Headache**, paraesthesia
Haematological	Lymphopenia
Liver/pancreas	**Elevated liver function tests**, hepatitis, hepatic failure
Musculoskeletal	**Myalgia**, rarely myolysis, arthralgia, elevated creatine phosphokinase
Urology	Elevated creatinine, renal failure

Rash (81% vs 67% respectively) and gastrointestinal manifestations (70% vs 54% respectively) were more frequently reported in children compared to adults.

Some patients with hypersensitivity reactions were initially thought to have gastroenteritis, respiratory disease (pneumonia, bronchitis, pharyngitis) or a flu-like illness. This delay in diagnosis of hypersensitivity has resulted in Ziagen being continued or re-introduced, leading to more severe hypersensitivity reactions or death. Therefore, the diagnosis of hypersensitivity reaction should be carefully considered for patients presenting with symptoms of these diseases.

Symptoms usually appeared within the first six weeks (median time to onset 11 days) of initiation of treatment with abacavir, although these reactions may occur at any time during therapy. Close medical supervision is necessary during the first two months, with consultations every two weeks.

It is likely that intermittent therapy may increase the risk of developing sensitisation and therefore occurrence of clinically significant hypersensitivity reactions. Consequently, patients should be advised of the importance of taking Ziagen regularly.

Restarting Ziagen following a hypersensitivity reaction results in a prompt return of symptoms within hours. This recurrence of the hypersensitivity reaction was usually more severe than on initial presentation, and may include life-threatening hypotension and death. **Patients who develop this hypersensitivity reaction must discontinue Ziagen and must never be rechallenged with Ziagen, or any other medicinal product containing abacavir (e.g. Kivexa, Trizivir).**

To avoid a delay in diagnosis and minimise the risk of a life-threatening hypersensitivity reaction, Ziagen must be permanently discontinued if hypersensitivity cannot be ruled out, even when other diagnoses are possible (respiratory diseases, flu-like illness, gastroenteritis or reactions to other medications).

Hypersensitivity reactions with rapid onset, including life-threatening reactions have occurred after restarting Ziagen in patients who had only one of the key symptoms of hypersensitivity (skin rash, fever, gastrointestinal, respiratory or constitutional symptoms such as lethargy and malaise) prior to stopping Ziagen. The most common isolated symptom of a hypersensitivity reaction was a skin rash. Moreover, on very rare occasions hypersensitivity reactions have been reported in patients who have restarted therapy and who had no preceding symptoms of a hypersensitivity reaction.

In both cases, if a decision is made to restart Ziagen this must be done in a setting where medical assistance is readily available.

Each patient must be warned about this hypersensitivity reaction to abacavir.

selection in the presence of abacavir (with zidovudine: 0/40, without zidovudine: 15/192, 8%).

(see Table 3 opposite)

TAMs might be selected when thymidine analogs are associated with abacavir. In a meta-analysis of six clinical trials, TAMs were not selected by regimens containing abacavir without zidovudine (0/127), but were selected by regimens containing abacavir and the thymidine analogue zidovudine (22/86, 26%).

In vivo resistance (Therapy experienced patients): Clinically significant reduction of susceptibility to abacavir has been demonstrated in clinical isolates of patients with uncontrolled viral replication, who have been pre-treated with and are resistant to other nucleoside inhibitors. In a meta-analysis of five clinical trials where abacavir was added to intensify therapy, of 166 subjects, 123 (74%) had M184V/I, 50 (30%) had T215Y/F, 45 (27%) had M41L, 30 (18%) had K70R and 25 (15%) had D67N. K65R was absent and L74V and Y115F were uncommon (≤3%). Logistic regression modelling of the predictive value for genotype (adjusted for baseline plasma HIV-1 RNA [vRNA], CD4+ cell count, number and duration of prior antiretroviral therapies), showed that the presence of 3 or more NRTI resistance-associated mutations was associated with reduced response at Week 4 (p=0.015) or 4 or more mutations at median Week 24 (p≤0.012). In addition, the 69 insertion complex or the Q151M mutation, usually found in combination with A62V, V75I, F77L and F116Y, cause a high level of resistance to abacavir.

(see Table 4 on next page)

Phenotypic resistance and cross-resistance: Phenotypic resistance to abacavir requires M184V with at least one other abacavir-selected mutation, or M184V with multiple TAMs. Phenotypic cross-resistance to other NRTIs with M184V or M184I mutation alone is limited. Zidovudine, didanosine, stavudine and tenofovir maintain their antiretroviral activities against such HIV-1 variants. The presence of M184V with K65R does give rise to cross-resistance between abacavir, tenofovir, didanosine and lamivudine, and M184V with L74V gives rise to cross-resistance between abacavir, didanosine and lamivudine. The presence of M184V with Y115F gives rise to cross-resistance between abacavir and lamivudine. Appropriate use of abacavir can be guided using currently recommended resistance algorithms.

Cross-resistance between abacavir and antiretrovirals from other classes (e.g. PIs or NNRTIs) is unlikely.

Clinical Experience

The demonstration of the benefit of Ziagen is mainly based on results of studies performed in adult treatment-naïve patients using a regimen of Ziagen 300 mg twice daily in combination with zidovudine and lamivudine.

Twice daily (300 mg) administration:

• *Therapy naïve adults*

In adults treated with abacavir in combination with lamivudine and zidovudine the proportion of patients with undetectable viral load (<400 copies/ml) was approximately 70% (intention to treat analysis at 48 weeks) with corresponding rise in CD4 cells.

One randomised, double blind, placebo controlled clinical study in adults has compared the combination of abacavir, lamivudine and zidovudine to the combination of indinavir, lamivudine and zidovudine. Due to the high proportion of premature discontinuation (42% of patients discontinued randomised treatment by week 48), no definitive conclusion can be drawn regarding the equivalence between the treatment regimens at week 48. Although a similar antiviral effect was observed between the abacavir and indinavir containing regimens in terms of proportion of patients with undetectable viral load (≤400 copies/ml; intention to treat analysis (ITT), 47% versus 49%; as treated analysis (AT), 86% versus 94% for abacavir and indinavir combinations respectively), results favoured the indinavir combination, particularly in the subset of patients with high viral load (>100,000 copies/ml at baseline; ITT, 46% versus 55%; AT, 84% versus 93% for abacavir and indinavir respectively).

In a multicentre, double-blind, controlled study (CNA30024), 654 HIV-infected, antiretroviral therapy-naïve patients were randomised to receive either abacavir 300 mg twice daily or zidovudine 300 mg twice daily, both in combination with lamivudine 150 mg twice daily and efavirenz 600 mg once daily. The duration of double-blind treatment was at least 48 weeks. In the intent-to-treat (ITT) population, 70% of patients in the abacavir group, compared to 69% of patients in the zidovudine group, achieved a virologic response of plasma HIV-1 RNA ≤50 copies/ml by Week 48 (point estimate for treatment difference: 0.8, 95% CI -6.3, 7.9). In the as treated (AT) analysis the difference between both treatment arms was more noticeable (88% of patients in the abacavir group, compared to 95% of patients in the zidovudine group (point estimate for treatment difference: -6.8, 95% CI -11.8; -1.7). However, both analyses were compatible with a conclusion of non-inferiority between both treatment arms.

ACTG5095 was a randomised (1:1:1), double-blind, placebo-controlled trial performed in 1147 antiretroviral naïve HIV-1 infected adults, comparing 3 regimens: zidovudine (ZDV), lamivudine (3TC), abacavir (ABC), efavirenz (EFV) vs ZDV/3TC/EFV vs ZDV/3TC/ABC. After a median follow-up of 32 weeks, the tritherapy with the three nucleosides ZDV/3TC/ABC was shown to be virologically inferior to the two other arms regardless of baseline viral load (< or > 100 000 copies/ml) with 26% of subjects on the ZDV/3TC/ABC arm, 16% on the ZDV/3TC/EFV arm and 13% on the 4 drug arm categorised as having virological failure (HIV RNA>200 copies/ml). At week 48 the proportion of subjects with HIV RNA <50 copies/ml were 63%, 80% and 86% for the ZDV/3TC/ABC, ZDV/3TC/EFV and ZDV/3TC/ABC/EFV arms, respectively. The study Data Safety

Table 3

Therapy	Abacavir + Combivir[1]	Abacavir + lamivudine + NNRTI	Abacavir + lamivudine + PI (or PI/ritonavir)	Total
Number of Subjects	282	1094	909	2285
Number of Virological Failures	43	90	158	306
Number of On-Therapy Genotypes	40 (100%)	51 (100%)[2]	141 (100%)	232 (100%)
K65R	0	1 (2%)	2 (1%)	3 (1%)
L74V	0	9 (18%)	3 (2%)	12 (5%)
Y115F	0	2 (4%)	0	2 (1%)
M184V/I	34 (85%)	22 (43%)	70 (50%)	126 (54%)
TAMs[3]	3 (8%)	2 (4%)	4 (3%)	9 (4%)

1. Combivir is a fixed dose combination of lamivudine and zidovudine
2. Includes three non-virological failures and four unconfirmed virological failures.
3. Number of subjects with ≥1 Thymidine Analogue Mutations (TAMs).

Table 4

Baseline Reverse Transcriptase Mutation	Week 4 (n = 166)		
	n	Median Change vRNA (log_{10} c/mL)	Percent with $<$400 copies/mL vRNA
None	15	-0.96	40%
M184V alone	75	-0.74	64%
Any one NRTI mutation	82	-0.72	65%
Any two NRTI-associated mutations	22	-0.82	32%
Any three NRTI-associated mutations	19	-0.30	5%
Four or more NRTI-associated mutations	28	-0.07	11%

Table 5

		ZDV/3TC/ABC	ZDV/3TC/EFV	ZDV/3TC/ABC/EFV
Virologic failure (HIV RNA > 200 copies/ml)	32 weeks	26%	16%	13%
	144 weeks	-	26%	25%
Virologic success (48 weeks HIV RNA < 50 copies/ml)		63%	80%	86%

Monitoring Board stopped the ZDV/3TC/ABC arm at this time based on the higher proportion of patients with virologic failure. The remaining arms were continued in a blinded fashion. After a median follow-up of 144 weeks, 25% of subjects on the ZDV/3TC/ABC/EFV arm and 26% on the ZDV/3TC/EFV arm were categorised as having virological failure. There was no significant difference in the time to first virologic failure (p=0.73, log-rank test) between the 2 arms. In this study, addition of ABC to ZDV/3TC/EFV did not significantly improve efficacy.

(see Table 5 above)

- *Therapy naïve children*

In a study comparing the unblinded NRTI combinations (with or without blinded nelfinavir) in children, a greater proportion treated with abacavir and lamivudine (71%) or abacavir and zidovudine (60%) had HIV-1 RNA ⩽400 copies/ml at 48 weeks, compared with those treated with lamivudine and zidovudine (47%)[p=0.09, intention to treat analysis]. Similarly, greater proportions of children treated with the abacavir containing combinations had HIV-1 RNA ⩽50 copies/ml at 48 weeks (53%, 42% and 28% respectively, p=0.07).

- *Therapy experienced patients*

In adults moderately exposed to antiretroviral therapy the addition of abacavir to combination antiretroviral therapy provided modest benefits in reducing viral load (median change 0.44 log_{10} copies/ml at 16 weeks).

In heavily NRTI pretreated patients the efficacy of abacavir is very low. The degree of benefit as part of a new combination regimen will depend on the nature and duration of prior therapy which may have selected for HIV-1 variants with cross-resistance to abacavir.

Once daily (600 mg) administration:

- *Therapy naïve adults*

The once daily regimen of abacavir is supported by a 48 weeks multi-centre, double-blind, controlled study (CNA30021) of 770 HIV-infected, therapy-naïve adults. These were primarily asymptomatic HIV infected patients (CDC stage A). They were randomised to receive either abacavir 600 mg once daily or 300 mg twice daily, in combination with efavirenz and lamivudine given once daily. Similar clinical success (point estimate for treatment difference -1.7, 95% CI -8.4, 4.9) was observed for both regimens. From these results, it can be concluded with 95% confidence that the true difference is no greater than 8.4% in favour of the twice daily regimen. This potential difference is sufficiently small to draw an overall conclusion of non-inferiority of abacavir once daily over abacavir twice daily.

There was a low, similar overall incidence of virologic failure (viral load >50 copies/ml) in both the once and twice daily treatment groups (10% and 8% respectively). In the small sample size for genotypic analysis, there was a trend toward a higher rate of NRTI-associated mutations in the once daily versus the twice daily abacavir regimens. No firm conclusion could be drawn due to the limited data derived from this study. Long term data with abacavir used as a once daily regimen (beyond 48 weeks) are currently limited.

- *Therapy experienced patients*

In study CAL30001, 182 treatment-experienced patients with virologic failure were randomised and received treatment with either the fixed-dose combination of abacavir/lamivudine (FDC) once daily or abacavir 300 mg twice daily plus lamivudine 300 mg once daily, both in combination with tenofovir and a PI or an NNRTI for 48 weeks. Results indicate that the FDC group was non-inferior to the abacavir twice daily group, based on similar reductions in HIV-1 RNA as measured by average area under the curve minus baseline (AAUCMB, -1.65 log_{10} copies/ml versus -1.83 log_{10} copies/ml respectively, 95% CI -0.13, 0.38). Proportions with HIV-1 RNA < 50 copies/ml (50% versus 47%) and < 400 copies/ml (54% versus 57%) were also similar in each group (ITT population). However, as there were only moderately experienced patients included in this study with an imbalance in baseline viral load between the arms, these results should be interpreted with caution.

In study ESS30008, 260 patients with virologic suppression on a first line therapy regimen containing abacavir 300 mg plus lamivudine 150 mg, both given twice daily and a PI or NNRTI, were randomised to continue this regimen or switch to abacavir/lamivudine FDC plus a PI or NNRTI for 48 weeks. Results indicate that the FDC group was associated with a similar virologic outcome (non-inferior) compared to the abacavir plus lamivudine group, based on proportions of subjects with HIV-1 RNA < 50 copies/ml (90% and 85% respectively, 95% CI -2.7, 13.5).

Additional information:

The safety and efficacy of Ziagen in a number of different multidrug combination regimens is still not completely assessed (particularly in combination with NNRTIs).

Abacavir penetrates the cerebrospinal fluid (CSF) (see section 5.2), and has been shown to reduce HIV-1 RNA levels in the CSF. However, no effects on neuropsychological performance were seen when it was administered to patients with AIDS dementia complex.

5.2 Pharmacokinetic properties

Absorption: abacavir is rapidly and well absorbed following oral administration. The absolute bioavailability of oral abacavir in adults is about 83%. Following oral administration, the mean time (t_{max}) to maximal serum concentrations of abacavir is about 1.5 hours for the tablet formulation and about 1.0 hour for the solution formulation.

At therapeutic dosages a dosage of 300 mg twice daily, the mean (CV) steady state C_{max} and C_{min} of abacavir are approximately 3.00 µg/ml (30%) and 0.01 µg/ml (99%), respectively. The mean (CV) AUC over a dosing interval of 12 hours was 6.02 µg.h/ml (29%), equivalent to a daily AUC of approximately 12.0 µg.h/ml. The C_{max} value for the oral solution is slightly higher than the tablet. After a 600 mg abacavir tablet dose, the mean (CV) abacavir C_{max} was approximately 4.26 µg/ml (28%) and the mean (CV) AUC_{∞} was 11.95 µg.h/ml (21%).

Food delayed absorption and decreased C_{max} but did not affect overall plasma concentrations (AUC). Therefore Ziagen can be taken with or without food.

Administration of crushed tablets with a small amount of semi-solid food or liquid would not be expected to have an impact on the pharmaceutical quality, and would therefore not be expected to alter the clinical effect. This conclusion is based on the physiochemical and pharmacokinetic data, assuming that the patient crushes and transfers 100% of the tablet and ingests immediately.

Distribution: following intravenous administration, the apparent volume of distribution was about 0.8 l/kg, indicating that abacavir penetrates freely into body tissues.

Studies in HIV infected patients have shown good penetration of abacavir into the cerebrospinal fluid (CSF), with a CSF to plasma AUC ratio of between 30 to 44%. The observed values of the peak concentrations are 9 fold greater than the IC_{50} of abacavir of 0.08 µg/ml or 0.26 µM when abacavir is given at 600 mg twice daily.

Plasma protein binding studies *in vitro* indicate that abacavir binds only low to moderately (~49%) to human plasma proteins at therapeutic concentrations. This indicates a low likelihood for interactions with other medicinal products through plasma protein binding displacement.

Metabolism: abacavir is primarily metabolised by the liver with approximately 2% of the administered dose being renally excreted, as unchanged compound. The primary pathways of metabolism in man are by alcohol dehydrogenase and by glucuronidation to produce the 5'-carboxylic acid and 5'-glucuronide which account for about 66% of the administered dose. The metabolites are excreted in the urine.

Elimination: the mean half-life of abacavir is about 1.5 hours. Following multiple oral doses of abacavir 300 mg twice a day there is no significant accumulation of abacavir. Elimination of abacavir is via hepatic metabolism with subsequent excretion of metabolites primarily in the urine. The metabolites and unchanged abacavir account for about 83% of the administered abacavir dose in the urine. The remainder is eliminated in the faeces.

Intracellular pharmacokinetics

In a study of 20 HIV-infected patients receiving abacavir 300 mg twice daily, with only one 300 mg dose taken prior to the 24 hour sampling period, the geometric mean terminal carbovir-TP intracellular half-life at steady-state was 20.6 hours, compared to the geometric mean abacavir plasma half-life in this study of 2.6 hours. In a crossover study in 27 HIV-infected patients, intracellular carbovir-TP exposures were higher for the abacavir 600 mg once daily regimen ($AUC_{24,ss}$ + 32 %, $C_{max24,ss}$ + 99 % and C_{trough} + 18 %) compared to the 300 mg twice daily regimen. Overall, these data support the use of abacavir 600 mg once daily for the treatment of HIV infected patients. Additionally, the efficacy and safety of abacavir given once daily has been demonstrated in a pivotal clinical study (CNA30021- See section 5.1 Clinical experience).

Special populations

Hepatically impaired: abacavir is metabolised primarily by the liver. The pharmacokinetics of abacavir have been studied in patients with mild hepatic impairment (Child-Pugh score 5-6) receiving a single 600 mg dose. The results showed that there was a mean increase of 1.89 fold [1.32; 2.70] in the abacavir AUC, and 1.58 [1.22; 2.04] fold in the elimination half-life. No recommendation on dosage reduction is possible in patients with mild hepatic impairment due to the substantial variability of abacavir exposure.

Renally impaired: abacavir is primarily metabolised by the liver with approximately 2% of abacavir excreted unchanged in the urine. The pharmacokinetics of abacavir in patients with end-stage renal disease is similar to patients with normal renal function. Therefore no dosage reduction is required in patients with renal impairment. Based on limited experience Ziagen should be avoided in patients with end-stage renal disease.

Children: according to clinical trials performed in children abacavir is rapidly and well absorbed from an oral solution administered to children. The overall pharmacokinetic parameters in children are comparable to adults, with greater variability in plasma concentrations. The recommended dose for children from three months to 12 years is 8 mg/kg twice daily. This will provide slightly higher mean plasma concentrations in children, ensuring that the majority will achieve therapeutic concentrations equivalent to 300 mg twice daily in adults.

There are insufficient safety data to recommend the use of Ziagen in infants less than three months old. The limited data available indicate that a dose of 2 mg/kg in neonates less than 30 days old provides similar or greater AUCs, compared to the 8 mg/kg dose administered to older children.

Elderly: the pharmacokinetics of abacavir have not been studied in patients over 65 years of age.

5.3 Preclinical safety data

Abacavir was not mutagenic in bacterial tests but showed activity *in vitro* in the human lymphocyte chromosome aberration assay, the mouse lymphoma assay, and the *in vivo* micronucleus test. This is consistent with the known activity of other nucleoside analogues. These results indicate that abacavir has a weak potential to cause chromosomal damage both *in vitro* and *in vivo* at high test concentrations.

Carcinogenicity studies with orally administered abacavir in mice and rats showed an increase in the incidence of malignant and non-malignant tumours. Malignant tumours occurred in the preputial gland of males and the clitoral gland of females of both species, and in rats in the thyroid gland of males and the liver, urinary bladder, lymph nodes and the subcutis of females.

The majority of these tumours occurred at the highest abacavir dose of 330 mg/kg/day in mice and 600 mg/kg/day in rats. The exception was the preputial gland tumour which occurred at a dose of 110 mg/kg in mice. The systemic exposure at the no effect level in mice and rats was equivalent to 3 and 7 times the human systemic exposure during therapy. While the carcinogenic potential in humans is unknown, these data suggest that a carcinogenic risk to humans is outweighed by the potential clinical benefit.

In pre-clinical toxicology studies, abacavir treatment was shown to increase liver weights in rats and monkeys. The clinical relevance of this is unknown. There is no evidence from clinical studies that abacavir is hepatotoxic. Additionally, autoinduction of abacavir metabolism or induction of the metabolism of other medicinal products hepatically metabolised has not been observed in man.

Mild myocardial degeneration in the heart of mice and rats was observed following administration of abacavir for two years. The systemic exposures were equivalent to 7 to 24 times the expected systemic exposure in humans. The clinical relevance of this finding has not been determined.

In reproductive toxicity studies, embryo and foetal toxicity have been observed in rats but not in rabbits. These findings included decreased foetal body weight, foetal oedema, and an increase in skeletal variations/malformations, early intra-uterine deaths and still births. No conclusion can be drawn with regard to the teratogenic potential of abacavir because of this embryo-foetal toxicity.

A fertility study in the rat has shown that abacavir had no effect on male or female fertility.

6. PHARMACEUTICAL PARTICULARS

6.1 List of excipients

Core:

Microcrystalline cellulose

Sodium starch glycollate

Magnesium stearate

Colloidal anhydrous silica

Coating:

Triacetin

Methylhydroxypropylcellulose

Titanium dioxide

Polysorbate 80

Iron oxide yellow

6.2 Incompatibilities

Not applicable

6.3 Shelf life

3 years

6.4 Special precautions for storage

Do not store above 30°C

6.5 Nature and contents of container

Polyvinyl chloride/foil blister packs containing 60 tablets.

6.6 Special precautions for disposal and other handling

No special requirements

7. MARKETING AUTHORISATION HOLDER

Glaxo Group Ltd

Greenford

Middlesex UB6 0NN

United Kingdom

8. MARKETING AUTHORISATION NUMBER(S)

EU/1/99/112/001

9. DATE OF FIRST AUTHORISATION/RENEWAL OF THE AUTHORISATION

Date of first authorisation: 8 July 1999

Date of latest renewal: 8 July 2004

10. DATE OF REVISION OF THE TEXT

08 June 2009

Detailed information on this medicinal product is available on the website of the European Medicines Agency (EMEA) http://www.emea.europa.eu

Zimovane 7.5mg & Zimovane LS 3.75mg film-coated tablets

(sanofi-aventis)

1. NAME OF THE MEDICINAL PRODUCT

Zimovane 7.5mg film-coated tablets

Zimovane LS 3.75mg film-coated tablets

2. QUALITATIVE AND QUANTITATIVE COMPOSITION

Zopiclone 7.5 mg or 3.75mg.

For full list of excipients, see section 6.1.

3. PHARMACEUTICAL FORM

Film-coated tablet (tablet)

Zimovane LS: White, round, biconvex, film-coated tablets

Zimonvane: White, elliptical, biconvex film-coated tablets with a score-line on one side. The tablet can be divided into equal halves.

4. CLINICAL PARTICULARS

4.1 Therapeutic indications

Short term treatment of insomnia, including difficulties in falling asleep, nocturnal awakening and early awakening, transient, situational or chronic insomnia, and insomnia secondary to psychiatric disturbances, in situations where the insomnia is debilitating or is causing severe distress for the patient. Long term continuous use is not recommended. A course of treatment should employ the lowest effective dose.

4.2 Posology and method of administration

Adults: The recommended dose is 7.5mg zopiclone by the oral route shortly before retiring.

Elderly: A lower dose of 3.75mg zopiclone should be employed to start treatment in the elderly. Depending on effectiveness and acceptability, the dosage subsequently may be increased if clinically necessary.

Children and young adults less than 18 years: The safe and effective dose has not been established.

Patients with hepatic insufficiency: As elimination of zopiclone may be reduced in patients with hepatic dysfunction, a lower dose of 3.75mg zopiclone nightly is recommended. The standard dose of 7.5mg zopiclone may be used with caution in some cases, depending on effectiveness and acceptability.

Renal insufficiency: Accumulation of zopiclone or its metabolites has not been seen during treatment of insomnia in patients with renal insufficiency. However, it is recommended that patients with impaired renal function should start treatment with 3.75mg.

Treatment duration

Transient insomnia 2 - 5 days. Short term insomnia 2 - 3 weeks. A single course of treatment should not continue for longer than 4 weeks including any tapering off.

Route of administration

For oral use. Each tablet should be swallowed without sucking, chewing or breaking (3.75mg only).

4.3 Contraindications

Zimovane is contraindicated in patients with myasthenia gravis, respiratory failure, severe sleep apnoea syndrome, severe hepatic insufficiency and those people with a hypersensitivity to zopiclone or to any of the excipients. As with all hypnotics Zimovane should not be used in children.

4.4 Special warnings and precautions for use

Use in hepatic insufficiency: A reduced dosage is recommended, see Posology.

Use in renal insufficiency: A reduced dosage is recommended, see Posology.

Risk of dependence: Clinical experience to date with Zimovane suggests that the risk of dependence is minimal when the duration of treatment is limited to not more than 4 weeks.

Use of benzodiazepines and benzodiazepine-like agents (even at therapeutic doses) may lead to the development of physical and psychological dependence upon these products. The risk of dependence increases with dose and duration of treatment; it is also greater in patients with a history of alcohol and or drug abuse, or those who have marked personality disorders. The decision to use a hypnotic in such patients should be taken only with this clearly in mind. If physical dependence has developed, abrupt termination of treatment will be accompanied by withdrawal symptoms (see warnings and precautions). These may consist of headaches, muscle pain, extreme anxiety, tension, restlessness, confusion and irritability. In severe cases the following symptoms may occur: derealisation, depersonalisation, hyperacusis, numbness and tingling of the extremities, hypersensitivity to light, noise and physical contact, hallucinations or epileptic seizures. Rare cases of abuse have been reported.

Withdrawal: The termination of treatment with Zimovane is unlikely to be associated with withdrawal effects when duration of treatment is limited to 4 weeks. Patients may benefit from tapering of the dose before discontinuation. (See also section 4.8. Undesirable Effects).

Depression: Zopiclone does not constitute a treatment for depression. Any underlying cause of the insomnia should also be addressed before symptomatic treatment to avoid under treating potentially serious effects of depression.

Tolerance: Some loss of efficacy to the hypnotic effect of benzodiazepines and benzodiazepine-like agents may develop after repeated use for a few weeks. However, with Zimovane there is an absence of any marked tolerance during treatment periods of up to 4 weeks.

Rebound insomnia is a transient syndrome where the symptoms which led to treatment with a benzodiazepine or benzodiazepine-like agent recur in an enhanced form on discontinuation of therapy. It may be accompanied by other reactions including mood changes, anxiety and restlessness. Since the risk of withdrawal/rebound phenomena may be increased after prolonged treatment, or abrupt discontinuation of therapy, decreasing the dosage in a stepwise fashion may be helpful.

A course of treatment should employ the lowest effective dose for the minimum length of time necessary for effective treatment. See Posology for guidance on possible treatment regimen. A course of treatment should not continue for longer than 4 weeks including any tapering off. (See also section 4.8 Undesirable Effects).

Amnesia: Amnesia is rare, but anterograde amnesia may occur, especially when sleep is interrupted or when retiring to bed is delayed after taking the tablet. Therefore, patients should ensure that they take the tablet when certain of retiring for the night and they are able to have a full night's sleep.

Driving: It has been reported that the risk that zopiclone adversely affects driving ability is increased by the concomitant intake of alcohol. Therefore, it is recommended not to drive while taking zopiclone and alcohol concomitantly.

Other psychiatric and paradoxical reactions:

Other psychiatric and paradoxical reactions have been reported (see Section 4.8 Undesireable effects)

Somnambulism and associated behaviours:

Sleep walking and other associated behaviours such as "sleep driving", preparing and eating food, or making phone calls, with amnesia for the event, have been reported in patients who have taken zopiclone and were not fully awake. The use of alcohol and other CNS-depressants with zopiclone appears to increase the risk of such behaviours, as does the use of zopiclone at doses exceeding the maximum recommended dose. Discontinuation of zopiclone should be strongly considered for patients who report such behaviours (see Section 4.5 Interactions with other medicinal products and other forms of interactions).

Excipients:

Patients with rare hereditary problems of galactose intolerance, the Lapp lactase deficiency or glucose-galactose malabsorption should not take this medicine.

4.5 Interaction with other medicinal products and other forms of interaction

The sedative effect of zopiclone may be enhanced when used in combination with alcohol, concomitant use is therefore not recommended. In particular this could affect the patient's ability to drive or use machines.

In combination with CNS depressants an enhancement of the central depressive effect may occur. The therapeutic benefit of co-adminstration with antipsychotics (neuroleptics), hypnotics, anxiolytics/sedatives, antidepressant agents, narcotic analgesics, anti-epileptic drugs, anaesthetics and sedative antihistamines should therefore be carefully weighed. Concomitant use of benzodiazepines or benzodiazepine-like agents with narcotic analgesics may enhance their euphoric effect and could lead to an increase in psychic dependence. Compounds which inhibit certain hepatic enzymes (particularly cytochrome P450) may enhance the activity of benzodiazepines and benzodiazepine-like agents.

The effect of erythromycin on the pharmacokinetics of zopiclone has been studied in 10 healthy subjects. The AUC of zopiclone is increased by 80% in presence of erythromycin which indicates that erythromycin can inhibit the metabolism of drugs metabolised by CYP 3A4. As a consequence, the hypnotic effect of zopiclone may be enhanced.

Since zopiclone is metabolised by the cytochrome P450 (CYP) 3A4 isoenzyme (see section 5.2 Pharmacokinetic properties), plasma levels of zopiclone may be increased when co-adminsterd with CYP3A4 inhibitors such as erythromycin, clarithromycin, ketoconazole, itraconazole and ritonavir. A dose reduction for zopiclone may be required when it is co-adminstered with CYP3A4 inhibitors.

Conversely, plasma levels of zopiclone may be decreased when co-administered with CYP3A4 inducers such as rifampicin, carbamazepine, phenobarbital, phenytoin and St. John's wort. A dose increase for zopiclone may be required when it is co-adminstered with CYP3A4 inducers.

4.6 Pregnancy and lactation

Use during pregnancy: Experience of use of zopiclone during pregnancy in humans is limited although there have been no adverse findings in animals. Use in pregnancy is therefore not recommended. If the product is prescribed to a woman of child bearing potential, she should be advised to contact her physician about stopping the product if she intends to become pregnant, or suspects that she is pregnant.

Moreover, if zopiclone is used during the last three months of pregnancy or during labour, due to the pharmacological action of the product, effects on the neonate, such as hypothermia, hypnotic and respiratory depression can be expected.

Infants born to mothers who took benzodiazepines or benzodiazepine-like agents chronically during the latter stages of pregnancy may have developed physical dependence and may be at some risk of developing withdrawal symptoms in the postnatal period.

Use during lactation: Zopiclone is excreted in breast milk and use in nursing mothers must be avoided.

4.7 Effects on ability to drive and use machines

Although residual effects are rare and generally of minor significance, patients should be advised not to drive or operate machinery the day after treatment until it is established that their performance is unimpaired. The risk is increased by concomitant intake of alcohol (see section 4.4 Special Warnings and Precautions for Use).

4.8 Undesirable effects

A mild bitter or metallic after-taste is the most frequently reported adverse effect. Less commonly, mild gastrointestinal disturbances, including nausea and vomiting, dizziness, headache, drowsiness and dry mouth have occurred.

Psychological and behavioural disturbances, such as irritability, aggressiveness, confusion, depressed mood, anterograde amnesia, sleep walking (see Section 4.4 Special warnings and precautions for use), hallucinations and nightmares have been reported. Rarely these reactions may be severe and may be more likely to occur in the elderly. Rarely allergic and allied manifestations such as urticaria or rashes have been observed and, more rarely, light headedness and incoordination. Angiodema and/or anaphylactic reactions have been reported very rarely.

Withdrawal syndrome has been reported upon discontinuation of zopiclone. (See section 4.4. Special Warnings and Precautions for Use). Withdrawal symptoms vary and may include rebound insomnia, anxiety, tremor, sweating, agitation, confusion, headache, palpitations, tachycardia, delirium, nightmares, hallucinations, panic attacks, muscle aches/cramps, gastrointestinal disturbances and irritability. In very rare cases, seizures may occur.

Mild to moderate increases in serum transaminases and/or alkaline phosphatase have been reported very rarely.

4.9 Overdose
Fatal dose not known.

Symptoms

In the cases of overdosage reported, the main effects are drowsiness, lethargy and ataxia.

Management

Consider activated charcoal if an adult has ingested more than 150 mg or a child more than 1.5 mg/kg within one hour. Alternatively, consider gastric lavage in adults within one hour of a potentially life-threatening overdose. If CNS depression is severe consider the use of flumazenil. It has a short half-life (about an hour). NOT TO BE USED IN MIXED OVERDOSE OR AS A "DIAGNOSTIC" TEST. Management should include general symptomatic and supportive measures including a clear airway and monitoring cardiac and vital signs until stable.

5. PHARMACOLOGICAL PROPERTIES

5.1 Pharmacodynamic properties
ATC Code: N05C F01

Zopiclone is an hypnotic agent, and a member of the cyclopyrrolone group of compounds. It rapidly initiates and sustains sleep without reduction of total REM sleep and with preservation of slow wave sleep. Negligible residual effects are seen the following morning. Its pharmacological properties include hypnotic, sedative, anxiolytic, anticonvulsant and muscle-relaxant actions. These are related to its high affinity and specific agonist action at central receptors belonging to the 'GABA' macromolecular receptor complex modulating the opening of the chloride ion channel. However, it has been shown that zopiclone and other cyclopyrrolones act on a different site to those of benzodiazepines including different conformational changes in the receptor complex.

5.2 Pharmacokinetic properties

Absorption: Zopiclone is absorbed rapidly. Peak concentrations are reached within 1.5 - 2 hours and they are approximately 30 ng/ml and 60 ng/ml after administration of 3.75mg and 7.5mg respectively. Absorption is not modified by gender, food or repetition of doses.

Distribution: The product is rapidly distributed from the vascular compartment. Plasma protein binding is weak (approximately 45%) and non saturable. There is very little risk of drug interactions due to protein binding. The volume of distribution is 91.8 - 104.6 litres.

At doses between 3.75 - 15mg, plasma clearance does not depend on dose. The elimination half life is approximately 5 hours. After repeated administration, there is no accumulation, and inter-individual variations appear to be very small.

Metabolism: Zopiclone is exensively metabolised in humans to two major metabolites, N-oxide zopiclone (pharmacologically active in animals) and N-desmethyl zopiclone (pharmacologically inactive in animals). An *in-vitro* study indicates that cytochrome P450 (CYP) 3A4 is the major isoenzyme involved in the metabolism of zopiclone to both metabolites, and that CYP2C8 is also involved with N-desmethyl zopiclone formation. Their apparent half-lives (evaluated from the urinary data) are approximately 4.5 hours and 1.5 hours respectively. No significant accumulation is seen on repeated dosing (15mg) for 14 days. In animals, no enzyme induction has been observed even at high doses.

Excretion: The low renal clearance value of unchanged zopiclone (mean 8.4ml/min) compared with the plasma clearance (232ml/min) indicates that zopiclone clearance is mainly metabolic. The product is eliminated by the urinary route (approximately 80%) in the form of free metabolites (n-oxide and n-desmethyl derivatives) and in the faeces (approximately 16%).

Special patient groups: In elderly patients, notwithstanding a slight decrease in hepatic metabolism and lengthening of elimination half-life to approximately 7 hours, various studies have shown no plasma accumulation of drug substance on repeated dosing. In renal insufficiency, no accumulation of zopiclone or of its metabolites has been detected after prolonged administration. Zopiclone crosses dialysis membranes. In cirrhotic patients, the plasma clearance of zopiclone is clearly reduced by the slowing of the desmethylation process: dosage will therefore have to be modified in these patients.

5.3 Preclinical safety data
There are no preclinical data of relevance to the prescriber which are additional to that already included in other sections of the SPC.

6. PHARMACEUTICAL PARTICULARS

6.1 List of excipients

Zimovane:

Tablet Core:
Lactose monohydrate
calcium hydrogen phosphate dihydrate
wheat starch
sodium starch glycollate
magnesium stearate

Film-coating:
hypromellose
titanium dioxide
macrogol 6000
purified water
Or
Opadry OY-S-38906
purified water

Zimovane LS:

Tablet Core:
Lactose monohydrate
calcium hydrogen phosphate dihydrate
wheat starch
sodium starch glycollate
magnesium stearate

Film-coating:
hypromellose
titanium dioxide
macrogol 6000
purified water

6.2 Incompatibilities
Not applicable

6.3 Shelf life
24 months.

6.4 Special precautions for storage
Store below 30°C.

Keep the blister in the outer carton in order to protect from light and moisture.

6.5 Nature and contents of container
PVC/aluminium foil blisters containing 28 film-coated tablets

6.6 Special precautions for disposal and other handling
No special requirements

7. MARKETING AUTHORISATION HOLDER
Sanofi-aventis
One Onslow Street
Guildford
Surrey, GU1 4YS, UK

8. MARKETING AUTHORISATION NUMBER(S)

Zimovane: PL 04425/0624
Zimovane LS: PL 04425/0625

9. DATE OF FIRST AUTHORISATION/RENEWAL OF THE AUTHORISATION

Zimovane: 27 January 2009
Zimovane LS: 28 January 2009

10. DATE OF REVISION OF THE TEXT
10 August 2009

Legal category: POM

Zinacef

(GlaxoSmithKline UK)

1. NAME OF THE MEDICINAL PRODUCT
Zinacef®

Cefuroxime (as sodium) INN for Injection or Infusion.

2. QUALITATIVE AND QUANTITATIVE COMPOSITION
Vials contain either 250mg, 750mg or 1.5g cefuroxime (as sodium).

3. PHARMACEUTICAL FORM
Cefuroxime is a white to cream powder to which appropriate amounts of water are added to prepare an off-white suspension for intramuscular use or a yellowish solution for intravenous administration.

4. CLINICAL PARTICULARS

4.1 Therapeutic indications
Zinacef is a bactericidal cephalosporin antibiotic which is resistant to most beta-lactamases and is active against a wide range of Gram-positive and Gram-negative organisms. It is indicated for the treatment of infections before the infecting organism has been identified or when caused by sensitive bacteria. In addition, it is an effective prophylactic against post-operative infection in a variety of operations. Usually Zinacef will be effective alone, but when appropriate it may be used in combination with an aminoglycoside antibiotic, or in conjunction with metronidazole, orally or by suppository or injection, (see Pharmaceutical precautions).

In situations where mixed aerobic and anaerobic infections are encountered or suspected (e.g. peritonitis, aspiration pneumonia, abscesses in the lung, pelvis and brain), or are likely to occur (e.g. in association with colorectal or gynaecological surgery) it is appropriate to administer Zinacef in combination with metronidazole.

Most of these infections will respond to an i.v. regimen of Zinacef (750mg) plus metronidazole injection (500mg/100ml) administered eight-hourly. In more severe or well established mixed infections, an i.v. regimen of Zinacef (1.5g) plus metronidazole injection (500mg/100ml) eight-hourly may be indicated. For the prophylaxis of infection in surgery (e.g. colorectal and gynaecological) a single dose of 1.5g Zinacef plus metronidazole injection (500mg/100ml) is appropriate.

Alternatively this may be followed by two 750mg doses of Zinacef plus metronidazole.

Indications include:

Respiratory tract infections for example, acute and chronic bronchitis, infected bronchiectasis, bacterial pneumonia, lung abscess and post operative chest infections.

Ear, nose and throat infections for example, sinusitis, tonsillitis and pharyngitis.

Urinary tract infections for example acute and chronic pyelonephritis, cystitis and asymptomatic bacteriuria.

Soft-tissue infections for example cellulitis, erysipelas, peritonitis and wound infections.

Bone and joint infections for example, osteomyelitis and septic arthritis.

Obstetric and gynaecological infections pelvic inflammatory diseases.

Gonorrhoea particularly when penicillin is unsuitable.

Other infections including septicaemia and meningitis.

Prophylaxis against infection in abdominal, pelvic, orthopaedic, cardiac, pulmonary, oesophageal and vascular surgery where there is increased risk from infection.

Cefuroxime is also available as the axetil ester (Zinnat) for oral administration.

This permits the use of sequential therapy with the same antibiotic, when a change from parenteral to oral therapy is clinically indicated. Where appropriate Zinacef is effective when used prior to oral therapy with Zinnat (cefuroxime axetil) in the treatment of pneumonia and acute exacerbations of chronic bronchitis.

4.2 Posology and method of administration

Intramuscular

Add 1ml water for injections to 250mg Zinacef or 3ml water for injections to 750mg Zinacef. Shake gently to produce an opaque suspension.

Intravenous

Dissolve Zinacef in water for injections using at least 2ml for 250mg, at least 6ml for 750mg or 15ml for 1.5g. For short intravenous infusion (e.g. up to 30 minutes), 1.5g may be dissolved in 50ml water for injections. These solutions may be given directly into the vein or introduced into the tubing of the giving set if the patient is receiving parenteral fluids.

General Recommendations

Adults: Many infections will respond to 750mg t.i.d. by im or iv injection. For more severe infections, this dose should be increased to 1.5g t.i.d. iv. The frequency of im or iv injection can be increased to six-hourly if necessary, giving total doses of 3g to 6g daily.

Where clinically indicated adults with pneumonia and acute exacerbations of chronic bronchitis have been shown to respond to 750mg or 1.5g bd, followed by oral therapy with Zinnat (see Sequential therapy).

Infants and Children: Doses of 30 to 100mg/kg/day given as three or four divided doses. A dose of 60mg/kg/day will be appropriate for most infections.

Neonates: Doses of 30 to 100mg/kg/day given as two or three divided doses. In the first weeks of life the serum half-life of cefuroxime can be three to five times that in adults.

Elderly: See dosage in adults.

Other Recommendations

Gonorrhoea: 1.5g should be given as a single dose. This may be given as 2 × 750mg injections into different sites eg each buttock.

Meningitis: Zinacef is suitable for sole therapy of bacterial meningitis due to sensitive strains. The following dosages are recommended.

Infants and Children: 200 to 240mg/kg/day iv in three or four divided doses. This dosage may be reduced to 100mg/kg/day iv after three days or when clinical improvement occurs.

Neonates: The initial dosage should be 100mg/kg/day iv. A reduction to 50mg/kg/day iv may be made when clinically indicated.

Adults: 3g iv every eight hours. Data are not yet sufficient to recommend a dose for intrathecal administration.

Prophylaxis: The usual dose is 1.5g iv with induction of anaethesia for abdominal, pelvic and orthopaedic operations, but may be supplemented with two 750mg im doses eight and sixteen hours later. In cardiac pulmonary oesophageal and vascular operations, the usual dose is 1.5g iv with induction of anaesthesia continuing with 750mg im t.d.s. for a further 24 to 48 hours.

In total joint replacement, 1.5g cefuroxime powder may be mixed dry with each pack of methyl methacrylate cement polymer before adding the liquid monomer.

Sequential therapy:

Pneumonia:

1.5g bd (iv or im) for 48-72 hours, followed by 500mg bd Zinnat (cefuroxime axetil) oral therapy for 7 days.

Acute exacerbations of chronic bronchitis:

750mg bd (iv or im) for 48-72 hours, followed by 500mg bd Zinnat (cefuroxime axetil) oral therapy for 5-7 days.

Duration of both parenteral and oral therapy is determined by the severity of the infection and the clinical status of the patient.

Dosage in impaired renal function

Cefuroxime is excreted by the kidneys. Therefore, as with all such antibiotics, in patients with markedly impaired renal function it is recommended that the dosage of Zinacef should be reduced to compensate for its slower excretion. However, it is not necessary to reduce the dose until the creatinine clearance falls below 20ml/min. In adults with marked impairment (creatinine clearance 10-20ml/min) 750mg bd is recommended and with severe impairment (creatinine clearance <10ml/min) 750mg once daily is adequate. For patients on haemodialysis a further 750mg dose should be given at the end of each dialysis. When continuous peritoneal dialysis is being used, a suitable dosage is usually 750mg twice daily.

For patients in renal failure on continuous arteriovenous haemodialysis or high-flux haemofiltration in intensive therapy units a suitable dosage is 750mg twice daily. For low-flux haemofiltration follow the dosage recommended under impaired renal function.

Cefuroxime is also available as the axetil ester (Zinnat) for oral administration. This permits parenteral therapy with cefuroxime to be followed by oral therapy in situations where a change from parenteral to oral is clinically indicated.

4.3 Contraindications

Hypersensitivity to cephalosporin antibiotics

4.4 Special warnings and precautions for use

Special care is indicated in patients who have experienced an allergic reaction to penicillins or beta-lactams.

Cephalosporin antibiotics at high dosage should be given with caution to patients receiving concurrent treatment with potent diuretics such as furosemide or aminoglycosides, as renal impairment has been reported with these combinations. Renal function should be monitored in these patients, the elderly, and those with pre-existing renal impairment (See section 4.2) Clinical experience with Zinacef has shown that this is not likely to be a problem at the recommended dose levels.

There may be some variation on the results of biochemical tests of renal function, but these do not appear to be of clinical importance. As a precaution, renal function should be monitored if this is already impaired.

Delayed sterilisation of the CSF in patients with Haemophilus influenzae meningitis may result in an adverse outcome such as deafness and /or neurological sequelae. Persistence of positive CSF cultures of *H. influenzae* at 18-36 hours has been noted in some patients treated with cefuroxime sodium injection and, as with other therapeutic regimens used in the treatment of meningitis, hearing loss has been reported in some children.

With a sequential therapy regime the timing of change to oral therapy is determined by severity of the infection, clinical status of the patient and susceptibility of the pathogens involved. The change to oral therapy should only be made once there is a clear clinical improvement. If there has been no clinical improvement after 72 hours of parenteral treatment, then the patient's treatment should be reviewed. Please refer to the relevant prescribing information for cefuroxime axetil before initiating sequential therapy.

As with other antibiotics, prolonged use of cefuroxime may result in the overgrowth of non-susceptible organisms (e.g. *Candida*, enterococci, *Clostridium difficile*), which may require interruption of treatment.

4.5 Interaction with other medicinal products and other forms of interaction

In common with other antibiotics, Zinacef may affect the gut flora, leading to lower oestrogen reabsorption and reduced efficacy of combined oral contraceptives.

As with other cephalosporin antibiotics in combination with potent diuretics such as furosemide or aminoglycosides, Zinacef may adversely affect renal function (See section 4.4).

Zinacef does not interfere in enzyme-based tests for glycosuria. Slight interference with copper reduction methods (Benedict's, Fehling's, Clinitest) may be observed. However, this should not lead to false-positive results, as may be experienced with some other cephalosporins.

It is recommended that either the glucose oxidase or hexokinase methods are used to determine blood/plasma glucose levels in patients receiving Zinacef. This antibiotic does not interfere in the alkaline picrate assay for creatinine.

4.6 Pregnancy and lactation

There is no experimental evidence of embryopathic or teratogenic effects attributable to Zinacef but, as with all drugs, it should be administered with caution during the early months of pregnancy.

Cefuroxime is excreted in human milk, and consequently caution should be exercised when Zinacef is administered to a nursing mother.

4.7 Effects on ability to drive and use machines

None reported.

4.8 Undesirable effects

Adverse drug reactions are very rare (<1/10,000) and are generally mild and transient in nature.

The frequency categories assigned to the adverse reactions below are estimates, as for most reactions suitable data for calculating incidence are not available. In addition the incidence of adverse reactions associated with cefuroxime sodium may vary according to the indication.

Data from clinical trials were used to determine the frequency of very common to rare undesirable effects. The frequencies assigned to all other undesirable effects (i.e., those occurring at <1/1000) were mainly determined using post-marketing data, and refer to a reporting rate rather than a true frequency.

The following convention has been used for the classification of frequency:

very common ≥1/10, common ≥1/100 and <1/10, uncommon ≥1/1000 and <1/100, rare ≥1/10,000 and <1/1000, very rare <1/10,000.

Infections and infestations	
Rare	Candida overgrowth from prolonged use.

Blood and lymphatic system disorders	
Common	Neutropenia, eosinophilia.
Uncommon	Leukopenia, decreased haemoglobin concentration, positive Coomb's test.
Rare	Thrombocytopenia.
Very rare	Haemolytic anaemia.

Cephalosporins as a class tend to be absorbed onto the surface of red cell membranes and react with antibodies directed against the drug to produce a positive Coomb's Test (which can interfere with cross matching of blood) and very rarely haemolytic anaemia.

Immune system disorders Hypersensitivity reactions including	
Uncommon	Skin rash, urticaria and pruritus.
Rare	Drug fever.
Very rare	Interstitial nephritis, anaphylaxis, cutaneous vasculitis

See also Skin and subcutaneous tissue disorders and Renal and urinary disorders.

Gastrointestinal disorders	
Uncommon	Gastrointestinal disturbance.
Very rare	Pseudomembranous colitis.
Hepatobiliary disorders	
Common	Transient rise in liver enzymes.
Uncommon	Transient rise in bilirubin.

Transient rises in serum liver enzymes or bilirubin occur, particularly in patients with pre-existing liver disease, but there is no evidence of harm to the liver.

Skin and subcutaneous tissue disorders	
Very rare	Erythema multiforme, toxic epidermal necrolysis and Stevens Johnson Syndrome.

See also Immune system disorders.

Renal and urinary disorders	
Very rare	Elevations in serum creatinine, elevations in blood urea nitrogen and decreased creatinine clearance (*See Section 4.4 Special Warnings and Precautions for use*).

See also Immune system disorders.

General disorders and administration site conditions	
Common	Injection site reactions which may include pain and thrombophlebitis

Pain at the intramuscular injection site is more likely at higher doses. However it is unlikely to be a cause for discontinuation of treatment.

4.9 Overdose

Overdosage of cephalosporins can cause cerebral irritation leading to convulsions. Serum levels of cefuroxime can be reduced by haemodialysis or peritoneal dialysis.

5. PHARMACOLOGICAL PROPERTIES

5.1 Pharmacodynamic properties

Cefuroxime is a bactericidal cephalosporin antibiotic which is resistant to most beta-lactamases and is active against a wide range of Gram-positive and Gram-negative organisms.

It is highly active against *Staphylococcus aureus*, including strains which are resistant to penicillin (but not the rare methicillin-resistant strains), *Staph. epidermidis, Haemophilus influenzae,* Klebsiella spp., Enterobacter spp., *Streptococcus pyogenes, Escherichia coli, Str. mitis (viridans group)*, Clostridium spp., *Proteus mirabilis*, Pr. rettgeri, *Salmonella typhi, S. typhimurium* and other Salmonella spp., Shigella spp., Neisseria spp. (including beta-lactamase producing strains of *N. gonorrhoea*) and *Bordetella pertussis*. It is also moderately active against strains of *Pr. vulgaris*, *Morganella morganii* (formerly *Proteus morganii*) and *Bacteroides fragilis*.

The following organisms are not susceptible to cefuroxime: *Clostridium difficile*, Pseudomonas spp., Campylobacter spp., *Acinetobacter calcoaceticus,* Legionella spp. and methicillin-resistant strains of *Staph. aureus* and *Staph. epidermidis*.

Some strains of the following genera have also been found not to be susceptible to Zinacef:

Strep. faecalis, Morganella morganii, Proteus vulgaris, Enterobacter spp., Citrobacter spp., Serratia spp. and *Bacteroides fragilis*.

In vitro the activities of Zinacef and aminoglycoside antibiotics in combination have been shown to be at least additive with occasional evidence of synergy.

5.2 Pharmacokinetic properties

Peak levels of cefuroxime are achieved within 30 to 45 minutes after intramuscular administration. The serum half-life after either intramuscular or intravenous injection is approximately 70 minutes. Concurrent administration of probenecid prolongs the excretion of the antibiotic and produces an elevated peak serum level. There is almost complete recovery of unchanged cefuroxime in the urine within 24 hours of administration, the major part being eliminated in the first six hours. Approximately 50% is excreted through the renal tubules and approximately 50% by glomerular filtration. Concentrations of cefuroxime in excess of the minimum inhibitory levels for common pathogens can be achieved in bone, synovial fluid and aqueous humor. Cefuroxime passes the blood-brain barrier when the meninges are inflamed.

5.3 Preclinical safety data

None stated

6. PHARMACEUTICAL PARTICULARS

6.1 List of excipients

None.

6.2 Incompatibilities

Cefuroxime is compatible with most commonly used intravenous fluids and electrolyte solutions.

The pH of 2.74% w/v sodium bicarbonate injection BP considerably affects the colour of solutions and therefore this solution is not recommended for the dilution of Zinacef. However, if required, for patients receiving sodium bicarbonate injection by infusion the Zinacef may be introduced into the tube of the giving set.

Zinacef should not be mixed in the syringe with aminoglycoside antibiotics.

6.3 Shelf life

Two years when stored below 25°C and protected from light.

6.4 Special precautions for storage

Store below 25°C and protect from light.

After constitution, Zinacef should be stored at 2 - 8°C for no longer than 24 hours.

6.5 Nature and contents of container

1) Moulded glass (type 1 or III) vials with bromobutyl or fluoro-resin laminated butyl rubber plug, overseal and flip-off cap containing either 250mg, 750mg or 1.5g Zinacef.

2) A bulk pack of 100 vials.

3) Monovial containing either 750mg or 1.5g Zinacef with transfer needle.

*Only the 1.5g injection pack is marketed (the infusion pack is not)

6.6 Special precautions for disposal and other handling
None.

Administrative Data

7. MARKETING AUTHORISATION HOLDER
Glaxo Operations UK Limited, Greenford, Middlesex UB6 0HE

Trading as

GlaxoSmithKline UK, Stockley Park West, Uxbridge, Middlesex UB11 1BT

8. MARKETING AUTHORISATION NUMBER(S)
PL 00004/0263.

9. DATE OF FIRST AUTHORISATION/RENEWAL OF THE AUTHORISATION
28 April 2002

10. DATE OF REVISION OF THE TEXT
17th November 2008

11. Legal Status
POM

Zineryt

(Astellas Pharma Ltd)

1. NAME OF THE MEDICINAL PRODUCT
Zineryt.

2. QUALITATIVE AND QUANTITATIVE COMPOSITION
Erythromycin 40 mg and zinc acetate 12 mg per ml on constitution.

3. PHARMACEUTICAL FORM
Dry powder bottle and solvent bottle to be admixed on dispensing.

4. CLINICAL PARTICULARS

4.1 Therapeutic indications
Topical treatment of acne vulgaris.

4.2 Posology and method of administration
For children, adults, and the elderly. Apply twice daily over the whole of the affected area for a period of 10 to 12 weeks.

4.3 Contraindications
Zineryt is contraindicated in patients who are hypersensitive to erythromycin or other macrolide antibiotics, or to zinc, di-isopropyl sebacate or ethanol.

4.4 Special warnings and precautions for use
Cross resistance may occur with other antibiotics of the macrolide group and also with lincomycin and clindamycin. Contact with the eyes or the mucous membranes of the nose and mouth should be avoided.

4.5 Interaction with other medicinal products and other forms of interaction
None known.

4.6 Pregnancy and lactation
There is no contraindication to the use of Zineryt in pregnancy or lactation.

4.7 Effects on ability to drive and use machines
None.

4.8 Undesirable effects

System Organ Class	Rare ≥1/10,000, <1/1000	Very rare <1/10,000, Not known (cannot be estimated from the available data)
Immune system disorders		Hypersensitivity
Skin and subcutaneous tissue disorders	Pruritus Erythema Skin irritation Skin burning sensation Dry skin Skin exfoliation	

4.9 Overdose
It is not expected that overdosage would occur in normal use. Patients showing idiosyncratic hypersensitivity should wash the treated area with copious water and simple soap.

5. PHARMACOLOGICAL PROPERTIES

5.1 Pharmacodynamic properties
Erythromycin is known to be efficacious, at 4%, in the topical treatment of acne vulgaris. Zinc, topically, is established as an aid to wound healing. The zinc acetate is solubilised by complexing with the erythromycin, and delivery of the complex is enhanced by the chosen vehicle.

5.2 Pharmacokinetic properties
The complex does not survive in the skin, and erythromycin and zinc penetrate independently. The erythromycin penetrates, and is partially systemically absorbed (0 - 10% in vitro, 40 - 50% in animal studies); that portion absorbed is excreted in 24 - 72 hours. The zinc is not absorbed systemically.

5.3 Preclinical safety data
No relevant pre-clinical safety data has been generated.

6. PHARMACEUTICAL PARTICULARS

6.1 List of excipients
Di-isopropyl sebacate, ethanol.

6.2 Incompatibilities
None known.

6.3 Shelf life
2 years; 5 weeks after constitution.

6.4 Special precautions for storage
Do not store above 25°C.

6.5 Nature and contents of container
Screw-capped HDPE bottles; an applicator assembly is fitted when dispensed. When constituted packs are of 30 ml and 90 ml.

6.6 Special precautions for disposal and other handling
None

Administrative Data

7. MARKETING AUTHORISATION HOLDER
Astellas Pharma Ltd

Lovett House

Lovett Road

Staines

TW18 3AZ

United Kingdom

8. MARKETING AUTHORISATION NUMBER(S)
0166/0109.

9. DATE OF FIRST AUTHORISATION/RENEWAL OF THE AUTHORISATION
First authorisation granted 7 March 1990/ 29 March 2001

10. DATE OF REVISION OF THE TEXT
21 May 2008

11. Legal category
POM

Zinnat Suspension

(GlaxoSmithKline UK)

1. NAME OF THE MEDICINAL PRODUCT
Zinnat Suspension 125mg/5ml

2. QUALITATIVE AND QUANTITATIVE COMPOSITION
Cefuroxime 125mg/5ml (as 150 mg cefuroxime axetil)

3. PHARMACEUTICAL FORM
Granules for constitution with water to form a suspension for oral administration.

4. CLINICAL PARTICULARS

4.1 Therapeutic indications
Cefuroxime axetil is an oral prodrug of the bactericidal cephalosporin antibiotic cefuroxime, which is resistant to most β-lactamases and is active against a wide range of Gram-positive and Gram-negative organisms.

It is indicated for the treatment of infections caused by sensitive bacteria.

Indications include: Lower respiratory tract infections for example, acute bronchitis, acute exacerbations of chronic bronchitis and pneumonia.

Upper respiratory tract infections for example, ear, nose, throat infections, such as otitis media, sinusitis, tonsillitis and pharyngitis.

Genito-urinary tract infections for example, pyelonephritis, cystitis and urethritis.

Skin and soft tissue infections for example, furunculosis, pyoderma and impetigo.

Gonorrhoea acute uncomplicated gonococcal urethritis, and cervicitis.

Treatment of early Lyme disease and subsequent prevention of late Lyme disease in adults and children over 12 years old.

Cefuroxime is also available as the sodium salt (Zinacef) for parenteral administration. This permits the use of sequential therapy with the same antibiotic, when a change from parenteral to oral therapy is clinically indicated.

Where appropriate Zinnat is effective when used following initial parenteral Zinacef (cefuroxime sodium) in the treatment of pneumonia and acute exacerbations of chronic bronchitis.

4.2 Posology and method of administration
Adults: Most infections will respond to 250mg b.d. In mild to moderate lower respiratory tract infections e.g. bronchitis 250mg b.d. should be given. For more severe lower respiratory tract infections, or if pneumonia is suspected then 500mg b.d. should be given. For urinary tract infections a dose of 125mg b.d. is usually adequate; in pyelonephritis the recommended dose is 250mg b.d. A single dose of one gram is recommended for the treatment of uncomplicated gonorrhoea.

Lyme disease in adults and children over the age of 12 years: the recommended dose is 500mg b.d. for 20 days.

Sequential therapy:

Pneumonia:

1.5g Zinacef bd (iv or im) for 48-72 hours, followed by 500mg bd Zinnat (cefuroxime axetil) oral therapy for 7 days.

Acute exacerbations of chronic bronchitis:

750mg Zinacef bd (iv or im) for 48-72 hours, followed by 500mg Zinnat (cefuroxime axetil) oral therapy for 5-7 days.

Duration of both parenteral and oral therapy is determined by the severity of the infection and the clinical status of the patient.

Children: The usual dose is 125mg b.d. (1 × 125mg tablet or 5ml of suspension or 1 × 125mg sachet), or 10mg/kg b.d. to a maximum of 250mg daily. For otitis media, in children less than 2 years of age the usual dosage is 125mg b.d. (1 × 125mg tablet or 5ml of suspension or 1 × 125mg sachet), or 10mg/kg b.d. to a maximum of 250mg daily and in children over 2 years of age, 250mg b.d. (1 × 250mg tablet or 10ml of suspension or 2 × 125mg sachets), or 15mg/kg b.d. to a maximum of 500mg daily. There is no experience in children under 3 months of age.

Zinnat Tablets should not be crushed, therefore in younger children the suspension is more appropriate.

Elderly and Patients with Renal Impairment: No special precautions are necessary in patients with renal impairment or on renal dialysis or in the elderly at dosages up to the normal maximum of 1g per day.

The usual course of therapy is seven days.

Zinnat should be taken after food for optimum absorption.

4.3 Contraindications
Hypersensitivity to cephalosporin antibiotics.

4.4 Special warnings and precautions for use
Special care is indicated in patients who have experienced an allergic reaction to penicillins or other beta-lactams.

As with other antibiotics, use of cefuroxime axetil may result in the overgrowth of *Candida*. Prolonged use may also result in the overgrowth of non-susceptible organisms (e.g. *Enterococci* and *Clostridium difficile*), which may require interruption of treatment.

Pseudomembranous colitis has been reported with the use of broad-spectrum antibiotics, therefore, it is important to consider its diagnosis in patients who develop serious diarrhoea during or after antibiotic use.

The Jarisch-Herxheimer reaction has been seen following Zinnat treatment of Lyme disease. It results from the bactericidal activity of Zinnat on the causative organism of Lyme disease, the spirochaete *Borrelia burgdorferi*. Patients should be reassured that this is a common and usually self-limited consequence of antibiotic treatment of Lyme disease.

With a sequential therapy regime the timing of change to oral therapy is determined by severity of the infection, clinical status of the patient and susceptibility of the pathogens involved. The change to oral therapy should only be made once there is a clear clinical improvement. If there has been no clinical improvement after 72 hours of parenteral treatment, then the patient's treatment should be reviewed. Please refer to the relevant prescribing information for cefuroxime sodium before initiating sequential therapy.

The sucrose content of Zinnat Suspension and granules (see section 6.1 List of Excipients) should be taken into account when treating diabetic patients, and appropriate advice provided.

Zinnat suspension contains aspartame, which is a source of phenylalanine and so should be used with caution in patients with phenylketonuria.

4.5 Interaction with other medicinal products and other forms of interaction
In common with other antibiotics, Zinnat may affect the gut flora, leading to lower oestrogen reabsorption and reduced efficacy of combined oral contraceptives.

As a false negative result may occur in the ferricyanide test, it is recommended that either the glucose oxidase or hexokinase methods are used to determine blood/plasma glucose levels in patients receiving cefuroxime axetil. This antibiotic does not interfere in the alkaline picrate assay for creatinine.

4.6 Pregnancy and lactation
There is no experimental evidence of embryopathic or teratogenic effects attributable to cefuroxime axetil but, as with all drugs, it should be administered with caution during early months of pregnancy. Cefuroxime is excreted in human milk, and consequently caution should be exercised when cefuroxime axetil is administered to a nursing mother.

4.7 Effects on ability to drive and use machines
As this medicine may cause dizziness, patients should be warned to be cautious when driving or operating machinery.

4.8 Undesirable effects
Adverse drug reactions to cefuroxime axetil are generally mild and transient in nature.

The following convention has been used for the classification of undesirable effects:- very common (≥1/10), common (≥1/100, <1/10), uncommon, (≥1/1000, <1/100,) rare(≥1/10,000, <1/1000), very rare (<1/10,000).

Infections and infestations

Common: Candida overgrowth

Blood and lymphatic system disorders

Common: Eosinophilia

Uncommon: Positive Coombs' test, thrombocytopenia, leukopenia (sometimes profound)

Very rare: Haemolytic anaemia

Cephalosporins as a class tend to be absorbed onto the surface of red cells membranes and react with antibodies directed against the drug to produce a positive Coombs' test (which can interfere with cross-matching of blood) and very rarely haemolytic anaemia.

Immune system disorders

Hypersensitivity reactions including

Uncommon: Skin rashes

Rare: Urticaria, pruritus

Very rare: Drug fever, serum sickness, anaphylaxis

Nervous system disorders

Common: Headache, dizziness

Gastrointestinal disorders

Common: Gastrointestinal disturbances including diarrhoea, nausea, abdominal pain

Uncommon: Vomiting

Rare: Pseudomembranous colitis

Hepatobiliary disorders

Common: Transient increasesof hepatic enzyme levels, [ALT (SGPT), AST (SGOT), LDH]

Very rare: Jaundice (predominantly cholestatic), hepatitis

Skin and subcutaneous tissue disorders

Very rare: Erythema multiforme, Stevens-Johnson syndrome, toxic epidermal necrolysis (exanthematic necrolysis)

Renal and Urinary tract disorders

Very Rare: interstitial nephritis

4.9 Overdose

Overdosage of cephalosporins can cause cerebral irritancy leading to convulsions.

Serum levels of cefuroxime can be reduced by haemodialysis or peritoneal dialysis.

5. PHARMACOLOGICAL PROPERTIES

5.1 Pharmacodynamic properties

Cefuroxime axetil is an oral prodrug of the bactericidal cephalosporin antibiotic cefuroxime, which is resistant to most beta-lactamases and is active against a wide range of gram-positive and gram-negative organisms.

Microbiology:

Cefuroxime axetil owes its *in vivo* bactericidal activity to the parent compound, cefuroxime. Cefuroxime is a well-characterized and effective antibacterial agent which has broad-spectrum bactericidal activity against a wide range of common pathogens, including beta-lactamase-producing strains. Cefuroxime has good stability to bacterial beta-lactamase and consequently, is active against many ampicillin-resistant and amoxicillin-resistant strains. The bactericidal action of cefuroxime results from inhibition of cell-wall synthesis by binding to essential target proteins.

Cefuroxime is usually active against the following organisms *in vitro*:

Aerobes, Gram-negative: *Haemophilus influenzae* (including ampicillin-resistant strains); *Haemophilus parainfluenzae; Moraxella catarrhalis; Escherichia coli;* Klebsiella species; *Proteus mirabilis; Proteus inconstans;* Providencia species; *Proteus rettgeri* and *Neisseria gonorrhoea* (including penicillinase and non-penicillinase-producing strains).

Some strains of *Morganella morganii*, Enterobacter species and Citrobacter species have been shown by *in vitro* tests to be resistant to cefuroxime and other beta-lactam antibiotics.

Aerobes, Gram-positive: *Staphylococcus aureus* (including penicillinase-producing strains but excluding methicillin-resistant strains); *Staphylococcus epidermidis*, (including penicillinase producing strains but excluding methicillin-resistant strains); *Streptococcus pyogenes* (and betahaemolytic streptococci), *Streptococcus pneumoniae;* Streptococcus Group B (*Streptococcus agalactiae*) and Propionibacterium species.

Certain strains of enterococci, eg. *Streptococcus faecalis*, are resistant.

Anaerobes, Gram-positive and Gram-negative cocci (including Peptococcus and Peptostreptococcus species); Gram-positive bacilli (including Clostridium species) and Gram-negative bacilli (including Bacteroides and Fusobacterium species). Most strains of *Bacteroides fragilis* are resistant.

Other organisms, *Borrelia burgdorferi*.

Pseudomonas species, Campylobacter species, *Acinetobacter calcoaceticus, Listeria monocytogenes,* Legionella species and most strains of Serratia and *Proteus vulgaris* and *Clostridium difficile* are resistant to many cephalosporins including cefuroxime.

5.2 Pharmacokinetic properties

After oral administration, cefuroxime axetil is absorbed from the gastrointestinal tract and rapidly hydrolysed in the intestinal mucosa and blood to release cefuroxime into the circulation. Optimum absorption occurs when it is administered after a meal. Peak serum cefuroxime levels occur approximately two to three hours after oral dosing. The serum half life is about 1.2 hours. Approximately 50% of serum cefuroxime is protein bound. Cefuroxime is not metabolised and is excreted by glomerular filtration and tubular secretion.

Concurrent administration of probenecid increases the area under the mean serum concentration time curve by 50%. Serum levels of cefuroxime are reduced by dialysis.

5.3 Preclinical safety data

No additional data of relevance.

6. PHARMACEUTICAL PARTICULARS

6.1 List of excipients

Aspartame

Xanthan gum

Acesulfame potassium

Povidone K30

Stearic Acid

Sucrose

Tutti Frutti Flavour

Purified Water

Sucrose Quantities:

125 mg/5ml Suspension 3.062 g/5ml	125 mg Sachet 3.062 g

6.2 Incompatibilities

None.

6.3 Shelf life

The shelf life of unconstituted Zinnat Suspension from date of manufacture is 24 months stored below 30°C. The reconstituted suspension, when refrigerated between 2 and 8°C can be kept for up to 10 days.

6.4 Special precautions for storage

Zinnat Suspension granules should be stored below 30°C.

Multidose Bottles: The reconstituted suspension must be refrigerated as soon as possible at between 2 and 8°C.

Sachets: Reconstituted suspension should be taken immediately.

6.5 Nature and contents of container

Zinnat Suspension 125mg/5ml, granules for oral suspension are supplied in multidose bottles* *of 50, 70, 100, 140 and 200ml (Delete as appropriate) and in 125 and 250mg sachets (heat-sealed laminate of paper/polyethylene/foil/ethylene-methacrylic acid ionomer).

125mg sachets are packed as either 1 duplex sachet in a carton or 7 duplex sachets in a carton (i.e. 2 or 14 doses).

250mg sachets are packed as 7 duplex sachets in a carton (i.e. 14 doses).

*Ph Eur Type III amber glass multiple unit bottles with a closure containing a heat-sealed induction membrane and a re-seal liner.

6.6 Special precautions for disposal and other handling

The bottle should always be shaken vigorously before administration.

The reconstituted suspension in multidose bottles when refrigerated between 2 and 8°C can be kept for up to 10 days.

If desired, Zinnat Suspension from multidose bottles can be further diluted in cold fruit juices, or milk drinks and should be taken immediately.

The reconstituted suspension or granules should not be mixed with hot liquids.

Directions for reconstituting suspension in multidose bottles: -

1. Shake the bottle to loosen the granules. Remove the cap and the heat-seal membrane. If the latter is damaged or not present, the product should be returned to the pharmacist.
2. Add the total amount of water to the bottle as stated on its label. Replace the cap.
3. Invert the bottle and rock vigorously (for at least 15 seconds) as shown below.

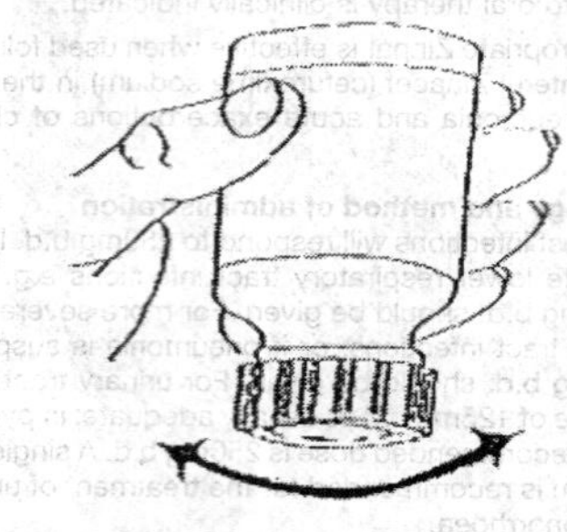

4. Turn the bottle into an upright position and shake vigorously.
5. Refrigerate as soon as possible at between 2 and 8°C.

Directions for reconstituting suspension from sachets: -

1. Empty granules from sachet into a glass.
2. Add a small volume of water.
3. Stir well and drink immediately.

Administrative Data

7. MARKETING AUTHORISATION HOLDER

Glaxo Wellcome UK Limited

t/a Glaxo Laboratories

Stockley Park West

Uxbridge

Middlesex UB11 1BT

8. MARKETING AUTHORISATION NUMBER(S)

PL10949/0094

9. DATE OF FIRST AUTHORISATION/RENEWAL OF THE AUTHORISATION

1 July 1993

10. DATE OF REVISION OF THE TEXT

3 July 2008

11. Legal Status

POM

Zinnat Tablets 125mg

(GlaxoSmithKline UK)

1. NAME OF THE MEDICINAL PRODUCT

Zinnat Tablets 125mg

2. QUALITATIVE AND QUANTITATIVE COMPOSITION

Each tablet contains 125mg cefuroxime (as cefuroxime axetil).

3. PHARMACEUTICAL FORM

White, film-coated, capsule-shaped tablet plain on one side and engraved with 'GXES5' on the other.

4. CLINICAL PARTICULARS

4.1 Therapeutic indications

Cefuroxime axetil is indicated for the treatment of infections caused by sensitive bacteria.

Lower respiratory tract infections for example, acute bronchitis, acute exacerbations of chronic bronchitis, and pneumonia.

Upper respiratory tract infections for example, ear, nose, throat infections, such as otitis media, sinusitis, tonsillitis and pharyngitis.

Genito-urinary tract infections for example, pyelonephritis, cystitis and urethritis.

Skin and soft tissue infections for example, furunculosis, pyoderma and impetigo.

Treatment of early Lyme disease and subsequent prevention of late Lyme disease in adults and children over 12 years old.

Gonorrhoea acute uncomplicated gonococcal urethritis, and cervicitis.

Cefuroxime is also available as the sodium salt (Zinacef) for parenteral administration. This permits the use of sequential therapy with the same antibiotic, when a change from parenteral to oral therapy is clinically indicated.

Where appropriate Zinnat is effective when used following initial parenteral Zinacef (cefuroxime sodium) in the treatment of pneumonia and acute exacerbations of chronic bronchitis.

4.2 Posology and method of administration

Route of administration: oral

Dosage in adults

Most infections will respond to 250mg bd. In mild to moderate lower respiratory tract infections e.g. bronchitis 250mg bd should be given. For more severe lower respiratory tract infections, or if pneumonia is suspected then 500mg bd should be given. For urinary tract infections a dose of 125mg bd is usually adequate; in pyelonephritis the recommended dose is 250mg bd. A single dose of one gram is recommended for the treatment of uncomplicated gonorrhoea. Lyme disease in adults and children over the age of 12 years: the recommended dose is 500mg bd for 20 days.

Sequential therapy:

Pneumonia:

1.5g Zinacef bd (iv or im) for 48-72 hours, followed by 500mg bd Zinnat (cefuroxime axetil) oral therapy for 7 days.

Acute exacerbations of chronic bronchitis:

750mg Zinacef bd (iv or im) for 48-72 hours, followed by 500mg bd Zinnat (cefuroxime axetil) oral therapy for 5-7 days.

Duration of both parenteral and oral therapy is determined by the severity of the infection and the clinical status of the patient.

Dosage in children

The usual dose is 125mg bd or 10mg/kg bd to a maximum of 250mg daily. For otitis media, in children less than

2 years of age the usual dosage is 125mg bd or 10mg/kg bd to a maximum of 250mg daily and in children over 2 years of age, 250mg bd or 15mg/kg bd to a maximum of 500mg daily. There is no experience in children under 3 months of age.

Zinnat Tablets should not be crushed, therefore in younger children the suspension is more appropriate.

Elderly and patients with renal impairment

No special precautions are necessary in patients with renal impairment or on renal dialysis or in the elderly at dosages up to the normal maximum of 1g per day.

The usual course of therapy is seven days.

Zinnat should be taken after food for optimum absorption.

4.3 Contraindications

Hypersensitivity to cephalosporin antibiotics.

4.4 Special warnings and precautions for use

Special care is indicated in patients who have experienced an allergic reaction to penicillins or other beta-lactams.

As with other antibiotics, use of cefuroxime axetil may result in the overgrowth of *Candida*. Prolonged use may also result in the overgrowth of non-susceptible organisms (e.g. *Enterococci* and *Clostridium difficile*), which may require interruption of treatment.

Pseudomembranous colitis has been reported with the use of broad-spectrum antibiotics, therefore, it is important to consider its diagnosis in patients who develop serious diarrhoea during or after antibiotic use.

The Jarisch-Herxheimer reaction has been seen following Zinnat treatment of Lyme disease. It results from the bactericidal activity of Zinnat on the causative organism of Lyme disease, the spirochaete *Borrelia burgdorferi*. Patients should be reassured that this is common and usually self-limited consequence of antibiotic treatment of Lyme disease.

With a sequential therapy regime the timing of change to oral therapy is determined by severity of the infection, clinical status of the patient and susceptibility of the pathogens involved. The change to oral therapy should only be made once there is a clear clinical improvement. If there has been no clinical improvement after 72 hours of parenteral treatment, then the patient's treatment should be reviewed. Please refer to the relevant prescribing information for cefuroxime sodium before initiating sequential therapy.

4.5 Interaction with other medicinal products and other forms of interaction

In common with other antibiotics, Zinnat may affect the gut flora, leading to lower oestrogen reabsorption and reduced efficacy of combined oral contraceptives.

As a false negative result may occur in the ferricyanide test, it is recommended that either the glucose oxidase or hexokinase methods are used to determine blood/plasma glucose levels in patients receiving cefuroxime axetil. This antibiotic does not interfere in the alkaline picrate assay for creatinine.

Concurrent administration of probenecid increases the area under the mean serum concentration time curve by 50%. Serum levels of cefuroxime are reduced by dialysis.

A positive Coomb's test has been reported during treatment with cephalosporins. This phenomenon can interfere with cross matching of blood.

4.6 Pregnancy and lactation

There is no experimental evidence of embryopathic or teratogenic effects attributable to cefuroxime axetil but, as with all drugs, it should be administered with caution during early months of pregnancy. Cefuroxime is excreted in human milk, and consequently caution should be exercised when cefuroxime axetil is administered to a nursing mother.

4.7 Effects on ability to drive and use machines

As this medicine may cause dizziness, patients should be warned to be cautious when driving or operating machinery.

4.8 Undesirable effects

Adverse drug reactions to cefuroxime axetil are generally mild and transient in nature.

The following convention has been used for the classification of frequency:

very common ($\geqslant$1/10), common ($\geqslant$1/100, <1/10), uncommon ($\geqslant$1/1000, <1/100), rare ($\geqslant$1/10,000 and <1/1000), very rare (<1/10,000).

Infections and infestations

Common: Candida overgrowth

Blood and lymphatic system disorders

Common: Eosinophilia

Uncommon: Positive Coombs' test, thrombocytopenia, leukopenia (sometimes profound)

Very rare: Haemolytic anaemia

Cephalosporins as a class tend to be absorbed onto the surface of red cells membranes and react with antibodies directed against the drug to produce a positive Coombs' test (which can interfere with cross-matching of blood) and very rarely haemolytic anaemia.

Immune system disorders

Hypersensitivity reactions including

Uncommon: Skin rashes

Rare: Urticaria, pruritus

Very rare: Drug fever, serum sickness, anaphylaxis

Nervous system disorders

Common: Headache, dizziness

Gastrointestinal disorders

Common: Gastrointestinal disturbances including diarrhoea, nausea, abdominal pain

Uncommon: Vomiting

Rare: Pseudomembranous colitis

Hepatobiliary disorders

Common: Transient increases of hepatic enzyme levels, [ALT (SGPT), AST (SGOT), LDH]

Very rare: Jaundice (predominantly cholestatic), hepatitis

Skin and subcutaneous tissue disorders

Very rare: Erythema multiforme, Stevens-Johnson syndrome, toxic epidermal necrolysis (exanthematic necrolysis)

4.9 Overdose

Overdosage of cephalosporins can cause cerebral irritancy leading to convulsions.

Serum levels of cefuroxime can be reduced by haemodialysis or peritoneal dialysis.

5. PHARMACOLOGICAL PROPERTIES

5.1 Pharmacodynamic properties

Cefuroxime axetil is an oral prodrug of the bactericidal cephalosporin antibiotic cefuroxime, which is resistant to most beta-lactamases and is active against a wide range of gram-positive and gram-negative organisms.

Microbiology

Cefuroxime axetil owes its *in vivo* bactericidal activity to the parent compound, cefuroxime. Cefuroxime is a well-characterized and effective antibacterial agent which has broad-spectrum bactericidal activity against a wide range of common pathogens, including beta-lactamase-producing strains.

Cefuroxime has good stability to bacterial beta-lactamase and consequently, is active against many ampicillin-resistant and amoxicillin-resistant strains. The bactericidal action of cefuroxime results from inhibition of cell-wall synthesis by binding to essential target proteins.

Cefuroxime is usually active against the following organisms *in vitro*:

Aerobes, Gram-negative: *Haemophilus influenzae* (including ampicillin-resistant strains); *Haemophilus parainfluenzae; Moraxella catarrhalis; Escherichia coli;* Klebsiella species; *Proteus mirabilis; Proteus inconstans;* Providencia species; *Proteus rettgeri* and *Neisseria gonorrhoea* (including penicillinase and non-penicillinase-producing strains).

Some strains of *Morganella morganii*, Enterobacter species and Citrobacter species have been shown by *in vitro* tests to be resistant to cefuroxime and other beta-lactam antibiotics.

Aerobes, Gram-positive: *Staphylococcus aureus* (including penicillinase-producing strains but excluding methicillin-resistant strains); *Staphylococcus epidermis,* (including penicillinase - producing strains but excluding methicillin-resistant strains); *Streptococcus pyogenes* (and other betahaemolytic streptococci); *Streptococcus pneumonia* Streptococcus Group B (*Streptococcus agalactiae)* and Propionibacterium species. Certain strains of enterococci, eg. *Streptococcus faecalis,* are resistant.

Anaerobes, Gram-positive and Gram-negative cocci (including Peptococcus and Peptostreptococcus species); Gram-positive bacilli (including Clostridium species) and Gram-negative bacilli (including Bacteroides and Fusobacterium species). Most strains of Bacteroides fragilis are resistant.

Other organisms, *Borrelia burgdorferi.*

Pseudomonas species, Campylobacter species, Acinetobacter calcoaceticus, Listeria monocytogenes, Legionella species and most strains of Serratia and Proteus vulgaris and Clostridium difficile are resistant to many cephalosporins including cefuroxime.

5.2 Pharmacokinetic properties

After oral administration, cefuroxime axetil is absorbed from the gastro-intestinal tract and rapidly hydrolysed in the intestinal mucosa and blood to release cefuroxime into the circulation. Optimum absorption occurs when it is administered after a meal. Peak serum cefuroxime levels occur approximately two to three hours after oral dosing. The serum half life is about 1.2 hours. Approximately 50% of serum cefuroxime is protein bound. Cefuroxime is not metabolised and is excreted by glomerular filtration and tubular secretion. Concurrent administration of probenecid increases the area under the mean serum concentration time curve by 50%.

5.3 Preclinical safety data

No additional data of relevance.

6. PHARMACEUTICAL PARTICULARS

6.1 List of excipients

Microcrystalline cellulose

Croscarmellose sodium, Type A

Sodium lauryl sulphate

Hydrogenated vegetable oil

Silica Colloidal Anhydrous

Methylhydroxypropyl cellulose

Propylene glycol

Methyl parahydroxybenzoate

Propyl parahydroxybenzoate

Opaspray white M-1-7120J

6.2 Incompatibilities

A positive Coombs' test has been reported during treatment with cephalosporins - this phenomenon can interfere with cross-matching of blood.

6.3 Shelf life

36 months in aluminium foil strips or blister packs.

24 months in HDPE bottles (not marketed in the UK)

6.4 Special precautions for storage

Cefuroxime axetil tablets in foil strips or blisters should be stored below 30°C.

Cefuroxime axetil tablets in HDPE bottles should be stored below 25°C (not marketed in the UK)

6.5 Nature and contents of container

Aluminium foil blister pack with an aluminium lid.

Pack size: 2, 4, 14 and 50

(2 and 4 not marketed in the UK)

Aluminium foil strips coated with surlyn polymer.

Pack size: 14 and 50

(not marketed in the UK)

White opaque, high density polyethylene bottles fitted with a clic-loc child resistant closure containing a pulp board wad to which is wax-bonded a 'lectraseal' membrane.

Pack size: 14 and 60

(not marketed in the UK)

6.6 Special precautions for disposal and other handling

None stated.

Administrative Data

7. MARKETING AUTHORISATION HOLDER

Glaxo Wellcome UK Limited trading as GlaxoSmithKline UK

Stockley Park West

Uxbridge

Middlesex

UB11 1BT

8. MARKETING AUTHORISATION NUMBER(S)

PL 10949/0095

9. DATE OF FIRST AUTHORISATION/RENEWAL OF THE AUTHORISATION

15 October 1998

10. DATE OF REVISION OF THE TEXT

3 July 2008

11. Legal Status

POM

Zinnat Tablets 250mg

(GlaxoSmithKline UK)

1. NAME OF THE MEDICINAL PRODUCT

Zinnat Tablets 250mg

2. QUALITATIVE AND QUANTITATIVE COMPOSITION

Each tablet contains 250mg cefuroxime (as cefuroxime axetil).

3. PHARMACEUTICAL FORM

White, film-coated, capsule-shaped tablet plain on one side and engraved with 'GXES7' on the other.

4. CLINICAL PARTICULARS

4.1 Therapeutic indications

Cefuroxime axetil is indicated for the treatment of infections caused by sensitive bacteria.

Lower respiratory tract infections for example, acute bronchitis, acute exacerbations of chronic bronchitis, and pneumonia.

Upper respiratory tract infections for example, ear, nose, throat infections, such as otitis media, sinusitis, tonsillitis and pharyngitis.

Genito-urinary tract infections for example, pyelonephritis, cystitis and urethritis.

Skin and soft tissue infections for example, furunculosis, pyoderma and impetigo.

Treatment of early Lyme disease and subsequent prevention of late Lyme disease in adults and children over 12 years old.

Gonorrhoea acute uncomplicated gonococcal urethritis, and cervicitis.

Cefuroxime is also available as the sodium salt (Zinacef) for parenteral administration. This permits the use of sequential therapy with the same antibiotic, when a change from parenteral to oral therapy is clinically indicated.

Where appropriate Zinnat is effective when used following initial parenteral Zinacef (cefuroxime sodium) in the treatment of pneumonia and acute exacerbations of chronic bronchitis.

4.2 Posology and method of administration
Route of administration: oral

Dosage in adults

Most infections will respond to 250mg bd. In mild to moderate lower respiratory tract infections e.g. bronchitis 250mg bd should be given. For more severe lower respiratory tract infections, or if pneumonia is suspected then 500mg bd should be given. For urinary tract infections a dose of 125mg bd is usually adequate; in pyelonephritis the recommended dose is 250mg bd. A single dose of one gram is recommended for the treatment of uncomplicated gonorrhoea. Lyme disease in adults and children over the age of 12 years: the recommended dose is 500mg bd for 20 days.

Sequential therapy:

Pneumonia:

1.5g Zinacef bd (iv or im) for 48-72 hours, followed by 500mg bd Zinnat (cefuroxime axetil) oral therapy for 7 days.

Acute exacerbations of chronic bronchitis:

750mg Zinacef bd (iv or im) for 48-72 hours, followed by 500mg bd Zinnat (cefuroxime axetil) oral therapy for 5-7 days.

Duration of both parenteral and oral therapy is determined by the severity of the infection and the clinical status of the patient.

Dosage in children

The usual dose is 125mg bd or 10mg/kg bd to a maximum of 250mg daily. For otitis media, in children less than 2 years of age the usual dosage is 125mg bd or 10mg/kg bd to a maximum of 250mg daily and in children over 2 years of age, 250mg bd or 15mg/kg bd to a maximum of 500mg daily. There is no experience in children under 3 months of age.

Zinnat Tablets should not be crushed, therefore in younger children the suspension is more appropriate.

Elderly and patients with renal impairment

No special precautions are necessary in patients with renal impairment or on renal dialysis or in the elderly at dosages up to the normal maximum of 1g per day.

The usual course of therapy is seven days.

Zinnat should be taken after food for optimum absorption.

4.3 Contraindications
Hypersensitivity to cephalosporin antibiotics.

4.4 Special warnings and precautions for use
Special care is indicated in patients who have experienced an allergic reaction to penicillins or other beta-lactams.

As with other antibiotics, use of cefuroxime axetil may result in the overgrowth of *Candida*. Prolonged use may also result in the overgrowth of non-susceptible organisms (e.g. *Enterococci* and *Clostridium difficile*), which may require interruption of treatment.

Pseudomembranous colitis has been reported with the use of broad-spectrum antibiotics, therefore, it is important to consider its diagnosis in patients who develop serious diarrhoea during or after antibiotic use.

The Jarisch-Herxheimer reaction has been seen following Zinnat treatment of Lyme disease. It results from the bactericidal activity of Zinnat on the causative organism of Lyme disease, the spirochaete *Borrelia burgdorferi*. Patients should be reassured that this is common and usually self-limited consequence of antibiotic treatment of Lyme disease.

With a sequential therapy regime the timing of change to oral therapy is determined by severity of the infection, clinical status of the patient and susceptibility of the pathogens involved. The change to oral therapy should only be made once there is a clear clinical improvement. If there has been no clinical improvement after 72 hours of parenteral treatment, then the patient's treatment should be reviewed. Please refer to the relevant prescribing information for cefuroxime sodium before initiating sequential therapy.

4.5 Interaction with other medicinal products and other forms of interaction
In common with other antibiotics, Zinnat may affect the gut flora, leading to lower oestrogen reabsorption and reduced efficacy of combined oral contraceptives.

As a false negative result may occur in the ferricyanide test, it is recommended that either the glucose oxidase or hexokinase methods are used to determine blood/plasma glucose levels in patients receiving cefuroxime axetil. This antibiotic does not interfere in the alkaline picrate assay for creatinine.

Concurrent administration of probenecid increases the area under the mean serum concentration time curve by 50%. Serum levels of cefuroxime are reduced by dialysis.

A positive Coomb's test has been reported during treatment with cephalosporins. This phenomenon can interfere with cross matching of blood.

4.6 Pregnancy and lactation
There is no experimental evidence of embryopathic or teratogenic effects attributable to cefuroxime axetil but, as with all drugs, it should be administered with caution during early months of pregnancy. Cefuroxime is excreted in human milk, and consequently caution should be exercised when cefuroxime axetil is administered to a nursing mother.

4.7 Effects on ability to drive and use machines
As this medicine may cause dizziness, patients should be warned to be cautious when driving or operating machinery.

4.8 Undesirable effects
Adverse drug reactions to cefuroxime axetil are generally mild and transient in nature.

The following convention has been used for the classification of frequency:

very common($\geqslant$1/10), common ($\geqslant$1/100, <1/10), uncommon($\geqslant$1/1000, <1/100), rare($\geqslant$1/10,000, <1/1000,) very rare (<1/10,000).

Infections and infestations

Common: Candida overgrowth

Blood and lymphatic system disorders

Common: Eosinophilia

Uncommon: Positive Coombs' test, thrombocytopenia, leukopenia (sometimes profound)

Very rare: Haemolytic anaemia

Cephalosporins as a class tend to be absorbed onto the surface of red cells membranes and react with antibodies directed against the drug to produce a positive Coombs' test (which can interfere with cross-matching of blood) and very rarely haemolytic anaemia.

Immune system disorders

Hypersensitivity reactions including

Uncommon: Skin rashes

Rare: Urticaria, pruritus

Very rare: Drug fever, serum sickness, anaphylaxis

Nervous system disorders

Common: Headache, dizziness

Gastrointestinal disorders

Common: Gastrointestinal disturbances including diarrhoea, nausea, abdominal pain

Uncommon: Vomiting

Rare: Pseudomembranous colitis

Hepatobiliary disorders

Common: Transient increases of hepatic enzyme levels, [ALT (SGPT), AST (SGOT), LDH]

Very rare: Jaundice (predominantly cholestatic), hepatitis

Skin and subcutaneous tissue disorders

Very rare: Erythema multiforme, Stevens-Johnson syndrome, toxic epidermal necrolysis (exanthematic necrolysis)

4.9 Overdose
Overdosage of cephalosporins can cause cerebral irritancy leading to convulsions.

Serum levels of cefuroxime can be reduced by haemodialysis or peritoneal dialysis.

5. PHARMACOLOGICAL PROPERTIES

5.1 Pharmacodynamic properties
Cefuroxime axetil is an oral prodrug of the bactericidal cephalosporin antibiotic cefuroxime, which is resistant to most beta-lactamases and is active against a wide range of gram-positive and gram-negative organisms.

Microbiology

Cefuroxime axetil owes its *in vivo* bactericidal activity to the parent compound, cefuroxime. Cefuroxime is a well-characterized and effective antibacterial agent which has broad-spectrum bactericidal activity against a wide range of common pathogens, including beta-lactamase-producing strains.

Cefuroxime has good stability to bacterial beta-lactamase and consequently, is active against many ampicillin-resistant and amoxicillin-resistant strains. The bactericidal action of cefuroxime results from inhibition of cell-wall synthesis by binding to essential target proteins.

Cefuroxime is usually active against the following organisms *in vitro*:

Aerobes, Gram-negative: *Haemophilus influenzae* (including ampicillin-resistant strains); *Haemophilus parainfluenzae; Moraxella catarrhalis; Escherichia coli;* Klebsiella species; *Proteus mirabilis; Proteus inconstans;* Providencia species; *Proteus rettgeri* and *Neisseria gonorrhoea* (including penicillinase and non-penicillinase-producing strains).

Some strains of *Morganella morganii,* Enterobacter species and Citrobacter species have been shown by *in vitro* tests to be resistant to cefuroxime and other beta-lactam antibiotics.

Aerobes, Gram-positive: *Staphylococcus aureus* (including penicillinase-producing strains but excluding methicillin-resistant strains); *Staphylococcus epidermis,* (including penicillinase-producing strains but excluding methicillin-resistant strains); *Streptococcus pyogenes (*and other betahaemolytic streptococci); *Streptococcus pneumonia* Streptococcus Group B (*Streptococcus agalactiae)* and Propionibacterium species. Certain strains of enterococci, eg. *Streptococcus faecalis,* are resistant.

Anaerobes, Gram-positive and Gram-negative cocci (including Peptococcus and Peptostreptococcus species); Gram-positive bacilli (including Clostridium species) and Gram-negative bacilli (including Bacteroides and Fusobacterium species). Most strains of Bacteroides fragilis are resistant.

Other organisms, *Borrelia burgdorferi*.

Pseudomonas species, *Campylobacter* species, *Acinetobacter calcoaceticus, Listeria monocytogenes, Legionella species* and most strains of Serratia and *Proteus vulgaris* and *Clostridium difficile* are resistant to many cephalosporins including cefuroxime.

5.2 Pharmacokinetic properties
After oral administration, cefuroxime axetil is absorbed from the gastro-intestinal tract and rapidly hydrolysed in the intestinal mucosa and blood to release cefuroxime into the circulation. Optimum absorption occurs when it is administered after a meal. Peak serum cefuroxime levels occur approximately two to three hours after oral dosing. The serum half life is about 1.2 hours. Approximately 50% of serum cefuroxime is protein bound. Cefuroxime is not metabolised and is excreted by glomerular filtration and tubular secretion. Concurrent administration of probenecid increases the area under the mean serum concentration time curve by 50%.

5.3 Preclinical safety data
No additional data of relevance.

6. PHARMACEUTICAL PARTICULARS

6.1 List of excipients
Microcrystalline cellulose
Croscarmellose sodium, Type A
Sodium lauryl sulphate
Hydrogenated vegetable oil
Silica Colloidal Anhydrous
Methylhydroxypropyl cellulose
Propylene glycol
Methyl parahydroxybenzoate
Propyl parahydroxybenzoate
Opaspray white M-1-7120J

6.2 Incompatibilities
A positive Coombs' test has been reported during treatment with cephalosporins - this phenomenon can interfere with cross-matching of blood.

6.3 Shelf life
36 months in aluminium foil strips or blister packs.
24 months in HDPE bottles (not marketed in the UK)

6.4 Special precautions for storage
Cefuroxime axetil tablets in foil strips or blisters should be stored below 30°C.

Cefuroxime axetil tablets in HDPE bottles should be stored below 25°C (not marketed in the UK)

6.5 Nature and contents of container
Aluminium foil blister pack with an aluminium lid.

Pack size: 2, 4, 14 and 50

(2 and 4 not marketed in the UK)

Aluminium foil strips coated with surlyn polymer.

Pack size: 14 and 50

(not marketed in the UK)

White opaque, high density polyethylene bottles fitted with a clic-loc child resistant closure containing a pulp board wad to which is wax-bonded a 'lectraseal' membrane.

Pack size: 14 and 60

(not marketed in the UK)

6.6 Special precautions for disposal and other handling
None stated

Administrative Data

7. MARKETING AUTHORISATION HOLDER
Glaxo Wellcome UK Limited trading as GlaxoSmithKline UK
Stockley Park West
Uxbridge
Middlesex
UB11 1BT

8. MARKETING AUTHORISATION NUMBER(S)
PL10949/0096

9. DATE OF FIRST AUTHORISATION/RENEWAL OF THE AUTHORISATION
15 October 1998

10. DATE OF REVISION OF THE TEXT
3 July 2008

11. Legal Status
POM

Zirtek Allergy Relief

(UCB Pharma Limited)

1. NAME OF THE MEDICINAL PRODUCT
Zirtek Allergy Relief

2. QUALITATIVE AND QUANTITATIVE COMPOSITION
Cetirizine hydrochloride: 10 mg per tablet.

3. PHARMACEUTICAL FORM
Film-coated tablet.

4. CLINICAL PARTICULARS

4.1 Therapeutic indications
Cetirizine is indicated for the symptomatic treatment of perennial rhinitis, seasonal allergic rhinitis and chronic idiopathic urticaria.

4.2 Posology and method of administration
Adults and Children aged 12 years and over: 10 mg once daily.

At present there are insufficient clinical data to recommend use of cetirizine tablets in children under the age of 6.

For the time being, there is no data to suggest that the dose needs to be reduced in elderly patients.

In patients with renal insufficiency the dosage should be reduced to half the usual recommended daily dose.

4.3 Contraindications
A history of hypersensitivity to any of the constituents of the formulation.

4.4 Special warnings and precautions for use
Do not exceed the stated dose. If symptoms persist consult your doctor.

Patients with rare hereditary problems of galactose intolerance, the Lapp lactase deficiency or glucose-galactose malabsorption should not take this medicine.

4.5 Interaction with other medicinal products and other forms of interaction
To date, there are no known interactions with other drugs. Studies with diazepam and cimetidine have revealed no evidence of interactions. As with other antihistamines it is advisable to avoid excessive alcohol consumption.

4.6 Pregnancy and lactation
No adverse effects have been reported from animal studies. There has been little or no clinical experience of cetirizine in pregnancy. As with other drugs, the use of cetirizine in pregnancy should be avoided.

Cetirizine is contraindicated in lactating women since it is excreted in breast milk.

4.7 Effects on ability to drive and use machines
Antihistamines can cause drowsiness in some patients. Although this has not been reported with cetirizine at the recommended dose please be cautious whilst driving or operating machinery.

4.8 Undesirable effects
In objective tests of psychomotor function the incidence of sedation with cetirizine was similar to that of placebo. There have been occasional reports of mild and transient side effects such as drowsiness, fatigue, headache, dizziness, agitation, dry mouth and gastro-intestinal discomfort. If desired the dose might be taken as 5mg in the morning and 5 mg in the evening.

Undesirable effects reported from post-marketing experience are listed in the following table per System Organ Class and per frequency. The frequency has been defined as: very common ($>10\,\%$); common ($\leqslant 10\,\%$ and $>1\,\%$); uncommon ($\leqslant 1\,\%$ and $>0.1\,\%$); rare ($\leqslant 0.1\,\%$ and $>0.01\,\%$); very rare ($\leqslant 0.01\,\%$, including isolated reports).

Blood and lymphatic disorders: Very rare: thrombocytopenia.

Cardiac disorders: Rare: tachycardia.

Eye disorders: Very rare: accommodation disorder, blurred vision.

Gastro-intestinal disorders: Uncommon: diarrhoea.

General disorders and administration site conditions: Uncommon: asthenia, malaise; Rare: oedema.

Immune system disorders: Rare: hypersensitivity; Very rare: anaphylactic shock

Hepatobiliary disorders: Rare: abnormal hepatic function (increased transaminases, alkaline, phosphatase, γ-GT and bilirubin).

Investigations: Rare: weight increase.

Nervous system disorders: Uncommon: paraesthesia; Rare: convulsions, movement disorders; Very rare: dysgeusia, syncope.

Psychiatric disorders: uncommon: agitation; rare: aggression, confusion, depression, hallucination, insomnia.

Renal and urinary disorders: Very rare: dysuria, enuresis, micturition difficulties.

Skin and subcutaneous tissue disorders: Uncommon: pruritus, rash, Rare: urticaria, Very rare: angioneurotic oedema, erythema multiforme.

4.9 Overdose

a) Symptoms
Symptoms observed after an important overdose of cetirizine are mainly associated with CNS effects or with effects that could suggest an anticholinergic effect.

Adverse events reported after an intake of at least 5 times the recommended daily dose are: confusion, diarrhoea, dizziness, fatigue, headache, malaise, mydriasis, pruritus, restlessness, sedation, somnolence, stupor, tachycardia, tremor and urinary retention.

b) Management
Should overdose occur, symptomatic or supportive measures are recommended. The patient should be kept under clinical observation for at least 4 hours after ingestion, and his blood pressure, heart rate and vital signs monitored until stable. In symptomatic cases, ECG should be performed.

The benefit of gastric lavage is uncertain. Oral activated charcoal (50g for an adult, 10-15 g for a child) should be considered if more than 2.5 mg/kg cetirizine has been ingested within 1 hour.

There is no known specific antidote to cetirizine.

Cetirizine is not effectively removed by dialysis.

5. PHARMACOLOGICAL PROPERTIES

5.1 Pharmacodynamic properties
Cetirizine is a potent antihistamine with a low potential for drowsiness at normal therapeutic doses which has additional anti-allergic properties. It is a selective H_1 antagonist with negligible effects on other receptors and so is virtually free from anti-cholinergic and anti-serotonin effects. Cetirizine inhibits the histamine-mediated early phase of the allergic reaction and also reduces the migration of certain inflammatory cells and the release of certain mediators associated with the late allergic response.

5.2 Pharmacokinetic properties
Peak blood levels of the order of 0.3 micrograms/ml are reached between 30 and 60 minutes after the oral administration of a 10 mg dose of cetirizine. The terminal half-life is approximately ten hours in adults, approximately six hours in children aged between 6 to 12 years and approximately 5 hours in children 2-6 years.

This is consistent with the urinary excretion half-life of the drug. The cumulative urinary excretion represents about two thirds of the administered dose for both adults and children.

The apparent plasma clearance in children is higher than that measured in adults. A high proportion of cetirizine is bound to human plasma proteins.

5.3 Preclinical safety data
None stated.

6. PHARMACEUTICAL PARTICULARS

6.1 List of excipients
Tablet core:
Microcrystalline cellulose
Lactose
Colloidal anhydrous silica
Magnesium stearate
Film coating:
Opadry Y-1-7000
- Hydroxypropylmethylcellulose (E464)
- Titanium dioxide (E 171)
- Polyethlene glycol

6.2 Incompatibilities
None.

6.3 Shelf life
60 months

6.4 Special precautions for storage
No special precautions for storage.

6.5 Nature and contents of container
Aluminium / PVC blister packs: containing 4, 5, or 7 tablets.

6.6 Special precautions for disposal and other handling
No special requirements

7. MARKETING AUTHORISATION HOLDER
UCB Pharma Limited,
208 Bath Road
Slough
Berkshire
SL1 3WE

8. MARKETING AUTHORISATION NUMBER(S)
PL 00039/0561

9. DATE OF FIRST AUTHORISATION/RENEWAL OF THE AUTHORISATION
12 December 2005

10. DATE OF REVISION OF THE TEXT

Zirtek allergy relief for children

(UCB Pharma Limited)

1. NAME OF THE MEDICINAL PRODUCT
Zirtek Allergy Relief for Children

2. QUALITATIVE AND QUANTITATIVE COMPOSITION
Cetirizine hydrochloride 1 mg / ml
For excipients, see 6.1

3. PHARMACEUTICAL FORM
Oral solution.

Clear, colourless solution with a banana flavour.

4. CLINICAL PARTICULARS

4.1 Therapeutic indications
Adults and children aged 6 years and over.

Symptomatic treatment of allergic rhinitis (seasonal and perennial), and chronic idiopathic urticaria.

4.2 Posology and method of administration
For oral use only.

Adults and children aged 6 year and over: 2 × 5ml once daily or 5 ml taken twice daily (morning and evening).

Children under 6 years: Not recommended.

There is no data to suggest that the dose should be reduced in elderly patients.

In patients with renal insufficiency the dosage should be reduced to half the normal recommended daily dose.

4.3 Contraindications
A history of hypersensitivity to any of the constituents of the formulation.

4.4 Special warnings and precautions for use
Do not exceed the recommended dose.

In patients with renal insufficiency the dosage should be reduced to half the recommended dose.

For patients whose symptoms persist, it is advised to consult a doctor or pharmacist.

Patients with rare hereditary problems of fructose intolerance should not take this medicine.

Methylparahydroxybenzoate and propylparahydroxybenzoate may cause allergic reactions (possibly delayed).

4.5 Interaction with other medicinal products and other forms of interaction
To date there are no known interactions with other drugs. Studies with diazepam and cimetidine have revealed no evidence of interactions. As with other antihistamines it is advisable to avoid excessive alcohol consumption.

4.6 Pregnancy and lactation
No adverse effects have been reported from animal studies. There has been little or no use of cetirizine during pregnancy. As with other drugs the use of cetirizine in pregnancy should be avoided.

Cetirizine is contraindicated in lactating women as it is excreted in breast milk.

4.7 Effects on ability to drive and use machines
At the recommended dose cetirizine does not cause drowsiness in the majority of people however rare cases have been reported. If affected do not drive or operate machinery.

4.8 Undesirable effects
In objective tests of psychomotor function the incidence of sedation with cetirizine was similar to that of placebo. There have been occasional reports of mild and transient side effects such as drowsiness, fatigue, headache, dizziness, agitation, dry mouth and gastro-intestinal discomfort. If desired the dose might be taken as 5mg in the morning and 5 mg in the evening.

Undesirable effects reported from post-marketing experience are listed in the following table per System Organ Class and per frequency. The frequency has been defined as: very common ($>10\,\%$); common ($\leqslant 10\,\%$ and $>1\,\%$); uncommon ($\leqslant 1\,\%$ and $>0.1\,\%$); rare ($\leqslant 0.1\,\%$ and $>0.01\,\%$); very rare ($\leqslant 0.01\,\%$, including isolated reports).

Blood and lymphatic disorders: Very rare: thrombocytopenia.

Cardiac disorders: Rare: tachycardia.

Eye disorders: Very rare: accommodation disorder, blurred vision.

Gastro-intestinal disorders: Uncommon: diarrhea.

General disorders and administration site conditions: Uncommon: asthenia, malaise; Rare: oedema.

Immune system disorders: Rare: hypersensitivity; Very rare: anaphylactic shock.

Hepatobiliary disorders: Rare: abnormal hepatic function (increased transaminases, alkaline, phosphatase, γ-GT and bilirubin).

Investigations: Rare: weight increase.

Nervous system disorders: Uncommon: paraesthesia; Rare: convulsions, movement disorders; Very rare: dysgeusia, syncope.

Psychiatric disorders: uncommon: agitation; rare: aggression, confusion, depression, hallucination, insomnia.

Renal and urinary disorders: Very rare: dysuria, enuresis, *micturition difficulties*.

Skin and subcutaneous tissue disorders: Uncommon: pruritus, rash, Rare: urticaria, Very rare: angioneurotic oedema, erythema multiforme.

4.9 Overdose

a) Symptoms

Symptoms observed after an important overdose of cetirizine are mainly associated with CNS effects or with effects that could suggest an anticholinergic effect.

Adverse events reported after an intake of at least 5 times the recommended daily dose are: confusion, diarrhoea, dizziness, fatigue, headache, malaise, mydriasis, pruritus, restlessness, sedation, somnolence, stupor, tachycardia, tremor and urinary retention.

b) Management

Should overdose occur, symptomatic or supportive measures are recommended. The patient should be kept under clinical observation for at least 4 hours after ingestion, and his blood pressure, heart rate and vital signs monitored until stable. In symptomatic cases, ECG should be performed.

The benefit of gastric lavage is uncertain. Oral activated charcoal (50g for an adult, 10-15 g for a child) should be considered if more than 2.5 mg/kg cetirizine has been ingested within 1 hour.

There is no known specific antidote to cetirizine.

Cetirizine is not effectively removed by dialysis.

5. PHARMACOLOGICAL PROPERTIES

5.1 Pharmacodynamic properties

ATC Code: R06AE07

Pharmacotherapeutic Group: Antihistamine for systemic use

Cetirizine is a potent antihistamine with a low potential for drowsiness at pharmacologically active doses and which has additional anti-allergic properties. It is a selective H1 - antagonist with negligible effects on other receptors and so is virtually free from anti-cholinergic and anti-serotonin effects. Cetirizine inhibits the histamine-mediated "early" phase of the allergic reaction and also reduces the migration of inflammatory cells and the release of certain mediators associated with the "late" allergic response.

5.2 Pharmacokinetic properties

Peak blood levels in the order of 0.3 micrograms / ml are attained between 30 and 60 minutes following the administration of a 10 mg oral dose of cetirizine.

The terminal half-life is approximately ten hours in adults, approximately six hours in children aged between 6 to 12 years and approximately 5 hours in children 2-6 years. This is consistent with the urinary excretion half-life of the drug. The cumulative urinary excretion represents about two thirds of the dose given for both adults and children.

The apparent plasma clearance in children is higher than that measured in adults. A high proportion of cetirizine is bound to human plasma proteins.

5.3 Preclinical safety data

There are no preclinical data of relevance to the prescriber, which are additional to that already included in other sections of the SPC.

6. PHARMACEUTICAL PARTICULARS

6.1 List of excipients

Sorbitol solution (E420)

Glycerol (E422)

Propylene glycol

Saccharin sodium

Methyl parahydroxybenzoate (E218)

Propyl parahydroxybenzoate (E216)

Banana flavouring

Sodium acetate

Acetic acid

Purified water.

6.2 Incompatibilities

None

6.3 Shelf life

3 years.

6.4 Special precautions for storage

Store below 30°C.

6.5 Nature and contents of container

70ml in a type III amber glass bottle with a child resistant polypropylene cap.

6.6 Special precautions for disposal and other handling

No special requirements

7. MARKETING AUTHORISATION HOLDER

UCB Pharma Limited,

208 Bath Road

Slough

Berkshire

SL1 3WE

8. MARKETING AUTHORISATION NUMBER(S)

PL 00039/0541

9. DATE OF FIRST AUTHORISATION/RENEWAL OF THE AUTHORISATION

12 December 2005

10. DATE OF REVISION OF THE TEXT

Zirtek Allergy Solution

(UCB Pharma Limited)

1. NAME OF THE MEDICINAL PRODUCT

Zirtek Allergy Solution 1mg/ml.

2. QUALITATIVE AND QUANTITATIVE COMPOSITION

Cetirizine hydrochloride 1 mg / ml

3. PHARMACEUTICAL FORM

Solution for oral administration.

4. CLINICAL PARTICULARS

4.1 Therapeutic indications

Cetirizine is indicated for the symptomatic treatment of seasonal allergic rhinitis, perennial rhinitis and chronic idiopathic urticaria in adults and children aged two years and over. Efficacy in children below 2 years has not been demonstrated.

4.2 Posology and method of administration

Adults and children 6 years and above: 10mg daily.

Adults and children aged 12 years and above: 10ml once daily.

Children aged between 6 to 11 years: Either 5ml twice daily or 10ml once daily.

Children aged between 2-5 years: 5mg daily.

Either 5ml once daily or 2.5ml twice daily.

At present there is insufficient clinical data to recommend the use of cetirizine in children under 2 years of age.

There is no data to suggest that the dose should be reduced in elderly patients.

In patients with renal insufficiency the dosage should be reduced to half the normal recommended daily dose.

4.3 Contraindications

A history of hypersensitivity to any of the constituents of the formulation.

4.4 Special warnings and precautions for use

Do not exceed the recommended dose.

In patients with renal insufficiency the dosage should be reduced to half the usual recommended dose.

For patients whose symptoms persist, it is advised to consult a doctor or pharmacist.

Patients with rare hereditary problems of fructose intolerance should not take this medicine.

Methylparahydroxybenzoate and propylparahydroxybenzoate may cause allergic reactions (possibly delayed).

4.5 Interaction with other medicinal products and other forms of interaction

To date there are no known interactions with other drugs. Studies with diazepam and cimetidine have revealed no evidence of interactions. As with other antihistamines it is advisable to avoid excessive alcohol consumption.

4.6 Pregnancy and lactation

No adverse effects have been reported from animal studies. There has been little or no use of cetirizine during pregnancy. As with other drugs the use of cetirizine in pregnancy should be avoided.

Cetirizine is contraindicated in lactating women as it is excreted in breast milk.

4.7 Effects on ability to drive and use machines

Studies in healthy volunteers at 20 and 25 mg/day have not revealed effects on alertness or reaction time; however patients are advised not to exceed the recommended dose if driving or operating machinery.

4.8 Undesirable effects

In objective tests of psychomotor function the incidence of sedation with cetirizine was similar to that of placebo. There have been occasional reports of mild and transient side effects such as drowsiness, fatigue, headache, dizziness, agitation, dry mouth and gastro-intestinal discomfort. If desired the dose might be taken as 5mg in the morning and 5 mg in the evening.

Undesirable effects reported from post-marketing experience are listed in the following table per System Organ Class and per frequency. The frequency has been defined as: very common (> 10 %); common ($\leqslant 10$ % and > 1 %); uncommon ($\leqslant 1$ % and > 0.1 %); rare ($\leqslant 0.1$ % and > 0.01 %); very rare ($\leqslant 0.01$ %, including isolated reports).

Blood and lymphatic disorders: Very rare: thrombocytopenia.

Cardiac disorders: Rare: tachycardia.

Eye disorders: Very rare: accommodation disorder, blurred vision.

Gastro-intestinal disorders: Uncommon: diarrhea.

General disorders and administration site conditions: Uncommon: asthenia, malaise; Rare: oedema.

Immune system disorders: Rare: hypersensitivity; Very rare: anaphylactic shock.

Hepatobiliary disorders: Rare: abnormal hepatic function (increased transaminases, alkaline, phosphatase, γ-GT and bilirubin).

Investigations: Rare: weight increase.

Nervous system disorders: Uncommon: paraesthesia; Rare: convulsions, movement disorders; Very rare: dysgeusia, syncope.

Psychiatric disorders: uncommon: agitation; rare: aggression, confusion, depression, hallucination, insomnia.

Renal and urinary disorders: Very rare: dysuria, enuresis, micturition difficulties.

Skin and subcutaneous tissue disorders: Uncommon: pruritus, rash, Rare: urticaria, Very rare: angioneurotic oedema, erythema multiforme.

4.9 Overdose

a) Symptoms

Symptoms observed after an important overdose of cetirizine are mainly associated with CNS effects or with effects that could suggest an anticholinergic effect.

Adverse events reported after an intake of at least 5 times the recommended daily dose are: confusion, diarrhoea, dizziness, fatigue, headache, malaise, mydriasis, pruritus, restlessness, sedation, somnolence, stupor, tachycardia, tremor and urinary retention.

b) Management

Should overdose occur, symptomatic or supportive measures are recommended. The patient should be kept under clinical observation for at least 4 hours after ingestion, and his blood pressure, heart rate and vital signs monitored until stable. In symptomatic cases, ECG should be performed.

The benefit of gastric lavage is uncertain. Oral activated charcoal (50g for an adult, 10-15 g for a child) should be considered if more than 2.5 mg/kg cetirizine has been ingested within 1 hour.

There is no known specific antidote to cetirizine.

Cetirizine is not effectively removed by dialysis.

5. PHARMACOLOGICAL PROPERTIES

5.1 Pharmacodynamic properties

Cetirizine is a potent antihistamine with a low potential for drowsiness at pharmacologically active doses and which has additional anti-allergic properties. It is a selective H1 - antagonist with negligible effects on other receptors and so is virtually free from anti-cholinergic and anti-serotonin effects. Cetirizine inhibits the histamine-mediated "early" phase of the allergic reaction and also reduces the migration of inflammatory cells and the release of certain mediators associated with the "late" allergic response.

5.2 Pharmacokinetic properties

Peak blood levels in the order of 0.3 micrograms / ml are attained between 30 and 60 minutes following the administration of a 10 mg oral dose of cetirizine.

The terminal half-life is approximately ten hours in adults, approximately six hours in children aged between 6 to 12 years and approximately 5 hours in children 2-6 years. This is consistent with the urinary excretion half-life of the drug. The cumulative urinary excretion represents about two thirds of the dose given for both adults and children.

The apparent plasma clearance in children is higher than that measured in adults. A high proportion of cetirizine is bound to human plasma proteins.

5.3 Preclinical safety data

None Stated.

6. PHARMACEUTICAL PARTICULARS

6.1 List of excipients

Sorbitol solution, glycerol, propylene glycol, saccharin sodium, methyl parahydroxybenzoate, propyl parahydroxybenzoate, banana flavouring, sodium acetate, acetic acid and purified water.

6.2 Incompatibilities

None

6.3 Shelf life

3 years.

6.4 Special precautions for storage

Store below 30°C.

6.5 Nature and contents of container

75 ml, 100 ml, 150ml or 200 ml in a type III amber glass bottle.

6.6 Special precautions for disposal and other handling

No special requirements

7. MARKETING AUTHORISATION HOLDER

UCB Pharma Limited,

208 Bath Road

Slough

Berkshire

SL1 3WE

8. MARKETING AUTHORISATION NUMBER(S)

PL 00039/0540

9. DATE OF FIRST AUTHORISATION/RENEWAL OF THE AUTHORISATION

12 December 2005

10. DATE OF REVISION OF THE TEXT

Zirtek Allergy Tablets

(UCB Pharma Limited)

1. NAME OF THE MEDICINAL PRODUCT

Zirtek Allergy

2. QUALITATIVE AND QUANTITATIVE COMPOSITION

Cetirizine hydrochloride: 10 mg per tablet.

3. PHARMACEUTICAL FORM

Film-coated tablet.

4. CLINICAL PARTICULARS

4.1 Therapeutic indications

Cetirizine is indicated for the symptomatic treatment of perennial rhinitis, seasonal allergic rhinitis and chronic idiopathic urticaria.

4.2 Posology and method of administration

Adults and children aged 6 years and over: 10 mg daily.

Adults 10 mg once daily

Children between 6 to 12 years of age: either 5 mg twice daily or 10 mg once daily.

At present there are insufficient clinical data to recommend use of cetirizine tablets in children under the age of 6.

For the time being, there is no data to suggest that the dose needs to be reduced in elderly patients.

In patients with renal insufficiency the dosage should be reduced to half the usual recommended daily dose.

4.3 Contraindications

A history of hypersensitivity to any of the constituents of the formulation.

4.4 Special warnings and precautions for use

Do not exceed the stated dose. If symptoms persist consult your doctor.

Patients with rare hereditary problems of galactose intolerance, the Lapp lactase deficiency or glucose-galactose malabsorption should not take this medicine.

4.5 Interaction with other medicinal products and other forms of interaction

To date, there are no known interactions with other drugs. Studies with diazepam and cimetidine have revealed no evidence of interactions. As with other antihistamines it is advisable to avoid excessive alcohol consumption.

4.6 Pregnancy and lactation

No adverse effects have been reported from animal studies. There has been little or no clinical experience of cetirizine in pregnancy. As with other drugs, the use of cetirizine in pregnancy should be avoided.

Cetirizine is contraindicated in lactating women since it is excreted in breast milk.

4.7 Effects on ability to drive and use machines

Antihistamines can cause drowsiness in some patients. Although this has not been reported with cetirizine at the recommended dose please be cautious whilst driving or operating machinery.

4.8 Undesirable effects

In objective tests of psychomotor function the incidence of sedation with cetirizine was similar to that of placebo. There have been occasional reports of mild and transient side effects such as drowsiness, fatigue, headache, dizziness, agitation, dry mouth and gastro-intestinal discomfort. If desired the dose might be taken as 5mg in the morning and 5 mg in the evening.

Undesirable effects reported from post-marketing experience are listed in the following table per System Organ Class and per frequency. The frequency has been defined as: very common > 10 %); common (⩽ 10 % and > 1 %); uncommon (⩽ 1 % and > 0.1 %); rare (⩽ 0.1 % and > 0.01 %); very rare (⩽ 0.01 %, including isolated reports).

Blood and lymphatic disorders: Very rare: thrombocytopenia.

Cardiac disorders: Rare: tachycardia.

Eye disorders: Very rare: accommodation disorder, blurred vision.

Gastro-intestinal disorders: Uncommon: diarrhoea.

General disorders and administration site conditions: Uncommon: asthenia, malaise; Rare: oedema.

Immune system disorders: Rare: hypersensitivity; Very rare: anaphylactic shock

Hepatobiliary disorders: Rare: abnormal hepatic function (increased transaminases, alkaline, phosphatase, γ-GT and bilirubin).

Investigations: Rare: weight increase.

Nervous system disorders: Uncommon: paraesthesia; Rare: convulsions, movement disorders; Very rare: dysgeusia, syncope.

Psychiatric disorders: uncommon: agitation; rare: aggression, confusion, depression, hallucination, insomnia.

Renal and urinary disorders: Very rare: dysuria, enuresis, micturition difficulties.

Skin and subcutaneous tissue disorders: Uncommon: pruritus, rash, Rare: urticaria, Very rare: angioneurotic oedema, erythema multiforme.

4.9 Overdose

a) Symptoms

Symptoms observed after an important overdose of cetirizine are mainly associated with CNS effects or with effects that could suggest an anticholinergic effect.

Adverse events reported after an intake of at least 5 times the recommended daily dose are: confusion, diarrhoea, dizziness, fatigue, headache, malaise, mydriasis, pruritus, restlessness, sedation, somnolence, stupor, tachycardia, tremor and urinary retention.

b) Management

Should overdose occur, symptomatic or supportive measures are recommended. The patient should be kept under clinical observation for at least 4 hours after ingestion, and his blood pressure, heart rate and vital signs monitored until stable. In symptomatic cases, ECG should be performed.

The benefit of gastric lavage is uncertain. Oral activated charcoal (50g for an adult, 10-15 g for a child) should be considered if more than 2.5 mg/kg cetirizine has been ingested within 1 hour.

There is no known specific antidote to cetirizine.

Cetirizine is not effectively removed by dialysis.

5. PHARMACOLOGICAL PROPERTIES

5.1 Pharmacodynamic properties

Cetirizine is a potent antihistamine with a low potential for drowsiness at normal therapeutic doses which has additional anti-allergic properties. It is a selective H_1 antagonist with negligible effects on other receptors and so is virtually free from anti-cholinergic and anti-serotonin effects. Cetirizine inhibits the histamine-mediated early phase of the allergic reaction and also reduces the migration of certain inflammatory cells and the release of certain mediators associated with the late allergic response.

5.2 Pharmacokinetic properties

Peak blood levels of the order of 0.3 micrograms/ml are reached between 30 and 60 minutes after the oral administration of a 10 mg dose of cetirizine. The terminal half-life is approximately ten hours in adults, approximately six hours in children aged between 6 to 12 years and approximately 5 hours in children 2-6 years.

This is consistent with the urinary excretion half-life of the drug. The cumulative urinary excretion represents about two thirds of the administered dose for both adults and children.

The apparent plasma clearance in children is higher than that measured in adults. A high proportion of cetirizine is bound to human plasma proteins.

5.3 Preclinical safety data

None stated.

6. PHARMACEUTICAL PARTICULARS

6.1 List of excipients

Tablet core:

Microcrystalline cellulose

Lactose

Colloidal anhydrous silica

Magnesium stearate

Film coating:

Opadry Y-1-7000

- Hydroxypropylmethylcellulose (E464)
- Titanium dioxide (E 171)
- Polyethlene glycol

6.2 Incompatibilities

None.

6.3 Shelf life

60 months

6.4 Special precautions for storage

No special precautions for storage.

6.5 Nature and contents of container

Aluminium / PVC blister packs: containing 7, 14, 21, 28, 30 or 60 tablets.

6.6 Special precautions for disposal and other handling

No special requirements

7. MARKETING AUTHORISATION HOLDER

UCB Pharma Limited,

208 Bath Road

Slough

Berkshire

SL1 3WE

8. MARKETING AUTHORISATION NUMBER(S)

PL 00039/0542

9. DATE OF FIRST AUTHORISATION/RENEWAL OF THE AUTHORISATION

12 December 2005

10. DATE OF REVISION OF THE TEXT

Zithromax Capsules, Suspension

(Pfizer Limited)

1. NAME OF THE MEDICINAL PRODUCT

ZITHROMAX® CAPSULES

ZITHROMAX® SUSPENSION

2. QUALITATIVE AND QUANTITATIVE COMPOSITION

Active ingredient: azithromycin.

Zithromax Capsules contain azithromycin dihydrate 262.05mg equivalent to 250mg azithromycin base.

Zithromax Powder for Oral Suspension is a dry blend of azithromycin dihydrate 209.64mg/5ml containing the equivalent of 200mg azithromycin base per 5ml on reconstitution with water.

3. PHARMACEUTICAL FORM

Zithromax Capsules are white, hard gelatin capsules marked Pfizer and ZTM 250.

Zithromax Powder for Oral Suspension is a dry powder which reconstitutes with water to give a cherry/banana flavoured suspension with a slight vanilla odour.

4. CLINICAL PARTICULARS

4.1 Therapeutic indications

Azithromycin is indicated for the treatment of the following infections when known or likely to be due to one or more susceptible microorganisms (see Section 5.1 Pharmacodynamic properties):

- bronchitis
- community-acquired pneumonia
- sinusitis
- pharyngitis/tonsillitis (see Section 4.4 regarding streptococcal infections)
- otitis media
- skin an dsoft tissue infections
- uncomplicated genital infections due to *Chlamydia trachomatis*.

Considerations should be given to official guidance regarding the appropriate use of antibacterial agents.

4.2 Posology and method of administration

Method of administration:

Zithromax should be given as a single daily dose. In common with many other antibiotics Zithromax Capsules should be taken at least 1 hour before or 2 hours after food.

Zithromax Suspension can be taken with food.

Children over 45kg body weight and adults, including elderly patients: The total dose of azithromycin is 1500mg which should be given over three days (500mg once daily). In uncomplicated genital infections due to *Chlamydia trachomatis*, the dose is 1000mg as a single oral dose.

In children under 45kg body weight: Zithromax Capsules are not suitable for Children under 45kg. Zithromax Suspension should be used for children under 45kg. There is no information on children less than 6 months of age. The dose in children is 10mg/kg as a single daily dose for 3 days:

Up to 15kg (less than 3 years): Measure the dose as closely as possible using the 10ml oral dosing syringe provided. The syringe is graduated in 0.25ml divisions, providing 10mg of azithromycin in every graduation.

For children weighing more than 15kg, Zithromax Suspension should be administered using the spoon provided according to the following guidance:

15-25 kg (3-7 years): 5ml (200mg) given as 1 × 5ml spoonful, once daily for 3 days.

26-35 kg (8-11 years): 7.5ml (300mg) given as 1 × 7.5ml spoonful, once daily for 3 days.

36-45 kg (12-14 years): 10ml (400mg) given as 1 × 10ml spoonful, once daily for 3 days.

Over 45 kg: Dose as per adults.

See Nature and contents of container, Section 6.5, for appropriate pack size to use depending on age/body weight of child.

The specially supplied measure should be used to administer Zithromax suspension to children.

Renal failure:

No dose adjustment is necessary in patients with mild to moderate renal impairment (GFR 10 - 80 ml/min). Caution should be exercised when azithromycin is administered to patients with severe renal impairment (GFR < 10 ml/min) (see section 4.4 - Special warnings and precautions for use).

Hepatic failure:

Since azithromycin is metabolised in the liver and excreted in the bile, the drug should not be given to patients suffering from severe liver disease. No studies have been conducted regarding treatment of such patients with azithromycin.

Zithromax Suspension is for oral administration only.

Zithromax Capsules are for oral Administration only.

4.3 Contraindications

Zithromax is contra-indicated in patients with a known hypersensitivity to azithromycin or any of the macrolide or ketolide antibiotics, erythromycin or to any excipients thereof as (for example) listed in Section 6.1 List of excipients.

Because of the theoretical possibility of ergotism, Zithromax and ergot derivatives should not be coadministered.

4.4 Special warnings and precautions for use

As with erythromycin and other macrolides, rare serious allergic reactions including angioneurotic oedema and anaphylaxis (rarely fatal), have been reported. Some of these reactions with Zithromax have resulted in recurrent symptoms and required a longer period of observation and treatment.

Prolonged cardiac repolarisation and QT interval, imparting a risk of developing cardiac arrhythmia and torsades de pointes, have been seen in treatment with other macrolides. A similar effect with azithromycin cannot be completely ruled out in patients at increased risk for prolonged cardiac repolarisation (see Section 4.8 Undesirable effects).

As with any antibiotic preparation, observation of signs of superinfection with non-susceptible organisms, including fungi is recommended. there is a possibility that superinfections could occur (e.g. fungal infections).

Streptococcal infections: Penicillin is usually the first choice for treatment of pharyngitis/tonsillitis due to *Streptococcus pyogenes* and also for prophylaxis of acute rheumatic fever. Azithromycin is in general effective against streptococcus in the oropharynx, but no data are available that demonstrate the efficacy of azithromycin in preventing acute rheumatic fever.

Use in renal impairment: In patients with severe renal impairment (GFR <10 ml/min) a 33% increase in systemic exposure to azithromycin was observed (see Section 5.2. Pharmacokinetic properties).

Zithromax capsules and suspension are for oral administration only.

4.5 Interaction with other medicinal products and other forms of interaction

Antacids: In patients receiving Zithromax and antacids, Zithromax should be taken at least 1 hour before or 2 hours after the antacid.

Carbamazepine: In a pharmacokinetic interaction study in healthy volunteers, no significant effect was observed on the plasma levels of carbamazepine or its active metabolite.

Cimetidine: A single dose of cimetidine administered 2 hours before Zithromax had no effect on the pharmacokinetics of azithromycin.

Cyclosporin: In a pharmacokinetic study with healthy volunteers that were administered a 500 mg/day oral dose of azithromycin for 3 days and were then administered a single 10 mg/kg oral dose of cyclosporin, the resulting cyclosporin C_{max} and AUC_{0-5} were found to be significantly elevated (by 24% and 21% respectively), however no significant changes were seen in $AUC_{0-\infty}$. Consequently, caution should be exercised before considering coadministration of these two drugs. If coadministration is necessary, cyclosporin levels should be monitored and the dose adjusted accordingly.

Digoxin: Some of the macrolide antibiotics have been reported to impair the metabolism of digoxin (in the gut) in some patients. Therefore, in patients receiving concomitant Zithromax and digoxin the possibility of raised digoxin levels should be borne in mind, and digoxin levels monitored.

Ergot derivatives: Because of the theoretical possibility of ergotism, Zithromax and ergot derivatives should not be coadministered.

Methylprednisolone: In a pharmacokinetic interaction study in healthy volunteers, Zithromax had no significant effect on the pharmacokinetics of methylprednisolone.

Nelfinavir: A study based on 12 healthy volunteers receiving co-administration of azithromycin (1200mg) and nelfinavir at a steady state (750mg three times daily) resulted in a 100% increase in azithromycin absorption and bioavailability. There was no significant effect upon the rate of absorption or the rate of clearance. The clinical consequences of this interaction are unknown, caution should be exercised when prescribing azithromycin to patients taking nelfinavir.

Terfenadine: Because of the occurrence of serious dysrhythmias secondary to prolongation of the QTc interval in patients receiving other anti-infectives in conjunction with terfenadine, pharmacokinetic interaction studies have been performed. These studies have reported no evidence of an interaction between azithromycin and terfenadine. There have been rare cases reported where the possibility of such an interaction could not be entirely excluded; however there was no specific evidence that such an interaction had occurred. As with other macrolides, Zithromax should be administered with caution in combination with terfenadine.

Theophylline: Theophylline levels may be increased in patients taking Zithromax.

Coumarin-Type Oral Anticoagulants: In a pharmacodynamic interaction study, Zithromax did not alter the anticoagulant effect of a single 15mg dose of warfarin administered to healthy volunteers. There have been reports received in the post-marketing period of potentiated anticoagulation subsequent to coadministration of azithromycin and coumarin-type oral anticoagulants. Although a causal relationship has not been established, consideration should be given to the frequency of monitoring prothrombin time when azithromycin is used in patients receiving coumarin-type oral anticoagulants.

Zidovudine: Single 1000mg doses and multiple 1200mg or 600mg doses of azithromycin did not affect the plasma pharmacokinetics or urinary excretion of zidovudine or its glucuronide metabolite. However, administration of azithromycin increased the concentrations of phosphorylated zidovudine, the clinically active metabolite, in peripheral blood mononuclear cells. The clinical significance of this finding is unclear, but it may be of benefit to patients.

Didanosine: Coadministration of daily doses of 1200mg azithromycin with didanosine in 6 subjects did not appear to affect the pharmacokinetics of didanosine as compared with placebo.

Rifabutin: Coadministration of azithromycin and rifabutin did not affect the serum concentrations of either drug.

Neutropenia was observed in subjects receiving concomitant treatment of azithromycin and rifabutin. Although neutropenia has been associated with the use of rifabutin, a causal relationship to combination with azithromycin has not been established (see Section 4.8. Undesirable effects).

4.6 Pregnancy and lactation

Use in pregnancy: Animal reproduction studies are insufficient with respect to effects on pregnancy, embryonal/ foetal development, parturition and post natal development (see Section 5.3 Preclinical safety data). The potential risks for humans is unknown. Zithromax should not be used during pregnancy unless clearly necessary.

Use in lactation: There is insufficient/ limited information on the excretion of azithromycin in human or animal breast milk. A risk to the suckling child cannot be excluded. A decision on whether to continue/ discontinue breast-feeding or to continue/ discontinue therapy with Zithromax should be made taking into account the benefit of breast-feeding to the child and the benefit of Zithromax therapy to the woman.

4.7 Effects on ability to drive and use machines

There is no evidence to suggest that Zithromax may have an effect on a patient's ability to drive or operate machinery.

4.8 Undesirable effects

Zithromax is well tolerated with a low incidence of side effects.

Blood and lymphatic system disorders

Rare (> 1/10000, < 1/1000)

Thrombocytopenia

In clinical trials there have been occasional reports of periods of transient, mild neutropenia. However, a causal relationship with azithromycin treatment has not been confirmed.

Psychiatric disorders

Rare (> 1/10000, < 1/1000)

Aggressiveness, agitation, anxiety and nervousness

Nervous system disorders

Uncommon (> 1/1000, < 1/100)

Dizziness/vertigo, somnolence, headache, convulsions (which have also been found to be caused by other macrolides), taste perversion, syncope

Rare (> 1/10000, < 1/1000)

Paraesthesia and asthenia

Insomnia and hyperactivity

Ear and labyrinth disorders

Rare (> 1/10000, < 1/1000)

Macrolide antibiotics have been reported to have caused hearing damage. In some patients receiving azithromycin impaired hearing, deafness and ringing in the ears have been reported. Many of these cases relate to experimental studies in which azithromycin was used at large doses over prolonged periods. According to available follow-up reports, the majority of these problems however were reversible.

Cardiac disorders

Rare (> 1/10000, < 1/1000)

Palpitations and arrhythmias including ventricular tachycardia (as seen with macrolides) have been reported. There have been rare reports of QT prolongation and torsades de pointes (see section 4.4 Special warnings and special precautions for use).

Vascular disorders

Rare (> 1/10000, < 1/1000)

Hypotension

Gastrointestinal disorders

Common (> 1/100, < 1/10)

Nausea, vomiting, diarrhoea, abdominal discomfort (pain/ cramps)

Uncommon (> 1/1000, < 1/100)

Loose stools, flatulence, digestive disorders, anorexia, dyspepsia

Rare (> 1/10000, < 1/1000)

Constipation, discoloration of the tongue, pancreatitis

Pseudomembranous colitis has been reported

Hepato-biliary disorders

Rare (> 1/10000, < 1/1000)

Hepatitis and cholestatic jaundice have been reported, including abnormal liver function test values, as well as rare cases of hepatic necrosis and hepatic dysfunction, which in rare instances have resulted in death

Skin and subcutaneous tissue disorders

Uncommon (> 1/1000, < 1/100)

Allergic reactions including pruritus and rash

Rare (> 1/10000, < 1/1000)

Allergic reactions including angioneurotic oedema, urticaria and photosensitivity; serious skin reactions such as erythema multiforme, Stevens-Johnson syndrome and toxic epidermal necrolysis

Musculoskeletal, connective tissue and bone disorders

Uncommon (> 1/1000, < 1/100)

Arthralgia

Renal and urinary disorders

Rare (> 1/10000, < 1/1000)

Interstitial nephritis and acute renal failure

Reproductive system and breast disorders

Uncommon (> 1/1000, < 1/100)

Vaginitis

General disorders

Rare (> 1/10000, < 1/1000)

Anaphylaxis including oedema (leads in rare cases to death, see section 4.4 Special warnings and precautions for use), candidiasis, fatigue, malaise

4.9 Overdose

Adverse events experienced in higher than recommended doses were similar to those seen at normal doses. The typical symptoms of an overdose with macrolide antibiotics include reversible loss of hearing, severe nausea, vomiting and diarrhoea. In the event of overdose, the administration of medicinal charcoal and general symptomatic treatment and supportive measures are indicated as required.

5. PHARMACOLOGICAL PROPERTIES

5.1 Pharmacodynamic properties

General properties

Antibacterials for systemic use. ATC code: J01FA10

Mode of action:

Zithromax is a macrolide antibiotic belonging to the azalide group. The molecule is constructed by adding a nitrogen atom to the lactone ring of erythromycin A. The chemical name of azithromycin is 9-deoxy-9a-aza-9a-methyl-9a-homoerythromycin A. The molecular weight is 749.0. The mechanism of action of azithromycin is based upon the suppression of bacterial protein synthesis by means of binding to the ribosomal 50s sub-unit and inhibition of peptide translocation.

Mechanism of resistance:

Resistance to azithromycin may be inherent or acquired. There are three main mechanisms of resistance in bacteria: target site alteration, alteration in antibiotic transport and modification of the antibiotic.

Complete cross resistance exists among *Streptococcus pneumoniae*, betahaemolytic streptococcus of group A, *Enterococcus faecalis* and *Staphylococcus aureus*, including methicillin resistant S. *aureus* (MRSA) to erythromycin, azithromycin, other macrolides and lincosamides.

Breakpoints

Azithromycin susceptibility breakpoints for typical bacterial pathogens are:

NCCLS:

- Susceptible ≤ 2mg/l; resistant ≥ 8mg/l
- *Haemophilus* spp.: susceptible ≤ 4mg/l
- *Streptococcus pneumoniae* and *Streptococcus pyogenes:*

Susceptible ≤ 0.5 mg/l; resistant ≥ 2 mg/l

Susceptibility

The prevalence of acquired resistance may vary geographically and with time for selected species and local information on resistance is desirable, particularly when treating severe infections. As necessary, expert advice should be sought when the local prevalence of resistance is such that the utility of the agent in at least some types of infections is questionable.

Table: Antibacterial spectrum of Azithromycin

Commonly susceptible species
Aerobic Gram-positive microorganisms
Staphylococcus aureus Methycillin-susceptible
Streptococcus pneumoniae Penicillin-susceptible
Streptococcus pyogenes **(Group A)**
Aerobic Gram-negative microorganisms
Haemophilus influenzae *Haemophilus parainfluenzae*
Legionella pneumophila
Moraxella catarrhalis
Pasteurella multocida
Anaerobic microorganisms
Clostridium perfringens
Fusobacterium spp.
Prevotella spp.
Porphyromonas spp.
Other microorganisms
Chlamydia trachomatis
Species for which acquired resistance may be a problem
Aerobic Gram-positive microorganisms
Streptococcus pneumoniae Penicillin-intermediate Penicillin-resistant
Inherently resistant organisms
Aerobic Gram-positive microorganisms
Enterococcus faecalis
Staphylococci **MRSA, MRSE***
Anaerobic microorganisms
Bacteroides fragilis group

* Methycillin-resistant staphylococci have a very high prevalence of acquired resistance to macrolides and have been placed here because they are rarely susceptible to azithromycin.

5.2 Pharmacokinetic properties

Absorption

Bioavailability after oral administration is approximately 37%. Peak plasma concentrations are attaned 2-3 hours after taking the medicinal product.

Distribution

Orally administered azithromycin is widely distributed throughout the body. In pharmacokinetic studies it has been demonstrated that the concentrations of azithromycin measured in tissues are noticeably higher (as much as 50 times) than those measured in plasma, which indicates that the agent strongly binds to tissues.

Binding to serum proteins varies according to plasma concentration and ranges from 12% at 0.5 microgram/ml up to 52% at 0.05 microgram azithromycin/ml serum. The mean volume of distribution at steady state (VVss) has been calculated to be 31.1 l/kg.

Elimination

The terminal plasma elimination half-life closely reflects the elimination half-life from tissues of 2-4 days.

Approximately 12% of an intravenously administered dose of azithromycin is excreted unchanged in urine within the following three days. Particularly high concentrations of unchanged azithromycin have been found in human bile. Also in bile, ten metabolites were detected, which were formed through N- and O- demethylation, hydroxylation of desosamine – and aglycone rings and cleavage of cladinose conjugate. Comparison of the results of liquid chromatography and microbiological analyses has shown that the metabolites of azithromycin are not microbiologically active.

In animal tests, high concentrations of azithromycin have been found in phagocytes. It has also been established that during active phagocytosis higher concentrations of azithromycin are released from inactive phagocytes. In animal models this results in high concentrations of azithromycin being delivered to the site of infection.

5.3 Preclinical safety data

In animal tests in which the doses used amounted to 40 times the clinical therapeutic dose, azithromycin caused reversible phospholipidosis but, as a rule, no true toxicological consequences were observed in association with this. Azithromycin has not been found to cause toxic reactions in patients when administered in accordance with the recommendations.

Carcinogenic potential:

Long-term studies in animals have not been performed to evaluate carcinogenic potential as the drug is indicated for short-term treatment only and there were no signs indicative of carcinogenic activity.

Mutagenic potential:

There was no evidence of a potential for genetic and chromosome mutations in in-vivo and in-vitro test models.

Reproductive toxicity:

In animal studies for embryotoxic effects of the substance, no teratogenic effect was observed in mice and rats. In rats, azithromycin doses of 100 and 200 mg/kg bodyweight/day led to mild retardation of fetal ossification and in maternal weight gain. In peri- and postnatal studies in rats, mild retardation following treatment with 50 mg/kg/day azithromycin and above was observed.

6. PHARMACEUTICAL PARTICULARS

6.1 List of excipients

Zithromax Capsules contain: Lactose, magnesium stearate, maize starch, and sodium lauryl sulphate. The capsule shells contain: Gelatin, iron oxide-black (E172), shellac, sulphur dioxide and titanium dioxide.

Zithromax Powder for Oral Suspension contains: Hydroxypropylcellulose, sodium phosphate tribasic anhydrous, sucrose, xanthan gum. Flavours: artificial banana, artificial cherry, artificial creme de vanilla.

6.2 Incompatibilities

None known

6.3 Shelf life

Zithromax Capsules 60 months.

Powder for Oral Suspension 3 years.

Once reconstituted with water, Zithromax Suspension has a shelf-life of 5 days.

6.4 Special precautions for storage

No special storage conditions required.

6.5 Nature and contents of container

Zithromax Capsules are available as:

Packs of 4 capsules. Aluminium/PVC blister strips, 4 capsules per strip, 1 strip in a carton box.

Pack of 6 capsules. Aluminium/PVC blister strips, 6 capsules per strip, 1 strip in a carton box.

Zithromax Powder for Oral Suspension is available as:

600mg (15ml) Pack: (Recommended for use in children up to 7 years (25kg)).

Packs of powder equivalent to 600mg azithromycin in a polypropylene container with child resistant screw cap (with or without a tamper evident seal), in a carton box. Pack contains a double-ended multi-dosing spoon and 10ml oral dosing syringe with detachable adaptor. A sticker for the syringe is appended to the bottle label. Reconstitute with 9ml of water to give 15ml suspension.

900mg (22.5ml) Pack: (Recommended for use in children aged from 8-11 years (26-35kg)). Packs of powder equivalent to 900mg azithromycin in a polypropylene container with child resistant screw cap (with or without a tamper evident seal), in a carton box. Pack contains a double-ended multi-dosing spoon. Reconstitute with 12ml of water to give 22.5ml suspension.

1200mg (30ml) Pack:(Recommended for use in children aged from 12-14 years (36-45kg)). Packs of powder equivalent to 1200mg azithromycin in a polypropylene container with child resistant screw cap (with or without a tamper evident seal), in a carton box. Pack contains a double-ended multi-dosing spoon. Reconstitute with 15ml of water to give 30ml suspension.

Multi-dosing spoon delivers doses as follows:

Small end	to graduation	2.5ml (100mg)
	brimful	5ml (200mg)
Large end	to graduation	7.5ml (300mg)
	brimful	10ml (400mg)

Each pack contains a Patient information/instruction leaflet.

6.6 Special precautions for disposal and other handling

When dispensing the 15ml pack, advice should be given as to whether the dose should be measured using the oral dosing syringe or the spoon provided and on correct usage.

If the dose is to be given using the oral dosing syringe, before dispensing, the syringe adaptor should be detached from the syringe and inserted into the bottle neck and the cap replaced.

The sticker provided should be used to mark the syringe at the appropriate level once the correct daily dosage has been calculated.

When dispensing 22.5ml and 30ml packs, advice should be given as to the correct usage of the multi-dosing spoon.

Zithromax Capsules should be swallowed whole.

7. MARKETING AUTHORISATION HOLDER

Pfizer Limited

Ramsgate Road

Sandwich

Kent CT13 9NJ

United Kingdom

8. MARKETING AUTHORISATION NUMBER(S)

Zithromax Capsules 250mg PL0057/0335

Zithromax Powder for Oral Suspension 200mg/5ml PL0057/0336

9. DATE OF FIRST AUTHORISATION/RENEWAL OF THE AUTHORISATION

Zithromax Capsules 250mg: 22 December 2005

Zithromax Powder for Oral Suspension 200mg/5ml: 22 December 2005

10. DATE OF REVISION OF THE TEXT

March 2008

ZX_11_0

Zocor 10mg, 20mg, 40mg and 80mg film-coated tablets

(Merck Sharp & Dohme Limited)

1. NAME OF THE MEDICINAL PRODUCT

Zocor 10 mg, film-coated tablets.

Zocor 20 mg, film-coated tablets.

Zocor 40 mg, film-coated tablets.

Zocor 80 mg, film-coated tablets.

2. QUALITATIVE AND QUANTITATIVE COMPOSITION

Each tablet contains 10 mg of simvastatin.

Each tablet contains 20 mg of simvastatin.

Each tablet contains 40 mg of simvastatin.

Each tablet contains 80 mg of simvastatin.

For a full list of excipients, see section 6.1.

Each 10 mg tablet contains 70.7 mg of lactose monohydrate.

Each 20 mg tablet contains 141.5 mg of lactose monohydrate.

Each 40 mg tablet contains 283.0 mg of lactose monohydrate.

Each 80 mg tablet contains 565.8 mg of lactose monohydrate.

3. PHARMACEUTICAL FORM

Film-coated tablet.

The peach-coloured, oval-shaped tablets marked 'MSD 735' contain 10 mg simvastatin. The tan-coloured, oval-shaped tablets marked 'MSD 740' contain 20 mg simvastatin. The brick-red coloured, oval-shaped tablets marked 'MSD 749' contain 40 mg simvastatin. The brick-red coloured, capsule-shaped tablets marked '543' on one side and '80' on the other contain 80 mg simvastatin.

4. CLINICAL PARTICULARS

4.1 Therapeutic indications

Hypercholesterolaemia

Treatment of primary hypercholesterolaemia or mixed dyslipidaemia, as an adjunct to diet, when response to diet and other non-pharmacological treatments (e.g. exercise, weight reduction) is inadequate.

Treatment of homozygous familial hypercholesterolaemia as an adjunct to diet and other lipid-lowering treatments (e.g. LDL apheresis) or if such treatments are not appropriate.

Cardiovascular prevention

Reduction of cardiovascular mortality and morbidity in patients with manifest atherosclerotic cardiovascular disease or diabetes mellitus, with either normal or increased cholesterol levels, as an adjunct to correction of other risk factors and other cardioprotective therapy (see section 5.1).

4.2 Posology and method of administration

The dosage range is 5-80 mg/day given orally as a single dose in the evening. Adjustments of dosage, if required, should be made at intervals of not less than 4 weeks, to a maximum of 80 mg/day given as a single dose in the evening. The 80-mg dose is only recommended in patients with severe hypercholesterolaemia and high risk for cardiovascular complications.

Hypercholesterolaemia

The patient should be placed on a standard cholesterol-lowering diet, and should continue on this diet during treatment with 'Zocor'. The usual starting dose is 10-20 mg/day given as a single dose in the evening. Patients who require a large reduction in LDL-C (more than 45 %) may be started at 20-40 mg/day given as a single dose in the evening. Adjustments of dosage, if required, should be made as specified above.

Homozygous familial hypercholesterolaemia

Based on the results of a controlled clinical study, the recommended dosage is 'Zocor' 40 mg/day in the evening or 80 mg/day in 3 divided doses of 20 mg, 20 mg, and an evening dose of 40 mg. 'Zocor' should be used as an adjunct to other lipid-lowering treatments (e.g., LDL apheresis) in these patients or if such treatments are unavailable.

Cardiovascular prevention

The usual dose of 'Zocor' is 20 to 40 mg/day given as a single dose in the evening in patients at high risk of coronary heart disease (CHD, with or without hyperlipidaemia). Drug therapy can be initiated simultaneously with diet and exercise. Adjustments of dosage, if required, should be made as specified above.

Concomitant therapy

'Zocor' is effective alone or in combination with bile acid sequestrants. Dosing should occur either > 2 hours before or > 4 hours after administration of a bile acid sequestrant.

In patients taking ciclosporin, danazol, gemfibrozil, or other fibrates (except fenofibrate) concomitantly with 'Zocor', the dose of 'Zocor' should not exceed 10 mg/day. In patients taking amiodarone or verapamil concomitantly with 'Zocor', the dose of 'Zocor' should not exceed 20 mg/day. (See sections 4.4 and 4.5.)

Dosage in renal insufficiency

No modification of dosage should be necessary in patients with moderate renal insufficiency.

In patients with severe renal insufficiency (creatinine clearance < 30 ml/min), dosages above 10 mg/day should be carefully considered and, if deemed necessary, implemented cautiously.

Use in the elderly

No dosage adjustment is necessary.

Use in children and adolescents

The experience in children is limited. Zocor is not recommended for paediatric use.

4.3 Contraindications

- Hypersensitivity to simvastatin or to any of the excipients
- Active liver disease or unexplained persistent elevations of serum transaminases
- Pregnancy and lactation (see section 4.6)
- Concomitant administration of potent CYP3A4 inhibitors (e.g. itraconazole, ketoconazole, HIV protease inhibitors, erythromycin, clarithromycin, telithromycin and nefazodone) (see section 4.5).

4.4 Special warnings and precautions for use

Myopathy/Rhabdomyolysis

Simvastatin, like other inhibitors of HMG-CoA reductase, occasionally causes myopathy manifested as muscle pain, tenderness or weakness with creatine kinase (CK) above ten times the upper limit of normal (ULN). Myopathy sometimes takes the form of rhabdomyolysis with or without acute renal failure secondary to myoglobinuria, and very rare fatalities have occurred. The risk of myopathy is increased by high levels of HMG-CoA reductase inhibitory activity in plasma.

As with other HMG-CoA reductase inhibitors, the risk of myopathy/rhabdomyolysis is dose related. In a clinical trial database in which 41,050 patients were treated with Zocor with 24,747 (approximately 60%) treated for at least 4 years, the incidence of myopathy was approximately 0.02%, 0.08% and 0.53% at 20, 40 and 80 mg/day, respectively. In these trials, patients were carefully monitored and some interacting medicinal products were excluded.

Creatine Kinase measurement

Creatine Kinase (CK) should not be measured following strenuous exercise or in the presence of any plausible alternative cause of CK increase as this makes value interpretation difficult. If CK levels are significantly elevated at baseline (> 5 × ULN), levels should be re-measured within 5 to 7 days later to confirm the results.

Before the treatment

All patients starting therapy with simvastatin, or whose dose of simvastatin is being increased, should be advised of the risk of myopathy and told to report promptly any unexplained muscle pain, tenderness or weakness.

Caution should be exercised in patients with pre-disposing factors for rhabdomyolysis. In order to establish a reference baseline value, a CK level should be measured before starting a treatment in the following situations:

- Elderly (age > 70 years)
- Renal impairment
- Uncontrolled hypothyroidism
- Personal or familial history of hereditary muscular disorders
- Previous history of muscular toxicity with a statin or fibrate
- Alcohol abuse.

In such situations, the risk of treatment should be considered in relation to possible benefit, and clinical monitoring is recommended. If a patient has previously experienced a muscle disorder on a fibrate or a statin, treatment with a different member of the class should only be initiated with caution. If CK levels are significantly elevated at baseline (> 5 × ULN), treatment should not be started.

Whilst on treatment

If muscle pain, weakness or cramps occur whilst a patient is receiving treatment with a statin, their CK levels should be measured. If these levels are found, in the absence of strenuous exercise, to be significantly elevated (> 5 × ULN), treatment should be stopped. If muscular symptoms are severe and cause daily discomfort, even if CK levels are < 5 × ULN, treatment discontinuation may be considered. If myopathy is suspected for any other reason, treatment should be discontinued.

If symptoms resolve and CK levels return to normal, then re-introduction of the statin or introduction of an alternative statin may be considered at the lowest dose and with close monitoring.

Therapy with simvastatin should be temporarily stopped a few days prior to elective major surgery and when any major medical or surgical condition supervenes.

Measures to reduce the risk of myopathy caused by medicinal product interactions (see also section 4.5)

The risk of myopathy and rhabdomyolysis is significantly increased by concomitant use of simvastatin with potent inhibitors of CYP3A4 (such as itraconazole, ketoconazole, erythromycin, clarithromycin, telithromycin, HIV protease inhibitors, nefazodone), as well as gemfibrozil, ciclosporin and danazol (see section 4.2).

The risk of myopathy and rhabdomyolysis is also increased by concomitant use of other fibrates, or by concomitant use of amiodarone or verapamil with higher doses of simvastatin (see sections 4.2 and 4.5). There is also a slight increase in risk when diltiazem is used with simvastatin 80 mg. The risk of myopathy including rhabdomyolysis may be increased by concomitant administration of fusidic acid with statins (see section 4.5).

Consequently, regarding CYP3A4 inhibitors, the use of simvastatin concomitantly with itraconazole, ketoconazole, HIV protease inhibitors, erythromycin, clarithromycin, telithromycin and nefazodone is contraindicated (see sections 4.3 and 4.5). If treatment with itraconazole, ketoconazole, erythromycin, clarithromycin or telithromycin is unavoidable, therapy with simvastatin must be suspended during the course of treatment. Moreover, caution should be exercised when combining simvastatin with certain other less potent CYP3A4 inhibitors: ciclosporin, verapamil, diltiazem (see sections 4.2 and 4.5). Concomitant intake of grapefruit juice and simvastatin should be avoided.

The dose of simvastatin should not exceed 10 mg daily in patients receiving concomitant medication with ciclosporin, danazol, or gemfibrozil. The combined use of simvastatin with gemfibrozil should be avoided, unless the benefits are likely to outweigh the increased risks of this drug combination. The benefits of the combined use of simvastatin 10 mg daily with other fibrates (except fenofibrate), ciclosporin or danazol should be carefully weighed against the potential risks of these combinations. (See sections 4.2 and 4.5.)

Caution should be used when prescribing fenofibrate or niacin (≥ 1g/day) with simvastatin, as either agent can cause myopathy when given alone.

The combined use of simvastatin at doses higher than 20 mg daily with amiodarone or verapamil should be avoided unless the clinical benefit is likely to outweigh the increased risk of myopathy (see sections 4.2 and 4.5).

If the combination proves necessary, patients on fusidic acid and simvastatin should be closely monitored (see section 4.5). Temporary suspension of simvastatin treatment may be considered.

Hepatic effects

In clinical studies, persistent increases (to > 3 × ULN) in serum transaminases have occurred in a few adult patients who received simvastatin. When simvastatin was interrupted or discontinued in these patients, the transaminase levels usually fell slowly to pre-treatment levels.

It is recommended that liver function tests be performed before treatment begins and thereafter when clinically indicated. Patients titrated to the 80-mg dose should receive an additional test prior to titration, 3 months after titration to the 80-mg dose, and periodically thereafter (e.g., semi-annually) for the first year of treatment. Special attention should be paid to patients who develop elevated serum transaminase levels, and in these patients, measurements should be repeated promptly and then performed more frequently. If the transaminase levels show evidence of progression, particularly if they rise to 3 × ULN and are persistent, simvastatin should be discontinued.

The product should be used with caution in patients who consume substantial quantities of alcohol.

As with other lipid-lowering agents, moderate (< 3 × ULN) elevations of serum transaminases have been reported following therapy with simvastatin. These changes appeared soon after initiation of therapy with simvastatin, were often transient, were not accompanied by any symptoms and interruption of treatment was not required.

Excipient

This product contains lactose. Patients with rare hereditary problems of galactose intolerance, the Lapp lactase deficiency or glucose-galactose malabsorption should not take this medicine.

4.5 Interaction with other medicinal products and other forms of interaction

Interaction studies have only been performed in adults.

Pharmacodynamic interactions

Interactions with lipid-lowering medicinal products that can cause myopathy when given alone

The risk of myopathy, including rhabdomyolysis, is increased during concomitant administration with fibrates and niacin (nicotinic acid) (≥ 1 g/day). Additionally, there is a pharmacokinetic interaction with gemfibrozil resulting in increased simvastatin plasma levels (see below *Pharmacokinetic interactions* and sections 4.2 and 4.4). When simvastatin and fenofibrate are given concomitantly, there is no evidence that the risk of myopathy exceeds the sum of the individual risks of each agent. Adequate pharmacovigilance and pharmacokinetic data are not available for other fibrates.

Pharmacokinetic interactions

Prescribing recommendations for interacting agents are summarised in the table below (further details are provided in the text; see also sections 4.2, 4.3 and 4.4).

Drug Interactions Associated with Increased Risk of Myopathy/Rhabdomyolysis

Interacting agents	Prescribing recommendations
Potent CYP3A4 inhibitors: Itraconazole Ketoconazole Erythromycin Clarithromycin Telithromycin HIV protease inhibitors Nefazodone	**Contraindicated with simvastatin**
Gemfibrozil	Avoid but if necessary, do not exceed 10 mg simvastatin daily
Ciclosporin Danazol Other fibrates (except fenofibrate)	Do not exceed 10 mg simvastatin daily
Amiodarone Verapamil	Do not exceed 20 mg simvastatin daily
Diltiazem	Do not exceed 40 mg simvastatin daily
Fusidic acid	Patients should be closely monitored. Temporary suspension of simvastatin treatment may be considered.
Grapefruit juice	Avoid grapefruit juice when taking simvastatin

Effects of other medicinal products on simvastatin

Interactions involving CYP3A4

Simvastatin is a substrate of cytochrome P450 3A4. Potent inhibitors of cytochrome P450 3A4 increase the risk of myopathy and rhabdomyolysis by increasing the concentration of HMG-CoA reductase inhibitory activity in plasma during simvastatin therapy. Such inhibitors include itraconazole, ketoconazole, erythromycin, clarithromycin, telithromycin, HIV protease inhibitors, and nefazodone. Concomitant administration of itraconazole resulted in a more than 10-fold increase in exposure to simvastatin acid (the active beta-hydroxyacid metabolite). Telithromycin caused an 11-fold increase in exposure to simvastatin acid.

Therefore, combination with itraconazole, ketoconazole, HIV protease inhibitors, erythromycin, clarithromycin, telithromycin and nefazodone is contraindicated. If treatment with itraconazole, ketoconazole, erythromycin, clarithromycin or telithromycin is unavoidable, therapy with simvastatin must be suspended during the course of treatment. Caution should be exercised when combining simvastatin with certain other less potent CYP3A4 inhibitors: ciclosporin, verapamil, diltiazem (see sections 4.2 and 4.4).

Ciclosporin

The risk of myopathy/rhabdomyolysis is increased by concomitant administration of ciclosporin particularly with higher doses of simvastatin (see sections 4.2 and 4.4). Therefore, the dose of simvastatin should not exceed 10 mg daily in patients receiving concomitant medication with ciclosporin. Although the mechanism is not fully understood, ciclosporin increases the AUC of HMG-CoA reductase inhibitors. The increase in AUC for simvastin is presumably due, in part, to inhibition of CYP3A4.

Danazol

The risk of myopathy and rhabdomyolysis is increased by concomitant administration of danazol with higher doses of simvastatin (see sections 4.2 and 4.4).

Gemfibrozil

Gemfibrozil increases the AUC of simvastatin acid by 1.9-fold, possibly due to inhibition of the glucuronidation pathway (see sections 4.2 and 4.4).

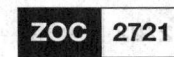

Amiodarone and verapamil

The risk of myopathy and rhabdomyolysis is increased by concomitant administration of amiodarone or verapamil with higher doses of simvastatin (see section 4.4). In an ongoing clinical trial, myopathy has been reported in 6 % of patients receiving simvastatin 80 mg and amiodarone.

An analysis of the available clinical trials showed an approximately 1 % incidence of myopathy in patients receiving simvastatin 40 mg or 80 mg and verapamil. In a pharmacokinetic study, concomitant administration with verapamil resulted in a 2.3-fold increase in exposure of simvastatin acid, presumably due, in part, to inhibition of CYP3A4. Therefore, the dose of simvastatin should not exceed 20 mg daily in patients receiving concomitant medication with amiodarone or verapamil, unless the clinical benefit is likely to outweigh the increased risk of myopathy and rhabdomyolysis.

Diltiazem

An analysis of the available clinical trials showed a 1 % incidence of myopathy in patients receiving simvastatin 80 mg and diltiazem. The risk of myopathy in patients taking simvastatin 40 mg was not increased by concomitant diltiazem (see section 4.4). In a pharmacokinetic study, concomitant administration of diltiazem caused a 2.7-fold increase in exposure of simvastatin acid, presumably due to inhibition of CYP3A4. Therefore, the dose of simvastatin should not exceed 40 mg daily in patients receiving concomitant medication with diltiazem, unless the clinical benefit is likely to outweigh the increased risk of myopathy and rhabdomyolysis.

Fusidic acid

The risk of myopathy may be increased by concomitant administration of fusidic acid with statins, including simvastatin. Isolated cases of rhabdomyolysis have been reported with simvastatin. Temporary suspension of simvastatin treatment may be considered. If it proves necessary, patients on fusidic acid and simvastatin should be closely monitored (see section 4.4).

Grapefruit juice

Grapefruit juice inhibits cytochrome P450 3A4. Concomitant intake of large quantities (over 1 litre daily) of grapefruit juice and simvastatin resulted in a 7-fold increase in exposure to simvastatin acid. Intake of 240 ml of grapefruit juice in the morning and simvastatin in the evening also resulted in a 1.9-fold increase. Intake of grapefruit juice during treatment with simvastatin should therefore be avoided.

Effects of simvastatin on the pharmacokinetics of other medicinal products

Simvastatin does not have an inhibitory effect on cytochrome P450 3A4. Therefore, simvastatin is not expected to affect plasma concentrations of substances metabolised via cytochome P450 3A4.

Oral anticoagulants

In two clinical studies, one in normal volunteers and the other in hypercholesterolaemic patients, simvastatin 20-40 mg/day modestly potentiated the effect of coumarin anticoagulants: the prothrombin time, reported as International Normalized Ratio (INR), increased from a baseline of 1.7 to 1.8 and from 2.6 to 3.4 in the volunteer and patient studies, respectively. Very rare cases of elevated INR have been reported. In patients taking coumarin anticoagulants, prothrombin time should be determined before starting simvastatin and frequently enough during early therapy to ensure that no significant alteration of prothrombin time occurs. Once a stable prothrombin time has been documented, prothrombin times can be monitored at the intervals usually recommended for patients on coumarin anticoagulants. If the dose of simvastatin is changed or discontinued, the same procedure should be repeated. Simvastatin therapy has not been associated with bleeding or with changes in prothrombin time in patients not taking anticoagulants.

4.6 Pregnancy and lactation

Pregnancy

'Zocor' is contraindicated during pregnancy (see section 4.3).

Safety in pregnant women has not been established. No controlled clinical trials with simvastatin have been conducted in pregnant women. Rare reports of congenital anomalies following intrauterine exposure to HMG-CoA reductase inhibitors have been received. However, in an analysis of approximately 200 prospectively followed pregnancies exposed during the first trimester to 'Zocor' or another closely related HMG-CoA reductase inhibitor, the incidence of congenital anomalies was comparable to that seen in the general population. This number of pregnancies was statistically sufficient to exclude a 2.5-fold or greater increase in congenital anomalies over the background incidence.

Although there is no evidence that the incidence of congenital anomalies in offspring of patients taking 'Zocor' or another closely related HMG-CoA reductase inhibitor differs from that observed in the general population, maternal treatment with 'Zocor' may reduce the foetal levels of mevalonate which is a precursor of cholesterol biosynthesis. Atherosclerosis is a chronic process, and ordinarily discontinuation of lipid-lowering medicinal products during pregnancy should have little impact on the long-term risk associated with primary hypercholesterolaemia. For these reasons, 'Zocor' must not be used in women who are pregnant, trying to become pregnant or suspect they are pregnant. Treatment with 'Zocor' must be suspended for the duration of pregnancy or until it has been determined that the woman is not pregnant. (See section 4.3.)

Lactation

It is not known whether simvastatin or its metabolites are excreted in human milk. Because many medicinal products are excreted in human milk and because of the potential for serious adverse reactions, women taking 'Zocor' must not breast-feed their infants (see section 4.3).

4.7 Effects on ability to drive and use machines

'Zocor' has no or negligible influence on the ability to drive and use machines. However, when driving vehicles or operating machines, it should be taken into account that dizziness has been reported rarely in post-marketing experiences.

4.8 Undesirable effects

The frequencies of the following adverse events, which have been reported during clinical studies and/or post-marketing use, are categorized based on an assessment of their incidence rates in large, long-term, placebo-controlled, clinical trials including HPS and 4S with 20,536 and 4,444 patients, respectively (see section 5.1). For HPS, only serious adverse events were recorded as well as myalgia, increases in serum transaminases and CK. For 4S, all the adverse events listed below were recorded. If the incidence rates on simvastatin were less than or similar to that of placebo in these trials, and there were similar reasonably causally related spontaneous report events, these adverse events are categorized as "rare".

In HPS (see section 5.1) involving 20,536 patients treated with 40 mg/day of 'Zocor' (n = 10,269) or placebo (n = 10,267), the safety profiles were comparable between patients treated with 'Zocor' 40 mg and patients treated with placebo over the mean 5 years of the study. Discontinuation rates due to side effects were comparable (4.8 % in patients treated with 'Zocor' 40 mg compared with 5.1 % in patients treated with placebo). The incidence of myopathy was < 0.1 % in patients treated with 'Zocor' 40 mg. Elevated transaminases ($> 3 \times$ ULN confirmed by repeat test) occurred in 0.21 % (n = 21) of patients treated with 'Zocor' 40 mg compared with 0.09 % (n = 9) of patients treated with placebo.

The frequencies of adverse events are ranked according to the following: Very common ($> 1/10$), Common ($\geq 1/100$, $< 1/10$), Uncommon ($\geq 1/1000$, $< 1/100$), Rare ($\geq 1/10,000$, $< 1/1000$), Very Rare ($< 1/10,000$) including isolated reports.

<u>Blood and lymphatic system disorders:</u>

Rare: anaemia

<u>Nervous system disorders:</u>

Rare: headache, paresthesia, dizziness, peripheral neuropathy

<u>Gastrointestinal disorders:</u>

Rare: constipation, abdominal pain, flatulence, dyspepsia, diarrhoea, nausea, vomiting, pancreatitis

<u>Hepato-biliary disorders:</u>

Rare: hepatitis/jaundice

Very rare: hepatic failure

<u>Skin and subcutaneous tissue disorders:</u>

Rare: rash, pruritus, alopecia

<u>Musculoskeletal, connective tissue and bone disorders:</u>

Rare: myopathy, rhabdomyolysis (see section 4.4), myalgia, muscle cramps

<u>General disorders and administration site conditions:</u>

Rare: asthenia

An apparent hypersensitivity syndrome has been reported rarely which has included some of the following features: angioedema, lupus-like syndrome, polymyalgia rheumatica, dermatomyositis, vasculitis, thrombocytopenia, eosinophilia, ESR increased, arthritis and arthralgia, urticaria, photosensitivity, fever, flushing, dyspnoea and malaise.

<u>Investigations:</u>

Rare: increases in serum transaminases (alanine aminotransferase, aspartate aminotransferase, γ-glutamyl transpeptidase) (see section 4.4 *Hepatic effects*), elevated alkaline phosphatase; increase in serum CK levels (see section 4.4).

4.9 Overdose

To date, a few cases of over-dosage have been reported; the maximum dose taken was 3.6 g. All patients recovered without sequelae. There is no specific treatment in the event of overdose. In this case, symptomatic and supportive measures should be adopted.

5. PHARMACOLOGICAL PROPERTIES

5.1 Pharmacodynamic properties

Pharmacotherapeutic group: HMG-CoA reductase inhibitor

ATC-Code: C10A A01

After oral ingestion, simvastatin, which is an inactive lactone, is hydrolyzed in the liver to the corresponding active beta-hydroxyacid form which has a potent activity in inhibiting HMG-CoA reductase (3 hydroxy – 3 methylglutaryl CoA reductase). This enzyme catalyses the conversion of HMG-CoA to mevalonate, an early and rate-limiting step in the biosynthesis of cholesterol.

'Zocor' has been shown to reduce both normal and elevated LDL-C concentrations. LDL is formed from very-low-density protein (VLDL) and is catabolised predominantly by the high affinity LDL receptor. The mechanism of the LDL-lowering effect of 'Zocor' may involve both reduction of VLDL-cholesterol (VLDL-C) concentration and induction of the LDL receptor, leading to reduced production and increased catabolism of LDL-C. Apolipoprotein B also falls substantially during treatment with 'Zocor'. In addition, 'Zocor' moderately increases HDL-C and reduces plasma TG. As a result of these changes the ratios of total- to HDL-C and LDL- to HDL-C are reduced.

<u>High Risk of Coronary Heart Disease (CHD) or Existing Coronary Heart Disease</u>

In the Heart Protection Study (HPS), the effects of therapy with 'Zocor' were assessed in 20,536 patients (age 40-80 years), with or without hyperlipidaemia, and with coronary heart disease, other occlusive arterial disease or diabetes mellitus. In this study, 10,269 patients were treated with 'Zocor' 40 mg/day and 10,267 patients were treated with placebo for a mean duration of 5 years. At baseline, 6,793 patients (33 %) had LDL-C levels below 116 mg/dL; 5,063 patients (25 %) had levels between 116 mg/dL and 135 mg/dL; and 8,680 patients (42 %) had levels greater than 135 mg/dL.

Treatment with 'Zocor' 40 mg/day compared with placebo significantly reduced the risk of all cause mortality (1328 [12.9 %] for simvastatin-treated patients versus 1507 [14.7 %] for patients given placebo; p = 0.0003), due to an 18 % reduction in coronary death rate (587 [5.7 %] versus 707 [6.9 %]; p = 0.0005; absolute risk reduction of 1.2 %). The reduction in non-vascular deaths did not reach statistical significance. 'Zocor' also decreased the risk of major coronary events (a composite endpoint comprised of non-fatal MI or CHD death) by 27 % ($p < 0.0001$). 'Zocor' reduced the need for undergoing coronary revascularization procedures (including coronary artery bypass grafting or percutaneous transluminal coronary angioplasty) and peripheral and other non-coronary revascularization procedures by 30 % ($p < 0.0001$) and 16 % (p = 0.006), respectively. 'Zocor' reduced the risk of stroke by 25 % ($p < 0.0001$), attributable to a 30 % reduction in ischemic stroke ($p < 0.0001$). In addition, within the subgroup of patients with diabetes, 'Zocor' reduced the risk of developing macrovascular complications, including peripheral revascularization procedures (surgery or angioplasty), lower limb amputations, or leg ulcers by 21 % (p = 0.0293). The proportional reduction in event rate was similar in each subgroup of patients studied, including those without coronary disease but who had cerebrovascular or peripheral artery disease, men and women, those aged either under or over 70 years at entry into the study, presence or absence of hypertension, and notably those with LDL cholesterol below 3.0 mmol/l at inclusion.

In the Scandinavian Simvastatin Survival Study (4S), the effect of therapy with 'Zocor' on total mortality was assessed in 4,444 patients with CHD and baseline total cholesterol 212-309 mg/dL (5.5-8.0 mmol/L). In this multicenter, randomised, double-blind, placebo-controlled study, patients with angina or a previous myocardial infarction (MI) were treated with diet, standard care, and either 'Zocor' 20-40 mg/day (n = 2,221) or placebo (n = 2,223) for a median duration of 5.4 years. 'Zocor' reduced the risk of death by 30 % (absolute risk reduction of 3.3 %). The risk of CHD death was reduced by 42 % (absolute risk reduction of 3.5 %). 'Zocor' also decreased the risk of having major coronary events (CHD death plus hospital-verified and silent nonfatal MI) by 34 %. Furthermore, 'Zocor' significantly reduced the risk of fatal plus nonfatal cerebrovascular events (stroke and transient ischemic attacks) by 28 %. There was no statistically significant difference between groups in non-cardiovascular mortality.

<u>Primary Hypercholesterolaemia and Combined Hyperlipidaemia</u>

In studies comparing the efficacy and safety of simvastatin 10, 20, 40 and 80 mg daily in patients with hypercholesterolemia, the mean reductions of LDL-C were 30, 38, 41 and 47 %, respectively. In studies of patients with combined (mixed) hyperlipidaemia on simvastatin 40 mg and 80 mg, the median reductions in triglycerides were 28 and 33 % (placebo: 2 %), respectively, and mean increases in HDL-C were 13 and 16 % (placebo: 3 %), respectively.

5.2 Pharmacokinetic properties

Simvastatin is an inactive lactone which is readily hydrolyzed *in vivo* to the corresponding beta-hydroxyacid, a potent inhibitor of HMG-CoA reductase. Hydrolysis takes place mainly in the liver; the rate of hydrolysis in human plasma is very slow.

Absorption

In man simvastatin is well absorbed and undergoes extensive hepatic first-pass extraction. The extraction in the liver is dependent on the hepatic blood flow. The liver is the primary site of action of the active form. The availability of the beta-hydroxyacid to the systemic circulation following an oral dose of simvastatin was found to be less than 5 % of the dose. Maximum plasma concentration of active inhibitors is reached approximately 1-2 hours after administration of simvastatin. Concomitant food intake does not affect the absorption.

The pharmacokinetics of single and multiple doses of simvastatin showed that no accumulation of medicinal product occurred after multiple dosing.

Distribution

The protein binding of simvastatin and its active metabolite is > 95 %.

Elimination

Simvastatin is a substrate of CYP3A4 (see sections 4.3 and 4.5). The major metabolites of simvastatin present in human plasma are the beta-hydroxyacid and four additional active metabolites. Following an oral dose of radioactive simvastatin to man, 13 % of the radioactivity was excreted in the urine and 60 % in the faeces within 96 hours. The amount recovered in the faeces represents absorbed medicinal product equivalents excreted in bile as well as unabsorbed medicinal product. Following an intravenous injection of the beta-hydroxyacid metabolite, its half-life averaged 1.9 hours. An average of only 0.3 % of the IV dose was excreted in urine as inhibitors.

5.3 Preclinical safety data

Based on conventional animal studies regarding pharmacodynamics, repeated dose toxicity, genotoxicity and carcinogenicity, there are no other risks for the patient than may be expected on account of the pharmacological mechanism. At maximally tolerated doses in both the rat and the rabbit, simvastatin produced no foetal malformations, and had no effects on fertility, reproductive function or neonatal development.

6. PHARMACEUTICAL PARTICULARS

6.1 List of excipients

Tablet core

butylated hydroxyanisole (E320)

ascorbic acid (E300)

citric acid monohydrate (E330)

microcrystalline cellulose (E460)

pregelatinized starch

magnesium stearate (E572)

lactose monohydrate

Tablet coating

hypromellose (E464)

hydroxypropylcellulose (E463)

titanium dioxide (E171)

talc (E553b)

yellow ferric oxide (E172) (5, 10, and 20 mg tablets)

red ferric oxide (E172) (10, 20, 40, and 80 mg tablets)

6.2 Incompatibilities

Not applicable

6.3 Shelf life

24 months.

6.4 Special precautions for storage

Do not store above 30°C.

6.5 Nature and contents of container

High Density Polyethylene (HDPE) bottles in packs of 30 or 50 tablets.

'Zocor' 10 mg

Blister packages of a trilaminate film composed of polyvinyl chloride (PVC)/Polyethylene (PE)/Polyvinylidene chloride (PVDC) with aluminium foil lidding in packs of 1,4, 10, 14, 15, 20, 28, 30, 50, 60, 98, or 100 tablets.

Blister packages composed of polyvinyl chloride (PVC) with aluminium foil lidding in packs of 4, 10, or 28, or 30 tablets.

Amber glass bottles with metal closures in packs of 30 or 50 tablets.

Polypropylene bottles in packs of 50 tablets.

High Density Polyethylene (HDPE) bottles in packs of 30, 50 or 100 tablets.

Unit dose blisters containing the trilaminate film composed of polyvinyl chloride (PVC)/Polyethylene (PE)/Polyvinylidene chloride (PVDC) with aluminium foil lidding in packs of 49 or 500 tablets.

'Zocor' 20 mg

Blister packages of a trilaminate film composed of polyvinyl chloride (PVC)/Polyethylene (PE)/Polyvinylidene chloride (PVDC) with aluminium foil lidding in packs of 1,4,10, 14, 15, 20, 28, 30, 50, 56, 60, 84, 90, 98, 100, or 168 tablets.

Blister packages composed of polyvinyl chloride (PVC) with aluminium foil lidding in packs of 14, 28, 30, 50, or 90 tablets.

Amber glass bottles with metal closures in packs of 30 or 50 tablets.

Polypropylene bottles in packs of 50 tablets.

High Density Polyethylene (HDPE) bottles in packs of 30, 50 or 100 tablets.

Unit dose blisters containing the trilaminate film composed of polyvinyl chloride (PVC)/Polyethylene (PE)/Polyvinylidene chloride (PVDC) with aluminium foil lidding in packs of 28, 49, 84, 98, or 500 tablets.

'Zocor' 40 mg

Blister packages of a trilaminate film composed of polyvinyl chloride (PVC)/Polyethylene (PE)/Polyvinylidene chloride (PVDC) with aluminium foil lidding in packs of 1,4, 7, 10, 14, 15, 20, 28, 30, 49, 50, 56, 60, 84, 90, 98, 100, or 168 tablets.

Blister packages composed of polyvinyl chloride (PVC) with aluminium foil lidding in packs of 7, 14, 28, 30, 49, 50, or 90 tablets.

Amber glass bottles with metal closures in packs of 30 or 50 tablets.

Polypropylene bottles in packs of 50 tablets.

High Density Polyethylene (HDPE) bottles in packs of 30, 50 or 100 tablets.

Unit dose blisters containing the trilaminate film composed of polyvinyl chloride (PVC)/Polyethylene (PE)/Polyvinylidene chloride (PVDC) with aluminium foil lidding in packs of 28, 49, 98, or 100 tablets.

'Zocor' 80 mg

Blister packages of a trilaminate film composed of polyvinyl chloride (PVC)/Polyethylene (PE)/Polyvinylidene chloride (PVDC) with aluminium foil lidding in packs of 7, 10, 14, 20, 28, 30, 49, 50, 56, 98, or 100 tablets.

High Density Polyethylene (HDPE) bottles in packs of 100 tablets.

Unit dose blisters containing the trilaminate film composed of polyvinyl chloride (PVC)/Polyethylene (PE)/Polyvinylidene chloride (PVDC) with aluminium foil lidding in packs of 28, 49, 56, or 98 tablets.

Not all pack sizes may be marketed.

6.6 Special precautions for disposal and other handling

No special requirements.

7. MARKETING AUTHORISATION HOLDER

Merck Sharp & Dohme Limited,

Hertford Road, Hoddesdon,

Hertfordshire

EN11 9BU, UK.

8. MARKETING AUTHORISATION NUMBER(S)

10 mg Tablet: PL0025/0241

20 mg Tablet: PL0025/0242

40 mg Tablet: PL0025/0243

80 mg Tablet: PL0025/0366.

9. DATE OF FIRST AUTHORISATION/RENEWAL OF THE AUTHORISATION

10 mg, 20 mg, 40 mg: Licence first granted April 1989.

80 mg: Licence first granted March 2000. Last renewed 1 September 2005

10. DATE OF REVISION OF THE TEXT

April 2009

LEGAL CATEGORY

POM

® denotes registered trademark of Merck & Co., Inc., Whitehouse Station, NJ, USA.

SPC.ZCR.09.UK.3056

Zofran Injection, Flexi-Amp Injection

(GlaxoSmithKline UK)

1. NAME OF THE MEDICINAL PRODUCT

Zofran Injection 2mg/ml. Zofran Flexi-amp Injection 2mg/ml.

2. QUALITATIVE AND QUANTITATIVE COMPOSITION

Zofran Injection 2mg/ml: 2ml glass ampoules each containing 4mg ondansetron (as hydrochloride dihydrate) in aqueous solution for intramuscular or intravenous administration. 4ml glass ampoules each containing 8mg ondansetron (as hydrochloride dihydrate) in aqueous solution for intravenous or intramuscular administration.

Zofran Flexi-amp Injection 2mg/ml: 2ml plastic ampoules each containing 4 mg ondansetron (as hydrochloride dihydrate) in aqueous solution for intramuscular or intravenous administration. 4ml plastic ampoules each containing 8 mg ondansetron (as hydrochloride dihydrate) in aqueous solution for intravenous or intramuscular administration.

3. PHARMACEUTICAL FORM

Injection (aqueous solution).

4. CLINICAL PARTICULARS

4.1 Therapeutic indications

Zofran is indicated for the management of nausea and vomiting induced by cytotoxic chemotherapy and radiotherapy, and for the prevention and treatment of post-operative nausea and vomiting (PONV).

4.2 Posology and method of administration
Chemotherapy and radiotherapy:

Adults: The emetogenic potential of cancer treatment varies according to the doses and combinations of chemotherapy and radiotherapy regimens used. The route of administration and dose of Zofran should be flexible in the range of 8-32mg a day and selected as shown below.

Emetogenic chemotherapy and radiotherapy: Zofran can be given either by rectal, oral (tablets or syrup), intravenous or intramuscular administration.

For most patients receiving emetogenic chemotherapy or radiotherapy, Zofran 8mg should be administered as a slow intravenous or intramuscular injection immediately before treatment, followed by 8mg orally twelve hourly.

To protect against delayed or prolonged emesis after the first 24 hours, oral or rectal treatment with Zofran should be continued for up to 5 days after a course of treatment.

Highly emetogenic chemotherapy: For patients receiving highly emetogenic chemotherapy, e.g. high-dose cisplatin, Zofran can be given either by rectal, intravenous or intramuscular administration. Zofran has been shown to be equally effective in the following dose schedules over the first 24 hours of chemotherapy:

A single dose of 8mg by slow intravenous or intramuscular injection immediately before chemotherapy.

A dose of 8mg by slow intravenous or intramuscular injection immediately before chemotherapy, followed by two further intravenous or intramuscular doses of 8mg two to four hours apart, or by a constant infusion of 1mg/hour for up to 24 hours.

A single dose of 32mg diluted in 50-100ml of saline or other compatible infusion fluid *(see Pharmaceutical Precautions)* and infused over not less than 15 minutes immediately before chemotherapy.

The selection of dose regimen should be determined by the severity of the emetogenic challenge.

The efficacy of Zofran in highly emetogenic chemotherapy may be enhanced by the addition of a single intravenous dose of dexamethasone sodium phosphate, 20mg administered prior to chemotherapy.

To protect against delayed or prolonged emesis after the first 24 hours, oral or rectal treatment with Zofran should be continued for up to 5 days after a course of treatment.

Children: Zofran may be administered as a single intravenous dose of 5mg/m^2 immediately before chemotherapy, followed by 4mg orally twelve hours later. 4mg orally twice daily should be continued for up to 5 days after a course of treatment.

Elderly: Zofran is well tolerated by patients over 65 years and no alteration of dosage, dosing frequency or route of administration are required.

Patients with Renal Impairment:

No alteration of daily dosage or frequency of dosing, or route of administration are required.

Patients with hepatic Impairment:

Clearance of Zofran is significantly reduced and serum half-life significantly prolonged in subjects with moderate or severe impairment of hepatic function. In such patients a total daily dose of 8mg should not be exceeded.

Post-operative nausea and vomiting (PONV):

Adults: For the prevention of PONV Zofran can be administered orally or by intravenous or intramuscular injection.

Zofran may be administered as a single dose of 4mg given by intramuscular or slow intravenous injection at induction of anaesthesia.

For treatment of established PONV a single dose of 4mg given by intramuscular or slow intravenous injection is recommended.

Children (aged 2 years and over): For prevention of PONV in paediatric patients having surgery performed under general anaesthesia, ondansetron may be administered by slow intravenous injection at a dose of 0.1mg/kg up to a maximum of 4mg either prior to, at or after induction of anaesthesia.

For treatment of established PONV in paediatric patients, ondansetron may be administered by slow intravenous injection at a dose of 0.1mg/kg up to a maximum of 4mg.

There is limited data on the use of Zofran in the prevention and treatment of PONV in children under 2 years of age.

Elderly: There is limited experience in the use of Zofran in the prevention and treatment of PONV in the elderly, however Zofran is well tolerated in patients over 65 years receiving chemotherapy.

Patients with renal impairment: No alteration of daily dosage or frequency of dosing, or route of administration are required.

Patients with hepatic impairment: Clearance of Zofran is significantly reduced and serum half life significantly prolonged in subjects with moderate or severe impairment of hepatic function. In such patients a total daily dose of 8mg should not be exceeded.

Patients with poor sparteine/debrisoquine metabolism: The elimination half-life of ondansetron is not altered in subjects classified as poor metabolisers of sparteine and debrisoquine. Consequently in such patients repeat dosing will give drug exposure levels no different from those of the general population. No alteration of daily dosage or frequency of dosing are required.

4.3 Contraindications

Hypersensitivity to any component of the preparation.

4.4 Special warnings and precautions for use

Hypersensitivity reactions have been reported in patients who have exhibited hypersensitivity to other selective $5HT_3$ receptor antagonists.

Very rarely and predominantly with intravenous Zofran, transient ECG changes including QT interval prolongation have been reported. Therefore caution should be exercised in patients with cardiac rhythm or conduction disturbances, in patients treated with anti-arrhythmic agents or beta-adrenergic blocking agents and in patients with significant electrolyte disturbances.

As ondansetron is known to increase large bowel transit time, patients with signs of subacute intestinal obstruction should be monitored following administration

4.5 Interaction with other medicinal products and other forms of interaction

There is no evidence that ondansetron either induces or inhibits the metabolism of other drugs commonly co-administered with it. Specific studies have shown that there are no pharmacokinetic interactions when ondansetron is administered with alcohol, temazepan, furosemide, tramadol or propofol.

Ondansetron is metabolised by multiple hepatic cytochrome P-450 enzymes: CYP3A4, CYP2D6 and CYP1A2. Due to the multiplicity of metabolic enzymes capable of metabolising ondansetron, enzyme inhibition or reduced activity of one enzyme (e.g. CYP2D6 genetic deficiency) is normally compensated by other enzymes and should result in little or no significant change in overall ondansetron clearance or dose requirement.

Phenytoin, Carbamazepine and Rifampicin: In patients treated with potent inducers of CYP3A4 (i.e. phenytoin, carbamazepine, and rifampicin), the oral clearance of ondansetron was increased and ondansetron blood concentrations were decreased.

Tramadol: Data from small studies indicate that ondansetron may reduce the analgesic effect of tramadol.

4.6 Pregnancy and lactation

The safety of ondansetron for use in human pregnancy has not been established. Evaluation of experimental animal studies does not indicate direct or indirect harmful effects with respect to the development of the embryo, or foetus, the course of gestation and peri- and post-natal development. However as animal studies are not always predictive of human response the use of ondansetron in pregnancy is not recommended.

Tests have shown that ondansetron passes into the milk of lactating animals. It is therefore recommended that mothers receiving Zofran should not breast-feed their babies.

4.7 Effects on ability to drive and use machines

In psychomotor testing ondansetron does not impair performance nor cause sedation.

4.8 Undesirable effects

Adverse events are listed below by system organ class and frequency. Frequencies are defined as: very common (≥1/10), common (≥1/100 and <1/10), uncommon (≥1/1000 and <1/100), rare (≥1/10,000 and <1/1000) and very rare (<1/10,000) including isolated reports. Very common, common and uncommon events were generally determined from clinical trial data. The incidence in placebo was taken into account. Rare and very rare events were generally determined from post-marketing spontaneous data.

The following frequencies are estimated at the standard recommended doses of ondansetron according to indication and formulation.

Immune system disorders

Rare: Immediate hypersensitivity reactions sometimes severe, including anaphylaxis.

Nervous system disorders

Very common: Headache.

Uncommon: Seizures, movement disorders including extrapyramidal reactions such as dystonic reactions, oculogyric crisis and dyskinesia have been observed without definitive evidence of persistent clinical sequelae.

Rare: Dizziness during i.v. administration, which in most cases is prevented or resolved by lengthening the infusion period.

Eye disorders

Rare: Transient visual disturbances (eg. blurred vision) during i.v. administration.

Very rare: Transient blindness predominantly during intravenous administration

The majority of the blindness cases reported resolved within 20 minutes. Most patients had received chemotherapeutic agents, which included cisplatin. Some cases of transient blindness were reported as cortical in origin.

Cardiac disorders

Uncommon: Arrhythmias, chest pain with or without ST segment depression, bradycardia.

Vascular disorders

Common: Sensation of warmth or flushing.

Uncommon: Hypotension.

Respiratory, thoracic and mediastinal disorders

Uncommon: Hiccups.

Gastrointestinal disorders

Common: Constipation.

Hepatobiliary disorders

Uncommon: Asymptomatic increases in liver function tests#.

#These events were observed commonly in patients receiving chemotherapy with cisplatin.

General disorders and administration site conditions

Common: Local i.v. injection site reactions.

4.9 Overdose

Little is known at present about overdosage with ondansetron, however, a limited number of patients received overdoses. Manifestations that have been reported include visual disturbances, severe constipation, hypotension and a vasovagal episode with transient second degree AV block. In all instances, the events resolved completely. There is no specific antidote for ondansetron, therefore in all cases of suspected overdose, symptomatic and supportive therapy should be given as appropriate.

5. PHARMACOLOGICAL PROPERTIES

5.1 Pharmacodynamic properties

Ondansetron is a potent, highly selective 5HT3 receptor-antagonist. Its precise mode of action in the control of nausea and vomiting is not known. Chemotherapeutic agents and radiotherapy may cause release of 5HT in the small intestine initiating a vomiting reflex by activating vagal afferents via 5HT3 receptors. Ondansetron blocks the initiation of this reflex. Activation of vagal afferents may also cause a release of 5HT in the area postrema, located on the floor of the fourth ventricle, and this may also promote emesis through a central mechanism. Thus, the effect of ondansetron in the management of the nausea and vomiting induced by cytotoxic chemotherapy and radiotherapy is probably due to antagonism of 5HT3 receptors on neurons located both in the peripheral and central nervous system. The mechanisms of action in post-operative nausea and vomiting are not known but there may be common pathways with cytotoxic induced nausea and vomiting.

Ondansetron does not alter plasma prolactin concentrations.

The role of ondansetron in opiate-induced emesis is not yet established.

5.2 Pharmacokinetic properties

Following oral administration, ondansetron is passively and completely absorbed from the gastrointestinal tract and undergoes first pass metabolism. Peak plasma concentrations of about 30ng/ml are attained approximately 1.5 hours after an 8mg dose. For doses above 8mg the increase in ondansetron systemic exposure with dose is greater than proportional; this may reflect some reduction in first pass metabolism at higher oral doses. Bioavailability, following oral administration, is slightly enhanced by the presence of food but unaffected by antacids. Studies in healthy elderly volunteers have shown slight, but clinically insignificant, age-related increases in both oral bioavailability (65%) and half-life (5 hours) of ondansetron. Gender differences were shown in the disposition of ondansetron, with females having a greater rate and extent of absorption following an oral dose and reduced systemic clearance and volume of distribution (adjusted for weight).

The disposition of ondansetron following oral, intramuscular(IM) and intravenous(IV) dosing is similar with a terminal half life of about 3 hours and steady state volume of distribution of about 140L. Equivalent systemic exposure is achieved after IM and IV administration of ondansetron.

A 4mg intravenous infusion of ondansetron given over 5 minutes results in peak plasma concentrations of about 65ng/ml. Following intramuscular administration of ondansetron, peak plasma concentrations of about 25ng/ml are attained within 10 minutes of injection.

Following administration of ondansetron suppository, plasma ondansetron concentrations become detectable between 15 and 60 minutes after dosing. Concentrations rise in an essentially linear fashion, until peak concentrations of 20-30 ng/ml are attained, typically 6 hours after dosing. Plasma concentrations then fall, but at a slower rate than observed following oral dosing due to continued absorption of ondansetron. The absolute bioavailability of ondansetron from the suppository is approximately 60% and is not affected by gender. The half life of the elimination phase following suppository administration is determined by the rate of ondansetron absorption, not systemic clearance and is approximately 6 hours. Females show a small, clinically insignificant, increase in half-life in comparison with males.

Ondansetron is not highly protein bound (70-76%). Ondansetron is cleared from the systemic circulation predominantly by hepatic metabolism through multiple enzymatic pathways. Less than 5% of the absorbed dose is excreted unchanged in the urine. The absence of the enzyme CYP2D6 (the debrisoquine polymorphism) has no effect on ondansetron's pharmacokinetics. The pharmacokinetic properties of ondansetron are unchanged on repeat dosing.

In a study of 21 paediatric patients aged between 3 and 12 years undergoing elective surgery with general anaesthesia, the absolute values for both the clearance and volume of distribution of ondansetron following a single intravenous dose of 2mg (3-7 years old) or 4mg (8-12 years old) were reduced. The magnitude of the change was age-related, with clearance falling from about 300mL/min at 12 years of age to 100mL/min at 3 years. Volume of distribution fell from about 75L at 12 years to 17L at 3 years. Use of weight-based dosing (0.1mg/kg up to 4mg maximum) compensates for these changes and is effective in normalising systemic exposure in paediatric patients.

In patients with renal impairment (creatinine clearance 15-60 ml/min), both systemic clearance and volume of distribution are reduced following IV administration of ondansetron, resulting in a slight, but clinically insignificant, increase in elimination half-life (5.4h). A study in patients with severe renal impairment who required regular haemodialysis (studied between dialyses) showed ondansetron's pharmacokinetics to be essentially unchanged following IV administration.

Specific studies in the elderly or patients with renal impairment have been limited to IV and oral administration. However, it is anticipated that the half-life of ondansetron after rectal administration in these populations will be similar to that seen in healthy volunteers, since the rate of elimination of ondansetron following rectal administration is not determined by systemic clearance.

Following oral, intravenous or intramuscular dosing in patients with severe hepatic impairment, ondansetron's systemic clearance is markedly reduced with prolonged elimination half-lives (15-32 h) and an oral bioavailability approaching 100% due to reduced pre-systemic metabolism. The pharmacokinetics of ondansetron following administration as a suppository have not been evaluated in patients with hepatic impairment.

5.3 Preclinical safety data

No additional data of relevance.

6. PHARMACEUTICAL PARTICULARS

6.1 List of excipients

Citric acid monohydrate, sodium citrate, sodium chloride, Water for Injections.

6.2 Incompatibilities

Zofran injection should not be administered in the same syringe or infusion as any other medication.

6.3 Shelf life

36 months (unopened). 24 hours (dilutions stored 2 - 8°C).

6.4 Special precautions for storage

Protect from light. Store below 30°C.

Dilutions of Zofran injection in compatible intravenous infusion fluids are stable under normal room lighting conditions or daylight for at least 24 hours, thus no protection from light is necessary while infusion takes place.

6.5 Nature and contents of container

Zofran Injection: Type I clear glass snap-ring ampoules.

Zofran Flexi-amp injection: Polypropylene blow-fill-sealed ampoules with a twist-off top and overwrapped in a double foil blister.

5 ampoules are packed in a carton.

6.6 Special precautions for disposal and other handling

Zofran Injection and Zofran Flexi-amp injection should not be autoclaved.

Compatibility with intravenous fluids

Zofran injection should only be admixed with those infusion solutions which are recommended:

Sodium Chloride Intravenous Infusion BP 0.9%w/v

Glucose Intravenous Infusion BP 5%w/v

Mannitol Intravenous Infusion BP 10%w/v

Ringers Intravenous Infusion

Potassium Chloride 0.3%w/v and Sodium Chloride 0.9%w/v Intravenous Infusion BP

Potassium Chloride 0.3%w/v and Glucose 5%w/v Intravenous Infusion BP

In keeping with good pharmaceutical practice dilutions of Zofran injection in intravenous fluids should be prepared at the time of infusion or stored at 2-8°C for no more than 24 hours before the start of administration.

Compatibility studies have been undertaken in polyvinyl chloride infusion bags and polyvinyl chloride administration sets. It is considered that adequate stability would also be conferred by the use of polyethylene infusion bags or Type 1 glass bottles. Dilutions of Zofran in sodium chloride 0.9%w/v or in glucose 5%w/v have been demonstrated to be stable in polypropylene syringes. It is considered that Zofran injection diluted with other compatible infusion fluids would be stable in polypropylene syringes.

Compatibility with other drugs: Zofran may be administered by intravenous infusion at 1mg/hour, e.g. from an infusion bag or syringe pump. The following drugs may be administered via the Y-site of the Zofran giving set for ondansetron concentrations of 16 to 160 micrograms/ml (e.g. 8 mg/500 ml and 8 mg/50 ml respectively);

Cisplatin: Concentrations up to 0.48 mg/ml (e.g. 240 mg in 500 ml) administered over one to eight hours.

5 -Fluorouracil:

Concentrations up to 0.8 mg/ml (e.g. 2.4g in 3 litres or 400mg in 500ml) administered at a rate of at least 20 ml per hour (500 ml per 24 hours). Higher concentrations of 5-fluorouracil may cause precipitation of ondansetron.

The 5-fluorouracil infusion may contain up to 0.045%w/v magnesium chloride in addition to other excipients shown to be compatible.

Carboplatin: Concentrations in the range 0.18 mg/ml to 9.9 mg/ml (e.g. 90 mg in 500 ml to 990 mg in 100 ml), administered over ten minutes to one hour.

Etoposide: Concentrations in the range 0.14 mg/ml to 0.25 mg/ml (e.g. 72 mg in 500 ml to 250 mg in 1 litre), administered over thirty minutes to one hour.

Ceftazidime: Doses in the range 250 mg to 2000 mg reconstituted with Water for Injections BP as recommended by the manufacturer (e.g. 2.5 ml for 250 mg and 10 ml for 2g ceftazidime) and given as an intravenous bolus injection over approximately five minutes.

Cyclophosphamide: Doses in the range 100 mg to 1g, reconstituted with Water for Injections BP, 5 ml per 100 mg cyclophosphamide, as recommended by the manufacturer and given as an intravenous bolus injection over approximately five minutes.

Doxorubicin: Doses in the range 10-100mg reconstituted with Water for Injections BP, 5 ml per 10 mg doxorubicin, as recommended by the manufacturer and given as an intravenous bolus injection over approximately 5 minutes.

Dexamethasone: Dexamethasone sodium phosphate 20mg may be administered as a slow intravenous injection over 2-5 minutes via the Y-site of an infusion set delivering 8 or 32mg of ondansetron diluted in 50-100ml of a compatible infusion fluid over approximately 15 minutes. Compatibility between dexamethasone sodium phosphate and ondansetron has been demonstrated supporting administration of these drugs through the same giving set resulting in concentrations in line of 32 microgram - 2.5mg/ml for dexamethasone sodium phosphate and 8 microgram - 1mg/ml for ondansetron.

Administrative Data

7. MARKETING AUTHORISATION HOLDER

Glaxo Operations UK Limited,

Greenford Road,

Greenford,

Middlesex, UB6 0HE

Trading as

GlaxoSmithKline UK

Stockley Park West

Uxbridge

Middlesex UB11 1BT

8. MARKETING AUTHORISATION NUMBER(S)

PL 00004/0375

9. DATE OF FIRST AUTHORISATION/RENEWAL OF THE AUTHORISATION

23rd October 2001

10. DATE OF REVISION OF THE TEXT

17 October 2006

11. Legal Status

POM

Zofran Melt 4mg

(GlaxoSmithKline UK)

1. NAME OF THE MEDICINAL PRODUCT

Zofran Melt 4mg

2. QUALITATIVE AND QUANTITATIVE COMPOSITION

White, round, plano-convex, freeze dried, fast dispersing oral dosage form.

Each Melt contains ondansetron 4mg.

3. PHARMACEUTICAL FORM

Oral lyophilisate.

4. CLINICAL PARTICULARS

4.1 Therapeutic indications

The management of nausea and vomiting induced by cytotoxic chemotherapy and radiotherapy, and for the prevention of post-operative nausea and vomiting in adults.

4.2 Posology and method of administration

Place the Melt on top of the tongue, where it will disperse within seconds, then swallow

Chemotherapy and radiotherapy induced nausea and vomiting.

Adults:

The emetogenic potential of cancer treatment varies according to the doses and combinations of chemotherapy and radiotherapy regimens used. The route of administration and dose of Zofran should be flexible and selected as shown below.

Emetogenic chemotherapy and radiotherapy: Zofran can be given either by rectal, oral (as Melt, tablets or syrup) intravenous or intramuscular administration.

For oral administration: 8mg 1-2 hours before treatment, followed by 8mg 12 hours later.

To protect against delayed or prolonged emesis after the first 24 hours, oral or rectal treatment with Zofran should be continued for up to 5 days after a course of treatment.

The recommended dose for oral administration is 8mg twice daily.

Highly emetogenic chemotherapy (e.g. high dose cisplatin): Zofran can be given either by rectal, intravenous or intramuscular administration.

To protect against delayed or prolonged emesis after the first 24 hours, oral or rectal treatment with Zofran should be continued for up to 5 days after a course of treatment.

The recommended dose for oral administration is 8mg twice daily.

Children:

Zofran may be administered as a single intravenous dose of 5mg/m^2 immediately before chemotherapy, followed by 4mg orally twelve hours later. 4mg orally twice daily should be continued for up to 5 days after a course of treatment.

Elderly:

Zofran is well tolerated by patients over 65 years and no alteration of dosage, dosing frequency or route of administration are required.

Post operative nausea and vomiting (PONV)

Adults:

For the prevention of PONV: Zofran may be administered either orally (as Melt, tablets or syrup) or by intravenous or intramuscular injection.

For oral administration: 16mg one hour prior to anaesthesia. Alternatively, 8mg one hour prior to anaesthesia followed by two further doses of 8mg at eight hourly intervals.

For the treatment of established PONV: Intravenous or intramuscular administration is recommended.

Children (aged 2 years and over):

For the prevention and treatment of PONV: Slow intravenous injection is recommended.

Elderly:

There is limited experience in the use of Zofran in the prevention and treatment of PONV in the elderly, however Zofran is well tolerated in patients over 65 years receiving chemotherapy.

For both indications

Patients with renal impairment:

No alteration of daily dosage or frequency of dosing, or route of administration are required.

Patients with hepatic impairment:

Clearance of Zofran is significantly reduced and serum half life significantly prolonged in subjects with moderate or severe impairment of hepatic function. In such patients a total daily dose of 8mg should not be exceeded.

Patients with poor sparteine/debrisoquine metabolism:

The elimination half-life of ondansetron is not altered in subjects classified as poor metabolisers of sparteine and debrisoquine. Consequently in such patients repeat dosing will give drug exposure levels no different from those of the general population. No alteration of daily dosage or frequency of dosing are required.

4.3 Contraindications

Hypersensitivity to any component of the preparation.

4.4 Special warnings and precautions for use

Hypersensitivity reactions have been reported in patients who have exhibited hypersensitivity to other selective $5HT_3$ receptor antagonists.

Very rarely and predominantly with intravenous Zofran, transient ECG changes including QT interval prolongation have been reported. Therefore caution should be exercised in patients with cardiac rhythm or conduction disturbances, in patients treated with anti-arrhythmic agents or beta-adrenergic blocking agents and in patients with significant electrolyte disturbances.

As ondansetron is known to increase large bowel transit time, patients with signs of subacute intestinal obstruction should be monitored following administration.

Caution in patients with phenylketonuria.

4.5 Interaction with other medicinal products and other forms of interaction

There is no evidence that ondansetron either induces or inhibits the metabolism of other drugs commonly co-administered with it. Specific studies have shown that there are no pharamcokinetic interactions when ondansetron is administered with alcohol, temazepam, furosemide, tramadol or propofol.

Ondansetron is metabolised by multiple hepatic cytochrome P-450 enzymes: CYP3A4, CYP2D6 and CYP1A2. Due to the multiplicity of metabolic enzymes capable of metabolising ondansetron, enzyme inhibition or reduced activity of one enzyme (e.g. CYP2D6 genetic deficiency) is normally compensated by other enzymes and should result in little or no significant change in overall ondansetron clearance or dose requirement.

Phenytoin, Carbamazepine and Rifampicin: In patients treated with potent inducers of CYP3A4 (i.e. phenytoin, carbamazepine, and rifampicin), the oral clearance of ondansetron was increased and ondansetron blood concentrations were decreased.

Tramadol: Data from small studies indicate that ondansetron may reduce the analgesic effect of tramadol.

4.6 Pregnancy and lactation

The safety of ondansetron for use in human pregnancy has not been established. Evaluation of experimental animal studies does not indicate direct or indirect harmful effects with respect to the development of the embryo, or the foetus, the course of gestation and peri- and post-natal development. However, as animal studies are not always predictive of human response the use of ondansetron in pregnancy is not recommended.

Tests have shown that ondansetron passes into the milk of lactating animals. It is therefore recommended that mothers receiving Zofran should not breast-feed their babies.

4.7 Effects on ability to drive and use machines

In psychomotor testing ondansetron does not impair performance nor cause sedation.

4.8 Undesirable effects

Adverse events are listed below by system organ class and frequency. Frequencies are defined as: very common (≥1/10), common (≥1/100 and <1/10), uncommon (≥1/1000 and <1/100), rare (≥1/10,000 and <1/1000) and very rare (<1/10,000) including isolated reports. Very common, common and uncommon events were generally determined from clinical trial data. The incidence in placebo was taken into account. Rare and very rare events were generally determined from post-marketing spontaneous data.

The following frequencies are estimated at the standard recommended doses of ondansetron according to indication and formulation.

Immune system disorders

Rare: Immediate hypersensitivity reactions sometimes severe, including anaphylaxis.

Nervous system disorders

Very common: Headache.

Uncommon: Seizures, movement disorders including extrapyramidal reactions such as dystonic reactions, oculogyric crisis and dyskinesia have been observed without definitive evidence of persistent clinical sequelae.

Rare: Dizziness during i.v. administration, which in most cases is prevented or resolved by lengthening the infusion period.

Eye disorders

Rare: Transient visual disturbances (eg. blurred vision) during i.v. administration.

Very rare: Transient blindness predominantly during intravenous administration

The majority of the blindness cases reported resolved within 20 minutes. Most patients had received chemotherapeutic agents, which included cisplatin. Some cases of transient blindness were reported as cortical in origin.

Cardiac disorders

Uncommon: Arrhythmias, chest pain with or without ST segment depression, bradycardia.

Vascular disorders

Common: Sensation of warmth or flushing.

Uncommon: Hypotension.

Respiratory, thoracic and mediastinal disorders

Uncommon: Hiccups.

Gastrointestinal disorders

Common: Constipation.

Hepatobiliary disorders

Uncommon: Asymptomatic increases in liver function tests#.

#These events were observed commonly in patients receiving chemotherapy with cisplatin.

4.9 Overdose

Little is known at present about overdosage with ondansetron, however, a limited number of patients received overdoses. Manifestations that have been reported include visual disturbances, severe constipation, hypotension and a vasovagal episode with transient second degree AV block. In all instances, the events resolved completely. There is no specific antidote for ondansetron, therefore in all cases of suspected overdose, symptomatic and supportive therapy should be given as appropriate.

5. PHARMACOLOGICAL PROPERTIES

5.1 Pharmacodynamic properties

Ondansetron is a potent, highly selective 5HT3 receptor-antagonist. Its precise mode of action in the control of nausea and vomiting is not known. Chemotherapeutic agents and radiotherapy may cause release of 5HT in the small intestine initiating a vomiting reflex by activating vagal afferents via 5HT3 receptors. Ondansetron blocks the initiation of this reflex. Activation of vagal afferents may also cause a release of 5HT in the area postrema, located on the floor of the fourth ventricle, and this may also promote emesis through a central mechanism. Thus, the effect of ondansetron in the management of the nausea and vomiting induced by cytotoxic chemotherapy and radiotherapy is probably due to antagonism of 5HT3 receptors on neurons located both in the peripheral and central nervous system. The mechanisms of action in post-operative nausea and vomiting are not known but there may be common pathways with cytotoxic induced nausea and vomiting.

Ondansetron does not alter plasma prolactin concentrations.

The role of ondansetron in opiate-induced emesis is not yet established.

5.2 Pharmacokinetic properties

Following oral administration of ondansetron, absorption is rapid with maximum peak plasma concentrations of about 30ng/ml being attained and achieved in approximately 1.5 hours after an 8mg dose. The syrup and tablet formulations are bioequivalent and have an absolute oral bioavailability of 60%. The disposition of ondansetron following oral, intravenous and intramuscular dosing is similar with a terminal elimination half-life of approximately 3 hours and a steady-state volume of distribution of about 140L. Ondansetron is not highly protein bound (70-76%) and is cleared from the systemic circulation predominantly by hepatic metabolism through multiple enzymatic pathways. Less than 5% of the absorbed dose is excreted unchanged in the urine. The absence of the enzyme CYP2D6 (the debrisoquine polymorphism) has no effect on the pharmacokinetics of ondansetron. The pharmacokinetic properties of ondansetron are unchanged on repeat dosing.

Studies in healthy elderly volunteers have shown a slight but clinically insignificant, age-related increases in both oral bioavailability (65%) and half-life (5h) of ondansetron. Gender differences were shown in the disposition of ondansetron, with females having a greater rate and extent of absorption following an oral dose and reduced systemic clearance and volume of distribution (adjusted for weight).

In a study of 21 paediatric patients aged between 3 and 12 years undergoing elective surgery with general anaesthesia, the absolute values for both the clearance and volume of distribution of ondansetron following a single intravenous dose of 2mg (3-7 years old) or 4mg (8-12 years old) were reduced. The magnitude of the change was age-related, with clearance falling from about 300ml/min at 12 years of age to 100ml/min at 3 years. Volume of distribution fell from about 75L at 12 years to 17L at 3 years. Use of weight-based dosing (0.1mg/kg up to 4mg maximum) compensates for these changes and is effective in normalising systemic exposure in paediatric patients.

In patients with renal impairment (creatinine clearance >15 ml/min), systemic clearance and volume of distribution are reduced, resulting in a slight, but clinically insignificant increase in elimination half-life (5.4h). A study in patients with severe renal impairment who required regular haemodialysis (studied between dialyses) showed ondansetron's pharmacokinetics to be essentially unchanged.

In patients with severe hepatic impairment, systemic clearance is markedly reduced with prolonged elimination half-lives (15-32h) and an oral bioavailability approaching 100% because of reduced pre-systemic metabolism.

5.3 Preclinical safety data

No additional data of relevance.

6. PHARMACEUTICAL PARTICULARS

6.1 List of excipients

Gelatin

Mannitol

Aspartame

Sodium methyl hydroxybenzoate

Sodium propyl hydroxybenzoate

Strawberry flavour

6.2 Incompatibilities

None reported.

6.3 Shelf life

3 years.

6.4 Special precautions for storage

Store below 30°C.

6.5 Nature and contents of container

Double aluminium foil blister strip containing 10 tablets

6.6 Special precautions for disposal and other handling

Do not attempt to push Zofran Melt through the lidding foil.

Peel back the lidding foil of one blister and gently remove the Zofran Melt.

Place the Melt on top of the tongue, where it will disperse within seconds then swallow.

Administrative Data

7. MARKETING AUTHORISATION HOLDER

Glaxo Wellcome UK Limited trading as GlaxoSmithKline UK

Stockley Park West

Uxbridge

Middlesex, UB11 1BT

8. MARKETING AUTHORISATION NUMBER(S)

PL 10949/0263

9. DATE OF FIRST AUTHORISATION/RENEWAL OF THE AUTHORISATION

3 April 1998

10. DATE OF REVISION OF THE TEXT

17 October 2006

11. Legal Status

POM

Zofran Melt 8mg

(GlaxoSmithKline UK)

1. NAME OF THE MEDICINAL PRODUCT

Zofran Melt 8mg

2. QUALITATIVE AND QUANTITATIVE COMPOSITION

White, round, plano-convex, freeze dried, fast dispersing oral dosage form.

Each Melt contains ondansetron 8mg.

3. PHARMACEUTICAL FORM

Oral lyophilisate.

4. CLINICAL PARTICULARS

4.1 Therapeutic indications

The management of nausea and vomiting induced by cytotoxic chemotherapy and radiotherapy, and for the prevention of post-operative nausea and vomiting in adults.

4.2 Posology and method of administration

Place the Melt on top of the tongue, where it will disperse within seconds, then swallow

Chemotherapy and radiotherapy induced nausea and vomiting.

Adults:

The emetogenic potential of cancer treatment varies according to the doses and combinations of chemotherapy and radiotherapy regimens used. The route of administration and dose of Zofran should be flexible and selected as shown below.

Emetogenic chemotherapy and radiotherapy: Zofran can be given either by rectal, oral (as Melt, tablets or syrup) intravenous or intramuscular administration.

For oral administration: 8mg 1-2 hours before treatment, followed by 8mg 12 hours later.

To protect against delayed or prolonged emesis after the first 24 hours, oral or rectal treatment with Zofran should be continued for up to 5 days after a course of treatment.

The recommended dose for oral administration is 8mg twice daily.

Highly emetogenic chemotherapy (e.g. high dose cisplatin): Zofran can be given either by rectal, intravenous or intramuscular administration.

To protect against delayed or prolonged emesis after the first 24 hours, oral or rectal treatment with Zofran should be continued for up to 5 days after a course of treatment.

The recommended dose for oral administration is 8mg twice daily.

Children:

Zofran may be administered as a single intravenous dose of 5mg/m^2 immediately before chemotherapy, followed by 4mg orally twelve hours later. 4mg orally twice daily should be continued for up to 5 days after a course of treatment.

Elderly:

Zofran is well tolerated by patients over 65 years and no alteration of dosage, dosing frequency or route of administration are required.

Post operative nausea and vomiting (PONV)

Adults:

For the prevention of PONV: Zofran may be administered either orally (as Melt, tablets or syrup) or by intravenous or intramuscular injection.

For oral administration: 16mg one hour prior to anaesthesia. Alternatively, 8mg one hour prior to anaesthesia followed by two further doses of 8mg at eight hourly intervals.

For the treatment of established PONV: Intravenous or intramuscular administration is recommended.

Children (aged 2 years and over):

For the prevention and treatment of PONV: Slow intravenous injection is recommended.

Elderly:

There is limited experience in the use of Zofran in the prevention and treatment of PONV in the elderly, however Zofran is well tolerated in patients over 65 years receiving chemotherapy.

For both indications

Patients with renal impairment:

No alteration of daily dosage or frequency of dosing, or route of administration are required.

Patients with hepatic impairment:

Clearance of Zofran is significantly reduced and serum half life significantly prolonged in subjects with moderate or severe impairment of hepatic function. In such patients a total daily dose of 8mg should not be exceeded.

Patients with poor sparteine/debrisoquine metabolism:

The elimination half-life of ondansetron is not altered in subjects classified as poor metabolisers of sparteine and debrisoquine. Consequently in such patients repeat dosing will give drug exposure levels no different from those of the general population. No alteration of daily dosage or frequency of dosing are required.

4.3 Contraindications

Hypersensitivity to any component of the preparation.

4.4 Special warnings and precautions for use

Hypersensitivity reactions have been reported in patients who have exhibited hypersensitivity to other selective $5HT_3$ receptor antagonists.

Very rarely and predominantly with intravenous Zofran, transient ECG changes including QT interval prolongation have been reported. Therefore caution should be exercised in patients with cardiac rhythm or conduction disturbances, in patients treated with anti-arrhythmic agents or beta-adrenergic blocking agents and in patients with significant electrolyte disturbances.

As ondansetron is known to increase large bowel transit time, patients with signs of subacute intestinal obstruction should be monitored following administration.

Caution in patients with phenylketonuria.

4.5 Interaction with other medicinal products and other forms of interaction

There is no evidence that ondansetron either induces or inhibits the metabolism of other drugs commonly co-administered with it. Specific studies have shown that there are no pharamcokinetic interactions when ondansetron is administered with alcohol, temazepam, furosemide, tramadol or propofol.

Ondansetron is metabolised by multiple hepatic cytochrome P-450 enzymes: CYP3A4, CYP2D6 and CYP1A2. Due to the multiplicity of metabolic enzymes capable of metabolising ondansetron, enzyme inhibition or reduced activity of one enzyme (e.g. CYP2D6 genetic deficiency) is normally compensated by other enzymes and should result in little or no significant change in overall ondansetron clearance or dose requirement.

Phenytoin, Carbamazepine and Rifampicin: In patients treated with potent inducers of CYP3A4 (i.e. phenytoin, carbamazepine, and rifampicin), the oral clearance of ondansetron was increased and ondansetron blood concentrations were decreased.

Tramadol: Data from small studies indicate that ondansetron may reduce the analgesic effect of tramadol.

4.6 Pregnancy and lactation

The safety of ondansetron for use in human pregnancy has not been established. Evaluation of experimental animal studies does not indicate direct or indirect harmful effects with respect to the development of the embryo, or the foetus, the course of gestation and peri- and post-natal development. However, as animal studies are not always predictive of human response the use of ondansetron in pregnancy is not recommended.

Tests have shown that ondansetron passes into the milk of lactating animals. It is therefore recommended that mothers receiving Zofran should not breast-feed their babies.

4.7 Effects on ability to drive and use machines

In psychomotor testing ondansetron does not impair performance nor cause sedation.

4.8 Undesirable effects

Adverse events are listed below by system organ class and frequency. Frequencies are defined as: very common (≥1/10), common (≥1/100 and <1/10), uncommon (≥1/1000 and <1/100), rare (≥1/10,000 and <1/1000) and very rare (<1/10,000) including isolated reports. Very common, common and uncommon events were generally determined from clinical trial data. The incidence in placebo was taken into account. Rare and very rare events were generally determined from post-marketing spontaneous data.

The following frequencies are estimated at the standard recommended doses of ondansetron according to indication and formulation.

Immune system disorders

Rare: Immediate hypersensitivity reactions sometimes severe, including anaphylaxis.

Nervous system disorders

Very common: Headache.

Uncommon: Seizures, movement disorders including extrapyramidal reactions such as dystonic reactions, oculogyric crisis and dyskinesia have been observed without definitive evidence of persistent clinical sequelae.

Rare: Dizziness during i.v. administration, which in most cases is prevented or resolved by lengthening the infusion period.

Eye disorders

Rare: Transient visual disturbances (eg. blurred vision) during i.v. administration.

Very rare: Transient blindness predominantly during intravenous administration

The majority of the blindness cases reported resolved within 20 minutes. Most patients had received chemotherapeutic agents, which included cisplatin. Some cases of transient blindness were reported as cortical in origin.

Cardiac disorders

Uncommon: Arrhythmias, chest pain with or without ST segment depression, bradycardia.

Vascular disorders

Common: Sensation of warmth or flushing.

Uncommon: Hypotension.

Respiratory, thoracic and mediastinal disorders

Uncommon: Hiccups.

Gastrointestinal disorders

Common: Constipation.

Hepatobiliary disorders

Uncommon: Asymptomatic increases in liver function tests#.

#These events were observed commonly in patients receiving chemotherapy with cisplatin.

4.9 Overdose

Little is known at present about overdosage with ondansetron, however, a limited number of patients received overdoses. Manifestations that have been reported include visual disturbances, severe constipation, hypotension and a vasovagal episode with transient second degree AV block. In all instances, the events resolved completely. There is no specific antidote for ondansetron, therefore in all cases of suspected overdose, symptomatic and supportive therapy should be given as appropriate.

5. PHARMACOLOGICAL PROPERTIES

5.1 Pharmacodynamic properties

Ondansetron is a potent, highly selective 5HT3 receptor-antagonist. Its precise mode of action in the control of nausea and vomiting is not known. Chemotherapeutic agents and radiotherapy may cause release of 5HT in the small intestine initiating a vomiting reflex by activating vagal afferents via 5HT3 receptors. Ondansetron blocks the initiation of this reflex. Activation of vagal afferents may also cause a release of 5HT in the area postrema, located on the floor of the fourth ventricle, and this may also promote emesis through a central mechanism. Thus, the effect of ondansetron in the management of the nausea and vomiting induced by cytotoxic chemotherapy and radiotherapy is probably due to antagonism of 5HT3 receptors on neurons located both in the peripheral and central nervous system. The mechanisms of action in post-operative nausea and vomiting are not known but there may be common pathways with cytotoxic induced nausea and vomiting.

Ondansetron does not alter plasma prolactin concentrations.

The role of ondansetron in opiate-induced emesis is not yet established.

5.2 Pharmacokinetic properties

Following oral administration of ondansetron, absorption is rapid with maximum peak plasma concentrations of about 30ng/ml being attained and achieved in approximately 1.5 hours after an 8mg dose. The syrup and tablet formulations are bioequivalent and have an absolute oral bioavailability of 60%. The disposition of ondansetron following oral, intravenous and intramuscular dosing is similar with a terminal elimination half-life of approximately 3 hours and a steady-state volume of distribution of about 140L. Ondansetron is not highly protein bound (70-76%) and is cleared from the systemic circulation predominantly by hepatic metabolism through multiple enzymatic pathways. Less than 5% of the absorbed dose is excreted unchanged in the urine. The absence of the enzyme CYP2D6 (the debrisoquine polymorphism) has no effect on the pharmacokinetics of ondansetron. The pharmacokinetic properties of ondansetron are unchanged on repeat dosing.

Studies in healthy elderly volunteers have shown a slight but clinically insignificant, age-related increases in both oral bioavailability (65%) and half-life (5h) of ondansetron. Gender differences were shown in the disposition of ondansetron, with females having a greater rate and extent of absorption following an oral dose and reduced systemic clearance and volume of distribution (adjusted for weight).

In a study of 21 paediatric patients aged between 3 and 12 years undergoing elective surgery with general anaesthesia, the absolute values for both the clearance and volume of distribution of ondansetron following a single intravenous dose of 2mg (3-7 years old) or 4mg (8-12 years old) were reduced. The magnitude of the change was age-related, with clearance falling from about 300ml/min at 12 years of age to 100ml/min at 3 years. Volume of distribution fell from about 75L at 12 years to 17L at 3 years. Use of weight-based dosing (0.1mg/kg up to 4mg maximum) compensates for these changes and is effective in normalising systemic exposure in paediatric patients.

In patients with renal impairment (creatinine clearance >15 ml/min), systemic clearance and volume of distribution are reduced, resulting in a slight, but clinically insignificant increase in elimination half-life (5.4h). A study in patients with severe renal impairment who required regular haemodialysis (studied between dialyses) showed ondansetron's pharmacokinetics to be essentially unchanged.

In patients with severe hepatic impairment, systemic clearance is markedly reduced with prolonged elimination half-lives (15-32h) and an oral bioavailability approaching 100% because of reduced pre-systemic metabolism.

5.3 Preclinical safety data

No additional data of relevance.

6. PHARMACEUTICAL PARTICULARS

6.1 List of excipients

Gelatin

Mannitol

Aspartame

Sodium methyl hydroxybenzoate

Sodium propyl hydroxybenzoate

Strawberry flavour

6.2 Incompatibilities

None reported.

6.3 Shelf life

3 years.

6.4 Special precautions for storage

Store below 30°C.

6.5 Nature and contents of container

Double aluminium foil blister strip containing 10 tablets

6.6 Special precautions for disposal and other handling

Do not attempt to push Zofran Melt through the lidding foil.

Peel back the lidding foil of one blister and gently remove the Zofran Melt.

Place the Melt on top of the tongue, where it will disperse within seconds then swallow.

Administrative Data

7. MARKETING AUTHORISATION HOLDER

Glaxo Wellcome UK Limited trading as GlaxoSmithKline UK

Stockley Park West

Uxbridge

Middlesex, UB11 1BT

8. MARKETING AUTHORISATION NUMBER(S)

PL 10949/0264

9. DATE OF FIRST AUTHORISATION/RENEWAL OF THE AUTHORISATION

3 April 1998

10. DATE OF REVISION OF THE TEXT

17 October 2006

11. Legal Status

POM

Zofran Suppositories 16mg

(GlaxoSmithKline UK)

1. NAME OF THE MEDICINAL PRODUCT

Zofran Suppositories 16mg

2. QUALITATIVE AND QUANTITATIVE COMPOSITION

White torpedo shaped suppositories containing 16mg of ondansetron.

3. PHARMACEUTICAL FORM

Suppositories.

4. CLINICAL PARTICULARS

4.1 Therapeutic indications

The management of nausea and vomiting induced by cytotoxic chemotherapy and radiotherapy.

4.2 Posology and method of administration

Adults (including the elderly):

The emetogenic potential of cancer treatment varies according to the doses and combinations of chemotherapy and radiotherapy regimens used. The route of administration and dose of Zofran should be flexible and selected as shown below.

Emetogenic chemotherapy and radiotherapy: Zofran can be given either by rectal, oral (tablets or syrup), intravenous or intramuscular administration.

For rectal administration: One suppository (16mg ondansetron) 1-2 hours before treatment.

To protect against delayed or prolonged emesis after the first 24 hours, oral or rectal treatment with Zofran should be continued for up to 5 days after a course of treatment. The recommended dose for rectal administration is one suppository daily.

Highly emetogenic chemotherapy (e.g. high dose cisplatin): Zofran can be given either by rectal, intravenous or intramuscular administration.

For rectal administration: One suppository (16mg ondansetron) 1-2 hours before treatment.

The efficacy of Zofran in highly emetogenic chemotherapy may be enhanced by the addition of a single intravenous dose of dexamethasone sodium phosphate 20mg, administered prior to chemotherapy.

To protect against delayed or prolonged emesis after the first 24 hours, oral or rectal treatment with Zofran should be continued for up to 5 days after a course of treatment. The recommended dose for rectal administration is one suppository daily.

Children:

The use of Zofran Suppositories in children is not recommended.

Zofran may be administered as a single intravenous dose of 5mg/m^2 immediately before chemotherapy, followed by 4mg orally twelve hours later. 4mg orally twice daily should be continued for up to 5 days after a course of treatment.

Patients with renal impairment:

No special requirements.

Patients with hepatic impairment:

Clearance of Zofran is significantly reduced and serum half-life significantly prolonged in subjects with moderate or severe impairment of hepatic function. In such patients a total daily dose of 8mg should not be exceeded and therefore intravenous or oral administration is recommended.

Patients with poor sparteine/debrisoquine metabolism:

The elimination half-life of ondansetron is not altered in subjects classified as poor metabolisers of sparteine and debrisoquine. Consequently in such patients repeat dosing will give drug exposure levels no different from those of the general population. No alteration of daily dosage or frequency of dosing are required.

4.3 Contraindications

Hypersensitivity to any ingredient.

4.4 Special warnings and precautions for use

Hypersensitivity reactions have been reported in patients who have exhibited hypersensitivity to other selective $5HT_3$ receptor antagonists.

Very rarely and predominantly with intravenous Zofran, transient ECG changes including QT interval prolongation have been reported. Therefore caution should be exercised in patients with cardiac rhythm or conduction disturbances, in patients treated with anti-arrhythmic agents or beta-adrenergic blocking agents and in patients with significant electrolyte disturbances.

As ondansetron is known to increase large bowel transit time, patients with signs of subacute intestinal obstruction should be monitored following administration.

4.5 Interaction with other medicinal products and other forms of interaction

There is no evidence that ondansetron either induces or inhibits the metabolism of other drugs commonly co-administered with it. Specific studies have shown that there are no pharmacokinetic interactions when ondansetron is administered with alcohol, temazepam, furosemide, tramadol or propofol.

Ondansetron is metabolised by multiple hepatic cytochrome P-450 enzymes: CYP3A4, CYP2D6 and CYP1A2. Due to the multiplicity of metabolic enzymes capable of metabolising ondansetron, enzyme inhibition or reduced activity of one enzyme (e.g. CYP2D6 genetic deficiency) is normally compensated by other enzymes and should result in little or no significant change in overall ondansetron clearance or dose requirement.

Phenytoin, Carbamazepine and Rifampicin: In patients treated with potent inducers of CYP3A4 (i.e. phenytoin, carbamazepine, and rifampicin), the oral clearance of ondansetron was increased and ondansetron blood concentrations were decreased.

Tramadol: Data from small studies indicate that ondansetron may reduce the analgesic effect of tramadol.

4.6 Pregnancy and lactation

The safety of ondansetron for use in human pregnancy has not been established. Evaluation of experimental animal studies does not indicate direct or indirect harmful effects with respect to the development of the embryo, or foetus, the course of gestation and peri- and post-natal development. However as animal studies are not always predictive of human response the use of ondansetron in pregnancy is not recommended.

Tests have shown that ondansetron passes into the milk of lactating animals. It is therefore recommended that mothers receiving Zofran should not breast-feed their babies.

4.7 Effects on ability to drive and use machines

None reported.

4.8 Undesirable effects

Adverse events are listed below by system organ class and frequency. Frequencies are defined as: very common ($\geqslant$1/10), common ($\geqslant$1/100 and <1/10), uncommon ($\geqslant$1/1000 and <1/100), rare ($\geqslant$1/10,000 and <1/1000) and very rare (<1/10,000) including isolated reports. Very common, common and uncommon events were generally determined from clinical trial data. The incidence in placebo was taken into account. Rare and very rare events were generally determined from post-marketing spontaneous data.

The following frequencies are estimated at the standard recommended doses of ondansetron according to indication and formulation.

Immune system disorders

Rare: Immediate hypersensitivity reactions sometimes severe, including anaphylaxis.

Nervous system disorders

Very common: Headache.

Uncommon: Seizures, movement disorders including extrapyramidal reactions such as dystonic reactions, oculogyric crisis and dyskinesia have been observed without definitive evidence of persistent clinical sequelae.

Rare: Dizziness during i.v. administration, which in most cases is prevented or resolved by lengthening the infusion period.

Eye disorders

Rare: Transient visual disturbances (eg. blurred vision) during i.v. administration.

Very rare: Transient blindness predominantly during intravenous administration

The majority of the blindness cases reported resolved within 20 minutes. Most patients had received chemotherapeutic agents, which included cisplatin. Some cases of transient blindness were reported as cortical in origin.

Cardiac disorders

Uncommon: Arrhythmias, chest pain with or without ST segment depression, bradycardia.

Vascular disorders

Common: Sensation of warmth or flushing.

Uncommon: Hypotension.

Respiratory, thoracic and mediastinal disorders

Uncommon: Hiccups.

Gastrointestinal disorders

Common: Constipation.

Hepatobiliary disorders

Uncommon: Asymptomatic increases in liver function tests#.

#These events were observed commonly in patients receiving chemotherapy with cisplatin.

General disorders and administration site conditions

Local burning sensation following insertion of suppositories.

4.9 Overdose

Little is known at present about overdosage with ondansetron, however, a limited number of patients received overdoses. Manifestations that have been reported include visual disturbances, severe constipation, hypotension and a vasovagal episode with transient second degree AV block. In all instances, the events resolved completely. There is no specific antidote for ondansetron, therefore in all cases of suspected overdose, symptomatic and supportive therapy should be given as appropriate.

5. PHARMACOLOGICAL PROPERTIES

5.1 Pharmacodynamic properties

Ondansetron is a potent, highly selective $5HT_3$ receptor-antagonist. The precise mode of action in the control of nausea and vomiting is not known. Chemotherapeutic agents and radiotherapy may cause release of 5HT in the small intestine initiating a vomiting reflex by activating vagal afferents via $5HT_3$ receptors. Ondansetron blocks the initiation of this reflex. Activation of vagal afferents may also cause a release of 5HT in the area postrema, located on the floor of the fourth ventricle, and this may also promote emesis through a central mechanism. Thus, the effect of ondansetron in the management of the nausea and vomiting induced by cytotoxic chemotherapy and radiotherapy is probably due to antagonism of $5HT_3$ receptors on neurons located both in the peripheral and central nervous system. The mechanisms of action in post-operative nausea and vomiting are not known but there may be common pathways with cytotoxic induced nausea and vomiting.

Ondansetron does not alter plasma prolactin concentrations.

The role of ondansetron in opiate-induced emesis is not yet established.

5.2 Pharmacokinetic properties

Following oral administration, ondansetron is passively and completely absorbed from the gastrointestinal tract and undergoes first pass metabolism. Peak plasma concentrations of about 30ng/ml are attained approximately 1.5 hours after an 8mg dose. For doses above 8mg the increase in ondansetron systemic exposure with dose is greater than proportional; this may reflect some reduction in first pass metabolism at higher oral doses. Bioavailability, following oral administration, is slightly enhanced by the presence of food but unaffected by antacids. Studies in healthy elderly volunteers have shown slight, but clinically insignificant, age-related increases in both oral bioavailability (65%) and half-life (5 hours) of ondansetron. Gender differences were shown in the disposition of ondansetron, with females having a greater rate and extent of absorption following an oral dose and reduced systemic clearance and volume of distribution (adjusted for weight).

The disposition of ondansetron following oral, intramuscular(IM) and intravenous(IV) dosing is similar with a terminal half life of about 3 hours and steady state volume of distribution of about 140L. Equivalent systemic exposure is achieved after IM and IV administration of ondansetron.

A 4mg intravenous infusion of ondansetron given over 5 minutes results in peak plasma concentrations of about 65ng/ml. Following intramuscular administration of ondansetron, peak plasma concentrations of about 25ng/ml are attained within 10 minutes of injection.

Following administration of ondansetron suppository, plasma ondansetron concentrations become detectable between 15 and 60 minutes after dosing. Concentrations rise in an essentially linear fashion, until peak concentrations of 20-30 ng/ml are attained, typically 6 hours after dosing. Plasma concentrations then fall, but at a slower rate than observed following oral dosing due to continued absorption of ondansetron. The absolute bioavailability of ondansetron from the suppository is approximately 60% and is not affected by gender. The half life of the elimination phase following suppository administration is determined by the rate of ondansetron absorption, not systemic clearance and is approximately 6 hours. Females show a small, clinically insignificant, increase in half-life in comparison with males.

Ondansetron is not highly protein bound (70-76%). Ondansetron is cleared from the systemic circulation predominantly by hepatic metabolism through multiple enzymatic pathways. Less than 5% of the absorbed dose is excreted unchanged in the urine. The absence of the enzyme CYP2D6 (the debrisoquine polymorphism) has no effect on ondansetron's pharmacokinetics. The pharmacokinetic properties of ondansetron are unchanged on repeat dosing.

In a study of 21 paediatric patients aged between 3 and 12 years undergoing elective surgery with general anaesthesia, the absolute values for both the clearance and volume of distribution of ondansetron following a single intravenous dose of 2mg (3-7 years old) or 4mg (8-12 years old) were reduced. The magnitude of the change was age-related, with clearance falling from about 300mL/min at 12 years of age to 100mL/min at 3 years. Volume of distribution fell from about 75L at 12 years to 17L at 3 years. Use of weight-based dosing (0.1mg/kg up to 4mg maximum) compensates for these changes and is effective in normalising systemic exposure in paediatric patients.

In patients with renal impairment (creatinine clearance 15-60 ml/min), both systemic clearance and volume of distribution are reduced following IV administration of ondansetron, resulting in a slight, but clinically insignificant, increase in elimination half-life (5.4h). A study in patients with severe renal impairment who required regular haemodialysis (studied between dialyses) showed ondansetron's pharmacokinetics to be essentially unchanged following IV administration.

Specific studies in the elderly or patients with renal impairment have been limited to IV and oral administration. However, it is anticipated that the half-life of ondansetron after rectal administration in these populations will be similar to that seen in healthy volunteers, since the rate of elimination of ondansetron following rectal administration is not determined by systemic clearance.

Following oral, intravenous or intramuscular dosing in patients with severe hepatic impairment, ondansetron's systemic clearance is markedly reduced with prolonged elimination half-lives (15-32 h) and an oral bioavailability approaching 100% due to reduced pre-systemic metabolism. The pharmacokinetics of ondansetron following administration as a suppository have not been evaluated in patients with hepatic impairment.

5.3 Preclinical safety data

No additional data of relevance.

6. PHARMACEUTICAL PARTICULARS

6.1 List of excipients

Witepsol S58.

6.2 Incompatibilities

None reported.

6.3 Shelf life

3 years.

6.4 Special precautions for storage

Store below 30°C.

6.5 Nature and contents of container

Each suppository is in an individually sealed cavity enclosed in a perforated cardboard mount and packed into a carton.

6.6 Special precautions for disposal and other handling

Insert into the rectum.

For detailed instructions see the patient information leaflet included in every pack.

Administrative Data

7. MARKETING AUTHORISATION HOLDER

Glaxo Wellcome UK Limited trading as GlaxoSmithKline UK

Stockley Park West

Uxbridge

Middlesex, UB11 1BT

8. MARKETING AUTHORISATION NUMBER(S)

PL10949/0247

9. DATE OF FIRST AUTHORISATION/RENEWAL OF THE AUTHORISATION

15th January 2002

10. DATE OF REVISION OF THE TEXT

17 October 2006

11. Legal Status

POM

Zofran Syrup

(GlaxoSmithKline UK)

1. NAME OF THE MEDICINAL PRODUCT

Zofran™ Syrup

2. QUALITATIVE AND QUANTITATIVE COMPOSITION

Sugar-free strawberry flavoured liquid.

Each 5ml contains 4mg of ondansetron as the hydrochloride dihydrate.

3. PHARMACEUTICAL FORM

Oral solution.

4. CLINICAL PARTICULARS

4.1 Therapeutic indications

The management of nausea and vomiting induced by cytotoxic chemotherapy and radiotherapy, and for the prevention of post-operative nausea and vomiting in adults.

4.2 Posology and method of administration

Chemotherapy and radiotherapy induced nausea and vomiting

Adults (including the elderly):

The emetogenic potential of cancer treatment varies according to the doses and combinations of chemotherapy and radiotherapy regimens used. The route of administration and dose of Zofran should be flexible and selected as shown below.

Emetogenic chemotherapy and radiotherapy: Zofran can be given either by rectal, oral (tablets or syrup), intravenous or intramuscular administration.

For oral administration: 8mg 1-2 hours before treatment, followed by 8mg 12 hours later.

To protect against delayed or prolonged emesis after the first 24 hours, oral or rectal treatment with Zofran should be continued for up to 5 days after a course of treatment.

The recommended dose for oral administration is 8mg twice daily.

Highly emetogenic chemotherapy (e.g. high dose cisplatin): Zofran can be given either by rectal, intravenous or intramuscular administration.

To protect against delayed or prolonged emesis after the first 24 hours, oral or rectal treatment with Zofran should be continued for up to 5 days after a course of treatment.

The recommended dose for oral administration is 8mg twice daily.

Children:

Zofran may be administered as a single intravenous dose of $5mg/m^2$ immediately before chemotherapy, followed by 4mg orally twelve hours later. 4mg orally twice daily should be continued for up to 5 days after a course of treatment.

Post operative nausea and vomiting (ponv).

Adults:

For the prevention of PONV: Zofran can be administered orally or by intravenous or intramuscular injection.

For oral administration: 16mg one hour prior to anaesthesia. Alternatively, 8mg one hour prior to anaesthesia followed by two further doses of 8mg at eight hourly intervals.

For the treatment of established PONV: Intravenous or intramuscular administration is recommended.

Children (aged 2 years and over):

For the prevention and treatment of PONV: Slow intravenous injection is recommended.

Elderly:

There is limited experience in the use of Zofran in the prevention and treatment of PONV in the elderly, however Zofran is well tolerated in patients over 65 years receiving chemotherapy.

For both indications

Patients with renal impairment:

No special requirements.

Patients with hepatic impairment:

Clearance of Zofran is significantly reduced and serum half life significantly prolonged in subjects with moderate or severe impairment of hepatic function. In such patients a total daily dose of 8mg should not be exceeded.

Patients with poor sparteine/debrisoquine metabolism:

The elimination half-life of ondansetron is not altered in subjects classified as poor metabolisers of sparteine and debrisoquine. Consequently in such patients repeat dosing will give drug exposure levels no different from those of the general population. No alteration of daily dosage or frequency of dosing are required.

4.3 Contraindications

Hypersensitivity to any ingredient.

4.4 Special warnings and precautions for use

Hypersensitivity reactions have been reported in patients who have exhibited hypersensitivity to other selective $5HT_3$ receptor antagonists.

Very rarely and predominantly with intravenous Zofran, transient ECG changes including QT interval prolongation have been reported. Therefore caution should be exercised in patients with cardiac rhythm or conduction disturbances, in patients treated with anti-arrhythmic agents or beta-adrenergic blocking agents and in patients with significant electrolyte disturbances.

As ondansetron is known to increase large bowel transit time, patients with signs of subacute intestinal obstruction should be monitored following administration.

4.5 Interaction with other medicinal products and other forms of interaction

There is no evidence that ondansetron either induces or inhibits the metabolism of other drugs commonly co-administered with it. Specific studies have shown that there are no pharamcokinetic interactions when ondansetron is administered with alcohol, temazepam, furosemide, tramadol or propofol.

Ondansetron is metabolised by multiple hepatic cytochrome P-450 enzymes: CYP3A4, CYP2D6 and CYP1A2. Due to the multiplicity of metabolic enzymes capable of metabolising ondansetron, enzyme inhibition or reduced activity of one enzyme (e.g. CYP2D6 genetic deficiency) is normally compensated by other enzymes and should result in little or no significant change in overall ondansetron clearance or dose requirement.

Phenytoin, Carbamazepine and Rifampicin: In patients treated with potent inducers of CYP3A4 (i.e. phenytoin, carbamazepine, and rifampicin), the oral clearance of ondansetron was increased and ondansetron blood concentrations were decreased.

Tramadol: Data from small studies indicate that ondansetron may reduce the analgesic effect of tramadol.

4.6 Pregnancy and lactation

The safety of ondansetron for use in human pregnancy has not been established. Evaluation of experimental animal studies does not indicate direct or indirect harmful effects with respect to the development of the embryo, or foetus, the course of gestation and peri- and post-natal development. However as animal studies are not always predictive of human response the use of ondansetron in pregnancy is not recommended.

Tests have shown that ondansetron passes into the milk of lactating animals. It is therefore recommended that mothers receiving Zofran should not breast-feed their babies.

4.7 Effects on ability to drive and use machines

None reported

4.8 Undesirable effects

Adverse events are listed below by system organ class and frequency. Frequencies are defined as: very common ($\geq$1/10), common ($\geq$1/100 and $<$1/10), uncommon ($\geq$1/1000 and $<$1/100), rare ($\geq$1/10,000 and $<$1/1000) and very rare ($<$1/10,000) including isolated reports. Very common, common and uncommon events were generally determined from clinical trial data. The incidence in placebo was taken into account. Rare and very rare events were generally determined from post-marketing spontaneous data.

The following frequencies are estimated at the standard recommended doses of ondansetron according to indication and formulation.

Immune system disorders

Rare: Immediate hypersensitivity reactions sometimes severe, including anaphylaxis.

Nervous system disorders

Very common: Headache.

Uncommon: Seizures, movement disorders including extrapyramidal reactions such as dystonic reactions, oculogyric crisis and dyskinesia have been observed without definitive evidence of persistent clinical sequelae.

Rare: Dizziness during i.v. administration, which in most cases is prevented or resolved by lengthening the infusion period.

Eye disorders

Rare: Transient visual disturbances (eg. blurred vision) during i.v. administration.

Very rare: Transient blindness predominantly during intravenous administration

The majority of the blindness cases reported resolved within 20 minutes. Most patients had received chemotherapeutic agents, which included cisplatin. Some cases of transient blindness were reported as cortical in origin.

Cardiac disorders

Uncommon: Arrhythmias, chest pain with or without ST segment depression, bradycardia.

Vascular disorders

Common: Sensation of warmth or flushing.

Uncommon: Hypotension.

Respiratory, thoracic and mediastinal disorders

Uncommon: Hiccups.

Gastrointestinal disorders

Common: Constipation.

Hepatobiliary disorders

Uncommon: Asymptomatic increases in liver function tests#.

#These events were observed commonly in patients receiving chemotherapy with cisplatin.

4.9 Overdose

Little is known at present about overdosage with ondansetron, however, a limited number of patients received overdoses. Manifestations that have been reported include visual disturbances, severe constipation, hypotension and a vasovagal episode with transient second degree AV block. In all instances, the events resolved completely. There is no specific antidote for ondansetron, therefore in all cases of suspected overdose, symptomatic and supportive therapy should be given as appropriate.

5. PHARMACOLOGICAL PROPERTIES

5.1 Pharmacodynamic properties

Ondansetron is a potent, highly selective 5HT3 receptor-antagonist. Its precise mode of action in the control of nausea and vomiting is not known. Chemotherapeutic agents and radiotherapy may cause release of 5HT in the small intestine initiating a vomiting reflex by activating vagal afferents via 5HT3 receptors. Ondansetron blocks the initiation of this reflex. Activation of vagal afferents may also cause a release of 5HT in the area postrema, located on the floor of the fourth ventricle, and this may also promote emesis through a central mechanism. Thus, the effect of ondansetron in the management of the nausea and vomiting induced by cytotoxic chemotherapy and radiotherapy is probably due to antagonism of 5HT3 receptors on neurons located both in the peripheral and central nervous system. The mechanisms of action in post-operative nausea and vomiting are not known but there may be common pathways with cytotoxic induced nausea and vomiting.

Ondansetron does not alter plasma prolactin concentrations.

The role of ondansetron in opiate-induced emesis is not yet established.

5.2 Pharmacokinetic properties

Following oral administration, ondansetron is passively and completely absorbed from the gastrointestinal tract and undergoes first pass metabolism. Peak plasma concentrations of about 30ng/ml are attained approximately 1.5 hours after an 8mg dose. For doses above 8mg the increase in ondansetron systemic exposure with dose is greater than proportional; this may reflect some reduction in first pass metabolism at higher oral doses. Bioavailability, following oral administration, is slightly enhanced by the presence of food but unaffected by antacids. Studies in healthy elderly volunteers have shown slight, but clinically insignificant, age-related increases in both oral bioavailability (65%) and half-life (5 hours) of ondansetron. Gender differences were shown in the disposition of ondansetron, with females having a greater rate and extent of absorption following an oral dose and reduced systemic clearance and volume of distribution (adjusted for weight).

The disposition of ondansetron following oral, intramuscular(IM) and intravenous(IV) dosing is similar with a terminal half life of about 3 hours and steady state volume of distribution of about 140L. Equivalent systemic exposure is achieved after IM and IV administration of ondansetron.

A 4mg intravenous infusion of ondansetron given over 5 minutes results in peak plasma concentrations of about 65ng/ml. Following intramuscular administration of ondansetron, peak plasma concentrations of about 25ng/ml are attained within 10 minutes of injection.

Following administration of ondansetron suppository, plasma ondansetron concentrations become detectable between 15 and 60 minutes after dosing. Concentrations rise in an essentially linear fashion, until peak concentrations of 20-30 ng/ml are attained, typically 6 hours after dosing. Plasma concentrations then fall, but at a slower rate than observed following oral dosing due to continued absorption of ondansetron. The absolute bioavailability of ondansetron from the suppository is approximately 60% and is not affected by gender. The half life of the elimination phase following suppository administration is determined by the rate of ondansetron absorption, not systemic clearance and is approximately 6 hours. Females show a small, clinically insignificant, increase in half-life in comparison with males.

Ondansetron is not highly protein bound (70-76%). Ondansetron is cleared from the systemic circulation predominantly by hepatic metabolism through multiple enzymatic pathways. Less than 5% of the absorbed dose is excreted unchanged in the urine. The absence of the enzyme CYP2D6 (the debrisoquine polymorphism) has no effect on ondansetron's pharmacokinetics. The pharmacokinetic properties of ondansetron are unchanged on repeat dosing.

In a study of 21 paediatric patients aged between 3 and 12 years undergoing elective surgery with general anaesthesia, the absolute values for both the clearance and volume of distribution of ondansetron following a single intravenous dose of 2mg (3-7 years old) or 4mg (8-12 years old) were reduced. The magnitude of the change was age-related, with clearance falling from about 300mL/min at 12 years of age to 100mL/min at 3 years. Volume of distribution fell from about 75L at 12 years to 17L at 3 years. Use of weight-based dosing (0.1mg/kg up to 4mg maximum) compensates for these changes and is effective in normalising systemic exposure in paediatric patients.

In patients with renal impairment (creatinine clearance 15-60 ml/min), both systemic clearance and volume of distribution are reduced following IV administration of ondansetron, resulting in a slight, but clinically insignificant, increase in elimination half-life (5.4h). A study in patients with severe renal impairment who required regular haemodialysis (studied between dialyses) showed ondansetron's pharmacokinetics to be essentially unchanged following IV administration.

Specific studies in the elderly or patients with renal impairment have been limited to IV and oral administration. However, it is anticipated that the half-life of ondansetron after rectal administration in these populations will be similar to that seen in healthy volunteers, since the rate of elimination of ondansetron following rectal administration is not determined by systemic clearance.

Following oral, intravenous or intramuscular dosing in patients with severe hepatic impairment, ondansetron's systemic clearance is markedly reduced with prolonged elimination half-lives (15-32 h) and an oral bioavailability approaching 100% due to reduced pre-systemic metabolism. The pharmacokinetics of ondansetron following administration as a suppository have not been evaluated in patients with hepatic impairment.

5.3 Preclinical safety data

No additional data of relevance.

6. PHARMACEUTICAL PARTICULARS

6.1 List of excipients

Citric acid

Sodium citrate dihydrate

Sodium benzoate

Sorbitol solution

Strawberry flavour

Purified water

6.2 Incompatibilities

None reported.

6.3 Shelf life

3 years.

6.4 Special precautions for storage

Store upright below 30°C. Do not refrigerate.

6.5 Nature and contents of container

60ml amber glass bottle with a child resistant cap containing 50ml of Zofran Syrup.

6.6 Special precautions for disposal and other handling

For oral administration. For detailed information see the patient information leaflet included in every pack.

Administrative Data

7. MARKETING AUTHORISATION HOLDER

Glaxo Wellcome UK Limited trading as GlaxoSmithKline UK

Stockley Park West

Uxbridge

Middlesex, UB11 1BT

8. MARKETING AUTHORISATION NUMBER(S)

PL 10949/0246

9. DATE OF FIRST AUTHORISATION/RENEWAL OF THE AUTHORISATION

17th August 2001

10. DATE OF REVISION OF THE TEXT

17 October 2006

11. Legal Status

POM

Zofran Tablets 4mg

(GlaxoSmithKline UK)

1. NAME OF THE MEDICINAL PRODUCT

Zofran Tablets 4mg

2. QUALITATIVE AND QUANTITATIVE COMPOSITION

Each Zofran Tablet 4mg is a yellow, oval, film coated tablet engraved "GLAXO" on one face and "4" on the other. Each tablet contains ondansetron 4mg (as hydrochloride dihydrate).

3. PHARMACEUTICAL FORM

Film coated tablet.

4. CLINICAL PARTICULARS

4.1 Therapeutic indications

Zofran is indicated for the management of nausea and vomiting induced by cytotoxic chemotherapy and radiotherapy, and for the prevention and treatment of post-operative nausea and vomiting.

4.2 Posology and method of administration

Chemotherapy and radiotherapy induced nausea and vomiting.

Adults:

The emetogenic potential of cancer treatment varies according to the doses and combinations of chemotherapy and radiotherapy regimens used. The route of administration and dose of Zofran should be flexible in the range of 8-32mg a day and selected as shown below.

Emetogenic Chemotherapy and Radiotherapy: Zofran can be given either by rectal, oral (tablets or syrup), intravenous or intramuscular administration.

For oral administration: 8mg 1-2 hours before treatment, followed by 8mg 12 hours later.

To protect against delayed or prolonged emesis after the first 24 hours, oral or rectal treatment with Zofran should be continued for up to 5 days after a course of treatment.

The recommended dose for oral administration is 8mg twice daily.

Highly Emetogenic Chemotherapy: For patients receiving highly emetogenic chemotherapy, eg. high-dose cisplatin, Zofran can be given either by rectal, intravenous or intramuscular administration.

To protect against delayed or prolonged emesis after the first 24 hours, oral or rectal treatment with Zofran should be continued for up to 5 days after a course of treatment.

The recommended dose for oral administration is 8mg twice daily.

Children:

Zofran may be administered as a single intravenous dose of 5mg/m^2 immediately before chemotherapy, followed by 4mg orally twelve hours later. 4mg orally twice daily should be continued for up to 5 days after a course of treatment.

Elderly:

Zofran is well tolerated by patients over 65 years and no alteration of dosage, dosing frequency or route of administration are required.

Patients with Renal Impairment:

No alteration of daily dosage or frequency of dosing, or route of administration are required.

Patients with hepatic Impairment:

Clearance of Zofran is significantly reduced and serum half-life significantly prolonged in subjects with moderate or severe impairment of hepatic function. In such patients a total daily dose of 8mg should not be exceeded.

Post operative nausea and vomiting:

Adults:

For the prevention of PONV: Zofran can be administered orally or by intravenous or intramuscular injection.

For oral administration: 16mg one hour prior to anaesthesia. Alternatively, 8mg one hour prior to anaesthesia followed by two further doses of 8mg at eight hourly intervals.

For the treatment of established PONV: Intravenous or intramuscular administration is recommended.

Children (aged 2 years and over):

For the prevention and treatment of PONV: Slow intravenous injection is recommended.

Elderly:

There is limited experience in the use of Zofran in the prevention and treatment of post-operative nausea and vomiting in the elderly, however Zofran is well tolerated in patients over 65 years receiving chemotherapy.

Patients with renal impairment:

No alteration of daily dosage or frequency of dosing, or route of administration are required.

Patients with hepatic impairment:

Clearance of Zofran is significantly reduced and serum half life significantly prolonged in subjects with moderate or severe impairment of hepatic function. In such patients a total daily dose of 8mg should not be exceeded.

Patients with poor sparteine/debrisoquine metabolism:

The elimination half-life of ondansetron is not altered in subjects classified as poor metabolisers of sparteine and debrisoquine. Consequently in such patients repeat dosing will give drug exposure levels no different from those of the general population. No alteration of daily dosage or frequency of dosing are required.

4.3 Contraindications

Hypersensitivity to any component of the preparation.

4.4 Special warnings and precautions for use

Hypersensitivity reactions have been reported in patients who have exhibited hypersensitivity to other selective $5HT_3$ receptor antagonists.

Very rarely and predominantly with intravenous Zofran, transient ECG changes including QT interval prolongation have been reported. Therefore caution should be exercised in patients with cardiac rhythm or conduction disturbances, in patients treated with anti-arrhythmic agents or beta-adrenergic blocking agents and in patients with significant electrolyte disturbances.

As ondansetron is known to increase large bowel transit time, patients with signs of subacute intestinal obstruction should be monitored following administration.

4.5 Interaction with other medicinal products and other forms of interaction

There is no evidence that ondansetron either induces or inhibits the metabolism of other drugs commonly coadministered with it. Specific studies have shown that there are no pharamcokinetic interactions when ondansetron is administered with alcohol, temazepam, furosemide, tramadol or propofol.

Ondansetron is metabolised by multiple hepatic cytochrome P-450 enzymes: CYP3A4, CYP2D6 and CYP1A2. Due to the multiplicity of metabolic enzymes capable of metabolising ondansetron, enzyme inhibition or reduced activity of one enzyme (e.g. CYP2D6 genetic deficiency) is normally compensated by other enzymes and should result in little or no significant change in overall ondansetron clearance or dose requirement.

Phenytoin, Carbamazepine and Rifampicin: In patients treated with potent inducers of CYP3A4 (i.e. phenytoin, carbamazepine, and rifampicin), the oral clearance of ondansetron was increased and ondansetron blood concentrations were decreased.

Tramadol: Data from small studies indicate that ondansetron may reduce the analgesic effect of tramadol.

4.6 Pregnancy and lactation

The safety of ondansetron for use in human pregnancy has not been established. Evaluation of experimental animal studies does not indicate direct or indirect harmful effects with respect to the development of the embryo, or foetus, the course of gestation and peri- and post-natal development. However as animal studies are not always predictive of human response the use of ondansetron in pregnancy is not recommended.

Tests have shown that ondansetron passes into the milk of lactating animals. It is therefore recommended that mothers receiving Zofran should not breast-feed their babies.

4.7 Effects on ability to drive and use machines

In psychomotor testing ondansetron does not impair performance nor cause sedation.

4.8 Undesirable effects

Adverse events are listed below by system organ class and frequency. Frequencies are defined as: very common (≥1/10), common (≥1/100 and <1/10), uncommon (≥1/1000 and <1/100), rare (≥1/10,000 and <1/1000) and very rare (<1/10,000) including isolated reports. Very common, common and uncommon events were generally determined from clinical trial data. The incidence in placebo was taken into account. Rare and very rare events were generally determined from post-marketing spontaneous data.

The following frequencies are estimated at the standard recommended doses of ondansetron according to indication and formulation.

Immune system disorders

Rare: Immediate hypersensitivity reactions sometimes severe, including anaphylaxis.

Nervous system disorders

Very common: Headache.

Uncommon: Seizures, movement disorders including extrapyramidal reactions such as dystonic reactions, oculogyric crisis and dyskinesia have been observed without definitive evidence of persistent clinical sequelae.

Rare: Dizziness during i.v. administration, which in most cases is prevented or resolved by lengthening the infusion period.

Eye disorders

Rare: Transient visual disturbances (eg. blurred vision) during i.v. administration.

Very rare: Transient blindness predominantly during intravenous administration

The majority of the blindness cases reported resolved within 20 minutes. Most patients had received chemotherapeutic agents, which included cisplatin. Some cases of transient blindness were reported as cortical in origin.

Cardiac disorders

Uncommon: Arrhythmias, chest pain with or without ST segment depression, bradycardia.

Vascular disorders

Common: Sensation of warmth or flushing.

Uncommon: Hypotension.

Respiratory, thoracic and mediastinal disorders

Uncommon: Hiccups.

Gastrointestinal disorders

Common: Constipation.

Hepatobiliary disorders

Uncommon: Asymptomatic increases in liver function tests[#].

[#]These events were observed commonly in patients receiving chemotherapy with cisplatin.

4.9 Overdose

Little is known at present about overdosage with ondansetron, however, a limited number of patients received overdoses. Manifestations that have been reported include visual disturbances, severe constipation, hypotension and a vasovagal episode with transient second degree AV block. In all instances, the events resolved completely. There is no specific antidote for ondansetron, therefore in all cases of suspected overdose, symptomatic and supportive therapy should be given as appropriate.

5. PHARMACOLOGICAL PROPERTIES

5.1 Pharmacodynamic properties

Ondansetron is a potent, highly selective 5HT3 receptor-antagonist. Its precise mode of action in the control of nausea and vomiting is not known. Chemotherapeutic agents and radiotherapy may cause release of 5HT in the small intestine initiating a vomiting reflex by activating vagal afferents via 5HT3 receptors. Ondansetron blocks the initiation of this reflex. Activation of vagal afferents may also cause a release of 5HT in the area postrema, located on the floor of the fourth ventricle, and this may also promote emesis through a central mechanism. Thus, the effect of ondansetron in the management of the nausea and vomiting induced by cytotoxic chemotherapy and radiotherapy is probably due to antagonism of 5HT3 receptors on neurons located both in the peripheral and central nervous system. The mechanisms of action in post-operative nausea and vomiting are not known but there may be common pathways with cytotoxic induced nausea and vomiting.

Ondansetron does not alter plasma prolactin concentrations.

5.2 Pharmacokinetic properties

Following oral administration, ondansetron is passively and completely absorbed from the gastrointestinal tract and undergoes first pass metabolism. Peak plasma concentrations of about 30ng/ml are attained approximately 1.5 hours after an 8mg dose. For doses above 8mg the increase in ondansetron systemic exposure with dose is greater than proportional; this may reflect some reduction in first pass metabolism at higher oral doses. Bioavailability, following oral administration, is slightly enhanced by the presence of food but unaffected by antacids. Studies in healthy elderly volunteers have shown slight, but clinically insignificant, age-related increases in both oral bioavailability (65%) and half-life (5 hours) of ondansetron. Gender differences were shown in the disposition of ondansetron, with females having a greater rate and extent of absorption following an oral dose and reduced systemic clearance and volume of distribution (adjusted for weight).

The disposition of ondansetron following oral, intramuscular(IM) and intravenous(IV) dosing is similar with a terminal half life of about 3 hours and steady state volume of distribution of about 140L. Equivalent systemic exposure is achieved after IM and IV administration of ondansetron.

A 4mg intravenous infusion of ondansetron given over 5 minutes results in peak plasma concentrations of about 65ng/ml. Following intramuscular administration of ondansetron, peak plasma concentrations of about 25ng/ml are attained within 10 minutes of injection.

Following administration of ondansetron suppository, plasma ondansetron concentrations become detectable between 15 and 60 minutes after dosing. Concentrations rise in an essentially linear fashion, until peak concentrations of 20-30 ng/ml are attained, typically 6 hours after dosing. Plasma concentrations then fall, but at a slower rate than observed following oral dosing due to continued absorption of ondansetron. The absolute bioavailability of ondansetron from the suppository is approximately 60% and is not affected by gender. The half life of the elimination phase following suppository administration is determined by the rate of ondansetron absorption, not systemic clearance and is approximately 6 hours. Females show a small, clinically insignificant, increase in half-life in comparison with males.

Ondansetron is not highly protein bound (70-76%). Ondansetron is cleared from the systemic circulation predominantly by hepatic metabolism through multiple enzymatic pathways. Less than 5% of the absorbed dose is excreted unchanged in the urine. The absence of the enzyme CYP2D6 (the debrisoquine polymorphism) has no effect on ondansetron's pharmacokinetics. The pharmacokinetic properties of ondansetron are unchanged on repeat dosing.

In a study of 21 paediatric patients aged between 3 and 12 years undergoing elective surgery with general anaesthesia, the absolute values for both the clearance and volume of distribution of ondansetron following a single intravenous dose of 2mg (3-7 years old) or 4mg (8-12 years old) were reduced. The magnitude of the change was age-related, with clearance falling from about 300mL/min at 12 years of age to 100mL/min at 3 years. Volume of distribution fell from about 75L at 12 years to 17L at 3 years. Use of weight-based dosing (0.1mg/kg up to 4mg maximum) compensates for these changes and is effective in normalising systemic exposure in paediatric patients.

In patients with renal impairment (creatinine clearance 15-60 ml/min), both systemic clearance and volume of distribution are reduced following IV administration of ondansetron, resulting in a slight, but clinically insignificant, increase in elimination half-life (5.4h). A study in patients with severe renal impairment who required regular haemodialysis (studied between dialyses) showed ondansetron's pharmacokinetics to be essentially unchanged following IV administration.

Specific studies in the elderly or patients with renal impairment have been limited to IV and oral administration. However, it is anticipated that the half-life of ondansetron after rectal administration in these populations will be similar to that seen in healthy volunteers, since the rate of elimination of ondansetron following rectal administration is not determined by systemic clearance.

Following oral, intravenous or intramuscular dosing in patients with severe hepatic impairment, ondansetron's systemic clearance is markedly reduced with prolonged elimination half-lives (15-32 h) and an oral bioavailability approaching 100% due to reduced pre-systemic metabolism. The pharmacokinetics of ondansetron following administration as a suppository have not been evaluated in patients with hepatic impairment.

5.3 Preclinical safety data

No additional data of relevance.

6. PHARMACEUTICAL PARTICULARS

6.1 List of excipients

Lactose, microcrystalline cellulose, pregelatinised maize starch, magnesium stearate, methylhydroxypropylcellulose, titanium dioxide (E171), iron oxide (E172).

6.2 Incompatibilities

None reported.

6.3 Shelf life

36 months

6.4 Special precautions for storage

Store below 30°C.

6.5 Nature and contents of container

Blister packs of 10 or 30 tablets comprising aluminium/PVC blister film and aluminium foil lidding.

Securitainer packs of 30 or 100 tablets.

Not all pack sizes may be marketed.

6.6 Special precautions for disposal and other handling

None stated.

Administrative Data

7. MARKETING AUTHORISATION HOLDER

Glaxo Wellcome UK Limited

Trading as GlaxoSmithKline UK

Stockley Park West

Uxbridge

Middlesex UB11 1BT

8. MARKETING AUTHORISATION NUMBER(S)

PL 10949/0110

9. DATE OF FIRST AUTHORISATION/RENEWAL OF THE AUTHORISATION

9 January 2002

10. DATE OF REVISION OF THE TEXT

17 October 2006

11. Legal Status

POM

Zofran Tablets 8mg

(GlaxoSmithKline UK)

1. NAME OF THE MEDICINAL PRODUCT

Zofran Tablets 8mg.

2. QUALITATIVE AND QUANTITATIVE COMPOSITION

Each Zofran Tablet 8mg is a yellow, oval, film coated tablet engraved "GLAXO" on one face and "8" on the other. Each tablet contains ondansetron 8mg (as hydrochloride dihydrate).

3. PHARMACEUTICAL FORM

Film coated tablet.

4. CLINICAL PARTICULARS

4.1 Therapeutic indications

Zofran is indicated for the management of nausea and vomiting induced by cytotoxic chemotherapy and radiotherapy, and for the prevention and treatment of post-operative nausea and vomiting.

4.2 Posology and method of administration

Chemotherapy and radiotherapy induced nausea and vomiting

Adults:

The emetogenic potential of cancer treatment varies according to the doses and combinations of chemotherapy and radiotherapy regimens used. The route of administration and dose of Zofran should be flexible in the range of 8-32mg a day and selected as shown below.

Emetogenic Chemotherapy and Radiotherapy: Zofran can be given either by rectal, oral (tablets or syrup), intravenous or intramuscular administration.

For oral administration: 8mg 1-2 hours before treatment, followed by 8mg 12 hours later.

To protect against delayed or prolonged emesis after the first 24 hours, oral or rectal treatment with Zofran should be continued for up to 5 days after a course of treatment.

The recommended dose for oral administration is 8mg twice daily.

Highly Emetogenic Chemotherapy: For patients receiving highly emetogenic chemotherapy, eg. high-dose cisplatin, Zofran can be given either by rectal, intravenous or intramuscular administration.

To protect against delayed or prolonged emesis after the first 24 hours, oral or rectal treatment with Zofran should be continued for up to 5 days after a course of treatment.

The recommended dose for oral administration is 8mg twice daily.

Children:

Zofran may be administered as a single intravenous dose of 5mg/m^2 immediately before chemotherapy, followed by 4mg orally twelve hours later. 4mg orally twice daily should be continued for up to 5 days after a course of treatment.

Elderly:

Zofran is well tolerated by patients over 65 years and no alteration of dosage, dosing frequency or route of administration are required.

Patients with Renal Impairment:

No alteration of daily dosage or frequency of dosing, or route of administration are required.

Patients with hepatic Impairment:

Clearance of Zofran is significantly reduced and serum half-life significantly prolonged in subjects with moderate or severe impairment of hepatic function. In such patients a total daily dose of 8mg should not be exceeded.

Post operative nausea and vomiting:

Adults:

For the prevention of PONV: Zofran can be administered orally or by intravenous or intramuscular injection.

For oral administration: 16mg one hour prior to anaesthesia. Alternatively, 8mg one hour prior to anaesthesia followed by two further doses of 8mg at eight hourly intervals.

For the treatment of established PONV: Intravenous or intramuscular administration is recommended.

Children (aged 2 years and over):

For the prevention and treatment of PONV: Slow intravenous injection is recommended.

Elderly:

There is limited experience in the use of Zofran in the prevention and treatment of post-operative nausea and vomiting in the elderly, however Zofran is well tolerated in patients over 65 years receiving chemotherapy.

Patients with renal impairment:

No alteration of daily dosage or frequency of dosing, or route of administration are required.

Patients with hepatic impairment:

Clearance of Zofran is significantly reduced and serum half life significantly prolonged in subjects with moderate or severe impairment of hepatic function. In such patients a total daily dose of 8mg should not be exceeded.

Patients with poor sparteine/debrisoquine metabolism:

The elimination half-life of ondansetron is not altered in subjects classified as poor metabolisers of sparteine and debrisoquine. Consequently in such patients repeat dosing will give drug exposure levels no different from those of the general population. No alteration of daily dosage or frequency of dosing are required.

4.3 Contraindications

Hypersensitivity to any component of the preparation.

4.4 Special warnings and precautions for use

Hypersensitivity reactions have been reported in patients who have exhibited hypersensitivity to other selective $5HT_3$ receptor antagonists.

Very rarely and predominantly with intravenous Zofran, transient ECG changes including QT interval prolongation have been reported. Therefore caution should be exercised in patients with cardiac rhythm or conduction disturbances, in patients treated with anti-arrhythmic agents or beta-adrenergic blocking agents and in patients with significant electrolyte disturbances.

As ondansetron is known to increase large bowel transit time, patients with signs of subacute intestinal obstruction should be monitored following administration.

4.5 Interaction with other medicinal products and other forms of interaction

There is no evidence that ondansetron either induces or inhibits the metabolism of other drugs commonly coadministered with it. Specific studies have shown that there are no pharamcokinetic interactions when ondansetron is administered with alcohol, temazepam, furosemide, tramadol or propofol.

Ondansetron is metabolised by multiple hepatic cytochrome P-450 enzymes: CYP3A4, CYP2D6 and CYP1A2. Due to the multiplicity of metabolic enzymes capable of metabolising ondansetron, enzyme inhibition or reduced activity of one enzyme (e.g. CYP2D6 genetic deficiency) is normally compensated by other enzymes and should result in little or no significant change in overall ondansetron clearance or dose requirement.

Phenytoin, Carbamazepine and Rifampicin: In patients treated with potent inducers of CYP3A4 (i.e. phenytoin, carbamazepine, and rifampicin), the oral clearance of ondansetron was increased and ondansetron blood concentrations were decreased.

Tramadol: Data from small studies indicate that ondansetron may reduce the analgesic effect of tramadol.

4.6 Pregnancy and lactation

The safety of ondansetron for use in human pregnancy has not been established. Evaluation of experimental animal studies does not indicate direct or indirect harmful effects with respect to the development of the embryo, or foetus, the course of gestation and peri- and post-natal development. However as animal studies are not always predictive of human response the use of ondansetron in pregnancy is not recommended.

Tests have shown that ondansetron passes into the milk of lactating animals. It is therefore recommended that mothers receiving Zofran should not breast-feed their babies.

4.7 Effects on ability to drive and use machines

In psychomotor testing ondansetron does not impair performance nor cause sedation.

4.8 Undesirable effects

Adverse events are listed below by system organ class and frequency. Frequencies are defined as: very common (≥1/10), common (≥1/100 and <1/10), uncommon (≥1/1000 and <1/100), rare (≥1/10,000 and <1/1000) and very rare (<1/10,000) including isolated reports. Very common, common and uncommon events were generally determined from clinical trial data. The incidence in placebo was taken into account. Rare and very rare events were generally determined from post-marketing spontaneous data.

The following frequencies are estimated at the standard recommended doses of ondansetron according to indication and formulation.

Immune system disorders

Rare: Immediate hypersensitivity reactions sometimes severe, including anaphylaxis.

Nervous system disorders

Very common: Headache.

Uncommon: Seizures, movement disorders including extrapyramidal reactions such as dystonic reactions, oculogyric crisis and dyskinesia have been observed without definitive evidence of persistent clinical sequelae.

Rare: Dizziness during i.v. administration, which in most cases is prevented or resolved by lengthening the infusion period.

Eye disorders

Rare: Transient visual disturbances (eg. blurred vision) during i.v. administration.

Very rare: Transient blindness predominantly during intravenous administration

The majority of the blindness cases reported resolved within 20 minutes. Most patients had received chemotherapeutic agents, which included cisplatin. Some cases of transient blindness were reported as cortical in origin.

Cardiac disorders

Uncommon: Arrhythmias, chest pain with or without ST segment depression, bradycardia.

Vascular disorders

Common: Sensation of warmth or flushing.

Uncommon: Hypotension.

Respiratory, thoracic and mediastinal disorders

Uncommon: Hiccups.

Gastrointestinal disorders

Common: Constipation.

Hepatobiliary disorders

Uncommon: Asymptomatic increases in liver function tests#.

#These events were observed commonly in patients receiving chemotherapy with cisplatin.

4.9 Overdose

Little is known at present about overdosage with ondansetron, however, a limited number of patients received overdoses. Manifestations that have been reported include visual disturbances, severe constipation, hypotension and a vasovagal episode with transient second degree AV block. In all instances, the events resolved completely. There is no specific antidote for ondansetron, therefore in all cases of suspected overdose, symptomatic and supportive therapy should be given as appropriate.

5. PHARMACOLOGICAL PROPERTIES

5.1 Pharmacodynamic properties

Ondansetron is a potent, highly selective 5HT3 receptor-antagonist. Its precise mode of action in the control of nausea and vomiting is not known. Chemotherapeutic agents and radiotherapy may cause release of 5HT in the small intestine initiating a vomiting reflex by activating vagal afferents via 5HT3 receptors. Ondansetron blocks the initiation of this reflex. Activation of vagal afferents may also cause a release of 5HT in the area postrema, located on the floor of the fourth ventricle, and this may also promote emesis through a central mechanism. Thus, the effect of ondansetron in the management of the nausea and vomiting induced by cytotoxic chemotherapy and radiotherapy is probably due to antagonism of 5HT3 receptors on neurons located both in the peripheral and central nervous system. The mechanisms of action in post-operative nausea and vomiting are not known but there may be common pathways with cytotoxic induced nausea and vomiting.

Ondansetron does not alter plasma prolactin concentrations.

5.2 Pharmacokinetic properties

Following oral administration, ondansetron is passively and completely absorbed from the gastrointestinal tract and undergoes first pass metabolism. Peak plasma concentrations of about 30ng/ml are attained approximately 1.5 hours after an 8mg dose. For doses above 8mg the increase in ondansetron systemic exposure with dose is greater than proportional; this may reflect some reduction in first pass metabolism at higher oral doses. Bioavailability, following oral administration, is slightly enhanced by the presence of food but unaffected by antacids. Studies in healthy elderly volunteers have shown slight, but clinically insignificant, age-related increases in both oral bioavailability (65%) and half-life (5 hours) of ondansetron. Gender differences were shown in the disposition of ondansetron, with females having a greater rate and extent of absorption following an oral dose and reduced systemic clearance and volume of distribution (adjusted for weight).

The disposition of ondansetron following oral, intramuscular(IM) and intravenous(IV) dosing is similar with a terminal half life of about 3 hours and steady state volume of distribution of about 140L. Equivalent systemic exposure is achieved after IM and IV administration of ondansetron.

A 4mg intravenous infusion of ondansetron given over 5 minutes results in peak plasma concentrations of about 65ng/ml. Following intramuscular administration of ondansetron, peak plasma concentrations of about 25ng/ml are attained within 10 minutes of injection.

Following administration of ondansetron suppository, plasma ondansetron concentrations become detectable between 15 and 60 minutes after dosing. Concentrations rise in an essentially linear fashion, until peak concentrations of 20-30 ng/ml are attained, typically 6 hours after dosing. Plasma concentrations then fall, but at a slower rate than observed following oral dosing due to continued absorption of ondansetron. The absolute bioavailability of ondansetron from the suppository is approximately 60% and is not affected by gender. The half life of the elimination phase following suppository administration is determined by the rate of ondansetron absorption, not systemic clearance and is approximately 6 hours. Females show a small, clinically insignificant, increase in half-life in comparison with males.

Ondansetron is not highly protein bound (70-76%). Ondansetron is cleared from the systemic circulation predominantly by hepatic metabolism through multiple enzymatic pathways. Less than 5% of the absorbed dose is excreted unchanged in the urine. The absence of the enzyme CYP2D6 (the debrisoquine polymorphism) has no effect on ondansetron's pharmacokinetics. The pharmacokinetic properties of ondansetron are unchanged on repeat dosing.

In a study of 21 paediatric patients aged between 3 and 12 years undergoing elective surgery with general anaesthesia, the absolute values for both the clearance and volume of distribution of ondansetron following a single intravenous dose of 2mg (3-7 years old) or 4mg (8-12 years old) were reduced. The magnitude of the change was age-related, with clearance falling from about 300mL/min at 12 years of age to 100mL/min at 3 years. Volume of distribution fell from about 75L at 12 years to 17L at 3 years. Use of weight-based dosing (0.1mg/kg up to 4mg maximum) compensates for these changes and is effective in normalising systemic exposure in paediatric patients.

In patients with renal impairment (creatinine clearance 15-60 ml/min), both systemic clearance and volume of distribution are reduced following IV administration of ondansetron, resulting in a slight, but clinically insignificant, increase in elimination half-life (5.4h). A study in patients with severe renal impairment who required regular haemodialysis (studied between dialyses) showed ondansetron's pharmacokinetics to be essentially unchanged following IV administration.

Specific studies in the elderly or patients with renal impairment have been limited to IV and oral administration. However, it is anticipated that the half-life of ondansetron after rectal administration in these populations will be similar to that seen in healthy volunteers, since the rate of elimination of ondansetron following rectal administration is not determined by systemic clearance.

Following oral, intravenous or intramuscular dosing in patients with severe hepatic impairment, ondansetron's systemic clearance is markedly reduced with prolonged elimination half-lives (15-32 h) and an oral bioavailability approaching 100% due to reduced pre-systemic metabolism. The pharmacokinetics of ondansetron following administration as a suppository have not been evaluated in patients with hepatic impairment.

5.3 Preclinical safety data

No additional data of relevance.

6. PHARMACEUTICAL PARTICULARS

6.1 List of excipients

Lactose, microcrystalline cellulose, pregelatinised maize starch, magnesium stearate, methylhydroxypropylcellulose, titanium dioxide (E171), iron oxide (E172).

6.2 Incompatibilities

None reported.

6.3 Shelf life

36 months

6.4 Special precautions for storage

Store below 30C.

6.5 Nature and contents of container

Blister packs of 10, 15, or 30 tablets comprising aluminium/PVC blister film and aluminium foil lidding.

Securitainer packs of 30 or 100 tablets.

Not all pack sizes may be marketed.

6.6 Special precautions for disposal and other handling

None stated.

Administrative Data

7. MARKETING AUTHORISATION HOLDER

Glaxo Wellcome UK Limited
Trading as GlaxoSmithKline UK
Stockley Park West
Uxbridge
Middlesex UB11 1BT

8. MARKETING AUTHORISATION NUMBER(S)

PL 10949/0111

9. DATE OF FIRST AUTHORISATION/RENEWAL OF THE AUTHORISATION

9 January 2002

10. DATE OF REVISION OF THE TEXT

17 October 2006

11. Legal Status

POM

Zoladex 3.6mg Implant

(AstraZeneca UK Limited)

1. NAME OF THE MEDICINAL PRODUCT

Zoladex® 3.6 mg Implant

2. QUALITATIVE AND QUANTITATIVE COMPOSITION

Goserelin acetate (equivalent to 3.6 mg goserelin).

For excipients, see 6.1.

3. PHARMACEUTICAL FORM

Implant, in pre-filled syringe.

4. CLINICAL PARTICULARS

4.1 Therapeutic indications

(i) Treatment of prostate cancer in the following settings (see also section 5.1):

• In the treatment of metastatic prostate cancer where Zoladex has demonstrated comparable survival benefits to surgical castrations (see section 5.1)

• In the treatment of locally advanced prostate cancer, as an alternative to surgical castration where Zoladex has demonstrated comparable survival benefits to an anti-androgen (see section 5.1)

• As adjuvant treatment to radiotherapy in patients with high-risk localised or locally advanced prostate cancer where Zoladex has demonstrated improved disease-free survival and overall survival (see section 5.1)

• As neo-adjuvant treatment prior to radiotherapy in patients with high-risk localised or locally advanced prostate cancer where Zoladex has demonstrated improved disease-free survival (see section 5.1)

• As adjuvant treatment to radical prostatectomy in patients with locally advanced prostate cancer at high risk of disease progression where Zoladex has demonstrated improved disease-free survival (see section 5.1)

(ii) Advanced breast cancer in pre and perimenopausal women suitable for hormonal manipulation.

(iii) Zoladex 3.6 mg is indicated as an alternative to chemotherapy in the standard of care for pre/perimenopausal women with oestrogen receptor (ER) positive early breast cancer.

(iv) Endometriosis: In the management of endometriosis, Zoladex alleviates symptoms, including pain, and reduces the size and number of endometrial lesions.

(v) Endometrial thinning: Zoladex is indicated for the prethinning of the uterine endometrium prior to endometrial ablation or resection.

(vi) Uterine fibroids: In conjunction with iron therapy in the haematological improvement of anaemic patients with fibroids prior to surgery.

(vii) Assisted reproduction: Pituitary downregulation in preparation for superovulation.

4.2 Posology and method of administration

Adults

One 3.6 mg depot of Zoladex injected subcutaneously into the anterior abdominal wall, every 28 days. No dosage adjustment is necessary for patients with renal or hepatic impairment, or in the elderly.

Endometriosis should be treated for a period of six months only, since at present there are no clinical data for longer treatment periods. Repeat courses should not be given due to concern about loss of bone mineral density. In patients receiving Zoladex for the treatment of endometriosis, the addition of hormone replacement therapy (a daily oestrogenic agent and a progestogenic agent) has been shown to reduce bone mineral density loss and vasomotor symptoms.

For use in endometrial thinning: four or eight weeks treatment. The second depot may be required for the patient with a large uterus or to allow flexible surgical timing.

For women who are anaemic as a result of uterine fibroids: Zoladex 3.6 mg depot with supplementary iron may be administered for up to three months before surgery.

Assisted reproduction: Zoladex 3.6 mg is administered to downregulate the pituitary gland, as defined by serum estradiol levels similar to those observed in the early follicular phase (approximately 150 pmol/l). This will usually take between 7 and 21 days.

When downregulation is achieved, superovulation (controlled ovarian stimulation) with gonadotrophin is commenced. The downregulation achieved with a depot agonist is more consistent suggesting that, in some cases, there may be an increased requirement for gonadotrophin. At the appropriate stage of follicular development, gonadotrophin is stopped and human chorionic gonadotrophin (hCG) is administered to induce ovulation. Treatment monitoring, oocyte retrieval and fertilisation techniques are performed according to the normal practice of the individual clinic.

Children

Zoladex is not indicated for use in children.

For correct administration of Zoladex, see instructions on the instruction card.

4.3 Contraindications

Zoladex should not be given to patients with a known hypersensitivity to the active substance, to other LHRH analogues, or to any of the excipients of this product.

Zoladex should not be used in pregnancy (see section 4.6).

4.4 Special warnings and precautions for use

Zoladex is not indicated for use in children, as safety and efficacy have not been established in this group of patients.

Males

The use of Zoladex in men at particular risk of developing ureteric obstruction or spinal cord compression should be considered carefully, and the patients monitored closely during the first month of therapy. Consideration should be given to the initial use of an anti-androgen (e.g. cyproterone acetate 300 mg daily for three days before and three weeks after commencement of Zoladex) at the start of LHRH analogue therapy since this has been reported to prevent the possible sequelae of the initial rise in serum testosterone. If spinal cord compression or renal impairment due to ureteric obstruction are present or develop, specific standard treatment of these complications should be instituted.

The use of LHRH agonists in men may cause a reduction in bone mineral density.

A reduction in glucose tolerance has been observed in males receiving LHRH agonists. This may manifest as diabetes or loss of glycaemic control in those with pre-existing diabetes mellitus. Consideration should therefore be given to monitoring blood glucose.

Females

The use of LHRH agonists in women may cause a reduction in bone mineral density. Following two years treatment for early breast cancer, the average loss of bone mineral density was 6.2% and 11.5% at the femoral neck and lumbar spine respectively. This loss has been shown to be partially reversible at the one year off treatment follow-up with recovery to 3.4% and 6.4% relative to baseline at the femoral neck and lumbar spine respectively, although this recovery is based on very limited data.

In patients receiving Zoladex for the treatment of endometriosis, the addition of hormone replacement therapy (a daily oestrogenic agent and a progestogenic agent), has been shown to reduce bone mineral density loss and vasomotor symptoms.

Zoladex should be used with caution in women with known metabolic bone disease.

Zoladex may cause an increase in uterine cervical resistance, which may result in difficulty in dilating the cervix.

Currently, there are no clinical data on the effect of treating benign gynaecological conditions with Zoladex for periods in excess of six months.

Zoladex should only be administered as part of a regimen for assisted reproduction under the supervision of a specialist experienced in the area.

As with other LHRH agonists, there have been reports of ovarian hyperstimulation syndrome (OHSS), associated with the use of Zoladex 3.6 mg in combination with gonadotrophin. It has been suggested that the downregulation achieved with a depot agonist may lead, in some cases, to an increased requirement for gonadotrophin. The stimulation cycle should be monitored carefully to identify patients at risk of developing OHSS because its severity and incidence may be dependent on the dose regimen of gonadotrophin. Human chorionic gonadotrophin (hCG) should be withheld, if appropriate.

It is recommended that Zoladex is used with caution in assisted reproduction regimens in patients with polycystic ovarian syndrome as follicle recruitment may be increased.

4.5 Interaction with other medicinal products and other forms of interaction

None known.

4.6 Pregnancy and lactation

Pregnancy: Although reproductive toxicity in animals gave no evidence of teratogenic potential, Zoladex should not be used in pregnancy as there is a theoretical risk of abortion or foetal abnormality if LHRH agonists are used during pregnancy. Potentially fertile women should be examined carefully before treatment to exclude pregnancy. Non-hormonal methods of contraception should be employed during therapy and in the case of endometriosis should be continued until menses are resumed.

Pregnancy should be excluded before Zoladex is used for assisted reproduction. The clinical data from use in this setting are limited but the available evidence suggests there is no causal association between Zoladex and any subsequent abnormalities of oocyte development or pregnancy and outcome.

Lactation: The use of Zoladex during breast-feeding is not recommended.

4.7 Effects on ability to drive and use machines

There is no evidence that Zoladex results in impairment of these activities.

4.8 Undesirable effects

General

Rare incidences of hypersensitivity reactions, which may include some manifestations of anaphylaxis, have been reported.

Arthralgia has been reported. Non-specific paraesthesias have been reported. Skin rashes have been reported which are generally mild, often regressing without discontinuation of therapy.

Changes in blood pressure, manifest as hypotension or hypertension, have been occasionally observed in patients administered Zoladex. The changes are usually transient, resolving either during continued therapy or after cessation of therapy with Zoladex. Rarely, such changes have been sufficient to require medical intervention including withdrawal of treatment from Zoladex.

As with other agents in this class, very rare cases of pituitary apoplexy have been reported following initial administration.

Occasional local reactions include mild bruising at the subcutaneous injection site.

The use of LHRH agonists may cause a reduction in bone mineral density (see section 4.4).

Males

Pharmacological effects in men include hot flushes and sweating and a decrease in libido, seldom requiring withdrawal of therapy. Breast swelling and tenderness have been noted infrequently. Initially, prostate cancer patients may experience a temporary increase in bone pain, which can be managed symptomatically. Isolated cases of ureteric obstruction and spinal cord compression have been recorded.

A reduction in glucose tolerance has been observed in males receiving LHRH agonists. This may manifest as diabetes or loss of glycaemic control in those with pre-existing diabetes mellitus.

Females

Pharmacological effects in women include hot flushes and sweating, and loss in libido, seldom requiring withdrawal of therapy. Headaches, mood changes including depression, vaginal dryness and change in breast size have been noted. During early treatment with Zoladex some women may experience vaginal bleeding of variable duration and intensity. If vaginal bleeding occurs it is usually in the first month after starting treatment. Such bleeding probably represents oestrogen withdrawal bleeding and is expected to stop spontaneously.

Initially, breast cancer patients may experience a temporary increase in signs and symptoms, which can be managed symptomatically. In women with fibroids, degeneration of fibroids may occur.

Rarely, breast cancer patients with metastases have developed hypercalcaemia on initiation of therapy.

Rarely, some women may enter the menopause during treatment with LHRH analogues and not resume menses on cessation of therapy. This may simply be a physiological change.

In assisted reproduction: As with other LHRH agonists, there have been reports of ovarian hyperstimulation syndrome (OHSS), associated with the use of Zoladex 3.6 mg in combination with gonadotrophin. It has been suggested that the downregulation achieved with a depot agonist may lead, in some cases, to an increased requirement for gonadotrophin. The stimulation cycle should be monitored carefully to identify patients at risk of developing OHSS because its severity and incidence may be dependent on the dose regimen of gonadotrophin. Human chorionic gonadotrophin (hCG) should be withheld, if appropriate.

Follicular and luteal ovarian cysts have been reported to occur following LHRH therapy. Most cysts are asymptomatic, non functional, varying in size and resolve spontaneously.

4.9 Overdose

There is limited experience of overdosage in humans. In cases where Zoladex has unintentionally been re-administered early or given at a higher dose, no clinically relevant adverse effects have been seen. Animal tests suggest that no effect other than the intended therapeutic effects on sex hormone concentrations and on the reproductive tract will be evident with higher doses of Zoladex. If overdosage occurs, this should be managed symptomatically.

5. PHARMACOLOGICAL PROPERTIES

5.1 Pharmacodynamic properties

Zoladex (D-Ser(Bu^t)^6 Azgly^{10} LHRH) is a synthetic analogue of naturally occurring LHRH. On chronic administration Zoladex results in inhibition of pituitary LH secretion leading to a fall in serum testosterone concentrations in males and serum estradiol concentrations in females. This effect is reversible on discontinuation of therapy. Initially, Zoladex, like other LHRH agonists, may transiently increase serum testosterone concentration in men and serum estradiol concentration in women.

In men, by around 21 days after the first depot injection, testosterone concentrations have fallen to within the castrate range and remain suppressed with continuous treatment every 28 days. This inhibition leads to prostate tumour regression and symptomatic improvement in the majority of patients.

In the management of patients with metastatic prostate cancer, Zoladex has been shown in comparative clinical trials to give similar survival outcomes to those obtained with surgical castrations.

In a combined analysis of 2 randomised controlled trials comparing bicalutamide 150 mg monotherapy versus castration (predominantly in the form of Zoladex), there was no significant difference in overall survival between bicalutamide-treated patients and castration-treated patients (hazard ratio = 1.05 [CI 0.81 to 1.36]) with locally advanced prostate cancer. However, equivalence of the two treatments could not be concluded statistically.

In comparative trials, Zoladex has been shown to improve disease-free survival and overall survival when used as an adjuvant therapy to radiotherapy in patients with high-risk localised (T_1-T_2 and PSA of at least 10 ng/mL or a Gleason score of at least 7), or locally advanced (T_3-T_4) prostate cancer. The optimum duration of adjuvant therapy has not been established; a comparative trial has shown that 3 years of adjuvant Zoladex gives significant survival improvement compared with radiotherapy alone. Neo-adjuvant Zoladex prior to radiotherapy has been shown to improve disease-free survival in patients with high risk localised or locally advanced prostate cancer.

After prostatectomy, in patients found to have extra-prostatic tumour spread, adjuvant Zoladex may improve disease-free survival periods, but there is no significant survival improvement unless patients have evidence of nodal involvement at time of surgery. Patients with pathologically staged locally advanced disease should have additional risk factors such as PSA of at least 10 ng/mL or a Gleason score of at least 7 before adjuvant Zoladex should be considered. There is no evidence of improved clinical outcomes with use of neo-adjuvant Zoladex before radical prostatectomy.

In women, serum estradiol concentrations are suppressed by around 21 days after the first depot injection and, with continuous treatment every 28 days, remain suppressed at levels comparable with those observed in postmenopausal women. This suppression is associated with a response in hormone-dependent advanced breast cancer, uterine fibroids, endometriosis and suppression of follicular development within the ovary. It will produce endometrial thinning and will result in amenorrhoea in the majority of patients.

During treatment with LHRH analogues patients may enter the menopause. Rarely, some women do not resume menses on cessation of therapy.

Zoladex in combination with iron has been shown to induce amenorrhoea and improve haemoglobin concentrations and related haematological parameters in women with fibroids who are anaemic. The combination produced a mean haemoglobin concentration 1 g/dl above that achieved by iron therapy alone.

5.2 Pharmacokinetic properties

The bioavailability of Zoladex is almost complete. Administration of a depot every four weeks ensures that effective concentrations are maintained with no tissue accumulations. Zoladex is poorly protein bound and has a serum elimination half-life of two to four hours in subjects with normal renal function. The half-life is increased in patients with impaired renal function. For the compound given monthly in a depot formulation, this change will have minimal effect. Hence, no change in dosing is necessary in these patients. There is no significant change in pharmacokinetics in patients with hepatic failure.

5.3 Preclinical safety data

Following long-term repeated dosing with Zoladex, an increased incidence of benign pituitary tumours has been observed in male rats. Whilst this finding is similar to that previously noted in this species following surgical castration, any relevance to man has not been established.

In mice, long-term repeated dosing with multiples of the human dose, produced histological changes in some regions of the digestive system manifested by pancreatic islet cell hyperplasia and a benign proliferative condition in the pyloric region of the stomach, also reported as a spontaneous lesion in this species. The clinical relevance of these findings is unknown.

6. PHARMACEUTICAL PARTICULARS

6.1 List of excipients

Lactide/glycolide copolymer.

6.2 Incompatibilities

None known.

6.3 Shelf life

36 months.

6.4 Special precautions for storage

Do not store above 25°C.

6.5 Nature and contents of container

Single dose Safe System㊗ syringe applicator with a protective sleeve.

6.6 Special precautions for disposal and other handling

Use as directed by the prescriber. Use only if pouch is undamaged. Use immediately after opening pouch. Dispose of the syringe in an approved sharps collector.

7. MARKETING AUTHORISATION HOLDER

AstraZeneca UK Limited,

600 Capability Green,

Luton, LU1 3LU, UK.

8. MARKETING AUTHORISATION NUMBER(S)

PL 17901/0064

9. DATE OF FIRST AUTHORISATION/RENEWAL OF THE AUTHORISATION

1st May 2001 (formerly 13.05.1993)

10. DATE OF REVISION OF THE TEXT

4th July 2008

Zoladex LA 10.8mg

(AstraZeneca UK Limited)

1. NAME OF THE MEDICINAL PRODUCT

Zoladex® LA 10.8 mg Implant

2. QUALITATIVE AND QUANTITATIVE COMPOSITION

Goserelin acetate (equivalent to 10.8 mg goserelin).

For excipients, see 6.1.

3. PHARMACEUTICAL FORM

Implant, in pre-filled syringe.

4. CLINICAL PARTICULARS

4.1 Therapeutic indications

Zoladex is indicated (see also section 5.1):

- In the treatment of metastatic prostate cancer where Zoladex has demonstrated comparable survival benefits to surgical castrations (see section 5.1)
- In the treatment of locally advanced prostate cancer, as an alternative to surgical castration where Zoladex has demonstrated comparable survival benefits to an anti-androgen (see section 5.1)
- As adjuvant treatment to radiotherapy in patients with high-risk localised or locally advanced prostate cancer where Zoladex has demonstrated improved disease-free survival and overall survival (see section 5.1)
- As neo-adjuvant treatment prior to radiotherapy in patients with high-risk localised or locally advanced prostate cancer where Zoladex has demonstrated improved disease-free survival (see section 5.1)
- As adjuvant treatment to radical prostatectomy in patients with locally advanced prostate cancer at high risk of disease progression where Zoladex has demonstrated improved disease-free survival (see section 5.1)

4.2 Posology and method of administration

Adult males (including the elderly): one depot of Zoladex LA injected subcutaneously into the anterior abdominal wall every 12 weeks.

Children: Zoladex LA is not indicated for use in children.

Renal impairment: no dosage adjustment is necessary for patients with renal impairment.

Hepatic impairment: no dosage adjustment for patients with hepatic impairment.

For correct administration of Zoladex, see instructions on the instruction card.

4.3 Contraindications
Zoladex LA should not be given to patients with a known hypersensitivity to the active substance, to other LHRH analogues, or to any of the excipients of this product.

4.4 Special warnings and precautions for use
Zoladex LA is not indicated for use in females, since there is insufficient evidence of reliable suppression of serum estradiol. For female patients requiring treatment with goserelin, refer to the prescribing information for Zoladex 3.6 mg.

Zoladex LA is not indicated for use in children, as safety and efficacy have not been established in this group of patients.

The use of Zoladex LA in patients at particular risk of developing ureteric obstruction or spinal cord compression should be considered carefully and the patients monitored closely during the first month of therapy. Consideration should be given to the initial use of an antiandrogen (e.g. cyproterone acetate 300 mg daily for three days before, and three weeks after commencement of Zoladex) at the start of LHRH analogue therapy since this has been reported to prevent the possible sequelae of the initial rise in serum testosterone.

If spinal cord compression or renal impairment due to ureteric obstruction are present or develop, specific standard treatment of these complications should be instituted.

The use of LHRH agonists in men may cause a reduction in bone mineral density.

A reduction in glucose tolerance has been observed in males receiving LHRH agonists. This may manifest as diabetes or loss of glycaemic control in those with pre-existing diabetes mellitus. Consideration should therefore be given to monitoring blood glucose.

4.5 Interaction with other medicinal products and other forms of interaction
None known.

4.6 Pregnancy and lactation
Zoladex LA is not indicated for use in females.

4.7 Effects on ability to drive and use machines
There is no evidence that Zoladex LA results in impairment of ability to drive or operate machinery.

4.8 Undesirable effects
Rare incidences of hypersensitivity reactions, which may include some manifestations of anaphylaxis, have been reported.

Arthralgia has been reported. Non-specific paraesthesias have been reported. Skin rashes have also been reported which are generally mild, often regressing without discontinuation of therapy.

Pharmacological effects in men include hot flushes and sweating and a decrease in libido, seldom requiring withdrawal of therapy. Breast swelling and tenderness have been noted infrequently. Initially, prostate cancer patients may experience a temporary increase in bone pain, which can be managed symptomatically. Isolated cases of spinal cord compression have been recorded.

A reduction in glucose tolerance has been observed in males receiving LHRH agonists. This may manifest as diabetes or loss of glycaemic control in those with pre-existing diabetes mellitus.

The use of LHRH agonists in men may cause a reduction in bone mineral density.

Changes in blood pressure, manifest as hypotension or hypertension, have been occasionally observed in patients administered Zoladex. The changes are usually transient, resolving either during continued therapy or after cessation of therapy with Zoladex. Rarely, such changes have been sufficient to require medical intervention including withdrawal of treatment from Zoladex.

As with other agents in this class, very rare cases of pituitary apoplexy have been reported following initial administration of Zoladex 3.6 mg.

Following the administration of Zoladex 3.6 mg isolated cases of ureteric obstruction have been recorded.

4.9 Overdose
There is limited experience of overdosage in humans. In cases where Zoladex has unintentionally been readministered early or given at a higher dose, no clinically relevant adverse effects have been seen. Animal tests suggest that no effect other than the intended therapeutic effects on sex hormone concentrations and on the reproductive tract will be evident with higher doses of Zoladex LA. If overdosage occurs, this should be managed symptomatically.

5. PHARMACOLOGICAL PROPERTIES

5.1 Pharmacodynamic properties
Zoladex (D-Ser(Bu^t)^{6}Azgly^{10} LHRH) is a synthetic analogue of naturally occurring luteinising-hormone releasing hormone (LHRH). On chronic administration Zoladex LA results in inhibition of pituitary luteinising hormone secretion leading to a fall in serum testosterone concentrations in males. Initially, Zoladex LA like other LHRH agonists transiently increases serum testosterone concentrations.

In men by around 21 days after the first depot injection, testosterone concentrations have fallen to within the castrate range and remain suppressed with treatment every 12 weeks.

In the management of patients with metastatic prostate cancer, Zoladex has been shown in comparative clinical trials to give similar survival outcomes to those obtained with surgical castrations.

In a combined analysis of 2 randomised controlled trials comparing bicalutamide 150 mg monotherapy versus castration (predominantly in the form of Zoladex), there was no significant difference in overall survival between bicalutamide-treated patients and castration-treated patients (hazard ratio = 1.05 [CI 0.81 to 1.36]) with locally advanced prostate cancer. However, equivalence of the two treatments could not be concluded statistically.

In comparative trials, Zoladex has been shown to improve disease-free survival and overall survival when used as an adjuvant therapy to radiotherapy in patients with high-risk localised (T_1-T_2 and PSA of at least 10 ng/mL or a Gleason score of at least 7), or locally advanced (T_3-T_4) prostate cancer. The optimum duration of adjuvant therapy has not been established; a comparative trial has shown that 3 years of adjuvant Zoladex gives significant survival improvement compared with radiotherapy alone. Neo-adjuvant Zoladex prior to radiotherapy has been shown to improve disease-free survival in patients with high risk localised or locally advanced prostate cancer.

After prostatectomy, in patients found to have extra-prostatic tumour spread, adjuvant Zoladex may improve disease-free survival periods, but there is no significant survival improvement unless patients have evidence of nodal involvement at time of surgery. Patients with pathologically staged locally advanced disease should have additional risk factors such as PSA of at least 10 ng/mL or a Gleason score of at least 7 before adjuvant Zoladex should be considered. There is no evidence of improved clinical outcomes with use of neo-adjuvant Zoladex before radical prostatectomy.

5.2 Pharmacokinetic properties
Administration of Zoladex LA every 12 weeks ensures that exposure to goserelin is maintained with no clinically significant accumulation. Zoladex is poorly protein bound and has a serum elimination half-life of two to four hours in subjects with normal renal function. The half-life is increased in patients with impaired renal function. For the compound given in a 10.8 mg depot formulation every 12 weeks this change will not lead to any accumulation. Hence, no change in dosing is necessary in these patients. There is no significant change in pharmacokinetics in patients with hepatic failure.

5.3 Preclinical safety data
Following long-term repeated dosing with Zoladex, an increased incidence of benign pituitary tumours has been observed in male rats. Whilst this finding is similar to that previously noted in this species following surgical castration, any relevance to humans has not been established.

In mice, long-term repeated dosing with multiples of the human dose produced histological changes in some regions of the digestive system. This is manifested by pancreatic islet cell hyperplasia and a benign proliferative condition in the pyloric region of the stomach, also reported as a spontaneous lesion in this species. The clinical relevance of these findings is unknown.

6. PHARMACEUTICAL PARTICULARS

6.1 List of excipients
A blend of high and low molecular weight lactide/glycolide copolymers.

6.2 Incompatibilities
None known.

6.3 Shelf life
36 months.

6.4 Special precautions for storage
Do not store above 25°C.

6.5 Nature and contents of container
Zoladex LA is supplied as a single dose SafeSystem™ syringe applicator with a protective sleeve in a sealed pouch which contains a desiccant.

6.6 Special precautions for disposal and other handling
Use as directed by the prescriber. Use only if pouch is undamaged. Use immediately after opening pouch. Dispose of the syringe in an approved sharps collector.

7. MARKETING AUTHORISATION HOLDER
AstraZeneca UK Limited,
600 Capability Green,
Luton, LU1 3LU, UK.

8. MARKETING AUTHORISATION NUMBER(S)
PL 17901/0065

9. DATE OF FIRST AUTHORISATION/RENEWAL OF THE AUTHORISATION
1st May 2001

10. DATE OF REVISION OF THE TEXT
4th July 2008

Zolvera 40mg/5ml Oral Solution

(Rosemont Pharmaceuticals Limited)

1. NAME OF THE MEDICINAL PRODUCT
ZOLVERA 40mg/5ml Oral Solution

2. QUALITATIVE AND QUANTITATIVE COMPOSITION
Verapamil Hydrochloride 40mg/5ml
For excipients see Section 6.1

3. PHARMACEUTICAL FORM
Oral Solution

4. CLINICAL PARTICULARS

4.1 Therapeutic indications
1. Treatment of mild to moderate hypertension.
2. Treatment and prophylaxis of chronic stable angina, vasospastic angina and unstable angina.
3. Treatment and prophylaxis of paroxysmal supraventricular tachycardia and the reduction of ventricular rate in atrial flutter/fibrillation. Verapamil should not be used when atrial flutter/fibrillation complicates Wolff-Parkinson-White syndrome (see Contraindications).

4.2 Posology and method of administration
Adults:
Hypertension: Initially 120mg b.d. increasing to 160mg b.d. when necessary. In some cases, dosages of up to 480mg daily, in divided doses, have been used. A further reduction in blood pressure may be obtained by combining verapamil with other antihypertensive agents, in particular diuretics. For concomitant administration with beta-blockers see Precautions.

Angina: 120mg t.d.s. is recommended. 80mg t.d.s. can be completely satisfactory in some patients with angina of effort. Less than 120mg t.d.s is not likely to be effective in variant angina.

Supraventricular tachycardias: 40-120mg, t.d.s. according to the severity of the condition.

Children:
Up to 2 years: 20mg, 2-3 times a day.
2 years and above: 40-120mg, 2-3 times a day, according to age and effectiveness.

Elderly:
The adult dose is recommended unless liver or renal function is impaired (see Precautions).

4.3 Contraindications
Hypersensitivity to verapamil or any of the ingredients
Cardiogenic shock
Acute myocardial infarction complicated by bradycardia, hypotension or left ventricular failure
Second or third degree atrioventricular block
Sino-atrial block
Sick sinus syndrome
Uncompensated heart failure
Bradycardia of less than 50 beats/minute
Hypotension of less than 90mmHg systolic
Atrial flutter or fibrillation associated with an accessory pathway (e.g. Wolff-Parkinson-White syndrome, Lown-Ganong-Levine syndrome)
Porphyria
Concomitant ingestion of grapefruit juice.

4.4 Special warnings and precautions for use
Since verapamil is extensively metabolised in the liver, careful dose titration of verapamil is required in patients with liver disease. The disposition of verapamil in patients with renal impairment has not been fully established and therefore careful patient monitoring is recommended. Verapamil is not removed during dialysis.

Verapamil may affect impulse conduction and therefore verapamil solution should be used with caution in patients with first degree AV block. Patients with atrial flutter/fibrillation in association with an accessory pathway (e.g. WPW syndrome) may develop increased conduction across the anomalous pathway and ventricular tachycardia may be precipitated.

Verapamil may affect left ventricular contractility; this effect is small and normally not important but cardiac failure may be precipitated or aggravated.

In patients with incipient cardiac failure, therefore, verapamil should be given only after such cardiac failure has been controlled with appropriate therapy, e.g. digitalis.

When treating hypertension with verapamil, monitoring of the patient's blood pressure at regular intervals is required.

This preparation contains benzoic acid which can irritate skin, eyes and mucous membranes. It may also increase the risk of jaundice in newborn babies.

It also contains liquid maltitol which may cause diarrhoea.

This product also contains liquid maltitol. Patients with rare hereditary problems of fructose should not take this medicine.

4.5 Interaction with other medicinal products and other forms of interaction

Interactions between verapamil and the following medications have been reported:

Digoxin: Verapamil has been shown to increase the serum concentration of digoxin and caution should be exercised with regard to digitalis toxicity. The digitalis level should be determined and the glycoside dose reduced, if required.

Beta-blockers, anti-arrhythmic agents or inhaled anaesthetics: The combination with verapamil may lead to additive cardiovascular effects (e.g. AV block, bradycardia, hypotension, heart failure). Intravenous beta-blockers should not be given to patients under treatment with verapamil.

Carbamazepine, ciclosporin, midazolam, and theophylline: Use of verapamil has resulted in increased serum levels of these medications, which could lead to increased side effects.

Rifampicin, phenytoin and phenobarbital: Serum levels of verapamil are reduced.

Lithium: Serum levels of lithium may be reduced (pharmacokinetic effect); there may be increased sensitivity to lithium causing enhanced neurotoxicity (pharmacodynamic effect).

Cimetidine: Increase in verapamil serum level is possible.

Neuromuscular blocking agents employed in anaesthesia: The effects may be potentiated.

The effects of verapamil may be additive to other hypotensive agents.

Simvastatin: Increased risk of myopathy, and therefore caution should be exercised when combining verapamil with simvastatin.

Sirolimus: Plasma concentration of both drugs may be increased.

Intravenous dantrolene: The combination of verapamil and intravenous dantrolene has been reported to cause hypotension, myocardial depression and hyperkalaemia (in animals). It is recommended that this combination is not used until the relevance of these findings to humans is established.

Alcohol: Plasma concentration may be increased (see Effects on ability to drive and use machines)

Grapefruit Juice: An increase in verapamil levels has been reported.

4.6 Pregnancy and lactation

Although animal studies have not shown any teratogenic effects, verapamil should not be given during the first trimester of pregnancy unless, in the clinician's judgement, it is essential for the welfare of the patient.

Verapamil is excreted into the breast milk in small amounts and is unlikely to be harmful. However, rare hypersensitivity reactions have been reported with verapamil and, therefore, it should only be used during lactation if, in the clinician's judgement, it is essential for the welfare of the patient.

4.7 Effects on ability to drive and use machines

Depending on individual susceptibility, the patient's ability to drive a vehicle or operate machinery may be impaired. This is particularly true in the initial stages of treatment, or when changing over from another medication. Like many other common medicines, verapamil has been shown to increase the blood levels of alcohol and slow its elimination. Therefore, the effects of alcohol may be exaggerated.

4.8 Undesirable effects

Verapamil is generally well tolerated. Side effects are usually mild and transient and discontinuation of therapy is rarely necessary.

Endocrine: On very rare occasions, gynaecomastia has been observed in elderly male patients under long-term verapamil treatment, which was fully reversible in all cases when the drug was discontinued.

Rises in prolactin levels have been reported.

Cardiac: Particularly when given in high doses or in the presence of previous myocardial damage, some cardiovascular effects of verapamil may occasionally be greater than therapeutically desired: bradycardic arrhythmias, such as sinus bradycardia, sinus arrest with asystole, second and third degree AV block, bradyarrhythmia in atrial fibrillation, hypotension, development or aggravation of heart failure.

Hepato-biliary: A reversible impairment of liver function, characterised by an increase in transaminase and/or alkaline phosphatase may occur on very rare occasions during verapamil treatment and is most probably a hypersensitivity reaction.

General: Constipation may occur. Flushing is observed occasionally and headaches, nausea, vomiting, dizziness, fatigue and ankle oedema have been reported rarely.

Allergic reactions (e.g. erythema, pruritus, urticaria, Quincke's oedema, Stevens-Johnson syndrome) are very rarely seen.

Gingival hyperplasia may very rarely occur when the drug is administered over prolonged periods, and is fully reversible when the drug is discontinued. Erythromelalgia and paraesthesia may occur. In very rare cases, there may be myalgia and arthralgia.

4.9 Overdose

The course of symptoms in verapamil intoxication depends on the amount taken, the point in time at which detoxification measures are taken and myocardial contractility (age-related). The main symptoms are as follows: blood pressure fall (at times to values not detectable), shock symptoms, loss of consciousness, first and second degree AV block (frequently as Wenckebach's phenomenon with or without escape rhythms), total AV block with total AV dissociation, escape rhythm, asystole, sinus bradycardia, sinus arrest. The therapeutic measures to be taken depend on the point in time at which verapamil was taken and the type and severity of intoxication symptoms. Gastric lavage, taking the usual precautionary measures may be appropriate. The usual intensive resuscitation measures, such as extrathoracic heart massage, respiration, defibrillation and/or pacemaker therapy. Specific measures to be taken: Elimination of cardiodepressive effects, hypotension or bradycardia. The specific antidote is calcium, e.g. 10-20ml of a 10% calcium gluconate solution administered intravenously (2.25 - 4.5mmol), repeated if necessary or given as a continuous drip infusion (e.g. 5mmol/hour). The following measures may also be necessary: In case of second and third degree AV block, sinus bradycardia, asystole: atropine, isoprenaline, orciprenaline or pacemaker therapy. In case of hypotension after appropriate positioning of the patient: dopamine, dobutamine, noradrenaline. If there are signs of continuing myocardial failure: dopamine, dobutamine, cardiac glycosides or if necessary, repeated calcium gluconate injections.

5. PHARMACOLOGICAL PROPERTIES

5.1 Pharmacodynamic properties

Verapamil is a calcium antagonist which blocks the inward movement of calcium ions in cardiac muscle cells, in smooth muscle cells of the coronary and systemic arteries and in the cells of the intracardiac conduction system. Verapamil lowers peripheral vascular resistance with no reflex tachycardia. Its efficacy in reducing both raised systolic and diastolic blood pressure is thought to be due to this mode of action. The decrease in systemic and coronary vascular resistance and the sparing effect on intracellular oxygen consumption appear to explain the anti-anginal properties of the drug. Because of its effect on the movement of calcium in the intracardiac conduction system, verapamil reduces automaticity, decreases conduction velocity and increases the refractory period.

5.2 Pharmacokinetic properties

Over 90% of verapamil is absorbed following administration with peak plasma concentrations occurring between 1 and 2 hours and does not appear to be affected markedly by food.

Verapamil is subject to pre-systemic hepatic metabolism with up to 80% of the dose eliminated this way. Because of rapid biotransformation of verapamil during its first pass through the portal circulation, absolute bioavailability ranges from 20-35%. Verapamil is widely distributed throughout the body with a distribution half-life of 15-30 mins. Verapamil is 90% bound to plasma proteins, mainly to albumin and α1 glycoprotein. The half life of verapamil after a single oral dose is between 2 and 7h. However, after repeated administration it increases to 4.5 to 12h resulting in accumulation of the drug.

5.3 Preclinical safety data

Verapamil is a drug on which extensive clinical experience has been obtained. Relevant information for the prescriber is provided elsewhere in the Summary of Product Characteristics.

6. PHARMACEUTICAL PARTICULARS

6.1 List of excipients

Propylene glycol, benzoic acid, liquid maltitol, dill water concentrate, liquorice flavour, citric acid monohydrate, sodium citrate and purified water.

6.2 Incompatibilities

Not applicable.

6.3 Shelf life

36 months

3 months once open

6.4 Special precautions for storage

Do not store above 25°C.

6.5 Nature and contents of container

Bottle: Amber (Type III) glass

Closures:

a) Aluminium, EPE wadded, roll-on pilfer proof screw cap.

b) HDPE, EPE wadded, tamper evident screw cap.

c) HDPE, EPE wadded, tamper evident, child resistant closure.

Pack Size: 150ml

6.6 Special precautions for disposal and other handling

Not applicable.

7. MARKETING AUTHORISATION HOLDER

Rosemont Pharmaceuticals Ltd, Rosemont House, Yorkdale Industrial Park, Braithwaite Street, Leeds, LS11 9XE, UK.

8. MARKETING AUTHORISATION NUMBER(S)

PL 00427/0130

9. DATE OF FIRST AUTHORISATION/RENEWAL OF THE AUTHORISATION

23/02/2007

10. DATE OF REVISION OF THE TEXT

23/02/2007

Zomacton 10mg Injection

(Ferring Pharmaceuticals Ltd)

1. NAME OF THE MEDICINAL PRODUCT

ZOMACTON 10 mg/ml, powder and solvent for solution for injection in pre-filled syringe.

2. QUALITATIVE AND QUANTITATIVE COMPOSITION

Somatropin*.10mg

(10mg/ml after reconstitution for one vial)

* Produced in *Escherichia coli* cells using recombinant DNA technology

For full list of excipients, see section 6.1.

3. PHARMACEUTICAL FORM

Powder and solvent for solution for injection in pre-filled syringe.

Zomacton is a white to off-white lyophilised powder. The solvent in prefilled syringe is clear and colourless.

4. CLINICAL PARTICULARS

4.1 Therapeutic indications

Zomacton is indicated for:

- the long-term treatment of children who have growth failure due to inadequate secretion of growth hormone

- the long-term treatment of growth retardation due to Turner's Syndrome confirmed by chromosome analysis.

4.2 Posology and method of administration

Zomacton therapy should be used only under the supervision of a qualified physician experienced in the management of patients with growth hormone deficiency.

The dosage of administration of Zomacton should be individualised for each patient.

The duration of treatment, usually a period of several years will depend on maximum achievable therapeutic benefit.

The subcutaneous administration of growth hormone may lead to loss or increase of adipose tissue at the injection site. Therefore, injection sites should be alternated.

GROWTH HORMONE DEFICIENCY

Generally a dose of 0.17 – 0.23 mg/kg bodyweight (approximating to 4.9 mg/m^2– 6.9 mg/m^2 body surface area) per week divided into 6 - 7 s.c. injections is recommended (corresponding to a daily injection of 0.02 – 0.03 mg/kg bodyweight or 0.7 – 1.0 mg/m^2 body surface area).

The total weekly dose of 0.27 mg/kg or 8 mg/m^2 body surface area should not be exceeded (corresponding to daily injections of up to about 0.04 mg/kg).

TURNER'S SYNDROME

Generally a dose of 0.33 mg/kg/bodyweight (approximating to 9.86 mg/m^2/body surface area) per week divided into 6 - 7 s.c. injections are recommended (corresponding to daily injection of 0.05 mg/kg/bodyweight or 1.40-1.63 mg/m^2/body surface area).

Instructions for preparation, see section 6.6.

Administration

The required dose of ZOMACTON 10 mg/ml is administered with a ZOMAJET VISION X needle-free device or with an ordinary syringe.

Specific instructions for the use of the ZOMAJET VISION X device are given in a booklet supplied with the device.

4.3 Contraindications

Zomacton should not be used in children with closed epiphyses.

Patients with evidence of progression of an underlying intra-cranial lesion or other active neoplasms should not receive Zomacton, since the possibility of a tumor growth promoting effect cannot be excluded. Prior to the initiation of therapy with Zomacton, neoplasms must be inactive and anti-tumor therapy completed.

Pregnancy and lactation (see section 4.6).

Hypersensitivity to somatropin or to any of the excipients.

Patients with acute critical illness suffering complications following open heart surgery, abdominal surgery, multiple accidental trauma, acute respiratory failure, or similar conditions should not be treated with Zomacton (see section 4.4).

4.4 Special warnings and precautions for use

Very rare cases of myositis have been observed and may be due to the metacresol used as preservative. In the case of myalgia or disproportionate pain at the injection site, myositis should be considered and, if confirmed, a Zomacton presentation without metacresol should be used.

Patients should be observed for evidence of glucose intolerance because growth hormone may induce a state of insulin resistance. Zomacton should be used with caution in patients with diabetes mellitus or with a family history predisposing for the disease. Strict monitoring of urine and blood glucose is necessary in these patients. In children with diabetes, the dose of insulin may need to be increased to maintain glucose control during Zomacton therapy.

In patients with growth hormone deficiency secondary to an intra-cranial lesion, frequent monitoring for progression or recurrence of the underlying disease process is advised.

Discontinue Zomacton therapy if progression or recurrence of the lesion occurs. In patients with previous malignant diseases special attention should be given to signs and symptoms of relapse.

Zomacton is not indicated for the long term treatment of paediatric patients who have growth failure due to genetically confirmed Prader-Willi syndrome, unless they also have a diagnosis of GH deficiency. There have been reports of sleep apnoea and sudden death associated with the use of growth hormone in paediatric patients with Prader-Willi syndrome who had one or more of the following risk factors: severe obesity, history of respiratory impairment or unidentified respiratory infection.

Scoliosis may progress in any child during rapid growth. Signs of scoliosis should be monitored during somatropin treatment.

Treatment with Zomacton should be discontinued at renal transplantation.

Rare cases of benign intra-cranial hypertension have been reported. In the event of severe or recurring headache, visual problems, and nausea/vomiting, a funduscopy for papilla edema is recommended. If papilla edema is confirmed, diagnosis of benign intra-cranial hypertension should be considered and if appropriate growth hormone treatment should be discontinued (see also section 4.8).

During treatment with somatropin an enhanced T4 to T3 conversion has been found which may result in a reduction in serum T4 and an increase in serum T3 concentrations. In general, the peripheral thyroid hormone levels have remained within the reference ranges for healthy subjects. The effects of somatropin on thyroid hormone levels may be of clinical relevance in patients with central subclinical hypothyroidism in whom hypothyroidism theoretically may develop. Conversely, in patients receiving replacement therapy with thyroxin mild hyperthyroidism may occur. It is therefore particularly advisable to test thyroid function after starting treatment with somatropin and after dose adjustments.

Leukaemia has been reported in a small number of growth hormone deficient patients treated with Somatropin as well as in untreated patients. Based on clinical experience of more than 10 years, the incidence of leukaemia in GH-treated patients without risk factors is not greater than that in the general population.

Slipped capital femoral epiphysis may occur more frequently in patients with endocrine disorders. A patient treated with Zomacton who develops a limp or complains of hip or knee pain should be evaluated by a physician.

The effects of treatment with growth hormone on recovery were studied in two placebo controlled trials involving 522 critically ill adult patients suffering complications following open heart surgery, abdominal surgery, multiple accidental trauma, or acute respiratory failure.

Mortality was higher (42 % vs. 19 %) among patients treated with growth hormones (doses 5.3 to 8 mg/day) compared to those receiving placebo. Based on this information, such patients should not be treated with growth hormones. As there is no information available on the safety of growth hormone substitution therapy in acutely critically ill patients, the benefits of continued treatment in this situation should be weighed against the potential risks involved.

Experience of local tolerability to administration of ZOMACTON 10 mg/ml with Zomajet Vision X needle-free device has been studied before marketing authorisation in a 12 week study including only Caucasian children.

In all patients developing other or similar acute critical illness, the possible benefit of treatment with growth hormone must be weighed against the possible risk involved.

4.5 Interaction with other medicinal products and other forms of interaction

Glucocorticoid therapy may inhibit the growth promoting effect of Zomacton. Patients with coexisting ACTH deficiency should have their glucocorticoid replacement dose carefully adjusted to avoid impairment of the growth promoting effect of Zomacton.

High doses of androgens, oestrogens, or anabolic steroids can accelerate bone maturation and may, therefore, diminish gain in final height.

Because somatropin can induce a state of insulin resistance, insulin dose may have to be adjusted in diabetic patients receiving concomitant Zomacton.

Data from an interaction study performed in GH deficient adults suggests that somatropin administration may increase the clearance of compounds known to be metabolised by cytochrome P450 isoenzymes. The clearance of compounds metabolised by cytochrome P450 3A4 (e.g. sex steroids, corticosteroids, anticonvulsants and cyclosporin) may be especially increased resulting in lower plasma levels of these compounds. The clinical significance of this is unknown.

4.6 Pregnancy and lactation

For Zomacton no clinical data on exposed pregnancies are available. Thus, the risk for humans is unknown. Although animal studies do not point to a potential risk of somatropin applied during pregnancy, Zomacton should be discontinued if pregnancy occurs. During pregnancy, maternal somatropin will largely be replaced by placental growth hormone.

It is not known whether somatropin is excreted in human milk, however, absorption of intact protein from the gastro-intestinal tract of the infant is unlikely.

4.7 Effects on ability to drive and use machines

Zomacton has no influence on the ability to drive and use machines.

4.8 Undesirable effects

The subcutaneous administration of growth hormone may lead to loss or increase of adipose tissue as well as punctual haemorrhage and bruising at the injection site. On rare occasions patients have developed pain and an itchy rash at the site of injection.

Somatropin has given rise to the formation of antibodies in approximately 1% of the patients. The binding capacity of these antibodies has been low and no clinical changes have been associated with their formation.

Rare cases of benign intra-cranial hypertension have been reported with somatropin (see section 4.4).

Very rare cases of leukaemia have been reported in growth hormone deficient children treated with somatropin, but the incidence appears to be similar to that in children without growth hormone deficiency.

(see Table 1 below)

4.9 Overdose

The recommended dose of Zomacton should not be exceeded.

Although there have been no reports of overdose with Zomacton, acute overdose may result in an initial hypoglycaemia followed by a subsequent hyperglycaemia.

The effects of long-term, repeated use of Zomacton in doses exceeding those recommended, are unknown. However, it is possible that such use might produce signs and symptoms consistent with the known effects of excess human growth hormone (e.g. acromegaly).

Table 1

	Common >1/100, <1/10	Uncommon >1/1000, <1/100	Rare >1/10 000, <1/1000	Very rare <1/10 000
Neoplasms, benign and malignant				Leukaemia
Immune system disorders	Formation of antibodies			
Endocrine disorders	Hypoglycaemia		Diabetes mellitus type II	
Nervous system disorders		Paraesthesia	Benign intracranial Hypertension Transient headache	
Skin and subcutaneous tissue disorders	Transient local skin reactions			
Musculoskeletal, connective tissue and bone disorders		Stiffness in the extremities, arthralgia, myalgia		
General disorders and administration site disorders		Peripheral oedema		

5. PHARMACOLOGICAL PROPERTIES

5.1 Pharmacodynamic properties

Pharmacotherapeutic group: Somatropin and somatropin agonists

ATC code: H 01 AC 01

Pharmacodynamic properties:

Identical to pituitary-derived human growth hormone (pit-hGH) in amino acid sequence, chain length (191 amino acids) and pharmacokinetic profile. Zomacton can be expected to produce the same pharmacological effects as the endogenous hormone.

Skeletal system:

Growth hormone produces a generally proportional growth of the skeletal bone in man. Increased linear growth in children with confirmed deficiency of pit-hGH has been demonstrated after exogenous administration of Zomacton. The measurable increase in height after administration of Zomacton results from an effect on the epiphyseal plates of long bones. In children who lack adequate amounts of pit-hGH, Zomacton produces increased growth rates and increased IGF-1 (Insulin-like Growth Factor/Somatomedin-C) concentrations that are similar to those seen after therapy with pit- hGH. Elevations in mean serum alkaline phosphatase concentrations are also involved.

Other organs and tissues:

An increase in size, proportional to total increase in body weight, occurs in other tissues in response to growth hormone, as well. Changes include: increased growth of connective tissues, skin and appendages; enlargement of skeletal muscle with increase in number and size of cells; growth of the thymus; liver enlargement with increased cellular proliferation; and a slight enlargement of the gonads, adrenals, and thyroid.

Disproportionate growth of the skin and flat bones, and accelerated sexual maturation have not been reported in association with the growth hormone replacement therapy.

Protein, carbohydrate and lipid metabolism:

Growth hormone exerts a nitrogen retaining effect and increases the transport of amino acids into tissue. Both processes augment the synthesis of protein. Carbohydrate use and lipogenesis are depressed by growth hormone. With large doses or in the absence of insulin, growth hormone acts as a diabetogenic agent, producing effects seen typically during fasting (i.e. intolerance to carbohydrate, inhibition of lipogenesis, mobilisation of fat and ketosis).

Mineral metabolism:

Conservation of sodium, potassium, and phosphorous occurs after treatment with growth hormone. Increased calcium loss by the kidney is offset by increased absorption in the gut. Serum calcium concentrations are not significantly altered in patients treated with Zomacton or with pit-hGH. Increased serum concentrations of inorganic phosphates have been shown to occur both after Zomacton and pit-hGH. Accumulation of these minerals signals an increased demand during tissue synthesis.

5.2 Pharmacokinetic properties

Twenty-four (24) healthy adult subjects received 1.67 mg somatropin either by conventional s.c. injection or by ZomaJet Vision needle free device. Peak plasma levels of around 20 ng/ml were observed 3.5 to 4 hours after administration of the medicinal product.

A terminal half-life 2.6 hours was observed when the compound was administered with Zomajet vision needle-free device which is likely to be due to a rate limiting absorption process.

Data from other somatropin containing products suggest that the bioavailability subcutaneously administered somatropin is approximately 80% in healthy adults and that both liver and kidney have been shown to be important protein catabolism organs eliminating the compound.

5.3 Preclinical safety data

Non-clinical data reveal no special hazard for humans based on conventional studies of repeated-dose toxicity and genotoxicity.

Genetically engineered somatropin is identical to endogenous human pituitary growth hormone. It has the same biological properties and it is usually administered in physiological doses. Therefore, studies on safety pharmacology, toxicity to reproduction and carcinogenicity have not been conducted as no such effects are anticipated.

6. PHARMACEUTICAL PARTICULARS

6.1 List of excipients

Powder

Mannitol

Disodium phosphate dodecahydrate

Sodium dihydrogen phosphate dihydrate

Solvent

Metacresol

Water for injections

6.2 Incompatibilities

In the absence of compatibility studies, this medicinal product must not be mixed with other medicinal products.

6.3 Shelf life

2 years

After reconstitution, the solution must be stored for a maximum of 28 days in a refrigerator at 2°C - 8°C.

After reconstitution, store vials in an upright position.

6.4 Special precautions for storage

Store in a refrigerator (2°C to - 8°C); keep in the outer carton in order to protect from light.

For storage condition of the reconstituted medicinal product, see section 6.3.

6.5 Nature and contents of container

Zomacton is supplied in various packs subject to national approvals:

a) Sets for use for needle injection:

Powder: Vial (type I glass) with closure (rubber, halobutyl polymer) in combination with an aluminium seal and "Flip-off" cap (plastic).

Solvent: Pre-filled syringe (type I glass) with tip cap (rubber, halobutyl polymer), plunger stopper (rubber, halobutyl polymer) and a solvent transfer connector (polycarbonate).

Packs: 1, 3 and 5

b) Sets for use with the needle free device Zomajet Vision X:

Powder: Vial (type I glass) with closure (rubber, halobutyl polymer) in combination with an aluminium seal and "Flip-off" cap (plastic).

Solvent: Pre-filled syringe (type I glass) with tip cap (rubber, halobutyl polymer), plunger stopper (rubber, halobutyl polymer) and vial adaptor (polycarbonate and silicone rubber).

Packs: 1, 3 and 5

Not all pack sizes may be marketed.

6.6 Special precautions for disposal and other handling

Reconstitution

The powder should be reconstituted only by introducing the provided solvent contained in the prefilled syringe into the vial.

See the package leaflet for detailed instructions for reconstitution.

The following is a general description of the reconstitution and administration process. Reconstitution should be performed in accordance with good practice rules, particularly in the respect of asepsis.

1. Hands should be washed.
2. Flip off the yellow plastic protective caps from the vial.
3. The top of the vial should be wiped with an antiseptic solution to prevent contamination of the content.
4. Place the vial adaptor or the solvent transfer connector over the centre of the vial with the spike facing downwards then push down firmly until it clicks into place. Remove the adaptor cap.
5. Take the prefilled syringe. Remove the grey cap. Place the syringe into the adaptor / connector of the vial and inject the solvent slowly into the vial aiming the stream of liquid against the glass wall in order to avoid foam.
6. Place the adaptor cap / connector cap back on the adaptor / connector.
7. Gently swirl the vial a few times until the content is completely dissolved. Do not shake; this may cause denaturation of the active substance.
8. If the solution is cloudy or contains particulate matter, it should not be used. In the case of cloudiness after refrigeration, the product should be allowed to warm to room temperature. If cloudiness persists, discard the vial and its contents. The content must be clear and colourless after reconstitution.

Any unused product or waste material should be disposed of in accordance with local requirements.

7. MARKETING AUTHORISATION HOLDER

Ferring Pharmaceuticals Ltd

The Courtyard,

Waterside Drive

Langley

Berkshire SL3 6EZ

8. MARKETING AUTHORISATION NUMBER(S)

PL 03194/0104

9. DATE OF FIRST AUTHORISATION/RENEWAL OF THE AUTHORISATION

21st November 2008

10. DATE OF REVISION OF THE TEXT

21st November 2008

Zomacton 4mg Injection

(Ferring Pharmaceuticals Ltd)

1. NAME OF THE MEDICINAL PRODUCT

Zomacton 4mg, powder and solvent for solution for injection

2. QUALITATIVE AND QUANTITATIVE COMPOSITION

Somatropin* 4mg

(1.3mg/ml or 3.3mg/ml after reconstitution)

* Produced in Escherichia coli cells by recombinant DNA technology

For a full list of excipients, see section 6.1.

3. PHARMACEUTICAL FORM

Powder and solvent for solution for injection.

Zomacton is a white to off-white lyophilised powder in a vial. The solvent in ampoule is clear and colorless.

4. CLINICAL PARTICULARS

4.1 Therapeutic indications

Zomacton is indicated for the long-term treatment of children who have growth failure due to inadequate secretion of growth hormone and for the long-term treatment of growth retardation due to Turner's Syndrome confirmed by chromosome analysis.

4.2 Posology and method of administration

Zomacton therapy should be used only under the supervision of a qualified physician experienced in the management of patients with growth hormone deficiency.

The dosage and schedule of administration of Zomacton should be individualized for each patient.

The duration of treatment, usually a period of several years, will depend on maximum achievable therapeutic benefit.

The subcutaneous administration of growth hormone may lead to loss or increase of adipose tissue at the injection site. Therefore, injection sites should be alternated.

Growth Hormone Deficiency

Generally a dose of 0.17 - 0.23mg/kg bodyweight (approximating to 4.9mg/m^2– 6.9mg/m^2 body surface area) per week divided into 6 - 7 s.c. injections is recommended (corresponding to a daily injection of 0.02 – 0.03mg/kg bodyweight or 0.7 - 1.0mg/m^2 body surface area). The total weekly dose of 0.27mg/kg or 8mg/m^2 body surface area should not be exceeded (corresponding to daily injections of up to about 0.04mg/kg).

Turner's Syndrome

Generally a dose of 0.33mg/kg/bodyweight (approximating to 9.86mg/m^2/body surface area) per week divided into 6 - 7 s.c. injections are recommended (corresponding to daily injection of 0.05mg/kg/bodyweight or 1.40-1.63mg/m^2/body surface area).

4.3 Contraindications

Zomacton should not be used in children with closed epiphyses.

Patients with evidence of progression of an underlying intra-cranial lesion or other active neoplasms should not receive Zomacton, since the possibility of a tumor growth promoting effect cannot be excluded. Prior to the initiation of therapy with Zomacton, neoplasms must be inactive and anti-tumor therapy completed.

Pregnancy and lactation (see section 4.6).

Hypersensitivity to somatropin or to any of the excipients. Zomacton must not be given to premature babies or neonates as the solvent contains benzyl alcohol.

Patients with acute critical illness suffering complications following open heart surgery, abdominal surgery, multiple accidental trauma, acute respiratory failure, or similar conditions should not be treated with Zomacton (see section 4.4).

4.4 Special warnings and precautions for use

Due to the presence of benzyl alcohol as excipient, Zomacton may cause toxic reactions and anaphylactoid reactions in infants and children up to 3 years old and must not be given to premature babies or neonates.

Patients should be observed for evidence of glucose intolerance because growth hormone may induce a state of insulin resistance. Zomacton should be used with caution in patients with diabetes mellitus or with a family history predisposition for the disease. Strict monitoring of urine and blood glucose is necessary in these patients. In children with diabetes, the dose of insulin may need to be increased to maintain glucose control during Zomacton therapy.

In patients with growth hormone deficiency secondary to an intra-cranial lesion, frequent monitoring for progression or recurrence of the underlying disease process is advised.

Discontinue Zomacton therapy if progression or recurrence of the lesion occurs.

In patients with previous malignant diseases special attention should be given to signs and symptoms of relapse.

Zomacton is not indicated for the long term treatment of paediatric patients who have growth failure due to genetically confirmed Prader-Willi syndrome, unless they also have a diagnosis of GH deficiency. There have been reports of sleep apnoea and sudden death associated with the use of growth hormone in paediatric patients with Prader-Willi syndrome who had one or more of the following risk factors: severe obesity, history of respiratory impairment or unidentified respiratory infection.

Scoliosis may progress in any child during rapid growth. Signs of scoliosis should be monitored during somatropin treatment.

Treatment with Zomacton should be discontinued at renal transplantation.

Rare cases of benign intra-cranial hypertension have been reported. In the event of severe or recurring headache, visual problems, and nausea/vomiting, a funduscopy for papilla edema is recommended. If papilla edema is confirmed, diagnosis of benign intra-cranial hypertension should be considered and if appropriate growth hormone treatment should be discontinued (see also section 4.8).

During treatment with somatropin an enhanced T4 to T3 conversion has been found which may result in a reduction in serum T4 and an increase in serum T3 concentrations. In general, the peripheral thyroid hormone levels have remained within the reference ranges for healthy subjects. The effects of somatropin on thyroid hormone levels may be of clinical relevance in patients with central subclinical hypothyroidism in whom hypothyroidism theoretically may develop. Conversely, in patients receiving replacement therapy with thyroxin mild hyperthyroidism may occur. It is therefore particularly advisable to test thyroid function after starting treatment with somatropin and after dose adjustments.

Leukaemia has been reported in a small number of growth hormone deficient patients treated with somatropin as well as in untreated patients. Based on clinical experience of more than 10 years, the incidence of leukaemia in GH-treated patients without risk factors is not greater than that in the general population.

Slipped capital femoral epiphysis may occur more frequently in patients with endocrine disorders. A patient treated with Zomacton who develops a limp or complains of hip or knee pain should be evaluated by a physician.

The effects of treatment with growth hormone on recovery were studied in two placebo controlled trials involving 522 critically ill adult patients suffering complications following open heart surgery, abdominal surgery, multiple accidental trauma, or acute respiratory failure.

Mortality was higher (42% vs. 19%) among patients treated with growth hormones (doses 5.3 to 8mg/day) compared to those receiving placebo. Based on this information, such patients should not be treated with growth hormones. As there is no information available on the safety of growth hormone substitution therapy in acutely critically ill patients, the benefits of continued treatment in this situation should be weighed against the potential risks involved.

In all patients developing other or similar acute critical illness, the possible benefit of treatment with growth hormone must be weighed against the possible risk involved.

4.5 Interaction with other medicinal products and other forms of interaction

Glucocorticoid therapy may inhibit the growth promoting effect of Zomacton. Patients with coexisting ACTH deficiency should have their glucocorticoid replacement dose carefully adjusted to avoid impairment of the growth promoting effect of Zomacton.

High doses of androgens, oestrogens, or anabolic steroids can accelerate bone maturation and may, therefore, diminish gain in final height.

Because somatropin can induce a state of insulin resistance, insulin dose may have to be adjusted in diabetic patients receiving concomitant Zomacton.

Data from an interaction study performed in GH deficient adults suggests that somatropin administration may increase the clearance of compounds known to be metabolised by cytochrome P450 isoenzymes. The clearance of compounds metabolised by cytochrome P450 3A4 (e.g. sex steroids, corticosteroids, anticonvulsants and cyclosporin) may be especially increased resulting in lower plasma levels of these compounds. The clinical significance of this is unknown.

4.6 Pregnancy and lactation

For Zomacton no clinical data on exposed pregnancies are available. Thus, the risk for humans is unknown. Although animal studies do not point to a potential risk of somatropin applied during pregnancy, Zomacton should be discontinued if pregnancy occurs. During pregnancy, maternal somatropin will largely be replaced by placental growth hormone.

It is not known whether somatropin is excreted in human milk, however, absorption of intact protein from the gastrointestinal tract of the infant is unlikely.

4.7 Effects on ability to drive and use machines

No effects on the ability to drive and use machines have been observed.

4.8 Undesirable effects

The subcutaneous administration of growth hormone may lead to loss or increase of adipose tissue at the injection site. On rare occasions patients have developed pain and an itchy rash at the site of injection.

Somatropin has given rise to the formation of antibodies in approximately 1% of the patients. The binding capacity of these antibodies has been low and no clinical changes have been associated with their formation.

Rare cases of benign intra-cranial hypertension have been reported with somatropin (see section 4.4).

Very rare cases of leukaemia have been reported in growth hormone deficient children treated with somatropin, but the incidence appears to be similar to that in children without growth hormone deficiency.

(see Table 1 below)

4.9 Overdose

The recommended dose of Zomacton should not be exceeded.

Although there have been no reports of overdosage with Zomacton, acute overdosage may result in an initial hypoglycaemia followed by a subsequent hyperglycaemia.

The effects of long-term, repeated use of Zomacton in doses exceeding those recommended, are unknown. However, it is possible that such use might produce signs and symptoms consistent with the known effects of excess human growth hormone (e.g. acromegaly).

5. PHARMACOLOGICAL PROPERTIES

5.1 Pharmacodynamic properties

Pharmacotherapeutic group: Somatropin and somatropin agonists

ATC code: H 01 AC 01

Identical to pituitary-derived human growth hormone (pit-hGH) in amino acid sequence, chain length (191 amino acids) and pharmacokinetic profile. Zomacton can be expected to produce the same pharmacological effects as the endogenous hormone.

Skeletal system:

Growth hormone produces a generally proportional growth of the skeletal bone in man. Increased linear growth in children with confirmed deficiency of pit-hGH has been demonstrated after exogenous administration of Zomacton. The measurable increase in height after administration of Zomacton results from an effect on the epiphyseal plates of long bones. In children who lack adequate amounts of pit-hGH, Zomacton produces increased growth rates and increased IGF-1 (Insulin-like Growth Factor/Somatomedin-C) concentrations that are similar to those seen after therapy with pit- hGH. Elevations in mean serum alkaline phosphatase concentrations are also involved.

Other organs and tissues:

An increase in size, proportional to total increase in body weight, occurs in other tissues in response to growth hormone, as well. Changes include: increased growth of connective tissues, skin and appendages; enlargement of skeletal muscle with increase in number and size of cells; growth of the thymus; liver enlargement with increased cellular proliferation; and a slight enlargement of the gonads, adrenals, and thyroid. Disproportionate growth of the skin and flat bones, and accelerated sexual maturation have not been reported in association with the growth hormone replacement therapy.

Protein, carbohydrate and lipid metabolism:

Growth hormone exerts a nitrogen-retaining effect and increases the transport of amino acids into tissue. Both processes augment the synthesis of protein. Carbohydrate use and lipogenesis are depressed by growth hormone. With large doses or in the absence of insulin, growth hormone acts as a diabetogenic agent, producing effects seen typically during fasting (i.e. intolerance to carbohydrate, inhibition of lipogenesis, mobilisation of fat and ketosis).

Mineral metabolism:

Conservation of sodium, potassium, and phosphorous occurs after treatment with growth hormone. Increased calcium loss by the kidney is offset by increased absorption in the gut. Serum calcium concentrations are not significantly altered in patients treated with Zomacton or with pit-hGH. Increased serum concentrations of inorganic phosphates have been shown to occur both after Zomacton and pit-hGH. Accumulation of these minerals signals an increased demand during tissue synthesis.

5.2 Pharmacokinetic properties

Eight healthy subjects received 0.1mg somatropin/kg body weight. Peak plasma levels of about 64ng/ml were found 6 hours after administration.

5.3 Preclinical safety data

Single dose toxicity:

Single dose toxicity studies were performed in rats (intramuscular application of 10mg/kg), dogs and monkeys (intramuscular dose of 5mg/kg, corresponding to the 50 - 100 fold of the human therapeutic dose). There was no evidence of drug-related toxicity in any of these species.

Repeated dose toxicity:

No relevant toxicological signs were observed in a rat study in which doses of 1.10mg/kg/day for 30 days and 0.37mg/kg/day for 90 days were administered to the animals.

Reproduction toxicology, mutagenic and carcinogenic potential

Genetically engineered somatropin is identical to endogenous human pituitary growth hormone. It has the same biological properties and it is usually administered in physiological doses. Therefore, it was not deemed necessary to perform the full range of such toxicological studies. Untoward effects on reproduction organs, on pregnancy and lactation are unlikely and also no carcinogenic potential has to be expected. A mutagenicity study showed the absence of mutagenic potential.

6. PHARMACEUTICAL PARTICULARS

6.1 List of excipients

The solution contains benzyl alcohol 9mg/ml.

Powder

Mannitol

Solvent

Sodium chloride

Benzyl alcohol

Water for injections

6.2 Incompatibilities

In the absence of compatibility studies, this medicinal product must not be mixed with other medicinal products.

6.3 Shelf life

3 years

After reconstitution, may be stored for a maximum of 14 days in a refrigerator at 2 °C-8 °C.

Store vials in an upright position.

6.4 Special precautions for storage

Unopened vial: Store in a refrigerator (2°C - 8°C); keep in the outer carton in order to protect from light.

For storage condition of the reconstituted medicinal product, see section 6.3.

6.5 Nature and contents of container

Zomacton is supplied in various packs subject to national approvals:

a) Powder in a vial (type I glass) with a stopper (grey halobutyl rubber), a seal and a "flip-off" top + 3.5 ml solvent in ampoule (type I glass): Pack size of 1, 5 and 10

b) Sets including powder in vial (type I glass) with a stopper (grey halobutyl rubber), a seal and a "flip-off" top + 3.5 ml solvent in ampoule (type I glass), a CE-marked syringe (polypropylene) with a plunger (polypropylene), a seal, and CE-marked needle (stainless steel) Pack size of 5

c) Sets for use with the needle free device ZomaJet 2 Vision including: powder in a vial (type I glass) with a stopper(grey halobutyl rubber), a seal and a "flip-off" top + 3.5 ml solvent in ampoule (type I glass), a CE-marked syringe (polypropylene) with a plunger (polypropylene), a seal, a CE-marked needle (stainless steel), and an CE-marked adapter (polycarbonate resin with silicone rubber membrane/seal)

Pack size of 1, 5 and 10

Not all pack sizes may be marketed.

6.6 Special precautions for disposal and other handling

Reconstitution

Zomacton powder is reconstituted by introducing the benzyl alcohol preserved isotonic saline solvent into the vial. After reconstitution the solvent forms a clear and colorless solution for injection.

Two concentrations can be prepared: 3.3mg/ml for use with the ZomaJet 2 Vision or conventional syringes and 1.3mg/ml for conventional syringes only.

The solution for injection 3.3mg/ml is prepared by reconstituting the Zomacton powder with 1.3ml benzyl alcohol preserved saline solvent using a graduated disposable syringe.

The solution for injection 1.3mg/ml is prepared by reconstituting Zomacton powder with 3.2ml of benzyl alcohol preserved saline solvent using a disposable syringe.

To prevent foaming of the solution, the stream of solvent should be aimed against the side of the vial. The vial must then be swirled with a gentle rotary motion until the contents are completely dissolved and a clear, colorless solution is produced. Since Zomacton is a protein, shaking or vigorous mixing is not recommended. If after mixing, the solution is cloudy or contains particulate matter, the contents must be discarded. In the case of cloudiness after refrigeration, the product should be allowed to warm to room temperature. If cloudiness persists or coloration appears, discard the vial and its contents.

Administration

The required Zomacton dose is administered by using the ZomaJet 2 Vision, a needle free device or alternatively a conventional syringe.

Specific instructions for use of the ZomaJet 2 Vision are given in a brochure supplied with the device.

Any unused product or waste material should be disposed of in accordance with local requirements.

7. MARKETING AUTHORISATION HOLDER

Ferring Pharmaceuticals Ltd

The Courtyard

Waterside Drive

Langley

Berkshire

SL3 6EZ

8. MARKETING AUTHORISATION NUMBER(S)

PL 03194/0052

9. DATE OF FIRST AUTHORISATION/RENEWAL OF THE AUTHORISATION

17/03/1995

10. DATE OF REVISION OF THE TEXT

April 2009

Table 1

	Common >1/100, <1/10	Uncommon >1/1000, <1/100	Rare >1/10 000, <1/1000	Very rare <1/10 000
Neoplasms, benign and malignant				Leukaemia
Immune system disorders	Formation of antibodies			
Endocrine disorders			Diabetes mellitus type II	
Nervous system disorders		Paraesthesia	Benign intracranial hypertension	
Skin and subcutaneous tissue disorders	transient local skin reactions			
Musculoskeletal, connective tissue and bone disorders		Stiffness in the extremities, arthralgia, myalgia		
General disorders and administration site disorders		Peripheral oedema		

Zomig Tablets 2.5mg

(AstraZeneca UK Limited)

1. NAME OF THE MEDICINAL PRODUCT

'Zomig'

2. QUALITATIVE AND QUANTITATIVE COMPOSITION

Tablets for oral administration containing 2.5 mg of zolmitriptan.

For excipients see 6.1.

3. PHARMACEUTICAL FORM

Tablets.

4. CLINICAL PARTICULARS

4.1 Therapeutic indications

'Zomig' is indicated for the acute treatment of migraine with or without aura.

4.2 Posology and method of administration

The recommended dose of 'Zomig' to treat a migraine attack is 2.5 mg.

If symptoms persist or return within 24 hours, a second dose has been shown to be effective. If a second dose is required, it should not be taken within 2 hours of the initial dose.

If a patient does not achieve satisfactory relief with 2.5 mg doses, subsequent attacks can be treated with 5 mg doses of 'Zomig'.

In those patients who respond, significant efficacy is apparent within 1 hour of dosing.

'Zomig' is equally effective whenever the tablets are taken during a migraine attack; although it is advisable that 'Zomig' tablets are taken as early as possible after the onset of migraine headache.

In the event of recurrent attacks, it is recommended that the total intake of 'Zomig' in a 24 hour period should not exceed 10 mg.

'Zomig' is not indicated for prophylaxis of migraine.

Use in Children (under 12 years of age)

Safety and efficacy of zolmitriptan tablets in paediatric patients have not been evaluated. Use of Zomig in children is therefore not recommended.

Adolescents (12 - 17 years of age)

The efficacy of Zomig tablets was not demonstrated in a placebo controlled clinical trial for patients aged 12 to

17 years. Use of Zomig tablets in adolescents is therefore not recommended.

Use in Patients Aged Over 65 years

Safety and efficacy of 'Zomig' in individuals aged over 65 years have not been systematically evaluated.

Patients with Hepatic Impairment

Metabolism is reduced in patients with hepatic impairment (See Section 5.2 Pharmacokinetic properties). Therefore for patients with moderate or severe hepatic impairment a maximum dose of 5 mg in 24 hours is recommended.

Patients with Renal Impairment

No dosage adjustment required (see Section 5.2 Pharmacokinetic Properties).

4.3 Contraindications

'Zomig' is contraindicated in patients with:

- Known hypersensitivity to any component of the product
- Uncontrolled hypertension
- Ischaemic heart disease
- Coronary vasospasm/Prinzmetal's angina
- A history of cerebrovascular accident (CVA) or transient ischaemic attack (TIA)
- Concomitant administration of Zomig with ergotamine or ergotamine derivatives or other 5-HT_1 receptor agonists.

4.4 Special warnings and precautions for use

'Zomig' should only be used where a clear diagnosis of migraine has been established. Care should be taken to exclude other potentially serious neurological conditions. There are no data on the use of 'Zomig' in hemiplegic or basilar migraine. Migraneurs may be at risk of certain cerebrovascular events. Cerebral haemorrhage, subarachnoid haemorrhage, stroke, and other cerebrovascular events have been reported in patients treated with $5\text{HT}_{1B/1D}$ agonists.

'Zomig' should not be given to patients with symptomatic Wolff-Parkinson-White syndrome or arrhythmias associated with other cardiac accessory conduction pathways.

In very rare cases, as with other $5\text{HT}_{1B/1D}$ agonists, coronary vasopasm, angina pectoris and myocardial infarction have been reported. In patients with risk factors for ischaemic heart disease, cardiovascular evaluation prior to commencement of treatment with this class of compounds, including 'Zomig'', is recommended (see Section 4.3 Contraindications). These evaluations, however, may not identify every patient who has cardiac disease, and in very rare cases, serious cardiac events have occurred in patients without underlying cardiovascular disease.

As with other $5\text{HT}_{1B/1D}$ agonists, atypical sensations over the precordium (see Section 4.8 Undesirable Effects) have been reported after the administration of zolmitriptan. If chest pain or symptoms consistent with ischaemic heart disease occur, no further doses of zolmitriptan should be taken until after appropriate medical evaluation has been carried out.

As with other $5\text{HT}_{1B/1D}$ agonists transient increases in systemic blood pressure have been reported in patients with and without a history of hypertension; very rarely these increases in blood pressure have been associated with significant clinical events.

As with other $5\text{HT}_{1B/1D}$ agonists, there have been rare reports of anaphylaxis/anaphylactoid reactions in patients receiving Zomig.

Excessive use of an acute anti-migraine medicinal product may lead to an increased frequency of headache, potentially requiring withdrawal of treatment.

Serotonin Syndrome has been reported with combined use of triptans, and Selective Serotonin Reuptake Inhibitors (SSRIs) and Serotonin Norepinephrine Reuptake Inhibitors (SNRIs). Serotonin Syndrome is a potentially life-threatening condition, and it may include signs and symptoms such as: mental status changes (e.g. agitation, hallucinations, coma), autonomic instability, (e.g. tachycardia, labile blood-pressure, hyperthermia), neuromuscular aberrations (e.g. hyperreflexia, in-coordination), and/or gastrointestinal symptoms (e.g. nausea, vomiting, diarrhoea). Careful observation of the patient is advised, if concomitant treatment with Zomig and an SSRI or SNRI is clinically warranted, particularly during treatment initiation and dosage increases (See section 4.5).

4.5 Interaction with other medicinal products and other forms of interaction

There is no evidence that concomitant use of migraine prophylactic medications has any effect on the efficacy or unwanted effects of 'Zomig' (for example beta blockers, oral dihydroergotamine, and pizotifen).

The pharmacokinetics and tolerability of 'Zomig' were unaffected by acute symptomatic treatments such as paracetamol, metoclopramide and ergotamine. Concomitant administration of other $5\text{HT}_{1B/1D}$ agonists within 12 hours of 'Zomig' treatment should be avoided.

Data from healthy subjects suggest there are no pharmacokinetic or clinically significant interactions between Zomig and ergotamine, however, the increased risk of coronary vasospasm is a theoretical possibility. Therefore, it is advised to wait at least 24 hours following the use of ergotamine containing preparations before administering Zomig. Conversely it is advised to wait at least six hours following use of Zomig before administering any ergotamine preparation (see Section 4.3 Contraindications).

Following administration of moclobemide, a specific MAO-A inhibitor, there was a small increase (26%) in AUC for zolmitriptan and a 3-fold increase in AUC of the active metabolite. Therefore, a maximum intake of 5 mg 'Zomig' in 24 hours is recommended in patients taking an MAO-A inhibitor.

Following the administration of cimetidine, a general P450 inhibitor, the half life of zolmitriptan was increased by 44% and the AUC increased by 48%. In addition the half life and AUC of the active N-desmethylated metabolite (183C91) were doubled. A maximum dose of 5 mg 'Zomig' in 24 hours is recommended in patients taking cimetidine. Based on the overall interaction profile, an interaction with inhibitors of the cytochrome P450 isoenzyme CYP1A2 cannot be excluded. Therefore, the same dosage reduction is recommended with compounds of this type, such as fluvoxamine and the quinolone antibiotics (eg, ciprofloxacin).

Fluoxetine does not affect the pharmacokinetic parameters of zolmitriptan. Therapeutic doses of the specific serotonin reuptake inhibitors, fluoxetine, sertraline, paroxetine and citalopram do not inhibit CYP1A2. However, Serotonin Syndrome has been reported during combined use of triptans, and SSRIs (e.g. fluoxetine, paroxetine, sertraline) and SNRIs (e.g. venlafaxine, duloxetine) (See section 4.4).

As with other $5\text{HT}_{IB/ID}$ agonists, there is the potential for dynamic interactions with the herbal remedy St John's wort (Hypericum perforatum) which may result in an increase in undesirable effects.

4.6 Pregnancy and lactation

Pregnancy

'Zomig' should be used in pregnancy only if the benefits to the mother justify potential risk to the foetus. There are no studies in pregnant women, but there is no evidence of teratogenicity in animal studies. (See Section 5.3 Preclinical Safety Data).

Lactation

Studies have shown that zolmitriptan passes into the milk of lactating animals. No data exist for passage of zolmitriptan into human breast milk. Therefore, caution should be exercised when administering 'Zomig' to women who are breast-feeding.

4.7 Effects on ability to drive and use machines

There was no significant impairment of performance of psychomotor tests with doses up to 20 mg 'Zomig'. Use is unlikely to result in an impairment of the ability of patients to drive or operate machinery. However it should be taken into account that somnolence may occur.

4.8 Undesirable effects

Zomig is well tolerated. Adverse reactions are typically mild/moderate, transient, not serious and resolve spontaneously without additional treatment.

Possible adverse reactions tend to occur within 4 hours of dosing and are no more frequent following repeated dosing.

The incidences of ADRs associated with ZOMIG therapy are tabulated below according to the format recommended by the Council for International Organizations of Medical Sciences (CIOMS III Working Group; 1995).

Frequency	System organ class	Event
Common (≥1% - <10%)	Nervous System Disorders	Abnormalities or disturbances of sensation Dizziness Headache Hyperaesthesia Paraesthesia Somnolence Warm sensation
	Cardiac Disorders	Palpitations
	Gastrointestinal Disorders	Abdominal Pain Dry mouth Nausea Vomiting
	Musculoskeletal and Connective Tissue Disorders	Muscle weakness Myalgia
	General Disorders	Asthenia Heaviness, tightness, pain or pressure in throat, neck limbs or chest
Uncommon (≥0.1% - < 1.0%)	Cardiac Disorders	Tachycardia
	Vascular Disorders	Transient increases in systemic blood pressure
	Renal and Urinary disorders	Polyuria Increased Urinary frequency
Rare (≥0.01% - <0.1%)	Immune System Disorders	Anaphylaxis/ Anaphylactoid Reactions Hypersensitivity reactions
	Skin and Subcutaneous Tissue Disorders	Angioedema Urticaria
Very rare (<0.01%)	Cardiac Disorders	Angina pectoris Coronary Vasospasm Myocardial Infarction
	Gastrointestinal Disorders	Bloody diarrhoea Gastrointestinal infarction or necrosis Gastrointestinal ischaemic events Ischaemic colitis Splenic Infarction
	Renal and Urinary Disorders	Urinary Urgency

4.9 Overdose

Volunteers receiving single oral doses of 50 mg commonly experienced sedation.

The elimination half-life of zolmitriptan tablets is 2.5 to 3 hours, (see Section 5.2 Pharmacokinetic Properties) and therefore monitoring of patients after overdose with 'Zomig' tablets should continue for at least 15 hours or while symptoms or signs persist.

There is no specific antidote to zolmitriptan. In cases of severe intoxication, intensive care procedures are recommended, including establishing and maintaining a patent airway, ensuring adequate oxygenation and ventilation, and monitoring and support of the cardiovascular system.

It is unknown what effect haemodialysis or peritoneal dialysis has on the serum concentrations of zolmitriptan.

5. PHARMACOLOGICAL PROPERTIES

5.1 Pharmacodynamic properties

In pre-clinical studies, zolmitriptan has been demonstrated to be a selective agonist for the vascular human recombinant 5HT_{1B} and 5HT_{1D} receptor subtypes. Zolmitriptan is a high affinity $5\text{HT}_{1B/1D}$ receptor agonist with modest affinity for 5HT_{1A} receptors. Zolmitriptan has no significant affinity (as measured by radioligand binding assays) or pharmacological activity at 5HT_2-, 5HT_3-, 5HT_4-, alpha$_1$-, alpha$_2$-, or beta$_1$-, adrenergic; H_1-, H_2-, histaminic; muscarinic; dopaminergic$_1$, or dopaminergic$_2$ receptors. The 5HT_{1D} receptor is predominately located presynaptically at both the peripheral and central synapses of the trigeminal nerve and preclinical studies have shown that zolmitriptan is able to act at both these sites.

One controlled clinical trial in 696 adolescents with migraine failed to demonstrate superiority of zolmitriptan tablets at doses of 2.5 mg, 5 mg and 10 mg over placebo. Efficacy was not demonstrated.

5.2 Pharmacokinetic properties

Zolmitriptan is rapidly and well absorbed (at least 64%) after oral administration to man. The mean absolute bioavailability of the parent compound is approximately 40%. There is an active metabolite (183C91, the N-desmethyl metabolite) which is also a $5\text{HT}_{1B/1D}$ agonist and is 2 to 6 times as potent, in animal models, as zolmitriptan.

In healthy subjects, when given as a single dose, zolmitriptan and its active metabolite 183C91, display dose-proportional AUC and C_{max} over the dose range 2.5 to 50 mg. Absorption is rapid with 75% of C_{max} achieved within 1 hour and plasma concentrations are sustained subsequently for 4 to 6 hours. Zolmitriptan absorption is unaffected by the presence of food. There is no evidence of accumulation on multiple dosing of zolmitriptan.

Zolmitriptan is eliminated largely by hepatic biotransformation followed by urinary excretion of the metabolites. There are three major metabolites: the indole acetic acid, (the major metabolite in plasma and urine), the N-oxide and N-desmethyl analogues. The N-desmethylated metabolite (183C91) is active whilst the others are not. Plasma concentrations of 183C91 are approximately half those of the parent drug, hence it would therefore be expected to contribute to the therapeutic action of 'Zomig'. Over 60% of a single oral dose is excreted in the urine (mainly as the indole acetic acid metabolite) and about 30% in faeces, mainly as unchanged parent compound.

A study to evaluate the effect of liver disease on the pharmacokinetics of zolmitriptan showed that the AUC and C_{max} were increased by 94% and 50% respectively in patients with moderate liver disease and by 226% and 47% in patients with severe liver disease compared with healthy volunteers. Exposure to the metabolites, including the active metabolite, was decreased. For the 183C91 metabolite, AUC and Cmax were reduced by 33% and

44% in patients with moderate liver disease and by 82% and 90% in patients with severe liver disease.

The plasma half-life ($T_{1/2}$) of Zolmitriptan was 4.7 hours in healthy volunteers, 7.3 hours in patients with moderate liver disease and 12 hours in those with severe liver disease. The corresponding $T_{1/2}$ values for the 183C91 metabolite were 5.7 hours, 7.5 hours and 7.8 hours respectively.

Following intravenous administration, the mean total plasma clearance is approximately 10 ml/min/kg, of which one third is renal clearance. Renal clearance is greater than glomerular filtration rate suggesting renal tubular secretion. The volume of distribution following intravenous administration is 2.4 L/kg. Plasma protein binding is low (approximately 25%). The mean elimination half-life of zolmitriptan is 2.5 to 3 hours. The half-lives of its metabolites are similar, suggesting their elimination is formation-rate limited.

Renal clearance of zolmitriptan and all its metabolites is reduced (7 to 8 fold) in patients with moderate to severe renal impairment compared to healthy subjects, although the AUC of the parent compound and the active metabolite were only slightly higher (16 and 35% respectively) with a 1 hour increase in half-life to 3 to 3.5 hours. These parameters are within the ranges seen in healthy volunteers.

In a small group of healthy individuals there was no pharmacokinetic interaction with ergotamine. Concomitant administration of 'Zomig' with ergotamine/caffeine was well tolerated and did not result in any increase in adverse events or blood pressure changes as compared with 'Zomig' alone.

Following the administration of rifampicin, no clinically relevant differences in the pharmacokinetics of zolmitriptan or its active metabolite were observed.

Selegiline, an MAO-B inhibitor, and fluoxetine (a selective serotonin reuptake inhibitor; SSRI) had no effect on the pharmacokinetic parameters of zolmitriptan.

The pharmacokinetics of zolmitriptan in healthy elderly subjects were similar to those in healthy young volunteers.

5.3 Preclinical safety data

An oral teratology study of 'Zomig' has been conducted. At the maximum tolerated doses of 'Zomig', 1200 mg/kg/day (AUC 605 μg/ml.h: approx. 3700 × AUC of the human maximum recommended daily intake of 15 mg) and 30 mg/kg/day (AUC 4.9 μg/ml.h: approx. 30 × AUC of the human maximum recommended daily intake of 15 mg) in rats and rabbits, respectively, no signs of teratogenicity were apparent.

Five genotoxicity tests have been performed. It was concluded that 'Zomig' is not likely to pose any genetic risk in humans.

Carcinogenicity studies in rats and mice were conducted at the highest feasible doses and gave no suggestion of tumorogenicity.

Reproductive studies in male and female rats, at dose levels limited by toxicity, revealed no effect on fertility.

6. PHARMACEUTICAL PARTICULARS

6.1 List of excipients

The following excipients are contained in each tablet as indicated:

Hydroxypropyl methylcellulose

Iron oxide - yellow

Lactose

Magnesium stearate

Microcrystalline cellulose

Polyethylene glycol (400 and 8000)

Sodium starch glycollate

Titanium dioxide

6.2 Incompatibilities

None known

6.3 Shelf life

3 years.

6.4 Special precautions for storage

Do not store above 30°C.

6.5 Nature and contents of container

Tablet strength	Carton (pack) contents	Total number of tablets
2.5mg	1 strip of 3 tablets	3
	2 strips of 3 tablets	6
	2 strips of 3 tablets (with wallet)	6
	2 strips of 6 tablets	12
	4 strips of 3 tablets	12
	6 strips of 3 tablets	18

6.6 Special precautions for disposal and other handling

No specific instructions.

7. MARKETING AUTHORISATION HOLDER

AstraZeneca UK Limited

600 Capability Green

Luton LU1 3LU

United Kingdom

8. MARKETING AUTHORISATION NUMBER(S)

PL 17901/0066

9. DATE OF FIRST AUTHORISATION/RENEWAL OF THE AUTHORISATION

8th June 2000

10. DATE OF REVISION OF THE TEXT

28th January 2008

Zomig 5mg Nasal Spray

(AstraZeneca UK Limited)

1. NAME OF THE MEDICINAL PRODUCT

Zomig 5 mg Nasal Spray.

2. QUALITATIVE AND QUANTITATIVE COMPOSITION

Zomig Nasal Spray is an aqueous solution containing 50 mg/ml zolmitriptan, buffered to pH 5.0. The device delivers a unit dose of 5 mg and is intended for a single use only.

For excipients see 6.1.

3. PHARMACEUTICAL FORM

Nasal Spray.

4. CLINICAL PARTICULARS

4.1 Therapeutic indications

Zomig is indicated for the acute treatment of migraine with or without aura.

4.2 Posology and method of administration

The recommended dose of Zomig Nasal Spray to treat a migraine attack is 5 mg.

Zomig Nasal Spray is administered as a single dose into one nostril. Zomig Nasal Spray provides particularly rapid onset of relief of migraine with the first signs of efficacy apparent within 15 minutes of dosing.

Zomig Nasal Spray provides an alternative non–oral formulation of zolmitriptan to that of Zomig oral tablets and orodispersible tablets. This formulation may also be beneficial where a non–oral route of treatment is either needed or preferred.

If symptoms persist or return within 24 hours a second dose has been shown to be effective. If a second dose is required, it should not be taken within 2 hours of the initial dose.

Zomig is effective whenever the nasal spray is administered during a migraine attack; although it is advisable that Zomig Nasal Spray is taken as early as possible after the onset of migraine headache.

In the event of recurrent attacks, it is recommended that the total intake of Zomig in a 24 hour period should not exceed 10 mg.

Zomig is not indicated for prophylaxis of migraine.

Use in children (under 12 years of age)

Safety and efficacy of Zomig Nasal Spray in paediatric patients have not been evaluated. Use of Zomig Nasal Spray in children is therefore not recommended.

Adolescents (12-17 years of age)

Safety and efficacy of Zomig Nasal Spray in adolescents have not been evaluated. Use of Zomig Nasal Spray in adolescents is therefore not recommended.

Use in Patients Aged Over 65 years

Safety and efficacy of Zomig in individuals aged over 65 years have not been systematically evaluated.

Patients with Hepatic Impairment

The effect of hepatic disease on the pharmacokinetics of zolmitriptan nasal spray has not been evaluated. However, for patients with moderate or severe hepatic impairment metabolism after oral dosing is reduced and a maximum dose of 5 mg oral zolmitriptan in 24 hours is recommended (see Section 5.2 Pharmacokinetic Properties).

Patients with Renal Impairment

No dosage adjustment required (see Section 5.2 Pharmacokinetic Properties).

4.3 Contraindications

Zomig is contraindicated in patients with:

– known hypersensitivity to any component of the product

– uncontrolled hypertension

– ischaemic heart disease

– coronary vasospasm/Prinzmetal's angina

– A history of cerebrovascular accident (CVA) or transient ischaemic attack (TIA)

– Concomitant administration of Zomig with ergotamine or ergotamine derivatives or other 5-HT_1 receptor agonists.

4.4 Special warnings and precautions for use

Zomig should only be used where a clear diagnosis of migraine has been established. Care should be taken to exclude other potentially serious neurological conditions. There are no data on the use of Zomig in hemiplegic or basilar migraine. Migraneurs may be at risk of certain cerebrovascular events. Cerebral haemorrhage, subarachnoid haemorrhage, stroke, and other cerebrovascular events have been reported in patients treated with $5HT_{1B/1D}$ agonists.

Zomig should not be given to patients with symptomatic Wolff-Parkinson-White syndrome or arrhythmias associated with other cardiac accessory conduction pathways.

In very rare cases, as with other $5HT_{1B/1D}$ agonists, coronary vasospasm, angina pectoris and myocardial infarction have been reported. In patients with risk factors for ischaemic heart disease, cardiovascular evaluation prior to commencement of treatment with this class of compounds, including Zomig, is recommended (see Section 4.3 Contraindications). These evaluations, however, may not identify every patient who has cardiac disease, and in very rare cases, serious cardiac events have occurred in patients without underlying cardiovascular disease.

As with other $5HT_{1B/1D}$ agonists, atypical sensations over the precordium (see Section 4.8 Undesirable Effects) have been reported after the administration of zolmitriptan.

If chest pain or symptoms consistent with ischaemic heart disease occur, no further doses of zolmitriptan should be taken until after appropriate medical evaluation has been carried out.

As with other 5HT $_{1B/1D}$ agonists transient increases in systemic blood pressure have been reported in patients with and without a history of hypertension; very rarely these increases in blood pressure have been associated with significant clinical events.

As with other 5HT $_{1B/1D}$ agonists, there have been rare reports of anaphylaxis/anaphylactoid reactions in patients receiving Zomig.

Excessive use of an acute anti-migraine medicinal product may lead to an increased frequency of headache, potentially requiring withdrawal of treatment.

Serotonin Syndrome has been reported with combined use of triptans, and Selective Serotonin Reuptake Inhibitors (SSRIs) and Serotonin Norepinephrine Reuptake Inhibitors (SNRIs). Serotonin Syndrome is a potentially life-threatening condition, and it may include signs and symptoms such as: mental status changes (e.g. agitation, hallucinations, coma), autonomic instability, (e.g. tachycardia, labile blood-pressure, hyperthermia), neuromuscular aberrations (e.g. hyperreflexia, in-coordination), and/or gastrointestinal symptoms (e.g. nausea, vomiting, diarrhoea). Careful observation of the patient is advised, if concomitant treatment with Zomig and an SSRI or SNRI is clinically warranted, particularly during treatment initiation and dosage increases (See section 4.5).

4.5 Interaction with other medicinal products and other forms of interaction

From studies using oral zolmitriptan tablets, there is no evidence that concomitant use of migraine prophylactic medications has any effect on the efficacy or unwanted effects of Zomig (for example beta-blockers, oral dihydroergotamine, pizotifen).

The pharmacokinetics and tolerability of Zomig oral tablets were unaffected by acute symptomatic treatments such as paracetamol, metoclopramide and ergotamine.

Concomitant administration of other $5HT_{1B/1D}$ agonists within 12 hours of Zomig treatment should be avoided.

Data from healthy subjects suggest that there are no pharmacokinetic or clinically significant interactions between Zomig and ergotamine, however, the increased risk of coronary vasospasm is a theoretical possibility. Therefore, it is advised to wait at least 24 hours following the use of ergotamine containing preparations before administering Zomig. Conversely it is advised to wait at least six hours following use of Zomig before administering any ergotamine preparation (see Section 4.3 Contraindications).

Following co-administration of moclobemide, a specific MAO-A inhibitor, and Zomig oral tablets, there was a small increase (26%) in AUC for zolmitriptan and a 3-fold increase in AUC of the active metabolite. Therefore, a maximum intake of 5 mg Zomig nasal spray in 24 hours is recommended in patients taking an MAO-A inhibitor.

Following the co-administration of cimetidine, a general P450 inhibitor, and Zomig oral tablets, the half-life of zolmitriptan was increased by 44% and the AUC increased by 48%. In addition the half-life and AUC of the active N-desmethylated metabolite (183C91) were doubled. A maximum dose of 5 mg Zomig Nasal Spray in 24 hours is recommended in patients taking cimetidine. Based on the overall interaction profile, an interaction with inhibitors of the cytochrome P450 isoenzyme CYP1A2 cannot be excluded. Therefore, the same dosage reduction is recommended with compounds of this type, such as fluvoxamine and the quinolone antibiotics (e.g. ciprofloxacin).

Fluoxetine did not affect the pharmacokinetic parameters of zolmitriptan in a study using oral zolmitriptan tablets. Therapeutic doses of the specific serotonin reuptake inhibitors, fluoxetine, sertraline, paroxetine and citalopram do not inhibit CYP1A2. However, Serotonin Syndrome has been reported during combined use of triptans, and SSRIs (e.g. fluoxetine, paroxetine, sertraline) and SNRIs (e.g. venlafaxine, duloxetine) (See section 4.4).

As with other $5HT_{1b/1d}$ agonists, there is the potential for dynamic interactions with the herbal remedy St John's wort (Hypericum perforatum) which may result in an increase in undesirable effects.

The absorption and pharmacokinetics of Zomig Nasal Spray is unaltered by prior administration of the sympathomimetic vasoconstrictor, xylometazoline.

4.6 Pregnancy and lactation

Pregnancy

Zomig should be used in pregnancy only if the benefits to the mother justify potential risk to the foetus. There are no studies in pregnant women, but there is no evidence of teratogenicity in animal studies. (See Section 5.3 Preclinical Safety Data).

Lactation

Studies have shown that zolmitriptan passes into the milk of lactating animals. No data exist for passage of zolmitriptan into human breast milk. Therefore, caution should be exercised when administering Zomig to women who are breast-feeding.

4.7 Effects on ability to drive and use machines

There was no significant impairment of performance of psychomotor tests with doses up to 20 mg oral Zomig. Use is unlikely to result in an impairment of the ability of patients to drive or operate machinery. However it should be taken into account that somnolence may occur.

4.8 Undesirable effects

Zomig is well tolerated. Adverse reactions are typically mild/moderate, transient, not serious and resolve spontaneously without additional treatment.

Possible adverse reactions tend to occur within 4 hours of dosing and are no more frequent following repeated dosing.

The incidences of ADRs associated with ZOMIG therapy are tabulated below according to the format recommended by the Council for International Organizations of Medical Sciences (CIOMS III Working Group; 1995).

Frequency	System organ class	Event
Very common ($\geq$10%)	Nervous system disorders	Taste Disturbance[1]
Common ($\geq$1% - <10%)	Nervous System Disorders	Abnormalities or disturbances of sensation Dizziness Headache Hyperaesthesia Paraesthesia Somnolence Warm sensation
	Cardiac Disorders	Palpitations
	Respiratory System Disorders	Epistaxis[1] Discomfort of Nasal Cavity[1]
	Gastrointestinal Disorders	Abdominal Pain Dry mouth Nausea Vomiting
	Musculoskeletal and Connective Tissue Disorders	Muscle weakness Myalgia
	General Disorders	Asthenia Heaviness, tightness, pain or pressure in throat, neck limbs or chest
Uncommon ($\geq$0.1% - < 1.0%)	Cardiac Disorders	Tachycardia
	Vascular Disorders	Transient increases in systemic blood pressure
	Renal and Urinary disorders	Polyuria Increased Urinary frequency
Rare ($\geq$0.01% - <0.1%)	Immune System Disorders	Anaphylaxis/ Anaphylactoid Reactions Hypersensitivity reactions
	Skin and Subcutaneous Tissue Disorders	Angioedema Urticaria
Very rare (<0.01%)	Cardiac Disorders	Angina pectoris Coronary Vasospasm Myocardial Infarction
	Gastrointestinal Disorders	Bloody diarrhoea Gastrointestinal infarction or necrosis Gastrointestinal ischaemic events Ischaemic colitis Splenic Infarction
	Renal and Urinary Disorders	Urinary Urgency

1 ZOMIG NASAL SPRAY only

4.9 Overdose

There has been no experience of overdose with zolmitriptan nasal spray. Volunteers receiving single oral doses of 50 mg commonly experienced sedation.

The elimination half-life of zolmitriptan following intranasal administration is 3 hours, (see Section 5.2 Pharmacokinetic Properties) and therefore monitoring of patients after overdose with Zomig Nasal Spray should continue for at least 15 hours or while symptoms or signs persist.

There is no specific antidote to zolmitriptan. In cases of severe intoxication, intensive care procedures are recommended, including establishing and maintaining a patent airway, ensuring adequate oxygenation and ventilation, and monitoring and support of the cardiovascular system.

5. PHARMACOLOGICAL PROPERTIES

5.1 Pharmacodynamic properties

In pre-clinical studies, zolmitriptan has been demonstrated to be a selective agonist for the vascular human recombinant $5HT_{1B}$ and $5HT_{1D}$ receptor subtypes. Zolmitriptan is a high affinity $5HT_{1B/1D}$ receptor agonist with modest affinity for $5HT_{1A}$ receptors. Zolmitriptan has no significant affinity (as measured by radioligand binding assays) or pharmacological activity at $5HT_2$-, $5HT_3$-, $5HT_4$-, alpha$_1$-, alpha$_2$-, or beta$_1$-, adrenergic; H_1-, H_2-, histaminic; muscarinic; dopaminergic$_1$, or dopaminergic$_2$ receptors.

The $5HT_{1B/1D}$ receptor is predominantly located presynaptically at both the peripheral and central synapses of the trigeminal nerve and preclinical studies have shown that zolmitriptan is able to act at both these sites.

One controlled clinical trial in 696 adolescents with migraine failed to demonstrate superiority of zolmitriptan tablets at doses of 2.5 mg, 5 mg and 10 mg over placebo. Efficacy was not demonstrated.

5.2 Pharmacokinetic properties

Zolmitriptan, following intranasal administration, is rapidly absorbed with detectable levels in the plasma within 5 minutes of dosing. A proportion of the dose seems to be directly absorbed in the naso-pharynx. On average 40% of C_{max} of the parent compound, zolmitriptan, is achieved within 15 minutes. The appearance in plasma of the active metabolite, 183C91, which is partly formed through first-pass metabolism, is delayed by 15 to 60 minutes post-dose. C_{max} of the parent compound, zolmitriptan is achieved after 3 hours. Plasma concentrations are sustained for up to 4 to 6 hours. Elimination of zolmitriptan and the active metabolite 183C91 after oral and intranasal delivery appear similar; the mean elimination half-life ($t\frac{1}{2}$) for both zolmitriptan and 183C91 are approximately 3 hours. The bioavailability of intranasal relative to oral administration is 102%. In healthy volunteers after single and multiple intranasal doses, zolmitriptan and its active metabolite 183C91 display dose proportional AUC and C_{max} over the range 1 to 5 mg. There is no evidence of accumulation of zolmitriptan after multiple intranasal dosing.

The plasma concentrations and elimination pharmacokinetics of zolmitriptan and the three major metabolites for the nasal spray and conventional tablet formulations are similar.

Following oral administration of Zomig conventional tablets, zolmitriptan is rapidly and well absorbed (at least 64%). The mean absolute bioavailability of the parent compound is approximately 40%.

Absorption is rapid with 75% of C_{max} achieved within 1 hour and plasma concentrations are sustained subsequently for 4 to 6 hours. After oral administration zolmitriptan absorption is unaffected by the presence of food.

Zolmitriptan is eliminated largely by hepatic biotransformation followed by urinary excretion of the metabolites. There are three major metabolites: the indole acetic acid, (the major metabolite in plasma and urine), the N-oxide and N-desmethyl analogues. The N-desmethyl metabolite (183C91) is an active metabolite which is also a $5H_{1B/1D}$ agonist and is 2 to 6 times as potent, in animal models, as zolmitriptan. Plasma concentrations of 183C91 are approximately half those of the parent drug, hence it would therefore be expected to contribute to the therapeutic action of Zomig. Over 60% of a single oral dose is excreted in the urine (mainly as the indole acetic acid metabolite) and about 30% in faeces, mainly as unchanged parent compound.

A study using oral zolmitriptan to evaluate the effect of liver disease on the pharmacokinetics of zolmitriptan showed that the AUC and C_{max} were increased by 94% and 50% respectively in patients with moderate liver disease and by 226% and 47% in patients with severe liver disease compared with healthy volunteers. Exposure to the metabolites, including the active metabolite, was decreased. For the 183C91 metabolite, AUC and C_{max} were reduced by 33% and 44% in patients with moderate liver disease and by 82% and 90% in patients with severe liver disease.

The plasma half-life ($T\frac{1}{2}$) of zolmitriptan was 4.7 hours in healthy volunteers, 7.3 hours in patients with moderate liver disease and 12 hours in those with severe liver disease. The corresponding $T\frac{1}{2}$ values for the 183C91 metabolite were 5.7 hours, 7.5 hours and 7.8 hours respectively. No studies have been undertaken to characterise the pharmacokinetics of intranasally administered zolmitriptan in patients with hepatic impairment.

Following intravenous administration, the mean total plasma clearance is approximately 10 ml/min/kg, of which one third is renal clearance. Renal clearance is greater than glomerular filtration rate suggesting renal tubular secretion. The volume of distribution following intravenous administration is 2.4 L/kg. Plasma protein binding is low (approximately 25%). The mean elimination half-life of zolmitriptan is 2.5 to 3 hours. The half-lives of its metabolites are similar, suggesting their elimination is formation-rate limited.

Renal clearance of zolmitriptan and all its metabolites is reduced (7 to 8 fold) in patients with moderate to severe renal impairment compared to healthy subjects, although the AUC of the parent compound and the active metabolite were only slightly higher (16 and 35% respectively) with a 1 hour increase in half-life to 3 to 3.5 hours. These parameters are within the ranges seen in healthy volunteers. These findings originate from studies with zolmitriptan tablets.

In a small group of healthy individuals there was no pharmacokinetic interaction with ergotamine. Concomitant administration of Zomig with ergotamine/caffeine was well tolerated and did not result in any increase in adverse events or blood pressure changes as compared with Zomig alone. These findings originate from studies with zolmitriptan tablets.

Selegiline, an MAO-B inhibitor, and fluoxetine (a selective serotonin reuptake inhibitor; SSRI) had no effect on the pharmacokinetic parameters of zolmitriptan. These findings originate from studies with zolmitriptan tablets.

Following the administration of rifampicin, no clinically relevant differences in the pharmacokinetics of zolmitriptan or its active metabolite were observed. The findings originate from studies with zolmitriptan tablets.

The pharmacokinetics of zolmitriptan in healthy elderly subjects were similar to those in healthy young volunteers. These findings originate from studies with zolmitriptan tablets.

The absorption of zolmitriptan nasal spray in healthy volunteers was found unaltered when administered concomitantly with the sympathomimetic nasal decongestant, xylometazoline.

5.3 Preclinical safety data

An oral teratology study of Zomig has been conducted. At the maximum tolerated doses of Zomig, 1200 mg/kg/day (AUC 605 µg/ml.h: approx. 3700 × AUC of the human maximum recommended daily intake of 15 mg) and 30 mg/kg/day (AUC 4.9 µg/ml.h: approx. 30 × AUC of the human maximum recommended daily intake of 15 mg) in rats and rabbits, respectively, no signs of teratogenicity were apparent.

A number of genotoxicity tests have been performed. It was concluded that Zomig is not likely to pose any genetic risk in humans.

Carcinogenicity studies in rats and mice were conducted at the highest feasible doses and gave no suggestion of tumorogenicity.

Reproductive studies in male and female rats, at dose levels limited by toxicity, revealed no effect on fertility.

6. PHARMACEUTICAL PARTICULARS

6.1 List of excipients

Each Zomig Nasal Spray vial contains the following excipients:

Citric acid

Disodium phosphate

Purified Water

6.2 Incompatibilities

None known.

6.3 Shelf life

30 months.

6.4 Special precautions for storage

Do not store above 25°C.

6.5 Nature and contents of container

Ph Eur Type I glass vials which are closed with chlorobutyl rubber stoppers. The vials are assembled into a unit dose nasal spray device, comprising of a vial holder, an actuation device and a protection cover.

Packs containing 1, 2, or 6 single use devices.

6.6 Special precautions for disposal and other handling

The protection cover must not be removed until immediately before use. For instructions for use see the patient information leaflet.

7. MARKETING AUTHORISATION HOLDER

AstraZeneca UK Limited

600 Capability Green

Luton

LU1 3LU

UK

8. MARKETING AUTHORISATION NUMBER(S)

PL 17901/0095

9. DATE OF FIRST AUTHORISATION/RENEWAL OF THE AUTHORISATION

19th September 2002/18th June 2008

10. DATE OF REVISION OF THE TEXT

18th June 2008

Zomig Rapimelt 2.5mg

(AstraZeneca UK Limited)

1. NAME OF THE MEDICINAL PRODUCT

'Zomig Rapimelt'

2. QUALITATIVE AND QUANTITATIVE COMPOSITION

Oro-dispersible tablets containing 2.5 mg of zolmitriptan.

For excipients, see Section 6.1.

3. PHARMACEUTICAL FORM

Oro-dispersible tablets.

4. CLINICAL PARTICULARS

4.1 Therapeutic indications

'Zomig Rapimelt' is indicated for the acute treatment of migraine with or without aura.

4.2 Posology and method of administration

The recommended dose of 'Zomig Rapimelt' to treat a migraine attack is 2.5mg. 'Zomig Rapimelt' rapidly dissolves when placed on the tongue and is swallowed with the patient's saliva. A drink of water is not required when taking 'Zomig Rapimelt'. 'Zomig Rapimelt' can be taken when water is not available thus allowing early administration of treatment for a migraine attack. This formulation may also be beneficial for patients who suffer from nausea and are unable to drink during a migraine attack, or for patients who do not like swallowing conventional tablet.

If symptoms persist or return within 24 hours, a second dose of zolmitriptan has been shown to be effective. If a second dose is required, it should not be taken within 2 hours of the initial dose.

If a patient does not achieve satisfactory relief with 2.5 mg doses, subsequent attacks can be treated with 5 mg doses of 'Zomig Rapimelt'. In those patients who respond, significant efficacy is apparent within 1 hour of dosing with zolmitriptan.

Zolmitriptan is equally effective whenever the tablets are taken during a migraine attack; although it is advisable that 'Zomig Rapimelt' is taken as early as possible after the onset of migraine headache.

In the event of recurrent attacks, it is recommended that the total intake of 'Zomig Rapimelt' in a 24 hour period should not exceed 10 mg.

'Zomig Rapimelt' is not indicated for prophylaxis of migraine.

Use in Children (under 12 years of age)

Safety and efficacy of zolmitriptan tablets in paediatric patients have not been evaluated. Use of Zomig Rapimelt in children is therefore not recommended.

Adolescents (12 - 17 years of age)

The efficacy of Zomig tablets was not demonstrated in a placebo controlled clinical trial for patients aged 12 to 17 years. Use of Zomig Rapimelt tablets in adolescents is therefore not recommended.

Use in Patients Aged Over 65 years

Safety and efficacy of 'Zomig Rapimelt' in individuals aged over 65 years have not been established.

Patients with Hepatic Impairment

Metabolism is reduced in patients with hepatic impairment (See Section 5.2 Pharmacokinetic properties). Therefore for patients with moderate or severe hepatic impairment a maximum dose of 5 mg in 24 hours is recommended.

Patients with Renal Impairment

No dosage adjustment required (see Section 5.2 Pharmacokinetic Properties).

4.3 Contraindications

'Zomig Rapimelt' is contraindicated in patients with:

- Known hypersensitivity to any component of the product.
- Uncontrolled hypertension.
- Ischaemic heart disease.
- Coronary vasospasm/Prinzmetal's angina.
- A history of cerebrovascular accident (CVA) or transient ischaemic attack (TIA)
- Concomitant administration of Zomig with ergotamine or ergotamine derivatives or other 5-HT_1 receptor agonists.

4.4 Special warnings and precautions for use

'Zomig Rapimelt' should only be used where a clear diagnosis of migraine has been established. Care should be taken to exclude other potentially serious neurological conditions. There are no data on the use of 'Zomig Rapimelt' in hemiplegic or basilar migraine. Migraineurs may be at risk of certain cerebrovascular events. Cerebral haemorrhage, subarachnoid haemorrhage, stroke, and other cerebrovascular events have been reported in patients treated with $5HT_{1B/1D}$ agonists.

'Zomig Rapimelt' should not be given to patients with symptomatic Wolff-Parkinson-White syndrome or arrhythmias associated with other cardiac accessory conduction pathways.

In very rare cases, as with other $5HT_{1B/1D}$ agonists, coronary vasospasm, angina pectoris and myocardial infarction have been reported. In patients with risk factors for ischaemic heart disease, cardiovascular evaluation prior to commencement of treatment with this class of compounds, including 'Zomig Rapimelt', is recommended (see Section 4.3 Contraindications). These evaluations, however, may not identify every patient who has cardiac disease, and in very rare cases, serious cardiac events have occurred in patients without underlying cardiovascular disease.

As with other $5HT_{1B/1D}$ agonists, atypical sensations over the precordium (see Section 4.8 Undesirable Effects) have been reported after the administration of zolmitriptan. If chest pain or symptoms consistent with ischaemic heart disease occur, no further doses of zolmitriptan should be taken until after appropriate medical evaluation has been carried out.

As with other $5HT_{1B/1D}$ agonists transient increases in systemic blood pressure have been reported in patients with and without a history of hypertension; very rarely these increases in blood pressure have been associated with significant clinical events.

As with other $5HT_{1B/1D}$ agonists, there have been rare reports of anaphylaxis/anaphylactoid reactions in patients receiving Zomig.

Patients with phenylketonuria should be informed that 'Zomig Rapimelt' contains phenylalanine (a component of aspartame). Each 2.5 mg orally dispersible tablet contains 2.81 mg of phenylalanine.

Excessive use of an acute anti-migraine medicinal product may lead to an increased frequency of headache, potentially requiring withdrawal of treatment.

Serotonin Syndrome has been reported with combined use of triptans, and Selective Serotonin Reuptake Inhibitors (SSRIs) and Serotonin Norepinephrine Reuptake Inhibitors (SNRIs). Serotonin Syndrome is a potentially life-threatening condition, and it may include signs and symptoms such as: mental status changes (e.g. agitation, hallucinations, coma), autonomic instability, (e.g. tachycardia, labile blood-pressure, hyperthermia), neuromuscular aberrations (e.g. hyperreflexia, in-coordination), and/or gastrointestinal symptoms (e.g. nausea, vomiting, diarrhoea). Careful observation of the patient is advised, if concomitant treatment with Zomig and an SSRI or SNRI is clinically warranted, particularly during treatment initiation and dosage increases (See section 4.5).

4.5 Interaction with other medicinal products and other forms of interaction

There is no evidence that concomitant use of migraine prophylactic medications has any effect on the efficacy or unwanted effects of zolmitriptan (for example beta blockers, oral dihydroergotamine, pizotifen).

The pharmacokinetics and tolerability of 'Zomig', when administered as the conventional tablet, were unaffected by acute symptomatic treatments such as paracetamol, metoclopramide and ergotamine. Concomitant administration of other $5HT_{1B/1D}$ agonists within 12 hours of 'Zomig Rapimelt' treatment should be avoided.

Data from healthy subjects suggest there are no pharmacokinetic or clinically significant interactions between Zomig and ergotamine, however, the increased risk of coronary vasospasm is a theoretical possibility. Therefore, it is advised to wait at least 24 hours following the use of ergotamine containing preparations before administering Zomig. Conversely it is advised to wait at least six hours following use of Zomig before administering any ergotamine preparation (see Section 4.3 Contraindications).

Following administration of moclobemide, a specific MAO-A inhibitor, there was a small increase (26%) in AUC for zolmitriptan and a 3-fold increase in AUC of the active metabolite. Therefore, a maximum intake of 5 mg 'Zomig Rapimelt' in 24 hours is recommended in patients taking an MAO-A inhibitor.

Following the administration of cimetidine, a general P450 inhibitor, the half life of zolmitriptan was increased by 44% and the AUC increased by 48%. In addition the half life and AUC of the active N-desmethylated metabolite (183C91) were doubled. A maximum dose of 5 mg 'Zomig Rapimelt' in 24 hours is recommended in patients taking cimetidine. Based on the overall interaction profile, an interaction with inhibitors of the cytochrome P450 isoenzyme CYP1A2 cannot be excluded. Therefore, the same dosage reduction is recommended with compounds of this type, such as fluvoxamine and the quinolone antibiotics (eg ciprofloxacin).

Fluoxetine does not affect the pharmacokinetic parameters of zolmitriptan. Therapeutic doses of the specific serotonin reuptake inhibitors, fluoxetine, sertraline, paroxetine and citalopram do not inhibit CYP1A2. However, Serotonin Syndrome has been reported during combined use of triptans, and SSRIs (e.g. fluoxetine, paroxetine, sertraline) and SNRIs (e.g. venlafaxine, duloxetine) (See section 4.4).

As with other $5HT_{1b/1d}$ agonists, there is the potential for dynamic interactions with the herbal remedy St John's wort (Hypericum perforatum) which may result in an increase in undesirable effects.

4.6 Pregnancy and lactation

Pregnancy

'Zomig Rapimelt' should be used in pregnancy only if the benefits to the mother justify potential risk to the foetus. There are no studies in pregnant women, but there is no evidence of teratogenicity in animal studies. (See Section 5.3 Preclinical Safety Data).

Lactation

Studies have shown that zolmitriptan passes into the milk of lactating animals. No data exist for passage of zolmitriptan into human breast milk. Therefore, caution should be exercised when administering 'Zomig Rapimelt' to women who are breast-feeding.

4.7 Effects on ability to drive and use machines

There was no significant impairment of performance of psychomotor tests with doses up to 20 mg zolmitriptan. Use is unlikely to result in an impairment of the ability of patients to drive or operate machinery. However it should be taken into account that somnolence may occur.

4.8 Undesirable effects

Zomig is well tolerated. Adverse reactions are typically mild/moderate, transient, not serious and resolve spontaneously without additional treatment.

Possible adverse reactions tend to occur within 4 hours of dosing and are no more frequent following repeated dosing.

The incidences of ADRs associated with ZOMIG therapy are tabulated below according to the format recommended by the Council for International Organizations of Medical Sciences (CIOMS III Working Group; 1995).

Frequency	System organ class	Event
Common ($\geq$1% - <10%)	Nervous System Disorders	Abnormalities or disturbances of sensation Dizziness Headache Hyperaesthesia Paraesthesia Somnolence Warm sensation
	Cardiac Disorders	Palpitations
	Gastrointestinal Disorders	Abdominal Pain Dry mouth Nausea Vomiting
	Musculoskeletal and Connective Tissue Disorders	Muscle weakness Myalgia
	General Disorders	Asthenia Heaviness, tightness, pain or pressure in throat, neck limbs or chest
Uncommon ($\geq$0.1% - < 1.0%)	Cardiac Disorders	Tachycardia
	Vascular Disorders	Transient increases in systemic blood pressure
	Renal and Urinary disorders	Polyuria Increased Urinary frequency
Rare ($\geq$0.01% - <0.1%)	Immune System Disorders	Anaphylaxis/Anaphylactoid Reactions Hypersensitivity reactions
	Skin and Subcutaneous Tissue Disorders	Angioedema Urticaria
Very rare (<0.01%)	Cardiac Disorders	Angina pectoris Coronary Vasospasm Myocardial Infarction
	Gastrointestinal Disorders	Bloody diarrhoea Gastrointestinal infarction or necrosis Gastrointestinal ischaemic events Ischaemic colitis Splenic Infarction
	Renal and Urinary Disorders	Urinary Urgency

4.9 Overdose

Volunteers receiving single oral doses of 50 mg commonly experienced sedation. The elimination half-life of zolmitriptan is 2.5 to 3 hours, (see Section 5.2 Pharmacokinetic Properties) and therefore monitoring of patients after overdose with 'Zomig Rapimelt' should continue for at least 15 hours or while symptoms or signs persist.

There is no specific antidote to zolmitriptan. In cases of severe intoxication, intensive care procedures are recommended, including establishing and maintaining a patent airway, ensuring adequate oxygenation and ventilation, and monitoring and support of the cardiovascular system.

It is unknown what effect haemodialysis or peritoneal dialysis has on the serum concentrations of zolmitriptan.

5. PHARMACOLOGICAL PROPERTIES

5.1 Pharmacodynamic properties

In pre-clinical studies, zolmitriptan has been demonstrated to be a selective agonist for the vascular human recombinant $5HT_{1B}$ and $5HT_{1D}$ receptor subtypes. Zolmitriptan is a high affinity $5HT_{1B/1D}$ receptor agonist with modest affinity for $5HT_{1A}$ receptors. Zolmitriptan has no significant affinity (as measured by radioligand binding assays) or pharmacological activity at $5HT_2$-, $5HT_3$-, $5HT_4$-, alpha$_1$-, alpha$_2$-, or beta$_1$-, adrenergic; H_1-, H_2-, histaminic; muscarinic; dopaminergic$_1$, or dopaminergic$_2$ receptors. The $5HT_{1D}$ receptor is predominately located presynaptically at both the peripheral and central synapses of the trigeminal nerve and preclinical studies have shown that zolmitriptan is able to act at both these sites.

One controlled clinical trial in 696 adolescents with migraine failed to demonstrate superiority of zolmitriptan tablets at doses of 2.5 mg, 5 mg and 10 mg over placebo. Efficacy was not demonstrated.

5.2 Pharmacokinetic properties

Following oral administration of 'Zomig' conventional tablets zolmitriptan is rapidly and well absorbed (at least 64%) in man. The mean absolute bioavailability of the parent compound is approximately 40%. There is an active metabolite (183C91, the N-desmethyl metabolite) which is also a $5HT_{1B/1D}$ agonist and is 2 to 6 times as potent, in animal models, as zolmitriptan.

In healthy subjects, when given as a single dose, zolmitriptan and its active metabolite 183C91, display dose-proportional AUC and C_{max} over the dose range 2.5 to 50 mg. Absorption is rapid with 75% of C_{max} achieved within 1 hour and plasma concentrations are sustained subsequently for 4 to 6 hours. Zolmitriptan absorption is unaffected by the presence of food. There is no evidence of accumulation on multiple dosing of zolmitriptan.

Zolmitriptan is eliminated largely by hepatic biotransformation followed by urinary excretion of the metabolites. There are three major metabolites: the indole acetic acid, (the major metabolite in plasma and urine), the N-oxide and N-desmethyl analogues. The N-desmethylated metabolite (183C91) is active whilst the others are not. Plasma concentrations of 183C91 are approximately half those of the parent drug, hence it would therefore be expected to contribute to the therapeutic action of 'Zomig Rapimelt'. Over 60% of a single oral dose is excreted in the urine (mainly as the indole acetic acid metabolite) and about 30% in faeces, mainly as unchanged parent compound.

A study to evaluate the effect of liver disease on the pharmacokinetics of zolmitriptan showed that the AUC and C_{max} were increased by 94% and 50% respectively in patients with moderate liver disease and by 226% and 47% in patients with severe liver disease compared with healthy volunteers. Exposure to the metabolites, including the active metabolite, was decreased. For the 183C91 metabolite, AUC and C_{max} were reduced by 33% and 44% in patients with moderate liver disease and by 82% and 90% in patients with severe liver disease.

The plasma half-life ($t_{½}$) of zolmitriptan was 4.7 hours in healthy volunteers, 7.3 hours in patients with moderate liver disease and 12 hours in those with severe liver disease. The corresponding $t_{½}$ values for the 183C91 metabolite were 5.7 hours, 7.5 hours and 7.8 hours respectively.

Following intravenous administration, the mean total plasma clearance is approximately 10 ml/min/kg, of which one third is renal clearance. Renal clearance is greater than glomerular filtration rate suggesting renal tubular secretion. The volume of distribution following intravenous administration is 2.4 L/kg. Plasma protein binding is low (approximately 25%). The mean elimination half-life of zolmitriptan is 2.5 to 3 hours. The half-lives of its metabolites are similar, suggesting their elimination is formation-rate limited.

Renal clearance of zolmitriptan and all its metabolites is reduced (7 to 8 fold) in patients with moderate to severe renal impairment compared to healthy subjects, although the AUC of the parent compound and the active metabolite were only slightly higher (16 and 35% respectively) with a 1 hour increase in half-life to 3 to 3.5 hours. These parameters are within the ranges seen in healthy volunteers.

In a small group of healthy individuals there was no pharmacokinetic interaction with ergotamine. Concomitant administration of zolmitriptan with ergotamine/caffeine was well tolerated and did not result in any increase in adverse events or blood pressure changes as compared with zolmitriptan alone.

Following the administration of rifampicin, no clinically relevant differences in the pharmacokinetics of zolmitriptan or its active metabolite were observed.

Selegiline, an MAO-B inhibitor, and fluoxetine (a selective serotonin reuptake inhibitor; SSRI) had no effect on the pharmacokinetic parameters of zolmitriptan.

The pharmacokinetics of zolmitriptan in healthy elderly subjects were similar to those in healthy young volunteers.

'Zomig Rapimelt' was demonstrated to be bioequivalent with the conventional tablet in terms of AUC and C_{max} for zolmitriptan and its active metabolite 183C91. Clinical pharmacology data show that the t_{max} for zolmitriptan can be later for the orally dispersible tablet (range 0.6 to 5h, median 3h) compared to the conventional tablet (range 0.5 to 3h, median 1.5h). The t_{max} for the active metabolite was similar for both formulations (median 3h).

5.3 Preclinical safety data

An oral teratology study of zolmitriptan has been conducted. At the maximum tolerated doses, 1200 mg/kg/day (AUC 605 µg/ml.h: approx. 3700 × AUC of the human maximum recommended daily intake of 15 mg) and 30 mg/kg/day (AUC 4.9 µg/ml.h: approx. 30 × AUC of the human maximum recommended daily intake of 15 mg) in rats and rabbits, respectively, no signs of teratogenicity were apparent.

Five genotoxicity tests have been performed. It was concluded that 'Zomig Rapimelt' is not likely to pose any genetic risk in humans.

Carcinogenicity studies in rats and mice were conducted at the highest feasible doses and gave no suggestion of tumorogenicity.

Reproductive studies in male and female rats, at dose levels limited by toxicity, revealed no effect on fertility.

6. PHARMACEUTICAL PARTICULARS

6.1 List of excipients

Each 'Zomig Rapimelt' orodispersible tablet contains the following excipients:

Aspartame

Citric Acid Anhydrous

Silica Colloidal Anhydrous

Crospovidone

Magnesium Stearate

Mannitol

Microcrystalline Cellulose

Orange Flavour SN027512

Sodium Hydrogen Carbonate

6.2 Incompatibilities

None known.

6.3 Shelf life

3 years.

6.4 Special precautions for storage

Do not store above 30°C.

6.5 Nature and contents of container

PVC aluminium/aluminium blister pack of 2 tablets (sample pack)* or 6 tablets (3 strips of 2 tablets) with a plastic re-usable wallet.

6.6 Special precautions for disposal and other handling

The blister pack should be peeled open as shown on the foil (tablets should not be pushed through the foil). The 'Zomig Rapimelt' tablet should be placed on the tongue, where it will dissolve and be swallowed with the saliva.

7. MARKETING AUTHORISATION HOLDER

AstraZeneca UK Ltd

600 Capability Green

Luton LU1 3LU

United Kingdom

8. MARKETING AUTHORISATION NUMBER(S)

PL 17901/0076

9. DATE OF FIRST AUTHORISATION/RENEWAL OF THE AUTHORISATION

20 June 2001

10. DATE OF REVISION OF THE TEXT

28 January 2008

'Zomig Rapimelt' is a trademark property of the AstraZeneca Group of Companies.

Zomig Rapimelt 5 mg Orodispersible Tablets

(AstraZeneca UK Limited)

1. NAME OF THE MEDICINAL PRODUCT

'Zomig Rapimelt'5 mg Orodispersible Tablets

2. QUALITATIVE AND QUANTITATIVE COMPOSITION

Orodispersible tablets containing 5 mg of zolmitriptan.

For excipients, see Section 6.1.

3. PHARMACEUTICAL FORM

Orodispersible tablet.

4. CLINICAL PARTICULARS

4.1 Therapeutic indications

'Zomig Rapimelt' is indicated for the acute treatment of migraine with or without aura.

4.2 Posology and method of administration

The recommended dose of 'Zomig Rapimelt' to treat a migraine attack is 2.5 mg. 'Zomig Rapimelt' rapidly dissolves when placed on the tongue and is swallowed with the patient's saliva. A drink of water is not required when taking 'Zomig Rapimelt'. 'Zomig Rapimelt' can be taken when water is not available thus allowing early administration of treatment for a migraine attack. This formulation may also be beneficial for patients who suffer from nausea and are unable to drink during a migraine attack, or for patients who do not like swallowing conventional tablets.

If symptoms persist or return within 24 hours, a second dose of zolmitriptan has been shown to be effective. If a second dose is required, it should not be taken within 2 hours of the initial dose.

If a patient does not achieve satisfactory relief with 2.5 mg doses, subsequent attacks can be treated with 5 mg doses of 'Zomig Rapimelt'. In those patients who respond, significant efficacy is apparent within 1 hour of dosing with zolmitriptan.

Zolmitriptan is equally effective whenever the tablets are taken during a migraine attack; although it is advisable that 'Zomig Rapimelt' is taken as early as possible after the onset of migraine headache.

In the event of recurrent attacks, it is recommended that the total intake of 'Zomig Rapimelt' in a 24 hour period should not exceed 10 mg.

'Zomig Rapimelt' is not indicated for prophylaxis of migraine.

Use in Children (under 12 years of age)

Safety and efficacy of zolmitriptan tablets in paediatric patients have not been evaluated. Use of Zomig Rapimelt in children is therefore not recommended.

Adolescents (12 - 17 years of age)

The efficacy of Zomig tablets was not demonstrated in a placebo controlled clinical trial for patients aged 12 to 17 years. Use of Zomig Rapimelt tablets in adolescents is therefore not recommended.

Use in Patients Aged Over 65 years

Safety and efficacy of 'Zomig Rapimelt' in individuals aged over 65 years have not been established.

Patients with Hepatic Impairment

Metabolism is reduced in patients with hepatic impairment (See Section 5.2 Pharmacokinetic properties). Therefore for patients with moderate or severe hepatic impairment a maximum dose of 5 mg in 24 hours is recommended.

Patients with Renal Impairment

No dosage adjustment required (see Section 5.2 Pharmacokinetic Properties).

4.3 Contraindications

'Zomig Rapimelt' is contraindicated in patients with:

- Known hypersensitivity to any component of the product.
- Uncontrolled hypertension.
- Ischaemic heart disease.
- Coronary vasospasm/Prinzmetal's angina.
- A history of cerebrovascular accident (CVA) or transient ischaemic attack (TIA).
- Concomitant administration of Zomig with ergotamine or ergotamine derivatives or other $5\text{-}HT_1$ receptor agonists.

4.4 Special warnings and precautions for use

'Zomig Rapimelt' should only be used where a clear diagnosis of migraine has been established. Care should be taken to exclude other potentially serious neurological conditions. There are no data on the use of 'Zomig Rapimelt' in hemiplegic or basilar migraine. Migraneurs may be at risk of certain cerebrovascular events. Cerebral haemorrhage, subarachnoid haemorrhage, stroke, and other cerebrovascular events have been reported in patients treated with $5HT_{1B/1D}$ agonists.

'Zomig Rapimelt' should not be given to patients with symptomatic Wolff-Parkinson-White syndrome or arrhythmias associated with other cardiac accessory conduction pathways.

In very rare cases, as with other $5HT_{1B/1D}$ agonists, coronary vasospasm, angina pectoris and myocardial infarction have been reported. In patients with risk factors for ischaemic heart disease, cardiovascular evaluation prior to commencement of treatment with this class of compounds, including 'Zomig Rapimelt', is recommended (see Section 4.3 Contraindications). These evaluations, however, may not identify every patient who has cardiac disease, and in very rare cases, serious cardiac events have occurred in patients without underlying cardiovascular disease.

As with other $5HT_{1B/1D}$ agonists, atypical sensations over the precordium (see Section 4.8 Undesirable Effects) have been reported after the administration of zolmitriptan. If chest pain or symptoms consistent with ischaemic heart disease occur, no further doses of zolmitriptan should be taken until after appropriate medical evaluation has been carried out.

As with other $5HT_{1B/1D}$ agonists transient increases in systemic blood pressure have been reported in patients with and without a history of hypertension; very rarely these increases in blood pressure have been associated with significant clinical events.

As with other $5HT_{1B/1D}$ agonists, there have been rare reports of anaphylaxis/anaphylactoid reactions in patients receiving Zomig.

Patients with phenylketonuria should be informed that 'Zomig Rapimelt' contains phenylalanine (a component of aspartame). Each 5 mg orally dispersible tablet contains 5.62 mg of phenylalanine.

Excessive use of an acute anti-migraine medicinal product may lead to an increased frequency of headache, potentially requiring withdrawal of treatment.

Serotonin Syndrome has been reported with combined use of triptans, and Selective Serotonin Reuptake Inhibitors (SSRIs) and Serotonin Norepinephrine Reuptake Inhibitors (SNRIs). Serotonin Syndrome is a potentially life-threatening condition, and it may include signs and symptoms such as: mental status changes (e.g. agitation, hallucinations, coma), autonomic instability, (e.g. tachycardia, labile blood-pressure, hyperthermia), neuromuscular aberrations (e.g. hyperreflexia, in-coordination), and/or gastrointestinal symptoms (e.g. nausea, vomiting, diarrhoea). Careful observation of the patient is advised, if concomitant treatment with Zomig and an SSRI or SNRI is clinically warranted, particularly during treatment initiation and dosage increases (See section 4.5).

4.5 Interaction with other medicinal products and other forms of interaction

There is no evidence that concomitant use of migraine prophylactic medications has any effect on the efficacy or unwanted effects of zolmitriptan (for example beta blockers, oral dihydroergotamine, pizotifen).

The pharmacokinetics and tolerability of 'Zomig', when administered as the conventional tablet, were unaffected by acute symptomatic treatments such as paracetamol, metoclopramide and ergotamine. Concomitant administration of other $5HT_{1B/1D}$ agonists within 12 hours of 'Zomig Rapimelt' treatment should be avoided.

Data from healthy subjects suggest there are no pharmacokinetic or clinically significant interactions between Zomig and ergotamine, however, the increased risk of coronary vasospasm is a theoretical possibility. Therefore, it is advised to wait at least 24 hours following the use of ergotamine containing preparations before administering Zomig. Conversely it is advised to wait at least six hours following use of Zomig before administering any ergotamine preparation (see Section 4.3 Contraindications).

Following administration of moclobemide, a specific MAO-A inhibitor, there was a small increase (26%) in AUC for zolmitriptan and a 3-fold increase in AUC of the active metabolite. Therefore, a maximum intake of 5 mg 'Zomig Rapimelt' in 24 hours is recommended in patients taking an MAO-A inhibitor.

Following the administration of cimetidine, a general P450 inhibitor, the half life of zolmitriptan was increased by 44% and the AUC increased by 48%. In addition the half life and AUC of the active N-desmethylated metabolite (183C91) were doubled. A maximum dose of 5 mg 'Zomig Rapimelt' in 24 hours is recommended in patients taking cimetidine. Based on the overall interaction profile, an interaction with inhibitors of the cytochrome P450 isoenzyme CYP1A2 cannot be excluded. Therefore, the same dosage reduction is recommended with compounds of this type, such as fluvoxamine and the quinolone antibiotics (e.g. ciprofloxacin).

Fluoxetine does not affect the pharmacokinetic parameters of zolmitriptan. Therapeutic doses of the specific serotonin reuptake inhibitors, fluoxetine, sertraline, paroxetine and citalopram do not inhibit CYP1A2. However, Serotonin Syndrome has been reported during combined use of triptans, and SSRIs (e.g. fluoxetine, paroxetine, sertraline) and SNRIs (e.g. venlafaxine, duloxetine) (See section 4.4).

As with other $5HT_{1b/1d}$ agonists, there is the potential for dynamic interactions with the herbal remedy St John's wort (Hypericum perforatum) which may result in an increase in undesirable effects.

4.6 Pregnancy and lactation

Pregnancy

'Zomig Rapimelt' should be used in pregnancy only if the benefits to the mother justify potential risk to the foetus. There are no studies in pregnant women, but there is no evidence of teratogenicity in animal studies. (See Section 5.3 Preclinical Safety Data).

Lactation

Studies have shown that zolmitriptan passes into the milk of lactating animals. No data exist for passage of zolmitriptan into human breast milk. Therefore, caution should be exercised when administering 'Zomig Rapimelt' to women who are breast-feeding.

4.7 Effects on ability to drive and use machines

There was no significant impairment of performance of psychomotor tests with doses up to 20 mg zolmitriptan. Use is unlikely to result in an impairment of the ability of patients to drive or operate machinery. However it should be taken into account that somnolence may occur.

4.8 Undesirable effects

Zomig is well tolerated. Adverse reactions are typically mild/moderate, transient, not serious and resolve spontaneously without additional treatment.

Possible adverse reactions tend to occur within 4 hours of dosing and are no more frequent following repeated dosing.

The incidences of ADRs associated with ZOMIG therapy are tabulated below according to the format recommended by the Council for International Organizations of Medical Sciences (CIOMS III Working Group; 1995).

Frequency	System organ class	Event
Common ($\geqslant$1% - <10%)	Nervous System Disorders	Abnormalities or disturbances of sensation Dizziness Headache Hyperaesthesia Paraesthesia Somnolence Warm sensation
	Cardiac Disorders	Palpitations
	Gastrointestinal Disorders	Abdominal Pain Dry mouth Nausea Vomiting
	Musculoskeletal and Connective Tissue Disorders	Muscle weakness Myalgia
	General Disorders	Asthenia Heaviness, tightness, pain or pressure in throat, neck limbs or chest
Uncommon ($\geqslant$0.1% - < 1.0%)	Cardiac Disorders	Tachycardia
	Vascular Disorders	Transient increases in systemic blood pressure
	Renal and Urinary disorders	Polyuria Increased Urinary frequency
Rare ($\geqslant$0.01% - <0.1%)	Immune System Disorders	Anaphylaxis/ Anaphylactoid Reactions Hypersensitivity reactions
	Skin and Subcutaneous Tissue Disorders	Angioedema Urticaria
Very rare (<0.01%)	Cardiac Disorders	Angina pectoris Coronary Vasospasm Myocardial Infarction
	Gastrointestinal Disorders	Bloody diarrhoea Gastrointestinal infarction or necrosis Gastrointestinal ischaemic events Ischaemic colitis Splenic Infarction
	Renal and Urinary Disorders	Urinary Urgency

4.9 Overdose

Volunteers receiving single oral doses of 50 mg commonly experienced sedation.

The elimination half-life of zolmitriptan is 2.5 to 3 hours, (see Section 5.2 Pharmacokinetic Properties) and therefore monitoring of patients after overdose with 'Zomig Rapimelt' should continue for at least 15 hours or while symptoms or signs persist.

There is no specific antidote to zolmitriptan. In cases of severe intoxication, intensive care procedures are recommended, including establishing and maintaining a patent airway, ensuring adequate oxygenation and ventilation, and monitoring and support of the cardiovascular system.

It is unknown what effect haemodialysis or peritoneal dialysis has on the serum concentrations of zolmitriptan.

5. PHARMACOLOGICAL PROPERTIES

5.1 Pharmacodynamic properties

Pharmacotherapeutic group: Selective serotonin ($5HT_1$) agonists

Therapeutic classification: N02CC03

In pre-clinical studies, zolmitriptan has been demonstrated to be a selective agonist for the vascular human recombinant $5HT_{1B}$ and $5HT_{1D}$ receptor subtypes. Zolmitriptan is a high affinity $5HT_{1B/1D}$ receptor agonist with modest affinity for $5HT_{1A}$ receptors. Zolmitriptan has no significant affinity (as measured by radioligand binding assays) or pharmacological activity at $5HT_2$-, $5HT_3$-, $5HT_4$-, alpha$_1$-, alpha$_2$-, or beta$_1$-, adrenergic; H_1-, H_2-, histaminic; muscarinic; dopaminergic$_1$, or dopaminergic$_2$ receptors. The $5HT_{1D}$ receptor is predominately located presynaptically at both the peripheral and central synapses of the trigeminal nerve and preclinical studies have shown that zolmitriptan is able to act at both these sites.

One controlled clinical trial in 696 adolescents with migraine failed to demonstrate superiority of zolmitriptan tablets at doses of 2.5 mg, 5 mg and 10 mg over placebo. Efficacy was not demonstrated.

5.2 Pharmacokinetic properties

Following oral administration of 'Zomig' conventional tablets zolmitriptan is rapidly and well absorbed (at least 64%) in man. The mean absolute bioavailability of the parent compound is approximately 40%. There is an active metabolite (183C91, the N-desmethyl metabolite) which is also a $5HT_{1B/1D}$ agonist and is 2 to 6 times as potent, in animal models, as zolmitriptan.

In healthy subjects, when given as a single dose, zolmitriptan and its active metabolite 183C91, display dose-proportional AUC and C_{max} over the dose range 2.5 to 50 mg. Absorption is rapid with 75% of C_{max} achieved within 1 hour and plasma concentrations are sustained subsequently for 4 to 6 hours. Zolmitriptan absorption is unaffected by the presence of food. There is no evidence of accumulation on multiple dosing of zolmitriptan.

Zolmitriptan is eliminated largely by hepatic biotransformation followed by urinary excretion of the metabolites. There are three major metabolites: the indole acetic acid, (the major metabolite in plasma and urine), the N-oxide and N-desmethyl analogues. The N-desmethylated metabolite (183C91) is active whilst the others are not. Plasma concentrations of 183C91 are approximately half those of the parent drug, hence it would therefore be expected to contribute to the therapeutic action of 'Zomig Rapimelt'. Over 60% of a single oral dose is excreted in the urine (mainly as the indole acetic acid metabolite) and about 30% in faeces, mainly as unchanged parent compound.

A study to evaluate the effect of liver disease on the pharmacokinetics of zolmitriptan showed that the AUC and C_{max} were increased by 94% and 50% respectively in patients with moderate liver disease and by 226% and 47% in patients with severe liver disease compared with healthy volunteers. Exposure to the metabolites, including the active metabolite, was decreased. For the 183C91 metabolite, AUC and C_{max} were reduced by 33% and 44% in patients with moderate liver disease and by 82% and 90% in patients with severe liver disease.

The plasma half-life ($t\frac{1}{2}$) of zolmitriptan was 4.7 hours in healthy volunteers, 7.3 hours in patients with moderate liver disease and 12 hours in those with severe liver disease. The corresponding $t\frac{1}{2}$ values for the 183C91 metabolite were 5.7 hours, 7.5 hours and 7.8 hours respectively.

Following intravenous administration, the mean total plasma clearance is approximately 10 ml/min/kg, of which one third is renal clearance. Renal clearance is greater than glomerular filtration rate suggesting renal tubular secretion. The volume of distribution following intravenous administration is 2.4 L/kg. Plasma protein binding is low (approximately 25%). The mean elimination half-life of zolmitriptan is 2.5 to 3 hours. The half-lives of its metabolites are similar, suggesting their elimination is formation-rate limited.

Renal clearance of zolmitriptan and all its metabolites is reduced (7 to 8 fold) in patients with moderate to severe renal impairment compared to healthy subjects, although the AUC of the parent compound and the active metabolite were only slightly higher (16 and 35% respectively) with a 1 hour increase in half-life to 3 to 3.5 hours. These parameters are within the ranges seen in healthy volunteers.

In a small group of healthy individuals there was no pharmacokinetic interaction with ergotamine. Concomitant administration of zolmitriptan with ergotamine/caffeine was well tolerated and did not result in any increase in adverse events or blood pressure changes as compared with zolmitriptan alone.

Following the administration of rifampicin, no clinically relevant differences in the pharmacokinetics of zolmitriptan or its active metabolite were observed.

Selegiline, an MAO-B inhibitor, and fluoxetine (a selective serotonin reuptake inhibitor; SSRI) had no effect on the pharmacokinetic parameters of zolmitriptan.

The pharmacokinetics of zolmitriptan in healthy elderly subjects were similar to those in healthy young volunteers.

'Zomig Rapimelt' was demonstrated to be bioequivalent with the conventional tablet in terms of AUC and C_{max} for zolmitriptan and its active metabolite 183C91. Clinical pharmacology data show that the t_{max} for zolmitriptan can be later for the orally dispersible tablet (range 0.6 to 5h, median 3h) compared to the conventional tablet (range 0.5 to 3h, median 1.5h). The t_{max} for the active metabolite was similar for both formulations (median 3h).

5.3 Preclinical safety data

An oral teratology study of zolmitriptan has been conducted. At the maximum tolerated doses, 1200 mg/kg/day (AUC 605 μg/ml.h: approx. 3700 × AUC of the human maximum recommended daily intake of 15 mg) and 30 mg/kg/day (AUC 4.9 μg/ml.h: approx. 30 × AUC of the human maximum recommended daily intake of 15 mg) in rats and rabbits, respectively, no signs of teratogenicity were apparent.

Five genotoxicity tests have been performed. It was concluded that 'Zomig Rapimelt' is not likely to pose any genetic risk in humans.

Carcinogenicity studies in rats and mice were conducted at the highest feasible doses and gave no suggestion of tumorogenicity.

Reproductive studies in male and female rats, at dose levels limited by toxicity, revealed no effect on fertility.

6. PHARMACEUTICAL PARTICULARS

6.1 List of excipients

Each 'Zomig Rapimelt' orodispersible tablet contains the following excipients:

Aspartame

Citric Acid Anhydrous

Silica Colloidal Anhydrous

Crospovidone

Magnesium Stearate

Mannitol

Microcrystalline Cellulose

Orange Flavour SN027512

Sodium Hydrogen Carbonate

6.2 Incompatibilities

None known

6.3 Shelf life

2 years

6.4 Special precautions for storage

Do not store above 30°C.

6.5 Nature and contents of container

PVC aluminium/aluminium blister pack of 6 tablets (1 strip of 6 tablets) with a plastic re-usable wallet.

6.6 Special precautions for disposal and other handling

The blister pack should be peeled open as shown on the foil (tablets should not be pushed through the foil). The 'Zomig Rapimelt' tablet should be placed on the tongue, where it will dissolve and be swallowed with the saliva.

7. MARKETING AUTHORISATION HOLDER

AstraZeneca UK Ltd

600 Capability Green

Luton LU1 3LU

United Kingdom.

8. MARKETING AUTHORISATION NUMBER(S)

PL 17901/0230

9. DATE OF FIRST AUTHORISATION/RENEWAL OF THE AUTHORISATION

21st September 2004/18th June 2008

10. DATE OF REVISION OF THE TEXT

18th June 2008

'Zomig Rapimelt' is a trademark property of the AstraZeneca Group of Companies.

Zonegran capsules

(Eisai Ltd)

1. NAME OF THE MEDICINAL PRODUCT

25 mg: Zonegran▼ 25 mg hard capsules.

50 mg: Zonegran▼ 50 mg hard capsules.

100 mg: Zonegran▼ 100 mg hard capsules.

2. QUALITATIVE AND QUANTITATIVE COMPOSITION

25 mg: Each Zonegran hard capsule contains 25 mg of zonisamide.

50 mg: Each Zonegran hard capsule contains 50 mg of zonisamide.

100 mg: Each Zonegran hard capsule contains 100 mg of zonisamide.

For a full list of excipients, see section 6.1.

3. PHARMACEUTICAL FORM

Hard capsule.

25 mg: A white opaque body and a white opaque cap printed with a logo and "ZONEGRAN 25" in black.

50 mg: A white opaque body and a grey opaque cap printed with a logo and "ZONEGRAN 50" in black.

100 mg: A white opaque body and a red opaque cap printed with a logo and "ZONEGRAN 100" in black.

4. CLINICAL PARTICULARS

4.1 Therapeutic indications

Zonegran is indicated as adjunctive therapy in the treatment of adult patients with partial seizures, with or without secondary generalisation.

4.2 Posology and method of administration

Zonegran hard capsules are for oral use.

<u>Adults</u>

Zonegran must be added to existing therapy and the dose should be titrated on the basis of clinical effect. Doses of 300 mg to 500 mg per day have been shown to be effective, though some patients, especially those not taking CYP3A4-inducing agents, may respond to lower doses.

The recommended initial daily dose is 50 mg in two divided doses. After one week the dose may be increased to 100 mg daily and thereafter the dose may be increased at one weekly intervals, in increments of up to 100 mg.

Use of two weekly intervals should be considered for patients with renal or hepatic impairment and patients not receiving CYP3A4-inducing agents (see Section 4.5).

Zonegran can be administered once or twice daily after the titration phase.

<u>Elderly</u>

Caution should be exercised at initiation of treatment in elderly patients as there is limited information on the use of Zonegran in these patients. Prescribers should also take account of the safety profile of Zonegran (see Section 4.8).

<u>Children and adolescents</u>

The safety and effectiveness in children and adolescents under 18 years have not been established. Therefore use in these patients is not recommended.

<u>Patients with renal impairment</u>

Caution must be exercised in treating patients with renal impairment, as there is limited information on use in such patients and a slower titration of Zonegran might be required. Since zonisamide and its metabolites are excreted renally, it should be discontinued in patients who develop acute renal failure or where a clinically significant sustained increase in serum creatinine is observed.

In subjects with renal impairment, renal clearance of single doses of zonisamide was positively correlated with creatinine clearance. The plasma AUC of zonisamide was increased by 35% in subjects with creatinine clearance < 20 ml/min.

<u>Patients with hepatic impairment</u>

Use in patients with hepatic impairment has not been studied. Therefore use in patients with severe hepatic impairment is not recommended. Caution must be exercised in treating patients with mild to moderate hepatic impairment, and a slower titration of Zonegran may be required.

<u>Effect of food</u>

Zonegran may be taken with or without food (see Section 5.2).

<u>Withdrawal of Zonegran</u>

When Zonegran treatment is to be discontinued, it should be withdrawn gradually. In clinical studies, dose reductions of 100 mg at weekly intervals have been used with concurrent adjustment of other anti-epileptic drug doses.

4.3 Contraindications

Hypersensitivity to zonisamide, to any of the excipients or to sulphonamides.

4.4 Special warnings and precautions for use

Serious rashes occur in association with Zonegran therapy, including cases of Stevens-Johnson syndrome.

Consideration must be given to discontinuing Zonegran in patients who develop an otherwise unexplained rash. All patients who develop a rash while taking Zonegran must be closely supervised, with additional levels of caution applied to those patients receiving concomitant antiepileptic agents that may independently induce skin rashes.

In accordance with current clinical practice, discontinuation of Zonegran in patients with epilepsy must be accomplished by gradual dose reduction, to reduce the possibility of seizures on withdrawal. There are insufficient data for the withdrawal of concomitant anti-epileptic medications once seizure control with Zonegran has been achieved in the add-on situation, in order to reach monotherapy with Zonegran. Therefore withdrawal of concomitant anti-epileptic agents must be undertaken with caution.

Zonegran is a benzisoxazole derivative, which contains a sulphonamide group. Serious immune based adverse reactions that are associated with medicinal products containing a sulphonamide group include rash, allergic reaction and major haematological disturbances including aplastic anaemia, which very rarely can be fatal.

Cases of agranulocytosis, thrombocytopenia, leukopenia, aplastic anaemia, pancytopenia and leucocytosis have been reported. There is inadequate information to assess the relationship, if any, between dose and duration of treatment and these events.

Suicidal ideation and behaviour have been reported in patients treated with anti-epileptic agents in several indications. A meta-analysis of randomised placebo-controlled trials of anti-epileptic drugs has also shown a small increased risk of suicidal ideation and behaviour. The mechanism of this risk is not known and the available data do not exclude the possibility of an increased risk for Zonegran.

Therefore patients should be monitored for signs of suicidal ideation and behaviours and appropriate treatment should be considered. Patients (and caregivers of patients) should be advised to seek medical advice should signs of suicidal ideation or behaviour emerge.

Kidney stones have occurred in patients treated with Zonegran. Zonegran should be used with caution in patients who have risk factors for nephrolithiasis, including prior stone formation, a family history of nephrolithiasis and hypercalcuria. Such patients may be at increased risk for renal stone formation and associated signs and symptoms such as renal colic, renal pain or flank pain. In addition, patients taking other medications associated with nephrolithiasis may be at increased risk. Increasing fluid intake and urine output may help reduce the risk of stone formation, particularly in those with predisposing risk factors.

Hyperchloraemic, non-anion gap, metabolic acidosis (i.e. decreased serum bicarbonate below the normal reference range in the absence of chronic respiratory alkalosis) is associated with Zonegran treatment. This metabolic acidosis is caused by renal bicarbonate loss due to the inhibitory effect of zonisamide on carbonic anhydrase. Such electrolyte imbalance has been observed with the use of Zonegran in placebo-controlled clinical trials and in the post-marketing period. Generally, zonisamide-induced metabolic acidosis occurs early in treatment although cases can occur at any time during treatment. The amounts by which bicarbonate is decreased are usually small – moderate (average decrease of approximately 3.5 mEq/ L at daily doses of 300 mg in adults); rarely patients can experience more severe decreases. Conditions or therapies that predispose to acidosis (such as renal disease, severe respiratory disorders, status epilepticus, diarrhoea, surgery, ketogenic diet, or drugs) may be additive to the bicarbonate lowering effects of zonisamide.

The risk of zonisamide induced metabolic acidosis appears to be more frequent and severe in younger patients. Appropriate evaluation and monitoring of serum bicarbonate levels should be carried out in patients taking zonisamide who have underlying conditions which might increase the risk of acidosis, in patients who are at an increased risk of adverse consequences of metabolic acidosis and in patients with symptoms suggestive of metabolic acidosis. If metabolic acidosis develops and persists, consideration should be given to reducing the dose or discontinuing Zonegran (by gradual discontinuation or reduction of a therapeutic dose). If the decision is made to continue patients on Zonegran in the face of persistent acidosis, alkali treatment should be considered.

Zonegran should be used with caution in patients being treated concomitantly with carbonic anhydrase inhibitors such as topiramate, as there are insufficient data to rule out a pharmacodynamic interaction (see Section 4.5).

Cases of decreased sweating and elevated body temperature have been reported mainly in paediatric patients. Heat stroke requiring hospital treatment was diagnosed in some cases. Most reports occurred during periods of warm weather. Patients or their carers must be warned to take care to maintain hydration and avoid exposure to excessive temperatures. Caution should be used when Zonegran is prescribed with other medicinal products that predispose patients to heat related disorders; these include carbonic anhydrase inhibitors and medicinal products with anticholinergic activity.

In patients taking Zonegran who develop the clinical signs and symptoms of pancreatitis, it is recommended that pancreatic lipase and amylase levels are monitored. If pancreatitis is evident, in the absence of another obvious cause, it is recommended that discontinuation of Zonegran be considered and appropriate treatment initiated.

In patients taking Zonegran, in whom severe muscle pain and/or weakness develop either in the presence or absence of a fever, it is recommended that markers of muscle damage be assessed, including serum creatine phosphokinase and aldolase levels. If elevated, in the absence of another obvious cause such as trauma or grand mal seizures, it is recommended that Zonegran discontinuation be considered and appropriate treatment initiated.

Women of child-bearing potential must use adequate contraception during treatment with Zonegran and for one month after discontinuation (see section 4.6). Physicians treating patients with Zonegran should try to ensure that appropriate contraception is used, and should use clinical judgement when assessing whether OCs, or the doses of the OC components, are adequate based on the individual patient's clinical situation.

Zonegran 100 mg hard capsules contain a yellow colour called sunset yellow FCF (E110), which may cause allergic reactions.

There is limited data from clinical studies in patients with a body weight of less than 40 kg. Therefore these patients should be treated with caution.

Zonegran may cause weight loss. A dietary supplement or increased food intake may be considered if the patient is losing weight or is underweight whilst on this medication. If substantial undesirable weight loss occurs, discontinuation of Zonegran should be considered.

4.5 Interaction with other medicinal products and other forms of interaction

<u>Effect of Zonegran on cytochrome P450 enzymes</u>

In vitro studies using human liver microsomes show no or little (<25%) inhibition of cytochrome P450 isozymes 1A2, 2A6, 2B6, 2C8, 2C9, 2C19, 2D6, 2E1 or 3A4 at zonisamide levels approximately two-fold or greater than clinically relevant unbound serum concentrations. Therefore Zonegran is not expected to affect the pharmacokinetics of other medicinal products via cytochrome P450-mediated mechanisms, as demonstrated for carbamazepine, phenytoin, ethinylestradiol and desipramine *in vivo*.

Potential for Zonegran to affect other medicinal products

Anti-epileptic drugs

In epileptic patients, steady-state dosing with Zonegran resulted in no clinically relevant pharmacokinetic effects on carbamazepine, lamotrigine, phenytoin, or sodium valproate.

Oral contraceptives

In clinical studies in healthy subjects, steady-state dosing with Zonegran did not affect serum concentrations of ethinylestradiol or norethisterone in a combined oral contraceptive.

Carbonic anhydrase inhibitors

There are insufficient data to rule out possible pharmacodynamic interactions with carbonic anhydrase inhibitors such as topiramate.

P-gp substrate

An *in vitro* study shows that zonisamide is a weak inhibitor of P-gp (MDR1) with an IC_{50} of 267 μmol/L and there is the theoretical potential for zonisamide to affect the pharmacokinetics of drugs which are P-gp substrates. Caution is advised when starting or stopping zonisamide treatment or changing the zonisamide dose in patients who are also receiving drugs which are P-gp substrates (e.g. digoxin, quinidine).

Potential medicinal product interactions affecting Zonegran

In clinical studies co-administration of lamotrigine had no apparent effect on zonisamide pharmacokinetics. The combination of Zonegran with other medicinal products that may lead to urolithiasis may enhance the risk of developing kidney stones; therefore the concomitant administration of such medicinal products should be avoided.

Zonisamide is metabolised partly by CYP3A4 (reductive cleavage), and also by N-acetyl-transferases and conjugation with glucuronic acid; therefore, substances that can induce or inhibit these enzymes may affect the pharmacokinetics of zonisamide:

- Enzyme Induction: Exposure to zonisamide is lower in epileptic patients receiving CYP3A4-inducing agents such as phenytoin, carbamazepine, and phenobarbitone. These effects are unlikely to be of clinical significance when Zonegran is added to existing therapy; however, changes in zonisamide concentrations may occur if concomitant CYP3A4-inducing anti-epileptic or other medicinal products are withdrawn, dose adjusted or introduced, and an adjustment of the Zonegran dose may be required. Rifampicin is a potent CYP3A4 inducer. If co-administration is necessary, the patient should be closely monitored and the dose of Zonegran and other CYP3A4 substrates adjusted as needed.

- CYP3A4 Inhibition: Based upon clinical data, known specific and non-specific CYP3A4 inhibitors appear to have no clinically relevant effect on zonisamide pharmacokinetic exposure parameters. Steady-state dosing of either ketoconazole (400 mg/day) or cimetidine (1200 mg/day) had no clinically relevant effects on the single-dose pharmacokinetics of zonisamide given to healthy subjects. Therefore, modification of Zonegran dosing should not be necessary when co-administered with known CYP3A4 inhibitors.

4.6 Pregnancy and lactation

Zonegran must not be used during pregnancy unless clearly necessary, in the opinion of the physician, and only if the potential benefit is considered to justify the risk to the foetus. The need for anti-epileptic treatment should be reviewed in patients planning to become pregnant. If Zonegran is prescribed, careful monitoring is recommended.

Specialist advice should be given to women who are likely to become pregnant in order to consider the optimal treatment during pregnancy. Women of childbearing potential should be given specialist advice regarding possible effects of Zonegran on the foetus and the risk should be discussed with the patient in relation to the benefits before starting treatment. The risk of birth defect is increased by factor 2 to 3 in the offspring of mothers treated with an antiepileptic medication. The most frequently reported are cleft lip, cardiovascular malformations and neural tube defect. Multiple antiepileptic drug therapy may be associated with a higher risk of congenital malformations than monotherapy. Women of childbearing potential must use adequate contraception during treatment with Zonegran, and for one month after discontinuation

There are no adequate data from the use of Zonegran in pregnant women. Studies in animals have shown reproductive toxicity (see Section 5.3). The potential risk for humans is unknown.

No sudden discontinuation of anti-epileptic therapy should be undertaken as this may lead to breakthrough seizures which could have serious consequences for both mother and child.

Zonisamide is excreted in human milk; the concentration in breast milk is similar to maternal plasma. A decision must be made whether to discontinue breast-feeding or to discontinue/abstain from Zonegran therapy. Due to the long retention time of zonisamide in the body, breast-feeding must not be resumed until one month after Zonegran therapy is completed.

4.7 Effects on ability to drive and use machines

Some patients may experience drowsiness or difficulty with concentration, particularly early in treatment or after a dose increase. Patients must be advised to exercise caution during activities requiring a high degree of alertness, e.g., driving or operating machinery.

4.8 Undesirable effects

Zonegran has been administered to over 1,200 patients in clinical studies, more than 400 of whom received Zonegran for at least 1 year. In addition there has been extensive post-marketing experience with zonisamide in Japan since 1989 and in the USA since 2000.

It should be noted that Zonegran is a benzisoxazole derivative, which contains a sulphonamide group. Serious immune based adverse reactions that are associated with medicinal products containing a sulphonamide group include rash, allergic reaction and major haematological disturbances including aplastic anaemia, which very rarely can be fatal (see Section 4.4).

The most common adverse reactions in controlled adjunctive-therapy studies were somnolence, dizziness and anorexia. Adverse reactions associated with Zonegran obtained from clinical studies and post-marketing surveillance are tabulated below. The frequencies are arranged according to the following scheme:

very common	⩾ 1/10
common	⩾ 1/100 < 1/10
uncommon	⩾ 1/1,000 < 1/100
rare	⩾ 1/10,000 < 1/1,000
very rare	< 1/10,000 including isolated reports

(see Table 1 on next page)

In addition there have been isolated cases of Sudden Unexplained Death in Epilepsy Patients (SUDEP) receiving Zonegran.

Additional information on special populations:

Review of post-marketing data suggests that patients aged 65 years or older report a higher frequency than the general population of the following events: Stevens-Johnson syndrome (SJS) and Drug Induced Hypersensitivity syndrome (DIHS).

4.9 Overdose

There have been cases of accidental and intentional overdose in adult and paediatric patients. In some cases, the overdoses were asymptomatic, particularly where emesis or lavage was prompt. In other cases, the overdose was followed by symptoms such as somnolence, nausea, gastritis, nystagmus, myoclonus, coma, bradycardia, reduced renal function, hypotension and respiratory depression. A very high plasma concentration of 100.1 μg/ml zonisamide was recorded approximately 31 hours after a patient took an overdose of Zonegran and clonazepam; the patient became comatose and had respiratory depression, but recovered consciousness five days later and had no sequelae.

Treatment

No specific antidotes for Zonegran overdose are available. Following a suspected recent overdose, emptying the stomach by gastric lavage or by induction of emesis may be indicated with the usual precautions to protect the airway. General supportive care is indicated, including frequent monitoring of vital signs and close observation. Zonisamide has a long elimination half-life so its effects may be persistent. Although not formally studied for the treatment of overdose, haemodialysis reduced plasma concentrations of zonisamide in a patient with reduced renal function, and may be considered as treatment of overdose if clinically indicated.

5. PHARMACOLOGICAL PROPERTIES

Zonisamide is benzisoxazole derivative. It is an anti-epileptic medicine with weak carbonic anhydrase activity *in-vitro*. It is chemically unrelated to other anti-epileptic agents.

5.1 Pharmacodynamic properties

Pharmacotherapeutic group: Anti-epileptics, ATC code: N03A X15

Efficacy has been demonstrated with Zonegran in 4 double-blind, placebo-controlled studies of periods of up to 24 weeks with either once or twice daily dosing. These studies show that the median reduction in partial seizure frequency is related to Zonegran dose with sustained efficacy at doses of 300-500 mg per day.

The anticonvulsant activity of zonisamide has been evaluated in a variety of models, in several species with induced or innate seizures, and zonisamide appears to act as a broad-spectrum anti-epileptic in these models. Zonisamide prevents maximal electroshock seizures and restricts seizure spread, including the propagation of seizures from cortex to sub-cortical structures and suppresses epileptogenic focus activity. Unlike phenytoin and carbamazepine however, zonisamide acts preferentially on seizures originating in the cortex.

The mechanism of action of zonisamide is not fully elucidated, but it appears to act on voltage-sensitive sodium and calcium channels, thereby disrupting synchronised neuronal firing, reducing the spread of seizure discharges and disrupting subsequent epileptic activity. Zonisamide also has a modulatory effect on GABA-mediated neuronal inhibition.

5.2 Pharmacokinetic properties

Absorption

Zonisamide is almost completely absorbed after oral administration, generally reaching peak serum or plasma concentrations within 2 to 5 hours of dosing. The first-pass metabolism is believed to be negligible. Absolute bioavailability is estimated to be approximately 100%. Oral bioavailability is not affected by food, although peak plasma and serum concentrations may be delayed.

Zonisamide AUC and C_{max} values increased almost linearly after single dose over the dose range of 100-800 mg and after multiple doses over the dose range of 100-400 mg once daily. The increase at steady state was slightly more than expected on the basis of dose, probably due to the saturable binding of zonisamide to erythrocytes. Steady state was achieved within 13 days. Slightly greater than expected accumulation occurs relative to single dosing.

Distribution

Zonisamide is 40 - 50 % bound to human plasma proteins, with *in vitro* studies showing that this is unaffected by the presence of various anti-epileptic medicinal products (i.e., phenytoin, phenobarbitone, carbamazepine, and sodium valproate). The apparent volume of distribution is about 1.1 – 1.7 l/kg in adults indicating that zonisamide is extensively distributed to tissues. Erythrocyte/plasma ratios are about 15 at low concentrations and about 3 at higher concentrations.

Metabolism

Zonisamide is metabolised primarily through reductive cleavage of the benzisoxazole ring of the parent drug by CYP3A4 to form 2-sulphamoylacetylphenol (SMAP) and also by N-acetylation. Parent drug and SMAP can additionally be glucuronidated. The metabolites, which could not be detected in plasma, are devoid of anticonvulsant activity. There is no evidence that zonisamide induces its own metabolism.

Elimination

Apparent clearance of zonisamide at steady-state after oral administration is about 0.70 l/h and the terminal elimination half-life is about 60 hours in the absence of CYP3A4 inducers. The elimination half-life was independent of dose and not affected by repeat administration. Fluctuation in serum or plasma concentrations over a dosing interval is low (< 30 %). The main route of excretion of zonisamide metabolites and unchanged drug is via the urine. Renal clearance of unchanged zonisamide is relatively low (approximately 3.5 ml/min); about 15 - 30 % of the dose is eliminated unchanged.

Special patient groups

In subjects with renal impairment, renal clearance of single doses of zonisamide was positively correlated with creatinine clearance. The plasma AUC of zonisamide was increased by 35% in subjects with creatinine clearance <20 ml/min (see also section 4.2.).

Patients with an impaired liver function: The pharmacokinetics of zonisamide in patients with impaired liver function have not been adequately studied.

Elderly: No clinically significant differences were observed in the pharmacokinetics between young (aged 21-40 years) and elderly (65-75 years).

Adolescents (12-18 years): Limited data indicate that pharmacokinetics in adolescents dosed to steady state at 1, 7 or 12 mg/kg daily, in divided doses, are similar to those observed in adults, after adjustment for bodyweight.

Other characteristics

No clear Zonegran dose-concentration-response relationship has been defined. When comparing the same dose level, subjects of higher total body weight appear to have lower steady-state serum concentrations, but this effect appears to be relatively modest. Age (⩾ 12 years) and gender, after adjustment for body weight effects, have no apparent effect on zonisamide exposure in epileptic patients during steady-state dosing.

5.3 Preclinical safety data

Findings not observed in clinical studies, but seen in the dog at exposure levels similar to clinical use, were liver changes (enlargement, dark-brown discolouration, mild hepatocyte enlargement with concentric lamellar bodies in the cytoplasm and cytoplasmic vacuolation) associated with increased metabolism.

Zonisamide was not genotoxic and has no carcinogenic potential.

Zonisamide caused developmental abnormalities in mice, rats, and dogs, and was embryolethal in monkeys, when administered during the period of organogenesis at zonisamide dosage and maternal plasma levels similar to or lower than therapeutic levels in humans.

6. PHARMACEUTICAL PARTICULARS

6.1 List of excipients

Capsule contents:

Microcrystalline cellulose

Hydrogenated vegetable oil

Sodium laurilsulfate.

Table 1

System Organ Class (MedDRA terminology)	Very Common	Common	Uncommon	Very Rare
Infections and infestation			Pneumonia Urinary tract infection	
Blood and lymphatic system disorders		Ecchymosis		Agranulocytosis Aplastic anaemia Leucocytosis Leucopenia Lymphadenopathy Pancytopenia, Thrombocytopenia
Immune system disorders		Hypersensitivity		
Metabolism and nutrition disorders	Anorexia		Hypokalaemia	Metabolic acidosis Renal tubular acidosis
Psychiatric Disorders	Agitation Irritability Confusional state Depression	Affect lability Anxiety Insomnia Psychotic disorder	Anger Aggression Suicidal ideation Suicide attempt	Hallucination
Nervous system disorders	Ataxia Dizziness Memory impairment Somnolence	Bradyphrenia Disturbance in attention Nystagmus Paraesthesia Speech disorder Tremor	Convulsion	Amnesia Coma Grand mal seizure Myasthenic syndrome Neuroleptic malignant syndrome Status epilepticus
Eye disorders	Diplopia			
Respiratory, thoracic and mediastinal disorders				Dyspnoea Pneumonia aspiration Respiratory disorder
Gastrointestinal disorders		Abdominal pain Constipation Diarrhoea Dyspepsia Nausea	Vomiting	Pancreatitis
Hepatobiliary disorders			Cholecystitis Cholelithiasis	Hepatocellular damage
Skin and subcutaneous tissue disorders		Rash		Anhidrosis Erythema multiforme Pruritis Stevens-Johnson syndrome Toxic epidermal necrolysis
Musculoskeletal and connective tissue disorders				Rhabdomyolysis
Renal and urinary disorders		Nephrolithiasis	Calculus urinary	Hydronephrosis Renal failure Urine abnormality
General disorders and administration site conditions		Fatigue Influenza-like illness Pyrexia		
Investigations	Decreased bicarbonate	Weight decreased		Blood creatine phosphokinase increased Blood creatinine increased Blood urea increased Liver function tests abnormal
Injury, poisoning and procedural complications				Heat stroke

The capsule shells contain:

Gelatin

Titanium dioxide (E171)

Shellac

Propylene glycol

Potassium hydroxide

Black iron oxide (E172).

Additionally the 100 mg capsule shells contain:

Allura red AC (E129)

Sunset yellow FCF (E110)

6.2 Incompatibilities

Not applicable.

6.3 Shelf life

3 years.

6.4 Special precautions for storage

Do not store above 30°C.

6.5 Nature and contents of container

25 mg: PVC/PVDC/Aluminium foil blisters, packs of 14, 28, 56 and 84 hard capsules.

50 mg: PVC/PVDC/Aluminium foil blisters, packs of 14, 28, 56 and 84 hard capsules.

100 mg: PVC/PVDC/aluminium foil blisters, packs of 28, 56, 84, 98 and 196 hard capsules.

Not all pack sizes may be marketed.

6.6 Special precautions for disposal and other handling

No special requirements.

7. MARKETING AUTHORISATION HOLDER

Eisai Limited

European Knowledge Centre

Mosquito Way

Hatfield

Hertfordshire AL10 9SN

United Kingdom

8. MARKETING AUTHORISATION NUMBER(S)

25 mg 14 capsules: EU/1/04/307/001

25 mg 28 capsules: EU/1/04/307/005

25 mg 56 capsules: EU/1/04/307/002

25 mg 84 capsules EU/1/04/307/013

50 mg 14 capsules: EU/1/04/307/010

50 mg 28 capsules: EU/1/04/307/009

50 mg 56 capsules: EU/1/04/307/003

50 mg 84 capsules EU/1/04/307/012

100 mg 28 capsules: EU/1/04/307/006

100 mg 56 capsules: EU/1/04/307/004

100 mg 84 capsules EU/1/04/307/011

100 mg 98 capsules: EU/1/04/307/007

100 mg 196 capsules: EU/1/04/307/008

9. DATE OF FIRST AUTHORISATION/RENEWAL OF THE AUTHORISATION

10 March 2005

10. DATE OF REVISION OF THE TEXT

July 2009

11. LEGAL CATEGORY

POM - Medicinal product subject to medical prescription

Zorac 0.05% Gel

(Allergan Ltd)

1. NAME OF THE MEDICINAL PRODUCT

ZORAC 0.05%, gel

2. QUALITATIVE AND QUANTITATIVE COMPOSITION

Active substance:

Tazarotene .... 0.05 g

Excipients with a well known effect:

Butylhydroxyanisole........................ 0.05 g

Butylhydroxytoluene........................ 0.05 g

For 100 g of gel

For a full list of excipients, see section 6.1.

3. PHARMACEUTICAL FORM

Gel.

Colourless to light yellow, translucent to homogeneous cloudy gel.

4. CLINICAL PARTICULARS

4.1 Therapeutic indications

For the topical treatment of mild to moderate plaque psoriasis involving up to 10% body surface area.

4.2 Posology and method of administration
Zorac gel is available in two concentrations.

To initiate a treatment with Zorac, it is advisable to start with Zorac 0.05% in order to evaluate the skin response and tolerance before progressing to Zorac 0.1% if necessary.

Treatment with the lower concentration gel is associated with a somewhat lower incidence of local adverse events (see sections 4.8 Undesirable effects and 5. Pharmacological Properties).

Treatment with the higher concentration gel gives a faster and numerically higher response rate. The physician should choose the concentration to be used based on clinical circumstances and the principle of using the least concentration of drug to achieve the desired effect.

Individual variations with respect to efficacy and tolerability are possible. It is thus advisable for patients to consult their physician on a weekly basis when initiating therapy.

A thin film of the gel should be applied once daily in the evening; care should be taken to apply it only to areas of affected skin, avoiding application to healthy skin or in skin folds. Treatment is limited to 10% body surface area (approximately equivalent to the total skin area of one arm).

If the patient experiences more drying or irritation, an effective greasy emollient (without pharmaceutically active ingredients) can be applied to the areas of the skin to be treated to improve tolerability. Healthy skin around the psoriatic plaques can be covered by using zinc paste, for example, to prevent irritation.

Usually, the treatment period is up to 12 weeks. Clinical experience, particularly on tolerability, is available on periods of use of up to 12 months.

4.3 Contraindications
- Hypersensitivity to any ingredient of the medication(s)
- Pregnancy or in women planning a pregnancy (see section 4.6 Pregnancy and lactation)
- Breast-feeding mothers
- Since there is, as yet, no clinical experience, Zorac should not be used in the treatment of psoriasis pustulosa and psoriasis exfoliativa, and the gel should not be applied to intertriginous areas, to the face or to hair-covered scalp.

4.4 Special warnings and precautions for use
Care should be taken to ensure that Zorac is applied only to psoriatic lesions, as application to normal, eczematous or inflamed skin or skin affected by other pathologies may cause irritation.

Patients should be advised to wash their hands after application of the gel to avoid accidental transfer to the eyes.

If psoriatic areas on the skin of the hands are being treated, particular care should be taken to ensure that no gel is transferred to facial skin or the eyes.

If skin irritation develops, treatment with Zorac should be interrupted.

The safety of use on more than 10% of the body surface area has not been established. There is limited experience of application to up to 20% of the body surface area.

Patients should be advised to avoid excessive exposure to UV light (including sunlight, use of a solarium, PUVA or UVB therapy) during treatment with Zorac (see section 5.3 Preclinical safety data).

No therapeutic studies using Zorac under occlusion or concomitantly with other antipsoriatic agents (including tar shampoos) have been carried out. To minimise interference with absorption and to avoid unnecessary spreading of the medication, topical application of emollients and cosmetics should not be applied within 1 hour of applying Zorac.

The safety and efficacy of Zorac have not been established in patients under the age of 18 years.

This medicinal product contains butylhydroxyanisole and butylhydroxytoluene and therefore may cause local skin reactions (e.g. contact dermatitis) or irritation to the eyes and mucous membranes.

4.5 Interaction with other medicinal products and other forms of interaction
Concomitant use of pharmaceutical and cosmetic preparations which cause irritation or have a strong drying effect should be avoided.

4.6 Pregnancy and lactation
Pregnancy
Zorac gel is contraindicated in women who are or may become pregnant (see 4.3). If this drug is used during pregnancy, or if the patient becomes pregnant while taking this drug, treatment should be discontinued and the patient apprised of the potential hazard to the foetus. Women of child-bearing potential should be warned of the potential risk and use adequate birthcontrol measures when Zorac gel is used. The possibility that a woman of childbearing potential is pregnant at the time of institution of therapy should be considered. A negative result for pregnancy test having a sensitivity down to at least 50 mIU/mL for human chorionic gonadotropin (hCG) should be obtained within 2 weeks prior to Zorac gel therapy, which should begin during a normal menstrual period.

Although in animals no malformations were observed after dermal application, skeletal alterations were seen in the foetuses, which may be attributable to systemic retinoid effects. Teratogenic effects were observed after oral administration.

Lactation
Although no data are available on the excretion of tazarotene in human milk, animal data indicate that excretion into milk is possible. For that reason Zorac gel should not be used during breast-feeding.

4.7 Effects on ability to drive and use machines
None known.

4.8 Undesirable effects
The most frequently reported adverse reactions in controlled clinical trials of Zorac in the treatment of psoriasis were pruritus (incidence 20-25%), burning, erythema, and irritation (10-20%), desquamation, non-specific rash, irritant contact dermatitis, skin pain, and a worsening of psoriasis (5-10 %).

More rarely observed were stinging and inflamed and dry skin (1-3 %).

The incidence of adverse reactions appears to be concentration-related and dependent on duration of use.

The higher concentration gel (0.1%) may cause up to 5% more cases of severe skin irritation than the lower concentration gel (0.05%), especially during the first 4 weeks of use.

Furthermore skin discoloration might occur.

4.9 Overdose
Excessive dermal use of Zorac may result in marked redness, peeling, or local discomfort.

Inadvertent ingestion of Zorac is a theoretical possibility. In such a case, the signs and symptoms associated with hypervitaminosis A (severe headache, nausea, vomiting, drowsiness, irritability, and pruritus) may occur. However, it is likely that these symptoms would prove to be reversible.

5. PHARMACOLOGICAL PROPERTIES
Both gels have demonstrated therapeutic effects as early as 1 week after commencement of a course of treatment. A good clinical response was seen in up to 65% of the patients after 12 weeks of treatment.

The therapeutic effect of the higher concentration gel is more rapidly apparent and the efficacy more marked.

In various studies in which patients were also evaluated for 12 weeks following cessation of therapy, it was found that patients continued to show a certain clinical benefit, however, no difference between the higher and lower concentrations with regard to this effect was observed.

5.1 Pharmacodynamic properties
Pharmacotherapeutic group: {group TOPICAL ANTIPSORIATIC AGENT, ATC-code: D05AX05}

Tazarotene, a member of the acetylenic class of retinoids, is a prodrug which is converted to its active free form, tazarotenic acid, by de-esterification in the skin area.

Tazarotenic acid is the only known metabolite of tazarotene to have retinoid activity.

The active metabolite specifically regulates gene expression, thus modulating cell proliferation, hyperplasia, and differentiation in a wide range of tissues, as has been demonstrated in *in vitro* and *in vivo* trials.

The exact mechanism of action of tazarotene in psoriasis is, as yet, unknown. Improvement in psoriatic patients occurs in association with restoration of normal cutaneous morphology, and reduction of the inflammatory markers ICAM-1 and HLA-DR, and of markers of epidermal hyperplasia and abnormal differentiation, such as elevated keratinocyte transglutaminase, involucrin, and keratin 16.

5.2 Pharmacokinetic properties
a) General characteristics

Absorption
Results of a pharmacokinetic study of single topical application of 0.1% ^{14}C-tazarotene gel show that approximately 5% is absorbed when applied to normal skin under occlusion.

After a single topical application of tazarotene gel to 20% body surface area for 10 hours in healthy volunteers, tazarotene was not detectable in the plasma. Maximum plasma levels for the active metabolite tazarotenic acid of 0.3 ± 0.2 ng/ml (for the 0.05% strength) and 0.5 ± 0.3 ng/ml (0.1% gel) were measured after approximately 15 hours. The AUC was 40% higher for the 0.1% gel compared with the 0.05% gel. Thus, the two strengths of the gel are not strictly dose proportional with respect to systemic absorption.

Repeated topical application of the 0.1% gel over 7 days led to maximum plasma levels for tazarotenic acid of 0.7 ± 0.6 ng/ml after 9 hours.

Biotransformation
After dermal application, tazarotene undergoes esterase hydrolysis to form its free acid, tazarotenic acid, and oxidative metabolism to form inactive sulphoxide and sulphone derivatives.

Elimination
Secondary metabolites of tazarotenic acid (the sulphoxide, the sulphone and an oxygenated derivative of tazarotenic acid) have been detected in human urine and faeces. The elimination half-life of tazarotenic acid after dermal application of tazarotene is approximately 18 hours in normal and psoriatic subjects.

After intravenous administration, the half-life of tazarotene was approximately 6 hours and that of tazarotenic acid 14 hours.

b) Characteristics after use in patients

After single topical application of 0.1% ^{14}C-tazarotene gel for 10 hours to psoriatic lesions (without occlusion), 4.5% of the dose was recovered in the stratum corneum and 2.4% in the epidermal/dermal layers. Less than 1% of the dose was absorbed systemically. More than 75% of drug elimination was completed within 72 hours.

In a small five patient study, repeated topical application of tazarotene 0.1% gel over 13 days results in a mean peak plasma level of tazarotenic acid of 12 ± 8 ng/ml. These patients had psoriatic lesions on 8-18% of body surface area. In a larger 24 psoriatic patient study, tazarotene 0.05% and 0.1% gels were applied for 3 months and yielded a Cmax of 0.45 ± 0.78 ng/ml and 0.83 ± 1.22 ng/ml, respectively.

In a 1 year clinical study with 0.05% and 0.1% tazarotene gel, tazarotene was detected in 3 out of 112 patients at plasma concentrations below 1 ng/ml, while its active metabolite tazarotenic acid was found in 31 patients. Only four patients had plasma concentrations of tazarotenic acid greater than or equal to 1 ng/ml (maximum 2.8 ng/ml).

5.3 Preclinical safety data
Subacute / Chronic toxicity

The safety of daily dermal application of tazarotene gel was tested in mouse, rat and mini-pig over periods of up to one year. The main observation was reversible skin irritation. In the case of the mini-pig, an incomplete healing of the dermal irritation was observed after an 8 week recovery period. The rat appears to be the most sensitive species to tazarotene, as is the case with other retinoids. Here, dermal application induced severe skin reactions and clinically significant retinoid-like systemic effects. No adverse systemic effects were observed in the other species.

After oral administration of 0.025 mg/kg/day for 1 year in the cynomolgus monkey, no toxic effects were observed. At higher doses, typical symptoms of retinoid toxicity were seen.

Reproductive toxicity

Safety of use during pregnancy has not been established. Teratogenic and embryotoxic effects were observed after oral administration in the rat and rabbit. In dermal application studies during foetal development, skeletal alterations and decreased pup weight at birth and at the end of the lactation period were observed.

Animal tests suggest that tazarotene or its active metabolite is excreted in breast milk and passes the placenta barrier.

No effects on fertility are reported after topical application in the male and female rat.

Mutagenicity / carcinogenicity

No evidence of a mutagenic potential of tazarotene has been reported in *in vitro* and *in vivo* trials.

In long term investigations of the effects of dermal and oral administration in animals, no carcinogenic effects were observed.

There was an increased incidence of photocarcinogenic effects in the hairless mouse when exposed to UV light after topical application of tazarotene.

Local tolerability

Tazarotene gel has a considerable irritative potential on skin in all animal species investigated.

Instillation of tazarotene gel in the eye of the rabbit resulted in irritation with marked hyperaemia of the conjunctiva, but there was no corneal damage.

6. PHARMACEUTICAL PARTICULARS
6.1 List of excipients
Benzyl alcohol
Macrogol 400
Hexylene glycol
Carbomer 974P
Trometamol
Poloxamer 407
Polysorbate 40
Ascorbic acid
Butylhydroxyanisole (E320)
Butylhydroxytoluene (E321)
Disodium edetate
Purified water.

6.2 Incompatibilities
Tazarotene is susceptible to oxidising agents and may undergo ester hydrolysis when in contact with bases.

6.3 Shelf life
3 years.
After first opening of the container: 6 months.

6.4 Special precautions for storage
Do not store above 30°C.

6.5 Nature and contents of container
10 g, 15 g, 30 g, 50 g, 60 g and 100 g in tube (aluminium, internally lacquered epoxyphenolic) with white polypropylene cap.

6.6 Special precautions for disposal and other handling
No special requirements.

7. MARKETING AUTHORISATION HOLDER
Allergan Pharmaceuticals Ireland
Castlebar Road
Westport
County Mayo
Ireland

8. MARKETING AUTHORISATION NUMBER(S)
PL 05179/0003

9. DATE OF FIRST AUTHORISATION/RENEWAL OF THE AUTHORISATION
30th July 1997 / 3rd December 2006

10. DATE OF REVISION OF THE TEXT
21st May 2009

Zorac 0.1% Gel

(Allergan Ltd)

1. NAME OF THE MEDICINAL PRODUCT
ZORAC 0.1%, gel

2. QUALITATIVE AND QUANTITATIVE COMPOSITION
Active substance:
Tazarotene .... 0.1 g
Excipients with a well known effect:
Butylhydroxyanisole.................................. 0.05 g
Butylhydroxytoluene .... 0.05 g
For 100 g of gel
For a full list of excipients, see section 6.1.

3. PHARMACEUTICAL FORM
Gel.

Colourless to light yellow, translucent to homogeneous cloudy gel.

4. CLINICAL PARTICULARS

4.1 Therapeutic indications
For the topical treatment of mild to moderate plaque psoriasis involving up to 10% body surface area.

4.2 Posology and method of administration
Zorac gel is available in two concentrations.

To initiate a treatment with Zorac, it is advisable to start with Zorac 0.05% in order to evaluate the skin response and tolerance before progressing to Zorac 0.1% if necessary.

Treatment with the lower concentration gel is associated with a somewhat lower incidence of local adverse events (see sections 4.8 Undesirable effects and 5. Pharmacological Properties).

Treatment with the higher concentration gel gives a faster and numerically higher response rate. The physician should choose the concentration to be used based on clinical circumstances and the principle of using the least concentration of drug to achieve the desired effect.

Individual variations with respect to efficacy and tolerability are possible. It is thus advisable for patients to consult their physician on a weekly basis when initiating therapy.

A thin film of the gel should be applied once daily in the evening; care should be taken to apply it only to areas of affected skin, avoiding application to healthy skin or in skin folds. Treatment is limited to 10% body surface area (approximately equivalent to the total skin area of one arm).

If the patient experiences more drying or irritation, an effective greasy emollient (without pharmaceutically active ingredients) can be applied to the areas of the skin to be treated to improve tolerability. Healthy skin around the psoriatic plaques can be covered by using zinc paste, for example, to prevent irritation.

Usually, the treatment period is up to 12 weeks. Clinical experience, particularly on tolerability, is available on periods of use of up to 12 months.

4.3 Contraindications
- Hypersensitivity to any ingredient of the medication(s)
- Pregnancy or in women planning a pregnancy (see section 4.6 Pregnancy and lactation)
- Breast-feeding mothers
- Since there is, as yet, no clinical experience, Zorac should not be used in the treatment of psoriasis pustulosa and psoriasis exfoliativa, and the gel should not be applied to intertriginous areas, to the face or to hair-covered scalp.

4.4 Special warnings and precautions for use
Care should be taken to ensure that Zorac is applied only to psoriatic lesions, as application to normal, eczematous or inflamed skin or skin affected by other pathologies may cause irritation.

Patients should be advised to wash their hands after application of the gel to avoid accidental transfer to the eyes.

If psoriatic areas on the skin of the hands are being treated, particular care should be taken to ensure that no gel is transferred to facial skin or the eyes.

If skin irritation develops, treatment with Zorac should be interrupted.

The safety of use on more than 10% of the body surface area has not been established. There is limited experience of application to up to 20% of the body surface area.

Patients should be advised to avoid excessive exposure to UV light (including sunlight, use of a solarium, PUVA or UVB therapy) during treatment with Zorac (see section 5.3 Preclinical safety data).

No therapeutic studies using Zorac under occlusion or concomitantly with other antipsoriatic agents (including tar shampoos) have been carried out. To minimise interference with absorption and to avoid unnecessary spreading of the medication, topical application of emollients and cosmetics should not be applied within 1 hour of applying Zorac.

The safety and efficacy of Zorac have not been established in patients under the age of 18 years.

This medicinal product contains butylhydroxyanisole and butylhydroxytoluene and therefore may cause local skin reactions (e.g. contact dermatitis) or irritation to the eyes and mucous membranes.

4.5 Interaction with other medicinal products and other forms of interaction
Concomitant use of pharmaceutical and cosmetic preparations which cause irritation or have a strong drying effect should be avoided.

4.6 Pregnancy and lactation
Pregnancy
Zorac gel is contraindicated in women who are or may become pregnant (see 4.3). If this drug is used during pregnancy, or if the patient becomes pregnant while taking this drug, treatment should be discontinued and the patient apprised of the potential hazard to the foetus. Women of child-bearing potential should be warned of the potential risk and use adequate birthcontrol measures when Zorac gel is used. The possibility that a woman of childbearing potential is pregnant at the time of institution of therapy should be considered. A negative result for pregnancy test having a sensitivity down to at least 50 mIU/mL for human chorionic gonadotropin (hCG) should be obtained within 2 weeks prior to Zorac gel therapy, which should begin during a normal menstrual period.

Although in animals no malformations were observed after dermal application, skeletal alterations were seen in the foetuses, which may be attributable to systemic retinoid effects. Teratogenic effects were observed after oral administration.

Lactation
Although no data are available on the excretion of tazarotene in human milk, animal data indicate that excretion into milk is possible. For that reason Zorac gel should not be used during breast-feeding.

4.7 Effects on ability to drive and use machines
None known.

4.8 Undesirable effects
The most frequently reported adverse reactions in controlled clinical trials of Zorac in the treatment of psoriasis were pruritus (incidence 20-25%), burning, erythema, and irritation (10-20%), desquamation, non-specific rash, irritant contact dermatitis, skin pain, and a worsening of psoriasis (5-10 %).

More rarely observed were stinging and inflamed and dry skin (1-3 %).

The incidence of adverse reactions appears to be concentration-related and dependent on duration of use.

The higher concentration gel (0.1%) may cause up to 5% more cases of severe skin irritation than the lower concentration gel (0.05%), especially during the first 4 weeks of use.

Furthermore skin discoloration might occur.

4.9 Overdose
Excessive dermal use of Zorac may result in marked redness, peeling, or local discomfort.

Inadvertent ingestion of Zorac is a theoretical possibility. In such a case, the signs and symptoms associated with hypervitaminosis A (severe headache, nausea, vomiting, drowsiness, irritability, and pruritus) may occur. However, it is likely that these symptoms would prove to be reversible.

5. PHARMACOLOGICAL PROPERTIES
Both gels have demonstrated therapeutic effects as early as 1 week after commencement of a course of treatment. A good clinical response was seen in up to 65% of the patients after 12 weeks of treatment.

The therapeutic effect of the higher concentration gel is more rapidly apparent and the efficacy more marked.

In various studies in which patients were also evaluated for 12 weeks following cessation of therapy, it was found that patients continued to show a certain clinical benefit, however, no difference between the higher and lower concentrations with regard to this effect was observed.

5.1 Pharmacodynamic properties
Pharmacotherapeutic group: {group TOPICAL ANTIPSORIATIC AGENT, ATC-code: D05AX05}

Tazarotene, a member of the acetylenic class of retinoids, is a prodrug which is converted to its active free form, tazarotenic acid, by de-esterification in the skin area.

Tazarotenic acid is the only known metabolite of tazarotene to have retinoid activity.

The active metabolite specifically regulates gene expression, thus modulating cell proliferation, hyperplasia, and differentiation in a wide range of tissues, as has been demonstrated in *in vitro* and *in vivo* trials.

The exact mechanism of action of tazarotene in psoriasis is, as yet, unknown. Improvement in psoriatic patients occurs in association with restoration of normal cutaneous morphology, and reduction of the inflammatory markers ICAM-1 and HLA-DR, and of markers of epidermal hyperplasia and abnormal differentiation, such as elevated keratinocyte transglutaminase, involucrin, and keratin 16.

5.2 Pharmacokinetic properties
a) General characteristics

Absorption
Results of a pharmacokinetic study of single topical application of 0.1% ^{14}C-tazarotene gel show that approximately 5% is absorbed when applied to normal skin under occlusion.

After a single topical application of tazarotene gel to 20% body surface area for 10 hours in healthy volunteers, tazarotene was not detectable in the plasma. Maximum plasma levels for the active metabolite tazarotenic acid of 0.3 ± 0.2 ng/ml (for the 0.05% strength) and 0.5 ± 0.3 ng/ml (0.1% gel) were measured after approximately 15 hours. The AUC was 40% higher for the 0.1% gel compared with the 0.05% gel. Thus, the two strengths of the gel are not strictly dose proportional with respect to systemic absorption.

Repeated topical application of the 0.1% gel over 7 days led to maximum plasma levels for tazarotenic acid of 0.7 ± 0.6 ng/ml after 9 hours.

Biotransformation
After dermal application, tazarotene undergoes esterase hydrolysis to form its free acid, tazarotenic acid, and oxidative metabolism to form inactive sulphoxide and sulphone derivatives.

Elimination
Secondary metabolites of tazarotenic acid (the sulphoxide, the sulphone and an oxygenated derivative of tazarotenic acid) have been detected in human urine and faeces. The elimination half-life of tazarotenic acid after dermal application of tazarotene is approximately 18 hours in normal and psoriatic subjects.

After intravenous administration, the half-life of tazarotene was approximately 6 hours and that of tazarotenic acid 14 hours.

b) Characteristics after use in patients

After single topical application of 0.1% ^{14}C-tazarotene gel for 10 hours to psoriatic lesions (without occlusion), 4.5% of the dose was recovered in the stratum corneum and 2.4% in the epidermal/dermal layers. Less than 1% of the dose was absorbed systemically. More than 75% of drug elimination was completed within 72 hours.

In a small five patient study, repeated topical application of tazarotene 0.1% gel over 13 days results in a mean peak plasma level of tazarotenic acid of 12 ± 8 ng/ml. These patients had psoriatic lesions on 8-18% of body surface area. In a larger 24 psoriatic patient study, tazarotene 0.05% and 0.1% gels were applied for 3 months and yielded a Cmax of 0.45 ± 0.78 ng/ml and 0.83 ± 1.22 ng/ml, respectively.

In a 1 year clinical study with 0.05% and 0.1% tazarotene gel, tazarotene was detected in 3 out of 112 patients at plasma concentrations below 1 ng/ml, while its active metabolite tazarotenic acid was found in 31 patients. Only four patients had plasma concentrations of tazarotenic acid greater than or equal to 1 ng/ml (maximum 2.8 ng/ml).

5.3 Preclinical safety data
Subacute / Chronic toxicity

The safety of daily dermal application of tazarotene gel was tested in mouse, rat and mini-pig over periods of up to one year. The main observation was reversible skin irritation. In the case of the mini-pig, an incomplete healing of the dermal irritation was observed after an 8 week recovery period. The rat appears to be the most sensitive species to tazarotene, as is the case with other retinoids. Here, dermal application induced severe skin reactions and clinically significant retinoid-like systemic effects. No adverse systemic effects were observed in the other species.

After oral administration of 0.025 mg/kg/day for 1 year in the cynomolgus monkey, no toxic effects were observed. At higher doses, typical symptoms of retinoid toxicity were seen.

Reproductive toxicity

Safety of use during pregnancy has not been established. Teratogenic and embryotoxic effects were observed after oral administration in the rat and rabbit. In dermal application studies during foetal development, skeletal alterations and decreased pup weight at birth and at the end of the lactation period were observed.

Animal tests suggest that tazarotene or its active metabolite is excreted in breast milk and passes the placenta barrier.

No effects on fertility are reported after topical application in the male and female rat.

Mutagenicity / carcinogenicity

No evidence of a mutagenic potential of tazarotene has been reported in *in vitro* and *in vivo* trials.

In long term investigations of the effects of dermal and oral administration in animals, no carcinogenic effects were observed.

There was an increased incidence of photocarcinogenic effects in the hairless mouse when exposed to UV light after topical application of tazarotene.

Local tolerability

Tazarotene gel has a considerable irritative potential on skin in all animal species investigated.

Instillation of tazarotene gel in the eye of the rabbit resulted in irritation with marked hyperaemia of the conjunctiva, but there was no corneal damage.

6. PHARMACEUTICAL PARTICULARS

6.1 List of excipients

Benzyl alcohol

Macrogol 400

Hexylene glycol

Carbomer 974P

Trometamol

Poloxamer 407

Polysorbate 40

Ascorbic acid

Butylhydroxyanisole (E320)

Butylhydroxytoluene (E321)

Disodium edetate

Purified water.

6.2 Incompatibilities

Tazarotene is susceptible to oxidising agents and may undergo ester hydrolysis when in contact with bases.

6.3 Shelf life

3 years.

After first opening of the container: 6 months.

6.4 Special precautions for storage

Do not store above 30°C.

6.5 Nature and contents of container

10 g, 15 g, 30 g, 50 g, 60 g and 100 g in tube (aluminium, internally lacquered epoxyphenolic) with white polypropylene cap.

6.6 Special precautions for disposal and other handling

No special requirements.

7. MARKETING AUTHORISATION HOLDER

Allergan Pharmaceuticals Ireland

Castlebar Road

Westport

County Mayo

Ireland

8. MARKETING AUTHORISATION NUMBER(S)

PL 05179/0002

9. DATE OF FIRST AUTHORISATION/RENEWAL OF THE AUTHORISATION

30th July 1997 / 3rd December 2006

10. DATE OF REVISION OF THE TEXT

21st May 2009

Zoton FasTab

(Wyeth Pharmaceuticals)

1. NAME OF THE MEDICINAL PRODUCT

Zoton FasTab* 15 mg oro-dispersible tablets

Zoton FasTab* 30 mg oro-dispersible tablets

2. QUALITATIVE AND QUANTITATIVE COMPOSITION

Each oro-dispersible tablet contains 15 mg of lansoprazole

Each oro-dispersible tablet contains 30 mg of lansoprazole

Excipient(s): Each 15 mg oro-dispersible tablet contains 15 mg of lactose and 4.5 mg of aspartame

Each 30 mg oro-dispersible tablet contains 30 mg of lactose and 9.0 mg of aspartame

For a full list of excipients, see section 6.1.

3. PHARMACEUTICAL FORM

Zoton FasTab 15 mg: White to yellowish white, circular flat beveled-edge oro-dispersible tablet with "15" debossed on one side. Each oro-dispersible tablet contains orange to dark brown microgranules.

Zoton FasTab 30 mg: White to yellowish white, circular flat beveled-edge oro-dispersible tablet with "30" debossed on one side. Each oro-dispersible tablet contains orange to dark brown microgranules.

4. CLINICAL PARTICULARS

4.1 Therapeutic indications

- Treatment of duodenal and gastric ulcer
- Treatment of reflux oesophagitis
- Prophylaxis of reflux oesophagitis
- Eradication of *Helicobacter pylori* (*H. pylori*) concurrently given with appropriate antibiotic therapy for treatment of *H. pylori*-associated ulcers
- Treatment of NSAID-associated benign gastric and duodenal ulcers in patients requiring continued NSAID treatment
- Prophylaxis of NSAID-associated gastric ulcers and duodenal ulcers in patients at risk (see section 4.2) requiring continued therapy
- Symptomatic gastroesophageal reflux disease
- Zollinger-Ellison syndrome.

4.2 Posology and method of administration

For optimal effect, Zoton FasTab should be taken once daily in the morning, except when used for *H. pylori* eradication when treatment should be twice a day, once in the morning and once in the evening. Zoton FasTab should be taken at least 30 minutes before food (see section 5.2). Zoton FasTab is strawberry flavoured and should be placed on the tongue and gently sucked. The tablet rapidly disperses in the mouth, releasing gastro-resistant microgranules which are swallowed with the patient's saliva. Alternatively, the tablet can be swallowed whole with a drink of water.

The orodispersible tablets can be dispersed in a small amount of water and administered via a naso-gastric tube or oral syringe.

Treatment of duodenal ulcer:

The recommended dose is 30 mg once daily for 2 weeks. In patients not fully healed within this time, the medication is continued at the same dose for another two weeks.

Treatment of gastric ulcer:

The recommended dose is 30 mg once daily for 4 weeks. The ulcer usually heals within 4 weeks, but in patients not fully healed within this time, the medication may be continued at the same dose for another 4 weeks.

Reflux oesophagitis:

The recommended dose is 30 mg once daily for 4 weeks. In patients not fully healed within this time, the treatment may be continued at the same dose for another 4 weeks.

Prophylaxis of reflux oesophagitis:

15 mg once daily. The dose may be increased up to 30 mg daily as necessary.

Eradication of *Helicobacter pylori:*

When selecting appropriate combination therapy consideration should be given to official local guidance regarding bacterial resistance, duration of treatment, (most commonly 7 days but sometimes up to 14 days), and appropriate use of antibacterial agents.

The recommended dose is 30 mg of Zoton FasTab twice daily for 7 days in combination with one of the following:

clarithromycin 250-500 mg twice daily + amoxicillin 1 g twice daily

clarithromycin 250 mg twice daily + metronidazole 400-500 mg twice daily

The *H. pylori* eradication results obtained when clarithromycin is combined with either amoxicillin or metronidazole give rates of up to 90%, when used in combination with Zoton FasTab.

Six months after successful eradication treatment, the risk of re infection is low and relapse is therefore unlikely.

Use of a regimen including lansoprazole 30 mg twice daily, amoxicillin 1 g twice daily and metronidazole 400-500 mg twice daily has also been examined. Lower eradication rates were seen using this combination than in regimens involving clarithromycin. It may be suitable for those who are unable to take clarithromycin as part of an eradication therapy, when local resistance rates to metronidazole are low.

Treatment of NSAID associated benign gastric and duodenal ulcers in patients requiring continued NSAID treatment:

30 mg once daily for four weeks. In patients not fully healed the treatment may be continued for another four weeks. For patients at risk or with ulcers that are difficult to heal, a longer course of treatment and/or a higher dose should probably be used.

Prophylaxis of NSAID associated gastric and duodenal ulcers in patients at risk (such as age ⩾ 65 or history of gastric or duodenal ulcer) requiring prolonged NSAID treatment:

15 mg once daily. If the treatment fails the dose 30 mg once daily should be used.

Symptomatic gastro-oesophageal reflux disease:

The recommended dose is 15 mg or 30 mg daily. Relief of symptoms is obtained rapidly. Individual adjustment of dosage should be considered. If the symptoms are not relieved within 4 weeks with a daily dose of 30 mg, further examinations are recommended.

Zollinger-Ellison syndrome:

The recommended initial dose is 60 mg once daily. The dose should be individually adjusted and the treatment should be continued for as long as necessary. Daily doses of up to 180 mg have been used. If the required daily dose exceeds 120 mg, it should be given in two divided doses.

Impaired hepatic or renal function:

There is no need for a dose adjustment in patients with impaired renal function.

Patients with moderate or severe liver disease should be kept under regular supervision and a 50% reduction of the daily dose is recommended (see section 4.4 and 5.2).

Elderly:

Due to reduced clearance of lansoprazole in the elderly an adjustment of dose may be necessary based on individual requirements. A daily dose of 30 mg should not be exceeded in the elderly unless there are compelling clinical indications.

Children:

The use of Zoton FasTab is not recommended in children as clinical data are limited (see also section 5.2).

4.3 Contraindications

Hypersensitivity to the active substance or to any of the excipients.

Lansoprazole should not be administered with atazanavir (see section 4.5).

4.4 Special warnings and precautions for use

In common with other anti-ulcer therapies, the possibility of malignant gastric tumour should be excluded when treating a gastric ulcer with lansoprazole because lansoprazole can mask the symptoms and delay the diagnosis.

Lansoprazole should be used with caution in patients with moderate and severe hepatic dysfunction (see sections 4.2 and 5.2).

Decreased gastric acidity due to lansoprazole might be expected to increase gastric counts of bacteria normally present in the gastrointestinal tract. Treatment with lansoprazole may lead to a slightly increased risk of gastrointestinal infections such as *Salmonella* and *Campylobacter*.

In patients suffering from gastro-duodenal ulcers, the possibility of *H.pylori* infection as an etiological factor should be considered.

If lansoprazole is used in combination with antibiotics for eradication therapy of *H.pylori*, then the instructions for the use of these antibiotics should also be followed.

Because of limited safety data for patients on maintenance treatment for longer than 1 year, regular review of the treatment and a thorough risk/benefit assessment should regularly be performed in these patients.

Very rarely cases of colitis have been reported in patients taking lansoprazole. Therefore, in the case of severe and/or persistent diarrhoea, discontinuation of therapy should be considered.

The treatment for the prevention of peptic ulceration of patients in need of continuous NSAID treatment should be restricted to high risk patients (e.g. previous gastrointestinal bleeding, perforation or ulcer, advanced age, concomitant use of medication known to increase the likelihood of upper GI adverse events [e.g. corticosteroids or anticoagulants], the presence of a serious co-morbidity factor or the prolonged use of NSAID maximum recommended doses).

As Zoton FasTab contains lactose, patients with rare hereditary problems of galactose intolerance, the Lapp lactase deficiency or glucose-galactose malabsorption should not take this medicine.

4.5 Interaction with other medicinal products and other forms of interaction

Effects of lansoprazole on other drugs

Medicinal products with pH dependent absorption

Lansoprazole may interfere with the absorption of drugs where gastric pH is critical to bioavailability.

Atazanavir:

A study has shown that co-administration of lansoprazole (60 mg once daily) with atazanavir 400 mg to healthy volunteers resulted in a substantial reduction in atazanavir exposure (approximately 90% decrease in AUC and Cmax). Lansoprazole should not be co-administered with atazanavir (see section 4.3).

Ketoconazole and itraconazole:

The absorption of ketoconazole and itraconazole from the gastrointestinal tract is enhanced by the presence of gastric acid. Administration of lansoprazole may result in subtherapeutic concentrations of ketoconazole and itraconazole and the combination should be avoided.

Digoxin:

Co-administration of lansoprazole and digoxin may lead to increased digoxin plasma levels. The plasma levels of digoxin should therefore be monitored and the dose of digoxin adjusted if necessary when initiating and ending lansoprazole treatment.

Medicinal products metabolised by P450 enzymes

Lansoprazole may increase plasma concentrations of drugs that are metabolised by CYP3A4. Caution is advised when combining lansoprazole with drugs which are metabolised by this enzyme and have a narrow therapeutic window.

Theophylline:

Lansoprazole reduces the plasma concentration of theophylline, which may decrease the expected clinical effect at the dose. Caution is advised when combining the two drugs.

Tacrolimus:

Co-administration of lansoprazole increases the plasma concentrations of tacrolimus (a CYP3A and P-gp substrate). Lansoprazole exposure increased the mean exposure of tacrolimus by up to 81%. Monitoring of tacrolimus plasma concentrations is advised when concomitant treatment with lanzoprazole is initiated or ended.

Medicinal products transported by P-glycoprotein

Lansoprazole has been observed to inhibit the transport protein, P-glycoprotein (P-gp) *in vitro*. The clinical relevance of this is unknown.

Effects of other drugs on lansoprazole

Drugs which inhibit CYP2C19

Fluvoxamine:

A dose reduction may be considered when combining lansoprazole with the CYP2C19 inhibitor fluvoxamine. A study shows that the plasma concentrations of lansoprazole increase up to 4-fold.

Drugs which induces CYP2C19 and CYP3A4

Enzyme inducers affecting CYP2C19 and CYP3A4 such as rifampicin, and St John's wort (*Hypericum perforatum*) can markedly reduce the plasma concentrations of lansoprazole.

Others

Sucralfate/Antacids:

Sucralfate/Antacids may decrease the bioavailability of lansoprazole. Therefore lansoprazole should be taken at least 1 hour after taking these drugs.

No clinically significant interactions of lansoprazole with nonsteroidal anti-inflammatory drugs have been demonstrated, although no formal interactions studies have been performed.

4.6 Pregnancy and lactation

Pregnancy:

For lansoprazole no clinical data on exposed pregnancies are available. Animal studies do not indicate direct or indirect harmful effects with respect to pregnancy, embryonal/foetal development, parturition or postnatal development.

Therefore, the use of lansoprazole during pregnancy is not recommended.

Lactation:

It is not known whether lansoprazole is excreted in human breast milk. Animal studies have shown excretion of lansoprazole in milk.

A decision on whether to continue/discontinue breastfeeding or to continue/discontinue therapy with lansoprazole should be made taking into account the benefit of breastfeeding to the child and the benefit of lansoprazole therapy to the woman.

4.7 Effects on ability to drive and use machines

Adverse drug reactions such as dizziness, vertigo, visual disturbances and somnolence may occur (see section 4.8). Under these conditions the ability to react may be decreased.

4.8 Undesirable effects

Frequencies are defined as common (> 1/100, < 1/10); uncommon (> 1/1,000, < 1/100); rare (>1/10,000, <1/1,000); very rare (<1/10,000).

(see Table 1 above)

Table 1

	Common	Uncommon	Rare	Very rare
Blood and lymphatic system disorders		Thrombocytopenia, eosinophilia, leucopenia	Anaemia	Agranulocytosis, pancytopenia
Psychiatric disorders		Depression	Insomnia, hallucination, confusion	
Nervous system disorders	Headache, dizziness		Restlessness, vertigo, paresthesia, somnolence, tremor	
Eye disorders			Visual disturbances	
Gastrointestinal disorders	Nausea, diarrhoea, stomach ache, constipation, vomiting, flatulence, dry mouth or throat		Glossitis, candidiasis of the oesophagus, pancreatitis, taste disturbances	Colitis, stomatitis
Hepatobiliary disorders	Increase in liver enzyme levels		Hepatitis, jaundice	
Skin and subcutaneous tissue disorders	Urticaria, itching, rash		Petechiae, purpura, hair loss, erythema multiforme, photosensitivity	Steven-Johnson syndrome, toxic epidermal necrolysis
Musculoskeletal and connective tissue disorders		Arthralgia, myalgia		
Renal and urinary disorders			Interstitial nephritis	
Reproductive system and breast disorders			Gynaecomastia	
General disorders and administration site conditions	Fatigue	Oedema	Fever, hyperhidrosis, angioedema, anorexia, impotence	Anaphylactic shock
Investigations				Increase in cholesterol and triglyceride levels, hyponatremia

4.9 Overdose

The effects of overdose on lansoprazole in humans are not known (although the acute toxicity is likely to be low) and, consequently, instruction for treatment cannot be given. However, daily doses of up to 180 mg of lansoprazole orally and up to 90 mg of lansoprazole intravenously have been administered in trials without significant undesirable effects.

Please refer to section 4.8 for possible symptoms of lansoprazole overdose.

In the case of suspected overdose the patient should be monitored. Lansoprazole is not significantly eliminated by haemodialysis. If necessary, gastric emptying, charcoal and symptomatic therapy is recommended.

5. PHARMACOLOGICAL PROPERTIES

5.1 Pharmacodynamic properties

Pharmacotherapeutic group: Proton pump inhibitors, ATC code: A02BC03

Lansoprazole is a gastric proton pump inhibitor. It inhibits the final stage of gastric acid formation by inhibiting the activity of H^+/K^+ ATPase of the parietal cells in the stomach. The inhibition is dose-dependent and reversible, and the effect applies to both basal and stimulated secretion of gastric acid. Lansoprazole is concentrated in the parietal cells and becomes active in their acidic environment, whereupon it reacts with the sulphydryl group of H^+/K^+ATPase causing inhibition of the enzyme activity.

Effect on gastric acid secretion:

Lansoprazole is a specific inhibitor of the parietal cell proton pump. A single oral 30 mg dose of lansoprazole inhibits pentagastrin-stimulated gastric acid secretion by about 80%. After repeated daily administration for seven days, about 90% inhibition of gastric acid secretion is achieved. It has a corresponding effect on the basal secretion of gastric acid. A single oral dose of 30 mg reduces basal secretion by about 70%, and the patients' symptoms are consequently relieved starting from the very first dose. After eight days of repeated administration the reduction is about 85%. A rapid relief of symptoms is obtained by one oro-dispersible tablet (30 mg) daily, and most patients with duodenal ulcer recover within 2 weeks, patients with gastric ulcer and reflux oesophagitis within 4 weeks. By reducing gastric acidity, lansoprazole creates an environment in which appropriate antibiotics can be effective against *H. pylori*.

5.2 Pharmacokinetic properties

Lansoprazole is a racemate of two active enantiomers that are biotransformed into the active form in the acidic environment of the parietal cells. As lansoprazole is rapidly inactivated by gastric acid, it is administered orally in enteric-coated form(s) for systemic absorption.

Absorption and distribution

Lansoprazole exhibits high (80-90%) bioavailability with a single dose. Peak plasma levels occur within 1.5 to 2.0 hours. Intake of food slows the absorption rate of lansoprazole and reduces the bioavailabilty by about 50%. The plasma protein binding is 97%.

Studies have shown that oro-dispersible tablets dispersed in a small amount of water and given via syringe directly into the mouth or administered via naso-gastric tube result in equivalent AUC compared to the usual mode of administration.

Metabolism and elimination

Lansoprazole is extensively metabolised by the liver and the metabolites are excreted by both the renal and biliary route. The metabolism of lansoprazole is mainly catalysed by the enzyme CYP2C19. The enzyme CYP3A4 also contributes to the metabolism. The plasma elimination half-life ranges from 1 to 2 hours following single or multiple doses in healthy subjects. There is no evidence of accumulation following multiple doses in healthy subjects. Sulphone, sulphide and 5-hydroxyl derivatives of lansoprazole have been identified in plasma. These metabolites have very little or no antisecretory activity.

A study with ^{14}C labelled lansoprazole indicated that approximately one-third of the administered radiation was excreted in the urine and two-thirds was recovered in the faeces.

Pharmacokinetics in elderly patients

The clearance of lansoprazole is decreased in the elderly, with elimination half-life increased approximately 50% to 100%. Peak plasma levels were not increased in the elderly.

Pharmacokinetics in paediatric patients

The evaluation of the pharmacokinetics in children aged 1 – 17 years of age showed a similar exposure as compared to adults with doses of 15 mg for those below 30 kg of weight and 30 mg for those above. The investigation of a dose of 17 mg/m² body surface or 1 mg/kg body weight also resulted in comparable exposure of lansoprazole in children aged 2-3 months up to one year of age compared to adults.

Higher exposure to lansoprazole in comparison to adults has been seen in infants below the age of 2-3 months with doses of both 1.0 mg/kg and 0.5 mg/kg body weight given as a single dose.

Pharmacokinetics in hepatic insufficiency

The exposure of lansoprazole is doubled in patients with mild hepatic impairment and much more increased in patients with moderate and severe hepatic impairment.

CYP2C19 poor metabolisers

CYP2C19 is subject to genetic polymorphism and 2-6 % of the population, called poor metabolisers (PMs), are homozygote for a mutant CYP2C19 allele and therefore lacks a functional CYP2C19 enzyme. The exposure of lansoprazole is several-fold higher in PMs than in extensive metabolisers (EMs).

5.3 Preclinical safety data

Preclinical data reveal no special hazards for humans based on conventional studies of safety pharmacology, repeated dose toxicity, toxicity to reproduction or genotoxicity.

In two rat carcinogenicity studies, lansoprazole produced dose-related gastric ECL cell hyperplasia and ECL cell carcinoids associated with hypergastrinaemia due to inhibition of acid secretion. Intestinal metaplasia was also observed, as were Leydig cell hyperplasia and benign Leydig cell tumours. After 18 months of treatment retinal atrophy was observed. This was not seen in monkeys, dogs or mice.

In mouse carcinogenicity studies dose-related gastric ECL cell hyperplasia developed as well as liver tumours and adenoma of rete testis.

The clinical relevance of these findings is unknown.

6. PHARMACEUTICAL PARTICULARS

6.1 List of excipients

Gastro-resistant microgranules: Lactose monohydrate, microcrystalline cellulose, heavy magnesium carbonate, low-substituted hydroxypropylcellulose, hydroxypropyl cellulose, hypromellose, titanium dioxide, talc, mannitol, methacrylic acid – ethyl acrylate copolymer (1:1) 30 per cent, polyacrylate dispersion 30 per cent, macrogol 8000, citric acid anhydrous, glyceryl monostearate, polysorbate 80, mannitol, iron oxide yellow (E172) and iron oxide red (E172).

Other excipients: Mannitol, microcrystalline cellulose, low-substituted hydroxypropylcellulose, citric acid anhydrous, crospovidone, magnesium stearate, strawberry flavour and aspartame.

6.2 Incompatibilities

Not applicable.

6.3 Shelf life

3 years.

6.4 Special precautions for storage

Do not store above 25°C. Store in the original package.

6.5 Nature and contents of container

Zoton FasTab 15 mg: Aluminium blister packs of 28 or 56 Tablets.

Zoton FasTab 30 mg: Aluminium blister packs of 2, 7, 14 or 28 Tablets.

Not all pack sizes may be marketed.

6.6 Special precautions for disposal and other handling

No special requirements.

7. MARKETING AUTHORISATION HOLDER

John Wyeth & Brother Limited

Trading as Wyeth Pharmaceuticals

Huntercombe Lane South

Taplow

Maidenhead

Berkshire SL6 0PH

UK

8. MARKETING AUTHORISATION NUMBER(S)

Zoton FasTab 15 mg: PL 00011/0290

Zoton FasTab 30 mg: PL 00011/0289

9. DATE OF FIRST AUTHORISATION/RENEWAL OF THE AUTHORISATION

Zoton FasTab 15 mg: 26 January 2004 / 11 March 2005

Zoton FasTab 30 mg: 26 January 2004 / 11 March 2005

10. DATE OF REVISION OF THE TEXT

9 August 2007

* Trademark of, and under licence agreement with, Takeda Pharmaceutical Company Limited, Japan.

Zovirax 200mg Tablets

(GlaxoSmithKline UK)

1. NAME OF THE MEDICINAL PRODUCT

Zovirax Tablets 200 mg.

2. QUALITATIVE AND QUANTITATIVE COMPOSITION

Aciclovir BP 200 mg

3. PHARMACEUTICAL FORM

Dispersible film-coated tablet.

4. CLINICAL PARTICULARS

4.1 Therapeutic indications

Zovirax Tablets are indicated for the treatment of herpes simplex virus infections of the skin and mucous membranes including initial and recurrent genital herpes.

Zovirax Tablets are indicated for the suppression (prevention of recurrences) of recurrent herpes simplex infections in immunocompetent patients.

Zovirax Tablets are indicated for the prophylaxis of herpes simplex infections in immunocompromised patients.

Zovirax Tablets are indicated for the treatment of varicella (chickenpox) and herpes zoster (shingles) infections.

Route of administration: Oral.

4.2 Posology and method of administration

Zovirax tablets may be dispersed in a minimum of 50 ml of water or swallowed whole with a little water. Ensure that patients on high doses of aciclovir are adequately hydrated.

Dosage in adults

Treatment of herpes simplex infections: 200 mg Zovirax should be taken five times daily at approximately four hourly intervals omitting the night time dose. Treatment should continue for 5 days, but in severe initial infections this may have to be extended.

In severely immunocompromised patients (e.g. after marrow transplant) or in patients with impaired absorption from the gut the dose can be doubled to 400 mg Zovirax or alternatively intravenous dosing could be considered.

Dosing should begin as early as possible after the start of an infection; for recurrent episodes this should preferably be during the prodromal period or when lesions first appear.

Suppression of herpes simplex infections in immunocompetent patients: 200 mg Zovirax should be taken four times daily at approximately six-hourly intervals.

Many patients may be conveniently managed on a regimen of 400 mg Zovirax twice daily at approximately twelve-hourly intervals.

Dosage titration down to 200 mg Zovirax taken thrice daily at approximately eight-hourly intervals or even twice daily at approximately twelve-hourly intervals may prove effective.

Some patients may experience break-through infection on total daily doses of 800 mg Zovirax.

Therapy should be interrupted periodically at intervals of six to twelve months, in order to observe possible changes in the natural history of the disease.

Prophylaxis of herpes simplex infections in immunocompromised patients: 200 mg Zovirax should be taken four times daily at approximately six-hourly intervals.

In severely immunocompromised patients (e.g. after marrow transplant) or in patients with impaired absorption from the gut, the dose can be doubled to 400 mg Zovirax, or alternatively, intravenous dosing could be considered.

The duration of prophylactic administration is determined by the duration of the period at risk.

Treatment of varicella and herpes zoster infections: 800 mg Zovirax should be taken five times daily at approximately four-hourly intervals, omitting the night time dose. Treatment should continue for seven days.

In severely immunocompromised patients (e.g. after marrow transplant) or in patients with impaired absorption from the gut, consideration should be given to intravenous dosing.

Dosing should begin as early as possible after the start of an infection: Treatment of herpes zoster yields better results if initiated as soon as possible after the onset of the rash. Treatment of chickenpox in immunocompetent patients should begin within 24 hours after onset of the rash.

Dosage in children

Treatment of herpes simplex infections, and prophylaxis of herpes simplex infections in the immunocompromised: Children aged two years and over should be given adult dosages and children below the age of two years should be given half the adult dose.

Treatment of varicella infection

6 years and over:	800 mg Zovirax four times daily.
2 - 5 years:	400mg Zovirax four times daily.
Under 2 years:	200mg Zovirax four times daily.

Treatment should continue for five days.

Dosing may be more accurately calculated as 20 mg/kg bodyweight (not to exceed 800 mg) Zovirax four times daily.

No specific data are available on the suppression of herpes simplex infections or the treatment of herpes zoster infections in immunocompetent children.

Dosage in the elderly:

The possibility of renal impairment in the elderly must be considered and the dosage should be adjusted accordingly (see Dosage in renal impairment below).

Adequate hydration of elderly patients taking high oral doses of aciclovir should be maintained.

Dosage in renal impairment:

Caution is advised when administering aciclovir to patients with impaired renal function. Adequate hydration should be maintained.

In the management of herpes simplex infections in patients with impaired renal function, the recommended oral doses will not lead to accumulation of aciclovir above levels that have been established safe by intravenous infusion. However for patients with severe renal impairment (creatinine clearance less than 10 ml/minute) an adjustment of dosage to 200 mg aciclovir twice daily at approximately twelve-hourly intervals is recommended.

In the treatment of herpes zoster infections it is recommended to adjust the dosage to 800 mg aciclovir twice daily at approximately twelve - hourly intervals for patients with severe renal impairment (creatinine clearance less than 10 ml/minute), and to 800 mg aciclovir three times daily at intervals of approximately eight hours for patients with moderate renal impairment (creatinine clearance in the range 10 – 25 ml/minute).

4.3 Contraindications

Zovirax tablets are contra-indicated in patients known to be hypersensitive to aciclovir or valaciclovir.

4.4 Special warnings and precautions for use

Use in patients with renal impairment and in elderly patients:

Aciclovir is eliminated by renal clearance, therefore the dose must be adjusted in patients with renal impairment (see 4.2 Posology and Method of Administration). Elderly patients are likely to have reduced renal function and therefore the need for dose adjustment must be considered in this group of patients. Both elderly patients and patients with renal impairment are at increased risk of developing neurological side effects and should be closely monitored for evidence of these effects. In the reported cases, these reactions were generally reversible on discontinuation of treatment (see 4.8 Undesirable Effects).

Hydration status: Care should be taken to maintain adequate hydration in patients receiving high oral doses of aciclovir.

The data currently available from clinical studies is not sufficient to conclude that treatment with aciclovir reduces the incidence of chickenpox-associated complications in immunocompetent patients.

4.5 Interaction with other medicinal products and other forms of interaction

No clinically significant interactions have been identified.

Aciclovir is eliminated primarily unchanged in the urine via active renal tubular secretion. Any drugs administered concurrently that compete with this mechanism may increase aciclovir plasma concentrations. Probenecid and cimetidine increase the AUC of aciclovir by this mechanism, and reduce aciclovir renal clearance. Similarly increases in plasma AUCs of aciclovir and of the inactive metabolite of mycophenolate mofetil, an immunosuppresant agent used in transplant patients have been shown when the drugs are coadministered. However no dosage adjustment is necessary because of the wide therapeutic index of aciclovir.

4.6 Pregnancy and lactation

A post-marketing aciclovir pregnancy registry has documented pregnancy outcomes in women exposed to any formulation of Zovirax. The birth defects described amongst Zovirax exposed subjects have not shown any uniqueness or consistent pattern to suggest a common cause.

Caution should however be exercised by balancing the potential benefits of treatment against any possible hazard. Findings from reproduction toxicology studies are included in Section 5.3.

Following oral administration of 200 mg Zovirax five times a day, aciclovir has been detected in breast milk at concentrations ranging from 0.6 to 4.1 times the corresponding plasma levels. These levels would potentially expose nursing infants to aciclovir dosages of up to 0.3 mg/kg/day. Caution is therefore advised if aciclovir is to be administered to a nursing woman.

Fertility:

There is no information on the effect of aciclovir on human female fertility.

In a study of 20 male patients with normal sperm count, oral aciclovir administered at doses of up to 1g per day for up to six months has been shown to have no clinically significant effect on sperm count, motility or morphology.

4.7 Effects on ability to drive and use machines

There have been no studies to investigate the effect of aciclovir on driving performance or the ability to operate machinery. A detrimental effect on such activities cannot be predicted from the pharmacology of the active substance, but the adverse event profile should be borne in mind.

4.8 Undesirable effects

The frequency categories associated with the adverse events below are estimates. For most events, suitable data for estimating incidence were not available. In addition, adverse events may vary in their incidence depending on the indication.

The following convention has been used for the classification of undesirable effects in terms of frequency:- Very common $\geqslant 1/10$, common $\geqslant 1/100$ and $< 1/10$, uncommon $\geqslant 1/1000$ and $< 1/100$, rare $\geqslant 1/10,000$ and $< 1/1000$, very rare $< 1/10,000$.

Blood and lymphatic system disorders:

Very rare: Anaemia, leukopenia, thrombocytopenia.

Immune system disorders:

Rare: Anaphylaxis.

Psychiatric and nervous system disorders:

Common: Headache, dizziness.

Very rare: Agitation, confusion, tremor, ataxia, dysarthria, hallucinations, psychotic symptoms, convulsions, somnolence, encephalopathy, coma.

The above events are generally reversible and usually reported in patients with renal impairment or with other predisposing factors (see 4.4 Special Warnings and Precautions for Use).

Respiratory, thoracic and mediastinal disorders:

Rare: Dyspnoea.

Gastrointestinal disorders:

Common: Nausea, vomiting, diarrhoea, abdominal pains.

Hepato-biliary disorders:

Rare: Reversible rises in bilirubin and liver related enzymes.

Very rare: Hepatitis, jaundice.

Skin and subcutaneous tissue disorders:

Common: Pruritus, rashes (including photosensitivity).

Uncommon: Urticaria. Accelerated diffuse hair loss. Accelerated diffuse hair loss has been associated with a wide variety of disease processes and medicines, the relationship of the event to aciclovir therapy is uncertain.

Rare: Angioedema.

Renal and urinary disorders:

Rare: Increases in blood urea and creatinine.

Very rare: Acute renal failure, renal pain.

Renal pain may be associated with renal failure and crystalluria.

General disorders and administration site conditions:

Common: Fatigue, fever.

4.9 Overdose

Symptoms and signs:- Aciclovir is only partly absorbed in the gastrointestinal tract. Patients have ingested overdoses of up to 20g aciclovir on a single occasion, usually without toxic effects. Accidental, repeated overdoses of oral aciclovir over several days have been associated with gastrointestinal effects (such as nausea and vomiting) and neurological effects (headache and confusion).

Overdosage of intravenous aciclovir has resulted in elevations of serum creatinine, blood urea nitrogen and subsequent renal failure. Neurological effects including confusion, hallucinations, agitation, seizures and coma have been described in association with intravenous overdosage.

Management:- Patients should be observed closely for signs of toxicity. Haemodialysis significantly enhances the removal of aciclovir from the blood and may, therefore, be considered a management option in the event of symptomatic overdose.

5. PHARMACOLOGICAL PROPERTIES

5.1 Pharmacodynamic properties

Aciclovir is a synthetic purine nucleoside analogue with *in vitro* and *in vivo* inhibitory activity against human herpes viruses, including herpes simplex virus (HSV) types I and II and varicella zoster virus (VZV).

The inhibitory activity of aciclovir for HSV I, HSV II and VZV is highly selective. The enzyme thymidine kinase (TK) of normal, uninfected cells does not use aciclovir effectively as a substrate, hence toxicity of mammalian host cells is low; however, TK encoded by HSV and VZV converts aciclovir to aciclovir monophosphate, a nucleoside analogue which is further converted to the diphosphate and finally to the triphosphate by cellular enzymes. Aciclovir triphosphate interferes with the viral DNA polymerase and inhibits viral DNA replication with resultant chain termination following its incorporation into the viral DNA.

Prolonged or repeated courses of aciclovir in severely immune-compromised individuals may result in the selection of virus strains with reduced sensitivity, which may not respond to continued aciclovir treatment. Most of the clinical isolates with reduced sensitivity have been relatively deficient in viral TK, however, strains with altered viral TK or viral DNA polymerase have also been reported. *In vitro* exposure of HSV isolates to aciclovir can also lead to the emergence of less sensitive strains. The relationship between the *in vitro* determined sensitivity of HSV isolates and clinical response to aciclovir therapy is not clear.

5.2 Pharmacokinetic properties

Aciclovir is only partially absorbed from the gut. Mean steady state peak plasma concentrations ($C^{ss}max$) following doses of 200 mg administered four-hourly were 3.1 microMol (0.7 micrograms/ml) and equivalent trough plasma levels ($C^{ss}min$) were 1.8 microMol (0.4 micrograms/ml). Corresponding $C^{ss}max$ levels following doses of 400 mg and 800 mg administered four-hourly were 5.3 microMol (1.2 micrograms/ml) and 8 microMol (1.8 micrograms/ml) respectively and equivalent $C^{ss}min$ levels were 2.7 microMol (0.6 micrograms/ml) and 4 microMol (0.9 micrograms/ml).

In adults the terminal plasma half-life of aciclovir after administrations of intravenous aciclovir is about 2.9 hours. Most of the drug is excreted unchanged by the kidney. Renal clearance of aciclovir is substantially greater than creatinine clearance, indicating that tubular secretion, in addition to glomerular filtration contributes to the renal elimination of the drug. 9-carboxymethoxymethylguanine is the only significant metabolite of aciclovir, and accounts for approximately 10 - 15% of the administered dose recovered from the urine. When aciclovir is given one hour after 1 gram of probenecid the terminal half-life and the area under the plasma concentration time curve is extended by 18% and 40%, respectively.

In adults, mean steady state peak plasma concentrations ($C^{ss}max$) following a one hour infusion of 2.5 mg/kg, 5 mg/kg and 10 mg/kg were 22.7 microMol (5.1 micrograms/ml), 43.6 microMol (9.8 micrograms/ml) and 92 microMol (20.7 micrograms/ml), respectively. The corresponding trough levels ($C^{ss}min$) 7 hours later were 2.2 microMol (0.5 micrograms/ml), 3.1 microMol (0.7 micrograms/ml), and 10.2 microMol (2.3 micrograms/ml), respectively.

In children over 1 year of age similar peak ($C^{ss}max$) and trough ($C^{ss}min$) levels were observed when a dose of 250 mg/m^2 was substituted for 5 mg/kg and a dose of 500 mg/m^2 was substituted for 10 mg/kg. In neonates and young infants (0 to 3 months of age) treated with doses of 10 mg/kg administered by infusion over a one-hour period every 8 hours the $C^{ss}max$ was found to be 61.2 microMol (13.8 micrograms/ml) and $C^{ss}min$ to be 10.1 microMol (2.3 micrograms/ml). The terminal plasma half-life in these patients was 3.8 hours. In the elderly, total body clearance falls with increasing age associated with decreases in creatinine clearance although there is little change in the terminal plasma half-life.

In patients with chronic renal failure the mean terminal half-life was found to be 19.5 hours. The mean aciclovir half-life during haemodialysis was 5.7 hours. Plasma aciclovir levels dropped approximately 60% during dialysis.

Cerebrospinal fluid levels are approximately 50% of corresponding plasma levels. Plasma protein binding is relatively low (9 to 33%) and drug interactions involving binding site displacement are not anticipated.

5.3 Preclinical safety data

Mutagenicity:- The results of a wide range of mutagenicity tests *in vitro* and *in vivo* indicate that aciclovir is unlikely to pose a genetic risk to man.

Carcinogenicity:- Aciclovir was not found to be carcinogenic in long term studies in the rat and the mouse.

Teratogenicity:- Systemic administration of aciclovir in internationally accepted standard tests did not produce embryotoxic or teratogenic effects in rats, rabbits or mice.

In a non-standard test in rats, foetal abnormalities were observed, but only following such high subcutaneous doses that maternal toxicity was produced. The clinical relevance of these findings is uncertain.

Fertility:- Largely reversible adverse effects on spermatogenesis in association with overall toxicity in rats and dogs have been reported only at doses of aciclovir greatly in excess of those employed therapeutically. Two generation studies in mice did not reveal any effect of aciclovir on fertility.

6. PHARMACEUTICAL PARTICULARS

6.1 List of excipients

Core:

Microcrystalline cellulose

Aluminium magnesium silicate

Sodium starch glycollate

Povidone K30

Magnesium stearate

Purified water

Industrial methylated spirit

Or

Ethanol

Or

Absolute alcohol

Film coat*:

Colour concentrate Y-1-7000, White

Purified water

* *Coating concentrate contains:*

Hypromellose

Polyethylene glycol 400

Titanium dioxide

Polish:

Polyethylene glycol 8000

Purified water

6.2 Incompatibilities

None known.

6.3 Shelf life

36 months.

6.4 Special precautions for storage

Do not store above 30°C.

Store in the original package.

6.5 Nature and contents of container

Amber glass bottles with polyethylene snap fitting caps.

PVC/PVDC/Aluminium foil blister packs.

Pack size: 25 tablets.

6.6 Special precautions for disposal and other handling

No special instructions

Administrative Data

7. MARKETING AUTHORISATION HOLDER

The Wellcome Foundation Limited

Glaxo Wellcome House

Berkeley Avenue

Greenford

Middlesex

UB6 0NN

Trading as

GlaxoSmithKline UK

Stockley Park West

Uxbridge

Middlesex UB11 1BT

8. MARKETING AUTHORISATION NUMBER(S)

PL 00003/0344

9. DATE OF FIRST AUTHORISATION/RENEWAL OF THE AUTHORISATION

13 September 2001

10. DATE OF REVISION OF THE TEXT

09 December 2008

Zovirax 400mg Tablets

(GlaxoSmithKline UK)

1. NAME OF THE MEDICINAL PRODUCT

Zovirax Tablets 400 mg

2. QUALITATIVE AND QUANTITATIVE COMPOSITION

Aciclovir BP 400 mg

3. PHARMACEUTICAL FORM

Dispersible film-coated tablet.

4. CLINICAL PARTICULARS

4.1 Therapeutic indications

Zovirax dispersible tablets are indicated for the treatment of herpes simplex virus infections of the skin and mucous membranes including initial and recurrent genital herpes.

Zovirax dispersible tablets are indicated for the suppression (prevention of recurrences) of recurrent herpes simplex infections in immunocompetent patients.

Zovirax dispersible tablets are indicated for the prophylaxis of herpes simplex infections in immunocompromised patients.

Zovirax dispersible tablets are indicated for the treatment of varicella (chickenpox) and herpes zoster (shingles) infections.

4.2 Posology and method of administration

Route of administration: Oral

Zovirax dispersible tablets may be dispersed in a minimum of 50 ml of water or swallowed whole with a little water. Ensure that patients on high doses of aciclovir are adequately hydrated.

Dosage in adults

Treatment of herpes simplex infections: 200 mg Zovirax should be taken five times daily at approximately four hourly intervals omitting the night time dose. Treatment should continue for 5 days, but in severe initial infections this may have to be extended.

In severe immunocompromised patients (e.g. after marrow transplant) or in patients with impaired absorption from the gut the dose can be doubled to 400 mg Zovirax or alternatively intravenous dosing could be considered.

Dosing should begin as early as possible after the start of an infection: for recurrent episodes this should preferably be during the prodromal period or when lesions first appear.

Suppression of herpes infections in immunocompetent patients: 200 mg Zovirax should be taken four times daily at approximately six-hourly intervals.

Many patients may be conveniently managed on a regimen of 400 mg Zovirax twice daily at approximately twelve-hourly intervals.

Dosage titration down to 200 mg Zovirax taken thrice daily at approximately eight-hourly intervals or even twice daily at approximately twelve-hourly intervals may prove, effective.

Some patients may experience break-through infection on total daily doses of 800 mg Zovirax.

Therapy should be interrupted periodically at intervals of six to twelve months, in order to observe possible changes in the natural history of the disease.

Prophylaxis of herpes simplex infections in immunocompromised patients: 200 mg Zovirax should be taken four times daily at approximately six-hourly intervals.

In severely immunocompromised patients (e.g. after marrow transplant) or in patients with impaired absorption from the gut, the dose can be doubled to 400 mg Zovirax or alternatively, intravenous dosing could be considered.

The duration of prophylactic administration is determined by the duration of the period at risk.

Treatment of varicella and herpes zoster infections 800 mg Zovirax should be taken five times daily at approximately four-hourly intervals, omitting the night time dose. Treatment should continue for seven days.

In severely, immunocompromised patients (e.g. after marrow transplant) or in patients with impaired absorption from the gut, consideration should be given to intravenous dosing.

Dosing should begin as early as possible after the start of an infection: Treatment of herpes zoster yields better results if initiated as soon as possible after the onset of the rash. Treatment of chickenpox in immunocompetent patients should begin within 24 hours after onset of the rash.

Dosage in children

Treatment of herpes simplex infections and prophylaxis of herpes simplex infections in the immunocompromised: Children aged two years and over should be given adult dosages and children below the age of two years should be given half the adult dose.

Treatment of varicella infection

6 years and over; 800 mg Zovirax four times daily

2-5 years; 400 mg Zovirax four times daily

Under 2 years; 200 mg Zovirax four times daily

Treatment should continue for five days.

No specific data are available on the suppression of herpes simplex infections or the treatment of herpes zoster infections in immunocompetent children.

Dosage in the elderly

The possibility of renal impairment in the elderly must be considered and the dosage should be adjusted accordingly (see Dosage in renal impairment below).

Adequate hydration of elderly patients taking high oral doses of aciclovir should be maintained.

Dosage in renal impairment:

Caution is advised when administering aciclovir to patients with impaired renal function. Adequate hydration should be maintained.

In the management of herpes simplex infections in patients with impaired renal function, the recommended oral doses will not lead to accumulation of aciclovir above levels that have been established safe by intravenous infusion. However for patients with severe renal impairment (creatinine clearance less than 10ml/minute) an adjustment of dosage to 200 mg aciclovir twice daily at approximately twelve-hourly intervals is recommended.

In the treatment of herpes zoster infections it is recommended to adjust the dosage to 800 mg aciclovir twice daily at approximately twelve hourly intervals for patients with severe renal impairment (creatinine clearance less than 10ml/minute), and to 800 mg aciclovir three times daily at intervals of approximately eight hours for patients with moderate renal impairment (creatinine clearance in the range 10-25ml/minute).

4.3 Contraindications

Aciclovir tablets are contra-indicated in patients known to be hypersensitive to aciclovir or valaciclovir.

4.4 Special warnings and precautions for use

Use in patients with renal impairment and in elderly patients:

Aciclovir is eliminated by renal clearance, therefore the dose must be adjusted in patients with renal impairment (see 4.2 Posology and Method of Administration). Elderly patients are likely to have reduced renal function and therefore the need for dose adjustment must be considered in this group of patients. Both elderly patients and patients with renal impairment are at increased risk of developing neurological side effects and should be closely monitored for evidence of these effects. In the reported cases, these reactions were generally reversible on discontinuation of treatment (see 4.8 Undesirable Effects).

Hydration status: Care should be taken to maintain adequate hydration in patients receiving higher oral doses of aciclovir.

The data currently available from clinical studies is not sufficient to conclude that treatment with aciclovir reduces the incidence of chickenpox-associated complications in immunocompetent patients.

4.5 Interaction with other medicinal products and other forms of interaction

No clinically significant interactions have been identified.

Aciclovir is eliminated primarily unchanged in the urine via active renal tubular secretion. Any drugs administered concurrently that compete with this mechanism may increase aciclovir plasma concentrations. Probenecid and cimetidine increase the AUC of aciclovir by this mechanism, and reduce aciclovir renal clearance. Similarly increases in plasma AUCs of aciclovir and of the inactive metabolite of mycophenolate mofetil, an immunosuppressant agent used in transplant patients have been shown when the drugs are coadministered. However no dosage adjustment is necessary because of the wide therapeutic index of aciclovir.

4.6 Pregnancy and lactation

A post-marketing aciclovir pregnancy registry has documented pregnancy outcomes in women exposed to any formulation of Zovirax. The birth defects described amongst Zovirax exposed subjects have not shown any uniqueness or consistent pattern to suggest a common cause.

Caution should however be exercised by balancing the potential benefits of treatment against any possible hazard. Findings from reproduction toxicology studies are included in Section 5.3.

Following oral administration of 200 mg Zovirax five times a day, aciclovir has been detected in breast milk at concentrations ranging from 0.6 to 4.1 times the corresponding plasma levels. These levels would potentially expose nursing infants to aciclovir dosages of up to 0.3 mg/kg/day. Caution is therefore advised if Zovirax is to be administered to a nursing woman.

Fertility:

There is no information on the effect of aciclovir on human female fertility.

In a study of 20 male patients with normal sperm count, oral aciclovir administered at doses of up to 1g per day for up to six months has been shown to have no clinically significant effect on sperm count, motility or morphology.

4.7 Effects on ability to drive and use machines

There have been no studies to investigate the effect of aciclovir on driving performance or the ability to operate machinery. A detrimental effect on such activities cannot be predicted from the pharmacology of the active substance, but the adverse event profile should be borne in mind.

4.8 Undesirable effects

The frequency categories associated with the adverse events below are estimates. For most events, suitable data for estimating incidence were not available. In addition, adverse events may vary in their incidence depending on the indication.

The following convention has been used for the classification of undesirable effects in terms of frequency:- Very common $\geqslant 1/10$, common $\geqslant 1/100$ and $< 1/10$, uncommon $\geqslant 1/1000$ and $< 1/100$, rare $\geqslant 1/10{,}000$ and $< 1/1000$, very rare $< 1/10{,}000$.

Blood and lymphatic system disorders:

Very rare: Anaemia, leukopenia, thrombocytopenia.

Immune system disorders:

Rare: Anaphylaxis.

Psychiatric and nervous system disorders:

Common: Headache, dizziness.

Very rare: Agitation, confusion, tremor, ataxia, dysarthria, hallucinations, psychotic symptoms, convulsions, somnolence, encephalopathy, coma.

The above events are generally reversible and usually reported in patients with renal impairment or with other predisposing factors (see 4.4 Special Warnings and Precautions for Use).

Respiratory, thoracic and mediastinal disorders:

Rare: Dyspnoea.

Gastrointestinal disorders:

Common: Nausea, vomiting, diarrhoea, abdominal pains.

Hepato-biliary disorders:

Rare: Reversible rises in bilirubin and liver related enzymes.

Very rare: Hepatitis, jaundice.

Skin and subcutaneous tissue disorders:

Common: Pruritus, rashes (including photosensitivity).

Uncommon: Urticaria. Accelerated diffuse hair loss. Accelerated diffuse hair loss has been associated with a wide variety of disease processes and medicines, the relationship of the event to aciclovir therapy is uncertain.

Rare: Angioedema

Renal and urinary disorders:

Rare: Increases in blood urea and creatinine.

Very rare: Acute renal failure, renal pain.

Renal pain may be associated with renal failure and crystalluria.

General disorders and administration site conditions:

Common: Fatigue, fever.

4.9 Overdose

Symptoms & signs:- Aciclovir is only partly absorbed in the gastrointestinal tract. Patients have ingested overdoses of up to 20g aciclovir on a single occasion, usually without toxic effects. Accidental, repeated overdoses of oral aciclovir over several days have been associated with gastrointestinal effects (such as nausea and vomiting) and neurological effects (headache and confusion).

Overdosage of intravenous aciclovir has resulted in elevations of serum creatinine, blood urea nitrogen and subsequent renal failure. Neurological effects including confusion, hallucinations, agitation, seizures and coma have been described in association with intravenous overdosage.

Management: patients should be observed closely for signs of toxicity. Haemodialysis significantly enhances the removal of aciclovir from the blood and may, therefore, be considered a management option in the event of symptomatic overdose.

5. PHARMACOLOGICAL PROPERTIES

5.1 Pharmacodynamic properties

Aciclovir is a synthetic purine nucleoside analogue with in vitro and in vivo inhibitory activity against human herpes viruses, including herpes simplex virus (HSV) types I and II and varicella zoster virus (VZV). The inhibitory activity of aciclovir for HSV I, HSV II and VZV is highly selective. The enzyme thymidine kinase (TK) of normal uninfected cells does not use aciclovir effectively as a substrate, hence toxicity of mammalian host cells is low. However, TK encoded by HSV and VZV converts aciclovir to aciclovir monophosphate, a nucleoside, analogue which is further converted to the diphosphate and finally to the triphosphate by cellular enzymes. Aciclovir triphosphate interferes with the viral DNA polymerase and inhibits viral DNS replication with resultant chain termination following its incorporation into the viral DNA.

Prolonged or repeated courses of aciclovir in severely immune-compromised individuals may result in the selective of virus strains with reduced sensitivity, which may not respond to continued aciclovir treatment. Most of the clinical isolates with reduced sensitivity have been relatively deficient in viral TK. However, strains with altered viral TK or DNA polymerase have also been reported. In vitro exposure of HSV isolates to aciclovir can also lead to the emergence of less sensitive strains. The relationship between the in vitro determined sensitivity of HSV isolate and clinical response to aciclovir therapy is not clear.

5.2 Pharmacokinetic properties

Aciclovir is only partially absorbed from the gut. Mean steady state peak plasma concentration ($C^{ss}Max$) following doses of 200 mg administered four-hourly were 3.1 micromol (0.7 micrograms/ml) and equivalent trough plasma levels ($C^{ss}Min$) were 1.8 micromol (0.4 micrograms/ml). Corresponding $C^{ss}Max$ levels following doses of 400 mg and 800 mg administered four-hourly were 5.3 micromol (1.2 micrograms/ml) and 8 micromol (1.8 micrograms/ml) respectively and equivalent $C^{ss}Min$ levels were 2.7 micromol (0.6 micrograms/ml) and 4 microMol (0.9 micrograms/ml).

In adults the terminal plasma half life after administration of intravenous aciclovir is about 2.9 hours. Most of the drug is excreted unchanged by the kidney. Renal clearance of aciclovir is substantially greater than creatinine clearance, indicating that tubular secretion in addition to glomerular filtration contributes to the renal elimination of the drug. 9-carboxymethoxymethyl-guanine is the only significant metabolite of aciclovir and accounts for approximately 10-15% of the administered dose recovered from the urine. When aciclovir is given one hour after 1 gram of probenecid the terminal half life and the area under the plasma concentration time curve is extended by 18% and 40% respectively.

In adults, mean steady state peak plasma concentrations ($C^{ss}max$) following a one hour infusion of 2.5mg/kg, 5mg/kg and 10mg/kg were 22.7 microMol (5.1 micrograms/ml), 43.6 microMol (9.8 micrograms/ml) and 92 microMol (20.7 micrograms/ml), respectively. The corresponding trough levels ($C^{ss}min$) 7 hours later were 2.2 microMol (0.5 micrograms/ml), 3.1 microMol (0.7 micrograms/ml), and 10.2 microMol (2.3 micrograms/ml), respectively.

In children over 1 year of age similar mean peak ($C^{ss}max$) and trough ($C^{ss}min$) levels were observed when a dose of 250 mg/m^2 was substituted for 5 mg/kg and a dose of 500 mg/m^2 was substituted for 10 mg/kg. In neonates and young infants (0-3 months of age) treated with doses of 10mg/kg administered by infusion over a one-hour period every 8 hours the $C^{ss}max$ was found to be 61.2 microMol (13.8 micrograms/ml) and $C^{ss}min$ to be 10.1 microMol (2.3 micrograms/ml). The terminal plasma half life in these patients was 3.8 hours. In the elderly total body clearance falls with increasing age associated with decreases in creatinine clearance although there is little changes in the terminal plasma half life.

In patients with chronic renal failure the mean terminal half life was found to be 19.5 hours. The mean aciclovir half life during haemodialysis was 5.7 hours. Plasma aciclovir levels dropped approximately 60% during dialysis.

Cerebrospinal fluid levels are approximately 50% of corresponding plasma levels. Plasma protein binding is relatively low (9 to 33%) and drug interactions involving binding site displacement are not anticipated.

5.3 Preclinical safety data

Mutagenicity:- The results of a wide range of mutagenicity tests *in vitro* and *in vivo* indicate that aciclovir is unlikely to pose a genetic risk to man.

Carcinogenicity:- Aciclovir was not found to be carcinogenic in long term studies in the rat and the mouse.

Teratogenicity:- Systemic administration of aciclovir in internationally accepted standard tests did not produce embryotoxic or teratogenic effects in rats, rabbits or mice.

In a non-standard test in rats, foetal abnormalities were observed, but only following such high subcutaneous doses that maternal toxicity was produced. The clinical relevance of these findings is uncertain.

Fertility:- Largely reversible adverse effects on spermatogenesis in association with overall toxicity in rats and dogs have been reported only at doses of aciclovir greatly in excess of those employed therapeutically. Two generation studies in mice did not reveal any effect of aciclovir on fertility.

6. PHARMACEUTICAL PARTICULARS

6.1 List of excipients

Core:

Microcrystalline cellulose

Aluminium magnesium silicate

Sodium starch glycollate

Povidone, K30

Magnesium stearate

Iron oxide, red E172

Industrial methylated spirit

Purified water

* Ethanol (96 per cent) or Absolute alcohol may be used as an alternative to industrial methylated spirit

Film coat:

Colour concentrate Y-1-7000, White*

Purified water

Methylated spirit

* The coating concentrate contains:

Hypromellose

Titanium dioxide

Polyethylene glycol 400

Polish:

Polyethylene glycol 8000

Purified water

6.2 Incompatibilities
None known.

6.3 Shelf life
36 months.

6.4 Special precautions for storage
Do not store above 30°C.

Store in the original package.

6.5 Nature and contents of container
Amber glass bottles with polyethylene snap fitting caps.

PVC/PVDC/Aluminium foil blister packs.

Pack size: 56 tablets

6.6 Special precautions for disposal and other handling
Not applicable.

Administrative Data

7. MARKETING AUTHORISATION HOLDER
The Wellcome Foundation Limited

Glaxo Wellcome House

Berkeley Avenue

Greenford

Middlesex

UB6 ONN

Trading as:

GlaxoSmithKline UK

Stockley Park West

Uxbridge

Middlesex UB11 1BT

8. MARKETING AUTHORISATION NUMBER(S)
PL 00003/0345

9. DATE OF FIRST AUTHORISATION/RENEWAL OF THE AUTHORISATION
04 June 2003

10. DATE OF REVISION OF THE TEXT
09 December 2008

Zovirax 800mg Tablets

(GlaxoSmithKline UK)

1. NAME OF THE MEDICINAL PRODUCT
Zovirax Tablets BP 800mg

2. QUALITATIVE AND QUANTITATIVE COMPOSITION
Aciclovir 800mg BP

3. PHARMACEUTICAL FORM
Dispersible film coated tablet

4. CLINICAL PARTICULARS

4.1 Therapeutic indications
Zovirax tablets 800 mg are indicated for the treatment of varicella (chickenpox) and herpes zoster (shingles) infections.

4.2 Posology and method of administration
Dosage in adults:

Treatment of varicella and herpes zoster infections: 800 mg Zovirax should be taken five times daily at approximately four-hourly intervals, omitting the night time dose. Treatment should continue for seven days.

In severely immunocompromised patients (e.g. after marrow transplant) or in patients with impaired absorption from the gut, consideration should be given to intravenous dosing.

Dosing should begin as early as possible after the start of an infection: Treatment of herpes zoster yields better results if initiated as soon as possible after the onset of the rash. Treatment of chickenpox in immunocompetent patients should begin within 24 hours after the onset of the rash.

Dosage in children:

Treatment of varicella infections:

6 years and over: 800 mg Zovirax four times daily.

Treatment should continue for five days.

No specific data are available on the treatment of herpes zoster infections in immunocompetent children.

Dosage in the elderly:

The possibility of renal impairment in the elderly must be considered and the dosage should be adjusted accordingly (see Dosage in renal impairment below).

Adequate hydration of elderly patients taking high oral doses of aciclovir should be maintained.

Dosage in renal impairment:

Caution is advised when administering aciclovir to patients with impaired renal function. Adequate hydration should be maintained.

In the treatment of herpes zoster infections it is recommended to adjust the dosage to 800 mg Aciclovir twice daily at approximately twelve-hourly intervals for patients with severe renal impairment (creatinine clearance less than 10 ml/minute) and to 800 mg Aciclovir three times daily at intervals of approximately eight hours for patients with moderate renal impairment (creatinine clearance in the range of 10-25 ml/minute).

Administration

Zovirax tablets are for oral administration and may be dispersed in a minimum of 50 ml of water or swallowed whole with a little water. Ensure that patients on high doses of aciclovir are adequately hydrated.

4.3 Contraindications
Zovirax tablets are contra-indicated in patients known to be hypersensitive to aciclovir or valaciclovir.

4.4 Special warnings and precautions for use
Use in patients with renal impairment and in elderly patients:

Aciclovir is eliminated by renal clearance, therefore the dose must be adjusted in patients with renal impairment (see 4.2 Posology and Method of Administration). Elderly patients are likely to have reduced renal function and therefore the need for dose adjustment must be considered in this group of patients. Both elderly patients and patients with renal impairment are at increased risk of developing neurological side effects and should be closely monitored for evidence of these effects. In the reported cases, these reactions were generally reversible on discontinuation of treatment (see 4.8 Undesirable Effects).

Hydration status: Care should be taken to maintain adequate hydration in patients receiving high doses of aciclovir.

The data currently available from clinical studies is not sufficient to conclude that treatment with aciclovir reduces the incidence of chickenpox-associated complications in immunocompetent patients.

4.5 Interaction with other medicinal products and other forms of interaction
No clinically significant interactions have been identified.

Aciclovir is eliminated primarily unchanged in the urine via active renal tubular secretion. Any drugs administered concurrently that compete with this mechanism may increase aciclovir plasma concentrations. Probenecid and cimetidine increase the AUC of aciclovir by this mechanism, and reduce aciclovir renal clearance. Similarly increases in plasma AUCs of aciclovir and of the inactive metabolite of mycophenolate mofetil, an immunosuppressant agent used in transplant patients have been shown when the drugs are coadministered. However no dosage adjustment is necessary because of the wide therapeutic index of aciclovir.

4.6 Pregnancy and lactation
A post-marketing aciclovir pregnancy registry has documented pregnancy outcomes in women exposed to any formulation of Zovirax. The birth defects described amongst Zovirax exposed subjects have not shown any uniqueness or consistent pattern to suggest a common cause.

Caution should however be exercised by balancing the potential benefits of treatment against any possible hazard. Findings from reproduction toxicology studies are included in Section 5.3.

Following oral administration of 200 mg Zovirax five times a day, Aciclovir has been detected in breast milk at concentrations ranging from 0.6 to 4.1 times the corresponding plasma levels. These levels would potentially expose nursing infants to Aciclovir dosages of up to 0.3 mg/kg/day. Caution is therefore advised if Zovirax is to be administered to a nursing woman.

Fertility:

There is no information on the effect of aciclovir on human female fertility.

In a study of 20 male patients with normal sperm count, oral aciclovir administered at doses of up to 1g per day for up to six months has been shown to have no clinically significant effect on sperm count, motility or morphology.

4.7 Effects on ability to drive and use machines
There have been no studies to investigate the effect of aciclovir on driving performance or the ability to operate machinery. A detrimental effect on such activities cannot be predicted from the pharmacology of the active substance, but the adverse event profile should be borne in mind.

4.8 Undesirable effects
The frequency categories associated with the adverse events below are estimates. For most events, suitable data for estimating incidence were not available. In addition, adverse events may vary in their incidence depending on the indication.

The following convention has been used for the classification of undesirable effects in terms of frequency:- Very common ⩾1/10, common ⩾1/100 and <1/10, uncommon ⩾1/1000 and <1/100, rare ⩾1/10,000 and <1/1000, very rare <1/10,000.

Blood and lymphatic system disorders:

Very rare: Anaemia, leukopenia, thrombocytopenia.

Immune system disorders:

Rare: Anaphylaxis.

Psychiatric and nervous system disorders:

Common: Headache, dizziness.

Very rare: Agitation, confusion, tremor, ataxia, dysarthria, hallucinations, psychotic symptoms, convulsions, somnolence, encephalopathy, coma.

The above events are generally reversible and usually reported in patients with renal impairment or with other predisposing factors (see 4.4 Special Warnings and Precautions for Use).

Respiratory, thoracic and mediastinal disorders:

Rare: Dyspnoea.

Gastrointestinal disorders:

Common: Nausea, vomiting, diarrhoea, abdominal pains.

Hepato-biliary disorders:

Rare: Reversible rises in bilirubin and liver related enzymes.

Very rare: Hepatitis, jaundice.

Skin and subcutaneous tissue disorders:

Common: Pruritus, rashes (including photosensitivity).

Uncommon: Urticaria. Accelerated diffuse hair loss. Accelerated diffuse hair loss has been associated with a wide variety of disease processes and medicines, the relationship of the event to aciclovir therapy is uncertain.

Rare: Angioedema

Renal and urinary disorders:

Rare: Increases in blood urea and creatinine.

Very rare: Acute renal failure, renal pain.

Renal pain may be associated with renal failure and crystalluria.

General disorders and administration site conditions:

Common: Fatigue, fever.

4.9 Overdose
Aciclovir is only partly absorbed in the gastrointestinal tract.

Patients have ingested overdoses of up to 20g aciclovir on a single occasion, usually without toxic effects. Accidental, repeated overdoses of oral aciclovir over several days have been associated with gastrointestinal effects (such as nausea and vomiting) and neurological effects (headache and confusion).

Overdosage of intravenous aciclovir has resulted in elevations of serum creatinine, blood urea nitrogen and subsequent renal failure. Neurological effects including confusion, hallucinations, agitation, seizures and coma have been described in association with intravenous overdosage.

Management: patients should be observed closely for signs of toxicity. Haemodialysis significantly enhances the removal of aciclovir from the blood and may, therefore, be considered a management option in the event of symptomatic overdose.

5. PHARMACOLOGICAL PROPERTIES

5.1 Pharmacodynamic properties
Aciclovir is a synthetic purine nucleoside analogue with *in vitro* and *in vivo* inhibitory activity against human herpes viruses, including herpes simplex virus (HSV) types I and II and varicella zoster virus (VZV). The inhibitory activity of Aciclovir for HSV I and HSV II and VZV is highly selective. The enzyme thymidine kinase (TK) of normal, uninfected cells does not use Aciclovir effectively as a substrate, hence toxicity to mammalian host cells is low; however, TK encoded by HSV and VZV converts Aciclovir to Aciclovir monophosphate, a nucleoside analogue which is further converted to the diphosphate and finally to the triphosphate by cellular enzymes. Aciclovir triphosphate interferes with the viral DNA polymerase and inhibits viral DNA replication with resultant chain termination following its incorporation into the viral DNA.

Prolonged or repeated courses of Aciclovir in severely immuno-compromised individuals may result in the selection of virus strains with reduced sensitivity, which may not respond to continued Aciclovir treatment. Most of the clinical isolates with reduced sensitivity have been relatively deficient in viral TK, however, strains with altered viral TK or viral DNA polymerase have also been reported. *In vitro* exposure of HSV isolates to Aciclovir can also lead to the emergence of less sensitive strains. The relationship between the *in vitro*-determined sensitivity of HSV isolates and clinical response to Aciclovir therapy is not clear.

5.2 Pharmacokinetic properties
Aciclovir is only partially absorbed from the gut. Mean steady state peak plasma concentrations ($C^{ss}max$) following doses of 800 mg Aciclovir administered four-hourly were 8 microMol (1.8 micrograms/ml) and equivalent trough plasma levels were 4 microMol (0.9 micrograms/ml).

In adults the terminal plasma half-life after administration of intravenous Aciclovir is about 2.9 hours. Most of the drug is excreted unchanged by the kidney. Renal clearance of Aciclovir is substantially greater than creatinine clearance, indicating that tubular secretion, in addition to glomerular filtration, contributes to the renal elimination of the drug. 9-carboxymethoxymethyl-guanine is the only significant metabolite of Aciclovir, and accounts for 10-15% of the dose excreted in the urine. When Aciclovir is given one hour after 1 gram of probenecid the terminal half-life and the area under the plasma concentration time curve is extended by 18% and 40% respectively.

In adults, mean steady state peak plasma concentrations ($C^{ss}max$) following a one hour infusion of 2.5 mg/kg, 5 mg/kg and 10 mg/kg were 22.7 microMol (5.1 micrograms/ml), 43.6 microMol (9.8 micrograms/ml) and 92 microMol (20.7 micrograms/ml), respectively. The corresponding trough levels ($C^{ss}min$) 7 hours later were 2.2 microMol (0.5 micrograms/ml), 3.1 microMol (0.7 micrograms/ml) and 10.2 microMol (2.3 micrograms/ml), respectively. In children over 1 year of age similar mean peak ($C^{ss}max$) and trough ($C^{ss}min$) levels were observed when a dose of 250 mg/m^2 was substituted for 5 mg/kg and a dose of 500 mg/m^2 was substituted for 10 mg/kg. In neonates and young infants (0 to 3 months of age) treated with doses of 10 mg/kg administered by infusion over a one-hour period every 8 hours the $C^{ss}max$ was found to be 61.2 microMol (13.8 micrograms/ml) and $C^{ss}min$ to be 10.1 microMol (2.3 micrograms/ml). The terminal plasma half-life in these patients was 3.8 hours. In the elderly, total body clearance falls with increasing age associated with decreases in creatinine clearance although there is little change in the terminal plasma half-life.

In patients with chronic renal failure the mean terminal half-life was found to be 19.5 hours. The mean Aciclovir half-life during haemodialysis was 5.7 hours. Plasma Aciclovir levels dropped approximately 60% during dialysis.

Cerebrospinal fluid levels are approximately 50% of corresponding plasma levels. Plasma protein binding is relatively low (9 to 33%) and drug interactions involving binding site displacement are not anticipated.

5.3 Preclinical safety data

Mutagenicity:- The results of a wide range of mutagenicity tests *in vitro* and *in vivo* indicate that aciclovir is unlikely to pose a genetic risk to man.

Carcinogenicity:- Aciclovir was not found to be carcinogenic in long term studies in the rat and the mouse.

Teratogenicity:- Systemic administration of aciclovir in internationally accepted standard tests did not produce embryotoxic or teratogenic effects in rats, rabbits or mice.

In a non-standard test in rats, foetal abnormalities were observed, but only following such high subcutaneous doses that maternal toxicity was produced. The clinical relevance of these findings is uncertain.

Fertility:- Largely reversible adverse effects on spermatogenesis in association with overall toxicity in rats and dogs have been reported only at doses of aciclovir greatly in excess of those employed therapeutically. Two generation studies in mice did not reveal any effect of aciclovir on fertility.

6. PHARMACEUTICAL PARTICULARS

6.1 List of excipients

Microcrystalline Cellulose Ph Eur

Aluminium Magnesium Silicate BP

Sodium Starch Glycollate BP

Povidone (K30) Ph Eur

Magnesium Stearate Ph Eur

Filmcoat

Hypromellose HSE

Titanium Dioxide HSE

Polyethylene glycol 400 HSE

Polish

Polyethylene Glycol 8000 NF

6.2 Incompatibilities

None known

6.3 Shelf life

36 months

6.4 Special precautions for storage

Do not store above 30°C.

Store in the original package.

6.5 Nature and contents of container

PVC/Aluminium foil blisterpack (5 tablets per blister strip)

Pack size: 35 tablets (marketed).

Polypropylene container with polyethylene snap-on lid.

Pack size: 35 and 800 tablets (non-marketed)

PVC/Aluminium foil blister sample pack.

Pack size: 5 and 2 tablets(non-marketed).

Polyethylene bag in a rigid polypropylene container with a polypropylene lid.

Pack size: 8000 tablets (non-marketed).

6.6 Special precautions for disposal and other handling

No special instructions for use.

Administrative Data

7. MARKETING AUTHORISATION HOLDER

The Wellcome Foundation Ltd

Glaxo Wellcome House

Berkeley Avenue

Greenford

Middlesex UB6 ONN

Trading as

GlaxoSmithKline UK

Stockley Park West

Uxbridge

Middlesex UB11 1BT

8. MARKETING AUTHORISATION NUMBER(S)

PL 00003/0299

9. DATE OF FIRST AUTHORISATION/RENEWAL OF THE AUTHORISATION

16 April 1997

10. DATE OF REVISION OF THE TEXT

09 December 2008

Zovirax Cream

(GlaxoSmithKline UK)

1. NAME OF THE MEDICINAL PRODUCT

Zovirax Cream

2. QUALITATIVE AND QUANTITATIVE COMPOSITION

Aciclovir BP 5.0% w/w

3. PHARMACEUTICAL FORM

Topical Cream

4. CLINICAL PARTICULARS

4.1 Therapeutic indications

Zovirax Cream is indicated for the treatment of Herpes Simplex virus infections of the skin including initial and recurrent genital herpes and herpes labialis.

Route of administration: topical.

Do not use in eyes.

4.2 Posology and method of administration

Adults and Children: Zovirax Cream should be applied five times daily at approximately four hourly intervals, omitting the night time application.

Zovirax Cream should be applied to the lesions or impending lesions as soon as possible, preferably during the early stages (prodrome or erythema). Treatment can also be started during the later (papule or blister) stages.

Treatment should be continued for at least 4 days for herpes labialis and for 5 days for genital herpes. If healing has not occurred then treatment may be continued for up to an additional 5 days.

Use in the elderly: No special comment

4.3 Contraindications

Zovirax Cream is contraindicated in patients known to be hypersensitive to aciclovir, valaciclovir, propylene glycol or any of the excipients of Zovirax Cream.

4.4 Special warnings and precautions for use

Zovirax Cream is not recommended for application to mucous membranes such as in the mouth, eye or vagina, as it may be irritant.

Particular care should be taken to avoid accidental introduction into the eye.

In severely immunocompromised patients (eg AIDS patients or bone marrow transplant recipients) oral Zovirax dosing should be considered. Such patients should be encouraged to consult a physician concerning the treatment of any infection.

Zovirax Cream contains a specially formulated base and should not be diluted or used as a base for the incorporation of other medicaments.

4.5 Interaction with other medicinal products and other forms of interaction

No clinically significant interactions have been identified.

4.6 Pregnancy and lactation

Pregnancy:

A post-marketing aciclovir pregnancy registry has documented pregnancy outcomes in women exposed to any formulation of Zovirax. The birth defects described amongst Zovirax exposed subjects have not shown any uniqueness or consistent pattern to suggest a common cause.

The use of Zovirax Cream should be considered only when the potential benefits outweigh the possibility of unknown risks.

Teratogenicity:

Effects in non-clinical studies were observed only at exposures considered sufficiently in excess of the maximum human exposure to indicate little relevance to clinical use (see section 5.3)

Lactation:

Limited human data show that the drug does pass into breast milk following systemic administration. However, the dosage received by a nursing infant following maternal use of Zovirax Cream would be insignificant.

Fertility:

There is no information on the effect of aciclovir on human female fertility.

In a study of 20 male patients with normal sperm count, oral aciclovir administered at doses of up to 1g per day for up to six months has been shown to have no clinically significant effect on sperm count, motility or morphology.

4.7 Effects on ability to drive and use machines

Not applicable

4.8 Undesirable effects

The following convention has been used for the classification of undesirable effects in terms of frequency: very common $\geqslant$1/10, common $\geqslant$1/100 and $<$1/10, uncommon $\geqslant$1/1000 and $<$1/100, rare $\geqslant$1/10,000 and $<$1/1000, very rare $<$1/10,000.

Immune system disorders:

Very rare

- Immediate hypersensitivity reactions including angioedema.

Skin and subcutaneous tissue disorders:

Uncommon

- Transient burning or stinging following application of Zovirax Cream
- Mild drying or flaking of the skin
- Itching

Rare

- Erythema
- Contact dermatitis following application. Where sensitivity tests have been conducted, the reactive substances have most often been shown to be components of the cream rather than aciclovir.

4.9 Overdose

No untoward effects would be expected if the entire contents of a 10 gram tube of Zovirax Cream containing 500 mg of aciclovir were ingested orally. However the accidental, repeated overdose of oral aciclovir, over several days has resulted in gastrointestinal effects (nausea and vomiting) and neurological effects (headache and confusion). Aciclovir is dialysable by haemodialysis.

5. PHARMACOLOGICAL PROPERTIES

5.1 Pharmacodynamic properties

Aciclovir is an antiviral agent which is highly active *in vitro* against herpes simplex virus (HSV) types I and II and varicella zoster virus. Toxicity to mammalian host cells is low.

Aciclovir is phosphorylated after entry into herpes infected cells to the active compound aciclovir triphosphate. The first step in this process is dependent on the presence of the HSV-coded thymidine kinase. Aciclovir triphosphate acts as an inhibitor of, and substrate for, the herpes-specified DNA polymerase, preventing further viral DNA synthesis without affecting normal cellular processes

In two large, double blind, randomised clinical studies involving 1,385 subjects treated over 4 days for recurrent herpes labialis, Zovirax Cream 5% was compared to vehicle cream. In these studies, time from start of treatment to healing was 4.6 days using Zovirax Cream and 5.0 days using vehicle cream ($p<0.001$). Duration of pain was 3.0 days after start of treatment in the Zovirax Cream group and 3.4 days in the vehicle group ($p=0.002$). Overall, approximately 60% of patients started treatment at an early lesion stage (prodrome or erythema) and 40% at a late stage (papule or blister). The results were similar in both groups of patients.

5.2 Pharmacokinetic properties

Pharmacology studies have shown only minimal systemic absorption of aciclovir following repeated topical administration of Zovirax Cream.

5.3 Preclinical safety data

The results of a wide range of mutagenicity tests *in vitro* and *in vivo* indicate that aciclovir does not pose a genetic risk to man.

Aciclovir was not found to be carcinogenic in long term studies in the rat and the mouse.

Largely reversible adverse effects on spermatogenesis in association with overall toxicity in rats and dogs have been reported only at doses of aciclovir greatly in excess of those employed therapeutically. Two generation studies in mice did not reveal any effect of orally administered aciclovir on fertility.

Systemic administration of aciclovir in internationally accepted standard tests did not produce embryotoxic or teratogenic effects in rats, rabbits or mice.

In a non-standard test in rats, foetal abnormalities were observed, but only following such high subcutaneous doses that maternal toxicity was produced. The clinical relevance of these findings is uncertain.

6. PHARMACEUTICAL PARTICULARS

6.1 List of excipients

Poloxamer 407

Cetostearyl alcohol

Sodium lauryl sulphate

White soft paraffin

Liquid paraffin

Propylene glycol

Purified water

Arlacel 165 (containing glycerol monostearate and polyoxyethylene stearate)

Dimeticone 20

6.2 Incompatibilities

None known.

6.3 Shelf life

3 years

6.4 Special precautions for storage

Store below 25°C. Do not refrigerate.

6.5 Nature and contents of container

Collapsible aluminium tubes with plastic screw caps

Pack size: 2g or 10g tubes

6.6 Special precautions for disposal and other handling

No special instructions.

Administrative Data

7. MARKETING AUTHORISATION HOLDER

The Wellcome Foundation

Glaxo Wellcome House

Berkeley Avenue

Greenford

Middlesex UB6 0NN

Trading as

GlaxoSmithKline UK

Stockley Park West

Uxbridge

Middlesex UB11 1BT

8. MARKETING AUTHORISATION NUMBER(S)

PL 00003/0180

9. DATE OF FIRST AUTHORISATION/RENEWAL OF THE AUTHORISATION

28 October 1999/ 28 October 2004

10. DATE OF REVISION OF THE TEXT

27 August 2008

11. LEGAL STATUS

POM

Zovirax Double-Strength Suspension

(GlaxoSmithKline UK)

1. NAME OF THE MEDICINAL PRODUCT

Zovirax Double Strength Suspension

2. QUALITATIVE AND QUANTITATIVE COMPOSITION

Aciclovir BP 400mg/5ml

3. PHARMACEUTICAL FORM

Suspension

4. CLINICAL PARTICULARS

4.1 Therapeutic indications

Zovirax Double Strength Suspension is indicated for the treatment of herpes simplex virus infections of the skin and mucous membranes including initial and recurrent genital herpes.

Zovirax Double Strength Suspension is indicated for the suppression (prevention of recurrences) of recurrent herpes simplex infections in immunocompetent patients.

Zovirax Double Strength Suspension is indicated for the prophylaxis of herpes simplex infections in immunocompromised patients.

Zovirax Double Strength Suspension is indicated for the treatment of varicella (chickenpox) and herpes zoster (shingles) infections.

Route of Administration: Oral

4.2 Posology and method of administration

Dosage in Adults

Treatment of herpes simplex infections: 200mg Zovirax should be taken five times daily at approximately four hourly intervals omitting the night time dose. Treatment should continue for 5 days, but in severe initial infections this may have to be extended.

In severely immunocompromised patients (eg after marrow transplant) or in patients with impaired absorption from the gut the dose can be doubled to 400mg Zovirax or alternatively intravenous dosing could be considered.

Dosing should begin as early as possible after the start of an infection; for recurrent episodes this should preferably be during the prodromal period or when lesions first appear.

Suppression of herpes simplex infections in immunocompetent patients:

200mg Zovirax should be taken four times daily at approximately six-hourly intervals.

Many patients may be conveniently managed on a regimen of 400mg Zovirax twice daily at approximately twelve-hourly intervals.

Dosage titration down to 200mg Zovirax taken thrice daily at approximately eight-hourly intervals or even twice daily at approximately twelve-hourly intervals, may prove effective.

Some patients may experience break-through infection on total daily doses of 800mg Zovirax.

Therapy should be interrupted periodically at intervals of six to twelve months, in order to observe possible changes in the natural history of the disease.

Prophylaxis of herpes simplex infections in immunocompromised patients:

200mg Zovirax should be taken four times daily at approximately six hourly intervals.

In severely immunocompromised patients (eg after marrow transplant) or in patients with impaired absorption from the gut, the dose can be doubled to 400mg Zovirax or, alternatively, intravenous dosing could be considered.

The duration of prophylactic administration is determined by the duration of the period at risk.

Treatment of varicella and herpes zoster infections: 800mg Zovirax should be taken five times daily at approximately four-hourly intervals, omitting the night time dose. Treatment should continue for seven days.

In severely immunocompromised patients (eg after marrow transplant) or in patients with impaired absorption from the gut, consideration should be given to intravenous dosing.

Dosing should begin as early as possible after the start of an infection: treatment of herpes zoster yields better results if initiated as soon as possible after the onset of the rash. Treatment of chickenpox in immunocompetent patients should begin within 24 hours after onset of the rash.

Dosage in Children

Treatment of herpes simplex infections, and prophylaxis of herpes simplex infections in the immunocompromised: Children aged two years and over should be given adult dosages and children below the age of two years should be given half the adult dose.

Treatment of varicella infections:

6 years and over: 800mg Zovirax four times daily.

2 - 6 years: 400mg Zovirax four times daily.

Under 2 years: 200mg Zovirax four times daily.

Treatment should continue for five days.

Dosing may be more accurately calculated as 20mg/kg body weight (not to exceed 800mg) Zovirax four times daily.

No specific data are available on the *suppression* of *herpes simplex* infections or the treatment of herpes *zoster* infections in immunocompetent children.

Zovirax Double Strength Suspension may be diluted with an equal volume of either Syrup BP or Sorbitol Solution (70%) (non-crystallising) BP. The diluted product is stable for 4 weeks at 25°C but it is recommended that all dilutions are freshly prepared.

Dosage in the Elderly

The possibility of renal impairment in the elderly must be considered and the dosage should be adjusted accordingly (see Dosage in Renal Impairment below).

Adequate hydration of elderly patients taking high oral doses of aciclovir should be maintained.

Dosage in Renal Impairment

Caution is advised when administering aciclovir to patients with impaired renal function. Adequate hydration should be maintained.

In the management of herpes simplex infections in patients with impaired renal function, the recommended oral doses will not lead to accumulation of aciclovir above levels that have been established safe by intravenous infusion. However, for patients with severe renal impairment (creatinine clearance less than 10ml/minute) an adjustment of dosage to 200mg aciclovir twice daily at approximately twelve-hourly intervals is recommended.

In the treatment of herpes zoster infections it is recommended to adjust the dosage to 800mg aciclovir twice daily at approximately twelve-hourly intervals for patients with severe renal impairment (creatinine clearance less than 10ml/minute), and to 800mg aciclovir three times daily at intervals of approximately eight hours for patients with moderate renal impairment (creatinine clearance in the range 10 to 25ml/minute).

4.3 Contraindications

Zovirax Double Strength Suspension is contra-indicated in patients known to be hypersensitive to aciclovir or valaciclovir.

4.4 Special warnings and precautions for use

Use in patients with renal impairment and in elderly patients:

Aciclovir is eliminated by renal clearance, therefore the dose must be adjusted in patients with renal impairment (see 4.2 Posology and Method of Administration). Elderly patients are likely to have reduced renal function and therefore the need for dose adjustment must be considered in this group of patients. Both elderly patients and patients with renal impairment are at increased risk of developing neurological side effects and should be closely monitored for evidence of these effects. In the reported cases, these reactions were generally reversible on discontinuation of treatment (see 4.8 Undesirable Effects).

Hydration status: Care should be taken to maintain adequate hydration in patients receiving high oral doses of aciclovir.

The data currently available from clinical studies is not sufficient to conclude that treatment with aciclovir reduces the incidence of chickenpox-associated complications in immunocompetent patients.

4.5 Interaction with other medicinal products and other forms of interaction

No clinically significant interactions have been identified.

Aciclovir is eliminated primarily unchanged in the urine via active renal tubular secretion. Any drugs administered concurrently that compete with this mechanism may increase aciclovir plasma concentrations. Probenecid and cimetidine increase the AUC of aciclovir by this mechanism, and reduce aciclovir renal clearance. Similarly increases in plasma AUCs of aciclovir and of the inactive metabolite of mycophenolate mofetil, an immunosuppressant agent used in transplant patients have been shown when the drugs are coadministered. However no dosage adjustment is necessary because of the wide therapeutic index of aciclovir.

4.6 Pregnancy and lactation

A post-marketing aciclovir pregnancy registry has documented pregnancy outcomes in women exposed to any formulation of Zovirax. The birth defects described amongst Zovirax exposed subjects have not shown any uniqueness or consistent pattern to suggest a common cause.

Caution should however be exercised by balancing the potential benefits of treatment against any possible hazard. Findings from reproduction toxicology studies are included in section 5.3.

Following oral administration of 200mg Zovirax five times a day, aciclovir has been detected in breast milk at concentrations ranging from 0.6 to 4.1 times the corresponding plasma levels. These levels would potentially expose nursing infants to aciclovir dosages of up to 0.3mg/kg/day. Caution is therefore advised if Zovirax is to be administered to a nursing woman.

Fertility

There is no information on the effect of aciclovir on human female fertility.

In a study of 20 male patients with normal sperm count, oral aciclovir administered at doses of up to 1g per day for up to six months has been shown to have no clinically significant effect on sperm count, motility or morphology.

4.7 Effects on ability to drive and use machines

No studies on the effects on the ability to drive and use machines have been performed.

4.8 Undesirable effects

The frequency categories associated with the adverse events below are estimates. For most events, suitable data for estimating incidence were not available. In addition, adverse events may vary in their incidence depending on the indication.

The following convention has been used for the classification of undesirable effects in terms of frequency:- Very common ⩾1/10, common ⩾1/100 and <1/10, uncommon ⩾1/1000 and <1/100, rare ⩾1/10,000 and <1/1000, very rare <1/10,000.

Blood and lymphatic system disorders:

Very rare: Anaemia, leukopenia, thrombocytopenia

Immune system disorders:

Rare: Anaphylaxis

Psychiatric and nervous system disorders:

Common: Headache, dizziness

Very rare: Agitation, confusion, tremor, ataxia, dysarthria, hallucinations, psychotic symptoms, convulsions, somnolence, encephalopathy, coma.

The above events are generally reversible and are usually reported in patients with renal impairment, or with other predisposing factors (see 4.4 Special Warnings and Precautions for Use).

Respiratory, thoracic and mediastinal disorders:

Rare: Dyspnoea

Gastrointestinal disorders

Common: Nausea, vomiting, diarrhoea, abdominal pains

Hepato-biliary disorders

Rare: Reversible rises in bilirubin and liver related enzymes

Very rare: Hepatitis, jaundice

Skin and subcutaneous tissue disorders:

Common: Pruritus, rashes (including photosensitivity)

Uncommon: Urticaria. Accelerated diffuse hair loss.

Accelerated diffuse hair loss has been associated with a wide variety of disease processes and medicines, the relationship of the event to aciclovir therapy is uncertain.

Rare: Angioedema

Renal and urinary disorders:

Rare: Increases in blood urea and creatinine

Very rare: Acute renal failure, renal pain.

Renal pain may be associated with renal failure and crystalluria.

General disorders and administration site conditions:

Common: Fatigue, fever

4.9 Overdose

Symptoms & signs: - Aciclovir is only partly absorbed in the gastrointestinal tract. Patients have ingested overdoses of up to 20g aciclovir on a single occasion, usually without toxic effects. Accidental, repeated overdoses of oral aciclovir over several days have been associated with gastrointestinal effects (such as nausea and vomiting) and neurological effects (headache and confusion).

Overdosage of intravenous aciclovir has resulted in elevations of serum creatinine, blood urea nitrogen and subsequent renal failure. Neurological effects including confusion, hallucinations, agitation, seizures and coma have been described in association with intravenous overdosage.

Management: - Patients should be observed closely for signs of toxicity. Haemodialysis significantly enhances the removal of aciclovir from the blood and may, therefore, be considered a management option in the event of symptomatic overdose.

5. PHARMACOLOGICAL PROPERTIES

5.1 Pharmacodynamic properties

Aciclovir is a synthetic purine nucleoside analogue with *in vitro* and *in vivo* inhibitory activity against human herpes viruses, including herpes simplex virus (HSV) types I and II and varicella zoster virus (VSV).

The inhibitory activity of aciclovir for HSV I, HSV II, and VZV is highly selective. The enzyme thymidine kinase (TK) of normal, uninfected cells does not use aciclovir effectively as a substrate, hence toxicity to mammalian host cells is low; however, TK encoded by HSV and VZV converts aciclovir to aciclovir monophosphate, a nucleoside analogue which is further converted to the diphosphate and finally to the triphosphate by cellular enzymes. Aciclovir triphosphate interferes with the viral DNA polymerase and inhibits viral DNA replication with the resultant chain termination following its incorporation into the viral DNA.

Prolonged or repeated courses of aciclovir in severely immunocompromised individuals may result in the selection of virus strains with reduced sensitivity, which may not respond to continued aciclovir treatment. Most of the clinical isolates with reduced sensitivity have been relatively deficient in viral TK, however, strains with altered viral TK or viral DNA polymerase have also been reported. *In vitro* exposure of HSV isolates to aciclovir can also lead to the emergence of less sensitive strains. The relationship between the *in vitro* determined sensitivity of HSV isolates and clinical response to aciclovir therapy is not clear.

5.2 Pharmacokinetic properties

Aciclovir is only partially absorbed from the gut. Mean steady state peak plasma concentrations ($C^{SS}max$) following doses of 200mg aciclovir administered four-hourly were 3.1 microMol (0.7 microgram/ml) and the equivalent trough plasma levels ($C^{SS}min$) were 1.8 microMol (0.4 microgram/ml). Corresponding steady-state plasma concentrations following doses of 400mg and 800mg aciclovir administered four-hourly were 5.3 microMol (1.2 microgram/ml) and 8 microMol (1.8 microgram/ml) respectively, and equivalent trough plasma levels were 2.7 microMol (0.6 microgram/ml) and 4 microMol (0.9 microgram/ml).

In adults the terminal plasma half-life after administration of intravenous aciclovir is about 2.9 hours. Most of the drug is excreted unchanged by the kidney. Renal clearance of aciclovir is substantially greater than creatinine clearance, indicating that tubular secretion, in addition to glomerular filtration, contributes to the renal elimination of the drug.

9-carboxymethoxymethylguanine is the only significant metabolite of aciclovir, and accounts for 10-15% of the dose excreted in the urine. When aciclovir is given one hour after 1 gram of probenecid the terminal half-life and the area under the plasma concentration time curve is extended by 18% and 40% respectively.

In adults, mean steady state peak plasma concentrations ($C^{SS}max$) following a one hour infusion of 2.5mg/kg, 5mg/kg and 10mg/kg were 22.7 microMol (5.1 microgram/ml), 43.6 microMol (9.8 microgram/ml) and 92 microMol (20.7 microgram/ml), respectively. The corresponding trough levels ($C^{SS}min$) 7 hours later were 2.2 microMol (0.5 microgram/ml), 3.1 microMol (0.7 microgram/ml) and 10.2 microMol (2.3 microgram/ml), respectively.

In children over 1 year of age similar mean peak ($C^{SS}max$) and trough ($C^{SS}min$) levels were observed when a dose of 250mg/m^2 was substituted for 5mg/kg and a dose of 500mg/m^2 was substituted for 10mg/kg. In neonates (0 to 3 months of age) treated with doses of 10mg/kg administered by infusion over a one-hour period every 8 hours the $C^{SS}max$ was found to be 61.2 microMol (13.8 microgram/ml) and $C^{SS}min$ to be 10.1 microMol (2.3 microgram/ml). The terminal plasma half-life in these patients was 3.8 hours.

In the elderly total body clearance falls with increasing age associated with decreases in creatinine clearance although there is little change in the terminal plasma half-life.

In patients with chronic renal failure the mean terminal half-life was found to be 19.5 hours. The mean aciclovir half-life during haemodialysis was 5.7 hours. Plasma aciclovir levels dropped approximately 60% during dialysis.

Cerebrospinal fluid levels are approximately 50% of corresponding plasma levels. Plasma protein binding is relatively low (9 to 33%) and drug interactions involving binding site displacement are not anticipated.

5.3 Preclinical safety data

Mutagenicity: - The results of a wide range of mutagenicity tests *in vitro* and *in vivo* indicate that aciclovir is unlikely to pose a genetic risk to man.

Carcinogenicity: - Aciclovir was not found to be carcinogenic in long term studies in the rat and the mouse.

Teratogenicity: - Systemic administration of aciclovir in internationally accepted standard tests did not produce embryotoxic or teratogenic effects in rats, rabbits or mice.

In a non-standard test in rats, foetal abnormalities were observed, but only following such high subcutaneous doses that maternal toxicity was produced. The clinical relevance of these findings is uncertain.

Fertility: - Largely reversible adverse effects on spermatogenesis in association with overall toxicity in rats and dogs have been reported only at doses of aciclovir greatly in excess of those employed therapeutically. Two generation studies in mice did not reveal any effect of aciclovir on fertility.

6. PHARMACEUTICAL PARTICULARS

6.1 List of excipients

Sorbitol Solution, 70%, non-crystallising EP

Glycerol EP

Dispersible cellulose BP

Methyl parahydroxybenzoate EP

Propyl parahydroxybenzoate EP

Flavour, orange, 52.570/T HSE

Purified water EP

6.2 Incompatibilities

None Known.

6.3 Shelf life

3 years.

6.4 Special precautions for storage

Store below 30°C

6.5 Nature and contents of container

Amber glass bottles fitted with white, child resistant caps with an EPE/Saranex liner or metal roll-on closures lined with PVDC-faced wads.

Pack sizes: 50ml[1], 100ml, 175ml[2], 350ml[3]

The 100ml pack contains a double-ended measuring spoon.

6.6 Special precautions for disposal and other handling

No special instructions.

7. MARKETING AUTHORISATION HOLDER

The Wellcome Foundation Ltd

Glaxo Wellcome House

Berkeley Avenue

Greenford

Middlesex

UB6 ONN

Trading as

GlaxoSmithKline UK

Stockley Park West

Uxbridge

Middlesex UB11 1BT

8. MARKETING AUTHORISATION NUMBER(S)

PL 00003/0264

9. DATE OF FIRST AUTHORISATION/RENEWAL OF THE AUTHORISATION

26 April 2001

10. DATE OF REVISION OF THE TEXT

31 July 2008

[1] Non-marketed pack size

[2] Non-marketed pack size

[3] Non-marketed pack size

Zovirax Eye Ointment

(GlaxoSmithKline UK)

1. NAME OF THE MEDICINAL PRODUCT

Zovirax Eye Ointment

2. QUALITATIVE AND QUANTITATIVE COMPOSITION

Aciclovir 3.0% W/W

3. PHARMACEUTICAL FORM

Ophthalmic Ointment

4. CLINICAL PARTICULARS

4.1 Therapeutic indications

Treatment of herpes simplex keratitis.

4.2 Posology and method of administration

Topical administration to the eye.

Adults: 1cm ribbon of ointment should be placed inside the lower conjunctival sac five times a day at approximately four hourly intervals, omitting the night time application. Treatment should continue for at least 3 days after healing is complete.

Children: As for adults

Use in the elderly: As for adults.

4.3 Contraindications

Zovirax eye ointment is contra-indicated in patients with a known hypersensitivity to aciclovir or valaciclovir.

4.4 Special warnings and precautions for use

Patients should avoid wearing contact lenses when using Zovirax Eye Ointment.

4.5 Interaction with other medicinal products and other forms of interaction

No clinically significant interactions have been identified.

4.6 Pregnancy and lactation

Pregnancy

A post-marketing aciclovir pregnancy registry has documented pregnancy outcomes in women exposed to any formulation of Zovirax. The birth defects described amongst Zovirax exposed subjects have not shown any uniqueness or consistent pattern to suggest a common cause.

The use of Zovirax Eye Ointment should be considered only when the potential benefits outweigh the possibility of unknown risks.

Lactation

Limited human data show that the drug does pass into breast milk following systemic administration. However, the dosage received by the nursing infant following maternal use of Zovirax Eye Ointment are likely to be insignificant.

Fertility

There is no information on the effect of aciclovir on human female fertility.

In a study of 20 male patients with normal sperm count, oral aciclovir administered at doses of up to 1g per day for up to six months has been shown to have no clinically significant effect on sperm count, motility or morphology.

4.7 Effects on ability to drive and use machines

Not applicable

4.8 Undesirable effects

Adverse reactions are listed below by MedDRA body system organ class and by frequency.

The frequency categories used are:

Very common ≥ 1/10,

Common ≥ 1/100 and < 1/10,

Uncommon ≥ 1/1,000 and < 1/100,

Rare ≥ 1/10,000 and < 1/1,000,

Very rare < 1/10,000.

Clinical trial data have been used to assign frequency categories to adverse reactions observed during clinical trials with aciclovir 3% ophthalmic ointment. Due to the nature of the adverse events observed, it is not possible to determine which events were related to the administration of the drug and which were related to the disease. Spontaneous reporting data has been used as a basis for allocating frequency for those events observed post-marketing.

Immune system disorders:

Very rare: Immediate hypersensitivity reactions including angioedema.

Eye disorders:

Very common: Superficial punctate keratopathy.

This did not necessitate an early termination of therapy and healed without apparent sequelae.

Common: Transient mild stinging of the eye occurring immediately following application, conjunctivitis.

Rare: Blepharitis.

4.9 Overdose

No untoward effects would be expected if the entire contents of the tube containing 135 mg of aciclovir were ingested orally. However, the accidental, repeated overdose of oral aciclovir, over several days, has resulted in gastrointestinal effects (nausea and vomiting) and neurological effects (headache and confusion). Aciclovir is dialysable by haemodialysis.

5. PHARMACOLOGICAL PROPERTIES

5.1 Pharmacodynamic properties

Aciclovir is an antiviral agent which is highly active *in vitro* against herpes simplex (HSV) types I and II, but its toxicity to mammalian cells is low.

Aciclovir is phosphorylated to the active compound aciclovir triphosphate after entry into a herpes infected cell. The first step in this process requires the presence of the HSV coded thymidine kinase. Aciclovir triphosphate acts as an inhibitor of, and substrate for, herpes specified DNA polymerase, preventing further viral DNA synthesis without affecting normal cellular processes

5.2 Pharmacokinetic properties

Aciclovir is rapidly absorbed from the ophthalmic ointment through the corneal epithelium and superficial ocular tissues, achieving antiviral concentrations in the aqueous humor. It has not been possible by existing methods to detect aciclovir in the blood after topical application to the eye. However, trace quantities are detectable in the urine. These levels are not therapeutically significant.

5.3 Preclinical safety data

The results of a wide range of mutagenicity tests *in vitro* and *in vivo* indicate that aciclovir does not pose a genetic risk to man.

Aciclovir was not found to be carcinogenic in long-term studies in the rat and the mouse.

Largely reversible adverse effects on spermatogenesis in association with overall toxicity in rats and dogs have been reported only at doses of aciclovir greatly in excess of those employed therapeutically. Two-generation studies in mice did not reveal any effect of orally administered aciclovir on fertility.

Systemic administration of aciclovir in internationally accepted standard tests did not produce embryotoxic or teratogenic effects in rats, rabbits or mice.

In a non-standard test in rats, foetal abnormalities were observed, but only following such high subcutaneous doses that maternal toxicity was produced. The clinical relevance of these findings is uncertain.

6. PHARMACEUTICAL PARTICULARS

6.1 List of excipients

White petrolatum USP

6.2 Incompatibilities

None known

6.3 Shelf life

5 years

6.4 Special precautions for storage

Store below 25°C

6.5 Nature and contents of container

Laminate ophthalmic ointment tubes closed with high-density polyethylene screw caps or tamper evident screw caps.

Pack size: 4.5G

6.6 Special precautions for disposal and other handling

No special instructions

Administrative Data

7. MARKETING AUTHORISATION HOLDER

The Wellcome Foundation Ltd
Glaxo Wellcome House
Berkeley Avenue
Greenford
Middlesex
UB6 ONN
Trading as
GlaxoSmithKline UK
Stockley Park West
Uxbridge
Middlesex UB11 1BT

8. MARKETING AUTHORISATION NUMBER(S)

PL 00003/0150

9. DATE OF FIRST AUTHORISATION/RENEWAL OF THE AUTHORISATION

16 October 1996

10. DATE OF REVISION OF THE TEXT

30 July 2008

Zovirax IV 250mg, 500mg

(GlaxoSmithKline UK)

1. NAME OF THE MEDICINAL PRODUCT

Zovirax I.V. 250 mg
Zovirax I.V. 500 mg

2. QUALITATIVE AND QUANTITATIVE COMPOSITION

250 mg aciclovir or 500 mg aciclovir in each vial

3. PHARMACEUTICAL FORM

Intravenous injection

4. CLINICAL PARTICULARS

4.1 Therapeutic indications

Zovirax I.V. is indicated for the treatment of *Herpes simplex* infections in immunocompromised patients and severe initial genital herpes in the non-immunocompromised.

Zovirax I.V. is indicated for the prophylaxis of *Herpes simplex* infections inimmunocompromised patients.

Zovirax I.V. is indicated for the treatment of *Varicella zoster* infections.

Zovirax I.V. is indicated for the treatment of herpes encephalitis.

Zovirax I.V. is indicated for the treatment of *Herpes simplex* infections in the neonate and infant up to 3 months of age.

4.2 Posology and method of administration

Route of administration: Slow intravenous infusion

A course of treatment with Zovirax I.V. usually lasts 5 days, but this may be adjusted according to the patient's condition and response to therapy. Treatment for herpes encephalitis and neonatal *Herpes simplex* infections usually lasts 10 days.

The duration of prophylactic administration of Zovirax I.V. is determined by the duration of the period at risk.

Dosage in adults:

Patients with *Herpes simplex* (except herpes encephalitis) or *Varicella zoster* infections should be given Zovirax I.V. in doses of 5 mg/kg body weight every 8 hours.

Immunocompromised patients with *Varicella zoster* infections or patients with herpes encephalitis should be given Zovirax I.V. in doses of 10 mg/kg body weight every 8 hours provided renal function is not impaired (see Dosage in renal impairment).

In obese patients dosed with intravenous aciclovir based on their actual body weight, higher plasma concentrations may be obtained (see 5.2 Pharmacokinetic properties). Consideration should therefore be given to dosage reduction in obese patients and especially in those with renal impairment or the elderly.

Dosage in children:

The dose of Zovirax I.V. for children aged between 3 months and 12 years is calculated on the basis of body surface area.

Children with *Herpes simplex* (except herpes encephalitis) or *Varicella zoster* infections should be given Zovirax I.V. in doses of 250 mg per square metre of body surface area every 8 hours.

In immunocompromised children with *Varicella zoster* infections or children with herpes encephalitis, Zovirax I.V. should be given in doses of 500 mg per square metre body surface area every 8 hours if renal function is not impaired.

Children with impaired renal function require an appropriately modified dose, according to the degree of impairment.

The dosage of Zovirax I.V. in neonates and infants up to 3 months of age is calculated on the basis of body weight.

Neonates and infants up to 3 months of age with *Herpes simplex* infections should be given Zovirax I.V. in doses of 10 mg/kg body weight every 8 hours. Treatment for neonatal herpes simplex infections usually lasts 10 days.

Dosage in the elderly:

The possibility of renal impairment in the elderly must be considered and dosage should be adjusted accordingly (see *Dosage in renal impairment* below).

Adequate hydration should be maintained.

Dosage in renal impairment:

Caution is advised when administering Zovirax I.V. to patients with impaired renal function. Adequate hydration should be maintained.

The following adjustments in dosage are suggested:

Creatinine Clearance	Dosage
25 to 50 ml/min	The dose recommended above (5 or 10 mg/kg body weight) should be given every 12 hours.
10 to 25 ml/min	The dose recommended above (5 or 10 mg/kg body weight) should be given every 24 hours.
0 (anuric) to 10 ml/min	In patients receiving continuous ambulatory peritoneal dialysis (CAPD) the dose recommended above (5 or 10 mg/kg body weight) should be halved and administered every 24 hours.
	In patients receiving haemodialysis the dose recommended above (5 or 10 mg/kg body weight) should be halved and administered every 24 hours and after dialysis.

4.3 Contraindications

Zovirax I.V. is contra-indicated in patients known to be previously hypersensitive to aciclovir or valaciclovir.

4.4 Special warnings and precautions for use

Use in patients with renal impairment and in elderly patients:

Aciclovir is eliminated by renal clearance, therefore the dose must be adjusted in patients with renal impairment (see section 4.2 Posology and method of administration). Elderly patients are likely to have reduced renal function and therefore the need for dose adjustment must be considered in this group of patients. Both elderly patients and patients with renal impairment are at increased risk of developing neurological side effects and should be closely monitored for evidence of these effects. In the reported cases, these reactions were generally reversible on discontinuation of treatment (see section 4.8 Undesirable effects).

In patients receiving Zovirax I.V. at higher doses (e.g. for herpes encephalitis) specific care regarding renal function should be taken, particularly when patients are dehydrated or have any renal impairment.

Reconstituted Zovirax I.V. has a pH of approximately 11 and should not be administered by mouth.

Zovirax I.V. contains no antimicrobial preservative. Reconstitution and dilution should therefore be carried out under full aseptic conditions immediately before use and any unused solution discarded. The reconstituted or diluted solutions should not be refrigerated.

Other warnings and precautions

The labels shall contain the following statements:

For intravenous infusion only

Keep out of the reach and sight of children

Store below 25°C

Prepare immediately prior to use

Discard unused solution

4.5 Interaction with other medicinal products and other forms of interaction

No clinically significant interactions have been identified.

Aciclovir is eliminated primarily unchanged in the urine via active renal tubular secretion. Any drugs administered concurrently that compete with this mechanism may increase aciclovir plasma concentrations. Probenecid and cimetidine increase the AUC of aciclovir by this mechanism and reduce aciclovir renal clearance. However no dosage adjustment is necessary because of the wide therapeutic index of aciclovir.

In patients receiving intravenous Zovirax caution is required during concurrent administration with drugs which compete with aciclovir for elimination, because of the potential for increased plasma levels of one or both drugs or their metabolites. Increases in plasma AUCs of aciclovir and of the inactive metabolite of mycophenolate mofetil, an immunosuppressant agent used in transplant patients, have been shown when the drugs are coadministered.

Care is also required (with monitoring for changes in renal function) if administering intravenous Zovirax with drugs which affect other aspects of renal physiology (e.g. ciclosporin, tacrolimus).

4.6 Pregnancy and lactation

A post-marketing aciclovir pregnancy registry has documented pregnancy outcomes in women exposed to any formulation of Zovirax. The birth defects described amongst Zovirax exposed subjects have not shown any uniqueness or consistent pattern to suggest a common cause.

Caution should therefore be exercised by balancing the potential benefits of treatment against any possible hazard. Findings from reproduction toxicology studies are included in Section 5.3.

Following oral administration of 200 mg five times a day, aciclovir has been detected in human breast milk at concentrations ranging from 0.6 to 4.1 times the corresponding plasma levels. These levels would potentially expose nursing infants to aciclovir dosages of up to 0.3 mg/kg body weight/day. Caution is therefore advised if Zovirax is to be administered to a nursing woman.

Fertility:

There is no information on the effect of aciclovir on human female fertility.

In a study of 20 male patients with normal sperm count, oral aciclovir administered at doses of up to 1g per day for up to six months has been shown to have no clinically significant effect on sperm count, motility or morphology.

4.7 Effects on ability to drive and use machines

No studies on the effects on the ability to drive and use machines have been performed.

4.8 Undesirable effects

The frequency categories associated with the adverse events below are estimates. For most events, suitable data for estimating incidence were not available. In addition, adverse events may vary in their incidence depending on the indication.

The following convention has been used for the classification of undesirable effects in terms of frequency:– Very common $\geqslant 1/10$, common $\geqslant 1/100$ and $< 1/10$, uncommon $\geqslant 1/1{,}000$ and $< 1/100$, rare $\geqslant 1/10{,}000$ and $< 1/1{,}000$, very rare $< 1/10{,}000$.

Blood and lymphatic system disorders:

Uncommon: decreases in haematological indices (anaemia, thrombocytopenia, leukopenia).

Immune system disorders:

Very rare: anaphylaxis.

Psychiatric and nervous system disorders:

Very rare: headache, dizziness, agitation, confusion, tremor, ataxia, dysarthria, hallucinations, psychotic symptoms, convulsions, somnolence, encephalopathy, coma.

The above events are generally reversible and usually reported in patients with renal impairment or with other predisposing factors (see 4.4 Special Warnings and Precautions for Use).

Vascular disorders:

Common: phlebitis.

Respiratory, thoracic and mediastinal disorders:

Very rare: dyspnoea.

Gastrointestinal disorders:

Common: nausea, vomiting.

Very rare: diarrhoea, abdominal pain.

Hepato-biliary disorders:

Common: reversible increases in liver-related enzymes.

Very rare: reversible increases in bilirubin, jaundice, hepatitis.

Skin and subcutaneous tissue disorders:

Common: pruritus, urticaria, rashes (including photosensitivity).

Very rare: angioedema.

Renal and urinary disorders:

Common: increases in blood urea and creatinine.

Rapid increases in blood urea and creatinine levels are believed to be related to the peak plasma levels and the state of hydration of the patient. To avoid this effect the drug should not be given as an intravenous bolus injection but by slow infusion over a one-hour period.

Very rare: renal impairment, acute renal failure and renal pain.

Adequate hydration should be maintained. Renal impairment usually responds rapidly to rehydration of the patient and/or dosage reduction or withdrawal of the drug. Progression to acute renal failure however, can occur in exceptional cases.

Renal pain may be associated with renal failure and crystalluria.

General disorders and administration site conditions:

Very rare: fatigue, fever, local inflammatory reactions

Severe local inflammatory reactions sometimes leading to breakdown of the skin have occurred when Zovirax I.V. has been inadvertently infused into extracellular tissues.

4.9 Overdose

Overdosage of intravenous aciclovir has resulted in elevations of serum creatinine, blood urea nitrogen and subsequent renal failure. Neurological effects including confusion, hallucinations, agitation, seizures and coma have been described in association with overdosage. Haemodialysis significantly enhances the removal of aciclovir from the blood and may, therefore, be considered an option in the management of overdose of this drug.

5. PHARMACOLOGICAL PROPERTIES

5.1 Pharmacodynamic properties

Aciclovir is a synthetic purine nucleoside analogue with in vitro and in vivo inhibitory activity against human herpes viruses, including Herpes simplex virus types 1 and 2 and Varicella zoster virus (VZV), Epstein Barr virus (EBV) and Cytomegalovirus (CMV). In cell culture aciclovir has the greatest antiviral activity against HSV-1, followed (in decreasing order of potency) by HSV-2, VZV, EBV and CMV.

The inhibitory activity of aciclovir for HSV-1, HSV-2, VZV and EBV is highly selective. The enzyme thymidine kinase (TK) of normal, uninfected cells does not use aciclovir effectively as a substrate, hence toxicity to mammalian host cells is low; however, TK encoded by HSV, VZV and EBV converts aciclovir to aciclovir monophosphate, a nucleoside analogue, which is further converted to the diphosphate and finally to the triphosphate by cellular enzymes. Aciclovir triphosphate interferes with the viral DNA polymerase and inhibits viral DNA replication with resultant chain termination following its incorporation into the viral DNA.

5.2 Pharmacokinetic properties

In adults, the terminal plasma half-life of aciclovir after administration of Zovirax I.V. is about 2.9 hours. Most of the drug is excreted unchanged by the kidney. Renal clearance of aciclovir is substantially greater than creatinine clearance, indicating that tubular secretion, in addition to glomerular filtration, contributes to the renal elimination of the drug. 9-carboxymethoxy-methylguanine is the only significant metabolite of aciclovir and accounts for 10 to 15% of the dose excreted in the urine.

When aciclovir is given one hour after 1 gram of probenecid, the terminal half-life and the area under the plasma concentration time curve, are extended by 18% and 40% respectively.

In adults, mean steady state peak plasma concentrations ($C^{ss}max$) following a one-hour infusion of 2.5 mg/kg, 5 mg/kg and 10 mg/kg were 22.7 micromolar (5.1 microgram/ml), 43.6 micromolar (9.8 microgram/ml) and 92 micromolar (20.7 microgram/ml) respectively. The corresponding trough levels ($C^{ss}min$) 7 hours later were 2.2 micromolar (0.5 microgram/ml), 3.1 micromolar (0.7 microgram/ml) and 10.2 micromolar (2.3 microgram/ml) respectively. In children over 1 year of age similar mean peak ($C^{ss}max$) and trough ($C^{ss}min$) levels were observed when a dose of 250 mg/m^2 was substituted for 5 mg/kg and a dose of 500 mg/m^2 was substituted for 10 mg/kg. In neonates (0 to 3 months of age) treated with doses of 10 mg/kg administered by infusion over a one-hour period every 8 hours the $C^{ss}max$ was found to be 61.2 micromolar (13.8 microgram/ml) and the $C^{ss}min$ to be 10.1 micromolar (2.3 microgram/ml).

The terminal plasma half-life in these patients was 3.8 hours. In the elderly, total body clearance falls with increasing age and is associated with decreases in creatinine clearance although there is little change in the terminal plasma half-life.

In patients with chronic renal failure the mean terminal half-life was found to be 19.5 hours. The mean aciclovir half-life during haemodialysis was 5.7 hours. Plasma aciclovir levels dropped approximately 60% during dialysis.

In a clinical study in which morbidly obese female patients (n=7) were dosed with intravenous aciclovir based on their actual body weight, plasma concentrations were found to be approximately twice that of normal weight patients (n=5), consistent with the difference in body weight between the two groups.

Cerebrospinal fluid levels are approximately 50% of corresponding plasma levels.

Plasma protein binding is relatively low (9 to 33%) and drug interactions involving binding site displacement are not anticipated.

5.3 Preclinical safety data

Mutagenicity:

The results of a wide range of mutagenicity tests *in vitro* and *in vivo* indicate that aciclovir is unlikely to pose a genetic risk to man.

Carcinogenicity:

Aciclovir was not found to be carcinogenic in long-term studies in the rat and the mouse.

Teratogenicity:

Systemic administration of aciclovir in internationally accepted standard tests did not produce embryotoxic or teratogenic effects in rabbits, rats or mice

In a non-standard test in rats, foetal abnormalities were observed but only following such high subcutaneous doses that maternal toxicity was produced. The clinical relevance of these findings is uncertain.

Fertility:

Largely reversible adverse effects on spermatogenesis in association with overall toxicity in rats and dogs have been reported only at doses of aciclovir greatly in excess of those employed therapeutically. Two-generation studies in mice did not reveal any effect of (orally administered) aciclovir on fertility.

6. PHARMACEUTICAL PARTICULARS

6.1 List of excipients

Sodium hydroxide (used to adjust pH)

6.2 Incompatibilities

None known

6.3 Shelf life

60 months

6.4 Special precautions for storage

Store below 25°C

6.5 Nature and contents of container

Type I glass vials closed with butyl or bromobutyl rubber stoppers secured by aluminium collars.

17 ml-nominal capacity of vial containing 250 mg aciclovir.

25 ml-nominal capacity of vial containing 500 mg aciclovir.

6.6 Special precautions for disposal and other handling

Reconstitution: Zovirax I.V. should be reconstituted using the following volumes of either Water for Injections BP or Sodium Chloride Intravenous Injection BP (0.9% w/v) to provide a solution containing 25 mg aciclovir per ml:

Formulation	*Volume of fluid for reconstitution*
250 mg vial	10 ml
500 mg vial	20 ml

From the calculated dose, determine the appropriate number and strength of vials to be used. To reconstitute each vial add the recommended volume of infusion fluid and shake gently until the contents of the vial have dissolved completely.

Administration:

The required dose of Zovirax I.V. should be administered by slow intravenous infusion over a one-hour period.

After reconstitution Zovirax I.V. may be administered by a controlled-rate infusion pump.

Alternatively, the reconstituted solution may be further diluted to give an aciclovir concentration of not greater than 5 mg/ml (0.5% w/v) for administration by infusion:

Add the required volume of reconstituted solution to the chosen infusion solution, as recommended below, and shake well to ensure adequate mixing occurs.

For children and neonates, where it is advisable to keep the volume of infusion fluid to a minimum, it is recommended that dilution is on the basis of 4 ml reconstituted solution (100 mg aciclovir) added to 20 ml of infusion fluid.

For adults, it is recommended that infusion bags containing 100 ml of infusion fluid are used, even when this would give an aciclovir concentration substantially below 0.5% w/v. Thus one 100 ml infusion bag may be used for any dose between 250 mg and 500 mg aciclovir (10 and 20 ml of reconstituted solution) but a second bag must be used for doses between 500 mg and 1000 mg.

When diluted in accordance with the recommended schedules, Zovirax I.V. is known to be compatible with the following infusion fluids and stable for up to 12 hours at room temperature (15°C to 25°C):

Sodium Chloride Intravenous Infusion BP (0.45% and 0.9% w/v)

Sodium Chloride (0.18% w/v) and Glucose (4% w/v) Intravenous Infusion BP

Sodium Chloride (0.45% w/v) and Glucose (2.5% w/v) Intravenous Infusion BP

Compound Sodium Lactate Intravenous Infusion BP (Hartmann's Solution).

Zovirax I.V. when diluted in accordance with the above schedule will give an aciclovir concentration not greater than 0.5% w/v.

Since no antimicrobial preservative is included, reconstitution and dilution must be carried out under full aseptic conditions, immediately before use, and any unused solution discarded.

Should any visible turbidity or crystallisation appear in the solution before or during infusion, the preparation should be discarded.

7. MARKETING AUTHORISATION HOLDER

The Wellcome Foundation Ltd., trading as GlaxoSmithKline UK, Stockley Park West, Uxbridge, Middlesex UB11 1BT

8. MARKETING AUTHORISATION NUMBER(S)

PL 00003/0159

9. DATE OF FIRST AUTHORISATION/RENEWAL OF THE AUTHORISATION

Date of first authorisation: 6 April 1982

Date of last renewal: 9th June 1997

10. DATE OF REVISION OF THE TEXT

31 July 2008

Zovirax Suspension

(GlaxoSmithKline UK)

1. NAME OF THE MEDICINAL PRODUCT

Zovirax Suspension

2. QUALITATIVE AND QUANTITATIVE COMPOSITION

Aciclovir 200mg/5ml

3. PHARMACEUTICAL FORM

Suspension

4. CLINICAL PARTICULARS

4.1 Therapeutic indications

Zovirax Suspension is indicated for the treatment of herpes simplex virus infections of the skin and mucous membranes including initial and recurrent genital herpes.

Zovirax Suspension is indicated for the suppression (prevention of recurrences) of recurrent herpes simplex infections in immunocompetent patients.

Zovirax Suspension is indicated for the prophylaxis of herpes simplex infections in immunocompromised patients.

Zovirax Suspension is indicated for the treatment of varicella (chickenpox) and herpes zoster (shingles) infections.

4.2 Posology and method of administration

Dosage in Adults

Treatment of herpes simplex infections: 200mg Zovirax should be taken five times daily at approximately four hourly intervals omitting the night time dose. Treatment should continue for 5 days, but in severe initial infections this may have to be extended.

In severely immunocompromised patients (e.g. after marrow transplant) or in patients with impaired absorption from the gut the dose can be doubled to 400mg Zovirax or alternatively intravenous dosing could be considered.

Dosing should begin as early as possible after the start of an infection; for recurrent episodes this should preferably be during the prodromal period or when lesions first appear.

Suppression of herpes simplex infections in immunocompetent patients:

200mg Zovirax should be taken four times daily at approximately six-hourly intervals.

Many patients may be conveniently managed on a regimen of 400mg Zovirax twice daily at approximately twelve-hourly intervals.

Dosage titration down to 200mg Zovirax taken thrice daily at approximately eight-hourly intervals or even twice daily at approximately twelve-hourly intervals, may prove effective.

Some patients may experience break-through infection on total daily doses of 800mg Zovirax.

Therapy should be interrupted periodically at intervals of six to twelve months, in order to observe possible changes in the natural history of the disease.

Prophylaxis of herpes simplex infections in immunocompromised patients:

200mg Zovirax should be taken four times daily at approximately six hourly intervals.

In severely immunocompromised patients (e.g. after marrow transplant) or in patients with impaired absorption from the gut, the dose can be doubled to 400mg Zovirax or, alternatively, intravenous dosing could be considered.

The duration of prophylactic administration is determined by the duration of the period at risk.

Treatment of varicella and herpes zoster infections: 800mg Zovirax should be taken five times daily at approximately four-hourly intervals, omitting the night time dose. Treatment should continue for seven days.

In severely immunocompromised patients (e.g. after marrow transplant) or in patients with impaired absorption from the gut, consideration should be given to intravenous dosing.

Dosing should begin as early as possible after the start of an infection: treatment of herpes zoster yields better results if initiated as soon as possible after the onset of the rash. Treatment of chickenpox in immunocompetent patients should begin within 24 hours after onset of the rash.

Dosage in Children

Treatment of herpes simplex infections, and prophylaxis of herpes simplex infections in the immunocompromised: Children aged two years and over should be given adult dosages and children below the age of two years should be given *half* the adult dose.

Treatment of varicella infections:

6 years and over: 800mg Zovirax four times daily.

2 to 5 years: 400mg Zovirax four times daily.

Under 2 years: 200mg Zovirax four times daily.

Treatment should continue for five days.

Dosing may be more accurately calculated as 20mg/kg body weight (not to exceed 800mg) Zovirax four times daily.

No specific data are available on the *suppression* of *herpes simplex* infections or the treatment of herpes *zoster* infections in immunocompetent children.

Zovirax Suspension may be diluted with an equal volume of either Syrup BP or Sorbitol Solution (70%) (non-crystallising) BP. The diluted product is stable for 4 weeks at 25°C but it is recommended that all dilutions are freshly prepared.

Dosage in the Elderly

The possibility of renal impairment in the elderly must be considered and the dosage should be adjusted accordingly (see Dosage in Renal Impairment below).

Adequate hydration of elderly patients taking high oral doses of aciclovir should be maintained.

Dosage in Renal Impairment

Caution is advised when administering aciclovir to patients with impaired renal function. Adequate hydration should be maintained.

In the management of herpes simplex infections in patients with impaired renal function, the recommended oral doses will not lead to accumulation of aciclovir above levels that have been established safe by intravenous infusion. However, for patients with severe renal impairment (creatinine clearance less than 10ml/minute) an adjustment of dosage to 200mg aciclovir twice daily at approximately twelve-hourly intervals is recommended.

In the treatment of herpes zoster infections it is recommended to adjust the dosage to 800mg aciclovir twice daily at approximately twelve-hourly intervals for patients with severe renal impairment (creatinine clearance less than 10ml/minute), and to 800mg aciclovir three times daily at intervals of approximately eight hours for patients with moderate renal impairment (creatinine clearance in the range 10 to 25ml/minute).

4.3 Contraindications

Zovirax Suspension is contra-indicated in patients known to be hypersensitive to aciclovir or valaciclovir.

4.4 Special warnings and precautions for use

Use in patients with renal impairment and in elderly patients:

Aciclovir is eliminated by renal clearance, therefore the dose must be adjusted in patients with renal impairment (see 4.2 Posology and Method of Administration) Elderly patients are likely to have reduced renal function and therefore the need for dose adjustment must be considered in this group of patients. Both elderly patients and patients with renal impairment are at increased risk of developing neurological side effects and should be closely monitored for evidence of these effects. In the reported cases, these reactions were generally reversible on discontinuation of treatment (see 4.8 Undesirable Effects).

Hydration status: Care should be taken to maintain adequate hydration in patients receiving high oral doses of aciclovir.

The data currently available from clinical studies is not sufficient to conclude that treatment with aciclovir reduces the incidence of chickenpox-associated complications in immunocompetent patients.

4.5 Interaction with other medicinal products and other forms of interaction

No clinically significant interactions have been identified.

Aciclovir is eliminated primarily unchanged in the urine via active renal tubular secretion. Any drugs administered concurrently that compete with this mechanism may increase aciclovir plasma concentrations. Probenecid and cimetidine increase the AUC of aciclovir by this mechanism, and reduce aciclovir renal clearance. Similarly increases in plasma AUCs of aciclovir and of the inactive metabolite of mycophenolate mofetil, an immunosuppressant agent used in transplant patients have been shown when the drugs are coadministered. However no dosage adjustment is necessary because of the wide therapeutic index of aciclovir.

4.6 Pregnancy and lactation

A post-marketing aciclovir pregnancy registry has documented pregnancy outcomes in women exposed to any formulation of Zovirax. The birth defects described amongst Zovirax exposed subjects have not shown any uniqueness or consistent pattern to suggest a common cause.

Caution should however be exercised by balancing the potential benefits of treatment against any possible hazard. Findings from reproduction toxicology studies are included in Section 5.3.

Following oral administration of 200mg Zovirax five times a day, aciclovir has been detected in breast milk at concentrations ranging from 0.6 to 4.1 times the corresponding plasma levels. These levels would potentially expose nursing infants to aciclovir dosages of up to 0.3mg/kg/day. Caution is therefore advised if Zovirax is to be administered to a nursing woman.

Fertility:

There is no information on the effect of aciclovir on human female fertility.

In a study of 20 male patients with normal sperm count, oral aciclovir administered at doses of up to 1g per day for up to six months has been shown to have no clinically significant effect on sperm count, motility or morphology.

4.7 Effects on ability to drive and use machines

No studies on the effects on the ability to drive and use machines have been performed.

4.8 Undesirable effects

The frequency categories associated with the adverse events below are estimates. For most events, suitable data for estimating incidence were not available. In addition, adverse events may vary in their incidence depending on the indication.

The following convention has been used for the classification of undesirable effects in terms of frequency:- Very common $\geqslant 1/10$, common $\geqslant 1/100$ and $< 1/10$, uncommon $\geqslant 1/1000$ and $< 1/100$, rare $\geqslant 1/10{,}000$ and $< 1/1000$, very rare $< 1/10{,}000$.

Blood and lymphatic system disorders:

Very rare: Anaemia, leukopenia, thrombocytopenia

Immune system disorders:

Rare: Anaphylaxis

Psychiatric and nervous system disorders:

Common: Headache, dizziness

Very rare: Agitation, confusion, tremor, ataxia, dysarthria, hallucinations, psychotic symptoms, convulsions, somnolence, encephalopathy, coma.

The above events are generally reversible and are usually reported in patients with renal impairment, or with other predisposing factors (see 4.4 Special Warnings & Precautions for Use).

Respiratory, thoracic and mediastinal disorders:

Rare: Dyspnoea

Gastrointestinal disorders

Common: Nausea, vomiting, diarrhoea, abdominal pains

Hepato-biliary disorders

Rare: Reversible rises in bilirubin and liver related enzymes

Very rare: Hepatitis, jaundice

Skin and subcutaneous tissue disorders:

Common: Pruritus, rashes (including photosensitivity)

Uncommon: Urticaria. Accelerated diffuse hair loss.

Accelerated diffuse hair loss has been associated with a wide variety of disease processes and medicines, the relationship of the event to aciclovir therapy is uncertain.

Rare: Angioedema

Renal and urinary disorders:

Rare: Increases in blood urea and creatinine

Very rare: Acute renal failure, renal pain.

Renal pain may be associated with renal failure and crystalluria.

General disorders and administration site conditions:

Common: Fatigue, fever

4.9 Overdose

Symptoms & signs:- Aciclovir is only partly absorbed in the gastrointestinal tract. Patients have ingested overdoses of up to 20g aciclovir on a single occasion, usually without toxic effects. Accidental, repeated overdoses of oral aciclovir over several days have been associated with gastrointestinal effects (such as nausea and vomiting) and neurological effects (headache and confusion).

Overdosage of intravenous aciclovir has resulted in elevations of serum creatinine, blood urea nitrogen and subsequent renal failure. Neurological effects including confusion, hallucinations, agitation, seizures and coma have been described in association with intravenous overdosage.

Management:- Patients should be observed closely for signs of toxicity. Haemodialysis significantly enhances the removal of aciclovir from the blood and may, therefore, be considered a management option in the event of symptomatic overdose.

5. PHARMACOLOGICAL PROPERTIES

5.1 Pharmacodynamic properties

Aciclovir is a synthetic purine nucleoside analogue with *in vitro* and *in vivo* inhibitory activity against human herpes viruses, including herpes simplex virus (HSV) types I and II and varicella zoster virus (VZV).

The inhibitory activity of aciclovir for HSV I, HSV II, and VZV is highly selective. The enzyme thymidine kinase (TK) of normal, uninfected cells does not use aciclovir effectively as a substrate, hence toxicity to mammalian host cells is low; however, TK encoded by HSV and VZV converts aciclovir to aciclovir monophosphate, a nucleoside analogue which is further converted to the diphosphate and finally to the triphosphate by cellular enzymes. Aciclovir triphosphate interferes with the viral DNA polymerase and inhibits viral DNA replication with the resultant chain termination following its incorporation into the viral DNA.

Prolonged or repeated courses of aciclovir in severely immunocompromised individuals may result in the selection of virus strains with reduced sensitivity, which may not respond to continued aciclovir treatment. Most of the clinical isolates with reduced sensitivity have been relatively deficient in viral TK, however, strains with altered viral TK or viral DNA polymerase have also been reported. *In vitro* exposure of HSV isolates to aciclovir can also lead to the emergence of less sensitive strains. The relationship between the *in vitro* determined sensitivity of HSV isolates and clinical response to aciclovir therapy is not clear.

5.2 Pharmacokinetic properties

Aciclovir is only partially absorbed from the gut. Mean steady state peak plasma concentrations ($C^{SS}max$) following doses of 200mg aciclovir administered four-hourly were 3.1 microMol (0.7 microgram/ml) and the equivalent trough plasma levels ($C^{SS}min$) were 1.8 microMol (0.4 microgram/ml). Corresponding steady-state plasma concentrations following doses of 400mg and 800mg aciclovir administered four-hourly were 5.3 microMol (1.2 microgram/ml) and 8 microMol (1.8 microgram/ml) respectively, and equivalent trough plasma levels were 2.7 microMol (0.6 microgram/ml) and 4 microMol (0.9 microgram/ml).

In adults the terminal plasma half-life after administration of intravenous aciclovir is about 2.9 hours. Most of the drug is excreted unchanged by the kidney. Renal clearance of aciclovir is substantially greater than creatinine clearance, indicating that tubular secretion, in addition to glomerular filtration, contributes to the renal elimination of the drug.

9-carboxymethoxymethylguanine is the only significant metabolite of aciclovir, and accounts for 10-15% of the dose excreted in the urine. When aciclovir is given one hour after 1 gram of probenecid the terminal half-life and the area under the plasma concentration time curve is extended by 18% and 40% respectively.

In adults, mean steady state peak plasma concentrations ($C^{SS}max$) following a one hour infusion of 2.5mg/kg, 5mg/kg and 10mg/kg were 22.7 microMol (5.1 microgram/ml), 43.6 microMol (9.8 microgram/ml) and 92 microMol (20.7 microgram/ml), respectively. The corresponding trough levels ($C^{SS}min$) 7 hours later were 2.2 microMol (0.5 microgram/ml), 3.1 microMol (0.7 microgram/ml) and 10.2 microMol (2.3 microgram/ml), respectively.

In children over 1 year of age similar mean peak ($C^{SS}max$) and trough ($C^{SS}min$) levels were observed when a dose of 250mg/m^2 was substituted for 5mg/kg and a dose of 500mg/m^2 was substituted for 10mg/kg. In neonates (0 to 3 months of age) treated with doses of 10mg/kg administered by infusion over a one-hour period every 8 hours the $C^{SS}max$ was found to be 61.2 microMol (13.8 microgram/ml) and $C^{SS}min$ to be 10.1 microMol (2.3 microgram/ml). The terminal plasma half-life in these patients was 3.8 hours.

In the elderly total body clearance falls with increasing age associated with decreases in creatinine clearance although there is little change in the terminal plasma half-life.

In patients with chronic renal failure the mean terminal half-life was found to be 19.5 hours. The mean aciclovir half-life during haemodialysis was 5.7 hours. Plasma aciclovir levels dropped approximately 60% during dialysis.

Cerebrospinal fluid levels are approximately 50% of corresponding plasma levels. Plasma protein binding is relatively low (9 to 33%) and drug interactions involving binding site displacement are not anticipated.

5.3 Preclinical safety data

Mutagenicity:- The results of a wide range of mutagenicity tests *in vitro* and *in vivo* indicate that aciclovir is unlikely to pose a genetic risk to man.

Carcinogenicity:- Aciclovir was not found to be carcinogenic in long term studies in the rat and the mouse.

Teratogenicity:-Systemic administration of aciclovir in internationally accepted standard tests did not produce embryotoxic or teratogenic effects in rats, rabbits or mice.

In a non-standard test in rats, foetal abnormalities were observed, but only following such high subcutaneous doses that maternal toxicity was produced. The clinical relevance of these findings is uncertain.

Fertility:- Largely reversible adverse effects on spermatogenesis in association with overall toxicity in rats and dogs have been reported only at doses of aciclovir greatly in excess of those employed therapeutically. Two generation studies in mice did not reveal any effect of aciclovir on fertility.

6. PHARMACEUTICAL PARTICULARS

6.1 List of excipients

Sorbitol Solution, 70%, non-crystallising

Glycerol

Dispersible cellulose

Methyl parahydroxybenzoate

Propyl parahydroxybenzoate

Flavour, banana 5708023

Vanillin

Purified water

6.2 Incompatibilities

None Known.

6.3 Shelf life

3 years.

6.4 Special precautions for storage

Store below 25°C

6.5 Nature and contents of container

Neutral amber glass bottles sealed with white, child resistant caps with an EPE/Saranex liner, polyolefin screw caps or metal roll-on closures fitted with sealing wads of agglomerate cork faced with saran-coated paper or saran-coated expanded polyethylene wads.

This container and these closures are applicable to both pack sizes 25ml and 125ml.

The 25ml pack is a starter pack.

The 125ml pack contains a double-ended measuring spoon.

6.6 Special precautions for disposal and other handling

No special instructions.

7. MARKETING AUTHORISATION HOLDER

The Wellcome Foundation Ltd

Glaxo Wellcome House

Berkeley Avenue

Greenford

Middlesex

UB6 ONN

Trading as

GlaxoSmithKline UK

Stockley Park West

Uxbridge

Middlesex UB11 1BT

8. MARKETING AUTHORISATION NUMBER(S)

PL 00003/0202

9. DATE OF FIRST AUTHORISATION/RENEWAL OF THE AUTHORISATION

30 April 2001

10. DATE OF REVISION OF THE TEXT

31 July 2008

Zumenon 1mg

(Solvay Healthcare Limited)

1. NAME OF THE MEDICINAL PRODUCT

Zumenon® 1mg Film-coated Tablets

2. QUALITATIVE AND QUANTITATIVE COMPOSITION

Each tablet contains 1 mg estradiol (as hemihydrate)

For excipients, see 6.1

3. PHARMACEUTICAL FORM

Film-coated tablets.

Round, biconvex, white tablets with inscription 'S' and '379'.

4. CLINICAL PARTICULARS

4.1 Therapeutic indications

Hormone replacement therapy (HRT) for estrogen deficiency symptoms in peri- and postmenopausal women.

The experience treating women older than 65 years is limited.

4.2 Posology and method of administration

Zumenon is an estrogen only continuous HRT for women with or without a uterus.

In women with a uterus, a progestagen such as Dydrogesterone 10mg, should be added to Zumenon for 12-14 days each month to reduce the risk to the endometrium. Unless there is a previous diagnosis of endometriosis, it is not recommended to add a progestagen in hysterectomised women.

For initiation and continuation of treatment of postmenopausal symptoms, the lowest effective dose for the shortest duration (see also section 4.4) should be used.

In general, treatment should start with Zumenon 1mg. Depending on the clinical response, the dosage can afterwards be adjusted to individual need. If the complaints linked to estrogen deficiency are not ameliorated the dosage can be increased by using Zumenon 2mg.

Starting Zumenon

In women who are not taking hormone replacement therapy and who are amenorrhoeic, are hysterectomised, or women who switch from a continuous combined hormone replacement therapy, treatment may be started on any convenient day. In women transferring from a cyclic or continuous sequential HRT regimen, treatment should begin the day following completion of the prior regimen. If the patient has regular menstruation periods, treatment is started within five days of the start of bleeding.

Administration

The dosage is one tablet per day. Zumenon should be taken continuously without a break between packs. Zumenon can be taken with or without food.

If a dose has been forgotten, it should be taken as soon as possible. When more than 12 hours have elapsed, it is recommended to continue with the next dose without taking the forgotten tablet. In the case of a missed or delayed dose the likelihood of breakthrough bleeding or spotting may be increased.

4.3 Contraindications

Known, past or suspected breast cancer;

Known or suspected estrogen-dependent malignant tumours (e.g. endometrial cancer);

Undiagnosed genital bleeding;

Untreated endometrial hyperplasia;

Previous idiopathic or current venous thromboembolism (deep vein thrombosis, pulmonary embolism);

Active or recent arterial thromboembolic disease (e.g. angina, myocardial infarction);

Acute liver disease, or a history of liver disease as long as liver function tests have failed to return to normal;

Known hypersensitivity to the active substance or to any of the excipients;

Porphyria

4.4 Special warnings and precautions for use

For the treatment of postmenopausal symptoms, HRT should only be initiated for symptoms that adversely affect quality of life. In all cases, a careful appraisal of the risks and benefits should be undertaken at least annually and HRT should only be continued as long as the benefit outweighs the risk.

Medical examination/follow up

Before initiating or reinstituting HRT, a complete personal and family medical history should be taken. Physical (including pelvic and breast) examination should be guided by this and by the contraindications and warnings for use. During treatment, periodic check-ups are recommended of a frequency and nature adapted to the individual woman. Women should be advised what changes in their breasts should be reported to their doctor or nurse (See "breast cancer" below). Investigations, including mammography, should be carried out in accordance with currently accepted screening practices, modified to the clinical needs of the individual.

Conditions which need supervision

If any of the following conditions are present, have occurred previously, and/or have been aggravated during pregnancy or previous hormone treatment, the patient should be closely supervised. It should be taken into account that these conditions may recur or be aggravated during treatment with Zumenon, in particular:

- Leiomyoma (uterine fibroids) or endometriosis
- A history of, or risk factors for, thromboembolic disorders (see below)
- Risk factors for estrogen dependent tumours, e.g. 1st degree heredity for breast cancer
- Hypertension
- Liver disorders (e.g. liver adenoma)
- Diabetes mellitus with or without vascular involvement
- Cholelithiasis
- Migraine or (severe) headache
- Systemic lupus erythematosus
- A history of endometrial hyperplasia (see below)
- Epilepsy
- Asthma
- Otosclerosis

Reasons for immediate withdrawal of therapy:

-Therapy should be discontinued in cases where a contra-indication is discovered and in the following situations:

- Jaundice or deterioration in liver function
- Significant increase in blood pressure
- New onset of migraine-type headache
- Pregnancy

Endometrial hyperplasia

The risk of endometrial hyperplasia and carcinoma is increased when estrogens are administered alone for prolonged periods (see section 4.8). The addition of a progestagen for at least 12 days of the cycle in non-hysterectomised women greatly reduces this risk.

Break-through bleeding and spotting may occur during the first few months of treatment. If break-through bleeding or spotting appears after some time on therapy, or continues after treatment has been discontinued, the reason should be investigated, which may include endometrial biopsy to exclude endometrial malignancy.

Unopposed estrogen stimulation may lead to premalignant or malignant transformation in the residual foci of endometriosis. Therefore, the addition of progestagens to estrogen replacement therapy should be considered in women who have undergone hysterectomy because of endometriosis, if they are known to have residual endometriosis.

Breast cancer

A randomised placebo-controlled trial, the Womens Health Initiative study (WHI) and epidemiological studies, including the Million Women Study (MWS), have reported an increased risk of breast cancer in women taking estrogens, estrogen-progestagen combinations or tibolone for HRT for several years (see Section 4.8).

For all HRT, an excess risk becomes apparent within a few years of use and increases with duration of intake but returns to baseline within a few (at most five) years after stopping treatment.

In the MWS, the relative risk of breast cancer with conjugated equine estrogens (CEE) or estradiol (E2) was greater when a progestagen was added, either sequentially or continuously, and regardless of type of progestagen. There was no evidence of a difference in risk between the different routes of administration.

In the WHI study, the continuous combined conjugated equine estrogen and medroxyprogesterone acetate (CEE + MPA) product used was associated with breast cancers that were slightly larger in size and more frequently had local lymph node metastases compared to placebo.

HRT, especially estrogen-progestagen combined treatment, increases the density of mammographic images which may adversely affect the radiological detection of breast cancer.

Venous thromboembolism

HRT is associated with a higher relative risk of developing venous thromboembolism (VTE), i.e. deep vein thrombosis or pulmonary embolism. One randomised controlled trial and epidemiological studies found a two-to threefold higher risk for users compared with non-users. For non-users, it is estimated that the number of cases of VTE that will occur over a 5 year period is about 3 per 1000 women aged 50-59 years and 8 per 1000 women aged between 60-69 years. It is estimated that in healthy women who use HRT for 5 years, the number of additional cases of VTE over a 5 year period will be between 2 and 6 (best estimate=4) per 1000 women aged 50-59 years and between 5 and 15 (best estimate = 9) per 1000 women aged 60-69 years. The occurrence of such an event is more likely in the first year of HRT than later.

● Generally recognised risk factors for VTE include a personal or family history, severe obesity (BMI >30 kg/m^2) and systemic lupus erythematosus (SLE). There is no consensus about the possible role of varicose veins in VTE.

● Patients with a history of VTE or known thrombophilic states have an increased risk of VTE. HRT may add to this risk. Personal or strong family history of thromboembolism or recurrent spontaneous abortion should be investigated in order to exclude a thrombophilic predisposition. Until a thorough evaluation of thrombophilic factors has been made or anticoagulant treatment initiated, use of HRT in such patients should be viewed as contraindicated. Those women already on anticoagulant treatment require careful consideration of the benefit-risk of use of HRT.

● The risk of VTE may be temporarily increased with prolonged immobilisation, major trauma or major surgery. As in all postoperative patients, scrupulous attention should be given to prophylactic measures to prevent VTE following surgery. Where prolonged immobilisation is liable to follow elective surgery, particularly abdominal or orthopaedic surgery to the lower limbs, consideration should be given to temporarily stopping HRT 4 to 6 weeks earlier, if possible. Treatment should not be restarted until the woman is completely mobilised.

• If VTE develops after initiating therapy, the drug should be discontinued. Patients should be told to contact their doctors immediately when they are aware of a potential thromboembolic symptom (e.g. painful swelling of a leg, sudden pain in the chest, dyspnea).

Coronary artery disease (CAD)

There is no evidence from randomised controlled trials of cardiovascular benefit with continuous combined conjugated estrogens and medroxyprogesterone acetate (MPA). Two large clinical trials (WHI and HERS i.e. Heart and Estrogen/progestin Replacement Study) showed a possible increased risk of cardiovascular morbidity in the first year of use and no overall benefit. For other HRT products there are only limited data from randomised controlled trials examining effects in cardiovascular morbidity or mortality. Therefore, it is uncertain whether these findings also extend to other HRT products.

Stroke

One large randomised clinical trial (WHI-trial) found, as a secondary outcome, an increased risk of ischaemic stroke in healthy women during treatment with continuous combined conjugated estrogens and MPA. For women who do not use HRT, it is estimated that the number of cases of stroke that will occur over a 5 year period is about 3 per 1000 women aged 50-59 and 11 per 1000 women aged 60-69 years. It is estimated that for women who use conjugated estrogens and MPA for 5 years, the number of additional cases will be between 0 and 3 (best estimate = 1) per 1000 users aged 50-59 years and between 1 and 9 (best estimate = 4) per 1000 users aged 60-69 years. It is unknown whether the increased risk also extends to other HRT products.

Ovarian cancer

Long-term (at least 5 to 10 years) use of estrogen-only HRT products in hysterectomised women has been associated with an increased risk of ovarian cancer in some epidemiological studies. It is uncertain whether long term use of combined HRT confers a different risk than estrogen-only products.

Other conditions

• Estrogens may cause fluid retention, and therefore patients with cardiac or renal dysfunction should be carefully observed. Patients with terminal renal insufficiency should be closely observed, since it is expected that the level of circulating active ingredients in Zumenon is increased.

• Women with pre-existing hypertriglyceridemia should be followed closely during estrogen replacement or hormone replacement therapy, since rare cases of large increases of plasma triglycerides leading to pancreatitis have been reported with estrogen therapy in this condition.

• Estrogens increase thyroid binding globulin (TBG), leading to increased circulating total thyroid hormone, as measured by protein-bound iodine (PBI), T4 levels (by column or by radio-immunoassay) or T3 levels (by radio-immunoassay). T3 resin uptake is decreased, reflecting the elevated TBG. Free T4 and free T3 concentrations are unaltered. Other binding proteins may be elevated in serum, i.e. corticoid binding globulin (CBG), sex-hormone-binding globulin (SHBG) leading to increased circulating corticosteroids and sex steroids, respectively. Free or biological active hormone concentrations are unchanged. Other plasma proteins may be increased (angiotensinogen/renin substrate, alpha-1-antitrypsin, ceruloplasmin).

• There is no conclusive evidence for improvement of cognitive function. There is some evidence from the WHI trial of increased risk of probable dementia in women who start using continuous combined CEE and MPA after the age of 65. It is unknown whether the findings apply to younger post-menopausal women or other HRT products.

• Patients with rare hereditary problems of galactose intolerance, the Lapp lactase deficiency or glucose-galactose malabsorption should not take this medicine.

• Women who may be at risk of pregnancy should be advised to adhere to non-hormonal contraceptive methods.

Table 1

MedDRA system organ class	Common >1/100, <1/10	Uncommon >1/1,000, <1/100	Rare >1/10,000, <1/1,000	Very rare <1/10,000 incl. isolated reports
Infections and infestations		Cystitis-like syndrome, Vaginal candidiasis		
Neoplasms benign, malignant and unspecified		Increase in size of leiomyoma		
Blood and the lymphatic system disorders				Haemolytic anaemia
Psychiatric disorders		Depression, Change in libido, Nervousness		
Nervous system disorders	Headache, Migraine	Dizziness		Chorea
Eye disorders			Intolerance to contact lenses, Steepening of corneal curvature	
Cardiac disorders				Myocardial infarction
Vascular disorders		Hypertension, Peripheral vascular disease, Varicose vein, Venous thromboembolism		Stroke
Gastrointestinal disorders	Nausea, Abdominal pain, Flatulence	Dyspepsia		Vomiting
Hepatobiliary disorders	Gall bladder disease		Alterations in liver function, sometimes with Asthenia or Malaise, Jaundice and Abdominal pain	
Skin and subcutaneous tissue disorders		Allergic skin reactions, Rash, Urticaria, Pruritus		Chloasma or melasma, which may persist when drug is discontinued, Erythema multiforme, Erythema nodosum, Vascular purpura, Angioedema
Musculoskeletal and connective tissue disorders	Leg cramps	Back pain		
Reproductive system and breast disorders	Breast pain/ tenderness, Breakthrough bleeding and spotting, Pelvic pain	Change in cervical erosion, Change in cervical secretion, Dysmenorrhoea, Menorrhagia, Metrorrhagia	Breast enlargement, Premenstrual-like symptoms	
Congenital and familial/genetic disorders				Aggravation of porphyria
General disorders and administration site reactions	Asthenia	Peripheral oedema		
Investigations	Increase/decrease in weight			

4.5 Interaction with other medicinal products and other forms of interaction

- The metabolism of estrogens may be increased by concomitant use of substances known to induce drug-metabolising enzymes, specifically cytochrome P450 enzymes, such as anticonvulsants (eg. phenobarbital, phenytoin, carbamezapine) and anti-infectives (e.g. rifampicin, rifabutin, nevirapine, efavirenz).

- Ritonavir and nelfinavir, although known as strong inhibitors, by contrast exhibit inducing properties when used concomitantly with steroid hormones.

- Herbal preparations containing St John's wort (Hypericum perforatum) may induce the metabolism of estrogens and progestagens.

- Clinically an increased metabolism of estrogens and progestagens may lead to decreased effect and changes in the uterine bleeding profile.

4.6 Pregnancy and lactation

Pregnancy

Zumenon is not indicated during pregnancy. If pregnancy occurs during medication with Zumenon, treatment should be withdrawn immediately.

The results of most epidemiological studies to date relevant to inadvertent foetal exposure to estrogens indicate no teratogenic or foetotoxic effects.

Lactation:

Zumenon is not indicated during lactation.

4.7 Effects on ability to drive and use machines

Zumenon does not affect the ability to drive or use machines.

4.8 Undesirable effects

The following undesirable effects have been reported in clinical trials with Zumenon 1mg and/or with other estrogen/progestagen therapy and in postmarketing experience:

(see Table 1 opposite)

Breast Cancer

According to evidence from a large number of epidemiological studies and one randomised placebo-controlled trial, the Women's Health Initiative (WHI), the overall risk of breast cancer increases with increasing duration of HRT use in current or recent HRT users.

For *estrogen-only* HRT, estimates of relative risk (RR) from a reanalysis of original data from 51 epidemiological studies (in which >80% of HRT use was estrogen-only HRT) and from the epidemiological Million Women Study (MWS) are similar at 1.35 (95%CI 1.21 – 1.49) and 1.30 (95%CI 1.21 – 1.40), respectively.

For *estrogen plus progestagen* combined HRT, several epidemiological studies have reported an overall higher risk for breast cancer than with estrogens alone.

The MWS reported that, compared to never users, the use of various types of estrogen-progestagen combined HRT was associated with a higher risk of breast cancer (RR = 2.00, 95%CI: 1.88 – 2.12) than use of estrogens alone (RR = 1.30, 95%CI: 1.21 – 1.40) or use of tibolone (RR=1.45; 95%CI 1.25-1.68).

The WHI trial reported a risk estimate of 1.24 (95%CI 1.01 – 1.54) after 5.6 years of use of estrogen-progestagen combined HRT (CEE + MPA) in all users compared with placebo.

The absolute risks calculated from the MWS and the WHI trials are presented below:

The MWS has estimated, from the known average incidence of breast cancer in developed countries, that:

– For women not using HRT, about 32 in every 1000 are expected to have breast cancer diagnosed between the ages of 50 and 64 years.

- For 1000 current or recent users of HRT, the number of *additional* cases during the corresponding period will be

- For users of *estrogen-only* replacement therapy

• between 0 and 3 (best estimate = 1.5) for 5 years' use

• between 3 and 7 (best estimate = 5) for 10 years' use.

- For users of *estrogen plus progestagen* combined HRT,

• between 5 and 7 (best estimate = 6) for 5 years' use

• between 18 and 20 (best estimate = 19) for 10 years' use.

The WHI trial estimated that after 5.6 years of follow-up of women between the ages of 50 and 79 years, an *additional* 8 cases of invasive breast cancer would be due to *estrogen-progestagen combined* HRT (CEE + MPA) per 10,000 women years.

According to calculations from the trial data, it is estimated that:

- For 1000 women in the placebo group,

• about 16 cases of invasive breast cancer would be diagnosed in 5 years.

- For 1000 women who used estrogen + progestagen combined HRT (CEE + MPA), the number of *additional* cases would be

• between 0 and 9 (best estimate = 4) for 5 years' use.

The number of additional cases of breast cancer in women who use HRT is broadly similar for women who start HRT irrespective of age at start of use (between the ages of 45-65) (see section 4.4).

Endometrial cancer

In women with an intact uterus, the risk of endometrial hyperplasia and endometrial cancer increases with increasing duration of use of unopposed estrogens. According to data from epidemiological studies, the best estimate of the risk is that for women not using HRT, about 5 in every 1000 are expected to have endometrial cancer diagnosed between the ages of 50 and 65. Depending on the duration of treatment and estrogen dose, the reported increase in endometrial cancer risk among unopposed estrogen users varies from 2-to 12-fold greater compared with non-users. Adding a progestagen to estrogen-only therapy greatly reduces this increased risk.

Other adverse reactions have been reported in association with estrogen/progestagen treatment:

- Estrogen-dependent neoplasms benign and malignant, e.g. endometrial cancer.

- Venous thromboembolism, i.e. deep leg or pelvic venous thrombosis and pulmonary embolism, is more frequent among hormone replacement therapy users than among non-users. For further information, see section 4.3 Contraindications and 4.4 Special warnings and precautions for use.

- Probable dementia (see section 4.4)

4.9 Overdose

Estradiol is a substance with low toxicity. Theoretically, symptoms such as nausea, vomiting, sleepiness and dizziness could occur in cases of overdosing. It is unlikely that any specific or symptomatic treatment will be necessary. Aforementioned information is applicable for overdosing by children also.

5. PHARMACOLOGICAL PROPERTIES

5.1 Pharmacodynamic properties

Estradiol

The active ingredient, synthetic 17β-estradiol, is chemically and biologically identical to endogenous human estradiol. It substitutes for the loss of estrogen production in menopausal women, and alleviates menopausal symptoms.

Combined therapy with progestagens is also recommended in hysterectomised women with a history of endometriosis as cancer development in extra-uterine endometriotic implants in women on estrogen-only therapy has been reported (see section 4.4 Special warnings and precautions).

Clinical trial information

• Relief of estrogen-deficiency symptoms and bleeding patterns

- Relief of menopausal symptoms was achieved during the first few weeks of treatment.

- Regular withdrawal bleeding in women treated with Zumenon 1mg daily for 28 days and Dydrogesterone 10mg daily for the last 12-14 days of a 28 day cycle, occurred in approximately 75-80% of women with a mean duration of 5 days. Withdrawal bleeding usually started on the day of the last pill of the progestagen phase. Breakthrough bleeding and/or spotting occurred in approximately 10% of the women; amenorrhoea occurred in 21-25% of the women for months 10 to 12 of treatment.

- In women treated with Zumenon 2mg daily for 28 days and Dydrogesterone 10mg daily for the last 12-14 days of a 28 day cycle, approximately 90% of women had regular withdrawal bleeding. The start day and duration of bleeding, and the number of women with intermittent bleeding was the same as with Zumenon 1mg, amenorrhoea (no bleeding or spotting) occurred in 7-11% of the women for months 10 to 12 of treatment.

5.2 Pharmacokinetic properties

Orally administered estradiol, comprising particles whose size has been reduced to less than 5 μm, is quickly and efficiently absorbed from the gastrointestinal tract. The primary unconjugated and conjugated metabolites are estrone and estrone sulphate. These metabolites can contribute to the estrogen effect, both directly and after conversion to estradiol. Estrogens are excreted in the bile and reabsorbed from the intestine. During this enterohepatic cycle the estrogens are broken down. Estrogens are excreted in the urine as biologically inactive glucuronide and sulphate compounds (90 to 95%), or in the faeces (5 to 10%), mostly unconjugated. Estrogens are secreted in the milk of nursing mothers.

During the administration of oral estradiol to post-menopausal women at 1 mg once a day, the $C_{average}$ is 28 pg/ml, the C_{min} is 20 pg/ml and the C_{max} is 54 pg/ml. The E1/E2 (Estrone/Estradiol) ratio is 7.0.

5.3 Preclinical safety data

Supraphysiological doses (prolonged overdoses) of estradiol have been associated with the induction of tumours in estrogen-dependent target organs for all rodent species tested

6. PHARMACEUTICAL PARTICULARS

6.1 List of excipients

Tablets core: Lactose

Hypromellose

Maize Starch

Colloidal anhydrous silica

Magnesium stearate

Film-coat: Hypromellose

Macrogol 400

Titanium dioxide (E171)

6.2 Incompatibilities

Not applicable.

6.3 Shelf life

3 years.

6.4 Special precautions for storage

Do not store above 30°C.

6.5 Nature and contents of container

The tablets are packed in blister strips of 28. The blister strips are made of PVC film with covering Aluminium foil. Each carton contains 84 tablets.

6.6 Special precautions for disposal and other handling

Not applicable.

7. MARKETING AUTHORISATION HOLDER

Solvay Healthcare Ltd

Mansbridge Road

West End

Southampton

SO18 3JD

8. MARKETING AUTHORISATION NUMBER(S)

PL 00512/0141

9. DATE OF FIRST AUTHORISATION/RENEWAL OF THE AUTHORISATION

01 August 1996/16 August 2001

10. DATE OF REVISION OF THE TEXT

January 2006

Legal category

POM

Zumenon 2mg

(Solvay Healthcare Limited)

1. NAME OF THE MEDICINAL PRODUCT

Zumenon® 2mg Film-coated Tablets

2. QUALITATIVE AND QUANTITATIVE COMPOSITION

Each tablet contains 2 mg estradiol (as hemihydrate)

For excipients, see 6.1

3. PHARMACEUTICAL FORM

Brick-red, round, biconvex, film-coated tablets imprinted '$' on one side and '379' on the other.

4. CLINICAL PARTICULARS

4.1 Therapeutic indications

Hormone replacement therapy (HRT) for estrogen deficiency symptoms in peri- and postmenopausal women.

Prevention of osteoporosis in postmenopausal women at high risk of future fractures who are intolerant of, or contra-indicated for, other medicinal products approved for the prevention of osteoporosis.

(See also section 4.4)

The experience of treating women older than 65 years is limited.

4.2 Posology and method of administration

Zumenon is an estrogen only continuous HRT for women with or without a uterus.

In women with a uterus, a progestagen such as Dydrogesterone 10mg, should be added to Zumenon for 12-14 days each month to reduce the risk to the endometrium. Unless there is a previous diagnosis of endometriosis, it is not recommended to add a progestagen in hysterectomised women.

For initiation and continuation of treatment of postmenopausal symptoms, the lowest effective dose for the shortest duration (see also section 4.4) should be used.

In general, treatment should start with Zumenon 1mg. Depending on the clinical response, the dosage can afterwards be adjusted to individual need. If the complaints linked to estrogen deficiency are not ameliorated the dosage can be increased by using Zumenon 2mg.

For the prevention of osteoporosis Zumenon 2 mg should be used.

Starting Zumenon

In women who are not taking hormone replacement therapy and who are amenorrhoeic, are hysterectomised, or women who switch from a continuous combined hormone replacement therapy, treatment may be started on any convenient day. In women transferring from a cyclic or continuous sequential HRT regimen, treatment should begin the day following completion of the prior regimen. If the patient has regular menstruation periods, treatment is started within five days of the start of bleeding

Administration

The dosage is one tablet per day. Zumenon should be taken continuously without a break between packs. Zumenon can be taken with or without food.

If a dose has been forgotten, it should be taken as soon as possible. When more than 12 hours have elapsed, it is recommended to continue with the next dose without taking the forgotten tablet. In the case of a missed or delayed dose the likelihood of breakthrough bleeding or spotting may be increased.

4.3 Contraindications

Known, past or suspected breast cancer;

Known or suspected estrogen-dependent malignant tumours (e.g. endometrial cancer);

Undiagnosed genital bleeding;

Untreated endometrial hyperplasia;

Previous idiopathic or current venous thromboembolism (deep vein thrombosis, pulmonary embolism);

Active or recent arterial thromboembolic disease (e.g. angina, myocardial infarction);

Acute liver disease, or a history of liver disease as long as liver function tests have failed to return to normal;

Known hypersensitivity to the active substance or to any of the excipients;

Porphyria

4.4 Special warnings and precautions for use

For the treatment of postmenopausal symptoms, HRT should only be initiated for symptoms that adversely affect quality of life. In all cases, a careful appraisal of the risks and benefits should be undertaken at least annually and HRT should only be continued as long as the benefit outweighs the risk.

Medical examination/follow up

Before initiating or reinstituting HRT, a complete personal and family medical history should be taken. Physical (including pelvic and breast) examination should be guided by this and by the contraindications and warnings for use. During treatment, periodic check-ups are recommended of a frequency and nature adapted to the individual woman. Women should be advised what changes in their breasts should be reported to their doctor or nurse (See "breast cancer" below). Investigations, including mammography, should be carried out in accordance with currently accepted screening practices, modified to the clinical needs of the individual.

Conditions which need supervision

If any of the following conditions are present, have occurred previously, and/or have been aggravated during pregnancy or previous hormone treatment, the patient should be closely supervised. It should be taken into account that these conditions may recur or be aggravated during treatment with Zumenon, in particular:

- Leiomyoma (uterine fibroids) or endometriosis

- A history of, or risk factors for, thromboembolic disorders (see below)

- Risk factors for estrogen dependent tumours, e.g. 1st degree heredity for breast cancer

- Hypertension

- Liver disorders (e.g. liver adenoma)

- Diabetes mellitus with or without vascular involvement

- Cholelithiasis

- Migraine or (severe) headache

- Systemic lupus erythematosus

- A history of endometrial hyperplasia (see below)

- Epilepsy

- Asthma

- Otosclerosis

Reasons for immediate withdrawal of therapy:

Therapy should be discontinued in cases where a contra-indication is discovered and in the following situations:

- Jaundice or deterioration in liver function

- Significant increase in blood pressure

- New onset of migraine-type headache

- Pregnancy

Endometrial hyperplasia

The risk of endometrial hyperplasia and carcinoma is increased when estrogens are administered alone for prolonged periods (see section 4.8). The addition of a progestagen for at least 12 days of the cycle in non-hysterectomised women greatly reduces this risk.

Break-through bleeding and spotting may occur during the first few months of treatment. If break-through bleeding or spotting appears after some time on therapy, or continues after treatment has been discontinued, the reason should be investigated, which may include endometrial biopsy to exclude endometrial malignancy.

Unopposed estrogen stimulation may lead to premalignant or malignant transformation in the residual foci of endometriosis. Therefore, the addition of progestagens to estrogen replacement therapy should be considered in women who have undergone hysterectomy because of endometriosis, if they are known to have residual endometriosis.

Breast Cancer

A randomised placebo-controlled trial, the Womens Health Initiative study (WHI) and epidemiological studies, including the Million Women Study (MWS), have reported an increased risk of breast cancer in women taking estrogens, estrogen-progestagen combinations or tibolone for HRT for several years (see Section 4.8).

For all HRT, an excess risk becomes apparent within a few years of use and increases with duration of intake but returns to baseline within a few (at most five) years after stopping treatment.

In the MWS, the relative risk of breast cancer with conjugated equine estrogens (CEE) or estradiol (E2) was greater when a progestagen was added, either sequentially or continuously, and regardless of type of progestagen. There was no evidence of a difference in risk between the different routes of administration.

In the WHI study, the continuous combined conjugated equine estrogen and medroxyprogesterone acetate (CEE + MPA) product used was associated with breast cancers that were slightly larger in size and more frequently had local lymph node metastases compared to placebo.

HRT, especially estrogen-progestagen combined treatment, increases the density of mammographic images which may adversely affect the radiological detection of breast cancer.

Venous thromboembolism

HRT is associated with a higher relative risk of developing venous thromboembolism (VTE), i.e. deep vein thrombosis or pulmonary embolism. One randomised controlled trial and epidermiological studies found a two-to threefold higher risk for users compared with non-users. For non-users, it is estimated that the number of cases of VTE that will occur over a 5 year period is about 3 per 1000 women aged 50-59 years and 8 per 1000 women aged between 60-69 years. It is estimated that in healthy women who use HRT for 5 years, the number of additional cases of VTE over a 5 year period will be between 2 and 6 (best estimate=4) per 1000 women aged 50-59 years and between 5 and 15 (best estimate = 9) per 1000 women aged 60-69 years. The occurrence of such an event is more likely in the first year of HRT than later.

• Generally recognised risk factors for VTE include a personal or family history, severe obesity (BMI >30 kg/m^2) and systemic lupus erythematosus (SLE). There is no consensus about the possible role of varicose veins in VTE.

• Patients with a history of VTE or known thrombophilic states have an increased risk of VTE. HRT may add to this risk. Personal or strong family history of thromboembolism or recurrent spontaneous abortion should be investigated in order to exclude a thrombophilic predisposition. Until a thorough evaluation of thrombophilic factors has been made or anticoagulant treatment initiated, use of HRT in such patients should be viewed as contraindicated. Those women already on anticoagulant treatment require careful consideration of the benefit-risk of use of HRT.

• The risk of VTE may be temporarily increased with prolonged immobilisation, major trauma or major surgery. As in all postoperative patients, scrupulous attention should be given to prophylactic measures to prevent VTE following surgery. Where prolonged immobilisation is liable to follow elective surgery, particularly abdominal or orthopaedic surgery to the lower limbs, consideration should be given to temporarily stopping HRT 4 to 6 weeks earlier, if possible. Treatment should not be restarted until the woman is completely mobilised.

• If VTE develops after initiating therapy, the drug should be discontinued. Patients should be told to contact their doctors immediately when they are aware of a potential thromboembolic symptom (e.g. painful swelling of a leg, sudden pain in the chest, dyspnea).

Coronary artery disease (CAD)

There is no evidence from randomised controlled trials of cardiovascular benefit with continuous combined conjugated estrogens and medroxyprogesterone acetate (MPA). Two large clinical trials (WHI and HERS i.e. Heart and Estrogen/progestin Replacement Study) showed a possible increased risk of cardiovascular morbidity in the first year of use and no overall benefit. For other HRT products there are only limited data from randomised controlled trials examining effects in cardiovascular morbidity or mortality. Therefore, it is uncertain whether these findings also extend to other HRT products.

Stroke

One large randomised clinical trial (WHI-trial) found, as a secondary outcome, an increased risk of ischaemic stroke in healthy women during treatment with continuous combined conjugated estrogens and MPA. For women who do not use HRT, it is estimated that the number of cases of stroke that will occur over a 5 year period is about 3 per 1000 women aged 50-59 and 11 per 1000 women aged 60-69 years. It is estimated that for women who use conjugated estrogens and MPA for 5 years, the number of additional cases will be between 0 and 3 (best estimate = 1) per 1000 users aged 50-59 years and between 1 and 9 (best estimate = 4) per 1000 users aged 60-69 years. It is unknown whether the increased risk also extends to other HRT products.

Ovarian cancer

Long-term (at least 5 to 10 years) use of estrogen-only HRT products in hysterectomised women has been associated with an increased risk of ovarian cancer in some epidemiological studies. It is uncertain whether long term use of combined HRT confers a different risk than estrogen-only products

Other conditions

• Estrogens may cause fluid retention, and therefore patients with cardiac or renal dysfunction should be carefully observed. Patients with terminal renal insufficiency should be closely observed, since it is expected that the level of circulating active ingredients in Zumenon is increased.

• Women with pre-existing hypertriglyceridemia should be followed closely during estrogen replacement or hormone replacement therapy, since rare cases of large increases of plasma triglycerides leading to pancreatitis have been reported with estrogen therapy in this condition.

• Estrogens increase thyroid binding globulin (TBG), leading to increased circulating total thyroid hormone, as measured by protein-bound iodine (PBI), T4 levels (by column or by radio-immunoassay) or T3 levels (by radio-immunoassay). T3 resin uptake is decreased, reflecting the elevated TBG. Free T4 and free T3 concentrations are unaltered. Other binding proteins may be elevated in serum, i.e. corticoid binding globulin (CBG), sex-hormone-binding globulin (SHBG) leading to increased circulating corticosteroids and sex steroids, respectively. Free or biological active hormone concentrations are unchanged. Other plasma proteins may be increased (angiotensinogen/renin substrate, alpha-1-antitrypsin, ceruloplasmin).

• There is no conclusive evidence for improvement of cognitive function. There is some evidence from the WHI trial of increased risk of probable dementia in women who start using continuous combined CEE and MPA after the age of 65. It is unknown whether the findings apply to younger post-menopausal women or other HRT products.

• Patients with rare hereditary problems of galactose intolerance, the Lapp lactase deficiency or glucose-galactose malabsorption should not take this medicine.

• Women who may be at risk of pregnancy should be advised to adhere to non-hormonal contraceptive methods.

4.5 Interaction with other medicinal products and other forms of interaction

- The metabolism of estrogens may be increased by concomitant use of substances known to induce drug-metabolising enzymes, specifically cytochrome P450 enzymes, such as anticonvulsants (eg. phenobarbital, phenytoin, carbamezapine) and anti-infectives (e.g. rifampicin, rifabutin, nevirapine, efavirenz).

- Ritonavir and nelfinavir, although known as strong inhibitors, by contrast exhibit inducing properties when used concomitantly with steroid hormones.

- Herbal preparations containing St John's wort (Hypericum perforatum) may induce the metabolism of estrogens and progestagens.

- Clinically an increased metabolism of estrogens and progestagens may lead to decreased effect and changes in the uterine bleeding profile.

4.6 Pregnancy and lactation

Pregnancy

Zumenon is not indicated during pregnancy. If pregnancy occurs during medication with Zumenon, treatment should be withdrawn immediately.

The results of most epidemiological studies to date relevant to inadvertent foetal exposure to estrogens indicate no teratogenic or foetotoxic effects.

Lactation:

Zumenon is not indicated during lactation.

4.7 Effects on ability to drive and use machines

Zumenon does not affect the ability to drive or use machines.

4.8 Undesirable effects

The following undesirable effects have been reported in clinical trials with Zumenon 2mg and/or with other estrogen/progestagen therapy and in postmarketing experience

(see Table 1 on next page)

Breast Cancer

According to evidence from a large number of epidemiological studies and one randomised placebo-controlled trial, the Women's Health Initiative (WHI), the overall risk of breast cancer increases with increasing duration of HRT use in current or recent HRT users.

For *estrogen-only* HRT, estimates of relative risk (RR) from a reanalysis of original data from 51 epidemiological studies (in which $>80\%$ of HRT use was estrogen-only HRT) and from the epidemiological Million Women Study (MWS) are similar at 1.35 (95%CI 1.21 – 1.49) and 1.30 (95%CI 1.21 – 1.40), respectively.

For *estrogen plus progestagen* combined HRT, several epidemiological studies have reported an overall higher risk for breast cancer than with estrogens alone.

The MWS reported that, compared to never users, the use of various types of estrogen-progestagen combined HRT was associated with a higher risk of breast cancer (RR = 2.00, 95%CI: 1.88 – 2.12) than use of estrogens alone (RR = 1.30, 95%CI: 1.21 – 1.40) or use of tibolone (RR=1.45; 95%CI 1.25-1.68).

The WHI trial reported a risk estimate of 1.24 (95%CI 1.01 – 1.54) after 5.6 years of use of estrogen-progestagen combined HRT (CEE + MPA) in all users compared with placebo.

The absolute risks calculated from the MWS and the WHI trials are presented below:

The MWS has estimated, from the known average incidence of breast cancer in developed countries, that:

- For women not using HRT, about 32 in every 1000 are expected to have breast cancer diagnosed between the ages of 50 and 64 years.

- For 1000 current or recent users of HRT, the number of *additional* cases during the corresponding period will be

- For users of *estrogen-only* replacement therapy

• between 0 and 3 (best estimate = 1.5) for 5 years' use

• between 3 and 7 (best estimate = 5) for 10 years' use.

- For users of *estrogen plus progestagen* combined HRT,

• between 5 and 7 (best estimate = 6) for 5 years' use

• between 18 and 20 (best estimate = 19) for 10 years' use.

The WHI trial estimated that after 5.6 years of follow-up of women between the ages of 50 and 79 years, an *additional* 8 cases of invasive breast cancer would be due to *estrogen-progestagen combined* HRT (CEE + MPA) per 10,000 women years.

According to calculations from the trial data, it is estimated that:

- For 1000 women in the placebo group,

• about 16 cases of invasive breast cancer would be diagnosed in 5 years.

- For 1000 women who used estrogen + progestagen combined HRT (CEE + MPA), the number of *additional* cases would be

• between 0 and 9 (best estimate = 4) for 5 years' use.

The number of additional cases of breast cancer in women who use HRT is broadly similar for women who start HRT irrespective of age at start of use (between the ages of 45-65) (see section 4.4).'

Endometrial cancer

In women with an intact uterus, the risk of endometrial hyperplasia and endometrial cancer increases with increasing duration of use of unopposed estrogens. According to data from epidemiological studies, the best estimate of the risk is that for women not using HRT, about 5 in every 1000 are expected to have endometrial cancer diagnosed between the ages of 50 and 65. Depending on the duration of treatment and estrogen dose, the reported increase in endometrial cancer risk among unopposed estrogen users varies from 2-to 12-fold greater compared with non-users. Adding a progestagen to estrogen-only therapy greatly reduces this increased risk.

Other adverse reactions have been reported in association with estrogen/progestagen treatment:

- Estrogen-dependent neoplasms benign and malignant, e.g. endometrial cancer.

- Venous thromboembolism, i.e. deep leg or pelvic venous thrombosis and pulmonary embolism, is more frequent among hormone replacement therapy users than among non-users. For further information, see section 4.3 Contra-indications and 4.4 Special warnings and precautions for use.

- Probable dementia (see section 4.4).

4.9 Overdose

Estradiol is a substance with low toxicity. Theoretically, symptoms such as nausea, vomiting, sleepiness and dizziness could occur in cases of overdosing. It is unlikely that any specific or symptomatic treatment will be necessary. Aforementioned information is applicable for overdosing by children also.

5. PHARMACOLOGICAL PROPERTIES

5.1 Pharmacodynamic properties

Estradiol

The active ingredient, synthetic 17β-estradiol, is chemically and biologically identical to endogenous human estradiol. It substitutes for the loss of estrogen production

Table 1

MedDRA system organ class	Common >1/100, <1/10	Uncommon >1/1,000, <1/100	Rare >1/10,000, <1/1,000	Very rare <1/10,000 incl. isolated reports
Infections and infestations		Cystitis-like syndrome, Vaginal candidiasis		
Neoplasms benign, malignant and unspecified		Increase in size of leiomyoma		
Blood and the lymphatic system disorders				Haemolytic anaemia
Psychiatric disorders		Depression, Change in libido, Nervousness		
Nervous system disorders	Headache, Migraine	Dizziness		Chorea
Eye disorders			Intolerance to contact lenses, Steepening of corneal curvature	
Cardiac disorders				Myocardial infarction
Vascular disorders		Hypertension, Peripheral vascular disease, Varicose vein, Venous thromboembolism		Stroke
Gastrointestinal disorders	Nausea, Abdominal pain, Flatulence	Dyspepsia		Vomiting
Hepatobiliary disorders		Gall bladder disease	Alterations in liver function, sometimes with Asthenia or Malaise, Jaundice and Abdominal pain	
Skin and subcutaneous tissue disorders		Allergic skin reactions, Rash, Urticaria, Pruritus		Chloasma or melasma, which may persist when drug is discontinued, Erythema multiforme, Erythema nodosum, Vascular purpura, Angioedema
Musculoskeletal and connective tissue disorders	Leg cramps	Back pain		
Reproductive system and breast disorders	Breast pain/ tenderness, Breakthrough bleeding and spotting, Pelvic pain	Change in cervical erosion, Change in cervical secretion, Dysmenorrhoea, Menorrhagia, Metrorrhagia	Breast enlargement, Premenstrual-like symptoms	
Congenital and familial/genetic disorders				Aggravation of porphyria
General disorders and administration site reactions	Asthenia	Peripheral oedema		
Investigations	Increase/decrease in weight			

in menopausal women, and alleviates menopausal symptoms. Estrogens prevent bone loss following menopause or ovariectomy.

Combined therapy with progestagens is also recommended in hysterectomised women with a history of endometriosis as cancer development in extra-uterine endometriotic implants in women on estrogen-only therapy has been reported (see section 4.4 Special warnings and precautions).

Clinical trial information

- Relief of estrogen-deficiency symptoms and bleeding patterns

- Relief of menopausal symptoms was achieved during the first few weeks of treatment.

- Regular withdrawal bleeding in women treated with Zumenon 1mg daily for 28 days and Dydrogesterone 10mg daily for the last 12-14 days of a 28 day cycle, occurred in approximately 75-80% of women with a mean duration of 5 days. Withdrawal bleeding usually started on the day of the last pill of the progestagen phase. Breakthrough bleeding and/or spotting occurred in approximately 10% of the women; amenorrhoea occurred in 21-25% of the women for months 10 to 12 of treatment.

- In women treated with Zumenon 2mg daily for 28 days and Dydrogesterone 10mg daily for the last 12-14 days of a 28 day cycle, approximately 90% of women had regular withdrawal bleeding. The start day and duration of bleeding, and the number of women with intermittent bleeding was the same as with Zumenon 1mg, amenorrhoea (no bleeding or spotting) occurred in 7-11% of the women for months 10 to 12 of treatment.

- Prevention of osteoporosis

- Estrogen deficiency at menopause is associated with an increasing bone turnover and decline in bone mass. The effect of estrogens on the bone mineral density is dose-dependent. Protection appears to be effective for as long as treatment is continued. After discontinuation of HRT, bone mass is lost at a rate similar to that in untreated women.

- Evidence from the WHI trial and meta-analysed trials shows that current use of HRT, alone or in combination with a progestagen – given to predominantly healthy women – reduces the risk of hip, vertebral, and other osteoporotic fractures. HRT may also prevent fractures in women with low bone density and/or established osteoporosis, but the evidence for that is limited.

- After two years of treatment with Zumenon 2mg, the increase in lumbar spine bone mineral density (BMD) was 6.7% ± 3.9% (mean ± SD). The percentage of women who maintained or gained BMD in lumbar zone during treatment was 94.5%.

- Zumenon 2mg also had an effect on hip BMD. The increase after two years of treatment with 2mg estradiol was 2.6% ± 5.0% (mean ± SD) at femoral neck, 4.6% ± 5.0% (mean ± SD) at trochanter and 4.1%±7.4% (mean ± SD) at Wards triangle. The percentage of women who maintained or gained BMD in the 3 hip areas after treatment with 2mg estradiol was 71-88%.

5.2 Pharmacokinetic properties

Orally administered estradiol, comprising particles whose size has been reduced to less than 5 μm, is quickly and efficiently absorbed from the gastrointestinal tract. The primary unconjugated and conjugated metabolites are estrone and estrone sulphate. These metabolites can contribute to the estrogen effect, both directly and after conversion to estradiol. Estrogens are excreted in the bile and reabsorbed from the intestine. During this enterohepatic cycle the estrogens are broken down. Estrogens are excreted in the urine as biologically inactive glucuronide and sulphate compounds (90 to 95%), or in the faeces (5 to 10%), mostly unconjugated. Estrogens are secreted in the milk of nursing mothers.

During the administration of oral estradiol to post-menopausal women at 2 mg once a day, the $C_{average}$ is 58 pg/ml, the C_{min} is 44 pg/ml and the C_{max} is 93 pg/ml. The E1/E2 (Estrone/Estradiol) ratio is 5.8

5.3 Preclinical safety data

Supraphysiological doses (prolonged overdoses) of estradiol have been associated with the induction of tumours in estrogen-dependent target organs for all rodent species tested.

6. PHARMACEUTICAL PARTICULARS

6.1 List of excipients

Tablets core:

Lactose

Hypromellose

Maize Starch

Colloidal andydrous silica

Magnesium stearate

Film-coat:

Hypromellose

Talc

Macrogol 400

Titanium dioxide E171

Iron oxide red E172

Iron oxide black E172

Iron oxide yellow E172

6.2 Incompatibilities

Not applicable.

6.3 Shelf life

3 years.

6.4 Special precautions for storage

Do not store above 30°C.

6.5 Nature and contents of container

The tablets are packed in blister strips of 28. The blister strips are made of PVC film with covering Aluminium foil. Each carton contains 84 tablets.

6.6 Special precautions for disposal and other handling

Not applicable.

7. MARKETING AUTHORISATION HOLDER

Solvay Healthcare Ltd

Mansbridge Road

West End

Southampton

SO18 3JD

8. MARKETING AUTHORISATION NUMBER(S)

PL 00512/0100

9. DATE OF FIRST AUTHORISATION/RENEWAL OF THE AUTHORISATION

14 May 1997

10. DATE OF REVISION OF THE TEXT

January 2006

Legal Category

POM

Zyban 150 mg prolonged release film-coated tablets

(GlaxoSmithKline UK)

1. NAME OF THE MEDICINAL PRODUCT

Zyban 150 mg prolonged release film-coated tablets.

2. QUALITATIVE AND QUANTITATIVE COMPOSITION

Each tablet contains bupropion hydrochloride 150 mg.

For a full list of excipients, see section 6.1.

3. PHARMACEUTICAL FORM

Prolonged release film-coated tablet.

White, film-coated, biconvex, round tablet printed on one side with GX CH7 and plain on the other side.

4. CLINICAL PARTICULARS

4.1 Therapeutic indications

Zyban tablets are indicated as an aid to smoking cessation in combination with motivational support in nicotine-dependent patients.

4.2 Posology and method of administration

Zyban should be used in accordance with smoking cessation guidelines.

Prescribers should assess the patient's motivation to quit. Smoking cessation therapies are more likely to succeed in those patients whom are motivated to quit and have motivational support.

Zyban tablets should be swallowed whole. The tablets should not be crushed or chewed as this may lead to an increased risk of adverse effects including seizures.

Zyban can be taken with or without food (see sections 4.5 and 5.2).

Patients should be treated for 7-9 weeks.

Although discontinuation reactions are not expected with Zyban, a tapering-off period may be considered.

If at seven weeks no effect is seen, treatment should be discontinued.

Use in Adults

It is recommended that treatment is started while the patient is still smoking and a "target stop date" set within the first two weeks of treatment with Zyban, preferably in the second week.

The initial dose is 150mg to be taken daily for six days, increasing on day seven to 150mg twice daily.

There should be an interval of at least 8 hours between successive doses.

The maximum single dose must not exceed 150mg and the maximum total daily dose must not exceed 300mg.

Insomnia is a very common adverse event which can be reduced by avoiding bedtime doses of Zyban (provided there is at least 8 hours between doses).

Use in Children and Adolescents

Use in patients under 18 years of age is not recommended as the safety and efficacy of Zyban tablets have not been evaluated in these patients.

Use in Elderly Patients

Zyban should be used with caution in elderly patients. Greater sensitivity in some elderly individuals cannot be ruled out. The recommended dose in the elderly is 150mg once a day (see section 4.4).

Use in Patients with Hepatic Insufficiency

Zyban should be used with caution in patients with hepatic impairment. Because of increased variability in the pharmacokinetics in patients with mild to moderate impairment the recommended dose in these patients is 150mg once a day.

Use in Patients with Renal Insufficiency

Zyban should be used with caution in patients with renal insufficiency. The recommended dose in these patients is 150mg once a day (see section 4.4).

4.3 Contraindications

Zyban is contraindicated in patients with hypersensitivity to bupropion or any of the excipients.

Zyban is contraindicated in patients with a current seizure disorder or any history of seizures.

Zyban is contraindicated in patients with a known central nervous system (CNS) tumour.

Zyban is contraindicated in patients who, at any time during treatment, are undergoing abrupt withdrawal from alcohol or any medicinal product known to be associated with risk of seizures on withdrawal (in particular benzodiazepines and benzodiazepine-like agents).

Zyban is contraindicated in patients with a current or previous diagnosis of bulimia or anorexia nervosa.

Zyban is contraindicated for use in patients with severe hepatic cirrhosis.

Concomitant use of Zyban and monoamine oxidase inhibitors (MAOIs) is contraindicated. At least 14 days should elapse between discontinuation of irreversible MAOIs and initiation of treatment with Zyban. For reversible MAOIs, a 24 hour period is sufficient.

Zyban is contraindicated in patients with a history of bipolar disorder as it may precipitate a manic episode during the depressed phase of their illness.

Zyban should not be administered to patients being treated with any other medicinal product containing bupropion as the incidence of seizures is dose dependent.

4.4 Special warnings and precautions for use

Seizures

The recommended dose of Zyban must not be exceeded, since bupropion is associated with a dose-related risk of seizure. At doses up to the maximum recommended daily dose (300mg of Zyban daily), the incidence of seizures is approximately 0.1% (1/1,000).

There is an increased risk of seizures occurring with the use of Zyban in the presence of predisposing risk factors which lower the seizure threshold. Zyban must not be used in patients with predisposing risk factors unless there is a compelling clinical justification for which the potential medical benefit of smoking cessation outweighs the potential increased risk of seizure. In these patients, a maximum dose of 150mg daily should be considered for the duration of treatment.

All patients should be assessed for predisposing risk factors, which include:

- concomitant administration of other medicinal products known to lower the seizure threshold (e.g., antipsychotics, antidepressants, antimalarials, tramadol, theophylline, systemic steroids, quinolones and sedating antihistamines). For patients prescribed such medicinal products whilst taking Zyban, a maximum dose of 150mg daily for the remainder of their treatment should be considered.
- alcohol abuse (see also section 4.3)
- history of head trauma
- diabetes treated with hypoglycaemics or insulin
- use of stimulants or anorectic products.

Zyban should be discontinued and not recommenced in patients who experience a seizure while on treatment.

Interactions (see section 4.5)

Due to pharmacokinetic interactions plasma levels of bupropion or its metabolites may be altered, which may increase the potential for undesirable effects (e.g. dry mouth, insomnia, seizures). Therefore care should be taken when bupropion is given concomitantly with medicinal products which can induce or inhibit the metabolism of bupropion.

Bupropion inhibits metabolism by cytochrome P450 2D6. Caution is advised when medicinal products metabolised by this enzyme are administered concomitantly.

Neuropsychiatry

Zyban is a centrally-acting noradrenaline/dopamine reuptake inhibitor. Neuropsychiatric reactions have been reported (see section 4.8). In particular, psychotic and manic symptomatology have been reported mainly in patients with a known history of psychiatric illness.

Depressed mood may be a symptom of nicotine withdrawal. Depression, rarely including suicidal ideation and behaviour (including suicide attempt), has been reported in patients undergoing a smoking cessation attempt. These symptoms have also been reported during Zyban treatment, and generally occurred early during the treatment course.

Bupropion is indicated for the treatment of depression in some countries. A meta-analysis of placebo controlled clinical trials of antidepressant drugs in adults with major depressive disorder and other psychiatric disorders showed an increased risk of suicidal thinking and behaviour associated with antidepressant use compared to placebo in patients less than 25 years old.

Clinicians should be aware of the possible emergence of significant depressive symptomatology in patients undergoing a smoking cessation attempt, and should advise patients accordingly.

Data in animals suggest a potential for drug abuse. However, studies on abuse liability in humans and extensive clinical experience show that bupropion has low abuse potential.

Hypersensitivity

Zyban should be discontinued if patients experience hypersensitivity reactions during treatment. Clinicians should be aware that symptoms may progress or recur following the discontinuation of Zyban and should ensure symptomatic treatment is administered for an adequate length of time (at least one week). Symptoms typically include skin rash, pruritus, urticaria or chest pain but more severe reactions may include angioedema, dyspnoea/bronchospasm, anaphylactic shock, erythema multiforme or Stevens-Johnson Syndrome. Arthralgia, myalgia and fever have also been reported in association with rash and other symptoms suggestive of delayed hypersensitivity. These symptoms may resemble serum sickness (See section 4.8). In most patients symptoms improved after stopping bupropion and initiating treatment with antihistamine or corticosteroids, and resolved over time.

Hypertension

In clinical practice, hypertension, which in some cases may be severe (see section 4.8) and require acute treatment, has been reported in patients receiving bupropion alone and in combination with nicotine replacement therapy. This has been observed in patients with and without pre-existing hypertension. A baseline blood pressure should be obtained at the start of treatment with subsequent monitoring, especially in patients with pre-existing hypertension. Consideration should be given to discontinuation of Zyban if a clinically significant increase in blood pressure is observed.

Limited clinical trial data suggest that higher smoking cessation rates may be achieved by the combination use of Zyban together with Nicotine Transdermal System (NTS). However, a higher rate of treatment-emergent hypertension was noted in the combination therapy group. If combination therapy with a NTS is used, caution must be exercised and weekly monitoring of blood pressure is recommended. Prior to initiation of combination therapy prescribers should consult the prescribing information of the relevant NTS.

Specific patient groups

Elderly – Clinical experience with bupropion has not identified any differences in tolerability between elderly and other adult patients. However, greater sensitivity of some elderly individuals cannot be ruled out. Elderly patients are more likely to have decreased renal function, hence 150 mg once a day is the recommended dose in these patients (see sections 4.2 and 5.2).

Hepatically-impaired - Bupropion is extensively metabolised in the liver to active metabolites, which are further metabolised. No statistically significant differences in the pharmacokinetics of bupropion were observed in patients with mild to moderate hepatic cirrhosis compared with healthy volunteers, but bupropion plasma levels showed a higher variability between individual patients. Therefore Zyban should be used with caution in patients with mild to moderate hepatic impairment and 150 mg once a day is the recommended dose in these patients.

All patients with hepatic impairment should be closely monitored for possible undesirable effects (e.g., insomnia, dry mouth) that could indicate high drug or metabolite levels.

Renally-impaired - Bupropion is mainly excreted into urine as its metabolites. Therefore 150 mg once a day is the recommended dose in patients with renal impairment, as bupropion and its active metabolites may accumulate to a greater extent than usual (see sections 4.2 and 5.2). The patient should be closely monitored for possible undesirable effects that could indicate high drug or metabolite levels.

4.5 Interaction with other medicinal products and other forms of interaction

In patients receiving medicinal products known to lower the seizure threshold, Zyban must only be used if there is a compelling clinical justification for which the potential medical benefit of smoking cessation outweighs the increased risk of seizure (see section 4.4).

The effect of bupropion on other medicinal products:

Although not metabolised by the CYP2D6 isoenzyme, bupropion and its main metabolite, hydroxybupropion, inhibit the CYP2D6 pathway. Co-administration of bupropion hydrochloride and desipramine to healthy volunteers known to be extensive metabolisers of the CYP2D6 isoenzyme resulted in large (2- to 5-fold) increases in the C_{max} and AUC of desipramine. Inhibition of CYP2D6 was present for at least 7 days after the last dose of bupropion hydrochloride.

Concomitant therapy with medicinal products with narrow therapeutic indices that are predominantly metabolised by CYP2D6 should be initiated at the lower end of the dose range of the concomitant medicinal product. Such medicinal products include certain antidepressants (e.g. desipramine, imipramine, paroxetine), antipsychotics (e.g. risperidone, thioridazine), beta-blockers (e.g. metoprolol), and Type 1C antiarrhythmics (e.g. propafanone, flecainide). If Zyban is added to the treatment regimen of a patient already receiving such a medicinal product, the need to decrease the dose of the original medicinal product should be considered. In these cases the expected benefit of treatment with Zyban should be carefully considered compared with the potential risks.

Although citalopram is not primarily metabolised by CYP2D6, in one study, bupropion increased the Cmax and AUC of citalopram by 30% and 40%, respectively.

The effect of other medicinal products on bupropion:

Bupropion is metabolised to its major active metabolite hydroxybupropion primarily by the cytochrome P450 CYP2B6 (see section 5.2). Co-administration of medicinal products that may affect the CYP2B6 isoenzyme (e.g. CYP2B6 substrates: cyclophosphamide, ifosfamide, and CYP2B6 inhibitors: orphenadrine, ticlopidine, clopidogrel), may result in increased bupropion plasma levels and lower levels of active metabolite hydroxy-bupropion. The clinical consequences of the interaction with CYP2B6 enzyme and the consequent changes in the bupropion-hydroxybupropion ratio are currently unknown.

Since bupropion is extensively metabolised, caution is advised when bupropion is co-administered with medicinal products known to induce metabolism (e.g. carbamazepine, phenytoin) or inhibit metabolism (e.g. valproate), as these may affect its clinical efficacy and safety.

In a series of studies in healthy volunteers, ritonavir (100 mg twice daily or 600 mg twice daily) or ritonavir 100 mg plus lopinavir 400 mg (Kaletra®) twice daily reduced the exposure of bupropion and its major metabolites in a dose dependent manor by approximately 20 to 80% (see section 5.2). This effect is thought to be due to the induction of bupropion metabolism. Patients receiving ritonavir may need increased doses of bupropion but the maximum recommended dose of bupropion should not be exceeded.

Nicotine, administered transdermally by patches, did not affect the pharmacokinetics of bupropion and its metabolites.

Other interactions:

Smoking is associated with an increase in CYP1A2 activity. After cessation of smoking, reduced clearance of medicinal products metabolised by this enzyme, with subsequent increases in plasma levels, may occur. This may be particularly important for those medicinal products primarily metabolised by CYP1A2 with narrow therapeutic windows (e.g. theophylline, tacrine and clozapine). The clinical consequences of smoking cessation on other medicinal products that are partially metabolised by CYP1A2 (e.g., imipramine, olanzapine, clomipramine, and fluvoxamine) are unknown. In addition, limited data indicate that the metabolism of flecainide or pentazocine may also be induced by smoking.

Administration of Zyban to patients receiving either levodopa or amantadine concurrently should be undertaken with caution. Limited clinical data suggest a higher incidence of undesirable effects (e.g. nausea, vomiting, and neuropsychiatric events – see section 4.8) in patients receiving bupropion concurrently with either levodopa or amantadine.

Although clinical data do not identify a pharmacokinetic interaction between bupropion and alcohol, there have been rare reports of adverse neuropsychiatric events or reduced alcohol tolerance in patients drinking alcohol during Zyban treatment. The consumption of alcohol during Zyban treatment should be minimised or avoided.

Since monoamine oxidase A and B inhibitors also enhance the catecholaminergic pathways, by a different mechanism from bupropion, concomitant use of Zyban and monoamine oxidase inhibitors (MAOIs) is contraindicated (see section 4.3) as there is an increased possibility of adverse reactions from their co-administration. At least 14 days should elapse between discontinuation of irreversible MAOIs and initiation of treatment with Zyban. For reversible MAOIs, a 24 hour period is sufficient.

Studies suggest that exposure to bupropion may be increased when sustained release bupropion tablets are taken with a high fat meal (see section 5.2).

4.6 Pregnancy and lactation

The safety of Zyban for use in human pregnancy has not been established.

In a retrospective study, there was no greater proportion of congenital malformations or cardiovascular malformations amongst more than a thousand first trimester exposures to bupropion compared with the use of other antidepressants.

Evaluation of experimental animal studies does not indicate direct or indirect harmful effects with respect to the development of the embryo or foetus, the course of gestation and peri-natal or post-natal development. Exposure in animals was, however, similar to the systemic exposure achieved in humans at the maximum recommended dose. The potential risk in humans is unknown.

Pregnant women should be encouraged to quit smoking without the use of pharmacotherapy. Zyban should not be used in pregnancy.

As bupropion and its metabolites are excreted in human breast milk mothers should be advised not to breast feed while taking Zyban.

4.7 Effects on ability to drive and use machines

As with other CNS acting drugs bupropion may affect ability to perform tasks that require judgement or motor and cognitive skills. Zyban has also been reported to cause dizziness and lightheadedness. Patients should therefore exercise caution before driving or use of machinery until they are reasonably certain Zyban does not adversely affect their performance.

4.8 Undesirable effects

The list below provides information on the undesirable effects identified from clinical experience, categorised by incidence and System Organ Class body system. It is important to note that smoking cessation is often associated with nicotine withdrawal symptoms (e.g. agitation, insomnia, tremor, sweating), some of which are also recognised as adverse events associated with Zyban.

Undesirable effects are ranked under headings of frequency using the following convention; very common (>1/10); common (>1/100, <1/10); uncommon (>1/1,000, <1/100); rare (>1/10000, <1/1,000); very rare (<1/10000).

(see Table 2 above)

Table 2

Immune system disorders*	Common	Hypersensitivity reactions such as urticaria.
	Rare	More severe hypersensitivity reactions including angioedema, dyspnoea/bronchospasm and anaphylactic shock. Arthralgia, myalgia and fever have also been reported in association with rash and other symptoms suggestive of delayed hypersensitivity. These symptoms may resemble serum sickness.
Metabolism and nutrition disorders	Uncommon	Anorexia.
	Rare	Blood glucose disturbances
Psychiatric disorders	Very common	Insomnia (see section 4.2)
	Common	Depression (see section 4.4), agitation, anxiety
	Uncommon	Confusion
	Rare	Irritability, hostility, hallucinations, depersonalization, abnormal dreams including nightmares
	Very rare	Delusions, paranoid ideation, restlessness, aggression
	Not known	Suicidal ideation and suicidal behaviour***
Nervous system disorders	Common	Tremor, concentration disturbance, headache, dizziness, taste disorders
	Rare	Seizures (see below)**, dystonia, ataxia, Parkinsonism, incoordination, memory impairment, paraesthesia, syncope
Eye disorders	Uncommon	Visual disturbance
Ear and labyrinth disorders	Uncommon	Tinnitus
Cardiac disorders	Uncommon	Tachycardia
	Rare	Palpitations
Vascular disorders	Uncommon	Increased blood pressure (sometimes severe), flushing
	Rare	Vasodilation, postural hypotension
Gastrointestinal disorders	Common	Dry mouth, gastrointestinal disturbance including nausea and vomiting, abdominal pain, constipation
Hepatobiliary disorders	Rare	Elevated liver enzymes, jaundice, hepatitis
Skin and subcutaneous tissue disorders*	Common	Rash, pruritus, sweating.
	Rare	Erythema multiforme and Stevens Johnson syndrome have also been reported. Exacerbation of psoriasis
Musculoskeletal and connective tissue disorders	Rare	Twitching
Renal and urinary disorders	Rare	Urinary frequency and/or retention
General disorders and administration site conditions	Common	Fever
	Uncommon	Chest pain, asthenia

* Hypersensitivity may manifest as skin reactions. See "Immune system disorders" and "Skin and subcutaneous tissue disorders".

**The incidence of seizures is approximately 0.1% (1/1,000). The most common type of seizures is generalised tonic-clonic seizures, a seizure type which can result in some cases in post-ictal confusion or memory impairment. (see section 4.4).

***Cases of suicidal ideation and suicidal behaviour have been reported during bupropion therapy (see section 4.4).

4.9 Overdose

Acute ingestion of doses in excess of 10 times the maximum therapeutic dose has been reported. In addition to those events reported as Undesirable Effects, overdose has resulted in symptoms including drowsiness, loss of consciousness and/or ECG changes such as conduction disturbances (including QRS prolongation), arrhythmias and tachycardia. QTc prolongation has also been reported but was generally seen in conjunction with QRS prolongation and increased heart rate. Although most patients recovered without sequelae, deaths associated with bupropion have been reported rarely in patients ingesting large overdoses of the drug.

<u>Treatment</u>: In the event of overdose, hospitalisation is advised. ECG and vital signs should be monitored.

Ensure an adequate airway, oxygenation and ventilation. The use of activated charcoal is recommended. No specific antidote for bupropion is known. Further management should be as clinically indicated.

5. PHARMACOLOGICAL PROPERTIES

5.1 Pharmacodynamic properties

Pharmacotherapeutic group: Other antidepressants, ATC code: N06 AX12.

Bupropion is a selective inhibitor of the neuronal re-uptake of catecholamines (noradrenaline and dopamine) with minimal effect on the re-uptake of indolamines (serotonin) and does not inhibit either monoamine oxidase. The mechanism by which bupropion enhances the ability of patients to abstain from smoking is unknown. However, it is presumed that this action is mediated by noradrenergic and/or dopaminergic mechanisms.

5.2 Pharmacokinetic properties

Absorption

After oral administration of 150 mg bupropion hydrochloride as a prolonged release tablet to healthy volunteers, maximum plasma concentrations (C_{max}) of approximately 100 nanograms per ml are observed after about 2.5 to 3 hours. The AUC and C_{max} values of bupropion and its active metabolites hydroxybupropion and threohydrobupropion increase dose proportionally over a dose range of 50-200 mg following single dosing and over a dose range of 300-450 mg/day following chronic dosing. The C_{max} and AUC values of hydroxybupropion are approximately 3 and 14 times higher, respectively, than bupropion C_{max} and AUC values. The C_{max} of threohydrobupropion is comparable with the C_{max} of bupropion, while the AUC of threohydrobupropion is approximately 5 times higher than that of bupropion. Peak plasma levels of hydroxybupropion and threohydrobupropion are reached after about 6 hours following administration of a single dose of bupropion. Plasma levels of erythrohydrobupropion (an isomer of threohydrobupropion, which is also active) are not quantifiable after single dosing with bupropion.

After chronic dosing with bupropion 150 mg bid, the C_{max} of bupropion is similar to values reported after single dosing. For hydroxybupropion and threohydrobupropion, the C_{max} values are higher (about 4 and 7 times respectively) at steady-state than after a single dosing. Plasma levels of erythrohydrobupropion are comparable to steady-state plasma levels of bupropion. Steady-state of bupropion and its metabolites is reached within 5-8 days. The absolute bioavailability of bupropion is not known; excretion data in urine, however, show that at least 87% of the dose of bupropion is absorbed.

Two studies with bupropion SR 150mg tablets in healthy volunteers suggest that exposure to bupropion may be increased when Zyban tablets are taken with food. When taken following a high fat breakfast, peak plasma concentration of bupropion (C_{max}) increased by 11% and 35% in the two studies, while the overall exposure to bupropion (AUC) increased by 16% and 19%.

Distribution

Bupropion is widely distributed with an apparent volume of distribution of approximately 2000 L.

Bupropion, hydroxybupropion and threohydrobupropion bind moderately to plasma proteins (84%, 77% and 42%, respectively).

Bupropion and its active metabolites are excreted in human breast milk. Animal studies show that bupropion and its active metabolites pass the blood-brain barrier and the placenta.

Metabolism

Bupropion is extensively metabolised in humans. Three pharmacologically active metabolites have been identified in plasma: hydroxybupropion and the amino-alcohol isomers, threohydrobupropion and erythrohydrobupropion. These may have clinical importance, as their plasma concentrations are as high or higher than those of bupropion. The active metabolites are further metabolised to inactive metabolites (some of which have not been fully characterised but may include conjugates) and excreted in the urine.

In vitro studies indicate that bupropion is metabolised to its major active metabolite hydroxybupropion primarily by the CYP2B6, while CYP1A2, 2A6, 2C9, 3A4 and 2E1 are less involved. In contrast, formation of threohydrobupropion involves carbonyl reduction but does not involve cytochrome P450 isoenzymes. (See section 4.5)

The inhibition potential of threohydrobupropion and erythrohydrobupropion towards cytochrome P450 has not been studied.

Bupropion and hydroxybupropion are both inhibitors of the CYP2D6 isoenzyme with K_i values of 21 and 13.3μM, respectively (See section 4.5).

Following oral administration of a single 150-mg dose of bupropion, there was no difference in C_{max}, half-life, T_{max}, AUC, or clearance of bupropion or its major metabolites between smokers and non-smokers.

Bupropion has been shown to induce its own metabolism in animals following sub-chronic administration. In humans, there is no evidence of enzyme induction of bupropion or hydroxybupropion in volunteers or patients receiving recommended doses of bupropion hydrochloride for 10 to 45 days.

Elimination

Following oral administration of 200mg of ^{14}C-bupropion in humans, 87% and 10% of the radioactive dose were recovered in the urine and faeces, respectively. The fraction of the dose of bupropion excreted unchanged was only 0.5%, a finding consistent with the extensive metabolism of bupropion. Less than 10% of this ^{14}C dose was accounted for in the urine as active metabolites.

The mean apparent clearance following oral administration of bupropion hydrochloride is approximately 200 L/hr and the mean elimination half-life of bupropion is approximately 20 hours.

The elimination half-life of hydroxybupropion is approximately 20 hours. The elimination half-lives for threohydrobupropion and erythrohydrobupropion are longer (37 and 33 hours, respectively).

Special Patient Groups:

Patients with renal impairment

The elimination of bupropion and its active major metabolites may be reduced in patients with impaired renal function. Limited data in patients with end-stage renal failure or moderately to severely impaired renal function indicate that exposure to bupropion and/or its metabolites was increased (see section 4.4).

Patients with hepatic impairment

The pharmacokinetics of bupropion and its active metabolites were not statistically significantly different in patients with mild to moderate cirrhosis when compared to healthy volunteers, although more variability was observed between individual patients. (see section 4.4) For patients with severe hepatic cirrhosis, the bupropion Cmax and AUC were substantially increased (mean difference approximately 70% and 3-fold, respectively) and more variable when compared to the values in healthy volunteers; the mean half-life was also longer (by approximately 40%). For hydroxybupropion, the mean Cmax was lower (by approximately 70%), the mean AUC tended to be higher (by approximately 30%), the median Tmax was later (by approximately 20 hrs), and the mean half-lives were longer (by approximately 4-fold) than in healthy volunteers. For threohydrobupropion and erythrohydrobupropion, the mean Cmax tended to be lower (by approximately 30%), the mean AUC tended to be higher (by approximately 50%), the median Tmax was later (by approximately 20 hrs), and the mean half-life was longer (by approximately 2-fold) than in healthy volunteers. (see section 4.3)

Elderly patients

Pharmacokinetic studies in the elderly have shown variable results. A single dose study showed that the pharmacokinetics of bupropion and its metabolites in the elderly do not differ from those in the younger adults. Another pharmacokinetic study, single and multiple dose, has suggested that accumulation of bupropion and its metabolites may occur to a greater extent in the elderly. Clinical experience has not identified differences in tolerability between elderly and younger patients, but greater sensitivity in older patients cannot be ruled out. (see section 4.4)

5.3 Preclinical safety data

In animal experiments bupropion doses several times higher than therapeutic doses in humans caused, amongst others, the following dose-related symptoms: ataxia and convulsions in rats, general weakness, trembling and emesis in dogs and increased lethality in both species. Due to enzyme induction in animals but not in humans, systemic exposures in animals were similar to the systemic exposures seen in humans at the maximum recommended dose.

Liver changes are seen in animal studies but these reflect the action of a hepatic enzyme inducer. At recommended doses in humans, bupropion does not induce its own metabolism. This suggests that the hepatic findings in laboratory animals have only limited importance in the evaluation and risk assessment of bupropion.

Genotoxicity data indicate that bupropion is a weak bacterial mutagen, but not a mammalian mutagen, and therefore is of no concern as a human genotoxic agent. Mouse and rat studies confirm the absence of carcinogenicity in these species.

6. PHARMACEUTICAL PARTICULARS

6.1 List of excipients

Tablet core

Microcrystalline cellulose

Hypromellose

Cysteine hydrochloride monohydrate

Magnesium stearate

Film coat

Hypromellose

Macrogol 400

Titanium dioxide (E171)

Carnauba wax

Printing ink

Iron oxide black (E172)

Hypromellose

6.2 Incompatibilities

Not applicable

6.3 Shelf life

2 years.

6.4 Special precautions for storage

Do not store above 25°C. Store in the original package.

6.5 Nature and contents of container

Cartons containing cold form foil / foil blister packs (PA-Alu-PVC / Alu).

30, 40, 50, 60 or 100 tablets are supplied in each pack. Each blister strip contains 10 tablets. Not all pack sizes may be marketed.

6.6 Special precautions for disposal and other handling

No special requirements.

7. MARKETING AUTHORISATION HOLDER

Glaxo Wellcome UK Ltd. trading as GlaxoSmithKline UK.

Stockley Park West

Uxbridge

Middlesex. UB11 1BT

UK

8. MARKETING AUTHORISATION NUMBER(S)

PL 10949/0340

9. DATE OF FIRST AUTHORISATION/RENEWAL OF THE AUTHORISATION

7 June 2000/1 Dec 2004

10. DATE OF REVISION OF THE TEXT

6 January 2009

Zyloric Tablets 100mg, 300mg

(GlaxoSmithKline UK)

1. NAME OF THE MEDICINAL PRODUCT

Zyloric 100 mg Tablets

Zyloric 300 mg Tablets

2. QUALITATIVE AND QUANTITATIVE COMPOSITION

Allopurinol 100 mg (Zyloric Tablets)

Allopurinol 300 mg (Zyloric-300 Tablets)

3. PHARMACEUTICAL FORM

Tablet

4. CLINICAL PARTICULARS

4.1 Therapeutic indications

Zyloric is indicated for reducing urate/uric acid formation in conditions where urate/uric acid deposition has already occurred (e.g. gouty arthritis, skin tophi, nephrolithiasis) or is a predictable clinical risk (e.g. treatment of malignancy potentially leading to acute uric acid nephropathy). The main clinical conditions where urate/uric acid deposition may occur are: idiopathic gout; uric acid lithiasis; acute uric acid nephropathy; neoplastic disease and myeloproliferative disease with high cell turnover rates, in which high urate levels occur either spontaneously, or after cytotoxic therapy; certain enzyme disorders which lead to overproduction of urate, for example: hypoxanthine-guanine phosphoribosyltransferase, including Lesch-Nyhan syndrome; glucose-6-phosphatase including glycogen storage disease; phosphoribosylpyrophosphate synthetase, phosphoribosylpyrophosphate amidotransferase; adenine phosphoribosyltransferase. Zyloric is indicated for management of 2,8-dihydroxyadenine (2,8-DHA) renal stones related to deficient activity of adenine phosphoribosyltransferase.

Zyloric is indicated for the management of recurrent mixed calcium oxalate renal stones in the presence of hyperuricosuria, when fluid, dietary and similar measures have failed.

4.2 Posology and method of administration

Dosage in Adults: Zyloric should be introduced at low dosage e.g. 100mg/day to reduce the risk of adverse reactions and increased only if the serum urate response is unsatisfactory. Extra caution should be exercised if renal function is poor (*see Dosage in renal impairment*). The following dosage schedules are suggested:

100 to 200 mg daily in mild conditions,

300 to 600 mg daily in moderately severe conditions,

700 to 900 mg daily in severe conditions.

If dosage on a mg/kg bodyweight basis is required, 2 to 10 mg/kg bodyweight/day should be used.

Dosage in children: Children under 15 years: 10 to 20 mg/kg bodyweight/day up to a maximum of 400 mg daily. Use in children is rarely indicated, except in malignant conditions (especially leukaemia) and certain enzyme disorders such as Lesch-Nyhan syndrome.

Dosage in the elderly: In the absence of specific data, the lowest dosage which produces satisfactory urate reduction should be used. Particular attention should be paid to advice in *Dosage in renal impairment* and *Precautions and Warnings*.

Dosage in renal impairment: Since allopurinol and its metabolites are excreted by the kidney, impaired renal function may lead to retention of the drug and/or its metabolites with consequent prolongation of plasma half-lives. In severe renal insufficiency, it may be advisable to use less than 100 mg per day or to use single doses of 100mg at longer intervals than one day.

If facilities are available to monitor plasma oxipurinol concentrations, the dose should be adjusted to maintain plasma oxipurinol levels below 100 micromol/litre (15.2 mg/litre).

Allopurinol and its metabolites are removed by renal dialysis. If dialysis is required two to three times a week consideration should be given to an alternative dosage schedule of 300-400 mg Zyloric immediately after each dialysis with none in the interim.

Dosage in hepatic impairment: Reduced doses should be used in patients with hepatic impairment. Periodic liver function tests are recommended during the early stages of therapy.

Treatment of high urate turnover conditions, e.g. neoplasia, Lesch-Nyhan syndrome: It is advisable to correct existing hyperuricaemia and/or hyperuricosuria with Zyloric before starting cytotoxic therapy. It is important to ensure adequate hydration to maintain optimum diuresis and to attempt alkalinisation of urine to increase solubility of urinary urate/uric acid. Dosage of Zyloric should be at the lower end of the recommended dosage schedule.

If urate nephropathy or other pathology has compromised renal function, the advice given in *Dosage in renal impairment* should be followed.

These steps may reduce the risk of xanthine and/or oxipurinol deposition complicating the clinical situation. See also *Drug Interactions And Adverse Reactions*.

Monitoring Advice: The dosage should be adjusted by monitoring serum urate concentrations and urinary urate/uric acid levels at appropriate intervals.

Instructions for Use: Zyloric may be taken orally once a day after a meal. It is well tolerated, especially after food. Should the daily dosage exceed 300 mg and gastrointestinal intolerance be manifested, a divided doses regimen may be appropriate.

4.3 Contraindications

Zyloric should not be administered to individuals known to be hypersensitive to allopurinol or to any of the components of the formulation.

4.4 Special warnings and precautions for use

Zyloric should be withdrawn *immediately* when a skin rash or other evidence of sensitivity occurs. Reduced doses should be used in patients with hepatic or renal impairment. Patients under treatment for hypertension or cardiac insufficiency, for example with diuretics or ACE inhibitors, may have some concomitant impairment of renal function and allopurinol should be used with care in this group.

Asymptomatic hyperuricaemia per se is generally not considered an indication for use of Zyloric. Fluid and dietary modification with management of the underlying cause may correct the condition.

Acute gouty attacks: Allopurinol treatment should not be started until an acute attack of gout has completely subsided, as further attacks may be precipitated.

In the early stages of treatment with Zyloric, as with uricosuric agents, an acute attack of gouty arthritis may be precipitated. Therefore it is advisable to give prophylaxis with a suitable anti-inflammatory agent or colchicine for at least one month. The literature should be consulted for details of appropriate dosage and precautions and warnings.

If acute attacks develop in patients receiving allopurinol, treatment should continue at the same dosage while the acute attack is treated with a suitable anti-inflammatory agent.

Xanthine deposition: In conditions where the rate of urate formation is greatly increased (e.g. malignant disease and its treatment, Lesch-Nyhan syndrome) the absolute concentration of xanthine in urine could, in rare cases, rise sufficiently to allow deposition in the urinary tract. This risk may be minimised by adequate hydration to achieve optimal urine dilution.

Impaction of uric acid renal stones: Adequate therapy with Zyloric will lead to dissolution of large uric acid renal pelvic stones, with the remote possibility of impaction in the ureter.

Lactose intolerance: Zyloric tablets contain lactose and therefore should not be administered to patients with rare hereditary problems of galactose intolerance, the Lapp lactase deficiency or glucose-galactose malabsorption.

4.5 Interaction with other medicinal products and other forms of interaction

6 -mercaptopurine and azathioprine: Azathioprine is metabolised to 6-mercaptopurine which is inactivated by the action of xanthine oxidase. When 6-mercaptopurine or azathioprine is given concurrently with Zyloric, only one-quarter of the usual dose of 6-mercaptopurine or azathioprine should be given because inhibition of xanthine oxidase will prolong their activity.

Vidarabine (Adenine Arabinoside): Evidence suggests that the plasma half-life of vidarabine is increased in the presence of allopurinol. When the two products are used concomitantly extra vigilance is necessary, to recognise enhanced toxic effects.

Salicylates and uricosuric agents: oxipurinol, the major metabolite of allopurinol and itself therapeutically active, is excreted by the kidney in a similar way to urate. Hence, drugs with uricosuric activity such as probenecid or large doses of salicylate may accelerate the excretion of oxipurinol. This may decrease the therapeutic activity of Zyloric, but the significance needs to be assessed in each case.

Chlorpropamide: If Zyloric is given concomitantly with chlorpropamide when renal function is poor, there may be an increased risk of prolonged hypoglycaemic activity because allopurinol and chlorpropamide may compete for excretion in the renal tubule.

Coumarin anticoagulants

There have been rare reports of increased effect of warfarin and other coumarin anticoagulants when co-administered with allopurinol, therefore, all patients receiving anticoagulants must be carefully monitored.

Phenytoin: Allopurinol may inhibit hepatic oxidation of phenytoin but the clinical significance has not been demonstrated.

Theophylline: Inhibition of the metabolism of theophylline has been reported. The mechanism of the interaction may be explained by xanthine oxidase being involved in the biotransformation of theophylline in man. Theophylline levels should be monitored in patients starting or increasing allopurinol therapy.

Ampicillin/Amoxicillin: An increase in frequency of skin rash has been reported among patients receiving ampicillin or amoxicillin concurrently with allopurinol compared to patients who are not receiving both drugs. The cause of the reported association has not been established. However, it is recommended that in patients receiving allopurinol an alternative to ampicillin or amoxicillin is used where available.

Cyclophosphamide, doxorubicin, bleomycin, procarbazine, mechloroethamine: Enhanced bone marrow suppression by cyclophosphamide and other cytotoxic agents has been reported among patients with neoplastic disease (other than leukaemia), in the presence of allopurinol. However, in a well-controlled study of patients treated with cyclophosphamide, doxorubicin, bleomycin, procarbazine and/or mechloroethamine (chlormethine hydrochloride) allopurinol did not appear to increase the toxic reaction of these cytotoxic agents.

Ciclosporin: Reports suggest that the plasma concentration of ciclosporin may be increased during concomitant treatment with allopurinol. The possibility of enhanced ciclosporin toxicity should be considered if the drugs are co-administered.

Didanosine: In healthy volunteers and HIV patients receiving didanosine, plasma didanosine C_{max} and AUC values were approximately doubled with concomitant allopurinol treatment (300 mg daily) without affecting terminal half life. Co-administration of these 2 drugs is generally not recommended. If concomitant use is unavoidable, a dose reduction of didanosine may be required, and patients should be closely monitored.

4.6 Pregnancy and lactation

There is inadequate evidence of safety of Zyloric in human pregnancy, although it has been in wide use for many years without apparent ill consequence.

Use in pregnancy only when there is no safer alternative and when the disease itself carries risk for the mother or unborn child.

Reports indicate that allopurinol and oxipurinol are excreted in human breast milk. Concentrations of 1.4mg/litre allopurinol and 53.7 mg/litre oxipurinol have been demonstrated in breast milk from woman taking Zyloric 300 mg/day. However, there are no data concerning the effects of allopurinol or its metabolites on the breast-fed baby.

4.7 Effects on ability to drive and use machines

Since adverse reactions such as somnolence, vertigo and ataxia have been reported in patients receiving allopurinol, patients should exercise caution before driving, using machinery or participating in dangerous activities until they are reasonably certain that allopurinol does not adversely affect performance.

4.8 Undesirable effects

For this product there is no modern clinical documentation which can be used as support for determining the frequency of undesirable effects. Undesirable effects may vary in their incidence depending on the dose received and also when given in combination with other therapeutic agents.

The frequency categories assigned to the adverse drug reactions below are estimates: for most reactions, suitable data for calculating incidence are not available. Adverse drug reactions identified through post-marketing surveillance were considered to be rare or very rare. The following convention has been used for the classification of frequency:

Very common ⩾1/10 (⩾10%)

Common ⩾1/100 and <1/10 (⩾1% and <10%)

Uncommon ⩾1/1000 and <1/100 (⩾0.1% and <1%)

Rare ⩾1/10,000 and <1/1000 (⩾0.01% and <0.1%)

Very rare <1/10,000 (<0.01%)

Adverse reactions in association with Zyloric are rare in the overall treated population and mostly of a minor nature. The incidence is higher in the presence of renal and/or hepatic disorder.

Infections and infestations

Very rare Furunculosis

Blood and lymphatic system disorders

Very rare Agranulocytosis, aplastic anaemia, thrombocytopenia

Very rare reports have been received of thrombocytopenia, agranulocytosis and aplastic anaemia, particularly in individuals with impaired renal and/or hepatic function, reinforcing the need for particular care in this group of patients.

Immune system disorders

Uncommon Hypersensitivity reactions

Very rare Angioimmunoblastic lymphadenopathy

Serious hypersensitivity reactions, including skin reactions associated with exfoliation, fever, lymphadenopathy, arthralgia and/or eosinophilia including Stevens-Johnson Syndrome and Toxic Epidermal Necrolysis occur rarely (see Skin and subcutaneous tissue disorders). Associated vasculitis and tissue response may be manifested in various ways including hepatitis, renal impairment and very rarely, seizures. Very rarely acute anaphylactic shock has been reported. If such reactions do occur, it may be at any time during treatment, Zyloric should be withdrawn *immediately and permanently*.

Corticosteroids may be beneficial in overcoming hypersensitivity skin reactions. When generalised hypersensitivity reactions have occurred, renal and/or hepatic disorder has usually been present particularly when the outcome has been fatal.

Angioimmunoblastic lymphadenopathy has been described very rarely following biopsy of a generalised lymphadenopathy. It appears to be reversible on withdrawal of Zyloric.

Metabolism and nutrition disorders

Very rare Diabetes mellitus, hyperlipidaemia

Psychiatric disorders

Very rare Depression

Nervous system disorders

Very rare Coma, paralysis, ataxia, neuropathy, paraesthesiae, somnolence, headache, taste perversion

Eye disorders

Very rare Cataract, visual disorder, macular changes

Ear and labyrinth disorders

Very rare Vertigo

Cardiac disorders

Very rare Angina, bradycardia

Vascular disorders

Very rare Hypertension

Gastrointestinal disorders

Uncommon Vomiting, nausea

Very rare Recurrent haematemesis, steatorrhoea, stomatitis, changed bowel habit

In early clinical studies, nausea and vomiting were reported. Further reports suggest that this reaction is not a significant problem and can be avoided by taking Zyloric after meals.

Hepatobiliary disorders

Uncommon Asymptomatic increases in liver function tests

Rare Hepatitis (including hepatic necrosis and granulomatous hepatitis)

Hepatic dysfunction has been reported without overt evidence of more generalised hypersensitivity.

Skin and subcutaneous tissue disorders

Common Rash

Very rare Angioedema, fixed drug eruption, alopecia, discoloured hair

Skin reactions are the most common reactions and may occur at any time during treatment. They may be pruritic, maculopapular, sometimes scaly, sometimes purpuric and rarely exfoliative. Zyloric should be withdrawn *immediately* should such reactions occur. After recovery from mild reactions, Zyloric may, if desired, be re-introduced at a small dose (e.g. 50mg/day) and gradually increased. If the rash recurs, Zyloric should be *permanently* withdrawn as more severe hypersensitivity may occur (see Immune system disorders).

Angioedema has been reported to occur with and without signs and symptoms of a more generalised hypersensitivity reaction.

Renal and urinary disorders

Very rare Haematuria, uraemia

Reproductive system and breast disorders

Very rare Male infertility, erectile dysfunction, gynaecomastia

General disorders and administration site conditions

Very rare Oedema, general malaise, asthenia, fever

Fever has been reported to occur with and without signs and symptoms of a more generalised Zyloric hypersensitivity reaction (see Immune system disorders).

4.9 Overdose

Ingestion of up to 22.5 g allopurinol without adverse effect has been reported. Symptoms and signs including nausea, vomiting, diarrhoea and dizziness have been reported in a patient who ingested 20 g allopurinol. Recovery followed general supportive measures. Massive absorption of Zyloric may lead to considerable inhibition of xanthine oxidase activity, which should have no untoward effects unless affecting concomitant medication, especially with 6-mercaptopurine and/or azathioprine. Adequate hydration to maintain optimum diuresis facilitates excretion of allopurinol and its metabolites. If considered necessary haemodialysis may be used.

5. PHARMACOLOGICAL PROPERTIES

5.1 Pharmacodynamic properties

Allopurinol is a xanthine-oxidase inhibitor. Allopurinol and its main metabolite oxipurinol lower the level of uric acid in plasma and urine by inhibition of xanthine oxidase, the enzyme catalyzing the oxidation of hypoxanthine to xanthine and xanthine to uric acid. In addition to the inhibition of purine catabolism in some but not all hyperuricaemic patients, de novo purine biosynthesis is depressed via feedback inhibition of hypoxanthine-guanine phosphoribosyltransferase. Other metabolites of allopurinol include allopurinol-riboside and oxipurinol-7 riboside.

5.2 Pharmacokinetic properties

Allopurinol is active when given orally and is rapidly absorbed from the upper gastrointestinal tract. Studies have detected allopurinol in the blood 30-60 minutes after dosing. Estimates of bioavailability vary from 67% to 90%. Peak plasma levels of allopurinol generally occur approximately 1.5 hours after oral administration of Zyloric, but fall rapidly and are barely detectable after 6 hours. Peak levels of oxipurinol generally occur after 3-5 hours after oral administration of Zyloric and are much more sustained.

Allopurinol is negligibly bound by plasma proteins and therefore variations in protein binding are not thought to significantly alter clearance. The apparent volume of distribution of allopurinol is approximately 1.6 litre/kg which suggests relatively extensive uptake by tissues. Tissue concentrations of allopurinol have not been reported in humans, but it is likely that allopurinol and oxipurinol will be present in the highest concentrations in the liver and intestinal mucosa where xanthine oxidase activity is high.

Approximately 20% of the ingested allopurinol is excreted in the faeces. Elimination of allopurinol is mainly by metabolic conversion to oxipurinol by xanthine oxidase and aldehyde oxidase, with less than 10% of the unchanged drug excreted in the urine. Allopurinol has a plasma half-life of about 1 to 2 hours.

Oxipurinol is a less potent inhibitor of xanthine oxidase than allopurinol, but the plasma half-life of oxipurinol is far more prolonged. Estimates range from 13 to 30 hours in man. Therefore effective inhibition of xanthine oxidase is maintained over a 24 hour period with a single daily dose of Zyloric. Patients with normal renal function will gradually accumulate oxipurinol until a steady-state plasma oxipurinol concentration is reached. Such patients, taking 300 mg of allopurinol per day will generally have plasma oxipurinol concentrations of 5-10 mg/litre.

Oxipurinol is eliminated unchanged in the urine but has a long elimination half-life because it undergoes tubular reabsorption. Reported values for the elimination half-life range from 13.6 hours to 29 hours. The large discrepancies in these values may be accounted for by variations in study design and/or creatinine clearance in the patients.

Pharmacokinetics in patients with renal impairment.

Allopurinol and oxipurinol clearance is greatly reduced in patients with poor renal function resulting in higher plasma levels in chronic therapy. Patients with renal impairment, where creatinine clearance values were between 10 and 20ml/min, showed plasma oxipurinol concentrations of approximately 30mg/litre after prolonged treatment with 300 mg allopurinol per day. This is approximately the concentration which would be achieved by doses of 600 mg/day in those with normal renal function. A reduction in the dose of Zyloric is therefore required in patients with renal impairment.

Pharmacokinetics in elderly patients.

The kinetics of the drug are not likely to be altered other than due to deterioration in renal function (see Pharmacokinetics in patients with renal impairment).

5.3 Preclinical safety data

A. Mutagenicity

Cytogenetic studies show that allopurinol does not induce chromosome aberrations in human blood cells *in vitro* at concentrations up to 100 micrograms/ml and *in vivo* at doses up to 600 mg/day for mean period of 40 months.

Allopurinol does not produce nitraso compounds *in vitro* or affect lymphocyte transformation *in vitro*.

Evidence from biochemical and other cytological investigations strongly suggests that allopurinol has no deleterious effects on DNA at any stage of the cell cycle and is not mutagenic.

B. Carcinogenicity

No evidence of carcinogenicity has been found in mice and rats treated with allopurinol for up to 2 years.

C. Teratogenicity

One study in mice receiving intraperitoneal doses of 50 or 100 mg/kg on days 10 or 13 of gestation resulted in foetal abnormalities, however in a similar study in rats at 120 mg/kg on day 12 of gestation no abnormalities were observed. Extensive studies of high oral doses of allopurinol in mice up to 100 mg/kg/day, rats up to 200 mg/kg/day and rabbits up to 150 mg/kg/day during days 8 to 16 of gestation produced no teratogenic effects.

An *in vitro* study using foetal mouse salivary glands in culture to detect embryotoxicity indicated that allopurinol would not be expected to cause embryotoxicity without also causing maternal toxicity.

6. PHARMACEUTICAL PARTICULARS

6.1 List of excipients

Lactose

Maize Starch

Povidone

Magnesium Stearate

Purified Water

6.2 Incompatibilities

None known.

6.3 Shelf life

5 years.

6.4 Special precautions for storage

Do not store above 25°C. Store in the original package

6.5 Nature and contents of container

Zyloric 100mg Tablets

PVC/aluminium foil blister pack

Zyloric-300 Tablets

PVC/aluminium foil blister pack

6.6 Special precautions for disposal and other handling

No special instructions.

Administrative Data

7. MARKETING AUTHORISATION HOLDER

The Wellcome Foundation Ltd

Glaxo Wellcome House

Berkeley Avenue

Greenford

Middlesex

Trading as GlaxoSmithKline UK

Stockley Park West

Uxbridge

Middlesex

UB11 1BT

8. MARKETING AUTHORISATION NUMBER(S)

PL 00003/5207R – Zyloric 100mg Tablets

PL 00003/0092R – Zyloric-300 Tablets

9. DATE OF FIRST AUTHORISATION/RENEWAL OF THE AUTHORISATION

Zyloric 100mg Tablets	Zyloric-300 Tablets
MAA: 20.03.80	14.07.80
Renewal: 06.06.90	18.02.91
Renewal: 14.11.95	25.11.98

10. DATE OF REVISION OF THE TEXT

4 June 2009

11. Legal Status

POM

ZYPADHERA 210 mg, 300 mg, and 405 mg, powder and solvent for prolonged release suspension for injection

(Eli Lilly and Company Limited)

1. NAME OF THE MEDICINAL PRODUCT

ZYPADHERA*▼ 210 mg, 300 mg, and 405 mg, powder and solvent for prolonged release suspension for injection.

2. QUALITATIVE AND QUANTITATIVE COMPOSITION

Each 210 mg vial contains olanzapine pamoate monohydrate equivalent to 210 mg olanzapine. After reconstitution each ml of suspension contains 150 mg olanzapine.

Each 300 mg vial contains olanzapine pamoate monohydrate equivalent to 300 mg olanzapine. After reconstitution each ml of suspension contains 150 mg olanzapine.

Each 405 mg vial contains olanzapine pamoate monohydrate equivalent to 405 mg olanzapine. After reconstitution each ml of suspension contains 150 mg olanzapine.

For a full list of excipients see section 6.1.

3. PHARMACEUTICAL FORM

Powder and solvent for prolonged release suspension for injection.

Powder: yellow solid

Solvent: clear, colourless to slightly yellow solution.

4. CLINICAL PARTICULARS

4.1 Therapeutic indications

Maintenance treatment of adult patients with schizophrenia sufficiently stabilised during acute treatment with oral olanzapine.

4.2 Posology and method of administration

FOR INTRAMUSCULAR USE ONLY. DO NOT ADMINISTER INTRAVENOUSLY OR SUBCUTANEOUSLY. (See section 4.4.)

ZYPADHERA should only be administered by deep intramuscular gluteal injection by a healthcare professional trained in the appropriate injection technique and in locations where post-injection observation and access to appropriate medical care in the case of overdose can be assured.

After each injection, patients should be observed in a healthcare facility by appropriately qualified personnel for at least 3 hours for signs and symptoms consistent with olanzapine overdose. It should be confirmed that the patient is alert, oriented, and absent of any signs and symptoms of overdose. If an overdose is suspected, close medical supervision and monitoring should continue until examination indicates that signs and symptoms have resolved (see section 4.4).

Patients should be treated initially with oral olanzapine before administering ZYPADHERA, to establish tolerability and response.

For Instructions for Use, see section 6.6.

Do not confuse ZYPADHERA 210 mg, 300 mg, and 405 mg, powder and solvent for prolonged release suspension for injection with olanzapine 10 mg powder for solution for injection.

In order to identify the first ZYPADHERA dose for all patients the scheme in Table 1 should be considered.

Table 1. Recommended dose scheme between oral olanzapine and ZYPADHERA

Target oral olanzapine dose	Recommended starting dose of ZYPADHERA	Maintenance dose after 2 months of ZYPADHERA treatment
10 mg/day	210 mg/2 weeks or 405 mg/4 weeks	150 mg/2 weeks or 300 mg/4 weeks
15 mg/day	300 mg/2 weeks	210 mg/2 weeks or 405 mg/4 weeks
20 mg/day	300 mg/2 weeks	300 mg/2 weeks

Dose adjustment

Patients should be monitored carefully for signs of relapse during the first one to two months of treatment. During antipsychotic treatment, improvement in the patient's clinical condition may take several days to some weeks. Patients should be closely monitored during this period. During treatment, dose may subsequently be adjusted on the basis of individual clinical status. After clinical reassessment, dose may be adjusted within the range 150 mg to 300 mg every 2 weeks or 300 to 405 mg every 4 weeks. (Table 1.)

Supplementation

Supplementation with oral olanzapine was not authorised in double-blind clinical studies. If oral olanzapine supplementation is clinically indicated, then the combined total dose of olanzapine from both formulations should not exceed the corresponding maximum oral olanzapine dose of 20 mg/day.

Switching to other antipsychotic medicinal products

There are no systematically collected data to specifically address switching patients from ZYPADHERA to other antipsychotic medicinal products. Due to the slow dissolution of the olanzapine pamoate salt which provides a slow continuous release of olanzapine that is complete approximately six to eight months after the last injection, supervision by a clinician, especially during the first 2 months after discontinuation of ZYPADHERA, is needed when switching to another antipsychotic product, and is considered medically appropriate.

Elderly patients

ZYPADHERA has not been systematically studied in elderly patients (> 65 years). ZYPADHERA is not recommended for treatment in the elderly population unless a well-tolerated and effective dose regimen using oral olanzapine has been established. A lower starting dose (150 mg/4 weeks) is not routinely indicated, but should be considered for those 65 and over when clinical factors warrant. ZYPADHERA is not recommended to be started in patients >75 years (see section 4.4).

Patients with renal and/or hepatic impairment

Unless a well-tolerated and effective dose regimen using oral olanzapine has been established in such patients, ZYPADHERA should not be used. A lower starting dose (150 mg every 4 weeks) should be considered for such patients. In cases of moderate hepatic insufficiency (cirrhosis, Child-Pugh class A or B), the starting dose should be 150 mg every 4 weeks and only increased with caution.

Gender

The starting dose and dose range need not be routinely altered for female patients relative to male patients.

Smokers

The starting dose and dose range need not be routinely altered for non-smokers relative to smokers.

When more than one factor is present which might result in slower metabolism (female gender, geriatric age, non-smoking status), consideration should be given to decreasing the dose. When indicated, dose escalation should be performed with caution in these patients.

Paediatric patients

ZYPADHERA is not recommended for use in children and adolescents below 18 years due to a lack of data on safety and efficacy.

4.3 Contraindications

Hypersensitivity to the active substance or to any of the excipients.

Patients with known risk of narrow-angle glaucoma.

4.4 Special warnings and precautions for use

Special care must be taken to apply appropriate injection technique to avoid inadvertent intravascular or subcutaneous injection (see section 6.6).

Use in patients who are in an acutely agitated or severely psychotic state

ZYPADHERA should not be used to treat patients with schizophrenia who are in an acutely agitated or severely psychotic state such that immediate symptom control is warranted.

Post-injection syndrome

During pre-marketing clinical studies, reactions that presented with signs and symptoms consistent with olanzapine overdose were reported in patients following an injection of ZYPADHERA. These reactions occurred in <0.1% of injections and approximately 1.4% of patients. Most of these patients have developed symptoms of sedation (ranging from mild in severity up to coma) and/or delirium (including confusion, disorientation, agitation, anxiety and other cognitive impairment). Other symptoms noted include extrapyramidal symptoms, dysarthria, ataxia, aggression, dizziness, weakness, hypertension and convulsion. In most cases, initial signs and symptoms related to this reaction have appeared within 1 hour following injection, and in all cases full recovery was reported to have occurred within 24 - 72 hours after injection. Reactions occurred rarely (<1 in 1,000 injections) between 1 and 3 hours, and very rarely (<1 in 10,000 injections) after 3 hours. Patients should be advised about this potential risk and the need to be observed for 3 hours in a healthcare facility each time ZYPADHERA is administered.

Prior to giving the injection, the healthcare professional should determine that the patient will not travel alone to their destination. After each injection, patients should be observed in a healthcare facility by appropriately qualified personnel for at least 3 hours for signs and symptoms consistent with olanzapine overdose.

It should be confirmed that the patient is alert, oriented, and absent of any signs and symptoms of overdose. If an overdose is suspected, close medical supervision and monitoring should continue until examination indicates that signs and symptoms have resolved.

For the remainder of the day after injection, patients should be advised to be vigilant for signs and symptoms of overdose secondary to post-injection adverse reactions, be able to obtain assistance if needed, and should not drive or operate machinery (see section 4.7).

If parenteral benzodiazepines are essential for management of post-injection adverse reactions, careful evaluation of clinical status for excessive sedation and cardiorespiratory depression is recommended (see section 4.5).

Injection site-related adverse events

The most commonly reported injection site-related adverse reaction was pain. The majority of these reactions were reported to be of "mild" to "moderate" severity. In the event of an injection site-related adverse reaction occurring, appropriate measures to manage these events should be taken (see section 4.8).

Dementia-related psychosis and/or behavioural disturbances

Olanzapine is not approved for the treatment of dementia-related psychosis and/or behavioural disturbances and is not recommended for use in this particular group of patients because of an increase in mortality and the risk of cerebrovascular accident. In placebo-controlled clinical trials (6-12 weeks duration) of elderly patients (mean age 78 years) with dementia-related psychosis and/or disturbed behaviours, there was a 2-fold increase in the incidence of death in oral olanzapine-treated patients compared to patients treated with placebo (3.5% vs. 1.5%, respectively). The higher incidence of death was not associated with olanzapine dose (mean daily dose 4.4 mg) or duration of treatment. Risk factors that may predispose this patient population to increased mortality include age > 65 years, dysphagia, sedation, malnutrition and dehydration, pulmonary conditions (e.g., pneumonia, with or without aspiration), or concomitant use of benzodiazepines. However, the incidence of death was higher in oral olanzapine-treated than in placebo-treated patients independent of these risk factors.

In the same clinical trials, cerebrovascular adverse reactions (CVAE's e.g., stroke, transient ischaemic attack), including fatalities, were reported. There was a 3-fold increase in CVAE in patients treated with oral olanzapine compared to patients treated with placebo (1.3% vs. 0.4%, respectively). All oral olanzapine- and placebo-treated patients who experienced a cerebrovascular event had pre-existing risk factors. Age > 75 years and vascular/mixed type dementia were identified as risk factors for CVAE in association with olanzapine treatment. The efficacy of olanzapine was not established in these trials.

Parkinson's disease

The use of olanzapine in the treatment of dopamine agonist associated psychosis in patients with Parkinson's disease is not recommended. In clinical trials, worsening of Parkinsonian symptomatology and hallucinations were reported very commonly and more frequently than with placebo (see section 4.8), and oral olanzapine was not more effective than placebo in the treatment of psychotic symptoms. In these trials, patients were initially required to be stable on the lowest effective dose of anti-Parkinsonian medicinal products (dopamine agonist) and to remain on the same anti-Parkinsonian medicinal products and dosages throughout the study. Oral olanzapine was started at 2.5 mg/day and titrated to a maximum of 15 mg/day based on investigator judgement.

Neuroleptic Malignant Syndrome (NMS)

NMS is a potentially life-threatening condition associated with antipsychotic medicinal products. Rare cases reported as NMS have also been received in association with oral olanzapine. Clinical manifestations of NMS are hyperpyrexia, muscle rigidity, altered mental status, and evidence of autonomic instability (irregular pulse or blood pressure, tachycardia, diaphoresis, and cardiac dysrhythmia). Additional signs may include elevated creatine phosphokinase, myoglobinuria (rhabdomyolysis), and acute renal failure. If a patient develops signs and symptoms indicative of NMS, or presents with unexplained high fever without additional clinical manifestations of NMS, all antipsychotic medicines, including olanzapine must be discontinued.

Hyperglycaemia and diabetes

Hyperglycaemia and/or development or exacerbation of diabetes occasionally associated with ketoacidosis or coma has been reported rarely, including some fatal cases (see section 4.8). In some cases, a prior increase in body weight has been reported which may be a predisposing factor. Appropriate clinical monitoring is advisable in accordance with utilised antipsychotic guidelines. Patients treated with any antipsychotic agents, including ZYPADHERA, should be observed for signs and symptoms of hyperglycaemia (such as polydipsia, polyuria, polyphagia, and weakness) and patients with diabetes mellitus or with risk factors for diabetes mellitus should be monitored regularly for worsening of glucose control. Weight should be monitored regularly.

Lipid alterations

Undesirable alterations in lipids have been observed in olanzapine-treated patients in placebo-controlled clinical trials (see section 4.8). Lipid alterations should be managed as clinically appropriate, particularly in dyslipidemic patients and in patients with risk factors for the development of lipids disorders. Patients treated with any antipsychotic agents, including ZYPADHERA, should be monitored regularly for lipids in accordance with utilised antipsychotic guidelines.

Anticholinergic activity

While olanzapine demonstrated anticholinergic activity *in vitro*, experience during the clinical trials revealed a low incidence of related events. However, as clinical experience with olanzapine in patients with concomitant illness is limited, caution is advised when prescribing for patients with prostatic hypertrophy, or paralytic ileus and related conditions.

Hepatic function

Transient, asymptomatic elevations of hepatic transaminases, ALT, AST have been seen commonly, especially in early treatment. Caution should be exercised in patients with elevated ALT and/or AST, in patients with signs and symptoms of hepatic impairment, in patients with pre-existing conditions associated with limited hepatic functional reserve, and in patients who are being treated with potentially hepatotoxic medicines. In the event of elevated ALT and/or AST during treatment, follow-up should be organised and dose reduction should be considered. In cases where hepatitis (including hepatocellular, cholestatic or mixed liver injury) has been diagnosed, olanzapine treatment should be discontinued.

Neutropenia

Caution should be exercised in patients with low leukocyte and/or neutrophil counts for any reason, in patients receiving medicines known to cause neutropenia, in patients with a history of drug-induced bone marrow depression/toxicity, in patients with bone marrow depression caused by concomitant illness, radiation therapy or chemotherapy and in patients with hypereosinophilic conditions or with myeloproliferative disease. Neutropenia has been reported commonly when olanzapine and valproate are used concomitantly (see section 4.8).

Discontinuation of treatment

Acute symptoms such as sweating, insomnia, tremor, anxiety, nausea, or vomiting have been reported very rarely (<0.01%) when oral olanzapine is stopped abruptly.

QT interval

In clinical trials with oral olanzapine, clinically meaningful QTc prolongations (Fridericia QT correction [QTcF] ⩾ 500 milliseconds [msec] at any time post-baseline in patients with baseline QTcF < 500 msec) were uncommon (0.1% to 1%) in patients treated with olanzapine, with no significant differences in associated cardiac events compared to placebo. In clinical trials with olanzapine powder for solution for injection or ZYPADHERA, olanzapine was not associated with a persistent increase in absolute QT or in QTc intervals. However, as with other antipsychotics, caution should be exercised when olanzapine is prescribed with medicines known to increase QTc interval, especially in the elderly, in patients with congenital long QT syndrome, congestive heart failure, heart hypertrophy, hypokalaemia or hypomagnesaemia.

Thromboembolism

Temporal association of olanzapine treatment and venous thromboembolism has very rarely (< 0.01%) been reported. A causal relationship between the occurrence of venous thromboembolism and treatment with olanzapine has not been established. However, since patients with schizophrenia often present with acquired risk factors for venous thromboembolism all possible risk factors of VTE e.g., immobilisation of patients, should be identified and preventive measures undertaken.

General CNS activity

Given the primary CNS effects of olanzapine, caution should be used when it is taken in combination with other centrally acting medicines and alcohol. As it exhibits *in vitro* dopamine antagonism, olanzapine may antagonise the effects of direct and indirect dopamine agonists.

Seizures

Olanzapine should be used cautiously in patients who have a history of seizures or are subject to factors which may lower the seizure threshold. Seizures have been reported to occur rarely in patients when treated with olanzapine. In most of these cases, a history of seizures or risk factors for seizures were reported.

Tardive Dyskinesia

In comparator studies of one year or less duration, olanzapine was associated with a statistically significant lower incidence of treatment emergent dyskinesia. However, the risk of tardive dyskinesia increases with long-term exposure, and therefore if signs or symptoms of tardive dyskinesia appear in a patient on olanzapine, a dose reduction or discontinuation should be considered. These symptoms can temporally deteriorate or even arise after discontinuation of treatment.

Postural hypotension

Postural hypotension was infrequently observed in the elderly in olanzapine clinical trials. As with other antipsychotics, it is recommended that blood pressure is measured periodically in patients over 65 years.

Use in children and adolescents under 18 years of age

Olanzapine is not indicated for use in the treatment of children and adolescents. Studies in patients aged 13-17 years showed various adverse reactions, including weight gain, changes in metabolic parameters and increases in prolactin levels. Long-term outcomes associated with these events have not been studied and remain unknown (see sections 4.8 and 5.1).

Use in elderly patients (>75 years)

No information on the use of ZYPADHERA in patients >75 years is available. Due to biochemical and physiological modification and reduction of muscular mass, this formulation is not recommended to be started in this sub-group of patients.

4.5 Interaction with other medicinal products and other forms of interaction

Interaction studies have only been performed in adults.

Caution should be exercised in patients who receive medicinal products that can induce hypotension or sedation.

Potential interactions affecting olanzapine

Since olanzapine is metabolised by CYP1A2, substances that can specifically induce or inhibit this isoenzyme may affect the pharmacokinetics of olanzapine.

Induction of CYP1A2

The metabolism of olanzapine may be induced by smoking and carbamazepine, which may lead to reduced olanzapine concentrations. Only slight to moderate increase in olanzapine clearance has been observed. The clinical consequences are likely to be limited, but clinical monitoring is recommended and an increase of olanzapine dose may be considered if necessary (see section 4.2).

Inhibition of CYP1A2

Fluvoxamine, a specific CYP1A2 inhibitor, has been shown to significantly inhibit the metabolism of olanzapine. The mean increase in olanzapine C_{max} following fluvoxamine was 54% in female non-smokers and 77% in male smokers. The mean increase in olanzapine AUC was 52% and 108% respectively. A lower starting dose of olanzapine should be considered in patients who are using fluvoxamine or any other CYP1A2 inhibitors, such as ciprofloxacin. A decrease in the dose of olanzapine should be considered if treatment with an inhibitor of CYP1A2 is initiated.

Fluoxetine (a CYP2D6 inhibitor), single doses of antacid (aluminium, magnesium) or cimetidine have not been found to significantly affect the pharmacokinetics of olanzapine.

Potential for olanzapine to affect other medicinal products

Olanzapine may antagonise the effects of direct and indirect dopamine agonists.

Olanzapine does not inhibit the main CYP450 isoenzymes *in vitro* (e.g., 1A2, 2D6, 2C9, 2C19, 3A4). Thus no particular interaction is expected as verified through *in vivo* studies where no inhibition of metabolism of the following active substances was found: tricyclic antidepressant (representing mostly CYP2D6 pathway), warfarin (CYP2C9), theophylline (CYP1A2) or diazepam (CYP3A4 and 2C19).

Olanzapine showed no interaction when co-administered with lithium or biperiden.

Therapeutic monitoring of valproate plasma levels did not indicate that valproate dosage adjustment is required after the introduction of concomitant olanzapine.

General CNS activity

Caution should be exercised in patients who consume alcohol or receive medicinal products that can cause central nervous system depression.

The concomitant use of olanzapine with anti-Parkinsonian medicinal products in patients with Parkinson's disease and dementia is not recommended (see section 4.4).

QTc interval

Caution should be used if olanzapine is being administered concomitantly with medicinal products known to increase QTc interval (see section 4.4).

4.6 Pregnancy and lactation

There are no adequate and well-controlled studies in pregnant women. Patients should be advised to notify their physician if they become pregnant or intend to become pregnant during treatment with olanzapine. Nevertheless, because human experience is limited, olanzapine should be used in pregnancy only if the potential benefit justifies the potential risk to the foetus.

Spontaneous reports have been very rarely received on tremor, hypertonia, lethargy and sleepiness, in infants born to mothers who had used olanzapine during the 3rd trimester.

In a study of oral olanzapine in breast-feeding, healthy women, olanzapine was excreted in breast milk. Mean infant exposure (mg/kg) at steady state was estimated to be 1.8% of the maternal olanzapine dose (mg/kg). Patients should be advised not to breast-feed an infant if they are taking olanzapine.

4.7 Effects on ability to drive and use machines

No studies on the effects on the ability to drive and use machines have been performed. As olanzapine may cause somnolence and dizziness, patients should be cautioned about operating machinery, including motor vehicles.

Patients should be advised not to drive or operate machinery for the remainder of the day after each injection due to the possibility of a post-injection syndrome event leading to symptoms consistent with olanzapine overdose (see section 4.4).

4.8 Undesirable effects

Post-injection syndrome reactions have occurred with ZYPADHERA leading to symptoms consistent with olanzapine overdose (see sections 4.2 and 4.4). Clinical signs and symptoms included symptoms of sedation (ranging from mild in severity up to coma) and/or delirium (including confusion, disorientation, agitation, anxiety and other cognitive impairment). Other symptoms noted include extrapyramidal symptoms, dysarthria, ataxia, aggression, dizziness, weakness, hypertension and convulsion.

Other adverse reactions observed in patients treated with ZYPADHERA were similar to those seen with oral olanzapine. In clinical trials with ZYPADHERA, the only adverse reaction reported at a statistically significantly higher rate in the ZYPADHERA group than in the placebo group was sedation (ZYPADHERA 8.2%, placebo 2.0%). Among all ZYPADHERA-treated patients, sedation was reported by 4.7% of patients.

In clinical trials with ZYPADHERA the incidence of injection site-related adverse reactions was approximately 8%. The most commonly reported injection site-related adverse reaction was pain (5%); some other injection site adverse reactions reported were (in decreasing frequency): nodule type reactions, erythema type reactions, non-specific injection site reactions, irritation, oedema type reactions, bruising, haemorrhage, and anaesthesia. These events occurred in about 0.1 to 1.1% of patients.

Table 2

Very common	Common	Uncommon	Not known
Blood and the lymphatic system disorders			
	Eosinophilia	Leukopenia Neutropenia	Thrombocytopenia
Immune system disorders			
			Allergic reaction
Metabolism and nutrition disorders			
Weight gain[1]	Elevated cholesterol levels[2,3] Elevated glucose levels[4] Elevated triglyceride levels[2,5] Glucosuria Increased appetite		Development or exacerbation of diabetes occasionally associated with ketoacidosis or coma, including some fatal cases (see section 4.4) Hypothermia
Nervous system disorders			
Somnolence	Dizziness Akathisia[6] Parkinsonism[6] Dyskinesia[6]		Seizures where in most cases a history of seizures or risk factors for seizures were reported Neuroleptic malignant syndrome (see section 4.4) Dystonia (including oculogyration) Tardive dyskinesia Discontinuation symptoms[7]
Cardiac disorders			
		Bradycardia QT_c prolongation (see section 4.4)	Ventricular tachycardia/fibrillation, sudden death (see section 4.4)
Vascular disorders			
	Orthostatic hypotension		Thromboembolism (including pulmonary embolism and deep vein thrombosis)
Gastro-intestinal disorders			
	Mild, transient anticholinergic effects including constipation and dry mouth		Pancreatitis
Hepato-biliary disorders			
	Transient, asymptomatic elevations of hepatic transaminases (ALT, AST), especially in early treatment (see section 4.4)		Hepatitis (including hepatocellular, cholestatic or mixed liver injury)
Skin and subcutaneous tissue disorders			
	Rash	Photosensitivity reaction Alopecia	
Musculoskeletal and connective tissue disorders			
			Rhabdomyolysis
Renal and urinary disorders			
			Urinary hesitation
Reproductive system and breast disorders			
			Priapism
General disorders and administration site conditions			
	Asthenia Fatigue Oedema		
Investigations			
Elevated plasma prolactin levels[8]		High creatine phosphokinase Increased total bilirubin	Increased alkaline phosphatase

[1] Clinically significant weight gain was observed across all baseline Body Mass Index (BMI) categories. Following short-term treatment (median duration 47 days), weight gain ⩾ 7% of baseline body weight was very common (22.2%), ⩾ 15% was common (4.2%) and ⩾ 25% was uncommon (0.8%). Patients gaining ⩾ 7%, ⩾ 15% and ⩾ 25% of their baseline body weight with long-term exposure (at least 48 weeks) were very common (64.4%, 31.7% and 12.3% respectively).

[2] Mean increases in fasting lipid values (total cholesterol, LDL cholesterol, and triglycerides) were greater in patients without evidence of lipid dysregulation at baseline.

[3] Observed for fasting normal levels at baseline (< 5.17 mmol/l) which increased to high (⩾ 6.2 mmol/l). Changes in total fasting cholesterol levels from borderline at baseline (⩾ 5.17 - < 6.2 mmol) to high (⩾ 6.2 mmol) were very common.

[4] Observed for fasting normal levels at baseline (< 5.56 mmol/l) which increased to high (⩾ 7 mmol/l). Changes in fasting glucose from borderline at baseline (⩾ 5.56 - < 7 mmol/l) to high (⩾ 7 mmol/l) were very common.

[5] Observed for fasting normal levels at baseline (< 1.69 mmol/l) which increased to high (⩾ 2.26 mmol/l). Changes in fasting triglycerides from borderline at baseline (⩾ 1.69 mmol/l - < 2.26 mmol/l) to high (⩾ 2.26 mmol/l) were very common.

[6] In clinical trials, the incidence of parkinsonism and dystonia in olanzapine-treated patients was numerically higher, but not statistically significantly different from placebo. Olanzapine-treated patients had a lower incidence of parkinsonism, akathisia and dystonia compared with titrated doses of haloperidol. In the absence of detailed information on the pre-existing history of individual acute and tardive extrapyramidal movement disorders, it can not be concluded at present that olanzapine produces less tardive dyskinesia and/or other tardive extrapyramidal syndromes.

[7] Acute symptoms such as sweating, insomnia, tremor, anxiety, nausea and vomiting have been reported when olanzapine is stopped abruptly.

[8] Associated clinical manifestations (e.g., gynaecomastia, galactorrhoea, and breast enlargement) were rare. In most patients, levels returned to normal ranges without cessation of treatment.

The undesirable effects listed below have been observed following administration of oral olanzapine but may occur following administration of ZYPADHERA.

Adults

The most frequently (seen in ⩾ 1% of patients) reported adverse reactions associated with the use of olanzapine in clinical trials were somnolence, weight gain, eosinophilia, elevated prolactin, cholesterol, glucose and triglyceride levels (see section 4.4), glucosuria, increased appetite, dizziness, akathisia, parkinsonism (see section 4.4), dyskinesia, orthostatic hypotension, anticholinergic effects, transient asymptomatic elevations of hepatic transaminases (see section 4.4), rash, asthenia, fatigue and oedema.

The following table lists the adverse reactions and laboratory investigations observed from spontaneous reporting and in clinical trials. Within each frequency grouping, adverse reactions are presented in order of decreasing seriousness. The frequency terms listed are defined as follows: Very common (⩾10%), common (⩾ 1% and < 10%), uncommon (⩾ 0.1% and < 1%), rare (⩾ 0.01% and < 0.1%), very rare (< 0.01%), not known (cannot be estimated from the data available).

(see Table 2 opposite)

Long-term exposure (at least 48 weeks)

The proportion of patients who had adverse, clinically significant changes in weight gain, glucose, total/LDL/HDL cholesterol or triglycerides increased over time. In adult patients who completed 9-12 months of therapy, the rate of increase in mean blood glucose slowed after approximately 6 months.

Additional information on special populations

In clinical trials in elderly patients with dementia, olanzapine treatment was associated with a higher incidence of death and cerebrovascular adverse reactions compared to placebo (see also section 4.4). Very common adverse reactions associated with the use of olanzapine in this patient group were abnormal gait and falls. Pneumonia, increased body temperature, lethargy, erythema, visual hallucinations and urinary incontinence were observed commonly.

In clinical trials in patients with drug-induced (dopamine agonist) psychosis associated with Parkinson's disease, worsening of Parkinsonian symptomatology and hallucinations were reported very commonly and more frequently than with placebo.

In one clinical trial in patients with bipolar mania, valproate combination therapy with olanzapine resulted in an incidence of neutropenia of 4.1%; a potential contributing factor could be high plasma valproate levels. Olanzapine administered with lithium or valproate resulted in increased levels (⩾10%) of tremor, dry mouth, increased appetite, and weight gain. Speech disorder was also reported commonly. During treatment with olanzapine in combination with lithium or divalproex, an increase of ⩾ 7% from baseline body weight occurred in 17.4% of patients during acute treatment (up to 6 weeks). Long-term olanzapine treatment (up to 12 months) for recurrence prevention in patients with bipolar disorder was associated with an increase of ⩾7% from baseline body weight in 39.9% of patients.

Children and adolescents

Olanzapine is not indicated for the treatment of children and adolescent patients below 18 years. Although no clinical studies designed to compare adolescents to adults have been conducted, data from the adolescent trials were compared to those of the adult trials.

The following table summarises the adverse reactions reported with a greater frequency in adolescent patients (aged 13-17 years) than in adult patients or adverse reactions only identified during short-term clinical trials in adolescent patients. Clinically significant weight gain (⩾ 7%) appears to occur more frequently in the adolescent population compared to adults with comparable exposures. The magnitude of weight gain and the proportion of adolescent patients who had clinically significant weight gain were greater with long-term exposure (at least 24 weeks) than with short-term exposure.

Within each frequency grouping, adverse reactions are presented in order of decreasing seriousness. The frequency terms listed are defined as follows: Very common (⩾ 10%), common (⩾ 1% and < 10%).

Metabolism and nutrition disorders *Very common:* Weight gain[9], elevated triglyceride levels[10], increased appetite. *Common:* Elevated cholesterol levels[11].
Nervous system disorders *Very common:* Sedation (including: hypersomnia, lethargy, somnolence).
Gastro-intestinal disorders *Common:* Dry mouth.
Hepato-biliary disorders *Very common:* Elevations of hepatic transaminases (ALT/AST; see section 4.4).

Investigations
Very common: Decreased total bilirubin, increased GGT, elevated plasma prolactin levels[12].

[9] Following short-term treatment (median duration 22 days), weight gain $\geqslant$ 7% of baseline body weight (kg) was very common (40.6%), $\geqslant$ 15% of baseline body weight was common (7.1%) and $\geqslant$ 25% was common (2.5%). With long-term exposure (at least 24 weeks), 89.4% gained $\geqslant$ 7%, 55.3% gained $\geqslant$ 15% and 29.1% gained $\geqslant$ 25% of their baseline body weight.

[10] Observed for fasting normal levels at baseline (< 1.016 mmol/l) which increased to high ($\geqslant$ 1.467 mmol/l) and changes in fasting triglycerides from borderline at baseline ($\geqslant$ 1.016 mmol/l - < 1.467 mmol/l) to high ($\geqslant$ 1.467 mmol/l).

[11] Changes in total fasting cholesterol levels from normal at baseline (< 4.39 mmol/l) to high ($\geqslant$ 5.17 mmol/l) were observed commonly. Changes in total fasting cholesterol levels from borderline at baseline ($\geqslant$ 4.39 - < 5.17 mmol/l) to high ($\geqslant$ 5.17 mmol/l) were very common.

[12] Elevated plasma prolactin levels were reported in 47.4% of adolescent patients.

4.9 Overdose

If signs and symptoms of overdose consistent with post-injection syndrome are observed, appropriate supportive measures should be taken (see section 4.4).

While overdose is less likely with parenteral than oral medicinal products, reference information for oral olanzapine overdose is presented below:

Signs and symptoms

Very common symptoms in overdose (>10% incidence) include tachycardia, agitation/ aggressiveness, dysarthria, various extrapyramidal symptoms, and reduced level of consciousness ranging from sedation to coma.

Other medically significant sequelae of overdose include delirium, convulsion, coma, possible neuroleptic malignant syndrome, respiratory depression, aspiration, hypertension or hypotension, cardiac arrhythmias (< 2% of overdose cases) and cardiopulmonary arrest. Fatal outcomes have been reported for acute oral overdoses as low as 450 mg but survival has also been reported following acute overdose of approximately 2 g of oral olanzapine.

Management of overdose

There is no specific antidote for olanzapine. Symptomatic treatment and monitoring of vital organ function should be instituted according to clinical presentation, including treatment of hypotension and circulatory collapse and support of respiratory function. Do not use epinephrine, dopamine, or other sympathomimetic agents with beta-agonist activity since beta stimulation may worsen hypotension. Cardiovascular monitoring is necessary to detect possible arrhythmias. Close medical supervision and monitoring should continue until the patient recovers.

5. PHARMACOLOGICAL PROPERTIES

5.1 Pharmacodynamic properties

Pharmacotherapeutic group: Diazepines, oxazepines and thiazepines. *ATC code:* N05AH03.

Olanzapine is an antipsychotic, antimanic and mood stabilising agent that demonstrates a broad pharmacologic profile across a number of receptor systems.

In preclinical studies, olanzapine exhibited a range of receptor affinities (Ki; < 100 nM) for serotonin 5-$HT_{2A/2C}$, 5-HT_3, 5-HT_6; dopamine D_1, D_2, D_3, D_4, D_5; cholinergic muscarinic receptors m_1-m_5; α_1-adrenergic; and histamine H_1 receptors. Animal behavioural studies with olanzapine indicated 5HT, dopamine, and cholinergic antagonism, consistent with the receptor-binding profile. Olanzapine demonstrated a greater *in vitro* affinity for serotonin 5-HT_2 than dopamine D_2 receptors and greater 5-HT_2 than D_2 activity in *in vivo* models. Electrophysiological studies demonstrated that olanzapine selectively reduced the firing of mesolimbic (A10) dopaminergic neurons, while having little effect on the striatal (A9) pathways involved in motor function. Olanzapine reduced a conditioned avoidance response, a test indicative of antipsychotic activity, at doses below those producing catalepsy, an effect indicative of motor side-effects. Unlike some other antipsychotic agents, olanzapine increases responding in an "anxiolytic" test.

The effectiveness of ZYPADHERA in the treatment and maintenance treatment of schizophrenia is consistent with the established effectiveness of the oral formulation of olanzapine.

In a Positron Emission Tomography (PET) study in patients treated with ZYPADHERA (300 mg/4 weeks), mean D_2 receptor occupancy was 60% or higher at the end of a 6-month period, a level consistent with that found during treatment with oral olanzapine.

A total of 1469 patients with schizophrenia were included in 2 pivotal trials:

The first, an 8-week, placebo-controlled trial conducted in adult patients (n=404) who were experiencing acute psychotic symptoms. Patients were randomized to receive injections of ZYPADHERA 405 mg every 4 weeks, 300 mg every 2 weeks, 210 mg every 2 weeks, or placebo every 2 weeks. No oral antipsychotic supplementation was allowed. Total Positive and Negative Symptom Scores (PANSS) showed significant improvement from baseline (baseline mean Total PANSS Score 101) to endpoint (mean changes -22.57, -26.32, -22.49 respectively) with each dose of ZYPADHERA (405 mg every 4 weeks, 300 mg every 2 weeks, and 210 mg every 2 weeks) as compared to placebo (mean change -8.51). Visitwise mean change from baseline to endpoint in PANSS Total Score indicated that by Day 3, patients in the 300 mg/2 weeks and 405 mg/4 weeks treatment groups had statistically significantly greater reductions in PANSS Total Score compared to placebo (-8.6, -8.2, and -5.2, respectively). All 3 ZYPADHERA treatment groups showed statistically significantly greater improvement than placebo beginning by end of Week 1. These results support efficacy for ZYPADHERA over 8 weeks of treatment and a drug effect that was observed as early as 1 week after starting treatment with ZYPADHERA.

The second, a long-term study in clinically stable patients (n=1065) (baseline mean Total PANSS Score 54.33 to 57.75) who were initially treated with oral olanzapine for 4 to 8 weeks and then switched to continue on oral olanzapine or to ZYPADHERA for 24 weeks. No oral antipsychotic supplementation was allowed. ZYPADHERA treatment groups of 150 mg and 300 mg given every 2 weeks (doses pooled for analysis) and 405 mg given every 4 weeks were non-inferior to the combined doses of 10, 15 and 20 mg of oral olanzapine (doses pooled for analysis) as measured by rates of exacerbation of symptoms of schizophrenia (respective exacerbation rates, 10%, 10%, 7%). Exacerbation was measured by worsening of items on the PANSS derived BPRS Positive scale and hospitalisation due to worsening of positive psychotic symptoms. The combined 150 mg and 300 mg/2 week treatment group was non-inferior to the 405 mg/4 week treatment group (exacerbation rates 10% for each group) at 24 weeks after randomisation.

Paediatric population

ZYPADHERA has not been studied in the paediatric population. The experience in adolescents (ages 13 to 17 years) is limited to short-term oral olanzapine efficacy data in schizophrenia (6 weeks) and mania associated with bipolar I disorder (3 weeks), involving less than 200 adolescents. Oral olanzapine was used as a flexible dose starting with 2.5 and ranging up to 20 mg/day. During treatment with oral olanzapine, adolescents gained significantly more weight compared with adults. The magnitude of changes in fasting total cholesterol, LDL cholesterol, triglycerides, and prolactin (see sections 4.4 and 4.8) were greater in adolescents than in adults. There are no data on maintenance of effect and limited data on long-term safety (see sections 4.4 and 4.8).

5.2 Pharmacokinetic properties

Olanzapine is metabolised in the liver by conjugative and oxidative pathways. The major circulating metabolite is the 10-N-glucuronide. Cytochromes P450-CYP1A2 and P450-CYP2D6 contribute to the formation of the N-desmethyl and 2-hydroxymethyl metabolites; both exhibited significantly less *in vivo* pharmacological activity than olanzapine in animal studies. The predominant pharmacologic activity is from the parent, olanzapine.

After a single IM injection with ZYPADHERA the slow dissolution of the olanzapine pamoate salt in muscle tissue begins immediately and provides a slow continuous release of olanzapine for more than four weeks. The release becomes diminishingly smaller within eight to twelve weeks. Antipsychotic supplementation is not required at the initiation of ZYPADHERA treatment (see section 4.2).

The combination of the release profile and the dosage regimen (IM injection every two or four weeks) result in sustained olanzapine plasma concentrations. Plasma concentrations remain measurable for several months after each ZYPADHERA injection. The half-life of olanzapine after ZYPADHERA is 30 days compared to 30 hours following oral administration. The absorption and elimination are complete approximately six to eight months after the last injection.

Oral olanzapine is rapidly distributed. The plasma protein binding of olanzapine is about 93% over the concentration range of 7 to about 1000 ng/mL. In plasma, olanzapine is bound to albumin and α_1-acid glycoprotein.

Olanzapine plasma clearance after oral olanzapine is lower in females (18.9 l/hr) versus males (27.3 l/hr), and in non-smokers (18.6 l/hr) versus smokers (27.7 l/hr). Similar pharmacokinetic differences between males and females and smokers and non-smokers were observed in ZYPADHERA clinical trials. However, the magnitude of the impact of gender, or smoking on olanzapine clearance is small in comparison to the overall variability between individuals.

After repeated IM injections with 150 to 300 mg ZYPADHERA every two weeks, the 10th to 90th percentile of steady-state plasma concentrations of olanzapine were between 4.2 and 73.2 ng/ml. The plasma concentrations of olanzapine observed across the dose range of 150mg every 4 weeks to 300mg every 2 weeks illustrate increased systemic olanzapine exposure with increased ZYPADHERA doses. During the initial three months of treatment with ZYPADHERA, accumulation of olanzapine was observed but there was no additional accumulation during long-term use (12 months) in patients who were injected with up to 300 mg every two weeks.

No specific investigations have been conducted in the elderly with ZYPADHERA. ZYPADHERA is not recommended for treatment in the elderly population (65 years and over) unless a well-tolerated and effective dosage regimen using oral olanzapine has been established. In healthy elderly (65 and over) versus non-elderly subjects, the mean elimination half-life was prolonged (51.8 versus 33.8 hours) and the clearance was reduced (17.5 versus 18.2 l/hr). The pharmacokinetic variability observed in the elderly is within the range for the non-elderly. In 44 patients with schizophrenia >65 years of age, dosing from 5 to 20 mg/day was not associated with any distinguishing profile of adverse events.

In renally impaired patients (creatinine clearance < 10 ml/min) versus healthy subjects, there was no significant difference in mean elimination half-life (37.7 versus 32.4 hours) or clearance (21.2 versus 25.0 l/hr). A mass balance study showed that approximately 57% of radiolabelled olanzapine appeared in urine, principally as metabolites. Although patients with renal impairment were not studied with ZYPADHERA, it is recommended that a well-tolerated and effective dosage regimen using oral olanzapine is established in patients with renal impairment before treatment with ZYPADHERA is initiated (see section 4.2).

In smoking subjects with mild hepatic dysfunction, mean elimination half-life (39.3 hours) of orally administered olanzapine was prolonged and clearance (18.0 l/hr) was reduced analogous to non-smoking healthy subjects (48.8 hours and 14.1 l/hr, respectively). Although patients with hepatic impairment were not studied with ZYPADHERA, it is recommended that a well-tolerated and effective dosage regimen using oral olanzapine is established in patients with hepatic impairment before treatment with ZYPADHERA is initiated (see section 4.2).

In a study of oral olanzapine given to Caucasians, Japanese, and Chinese subjects, there were no differences in the pharmacokinetic parameters among the three populations.

5.3 Preclinical safety data

Preclinical safety studies were performed using olanzapine pamoate monohydrate. The main findings found in repeat-dose toxicity studies (rat, dog), in a 2-year rat carcinogenicity study, and in toxicity to reproduction studies (rat, rabbit) were limited to injection-site reactions for which no NOAEL could be determined. No new toxic effect resulting from systemic exposure to olanzapine could be identified. However, systemic concentrations in these studies were generally less than that seen at effect levels in the oral studies; thus the information on oral olanzapine is provided below for reference.

Acute (single-dose) toxicity

Signs of oral toxicity in rodents were characteristic of potent antipsychotic compounds: hypoactivity, coma, tremors, clonic convulsions, salivation, and depressed weight gain. The median lethal doses were approximately 210 mg/kg (mice) and 175 mg/kg (rats). Dogs tolerated single oral doses up to 100 mg/kg without mortality. Clinical signs included sedation, ataxia, tremors, increased heart rate, laboured respiration, miosis, and anorexia. In monkeys, single oral doses up to 100 mg/kg resulted in prostration and, at higher doses, semi-consciousness.

Repeated-dose toxicity

In studies up to 3 months duration in mice and up to 1 year in rats and dogs, the predominant effects were CNS depression, anticholinergic effects, and peripheral haematological disorders. Tolerance developed to the CNS depression. Growth parameters were decreased at high doses. Reversible effects consistent with elevated prolactin in rats included decreased weights of ovaries and uterus and morphologic changes in vaginal epithelium and in mammary gland.

Haematologic toxicity: Effects on haematology parameters were found in each species, including dose-related reductions in circulating leukocytes in mice and non-specific reductions of circulating leukocytes in rats; however, no evidence of bone marrow cytotoxicity was found. Reversible neutropenia, thrombocytopenia, or anaemia developed in a few dogs treated with 8 or 10 mg/kg/day (total olanzapine exposure [AUC] is 12- to 15-fold greater than that of a man given a 12 mg dose). In cytopenic dogs, there were no undesirable effects on progenitor and proliferating cells in the bone marrow.

Reproductive toxicity

Olanzapine had no teratogenic effects. Sedation affected mating performance of male rats. Oestrous cycles were affected at doses of 1.1 mg/kg (3-times the maximum human dose) and reproduction parameters were influenced in rats given 3 mg/kg (9-times the maximum human dose). In the offspring of rats given olanzapine, delays in foetal development and transient decreases in offspring activity levels were seen.

Mutagenicity

Olanzapine was not mutagenic or clastogenic in a full range of standard tests, which included bacterial mutation tests and *in vitro* and oral *in vivo* mammalian tests.

Carcinogenicity

Based on the results of oral studies in mice and rats, it was concluded that olanzapine is not carcinogenic.

6. PHARMACEUTICAL PARTICULARS

6.1 List of excipients

Powder

No excipients.

Solvent

Croscarmellose sodium

Mannitol

Polysorbate 80

Water for injections

Hydrochloric acid (for pH adjustment)

Sodium hydroxide (for pH adjustment)

6.2 Incompatibilities

This medicinal product must not be mixed with other medicinal products except those mentioned in section 6.6.

6.3 Shelf life

2 years.

After reconstitution in the vial: 24 hours. If the product is not used right away, it should be shaken vigorously to re-suspend. Once withdrawn from vial into syringe, the suspension should be used immediately.

Chemical and physical stability of the suspension in the vials has been demonstrated for 24 hours at 20-25°C. From a microbiological point of view, the product should be used immediately. If not used immediately, in-use storage times and conditions prior to use are the responsibility of the user and would normally not be longer than 24 hours at 20-25°C.

6.4 Special precautions for storage

Do not refrigerate or freeze.

6.5 Nature and contents of container

210 mg powder: Type I glass vial. Bromobutyl stopper with rust-colour seal.

300 mg powder: Type I glass vial. Bromobutyl stopper with olive-colour seal.

405 mg powder: Type I glass vial. Bromobutyl stopper with steel blue-colour seal.

3 ml solvent: Type I glass vial. Butyl stopper with purple seal.

One carton contains one vial of powder and one vial of solvent, one Hypodermic Needle-Pro 3ml syringe with pre-attached 19-gauge, 38 mm safety needle, one 19-gauge, 38 mm Hypodermic Needle-Pro safety needle and one 19-gauge, 50 mm Hypodermic Needle-Pro safety needle.

6.6 Special precautions for disposal and other handling

FOR DEEP INTRAMUSCULAR GLUTEAL INJECTION ONLY. DO NOT ADMINISTER INTRAVENOUSLY OR SUBCUTANEOUSLY.

Any unused product or waste material should be disposed of in accordance with local requirements.

<u>**Reconstitution**</u>

STEP 1: Preparing materials

It is recommended that gloves are used as ZYPADHERA may irritate the skin.

Reconstitute ZYPADHERA powder for prolonged release suspension for injection only with the solvent provided in the pack using standard aseptic techniques for reconstitution of parenteral products.

STEP 2: Determining solvent volume for reconstitution

This table provides the amount of solvent required to reconstitute ZYPADHERA powder for prolonged release suspension for injection.

ZYPADHERA vial strength (mg)	Volume of solvent to add (ml)
210	1.3
300	1.8
405	2.3

It is important to note that there is more solvent in the vial than is needed to reconstitute.

STEP 3: Reconstituting ZYPADHERA

1. Loosen the powder by lightly tapping the vial.

2. Open the pre-packaged Hypodermic Needle-Pro syringe and needle with needle protection device. Peel blister pouch and remove device. Insure needle is firmly seated on the Needle-Pro device with a push and a clockwise twist, then pull the needle cap straight away from the needle. Failure to follow these instructions may result in a needle-stick injury.

3. Withdraw the pre-determined solvent volume (Step 2) into the syringe.

4. Inject the solvent volume into the powder vial.

5. Withdraw air to equalize the pressure in the vial.

6. Remove the needle, holding the vial upright to prevent any loss of solvent.

7. Engage the needle safety device. Press the needle into the sheath using a one-handed technique. Perform a one-handed technique by GENTLY pressing the sheath against a flat surface. AS THE SHEATH IS PRESSED, THE NEEDLE IS FIRMLY ENGAGED INTO THE SHEATH (Figure 1 and 2).

8. Visually confirm that the needle is fully engaged into the needle protection sheath (Figure 3). Only remove the Needle-Pro device with the engaged needle from the syringe when required by a specific medical procedure. Remove by grasping the Luer hub of the needle protection device with thumb and forefinger, keeping the free fingers clear of the end of the device containing the needle point.

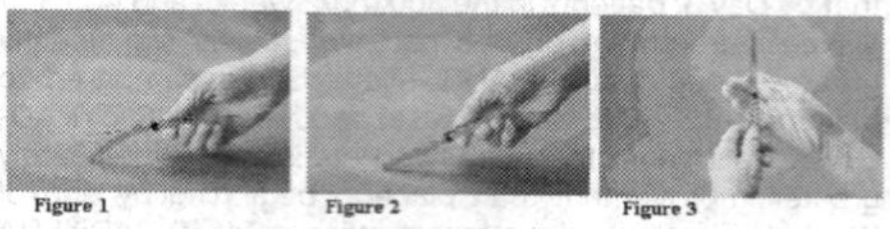

Figure 1 Figure 2 Figure 3

9. Tap the vial firmly and repeatedly on a hard surface until no powder is visible. Protect the surface to cushion impact (see Figure A).

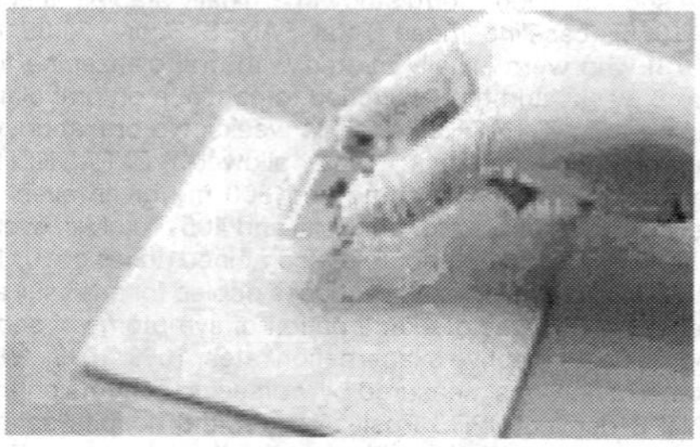

Figure A: Tap firmly to mix

10. Visually check the vial for clumps. Unsuspended powder appears as yellow, dry clumps clinging to the vial. Additional tapping may be required if clumps remain (see Figure B).

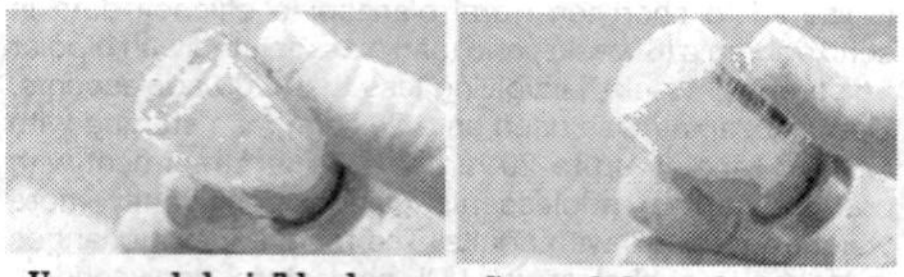

Unsuspended: visible clumps **Suspended: no clumps**

Figure B: Check for unsuspended powder and repeat tapping if needed.

11. Shake the vial vigorously until the suspension appears smooth and is consistent in colour and texture. The suspended product will be yellow and opaque (see Figure C).

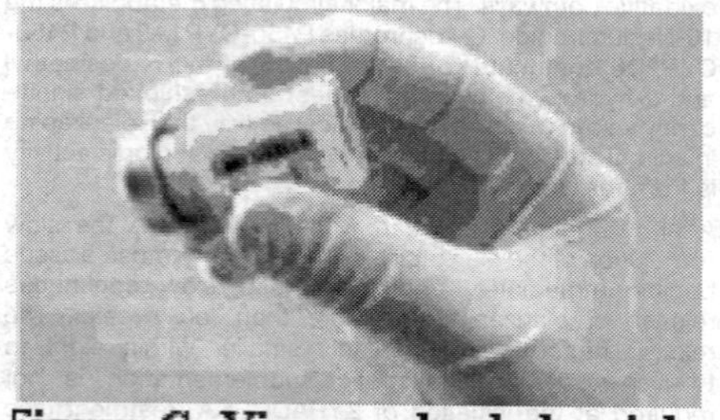

Figure C: Vigorously shake vial

If foam forms, let vial stand to allow foam to dissipate. If the product is not used immediately, it should be shaken vigorously to re-suspend. Reconstituted ZYPADHERA remains stable for up to 24 hours in the vial.

Administration

STEP 1: Injecting ZYPADHERA

This table confirms the final ZYPADHERA suspension volume to inject. Suspension concentration is 150 mg/ml olanzapine.

Dose (mg)	Final volume to inject (ml)
150	1.0
210	1.4
300	2.0
405	2.7

1. Determine which needle will be used to administer the injection to the patient. For obese patients, the 50 mm needle is recommended for injection:

• If the 50 mm needle is to be used for injection, attach the 38 mm safety needle to the syringe to withdraw the required suspension volume.

• If the 38 mm needle is to be used for the injection, attach the 50 mm safety needle to withdraw the required suspension volume.

2. Slowly withdraw the desired amount. Some excess product will remain in the vial.

3. Engage the needle safety device and remove needle from syringe.

4. Attach the remaining safety needle to the syringe prior to injection. Once the suspension has been removed from the vial, it should be injected immediately.

5. Select and prepare a site for injection in the gluteal area. DO NOT INJECT INTRAVENOUSLY OR SUBCUTANEOUSLY.

6. After insertion of the needle, aspirate for several seconds to ensure no blood appears. If any blood is drawn into the syringe, discard the syringe and the dose and begin reconstitution and administration procedure again. The injection should be performed with steady, continuous pressure.

DO NOT MASSAGE THE INJECTION SITE.

7. Engage the needle safety device (Figure 1 and 2).

8. Discard the vials, syringe, needles and any unused solvent in accordance with appropriate clinical procedures. The vial is for single use only.

7. MARKETING AUTHORISATION HOLDER

Eli Lilly Nederland BV, Grootslag 1 – 5, NL-3991 RA, Houten, The Netherlands.

8. MARKETING AUTHORISATION NUMBER(S)

EU/1/08/479/001 ZYPADHERA 210 mg - 1 vial + 1 vial

EU/1/08/479/002 ZYPADHERA 300 mg - 1 vial + 1 vial

EU/1/08/479/003 ZYPADHERA 405 mg - 1 vial + 1 vial

9. DATE OF FIRST AUTHORISATION/RENEWAL OF THE AUTHORISATION

Date of first authorisation: 19 November 2008

10. DATE OF REVISION OF THE TEXT

27 July 2009

LEGAL CATEGORY

POM

*ZYPADHERA (olanzapine pamoate monohydrate) is a trademark of Eli Lilly and Company. ZYA3M

Zyprexa 2.5mg, 5mg, 7.5mg, 10mg, 15mg, and 20mg coated tablets. Zyprexa Velotab 5mg, 10mg, 15mg, and 20mg orodispersible tablets

(Eli Lilly and Company Limited)

1. NAME OF THE MEDICINAL PRODUCT

ZYPREXA* 2.5 mg, 5 mg, 7.5 mg, 10 mg, 15 mg, and 20 mg coated tablets.

ZYPREXA VELOTAB* 5 mg, 10 mg, 15 mg, and 20 mg orodispersible tablets.

2. QUALITATIVE AND QUANTITATIVE COMPOSITION

Each coated tablet contains 2.5 mg olanzapine.

Excipient: 102 mg lactose monohydrate.

Each coated tablet contains 5 mg olanzapine.

Excipient: 156 mg lactose monohydrate.

Each coated tablet contains 7.5 mg olanzapine.

Excipient: 234 mg lactose monohydrate.

Each coated tablet contains 10 mg olanzapine.

Excipient: 312 mg lactose monohydrate.

Each coated tablet contains 15 mg olanzapine.

Excipient: 178 mg lactose monohydrate.

Each coated tablet contains 20 mg olanzapine.

Excipient: 238 mg lactose monohydrate.

Each orodispersible tablet contains 5 mg olanzapine.

Excipients: Each orodispersible tablet contains

0.60 mg aspartame

0.1125 mg sodium methyl parahydroxybenzoate

0.0375 mg sodium propyl parahydroxybenzoate

Each orodispersible tablet contains 10 mg olanzapine.

Excipients: Each orodispersible tablet contains

0.80 mg aspartame

0.15 mg sodium methyl parahydroxybenzoate

0.05 mg sodium propyl parahydroxybenzoate

Each orodispersible tablet contains 15 mg olanzapine.

Excipients: Each orodispersible tablet contains

1.20 mg aspartame

0.225 mg sodium methyl parahydroxybenzoate

0.075 mg sodium propyl parahydroxybenzoate

Each orodispersible tablet contains 20 mg olanzapine.

Excipients: Each orodispersible tablet contains

1.60 mg aspartame

0.30 mg sodium methyl parahydroxybenzoate

0.10 mg sodium propyl parahydroxybenzoate

For a full list of excipients, see section 6.1.

3. PHARMACEUTICAL FORM

Coated Tablets

ZYPREXA 2.5 mg tablets: Round, white, coated tablets imprinted with 'LILLY' and a numeric identicode '4112'.

ZYPREXA 5 mg tablets: Round, white, coated tablets imprinted with 'LILLY' and a numeric identicode '4115'.

ZYPREXA 7.5 mg tablets: Round, white, coated tablets imprinted with 'LILLY' and a numeric identicode '4116'.

ZYPREXA 10 mg tablets: Round, white, coated tablets imprinted with 'LILLY' and a numeric identicode '4117'.

ZYPREXA 15 mg tablets: Elliptical, blue, coated tablets debossed with 'LILLY' and a numeric identicode '4415'.

ZYPREXA 20 mg tablets: Pink, elliptical, coated tablets debossed with 'LILLY' and a numeric identicode '4420'.

Orodispersible Tablets

ZYPREXA VELOTAB 5 mg, 10 mg, 15 mg, and 20 mg orodispersible tablet is a yellow, round, freeze-dried, rapid-dispersing preparation to be placed in the mouth or alternatively to be dispersed in water or other suitable beverage for administration.

4. CLINICAL PARTICULARS

4.1 Therapeutic indications

Adults

Olanzapine is indicated for the treatment of schizophrenia.

Olanzapine is effective in maintaining the clinical improvement during continuation therapy in patients who have shown an initial treatment response.

Olanzapine is indicated for the treatment of moderate to severe manic episode.

In patients whose manic episode has responded to olanzapine treatment, olanzapine is indicated for the prevention of recurrence in patients with bipolar disorder (see section 5.1).

4.2 Posology and method of administration

Adults

Schizophrenia: The recommended starting dose for olanzapine is 10 mg/day.

Manic episode: The starting dose is 15 mg as a single daily dose in monotherapy or 10 mg daily in combination therapy (see section 5.1).

Preventing recurrence in bipolar disorder: The recommended starting dose is 10 mg/day. For patients who have been receiving olanzapine for treatment of manic episode, continue therapy for preventing recurrence at the same dose. If a new manic, mixed, or depressive episode occurs, olanzapine treatment should be continued (with dose optimisation as needed), with supplementary therapy to treat mood symptoms, as clinically indicated.

During treatment for schizophrenia, manic episode, and recurrence prevention in bipolar disorder, daily dosage may subsequently be adjusted on the basis of individual clinical status within the range 5-20 mg/day. An increase to a dose greater than the recommended starting dose is advised only after appropriate clinical reassessment and should generally occur at intervals of not less than 24 hours.

Olanzapine can be given without regard for meals, as absorption is not affected by food. Gradual tapering of the dose should be considered when discontinuing olanzapine.

ZYPREXA VELOTAB orodispersible tablet should be placed in the mouth, where it will rapidly disperse in saliva, so it can be easily swallowed. Removal of the intact orodispersible tablet from the mouth is difficult. Since the orodispersible tablet is fragile, it should be taken immediately on opening the blister. Alternatively, it may be dispersed in a full glass of water or other suitable beverage (orange juice, apple juice, milk, or coffee) immediately before administration.

Olanzapine orodispersible tablet is bioequivalent to olanzapine coated tablets, with a similar rate and extent of absorption. It has the same dosage and frequency of administration as olanzapine coated tablets. Olanzapine orodispersible tablets may be used as an alternative to olanzapine coated tablets.

Children and adolescents

Olanzapine is not recommended for use in children and adolescents below 18 years of age due to a lack of data on safety and efficacy. A greater magnitude of weight gain, lipid and prolactin alterations has been reported in short-term studies of adolescent patients than in studies of adult patients (see sections 4.4, 4.8, 5.1 and 5.2).

Elderly

A lower starting dose (5 mg/day) is not routinely indicated but should be considered for those 65 and over when clinical factors warrant (see section 4.4).

Renal and/or hepatic impairment

A lower starting dose (5 mg) should be considered for such patients. In cases of moderate hepatic insufficiency (cirrhosis, Child-Pugh class A or B), the starting dose should be 5 mg and only increased with caution.

Gender

The starting dose and dose range need not be routinely altered for female patients relative to male patients.

Smokers

The starting dose and dose range need not be routinely altered for non-smokers relative to smokers.

When more than one factor is present which might result in slower metabolism (female gender, geriatric age, non-smoking status), consideration should be given to decreasing the starting dose. Dose escalation, when indicated, should be conservative in such patients.

In cases where dose increments of 2.5 mg are considered necessary, ZYPREXA coated tablets should be used.

(See sections 4.5 and 5.2.)

4.3 Contraindications

Hypersensitivity to the active substance or to any of the excipients. Patients with known risk of narrow-angle glaucoma.

4.4 Special warnings and precautions for use

During antipsychotic treatment, improvement in the patient's clinical condition may take several days to some weeks. Patients should be closely monitored during this period.

Dementia-related psychosis and/or behavioural disturbances

Olanzapine is not approved for the treatment of dementia-related psychosis and/or behavioural disturbances and is not recommended for use in this particular group of patients because of an increase in mortality and the risk of cerebrovascular accident. In placebo-controlled clinical trials (6-12 weeks duration) of elderly patients (mean age 78 years) with dementia-related psychosis and/or disturbed behaviours, there was a 2-fold increase in the incidence of death in olanzapine-treated patients compared to patients treated with placebo (3.5% vs. 1.5%, respectively). The higher incidence of death was not associated with olanzapine dose (mean daily dose 4.4 mg) or duration of treatment. Risk factors that may predispose this patient population to increased mortality include age > 65 years, dysphagia, sedation, malnutrition and dehydration, pulmonary conditions (e.g., pneumonia, with or without aspiration), or concomitant use of benzodiazepines. However, the incidence of death was higher in olanzapine-treated than in placebo-treated patients independent of these risk factors.

In the same clinical trials, cerebrovascular adverse events (CVAE e.g., stroke, transient ischaemic attack), including fatalities, were reported. There was a 3-fold increase in CVAE in patients treated with olanzapine compared to patients treated with placebo (1.3% vs. 0.4%, respectively). All olanzapine- and placebo-treated patients who experienced a cerebrovascular event had pre-existing risk factors. Age > 75 years and vascular/mixed type dementia were identified as risk factors for CVAE in association with olanzapine treatment. The efficacy of olanzapine was not established in these trials.

Parkinson's disease

The use of olanzapine in the treatment of dopamine agonist associated psychosis in patients with Parkinson's disease is not recommended. In clinical trials, worsening of Parkinsonian symptomatology and hallucinations were reported very commonly and more frequently than with placebo (see section 4.8), and olanzapine was not more effective than placebo in the treatment of psychotic symptoms. In these trials, patients were initially required to be stable on the lowest effective dose of anti-Parkinsonian medicinal products (dopamine agonist) and to remain on the same anti-Parkinsonian medicinal products and dosages throughout the study. Olanzapine was started at 2.5 mg/day and titrated to a maximum of 15 mg/day based on investigator judgement.

Neuroleptic Malignant Syndrome (NMS)

NMS is a potentially life-threatening condition associated with antipsychotic medicinal product. Rare cases reported as NMS have also been received in association with olanzapine. Clinical manifestations of NMS are hyperpyrexia, muscle rigidity, altered mental status, and evidence of autonomic instability (irregular pulse or blood pressure, tachycardia, diaphoresis, and cardiac dysrhythmia). Additional signs may include elevated creatine phosphokinase, myoglobinuria (rhabdomyolysis), and acute renal failure. If a patient develops signs and symptoms indicative of NMS, or presents with unexplained high fever without additional clinical manifestations of NMS, all antipsychotic medicines, including olanzapine must be discontinued.

Hyperglycaemia and diabetes

Hyperglycaemia and/or development or exacerbation of diabetes, occasionally associated with ketoacidosis or coma, has been reported rarely, including some fatal cases (see section 4.8). In some cases, a prior increase in body weight has been reported, which may be a predisposing factor. Appropriate clinical monitoring is advisable in accordance with utilised antipsychotic guidelines. Patients treated with any antipsychotic agents, including ZYPREXA/ZYPREXA VELOTAB, should be observed for signs and symptoms of hyperglycaemia (such as polydipsia, polyuria, polyphagia, and weakness) and patients with diabetes mellitus or with risk factors for diabetes mellitus should be monitored regularly for worsening of glucose control. Weight should be monitored regularly.

Lipid alterations

Undesirable alterations in lipids have been observed in olanzapine-treated patients in placebo-controlled clinical trials (see section 4.8). Lipid alterations should be managed as clinically appropriate, particularly in dyslipidemic patients and in patients with risk factors for the development of lipids disorders. Patients treated with any antipsychotic agents, including ZYPREXA/ZYPREXA VELOTAB, should be monitored regularly for lipids in accordance with utilised antipsychotic guidelines.

Anticholinergic activity

While olanzapine demonstrated anticholinergic activity *in vitro*, experience during the clinical trials revealed a low incidence of related events. However, as clinical experience with olanzapine in patients with concomitant illness is limited, caution is advised when prescribing for patients with prostatic hypertrophy, or paralytic ileus and related conditions.

Hepatic function

Transient, asymptomatic elevations of hepatic transaminases, alanine transferase (ALT), aspartate transferase (AST) have been seen commonly, especially in early treatment. Caution should be exercised in patients with elevated ALT and/or AST, in patients with signs and symptoms of hepatic impairment, in patients with pre-existing conditions associated with limited hepatic functional reserve, and in patients who are being treated with potentially hepatotoxic medicines. In the event of elevated ALT and/or AST during treatment, follow-up should be organised and dose reduction should be considered. In cases where hepatitis (including hepatocellular, cholestatic or mixed liver injury) has been diagnosed, olanzapine treatment should be discontinued.

Neutropenia

Caution should be exercised in patients with low leucocyte and/or neutrophil counts for any reason, in patients receiving medicines known to cause neutropenia, in patients with a history of drug-induced bone marrow depression/toxicity, in patients with bone marrow depression caused by concomitant illness, radiation therapy or chemotherapy and in patients with hypereosinophilic conditions or with myeloproliferative disease. Neutropenia has been reported commonly when olanzapine and valproate are used concomitantly (see section 4.8).

Discontinuation of treatment

Acute symptoms such as sweating, insomnia, tremor, anxiety, nausea, or vomiting have been reported very rarely (<0.01%) when olanzapine is stopped abruptly.

QT interval

In clinical trials, clinically meaningful QTc prolongations (Fridericia QT correction [QTcF] ⩾ 500 milliseconds [msec] at any time post-baseline in patients with baseline QTcF < 500 msec) were uncommon (0.1% to 1%) in patients treated with olanzapine, with no significant differences in associated cardiac events compared to placebo. However, as with other antipsychotics, caution should be exercised when olanzapine is prescribed with medicines known to increase QTc interval, especially in the elderly, in patients with congenital long QT syndrome, congestive heart failure, heart hypertrophy, hypokalaemia or hypomagnesaemia.

Thromboembolism

Temporal association of olanzapine treatment and venous thromboembolism has very rarely (< 0.01%) been reported. A causal relationship between the occurrence of venous thromboembolism and treatment with olanzapine has not been established. However, since patients with schizophrenia often present with acquired risk factors for venous thromboembolism, all possible risk factors of VTE e.g., immobilisation of patients, should be identified and preventive measures undertaken.

General CNS activity

Given the primary CNS effects of olanzapine, caution should be used when it is taken in combination with other centrally acting medicines and alcohol. As it exhibits *in vitro* dopamine antagonism, olanzapine may antagonise the effects of direct and indirect dopamine agonists.

Seizures

Olanzapine should be used cautiously in patients who have a history of seizures or are subject to factors which may lower the seizure threshold. Seizures have been reported to occur rarely in patients when treated with olanzapine. In most of these cases, a history of seizures or risk factors for seizures were reported.

Tardive dyskinesia

In comparator studies of one year or less duration, olanzapine was associated with a statistically significant lower incidence of treatment-emergent dyskinesia. However, the risk of tardive dyskinesia increases with long-term exposure, and therefore if signs or symptoms of tardive dyskinesia appear in a patient on olanzapine, a dose reduction or discontinuation should be considered. These symptoms can temporally deteriorate or even arise after discontinuation of treatment.

Postural hypotension

Postural hypotension was infrequently observed in the elderly in olanzapine clinical trials. As with other antipsychotics, it is recommended that blood pressure is measured periodically in patients over 65 years.

Use in children and adolescents under 18 years of age

Olanzapine is not indicated for use in the treatment of children and adolescents. Studies in patients aged 13-17 years showed various adverse reactions, including weight gain, changes in metabolic parameters and increases in prolactin levels. Long-term outcomes associated with

Table 1

Very common	Common	Uncommon	Not known
Blood and the lymphatic system disorders			
	Eosinophilia	Leucopenia Neutropenia	Thrombocytopenia
Immune system disorders			
			Allergic reaction
Metabolism and nutrition disorders			
Weight gain[1]	Elevated cholesterol levels[2,3] Elevated glucose levels[4] Elevated triglyceride levels[2,5] Glucosuria Increased appetite		Development or exacerbation of diabetes occasionally associated with ketoacidosis or coma, including some fatal cases (see section 4.4) Hypothermia
Nervous system disorders			
Somnolence	Dizziness Akathisia[6] Parkinsonism[6] Dyskinesia[6]		Seizures where in most cases a history of seizures or risk factors for seizures were reported Neuroleptic malignant syndrome (see section 4.4) Dystonia (including oculogyration) Tardive dyskinesia Discontinuation symptoms[7]
Cardiac disorders			
		Bradycardia QTc prolongation (see section 4.4)	Ventricular tachycardia/fibrillation, sudden death (see section 4.4)
Vascular disorders			
	Orthostatic hypotension		Thromboembolism (including pulmonary embolism and deep vein thrombosis)
Gastrointestinal disorders			
	Mild, transient anticholinergic effects including constipation and dry mouth		Pancreatitis
Hepato-biliary disorders			
	Transient, asymptomatic elevations of hepatic transaminases (ALT, AST), especially in early treatment (see section 4.4)		Hepatitis (including hepatocellular, cholestatic or mixed liver injury)
Skin and subcutaneous tissue disorders			
	Rash	Photosensitivity reaction Alopecia	
Musculoskeletal and connective tissue disorders			
			Rhabdomyolysis
Renal and urinary disorders			
			Urinary hesitation
Reproductive system and breast disorders			
			Priapism
General disorders and administration site conditions			
	Asthenia Fatigue Oedema		
Investigations			
Elevated plasma prolactin levels[8]		High creatine phosphokinase Increased total bilirubin	Increased alkaline phosphatase

[1] Clinically significant weight gain was observed across all baseline Body Mass Index (BMI) categories. Following short-term treatment (median duration 47 days), weight gain ≥ 7% of baseline body weight was very common (22.2 %), ≥ 15 % was common (4.2 %) and ≥ 25 % was uncommon (0.8 %). Patients gaining ≥ 7 %, ≥ 15 % and ≥ 25 % of their baseline body weight with long-term exposure (at least 48 weeks) were very common (64.4 %, 31.7 % and 12.3 % respectively).

[2] Mean increases in fasting lipid values (total cholesterol, LDL cholesterol, and triglycerides) were greater in patients without evidence of lipid dysregulation at baseline.

[3] Observed for fasting normal levels at baseline (< 5.17 mmol/l) which increased to high (≥ 6.2 mmol/l). Changes in total fasting cholesterol levels from borderline at baseline (≥ 5.17 - < 6.2 mmol/l) to high (≥ 6.2 mmol/l) were very common.

[4] Observed for fasting normal levels at baseline (< 5.56 mmol/l) which increased to high (≥ 7 mmol/l). Changes in fasting glucose from borderline at baseline (≥ 5.56 - < 7 mmol/l) to high (≥ 7 mmol/l) were very common.

[5] Observed for fasting normal levels at baseline (< 1.69 mmol/l) which increased to high (≥ 2.26 mmol/l). Changes in fasting triglycerides from borderline at baseline (≥ 1.69 mmol/l - < 2.26 mmol/l) to high (≥ 2.26 mmol/l) were very common.

[6] In clinical trials, the incidence of parkinsonism and dystonia in olanzapine-treated patients was numerically higher, but not statistically significantly different from placebo. Olanzapine-treated patients had a lower incidence of parkinsonism, akathisia and dystonia compared with titrated doses of haloperidol. In the absence of detailed information on the pre-existing history of individual acute and tardive extrapyramidal movement disorders, it can not be concluded at present that olanzapine produces less tardive dyskinesia and/or other tardive extrapyramidal syndromes.

[7] Acute symptoms such as sweating, insomnia, tremor, anxiety, nausea and vomiting have been reported when olanzapine is stopped abruptly.

[8] Associated clinical manifestations (e.g., gynaecomastia, galactorrhoea, and breast enlargement) were rare. In most patients, levels returned to normal ranges without cessation of treatment.

these events have not been studied and remain unknown (see sections 4.8 and 5.1).

Phenylalanine

ZYPREXA VELOTAB orodispersible tablet contains aspartame, which is a source of phenylalanine. May be harmful for people with phenylketonuria.

Mannitol

ZYPREXA VELOTAB orodispersible tablet contains mannitol.

Sodium methyl parahydroxybenzoate and sodium propyl parahydroxybenzoate

Olanzapine orodispersible tablet contains sodium methyl parahydroxybenzoate and sodium propyl parahydroxybenzoate. These preservatives are known to cause urticaria. Generally, delayed type reactions such as contact dermatitis may occur, but rarely immediate reactions with bronchospasm may occur.

Lactose

ZYPREXA tablets contain lactose. Patients with rare hereditary problems of galactose intolerance, the Lapp lactase deficiency or glucose-galactose malabsorption should not take this medicine.

4.5 Interaction with other medicinal products and other forms of interaction

Interaction studies have only been performed in adults.

Potential Interactions Affecting Olanzapine

Since olanzapine is metabolised by CYP1A2, substances that can specifically induce or inhibit this isoenzyme may affect the pharmacokinetics of olanzapine.

Induction of CYP1A2

The metabolism of olanzapine may be induced by smoking and carbamazepine, which may lead to reduced olanzapine concentrations. Only slight to moderate increase in olanzapine clearance has been observed. The clinical consequences are likely to be limited, but clinical monitoring is recommended and an increase of olanzapine dose may be considered if necessary (see section 4.2).

Inhibition of CYP1A2

Fluvoxamine, a specific CYP1A2 inhibitor, has been shown to significantly inhibit the metabolism of olanzapine. The mean increase in olanzapine C_{max} following fluvoxamine was 54% in female non-smokers and 77% in male smokers. The mean increase in olanzapine AUC was 52% and 108%, respectively. A lower starting dose of olanzapine should be considered in patients who are using fluvoxamine or any other CYP1A2 inhibitors, such as ciprofloxacin. A decrease in the dose of olanzapine should be considered if treatment with an inhibitor of CYP1A2 is initiated.

Decreased bioavailability

Activated charcoal reduces the bioavailability of oral olanzapine by 50 to 60% and should be taken at least 2 hours before or after olanzapine.

Fluoxetine (a CYP2D6 inhibitor), single doses of antacid (aluminium, magnesium) or cimetidine have not been found to significantly affect the pharmacokinetics of olanzapine.

Potential for Olanzapine to Affect Other Medicinal Products

Olanzapine may antagonise the effects of direct and indirect dopamine agonists.

Olanzapine does not inhibit the main CYP450 isoenzymes *in vitro* (e.g., 1A2, 2D6, 2C9, 2C19, 3A4). Thus, no particular interaction is expected, as verified through *in vivo* studies, where no inhibition of metabolism of the following active substances was found: tricyclic antidepressant (representing mostly CYP2D6 pathway), warfarin (CYP2C9), theophylline (CYP1A2), or diazepam (CYP3A4 and 2C19).

Olanzapine showed no interaction when co-administered with lithium or biperiden.

Therapeutic monitoring of valproate plasma levels did not indicate that valproate dosage adjustment is required after the introduction of concomitant olanzapine.

General CNS activity

Caution should be exercised in patients who consume alcohol or receive medicinal products that can cause central nervous system depression.

The concomitant use of olanzapine with anti-Parkinsonian medicinal products in patients with Parkinson's disease and dementia is not recommended (see section 4.4).

QTc interval

Caution should be used if olanzapine is being administered concomitantly with medicinal products known to increase QTc interval (see section 4.4).

4.6 Pregnancy and lactation

There are no adequate and well-controlled studies in pregnant women. Patients should be advised to notify their physician if they become pregnant or intend to become pregnant during treatment with olanzapine. Nevertheless, because human experience is limited, olanzapine should be used in pregnancy only if the potential benefit justifies the potential risk to the foetus.

Spontaneous reports have been very rarely received on tremor, hypertonia, lethargy and sleepiness, in infants born to mothers who had used olanzapine during the 3rd trimester.

In a study in breast-feeding, healthy women, olanzapine was excreted in breast milk. Mean infant exposure (mg/kg) at steady-state was estimated to be 1.8% of the maternal olanzapine dose (mg/kg). Patients should be advised not to breast-feed an infant if they are taking olanzapine.

4.7 Effects on ability to drive and use machines

No studies on the effects on the ability to drive and use machines have been performed. Because olanzapine may cause somnolence and dizziness, patients should be cautioned about operating machinery, including motor vehicles.

4.8 Undesirable effects

Adults

The most frequently (seen in ⩾ 1% of patients) reported adverse reactions associated with the use of olanzapine in clinical trials were somnolence, weight gain, eosinophilia, elevated prolactin, cholesterol, glucose and triglyceride levels (see section 4.4), glucosuria, increased appetite, dizziness, akathisia, parkinsonism (see section 4.4), dyskinesia, orthostatic hypotension, anticholinergic effects, transient asymptomatic elevations of hepatic transaminases (see section 4.4), rash, asthenia, fatigue and oedema.

The following table lists the adverse reactions and laboratory investigations observed from spontaneous reporting and in clinical trials. Within each frequency grouping, adverse reactions are presented in order of decreasing seriousness. The frequency terms listed are defined as follows: Very common (⩾10%), common (⩾ 1% and < 10%), uncommon (⩾ 0.1% and < 1%), rare (⩾ 0.01% and < 0.1%), very rare (< 0.01%), not known (cannot be estimated from the data available).

(see Table 1 on previous page)

Long-term exposure (at least 48 weeks)

The proportion of patients who had adverse, clinically significant changes in weight gain, glucose, total/LDL/HDL cholesterol or triglycerides increased over time. In adult patients who completed 9-12 months of therapy, the rate of increase in mean blood glucose slowed after approximately 6 months.

Additional information on special populations

In clinical trials in elderly patients with dementia, olanzapine treatment was associated with a higher incidence of death and cerebrovascular adverse reactions compared to placebo (see section 4.4). Very common adverse reactions associated with the use of olanzapine in this patient group were abnormal gait and falls. Pneumonia, increased body temperature, lethargy, erythema, visual hallucinations and urinary incontinence were observed commonly.

In clinical trials in patients with drug-induced (dopamine agonist) psychosis associated with Parkinson's disease, worsening of Parkinsonian symptomatology and hallucinations were reported very commonly and more frequently than with placebo.

In one clinical trial in patients with bipolar mania, valproate combination therapy with olanzapine resulted in an incidence of neutropenia of 4.1%; a potential contributing factor could be high plasma valproate levels. Olanzapine administered with lithium or valproate resulted in increased levels (⩾10%) of tremor, dry mouth, increased appetite, and weight gain. Speech disorder was also reported commonly. During treatment with olanzapine in combination with lithium or divalproex, an increase of ⩾ 7% from baseline body weight occurred in 17.4% of patients during acute treatment (up to 6 weeks). Long-term olanzapine treatment (up to 12 months) for recurrence prevention in patients with bipolar disorder was associated with an increase of ⩾7% from baseline body weight in 39.9% of patients.

Children and adolescents

Olanzapine is not indicated for the treatment of children and adolescent patients below 18 years. Although no clinical studies designed to compare adolescents to adults have been conducted, data from the adolescent trials were compared to those of the adult trials.

The following table summarises the adverse reactions reported with a greater frequency in adolescent patients (aged 13-17 years) than in adult patients or adverse reactions only identified during short-term clinical trials in adolescent patients. Clinically significant weight gain (⩾ 7%) appears to occur more frequently in the adolescent population compared to adults with comparable exposures. The magnitude of weight gain and the proportion of adolescent patients who had clinically significant weight gain were greater with long-term exposure (at least 24 weeks) than with short-term exposure.

Within each frequency grouping, adverse reactions are presented in order of decreasing seriousness. The frequency terms listed are defined as follows: Very common (⩾ 10%), common (⩾ 1% and < 10%).

Metabolism and nutrition disorders *Very common:* Weight gain[9], elevated triglyceride levels[10], increased appetite. *Common:* Elevated cholesterol levels[11].
Nervous system disorders *Very common:* Sedation (including: hypersomnia, lethargy, somnolence).
Gastrointestinal disorders *Common:* Dry mouth.
Hepato-biliary disorders *Very common:* Elevations of hepatic transaminases (ALT/AST; see section 4.4).
Investigations *Very common:* Decreased total bilirubin, increased GGT, elevated plasma prolactin levels[12].

[9]Following short-term treatment (median duration 22 days), weight gain ⩾ 7 % of baseline body weight (kg) was very common (40.6 %), ⩾ 15 % of baseline body weight was common (7.1 %) and ⩾ 25 % was common (2.5 %). With long-term exposure (at least 24 weeks), 89.4 % gained ⩾ 7 %, 55.3 % gained ⩾ 15 % and 29.1 % gained ⩾ 25% of their baseline body weight.

[10]Observed for fasting normal levels at baseline (< 1.016 mmol/l) which increased to high (⩾ 1.467 mmol/l) and changes in fasting triglycerides from borderline at baseline (⩾ 1.016 mmol/l - < 1.467 mmol/l) to high (⩾ 1.467 mmol/l).

[11]Changes in total fasting cholesterol levels from normal at baseline (< 4.39 mmol/l) to high (⩾ 5.17 mmol/l) were observed commonly. Changes in total fasting cholesterol levels from borderline at baseline (⩾ 4.39 - < 5.17 mmol/l) to high (⩾ 5.17 mmol/l) were very common.

[12]Elevated plasma prolactin levels were reported in 47.4% of adolescent patients.

4.9 Overdose

Signs and Symptoms

Very common symptoms in overdose (>10% incidence) include tachycardia, agitation/aggressiveness, dysarthria, various extrapyramidal symptoms, and reduced level of consciousness ranging from sedation to coma.

Other medically significant sequelae of overdose include delirium, convulsion, coma, possible neuroleptic malignant syndrome, respiratory depression, aspiration, hypertension or hypotension, cardiac arrhythmias (<2% of overdose cases), and cardiopulmonary arrest. Fatal outcomes have been reported for acute overdoses as low as 450 mg, but survival has also been reported following acute overdose of approximately 2 g of oral olanzapine.

Management of Overdose

There is no specific antidote for olanzapine. Induction of emesis is not recommended. Standard procedures for management of overdose may be indicated (i.e., gastric lavage, administration of activated charcoal). The concomitant administration of activated charcoal was shown to reduce the oral bioavailability of olanzapine by 50 to 60%.

Symptomatic treatment and monitoring of vital organ function should be instituted according to clinical presentation, including treatment of hypotension and circulatory collapse and support of respiratory function. Do not use epinephrine, dopamine, or other sympathomimetic agents with beta-agonist activity, since beta stimulation may worsen hypotension. Cardiovascular monitoring is necessary to detect possible arrhythmias. Close medical supervision and monitoring should continue until the patient recovers.

5. PHARMACOLOGICAL PROPERTIES

5.1 Pharmacodynamic properties

Pharmacotherapeutic group: Diazepines, oxazepines and thiazepines. *ATC code:* N05A H03.

Olanzapine is an antipsychotic, antimanic, and mood stabilising agent that demonstrates a broad pharmacologic profile across a number of receptor systems.

In preclinical studies, olanzapine exhibited a range of receptor affinities (Ki; <100nM) for serotonin $5HT_{2A/2C}$, $5HT_3$, $5HT_6$; dopamine D_1, D_2, D_3, D_4, D_5; cholinergic muscarinic receptors m_1-m_5; α_1 adrenergic; and histamine H_1 receptors. Animal behavioural studies with olanzapine indicated 5HT, dopamine, and cholinergic antagonism, consistent with the receptor-binding profile. Olanzapine demonstrated a greater *in vitro* affinity for serotonin $5HT_2$ than dopamine D_2 receptors and greater $5HT_2$ than D_2 activity in *in vivo* models. Electrophysiological studies demonstrated that olanzapine selectively reduced the firing of mesolimbic (A10) dopaminergic neurons, while having little effect on the striatal (A9) pathways involved in motor function. Olanzapine reduced a conditioned avoidance response, a test indicative of antipsychotic activity, at doses below those producing catalepsy, an effect indicative of motor side-effects. Unlike some other antipsychotic agents, olanzapine increases responding in an 'anxiolytic' test.

In a single oral dose (10 mg) Positron Emission Tomography (PET) study in healthy volunteers, olanzapine produced a higher $5HT_{2A}$ than dopamine D_2 receptor occupancy. In addition, a Single Photon Emission Computed Tomography (SPECT) imaging study in schizophrenic patients revealed that olanzapine-responsive patients had lower striatal D_2 occupancy than some other antipsychotic- and risperidone-responsive patients, while being comparable to clozapine-responsive patients.

In two of two placebo- and two of three comparator-controlled trials with over 2,900 schizophrenic patients presenting with both positive and negative symptoms, olanzapine was associated with statistically significantly greater improvements in negative as well as positive symptoms.

In a multinational, double-blind, comparative study of schizophrenia, schizoaffective and related disorders, which included 1,481 patients with varying degrees of associated depressive symptoms (baseline mean of 16.6 on the Montgomery-Asberg Depression Rating Scale), a prospective secondary analysis of baseline to endpoint mood score change demonstrated a statistically significant improvement (P = 0.001) favouring olanzapine (-6.0) versus haloperidol (-3.1).

In patients with a manic or mixed episode of bipolar disorder, olanzapine demonstrated superior efficacy to placebo and valproate semisodium (divalproex) in reduction of manic symptoms over 3 weeks. Olanzapine also demonstrated comparable efficacy results to haloperidol in terms of the proportion of patients in symptomatic remission from mania and depression at 6 and 12 weeks. In a co-therapy study of patients treated with lithium or valproate for a minimum of 2 weeks, the addition of olanzapine 10 mg (co-therapy with lithium or valproate) resulted in a greater reduction in symptoms of mania than lithium or valproate monotherapy after 6 weeks.

In a 12-month recurrence prevention study in manic episode patients who achieved remission on olanzapine and were then randomised to olanzapine or placebo, olanzapine demonstrated statistically significant superiority over placebo on the primary endpoint of bipolar recurrence. Olanzapine also showed a statistically significant advantage over placebo in terms of preventing either recurrence into mania or recurrence into depression.

In a second 12-month recurrence prevention study in manic episode patients who achieved remission with a combination of olanzapine and lithium and were then randomised to olanzapine or lithium alone, olanzapine was statistically non-inferior to lithium on the primary endpoint of bipolar recurrence (olanzapine 30.0%, lithium 38.3%; P = 0.055).

In an 18-month co-therapy study in manic or mixed episode patients stabilised with olanzapine plus a mood stabiliser (lithium or valproate), long-term olanzapine co-therapy with lithium or valproate was not statistically significantly superior to lithium or valproate alone in delaying bipolar recurrence, defined according to syndromic (diagnostic) criteria.

Paediatric population

The experience in adolescents (ages 13 to 17 years) is limited to short-term efficacy data in schizophrenia (6 weeks) and mania associated with bipolar I disorder (3 weeks), involving less than 200 adolescents. Olanzapine was used as a flexible dose starting with 2.5 and ranging up to 20 mg/day. During treatment with olanzapine, adolescents gained significantly more weight compared with adults. The magnitude of changes in fasting total cholesterol, LDL cholesterol, triglycerides, and prolactin (see sections 4.4 and 4.8) were greater in adolescents than in adults. There are no data on maintenance of effect and limited data on long-term safety (see sections 4.4 and 4.8).

5.2 Pharmacokinetic properties

Olanzapine orodispersible tablet is bioequivalent to olanzapine coated tablets, with a similar rate and extent of absorption. Olanzapine orodispersible tablets may be used as an alternative to olanzapine coated tablets.

Olanzapine is well absorbed after oral administration, reaching peak plasma concentrations within 5 to 8 hours. The absorption is not affected by food. Absolute oral bioavailability relative to intravenous administration has not been determined.

Olanzapine is metabolised in the liver by conjugative and oxidative pathways. The major circulating metabolite is the 10-N-glucuronide, which does not pass the blood brain barrier. Cytochromes P450-CYP1A2 and P450-CYP2D6 contribute to the formation of the N-desmethyl and 2-hydroxymethyl metabolites; both exhibited significantly less *in vivo* pharmacological activity than olanzapine in animal studies. The predominant pharmacologic activity is from the parent, olanzapine. After oral administration, the mean terminal elimination half-life of olanzapine in healthy subjects varied on the basis of age and gender.

In healthy elderly (65 and over) versus non-elderly subjects, the mean elimination half-life was prolonged (51.8 versus 33.8 hours) and the clearance was reduced (17.5 versus 18.2 l/hr). The pharmacokinetic variability observed in the elderly is within the range for the non-elderly. In 44 patients with schizophrenia >65 years of age, dosing from 5 to 20 mg/day was not associated with any distinguishing profile of adverse events.

In female versus male subjects, the mean elimination half-life was somewhat prolonged (36.7 versus 32.3 hours) and the clearance was reduced (18.9 versus 27.3 l/hr). However, olanzapine (5-20 mg) demonstrated a comparable safety profile in female (n = 467) as in male patients (n = 869).

In renally impaired patients (creatinine clearance <10ml/min) versus healthy subjects, there was no significant difference in mean elimination half-life (37.7 versus 32.4 hours) or clearance (21.2 versus 25.0 l/hr). A mass balance study showed that approximately 57% of radiolabelled olanzapine appeared in urine, principally as metabolites.

In smoking subjects with mild hepatic dysfunction, mean elimination half-life (39.3 hours) was prolonged and clearance (18.0 l/hr) was reduced analogous to non-smoking healthy subjects (48.8 hours and 14.1 l/hr, respectively).

In non-smoking versus smoking subjects (males and females), the mean elimination half-life was prolonged (38.6 versus 30.4 hours) and the clearance was reduced (18.6 versus 27.7 l/hr).

The plasma clearance of olanzapine is lower in elderly versus young subjects, in females versus males, and in non-smokers versus smokers. However, the magnitude of the impact of age, gender, or smoking on olanzapine clearance and half-life is small in comparison to the overall variability between individuals.

In a study of Caucasians, Japanese, and Chinese subjects, there were no differences in the pharmacokinetic parameters among the three populations.

The plasma protein binding of olanzapine was about 93% over the concentration range of about 7 to about 1,000ng/ml. Olanzapine is bound predominantly to albumin and α_1-acid-glycoprotein.

Paediatric population

Adolescents (ages 13 to 17 years): The pharmacokinetics of olanzapine are similar between adolescents and adults. In clinical studies, the average olanzapine exposure was approximately 27% higher in adolescents. Demographic differences between the adolescents and adults include a lower average body weight and fewer adolescents were smokers. Such factors possibly contribute to the higher average exposure observed in adolescents.

5.3 Preclinical safety data

Acute (Single-Dose) Toxicity

Signs of oral toxicity in rodents were characteristic of potent neuroleptic compounds: hypoactivity, coma, tremors, clonic convulsions, salivation, and depressed weight gain. The median lethal doses were approximately 210 mg/kg (mice) and 175 mg/kg (rats). Dogs tolerated single oral doses up to 100 mg/kg without mortality. Clinical signs included sedation, ataxia, tremors, increased heart rate, laboured respiration, miosis, and anorexia. In monkeys, single oral doses up to 100 mg/kg resulted in prostration and, at higher doses, semi-consciousness.

Repeated-Dose Toxicity

In studies up to 3 months duration in mice and up to 1 year in rats and dogs, the predominant effects were CNS depression, anticholinergic effects, and peripheral haematological disorders. Tolerance developed to the CNS depression. Growth parameters were decreased at high doses. Reversible effects consistent with elevated prolactin in rats included decreased weights of ovaries and uterus and morphologic changes in vaginal epithelium and in mammary gland.

Haematologic Toxicity

Effects on haematology parameters were found in each species, including dose-related reductions in circulating leucocytes in mice and non-specific reductions of circulating leucocytes in rats; however, no evidence of bone marrow cytotoxicity was found. Reversible neutropenia, thrombocytopenia, or anaemia developed in a few dogs treated with 8 or 10 mg/kg/day (total olanzapine exposure [area under the curve - AUC] is 12- to 15-fold greater than that of a man given a 12 mg dose). In cytopenic dogs, there were no adverse effects on progenitor and proliferating cells in the bone marrow.

Reproductive Toxicity

Olanzapine had no teratogenic effects. Sedation affected mating performance of male rats. Oestrous cycles were affected at doses of 1.1 mg/kg (3-times the maximum human dose) and reproduction parameters were influenced in rats given 3 mg/kg (9-times the maximum human dose). In the offspring of rats given olanzapine, delays in foetal development and transient decreases in offspring activity levels were seen.

Mutagenicity

Olanzapine was not mutagenic or clastogenic in a full range of standard tests, which included bacterial mutation tests and *in vitro* and *in vivo* mammalian tests.

Carcinogenicity

Based on the results of studies in mice and rats, it was concluded that olanzapine is not carcinogenic.

6. PHARMACEUTICAL PARTICULARS

6.1 List of excipients

ZYPREXA tablet

Tablet core

Lactose monohydrate

Hyprolose

Crospovidone

Microcrystalline cellulose

Magnesium stearate

Tablet coat

2.5 mg, 5 mg, 7.5 mg, and 10 mg tablets:

Hypromellose

Colour mixture white (hypromellose, titanium dioxide [E171], macrogol, polysorbate 80)

Carnauba wax

Edible blue ink (shellac, macrogol, propylene glycol, indigo carmine [E132])

15 mg tablets:

Hypromellose

Colour mixture light blue (titanium dioxide [E171], lactose monohydrate, hypromellose, triacetin, indigo carmine [E132])

Carnauba wax

20 mg tablets:

Hypromellose

Colour mixture pink (titanium dioxide [E171], macrogol, lactose monohydrate, hypromellose, synthetic red iron oxide)

Carnauba wax

ZYPREXA VELOTAB

Gelatin

Mannitol (E421)

Aspartame (E951)

Sodium methyl parahydroxybenzoate (E219)

Sodium propyl parahydroxybenzoate (E217)

6.2 Incompatibilities

Not applicable.

6.3 Shelf life

ZYPREXA tablets: Three years (5 mg, 7.5 mg, 10 mg, 15 mg, and 20 mg).

ZYPREXA tablets: Two years (2.5 mg).

ZYPREXA VELOTABS: Three years.

6.4 Special precautions for storage

ZYPREXA tablets: Store in the original package in order to protect from light and moisture.

ZYPREXA VELOTABS: Store in the original package in order to protect from light and moisture.

6.5 Nature and contents of container

ZYPREXA 2.5 mg tablets are available in cold-formed aluminium blister strips in cartons of 28, 35, 56 or 70 tablets per carton.

ZYPREXA 5 mg tablets are available in cold-formed aluminium blister strips in cartons of 28, 35, 56 or 70 tablets per carton.

ZYPREXA 7.5 mg tablets are available in cold-formed aluminium blister strips in cartons of 28, 35, 56 or 70 tablets per carton.

ZYPREXA 10 mg tablets are available in cold-formed aluminium blister strips in cartons of 7, 28, 35, 56 or 70 tablets per carton.

ZYPREXA 15 mg tablets are available in cold-formed aluminium blister strips in cartons of 28, 35, 56 or 70 tablets per carton.

ZYPREXA 20 mg tablets are available in cold-formed aluminium blister strips in cartons of 28, 35, 56 or 70 tablets per carton.

ZYPREXA VELOTAB 5 mg, 10 mg, 15 mg, and 20 mg is supplied in aluminium blister strips in cartons of 28, 35, 56 or 70 orodispersible tablets per carton.

Not all pack sizes may be marketed.

6.6 Special precautions for disposal and other handling

No special requirements.

7. MARKETING AUTHORISATION HOLDER

Eli Lilly Nederland BV, Grootslag 1-5, NL-3991 RA Houten, The Netherlands.

8. MARKETING AUTHORISATION NUMBER(S)

EU/1/96/022/002: ZYPREXA 2.5 mg coated tablets - 28 tablets per box

EU/1/96/022/019: ZYPREXA 2.5 mg coated tablets - 56 tablets per box

EU/1/96/022/023: ZYPREXA 2.5 mg coated tablets - 35 tablets per box

EU/1/96/022/029: ZYPREXA 2.5 mg coated tablets - 70 tablets per box

EU/1/96/022/004: ZYPREXA 5 mg coated tablets - 28 tablets per box

EU/1/96/022/020: ZYPREXA 5 mg coated tablets - 56 tablets per box

EU/1/96/022/024: ZYPREXA 5 mg coated tablets - 35 tablets per box

EU/1/96/022/030: ZYPREXA 5 mg coated tablets - 70 tablets per box

EU/1/96/022/011: ZYPREXA 7.5 mg coated tablets - 28 tablets per box

EU/1/96/022/006: ZYPREXA 7.5 mg coated tablets - 56 tablets per box

EU/1/96/022/025: ZYPREXA 7.5 mg coated tablets - 35 tablets per box

EU/1/96/022/031: ZYPREXA 7.5 mg coated tablets - 70 tablets per box

EU/1/96/022/008: ZYPREXA 10 mg coated tablets - 7 tablets per box

EU/1/96/022/009: ZYPREXA 10 mg coated tablets - 28 tablets per box

EU/1/96/022/010: ZYPREXA 10 mg coated tablets - 56 tablets per box

EU/1/96/022/026: ZYPREXA 10 mg coated tablets - 35 tablets per box

EU/1/96/022/032: ZYPREXA 10 mg coated tablets - 70 tablets per box

EU/1/96/022/012: ZYPREXA 15 mg coated tablets - 28 tablets per box

EU/1/96/022/021: ZYPREXA 15 mg coated tablets - 56 tablets per box

EU/1/96/022/027: ZYPREXA 15 mg coated tablets - 35 tablets per box

EU/1/96/022/033: ZYPREXA 15 mg coated tablets - 70 tablets per box

EU/1/96/022/014: ZYPREXA 20 mg coated tablets - 28 tablets per box

EU/1/96/022/022: ZYPREXA 20 mg coated tablets - 56 tablets per box

EU/1/96/022/028: ZYPREXA 20 mg coated tablets - 35 tablets per box

EU/1/96/022/034: ZYPREXA 20 mg coated tablets - 70 tablets per box

EU/1/99/125/001: 5 mg × 28 Velotabs

EU/1/99/125/005: 5 mg × 56 Velotabs

EU/1/99/125/009: 5 mg × 35 Velotabs

EU/1/99/125/013: 5 mg × 70 Velotabs

EU/1/99/125/002: 10 mg × 28 Velotabs

EU/1/99/125/006: 10 mg × 56 Velotabs

EU/1/99/125/010: 10 mg × 35 Velotabs

EU/1/99/125/014: 10 mg × 70 Velotabs

EU/1/99/125/003: 15 mg × 28 Velotabs

EU/1/99/125/007: 15 mg × 56 Velotabs

EU/1/99/125/011: 15 mg × 35 Velotabs

EU/1/99/125/015: 15 mg × 70 Velotabs

EU/1/99/125/004: 20 mg × 28 Velotabs

EU/1/99/125/008: 20 mg × 56 Velotabs

EU/1/99/125/012: 20 mg × 35 Velotabs

EU/1/99/125/016: 20 mg × 70 Velotabs

9. DATE OF FIRST AUTHORISATION/RENEWAL OF THE AUTHORISATION

2.5 mg, 5 mg, 7.5 mg, 10 mg, 15 mg, and 20 mg ZYPREXA tablets:

Date of first authorisation: 27 September 1996

Date of last renewal of the authorisation: 27 September 2006

ZYPREXA VELOTABS:

Date of first authorisation: 3 February 2000

Date of latest renewal: 27 September 2006

10. DATE OF REVISION OF THE TEXT

ZYPREXA tablets: 03 July 2009

ZYPREXA VELOTABS: 07 July 2009

LEGAL CATEGORY

POM

*ZYPREXA (olanzapine) and VELOTAB are trademarks of Eli Lilly and Company. ZY47M

Zyprexa Powder for Solution for Injection

(Eli Lilly and Company Limited)

1. NAME OF THE MEDICINAL PRODUCT

ZYPREXA*▼ 10 mg Powder for Solution for Injection.

2. QUALITATIVE AND QUANTITATIVE COMPOSITION

Each vial contains 10 mg olanzapine. After reconstitution each ml of the solution contains 5 mg olanzapine.

For a full list of excipients, see section 6.1.

3. PHARMACEUTICAL FORM

Powder for solution for injection.

Yellow lyophilised powder.

4. CLINICAL PARTICULARS

4.1 Therapeutic indications

Adults

ZYPREXA powder for solution for injection is indicated for the rapid control of agitation and disturbed behaviours in patients with schizophrenia or manic episode, when oral therapy is not appropriate. Treatment with ZYPREXA powder for solution for injection should be discontinued and the use of oral olanzapine should be initiated, as soon as clinically appropriate.

4.2 Posology and method of administration

Adults

For intramuscular use. Do not administer intravenously or subcutaneously. ZYPREXA powder for solution for injection is intended for short-term use only, for up to a maximum of three consecutive days.

The maximum daily dose of olanzapine (including all formulations of olanzapine) is 20 mg.

The recommended initial dose for olanzapine injection is 10 mg, administered as a single intramuscular injection. A lower dose (5 mg or 7.5 mg) may be given, on the basis of individual clinical status, which should also include consideration of medicinal products already administered either for maintenance or acute treatment (see section 4.4). A second injection, 5-10 mg, may be administered 2 hours after the first injection, on the basis of individual clinical status.

Not more than three injections should be given in any 24-hour period and the maximum daily dose of olanzapine of 20 mg (including all formulations) should not be exceeded.

ZYPREXA powder for solution for injection should be reconstituted in accordance with the recommendation in section 6.6.

For further information on continued treatment with oral olanzapine (5 to 20 mg daily), see the Summary of Product Characteristics for ZYPREXA coated tablets or ZYPREXA VELOTAB orodispersible tablets.

Children and adolescents

There is no experience in children. ZYPREXA powder for solution for injection is not recommended for use in children and adolescents due to a lack of data on safety and efficacy.

Elderly

The recommended starting dose in elderly patients (>60 years) is 2.5-5 mg. Depending on the patient's clinical status (see section 4.4), a second injection, 2.5-5 mg, may be administered 2 hours after the first injection. Not more than 3 injections should be given in any 24-hour period and the maximum daily dose of 20 mg (including all formulations) of olanzapine should not be exceeded.

Renal and/or hepatic impairment

A lower starting dose (5 mg) should be considered for such patients. In cases of moderate hepatic insufficiency (cirrhosis, Child-Pugh class A or B), the starting dose should be 5 mg and only increased with caution.

Gender

The dose and dose range need not be routinely altered for female patients relative to male patients.

Smokers

The dose and dose range need not be routinely altered for non-smokers relative to smokers.

When more than one factor is present which might result in slower metabolism (female gender, geriatric age, non-smoking status), consideration should be given to decreasing the dose. Additional injections, when indicated, should be conservative in such patients.

(See sections 4.5 and 5.2.)

4.3 Contraindications

Hypersensitivity to the active substance or to any of the excipients. Patients with known risk of narrow-angle glaucoma.

4.4 Special warnings and precautions for use

The efficacy of IM olanzapine has not been established in patients with agitation and disturbed behaviours related to conditions other than schizophrenia or manic episode.

Unstable medical conditions

IM olanzapine should not be administered to patients with unstable medical conditions, such as acute myocardial infarction, unstable angina pectoris, severe hypotension and/or bradycardia, sick sinus syndrome, or following heart surgery. If the patient's medical history with regard to these unstable medical conditions cannot be determined, the risks and benefits of IM olanzapine should be considered in relation to other alternative treatments.

Concomitant use of benzodiazepines and other medicinal products

Special caution is necessary in patients who have received treatment with other medicinal products having haemodynamic properties similar to those of intramuscular olanzapine including other antipsychotics (oral and/or intramuscular) and benzodiazepines (see section 4.5). Temporal association of treatment with IM olanzapine with hypotension, bradycardia, respiratory depression and death has been very rarely (< 0.01%) reported, particularly in patients who have received benzodiazepines and/or other antipsychotics (see section 4.8).

Simultaneous injection of intramuscular olanzapine and parenteral benzodiazepine is not recommended (see sections 4.5 and 6.2). If the patient is considered to need parenteral benzodiazepine treatment, this should not be given until at least one hour after IM olanzapine administration. If the patient has received parenteral benzodiazepine, IM olanzapine administration should only be considered after careful evaluation of clinical status, and the patient should be closely monitored for excessive sedation and cardiorespiratory depression.

Hypotension

It is extremely important that patients receiving intramuscular olanzapine should be closely observed for hypotension, including postural hypotension, bradyarrhythmia, and/or hypoventilation, particularly for the first 4 hours following injection, and close observation should be continued after this period if clinically indicated. Blood pressure, pulse, respiratory rate, and level of consciousness should be observed regularly and remedial treatment provided if required. Patients should remain recumbent if dizzy or drowsy after injection until examination indicates that they are not experiencing hypotension, including postural hypotension, bradyarrhythmia, and/or hypoventilation.

The safety and efficacy of IM olanzapine has not been evaluated in patients with alcohol or drug intoxication (either with prescribed or illicit drugs) (see section 4.5).

Dementia-related psychosis and/or behavioural disturbances

Olanzapine is not approved for the treatment of dementia-related psychosis and/or behavioural disturbances and is not recommended for use in this particular group of patients because of an increase in mortality and the risk of cerebrovascular accident. In placebo-controlled clinical trials (6-12 weeks duration) of elderly patients (mean age 78 years) with dementia-related psychosis and/or disturbed behaviours, there was a 2-fold increase in the incidence of death in olanzapine-treated patients compared to patients treated with placebo (3.5% vs. 1.5%, respectively). The higher incidence of death was not associated with olanzapine dose (mean daily dose 4.4 mg) or duration of treatment. Risk factors that may predispose this patient population to increased mortality include age > 65 years, dysphagia, sedation, malnutrition and dehydration, pulmonary conditions (e.g., pneumonia, with or without aspiration), or concomitant use of benzodiazepines. However, the incidence of death was higher in olanzapine-treated than in placebo-treated patients independent of these risk factors.

In the same clinical trials, cerebrovascular adverse events (CVAE e.g., stroke, transient ischaemic attack), including fatalities, were reported. There was a 3-fold increase in CVAE in patients treated with olanzapine compared to patients treated with placebo (1.3% vs. 0.4%, respectively). All olanzapine- and placebo-treated patients who experienced a cerebrovascular event had pre-existing risk factors. Age > 75 years and vascular/mixed type dementia were identified as risk factors for CVAE in association with olanzapine treatment. The efficacy of olanzapine was not established in these trials.

Parkinson's disease

The use of olanzapine in the treatment of dopamine agonist associated psychosis in patients with Parkinson's disease is not recommended. In clinical trials, worsening of Parkinsonian symptomatology and hallucinations were reported very commonly and more frequently than with placebo (see section 4.8), and olanzapine was not more effective than placebo in the treatment of psychotic symptoms. In these trials, patients were initially required to be stable on the lowest effective dose of anti-Parkinsonian medicinal products (dopamine agonist) and to remain on the same anti-Parkinsonian medicinal products and dosages throughout the study. Olanzapine was started at 2.5 mg/day and titrated to a maximum of 15 mg/day based on investigator judgement.

Neuroleptic Malignant Syndrome (NMS)

NMS is a potentially life-threatening condition associated with antipsychotic medicinal product. Rare cases reported as NMS have also been received in association with olanzapine. Clinical manifestations of NMS are hyperpyrexia, muscle rigidity, altered mental status, and evidence of autonomic instability (irregular pulse or blood pressure, tachycardia, diaphoresis, and cardiac dysrhythmia). Additional signs may include elevated creatine phosphokinase, myoglobinuria (rhabdomyolysis), and acute renal failure. If a patient develops signs and symptoms indicative of NMS, or presents with unexplained high fever without additional clinical manifestations of NMS, all antipsychotic medicines, including olanzapine must be discontinued.

Hyperglycaemia and diabetes

Hyperglycaemia and/or development or exacerbation of diabetes occasionally associated with ketoacidosis or coma has been reported rarely, including some fatal cases (see section 4.8). In some cases, a prior increase in body weight has been reported which may be a predisposing factor. Appropriate clinical monitoring is advisable in accordance with utilised antipsychotic guidelines. Patients treated with any antipsychotic agents, including ZYPREXA, should be observed for signs and symptoms of hyperglycaemia (such as polydipsia, polyuria, polyphagia, and weakness) and patients with diabetes mellitus or with risk factors for diabetes mellitus should be monitored regularly for worsening of glucose control. Weight should be monitored regularly.

Lipid alterations

Undesirable alterations in lipids have been observed in olanzapine-treated patients in placebo-controlled clinical trials (see section 4.8). Lipid alterations should be managed as clinically appropriate, particularly in dyslipidemic patients and in patients with risk factors for the development of lipids disorders. Patients treated with any antipsychotic agents, including ZYPREXA, should be monitored regularly for lipids in accordance with utilised antipsychotic guidelines.

Anticholinergic activity

While olanzapine demonstrated anticholinergic activity *in vitro*, experience during oral clinical trials revealed a low incidence of related events. However, as clinical experience with olanzapine in patients with concomitant illness is limited, caution is advised when prescribing for patients with prostatic hypertrophy, or paralytic ileus and related conditions.

Hepatic function

Transient, asymptomatic elevations of hepatic transaminases, ALT, AST have been seen commonly, especially in early treatment. Caution should be exercised in patients with elevated ALT and/or AST, in patients with signs and symptoms of hepatic impairment, in patients with pre-existing conditions associated with limited hepatic functional reserve, and in patients who are being treated with potentially hepatotoxic medicines. In the event of elevated ALT and/or AST during treatment, follow-up should be organised and dose reduction should be considered. In cases where hepatitis (including hepatocellular, cholestatic or mixed liver injury) has been diagnosed, olanzapine treatment should be discontinued.

Neutropenia

Caution should be exercised in patients with low leucocyte and/or neutrophil counts for any reason, in patients receiving medicines known to cause neutropenia, in patients with a history of drug-induced bone marrow depression/toxicity, in patients with bone marrow depression caused by concomitant illness, radiation therapy or chemotherapy and in patients with hypereosinophilic conditions or with myeloproliferative disease. Neutropenia has been reported commonly when olanzapine and valproate are used concomitantly (see section 4.8).

Discontinuation of treatment

Acute symptoms such as sweating, insomnia, tremor, anxiety, nausea, or vomiting have been reported very rarely (<0.01%) when olanzapine is stopped abruptly.

QT interval

In clinical trials with oral administration, clinically meaningful QTc prolongations (Fridericia QT correction [QTcF] ⩾500 milliseconds [msec] at any time post-baseline in patients with baseline QTcF<500 msec) were uncommon (0.1% to 1%) in patients treated with olanzapine, with no significant differences in associated cardiac events compared to placebo. In clinical trials with ZYPREXA powder for solution for injection, olanzapine was not associated with a persistent increase in absolute QT or in QTc intervals. However, as with other antipsychotics, caution should be exercised when olanzapine is prescribed with medicines known to increase QTc interval, especially in the elderly, in patients with congenital long QT syndrome, congestive heart failure, heart hypertrophy, hypokalaemia or hypomagnesaemia.

Thromboembolism

Temporal association of olanzapine treatment and venous thromboembolism has very rarely (< 0.01%) been reported. A causal relationship between the occurrence of venous thromboembolism and treatment with olanzapine has not been established. However, since patients with schizophrenia often present with acquired risk factors for venous thromboembolism, all possible risk factors of VTE e.g., immobilisation of patients, should be identified and preventive measures undertaken.

General CNS activity

Given the primary CNS effects of olanzapine, caution should be used when it is taken in combination with other centrally acting medicines and alcohol. As it exhibits *in vitro* dopamine antagonism, olanzapine may antagonise the effects of direct and indirect dopamine agonists.

Seizures

Olanzapine should be used cautiously in patients who have a history of seizures or are subject to factors which may lower the seizure threshold. Seizures have been reported to occur rarely in patients when treated with olanzapine. In most of these cases, a history of seizures or risk factors for seizures were reported.

Tardive dyskinesia

In comparator oral studies of one year or less duration, olanzapine was associated with a statistically significant lower incidence of treatment-emergent dyskinesia. However, the risk of tardive dyskinesia increases with long-term exposure, and therefore if signs or symptoms of tardive dyskinesia appear in a patient on olanzapine, a dose reduction or discontinuation should be considered. These symptoms can temporally deteriorate or even arise after discontinuation of treatment.

Postural hypotension

Postural hypotension was infrequently observed in the elderly in oral olanzapine clinical trials. As with other antipsychotics, it is recommended that blood pressure is measured periodically in patients over 65 years.

4.5 Interaction with other medicinal products and other forms of interaction

IM olanzapine has not been studied in patients with alcohol or drug intoxication (see section 4.4).

Caution should be exercised in patients who consume alcohol or receive medicinal products that can induce hypotension, bradycardia, respiratory or central nervous system depression (see section 4.4).

Potential for Interaction, Following Intramuscular Injection

In a single dose intramuscular study of olanzapine 5 mg, administered 1 hour before intramuscular lorazepam 2 mg (metabolised by glucuronidation), the pharmacokinetics of both medicines were unchanged. However, the combination added to the somnolence observed with either medicine alone. Concomitant injection of olanzapine and parenteral benzodiazepine is not recommended (see sections 4.4 and 6.2).

Potential Interactions Affecting Olanzapine

Since olanzapine is metabolised by CYP1A2, substances that can specifically induce or inhibit this isoenzyme may affect the pharmacokinetics of olanzapine.

Induction of CYP1A2

The metabolism of olanzapine may be induced by smoking and carbamazepine, which may lead to reduced olanzapine concentrations. Only slight to moderate increase in olanzapine clearance has been observed. The clinical consequences are likely to be limited, but clinical monitoring is recommended and an increase of olanzapine dose may be considered if necessary (see section 4.2).

Inhibition of CYP1A2

Fluvoxamine, a specific CYP1A2 inhibitor, has been shown to significantly inhibit the metabolism of olanzapine. The mean increase in olanzapine C_{max} following fluvoxamine was 54% in female non-smokers and 77% in male smokers. The mean increase in olanzapine AUC was 52% and 108%, respectively. A lower starting dose of olanzapine should be considered in patients who are using fluvoxamine or any other CYP1A2 inhibitors, such as ciprofloxacin. A decrease in the dose of olanzapine should be considered if treatment with an inhibitor of CYP1A2 is initiated.

Decreased bioavailability

Activated charcoal reduces the bioavailability of oral olanzapine by 50 to 60% and should be taken at least 2 hours before or after olanzapine.

Fluoxetine (a CYP2D6 inhibitor), single doses of antacid (aluminium, magnesium) or cimetidine have not been found to significantly affect the pharmacokinetics of olanzapine.

Potential for Olanzapine to Affect Other Medicinal Products

Olanzapine may antagonise the effects of direct and indirect dopamine agonists (see section 6.2).

Olanzapine does not inhibit the main CYP450 isoenzymes *in vitro* (e.g., 1A2, 2D6, 2C9, 2C19, 3A4). Thus, no particular interaction is expected, as verified through *in vivo* studies, where no inhibition of metabolism of the following active substances was found: tricyclic antidepressant (representing mostly CYP2D6 pathway), warfarin (CYP2C9), theophylline (CYP1A2), or diazepam (CYP3A4 and 2C19).

Olanzapine showed no interaction when co-administered with lithium or biperiden.

Therapeutic monitoring of valproate plasma levels did not indicate that valproate dosage adjustment is required after the introduction of concomitant olanzapine.

The concomitant use of olanzapine with anti-Parkinsonian medicinal products in patients with Parkinson's disease and dementia is not recommended (see section 4.4).

QTc interval

Caution should be used if olanzapine is being administered concomitantly with medicinal products known to increase QTc interval (see section 4.4).

4.6 Pregnancy and lactation

There are no adequate and well-controlled studies in pregnant women. Patients should be advised to notify their physician if they become pregnant or intend to become pregnant during treatment with olanzapine. Nevertheless, because human experience is limited, olanzapine should be used in pregnancy only if the potential benefit justifies the potential risk to the foetus.

Spontaneous reports have been very rarely received on tremor, hypertonia, lethargy, and sleepiness, in infants born to mothers who had used olanzapine during the 3rd trimester.

In a study in breast-feeding, healthy women, olanzapine was excreted in breast milk. Mean infant exposure (mg/kg) at steady-state was estimated to be 1.8% of the maternal olanzapine dose (mg/kg). Patients should be advised not to breast-feed an infant if they are taking olanzapine.

4.7 Effects on ability to drive and use machines

No studies on the effects on the ability to drive and use machines have been performed. Because olanzapine may cause somnolence and dizziness, patients should be cautioned about operating machinery, including motor vehicles.

4.8 Undesirable effects

A common (1-10%) undesirable effect associated with the use of intramuscular olanzapine in clinical trials was somnolence.

In post-marketing reports, temporal association of treatment with IM olanzapine with cases of respiratory depression, hypotension or bradycardia, and death have been very rarely reported, mostly in patients who concomitantly received benzodiazepines and/or other antipsychotic medicinal products, or who were treated in excess of olanzapine recommended daily doses (see sections 4.4 and 4.5).

The following table is based on the undesirable effects and laboratory investigations from clinical trials with ZYPREXA powder for solution for injection rather than oral olanzapine.

Cardiac disorders *Common (1-10%):* Bradycardia, with or without hypotension or syncope, tachycardia. *Uncommon (0.1-1%):* Sinus pause.
Vascular disorders *Common (1-10%):* Postural hypotension, hypotension.
Respiratory disorders *Uncommon (0.1-1%):* Hypoventilation.
General disorders and administration site conditions *Common (1-10%):* Injection site discomfort.

The undesirable effects listed below have been observed following administration of oral olanzapine, but may also occur following administration of ZYPREXA powder for solution for injection.

Adults

The most frequently (seen in ⩾ 1% of patients) reported adverse reactions associated with the use of olanzapine in clinical trials were somnolence, weight gain, eosinophilia, elevated prolactin, cholesterol, glucose and triglyceride levels (see section 4.4), glucosuria, increased appetite, dizziness, akathisia, parkinsonism (see section 4.4), dyskinesia, orthostatic hypotension, anticholinergic effects, transient asymptomatic elevations of hepatic transaminases (see section 4.4), rash, asthenia, fatigue and oedema.

The following table lists the adverse reactions and laboratory investigations observed from spontaneous reporting and in clinical trials. Within each frequency grouping, adverse reactions are presented in order of decreasing seriousness. The frequency terms listed are defined as follows: Very common (⩾ 10%), common (⩾ 1% and < 10%), uncommon (⩾ 0.1% and < 1%), rare (⩾ 0.01% and < 0.1%), very rare (< 0.01%), not known (cannot be estimated from the data available).

(see Table 1 on next page)

Long-term exposure (at least 48 weeks)

The proportion of patients who had adverse, clinically significant changes in weight gain, glucose, total/LDL/HDL cholesterol or triglycerides increased over time. In adult patients who completed 9-12 months of therapy, the rate of increase in mean blood glucose slowed after approximately 6 months.

Additional information on special populations

In clinical trials in elderly patients with dementia, olanzapine treatment was associated with a higher incidence of death and cerebrovascular adverse reactions compared to placebo (see also section 4.4). Very common adverse reactions associated with the use of olanzapine in this patient group were abnormal gait and falls. Pneumonia, increased body temperature, lethargy, erythema, visual hallucinations and urinary incontinence were observed commonly.

In clinical trials in patients with drug-induced (dopamine agonist) psychosis associated with Parkinson's disease, worsening of Parkinsonian symptomatology and hallucinations were reported very commonly and more frequently than with placebo.

In one clinical trial in patients with bipolar mania, valproate combination therapy with olanzapine resulted in an incidence of neutropenia of 4.1%; a potential contributing factor could be high plasma valproate levels. Olanzapine administered with lithium or valproate resulted in increased levels (⩾ 10%) of tremor, dry mouth, increased appetite, and weight gain. Speech disorder was also reported commonly. During treatment with olanzapine in combination with lithium or divalproex, an increase of ⩾ 7% from baseline body weight occurred in 17.4% of patients during acute treatment (up to 6 weeks). Long-term olanzapine treatment (up to 12 months) for recurrence prevention in patients with bipolar disorder was associated with an increase of ⩾ 7% from baseline body weight in 39.9% of patients.

4.9 Overdose

Signs and Symptoms

Very common symptoms in overdose (>10% incidence) include tachycardia, agitation/aggressiveness, dysarthria, various extrapyramidal symptoms, and reduced level of consciousness, ranging from sedation to coma.

Other medically significant sequelae of overdose include delirium, convulsion, coma, possible neuroleptic malignant syndrome, respiratory depression, aspiration, hypertension or hypotension, cardiac arrhythmias (<2% of overdose cases), and cardiopulmonary arrest. Fatal outcomes have been reported for acute overdoses as low as 450mg, but survival has also been reported following acute overdose of approximately 2 g of oral olanzapine.

Management of Overdose

There is no specific antidote for olanzapine. Induction of emesis is not recommended. Standard procedures for management of overdose may be indicated (i.e., gastric lavage, administration of activated charcoal). The concomitant administration of activated charcoal was shown to reduce the oral bioavailability of olanzapine by 50 to 60%.

Symptomatic treatment and monitoring of vital organ function should be instituted according to clinical presentation, including treatment of hypotension and circulatory collapse, and support of respiratory function. Do not use epinephrine, dopamine, or other sympathomimetic agents with beta-agonist activity, since beta stimulation may worsen hypotension. Cardiovascular monitoring is necessary to detect possible arrhythmias. Close medical supervision and monitoring should continue until the patient recovers.

5. PHARMACOLOGICAL PROPERTIES

5.1 Pharmacodynamic properties

Pharmacotherapeutic group: Diazepines, oxazepines and thiazepines. *ATC code:* N05A H03.

Olanzapine is an antipsychotic, antimanic, and mood stabilising agent that demonstrates a broad pharmacologic profile across a number of receptor systems.

In preclinical studies, olanzapine exhibited a range of receptor affinities (Ki; <100nM) for serotonin $5\text{-}HT_{2A/2C}$, $5\text{-}HT_3$, $5\text{-}HT_6$; dopamine D_1, D_2, D_3, D_4, D_5; cholinergic muscarinic receptors m_1-m_5; α_1-adrenergic; and histamine H_1 receptors. Animal behavioural studies with olanzapine indicated 5HT, dopamine, and cholinergic antagonism, consistent with the receptor-binding profile. Olanzapine demonstrated a greater *in vitro* affinity for serotonin $5\text{-}HT_2$ than dopamine D_2 receptors and greater $5\text{-}HT_2$ than D_2 activity in *in vivo* models. Electrophysiological studies demonstrated that olanzapine selectively reduced the firing of mesolimbic (A10) dopaminergic neurons, while having little effect on the striatal (A9) pathways involved in motor function. Olanzapine reduced a conditioned avoidance response, a test indicative of antipsychotic activity, at doses below those producing catalepsy, an effect indicative of motor side-effects. Unlike some other antipsychotic agents, olanzapine increases responding in an 'anxiolytic' test.

In a single oral dose (10 mg) Positron Emission Tomography (PET) study in healthy volunteers, olanzapine produced a higher $5\text{-}HT_{2A}$ than dopamine D_2 receptor occupancy. In addition, a SPECT imaging study in schizophrenic patients revealed that olanzapine-responsive patients had lower striatal D_2 occupancy than some other antipsychotic- and risperidone-responsive patients, while being comparable to clozapine-responsive patients.

In two of two placebo- and two of three comparator-controlled trials with oral olanzapine, in over 2,900 schizophrenic patients presenting with both positive and negative symptoms, olanzapine was associated with statistically significantly greater improvements in negative as well as positive symptoms.

In a multinational, double-blind, comparative study of schizophrenia, schizoaffective and related disorders, which included 1,481 patients with varying degrees of associated depressive symptoms (baseline mean of 16.6 on the Montgomery-Asberg Depression Rating Scale), a prospective secondary analysis of baseline to endpoint mood score change demonstrated a statistically significant improvement (P = 0.001) favouring oral olanzapine (-6.0) versus haloperidol (-3.1).

In patients with manic or mixed episode of bipolar disorder, oral olanzapine demonstrated superior efficacy to placebo and valproate semisodium (divalproex) in reduction of manic symptoms over 3 weeks. Oral olanzapine also demonstrated comparable efficacy results to haloperidol in terms of the proportion of patients in symptomatic remission from mania and depression at 6 and 12 weeks. In a co-therapy study of patients treated with lithium or valproate for a minimum of 2 weeks, the addition of oral olanzapine 10 mg (co-therapy with lithium or valproate) resulted in a greater reduction in symptoms of mania than lithium or valproate monotherapy after 6 weeks.

In a 12-month recurrence prevention study in manic episode patients who achieved remission on olanzapine and were then randomised to olanzapine or placebo, olanzapine demonstrated statistically significant superiority over placebo on the primary endpoint of bipolar recurrence. Olanzapine also showed a statistically significant advantage over placebo in terms of preventing either recurrence into mania or recurrence into depression.

In a second 12-month recurrence prevention study in manic episode patients who achieved remission with a combination of olanzapine and lithium and were then randomised to olanzapine or lithium alone, olanzapine was statistically non-inferior to lithium on the primary endpoint of bipolar recurrence (olanzapine 30.0%, lithium 38.3%; P = 0.055).

In an 18-month co-therapy study in manic or mixed episode patients stabilised with olanzapine plus a mood stabiliser (lithium or valproate), long-term olanzapine co-therapy with lithium or valproate was not statistically significantly superior to lithium or valproate alone in delaying bipolar recurrence, defined according to syndromic (diagnostic) criteria.

5.2 Pharmacokinetic properties

In a pharmacokinetic study in healthy volunteers, a dose of 5 mg of ZYPREXA powder for solution for injection produced a maximum plasma concentration (C_{max}) approximately 5-times higher than that seen with the same dose of olanzapine administered orally. The C_{max} occurs earlier after intramuscular compared to oral use (15 to 45 minutes versus 5 to 8 hours). As with oral use, C_{max} and area under the curve after intramuscular use are directly proportional to the dose administered. For the same dose of olanzapine

Table 1

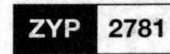

Very common	Common	Uncommon	Not known
Blood and the lymphatic system disorders			
	Eosinophilia	Leucopenia Neutropenia	Thrombocytopenia
Immune system disorders			
			Allergic reaction
Metabolism and nutrition disorders			
Weight gain[1]	Elevated cholesterol levels[2,3] Elevated glucose levels[4] Elevated triglyceride levels[2,5] Glucosuria Increased appetite		Development or exacerbation of diabetes occasionally associated with ketoacidosis or coma, including some fatal cases (see section 4.4) Hypothermia
Nervous system disorders			
Somnolence	Dizziness Akathisia[6] Parkinsonism[6] Dyskinesia[6]		Seizures where in most cases a history of seizures or risk factors for seizures were reported Neuroleptic malignant syndrome (see section 4.4) Dystonia (including oculogyration) Tardive dyskinesia Discontinuation symptoms[7]
Cardiac disorders			
		Bradycardia QTc prolongation (see section 4.4)	Ventricular tachycardia/fibrillation, sudden death (see section 4.4)
Vascular disorders			
	Orthostatic hypotension		Thromboembolism (including pulmonary embolism and deep vein thrombosis)
Gastrointestinal disorders			
	Mild, transient anticholinergic effects including constipation and dry mouth		Pancreatitis
Hepato-biliary disorders			
	Transient, asymptomatic elevations of hepatic transaminases (ALT, AST), especially in early treatment (see section 4.4)		Hepatitis (including hepatocellular, cholestatic or mixed liver injury)
Skin and subcutaneous tissue disorders			
	Rash	Photosensitivity reaction Alopecia	
Musculoskeletal and connective tissue disorders			
			Rhabdomyolysis
Renal and urinary disorders			
			Urinary hesitation
Reproductive system and breast disorders			
			Priapism
General disorders and administration site conditions			
	Asthenia Fatigue Oedema		
Investigations			
Elevated plasma prolactin levels[8]		High creatine phosphokinase Increased total bilirubin	Increased alkaline phosphatase

[1] Clinically significant weight gain was observed across all baseline Body Mass Index (BMI) categories. Following short-term treatment (median duration 47 days), weight gain ⩾ 7 % of baseline body weight was very common (22.2 %), ⩾ 15% was common (4.2 %) and ⩾ 25 % was uncommon (0.8 %). Patients gaining ⩾ 7 %, ⩾ 15 % and ⩾ 25 % of their baseline body weight with long-term exposure (at least 48 weeks) were very common (64.4 %, 31.7 % and 12.3 % respectively).

[2] Mean increases in fasting lipid values (total cholesterol, LDL cholesterol, and triglycerides) were greater in patients without evidence of lipid dysregulation at baseline.

[3] Observed for fasting normal levels at baseline (< 5.17 mmol/l) which increased to high (⩾ 6.2 mmol/l). Changes in total fasting cholesterol levels from borderline at baseline (⩾ 5.17-< 6.2 mmol/l) to high (⩾ 6.2 mmol/l) were very common.

[4] Observed for fasting normal levels at baseline (< 5.56 mmol/l) which increased to high (⩾ 7 mmol/l). Changes in fasting glucose from borderline at baseline (⩾ 5.56 - < 7 mmol/l) to high (⩾ 7 mmol/l) were very common.

[5] Observed for fasting normal levels at baseline (< 1.69 mmol/l) which increased to high (⩾ 2.26 mmol/l). Changes in fasting triglycerides from borderline at baseline (⩾ 1.69 mmol/l - < 2.26 mmol/l) to high (⩾ 2.26 mmol/l) were very common.

[6] In clinical trials, the incidence of parkinsonism and dystonia in olanzapine-treated patients was numerically higher, but not statistically significantly different from placebo. Olanzapine-treated patients had a lower incidence of parkinsonism, akathisia and dystonia compared with titrated doses of haloperidol. In the absence of detailed information on the pre-existing history of individual acute and tardive extrapyramidal movement disorders, it can not be concluded at present that olanzapine produces less tardive dyskinesia and/or other tardive extrapyramidal syndromes.

[7] Acute symptoms such as sweating, insomnia, tremor, anxiety, nausea and vomiting have been reported when olanzapine is stopped abruptly.

[8] Associated clinical manifestations (e.g., gynaecomastia, galactorrhoea, and breast enlargement) were rare. In most patients, levels returned to normal ranges without cessation of treatment.

administered intramuscularly and orally, the associated area under the curve, half-life, clearance, and volume of distribution are similar. The metabolic profiles following intramuscular and oral use are similar.

In non-smoking versus smoking subjects (males and females) administered olanzapine intramuscularly, the mean elimination half-life was prolonged (38.6 versus 30.4 hours) and the clearance was reduced (18.6 versus 27.7 l/hr).

Additional pharmacokinetic data following administration of oral olanzapine are described below.

Olanzapine is metabolised in the liver by conjugative and oxidative pathways. The major circulating metabolite is the 10-N-glucuronide, which does not pass the blood brain barrier. Cytochromes P450-CYP1A2 and P450-CYP2D6 contribute to the formation of the N-desmethyl and 2-hydroxymethyl metabolites; both exhibited significantly less *in vivo* pharmacological activity than olanzapine in animal studies. The predominant pharmacologic activity is from the parent, olanzapine. After oral administration, the mean terminal elimination half-life of olanzapine in healthy subjects varied on the basis of age and gender.

In healthy elderly (65 and over) versus non-elderly subjects administered oral olanzapine, the mean elimination half-life was prolonged (51.8 versus 33.8 hours) and the clearance was reduced (17.5 versus 18.2 l/hr). The pharmacokinetic variability observed in the elderly is within the range for the non-elderly. In 44 patients with schizophrenia > 65 years of age, dosing from 5 to 20 mg/day was not associated with any distinguishing profile of adverse events.

In female versus male subjects administered oral olanzapine, the mean elimination half-life was somewhat prolonged (36.7 versus 32.3 hours) and the clearance was reduced (18.9 versus 27.3 l/hr). However, olanzapine (5-20 mg) demonstrated a comparable safety profile in female (n = 467) as in male patients (n = 869).

In renally impaired patients (creatinine clearance < 10ml/min) versus healthy subjects administered oral olanzapine, there was no significant difference in mean elimination half-life (37.7 versus 32.4 hours) or clearance (21.2 versus 25.0 l/hr). A mass balance study showed that approximately 57% of radiolabelled olanzapine appeared in urine, principally as metabolites.

In smoking subjects with mild hepatic dysfunction administered olanzapine orally, mean elimination half-life (39.3 hours) was prolonged and clearance (18.0 l/hr) was reduced analogous to non-smoking healthy subjects (48.8 hours and 14.1 l/hr, respectively).

The plasma clearance of olanzapine is lower in elderly versus young subjects, in females versus males, and in non-smokers versus smokers. However, the magnitude of the impact of age, gender, or smoking on olanzapine clearance and half-life is small in comparison to the overall variability between individuals.

In a study of Caucasians, Japanese, and Chinese subjects, there were no differences in the pharmacokinetic parameters among the three populations.

The plasma protein binding of olanzapine was about 93% over the concentration range of about 7 to about 1,000ng/ml. Olanzapine is bound predominantly to albumin and α_1-acid-glycoprotein.

5.3 Preclinical safety data

Acute (Single-Dose) Toxicity

Signs of oral toxicity in rodents were characteristic of potent antipsychotic compounds: hypoactivity, coma, tremors, clonic convulsions, salivation, and depressed weight gain. The median lethal doses were approximately 210 mg/kg (mice) and 175 mg/kg (rats). Dogs tolerated single oral doses up to 100 mg/kg without mortality. Clinical signs included sedation, ataxia, tremors, increased heart rate, laboured respiration, miosis, and anorexia. In monkeys, single oral doses up to 100 mg/kg resulted in prostration and, at higher doses, semi-consciousness.

Repeated-Dose Toxicity

In studies up to 3 months duration in mice and up to 1 year in rats and dogs, the predominant effects were CNS depression, anticholinergic effects, and peripheral haematological disorders. Tolerance developed to the CNS depression. Growth parameters were decreased at high doses. Reversible effects consistent with elevated prolactin in rats included decreased weights of ovaries and uterus, and morphologic changes in vaginal epithelium and in mammary gland.

Haematologic Toxicity

Effects on haematology parameters were found in each species, including dose-related reductions in circulating leucocytes in mice and non-specific reductions of circulating leucocytes in rats; however, no evidence of bone marrow cytotoxicity was found. Reversible neutropenia, thrombocytopenia, or anaemia developed in a few dogs treated with 8 or 10 mg/kg/day (total olanzapine exposure [AUC] is 12- to 15-fold greater than that of a man given a 12 mg dose). In cytopenic dogs, there were no undesirable effects on progenitor and proliferating cells in the bone marrow.

Reproductive Toxicity

Olanzapine had no teratogenic effects. Sedation affected mating performance of male rats. Oestrous cycles were affected at doses of 1.1 mg/kg (3-times the maximum human dose) and reproduction parameters were influenced in rats given 3 mg/kg (9-times the maximum human dose). In the offspring of rats given olanzapine, delays in foetal development and transient decreases in offspring activity levels were seen.

Mutagenicity

Olanzapine was not mutagenic or clastogenic in a full range of standard tests, which included bacterial mutation tests and *in vitro* and oral *in vivo* mammalian tests.

Carcinogenicity

Based on the results of oral studies in mice and rats, it was concluded that olanzapine is not carcinogenic.

6. PHARMACEUTICAL PARTICULARS

6.1 List of excipients

Lactose monohydrate

Tartaric acid (E334)

Hydrochloric acid

Sodium hydroxide

6.2 Incompatibilities

This medicinal product must not be mixed with other medicinal products except those mentioned in section 6.6.

Olanzapine for injection should not be combined in a syringe with diazepam injection because precipitation occurs when these products are mixed.

Lorazepam injection should not be used to reconstitute olanzapine for injection as this combination results in a delayed reconstitution time.

Olanzapine for injection should not be combined in a syringe with haloperidol injection because the resulting low pH has been shown to degrade olanzapine over time.

6.3 Shelf life

Powder: 3 years.

Solution (after reconstitution): 1 hour. Do not freeze.

6.4 Special precautions for storage

Do not store above 25°C. Store in the original package in order to protect from light. For storage conditions of the reconstituted medicinal product, see section 6.3.

6.5 Nature and contents of container

ZYPREXA 10 mg Powder for Solution for Injection: Type I, 5 ml glass vial.

One carton contains 1 or 10 vial(s).

Not all pack sizes may be marketed.

6.6 Special precautions for disposal and other handling

Reconstitute ZYPREXA only with water for injections, using standard aseptic techniques for reconstitution of parenteral products. No other solutions should be used for reconstitution (see section 6.2).

1. Withdraw 2.1ml of water for injection into a sterile syringe. Inject into a vial of ZYPREXA.

2. Rotate the vial until the contents have completely dissolved, giving a yellow-coloured solution. The vial contains 11.0 mg olanzapine as a solution of 5 mg/ml (1 mg olanzapine is retained in the vial and syringe, thus allowing delivery of 10 mg olanzapine).

3. The following table provides injection volumes for delivering various doses of olanzapine:

Dose (mg)	Volume of Injection (ml)
10	2.0
7.5	1.5
5	1.0
2.5	0.5

4. Administer the solution intramuscularly. Do not administer intravenously or subcutaneously.

5. Discard the syringe and any unused solution in accordance with appropriate clinical procedures.

6. Use the solution immediately within 1 hour of reconstitution.

Parenteral medicines should be inspected visually for particulate matter prior to administration.

7. MARKETING AUTHORISATION HOLDER

Eli Lilly Nederland BV, Grootslag 1-5, NL-3991 RA, Houten, The Netherlands.

8. MARKETING AUTHORISATION NUMBER(S)

EU/1/96/022/016: ZYPREXA - Powder for solution for injection, 1 Vial.

EU/1/96/022/017: ZYPREXA - Powder for solution for injection, 10 Vials.

9. DATE OF FIRST AUTHORISATION/RENEWAL OF THE AUTHORISATION

Date of first authorisation: 27 September 1996

Date of latest renewal: 27 September 2006

10. DATE OF REVISION OF THE TEXT

03 July 2009

LEGAL CATEGORY

POM

*ZYPREXA (olanzapine) and VELOTAB are trademarks of Eli Lilly and Company. ZY48M

Zyvox 600 mg Film-Coated Tablets, 100 mg/5 ml Granules for Oral Suspension, 2 mg/ml Solution for Infusion

(Pharmacia Limited)

1. NAME OF THE MEDICINAL PRODUCT

Zyvox ▼ 600 mg Film-Coated Tablets

Zyvox ▼ 100 mg/5 ml Granules for Oral Suspension

Zyvox ▼ 2 mg/ml Solution for Infusion

2. QUALITATIVE AND QUANTITATIVE COMPOSITION

Zyvox 600 mg Film-Coated Tablets

Each tablet contains 600 mg linezolid.

Zyvox 100 mg/5 ml Granules for Oral Suspension

Following reconstitution with 123 ml water, each 5 ml contains 100 mg linezolid.

Zyvox 2 mg/ml Solution for Infusion

1 ml contains 2 mg linezolid. 300 ml infusion bags contain 600 mg linezolid.

For excipients, see section 6.1.

3. PHARMACEUTICAL FORM

Zyvox 600 mg Film-Coated Tablets

Film-coated tablet.

White, ovaloid tablet with "ZYVOX 600 mg" printed on one side.

Zyvox 100 mg/5 ml Granules for Oral Suspension

Granules for oral suspension.

White to light-yellow, orange flavoured granules.

Zyvox 2 mg/ml Solution for Infusion

Solution for infusion.

Isotonic, clear, colourless to yellow solution.

4. CLINICAL PARTICULARS

4.1 Therapeutic indications

Nosocomial pneumonia

Community acquired pneumonia

Zyvox is indicated for the treatment of community acquired pneumonia and nosocomial pneumonia when known or suspected to be caused by susceptible Gram positive bacteria. In determining whether Zyvox is an appropriate treatment, the results of microbiological tests or information on the prevalence of resistance to antibacterial agents among Gram positive bacteria should be taken into consideration. (See section 5.1 for the appropriate organisms).

Linezolid is not active against infections caused by Gram negative pathogens. Specific therapy against Gram negative organisms must be initiated concomitantly if a Gram negative pathogen is documented or suspected.

Complicated skin and soft tissue infections (see section 4.4)

Zyvox is indicated for the treatment of complicated skin and soft tissue infections **only** when microbiological testing has established that the infection is known to be caused by susceptible Gram positive bacteria.

Linezolid is not active against infections caused by Gram negative pathogens. Linezolid should only be used in patients with complicated skin and soft tissue infections with known or possible co-infection with Gram negative organisms if there are no alternative treatment options available (see section 4.4). In these circumstances treatment against Gram negative organisms must be initiated concomitantly.

Linezolid should only be initiated in a hospital environment and after consultation with a relevant specialist such as a microbiologist or infectious diseases specialist.

Consideration should be given to official guidance on the appropriate use of antibacterial agents.

4.2 Posology and method of administration

Zyvox solution for infusion, film-coated tablets or oral suspension may be used as initial therapy. Patients who commence treatment on the parenteral formulation may be switched to either oral presentation when clinically indicated. In such circumstances, no dose adjustment is required as linezolid has an oral bioavailability of approximately 100%.

Recommended dosage and duration of treatment for adults: The duration of treatment is dependent on the pathogen, the site of infection and its severity, and on the patient's clinical response.

The following recommendations for duration of therapy reflect those used in the clinical trials. Shorter treatment regimens may be suitable for some types of infection but have not been evaluated in clinical trials.

The maximum treatment duration is 28 days. The safety and effectiveness of linezolid when administered for periods longer than 28 days have not been established (see section 4.4).

No increase in the recommended dosage or duration of treatment is required for infections associated with concurrent bacteraemia.

The dose recommendation for the solution for infusion and the tablets/granules for oral suspension are identical and are as follows:

Infections	Dosage	Duration of treatment
Nosocomial pneumonia	600 mg twice daily	10-14 Consecutive days
Community acquired pneumonia	600 mg twice daily	10-14 Consecutive days
Complicated skin and soft tissue infections	600 mg twice daily	10-14 Consecutive days

Children: There are insufficient data on the safety and efficacy of linezolid in children and adolescents (< 18 years old) to establish dosage recommendations (see sections 5.1 and 5.2). Therefore, until further data are available, use of linezolid in this age group is not recommended.

Elderly patients: No dose adjustment is required.

Patients with renal insufficiency: No dose adjustment is required (see sections 4.4 and 5.2).

Patients with severe renal insufficiency (i.e. $CL_{CR} < 30$ ml/min): No dose adjustment is required. Due to the unknown clinical significance of higher exposure (up to 10 fold) to the two primary metabolites of linezolid in patients with severe renal insufficiency, linezolid should be used with special caution in these patients and only when the anticipated benefit is considered to outweigh the theoretical risk.

As approximately 30% of a linezolid dose is removed during 3 hours of haemodialysis, linezolid should be given after dialysis in patients receiving such treatment. The primary metabolites of linezolid are removed to some extent by haemodialysis, but the concentrations of these metabolites are still very considerably higher following dialysis than those observed in patients with normal renal function or mild to moderate renal insufficiency.

Therefore, linezolid should be used with special caution in patients with severe renal insufficiencies that are undergoing dialysis and only when the anticipated benefit is considered to outweigh the theoretical risk.

To date, there is no experience of linezolid administration to patients undergoing continuous ambulatory peritoneal dialysis (CAPD) or alternative treatments for renal failure (other than haemodialysis).

Patients with hepatic insufficiency: No dose adjustment is required. However, there are limited clinical data and it is recommended that linezolid should be used in such patients only when the anticipated benefit is considered to outweigh the theoretical risk (see sections 4.4 and 5.2).

Method of administration: The recommended linezolid dosage should be administered intravenously or orally twice daily.

Zyvox 600 mg Film-Coated Tablets

Route of administration: Oral use.

The film-coated tablets may be taken with or without food.

Zyvox 100 mg/5 ml Granules for Oral Suspension

Route of administration: Oral use.

The oral suspension may be taken with or without food.

A 600 mg dose is provided by 30 ml of reconstituted suspension (i.e. six 5 ml spoonfuls).

Zyvox 2 mg/ml Solution for Infusion

Route of administration: Intravenous use.

The solution for infusion should be administered over a period of 30 to 120 minutes.

4.3 Contraindications

Patients hypersensitive to linezolid or any of the excipients (see section 6.1).

Linezolid should not be used in patients taking any medicinal product which inhibits monoamine oxidases A or B (e.g. phenelzine, isocarboxazid, selegiline, moclobemide) or within two weeks of taking any such medicinal product.

Unless there are facilities available for close observation and monitoring of blood pressure, linezolid should not be administered to patients with the following underlying clinical conditions or on the following types of concomitant medications:

- Patients with uncontrolled hypertension, phaeochromocytoma, carcinoid, thyrotoxicosis, bipolar depression, schizoaffective disorder, acute confusional states.

- Patients taking any of the following medications: serotonin re-uptake inhibitors (see section 4.4), tricyclic antidepressants, serotonin 5-HT_1 receptor agonists (triptans), directly and indirectly acting sympathomimetic agents (including the adrenergic bronchodilators, pseudoephedrine and phenylpropanolamine), vasopressive agents (e.g. epinephrine, norepinephrine), dopaminergic agents (e.g. dopamine, dobutamine), pethidine or buspirone.

Animal data suggest that linezolid and its metabolites may pass into breast milk and, accordingly, breastfeeding should be discontinued prior to and throughout administration (see section 4.6).

4.4 Special warnings and precautions for use

Linezolid is a reversible, non-selective inhibitor of monoamine oxidase (MAOI); however, at the doses used for antibacterial therapy, it does not exert an anti-depressive effect. There are very limited data from drug interaction studies and on the safety of linezolid when administered to patients with underlying conditions and/or on concomitant medications which might put them at risk from MAO inhibition. Therefore, linezolid is not recommended for use in these circumstances unless close observation and monitoring of the recipient is possible (see sections 4.3 and 4.5).

Patients should be advised against consuming large amounts of tyramine rich foods (see section 4.5).

Zyvox 100 mg/5 ml Granules for Oral Suspension

The reconstituted oral suspension contains a source of phenylalanine (aspartame) equivalent to 20 mg/5 ml. Therefore, this formulation may be harmful for people with phenylketonuria. For patients with phenylketonuria, Zyvox solution for infusion or tablets is recommended.

The suspension also contains sucrose, mannitol and sodium equivalent to 1.7 mg/ml.

Therefore, it should not be administered to patients with rare hereditary problems of fructose intolerance, glucose-galactose malabsorption or sucrase-isomaltase insufficiency. Due to its mannitol content, the oral suspension may have a mild laxative effect. The product contains 8.5 mg sodium per 5 ml dose. The sodium content should be taken into account in patients on a controlled sodium diet.

Zyvox 2 mg/ml Solution for Infusion

Each ml of the solution contains 45.7 mg (i.e. 13.7 g/300 ml) glucose. This should be taken into account in patients with diabetes mellitus or other conditions associated with glucose intolerance. Each ml of solution also contains 0.38 mg (114 mg/300 ml) sodium.

Myelosuppression (including anaemia, leucopenia, pancytopenia and thrombocytopenia) has been reported in patients receiving linezolid. In cases where the outcome is known, when linezolid was discontinued, the affected haematologic parameters have risen toward pre-treatment levels. The risk of these effects appears to be related to the duration of treatment. Thrombocytopenia may occur more commonly in patients with severe renal insufficiency, whether or not on dialysis. Therefore, close monitoring of blood counts is recommended in patients who: have pre-existing anaemia, granulocytopenia or thrombocytopenia; are receiving concomitant medications that may decrease haemoglobin levels, depress blood counts or adversely affect platelet count or function; have severe renal insufficiency; receive more than 10-14 days of therapy. Linezolid should be administered to such patients only when close monitoring of haemoglobin levels, blood counts and platelet counts is possible.

If significant myelosuppression occurs during linezolid therapy, treatment should be stopped unless it is considered absolutely necessary to continue therapy, in which case intensive monitoring of blood counts and appropriate management strategies should be implemented.

In addition, it is recommended that complete blood counts (including haemoglobin levels, platelets, and total and differentiated leucocyte counts) should be monitored weekly in patients who receive linezolid regardless of baseline blood count.

In compassionate use studies, a higher incidence of serious anaemia was reported in patients receiving linezolid for more than the maximum recommended duration of 28 days. These patients more often required blood transfusion. Cases of anaemia requiring blood transfusion have also been reported post marketing, with more cases occurring in patients who received linezolid therapy for more than 28 days.

Lactic acidosis has been reported with the use of linezolid. Patients who develop signs and symptoms of metabolic acidosis including recurrent nausea or vomiting, abdominal pain, a low bicarbonate level, or hyperventilation while receiving linezolid should receive immediate medical attention.

Excess mortality was seen in patients treated with linezolid, relative to vancomycin/dicloxacillin/oxacillin, in an open-label study in seriously ill patients with intravascular catheter-related infections [78/363 (21.5%) vs 58/363 (16.0%)]. The main factor influencing the mortality rate was the Gram positive infection status at baseline. Mortality rates were similar in patients with infections caused purely by Gram positive organisms (odds ratio 0.96; 95% confidence interval: 0.58-1.59) but were significantly higher (p=0.0162) in the linezolid arm in patients with any other pathogen or no pathogen at baseline (odds ratio 2.48; 95% confidence interval: 1.38-4.46). The greatest imbalance occurred during treatment and within 7 days following discontinuation of study drug. More patients in the linezolid arm acquired Gram negative pathogens during the study and died from infection caused by Gram negative pathogens and polymicrobial infections. Therefore, in complicated skin and soft tissue infections linezolid should only be used in patients with known or possible co-infection with Gram negative organisms if there are no alternative treatment options available (see section 4.1). In these circumstances treatment against Gram negative organisms must be initiated concomitantly.

Controlled clinical trials did not include patients with diabetic foot lesions, decubitus or ischaemic lesions, severe burns or gangrene. Therefore, experience in the use of linezolid in the treatment of these conditions is limited.

Linezolid should be used with special caution in patients with severe renal insufficiency and only when the anticipated benefit is considered to outweigh the theoretical risk (see sections 4.2 and 5.2).

It is recommended that linezolid should be given to patients with severe hepatic insufficiency only when the perceived benefit outweighs the theoretical risk (see sections 4.2 and 5.2).

Pseudomembranous colitis has been reported with nearly all antibacterial agents, including linezolid. Therefore, it is important to consider this diagnosis in patients who present with diarrhoea subsequent to the administration of any antibacterial agent. In cases of suspected or verified antibiotic-associated colitis, discontinuation of linezolid may be warranted. Appropriate management measures should be instituted.

Antibiotic-associated diarrhoea and antibiotic-associated colitis, including pseudomembranous colitis and Clostridium difficile-associated diarrhoea, has been reported in association with the use of nearly all antibiotics including linezolid and may range in severity from mild diarrhoea to fatal colitis. Therefore, it is important to consider this diagnosis in patients who develop serious diarrhoea during or after the use of linezolid. If antibiotic-associated diarrhoea or antibiotic-associated colitis is suspected or confirmed, ongoing treatment with antibacterial agents, including linezolid, should be discontinued and adequate therapeutic measures should be initiated immediately. Drugs inhibiting peristalsis are contraindicated in this situation.

The effects of linezolid therapy on normal flora have not been evaluated in clinical trials.

The use of antibiotics may occasionally result in an overgrowth of non-susceptible organisms. For example, approximately 3% of patients receiving the recommended linezolid doses experienced drug-related candidiasis during clinical trials. Should superinfection occur during therapy, appropriate measures should be taken.

The safety and effectiveness of linezolid when administered for periods longer than 28 days have not been established.

Peripheral neuropathy and optic neuropathy, sometimes progressing to loss of vision, have been reported in patients treated with Zyvox; these reports have primarily been in patients treated for longer than the maximum recommended duration of 28 days.

All patients should be advised to report symptoms of visual impairment, such as changes in visual acuity, changes in colour vision, blurred vision, or visual field defect. In such cases, prompt evaluation is recommended with referral to an ophthalmologist as necessary. If any patients are taking Zyvox for longer than the recommended 28 days, their visual function should be regularly monitored.

If peripheral or optic neuropathy occurs, the continued use of Zyvox should be weighed against the potential risks.

Convulsions have been reported to occur in patients when treated with Zyvox. In most of these cases, a history of seizures or risk factors for seizures was reported. Patients should be advised to inform their physician if they have a history of seizures.

Spontaneous reports of serotonin syndrome associated with the co-administration of linezolid and serotonergic agents, including antidepressants such as selective serotonin reuptake inhibitors (SSRIs) have been reported. Co-administration of linezolid and serotonergic agents is therefore contraindicated (see section 4.3) except where administration of linezolid and concomitant serotonergic agents is essential. In those cases patients should be closely observed for signs and symptoms of serotonin syndrome such as cognitive dysfunction, hyperpyrexia, hyperreflexia and incoordination. If signs or symptoms occur physicians should consider discontinuing either one or both agents; if the concomitant serotonergic agent is withdrawn, discontinuation symptoms can occur.

Linezolid reversibly decreased fertility and induced abnormal sperm morphology in adult male rats at exposure levels approximately equal to those expected in humans; possible effects of linezolid on the human male reproductive system are not known (see section 5.3).

4.5 Interaction with other medicinal products and other forms of interaction

Linezolid is a reversible, non-selective inhibitor of monoamine oxidase (MAOI). There are very limited data from drug interaction studies and on the safety of linezolid when administered to patients on concomitant medications that might put them at risk from MAO inhibition. Therefore, linezolid is not recommended for use in these circumstances unless close observation and monitoring of the recipient is possible (see sections 4.3 and 4.4).

In normotensive healthy volunteers, linezolid enhanced the increases in blood pressure caused by pseudoephedrine and phenylpropanolamine hydrochloride. Co-administration of linezolid with either pseudoephedrine or phenylpropanolamine resulted in mean increases in systolic blood pressure of the order of 30-40 mmHg, compared with 11-15 mmHg increases with linezolid alone, 14-18 mmHg with either pseudoephedrine or phenylpropanolamine alone and 8-11 mmHg with placebo. Similar studies in hypertensive subjects have not been conducted. It is recommended that doses of drugs with a vasopressive action, including dopaminergic agents, should be carefully titrated to achieve the desired response when co-administered with linezolid.

The potential drug-drug interaction with dextromethorphan was studied in healthy volunteers. Subjects were administered dextromethorphan (two 20 mg doses given 4 hours apart) with or without linezolid. No serotonin syndrome effects (confusion, delirium, restlessness, tremors, blushing, diaphoresis, hyperpyrexia) have been observed in normal subjects receiving linezolid and dextromethorphan.

Post marketing experience: there has been one report of a patient experiencing serotonin syndrome-like effects while taking linezolid and dextromethorphan which resolved on discontinuation of both medications.

During clinical use of linezolid with serotonergic agents, including antidepressants such as selective serotonin reuptake inhibitors (SSRIs), cases of serotonin syndrome have been reported. Therefore, while co-administration is contraindicated (see section 4.3), management of patients for whom treatment with linezolid and serotonergic agents is essential, is described in section 4.4.

No significant pressor response was observed in subjects receiving both linezolid and less than 100 mg tyramine. This suggests that it is only necessary to avoid ingesting excessive amounts of food and beverages with a high tyramine content (e.g. mature cheese, yeast extracts, undistilled alcoholic beverages and fermented soya bean products such as soy sauce).

Linezolid is not detectably metabolised by the cytochrome P450 (CYP) enzyme system and it does not inhibit any of the clinically significant human CYP isoforms (1A2, 2C9, 2C19, 2D6, 2E1, 3A4). Similarly, linezolid does not induce P450 isoenzymes in rats. Therefore, no CYP450-induced drug interactions are expected with linezolid.

The effect of rifampicin on the pharmacokinetics of linezolid was studied in sixteen healthy adult male volunteers administered linezolid 600 mg twice daily for 2.5 days with and without rifampicin 600 mg once daily for 8 days. Rifampicin decreased the linezolid C_{max} and AUC by a mean 21% [90% CI, 15, 27] and a mean 32% [90% CI, 27, 37], respectively. The mechanism of this interaction and its clinical significance are unknown.

When warfarin was added to linezolid therapy at steady-state, there was a 10% reduction in mean maximum INR on co-administration with a 5% reduction in AUC INR. There are insufficient data from patients who have received warfarin and linezolid to assess the clinical significance, if any, of these findings.

4.6 Pregnancy and lactation

There are no adequate data from the use of linezolid in pregnant women. Studies in animals have shown reproductive toxicity (see section 5.3). A potential risk for humans exists.

Linezolid should not be used during pregnancy unless clearly necessary i.e. only if the potential benefit outweighs the theoretical risk.

Animal data suggest that linezolid and its metabolites may pass into breast milk and, accordingly, breastfeeding should be discontinued prior to and throughout administration.

4.7 Effects on ability to drive and use machines

Patients should be warned about the potential for dizziness whilst receiving linezolid and should be advised not to drive or operate machinery if dizziness occurs.

4.8 Undesirable effects

The information provided is based on data generated from clinical studies in which more than 2,000 adult patients received the recommended linezolid doses for up to 28 days.

Approximately 22% of patients experienced adverse reactions; those most commonly reported were headache (2.1%), diarrhoea (4.2%), nausea (3.3%) and candidiasis (particularly oral [0.8%] and vaginal [1.1%] candidiasis, see table below).

The most commonly reported drug-related adverse events which led to discontinuation of treatment were headache, diarrhoea, nausea and vomiting. About 3% of patients discontinued treatment because they experienced a drug-related adverse event.

(see Table 1 on next page)

The following adverse reactions to linezolid were considered to be serious in isolated cases: localised abdominal pain, transient ischaemic attacks, hypertension, pancreatitis and renal failure.

During clinical trials, a single case of arrhythmia (tachycardia) was reported as drug related.

Table 1

Adverse drug reactions occurring at frequencies > 0.1%		
Infections and infestations	Common	Candidiasis (particularly oral and vaginal candidiasis) or fungal infections.
	Uncommon	Vaginitis.
Blood and the lymphatic system disorders	Uncommon	(Frequency as reported by clinician): Eosinophilia, leucopenia, neutropenia, thrombocytopenia.
Psychiatric disorders	Uncommon	Insomnia
Nervous system disorders	Common:	Headache, Taste perversion (metallic taste)
	Uncommon:	Dizziness, hypoaesthesia, paraesthesia.
Eye disorders	Uncommon:	Blurred vision
Ear and labyrinth disorders	Uncommon:	Tinnitus
Vascular disorders	Uncommon:	Hypertension, phlebitis/thrombophlebitis.
Gastrointestinal disorders	Common:	Diarrhoea, nausea, vomiting.
	Uncommon:	Localised or general abdominal pain, constipation, dry mouth, dyspepsia, gastritis, glossitis, loose stools, pancreatitis, stomatitis, tongue discolouration or disorder.
Hepato-biliary disorders	Common:	Abnormal liver function test.
Skin and subcutaneous tissue disorders	Uncommon:	Dermatitis, diaphoresis, pruritus, rash, urticaria.
Renal and urinary disorders	Uncommon:	Polyuria.
Reproductive system and breast disorders	Uncommon:	Vulvovaginal disorder
General disorders and administration site conditions	Uncommon:	Chills, fatigue, fever, injection site pain, increased thirst, localised pain.
Investigations		
Chemistry	Common:	Increased AST, ALT, LDH, alkaline phosphatase, BUN, creatine kinase, lipase, amylase or non fasting glucose. Decreased total protein, albumin, sodium or calcium. Increased or decreased potassium or bicarbonate.
	Uncommon:	Increased total bilirubin, creatinine, sodium or calcium. Decreased non fasting glucose. Increased or decreased chloride.
Haematology	Common:	Increased neutrophils or eosinophils. Decreased haemoglobin, haematocrit or red blood cell count. Increased or decreased platelet or white blood cell counts.
	Uncommon:	Increased reticulocyte count. Decreased neutrophils.
Common	> 1/100 and < 1/10 or > 1% and < 10%	
Uncommon	> 1/1,000 and < 1/100 or > 0.1% and < 1%	

In controlled clinical trials where linezolid was administered for up to 28 days, less than 0.1% of the patients reported anaemia. In a compassionate use program of patients with life-threatening infections and underlying co-morbidities, the percentage of patients who developed anaemia when receiving linezolid for ⩽ 28 days was 2.5% (33/1326) as compared with 12.3% (53/430) when treated for >28 days. The proportion of cases reporting drug-related serious anaemia and requiring blood transfusion was 9% (3/33) in patients treated for ⩽ 28 days and 15% (8/53) in those treated for >28 days.

Safety data from clinical studies based on more than 500 paediatric patients (from birth to 17 years) do not indicate that the safety profile of linezolid for paediatric patients differs from that for adult patients.

Post-marketing experience

Infections and infestations: antibiotic-associated colitis, including pseudomembranous colitis, potentially associated with life-threatening complications (see section 4.4).

Blood and lymphatic system disorders: Anaemia, leucopenia, neutropenia, thrombocytopenia, pancytopenia and myelosupression (see section 4.4). Of the cases reporting anaemia, more patients required blood transfusion when treated with linezolid for longer than the maximum recommended duration of 28 days (see section 4.4).

Immune system disorders: Anaphylaxis.

Metabolism and nutrition disorders: Lactic acidosis (see section 4.4).

Nervous system disorders: Peripheral neuropathy, convulsions, serotonin syndrome. Peripheral neuropathy has been reported in patients treated with Zyvox; these reports have primarily been in patients treated for longer than the maximum recommended duration of 28 days (see section 4.4)

Convulsions have been reported in patients when treated with Zyvox. In most of these cases, a history or seizures or risk factors for seizures was reported (see section 4.4)

Cases of serotonin syndrome have been reported (see sections 4.3, 4.4 and 4.5).

Eye disorders: Optic neuropathy

Optic neuropathy, sometimes progressing to loss of vision, has been reported in patients treated with Zyvox; these reports have primarily been in patients treated for longer than the maximum recommended duration of 28 days (see section 4.4)

Gastrointestinal disorders: Superficial tooth discolouration.

Skin and subcutaneous tissue disorders: Angioedema, bullous skin disorders such as those described as Stevens-Johnson syndrome have been received.

4.9 Overdose

No specific antidote is known.

No cases of overdose have been reported. However, the following information may prove useful:

Supportive care is advised together with maintenance of glomerular filtration. Approximately 30% of a linezolid dose is removed during 3 hours of haemodialysis, but no data are available for the removal of linezolid by peritoneal dialysis or haemoperfusion. The two primary metabolites of linezolid are also removed to some extent by haemodialysis.

Signs of toxicity in rats following doses of 3000 mg/kg/day linezolid were decreased activity and ataxia whilst dogs treated with 2000 mg/kg/day experienced vomiting and tremors.

5. PHARMACOLOGICAL PROPERTIES

5.1 Pharmacodynamic properties

Pharmacotherapeutic group: Other antibacterials.

ATC code: J 01 X X 08

General Properties

Linezolid is a synthetic, antibacterial agent that belongs to a new class of antimicrobials, the oxazolidinones. It has in vitro activity against aerobic Gram positive bacteria and anaerobic micro-organisms. Linezolid selectively inhibits bacterial protein synthesis via a unique mechanism of action. Specifically, it binds to a site on the bacterial ribosome (23S of the 50S subunit) and prevents the formation of a functional 70S initiation complex which is an essential component of the translation process.

The in vitro postantibiotic effect (PAE) of linezolid for *Staphylococcus aureus* was approximately 2 hours. When measured in animal models, the in vivo PAE was 3.6 and 3.9 hours for *Staphylococcus aureus* and *Streptococcus pneumoniae*, respectively. In animal studies, the key pharmacodynamic parameter for efficacy was the time for which the linezolid plasma level exceeded the minimum inhibitory concentration (MIC) for the infecting organism.

Breakpoints

Minimum inhibitory concentration (MIC) breakpoints established by the European Committee on Antimicrobial Susceptibility Testing (EUCAST) for staphylococci and enterococci are Susceptible ⩽ 4mg/L and Resistant >4 mg/L. For streptococci (including *S. pneumoniae*) the breakpoints are Susceptible ⩽ 2 mg/L and Resistant >4 mg/L.

Non-species related MIC breakpoints are Susceptible ⩽ 2 mg/L and Resistant > 4 mg/L. Non-species related breakpoints have been determined mainly on the basis of PK/PD data and are independent of MIC distributions of specific species. They are for use only for organisms that have not been given a specific breakpoint and not for those species where susceptibility testing is not recommended.

Susceptibility

The prevalence of acquired resistance may vary geographically and with time for selected species and local information on resistance is desirable, particularly when treating severe infections. As necessary, expert advice should be sought when local prevalence of resistance is such that the utility of the agent in at least some types of infections is questionable.

Category
Susceptible organisms
Gram positive aerobes:
Enterococcus faecalis
*Enterococcus faecium**
*Staphylococcus aureus**
Coagulase negative staphylococci
*Streptococcus agalactiae**
Streptococcus pneumoniae*
*Streptococcus pyogenes**
Group C streptococci
Group G streptococci
Gram positive anaerobes:
Clostridium perfringens
Peptostreptococcus anaerobius
Peptostreptococcus species
Resistant organisms
Haemophilus influenzae
Moraxella catarrhalis
Neisseria species
Enterobacteriaceae
Pseudomonas species

*Clinical efficacy has been demonstrated for susceptible isolates in approved clinical indications.

Whereas linezolid shows some in vitro activity against *Legionella*, *Chlamydia pneumoniae* and *Mycoplasma pneumoniae*, there are insufficient data to demonstrate clinical efficacy.

Resistance

Cross resistance

Linezolid's mechanism of action differs from those of other antibiotic classes. In vitro studies with clinical isolates (including methicillin-resistant staphylococci, vancomycin-resistant enterococci, and penicillin- and erythromycin-resistant streptococci) indicate that linezolid is usually active against organisms which are resistant to one or more other classes of antimicrobial agents.

Resistance to linezolid is associated with point mutations in the 23S rRNA. As documented with other antibiotics when used in patients with difficult to treat infections and/or for prolonged periods, emergent decreases in susceptibility have been observed with linezolid. Resistance to linezolid has been reported in enterococci, Staphylococcus aureus and coagulase negative staphylococci. This generally has been associated with prolonged courses of therapy and the presence of prosthetic materials or undrained abscesses. When antibiotic-resistant organisms are encountered in the hospital it is important to emphasize infection control policies.

Information from clinical trials

Studies in the paediatric population:

In an open study, the efficacy of linezolid (10 mg/kg q8h) was compared to vancomycin (10- 15mg/kg q6- 24h) in treating infections due to suspected or proven resistant gram-positive pathogens(including nosocomial pneumonia, complicated skin and skin structure infections, catheter related bacteraemia, bacteraemia of unknown source, and other infections), in children from birth to 11 years. Clinical cure rates in the clinically evaluable population were 89.3% (134/150) and 84.5%(60/71) for linezolid and vancomycin, respectively (95%CI: -4.9, 14.6).

5.2 Pharmacokinetic properties

Zyvox primarily contains (s)-linezolid which is biologically active and is metabolised to form inactive derivatives.

Absorption

Linezolid is rapidly and extensively absorbed following oral dosing. Maximum plasma concentrations are reached within 2 hours of dosing. Absolute oral bioavailability of linezolid (oral and intravenous dosing in a crossover study) is complete (approximately 100%). Absorption is not significantly affected by food and absorption from the oral suspension is similar to that achieved with the film-coated tablets.

Plasma linezolid C_{max} and C_{min} (mean and [SD]) at steady-state following twice daily intravenous dosing of 600 mg have been determined to be 15.1 [2.5] mg/l and 3.68 [2.68] mg/l, respectively.

In another study following oral dosing of 600 mg twice daily to steady-state, C_{max} and C_{min} were determined to be 21.2 [5.8] mg/l and 6.15 [2.94] mg/l, respectively. Steady-state conditions are achieved by the second day of dosing.

Distribution

Volume of distribution at steady-state averages at about 40-50 litres in healthy adults and approximates to total body water. Plasma protein binding is about 31% and is not concentration dependent.

Linezolid concentrations have been determined in various fluids from a limited number of subjects in volunteer studies following multiple dosing. The ratio of linezolid in saliva and sweat relative to plasma was 1.2:1.0 and 0.55:1.0, respectively. The ratio for epithelial lining fluid and alveolar cells of the lung was 4.5:1.0 and 0.15:1.0, when measured at steady-state C_{max}, respectively. In a small study of subjects with ventricular-peritoneal shunts and essentially non-inflamed meninges, the ratio of linezolid in cerebrospinal fluid to plasma at C_{max} was 0.7:1.0 after multiple linezolid dosing.

Metabolism

Linezolid is primarily metabolised by oxidation of the morpholine ring resulting mainly in the formation of two inactive open-ring carboxylic acid derivatives; the aminoethoxyacetic acid metabolite (PNU-142300) and the hydroxyethyl glycine metabolite (PNU-142586). The hydroxyethyl glycine metabolite (PNU-142586) is the predominant human metabolite and is believed to be formed by a non-enzymatic process. The aminoethoxyacetic acid metabolite (PNU-142300) is less abundant. Other minor, inactive metabolites have been characterised.

Elimination

In patients with normal renal function or mild to moderate renal insufficiency, linezolid is primarily excreted under steady-state conditions in the urine as PNU-142586 (40%), parent drug (30%) and PNU-142300 (10%). Virtually no parent drug is found in the faeces whilst approximately 6% and 3% of each dose appears as PNU-142586 and PNU-142300, respectively. The elimination half-life of linezolid averages at about 5-7 hours.

Non-renal clearance accounts for approximately 65% of the total clearance of linezolid. A small degree of non-linearity in clearance is observed with increasing doses of linezolid. This appears to be due to lower renal and non-renal clearance at higher linezolid concentrations. However, the difference in clearance is small and is not reflected in the apparent elimination half-life.

Special Populations

Patients with renal insufficiency: After single doses of 600 mg, there was a 7-8 fold increase in exposure to the two primary metabolites of linezolid in the plasma of patients with severe renal insufficiency (i.e. creatinine clearance < 30 ml/min). However, there was no increase in AUC of parent drug. Although there is some removal of the major metabolites of linezolid by haemodialysis, metabolite plasma levels after single 600 mg doses were still considerably higher following dialysis than those observed in patients with normal renal function or mild to moderate renal insufficiency.

In 24 patients with severe renal insufficiency, 21 of whom were on regular haemodialysis, peak plasma concentrations of the two major metabolites after several days dosing were about 10 fold those seen in patients with normal renal function. Peak plasma levels of linezolid were not affected.

The clinical significance of these observations has not been established as limited safety data are currently available (see sections 4.2 and 4.4).

Patients with hepatic insufficiency: Limited data indicate that the pharmacokinetics of linezolid, PNU-142300 and PNU-142586 are not altered in patients with mild to moderate hepatic insufficiency (i.e. Child-Pugh class A or B). The pharmacokinetics of linezolid in patients with severe hepatic insufficiency (i.e. Child-Pugh class C) have not been evaluated. However, as linezolid is metabolised by a non-enzymatic process, impairment of hepatic function would not be expected to significantly alter its metabolism (see sections 4.2 and 4.4).

Children and adolescents (< 18 years old): There are insufficient data on the safety and efficacy of linezolid in children and adolescents (< 18 years old) and therefore, use of linezolid in this age group is not recommended. (See section 4.2). Further studies are needed to establish safe and effective dosage recommendations. Pharmacokinetic studies indicate that after single and multiple doses in children (1 week to 12 years), linezolid clearance (based on kg body weight) was greater in paediatric patients than in adults, but decreased with increasing age.

In children 1 week to 12 years old, administration of 10 mg/kg every 8 hours daily gave exposure approximating to that achieved with 600 mg twice daily in adults.

In neonates up to 1 week of age, the systemic clearance of linezolid (based on kg body weight) increases rapidly in the first week of life. Therefore, neonates given 10 mg/kg every 8 hours daily will have the greatest systemic exposure on the first day after delivery. However, excessive accumulation is not expected with this dosage regimen during the first week of life as clearance increases rapidly over that period.

In adolescents (12 to 17 years old), linezolid pharmacokinetics were similar to that in adults following a 600mg dose. Therefore, adolescents administered 600 mg every 12 hours daily will have similar exposure to that observed in adults receiving the same dosage.

In paediatric patients with ventriculoperitoneal shunts who were administered linezolid 10mg/kg either 12 hourly or 8 hourly, variable cerebrospinal fluid (CSF) linezolid concentrations were observed following either single or multiple dosing of linezolid. Therapeutic concentrations were not consistently achieved or maintained in the CSF. Therefore, the use of linezolid for the empirical treatment of paediatric patients with central nervous system infections is not recommended.

Elderly patients: The pharmacokinetics of linezolid are not significantly altered in elderly patients aged 65 and over.

Female patients: Females have a slightly lower volume of distribution than males and the mean clearance is reduced by approximately 20% when corrected for body weight. Plasma concentrations are higher in females and this can partly be attributed to body weight differences. However, because the mean half life of linezolid is not significantly different in males and females, plasma concentrations in females are not expected to substantially rise above those known to be well tolerated and, therefore, dose adjustments are not required.

5.3 Preclinical safety data

Linezolid decreased fertility and reproductive performance of male rats at exposure levels approximately equal to those expected in humans. In sexually mature animals these effects were reversible. However, these effects did not reverse in juvenile animals treated with linezolid for nearly the entire period of sexual maturation. Abnormal sperm morphology in testis of adult male rats, and epithelial cell hypertrophy and hyperplasia in the epididymis were noted. Linezolid appeared to affect the maturation of rat spermatozoa. Supplementation of testosterone had no effect on linezolid-mediated fertility effects. Epididymal hypertrophy was not observed in dogs treated for 1 month, although changes in the weights of prostate, testes and epididymis were apparent.

Reproductive toxicity studies in mice and rats showed no evidence of a teratogenic effect at exposure levels 4 times or equivalent, respectively, to those expected in humans. The same linezolid concentrations caused maternal toxicity in mice and were related to increased embryo death including total litter loss, decreased foetal body weight and an exacerbation of the normal genetic predisposition to sternal variations in the strain of mice. In rats, slight maternal toxicity was noted at exposures lower than expected clinical exposures. Mild foetal toxicity, manifested as decreased foetal body weights, reduced ossification of sternebrae, reduced pup survival and mild maturational delays were noted. When mated, these same pups showed evidence of a reversible dose-related increase in pre-implantation loss with a corresponding decrease in fertility. In rabbits, reduced foetal body weight occurred only in the presence of maternal toxicity (clinical signs, reduced body weight gain and food consumption) at low exposure levels 0.06 times compared to the expected human exposure based on AUCs. The species is known to be sensitive to the effects of antibiotics.

Linezolid and its metabolites are excreted into the milk of lactating rats and the concentrations observed were higher than those in maternal plasma.

Linezolid produced reversible myelosuppression in rats and dogs.

In rats administered linezolid orally for 6 months, non-reversible, minimal to mild axonal degeneration of sciatic nerves was observed at 80 mg/kg/day; minimal degeneration of the sciatic nerve was also observed in 1 male at this dose level at a 3-month interim necropsy. Sensitive morphologic evaluation of perfusion-fixed tissues was conducted to investigate evidence of optic nerve degeneration. Minimal to moderate optic nerve degeneration was evident in 2 of 3 male rats after 6 months of dosing, but the direct relationship to drug was equivocal because of the acute nature of the finding and its asymmetrical distribution. The optic nerve degeneration observed was microscopically comparable to spontaneous unilateral optic nerve degeneration reported in aging rats and may be an exacerbation of common background change.

Preclinical data, based on conventional studies of repeated-dose toxicity and genotoxicity, revealed no special hazard for humans beyond those addressed in other sections of this Summary of Product Characteristics. Carcinogenicity / oncogenicity studies have not been conducted in view of the short duration of dosing and lack of genotoxicity in the standard battery of studies.

6. PHARMACEUTICAL PARTICULARS

6.1 List of excipients

Zyvox 600 mg Film-Coated Tablets

Tablet core:

Microcrystalline cellulose (E460)

Maize starch

Sodium starch glycollate type A

Hydroxypropylcellulose (E463)

Magnesium stearate (E572)

Film coat:

Hypromellose (E464)

Titanium dioxide (E171)

Macrogol 400

Carnauba wax (E903)

Red ink

Red iron oxide (E172)

Zyvox 100 mg/5 ml Granules for Oral Suspension

Sucrose

Mannitol (E421)

Microcrystalline cellulose (E460)

Carboxymethylcellulose sodium (E466)

Aspartame (E951)

Anhydrous colloidal silica (E551)

Sodium citrate (E331)

Xanthan gum (E415)

Sodium benzoate (E211)

Citric acid anhydrous (E330)

Sodium chloride

Sweeteners (fructose, maltodextrin, monoammonium glycyrrhizinate, sorbitol)

Orange, Orange Cream, Peppermint, Vanilla flavourings (acetoin, alpha tocopherols acetaldehyde, anisic aldehyde, beta-caryophyllene, n-butyric acid, butyl butyryl lactate, decalactone delta, dimethyl benzyl carb acetate, ethyl alcohol, ethyl butyrate, ethyl maltol, ethyl vanillin, furaneol, grapefruit terpenes, heliotropin, maltodextrin, modified food starch, monomethyl succinate, orange aldehyde, orange oil FLA CP, orange oil Valencia 2X, orange oil 5X Valencia, orange essence oil, orange juice carbonyls, orange terpenes, peppermint essential oil, propylene glycol, tangerine oil, vanilla extract, vanillin, water)

Zyvox 2 mg/ml Solution for Infusion

Glucose monohydrate

Sodium citrate (E331)

Citric acid anhydrous (E330)

Hydrochloric acid (E507)

Sodium hydroxide (E524)

Water for injections

6.2 Incompatibilities

Zyvox 600 mg Film-Coated Tablets and Zyvox 100 mg/5 ml Granules for Oral Suspension

Not applicable.

Zyvox 2 mg/ml Solution for Infusion

Additives should not be introduced into this solution. If linezolid is to be given concomitantly with other drugs, each drug should be given separately in accordance with its own directions for use. Similarly, if the same intravenous line is to be used for sequential infusion of several drugs, the line should be flushed prior to and following linezolid administration with a compatible infusion solution (see section 6.6).

Zyvox solution for infusion is known to be physically incompatible with the following compounds: amphotericin B, chlorpromazine hydrochloride, diazepam, pentamidine isethionate, erythromycin lactobionate, phenytoin sodium and sulphamethoxazole / trimethoprim. Additionally, it is chemically incompatible with ceftriaxone sodium.

6.3 Shelf life

Zyvox 600 mg Film-Coated Tablets

3 years.

Zyvox 100 mg/5 ml Granules for Oral Suspension

Before reconstitution:	2 years.
After reconstitution:	3 weeks.

Zyvox 2 mg/ml Solution for Infusion

Before opening: 3 years.

After opening: From a microbiological point of view, unless the method of opening precludes the risk of microbial contamination, the product should be used immediately. If not used immediately, in-use storage times and conditions are the responsibility of the user.

6.4 Special precautions for storage

Zyvox 600 mg Film-Coated Tablets

No special precautions for storage.

Zyvox 100 mg/5 ml Granules for Oral Suspension

Before reconstitution: Keep the container tightly closed.

After reconstitution: Keep the container in the outer carton.

Zyvox 2 mg/ml Solution for Infusion

Store in the original package (overwrap and carton) until ready to use.

6.5 Nature and contents of container

Zyvox 600 mg Film-Coated Tablets

White, HDPE bottle with a polypropylene screw cap containing either 10*, 14*, 20*, 24, 30, 50 or 60 tablets.

White, HDPE bottle with a polypropylene screw cap containing 100 tablets (for hospital use only).

Note:

*The above bottles may also be supplied in "hospital packs" of 5 or 10.

Polyvinylchloride (PVC)/foil blisters of 10 tablets packaged in a box. Each box contains either 10*, 20*, 30, 50 or 60 tablets.

Polyvinylchloride (PVC)/foil blisters of 10 tablets packaged in a box. Each box contains 100 tablets (for hospital use only).

Note:

*The above boxes may also be supplied in "hospital packs" of 5 or 10.

Not all package sizes may be marketed.

Zyvox 100 mg/5 ml Granules for Oral Suspension

Amber, Type III glass bottles with a nominal volume of 240 ml containing 66 g granules for oral suspension. Each bottle has a polypropylene, child resistant screw cap and is packaged in a box with a 2.5 ml/5 ml measuring spoon.

Note:

The above bottles may also be supplied in "hospital packs" of 5 or 10.

Not all package sizes may be marketed.

Zyvox 2 mg/ml Solution for Infusion

Single use, ready-to-use, latex-free, multilayered (inner layer: ethylene propylene copolymer and styrene/ethylene butylene/styrene copolymer; middle layer: styrene/ethylene butylene/styrene copolymer; outer layer: copolyester) film infusion bags sealed inside a foil laminate overwrap. The bag holds 300 ml solution and is packaged in a box. Each box contains 1*, 2**, 5, 10, 20 or 25 infusion bags.

Note:

The above boxes may also be supplied in "hospital" packs of:

* 5, 10 or 20

** 3, 6 or 10

Not all package sizes may be marketed.

6.6 Special precautions for disposal and other handling

Zyvox 600 mg Film-Coated Tablets

No special requirements.

Zyvox 100 mg/5 ml Granules for Oral Suspension

Loosen the granules and reconstitute using 123 ml water in two approximately equal aliquots to produce 150 ml oral suspension. The suspension should be vigorously shaken between each addition of water.

Before use, gently invert the bottle a few times. Do not shake.

Zyvox 2 mg/ml Solution for Infusion

For single use only. Remove overwrap only when ready to use, then check for minute leaks by squeezing the bag firmly. If the bag leaks, do not use as sterility may be impaired. The solution should be visually inspected prior to use and only clear solutions, without particles should be used. Do not use these bags in series connections. Any unused solution must be discarded. Do not reconnect partially used bags.

Zyvox solution for infusion is compatible with the following solutions: 5% glucose intravenous infusion, 0.9% sodium chloride intravenous infusion, Ringer-lactate solution for injection (Hartmann's solution for injection).

7. MARKETING AUTHORISATION HOLDER

Pharmacia Limited

Ramsgate Road

Sandwich

Kent

CT13 9NJ

8. MARKETING AUTHORISATION NUMBER(S)

Zyvox 600 mg Film-Coated Tablets - PL 00032/0261

Zyvox 100 mg/5 ml Granules for Oral Suspension - PL 00032/0262

Zyvox 2 mg/ml Solution for Infusion - PL 00032/0259

9. DATE OF FIRST AUTHORISATION/RENEWAL OF THE AUTHORISATION

5 January 2001/4 January 2006

10. DATE OF REVISION OF THE TEXT

24th June 2009

REF: ZY 10_1 UK

CODE OF PRACTICE for the PHARMACEUTICAL INDUSTRY

The pharmaceutical industry in the UK is committed to benefiting patients by operating in a professional, ethical and transparent manner to ensure the appropriate use of medicines and support the provision of high quality healthcare. The Association of the British Pharmaceutical Industry (ABPI), which represents the UK industry, decided that certain activities should be covered in detail and thus agreed the first ABPI Code of Practice in 1958. The Code is regularly updated. It reflects and extends beyond the relevant UK law.

The Prescription Medicines Code of Practice Authority (PMCPA) was established by the ABPI in 1993 to operate the Code of Practice for the Pharmaceutical Industry at arm's length from the ABPI itself. Compliance with the Code is obligatory for ABPI member companies and, in addition, over fifty non member companies voluntarily agree to comply with the Code and to accept the jurisdiction of the PMCPA.

The Code covers the promotion of medicines to, and interactions with, health professionals and administrative staff. It also covers information about prescription only medicines made available to the public and relationships with patient organisations.

Complaints submitted under the Code are considered by the Code of Practice Panel which consists of the three members of the PMCPA. Both complainants and respondents may appeal to the Code of Practice Appeal Board against rulings made by the Panel. The Code of Practice Appeal Board is chaired by an independent legally qualified Chairman, Mr William Harbage QC, and includes independent members from outside the industry.

In each case where a breach of the Code is ruled, the company concerned must give an undertaking that the practice in question has ceased forthwith and that all possible steps have been taken to avoid a similar breach in the future. An undertaking must be accompanied by details of the action taken to implement the ruling. Additional sanctions are imposed in serious cases.

Complaints about the promotion of medicines, or the provision of information to the public, should be sent to the Director of the Prescription Medicines Code of Practice Authority, 12 Whitehall, London, SW1A 2DY or emailed to complaints@pmcpa.org.uk.

A copy of the Code and further information about the PMCPA including details about ongoing and completed cases can be found at www.pmcpa.org.uk.

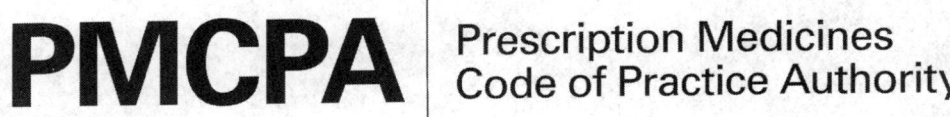

PMCPA | Prescription Medicines Code of Practice Authority

For additional & updated information visit www.emc.medicines.org.uk

DIRECTORY of PARTICIPANTS

This directory is included in the Compendium so that doctors and other healthcare professionals may obtain additional information about products from the participating pharmaceutical companies.

A.MENARINI PHARMA U.K. S.R.L.
Menarini House
Mercury Park
Wycombe Lane
Buckinghamshire HP10 0HH
Tel: +44 (0) 1628 856400
Fax: +44 (0)1628 856 402
Careline: 0800 085 8678
email: menarini@medinformation.co.uk

ABBOTT LABORATORIES LIMITED
Abbott House
Vanwall Business Park
Vanwall Road
Berkshire SL6 4XE
UK
Tel: +44 (0)1628 773 355
Fax: +44 (0)1628 644 185
email: ukmedinfo@abbott.com
Website: http://www.abbottuk.com

ABRAXIS BIOSCIENCE LIMITED
Rosanne House
Parkway
Welwyn Garden City
Herts
AL8 6HG
Tel: +44 (0) 207 081 0850
Careline: +44 (0) 5603 141 956
email: abraxismedical@idispharma.com

ACTAVIS UK LTD
Whiddon Valley
Devon EX32 8NS
UK
Tel: +44 (0)1271 311 200
Fax: +44 (0)1271 346 106
Medical Information only: +44 (0)1271 311 257
email: medinfo@actavis.co.uk
Website: http://www.actavis.co.uk

ALK-ABELLO LTD
1 Tealgate
Berkshire RG17 0YT
UK
Tel: +44 (0)1488 686 016
Fax: +44 (0)1488 685 423
Medical Information only: +44 (0)1488 686 016
Medical Information fax: +44 (0)1488 685 423
Careline: +44 (0)1488 686 016
email: medinfo@uk.alk-abello.com

ALLEN & HANBURYS
Stockley Park West
Middlesex UB11 1BT
Tel: +44 (0)800 221 441
Fax: +44 (0)208 990 4328
email: customercontactuk@gsk.com

ALLERGAN LTD
Marlow International
The Parkway
Bucks SL7 1YL
UK
Tel: +44 (0)1628 494444
Fax: +44 (0)1628 494449
Medical Information only: +44 (0)1628 494026
email: UK_MedInfo@Allergan.com
Website: http://www.allergan.co.uk

ALLIANCE PHARMACEUTICALS
Avonbridge House
Bath Road
Wiltshire SN15 2BB
Tel: +44 (0)1249 466 966
Fax: +44 (0)1249 466 977
email: medinfo@alliancepharma.co.uk
Website: http://www.alliancepharma.co.uk

ASTELLAS PHARMA LTD
Lovett House
Lovett Road
Middlesex TW18 3AZ
Tel: +44 (0)1784 419615
Fax: +44 (0)1784 419 401

ASTRAZENECA UK LIMITED
Horizon Place
600 Capability Green
Bedfordshire LU1 3LU
Tel: +44 (0)1582 836 000
Fax: +44 (0)1582 838 000
Medical Information only: +44 (0)1582 836 836
Medical Information fax: +44 (0)1582 838 003
Careline: +44 (0)1582 837 837
email: medical.informationuk@astrazeneca.com

BASILEA PHARMACEUTICALS LTD
14/16 Frederick Sanger Road
The Surrey Research Park
Surrey GU2 7YD
Tel: +44 (0)1483 600095
Fax: +44 (0)1483 505365
Medical Information only: +44 (0)1483 790023
email: ukmedinfo@basilea.com
Website: http://www.basilea.com

BEACON PHARMACEUTICALS
85 High Street
TN1 1YG
Tel: +44 (0)1892 600 930
Fax: +44 (0)1892 600 937
email: info@beaconpharma.co.uk
Website: http://www.beaconpharma.co.uk

BIOGEN IDEC LTD
Innovation House
70 Norden Road
Berkshire SL6 4AY
UK
Tel: +44 (0)1628 501 000
Fax: +44 (0)1628 501 010
Medical Information only: 0800 008 7401
Medical Information fax: +44(0)1748 828801

BOEHRINGER INGELHEIM LIMITED
Ellesfield Avenue
Berkshire RG12 8YS
Tel: +44 (0)1344 424 600
Fax: +44 (0)1344 741 298
Medical Information only: +44 (0)1344 741 286
email: medinfo@bra.boehringer-ingelheim.com
Website: http://www.boehringer-ingelheim.co.uk

BRACCO UK LIMITED
Bracco House
Mercury Park
Wycombe Lane
Wooburn Green
Bucks HP10 0HH
Tel: +44 (0)1628 851 500
Fax: +44 (0)1628 819 317

BRITANNIA PHARMACEUTICALS
Park View House
65 London Road
Berkshire RG14 1JN
Tel: +44 (0) 1635 568 400
Fax: +44 (0) 1635 568 401
Medical Information only: +44 (0)870 851 0207
email: enquiries@medinformation.co.uk
Website: http://www.britannia-pharm.co.uk/

CAMBRIDGE LABORATORIES
Deltic House
Kingfisher Way
Silverlink Business Park
Tyne & Wear NE28 9NX
Tel: +44 (0)191 296 9369
Fax: +44 (0)191 296 9368
Medical Information only: +44 (0)191 296 9339
Careline: +44 (0)191 296 9300
email: medicines.information@camb-labs.com

CEPHALON (UK) LIMITED
1 Albany Place
Hyde Way
Welwyn Garden City
Hertfordshire AL7 3BT
Tel: +44 (0) 1707 385800
Fax: +44 (0) 1707 385801
Medical Information only: 0800 783 4869
Medical Information fax: +44 (0) 1707 385802
email: ukmedinfo@cephalon.com
Website: http://www.cephalon.co.uk

CEPHALON LIMITED
1 Albany Place
Hyde Way
Hertfordshire AL7 3BT
UK
Tel: +44 (0)1707 385800
Fax: +44 (0)1707 385801
Medical Information only: 0800 783 4869
email: ukmedinfo@cephalon.com
Website: http://www.cephalon.co.uk

CHUGAI PHARMA UK LIMITED
Mulliner House
Flanders Road
London W4 1NN
Tel: +44 (0)208 987 5600
Fax: +44 (0)208 987 5660

CSL BEHRING UK LIMITED
Hayworth House
Market Place
West Sussex RH16 1DB
UK
Tel: +44 (0)1444 447 400
Fax: +44 (0)1444 447 403
Medical Information only: +44 (0)1444 447 405
Careline: +44 (0)1444 447 402
email: medinfo@cslbehring.com

DAIICHI SANKYO UK LIMITED
Chiltern Place
Chalfont Park
Buckinghamshire SL9 0BG
UK
Tel: +44 (0)1753 482 771
Medical Information only: +44 (0)1753 482 771
Medical Information fax: +44 (0)1753 893 894
Careline: +44 (0)1753 482 771
email: medinfo@daiichi-sankyo.co.uk

DDD LIMITED
94 Rickmansworth Road
Watford
Hertfordshire
WD18 7JJ
Tel: +44 1923 22 9251
Fax: +44 1923 22 0728
Medical Information only: +44 1923 22 9251
+44 7977 98 9686
Medical Information fax: +44 1923 220 728
Careline: +44 1923 22 9251
email: info@dentinox.co.uk
Website: www.dddgroup.co.uk

DERMAL LABORATORIES LIMITED
Tatmore Place
Gosmore
Herts SG4 7QR
Tel: +44 (0)1462 458 866
Fax: +44 (0)1462 420 565
Website: http://www.dermal.co.uk

DR. FALK PHARMA UK LTD
Bourne End Business Park
Cores End Road
Buckinghamshire SL8 5AS
Tel: +44 (0)1628 536 600
Fax: +44 (0)1628 536 601
Medical Information only: +44 (0)1628 536 616
Medical Information fax: +44 (0)1628 536 601
Careline: +44 (0)1628 536 600

EISAI LTD
European Knowledge Centre
Mosquito Way
Hertfordshire AL10 9SN
Tel: +44 (0)845 676 1400
Fax: +44 (0)845 676 1486
email: Lmedinfo@eisai.net

ELI LILLY AND COMPANY LIMITED
Lilly House
Priestley Road
Hampshire RG24 9NL
Tel: +44 (0)1256 315 000
Fax: +44 (0)1256 775 858
Medical Information fax: +44 (0)1256 775 569
Careline: +44 (0)1256 315 999
email: ukmedinfo@lilly.com
Website: http://www.lilly.co.uk

ENTURIA
Reigate Place
43 London Road
Surrey RH2 9PW
Tel: +44 1737 237 940
Fax: +44 1737 237 950
Careline: 0800 043 7546
Careline: +44 1737 237 940
email: enquires@enturia.co.uk
Website: www.enturia.co.uk

EUSA PHARMA (EUROPE) LIMITED
Building 3
Arlington Business Park
Whittle Way
Stevenage
SG1 2FP
Tel: +44 (0) 1438 740720
Fax: +44 (0) 1438 735740
Medical Information only: +44 (0) 1438 740720
Medical Information fax: +44 (0) 1438 735740
Careline: +44 (0) 1438 740720
email: Medinfo-uk@eusapharma.com
Website: http://www.eusapharma.com

FERRING PHARMACEUTICALS LTD
The Courtyard
Waterside Drive
Berkshire SL3 6EZ
Tel: +44 (0)1753 214 800
Fax: +44 (0)1753 214 802
Medical Information only: +44 (0)1753 214 845
Medical Information fax: +44 (0)1753 214 801
email: medical@ferring.com
Website: http://www.ferring.co.uk

FOREST LABORATORIES UK LIMITED
Riverbridge House
Anchor Boulevard
Crossways Business Park
Kent DA2 6SL
Tel: +44 (0)1322 421 800
Fax: +44 (0)1322 291 306
email: medinfo@forest-labs.co.uk
Website: http://www.forestlabs.com

GALDERMA (U.K) LTD
Meridien House
69-71 Clarendon Road
Hertfordshire WD17 1DS
UK
Tel: +44 (0)1923 208950
Fax: +44 (0)1923 208998

GALEN LIMITED
Seagoe Industrial Estate
Craigavon
Northern Ireland BT63 5UA
Ireland
Tel: +44 (0)28 3833 4974
Fax: +44 (0)28 3835 0206
email: customer.services@galen.co.uk
Website: http://www.galen.co.uk

GENUS PHARMACEUTICALS
Park View House
65 London Road
Berkshire RG14 1JN
Tel: +44 (0)1635 568 400
Fax: +44 (0)1635 568 401
Medical Information only: +44 (0)870 851 0207
Medical Information fax: +44 (0)1793 710 387
Careline: +44 (0)1635 568 445
email: genus@medinformation.co.uk

GILEAD SCIENCES LTD
Flowers Building
Granta Park
Abington
Cambridge CB21 6GT
UK
Tel: +44 (0)1223 897 300
Fax: +44 (0)1223 897 291
Medical Information only: +44 (0)1223 897 555
Medical Information fax: +44 (0)1223 897 281
Careline: +44 (0)1223 897 400
email: ukmedinfo@gilead.com

GLAXOSMITHKLINE UK
Stockley Park West
Middlesex UB11 1BT
Tel: +44 (0)800 221 441
Fax: +44 (0)208 990 4328
email: customercontactuk@gsk.com

GRUNENTHAL LTD
2 Beacon Heights Business Park
Ibstone Road
Stokenchurch
Buckinghamshire HP14 3XR
UK
Tel: +44 (0)870 351 8960
Fax: +44 (0)870 351 8961
Medical Information only: +44 (0)870 351 8960
Medical Information fax: +44 (0)1494 486298
email: medicalinformationuk@grunenthal.com
Website: http://www.grunenthal.co.uk

HK PHARMA LIMITED
PO Box 105
Herts SG5 2GG
Tel: +44(0)1462 433 993
Fax: +44 (0)1462 450 755

INTERNATIONAL MEDICATION SYSTEMS (UK) LTD
208 Bath Road
Berkshire SL1 3WE
Tel: +44 (0)1753 534 655
Fax: +44 (0)1753 536 632
Medical Information only: +44 (0)1753 447 690
Medical Information fax: +44 (0)1753 447 647
Careline: +44 (0)800 953 0183
email: Medicalinformationuk@ucb.com

INTRAPHARM LABORATORIES LTD
60 Boughton Lane
Kent ME15 9QS
Tel: +44 (0)1622 749 222
Medical Information fax: +44 (0)1622 743 816
email: sales@intrapharmlabs.com

IPSEN LTD
190 Bath Road
Berkshire SL1 3XE
Tel: +44 (0)1753 627 777
Fax: +44 (0)1753 627 778
Medical Information only: +44 (0)1753 627 777
Careline: +44 (0)1753 627 627
email: medical.information.uk@ipsen.com

JANSSEN-CILAG LTD
50 - 100 Holmers Farm Way
Bucks HP12 4EG
Tel: +44 (0)1494 567 567
Fax: +44 (0)1494 567 568
Medical Information only: +44 (0)800 731 8450
Careline: +44 (0)800 731 5550
email: medinfo@janssen-cilag.co.uk
Website: http://www.janssen-cilag.co.uk

KING PHARMACEUTICALS LTD
Donegal Street
County Donegal
Medical Information only: +44 (0)1462 434 366
Medical Information fax: +44 (0)1462 450 755

KYOWA HAKKO KIRIN UK LTD
258 Bath Road
Berkshire SL1 4DX
Tel: +44 (0)1753 566 020
Fax: +44 (0)1753 566 030
Medical Information fax: +44 (0)1753 566 030
email: medinfo@kyowa-uk.co.uk

LABORATORIOS CASEN FLEET S.L.U
Autovia De Logrono KM 13
3 Utebo-Zaragoza
50180
Spain
Tel: +34976462626
Fax: +34976771560
Medical Information only: +34913517964
Medical Information fax: +34913518799
Careline: +34913518800
email: centrodeinformacion@casenfleet.com
Website: http://www.casenfleet.com

LEO LABORATORIES LIMITED
Longwick Road
Bucks. HP27 9RR
Tel: +44 (0)1844 347 333
Fax: +44 (0)1844 342 278
email: medical-info.uk@leo-pharma.com

LUNDBECK LIMITED
Lundbeck House
Caldecotte Lake Business Park
Milton Keynes MK7 8LG
Tel: +44 (0)1908 649 966
Fax: +44 (0)1908 647 888
Medical Information only: +44 (0)1908 638 972
Careline: +44 (0)1908 638 935
email: ukmedicalinformation@lundbeck.com
Website: http://www.lundbeck.co.uk

MANX HEALTHCARE
Taylor Group House
Wedgnock Lane
Warwickshire CV34 5YA
Tel: +44 (0)1926 482 511
Fax: +44 (0)1926 498 711

MEDAC GMBH
Fehlandtstrasse 3
Germany
Tel: +44 (0)1786 458086
Fax: +44 (0)1786 458032
email: info@medac-uk.co.uk

MERCK SERONO
Bedfont Cross
Stanwell Road
Middlesex TW14 8NX
UK
Tel: +44 (0)208 818 7200
Fax: +44 (0)208 818 7267
Medical Information only: +44 (0)208 818 7373
Medical Information fax: +44 (0)208 818 7274
email: medinfo.uk@merckserono.net

MERCK SHARP & DOHME LIMITED
Hertford Road
Hertfordshire EN11 9BU
Tel: +44 (0)1992 467 272
Fax: +44 (0)1992 451 066

MERZ PHARMA UK LTD
260 Centennial Park
Elstree Hill
South Elstree
Herts WD6 3SR
Tel: +44 (0)208 236 0000
Fax: +44 (0)208 236 3501
Medical Information only: +44 (0)845 009 0110
Medical Information fax: +44 (0)845 009 0330
Careline: +44 (0)208 236 3516
email: medical.information@merz.com
Website: http://www.merzpharma.co.uk

MSD-SP LTD
Hertford Road
Hertfordshire EN11 9BU
Tel: +44 (0)1992 467 272
Fax: +44 (0)1992 451 066
Medical Information fax: +44 (0)1707 363 763

NAPP PHARMACEUTICALS LIMITED
Cambridge Science Park
Milton Road
Cambridgeshire CB4 0GW
Tel: +44 (0)1223 424 444
Fax: +44 (0)1223 424 441
Medical Information fax: +44 (0)1223 424 912
Website: http://www.napp.co.uk

NORGINE LIMITED
Chaplin House
Widewater Place
Moorhall Road
Middlesex UB9 6NS
Tel: +44 (0)1895 826 600
Fax: +44 (0)1895 825 865
email: medinfo@norgine.com

NOVARTIS CONSUMER HEALTH
Wimblehurst Road
West Sussex RH12 5AB
Tel: +44 (0)1403 210 211
Fax: +44 (0)1403 323 919
Medical Information only: +44 (0)1403 323 046
Medical Information fax: +44 (0)1403 324 024
Careline: +44 (0)1403 218 111
email: medicalaffairs.uk@novartis.com

NOVARTIS VACCINES
Frimley Business Park
Frimley
Surrey GU16 7SR
Tel: +44 (0)1276 694 490
Fax: +44 (0)1276 698 460
Medical Information only: +44 (0)8457 451 500
Medical Information fax: +44 (0)1517 055 669
email: serviceuk@novartis.com
Website: http://www.novartis.com

NOVO NORDISK LIMITED
Broadfield Park
Brighton Road
West Sussex RH11 9RT
Tel: +44 (0)1293 613555
Fax: +44 (0)1293 613535
Medical Information only: +44 (0)845 600 5055
Medical Information fax: +44 (0)1293 613211
Careline: +44 (0)845 600 5055
email: ukmedicalinfo@novonordisk.com

NYCOMED UK LTD
Nycomed UK Ltd
3 Globeside Business Park
Fieldhouse Lane
Buckinghamshire SL7 1HZ
UK
Tel: +44 (0)1628 646 400
Fax: +44 (0)1628 646 401
Medical Information only: +44 (0) 800 633 5797
Medical Information fax: +44 (0)1628 646534
email: medinfo@nycomed.com
Website: http://www.nycomed.com

ORION PHARMA (UK) LIMITED
Oaklea Court
22 Park Street
Berkshire RG14 1EA
Tel: +44 (0)1635 520 300
Fax: +44 (0)1635 580 180
email: medicalinformation@orionpharma.com

OTSUKA PHARMACEUTICALS (UK) LTD
3 Furzeground Way
Stockley Park
Middlesex UB11 1EZ
UK
Tel: +44 (0)20 8742 4300
Fax: +44 (0)20 8848 0529
email: otsuka@medinformation.co.uk
Website: http://www.otsuka-europe.com

PAINES & BYRNE LIMITED
Lovett House
Lovett Road
Middlesex TW18 3AZ
UK
Tel: +44 (0)1784 419 620
Fax: +44 (0)1784 419 583

PFIZER LIMITED
Ramsgate Road
Kent CT13 9NJ
Tel: +44 (0)1304 616 161
Fax: +44 (0)1304 656 221

PHARMA MAR, S.A.
Avda. de Los Reyes 1
Poligono Industrial La Mina
Madrid 28770
Spain
Tel: +44 (0)1932 824100
Fax: +44 (0)1932 842300
Medical Information only: +44 (0)1932 824026
Medical Information fax: +44 (0)1932 824 226
Careline: +44 (0)1932 824100
email: mpenas@pharmamar.com

PHARMACIA LIMITED
Ramsgate Road
Kent CT13 9NJ
Tel: +44 (0)1304 616 161
Fax: +44 (0)1304 656 221

PIERRE FABRE LIMITED
Hyde Abbey House
23 Hyde Street
Hampshire SO23 7DR
Tel: +44 (0)1962 874 400
Fax: +44 (0)1962 844 014
Medical Information only: +44 (0)1962 874 435
Medical Information fax: +44 (0)1962 874 413
Careline: +44 (0)1962 874 402
email: medicalinformation@pierre-fabre.co.uk

PROCTER & GAMBLE PHARMACEUTICALS UK LIMITED
Rusham Park Technical Centre
Whitehall Lane
Surrey TW20 9NW
Tel: +44 (0)1784 474 900
Fax: +44 (0)1784 474 705

PROFILE PHARMA LIMITED
Chichester Business Park
City Fields Way
Tangmere
West Sussex PO20 2FT
Tel: +44 (0)800 1300 855
Fax: +44 (0)800 1300 856
Medical Information only: +44 (0)870 423 1475
email: info@profilepharma.com
Website: http://www.profilepharma.com

PROSTRAKAN
Galabank Business Park
TD1 1QH
Tel: +44 (0)1896 664 000
Fax: +44 (0)1896 664 001
email: medinfo@prostrakan.com
Website: http://www.ProStrakan.com

ROCHE PRODUCTS LIMITED
Hexagon Place
6 Falcon Way
Shire Park
Hertfordshire AL7 1TW
Tel: +44 (0)1707 366 000
Fax: +44 (0)1707 338 297
Medical Information only: +44 (0)800 328 1629
Medical Information fax: +44 (0)1707 384555
Careline: +44 (0)800 731 5711
email: medinfo.uk@roche.com
Website: http://www.rocheuk.com

ROSEMONT PHARMACEUTICALS LIMITED
Rosemont House
Yorkdale Industrial Park
Braithwaite Street
Yorkshire LS11 9XE
Tel: +44 (0)113 244 1400
Fax: +44 (0)113 246 0738
Careline: +44 (0)800 919 312
Website: http://www.rosemontpharma.com

SANDOZ LIMITED
37 Woolmer Way
Hants GU35 9QE
UK
Tel: +44 (0) 1420 478301
Fax: +44 (0) 1420 487073
email: uk.drugsafety@sandoz.com
Website: www.sandoz.com

SANOFI-AVENTIS
1 Onslow Street
Surrey GU1 4YS
UK
Tel: +44 (0)1483 505 515
Fax: +44 (0)1483 535 432
email: uk-medicalinformation@sanofi-aventis.com

SERVIER LABORATORIES LIMITED
Gallions
Wexham Springs
Framewood Road
Wexham
SL3 6RJ
Tel: +44 (0)1753 662744
Fax: +44 (0)1753 663456
Medical Information only: +44 (0)1753 666409
email: medical.information@uk.netgrs.com

SHIRE HUMAN GENETIC THERAPIES
Hampshire International Business Park
Chineham
Hampshire RG24 8EP
UK
Tel: +44 (0)1256 894000
Medical Information only: +44 (0)800 055 6614
email: medinfouk@shire.com

SHIRE PHARMACEUTICALS LIMITED
Hampshire International Business Park
Chineham
Hampshire RG24 8EP
Tel: +44 (0)1256 894 000
Medical Information only: 0800 055 6614
Careline: +44 (0)1256 894 107
email: medinfoglobal@shire.com
Website: http://www.shire.com

SIGMA-TAU PHARMA LIMITED UK
Abbey House
1650 Arlington Business Park
Berkshire RG7 4SA
UK
Tel: +44 (0)118 929 8075
Fax: +44 (0) 118 929 8076
Medical Information only: +44 (0) 8000431268
email: medical.information@sigma-tau.co.uk

SOLVAY HEALTHCARE LIMITED
Mansbridge Road
West End
SO18 3JD
Tel: +44 (0)2380 467 000
Fax: +44 (0)2380 465 350
Medical Information fax: +44 (0)2380 474518
email: medinfo.shl@solvay.com

SPECIALITY EUROPEAN PHARMA
16 John Street
London
WC1N 2DL
Tel: 0800 118 5171
Fax: 0207 421 7401
Medical Information only: 0800 118 517
Medical Information fax: 0207 421 7401
Careline: 0800 118 5171
email: info@spepharma.com
Website: www.specialityeuropeanpharma.com

SPEPHARM UK LTD
2B Bankside
Hanborough Business Park
Long Hanborough
Oxfordshire OX29 1LJ
UK
Tel: +44 (0) 844 800 7335
Fax: +44 (0) 844 800 7341
Medical Information only: 0844 800 7579
Medical Information fax: 0844 800 7336
Website: http://www.spepharm.com

SSL INTERNATIONAL PLC
Venus
1 Old Park Lane
Trafford Park
Manchester M41 7HA
UK
Tel: +44 (0)8701 222 690
Fax: +44 (0)8701 222 696
Medical Information only: +44 (0)161 638 2027
Medical Information fax: +44 (0)161 615 8819
Careline: +44 (0)161 638 2399
email: medical.information@ssl-international.com
Website: http://www.ssl-international.com

STD PHARMACEUTICAL PRODUCTS LTD
Plough Lane
Herefordshire HR4 0EL
Tel: +44 (0)1432 373 555
Fax: +44 (0)1432 373 556
Website: http://www.stdpharm.co.uk

STIEFEL LABORATORIES (UK) LIMITED
Eurasia Headquarters
Concorde Road
Berkshire SL6 4BY
UK
Tel: +44 (0)1628 612 000
Fax: +44 (0)1628 612 001

SYNER-MED (PHARMACEUTICAL PRODUCTS) LTD
Beech House
840 Brighton Road
Surrey CR8 2BH
Tel: +44 (0)845 634 2100
Fax: +44 (0)845 634 2101

THE MEDICINES COMPANY
The Medicines Company
Suite B
Park House
11 Milton Park
Oxfordshire OX14 4RS
UK
Tel: + 44 (0) 1235 438 250
Fax: + 44 (0) 1235 438 251
Medical Information only: + (00) 800 843 633 26
Careline: + (00) 800 843 633 26
email: medical.information@themedco.com
Website: http://www.themedicinescompany.com

UCB PHARMA LIMITED
208 Bath Road
Berkshire SL1 3WE
Tel: +44 (0)1753 534 655
Fax: +44 (0) 1773 810644
Medical Information only: +44 (0)1753 447 690
Careline: +44 (0) 1773 510123
email: Medicalinformationuk@ucb.com

WYETH PHARMACEUTICALS
Huntercombe Lane South
Taplow
Berks SL6 0PH
Tel: +44 (0)1628 604 377
Fax: +44 (0)1628 666 368
Medical Information only: +44 (0)845 367 0098
Medical Information fax: +44 (0)845 367 0777
email: ukmedinfo@wyeth.com

INDEX by COMPANY

AstraZeneca UK Limited

Basilea Pharmaceuticals Ltd

Beacon Pharmaceuticals

Biogen Idec Ltd

Boehringer Ingelheim Limited

Bracco UK Limited

Britannia Pharmaceuticals

Cambridge Laboratories

Cephalon (UK) Limited

Cephalon Limited

Chugai Pharma UK Limited

CSL Behring UK Limited

Daiichi Sankyo UK Limited

DDD Limited

Dermal Laboratories Limited

Dr. Falk Pharma UK Ltd

Eisai Ltd

Eli Lilly and Company Limited

Enturia

EUSA Pharma (Europe) Limited

Ferring Pharmaceuticals Ltd

Forest Laboratories UK Limited

Galderma (U.K) Ltd

Galen Limited

Genus Pharmaceuticals

Gilead Sciences Ltd

GlaxoSmithKline UK

Grunenthal Ltd

HK Pharma Limited

International Medication Systems (UK) Ltd

Intrapharm Laboratories Ltd

Ipsen Ltd

Janssen-Cilag Ltd

King Pharmaceuticals Ltd

Kyowa Hakko Kirin UK Ltd

Laboratorios Casen Fleet S.L.U

Leo Laboratories Limited

Lundbeck Limited

Manx Healthcare

medac GmbH

Merck Serono

Merck Sharp & Dohme Limited

Merz Pharma UK Ltd

MSD-SP LTD

Napp Pharmaceuticals Limited

Norgine Limited

Novartis Consumer Health

Novartis Vaccines

Novo Nordisk Limited

Nycomed UK Ltd

Orion Pharma (UK) Limited

Otsuka Pharmaceuticals (UK) Ltd

Rosemont Pharmaceuticals Limited

Sandoz Limited

sanofi-aventis

Servier Laboratories Limited

Shire Human Genetic Therapies

Shire Pharmaceuticals Limited

sigma-tau Pharma Limited UK

Solvay Healthcare Limited

Speciality European Pharma

SpePharm UK Ltd

SSL International plc

STD Pharmaceutical Products Ltd

Stiefel Laboratories (UK) Limited

Syner-Med (Pharmaceutical Products) Ltd

The Medicines Company

UCB Pharma Limited

Wyeth Pharmaceuticals

INDEX by PRODUCT

Proprietary names are in ordinary type, generic names in *italics*. It should be noted that although different products may contain the same active ingredients this does not imply that they are equivalent in regard to bio-availability or therapeutic activity.

UK POISONS INFORMATION UNITS

The National Poisons Information Service (NPIS) Centres provide a year-round 24-hour-a-day service for healthcare professionals on the diagnosis, treatment and management of patients who may have been poisoned.

For assistance, advice or further information:

Telephone: 0844 892 0111

UK REGIONAL MEDICINES INFORMATION UNITS

The Medicines Information (MI) service in the United Kingdom (UKMi) is provided on a national basis by specialist pharmacists and technicians, the majority of whom are based within hospital trusts located across the UK. Their work is supported by regional MI centres which provide additional resources and support to local centres.

For details of your nearest regional centre, please see below:

England

East Anglia

East Anglia Medicines Information Service
Ipswich Hospital NHS Trust
Heath Road
Ipswich
Suffolk
IP4 5PD

Tel:	01473 704 431
Fax:	01473 704 433
eMail:	eastanglia.mis@ipswichhospital.nhs.uk

London – North-Thames

Medicines Information
Pharmacy Department
Northwick Park Hospital
Watford Road
Harrow
Middlesex
HA1 3UJ

Tel:	0208 869 3973 0208 869 2761/2762
Fax:	0208 869 2764
eMail:	med.info@nwlh.nhs.uk

London and South East

Medicines Information
Pharmacy Department
Guy's Hospital
St Thomas' Street
London
SE1 9RT

Tel:	0207 188 8750
Fax:	0207 188 3857
eMail:	medicinesinformation@gstt.nhs.uk

North West

North West Medicines Information Centre
Pharmacy Practice Unit
70 Pembroke Place
Liverpool
L69 3GF

Tel:	0151 794 8117
Fax:	0151 794 8118
eMail:	druginfo@liv.ac.uk

Northern & Yorkshire (Leeds)
Pharmacy Department
Leeds General Infirmary
Great George Street
Leeds
LS1 3EX

Tel:	0113 392 3547
Fax:	0113 244 5849
eMail:	medicines.information@leedsth.nhs.uk

Northern & Yorkshire (Newcastle)
Wolfson Unit
Regional Drug & Therapeutics Centre
24 Claremont Place
Newcastle upon Tyne
NE2 4HH

Tel:	0191 232 1525
Fax:	0191 260 6192
eMail:	nyrdtc.di@ncl.ac.uk

South West
South West Medicines Information & Training
Bristol Royal Infirmary
Marlborough Street
Bristol
BS2 8HW

Tel:	0117 342 2867
Fax:	0117 342 3818
eMail:	swmi@UHBristol.nhs.uk

Trent
Trent Medicines Information Service
Leicester Royal Infirmary
Leicester
LE1 5WW

Tel:	0116 258 6491
Fax:	0116 258 5680
eMail:	medicines.info@uhl-tr.nhs.uk

Wessex
Wessex Medicines Information Centre
Mailpoint 31
Southampton General Hospital
Tremona Road
Southampton
SO16 6YD

Tel:	023 8079 6908
	023 8079 6909
Fax:	023 8079 4467
eMail:	medicinesinformation@suht.swest.nhs.uk

West Midlands
West Midlands Medicines Information Service
Heart of England NHS Foundation Trust
Good Hope Hospital
Sutton Coldfield
B75 7RR

Tel:	0121 242 7298
Fax:	0121 378 1594
eMail:	wmmis@heartofengland.nhs.uk

Northern Ireland

Belfast

Regional Medicines & Poisons Information Service
The Royal Hospitals
Grosvenor Road
Belfast
BT12 6BA

Tel:	028 90 632 032
	028 90 633 847
Fax:	028 90 248 030
eMail:	nirdic.nirdic@belfasttrust.hscni.net

Scotland

Aberdeen

Grampian Medicines Information Centre
Aberdeen Royal Infirmary
Pharmacy Department
Foresterhill Site
Aberdeen
AB25 2ZN

Tel:	01224 552 316
Fax:	01224 553 371
eMail:	grampian.medinfo@nhs.net

Dundee

Ninewells Hospital & Medical School
Pharmacy Department
Dundee
DD1 9SY

Tel:	01382 632 351
Fax:	01382 632 599
eMail:	Tay-UHB.medinfo@nhs.net

Edinburgh

Royal Infirmary of Edinburgh
NHS Lothian – University Hospitals Division
51 Little France Crescent
Old Dalkeith Road
Edinburgh
EH16 4SA

Tel:	0131 242 2920
	0131 536 1000 Ext: 22920
Fax:	0131 242 2925
eMail:	medicines.information@luht.scot.nhs.uk

Glasgow

Glasgow Royal Infirmary
Pharmacy Department
84 Castle Street
Glasgow
G4 0SF

Tel:	0141 211 4407
Fax:	0141 552 8170
eMail:	med.info@ggc.scot.nhs.uk

Wales

Cardiff

Welsh Medicines Information Centre
University Hospital of Wales
Heath Park
Cardiff
CF14 4XW

Tel:	02920 742 979
	02920 743 877
Fax:	02920 743 879
eMail:	welshmedicines.information@cardiffandvale.wales.nhs.uk

Notes

Notes

Notes

Notes

Notes

Notes

Notes

Notes

Notes

Notes

In Confidence

COMPENDIUM

YellowCard

COMMISSION ON HUMAN MEDICINES (CHM)

MHRA

SUSPECTED ADVERSE DRUG REACTIONS

If you are suspicious that an adverse reaction may be related to a drug or combination of drugs please complete this Yellow Card. For reporting advice please see over. Do not be put off reporting because some details are not known.

PATIENT DETAILS Patient Initials: Sex: M / F Weight if known (kg):

Age (at time of reaction): ______ Identification number (Your Practice / Hospital Ref.)*: ______

SUSPECTED DRUG(S)

Give brand name of drug and batch number if known	Route	Dosage	Date started	Date stopped	Prescribed for

SUSPECTED REACTION(S)

Please describe the reaction(s) and any treatment given:

Outcome

Recovered ☐
Recovering ☐
Continuing ☐
Other ☐

Date reaction(s) started: ______ Date reaction(s) stopped: ______

Do you consider the reactions to be serious? Yes / No

If yes, please indicate why the reaction is considered to be serious (please tick all that apply):

Patient died due to reaction ☐ Involved or prolonged inpatient hospitalisation ☐
Life threatening ☐ Involved persistent or significant disability or incapacity ☐
Congenital abnormality ☐ Medically significant; please give details: ______

In Confidence

COMPENDIUM

YellowCard

COMMISSION ON HUMAN MEDICINES (CHM)

MHRA

SUSPECTED ADVERSE DRUG REACTIONS

If you are suspicious that an adverse reaction may be related to a drug or combination of drugs please complete this Yellow Card. For reporting advice please see over. Do not be put off reporting because some details are not known.

PATIENT DETAILS Patient Initials: ______ Sex: M / F Weight if known (kg): ______

Age (at time of reaction): ______ Identification number (Your Practice / Hospital Ref.)*: ______

SUSPECTED DRUG(S)

Give brand name of drug and batch number if known	Route	Dosage	Date started	Date stopped	Prescribed for

SUSPECTED REACTION(S)

Please describe the reaction(s) and any treatment given:

Outcome

Recovered ☐
Recovering ☐
Continuing ☐
Other ☐

Date reaction(s) started: ______ Date reaction(s) stopped: ______

Do you consider the reactions to be serious? Yes / No

If yes, please indicate why the reaction is considered to be serious (please tick all that apply):

Patient died due to reaction ☐ Involved or prolonged inpatient hospitalisation ☐
Life threatening ☐ Involved persistent or significant disability or incapacity ☐
Congenital abnormality ☐ Medically significant; please give details: ______

OTHER DRUGS (including self-medication & herbal remedies)

Did the patient take any other drugs in the last 3 months prior to the reaction? Yes / No

If yes, please give the following information if known:

Drug (Brand, if known)	Route	Dosage	Date started	Date stopped	Prescribed for

Additional relevant information e.g. medical history, test results, known allergies, rechallange (if performed), suspect drug interactions. For congenital abnormalities please state all other drugs taken during pregnancy and the last menstrual period.

REPORTER DETAILS

Name and Professional Address: ____________________

Post code: __________ Tel No: __________

Speciality: __________

Signature: __________ Date: __________

CLINICIAN (if not the reporter)

Name and Professional Address: ____________________

Post code: __________

Tel No: __________ Speciality: __________

If you report from an area served by a Yellow Card Centre (YCC), MHRA may ask the Centre to communicate with you, on its behalf, about your report. If you want only MHRA to contact you, please tick this box. ☐
See page 10 of BNF for details on YCCs.

* This is to enable you to identify the patient in any future correspondence concerning this report

Please attach additional pages if necessary

OTHER DRUGS (including self-medication & herbal remedies)

Did the patient take any other drugs in the last 3 months prior to the reaction? Yes / No

If yes, please give the following information if known:

Drug (Brand, if known)	Route	Dosage	Date started	Date stopped	Prescribed for

Additional relevant information e.g. medical history, test results, known allergies, rechallange (if performed), suspect drug interactions. For congenital abnormalities please state all other drugs taken during pregnancy and the last menstrual period.

REPORTER DETAILS

Name and Professional Address: ____________________

Post code: __________ Tel No: __________

Speciality: __________

Signature: __________ Date: __________

CLINICIAN (if not the reporter)

Name and Professional Address: ____________________

Post code: __________

Tel No: __________ Speciality: __________

If you report from an area served by a Yellow Card Centre (YCC), MHRA may ask the Centre to communicate with you, on its behalf, about your report. If you want only MHRA to contact you, please tick this box. ☐
See page 10 of BNF for details on YCCs.

* This is to enable you to identify the patient in any future correspondence concerning this report

Please attach additional pages if necessary

In Confidence

COMPENDIUM

YellowCard

COMMISSION ON HUMAN MEDICINES (CHM)

MHRA

SUSPECTED ADVERSE DRUG REACTIONS

If you are suspicious that an adverse reaction may be related to a drug or combination of drugs please complete this Yellow Card. For reporting advice please see over. Do not be put off reporting because some details are not known.

PATIENT DETAILS Patient Initials: ______ Sex: M / F Weight if known (kg): ______

Age (at time of reaction): ______ Identification number (Your Practice / Hospital Ref.)*: ______

SUSPECTED DRUG(S)

Give brand name of drug and batch number if known	Route	Dosage	Date started	Date stopped	Prescribed for

SUSPECTED REACTION(S)

Please describe the reaction(s) and any treatment given:

Outcome

Recovered ☐
Recovering ☐
Continuing ☐
Other ☐

Date reaction(s) started: ______ Date reaction(s) stopped: ______

Do you consider the reactions to be serious? Yes / No

If yes, please indicate why the reaction is considered to be serious (please tick all that apply):

Patient died due to reaction ☐
Life threatening ☐
Congenital abnormality ☐
Involved or prolonged inpatient hospitalisation ☐
Involved persistent or significant disability or incapacity ☐
Medically significant; please give details: ______

In Confidence

COMPENDIUM

YellowCard

COMMISSION ON HUMAN MEDICINES (CHM)

MHRA

SUSPECTED ADVERSE DRUG REACTIONS

If you are suspicious that an adverse reaction may be related to a drug or combination of drugs please complete this Yellow Card. For reporting advice please see over. Do not be put off reporting because some details are not known.

PATIENT DETAILS Patient Initials: ______ Sex: M / F Weight if known (kg): ______

Age (at time of reaction): ______ Identification number (Your Practice / Hospital Ref.)*: ______

SUSPECTED DRUG(S)

Give brand name of drug and batch number if known	Route	Dosage	Date started	Date stopped	Prescribed for

SUSPECTED REACTION(S)

Please describe the reaction(s) and any treatment given:

Outcome

Recovered ☐
Recovering ☐
Continuing ☐
Other ☐

Date reaction(s) started: ______ Date reaction(s) stopped: ______

Do you consider the reactions to be serious? Yes / No

If yes, please indicate why the reaction is considered to be serious (please tick all that apply):

Patient died due to reaction ☐
Life threatening ☐
Congenital abnormality ☐
Involved or prolonged inpatient hospitalisation ☐
Involved persistent or significant disability or incapacity ☐
Medically significant; please give details: ______

OTHER DRUGS (including self-medication & herbal remedies)

Did the patient take any other drugs in the last 3 months prior to the reaction? Yes / No

If yes, please give the following information if known:

Drug (Brand, if known)	Route	Dosage	Date started	Date stopped	Prescribed for

Additional relevant information e.g. medical history, test results, known allergies, rechallange (if performed), suspect drug interactions. For congenital abnormalities please state all other drugs taken during pregnancy and the last menstrual period.

REPORTER DETAILS

Name and Professional Address: ____________

Post code: ____________ Tel No: ____________

Speciality: ____________

Signature: ____________ Date: ____________

CLINICIAN (if not the reporter)

Name and Professional Address: ____________

Post code: ____________

Tel No: ____________ Speciality: ____________

If you report from an area served by a Yellow Card Centre (YCC), MHRA may ask the Centre to communicate with you, on its behalf, about your report. If you want only MHRA to contact you, please tick this box. ☐

See page 10 of BNF for details on YCCs.

* This is to enable you to identify the patient in any future correspondence concerning this report

Please attach additional pages if necessary

OTHER DRUGS (including self-medication & herbal remedies)

Did the patient take any other drugs in the last 3 months prior to the reaction? Yes / No

If yes, please give the following information if known:

Drug (Brand, if known)	Route	Dosage	Date started	Date stopped	Prescribed for

Additional relevant information e.g. medical history, test results, known allergies, rechallange (if performed), suspect drug interactions. For congenital abnormalities please state all other drugs taken during pregnancy and the last menstrual period.

REPORTER DETAILS

Name and Professional Address: ____________

Post code: ____________ Tel No: ____________

Speciality: ____________

Signature: ____________ Date: ____________

CLINICIAN (if not the reporter)

Name and Professional Address: ____________

Post code: ____________

Tel No: ____________ Speciality: ____________

If you report from an area served by a Yellow Card Centre (YCC), MHRA may ask the Centre to communicate with you, on its behalf, about your report. If you want only MHRA to contact you, please tick this box. ☐

See page 10 of BNF for details on YCCs.

* This is to enable you to identify the patient in any future correspondence concerning this report

Please attach additional pages if necessary

In Confidence

COMPENDIUM

YellowCard

COMMISSION ON HUMAN MEDICINES (CHM)

MHRA

SUSPECTED ADVERSE DRUG REACTIONS

If you are suspicious that an adverse reaction may be related to a drug or combination of drugs please complete this Yellow Card. For reporting advice please see over. Do not be put off reporting because some details are not known.

PATIENT DETAILS Patient Initials: ______ Sex: M / F Weight if known (kg): ______

Age (at time of reaction): ______ Identification number (Your Practice / Hospital Ref.)*: ______

SUSPECTED DRUG(S)

Give brand name of drug and batch number if known	Route	Dosage	Date started	Date stopped	Prescribed for

SUSPECTED REACTION(S)

Please describe the reaction(s) and any treatment given:

Outcome

- Recovered ☐
- Recovering ☐
- Continuing ☐
- Other ☐

Date reaction(s) started: ______ Date reaction(s) stopped: ______

Do you consider the reactions to be serious? Yes / No

If yes, please indicate why the reaction is considered to be serious (please tick all that apply):

- Patient died due to reaction ☐
- Life threatening ☐
- Congenital abnormality ☐
- Involved or prolonged inpatient hospitalisation ☐
- Involved persistent or significant disability or incapacity ☐
- Medically significant; please give details: ______

In Confidence

COMPENDIUM

YellowCard

COMMISSION ON HUMAN MEDICINES (CHM)

MHRA

SUSPECTED ADVERSE DRUG REACTIONS

If you are suspicious that an adverse reaction may be related to a drug or combination of drugs please complete this Yellow Card. For reporting advice please see over. Do not be put off reporting because some details are not known.

PATIENT DETAILS Patient Initials: ______ Sex: M / F Weight if known (kg): ______

Age (at time of reaction): ______ Identification number (Your Practice / Hospital Ref.)*: ______

SUSPECTED DRUG(S)

Give brand name of drug and batch number if known | Route | Dosage | Date started | Date stopped | Prescribed for

SUSPECTED REACTION(S)

Please describe the reaction(s) and any treatment given:

Outcome

- Recovered ☐
- Recovering ☐
- Continuing ☐
- Other ☐

Date reaction(s) started: ______ Date reaction(s) stopped: ______

Do you consider the reactions to be serious? Yes / No

If yes, please indicate why the reaction is considered to be serious (please tick all that apply):

- Patient died due to reaction ☐
- Life threatening ☐
- Congenital abnormality ☐
- Involved or prolonged inpatient hospitalisation ☐
- Involved persistent or significant disability or incapacity ☐
- Medically significant; please give details: ______

OTHER DRUGS **(including self-medication & herbal remedies)**

Did the patient take any other drugs in the last 3 months prior to the reaction? Yes / No

If yes, please give the following information if known:

Drug (Brand, if known)	Route	Dosage	Date started	Date stopped	Prescribed for

Additional relevant information e.g. medical history, test results, known allergies, rechallange (if performed), suspect drug interactions. For congenital abnormalities please state all other drugs taken during pregnancy and the last menstrual period.

REPORTER DETAILS

Name and Professional Address: ____________

Post code: ____________ Tel No: ____________

Speciality: ____________

Signature: ____________ Date: ____________

CLINICIAN (if not the reporter)

Name and Professional Address: ____________

Post code: ____________

Tel No: ____________ Speciality: ____________

If you report from an area served by a Yellow Card Centre (YCC), MHRA may ask the Centre to communicate with you, on its behalf, about your report. If you want only MHRA to contact you, please tick this box. ☐
See page 10 of BNF for details on YCCs.

* This is to enable you to identify the patient in any future correspondence concerning this report

Please attach additional pages if necessary

OTHER DRUGS **(including self-medication & herbal remedies)**

Did the patient take any other drugs in the last 3 months prior to the reaction? Yes / No

If yes, please give the following information if known:

Drug (Brand, if known)	Route	Dosage	Date started	Date stopped	Prescribed for

Additional relevant information e.g. medical history, test results, known allergies, rechallange (if performed), suspect drug interactions. For congenital abnormalities please state all other drugs taken during pregnancy and the last menstrual period.

REPORTER DETAILS

Name and Professional Address: ____________

Post code: ____________ Tel No: ____________

Speciality: ____________

Signature: ____________ Date: ____________

CLINICIAN (if not the reporter)

Name and Professional Address: ____________

Post code: ____________

Tel No: ____________ Speciality: ____________

If you report from an area served by a Yellow Card Centre (YCC), MHRA may ask the Centre to communicate with you, on its behalf, about your report. If you want only MHRA to contact you, please tick this box. ☐
See page 10 of BNF for details on YCCs.

* This is to enable you to identify the patient in any future correspondence concerning this report

Please attach additional pages if necessary

In Confidence

COMPENDIUM

YellowCard

COMMISSION ON HUMAN MEDICINES (CHM)

MHRA

SUSPECTED ADVERSE DRUG REACTIONS

If you are suspicious that an adverse reaction may be related to a drug or combination of drugs please complete this Yellow Card. For reporting advice please see over. Do not be put off reporting because some details are not known.

PATIENT DETAILS Patient Initials: ________ Sex: M / F Weight if known (kg): ________

Age (at time of reaction): ________ Identification number (Your Practice / Hospital Ref.)*: ________

SUSPECTED DRUG(S)

Give brand name of drug and batch number if known	Route	Dosage	Date started	Date stopped	Prescribed for

SUSPECTED REACTION(S)

Please describe the reaction(s) and any treatment given:

Outcome

- Recovered ☐
- Recovering ☐
- Continuing ☐
- Other ☐

Date reaction(s) started: ________ Date reaction(s) stopped: ________

Do you consider the reactions to be serious? Yes / No

If yes, please indicate why the reaction is considered to be serious (please tick all that apply):

- Patient died due to reaction ☐
- Life threatening ☐
- Congenital abnormality ☐
- Involved or prolonged inpatient hospitalisation ☐
- Involved persistent or significant disability or incapacity ☐
- Medically significant; please give details: ________

In Confidence

COMPENDIUM

YellowCard

COMMISSION ON HUMAN MEDICINES (CHM)

MHRA

SUSPECTED ADVERSE DRUG REACTIONS

If you are suspicious that an adverse reaction may be related to a drug or combination of drugs please complete this Yellow Card. For reporting advice please see over. Do not be put off reporting because some details are not known.

PATIENT DETAILS Patient Initials: ________ Sex: M / F Weight if known (kg): ________

Age (at time of reaction): ________ Identification number (Your Practice / Hospital Ref.)*: ________

SUSPECTED DRUG(S)

Give brand name of drug and batch number if known | Route | Dosage | Date started | Date stopped | Prescribed for

SUSPECTED REACTION(S)

Please describe the reaction(s) and any treatment given:

Outcome

Recovered ☐
Recovering ☐
Continuing ☐
Other ☐

Date reaction(s) started: ________ Date reaction(s) stopped: ________

Do you consider the reactions to be serious? Yes / No

If yes, please indicate why the reaction is considered to be serious (please tick all that apply):

Patient died due to reaction ☐
Life threatening ☐
Congenital abnormality ☐
Involved or prolonged inpatient hospitalisation ☐
Involved persistent or significant disability or incapacity ☐
Medically significant; please give details: ________

OTHER DRUGS (including self-medication & herbal remedies)

Did the patient take any other drugs in the last 3 months prior to the reaction? Yes / No

If yes, please give the following information if known:

Drug (Brand, if known)	Route	Dosage	Date started	Date stopped	Prescribed for

Additional relevant information e.g. medical history, test results, known allergies, rechallange (if performed), suspect drug interactions. For congenital abnormalities please state all other drugs taken during pregnancy and the last menstrual period.

REPORTER DETAILS

Name and Professional Address: ____

Post code: ____ Tel No: ____

Speciality: ____

Signature: ____ Date: ____

CLINICIAN (if not the reporter)

Name and Professional Address: ____

Post code: ____

Tel No: ____ Speciality: ____

If you report from an area served by a Yellow Card Centre (YCC), MHRA may ask the Centre to communicate with you, on its behalf, about your report. If you want only MHRA to contact you, please tick this box. ☐
See page 10 of BNF for details on YCCs.

* This is to enable you to identify the patient in any future correspondence concerning this report

Please attach additional pages if necessary

OTHER DRUGS (including self-medication & herbal remedies)

Did the patient take any other drugs in the last 3 months prior to the reaction? Yes / No

If yes, please give the following information if known:

Drug (Brand, if known)	Route	Dosage	Date started	Date stopped	Prescribed for

Additional relevant information e.g. medical history, test results, known allergies, rechallange (if performed), suspect drug interactions. For congenital abnormalities please state all other drugs taken during pregnancy and the last menstrual period.

REPORTER DETAILS

Name and Professional Address: ____

Post code: ____ Tel No: ____

Speciality: ____

Signature: ____ Date: ____

CLINICIAN (if not the reporter)

Name and Professional Address: ____

Post code: ____

Tel No: ____ Speciality: ____

If you report from an area served by a Yellow Card Centre (YCC), MHRA may ask the Centre to communicate with you, on its behalf, about your report. If you want only MHRA to contact you, please tick this box. ☐
See page 10 of BNF for details on YCCs.

* This is to enable you to identify the patient in any future correspondence concerning this report

Please attach additional pages if necessary